Be sure to complete your 1990 PDR® Library with these must-have volumes and electronic reference sources!

Ask for them wherever PDR® is sold.

PDR ®
44 EDITION 1990

PHYSICIANS' DESK REFERENCE ®

Publisher ● EDWARD R. BARNHART

Production Manager
CARRIE HENWOOD

Manager of Production Services
ELIZABETH H. CARUSO

Index Editor
ADELE L. DOWD

Medical Consultant
GERALD F. DEDERICK JR.

Art Associate
JOAN AKERLIND

Editorial Assistants
CATHLEEN C. BUNNELL
JANE T. PASINSKI

Editorial Consultant
DAVID W. SIFTON

Senior Research Analyst
PATRICIA DeSIMONE

Promotion Manager
RONALD YOUNG

Assistant Circulation Director
ANNETTE G. VERNON

Fulfillment Manager
ANITA H. MOORE

Professional Relations Manager
ANNA E. BARBAGALLO

Marketing Administrator
DAWN TERRANOVA

Circulation Coordinator
MARY J. CADLEY

Account Managers
JEFFERY J. BONISTALLI
CHARLIE J. MEITNER
JOANNE C. TERZIDES

Administrative Assistants
SONIA C. RYAN
HELENE WATTMAN

ISBN 0-87489-709-2

Foreword to the Forty-fourth Edition

The 1990 PHYSICIANS' DESK REFERENCE® represents the 44th edition of the publication. Product overviews for selected drugs have been included to give abbreviated information about the product's use. These appear immediately before the full product labeling. An explanation for pregnancy categories used in drug labeling is included, along with definitions for the various classes of controlled drug substances (see contents page). Information on inactive ingredients, educational materials (for you and your patients), bibliographies and phonetic spellings in the Product Information Section join to make the reference more valuable. Special features also include . . . Guide to the Management of Drug Overdose and a listing of Poison Control Centers.

PHYSICIANS' DESK REFERENCE® is published annually by Medical Economics Company Inc. with the cooperation of the manufacturers whose products appear in the Product Identification (Gray Section), the Product Information (White Section), and the Diagnostic Product Information (Green Section). Intended primarily for physicians, PDR's purpose is to make available essential information on major pharmaceutical and diagnostic products. In addition to this volume, three other editions of PHYSICIANS' DESK REFERENCE will be published in 1990: PDR DRUG INTERACTIONS AND SIDE EFFECTS INDEX™, PDR FOR NONPRESCRIPTION DRUGS® and PDR FOR OPHTHALMOLOGY®. The PDR Drug Interactions and Side Effects Index is available on Computer Diskettes. All the volumes are included on a compact disc—PDR® on CD-ROM.

This edition of PHYSICIANS' DESK REFERENCE® includes, the latest available information on over 2000 products. During the year as important new or revised information about these products becomes available to us, it will be published periodically in a PDR® Supplement. Retain the Supplement with PDR and before prescribing or administering any product described in PHYSICIANS' DESK REFERENCE, consult the latest PDR Supplement to determine if new information about the product has been published.

The function of the Publisher is the compilation, organization and distribution of this information. Product descriptions have been prepared by manufacturers, edited and approved by their medical department and/or medical consultant. Manufacturers suggest headings under which products should appear in the Product Category Index (Blue Section) and the Generic and Chemical Name Index (Yellow Section).

Under the federal Food, Drug & Cosmetic (FD&C) Act, a drug approved for marketing may be labeled, promoted, and advertised by the manufacturer only for those uses for which the drug's safety and effectiveness have been established. The Code of Federal Regulations 201.100 (d) (1) pertaining to labeling for prescription products require that for PDR content, "indications, effects, dosages, routes, methods, and frequency and duration of administration and any relevant warnings, hazards, contraindications, side effects, and precautions" must be the *"same in language and emphasis"* as the approved labeling for the product. FDA regards the words *"same in language and emphasis"* as requiring VERBATIM use of the approved labeling providing such information. Furthermore, information in the approved labeling that is emphasized by the use of type set in a box or in capitals, bold face, or italics must also be given the same emphasis in PDR.

The FDA has also announced that the FD&C Act "does not, however, limit the manner in which a physician may use an approved drug. Once a product has been approved for marketing, a physician may prescribe it for uses or in treatment regimens or patient populations that are not included in approved labeling." Thus the FDA states also that "accepted medical practice" often includes drug use that is not reflected in approved drug labeling.

For products which do not have official package circulars, the Publisher has emphasized to manufacturers the necessity of describing such products comprehensively so that physicians would have access to all information essential for intelligent and informed prescribing. In organizing and presenting the material in PHYSICIANS' DESK REFERENCE®, the Publisher is providing all the information made available to PDR® by manufacturers. In making this material available, it should be understood that the Publisher is not advocating the use of any product described herein. Additional information on any product may be obtained from the manufacturer.

EDWARD R. BARNHART
Publisher

Contents

SECTION 1

Manufacturers' Index

The manufacturers appearing in this index (white pages) have provided information concerning their pharmaceutical products in either the Product Information or Diagnostic Product Information Section. It is through their patronage that PHYSICIANS' DESK REFERENCE® is made available to you.

Included in this index are the names and addresses of manufacturers, individuals or departments to whom you may address inquiries, a partial list of products as well as emergency telephone numbers wherever available. The symbol ◆ indicates the product is shown in the Product Identification Section. The symbol ▣▫ indicates the product is described in PDR FOR NONPRESCRIPTION DRUGS®.

Italic page number indicates a brief listing.

ABBOTT LABORATORIES   403, 502
For Medical Information
  Pharmaceutical Products Division
    (708) 937-7069
  Hospital Products Division
    (708) 937-3806
Order Entry/Customer
Service Inquiries
  Pharmaceutical Products Division
    (800) 255-5162
  Hospital Products Division
    (800) 222-6883
Products Described
Abbokinase 502
Abbokinase Open-Cath 504
Abbo-Pac *502*
Sterile A-hydroCort 505
Sterile A-methaPred 507
Butesin Picrate Ointment..................509
Calcidrine Syrup 509
Calcijex Injection 509
◆ Cartrol Tablets....................... 403, 510
◆ Cefol Filmtab 403, 512
◆ Chlorthalidone Tablets 403, *512*
◆ Cylert Chewable Tablets 403, 512
◆ Cylert Tablets 403, 512
Dayalets Filmtab...............................▣▫
Dayalets Plus Iron Filmtab ....▣▫
◆ Depakene Capsules & Syrup .. 403, 513
◆ Depakote Tablets 403, 515
◆ Desoxyn Gradumet Tablets 403, 517
Desoxyn Tablets...................................517
Dical-D Tablets & Wafers..................518
◆ Dicumarol Tablets 403, 518
◆ E.E.S. 400 Filmtab 403, 524
E.E.S. Granules 524
E.E.S. 200 Liquid 524
E.E.S. 400 Liquid 524
◆ Enduron Tablets 403, 519
◆ Enduronyl Forte Tablets 403, 521
◆ Enduronyl Tablets 403, 521
EryDerm 2% Solution.........................522
◆ EryPed Drops and Chewable
  Tablets 403, 522
◆ EryPed 200 & EryPed 400 .... 403, 522
◆ Ery-Tab Delayed-Release
  Tablets 403, 523
Erythrocin Lactobionate-I.V. 525
Erythrocin Piggyback..........................527
◆ Erythrocin Stearate Filmtab...... 403, 528
◆ Erythromycin Base Filmtab ... 403, 529
◆ Erythromycin Delayed-Release
  Capsules, USP..................... 403, 530
◆ Eutonyl Filmtab.................................403
◆ Eutron Filmtab..................................403
◆ Fero-Folic-500 Filmtab 403, 531
◆ Fero-Grad-500 Filmtab 403, 532
Fero-Gradumet Filmtab......................532
H-BIG *532*

Harmonyl Tablets 533
◆ Hytrin Tablets 403, 533
Iberet Filmtab 535
◆ Iberet-500 Filmtab 403, 535
Iberet-500 Liquid 536
◆ Iberet-Folic-500 Filmtab 403, 531
Iberet-Liquid 536
◆ Janimine Filmtab Tablets 403, *536*
◆ K-Lor Powder Packets 403, 536
◆ K-Tab Filmtab 403, 537
Lidocaine Hydrochloride
  Injection, U.S.P. 538
◆ Nembutal Sodium Capsules 403, 540
Nembutal Sodium Solution 543
Nembutal Sodium
  Suppositories 545
Nitropress 547
Norisodrine Aerotrol...........................548
Norisodrine with Calcium
  Iodide Syrup *549*
◆ Ogen Tablets 403, 549
◆ Ogen Vaginal Cream 403, 549
◆ Optilets-500 Filmtab 403
◆ Optilets-M-500 Filmtab 403
◆ Oretic Tablets 403, 552
Oretic Forte Tablets 553
Oreticyl Tablets 553
◆ PCE Dispertab Tablets........... 403, 558
Panhematin 555
◆ Panwarfin Tablets 403, 555
◆ Paradione Capsules & Oral
  Solution 403, 557
◆ Peganone Tablets 403, 559
Penthrane 560
Pentothal Kit 562
Pentothal RTM Syringe 562
Pentothal (Sterile Powder) 562
Pentothal (Thiopental Sodium
  for Injection) 562
Phenurone Tablets 564
◆ Placidyl Capsules 403, 565
Quelidrine Syrup 566
Selsun Lotion 566
Surbex...▣▫
Surbex with C ....▣▫
◆ Surbex-750 with Iron Filmtab 403
◆ Surbex-750 with Zinc Filmtab...........403
◆ Surbex-T Filmtab..............................403
◆ Tranxene T-TAB Tablets 403, 567
◆ Tranxene-SD Half Strength
  Tablets 403, 567
◆ Tranxene-SD Tablets 403, 567
◆ Tridione Capsules 403, 568
◆ Tridione Dulcet Tablets 403, 568
Tridione Solution 568
Tronothane Hydrochloride Cream 569
Other Products Available
0.25% Acetic Acid Irrigation, USP
(Aqualite)

5% Alcohol & 5% Dextrose Injection
Amidate (Etomidate Injection) Ampul,
  Abboject
Aminophylline 250 mg., 10 ml., Ampul
  & Vial
Aminophylline 500 mg., 20 ml., Ampul
  & Vial
Aminosyn 3.5% M
Aminosyn 5%
Aminosyn 7%
Aminosyn II 7%
Aminosyn 7% TPN Kit
Aminosyn 7% with Electrolytes
Aminosyn 7% with Electrolytes TPN Kit
Aminosyn 8.5%
Aminosyn II 8.5%
Aminosyn 8.5% TPN Kit
Aminosyn 8.5% with Electrolytes
Aminosyn 10%
Aminosyn II 10%
Aminosyn 10% TPN Kit
Aminosyn (pH6) 7%, 8.5% and 10%
Aminosyn with Dextrose, Nutrimix Dual
  Chamber
Aminosyn II in Dextrose, Nutrimix
  Dual Chamber
Aminosyn-HBC 7%
Aminosyn-PF 7% and 10%
Ammonium Chloride
Anticoagulant Citrate Phosphate
  Dextrose Solution, USP
Atropine 0.1 mg./ml., 5 ml., Abboject
  Syringe
Atropine 0.1 mg./ml., 10 ml., Abboject
  Syringe
Balanced Salt Solution
Bretylium Tosylate in 5% Dextrose
  Injection (2 mg/mL and 4 mg/mL)
Bupivacaine Hydrochloride Injection,
  USP, 0.25%, 0.5%, 0.75%, Ampul,
  Abboject Syringe
Butyn Dental Ointment
Calcijex (calcitriol injection)
Calcium Chloride 10%, Abboject
Calcium Glucepate Injection Ampul &
  Abboject
Cecon Solution
Cenolate Ampules
Chromium 10 mL (4 mg/mL)
Colchicine Tablets
Copper 10 mL (4 mg/mL)
Covicone Cream
Cysteine Hydrochloride Injection
Dehydrated Alcohol Injection, USP
6% Dextran 75 w/v & 5% Dextrose
  Injection
6% Dextran 75 w/v & 0.9% Sodium
  Chloride Injection

2.5% Dextrose & ½ Str Lactated
  Ringer's Injection
5% Dextrose & Lactated Ringer's
  Injection
5% Dextrose & Ringer's Injection
2.5% Dextrose & 0.45% Sodium
  Chloride Injection, USP
5% Dextrose & 0.225% Sodium
  Chloride Injection, USP
5% Dextrose & 0.3% Sodium Chloride
  Injection, USP
5% Dextrose & 0.45% Sodium
  Chloride Injection, USP
5% Dextrose & 0.9% Sodium Chloride
  Injection, USP
10% Dextrose & 0.9% Sodium
  Chloride Injection, USP
2.5% Dextrose Injection, USP
5% Dextrose Injection, USP
5% Dextrose Injection, USP
  (ADD-Vantage)
5% Dextrose Injection, USP (Partial fill)
10% Dextrose Injection, USP
20% Dextrose Injection, USP
50% Dextrose Injection, USP
5% Dextrose & 0.15% Pot Chl
  Injection (20 mEq)
5% Dextrose & 0.224% Pot Chl
  Injection (30 mEq)
5% Dextrose & 0.3% Pot Chl Injection
  (40 mEq)
5% Dextrose & 0.225% Sodium
  Chloride with 0.075% Potassium
  Chloride Injection (10 mEq)
5% Dextrose & 0.225% Sodium
  Chloride with 0.15% Potassium
  Chloride Injection (20 mEq)
5% Dextrose & 0.225% Sodium
  Chloride with 0.224% Potassium
  Chloride Injection (30 mEq)
5% Dextrose & 0.225% Sodium
  Chloride with 0.3% Potassium
  Chloride Injection (40 mEq)
5% Dextrose & 0.3% Sodium Chloride
  with 0.075% Potassium Chloride
  Injection (10 mEq)
5% Dextrose & 0.3% Sodium Chloride
  with 0.15% Potassium Chloride
  Injection (20 mEq)
5% Dextrose & 0.3% Sodium Chloride
  with 0.224% Potassium Chloride
  Injection (30 mEq)
5% Dextrose & 0.45% Sodium
  Chloride with 0.075% Potassium
  Chloride Injection (10 mEq)

5% Dextrose & 0.45% Sodium Chloride with 0.15% Potassium Chloride Injection (20 mEq)
5% Dextrose & 0.45% Sodium Chloride with 0.224% Potassium Chloride Injection (30 mEq)
5% Dextrose & 0.45% Sodium Chloride with 0.3% Potassium Chloride Injection (40 mEq)
10% Dextrose Injection, USP
20% Dextrose Injection, USP
30% Dextrose Injection, USP
40% Dextrose Injection, USP
50% Dextrose Injection, USP
60% Dextrose Injection, USP
70% Dextrose Injection, USP
Dopamine Hydrochloride in 5% Dextrose Injection (800, 1600, 3200 mcg/mL)
Empty Evacuated Container
Endrate Solution, Ampoules
Ephedrine Sulfate, Injection
Epinephrine 1:10,000, 10 ml., Abboject
Erythrocin ADD-Vantage Kits
Erythrocin-I.V.
Fentanyl Injection, Ampul, Vial
Gentamicin Premix ADD-Vantage Products
Gentamicin Sulfate in 0.9% Sodium Chloride Injection (0.8, 0.9, 1.0, 1.2, 1.4 mg/mL)
Gerilets Filmtab
Gerix Elixir
1.5% Glycine Irrigation/Aqualite
1.5% Glycine Irrigation, USP (Flex & Aqualite)
Glycopyrrolate Injection
Halothane
Heparin Sodium in 5% Dextrose Injection (50 & 100 Units/mL)
Heparin Sodium in 0.45% Sodium Chloride Injection (50 & 100 Units/mL)
Hydroxyzine HCl Injection, Abbojects, Ampuls, Vials, Syringes
Iberol Filmtab
Iberol-F Filmtab
Inpersol & 1.5% Dextrose
Inpersol & 2.5% Dextrose
Inpersol & 4.25% Dextrose
Inpersol-LM with 1.5% Dextrose
Inpersol-LM with 2.5% Dextrose
Inpersol-LM with 4.25% Dextrose
Isoproterenol HCl 1:5,000 5 mL, Universal Add Syringe
Isoproterenol HCl 1:5,000 10 mL, Universal Add Syringe
Isoproterenol HCl 1:50,000, 10 mL, Abboject
10% LMD w/v and 5% Dextrose Injection
10% LMD w/v and 0.9% Sodium Chloride Injection
LTA Kit, Preattached
LTA II Kit
LTA Pediatric Kit
Lactated Ringers for Irrigation (Flex)
Lactated Ringer's Injection, USP
Lidocaine HCl Injection, 0.2% in 5% Dextrose
Lidocaine HCl Injection, 0.4% in 5% Dextrose
Lidocaine HCl Injection, 0.8% in 5% Dextrose
Lidocaine HCl Injection, USP, 1%, 5 mL, Abboject
Lidocaine HCl Injection, USP, 1%, 5 mL, Sterile Pack Abboject
Lidocaine HCl Injection, USP, 2%, 5 mL, Abboject
Lidocaine HCl Injection, USP, 2%, 5 mL, Sterile Pack Abboject
Lidocaine HCl Injection, USP, 20%, 5 mL, 1 gram-Pintop, U.A.S.
Lidocaine HCl Injection, USP, 20%, 10 mL, 2 gram-Pintop, U.A.S.
Lidocaine HCl Injection, USP, 5% with 7.5% Dextrose
Liposyn II 10% and 20%
Magnesium Sulfate 12.5%, 8 mL, Pintop
Magnesium Sulfate 50% w/v Ampoules & Abboject
Mammol Ointment
Manganese 10 mL (1 mg/mL)
5% Mannitol Injection, USP
10% Mannitol Injection, USP
15% Mannitol Injection, USP
20% Mannitol Injection, USP
25% Mannitol Injection, USP
Meperidine HCl Injection (10 mg/mL, PCA Vials)
Metronidazole Injection, USP (5 mg/mL)
Morphine Sulfate Injection, USP (1 & 5 mg/mL, PCA Vials)
Nalbuphine Hydrochloride Injection, USP
Nembutal Elixir
Neut Abbo-Vial & Pintop
Normosol-M 900 CAL
Normosol-M & 5% Dextrose Injection
Normosol-M & Surbex-T & 5% Dextrose Injection
Normosol-R
Normosol-R pH 7.4
Normosol-R & 5% Dextrose Injection
Normosol-R/K +& 5% Dextrose Injection
Pentothal Rectal Suspension in Syringe
Phenobarbital Sodium Ampoules

Physiosol Irrigation (Aqualite)
Plegisol
Potassium Acetate 40 mEq Vial, Pintop & Fliptop
Potassium Chloride Injection Ampoules & Vials, Pintop & Universal Additive Syringe
Potassium Chloride 20 mEq. in D-5 W in Abbo-Vac
Potassium Phosphate 15 mM Vial, Pintop & Fliptop
Potassium Phosphate 45 mM Vial
Procainamide Hydrochloride Injection, USP
Procaine Hydrochloride Injection 1% & 2% Vial
Quelicin (Succinylcholine Chloride Injection) Ampul & Vial, Pintop
Ringer's Injection, USP
Ringer's Irrigation, USP (Aqualite)
Selsun Suspension
Sodium Acetate 40 mEq Vial
5% Sodium Bicarbonate Injection, USP
4.2% Sodium Bicarbonate Injection, 10 mEq in 10 mL Abboject (Neonatal)
7.5% Sodium Bicarbonate Injection, 44.6 mEq in 50 mL ampul or Abboject
8.4% Sodium Bicarbonate Injection, 50 mEq in 50 mL Abboject or Fliptop Vial
8.4% Sodium Bicarbonate Injection, 10 mEq in 10 mL Abboject (Pediatric)
0.45% Sodium Chloride Injection, USP
5% Sodium Chloride
20% Sodium Chloride
0.9% Sodium Chloride Injection
0.9% Sodium Chloride Injection, USP (ADD-Vantage)
0.9% Sodium Chloride Injection, USP (Partial Fill)
0.9% Sodium Chloride Irrigation, USP (Flex and Aqualite)
0.45% Sodium Chloride Irrigation, USP (Aqualite)
Sodium Lactate Injection, USP, 1/6 Molar
Sodium Phosphate 45 mg/15 mL
Sorbitol-Mannitol Irrigation (Flex & Aqualite)
Sterile Urea
TPN Electrolytes
Tham-E
Tham Solution
Theophylline in 5% Dextrose Injection (0.4, 0.8, 1.6, 2, 4 mg/mL)
Tubocurarine Chloride Injection, USP
Ureaphil
Urologic G Irrigation (Aqualite)
Vercyte Tablets
Vita-Kaps Filmtab
Vita-Kaps M Filmtab
Vitamin C Filmtab
Water for Injection, Ampoules, Vial
Water for Injection Bacteriostatic 30 mL Fliptop
Water for Injection, Sterile, USP
Water, for Irrigation, Sterile, USP (Flex and Aqualite)
Water for Respiratory Therapy, Sterile (Flex)
Zinc 10 mL (1 mg/1 mL)

ADAMS LABORATORIES, INC. 569
P.O. Box 487
7450 Whitehall Street
Ft. Worth, TX 76118
Address inquiries to:
John Q. Adams   (817) 589-1188
For Medical Emergencies Contact:
John Q. Adams   (817) 589-1188
Products Described
Atrohist L.A. Tablets *569*
Atrohist Sprinkle Capsules 569
Deconsal L.A. Tablets 571
Deconsal Sprinkle Capsules 570
Deconsal II Tablets 570
Humibid DM Tablets 571
Humibid L.A. Tablets 571
Humibid Sprinkle Capsules 571

ADRIA LABORATORIES   404, 572
Division of Erbamont Inc.
Administrative Offices:
7001 Post Road
Dublin, OH 43017
Mailing Address:
P. O. Box 16529
Columbus, OH 43216
Address inquiries to:
Medical Department
                        (614) 764-8100
Products Described
Adriamycin PFS 572
Adriamycin RDF 573
Axotal 575
◆ Emetrol 404, 575
Evac-Q-Kit 575
Evac-Q-Kwik 576
Ilopan Injection (ampules) 577
Ilopan Stat-Pak (Disposable Syringe) 577
Kaochlor 10% Liquid 577
Kaochlor S-F 10% Liquid 577
◆ Kaon Cl 404, 579
◆ Kaon Cl-10 Tablets 404, 579
Kaon Elixir, Grape Flavor 578
Kaon-Cl 20% Liquid 577

Magan Tablets 580
Modane Mild Tablets 581
Modane Plus Tablets 581
Modane Soft Capsules 581
Modane Tablets 581
Neosar for Injection 582
◆ Nitrol Ointment 404, 583
Octamide PFS 584
Tympagesic Otic Solution 586
Vancor Intravenous 586
Other Products Available
Adrucil
Chymex
Folex for Injection
Folex PFS Injection, USP
Ilopan-Choline Tablets
Ilozyme Tablets
Kaochlor-Eff Tablets
Kaon Elixir, Lemon-Lime Flavor
Kaon Tablets
Modane Bulk
Modane Versabran
Nitrol Ointment
Octamide
Taloin Ointment
Velsar
Vincasar PFS
Xylo-Pfan

ADVANCED NUTRITIONAL   404, 588
TECHNOLOGY, INC.
1111 Jefferson Avenue
P.O. Box 3225
Elizabeth, NJ 07207-3225
Address inquiries to:
Wayne L. Phillips   (201) 354-2740
                        (201) 354-2741
Products Described
Lactase Enzyme Softgels *588*
Liqui-Cal Softgels *588*
N'Odor Softgels *588*
PhosChol Concentrate *588*
◆ PhosChol 565 Softgels 404, *588*
◆ PhosChol 900 Softgels 404, *588*
Precorsin Softgels *588*
◆ SuperEPA 1200 Softgels 404, *588*

AKORN, INC.   588
100 Akorn Drive
Abita Springs, LA 70420
Address inquiries to:
David Turner
Vice President, Sales & Marketing
                        (504) 893-9300
Products Described
Please consult PDR FOR OPHTHALMOLOGY

ALCON LABORATORIES, INC.   589
Alcon Laboratories, Inc.
And its affiliates Inc.
Corporate Headquarters
P.O. Box 6600
6201 South Freeway
Fort Worth, TX 76134
Address inquiries to:
Sales Services   (817) 293-0450
Products Described
Betoptic Sterile Ophthalmic Solution 589
Naphcon-A Ophthalmic Solution 590
Tears Naturale II Lubricant Eye Drops 590
Tobrex Ophthalmic Ointment and Solution 590
Other Products Available
A-OK Ophthalmic Knife
Alcon Surgical System (Irrigation/Aspiration Kits; Phacoemulsification Kits)
BSS Irrigation Solution (15mL, 30mL, 250mL, 500mL)
BSS Plus Irrigation Solution (30mL, 500mL)
BSS and BSS Plus Irrigation Solution Administration Set
Cetamide Ointment
Cetapred Ointment
Cryophake Sterile, Disposable Cryoextractor
Cyclogyl Ophthalmic Solution
Cyclomydril Ophthalmic Solution
Cystitomes & Cannulas
Duratears Naturale Lubricant Eye Ointment
Enuclene Ophthalmic Solution
Epinal Ophthalmic Solution
Eye Pak Surgical Drape
Eye Stream Eye Irrigating Solution
Fluorescite Injection
Gonioscopic Prism Solution
I-Knife Ophthalmic Knife
Intraocular Lenses
Iopidine Ophthalmic Solution
Ismotic Solution
Maxidex Ointment
Maxitrol Ointment
Microphake Sterile Disposable Cryoextractor
Microsponge Miniature Surgical Sponge
Miostat Intraocular Solution
Natacyn Ophthalmic Suspension
Optemp Sterile Disposable Cautery
Osmoglyn Oral Osmotic Agent
PTG, Alcon Applanation Pneumatonograph
Pilopine HS Gel
Post-Operative Kits

Procedure Packs
Steri-Units Sterile Ophthalmic Units for Single Use Only
Zolyse Ophthalmic Solution

ALCON (PUERTO RICO) INC.
P.O. Box 3000
Humacao, Puerto Rico 00661
Address inquiries to:
Medical Department
P.O. Box 6380
Fort Worth, TX 76115
                        (817) 293-0450

Products Available
Adsorbocarpine
Adsorbonac
Adsorbotear
Alcaine
Econopred
Econopred Plus
Glaucon
Isopto Atropine
Isopto Carbachol
Isopto Carpine
Isopto Cetamide
Isopto Cetapred
Isopto Homatropine
Isopto Hyoscine
Maxidex Suspension
Maxitrol Suspension
Mydfrin 2.5%
Mydrapred
Mydriacyl
Naphcon
Naphcon Forte
Zincfrin

ALLEN & HANBURYS   404, 591
Division of Glaxo Inc.
Five Moore Drive
Research Triangle Park
North Carolina 27709
                        (919) 248-2100
Address inquiries to:
Medical Services Department
For Medical Emergencies Contact:
                        (919) 248-2100
Products Described
◆ Beclovent Inhalation Aerosol.... 404, 591
◆ Beclovent Inhalation Aerosol Refill 404, 591
◆ Beconase AQ Nasal Spray 404, 592
◆ Beconase Inhalation Aerosol & Refill 404, 592
◆ Ceftin Tablets 404, 594
Corticaine Cream 595
Ethatab Tablets 596
◆ Theobid Duracap Capsules 404, 596
◆ Theobid Jr. Duracap Capsules 404, 596
◆ Trandate HCT Tablets 404, 600
◆ Trandate Injection 404, 598
◆ Trandate Tablets 404, 600
◆ Trinsicon/Trinsicon M Capsules 404, 603
◆ Ventolin Inhalation Aerosol ... 404, 604
◆ Ventolin Inhalation Aerosol Refill 404, 604
◆ Ventolin Rotacaps for Inhalation 404, 604
◆ Ventolin Solution for Inhalation 404, 604
◆ Ventolin Syrup 404, 604
◆ Ventolin Tablets 404, 604
◆ Vicon Forte Capsules 404, 607
◆ Vicon Plus Capsules 404, 607
◆ Vicon-C Capsules 404, 607
◆ Vi-Zac Capsules.....................404, 607
Other Products Available
Amesec Capsules
Atrocholin Tablets
Dionosil Oily

ALLERGAN OPTICAL   607
A Division of Allergan, Inc.
2525 Dupont Drive
Irvine, CA 92715-1599
Address inquiries to:
                        (714) 752-4500
Products Available
Allergan Enzymatic Contact Lens Cleaner
Allergan Hydrocare Cleaning & Disinfecting Solution
Allergan Hydrocare Preserved Saline Solution
Allergan Sorbi-Care Saline Solution
Blink-N-Clean Hard Contact Lens Solution
Clean-N-Soak Hard Contact Lens Cleaning & Soaking Solution
Clean-N-Soakit Hard Contact Lens Storage Case
Clean-N-Stow Hard Contact Lens Storage Case
EasyClean/GP Daily Cleaner
Extenzyme Protein Cleaner
LC-65 Daily Contact Lens Cleaner
Lens Clear Soft Contact Lens Cleaner
Lens Fresh Lubricating & Rewetting Drops
LensKeeper Contact Lens Carrying Case
Lens Plus Daily Cleaner
Lens Plus Oxysept 1 Disinfecting Solution
Lens Plus Oxysept 2 Rinse & Neutralizer
Lens Plus Rewetting Drops

Lens Plus Sterile Saline Solution
Lensrins Preserved Saline Solution
Lens-Wet Lubricating & Rewetting
Solution
Liquifilm Wetting Solution
OxyCup Lens Case
ProFree/GP Weekly Enzymatic Cleaner
Resolve/GP Daily Cleaner
Soakare Hard Contact Lens Soaking
Solution
Style Keeper Contact Lens Carrying
Case
Total The All-in-one Hard Contact Lens
Solution
Ultrazyme Enzymatic Cleaner
Wet-N-Soak Wetting and Soaking
Solution
Wet-N-Soak PLUS Wetting and Soaking
Solution

ALLERGAN PHARMACEUTICALS 607
A Division of Allergan, Inc.
2525 Dupont Drive
Irvine, CA 92715-1599
Address inquiries to:
(714) 752-4500
(See also Herbert Laboratories)
Products Available
Celluvisc Lubricant
Ophthalmic Solution .... ⊡□
Lacril Lubricant Ophthalmic
Solution .... ⊡□
Lacri-Lube S.O.P. Lubricant
Ophthalmic Ointment .... ⊡□
Liquifilm Forte Lubricant
Ophthalmic Solution .... ⊡□
Liquifilm Tears Lubricant
Ophthalmic Solution .... ⊡□
Prefrin Liquifilm
Vasoconstrictor (Redness
Reliever) and Lubricant Eye
Drops .... ⊡□
Refresh Lubricant Ophthalmic
Solution .... ⊡□
Refresh P.M. Lubricant
Ophthalmic Ointment .... ⊡□
Relief Vasoconstrictor
(Redness Reliever) and
Lubricant Eye Drops .... ⊡□
Tears Plus Lubricant
Ophthalmic Solution .... ⊡□
Other Products Available
Albalon with Liquifilm
Albalon-A Liquifilm Sterile Ophthalmic
Solution
Atropine Sulfate ½% S.O.P. Sterile
Ophthalmic Ointment
Atropine Sulfate 1.0% S.O.P. Sterile
Ophthalmic Ointment
Atropine Sulfate 1% Sterile Ophthalmic
Solution
Betagan Liquifilm Sterile Ophthalmic
Solution with C Cap Compliance Q.D.
and B.I.D.
Bleph-10 Sterile Ophthalmic Ointment
Bleph-10 with Liquifilm
Blephamide Liquifilm Sterile Ophthalmic
Suspension
Blephamide S.O.P. Sterile Ophthalmic
Ointment
Chloroptic Liquifilm Sterile Ophthalmic Solution
Chloroptic S.O.P. Sterile Ophthalmic
Ointment
Epifrin Sterile Ophthalmic Solution
FML Forte Liquifilm Sterile Ophthalmic
Suspension
FML Liquifilm Sterile Ophthalmic
Suspension
FML S.O.P. Sterile Ophthalmic Ointment
Genoptic Liquifilm Sterile Ophthalmic
Solution
Genoptic S.O.P. Sterile Ophthalmic
Ointment
HMS Liquifilm Sterile Ophthalmic
Suspension
Herplex Liquifilm Sterile Ophthalmic
Solution
Lacri-Lube NP Lubricant Ophthalmic
Ointment
Ocufen Liquifilm Sterile Ophthalmic
Solution
Ophthetic Sterile Ophthalmic Solution
Pilagan Liquifilm Sterile Ophthalmic
Solution with C Cap Compliance Cap
Poly-Pred Liquifilm Sterile Ophthalmic
Suspension
Pred Forte Sterile Ophthalmic
Suspension
Pred Mild Sterile Ophthalmic
Suspension
Pred-G Liquifilm Sterile Ophthalmic
Suspension
Prefrin-A Sterile Ophthalmic Solution
Propine Ophthalmic Solution, USP,
0.1% with C Cap Compliance Cap
B.I.D.

ALPHA THERAPEUTIC 608
CORPORATION
5555 Valley Boulevard
Los Angeles, CA 90032
Address inquires to:
(213) 227-7526
(800) 421-0008
CA (800) 851-8891
For Medical Emergencies Contact:
C. McAuley, M.D., Medical Director
(213) 227-7419

After hours emergency orders
(818) 304-6860
Products Described
Albutein 5% 608
Albutein 25% 608
Monoclate 608
Plasmatein 5% 608
Profilate HP 608
Profilate SD 608
Profilnine Heat-Treated 608
Soyacal 10% 608
Soyacal 20% 608
Venoglobulin-I 608

ALRA LABORATORIES, INC. 608
3850 Clearview Court
Gurnee, IL 60031
Address inquiries to:
Professional Services
(312) 244-9440
(800) 248-ALRA
Products Described
Alramucil Instant Mix, Orange 608
Alramucil Instant Mix, Regular 608
Cholac Lactulose Syrup, USP.............608
Constilac Lactulose Syrup,
USP 608
Eryzole Oral Suspension, USP 608
Gelpirin Tablets 608
Gelpirin-CCF Tablets 608
Gen-XENE Tablets 608
IBU-TAB Ibuprofen Tablets,
USP 608
K+ Care 609
K+ Care ET 609
K+ 10 Tablets 609
Methalgen Cream 609

ALZA CORPORATION 404, 609
950 Page Mill Road
P.O. Box 10950
Palo Alto, California 94303-0802
Address inquiries to:
Carol A. Christopher
Group Product Manager
(415) 496-8073
For Medical Emergencies Contact:
Jonathan Parmer, M.D.
Medical Director, ALZA Pharmaceuticals
(415) 496-8807
*To order product or
request literature, call:*
(800) 227-9953
In CA call collect (415) 494-5067
*For medical or technical
questions, call:*
(800) 634-8977
Products Described
◆ Progestasert Intrauterine
Contraceptive System 404, 609
Other Products Available
Ocusert Ocular Therapeutic Systems
Pilo-20
Pilo-40

AMERICAN DERMAL 615
CORPORATION
Bedminster Industrial Park
P.O. Box 900
Plumsteadville, PA 18949
Address Inquiries to:
Professional Services Department
(800) 526-0199
In PA call: (215) 766-2110
Products Described
Drithocreme 615
Dritho-Scalp 615
Viranol Gel 615
Viranol Solution 616

AMGEN INC. 405, 616
1900 Oak Terrace Lane
Thousand Oaks, CA 91320
Address inquiries to:
Ellen E. Nichols (805) 499-5725
Products Described
◆ Epogen for Injection 405, 616

ANAQUEST 405, 619
2005 West Beltline Highway
Madison, WI 53713-2318
Address inquiries to:
"(800) ANA-DRUG"
For Product Orders:
"(800) CALL4RX"
Sales Offices
SOUTHEAST
4565 Winters Chapel Road
Atlanta, GA 30360
(404) 242-7673
EASTERN
1 Executive Drive
Fort Lee Executive Park
Fort Lee, NJ 07024
(201) 947-5556
MIDWEST
7 Salt Creek Lane
Hinsdale, IL 60521
(312) 986-7800
PACIFIC
5635 West Las Positas Blvd.
Suite 406
Pleasanton, CA 94566
(415) 463-2133
SOUTHWEST
831 Greenview Drive
Grand Prairie, TX 75050
(214) 988-6639
CANADA
2000 Argentia Road, Plaza II

Suite 407
Mississauga, Ontario L5N 1V8
(416) 821-7785
Products Described
◆ Enlon Injection 405, 619
◆ Ethrane 405, 619
◆ Forane 405, 621

ARCO PHARMACEUTICALS, INC. 622
105 Orville Drive
Bohemia, NY 11716
Address inquiries to:
Professional Service Dept.
(516) 567-9500
Products Described
Arco-Lase Plus Tablets 622
Arco-Lase Tablets 622
Mega-B 622
Megadose 622
Other Products Available
Arco-Cee Tablets
Arcoret Tablets
Arcoret w/Iron Tablets
Arcotinic Liquid
Arcotinic Tablets
C-B Time Capsules
C-B Time 500 Tablets
C-B Time Liquid
Co-Gel Tablets
Mega-B with C
Spantuss Liquid
Spantuss Tablets

ARMOUR PHARMACEUTICAL 622
COMPANY
Executive Office
Suite 200
920A Harvest Drive
Blue Bell, PA 19422
(215) 540-8100
Order Entry
P.O. Box 511
Kankakee, IL 60901
Illinois customers (800) 892-1865
All Other customers
(800) 435-1852
Customer Service (815) 932-6771
Products Described
Albuminar-5, Albumin
(Human) U.S.P. 5% 622
Albuminar-25, Albumin
(Human) U.S.P. 25% 622
Gammar, Immune Globulin
(Human) U.S.P. 622
Gamulin Rh, Rh_0(D) Immune
Globulin (Human) 622
Humate P, Antihemophilic
Factor (Human),
Pasteurized 622
Mini-Gamulin Rh, Rh_0(D)
Immune Globulin (Human) 623
Monoclate Factor VIII:C,
Heat-Treated,
Antihemophilic Factor
(Human) 623
Plasma-Plex Plasma Protein
Fraction (Human) 623
Other Products Available
Plasma Derivative Products
Albuminar-5, Albumin (Human) U.S.P.
5%
Albuminar-25, Albumin (Human)
U.S.P. 25%
Gammar, Immune Globulin (Human)
U.S.P.
Gamulin Rh, Rh_0(D) Immune Globulin
(Human)
Humate-P, Antihemophilic Factor
(Human), Pasteurized
Mini-Gamulin Rh, Rh_0(D) Immune
Globulin (Human)
Monoclate, Factor VIII:C,
Heat-Treated,
Antihemophilic Factor (Human)
Plasma Plex Plasma Protein Fraction
(Human)

ARTHER, INC. 623
P.O. Box 1455
West Caldwell, NJ 07007-1455
Address inquiries to:
A. Arthur Lowenthal, President
(800) 327-7914
(201) 226-5288
Products Described
Tryptacin 623

B. F. ASCHER & COMPANY, INC. 623
15501 W 109th St.
Lenexa, KS 66219
Address inquiries to:
Product Information Dept.
(913) 888-1880
Products Described
Adipost Capsules 623
Allent Capsules 623
Anaspaz Tablets 623
Ayr Saline Nasal Drops .... ⊡□
Ayr Saline Nasal Mist .... ⊡□
Drize Capsules 623
Hy-Phen Tablets (formerly
Hycodaphen) 623
Kwelcof Liquid 623
Mobigesic Analgesic Tablets .... ⊡□
Mobisyl Analgesic Creme .... ⊡□
Pen•Kera Creme .... ⊡□
Tolfrinic Tablets 623
Unilax Stool Softener/Laxative
Softgel Capsules .... ⊡□

Other Products Available
Drotic Ear Drops
Ethaquin Tablets
Mobidin Tablets
Niloric Tablets
Soft 'N Soothe Creme

ASTRA PHARMACEUTICAL 624
PRODUCTS INC.
50 Otis Street
Westboro, MA 01581-4428
Address inquiries to:
Professional Information Department
(508) 366-1100
Products Described
Astramorph PF Injection, USP
(Preservative-Free) 624
Atropine Sulfate Injection,
USP 625
Bretylium Tosylate Injection,
USP 625
Calcium Chloride 10%
Injection, USP 625
Calcium Gluconate 10%
Injection, USP 625
Clindamycin Phosphate
Injection, USP 625
Dextrose 50% Injection, USP 626
Dopamine Hydrochloride
Injection, USP 626
Droperidol Injection, USP 626
Duranest Injections 626
Dyclone 0.5% and 1%
Topical Solutions, USP 628
Epinephrine Injection, USP 629
Fentanyl Citrate and
Droperidol Injection 629
Furosemide Injection, USP 629
Hemopad Absorbable
Collagen Hemostat 629
Hydromorphone HCl Injection 630
Magnesium Sulfate Injection,
USP 630
Mannitol Injection, USP, 25% 630
Meperidine Hydrochloride
Injection 630
Methotrexate Sodium
Injection, USP 630
Morphine Sulfate Injection,
USP 630
Nalbuphine Hydrochloride
Injection 631
Naloxone Hydrochloride
Injection, USP 631
Nesacaine Injections 631
Nesacaine-MPF Injection 631
Pancuronium Bromide
Injection 633
Polocaine Injection, USP 633
Sensorcaine with Epinephrine
Injection 633
Sensorcaine Injection 633
Sensorcaine Spinal 636
Sodium Bicarbonate Injection,
USP 636
Xylocaine Injections 637
Xylocaine Injections for
Ventricular
Arrhythmias-Intravenous
Injection or Continuous
Infusion; Intramuscular
Injection 639
Xylocaine 2% Jelly 643
Xylocaine Ointment 2.5% .... ⊡□
Xylocaine 5% Ointment 644
Xylocaine 10% Oral Spray 645
Xylocaine 1.5% Solution with
Dextrose 7.5% 642
Xylocaine 5% Solution with
Glucose 7.5% 643
Xylocaine 4% Sterile Solution 641
Xylocaine 4% Topical
Solution 642
Xylocaine 2% Viscous
Solution 646
Yutopar Intravenous Injection 647
Yutopar Tablets 647
Other Products Available
Citanest Solutions

AYERST LABORATORIES 649
Division of American Home Products
Corporation
685 Third Avenue
New York, NY 10017-4071
See WYETH-AYERST LABORATORIES
for prescription drugs and WHITEHALL
LABORATORIES INC. for
nonprescription drugs.

BAKER CUMMINS 649
PHARMACEUTICALS, INC.
8800 N.W. 36th Street
Miami, FL 33178
Address inquiries to:
Orders (800) 347-4774
Professional Services
(305) 590-2200
For Medical Emergencies Contact:
Charles Dunn, M.D.
(305) 590-2254
Products Described
Acno Cleanser .... ⊡□
Acno Lotion .... ⊡□
Aqua-A Cream .... ⊡□
Aquaderm Combination
Treatment/Moisturizer .... ⊡□
Aquaderm Therapeutic Lotion
and Cream .... ⊡□

(◆ Shown in Product Identification Section)   *Italic Page Number* Indicates Brief Listing   (▣ Described in PDR For Nonprescription Drugs)

Liquid Dial Antibacterial Soap
Lurodine Iodine Antiseptic Skin Cleanser
Lurosep Antiseptic Lotion Hand
  Cleanser
Lurosoothe Hand Cream
MD #1 Dry Sterile Brush/Sponge
MD #2 Brush/Sponge with
  Chlorhexidine Gluconate
MD #3 Brush/Sponge with PCMX
MD #4 Brush/Sponge with
  Povidone-Iodine
Pure & Natural Soap
Tone Soap

DISTA PRODUCTS COMPANY   409, 894
Division of Eli Lilly and Company
For Medical Information, Write:
Lilly Research Laboratories
Lilly Corporate Center
Indianapolis, IN 46285
                    (317) 276-3714
For Other Inquiries:
Dista Products Company
Lilly Corporate Center
Indianapolis, IN 46285
                    (317) 276-4000
Regional Sales Offices
Atlanta, GA 30328
  Northpark Town Center
  Building 500, Suite 710
  1100 Abernathy Road, NE
                    (404) 551-5383
Chicago, IL 60631
  Suite 270, O'Hare Plaza
  8735 West Higgins Road
                    (312) 693-8360
Pasadena, CA 91101
  811 Mutual Savings Building
  301 East Colorado Blvd.
                    (818) 792-3197
Stamford, CT 06902
  300 First Stamford Place
                    (203) 357-8872
Products Described
◆ Cinobac Pulvules 409, 895
Cordran Ointment & Lotion 896
Cordran SP Cream 896
Cordran Tape 897
Cordran-N Cream and
  Ointment 896
Ilosone Chewable Tablets 898
Ilosone Liquids, Oral
  Suspensions 898
◆ Ilosone Pulvules & Tablets........ 409, 898
Ilosone Ready-Mixed Drops...........898
Ilotycin Gluceptate, IV, Vials 901
Ilotycin Ophthalmic Ointment 899
Ilotycin Tablets 899
Keflet Tablets 901
◆ Keflex, Pulvules & Tablets 409
◆ Keftab, Tablets 409, 902
◆ Nalfon 200 Pulvules................. 409, 903
◆ Nalfon Pulvules & Tablets 409, 903
◆ Prozac Pulvules...................... 409, 905
◆ Valmid Pulvules...................... 409, 908
Other Products Available
Becotin Pulvules
Becotin with Vitamin C Pulvules
Becotin-T Tablets
Co-Pyronil 2, Pulvules and Liquid
Keflex, for Oral Suspension
Keflex, for Pediatric Drops
Mi-Cebrin Tablets
Mi-Cebrin T Tablets

DOCTORS' RECOMMENDED   409, 908
PHARMACEUTICAL
PRODUCTS
9400 Brighton Way
Suite 414
Beverly Hills, CA 90210
Address inquiries to:
John Mir, Vice President
                    (213) 276-6255
Products Described
Doctors' Recommended Best
  Multivitamins and Minerals 908
◆ Doctors' Recommended High
  Potency
  Therapeutic MultiVitamins
  and Minerals 409, 909

DORSEY LABORATORIES
See SANDOZ
PHARMACEUTICALS/CONSUMER
DIVISION

DORSEY PHARMACEUTICALS   909
See SANDOZ PHARMACEUTICALS
CORPORATION, DORSEY DIVISION

DU PONT PHARMACEUTICALS   409, 909
E.I. du Pont de Nemours & Company
Wilmington, Delaware 19898

DU PONT PHARMACEUTICALS
CARIBE, INC.
Subsidiary of E.I. du Pont de Nemours
& Company
Post Office Box 12
Manati, Puerto Rico 00701

DU PONT
PHARMACEUTICALS
E.I. du Pont de Nemours & Company
Wilmington, DE 19898

For Pharmaceutical Product-Related
Inquiries
Write:
Professional Services
Du Pont Pharmaceuticals
P.O. Box 80026
Wilmington, DE 19880-0026
Business hours only (8:00 AM to 4:30
PM)
      Eastern Time (302) 992-4240
For Adverse Experience Reporting:
Call: (302) 892-1979
                Business Hours Only
For Medical Emergency
Information Only
After hours or on weekends
Call: (302) 892-1980
Products Described
Bretylol Injection 909
Brevibloc Injection...........................910
Calciparine Injection 912
◆ Coumadin Injection & Tablets 409, 914
Hespan Injection 916
◆ Hycodan Syrup, Tablets 409, 917
Hycomine Compound Tablets 919
Hycomine Pediatric Syrup 918
Hycomine Syrup 918
Hycotuss Expectorant Syrup 920
Intropin Injection 921
◆ Moban Tablets & Concentrate 409, 922
◆ Narcan Injection 409, 924
◆ Nubain Injection 409, 925
Numorphan Hydrochloride
  Injection 925
◆ Numorphan Suppositories 409, 926
Pentaspan Injection 926
◆ Percocet Tablets 409, 927
◆ Percodan Tablets 409, 928
◆ Percodan-Demi Tablets 409, 928
◆ Symmetrel Capsules & Syrup... 410, 929
◆ Trexan Tablets 410, 930
Tridil 932
Valpin 50 Tablets 933
◆ Zydone Capsules 410, 934
Other Products Available
Aminocaproic Acid Injection, USP
Doxycycline Hyclate for Injection, USP
Droperidol Injection, USP
Sterile Erythromycin Lactobionate
Fluphenazine Decanoate Injection
Haloperidol Injection, USP
Kanamycin Sulfate Injection, USP
Methyldopate HCl Injection, USP
Methotrexate Sodium Injection, USP
Nalbuphine HCl Injection
Procainamide HCl Injection, USP
Protamine Sulfate Injection, USP
Ritodrine HCl, USP
Sulfamethoxazole & Trimethoprim
  Concentrate for Injection, USP
Verapamil HCl, USP
Vincristine Sulfate Injection, USP

DURA PHARMACEUTICALS, INC   935
P.O. Box 2209
Ramona, CA 92065-0938
Address inquiries to:
Same as above   (619) 789-6840
For Medical Emergencies Contact:
Craig Wheeler   (619) 789-6840
Tom Evangelisti
Products Described
Dura-Gest Capsules 935
Dura-Tap/PD Capsules 935
Dura-Vent/A Capsules 935
Dura-Vent/DA Tablets 935
Dura-Vent Tablets...........................935
Fenesin Tablets...............................936

DURAMED PHARACEUTICALS,   936
INC.
5040 Lester Road
Cincinnati, OH 45213
Address inquiries to:
                    (513) 731-9900
  Outside OH (800) 543-8338
  Telecopier (513) 791-5785
Products Described
Aminophylline Tablets 936
Chlorpropamide Tablets 936
Chlorzoxazone with APAP
  Tablets 936
Clonidine HCl Tablets 936
Conjugated Estrogens Tablets,
  USP 936
Cyproheptadine HCl Tablets 936
Diazepam Tablets............................936
Dipyridamole Tablets 936
Haloperidol Tablets 936
Hydroxyzine Pamoate
  Capsules 936
Indomethacin Capsules 936
Isoniazid Tablets 936
Methyldopa Tablets 936
Methylprednisolone Tablets 936
Phentermine HCl Capsules 936
Phenylpropanolamine HCl &
  Guaifenesin Long-Acting
  Tablets 936
Prednisone Tablets 936
Prochlorperazine Maleate
  Tablets 936
Propranolol HCl and
  Hydrochlorothiazide Tablets 936
Propranolol HCl Tablets 936
Temazepam Capsules 936
Tolazamide Tablets 936
Trifluoperazine HCl Tablets 936

Other Products Available
Duratex Capsules
Iodur DM Liquid
Iodur Elixir Liquid
Iodur with Codeine Liquid

ELDER PHARMACEUTICALS, INC.   936
ICN Plaza
3300 Hyland Avenue
Costa Mesa, CA 92626
See ICN PHARMACEUTICALS, INC.

ELKINS-SINN, INC.   936
A subsidiary of A.H. Robins Company
2 Esterbrook Lane
Cherry Hill, NJ 08003-4099
                    (800) 257-8349
Address price and packaging
inquiries to:
Marketing Department
Address scientific information
inquiries to:
Professional Services Department
Products Described
Aminocaproic Acid Injection 936
Aminophylline Injection
  (Preservative-Free) 936
Ampicillin Sodium, Sterile
  (Preservative-Free) 936
Atropine Sulfate Injection 936
Bretylium Tosylate Injection
  (Preservative-Free) 936
Calcium Gluconate Injection 936
Chlorpromazine Hydrochloride
  Injection 936
Clindamycin Phosphate
  Injection 936
Codeine Phosphate Injection 936
Cyanocobalamin (Vit. B_{12})
  Injection 936
Cyclophosphamide for
  Injection (Preservative-Free) 936
Dexamethasone Sodium
  Phosphate Injection 936
Dextrose Injection 936
Diazepam Injection 936
Digoxin Injection 936
Diphenhydramine
  Hydrochloride Injection 936
Dopamine Hydrochloride
  Injection 936
Doxycycline Hyclate for
  Injection 936
Duramorph 937
Epinephrine Injection 936
Erythromycin Lactobionate for
  Injection 936
Fentanyl Citrate Injection
  (Preservative-Free) 936
Furosemide Injection
  (Preservative-Free) 936
Gentamicin Sulfate Injection 936
Heparin Sodium Injection 936
Hep-Lock (Heparin Lock Flush
  Solution) 936
Hep-Lock U/P
  (Preservative-Free Heparin
  Lock Flush Solution) 936
Hydromorphone
  Hydrochloride Injection 936
Hydroxyzine Hydrochloride
  Injection 936
Isoproterenol Hydrochloride
  Injection 936
Leucovorin Calcium for
  Injection (Preservative-Free) 936
Lidocaine Hydrochloride
  Injection 936
Lidocaine Hydrochloride
  Injection (Preservative-Free) 936
Lidocaine Hydrochloride &
  Epinephrine Injection 936
Meperidine Hydrochloride
  Injection 936
Methyldopate Hydrochloride
  Injection 936
Metronidazole Redi-Infusion
  (Preservative-Free) 936
Morphine Sulfate Injection 936
Naloxone Hydrochloride
  Injection 936
Neostigmine Methylsulfate
  Injection 936
Pancuronium Bromide
  Injection 936
Phenobarbital Sodium
  Injection 936
Phenylephrine Hydrochloride
  Injection 936
Phenytoin Sodium Injection 936
Procainamide Hydrochloride
  Injection 936
Prochlorperazine Edisylate
  Injection 936
Promethazine Hydrochloride
  Injection 936
Protamine Sulfate Injection
  (Preservative-Free) 936
Sodium Chloride Injection,
  Bacteriostatic 936
Sodium Chloride Injection
  (Preservative-Free) 936
Sodium Nitroprusside, Sterile 936
Sotradecol (Sodium
  Tetradecyl Sulfate Injection) 939

Sulfamethoxazole &
  Trimethoprim Concentrate
  for Injection 936
Thiamine Hydrochloride
  Injection 936
Vancomycin Hydrochloride,
  Sterile 936
Water For Injection,
  Bacteriostatic 936
Water for Injection, Sterile
  (Preservative-Free) 936
Other Products Available
Sterile Empty Vial

EVERETT LABORATORIES, INC.   939
76 Franklin Street
East Orange, NJ 07017
Address inquiries to:
Professional Service Department
                    (201) 674-8455
          FAX (201) 674-0933
Products Described
Florvite Chewable Tablets 0.5
  mg & 1 mg 939
Florvite Drops 0.25 mg & 0.5
  mg 939
Florvite + Iron Chewable
  Tablets 1 mg and 0.5 mg 939
Florvite + Iron Drops 0.25
  mg 939
Libidinal ZE Caps Soft Gel
  Capsules 940
Repan Tablets and Capsules 940
Strovite Plus Tablets 940
Tussafed Drops & Syrup 940
Vitafol Syrup 940
Vitafol Tablets 940
Other Products Available
Bemot Capsules 10 mg & Tablets 20
  mg
Hycort Cream & Ointment 1%
Pavatym 150 mg T.R. Capsules
Strovite Tablet

FERNDALE LABORATORIES, INC.   940
780 W. Eight Mile Road
Ferndale, MI 48220
Address inquiries to:
Professional Service Dept.
                    (313) 548-0900
                    (800) 621-6003
Products Described
Analpram-HC Rectal Cream 940
Kronofed-A Kronocaps 940
Kronofed-A-Jr. Kronocaps 940
Pramosone Cream, Lotion &
  Ointment 940
Prax Cream & Lotion 940
Other Products Available
Adphen Tablets
Aquaphyllin Syrup
Benase Tablets
Betuline Liniment
Dapa Tablets
Dapacin Capsules
Dapex 37.5 mg Capsules
Delaxin Tablets
Detachol Adhesive Remover
Fastamine Tablets
Liqui-Doss
Maigret-50 Tablets
Mastisol Liquid Adhesive
Obestin-30 Capsules
Oxychinol Tablets
Procute Cream & Lotion
Rhinocaps Capsules
Salatin Capsules
Strifon Forte DSC Tablets
Synabrom Capsules
Tin-Ben Dispenser
Tin-Co-Ben Dispenser
Tri-Pain Tablets
Vio-Pramosone Cream

FERRING LABORATORIES, INC.   941
75 Montebello Road
Suffern, NY 10901
Address inquires to:
                    (914) 368-2244
For Medical Emergencies Contact:
                    (914) 368-2244
Products Described
Secretin-Ferring 75 CU....................941

THE FIELDING COMPANY   941
2384 Centerline Industrial Drive
St. Louis, MO 63146
Address inquiries to:
Professional Services Dept.
                    (314) 567-5462
For Medical Emergencies Contact:
                    (314) 567-5462
Products Described
Gerimed Tablets..............................941
Irospan Capsules 941
Irospan Tablets 941
Lurline PMS Tablets 941
Metric 21 Tablets 941
Nestabs FA Tablets 941
Other Products Available
Duracid
Nestabs Tablets
Nestrex Tablets

FISONS CONSUMER HEALTH   941
PHARMACRAFT
Fisons Corporation
P.O. Box 1212
Rochester, NY 14603

Address inquiries to:
Professional Service Department
P.O. Box 1212
Rochester, NY 14603
(716) 475-9000
Products Described
Allerest Allergy Tablets .... ⊞
Allerest Children's Chewable
Tablets .... ⊞
Allerest Headache Strength
Tablets .... ⊞
Allerest 12 Hour Caplets .... ⊞
Allerest No Drowsiness
Tablets .... ⊞
Allerest Sinus Pain Formula .... ⊞
Americaine Hemorrhoidal
Ointment .... ⊞
Americaine Topical Anesthetic
Ointment .... ⊞
Americaine Topical Anesthetic
Spray .... ⊞
CaldeCORT Anti-Itch
Hydrocortisone Cream .... ⊞
CaldeCORT Anti-Itch
Hydrocortisone Spray .... ⊞
CaldeCORT Light Creme .... ⊞
Caldesene Medicated
Ointment .... ⊞
Caldesene Medicated Powder .... ⊞
Cruex Antifungal Powder,
Spray Powder & Cream .... ⊞
Desenex Antifungal Cream .... ⊞
Desenex Antifungal Foam .... ⊞
Desenex Antifungal Liquid .... ⊞
Desenex Antifungal Ointment .... ⊞
Desenex Antifungal Powder .... ⊞
Desenex Antifungal Spray
Powder .... ⊞
Desenex Foot & Sneaker
Spray .... ⊞
Desenex Soap .... ⊞
Sinarest No Drowsiness
Tablets .... ⊞
Sinarest Tablets & Extra
Strength Tablets .... ⊞

FISONS CORPORATION   **941**
PRESCRIPTION PRODUCTS
755 Jefferson Road
Rochester NY 14623
Address inquiries to:
Professional Services Department
(716) 475-9000
Distribution Centers
ATLANTA
James M. Hogan Co., Inc.
P.O. Box 1104
Tucker, GA 30084
(404) 938-7901
ROCHESTER
Fisons Corporation
P.O. Box 1710
Rochester, NY 14603
(716) 475-9000
(800) BUY FISN
LOS ANGELES
Obergfel Brothers
2660 East 37th Street
Vernon, CA 90058
(213) 583-8981
Products Described
Adapin Capsules *941*
Americaine Anesthetic
Lubricant *941*
Americaine Otic Topical
Anesthetic Ear Drops *942*
Biphetamine Capsules *941*
Ergomar Sublingual Tablets *941*
Hylorel Tablets *941*
Imferon *942*
Intal Capsules *944*
Intal Inhaler *944*
Ionamin Capsules *941*
K-Norm Capsules *941*
Kolyum Liquid and Powder *941*
Mykrox ½ mg Tablets *945*
Nasalcrom Nasal Solution *946*
Opticrom 4% *947*
Pediapred Oral Liquid *947*
Penntuss Suspension *949*
Somophyllin CRT Capsules *941*
Somophyllin DF Oral Liquid *941*
Somophyllin Oral Liquid *941*
Somophyllin Rectal Solution *941*
Somophyllin-T Capsules *941*
Tussionex Pennkinetic
Extended-Release
Suspension *949*
Zaroxolyn Tablets *941*

C. B. FLEET CO., INC.   **950**
4615 Murray Place
Lynchburg, VA 24502-2235
Address inquiries to:
Fran Clements   (804) 528-4000
Products Described
Fleet Babylax 950
Fleet Bisacodyl Enema 950
Fleet Children's Enema 950
Fleet Enema 950
Fleet Flavored Castor Oil
Emulsion 952
Fleet Mineral Oil Enema 951
Fleet Phospho-Soda 951
Fleet Prep Kits 951
Fleet Relief 952
Summer's Eve Medicated
Douche 952

FLEMING & COMPANY   **952**
1600 Fenpark Dr.
Fenton, MO 63026
Address inquiries to:
John J. Roth, M.D.   (314) 343-8200
Products Described
Aerolate Jr. T.D. Capsules 952
Aerolate Liquid 952
Aerolate Sr. T.D. Capsules 952
Aerolate III T.D. Capsules 952
Chlor-3 Condiment 952
Congess Jr. T.D. Capsules 953
Congess Sr. T.D. Capsules 953
Extendryl Chewable Tablets 953
Extendryl Sr. & Jr. T.D.
Capsules 953
Extendryl Syrup 953
Impregon Concentrate 953
Magonate Liquid 953
Magonate Tablets .... ⊞
Marblen Suspension
Peach/Apricot .... ⊞
Marblen Suspension
Unflavored .... ⊞
Marblen Tablets .... ⊞
Nephrocaps 953
Nephrox Suspension .... ⊞
Nicotinex Elixir .... ⊞
Ocean Nasal Mist .... ⊞
Ocean-A/S Nasal Spray 953
Pima Syrup 953
Purge Concentrate 953
Rum-K Syrup 953
S-P-T "Liquid" Capsules 953
Other Products Available
Alumadrine Tablets
Deter T.D. Capsules
Ectasule Minus III T.D. Capsules
Ectasule Minus Jr. T.D. Capsules
Ectasule Minus Sr. T.D. Capsules
Ectasule III T.D. Capsules
Ectasule Jr. T.D. Capsules
Ectasule Sr. T.D. Capsules
Ocean-Plus Mist

FLUORITAB CORPORATION   **954**
P.O. Box 507
Temperance, MI 48182-0507
Address inquiries to:
Keith Andres, President
(313) 847-3985
Products Described
Fluoritab Liquid 954
Fluoritab Tablets 954

FOREST LABORATORIES   **410**
150 East 58th Street
New York, NY 10155
**Address ordering and
product information to:**
INWOOD LABORATORIES
300 Prospect Street
Inwood, NY 11696
(718) 471-8000
See Inwood Laboratories for Theochron
Controlled Release Tablets

FOREST PHARMACEUTICALS,   **410, 954**
INC.
Subsidiary of FOREST LABORATORIES,
INC.
2510 Metro Blvd.
St. Louis, MO 63043
Address inquiries to:
Professional Services Department
(314) 569-3610
Products Described
◆ AeroBid Inhaler System 410, 954
◆ AeroChamber 410, 955
◆ AeroChamber with Mask 410, 956
Ambenyl Cough Syrup 957
Ambenyl-D Decongestant
Cough Formula 958
Antilirium Injectable 958
◆ Bancap HC Capsules 410, 958
Dalalone D.P. Injectable 959
Duraphyl Controlled Release
Tablets 961
Elixophyllin Dye-Free Capsules 961
Elixophyllin Elixir 961
Elixophyllin SR Capsules 961
Elixophyllin-GG Oral Solution 963
Elixophyllin-KI Elixir 965
◆ Esgic with Codeine Capsules .. 410, 966
◆ Esgic Tablets & Capsules 410, 965
Feostat Drops 968
Feostat Suspension 968
Feostat Tablets 968
Iodo-Niacin Tablets 968
Kay Ciel Oral Solution 10% 968
Kay Ciel Powder 968
Pedameth Capsules 968
Pedameth Liquid 968
Pyocidin-Otic Solution 968
Sus-Phrine Injection 968
◆ Tessalon Perles 410, 969
Other Products Available
Almora Tablets
Amonidrin Tablets
Anaids Tablets
Andro L.A. "200" Injectable
Andro "100" Injectable
Androgyn L.A. Injectable
Anergan "25" & "50" Injectable
Anodynos-DHC Tablets 100's
Arbon Plus Tablets
Arbon Tablets
Banalg Hospital Strength Arthritic Pain
Reliever
Banalg Liniment
Bancap Capsules
Banesin Tablets
Banflex Injectable
Beesix Injectable
Belfer Tablets
Betaprone Liquid
Biamine Injectable
Cebocap Capsules
Cetane Injection (w/o preservative)
Cetane Timed Capsules
Choron "10" Injectable Pak
Codroxomin Injectable
Conex DA Tablet
Conex Liquid
Conex Lozenges
Conex Plus Tablets
Conex c̄ Codeine Liquid
Cyomin Injectable
Dalalone Injectable
Dalalone L.A. Injectable
Dehist Capsules
Dehist Injectable
depAndro "100" & "200" Injectable
depAndrogyn Injectable
depGynogen Injectable
depMedalone "40" Injectable
depMedalone "80" Injectable
Diabismul Suspension
Diabismul Tablets
Disotate Injectable
Dommanate Injectable
Duradyne DHC Tablets
Duradyne Tablets
E Vitamin Ointment
E Vitamin Succinate Capsules
G.B.S. Tablets
Gesterol "50" Injectable
Gesterol L.A. "250" Injectable
Glycate Tablets
Gynogen Injectable
Gynogen L.A. "10", "20" & "40"
Injectable
Lidocaine 1% & 2% Injectable
Livroben Injectable
Magnesium Sulfate Injectable
Metra Tablets
N.B.P. Ointment
Nandrobolic Injectable
Neoquess Injectable
Neoquess Tablets
Niac Capsules
Paral Liquid
Predalone 50 Injectable
Predalone T.B.A. Injectable
Queltuss Tablets
Quiess Injectable
Rogenic Injectable
Rogenic Tablets
Solu-Eze Solvent
Triamolone "40" Injectable
Triamonide "40" Injectable
Verazinc Capsules

FUJISAWA SMITHKLINE   **969**
CORPORATION
401 City Avenue, Suite 300
Bala Cynwyd, PA 19004
For Medical Emergencies Contact:
Richard D. Leavitt, M.D.
(215) 751-6785
Products Described
Cefizox Injection 969
Vagistat 972

GEBAUER CHEMICAL COMPANY   **972**
9410 St. Catherine Avenue
Cleveland, OH 44104
Address inquiries to:
Denise Bodkin, Laboratory Manager
(800) 321-9348
OH (216) 271-5252
For Medical Emergencies Contact:
(800) 321-9348
OH (216) 271-5252
After Hours Emergency call:
Chemtrec   (800) 424-9300
Products Described
Ethyl Chloride, U.S.P. 972
Fluori-Methane 973
Fluro-Ethyl 973

GEIGY PHARMACEUTICALS   **410, 973**
Division of CIBA-GEIGY Corporation
Ardsley, NY 10502
Address inquiries to:
Medical Services Department
556 Morris Avenue
Summit, NJ 07901
(201) 277-5000
Warehouse Offices & Shipping Branches
Eastern
14 Henderson Drive
West Caldwell, NJ 07006
(201) 882-4700
Central
900 Corporate Grove Drive
Buffalo Grove, IL 60089
Buffalo Grove (312) 520-7770
Western
12850 Moore Street
P.O. Box 6300
Cerritos, CA 90701
Cerritos (213) 404-2651
Products Described
◆ Brethaire Inhaler 410, 974
◆ Brethancer Inhaler 410, 975
◆ Brethine Ampuls 410, 976
◆ Brethine Tablets 410, 976

◆ Butazolidin Capsules &
Tablets 410, 977
◆ Constant-T Tablets 410, 979
◆ Lamprene Capsules 410, 980
◆ Lioresal Tablets 410, 981
Lopressor Ampuls 982
◆ Lopressor HCT Tablets 410, 984
Lopressor Prefilled Syringes 982
◆ Lopressor Tablets 410, 982
Otrivin Nasal Solution 986
Otrivin Nasal Spray and Nasal
Drops 986
Otrivin Pediatric Nasal Drops 986
◆ PBZ Tablets & Elixir 410, 987
◆ PBZ-SR Tablets 410, 986
◆ Tegretol Chewable Tablets 410, 988
◆ Tegretol Suspension 410, 990
◆ Tegretol Tablets 410, 988
◆ Tofranil Ampuls 410, 992
◆ Tofranil Tablets 410, 993
◆ Tofranil-PM Capsules 410, 995
◆ Voltaren Tablets 410, 996

GENDERM CORPORATION   **998**
425 Huehl Road
Northbrook, IL 60062
Address inquiries to:
Professional Services Department
(312) 564-5435
Products Described
Occlusal 998
Occlusal-HP 999
Ovide Lotion 999
Pentrax Tar Shampoo with
Fractar 999
PrameGel 999
SalAc 999
Zostrix 1000
Other Products Available
A-Fil
Maxafil
Meted Shampoo
Packer's Pine Tar Shampoo
Packer's Pine Tar Soap
Texacort Scalp Solution

GENENTECH, INC.   **410, 1000**
460 Point San Bruno Blvd.
South San Francisco, CA 94080
(415) 266-1000
**For Medical Information,
24 Hours a Day**
Call: Professional Services Dept.
(800) 821-8590
(415) 266-1000
Or write:
Professional Services Dept.
Genentech, Inc.
460 Point San Bruno Blvd.
South San Francisco, CA 94080
Area Offices
WESTERN AREA OFFICE
6785 Telegraph Road, #330
Birmingham, MI 48010
(313) 647-2107
(313) 647-7830 (Panafax)
Western Area Manager:
Mr. Ed Jennings
EASTERN AREA OFFICE
19 Compo Road South
Westport, CT 06880
(203) 454-2625
(203) 454-7419 (Panafax)
Eastern Area Manager:
Mr. F. Ken Andrews
Products Described
◆ Activase 410, 1000
◆ Protropin 410, 1002

GENEVA GENERICS, INC.   **1003**
2599 West Midway Blvd.
Broomfield, CO 80020
Products Described
Acetaminophen/Codeine
Tablets *1003*
Allopurinol Tablets *1003*
Aminophylline Tablets *1003*
Amitriptyline HCl Tablets *1003*
Butalbital Compound Tablets *1003*
Carisoprodol and
Carisoprodol Compound
Tablets *1003*
Cefadroxil Capsules and Oral
Suspension *1003*
Cephalexin Capsules and
Suspension *1003*
Chlordiazepoxide HCl
Capsules *1003*
Chlorpheniramine Maleate
Capsules and Tablets *1003*
Chlorpromazine HCl Tablets
and Liquids *1003*
Chlorpropamide Tablets *1003*
Clonidine HCl Tablets *1003*
Conjugated Estrogens Tablets *1003*
Diazepam Tablets *1003*
Dicyclomine Capsules and
Tablets *1003*
Diphenhydramine HCl
Capsules *1003*
Dipyridamole Tablets *1003*
Doxepin HCl Capsules *1003*
Ergoloid Mesylates Tablets *1003*
Furosemide Tablets and Oral
Solution *1003*
H-H-R (Hydralazine
HCl/Hydrochlorothiazide/Re-
serpine) Tablets *1003*
Hydralazine Tablets *1003*

HOLLISTER-STIER   1052
See MILES INC.,
PHARMACEUTICAL DIVISION

HYLAND DIVISION   1052
Baxter Healthcare Corporation
444 W. Glenoaks Blvd.
Glendale, CA 91202-2936
   Address inquiries to:
Product Management
   (toll free) (800) 423-2090
   For Medical Emergencies Contact:
Medical Director,
Baxter Hyland Division
         (818) 956-3200
Coagulation Products Distributed By:
Baxter Hyland Division
Glendale, CA 91202
        (800) 423-2090
Plasma Extenders & Gamma Globulin
Products Distributed By:
Baxter Hyland Division
Glendale, CA 91202
        (800) 423-2090
   Products Described
Autoplex T, Anti-Inhibitor
  Coagulant Complex, Heat
  Treated *1052*
Buminate 5%, Albumin
  (Human), USP, 5% Solution *1052*
Buminate 25%, Albumin
  (Human), USP, 25%
  Solution *1052*
Hemofil M, Antihemophilic
  Factor (Human), Method M,
  Monoclonal Purified *1053*
Immune Globulin, Intravenous
  (Human), Gammagard *1052*
Proplex T, Factor IX Complex,
  Heat Treated *1053*
Protenate 5%, Plasma
  Protein Fraction (Human),
  USP, 5% Solution *1053*

HYNSON, WESTCOTT   1053
& DUNNING PRODUCTS
Becton Dickinson Microbiology Systems
Division of Becton Dickinson and
Company
P.O. Box 243
Cockeysville, MD 21030
        (800) 638-8663
   Products Described
BAL in Oil Ampules 1053
Lactinex Tablets & Granules .... ⬛
   Other Products Available
Cardio-Green Vials
Indigo Carmine Solution Ampules

ICI PHARMA   412, 1053
A business unit of ICI Americas Inc.
Wilmington, DE 19897 USA
   Address Pharmaceutical
   product-related inquiries to:
Yvonne Graham, Manager
  Professional Services
        (302) 886-2231
   For Medical Emergencies Contact:
After Hours or On Weekends, call
        (302) 886-3000
   Products Described
◆ Nolvadex Tablets 412, 1053
◆ Sorbitrate Chewable Tablets 412, 1055
◆ Sorbitrate Oral Tablets 412, 1055
◆ Sorbitrate Sublingual Tablets .. 412, 1055
◆ Sorbitrate Sustained Action
  Tablets 412, 1055
◆ Tenoretic Tablets 412, 1056
◆ Tenormin Tablets 412, 1058

ICN PHARMACEUTICALS,   412, 1060
INC.
ICN Plaza
3300 Hyland Avenue
Costa Mesa, CA 92626
   Address inquiries to:
Professional Service Dept.
        (800) 556-1937
    In CA (800) 331-2331
        (714) 545-0100
   Products Described
Android-5 Buccal 1060
Android-10 Tablets 1060
Android-25 Tablets 1060
Benoquin Cream 20% 1061
Eldopaque Forte 4% Cream 1061
Eldoquin Forte 4% Cream 1062
Fototar Cream 1062
Kato Potassium Supplement 1063
Lipo-Nicin/300 mg. Capsules 1063
Lipo-Nicin/100 mg. Tablets 1063
Lipo-Nicin/250 mg. Tablets 1063
Mestinon Injectable 1063
Mestinon Syrup 1064
Mestinon Tablets 1064
Mestinon Timespan Tablets 1064
Oxsoralen Lotion 1% 1065
◆ Oxsoralen-Ultra Capsule 412, 1065
Precef Injection 1068
Prostigmin Injectable 1070
Prostigmin Tablets 1071

Solaquin Forte 4% Cream 1071
Solaquin Forte 4% Gel 1072
Tensilon Injectable 1072
◆ Testred Capsules 412, 1073
◆ Trisoralen Tablets 412, 1075
Virazole 1075
   Other Products Available
Eldopaque 2% Cream
Eldoquin 2% Cream
Eldoquin 2% Lotion
RVP Ointment
RVPaba Lip Stick
RVPaque Ointment
Solaquin 2% Cream
Vitadye Lotion

INWOOD LABORATORIES   410, 1076
Subsidiary of Forest Laboratories
300 Prospect Street
Inwood, NY 11696
   Address inquiries to:
        (718) 471-8000
   Products Described
Carbamazepine Tablets 1076
Indomethacin E.R. Capsules 1076
Isosorbide Dinitrate E.R.
  Tablets 1076
Propranolol Hydrochloride
  E.R. Capsules 1076
◆ Theochron Controlled Release
  Tablets 410, 1076

JACOBUS PHARMACEUTICAL   1079
CO., INC.
37 Cleveland Lane
P.O. Box 5290
Princeton, NJ 08540
   Address inquiries to:
Professional Services
   For Medical Emergencies Contact:
Medical Department
        (609) 921-7447
   Products Described
Dapsone USP 1079

JAMOL LABORATORIES INC.   1080
13 Ackerman Avenue
Emerson, NJ 07630
   Address inquiries to:
        (201) 262-6363
   Products Described
Ponaris Nasal Mucosal
  Emollient 1080
   Other Products Available
Bahim Foot-Aide
Bahim Oil
Otide
Prep-Aide
Roma-Nol Antiseptic

JANSSEN PHARMACEUTICA   412, 1080
INC.
40 Kingsbridge Road
Piscataway, NJ 08854
        (201) 524-9591
   Address medical/pharmacy inquiries to:
Janssen Research Foundation
Department of Medical Affairs
        (800) 253-3682
After 5PM EST or on weekends:
        (800) 253-3682
   Products Described
◆ Alfenta Injection 412, 1080
◆ Hismanal Tablets 412, 1082
◆ Imodium Capsules 412, 1083
◆ Inapsine Injection 412, 1084
◆ Innovar Injection 412, 1085
◆ Monistat I.V. 412, 1086
◆ Nizoral 2% Cream 412, 1087
◆ Nizoral Tablets 412, 1088
◆ Sublimaze Injection 412, 1089
◆ Sufenta Injection 412, 1090
◆ Vermox Chewable Tablets 412, 1092

JOHNSON & JOHNSON PATIENT   1093
CARE, INC.
410 George Street
New Brunswick, NJ 08901-2023
        (800) 524-JJPC
   Products Described
Debrisan Wound Cleaning
  Beads 1093
Debrisan Wound Cleaning
  Paste 1093
Instat Collagen Absorbable
  Hemostat 1094
Surgicel Absorbable Hemostat 1094
Surgicel Nu-Knit Absorbable
  Hemostat 1094
Thrombin, Topical USP
  Thrombogen Spray Kit 1095
Thrombin, Topical USP
  Thrombogen Transfer
  Needle 1096

JOHNSON & JOHNSON   1097
PROFESSIONAL DIAGNOSTICS
INC.
Route 202
Raritan, NJ 08869
   Address inquiries to:
Customer Service Division
        (800) 932-0149
Products Manufactured by ORTHO
DIAGNOSTIC SYSTEMS, Raritan, NJ
08869
   Products Described
MICRhoGAM Rh₀(D) Immune
  Globulin (Human) 1097

RhoGAM Rh₀(D) Immune
  Globulin (Human) 1097

JONES MEDICAL INDUSTRIES,   1098
INC.
Corporate Offices and Distribution
11710 Lackland Industrial Drive
St. Louis, MO 63146
(314) 432-7557
   Manufacturing
119 Schroyer Avenue, S.W.
Canton, OH 44702
405 South Siesta Lane
Tempe, AZ 85281
   Products Described
Liqui-Char Unit-Dose
  Antidotes *1098*
Nico-400 Capsule *1098*
Therevac Plus Mini Enema *1098*
Therevac S.B. Mini Enema *1098*
Thyroid Strong Tablets *1098*
   Other Products Available
B-Plex Plus Injection
Bowman's Poison Antidote Kit
Cari-Tab Tablet
Decasone R.P. Injection
Duotrate Capsule
Duotrate 45 Capsule
Ivy-Chex Spray
KCL-20 Powder
Lano-Vera Lotion
Muslax Capsule
Obezine Tablets
Phentride Capsules
Quic-K Tablet
Superwestvite Tablet
T-Circ Capsule
T-Diet Capsule
T-Dry Capsule
T-Dry Jr. Capsule
T-Moist Tablet
Westhroid Tablets

KABIVITRUM, INC.   1099
160 Industrial Drive
Franklin, OH 45005
   Order Information for
   Pharmaceuticals:
        (800) 526-5224
   Product Information for
   Pharmaceuticals
        (800) 447-3846
KABIVITRUM, INC.
P.O. Box 597
Clayton, NC 27520
Order Information for Nutritional
  Products should be addressed to:
Clintec Nutrition Company
1425 Lake Cook Road
Deerfield, IL 60015
        (800) 422-2752 015
Order Information for Diagnostic
Product: (800) 526-5224
   Pharmaceutical Products Available
Cyklokapron Tablets and
  Injection *1099*
Kabikinase (Streptokinase) *1099*
   Nutritional Products Available
Aminess 5.2% Injection *1099*
Aminess Tablets *1099*
Intralipid 10% *1099*
Intralipid 20% *1099*
Novamine 11.4% Injection *1099*
Novamine 15% Injection *1099*
   Diagnostic Product Available
R-Gene 10 Injection *1099*

KENWOOD LABORATORIES   1099
a division of BRADLEY
PHARMACEUTICALS, INC.
383 Route 46 West
Fairfield, NJ 07006-2402
   Address inquiries to:
        (201) 882-1505
   Products Described
Apatate Liquid/Tablets *1099*
Bonacal Plus Tablets *1099*
Glutofac Tablets *1099*
I.L.X. B₁₂ Elixir Crystalline *1099*
I.L.X. B₁₂ Tablets Crystalline *1099*
I.L.X. Elixir *1099*
Ipsatol Expectorant Syrup *1099*
Ircon Tablets *1099*
Ircon-FA Tablets *1099*
Kenwood Therapeutic Liquid *1099*
Nitroglyn Sustained Release
  Capsules *1099*
Posterisan Hemorrhoidal
  Ointment/Suppositories *1099*
Tyzine Nasal Solution/Nasal
  Spray/Pediatric Nasal
  Drops *1099*

KEY PHARMACEUTICALS,   412, 1100
INC.
Galloping Hill Road
Kenilworth, NJ 07033
        (201) 298-4000
   Address inquiries to:
Professional Services Department
9:00 AM to 5:00 PM EST:
        (800) 526-4099
After regular hours and on weekends:
        (201) 298-4000

   Products Described
Genapax Tampons 1100
◆ K-Dur Microburst Release
  System (potassium
  chloride, USP) E.R. Tablets .. 412, 1100
◆ Nitro-Dur (nitroglycerin)
  Transdermal Infusion
  System 412, 1101
Quinora (quinidine sulfate
  tablets, USP) 1102
◆ Theo-Dur Sprinkle 412, 1106
◆ Theo-Dur Tablets 412, 1104
   Other Products Available
Diasorb Tablets/Liquid
Guanidine Hydrochloride Tablets

KNOLL PHARMACEUTICALS   413, 1108
A Unit of BASF K&F Corporation
30 North Jefferson Road
Whippany, NJ 07981
General Number   (201) 887-8300
Customer Service   (800) 526-0710
Medical Information   (800) 526-0221
        NJ (201) 428-8250
   Products Described
Akineton Injection 1108
◆ Akineton Tablets 413, 1108
◆ Collagenase Santyl Ointment .. 413, 1109
◆ Dilaudid Cough Syrup 1110
◆ Dilaudid Hydrochloride
  Ampules 413, 1109
Dilaudid Injection 1109
Dilaudid Multiple Dose Vials
  (Sterile Solution) 1109
Dilaudid Powder 1109
Dilaudid Rectal Suppositories 1109
◆ Dilaudid Tablets 413, 1109
◆ Dilaudid-HP Injection 413, 1111
◆ Isoptin Ampules 413, 1113
◆ Isoptin for Intravenous
  Injection 413, 1113
◆ Isoptin Oral Tablets 413, 1115
◆ Isoptin SR Sustained Release
  Tablets 413, 1117
◆ Quadrinal Tablets 413, 1119
◆ Vicodin Tablets 413, 1121
◆ Vicodin ES 413, 1122
   Other Products Available
Codeine Sulfate Tablets

KRAMER LABORATORIES INC.   1123
8778 S.W. 8th Street
Miami, FL 33174
   Address inquiries to:
8778 S.W. 8th Street
Miami, FL 33174   1 (800) 824-4894
   For Medical Emergencies Contact:
Professional Director
       1 (800) 824-4894
   Products Described
Charcoal Plus Tablets 1123
Fungi-Nail Tincture 1123
Yohimex Tablets 1123

KREMERS URBAN COMPANY   1124
See SCHWARZ PHARMA

LACTAID INC.   413, 1124
P.O. Box 111
Pleasantville, NJ 08232-0111
   Address inquiries to:
Alan E. Kligerman   (609) 653-6100
   Products Described
◆ Lactaid brand lactase enzyme
  caplets 413, 1124
◆ Lactaid brand lactase liquid
  enzyme drops 413, 1124

LAKESIDE   413, 1124
PHARMACEUTICALS
Division of Merrell Dow Pharmaceuticals
Inc.
2110 E. Galbraith Road
Cincinnati, OH 45215
   Address inquiries to:
Professional Information Department
Business hours only 9:00 AM to 4:30
PM EST)
        (800) 552-3656
For Medical Emergency Information
After hours or on weekends only,
        (513) 948-9111
   Products Described
◆ Bentyl 10 mg Capsules 413, 1124
Bentyl Injection 1124
Bentyl Syrup 1124
◆ Bentyl 20 mg Tablets 413, 1124
◆ Bricanyl Injection 413, 1126
◆ Bricanyl Tablets 413, 1126
Cepacol Anesthetic Lozenges
  (Troches) .... ⬛
Cepacol/Cepacol Mint
  Mouthwash/Gargle .... ⬛
Cepacol Throat Lozenges .... ⬛
CEPASTAT Cherry Flavor Sore
  Throat Lozenges .... ⬛
CEPASTAT Sore Throat
  Lozenges .... ⬛
◆ Nicorette 413, 1127
◆ Novafed A Capsules 413, 1130
◆ Novafed Capsules 413, 1130
◆ Novahistine DH 413, 1131
Novahistine DMX .... ⬛
Novahistine Elixir .... ⬛
◆ Novahistine Expectorant 413, 1131
Singlet Tablets .... ⬛
◆ Tenuate Dospan
  Controlled-release Tablets 413, 1132
◆ Tenuate Immediate-release
  Tablets 413, 1132

LANNETT COMPANY, INC.   **1133**
9000 State Road
Philadelphia, PA 19136
Address inquiries to:
Medical Service Dept.
(215) 333-9000
Products Described
Acnederm Lotion & Soap...................... ⊡
Codalan Tablets *1133*
Disonate Capsules, Liquid &
Syrup *1133*
Laniazid Tablets & Syrup *1133*
Magnatril Suspension &
Tablets .... ⊡
Quinalan Sustained Release
Tablets *1133*
Other Products Available
Acetazolamide Tablets
Adalan Lanatabs
Alphamul Suspension
Amtren Tablets
Arithmin Tablets
Baroflave Powder
Bellafedrol AH Tablets
Bethanechol Chloride Tablets
Bisacodyl Suppositories & Tablets
Brompheniramine Maleate Tablets
Castaderm
Chlorpromazine Tablets
Chlorulan Tablets
Dicalsonate Capsules
Diphenoxylate & Atropine Tablets
Disanthrol Capsules
Disolan Capsules
Efricon Expectorant
Glutethimide Tablets
Hydrochlorulan Tablets
Isoniazid Tablets & Syrup
Kaylixir
Lanacillin "400"
Lanahex Liquid
Lanamin Capsules
Lanatuss Expectorant
Lanorinal Capsules & Tablets
Lanvisone Cream
Lofene Tablets
Lycolan Elixir
Neocastaderm
Nitrofurantoin Tablets
Obalan Tablets
Orcophen Capsules
Paverolan Lanacaps
Potasalan Elixir
Primidone Tablets
Probenecid Tablets
Promethazine Syrup
Promethazine Tablets
Pyrralan Expectorant DM
Rufolex Capsules
S-A-C Tablets
Salatar Cream
Sedragesic Tablets
Trichlorex Tablets
Trichlormethiazide Tablets
Veltane Tablets & Expectorant

LASER, INC.   **1133**
2000 N. Main Street,
P.O. Box 905
Crown Point, IN 46307
Address inquiries to:
Donald A. Laser   (219) 663-1165
Products Described
Dallergy Capsules, Tablets,
Syrup *1133*
Dallergy-JR Capsules *1133*
Donatussin DC Syrup *1133*
Donatussin Drops *1133*
Lactocal-F Tablets *1133*
Respaire-SR Capsules 60,
120 .... *1133*
Theospan-SR Capsules 130
mg., 260 mg. *1133*
Theostat 80 Syrup *1133*
Trimstat Tablets *1133*
Other Products Available
Dallergy-D Capsules
Dallergy-D Syrup
Donatussin Syrup
Fumatinic Capsules
Fumerin Tablets
Kie Syrup

LEDERLE   **413, 1134, 2460**
LABORATORIES
Division of American Cyanamid Co.
One Cyanamid Plaza
Wayne, NJ 07470
LEDERLE PARENTERALS, INC.
Carolina, Puerto Rico 00630
LEDERLE PIPERACILLIN, INC.
Carolina, Puerto Rico 00630
*Address medical/pharmacy inquiries on
marketed products only to:*
Professional Services Department
Lederle Laboratories
Pearl River, NY 10965
During business hours (8 AM to 4:30
PM E.S.T.):
(914) 735-2815
All other inquiries and
after hours emergencies:
(914) 732-5000
Distribution Centers
ATLANTA
Contact EASTERN (Philadelphia)
Distribution Center

CHICAGO
Bulk Address
1100 E. Business Center Drive
Mt. Prospect, IL 60056
Mail Address
P.O. Box 7614
Mt. Prospect, IL 60056-7614
(800) 533-3753
(312) 827-8871
DALLAS
Bulk Address
7611 Carpenter Freeway
Dallas, TX 75247
Mail Address
P.O. Box 655731
Dallas, TX 76265   (800) 533-3753
(214) 631-2130
LOS ANGELES
Bulk Address
2300 S. Eastern Avenue
Los Angeles, CA 90040
Mail Address
T.A. Box 2202
Los Angeles, CA 90051   (800) 533-3753
(213) 726-1016
EASTERN (Philadelphia)
Bulk Address
202 Precision Drive
Horsham, PA 19044
Mail Address
P.O. Box 993
Horsham, PA 19044   (800) 533-3753
(215) 672-5400
Products Described
Acetaminophen Capsules,
Tablets, Liquid, Elixir *1134*
Acetaminophen w/Codeine
Tablets *1134*
Aches-N-Pain *1134*
◆ Achromycin V Capsules 413, *1137*
Achromycin Intramuscular *1135*
Achromycin Intravenous *1135*
Achromycin 3% Ointment *1138*
Achromycin Ophthalmic
Ointment 1% (See PDR for
Ophthalmology) *1138*
◆ Achromycin Ophthalmic
Suspension 1% (See PDR
For Ophthalmology) 413, *1137*
Achromycin V Oral
Suspension *1137*
Allopurinol Tablets *1134*
◆ Amicar Intravenous, Syrup &
Tablets 413, *1138*
Amiloride Hydrochlorothiazide
Tablets, USP *1134*
Amitriptyline HCl Tablets *1134*
Amoxicillin Capsules, Oral
Suspension *1134*
Ampicillin Trihydrate
Capsules, Oral Suspension *1134*
◆ Aristocort A Topical Cream 414, *1144*
◆ Aristocort A Topical Ointment 414, *1144*
◆ Aristocort Forte Parenteral 414, *1142*
◆ Aristocort Intralesional 414, *1142*
◆ Aristocort Syrup *1139*
◆ Aristocort Tablets 414, *1139*
◆ Aristocort Topical Cream 413, *1141*
◆ Aristocort Topical Ointment 413, *1141*
◆ Aristocort Topical Products...... 413, *1141*
◆ Aristo-Pak *414*
◆ Aristospan Suspension
(Intra-articular) 414, *1145*
◆ Aristospan Suspension
(Intralesional) 414, *1145*
◆ Artane Elixir 414, *1146*
◆ Artane Sequels 414, *1146*
◆ Artane Tablets 414, *1146*
◆ Asendin Tablets 414, *1147*
Aureomycin Ophthalmic
Ointment 1.0% *1134*
Benztropine Mesylate Tablets *1134*
◆ Caltrate 600 Tablets 414, *1149*
◆ Caltrate 600 + Iron 414, *1149*
◆ Caltrate, Jr. Tablets 414, *1149*
◆ Caltrate 600 + Vitamin D 414, *1149*
Carbamazepine Tablets *1134*
Centrum Tablets .... ⊡
Centrum, Jr. (Children's
Chewable) + Extra C .... ⊡
Centrum, Jr. (Children's
Chewable) + Extra Calcium ...... ⊡
Centrum, Jr. (Children's
Chewable) + Iron .... ⊡
Cephalexin Capsules, Tablets,
Oral Suspension *1134*
Cephradine Capsules *1134*
Chlordiazepoxide &
Amitriptyline HCl Tablets *1134*
Chlorpheniramine Maleate
Tablets & T.D. Capsules *1134*
Chlorpromazine HCl Liquid
Concentrate *1134*
Chlorpropamide Tablets *1134*
Chlorthalidone Tablets *1134*
Clindamycin Phosphate
Injection *1134*
Clonidine HCl Tablets *1134*
Clorazepate Dipotassium
Capsules, Tablets *1134*
Cloxacillin Sodium Capsules *1134*
◆ Cyclocort Cream 414, *1149*
◆ Cyclocort Lotion 414, *1149*
◆ Cyclocort Ointment 414, *1149*
◆ Declomycin Capsules and
Tablets 414, *1150*

Diamox Parenteral-See PDR
For Ophthalmology *1151*
◆ Diamox Sequels-Sustained
Release-See PDR For
Ophthalmology 414, *1151*
◆ Diamox Tablets-See PDR For
Ophthalmology 414, *1151*
Diazepam Injection, Tablets *1134*
Dicloxacillin Sodium Capsules *1134*
Dicyclomine HCl Capsules,
Tablets *1134*
Diphenhydramine HCl Cough
Syrup and Elixir *1134*
Diphenoxylate HCl 2.5 mg &
Atropine Sulfate 0.025 mg
Tablets *1134*
Diphtheria & Tetanus Toxoids,
Adsorbed Purogenated *1151*
Dipyridamole Tablets *1134*
Disopyramide Phosphate
Capsules *1134*
Divalproex Sodium
Enteric-Coated Tablets *1134*
Docusate Sodium (DSS)
Capsules, Syrup *1134*
Docusate Sodium (DSS)
w/Casanthranol Capsules,
Syrup *1134*
Dolene AP-65 Tablets *1134*
Dolene Propoxyphene HCl
Capsules *1134*
Doxepin HCl Capsules *1134*
Doxycycline Hyclate Capsules,
Tablets *1134*
Ergoloid Mesylates Oral
Tablets *1134*
Erythromycin Estolate Oral
Suspension *1134*
Erythromycin Ethylsuccinate
Oral Suspension & Tablets *1134*
Erythromycin Ethylsuccinate/
Sulfisoxazole Acetyl Oral
Suspension *1134*
Sterile Erythromycin
Lactobionate for Injection *1134*
Erythromycin Stearate Tablets *1134*
Fenoprofen Calcium Tablets.......... *1134*
◆ Ferro-Sequels 414, *1152*
Ferrous Gluconate Iron
Supplement Tablets *1134*
Ferrous Sulfate Elixir, Tablets *1134*
◆ FiberCon Tablets 414, *1153*
Filibon F.A. Prenatal Vitamin
Tablets *414*
◆ Filibon Forte Tablets *414*
◆ Filibon Prenatal Vitamin
Tablets *414*
Flu-Imune Influenza Virus
Vaccine *1153*
Flurazepam HCl Capsules *1134*
Furosemide Tablets *1134*
Gevrabon Liquid .... ⊡
Gevral T Tablets .... ⊡
Gevral Tablets .... ⊡
Guaifenesin w/D-Methorphan
Hydrobromide Syrup *1134*
Guaifenesin Syrup *1134*
Haloperidol Oral Solution,
Tablets *1134*
Hydralazine HCl Tablets *1134*
Hydrochlorothiazide Tablets *1134*
◆ Hydromox R Tablets 414, *1156*
◆ Hydromox Tablets 414, *1155*
Hydroxyzine HCl Tablets *1134*
Ibuprofen Tablets *1134*
Imipramine HCl Tablets *1134*
Incremin w/Iron Syrup .... ⊡
Indomethacin Capsules *1134*
Isosorbide Dinitrate S.A.
Tablets *1134*
Isosorbide Dinitrate Tablets *1134*
Ledercillin VK Oral Solution &
Tablets *1134*
Lederplex Capsules and
Liquid .... ⊡
◆ Leucovorin Calcium Injection .. 414, *1157*
◆ Leucovorin Calcium Tablets 414, *1158*
Levothyroxine Sodium Tablets *1134*
Lorazepam Tablets *1134*
◆ Loxitane C Oral Concentrate 414, *1159*
◆ Loxitane Capsules 414, *1159*
◆ Loxitane IM 414, *1159*
◆ Materna Tablets 414, *1161*
◆ Maxzide Tablets 415, *1161*
◆ Maxzide-25 MG Tablets 415, *1161*
Meclizine HCl Tablets *1134*
Meclofenamate Sodium
Capsules *1134*
Medroxyprogesterone Acetate
Tablets *1134*
Methenamine Mandelate
Suspension Forte *1134*
Methocarbamol Tablets *1134*
◆ Methotrexate Tablets,
Parenteral and LPF
Parenteral 415, *1163*
Methyclothiazide Tablets *1134*
Methyldopa &
Hydrochlorothiazide Tablets *1134*
Methyldopa Tablets *1134*
Metoclopramide HCl Tablets *1134*
Metronidazole Tablets *1134*
◆ Minocin Capsules 415, *1169*
◆ Minocin Intravenous 415, *1167*
Minocin Oral Suspension *1134*
◆ Minocin Tablets 415, *1169*
◆ Myambutol Tablets 415, *1170*
Neoloid Emulsified Castor Oil *1171*
Neomycin Sulfate Tablets *1134*

◆ Neptazane Tablets (See PDR
For Ophthalmology) 415, *1172*
◆ Nilstat for Preparation of Oral
Suspension *415*
◆ Nilstat Oral Suspension *415*
Nitrofurantoin Macrocrystals
Capsules *1134*
Nitroglycerin S.R. Capsules *1134*
◆ Novantrone 415, *1172*
Occucoat (See PDR For
Ophthalmology) *1173*
Orimune Poliovirus Vaccine,
Live Oral Trivalent *1173*
Papaverine HCl Tablets *1134*
Papaverine HCl T.R. Capsules *1134*
Peritinic Tablets *1175*
Perphenazine and
Amitriptyline HCl
Tablets *1134*
Phenobarbital Tablets *1134*
Phenytoin Sodium (Extended)
Capsules *1134*
◆ Pipracil 415, *1175*
Pnu-Imune 23 Pneumococcal
Vaccine Polyvalent *1178*
Potassium Chloride Extended
Release Tablets, Liquid,
Liquid Concentrate *1134*
Prazosin HCl Capsules *1134*
Prednisone Tablets *1134*
Probenecid with Colchicine
Tablets *1134*
Probenecid Tablets *1134*
Procainamide HCl Capsules *1134*
Procainamide HCl S.R.
Tablets *1134*
Promethazine HCl Syrup
w/Codeine *1134*
Promethazine HCl Syrup Plain *1134*
Promethazine HCl Syrup VC
w/Codeine *1134*
Promethazine HCl Syrup VC
Plain *1134*
Propoxyphene HCl Capsules *1134*
Propoxyphene HCl &
Acetaminophen Tablets *1134*
Propoxyphene Napsylate with
Acetaminophen Tablets *1134*
Propranolol HCl Tablets *1134*
Propylthiouracil Tablets *1134*
Pseudoephedrine HCl Syrup &
Tablets *1134*
Pyrazinamide Tablets *1134*
Quinidine Gluconate S.R.
Tablets *1134*
Quinidine Sulfate Tablets *1134*
Quinine Sulfate Capsules *1134*
Reserpine,
Hydrochlorothiazide &
Hydralazine HCl Tablets *1134*
◆ Rheumatrex Methotrexate
Dose Pack 415, *1163*
Spironolactone with
Hydrochlorothiazide Tablets *1134*
Spironolactone Tablets *1134*
Stresscaps Capsules .... ⊡
Stresstabs .... ⊡
Stresstabs + Iron, Advanced
Formula .... ⊡
Stresstabs + Zinc .... ⊡
Sulfamethoxazole &
Trimethoprim Pediatric
Suspension & Tablets *1134*
Sulfasalazine Tablets *1134*
Suprax 415, *1180*
Temazepam Capsules *1134*
Tetanus & Diphtheria Toxoids,
Adsorbed Purogenated *1182*
Tetanus Toxoid, Adsorbed
Purogenated *1183*
Tetanus Toxoid Purogenated *1185*
Theophylline Controlled
Release Tablets *1134*
Thioridazine HCl Tablets *1134*
◆ Thiotepa Parenteral 415, *1186*
Timolol Maleate Tablets *1134*
Tobramycin Sulfate Injection *1134*
Tolazamide Tablets *1134*
Tolbutamide Tablets *1134*
Trazodone HCl Tablets *1134*
Tri-Immunol Diphtheria &
Tetanus Toxoids &
Pertussis Vaccine,
Adsorbed *1187*
Triprolidine HCl with
Pseudoephedrine HCl Syrup
& Tablets *1134*
Tuberculin, Old, Tine Test *2460*
Tuberculin Purified Protein
Derivative Tine Test (PPD) *2460*
Vancoled *1134*
Verapamil HCl Tablets *1134*
Zincon Dandruff Shampoo .... ⊡
Other Products Available
Folvite Parenteral & Tablets
Nilstat Oral Tablets
Nilstat Topical Cream
Nilstat Topical Ointment
Nilstat Vaginal Tablets

LEEMING DIVISION   **1190**
Pfizer Inc.
100 Jefferson Rd.
Parsippany, NJ 07054
Address inquiries to:
Research and Development Dept.
(201) 887-2100

(◆ Shown in Product Identification Section)   *Italic Page Number* Indicates Brief Listing   (⊡ Described in PDR For Nonprescription Drugs)

Soda Mint Tablets
Sodium Bicarbonate Tablets
Sodium Chloride Vials, Enseals &
Tablets
Sodium Salicylate Enseals
Streptomycin Sulfate Vials
Sulfadiazine Tablets
Sulfapyridine Tablets
Sulfur Ointment
Surfadil Lotion
Tapazole Tablets
Terpin Hydrate & Codeine Elixir
Terpin Hydrate Elixir
Testosterone Propionate Vials
Theracebrin Pulvules
Thiamine Hydrochloride Ampoules,
Tablets, & Vials
Thyroid Enseals & Tablets
Trikates Oral Solution
Tubocurarine Chloride Vials
Tuinal Pulvules
V-Cillin K for Oral Solution & Tablets
Vitamin B Complex, Elixir & Pulvules
Vitamin C, Tablets
Vitamin D, Gelseals
Vitamin E, Gelseals
Whitfield's Ointment (Double Strength)
Wild Cherry Syrup
Zentinic Pulvules
Zentron Chewable Tablets
Zentron Liquid
Zinc Oxide Ointments
Zinc Oxide Paste Ointment

LUNSCO, INC. 1248
Route 2, Box 62
Pulaski, VA 24301
Address inquiries to:
(703) 980-4358
For Medical Emergencies Contact:
(703) 980-4358
Products Described
Appecon Capsules 1248
Dytuss 1248
Fetrin Capsules 1248
Hyco-Pap Capsules 1248
Pacaps Capsules 1248
Protid Tablets 1248

LYPHOMED, INC. 1248
10401 W. Touhy Ave.
Rosemont, IL 60018
(312) 390-6500
(800) 888-7704
Lyphomed Product Emergency Hotline
(312) 345-9746
NebuPent Hotline (800) 727-7003
*Address medical or scientific
inquiries to:*
Department of Professional Relations
Distribution Centers
ILLINOIS
10401 West Touhy
Rosemont, IL 60018
NEW JERSEY
47 Brunswick Lane
Edison, NJ 08817
CALIFORNIA
2660 East 37th Street
Vernon, CA 90058
TEXAS
1625 Vantage Way
Dallas, TX 75006
GEORGIA
5356 East Ponce de Leon Ave.
Stone Mountain, GA 30083
Products Described
NebuPent for Inhalation
Solution 1248
Pentam 300 1249
Other Products Available
Aminocaproic Acid 250mg/mL
Aminophylline Injection, USP, 25mg/mL
Amphotericin B for Injection, USP 50mg
Atropine Sulfate Injection, USP,
0.3/0.4/0.5/1.0mg per mL
B Complex Injection with Ascorbic Acid
+B₁₂- 10,000 units
Bretylium Tosylate 50mg/mL
Bristoject Emergency Syringe System
Aminophylline 25mg/mL
Atropine 0.5mg, 1mg
Calcium Chloride 10%
Dexamethasone Sodium Phosphate
4mg/mL
Dextrose 50%
Diphenhydramine 50mg
Dopamine 40mg/mL
Ephedrine 500mg
Epinephrine 1mg
Lidocaine 1, 2, 4%
Magnesium Sulfate 50%
Metaraminol Bitartrate 1%
Sodium Bicarbonate 4.2, 7.5, 8.4%
Calcium Chloride Injection, USP, 10%
Calcium Gluconate Injection, USP, 10%
Cefazolin Sodium for Injection, USP,
500mg, 1gm, 10gm, 20gm
Cephalothin Sodium for Injection, USP,
1gm, 2gm, 20gm
Cephapirin Sodium, USP, 1g, 2g, 20g
Chloramphenicol Sodium Succinate,
USP, 1 gm
Chorionic Gonadotropin for Injection,
USP, 5,000/10,000/20,000 USP
units

Chromic Chloride Injection, USP,
4mcg/mL
Clindamycin Phosphate
Cupric Sulfate Injection, USP,
0.4mg/mL
Cyanocobalamin Injection, USP,
100mcg/1,000mcg
Dacarbazine 100mg/200mg per vial
Dehydrated Alcohol Injection, USP, 1mL,
5mL
Dexamethasone Sodium Phosphate
Injection, USP, 4mg/mL, 10mg/mL
Dextrose Injection, USP, 50%
Diazepam Injection, USP, 10, 50mg
Diazoxide Injection, USP, 300mg
Dopamine HCl Injection, USP, 200, 400
& 800mg
Doxy-100 & Doxy-200 (Doxycycline
Hyclate for Injection, USP)
Droperidol Injection, USP, 5, 12.5, 25mg
Erythromycin Lactobionate Injection,
USP, 500mg/1,000mg per vial
Fluorouracil Injection, USP, 50mg/mL
Fluphenazine Decanoate Injection,
25mg/mL
Fluphenazine HCl Injection, USP,
2.5mg/mL
Folic Acid Injection, USP, 5mg/mL
Furosemide Injection, USP, 10mg/mL
Gentamicin Sulfate Injection, USP,
10mg/mL, 40mg/mL
Glycopyrrolate Injection, USP,
0.2mg/mL
Haloperidol Injection, USP, 5, 50mg/vial
Heparin Lock Flush Solution, USP,
100u/mL
Heparin Sodium Injection, USP,
1,000u/mL Preservative Free
Heparin Sodium Injection, USP,
1,000/5,000/10,000/20,000 units
per mL
Heparin Sodium Injection, USP (Beef
Lung Origin) 1,000, 10,000 units
per mL
HepFlush Kit (Heparin Lock Flush
Solution, USP, 10u/mL, 100u/mL
HepFlush-10 (Heparin Lock Flush
Solution, USP, 10u/mL)
Hydralazine HCl Injection, USP, 20mg
Hydrocortisone Sodium Succinate for
Injection, USP, 100, 250, 500 &
1,000mg
Hydroxyzine Hydrochloride Injection,
USP, 25mg/mL, 50mg/mL
I.V. Transfer Spikes
Iodopen (Sodium Iodide Injection)
100mcg/mL
Kanamycin Sulfate Injection, USP,
500mg/2mL, 1gm/3mL
Leucovorin Calcium Injection, USP
50mg
Levothyroxine Sodium for Injection,
200, 500mcg
Lidocaine Hydrochloride Injection, USP,
1%, 2%, 4%, 20%
Lyphocin (Vanomycin Hydrochloride
USP) 500mg, 1g, 5g
LyphoLyte & LyphoLyte-II
(Multielectrolyte Concentrate)
MTE-4 & MTE-4 Concentrated (Multiple
Trace Elements)
MTE-5 & MTE-5 Concentrated (Multiple
Trace Elements)
MTE-6 & MTE-6 Concentrated (Multiple
Trace Elements)
MTE 7 (Multiple Trace Elements)
MVC 9+3 and MVC 9+3 VitaGard
MVC 10+3 Pediatric
Magnesium Sulfate Injection, USP, 10%
& 50%
Manganese Sulfate Injection, USP,
0.1mg/mL
Mannitol Injection, USP, 25%
Maxifill Transfer Set
Metaraminol Bitartrate Injection 1%
Methotrexate Sodium for Injection, USP,
5, 50, 100, 200, 250mg/vial
Methyldopate Hydrochloride Injection
250, 500mg
Methylprednisolone Sodium Succinate
for Injection, USP, 40, 125, 500,
1000mg
Metoclopramide Injection 5mg/mL
Metronidazole Injection 500mg PB
Molypen (Ammonium Molybdate
Injection, USP) 25mcg/mL
Multilyte-20, -40 (Multi-Electrolyte
Concentrate)
Multivitamin Concentrate
Muri-Lube (mineral oil, sterile, light)
Nalbuphine Injection 10mg/mL,
20mg/mL
Naloxone Hydrochloride Injection, USP,
0.4, 0.02mg/mL
Nandrolone Decanoate Injection, USP,
100 mg/mL, 200mg/mL
Neostigmine Methylsulfate Injection,
USP, 1:1000, 1:2000
NeoTrace-4 (neonatal multiple trace
elements)
Nitroglycerin Injection 25, 50, 100mg
Oxytocin Injection, USP, Synthetic, 10
USP Units/mL
PTE-4 (pediatric multiple trace
elements)
PTE-5 (pediatric multiple trace
elements)
PedTrace-4 (pediatric multiple trace
elements)

Phenytoin Sodium Injection, USP,
50mg/mL
Potassium Acetate Injection, USP, 2,
4mEq/mL
Potassium Chloride Injection, USP, 2,
3mEq/mL
Potassium Phosphates Injection, USP,
3mM phosphate/mL
Procainamide Hydrochloride Injection,
100mg/mL, 500mg/mL
Protamine Sulfate Injection, USP, 50,
250mg
Pyridoxine Hydrochloride Injection, USP,
100mg/mL
Ritodrine HCl Injection, USP, 50,
150mg
Scopolamine Hydrobromide Injection,
USP, 0.3mg/mL, 0.4mg/mL,
1.0mg/mL
Selepen (Selenious Acid Injection)
40mcg/mL
Sodium Acetate Injection, USP, 2,
4mEq/mL
Sodium Bicarbonate Injection, USP,
4.2%, 7.5%, 8.4%
Sodium Chloride Injection, USP, 0.9%,
14.6%, 23.4%
Sodium Lactate Injection, USP 50mEq
Sodium Nitroprusside Injection, USP,
50mg
Sodium Phosphates Injection, USP,
3mM/phosphate/mL
Sodium Thiosulfate Injection, USP, 25%
Soyacal 10%, 20% (intravenous lipids)
Spark Kit (Systemic Pulmonary/Cardiac
Anaphylaxis Resuscitation Kit)
Sterile Empty Vials 5, 10, 30mL
Sterile Water for Injection, USP
Sulfamethoxazole & Trimethoprim for
Injection, USP 80mg, SMX, 16mg
TMP/mL)
Thiamine Hydrochloride Injection, USP,
100mg/mL
TraceLyte & TraceLyte-II (Trace
elements & electrolytes additive)
TraceLyte with Double Electrolytes &
TraceLyte-II with Double Electrolytes
Transfer Needles, thin wall, 19 gauge
Vasopressin Injection, USP, 10 units,
20 units
Verapamil Hydrochloride Injection 2.5
mg/mL
Vinblastine Sulfate Injection 10mg,
30mg
Vincristine Sulfate Injection, USP,
1mg/2mg/5mg per vial
Water (Bacteriostatic) for Injection, USP
Zinc Sulfate Injection, USP, 1, 5mg/mL

3M RIKER 415, 1250
3M HEALTH CARE
225-1S-07 3M Center
St. Paul, MN 55144
For Medical Information:
Write:
Medical Services Department
3M Riker
225-1N-07 3M Center
St. Paul, MN 55144
Call (612) 736-4930
For Medical Emergencies:
Call: (612) 736-4930 (all hours)
*Customer Service and
other services:*
Call: (800) 423-5197
(Outside of CA) (800) 423-5146
(CA Residents) (818) 341-1300
Products Described
Alu-Cap Capsules 1250
Alu-Tab Tablets 1250
Calcium Disodium Versenate
Injection 1250
◆ Disalcid Capsules 415, 1251
◆ Disalcid Tablets 415, 1251
Duo-Medihaler Aerosol 1252
◆ Maxair Inhaler 416, 1252
◆ Medihaler Ergotamine Aerosol 416, 1253
Medihaler-Epi Aerosol 1253
Medihaler-Iso Aerosol 1253
◆ Minitran Transdermal Delivery
System 416, 1253
◆ Norflex Injectable 416, 1254
◆ Norflex Sustained-Release
Tablets 416, 1254
◆ Norgesic Forte Tablets 416, 1254
◆ Norgesic Tablets 416, 1254
Tambocor Tablets 1255
Tepanil Tablets 1257
◆ Tepanil Ten-tab Tablets 416, 1257
Theolair Liquid 1257
◆ Theolair Tablets 416, 1257
◆ Theolair-SR Tablets 416, 1257
Urex Tablets 1257

MDR FITNESS CORPORATION 1258
5207 N.W. 163rd Street
Miami, FL 33014
Address inquiries to:
(800) MDR TABS
Or (800) 837-8227
Or (305) 624-4466
Products Described
M.D.R. High Performance
Tabs 1258
MDR Fitness Tabs for Men
and Women 1258

MACSIL, INC. 1258
1326 Frankford Avenue
Philadelphia, PA 19125
(215) 739-7300
Products Described
Balmex Baby Powder .... ⊞
Balmex Emollient Lotion .... ⊞
Balmex Ointment .... ⊞

MARION LABORATORIES, 416, 1258
INC.
Marion Park Drive
Kansas City, MO 64137
Address inquiries to:
Product Surveillance Dept.
P.O. Box 9627
Kansas City, MO 64134
(816) 966-5000
Products Described
◆ Carafate Tablets 416, 1258
◆ Cardizem 30-mg Tablets 416, 1259
◆ Cardizem 60-mg Tablets 416, 1259
◆ Cardizem 90-mg Tablets 416, 1259
◆ Cardizem 120-mg Tablets 416, 1259
◆ Cardizem SR
Capsules-60-mg, 90-mg
and 120-mg 416, 1260
◆ Debrox Drops 416, 1262
Ditropan Syrup 1262
◆ Ditropan Tablets 416, 1262
Enviclusive Semi-occlusive
Adhesive Film Dressing 1263
Envinet Nylon Net for Envisan
Treatment 1263
Envisan Wound Cleaning Pad 1263
Envisan Wound Cleaning
Paste 1264
◆ Gaviscon Antacid Tablets 416, 1265
◆ Gaviscon Extra Strength
Relief Formula Liquid
Antacid 416, 1265
◆ Gaviscon Extra Strength
Relief Formula Antacid
Tablets 416, 1265
◆ Gaviscon Liquid Antacid 416, 1265
◆ Gly-Oxide Liquid 416, 1265
Nitro-Bid IV 1266
Nitro-Bid Ointment 1267
◆ Nitro-Bid 2.5 Plateau Caps 416, 1266
◆ Nitro-Bid 6.5 Plateau Caps 416, 1266
◆ Nitro-Bid 9 Plateau Caps 416, 1266
◆ Os-Cal 500 Chewable Tablets 416, 1268
◆ Os-Cal 250+D Tablets 416, 1268
◆ Os-Cal 500+D Tablets 416, 1268
◆ Os-Cal Fortified Tablets 416, 1268
◆ Os-Cal Plus Tablets 416, 1269
◆ Os-Cal 500 Tablets 416, 1268
◆ Pavabid Capsules 416, 1269
◆ Pavabid HP Capsulets 416, 1269
◆ Silvadene Cream 1% 416, 1269
◆ Throat Discs Throat Lozenges 416, 1270

MARLYN HEALTH CARE 1270
6324 Ferris Square
San Diego, CA 92121
(619) 453-5600
Address inquiries to:
Professioinal Services Department
6324 Ferris Square
San Diego, CA 92121
Toll Free (800) 4 MARLYN
In CA call (619) 453-5600
Products Described
Hep-Forte Capsules 1270
Marlyn Formula 50 Capsules 1270
Marlyn Formula 50 Mega
Forte Capsules 1271
Pro-Hepatone Capsules 1271
Other Products Available
Albumin 500 Tablets
Daily Nutritional Paks
Care-4
Pro-Formance
Soft Stress
Marlyn PMS
Marlyn Daily Multi Vitamin-Mineral
Supplements
4-Hair
4-Nails
Family Vita Health
Hi-Vita
Kiddy Bees (children vitamins)
Marbec Tablets
Omega 3
Osteo-Fem
Royal Energy B-12
Vitamin E 400 IU
Vitamin E 1000 IU

MASON PHARMACEUTICALS, 416, 1271
INC.
5000 Birch, Suite 6100
Newport Beach, CA 92660
(714) 851-6860
Products Described
◆ Damason-P 416, 1271
◆ DuoCet 416, 1272

MATRIX TECHNOLOGIES, INC. 1273
1020 Bay Area Boulevard
Houston, TX 77058
Address inquiries to:
Gary Bell (800) 345-8912
For Medical Emergencies Contact:
Michael C. Trachtenberg, Ph.D.
(800) 345-8912
Products Described
Saave 1273
Tropamine 1273

MAYRAND, INC. 1274
P.O. Box 8869
4 Dundas Circle
Greensboro, NC 27419
(919) 292-5347
Products Described
B-A-C Tablets *1274*
Eldercaps *1274*
Eldertonic *1274*
May-Vita Elixir *1274*
Nu-Iron 150 Caps *1274*
Nu-Iron Elixir *1274*
Sedapap Tablets *1274*
Sterapred DS Unipak *1275*
Sterapred Unipak *1275*
Other Products Available
ACTH 40 & ACTH 80
Anamine Syrup
Anamine HD Syrup
Anamine T. D. Caps
Anatuss Tablets & Syrup
Anatuss with Codeine Syrup
Asproject
Becomject
Benoject-10
Benoject-50
Corgonject-5
Cyanoject
Decaject
Decaject-L.A.
Depoject-40 & Depoject-80
Dramoject
Estroject-2
Estroject-LA
Flexoject
Glytuss Tabs
Histaject
Kenaject-40
Lidoject-1 & Lidoject-2
Lifoject
Menoject-LA
Nu-Iron Plus Elixir
Nu-Iron-V Tablets
Phenoject-50
Predaject-50
Progestaject-50
Selestoject
Spasmoject
Sterapred DS 12 Day Unipak
Sulfa-Gyn
Testoject-50
Testoject-100 L.A. & Testoject-200 L.A.
Tiject-20
Trimtabs
Tristoject
Vistaject-25 & Vistaject-50

McGREGOR PHARMACEUTICALS 1275
INC.
32580 Grand River Avenue
Farmington, MI 48024
Address inquiries to:
Mr. Edward McGregor
(313) 474-8727
Products Described
Rhindecon Capsules *1275*
Rhinolar Capsules *1275*
Rhinolar-EX Capsules *1275*
Rhinolar-EX 12 Capsules *1275*

McNEIL CONSUMER 416, 1275
PRODUCTS CO.
Division of McNeil-PPC, Inc.
Camp Hill Road
Fort Washington, PA 19034
(215) 233-7000
Address inquiries to:
Consumer Affairs Department
Fort Washington, PA 19034
Manufacturing Divisions
Fort Washington, PA 19034
Southwest Manufacturing Plant
4001 N. I-35
Round Rock, TX 78664
Distribution Centers
Customer Service
Fort Washington, PA 19034
Camp Hill Road
Local Area   (215) 233-7000
Ontario, CA 91761
McNeil CPC
c/o Morgan & Sampson
(714) 923-2322
Montgomeryville, PA 18936
1390 Welsh Road (215) 641-1420
Products Described
◆ Delsym Cough Suppressant
   Syrup 417, 1275
◆ Imodium A-D Caplets and
   Liquid 417, 1275
◆ Medipren ibuprofen Caplets
   and Tablets 416, 1276
◆ Pediacare Cold Formula
   Liquid 417, 1276
◆ Pediacare Cough-Cold
   Formula Liquid and
   Chewable Tablets 417, 1276
◆ Pediacare Infants' Oral
   Decongestant Drops 417, 1276
◆ Pediacare Night Rest
   Cough-Cold Formula Liquid 417, 1276
◆ Sine-Aid Maximum Strength
   Sinus Headache Caplets 417, 1277

◆ Sine-Aid Maximum Strength
   Sinus Headache Tablets 417, 1277
◆ Tylenol acetaminophen
   Children's Chewable Tablets
   & Elixir 416, 1277
◆ Tylenol Allergy Sinus
   Medication, Maximum
   Strength, Caplets and
   Tablets 417, 1281
◆ Tylenol Cold Medication
   Caplets and Tablets 417, 1280
◆ Children's Tylenol Liquid Cold
   Formula and Chewable Cold
   Tablets 417, 1279
◆ Tylenol Cold Medication
   Liquid 417, 1280
◆ Tylenol Cold Medication No
   Drowsiness Formula Caplets 417, 1281
   Tylenol, Extra-Strength,
   acetaminophen Adult Liquid
   Pain Reliever 1279
   Tylenol, Extra-Strength,
   acetaminophen Caplets,
   Gelcaps, Tablets 416, 1278
   Tylenol, Infants' Drops 416, 1277
◆ Tylenol, Junior Strength,
   acetaminophen Coated
   Caplets 416, 1278
◆ Tylenol Sinus Medication,
   Maximum Strength, Tablets
   and Caplets 417, 1282
◆ Tylenol, Regular Strength,
   acetaminophen Tablets and
   Caplets 416, 1278

McNEIL PHARMACEUTICAL 417, 1282
McNEILAB, INC.
Spring House, PA 19477
Address inquiries to:
Medical Services Division
Spring House, PA 19477
Or call:
(800) 542-5365 (business hours)
For all other inquiries call:
(215) 628-5000
Manufacturing Affiliate
Dorado, Puerto Rico 00646
P.O. Box 710
Distribution Divisions
Burr Ridge, IL 60521
261 Shore Drive
Glendale, CA 91201
1220 Air Way
Montgomeryville, PA 18936
101 Park Drive
Products Described
◆ Haldol Decanoate Injection ... 417, 1284
◆ Haldol Injection, Tablets and
   Concentrate 417, 1282
◆ Haloperidol, see Haldol 417
◆ Pancrease 417, 1286
◆ Pancrease MT 417, 1286
   Paraflex Tablets 1287
◆ Parafon Forte DSC Caplets ... 417, 1287
◆ Tolectin (200, 400 and 600
   mg) 417, 1288
◆ Tolmetin Sodium, see Tolectin ...417
◆ Tylenol with Codeine
   Phosphate Elixir 417, 1289
◆ Tylenol with Codeine
   Phosphate Tablets 417, 1289
◆ Tylox Capsules 417, 1291
Other Products Available
Chlorzoxazone, see Paraflex

MEAD JOHNSON 417, 1292
LABORATORIES
A Bristol-Myers Company
2400 W. Lloyd Expressway
Evansville, IN 47721-0001
(812) 429-5000
Address inquiries to:
Scientific Information Section
Medical Department
Products Described
◆ Estrace 417, 1292
◆ Estrace Vaginal Cream 417, 1294
◆ Natalins Rx 417, 1297
◆ Natalins Tablets 417, 1297
◆ Ovcon 35 .... 417, 1297
◆ Ovcon 50 .... 417, 1297

MEAD JOHNSON NUTRITIONALS 1303
A Bristol-Myers Company
2400 W. Lloyd Expressway
Evansville, IN 47721-0001
(812) 429-5000
Address inquiries to:
Scientific Information Section
Medical Department
Products Described
Casec .... ▣
Ce-Vi-Sol .... ▣
Criticare HN .... ▣
Enfamil Concentrated Liquid,
   Powder, and Ready-To-Use ...... ▣
Enfamil w/Iron Concentrated
   Liquid, Powder and
   Ready-To-Use .... ▣
Enfamil Nursette .... ▣
Fer-In-Sol .... ▣
Isocal Complete Liquid Diet .... ▣
Isocal HCN .... ▣
Isocal HN .... ▣
Lonalac .... ▣
Lytren .... ▣
MCT Oil .... ▣

Nutramigen .... ▣
Poly-Vi-Flor 0.25 mg Vitamins
   with Fluoride Chewable
   Tablets 1303
Poly-Vi-Flor 0.5 mg Vitamins
   with Fluoride Chewable
   Tablets 1303
Poly-Vi-Flor 1.0 mg Vitamins
   with Fluoride Chewable
   Tablets 1303
Poly-Vi-Flor 0.25 mg Vitamins
   with Fluoride Drops 1304
Poly-Vi-Flor 0.5 mg Vitamins
   with Fluoride Drops 1304
Poly-Vi-Flor 0.25 mg Vitamins
   with Iron and Fluoride
   Chewable Tablets 1305
Poly-Vi-Flor 0.5 mg Vitamins
   with Iron and Fluoride
   Chewable Tablets 1305
Poly-Vi-Flor 1.0 mg Vitamins
   with Iron and Fluoride
   Chewable Tablets 1305
Poly-Vi-Flor 0.25 mg Vitamins
   with Iron and Fluoride
   Drops 1305
Poly-Vi-Flor 0.5 mg Vitamins
   with Iron and Fluoride
   Drops 1305
Poly-Vi-Sol Vitamins Chewable
   Tablets & Drops .... ▣
Poly-Vi-Sol Vitamins with Iron
   Chewable Tablets .... ▣
Poly-Vi-Sol Vitamins with Iron
   Drops .... ▣
Portagen .... ▣
Pregestimil .... ▣
ProSobee .... ▣
Sustacal HC .... ▣
Sustacal Liquid .... ▣
Sustacal Powder & Pudding .... ▣
Sustagen .... ▣
Tempra .... ▣
TraumaCal .... ▣
Trind .... ▣
Trind-DM .... ▣
Tri-Vi-Flor 1.0 mg Vitamins
   with Fluoride Chewable
   Tablets 1306
Tri-Vi-Flor 0.25 mg Vitamins
   with Fluoride Drops 1307
Tri-Vi-Flor 0.5 mg Vitamins
   with Fluoride Drops 1307
Tri-Vi-Flor 0.25 mg Vitamins
   with Iron and Fluoride
   Drops 1307
Tri-Vi-Sol Vitamins Drops .... ▣
Tri-Vi-Sol Vitamins w/Iron
   Drops .... ▣
Moducal
Other Products Available

MEAD JOHNSON 418, 1308
PHARMACEUTICALS
A Bristol-Myers Company
2400 W. Lloyd Expressway
Evansville, IN 47721-0001
(812) 429-5000
Address inquiries to:
Scientific Information Section
Medical Department
Products Described
◆ BuSpar 418, 1308
◆ Colace 418, 1310
◆ Desyrel and Desyrel Dividose .. 417, 1310
◆ Duricef 418, 1312
◆ Klotrix 418, 1313
◆ Peri-Colace 418, 1314

MEDICAL MARKET SPECIALTIES 1314
INC.
P.O. Box 150
Boonton, NJ 07005
Executive Offices   (201) 263-4243
Order Department   (201) 263-4243
After Hours   (201) 239-3915
Products Described
Proglycem Capsules 1314
Proglycem Suspension 1314

MEDICONE COMPANY 418, 1315
225 Varick St.
New York, NY 10014
Address inquiries to:
Professional Service Dept.
(212) 924-5166
Products Described
Medicone Derma Ointment .... ▣
◆ Medicone Derma-HC
   Ointment 418, 1315
Medicone Dressing Cream .... ▣
Medicone Rectal Ointment .... ▣
◆ Medicone Rectal
   Suppositories 418
Mediconet Cleansing Cloths .... ▣

MERCK SHARP & DOHME 418, 1316
Division of Merck & Co., Inc.
West Point, PA 19486
(215) 661-5000
For Product Information
Write: Professional Information
   West Point, PA 19486-9989
Call (215) 661-7300
Business hours only (8:30 a.m. to
   4:45 p.m. (EST)
Address other inquiries to:
Professional Services Department
West Point, PA 19486-9989

Branch Offices
Arlington, TX 76011
925-111th Street   (817) 640-5657
Atlanta Area:
   See Norcross, GA
Baltimore Area:
   see Columbia, MD
Boston Area:
   see Needham Heights, MA
Chicago Area:
   see Oak Brook, IL
Columbia, MD 21045
9199 Red Branch Rd.
(301) 730-8240
Columbus, OH 43228
4242 Janitrol Road
(614) 276-5308
Dallas/Ft. Worth Area:
   see Arlington, TX
Denver, CO 80216
4900 Jackson Street
(303) 355-1602
Kansas City Area:
   see Overland Park, KS
Kenner, LA 70062
1431 E. Airline Highway
(504) 464-0111
Los Angeles, CA 90040
6409 E. Gayhart Street
(213) 723-9661
Memphis, TN 38106
1980 Latham Street
(901) 948-8501
Minneapolis, MN 55441
12955 State Highway 55
(612) 559-4445
Needham Heights, MA 02194
40 A Street   (617) 444-5510
New Orleans Area:
   see Kenner, LA
New York Area:
   see Somerset, NJ
Norcross, GA 30071
2825 Northwoods Parkway
(404) 662-7200
Oak Brook, IL 60522
2010 Swift Drive   (312) 574-2160
Overland Park, KS 66215
9001 Quivira Rd.   (913) 888-1110
Portland, OR 97211
717 N.E. Lombard St.
(503) 285-2582
Somerset, NJ 08873
300 Franklin Square Drive
(201) 805-0300
Products Described
◆ Aldoclor Tablets 418, 1317
   Aldomet Ester HCl Injection 1321
   Aldomet Oral Suspension 1319
◆ Aldomet Tablets 418, 1319
◆ Aldoril Tablets 418, 1322
   Aminohippurate Sodium
   Injection 1325
   Antivenin (Black Widow
   Spider) 1325
   AquaMEPHYTON Injection 1326
   Aramine Injection 1327
   Attenuvax 1328
◆ Benemid Tablets 418, 1330
   Biavax ₌ 1331
◆ Blocadren Tablets 418, 1333
◆ Clinoril Tablets 418, 1335
   Cogentin Injection 1337
◆ Cogentin Tablets 418, 1337
◆ ColBENEMID Tablets 418, 1338
   Cortone Acetate Sterile
   Suspension 1339
◆ Cortone Acetate Tablets . 418, 1341
   Cosmegen Injection 1342
   Cuprid Capsules 1344
◆ Cuprimine Capsules 418, 1345
◆ Daranide Tablets 418, 1348
   Decaderm 0.1% Topical 1348
   Decadron Elixir 1349
   Decadron Phosphate Injection .. 1353
   Decadron Phosphate
   Respihaler 1358
   Decadron Phosphate Sterile
   Ophthalmic Ointment 1357
   Decadron Phosphate Sterile
   Ophthalmic Solution 1357
   Decadron Phosphate Topical
   Cream 1359
   Decadron Phosphate
   Turbinaire 1360
   Decadron Phosphate with
   Xylocaine Injection, Sterile ... 1355
◆ Decadron Tablets 418, 1351
   Decadron-LA Sterile
   Suspension 1361
   Decaspray Topical Aerosol 1363
◆ Demser Capsules 418, 1364
◆ Diupres Tablets 418, 1365
   Diuril Oral Suspension 1368
   Diuril Sodium Intravenous 1367
◆ Diuril Tablets 418, 1368
◆ Dolobid Tablets 418, 1369
   Edecrin Sodium Intravenous 1372
◆ Edecrin Tablets 418, 1372
◆ Elavil Injection 418, 1374
◆ Elavil Tablets 418, 1374
   Elspar 1375
◆ Flexeril Tablets 418, 1377
   Floropryl Sterile Ophthalmic
   Ointment 1378
   Hep-B-Gammagee 1379
   Heptavax-B 1380
   Humorsol Sterile Ophthalmic
   Solution 1382

MERICON INDUSTRIES, INC.   1465
8819 N. Pioneer Road
Peoria, IL 61615
Address inquiries to:
Thomas P. Morrissey
  (309) 693-2150
Products Described
Orazinc Capsules .... ⊞□
Orazinc Lozenges .... ⊞□

MERIEUX INSTITUTE, INC.   1465, 2462
P.O. Box 523980
Miami, FL 33152-3980
Address inquiries to:
P.O. Box 52-3980
Miami, FL 33152-3980
  (305) 593-9577
For Medical Emergencies Contact:
Merieux Institute, Inc.
  (800) 327-2842
  FL (305) 593-9577
Products Described
Imogam Rabies Immune
  Globulin (Human) 1465
Imovax Rabies I.D. 1465
Imovax Rabies Vaccine 1465
Mono-Vacc Test (O.T.) 1465
Multitest CMI Skin Test
  Antigens for Cellular
  Hypersensitivity 1466, 2462
Rabies Immune Globulin
  (Human), Imogam Rabies
  Vaccine 1465
Rabies Vaccine Human
  Diploid Cell, Imovax Rabies 1465
Rabies Vaccine Human
  Diploid Cell, Imovax Rabies
  I.D. 1465
Skin Test Antigens for
  Cellular Hypersensitivity,
  Multitest CMI 1466, 2462
Tuberculin, Mono-Vacc Test
  (O.T.) 2462

MERRELL DOW U.S.A.   419, 1466
Division of Merrell Dow Pharmaceuticals
Inc.
2110 E. Galbraith Road
Cincinnati, OH 45215
Address inquiries to:
Professional Information Department
Business hours only 9:00 AM to 4:30
PM EST
  (800) 552-3656

For Medical Emergency Information
After hours or on weekends only,
  (513) 948-9111
Products Described
AVC Cream 1466
AVC Suppositories 1466
◆ Cantil Tablets 419, 1466
◆ Cephulac Syrup 419, 1467
◆ Chronulac Syrup 419, 1468
◆ Clomid Tablets 419, *1469*
◆ Hiprex Tablets 419, 1469
◆ Lorelco Tablets 419, 1469
◆ Norpramin Tablets 419, 1471
◆ Quinamm Tablets 419, 1472
◆ Rifadin Capsules 419, 1473
  Rifadin I.V. 1473
◆ Rifamate Capsules 419, 1475
◆ Seldane Tablets 419, 1477
◆ TACE 12 mg Capsules 419, 1478
◆ TACE 25 mg Capsules 419, 1478
◆ TACE 72 mg Capsules 419, 1480
Other Products Available
Accurbron
DV Cream
Hesper Bitabs
Metahydrin
Metatensin

MILES INC.   1482
CONSUMER HEALTHCARE
DIVISION
1127 Myrtle Street
Elkhart, IN 46515
Address inquiries to:
Manager, Consumer Affairs Dept.
  (219) 264-8955
For Medical Emergencies Contact:
  (219) 264-8111
Products Described
Alka-Mints Chewable Antacid .... ⊞□
Alka-Seltzer Advanced
  Formula Effervescent
  Antacid & Non-Aspirin Pain
  Reliever .... ⊞□
Alka-Seltzer Effervescent
  Antacid....................................... 1484
Alka-Seltzer Effervescent
  Antacid and Pain Reliever 1482
Alka-Seltzer Extra Strength
  Effervescent Antacid and
  Pain Reliever 1484
Alka-Seltzer (Flavored)
  Effervescent Antacid and
  Pain Reliever 1483
Alka-Seltzer Plus Cold
  Medicine .... ⊞□
Alka-Seltzer Plus Night-Time
  Cold Medicine .... ⊞□
Bactine Antiseptic/Anesthetic
  First Aid Spray .... ⊞□
Bactine First Aid Antibiotic
  Ointment .... ⊞□
Bactine Hydrocortisone Skin
  Care Cream .... ⊞□
Biocal 500 mg Tablet
  Calcium Supplement .... ⊞□
Bugs Bunny Children's
  Chewable Vitamins +
  Minerals with Iron and
  Calcium (Sugar Free) .... ⊞□
Bugs Bunny Children's
  Chewable Vitamins (Sugar
  Free) .... ⊞□
Bugs Bunny With Extra C
  Children's Chewable
  Vitamins (Sugar Free) .... ⊞□
Bugs Bunny Plus Iron
  Children's Chewable
  Vitamins (Sugar Free) .... ⊞□
Flintstones Children's
  Chewable Vitamins .... ⊞□
Flintstones Children's
  Chewable Vitamins With
  Extra C .... ⊞□
Flintstones Children's
  Chewable Vitamins Plus
  Iron .... ⊞□
Flintstones Complete With
  Calcium, Iron & Minerals
  Children's Chewable
  Vitamins .... ⊞□
Miles Nervine Nighttime
  Sleep-Aid .... ⊞□
One-A-Day Essential Vitamins
  with Beta Carotene .... ⊞□
One-A-Day Maximum Formula
  Vitamins and Minerals with
  Beta Carotene .... ⊞□
One-A-Day Plus Extra C
  Vitamins with Beta
  Carotene .... ⊞□
One-A-Day Stressgard Stress
  Formula Vitamins with Beta
  Carotene .... ⊞□
One-A-Day Within Multivitamin
  for Women with Calcium,
  Extra Iron, Zinc and Beta
  Carotene .... ⊞□

MILES INC.   1485
CUTTER BIOLOGICAL
400 Morgan Lane
West Haven, CT 06516
Products Described
Alpha₁-Proteinase Inhibitor
  (Human) Prolastin 1488

Antihemophilic Factor
  (Human) Koāte-HS *1488*
Antihemophilic Factor
  (Human) Koāte-HT *1488*
Factor IX Complex Konȳne-HT *1488*
Hepatitis B Immune Globulin
  (Human) HyperHep *1486*
Immune Globulin (Human)
  Gamastan
Immune Globulin Intravenous
  (Human), Gamimune N 1485
Plague Vaccine *1488*
Rhₒ-D Immune Globulin
  (Human) HypRho-D *1487*
Rhₒ-D Immune Globulin
  (Human) HypRho-D
  Mini-Dose *1486*
Rabies Immune Globulin
  (Human) Hyperab *1486*
Tetanus Immune Globulin
  (Human) Hyper-Tet *1486*
Other Products Available
Albumin (Human) 5% Plasbumin-5
Albumin (Human) 25% Plasbumin-25
Plasma Protein Fraction (Human) 5%
  Plasmanate

MILES INC.   419, 1490
PHARMACEUTICAL DIVISION
400 Morgan Lane
West Haven, CT 06516
Address Inquiries to:
Director, Medical Services
  (800) 468-0894
  (203) 937-2000
Products Described
◆ Adalat Capsules (10 mg and
  20 mg) 419, 1490
  Ana-Kit Anaphylaxis
  Emergency Treatment Kit 1492
  Azlin 1493
◆ Biltricide 419, 1496
◆ Cipro Tablets 419, 1496
  DTIC-Dome 1499
◆ Decholin Tablets 419, 1499
◆ Domeboro Powder Packets,
  Effervescent Tablets 419, 1499
◆ Lithane Tablets 419, 1500
  Mezlin 1501
  Mezlin Pharmacy Bulk
  Package 1504
  Mithracin 1506
  Mycelex 1% Cream 1508
◆ Mycelex Troches 419, 1509
◆ Mycelex-G 1% Vaginal Cream 1510
◆ Mycelex-G 100 mg Vaginal
  Tablets 419, 1510
◆ Mycelex-G 500 mg Vaginal
  Tablets 419, 1510
◆ Niclocide Chewable Tablets .. 419, 1511
◆ Nimotop Capsules 419, 1512
  Otic Domeboro Solution 1513
  Otic Tridesilon Solution
  0.05% 1516
◆ Stilphostrol Tablets and
  Ampuls 419, 1513
  Tridesilon Creme 0.05% 1515
  Tridesilon Ointment 0.05% 1515
Other Products Available
Cort-Dome High Potency Suppositories
Cort-Dome ¼%, ½%, and 1% Creme
Cort-Dome ¼%, ½%, and 1% Lotion
Dome-Paste Bandage (Unna's Boot)
Domol Bath & Shower Oil
Mycelex 1% Solution
Mycelex Twin Pack
Neo Cort-Dome Creme

MILEX PRODUCTS, INC.   1517
5915 Northwest Highway
Chicago, IL 60631   (312) 631-6484
Shipping Offices
Milex Western
  Post Office Box 46305
  Los Angeles, CA 90046
  (213) 651-4301
Milex Puerto Rico
  GPO Box 554
  San Juan, PR 00936
  (809) 764-8602
Milex Hawaii
  Box 6337
  Honolulu, HI 96818
  (808) 422-9581
Milex Southeastern
  Post Office Drawer 4647
  Clearwater, FL 34618
  (813) 461-1949
Milex Southern
  Post Office Drawer "M"
  Weatherford, TX 76086
  (817) 599-7604
Milex Carolinas
  Post Office Box 23060
  Charlotte, NC 28212
  (704) 545-4567
Milex Delaware Valley
  350 White Horse Pike
  Atco, NJ 08004   (609) 767-4818
Products Described
Amino-Cerv 1517
Pro-Ception 1517
Other Products Available
Amniosac Finger Cot
Breast Biopsy Needle with Syringe
Breast Self-Examination Kit
Cannula Curette with Swivel Handle
Dilateria
Endometrial Suction Curettes

Fertility Cannula
Fertilo-Pak
Laminaria Japonica
Oligospermia Cups
Pessaries
Rectal Dilators (flexible)
Seminal Pouches
Shur-Seal Gel
Spatula
Spatula/Endo "C" Brush Combo
Tis-U-Trap
Trimo-San
Uterine Explora Curette
Vaginal Dilators (flexible)
Wide-Seal Diaphragm
Word Bartholin Gland Catheter

MINNETONKA MEDICAL   419, 1517
Minnetonka, Inc.
P.O. Box 1A
Minnetonka, MN 55343
Address inquiries to:
Minnetonka Medical
  (800) 328-5928
  (612) 448-4181
For Medical Emergencies Contact:
St. Paul Ramsey Poison Control
  (800) 228-5635
  (612) 221-2113
Products Described
◆ Trans-Plantar 419, 1517
◆ Trans-Ver-Sal 419, 1517

MISSION PHARMACAL COMPANY   1518
1325 E. Durango
San Antonio, TX 78210
Address inquiries to:
Professional Service Dept.
  (512) 533-7118
Post Office Box 1676
San Antonio, TX 78296
Products Described
Calcet 1518
Calcet Plus 1518
Calcibind *1519*
Citracal 1518
Citracal Liquitab 1518
Compete *1519*
Ferralet *1519*
Fosfree *1519*
Iromin-G *1519*
Lithostat *1519*
Medilax *1519*
Mission Prenatal 1520
Mission Prenatal F.A. 1520
Mission Prenatal H.P. 1520
Mission Prenatal RX 1520
Mission Surgical Supplement 1520
Prulet 1521
Supac 1521
Therabid 1521
Thera-Gesic 1521
Thiola Tablets 1520
Urocit-K 1520

MURO PHARMACEUTICAL, INC.   1521
890 East Street
Tewksbury, MA 01876-9987
Address inquiries to:
Professional Service Dept.
  1-(800) 225-0974
  (617) 851-5981
Products Described
Bromfed Capsules (Timed
  Release) 1521
Bromfed Syrup .... ⊞□
Bromfed Tablets 1521
Bromfed-DM Cough Syrup *1521*
Bromfed-PD Capsules (Timed
  Release) 1521
Guaifed Capsules (Timed
  Release) 1521
Guaifed-PD Capsules (Timed
  Release) 1521
IoTuss Liquid 1522
IoTuss-DM Liquid 1522
Liquid Pred Syrup 1522
Prelone Syrup 1522
Salinex Nasal Mist and Drops .... ⊞□

MYLAN PHARMACEUTICALS INC.   1522
781 Chestnut Ridge Road
P.O. Box 4310
Morgantown, WV 26505-4310
  (304) 599-2595
Address medical inquiries to:
Mr. Byron Witt
Quality Assurance Manager
  (304) 599-2595
Direct orders to:
Sales Department   (800) 82-MYLAN
Products Described
Allopurinol Tablets *1522*
Amitriptyline Hydrochloride
  Tablets *1522*
Amoxicillin Trihydrate
  Capsules & for Oral
  Suspension *1522*
Ampicillin Trihydrate Capsules
  & for Oral Suspension *1522*
Chlordiazepoxide &
  Amitriptyline Hydrochloride
  Tablets *1522*
Chlorothiazide Tablets *1522*
Chlorpropamide Tablets *1522*
Chlorthalidone Tablets *1522*

PORTON PRODUCTS, LTD. 1681
6625 Valjean Avenue
Van Nuys CA 91406
Address inquiries to:
Customer Services Department
(818) 989-5356
For Medical Emergencies Contact:
After business hours, during weekends
and holidays (818) 989-5393
Products Described
Hyate:C-Antihemophilic Factor
(Porcine) 1681

POYTHRESS LABORATORIES, 1682
INC.
16 N. 22nd St.
Post Office Box 26946
Richmond, VA 23261
(804) 644-8591
Address inquiries to:
Special Services Department
Products Described
Antrocol Tablets, Capsules &
Elixir 1682
Bensulfoid Tablets 1682
Mudrane GG Elixir 1682
Mudrane GG Tablets 1682
Mudrane GG-2 Tablets 1682
Mudrane Tablets 1682
Mudrane-2 Tablets 1682
Solfoton Tablets & Capsules 1682
Uro-Phosphate Tablets 1682

PRINCETON 422, 1682
PHARMACEUTICAL
PRODUCTS
(A Squibb Company)
P.O. Box 4500
Princeton, NJ 08543-4500
(609) 243-6000
Address inquiries to:
Squibb Professional Services Dept.
P.O. Box 4500
Princeton, NJ 08543-4500
(609) 243-6305
or (609) 243-6306
Adverse Drug Experience and Product
Defects Reporting During Business
Hours Only Call (201) 519-2020
Direct orders to:
E. R. Squibb and Sons, Inc.
(Local Distribution Center)
Products Described
◆ Corgard 422, 1682
◆ Corzide 422, 1684
Halog Cream, Ointment &
Solution 1686
Halog-E Cream 1686
◆ Naturetin Tablets 422, 1687
Prolixin Decanoate 1692
Prolixin Elixir 1691
Prolixin Enanthate 1694
Prolixin Injection 1688
Prolixin Oral Concentrate 1689
◆ Prolixin Tablets 422, 1691
◆ Pronestyl Capsules and
Tablets 422, 423,
Pronestyl Injection 1695
◆ Pronestyl-SR Tablets 423, 1699
◆ Raudixin Tablets 423, 1701
◆ Rauzide Tablets 423, 1702
Other Products Available
Vesprin Injection

PROCTER & GAMBLE 423, 1704
P.O. Box 171
Cincinnati, OH 45201
Also see Norwich Eaton
Pharmaceuticals, Inc. & Vicks Health
Care Products
Address inquiries to:
Arnold P. Austin (800) 358-8707
For Medical Emergencies Contact:
J. B. Lucas, M.D. (513) 530-3350
After Hours, call COLLECT
(513) 751-5525
Products Described
◆ Head & Shoulders 423, 1704
Metamucil Effervescent Sugar
Free, Lemon-Lime Flavor 1705
Metamucil Effervescent Sugar
Free, Orange Flavor 1706
Metamucil Powder, Orange
Flavor 1704
Metamucil Powder, Regular
Flavor 1704
Metamucil Powder,
Strawberry Flavor 1705
Metamucil Powder, Sugar
Free, Orange Flavor 1705
Metamucil Powder, Sugar
Free, Regular Flavor 1704
Maximum Strength
Pepto-Bismol Liquid 1706
Pepto-Bismol Liquid & Tablets 1706
Peridex 1706

THE PURDUE FREDERICK 423, 1707
COMPANY
100 Connecticut Avenue
Norwalk, CT 06856
(203) 853-0123
Address inquiries to:
Medical Department
Products Described
Betadine Cream 1707
Betadine Disposable
Medicated Douche 1708
Betadine Medicated Douche 1708

Betadine Medicated Gel 1708
Betadine Medicated Vaginal
Suppositories 1709
Betadine Ointment 1708
Betadine Skin Cleanser 1708
Betadine Solution 1708
Betadine Surgical Scrub 1708
◆ Cardioquin Tablets 423, 1709
Cerumenex Drops 1710
Fibermed High Fiber
Supplements 1710
Fibermed Miniatures 1710
◆ MS Contin Tablets 423, 1710
◆ MSIR Oral Solution 423, 1713
◆ MSIR Oral Solution
Concentrate 423, 1713
◆ MSIR Tablets 423, 1713
◆ Norzine Ampuls 423, 1714
◆ Norzine Tablets and
Suppositories 423, 1714
Senokot Granules 1715
Senokot Syrup 1715
Senokot Tablets 1715
SenokotXTRA Tablets 1715
Senokot-S Tablets 1716
◆ T-PHYL (Uniphyl) 200 mg
Tablets 423, 1716
Trilisate Liquid 1717
◆ Trilisate Tablets 423, 1717
◆ Uniphyl 400 mg Tablets 423, 1718
Other Products Available
Arthropan Liquid
Betadine Aerosol Spray
Betadine Antiseptic Gauze Pad
Betadine Antiseptic Lubricating Gel
Betadine Helafoam Solution
Betadine Medicated Douche Kit
Betadine Mouthwash/Gargle
Betadine Perineal Wash Concentrate Kit
Betadine Shampoo
Betadine Skin Cleanser Foam
Betadine Solution Swab Aid
Betadine Solution Swabsticks
Betadine Surgi-Prep Sponge-Brush
Betadine Viscous Formula Antiseptic
Gauze Pad
Betadine Whirlpool Concentrate
Phyllocontin
Senokot Suppositories
Senokot Tablets Unit Strip Pack

BLAIR LABORATORIES, INC.
Other Products Available
Calamatum Lotion
Calamatum Ointment
Calamatum Spray
Fungacetin Ointment
Gentlax B Granules
Gentlax S Tablets
Saratoga Ointment

QUAD PHARMACEUTICALS, INC. 1721
6340 LaPas Trail
Indianapolis, IN 46268
Address inquiries to:
Customer Service Department
(800) 222-6925
Products Described
Acetazolamide Sodium Sterile 1721
Acetylcysteine Solution 1721
Aminocaproic Acid Injection 1721
Aminohippurate Sodium
Injection 1721
Azathioprine Sodium 1721
B C G Vaccine 1721
Bacitracin Sterile 1721
Bethanechol Chloride Injection 1721
Caffeine Sodium Benzoate
Injection 1721
Chorionic Gonadotropin for
Injection 1721
Clindamycin Phosphate
Injection 1721
L-Cysteine Hydrochloride
Injection 1721
Cytarabine for Injection 1721
Dacarbazine for Injection 1721
Dexamethasone Sodium
Phosphate Injection 1721
Diazoxide Injection 1721
Droperidol Injection 1721
Estradiol Cypionate Injection 1721
Floxuridine Injection 1721
Floxuridine Sterile 1721
Fluorouracil Injection 1721
Fluphenazine Decanoate
Injection 1721
Fluphenazine Hydrochloride
Injection 1721
Glucagon for Injection 1721
Glycopyrrolate Injection 1721
Gold Sodium Thiomalate
Injection 1721
Haloperidol (as Lactate)
Injection 1721
Hydrocortisone Sodium
Phosphate Injection 1721
Hydroxyprogesterone
Caproate Injection 1721
Isoniazid Injection 1721
Kanamycin Sulfate Injection 1721
Ketamine Hydrochloride
Injection 1721
Leucovorin Calcium Injection
and Tablets 1721
Levothyroxine Sodium for
Injection 1721

Megestrol Acetate Tablets 1721
Metaproterenol Sulfate
Inhalation Solution 1721
Methotrexate Sodium Injection
and for Injection 1721
Methyldopate Hydrochloride
Injection 1721
Metoclopramide
Hydrochloride Injection 1721
Metocurine Iodide Injection 1721
Morrhuate Sodium Injection 1721
Nalbuphine Hydrochloride
Injection 1721
Naloxone Hydrochloride
Injection 1721
Neostigmine Methylsulfate
Injection 1721
Nitroglycerin Injection 1721
Pancuronium Bromide
Injection 1721
Phenylephrine Hydrochloride
Injection 1721
Physostigmine Salicylate 1721
Sterile Pralidoxime Chloride 1721
Procainamide Hydrochloride
Injection 1721
Prochlorperazine Edisylate
Injection 1721
Protamine Sulfate for
Injection 1721
Ritodrine Hydrochloride
Injection 1721
Sodium Iodide Injection 1721
Sodium Thiosulfate Injection 1721
Sulfamethoxazole &
Trimethoprim Concentrate
for Injection 1721
Testosterone Enanthate
Injection 1721
Trifluoperazine Hydrochloride
Injection 1721
Tubocurarine Chloride
Injection 1721
Vancomycin Hydrochloride
Sterile 1721
Vasopressin Injection 1721
Verapamil Hydrochloride
Injection 1721
Vinblastine Sulfate Injection 1721
Vincristine Sulfate Injection 1721
Other Products Available
Cyanide Antidote Package

RAM LABORATORIES 1722
CORPORATION
P. O. Box 559071
Miami, FL 33255
Address inquiries to:
In the United States
(305) 264-6620
In Puerto Rico (809) 792-2002
Products Described
Algisin Capsules 1722
Apetil Liquid 1722
Digepepsin Tablets 1722
Geroton Forte 1722
Hepacolin Capsules 1722
Neurochol Capsules 1722
Otisan Drops 1722
Pasmol Tablets 1722
Tricol Softgels 1722
Tusibron 1722
Tusibron-DM 1722
Zincvit Capsules 1722

REED & CARNRICK 423, 1722
1 New England Avenue
Piscataway, NJ 08855
Address inquiries to:
Professional Service Dept.
(201) 981-0070
Products Described
◆ Colyte 423, 1722
◆ Cortifoam 423, 1722
◆ Dilatrate-SR 423, 1723
◆ Epifoam 423, 1724
◆ Kwell Cream 423, 1725
◆ Kwell Lotion 423, 1726
◆ Kwell Shampoo 423, 1726
◆ Levatol 423, 1727
◆ Phazyme-125 Softgels
Maximum Strength 423, 1729
◆ Phazyme Tablets 423, 1729
◆ Phazyme-95 Tablets 423, 1729
◆ ProctoCream-HC 423, 1729
ProctoFoam/non-steroid 🅟🅓
◆ Proctofoam-HC 423, 1730
R&C Lice Treatment Kit 🅟🅓
R&C Shampoo 🅟🅓
R & C Spray III 🅟🅓
Other Products Available
Alphosyl Lotion, Cream
Proxigel
Trichotine Liquid, Vaginal Douche
Trichotine Powder, Vaginal Douche

REID-PROVIDENT LABORATORIES,
INC.
See REID-ROWELL

REID-ROWELL 423, 1731
901 Sawyer Road
Marietta, GA 30062
(404) 578-9000
Address inquiries to:
Laurence J. Downey, M.D.
(404) 578-9000
Orders may be placed by calling this
toll-free number: (800) 241-1643

Mail orders should be sent to:
Reid-Rowell
Order Entry Department
901 Sawyer Road
Marietta, GA 30062
Products Described
Balneol 🅟🅓
◆ Chenix 423, 1731
◆ Cortenema 423, 1733
◆ Creon Capsules 423, 1733
◆ Curretab Tablets 423, 1734
◆ Duphalac Syrup 424, 1734
◆ Estratab Tablets 0.3, 0.625,
1.25 and 2.5 424, 1735
◆ Estratest H.S. Tablets 424, 1738
◆ Estratest Tablets 424, 1738
Hydrocil Instant 🅟🅓
◆ Melfiat-105 Unicelles 424, 1741
P-V-Tussin Syrup 1741
P-V-Tussin Tablets 1741
◆ Proctocort 424
◆ Rowasa 424, 1741
◆ Zenate Tablets 424, 1743
Other Products Available
Cin-Quin
Colrex Compound Capsules
Compal Capsules
Dermacort Cream
Dermacort Lotion 1%
Dexone 0.5, 0.75, 1.5, 4
Histalet Forte Tablets
Histalet Syrup
Histalet X Syrup
Histalet X Tablets
Lithonate
Lithotabs
Multivitamins Rowell
Norlac RX
Orasone 1, 5, 10, 20, 50
Otoreid-HC Ear Drops
Procainamide SR 250, 500, 750
Tablets
Ru-Vert-M Tablets
Symadine Capsules
Unipres Tablets
Vio-Bec

RESEARCH INDUSTRIES 1743
CORPORATION
Pharmaceutical Division
1847 West 2300 South
Salt Lake City, UT 84119
Address inquiries to:
Medical Department
(800) 453-8432
(801) 972-5500
For Medical Emergencies Contact:
Medical Department
(800) 453-8432
(801) 972-5500
Products Described
Rimso-50 1743

RHONE-POULENC 1744
PHARMACEUTICALS
Division of Rhone-Poulenc, Inc.
117 Campus Drive
Princeton, NJ 08540
(609) 520-0880
Products Described
Nitrong Ointment 1744
Nitrong 2.6 mg. Tablets 1744
Nitrong 6.5 mg. Tablets 1744

RICHARDSON-VICKS INC 424, 1744
One Far Mill Crossing
Shelton, CT 06484
Address inquiries to:
Vicks Research Center
(203) 925-7610
For Medical Emergencies Contact
Medical Director
Vicks Research Center
(203) 925-7610
Products Described
Children's Chloraseptic
Lozenges 1744
Chloraseptic Liquid, Cherry,
Menthol or Cool Mint 1744
◆ Chloraseptic Liquid - Nitrogen
Propelled Spray 1744
Chloraseptic Lozenges, Cherry
or Menthol 1744
Chloraseptic Lozenges, Cool
Mint 1744
Dramamine Chewable Tablets 1745
Dramamine Liquid 1745
Dramamine Tablets 1745
Icy Hot Balm 🅟🅓
Icy Hot Cream 🅟🅓
Icy Hot Stick 🅟🅓
Percogesic Analgesic Tablets 1745
Vicks Children's Cough Syrup 🅟🅓
◆ Vicks Children's NyQuil 424, 1745
Vicks Cough Silencers Cough
Drops 🅟🅓
Vicks Daycare Colds Caplets 🅟🅓
Vicks Daycare Colds Liquid 🅟🅓
Vicks Formula 44 Cough
Control Discs 🅟🅓
Vicks Formula 44 Cough
Mixture 🅟🅓
Vicks Formula 44D
Decongestant Cough
Mixture 🅟🅓
Vicks Formula 44M
Multi-Symptom Cough
Mixture 🅟🅓
Vicks Inhaler 🅟🅓

(◆ Shown in Product Identification Section) *Italic Page Number* Indicates Brief Listing (🅟🅓 Described in PDR For Nonprescription Drugs)

Address inquiries to:
Squibb Professional Services Dept.
P.O. Box 4500
Princeton, NJ 08543-4500
(609) 243-6305
(609) 243-6306
Adverse Drug Experience and Product
Defects Reporting During Business
Hours Only Call (201) 519-2020
Squibb Diagnostics
P.O. Box 4500
Princeton, NJ 08543-4500
State of NJ Customers Call
(800) 582-5913
All others call (800) 257-5181

Distribution Centers
ATLANTA, GEORGIA
Post Office Box 16503
Atlanta, GA 30321
All Customers Call (800) 241-5364
CHICAGO, ILLINOIS
Post Office Box 788
Arlington Heights, IL 60006-0788
State of IL Customers Call
(800) 942-0674
All others call (800) 323-0665
IRVING, TEXAS
P.O. Box 152373
Irving, TX 75015
Mail or telephone orders and customer
service inquiries should be directed to
Atlanta, GA (see above)
All others call (800) 241-5364
LOS ANGELES, CALIFORNIA
Post Office Box 19618
Irvine, CA 92713-9618
State of CA Customers Call
(800) 422-4254
State of HI Customers Call
(714) 727-7200
All others call (800) 854-3050
SEATTLE, WASHINGTON
Mail or telephone orders and customer
service inquiries should be directed to
Los Angeles, CA (see above)
State of AK Customers Call
(714) 727-7200
State of CA Customers Call
(800) 422-4254
All others call (800) 854-3050
NEW YORK AREA
CN 5250
Princeton, NJ 08543-5250
State of NJ Customers Call
(800) 352-4865
All others call (800) 631-5244
For Radiopharmaceuticals call
(800) 447-6883
For listing of standard, purified, and
human insulins, see SQUIBB-NOVO, INC.

Products Described
Allopurinol Tablets 2124
Azactam for Injection 2124
Azactam Injection 2127
◆ Capoten 431, 2129
◆ Capozide 431, 2132
Cephalexin Capsules and for
Oral Suspension USP 2124
Chlorpropamide Tablets USP 2124
Chlorthalidone Tablets USP 2124
Clonidine Tablets 2124
Clorazepate Dipotassium
Tablets 2124
Cloxacillin Sodium Capsules
USP 2124
Diazepam Tablets USP 2124
Dicloxacillin Sodium Capsules
USP 2124
Doxycycline Hyclate Capsules
& Tablets USP 2124
Fenoprofen Calcium Tablets 2124
Fungizone Cream, Lotion and
Ointment 2135
Fungizone Intravenous 2135
Furosemide Tablets USP 2124
◆ Hydrea Capsules 431, 2137
Indomethacin Capsules USP &
Indomethacin Sustained
Release-Capsules 2124
Kenalog Cream, Lotion,
Ointment, Spray 2138
Kenalog-10 Injection 2141
Kenalog-40 Injection 2139
Kenalog in Orabase 2142
Lorazepam Tablets USP 2124
Loxapine Succinate Capsules 2124
Meclofenamate Capsules 2124
Methyldopa/Hydrochlorothi-
azide Tablets USP 2124
Methyldopa Tablets USP 2124
Metoclopramide
Hydrochloride Tablets USP 2124
Metronidazole Tablets USP 2124
Mycolog II Cream and
Ointment 2142
Mycostatin Cream, Ointment,
Topical Powder 2143
Mycostatin Oral Suspension 2143
◆ Mycostatin Oral Tablets 431, 2144
◆ Mycostatin Pastilles 431, 2144
◆ Mycostatin Vaginal Tablets 431, 2144
'Ora-Testryl'
(Fluoxymesterone) Tablets
USP 2124
Oxazepam Capsules USP 2124

Penicillin G Potassium for
Injection USP 2124
Penicillin G Sodium for
Injection USP 2124
Pentids for Syrup 2145
Pentids '400' for Syrup 2145
Pentids Tablets 2146
Pentids '400' & '800' Tablets 2146
Perphenazine & Amitriptyline
Hydrochloride Tablets 2124
Phenytoin Capsules 2124
◆ Principen Capsules '250' &
'500' 431, 2147
Principen for Oral Suspension
'125' & '250' 2147
Principen with Probenecid
Capsules 2148
Procainamide Hydrochloride
Sustained-Release Tablets 2124
Propranolol Hydrochloride
Tablets USP 2124
Quinidine Gluconate
Sustained-Release Tablets 2124
◆ Sumycin '250' & '500'
Capsules 432, 2149
Sumycin Syrup 2149
◆ Sumycin '250' and '500'
Tablets 432, 2149
Temazepam Capsules 2124
Teslac Tablets 2150
◆ Theragran Hematinic Tablets .. 432, 2151
Theragran Jr. Chewable
Tablets .... ▣
Theragran Jr. Chewable
Tablets with Extra Vitamin
C .... ▣
Theragran Jr. Chewable
Tablets with Iron .... ▣
Theragran Liquid .... ▣
Theragran Stress Formula .... ▣
Theragran Tablets .... ▣
Theragran-M Tablets .... ▣
Tolazamide Tablets USP 2124
Trazodone HCl Tablets 2124
Triamterene/Hydrochlorothi-
azide Tablets & Capsules 2124
◆ Trimox '250' & '500'
Capsules 432, 2152
Trimox 125 & 250 for Oral
Suspension 2152
Veetids '125' & '250' for
Oral Solution 2153
◆ Veetids '250' & '500' Tablets 432, 2153
◆ Velosef '250' & '500'
Capsules 432, 2155
Velosef for Injection 2156
◆ Velosef '125' & '250' for
Oral Suspension 2155

Other Products Available
Aspirin Tablets USP
B Complex Vitamin Tablets
Broxodent Automatic-Action Toothbrush
Calcium 500
Castor Oil USP
Cholografin Meglumine
Cholografin Meglumine for Infusion
Cod Liver Oil Capsules
Cod Liver Oil Plain & Mint Flavored
Cystografin
Cystografin Dilute
Deladumone
Deladumone OB
Delatestryl
Delestrogen
Diatrizoate Meglumine Injection USP
76%
Florinef Acetate Tablets
Follutein
Fungizone for Tissue Culture
Gastrografin
Iron and Vitamin C Tablets
Isovue 128
Isovue 200
Isovue 300
Isovue 370
Isovue-M 200
Isovue-M 300
Kenacort Diacetate Syrup
Kenacort Tablets
Kenalog-H Cream
Kinevac
Milk of Magnesia Liquid
Mineral Oil
Mycostatin Powder (for laboratory use)
Niacin Tablets USP
Nitrazine Paper
Noctec Capsules & Syrup
Nuclear Medicine Products
(Radiopharmaceuticals)
A-C-D Solution Modified
Choletec
Chromitope Sodium Diagnostic
Injection
Cobatope-57 Reference Standard
Solution
Hipputope I 131 Diagnostic Injection
Intrinsic Factor Concentrate Capsules
Iodotope I 131 Diagnostic Capsules
Iodotope I 131 Therapeutic Capsules
Iodotope I 131 Therapeutic Oral
Solution
MDP-Squibb
Macrotec
Minitec
Phosphotec

Rubratope-57 (Cyanocobalamin Co
57) Diagnostic Capsules
Rubratope-57 (Cyanocobalamin Co
57) Diagnostic Kit
Techneplex
Tesuloid
O-V Statin
Ophthaine Solution
Oragrafin Calcium Granules
Oragrafin Sodium Capsules
Renografin-60
Renografin-76
Reno-M-DIP
Reno-M-30
Reno-M-60
Renovist
Renovist II
Renovue-65
Renovue-DIP
SMZ-TMP Oral Solution
SMZ-TMP Tablets
Sinografin
Solution Administration Sets
Spec-T Sore Throat Anesthetic Lozenges
Spec-T Sore Throat/Cough Suppressant
Lozenges
Spec-T Sore Throat/Decongestant
Lozenges
Spectrocin Ointment
Suppositories, Glycerin, USP
Sweeta Liquid
Terfonyl Oral Suspension
Trigesic Tablets
Valadol Tablets, Liquid
Vigran Tablets
Vitamin C Tablets
Vitamin E Capsules
Zinc Oxide Ointment USP

SQUIBB DERM 2158
CN 5271
Princeton, NJ 08543-5271
Address inquiries to:
Professional Services
CN 5254
Princeton, NJ 08543-5254
(800) 422-8811
For Medical Emergencies Contact:
Professional Services
(800) 422-8811
Products Available
Fungizone Cream, Lotion and Ointment
Halog Cream, Ointment and Solution
Halog E Cream
Kenalog Cream, Lotion, Ointment and
Spray
Kenalog H-Cream
Mycolog II Cream and Ointment
Mycostatin Cream and Ointment
Mycostatin Topical Powder
Sumycin '250' and '500' Capsules
Sumycin '250' and '500' Tablets

See PRINCETON PHARMACEUTICAL
PRODUCTS and E.R. SQUIBB &
SONS, INC.

SQUIBB-NOVO, INC. 432, 2158
211 Carnegie Center
Princeton, NJ 08540-6213
Address inquiries to:
Professional Services
(609) 987-5800
For Medical Emergencies Contact:
Professional Services
(609) 987-5800
Products Described
Insulin Injection USP
(Regular) 2158
Lente Insulin 2158
Lente Purified Pork Insulin 2159
NPH Insulin (Isophane Insulin
Suspension USP) 2158
NPH Purified Pork Insulin 2159
◆ Novolin 70/30 .... 432, 2159
◆ Novolin L 432, 2159
◆ Novolin N 432, 2159
Novolin N PenFill 2159
Novolin 70/30 PenFill 2159
◆ Novolin R 432, 2159
Novolin R PenFill 2159
NovolinPen Assembly and
Injection 2160
NovolinPen (Dial-A-Dose
Insulin Delivery Device) 2160
NovoPen (Insulin Delivery Device).. 2160
PenNeedle Disposable Needle 2160
Regular Purified Pork Insulin
Injection 2158
Semilente Insulin 2158
Semilente Purified Pork
Insulin 2158
Ultralente Insulin 2158
Ultralente Purified Beef
Insulin 2159

STAR PHARMACEUTICALS, 432, 2163
INC.
1990 N.W. 44th Street
Pompano Beach, FL 33064-8712
Address inquiries to:
Scott L. Davidson, President
(305) 971-9704
Stellar Pharmacal Corp.
A Star Pharmaceutical Co.,
1990 N.W. 44th St.,
Pompano Beach, FL 33064-8712
FAX (305) 971-7718

For Medical Emergencies Contact:
Scott L. Davidson (305) 972-6060
Branch Office
Panamerican Pharmaceutical Inc.
Marina St., #300
P.O. Box 817
Aguada, PR 00602
Address inquiries to:
Luis Cardona, President
(809) 868-2415
Products Described
◆ Aphrodyne 432, 2163
Uro-KP-Neutral 2163
Urolene Blue 2163
◆ Virilon 432, 2163
◆ Virilon IM 432, 2163

STELLAR PHARMACAL 2163
CORPORATION
1990 N.W. 44th Street
Pompano Beach, FL 33064-8712

Address inquiries to:
Scott L. Davidson, President
(305) 972-6060
FAX (305) 971-7718
Branch Offices
Panamerican Pharmaceutical Inc.
Marina St., #300
P.O. Box 817
Aguada, PR 00602
(809) 868-2415

Products Described
Star-Otic Ear Solution .... ▣

STIEFEL LABORATORIES, INC. 2163
2801 Ponce de Leon Blvd.
Coral Gables, FL 33134
Address inquiries to:
Professional Services Department
(305) 443-3807
Branch Offices
GEORGIA
Post Office Box 47789
Doraville, GA 30362
(404) 455-1896
NEVADA
972 United Circle
Sparks, NV 89431
NEW YORK
Route 145
Oak Hill, NY 12460
(518) 239-6901
PUERTO RICO
P.O. Box 387
Mayaguez, PR 00708
(809) 832-1376
Products Described
Duofilm 2163
Duoplant 2163
LactiCare-HC Lotion, 1% 2163
LactiCare-HC Lotion, 2½% 2163
PanOxyl 5 Acne Gel 2164
PanOxyl 10 Acne Gel 2164
PanOxyl AQ 2½ Acne Gel 2164
PanOxyl AQ 5 Acne Gel 2164
PanOxyl AQ 10 Acne Gel 2164
Sulfoxyl Lotion Regular 2164
Sulfoxyl Lotion Strong 2164
Other Products Available
Acne-Aid Cleansing Bar
Acne-Aid Cream
Benoxyl-5 Lotion
Benoxyl-10 Lotion
Brasivol Base
Brasivol Fine
Brasivol Medium
Brasivol Rough
Epilyt Lotion
LactiCare Lotion
Lasan Ointment
Oilatum Soap (Scented)
Oilatum Soap (Unscented)
PanOxyl Bar 5
PanOxyl Bar 10
Polytar Bath
Polytar Shampoo
Polytar Soap
SFC Lotion
Salicylic Acid Soap
Salicylic Acid & Sulfur Soap
Saligel
Sarna Lotion
SAStid (AL)
SAStid (Plain)
SAStid Soap
Scabene Lotion
Scabene Shampoo
Sulfoxyl Lotion Regular
Sulfoxyl Lotion Strong
Sulfur Soap
Surfol Bath Oil
ZNP Bar
ZeaSORB Powder
ZeaSORB-AF Powder

STUART 432, 2164
PHARMACEUTICALS
A business unit of ICI Americas Inc.
Wilmington, DE 19897 USA
Address Pharmaceutical
product-related inquiries to:
Yvonne Graham, Manager
Professional Services
(302) 886-2231
FAX (302) 886-7895

For Medical Emergencies Contact:
After Hours or On Weekends, call
(302) 886-3000
Products Described
◆ ALternaGEL Liquid 432, 2164
◆ Bucladin-S Softab Chewable
   Tablets 432, 2164
◆ Cefotan 432, 2164
◆ Dialose Capsules 432, 2167
◆ Dialose Plus Capsules 432, 2167
◆ Effer-Syllium Natural Fiber
   Bulking Agent 432, 2167
◆ Ferancee Chewable Tablets 432, 2167
◆ Ferancee-HP Tablets 432, 2167
◆ Hibiclens Antimicrobial Skin
   Cleanser 432, 2167
◆ Hibiclens Sponge/Brush with
   Nail Cleaner 432
◆ Hibistat Germicidal Hand
   Rinse 432, 2168
◆ Hibistat Towelette 432, 2168
◆ Kasof Capsules 432, 2169
◆ Kinesed Tablets 432, 2169
◆ Mulvidren-F Softab Tablets 432, 2169
◆ Mylanta Liquid 432, 2170
◆ Mylanta Tablets 432, 2170
◆ Mylanta-II Liquid 432, 2170
◆ Mylanta-II Tablets 432, 2170
◆ Mylicon Drops 432, 2170
   Mylicon Tablets 2170
◆ Mylicon-80 Tablets 432, 2171
◆ Mylicon-125 Tablets 432, 2171
   Orexin Softab Tablets 2171
◆ Probec-T Tablets 432, 2171
◆ Stuart Prenatal Tablets 432, 2171
◆ The Stuart Formula Tablets 432, 2171
◆ Stuartinic Tablets 432, 2171
◆ Stuartnatal 1+1 Tablets 432, 2172
◆ Zestoretic 432, 2172
◆ Zestril Tablets 433, 2175

SUMMIT   433, 2178
PHARMACEUTICALS
Division of CIBA-Geigy Corporation
Summit, NJ 07901
  Address inquiries to:
Medical Services Department
556 Morris Avenue
Summit, NJ 07901
              (201) 277-5000
  Warehouse Offices and
    Shipping Branches
Eastern
14 Henderson Drive
West Caldwell, NJ 07006
              (201) 882-4700
Central
900 Corporate Grove Drive
Buffalo Grove, IL 60089
              (312) 520-7770
Western
12850 Moore Street, P.O. Box 6300
Cerrito, CA 90701
              (213) 404-2651
  Products Described
◆ Actigall Capsules 433, 2178
◆ Slow-K Tablets 433, 2179
◆ Ten-K Controlled-Release
   Tablets 433, 2180
◆ Transderm-Nitro Transdermal
   Therapeutic System 433, 2181

SWEEN CORPORATION   2183
1940 Commerce Drive
P.O. Box 8300
North Mankato, MN 56001
              (507) 345-6200
  Products Described
Atrac-Tain Moisturizing Cream 2183
Atrac-Tain Moisturizing Lotion 2183
Micro-Guard Cream 2183
Micro-Guard Powder 2183
Puri-Clens 2183
Sween Cream 2183
Sween Prep 2184
Sween-A-Peel 2183

SYNTEX (F.P.) INC.   433, 2184
Humacao, Puerto Rico 00661
  Address inquiries to:
Syntex Laboratories, Inc. (see below)

SYNTEX LABORATORIES,
INC.
3401 Hillview Ave.
P.O. Box 10850
Palo Alto, CA 94303
  Direct General/Sales/Order inquiries
    for U.S. marketed products to:
Marketing Information Department
(Specify product)   (415) 855-5050
  Direct Medical Inquiries on
    U.S. marketed products to:
Medical Information
Medical Services Department
  General Medical Inquiries
             (415) 855-5545
  Adverse Reaction Inquiries
             (415) 852-1386

SYNTEX PUERTO RICO, INC.
Humacao, Puerto Rico 00661
  Address Medical inquires to:
Syntex Laboratories, Inc. (see above)
  Products Described
◆ Anadrol-50 .... 433, 2184
◆ Anaprox and Anaprox DS
   Tablets 433, 2185
◆ Brevicon 21-Day Tablets 433, 2187
◆ Brevicon 28-Day Tablets 433, 2187

◆ Cardene 433, 2192
◆ Carmol 20 Cream .... ■□
◆ Carmol HC Cream 1% 2198
◆ Carmol 10 Lotion .... ■□
   Cytovene 2195
◆ Femstat Prefill Vaginal Cream
   2% 433, 2198
◆ Femstat Vaginal Cream 2% ... 433, 2197
   Lidex Cream 0.05% 2198
   Lidex Gel 0.05% 2198
   Lidex Ointment 0.05% 2198
   Lidex Topical Solution 0.05% 2198
   Lidex-E Cream 0.05% 2198
◆ Naprosyn Suspension 433, 2200
◆ Naprosyn Tablets 433, 2200
   Nasalide Nasal Solution
   0.025% 2202
   Neo-Synalar Cream 2198
◆ Norinyl 1+35 Tablets
   21-Day 433, 2187
◆ Norinyl 1+35 Tablets
   28-Day 433, 2187
◆ Norinyl 1+50 21-Day 433, 2187
◆ Norinyl 1+50 28-Day 433, 2187
◆ Nor-Q D Tablets 433, 2187
   Synacort Creams 1%, 2.5% 2198
   Synalar Creams 0.025%,
   0.01% 2198
   Synalar Ointment 0.025% 2198
   Synalar Topical Solution
   0.01% 2198
   Synalar-HP Cream 0.2% 2198
   Synemol Cream 0.025% 2198
◆ Tri-Norinyl 21-Day Tablets 433, 2187
◆ Tri-Norinyl 28-Day Tablets 433, 2187
◆ Wallette Pill Dispenser 433
  Other Products Available
Topic Gel

TAP PHARMACEUTICALS   2203
1401 Sheridan Road
North Chicago, IL 60064
  Address inquiries to:
Medical Dept.   1(800) 622-2011
  For Medical Emergencies Contact:
Medical Dept.   1(800) 622-2011
  Products Described
◆ Lupron Depot 2205
◆ Lupron Injection 2203

TOPPMED, INC.   2206
5015 Birch Street
Newport Beach, CA 92660
  Address inquiries to:
              (714) 752-7337
  Products Described
ToppFast 2206

TYSON and ASSOCIATES, INC.   2206
1661 Lincoln Blvd.
Suite 300
Santa Monica, CA 90404
  Address Inquiries to:
Professional Services Dept.
Call Collect within CA (213) 452-7844
            (800) 367-7744
  Products Described
Adenosine Triphosphate 2206
I-Alanine 2206
Alpha Plus Capsules 2206
Alphaketoglutaric Acid 2206
Aminolete Capsules 2206
Aminomine Capsules 2206
Aminoplex Capsules &
   Powder 2206
Aminosine Capsules 2206
Aminostasis Capsules &
   Powder 2206
Aminotate Capsules 2206
Aminoxin Tablets
   (Coenzymatic B₆) 2207
I-Arginine 2206
I-Aspartic Acid 2206
L-Carnitine Capsules 2207
Catemine 2207
L-Citrulline 2206
Complex-Cho 2207
L-Cysteine Mono HCl 2206
L-Cystine 2206
EFA Plus 2207
Endorphan 2207
Endorphenyl Capsules
   (d-Phenylalanine) 2207
L-Glutamic Acid 2206
L-Glutamine 2206
Glycine 2206
L-Histidine 2206
Iso-B 2207
L-Isoleucine 2206
L-Leucine 2206
L-Lysine 2206
MVM Capsules 2207
Maxovite Tablets 2207
L-Methionine 2206
Niaplus 2207
Nutrox 2207
L-Ornithine 2206
D-Phenylalanine 2206
L-Phenylalanine 2206
Proline 2206
Ribo-2 2207
Riboflavin 5' Phosphate 2206
L-Serine 2206
Taurine 2206
Thiamilate 2207
L-Threonine 2206
Threostat 2207
Trio-Dophilus 2207
I-Tryptophan 2206

Tryptoplex Capsules 2207
Trypto-Som 2207
L-Tyrosine 2206
UltraCholine (Phosphatide
   Complex) 2207
I-Valine 2206
  Other Products Available
GABA

UAD LABORATORIES, INC.   2207
8339 Highway 18
Jackson, MS 39209
  Address inquiries to:
Professional Services Department
             (601) 372-7773
  For Medical Emergencies Contact:
             (601) 372-7773
  Products Described
Bucet 2207
Lorcet Plus 2208
Lorcet-HD 2207
Zone-A Cream 1% 2208
Zone-A Lotion 1% 2208
  Other Products Available
Adbeon
Adlone 40 and 80
Cezin & Cezin-S
Desone & Desone-LA
Dital
E-Lor
Endafed
Endal
Endal Expectorant
Endal-HD
Enzone Cream 1%
Eudal-SR
UAD Cream & Cream Lotion
UAD Otic
UAD Pred
Vertab Capsules
Zone-A Forte

U. S. ETHICALS INC.
See RHONE-POULENC
PHARMACEUTICALS

U.S. PHARMACEUTICAL   2208
CORPORATION
2500 Park Central Blvd.
Decatur, GA 30035
             (404) 987-4745
  Mailing Address:
2500 Park Central Blvd.
Decatur, GA 30035
  Address inquiries to:
Raymond F. Meyer, R.Ph.
Marketing Director (404) 987-4745
  Products Described
Hemocyte Plus Tabules 2208
Hemocyte Tablets 2208
Hemocyte-F Tablets 2208
Isovex Capsules 2208
Magsal Tablets 2208
Medigesic Capsules/Tablets 2208

THE UPJOHN COMPANY   433, 2208
7000 Portage Road
Kalamazoo, MI 49001
             (616) 323-4000
  For Medical and Pharmaceutical
  Information, Including Emergencies
            (616) 329-8244
      or (616) 323-6615
  Address inquiries to:
Medical Information
The Upjohn Company
Kalamazoo, MI 49001
  Pharmaceutical Sales Areas
    and Distribution Centers
Atlanta (Chamblee),
  GA 30341-2626   (404) 451-4822
Boston (Wellesley), MA 02181
            (617) 431-7970
Buffalo (Amherst),
  NY 14221   (716) 632-5942
Chicago (Oak Brook Terrace),
  IL 60181   (312) 574-3300
Cincinnati, OH 45202
            (513) 723-1010
Dallas (Irving), TX 57062
            (214) 256-0022
Denver, CO 80216
            (303) 399-3113
Hartford (Enfield),
  CT 06082   (203) 741-3421
Honolulu, HI 96818
            (808) 422-2777
Kalamazoo, MI 49001
            (616) 323-4000
Kansas City, MO 64131
            (816) 361-2286
Los Angeles, CA 90038
            (213) 463-8101
Memphis, TN 38119
            (901) 685-8192
Minneapolis, MN 55422
            (612) 921-8484
New York (Uniondale),
  NY 11553   (516) 745-6100
Orlando, FL 32809
            (407) 859-4591
Philadelphia (Berwyn),
  PA 19312   (215) 993-0100
Pittsburgh, (Bridgeville),
  PA 15017   (412) 257-0200
Portland, OR 97232
            (503) 232-2133
St. Louis, MO 63146
            (314) 872-8626

San Francisco (Palo Alto),
  CA 94306-2117 (415) 493-8080
Shreveport, LA 71129
            (318) 688-3700
Washington, DC 20011
            (202) 882-6163
  Products Described
◆ Adeflor Chewable Tablets 433, 2209
   Adeflor Drops 2209
   Ansaid Tablets 433, 2209
   Baciguent Antibiotic Ointment .... ■□
   Cheracol D Cough Formula .... ■□
   Cheracol Plus Head
   Cold/Cough Formula .... ■□
   Citrocarbonate Antacid .... ■□
◆ Cleocin HCl Capsules 433, 2211
   Cleocin Pediatric Flavored
   Granules 2212
◆ Cleocin Phosphate Sterile
   Solution 433, 2213
◆ Cleocin T Topical Gel 433, 2216
◆ Cleocin T Topical Lotion 433, 2216
◆ Cleocin T Topical Solution 433, 2216
◆ Colestid Granules 433, 2216
   Cortaid Cream with Aloe .... ■□
   Cortaid Lotion .... ■□
   Cortaid Ointment with Aloe .... ■□
   Cortaid Spray .... ■□
   Cortef Feminine Itch Cream .... ■□
◆ Cytosar-U Sterile Powder 2218
◆ Deltasone Tablets 433, 2220
◆ Depo-Medrol Sterile Aqueous
   Suspension 433, 2220
   Depo-Provera Sterile Aqueous
   Suspension 2223
   DEPO-Testosterone Sterile
   Solution 2224
◆ Didrex Tablets 433, 2224
   Gelfoam Sterile Powder 2226
   Gelfoam Sterile Sponge 2225
◆ Halcion Tablets 433, 2226
◆ Halotestin Tablets 434, 2228
   Haltran Tablets .... ■□
   Heparin Sodium Injection,
   USP, Sterile Solution 2229
   Kaopectate Concentrated
   Anti-Diarrheal, Peppermint
   Flavor .... ■□
   Kaopectate Concentrated
   Anti-Diarrheal, Regular
   Flavor .... ■□
   Maximum Strength
   Kaopectate Tablets
   Anti-Diarrhea Medicine .... ■□
   Lincocin Capsules 2231
   Lincocin Pediatric Capsules 2231
   Lincocin Sterile Solution 2231
◆ Loniten Tablets 434, 2232
◆ Maolate Tablets 434, 2234
   Medrol Acetate Topical 2234
◆ Medrol Dosepak Unit of Use 434, 2234
◆ Medrol Tablets 434, 2234
◆ Micronase Tablets 434, 2236
◆ Motrin Tablets 434, 2238
   Motrin IB Tablets and Caplets .... ■□
   Myciguent Antibiotic Ointment .... ■□
   Mycitracin Triple Antibiotic
   Ointment .... ■□
◆ Orinase Tablets 434, 2240
   Pamine Tablets 2242
   Prostin VR Pediatric Sterile
   Solution 2242
◆ Provera Tablets 434, 2243
   Pyrroxate Capsules .... ■□
◆ Rogaine Topical Solution 434, 2244
   Sigtab Tablets .... ■□
   Solu-Cortef Sterile Powder 2247
◆ Solu-Medrol Act-O-Vial & Vials 434
◆ Solu-Medrol Sterile Powder 434, 2249
◆ Tolinase Tablets 434, 2250
   Trobicin Sterile Powder 2252
   Unicap Capsules & Tablets .... ■□
   Unicap Jr Chewable Tablets .... ■□
   Unicap M Tablets .... ■□
   Unicap Plus Iron Tablets .... ■□
   Unicap Sr. Tablets .... ■□
   Unicap T Tablets .... ■□
◆ Xanax Tablets 434, 2253
  Other Products Available
Adeflor M Tablets
Albamycin Capsules
Alkets Tablets
Atgam Sterile Solution
Bacitracin, USP, Sterile Powder
Calcium Chloride Injection, USP, Sterile
   Solution
Calcium Gluconate Injection, USP,
   Sterile Solution
Calcium Gluconate Tablets, USP
Calcium Lactate Tablets, USP
Cheracol Cough Syrup
Clocream Skin Cream
Cortef Acetate Ointment
Cortef Oral Suspension
Cortef Tablets
Cortisone Acetate Tablets, USP
Delta-Cortef Tablets
Depo-Estradiol Sterile Solution
Depo-Testadiol Sterile Solution
Diostate D Tablets
Erythromycin, USP (See E-Mycin)
Feminone Tablets
Gelfilm Sterile Film
Gelfilm Sterile Ophthalmic Film
Gelfoam Dental Packs
Gelfoam Packs
Gelfoam Prostatectomy Cones
Gelfoam Sterile Compressed Sponge
Halodrin Tablets

(◆ Shown in Product Identification Section)   *Italic Page Number* **Indicates Brief Listing**   (■□ Described in PDR For Nonprescription Drugs)

PreSun 15 Lotion Sunscreen 2287
PreSun 8, 15 and 39 Creamy
　　Sunscreens 2287
PreSun 15 and 29 Sensitive
　　Skin Sunscreen 2288
Sebulex Shampoo 2288
Sebulex Shampoo with
　　Conditioners 2288
Sebutone and Sebutone
　　Cream Shampoos 2288
T-Stat (erythromycin) 2.0%
　　Topical Solution and Pads 2289
◆ Tacaryl Chewable Tablets........ 435, 2288
◆ Tacaryl Syrup & Tablets 435, 2288
Westcort Cream 0.2% 2289
Westcort Ointment 0.2% 2289

WHARTON LABORATORIES INC
See RHONE-POULENC
PHARMACEUTICALS

WHITEHALL LABORATORIES　435, 2290
INC.
Division of American Home Products
Corporation
685 Third Avenue
New York, NY 10017
　　Address inquiries to:
Medical Department
　　　　　　　　　　　　(212) 878-5188
　　　Products Described
◆ Advil Ibuprofen Tablets and
　　Caplets 435, 2293
◆ Children's Advil Suspension 435, 2290
◆ Anacin Analgesic Coated
　　Caplets 435, 2293
◆ Anacin Analgesic Coated
　　Tablets 435, 2293
◆ Anacin-3 Children's
　　Acetaminophen Chewable
　　Tablets, Alcohol-Free Liquid,
　　and Infants' Drops 435, 2293
◆ Anacin-3 Maximum Strength
　　Acetaminophen Film Coated
　　Caplets 435, 2294
◆ Anacin-3 Maximum Strength
　　Acetaminophen Film Coated
　　Tablets 435, 2294
◆ Anacin Maximum Strength
　　Analgesic Coated Tablets...... 435, 2294
◆ Anacin-3 Regular Strength
　　Acetaminophen Film Coated
　　Tablets 435, 2294
◆ Anbesol Baby Teething Gel
　　Anesthetic 435, 2294
◆ Anbesol Gel
　　Antiseptic-Anesthetic 435, 2294
◆ Anbesol Gel
　　Antiseptic-Anesthetic -
　　Maximum Strength 435, 2294
◆ Anbesol Liquid
　　Antiseptic-Anesthetic 435, 2294
◆ Anbesol Liquid
　　Antiseptic-Anesthetic -
　　Maximum Strength 435, 2294
◆ Arthritis Pain Formula By the
　　Makers of Anacin Analgesic
　　Tablets and Caplets 435, 2294
◆ CoAdvil 435, 2295
　　Compound W Gel 2295
　　Compound W Solution 2295
◆ Denorex Medicated Shampoo
　　and Conditioner 435, 2295
◆ Denorex Medicated Shampoo,
　　Extra Strength 435, 2295
◆ Denorex Medicated Shampoo,
　　Regular & Mountain Fresh
　　Herbal Scent 435, 2295
　　Dermoplast Anesthetic Pain
　　Relief Lotion 2295
　　Dermoplast Anesthetic Pain
　　Relief Spray 2296
◆ Dristan Decongestant/
　　Antihistamine / Analgesic
　　Coated Caplets 435, 2296
◆ Dristan Decongestant/
　　Antihistamine / Analgesic
　　Coated Tablets 435, 2296
◆ Dristan Long Lasting Menthol
　　Nasal Spray 435, 2296
◆ Dristan Long Lasting Nasal
　　Spray, Regular 435, 2296
◆ Maximum Strength Dristan
　　Decongestant/Analgesic
　　Coated Caplets 435, 2296
◆ Dristan Nasal Spray, Regular
　　& Menthol 435, 2296
　　Posture 600 mg 2297
　　Posture-D 600 mg 2297
◆ Preparation H Hemorrhoidal
　　Cream 435, 2297
◆ Preparation H Hemorrhoidal
　　Ointment 435, 2297
◆ Preparation H Hemorrhoidal
　　Suppositories 435, 2297
◆ Primatene Mist 435, 2297
　　Primatene Mist Suspension 2297
◆ Primatene Tablets-M Formula .. 435, 2298
◆ Primatene Tablets-P Formula .. 435, 2298
◆ Primatene Tablets-Regular
　　Formula 435, 2298
◆ Riopan Antacid Chew Tablets . 435, 2298
　　Riopan Antacid Chew Tablets
　　in Rollpack 2298
　　Riopan Antacid Suspension 2298

◆ Riopan Antacid Swallow
　　Tablets 435, 2298
◆ Riopan Plus Chew Tablets 435, 2298
　　Riopan Plus Chew Tablets in
　　Rollpack 2298
◆ Riopan Plus 2 Chew Tablets ... 435, 2298
　　Riopan Plus Suspension 2298
　　Riopan Plus 2 Suspension 2298
◆ Semicid Vaginal Contraceptive
　　Inserts 435, 2299
◆ Today Vaginal Contraceptive
　　Sponge 435, 2299
　　　Other Products Available
Arthritis Pain Formula Aspirin-Free By
　　the Makers of Anacin Analgesic
　　Tablets
Beminal 500 Tablets
Bisodol Antacid Powder
Bisodol Antacid Tablets
Bronitin Asthma Tablets
Bronitin Mist
Clusivol Syrup
Denalan Denture Cleanser
Dristan Inhaler
Dristan Room Vaporizer
Dristan-AF Decongestant/Antihistamine/
　　Analgesic Tablets
Dry and Clear Acne Medication Lotion
Dry and Clear Double Strength Cream
Freezone Solution
Heather Feminine Deodorant Spray
Heet Analgesic Liniment
Heet Spray Analgesic
InfraRub Analgesic Cream
Medicated Cleansing Pads by the
　　Makers of Preparation H
　　Hemorrhoidal Remedies
Momentum Muscular Backache Formula
Neet Bikini Line Hair Remover Kit
Neet Depilatory Cream
Neet Depilatory Lotion
Outgro Solution
Oxipor VHC Lotion for Psoriasis
Quiet World Nighttime Pain Formula
Sleep-eze 3 Tablets
Sudden Beauty Hair Spray
Trendar Ibuprofen Tablets
Viro-Med Tablets
Youth Garde Moisturizer plus PABA

WILLEN DRUG COMPANY　　　2299
18 North High St.
Baltimore, MD 21202
　　Address inquiries to:
Professional Services Dept.
　　　　　　　　　　　　(800) 336-7000
　　　In MD (301) 752-1865
　　　Products Described
Bicitra—Sugar-Free 2299
Neutra-Phos Powder &
　　Capsules 2300
Neutra-Phos-K Powder &
　　Capsules 2300
Polycitra Syrup 2300
Polycitra-K Crystals 2301
Polycitra-K Oral Solution 2301
Polycitra-LC—Sugar-Free 2300

WINTHROP CONSUMER　　　　2301
PRODUCTS
Division of Sterling Drug Inc.
90 Park Avenue
New York, NY 10016
　　Address inquiries to:
Winthrop Consumer Products
　　For Medical Emergencies Contact:
Medical Department
　　　　　　　　　　　　(212) 907-3027
　　　Products Described
Bronkaid Mist 2301
Bronkaid Mist Suspension 2302
Bronkaid Tablets 2302
Campho-Phenique Cold Sore
　　Gel 2302
Campho-Phenique Liquid 2302
Campho-Phenique Triple
　　Antibiotic Ointment Plus
　　Pain Reliever 2302
Fergon Elixir 2302
Fergon Iron Plus Calcium
　　Caplets 2303
Fergon Tablets 2302
NTZ Long Acting Nasal Spray
　　& Drops 0.05% 2304
NāSal Saline Nasal Spray 2303
NāSal Saline Nose Drops 2303
Neo-Synephrine 12 Hour
　　Adult Nose Drops 2303
Neo-Synephrine 12 Hour
　　Nasal Spray 2303
Neo-Synephrine Jelly 2303
Neo-Synephrine Nasal Spray
　　(Mentholated) 2303
Neo-Synephrine Nasal Sprays 2303
Neo-Synephrine Nose Drops 2303
pHisoDerm For Baby 2304
pHisoDerm Skin Cleanser and
　　Conditioner - Regular and
　　Oily 2304
WinGel Liquid & Tablets 2304

WINTHROP　　　　435, 2304, 2464
PHARMACEUTICALS
90 Park Avenue
New York, NY 10016
　　　　　　　　　　　　(212) 907-2000
　　Professional Services Department
　　Call toll-free (800) 446-6267
　　　Products Described
Aralen Hydrochloride Injection 2304
Aralen Phosphate
　　w/Primaquine Phosphate
　　Tablets 2306
◆ Aralen Phosphate Tablets 435, 2305
◆ Atabrine Hydrochloride
　　Tablets 2307
◆ Bilopaque Sodium Capsules 435
　　Breonesin Capsules .... ▣▢
　　Bronkephrine Injection 2307
　　Bronkodyl Capsules 2307
　　Bronkolixir .... ▣▢
　　Bronkometer Aerosol 2308
　　Bronkosol 2308
　　Bronkotabs Tablets .... ▣▢
　　Carbocaine Hydrochloride
　　　Injection 2308
　　Carpuject Sterile
　　　Cartridge-Needle Unit 2311
◆ Danocrine 435, 2312
◆ Demerol APAP Tablets 435
　　Demerol Hydrochloride
　　　Carpuject 2312
　　Demerol Hydrochloride
　　　Injection 2312
　　Demerol Hydrochloride Syrup 2312
◆ Demerol Hydrochloride
　　Tablets 435, 2312
　　Demerol Hydrochloride
　　　Uni-Amp 2312
　　Inocor Lactate Injection 2314
　　Isuprel Hydrochloride
　　　Glossets 2318
　　Isuprel Hydrochloride
　　　Injection 1:5000 2315
　　Isuprel Hydrochloride
　　　Mistometer 2316
　　Isuprel Hydrochloride Solution
　　　1:200 & 1:100 2317
　　Kayexalate 2318
　　Levophed Bitartrate Injection 2319
　　Lotusate Caplets 2320
　　Marcaine Hydrochloride with
　　　Epinephrine 1:200,000 2320
　　Marcaine Hydrochloride
　　　Injection 2320
　　Marcaine Spinal 2323
　　Measurin Caplets .... ▣▢
◆ Mebaral Tablets 2325
◆ Modrastane Capsules 435
◆ NegGram Caplets 435, 2327
　　NegGram Suspension 2327
　　Neo-Synephrine Hydrochloride
　　　1% Carpuject 2328
　　Neo-Synephrine Hydrochloride
　　　1% Injection 2328
　　Neo-Synephrine Hydrochloride
　　　(Ophthalmic) 2329
　　Novocain Hydrochloride for
　　　Spinal Anesthesia 2330
　　Novocain Hydrochloride
　　　Injection 2330
　　Omnipaque 2464
　　pHisoDerm .... ▣▢
　　pHisoHex 2331
　　Pediacof Cough Syrup 2331
◆ Plaquenil Sulfate Tablets 435, 2332
　　Pontocaine Hydrochloride for
　　　Spinal Anesthesia 2333
　　Sulfamylon Cream 2335
◆ Talacen 435, 2335
　　Talwin Ampuls 2337
　　Talwin Carpuject 2337
　　Talwin Compound 2338
　　Talwin Injection 2337
◆ Talwin Nx 435, 2338
◆ Telepaque Tablets 435
◆ Tornalate 2339
◆ Trancopal Caplets 435, 2340
◆ Winstrol Tablets 435, 2341
　　Zephiran Chloride Aqueous
　　　Solution .... ▣▢
　　Zephiran Chloride
　　　Concentrate Solution .... ▣▢
　　Zephiran Chloride Spray .... ▣▢
　　Zephiran Chloride Tinted
　　　Tincture .... ▣▢
　　Zephiran Towelettes .... ▣▢
　　　Other Products Available
Amipaque
Anti-Rust Tablets
Atropine & Demerol Carpuject
BioBrane
Codeine Phosphate Carpuject
Dextrose Injection, 10%
Drisdol 50,000 Unit Capsules
Drisdol in Propylene Glycol
Empty Sterile Carpuject
Furosemide Injection Carpuject
Heparin Lock Flush Solution Carpuject
Heparin Sodium Carpuject
HEP-PAK Convenience Package
HEP-PAK CVC Convenience Package
HEP-PAK 2
Hydromorphone Carpuject
Hydroxyzine Carpuject
Hypaque Meglumine 30%
Hypaque Meglumine 60%
Hypaque Sodium Oral Powder
Hypaque Sodium Oral Solution

Hypaque Sodium 20%
Hypaque Sodium 25%
Hypaque Sodium 50% Injection
Hypaque-Cysto 30%
Hypaque-Cysto 30% Pediatric
Hypaque-M, 75% Injection
Hypaque-M, 90% Injection
Hypaque-76 Injection
Hytakerol Capsules & Liquid
Luminal Sodium Injection
Morphine Sulfate Carpuject
Mytelase Chloride Caplets
Phenytoin Sodium Injection Carpuject
Pontocaine Cream
Pontocaine Ointment
Pontocaine Hydrochloride Eye Ointment
Pontocaine Hydrochloride Topical
　　Solution
Pontocaine 0.2% with Dextrose 6%
Pontocaine 0.3% with Dextrose 6%
Primaquine Phosphate Tablets
Procainamide Hydrochloride Carpuject
Prochlorperazine Edisylate Injection
　　Carpuject
Sodium Chloride Carpuject
Trimethobenzamide Hydrochloride
　　Carpuject
Verapamil Hydrochloride Carpuject
Vitamins
　　Vitamin D, USP
　　　Drisdol 50,000 Unit Capsules
　　　Drisdol in Propylene Glycol

WYETH-AYERST　　　436, 2342, 2471
LABORATORIES
Division of American Home Products
Corporation
P.O. Box 8299
Philadelphia, PA 19101
　　Address inquiries to:
Professional Service
　　For General Information call:
　　　　　　　　　　　　(215) 688-4400
　　For Medical Emergency Information
Day or night call　　　(215) 688-4400
　　WYETH-AYERST DISTRIBUTION
　　　　　　CENTERS:
(Do not use freight addresses for
mailing of orders.)

Wyeth Distribution Centers:
Atlanta, GA— P.O. Box 1773
　　Paoli, PA 19301-1773
　　　　　　　　　　　(800) 666-7248
　　Freight address—221 Armour Drive
　　N.E.
　　Atlanta, GA 30324
Boston, MA—P.O. Box 1773
　　Paoli, PA 19301-1773
　　　　　　　　　　　(800) 666-7248
　　Freight address—7 Connector Road
　　Andover, MA 01810
Chicago, IL—P.O. Box 1773
　　Paoli, PA 19301-1773
　　　　　　　　　　　(800) 666-7248
　　Freight address—745 N. Gary
　　Avenue
　　Carol Stream, IL 60188
Dallas, TX—P.O. Box 1773
　　Paoli, PA 19301-1773
　　　　　　　　　　　(800) 666-7248
　　Freight address—11240 Petal Street
　　Dallas, TX 75238
Hawaii—96-1185 Waihona St., Unit C1
　　Pearl City, HI 96782
　　　　　　　　　　　(808) 456-4567
Kansas City, MO—P.O. Box 1773
　　Paoli, PA 19301-1773
　　　　　　　　　　　(800) 666-7248
　　Freight address—1340 Taney Street
　　N. Kansas City, MO 64116
Los Angeles, CA—P.O. Box 5000
　　Buena Park, CA 90622-5000
　　　　Buena Park (714) 523-5500
　　　　Los Angeles (213) 627-5374
　　　　　　In CA (800) 225-6802
　　　　Outside CA (800) 544-4400
　　Freight address—6530 Altura Blvd.
　　Buena Park, CA 90620
Philadelphia, PA—P.O. Box 1773
　　Paoli, PA 19301-1773
　　　　　　　　　　　(800) 666-7248
　　Freight address—31 Moorehall Rd.
　　Frazer, PA 19355
Seattle, WA—P.O. Box 1773
　　Paoli, PA 19301-1773
　　　　　　　　　　　(800) 666-7248
　　Freight address—19255 80th Ave.
　　So.
　　Kent, WA 98032

Ayerst Distribution Centers:
Chamblee, GA—3600 American Drive
　　Chamblee, GA 30341
　　　　　　　　　　　(404) 457-2518
　　　　　　In GA (800) 282-3523
　　　　Outside GA (800) 241-7360
Chicago, IL—P.O. Box 1773
　　Paoli, PA 19301-1773
　　　　　　　　　　　(800) 666-7248
　　Freight address—745 N. Gary Ave.
　　Carol Stream, IL 60188

(◆ Shown in Product Identification Section)　　　　*Italic Page Number* Indicates Brief Listing　　　　(▣▢ Described in PDR For Nonprescription Drugs)

Dallas, TX—P.O. Box 1773
Paoli, PA 19301-1773
    (800) 666-7248
Freight address—11240 Petal Street
Dallas, TX 75238
Foster City, CA—1147 Chess Drive
Foster City, CA 94404
    (415) 574-6061
In CA (800) 225-6886
Outside CA (800) 321-8151
Kansas City, MO—P.O. Box 1773
Paoli, PA 19301-1773
    (800) 666-7248
Freight address—1340 Taney Street
N. Kansas City, MO 64116
South Plainfield, NJ—4000 Hadley Rd.
South Plainfield, NJ 07080
In NJ (201) 754-6220
(212) 964-3903
In NJ (800) 272-1013
Outside NJ (800) 631-5331
Maine only (800) 631-5360

Products Described

A.P.L. 2346
Aludrox Oral Suspension 2343
Amphojel Suspension 2343
Amphojel Suspension without Flavor 2343
Amphojel Tablets 2343
◆ Antabuse 436, 2343
Antivenin (Crotalidae) Polyvalent 2344
Antivenin (Micrurus fulvius) 2345
Ativan Injection 2346
◆ Ativan Tablets 436, 2348
Ativan in Tubex 2346
◆ Atromid-S 436, 2349
Auralgan Otic Solution 2350
◆ Aygestin 436, 2351
Basaljel Capsules 2352
Basaljel Suspension 2352
Basaljel Tablets 2352
Bicillin C-R Injection 2352
Bicillin C-R in Tubex 2352
Bicillin C-R 900/300 Injection 2354
Bicillin C-R 900/300 in Tubex 2354
Bicillin L-A Injection 2355
Bicillin L-A in Tubex 2355
Cerose-DM 2357
Cerubidine 2357
Cholera Vaccine 2358
Codeine Phosphate in Tubex 2444
Collyrium for Fresh Eyes 2358
Collyrium Fresh 2359
◆ Cordarone Tablets 436, 2359
◆ Cyanocobalamin in Tubex 437, 2444
◆ Cycrin Tablets 436, 2362
◆ Dicloxacillin Sodium Monohydrate (see Pathocil) 437
Digoxin in Tubex 2444
Dimenhydrinate in Tubex 2444
Diphenhydramine HCl in Tubex 2444
Diphtheria & Tetanus Toxoids Adsorbed, Pediatric, in Tubex 2363
Diphtheria & Tetanus Toxoids Adsorbed, Ultrafined, Pediatric 2363
◆ Diucardin 436, 2363
Epinephrine in Tubex 2444
Epitrate 2364
◆ Equagesic Tablets 436, 2364
◆ Equanil Tablets 436, 2365
Estradurin 2365
◆ Factrel 436, 2471
Fluothane 2367
◆ Grisactin 436, 2367

◆ Grisactin Ultra 436, 2368
Heparin Flush Kits 2369
Heparin Lock Flush Solution 2369
◆ Heparin Lock Flush Solution in Tubex 436, 2369
Heparin Sodium Injection 2370
Heparin Sodium in Tubex 2370
Hydromorphone HCl in Tubex 2444
◆ Inderal Injectable 436, 2372
◆ Inderal LA Long Acting Capsules 436, 2374
◆ Inderal Tablets 436, 2372
◆ Inderide LA Long Acting Capsules 436, 2378
◆ Inderide Tablets 436, 2376
Influenza Virus Vaccine, Trivalent, Subvirion Type 2379
Influenza Virus Vaccine, Trivalent, Subvirion Type in Tubex 2379
◆ Isordil Sublingual Tablets 2.5 mg, 5 mg & 10 mg 437, 2380
◆ Isordil Tembids Capsules (40 mg) 436, 2380
◆ Isordil Tembids Tablets (40 mg) 436, 2380
◆ Isordil 5 Titradose Tablets, 5 mg 437, 2380
◆ Isordil 10 Titradose Tablets, 10 mg 437, 2380
◆ Isordil 20 Titradose Tablets, 20 mg 437, 2380
◆ Isordil 30 Titradose Tablets, 30 mg 437, 2380
◆ Isordil 40 Titradose Tablets, 40 mg 437, 2380
◆ Lo/Ovral Tablets 437, 2381
◆ Lo/Ovral-28 Tablets 437, 2387
◆ Mazanor Tablets 437, 2387
◆ Mediatric Capsules 437, 2388
◆ Mepergan Fortis Capsules 437
Mepergan Injection 2390
Mepergan in Tubex 2390
Meperidine HCl in Tubex 2444
Morphine Sulfate in Tubex 2444
Mysoline Suspension 2392
◆ Mysoline Tablets 437, 2392
◆ Nordette-21 Tablets 437, 2392
◆ Nordette-28 Tablets 437, 2396
◆ Nursoy, Soy Protein Formula for Infants, Concentrated, Liquid, Ready-to-Feed, and Powder 437, 2396
◆ Omnipen Capsules 437, 2397
Omnipen for Oral Suspension 2397
Omnipen-N Injection 2397
◆ Orudis Capsules 437, 2397
◆ Ovral Tablets 437, 2399
◆ Ovral-28 Tablets 437, 2400
Ovrette Tablets 2400
Oxytocin Injection 2401
Oxytocin in Tubex 2401
◆ PMB 200 and PMB 400 .... 437, 2414
◆ Pathocil Capsules 437, 2402
Pathocil for Oral Suspension 2402
Pen•Vee K for Oral Solution 2402
◆ Pen•Vee K Tablets 437, 2402
Pentobarbital Sodium in Tubex 2444
Peptavlon 2472
Phenergan with Codeine 2406
Phenergan with Dextromethorphan 2407
Phenergan Injection 2402
◆ Phenergan Suppositories 437, 2404
Phenergan Syrup Fortis 2403
Phenergan Syrup Plain 2403
◆ Phenergan Tablets 437, 2404
Phenergan in Tubex 2402
Phenergan VC 2410

Phenergan VC with Codeine 2411
◆ Phenergan-D Tablets 437, 2408
Phenobarbital Sodium in Tubex 2444
Phospholine Iodide 2414
◆ Plegine 437, 2414
Premarin Intravenous 2418
◆ Premarin with Methyltestosterone 437, 2425
◆ Premarin Tablets 437, 2420
◆ Premarin Vaginal Cream 437, 2422
Prochlorperazine Edisylate in Tubex 2444
Protopam Chloride for Injection 2428
Protopam Chloride Tablets 2428
◆ Resol Oral Electrolyte Rehydration & Maintenance Solution 437, 2430
◆ SMA Iron Fortified Infant Formula, Concentrated, Ready-To-Feed & Powder 437, 2434
◆ SMA lo-iron 437, 2434
Secobarbital Sodium in Tubex 2444
◆ Sectral Capsules 437, 2430
◆ Serax Capsules 437, 2432
◆ Serax Tablets 438, 2432
Sodium Chloride, Bacteriostatic in Tubex 2444
Sparine Injection in Tubex 2444
◆ Sparine Tablets 438
◆ Surmontil Capsules 438, 2434
◆ Synalgos-DC Capsules 438, 2435
Tetanus & Diphtheria Toxoids Adsorbed for Adult Use 2436
Tetanus & Diphtheria Toxoids Adsorbed for Adult Use in Tubex 2436
Tetanus Toxoid Adsorbed, Aluminum Phosphate Adsorbed, Ultrafined 2436
Tetanus Toxoid Adsorbed, Aluminum Phosphate Adsorbed, Ultrafined in Tubex 2436
Tetanus Toxoid Fluid, Purified, Ultrafined 2436
Tetanus Toxoid Fluid, Purified, Ultrafined in Tubex 2436
◆ Tetracycline HCl Capsules 438
Thiamine HCl in Tubex 2444
◆ Thiosulfil Forte Tablets 438, 2436
Trecator-SC Tablets 2437
◆ Triphasil-21 Tablets 438, 2437
◆ Triphasil-28 Tablets 438, 2444
◆ Tubex Closed Injection System Products 436, 2444
◆ Tubex Fast Trak Syringe 436
◆ Tubex Injector 436
◆ Tubex Metal Syringe 436
Typhoid Vaccine 2447
◆ Unipen Capsules 438, 2447
Unipen Powder for Oral Solution 2447
◆ Unipen Tablets 438, 2447
◆ Vitamin B₁₂ (Cyanocobalamin) in Tubex 436, 2444
◆ Vitamin B₁₂ Injection (see Cyanocobalamin) 436
◆ Wyamycin S Tablets 438, 2449
◆ Wyanoids Relief Factor Hemorrhoidal Suppositories 438, 2449
Wycillin Injection 2449
Wycillin Injection & Probenecid Tablets 2451
Wycillin in Tubex 2449
Wydase, Lyophilized 2452

◆ Wygesic Tablets 438, 2452
◆ Wymox Capsules 438, 2454
Wymox for Oral Suspension 2454
◆ Wytensin Tablets 438, 2454

Other Products Available

Antisnakebite Serum (see Antivenin)
Benzathine Penicillin G (see Bicillin)
Bicillin Tablets
CVC Heparin Flush Kits
Codeine Phosphate Injection
Codeine Sulfate Tablets, Redipak
Cyanocobalamin Injection
Digoxin Injection
Dimenhydrinate Injection
Diphenhydramine HCl Injection
Epinephrine Injection (1:1000)
Estrogenic Substance (estrone) In Aqueous Suspension
Fluor-I-Strip Applicators
Fluor-I-Strip A.T. Applicators
Hydromorphone HCl Injection
Largon Injection
Meperidine HCl Injection
Meperidine HCl Tablets, Redipak
Morphine Sulfate Injection
Naloxone HCl Injection
Ophthalgan
Opium & Belladonna Rectal Suppositories
Phenobarbital Tablets, Redipak
Phosphaljel
Prochlorperazine Edisylate Injection
Redipak Unit Dose Medications (Strip Pack and/or Individually Wrapped) Products:
Ativan Tablets
Codeine Sulfate Tablets
Isordil Sublingual Tablets, 2.5 mg
Isordil Sublingual Tablets, 5 mg
Isordil 5 Titradose Tablets, 5 mg
Isordil 10 Titradose Tablets, 10 mg
Isordil 20 Titradose Tablets, 20 mg
Isordil 30 Titradose Tablets, 30 mg
Isordil 40 Titradose Tablets, 40 mg
Meperidine HCl Tablets
Pen•Vee K Tablets
Phenergan Tablets
Phenobarbital Tablets
Sectral Capsules, 200 mg
Serax Capsules
Surmontil Capsules, 25 mg
Surmontil Capsules, 50 mg
Wygesic Tablets
Wytensin Tablets, 4 mg
Redipak (Respiratory Therapy Unit) Products:
Sodium Chloride 0.9%
RediTemp-C, Disposable Cold Pack
Saline Solution (see Sodium Chloride Injection)
Secobarbital Sodium Injection
Sodium Chloride Injection, Bacteriostatic
Sodium Chloride Solution, 0.9%
Sonacide
Sparine Injection
Testuria
Tubex Sterile Cartridge-Needle Unit Empty
Wyamine Sulfate Injection
Wydase, Stabilized Solution

YOUNG PHARMACEUTICALS INC. 2455
1840 Berlin Turnpike
Wethersfield, CT 06109
Address inquiries to:
Professional Services Department
Toll-free (800) 874-9686
(203) 529-7919

Products Described

PharmaCreme 2455

SECTION 2
Product Name Index

In this section products are listed in alphabetical sequence by brand name or (if described) generic name. Only described products have page numbers to assist you in locating additional information. For additional information on other products, you may wish to contact the manufacturer directly.

The symbol ◆ indicates the product is shown in the Product Identification Section. The symbol ⊞ indicates the product is described in PDR FOR NONPRESCRIPTION DRUGS®. Italic page number indicates a brief listing.

(◆ Shown in Product Identification Section)   *Italic Page Number* Indicates Brief Listing   (⬛ Described in PDR For Nonprescription Drugs)

SECTION 3

Product Category Index

Products described in the Product Information (White) or Diagnostic Product Information (Green) Sections are listed according to their classifications. The headings and sub-headings have been determined by the Publisher with the cooperation of the individual manufacturers. In cases where there were differences of opinion or where the manufacturer had no opinion, the Publisher made the final decision. A QUICK-REFERENCE INDEX of headings and sub-headings can be found below.

Product Category Quick-Reference

A

AIDS CHEMOTHERAPEUTIC AGENTS
AIDS RELATED COMPLEX (ARC) THERAPEUTIC AGENTS
ADRENAL CORTICAL STEROID INHIBITOR
ADRENAL CORTICOSTEROID
ALCOHOL ABUSE REDUCTION PREPARATIONS
ALLERGENS
ALLERGY RELIEF PRODUCTS
AMINO ACID PREPARATIONS
ANALGESICS
  Acetaminophen
  Acetaminophen & Combinations
  Aspirin
  Aspirin Combinations
  Aspirin with Antacids
  Aspirin with Codeine
  NSAIDS
  Narcotic Agonist-Antagonist
  Narcotics, Synthetics & Combinations
  Other Salicylates & Combinations
  Topical-Analgesic
  Topical-Counterirritant
  Other
ANESTHETICS
  Caudal
  Epidural
  Inhalation
  Injectable
  Rectal
  Retrobulbar
  Spinal
  Topical
ANORECTAL PRODUCTS
  Creams, Foams, Lotions, Ointments
  Suppositories
  Other
ANTACIDS
  Antacids
  Antacid Combinations
  Antacids with Antiflatulents
ANTIBACTERIALS & ANTISEPTICS
  Antibacterials
  Fungicides
  Ophthalmic
  Parenteral
  Quinolones
  Sulfonamide Combinations
  Sulfonamides
  Topical
  Urinary Antibacterial
  Urinary Antibacterial with Analgesics
ANTIBIOTICS
  Amebicides
  Broad & Medium Spectrum
  Cephalosporins
  Fungal Medications
  Monobactams
  Penicillin
  Tuberculosis
  Viral Agents
ANTICHOLINERGIC DRUG INHIBITOR

ANTICOAGULANT ANTAGONIST
ANTICOAGULANTS
ANTIDEPRESSANTS
  Aminoketones
  Monoamine Oxidase Inhibitors
  Phenothiazines & Combinations
  Serotonin Uptake Inhibitors
  Tetracyclics
  Tricyclics
ANTIDIURETICS
ANTIDOTES
  Anticholinesterase
  Digoxin
ANTIGLAUCOMATOUS AGENTS
  Beta Adrenergic Blocking Agent (Topical)
  Carbonic Anhydrase Inhibitors
  Miotic (Indirect Acting)
    Cholinesterase Inhibitor
ANTIHISTAMINES
ANTI-INFLAMMATORY AGENTS
  Enzymes
  Non-Steroidals
  Salicylates
  Steroids & Combinations
  Sulfonamides
  Other
ANTIMETABOLITES
ANTINEOPLASTICS
  Androgen Inhibitor
  Antibiotic Derivatives
  Antiestrogen
  Antimetabolites
  Cytotoxic Agents
  Hormones
  Nitrogen Mustard Derivatives
  Steroids & Combinations
  Other
ANTIOXIDANTS
ANTIPARASITICS
  Arthropods
    Lice
    Scabies
  Helminths
    Ascaris (roundworm)
    Enterobius (pinworm)
    Hookworm
    Strongyloids (threadworm)
    Taenia (tapeworm)
    Trematodes (schistosomes)
    Trichuris (whipworm)
  Protozoa
    Amebas, extraintestinal
    Amebas, intestinal
    Malaria
    Toxoplasma
    Trichomonas
ANTIPYRETICS
ANTISPASMODICS & ANTICHOLINERGICS
  Gastrointestinal
APPETITE SUPPRESSANTS
  Amphetamines
  Non-Amphetamines

ARTHRITIS MEDICATIONS
  Gold Compounds
  NSAIDS
  Salicylates
  Steroids
  Others
ASTHMA PREPARATIONS

B

BABY PRODUCTS
BIOLOGICALS
  Alpha$_1$-Antitrypsin
  Antigens
  Antiserum
  Antitoxin
  RH$_0$ (D) Immune Globulin (Human)
  Serum
  Toxoids
  Vaccines
  Vaccines (Live)
  Other
BISMUTH PREPARATIONS
BONE METABOLISM REGULATOR
  Heterotopic Ossification Agent
  Hypercalcemic Agent
  Pagetic Agent
BOWEL EVACUANTS
BRONCHIAL DILATORS
  Anticholinergic
  Beta Adrenergic Stimulator
  Devices
  Iodides & Combinations
  Sympathomimetics
  Sympathomimetics & Combinations
  Xanthine Derivatives & Combinations

C

CALCIUM PREPARATIONS
  Calcium Regulator
  Calcium Supplements
CARDIOVASCULAR PREPARATIONS
  Alpha Adrenoceptor Agonist
  Alpha Receptor Blocking Agent
  Alpha and Beta Receptor Blocking Agent
  Anginal Preparations
  Angiotensin Converting Enzyme Inhibitors
  Antihypertensives
  Antihypertensives with Diuretics
  Arrhythmia Medications
  Beta Blocking Agents
  Calcium Channel Blocker
  Cardiac Glycosides
  Hemorrheologic Agent
  Inotropic Agent
  Myocardial Infarction Prophylaxis
  Quinidine
  Vasodilators, Cerebral
  Vasodilators, Coronary
  Vasodilators, General
  Vasodilators, Peripheral
  Vasopressors
  Other Cardiovasculars
CATECHOLAMINE SYNTHESIS INHIBITOR
CENTRAL NERVOUS SYSTEM STIMULANTS

CEREBRAL METABOLIC ENHANCER
CERUMENOLYTICS
CHELATING AGENTS
CHOLINESTERASE INHIBITOR
COLD PREPARATIONS
  Decongestants
    Oral & Combinations
  Non-Narcotic
CONTRACEPTIVES
  Devices
  Devices, copper containing
  Oral
  Topical
CONVULSION MEDICATIONS
CORTICOSTEROIDS & COMBINATIONS, OPHTHALMIC
COSMETICS
COUGH PREPARATIONS
  Antitussives & Combinations
  Expectorants & Combinations
  Non-Narcotic
  With Narcotics
COUGH & COLD PREPARATIONS
  Non-Narcotic
  With Narcotics

D

DECONGESTANTS
  Oral
  Topical, Nasal
DECONGESTANTS, EXPECTORANTS & COMBINATIONS
DECONGESTANTS, OPHTHALMIC
DENTAL PREPARATIONS
DEODORANTS
  Internal
  Oral
  Topical
DERMATOLOGICALS
  Abradant
  Acne Preparations
  Analgesic
  Antibacterial
  Antibacterial, Antifungal & Combinations
  Antibiotic
  Anti-Inflammatory Agents
  Antiperspirants
  Astringents
  Burn Relief
  Coal Tar
  Coal Tar & Sulfur
  Conditioning Rinses
  Cradle Cap Agent
  Dandruff Medications
  Deodorants
  Depigmenting Agent
  Dermatitis Herpetiformis
  Dermatitis Relief
  Detergents
  Diaper Rash Relief
  Drying Agent
  Emollients
  Epidermal & Cellular Growth

Fungicides
  General
  Herpes Treatment
  Insect Bites & Stings
  Keratolytics
  Moisturizer
  Ovicide
  Pediculicides
  Photosensitizer
  Powders
  Pruritic Medications
  Psoriasis Agents
  Scabicides
  Seborrhea Treatment
  Shampoos
  Skin Bleaches
  Skin Protectant
  Soaps & Cleansers
  Steroids & Combinations
  Sulfur & Salicylic Acid
  Sunburn Preparations
  Sunscreens
  Tissue Granulation
  Vehicles, Compounding
  Wart Removers
  Wet Dressings
  Wound Cleanser
  Wound Dressings
  Other
DETOXIFYING AGENT
DIABETES AGENTS
  Intermediate Acting Insulins
  Intermediate Acting Insulins (Premixed)
  Long Acting Insulins
  Oral
  Rapid Acting Insulins
  Rapid Acting Insulins (Premixed)
DIAGNOSTICS
  ACTH Test
  Adrenocortical Function
  Allergy, Skin Tests
  Angiocardiography
  Angiography
  Aortography
  Arthrography
  Blood Glucose
  Bronchial Airway Hyperreactivity
  Cerebral Angiography
  Cisternography-CT
  CT Scan Enhancement
  Diabetes Tests
  Endoscopic Retrograde Pancreatography
  Excretory Urography
  Herniography
  Hypocalcemia Test
  Hysterosalpingography
  Hysteroscopic Fluid
  Intravenous Digital Arteriography
  Intravenous Venography
  Lymphography
  Myelography
  Myelography-CT
  Occult Blood in Feces
  Parathyroid Function Test
  Pediatric Angiocardiography
  Peripheral Angiography
  Peripheral Arteriography
  Phenochromocytoma Test
  Renal Function
  Thyroid Releasing Factor
  Tuberculin
    Tuberculin, Old
    Tuberculin, P.P.D.
  Urine Test
    Bilirubin
    Blood
    Glucose
    Ketones & Glucose
    Leukocytes
    Nitrite
    pH
    Protein
    Urobilinogen
  Urography
  Venography, Lower Extremity
DIAPER RASH RELIEF
DIARRHEA MEDICATIONS
DIETARY SUPPLEMENTS
DIURETICS
  Antihypertensive Saluretic
  Indoline Antihypertensives
  Loop Diuretics
    Bumetanide
    Ethracrynic Acid Derivatives
    Furosemide
  Monosulfamyl
  Potassium Sparing
  Thiazides and Combinations
DOPAMINE RECEPTOR AGONIST
DRUG DELIVERY SYSTEM
DUODENAL ULCER ADHERENT COMPLEX

E

ELECTROLYTES
  Alkalinizing Agents
  Concentrates
  Fluid Maintenance Therapy
  Fluid Replacement Therapy
  Magnesium Preparations
  Potassium Preparations
  Other
ENURESIS
ENZYMES & DIGESTANTS
  Collagenolytic
  Digestants
  Fibrinolytic & Proteolytic
  Proteolytic
  Topical
ERGOT PREPARATIONS
  Migraine Preparations
  Uterine Contractant
EYEWASHES

F

FERTILITY AGENTS
FIBER SUPPLEMENT
FIBRINOLYTIC AGENTS
FIBROTICS, SYSTEMIC
FLATULENCE RELIEF
FLUORIDE PREPARATIONS
FOODS
  Allergy Diet
  Carbohydrate
  Complete Therapeutic
  Enteral
  High Fat
  High Nitrogen
  Infant
  Lactose Free
  Low Fat
  Low Residue
  Medium Chain Triglycerides
  Metabolic Dysfunction
  Parenteral Hyperalimentation Kit
  Protein
FOOT CARE PRODUCTS
FUNGAL AGENTS
  Systemic
  Topical

G

GALACTOKINETIC
GALACTORRHEA INHIBITOR
GALL STONE DISSOLUTION AGENT
GASTRIC ACID SECRETION INHIBITOR
GASTROINTESTINAL MOTILITY FACTOR
GONADOTROPIN INHIBITORS

H

HAIR GROWTH STIMULANT
HEMATINICS
  Cyanocobalamin
  Folic Acid
  Iron & Combinations
  Liver
  Vitamin B$_{12}$
  Other
HEMOSTATICS
HERPES TREATMENT
HISTAMINE H$_2$ RECEPTOR ANTAGONIST
HORMONES
  ACTH
  Anabolics
  Androgen & Estrogen Combinations
  Androgens
  Corticoids & Analgesics
  Corticoids & Antibiotics, Topical
  Estrogens
  Glucocorticoid
  Gonadotropin
  Gonadotropin Releasing
  Human Growth Hormone
  Hypocalcemic
  Menotropins
  Parathyroid
  Progesterone
  Progestogen
  Progestogen & Estrogen Combinations
  Somatostatin-Like Compounds
  Urofollitropin
  Vasopressin
  Other
HYPERAMMONIA REDUCTION
HYPERGLYCEMIC AGENTS
HYPNOTICS
HYPOCALCEMIA MANAGEMENT
HYPOLIPIDEMICS

I

IMMUNOMODULATORS
IMMUNOSUPPRESSIVES

INFANT FORMULAS, REGULAR
  Liquid Concentrate
  Liquid Ready-to-feed
  Powder
INFANT FORMULAS, SPECIAL PURPOSE
  Hypo-Allergenic
    Liquid Concentrate
    Liquid Ready-to-feed
    Powder
  Iron Supplement
    Liquid Concentrate
    Liquid Ready-to-feed
    Powder
  Lactose Free
    Liquid Concentrate
    Liquid Ready-to-feed
    Powder
  Low Iron
    Liquid Ready-to-feed
  Medium Chain Triglycerides
    Liquid Ready-to-feed
  Metabolic Dysfunction
    Liquid Concentrate
    Powder
  Milk Free
    Liquid Concentrate
    Liquid Ready-to-feed
    Powder
  With Whey
    Liquid Ready-to-feed
  Other
INSECT STING EMERGENCY KIT
INSULIN DELIVERY DEVICE

L

LH-RH ANALOG
LAPROSTATICS
LAXATIVES
  Bulk
  Combinations
  Enemas
  Fecal Softeners
  Mineral oil
  Saline
  Stimulant
LEUKAPHERESIS ADJUNCT
LIP BALM
LIPOTROPICS
LUBRICANTS, OPHTHALMIC
  Ocular
  Ophthalmic

M

MAGNESIUM PREPARATIONS
MENSTRUAL PREPARATIONS
MIGRAINE PREPARATIONS
MINERALS
MOTION SICKNESS REMEDIES
MOUTHRINSE, ANTIMICROBIAL
MOUTHWASHES
MUCOLYTICS
MUSCLE RELAXANT ANTAGONIST
MUSCLE RELAXANTS
  Neuromuscular Blocking Agent
  Skeletal Muscle Relaxants
  Skeletal Muscle Relaxants with Analgesics
  Smooth Muscle Relaxants
MUSCULAR ENERGY PRODUCTION
MYDRIATIC

N

NARCOTIC ANTAGONISTS
NARCOTIC DETOXIFICATION
NASAL PREPARATIONS
NAUSEA MEDICATIONS
NEUROLEPTICS

O

OPHTHALMOLOGICALS
OSTEOPOROSIS PREPARATIONS
  Postmenopausal
OTIC PREPARATIONS
OXYTOCICS

P

PARASYMPATHOLYTICS
PARASYMPATHOMIMETICS
PARKINSONISM DRUGS
PENICILLIN ADJUVANT
PHOSPHOLIPIDS
PHOSPHORUS PREPARATIONS
PLASMA EXTENDERS & EXPANDERS
PLASMA FRACTIONS, HUMAN
  Albumin (Human)
  Antihemophilic Factor
  Factor IX Complex
  Immune Globulin (Human)
  Plasma Protein Fraction (Human)
  RH$_O$ (D) Immune Globulin (Human)
PLASMA FRACTIONS, PORCINE
PLATELET INHIBITORS

PORPHYRIA AGENT
PRIMARY SYSTEMIC CARNITINE DEFICIENCY
PROGESTAGLANDIN ANALOG
PROSTAGLANDINS
PROTOZOAL AGENTS
PRURITIS MEDICATIONS
PSYCHOSTIMULANTS
PSYCHOTIC MEDICATIONS
PYRETICS

Q

QUINIDINES

R

RESINS, ION EXCHANGE
RESPIRATORY STIMULANTS

S

SALT SUBSTITUTE
SCLEROSING AGENTS
SEDATIVES
  Barbiturates
  Non-Barbiturates
SHOCK EMERGENCY KIT
SKIN WOUND PREPARATIONS
  Cleansers
  Healing Agents
SLEEP AIDS
SMOKING CESSATION AID
SYMPATHOLYTICS
SYMPATHOMIMETICS & COMBINATIONS

T

TEETHING LOTIONS & GELS
THROAT LOZENGES
THROMBOLYTICS
THYROID PREPARATIONS
  Synthetic Thyroid Hormone
  Thyroid
  Thyroxine Sodium
TONICS
TOURETTES SYNDROME AGENT
TRANQUILIZERS
  Anxiety Agents
  Benzodiazepine
  Butyrophenones & Combinations
  Hydroxyzines
  Lithium Preparations
  Meprobamate & Combinations
  Phenothiazines & Combinations
  Rauwolfia Serpentina
  Reserpine
  Thioxanthenes
  Other
TREMOR PREPARATIONS
TUBERCULOSIS PREPARATIONS

U

UNIT DOSE SYSTEMS
UNNA BOOT
URICOSURIC AGENTS
URINARY TRACT AGENTS
  Acidifiers
  Alkalinizing
  Analgesics
  Antispasmodics
  Calcium Oxalate Stone Preventative
  Irrigants
UTERINE CONTRACTANTS
UTERINE RELAXANTS

V

VAGINAL PREPARATIONS
  Capsules, Tablets
  Cleansers, External
  Creams
  Douches
  Inserts, Suppositories
  Jellies, Ointments
  Lubricants
  Tampons
  Trichomonacides
VERTIGO AGENTS
VIRAL AGENTS
VIRAL AGENTS, OPHTHALMOLOGICAL
VITAMINS
  Anti-folic Acid Antagonist
  Geriatric
  Intranasal Application
  Multivitamins
  Multivitamins with Minerals
  Parenteral
  Pediatric
  Pediatric with Fluoride
  Prenatal
  Therapeutic
  Other

X

X-RAY CONTRAST MEDIA

Product Category Index

Italic Page Number **Indicates Brief Listing**

Italic Page Number **Indicates Brief Listing**

Italic Page Number **Indicates Brief Listing**

Italic Page Number Indicates Brief Listing

SECTION 4
Generic and Chemical Name Index

In this section the products described in the Product Information (White) and Diagnostic Product Information (Green) Sections are listed under generic and chemical name headings according to the principal ingredient(s). The headings under which products are listed have been determined by the Publisher with the cooperation of the individual manufacturers.

Italic Page Number **Indicates Brief Listing**

Sine-Aid Maximum Strength Sinus Headache Tablets (McNeil Consumer) 417, 1277
Sinulin (Carnrick) 408, 831
Spasgesic (Legere) 1192
Supac (Mission) 1521
Talacen (Winthrop Pharmaceuticals) 435, 2335
Tylenol acetaminophen Children's Chewable Tablets & Elixir (McNeil Consumer) 416, 1277
Tylenol Allergy Sinus Medication, Maximum Strength, Caplets and Tablets (McNeil Consumer) 417, 1281
Tylenol with Codeine Phosphate Elixir (McNeil Pharmaceutical) 417, 1289
Tylenol with Codeine Phosphate Tablets (McNeil Pharmaceutical) 417, 1289
Tylenol Cold Medication Caplets and Tablets (McNeil Consumer) 417, 1280
Children's Tylenol Liquid Cold Formula and Chewable Cold Tablets (McNeil Consumer) 417, 1279
Tylenol Cold Medication Liquid (McNeil Consumer) 417, 1280
Tylenol Cold Medication No Drowsiness Formula Caplets (McNeil Consumer) 417, 1281
Tylenol, Extra-Strength, acetaminophen Adult Liquid Pain Reliever (McNeil Consumer) 1279
Tylenol, Extra-Strength, acetaminophen Caplets, Gelcaps, Tablets (McNeil Consumer) 416, 1278
Tylenol, Infants' Drops (McNeil Consumer) 416, 1277
Tylenol, Junior Strength, acetaminophen Coated Caplets (McNeil Consumer) 416, 1278
Tylenol, Regular Strength, acetaminophen Tablets and Caplets (McNeil Consumer) 416, 1278
Tylenol Sinus Medication, Maximum Strength, Tablets and Caplets (McNeil Consumer) 417, 1282
Tylox Capsules (McNeil Pharmaceutical) 417, 1291
Unisom Dual Relief Nighttime Sleep Aid/Analgesic (Leeming) 1191
Vanquish Analgesic Caplets (Glenbrook) 411, 1021
Vicodin (Knoll) 413, 1121
Vicodin ES (Knoll) 413, 1122
Wygesic Tablets (Wyeth-Ayerst) 438, 2452
Zydone Capsules (DuPont Pharmaceuticals) 410, 934

ACETAZOLAMIDE
Acetazolamide Tablets (Rugby) 1914
Diamox Parenteral-See PDR For Ophthalmology (Lederle) 1151
Diamox Sequels-Sustained Release-See PDR For Ophthalmology (Lederle) 414, 1151
Diamox Tablets-See PDR For Ophthalmology (Lederle) 414, 1151

ACETAZOLAMIDE SODIUM
Acetazolamide Sodium Sterile (Quad) 1721

ACETIC ACID
Acetic Acid Otic Solution with Hydrocortisone (Rugby) 1914
Aci-Jel Therapeutic Vaginal Jelly (Ortho Pharmaceutical) 1549
Borofair Otic (Pharmafair) 1680
Fungi-Nail Tincture (Kramer) 1123
Fungoid Tincture (Pedinol) 1661
Otic Domeboro Solution (Miles Pharmaceutical) 1513
Otic Tridesilon Solution 0.05% (Miles Pharmaceutical) 1516
VōSoL HC Otic Solution (Wallace) 434, 2275
VōSoL Otic Solution (Wallace) .. 434, 2275

ACETOHYDROXAMIC ACID
Lithostat (Mission) 1519

ACETYL SULFISOXAZOLE
Gantrisin Pediatric Suspension (Roche) 1793
Gantrisin Syrup (Roche) 1793
Pediazole (Ross) 1896

ACETYLCYSTEINE
Acetylcysteine Solution (Quad) 1721
Mucomyst (Bristol-Myers Institutional) 739

**ACETYLSALICYLIC ACID
(see under ASPIRIN)**

ACIDOPHILUS
Trio-Dophilus (Tyson) 2207

**ACTH
(see under ADRENOCORTICOTROPIC HORMONE)**

ACYCLOVIR
Zovirax Capsules (Burroughs Wellcome) 408, 816
Zovirax Ointment 5% (Burroughs Wellcome) 818

ACYCLOVIR SODIUM
Zovirax Sterile Powder (Burroughs Wellcome) 819

ADENOSINE TRIPHOSPHATE
Adenosine Triphosphate (Tyson) 2206

ADENOSINE-5-MONOPHOSPHATE
Adenosine (Legere) 1192

ADRENOCORTICOTROPIC HORMONE
Acthar (Rorer Pharmaceuticals) 1860
Cortrophin-Zinc ACTH (Organon) 1545
Cortrosyn (Organon) 1545
HP Acthar Gel (Rorer Pharmaceuticals) 1860

L-ALANINE
l-Alanine (Tyson) 2206
Pros-Tech Capsules (Bio-Tech) 681

ALBUMIN (HUMAN)
Albuminar-5, Albumin (Human) U.S.P. 5% (Armour) 622
Albuminar-25, Albumin (Human) U.S.P. 25% (Armour) 622
Albutein 5% (Alpha Therapeutic) 608
Albutein 25% (Alpha Therapeutic) 608
Buminate 5%, Albumin (Human), USP, 5% Solution (Hyland Division) 1052
Buminate 25%, Albumin (Human), USP, 25% Solution (Hyland Division) 1052

ALBUTEROL
Proventil Inhaler (Schering) 428, 2013
Ventolin Inhalation Aerosol (Allen & Hanburys) 404, 604
Ventolin Inhalation Aerosol Refill (Allen & Hanburys) 404, 604

ALBUTEROL SULFATE
Albuterol Sulfate Tablets (Biocraft) 680
Proventil Repetabs Tablets (Schering) 428, 2016
Proventil Solutions for Inhalation 0.5% and 0.083% (Schering) 2014
Proventil Syrup (Schering) 2015
Proventil Tablets (Schering) 428, 2016
Ventolin Rotacaps for Inhalation (Allen & Hanburys) 404, 604
Ventolin Solution for Inhalation (Allen & Hanburys) 404, 604
Ventolin Syrup (Allen & Hanburys) 404, 604
Ventolin Tablets (Allen & Hanburys) 404, 604

ALCLOMETASONE DIPROPIONATE
Aclovate Cream (Glaxo Dermatology) 410, 1005
Aclovate Ointment (Glaxo Dermatology) 410, 1005

ALFENTANIL HYDROCHLORIDE
Alfenta Injection (Janssen) 412, 1080

ALLANTOIN
Herpecin-L Cold Sore Lip Balm (Campbell) 823

ALLOPURINOL
Allopurinol Tablets (Geneva) 1003
Allopurinol Tablets (Lederle) 1134
Allopurinol Tablets (Mylan) 1522
Allopurinol Tablets (Par) 1576
Allopurinol Tablets (Rugby) 1914
Allopurinol Tablets (Squibb) 2124
Zyloprim (Burroughs Wellcome) 408, 821

ALOE VERA
Dermaide Aloe Cream (Dermaide Research) 409, 888

**ALPHA TOCOPHERAL ACETATE
(see under VITAMIN E)**

ALPHAKETOGLUTARIC ACID
Alphaketoglutaric Acid (Tyson) 2206

ALPHA₁-PROTEINASE INHIBITOR (HUMAN)
Alpha₁-Proteinase Inhibitor (Human) Prolastin (Miles-Cutter) 1488

ALPRAZOLAM
Xanax Tablets (Upjohn) 434, 2253

ALPROSTADIL
Prostin VR Pediatric Sterile Solution (Upjohn) 2242

ALTEPLASE, RECOMBINANT
Activase (Genentech) 410, 1000

ALUMINA (FUSED)
Magnesia & Alumina Oral Suspension (Roxane) 1905

ALUMINUM ACETATE
Acid Mantle Creme (Sandoz Consumer) 1925
Osti-Derm Lotion (Pedinol) 1662
Otic Domeboro Solution (Miles Pharmaceutical) 1513

ALUMINUM CARBONATE GEL
Basaljel Capsules (Wyeth-Ayerst) 2352
Basaljel Suspension (Wyeth-Ayerst) 2352
Basaljel Tablets (Wyeth-Ayerst) 2352

ALUMINUM CHLORHYDROXIDE
Pedi-Dri Foot Powder (Pedinol) 1662
Pedi-Pro Foot Powder (Pedinol) 1662

ALUMINUM CHLORIDE
Drysol (Persón & Covey) 1663
Xerac AC (Persón & Covey) 1663

ALUMINUM CHLOROHYDRATE
Breezee Mist Foot Powder (Pedinol) 1661
Dr. Scholl's Super Deodorant Foot Powder (Aluminum Chlorhydrate 15%) (Scholl) .. 429, 2041

ALUMINUM HYDROXIDE
Aluminum & Magnesium Hydroxides with Simethicone I (Roxane) 1905
Aluminum & Magnesium Hydroxides with Simethicone II (Roxane) 1905
Gaviscon Extra Strength Relief Formula Liquid Antacid (Marion) 416, 1265
Gaviscon Extra Strength Relief Formula Antacid Tablets (Marion) 416, 1265
Gaviscon Liquid Antacid (Marion) 416, 1265
WinGel Liquid & Tablets (Winthrop Consumer Products) 2304

ALUMINUM HYDROXIDE GEL
ALternaGEL Liquid (Stuart) 432, 2164
Aludrox Oral Suspension (Wyeth-Ayerst) 2343
Aluminum Hydroxide Gel Concentrated (Roxane) 1905
Aluminum Hydroxide Gel & Tablets (Roxane) 1905
Amphojel Suspension (Wyeth-Ayerst) 2343
Amphojel Suspension without Flavor (Wyeth-Ayerst) 2343
Mylanta Liquid (Stuart) 432, 2170
Mylanta-II Liquid (Stuart) 432, 2170

ALUMINUM HYDROXIDE GEL, DRIED
Alu-Cap Capsules (3M Riker) 1250
Alu-Tab Tablets (3M Riker) 1250
Amphojel Tablets (Wyeth-Ayerst) 2343
Dolprn #3 Tablets (Bock) 681
Gaviscon Antacid Tablets (Marion) 416, 1265
Mylanta Tablets (Stuart) 432, 2170
Mylanta-II Tablets (Stuart) 432, 2170

ALUMINUM SULFATE
Domeboro Powder Packets & Tablets (Miles Pharmaceutical) 419, 1499
Pedi-Boro Soak Paks (Pedinol) 1662

AMANTADINE HYDROCHLORIDE
Amantadine HCl Capsules (Lemmon) 1193
Amantadine HCl Capsules (Warner Chilcott) 2276
Amantadine HCl SG Capsules (Rugby) 1914
Symmetrel (DuPont Pharmaceuticals) 410, 929

AMCINONIDE
Cyclocort Cream (Lederle) 414, 1149
Cyclocort Lotion (Lederle) 414, 1149
Cyclocort Ointment (Lederle) 414, 1149

AMIKACIN SULFATE
Amikin Injectable (Bristol Laboratories) 718
Amiloride Hydrochlorothiazide Tablets, USP (Lederle) 1134

AMILORIDE HYDROCHLORIDE
Amiloride HCl Tablets (Par) 1576

Amiloride HCl and Hydrochlorothiazide Tablets (Biocraft) 680
Amiloride with Hydrochlorothiazide (Par) 1576
Amiloride with Hydrochlorothiazide Tablets (Rugby) 1914
Midamor Tablets (Merck Sharp & Dohme) 418, 1415
Moduretic Tablets (Merck Sharp & Dohme) 418, 1417

AMINO ACID PREPARATIONS
Alpha Plus Capsules (Tyson) 2206
Aminess 5.2% Injection (KabiVitrum) 1099
Aminess Tablets (KabiVitrum) 1099
Amino-Cerv (Milex) 1517
Aminolete Capsules (Tyson) 2206
Aminomine Capsules (Tyson) 2206
Aminoplex Capsules & Powder (Tyson) 2206
Aminosine Capsules (Tyson) 2206
Aminostasis Capsules & Powder (Tyson) 2206
Aminotate Capsules (Tyson) 2206
Branched-Chain Amino Acids Capsules (Solgar) 2121
Marlyn Formula 50 Capsules (Marlyn) 1270
Marlyn Formula 50 Mega Forte Capsules (Marlyn) 1271
Novamine 11.4% Injection (KabiVitrum) 1099
Novamine 15% Injection (KabiVitrum) 1099
Saave (Matrix) 1273
Threonine 500 mg Capsules (Solgar) 2121
Tolerex (Norwich Eaton) 1541
Tropamine (Matrix) 1273
Tryptacin (Arther) 623
Vivonex T.E.N. (Norwich Eaton) 1542

2-AMINO-6-MERCAPTOPURINE
Thioguanine, Tabloid Brand (Burroughs Wellcome) 408, 807

5-AMINO-SALICYLIC ACID
Rowasa (Reid-Rowell) 424, 1741

AMINOBENZOATE POTASSIUM
Pabalate-SF Tablets (Robins) 424, 1757
Potaba (Glenwood) 411, 1021

AMINOBENZOIC ACID
PreSun 15 Lotion Sunscreen (Westwood) 2287

AMINOCAPROIC ACID
Amicar (Lederle) 413, 1138
Aminocaproic Acid Injection (Elkins-Sinn) 936
Aminocaproic Acid Injection (Quad) 1721

AMINOGLUTETHIMIDE
Cytadren (CIBA Pharmaceutical) 408, 848

AMINOHIPPURATE SODIUM
Aminohippurate Sodium Injection (Merck Sharp & Dohme) 1325
Aminophippurate Sodium Injection (Quad) 1721

AMINOPHYLLINE
Aminophyllin Tablets (Searle) 2050
Aminophylline Injection (Preservative-Free) (Elkins-Sinn) 936
Aminophylline Tablets (Duramed) 936
Aminophylline Tablets (Geneva) 1003
Aminophylline Tablets & Oral Solution (Roxane) 1905
Mudrane GG Tablets (Poythress) 1682
Mudrane GG-2 Tablets (Poythress) 1682
Mudrane Tablets (Poythress) 1682
Mudrane-2 Tablets (Poythress) 1682
Somophyllin DF Oral Liquid (Fisons Pharmaceuticals) 941
Somophyllin Oral Liquid (Fisons Pharmaceuticals) 941
Somophyllin Rectal Solution (Fisons Pharmaceuticals) 941

AMIODARONE HYDROCHLORIDE
Cordarone Tablets (Wyeth-Ayerst) 436, 2359

AMITRIPTYLINE HYDROCHLORIDE
Amitriptyline HCl Tablets (Biocraft) 680
Amitriptyline HCl Tablets (Geneva) 1003
Amitriptyline HCl Tablets (Lederle) 1134
Amitriptyline HCl Tablets (Lemmon) 1193
Amitriptyline HCl Tablets (Rugby) 1914

Italic Page Number **Indicates Brief Listing**

C

Italic Page Number **Indicates Brief Listing**

Anbesol Liquid
Antiseptic-Anesthetic
(Whitehall) **435, 2294**
Anbesol Liquid
Antiseptic-Anesthetic -
Maximum Strength
(Whitehall) **435, 2294**
Stri-Dex Regular Strength
Pads (Glenbrook) **1020**
Stri-Dex Regular Strength Big
Pads (Glenbrook) **1020**

ETHYL AMINOBENZOATE
Medicone Derma-HC
Ointment (Medicone) **418, 1315**

ETHYL CHLORIDE
Ethyl Chloride, U.S.P. (Gebauer
Chemical) **972**
Fluro-Ethyl (Gebauer Chemical) **973**

**ETHYLNOREPINEPHRINE
HYDROCHLORIDE**
Bronkephrine Hydrochloride
Injection (Winthrop
Pharmaceuticals) **2307**

ETHYLPAPAVERINE HYDROCHLORIDE
(see under ETHAVERINE
HYDROCHLORIDE)

ETHYNODIOL DIACETATE
Demulen 1/35-21 (Searle) **429, 2057**
Demulen 1/35-28 (Searle) **429, 2057**
Demulen 1/50-21 (Searle) **429, 2057**
Demulen 1/50-28 (Searle) **429, 2057**

ETIDOCAINE HYDROCHLORIDE
Duranest Injections (Astra) **626**

**ETIDRONATE DISODIUM
(DIPHOSPHONATE)**
Didronel (Norwich Eaton) **420, 1534**
Didronel I.V. Infusion (Norwich
Eaton) **1535**

ETOPOSIDE
VePesid Capsules and
Injection (Bristol-Myers
Oncology) **407, 757**

ETRETINATE
Tegison Capsules (Roche
Dermatologics) **425, 1773**

EUCALYPTOL
Ponaris Nasal Mucosal
Emollient (Jamol) **1080**

EUCERITE
Eucerin Cleansing Bar
(Beiersdorf) **669**

F

FACTOR IX COMPLEX
Factor IX Complex Konÿne-HT
(Miles-Cutter) *1488*
Proplex T, Factor IX Complex,
Heat Treated (Hyland
Division) *1053*

FACTOR IX COMPLEX (HUMAN)
Profilnine Heat-Treated (Alpha
Therapeutic) *608*

FAMOTIDINE
Pepcid I.V. (Merck Sharp &
Dohme) **1428**
Pepcid Oral Suspension
(Merck Sharp & Dohme) **1428**
Pepcid Tablets (Merck Sharp &
Dohme) **418, 1428**

FAT EMULSION, INTRAVENOUS
Soyacal 10% (Alpha
Therapeutic) *608*
Soyacal 20% (Alpha
Therapeutic) *608*

FATTY ACIDS
EFA Plus (Tyson) *2207*
Soyacal 10% (Alpha
Therapeutic) *608*
Soyacal 20% (Alpha
Therapeutic) *608*
SuperEPA 1200 Softgels
(Advanced Nutritional) **404, 588**

FENFLURAMINE HYDROCHLORIDE
Pondimin Tablets (Robins) **424, 1759**

FENOPROFEN CALCIUM
Fenoprofen Calcium Capsules
and Tablets (Lemmon) *1193*
Fenoprofen Calcium Capsules
& Tablets (Par) *1576*
Fenoprofen Calcium Capsules
and Tablets (Warner
Chilcott) *2276*
Fenoprofen Calcium Tablets
(Lederle) *1134*
Fenoprofen Calcium Tablets
(Mylan) *1522*
Fenoprofen Calcium Tablets
(Rugby) *1914*

Fenoprofen Calcium Tablets
(Squibb) *2124*
Nalfon 200 Pulvules (Dista) **409, 903**
Nalfon Pulvules & Tablets
(Dista) **409, 903**

FENTANYL CITRATE
Fentanyl Citrate Injection
(Preservative-Free)
(Elkins-Sinn) *936*
Fentanyl Citrate and
Droperidol Injection (Astra) *629*
Innovar Injection (Janssen) **412, 1085**
Sublimaze Injection (Janssen) ... **412, 1089**

FERROUS FUMARATE
Caltrate 600 + Iron (Lederle) **414, 1149**
Cevi-Fer Capsules (sustained
release) (Geriatric) *1004*
Chromagen Capsules (Savage).. **427, 1965**
Doctors' Recommended Best
Multivitamins and Minerals
(Doctors' Recommended) *908*
Doctors' Recommended High
Potency
Therapeutic MultiVitamins
and Minerals (Doctors'
Recommended) **409, 909**
Feostat Drops (Forest
Pharmaceuticals) *968*
Feostat Suspension (Forest
Pharmaceuticals) *968*
Feostat Tablets (Forest
Pharmaceuticals) *968*
Ferancee Chewable Tablets
(Stuart) **432, 2167**
Ferancee-HP Tablets (Stuart) **432, 2167**
Fergon Iron Plus Calcium
Caplets (Winthrop Consumer
Products) *2303*
Ferro-Sequels (Lederle) **414, 1152**
Fetrin Capsules (Lunsco) *1248*
Fumarcee Tablets (Legere) *1192*
Hemaspan Tablets (Bock) *681*
Hemocyte Plus Tabules (U.S.
Pharmaceutical) *2208*
Hemocyte Tablets (U.S.
Pharmaceutical) *2208*
Hemocyte-F Tablets (U.S.
Pharmaceutical) *2208*
Ircon Tablets (Kenwood) *1099*
Ircon-FA Tablets (Kenwood) *1099*
Natalins Rx (Mead Johnson
Laboratories) **417, 1297**
Natalins Tablets (Mead
Johnson Laboratories) **417, 1297**
Poly-Vi-Flor 0.25 mg Vitamins
with Iron and Fluoride
Chewable Tablets (Mead
Johnson Nutritionals) **1305**
Poly-Vi-Flor 0.5 mg Vitamins
with Iron and Fluoride
Chewable Tablets (Mead
Johnson Nutritionals) **1305**
Poly-Vi-Flor 1.0 mg Vitamins
with Iron and Fluoride
Chewable Tablets (Mead
Johnson Nutritionals) **1305**
Pramilet FA (Ross) **1897**
Prenate 90 Tablets (Bock) *681*
Span FF (Lexis) *1196*
Stuartinic Tablets (Stuart) **432, 2171**
Superkids Chewable Tablets
(Health Maintenance) *1036*
Tolfrinic Tablets (Ascher) *623*
Trinsicon/Trinsicon M
Capsules (Allen & Hanburys) **404, 603**
Zenate Tablets (Reid-Rowell).... **424, 1743**

FERROUS GLUCONATE
Fergon Elixir (Winthrop
Consumer Products) *2302*
Fergon Tablets (Winthrop
Consumer Products) *2302*
Ferralet (Mission) *1519*
Ferrous Gluconate Iron
Supplement Tablets
(Lederle) *1134*
Fosfree (Mission) *1519*
I.L.X. B₁₂ Tablets Crystalline
(Kenwood) *1099*
Iromin-G (Mission) *1519*
Megadose (Arco) *622*
Mission Prenatal (Mission) *1520*
Mission Prenatal F.A. (Mission) *1520*
Mission Prenatal H.P. (Mission) *1520*
Mission Surgical Supplement
(Mission) *1520*

FERROUS SULFATE
Feosol Capsules (SmithKline
Consumer) *2083*
Feosol Elixir (SmithKline
Consumer) *2083*
Feosol Tablets (SmithKline
Consumer) *2084*
Fero-Folic-500 (Abbott) **403, 531**
Fero-Grad-500 Filmtab
(Abbott) **403, 532**
Fero-Gradumet Filmtab
(Abbott) *532*
Ferrous Sulfate Elixir, Tablets
(Lederle) *1134*
Ferrous Sulfate Oral Solution
& Tablets (Roxane) *1905*
Heptuna Plus Capsules
(Roerig) **426, 1840**
Iberet (Abbott) *535*
Iberet-500 Filmtab (Abbott) **403, 535**

Iberet-500 Liquid (Abbott) **536**
Iberet-Folic-500 (Abbott) **403, 531**
Iberet-Liquid (Abbott) **536**
Irospan Capsules (Fielding) **941**
Irospan Tablets (Fielding) **941**
Mevanin-C Capsules (Beutlich) **680**
Pramet FA (Ross) **1897**
Slow Fe Tablets (CIBA
Consumer) **408, 839**

FIBER SUPPLEMENT
Complex-Cho (Tyson) *2207*
Enrich (Ross) **1892**
Fibermed High Fiber
Supplements (Purdue
Frederick) **1710**
Fibermed Miniatures (Purdue
Frederick) **1710**
Glucerna (Ross) **1893**
Unifiber (Hickam) **1040**

FIBRINOLYSIN
Elase (Parke-Davis) **421, 1608**
Elase Ointment (Parke-Davis) ... **421, 1608**
Elase-Chloromycetin Ointment
(Parke-Davis) **421, 1608**

FLAVOXATE HYDROCHLORIDE
Urispas Tablets (Smith Kline
&French) **431, 2119**

FLECAINIDE ACETATE
Tambocor Tablets (3M Riker) **1255**

FLOXURIDINE
FUDR Injectable (Roche) **1790**
Floxuridine Injection (Quad) *1721*
Floxuridine Sterile (Quad) *1721*

FLUCYTOSINE
Ancobon Capsules (Roche) **424, 1778**

FLUNISOLIDE
AeroBid Inhaler System
(Forest Pharmaceuticals) **410, 954**
Nasalide Nasal Solution
0.025% (Syntex) **2202**

FLUOCINOLONE ACETONIDE
Fluocinolone Acetate Topical
Solution (Rugby) *1914*
Fluocinolone Acetonide
Cream, Ointment &
Solution (Pharmafair) *1680*
Fluonid Topical Solution
(Herbert) *1037*
Neo-Synalar Cream (Syntex) **2198**
Synalar Creams 0.025%,
0.01% (Syntex) **2198**
Synalar Ointment 0.025%
(Syntex) **2198**
Synalar Topical Solution
0.01% (Syntex) **2198**
Synalar-HP Cream 0.2%
(Syntex) **2198**
Synemol Cream 0.025%
(Syntex) **2198**

FLUOCINONIDE
Fluocinonide Cream, Gel,
Topical Solution and Cream
(Emulsified Base) (Lemmon) *1193*
Fluocinonide Cream (Rugby) *1914*
Lidex Cream 0.05% (Syntex) **2198**
Lidex Gel 0.05% (Syntex) **2198**
Lidex Ointment 0.05%
(Syntex) **2198**
Lidex Topical Solution 0.05%
(Syntex) **2198**
Lidex-E Cream 0.05%
(Syntex) **2198**

FLUORINE & FLUORIDE PREPARATIONS
Adeflor Chewable Tablets
(Upjohn) **433, 2209**
Adeflor Drops (Upjohn) *2209*
Fluoritab Liquid (Fluoritab) **954**
Fluoritab Tablets (Fluoritab) **954**
Luride Drops (Colgate-Hoyt) **875**
Luride Lozi-Tabs Tablets
(Colgate-Hoyt) **409, 875**
Mulvidren-F Softab Tablets
(Stuart) **432, 2169**
Pediaflor Drops (Ross) **1895**
Phos-Flur Oral
Rinse/Supplement
(Colgate-Hoyt) **876**
Point-Two Dental Rinse
(Colgate-Hoyt) **877**
Poly-Vi-Flor 0.25 mg Vitamins
with Fluoride Chewable
Tablets (Mead Johnson
Nutritionals) **1303**
Poly-Vi-Flor 0.5 mg Vitamins
with Fluoride Chewable
Tablets (Mead Johnson
Nutritionals) **1303**
Poly-Vi-Flor 1.0 mg Vitamins
with Fluoride Chewable
Tablets (Mead Johnson
Nutritionals) **1303**
Poly-Vi-Flor 0.25 mg Vitamins
with Fluoride Drops (Mead
Johnson Nutritionals) **1304**
Poly-Vi-Flor 0.5 mg Vitamins
with Fluoride Drops (Mead
Johnson Nutritionals) **1304**

Poly-Vi-Flor 0.25 mg Vitamins
with Iron and Fluoride
Chewable Tablets (Mead
Johnson Nutritionals) **1305**
Poly-Vi-Flor 0.5 mg Vitamins
with Iron and Fluoride
Chewable Tablets (Mead
Johnson Nutritionals) **1305**
Poly-Vi-Flor 1.0 mg Vitamins
with Iron and Fluoride
Chewable Tablets (Mead
Johnson Nutritionals) **1305**
Poly-Vi-Flor 0.25 mg Vitamins
with Iron and Fluoride
Drops (Mead Johnson
Nutritionals) **1305**
Poly-Vi-Flor 0.5 mg Vitamins
with Iron and Fluoride
Drops (Mead Johnson
Nutritionals) **1305**
Poly-Vitamin Fluoride Tablets
(Rugby) *1914*
PreviDent Brush-On Gel
(Colgate-Hoyt) **877**
Thera-Flur Gel-Drops
(Colgate-Hoyt) **877**
Thera-Flur-N Topical
Gel-Drops (Colgate-Hoyt) **877**
Tri-Vi-Flor 0.25 mg Vitamins
with Iron and Fluoride
Drops (Mead Johnson
Nutritionals) **1307**
Tri-Vitamins with Fluoride
Drops (Rugby) *1914*
Vi-Daylin/F ADC Vitamins
Drops With Fluoride (Ross) **1903**
Vi-Daylin/F ADC Vitamins +
Iron Drops With Fluoride
(Ross) **1903**
Vi-Daylin/F Multivitamin
Drops With Fluoride (Ross) **1903**
Vi-Daylin/F Multivitamin +
Iron Drops With Fluoride
(Ross) **1903**
Vi-Daylin/F Multivitamin
Chewable Tablets With
Fluoride (Ross) **1904**
Vi-Daylin/F Multivitamin +
Iron Chewable Tablets With
Fluoride (Ross) **1904**

FLUOROURACIL
Efudex Cream (Roche
Dermatologics) **1772**
Efudex Solutions (Roche
Dermatologics) **1772**
Fluoroplex Topical Solution &
Cream 1% (Herbert) **1037**
Fluorouracil Injection (Quad) *1721*
Fluorouracil Injection (Roche) **1789**

FLUOXETINE HYDROCHLORIDE
Prozac Pulvules (Dista) **409, 905**

FLUOXYMESTERONE
Halotestin Tablets (Upjohn) **434, 2228**
'Ora-Testryl'
(Fluoxymesterone) Tablets
USP (Squibb) *2124*

FLUPHENAZINE
Fluphenazine Tablets (Warner
Chilcott) *2276*

FLUPHENAZINE DECANOATE
Fluphenazine Decanoate
Injection (Quad) *1721*
Prolixin Decanoate (Princeton) **1692**

FLUPHENAZINE ENANTHATE
Prolixin Enanthate (Princeton) **1694**

FLUPHENAZINE HYDROCHLORIDE
Fluphenazine Hydrochloride
Injection (Quad) *1721*
Fluphenazine Hydrochloride
Tablets (Mylan) *1522*
Fluphenazine HCl Tablets
(Rugby) *1914*
Permitil Oral Concentrate
(Schering) **2011**
Permitil Tablets (Schering) **428, 2011**
Prolixin Elixir (Princeton) **1691**
Prolixin Injection (Princeton) **1688**
Prolixin Oral Concentrate
(Princeton) **1689**
Prolixin Tablets (Princeton) **422, 1691**

FLURANDRENOLIDE
Cordran Ointment & Lotion
(Dista) **896**
Cordran SP Cream (Dista) **896**
Cordran Tape (Dista) **897**
Cordran-N Cream and
Ointment (Dista) **896**

FLURAZEPAM HYDROCHLORIDE
Dalmane Capsules (Roche
Products) **425, 1818**
Flurazepam HCl Capsules
(Lederle) *1134*
Flurazepam HCl Capsules
(Par) *1576*
Flurazepam HCl Capsules
(Rugby) *1914*
Flurazepam HCl Capsules
(Warner Chilcott) *2276*

Italic Page Number Indicates Brief Listing

Italic Page Number Indicates Brief Listing

Italic Page Number **Indicates Brief Listing**

Certified poison control centers

The poison control centers in the following list are certified by the American Association of Poison Control Centers. To receive certification, each center must meet certain criteria. It must, for example, serve a large geographic area; it must be open 24 hours a day and provide direct dialing or toll-free access; it must be supervised by a medical director; and it must have registered pharmacists or nurses available to answer questions from the public.

Staff members of these centers are trained to resolve toxicity situations in the home of the caller, but, in some instances, hospital referrals are given.

The centers have a wide variety of toxicology resources, including a computer capability covering some 350,000 substances that are updated quarterly. They also offer a range of educational services to the public as well as to the health-care professional. In some states, these large centers exist side by side with smaller poison control centers that provide more limited information.

AMERICAN ASSOCIATION OF POISON CONTROL CENTERS

ALABAMA

Alabama Poison Center
Alabama Poison Center
809 University Boulevard East
Tuscaloosa, AL 35401
Emergency Numbers
800/462-0800 AL only
205/345-0600
FAX: 205/759-7994
Director:Richard W.Looser, B.S.;
205/345-0938
Medical Director: Perry L.
Lovely, M.D.; 205/345-0600

Children's Hospital of Alabama Regional Poison Control Center
1600 7th Avenue South
Birmingham, AL 35233
Emergency Numbers
205/939-9201 AL only
800/292-6678
205/933-4050
Director: William D. King,
R. Ph., M.P.H.: 205/939-9720
Medical Director: Edward C.
Kohaut, M.D.; 205/939-9100

ARIZONA

Arizona Poison and Drug Information Center
Health Sciences Center,
Room 3204K
1501 North Campbell
Tucson, AZ 85724
Emergency Numbers
602/626-6016 (Tucson)
800/362-0101 (statewide)
FAX: 602/626-4063
Director: Theodore G. Tong,
Pharm. D.; 602/626-7899
Medical Director: John B.
Sullivan, Jr., M.D.;
602/626-6312

Samaritan Regional Poison Center
Good Samaritan Medical
Center
1130 East McDowell, Suite A5
Phoenix, AZ 85006
Emergency Numbers
602/253-3334
FAX: 602/239-4138
Director: Joyce M. Bradley,
R.N., M.S.; 602/253-0813
Medical Director: Donald B.
Kunkel, M.D.; 602/253-2314

CALIFORNIA

Fresno Regional Poison Control Center
Fresno Community Hospital
and Medical Center
Fresno and R Streets
Fresno, CA 93715
Emergency Numbers
209/445-1222
800/346-5922
FAX: 209/442-6483
Director: Brent R. Ekins,
Pharm. D.; 209/442-6479
Medical Director: Rick Geller,
M.D.; 209/442-6408

Los Angeles County Medical Association
Regional Poison Center
1925 Wilshire Bouevard
Los Angeles, CA 90057
Emergency Numbers
213/664-2121
213/484-5151
800/777-6476
FAX: 213/413-5255
Director: Corrine Ray, R.N.,
B.S; 213/664-2121
Medical Director: Marc J.
Bayer, M.D.; 818/364-3107

San Diego Regional Poison Center
UCSD Medical Center
225 Dickinson Street
San Diego, CA 92103-1990
Emergency Numbers
619/543-6000
800/876-4766
FAX: 619/692-1867
Director: Anthony S.
Manoguerra, Pharm. D.;
619/543-6010
Medical Director: George M.
Shumaik, M.D.; 619/543-3666

San Francisco Regional Poison Center
San Francisco General
Hospital
1001 Potrero Avenue, Room
IE86
San Francisco, CA 94110
Emergency Numbers
415/476-6600
800/523-2222
FAX: 415/821-8513
Director/Medical Director:
Kent R. Olson, M.D.;
415/821-5524

UC Davis Regional Poison Control Center
2315 Stockton Boulevard,
Room 1511
Sacramento, CA 95817
Emergency Numbers
916/453-3692
800/342-9293 (Northern
CA only)
FAX: 916/453-7796
Director: Judith Alsop,
Pharm. D.; 916/453-3414
Medical Director: Timothy
Albertson, M.D., Ph.D.;
916/453-5010

COLORADO

Rocky Mountain Poison and Drug Center
645 Bannock Street
Denver, CO 80204-4507
Emergency Numbers
303/629-1123 (CO)
FAX: 303/623-1119
Director: Barry H. Rumack,
M.D.; 303/893-7774
Medical Director: Kenneth
Kulig, M.D., F.A.C.E.P.;
303/893-7774

FLORIDA

Florida Poison Information Center
The Tampa General Hospital
Davis Islands
Post Office Box 1289
Tampa, FL 33601
Emergency Numbers
813/253-4444 (Tampa only)
800/282-3171 (Florida)
Director: Sven A. Normann,
Pharm.D.; 813/251-7044
Co-Medical Directors: James
V. Hilllman, M.D.; Gregory G.
Gaar, M.D.; 813/251-6911

GEORGIA

Georgia Regional Poison Control Center
80 Butler Street, S.E.
Atlanta, GA 30335-3801
Emergency Numbers
404/589-4400
800/282-5846 (GA only)
FAX: 404/525-2816
Director: Gaylord P. Lopez,
Pharm.D.; 404/589-4400
Medical Director: Robert J.
Geller, M.D.; 404/589-4400

KENTUCKY

Kentucky Regional Poison Center of Kosair Chidren's Hospital
224 East Broadway, Suite 305
Louisville, KY 40202
Emergency Numbers
502/589-8222
800/722-5725 (KY Toll free)
Director: Nancy J. Matyunas,
Pharm.D.; 502/562-7263
Medical Director: George C.
Rodgers Jr, M.D., Ph.D.;
502/562-8837

MARYLAND

Maryland Poison Center
20 North Pine Street
Baltimore, MD 21201
Emergency Numbers
301/528-7701
800/492-2414 (MD only)
FAX: 301/328-7184
Director: Gary M. Oderda,
Pharm.D., M.P.H.; 301/328-7604
Medical Director: Richard L.
Gorman, M.D; 301/328-7604

334

MASSACHUSETTS

Massachusetts Poison Control System
300 Longwood Avenue
Boston, MA 02115
Emergency Numbers
617/232-2120 Boston Area
800/682-9211 Toll Free in MA
Director/Medical Director:
Alan Woolf, M.D., M.P.H.;
617/735-6609

MICHIGAN

Blodgett Regional Poison Center
1840 Wealthy Street S.E.
Grand Rapids, MI 49506
Emergency Numbers
800/632-2727 MI only
FAX: 616/774-7204
Director: Daniel J. McCoy,
Ph.D.; 616/774-7851
Medical Director: John R.
Mauer, M.D.; 616/774-7851

Poison Control Center
Children's Hospital of
Michigan
3901 Beaubien Boulevard
Detroit, MI 48201
Emergency Numbers
313/745-5711 (Metro
Detroit)
800/462-6642 (Rest of MI)
FAX: 313/745-5602
Director/Medical Director:
Regine Aronow, M.D.;
313/745-5335
Administrative Manager:
Richard Dorsch, M.D.;
313/745-5329

MINNESOTA

Hennepin Regional Poison Center
Hennepin County Medical
Center
701 Park Avenue South
Minneapolis, MN 55415
Emergency Numbers
612/347-3141
FAX: 612/347-3968
Director: Michael J. Wieland,
R.Ph.; 612/347-3144
Medical Director: Louis J.
Ling, M.D.; 612/347-3174

Minnesota Regional Poison Center
St. Paul-Ramsey Medical
Center
640 Jackson Street
St. Paul, MN 55101
Emergency Numbers
612/221-2113
800/222-1222 MN only
Director: Leo Sioris,
Pharm.D.; 612/221-3192
Medical Director: Samuel
Hall, M.D., A.B.M.T.;
612/221-3470

MISSOURI

Cardinal Glennon Children's Hospital
Regional Poison Center
1465 South Grand Boulevard
St. Louis, MO 63104
Emergency Numbers
800/392-9111 (MI only)
314/772-5200
800/366-8888
FAX: 314/577-5355
Director: Michael W.
Thompson, B.S. Pharm.;
314/772-8300
Medical Director: Anthony J.
Scalzo, M.D.; 314/772-8300

NEW JERSEY

New Jersey Poison Information and Education System
201 Lyons Avenue
Newark, NJ 07112
Emergency Numbers
800/962-1253 (NJ only)
201/923-0764 (Outside of
NJ)
FAX: 201/926-0013
Director/Medical Director:
Steven M. Marcus, M.D;
201/926-7443

NEW MEXICO

New Mexico Poison and Drug Information Center
University of New Mexico
Albuquerque, NM 87131
Emergency Numbers
505/843-2551
800/432-6866 (NM only)
Director: William G.
Troutman, Pharm.D.;
505/277-4261
Medical Director: Dan
Tandberg, M.D.; 505/277-5064

NEW YORK

Long Island Regional Poison Control Center
2201 Hempstead Turnpike
East Meadow, NY 11554
Emergency Numbers
516/542-2323
Director/Medical Director:
Howard C. Mofenson, M.D.;
516/542-3707

New York City Poison Center
455 First Avenue, Room 123
New York, NY 10016
Emergency Numbers
212/340-4494
212/764-7667
FAX: 212/340-4525
Director: Richard S.
Weisman, Pharm.D.;
212/340-4497
Medical Director: Lewis
Goldfrank, M.D.; 212/561-3346

NORTH CAROLINA

Duke Regional Poison Control Center
Duke University Medical
Center
Box 3007
Durham, NC 27710
Emergency Numbers
800/672-1697 (NC only)
Medical Director: Shirley
Osterhout, M.D.; 919/684-4438
Assistant Director: Chris
Rudd, Pharm.D.;
919/681-4574

OHIO

Central Ohio Poison Center
700 Children's Drive
Columbus, OH 43205
Emergency Numbers
614/228-1323
800/682-7625
Director: Judith G. D'Orsi,
B.A. 614/461-2717
Medical Director: Mary Ellen
Mortensen, M.D.;
614/461-2256

Regional Poison Control System and Cincinnati Drug and Poison Information Center
231 Bethesda Avenue, M.L.,
#144
Cincinnati, OH 45267-0144
Emergency Numbers
513/558-5111
FAX: 513/558-5301
Director: Leonard T. Sigell,
Ph.D.; 513/558-9182
Medical Director: Clifford G.
Grulee, Jr., M.D.;
513/558-7336

OREGON

Oregon Poison Center
Oregon Health Sciences
University
3181 SW Sam Jackson Park
Road
Portland, OR 97201
Emergency Numbers
503/279-8968;
800/452-7165 OR only
Director: Terry Putman, R.N.;
503/279-7799
Medical Director: Brent T.
Burton, M.D.; 503/279-7799

PENNSYLVANIA

Delaware Valley Regional Poison Control Center
One Children's Center
34th & Civic Center
Boulevard
Philadelphia, PA 19104
Emergency Numbers
215/386-2100
FAX: 215/386-3692
Director: Thomas E.
Kearney, Pharm.D.; 215/823-
7203
Medical Director: Fred M.
Henretig, M.D.; 215/596-8454

Pittsburgh Poison Center
One Children's Place
3705 5th Avenue at DeSoto
Pittsburgh, PA 15213
Emergency Numbers
412/681-6669
FAX: 412/692-5868
Director: Edward P.
Krenzelok, Pharm.D.;
412/692-5600
Assistant Director: Bonnie S.
Dean, R.N., B.S.N.;
412/692-5600
Medical Director: Sandra M.
Schneider, M.D.;
412/648-6000, ext. 3669

RHODE ISLAND

593 Eddy Street
Providence, RI 02903
Emergency Numbers
401/277-5727
401/277-8062 (TDD)
Director: Philip N. Johnson,
Ph.D.; 401/277-5906
Medical Director: William J.
Lewander, M.D.; 401/277-5906

TEXAS

North Texas Poison Center
5201 Harry Hines Boulevard
Dallas, TX 75235
Emergency Numbers
214/590-5000
800/441-0040 (TX only)
FAX: 214/590-8096,
Attention: Poison Center
Director: Lena C. Day, R.N.,
B.S.N., C.S.P.I.; 214/590-5625
Medical Director: Gary Reed,
M.D.; 214/688-2992
Assistant Medical Director:
Tom Kurt, M.D.; 214/590-6625

Texas State Poison Center
University of Texas Medical
Branch
Galveston, TX 77550-2780
Emergency Numbers
409/765-1420 (Galveston)
800/392-8548 (TX only)
713/654-1701 (Houston)
512/478-4490 (Austin)
Director: Michael D. Ellis,
M.S.; 409/761-3332
Medical Director: Wayne R.
Snodgrass, M.D., Ph.D.;
409/761-1561

UTAH

Intermountain Regional Poison Control Center
50 North Medical Drive,
Building 528
Salt Lake City, UT 84132
Emergency Number
801/581-2151
Director: Joseph C. Veltri,
Pharm.D.; 801/581-7504
Medical Director: Douglas
Rollins, M.D., Ph.D.;
801/581-5117

WASHINGTON, D.C.

National Capital Poison Center
Georgetown University
Hospital
3800 Reservoir Road, N.W.
Washington, DC 20007
Business/Emergency
Numbers
202/625-3333
202/784-4660 (TTY)
FAX: 202/784-2530
Director/Medical Director:
Toby Litovitz, M.D.;
202/784-2088

WEST VIRGINIA

West Virginia Poison Center
3110 MacCorkle Avenue, S.E.
Charleston, WV 25304
Emergency Numbers
304/348-4211 (local)
800/642-3625 (intrastate)
FAX: 304/348-9560
Director: Gregory P. Wedin,
Pharm.D.; 304/347-1212
Medical Director: David E.
Seidler, M.D.; 304/347-1212

Conversion Tables

Metric Doses With Approximate Apothecary Equivalents

The approximate dose equivalents represent the quantities usually prescribed by physicians using, respectively, the metric and apothecary system of weights and measures. When prepared dosage forms such as tablets, capsules, etc. are prescribed in the metric system, the pharmacist may dispense the corresponding approximate equivalent in the apothecary system and vice versa. (Note: A milliliter [mL] is the approximate equivalent of a cubic centimeter [cc]). Exact equivalents, which appear in the United States Pharmacopeia and the National Formulary, must be used to calculate quantities in pharmaceutical formulas and prescription compounding:

Metric	LIQUID MEASURE Approximate Apothecary Equivalents	Metric	LIQUID MEASURE Approximate Apothecary Equivalents	Metric	LIQUID MEASURE Approximate Apothecary Equivalents	Metric	LIQUID MEASURE Approximate Apothecary Equivalents
1000 mL	1 quart	3 mL	45 minims	30 mL	1 fluid ounce	0.25 mL	4 minims
750 mL	1½ pints	2 mL	30 minims	15 mL	4 fluid drams	0.2 mL	3 minims
500 mL	1 pint	1 mL	15 minims	10 mL	2½ fluid drams	0.1 mL	1½ minims
250 mL	8 fluid ounces	0.75 mL	12 minims	8 mL	2 fluid drams	0.06 mL	1 minim
200 mL	7 fluid ounces	0.6 mL	10 minims	5 mL	1¼ fluid drams	0.05 mL	¾ minim
100 mL	3½ fluid ounces	0.5 mL	8 minims	4 mL	1 fluid dram	0.03 mL	½ minim
50 mL	1¾ fluid ounces	0.3 mL	5 minims				

Metric	WEIGHT Approximate Apothecary Equivalents	Metric	WEIGHT Approximate Apothecary Equivalents	Metric	WEIGHT Approximate Apothecary Equivalents	Metric	WEIGHT Approximate Apothecary Equivalents
30g	1 ounce	30mg	1/2 grain	500mg	7½ grains	1.2 mg	1/50 grain
15g	4 drams	25mg	3/8 grain	400mg	6 grains	1 mg	1/60 grain
10g	2½ drams	20mg	1/3 grain	300mg	5 grains	800 μg	1/80 grain
7.5g	2 drams	15mg	1/4 grain	250mg	4 grains	600 μg	1/100 grain
6g	90 grains	12mg	1/5 grain	200mg	3 grains	500 μg	1/120 grain
5g	75 grains	10mg	1/6 grain	150mg	2½ grains	400 μg	1/150 grain
4g	60 grains (1 dram)	8mg	1/8 grain	125mg	2 grains	300 μg	1/200 grain
3g	45 grains	6mg	1/10 grain	100mg	1½ grains	250 μg	1/250 grain
2g	30 grains (½ dram)	5mg	1/12 grain	75mg	1¼ grains	200 μg	1/300 grain
1.5g	22 grains	4mg	1/15 grain	60mg	1 grain	150 μg	1/400 grain
1g	15 grains	3mg	1/20 grain	50mg	¾ grain	120 μg	1/500 grain
750mg	12 grains	2mg	1/30 grain	40mg	⅔ grain	100 μg	1/600 grain
600mg	10 grains	1.5mg	1/40 grain				

Approximate Household Equivalents

For household purposes, an American Standard Teaspoon is defined by the American National Standards Institute as containing 4.93 ± 0.24 mL. The USP states that in view of the almost universal practice of employing teaspoons ordinarily available in the household for administration of medicine, the teaspoon may be regarded as representing 5 mL. Household units of measure often are used to inform patients of the size of a liquid dose. Because of difficulties involved in measuring liquids under normal conditions of use, household spoons are not appropriate when accurate measurement of a liquid dose is required. When accurate measurement of a liquid dose is required, the USP recommends that a calibrated oral syringe or dropper be used.

1 fluid dram = 1 teaspoonful = 5 mL
2 fluid drams = 1 dessertspoonful = 10 mL
4 fluid drams = 1 tablespoonful = 15 mL
2 fluid ounces = 1 wineglassful = 60 mL
4 fluid ounces = 1 teacupful = 120 mL
8 fluid ounces = 1 tumblerful = 240 mL

Pounds—Kilograms (kg) Conversion

1 pound = 0.453592 kg
1 kg = 2.2 pounds

Temperature Conversion Table:

$$9 \times °C = (5 \times °F) - 160$$
Centigrade to Fahrenheit = $(°C \times 9/5) + 32 = °F$
Fahrenheit to Centigrade = $(°F - 32) \times 5/9 = °C$

Milliequivalents per Liter (mEq/L)

$$mEq/L = \frac{\text{weight of salt (g)} \times \text{valence of ion} \times 1000}{\text{molecular weight of salt}}$$

$$\text{weight of salt (g)} = \frac{mEq/L \times \text{molecular weight of salt}}{\text{valence of ion} \times 1000}$$

Key to Controlled Substances Categories

Products listed with the symbols shown below are subject to the Controlled Substances Act of 1970. These drugs are categorized according to their potential for abuse. The greater the potential, the more severe the limitations on their prescription.

CATEGORY	INTERPRETATION
C II	**High potential for abuse.** Use may lead to severe physical or psychological dependence. Prescriptions must be written in ink, or typewritten and signed by the practitioner. Verbal prescriptions must be confirmed in writing within 72 hours, and may be given only in a genuine emergency. No renewals are permitted.
C III	**Some potential for abuse.** Use may lead to low-to-moderate physical dependence or high psychological dependence. Prescriptions may be oral or written. Up to 5 renewals are permitted within 6 months.
C IV	**Low potential for abuse.** Use may lead to limited physical or psychological dependence. Prescriptions may be oral or written. Up to 5 renewals are permitted within 6 months.
C V	**Subject to state and local regulation.** Abuse potential is low; a prescription may not be required.

Key to FDA Use-in-pregnancy Ratings

The Food and Drug Administration's Pregnancy Categories are based on the degree to which available information has ruled out risk to the fetus, balanced against the drug's potential benefits to the patient. Ratings range from "A," for drugs that have been tested for teratogenicity under controlled conditions without showing evidence of damage to the fetus, to "D" and "X" for drugs that are definitely teratogenic. The "D" rating is generally reserved for drugs with no safer alternatives. The "X" rating means there is absolutely no reason to risk using the drug in pregnancy.

CATEGORY	INTERPRETATION
A	**Controlled studies show no risk.** Adequate, well-controlled studies in pregnant women have failed to demonstrate risk to the fetus.
B	**No evidence of risk in humans.** Either animal findings show risk, but human findings do not; or, if no adequate human studies have been done, animal findings are negative.
C	**Risk cannot be ruled out.** Human studies are lacking, and animal studies are either positive for fetal risk, or lacking as well. However, potential benefits may justify the potential risk.
D	**Positive evidence of risk.** Investigational or post-marketing data show risk to the fetus. Nevertheless, potential benefits may outweigh the potential risk.
X	**Contraindicated in pregnancy.** Studies in animals or human, or investigational or post-marketing reports have shown fetal risk which clearly outweighs any possible benefit to the patient.

Product Identification Section

Designed to help you identify products, this section contains actual size, full-color reproductions of tablets, caplets and capsules selected for inclusion by participating manufacturers. Tubes, ampules, vials, bottles, etc. are reduced in size to fit space available.

Because tablets and capsules, for the most part, are shown here, you should not infer that these are the only dosage forms. Where other dosage forms are available, the product name is preceded by the † symbol. Refer to the product's description in the PRODUCT INFORMATION (White Section) or check directly with manufacturer.

Letters and/or numbers followed by an asterisk (*) accompanying a product photograph designate the manufacturers' identification code.

While every effort has been made to reproduce products faithfully, this section should be considered only as a quick reference identification aid.

INDEX BY MANUFACTURER

This section is made possible through the courtesy of the manufacturers whose products appear on the following pages. Page numbers of individual products included can be found in the Product Name, Generic and Product Category Indices.

ABBOTT

For description of Abbo-Code™ identifications, see Abbo-Code index at beginning of Abbott Product Information Section.

Abbott — AN* 25 mg, AO* 50 mg**
Dicumarol Tablets, USP

Abbott — EA* 250 mg, 500 mg
Erythromycin Base Filmtab®
(erythromycin tablets, USP)

Abbott — 10 mEq (750 mg)
K•Tab®
(potassium chloride extended-release tablets, USP)

Abbott — AD* 250 mg**, AE* 500 mg**
Peganone®
(ethotoin tablets)

Abbott — 1A* 2.5 mg, 1C* 5 mg
Cartrol® Filmtab® Tablet
(carteolol hydrochloride)

Abbott — 2.5 mg**, 5 mg**
Enduron®
(methyclothiazide tablets, USP)

Abbott — ER 250 mg
Erythromycin Delayed-Release Capsules, USP

Abbott — CF 50 mg, CH 100 mg
†Nembutal® Sodium
(pentobarbital sodium capsules, USP)

Abbott — 200 mg, PLACIDYL 500 mg, PLACIDYL 750 mg
Placidyl®
(ethchlorvynol capsules, USP)

Abbott — NJ*
Cefol® Filmtab®
(high potency B-complex, folic acid, vitamin E with 750 mg vitamin C)

Abbott — LS*, LT*
Enduronyl® **Enduronyl® Forte****
(methyclothiazide and deserpidine)

Abbott — NA*, NB* 10 mg, 25 mg
Eutonyl® Filmtab®
(pargyline hydrochloride tablets, USP)

Abbott — LU* Ogen .625, LV* Ogen 1.25, Ogen 2.5, LX* LY* Ogen 5
Ogen®
(estropipate tablets, USP)

Abbott — AA* 25 mg, AB* 50 mg
Chlorthalidone Tablets, USP

Abbott — CHEW EZ 200 mg
†EryPed® Chewable
(erythromycin ethylsuccinate tablets, USP)

Abbott — NK
Eutron® Filmtab®
(pargyline hydrochloride and methyclothiazide)

Abbott (Applicator and tube shown smaller than actual size)
OGEN® Vaginal Cream 1½ oz 1.5 mg/g
Ogen® Vaginal Cream
(estropipate vaginal cream, USP)

Abbott
Surbex-T® Filmtab®
Surbex®-750 With Iron Filmtab®
Surbex®-750 With Zinc Filmtab®
(high-potency B-complex vitamins)

Abbott — TH* 18.75 mg, TI* 37.5 mg, TJ* 75 mg
Cylert®
(pemoline)

Abbott — EE 400 mg
†E.E.S. 400® Filmtab®
(erythromycin ethylsuccinate tablets, USP)

Abbott
Fero-Folic-500® Filmtab®
(controlled-release Iron with Vitamin C and folic acid)
Fero-Grad-500® Filmtab®
(controlled-release Iron plus Vitamin C)

Abbott — TK* 37.5 mg chewable tablets
Cylert®
(pemoline)

Abbott (Shown smaller than actual size)
200 mg/5 ml **EryPed® 200**, 400 mg/5 ml **EryPed® 400**
100 mg/2.5 ml (dropperful) **EryPed® Drops**
(erythromycin ethylsuccinate for oral suspension, USP)

Abbott — DF* 1 mg, DH* 2 mg, DJ* 5 mg, DI* 10 mg
Hytrin®
(terazosin hydrochloride tablets)

Abbott
Optilets®-500 (high potency therapeutic vitamin formulation)
Optilets-M-500® (high potency therapeutic vitamin formulation with minerals)

Abbott — TX 11.25 mg **Tranxene®-SD Half Strength**, 22.5 mg **Tranxene®-SD**
(clorazepate dipotassium)

Abbott — 250 mg
†Depakene®
(valproic acid capsules, USP)

Abbott — AK
Iberet®-500 Filmtab®
(controlled-release Iron plus B-Complex and Vitamin C)
Iberet-Folic-500® Filmtab®
(controlled-release Iron with Vitamin C and B-Complex including folic acid)

Abbott — Oretic* 25 mg, Oretic* 50 mg**
Hydrochlorothiazide Tablets, USP
Oretic®

Abbott — TL* 3.75 mg**, TM* 7.5 mg**, TN* 15 mg**
Tranxene® T-Tab™ Tablets
(clorazepate dipotassium tablets)

Abbott — 125 mg, NR 250 mg, NS 500 mg
Depakote®
(divalproex sodium enteric-coated tablets)

Abbott — ND* 10 mg, NE* 25 mg, NL* 50 mg
Janimine® Filmtab®
(imipramine hydrochloride tablets, USP)

Abbott — LM* 2 mg, 2½ mg, 5 mg, LO*, LN* 7½ mg, 10 mg, LR* **Panwarfin®** LF*
Panwarfin®
(warfarin sodium tablets, USP)

Abbott — EC 250 mg, ED 500 mg, EH 333 mg
Ery-Tab®
(erythromycin delayed-release tablets, USP)

Abbott (Shown smaller than actual size)
NDC 0074-3611 **K-Lor™ 20 mEq** POTASSIUM CHLORIDE FOR ORAL SOLUTION, USP
K-LOR™ 20 mEq
(potassium chloride for oral solution, USP)

Abbott — 150 mg, 300 mg
†Paradione®
(paramethadione capsules, USP)

Abbott — AM 300 mg Capsules, USP, LE* 150 mg Dulcet® Tablet, USP
†Tridione®
(trimethadione)

Abbott — Gradumet® tablets MC* 5 mg, ME* 10 mg, MF* 15 mg
†Desoxyn®
(methamphetamine hydrochloride)

Abbott — ES* 250 mg, ET* 500 mg
Erythrocin® Stearate Filmtab®
(erythromycin stearate tablets, USP)

Abbott — PCE 333 mg
PCE®
(erythromycin particles in tablets)

While every effort has been made to reproduce products faithfully, this section is to be considered a quick-reference identification aid. In cases of suspected overdosage, etc., chemical analysis of the product should be done.

*Abbott Abbo-Code identification letters. Filmtab®—Film-sealed tablets, Abbott. **Grooved tablets.

ADRIA

Original Flavor

Cherry Flavor

Emetrol®
(phosphorated carbohydrate solution)

Adria

500 mg
(6.7 mEq)
(Both sides of tablet shown)

Kaon-Cl® (potassium chloride)
Extended-Release Tablets

Adria
(Both sides of tablet shown)

750 mg (10 mEq)
Kaon Cl®-10
Extended-Release Tablets
(potassium chloride)

Adria

Nitrol® Ointment
(2% nitroglycerin ointment)

ADVANCED NUTRITIONAL

PhosChol® 565 Softgel
(phosphatidylcholine, highly purified lecithin)

Advanced Nutritional

PhosChol® 900 Softgel
(phosphatidylcholine, highly purified lecithin)

Advanced Nutritional

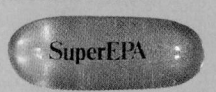

SuperEPA® 1200 Softgel
(omega-3 polyunsaturated fatty acids)

Because tablets and capsules are shown in this section, do not infer that these are the only dosage forms available. Where a product name is preceded by the symbol †, refer to the description in the Product Information (White Section) for other forms.

ALLEN & HANBURYS

(Shown smaller than actual size)

Beclovent® Inhalation Aerosol
(beclomethasone dipropionate, USP)
42 mcg of beclomethasone dipropionate per inhalation

Allen & Hanburys

(Shown smaller than actual size)

**Beclovent®/Beconase®
Inhalation Aerosol**
(beclomethasone dipropionate, USP)
42 mcg of beclomethasone dipropionate per inhalation

Allen & Hanburys
(Shown smaller than actual size)

Beconase® Inhalation Aerosol
(beclomethasone dipropionate, USP)
42 mcg of beclomethasone dipropionate per inhalation

Allen & Hanburys
(Shown smaller than actual size)

Beconase AQ® Nasal Spray, 0.042%
(beclomethasone dipropionate, monohydrate)
42 mcg of beclomethasone dipropionate per actuation

Allen & Hanburys
(Both sides of tablet shown)

125 mg

250 mg

500 mg

Ceftin® Tablets
(cefuroxime axetil)

Allen & Hanburys

130 mg
Theobid® Jr.

260 mg
Theobid®

(theophylline, anhydrous)

Allen & Hanburys

20 ml   40 ml

Trandate® Injection
(labetalol hydrochloride)

Allen & Hanburys

4 ml

8 ml

Prefilled, disposable syringes
(Shown smaller than actual size)
Trandate® Injection
(labetalol hydrochloride)

Allen & Hanburys
(Both sides of tablet shown)

100 mg

200 mg

300 mg
Trandate® Tablets
(labetalol hydrochloride)

Allen & Hanburys
(Both sides of tablet shown)

100/25

200/25

300/25

Trandate® HCT Tablets
(labetalol hydrochloride/
hydrochlorothiazide)

Allen & Hanburys

Trinsicon® Capsules
(hematinic concentrate with intrinsic factor)

Allen & Hanburys

Trinsicon® M
(hematinic concentrate modified)

Allen & Hanburys
(Shown smaller than actual size)

Ventolin® Inhalation Aerosol
(albuterol, USP)
90 mcg of albuterol per inhalation

Allen & Hanburys
(Shown smaller than actual size)

To be used only with Ventolin Actuator

Ventolin® Inhalation Aerosol Refill
(albuterol, USP)
90 mcg of albuterol per inhalation

Allen & Hanburys

**Ventolin
Rotacaps®
for Inhalation
Capsule**

Rotahaler®
(Shown smaller than actual size)

Ventolin Rotacaps® for Inhalation
(albuterol sulfate, USP)
200 mcg albuterol

Allen & Hanburys

20 ml, 5 mg/ml

**Ventolin®
Solution for Inhalation, 0.5%**
(albuterol sulfate, USP)

Allen & Hanburys
(Shown smaller than actual size)

Ventolin® Syrup
(albuterol sulfate)
2 mg/5 ml

Allen & Hanburys
(Both sides of tablets shown)

2 mg   4 mg
Ventolin® Tablets
(albuterol sulfate, USP)

Allen & Hanburys

Vicon-C®
(B-complex with Vitamin C, zinc and magnesium)

Allen & Hanburys

Vicon Forte® Capsules
(B-complex with Vitamins C, A, and E, zinc, magnesium, and manganese)

Allen & Hanburys

Vicon® Plus Capsules
(B-complex with Vitamins C, A, and E, zinc, magnesium, and manganese)

Allen & Hanburys

Vi-Zac® Capsules
(Vitamins A, C, and E with zinc)

ALZA
(Shown smaller than actual size)

Inserter

PROGESTASERT®
Intrauterine Progesterone
Contraceptive System

AMGEN

1 ml vials
2,000 units/ml, 4000 units/ml
& 10,000 units/ml

EPOGEN®
(Epoetin alfa)

ANAQUEST

15 mL (10 mg/mL)
multidose vials

Enlon®
(edrophonium chloride
injection, USP)

Anaquest

125 mL
also available: 250 mL

Ēthrane®
(enflurane, USP)

Anaquest

100 mL
Forane®
(isoflurane, USP)

BEACH

BEELITH

Beach

K-PHOS® M.F.   K-PHOS® No. 2**

Beach

K-PHOS® NEUTRAL**

Beach

500 mg.
K-PHOS® Original (Sodium Free)
(Potassium Acid Phosphate)

Beach

THIACIDE™**

Beach

UROQID®-Acid   UROQID®-Acid No. 2**

Beecham Laboratories

250 mg. amoxicillin trihydrate/
125 mg. clavulanate potassium

500 mg. amoxicillin trihydrate/
125 mg. clavulanate potassium
†Augmentin®
(amoxicillin/clavulanate potassium)

Beecham Laboratories

125 mg. amoxicillin trihydrate/
31.25 mg. clavulanate potassium

250 mg. amoxicillin trihydrate/
62.5 mg. clavulanate potassium
†Augmentin® Chewable Tablets

Beecham Laboratories

Available also as
oral suspension,
pediatric drops and
chewable tablets

250 mg.

500 mg.
†Amoxil®
(amoxicillin)

Beecham Laboratories

125 mg.

250 mg.
(Both sides of tablets shown)
†Amoxil® Chewable Tablets
(amoxicillin)

Beecham Laboratories

Anexsia® 5/500
(hydrocodone bitartrate 5 mg. and
acetaminophen 500 mg.)

Beecham Laboratories

Anexsia® 7.5/650
(hydrocodone bitartrate 7.5 mg. and
acetaminophen 650 mg.)

Beecham Laboratories

250 mg.
Bactocill®
(oxacillin)   500 mg.

Beecham Laboratories

Net Wt.
15 grams

Bactroban®
(mupirocin)   **Ointment 2%**

Beecham Laboratories

250 mg.
Cloxapen®   500 mg.
(cloxacillin)

Beecham Laboratories

250 mg.
Dycill®   500 mg.
(dicloxacillin)

Beecham Laboratories

30 mg.
Fastin®
(phentermine HCl)

Beecham Laboratories

†Nucofed®
(20 mg. codeine phosphate)
(60 mg. pseudoephedrine HCl)

Beecham Laboratories

100 mg.

250 mg.

†Tigan® Capsules
(trimethobenzamide HCl)

Beecham Laboratories

3.1 Gram Vial

3.1 Gram PB

31 Gram Pharmacy Bulk Package

31 Gm

Timentin®
(sterile ticarcillin disodium
and clavulanate potassium)

BEECHAM PRODUCTS USA

Special Comb
Included

4 fl. oz.

A200

**A-200™
Pediculicide Shampoo**
Also available:
A-200 Shampoo, 2 fl. oz.
A-200 Gel Concentrate, 1 oz.

BERLEX

scored
dye-free
tablet

†Deconamine® Tablets
(4 mg chlorpheniramine maleate
and 60 mg d-pseudoephedrine HCl)

(sustained release)
Deconamine® SR Capsules
(8 mg chlorpheniramine maleate and
120 mg d-pseudoephedrine HCl)

Berlex

**†Levlen® 28 Tablets
28-Day Regimen**
(Each light-orange tablet contains 0.15 mg
levonorgestrel and 0.03 mg ethinyl
estradiol. Each pink tablet is inert.)

Also available
in 21-day
regimen

Berlex

**†Tri-Levlen® 28 Tablets
28-Day Regimen**
(Each brown tablet contains 0.050 mg
levonorgestrel and 0.030 mg ethinyl
estradiol. Each white tablet contains
0.075 mg levonorgestrel and 0.040 mg
ethinyl estradiol. Each light-yellow tablet
contains 0.125 mg levonorgestrel and
0.030 mg ethinyl estradiol. Each light-
green tablet is inert.)

Also available
in 21-day
regimen

Berlex   (Both sides of tablet shown)

324 mg
**Quinaglute®
Dura-Tabs®
Tablets**

(quinidine gluconate sustained-release tablet)
The tablet designs are trademarks
of Berlex Laboratories, Inc.

Boehringer Ingelheim

†Alupent® Inhalation Aerosol
(metaproterenol sulfate USP)
0.65 mg per inhalation

Boehringer Ingelheim

74*   72*

10 mg   20 mg
†Alupent® Tablets
(metaproterenol sulfate USP)

Boehringer Ingelheim

Atrovent® Inhalation Aerosol
(ipratropium bromide)

18 mcg per inhalation

**The name BEACH appears on the reverse side of these tablets.

Boehringer Ingelheim
(Shown smaller than actual size)

TTS®-1
(0.1 mg clonidine per day, for one week)

TTS®-2
(0.2 mg clonidine per day, for one week)

TTS®-3
(0.3 mg clonidine per day, for one week)
Catapres-TTS®
(clonidine)
Transdermal Therapeutic System

Boehringer Ingelheim
6*   7*   11*
0.1 mg   0.2 mg   0.3 mg
Catapres® Tablets
(clonidine hydrochloride USP)

Boehringer Ingelheim
8*   9*   10*
0.1/15   0.2/15   0.3/15
Combipres® Tablets
(clonidine hydrochloride USP, 0.1, 0.2 or
0.3 mg and chlorthalidone USP, 15 mg)

Boehringer Ingelheim
12*
5 mg
Dulcolax® Tablets
(bisacodyl USP)

Boehringer Ingelheim
Dulcolax® Suppositories 10 mg
(bisacodyl USP)

Boehringer Ingelheim
150 mg
250 mg
200 mg
Mexitil® Capsules
(mexiletine hydrochloride)

Boehringer Ingelheim
17*   18*   19*
25 mg   50 mg   75 mg
Persantine® Tablets
(dipyridamole USP)

Boehringer Ingelheim
62*
75 mg
prolonged-action tablets
Preludin® Endurets®
(phenmetrazine hydrochloride USP)

Boehringer Ingelheim
BI 64
105 mg
timed-release capsules
Prelu-2®
(phendimetrazine tartrate)

Boehringer Ingelheim
250 mg   500 mg
sustained-release tablets
Respbid®
(anhydrous theophylline)

Boehringer Ingelheim
10 mg
†**Serentil® Tablets**
(mesoridazine besylate USP)
Also 25 mg, 50 mg, 100 mg

Boehringer Ingelheim
76*   Also
available:
15 mg
25 mg
†**Thalitone®**
(chlorthalidone)

BOLAR

Carisoprodol Compound Tablets
(325 mg. aspirin and 200 mg.
carisoprodol)

Bolar
100 mg.   150 mg.
**Disopyramide Phosphate
CR Capsules**

Bolar
100 mg.
**Extended Phenytoin
Sodium Capsules, USP**

Bolar
5 mg./24 hrs.
(10 cm²)
10 mg./24 hrs.
(20 cm²)
15 mg./24 hrs.
(30 cm²)
Nitroglycerin Transdermal System

Bolar
324 mg.
Quinidine Gluconate Tablets

Bolar
50 mg./25 mg.
**Triamterene and
Hydrochlorothiazide Capsules**

BOOTS

103*   3176*
250 mg   333 mg
E-Mycin® Tablets
(erythromycin delayed release) tablets

Boots
400 mg
600 mg
800 mg
RUFEN®
(ibuprofen)

BOOTS-FLINT

1 mg.   2 mg.
4 mg.   6 mg.
CHOLOXIN®
(dextrothyroxine sodium, USP)

Boots-Flint
1000 Grams
400 Grams
50 Grams
Flint SSD™
1% Silver Sulfadiazine Cream
For Topical Use Only

Boots-Flint
RU-TUSS® TABLETS
(antihistamine—decongestant)

Boots-Flint
RU-TUSS® II CAPSULES
(antihistamine-decongestant)

Boots-Flint
25 mcg.   50 mcg.   75 mcg.
0.025 mg.   0.05 mg.   0.075 mg.
100 mcg.   112 mcg.   125 mcg.
0.1 mg.   0.112 mg.   0.125 mg.
150 mcg.   175 mcg.
0.15 mg.   0.175 mg.
200 mcg.   300 mcg.
0.2 mg.   0.3 mg.
SYNTHROID®
(levothyroxine sodium, USP)

Boots-Flint
200 mcg.
500 mcg.
SYNTHROID® for Injection
(levothyroxine sodium, USP)

Boots-Flint
(Tube shown
smaller than
actual size)
TRAVASE® Ointment
(sutilains ointment, USP)

Boots-Flint (Both sides of tablet shown)
800 mg.
ZORPRIN®
(aspirin)
zero-order release

BRAINTREE
(Shown smaller
than actual size)
4 Liter
GoLYTELY®
PEG-3350 and Electrolytes for
Oral Solution

BRISTOL LABORATORIES
25 mg
35 mg
50 mg
Enkaid®
(encainide hydrochloride)

Bristol Laboratories
(Tablets shown smaller than actual size)
lime flavor   orange flavor
K-Lyte® & K-Lyte® DS
Effervescent Tablets
Potassium Supplement

citrus flavor   fruit punch flavor
K-Lyte/CL® & K-Lyte/CL® 50
Effervescent Tablets
Potassium Chloride Supplement

Bristol Laboratories
†**Naldecon®**
(antihistamines/decongestants)

Bristol Laboratories
†**Quibron® Capsules**
(theophylline-guaifenesin)

Bristol Laboratories
300 mg trisected
immediate-release tablet
Quibron®-T Dividose® Tablets
(theophylline anhydrous)

Bristol Laboratories

300 mg
sustained-release tablet
Quibron®-T/SR Dividose® Tablets
(theophylline anhydrous)

Bristol Laboratories

50 mg
Saluron®
(hydroflumethiazide)

Bristol Laboratories

Salutensin-Demi®

Salutensin®

(hydroflumethiazide, reserpine)

BRISTOL-MYERS

Oncology Division

100 mg.   200 mg.

500 mg.

1 gm.   2 gm.

Cytoxan® Injection
(cyclophosphamide for injection, USP)

Bristol-Myers Oncology Division

25 mg.   50 mg.
†Cytoxan® Tablets
(cyclophosphamide tablets, USP)

Bristol-Myers Oncology Division

10 mg.   100 mg.
40 mg.
CeeNu®
(lomustine [CCNU])

Bristol-Myers Oncology Division

500 mg.
Lysodren®
(mitotane tablets, USP)

Bristol-Myers Oncology Division

20 mg.   40 mg.
Megace® Tablets
(megestrol acetate tablets, USP)

Bristol-Myers Oncology Division

40 mg.
Mutamycin®
(mitomycin for injection, USP)

Bristol-Myers Oncology Division

50 mg.   100 mg.
Platinol®-AQ
(cisplatin injection)

Bristol-Myers Oncology Division

50 mg.
VePesid® Capsules
(etoposide)

Bristol-Myers Products

325 mg.
aspirin
**Tri-Buffered Bufferin® Coated
Analgesic Tablets & Caplets**
(aspirin with buffers)

Bristol-Myers Products

500 mg.
aspirin
**Arthritis Strength Tri-Buffered
Bufferin® Analgesic Caplets**
(aspirin with buffers)

Bristol-Myers Products

500 mg.
aspirin
**Extra-Strength Tri-Buffered
Bufferin® Analgesic Tablets**
(aspirin with buffers)

Bristol-Myers Products

**Comtrex®
Multi-Symptom Cold Reliever
Tablets & Caplets**
(acetaminophen, chlorpheniramine maleate,
pseudoephedrine HCl, dextromethorphan HBr)

Bristol-Myers Products
Bottles of 6 & 10 fl oz.
**Comtrex® Liquid
Multi-Symptom
Cold Reliever**
(acetaminophen,
chlorpheniramine maleate,
pseudoephedrine HCl,
dextromethorphan HBr)

Bristol-Myers Products
Liquid
Filled
Gelatin
Capsules
**Comtrex® Liqui-Gel
Multi-Symptom Cold Reliever**
(acetaminophen, chlorpheniramine
maleate, phenylpropanolamine HCl,
dextromethorphan HBr)

Bristol-Myers Products

**Allergy-Sinus Comtrex®
Tablets & Caplets**
(acetaminophen, chlorpheniramine maleate,
pseudoephedrine HCl, dextromethorphan HBr)

Bristol-Myers Products

500 mg.
**Extra-Strength Datril®
Analgesic Tablets & Caplets**
(acetaminophen)

Bristol-Myers Products

**Extra-Strength Excedrin®
Analgesic Tablets & Caplets**
(acetaminophen, aspirin and caffeine)

Bristol-Myers Products

3.5 oz. 8 oz., 16 oz.
**Therapeutic
Mineral Ice™
Topical Analgesic Gel**
(menthol)

Bristol-Myers Products

200 mg.
**Nuprin®
Analgesic Tablets & Caplets**
(ibuprofen)

BURROUGHS WELLCOME

2.5 mg
†ACTIDIL® tablets
(triprolidine hydrochloride)

Burroughs Wellcome

†ACTIFED® capsules
Safety sealed with orange bands.
(triprolidine hydrochloride 2.5 mg and
pseudoephedrine hydrochloride 60 mg)

Burroughs Wellcome

ACTIFED® 12-Hour capsules
Safety sealed with orange bands.
(triprolidine hydrochloride 5 mg and
pseudoephedrine hydrochloride 120 mg)

Burroughs Wellcome

†ACTIFED® tablets
(triprolidine hydrochloride 2.5 mg and
pseudoephedrine hydrochloride 60 mg)

Burroughs Wellcome

ACTIFED® PLUS tablets and caplets
(acetaminophen 500 mg,
pseudoephedrine hydrochloride 30 mg,
and triprolidine hydrochloride 1.25 mg)

Burroughs Wellcome

2 mg
ALKERAN® tablets
(melphalan)

Burroughs Wellcome

ALLERACT™
(triprolidine hydrochloride 2.5 mg)

Burroughs Wellcome

**ALLERACT™ Decongestant
tablets and caplets**
(triprolidine hydrochloride 2.5 mg and
pseudoephedrine hydrochloride 60 mg)

Burroughs Wellcome

10 mg
CARDILATE® tablets
(erythrityl tetranitrate)

Burroughs Wellcome

25 mg
DARAPRIM® tablets
(pyrimethamine)

Burroughs Wellcome

EMPIRIN® ASPIRIN tablets
(aspirin 325 mg)

Burroughs Wellcome

No. 2, 15 mg

No. 3, 30 mg

No. 4, 60 mg
EMPIRIN® With Codeine
(each tablet contains aspirin 325 mg
and codeine phosphate)

Burroughs Wellcome

50 mg
†IMURAN® tablets
(azathioprine)

Burroughs Wellcome

5 mg
KEMADRIN® tablets
(procyclidine hydrochloride)

Burroughs Wellcome

0.05 mg

0.1 mg

0.2 mg
LANOXICAPS®
(digoxin solution in capsules)

Burroughs Wellcome

0.125 mg

0.25 mg

0.5 mg
†LANOXIN® tablets
(digoxin)

Burroughs Wellcome

2 mg
LEUKERAN® tablets
(chlorambucil)

Burroughs Wellcome

50 mg
†MAREZINE® tablets
(cyclizine hydrochloride)

Burroughs Wellcome

2 mg
MYLERAN® tablets
(busulfan)

Burroughs Wellcome

100 mg   200 mg
PROLOPRIM®
(trimethoprim)

Burroughs Wellcome

50 mg
PURINETHOL® tablets
(mercaptopurine)

Burroughs Wellcome

100 mg
RETROVIR® capsules
(zidovudine)

Burroughs Wellcome
†SEPTRA® tablets
(trimethoprim 80 mg and sulfamethoxazole 400 mg)

Burroughs Wellcome
100 mg   300 mg
ZYLOPRIM® tablets
(allopurinol)

Carnrick
NOLEX™ LA
(phenylpropanolamine HCl 75 mg, guaifenesin 400 mg)

Central Pharmaceuticals
(Both sides of tablet shown)
CO-GESIC® Tablets
(hydrocodone bitartrate and acetaminophen)

CIBA
41*   168*
100 mg.   200 mg.
Anturane®
(sulfinpyrazone USP)

Burroughs Wellcome
†SEPTRA® DS
(trimethoprim 160 mg and sulfamethoxazole 800 mg)

CARNRICK
(Both sides of tablet shown)
AMEN®
(medroxyprogesterone acetate, USP 10 mg)

Carnrick
PHRENILIN®
(butalbital, USP 50 mg, acetaminophen, USP 325 mg)

Central Pharmaceuticals
(Both sides of tablets shown)
500 mg
750 mg
MONO-GESIC® Tablets
(salsalate)

CIBA
139*   149*
159*
25/25   50/50
100/50
Apresazide®
(hydralazine HCl and hydrochlorothiazide)

Burroughs Wellcome
30 mg   60 mg
†SUDAFED® tablets
(pseudoephedrine hydrochloride)

Carnrick
(Both sides of tablet shown)
35 mg
BONTRIL® PDM
(phendimetrazine tartrate, USP 35 mg)

Carnrick
8656
PHRENILIN® FORTE
(butalbital, USP 50 mg, acetaminophen, USP 650 mg)

CIBA
37*   39*
10 mg.   25 mg.
73*   101*
50 mg.   100 mg.
Apresoline® hydrochloride
(hydralazine hydrochloride USP)

Burroughs Wellcome
SUDAFED® 12 Hour
Safety sealed with blue bands.
120 mg
(pseudoephedrine hydrochloride)

Carnrick
8647
105 mg
BONTRIL® SLOW-RELEASE
(phendimetrazine tartrate 105 mg)

Carnrick
(Both sides of tablet shown)
PROPAGEST®
(phenylpropanolamine HCl 25 mg)

Central Pharmaceuticals
NIFEREX®-150 Capsules
(polysaccharide-iron complex)

Burroughs Wellcome
†SUDAFED® PLUS tablets
(each scored tablet contains pseudoephedrine hydrochloride 60 mg and chlorpheniramine maleate 4 mg)

Carnrick
CAPITAL® and CODEINE SUSPENSION
(acetaminophen 120 mg/5 mL codeine phosphate 12 mg/5 mL)

Carnrick
8671
500 mg
86 72
750 mg
SALFLEX®
(salsalate)

Central Pharmaceuticals
44
NIFEREX®-150 Forte Capsules
(polysaccharide-iron complex with folic acid and vitamin B₁₂)

CIBA
129*
Apresoline®-Esidrix®
(hydralazine hydrochloride and hydrochlorothiazide)

Burroughs Wellcome
SUDAFED® SINUS tablets and caplets
(acetaminophen 500 mg and pseudoephedrine hydrochloride 30 mg)

Carnrick
8657
HYDROCET®
(hydrocodone bitartrate, USP 5 mg acetaminophen, USP 500 mg)

Central Pharmaceuticals
131/05
NIFEREX®-PN Tablets
(prenatal vitamin)

CIBA
24*
250 mg.
Cytadren®
(aminoglutethimide tablets USP)

Burroughs Wellcome
40 mg
THIOGUANINE, TABLOID® brand tablets
(thioguanine)

Carnrick
MIDRIN®
(isometheptene mucate 65 mg, dichloralphenazone 100 mg, acetaminophen 325 mg)

Carnrick
8666
SINULIN®
(acetaminophen 650 mg, chlorpheniramine maleate 4 mg, phenylpropanolamine HCl 25 mg)

Central Pharmaceuticals
(Both sides of tablet shown)
NIFEREX®-PN Forte Tablets
(prenatal vitamin)

CIBA
22*   46*   192*
25 mg.   50 mg.   100 mg.
Esidrix®
(hydrochlorothiazide USP)

Burroughs Wellcome
75 mg   100 mg
WELLBUTRIN® tablets
(bupropion hydrochloride)

Carnrick
MOTOFEN®
(difenoxin 1 mg as the hydrochloride, atropine sulfate 0.025 mg)

Carnrick
86 62
SKELAXIN®
(metaxalone 400 mg)

Central Pharmaceuticals
130 mg   260 mg
THEOCLEAR® L.A.-130   THEOCLEAR® L.A.-260
(theophylline sustained release)

CIBA
47*
Esimil®
(guanethidine monosulfate and hydrochlorothiazide)

Burroughs Wellcome
5 mg   25 mg
†WELLCOVORIN® tablets
(leucovorin calcium)

Carnrick
NOLAHIST®
(phenindamine tartrate 25 mg)

CENTRAL
(Both sides of tablet shown)
AZDONE® Tablets
(hydrocodone bitartrate and aspirin)

CIBA CONSUMER
Available in packages of 30, 60 & 100 tablets
SLOW FE®
Slow Release Iron

CIBA
2310*   2320*
0.05 mg.   Estraderm®   0.1 mg.
(estradiol transdermal system)

Burroughs Wellcome
200 mg
†ZOVIRAX® capsules
(acyclovir)

Carnrick
NOLAMINE®
(chlorpheniramine maleate 4 mg, phenindamine tartrate 24 mg, phenylpropanolamine hydrochloride 50 mg)

Central Pharmaceuticals
CODIMAL®-L.A. Capsules
(chlorpheniramine maleate and pseudoephedrine hydrochloride)

See page 438 for Daniels Pharmaceuticals, Inc. color photos of Levoxine® and Tussigon®.

CIBA
49*   103*
10 mg.   25 mg.
Ismelin® sulfate
(guanethidine monosulfate)

CIBA
65* — CIBA 65 — 300 mg.
Lithobid®
(lithium carbonate USP)

CIBA
110* — 25 mg.
26* — 50 mg.
135* — 75 mg.
Ludiomil®
(maprotiline hydrochloride USP)

CIBA
30* — 10 mg.
32* — 25 mg.
Tablets
51* — 5 mg.
64* — 10 mg.
Linguets
Metandren®
(methyltestosterone USP)

CIBA
130* — 250 mg.
Metopirone®
(metyrapone USP)

CIBA
154* — CIBA 154 — 300 mg.
Rimactane®
(rifampin USP)

CIBA
16* — CIBA 16
20 mg. sustained-release tablets
Ritalin-SR®
(methylphenidate hydrochloride USP)

CIBA
7* — 5 mg.
3* — 10 mg.
34* — 20 mg.
Ritalin® hydrochloride
(methylphenidate hydrochloride USP)

CIBA
71*
Ser-Ap-Es®
(reserpine, hydralazine hydrochloride, and hydrochlorothiazide)

CIBA
35* — 0.1 mg.
36* — 0.25 mg.
Serpasil®
(reserpine USP)

CIBA
40* #1
104* #2
Serpasil®-Apresoline®
(reserpine and hydralazine hydrochloride)

CIBA
13* #1
97* #2
Serpasil®-Esidrix®
(reserpine and hydrochlorothiazide)

CIBA
4345*
Transderm Scōp®
(scopolamine)
Transdermal Therapeutic System
0.5 mg/3 days

Colgate-Hoyt Laboratories
*186 vanilla 0.25mgF
*014 grape 0.5mgF
*006 cherry 1.0mgF
*142 orange 1.0mgF
*141 lemon 1.0mgF
*140 lime 1.0mgF
*007 SF** (**Special Formula)
†LURIDE®
(sodium fluoride)

DERMAIDE
Dermaide® Aloe Cream

DISTA
For description of Dista Identi-Code® identifications, see Dista Identi-Code index at beginning of Dista Product Information Section.

Dista
DISTA 3056 CINOBAC 500 mg
500 mg
Cinobac®
(cinoxacin)

Dista
250 mg
†Ilosone®
(erythromycin estolate)

Dista
KEFLEX 250 mg
250 mg
KEFLEX 500 mg
500 mg
†Keflex®
(cephalexin)

Dista
KEFTAB 250
250 mg
KEFTAB 500
500 mg
Keftab®
(cephalexin hydrochloride)

Dista
DISTA H77 NALFON
300 mg
600 mg
Nalfon®
(fenoprofen calcium)

Dista
DISTA H76 NALFON 200
200 mg
Nalfon® 200
(fenoprofen calcium)

Dista
DISTA 3105 PROZAC 20 mg
20 mg
Prozac®
(fluoxetine hydrochloride)

Dista
DISTA H74 DISTA H74
500 mg
Valmid®
(ethinamate)

Doctors' Recommended
High Potency Therapeutic MultiVitamins and Minerals

Du Pont Pharmaceuticals
2 mg lavender
2½ mg green
5 mg peach
(Both sides of tablets shown)
7½ mg yellow
10 mg white
COUMADIN® Tablets
(crystalline warfarin sodium, USP)

Du Pont Pharmaceuticals
(Both sides of tablet shown)
†HYCODAN® Tablets
[hydrocodone bitartrate 5 mg (WARNING: May be habit forming), homatropine methylbromide 1.5 mg]

Du Pont Pharmaceuticals
0072 — 5 mg
0073 — 10 mg
0074 — 25 mg
0076 — 50 mg
0077 — 100 mg
†MOBAN®
(molindone HCl)

Du Pont Pharmaceuticals, Inc.
Manati, Puerto Rico
0.4 mg/ml 1 ml ampul (paraben-free)
1 mg/ml 10 ml vial
0.4 mg/ml 10 ml vial
NARCAN®
(naloxone HCl)
1 mg/ml 2 ml ampul
0.02 mg/ml 2 ml ampul
0.4 mg/ml 1 ml prefilled calibrated syringe

Du Pont Pharmaceuticals, Inc.
Manati, Puerto Rico
10 mg/ml 10 ml multiple dose vial
10 mg/ml 1 ml ampul
20 mg/ml 1 ml prefilled calibrated syringe
20 mg/ml 10 ml multiple dose vial
20 mg/ml 1 ml ampul
NUBAIN®
(nalbuphine HCl)
10 mg/ml and 20 mg/ml

Du Pont Pharmaceuticals
(Shown smaller than actual size)
5 mg
NUMORPHAN® SUPPOSITORIES
(oxymorphone HCl)
Also available:
NUMORPHAN® INJECTION
1 mg/ml and 1.5 mg/ml

Du Pont Pharmaceuticals Caribe, Inc.
Manati, Puerto Rico
0060-0127
PERCOCET® Tablets
[5 mg oxycodone HCl and 325 mg acetaminophen (USP)/tablet]
(Both sides of tablets shown)
0060-0135
PERCODAN® Tablets
[4.50 mg oxycodone HCl, 0.38 mg oxycodone terephthalate, 325 mg aspirin/tablet]
0060-0136
PERCODAN®-Demi Tablets
[2.25 mg oxycodone HCl, 0.19 mg oxycodone terephthalate, 325 mg aspirin/tablet]

Du Pont Pharmaceuticals
(Both sides of capsule shown)
Capsule

1 pint
50 mg/5 ml
syrup

†SYMMETREL®   100 mg
(amantadine HCl)

Du Pont Pharmaceuticals
(Both sides of tablet shown)

0056-0080

50 mg
TREXAN™
(naltrexone hydrochloride)

Du Pont Pharmaceuticals
ZYDONE

ZYDONE™ CAPSULES
(hydrocodone bitartrate
5 mg, and acetaminophen 500 mg)

FOREST

7g

100 metered
inhalations

AeroBid®
Inhaler System
(flunisolide)

Forest (Aerosol holding chambers for use
with metered-dose inhalers)

AeroChamber™   AeroChamber®
With Mask

Forest
: FOREST   610 :

Bancap HC®
(hydrocodone bitartrate, 5 mg and
acetaminophen, 500 mg)

Forest
(Both sides
of tablet
shown)
tablet

535-12
capsule
Esgic®
(acetaminophen 325 mg/butalbital
50 mg [Warning: May be habit forming]
/caffeine 40 mg)

Forest
: FOREST   677 :
Esgic® with Codeine
(butalbital 50 mg [Warning: May be habit
forming]/acetaminophen 325 mg/caffeine
40 mg/codeine phosphate 30 mg
[Warning: May be habit forming])

Forest
T
100 mg
TESSALON® Perles
(benzonatate USP)

Forest
See Product Information under
Inwood Laboratories—Subsidiary
of Forest Laboratories.

100 mg   200 mg

300 mg
Theochron™
(theophylline anhydrous)

GEIGY

(Shown smaller than
actual size)

557*

Brethaire®
(terbutaline sulfate USP
inhalation aerosol)

Geigy
Brethine
terbutaline sulfate USP
507*

1 mg./ml.
Ampul
(Shown smaller than
actual size)

Geigy
72*   105*

2.5 mg.   5 mg.
Tablets
†Brethine®
(terbutaline sulfate USP)

Geigy
14*

100 mg.
Butazolidin® Tablets
(phenylbutazone USP)

Geigy
44*
100 mg.   GEIGY 44
Butazolidin® Capsules
(phenylbutazone USP)

Geigy
42*   57*

200 mg.   300 mg.
Constant-T®
(theophylline [anhydrous] USP)

Geigy
108*   109*

50 mg.   100 mg.
Lamprene®
(clofazimine)

Geigy
23*   33*

10 mg.   20 mg.
Lioresal®
(baclofen USP)

Geigy
51*   71*

50 mg.   100 mg.
†Lopressor®
(metoprolol tartrate USP)

Geigy   35*   53*

50/25   100/25
73*   100/50
Lopressor HCT®
(metoprolol tartrate and hydrochlorothiazide)

Geigy
48*

100 mg.
PBZ-SR®
(tripelennamine HCl USP
sustained-release tablet)

Geigy
111*   117*

25 mg.   50 mg.
PBZ® Tablets
(tripelennamine HCl USP)

Geigy
7019*   27*

200 mg.
Tegretol®

52*

Tegretol®
Suspension
100 mg./5 ml.   100 mg.
Tegretol®
Chewable
(carbamazepine USP)

Geigy
32*   140*   136*

10 mg.   25 mg.   50 mg.
†Tofranil®
(imipramine hydrochloride USP)

Geigy
20*
Geigy 20
75 mg.**

45*
Geigy 45
125 mg.**

40*
Geigy 40
100 mg.**

22*
Geigy 22
150 mg.**

Tofranil-PM®
(imipramine pamoate)

**Capsules contain imipramine pamoate
equivalent to 75, 100, 125 or 150 mg. of
imipramine hydrochloride.

Geigy
58*   162*   164*

25   50   VOLTAREN

25 mg.   50 mg.   75 mg.
Voltaren®
(diclofenac sodium)

GENENTECH

20 mg
11.6 million IU

Packaged with
diluent

50 mg
29 million IU
Activase®
(Alteplase, recombinant)

Genentech

5 mg
approx. 13 IU

Protropin®
(somatrem for injection)

Packaged with 10 mL multiple dose
vial of bacteriostatic water
(benzyl alcohol preserved)

Glaxo Dermatology

15 g

45 g
Aclovate® Cream, 0.05%
(alclometasone dipropionate)

Glaxo Dermatology

15 g

45 g
Aclovate® Ointment, 0.05%
(alclometasone dipropionate)

Glaxo Dermatology

15 g

30 g
Oxistat® Cream, 1%
(oxiconazole nitrate)

Glaxo Dermatology

Also
available
in 15 g
& 45 g

Temovate® Cream, 0.05%
Temovate® Ointment, 0.05%
(clobetasol propionate)
15 g, 30 g, 45 g each

Glaxo Pharmaceuticals

(Shown smaller than actual size)

2 ml
Ethamolin® Injection, 5%
(ethanolamine oleate)

Glaxo Pharmaceuticals

(Shown smaller than
actual size)

1-g
IV infusion pack

2-g
IV infusion pack
Fortaz®
(ceftazidime for injection)

Glaxo Pharmaceuticals

(Shown smaller than actual size)

500-mg vial

1-g vial

2-g vial

Fortaz®
(ceftazidime for injection)

Glaxo Pharmaceuticals

(Shown smaller than actual size)

6-g pharmacy bulk package
Fortaz®
(ceftazidime for injection)

Glaxo Pharmaceuticals

(Both sides of tablet shown)

150 mg
Zantac® 150 Tablets
(ranitidine hydrochloride)

Glaxo Pharmaceuticals

(Both sides of tablet shown)

300 mg
Zantac® 300 Tablets
(ranitidine hydrochloride)

Glaxo Pharmaceuticals

(Shown smaller than actual size)

Also available:
2-ml vial
40-ml pharmacy bulk package
10-ml vial
25 mg/ml

2-ml prefilled syringe
Zantac® Injection
(ranitidine hydrochloride)

Glaxo Pharmaceuticals

(Shown smaller than actual size)

50 mg/100 ml
Zantac® Injection Premixed
(ranitidine hydrochloride)

Glaxo Pharmaceuticals

(Shown smaller than actual size)

15 mg/ml
Zantac® Syrup
(ranitidine hydrochloride)

Glaxo Pharmaceuticals

(Shown smaller than actual size)

750-mg vial   1.5-g vial

750-mg IV infusion pack   1.5-g IV infusion pack

7.5-g pharmacy bulk package
Zinacef®
(sterile cefuroxime sodium)

GLENBROOK

325 mg   500 mg
Genuine Bayer®   **Maximum Bayer®**
Patented Film Coated Aspirin Tablet   Patented Film Coated Aspirin Tablet

81 mg   650 mg
Bayer® Children's   **8-Hour Bayer®**
Flavored Chewable Aspirin Tablet   Timed-Release Aspirin Caplet

325 mg   500 mg
Genuine Bayer®   **Maximum Bayer®**
Patented Film Coated Caplet   Patented Film Coated Caplet

Glenbrook

Bayer® Children's Cold Tablets
[phenylpropanolamine HCl 3.125 mg, aspirin 1¼ gr (81 mg)]

Glenbrook

Each 5 ml (1 tsp) contains phenylpropanolamine HCl 9 mg and dextromethorphan hydrobromide 7.5 mg
Bayer® Children's Cough Syrup

Glenbrook

Regular Strength Midol®
(acetaminophen 325 mg, pyrilamine maleate 12.5 mg)

Maximum Strength Midol®
(acetaminophen 500 mg, pyrilamine maleate 15 mg)

Glenbrook

Maximum Strength Midol® PMS
(acetaminophen 500 mg, pamabrom 25 mg, pyrilamine maleate 15 mg)

Glenbrook

(Both sides of tablet shown)
Midol® 200
(ibuprofen)
200 mg per tablet

Glenbrook

80 mg acetaminophen
Children's Panadol®
Chewable Tablets

Glenbrook

80 mg acetaminophen per ½ teaspoonful
Children's Panadol® Liquid
Contains no alcohol or sugar

Glenbrook

80 mg acetaminophen per 0.8 ml dropper
Infant's Panadol® Drops
Contains no alcohol or sugar

Glenbrook

160 mg acetaminophen per caplet
Junior Strength Panadol®

Glenbrook

500 mg
Panadol®
Acetaminophen Tablet & Caplet

Glenbrook

Vanquish®
Analgesic Caplets
(aspirin 227 mg, acetaminophen 194 mg, caffeine 33 mg per caplet)

Glenbrook

Phillips'® LaxCaps®
(phenolphthalein 90 mg and docusate sodium 83 mg)

Glenbrook

Haley's M-O®
Milk of Magnesia Plus Mineral Oil
(magnesium hydroxide 304 mg, mineral oil 1.25 ml per teaspoonful)

Glenbrook

Phillips'® Milk of Magnesia
400 mg magnesium hydroxide per teaspoon (5 ml)
Available Regular and Mint Flavor

Glenbrook

Phillips'® Milk of Magnesia Tablets
311 mg magnesium hydroxide per tablet
(Mint Flavored. Used as a laxative or an antacid.)

GLENWOOD

500 mg   500 mg
Potaba® Tablet Potaba® Capsule

Glenwood

2.0 grams
Potaba® Envules

GYNOPHARMA

ParaGard™ T 380A
(Intrauterine Copper Contraceptive)

HOECHST-ROUSSEL

(Shown smaller than actual size)

60 mL
(with applicator)

2% Acne Topical Solution
A/T/S®
(erythromycin)

Hoechst-Roussel

5 mg

2.5 mg

1.25 mg
DIAβETA® Tablets
(glyburide)

Hoechst-Roussel

Doxidan®
DOXIDAN® Liquigels
Stimulant/Stool Softener Laxative
(phenolphthalein USP and docusate calcium USP)

Hoechst-Roussel

FESTAL® II Tablets
(digestive enzymes)

Hoechst-Roussel

Single-use Vials
2, 4 and 10 mL
(10 mg/mL)

Ampuls
2, 4 and 10 mL
(10 mg/mL)
LASIX® Injection
(furosemide)

2, 4 and 10 mL
(10 mg/mL)
LASIX® Prefilled Syringe
(furosemide)

(Shown smaller than actual size)

Hoechst-Roussel

60 mL
(with calibrated dropper)

Also available,
120 mL
(with dispensing spoon)

LASIX®
Oral Solution
(furosemide)

(Lasix Oral Solution shown smaller than actual size)

Hoechst-Roussel

20 mg   40 mg

80 mg

LASIX® Tablets
(furosemide)

Hoechst-Roussel

15, 30 and 90 g tubes
LOPROX® Cream 1%

30 mL

LOPROX® Lotion 1%

(Shown smaller than actual size)
(ciclopirox olamine)

Hoechst-Roussel

240 mg   50 mg

SURFAK® Liquigels
(docusate calcium USP)

Hoechst-Roussel
(Tubes shown smaller than actual size)

15 g, 60 g, and 4 oz. tubes
TOPICORT® Emollient Cream 0.25%
(desoximetasone)

15 and 60 g tubes
TOPICORT® Ointment 0.25%
(desoximetasone)

15 and 60 g tubes
TOPICORT® LP Emollient Cream 0.05%
(desoximetasone)

Hoechst-Roussel

15 and 60 g tubes
TOPICORT® Gel 0.05%
(desoximetasone)

Hoechst-Roussel

400 mg film-coated tablet
Trental®
(pentoxifylline)

ICI PHARMA

(Both sides of tablet shown)
NDC 310-600
10 mg
NOLVADEX® tablets
(tamoxifen citrate)

ICI Pharma
(Both sides of tablets shown)
NDC 310-853   NDC 310-760   NDC 310-761

2.5 mg   5 mg   10 mg
SORBITRATE® SUBLINGUAL tablets
(isosorbide dinitrate)

ICI Pharma   (Both sides of tablet shown)

5 mg   10 mg
NDC 310-770   NDC 310-780

20 mg
NDC 310-820

30 mg   40 mg
NDC 310-773   NDC 310-774

40 mg SA (Sustained Action)
NDC 310-880
SORBITRATE® ORAL tablets
(isosorbide dinitrate)

ICI Pharma   (Both sides of tablet shown)
NDC 310-810   NDC 310-815

5 mg   10 mg
CHEWABLE SORBITRATE® tablets
(isosorbide dinitrate)

ICI Pharma   (Both sides of tablet shown)

50 mg   100 mg
NDC 310-115   NDC 310-117
TENORETIC® tablets
(atenolol, chlorthalidone, 25 mg)

ICI Pharma   (Both sides of tablets shown)

50 mg   100 mg
NDC 310-105   NDC 310-101
TENORMIN® tablets
(atenolol)

ICN

10 mg.
Oxsoralen-Ultra®
Capsules
(methoxsalen)

ICN

10 mg
Testred® Capsules
(methyltestosterone USP)

ICN

5 mg.
Trisoralen® Tablets
(trioxsalen)

JANSSEN

10 mg tablets
HISMANAL®
(astemizole)

Janssen

2 mg capsules
IMODIUM®
(loperamide HCl)

Janssen

15 gm

30 gm

60 gm

NIZORAL® 2% Cream
(ketoconazole)

Janssen

200 mg tablets
NIZORAL®
(ketoconazole)

Janssen

100 mg tablet
VERMOX®
(mebendazole)

Janssen

20 ml ampoule
MONISTAT i.v.™
(miconazole)

Janssen

2 ml

5 ml

10 ml

20 ml

ampoules
ALFENTA® Injection
(alfentanil hydrochloride)

Janssen

1 ml   2 ml   5 ml   10 ml multiple-dose vial
ampoules
INAPSINE® Injection
(droperidol)

Janssen

2 ml ampoules 5 ml
INNOVAR® Injection
(fentanyl citrate/droperidol)

Janssen

2 ml   5 ml   10 ml   20 ml
ampoules
SUBLIMAZE® Injection
(fentanyl citrate)

Janssen

1 ml   2 ml   5 ml
ampoules
SUFENTA® Injection
(sufentanil citrate)

Key Pharmaceuticals

K-Dur® 10   **K-Dur® 20**
(potassium chloride USP)
Microburst Release System®

Key Pharmaceuticals
(Shown smaller than actual size)

0.1 mg/hr   0.2 mg/hr

0.3 mg/hr

0.4 mg/hr

0.6 mg/hr

Nitro-Dur®
(nitroglycerin)
Transdermal Infusion System

Key Pharmaceuticals

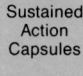

100 mg   200 mg

300 mg   450 mg

Theo-Dur®
(theophylline anhydrous)
Sustained Action Tablets

Key Pharmaceuticals

Sustained Action Capsules

50 mg   75 mg

125 mg   200 mg

Theo-Dur® Sprinkle
(theophylline anhydrous)

While every effort has been made to reproduce products faithfully, this section is to be considered a quick-reference identification aid. In cases of suspected overdosage, etc., chemical analysis of the product should be done.

KNOLL
(Both sides of tablet shown)

2 mg   11*

†Akineton®
(biperiden HCl)

Knoll (Both sides of tablets shown)

1 mg   2 mg   3 mg   4 mg

†Dilaudid®
(hydromorphone HCl)

Knoll

DILAUDID-HP
hydromorphone HCl
10 mg

10 mg/ml

Dilaudid-HP® Injection
(hydromorphone HCl)

Knoll

Dilaudid-HP
hydromorphone HCl
50 mg/5 ml

50 mg/5ml

Dilaudid-HP® Injection
(hydromorphone HCl)

Knoll

5 mg/2ml

10 mg/4ml

Single Dose Vials
Isoptin® I.V.
(verapamil HCl)

Knoll

ISOPTIN®
verapamil HCl

Isoptin® 5 mg/2ml Ampule
(verapamil HCl)

Knoll

ISOPTIN®
verapamil HCl
INTRAVENOUS
10 mg/4 ml

Isoptin® 10 mg/4ml Ampule
(verapamil HCl)

Knoll (Both sides of tablets shown)
Film-coated tablets

40 mg

80 mg

120 mg
Isoptin®
(verapamil HCl)

Knoll
(Both sides of tablet shown)
Film-coated tablet

ISOPTIN SR

240 mg

Isoptin® SR (verapamil HCl)
Sustained Release Oral Tablets

Knoll
(Both sides of tablet shown)

14*

†Quadrinal™

Knoll

Collagenase
Santyl► OINTMENT

15 Gm. and 30 Gm. Tubes
Collagenase Santyl►®
Ointment

Knoll
(Both sides of tablet shown)

VICODIN

24*

Vicodin®
(hydrocodone bitartrate 5 mg and
acetaminophen 500 mg)

Knoll
(Both sides of tablet shown)

VICODIN ES

Vicodin ES®
(hydrocodone bitartrate 7.5 mg and
acetaminophen 750 mg)

Because tablets and capsules are
shown in this section, do not infer
that these are the only dosage forms
available. Where a product name is
preceded by the symbol †, refer to the
description in the Product Information (White Section) for other forms.

LACTAID INC.

Lactaid
Lactaid
caplets
ENZYME
100 caplets

(Both sides of
caplet shown)

(Shown smaller than
actual size)

Lactaid® Caplets
(lactase enzyme tablets)

Lactaid Inc.

(Shown smaller than
actual size)

Gas – Bloat – Diarrhea?
...may be from the MILK you drink!
Lactaid
lactase enzyme
75
Makes milk
digestible

Lactaid
for milk

Lactaid
for milk

Lactaid®
(lactase enzyme)

Lakeside Pharmaceuticals

Division of Merrell Dow
Pharmaceuticals Inc.

BENTYL
10

10 mg

BENTYL
20

20 mg

†Bentyl®
(dicyclomine hydrochloride USP)

Lakeside Pharmaceuticals

2.5 mg   5 mg

Injection

Bricanyl®
(terbutaline sulfate)

Lakeside Pharmaceuticals

2 mg
Nicorette® (nicotine polacrilex)

Lakeside Pharmaceuticals

AFED
AFED
controlled-release
Novafed®
(pseudoephedrine HCl)

Lakeside Pharmaceuticals

AFED
AFED
controlled-release

Novafed® A
(120 mg pseudoephedrine
HCl and 8 mg
chlorpheniramine maleate)

Lakeside Pharmaceuticals

(Shown smaller
than actual
size)

Novahistine
DH

Novahistine
Expectorant

Novahistine® DH   **Novahistine®**
(antitussive-decon-   **Expectorant**
gestant-antihista-   (antitussive-deconges-
mine)   tant-expectorant)

Available 4 oz and pints

Lakeside Pharmaceuticals

TENUATE
25

25 mg

Tenuate®

TENUATE
75

75 mg

Tenuate Dospan®
(diethylpropion hydrochloride USP)

LEDERLE

**LEDERMARK® Product
Identification Code
Many Lederle tablets and capsules bear an
identification code, and these codes are listed
with each product pictured. A current listing
appears in the Product Information Section.

Lederle

A5**
A3**
500 mg.
250 mg.

†ACHROMYCIN® V Capsules
(tetracycline HCl)

Lederle
(Shown smaller than actual size)

ACHROMYCIN
Tetracycline Hydrochloride
OPHTHALMIC SUSPENSION 1.0%
STERILE

Unit-of-Use Dispenser
ACHROMYCIN®
Ophthalmic Suspension 1.0%
(tetracycline HCl)

Lederle   A10**

A10

500 mg.
(aminocaproic
acid tablet)

Amicar
Aminocaproic Acid
Intravenous
250 mg/ml

5 gram
(20 ml. vial)
(aminocaproic acid
intravenous
250 mg./ml.)

Amicar
Aminocaproic Acid
Syrup 25%

16 fl. oz.
(aminocaproic
acid syrup)

Amicar
Aminocaproic Acid
250 mg/ml
Intravenous

24 gram
(96 ml. vial)
(aminocaproic
acid intravenous
250 mg./ml.)

AMICAR®
(aminocaproic acid)

Lederle

Color Coding for
ARISTOCORT® (Triamcinolone Acetonide)
Dermatological Products

HP
0.5%
HIGH
POTENCY
CREAM

R
0.1%
REGULAR
POTENCY
CREAM

R
0.1%
REGULAR
POTENCY
OINTMENT

LP
0.025%
LOW
POTENCY
CREAM

HP
0.5%
HIGH
POTENCY
OINTMENT

Aristocort
Triamcinolone
Acetonide
Cream 0.5%
HP

Aristocort
Triamcinolone
Acetonide
Cream 0.1%
R

Aristocort
Triamcinolone
Acetonide
Ointment
0.1%
R

Aristocort
Triamcinolone
Acetonide
Cream 0.025%
LP

Aristocort
Triamcinolone
Acetonide
Ointment
0.5%
HP

(Tubes shown smaller than actual size)

15 Gm.
tubes
240 Gm. jar

15 and 60 Gm.
tubes
240 Gm. and
5¼ lb. jars

15 and 60 Gm.
tubes
240 Gm. and
5 lb. jars

15 and 60 Gm.
tubes
and
5¼ lb. jar

15 Gm.
tubes
240 Gm. jar

**Ledermark Product Identification Codes.

Lederle
A1** 1 mg. 2 mg. A2**
A4** 4 mg. 8 mg. A8**
†ARISTOCORT® Tablets
(triamcinolone)

Lederle
20 mg./ml.
ARISTOSPAN®
SUSPENSION
(triamcinolone hexacetonide)

Lederle
CYCLOCORT®
Amcinonide 0.1%
Lotion
with AQUATAIN™
Available in 20 ml.
and 60 ml. plastic
squeeze bottles

Lederle
F66**
Helps Maintain Regularity
for Good Digestive Health
FiberCon
Natural Action of Fiber
for Healthy Regularity
FIBERCON®
(calcium polycarbophil)

Lederle
Injection USP
3 mg./ml. For IM/IV
Use as Leucovorin
Leucovorin
Calcium 50 mg/
Injection
For Intramuscular Use
50 mg./vial
For Injection
For IM/IV Use

Lederle
Aristo-Pak®
Triamcinolone
Tablets 4 mg.
16 TABLETS
A4**
(Shown smaller
than actual size)
ARISTO-PAK®
(triamcinolone 4 mg.)
Six-Day Therapy Pack

Lederle
Artane®
1 pint
(473 ml.)
ARTANE®
(trihexyphenidyl hydrochloride)
A11** 2 mg.
A12** 5 mg.
Tablets
A9** 5 mg.
†Sequels®

Lederle
CYCLOCORT®
AMCINONIDE
OINTMENT 0.1%
15 Gm.
CYCLOCORT®
AMCINONIDE
OINTMENT 0.1%
30 Gm.
CYCLOCORT®
AMCINONIDE OINTMENT 0.1%
60 Gm.
CYCLOCORT®
Amcinonide Ointment 0.1%
(Shown smaller than actual size)

Lederle
F4** Supplied in
bottles of 100
F5**
FILIBON®
FILIBON® F.A.
F6**
FILIBON® Forte
Prenatal Tablets

Lederle
100 mg./vial
Leucovorin
350 mg.
Vial

Lederle
(Tubes shown smaller than
actual size)
Aristocort A
Cream 0.5%
15 Gm. tubes
Aristocort A
Cream 0.1%
15 and 60 Gm. tubes
and 240 Gm. jars
Aristocort A
Cream 0.025%
15 and 60 Gm.
tubes
ARISTOCORT A®
(triamcinolone acetonide with AQUATAIN™)

Lederle
A13** 25 mg.
A15** 50 mg.
A17** 100 mg.
A18** 150 mg.
ASENDIN®
(amoxapine)

Lederle
D9** 150 mg.
DECLOMYCIN® Capsules
(demeclocycline HCl)
D11** 150 mg.
D12** 300 mg.
DECLOMYCIN® Tablets
(demeclocycline HCl)

Lederle
H1** H2**
HYDROMOX®
Tablets
(quinethazone
50 mg.)
HYDROMOX® R
(quinethazone 50 mg.
with reserpine
0.125 mg.)

Lederle
Box of
25
50 mg./vial
Leucovorin Calcium
Injection
50 mg/vial
For IV/IM Use
LEUCOVORIN CALCIUM

Lederle
(Tube shown
smaller
than actual
size)
Aristocort A
Ointment 0.1%
15 and 60 Gm. tubes
ARISTOCORT A® Ointment
(triamcinolone acetonide with
propylene glycol)

Lederle
C360**
C 360
CALTRATE® JR.
C45**
CALTRATE® + IRON + VITAMIN D
C40**
C 40
CALTRATE® 600 + D
C600**
C 600
CALTRATE® 600
High Potency Calcium Supplement
(calcium carbonate)

Lederle
D1** D2**
125 mg. 250 mg.
†DIAMOX® Tablets
DIAMOX D3** 500 mg.
†DIAMOX® Sequels®
(acetazolamide)

Lederle
L1** 5 mg.
L2** 10 mg.
L3** 25 mg.
L4** 50 mg.
LOXITANE® Capsules
(loxapine succinate)

Lederle
C33** 5 mg.
C35** 15 mg.
C12** 10 mg.

Lederle
40 mg./ml.
Available in 1 ml.
and 5 ml.
Caltrate
600
ARISTOCORT® FORTE
(triamcinolone diacetate)

Lederle
F2**
DUAL-ACTION FORMULA
TIME-RELEASE IRON
Ferro-Sequels
DUAL ACTION
Ferro-Sequels
FERRO-SEQUELS® DUAL ACTION
High Potency Iron Supplement
(ferrous fumarate)

Lederle
(Shown smaller than actual size)
Loxitane IM
LOXAPINE
HYDROCHLORIDE
Intramuscular
50 mg base/ml.
50 mg. base/ml.
Also available in 10ml.
multidose vial
†LOXITANE® Intramuscular
(loxapine HCl)

Lederle
10-strip of 15 mg. unit dose
LEUCOVORIN CALCIUM Tablets

Lederle
25 mg./ml.
ARISTOCORT®
INTRALESIONAL
(triamcinolone diacetate)

Lederle
CYCLOCORT®
AMCINONIDE
CREAM 0.1%
15 Gm.
CYCLOCORT®
AMCINONIDE
CREAM 0.1%
30 Gm.
CYCLOCORT®
AMCINONIDE
CREAM 0.1%
60 Gm.
CYCLOCORT® Cream 0.1%
Amcinonide with AQUATAIN™
(Shown smaller than actual size)

Lederle
(Shown smaller than
actual size)
Loxitane C
Loxitane C
LOXAPINE HCl
HYDROCHLORIDE
Oral Concentrate
25 mg base/ml
25 mg./ml.
LOXITANE® C Oral Concentrate
(loxapine HCl)

Lederle
(Both sides of tablet shown)
M40**
MATERNA
MHO
MATERNA®
Prenatal Vitamin and Mineral Tablets
Supplied in bottles of 100

Lederle
5 mg./ml.
Aristospan
ARISTOSPAN®
INTRALESIONAL
(triamcinolone hexacetonide)

Designed to help you identify drugs,
this section contains actual size, full-
color reproductions of products selected for inclusion by participating
manufacturers.

**Ledermark Product Identification Codes.

Lederle (Both sides of tablet shown)

M8**

MAXZIDE®
(triamterene 75 mg./hydro-
chlorothiazide 50 mg./tablets)
®: Unique tablet shape is a trademark
of American Cyanamid Company.

Lederle (Both sides of tablet shown)

M9**

MAXZIDE® 25-MG
(triamterene 37.5 mg./hydro-
chlorothiazide 25 mg./tablets)
®: Unique tablet shape is a trademark
of American Cyanamid Company.

Lederle

M1**

2.5 mg.

METHOTREXATE Tablets
Bottle of 100

Lederle

20 mg.
(Low Sodium)
20 mg. vial

METHOTREXATE
Sodium Parenteral

50 mg. 2 ml. vial
25 mg./ml.*
Liquid preserva-
tive protected

METHOTREXATE
Sodium Parenteral

*Also available in LPF &
powder form & 100 mg. vials

250 mg. 10 ml. vial
25 mg./ml.
Liquid preserva-
tive protected

METHOTREXATE
Sodium Parenteral

250 mg., Liquid,
Preservative-Free
(isotonic solution)
10 ml. vial 25 mg./ml.

METHOTREXATE LPF®
Sodium Parenteral

200-250 mg.
vials—LPF®
Available in
boxes of 25

1 gram vial
freeze dried

METHOTREXATE
Sodium Parenteral

Lederle

M6**   M7**

100 mg.   400 mg.

MYAMBUTOL® Tablets
(ethambutol hydrochloride)

Lederle

M2**   M4**

50 mg.   100 mg.

M3**   M5**

50 mg.   100 mg

Intravenous
100 mg. vial

MINOCIN®
(minocycline HCl)

Lederle

60 ml.

Oral Suspension

Powder

NILSTAT®
(nystatin)

Lederle

20 mg.   25 mg.

30 mg.

NOVANTRONE®
(mitoxantrone hydrochloride)

Lederle

2 gram vial

3 gram vial

4 gram vial

40 gram bulk vial

Abbott ADD-Vantage®
Available in 2, 3 and
4 gram vials

Also available in 2, 3 & 4 gram
infusion bottles.

†PIPRACIL®
(piperacillin sodium)

Lederle

5 mg PER WEEK
4 WEEK DOSE PACK

5.0 mg.
Per Week

7.5 mg PER WEEK
4 WEEK DOSE PACK

7.5 mg.
Per Week

10 mg PER WEEK
4 WEEK DOSE PACK

10.0 mg.
Per Week

12.5 mg PER WEEK
4 WEEK DOSE PACK

12.5 mg.
Per Week

15 mg PER WEEK
4 WEEK DOSE PACK

15.0 mg.
Per Week

RHEUMATREX® Dose Packs
Methotrexate 2.5 mg. Tablets

Lederle

50 ml.
(100 mg. per 5 ml.)

Calibrated
Dropper

Powdered for
Oral Suspension

100 ml.
(100 mg. per 5 ml.)

400 mg. Tablet
SUPRAX®
(cefixime)

Lederle

Parenteral
15 mg./vial

THIOTEPA

LEMMON

(Both sides of tablet shown)

37.5 mg.
Adipex-P®
(phentermine hydrochloride)

Lemmon
(Both sides of tablet shown)

200 mg.
Epitol™
(carbamazepine tablets, USP)

Lemmon

2 mg.
Orap™
(pimozide)

LILLY

For description of Lilly
Identi-Code® identifications, see
Lilly Identi-Code index at
beginning of Lilly Product
Information Section.

Lilly

150 mg   300 mg

Axid®
(nizatidine)

Lilly

250 mg
†Ceclor®
(cefaclor)

Lilly

0.1 mg
Crystodigin®
(digitoxin)

Lilly

Darvocet-N® 50
(propoxyphene napsylate and
acetaminophen)

Lilly

Darvocet-N® 100
(propoxyphene napsylate and
acetaminophen)

Lilly

32 mg   65 mg

Darvon®
(propoxyphene hydrochloride)

Lilly

Darvon® Compound
(propoxyphene hydrochloride,
aspirin, and caffeine)

Lilly

Darvon® Compound-65
(propoxyphene hydrochloride,
aspirin, and caffeine)

Lilly

Darvon® with A.S.A.®
(propoxyphene hydrochloride and aspirin)

Lilly

†Darvon-N®
(propoxyphene napsylate)

Lilly

Darvon-N® with A.S.A.®
(propoxyphene napsylate and aspirin)

Lilly

Methadone HCl Disket®

Lilly
(Both sides of tablets shown)

0.05 mg

0.25 mg

1 mg
Permax®
(pergolide mesylate)

3M RIKER

500 mg.

750 mg.

500 mg.

Disalcid®
(salsalate)
Riker

3M Riker

0.2 mg. of pirbuterol per inhalation

Maxair® Inhaler
(pirbuterol acetate inhalation aerosol)

3M Riker

2.5 ml.

Medihaler Ergotamine®
(ergotamine tartrate)

3M Riker (Shown smaller than actual size)

2.5 mg./24 hr. patch   5 mg./24 hr. patch

10 mg./24 hr. patch   15 mg./24 hr. patch

Minitran™
(nitroglycerin)
Transdermal Delivery System

3M Riker

100 mg.
†Norflex®
(orphenadrine citrate)

3M Riker

60 mg./2 ml. ampule

Norflex® Injectable
(orphenadrine citrate)

3M Riker

Norgesic®   **Norgesic® Forte**

3M Riker

125 mg.   250 mg.
†Theolair™
(theophylline)
Regular-Release Tablets

500 mg.

250 mg.

200 mg.
Theolair™-SR   300 mg.
(theophylline)
Sustained-Release Tablets

3M Riker

75 mg.
Tepanil® Ten-Tab®
(diethylpropion hydrochloride, USP)

MARION

(Both sides of tablet shown)

CARAFATE

1 gm

CARAFATE® Tablets
(sucralfate)

Marion

ardizem 60 mg   ardizem 90 mg

60 mg   90 mg

ardizem 120 m

120 mg
CARDIZEM® SR
(diltiazem hydrochloride)
Sustained Release Capsules

Marion
(Both sides of tablets shown)

30 mg

60 mg

90 mg

120 mg

CARDIZEM® Tablets
(diltiazem hydrochloride)

Marion

Debrox   Debrox
½ fl oz   1 fl oz

DEBROX® Drops

Marion
(Both sides of tablet shown)

5 mg
DITROPAN® Tablets
(oxybutynin chloride)

Marion
(Both sides of tablets shown)

MARION   GAVISCON

GAVISCON® Antacid Tablets

MARION   GAVISCON ESR

GAVISCON® EXTRA STRENGTH RELIEF FORMULA Antacid Tablets

Marion

12 fl oz

6 fl oz

GAVISCON® Liquid Antacid

12 fl oz

GAVISCON® EXTRA STRENGTH RELIEF FORMULA Liquid Antacid

Marion

½ fl oz   2 fl oz

GLY-OXIDE® Liquid

Marion

2.5 mg
NITRO-BID® 2.5 PLATEAU CAPS®
(nitroglycerin)

6.5 mg
NITRO-BID® 6.5 PLATEAU CAPS®
(nitroglycerin)

9 mg
NITRO-BID® 9 PLATEAU CAPS®
(nitroglycerin)

Marion

MARION 1555
150 mg
PAVABID® PLATEAU CAPS®
(papaverine hydrochloride)

Marion (Both sides of tablet shown)

300 mg
PAVABID® HP Capsulets
(papaverine hydrochloride)

Marion

MARION OS-CAL 1650
OS-CAL® 250+D Tablets

OS-CAL® 500 Tablets

OS-CAL
OS-CAL® 500 CHEWABLE Tablets

OS-CAL® 500+D Tablets

MULTIVITAMIN & MINERALS OS-CAL FORTIFIED 100 TABLETS
OS-CAL® FORTIFIED Tablets

OS-CAL® PLUS Tablets

(OS-CAL® family of calcium supplements)

Marion

1000 gm   400 gm

85 gm   50 gm
20 gm
SILVADENE® Cream 1%
(silver sulfadiazine)

Marion

Box of 60 lozenges
THROAT DISCS®
Throat Lozenges

MASON PHARMACEUTICALS

DuoCet™
(hydrocodone bitartrate 5 mg; acetaminophen 500 mg)

Mason Pharmaceuticals

(Both sides of tablet shown)

Damason-P®
(hydrocodone bitartrate 5 mg; aspirin 224 mg; caffeine 32 mg)

McNeil Consumer Products

325 mg.
Regular Strength TYLENOL®
(acetaminophen)
Tablets and Caplets

McNeil Consumer Products

TYLENOL 500 mg.

TYLENOL 500

500 mg.

Extra-Strength TYLENOL®
(acetaminophen)
Caplets, Gelcaps, and Tablets

Also Available: Extra-Strength TYLENOL® Adult Liquid

McNeil Consumer Products

MEDIPREN   MEDIPREN

200 mg.
MEDIPREN®
(ibuprofen)
Tablets and Caplets

McNeil Consumer Products
(Shown smaller than actual size)

80 mg. per dropperful (0.8 ml.)
Infants' TYLENOL® Drops
(acetaminophen)

McNeil Consumer Products
(Shown smaller than actual size)
Cherry and Grape Flavors
80 mg. per ½ tsp.
Children's TYLENOL® Elixir
(acetaminophen)

McNeil Consumer Products

80 mg.
Available: Fruit and Grape Flavors
TYLENOL 80
Children's TYLENOL®
(acetaminophen)
Chewable Tablets

McNeil Consumer Products

160 mg.
Junior Strength TYLENOL®
(acetaminophen)
Easy-to-Swallow Coated Caplets

McNeil Consumer Products

Maximum Strength SINE-AID® Tablets

Maximum Strength SINE-AID® Caplets
(acetaminophen and pseudoephedrine hydrochloride)

McNeil Consumer Products

Maximum Strength TYLENOL® Sinus Medication Tablets and Caplets
(acetaminophen and pseudoephedrine hydrochloride)

McNeil Consumer Products

Maximum Strength TYLENOL® Allergy Sinus Caplets
(acetaminophen, chlorpheniramine maleate, pseudoephedrine hydrochloride)

McNeil Consumer Products

TYLENOL® Cold Medication Tablets and Caplets

TYLENOL® Cold Medication Liquid

McNeil Consumer Products

TYLENOL® Cold Medication No Drowsiness Formula Caplets

McNeil Consumer Products
(Dosage cup shown smaller than actual size)

Children's TYLENOL® Cold Chewable Tablets and Liquid Cold Medication

McNeil Consumer Products

Children's Liquid

PEDIACARE® NightRest Liquid
(dextromethorphan hydrobromide, pseudoephedrine hydrochloride, chlorpheniramine maleate)

McNeil Consumer Products

Oral Decongestant Drops

Chewable Tablets

(Dosage cup and dropper shown smaller than actual size)

Children's Liquid

PEDIACARE®

McNeil Consumer Products

15 mg. per 5 ml. teaspoon   Dosage Spoon

DELSYM® Cough Suppressant Syrup
(dextromethorphan polistirex)

McNeil Consumer Products

IMODIUM® A-D
(loperamide HCl)

Liquid (1 mg./5 mL)

McNeil Pharmaceutical

½ mg   1 mg   2 mg

5 mg   10 mg   20 mg

Concentrate 2 mg per mL   Injectable 5 mg per mL (1 mL/ampul)

HALDOL® (haloperidol)

McNeil Pharmaceutical

50 mg haloperidol/mL*

5 mL Vial

1 mL Ampul

HALDOL® Decanoate
(haloperidol decanoate)
*as 70.5 mg haloperidol decanoate

McNeil Pharmaceutical

PANCREASE® Capsules
(pancrelipase) enteric coated microspheres

McNeil Pharmaceutical

enteric coated microtablets

PANCREASE® MT 4
(pancrelipase)

McNeil Pharmaceutical

enteric coated microtablets

PANCREASE® MT 10
(pancrelipase)

McNeil Pharmaceutical

enteric coated microtablets

PANCREASE® MT 16
(pancrelipase)

McNeil Pharmaceutical

500 mg

PARAFON FORTE™ DSC Caplets
(chlorzoxazone)

McNeil Pharmaceutical

600 mg
TOLECTIN® 600
(tolmetin sodium) tablets

McNeil Pharmaceutical

400 mg
TOLECTIN® DS
(tolmetin sodium) capsules

McNeil Pharmaceutical

200 mg
TOLECTIN® 200
(tolmetin sodium) tablets

McNeil Pharmaceutical

Each 5 mL contains: 12 mg codeine phosphate and 120 mg acetaminophen

TYLENOL® with Codeine Elixir
(acetaminophen and codeine phosphate)

McNeil Pharmaceutical

5 mL   15 mL

TYLENOL® with Codeine Elixir Unit Dose
(acetaminophen and codeine phosphate)

McNeil Pharmaceutical

No. 1 7.5 mg

No. 2 15 mg

No. 3 30 mg

No. 4 60 mg

TYLENOL® with Codeine Tablets
(acetaminophen 300 mg and codeine phosphate)

McNeil Pharmaceutical

TYLOX®
(oxycodone and acetaminophen) capsules

Mead Johnson Laboratories

Scored Tablets

1 mg

2 mg

Estrace®
(estradiol)

Mead Johnson Laboratories

1½ oz tube

Applicator

Estrace® Vaginal Cream
(estradiol)

Mead Johnson Laboratories

Natalins® Tablets
Multivitamin and Multimineral Supplement

Mead Johnson Laboratories

Natalins® Rx Tablets
Multivitamin and Multimineral Supplement

Mead Johnson Laboratories

(Compact shown not actual size)

Ovcon® 50
(norethindrone and ethinyl estradiol)

Mead Johnson Laboratories

(Compact shown not actual size)

Ovcon® 35
(norethindrone and ethinyl estradiol)

(Cycle Pak shown not actual size)

While every effort has been made to reproduce products faithfully, this section is to be considered a quick-reference identification aid. In cases of suspected overdosage, etc., chemical analysis of the product should be done.

Because tablets and capsules are shown in this section, do not infer that these are the only dosage forms available. Where a product name is preceded by the symbol †, refer to the description in the Product Information (White Section) for other forms.

Mead Johnson Pharmaceuticals

BuSpar® Tablets
(buspirone HCl)
5 mg   10 mg

†Colace® Capsules
(docusate sodium)
50 mg   100 mg

Desyrel® Tablets
(trazodone HCl)
50 mg   100 mg

Desyrel® Dividose® Tablets
(trazodone HCl)
150 mg
300 mg

Duricef®
(cefadroxil monohydrate)
500 mg Capsules   1 g Tablets

Klotrix®
slow-release tablets, 10mEq
Potassium Chloride Supplement

†Peri-Colace® Capsules
(casanthranol and
docusate sodium)

MEDICONE

Medicone® Derma-HC 1%
(Topical Hydrocortisone Anesthetic Ointment)
20 Gm.
7 Gm.

Medicone

Medicone® Rectal Suppository
(Gold Foil Wrapped)   (OTC)

Merck Sharp & Dohme

ALDOCLOR®
(Methyldopa-Chlorothiazide | MSD)
612* 150   634* 250

†ALDOMET®
(Methyldopa | MSD)
135* 125 mg
401* 250 mg
516* 500 mg

ALDORIL®
(Methyldopa-Hydrochlorothiazide | MSD)
423* 15   456* 25
694* D30   935* D50

BENEMID®
(Probenecid | MSD)
501* 0.5 g

BLOCADREN®
(Timolol Maleate | MSD)
59* 5 mg   136* 10 mg
437* 20 mg

CLINORIL®
(Sulindac | MSD)
941* 150 mg   942* 200 mg

Merck Sharp & Dohme

†COGENTIN®
(Benztropine Mesylate | MSD)
21* 0.5 mg   635* 1 mg   60* 2 mg

ColBENEMID®
(Probenecid-Colchicine | MSD)
614*

†CORTONE® Acetate
(Cortisone Acetate | MSD)
219* 25 mg

CUPRIMINE®
(Penicillamine | MSD)
672* 125 mg   602* 250 mg

DARANIDE®
(Dichlorphenamide | MSD)
49* 50 mg

†DECADRON®
(Dexamethasone | MSD)
20* 0.25 mg   41* 0.5 mg   63* 0.75 mg
95* 1.5 mg   97* 4 mg   147* 6 mg

DEMSER®
(Metyrosine | MSD)
690* 250 mg

DIUPRES®
(Reserpine-Chlorothiazide | MSD)
230* 250   405* 500

†DIURIL®
(Chlorothiazide | MSD)
214* 250 mg   432* 500 mg

Merck Sharp & Dohme

DOLOBID®
(Diflunisal | MSD)
675* 250 mg   697* 500 mg

†EDECRIN®
(Ethacrynic Acid | MSD)
65* 25 mg   90* 50 mg

†ELAVIL®
(Amitriptyline HCl | MSD)
23* 10 mg   45* 25 mg   102* 50 mg
430* 75 mg   435* 100 mg   673* 150 mg

FLEXERIL®
(Cyclobenzaprine HCl | MSD)
931* 10 mg

HYDROCORTONE®
(Hydrocortisone | MSD)
619* 10 mg   625* 20 mg

HydroDIURIL®
(Hydrochlorothiazide | MSD)
42* 25 mg   105* 50 mg   410* 100 mg

HYDROPRES®
(Reserpine-Hydrochlorothiazide | MSD)
53* 25   127* 50

†INDOCIN®
(Indomethacin | MSD)
25* 25 mg   50* 50 mg

†INDOCIN® SR
(Indomethacin | MSD)
693* 75 mg

Merck Sharp & Dohme

†INDOCIN® Suppositories
(Indomethacin | MSD)
50 mg

INVERSINE®
(Mecamylamine HCl | MSD)
52* 2.5 mg

LOSEC®
(Omeprazole | MSD)
®AB Astra
727* 20 mg

MEPHYTON®
(Phytonadione | MSD)
43* 5 mg

MEVACOR®
(Lovastatin | MSD)
731* 20 mg   732* 40 mg

MIDAMOR®
(Amiloride HCl | MSD)
92* 5 mg

†MINTEZOL®
(Thiabendazole | MSD)
907* 500 mg

MODURETIC®
(Amiloride HCl-Hydrochlorothiazide | MSD)
5-50   917*

NOROXIN®
(Norfloxacin | MSD)
705* 400 mg

†PEPCID®
(Famotidine | MSD)
963* 20 mg   964* 40 mg

Merck Sharp & Dohme
62*
4 mg
†PERIACTIN®
(Cyproheptadine HCl | MSD)

Merck Sharp & Dohme
19* 106*
5 mg 10 mg
207* 237*
20 mg 40 mg
PRINIVIL®
(Lisinopril | MSD)

Merck Sharp & Dohme
140* 142*
12.5 25
PRINZIDE®
(Lisinopril-Hydrochlorothiazide | MSD)

Merck Sharp & Dohme
647* 654*
10-100 25-250
650*
25-100
SINEMET®
(Carbidopa-Levodopa | MSD)

Merck Sharp & Dohme
67*
10-25
TIMOLIDE®
(Timolol Maleate-Hydrochlorothiazide | MSD)

Merck Sharp & Dohme
707* 709*
400 mg 600 mg
Registered trademark
of Astra Pharm. TONOCARD®
Products, Inc. (Tocainide HCl | MSD)

Merck Sharp & Dohme
914* 921*
2-10 2-25
517*
934* 946*
4-10 4-25 4-50
TRIAVIL®
(Perphenazine-Amitriptyline HCl | MSD)

Merck Sharp & Dohme
403* 412*
5 mg 10 mg
457* 460*
25 mg 50 mg
†URECHOLINE®
(Bethanechol Chloride | MSD)

Merck Sharp & Dohme
720*
10-25
VASERETIC®
(Enalapril Maleate-
Hydrochlorothiazide | MSD)

Merck Sharp & Dohme
14* 712*
2.5 mg 5 mg
713* 714*
10 mg 20 mg
VASOTEC®
(Enalapril Maleate | MSD)

Merck Sharp & Dohme
26* 47*
5 mg 10 mg
VIVACTIL®
(Protriptyline HCl | MSD)

MERRELL DOW U.S.A.
See also
Lakeside Pharmaceuticals
Cantil®
(mepenzolate bromide
25 mg USP)

Merrell Dow U.S.A.
50 mg
Clomid®
(clomiphene citrate)

Merrell Dow U.S.A.
Cephulac®
(lactulose)
Syrup
(Shown smaller
than actual size)

Merrell Dow U.S.A.
Chronulac®
(lactulose)
Syrup
(Shown smaller
than actual size)

Merrell Dow U.S.A.
1.0 gm
Hiprex®
(methenamine hippurate)

Merrell Dow U.S.A.
250 mg 500 mg
Lorelco®
(probucol)

Merrell Dow U.S.A.
10 mg 25 mg 50 mg
75 mg
100 mg 150 mg
Norpramin®
(desipramine hydrochloride USP)

Merrell Dow U.S.A.
260 mg
Quinamm™
(quinine sulfate tablets)

Merrell Dow U.S.A.
150 mg
300 mg
Rifadin®
(rifampin)

**Merrell Dow
U.S.A.**
Rifamate®
(300 mg rifampin and 150 mg isoniazid)

Merrell Dow U.S.A.
60 mg
Seldane®
(terfenadine)

Merrell Dow U.S.A.
12 mg
25 mg
72 mg
TACE®
(chlorotrianisene USP)

MILES INC.
Miles Miles
811* 821*
10 mg Adalat® 20 mg
(nifedipine)

Pharmaceutical Division
Miles
521*
600 mg
Biltricide®
(praziquantel)

Pharmaceutical Division
Miles
512*
250 mg
Miles
513*
500 mg
Miles
514*
750 mg
Cipro™
(ciprofloxacin hydrochloride)

Pharmaceutical Division
Miles
121*
250 mg
Decholin®
(dehydrocholic acid)

Pharmaceutical Division
Miles
411*
Domeboro®
Effervescent
Tablets
(aluminum sulfate—calcium acetate)

Pharmaceutical Division
Miles
951
300 mg
Lithane®
(lithium carbonate)

Pharmaceutical Division
Miles
097*
500 mg
Mycelex®-G Vaginal Tablet
(clotrimazole)
Miles
093*
100 mg
Mycelex®-G Vaginal Tablet
(clotrimazole)

Pharmaceutical Division
Miles
095*
10 mg
Mycelex® Troche
(clotrimazole)

Pharmaceutical Division
Miles
721*
500 mg
Niclocide® Chewable Tablets
(niclosamide)

Pharmaceutical Division
Miles
855*
30 mg
Nimotop® Capsules
(nimodipine/Miles)

Pharmaceutical Division
Miles
132*
50 mg
Stilphostrol®
(diethyl stilbestrol diphosphate)

MINNETONKA
6mm
patch 12mm
patch
TRANS-VER-SAL®
(salicylic acid USP,
15% in karaya gum base)
Sizes Available: 6mm and 12mm
20mm
patch
TRANS-PLANTAR™
(salicylic acid USP,
21% in karaya gum base)
One Size Available: 20mm

NORWICH EATON

200 mg

400 mg

Didronel®
(etidronate disodium)

Norwich Eaton

scored tablet　　sustained release

Entex® LA Tablets
(guaifenesin 400 mg
phenylpropanolamine HCl 75 mg)

Norwich Eaton

25 mg　　50 mg

100 mg

Macrodantin® Capsules
(nitrofurantoin macrocrystals)

Norwich Eaton
(Shown smaller than actual size)

MACPAC 50 mg

Macrodantin
nitrofurantoin
macrocrystals

4 capsules (50 mg) for
breakfast, lunch, dinner
and bedtime

Macrodantin® Macpac™
(nitrofurantoin macrocrystals)

ORGANON

ORG 472　　ORG 474

20 mcg.　　50 mcg.

Calderol®
(calcifediol capsules, USP)

Organon

388*

Cotazym®-S
(pancrelipase, USP)
enteric coated spheres

Organon

381*

†Cotazym®
(pancrelipase capsules, USP)

Organon

795*

Hexadrol
Therapeutic Pack

(pack shown smaller
than actual size)

6 Hexadrol 1.5 mg. tablets and
8 Hexadrol 0.75 mg. tablets

Hexadrol® Therapeutic Pack
(dexamethasone tablets, USP)

Organon

792*　　791*

0.5 mg.　　0.75 mg.

790*　　798*

1.5 mg.　　4.0 mg.

†Hexadrol®
(dexamethasone tablets, USP)

Organon

542*

Wigraine®
(ergotamine tartrate and caffeine
tablets, USP)

Organon

WIGRAINE SUPP
ORGANON, INC.
9/90
WIGRAINE SUPP

Wigraine®
(ergotamine tartrate and caffeine
suppositories, USP)

Organon

393*

Zymase®
(pancrelipase, USP)
enteric coated spheres

ORTHO

Ortho
compacts
shown smaller
than actual
size

Also available
in 28-day
regimen
containing 7
inert green
tablets

**ORTHO-NOVUM™
7/7/7□21 Day Regimen**
(Each white tablet contains
0.5 mg of norethindrone and
0.035 mg of ethinyl estradiol)
(Each light peach tablet contains
0.75 mg of norethindrone and
0.035 mg of ethinyl estradiol)
(Each peach tablet contains
1 mg of norethindrone and
0.035 mg of ethinyl estradiol)

Ortho

Also
available
in 28-day
regimen con-
taining 7 inert
green tablets

**ORTHO-NOVUM™
10/11□21 Day Regimen**
(Each white tablet contains 0.5 mg of norethindrone with 0.035 mg of ethinyl estradiol)
(Each peach tablet contains 1 mg of norethindrone with 0.035 mg of ethinyl estradiol)

Ortho

**ORTHO-NOVUM™
1/35□21 Day Regimen**
(1 mg of norethindrone with
0.035 mg of ethinyl estradiol)

Also available in 28-day regimen
containing 7 inert green tablets

Ortho

**ORTHO-NOVUM™
1/50□21 Day Regimen**
(1 mg of norethindrone with
0.05 mg of mestranol)

Also available in 28-day regimen
containing 7 inert green tablets

Ortho

**ORTHO-NOVUM™
1/80□21 Day Regimen**
(1 mg of norethindrone with
0.08 mg of mestranol)

Also available in 28-day regimen
containing 7 inert green tablets

Ortho

MODICON™ 21 Day Regimen
(0.5 mg of norethindrone with
0.035 mg of ethinyl estradiol)

Also available in 28-day regimen
containing 7 inert green tablets

Ortho

MICRONOR™ 28 Day Regimen
(0.35 mg of norethindrone)

Ortho

**ORTHO-NOVUM™
2 mg□21 Day Regimen**
(2 mg of norethindrone with
0.10 mg of mestranol)

Ortho

MONISTAT™ 7 Vaginal Cream
(miconazole nitrate 2%)

Ortho

MONISTAT™ Dual-Pak™
(miconazole nitrate)

Ortho

Monistat 7　Monistat 3
istat 3　Monistat 3　Monistat
MONISTAT™ 3
Vaginal Suppositories
(200 mg miconazole nitrate)

Ortho

Monistat 7　Monistat 7
nistat 7　Monistat 7　Monis
MONISTAT™ 7
Vaginal Suppositories
(100 mg miconazole nitrate)

Ortho

NDC 0062-7102-01
6-5 ml Ampules
MUROMONAB-CD3
ORTHOCLONE OKT® 3
Sterile Solution
5mg (1mg/ml)
For Intravenous Use Only
ATTENTION: Filter Precaution
See Insert

ORTHOCLONE OKT® 3
(muromonab-CD 3)

Ortho

250 mg

500 mg

PROTOSTAT™
(metronidazole)
tablets

Ortho

Terazol 3　Terazol
zol*3　Terazol 3　Terazol
**TERAZOL® 3
Vaginal Suppositories**

With
Applicator

**TERAZOL® 7
Vaginal Cream**

(terconazole)

PALISADES

100 mg

PALS™
(chlorophyllin copper complex)

Palisades

5%　30 ML

Scleromate™
(morrhuate sodium
injection, USP)

Palisades

5.4 mg

Yocon®
(yohimbine hydrochloride)

Designed to help you identify drugs,
this section contains actual size, full-
color reproductions of products selected for inclusion by participating
manufacturers.

PARKE-DAVIS

PARCODE®
(Parke-Davis
Accurate Recognition Code)
For Prompt, Accurate Product
Identification

The imprinted P-D identifies
the product as manufactured
by Parke-Davis.
The imprinted number designates
the particular Parke-Davis Product.

A complete listing of PARCODE
numbers appears at the beginning
of Parke-Davis Product monographs
in the white section.

Effective July 1, 1987 all
Parke-Davis Generics are marketed under Warner Chilcott
Laboratories, a separate division
of Warner-Lambert Company.

Parke-Davis

†**Anusol-HC® Suppositories
w/Hydrocortisone**

Parke-Davis

(Shown smaller than actual size)

28.4 gram tube

†**Anusol-HC®**
(rectal cream with hydrocortisone acetate)

Parke-Davis

25 mg. 50 mg.
**Benadryl   †Benadryl®
Capsules   Kapseals®**
(diphenhydramine hydrochloride capsules, USP)

Parke-Davis

150 mg. 300 mg.
**Celontin®
Kapseals®**
(methsuximide capsules, USP)

Parke-Davis

5 mg. †**Centrax®** 20 mg.
10 mg.
(prazepam)

Parke-Davis

250 mg.
†**Chloromycetin® Kapseals®**
(chloramphenicol capsules, USP)

Parke-Davis

100 mg. 200 mg.
†**Choledyl®**
(oxtriphylline)

Parke-Davis

400 mg. 600 mg.
Choledyl® SA
(oxtriphylline)

Parke-Davis

Raspberry Flavored

Caramel Flavored
Cholybar®
(cholestyramine resin bar)

Parke-Davis

50 mg.
†**Dilantin® Infatabs®**
(phenytoin tablets, USP)

Parke-Davis

30 mg. 100 mg.
†**Dilantin® Kapseals®**

Parke-Davis

**Dilantin® (phenytoin sodium)
with ¼ gr. Phenobarbital
Kapseals®**

Parke-Davis

**Dilantin® (phenytoin sodium)
with ½ gr. Phenobarbital
Kapseals®**

Parke-Davis

100 mg.
Doryx®
(coated doxycycline hyclate pellets)

Parke-Davis

15 grain (975 mg.)
Easprin®
(Aspirin Tablets, USP)
Enteric Coated Tablets

Parke-Davis

Elase®
[fibrinolysin and desoxyribonuclease
combined (bovine)]

Parke-Davis

**Elase-Chloromycetin®
Ointment**
[fibrinolysin and desoxyribonuclease, combined (bovine)
with chloramphenicol ointment]
**Elase®
Ointment**
[fibrinolysin and desoxyribonuclease
combined (bovine) ointment]

Parke-Davis

Ergostat®
(ergotamine tartrate tablets)
Sublingual Tablets, 2 mg.

Parke-Davis

250 mg.
Eryc®
(erythromycin capsules)

Parke-Davis

-½ -1

-2 -3
Euthroid®
(liotrix tablets, USP)

Parke-Davis

100 mcg.
Estrovis®
(quinestrol)

Parke-Davis

Loestrin® 21 1/20
(1 mg. norethindrone acetate and
20 mcg. ethinyl estradiol tablets, USP)

Parke-Davis

"Credit Card"
in black
carrying case
Loestrin® Fe 1/20
(1 mg. norethindrone acetate and 20 mcg.
ethinyl estradiol tablets, USP)
Each brown tablet contains 75 mg.
ferrous fumarate, USP

Parke-Davis

Loestrin® 21 1.5/30
(1.5 mg. norethindrone acetate and
30 mcg. ethinyl estradiol tablets, USP)

Parke-Davis

"Credit Card"
in black
carrying case
Loestrin® Fe 1.5/30
(1.5 mg. norethindrone acetate and 30 mcg.
ethinyl estradiol tablets, USP)
Each brown tablet contains 75 mg. ferrous
fumarate, USP

Parke-Davis

300 mg.
Lopid®
(gemfibrozil)

Parke-Davis

600 mg.
Lopid®
(gemfibrozil)

Parke-Davis

½ gram 1 gram
†**Mandelamine®**
(methenamine mandelate)

Parke-Davis

50 mg. 100 mg.
Meclomen®
(meclofenamate sodium)

Parke-Davis

500 mg.
Milontin®
(phensuximide capsules, USP)

Parke-Davis

15 mg.
Nardil®
(phenelzine sulfate)

Parke-Davis

(Bottles shown smaller than actual size)

0.15 mg. 0.3 mg.

0.4 mg. 0.6 mg.
†**Nitrostat®**
(nitroglycerin tablets, USP)
Sublingual Tablets

Parke-Davis

8 mg./10 mL. 50 mg./10 mL. 100 mg./10 mL.
Nitrostat® IV
(nitroglycerin for infusion)

Parke-Davis

(Shown smaller than
actual size)

60 grams
†**Nitrostat®
Ointment 2%**
(nitroglycerin)

Parke-Davis

1 mg.

2 mg.

3 mg.
Nitrogard®
(transmucosal controlled-release
nitroglycerin tablets)

Parke-Davis

5 mg.

Norlutate®
(norethindrone acetate
tablets, USP)

Parke-Davis

5 mg.

Norlutin® Tablets
(norethindrone
tablets, USP)

Parke-Davis

Supplied in pale
green compact

Norlestrin® 21 1/50
(1 mg. norethindrone acetate and 50 mcg.
ethinyl estradiol tablets, USP)

Parke-Davis

Supplied in olive
green compact

Norlestrin® Fe 1/50
(1 mg. norethindrone acetate and
50 mcg. ethinyl estradiol tablets, USP)
Each brown tablet contains 75 mg.
ferrous fumarate, USP

Parke-Davis

Supplied in pale
lavender compact

Norlestrin® 21 2.5/50
(2.5 mg. norethindrone acetate and
50 mcg. ethinyl estradiol tablets, USP)

Parke-Davis

Supplied in deep
lavender compact

Norlestrin® Fe 2.5/50
(2.5 mg. norethindrone acetate and
50 mcg. ethinyl estradiol tablets, USP)
Each brown tablet contains 75 mg.
ferrous fumarate, USP

Parke-Davis

10 mg.   20 mg.   40 mg.

Peritrate®
(pentaerythritol tetranitrate)

Sustained Action
80 mg.

Peritrate® SA

Parke-Davis

250 mg.

500 mg.

750 mg.

1000 mg.

Procan® SR
(procainamide hydrochloride tablets)

Parke-Davis

½ grain   1 grain   1½ grain

2 grain   3 grain

Proloid®
(thyroglobulin)

Parke-Davis

P.D.
540

250 mg.

PONSTEL

Ponstel® Kapseals®
(mefenamic acid)

Parke-Davis

P.D.
183

100 mg.

P.D.
181

200 mg.

Pyridium®
(phenazopyridine hydrochloride)

Parke-Davis

P.D.
182

Pyridium® Plus

Parke-Davis

P.D.
237

250 mg.

†Zarontin® Capsules
(ethosuximide capsules, USP)

PFIZER LABORATORIES

393*

100 mg
(scored)

394*

250 mg
(scored)

Diabinese®
(chlorpropamide)

Pfizer Laboratories

322*   323*

FELDENE PFIZER   FELDENE PFIZER
322   323

10 mg   20 mg

Feldene®
(piroxicam)

Pfizer Laboratories

MINIPRESS   PFIZER
431

431*

1 mg

MINIPRESS   PFIZER
437

437*

2 mg

MINIPRESS   PFIZER
438

438*

5 mg

Minipress®
(prazosin HCl)

Pfizer Laboratories

MINIZIDE   PFIZER
430

430*

Minizide® 1
(1 mg prazosin + 0.5 mg polythiazide)

MINIZIDE   PFIZER
432

432*

Minizide® 2
(2 mg prazosin + 0.5 mg polythiazide)

MINIZIDE   PFIZER
436

436*

Minizide® 5
(5 mg prazosin + 0.5 mg polythiazide)

Minizide®
(prazosin HCl/polythiazide)

Pfizer Laboratories

441*   442*

PFIZER
441   PFIZER
442

0.25 mg   0.5 mg

Moderil®
(rescinnamine)

Pfizer Laboratories

             Reverse side:
             yellow
260*   261*

PROCARDIA   PROCARDIA
PFIZER 260   PFIZER 261

10 mg   20 mg

Procardia®
(nifedipine)

Pfizer Laboratories

375*

1 mg

376*

2 mg

377*

4 mg

Renese®
(polythiazide)

Pfizer Laboratories

446*

Renese®-R
(polythiazide 2.0 mg and
reserpine 0.25 mg)

Pfizer Laboratories

073*

TERRAMYCIN   PFIZER
073

250 mg

Terramycin®
(oxytetracycline HCl)

Pfizer Laboratories

641*

PFIZER
641

250 mg

Vansil™
(oxamniquine)

Pfizer Laboratories

VIBRA   PFIZER
094

094*

50 mg

VIBRA   PFIZER
095

095*

100 mg

Vibramycin® Hyclate
(doxycycline hyclate)

PFIZER
099

099*

100 mg film-coated

Reverse side imprinted: Vibra-Tab

Vibra-Tabs®
(doxycycline hyclate)

Pfizer Laboratories

PFIZER
541

541*

25 mg

PFIZER
542

542*

50 mg

PFIZER
543

543*

100 mg

Vistaril®
(hydroxyzine pamoate)

PHARMACIA

500 mg.

EN   102

Azulfidine EN-tabs®
(sulfasalazine, USP)
Enteric Coated

Pharmacia

Pharmacia   EMCYT®
132

140 mg.

Emcyt®
(estramustine phosphate
sodium/Pharmacia)

While every effort has been made to
reproduce products faithfully, this
section is to be considered a quick-
reference identification aid. In cases
of suspected overdosage, etc., chemical analysis of the product should
be done.

Princeton Pharm. Products

A Squibb Company

PPP 232   PPP 207

20 mg   40 mg
232**   207**

PPP 241   PPP 208

80 mg   120 mg
241**   208**

PPP 246

160 mg
246**

CORGARD®
(Nadolol Tablets USP)

Princeton Pharmaceutical Prod.

PPP 283   PPP 284

40 mg/5 mg   80 mg/5 mg
283**   284**

CORZIDE®
(Nadolol-Bendroflumethiazide Tablets)

Princeton Pharmaceutical Prod.

SQUIBB 605

5 mg
606**

PPP 618

10 mg
618**

NATURETIN®
(Bendroflumethiazide Tablets USP)

Princeton Pharmaceutical Prod.

PPP 863   PPP 864

1 mg   2.5 mg
863**   864**

PPP 877   PPP 956

5 mg   10 mg
877**   956**

†PROLIXIN®
(Fluphenazine Hydrochloride Tablets USP)

Princeton Pharmaceutical Prod.

PPP 758   PPP 758   PPP 756   PPP 756

250 mg   375 mg
758**   756**

PPP 757   PPP 757

500 mg
757**

†PRONESTYL®
(Procainamide Hydrochloride Capsules USP)

Parke-Davis

P.D. 202   PD 204

250 mg.

500 mg.

PD 205

750 mg.

1000 mg.

Princeton Pharmaceutical Prod.

250 mg
431**

375 mg
434**

500 mg
438**

†PRONESTYL®
(Procainamide Hydrochloride Tablets)

Princeton Pharmaceutical Prod.

500 mg
775**
†PRONESTYL-SR®
(Procainamide Hydrochloride Sustained-Release Tablets)

Princeton Pharmaceutical Prod.

50 mg
713**

100 mg
776**

RAUDIXIN®
(Rauwolfia Serpentina Tablets USP)

Princeton Pharmaceutical Prod.

769**
RAUZIDE®
(Powdered Rauwolfia Serpentina 50 mg
with Bendroflumethiazide 4 mg)

"SQUIBB" marking on
tablets will be
changed to "PPP"
during 1990.

PROCTER & GAMBLE

Head &
Shoulders
shampoo

Head &
Shoulders
concentrate
shampoo

Dandruff
Care Shampoo
Head & Shoulders®

Important Notice
Before prescribing or
administering any product
described in PHYSICIANS' DESK
REFERENCE always consult the
PDR Supplement for possible
new or revised information.

PURDUE FREDERICK

(Both sides of
tablet shown)

275 mg
Bottles of 100 and 500 tablets
CARDIOQUIN® Tablets
(quinidine polygalacturonate)

Purdue Frederick (Both sides of
tablet shown)

30 mg
Bottles of 50, 100,
250, and 500 tablets
and also in unit
dose packaging.

60 mg
Bottles of 100
tablets and also
in unit dose
packaging.

NOW
AVAILABLE
15 mg
Bottles of 100
tablets and also
in unit dose
packaging.

MS CONTIN® Tablets
(morphine sulfate controlled-release)

Purdue Frederick (Both sides of
tablets shown)

15 mg   30 mg

MSIR® Tablets
(morphine sulfate immediate-release)
Bottle of 50 tablets.

Purdue Frederick

MSIR
Oral Solution
MSIR Oral Solution
(pleasantly flavored)
10 mg/5 ml and
20 mg/5 ml in plastic
metered-dose bottles of
120 ml and 500 ml
Also available in 5 ml
unit dose cups.

Oral Solution
Concentrate
MSIR Oral Solution Concentrate (unflavored)
20 mg/1 ml in child-resistant plastic bottles
of 30 ml and 120 ml
with child-resistant
dropper.

MSIR®
(morphine sulfate immediate-release)

Purdue Frederick (Both sides of
tablet shown)

10 mg
Nz   PF
Bottles of 100
NORZINE® Tablets
(thiethylperazine maleate USP)

Purdue Frederick (Shown smaller
than actual size)
Boxes of 20

10 mg/ml
NORZINE® Ampuls
(thiethylperazine maleate USP)

Purdue Frederick (Shown smaller
than actual size)
Packages of 12
10 mg

NORZINE® Suppositories
(thiethylperazine maleate USP)

Purdue Frederick

(Both sides of tablets shown)
Trilisate Tablets 500 mg and 750 mg available in bottles of 100 and 500 tablets and
in unit dose packaging. Trilisate 1000 mg
available in bottles of 60 tablets. Trilisate
Liquid 500 mg available in bottles of 8 fluid
ounces.

500 mg

750 mg

1000 mg

TRILISATE® Tablets
(choline magnesium trisalicylate)

Purdue Frederick (Both sides of
tablets shown)

200 mg
Bottles of
100
T-Phyl® 200 mg
Controlled-Release Tablets
(theophylline, anhydrous)
(Formerly UNIPHYL® 200 mg tablets)

Purdue Frederick (Both sides of
tablet shown)

400 mg
Bottles of
100 and 500,
and Unit-Dose
Packaging
UNIPHYL® 400 mg
Controlled-Release Tablets
(theophylline, anhydrous)

REED & CARNRICK

4 liter
size

Colyte

(Shown smaller
than actual
size)

1 gallon
size

Colyte

Colyte®
Colon Electrolyte
Lavage Preparation
(PEG-3350 & electrolytes for
oral solution)

Reed & Carnrick

(Shown smaller
than actual
size)

Cortifoam

Cortifoam®
(hydrocortisone acetate) 10%

Reed & Carnrick

Sustained Release Capsules

40 mg.
Dilatrate®-SR
(isosorbide dinitrate)

Reed & Carnrick

(Shown smaller
than actual size)

Epifoam

Epifoam®
(hydrocortisone acetate 1%
and pramoxine hydrochloride
1% topical aerosol)

Reed & Carnrick
(Shown smaller than actual size)

KWELL
Cream

Kwell®
Cream
(lindane) 1%

Reed & Carnrick
(Shown smaller than actual size)

KWELL
Lotion

KWELL
Shampoo

Kwell®
Lotion

Kwell®
Shampoo
(lindane) 1%

Reed & Carnrick

20 mg.
Levatol®
(penbutolol sulfate)

Reed & Carnrick

Available in
bottles of 50
and 100

Phazyme®
Relieves Gas Pain

Reed & Carnrick
Bottles of
50 & 100

Available in
consumer
package
of 10

Phazyme®-95
Relieves Gas Pain

Reed & Carnrick

Bottles
of 50

Available in
consumer
package
of 10

Maximum Strength
Phazyme®-125
Relieves Gas Pain

Reed & Carnrick
(Shown smaller than actual size)

proctoCream-HC

ProctoCream™-HC
(hydrocortisone acetate 1%
and pramoxine hydrochloride 1%)

Reed & Carnrick

(Shown smaller
than actual
size)

PROCTOFOAM

Proctofoam®-HC
(hydrocortisone acetate 1%
and pramoxine hydrochloride
1% topical aerosol)

REID-ROWELL

*7720
7720

250 mg

Chenix®
(chenodiol)

Reid-Rowell

(Shown smaller
than actual
size)

*1904

Cortenema®
(hydrocortisone retention enema)

Reid-Rowell

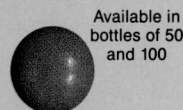

*1200

Creon®
(pancreatin, USP)

Reid-Rowell

*1007

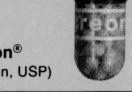

10 mg
Curretab®
(medroxyprogesterone acetate,
10 mg USP)

**Princeton, A Squibb Company, product identification number.

Reid-Rowell

*1602

DUPHALAC
(lactulose Syrup, USP)
10 g/15 mL

10 g/15 mL

Duphalac®
(lactulose syrup, USP)

Reid-Rowell

*1014 — RR 1014 — 0.3 mg
*1022 — RR 1022 — 0.625 mg
*1024 — RR 1024 — 1.25 mg
*1025 — RR 1025 — 2.5 mg

Estratab®
(esterified estrogens)

Reid-Rowell

*1026 — RR 1026

Estratest®
(esterified estrogens, USP 1.25 mg
and methyltestosterone, USP 2.5 mg)

Reid-Rowell

*1023 — RR 1023

Estratest® H.S.
(esterified estrogens, USP 0.625 mg
and methyltestosterone, USP 1.25 mg)

Reid-Rowell

*1082 — RR 1082

105 mg
Melfiat®-105 Unicelles®
(phendimetrazine tartrate 105 mg)

Reid-Rowell

(Shown smaller than
actual size)

PROCTOCORT
Hydrocortisone Cream USP, 1%

*1920

Proctocort™
(buffered 1% hydrocortisone
cream, USP, 1%)

Reid-Rowell

1924*

Rowasa®
(mesalamine, rectal suspension enema)
4g/60 mL Unit Dose

Reid-Rowell
(Both sides of tablet shown)

R R — 1146

Zenate®
(prenatal multivitamin/
mineral supplement)

RICHARDSON-VICKS

Health Care Products

**Vicks®
Children's NyQuil®**

Richardson-Vicks

Cough — Cough & Congestion — Cough & Cold
Pediatric Formula 44®

A. H. ROBINS

Pharmaceutical Division

Tablets

AHR 4207
Capsules

AHR DONNATAL EXTENTAB
Extentabs®
†Donnatal®

A. H. Robins

AHR 4649 — AHR 5049
Donnazyme® — **Entozyme®**

A. H. Robins

20 mL
20 mg./mL
Dopram® Injectable
(Doxapram Hydrochloride Injection, USP)

A. H. Robins

AHR ENTOLASE HP — AHR ENTOLASE
Entolase® HP
(Pancrelipase)
Entolase®
(Pancrelipase)

A. H. Robins

AHR 50 mg.
Exna®
(Benzthiazide Tablets, USP)

A. H. Robins

MICRO-K AHR 5720
600 mg. (8 mEq K)
Micro-K Extencaps®
(Potassium Chloride)

A. H. Robins

MICRO-K 10 AHR 5730
750 mg. (10 mEq K)
Micro-K 10 Extencaps®
(Potassium Chloride)

A. H. Robins

AHR 1535
Mitrolan®
(Calcium Polycarbophil)

A. H. Robins

AHR 5816 — AHR 5883
Pabalate® — **Pabalate®-SF**

A. H. Robins

AHR
Phenaphen® Caplets
(Acetaminophen Tablets, USP)

AHR 6242 — No. 2
AHR 6257 — No. 3
AHR 6274 — No. 4
Phenaphen® with Codeine

A. H. Robins

Phenaphen®-650 with Codeine

A. H. Robins

20 mg.
Pondimin®
(Fenfluramine Hydrochloride)

A. H. Robins

QUINIDEX AHR
Quinidex Extentabs®
(Quinidine Sulfate
Extended-Release Tablets, USP)

A. H. Robins

5 mg. — 10 mg.
†**Reglan®**
(Metoclopramide Hydrochloride)

A. H. Robins

2 mL Ampuls — 10 mL Ampuls
2 mL Vial — 10 mL Vial — 30 mL Vial
Reglan® Injectable
(Metoclopramide Hydrochloride)
5 mg. Metoclopramide Base/mL

A. H. Robins

500 mg. ROBAXIN AHR — 750 mg. ROBAXIN 750
†**Robaxin®** — **Robaxin®-750**
(Methocarbamol Tablets, USP)

A. H. Robins

10 mL
100 mg./mL
Robaxin® Injectable
(Methocarbamol Injection, USP)

A. H. Robins

Robaxisal®

A. H. Robins

1 mL — 2 mL — 5 mL — 20 mL
Robinul® Injectable
(Glycopyrrolate Injection, USP)

A. H. Robins

AHR 7824 — AHR 72
†**Robinul®** — **Robinul® Forte**
(Glycopyrrolate Tablets, USP)

A. H. Robins

1 mg.
Tenex®
(Guanfacine Hydrochloride)

A. H. Robins

VIOKASE AHR
Viokase® Tablets
(Pancrelipase, USP)

ROCHE

ACCUTANE 10 ROCHE — 10 mg
ACCUTANE 20 ROCHE — 20 mg
ACCUTANE 40 ROCHE — 40 mg
**Accutane®
(isotretinoin/Roche)

Roche

ANCOBON 250 ROCHE — 250 mg
ANCOBON 500 ROCHE — 500 mg
Ancobon®
(flucytosine/Roche)

Roche

Azo Gantanol®

Roche

Azo Gantrisin®

Roche

BACTRIM
†**Bactrim™**
(trimethoprim and sulfamethoxazole)

Roche

BACTRIM
†**Bactrim™ DS**
(trimethoprim and sulfamethoxazole)

Roche

BEROCCA ROCHE
Berocca® Tablets

Roche

BEROCCA PLUS
Berocca® Plus

Roche

0.5 mg

1 mg

2 mg

†Bumex®
(bumetanide/Roche)

Roche ©

0.5 mg   1 mg   2 mg

Klonopin™
(clonazepam/Roche)

Roche

Larobec®

Roche ©

5 mg   10 mg   25 mg

*Libritabs®
(chlordiazepoxide/Roche)

Roche ©

5 mg   10 mg   25 mg

*†Librium®
(chlordiazepoxide HCl/Roche)

Roche ©

200 mg

Noludar® Tablets
(methyprylon/Roche)

Roche

2.5 mg   5 mg

*Quarzan®
(clidinium bromide/Roche)

Roche ©
(Shown slightly smaller than actual size)

Scale in mg on both sides of barrel eases visibility during administration.

Prefilled disposable syringe with a 1½" needle to help insure deep administration into muscle.

Tel-E-Ject®
2 ml = 10 mg

Roche ©

15 mg

30 mg

*Dalmane®
(flurazepam HCl/Roche)

Roche

10 mg   25 mg

50 mg   75 mg

100 mg   150 mg

*Endep®
(amitriptyline HCl/Roche)

Roche

0.1 Gm Capsule

0.25 Gm Capsule

0.5 Gm Capsule

0.1 Gm Tablet   0.25 Gm Tablet

0.5 Gm Tablet

Larodopa®
(levodopa/Roche)

Roche

*Limbitrol®   *Limbitrol® DS

(chlordiazepoxide and amitriptyline HCl/Roche)

Roche

10 mg

Marplan®
(isocarboxazid/Roche)

Roche

50 mg

Matulane®
(procarbazine HCl/Roche)

Roche

0.25 mcg   0.5 mcg

Rocaltrol®
(calcitriol/Roche)

Roche

30 mg

Solatene®
(beta-carotene/Roche)

Roche

5 mg

†Synkayvite®
(menadiol sodium diphosphate/Roche)

†Valium Injectable
(diazepam/Roche)

Roche ©

2 mg

†Levo-Dromoran®
(levorphanol tartrate/Roche)

Roche

*Librax®

Roche ©

*Menrium®   *Menrium®   *Menrium®
5-2   5-4   10-4

Roche ©

300 mg

Noludar® 300
(methyprylon/Roche)

Roche

10 mg   25 mg

50 mg   100 mg

†Taractan®
(chlorprothixene/Roche)

Roche ©

15 mg

Valrelease™
(diazepam/Roche)

ROERIG

210*

12.5 mg.

Antivert®
(meclizine HCl)

Roche

Fansidar®
(sulfadoxine and pyrimethamine)

Roche

500 mg

†Gantanol®
(sulfamethoxazole/Roche)

Roche

500 mg

†Gantrisin®
(sulfisoxazole/Roche)

TEL-E-DOSE® ROCHE®
Example:

GANTANOL® 0.5 g
(sulfamethoxazole)
ROCHE, NUTLEY, N.J.
LOT 2230-1
EXP. 07-1-90

Gantanol®
(sulfamethoxazole/Roche)

Tel-E-Dose is a unit package designed by Roche for convenience in dispensing medications in the hospital and nursing home. Each unit, sealed against contamination and moisture, is clearly identified by product name and strength and carries the control number and expiration date.

Currently available in this package form are the following Roche products: Bactrim™ (80 mg trimethoprim and 400 mg sulfamethoxazole) tablets; Bactrim™ DS (160 mg trimethoprim and 800 mg sulfamethoxazole) tablets; Bumex® (bumetanide) tablets, 0.5 mg, 1 mg, 2 mg; Dalmane® (flurazepam HCl) capsules, 15 mg, 30 mg; Gantanol® (sulfamethoxazole) tablets, 0.5 Gm; Gantrisin® (sulfisoxazole) tablets, 0.5 Gm; Librax® (5 mg chlordiazepoxide HCl and 2.5 mg clidinium Br) capsules; Librium® (chlordiazepoxide HCl) capsules, 5 mg, 10 mg, 25 mg; Limbitrol® (5 mg chlordiazepoxide and 12.5 mg amitriptyline HCl) tablets; Limbitrol® DS (10 mg chlordiazepoxide and 25 mg amitriptyline HCl) tablets; Trimpex® (trimethoprim) tablets, 100 mg; and Valium® (diazepam) tablets, 2 mg, 5 mg, 10 mg.

Roche

10 mg   25 mg

**Tegison®
(etretinate/Roche)

Roche

100 mg

Trimpex®
(trimethoprim/Roche)

Roche ©

2 mg   5 mg   10 mg

*†Valium®
(diazepam/Roche)

Roerig

211*

25 mg.

Antivert®/25
(meclizine HCl)

Roerig

212*

25 mg.

Antivert®/25 Chewable Tablets
(meclizine HCl)

Roerig

214*

50 mg.

Antivert®/50
(meclizine HCl)

*Dalmane, Endep, Librax, Libritabs, Librium, Limbitrol, Menrium, Quarzan and Valium are products of Roche Products Inc., Manati, PR 00701.
**Accutane and Tegison are products of Roche Dermatologics, Little Falls, NJ 07424.

Roerig

10 mg. 560*
25 mg. 561*
50 mg. 562*
100 mg. 563*

†**Atarax®**
(hydroxyzine hydrochloride)

Roerig

143*

Geocillin® Tablets
(carbenicillin indanyl sodium)
equivalent to 382 mg. carbenicillin

Roerig

411*
5 mg.

412*
10 mg.

Glucotrol®
(glipizide)

Roerig

504*

Heptuna® Plus

Roerig (Both sides of tablet shown)

254*

†**Marax®**
(Each tablet contains ephedrine sulfate
25 mg., theophylline 130 mg., and Atarax
[hydroxyzine HCl], 10 mg.)

Roerig

1 mg. 571*
2 mg. 572*
5 mg. 573*
10 mg. 574*
20 mg. 577*

†**Navane®**
(thiothixene)

Roerig

035*
400 mg.
chemically equivalent to 280 mg. ampicillin

†**Spectrobid®**
(bacampicillin HCl)

Roerig

534* 10 mg.
535* 25 mg.
536* 50 mg.
539* 75 mg.
538* 100 mg.
537* 150 mg.

†**Sinequan®**
(doxepin HCl)

Roerig

159* 250 mg.

†**Tao®**
(troleandomycin)

Roerig

092*

Urobiotic®-250
(Each capsule contains oxytetracycline
HCl 250 mg., sulfamethizole 250 mg., and
phenazopyridine HCl 50 mg.)

**Rorer Pharmaceuticals

¼ gr.   ½ gr.   1 gr.   1½ gr.
2 gr.   3 gr.
4 gr.   5 gr.

Armour® Thyroid
(thyroid USP)

Rorer (Shown smaller than actual size)

60 mg

Azmacort™ Inhaler
(triamcinolone acetonide)

Rorer (Shown smaller than actual size)

200 I.U.
per mL

Calcimar® Injection, Synthetic
(calcitonin-salmon)

Rorer
(Shown smaller than
actual size)

0.1 mg/mL

DDAVP® Intranasal
(desmopressin acetate)

Rorer
(Shown smaller than
actual size)

0.1 mg/mL

DDAVP® Nasal Spray
(desmopressin acetate)

Rorer
(Shown smaller than
actual size)

4 mcg/mL
1 mL

4 mcg/mL
10 mL

DDAVP® Injection
(desmopressin acetate)

Rorer

22*   20*   21*
25 mg   50 mg   100 mg

Hygroton®
(chlorthalidone USP)

Rorer

25 mcg   50 mcg   75 mcg
100 mcg   125 mcg   150 mcg
175 mcg   200 mcg   300 mcg

Levothroid®
(levothyroxine sodium tablets, USP)

Rorer (Shown smaller than actual size)

200 mcg

500 mcg

Levothroid®
(levothyroxine sodium, USP injection)

Rorer

2.5 mg

Lozol®
(indapamide)

Rorer

2835* 125 mg
2840* 250 mg
2841* 500 mg

Timed-Release Nicotinic
Acid Tempules®

In the future, all strengths will
contain dye-free beads.

Nicobid®
(niacin, Rorer)

Rorer

500 mg

Nicolar®
(niacin tablets)

Rorer
(Shown smaller than)
actual size)

Nitrolingual® Spray
(nitroglycerin
lingual aerosol)

Rorer

Demi-Regroton®
(chlorthalidone USP 25 mg,
reserpine USP 0.125 mg)

Rorer

Regroton®
(chlorthalidone USP 50 mg,
reserpine USP 0.25 mg)

Rorer

WHR 1354 60 mg
WHR 1355 125 mg
WHR 1356 250 mg

(timed-release capsules)   Dye-
Free
Beads

†**Slo-Phyllin® Gyrocaps®**
(theophylline, anhydrous)

Rorer

100 mg   200 mg

†**Slo-Phyllin® Tablets**
(theophylline)

Rorer

50 mg
100 mg

Slo-bid 75   75 mg
Slo-bid 125   125 mg

WHR 200   200 mg
WHR 300   300 mg

(timed-release capsules)

Slo-bid™ Gyrocaps®
(theophylline, anhydrous)

Rorer

Thyrolar-¼   Thyrolar-½   Thyrolar-1
Thyrolar-2   Thyrolar-3

Each Thyrolar-1 tablet contains
50 mcg T₄ and 12.5 mcg T₃

Thyrolar®
(liotrix, Rorer) tablets

ROXANE

2.5 mg   5 mg   10 mg

Marinol®
(dronabinol)

Roxane

Roxanol™

Roxanol 100™

(morphine sulfate concentrated
oral solution)

Roxane

54 090 30 mg

Roxanol SR™
(morphine sulfate sustained release)

**During the next year, new Rorer identification will appear on the products.

RUGBY

GENORA® 1/35
21 Day Regimen
(1 mg of norethindrone and 0.035 mg of ethinyl estradiol)

Also available in 28-day regimen containing 7 inert peach tablets.

Rugby

GENORA® 1/50
21 Day Regimen
(1 mg of norethindrone and 0.05 mg of ethinyl estradiol)

Also available in 28-day regimen containing 7 inert peach tablets.

Rugby

GENORA® 0.5/35
28 Day Regimen
(0.5 mg of norethindrone and 0.035 mg of ethinyl estradiol)

The 28-day regimen contains 7 inert peach tablets.

RUSS

Lortab® 2.5/500   Lortab® 5/500

Lortab® 7.5/500

(Lortab 2.5: hydrocodone bitartrate 2.5 mg/acetaminophen 500 mg; Lortab 5: hydrocodone bitartrate 5 mg/acetaminophen 500 mg; Lortab 7.5: hydrocodone bitartrate 7.5 mg/acetaminophen 500 mg)

Russ

(Both sides of tablet shown)

Lortab® ASA
(hydrocodone bitartrate 5 mg/aspirin 500 mg)

Russ

Lortab® Liquid
(hydrocodone bitartrate 2.5 mg/acetaminophen 120 mg) per mL

SANDOZ

#78-31*
(other side: scored)
Bellergal-S®
Tablets

Sandoz

#78-34*
(other side: branded Ⓢ)
†Cafergot® Tablets
(ergotamine tartrate and caffeine) tablets, USP

Sandoz

#78-84*
(other side: branded Fioricet and Ⓢ)
Fioricet® Tablets

Sandoz

capsules
#78-103*
Fiorinal®

tablets
#78-104*
(other side: tablets branded SANDOZ)
Fiorinal®

Sandoz

F-C
#3
½ gram
(#3)
#78-107*
Fiorinal® with Codeine

Sandoz

#78-70*
1 mg
(other side: branded Ⓢ)
Hydergine® Tablets (oral)
(ergoloid mesylates)

#78-77*   #78-51*
1 mg   0.5 mg
(other side: 1 mg tablet branded 78-77 and 0.5 mg tablet branded Ⓢ)
Hydergine® Sublingual Tablets
(ergoloid mesylates)

Sandoz

#78-101*
HYDERGINE LC
1 mg
1 mg
(other side: branded Ⓢ)
Hydergine® LC
(ergoloid mesylate) liquid capsules

Designed to help you identify drugs, this section contains actual size, full-color reproductions of products selected for inclusion by participating manufacturers.

Sandoz

10 mg   15 mg   25 mg
#78-2*   #78-8*   #78-3*

50 mg   100 mg
#78-4*   #78-5*

150 mg   200 mg
#78-6*   #78-7*

(other side: branded Ⓢ)
†Mellaril® Tablets
(thioridazine HCl tablets, USP)

Sandoz

#78-86*   #78-87*
10 mg   25 mg

#78-78*   #78-79*
50 mg   75 mg

†Pamelor®
(nortriptyline HCl) capsules, USP

Sandoz

#78-102*
5 mg
Parlodel® Capsules
(bromocriptine mesylate) capsules

Sandoz

#78-17*
2½ mg
(other side: scored)
Parlodel® Snaptabs™
(bromocriptine mesylate) tablets, USP

Sandoz

15 mg   #78-98*
FOR SLEEP

30 mg   #78-99*
FOR SLEEP
Restoril®
(temazepam) capsules

Sandoz

#78-110

Oral Solution & Pipette
5 ml (250 mg)

#78-109
I.V. 5 ml (250 mg)
Sandimmune®
(cyclosporine)

Sandoz

#78-120   #78-122

1 gram lyophilized

3 grams lyophilized

#78-124

6 grams lyophilized
Sandoglobulin®
(immune globulin intravenous [Human])

Sandoz

#78-180   #78-181

#78-182

0.05 mg/ml injection   0.1 mg/ml injection

0.5 mg/ml injection
Sandostatin®
(octreotide acetate/Sandoz)

Sandoz

#78-75*
1.34 mg
(other side: branded 78-75)
Tavist-1® Tablets
(clemastine fumarate) tablets, USP

Sandoz

#78-72*
2.68 mg
(other side: branded 78-72)
Tavist® Tablets
(clemastine fumarate) tablets, USP

Sandoz

#78-221*
1.34 mg
(other side: branded 78-221)
Tavist-D® Tablets
(clemastine fumarate, USP phenylpropanolamine HCl, USP)

Sandoz

#78-111*   #78-73*
5 mg   10 mg
(other side: 5 mg scored and branded 78-111, 10 mg scored and branded 78-73)
Visken® Tablets
(pindolol)

SAVAGE

1934*
Brexin® L.A. Capsules

Savage

4285*
Chromagen® Capsules

Savage

1115*
Dilor®
(dyphylline)
200 mg

1116*
Dilor®-400
(dyphylline)
400 mg

Dilor® Injectable
(dyphylline)
2 ml-500 mg/ml
(Shown smaller than actual size)

Savage

1124*
Dilor®-G

Savage

60 grams
Mytrex® Cream and Ointment

12 x 1.5 grams
Mytrex® Foilpac®
(nystatin, 100,000 units/triamcinolone acetonide, 1 mg)

SCHERING

120 mg
(60 mg per layer)   AFRINOL
AFRINOL® REPETABS® Tablets
Long Acting Nasal Decongestant
(pseudoephedrine sulfate)

Schering

080
4 mg
CHLOR-TRIMETON®
ALLERGY Tablets
(chlorpheniramine maleate, USP)

Schering

374
8 mg
Long Acting CHLOR-TRIMETON®
Allergy REPETABS® Tablets
(chlorpheniramine maleate, USP)

Schering
009
12 mg
CHLOR-TRIMETON®
Antihistamine REPETABS®
Timed-Release Allergy Tablets
(chlorpheniramine maleate, USP)

Schering
901
CHLOR-TRIMETON®
Decongestant Tablets
(chlorpheniramine maleate, USP and
pseudoephedrine sulfate)

Schering
CTM SINUS
CHLOR-TRIMETON® SINUS Caplets
(chlorpheniramine maleate USP,
phenylpropanolamine HCl, and
acetaminophen)

LA CTM D
Long Acting CHLOR-TRIMETON®
Decongestant REPETABS® Tablets
(chlorpheniramine maleate, USP
and pseudoephedrine sulfate)

Schering/White Product Line
Cod Liver Oil Concentrate Capsules

Cod Liver Oil Concentrate Tablets

**Cod Liver Oil Concentrate Tablets
w/Vitamin C**

Schering
307
**CORICIDIN® 'D® Decongestant
Tablets**

Schering
**CORICIDIN®
DEMILETS®
Tablets**

Schering
522
CORICIDIN® Tablets

Schering
751
DEMAZIN® REPETABS® Tablets
(chlorpheniramine maleate, USP and
phenylpropanolamine hydrochloride, USP)

Schering
WBS
Tablets

Schering
555
Chronotab®
Tablets
DISOPHROL®
(dexbrompheniramine maleate, USP and
pseudoephedrine sulfate, USP)

Schering
DRIXORAL
DRIXORAL®
Sustained-Action Tablets
(dexbrompheniramine maleate, USP and
pseudoephedrine sulfate, USP)

Schering
DRIXORAL PLUS
**DRIXORAL® PLUS
Extended Release Tablets**

Schering
0.02 mg 298 | 0.5 mg 150 | 0.05 mg 070
ESTINYL® Tablets
(ethinyl estradiol, USP)

Schering
ANA or 287 | ANB or 119
**ETRAFON® 2-10
Tablets
(2-10)** | **ETRAFON-A
Tablets
(4-10)**

ANC or 598 | ANE or 720
**ETRAFON
Tablets
(2-25)** | **ETRAFON-FORTE
Tablets
(4-25)**
(perphenazine, USP and
amitriptyline hydrochloride, USP)

Schering
525
125 mg
EULEXIN® Capsules
(flutamide)

Schering
AUF or 948
250 mg

AUG or 496
500 mg
FULVICIN-U/F® Tablets
[griseofulvin (microsize), USP]

Schering
228 125 mg
507 250 mg
654 165 mg
352 330 mg
FULVICIN® P/G Tablets
(ultramicrosize griseofulvin, USP)

Schering
734 100 mg
GYNE-LOTRIMIN® Vaginal Tablets
(clotrimazole, USP)

Schering
396 500 mg
GYNE-LOTRIMIN® Vaginal Tablets
(clotrimazole, USP)

Schering/White Product Line
Tablets | with Vitamin C Tablets
MOL-IRON

Schering
244 100 mg | 752 200 mg
438 300 mg
NORMODYNE® Tablets
(labetalol hydrochloride)

Schering
235 | 227
100/25 | 200/25
391 | 300/25
NORMOZIDE® TABLETS
(labetalol HCl and hydrochlorothiazide, USP)

Schering
282 1 mg
OPTIMINE® Tablets
(azatadine maleate, USP)

Schering/White Product Line
WDR or 442 | WFF or 550
2.5 mg tablet | 5 mg tablet

WFG or 316
10 mg tablet
PERMITIL®
(fluphenazine hydrochloride, USP)

Schering
820 2 mg
POLARAMINE® Tablets
(dexchlorpheniramine maleate, USP)

Schering
095 4 mg | 148 6 mg
POLARAMINE® REPETABS® Tablets
(dexchlorpheniramine maleate, USP)

Schering
(Shown smaller than actual size)
17 g canister
PROVENTIL® Inhaler
(albuterol)

Schering
252 2 mg | 573 4 mg
4 mg | 431
REPETABS®
PROVENTIL® Tablets
(albuterol sulfate)

Schering
705 2 mg | 940 4 mg
313 8 mg | 077 16 mg
TRILAFON® Tablets
(perphenazine, USP)

Schering
703
**TRINALIN® Long-Acting
Antihistamine/Decongestant
REPETABS® Tablets**
(azatadine maleate, USP and
pseudoephedrine sulfate, USP)

Schering
25 g
**VANCENASE® AQ
NASAL SPRAY**
(beclomethasone
dipropionate, monohydrate)

Schering
(Shown smaller than actual size)
16.8 g canister
VANCENASE® Nasal Inhaler
(beclomethasone dipropionate, USP)

Schering
(Shown smaller than actual size)
16.8 g canister
VANCERIL® Inhaler
(beclomethasone dipropionate, USP)

Schiapparelli Searle

1847
500 mg
metronidazole
in 100-ml
ready-to-use
containers
(5 mg/ml)
(Container is
shown smaller
than actual size)
Flagyl I.V.™ RTU®
(metronidazole)

Schiapparelli Searle
1804
Sterile lyophilized
powder in
single-dose vials
(equivalent to 500 mg
metronidazole
(Vial shown smaller
than actual size)
Flagyl I.V.™
(metronidazole HCl)

SCHOLL, INC.

Dr. Scholl's Athlete's Foot
Spray Liquid
(tolnaftate 1%)

Cures Athlete's Foot — 4 oz

Scholl, Inc.

Dr. Scholl's Tritin™
Antifungal Powder

2 oz

Schwarz Pharma

Ku-Zyme®
(amylase, lipase, protease, cellulase)
Kutrase®
(Ku-Zyme® plus hyoscyamine sulfate/
phenyltoloxamine citrate)

Schwarz Pharma

Ku-Zyme® HP
(pancrelipase capsules USP)

G. D. Searle & Co.

Both sides of tablets shown

1771 — 1851 — 1861

40 mg — 80 mg — 120 mg

Calan®
(verapamil HCl)

G. D. Searle & Co.

1831 — 250 mg

1821 — 500 mg

Flagyl®
(metronidazole)

Scholl, Inc.

Dr. Scholl's Athlete's Foot
Spray Powder
(tolnaftate 1%)

Advanced Formula Super Moisture Absorption — Prevents & Cures Athlete's Foot — 3.5 oz

Scholl, Inc.

Dr. Scholl's Maximum
Strength Tritin™
Antifungal Spray Powder

3 oz

Schwarz Pharma

Lactrase®
(lactase) 250 mg

Schwarz Pharma

0.125 mg Sublingual
Levsin®/SL Tablets
0.125 mg Oral
Levsin® Tablets

0.375 mg Timed Release
Levsinex™ Timecaps™
Levsin®
(hyoscyamine sulfate USP)

G. D. Searle & Co.

Both sides of caplet shown

1891

240 mg

Calan® SR
(verapamil HCl)

Both sides of tablets shown

Flagyl®
(metronidazole)

G. D. Searle & Co.

Both sides of tablet shown

61

†Lomotil®
(diphenoxylate hydrochloride 2.5 mg/
atropine sulfate 0.025 mg)

Scholl, Inc.

Dr. Scholl's Smooth Touch®
Deep Moisturizing Cream

Penetrates extra-dry
and calloused skin

Smooth Touch — 2 oz

Scholl, Inc.

Dr. Scholl's Work Day®
Super Comfort Insoles

One size fits all

Work Day

G. D. SEARLE & CO.

Both sides of tablets shown

1011 — 25 mg/25 mg

1021 — 50 mg/50 mg

Aldactazide®
(spironolactone/hydrochlorothiazide)

G. D. Searle & Co.

Both sides of tablet shown

1461 — 200 mcg

Cytotec®
(misoprostol)

G. D. Searle & Co.

Both sides of tablet shown

151

Demulen® 1/35-21, -28
(ethynodiol diacetate 1 mg/
ethinyl estradiol 35 mcg)

The 28-day Compack® also contains 7 blue placebo tablets.

(Compack shown smaller than actual size)

G. D. Searle & Co.

(Discs shown smaller than actual size)

5 mg/24 hr — 2058

7.5 mg/24 hr — 2078

10 mg/24 hr — 2068

Nitrodisc®
(transdermal nitroglycerin system)

Scholl, Inc.

Dr. Scholl's Soap 'n Soak®
Instant Foot Bath

4 packets in a carton

1 oz each

SCHWARZ PHARMA

Deponit®
(nitroglycerin transdermal delivery system)

5 mg/24 hrs.
One System
(Shown smaller than actual size)

G. D. Searle & Co.

1001 — 25 mg

1041 — 50 mg

1031 — 100 mg

Both sides of tablets shown

Aldactone®
(spironolactone)

G. D. Searle & Co.

Both sides of tablet shown

71

Demulen® 1/50-21, -28
(ethynodiol diacetate 1 mg/
ethinyl estradiol 50 mcg)

The 28-day Compack® also contains 7 pink placebo tablets.

(Compack shown smaller than actual size)

Because tablets and capsules are
shown in this section, do not infer
that these are the only dosage forms
available. Where a product name is
preceded by the symbol †, refer to the
description in the Product Information (White Section) for other forms.

G. D. Searle & Co.

2752 — 100 mg
2762 — 150 mg

Norpace®
(disopyramide phosphate)

Scholl, Inc.

Dr. Scholl's Super Deodorant
Foot Powder
For Bromidrosis...
Excessive perspiration and
foot odor

2¾ oz

Schwarz Pharma

†Fedahist® Gyrocaps®
(65 mg pseudoephedrine HCl USP and
10 mg chlorpheniramine maleate USP)

timed release

Schwarz Pharma

†Fedahist® Timecaps™
(120 mg pseudoephedrine HCl USP and
8 mg chlorpheniramine maleate USP)

timed release

G. D. Searle & Co.

2732 — 100 mg
2742 — 150 mg

Norpace® CR
(disopyramide phosphate)

G. D. Searle & Co.

100 mg
2832

200 mg
2842

300 mg
2852

Theo-24®
(theophylline anhydrous)

SMITH KLINE &FRENCH

1 gram
Also 250 mg,
500 mg

1 gram
Also 500 mg

10 grams
Also 5 grams

1 gram
Also 500 mg

ANCEF®
(sterile cefazolin sodium, SK&F and
cefazolin sodium injection, SK&F)

Smith Kline &French

ANSPOR

250 mg

ANSPOR

500 mg

Also oral suspension 125 mg or
250 mg per 5 mL teaspoonful
(in 100 mL bottles).

ANSPOR® Capsules
(cephradine, SK&F)

FSK

1 gram
Also 2 grams

1 gram
Also 2 grams

10 gram

1 gram
Also 2 grams

CEFIZOX®
(sterile ceftizoxime sodium, FSK and
ceftizoxime sodium injection, FSK)

Smith Kline &French

C47
30 mg

Also 10 mg C44, 15 mg C46

†COMPAZINE® SPANSULE®
(prochlorperazine, SK&F)
Capsules

Smith Kline &French

C60
2½ mg

C61
5 mg

C62
25 mg

†COMPAZINE® Suppositories
(prochlorperazine, SK&F)

SMITH KLINE &FRENCH LABORATORIES
Division of SmithKline Beckman Corporation
TABLET & CAPSULE IDENTIFICATION

The unique "taper-end" shape of SK&F capsules is a trademark that quickly identifies them as products of Smith Kline &French Laboratories.

Product Identification Code: Each SK&F capsule and tablet bears a monogram consisting of a three-character code or the name of the specific product. A product-by-product listing of identification codes appears in SK&F's complete list of products in the Product Information section.

 OR

Capsule Shape: Trademark

The three-unit product identification codes or names that appear beside products in the photo blocks are the same as those imprinted on the pictured products because the codes may be difficult to read in the photo reproductions.

NOTE: Dyazide®, Dyrenium®, Stelazine® and Tagamet® are products of SK&F Lab Co., Cidra, P.R. 00639, a subsidiary of SmithKline Beckman Corporation. Cefizox® is manufactured for Fujisawa SmithKline by Fujisawa Pharmaceutical Co., Ltd., distributed by SK&F Laboratories, Division of SmithKline Beckman Corporation.

Smith Kline &French

C66
5 mg

Also 10 mg C67, 25 mg C69
†COMPAZINE® Tablets
(prochlorperazine, SK&F)

Smith Kline &French

†COMPAZINE®
(prochlorperazine, SK&F)
2 mL (5 mg/mL) **Ampuls**

Smith Kline &French

†COMPAZINE®
(prochlorperazine, SK&F)
10 mL (5 mg/mL)
Multiple-dose Vials

Smith Kline &French

4 fl oz

†COMPAZINE®
(prochlorperazine, SK&F)
Syrup
(5 mg/5 mL)

Smith Kline &French

†COMPAZINE®
(prochlorperazine, SK&F)
2 mL (5 mg/mL)
Prefilled Disposable Syringes

Smith Kline &French

D14   D16   D17

5 mcg   25 mcg   50 mcg

liothyronine as the sodium salt
CYTOMEL® Tablets
(liothyronine sodium, SK&F)

Smith Kline &French

D62

5 mg

DARBID® Tablets
(isopropamide iodide, SK&F)

Smith Kline &French

E14
15 mg

Also 5 mg E12, 10 mg E13

†DEXEDRINE® SPANSULE®
(dextroamphetamine sulfate, SK&F)
Capsules

Smith Kline &French

E19

5 mg

†DEXEDRINE® Tablets
(dextroamphetamine sulfate, SK&F)

Smith Kline &French

E33

10 mg

DIBENZYLINE® Capsules
(phenoxybenzamine
hydrochloride, SK&F)

SK&F Lab Co.

DYAZIDE

DYAZIDE® Capsules

SK&F Lab Co.

50 mg   100 mg

DYRENIUM® Capsules
(triamterene, SK&F)

Smith Kline &French

ESKALITH

300 mg

ESKALITH® Capsules
(lithium carbonate, SK&F)

Smith Kline &French

J09

300 mg

ESKALITH® Tablets
(lithium carbonate, SK&F)

Smith Kline &French

J10
450 mg

ESKALITH CR®
(lithium carbonate, SK&F)
Controlled Release Tablets

Smith Kline &French

500 mg

1 gram

1 gram

10 grams

MONOCID®
(sterile cefonicid sodium, SK&F)
(lyophilized)

Smith Kline &French

ORNADE

ORNADE® SPANSULE® Capsules

Smith Kline &French

PARNATE

10 mg

PARNATE® Tablets
(tranylcypromine sulfate, SK&F)

Smith Kline &French

RIDAURA

3 mg

RIDAURA® Capsules
(auranofin, SK&F)

SK&F Lab Co.

2 mg S04
Also 1 mg S03,
5 mg S06,
10 mg S07

†STELAZINE® Tablets
(trifluoperazine HCl, SK&F)

SK&F Lab Co.

10 mL
(2 mg/mL)
Multiple-dose Vials

†STELAZINE®
(trifluoperazine HCl, SK&F)

STELAZINE®
(trifluoperazine hydrochloride, SK&F)
Concentrate
(10 mg/mL)

SK&F Lab Co.

8 fl oz

Single-dose unit

Each 5 mL contains cimetidine
hydrochloride equivalent to
cimetidine, 300 mg
TAGAMET® LIQUID
(cimetidine hydrochloride, SK&F)

SK&F Lab Co.

TAGAMET
200 mg

TAGAMET
300 mg

TAGAMET
400 mg

TAGAMET® Tablets
(cimetidine, SK&F)

TAGAMET
800 mg

TAGAMET® TILTAB® Tablets
(cimetidine, SK&F)

2 mL
Single-dose

8 mL
Multiple-dose

Prefilled Disposable Syringe
TAGAMET® INJECTION
(cimetidine hydrochloride, SK&F)
300 mg/2 mL

300 mg/50 mL

TAGAMET® INJECTION
(cimetidine hydrochloride, SK&F)

300 mg/2 mL

TAGAMET® INJECTION
(cimetidine hydrochloride, SK&F
in ADD-Vantage® Vials)

Smith Kline &French

T64
75 mg

Also 30 mg T63, 150 mg T66,
200 mg T67, 300 mg T69
†THORAZINE® SPANSULE®
(chlorpromazine hydrochloride, SK&F)
Capsules

Smith Kline &French

T74
25 mg

Also 10 mg T73, 50 mg T76,
100 mg T77, 200 mg T79
†THORAZINE® Tablets
(chlorpromazine hydrochloride, SK&F)

Smith Kline &French

T70
25 mg

Also 100 mg T71
†THORAZINE® Suppositories
(chlorpromazine, SK&F)

Smith Kline &French

THORAZINE®
(chlorpromazine hydrochloride, SK&F)
Syrup
(10 mg/5 mL)

Smith Kline &French

1 mL

2 mL

THORAZINE®
(chlorpromazine hydrochloride, SK&F)
Ampuls
(25 mg/mL)

Smith Kline &French

THORAZINE®
(chlorpromazine hydrochloride, SK&F)
Multiple-dose Vials
10 mL (25 mg/mL)

Smith Kline &French

THORAZINE®
(chlorpromazine hydrochloride, SK&F)
Concentrate
(30 mg/mL)
(100 mg/mL)

Smith Kline &French

1 gram
Also 2 grams

1 gram
Also 2 grams

6 grams

TAZICEF®
(ceftazidime for injection, SK&F)

Smith Kline &French

TUSS-ORNADE

**†TUSS-ORNADE®
SPANSULE® Capsules**

Smith Kline &French

URISPAS

100 mg
URISPAS® Tablets
(flavoxate HCl, SK&F)

Smith Kline &French

25 mg
VONTROL® Tablets
(diphenidol as the hydrochloride, SK&F)

SOLGAR

Fish Oil
Concentrate

MaxEPA® 1000 mg. Softgels
(eicosapentaenoic acid and
docosahexaenoic acid)

While every effort has been made to
reproduce products faithfully, this
section is to be considered a quick-
reference identification aid. In cases
of suspected overdosage, etc., chemical analysis of the product should
be done.

E. R. SQUIBB & SONS

12.5 mg   25 mg
450**   452**

50 mg   100 mg
482**   485**

CAPOTEN®
(Captopril Tablets)

E. R. Squibb & Sons

25 mg/15 mg   25 mg/25 mg
338**   349**

50 mg/15 mg   50 mg/25 mg
384**   390**

CAPOZIDE®
(Captopril-Hydrochlorothiazide Tablets)

E. R. Squibb & Sons

500 mg
830**

HYDREA®
(Hydroxyurea Capsules USP)

E. R. Squibb & Sons

500,000 u
580**

†MYCOSTATIN®
(Nystatin Tablets USP)

E. R. Squibb & Sons

200,000 u

MYCOSTATIN® Pastilles
(Nystatin)

E. R. Squibb & Sons

100,000 u
457**

MYCOSTATIN® Vaginal Tablets
(Nystatin Vaginal Tablets USP)

E. R. Squibb & Sons

250 mg
971**

500 mg
974**

†PRINCIPEN®
(Ampicillin Capsules USP)

**Squibb product identification number.

E. R. Squibb & Sons

250 mg
655**

500 mg
763**

†SUMYCIN®
(Tetracycline Hydrochloride Capsules USP)

E. R. Squibb & Sons

250 mg
663**

500 mg
603**

†SUMYCIN®
(Tetracycline Hydrochloride Tablets USP)

E. R. Squibb & Sons

535**

THERAGRAN HEMATINIC®
(Therapeutic Formula Vitamin Tablets
with Hematinics)

E. R. Squibb & Sons

250 mg
230**

500 mg
231**

†TRIMOX®
(Amoxicillin Capsules USP)

E. R. Squibb & Sons

250 mg
684**

500 mg
648**

†VEETIDS®
(Penicillin V Potassium Tablets USP)

E. R. Squibb & Sons

250 mg
113**

500 mg
114**

†VELOSEF®
(Cephradine Capsules USP)

SQUIBB-NOVO

**Novolin® 10 ml/100 units/ml
Human Insulin**
(semi-synthetic)

STAR

5.4 mg.
Aphrodyne™ Caplets
(yohimbine hydrochloride)

Star

10 mg.
Virilon® Capsules
(macro-bead methyltestosterone USP)

200 mg./ml.
Virilon® IM
(testosterone cypionate)

STUART

12 oz   NDC 38-860

unit
dose

30 mL

5 oz

ALternaGEL® Liquid
(Each 5 mL contains aluminum
hydroxide, 600 mg)

Stuart

NDC 38-864

(Both sides of tablet shown)
BUCLADIN®-S Softab®
(buclizine hydrochloride, 50 mg)

Stuart

NDC 38-377   NDC 38-376

2 g in
20 mL vial

CEFOTAN
2 g

CEFOTAN
1 g

1 g in
10 mL vial

NDC 38-375

CEFOTAN
10 g

10 g bulk pharmacy package

CEFOTAN
2 g

CEFOTAN
1 g

2 g in 100 mL vial   1 g in 100 mL vial

CEFOTAN® IM/IV
(cefotetan disodium)

Stuart

NDC 38-470
DIALOSE® Capsules
(docusate potassium, 100 mg)

Stuart

NDC 38-475
DIALOSE® PLUS Capsules
(casanthranol, 30 mg; docusate
potassium, 100 mg)

Stuart   NDC 38-440

Available in
9 oz and 16 oz
bottles

EFFER-SYLLIUM

EFFER-SYLLIUM
NATURAL
FIBER
BULKING
AGENT
EFFERVESCENT
LEMON-LIME
TASTE

Convenience
Packets, 12's and 24's
EFFER-SYLLIUM® Instant Mix
Bulk Laxative containing
Natural Dietary Fiber

Stuart   (layered tablet)

NDC 38-650

FERANCEE® Chewable Tablets

Stuart

NDC 38-863
FERANCEE®-HP Tablets

Stuart

NDC 38-575

32 oz with
foot-operated
wall dispenser

packettes
15 mL

16 oz with hand-
operated wall
dispenser

4 oz,
8 oz,
and
1 gal

HIBICLENS®
(chlorhexidine gluconate)

Stuart

NDC 38-577
**HIBICLENS®
Sponge/Brush
with nail cleaner**
22 mL
(chlorhexidine
gluconate)

Stuart   NDC 38-587

HIBISTAT

Towelette
5 mL

HIBISTAT

NDC 38-585

8 oz   4 oz

HIBISTAT®
(chlorhexidine gluconate)

Stuart

240 mg   NDC 38-380
KASOF® Capsules
(docusate potassium)

Stuart   (Both sides of
tablet shown)

NDC 38-220

KINESED® Tablets
(belladonna alkaloids and phenobarbital)

Stuart   NDC 38-455

NDC 38-858

MYLICON®-80   **MYLICON®-125**
(simethicone)

Stuart

NDC 38-630

1 fl oz
MYLICON® Drops
(simethicone)

Stuart   NDC 38-620
(layered tablet)

12 oz and 5 oz

24 oz

12 tablet roll

NDC 38-610 (liquids)

5 oz
Hosp.
Pak

30 mL
Unit
Dose

MYLANTA® Liquid and Tablets
(Each 5 mL and each tablet contains
aluminum hydroxide, 200 mg; magnesium
hydroxide, 200 mg; simethicone, 20 mg)

Stuart

NDC 38-651
(layered tablet)

8 tablet roll

MYLANTA-II

12 oz
and 5 oz

24 oz

NDC 38-652 (liquids)

5 oz
Hosp.
Pak

30 mL
Unit
Dose

MYLANTA®-II Liquid and Tablets
(Each 5 mL and each tablet contains
aluminum hydroxide, 400 mg; magnesium
hydroxide, 400 mg; simethicone, 40 mg)

Stuart (Both sides of tablet shown)

NDC 38-710

**MULVIDREN®-F
Softab®**
(Fluoride with Multivitamins)

Stuart

NDC 38-840

PROBEC®-T Tablets

Stuart

NDC 38-866

STUART FORMULA® Tablets

Stuart

NDC 38-862

STUARTINIC® Tablets

Stuart

NDC 38-071

STUART PRENATAL® Tablets

Stuart

NDC 38-021

STUARTNATAL® 1+1 Tablets

Stuart
NDC 38-142   NDC 38-145

20-12.5   20-25

Zestoretic®
(lisinopril and hydrochlorothiazide)

Stuart

NDC 38-130

5 mg

NDC 38-131   NDC 38-132

10 mg   20 mg

NDC 38-134

40 mg

ZESTRIL®
(lisinopril)

SUMMIT

153*

300 mg.
Actigall™
(ursodiol)

Summit

165*

600 mg. (8 mEq)
Slow-K® slow-release tablets
(potassium chloride USP)

Summit

146*

750 mg.
(10 mEq)

Controlled-release tablets
Ten-K®
(potassium chloride USP)

Summit

902*

2.5 mg/24 hr

905*

5 mg/24 hr

910*   10 mg/24 hr

915*   15 mg/24 hr

Transderm-Nitro®
(nitroglycerin)
Transdermal Therapeutic System

SYNTEX

50 mg.   2902*

Anadrol®-50 tablets
(oxymetholone)

Syntex

274*

275 mg.
Anaprox®

276*

550 mg.
Anaprox® DS

tablets
(naproxen sodium)

Syntex

20 mg.   30 mg.

Cardene® capsules
(nicardipine hydrochloride)

Syntex

125 mg./5 ml.

Naprosyn® suspension
(naproxen)

Syntex

272*   273*

250 mg.   375 mg.

277*

500 mg.

Naprosyn® tablets
(naproxen)

Syntex

FEMSTAT PREFILL

Femstat® Prefill
(butoconazole nitrate)
vaginal cream 2%

Syntex

FEMSTAT

Femstat®
(butoconazole nitrate)
vaginal cream 2%

Applicator

Syntex
(inert tablet)   110*

Wallette® pill
dispenser in 21-
and 28-day regimens

Brevicon® tablets
(norethindrone with ethinyl estradiol)

Syntex
(inert tablet)   111*

Wallette® pill
dispenser in 21-
and 28-day
regimens

Norinyl® 1+35 tablets
(norethindrone with ethinyl estradiol)

Syntex
(inert tablet)   1*

Wallette® pill
dispenser in 21-
and 28-day
regimens

Norinyl® 1+50 tablets
(norethindrone with mestranol)

Syntex
110*   (inert tablet)   111*

Wallette® pill
dispenser in 21-
and 28-day
regimens

Tri-Norinyl® tablets
(norethindrone with ethinyl estradiol)

Syntex

0.35 mg.

NOR-QD® tablets
(norethindrone)

UPJOHN

170*   305*

50 mg   100 mg

Ansaid® Tablets
(flurbiprofen)

Upjohn
(Both sides of tablets shown)

81*
0.5 mg

92*
1 mg

†**Adeflor Chewable® Tablets**

Upjohn

Colestid

5 gram packet

500 gram bottle
Colestid® Granules
(colestipol hydrochloride for oral
suspension, USP)

Upjohn

870*   775*

2 ml vial
(300 mg)   4 ml vial
(600 mg)

(Shown
smaller
than
actual
size)

902*

6 ml vial (900 mg)
(also available:
60 ml pharmacy bulk pkg.)

Cleocin Phosphate® Sterile Solution
(clindamycin phosphate injection, USP)

Upjohn

75 mg   150 mg
331*   225*

300 mg
395*

Cleocin HCl® Capsules
(clindamycin hydrochloride
capsules, USP)

Upjohn (Shown smaller than actual size)

Cleocin T® 1%

30 gram tube
Cleocin T® Topical Gel
(clindamycin phosphate topical gel, USP)

Upjohn

Cleocin T® 1%
clindamycin phosphate, USP

10 mg/ml
60 ml bottle

Cleocin T® Topical Lotion
(clindamycin phosphate
topical lotion, USP)

Upjohn
(Shown
smaller
than
actual
size)

Cleocin T   Cleocin T

30 ml   60 ml

Cleocin T® Topical Solution
(clindamycin phosphate topical solution, USP)

Upjohn

(Shown smaller
than actual
size)

available:
20 mg/ml
(5 ml)
40 mg/ml
(1, 5, 10 ml)
80 mg/ml
(1, 5 ml)

Depo-Medrol

†**Depo-Medrol®**
Sterile Aqueous Suspension
(sterile methylprednisolone acetate
suspension, USP)

Upjohn

32*   45*

2.5 mg   5 mg

193*

10 mg

165*   388*

20 mg   50 mg

Deltasone® Tablets
(prednisone tablets, USP)

Upjohn

25 mg   50 mg
18*   24*

Didrex® Tablets
(benzphetamine hydrochloride)

Upjohn

10*   17*

0.125 mg   0.25 mg

Halcion® Tablets
(triazolam tablets, USP)

Upjohn

14* 2 mg   19* 5 mg   36* 10 mg

Halotestin® Tablets
(fluoxymesterone tablets, USP)

Upjohn

121*   2.5 mg
(Both sides of tablet shown)

137*   10 mg

Loniten® Tablets
(minoxidil tablets, USP)

Upjohn

412*

400 mg

Maolate® Tablets
(chlorphenesin carbamate)

Upjohn

2 mg 49*   4 mg 56*   8 mg 22*

16 mg 73*   24 mg 155*   32 mg 176*

†Medrol® Tablets
(methylprednisolone tablets, USP)

Upjohn

(Shown smaller than actual size)

56*

Medrol® Dosepak™ 4 mg

4 mg

Medrol® Dosepak™ Unit of Use
(methylprednisolone tablets, USP)

Upjohn

MOTRIN 300mg 733*   MOTRIN 400mg 750*

300 mg   400 mg

MOTRIN 600mg 742*

600 mg

MOTRIN 800mg 725*

800 mg

Motrin® Tablets
(ibuprofen tablets, USP)

Upjohn

131* 1.25 mg   141* 2.5 mg   171* 5 mg

Micronase® Tablets
(glyburide)

Upjohn

701*   100*

250 mg   500 mg

Orinase® Tablets
(tolbutamide tablets, USP)

Upjohn

2.5 mg 64*   5 mg 286*   10 mg 50*

Provera® Tablets
(medroxyprogesterone acetate tablets, USP)

Upjohn

Rogaine

60 ml bottle with applicators
Rogaine® Topical Solution
(minoxidil 2%)

Upjohn

40 mg Act-O-Vial®
125 mg Act-O-Vial®
500 mg vial
1 gram vial
2 gram vial

(Shown smaller than actual size)

1 gram with Intravenous Administration Set

Solu-Medrol® Sterile Powder
(methylprednisolone sodium succinate for injection, USP)

Upjohn

100 mg 70*   250 mg 114*

500 mg 477*

Tolinase® Tablets
(tolazamide tablets, USP)

Upjohn   Ⓒ

0.25 mg 29*   0.5 mg 55*   1.0 mg 90*

Xanax® Tablets
(alprazolam tablets, USP)

UPSHER-SMITH

KLOR-CON 8   Extended-release Tablets, U.S.P.   KLOR-CON 10

Klor-Con® 8/Klor-Con® 10
(potassium chloride)

WALLACE

Aquatensen®
(methyclothiazide 5 mg.)

Wallace   Ⓒ

15 mg.   30 mg.

†Butisol Sodium Tablets
(butabarbital)

Wallace

Diutensen®-R
(methyclothiazide, 2.5 mg. and reserpine, 0.1 mg.)

Wallace

200 mg. **†Lufyllin®**
(dyphylline)

400 mg. **Lufyllin®-400**
(dyphylline)

Wallace

LUFYLLIN DYPHYLLINE Injection 250 mg. per TRAMUSCUL ACE LABORA bury, N.J. 001 EXP

2 mL (250 mg./mL) Lufyllin® Injection
(dyphylline)
(Ampul shown slightly smaller than actual size)

Wallace

†Lufyllin®-GG
(dyphylline, 200 mg. and guaifenesin, 200 mg.)

Wallace   Ⓒ

200 mg.

400 mg.

WALLACE

600 mg.

Miltown
(meprobamate)

Wallace

30 mg. **†Organidin®**
(iodinated glycerol)

Organidin® Elixir
(iodinated glycerol)
per 5 mL-1.2%,
60 mg. Organidin

Organidin® Solution
(iodinated glycerol)
per mL-5%,
50 mg. Organidin

Organidin Elixir

Wallace   Ⓒ

WALLACE 37-107 300   WALLACE 37-108 150

300 mg.   150 mg.

†Rondomycin®
(methacycline HCl)

Wallace   (Both sides of tablet shown)

Rynatan®
(phenylephrine tannate, 25 mg., chlorpheniramine tannate, 8 mg. and pyrilamine tannate, 25 mg.)

Rynatan®-S*
Pediatric Suspension
(each teaspoonful 5mL contains: phenylephrine tannate, 5 mg.; chlorpheniramine tannate, 2 mg.; pyrilamine tannate, 12.5 mg.)

*Patent Pending. Rynatan®-S is the combination of Rynatan® Pediatric Suspension (4 fl. oz.) and a 10 mL calibrated, oral syringe.

Wallace

Rynatuss®
(carbetapentane tannate, 60 mg., chlorpheniramine tannate, 5 mg., ephedrine tannate, 10 mg. and phenylephrine tannate, 10 mg.)

**Rynatuss®
Pediatric Suspension**
(in 5 mL-carbetapentane tannate, 30 mg.; chlorpheniramine tannate, 4 mg.; ephedrine tannate, 5 mg.; phenylephrine tannate, 5 mg.)

Wallace

350 mg.

Soma®
(carisoprodol)

Wallace

Soma® Compound
(200 mg. carisoprodol + 325 mg. aspirin)

Wallace   Ⓒ

Soma® Compound with Codeine
(200 mg. carisoprodol + 325 mg. aspirin + 16 mg. codeine phosphate)

Wallace

Theo-Organidin Elixir

Theo-Organidin® Elixir
[15 mL contains: theophylline (anhydrous), 120 mg.; Organidin (iodinated glycerol containing 15 mg. organically bound iodine), 30 mg.; 15% alcohol by volume]

Wallace   Ⓒ

Tussi-Organidin   Tussi-Organidin DM Liquid

Tussi-Organidin®
[(per 5 mL)-Organidin (iodinated glycerol) containing 15 mg. organically bound iodine, 30 mg.; codeine phosphate, 10 mg.]

Tussi-Organidin® DM
[(per 5 mL)-Organidin (iodinated glycerol) containing 15 mg. organically bound iodine, 30 mg.; dextromethorphan hydrobromide, 10 mg.]

Wallace

(Shown smaller than actual size)

VōSol   15 mL   VōSol   10 mL

VōSol
(acetic acid-nonaqueous 2%)

VōSol HC
(hydrocortisone 1% acetic acid-nonaqueous 2%)

VōSol   30 mL

VōSol
(acetic acid-nonaqueous 2%)

WESTWOOD

3.6 mg. 8 mg.
†Tacaryl
(methdilazine base and hydrochloride)

WHITEHALL

Advil Advil
ADVIL® TABLETS AND CAPLETS
(ibuprofen)

Whitehall 100 mg/5mL
CHILDREN'S ADVIL® SUSPENSION
(ibuprofen suspension)

Whitehall
CoADVIL™ CAPLETS
(200 mg ibuprofen and 30 mg pseudo-ephedrine hydrochloride)

Whitehall
ANACIN
ANACIN®
Coated Tablets and Caplets

Whitehall
Front Back
MAXIMUM STRENGTH ANACIN®
Analgesic Tablets

Whitehall 80 mg
Front Back
CHILDREN'S ANACIN-3®
Acetaminophen Chewable Tablets

Whitehall (Shown smaller than actual size)
Liquid Drops
Liquid: 80 mg per ½ teaspoon
Drops: 80 mg per 0.8 mL
CHILDREN'S ANACIN-3®
Acetaminophen

Whitehall
A-3 500
ANACIN-3 Front Back
MAXIMUM STRENGTH ANACIN-3®
Acetaminophen Tablets and Caplets
(Film Coated)

Whitehall
A-3 325 mg
Front Back
REGULAR STRENGTH ANACIN-3®
Acetaminophen Tablets
(Film Coated)

Whitehall
Liquid Gel Baby Gel
ANBESOL®
Anesthetic For Topical Oral
Pain Relief

Whitehall
Liquid Gel
MAXIMUM STRENGTH ANBESOL®
Anesthetic for Topical Oral
Pain Relief

Whitehall
ARTHRITIS PAIN FORMULA
by the makers of ANACIN®
Analgesic Tablets

Whitehall
(Shown smaller than actual size)
Extra Strength Shampoo
Denorex Denorex Denorex
Regular Formula Mountain Fresh Herbal Scent Shampoo and Conditioner
DENOREX®
Medicated Shampoo

Whitehall (Shown smaller than actual size)
Long Lasting Regular
DRISTAN®
Nasal Sprays

Whitehall
Front Back
Front Back
DRISTAN® TABLETS AND CAPLETS
Decongestant/Antihistamine/Analgesic

Whitehall
Front Back
**MAXIMUM STRENGTH
DRISTAN® CAPLETS**
Decongestant/Analgesic
(500 mg acetaminophen and 30 mg
pseudoephedrine hydrochloride)

Whitehall Suppository
PREPARATION H®

Ointment

PREPARATION H HEMORRHOIDAL OINTMENT

Cream

PREPARATION H CREAM
(Shown smaller than actual size)
PREPARATION H®
Hemorrhoidal Ointment,
Suppositories and Cream

Whitehall
Regular
Front Back
P Formula
Front Back
M Formula
Front Back
PRIMATENE® TABLETS
Asthma Remedy

Whitehall (Shown smaller than actual size)
PRIMATENE® MIST
Asthma Remedy

Whitehall
Antacid
Swallow Tablet Chew Tablet
†RIOPAN®
(magaldrate)

Whitehall
Antacid/
Anti-Gas Chew Tablet
†RIOPAN PLUS®
(magaldrate and simethicone)

Whitehall
Front Back
**MAXIMUM STRENGTH
RIOPAN® PLUS® 2
DOUBLE STRENGTH**
(magaldrate and simethicone)

Whitehall (Shown smaller than actual size)
SEMICID®
Vaginal Contraceptive Inserts

Whitehall
Today
Available in Packages of 3, 6 and 12
Contraceptive Sponge
TODAY®
Vaginal Contraceptive Sponge

Winthrop Pharmaceuticals

A77* 500 mg
†Aralen® Phosphate
Brand of chloroquine phosphate tablets, USP

Winthrop Pharmaceuticals
B 34 B34*
750 mg
Bilopaque® Sodium Capsules
Brand of tyropanoate sodium, USP

Winthrop Pharmaceuticals
D03* D04*
50 mg 100 mg
D05*
200 mg
Danocrine® Capsules
Brand of danazol capsules, USP

Winthrop Pharmaceuticals
D35* D37*
50 mg 100 mg
scored tablet
†Demerol® Hydrochloride Tablets
Brand of meperidine hydrochloride
tablets, USP

Winthrop Pharmaceuticals
Demerol® APAP
Each tablet contains meperidine
hydrochloride, USP, 50 mg with
acetaminophen, USP, 300 mg

Winthrop Pharmaceuticals
M91* M90*
M-91 30 MG M-90
30 mg 60 mg
Modrastane®
Brand of trilostane

Winthrop Pharmaceuticals
N21* N22*
250 mg 500 mg
N23*
1 Gram
scored tablets
†NegGram® Caplets®
Brand of nalidixic acid tablets, USP

Winthrop Pharmaceuticals
P61*
200 mg
scored tablet
Plaquenil® Sulfate Tablets
Brand of hydroxychloroquine
sulfate tablets, USP

Winthrop Pharmaceuticals
Winthrop T37*
Talacen®
Each tablet contains pentazocine hydro-
chloride, USP, equivalent to 25 mg base
and acetaminophen, USP, 650 mg

Winthrop Pharmaceuticals
T51*
Talwin® Nx
Brand of pentazocine and naloxone
hydrochlorides tablets, USP

Winthrop Pharmaceuticals
T31*
500 mg
scored tablet
Telepaque®
Brand of iopanoic acid tablets, USP

Winthrop Pharmaceuticals
T100* T200*
100 mg 200 mg
scored tablets
Trancopal®
Brand of chlormezanone

Winthrop Pharmaceuticals
W53*
2 mg
scored tablet
Winstrol®
Brand of stanozolol tablets, USP

Because tablets and capsules are
shown in this section, do not infer
that these are the only dosage forms
available. Where a product name is
preceded by the symbol †, refer to the
description in the Product Information (White Section) for other forms.

WYETH-AYERST

As a result of the merger of Wyeth Laboratories and Ayerst Laboratories, all prescription products formerly of both companies are now products of Wyeth-Ayerst Laboratories. All nonprescription products formerly of Ayerst Laboratories are products of Whitehall Laboratories.

Wyeth-Ayerst

809*
250 mg.

810*
500 mg.

ANTABUSE®
(disulfiram)

Wyeth-Ayerst

81**
0.5 mg.

64**
1 mg.

65**
2 mg.

ATIVAN®
(lorazepam)
The appearances of these tablets are registered trademarks of Wyeth-Ayerst Laboratories.

Wyeth-Ayerst

243*   500 mg.
ATROMID-S 500

ATROMID-S®
(clofibrate)
The appearance of this capsule is a trademark of Wyeth-Ayerst Laboratories.

Wyeth-Ayerst

894*
5 mg.
(Packs shown smaller than actual size)

Cycle Pack
Cycle Pack of 10 tablets

AYGESTIN®
(norethindrone acetate tablets, USP)

Wyeth-Ayerst   (Both sides of tablet shown)

4188*
200 mg.

CORDARONE®
(amiodarone HCl)

Wyeth-Ayerst

(Shown smaller than actual size)

TUBEX® CLOSED INJECTION SYSTEM

Tubex® Injector ready for injection with Heparin Lock Flush Solution, USP, 10 USP units per ml

Tubex® Fast-Trak® Syringe

Cyanocobalamin Injection, USP (Vitamin B$_{12}$) 1000 mcg./ml; 1 ml fill in 2 ml size
Tubex® Sterile Cartridge-Needle Unit

Loaded Tubex® syringe ready for injection

Examples of Tubex® Sterile Cartridge-Needle Units and the Tubex® Injector, Tubex® Fast-Trak® Syringe, and the Tubex® Quick-Loading 2 ml size Syringe, components of the Tubex Closed Injection System, the most comprehensive line of small-volume unit-dose injectables. For a complete list of products available, consult TUBEX listing in the Product Information Section.

Wyeth-Ayerst

896*
10 mg.
(Pack shown smaller than actual size)

Cycle Pack of 10 Tablets

CYCRIN®
(medroxyprogesterone acetate tablets, USP)

Wyeth-Ayerst

702*
50 mg.

DIUCARDIN®
(hydroflumethiazide)

Wyeth-Ayerst

91*
EQUAGESIC®
(meprobamate 200 mg. and aspirin 325 mg.)
The appearance of this tablet is a trademark of Wyeth-Ayerst Laboratories.

Wyeth-Ayerst

2**
200 mg.

1**
400 mg.

†EQUANIL®
(meprobamate)

Wyeth-Ayerst

507*
100 mcg.

509*
500 mcg.

FACTREL®
(gonadorelin hydrochloride)
Synthetic Luteinizing Hormone Releasing Hormone (LH-RH)

Wyeth-Ayerst

442*
125 mg.

443*
250 mg.

444*
500 mg.

GRISACTIN®
[griseofulvin (microsize)]
The appearances of these capsules and tablet are trademarks of Wyeth-Ayerst Laboratories.

Wyeth-Ayerst

434*   435*
125 mg.   250 mg.

437*
330 mg.

GRISACTIN® ULTRA
[griseofulvin (ultramicrosize)]
The appearance of these tablets is a trademark of Wyeth-Ayerst Laboratories.

Wyeth-Ayerst
(Both sides of tablets shown)

484*
40/25

488*
80/25

INDERIDE®
[propranolol hydrochloride (Inderal®) and hydrochlorothiazide]
The appearance of these tablets is a trademark of Wyeth-Ayerst Laboratories.

Wyeth-Ayerst

455*   457*   459*
80/50   120/50   160/50

INDERIDE® LA
[propranolol hydrochloride (Inderal® LA) and hydrochlorothiazide]
Long Acting Capsules
The appearance of these capsules is a registered trademark of Wyeth-Ayerst Laboratories.

Wyeth-Ayerst
(Ampul shown smaller than actual size)
(Both sides of tablets shown)

421*
10 mg.

422*
20 mg.

424*
40 mg.

426*
60 mg.

428*
80 mg.

Tablets

3265*
Injectable

INDERAL®
(propranolol hydrochloride)
The appearance of these tablets is a registered trademark of Wyeth-Ayerst Laboratories.

Wyeth-Ayerst

470*   471*
60 mg.   80 mg.

473*   479*
120 mg.   160 mg.

INDERAL® LA
(propranolol hydrochloride)
Long Acting Capsules
The appearance of these capsules is a registered trademark of Wyeth-Ayerst Laboratories.

Wyeth-Ayerst

4140*
WYETH 4140
Tembids® Capsule

4125*
Tembids® Tablet
Sustained Action 40 mg.
(Both sides of tablet shown)

ISORDIL®
(isosorbide dinitrate)
The appearance of this capsule and this tablet are trademarks of Wyeth-Ayerst Laboratories.

Wyeth-Ayerst

4161* 4126* 4139*
10 mg. 5 mg. 2.5 mg.
Sublingual

Oral Titradose® Dosage Forms:
4152* 4153*
5 mg. Titradose® 10 mg. Titradose®
4154* 4159*
20 mg. Titradose® 30 mg. Titradose®
4192*
40 mg. Titradose®
Both sides of Titradose® tablets shown above

ISORDIL®
(isosorbide dinitrate)

Wyeth-Ayerst 261* ©
MEPERGAN® FORTIS
(each capsule contains 50 mg. meperidine HCl and 25 mg. promethazine HCl) The appearance of this capsule is a trademark of Wyeth-Ayerst Laboratories.

Wyeth-Ayerst 430*
431*
50 mg. 250 mg.
†MYSOLINE®
(primidone)

Wyeth-Ayerst 75**
(Dispenser shown smaller than actual size)
75*
Pilpak® Dispenser
NORDETTE®-21
(each tablet contains 0.15 mg. levonorgestrel with 0.03 mg. ethinyl estradiol)

Wyeth-Ayerst 78**
(Dispenser shown smaller than actual size)
78*
Pilpak® Dispenser
LO/OVRAL®
(each tablet contains 0.3 mg. norgestrel with 0.03 mg. ethinyl estradiol)

Wyeth-Ayerst 75**
(Dispenser shown smaller than actual size)
2533* 486**
Pilpak® Dispenser
NORDETTE®-28
(21 light-orange tablets each containing 0.15 mg. of levonorgestrel and 0.03 mg. of ethinyl estradiol and 7 pink inert tablets)

Wyeth-Ayerst 78**
(Dispenser shown smaller than actual size)
2514* 486**
Pilpak® Dispenser
LO/OVRAL®-28
(21 white tablets, each containing 0.3 mg. norgestrel with 0.03 mg. ethinyl estradiol, and 7 pink inert tablets)

Wyeth-Ayerst 71** ©
1 mg.
MAZANOR®
(mazindol)

Wyeth-Ayerst 252* ©
Ayerst 252
MEDIATRIC®
The appearance of this capsule is a trademark of Wyeth-Ayerst Laboratories.

Wyeth-Ayerst
4186*
25 mg.
4181* 4187*
50 mg. 75 mg.
ORUDIS®
(ketoprofen)
The appearances of these capsules are trademarks of Wyeth-Ayerst Laboratories.

Wyeth-Ayerst 56**
(Dispenser shown smaller than actual size)
56*
Pilpak® Dispenser
OVRAL®
(Each tablet contains 0.5 mg. norgestrel with 0.05 mg. ethinyl estradiol)

Wyeth-Ayerst 56**
(Dispenser shown smaller than actual size)
2511* 445**
Pilpak® Dispenser
OVRAL®-28
(21 white tablets each containing 0.5 mg. norgestrel with 0.05 mg. ethinyl estradiol and 7 pink inert tablets)

Wyeth-Ayerst
360* 593*
250 mg. 500 mg.
†PATHOCIL®
(dicloxacillin sodium monohydrate)
The appearance of these capsules is a trademark of Wyeth-Ayerst Laboratories.

Wyeth-Ayerst 390**
59**
250 mg. 500 mg.
†PEN-VEE® K
(penicillin V potassium)

Wyeth-Ayerst
19** 27* 227**
12.5 mg. 25 mg. 50 mg.
†PHENERGAN®
(promethazine hydrochloride)

Wyeth-Ayerst
434**
PHENERGAN®-D
(Each tablet contains 6.25 mg. promethazine hydrochloride and 60 mg. pseudoephedrine hydrochloride)
The appearance of this tablet is a trademark of Wyeth-Ayerst Laboratories.

Wyeth-Ayerst
498*
12.5 mg.
212*
25 mg.
229*
50 mg.
†PHENERGAN® Rectal Suppositories
(promethazine HCl)

Wyeth-Ayerst ©
755*
35 mg.
PLEGINE®
(phendimetrazine tartrate)

Wyeth-Ayerst
Premarin
872*
0.625 mg. per g Net Wt. 1½ oz. (42.5 g)
(Shown smaller than actual size)
PREMARIN® Vaginal Cream
(conjugated estrogens)

Wyeth-Ayerst
865* 866*
2.5 mg. 1.25 mg.
864*
867* 0.9 mg. 868*
0.625 mg. 0.3 mg.
0.625 mg.
Cycle Pack of 25 tablets
0.9 mg.
Cycle Pack of 25 tablets
1.25 mg.
Cycle Pack of 25 tablets
†PREMARIN®
(conjugated estrogens tablets, USP)
The appearance of these tablets is a trademark of Wyeth-Ayerst Laboratories.

Wyeth-Ayerst
879* 1.25 mg. with 10.0 mg. MT
878* 0.625 mg. with 5.0 mg. MT
PREMARIN®
(conjugated estrogens, USP) with Methyltestosterone (MT)
The appearance of these tablets is a trademark of Wyeth-Ayerst Laboratories.

Wyeth-Ayerst 880* 881*
PMB® 200 **PMB® 400**
[Premarin® (conjugated estrogens, USP) with meprobamate]
The appearance of these tablets is a trademark of Wyeth-Ayerst Laboratories.

Wyeth-Ayerst
Resol
Ready to Use 32 oz.
Ready to Use DO NOT ADD WATER
RESOL®
Oral Electrolyte Rehydration and Maintenance Solution

Wyeth-Ayerst
13 Fl. Oz.
S·M·A S·M·A
Lo-Iron Iron Fortified
S·M·A® INFANT FORMULA Concentrated Liquid
Also available in Ready-to-Feed Liquid and Powder

Wyeth-Ayerst 400 mg.
200 mg. SECTRAL
4177* **SECTRAL®** 4179*
(acebutolol hydrochloride)
The appearances of these capsules are trademarks of Wyeth-Ayerst Laboratories.

Wyeth-Ayerst ©
51*
10 mg.
6* 52*
15 mg. 30 mg.
†SERAX®
(oxazepam)
The appearance of these capsules is a registered trademark of Wyeth-Ayerst Laboratories.

Wyeth-Ayerst
Nursoy
13 fl. oz. Iron Fortified
(Shown smaller than actual size)
NURSOY®
SOY PROTEIN FORMULA Concentrated Liquid
Also Available in Ready-to-Feed Liquid and Powder

Wyeth-Ayerst
53*
250 mg.
309*
500 mg.
†OMNIPEN®
(ampicillin) ampicillin anhydrous
The appearance of these capsules is a trademark of Wyeth-Ayerst Laboratories.

Wyeth-Ayerst
PREMARIN® 12.5 mg. 25 mg. 50 mg.

**Product identification number on reverse side of tablet.

Wyeth-Ayerst Ⓒ
(Both sides of tablets shown)
317*
15 mg.
†**SERAX**®
(oxazepam)
The appearance of this tablet is a trademark of Wyeth-Ayerst Laboratories.

Wyeth-Ayerst
29*   28*
25 mg.   50 mg.
200*
100 mg.
†**SPARINE**®
(promazine hydrochloride)
The appearance of these tablets is a trademark of Wyeth-Ayerst Laboratories.

Wyeth-Ayerst
4132*   4133*
WYETH 4132   WYETH 4133
25 mg.   50 mg.
4158*
WYETH 4158
100 mg.
SURMONTIL®
(trimipramine maleate)
The appearances of these capsules are trademarks of Wyeth-Ayerst Laboratories.

Wyeth-Ayerst Ⓒ
WYETH 4191
4191*
SYNALGOS®-DC
(each capsule contains 16 mg. drocode [dihydrocodeine] bitartrate, 356.4 mg. aspirin, and 30 mg. caffeine)
The appearance of this capsule is a trademark of Wyeth-Ayerst Laboratories.

Wyeth-Ayerst
**   **   **
641   642   643
(Compact shown smaller than actual size)
2535*
TRIPHASIL®-21
(21 tablets containing the following: 6 brown tablets—0.050 mg. levonorgestrel + 0.030 mg. ethinyl estradiol; 5 white tablets—0.075 mg. levonorgestrel + 0.040 mg. ethinyl estradiol; 10 light-yellow tablets—0.125 mg. levonorgestrel + 0.030 mg. ethinyl estradiol)

Wyeth-Ayerst
**   **   **   **
641   642   643   650
(Compact shown smaller than actual size)
2536*
TRIPHASIL®-28
(28 tablets containing the following: 6 brown tablets—0.050 mg. levonorgestrel + 0.030 mg. ethinyl estradiol; 5 white tablets—0.075 mg. levonorgestrel + 0.040 mg. ethinyl estradiol; 10 light-yellow tablets—0.125 mg. levonorgestrel + 0.030 mg. ethinyl estradiol; 7 light-green tablets—inert)

Wyeth-Ayerst
WYETH 389   389*
                         471*
WYETH 471
250 mg.   500 mg.
TETRACYCLINE HCl CAPSULES, USP

Wyeth-Ayerst
786*
Ayerst
786
500 mg.
THIOSULFIL® **FORTE**
(sulfamethizole 500 mg.)

Wyeth-Ayerst
464**
WYETH
500 mg.
†**UNIPEN**®
(nafcillin sodium)

Wyeth-Ayerst
57*
WYETH 57
250 mg.
†**UNIPEN**®
(nafcillin sodium)
The appearance of this capsule is a trademark of Wyeth-Ayerst Laboratories.

Wyeth-Ayerst
576*
WYETH 576
250 mg.
578*
WYETH 578
500 mg.
WYAMYCIN® **S**
(erythromycin stearate)

Wyeth-Ayerst 659*
Wyanoids
Relief Factor
yanoids

Wyeth 77
Wyanoids
12 hemorrhoidal suppositories
Relief Factor
Prompt, temporary relief from pain and itching. Helps shrink swelling of hemorrhoidal tissues.
(Box shown smaller than actual size)
Box of 24 suppositories
WYANOIDS®
RELIEF FACTOR
Also available in boxes of 12

Wyeth-Ayerst 85** Ⓒ
WYETH
WYGESIC®
(each tablet contains 65 mg. propoxyphene HCl, USP, and 650 mg. acetaminophen, USP)

Wyeth-Ayerst
559*
WYETH 559
250 mg.
560*
WYETH 560
500 mg.
†**WYMOX**®
(amoxicillin)

Wyeth-Ayerst
73**   74**
4 mg.   8 mg.
WYTENSIN® (guanabenz acetate)
The appearance of these tablets is a registered trademark of Wyeth-Ayerst Laboratories.

Daniels Pharmaceuticals

dp ½   dp 25   dp 50
12½ mcg   25 mcg   50 mcg
(0.0125 mg) (0.025 mg) (0.05 mg)

dp 75   dp 100   dp 112
75 mcg   100 mcg   112 mcg
(0.075 mg) (0.1 mg)   (0.112 mg)

dp 125   dp 150   dp 175
125 mcg   150 mcg   175 mcg
(0.125 mg) (0.150 mg) (0.175 mg)

dp 200   dp 300
200 mcg   300 mcg
(0.2 mg)   (0.3 mg)
LEVOXINE®
(Levothyroxine Sodium USP)

Daniels Pharmaceuticals
TUSSIGON
TUSSIGON®
(5 mg hydrocodone bitartrate [WARNING: May be habit forming], 1.5 mg homatropine methylbromide)

Because tablets and capsules are shown in this section, do not infer that these are the only dosage forms available. Where a product name is preceded by the symbol †, refer to the description in the Product Information (White Section) for other forms.

SECTION 6

Product Information Section

This section is made possible through the courtesy of the manufacturers whose products appear on the following pages. The information concerning each product has been prepared, edited and approved by the medical department, medical director, and/or medical counsel of each manufacturer.

Products described in PHYSICIANS' DESK REFERENCE® which have official package circulars must be in full compliance with Food & Drug Administration regulations pertaining to labeling for prescription drugs. These regulations require that for PDR copy, "indications, effects, dosages, routes, methods, and frequency and duration of administration, and any relevant warnings, hazards, contraindications, side effects, and precautions" must be the "*same in language and emphasis*" as the approved labeling for the product. FDA regards the words "*same language and emphasis*" as requiring VERBATIM use of the approved labeling providing such information. Furthermore, information in the approved labeling that is emphasized by the use of type set in a box or in capitals, bold face, or italics must also be given the same emphasis in PDR. For products which do not have official package circulars, the Publisher has emphasized to manufacturers the necessity of describing such products comprehensively so that physicians would have access to all information essential for intelligent and informed prescribing. In organizing and presenting the material in PHYSICIANS' DESK REFERENCE, the Publisher is providing all the information made available to PDR by manufacturers.

This edition of PHYSICIANS' DESK REFERENCE contains the latest product information available at press-time. During the year, however, new and revised information about the products described herein may be furnished us. This information will be published in the PDR Supplement. Therefore, before prescribing or administering any product described in the following pages, you should first consult the PDR Supplement.

In presenting the following material to the medical profession, the Publisher is not necessarily advocating the use of any product listed.

Abbott Laboratories
Pharmaceutical Products Division
NORTH CHICAGO, IL 60064

ABBO–CODE™ INDEX

The Abbo-Code identification system provides positive identification of a drug and dosage strength. The following Abbott products are imprinted or debossed with an Abbo-Code designation:

PRODUCT	ABBO-CODE
Cartrol® (carteolol hydrochloride) Filmtab® Tablets	
2.5 mg	IA
5 mg	IC
Cefol® Filmtab® Tablets B-complex vitamins with folic acid, vitamin E, and vitamin C	NJ
Chlorthalidone Tablets, USP	
25 mg	AA
50 mg	AB
Colchicine Tablets, USP	
0.6 mg	AF
Cylert® Tablets Ⓒ (pemoline)	
18.75 mg	TH
37.5 mg	TI
75 mg	TJ
37.5 mg Chewable	TK
Depakene® Capsules (valproic acid capsules, USP)	
250 mg	DEPAKENE
Depakote® Tablets (divalproex sodium enteric-coated tablets)	
125 mg	NT
250 mg	NR
500 mg	NS
Desoxyn® Ⓒ (methamphetamine hydrochloride)	
5 mg Tablet	TE
5 mg Gradumet®	MC
10 mg Gradumet	ME
15 mg Gradumet	MF
Dicumarol Tablets, USP	
25 mg	AN
50 mg	AO
E.E.S.® Chewable Tablets (erythromycin ethylsuccinate tablets, USP)	
200 mg erythromycin activity	EF
E.E.S. 400® Filmtab® Tablets (erythromycin ethylsuccinate tablets, USP)	
400 mg erythromycin activity	EE
EryPed® Chewable Tablets (erythromycin ethylsuccinate tablets, USP)	EZ
Enduron® Tablets (methyclothiazide tablets, USP)	
2.5 mg	ENDURON
5 mg	ENDURON
Enduronyl® Tablets 5 mg methyclothiazide and 0.25 mg deserpidine	LS
Enduronyl® Forte Tablets 5 mg methyclothiazide and 0.5 mg deserpidine	LT
Ery-Tab® Enteric-Coated Tablets (erythromycin delayed release tablets, USP)	
250 mg	EC
333 mg	EH
500 mg	ED
Erythrocin® Stearate Filmtab® Tablets (erythromycin stearate tablets, USP)	
250 mg erythromycin activity	ES
500 mg erythromycin activity	ET
Erythromycin Base Filmtab® Tablets (erythromycin tablets, USP)	
250 mg	EB
500 mg	EA
Erythromycin Delayed-release Capsules, USP	
250 mg	ER
Fero-Folic-500® Filmtab® Tablets controlled-release iron, folic acid, and vitamin C	AJ
Harmonyl® Tablets (deserpidine tablets)	
0.25 mg	LK
Hytrin® Tablets (terazosin hydrochloride tablets)	
1 mg	DF
2 mg	DH
5 mg	DJ
10 mg	DI

Iberet-Folic-500® Filmtab® Tablets controlled-release iron, B-complex vitamins with folic acid, and vitamin C	AK
Janimine® Filmtab® Tablets (imipramine hydrochloride tablets, USP)	
10 mg	ND
25 mg	NE
50 mg	NL
K·Tab® Filmtab® Tablets (potassium chloride extended-release tablets, USP)	
10 mEq (750 mg)	NM
Nembutal® Sodium Capsules Ⓒ (pentobarbital sodium capsules, USP)	
50 mg	CF
100 mg	CH
Ogen® Tablets (estropipate tablets, USP)	
0.625 tablet (0.75 mg estropipate)	LU
1.25 tablet (1.5 mg estropipate)	LV
2.5 tablet (3 mg estropipate)	LX
5 tablet (6 mg estropipate)	LY
Oretic® Tablets (hydrochlorothiazide tablets, USP)	
25 mg	ORETIC
50 mg	ORETIC
Oreticyl® 25 Tablets 25 mg hydrochlorothiazide and 0.125 mg deserpidine	AH
Oreticyl® 50 Tablets 50 mg hydrochlorothiazide and 0.125 mg deserpidine	AI
Oreticyl® Forte Tablets 25 mg hydrochlorothiazide and 0.25 mg deserpidine	LL
Panwarfin® Tablets (warfarin sodium tablets, USP)	
2 mg	LM
2.5 mg	LN
5 mg	LO
7.5 mg	LR
10 mg	LF
PCE® Dispertab® Tablets (erythromycin particles in tablets)	
333 mg	PCE
Peganone® Tablets (ethotoin tablets)	
250 mg	AD
500 mg	AE
Phenurone® Tablets (phenacemide tablets, USP)	
500 mg	I I
Placidyl® Capsules Ⓒ (ethchlorvynol capsules, USP)	
500 mg	PLACIDYL 500
750 mg	PLACIDYL 750
Tranxene® T-Tab™ Tablets Ⓒ (clorazepate dipotassium)	
3.75 mg Tablet	TL
7.5 mg Tablet	TM
15 mg Tablet	TN
Tranxene-SD™ Ⓒ Single Dose Tablets (clorazepate dipotassium)	
22.5 mg	TY
11.25 mg Half Strength	TX
Tridione® Dulcet® Tablets (trimethadione tablets, USP)	
150 mg	LE
Tridione® Capsules (trimethadione capsules, USP)	
300 mg	AM
Vercyte® Tablets (pipobroman tablets)	
25 mg	AT

ABBO-PAC®
Unit Dose Packages

The Abbo-Pac unit dose system from Abbott Laboratories offers a wide range of drugs.
Each individual dose is clearly identified by generic name, Abbott trademark name, strength, NDC identification number, expiration date and lot number. Abbo-Pac unit dose containers are designed to accommodate virtually all hospital pharmacy storage racks and to provide maximum accessibility and ease of handling.
The following is a list of products which are now available:

PRODUCT	DOSAGE STRENGTH
Depakene® Capsules (valproic acid capsules, USP)	250 mg
Depakote® Tablets (divalproex sodium enteric-coated tablets)	125 mg
Depakote Tablets	250 mg
Depakote Tablets	500 mg

Enduron® Tablets (methyclothiazide tablets, USP)	5 mg
Enduronyl® Tablets (methyclothiazide 5 mg and deserpidine 0.25 mg)	
E.E.S. 400® Filmtab (erythromycin ethylsuccinate tablets, USP)	400 mg
EryPed® Chewable Tablets (erythromycin ethylsuccinate tablets, USP)	200 mg
E.E.S.® Granules (erythromycin ethylsuccinate for oral suspension, USP)	200 mg/5 ml
EryPed® 200 Granules (erythromycin ethylsuccinate for oral suspension, USP)	200 mg/5 ml
EryPed® 400 Granules (erythromycin ethylsuccinate for oral suspension, USP)	400 mg/5 ml
Ery-Tab® Enteric-Coated Tablets (erythromycin delayed-release tablets, USP)	250 mg
Ery-Tab® Tablets	333 mg
Ery-Tab® Tablets	500 mg
Erythrocin® Stearate Filmtab (erythromycin stearate tablets, USP)	250 mg
Erythromycin Base Filmtab® (erythromycin tablets, USP)	250 mg
Fero-Grad-500® Filmtab Controlled-Release Iron plus Vitamin C	
Hytrin® Tablets (terazosin hydrochloride tablets)	1 mg
Hytrin Tablets	2 mg
Hytrin Tablets	5 mg
Hytrin Tablets	10 mg
Iberet®-500 Filmtab Controlled-Release Iron plus B-Complex and Vitamin C	
K-Lor™ 20 mEq (potassium chloride for oral solution, USP)	20 mEq Potassium 20 mEq Chloride/Packet
K-Lor™ 15 mEq	15 mEq Potassium 15 mEq Chloride/Packet
K·Tab® Filmtab® (potassium chloride extended-release tablets, USP)	10 mEq (750 mg)
Nembutal® Sodium Capsules Ⓒ (pentobarbital sodium capsules, USP)	100 mg
Oretic® Tablets (hydrochlorothiazide tablets, USP)	25 mg
Oretic® Tablets	50 mg
Panwarfin® Tablets (warfarin sodium tablets, USP)	2 mg
Panwarfin Tablets	2.5 mg
Panwarfin Tablets	5 mg
Panwarfin Tablets	7.5 mg
Panwarfin Tablets	10 mg
Placidyl® Capsules Ⓒ (ethchlorvynol capsules, USP)	500 mg
Surbex-T® Filmtab High-Potency B-Complex Vitamins with Vitamin C	
Tranxene® T-Tab™ Tablets Ⓒ (clorazepate dipotassium)	3.75 mg
Tranxene® T-Tab™ Tablets Ⓒ	7.5 mg
Tranxene® T-Tab™ Tablets Ⓒ	15 mg

ABBOKINASE®
[ab-bo-kī′nāze]
Urokinase For Injection　　　　　　　　　　℞

PRODUCT OVERVIEW

KEY FACTS

ABBOKINASE is the human thrombolytic enzyme, urokinase, that activates the endogenous fibrinolytic system by directly converting plasminogen to plasmin. Fibrinolytic activity produced by urokinase disappears within a few hours of discontinuation of therapy. ABBOKINASE is intended for intravenous, intra-arterial and intracoronary administration. ABBOKINASE is available in vials containing 250,000 IU urokinase activity.

MAJOR USES

ABBOKINASE is indicated for the lysis of pulmonary emboli, coronary artery thrombosis, and peripheral arterial and graft thromboembolic occlusions. ABBOKINASE is also indicated for restoring patency to intravenous (including central venous) catheters. Heparin may be concomitantly administered during the intracoronary and intra-arterial administration of ABBOKINASE. Thrombolytic therapy with urokinase should be considered in all situations where the achievable benefits outweigh the risks of potentially serious bleeding. Baseline coagulation values including hematocrit, platelet count, and thrombin time, activated partial thromboplastin time, or prothrombin time should be obtained prior to instituting therapy.

SAFETY INFORMATION

ABBOKINASE is contraindicated in patients with active internal bleeding, severe uncontrolled hypertension, intracranial neoplasm or recent (within two months) cerebrovascular accident, intracranial or intraspinal surgery. In certain other situations the risks of bleeding may be increased and should be weighed against the anticipated benefits of therapy. In the event that serious bleeding occurs, ABBOKINASE should be discontinued. Blood loss and the reversal of bleeding can be effectively managed with appropriate replacement therapy if necessary.

PRESCRIBING INFORMATION

ABBOKINASE®

[ab-bo-ki'nāze]

Urokinase For Injection

℞

ABBOKINASE (urokinase for injection) should be used in hospitals where the recommended diagnostic and monitoring techniques are available. Thrombolytic therapy should be considered in all situations where the benefits to be achieved outweigh the risk of potentially serious hemorrhage. When internal bleeding does occur, it may be more difficult to manage than that which occurs with conventional anticoagulant therapy.

Urokinase treatment should be instituted as soon as possible after onset of pulmonary embolism, preferably no later than seven days after onset. Any delay in instituting lytic therapy to evaluate the effect of heparin decreases the potential for optimal efficacy.[1]

When urokinase is used for treatment of coronary artery thrombosis associated with evolving transmural myocardial infarction, therapy should be instituted within six hours of symptom onset.

DESCRIPTION

Urokinase is an enzyme (protein) produced by the kidney, and found in the urine. There are two forms of urokinase differing in molecular weight but having similar clinical effects. ABBOKINASE (urokinase for injection) is a thrombolytic agent obtained from human kidney cells by tissue culture techniques and is primarily the low molecular weight form. It is supplied as a sterile lyophilized white powder containing mannitol (25 mg/vial), albumin (human) (250 mg/vial), and sodium chloride (50 mg/vial).

Thin translucent filaments may occasionally occur in reconstituted ABBOKINASE vials, but do not indicate any decrease in potency of this product. No clinical problems have been associated with these filaments. See "Dosage and Administration" section.

Following reconstitution with 5 ml of Sterile Water for Injection, USP, it is a clear, slightly straw-colored solution; each ml contains 50,000 IU of urokinase activity, 0.5% mannitol, 5% albumin (human), and 1% sodium chloride. The pH is adjusted with sodium hydroxide and/or hydrochloric acid prior to lyophilization.

ABBOKINASE is for intravenous and intracoronary infusion only.

CLINICAL PHARMACOLOGY

Urokinase acts on the endogenous fibrinolytic system. It converts plasminogen to the enzyme plasmin. Plasmin degrades fibrin clots as well as fibrinogen and other plasma proteins.

Intravenous infusion of urokinase in doses recommended for lysis of pulmonary embolism is followed by increased fibrinolytic activity. This effect disappears within a few hours after discontinuation, but a decrease in plasma levels of fibrinogen and plasminogen and an increase in the amount of circulating fibrin (ogen) degradation products may persist for 12–24 hours.[3,4] There is a lack of correlation between embolus resolution and changes in coagulation and fibrinolytic assay results.

Information is incomplete about the pharmacokinetic properties in man. Urokinase administered by intravenous infusion is cleared rapidly by the liver. The serum half-life in man is 20 minutes or less. Patients with impaired liver function (e.g., cirrhosis) would be expected to show a prolongation in half-life. Small fractions of an administered dose are excreted in bile and urine.

INDICATIONS AND USAGE

Pulmonary Embolism: ABBOKINASE (urokinase for injection) is indicated in adults:

—For the lysis of acute massive pulmonary emboli, defined as obstruction of blood flow to a lobe or multiple segments.

—For the lysis of pulmonary emboli accompanied by unstable hemodynamics, i.e., failure to maintain blood pressure without supportive measures.

The diagnosis should be confirmed by objective means, such as pulmonary angiography via an upper extremity vein, or non-invasive procedures such as lung scanning.

Angiographic and hemodynamic measurements demonstrate a more rapid improvement with lytic therapy than with heparin therapy.[5,6,7,8,9]

Coronary Artery Thrombosis: ABBOKINASE has been reported to lyse acute thrombi obstructing coronary arteries, associated with evolving transmural myocardial infarction.[2] The majority of patients who received ABBOKINASE by intracoronary infusion within six hours following onset of symptoms showed recanalization of the involved vessel.

IT HAS NOT BEEN ESTABLISHED THAT INTRACORONARY ADMINISTRATION OF ABBOKINASE DURING EVOLVING TRANSMURAL MYOCARDIAL INFARCTION RESULTS IN SALVAGE OF MYOCARDIAL TISSUE, NOR THAT IT REDUCES MORTALITY. THE PATIENTS WHO MIGHT BENEFIT FROM THIS THERAPY CANNOT BE DEFINED.

I.V. Catheter Clearance: ABBOKINASE is indicated for the restoration of patency to intravenous catheters, including central venous catheters, obstructed by clotted blood or fibrin.[10,11] (See separate section at end of insert concerning I.V. catheter clearance for information regarding warnings, precautions, adverse reactions, and dosage and administration.)

CONTRAINDICATIONS

Because thrombolytic therapy increases the risk of bleeding, urokinase is contraindicated in the following situations: (See WARNINGS.)

—Active internal bleeding

—Recent (within two months) cerebrovascular accident, intracranial or intraspinal surgery

—Intracranial neoplasm

WARNINGS

Bleeding: The aim of urokinase is the production of sufficient amounts of plasmin for lysis of intravascular deposits of fibrin; however, fibrin deposits which provide hemostasis, for example, at sites of needle puncture, will also lyse, and bleeding from such sites may occur.

Intramuscular injections and nonessential handling of the patient must be avoided during treatment with urokinase. Venipunctures should be performed carefully and as infrequently as possible.

Should an arterial puncture be necessary (except for intracoronary administration), upper extremity vessels are preferable. Pressure should be applied for at least 30 minutes, a pressure dressing applied, and the puncture site checked frequently for evidence of bleeding.

In the following conditions, the risks of therapy may be increased and should be weighed against the anticipated benefits:

—Recent (within 10 days) major surgery, obstetrical delivery, organ biopsy, previous puncture of non-compressible vessels

—Recent (within 10 days) serious gastrointestinal bleeding

—Recent trauma including cardiopulmonary resuscitation

—Severe uncontrolled arterial hypertension

—High likelihood of a left heart thrombus, e.g., mitral stenosis with atrial fibrillation

—Subacute bacterial endocarditis

—Hemostatic defects including those secondary to severe hepatic or renal disease

—Pregnancy

—Cerebrovascular disease

—Diabetic hemorrhagic retinopathy

—Any other condition in which bleeding might constitute a significant hazard or be particularly difficult to manage because of its location

Should serious spontaneous bleeding (not controllable by local pressure) occur, the infusion of urokinase should be terminated immediately, and treatment instituted as described under ADVERSE REACTIONS.

Use of Anticoagulants: Concurrent use of anticoagulants with intravenous administration of ABBOKINASE is not recommended. However, concurrent use of heparin may be required during intracoronary administration of ABBOKINASE. A clinical study[2] with concurrent use of heparin and ABBOKINASE during intracoronary administration has demonstrated no tendency toward increased bleeding that would not be attributable to the procedure or ABBOKINASE alone. Nevertheless, careful monitoring for excessive bleeding is advised.

Arrhythmias: Rapid lysis of coronary thrombi has been reported occasionally to cause atrial or ventricular dysrhythmias as a result of reperfusion requiring immediate treatment. Careful monitoring for arrhythmias should be maintained during and immediately following intracoronary administration of ABBOKINASE.

PRECAUTIONS

Laboratory Tests: Before commencing thrombolytic therapy, obtain a hematocrit, platelet count, and a thrombin time (TT), activated partial thromboplastin time (APTT), or prothrombin time (PT). If heparin has been given, it should be discontinued unless it is to be used in conjunction with ABBOKINASE for intracoronary administration. TT or APTT should be less than twice the normal control value before thrombolytic therapy is started.

During the infusion, coagulation tests and/or measures of fibrinolytic activity may be performed if desired. Results do not, however, reliably predict either efficacy or a risk of bleeding. The clinical response should be observed frequently, and vital signs, i.e., pulse, temperature, respiratory rate and blood pressure, should be checked at least every four hours. The blood pressure should not be taken in the lower extremities to avoid dislodgement of possible deep vein thrombi.

Following the intravenous infusion, *before (re)instituting heparin*, the TT or APTT should be less than twice the upper limits of normal. Following intracoronary infusion of ABBOKINASE, blood coagulation parameters should be determined and heparin therapy continued as appropriate.

Drug Interactions: The interaction of urokinase with other drugs has not been studied. Drugs that alter platelet function should not be used. Common examples are: aspirin, indomethacin and phenylbutazone.

Although a bolus dose of heparin is recommended prior to intracoronary use of urokinase, oral anticoagulants or heparin should not be given concurrently with large doses of urokinase such as those used for pulmonary embolism. Concomitant use of intravenous urokinase and oral anticoagulants or heparin may increase the risk of hemorrhage. (See "WARNINGS" section.)

Carcinogenicity: Adequate data are not available on the long-term potential for carcinogenicity in animals or humans.

Pregnancy: Pregnancy category B. Reproduction studies have been performed in mice and rats at doses up to 1,000 times the human dose and have revealed no evidence of impaired fertility or harm to the fetus due to urokinase. There are, however, no adequate and well-controlled studies in pregnant women. Because animal reproduction studies are not always predictive of human response, this drug should be used during pregnancy only if clearly needed.

Nursing Mothers: It is not known whether this drug is excreted in human milk. Because many drugs are excreted in human milk, caution should be exercised when urokinase is administered to a nursing woman.

Pediatric Use: Safety and effectiveness in children have not been established.

ADVERSE REACTIONS

The following adverse reactions have been associated with intravenous therapy but may also occur with intracoronary artery infusion.

Bleeding: The type of bleeding associated with thrombolytic therapy can be placed into two broad categories:

—Superficial or surface bleeding, observed mainly at invaded or disturbed sites (e.g., venous cutdowns, arterial punctures, sites of recent surgical intervention, etc.).

—Internal bleeding, involving, e.g., the gastrointestinal tract, genitourinary tract, vagina, or intramuscular, retroperitoneal, or intracerebral sites.

Several fatalities due to cerebral or retroperitoneal hemorrhage have occurred during thrombolytic therapy.

Should serious bleeding occur, urokinase infusion should be discontinued and, if necessary, blood loss and reversal of the bleeding tendency can be effectively managed with whole blood (fresh blood preferable), packed red blood cells and cryoprecipitate or fresh frozen plasma. Dextran should not be used. Although the use of aminocaproic acid (ACA, AMICAR®) in humans as an antidote for urokinase has not been documented, it may be considered in an emergency situation.

Allergic Reactions: *In vitro* tests with urokinase, as well as intradermal tests in humans, gave no evidence of induced antibody formation. Relatively mild allergic type reactions, e.g., bronchospasm and skin rash, have been reported rarely. When such reactions occur, they usually respond to conventional therapy.

Fever: Febrile episodes have occurred in approximately 2–3% of treated patients. A cause and effect relationship has not been established. Symptomatic treatment with acetaminophen is usually sufficient to alleviate discomfort. Aspirin is not recommended.

DOSAGE AND ADMINISTRATION

ABBOKINASE IS INTENDED FOR INTRAVENOUS AND INTRACORONARY INFUSION ONLY.

A. Pulmonary Embolism:

Preparation: Reconstitute ABBOKINASE (urokinase for injection) by aseptically adding 5 ml of Sterile Water for Injection, USP, to the vial. (It is important that ABBOKINASE be reconstituted *only* with Sterile Water for Injection, USP, *without* preservatives. Bacteriostatic Water for Injection should *not* be used.) Each vial should be visually inspected for discoloration (slightly straw-colored solution) and for the presence of particulate material. Highly colored solutions should not be used. Because ABBOKINASE contains no preservatives, it should not be reconstituted until immediately before using. Any unused portion of the reconstituted material should be discarded.

Continued on next page

Abbott—Cont.

To minimize formation of filaments, avoid shaking the vial during reconstitution. Roll and tilt the vial to enhance reconstitution. The solution may be terminally filtered, e.g., through a 0.45 micron or smaller cellulose membrane filter. No other medication should be added to this solution. Reconstituted ABBOKINASE is diluted with 0.9% Sodium Chloride Injection, USP or 5% Dextrose Injection, USP, prior to intravenous infusion. (See Table I, **Dose Preparation.**)

Administration: Administer ABBOKINASE (urokinase for injection) by means of a constant infusion pump that is capable of delivering a total volume of 195 ml. The following table may be used as an aid in the preparation of ABBOKINASE (urokinase for injection) for administration.

A priming dose of 2,000 IU/lb (4,400 IU/kg) of ABBOKINASE is given as the ABBOKINASE -0.9% Sodium Chloride Injection or 5% Dextrose Injection admixture at a rate of 90 ml/hour over a period of 10 minutes. This is followed by a continuous infusion of 2,000 IU/lb/hr (4,400 IU/kg/hr) of ABBOKINASE at a rate of 15 ml/hour for 12 hours. Since some ABBOKINASE admixture will remain in the tubing at the end of an infusion pump delivery cycle, the following flush procedure should be performed to insure that the total dose of ABBOKINASE is administered. A solution of 0.9% Sodium Chloride Injection or 5% Dextrose Injection approximately equal in amount to the volume of the tubing in the infusion set should be administered via the pump to flush the ABBOKINASE admixture from the entire length of the infusion set. The pump should be set to administer the flush solution at the continuous infusion rate of 15 ml/hour.

Anticoagulation After Terminating Urokinase Treatment: At the end of urokinase therapy, treatment with heparin by continuous intravenous infusion is recommended to prevent recurrent thrombosis. Heparin treatment, without a loading dose, should not begin until the thrombin time has decreased to *less than twice* the normal control value (approximately 3 to 4 hours after completion of the infusion). See manufacturer's prescribing information for proper use of heparin. This should then be followed by oral anticoagulants in the conventional manner.

B. Lysis of Coronary Artery Thrombi:[2]
Preparation: Reconstitute three (3) 250,000 IU vials of ABBOKINASE by aseptically adding 5 ml of Sterile Water for Injection, USP, to each vial. (It is important that ABBOKINASE be reconstituted *only* with Sterile Water for Injection, USP, *without* preservatives. Bacteriostatic Water for Injection should *not* be used.) Each vial should be visually inspected for discoloration (slightly straw-colored solution) and for the presence of particulate material. Highly colored solutions should not be used. Because ABBOKINASE contains no preservatives, it should not be reconstituted until immediately before using. Any unused portion of the reconstituted material should be discarded.

To minimize formation of filaments, avoid shaking the vial during reconstitution. Roll and tilt the vial to enhance reconstitution. The solution may be terminally filtered, e.g., through a 0.45 micron or smaller cellulose membrane filter.

Add the contents of the three (3) reconstituted ABBOKINASE vials to 500 ml of 5% Dextrose Injection, USP. The resulting solution admixture will have a concentration of approximately 1500 IU per ml. No other medication should be added to the solution.

The admixture should be administered immediately as described under Administration. Any solution remaining after administration should be discarded.

NOTE: Adsorption of drug from dilute protein solutions to various materials has been reported in the literature. Therefore, the directions for Preparation and Administration must be followed to assure that significant drug loss does not occur.

Administration: Prior to the infusion of ABBOKINASE, a bolus dose of heparin ranging from 2500 to 10,000 units should be administered intravenously. Prior heparin administration should be considered when calculating the heparin dose for this procedure. Following the bolus dose of heparin, the prepared ABBOKINASE solution should be infused into the occluded artery at a rate of 4 ml per minute (6000 IU per minute) for periods up to 2 hours. In a clinical study, the average total dose of ABBOKINASE utilized for lysis of coronary artery thrombi was 500,000 IU.[2]

To determine response to ABBOKINASE therapy, periodic angiography during the infusion is recommended. It is suggested that the angiography be repeated at approximately 15 minute intervals. ABBOKINASE therapy should be continued until the artery is maximally opened, usually 15 to 30 minutes after the initial opening. Following the infusion, coagulation parameters should be determined. It is advisable to continue heparin therapy after the artery is opened by ABBOKINASE.

When ABBOKINASE was administered selectively into thrombosed coronary arteries via coronary catheter within 6 hours following onset of symptoms of acute transmural myocardial infarction, 60% of the occlusions were opened.[2]

I.V. Catheter Clearance:
Warnings: Excessive pressure should be avoided when ABBOKINASE is injected into the catheter. Such force could cause rupture of the catheter or expulsion of the clot into the circulation.

Precautions: Catheters may be occluded by substances other than blood products, such as drug precipitate. ABBOKINASE is not effective in such a case, and there is the possibility that the precipitate may be forced into the vascular system.

Adverse Reactions: Although there have been no adverse reactions reported as a result of using ABBOKINASE for the removal of clot obstruction from I.V. catheters, the possibility of reactions should nevertheless be considered.

Dosage and Administration:
Preparation: Reconstitute ABBOKINASE (urokinase for injection) by aseptically adding 5 ml of Sterile Water for Injection, USP, to the vial. (It is important that ABBOKINASE be reconstituted *only* with Sterile Water for Injection, USP, *without* preservatives. Bacteriostatic Water for Injection should *not* be used.) Add 1 ml of the reconstituted drug to 9 ml Sterile Water for Injection, USP, to make a final dilution equivalent to 5,000 IU/ml. One ml of this preparation is to be utilized for each catheter clearing procedure. BECAUSE ABBOKINASE CONTAINS NO PRESERVATIVES, IT SHOULD NOT BE RECONSTITUTED UNTIL IMMEDIATELY BEFORE USING.

Administration: NOTE: When the following procedure is used to clear a central venous catheter, the patient should be instructed to exhale and hold his breath any time the catheter is not connected to I.V. tubing or a syringe. This is to prevent air from entering the open catheter.

Aseptically disconnect the I.V. tubing connection at the catheter hub and attach a 10 ml syringe. Determine occlusion of the catheter by *gently* attempting to aspirate blood from the catheter with the 10 ml syringe. If aspiration is not possible, remove the 10 ml syringe and attach a 1 ml tuberculin syringe filled with prepared ABBOKINASE to the catheter. Slowly and gently inject an amount of ABBOKINASE equal to the volume of the catheter. Aseptically remove the tuberculin syringe and connect a 5 ml syringe to the catheter. Wait at least 5 minutes before attempting to aspirate the drug and residual clot with the 5 ml syringe. Repeat aspiration attempts every 5 minutes. If the catheter is not open within 30 minutes, the catheter may be capped allowing ABBOKINASE to remain in the catheter for 30 to 60 minutes before again attempting to aspirate. A second injection of ABBOKINASE may be necessary in resistant cases.

When patency is restored, aspirate 4 to 5 ml of blood to assure removal of all drug and clot residual. Remove the blood-filled syringe and replace it with a 10 ml syringe filled with 0.9% Sodium Chloride Injection, USP. The catheter should then be gently irrigated with this solution to assure patency of the catheter. After the catheter has been irrigated, remove the 10 ml syringe and aseptically reconnect sterile I.V. tubing to the catheter hub.
[See table below left].

HOW SUPPLIED

ABBOKINASE (urokinase for injection) is supplied as a sterile lyophilized preparation (NDC 0074-6109-05). Each vial contains 250,000 IU urokinase activity, 25 mg mannitol, 250 mg albumin (human), and 50 mg sodium chloride. Store ABBOKINASE powder at 2° to 8°C.

REFERENCES
1. Sherry, S., *et al:* Thrombolytic Therapy in Thrombosis: A National Institutes of Health Consensus Development Conference. Ann. Intern. Med. 93:141–144 (1980).
2. Tennant, S. N., Campbell, W.B., *et al:* Intracoronary Thrombolysis In Acute Myocardial Infarction: Comparison of the Efficacy of Urokinase to Streptokinase. Accepted for Publication, Circulation.
3. Bang, N. U.: Physiology and Biochemistry of Fibrinolysis in *Thrombosis and Bleeding Disorders* (Bang, N. U., Beller, F. K., Deutsch, E., Mammen, E. F., eds.). Academic Press (1971). pp. 292–327.
4. McNicol, G. P.: The Fibrinolytic Enzyme System. Postgrad. Med. J. (August Suppl. 5). 49:10–12 (1973).
5. Sasahara, A. A., Hyers, T. M., Cole, C. M., *et al.:* The Urokinase Pulmonary Embolism Trial Circulation, (Suppl. II) 47:1–108 (1973).
6. Urokinase pulmonary embolism trial study group: Urokinase-Streptokinase Embolism Trial. JAMA 229:1606-1613 (1974).
7. Sasahara, A. A., Bell, W. R., Simon, T. L., Stengle, J. M. and Sherry, S.: The Phase II Urokinase-Streptokinase Pulmonary Embolism Trial. Thrombos. Diathes, Haemorrh. (Stuttg.). 33:464–476 (1975).
8. Bell, W. R.: Thrombolytic Therapy: A Comparison Between Urokinase and Streptokinase. Sem. Thromb. Hemost. 2:1–13 (1975).
9. Fratantoni, J. C., Ness, P., Simon, T. L.: Thrombolytic Therapy: Current Status. N. Eng. J. Med., 293:1073–1078 (1975).
10. Lawson, M., *et al:* The Use of Urokinase to Restore the Patency of Occluded Central Venous Catheters. Am. J. Intravenous Therapy and Clinical Nutrition, 9:29–32 (Oct. 1982).
11. Glynn, M.F.X., *et al:* Therapy for Thrombotic Occlusion of Long-term Intravenous Alimentation Catheters, Journal of Parenteral and Enteral Nutrition, 4 (4):387–390 (July/Aug. 1980).

Abbott Laboratories
North Chicago, IL 60064
Ref. 01-2410-R7

ABBOKINASE® OPEN-CATH® ℞
[ab-bō-kī'nāze open-cath]
Urokinase for Catheter Clearance

PRODUCT OVERVIEW

KEY FACTS

ABBOKINASE OPEN-CATH contains the human thrombolytic enzyme, urokinase, that activates the endogenous fibrinolytic system by directly converting plasminogen to plasmin. When used for intravenous catheter clearance, only small amounts of urokinase may reach the circulation and, therefore, systemic fibrinolysis is not expected to occur. ABBOKI-

TABLE I
Dose Preparation–Pulmonary Embolism

Weight (pounds)	Total Dose* Urokinase (IU)	Number Vials ABBOKINASE (urokinase for injection)	Volume of ABBOKINASE After Reconstitution (ml)** +	Volume of Diluent (ml) =	Final Volume (ml)
81–90	2,250,000	9	45	150	195
91–100	2,500,000	10	50	145	195
101–110	2,750,000	11	55	140	195
111–120	3,000,000	12	60	135	195
121–130	3,250,000	13	65	130	195
131–140	3,500,000	14	70	125	195
141–150	3,750,000	15	75	120	195
151–160	4,000,000	16	80	115	195
161–170	4,250,000	17	85	110	195
171–180	4,500,000	18	90	105	195
181–190	4,750,000	19	95	100	195
191–200	5,000,000	20	100	95	195
201–210	5,250,000	21	105	90	195
211–220	5,500,000	22	110	85	195
221–230	5,750,000	23	115	80	195
231–240	6,000,000	24	120	75	195
241–250	6,250,000	25	125	70	195

Infusion Rate:	Priming Dose	Dose for 12-Hour Period
	15 ml/10 min***	15 ml/hr for 12 hrs

*Priming dose + dose administered during 12-hour period.
**After addition of 5 ml of Sterile Water for Injection, USP, per vial (See Preparation.)
***Pump rate = 90 ml/hr

NASE OPEN-CATH is available in single-dose Unival® packages (diluent in upper chamber) in 1 mL and 1.8 mL sizes containing 5,000 IU urokinase activity per mL.

MAJOR USES

ABBOKINASE OPEN-CATH is indicated for the restoration of patency to intravenous (including central venous) catheters obstructed by clotted blood or fibrin. Basically, the use of ABBOKINASE OPEN-CATH includes the instillation into the catheter a volume of prepared ABBOKINASE OPEN-CATH equal in volume to the internal volume of the occluded catheter. Aspiration attempts should then be made at 5 minute intervals. When patency is restored, aspirate 4 to 5 mL of blood and gently irrigate the catheter with 10 mL of 0.9% Sodium Chloride Injection, USP. A second instillation of ABBOKINASE OPEN-CATH may be required in resistant cases.

SAFETY INFORMATION

Avoid excessive pressure while injecting ABBOKINASE OPEN-CATH and vigorous suction when making aspiration attempts. To prevent air from entering the open catheter, the patient should be instructed to exhale and hold his breath during any time the catheter is not connected to intravenous tubing or a syringe. While thrombolytic therapy is contraindicated in patients with active internal bleeding, severe uncontrolled hypertension, intracranial neoplasm or recent (within two months) cerebrovascular accident, intracranial or intraspinal surgery, there have been no reports which would suggest a contraindication for the use of ABBOKINASE OPEN-CATH for intravenous catheter clearance.

PRESCRIBING INFORMATION

ABBOKINASE® OPEN-CATH®   ℞

[ab-bō-kī'nāze open-cath]
Urokinase for Catheter Clearance

DESCRIPTION

Urokinase is an enzyme (protein) produced by the kidney and found in the urine. There are two forms of urokinase differing in molecular weight but having similar clinical effects. Urokinase is a thrombolytic agent obtained from human kidney cells by tissue culture techniques and is primarily the low molecular weight form. It is supplied as a sterile lyophilized white powder. Following reconstitution ABBOKINASE OPEN-CATH is a clear, practically colorless solution.

Each ml of reconstituted ABBOKINASE OPEN-CATH contains 5000 IU of urokinase activity, 5 mg gelatin, 15 mg mannitol, 1.7 mg sodium chloride and 4.6 mg monobasic sodium phosphate anhydrous. The pH of ABBOKINASE is adjusted with sodium hydroxide and/or hydrochloric acid prior to lyophilization.

CLINICAL PHARMACOLOGY

Urokinase acts on the endogenous fibrinolytic system. It converts plasminogen to the enzyme plasmin. Plasmin degrades fibrin clots as well as fibrinogen and other plasma proteins.

When used as directed for I.V. catheter clearance, only small amounts of urokinase may reach the circulation; therefore, therapeutic serum levels are not expected to be achieved. Nevertheless, one should be aware of the clinical pharmacology of urokinase.

Intravenous infusion of urokinase in doses recommended for lysis of pulmonary embolism is followed by increased fibrinolytic activity. This effect disappears within a few hours after discontinuation, but a decrease in plasma levels of fibrinogen and plasminogen and an increase in the amount of circulating fibrin (ogen) degradation products may persist for 12–24 hours.[1,2] There is a lack of correlation between embolus resolution and changes in coagulation and fibrinolytic assay results.

Information is incomplete about the pharmacokinetic properties in man. Urokinase administered by intravenous infusion is cleared rapidly by the liver. The serum half-life in man is 20 minutes or less. Patients with impaired liver function (e.g., cirrhosis) would be expected to show a prolongation in half-life. Small fractions of an administered dose are excreted in bile and urine.

INDICATIONS AND USAGE

ABBOKINASE OPEN-CATH (urokinase for catheter clearance) is indicated for the restoration of patency to intravenous catheters, including central venous catheters, obstructed by clotted blood or fibrin.[3,4,5]

CONTRAINDICATIONS

Because thrombolytic therapy increases the risk of bleeding, urokinase is contraindicated in the following situations:
—Active internal bleeding
—Recent (within two months) cerebrovascular accident, intracranial or intraspinal surgery
—Intracranial neoplasm

There have been no reports, however, which would suggest a contraindication for the use of urokinase for I.V. catheter clearance.

WARNINGS

Excessive pressure should be avoided when ABBOKINASE is injected into the catheter. Such force could cause rupture of the catheter or expulsion of the clot into the circulation. During attempts to determine catheter occlusion, vigorous suction should not be applied due to possible damage to the vascular wall or collapse of soft-wall catheters.

Catheters may be occluded by substances other than fibrin clots, such as drug precipitates. ABBOKINASE is not effective in such cases and there is the possibility that the substances may be forced into the vascular system.

PRECAUTIONS

Carcinogenicity: Adequate data is not available on the long-term potential for carcinogenicity in animals or humans.

Pregnancy: Pregnancy category B. Reproduction studies have been performed in mice and rats at doses up to 1,000 times the human therapeutic dose and have revealed no evidence of impaired fertility or harm to the fetus due to urokinase. There are, however, no adequate and well-controlled studies in pregnant women. Because animal reproduction studies are not always predictive of human response, this drug should be used during pregnancy only if clearly needed.

Nursing Mothers: It is not known whether this drug is excreted in human milk. Because many drugs are excreted in human milk, caution should be exercised when urokinase is administered to a nursing woman.

Pediatric Use: Safety and effectiveness in children have not been established.

ADVERSE REACTIONS

Although there have been no adverse reactions reported as a result of using ABBOKINASE for the removal of clot obstruction from I.V. catheters, the possibility of reactions should nevertheless be considered. The following reactions have been associated with ABBOKINASE in doses recommended for lysis of pulmonary embolism.

Bleeding: The type of bleeding associated with thrombolytic therapy can be placed into two broad categories:
—Superficial or surface bleeding, observed mainly at invaded or disturbed sites (e.g., venous cutdowns, arterial punctures, sites of recent surgical intervention, etc.).
—Internal bleeding, involving, e.g., the gastrointestinal tract, genitourinary tract, vagina, or intramuscular, retroperitoneal, or intracerebral sites.

Several fatalities due to cerebral or retroperitoneal hemorrhage have occurred during thrombolytic therapy.

Should serious bleeding occur, urokinase infusion should be discontinued and, if necessary, blood loss and reversal of the bleeding tendency can be effectively managed with whole blood (fresh blood preferable), packed red blood cells and cryoprecipitate or fresh frozen plasma. Dextran should not be used. Although the use of aminocaproic acid (ACA, AMICAR®) in humans as an antidote for urokinase has not been documented, it may be considered in an emergency situation.

Allergic Reactions: *In vitro* tests with urokinase, as well as intradermal tests in humans, gave no evidence of induced antibody formation. Relatively mild allergic type reactions, e.g., bronchospasm and skin rash, have been reported rarely. When such reactions occur, they usually respond to conventional therapy.

Fever: Febrile episodes have occurred in approximately 2–3% of treated patients. A cause and effect relationship has not been established. Symptomatic treatment with acetaminophen is usually sufficient to alleviate discomfort. Aspirin is not recommended.

DOSAGE AND ADMINISTRATION

CONTAINS NO PRESERVATIVE.
USE IMMEDIATELY AFTER RECONSTITUTION. DISCARD ANY UNUSED PORTION.
Preparation of Solution: *Univial:*
1. Remove protective cap. Turn plunger-stopper a quarter turn and press to force diluent into lower chamber.
2. Roll and tilt to effect solution. Use only a clear, colorless solution.
3. Sterilize top of stopper with a suitable germicide.
4. Insert needle through the center of stopper until tip is barely visible. Withdraw dose.

It is recommended that vigorous shaking be avoided during reconstitution; roll and tilt to enhance reconstitution. Parenteral drug products should be inspected visually for particulate matter and discoloration prior to administration, whenever solution and container permit.

ADMINISTRATION

When the following procedure is used to clear a central venous catheter, the patient should be instructed to exhale and hold his breath any time the catheter is not connected to I.V. tubing or a syringe. This is to prevent air from entering the open catheter.

Aseptically disconnect the I.V. tubing connection at the catheter hub and attach an empty 10 ml syringe. Determine occlusion of the catheter by *gently* attempting to aspirate blood from the catheter with the 10 ml syringe. If aspiration is not possible, remove the 10 ml syringe and attach a tuberculin

syringe filled with an amount of prepared ABBOKINASE OPEN-CATH equal to the internal volume of the catheter. Slowly and gently inject the ABBOKINASE solution into the catheter. Aseptically remove the tuberculin syringe and connect an empty syringe (e.g., 5 ml) to the catheter. Wait at least 5 minutes before attempting to aspirate the drug and residual clot with the empty syringe. Repeat aspiration attempts every 5 minutes. If the catheter is not open within 30 minutes, the catheter may be capped allowing ABBOKINASE to remain in the catheter for 30 to 60 minutes before again attempting to aspirate. A second injection of ABBOKINASE may be necessary in resistant cases.

When patency is restored, aspirate 4 to 5 ml of blood to assure removal of all drug and clot residual. Remove the blood-filled syringe and replace it with a 10 ml syringe filled with 0.9% Sodium Chloride Injection, USP. The catheter should then be gently irrigated with this solution to assure patency of the catheter. After the catheter has been irrigated, remove the 10 ml syringe and aseptically reconnect sterile I.V. tubing to the catheter hub.

HOW SUPPLIED

ABBOKINASE OPEN-CATH (urokinase for catheter clearance) is supplied as a sterile lyophilized preparation in a 1 ml single dose Unival® package (NDC 0074-6111-01) and 1.8 ml (NDC 0074-6145-02). Store powder below 77°F (25°C). Avoid freezing.

REFERENCES

1. Bang, N. U.: Physiology and Biochemistry of Fibrinolysis In *Thrombosis and Bleeding Disorders* (Bang, N. U., Beller, F. K., Deutsch, E., Mammen, E. F., eds.). Academic Press (1971). pp. 292–327.
2. McNicol, G. P.: The Fibrinolytic Enzyme System. Postgrad. Med. J. (August Suppl. 5). 49:10–12 (1973).
3. Hurtubise, Michel R., M.D., Bottino, Joseph C., M.D., Lawson, Millie, R.N., McCredie, Kenneth B., M.D.: Restoring Patency of Occluded Central Venous Catheters. Arch. Surg. 115:212–213 (1980).
4. Glynn, M. F. X., *et al:* Therapy for Thrombotic Occlusion of Long-term Intravenous Alimentation Catheters. Journal of Parenteral and Enteral Nutrition. 4 (4):387–390 (July/Aug. 1980).
5. Lawson, M., Bottino, J. C., Hurtubise, M. R., McCredie, K. B.: The Use of Urokinase to Restore the Patency of Occluded Central Venous Catheters. Am. J. I.V. Ther. and Clin. Nutr., 9(9):29–30,32 (October, 1982).

Abbott Laboratories
North Chicago, IL 60064
Ref. 01-2429-R2

STERILE A-HYDROCORT™   ℞

[ā-hī'dro-cort"]
(Hydrocortisone Sodium Succinate for Injection, USP)
For Intravenous or Intramuscular Use

DESCRIPTION

Hydrocortisone Sodium Succinate, USP, an adrenocortical-like steroid, is the sodium succinate ester of hydrocortisone. It occurs as a white, or nearly white, odorless hygroscopic amorphous solid. Hydrocortisone sodium succinate is very soluble in water and in alcohol; it is insoluble in chloroform and is very slightly soluble in acetone.

Hydrocortisone sodium succinate is soluble in water and is especially well suited for intravenous use in situations in which high blood levels of hydrocortisone are required rapidly.

A-HYDROCORT (Hydrocortisone Sodium Succinate for Injection, USP) is available as:

100 mg Unival®—Each 2 mL (when mixed) contains hydrocortisone sodium succinate equivalent to 100 mg hydrocortisone; also 0.8 mg monobasic sodium phosphate anhydrous; 8.7 mg dibasic sodium phosphate anhydrous; and 18 mg benzyl alcohol.

250 mg Unival—Each 2 mL (when mixed) contains hydrocortisone sodium succinate equivalent to 250 mg hydrocortisone; also 2 mg monobasic sodium phosphate anhydrous; 21.8 mg dibasic sodium phosphate anhydrous; and 18 mg benzyl alcohol.

500 mg Unival—Each 4 mL (when mixed) contains hydrocortisone sodium succinate equivalent to 500 mg hydrocortisone; also 4 mg monobasic sodium phosphate anhydrous; 44 mg dibasic sodium phosphate anhydrous; and 36 mg benzyl alcohol.

1000 mg Unival—Each 8 mL (when mixed) contains hydrocortisone sodium succinate equivalent to 1000 mg hydrocortisone; also 8 mg monobasic sodium phosphate anhydrous;

Continued on next page

Abbott—Cont.

88 mg dibasic sodium phosphate anhydrous; and 72 mg benzyl alcohol.

May contain sodium hydroxide and/or hydrochloric acid for pH adjustment.

IMPORTANT

The solid contents of A-HYDROCORT should not be used with any diluent other than that provided. **Use within 3 days after mixing.**

When reconstituted as directed, the pH of the solutions ranges from 7–8 and the tonicities are, for the 100 mg per 2 mL solution, 0.36 osmolar; for the 250 mg per 2 mL, 500 mg per 4 mL, and 1000 mg per 8 mL solutions, 0.57 osmolar. [Isotonic saline (0.9% Sodium Chloride Injection, USP) = 0.28 osmolar.]

CLINICAL PHARMACOLOGY

Hydrocortisone sodium succinate has potent anti-inflammatory effects. Because it is an adrenocortical-like steroid, hydrocortisone sodium succinate may cause profound and varied metabolic effects in addition to modifying the body's immune response to diverse stimuli.

When given parenterally and in equimolar quantities, hydrocortisone sodium succinate and hydrocortisone are equivalent in biologic activity.

Following intravenous injection of hydrocortisone sodium succinate, demonstrable effects are evident within one hour and persist for a variable period. Excretion of the administered dose is nearly complete within 12 hours. Thus, if constantly high blood levels are required, injections should be made every four to six hours.

This preparation is also rapidly absorbed when administered intramuscularly and is excreted in a pattern similar to that observed after intravenous injection.

INDICATIONS

Sterile A-HYDROCORT (hydrocortisone sodium succinate) is indicated in situations requiring a rapid and intense hormonal effect.

Intravenous administration of A-HYDROCORT is most appropriate for the following indications:

1. **Endocrine disorders:**
   a. Acute adrenocortical insufficiency (hydrocortisone or cortisone is the drug of choice; mineralocorticoid supplementation may be necessary, particularly when synthetic analogs are used).
   b. Preoperatively and in the event of serious trauma or illness, in patients with known adrenal insufficiency or when adrenocortical reserve is doubtful.
   c. Shock unresponsive to conventional therapy if adrenocortical insufficiency exists or is suspected.
2. **Collagen diseases**—During an exacerbation or as maintenance therapy in selected cases of:
   a. Acute rheumatic carditis.
3. **Allergic states**—Control of severe or incapacitating allergic conditions intractable to adequate trials of conventional treatment in:
   a. Bronchial asthma.
   b. Serum sickness.
   c. Drug hypersensitivity reactions.
   d. Urticarial transfusion reactions.
   e. Acute noninfectious laryngeal edema (epinephrine is the drug of first choice).
4. **Hematologic disorders:**
   a. Idiopathic thrombocytopenic purpura in adults (I.M. administration is contraindicated).

Intramuscular administration of A-HYDROCORT is appropriate for the following indications:

1. **Endocrine disorders:**
   a. Primary or secondary adrenocortical insufficiency (hydrocortisone or cortisone is the drug of choice; synthetic analogs may be used in conjunction with mineralocorticoids where applicable; in infancy, mineralocorticoid supplementation is of particular importance).
   b. Acute adrenocortical insufficiency (hydrocortisone or cortisone is the drug of choice; mineralocorticoid supplementation may be necessary, particularly when synthetic analogs are used).
   c. Preoperatively and in the event of serious trauma or illness, in patients with known adrenal insufficiency or when adrenocortical reserve is doubtful.
   d. Shock unresponsive to conventional therapy if adrenocortical insufficiency exists or is suspected.
   e. Congenital adrenal hyperplasia.
   f. Nonsuppurative thyroiditis.
   g. Hypercalcemia associated with cancer.
2. **Rheumatic disorders**—As adjunctive therapy for short-term administration (to tide the patient over an acute episode or exacerbation) in:

a. Post-traumatic osteoarthritis.
b. Synovitis of osteoarthritis.
c. Rheumatoid arthritis, including juvenile rheumatoid arthritis (selected cases may require low-dose maintenance therapy).
d. Acute and subacute bursitis.
e. Epicondylitis.
f. Acute nonspecific tenosynovitis.
g. Acute gouty arthritis.
h. Psoriatic arthritis.
i. Ankylosing spondylitis.
3. **Collagen diseases**—During an exacerbation or as maintenance therapy in selected cases of:
   a. Systemic lupus erythematosus.
   b. Acute rheumatic carditis.
4. **Dermatologic diseases:**
   a. Severe erythema multiforme (Stevens-Johnson syndrome).
   b. Exfoliative dermatitis.
   c. Bullous dermatitis herpetiformis.
   d. Severe seborrheic dermatitis.
   e. Severe psoriasis.
   f. Pemphigus.
   g. Mycosis fungoides.
   h. Systemic dermatomyositis (polymyositis).
5. **Allergic states**—Control of severe or incapacitating allergic conditions intractable to adequate trials of conventional treatment in:
   a. Bronchial asthma.
   b. Contact dermatitis.
   c. Atopic dermatitis.
   d. Serum sickness.
   e. Seasonal or perennial allergic rhinitis.
   f. Drug hypersensitivity reactions.
   g. Urticarial transfusion reactions.
   h. Acute noninfectious laryngeal edema (epinephrine is the drug of first choice).
6. **Ophthalmic diseases**—Severe acute and chronic allergic and inflammatory processes involving the eye, such as:
   a. Herpes zoster ophthalmicus.
   b. Iritis, iridocyclitis.
   c. Chorioretinitis.
   d. Diffuse posterior uveitis and choroiditis.
   e. Optic neuritis.
   f. Sympathetic ophthalmia.
   g. Anterior segment inflammation.
   h. Allergic conjunctivitis.
   i. Allergic corneal marginal ulcers.
7. **Gastrointestinal diseases**—To tide the patient over a critical period of disease in:
   a. Ulcerative colitis—(Systemic therapy).
   b. Regional enteritis—(Systemic therapy).
8. **Respiratory diseases:**
   a. Symptomatic sarcoidosis.
   b. Berylliosis.
   c. Fulminating or disseminated pulmonary tuberculosis when concurrently accompanied by appropriate antituberculous chemotherapy.
   d. Aspiration pneumonitis.
   e. Loeffler's syndrome not manageable by other means.
9. **Hematologic disorders:**
   a. Acquired (autoimmune) hemolytic anemia.
   b. Secondary thrombocytopenia in adults.
   c. Erythroblastopenia (RBC anemia).
   d. Congenital (erythroid) hypoplastic anemia.
10. **Neoplastic diseases**—For palliative management of:
    a. Leukemias and lymphomas in adults.
    b. Acute leukemia of childhood.
11. **Edematous state**—To induce diuresis or remission of proteinuria in the nephrotic syndrome, without uremia, of the idiopathic type or that due to lupus erythematosus.
12. **Nervous system**—Acute exacerbations of multiple sclerosis.
13. **Miscellaneous:**
    a. Tuberculous meningitis with subarachnoid block or impending block when used concurrently with appropriate antituberculous chemotherapy.
    b. Trichinosis with neurologic or myocardial involvement.

CONTRAINDICATIONS

Systemic fungal infections.

Not for use in newborns. Benzyl alcohol, a preservative in the Bacteriostatic Water for Injection provided with these products, has been associated with toxicity in newborns. Data are unavailable on the toxicity of other preservatives in this age group.

WARNINGS

In patients on corticosteroid therapy subjected to any unusual stress, increased dosage of rapidly acting corticosteroids before, during, and after the stressful situation is indicated.

Corticosteroids may mask some signs of infection, and new infections may appear during their use. There may be decreased resistance and inability to localize infection when corticosteroids are used.

Prolonged use of corticosteroids may produce posterior subcapsular cataracts, glaucoma with possible damage to the optic nerves, and may enhance the establishment of secondary ocular infections due to fungi or viruses.

Average and large doses of cortisone or hydrocortisone can cause elevation of blood pressure, salt and water retention, and increased excretion of potassium. These effects are less likely to occur with the synthetic derivatives except when used in large doses. Dietary salt restriction and potassium supplementation may be necessary. All corticosteroids increase calcium excretion.

While on corticosteroid therapy patients should not be vaccinated against smallpox. Other immunization procedures should not be undertaken in patients who are on corticosteroids, especially on high dose, because of possible hazards of neurological complications and a lack of antibody response.

The use of A-HYDROCORT (hydrocortisone sodium succinate) in active tuberculosis should be restricted to those cases of fulminating or disseminated tuberculosis in which the corticosteroid is used for the management of the disease in conjunction with an appropriate antituberculous regimen.

If corticosteroids are indicated in patients with latent tuberculosis or tuberculin reactivity, close observation is necessary as reactivation of the disease may occur. During prolonged corticosteroid therapy, these patients should receive chemoprophylaxis.

Because rare instances of anaphylactoid reactions have occurred in patients receiving parenteral corticosteroid therapy, appropriate precautionary measures should be taken prior to administration, especially when the patient has a history of allergy to any drug.

USAGE IN PREGNANCY

Since adequate human reproduction studies have not been done with corticosteroids, the use of these drugs in pregnancy, nursing mothers, or women of childbearing potential requires that the possible benefits of the drug be weighed against the potential hazards to the mother and embryo or fetus. Infants born of mothers who have received substantial doses of corticosteroids during pregnancy should be carefully observed for signs of hypoadrenalism.

PRECAUTIONS

Drug-induced secondary adrenocortical insufficiency may be minimized by gradual reduction of dosage. This type of relative insufficiency may persist for months after discontinuation of therapy; therefore, in any situation of stress occurring during that period, hormone therapy should be reinstituted. Since mineralocorticoid secretion may be impaired, salt and/or a mineralocorticoid should be administered concurrently. There is an enhanced effect of corticosteroids in patients with hypothyroidism and in those with cirrhosis.

Corticosteroids should be used cautiously in patients with ocular herpes simplex because of possible corneal perforation.

The lowest possible dose of corticosteroid should be used to control the condition under treatment, and when reduction in dosage is possible, the reduction should be gradual.

Psychic derangements may appear when corticosteroids are used, ranging from euphoria, insomnia, mood swings, personality changes and severe depression, to frank psychotic manifestations. Also, existing emotional instability or psychotic tendencies may be aggravated by corticosteroids.

Aspirin should be used cautiously in conjunction with corticosteroids in hypoprothrombinemia.

Steroids should be used with caution in nonspecific ulcerative colitis, if there is a probability of impending perforation, abscess or other pyogenic infection; diverticulitis; fresh intestinal anastomoses; active or latent peptic ulcer; renal insufficiency; hypertension; osteoporosis; and myasthenia gravis.

Growth and development of infants and children on prolonged corticosteroid therapy should be carefully observed. Although controlled clinical trials have shown corticosteroids to be effective in speeding the resolution of acute exacerbations of multiple sclerosis they do not show that they affect the ultimate outcome or natural history of the disease. The studies do show that relatively high doses of corticosteroids are necessary to demonstrate a significant effect. (See "DOSAGE AND ADMINISTRATION" section).

Since complications of treatment with glucocorticoids are dependent on the size of the dose and the duration of treatment a risk/benefit decision must be made in each individual case as to dose and duration of treatment and as to whether daily or intermittent therapy should be used.

ADVERSE REACTIONS

Fluid and Electrolyte Disturbances
  Sodium retention
  Fluid retention
  Congestive heart failure in susceptible patients

Potassium loss
Hypokalemic alkalosis
Hypertension

Musculoskeletal
Muscle weakness
Steroid myopathy
Loss of muscle mass
Osteoporosis
Vertebral compression fractures
Aseptic necrosis of femoral and humeral heads
Pathologic fracture of long bones

Gastrointestinal
Peptic ulcer with possible perforation and hemorrhage
Pancreatitis
Abdominal distention
Ulcerative esophagitis

Dermatologic
Impaired wound healing
Thin fragile skin
Petechiae and ecchymoses
Facial erythema
Increased sweating
May suppress reactions to skin tests

Neurological
Increased intracranial pressure with papilledema (pseudo-tumor cerebri) usually after treatment
Convulsions
Vertigo
Headache

Endocrine
Development of Cushingoid state
Suppression of growth in children
Secondary adrenocortical and pituitary unresponsiveness, particularly in times of stress, as in trauma, surgery or illness
Menstrual irregularities
Decreased carbohydrate tolerance
Manifestations of latent diabetes mellitus
Increased requirements for insulin or oral hypoglycemic agents in diabetics

Ophthalmic
Posterior subcapsular cataracts
Increased intraocular pressure
Glaucoma
Exophthalmos

Metabolic
Negative nitrogen balance due to protein catabolism

The following additional adverse reactions are related to parenteral corticosteroid therapy:
Hyperpigmentation or hypopigmentation
Subcutaneous and cutaneous atrophy
Sterile abscess

DOSAGE AND ADMINISTRATION

This preparation may be administered by intravenous injection, by intravenous infusion or by intramuscular injection; the preferred method for initial emergency use being intravenous injection. Following the initial emergency period, consideration should be given to employing a longer acting injectable preparation or an oral preparation.

Therapy is initiated by administering hydrocortisone sodium succinate intravenously over a period of 30 seconds (e.g., 100 mg) to 10 minutes (e.g., 500 mg or more). In general, high dose corticosteroid therapy should be continued only until the patient's condition has stabilized—usually not beyond 48 to 72 hours. Although adverse effects associated with high dose, short-term corticoid therapy are uncommon, peptic ulceration may occur. Prophylactic antacid therapy may be indicated.

When high dose hydrocortisone therapy must be continued beyond 48 to 72 hours, hypernatremia may occur. Under such circumstances it may be desirable to replace hydrocortisone sodium succinate with a corticoid which causes little or no sodium retention.

The initial dose of hydrocortisone sodium succinate is 100 mg to 500 mg depending upon the severity of the condition. This dose may be repeated at intervals of 2, 4, or 6 hours as indicated by the patient's response and clinical condition. While the dose may be reduced for infants and children, it is governed more by the severity of the condition and response of the patient than by age or body weight but should not be less than 25 mg daily. Patients subjected to severe stress following corticosteroid therapy should be observed closely for signs and symptoms of adrenocortical insufficiency.

Corticoid therapy is an adjunct to, and not a replacement for, conventional therapy.

Multiple Sclerosis:
In the treatment of acute exacerbations of multiple sclerosis, daily doses of 200 mg of prednisolone for a week followed by 80 mg every other day for one month have been shown to be effective (20 mg of hydrocortisone is equivalent to 5 mg of prednisolone).

PREPARATION OF SOLUTIONS

Univial:
1. Remove protective cap, give the plunger-stopper a quarter turn and press to force diluent into lower compartment.
2. Gently agitate to effect solution. Use solution within 72 hours.
3. Sterilize top of plunger-stopper with a suitable germicide.
4. Insert needle squarely through center of plunger stopper until tip is just visible. Invert vial and withdraw dose.

Further dilution is not necessary for intravenous or intramuscular injection.

For Intravenous Infusion:
Prepare solution as described above. The 100 mg solution may then be added to 100 to 1000 mL (but not less than 100 mL) of 5% Dextrose Injection, (or 0.9% Sodium Chloride Injection, or 5% Dextrose and 0.9% Sodium Chloride Injection, if the patient is not on sodium restriction). The 250 mg solution may be added to 250 to 1000 mL (but not less than 250 mL), the 500 mg solution may be added to 500 to 1000 mL (but not less than 500 mL) and the 1000 mg solution to not less than 1000 mL of the same diluents.

Parenteral drug products should be inspected visually for particulate matter and discoloration prior to administration, whenever solution and container permit.

HOW SUPPLIED

Sterile A-HYDROCORT (hydrocortisone sodium succinate for injection, USP) is available in the following packages:
100 mg/2 mL Univial **NDC** 0074-5671-02;
250 mg/2 mL Univial **NDC** 0074-5672-02;
500 mg/4 mL Univial **NDC** 0074-5673-04;
1000 mg/8 mL Univial **NDC** 0074-5674-08.

Store at controlled room temperature 15° to 30° C (59° to 86°F). Protect from light.

Caution: Federal (USA) law prohibits dispensing without prescription.

Univial® - Sterile two-compartment vial, Abbott

Abbott Laboratories
North Chicago, IL 60064, USA
Ref. 01-2432-R3 - Rev. Aug., 1988

STERILE A-METHAPRED®   ℞
[ā-meth 'a-pred "]
(Methylprednisolone Sodium Succinate for Injection, USP)
For Intravenous or Intramuscular Use

DESCRIPTION

Methylprednisolone sodium succinate, USP, an adrenocortical-like steroid, is the sodium succinate ester of methylprednisolone.

It occurs as a white, or nearly white, odorless hygroscopic, amorphous solid.

Methylprednisolone sodium succinate is extremely soluble in water and is especially well suited for intravenous use in situations in which high blood levels of methylprednisolone are required rapidly.

A-METHAPRED (methylprednisolone sodium succinate for injection, USP) is available as:

40 mg Univial —Each 1 mL (when mixed) contains methylprednisolone sodium succinate equivalent to 40 mg methylprednisolone; also 1.6 mg monobasic sodium phosphate anhydrous; 17.5 mg dibasic sodium phosphate anhydrous; 25 mg lactose anhydrous; and 9 mg of benzyl alcohol.

125 mg Univial—Each 2 mL (when mixed) contains methylprednisolone sodium succinate equivalent to 125 mg methylprednisolone; also 1.6 mg monobasic sodium phosphate anhydrous; 17.4 mg dibasic sodium phosphate anhydrous; and 18 mg of benzyl alcohol.

500 mg Univial—Each 4 mL (when mixed) contains methylprednisolone sodium succinate equivalent to 500 mg methylprednisolone; also 6.4 mg monobasic sodium phosphate anhydrous; 69.6 mg dibasic sodium phosphate anhydrous; and 36 mg of benzyl alcohol.

1000 mg Univial—Each 8 mL (when mixed) contains methylprednisolone sodium succinate equivalent to 1000 mg methylprednisolone; also 12.8 mg monobasic sodium phosphate anhydrous; 139.2 mg dibasic sodium phosphate anhydrous; and 72 mg of benzyl alcohol.

May contain sodium hydroxide and/or hydrochloric acid for pH adjustment.

NOTE: The 40 mg and 125 mg Univial should be used within 48 hours after mixing. The 500 mg and 1000 mg Univial should be used within 72 hours after mixing.

CLINICAL PHARMACOLOGY

Methylprednisolone sodium succinate is a potent anti-inflammatory steroid. It has a greater anti-inflammatory potency than prednisolone and even less tendency than prednisolone to induce sodium and water retention. Like the adrenocortical steroids, methylprednisolone sodium succinate may cause profound and varied metabolic effects in addition to modifying the body's immune response to diverse stimuli. When given parenterally and in equimolar quantities, methylprednisolone sodium succinate and methylprednisolone are equivalent in biologic activity.

The relative potency of methylprednisolone sodium succinate and hydrocortisone sodium succinate, as indicated by depression of eosinophil count, following intravenous administration, is at least four to one. This is in good agreement with the relative oral potency of methylprednisolone and hydrocortisone.

INDICATIONS AND USAGE

When oral therapy is not feasible, and the strength, dosage form and route of administration of the drug reasonably lend the preparation to the treatment of the condition, A-METHAPRED (methylprednisolone sodium succinate) is indicated for intravenous or intramuscular use in the following conditions:

1. **Endocrine disorders:**
   a. Primary or secondary adrenocortical insufficiency (hydrocortisone or cortisone is the drug of choice, synthetic analogs may be used in conjunction with mineralocorticoids where applicable; in infancy, mineralocorticoid supplementation is of particular importance).
   b. Acute adrenocortical insufficiency (hydrocortisone or cortisone is the drug of choice; mineralocorticoid supplementation may be necessary, particularly when synthetic analogs are used).
   c. Preoperatively and in the event of serious trauma or illness, in patients with known adrenal insufficiency or when adrenocortical reserve is doubtful.
   d. Shock unresponsive to conventional therapy if adrenocortical insufficiency exists or is suspected.
   e. Congenital adrenal hyperplasia.
   f. Hypercalcemia associated with cancer.
   g. Nonsuppurative thyroiditis.

2. **Rheumatic disorders**—As adjunctive therapy for short-term administration (to tide the patient over an acute episode or exacerbation) in:
   a. Post-traumatic osteoarthritis.
   b. Synovitis of osteoarthritis.
   c. Rheumatoid arthritis, including juvenile rheumatoid arthritis (selected cases may require low-dose maintenance therapy).
   d. Acute and subacute bursitis.
   e. Epicondylitis.
   f. Acute nonspecific tenosynovitis.
   g. Acute gouty arthritis.
   h. Psoriatic arthritis.
   i. Ankylosing spondylitis.

3. **Collagen diseases** — During an exacerbation or as maintenance therapy in selected cases of:
   a. Systemic lupus erythematosus.
   b. Acute rheumatic carditis.
   c. Systemic dermatomyositis (polymyositis).

4. **Dermatologic diseases:**
   a. Severe erythema multiforme (Stevens-Johnson syndrome).
   b. Exfoliative dermatitis.
   c. Bullous dermatitis herpetiformis.
   d. Severe seborrheic dermatitis.
   e. Severe psoriasis.
   f. Pemphigus.
   g. Mycosis fungoides.

5. **Allergic states** — Control of severe or incapacitating allergic conditions intractable to adequate trials of conventional treatment in:
   a. Bronchial asthma.
   b. Contact dermatitis.
   c. Atopic dermatitis.
   d. Serum sickness.
   e. Seasonal or perennial allergic rhinitis.
   f. Drug hypersensitivity reactions.
   g. Urticarial transfusion reactions.
   h. Acute noninfectious laryngeal edema (epinephrine is the drug of first choice).

6. **Ophthalmic diseases** — Severe acute and chronic allergic and inflammatory processes involving the eye, such as:
   a. Herpes zoster ophthalmicus.
   b. Iritis, iridocyclitis.
   c. Chorioretinitis.
   d. Diffuse posterior uveitis and choroiditis.
   e. Optic neuritis.
   f. Sympathetic ophthalmia.
   g. Anterior segment inflammation.
   h. Allergic conjunctivitis.
   i. Allergic corneal marginal ulcers.
   j. Keratitis.

Continued on next page

Abbott—Cont.

7. **Gastrointestinal diseases** — To tide the patient over a critical period of disease in:
   a. Ulcerative colitis — (Systemic therapy).
   b. Regional enteritis — (Systemic therapy).
8. **Respiratory diseases:**
   a. Symptomatic sarcoidosis.
   b. Berylliosis.
   c. Fulminating or disseminated pulmonary tuberculosis when concurrently accompanied by appropriate antituberculous chemotherapy.
   d. Aspiration pneumonitis.
   e. Loeffler's syndrome not manageable by other means.
9. **Hematologic disorders:**
   a. Acquired (autoimmune) hemolytic anemia.
   b. Idiopathic thrombocytopenic purpura in adults (IV only; IM administration is contraindicated).
   c. Secondary thrombocytopenia in adults.
   d. Erythroblastopenia (RBC anemia).
   e. Congenital (erythroid) hypoplastic anemia.
10. **Neoplastic diseases** — For palliative management of:
    a. Leukemias and lymphomas in adults.
    b. Acute leukemia of childhood.
11. **Edematous state** — To induce diuresis or remission of proteinuria in the nephrotic syndrome, without uremia, of the idiopathic type or that due to lupus erythematosus.
12. **Nervous system:**
    a. Acute exacerbations of multiple sclerosis.
13. **Miscellaneous:**
    a. Tuberculous meningitis with subarachnoid block or impending block when used concurrently with appropriate antituberculous chemotherapy.
    b. Trichinosis with neurologic or myocardial involvement.

CONTRAINDICATIONS
Systemic fungal infections.
A-METHAPRED is contraindicated in the treatment of sepsis syndrome or septic shock.
Not for use in newborns. Benzyl alcohol, a preservative in the Bacteriostatic Water for Injection provided with these products, has been associated with toxicity in newborns. Data are unavailable on the toxicity of other preservatives in this age group.

WARNINGS
In patients on corticosteroid therapy subjected to any unusual stress, increased dosage of rapidly acting corticosteroids before, during, and after the stressful situation is indicated.
Corticosteroids may mask some signs of infection, and new infections may appear during their use. There may be decreased resistance and inability to localize infection when corticosteroids are used.
A-METHAPRED is contraindicated in the treatment of sepsis syndrome or septic shock. The use of A-METHAPRED in the treatment of sepsis syndrome or septic shock may cause an increased risk of mortality where there is an elevated creatinine level or in patients who develop secondary infections after treatment with A-METHAPRED has begun.
Prolonged use of corticosteroids may produce posterior subcapsular cataracts, glaucoma with possible damage to the optic nerves, and may enhance the establishment of secondary ocular infections due to fungi or viruses.
Average and large doses of cortisone or hydrocortisone can cause elevation of blood pressure, salt and water retention, and increased excretion of potassium. These effects are less likely to occur with the synthetic derivatives except when used in large doses. Dietary salt restriction and potassium supplementation may be necessary. All corticosteroids increase calcium excretion.
While on corticosteroid therapy patients should not be vaccinated against smallpox. Other immunization procedures should not be undertaken in patients who are on corticosteroids, especially on high dose, because of possible hazards of neurological complications and a lack of antibody response.
The use of A-METHAPRED (methylprednisolone sodium succinate) in active tuberculosis should be restricted to those cases of fulminating or disseminated tuberculosis in which the corticosteroid is used for the management of the disease in conjunction with appropriate antituberculous regimen. If corticosteroids are indicated in patients with latent tuberculosis or tuberculin reactivity, close observation is necessary as reactivation of the disease may occur. During prolonged corticosteroid therapy, these patients should receive chemoprophylaxis.
Because rare instances of anaphylactoid reactions have occurred in patients receiving parenteral corticosteroid therapy, appropriate precautionary measures should be taken prior to administration, especially when the patient has a history of allergy to any drug.

There are reports of cardiac arrhythmias and/or circulatory collapse and/or cardiac arrest following the rapid administration of large I.V. doses of methylprednisolone sodium succinate (greater than 0.5 gram administered over a period of less than 10 minutes).

USAGE IN PREGNANCY
Since adequate human reproduction studies have not been done with corticosteroids, the use of these drugs in pregnancy, nursing mothers, or women of childbearing potential requires that the possible benefits of the drug be weighed against the potential hazards to the mother and embryo or fetus. Infants born of mothers who have received substantial doses of corticosteroids during pregnancy should be carefully observed for signs of hypoadrenalism.

PRECAUTIONS
Drug-induced secondary adrenocortical insufficiency may be minimized by gradual reduction of dosage. This type of relative insufficiency may persist for months after discontinuation of therapy, therefore, in any situation of stress occurring during that period, hormone therapy should be reinstituted. Since mineralocorticoid secretion may be impaired, salt and/or a mineralocorticoid should be administered concurrently.
There is an enhanced effect of corticosteroids on patients with hypothyroidism and in those with cirrhosis.
Corticosteroids should be used cautiously in patients with ocular herpes simplex because of possible corneal perforation.
The lowest possible dose of corticosteroid should be used to control the condition under treatment, and when reduction in dosage is possible, the reduction should be gradual.
Psychic derangements may appear when corticosteroids are used, ranging from euphoria, insomnia, mood swings, personality changes and severe depression, to frank psychotic manifestations. Also, existing emotional instability or psychotic tendencies may be aggravated by corticosteroids.
Aspirin should be used cautiously in conjunction with corticosteroids in hypoprothrombinemia.
Steroids should be used with caution in nonspecific ulcerative colitis, if there is a probability of impending perforation, abscess or other pyogenic infection; diverticulitis; fresh intestinal anastomoses; active or latent peptic ulcer; renal insufficiency; hypertension; osteoporosis; and myasthenia gravis.
Growth and development of infants and children on prolonged corticosteroid therapy should be carefully observed.
Although controlled clinical trials have shown corticosteroids to be effective in speeding the resolution of acute exacerbations of multiple sclerosis, they do not show that corticosteroids affect the ultimate outcome or natural history of the disease. The studies do show that relatively high doses of corticosteroids are necessary to demonstrate a significant effect. (See "DOSAGE AND ADMINISTRATION" section).
Since complications of treatment with glucocorticoids are dependent on the size of the dose and the duration of treatment, a risk/benefit decision must be made in each individual case as to dose and duration of treatment and as to whether daily or intermittent therapy should be used.

ADVERSE REACTIONS
Fluid and Electrolyte Disturbances
  Sodium retention
  Fluid retention
  Congestive heart failure in susceptible patients
  Potassium loss
  Hypokalemic alkalosis
  Hypertension
Musculoskeletal
  Muscle weakness
  Steroid myopathy
  Loss of muscle mass
  Severe arthralgia
  Osteoporosis
  Vertebral compression fractures
  Aseptic necrosis of femoral and humeral heads
  Pathologic fracture of long bones
Gastrointestinal
  Peptic ulcer with possible perforation and hemorrhage
  Pancreatitis
  Abdominal distention
  Ulcerative esophagitis
Dermatologic
  Impaired wound healing
  Thin fragile skin
  Petechiae and ecchymoses
  Facial erythema
  Increased sweating
  May suppress reactions to skin tests
Neurological
  Increased intracranial pressure with papilledema (pseudo-tumor cerebri) usually after treatment

  Convulsions
  Vertigo
  Headache
Endocrine
  Development of Cushingoid state
  Suppression of growth in children
  Secondary adrenocortical and pituitary unresponsiveness, particularly in times of stress, as in trauma, surgery or illness
  Menstrual irregularities
  Decreased carbohydrate tolerance
  Manifestations of latent diabetes mellitus
  Increased requirements for insulin or oral hypoglycemic agents in diabetics
Ophthalmic
  Posterior subcapsular cataracts
  Increased intraocular pressure
  Glaucoma
  Exophthalmos
Metabolic
  Negative nitrogen balance due to protein catabolism
The following additional adverse reactions are related to parenteral corticosteroid therapy:
  Hyperpigmentation or hypopigmentation
  Subcutaneous and cutaneous atrophy
  Sterile abscess
  Anaphylactic reaction with or without circulatory collapse, cardiac arrest, bronchospasm
  Urticaria
  Nausea and vomiting
  Cardiac arrhythmias, hypotension or hypertension

DOSAGE AND ADMINISTRATION
When high dose therapy is desired, the recommended dose of methylprednisolone as the sodium succinate is 30 mg/kg administered intravenously over a 10 to 20-minute period. This dose may be repeated every 4 to 6 hours. In general, high dose corticosteroid therapy should be continued only until the patient's condition has stabilized, usually not beyond 48 to 72 hours.
Although adverse effects associated with high dose short-term corticoid therapy are uncommon, peptic ulceration may occur. Prophylactic antacid therapy may be indicated.
In other indications initial dosage will vary from 10 to 40 mg of methylprednisolone depending on the clinical problem being treated. The larger doses may be required for short-term management of severe, acute conditions. The initial dose usually should be given intravenously over a period of one to several minutes. Subsequent doses may be given intravenously or intramuscularly at intervals dictated by the patient's response and clinical condition. Corticoid therapy is an adjunct to, and not replacement for conventional therapy.
Dosage may be reduced for infants and children but should be governed more by the severity of the condition and response of the patient than by age or size. It should not be less than 0.5 mg/kg every 24 hours.
Dosage must be decreased or discontinued gradually when the drug has been administered for more than a few days. If a period of spontaneous remission occurs in a chronic condition, treatment should be discontinued. Routine laboratory studies, such as urinalysis, two-hour postprandial blood sugar, determination of blood pressure and body weight, and a chest X-ray should be made at regular intervals during prolonged therapy. Upper GI X-rays are desirable in patients with an ulcer history or significant dyspepsia.
Methylprednisolone may be administered intravenously by direct push, or by intermittent or continuous infusion; or by intramuscular injection. The preferred method for initial emergency use is either direct I.V. push or intermittent infusion. To administer by intravenous (or intramuscular) injection, prepare solution as directed. The desired dose may be administered intravenously over a period of one to several minutes (for doses of 40 mg or less).
Multiple Sclerosis
In treatment of acute exacerbations of multiple sclerosis, daily doses of 200 mg of prednisolone for a week followed by 80 mg every other day for 1 month have been shown to be effective (4 mg of methylprednisolone is equivalent to 5 mg of prednisolone).

PREPARATION OF UNIVIAL SOLUTIONS
1. Remove protective cap, give the plunger-stopper a quarter turn and press to force diluent into the lower compartment.
2. Agitate immediately to effect solution. With the 1000 mg Univial, for best results, shake continuously for a minimum of 45 seconds before inspecting solution. If necessary, continue shaking to effect complete solution. The Univial should be agitated in a manner which insures mixing throughout both compartments.

Abbott—Cont.

Calcijex should be given cautiously to patients on digitalis, because hypercalcemia in such patients may precipitate cardiac arrhythmias.

2. Information for The Patient

The patient and his or her parents should be informed about adherence to instructions about diet and calcium supplementation and avoidance of the use of unapproved non-prescription drugs, including magnesium-containing antacids. Patients should also be carefully informed about the symptoms of hypercalcemia (see ADVERSE REACTIONS).

3. Essential Laboratory Tests

Serum calcium, phosphorus, magnesium and alkaline phosphatase and 24-hour urinary calcium and phosphorus should be determined periodically. During the initial phase of the medication, serum calcium and phosphorus should be determined more frequently (twice weekly).

4. Drug Interactions

Magnesium-containing antacid and Calcijex should not be used concomitantly, because such use may lead to the development of hypermagnesemia.

5. Carcinogenesis, Mutagenesis, Impairment of Fertility

Long-term studies in animals have not been performed to evaluate the carcinogenic potential of Calcijex (calcitriol injection). There was no evidence of mutagenicity as studied by the Ames Method. No significant effects of calcitriol on fertility were reported using oral Calcitriol.

6. Use in Pregnancy: *Pregnancy Category C:* Calcitriol given

orally has been reported to be teratogenic in rabbits when given in doses 4 and 15 times the dose recommended for human use.
All 15 fetuses in 3 litters at these doses showed external and skeletal abnormalities. However, none of the other 23 litters (156 fetuses) showed significant abnormalities compared with controls.
Teratology studies in rats showed no evidence of teratogenic potential. There are no adequate and well-controlled studies in pregnant women. Calcijex should be used during pregnancy only if the potential benefit justifies the potential risk to the fetus.

7. Nursing Mothers

It is not known whether this drug is excreted in human milk. Because many drugs are excreted in human milk and because of the potential for serious adverse reactions in nursing infants from calcitriol, a decision should be made whether to discontinue nursing or to discontinue the drug, taking into account the importance of the drug to the mother.

8. Pediatric Use

Safety and efficacy of Calcijex in children have not been established.

ADVERSE REACTIONS

Adverse effects of Calcijex (calcitriol injection) are, in general, similar to those encountered with excessive vitamin D intake. The early and late signs and symptoms of vitamin D intoxication associated with hypercalcemia include:

1. Early

Weakness, headache, somnolence, nausea, vomiting, dry mouth, constipation, muscle pain, bone pain and metallic taste.

2. Late

Polyuria, polydipsia, anorexia, weight loss, nocturia, conjunctivitis (calcific), pancreatitis, photophobia, rhinorrhea, pruritus, hyperthermia, decreased libido, elevated BUN, albuminuria, hypercholesterolemia, elevated SGOT and SGPT, ectopic calcification, hypertension, cardiac arrhythmias and, rarely, overt psychosis.
Occasional mild pain on injection has been observed.

OVERDOSAGE

Administration of Calcijex (calcitriol injection) to patients in excess of their requirements can cause hypercalcemia, hypercalciuria and hyperphosphatemia. High intake of calcium and phosphate concomitant with Calcijex may lead to similar abnormalities.

1. Treatment of Hypercalcemia and Overdosage in Patients on Hemodialysis

General treatment of hypercalcemia (greater than 1 mg/dl above the upper limit of normal range) consists of immediate discontinuation of Calcijex therapy, institution of a low calcium diet and withdrawal of calcium supplements. Serum calcium levels should be determined daily until normocalcemia ensues. Hypercalcemia usually resolves in two to seven days. When serum calcium levels have returned to within normal limits, Calcijex therapy may be reinstituted at a dose 0.5 mcg less than prior therapy. Serum calcium levels should be obtained at least twice weekly after all dosage changes.
Persistent or markedly elevated serum calcium levels may be corrected by dialysis against a calcium-free dialysate.

2. Treatment of Accidental Overdosage of Calcitriol Injection

The treatment of acute accidental overdosage of Calcijex

should consist of general supportive measures. Serial serum electrolyte determinations (especially calcium), rate of urinary calcium excretion and assessment of electrocardiographic abnormalities due to hypercalcemia should be obtained. Such monitoring is critical in patients receiving digitalis. Discontinuation of supplemental calcium and low calcium diet are also indicated in accidental overdosage. Due to the relatively short duration of the pharmacological action of calcitriol, further measures are probably unnecessary. Should, however, persistent and markedly elevated serum calcium levels occur, there are a variety of therapeutic alternatives which may be considered, depending on the patients' underlying condition. These include the use of drugs such as phosphates and corticosteroids as well as measures to induce an appropriate forced diuresis. The use of peritoneal dialysis against a calcium-free dialysate has also been reported.

DOSAGE AND ADMINISTRATION

The optimal dose of Calcijex (calcitriol injection) must be carefully determined for each patient.
The effectiveness of Calcijex therapy is predicated on the assumption that each patient is receiving an adequate and appropriate daily intake of calcium. The RDA for calcium in adults is 800 mg. To ensure that each patient receives an adequate daily intake of calcium, the physician should either prescribe a calcium supplement or instruct the patient in proper dietary measures.
The recommended initial dose of Calcijex is 0.5 mcg (0.01 mcg/kg) administered three times weekly, approximately every other day. Calcijex can be administered as a bolus dose intravenously through the catheter at the end of hemodialysis. If a satisfactory response in the biochemical parameters and clinical manifestations of the disease state is not observed, the dose may be increased by 0.25 to 0.50 mcg at two to four week intervals. During this titration period, serum calcium and phosphorus levels should be obtained at least twice weekly, and if hypercalcemia is noted, the drug should be immediately discontinued until normocalcemia ensues. Most patients undergoing hemodialysis respond to doses between 0.5 and 3.0 mcg (0.01 to 0.05 mcg/kg) three times per week.
Parenteral drug products should be inspected visually for particulate matter and discoloration prior to administration, whenever solution and container permit.
Discard unused portion.

HOW SUPPLIED

Calcijex™ (calcitriol injection) is supplied in 1 mL ampuls containing 1 mcg (List No. 1200) and 2 mcg (List No. 1210).
Protect from light.
Exposure of pharmaceutical products to heat should be minimized. Avoid excessive heat. Protect from freezing. It is recommended that the product be stored at room temperature (25° C); however, brief exposure up to 40° C does not adversely affect the product.
Caution: Federal (USA) law prohibits dispensing without prescription.
© Abbott 1986
06-3887-R3 Rev. Oct., 1986

CARTROL®　　　　　　　　　　　　　　　　　℞

(carteolol hydrochloride)
Filmtab® Tablets

PRODUCT OVERVIEW

KEY FACTS

CARTROL (carteolol HCl) is a long-acting beta-blocker with ISA. It is a hydrophilic compound and has a favorable side-effect profile. CARTROL Filmtab tablets contain either 2.5 mg or 5 mg of careolol hydrochloride. Most patients are maintained on a dose of either 2.5 mg or 5 mg once-a-day.

MAJOR USES

CARTROL tablets are used for the management of hypertension. It may be utilized as monotherapy or in combination with other agents. CARTROL tablets are suitable for the entire age range of hypertensive patients.

SAFETY INFORMATION

CARTROL tablets are contraindicated only in patients who fall into one of several categories listed in the CONTRAINDICATION section of the package insert.

PRODUCT ILLUSTRATION

2.5 mg

5 mg

PRESCRIBING INFORMATION

CARTROL®　　　　　　　　　　　　　　　℞
(Carteolol Hydrochloride)
Filmtab® Tablets

DESCRIPTION

CARTROL (carteolol hydrochloride) is a synthetic, nonselective, beta-adrenergic receptor blocking agent with intrinsic sympathomimetic activity. It is chemically described as 5-[3-[(1,1-dimethylethyl) amino]-2-hydroxypropoxy]-3,4-dihydro-2(1H)-quinolinone monohydrochloride.
Carteolol hydrochloride is a stable, white crystalline powder which is soluble in water and slightly soluble in ethanol. The molecular weight is 328.84 and $C_{16}H_{24}N_2O_3 \cdot HCl$ is the empirical formula.
CARTROL (carteolol hydrochloride) is available as tablets containing either 2.5 mg or 5 mg of carteolol hydrochloride for oral administration.

INACTIVE INGREDIENTS

2.5 mg Tablet: Cellulosic polymers, corn starch, iron oxide, lactose, magnesium stearate, microcrystalline cellulose, polyethylene glycol, propylene glycol, and titanium dioxide.
5 mg Tablet: Cellulosic polymers, corn starch, lactose, magnesium stearate, microcrystalline cellulose, polyethylene glycol, propylene glycol, and titanium dioxide.

CLINICAL PHARMACOLOGY

CARTROL (carteolol hydrochloride) is a long-acting, nonselective, beta-adrenergic receptor blocking agent with intrinsic sympathomimetic activity (ISA) and without significant membrane stabilizing (local anesthetic) activity.
Pharmacodynamics:
Carteolol specifically competes with beta-adrenergic receptor agonists for both $beta_1$-receptors located principally in cardiac muscle and $beta_2$-receptors located in the bronchial and vascular musculature, blocking the chronotropic, inotropic, and vasodilator responses to beta-adrenergic stimulation proportionately. Because of its partial agonist activity, however, carteolol does not reduce resting beta-agonist activity as much as beta-adrenergic blockers lacking this activity. Thus, in clinical trials in man, the decreases in resting pulse rate produced by carteolol (2–5 beats per minute in various studies) were less than those produced by beta-blockers (nadolol and propranolol) without ISA (10–12 beats per minute). There are also equivocal effects on renin secretion, in contrast to beta-blockers without ISA, which inhibit renin secretion.
In controlled clinical trials carteolol at doses up to 20 mg as monotherapy or in combination with thiazide type diuretics, produced significantly greater reductions in blood pressure than did placebo, with the full effect seen between two and four weeks. The observed differences from placebo ranged from 3.1 to 6.7 mmHg for supine diastolic blood pressure. The antihypertensive effects of carteolol are smaller in black populations but do not seem to be affected by age or sex. Doses of carteolol greater than 10 mg once a day did not produce greater reductions in blood pressure. In fact, doses of 20 mg and above appeared to produce blood pressure reductions less than those produced by 10 mg and below. When carteolol was compared to nadolol and propranolol, although the differences were not statistically significant in relatively small studies, carteolol at doses up to 20 mg produced supine diastolic blood pressure changes consistently 2 mmHg less than that produced by either nadolol or propranolol.
Although the mechanism of the antihypertensive effect of beta-adrenergic blocking agents has not been established, multiple factors are thought to contribute to the lowering of blood pressure, including diminished response to sympathetic nerve outflow from vasomotor centers in the brain, diminished release of renin from the kidneys, and decreased cardiac output. Carteolol does not have a consistent effect on renin and other agents with ISA have been shown to have less effect than other beta-blockers on resting cardiac output (although they cause the usual decrease in exercise cardiac output so that the difference is of uncertain clinical importance), so that the mechanism of its action is particularly uncertain.
Beta-blockade interferes with endogenous adrenergic bronchodilator activity and diminishes the response to exogenous bronchodilators. This is especially important in patients subject to bronchospasm.
Single intravenous doses of carteolol (0.5 mg, 1 mg, 2.5 mg and 5 mg) produced statistically, but not clinically, significant increases from baseline in AV node conduction time and RR and PR intervals.
CARTROL (carteolol hydrochloride) induced no significant alteration in total serum cholesterol and triglycerides.
Following discontinuation of carteolol treatment in man, pharmacologic activity (evaluated by blockade of the tachycardia induced by isoproterenol or postural changes) is present for 2 to 21 days (median 14 days) after the last dose of carteolol. Following administration of recommended doses of

CARTROL (carteolol hydrochloride), both beta-blocking and antihypertensive effects persist for at least 24 hours.

Pharmacokinetics and Metabolism:
Following oral administration in man, peak plasma concentrations of carteolol usually occur within one to three hours. Carteolol is well absorbed when administered orally as CARTROL (carteolol hydrochloride) tablets. The presence of food in the gastrointestinal tract somewhat slows the rate of absorption, but the extent of absorption is not appreciably affected. Compared to intravenous administration, the absolute bioavailability of carteolol from CARTROL (carteolol hydrochloride) tablets is approximately 85%.

The plasma half-life of carteolol averages approximately six hours. Steady-state serum levels are achieved within one to two days after initiating therapeutic doses of carteolol in persons with normal renal function. Since approximately 50 to 70% of a carteolol dose is eliminated unchanged by the kidneys, the half-life is increased in patients with impaired renal function. Significant reductions in the rate of carteolol elimination (and prolongations of the half-life) occur in patients as creatinine clearance decreases. Therefore, a reduction in maintenance dose and/or prolongation in dosing interval is appropriate (see DOSAGE and ADMINISTRATION).

Carteolol is 23–30% bound to plasma proteins in humans. The major metabolic products of carteolol are 8-hydroxycarteolol and the glucuronic acid conjugates of both carteolol and 8-hydroxycarteolol. In man, 8-hydroxycarteolol is an active metabolite with a half-life of approximately 8 to 12 hours and represents approximately 5% of the administered dose excreted in the urine.

INDICATIONS AND USAGE

CARTROL (carteolol hydrochloride) is indicated in the management of hypertension. It may be used alone or in combination with other antihypertensive agents, especially thiazide diuretics. Preliminary data indicate that carteolol does not have a favorable effect on arrhythmias.

CONTRAINDICATIONS

CARTROL (carteolol hydrochloride) is contraindicated in patients with: 1) bronchial asthma, 2) severe bradycardia, 3) greater than first degree heart block, 4) cardiogenic shock, and 5) clinically evident congestive heart failure (see WARNINGS).

WARNINGS

Congestive Heart Failure:
Sympathetic stimulation may be a vital component supporting circulatory function in patients with congestive heart failure, and impairing that support by beta-blockade may precipitate more severe decompensation. Although CARTROL (carteolol hydrochloride) should be avoided in clinically evident congestive heart failure, it can be used with caution, if necessary, in patients with a history of failure who are well-compensated and are receiving digitalis and diuretics. Beta-adrenergic blocking agents do not abolish the inotropic action of digitalis on heart muscle.

IN PATIENTS WITHOUT A HISTORY OF CONGESTIVE HEART FAILURE, the use of beta-blockers can, in some instances, lead to congestive heart failure. Therefore, at the first sign or symptom of cardiac decompensation, discontinuation of beta-blocker therapy should be considered. The patient should be closely observed and treatment should include a diuretic and/or digitalization as necessary.

Exacerbation of Angina Pectoris Upon Withdrawal:
In patients with angina pectoris, exacerbation of angina and, in some cases, myocardial infarction have been reported following abrupt discontinuation of therapy with some beta-blockers. Therefore such patients should be cautioned against interruption of therapy without a physician's advice. The long persistence of beta-adrenergic blockade following abrupt discontinuation of CARTROL (carteolol hydrochloride), however, might be expected to minimize the possibility of this complication. When discontinuation of CARTROL (carteolol hydrochloride) is planned, dosage should be tapered gradually, as it is with other beta-blockers. If exacerbation of angina occurs when CARTROL (carteolol hydrochloride) therapy is interrupted, it is advisable to reinstitute CARTROL (carteolol hydrochloride) or other beta-blocker therapy, at least temporarily, and to take other measures appropriate for the management of unstable angina pectoris.

PATIENTS WITHOUT CLINICALLY RECOGNIZED ANGINA PECTORIS should be carefully monitored after withdrawal of CARTROL (carteolol hydrochloride) therapy, since coronary artery disease may be unrecognized.

Nonallergic Bronchospasm (e.g., chronic bronchitis, emphysema):
Patients with bronchospastic disease generally should not receive beta-blocker therapy and carteolol is contraindicated in patients with bronchial asthma. If use of CARTROL (carteolol hydrochloride) is essential, it should be administered with caution since it may block bronchodilation produced by endogenous catecholamine stimulation of beta$_2$-receptors or diminish response to therapy with a beta-receptor agonist.

Major Surgery:
The necessity, or desirability, of withdrawal of beta-blocking therapy prior to major surgery is controversial. Because beta-blockade impairs the ability of the heart to respond to reflex stimuli and may increase risks of general anesthesia and surgical procedures resulting in protracted hypotension or low cardiac output, and difficulty in restarting or maintaining a heartbeat, it has been suggested that beta-blocker therapy should be withdrawn several days prior to surgery. It is also recognized, however, that increased sensitivity to catecholamines of patients recently withdrawn from beta-blocker therapy could increase certain risks. Given the persistence of the beta-blocking activity of CARTROL (carteolol hydrochloride), effective withdrawal would take several weeks and would ordinarily be impractical. When beta-blocker therapy is not discontinued, anesthetic agents that depress the myocardium should be avoided. In one study using intravenous carteolol during surgery, recovery from anesthesia was somewhat delayed in three patients who received carteolol near the end of anesthesia, and respiratory arrest occurred in one of these patients immediately following administration of intravenous carteolol.

In the event that CARTROL (carteolol hydrochloride) treatment is not discontinued before surgery, the anesthesiologist should be informed that the patient is receiving CARTROL (carteolol hydrochloride). The effects on the heart of beta-adrenergic blocking agents, such as CARTROL (carteolol hydrochloride), may be reversed by cautious administration of isoproterenol or dobutamine.

Diabetes Mellitus and Hypoglycemia:
Beta-adrenergic blockade may prevent the appearance of premonitory signs and symptoms (e.g., tachycardia and blood pressure changes) of acute hypoglycemia, and it inhibits glycogenolysis, a normal compensatory mechanism for hypoglycemia. This is especially important for patients with labile diabetes mellitus. Beta-blockade also reduces the release of insulin in response to hyperglycemia; therefore, it may be necessary to adjust the dose of antidiabetic agents used to treat hyperglycemia.

Thyrotoxicosis:
Beta-adrenergic blockade may mask certain clinical signs of hyperthyroidism such as tachycardia. Patients suspected of having thyrotoxicosis should be managed carefully to avoid abrupt withdrawal of beta-adrenergic blockade which might precipitate a thyroid storm.

PRECAUTIONS

General:

Impaired Renal Function:
CARTROL (carteolol hydrochloride) should be used with caution in patients with impaired renal function. Patients with impaired renal function clear carteolol at a reduced rate, and dosage should be reduced accordingly (see Dosage and Administration).

Beta-adrenoreceptor blockade can cause reduction in intraocular pressure. Therefore, CARTROL (carteolol hydrochloride) may interfere with glaucoma testing. Withdrawal may lead to a return of increased intraocular pressure.

Information for Patients:
Patients, especially those with evidence of coronary artery insufficiency, should be warned against interruption or discontinuation of CARTROL (carteolol hydrochloride) therapy without the physician's advice. Although cardiac failure rarely occurs in properly selected patients, patients being treated with beta-adrenergic blocking agents should be advised to consult the physician at the first sign or symptom of impending failure (i.e., fatigue with exertion, difficulty breathing, cough or unusually fast heartbeat).

Drug Interactions:
Catecholamine-depleting drugs (e.g., reserpine) may have an additive effect when given with beta-blocking agents. Therefore, patients treated with CARTROL (carteolol hydrochloride) plus a catecholamine-depleting agent must be observed carefully for evidence of hypotension and/or excessive bradycardia, which may produce syncope or postural hypotension.

Concurrent administration of *general anesthetics* and beta-blocking agents may result in exaggeration of the hypotension induced by general anesthetics (see WARNINGS, Major Surgery).

Blunting of the antihypertensive effect of beta-adrenoreceptor blocking agents by *non-steroidal anti-inflammatory drugs* has been reported. When using these agents concomitantly, patients should be observed carefully to confirm that the desired therapeutic effect has been obtained.

Literature reports suggest that *oral calcium antagonists* may be used in combination with beta-adrenergic blocking agents when heart function is normal, but should be avoided in patients with impaired cardiac function. Hypotension, AV conduction disturbances, and left ventricular failure have been reported in some patients receiving beta-adrenergic blocking agents when an oral calcium antagonist was added to the treatment regimen. Hypotension was more likely to occur if the calcium antagonist were a dihydropyridine derivative, e.g., nifedipine, while left ventricular failure and AV conduc-

tion disturbances were more likely to occur with either verapamil or diltiazem.

Intravenous calcium antagonists should be used with caution in patients receiving beta-adrenergic blocking agents. The concomitant use of beta-adrenergic blocking agents with digitalis and either diltiazem or verapamil may have additive effects in prolonging AV conduction time.

Concomitant use of oral antidiabetic agents or insulin with beta-blocking agents may be associated with hypoglycemia or possibly hyperglycemia. Dosage of the antidiabetic agent should be adjusted accordingly (see WARNINGS, Diabetes Mellitus and Hypoglycemia).

Carcinogenesis, Mutagenesis, Impairment of Fertility:
CARTROL (carteolol hydrochloride) did not produce carcinogenic effects at doses 280 times the maximum recommended human dose (10 mg/70 kg/day) in two-year oral rat and mouse studies.

Tests of mutagenicity, including the Ames Test, recombinant (rec)-assay, *in vivo* cytogenetics and dominant lethal assay demonstrated no evidence for mutagenic potential. Fertility of male and female rats and male and female mice was unaffected by administration of CARTROL (carteolol hydrochloride) at dosages up to 150 mg/kg/day. This dosage is approximately 1052 times the maximum recommended human dose.

Pregnancy:
Teratogenic Effects: Pregnancy Category C. CARTROL (carteolol hydrochloride) increased resorptions and decreased fetal weights in rabbits and rats at maternally toxic doses approximately 1052 and 5264 times the maximum recommended human dose (10 mg/70 kg/day), respectively. A dose-related increase in wavy ribs was noted in the developing rat fetus when pregnant females received daily doses of approximately 212 times the maximum recommended human dose. No such effects were noted in pregnant mice subjected to up to 1052 times the maximum recommended human dose. There are no adequate and well-controlled studies in pregnant women. CARTROL (carteolol hydrochloride) should be used during pregnancy only if the potential benefit justifies the potential risk to the fetus.

Nursing Mothers:
Studies have not been conducted in lactating humans and, therefore, it is not known whether carteolol is excreted in human milk. Studies in lactating rats indicate that CARTROL (carteolol hydrochloride) is excreted in milk. Because many drugs are excreted in human milk, caution should be exercised when CARTROL (carteolol hydrochloride) is administered to a nursing woman.

Pediatric Use:
Safety and effectiveness in children have not been established.

ADVERSE REACTIONS

The prevalence of adverse reactions has been ascertained from clinical studies conducted primarily in the United States. All adverse experiences (events) reported during these studies were recorded as adverse reactions. The prevalence rates presented below are based on combined data from nineteen placebo-controlled studies of patients with hypertension, angina or dysrhythmias, using once-daily carteolol at doses up to 60 mg. Table 1 summarizes those adverse experiences reported for patients in these studies where the prevalence in the carteolol group is 1% or greater and exceeds the prevalence in the placebo group. Asthenia and muscle cramps were the only symptoms that were significantly more common in patients receiving carteolol than in patients receiving placebo. Patients in clinical trials were carefully selected to exclude those, such as patients with asthma or known bronchospasm, or congestive heart failure, who would be at high risk of experiencing beta-adrenergic blocker adverse effect (See WARNINGS and CONTRAINDICATIONS):

TABLE 1
Adverse Reactions During
Placebo-Controlled Studies

	Placebo (n=448) %	Carteolol (n=761) %
Body as a Whole		
†Asthenia	4.0	7.1*
Abdominal Pain	0.4	1.3
Back Pain	1.6	2.1
Chest Pain	1.8	2.2
Digestive System		
Diarrhea	2.0	2.1
Nausea	1.8	2.1
Metabolic/Nutritional Disorders		
Abnormal Lab Test	1.1	1.2
Peripheral Edema	1.1	1.7

Continued on next page

Abbott—Cont.

Musculoskeletal System		
Arthralgia	1.1	1.2
Muscle Cramps	0.2	2.6*
Lower Extremity Pain	0.2	1.2
Nervous System		
Insomnia	0.7	1.7
Paresthesia	1.1	2.0
Respiratory System		
Nasal Congestion	0.9	1.1
Pharyngitis	0.9	1.1
Skin and Appendages		
Rash	1.1	1.3

† Includes weakness, tiredness, lassitude and fatigue.
* Statistically significant at p=0.05 level.

The adverse experiences were usually mild or moderate in intensity and transient, but sometimes were serious enough to interrupt treatment. The adverse reactions that were most bothersome, as judged by their being reported as reasons for discontinuation of therapy by at least 0.4% of the carteolol group are shown in Table 2.

TABLE 2
Discontinuations During
Placebo-Controlled Studies

	Placebo (n=448) %	Carteolol (n=761) %
Body as a Whole		
Asthenia	0.2	0.5
Headache	0.7	0.7
Chest Pain	0.2	0.4
Skin and Appendages		
Rash	0.0	0.4
Sweating	0.2	0.4
Digestive System		
Nausea	0.0	0.4
Overall Adverse Reactions	4.2	3.3

Additional adverse reactions have been reported, but these are, in general, not distinguishable from symptoms that might have occurred in the absence of exposure to carteolol. The following additional adverse reactions were reported by at least 1% of 1568 patients who received carteolol in controlled or open, short- or long-term clinical studies, or represent less common, but potentially important, reactions reported in clinical studies or marketing experience (these rare reactions are shown in italics): *Body as a Whole:* fever, infection, injury, malaise, pain, neck pain, shoulder pain; *Cardiovascular System:* angina pectoris, arrhythmia, *heart failure,* palpitations, *second degree heart block,* vasodilation; *Digestive System: acute hepatitis with jaundice,* constipation, dyspepsia, flatulence, gastrointestinal disorder; *Metabolic/Nutritional Disorder:* gout, *Musculoskeletal System:* pain in extremity, joint disorder, arthritis; *Nervous System: abnormal dreams,* anxiety, depression, dizziness, nervousness, somnolence; *Respiratory System:* bronchitis, *bronchospasm,* cold symptoms, cough, dyspnea, flu symptoms, lung disorder, rhinitis, sinusitis, *wheezing; Skin and Appendages:* sweating; *Special Senses:* blurred vision, conjunctivitis, eye disorder, tinnitus; *Urogenital:* impotence, urinary frequency, urinary tract infection.

In studies of patients with hypertension or angina pectoris where carteolol and positive reference beta-adrenergic blocking agents [nadolol (n=82) and propranolol (n=50)] have been compared, the differences in prevalence rates between the carteolol group and the reference agent group were statistically significant (p ≤ 0.05) for the adverse reactions listed in Table 3.

TABLE 3
Adverse Reactions During
Positive-Controlled Studies

	Reference Agents (n=132) %	Carteolol (n=135) %
Body as a Whole		
Chest Pain	5.3	0.7
Cardiovascular System		
Bradycardia	4.5	0.0
Digestive System		
Diarrhea	11.4	4.4
Nervous System		
Somnolence	0.8	7.4
Skin and Appendages		
Sweating	5.3	0.7

POTENTIAL ADVERSE REACTIONS

In addition, other adverse reactions not listed above have been reported with other beta-adrenergic blocking agents and should be considered potential adverse reactions of CARTROL (carteolol hydrochloride).

Body as a Whole:
Fever combined with aching and sore throat.
Cardiovascular System:
Intensification of AV block. (See *CONTRAINDICATIONS.*)
Digestive System:
Mesenteric arterial thrombosis, ischemic colitis.
Hemic/Lymphatic System:
Agranulocytosis, thrombocytopenic and non-thrombocytopenic purpura.
Nervous System:
Reversible mental depression progressing to catatonia; an acute reversible syndrome characterized by disorientation to time and place, short-term memory loss, emotional lability, slightly clouded sensorium, and decreased performance on neuropsychometric testing.
Respiratory System:
Laryngospasm, respiratory distress.
Skin and Appendages:
Erythematous rash, reversible alopecia.
Urogenital System:
Peyronie's disease.

The oculomucocutaneous syndrome associated with the beta-adrenergic blocking agent practolol has not been reported with carteolol.

OVERDOSAGE

No specific information on emergency treatment of overdosage in humans is available. The most common effects expected with overdosage of a beta-adrenergic blocking agent are bradycardia, bronchospasm, congestive heart failure and hypotension.

In case of overdosage, treatment with CARTROL (carteolol hydrochloride) should be discontinued and gastric lavage considered. The patient should be closely observed and vital signs carefully monitored. The prolonged effects of carteolol must be considered when determining the duration of corrective therapy. On the basis of the pharmacologic profile, the following additional measures should be considered as appropriate.
Symptomatic Bradycardia:
Administer atropine. If there is no response to vagal blockade, administer isoproterenol cautiously.
Bronchospasm:
Administer a beta₂-stimulating agent such as isoproternol and/or a theophylline derivative.
Congestive Heart Failure:
Administer diuretics and digitalis glycosides as necessary.
Hypotension:
Administer vasopressors such as intravenous dopamine, epinephrine or norepinephrine bitartrate.

DOSAGE AND ADMINISTRATION

Dosage must be individualized. The initial dose of CARTROL (carteolol hydrochloride) is 2.5 mg given as a single daily oral dose either alone or added to diuretic therapy. If an adequate response is not achieved, the dose can be gradually increased to 5 mg and 10 mg as single daily doses. Increasing the dose above 10 mg per day is unlikely to produce further substantial benefits and, in fact, may decrease the response. The usual maintenance dose of carteolol is 2.5 or 5 mg once daily.
Dosage Adjustment in Renal Impairment:
Carteolol is excreted principally by the kidneys. When administering CARTROL (carteolol hydrochloride) to patients with renal impairment, the dosage regimen should be adjusted individually by the physician. Guidelines for dose interval adjustment are shown below:

Creatinine Clearance (mL/min)	Dosage Interval (hours)
>60	24
20–60	48
<20	72

HOW SUPPLIED

CARTROL (carteolol hydrochloride) is supplied as:
2.5 mg gray tablets:
Bottles of 100 .... (**NDC** 0074-1664-13)
5 mg white tablets:
Bottles of 100 .... (**NDC** 0074-1665-13).
Recommended storage: Avoid exposure to temperatures in excess of 104°F (40°C).
Abbott Laboratories
North Chicago IL 60064
07-5664-R1
Shown in Product Identification Section, page 403

CEFOL® Filmtab® Tablets   ℞
[*c'full*]
**(B-Complex, folic acid, vitamin E
with 750 mg vitamin C)**

DESCRIPTION

Each oral Cefol Filmtab vitamin tablet provides:

Ascorbic Acid (C)	.... 750 mg
Niacinamide	.... 100 mg
Calcium Pantothenate	.... 20 mg
Thiamine Mononitrate (B₁)	.... 15 mg
Riboflavin (B₂)	.... 10 mg
Pyridoxine Hydrochloride (B₆)	.... 5 mg
Folic Acid	.... 500 mcg
Cyanocobalamin (B₁₂)	.... 6 mcg
Vitamin E (as dl-alpha tocopheryl acetate)	.... 30 IU

Inactive Ingredients: Cellulosic polymers, colloidal silicon dioxide, corn starch, D&C Yellow No. 10, FD&C Blue No. 1, magnesium stearate, microcrystalline cellulose, polyethylene glycol, povidone, propylene glycol, titanium dioxide, and vanillin.

CLINICAL PHARMACOLOGY

The vitamin components of Cefol are absorbed by the active transport process. All but Vitamin E are rapidly eliminated and not stored in the body. Vitamin E is stored in body tissues.

INDICATIONS AND USAGE

Cefol is indicated in non-pregnant* adults for the treatment of Vitamin C deficiency states with an associated deficient intake or increased need for Vitamin B-Complex, Folic Acid, and Vitamin E.
*Pregnancy may require greater Folic Acid intake.

CONTRAINDICATIONS

Rare hypersensitivity to Folic Acid.

WARNINGS

Folic Acid alone is improper treatment of pernicious anemia and other megaloblastic anemias where Vitamin B₁₂ is deficient.

PRECAUTIONS

Folic Acid above 0.1 mg daily may obscure pernicious anemia (hematologic remission may occur while neurological manifestations remain progressive).

ADVERSE REACTIONS

Allergic sensitization has been reported following oral and parenteral administration of Folic Acid.

DOSAGE

Usual adult dose is one tablet daily.

HOW SUPPLIED

Cefol is supplied as green Filmtab tablets in bottles of 100 (NDC 0074-6089-13).
Filmtab—Film-sealed tablets, Abbott.
Abbott Pharmaceuticals, Inc.
North Chicago, IL 60064
Ref. 03-1577-2/R17
Shown in Product Identification Section, page 403

CHLORTHALIDONE Tablets, USP   ℞
[*clor-thal'i-done*]

HOW SUPPLIED

Abbott Chlorthalidone Tablets, USP are available as scored tablets in two dosage strengths:
25 mg, peach-colored:
Bottles of 100 (**NDC** 0074-4325-13).
50 mg, lavender-colored:
Bottles of 100 (**NDC** 0074-4338-13).
Bottles of 500 (**NDC** 0074-4338-53).
Inactive Ingredients
25 mg tablet: Corn starch, FD&C Yellow No. 6, lactose, magnesium stearate, povidone, pregelatinized starch (contains corn starch) and talc.
50 mg tablet: Corn starch, D&C Red No. 33, FD&C Blue No. 2, lactose, magnesium stearate, povidone, pregelatinized starch (contains corn starch) and talc.
Shown in Product Identification Section, page 403

CYLERT® Tablets   ℞ ©
[*ci'lert*]
(Pemoline)

DESCRIPTION

CYLERT (pemoline) is a central nervous system stimulant. Pemoline is structurally dissimilar to the amphetamines and methylphenidate.
It is an oxazolidine compound and is chemically identified as 2-amino-5-phenyl-2-oxazolin-4-one.
Pemoline is a white, tasteless, odorless powder, relatively insoluble (less than 1 mg/ml) in water, chloroform, ether, acetone, and benzene; its solubility in 95% ethyl alcohol is 2.2 mg/ml.
CYLERT (pemoline) is supplied as tablets containing 18.75 mg, 37.5 mg or 75 mg of pemoline for oral administration. CYLERT is also available as chewable tablets containing 37.5 mg of pemoline.
Inactive Ingredients
18.75 mg tablet: corn starch, gelatin, lactose, magnesium hydroxide, polyethylene glycol and talc.
37.5 mg tablet: corn starch, FD&C Yellow No. 6, gelatin, lactose, magnesium hydroxide, polyethylene glycol and talc.

Abbott—Cont.

TESTS SHOULD BE PERFORMED PRIOR TO THERAPY AND AT FREQUENT INTERVALS THEREAFTER. ESPECIALLY DURING THE FIRST SIX MONTHS.

DESCRIPTION

DEPAKENE (valproic acid) is a carboxylic acid designated as 2-propylpentanoic acid. It is also known as dipropylacetic acid.

Valproic acid (pKa 4.8) has a molecular weight of 144 and occurs as a colorless liquid with a characteristic odor. It is slightly soluble in water (1.3 mg/ml) and very soluble in organic solvents.

DEPAKENE is supplied as soft elastic capsules and syrup for oral administration. Each capsule contains 250 mg valproic acid. The syrup contains the equivalent of 250 mg valproic acid per 5 ml as the sodium salt.

Inactive Ingredients:

250 mg capsules: corn oil, FD&C Yellow No. 6, gelatin, glycerin, iron oxide, methylparaben, propylparaben and titanium dioxide.

Syrup: FD&C Red No. 40, glycerin, methylparaben, propylparaben, sorbitol, sucrose, water and natural and artificial flavors.

CLINICAL PHARMACOLOGY

DEPAKENE is an antiepileptic agent which is chemically unrelated to other drugs used to treat seizure disorders. It has no nitrogen or aromatic moiety characteristic of other antiepileptic drugs. The mechanism by which DEPAKENE exerts its antiepileptic effects has not been established. It has been suggested that its activity is related to increased brain levels of gamma-aminobutyric acid (GABA). The effect on the neuronal membrane is unknown.

DEPAKENE is rapidly absorbed after oral administration. Peak serum levels of valproic acid occur approximately one to four hours after a single oral dose of DEPAKENE. The serum half-life of the parent compound is typically in the range of six to sixteen hours. Half-lives in the lower part of the above range are usually found in patients taking other antiepileptic drugs. A slight delay in absorption occurs when the drug is administered with meals but this does not affect the total absorption.

Valproic acid is rapidly distributed and at therapeutic drug concentrations, drug is highly bound (90%) to human plasma proteins. Increases in dose may result in decreases in the extent of protein binding and variable changes in valproate clearance and elimination.

Elimination of DEPAKENE and its metabolites occurs principally in the urine, with minor amounts in the feces and expired air. Very little unmetabolized parent drug is excreted in the urine. The drug is primarily metabolized in the liver and is excreted as the glucuronide conjugate. Other metabolites in the urine are products of beta, omega-1, and omega oxidation (C-3, C-4, and C-5 positions). The major oxidative metabolite in the urine is 2-propyl-3-keto-pentanoic acid; minor metabolites are 2-propyl-glutaric acid, 2-propyl-5-hydroxypentanoic acid, 2-propyl-3-hydroxypentanoic acid and 2-propyl-4-hydroxypentanoic acid.

INDICATIONS

DEPAKENE (valproic acid) is indicated for use as sole and adjunctive therapy in the treatment of simple (petit mal) and complex absence seizures. DEPAKENE may also be used adjunctively in patients with multiple seizure types which include absence seizures.

In accordance with the International Classification of Seizures, simple absence is defined as very brief clouding of the sensorium or loss of consciousness (lasting usually 2–15 seconds), accompanied by certain generalized epileptic discharges without other detectable clinical signs. Complex absence is the term used when other signs are also present. SEE "WARNINGS" SECTION FOR STATEMENT REGARDING FATAL HEPATIC DYSFUNCTION.

CONTRAINDICATIONS

DEPAKENE (VALPROIC ACID) SHOULD NOT BE ADMINISTERED TO PATIENTS WITH HEPATIC DISEASE OR SIGNIFICANT DYSFUNCTION.

DEPAKENE is contraindicated in patients with known hypersensitivity to the drug.

WARNINGS

Hepatic failure resulting in fatalities has occurred in patients receiving DEPAKENE. These incidents usually have occurred during the first six months of treatment with DEPAKENE. Serious or fatal hepatotoxicity may be preceded by non-specific symptoms such as loss of seizure control, malaise, weakness, lethargy, facial edema, anorexia and vomiting. Patients should be monitored closely for appearance of these symptoms. Liver function tests should be performed prior to therapy and at frequent intervals thereafter, especially during the first six months. However, physicians should not rely

totally on serum biochemistry since these tests may not be abnormal in all instances, but should also consider the results of careful interim medical history and physical examination. Caution should be observed when administering DEPAKENE to patients with a prior history of hepatic disease. Patients on multiple anticonvulsants, children, those with congenital metabolic disorders, those with severe seizure disorders accompanied by mental retardation, and those with organic brain disease may be at particular risk. Experience has indicated that children under the age of two years are at considerably increased risk of developing fatal hepatotoxicity, especially those with the aforementioned conditions. When DEPAKENE is used in this patient group, it should be used with extreme caution and as a sole agent. The benefits of seizure control should be weighed against the risks. Above this age group, experience has indicated that the incidence of fatal hepatotoxicity decreases considerably in progressively older patient groups.

The drug should be discontinued immediately in the presence of significant hepatic dysfunction, suspected or apparent. In some cases, hepatic dysfunction has progressed in spite of discontinuation of drug.

The frequency of adverse effects (particularly elevated liver enzymes) may be dose-related. The benefit of improved seizure control which may accompany the higher doses should therefore be weighed against the possibility of a greater incidence of adverse effects.

Usage in Pregnancy: ACCORDING TO PUBLISHED AND UNPUBLISHED REPORTS DEPAKENE MAY PRODUCE TERATOGENIC EFFECTS IN THE OFFSPRING OF HUMAN FEMALES RECEIVING THE DRUG DURING PREGNANCY.

THERE ARE MULTIPLE REPORTS IN THE CLINICAL LITERATURE WHICH INDICATE THAT THE USE OF ANTIEPILEPTIC DRUGS DURING PREGNANCY RESULTS IN AN INCREASED INCIDENCE OF BIRTH DEFECTS IN THE OFFSPRING. ALTHOUGH DATA ARE MORE EXTENSIVE WITH RESPECT TO TRIMETHADIONE, PARAMETHADIONE, PHENYTOIN, AND PHENOBARBITAL, REPORTS INDICATE A POSSIBLE SIMILAR ASSOCIATION WITH THE USE OF OTHER ANTIEPILEPTIC DRUGS. THEREFORE, ANTIEPILEPTIC DRUGS SHOULD BE ADMINISTERED TO WOMEN OF CHILDBEARING POTENTIAL ONLY IF THEY ARE CLEARLY SHOWN TO BE ESSENTIAL IN THE MANAGEMENT OT THEIR SEIZURES.

THE INCIDENCE OF NEURAL TUBE DEFECTS IN THE FETUS MAY BE INCREASED IN MOTHERS RECEIVING VALPROATE DURING THE FIRST TRIMESTER OF PREGNANCY. THE CENTERS FOR DISEASE CONTROL (CDC) HAS ESTIMATED THE RISK OF VALPROIC ACID EXPOSED WOMEN HAVING CHILDREN WITH SPINA BIFIDA TO BE APPROXIMATELY 1 to 2%.[1] THIS RISK IS SIMILAR TO THAT FOR NONEPILEPTIC WOMEN WHO HAVE HAD CHILDREN WITH NEURAL TUBE DEFECTS (ANENCEPHALY AND SPINA BIFIDA).

ANIMAL STUDIES HAVE ALSO DEMONSTRATED DEPAKENE INDUCED TERATOGENICITY. Studies in rats and human females demonstrated placental transfer of the drug. Doses greater than 65 mg/kg/day given to pregnant rats and mice produced skeletal abnormalities in the offspring, primarily involving ribs and vertebrae; doses greater than 150 mg/kg/day given to pregnant rabbits produced fetal resorptions and (primarily) soft-tissue abnormalities in the offspring. In rats a dose-related delay in the onset of parturition was noted. Postnatal growth and survival of the progeny were adversely affected, particularly when drug administration spanned the entire gestation and early lactation period.

Antiepileptic drugs should not be discontinued in patients in whom the drug is administered to prevent major seizures because of the strong possibility of precipitating status epilepticus with attendant hypoxia and threat to life. In individual cases where the severity and frequency of the seizure disorder are such that the removal of medication does not pose a serious threat to the patient, discontinuation of the drug may be considered prior to and during pregnancy, although it cannot be said with any confidence that even minor seizures do not pose some hazard to the developing embryo or fetus.

The prescribing physician will wish to weigh these considerations in treating or counseling epileptic women of childbearing potential.

PRECAUTIONS

Hepatic dysfunction: See "Boxed Warning," "Contraindications" and "Warnings" sections.

General: Because of reports of thrombocytopenia, inhibition of the secondary phase of platelet aggregation, and abnormal coagulation parameters, platelet counts and coagulation tests are recommended before initiating therapy and at periodic intervals. It is recommended that patients receiving DEPAKENE be monitored for platelet count and coagulation parameters prior to planned surgery. Evidence of hemorrhage, bruising or a disorder of hemostasis/coagulation is an

indication for reduction of DEPAKENE dosage or withdrawal of therapy.

Hyperammonemia with or without lethargy or coma has been reported and may be present in the absence of abnormal liver function tests. If clinically significant elevation occurs, DEPAKENE should be discontinued.

Since DEPAKENE (valproic acid) may interact with concurrently administered antiepileptic drugs, periodic serum level determinations of concomitant antiepileptic drugs are recommended during the early course of therapy. (See "Drug Interactions" section.)

DEPAKENE is partially eliminated in the urine as a keto-metabolite which may lead to a false interpretation of the urine ketone test.

There have been reports of altered thyroid function tests associated with DEPAKENE. The clinical significance of these is unknown.

Information for Patients: Since DEPAKENE may produce CNS depression, especially when combined with another CNS depressant (e.g., alcohol), patients should be advised not to engage in hazardous occupations, such as driving an automobile or operating dangerous machinery, until it is known that they do not become drowsy from the drug.

Drug Interactions: DEPAKENE may potentiate the CNS depressant activity of alcohol.

The concomitant administration of valproic acid with drugs that exhibit extensive protein binding (e.g., aspirin, carbamazepine, and dicumarol) may result in alteration of serum drug levels.

THERE IS EVIDENCE THAT DEPAKENE CAN CAUSE AN INCREASE IN SERUM PHENOBARBITAL LEVELS BY IMPAIRMENT OF NONRENAL CLEARANCE. THIS PHENOMENON CAN RESULT IN SEVERE CNS DEPRESSION. THE COMBINATION OF DEPAKENE AND PHENOBARBITAL HAS ALSO BEEN REPORTED TO PRODUCE CNS DEPRESSION WITHOUT SIGNIFICANT ELEVATIONS OF BARBITURATE OR VALPROATE SERUM LEVELS. ALL PATIENTS RECEIVING CONCOMITANT BARBITURATE THERAPY SHOULD BE CLOSELY MONITORED FOR NEUROLOGICAL TOXICITY. SERUM BARBITURATE LEVELS SHOULD BE OBTAINED, IF POSSIBLE, AND THE BARBITURATE DOSAGE DECREASED, IF APPROPRIATE.

Primidone is metabolized into a barbiturate and, therefore, may also be involved in a similar or identical interaction. THERE HAVE BEEN REPORTS OF BREAKTHROUGH SEIZURES OCCURRING WITH THE COMBINATION OF DEPAKENE AND PHENYTOIN. MOST REPORTS HAVE NOTED A DECREASE IN TOTAL PLASMA PHENYTOIN CONCENTRATION. HOWEVER, INCREASES IN TOTAL PHENYTOIN SERUM CONCENTRATION HAVE BEEN REPORTED. AN INITIAL FALL IN TOTAL PHENYTOIN LEVELS WITH SUBSEQUENT INCREASE IN PHENYTOIN LEVELS HAS ALSO BEEN REPORTED. IN ADDITION, A DECREASE IN TOTAL SERUM PHENYTOIN WITH AN INCREASE IN THE FREE VS. PROTEIN BOUND PHENYTOIN LEVELS HAS BEEN REPORTED. THE DOSAGE OF PHENYTOIN SHOULD BE ADJUSTED AS REQUIRED BY THE CLINICAL SITUATION.

THE CONCOMITANT USE OF VALPROIC ACID AND CLONAZEPAM MAY PRODUCE ABSENCE STATUS.

There is inconclusive evidence regarding the effects of valproate on serum ethosuximide levels. Patients receiving valproate and ethosuximide, especially along with other anticonvulsants, should be monitored for alterations in serum concentrations of both drugs.

Caution is recommended when DEPAKENE (valproic acid) is administered with drugs affecting coagulation, e.g., aspirin and warfarin. (See "Adverse Reactions" section.)

Carcinogenesis: DEPAKENE was administered to Sprague Dawley rats and ICR (HA/ICR) mice at doses of 0, 80 and 170 mg/kg/day for two years. Although a variety of neoplasms were observed in both species, the chief findings were a statistically significant increase in the incidence of subcutaneous fibrosarcomas in high dose male rats receiving DEPAKENE and a statistically significant dose-related trend for benign pulmonary adenomas in male mice receiving DEPAKENE. The significance of these findings for man is unknown at present.

Mutagenesis: Studies on DEPAKENE have been performed using bacterial and mammalian systems. These studies have provided no evidence of a mutagenic potential for DEPAKENE.

Fertility: Chronic toxicity studies in juvenile and adult rats and dogs demonstrated reduced spermatogenesis and testicular atrophy at doses greater than 200 mg/kg/day in rats and greater than 90 mg/kg/day in dogs. Segment I fertility studies in rats have shown doses up to 350 mg/kg/day for 60 days to have no effect on fertility. THE EFFECT OF DEPAKENE (VALPROIC ACID) ON THE DEVELOPMENT OF THE TESTES AND ON SPERM PRODUCTION AND FERTILITY IN HUMANS IS UNKNOWN.

Pregnancy: See "WARNINGS" section.

Nursing Mothers: DEPAKENE is excreted in breast milk. Concentrations in breast milk have been reported to be 1–10% of serum concentrations. It is not known what effect this would have on a nursing infant. Caution should be exercised when DEPAKENE is administered to a nursing woman.

ADVERSE REACTIONS

Since DEPAKENE (valproic acid) has usually been used with other antiepileptic drugs, it is not possible, in most cases, to determine whether the following adverse reactions can be ascribed to DEPAKENE alone, or the combination of drugs.
Gastrointestinal: The most commonly reported side effects at the initiation of therapy are nausea, vomiting and indigestion. These effects are usually transient and rarely require discontinuation of therapy. Diarrhea, abdominal cramps and constipation have been reported. Both anorexia with some weight loss and increased appetite with weight gain have also been reported. Some patients experiencing gastrointestinal side effects may benefit by converting therapy from DEPAKENE to Depakote (divalproex sodium enteric-coated tablets).[2]
CNS Effects: Sedative effects have been noted in patients receiving valproic acid alone but are found most often in patients receiving combination therapy. Sedation usually disappears upon reduction of other antiepileptic medication. Tremor has been reported in patients receiving valproate and may be dose related. Ataxia, headache, nystagmus, diplopia, asterixis, "spots before eyes", dysarthria, dizziness, and incoordination have rarely been noted. Rare cases of coma have been noted in patients receiving valproic acid alone or in conjunction with phenobarbital.
Dermatologic: Transient increases in hair loss have been observed. Skin rash, erythema multiforme, and generalized pruritus have rarely been noted.
Psychiatric: Emotional upset, depression, psychosis, aggression, hyperactivity and behavioral deterioration have been reported.
Musculoskeletal: Weakness has been reported.
Hematologic: Thrombocytopenia has been reported. Valproic acid inhibits the secondary phase of platelet aggregation. (See "Drug Interactions" section.) This may be reflected in altered bleeding time. Petechiae, bruising, hematoma formation and frank hemorrhage have been reported. (see "Precautions" section.) Relative lymphocytosis and hypofibrinogenemia have been noted. Leukopenia and eosinophilia have also been reported. Anemia and bone marrow suppression have been reported.
Hepatic: Minor elevations of transaminases (e.g., SGOT and SGPT) and LDH are frequent and appear to be dose related. Occasionally, laboratory test results include, as well, increases in serum bilirubin and abnormal changes in other liver function tests. These results may reflect potentially serious hepatotoxicity. (See "Warnings" section.)
Endocrine: There have been reports of irregular menses and secondary amenorrhea, and rare reports of breast enlargement and galactorrhea occurring in patients receiving DEPAKENE.
Abnormal thyroid function tests have been reported. (see "Precautions" section.)
Pancreatic: There have been reports of acute pancreatitis, including rare fatal cases, occurring in patients receiving DEPAKENE.
Metabolic: Hyperammonemia. (See "Precautions" section.) Hyperglycinemia has been reported and has been associated with a fatal outcome in a patient with preexistent nonketotic hyperglycinemia.
Other: Edema of the extremities has been reported.

OVERDOSAGE

Overdosage with valproic acid may result in deep coma. Since DEPAKENE is absorbed very rapidly, the value of gastric evacuation will vary with the time since ingestion. General supportive measures should be applied with particular attention being given to the maintenance of adequate urinary output.
Naloxone has been reported to reverse the CNS depressant effects of DEPAKENE overdosage. Because naloxone could theoretically also reverse the antiepileptic effects of DEPAKENE it should be used with caution.

DOSAGE AND ADMINISTRATION

DEPAKENE (valproic acid) is administered orally. The recommended initial dose is 15 mg/kg/day, increasing at one week intervals by 5 to 10 mg/kg/day, until seizures are controlled or side effects preclude further increases. The maximum recommended dosage is 60 mg/kg/day. If the total daily dose exceeds 250 mg, it should be given in a divided regimen. The following table is a guide for the initial daily dose of DEPAKENE (valproic acid) (15 mg/kg/day):
[See table above].
The frequency of adverse effects (particularly elevated liver enzymes) may be dose-related. The benefit of improved seizure control which may accompany the higher doses should therefore be weighed against the possibility of a greater incidence of adverse reactions.
A good correlation has not been established between daily dose, serum level and therapeutic effect. However, therapeutic serum levels for most patients will range from 50 to 100 mcg/ml. Occasional patients may be controlled with serum levels lower or higher than this range.

Recommended Initial Dosages for DEPAKENE

Weight (kg)	Weight (lb)	Total Daily Dose (mg)	Number of Capsules or Teaspoonfuls of Syrup Dose 1	Dose 2	Dose 3
10—24.9	22— 54.9	250	0	0	1
25—39.9	55— 87.9	500	1	0	1
40—59.9	88—131.9	750	1	1	1
60—74.9	132—164.9	1,000	1	1	2
75—89.9	165—197.9	1,250	2	1	2

As the DEPAKENE dosage is titrated upward, blood levels of phenobarbital and/or phenytoin may be affected. (See "Precautions" section.)
Patients who experience G.I. irritation may benefit from administration of the drug with food or by slowly building up the dose from an initial low level.
THE CAPSULES SHOULD BE SWALLOWED WITHOUT CHEWING TO AVOID LOCAL IRRITATION OF THE MOUTH AND THROAT.

HOW SUPPLIED

DEPAKENE (valproic acid) is available as orange-colored soft gelatin capsules* of 250 mg valproic acid in bottles of 100 capsules (NDC 0074-5681-13), in ABBO-PAC® unit dose packages of 100 capsules (NDC 0074-5681-11), and as a red syrup containing the equivalent of 250 mg valproic acid per 5 ml as the sodium salt in bottles of 16 ounces (NDC 0074-5682-16).

REFERENCES

1. Centers for Disease Control, Valproate: A New Cause of Birth Defects—Report from Italy and Follow-Up from France, *Morbidity and Mortality Weekly Report*, 32(33): 438–439, August 26, 1983.
2. Wilder, B.J., et al, Gastrointestinal Tolerance of Divalproex Sodium, *Neurology* 33:808–811, June, 1983
Abbott Laboratories
North Chicago, IL 60064
Ref. 07-5479-R17   4/16/87
Capsules shown in Product Identification Section, page 403

DEPAKOTE®   ℞
[dep 'ă-cōat]
(Divalproex Sodium
Enteric–Coated Tablets)

> **WARNING**
> HEPATIC FAILURE RESULTING IN FATALITIES HAS OCCURRED IN PATIENTS RECEIVING VALPROIC ACID AND ITS DERIVATIVES. EXPERIENCE HAS INDICATED THAT CHILDREN UNDER THE AGE OF TWO YEARS ARE AT A CONSIDERABLY INCREASED RISK OF DEVELOPING FATAL HEPATOTOXICITY, ESPECIALLY THOSE ON MULTIPLE ANTICONVULSANTS, THOSE WITH CONGENITAL METABOLIC DISORDERS, THOSE WITH SEVERE SEIZURE DISORDERS ACCOMPANIED BY MENTAL RETARDATION, AND THOSE WITH ORGANIC BRAIN DISEASE. WHEN DEPAKOTE IS USED IN THIS PATIENT GROUP, IT SHOULD BE USED WITH EXTREME CAUTION AND AS A SOLE AGENT. THE BENEFITS OF SEIZURE CONTROL SHOULD BE WEIGHED AGAINST THE RISKS. ABOVE THIS AGE GROUP, EXPERIENCE HAS INDICATED THAT THE INCIDENCE OF FATAL HEPATOTOXICITY DECREASES CONSIDERABLY IN PROGRESSIVELY OLDER PATIENT GROUPS.
> THESE INCIDENTS USUALLY HAVE OCCURRED DURING THE FIRST SIX MONTHS OF TREATMENT. SERIOUS OR FATAL HEPATOTOXICITY MAY BE PRECEDED BY NON-SPECIFIC SYMPTOMS SUCH AS LOSS OF SEIZURE CONTROL, MALAISE, WEAKNESS, LETHARGY, FACIAL EDEMA, ANOREXIA AND VOMITING. PATIENTS SHOULD BE MONITORED CLOSELY FOR APPEARANCE OF THESE SYMPTOMS. LIVER FUNCTION TESTS SHOULD BE PERFORMED PRIOR TO THERAPY AND AT FREQUENT INTERVALS THEREAFTER, ESPECIALLY DURING THE FIRST SIX MONTHS.

DESCRIPTION

Divalproex sodium is a stable co-ordination compound comprised of sodium valproate and valproic acid in a 1:1 molar relationship and formed during the partial neutralization of valproic acid with 0.5 equivalent of sodium hydroxide. Chemically it is designated as sodium hydrogen bis (2-propylpentanoate).
Divalproex sodium has a molecular weight of 310.41 and occurs as a white powder with a characteristic odor.
DEPAKOTE is an oral antiepileptic supplied as enteric-coated tablets in three dosage strengths containing divalproex sodium equivalent to 125 mg, 250 mg or 500 mg of valproic acid.

Inactive Ingredients:

125 mg tablets: cellulosic polymers, diacetylated monoglycerides, FD&C Blue No. 1, FD&C Red No. 40, povidone, pregelatinized starch (contains corn starch), silica gel, talc, titanium dioxide and vanillin.
250 mg tablets: cellulosic polymers, diacetylated monoglycerides, FD&C Yellow No. 6, iron oxide, povidone, pregelatinized starch (contains corn starch), silica gel, talc, titanium dioxide and vanillin.
500 mg tablets: cellulosic polymers, diacetylated monoglycerides, D&C Red No. 30, FD&C Blue No. 2, iron oxide, povidone, pregelatinized starch (contains corn starch), silica gel, talc, titanium dioxide and vanillin.

CLINICAL PHARMACOLOGY

DEPAKOTE is an antiepileptic agent which is chemically related to valproic acid. It has no nitrogen or aromatic moiety characteristic of other antiepileptic drugs. The mechanism by which DEPAKOTE exerts its antiepileptic effects has not been established. It has been suggested that its activity is related to increased brain levels of gamma-aminobutyric acid (GABA). The effect on the neuronal membrane is unknown. DEPAKOTE dissociates into valproate in the gastrointestinal tract.
Because of the enteric coating of DEPAKOTE, absorption is delayed one hour following oral administration. Thereafter, DEPAKOTE is uniformly and reliably absorbed, as shown by studies in normal volunteers. Peak serum levels of valproate occur in 3 to 4 hours. Bioavailability of divalproex sodium tablets was found to be equivalent to that of DEPAKENE ® (valproic acid) capsules. Concomitant administration with food would be expected to slow absorption but not affect the extent of absorption. The serum half-life of valproate is typically in the range of six to sixteen hours. Half-lives in the lower part of the above range are usually found in patients taking other antiepileptic drugs capable of enzyme induction.
Enteric-coated divalproex sodium may reduce the incidence of the irritative gastrointestinal effects of valproate as compared to valproic acid capsules.
Valproate is rapidly distributed and at therapeutic drug concentrations, drug is highly bound (90%) to human plasma proteins. Increases in dose may result in decreases in the extent of protein binding and increased valproate clearance and elimination.
Elimination of DEPAKOTE and its metabolites occurs principally in the urine, with minor amounts in the feces and expired air. Very little unmetabolized parent drug is excreted in the urine. The drug is primarily metabolized in the liver and is excreted as the glucuronide conjugate. Other metabolites in the urine are products of beta, omega-1, and omega oxidation (C-3, C-4 and C-5 positions). The major oxidative metabolite in the urine is 2-propyl-3-keto-pentanoic acid; minor metabolites are 2-propyl-glutaric acid, 2-propyl-5-hydroxypentanoic acid, 2-propyl-3-hydroxypentanoic acid and 2-propyl-4-hydroxypentanoic acid.

INDICATIONS AND USAGE

DEPAKOTE (divalproex sodium) is indicated for use as sole and adjunctive therapy in the treatment of simple (petit mal) and complex absence seizures. DEPAKOTE may also be used adjunctively in patients with multiple seizure types which include absence seizures.
In accordance with the International Classification of Seizures, simple absence is defined as very brief clouding of the sensorium or loss of consciousness (lasting usually 2–15 seconds), accompanied by certain generalized epileptic discharges without other detectable clinical signs. Complex absence is the term used when other signs are also present.
SEE "WARNINGS" SECTION FOR STATEMENT REGARDING FATAL HEPATIC DYSFUNCTION.

CONTRAINDICATIONS

DEPAKOTE (DIVALPROEX SODIUM) SHOULD NOT BE ADMINISTERED TO PATIENTS WITH HEPATIC DISEASE OR SIGNIFICANT DYSFUNCTION.

Continued on next page

Abbott—Cont.

DEPAKOTE is contraindicated in patients with known hypersensitivity to the drug.

WARNINGS

Hepatic failure resulting in fatalities has occurred in patients receiving valproic acid. These incidents usually have occurred during the first six months of treatment. Serious or fatal hepatotoxicity may be preceded by nonspecific symptoms such as loss of seizure control, malaise, weakness, lethargy, facial edema, anorexia, and vomiting. Patients should be monitored closely for appearance of these symptoms. Liver function tests should be performed prior to therapy and at frequent intervals thereafter, especially during the first six months. However, physicians should not rely totally on serum biochemistry since these tests may not be abnormal in all instances, but should also consider the results of careful interim medical history and physical examination. Caution should be observed when administering DEPAKOTE to patients with a prior history of hepatic disease. Patients on multiple anticonvulsants, children, those with congenital metabolic disorders, those with severe seizure disorders accompanied by mental retardation, and those with organic brain disease may be at particular risk. Experience has indicated that children under the age of two years are at considerably increased risk of developing fatal hepatotoxicity, especially those with the aforementioned conditions. When DEPAKOTE is used in this patient group, it should be used with extreme caution and as a sole agent. The benefits of seizure control should be weighed against the risks. Above this age group, experience has indicated that the incidence of fatal hepatotoxicity decreases considerably in progressively older patient groups.

The drug should be discontinued immediately in the presence of significant hepatic dysfunction, suspected or apparent. In some cases, hepatic dysfunction has progressed in spite of discontinuation of drug.

The frequency of adverse effects (particularly elevated liver enzymes) may be dose-related. The benefit of improved seizure control which may accompany the higher doses should therefore be weighed against the possibility of a greater incidence of adverse effects.

Usage in Pregnancy: ACCORDING TO PUBLISHED AND UNPUBLISHED REPORTS, VALPROIC ACID MAY PRODUCE TERATOGENIC EFFECTS IN THE OFFSPRING OF HUMAN FEMALES RECEIVING THE DRUG DURING PREGNANCY.

THERE ARE MULTIPLE REPORTS IN THE CLINICAL LITERATURE WHICH INDICATE THAT THE USE OF ANTIEPILEPTIC DRUGS DURING PREGNANCY RESULTS IN AN INCREASED INCIDENCE OF BIRTH DEFECTS IN THE OFFSPRING. ALTHOUGH DATA ARE MORE EXTENSIVE WITH RESPECT TO TRIMETHADIONE, PARAMETHADIONE, PHENYTOIN, AND PHENOBARBITAL, REPORTS INDICATE A POSSIBLE SIMILAR ASSOCIATION WITH THE USE OF OTHER ANTIEPILEPTIC DRUGS. THEREFORE, ANTIEPILEPTIC DRUGS SHOULD BE ADMINISTERED TO WOMEN OF CHILDBEARING POTENTIAL ONLY IF THEY ARE CLEARLY SHOWN TO BE ESSENTIAL IN THE MANAGEMENT OF THEIR SEIZURES.

THE INCIDENCE OF NEURAL TUBE DEFECTS IN THE FETUS MAY BE INCREASED IN MOTHERS RECEIVING VALPROATE DURING THE FIRST TRIMESTER OF PREGNANCY. THE CENTERS FOR DISEASE CONTROL (CDC) HAS ESTIMATED THE RISK OF VALPROIC ACID EXPOSED WOMEN HAVING CHILDREN WITH SPINA BIFIDA TO BE APPROXIMATELY 1 to 2%.[1] THIS RISK IS SIMILAR TO THAT FOR NONEPILEPTIC WOMEN WHO HAVE HAD CHILDREN WITH NEURAL TUBE DEFECTS (ANENCEPHALY AND SPINA BIFIDA).

ANIMAL STUDIES HAVE ALSO DEMONSTRATED VALPROIC ACID INDUCED TERATOGENICITY. Studies in rats and human females demonstrated placental transfer of the drug. Doses greater than 65 mg/kg/day given to pregnant rats and mice produced skeletal abnormalities in the offspring, primarily involving ribs and vertebrae; doses greater than 150 mg/kg/day given to pregnant rabbits produced fetal resorptions and (primarily) soft-tissue abnormalities in the offspring. In rats a dose-related delay in the onset of parturition was noted. Postnatal growth and survival of the progeny were adversely affected, particularly when drug administration spanned the entire gestation and early lactation period.

Antiepileptic drugs should not be discontinued in patients in whom the drug is administered to prevent major seizures because of the strong possibility of precipitating status epilepticus with attendant hypoxia and threat to life. In individual cases where the severity and frequency of the seizure disorder are such that the removal of medication does not pose a serious threat to the patient, discontinuation of the drug may be considered prior to and during pregnancy, although it cannot be said with any confidence that even minor seizures do not pose some hazard to the developing embryo or fetus.

The prescribing physician will wish to weigh these considerations in treating or counseling epileptic women of childbearing potential.

PRECAUTIONS

Hepatic Dysfunction: See "Boxed Warning," "Contraindications" and "Warnings" sections.

General: Because of reports of thrombocytopenia, inhibition of the secondary phase of platelet aggregation, and abnormal coagulation parameters, platelet counts and coagulation tests are recommended before initiating therapy and at periodic intervals. It is recommended that patients receiving DEPAKOTE (divalproex sodium) be monitored for platelet count and coagulation parameters prior to planned surgery. Evidence of hemorrhage, bruising or a disorder of hemostasis/coagulation is an indication for reduction of DEPAKOTE dosage or withdrawal of therapy.

Hyperammonemia with or without lethargy or coma has been reported and may be present in the absence of abnormal liver function tests. If clinically significant elevation occurs, DEPAKOTE should be discontinued.

Since DEPAKOTE (divalproex sodium) may interact with concurrently administered antiepileptic drugs, periodic serum level determinations of concomitant antiepileptic drugs are recommended during the early course of therapy. (See "Drug Interactions" section).

Valproate is partially eliminated in the urine as a keto-metabolite which may lead to a false interpretation of the urine ketone test.

There have been reports of altered thyroid function tests associated with valproate. The clinical significance of these is unknown.

Information for Patients: Since DEPAKOTE may produce CNS depression, especially when combined with another CNS depressant (e.g., alcohol), patients should be advised not to engage in hazardous occupations, such as driving an automobile or operating dangerous machinery, until it is known that they do not become drowsy from the drug.

Drug Interactions: Valproic acid may potentiate the CNS depressant activity of alcohol.

The concomitant administration of valproic acid with drugs that exhibit extensive protein binding (e.g., aspirin, carbamazepine, and dicumarol) may result in alteration of serum drug levels.

THERE IS EVIDENCE THAT VALPROIC ACID CAN CAUSE AN INCREASE IN SERUM PHENOBARBITAL LEVELS BY IMPAIRMENT OF NONRENAL CLEARANCE. THIS PHENOMENON CAN RESULT IN SEVERE CNS DEPRESSION. THE COMBINATION OF VALPROIC ACID AND PHENOBARBITAL HAS ALSO BEEN REPORTED TO PRODUCE CNS DEPRESSION WITHOUT SIGNIFICANT ELEVATIONS OF BARBITURATE OR VALPROATE SERUM LEVELS. ALL PATIENTS RECEIVING CONCOMITANT BARBITURATE THERAPY SHOULD BE CLOSELY MONITORED FOR NEUROLOGICAL TOXICITY. SERUM BARBITURATE LEVELS SHOULD BE OBTAINED, IF POSSIBLE, AND THE BARBITURATE DOSAGE DECREASED, IF APPROPRIATE. Primidone is metabolized into a barbiturate and, therefore, may also be involved in a similar or identical interaction. THERE HAVE BEEN REPORTS OF BREAK-THROUGH SEIZURES OCCURRING WITH THE COMBINATION OF VALPROIC ACID AND PHENYTOIN. MOST REPORTS HAVE NOTED A DECREASE IN TOTAL PLASMA PHENYTOIN CONCENTRATION. HOWEVER, INCREASES IN TOTAL PHENYTOIN SERUM CONCENTRATION HAVE BEEN REPORTED. AN INITIAL FALL IN TOTAL PHENYTOIN LEVELS WITH SUBSEQUENT INCREASE IN PHENYTOIN LEVELS HAS ALSO BEEN REPORTED. IN ADDITION, A DECREASE IN TOTAL SERUM PHENYTOIN WITH AN INCREASE IN THE FREE VS. PROTEIN BOUND PHENYTOIN LEVELS HAS BEEN REPORTED. THE DOSAGE OF PHENYTOIN SHOULD BE ADJUSTED AS REQUIRED BY THE CLINICAL SITUATION. THE CONCOMITANT USE OF VALPROIC ACID AND CLONAZEPAM MAY PRODUCE ABSENCE STATUS.

There is inconclusive evidence regarding the effect of valproate on serum ethosuximide levels. Patients receiving valproate and ethosuximide, especially along with other anticonvulsants, should be monitored for alterations in serum concentrations of both drugs.

Caution is recommended when DEPAKOTE (divalproex sodium) is administered with drugs affecting coagulation, e.g., aspirin and warfarin. (See "Adverse Reactions" section).

Carcinogenesis: Valproic acid was administered to Sprague Dawley rats and ICR (HA /ICR) mice at doses of 0, 80 and 170 mg/kg/day for two years. Although a variety of neoplasms were observed in both species, the chief findings were a statistically significant increase in the incidence of subcutaneous fibrosarcomas in high dose male rats receiving valproic acid and a statistically significant dose-related trend for benign pulmonary adenomas in male mice receiving valproic acid. The significance of these findings for man is unknown at present.

Mutagenesis: Studies on valproic acid have been performed using bacterial and mammalian systems. These studies have provided no evidence of a mutagenic potential for DEPAKOTE.

Fertility: Chronic toxicity studies in juvenile and adult rats and dogs demonstrated reduced spermatogenesis and testicular atrophy at doses greater than 200 mg/kg/day in rats and greater than 90 mg/kg/day in dogs. Segment I fertility studies in rats have shown doses up to 350 mg/kg/day for 60 days to have no effect on fertility. THE EFFECT OF DEPAKOTE (DIVALPROEX SODIUM) ON THE DEVELOPMENT OF THE TESTES AND ON SPERM PRODUCTION AND FERTILITY IN HUMANS IS UNKNOWN.

Pregnancy: Pregnancy Category D: See "Warnings" section.

Nursing Mothers: Valproate is excreted in breast milk. Concentrations in breast milk have been reported to be 1–10% of serum concentrations. It is not known what effect this would have on a nursing infant. Caution should be exercised when DEPAKOTE is administered to a nursing woman.

ADVERSE REACTIONS

Since valproic acid and its derivatives have usually been used with other antiepileptic drugs, it is not possible, in most cases, to determine whether the following adverse reactions can be ascribed to valproic acid alone, or the combination of drugs.

Gastrointestinal: The most commonly reported side effects at the initiation of therapy are nausea, vomiting and indigestion. These effects are usually transient and rarely require discontinuation of therapy. Diarrhea, abdominal cramps and constipation have been reported. Both anorexia with some weight loss and increased appetite with weight gain have also been reported. The administration of enteric-coated divalproex sodium may result in reduction of gastrointestinal side effects in some patients.[2]

CNS Effects: Sedative effects have been noted in patients receiving valproic acid alone but are found most often in patients receiving combination therapy. Sedation usually disappears upon reduction of other antiepileptic medication. Tremor has been reported in patients receiving valproate and may be dose-related. Ataxia, headache, nystagmus, diplopia, asterixis, "spots before eyes," dysarthria, dizziness, and incoordination have rarely been noted. Rare cases of coma have been noted in patients receiving valproic acid alone or in conjunction with phenobarbital.

Dermatologic: Transient increases in hair loss have been observed. Skin rash, erythema multiforme, and generalized pruritus have rarely been noted.

Psychiatric: Emotional upset, depression, psychosis, aggression, hyperactivity and behavioral deterioration have been reported.

Musculoskeletal: Weakness has been reported.

Hematologic: Thrombocytopenia has been reported. Valproic acid inhibits the secondary phase of platelet aggregation. (See "Drug Interactions" section). This may be reflected in altered bleeding time. Petechiae, bruising, hematoma formation, and frank hemorrhage have been reported. (See "Precautions" section). Relative lymphocytosis and hypofibrinogenemia have been noted. Leukopenia and eosinophilia have also been reported. Anemia and bone marrow suppression have been reported.

Hepatic: Minor elevations of transaminases (e.g., SGOT and SGPT) and LDH are frequent and appear to be dose related. Occasionally, laboratory test results include, as well, increases in serum bilirubin and abnormal changes in other liver function tests. These results may reflect potentially serious hepatotoxicity. (See "Warnings" section).

Endocrine: There have been reports of irregular menses and secondary amenorrhea, and rare reports of breast enlargement and galactorrhea occurring in patients receiving valproic acid and its derivatives.

Abnormal thyroid function tests have been reported. (See "Precautions" section).

Pancreatic: There have been reports of acute pancreatitis, including rare fatal cases, occurring in patients receiving valproic acid and its derivatives.

Metabolic: Hyperammonemia. (See "Precautions" section). Hyperglycinemia has been reported and has been associated with a fatal outcome in a patient with preexistent nonketotic hyperglycinemia.

Other: Edema of the extremities has been reported.

OVERDOSAGE

Overdosage with valproic acid may result in deep coma. Since DEPAKOTE tablets are enteric-coated, the benefit of gastric lavage or emesis will vary with the time since ingestion. General supportive measures should be applied with particular attention being given to the maintenance of adequate urinary output.

Naloxone has been reported to reverse the CNS depressant effects of valproate overdosage. Because naloxone could theoretically also reverse the antiepileptic effects of DEPAKOTE it should be used with caution.

DOSAGE AND ADMINISTRATION

DEPAKOTE is administered orally. The recommended initial dose is 15 mg/kg/day, increasing at one week intervals by 5 to 10 mg/kg/day until seizures are controlled or side effects preclude further increases. The maximum recommended dosage is 60 mg/kg/day. If the total daily dose exceeds 250 mg, it should be given in a divided regimen.

Conversion from DEPAKENE to DEPAKOTE: In patients previously receiving DEPAKENE (valproic acid) therapy, DEPAKOTE should be initiated at the same total daily dose and dosing schedule.[3] After the patient is stabilized on DEPAKOTE, a twice-a-day or three-times-a-day schedule may be instituted in selected patients.

The frequency of adverse effects (particularly elevated liver enzymes) may be dose-related. The benefit of improved seizure control which may accompany higher doses should therefore be weighed against the possibility of a greater incidence of adverse reactions.

A good correlation has not been established between daily dose, serum level and therapeutic effect. However, therapeutic valproate serum levels for most patients will range from 50 to 100 mcg/ml. Occasional patients may be controlled with serum levels lower or higher than this range.

As the DEPAKOTE dosage is titrated upward, blood levels of phenobarbital and/or phenytoin may be affected. (See "Precautions" section).

Patients who experience G. I. irritation may benefit from administration of the drug with food or by slowly building up the dose from an initial low level.

HOW SUPPLIED

DEPAKOTE (divalproex sodium enteric-coated tablets) are supplied as:

125 mg salmon pink-colored tablets in bottles of 100 (**NDC** 0074-6212-13) and Abbo-Pac® unit dose packages of 100 (**NDC** 0074-6212-11).

250 mg peach-colored tablets in bottles of 100 (**NDC** 0074-6214-13) and Abbo-Pac® unit dose packages of 100 (**NDC** 0074-6214-11).

500 mg lavender-colored tablets in bottles of 100 (**NDC** 0074-6215-13) and Abbo-Pac® unit dose packages of 100 (**NDC** 0074-6215-11).

REFERENCES

1. Centers for Disease Control, Valproate: A New Cause of Birth Defects—Report from Italy and Follow-up from France, *Morbidity and Mortality Weekly Report* 32(33):438–439, August 26, 1983.
2. Wilder, B.J., et al, Gastrointestinal Tolerance of Divalproex Sodium, *Neurology* 33:808–811, June, 1983.
3. Wilder, B.J., et al, Twice-Daily Dosing of Valproate with Divalproex, *Clin Pharmacol Ther* 34(4): 501–504, 1983.

Abbott Laboratories
North Chicago, IL 60064
Ref. 03-4325-R11

Shown in Product Identification Section, page 403

DESOXYN®
(methamphetamine hydrochloride)
Tablets—Gradumet® Tablets   ℞ ©

METHAMPHETAMINE HAS A HIGH POTENTIAL FOR ABUSE. IT SHOULD THUS BE TRIED ONLY IN WEIGHT REDUCTION PROGRAMS FOR PATIENTS IN WHOM ALTERNATIVE THERAPY HAS BEEN INEFFECTIVE. ADMINISTRATION OF METHAMPHETAMINE FOR PROLONGED PERIODS OF TIME IN OBESITY MAY LEAD TO DRUG DEPENDENCE AND MUST BE AVOIDED. PARTICULAR ATTENTION SHOULD BE PAID TO THE POSSIBILITY OF SUBJECTS OBTAINING METHAMPHETAMINE FOR NON-THERAPEUTIC USE OR DISTRIBUTION TO OTHERS, AND THE DRUG SHOULD BE PRESCRIBED OR DISPENSED SPARINGLY.

DESCRIPTION

DESOXYN (methamphetamine hydrochloride), chemically known as (S)-N, α-dimethylbenzeneethanamine hydrochloride, is a member of the amphetamine group of sympathomimetic amines.

DESOXYN is available as Gradumet sustained-release tablets containing 5 mg, 10 mg or 15 mg of methamphetamine hydrochloride and as conventional tablets containing 5 mg methamphetamine hydrochloride, for oral administration. The Gradumet is an inert, porous, plastic matrix, which is impregnated with DESOXYN. The drug is leached slowly from the Gradumet as it passes through the gastrointestinal tract. The expended matrix is not absorbed and is excreted in the stool.

Inactive Ingredients: 5 mg Gradumet tablet: magnesium stearate, methyl acrylate-methyl methacrylate copolymer, povidone, talc and other ingredients.

10 mg Gradumet tablet: FD&C Yellow No. 6 (Sunset Yellow), magnesium stearate, methyl acrylate-methyl methacrylate copolymer, povidone, talc and other ingredients.

15 mg Gradumet tablet: FD&C Yellow No. 5 (tartrazine), magnesium stearate, methyl acrylate-methyl methacrylate copolymer, povidone, talc and other ingredients.

5 mg tablet: corn starch, lactose, sodium paraminobenzoate, stearic acid, talc and other ingredients.

CLINICAL PHARMACOLOGY

DESOXYN (methamphetamine hydrochloride) is a sympathomimetic amine with CNS stimulant activity. Peripheral actions include elevation of systolic and diastolic blood pressures and weak bronchodilator and respiratory stimulant action. Drugs of this class used in obesity are commonly known as "anorectics" or "anorexigenics." It has not been established, however, that the action of such drugs in treating obesity is primarily one of appetite suppression. Other central nervous system actions, or metabolic effects, may be involved, for example.

Adult obese subjects instructed in dietary management and treated with "anorectic" drugs, lose more weight on the average than those treated with placebo and diet, as determined in relatively short-term clinical trials.

The magnitude of increased weight loss of drug-treated patients over placebo-treated patients is only a fraction of a pound a week. The rate of weight loss is greatest in the first weeks of therapy for both drug and placebo subjects and tends to decrease in succeeding weeks. The origins of the increased weight loss due to the various possible drug effects are not established. The amount of weight loss associated with the use of an "anorectic" drug varies from trial to trial, and the increased weight loss appears to be related in part to variables other than the drug prescribed, such as the physician-investigator, the population treated, and the diet prescribed. Studies do not permit conclusions as to the relative importance of the drug and non-drug factors on weight loss. The natural history of obesity is measured in years, whereas the studies cited are restricted to a few weeks duration; thus, the total impact of drug-induced weight loss over that of diet alone must be considered clinically limited.

The mechanism of action involved in producing the beneficial behavioral changes seen in hyperkinetic children receiving DESOXYN is unknown.

In humans, methamphetamine is rapidly absorbed from the gastrointestinal tract. The primary site of metabolism is in the liver by aromatic hydroxylation, N-dealkylation and deamination. At least seven metabolites have been identified in the urine. The biological half-life has been reported in the range of 4 to 5 hours. Excretion occurs primarily in the urine and is dependent on urine pH. Alkaline urine will significantly increase the drug half-life. Approximately 62% of an oral dose is eliminated in the urine within the first 24 hours with about one-third as intact drug and the remainder as metabolites.

INDICATIONS AND USAGE

Attention Deficit Disorder with Hyperactivity—DESOXYN is indicated as an integral part of a total treatment program which typically includes other remedial measures (psychological, educational, social) for a stabilizing effect in children over 6 years of age with a behavioral syndrome characterized by the following group of developmentally inappropriate symptoms: moderate to severe distractibility, short attention span, hyperactivity, emotional lability, and impulsivity. The diagnosis of this syndrome should not be made with finality when these symptoms are only of comparatively recent origin. Nonlocalizing (soft) neurological signs, learning disability, and abnormal EEG may or may not be present, and a diagnosis of central nervous system dysfunction may or may not be warranted.

Exogenous Obesity—as a short-term (i.e., a few weeks) adjunct in a regimen of weight reduction based on caloric restriction, for patients in whom obesity is refractory to alternative therapy, e.g., repeated diets, group programs, and other drugs. The limited usefulness of DESOXYN (see "Clinical Pharmacology" section) should be weighed against possible risks inherent in use of the drug, such as those described below.

CONTRAINDICATIONS

DESOXYN is contraindicated during or within 14 days following the administration of monoamine oxidase inhibitors; hypertensive crises may result. It is also contraindicated in patients with glaucoma, advanced arteriosclerosis, symptomatic cardiovascular disease, moderate to severe hypertension, hyperthyroidism or known hypersensitivity or idiosyncrasy to sympathomimetic amines. Methamphetamine should not be given to patients who are in an agitated state or who have a history of drug abuse.

WARNINGS

Tolerance to the anorectic effect usually develops within a few weeks. When this occurs, the recommended dose should not be exceeded in an attempt to increase the effect; rather, the drug should be discontinued (see "Drug Abuse and Dependence" section).

Decrements in the predicted growth (i.e., weight gain and/or height) rate have been reported with the long-term use of

stimulants in children. Therefore, patients requiring long-term therapy should be carefully monitored.

Usage in Nursing Mothers: Amphetamines are excreted in human milk. Mothers taking amphetamines should be advised to refrain from nursing.

PRECAUTIONS

General: DESOXYN (methamphetamine hydrochloride) should be used with caution in patients with even mild hypertension.

Methamphetamine should not be used to combat fatigue or to replace rest in normal persons.

Prescribing and dispensing of methamphetamine should be limited to the smallest amount that is feasible at one time in order to minimize the possibility of overdosage.

The 15 mg dosage strength of DESOXYN Gradumet tablets contains FD&C Yellow No. 5 (tartrazine) which may cause allergic-type reactions (including bronchial asthma) in certain susceptible individuals. Although the overall incidence of FD&C Yellow No. 5 (tartrazine) sensitivity in the general population is low, it is frequently seen in patients who also have aspirin hypersensitivity.

Information for Patients: The patient should be informed that methamphetamine may impair the ability to engage in potentially hazardous activities, such as, operating machinery or driving a motor vehicle.

The patient should be cautioned not to increase dosage, except on advice of the physician.

Drug Interactions: Insulin requirements in diabetes mellitus may be altered in association with the use of methamphetamine and concomitant dietary regimen.

Methamphetamine may decrease the hypotensive effect of *guanethidine*.

DESOXYN should not be used concurrently with *monoamine oxidase inhibitors* (see "Contraindications" section).

Concurrent administration of *tricyclic antidepressants* and indirect-acting sympathomimetic amines such as amphetamines, should be closely supervised and dosage carefully adjusted.

Phenothiazines are reported in the literature to antagonize the CNS stimulant action of the amphetamines.

Drug/Laboratory Test Interactions: Literature reports suggest that amphetamines may be associated with significant elevation of plasma corticosteroids. This should be considered if determination of plasma corticosteroid levels is desired in a person receiving amphetamines.

Carcinogensis, Mutagenesis, Impairment of Fertility: Data are not available on long-term potential for carcinogenicity, mutagenicity, or impairment of fertility.

Pregnancy: Teratogenic effects: Pregnancy Category C. Methamphetamine has been shown to have teratogenic and embryocidal effects in mammals given high multiples of the human dose. There are no adequate and well-controlled studies in pregnant women. DESOXYN should not be used during pregnancy unless the potential benefit justifies the potential risk to the fetus.

Nonteratogenic effects: Infants born to mothers dependent on amphetamines have an increased risk of premature delivery and low birth weight. Also, these infants may experience symptoms of withdrawal as demonstrated by dysphoria, including agitation and significant lassitude.

Nursing Mothers: See "Warnings" section.

Pediatric Use: Safety and effectiveness for use as an anorectic agent in children below the age of 12 years have not been established.

Long-term effects of DESOXYN in children have not been established (see "Warnings" section).

Drug treatment is not indicated in all cases of the behavioral syndrome characterized by moderate to severe distractibility, short attention span, hyperactivity, emotional lability and impulsivity. It should be considered only in light of the complete history and evaluation of the child. The decision to prescribe DESOXYN should depend on the physician's assessment of the chronicity and severity of the child's symptoms and their appropriateness for his/her age. Prescription should not depend solely on the presence of one or more of the behavioral characteristics.

When these symptoms are associated with acute stress reaction, treatment with DESOXYN is usually not indicated.

Clinical experience suggests that in psychotic children, administration of DESOXYN may exacerbate symptoms of behavior disturbance and thought disorder.

Amphetamines have been reported to exacerbate motor and phonic tics and Tourette's syndrome. Therefore, clinical evaluation for tics and Tourette's syndrome in children and their families should precede use of stimulant medications.

Continued on next page

If desired, additional literature on any Abbott Product will be provided upon request to Abbott Laboratories.

Abbott—Cont.

ADVERSE REACTIONS

The following are adverse reactions in decreasing order of severity within each category that have been reported with DESOXYN:

Cardiovascular: Elevation of blood pressure, tachycardia and palpitation.

Central Nervous System: Psychotic episodes have been rarely reported at recommended doses. Dizziness, dysphoria, overstimulation, euphoria, insomnia, tremor, restlessness and headache. Exacerbation of motor and phonic tics and Tourette's syndrome.

Gastrointestinal: Diarrhea, constipation, dryness of mouth, unpleasant taste and other gastrointestinal disturbances.

Hypersensitivity: Urticaria.

Endocrine: Impotence and changes in libido.

Miscellaneous: Suppression of growth has been reported with the long-term use of stimulants in children (see "Warnings" section).

DRUG ABUSE AND DEPENDENCE

Controlled Substance: DESOXYN (methamphetamine hydrochloride) is subject to control under DEA schedule II.

Abuse: DESOXYN has been extensively abused. Tolerance, extreme psychological dependence, and severe social disability have occurred. There are reports of patients who have increased the dosage to many times that recommended. Abrupt cessation following prolonged high dosage administration results in extreme fatigue and mental depression; changes are also noted on the sleep EEG. Manifestations of chronic intoxication with DESOXYN include severe dermatoses, marked insomnia, irritability, hyperactivity, and personality changes. The most severe manifestation of chronic intoxication is psychosis, often clinically indistinguishable from schizophrenia.

OVERDOSAGE

Manifestations of acute overdosage with methamphetamine include restlessness, tremor, hyperreflexia, rapid respiration, confusion, assaultiveness, hallucinations, panic states, hyperpyrexia, and rhabdomyolysis. Fatigue and depression usually follow the central stimulation. Cardiovascular effects include arrhythmias, hypertension or hypotension, and circulatory collapse. Gastrointestinal symptoms include nausea, vomiting, diarrhea, and abdominal cramps. Fatal poisoning usually terminates in convulsions and coma.

Management of acute methamphetamine intoxication is largely symptomatic and includes gastric evacuation and sedation with a barbiturate. Experience with hemodialysis or peritoneal dialysis is inadequate to permit recommendations in this regard.

Acidification of urine increases methamphetamine excretion. Intravenous phentolamine (Regitine®) has been suggested for possible acute, severe hypertension, if this complicates methamphetamine overdosage. Usually a gradual drop in blood pressure will result when sufficient sedation has been achieved. Chlorpromazine has been reported to be useful in decreasing CNS stimulation and sympathomimetic effects.

Since the Gradumet tablet releases methamphetamine gradually, therapy should be directed at reversing the effects of the ingested drug and at supporting the patient until symptoms subside. Saline cathartics are useful for hastening the evacuation of the tablets that have not already released medication.

DOSAGE AND ADMINISTRATION

DESOXYN (methamphetamine hydrochloride) is given orally. Methamphetamine should be administered at the lowest effective dosage, and dosage should be individually adjusted. Late evening medication should be avoided because of the resulting insomnia.

Attention Deficit Disorder with Hyperactivity:

For treatment of children 6 years or older with a behavioral syndrome characterized by moderate to severe distractibility, short attention span, hyperactivity, emotional lability and impulsivity: an initial dose of 5 mg DESOXYN (methamphetamine hydrochloride) once or twice a day is recommended. Daily dosage may be raised in increments of 5 mg at weekly intervals until optimum clinical response is achieved. The usual effective dose is 20 to 25 mg daily. The total daily dose may be given as conventional tablets in two divided doses daily or once daily using the Gradumet tablet. The Gradumet form should not be utilized for initiation of dosage nor until the conventional titrated daily dosage is equal to or greater than the dosage provided in a Gradumet tablet. Where possible, drug administration should be interrupted occasionally to determine if there is a recurrence of behavioral symptoms sufficient to require continued therapy.

For obesity: one Gradumet tablet, 10 or 15 mg, once a day in the morning. When the conventional tablet form is prescribed, 5 mg should be taken one-half hour before each meal. Treatment should not exceed a few weeks in duration.

Methamphetamine is not recommended for use as an anorectic agent in children under 12 years of age.

HOW SUPPLIED

DESOXYN (methamphetamine hydrochloride) is supplied as follows:

Gradumet Tablets, 5 mg, white, in bottles of 100 (**NDC** 0074-6941-04); 10 mg, orange, in bottles of 100 (**NDC** 0074-6948-08) and 500 (**NDC** 0074-6948-09); and 15 mg, yellow, in bottles of 100 (**NDC** 0074-6959-07) and 500 (**NDC** 0074-6959-08).

Tablets, 5 mg, white, in bottles of 100 (**NDC** 0074-3377-04).

Abbott Pharmaceuticals Inc.

North Chicago, IL 60064

Ref. 03-4314-R9

Shown in Product Identification Section, page 403

DICAL-D® TABLETS—WAFERS

[*dī'cal-d*]

(Dibasic Calcium Phosphate with Vitamin D)

DESCRIPTION

Tablets

Daily dosage (three tablets) provides:

Vitamin D	399 IU	99% USRDA*
	(10 mcg)	
Calcium	0.35 g	35% USRDA
Phosphorus	0.27 g	27% USRDA

Each tablet contains:

Dibasic Calcium Phosphate, hydrous (as anhydrous form) .... 500 mg

Cholecalciferol .... 3.33 mcg (133 IU)

Microcrystalline cellulose, sodium starch glycolate, corn starch, hydrogenated vegetable oil wax, magnesium stearate and talc added.

Calcium to phosphorous ratio 1.3 to 1.

Wafers

Daily dosage (two wafers) provides:

Vitamin D	400 IU	100% USRDA
	(10 mcg)	
Calcium	0.464 g	46% USRDA
Phosphorous	0.36 g	36% USRDA

Each wafer contains:

Cholecalciferol .... 5 mcg (200 IU)

Dibasic Calcium Phosphate, hydrous .... 1 g

Added dextrose, sucrose, talc, stearic acid, mineral oil, salt, and natural and artificial flavorings.

Calcium to phosphorous ratio 1.29 to 1.

*% U.S. Recommended Daily Allowance for adults and children 4 or more years of age.

INDICATIONS

For those individuals who must restrict their intake of dairy products.

DOSAGE AND ADMINISTRATION

Usual dose for adults and children 4 years and older:

Wafers—Chew 1 wafer twice daily with meals, or as directed by the physician or dentist.

Tablets—1 tablet 3 times daily with meals, or as directed by the physician or dentist.

HOW SUPPLIED

Dical-D Tablets in bottles of 100 (NDC 0074-3741-13) and 500 (NDC 0074-3741-53).

Dical-D Wafers in box of 51 (NDC 0074-3589-01).

Abbott Laboratories/

Abbott Pharmaceuticals, Inc.

North Chicago, IL 60064

Ref. 03-1395-2/R1 & 09-5876-5/R9

DICUMAROL Tablets, USP   ℞

[*dīcoo'mu-rawl*]

DESCRIPTION

Dicumarol is a coumarin anticoagulant, chemically designated as 3,3'-methylenebis [4-hydroxycoumarin].

Inactive Ingredients:

25 mg tablets: corn starch, lactose, magnesium stearate, talc and other ingredients.

50 mg tablets: corn starch, D&C Red No. 30, lactose, stearic acid, talc and other ingredients.

ACTIONS

Dicumarol and other coumarin anticoagulants act by depressing synthesis in the liver of several factors which are known to be active in the coagulation mechanisms in a variety of diseases characterized by thromboembolic phenomena. The resultant *in vivo* effect is a sequential depression of Factors VII, IX, X and II. The degree of depression is dependent upon the dosage administered. Anticoagulants have no direct effect on an established thrombus, nor do they reverse ischemic tissue damage. However, once a thrombosis has occurred, anticoagulant treatment aims to prevent further extension of the formed clot and prevents secondary throm-

boembolic complications which may result in serious and possible fatal sequelae.

Maximal plasma concentrations are reached in 1 to 9 hours. Approximately 97% is bound to albumin within the plasma. Dicumarol usually induces hypoprothrombinemia in 36 to 48 hours, and its duration of action may persist for 5 to 6 days, thus producing a smooth, long lasting response curve. Little is known of the metabolic pathways involved in the biotransformation of oral anticoagulants in man. However, their metabolites appear to be eliminated principally in the urine.

INDICATIONS

Dicumarol is indicated for the prophylaxis and treatment of venous thrombosis and its extension, the treatment of atrial fibrillation with embolization, the prophylaxis and treatment of pulmonary embolism, and as an adjunct in the treatment of coronary occlusion.

CONTRAINDICATIONS

Anticoagulation is contraindicated in any localized or general physical condition or personal circumstance in which the hazard of hemorrhage might be greater than its potential clinical benefits, such as:

Pregnancy:

Dicumarol is contraindicated in pregnancy because the drug passes through the placental barrier and may cause fatal hemorrhage to the fetus in utero. Furthermore, there have been reports of birth malformations in children born to mothers who have been treated with dicumarol during pregnancy. Women of childbearing potential who are candidates for anticoagulant therapy should be carefully evaluated and the indications critically reviewed with the patient. If the patient becomes pregnant while taking this drug, she should be apprised of the potential risks to the fetus, and the possibility of termination of the pregnancy should be discussed in light of those risks.

Hemorrhagic tendencies or blood dyscrasias.

Recent or contemplated surgery of:

(1) central nervous system; (2) eye; (3) traumatic surgery resulting in large open surfaces.

Bleeding tendencies associated with active ulceration or overt bleeding of:

(1) gastrointestinal, genitourinary or respiratory tracts; (2) cerebrovascular hemorrhage; (3) aneurysms—cerebral, dissecting aorta; (4) pericarditis and pericardial effusions.

Threatened abortion, eclampsia and preeclampsia.

Inadequate laboratory facilities or unsupervised senility, alcoholism, psychosis; or lack of patient cooperation.

Spinal puncture and other diagnostic or therapeutic procedures with potential for uncontrollable bleeding.

Miscellaneous: major regional, lumbar block anesthesia, severe uncontrolled and/or malignant hypertension, subacute bacterial endocarditis, open wounds, visceral carcinoma, vitamin K deficiency, and severe liver or kidney disease.

WARNINGS

The most serious risks associated with anticoagulant therapy with dicumarol are hemorrhage in any tissue or organ and, less frequently, necrosis and/or gangrene of skin and other tissues. The risk of hemorrhage is related to the level of intensity and the duration of anticoagulant therapy. Hemorrhage and necrosis have in some cases been reported to result in death or permanent disability. Necrosis appears to be associated with local thrombosis and usually appears within a few days of the start of anticoagulant therapy. In severe cases of necrosis, treatment through debridement or amputation of the affected tissue, limb, breast or penis has been reported. Careful diagnosis is required to determine whether necrosis is caused by an underlying disease. Dicumarol therapy should be discontinued when dicumarol is suspected to be the cause of developing necrosis and heparin therapy may be considered for anticoagulation. Although various treatments have been attempted, no treatment for necrosis has been considered uniformly effective. See below for information on predisposing conditions. These and other risks associated with anticoagulant therapy must be weighed against the risk of thrombosis or embolization in untreated cases. Dicumarol is a potent drug with a half-life of 1 to 2 days; therefore its effects may become more pronounced as daily maintenance doses overlap. It cannot be emphasized too strongly that treatment of each patient is a highly individualized matter. Dosage should be controlled by periodic determinations of prothrombin time or other suitable coagulation tests. Determinations of whole blood clotting and bleeding times are not effective measures for control of therapy. Heparin prolongs the one-stage prothrombin time. Therefore, to obtain a valid prothrombin time when heparin and dicumarol are given together, a period of at least 5 hours should elapse after the last intravenous dose and 24 hours after the last subcutaneous dose of heparin, before blood is drawn. Caution should be observed when dicumarol is administered in any situation or in the presence of any predisposing condition where added risk of hemorrhage or necrosis is present. Administration of anticoagulants in the following conditions will be based upon clinical judgment in which the risks of anticoagulant therapy are weighed against the risk of thrombosis or embolization in untreated cases. The following may be associated with these increased risks:

Lactation—Coumarins may pass into the milk of mothers and cause a prothrombinopenic state in the nursing infant.

Mild to moderate hepatic or renal insufficiency.

Infectious diseases or disturbances of intestinal flora—sprue, antibiotic therapy.

Trauma which may result in internal bleeding.

Surgery or trauma resulting in large exposed raw surfaces.

Indwelling catheters and/or drainage tubes in any orifice.

Mild to moderate hypertension.

Known or suspected hereditary familial or clinical deficiency in protein C—This condition which should be suspected if there is a history of recurrent episodes of thromboembolic disorders in the patient or in the family, has been associated with an increased risk of developing necrosis following dicumarol administration. Skin necrosis may occur in the absence of protein C deficiency. It has been reported that initiation of anticoagulation therapy with heparin for 4 to 5 days before initiation of therapy with dicumarol may minimize the incidence of this reaction. Dicumarol therapy should be discontinued when dicumarol is suspected to be the cause of developing necrosis and heparin therapy may be considered for anticoagulation.

Miscellaneous: polycythemia vera, vasculitis, severe diabetes, severe allergic and anaphylactic disorders, active tuberculosis, history of ulcerative disease of the gastrointestinal tract and during the postpartum period.

Patients with congestive heart failure may become more sensitive to dicumarol, thereby requiring more frequent laboratory monitoring, and reduced doses of dicumarol.

Use of anticoagulants with streptokinase or urokinase may be hazardous and caution should be exercised when used concomitantly. (Please note recommendations accompanying these preparations.)

Abrupt cessation of anticoagulant therapy is not generally recommended; taper dose gradually over 3 to 4 weeks.

PRECAUTIONS
Periodic determination of prothrombin time or other suitable coagulation test is essential.

Numerous factors, alone or in combination, including travel, changes in diet, environment, physical state and medication may influence response of the patient to anticoagulants. It is generally good practice to monitor the patient's response with additional prothrombin time determinations in the period immediately after discharge from the hospital, and whenever other medications are initiated, discontinued or taken haphazardly. The following factors are listed for your reference; however, other factors may also affect the prothrombin response.

The following factors alone or in combination, may be responsible for increased prothrombin time response:
ENDOGENOUS FACTORS:
Carcinoma; collagen disease; congestive heart failure; diarrhea; elevated temperature; hepatic disorders—infectious hepatitis, hyperthyroidism, jaundice; poor nutritional state; vitamin K deficiency—steatorrhea.
EXOGENOUS FACTORS:
Alcohol†; allopurinol; aminosalicyclic acid; amiodarone; anabolic steroids; antibiotics; bromelains; chloral hydrate†; chloramphenicol; chlorpropamide; chymotrypsin; cimetidine; cinchophen; clofibrate; dicumarol overdosage; dextran; dextrothyroxine; diazoxide; dietary deficiencies; diflunisal; diuretics†; disulfiram; drugs affecting blood elements; ethacrynic acid; fenoprofen; glucagon; hepatotoxic drugs; ibuprofen; indomethacin; influenza virus vaccine; inhalation anesthetics; mefenamic acid; methyldopa; methylphenidate; methylthiouracil; metronidazole; miconazole; monoamine oxidase inhibitors; nalidixic acid; naproxen; nortriptyline; oxolinic acid; oxyphenbutazone; pentoxifylline; phenylbutazone; phenyramidol; phenytoin; prolonged hot weather; prolonged narcotics; propylthiouracil; pyrazolones; quinidine; quinine; ranitidine†; salicylates; sulfinpyrazone; sulfonamides, long acting; sulindac; thyroid drugs; tolbutamide; triclofos sodium; trimethoprim/sulfamethoxazole; unreliable prothrombin time determinations.

The following factors, alone or in combination, may be responsible for decreased prothrombin time response:
ENDOGENOUS FACTORS:
Edema; hereditary resistance to coumarin therapy; hyperlipemia; hypothyroidism.
EXOGENOUS FACTORS:
ACTH steroids: alcohol†; antacids; antihistamines; phenobarbital and other barbiturates; carbamazepine; chloral hydrate†; chlordiazepoxide; cholestyramine; dicumarol underdosage; diet high in vitamin K; diuretics†; ethchlorvynol; glutethimide; griseofulvin; haloperidol; meprobamate; oral contraceptives; paraldehyde; primidone; ranitidine†; rifampin; unreliable prothrombin time determinations; vitamin C.

A patient may be exposed to a combination of the above factors, some of which may increase and some decrease his sensitivity to dicumarol. Because the net effect on his prothrombin time response may be unpredictable under these circumstances, more frequent laboratory monitoring is advisable.

Drugs not yet shown to interact or not to interct with coumarins are best regarded with suspicion, and when their administration is started or stopped, the prothrombin time should be determined more often than usual.

Coumarins also affect the action of other drugs. Hypoglycemic agents (chlorpropamide and tolbutamide) and anticonvulsants (phenytoin and phenobarbital) may accumulate in the body as a result of interference with either their metabolism or excretion.

† Increased and decreased prothrombin time responses have been reported.

ADVERSE REACTIONS
Potential adverse reactions to dicumarol may include:
Hemorrhage from any tissue or organ. This is a consequence of the anticoagulant effect. The signs and symptoms will vary according to the location and degree or extent of the bleeding. Therefore, the possibility of hemorrhage should be considered in evaluating the condition of any anticoagulated patient with complaints which do not indicate an obvious diagnosis. Bleeding during anticoagulant therapy does not always correlate with prothrombin activity. (See **TREATMENT FOR OVERDOSAGE**.)

Adrenal hemorrhage with resultant acute adrenal insufficiency has occurred during anticoagulant therapy. Anticoagulant therapy should be discontinued in patients who develop signs and symptoms compatible with acute adrenal hemorrhage or insufficiency. Plasma cortisol levels should be measured immediately, and vigorous therapy with intravenous corticosteroids should be instituted promptly. Initiation of therapy should not depend upon laboratory confirmation of the diagnosis, since any delay in an acute situation may result in the patient's death.

Ovarian hemorrhage: Reports indicate that a women receiving short- or long-term therapy with heparin or warfarin sodium may be at risk of developing ovarian hemorrhage at the time of ovulation. Caution should be observed when dicumarol is administered since these compounds have similar actions.

Paralytic ileus and intestinal obstruction have been reported from submucosal or intramural hemorrhage.

Excessive uterine bleeding has occurred but menstrual flow is usually normal.

Bleeding which occurs when the prothrombin time is within the therapeutic range warrants diagnostic investigation since it may unmask a previously unsuspected lesion, e.g. tumor, ulcer, etc.

Necrosis of skin and other tissues. (See **WARNINGS**.)

Other adverse reactions are infrequent and consist of alopecia, urticaria, dermatitis, fever, nausea, diarrhea, abdominal cramping, a syndrome called "purple toes," hypersensitivity reactions, leukopenia, and vomiting.

Priapism has been associated with anticoagulant administration, however, a causal relationship has not been established.

DOSAGE AND LABORATORY CONTROL
The aim of anticoagulant therapy is to impede the coagulation or clotting mechanism to such an extent that thrombosis will not occur, but at the same time avoiding such extensive impairment as might produce spontaneous bleeding. Effective therapeutic levels with minimal complications can be achieved in cooperative and well-instructed patients, who keep the doctor informed of their status between visits.

The administration and dosage of dicumarol must be individualized for each patient according to the particular patient's sensitivity to the drug as indicated by the prothrombin time. The prothrombin time reflects the depression of vitamin K dependent Factors VII, X and II: These factors, in addition to Factor IX, are affected by coumarin anticoagulants. There are several modifications of the Quick one-stage prothrombin time and the physician should become familiar with the specific method used in his laboratory.

Administration of dicumarol should be gauged according to prothrombin time determinations by a suitable method. The blood prothrombin time should usually be determined daily after the administration of the initial dose until prothrombin time results stabilize in the therapeutic range. Intervals between subsequent prothrombin time determinations should be based upon the physician's judgment of the patient's reliability and response to dicumarol in order to maintain the individual within the therapeutic range. Acceptable intervals for prothrombin time determinations have usually fallen within the range of 1 to 4 weeks. Satisfactory levels for maintenance of therapeutic anticoagulation are $1\frac{1}{2}$ to $2\frac{1}{2}$ times the normal prothrombin time (e.g. 18 to 30 seconds, with a control of 12 seconds).

Induction
The dosage range for the average adult with normal prothrombin activity ranges from 200 to 300 mg the first day.

Maintenance
On subsequent days the dosage ranges from 25 to 200 mg. It is essential that prothrombin time be measured daily while establishing the correct maintenance dose. Once this has been determined, prothrombin times can be checked less frequently. Dicumarol tablets may not be interchangeable

with dicumarol capsules. Retitration of the dosage should be considered if the dosage form prescribed is changed.

Duration of therapy
The duration of therapy in each patient should be individualized. In general, anticoagulant therapy should be continued until the danger of thrombosis and embolism has passed.

Treatment during dentistry and surgery
The management of patients who undergo dental and surgical procedures requires close liaison between attending physicians and dentists. Interruption of anticoagulant therapy may precipitate thromboembolism, and conversely, if anticoagulants are maintained at full doses, some patients may hemorrhage excessively. If it is elected to administer anticoagulants prior to, during, or immediately following dental or surgical procedures, it is recommended that the dosage of dicumarol be adjusted to maintain the prothrombin time at approximately $1\frac{1}{2}$ to $2\frac{1}{2}$ times the control level. The operative site should be sufficiently limited to permit the effective use of local procedures for hemostasis including absorbable hemostatic agents, sutures, and pressure dressings if necessary. Under these conditions dental and surgical procedures may be performed without undue risk of hemorrhage.

DICUMAROL with HEPARIN
Since a delay intervenes between the administration of the initial dose and the therapeutic prolongation of prothrombin time, it may be advisable in emergency situations to administer sodium heparin initially along with dicumarol.

It should be noted that heparin may affect the prothrombin time, and therefore, when patients are receiving both heparin and dicumarol, the blood sample for prothrombin time determination should be drawn just prior to the next heparin dosage, at least 5 hours after the last intravenous injection or 24 hours after the last subcutaneous injection.

TREATMENT FOR OVERDOSAGE
Excessive prothrombinopenia, with or without bleeding, is readily controlled by discontinuing dicumarol, and if necessary, the oral or parenteral administration of vitamin K_1 The appearance of microscopic hematuria, excessive menstrual bleeding, melena, petechiae or oozing from nicks made while shaving are early manifestations of hyproprothrombinemia beyond a safe and satisfactory level.

In excessive prothrombinopenia with mild or no bleeding, omission of one or more doses of dicumarol may suffice; and if necessary, small doses of vitamin K_1 orally, $2\frac{1}{2}$ to 10 mg, will usually correct the problem.

If minor bleeding persists, or progresses to frank bleeding, vitamin K_1 in doses of 5 to 25 mg may be given parenterally. (Please note recommendations accompanying vitamin K preparations prior to use.)

Fresh whole blood tranfusions should be considered in cases of severe bleeding or prothrombinopenic states unresponsive to vitamin K_1.

Resumption of dicumarol administration reverses the effect of vitamin K_1, and a therapeutic hypoprothrombinemia level can again be obtained. A hypercoagulable state has been reported to occur following rapid reversal of a prolonged prothrombin time, therefore, caution must be used in determing the need for this vitamin.

HOW SUPPLIED
Dicumarol tablets, USP are supplied as:
25 mg tablets:
bottles of 100 (**NDC** 0074-3794-01)
bottles of 1000 (**NDC** 0074-3794-06)
50 mg tablets:
bottles of 100 (**NDC** 0074-3773-01)
bottles of 1000 (**NDC** 0074-3773-02)
Abbott Pharmaceuticals, Inc.
North Chicago, IL 60064
Ref. 03-4305-RI
Shown in Product Identification Section, page 403

ENDURON®　　　　　　　　　　　　　　　　℞
[en 'de-ron]
(methyclothiazide tablets, USP)

DESCRIPTION
Methyclothiazide is a member of the benzothiadiazine (thiazide) class of drugs. It is an analogue of hydrochlorothiazide and occurs as a white to practically white crystalline powder which is basically odorless. Methyclothiazide is very slightly soluble in water and chloroform, and slightly soluble in alcohol. Chemically, methyclothiazide is represented as 6-chloro-3-(chloromethyl)-3, 4-dihydro-2-methyl-2H-1,2,4-benzothiadiazine-7-sulfonamide 1,1-dioxide.

Clinically, ENDURON (methyclothiazide) is an oral diuretic-antihypertensive agent. ENDURON tablets are available in

Continued on next page

Abbott—Cont.

two dosage strengths containing 2.5 mg and 5 mg of methyclothiazide.

Inactive Ingredients:

2.5 mg tablets: corn starch, FD&C Yellow No. 6, lactose, magnesium stearate and talc.

5 mg tablets: corn starch, D&C Red No. 36, FD&C Red No. 3, lactose, magnesium stearate and talc.

CLINICAL PHARMACOLOGY

The diuretic and saluretic effects of methyclothiazide result from a drug-induced inhibition of the renal tubular reabsorption of electrolytes. The excretion of sodium and chloride is greatly enhanced. Potassium excretion is also enhanced to a variable degree, as it is with the other thiazides. Although urinary excretion of bicarbonate is increased slightly, there is usually no significant change in urinary pH. Methyclothiazide has a per mg natriuretic activity approximately 100 times that of the prototype thiazide, chlorothiazide. At maximal therapeutic dosages, all thiazides are approximately equal in their diuretic/natriuretic effects.

There is significant natriuresis and diuresis within two hours after administration of a single dose of methyclothiazide. These effects reach a peak in about six hours and persist for 24 hours following oral administration of a single dose. Like other benzothiadiazines, methylclothiazide also has antihypertensive properties, and may be used for this purpose either alone or to enhance the antihypertensive action of other drugs. The mechanism by which the benzothiadiazines, including methyclothiazide, produce a reduction of elevated blood pressure is not known. However, sodium depletion appears to be involved.

Methyclothiazide is rapidly absorbed and slowly eliminated by the kidneys as intact drug but primarily as an inactive metabolite. Additional information on the pharmacokinetics is not known at this time.

INDICATIONS AND USAGE

ENDURON (methyclothiazide) is indicated in the management of hypertension either as the sole therapeutic agent or to enhance the effect of other antihypertensive drugs in the more severe forms of hypertension.

ENDURON tablets are indicated as adjunctive therapy in edema associated with congestive heart failure, hepatic cirrhosis, and corticosteroid and estrogen therapy.

ENDURON tablets have also been found useful in edema due to various forms of renal dysfunction such as the nephrotic syndrome, acute glomerulonephritis, and chronic renal failure.

Usage in Pregnancy: The routine use of diuretics in an otherwise healthy pregnant woman is inappropriate and exposes mother and fetus to unnecessary hazard. Diuretics do not prevent development of toxemia of pregnancy, and there is no satisfactory evidence that they are useful in the treatment of developed toxemia.

Edema during pregnancy may arise from pathological causes or from the physiological and mechanical consequences of pregnancy. Thiazides are indicated in pregnancy when edema is due to pathological causes, just as they are in the absence of pregnancy (see PRECAUTIONS—Pregnancy). Dependent edema in pregnancy, resulting from restriction of venous return by the expanded uterus, is properly treated through elevation of the lower extremities and use of support hose; use of diuretics to lower intravascular volume in this case is illogical and unnecessary. There is hypervolemia during normal pregnancy that is harmful to neither the fetus nor the mother (in the absence of cardiovascular disease), but that is associated with edema, including generalized edema, in the majority of pregnant women. If this edema produces discomfort, increased recumbency will often provide relief. In rare instances, this edema may cause extreme discomfort that is not relieved by rest. In these cases, a short course of diuretics may provide relief and may be appropriate.

CONTRAINDICATIONS

Methyclothiazide is contraindicated in patients with anuria and in patients with a history of hypersensitivity to this compound or other sulfonamide-derived drugs.

WARNINGS

Methyclothiazide shares with other thiazides the propensity to deplete potassium reserves to an unpredictable degree. There have been isolated reports that certain non-edematous individuals developed severe fluid and electrolyte derangements after only brief exposure to normal doses of thiazide and non-thiazide diuretics.

Thiazides should be used with caution in patients with renal disease or significant impairment of renal function, since azotemia may be precipitated and cumulative drug effects may occur.

Thiazides should be used with caution in patients with impaired hepatic function or progressive liver disease, since minor alterations of fluid and electrolyte balance may precipitate hepatic coma.

Sensitivity reactions may occur in patients with a history of allergy or bronchial asthma.

The possibility of exacerbation or activation of systemic lupus erythematosus has been reported.

Hyperuricemia may occur or frank gout may be precipitated in certain patients receiving thiazide therapy.

PRECAUTIONS

Laboratory Tests: Initial and periodic determinations of serum electrolytes should be performed at appropriate intervals for the purpose of detecting possible electrolyte imbalances such as hyponatremia, hypochloremic alkalosis, and hypokalemia. Serum and urine electrolyte determinations are particularly important when a patient is vomiting excessively or receiving parenteral fluids.

General: All patients should be observed for clinical signs of electrolyte imbalances such as dryness of mouth, thirst, weakness, lethargy, drowsiness, restlessness, muscle pains or cramps, muscular fatigue, hypotension, oliguria, tachycardia, and gastrointestinal disturbances such as nausea and vomiting.

Hypokalemia may develop, especially with brisk diuresis, when severe cirrhosis is present, during concomitant use of corticosteroids or ACTH, or after prolonged therapy. Interference with adequate oral electrolyte intake will also contribute to hypokalemia. Hypokalemia may be avoided or treated by use of potassium supplements or foods with a high potassium content.

Any chloride deficit is generally mild and usually does not require specific treatment except under extraordinary circumstances (as in liver disease or renal disease). Dilutional hyponatremia may occur in edematous patients in hot weather; appropriate therapy is water restriction rather than administration of salt, except in rare instances when the hyponatremia is life threatening. In actual salt depletion, appropriate replacement is the therapy of choice.

Latent diabetes mellitus may become manifest during thiazide administration.

The antihypertensive effects of the drug may be enhanced in the postsympathectomy patient.

If progressive renal impairment becomes evident as indicated by a rising nonprotein nitrogen or blood urea nitrogen, a careful reappraisal of therapy is necessary with consideration given to withholding or discontinuing diuretic therapy. Thiazides may decrease urinary calcium excretion. Thiazides may cause intermittent and slight elevation of serum calcium in the absence of known disorders of calcium metabolism. Marked hypercalcemia may be evidence of hidden hyperparathyroidism. Thiazides should be discontinued before carrying out tests for parathyroid function.

Thiazides may cause increased concentrations of total serum cholesterol, total triglycerides, and low-density lipoproteins in some patients. Use thiazides with caution in patients with moderate or high cholesterol concentrations and in patients with elevated triglyceride levels.

Information for Patients: Patients should inform their doctor if they have: 1) had an allergic reaction to methyclothiazide or other diuretics 2) asthma 3) kidney disease 4) liver disease 5) gout 6) systemic lupus erythematosus, or 7) been taking other drugs such as cortisone, digitalis, lithium carbonate, or drugs for diabetes.

The physician should inform patients of possible side effects and caution the patient to report any of the following symptoms of electrolyte imbalance; dryness of mouth, thirst, weakness, tiredness, drowsiness, restlessness, muscle pains or cramps, nausea, vomiting or increased heart rate.

The physician should advise the patient to take this medication every day as directed. Physicians should also caution patients that drinking alcohol can increase the chance of dizziness.

Drug Interactions: Hypokalemia can sensitize or exaggerate the response of the heart to the toxic effects of *digitalis* (e.g., increased ventricular irritability).

Hypokalemia may develop during concomitant use of *steroids* or *ACTH*.

Insulin requirements in diabetic patients may be increased, decreased, or unchanged.

Thiazides may decrease arterial responsiveness to *norepinephrine*. This diminution is not sufficient to preclude effectiveness of the pressor agent for therapeutic use.

Thiazide drugs may increase the responsiveness to *tubocurarine*.

Lithium renal clearance is reduced by thiazides, increasing the risk of lithium toxicity.

Thiazides may add to or potentiate the action of *other antihypertensive drugs*. Potentiation occurs with ganglionic or peripheral adrenergic blocking drugs.

Drug/Laboratory Test Interactions: Thiazides may decrease serum PBI levels without signs of thyroid disturbance.

Thiazides should be discontinued before carrying out tests for parathyroid function.

Carcinogenesis, Mutagenesis, Impairment of Fertility: No data are available concerning the potential for carcinogenicity or mutagenicity in animals or humans. Methyclothiazide did not impair fertility in rats receiving up to 4 mg/kg/day (at least 20 times the maximum recommended human dose

of 10 mg, assuming patient weight equal to or greater than 50 kg).

Pregnancy—Teratogenic Effects: Pregnancy Category B. Reproduction studies performed in rats and rabbits at doses up to 4 mg/kg/day have revealed no evidence of harm to the fetus due to methyclothiazide. There are, however, no adequate and well-controlled studies in pregnant women. Because animal reproduction studies are not always predictive of human response, this drug should be used during pregnancy only if clearly needed.

Nonteratogenic Effects: Thiazides cross the placental barrier and appear in cord blood. The use of thiazides in pregnant women requires that the anticipated benefit be weighed against possible hazards to the fetus. These hazards include fetal or neonatal jaundice, thrombocytopenia and possible other adverse reactions that have occurred in the adult.

Nursing Mothers: Thiazides are excreted in breast milk. Because of the potential for serious adverse reactions in nursing infants, a decision should be made whether to discontinue nursing or to discontinue the drug taking into account the importance of the drug to the mother.

Pediatric Use: Safety and effectiveness in children have not been established.

ADVERSE REACTIONS

Adverse reactions are usually reversible upon reduction of dosage or discontinuation of ENDURON tablets. Whenever adverse reactions are moderate or severe, it may be necessary to discontinue the drug.

The following adverse reactions have been observed, but there has not been enough systematic collection of data to support an estimate of their frequency. Consequently the reactions are categorized by organ system and are listed in decreasing order of severity and not frequency.

Body as a Whole: Headache, cramping, weakness.

Cardiovascular System: Orthostatic hypotension (may be potentiated by alcohol, barbiturates, or narcotics).

Digestive System: Pancreatitis, jaundice (intrahepatic cholestatic), sialadenitis, vomiting, diarrhea, nausea, gastric irritation, constipation, anorexia.

Hemic and Lymphatic System: Aplastic anemia, hemolytic anemia, agranulocytosis, leukopenia, thrombocytopenia.

Hypersensitivity Reactions: Anaphylactic reactions, necrotizing angiitis (vasculitis, cutaneous vasculitis), Stevens-Johnson syndrome, respiratory distress including pneumonitis and pulmonary edema, fever, purpura, urticaria, rash, photosensitivity.

Metabolic and Nutritional Disorders: Hyperglycemia, hyperuricemia, electrolyte imbalance (see PRECAUTIONS section), hypercalcemia.

Nervous System: Vertigo, dizziness, paresthesias, muscle spasm, restlessness.

Special Senses: Transient blurred vision, xanthopsia.

Urogenital System: Glycosuria.

OVERDOSAGE

Symptoms of overdosage include electrolyte imbalance and signs of potassium deficiency such as confusion, dizziness, muscular weakness, and gastrointestinal disturbances. General supportive measures including replacement of fluids and electrolytes may be indicated in treatment of overdosage.

DOSAGE AND ADMINISTRATION

ENDURON (methyclothiazide) is administered orally. Therapy should be individualized according to patient response. This therapy should be titrated to gain maximal therapeutic response as well as the minimal dose possible to maintain that therapeutic response.

For edematous conditions: The usual adult dose ranges from 2.5 to 10 mg once daily. Maximum effective single dose is 10 mg; larger single doses do not accomplish greater diuresis, and are not recommended.

For the treatment of hypertension: The usual adult dose ranges from 2.5 to 5 mg once daily.

If control of blood pressure is not satisfactory after 8 to 12 weeks of therapy with 5 mg once daily, another antihypertensive drug should be added. Increasing the dosage of methyclothiazide will usually not result in further lowering of blood pressure.

Methyclothiazide may be either employed alone for mild to moderate hypertension or concurrently with other antihypertensive drugs in the management of more severe forms of hypertension. Combined therapy may provide adequate control of hypertension with lower dosage of the component drugs and fewer or less severe side effects. An enhanced response frequently follows its concurrent administration with Harmonyl® (deserpidine) so that dosage of both drugs may be reduced.

When other antihypertensive agents are to be added to the regimen, this should be accomplished gradually. Ganglionic blocking agents should be given at only half the usual dose since their effect is potentiated by pretreatment with ENDURON tablets.

HOW SUPPLIED

ENDURON (methyclothiazide tablets, USP) is provided in two dosage sizes as monogrammed, grooved, square-shaped tablets:

2.5 mg, orange-colored:
bottles of 100 (**NDC** 0074-6827-01),
bottles of 1000 (**NDC** 0074-6827-02).

5 mg, salmon-colored:
bottles of 100 (**NDC** 0074-6812-01),
bottles of 1000 (**NDC** 0074-6812-02),
bottles of 5000 (**NDC** 0074-6812-03),
Abbo-Pac® unit dose packages of 100 (**NDC** 0074-6812-10).

Dispense in a USP tight container.
Recommended storage: Protect from excessive heat.
Abbott Pharmaceuticals, Inc.
North Chicago, IL 60064
Ref. 03-4355-R7
Shown in Product Identification Section, page 403

ENDURONYL® Tablets ℞
[en-du're-nil]
(methyclothiazide and deserpidine)

Oral thiazide-rauwolfia therapy for hypertension.

WARNING

This fixed combination drug is not indicated for initial therapy of hypertension. Hypertension requires therapy titrated to the individual patient. If the fixed combination represents the dosage so determined, its use may be more convenient in patient management. The treatment of hypertension is not static, but must be reevaluated as conditions in each patient warrant.

DESCRIPTION

ENDURONYL is an orally-administered combination of Enduron® (methyclothiazide) and Harmonyl® (deserpidine). Methyclothiazide is an oral diuretic-antihypertensive of the benzothiadiazine (thiazide) class. Deserpidine is a purified rauwolfia alkaloid, chemically identified as 11-desmethoxyreserpine, which produces antihypertensive effects.

Inactive Ingredients:

Enduronyl tablets: corn starch, D&C Yellow No. 10, FD&C Yellow No. 6, lactose, magnesium stearate and talc.
Enduronyl Forte tablets: corn starch, iron oxide, lactose, magnesium stearate and talc.

ACTIONS

The combined antihypertensive actions of methyclothiazide and deserpidine result in a total clinical antihypertensive effect which is greater than can ordinarily be achieved by either drug given individually.

The diuretic and saluretic effects of methyclothiazide result from a drug-induced inhibition of the renal tubular reabsorption of electrolytes. The excretion of sodium and chloride is greatly enhanced. Potassium excretion is also enhanced to a variable degree, as it is with the other thiazides. Although urinary excretion of bicarbonate is increased slightly, there is usually no significant change in urinary pH. Methyclothiazide has a per mg natriuretic activity approximately 100 times that of the prototype thiazide, chlorothiazide. At maximal therapeutic dosages, all thiazides are approximately equal in their diuretic/natriuretic effects.

There is significant natriuresis and diuresis within two hours after administration of a single dose of methyclothiazide. These effects reach a peak in about six hours and persist for 24 hours following oral administration of a single dose. Like other benzothiadiazines, methyclothiazide also has antihypertensive properties, and may be used for this purpose either alone or to enhance the antihypertensive action of other drugs. The mechanism by which the benzothiadiazines, including methyclothiazide, produce a reduction of elevated blood pressure is not known. However, sodium depletion appears to be involved.

Methyclothiazide is rapidly absorbed and slowly eliminated by the kidney as both intact drug and as a metabolite showing no diuretic activity in a rat model.

The pharmacologic actions of Harmonyl (deserpidine) are essentially the same as those of other active rauwolfia alkaloids. Deserpidine probably produces its antihypertensive effects through depletion of tissue stores of catecholamines (epinephrine and norepinephrine) from peripheral sites. The antihypertensive effect is often accompanied by bradycardia. There is no significant alteration in cardiac output or renal blood flow. The carotid sinus reflex is inhibited, but postural hypotension is rarely seen with the use of conventional doses of Harmonyl alone.

Deserpidine, like other rauwolfia alkaloids, is characterized by slow onset of action and sustained effect which may persist following withdrawal of the drug.

INDICATIONS

ENDURONYL (methyclothiazide and deserpidine) is indicated in the treatment of mild to moderately severe hypertension (see boxed warning). In many cases ENDURONYL alone produces an adequate reduction of blood pressure. In resistant or unusually severe cases ENDURONYL also may be supplemented by more potent antihypertensive agents. When administered with ENDURONYL, more potent agents can be given at reduced dosage to minimize undesirable side effects.

CONTRAINDICATIONS

Methyclothiazide is contraindicated in patients with renal decompensation and in those who are hypersensitive to this or other sulfonamide-derived drugs.

Deserpidine is contraindicated in patients with known hypersensitivity, history of mental depression especially with suicidal tendencies, active peptic ulcer, and ulcerative colitis. It is also contraindicated in patients receiving electroconvulsive therapy.

WARNINGS

Methyclothiazide

Methyclothiazide shares with other thiazides the propensity to deplete potassium reserves to an unpredictable degree. Thiazides should be used with caution in patients with renal disease or significant impairment of renal function, since azotemia may be precipitated and cumulative drug effects may occur.

Thiazides should be used with caution in patients with impaired hepatic function or progressive liver disease, since minor alterations of fluid and electrolyte balance may precipitate hepatic coma.

Thiazides may be additive or potentiative of the action of other antihypertensive drugs. Potentiation occurs with ganglionic or peripheral adrenergic blocking drugs.

Sensitivity reactions may occur in patients with a history of allergy or bronchial asthma.

The possibility of exacerbation or activation of systemic lupus erythematosus has been reported.

Deserpidine

Deserpidine differs slightly in chemical structure from reserpine, however, its actions, indications, cautions and adverse reactions are common to the class of rauwolfia alkaloids. Reserpine may cause mental depression. Recognition of depression may be difficult because this condition may often be disguised by somatic complaints (Masked Depression). The drug should be discontinued at first signs of depression such as despondency, early morning insomnia, loss of appetite, impotence, or self-deprecation. Drug-induced depression may persist for several months after drug withdrawal and may be severe enough to result in suicide.

Usage in Pregnancy and Lactation:

Methyclothiazide

Thiazides cross the placental barrier and appear in cord blood. The use of thiazides in pregnant women requires that the anticipated benefit be weighed against possible hazards to the fetus. These hazards include fetal or neonatal jaundice, thrombocytopenia, and possible other adverse reactions that have occurred in the adult.

Thiazides appear in breast milk. If use of the drug is deemed essential, the patient should stop nursing.

Deserpidine

The safety of deserpidine for use during pregnancy or lactation has not been established; therefore, it should be used in pregnant women or in women of childbearing potential only when in the judgment of the physician its use is deemed essential to the welfare of the patient. Increased respiratory secretions, nasal congestion, cyanosis, and anorexia may occur in infants born to rauwolfia alkaloid-treated mothers, since these preparations are known to cross the placental barrier to enter the fetal circulation and appear in cord blood. They also are secreted by nursing mothers into breast milk.

Reproductive and teratology studies in rats reduced the mating index and neonatal survival indices; the no-effect dosage has not been established.

PRECAUTIONS

Periodic determinations of serum electrolytes should be performed at appropriate intervals for the purpose of detecting possible electrolyte imbalances such as hyponatremia, hypochloremic alkalosis, and hypokalemia. Serum and urine electrolyte determinations are particularly important when a patient is vomiting excessively or receiving parenteral fluids. All patients should be observed for other clinical signs of electrolyte imbalances such as dryness of mouth, thirst, weakness, lethargy, drowsiness, restlessness, muscle pains or cramps, muscular fatigue, hypotension, oliguria, tachycardia, and gastrointestinal disturbances such as nausea and vomiting.

Hypokalemia may develop with thiazides as with any other potent diuretic, especially when brisk diuresis occurs, severe cirrhosis is present, or when corticosteroids or ACTH are given concomitantly. Interference with the adequate oral intake of electrolytes will also contribute to the possible development of hypokalemia. Potassium depletion, even of a

mild degree, resulting from thiazide use, may sensitize a patient to the effects of cardiac glycosides such as digitalis. Any chloride deficit is generally mild and usually does not require specific treatment except under extraordinary circumstances (as in liver disease or renal disease). Dilutional hyponatremia may occur in edematous patients in hot weather; appropriate therapy is water restriction rather than administration of salt, except in rare instances when the hyponatremia is life threatening.

In actual salt depletion, appropriate replacement is the therapy of choice.

Hyperuricemia may occur or frank gout may be precipitated in certain patients receiving thiazide therapy.

Insulin requirements in diabetic patients may be increased, decreased, or unchanged. Latent diabetes mellitus may become manifest during thiazide administration.

Thiazide drugs may increase the responsiveness to tubocurarine.

The antihypertensive effects of the drug may be enhanced in the postsympathectomy patient.

Thiazides may decrease arterial responsiveness to norepinephrine. This diminution is not sufficient to preclude effectiveness of the pressor agent for therapeutic use.

If progressive renal impairment becomes evident as indicated by a rising nonprotein nitrogen or blood urea nitrogen, a careful reappraisal of therapy is necessary with consideration given to withholding or discontinuing diuretic therapy.

Thiazides may decrease serum PBI levels without signs of thyroid disturbance.

Thiazides have been reported, on rare occasions, to have elevated serum calcium to hypercalcemic levels. The serum calcium levels have returned to normal when the medication has been stopped. This phenomenon may be related to the ability of the thiazide diuretics to lower the amount of calcium excreted in the urine.

Because rauwolfia preparations increase gastrointestinal motility and secretion, this drug should be used cautiously in patients with a history of peptic ulcer, ulcerative colitis, or gallstones, where biliary colic may be precipitated.

Caution should be exercised when treating hypertensive patients with renal insufficiency since they adjust poorly to lowered blood pressure levels.

Use deserpidine cautiously with digitalis and quinidine since cardiac arrhythmias have occurred with rauwolfia preparations.

Preoperative withdrawal of deserpidine does not assure that circulatory instability will not occur. It is important that the anesthesiologist be aware of the patient's drug intake and consider this in the overall management, since hypotension has occurred in patients receiving rauwolfia preparations. Anticholinergic and/or adrenergic drugs (metaraminol, norepinephrine) have been employed to treat adverse vagocirculatory effects.

Animal tumorigenicity: There are no studies demonstrating that deserpidine is an animal tumorigen, although it is a prolactin stimulator and structurally related to reserpine. Rodent studies with reserpine, however, have shown that reserpine is an animal tumorigen, causing an increased incidence of mammary fibroadenomas in female mice, malignant tumors of the seminal vesicles in male mice, and malignant adrenal medullary tumors in male rats. These findings arose in 2 year studies in which the drug was administered in the feed at concentrations of 5 to 10 ppm—about 100 to 300 times the usual human dose. The breast neoplasms are thought to be related to reserpine's prolactin-elevating effect. Several other prolactin-elevating drugs have also been associated with an increased incidence of mammary neoplasia in rodents.

The extent to which these findings indicate a risk to humans is uncertain. Tissue culture experiments show that about one-third of human breast tumors are prolactin-dependent *in vitro,* a factor of considerable importance if the use of the drug is contemplated in a patient with previously detected breast cancer. The possibility of an increased risk of breast cancer in reserpine users has been studied extensively; however, no firm conclusion has emerged. Although a few epidemiologic studies have suggested a slightly increased risk (less than twofold in all studies except one) in women who have used reserpine, other studies of generally similar design have not confirmed this. Epidemiologic studies conducted using other drugs (neuroleptic agents) that, like reserpine, increase prolactin levels and, therefore, would be considered rodent mammary carcinogens, have not shown an association between chronic administration of the drug and human mammary tumorigenesis. While long-term clinical observation has not suggested such an association, the available evidence is considered too limited to be conclusive at this time. An association of reserpine intake with pheochromocytoma or tumors of the seminal vesicles has not been explored.

Continued on next page

Abbott—Cont.

ADVERSE REACTIONS

Methyclothiazide

Gastrointestinal System Reactions: Anorexia, gastric irritation, nausea, vomiting, cramping, diarrhea, constipation, jaundice (intrahepatic cholestatic jaundice), pancreatitis.

Central Nervous System Reactions: Dizziness, vertigo, paresthesias, headache, xanthopsia.

Hematologic Reactions: Leukopenia, agranulocytosis, thrombocytopenia, aplastic anemia.

Dermatologic — Hypersensitivity Reactions: Purpura, photosensitivity, rash, urticaria, necrotizing angiitis (vasculitis) (cutaneous vasculitis).

Cardiovascular Reaction: Orthostatic hypotension may occur and may be aggravated by alcohol, barbiturates, or narcotics.

Other: Hyperglycemia, glycosuria, hypercalcemia, hyperuricemia, muscle spasm, weakness, restlessness.

There have been isolated reports that certain nonedematous individuals developed severe fluid and electrolyte derangements after only brief exposure to normal doses of thiazide and non-thiazide diuretics. The condition is usually manifested as severe dilutional hyponatremia, hypokalemia, and hypochloremia. It has been reported to be due to inappropriately increased ADH secretion and appears to be idiosyncratic. Potassium replacement is apparently the most important therapy in the treatment of this syndrome along with removal of the offending drug.

Whenever adverse reactions are severe, treatment should be discontinued.

Deserpidine

The following adverse reactions have been reported with rauwolfia preparations. These reactions are usually reversible and disappear when the drug is discontinued.

Gastrointestinal: Including hypersecretion, anorexia, diarrhea, nausea, and vomiting.

Cardiovascular: Including angina-like symptoms, arrhythmias (particularly when used concurrently with digitalis or quinidine), and bradycardia.

Central Nervous System: Including drowsiness, depression, nervousness, paradoxical anxiety, nightmares, extrapyramidal tract symptoms, CNS sensitization manifested by dull sensorium, and deafness.

Dermatologic—Hypersensitivity: Including pruritus, rash, and asthma in asthmatic patients.

Ophthalmologic: Including glaucoma, uveitis, optic atrophy, and conjunctival injection.

Hematologic: Thrombocytopenic purpura.

Miscellaneous: Nasal congestion, weight gain, impotence or decreased libido, dysuria, dyspnea, muscular aches, dryness of mouth, dizziness, and headache.

DOSAGE AND ADMINISTRATION

Dosage should be determined by individual titration of ingredients (see boxed warning). Dosage of both components should be carefully adjusted to the needs of the individual patient. Since at least ten days to two weeks may elapse before the full effects of the drugs become manifest, the dosage of the drugs should not be adjusted more frequently.

Two tablet strengths, ENDURONYL (methyclothiazide 5 mg, deserpidine 0.25 mg) and ENDURONYL FORTE (methyclothiazide 5 mg, deserpidine 0.5 mg), each grooved, are provided to permit considerable latitude in meeting the dosage requirements of individual patients.*

The following table will help in determining which dose of ENDURONYL or ENDURONYL FORTE best represents the equivalent of the titrated dose.

Daily Dosage of ENDURONYL	methyclothiazide	deserpidine
½ tablet	2.5 mg	0.125 mg
1 tablet	5.0 mg	0.250 mg
1½ tablet	7.5 mg	0.375 mg
2 tablets	10.0 mg	0.500 mg

Daily Dosage of ENDURONYL FORTE	methyclothiazide	deserpidine
½ tablet	2.5 mg	0.250 mg
1 tablet	5.0 mg	0.500 mg
1½ tablet	7.5 mg	0.750 mg
2 tablets	10.0 mg	1.000 mg

The appropriate dose of ENDURONYL is administered orally, once daily. The usual adult dosage is one lower-strength ENDURONYL tablet daily.

There is no contraindication to combining the administration of ENDURONYL with other antihypertensive agents. When other antihypertensive agents are to be added to the regimen, this should be accomplished gradually. Ganglionic blocking agents should be given at only half the usual dose

since their effect is potentiated by pretreatment with ENDURONYL.

OVERDOSAGE

Symptoms of thiazide overdosage include electrolyte imbalance and signs of potassium deficiency such as confusion, dizziness, muscular weakness, and gastrointestinal disturbances. General supportive measures including replacement of fluids and electrolytes may be indicated in treatment of overdosage.

An overdosage of deserpidine is characterized by flushing of the skin, conjunctival injection, and pupillary constriction. Sedation ranging from drowsiness to coma may occur. Hypotension, hypothermia, central respiratory depression and bradycardia may develop in cases of severe overdosage. Treatment consists of the careful evacuation of stomach contents followed by the usual procedures for the symptomatic management of CNS depressant overdosage. If severe hypotension occurs it should be treated with a direct acting vasopressor such as norepinephrine bitartrate injection.

HOW SUPPLIED

ENDURONYL (methyclothiazide and deserpidine) is supplied as monogrammed, grooved, square-shaped tablets in the following dosage sizes and quantities:

ENDURONYL (5 mg of methyclothiazide and 0.25 mg of deserpidine) yellow tablets in bottles of 100 (**NDC** 0074-6838-01) and 1000 (**NDC** 0074-6838-02). Also available in ABBO-PAC® unit dose packages, 100 tablets (**NDC** 0074-6838-06), in strips of 10 tablets.

ENDURONYL FORTE (5 mg of methyclothiazide and 0.5 mg of deserpidine) gray-colored tablets in bottles of 100 (**NDC** 0074-6854-01) and 1000 (**NDC** 0074-6854-02).

---

*Each component is separately available as ENDURON (methyclothiazide) and HARMONYL (deserpidine).

Abbott Pharmaceuticals, Inc.
North Chicago, IL 60064
Ref. 03-4344-R8

Shown in Product Identification Section, page 403

ERYDERM® 2%   ℞
[e´ry-derm]
erythromycin topical solution, USP

DESCRIPTION

Erythromycin is an antibiotic produced from a strain of *Streptomyces erythraeus.* It is basic and readily forms salts with acids. Each ml of ERYDERM 2% (erythromycin topical solution) contains 20 mg of erythromycin base in a vehicle consisting of polyethylene glycol, acetone, and alcohol 77%.

ACTIONS

Although the mechanism by which ERYDERM acts in reducing inflammatory lesions of acne vulgaris is unknown, it is presumably due to its antibiotic action.

INDICATIONS

ERYDERM is indicated for the topical control of acne vulgaris.

CONTRAINDICATIONS

ERYDERM is contraindicated in persons who have shown hypersensitivity to any of its ingredients.

WARNINGS

The safe use of ERYDERM during pregnancy or lactation has not been established.

PRECAUTIONS

General: The use of antibiotic agents may be associated with the overgrowth of antibiotic-resistant organisms. If this occurs, administration of this drug should be discontinued and appropriate measures taken.

Information for Patients: ERYDERM is for external use only and should be kept away from the eyes, nose, mouth, and other mucous membranes. Concomitant topical acne therapy should be used with caution because a cumulative irritant effect may occur, especially with the use of peeling, desquamating, or abrasive agents.

Do not allow solution to contact clothing and furniture.

Carcinogenesis, Mutagenesis, Impairment of Fertility: Long-term (2-year) oral studies conducted in rats with erythromycin base did not provide evidence of tumorigenicity. Mutagenicity studies have not been conducted. There was no apparent effect on male or female fertility in rats fed erythromycin (base) at levels up to 0.25 percent of diet.

Pregnancy: Pregnancy Category B: There is no evidence of teratogenicity or any other adverse effect on reproduction in female rats fed erythromycin base (up to 0.25 percent of diet) prior to and during mating, during gestation, and through weaning of two successive litters. There are, however, no adequate and well-controlled studies in pregnant women. Because animal reproduction studies are not always predictive of human response, this drug should be used during pregnancy only if clearly needed. Erythromycin has been reported to cross the placental barrier in humans, but fetal plasma levels are generally low.

Nursing Mothers: Erythromycin is excreted in breast milk. Caution should be exercised when erythromycin is administered to a nursing woman.

ADVERSE REACTIONS

Adverse conditions reported include dryness, tenderness, pruritus, desquamation, erythema, oiliness, and burning sensation. Irritation of the eyes has also been reported. A case of generalized urticarial reaction, possibly related to the drug, which required the use of systemic steroid therapy has been reported.

DOSAGE AND ADMINISTRATION

ERYDERM should be applied with applicator or pad to the affected area twice a day after the skin is thoroughly washed with warm water and soap and patted dry. Acne lesions on the face, neck, shoulder, chest, and back may be treated in this manner. The solution should be applied with a dabbing action when the applicator is used. Use enough solution to cover the affected area lightly.

HOW SUPPLIED

ERYDERM 2% (erythromycin topical solution, USP) is supplied in 60 ml bottles with applicator (**NDC** 0074-2698-02). Store at temperatures below 86°F (30°C).

Abbott Laboratories
North Chicago, IL 60064
Ref. 09-6257-3/R4

ERYPED®   ℞
[erē´ped]
(erythromycin ethylsuccinate for oral suspension, USP)

DESCRIPTION

Erythromycin is produced by a strain of *Streptomyces erythraeus* and belongs to the macrolide group of antibiotics. It is basic and readily forms salts with acids. The base, the stearate salt, and the esters are poorly soluble in water. Erythromycin ethylsuccinate is an ester of erythromycin suitable for oral administration.

EryPed 200 and EryPed Drops (erythromycin ethylsuccinate for oral suspension) when reconstituted with water, forms a suspension containing erythromycin ethylsuccinate equivalent to 200 mg erythromycin per 5 ml (teaspoonful) or 100 mg per 2.5 ml (dropperful) with an appealing fruit flavor. EryPed 400 when reconstituted with water, forms a suspension containing erythromycin ethylsuccinate equivalent to 400 mg of erythromycin per 5 ml (teaspoonful) with an appealing banana flavor. After mixing, EryPed must be stored below 77°F (25°C) and used within 35 days; refrigeration is not required.

Fruit-flavored EryPed Chewable tablets are easily ingested and are particularly acceptable for the administration of antibiotic medication to young children who are unable to swallow regular tablets or in whom persuasion of a pleasant taste insures cooperation. Each chewable tablet contains the equivalent of 200 mg of erythromycin activity and is scored for division into half-dose (100 mg) portions.

These products are intended primarily for pediatric use but can also be used in adults.

Inactive Ingredients: EryPed 200, EryPed 400 and EryPed Drops: Caramel, polysorbate, sodium citrate, sucrose, xanthan gum and artificial flavors.

EryPed Chewable Tablets: Citric acid, confectioner's sugar (contains corn starch), magnesium aluminum silicate, magnesium stearate, sodium carboxymethyl cellulose, sodium citrate and artificial flavor.

ACTIONS

Microbiology: Biochemical tests demonstrate that erythromycin inhibits protein synthesis of the pathogen without directly affecting nucleic acid synthesis. Antagonism has been demonstrated between clindamycin and erythromycin. NOTE: Many strains of *Hemophilus influenzae* are resistant to erythromycin alone, but are susceptible to erythromycin and sulfonamides together. Staphylococci resistant to erythromycin may emerge during a course of erythromycin therapy. Culture and susceptibility testing should be performed.

Disc Susceptibility Tests: Quantitative methods that require measurement of zone diameters give the most precise estimates of antibiotic susceptibility. One recommended procedure (21 CFR section 460.1) uses erythromycin class discs for testing susceptibility; interpretations correlate zone diameters of this disc test with MIC values for erythromycin. With this procedure, a report from the laboratory of "susceptible" indicates that the infecting organism is likely to respond to therapy. A report of "resistant" indicates, that the infective organism is not likely to respond to therapy. A report of "intermediate susceptibility" suggests that the organism would be susceptible if higher doses were used.

Clinical Pharmacology: Erythromycin binds to the 50 S ribosomal subunits of susceptible bacteria and suppresses protein synthesis.

Orally administered erythromycin ethylsuccinate suspension is readily and reliably absorbed under both fasting and nonfasting conditions.

Erythromycin diffuses readily into most body fluids. Only low concentrations are normally achieved in the spinal fluid, but passage of the drug across the blood-brain barrier increases in meningitis. In the presence of normal hepatic function, erythromycin is concentrated in the liver and excreted in the bile; the effect of hepatic dysfunction on excretion of erythromycin by the liver into the bile is not known. Less than 5 percent of the orally administered dose of erythromycin is excreted in active form in the urine.

Erythromycin crosses the placental barrier and is excreted in breast milk.

INDICATIONS

Streptococcus pyogenes (Group A beta-hemolytic streptococcus): Upper and lower respiratory tract, skin, and soft tissue infections of mild to moderate severity.

Injectable benzathine penicillin G is considered by the American Heart Association to be the drug of choice in the treatment and prevention of streptococcal pharyngitis and in long-term prophylaxis of rheumatic fever.

When oral medication is preferred for treatment of the above conditions, penicillin G, V, or erythromycin are alternate drugs of choice.

When oral medication is given, the importance of strict adherence by the patient to the prescribed dosage regimen must be stressed. A therapeutic dose should be administered for at least 10 days.

Alpha-hemolytic streptococci (viridans group): Although no controlled clinical efficacy trials have been conducted, oral erythromycin has been suggested by the American Heart Association and American Dental Association for use in a regimen for prophylaxis against bacterial endocarditis in patients hypersensitive to penicillin who have congenital heart disease, or rheumatic or other acquired valvular heart disease when they undergo dental procedures and surgical procedures of the upper respiratory tract.[1] Erythromycin is not suitable prior to genitourinary or gastrointestinal tract surgery. NOTE: When selecting antibiotics for the prevention of bacterial endocarditis the physician or dentist should read the full joint statement of the American Heart Association and the American Dental Association.[1]

Staphylococcus aureus: Acute infections of skin and soft tissue of mild to moderate severity. Resistant organisms may emerge during treatment.

Streptococcus pneumoniae (Diplococcus pneumoniae): Upper respiratory tract infections (e.g., otitis media, pharyngitis) and lower respiratory tract infections (e.g., pneumonia) of mild to moderate degree.

Mycoplasma pneumoniae (Eaton agent, PPLO): For respiratory infections due to this organism.

Hemophilus influenzae: For upper respiratory tract infections of mild to moderate severity when used concomitantly with adequate doses of sulfonamides. (See sulfonamide labeling for appropriate prescribing information). The concomitant use of the sulfonamides is necessary since not all strains of *Hemophilus influenzae* are susceptible to erythromycin at the concentrations of the antibiotic achieved with usual therapeutic doses.

Chlamydia trachomatis: For the treatment of urethritis in adult males due to *Chlamydia trachomatis.*

Ureaplasma urealyticum: For the treatment of urethritis in adult males due to *Ureaplasma urealyticum.*

Treponema pallidum: Erythromycin is an alternate choice of treatment for primary syphilis in patients allergic to the penicillins. In treatment of primary syphilis, spinal fluid examinations should be done before treatment and as part of follow-up after therapy.

Corynebacterium diphtheriae: As an adjunct to antitoxin, to prevent establishment of carriers, and to eradicate the organism in carriers.

Corynebacterium minutissimum: For the treatment of erythrasma.

Entamoeba histolytica: In the treatment of intestinal amebiasis only. Extraenteric amebiasis requires treatment with other agents.

Listeria monocytogenes: Infections due to this organism.

Bordetella pertussis: Erythromycin is effective in eliminating the organism from the nasopharynx of infected individuals, rendering them non-infectious. Some clinical studies suggest that erythromycin may be helpful in the prophylaxis of pertussis in exposed susceptible individuals.

Legionnaires' Disease: Although no controlled clinical efficacy studies have been conducted, *in vitro* and limited preliminary clinical data suggest that erythromycin may be effective in treating Legionnaires' Disease.

CONTRAINDICATIONS

Erythromycin is contraindicated in patients with known hypersensitivity to this antibiotic.

PRECAUTIONS

Erythromycin is principally excreted by the liver. Caution should be exercised in administering the antibiotic to patients with impaired hepatic function. There have been re-

ports of hepatic dysfunction, with or without jaundice occurring in patients receiving oral erythromycin products.

Areas of localized infection may require surgical drainage in addition to antibiotic therapy.

Recent data from studies of erythromycin reveal that its use in patients who are receiving high doses of theophylline may be associated with an increase of serum theophylline levels and potential theophylline toxicity. In case of theophylline toxicity and/or elevated serum theophylline levels, the dose of theophylline should be reduced while the patient is receiving concomitant erythromycin therapy.

Usage during pregnancy and lactation: The safety of erythromycin for use during pregnancy has not been established. Erythromycin crosses the placental barrier. Erythromycin also appears in breast milk.

ADVERSE REACTIONS

The most frequent side effects of erythromycin preparations are gastrointestinal, such as abdominal cramping and discomfort, and are dose related. Nausea, vomiting, and diarrhea occur infrequently with usual oral doses.

During prolonged or repeated therapy, there is a possibility of overgrowth of nonsusceptible bacteria or fungi. If such infections occur, the drug should be discontinued and appropriate therapy instituted.

Allergic reactions ranging from urticaria and mild skin eruptions to anaphylaxis have occurred.

There have been isolated reports of reversible hearing loss occurring chiefly in patients with renal insufficiency and in patients receiving high doses of erythromycin.

DOSAGE AND ADMINISTRATION

EryPed (erythromycin ethylsuccinate for oral suspension) may be administered without regard to meals.

Children: Age, weight, and severity of the infection are important factors in determining the proper dosage. In mild to moderate infections the usual dosage of erythromycin ethylsuccinate for children is 30 to 50 mg/kg/day in equally divided doses every six hours. For more severe infections this dosage may be doubled. If twice-a-day dosage is desired, one-half of the total daily dose may be given every 12 hours. Doses may also be given three times daily by administering one-third of the total daily dose every 8 hours.

The following dosage schedule is suggested for mild to moderate infections:

Body Weight	Total Daily Dose
Under 10 lbs	30-50 mg/kg/day 15-25 mg/lb/day
10 to 15 lbs	200 mg
16 to 25 lbs	400 mg
26 to 50 lbs	800 mg
51 to 100 lbs	1200 mg
over 100 lbs	1600 mg

Adults: 400 mg erythromycin ethylsuccinate every 6 hours is the usual dose. Dosage may be increased up to 4 g per day according to the severity of the infection. If twice-a-day dosage is desired, one-half of the total daily dose may be given every 12 hours. Doses may also be given three times daily by administering one-third of the total daily dose every 8 hours.

For adult dosage calculation, use a ratio of 400 mg of erythromycin activity as the ethylsuccinate to 250 mg of erythromycin activity as the stearate, base or estolate.

In the treatment of streptococcal infections, a therapeutic dosage of erythromycin ethylsuccinate should be administered for at least 10 days. In continuous prophylaxis against recurrences of streptococcal infections in persons with a history of rheumatic heart disease, the usual dosage is 400 mg twice a day.

For prophylaxis against bacterial endocarditis[1] in patients with congenital heart disease, or rheumatic or other acquired valvular heart disease when undergoing dental procedures or surgical procedures of the upper respiratory tract, give 1.6 g (20 mg/kg for children) orally 1 ½ to 2 hours before the procedure, and then, 800 mg (10 mg/kg for children) orally every 6 hours for 8 doses.

For treatment of urethritis due to *C. trachomatis* or *U. urealyticum:* 800 mg three times a day for 7 days.

For treatment of primary syphilis: Adults: 48 to 64 g given in divided doses over a period of 10 to 15 days.

For intestinal amebiasis: Adults: 400 mg four times daily for 10 to 14 days. Children: 30 to 50 mg/kg/day in divided doses for 10 to 14 days.

For use in pertussis: Although optimal dosage and duration have not been established, doses of erythromycin utilized in reported clinical studies were 40 to 50 mg/kg/day, given in divided doses for 5 to 14 days.

For treatment of Legionnaires' Disease: Although optimal doses have not been established, doses utilized in reported clinical data were 1.6 to 4 g daily in divided doses.

HOW SUPPLIED

EryPed 200 (erythromycin ethylsuccinate for oral suspension, USP) is supplied in bottles of 100 ml (**NDC** 0074-6302-13), 200 ml (**NDC** 0074-6302-53), and 5 ml unit dose in ABBO-PAC® packages (**NDC** 0074-6302-05). Each 5 ml (teaspoonful) of reconstituted suspension contains activity equivalent to 200 mg erythromycin.

EryPed 400 (erythromycin ethylsuccinate for oral suspension, USP) is supplied in bottles of 60 ml (**NDC** 0074-6305-60). 100 ml (**NDC** 0074-6305-13), 200 ml (**NDC** 0074-6305-53), and 5 ml unit dose in ABBO-PAC packages (**NDC** 0074-6305-05). Each 5 ml (teaspoonful) of reconstituted suspension contains activity equivalent to 400 mg erythromycin.

EryPed Drops (erythromycin ethylsuccinate for oral suspension) is supplied in 50 ml bottles (**NDC** 0074-6303-50). Each 2.5 ml dropperful (½ teaspoonful of reconstituted suspension contains activity equivalent to 100 mg of erythromycin. After reconstitution, EryPed must be stored below 77°F (25°C) and used within 35 days; refrigeration not required.

EryPed Chewable (erythromycin ethylsuccinate tablets, USP) are fruit-flavored wafers containing activity equivalent to 200 mg of erythromycin and are available in packages of 40 (**NDC** 0074-6314-40). Each wafer is individually sealed in a blister package.

Reference: 1. American Heart Association. 1977. Prevention of bacterial endocarditis. Circulation 56:139A-143A.

Abbott Laboratories
North Chicago, IL 60064
Ref. 01-2441-R1

Shown in Product Identification Section, page 403

ERY-TAB®   ℞

[ĕrē'tab]
(erythromycin delayed-release tablets, USP)
ENTERIC-COATED

DESCRIPTION

Erythromycin is produced by a strain of *Streptomyces erythraeus* and belongs to the macrolide group of antibiotics. It is basic and readily forms salts with acids. The base is white to off-white crystals or powder slightly soluble in water, soluble in alcohol, in chloroform, and in ether. ERY-TAB (erythromycin delayed-release tablets) is specially enteric-coated to protect the contents from the inactivating effects of gastric acidity and to permit efficient absorption of the antibiotic in the small intestine.

ERY-TAB is available in three dosage strengths containing either 250 mg, 333 mg, or 500 mg of erythromycin as the free base.

Inactive Ingredients: 250 mg tablet: cellulosic polymers, corn starch, diacetylated monoglycerides, D&C red no. 30, iron oxide, magnesium hydroxide, magnesium stearate, sodium starch glycolate, titanium dioxide, vanillin and other ingredients.

333 mg tablet: cellulosic polymers, diacetylated monoglycerides, FD&C blue no. 1, magnesium stearate, microcrystalline cellulose, povidone, sodium citrate, soybean derivatives, talc, titanium dioxide, vanillin and other ingredients.

500 mg tablet: cellulosic polymers, diacetylated monoglycerides, FD&C red no. 40, iron oxide, magnesium stearate, microcrystalline cellulose, povidone, sodium citrate, soybean derivatives, talc, titanium dioxide, vanillin and other ingredients.

ACTIONS

The mode of action of erythromycin is inhibition of protein synthesis without affecting nucleic acid synthesis. Resistance to erythromycin of some strains of *Hemophilus influenzae* and staphylococci has been demonstrated. Culture and susceptibility testing should be done. If the Kirby-Bauer method of disc susceptibility is used, a 15 mcg erythromycin disc should give a zone diameter of at least 18 mm when tested against an erythromycin susceptible organism.

Bioavailability data are available from Abbott Laboratories, Dept. 355.

ERY-TAB is well absorbed and may be given without regard to meals.

After absorption, erythromycin diffuses readily into most body fluids. In the absence of meningeal inflammation, low concentrations are normally achieved in the spinal fluid but passage of the drug across the blood-brain barrier increases in meningitis. In the presence of normal hepatic function, erythromycin is concentrated in the liver and excreted in the bile; the effect of hepatic dysfunction on excretion of erythromycin by the liver into the bile is not known. After oral administration, less than 5 percent of the activity of the administered dose can be recovered in the urine.

Continued on next page

Abbott—Cont.

Erythromycin crosses the placental barrier but fetal plasma levels are low.

INDICATIONS

Streptococcus pyogenes (Group A beta-hemolytic streptococcus): For upper and lower respiratory tract, skin, and soft tissue infections of mild to moderate severity.

Injectable benzathine penicillin G is considered by the American Heart Association to be the drug of choice in the treatment and prevention of streptococcal pharyngitis and in long-term prophylaxis of rheumatic fever.

When oral medication is preferred for treatment of the above conditions, penicillin G, V, or erythromycin are alternate drugs of choice.

When oral medication is given, the importance of strict adherence by the patient to the prescribed dosage regimen must be stressed. A therapeutic dose should be administered for at least 10 days.

Alpha-hemolytic streptococci (viridans group): Although no controlled clinical efficacy trials have been conducted, oral erythromycin has been suggested by the American Heart Association and American Dental Association for use in a regimen for prophylaxis against bacterial endocarditis in patients hypersensitive to penicillin who have congenital heart disease, or rheumatic or other acquired valvular heart disease when they undergo dental procedures and surgical procedures of the upper respiratory tract.[1] Erythromycin is not suitable prior to genitourinary or gastrointestinal tract surgery. NOTE: When selecting antibiotics for the prevention of bacterial endocarditis the physician or dentist should read the full joint statement of the American Heart Association and the American Dental Association.[1]

Staphylococcus aureus: For acute infections of skin and soft tissue of mild to moderate severity. Resistant organisms may emerge during treatment.

Streptococcus pneumoniae (Diplococcus pneumoniae): For upper respiratory tract infections (e.g., otitis media, pharyngitis) and lower respiratory tract infections (e.g., pneumonia) of mild to moderate degree.

Mycoplasma pneumoniae (Eaton agent, PPLO): For respiratory infections due to this organism.

Hemophilus influenzae: For upper respiratory tract infections of mild to moderate severity when used concomitantly with adequate doses of sulfonamides. Not all strains of this organism are susceptible at the erythromycin concentrations ordinarily achieved (see appropriate sulfonamide labeling for prescribing information).

Chlamydia trachomatis: Erythromycin is indicated for treatment of the following infections caused by *Chlamydia trachomatis:* conjunctivitis of the newborn, pneumonia of infancy and urogenital infections during pregnancy. When tetracyclines are contraindicated or not tolerated, erythromycin is indicated for the treatment of uncomplicated urethral, endocervical, or rectal infections in adults due to *Chlamydia trachomatis.*[2]

Treponema pallidum: Erythromycin is an alternate choice of treatment for primary syphilis in patients allergic to the penicillins. In treatment of primary syphilis, spinal fluid examinations should be done before treatment and as part of follow-up after therapy.

Corynebacterium diphtheriae and C. minutissimum: As an adjunct to antitoxin, to prevent establishment of carriers, and to eradicate the organism in carriers. In the treatment of erythrasma.

Entamoeba histolytica: In the treatment of intestinal amebiasis only. Extra-enteric amebiasis requires treatment with other agents.

Listeria monocytogenes: Infections due to this organism.

Neisseria gonorrhoeae: Erythrocin® Lactobionate-I.V. (erythromycin lactobionate for injection, USP) in conjunction with erythromycin base orally, as an alternative drug in treatment of acute pelvic inflammatory disease caused by *N. gonorrhoeae* in female patients with a history of sensitivity to penicillin. Before treatment of gonorrhea, patients who are suspected of also having syphilis should have a microscopic examination for *T. pallidum* (by immunofluorescence or darkfield) before receiving erythromycin, and monthly serologic tests for a minimum of 4 months.

Bordetella pertussis: Erythromycin is effective in eliminating the organism from the nasopharynx of infected individuals, rendering them non-infectious. Some clinical studies suggest that erythromycin may be helpful in the prophylaxis of pertussis in exposed susceptible individuals.

Legionnaires' Disease: Although no controlled clinical efficacy studies have been conducted, *in vitro* and limited preliminary clinical data suggest that erythromycin can be effective in treating Legionnaires' Disease.

CONTRAINDICATIONS

Erythromycin is contraindicated in patients with known hypersensitivity to this antibiotic.

WARNING

Usage in pregnancy: Safety for use in pregnancy has not been established.

PRECAUTIONS

Erythromycin is principally excreted by the liver. Caution should be exercised in administering the antibiotic to patients with impaired hepatic function.

There have been reports of hepatic dysfunction, with or without jaundice, occurring in patients receiving oral erythromycin products.

Recent data from studies of erythromycin reveal that its use in patients who are receiving high doses of theophylline may be associated with an increase of serum theophylline levels and potential theophylline toxicity. In cases of theophylline toxicity and/or elevated serum theophylline levels, the dose of theophylline should be reduced while the patient is receiving concomitant erythromycin therapy.

Surgical procedures should be performed when indicated.

ADVERSE REACTIONS

The most frequent side effects of erythromycin preparations are gastrointestinal, such as abdominal cramping and discomfort, and are dose-related. Nausea, vomiting, and diarrhea occur infrequently with usual oral doses.

During prolonged or repeated therapy, there is a possibility of overgrowth of nonsusceptible bacteria or fungi. If such infections occur, the drug should be discontinued and appropriate therapy instituted.

Mild allergic reactions such as urticaria and other skin rashes have occurred. Serious allergic reactions, including anaphylaxis, have been reported. Allergic reactions should be handled in the usual manner.

There have been isolated reports of reversible hearing loss occurring chiefly in patients with renal insufficiency and in patients receiving high doses of erythromycin.

DOSAGE AND ADMINISTRATION

Ery-Tab (erythromycin delayed-release tablets) is well absorbed and may be given without regard to meals.

Adults: The usual dose is 250 mg four times daily in equally spaced doses. The 333 mg tablet is recommended if dosage is desired every 8 hours. If twice-a-day dosage is desired, the recommended dose is 500 mg every 12 hours.

Dosage may be increased up to 4 or more grams per day according to the severity of the infection. Twice-a-day dosing is not recommended when doses larger than 1 gram daily are administered.

Children: Age, weight, and severity of the infection are important factors in determining the proper dosage. 30 to 50 mg/kg/day, in divided doses, is the usual dose. For more severe infections, this dose may be doubled.

In the treatment of streptococcal infections, a therapeutic dosage of erythromycin should be administered for at least 10 days. In continuous prophylaxis of streptococcal infections in persons with a history of rheumatic heart disease, the dose is 250 mg twice a day.

For prophylaxis against bacterial endocarditis[1] in patients with congenital heart disease, or rheumatic or other acquired valvular heart disease when undergoing dental procedures or surgical procedures of the upper respiratory tract, give 1 g (20 mg/kg for children) orally 1½ to 2 hours before the procedure, and then, 500 mg (10 mg/kg in children) orally every 6 hours for 8 doses.

For conjunctivitis of the newborn caused by *Chlamydia trachomatis:* Oral erythromycin suspension 50 mg/kg/day in 4 divided doses for at least 2 weeks.[2]

For pneumonia of infancy caused by *Chlamydia trachomatis:* Although the optimal duration of therapy has not been established, the recommended therapy is oral erythromycin suspension 50 mg/kg/day in 4 divided doses for at least 3 weeks.[2]

For urogenital infections during pregnancy due to *Chlamydia trachomatis:* Although the optimal dose and duration of therapy have not been established, the suggested treatment is erythromycin 500 mg, by mouth, 4 times a day for at least 7 days. For women who cannot tolerate this regimen, a decreased dose of 250 mg, by mouth, 4 times a day should be used for at least 14 days.[2]

For adults with uncomplicated urethral, endocervical, or rectal infections caused by *Chlamydia trachomatis* in whom tetracyclines are contraindicated or not tolerated: 500 mg, by mouth, 4 times a day for at least 7 days.[2]

For treatment of primary syphilis: 30 to 40 grams given in divided doses over a period of 10 to 15 days.

For treatment of acute pelvic inflammatory disease caused by *N. gonorrhoeae:* After initial treatment with Erythrocin® Lactobionate-I.V. (erythromycin lactobionate for injection, USP) 500 mg every 6 hours for 3 days, the oral dosage recommendation is 250 mg every 6 hours for 7 days.

For dysenteric amebiasis: 250 mg four times daily for 10 to 14 days, for adults; 30 to 50 mg/kg/day in divided doses for 10 to 14 days, for children.

For use in pertussis: Although optimal dosage and duration have not been established, doses of erythromycin uti-

lized in reported clinical studies were 40 to 50 mg/kg/day, given in divided doses for 5 to 14 days.

For treatment of Legionnaires' Disease: Although optimal doses have not been established, doses utilized in reported clinical data were 1 to 4 grams erythromycin base daily in divided doses.

OVERDOSAGE

Gastrointestinal side effects of erythromycin are dose related. Some individuals may exhibit gastric intolerance to even therapeutic amounts.

Erythromycin serum levels are not appreciably affected by hemodialysis or peritoneal dialysis.

HOW SUPPLIED

Ery-Tab (erythromycin delayed-release tablets, USP), 250 mg, is supplied as pink tablets in bottles of 100 (NDC 0074-6304-13), bottles of 500 (NDC 0074-6304-53), and Abbo-Pac® unit dose packages of 100 (NDC 0074-6304-11).

Ery-Tab, 333 mg, is supplied as white tablets in bottles of 100 (NDC 0074-6320-13), bottles of 500 (NDC 0074-6320-53), and Abbo-Pac® unit dose packages of 100 (NDC 0074-6320-11).

Ery-Tab, 500 mg, is supplied as pink tablets in bottles of 100 (NDC 0074-6321-13) and Abbo-Pac® unit dose packages of 100 (NDC 0074-6321-11).

REFERENCES

1. American Heart Association. 1977. Prevention of bacterial endocarditis. Circulation 56:139A-143A.
2. CDC Sexually Transmitted Diseases Treatment Guidelines 1982.

333 mg and 500 mg tablets—U.S. Pat. No. 4,340,582.
Abbott Laboratories
North Chicago, IL 60064
Ref. 07-5626-R4
Shown in Product Identification Section, page 403

E.E.S.®   ℞
[*ē-ē-s*]
(erythromycin ethylsuccinate)

DESCRIPTION

Erythromycin is produced by a strain of *Streptomyces erythraeus* and belongs to the macrolide group of antibiotics. It is basic and readily forms salts with acids. The base, the stearate salt, and the esters are poorly soluble in water. Erythromycin ethylsuccinate is an ester of erythromycin suitable for oral administration.

The granules are intended for reconstitution with water. When reconstituted, they are palatable cherry-flavored suspensions.

The pleasant tasting, fruit-flavored liquids are supplied ready for oral administration.

Granules and ready-made suspensions are intended primarily for pediatric use but can also be used in adults.

The Filmtab® tablets are intended primarily for adults or older children.

Inactive Ingredients: E.E.S. 200 Liquid: FD&C Red No. 40, methylparaben, polysorbate 60, propylparaben, sodium citrate, sucrose, water, xanthan gum and natural and artificial flavors.

E.E.S. 400 Liquid: D&C Yellow No. 10, FD&C Yellow No. 6, methylparaben, polysorbate 60, propylparaben, sodium citrate, sucrose, water, xanthan gum and natural and artificial flavors.

E.E.S. Granules: Citric acid, FD&C Red No. 3, magnesium aluminum silicate, sodium carboxymethyl cellulose, sodium citrate, sucrose and artificial flavor.

E.E.S. 400 Filmtab Tablets: Cellulosic polymers, confectioner's sugar (contains corn starch), corn starch, D&C Red No. 30, D&C Yellow No. 10, FD&C Red No. 40, magnesium stearate, polacrilin potassium, polyethylene glycol, propylene glycol, sodium citrate, sorbic acid, sorbitan monooleate, titanium dioxide and vitamin E.

ACTIONS

Microbiology: Biochemical tests demonstrate that erythromycin inhibits protein synthesis of the pathogen without directly affecting nucleic acid synthesis. Antagonism has been demonstrated between clindamycin and erythromycin. NOTE: Many strains of *Hemophilus influenzae* are resistant to erythromycin alone, but are susceptible to erythromycin and sulfonamides together. Staphylococci resistant to erythromycin may emerge during a course of erythromycin therapy. Culture and susceptibility testing should be performed.

Disc Susceptibility Tests: Quantitative methods that require measurement of zone diameters give the most precise estimates of antibiotic susceptibility. One recommended procedure (21 CFR section 460.1) uses erythromycin class discs for testing susceptibility; interpretations correlate zone diameters of this disc test with MIC values for erythromycin. With this procedure, a report from the laboratory of "susceptible" indicates that the infecting organism is likely to respond to therapy. A report of "resistant" indicates that the infective organism is not likely to respond to therapy. A report of "intermediate susceptibility" suggests that the organism would be susceptible if higher doses were used.

Clinical Pharmacology: Erythromycin binds to the 50 S ribosomal subunits of susceptible bacteria and suppresses protein synthesis.

Orally administered erythromycin ethylsuccinate suspensions and Filmtab tablets are readily and reliably absorbed. Comparable serum levels of erythromycin are achieved in the fasting and nonfasting states.

Erythromycin diffuses readily into most body fluids. Only low concentrations are normally achieved in the spinal fluid, but passage of the drug across the blood-brain barrier increases in meningitis. In the presence of normal hepatic function, erythromycin is concentrated in the liver and excreted in the bile; the effect of hepatic dysfunction on excretion of erythromycin by the liver into the bile is not known. Less than 5 percent of the orally administered dose of erythromycin is excreted in active form in the urine.

Erythromycin crosses the placental barrier and is excreted in breast milk.

INDICATIONS

Streptococcus pyogenes (Group A beta-hemolytic streptococcus): Upper and lower respiratory tract, skin, and soft tissue infections of mild to moderate severity.

Injectable benzathine penicillin G is considered by the American Heart Association to be the drug of choice in the treatment and prevention of streptococcal pharyngitis and in long-term prophylaxis of rheumatic fever.

When oral medication is preferred for treatment of the above conditions, penicillin G, V, or erythromycin are alternate drugs of choice.

When oral medication is given, the importance of strict adherence by the patient to the prescribed dosage regimen must be stressed during treatment. A therapeutic dose should be administered for at least 10 days.

Alpha-hemolytic streptococci (viridans group): Although no controlled clinical efficacy trials have been conducted, oral erythromycin has been suggested by the American Heart Association and American Dental Association for use in a regimen for prophylaxis against bacterial endocarditis in patients hypersensitive to penicillin who have congenital heart disease, or rheumatic or other acquired valvular heart disease when they undergo dental procedures and surgical procedures of the upper respiratory tract.[1] Erythromycin is not suitable prior to genitourinary or gastrointestinal tract surgery. NOTE: When selecting antibiotics for the prevention of bacterial endocarditis the physician or dentist should read the full joint statement of the American Heart Association and the American Dental Association.[1]

Staphylococcus aureus: Acute infections of skin and soft tissue of mild to moderate severity. Resistant organisms may emerge during treatment.

Streptococcus pneumoniae (Diplococcus pneumoniae): Upper respiratory tract infections (e.g., otitis media, pharyngitis) and lower respiratory tract infections (e.g., pneumonia) of mild to moderate degree.

Mycoplasma pneumoniae (Eaton agent, PPLO): For respiratory infections due to this organism.

Hemophilus influenzae: For upper respiratory tract infections of mild to moderate severity when used concomitantly with adequate doses of sulfonamides. (See sulfonamide labeling for appropriate prescribing information.) The concomitant use of the sulfonamides is necessary since not all strains of *Hemophilus influenzae* are susceptible to erythromycin at the concentrations of the antibiotic achieved with usual therapeutic doses.

Chlamydia trachomatis: For the treatment of urethritis in adult males due to *Chlamydia trachomatis.*

Ureaplasma urealyticum: For the treatment of urethritis in adult males due to *Ureaplasma urealyticum.*

Treponema pallidum: Erythromycin is an alternate choice of treatment for primary syphilis in patients allergic to the penicillins. In treatment of primary syphilis, spinal fluid examinations should be done before treatment and as part of follow-up after therapy.

Corynebacterium diphtheriae: As an adjunct to antitoxin, to prevent establishment of carriers, and to eradicate the organism in carriers.

Corynebacterium minutissimum: For the treatment of erythrasma.

Entamoeba histolytica: In the treatment of intestinal amebiasis only. Extraenteric amebiasis requires treatment with other agents.

Listeria monocytogenes: Infections due to this organism.

Bordetella pertussis: Erythromycin is effective in eliminating the organism from the nasopharynx of infected individuals, rendering them non-infectious. Some clinical studies suggest that erythromycin may be helpful in the prophylaxis of pertussis in exposed susceptible individuals.

Legionnaires' Disease: Although no controlled clinical efficacy studies have been conducted, *in vitro* and limited preliminary clinical data suggest that erythromycin may be effective in treating Legionnaires' Disease.

CONTRAINDICATIONS

Erythromycin is contraindicated in patients with known hypersensitivity to this antibiotic.

PRECAUTIONS

Erythromycin is principally excreted by the liver. Caution should be exercised in administering the antibiotic to patients with impaired hepatic function. There have been reports of hepatic dysfunction, with or without jaundice occurring in patients receiving oral erythromycin products.

Areas of localized infection may require surgical drainage in addition to antibiotic therapy.

Recent data from studies of erythromycin reveal that its use in patients who are receiving high doses of theophylline may be associated with an increase of serum theophylline levels and potential theophylline toxicity. In case of theophylline toxicity and/or elevated serum theophylline levels, the dose of theophylline should be reduced while the patient is receiving concomitant erythromycin therapy.

Usage during pregnancy and lactation: The safety of erythromycin for use during pregnancy has not been established. Erythromycin crosses the placental barrier. Erythromycin also appears in breast milk.

ADVERSE REACTIONS

The most frequent side effects of erythromycin preparations are gastrointestinal, such as abdominal cramping and discomfort, and are dose related. Nausea, vomiting, and diarrhea occur infrequently with usual oral doses.

During prolonged or repeated therapy, there is a possibility of overgrowth of nonsusceptible bacteria or fungi. If such infections occur, the drug should be discontinued and appropriate therapy instituted.

Allergic reactions ranging from urticaria and mild skin eruptions to anaphylaxis have occurred.

There have been isolated reports of reversible hearing loss occurring chiefly in patients with renal insufficiency and in patients receiving high doses of erythromycin.

DOSAGE AND ADMINISTRATION

Erythromycin ethylsuccinate suspensions and Filmtab tablets may be administered without regard to meals.

Children: Age, weight, and severity of the infection are important factors in determining the proper dosage. In mild to moderate infections the usual dosage of erythromycin ethylsuccinate for children is 30 to 50 mg/kg/day in equally divided doses every 6 hours. For more severe infections this dosage may be doubled. If twice-a-day dosage is desired, one-half of the total daily dose may be given every 12 hours. Doses may also be given three times daily by administering one-third of the total daily dose every 8 hours.

The following dosage schedule is suggested for mild to moderate infections:

Body Weight	Total Daily Dose
Under 10 lbs	30–50 mg/kg/day 15–25 mg/lb/day
10 to 15 lbs	200 mg
16 to 25 lbs	400 mg
26 to 50 lbs	800 mg
51 to 100 lbs	1200 mg
over 100 lbs	1600 mg

Adults: 400 mg erythromycin ethylsuccinate every 6 hours is the usual dose. Dosage may be increased up to 4 g per day according to the severity of the infection. If twice-a-day dosage is desired, one-half of the total daily dose may be given every 12 hours. Doses may also be given three times daily by administering one-third of the total daily dose every 8 hours. For adult dosage calculation, use a ratio of 400 mg of erythromycin activity as the ethylsuccinate to 250 mg of erythromycin activity as the stearate, base or estolate.

In the treatment of streptococcal infections, a therapeutic dosage of erythromycin ethylsuccinate should be administered for at least 10 days. In continuous prophylaxis against recurrences of streptococcal infections in persons with a history of rheumatic heart disease, the usual dosage is 400 mg twice a day.

For prophylaxis against bacterial endocarditis[1] in patients with congenital heart disease, or rheumatic or other acquired valvular heart disease when undergoing dental procedures or surgical procedures of the upper respiratory tract, give 1.6 g (20 mg/kg for children) orally 1½ to 2 hours before the procedure, and then, 800 mg (10 mg/kg for children) orally every 6 hours for 8 doses.

For treatment of urethritis due to *C. trachomatis* or *U. urealyticum:* 800 mg three times a day for 7 days.

For treatment of primary syphilis: Adults: 48 to 64 g given in divided doses over a period of 10 to 15 days.

For intestinal amebiasis: Adults: 400 mg four times daily for 10 to 14 days. Children: 30 to 50 mg/kg/day in divided doses for 10 to 14 days.

For use in pertussis: Although optimal dosage and duration have not been established, doses of erythromycin utilized in reported clinical studies were 40 to 50 mg/kg/day, given in divided doses for 5 to 14 days.

For treatment of Legionnaires' Disease: Although optimal doses have not been established, doses utilized in reported clinical data were those recommended above (1.6 to 4 g daily in divided doses).

HOW SUPPLIED

E.E.S. 200 LIQUID (erythromycin ethylsuccinate oral suspension, USP) is supplied in 1 pint bottles (NDC 0074-6306-16) and in packages of six 100-ml bottles (NDC 0074-6306-13). Each 5-ml teaspoonful of fruit-flavored suspension contains activity equivalent to 200 mg of erythromycin.

E.E.S. 400® LIQUID (erythromycin ethylsuccinate oral suspension, USP) is supplied in 1 pint bottles (NDC 0074-6373-16) and in packages of six 100-ml bottles (NDC 0074-6373-13). Each 5-ml teaspoonful of orange, fruit-flavored suspension contains activity equivalent to 400 mg of erythromycin.

Both liquid products require refrigeration to preserve taste until dispensed. Refrigeration by patient is not required if used within 14 days.

E.E.S. GRANULES (erythromycin ethylsuccinate for oral suspension, USP) is supplied in 100-ml (NDC 0074-6369-02) and 200-ml (NDC 0074-6369-10) size bottles. Each 5-ml teaspoonful of reconstituted cherry-flavored suspension contains activity equivalent to 200 mg of erythromycin.

E.E.S. 400 Filmtab tablets (erythromycin ethylsuccinate tablets, USP) 400 mg, are available in bottles of 100 (NDC 0074-5729-13) and 500 (NDC 0074-5729-53), and in ABBO-PAC® unit dose strip packages of 100 (NDC 0074-5729-11). Tablets are pink in color.

REFERENCE

1. American Heart Association. 1977. Prevention of bacterial endocarditis. Circulation 56: 139A-143A.

Filmtab—Film-sealed tablets, Abbott.

Abbott Laboratories
North Chicago, IL 60064
Ref. 01-2446-R14
Shown in Product Identification Section, page 403

ERYTHROCIN® LACTOBIONATE-I.V.   ℞
[e-rith 'ro-sin lac-tō-bī"ō-nāte ĭ. v.]
(erythromycin lactobionate for injection, USP)
Vials For I.V. use only

DESCRIPTION

Erythromycin is produced by a strain of *Streptomyces erythraeus* and belongs to the macrolide group of antibiotics. It is basic and readily forms salts with acids.

Erythrocin Lactobionate (erythromycin lactobionate for injection, USP), is a soluble salt of erythromycin suitable for intravenous administration. It is available as a sterile, lyophilized powder in vials containing the equivalent of 500 mg of erythromycin activity with 90 mg benzyl alcohol or 1 g of erythromycin activity with 180 mg benzyl alcohol.

Erythromycin lactobionate is chemically known as erythromycin mono (4-0-β-D-galactopyran-osyl-D-gluconate) (salt). The structural formula is:

$\cdot C_{12}H_{22}O_{12}$

CLINICAL PHARMACOLOGY

Erythromycin diffuses readily into most body fluids. In the absence of meningeal inflammation, low concentrations are normally achieved in the spinal fluid but the passage of the drug across the blood-brain barrier increases in meningitis. Erythromycin crosses the placental barrier and is excreted in breast milk. Erythromycin is not removed by peritoneal dialysis or hemodialysis.

In the presence of normal hepatic function, erythromycin is concentrated in the liver and is excreted in the bile; the ef-

Continued on next page

Abbott—Cont.

fect of hepatic dysfunction on biliary excretion of erythromycin is not known. From 12 to 15 percent of intravenously administered erythromycin is excreted in active form in the urine.

Intravenous infusion of 500 mg of erythromycin lactobionate at a constant rate over 1 hour in fasting adults produced a mean serum erythromycin level of approximately 7 mcg/mL at 20 minutes, 10 mcg/mL at 1 hour, 2.6 mcg/mL at 2.5 hours, and 1 mcg/mL at 6 hours.

Microbiology:
Erythromycin acts by inhibition of protein synthesis by binding 50 S ribosomal subunits of susceptible organisms. It does not affect nucleic acid synthesis. Antagonism has been demonstrated in vitro between erythromycin and clindamycin, lincomycin and chloramphenicol.

Many strains of Haemophilus influenzae are resistant to erythromycin alone, but are susceptible to erythromycin and sulfonamides together.

Staphylococci resistant to erythromycin may emerge during a course of therapy. Culture and susceptibility testing should be performed.

Erythromycin is usually active against the following organisms in vitro (prior to use, refer to "INDICATIONS AND USAGE" section):

Gram-positive Bacteria: Staphylococcus aureus (resistant organisms may emerge during treatment), Streptococcus pyogenes (Group A beta-hemolytic streptococcus), Alpha-hemolytic streptococcus (viridans group), Streptococcus (diplococcus) pneumoniae, Corynebacterium diphtheriae, Corynebacterium minutissimum.

Gram-negative Bacteria: Neisseria gonorrhoeae, Legionella pneumophila, Bordetella pertussis.

Mycoplasma: Mycoplasma pneumoniae, Ureaplasma urealyticum.

Other Microorganisms: Chlamydia trachomatis, Entamoeba histolytica, Treponema pallidum, Listeria monocytogenes.

Susceptibility Testing:
Quantitative methods that require measurement of zone diameters give the most precise estimates of antibiotic susceptibility. One such standardized single-disc procedure has been recommended for use with discs to test susceptibility to erythromycin.[1] Interpretation involves correlation of the zone diameters obtained in the disc test with minimal inhibitory concentration (MIC) values for erythromycin.

Reports from the laboratory giving results of the standardized single-disc susceptibility test using a 15 mcg erythromycin disc should be interpreted according to the following criteria:

Susceptible organisms produce zones of 18 mm or greater, indicating that the tested organism is likely to respond to therapy.

Resistant organisms produce zones of 13 mm or less, indicating that other therapy should be selected.

Organisms of intermediate susceptibility produce zones of 14 to 17 mm. The "intermediate" category provides a "buffer zone" which should prevent small, uncontrolled technical factors from causing major discrepancies in interpretations; thus, when a zone diameter falls within the "intermediate" range, the results may be considered equivocal. If alternative drugs are not available, confirmation by dilution tests may be indicated.

Standardized procedures require the use of control organisms. The 15 mcg erythromycin disc should give zone diameters between 22 and 30 mm for the S. aureus ATCC 25923 control strain.

A bacterial isolate may be considered susceptible if the MIC value[2] for erythromycin is not more than 2 mcg/mL. Organisms are considered resistant if the MIC is 8 mcg/mL or higher. The MIC of erythromycin for S. aureus ATCC 29213 control strain should be between 0.12 and 0.5 mcg/mL.

INDICATIONS AND USAGE
Erythrocin Lactobionate I.V. (erythromycin lactobionate for injection, USP) is indicated in the treatment of infections caused by susceptible strains of the designated organisms in the diseases listed below when oral administration is not possible or when the severity of the infection requires immediate high serum levels of erythromycin. Intravenous therapy should be replaced by oral administration at the appropriate time.

Upper respiratory tract infections of mild to moderate degree caused by Streptococcus pyogenes (Group A beta-hemolytic streptococci); Streptococcus pneumoniae (Diplococcus pneumoniae); Haemophilus influenzae (when used concomitantly with adequate doses of sulfonamides, since many strains of H. influenzae are not susceptible to the erythromycin concentrations ordinarily achieved). (See appropriate sulfonamide labeling for prescribing information.)

Lower respiratory tract infections of mild to moderate severity caused by Streptococcus pyogenes (Group A beta-hemolytic streptococci); Streptococcus pneumoniae (Diplococcus pneumoniae).

Respiratory tract infections due to Mycoplasma pneumoniae. Skin and skin structure infections of mild to moderate severity caused by Streptococcus pyogenes and Staphylococcus aureus (resistant staphylococci may emerge during treatment).

Diphtheria: As an adjunct to antitoxin infections due to Corynebacterium diphtheriae to prevent establishment of carriers and to eradicate the organism in carriers.

Erythrasma: In the treatment of infections due to Corynebacterium minutissimum.

Acute pelvic inflammatory disease caused by Neisseria gonorrhoeae: Erythrocin Lactobionate-I.V. (erythromycin lactobionate for injection, USP) followed by erythromycin stearate of base orally, as an alternative drug in treatment of acute pelvic inflammatory disease caused by N. gonorrhoeae in female patients with a history of sensitivity to penicillin. Before treatment of gonorrhea, patients who are suspected of also having syphilis should have a microscopic examination for T. pallidum (by immunofluorescence or darkfield) before receiving erythromycin and monthly serologic tests for a minimum of 4 months thereafter.

Legionnaires' Disease caused by Legionella pneumophila. Although no controlled clinical efficacy studies have been conducted, in vitro and limited preliminary clinical data suggest that erythromycin may be effective in treating Legionnaires' Disease.

Prevention of Initial Attacks of Rheumatic Fever: Penicillin is considered by the American Heart Association to be the drug of choice in the prevention of initial attacks of rheumatic fever (treatment of Group A beta-hemolytic streptococcal infections of the upper respiratory tract e.g., tonsillitis, or pharyngitis).[3] Erythromycin is indicated for the treatment of penicillin-allergic patients. The therapeutic dose should be administered for ten days.

Prevention of Recurrent Attacks of Rheumatic Fever: Penicillin or sulfonamides are considered by the American Heart Association to be the drugs of choice in the prevention of recurrent attacks of rheumatic fever. In patients who are allergic to penicillin and sulfonamides, oral erythromycin is recommended by the American Heart Association in the long-term prophylaxis of streptococcal pharyngitis (for the prevention of recurrent attacks of rheumatic fever).[3]

Prevention of Bacterial Endocarditis: Although no controlled clinical efficacy trials have been conducted, oral erythromycin has been recommended by the American Heart Association for prevention of bacterial endocarditis in penicillin-allergic patients with prosthetic cardiac valves, most congenital cardiac malformations, surgically constructed systemic pulmonary shunts, rheumatic or other acquired valvular dysfunction, idiopathic hypertrophic subaortic stenosis (IHSS), previous history of bacterial endocarditis and mitral valve prolapse with insufficiency when they undergo dental procedures and surgical procedures of the upper respiratory tract.[4]

CONTRAINDICATIONS
Erythromycin is contraindicated in patients with known hypersensitivity to this antibiotic.

WARNINGS
There have been reports of hepatic dysfunction with or without jaundice occurring in patients receiving oral erythromycin products.

PRECAUTIONS
General: Since erythromycin is principally excreted by the liver, caution should be exercised when erythromycin is administered to patients with impaired hepatic function. (See "CLINICAL PHARMACOLOGY" and "WARNINGS" sections.)

Prolonged or repeated use of erythromycin may result in an overgrowth of non-susceptible bacteria or fungi. If superinfection occurs, erythromycin should be discontinued and appropriate therapy instituted.

When indicated, incision and drainage or other surgical procedures should be performed in conjunction with antibiotic therapy.

Laboratory Tests: Erythromycin interferes with the fluorometric determination of urinary catecholamines.

Drug Interactions: Erythromycin use in patients who are receiving high doses of theophylline may be associated with an increase of serum theophylline levels and potential theophylline toxicity. Serum theophylline levels should be monitored in patients receiving concomitant erythromycin. The theophylline dose may need to be reduced in some patients.

Erythromycin administration in patients receiving carbamazepine has been reported to cause increased serum levels of carbamazepine with subsequent development of signs of carbamazepine toxicity.

Concomitant administration of erythromycin and digoxin has been reported to result in elevated serum digoxin levels. There have been reports of increased anticoagulant effects when erythromycin and oral anticoagulants were used concomitantly.

Carcinogenesis, Mutagenesis, Impairment of Fertility: Long-term animal data with erythromycin lactobionate for use in determination of possible carcinogenic effects are not available. However, long-term oral studies in rats with erythromycin ethylsuccinate and erythromycin base did not provide evidence of tumorigenicity. Mutagenicity studies have not been conducted. There was no apparent effect on male or female fertility in rats fed erythromycin (base) at levels up to 0.25% of diet.

Pregnancy
Pregnancy Category B: There was no evidence of teratogenicity or any other adverse effect on reproduction in female rats fed erythromycin base (up to 0.25% of diet) prior to and during mating, during gestation, and through weaning of two successive litters. There are, however, no adequate and well-controlled studies in pregnant women. Because animal reproduction studies are not always predictive of human response, this drug should be used during pregnancy only if clearly needed. Erythromycin has been reported to cross the placental barrier in humans, but fetal plasma levels are generally low.

Labor and Delivery: The effect of erythromycin on labor and delivery is unknown.

Nursing Mothers: Erythromycin is excreted in breast milk. Caution should be exercised when erythromycin is administered to a nursing woman.

Pediatric Use: See "INDICATIONS AND USAGE" and "DOSAGE AND ADMINISTRATION" sections.

This product contains benzyl alcohol which has been associated with a fatal gasping syndrome in infants.

ADVERSE REACTIONS
Side effects following the use of intravenous erythromycin are rare. Occasional venous irritation has been encountered, but if the infusion is given slowly, in dilute solution, preferably by continuous intravenous infusion or intermittent infusion in no less than 20 to 60 minutes, pain and vessel trauma are minimized.

Occasional nausea, vomiting, abdominal cramping and abdominal pain have been reported.

Allergic reactions, ranging from urticaria and mild skin eruptions to anaphylaxis, have occurred with intravenously administered erythromycin.

There have been isolated reports of reversible hearing loss occurring chiefly in patients with renal insufficiency and in patients receiving high doses of erythromycin.

OVERDOSAGE
In the case of overdosage, erythromycin infusion should be discontinued and all other appropriate measures should be instituted.

Erythromycin is not removed by peritoneal dialysis or hemodialysis.

DOSAGE AND ADMINISTRATION
For the treatment of severe infections in adults and children, the recommended intravenous dose of erythromycin lactobionate is 15 to 20 mg/kg/day. Higher doses, up to 4 g/day, may be given for severe infections. Erythrocin Lactobionate-I.V. (erythromycin lactobionate for injection, USP) must be administered by continuous or intermittent intravenous infusion only. Due to the irritative properties of erythromycin, I.V. push is an unacceptable route of administration. Continuous infusion of erythromycin lactobionate is preferable due to the slower infusion rate and lower concentration of erythromycin; however, intermittent infusion at six hour intervals is also effective. Intravenous erythromycin should be replaced by oral erythromycin as soon as possible.

For slow continuous infusion: The final diluted solution of erythromycin lactobionate is prepared to give a concentration of 1 g per liter (1 mg/mL).

For intermittent infusion: Administer one-fourth the total daily dose of erythromycin lactobionate by intravenous infusion in 20 to 60 minutes at intervals not greater than every six hours. The final diluted solution of erythromycin lactobionate is prepared to give a concentration of 1 to 5 mg/mL. No less than 100 mL of I.V. diluent should be used. Infusion should be sufficiently slow to minimize pain along the vein. For treatment of acute pelvic inflammatory disease caused by N. gonorrhoeae, in female patients hypersensitive to penicillins, administer 500 mg erythromycin lactobionate every six hours for three days, followed by oral administration of 250 mg erythromycin stearate or base every six hours for seven days.

For treatment of Legionnaires' Disease: Although optimal doses have not been established, doses utilized in reported clinical data were 1 to 4 grams daily in divided doses.

In the treatment of Group A beta-hemolytic streptococcal infections of the upper respiratory tract (e.g., tonsillitis or pharyngitis), the therapeutic dosage of erythromycin should be administered for ten days. The American Heart Association suggests a dosage of 250 mg of erythromycin orally, twice a day in long-term prophylaxis of streptococcal upper respiratory tract infections for the prevention of recurring attacks of rheumatic fever in patients allergic to penicillin and sulfonamides[3].

In prophylaxis against bacterial endocarditis (see "INDICATIONS AND USAGE" section), the oral regimen for penicillin allergic patients is erythromycin 1 gram, 1 hour before the procedure followed by 500 mg six hours later.[4]

Preparation of Solution:

1. PREPARE THE INITIAL SOLUTION OF ERYTHRO-CIN® LACTOBIONATE-I.V. BY ADDING 10 ML OF STERILE WATER FOR INJECTION, USP, TO THE 500 MG VIAL OR 20 ML OF STERILE WATER FOR INJECTION, USP, TO THE 1 g VIAL. Use only Sterile Water for Injection, USP, as other diluents may cause precipitation during reconstitution. Do not use diluents containing preservatives or inorganic salts. Note: When the product is reconstituted as directed above, the resulting solution contains an effective antimicrobial preservative.

After reconstitution, each mL contains 50 mg of erythromycin activity. The initial solution is stable at refrigerator temperature for two weeks, or for 24 hours at room temperature.

2. ADD THE INITIAL DILUTION TO ONE OF THE FOLLOWING DILUENTS BEFORE ADMINISTRATION to give a concentration of 1 g of erythromycin activity per liter (1 mg/mL) for continuous infusion or 1 to 5 mg/mL for intermittent infusion:

0.9% SODIUM CHLORIDE INJECTION, USP LACTATED RINGER'S INJECTION, USP NORMOSOL®-R.

3. THE FOLLOWING SOLUTIONS MAY ALSO BE USED PROVIDING THEY ARE FIRST BUFFERED WITH NEUT® (4% SODIUM BICARBONATE, ABBOTT) by adding 1 mL of Neut per 100 mL of solution:

5% DEXTROSE INJECTION, USP
5% DEXTROSE AND LACTATED RINGER'S INJECTION
5% DEXTROSE AND 0.9% SODIUM CHLORIDE INJECTION, USP

Neut® (4% sodium bicarbonate, Abbott) must be added to these solutions so that their pH is in the optimum range for erythromycin lactobionate stability. Acidic solutions of erythromycin lactobionate are unstable and lose their potency rapidly. A pH of at least 5.5 is desirable for the final diluted solution of erythromycin lactobionate.

No drug or chemical agent should be added to an erythromycin lactobionate-I.V. fluid admixture unless its effect on the chemical and physical stability of the solution has first been determined.

Stability:

The final diluted solution of erythromycin lactobionate should be completely administered within 8 hours, since it is not suitable for storage.*

Parenteral drug products should be inspected visually for particulate matter and discoloration prior to administration, whenever solution and container permit.

HOW SUPPLIED

Erythrocin Lactobionate-I.V. (erythromycin lactobionate for injection, USP) is supplied as a sterile, lyophilized powder in packages of 10 vials (NDC 0074-6342-05), each vial containing the equivalent of 1 Gm of erythromycin with 180 mg benzyl alcohol added as preservative; and in packages of 10 vials (NDC 0074-6365-02), each vial containing the equivalent of 500 mg of erythromycin with 90 mg benzyl alcohol added as preservative.

Store at controlled room temperature 15° to 30° C (59° to 86° F).

REFERENCES

1. National Committee for Clinical Laboratory Standards, Approved Standard: *Performance Standards for Antimicrobial Disk Susceptibility Tests*, 3rd Edition, Vol. 4(16):M2-A3, Villanova, PA, December 1984.

2. Ericson, H.M., Sherris, J.C., Antibiotic Sensitivity Testing Report of an International Collaborative Study, *Acta Pathologica et Microbiologica Scandinavica* Section B. Suppl. 217:1-90, 1971.

3. Committee on Rheumatic Fever and Infective Endocarditis of the Council on Cardiovascular Disease of the Young: Prevention of Rheumatic Fever, *Circulation* 70(6):1118A-1122A, December 1984.

4. Committee on Rheumatic Fever and Infective Endocarditis of the Council on Cardiovascular Disease of the Young: Prevention of Bacterial Endocarditis, *Circulation* 70(6):1123A-1127A, December 1984.

Caution: Federal (USA) law prohibits dispensing without prescription.

*Contact Abbott Laboratories, Dept. 97H, for additional stability data.

Abbott Laboratories
North Chicago, IL 60064
Ref. 01-2417 R17-REV. JAN., 1988

ERYTHROCIN® PIGGYBACK   ℞

[e-rith'ro-sin pig'gy back]
(Erythromycin Lactobionate for Injection, USP)
Single Dose Dispensing Vial
For I.V. Use Only

DESCRIPTION

Erythromycin is produced by a strain of *Streptomyces erythraeus* and belongs to the macrolide group of antibiotics. It is basic and readily forms salts with acids.

Erythromycin Lactobionate is a soluble salt of erythromycin. ERYTHROCIN PIGGYBACK (erythromycin lactobionate for injection, USP), is a dosage form suitable for intermittent intravenous administration.

It is available as a sterile, lyophilized powder in single dose, dispensing vials containing the equivalent of 500 mg of erythromycin activity with 90 mg of benzyl alcohol.

Erythromycin lactobionate is chemically known as erythromycin mono (4-0-β-D-galactopyranosyl-D-gluconate) (salt). The structural formula is:

CLINICAL PHARMACOLOGY

Erythromycin diffuses readily into most body fluids. In the absence of meningeal inflammation, low concentrations are normally achieved in the spinal fluid but the passage of the drug across the blood-brain barrier increases in meningitis. Erythromycin crosses the placental barrier and is excreted in breast milk. Erythromycin is not removed by peritoneal dialysis or hemodialysis.

In the presence of normal hepatic function, erythromycin is concentrated in the liver and is excreted in the bile; the effect of hepatic dysfunction on biliary excretion of erythromycin is not known. From 12 to 15 percent of intravenously administered erythromycin is excreted in active form in the urine.

Intravenous infusion of 500 mg of erythromycin lactobionate at a constant rate over 1 hour in fasting adults produced a mean serum erythromycin level of approximately 7 mcg/mL at 20 minutes, 10 mcg/mL at 1 hour, 2.6 mcg/mL at 2.5 hours, and 1 mcg/mL at 6 hours.

Microbiology:

Erythromycin acts by inhibition of protein synthesis by binding 50 S ribosomal subunits of susceptible organisms. It does not affect nucleic acid synthesis. Antagonism has been demonstrated *in vitro* between erythromycin and clindamycin, lincomycin and chloramphenicol.

Many strains of *Haemophilus influenzae* are resistant to erythromycin alone, but are susceptible to erythromycin and sulfonamides together.

Staphylococci resistant to erythromycin may emerge during a course of therapy. Culture and susceptibility testing should be performed.

Erythromycin is usually active against the following organisms *in vitro* (prior to use, refer to "Indications and Usage" section):

Gram-positive Bacteria: Staphylococcus aureus (resistant organisms may emerge during treatment), Streptococcus pyogenes (Group A beta-hemolytic streptococcus), Alpha-hemolytic streptococcus (viridans group), Streptococcus (diplococcus) pneumoniae, Corynebacterium diphtheriae, Corynebacterium minutissimum.

Gram-negative Bacteria: Neisseria gonorrhoeae, Legionella pneumophila, Bordetella pertussis.

Mycoplasma: Mycoplasma pneumoniae, Ureaplasma urealyticum.

Other Microorganisms: Chlamydia trachomatis, Entamoeba histolytica, Treponema pallidum, Listeria monocytogenes.

Susceptibility Testing:

Quantitative methods that require measurement of zone diameters give the most precise estimates of antibiotic susceptibility. One such standardized single-disc procedure has been recommended for use with discs to test susceptibility to erythromycin.[1] Interpretation involves correlation of the zone diameters obtained in the disc test with minimal inhibitory concentration (MIC) values for erythromycin.

Reports from the laboratory giving results of the standardized single-disc susceptibility test using a 15 mcg erythromycin disc should be interpreted according to the following criteria:

Susceptible organisms produce zones of 18 mm or greater, indicating that the tested organism is likely to respond to therapy.

Resistant organisms produce zones of 13 mm or less, indicating that other therapy should be selected.

Organisms of intermediate susceptibility produce zones of 14 to 17 mm. The "intermediate" category provides a "buffer zone" which should prevent small, uncontrolled technical factors from causing major discrepancies in interpretations; thus, when a zone diameter falls within the "intermediate" range, the results may be considered equivocal. If alternative drugs are not available, confirmation by dilution tests may be indicated.

Standardized procedures require the use of control organisms. The 15 mcg erythromycin disc should give zone diameters between 22 and 30 mm for the S. aureus ATCC 25923 control strain.

A bacterial isolate may be considered susceptible if the MIC value[2] for erythromycin is not more than 2 mcg/mL. Organisms are considered resistant if the MIC is 8 mcg/mL or higher. The MIC of erythromycin for S. aureus ATCC 29213 control strain should be between 0.12 and 0.5 mcg/mL.

INDICATIONS AND USAGE

ERYTHROCIN PIGGYBACK (erythromycin lactobionate for injection, USP) is indicated in the treatment of infections caused by susceptible strains of the designated organisms in the diseases listed below when oral administration is not possible or when the severity of the infection requires immediate high serum levels of erythromycin. Intravenous therapy should be replaced by oral administration at the appropriate time.

Upper respiratory tract infections of mild to moderate degree caused by *Streptococcus pyogenes* (Group A beta-hemolytic streptococci); *Streptococcus pneumoniae (Diplococcus pneumoniae); Haemophilus influenzae* (when used concomitantly with adequate doses of sulfonamides, since many strains of *H. influenzae* are not susceptible to the erythromycin concentrations ordinarily achieved). (See appropriate sulfonamide labeling for prescribing information.)

Lower respiratory tract infections of mild to moderate severity caused by *Streptococcus pyogenes* (Group A beta-hemolytic streptococci); *Streptococcus pneumoniae (Diplococcus pneumoniae)*.

Respiratory tract infections due to *Mycoplasma pneumoniae*.

Skin and skin structure infections of mild to moderate severity caused by *Streptococcus pyogenes* and *Staphylococcus aureus* (resistant staphylococci may emerge during treatment).

Diphtheria: As an adjunct to antitoxin in infections due to *Corynebacterium diphtheriae* to prevent establishment of carriers and to eradicate the organism in carriers.

Erythrasma: In the treatment of infections due to *Corynebacterium minutissimum*.

Acute pelvic inflammatory disease caused by *Neisseria gonorrhoeae*: Erythrocin Piggyback (erythromycin lactobionate for injection, USP) followed by erythromycin stearate or base orally, as an alternative drug in treatment of acute pelvic inflammatory disease caused by N. gonorrhoeae in female patients with a history of sensitivity to penicillin.

Before treatment of gonorrhea, patients who are suspected of also having syphilis should have a microscopic examination for T. pallidum (by immunofluorescence or darkfield) before receiving erythromycin and monthly serologic tests for a minimum of 4 months thereafter.

Legionnaires' Disease caused by *Legionella pneumophila*: Although no controlled clinical efficacy studies have been conducted, *in vitro* and limited preliminary clinical data suggest that erythromycin may be effective in treating Legionnaires' Disease.

Prevention of Initial Attacks of Rheumatic Fever: Penicillin is considered by the American Heart Association to be the drug of choice in the prevention of initial attacks of rheumatic fever (treatment of Group A beta-hemolytic streptococcal infections of the upper respiratory tract e.g., tonsillitis, or pharyngitis).[3] Erythromycin is indicated for the treatment of penicillin-allergic patients. The therapeutic dose should be administered for ten days.

Prevention of Recurrent Attacks of Rheumatic Fever: Penicillin or sulfonamides are considered by the American Heart Association to be the drugs of choice in the prevention of recurrent attacks of rheumatic fever. In patients who are allergic to penicillin and sulfonamides, oral erythromycin is recommended by the American Heart Association in the long-term prophylaxis of streptococcal pharyngitis (for the prevention of recurrent attacks of rheumatic fever).[3]

Prevention of Bacterial Endocarditis: Although no controlled clinical efficacy trials have been conducted, oral erythromycin has been recommended by the American Heart Association for prevention of bacterial endocarditis in penicillin-allergic patients with prosthetic cardiac valves,

Continued on next page

If desired, additional literature on any Abbott Product will be provided upon request to Abbott Laboratories.

Abbott—Cont.

most congenital cardiac malformations, surgically constructed systemic pulmonary shunts, rheumatic or other acquired valvular dysfunction, idiopathic hypertrophic subaortic stenosis (IHSS), previous history of bacterial endocarditis and mitral valve prolapse with insufficiency when they undergo dental procedures and surgical procedures of the upper respiratory tract.[4]

CONTRAINDICATIONS

Erythromycin is contraindicated in patients with known hypersensitivity to this antibiotic.

WARNINGS

There have been reports of hepatic dysfunction, with or without jaundice occurring in patients receiving oral erythromycin products.

PRECAUTIONS

General:
Since erythromycin is principally excreted by the liver, caution should be exercised when erythromycin is administered to patients with impaired hepatic function. (See "CLINICAL PHARMACOLOGY" and "WARNINGS" sections.)
Prolonged or repeated use of erythromycin may result in an overgrowth of non-susceptible bacteria or fungi. If superinfection occurs, erythromycin should be discontinued and appropriate therapy instituted.
When indicated, incision and drainage or other surgical procedures should be performed in conjunction with antibiotic therapy.
Laboratory Tests: Erythromycin interferes with the fluorometric determination of urinary catecholamines.
Drug Interactions: Erythromycin use in patients who are receiving high doses of theophylline may be associated with an increase of serum theophylline levels and potential theophylline toxicity. Serum theophylline levels should be monitored in patients receiving concomitant erythromycin. The theophylline dose may need to be reduced in some patients.
Erythromycin administration in patients receiving carbamazepine has been reported to cause increased serum levels of carbamazepine with subsequent development of signs of carbamazepine toxicity.
Concomitant administration of erythromycin and digoxin has been reported to result in elevated serum digoxin levels.
There have been reports of increased anticoagulant effects when erythromycin and oral anticoagulants were used concomitantly.
Carcinogenesis, Mutagenesis, Impairment of Fertility: Long-term animal data with erythromycin lactobionate for use in determination of possible carcinogenic effects are not available. However, long-term oral studies in rats with erythromycin ethylsuccinate and erythromycin base did not provide evidence of tumorigenicity. Mutagenicity studies have not been conducted. There was no apparent effect on male or female fertility in rats fed erythromycin (base) at levels up to 0.25% of diet.
Pregnancy: *Pregnancy Category B:* There was no evidence of teratogenicity or any other adverse effect on reproduction in female rats fed erythromycin base (up to 0.25% of diet) prior to and during mating, during gestation, and through weaning of two successive litters. There are, however, no adequate and well-controlled studies in pregnant women. Because animal reproduction studies are not always predictive of human response, this drug should be used during pregnancy only if clearly needed. Erythromycin has been reported to cross the placental barrier in humans, but fetal plasma levels are generally low.
Labor and Delivery: The effect of erythromycin on labor and delivery is unknown.
Nursing Mothers: Erythromycin is excreted in breast milk. Caution should be exercised when erythromycin is administered to a nursing woman.
Pediatric Use: See "INDICATIONS AND USAGE" and "DOSAGE AND ADMINISTRATION" sections.
This product contains benzyl alcohol which has been associated with a fatal gasping syndrome in infants.

ADVERSE REACTIONS

Side effects following the use of intravenous erythromycin are rare. Occasional venous irritation has been encountered, but if the infusion is given slowly, in dilute solution, preferably by continuous intravenous infusion or intermittent infusion in no less than 20 to 60 minutes, pain and vessel trauma are minimized.
Occasional nausea, vomiting, abdominal cramping and abdominal pain have been encountered.
Allergic reactions, ranging from urticaria and mild skin eruptions to anaphylaxis, have occurred with intravenously administered erythromycin.
There have been isolated reports of reversible hearing loss occurring chiefly in patients with renal insufficiency and in patients receiving high doses of erythromycin.

OVERDOSAGE

In the case of overdosage, erythromycin infusion should be discontinued and all other appropriate measures should be instituted.
Erythromycin is not removed by peritoneal dialysis or hemodialysis.

DOSAGE AND ADMINISTRATION

For the treatment of severe infections in adults and children, the recommended intravenous dose of erythromycin lactobionate is 15 to 20 mg/kg/day. Higher doses, up to 4 g/day, may be given for severe infections. ERYTHROCIN PIGGYBACK (erythromycin lactobionate for injection, USP) should be administered by intravenous infusion. Due to the high concentration of erythromycin, I.V. push is not an acceptable route of administration. Intravenous erythromycin should be replaced by oral erythromycin as soon as possible.
After reconstitution each mL of ERYTHROCIN PIGGYBACK solution contains 5 mg of erythromycin activity (500 mg in 100 mL). The drug may be administered directly from the vial. When this preparation is administered by intermittent infusion one-fourth the total daily dose of erythromycin lactobionate should be administered in 20 to 60 minutes at intervals not greater than every six hours. The infusion should be sufficiently slow to minimize pain along the vein.
For treatment of acute pelvic inflammatory disease caused by *N. gonorrhoeae*, in female patients hypersensitive to penicillins, administer 500 mg erythromycin lactobionate every 6 hours for 3 days, followed by oral administration of 250 mg erythromycin stearate or base every 6 hours for 7 days.
For treatment of Legionnaires' Disease: Although optimal doses have not been established, doses utilized in reported clinical data were 1 to 4 grams daily in divided doses.
In the treatment of Group A beta-hemolytic streptococcal infections of the upper respiratory tract (e.g., tonsillitis or pharyngitis), the therapeutic dosage of erythromycin should be administered for ten days. The American Heart Association suggests a dosage of 250 mg of erythromycin orally, twice a day in long-term prophylaxis of streptococcal upper respiratory tract infections for the prevention of recurring attacks of rheumatic fever in patients allergic to penicillin and sulfonamides.[3]
In prophylaxis against bacterial endocarditis (see "Indications and Usage" section) the oral regimen for penicillin allergic patients is erythromycin 1 gram, 1 hour before the procedure followed by 500 mg six hours later.[4]
Preparation of solution:
Prepare the ERYTHROCIN PIGGYBACK (erythromycin lactobionate for injection, USP) solution by adding 100 mL of 0.9% Sodium Chloride Injection, USP, or Lactated Ringer's Injection, USP, or Normosol®-R Solution to the dispensing vial. Immediately after adding diluent, the product should be shaken well to aid dissolution. Lack of immediate agitation will greatly increase time required for complete dissolution.
Reconstitution may also be made using 100 mL of the following solutions to which 1 mL of Neut® (4% sodium bicarbonate, Abbott) has first been added:
  5% Dextrose Injection, USP
  5% Dextrose and Lactated Ringer's Injection
  5% Dextrose and 0.9% Sodium Chloride Injection, USP
  Normosol®-M and 5% Dextrose Injection
  Normosol®-R and 5% Dextrose Injection
Neut® (4% sodium bicarbonate, Abbott) must be added to these solutions so that their pH is in the optimum range for erythromycin lactobionate stability. Acidic solutions of erythromycin lactobionate are unstable and lose their potency rapidly. A pH of at least 5.5 is desirable.
No drug or chemical agent should be added to an erythromycin lactobionate-I.V. fluid admixture unless its effect on the chemical and physical stability of the solution has first been determined.
Stability:
The solution should be used within 8 hours if stored at room temperature and 24 hours if stored in the refrigerator. If the solution is to be frozen, it should be frozen (−10° C to −20° C) within 4 hours of preparation. Frozen solution may be stored for 30 days. Frozen solution should be thawed in the refrigerator and used within 8 hours after thawing is completed.
THAWED SOLUTION MUST NOT BE REFROZEN.
Parenteral drug products should be inspected visually for particulate matter and discoloration prior to administration, whenever solution and container permit.

HOW SUPPLIED

ERYTHROCIN PIGGYBACK (erythromycin lactobionate for injection, USP) is supplied as a sterile, lyophilized powder in packages of 5 single-dose dispensing vials (NDC 0074-6368-13). Each vial contains the equivalent of 500 mg of erythromycin with 90 mg of benzyl alcohol.
Store at controlled room temperature 15° to 30° C (59° to 86° F).

REFERENCES

1. National Committee for Clinical Laboratory Standards, Approved Standard: *Performance Standards for Antimicrobial Disk Susceptibility Tests*, 3rd Edition, Vol. 4(16):M2–A3, Villanova, PA, December 1984.
2. Ericson, H.M., Sherris, J.C., Antibiotic Sensitivity Testing Report of an International Collaborative Study, *Acta Pathologica et Microbiologica Scandinavica* Section B Suppl. 217:1–90, 1971.
3. Committee on Rheumatic Fever and Infective Endocarditis of the Council on Cardiovascular Disease of the Young: Prevention of Rheumatic Fever, *Circulation* 70(6):1118A–1122A, December 1984.
4. Committee on Rheumatic Fever and Infective Endocarditis of the Council on Cardiovascular Disease of the Young: Prevention of Bacterial Endocarditis, *Circulation* 70(6):1123A–1127A, December 1984.
Caution: Federal (USA) law prohibits dispensing without prescription.

Abbott Laboratories
North Chicago, IL 60064, USA
Ref. 01-2416-R-6-Rev. Jan., 1988

ERYTHROCIN® STEARATE   ℞
[e-ry'thrō-sin]
(erythromycin stearate tablets, USP)
Filmtab® Tablets

DESCRIPTION

Erythromycin is produced by a strain of *Streptomyces erythraeus* and belongs to the macrolide group of antibiotics. It is basic and readily forms salts with acids. The base, the stearate salt, and the esters are poorly soluble in water, and are suitable for oral administration.
ERYTHROCIN STEARATE Filmtab tablets contain the stearate salt of the antibiotic in a unique film coating.
Inactive Ingredients: 250 mg tablet: Cellulosic polymers, corn starch, D&C Red No. 7, polacrilin potassium, polyethylene glycol, povidone, propylene glycol, sodium carboxymethylcellulose, sodium citrate, sorbic acid, sorbitan monooleate and titanium dioxide.
500 mg tablet: Cellulosic polymers, corn starch, FD&C Red No. 3, magnesium hydroxide, polacrilin potassium, povidone, propylene glycol, sorbitan monooleate, titanium dioxide and vanillin.

ACTIONS

Microbiology: Biochemical tests demonstrate that erythromycin inhibits protein synthesis of the pathogen without directly affecting nucleic acid synthesis. Antagonism has been demonstrated between clindamycin and erythromycin.
NOTE: Many strains of *Hemophilus influenzae* are resistant to erythromycin alone, but are susceptible to erythromycin and sulfonamides together. Staphylococci resistant to erythromycin may emerge during a course of erythromycin therapy. Culture and susceptibility testing should be performed.
Disc Susceptibility Tests: Quantitative methods that require measurement of zone diameters give the most precise estimates of antibiotic susceptibility. One recommended procedure (21 CFR section 460.1) uses erythromycin class discs for testing susceptibility; interpretations correlate zone diameters of this disc test with MIC values for erythromycin. With this procedure, a report from the laboratory of "susceptible" indicates that the infecting organism is likely to respond to therapy. A report of "resistant" indicates that the infective organism is not likely to respond to therapy. A report of "intermediate susceptibility" suggests that the organism would be susceptible if higher doses were used.
Clinical Pharmacology: Erythromycin binds to the 50 S ribosomal subunits of susceptible bacteria and suppresses protein synthesis.
Orally administered ERYTHROCIN STEARATE tablets are readily and reliably absorbed. Optimal serum levels of erythromycin are reached when the drug is taken in the fasting state or immediately before meals.
Erythromycin diffuses readily into most body fluids. Only low concentrations are normally achieved in the spinal fluid, but passage of the drug across the blood-brain barrier increases in meningitis. In the presence of normal hepatic function, erythromycin is concentrated in the liver and excreted in the bile; the effect of hepatic dysfunction on excretion of erythromycin by the liver into the bile is not known. Less than 5 percent of the orally administered dose of erythromycin is excreted in active form in the urine.
Erythromycin crosses the placental barrier and is excreted in breast milk.

INDICATIONS

Streptococcus pyogenes (Group A beta-hemolytic streptococcus): Upper and lower respiratory tract, skin, and soft tissue infections of mild to moderate severity.
Injectable benzathine penicillin G is considered by the American Heart Association to be the drug of choice in the treatment and prevention of streptococcal pharyngitis and in long-term prophylaxis of rheumatic fever.
When oral medication is preferred for treatment of the above conditions, penicillin G, V, or erythromycin are alternate drugs of choice.

When oral medication is given, the importance of strict adherence by the patient to the prescribed dosage regimen must be stressed. A therapeutic dose should be administered for at least 10 days.

Alpha-hemolytic streptococci (viridans group):
Although no controlled clinical efficacy trials have been conducted, oral erythromycin has been suggested by the American Heart Association and American Dental Association for use in a regimen for prophylaxis against bacterial endocarditis in patients hypersensitive to penicillin who have congenital heart disease, or rheumatic or other acquired valvular heart disease when they undergo dental procedures and surgical procedures of the upper respiratory tract.[1] Erythromycin is not suitable prior to genitourinary or gastrointestinal tract surgery. NOTE: When selecting antibiotics for the prevention of bacterial endocarditis the physician or dentist should read the full joint statement of the American Heart Association and the American Dental Association.[1]

Staphylococcus aureus: Acute infections of skin and soft tissue of mild to moderate severity. Resistant organisms may emerge during treatment.

Streptococcus pneumoniae (Diplococcus pneumoniae): Upper respiratory tract infections (e.g., otitis media, pharyngitis) and lower respiratory tract infections (e.g., pneumonia) of mild to moderate degree.

Mycoplasma pneumoniae (Eaton agent, PPLO): For respiratory infections due to this organism.

Hemophilus influenzae: For upper respiratory tract infections of mild to moderate severity when used concomitantly with adequate doses of sulfonamides. (See sulfonamide labeling for appropriate prescribing information). The concomitant use of the sulfonamides is necessary since not all strains of *Hemophilus influenzae* are susceptible to erythromycin at the concentrations of the antibiotic achieved with usual therapeutic doses.

Chlamydia trachomatis: Erythromycin is indicated for treatment of the following infections caused by *Chlamydia trachomatis:* conjunctivitis of the newborn, pneumonia of infancy and urogenital infections during pregnancy. When tetracyclines are contraindicated or not tolerated, erythromycin is indicated for the treatment of uncomplicated urethral, endocervical, or rectal infections in adults due to *Chlamydia trachomatis.*[2]

Treponema pallidum: Erythromycin is an alternate choice of treatment for primary syphilis in patients allergic to the penicillins. In treatment of primary syphilis, spinal fluid examinations should be done before treatment and as part of follow-up after therapy.

Corynebacterium diphtheriae: As an adjunct to antitoxin, to prevent establishment of carriers, and to eradicate the organism in carriers.

Corynebacterium minutissimum: For the treatment of erythrasma.

Entamoeba histolytica: In the treatment of intestinal amebiasis only. Extra-enteric amebiasis requires treatment with other agents.

Listeria monocytogenes: Infections due to this organism.

Neisseria gonorrhoeae: Erythrocin Lactobionate-I.V. (erythromycin lactobionate for injection) in conjunction with erythromycin stearate orally, as an alternative drug in treatment of acute pelvic inflammatory disease caused by *N. gonorrhoeae* in female patients with a history of sensitivity to penicillin. Before treatment of gonorrhea, patients who are suspected of also having syphilis should have a microscopic examination for *T. pallidum* (by immunofluorescence or darkfield) before receiving erythromycin, and monthly serologic tests for a minimum of 4 months.

Bordetella pertussis: Erythromycin is effective in eliminating the organism from the nasopharynx of infected individuals, rendering them non-infectious. Some clinical studies suggest that erythromycin may be helpful in the prophylaxis of pertussis in exposed susceptible individuals.

Legionnaires' Disease: Although no controlled clinical efficacy studies have been conducted, *in vitro* and limited preliminary clinical data suggest that erythromycin may be effective in treating Legionnaires' Disease.

CONTRAINDICATIONS

Erythromycin is contraindicated in patients with known hypersensitivity to this antibiotic.

PRECAUTIONS

Erythromycin is principally excreted by the liver. Caution should be exercised in administering the antibiotic to patients with impaired hepatic function. There have been reports of hepatic dysfunction, with or without jaundice occurring in patients receiving oral erythromycin products.

Areas of localized infection may require surgical drainage in addition to antibiotic therapy.

Recent data from studies of erythromycin reveal that its use in patients who are receiving high doses of theophylline may be associated with an increase of serum theophylline levels and potential theophylline toxicity. In case of theophylline toxicity and/or elevated serum theophylline levels, the dose of theophylline should be reduced while the patient is receiving concomitant erythromycin therapy.

Usage during pregnancy and lactation: The safety of erythromycin for use during pregnancy has not been established. Erythromycin crosses the placental barrier. Erythromycin also appears in breast milk.

ADVERSE REACTIONS

The most frequent side effects of oral erythromycin preparations are gastrointestinal, such as abdominal cramping and discomfort, and are dose-related. Nausea, vomiting, and diarrhea occur infrequently with usual oral doses.

During prolonged or repeated therapy, there is a possibility of overgrowth of nonsusceptible bacteria or fungi. If such infections occur, the drug should be discontinued and appropriate therapy instituted.

Allergic reactions ranging from urticaria and mild skin eruptions to anaphylaxis have occurred.

There have been isolated reports of reversible hearing loss occurring chiefly in patients with renal insufficiency and in patients receiving high doses of erythromycin.

DOSAGE AND ADMINISTRATION

Optimal serum levels of erythromycin are reached when ERYTHROCIN STEARATE (erythromycin stearate) is taken in the fasting state or immediately before meals.

Adults: The usual dosage is 250 mg every 6 hours; or 500 mg every 12 hours, taken in the fasting state or immediately before meals. Up to 4 g per day may be administered, depending upon the severity of the infection.

Children: Age, weight, and severity of the infection are important factors in determining the proper dosage. For the treatment of mild to moderate infections, the usual dosage is 30 to 50 mg/kg/day in 3 or 4 divided doses. When dosage is desired on a twice-a-day schedule, one-half of the total daily dose may be taken every 12 hours in the fasting state or immediately before meals. For the treatment of more severe infections the total daily dose may be doubled.

In the treatment of streptococcal infections, a therapeutic dosage of erythromycin should be administered for at least 10 days. In continuous prophylaxis of streptococcal infections in persons with a history of rheumatic heart disease, the dose is 250 mg twice a day.

For prophylaxis against bacterial endocarditis[1] in patients with congenital heart disease, or rheumatic or other acquired valvular heart disease when undergoing dental procedures or surgical procedures of the upper respiratory tract, give 1 g (20 mg/kg for children) orally 1½ to 2 hours before the procedure, and then, 500 mg (10 mg/kg for children) orally every 6 hours for 8 doses.

For conjunctivitis of the newborn caused by *Chlamydia trachomatis:* Oral erythromycin suspension 50 mg/kg/day in 4 divided doses for at least 2 weeks.[2]

For pneumonia of infancy caused by *Chlamydia trachomatis:* Although the optimal duration of therapy has not been established, the recommended therapy is oral erythromycin suspension 50 mg/kg/day in 4 divided doses for at least 3 weeks.[2]

For urogenital infections during pregnancy due to *Chlamydia trachomatis:* Although the optimal dose and duration of therapy have not been established, the suggested treatment is erythromycin 500 mg, by mouth, 4 times a day on an empty stomach for at least 7 days. For women who cannot tolerate this regimen, a decreased dose of 250 mg, by mouth, 4 times a day should be used for at least 14 days.[2]

For adults with uncomplicated urethral, endocervical, or rectal infections caused by *Chlamydia trachomatis* in whom tetracyclines are contraindicated or not tolerated: 500 mg, by mouth, 4 times a day for at least 7 days.[2]

For treatment of primary syphilis: 30 to 40 g given in divided doses over a period of 10 to 15 days.

For treatment of acute pelvic inflammatory disease caused by *N. gonorrhoeae:* 500 mg Erythrocin Lactobionate-I.V. (erythromycin lactobionate for injection) every 6 hours for 3 days, followed by 250 mg ERYTHROCIN STEARATE every 6 hours for 7 days.

For intestinal amebiasis: Adults: 250 mg four times daily for 10 to 14 days. Children: 30 to 50 mg/kg/day in divided doses for 10 to 14 days.

For use in pertussis: Although optimal dosage and duration have not been established, doses of erythromycin utilized in reported clinical studies were 40 to 50 mg/kg/day, given in divided doses for 5 to 14 days.

For treatment of Legionnaires' Disease: Although optimal doses have not been established, doses utilized in reported clinical data were 1 to 4 g daily in divided doses.

HOW SUPPLIED

ERYTHROCIN STEARATE Filmtab Tablets (erythromycin stearate tablets, USP) are supplied as:

Erythrocin Stearate Filmtab, 250 mg

Bottles of 100 ....(NDC 0074-6346-20)
Bottles of 500 ....(NDC 0074-6346-53)
ABBO-PAC® unit dose strip packages of
100 tablets ....(NDC 0074-6346-38)

Erythrocin Stearate Filmtab, 500 mg

Bottles of 100 ....(NDC 0074-6316-13)

REFERENCES

1. American Heart Association. 1977. Prevention of bacterial endocarditis. Circulation 56: 139A-143A.
2. CDC Sexually Transmitted Diseases Treatment Guidelines 1982.
FILMTAB—Film-sealed tablets, Abbott
Abbott Laboratories
North Chicago, IL 60064
Ref. 07-5360-R10
Shown in Product Identification Section, page 403

ERYTHROMYCIN BASE FILMTAB®   ℞
[e-ri-thrō-mī'sin]
(erythromycin tablets, USP)

DESCRIPTION

Erythromycin is produced by a strain of *Streptomyces erythraeus* and belongs to the macrolide group of antibiotics. It is basic and readily forms salts with acids. The base, the stearate salt, and the esters are poorly soluble in water, and are suitable for oral administration.

ERYTHROMYCIN BASE FILMTAB tablets contain erythromycin, USP, in a unique, nonenteric film coating.

Inactive Ingredients: 250 mg tablet: Cellulosic polymers, corn starch, D&C Red No. 30, iron oxide, magnesium hydroxide, magnesium stearate, polyethylene glycol, propylene glycol, sodium starch glycolate, sorbic acid, sorbitan monooleate, titanium dioxide and other ingredients.

500 mg tablet: Cellulosic polymers, corn starch, D&C Red No. 30, magnesium hydroxide, magnesium stearate, microcrystalline cellulose, polyethylene glycol, propylene glycol, sodium starch glycolate, sorbic acid, sorbitan monooleate, titanium dioxide and other ingredients.

ACTIONS

Microbiology: Biochemical tests demonstrate that erythromycin inhibits protein synthesis of the pathogen without directly affecting nucleic acid synthesis. Antagonism has been demonstrated between clindamycin and erythromycin. NOTE: Many strains of *Hemophilus influenzae* are resistant to erythromycin alone, but are susceptible to erythromycin and sulfonamides together. Staphylococci resistant to erythromycin may emerge during a course of erythromycin therapy. Culture and susceptibility testing should be performed.

Disc Susceptibility Tests: Quantitative methods that require measurement of zone diameters give the most precise estimates of antibiotic susceptibility. One recommended procedure (21 CFR section 460.1) uses erythromycin class discs for testing susceptibility; interpretations correlate zone diameters of this disc test with MIC values for erythromycin. With this procedure, a report from the laboratory of "susceptible" indicates that the infecting organism is likely to respond to therapy. A report of "resistant" indicates that the infective organism is not likely to respond to therapy. A report of "intermediate susceptibility" suggests that the organism would be susceptible if higher doses were used.

Clinical Pharmacology: Erythromycin binds to the 50 S ribosomal subunits of susceptible bacteria and suppresses protein synthesis.

Orally administered erythromycin is readily absorbed by most patients, especially on an empty stomach, but patient variation is observed. Due to its formulation and nonenteric coating, this erythromycin tablet gives reliable blood levels in the average subject; however, the levels may vary with the individual.

Erythromycin diffuses readily into most body fluids. Only low concentrations are normally achieved in the spinal fluid, but passage of the drug across the blood-brain barrier increases in meningitis. In the presence of normal hepatic function, erythromycin is concentrated in the liver and excreted in the bile; the effect of hepatic dysfunction on excretion of erythromycin by the liver into the bile is not known. Less than 5 percent of the orally administered dose of erythromycin is excreted in active form in the urine.

Erythromycin crosses the placental barrier and is excreted in breast milk.

INDICATIONS

Streptococcus pyogenes (Group A beta-hemolytic streptococcus): Upper and lower respiratory tract, skin, and soft tissue infections of mild to moderate severity.

Injectable benzathine penicillin G is considered by the American Heart Association to be the drug of choice in the treatment and prevention of streptococcal pharyngitis and in long-term prophylaxis of rheumatic fever.

When oral medication is preferred for treatment of the above conditions, penicillin G, V, or erythromycin are alternate drugs of choice.

When oral medication is given, the importance of strict adherence by the patient to the prescribed dosage regimen

Continued on next page

If desired, additional literature on any Abbott Product will be provided upon request to Abbott Laboratories.

Abbott—Cont.

must be stressed. A therapeutic dose should be administered for at least 10 days.

Alpha-hemolytic streptococci (viridans group): Although no controlled clinical efficacy trials have been conducted, oral erythromycin has been suggested by the American Heart Association and American Dental Association for use in a regimen for prophylaxis against bacterial endocarditis in patients hypersensitive to penicillin who have congenital heart disease, or rheumatic or other acquired valvular heart disease when they undergo dental procedures and surgical procedures of the upper respiratory tract.[1] Erythromycin is not suitable prior to genitourinary or gastrointestinal tract surgery. NOTE: When selecting antibiotics for the prevention of bacterial endocarditis the physician or dentist should read the full joint statement of the American Heart Association and the American Dental Association.[1]

Staphylococcus aureus: Acute infections of skin and soft tissue of mild to moderate severity. Resistant organisms may emerge during treatment.

Streptococcus pneumoniae (Diplococcus pneumoniae): Upper respiratory tract infections (e.g., otitis media, pharyngitis) and lower respiratory tract infections (e.g., pneumonia) of mild to moderate degree.

Mycoplasma pneumoniae (Eaton agent, PPLO): For respiratory infections due to this organism.

Hemophilus influenzae: For upper respiratory tract infections of mild to moderate severity when used concomitantly with adequate doses of sulfonamides. (See sulfonamide labeling for appropriate prescribing information). The concomitant use of the sulfonamides is necessary since not all strains of *Hemophilus influenzae* are susceptible to erythromycin at the concentrations of the antibiotic achieved with usual therapeutic doses.

Chlamydia trachomatis: Erythromycin is indicated for treatment of the following infections caused by *Chlamydia trachomatis:* conjunctivitis of the newborn, pneumonia of infancy and urogenital infections during pregnancy. When tetracyclines are contraindicated or not tolerated, erythromycin is indicated for the treatment of uncomplicated urethral, endocervical, or rectal infections in adults due to *Chlamydia trachomatis.*[2]

Treponema pallidum: Erythromycin is an alternate choice of treatment for primary syphilis in patients allergic to the penicillins. In treatment of primary syphilis, spinal fluid examinations should be done before treatment and as part of follow-up after therapy.

Corynebacterium diphtheriae: As an adjunct to antitoxin, to prevent establishment of carriers, and to eradicate the organism in carriers.

Corynebacterium minutissimum: For the treatment of erythrasma.

Entamoeba histolytica: In the treatment of intestinal amebiasis only. Extra-enteric amebiasis requires treatment with other agents.

Listeria monocytogenes: Infections due to this organism.

Neisseria gonorrhoeae: Erythrocin® Lactobionate-I.V. (erythromycin lactobionate for injection) in conjunction with erythromycin base orally, as an alternative drug in treatment of acute pelvic inflammatory disease caused by *N. gonorrhoeae* in female patients with a history of sensitivity to penicillin. Before treatment of gonorrhea, patients who are suspected of also having syphilis should have a microscopic examination for *T. pallidum* (by immunofluorescence or darkfield) before receiving erythromycin, and monthly serologic tests for a minimum of 4 months.

Bordetella pertussis: Erythromycin is effective in eliminating the organism from the nasopharynx of infected individuals, rendering them non-infectious. Some clinical studies suggest that erythromycin may be helpful in the prophylaxis of pertussis in exposed susceptible individuals.

Legionnaires' Disease: Although no controlled clinical efficacy studies have been conducted, *in vitro* and limited preliminary clinical data suggest that erythromycin may be effective in treating Legionnaires' Disease.

CONTRAINDICATIONS

Erythromycin is contraindicated in patients with known hypersensitivity to this antibiotic.

PRECAUTIONS

Erythromycin is principally excreted by the liver. Caution should be exercised in administering the antibiotic to patients with impaired hepatic function. There have been reports of hepatic dysfunction, with or without jaundice occurring in patients receiving oral erythromycin products.

Areas of localized infection may require surgical drainage in addition to antibiotic therapy.

Recent data from studies of erythromycin reveal that its use in patients who are receiving high doses of theophylline may be associated with an increase of serum theophylline levels and potential theophylline toxicity. In case of theophylline toxicity and/or elevated serum theophylline levels, the dose of theophylline should be reduced while the patient is receiving concomitant erythromycin therapy.

Usage during pregnancy and lactation: The safety of erythromycin for use during pregnancy has not been established. Erythromycin crosses the placental barrier. Erythromycin also appears in breast milk.

ADVERSE REACTIONS

The most frequent side effects of oral erythromycin preparations are gastrointestinal, such as abdominal cramping and discomfort, and are dose-related. Nausea, vomiting, and diarrhea occur infrequently with usual oral doses.

During prolonged or repeated therapy, there is a possibility of overgrowth of nonsusceptible bacteria or fungi. If such infections occur, the drug should be discontinued and appropriate therapy instituted.

Allergic reactions ranging from urticaria and mild skin eruptions to anaphylaxis have occurred.

There have been isolated reports of reversible hearing loss occurring chiefly in patients with renal insufficiency and in patients receiving high doses of erythromycin.

DOSAGE AND ADMINISTRATION

Optimum blood levels are obtained when doses are given on an empty stomach.

Adults: 250 mg every 6 hours is the usual dose; or 500 mg every 12 hours one hour before meals. Dosage may be increased up to 4 g per day according to the severity of the infection.

Children: Age, weight, and severity of the infection are important factors in determining the proper dosage. 30 to 50 mg/kg/day, in divided doses, is the usual dose. For more severe infections this dose may be doubled. If dosage is desired on a twice-a-day schedule, one-half of the total daily dose may be given every 12 hours, one hour before meals.

For the treatment of streptococcal infections: a therapeutic dosage should be administered for at least 10 days. In continuous prophylaxis of streptococcal infections in persons with rheumatic heart disease history, the dose is 250 mg twice a day.

For prophylaxis against bacterial endocarditis[1] in patients with congenital heart disease, or rheumatic or other acquired valvular heart disease when undergoing dental procedures or surgical procedures of the upper respiratory tract, give 1 g (20 mg/kg for children) orally 1½ to 2 hours before the procedure, and then, 500 mg (10 mg/kg for children) orally every 6 hours for 8 doses.

For conjunctivitis of the newborn caused by *Chlamydia trachomatis:* Oral erythromycin suspension 50 mg/kg/day in 4 divided doses for at least 2 weeks.[2]

For pneumonia of infancy caused by *Chlamydia trachomatis:* Although the optimal duration of therapy has not been established, the recommended therapy is oral erythromycin suspension 50 mg/kg/day in 4 divided doses for at least 3 weeks.[2]

For urogenital infections during pregnancy due to *Chlamydia trachomatis:* Although the optimal dose and duration of therapy have not been established, the suggested treatment is erythromycin 500 mg, by mouth, 4 times a day on an empty stomach for at least 7 days. For women who cannot tolerate this regimen, a decreased dose of 250 mg, by mouth 4 times a day should be used for at least 14 days.[2]

For adults with uncomplicated urethral, endocervical, or rectal infections caused by *Chlamydia trachomatis* in whom tetracyclines are contraindicated or not tolerated: 500 mg, by mouth, 4 times a day for at least 7 days.[2]

For treatment of primary syphilis: 30 to 40 g given in divided doses over a period of 10 to 15 days.

For treatment of acute pelvic inflammatory disease caused by *N. gonorrhoeae:* 500 mg Erythrocin Lactobionate-I.V. (erythromycin lactobionate for injection) every 6 hours for 3 days, followed by 250 mg erythromycin base every 6 hours for 7 days.

For intestinal amebiasis: Adults: 250 mg four times daily for 10 to 14 days. Children: 30 to 50 mg/kg/day in divided doses for 10 to 14 days.

For use in pertussis: Although optimal dosage and duration have not been established, doses of erythromycin utilized in reported clinical studies were 40 to 50 mg/kg/day, given in divided doses for 5 to 14 days.

For treatment of Legionnaires' Disease: Although optimal doses have not been established, doses utilized in reported clinical data were 1 to 4 g daily in divided doses.

HOW SUPPLIED

ERYTHROMYCIN BASE FILMTAB tablets (erythromycin tablets, USP) are supplied as pink capsule-shaped tablets in two dosage strengths:

250 mg tablets:
Bottles of 100 ....(NDC 0074-6326-13)
Bottles of 500 ....(NDC 0074-6326-53)
ABBO-PAC® unit dose strip packages of
100 tablets ....(NDC 0074-6326-11)
500 mg tablets:
Bottles of 100 ....(NDC 0074-6227-13)

REFERENCES
1. American Heart Association. 1977. Prevention of bacterial endocarditis. Circulation. 56: 139A-143A.
2. CDC Sexually Transmitted Diseases Treatment Guidelines 1982.

FILMTAB—Film-sealed tablets, Abbott.
Abbott Laboratories
North Chicago, IL 60064
Ref: 07-5478-R1
Shown in Product Identification Section, page 403

ERYTHROMYCIN DELAYED-RELEASE CAPSULES, USP ℞

DESCRIPTION

Erythromycin Delayed-Release Capsules contain enteric-coated pellets of erythromycin base for oral administration. Erythromycin is produced by a strain of *Streptomyces erythraeus* and belongs to the macrolide group of antibiotics. It is basic and readily forms salts with acids, but it is the base which is microbiologically active. Each Erythromycin Delayed-Release Capsule contains 250 milligrams of erythromycin base.

Inactive Ingredients: Cellulosic polymers, citrate ester, D&C Red No. 30, D&C Yellow No. 10, magnesium stearate, povidone, and other ingredients. The capsule shell contains FD&C Blue No. 1, FD&C Red No. 3, gelatin, and titanium dioxide.

Erythromycin base is (3R*, 4S*, 5S*, 6R*, 7R*, 9R*, 11R*, 12R*, 13S*, 14R*)-4-[(2,6-Dideoxy-3-C-methyl-3-0-methyl-α-L-ribo-hexopyranosyl)oxy]-14-ethyl-7,12,13-trihydroxy-3, 5, 7, 9, 11, 13-hexamethyl-6-[[3, 4, 6-trideoxy-3-(dimethyl-amino)-β-D-xylo-hexopyranosyl]oxy]oxacyclotetradecane-2,10-dione.

CLINICAL PHARMACOLOGY

Orally administered erythromycin base and its salts are readily absorbed in the microbiologically active form. Interindividual variations in the absorption of erythromycin are, however, observed, and some patients do not achieve acceptable serum levels. Erythromycin is largely bound to plasma proteins, and the freely dissociating bound fraction after administration of erythromycin base represents 90% of the total erythromycin absorbed. After absorption, erythromycin diffuses readily into most body fluids. In the absence of meningeal inflammation, low concentrations are normally achieved in the spinal fluid, but the passage of the drug across the blood-brain barrier increases in meningitis. Erythromycin is excreted in breast milk. The drug crosses the placental barrier but plasma levels are low.

In the presence of normal hepatic function, erythromycin is concentrated in the liver and is excreted in the bile; the effect of hepatic dysfunction in biliary excretion of erythromycin is not known. After oral administration, less than 5% of the administered dose can be recovered in the active form in the urine.

The enteric coating of pellets in Erythromycin Delayed-Release Capsules protects the erythromycin base from inactivation by gastric acidity. Because of their small size and enteric coating, the pellets readily pass intact from the stomach to the small intestine and dissolve efficiently to allow absorption of erythromycin in a uniform manner. After administration of a single dose of a 250 mg Erythromycin Delayed-Release Capsule, peak serum levels in the range of 1.13 to 1.68 mcg/ml are attained in approximately 3 hours and decline to 0.30-0.42 mcg/ml in 6 hours. Optimal conditions for stability in the presence of gastric secretion and for complete absorption are attained when Erythromycin Delayed-Release Capsules are taken on an empty stomach.

Microbiology

Erythromycin acts by inhibition of protein synthesis by binding 50 S ribosomal subunits of susceptible organisms. It does not affect nucleic acid synthesis. Antagonism has been demonstrated between clindamycin and erythromycin. Resistance to erythromycin of many strains of *Haemophilus influenzae* and some strains of staphylococci has been demonstrated. Specimens should be obtained for culture and susceptibility testing.

Erythromycin is usually active against the following organisms *in vitro* and in clinical infections:

Streptococcus pyogenes
Alpha-hemolytic streptococci (viridans group)
Staphylococcus aureus (Resistant organisms may emerge during treatment.)
Streptococcus pneumoniae
Mycoplasma pneumoniae (Eaton's Agent)
Haemophilus influenzae (Many strains are resistant to erythromycin alone, but are susceptible to erythromycin and sulfonamides together.)
Treponema pallidum
Corynebacterium diphtheriae
Corynebacterium minutissimum
Entamoeba histolytica
Listeria monocytogenes
Neisseria gonorrhoeae

Bordetella pertussis
Legionella pneumophila (agent of Legionnaires' disease)

Susceptibility Testing

Quantitative methods that require measurement of zone diameters give the most precise estimates of antibiotic susceptibility. One such standardized single-disc procedure has been recommended for use with discs to test susceptibility to erythromycin.[1] Interpretation involves correlation of the zone diameters obtained in the disc test with minimal inhibitory concentration (MIC) values for erythromycin.

Reports from the laboratory giving results of the standardized single-disc susceptibility test using a 15 mcg erythromycin disc should be interpreted according to the following criteria:

Susceptible organisms produce zones of 18 mm or greater, indicating that the tested organism is likely to respond to therapy.

Resistant organisms produce zones of 13 mm or less, indicating that other therapy should be selected.

Organisms of intermediate susceptibility produce zones of 14 to 17 mm. The "intermediate" category provides a "buffer zone" which should prevent small, uncontrolled technical factors from causing major discrepancies in interpretations; thus, when a zone diameter falls within the "intermediate" range, the results may be considered equivocal. If alternative drugs are not available, confirmation by dilution tests may be indicated.

A bacterial isolate may be considered susceptible if the MIC value[2] (minimal inhibitory concentration) for erythromycin is not more than 2 mcg/ml. Organisms are considered resistant if the MIC is 8 mcg/ml or higher.

INDICATIONS AND USAGE

Erythromycin Delayed-Release Capsules are indicated in adults and children for treatment of the following conditions:

Upper respiratory tract infections of mild to moderate degree caused by *Streptococcus pyogenes* (Group A beta-hemolytic streptococci); *Streptococcus pneumoniae (Diplococcus pneumoniae); Haemophilus influenzae* (when used concomitantly with adequate doses of sulfonamides, since many strains of *H. influenzae* are not susceptible to the erythromycin concentrations ordinarily achieved). (See appropriate sulfonamide labeling for prescribing information.)

Lower respiratory tract infections of mild to moderate severity caused by *Streptococcus pyogenes* (Group A beta-hemolytic streptococci); *Streptococcus pneumoniae (Diplococcus pneumoniae).*

Respiratory tract infections due to *Mycoplasma pneumoniae* (Eaton's agent).

Pertussis (whooping cough) caused by *Bordetella pertussis.* Erythromycin is effective in eliminating the organism from the nasopharynx of infected individuals, rendering them noninfectious. Some clinical studies suggest that erythromycin may be helpful in the prophylaxis of pertussis in exposed susceptible individuals.

Diphtheria—As an adjunct to antitoxin in infections due to *Corynebacterium diphtheriae*, to prevent establishment of carriers and to eradicate the organism in carriers.

Erythrasma—In the treatment of infections due to *Corynebacterium minutissimum.*

Intestinal amebiasis caused by *Entamoeba histolytica* (oral erythromycins only). Extraenteric amebiasis requires treatment with other agents.

Infections due to *Listeria monocytogenes*

Skin and soft tissue infections of mild to moderate severity caused by *Streptococcus pyogenes* and *Staphylococcus aureus* (resistant staphylococci may emerge during treatment).

Primary syphilis caused by *Treponema pallidum.* Erythromycin (oral forms only) is an alternate choice of treatment for primary syphilis in patients allergic to the penicillins. In treatment of primary syphilis, spinal fluid should be examined before treatment and as part of the follow-up after therapy. The use of erythromycin for the treatment of *in utero* syphilis is not recommended. (See "CLINICAL PHARMACOLOGY" section.)

Erythromycins are indicated for treatment of the following infections caused by *Chlamydia trachomatis:* conjunctivitis of the newborn, pneumonia of infancy, and urogenital infections during pregnancy. When tetracyclines are contraindicated or not tolerated, erythromycin is indicated for the treatment of uncomplicated urethral, endocervical, or rectal infections in adults due to *Chlamydia trachomatis.*[3]

Legionnaires' disease caused by *Legionella pneumophila.* Although no controlled clinical efficacy studies have been conducted, *in vitro* and limited preliminary clinical data suggest that erythromycin may be effective in treating Legionnaires' disease.

Therapy with erythromycin should be monitored by bacteriological studies and by clinical response. (See "CLINICAL PHARMACOLOGY—Microbiology" section.)

Injectable benzathine penicillin G is considered by the American Heart Association to be the drug of choice in the treatment and prevention of streptococcal pharyngitis and in long-term prophylaxis of rheumatic fever. When oral medication is preferred for treatment of the above conditions,

penicillin G, V or erythromycin are alternate drugs of choice.

Although no controlled clinical efficacy trials have been conducted, erythromycin has been suggested by the American Heart Association and the American Dental Association for use in a regimen for prophylaxis against bacterial endocarditis in patients allergic to penicillin who have congenital and/or rheumatic or other acquired valvular heart disease when they undergo dental procedures and surgical procedures of the upper respiratory tract.[3] (Erythromycin is not suitable prior to genitourinary surgery where the organisms likely to lead to bacteremia are gram-negative bacilli or the enterococcal group of streptococci.)

NOTE: When selecting antibiotics for the prevention of bacterial endocarditis the physician or dentist should read the full joint 1984 statement of the American Heart Association and the American Dental Association.[3]

CONTRAINDICATION

Erythromycin is contraindicated in patients with known hypersensitivity to this antibiotic.

WARNING

There have been a few reports of hepatic dysfunction, with or without jaundice, occurring in patients receiving erythromycin ethylsuccinate, base and stearate products.

PRECAUTIONS

Caution should be exercised when erythromycin is administered to patients with impaired hepatic function. (See "CLINICAL PHARMACOLOGY" and "WARNING" sections.)

Erythromycin use in patients who are receiving high doses of theophylline may be associated with an increase in serum theophylline levels and potential theophylline toxicity. In case of theophylline toxicity and/or elevated serum theophylline levels, the dose of theophylline should be reduced while the patient is receiving concomitant erythromycin.

Erythromycin interferes with the fluorometric determination of urinary catecholamines.

Prolonged or repeated use of erythromycin may result in an overgrowth of nonsusceptible bacteria or fungi. If superinfection occurs, erythromycin should be discontinued and appropriate therapy instituted.

When indicated, incision and drainage or other surgical procedures should be performed in conjunction with antibiotic therapy.

Pregnancy Category B: Reproduction studies have been performed in rats, mice, and rabbits using erythromycin and its various salts and esters at doses which were several times the usual human dose. No evidence of impaired fertility or harm to the fetus that appeared related to erythromycin was reported in these studies. There are, however, no adequate and well-controlled studies in pregnant women. Because animal reproduction studies are not always predictive of human response, this drug should be used during pregnancy only if clearly needed.

Labor and Delivery: The effect of erythromycin on labor and delivery is unknown.

Nursing Mothers: Erythromycin is excreted in milk. (See "CLINICAL PHARMACOLOGY" section.)

Pediatric Use: See "INDICATIONS AND USAGE" and "DOSAGE AND ADMINISTRATION" sections.

ADVERSE REACTIONS

The most frequent side effects of oral erythromycin preparations are gastrointestinal and are dose-related. They include nausea, vomiting, abdominal pain, diarrhea and anorexia. Symptoms of hepatic dysfunction and/or abnormal liver function test results may occur (see "WARNING" section.)

Mild allergic reactions such as rashes with or without pruritus, urticaria, bullous fixed eruptions, and eczema have been reported with erythromycin. Serious allergic reactions, including anaphylaxis have been reported.

There have been isolated reports of reversible hearing loss occurring chiefly in patients with renal insufficiency and in patients receiving high doses of erythromycin.

DOSAGE AND ADMINISTRATION

Administration of a dose of Erythromycin Delayed-Release Capsules in the presence of food lowers the blood levels of systemically available erythromycin. Although the blood levels obtained upon administration of enteric-coated erythromycin products in the presence of food are still above minimum inhibitory concentrations (MICs) of most organisms for which erythromycin is indicated, optimum blood levels are obtained on a fasting stomach (administration at least $\frac{1}{2}$ hour and preferably two hours before or after a meal).

Adults: The usual dose is 250 mg every 6 hours taken one hour before meals. If twice-a-day dosage is desired, the recommended dose is 500 mg every 12 hours. Dosage may be increased up to 4 grams per day, according to the severity of infection. Twice-a-day dosing is not recommended when doses larger than 1 gram daily are administered.

Children: Age, weight, and severity of the infection are important factors in determining the proper dosage. The usual dosage is 30 to 50 mg/kg/day, in divided doses. For the

treatment of more severe infections this dosage may be doubled.

Streptococcal infections: A therapeutic dosage of oral erythromycin should be administered for at least 10 days. For continuous prophylaxis against recurrences of streptococcal infections in persons with a history of rheumatic heart disease, the dose is 250 mg twice a day.

For the prevention of bacterial endocarditis in penicillin-allergic patients with valvular heart disease who are to undergo dental procedures or surgical procedures of the upper respiratory tract, the adult dose is 1 gram orally (20 mg/kg for children) one hour prior to the procedure and then 500 mg (10 mg/kg for children) orally 6 hours later.[3] (See "INDICATIONS AND USAGE" section.)

Primary syphilis: 30 to 40 g given in divided doses over a period of 10 to 15 days.

Intestinal amebiasis: 250 mg every 6 hours for 10 to 14 days for adults; 30 to 50 mg/kg/day in divided doses for 10 to 14 days for children.

Legionnaires' disease: Although optimal doses have not been established, doses utilized in reported clinical data were those recommended above (1 to 4 g daily in divided doses).

Urogenital infections during pregnancy due to *Chlamydia trachomatis:* Although the optimal dose and duration of therapy have not been established, the suggested treatment is 500 mg by mouth four times a day on an empty stomach for at least 7 days. For women who cannot tolerate this regimen, a decreased dose of 250 mg by mouth four times a day should be used for at least 14 days.[4]

For adults with uncomplicated urethral, endocervical, or rectal infections caused by *Chlamydia trachomatis*, when tetracycline is contrainidicated or not tolerated, 500 mg of erythromycin by mouth four times a day for at least 7 days.[4]

Pertussis: Although optimum dosage and duration of therapy have not been established, doses of erythromycin utilized in reported clinical studies were 40 to 50 mg/kg/day, given in divided doses for 5 to 14 days.

HOW SUPPLIED

Erythromycin Delayed-Release Capsules, USP, are clear and opaque maroon capsules with pink and yellow particles containing 250 mg of erythromycin supplied in bottles of 100 (**NDC** 0074-6301-13) and 500 (**NDC** 0074-6301-53).

Storage Conditions: Protect from moisture and excessive heat. Store at room temperature below 86°F (30°C).

REFERENCES

1. Approved Standard ASM-2 "Performance Standards for Antimicrobial Disc Susceptibility Test." National Committee for Clinical Laboratory Standards, 771 East Lancaster Avenue, Villanova, PA 19085.
2. Ericson, H.M., Sherris, J.C.: "Antibiotic Sensitivity Testing Report of an International Collaborative Study." *Acta Pathologica et Microbiologica Scandinavica*, Section B, Supp. 217, 1971.
3. American Heart Assoc. and American Dental Assoc. "Prevention of Bacterial Endocarditis," *Circulation:* Vol. 70, No. 6, December, 1984, 1123A-1127A.
4. CDC Sexually Transmitted Diseases Treatment Guidelines 1982.

Caution—Federal (U.S.A.) law prohibits dispensing without prescription.

Ref. 01-2443-R1 Revised: January, 1989

Abbott Laboratories
North Chicago, IL 60064

Shown in Product Identification Section, page 403

FERO–FOLIC–500® Filmtab® Tablets   ℞
[fe 'ro fo-lic]
Controlled-Release Iron with Folic Acid and Vitamin C

IBERET–FOLIC–500® Filmtab®   ℞
Tablets
Controlled-Release Iron with Vitamin C, and B-Complex, including Folic Acid

DESCRIPTION

FERO-FOLIC-500 Filmtab is a hematinic for oral administration containing 525 mg of ferrous sulfate (equivalent to 105 mg of elemental iron) in a unique controlled-release vehicle, the Gradumet®. In addition, this product contains 800 mcg of folic acid and 500 mg of ascorbic acid present as sodium ascorbate.

Inactive Ingredients: Cellulosic polymers, D&C Red No. 30, FD&C Blue No. 1, magnesium stearate, methyl acrylate-methyl methacrylate copolymer, pregelatinized starch (contains corn starch), polyethylene glycol, povidone, propylene glycol, talc, titanium dioxide and vanillin.

Continued on next page

If desired, additional literature on any Abbott Product will be provided upon request to Abbott Laboratories.

Abbott—Cont.

IBERET-FOLIC-500 is an Abbott hematinic containing iron in the Gradumet® controlled-release vehicle; vitamin C for enhancement of iron absorption; and the B-Complex vitamins including folic acid. The IBERET-FOLIC-500 Filmtab is for oral use.

Each Filmtab tablet provides:

*Ferrous Sulfate	525 mg
(equivalent to 105 mg of elemental iron)	
Ascorbic Acid (present as sodium ascorbate) (C)	500 mg
Niacinamide	30 mg
Calcium Pantothenate	10 mg
Thiamine Mononitrate (B₁)	6 mg
Riboflavin (B₂)	6 mg
Pyridoxine Hydrochloride (B₆)	5 mg
Folic Acid	800 mcg
Cyanocobalamin (B₁₂)	25 mcg

*In controlled-release form (Gradumet)

Inactive Ingredients: Cellulosic polymers, corn starch, D&C Red No. 7, FD&C Blue No. 1, FD&C Blue No. 2, FD&C Red No. 3, magnesium stearate, methyl acrylate-methyl methacrylate copolymer, polyethylene glycol, povidone, propylene glycol, stearic acid, talc, titanium dioxide and vanillin.

Controlled-release of iron from the Gradumet protects against gastric side effects. The Gradumet is an inert, porous, plastic matrix which is impregnated with ferrous sulfate. Iron is leached from the Gradumet as it passes through the gastrointestinal tract, and the expended matrix is excreted harmlessly in the stool. Controlled-release iron is particularly helpful in patients who have demonstrated intolerance to oral iron preparations.

CLINICAL PHARMACOLOGY

Oral iron is absorbed most efficiently when it is administered between meals. Conventional iron preparations, however, frequently cause gastric irritation when taken on an empty stomach. Studies with iron in the Gradumet have indicated that relatively little of the iron is released in the stomach, gastric intolerance is seldom encountered, and hematologic response ranks with that obtained from plain ferrous sulfate. Iron is found in the body principally as hemoglobin. Storage in the form of ferritin occurs in the liver, spleen, and bone marrow. Concentrations of plasma iron and the total iron-binding capacity of plasma vary greatly in different physiological conditions and disease states.

Large amounts of ascorbic acid administered orally with ferrous sulfate have been shown to enhance iron absorption. Apparently this is due to the ability of ascorbic acid to prevent the oxidation of ferrous iron to the less effectively absorbed ferric form.

Folic acid and iron are absorbed in the proximal small intestine, particularly the duodenum. Folic acid is absorbed maximally and rapidly at this site, and iron is absorbed in a descending gradient from the duodenum distally.

After absorption folic acid is rapidly converted into its metabolically active forms. Approximately two-thirds is bound to plasma protein. Half of the folic acid stored in the body is found in the liver. Folic acid is also concentrated in spinal fluid.

Except for the folates ingested in liver, yeast, and egg yolk, the percentage of absorption of food folates averages about 10%.

The B-complex vitamins in IBERET-FOLIC-500 are absorbed by the active transport process. B-complex vitamins are rapidly eliminated and therefore are not stored in the body.

Calcium pantothenate is absorbed readily from the gastrointestinal tract and distributed to all body tissues.

INDICATIONS AND USAGE

FERO-FOLIC-500 is indicated for the treatment of iron deficiency and prevention of concomitant folic acid deficiency in nonpregnant adults. FERO-FOLIC-500 is also indicated in pregnancy for the prevention and treatment of iron deficiency and to supply a maintenance dosage of folic acid.

IBERET-FOLIC-500 is indicated in non-pregnant adults for the treatment of iron deficiency and prevention of concomitant folic acid deficiency where there is an associated deficient intake or increased need for the B-complex vitamins. IBERET-FOLIC-500 is also indicated in pregnancy for the prevention and treatment of iron deficiency where there is a concomitant deficient intake or increased need for the B-complex vitamins (including folic acid).

CONTRAINDICATIONS

FERO-FOLIC-500 and IBERET-FOLIC-500 are contraindicated in patients with pernicious anemia.

FERO-FOLIC-500 and IBERET-FOLIC-500 are also contraindicated in the rare instance of hypersensitivity to folic acid.

WARNINGS

Folic acid alone is improper therapy in the treatment of pernicious anemia and other megaloblastic anemias where vitamin B₁₂ is deficient.

PRECAUTIONS

Where anemia exists, its nature should be established and underlying causes determined.

FERO-FOLIC-500 and IBERET-FOLIC-500 contain 800 mcg of folic acid per tablet. Folic acid especially in doses above 0.1 mg daily may obscure pernicious anemia, in that hematologic remission may occur while neurological manifestations remain progresssive. Concomitant parenteral therapy with vitamin B₁₂ may be necessary in patients with deficiency of vitamin B₁₂. Pernicious anemia is rare in women of childbearing age, and the likelihood of its occurrence along with pregnancy is reduced by the impairment of fertility associated with vitamin B₁₂ deficiency.

Like other oral iron preparations, FERO-FOLIC-500 and IBERET-FOLIC-500 should be stored out of the reach of children to guard against accidental iron poisoning (see Overdosage).

Laboratory Tests: In older patients and those with conditions tending to lead to vitamin B₁₂ depletion, serum B₁₂ levels should be regularly assessed during treatment with FERO-FOLIC-500 or IBERET-FOLIC-500.

Drug Interactions: Absorption of iron is inhibited by *magnesium trisilicate* and *antacids containing carbonates.*

Ferrous sulfate may interfere with the absorption of *tetracyclines.*

The antiparkinsonism effects of *levodopa* may be reversed by pyridoxine.

Iron absorption is inhibited by the ingestion of eggs or milk.

Carcinogenesis: Adequate data are not available on long-term potential for carcinogenesis in animals or humans.

Pregnancy: Pregnancy Category A. Studies in pregnant women have not shown that FERO-FOLIC-500 or IBERET-FOLIC-500 increase the risk of fetal abnormalities if administered during pregnancy. If either of these drugs is used during pregnancy, the possibility of fetal harm appears remote. Because studies cannot rule out the possibility of harm, however, FERO-FOLIC-500 or IBERET-FOLIC-500 should be used during pregnancy only if clearly needed.

Nursing Mothers: Folic acid, ascorbic acid, and B-complex vitamins are excreted in breast milk.

ADVERSE REACTIONS

The likelihood of gastric intolerance to iron in the controlled-release Gradumet vehicle is remote. If such should occur, the tablet may be taken after a meal. Allergic sensitization has been reported following both oral and parenteral administration of folic acid.

OVERDOSAGE

Signs of serious toxicity may be delayed because the iron is in a controlled-release dose form. Increased capillary permeability, reduced plasma volume, increased cardiac output, and sudden cardiovascular collapse may occur in acute iron intoxication. In overdosage, efforts should be made to hasten the elimination of the Gradumet tablets ingested. An emetic should be administered as soon as possible, followed by gastric lavage if indicated. Immediately following emesis, a large dose of a saline cathartic should be used to speed passage through the intestinal tract. X-ray examination may then be considered to determine the position and number of Gradumet tablets remaining in the gastrointestinal tract.

DOSAGE AND ADMINISTRATION

FERO-FOLIC-500 is administered orally and may be taken on an empty stomach.

Adults: For treatment of iron deficiency and prevention of folic acid deficiency, the recommended dose is one tablet daily.

Pregnant Adults: For prevention and treatment of iron deficiency and to supply a maintenance dosage of folic acid, the recommended dose is one tablet daily.

IBERET-FOLIC-500 is administered orally and may be taken on an empty stomach.

Adults: For the treatment of iron deficiency and prevention of concomitant folic acid deficiency where there is an associated deficient intake or increased need for the B-complex vitamins, the recommended dose is one tablet daily.

Pregnant Adults: For the prevention and treatment of iron deficiency where there is a concomitant deficient intake or increased need for the B-complex vitamins including folic acid, the recommended dose is one tablet daily.

HOW SUPPLIED

FERO-FOLIC-500 is supplied as red Filmtab tablets in bottles of 100 (**NDC** 0074-7079-13) and 500 (**NDC** 0074-7079-53).

IBERET-FOLIC-500 is supplied as red Filmtab tablets in bottles of 60 (**NDC** 0074-7125-60).

Abbott Pharmaceuticals, Inc.
North Chicago, IL 60064
Ref. 03-4352-R6
Shown in Product Identification Section, page 403

FERO-GRAD-500® Filmtab® tablets
[*fe'ro-grad*]
IRON plus Vitamin C
Well-tolerated once-daily hematinic with controlled-release iron.
FERO-GRADUMET® Filmtab® tablets
Hematinic supplying controlled-release iron

DESCRIPTION

Each Fero-Gradumet and Fero-Grad-500 tablet contains the equivalent of 105 mg of elemental iron (525 mg of ferrous sulfate) in a unique controlled-release vehicle, the Gradumet®. In addition, each Fero-Grad-500 tablet contains 500 mg of vitamin C (as sodium ascorbate) to improve iron absorption.

The Gradumet, an inert, porous, plastic matrix, is impregnated with ferrous sulfate. Iron is leached from the Gradumet as it passes through the gastrointestinal tract, and the expended matrix is excreted harmlessly in the stool. Controlled-release iron is particularly helpful in patients who have demonstrated intolerance to other oral iron preparations.

Inactive Ingredients: Fero-Grad-500: Cellulosic polymers, D&C Red No. 7, FD&C Blue No. 1, magnesium stearate, methyl acrylate-methyl methacrylate copolymer, polyethylene glycol, povidone, pregelatinized starch (contains corn starch), propylene glycol, talc, titanium dioxide and vanillin.
Fero-Gradumet: Castor oil, cellulosic polymers, FD&C Red No. 40, FD&C Yellow No. 6, magnesium stearate, methyl acrylate-methyl methacrylate copolymer, polyethylene glycol, povidone, sorbitan monooleate, titanium dioxide and vanillin.

INDICATIONS

Fero-Grad-500: For the treatment of iron deficiency or iron deficiency anemia. Fero-Gradumet: For the prevention and treatment of iron deficiency.

PRECAUTIONS

Where anemia exists, its nature should be established and underlying cause determined.

Like other oral iron preparations Fero-Gradumet and Fero-Grad-500 should be stored out of the reach of children to protect against accidental iron poisoning (see Overdosage).

ADVERSE REACTIONS

The likelihood of gastric intolerance to iron in the controlled-release Gradumet vehicle is slight. If it should occur, the tablet may be taken after a meal.

DOSAGE AND ADMINISTRATION

Fero-Gradumet and Fero-Grad-500 are administered orally and may be taken on an empty stomach. The Gradumet controlled-release vehicle reduces the incidence of gastric side effects by delaying the release of almost all the iron until the tablet has passed the stomach.

Fero-Grad-500: Usual adult dose, including pregnant females: One tablet daily, or as directed by the physician.
Fero-Gradumet: Usual adult dose: Prevention: One tablet daily; Treatment: One tablet twice daily, or as directed by the physician. Pregnant females: Prevention: One tablet daily, or as directed by physician.

OVERDOSAGE

Signs of serious toxicity may be delayed because the iron is in a controlled-release dose form. Increased capillary permeability, reduced plasma volume, increased cardiac output, and sudden cardiovascular collapse may occur in acute iron intoxication. In overdosage, efforts should be made to hasten the elimination of the Gradumet tablets ingested. An emetic should be administered as soon as possible, followed by gastric lavage if indicated. Immediately following emesis, a large dose of a saline cathartic should be used to speed passage through the intestinal tract. X-ray examination may then be considered to determine the position and number of Gradumet tablets remaining in the gastrointestinal tract.

HOW SUPPLIED

Fero-Gradumet is supplied as red tablets in bottles of 100 (**NDC** 0074-6852-02); Fero-Grad-500 is supplied as red tablets in bottles of 30 (**NDC** 0074-7238-30), 100 (**NDC** 0074-7238-01) and 500 (**NDC** 0074-7238-02). The ingredients of these products are listed in one or more of the Medicare designated compendia.

Abbott Pharmaceuticals, Inc.
North Chicago, IL 60064
Ref. 03-1619-7/R26 and 03-1224-7/R29
Shown in Product Identification Section, page 403

H-BIG®
(Hepatitis B Immune Globulin [Human])

½ ml syringe	(NDC 0074-8399-11)
1 ml vial	(NDC 0074-8399-01)
4 ml vial	(NDC 0074-8399-04)
5 ml vial	(NDC 0074-8399-05)

HARMONYL® Tablets   ℞
[har'mō-nil]
(deserpidine)

DESCRIPTION

Harmonyl (deserpidine) is a purified rauwolfia alkaloid chemically identified as 11-desmethoxyreserpine.

Inactive Ingredients: Corn starch, D&C Red No. 36, lactose, magnesium stearate, stearic acid and talc.

ACTIONS

The pharmacologic actions of HARMONYL (deserpidine) are essentially the same as those of other active rauwolfia alkaloids. Deserpidine probably produces its antihypertensive effects through depletion of tissue stores of catecholamines (epinephrine and norepinephrine) from peripheral sites. By contrast, its sedative and tranquilizing properties are thought to be related to depletion of 5-hydroxytryptamine from the brain.

The antihypertensive effect is often accompanied by bradycardia. There is no significant alteration in cardiac output or renal blood flow. The carotid sinus reflex is inhibited, but postural hypotension is rarely seen with the use of conventional doses of HARMONYL alone.

Deserpidine, like other rauwolfia alkaloids, is characterized by slow onset of action and sustained effect which may persist following withdrawal of the drug.

INDICATIONS

HARMONYL (deserpidine) is indicated for the treatment of mild essential hypertension. It is also useful as adjunctive therapy with other antihypertensive agents in the more severe forms of hypertension.

The drug is also indicated for the relief of symptoms in agitated psychotic states, e.g., schizophrenia—primarily in those individuals unable to tolerate phenothiazine derivatives or those who also require antihypertensive medication.

CONTRAINDICATIONS

HARMONYL (deserpidine) is contraindicated in patients with known hypersensitivity, history of mental depression especially with suicidal tendencies, active peptic ulcer, and ulcerative colitis. It is also contraindicated in patients receiving electroconvulsive therapy.

WARNINGS

HARMONYL (deserpidine) differs slightly in chemical structure from reserpine, however, its actions, indications, cautions and adverse reactions are common to the class of rauwolfia alkaloids. Reserpine may cause mental depression. Recognition of depression may be difficult because this condition may often be disguised by somatic complaints (Masked Depression). The drug should be discontinued at first signs of depression such as despondency, early morning insomnia, loss of appetite, impotence, or self-deprecation. Drug-induced depression may persist for several months after drug withdrawal and may be severe enough to result in suicide.

Usage in Pregnancy and Lactation

The safety of deserpidine for use during pregnancy or lactation has not been established; therefore, it should be used in pregnant women or in women of childbearing potential only when, in the judgment of the physician, its use is deemed essential to the welfare of the patient. Increased respiratory secretions, nasal congestion, cyanosis, and anorexia may occur in infants born to rauwolfia alkaloid-treated mothers since these preparations are known to cross the placental barrier to enter the fetal circulation and appear in cord blood. They also are secreted by nursing mothers into breast milk.

Reproductive and teratology studies in rats reduced the mating index and neonatal survival indices; the no-effect dosage has not been established.

PRECAUTIONS

Because rauwolfia preparations increase gastrointestinal motility and secretion, this drug should be used cautiously in patients with a history of peptic ulcer, ulcerative colitis, or gallstones, where biliary colic may be precipitated.

Caution should be exercised when treating hypertensive patients with renal insufficiency since they adjust poorly to lowered blood pressure levels.

Use HARMONYL (deserpidine) cautiously with digitalis and quinidine since cardiac arrhythmias have occurred with rauwolfia preparations.

Preoperative withdrawal of deserpidine does not assure that circulatory instability will not occur. It is important that the anesthesiologist be aware of the patient's drug intake and consider this in the overall management, since hypotension has occurred in patients receiving rauwolfia preparations. Anticholinergic and/or adrenergic drugs (metaraminol, norepinephrine) have been employed to treat adverse vagocirculatory effects.

Animal tumorigenicity: There are no studies demonstrating that deserpidine is an animal tumorigen, although it is a prolactin stimulator and structurally related to reserpine. Rodent studies with reserpine, however, have shown that reserpine is an animal tumorigen, causing an increased inci-

dence of mammary fibroadenomas in female mice, malignant tumors of the seminal vesicles in male mice, and malignant adrenal medullary tumors in male rats. These findings arose in 2 year studies in which the drug was administered in the feed at concentrations of 5 and 10 ppm—about 100 to 300 times the usual human dose. The breast neoplasms are thought to be related to reserpine's prolactin-elevating effect. Several other prolactin-elevating drugs have also been associated with an increased incidence of mammary neoplasia in rodents.

The extent to which these findings indicate a risk to humans is uncertain. Tissue culture experiments show that about one-third of human breast tumors are prolactin-dependent *in vitro*, a factor of considerable importance if the use of the drug is contemplated in a patient with previously detected breast cancer. The possibility of an increased risk of breast cancer in reserpine users has been studied extensively; however, no firm conclusion has emerged. Although a few epidemiologic studies have suggested a slightly increased risk (less than twofold in all studies except one) in women who have used reserpine, other studies of generally similar design have not confirmed this. Epidemiologic studies conducted using other drugs (neuroleptic agents) that, like reserpine, increase prolactin levels and, therefore, would be considered rodent mammary carcinogens, have not shown an association between chronic administration of the drug and human mammary tumorigenesis. While long-term clinical observation has not suggested such an association, the available evidence is considered too limited to be conclusive at this time. An association of reserpine intake with pheochromocytoma or tumors of the seminal vesicles has not been explored.

ADVERSE REACTIONS

The following adverse reactions have been reported with rauwolfia preparations. These reactions are usually reversible and disappear when the drug is discontinued.

Gastrointestinal: Including hypersecretion, anorexia, diarrhea, nausea, and vomiting.

Cardiovascular: Including angina-like symptoms, arrhythmias (particularly when used concurrently with digitalis or quinidine), and bradycardia.

Central Nervous System: Including drowsiness, depression, nervousness, paradoxical anxiety, nightmares, extrapyramidal tract symptoms, CNS sensitization manifested by dull sensorium, and deafness.

Dermatologic-Hypersensitivity: Including pruritus, rash, and asthma in asthmatic patients.

Ophthalmologic: Including glaucoma, uveitis, optic atrophy, and conjunctival injection.

Hematologic: Thrombocytopenic purpura.

Miscellaneous: Nasal congestion, weight gain, impotence or decreased libido, dysuria, dyspnea, muscular aches, dryness of mouth, dizziness, and headache.

Water retention with edema in patients with hypertensive vascular disease may occur rarely, but the condition generally clears with cessation of therapy or with the administration of a diuretic agent.

DOSAGE AND ADMINISTRATION

HARMONYL (deserpidine) is administered orally. For the management of mild essential hypertension in the average patient not receiving other antihypertensive agents, the usual initial adult dose is 0.75 to 1 mg daily. Because 10 to 14 days are required to produce the full effects of the drug, adjustments in dosage should not be made more frequently. If the therapeutic response is not adequate, it is generally advisable to add another antihypertensive agent to the regimen. For maintenance, dosage should be reduced. A single daily dose of 0.25 mg of deserpidine may suffice for some patients.

Concomitant use of deserpidine with ganglionic blocking agents, guanethidine, veratrum, hydralazine, methyldopa, chlorthalidone, or thiazides necessitates careful titration of dosage with each agent.

For psychiatric disorders: The average initial oral dose is 0.5 mg daily with a range of 0.125 to 1 mg. Adjust dosage upward or downward according to the patient's response.

OVERDOSAGE

An overdosage of deserpidine is characterized by flushing of the skin, conjunctival injection, and pupillary constriction. Sedation ranging from drowsiness to coma may occur. Hypotension, hypothermia, central respiratory depression and bradycardia may develop in cases of severe overdosage. Treatment consists of the careful evacuation of stomach contents followed by the usual procedures for the symptomatic management of CNS depressant overdosage. If severe hypotension occurs, it should be treated with a direct acting vasopressor such as Levophed® (norepinephrine bitartrate injection, USP).

HOW SUPPLIED

HARMONYL (deserpidine tablets) grooved, salmon-pink, 0.25 mg tablets are supplied in bottles of 100 (**NDC** 0074-6906-07).

Abbott Laboratories
North Chicago, IL 60064
Ref. 01-2408-R3

HYTRIN®   ℞
(terazosin hydrochloride)

PRODUCT OVERVIEW

KEY FACTS

HYTRIN (terazosin HCl) is a quinazoline derivative that exerts its hypotensive effect by selectively blocking the postsynaptic alpha$_1$-adrenoceptors. Terazosin has a half-life of approximately 12 hours which allows for effective once-daily dosing, however, a twice-daily dosing regimen may be considered for some patients. HYTRIN tablets contain 1 mg, 2 mg, 5 mg or 10 mg of terazosin.

MAJOR USES

HYTRIN tablets are indicated for the treatment of hypertension. HYTRIN tablets may be prescribed as monotherapy or in combination with other antihypertensive agents such as diuretics or beta-adrenergic receptor blocking agents. The usual dose range is 1 mg to 10 mg daily; some patients may benefit from doses up to 20 mg daily. Clinical studies and available literature do not suggest any contraindication to the use of HYTRIN tablets.

SAFETY INFORMATION

HYTRIN therapy should be initiated with a 1 mg dose given at bedtime to minimize the potential for severe hypotensive effects or syncopal episodes. Caution should be observed when HYTRIN tablets are given concomitantly with other antihypertensive agents (eg, calcium antagonists) to avoid the possibility of significant hypotension. When adding a diuretic or other antihypertensive agent, dosage reduction and retitration may be necessary. Adverse events have generally been mild to moderate in intensity. The most commonly reported adverse events are: asthenia, blurred vision, dizziness, nasal congestion, nausea, peripheral edema, palpitations, and somnolence. HYTRIN tablets have been administered to patients on a wide variety of concomitant drug therapies without any apparent drug-drug interactions.

PRODUCT ILLUSTRATION

1 mg

2 mg

5 mg

10 mg

PRESCRIBING INFORMATION

HYTRIN®   ℞
(terazosin hydrochloride)

DESCRIPTION

HYTRIN (terazosin hydrochloride), an alpha-1-selective adrenoceptor blocking agent, is a quinazoline derivative represented by the following chemical name and structural formula: Piperazine, 1-(4-amino-6,7-dimethoxy-2-quinazolinyl) -4- [(tetrahydro-2-furanyl)carbonyl]-, monohydrochloride, dihydrate.

Terazosin hydrochloride is a white, crystalline substance, freely soluble in water and isotonic saline and has a molecular weight of 459.93. HYTRIN tablets (terazosin hydrochloride tablets) for oral ingestion are supplied in four dosage strengths containing terazosin hydrochloride equivalent to 1 mg, 2 mg, 5 mg, or 10 mg of terazosin.

Inactive Ingredients:

1 mg tablet: corn starch, lactose, magnesium stearate, povidone and talc.

2 mg tablet: corn starch, FD&C Yellow No. 6, lactose, magnesium stearate, povidone and talc.

5 mg tablet: corn starch, iron oxide, lactose, magnesium stearate, povidone and talc.

10 mg tablet: corn starch, D&C Yellow No. 10, FD&C Blue No. 2, lactose, magnesium stearate, povidone and talc.

CLINICAL PHARMACOLOGY

Pharmacodynamics:

In animals, terazosin causes a decrease in blood pressure by decreasing total peripheral vascular resistance. The

Continued on next page

Abbott—Cont.

vasodilatory hypotensive action of terazosin appears to be produced mainly by blockade of alpha-1-adrenoceptors. Terazosin decreases blood pressure gradually within 15 minutes following oral administration.

Clinical studies of terazosin in man used once daily (the great majority) and twice daily regimens with total doses usually in the range of 5–20 mg/day, in patients with mild (about 77%, diastolic pressure 95–105 mmHg) or moderate (23%, diastolic pressure 105–115 mmHg) hypertension. Because terazosin, like all alpha antagonists, can cause unusually large falls in blood pressure after the first dose or first few doses, the initial dose was 1 mg in virtually all studies, with subsequent titration to a specified fixed dose or titration to some specified blood pressure end point (usually a supine diastolic pressure of 90 mmHg).

Blood pressure responses were measured at the end of the dosing interval (usually 24 hours) and effects were shown to persist throughout the interval, with the usual supine responses 5–10 mmHg systolic and 3.5–8 mmHg diastolic greater than placebo. The responses in the standing position tended to be somewhat larger, by 1–3 mmHg, although this was not true in all studies. The magnitude of the blood pressure responses was similar to prazosin and less than hydrochlorothiazide (in a single study). In measurements 24 hours after dosing, heart rate was unchanged.

Limited measurements of peak response (2–3 hours after dosing) during chronic terazosin administration indicate that it is greater than about twice the trough (24 hour) response, suggesting some attenuation of response at 24 hours, presumably due to a fall in blood terazosin concentrations at the end of the dose interval. This explanation is not established with certainty, however, and is not consistent with the similarity of blood pressure response to once daily and twice daily dosing and with the absence of an observed dose-response relationship over a range of 5–20 mg, i.e., if concentrations had fallen to the point of providing less than full effect at 24 hours, a shorter dosing interval or larger dose should have led to increased response. Further dose response and dose duration studies are being carried out. Blood pressure should be measured at the end of the dose interval; if response is not satisfactory, patients may be tried on a larger dose or twice daily dosing regimen. The latter should also be considered if possibly blood pressure-related side effects, such as dizziness, palpitations, or orthostatic complaints, are seen within a few hours after dosing.

The greater blood pressure effect associated with peak plasma concentrations (first few hours after dosing) appears somewhat more position-dependent (greater in the erect position) than the effect of terazosin at 24 hours and in the erect position there is also a 6–10 beat per minute increase in heart rate in the first few hours after dosing. During the first 3 hours after dosing 12.5% of patients had a systolic pressure fall of 30 mmHg or more from supine to standing, or standing systolic pressure below 90 mmHg with a fall of at least 20 mmHg, compared to 4% of a placebo group.

There was a tendency for patients to gain weight during terazosin therapy. In placebo-controlled monotherapy trials, male and female patients receiving terazosin gained a mean of 1.7 and 2.2 pounds respectively, compared to losses of 0.2 and 1.2 pounds respectively, in the placebo group. Both differences were statistically significant.

During controlled clinical studies, patients receiving terazosin monotherapy had a small but statistically significant decrease (a 3% fall) compared to placebo in total cholesterol and the combined low-density and very-low-density lipoprotein fractions. No significant changes were observed in high-density lipoprotein fraction and triglycerides compared to placebo.

Analysis of clinical laboratory data following administration of terazosin suggested the possibility of hemodilution based on decreases in hematocrit, hemoglobin, white blood cells, total protein and albumin. Decreases in hematocrit and total protein have been observed with alpha-blockade and are attributed to hemodilution.

Pharmacokinetics:

Relative to solution, terazosin hydrochloride administered as HYTRIN tablets is essentially completely absorbed in man. Food had little or no effect on the bioavailability of terazosin. Terazosin has been shown to undergo minimal hepatic first-pass metabolism and nearly all of the circulating dose is in the form of parent drug. The plasma levels peak about one hour after dosing, and then decline with a half-life of approximately 12 hours. The drug is highly bound to plasma proteins and binding is constant over the clinically observed concentration range. Approximately 10% of an orally administered dose is excreted as parent drug in the urine and approximately 20% is excreted in the feces. The remainder is eliminated as metabolites. Overall, approximately 40% of the administered dose is excreted in the urine and approximately 60% in the feces. The disposition of the compound in animals is qualitatively similar to that in man.

INDICATIONS AND USAGE

HYTRIN (terazosin hydrochloride) is indicated for the treatment of hypertension. It can be used alone or in combination with other antihypertensive agents such as diuretics or beta-adrenergic blocking agents.

CONTRAINDICATIONS

Clinical studies and available literature do not suggest any contraindication to the use of HYTRIN.

WARNINGS

Syncope and "First-dose" Effect:

Terazosin, like other alpha-adrenergic blocking agents, can cause marked hypotension, especially postural hypotension, and syncope in association with the first dose or first few doses of therapy. A similar effect can be anticipated if therapy is interrupted for more than a few doses. Syncope has also been reported with other alpha-adrenergic blocking agents in association with rapid dosage increases or the introduction of another antihypertensive drug. Syncope is believed to be due to an excessive postural hypotensive effect, although occasionally the syncopal episode has been preceded by a bout of severe supraventricular tachycardia with heart rates of 120–160 beats per minute.

To decrease the likelihood of syncope or excessive hypotension, treatment should always be initiated with a 1 mg dose of terazosin, given at bedtime. The 2 mg, 5 mg and 10 mg tablets are not indicated as initial therapy. Dosage should then be increased slowly, according to recommendations in the Dosage and Administration section and additional antihypertensive agents should be added with caution. The patient should be cautioned to avoid situations where injury could result should syncope occur during initiation of therapy.

In early investigational studies, where increasing single doses up to 7.5 mg were given at 3 day intervals, tolerance to the first dose phenomenon did not necessarily develop and the "first dose" effect could be observed at all doses. Syncopal episodes occurred in 3 of the 14 subjects given terazosin at doses of 2.5, 5 and 7.5 mg, which are higher than the recommended initial dose; in addition, severe orthostatic hypotension (blood pressure falling to 50/0 mmHg) was seen in two others and dizziness, tachycardia, and lightheadedness occurred in most subjects. These adverse effects all occurred within 90 minutes of dosing.

In multiple dose clinical trials involving nearly 2000 patients, syncope was reported in about 1% of patients, in no case severe or prolonged, and was not necessarily associated with early doses.

If syncope occurs, the patient should be placed in a recumbent position and treated supportively as necessary. There is evidence that the orthostatic effect of terazosin is greater, even in chronic use, shortly after dosing.

PRECAUTIONS

General:

Orthostatic Hypotension

While syncope is the most severe orthostatic effect of terazosin (see Warnings), other symptoms of lowered blood pressure, such as dizziness, lightheadedness and palpitations, are more common, occurring in some 28% of patients in clinical trials. Patients with occupations in which such events represent potential problems should be treated with particular caution.

Information for Patients:

Patients should be made aware of the possibility of syncopal and orthostatic symptoms, especially at the initiation of therapy, and to avoid driving or hazardous tasks for 12 hours after the first dose, after a dosage increase, and after interruption of therapy when treatment is resumed. They should be cautioned to avoid situations where injury could result should syncope occur during initiation of terazosin therapy. They should also be advised of the need to sit or lie down when symptoms of lowered blood pressure occur, although these symptoms are not always orthostatic, and to be careful when rising from a sitting or lying position. If dizziness, lightheadedness, or palpitations are bothersome they should be reported to the physician, so that dose adjustment can be considered.

Patients should also be told that drowsiness or somnolence can occur with terazosin, requiring caution in people who must drive or operate heavy machinery.

Laboratory Tests:

Small but statistically significant decreases in hematocrit, hemoglobin, white blood cells, total protein and albumin were observed in controlled clinical trials. The magnitude of the decreases did not worsen with time. These laboratory findings suggested the possibility of hemodilution.

Drug Interactions:

In controlled trials, terazosin has been added to diuretics, and several beta-adrenergic blockers; no unexpected interactions were observed. Terazosin has also been used in patients on a variety of concomitant therapies; while these were not formal interaction studies, no interactions were observed. Terazosin has been used concomitantly in at least 50 patients on the following drugs or drug classes: 1) analgesic/anti-inflammatory (e.g., acetaminophen, aspirin, codeine, ibuprofen, indomethacin); 2) antibiotics (e.g., erythromycin, trimethoprim and sulfamethoxazole); 3) anticholinergic/sympathomimetics (e.g., phenylephrine hydrochloride, phenylpropanolamine hydrochloride, pseudoephedrine hydrochloride); 4) antigout (e.g., allopurinol); 5) antihistamines (e.g., chlorpheniramine); 6) cardiovascular agents (e.g., atenolol, hydrochlorothiazide, methylclothiazide, propranolol); 7) corticosteroids; 8) gastrointestinal agents (e.g., antacids); 9) hypoglycemics; 10) sedatives and tranquilizers (e.g., diazepam).

Carcinogenesis, Mutagenesis, Impairment of Fertility:

HYTRIN was devoid of mutagenic potential when evaluated *in vivo* and *in vitro* (the Ames test, *in vivo* cytogenetics, the dominant lethal test in mice, *in vivo* Chinese hamster chromosome aberration test and V79 forward mutation assay). HYTRIN, administered in the feed to rats at doses of 8, 40, and 250 mg/kg/day for two years, was associated with a statistically significant increase in benign adrenal medullary tumors of male rats exposed to the 250 mg/kg dose. This dose is 695 times the maximum recommended human dose of 20 mg/55 kg patient. Female rats were unaffected. HYTRIN was not oncogenic in mice when administered in feed for 2 years at a maximum tolerated dose of 32 mg/kg/day.

The absence of mutagenicity in a battery of tests, of tumorigenicity of any cell type in the mouse carcinogenicity assay, of increased total tumor incidence in either species, and of proliferative adrenal lesions in female rats, suggests a male rat species-specific event. Numerous other diverse pharmaceutical and chemical compounds have also been associated with benign adrenal medullary tumors in male rats without supporting evidence for carcinogenicity in man.

The effect of HYTRIN on fertility was assessed in a standard fertility/reproductive performance study in which male and female rats were administered oral doses of 8, 30 and 120 mg/kg/day. Four of 20 male rats given 30 mg/kg and five of 19 male rats given 120 mg/kg failed to sire a litter. Testicular weights and morphology were unaffected by treatment. Vaginal smears at 30 and 120 mg/kg/day, however, appeared to contain less sperm than smears from control matings and good correlation was reported between sperm count and subsequent pregnancy.

Oral administration of HYTRIN for one or two years elicited a statistically significant increase in the incidence of testicular atrophy in rats exposed to 40 and 250 mg/kg/day, but not in rats exposed to 8 mg/kg/day (> 20 times the maximum recommended human dose). Testicular atrophy was also observed in dogs dosed with 300 mg/kg/day (> 800 times the maximum recommended human dose) for three months but not after one year when dosed with 20 mg/kg/day. This lesion has also been seen with Minipress®, another (marketed) selective-alpha-1 blocking agent.

Pregnancy:

Teratogenic effects: Pregnancy Category C. HYTRIN was not teratogenic in either rats or rabbits when administered at oral doses up to 1330 and 165 times, respectively, the maximum recommended human dose. Fetal resorptions occurred in rats dosed with 480 mg/kg/day, approximately 1330 times the maximum recommended human dose. Increased fetal resorptions, decreased fetal weight and an increased number of supernumerary ribs were observed in offspring of rabbits dosed with 165 times the maximum recommended human dose. These findings (in both species) were most likely secondary to maternal toxicity. There are no adequate and well-controlled studies in pregnant women and the safety of terazosin in pregnancy has not been established. HYTRIN is not recommended during pregnancy unless the potential benefit justifies the potential risk to the mother and fetus. Nonteratogenic effects: In a peri- and post-natal development study in rats, significantly more pups died in the group dosed at 120 mg/kg/day (> 300 times the maximum recommended human dose) than in the control group during the three-week post-partum period.

Nursing Mothers:

It is not known whether terazosin is excreted in breast milk. Because many drugs are excreted in breast milk, caution should be exercised when terazosin is administered to a nursing woman.

Pediatric Use:

Safety and effectiveness in children have not been determined.

ADVERSE REACTIONS

The prevalence of adverse reactions has been ascertained from clinical studies conducted primarily in the United States. All adverse experiences (events) reported during these studies were recorded as adverse reactions. The prevalence rates presented below are based on combined data from fourteen placebo-controlled studies involving once-a-day administration of terazosin as monotherapy or in combination with other antihypertensive agents, at doses ranging from 1 to 40 mg. Table 1 summarizes those adverse experiences reported for patients in these studies where the prevalence rate in the terazosin group was at least 5%, where the prevalence rate for the terazosin group was at least 2% and was greater than the prevalence rate for the placebo group, or where the reaction is of particular interest. Asthenia, blurred vision, dizziness, nasal congestion, nausea, peripheral edema, palpitations and somnolence were the only symptoms that were significantly ($p < 0.05$) more common in patients receiving terazosin than in patients receiving placebo. Similar adverse reaction rates were observed in placebo-controlled monotherapy trials.

TABLE 1
ADVERSE REACTIONS DURING PLACEBO-CONTROLLED STUDIES

	Terazosin (N=859)	Placebo (N=506)
BODY AS A WHOLE		
†Asthenia	11.3%*	4.3%
Back Pain	2.4%	1.2%
Headache	16.2%	15.8%
CARDIOVASCULAR SYSTEM		
Palpitations	4.3%*	1.2%
Postural Hypotension	1.3%	0.4%
Tachycardia	1.9%	1.2%
DIGESTIVE SYSTEM		
Nausea	4.4%*	1.4%
METABOLIC/NUTRITIONAL DISORDERS		
Edema	0.9%	0.6%
Peripheral Edema	5.5%*	2.4%
Weight Gain	0.5%	0.2%
MUSCULOSKELETAL SYSTEM		
Pain-Extremities	3.5%	3.0%
NERVOUS SYSTEM		
Depression	0.3%	0.2%
Dizziness	19.3%*	7.5%
Libido Decreased	0.6%	0.2%
Nervousness	2.3%	1.8%
Paresthesia	2.9%	1.4%
Somnolence	5.4%*	2.6%
RESPIRATORY SYSTEM		
Dyspnea	3.1%	2.4%
Nasal Congestion	5.9%*	3.4%
Sinusitis	2.6%	1.4%
SPECIAL SENSES		
Blurred Vision	1.6%*	0.0%
UROGENITAL SYSTEM		
Impotence	1.2%	1.4%

† Includes weakness, tiredness, lassitude, and fatigue.
* Statistically significant at $p=0.05$ level.

The adverse reactions were usually mild or moderate in intensity but sometimes were serious enough to interrupt treatment. The adverse reactions that were most bothersome, as judged by their being reported as reasons for discontinuation of therapy by at least 0.5% of the terazosin group and being reported more often than in the placebo group are shown in Table 2.

TABLE 2
DISCONTINUATIONS DURING PLACEBO-CONTROLLED STUDIES

	Terazosin (N=859)	Placebo (N=506)
BODY AS A WHOLE		
Asthenia	1.6%	0.0%
Headache	1.3%	1.0%
CARDIOVASCULAR SYSTEM		
Palpitations	1.4%	0.2%
Postural Hypotension	0.5%	0.0%
Syncope	0.5%	0.2%
Tachycardia	0.6%	0.0%
DIGESTIVE SYSTEM		
Nausea	0.8%	0.0%
METABOLIC/NUTRITIONAL DISORDERS		
Peripheral Edema	0.6%	0.0%
NERVOUS SYSTEM		
Dizziness	3.1%	0.4%
Paresthesia	0.8%	0.2%
Somnolence	0.6%	0.2%
RESPIRATORY SYSTEM		
Dyspnea	0.9%	0.6%
Nasal Congestion	0.6%	0.0%
SPECIAL SENSES		
Blurred Vision	0.6%	0.0%

Additional adverse reactions have been reported, but these are, in general, not distinguishable from symptoms that might have occurred in the absence of exposure to terazosin. The following additional adverse reactions were reported by at least 1% of 1987 patients who received terazosin in controlled or open, short- or long-term clinical studies or have been reported during marketing experience: *Body as a Whole:* chest pain, facial edema, fever, abdominal pain, neck pain, shoulder pain; *Cardiovascular System:* arrhythmia, vasodilation; *Digestive System:* constipation, diarrhea, dry mouth, dyspepsia, flatulence, vomiting; *Metabolic/Nutritional Disorders:* gout; *Musculoskeletal System:* arthralgia, arthritis, joint disorder, myalgia; *Nervous System:* anxiety, insomnia; *Respiratory System:* bronchitis, cold symptoms, epistaxis, flu symptoms, increased cough, pharyngitis, rhinitis; *Skin and Appendages:* pruritus, rash, sweating; *Special Senses:* abnormal vision, conjunctivitis, tinnitus; *Urogenital System:* urinary frequency, urinary incontinence primarily reported in postmenopausal women, urinary tract infection.

OVERDOSAGE
Should overdosage of HYTRIN lead to hypotension, support of the cardiovascular system is of first importance. Restoration of blood pressure and normalization of heart rate may be accomplished by keeping the patient in the supine position. If this measure is inadequate, shock should first be treated with volume expanders. If necessary, vasopressors should then be used and renal function should be monitored and supported as needed. Laboratory data indicate that HYTRIN is highly protein bound; therefore, dialysis may not be of benefit.

DOSAGE AND ADMINISTRATION
The dose of HYTRIN and the dose interval (12 or 24 hours) should be adjusted according to the patient's individual blood pressure response. The following is a guide to its administration:

Initial Dose:
1 mg at bedtime is the starting dose for all patients, and this dose should not be exceeded. This initial dosing regimen should be strictly observed to minimize the potential for severe hypotensive effects.

Subsequent Doses:
The dose may be slowly increased to achieve the desired blood pressure response. The usual recommended dose range is 1 mg to 5 mg administered once a day; however, some patients may benefit from doses as high as 20 mg per day. Doses over 20 mg do not appear to provide further blood pressure effect and doses over 40 mg have not been studied. Blood pressure should be monitored at the end of the dosing interval to be sure control is maintained throughout the interval. It may also be helpful to measure blood pressure 2-3 hours after dosing to see if the maximum and minimum responses are similar, and to evaluate symptoms such as dizziness or palpitations which can result from excessive hypotensive response. If response is substantially diminished at 24 hours an increased dose or use of a twice daily regimen can be considered. **If terazosin administration is discontinued for several days or longer, therapy should be reinstituted using the initial dosing regimen.** In clinical trials, except for the initial dose, the dose was given in the morning.

Use With Other Drugs:
Caution should be observed when terazosin is administered concomitantly with other antihypertensive agents (e.g., calcium antagonists) to avoid the possibility of significant hypotension. When adding a diuretic or other antihypertensive agent, dosage reduction and retitration may be necessary.

HOW SUPPLIED
HYTRIN tablets (terazosin hydrochloride tablets) are available in four dosage strengths:

1 mg, white:
Bottles of 100 ....(NDC 0074-3322-13)
Abbo-Pac® unit dose strip packages of
100 tablets ....(NDC 0074-3322-11).
2 mg, orange:
Bottles of 100 ....(NDC 0074-3323-13)
Abbo-Pac® unit dose strip packages of
100 tablets ....(NDC 0074-3323-11).
5 mg, tan:
Bottles of 100 ....(NDC 0074-3324-13)
Abbo-Pac® unit dose strip packages of
100 tablets ....(NDC 0074-3324-11).
10 mg, green:
Bottles of 100 ....(NDC 0074-3325-13)
Abbo-Pac® unit dose strip packages of
100 tablets ....(NDC 0074-3325-11)

Recommended storage: Avoid exposure to temperatures in excess of 104° F (40° C).
Abbott Health Care Products, Inc.
North Chicago, IL 60064, U.S.A.
Ref. 03-4351-R4   Revised: March, 1989
Shown in Product Identification Section, page 403

IBERET®–500 Filmtab® tablets
[ī′be-ret]
IRON plus B-complex and Vitamin C
Well-tolerated once-daily hematinic with controlled-release iron.
IBERET® Filmtab® tablets
Hematinic Supplying Controlled-Release Iron, Vitamin C and Vitamin B-Complex

DESCRIPTION
Each Iberet-500 and Iberet Filmtab tablet contains 525 mg of ferrous sulfate (equivalent to 105 mg elemental iron) in the Gradumet® controlled-release vehicle. To enhance iron absorption, 500 mg of vitamin C has been added to each Iberet-500 Filmtab.
The Gradumet is an inert, porous, plastic matrix which is impregnated with ferrous sulfate. Iron is leached from the Gradumet as it passes through the gastrointestinal tract, and the expended matrix is excreted harmlessly in the stool. Controlled-release iron is particularly helpful in patients who have demonstrated intolerance to other oral iron preparations.
Each Iberet-500 Filmtab tablet contains:
Ferrous Sulfate.......................................525 mg
  (equivalent to 105 mg of elemental iron)
Vitamin C (as Sodium Ascorbate)..............500 mg
Niacinamide..30 mg
Calcium Pantothenate.............................10 mg
Vitamin B_1 (Thiamine Mononitrate)..........6 mg
Vitamin B_2 (Riboflavin)..........................6 mg
Vitamin B_6 (Pyridoxine Hydrochloride).......5 mg
Vitamin B_{12} (Cyanocobalamin)...............25 mcg
The formulation of Iberet differs from Iberet-500 only in that it contains a lesser amount of vitamin C, 150 mg per Filmtab tablet.

Inactive Ingredients:
Iberet Filmtab: Albumen, castor oil cellulosic polymers, corn starch, FD&C Red No. 40, FD&C Yellow No. 6, iron oxide, magnesium stearate, methyl acrylate-methyl methacrylate copolymer, polyethylene glycol, povidone, stearic acid, talc, titanium dioxide and vanillin.
Iberet-500 Filmtab: Cellulosic polymers, corn starch, FD&C Red No. 40, FD&C Yellow No. 6, iron oxide, magnesium stearate, methyl acrylate-methyl methacrylate copolymer, polyethylene glycol, povidone, propylene glycol, stearic acid, talc, titanium dioxide and vanillin.

INDICATIONS
Iberet-500: For the treatment of iron deficiency or iron deficiency anemia when there is a deficient intake or increased need for B-complex vitamins. Iberet: For conditions in which iron deficiency and vitamin C deficiency occur concomitantly with deficient intake or increased need for the B-complex vitamins.

PRECAUTIONS
Where anemia exists, its nature should be established and underlying cause determined.
Like other oral iron preparations, Iberet-500 and Iberet should be stored out of the reach of children to protect against accidental iron poisoning (see Overdosage).

ADVERSE REACTIONS
The likelihood of gastric intolerance to iron in the controlled-release Gradumet vehicle is slight. If it should occur, the tablet may be taken after a meal.

DOSAGE AND ADMINISTRATION
Iberet-500 and Iberet are administered orally and may be taken on an empty stomach. Usual Adult Dose, including pregnant females: One tablet daily, or as directed by the physician.

OVERDOSAGE
Signs of serious iron toxicity may be delayed because the iron is in a controlled-release dose form. Increased capillary permeability, reduced plasma volume, increased cardiac output, and sudden cardiovascular collapse may occur in acute iron intoxication. In overdosage, efforts should be made to hasten the elimination of the Gradumet tablets ingested. An emetic should be administered as soon as possible, followed by gastric lavage if indicated. Immediately following emesis, a saline cathartic should be administered to hasten passage through the intestinal tract. X-ray examination may then be considered to determine the position and number of Gradumet tablets remaining in the gastrointestinal tract.

HOW SUPPLIED
Iberet-500 is supplied as red, oval shaped tablets in bottles of 30 (NDC 0074-7235-30), 60 (NDC 0074-7235-01) and 500 (NDC 0074-7235-03), and in Abbo-Pac® unit dose packages

Continued on next page

Abbott—Cont.

of 100 (**NDC** 0074-7235-11); Iberet is supplied as red, round tablets in bottles of 60 (**NDC** 0074-6863-01).
Abbott Pharmaceuticals, Inc.
North Chicago, IL 60064
Ref. 03-1485-2/R29
Iberet-500 shown in Product Identification Section, page 403

IBERET–FOLIC–500®
Controlled-Release Iron with Vitamin C,
and B-Complex, including Folic Acid
Filmtab® Tablets

See combined listing under FERO-FOLIC-500.
Shown in Product Identification Section, page 403

IBERET®–500 LIQUID
[ī'bĕ-rĕt]
Hematinic Supplying Iron, Vitamin C
and Vitamin B-Complex
IBERET®–LIQUID
Hematinic Supplying Iron, Vitamin C
and Vitamin B-Complex

DESCRIPTION
Iberet-500 Liquid and Iberet-Liquid are hematinic preparations of ferrous sulfate, B-complex vitamins and ascorbic acid. Each teaspoonful (5 ml) of Iberet-500 Liquid provides:
Elemental Iron (as Ferrous Sulfate) ....26.25 mg
Vitamin C (Ascorbic Acid) ....125 mg
Niacinamide ....7.5 mg
Dexpanthenol ....2.5 mg
VitaminB_1 (Thiamine Hydrochloride) ....1.5 mg
Vitamin B_2 (Riboflavin) ....1.5 mg
Vitamin B_6 (Pyridoxine Hydrochloride) ....1.25 mg
Vitamin B_{12} (Cyanocobalamin) ....6.25 mcg
In a citrus-flavored vehicle.
Iberet-Liquid has a raspberry-mint flavored vehicle; Iberet-Liquid has a smaller amount of ascorbic acid: 37.5 mg per teaspoonful. Riboflavin 5' phosphate sodium is the source of riboflavin in Iberet Liquid.

INACTIVE INGREDIENTS
Iberet-Liquid: Alcohol 1%, methylparaben, propylparaben, sorbitol, water and natural and artificial flavors.
Iberet-500 Liquid: Glycerin, methylparaben, propylene glycol, propylparaben, sodium bicarbonate, sorbitol, sucrose, water and artificial flavor.

INDICATIONS
Iberet-500 Liquid: For conditions in which iron deficiency occurs concomitantly with deficient intake or increased need for the B-complex vitamins. Iberet-Liquid: For conditions in which iron deficiency and vitamin C deficiency occur concomitantly with deficient intake or increased need for the B-complex vitamins.

PRECAUTIONS
Where anemia exists, its nature should be established and underlying cause determined. Iberet-500 Liquid and Iberet-Liquid should be stored out of the reach of children because of the possibility of iron intoxication from accidental overdosage.

ADVERSE REACTIONS
If gastrointestinal symptoms appear as a sign of iron intolerance, smaller individual doses may be given at more frequent intervals to provide the desired daily amount. Administering Iberet-500 Liquid or Iberet-Liquid after meals may also reduce such effects.
Like other liquid iron preparations, Iberet-500 Liquid or Iberet-Liquid may stain the teeth on continued use. Stains may be prevented to a large extent by taking the dose through a straw, first mixing it with water or fruit juice, and by following the dose with a drink of plain water or juice. Brushing the teeth with sodium bicarbonate or hydrogen peroxide will usually remove existing stains.

DOSAGE AND ADMINISTRATION
Iberet-500 Liquid and Iberet-Liquid are administered orally, preferably after meals. Each has a fruit-flavored vehicle, and is suitable for pediatric patients who are unable to take tablets or capsules, and for patients who prefer or can better tolerate liquid medication. Iberet-500 Liquid and Iberet-Liquid may be administered by spoon or incorporated into infant formulas, water, or fruit juices. Iberet-500 Liquid: Usual dosage; Adults, including pregnant females and children 4 years of age and older—2 teaspoonfuls (10 ml) twice daily, after meals; Children 1–3 years of age—1 teaspoonful (5 ml) twice daily, after meals. Otherwise as directed by the physician. Iberet-Liquid: Usual dosage: Adults including pregnant females and children 4 years of age and older—2 teaspoonfuls (10 ml) three times daily, after meals; Children

1–3 years of age—1 teaspoonful (5 ml) three times daily, after meals. Otherwise as directed by the physician.

HOW SUPPLIED
Iberet-500 Liquid (**NDC** 0074-8422-02) and Iberet-Liquid (**NDC** 0074-7173-01) are supplied in 8 fl oz bottles.
Abbott Laboratories
North Chicago, IL 60064
Ref. 07-5452-4/R16 & 07-5781-4/R20

JANIMINE® Filmtab® Tablets   ℞
[ja-ni-mīne]
(imipramine hydrochloride tablets, USP)

HOW SUPPLIED
JANIMINE is provided as monogrammed tablets in three dosage strengths containing imipramine hydrochloride:
  10 mg, round-shaped, orange-colored, in bottles of 100 (**NDC** 0074-1897-13) and bottles of 1000 (**NDC** 0074-1897-19).
  25 mg, round-shaped, yellow, in bottles of 100 (**NDC** 0074-1898-13) and bottles of 1000 (**NDC** 0074-1898-19).
  50 mg, ovaloid-shaped, peach-colored, in bottles of 100 (**NDC** 0074-1899-13) and bottles of 1000 (**NDC** 0074-1899-19).
Inactive Ingredients: 10 mg tablet: Castor oil, cellulosic polymers, corn starch, FD&C Yellow No. 5 (tartrazine), FD&C Yellow No. 6, microcrystalline cellulose, propylene glycol, stearic acid, talc, titanium dioxide and vanillin.
25 mg tablet: Castor oil, cellulosic polymers, corn starch, FD&C Yellow No. 5 (tartrazine), microcrystalline cellulose, propylene glycol, stearic acid, talc, titanium dioxide and vanillin.
50 mg tablet: Castor oil, cellulosic polymers, corn starch, FD&C Yellow No. 6, microcrystalline cellulose, stearic acid, talc, titanium dioxide and vanillin.
Abbott Laboratories
North Chicago, IL 60064
Ref. 01-4479-R8 Revised: July, 1988
Shown in Product Identification Section, page 403

K-LOR™ Powder   ℞
[k'lor]
(potassium chloride for oral solution, USP)

DESCRIPTION
Natural fruit-flavored K-LOR (potassium chloride for oral solution, USP) is an oral potassium supplement offered in individual packets as a powder for reconstitution. Each packet of K-LOR 20 mEq powder contains potassium 20 mEq and chloride 20 mEq provided by potassium chloride 1.5 g. Each packet of K-LOR 15 mEq powder contains potassium 15 mEq and chloride 15 mEq provided by potassium chloride 1.125 g.
K-LOR powder is an electrolyte replenisher. The chemical name is potassium chloride, and the structural formula is KCl. Potassium chloride, USP, occurs as a white, granular powder or as colorless crystals. It is odorless and has a saline taste. Its solutions are neutral to litmus. It is freely soluble in water and insoluble in alcohol.
Inactive Ingredients: FD&C Yellow No. 6, maltodextrin (contains corn derivative), malic acid, saccharin, silica gel and natural flavoring.

CLINICAL PHARMACOLOGY
Potassium ion is the principal intracellular cation of most body tissues. Potassium ions participate in a number of essential physiological processes including the maintenance of intracellular tonicity, the transmission of nerve impulses, the contraction of cardiac, skeletal and smooth muscle, and the maintenance of normal renal function.
The intracellular concentration of potassium is approximately 150 to 160 mEq per liter. The normal adult plasma concentration is 3.5 to 5 mEq per liter. An active ion transport system maintains this gradient across the plasma membrane.
Potassium is a normal dietary constituent and under steady state conditions the amount of potassium absorbed from the gastrointestinal tract is equal to the amount excreted in the urine. The usual dietary intake of potassium is 50 to 100 mEq per day.
Potassium depletion will occur whenever the rate of potassium loss through renal excretion and/or loss from the gastrointestinal tract exceeds the rate of potassium intake. Such depletion usually develops as a consequence of therapy with diuretics, primary or secondary hyperaldosteronism, diabetic ketoacidosis, or inadequate replacement of potassium in patients on prolonged parenteral nutrition. Depletion can develop rapidly with severe diarrhea, especially if associated with vomiting. Potassium depletion due to these causes is usually accompanied by a concomitant loss of chloride and is manifested by hypokalemia and metabolic alkalosis. Potassium depletion may produce weakness, fatigue, disturbances of cardiac rhythm (primarily ectopic beats),

prominent U-waves in the electrocardiogram, and, in advanced cases, flaccid paralysis and/or impaired ability to concentrate urine.
If potassium depletion associated with metabolic alkalosis cannot be managed by correcting the fundamental cause of the deficiency, e.g., where the patient requires long term diuretic therapy, supplemental potassium in the form of high potassium food or potassium chloride may restore normal potassium levels.
In rare circumstances, (e.g., patients with renal tubular acidosis) potassium depletion may be associated with metabolic acidosis and hyperchloremia. In such patients potassium replacement should be accomplished with potassium salts other than the chloride, such as potassium bicarbonate, potassium citrate, potassium acetate, or potassium gluconate.

INDICATIONS AND USAGE
1. For the treatment of patients with hypokalemia with or without metabolic alkalosis, in digitalis intoxication, and in patients with hypokalemic familial periodic paralysis. If hypokalemia is the result of diuretic therapy, consideration should be given to the use of a lower dose of diuretic, which may be sufficient without leading to hypokalemia.
2. For the prevention of hypokalemia in patients who would be at particular risk if hypokalemia were to develop, e.g., digitalized patients or patients with significant cardiac arrhythmias.
The use of potassium salts in patients receiving diuretics for uncomplicated essential hypertension is often unnecessary when such patients have a normal dietary pattern, and when low doses of the diuretic are used. Serum potassium should be checked periodically, however, and, if hypokalemia occurs, dietary supplementation with potassium-containing foods may be adequate to control milder cases. In more severe cases, and if dose adjustment of the diuretic is ineffective or unwarranted, supplementation with potassium salts may be indicated.

CONTRAINDICATIONS
Potassium supplements are contraindicated in patients with hyperkalemia since a further increase in serum potassium concentration in such patients can produce cardiac arrest. Hyperkalemia may complicate any of the following conditions: chronic renal failure, systemic acidosis such as diabetic acidosis, acute dehydration, extensive tissue breakdown as in severe burns, adrenal insufficiency, or the administration of a potassium-sparing diuretic, e.g., spironolactone, triamterene, or amiloride, (see OVERDOSAGE).
K-LOR (potassium chloride for oral solution) is contraindicated in patients with known hypersensitivity to any ingredient in this product.

WARNINGS
Hyperkalemia: (See OVERDOSAGE): In patients with impaired mechanisms for excreting potassium, the administration of potassium salts can produce hyperkalemia and cardiac arrest. This occurs most commonly in patients given potassium intravenously, but may also occur in patients given potassium orally. Potentially fatal hyperkalemia can develop rapidly and can be asymptomatic. The use of potassium salts in patients with chronic renal disease, or any other condition which impairs potassium excretion, requires particularly careful monitoring of the serum potassium concentration and appropriate dosage adjustment.
Interaction with Potassium-Sparing Diuretics: Hypokalemia should not be treated by the concomitant administration of potassium salts and a potassium-sparing diuretic, e.g., spironolactone, triamterene or amiloride, since the simultaneous administration of these agents can produce severe hyperkalemia.
Interaction with Angiotensin Converting Enzyme Inhibitors: Angiotensin converting enzyme (ACE) inhibitors (e.g., captopril, enalapril) will produce some potassium retention by inhibiting aldosterone production. Potassium supplements should be given to patients receiving ACE inhibitors only with close monitoring.
Metabolic Acidosis: Hypokalemia in patients with metabolic acidosis should be treated with an alkalinizing potassium salt such as potassium bicarbonate, potassium citrate, potassium acetate or potassium gluconate.

PRECAUTIONS
General: The diagnosis of potassium depletion is ordinarily made by demonstrating hypokalemia in a patient with a clinical history suggesting some cause for potassium depletion. In interpreting the serum potassium level, the physician should bear in mind that acute alkalosis *per se* can produce hypokalemia in the absence of a deficit in total body potassium, while acute acidosis *per se* can increase the serum potassium concentration to within the normal range even in the presence of a reduced total body potassium. The treatment of potassium depletion, particularly in the presence of cardiac disease, renal disease, or acidosis, requires careful attention to acid-base balance and appropriate monitoring of serum electrolytes, the electrocardiogram, and the clinical status of the patient.
Information for Patients: Physicians should consider reminding the patient of the following:

To dilute each packet of powder in ½ glassful of water or other liquid and take each dose after a meal.

To take this medicine following the frequency and amount prescribed by the physician. This is especially important if the patient is also taking diuretics and/or digitalis preparations.

Laboratory Tests: When blood is drawn for analysis of plasma potassium it is important to recognize that artifactual elevations can occur after improper venipuncture technique or as a result of *in vitro* hemolysis of the sample.

Drug Interactions: Potassium-sparing diuretics, angiotensin converting enzyme inhibitors (see WARNINGS).

Carcinogenesis, Mutagenesis, Impairment of Fertility: Carcinogenicity, mutagenicity and fertility studies in animals have not been performed. Potassium is a normal dietary constituent.

Pregnancy Category C: Animal reproduction studies have not been conducted with K-LOR powder. It is unlikely that potassium supplementation that does not lead to hyperkalemia would have an adverse effect on the fetus or would affect reproductive capacity.

Nursing Mothers: The normal potassium ion content of human milk is about 13 mEq per liter. Since oral potassium becomes part of the body potassium pool, as long as body potassium is not excessive, the contribution of potassium chloride supplementation should have little or no effect on the level in human milk.

Pediatric Use: Safety and effectiveness in children have not been established.

ADVERSE REACTIONS

One of the most severe adverse effects is hyperkalemia (see CONTRAINDICATIONS, WARNINGS and OVERDOSAGE).

The most common adverse reactions to oral potassium salts are nausea, vomiting, flatulence, abdominal pain/discomfort, and diarrhea. These symptoms are due to irritation of the gastrointestinal tract and are best managed by diluting the preparation further, taking the dose with meals, or reducing the amount taken at one time.

Skin rash has been reported rarely.

OVERDOSAGE

The administration of oral potassium salts to persons with normal excretory mechanisms for potassium rarely causes serious hyperkalemia. However, if excretory mechanisms are impaired or if intravenous administration is too rapid, potentially fatal hyperkalemia can result (see CONTRAINDICATIONS and WARNINGS). It is important to recognize that hyperkalemia is usually asymptomatic and may be manifested only by an increased serum potassium concentration (6.5–8 mEq/L) and characteristic electrocardiographic changes (peaking of T-waves, loss of P-waves, depression of S-T segments, and prolongation of the QT intervals). Late manifestations include muscle paralysis and cardiovascular collapse from cardiac arrest (9–12 mEq/L).

Treatment measures for hyperkalemia include the following:

1. Elimination of foods and medications containing potassium and of any agents with potassium-sparing properties;
2. Intravenous administration of 300 to 500 ml/hr of 10% dextrose solution containing 10–20 units of crystalline insulin per 1,000 ml;
3. Correction of acidosis, if present, with intravenous sodium bicarbonate;
4. Use of exchange resins, hemodialysis, or peritoneal dialysis.

In treating hyperkalemia, it should be recalled that in patients who have been stabilized on digitalis, lowering the serum potassium concentration too rapidly can produce digitalis toxicity.

DOSAGE AND ADMINISTRATION

The usual dietary potassium intake by the average adult is 50 to 100 mEq per day. Potassium depletion sufficient to cause hypokalemia usually requires the loss of 200 or more mEq of potassium from the total body store.

Dosage must be adjusted to the individual needs of each patient. The dose for the prevention of hypokalemia is typically in the range of 20 mEq per day. Doses of 40–100 mEq per day or more are used for the treatment of potassium depletion. Dosage should be divided if more than 20 mEq per day is given such that no more than 20 mEq is given in a single dose. The dose should be taken after a meal.

K-LOR 20 mEq powder provides 20 mEq and K-LOR 15 mEq powder provides 15 mEq of potassium chloride.

Each 20 mEq (one K-LOR mEq packet) of potassium should be dissolved in at least 4 oz (approximately ½ glassful) cold water or juice. Each 15 mEq (One K-LOR 15 mEq packet) of potassium should be dissolved in at least 3 oz (approximately ½ glassful) cold water or juice. These preparations, like other potassium supplements, must be properly diluted to avoid the possibility of gastrointestinal irritation.

HOW SUPPLIED

K-LOR 20 mEq (potassium chloride for oral solution, USP) is supplied in cartons of 30 packets (NDC 0074-3611-01), and

cartons of 100 packets (**NDC** 0074-3611-02). Each packet contains potassium, 20 mEq, and chloride, 20 mEq, provided by potassium chloride, 1.5 g.

K-LOR 15 mEq (potassium chloride for oral solution, USP) is supplied in cartons of 100 packets (**NDC** 0074-3633-11). Each packet contains potassium, 15 mEq, and chloride, 15 mEq, provided by potassium chloride, 1.125 g.

Recommended storage: Avoid excessive heat (104°F).

Caution: Federal law prohibits dispensing without prescription.

Abbott Laboratories
North Chicago, IL 60064
TM—Trademark
Ref. 09-6334-5/R22 Revised: November, 1988
Shown in Product Identification Section, page 403

K•Tab®   ℞
[k 'tăb]
(Potassium Chloride Extended-Release Tablets, USP)

DESCRIPTION

K-TAB (potassium chloride extended-release tablets) is a solid oral dosage form of potassium chloride containing 750 mg of potassium chloride, USP, equivalent to 10 mEq of potassium in a film-coated (not enteric-coated), wax matrix tablet. This formulation is intended to slow the release of potassium so that the likelihood of a high localized concentration of potassium chloride within the gastrointestinal tract is reduced. The expended inert, porous, wax/polymer matrix is not absorbed and may be excreted intact in the stool.

K-TAB tablets are an electrolyte replenisher. The chemical name is potassium chloride, and the structural formula is KCl. Potassium chloride, USP, occurs as a white, granular powder or as colorless crystals. It is odorless and has a saline taste. Its solutions are neutral to litmus. It is freely soluble in water and insoluble in alcohol.

Inactive Ingredients
Castor oil, cellulosic polymers, colloidal silicon dioxide, D&C Yellow No. 10, magnesium stearate, paraffin, polyvinyl acetate, titanium dioxide, vanillin and vitamin E.

CLINICAL PHARMACOLOGY

Potassium ion is the principal intracellular cation of most body tissues. Potassium ions participate in a number of essential physiological processes including the maintenance of intracellular tonicity, the transmission of nerve impulses, the contraction of cardiac, skeletal, and smooth muscle, and the maintenance of normal renal function.

The intracellular concentration of potassium is approximately 150 to 160 mEq per liter. The normal adult plasma concentration is 3.5 to 5 mEq per liter. An active ion transport system maintains this gradient across the plasma membrane.

Potassium is a normal dietary constituent and under steady state conditions the amount of potassium absorbed from the gastrointestinal tract is equal to the amount excreted in the urine. The usual dietary intake of potassium is 50 to 100 mEq per day.

Potassium depletion will occur whenever the rate of potassium loss through renal excretion and/or loss from the gastrointestinal tract exceeds the rate of potassium intake. Such depletion usually develops as a consequence of therapy with diuretics, primary or secondary hyperaldosteronism, diabetic ketoacidosis, or inadequate replacement of potassium in patients on prolonged parenteral nutrition. Depletion can develop rapidly with severe dairrhea, expecially if associated with vomiting. Potassium depletion due to these causes is usually accompanied by a concomitant loss of chloride and is manifested by hypokalemia and metabolic alkalosis. Potassium depletion may produce weakness, fatigue, disturbances of cardiac rhythm (primarily ectopic beats), prominent U-waves in the electrocardiogram, and in advanced cases, flaccid paralysis and/or impaired ability to concentrate urine.

If potassium depletion associated with metabolic alkalosis cannot be managed by correcting the fundamental causes of the deficiency, e.g., where the patient requires long term diuretic therapy, supplemental potassium in the form of high potassium food or potassium chloride may restore normal levels.

In rare circumstances, (e.g., patients with renal tubular acidosis) potassium depletion may be associated with metabolic acidosis and hyperchloremia. In such patients potassium replacement should be accomplished with potassium salts other than the chloride, such as potassium bicarbonate, potassium citrate, potassium acetate, or potassium gluconate.

INDICATIONS AND USAGE

BECAUSE OF REPORTS OF INTESTINAL AND GASTRIC ULCERATION AND BLEEDING WITH CONTROLLED-RELEASE POTASSIUM CHLORIDE PREPARATIONS, THESE DRUGS SHOULD BE RESERVED FOR THOSE PATIENTS WHO CANNOT TOLERATE OR REFUSE TO TAKE LIQUID OR EFFERVESCENT POTASSIUM PREPARATIONS, OR

FOR PATIENTS WITH WHOM THERE IS A PROBLEM OF COMPLIANCE WITH THESE PREPARATIONS.

1. For the treatment of patients with hypokalemia with or without metabolic alkalosis, in digitalis intoxication, and in patients with hypokalemic familial periodic paralysis. If hypokalemia is the result of diuretic therapy, consideration should be given to the use of a lower dose of diuretic, which may be sufficient without leading to hypokalemia.
2. For the prevention of hypokalemia in patients who would be at particular risk if hypokalemia were to develop, e.g., digitalized patients or patients with significant cardiac arrhythmias.

The use of potassium salts in patients receiving diuretics for uncomplicated essential hypertension is often unnecessary when such patients have a normal dietary pattern, and when low doses of the diuretic are used. Serum potassium should be checked periodically, however, and, if hypokalemia occurs, dietary supplementation with potassium-containing foods may be adequate to control milder cases. In more severe cases, and if dose adjustment of the diuretic is ineffective or unwarranted, supplementation with potassium salts may be indicated.

CONTRAINDICATIONS

Potassium supplements are contraindicated in patients with hyperkalemia since a further increase in serum potassium concentration in such patients can produce cardiac arrest. Hyperkalemia may complicate any of the following conditions: chronic renal failure, systemic acidosis such as diabetic acidosis, acute dehydration, extensive tissue breakdown as in severe burns, adrenal insufficiency, or the administration of potassium-sparing diuretic, e.g., spironolactone, triamterene, or amiloride, (see OVERDOSAGE).

K-TAB tablets are contraindicated in patients with known hypersensitivity to any ingredient in this product.

Controlled-release formulations of potassium chloride have produced esophageal ulceration in certain cardiac patients with esophageal compression due to an enlarged left atrium. Potassium supplementation, when indicated in such patients, should be given as a liquid preparation.

All solid dosage forms of potassium supplements are contraindicated in any patient in whom there is structural, pathological, e.g., diabetic gastroparesis, or pharmacologic (use of anticholinergic agents or other agents with anticholinergic properties at sufficient doses to exert anticholinergic effects) cause for arrest or delay in tablet passage through the gastrointestinal tract.

WARNINGS

Hyperkalemia (see OVERDOSAGE)

In patients with impaired mechanisms for excreting potassium, the administration of potassium salts can produce hyperkalemia and cardiac arrest. This occurs most commonly in patients given potassium intravenously, but may also occur in patients given potassium orally. Potentially fatal hyperkalemia can develop rapidly and can be asymptomatic. The use of potassium salts in patients with chronic renal disease, or any other condition which impairs potassium excretion, requires particularly careful monitoring of the serum potassium concentration and appropriate dosage adjustment.

Interaction with Potassium-Sparing Diuretics

Hypokalemia should not be treated by the concomitant administration of potassium salts and a potassium-sparing diuretic e.g., spironolactone, triamterene, or amiloride, since the simultaneous administration of these agents can produce severe hyperkalemia.

Interaction with Angiotensin Converting Enzyme Inhibitors

Angiotensin converting enzyme (ACE) inhibitors (e.g., captopril, enalapril) will produce some potassium retention by inhibiting aldosterone production. Potassium supplements should be given to patients receiving ACE inhibitors only with close monitoring.

Gastrointestinal Lesions

Solid oral dosage forms of potassium chloride can produce ulcerative and/or stenotic lesions of the gastrointestinal tract. Based on spontaneous adverse reaction reports, enteric-coated preparations of potassium chloride are associated with an increased frequency of small bowel lesions (40-50 per 100,000 patient years) compared to sustained-release wax matrix formulations (less than one per 100,000 patient years). Because of the lack of extensive marketing experience with microencapsulated products, a comparison between such products and wax matrix or enteric-coated products is not available. K-TAB tablets consist of a wax matrix formulated to provide a controlled rate of release of potassium chloride and thus to minimize the possibility of a high local concentration of potassium near the gastrointestinal wall.

Continued on next page

Abbott—Cont.

Prospective trials have been conducted in normal human volunteers in which the upper gastrointestinal tract was evaluated by endoscopic inspection before and after one week of solid oral potassium chloride therapy. The ability of this model to predict events occuring in usual clinical practice is unknown. Trials which approximated usual clinical practice did not reveal any clear differences between the wax matrix and microencapsulated dosage forms. In contrast, there was a higher incidence of gastric and duodenal lesions in subjects receiving a high dose of a wax matrix controlled-release formulation under conditions which did not resemble usual or recommended clinical practice, i.e., 96 mEq per day in divided doses of potassium chloride administered to fasted patients in the presence of an anticholinergic drug to delay gastric emptying. The upper gastrointestinal lesions observed by endoscopy were asymptomatic and were not accompanied by evidence of bleeding (hemoccult testing). The relevance of these findings to the usual conditions, i.e., non-fasting, no anticholinergic agent, and smaller doses, under which controlled-release potassium chloride products are used is uncertain. Epidemiologic studies have not identified an elevated risk, compared to microencapsulated products, for upper gastrointestinal lesions in patients receiving wax matrix formulations. K-TAB tablets should be discontinued immediately and the possibility of ulceration, obstruction or perforation considered if severe vomiting, abdominal pain, distention, or gastrointestinal bleeding occurs.

Metabolic Acidosis
Hypokalemia in patients with metabolic acidosis should be treated with an alkalinizing potassium salt such as potassium bicarbonate, potassium citrate, potassium acetate, or potassium gluconate.

PRECAUTIONS

General: The diagnosis of potassium depletion is ordinarily made by demonstrating hypokalemia in a patient with a clinical history suggesting some cause for potassium depletion. In interpreting the serum potassium level, the physician should bear in mind that acute alkalosis *per se* can produce hypokalemia in the absence of a deficit in total body potassium, while acute acidosis *per se* can increase the serum potassium concentration to within the normal range even in the presence of a reduced total body potassium. The treatment of potassium depletion, particularly in the presence of cardiac disease, renal disease, or acidosis, requires careful attention to acid-base balance and appropriate monitoring of serum electrolytes, the electrocardiogram, and the clinical status of the patient.

Information for Patients: Physicians should consider reminding the patient of the following:
To take each dose with meals and with a full glass of water or other liquid.
To take this medicine following the frequency and amount prescribed by the physician. This is especially important if the patient is also taking diuretics and/or digitalis preparations.
To check with the physician if there is trouble swallowing tablets or if the tablets seem to stick in the throat.
To check with the physician at once if tarry stools or other evidence of gastrointestinal bleeding is noticed.
To take each dose without crushing, chewing or sucking the tablets.

Laboratory Tests: When blood is drawn for analysis of plasma potassium it is important to recognize that artifactual elevations can occur after improper venipuncture technique or as a result of *in vitro* hemolysis of the sample.

Drug Interactions: Potassium-sparing diuretics, angiotensin converting enzyme inhibitors (see WARNINGS).

Carcinogenesis, Mutagenesis, Impairment of Fertility: Carcinogenicity, mutagenicity and fertility studies in animals have not been performed. Potassium is a normal dietary constituent.

Pregnancy Category C: Animal reproduction studies have not been conducted with K-TAB tablets. It is unlikely that potassium supplementation that does not lead to hyperkalemia would have an adverse effect on the fetus or would affect reproductive capacity.

Nursing Mothers: The normal potassium ion content of human milk is about 13 mEq per liter. Since oral potassium becomes part of the body potassium pool, as long as body potassium is not excessive, the contribution of potassium chloride supplementation should have little or no effect on the level in human milk.

Pediatric Use: Safety and effectiveness in children have not been established.

ADVERSE REACTIONS

One of the most severe adverse effects is hyperkalemia (see CONTRAINDICATIONS, WARNINGS, and OVERDOSAGE). There also have been reports of upper and lower gastrointestinal conditions including obstruction, bleeding, ulceration, and perforation (see CONTRAINDICATIONS and WARNINGS).

The most common adverse reactions to oral potassium salts are nausea, vomiting, flatulence, abdominal pain/discomfort, and diarrhea. These symptoms are due to irritation of the gastrointestinal tract and are best managed by taking the dose with meals, or reducing the amount taken at one time.
Skin rash has been reported rarely.

OVERDOSAGE

The administration of oral potassium salts to persons with normal excretory mechanisms for potassium rarely causes serious hyperkalemia. However, if excretory mechanisms are impaired or if intravenous administration is too rapid, potentially fatal hyperkalemia can result (see CONTRAINDICATIONS and WARNINGS). It is important to recognize that hyperkalemia is usually asymptomatic and may be manifested only by an increased serum potassium concentration (6.5-8.0 mEq/L) and characteristic electrocardiographic changes (peaking of T-waves, loss of P-waves, depression of S-T segments, and prolongation of QT intervals). Late manifestations include muscle paralysis and cardiovascular collapse from cardiac arrest. (9-12 mEq/L).
Treatment measures for hyperkalemia include the following:
1. Elimination of foods and medications containing potassium and of any agents with potassium-sparing properties;
2. Intravenous administration of 300 to 500 mL/hr of 10% dextrose solution containing 10-20 units of crystalline insulin per 1,000 mL;
3. Correction of acidosis, if present, with intravenous sodium bicarbonate;
4. Use of exchange resins, hemodialysis, or peritoneal dialysis.
In treating hyperkalemia, it should be recalled that in patients who have been stabilized on digitalis, lowering the serum potassium concentration too rapidly can produce digitalis toxicity.

DOSAGE AND ADMINISTRATION

The usual dietary potassium intake by the average adult is 50 to 100 mEq per day. Potassium depletion sufficient to cause hypokalemia usually requires the loss of 200 or more mEq of potassium from the total body store.
Dosage must be adjusted to the individual needs of each patient. The dose for the prevention of hypokalemia is typically in the range of 20 mEq per day. Doses of 40-100 mEq per day or more are used for the treatment of potassium depletion. Dosage should be divided if more than 20 mEq per day is given such that no more than 20 mEq is given in a single dose.
K-TAB tablets provide 10 mEq of potassium chloride.
K-TAB tablets should be taken with meals and with a glass of water or other liquid. This product should not be taken on an empty stomach because of its potential for gastric irritation (see WARNINGS).
NOTE: K-TAB tablets are to be swallowed whole without crushing, chewing or sucking the tablets.

HOW SUPPLIED

K-TAB (potassium chloride extended-release tablets, USP) contains 750 mg of potassium chloride (equivalent to 10 mEq). K-TAB tablets are provided as yellow, ovaloid, extended-release Filmtab® tablets in bottles of 100 (NDC 0074-7804-13), 1000 (NDC 0074-7804-19) and 5000 (NDC 0074-7804-59) and in ABBO-PAC® unit dose packages of 100 (NDC 0074-7804-11).

Filmtab—Film-sealed tablets, Abbott
Abbott Pharmaceuticals, Inc.
North Chicago, IL 60064
Ref. 03-4346-R12 Revised: March, 1989
Shown in Product Identification Section, page 403

LIDOCAINE HYDROCHLORIDE INJECTION, USP   ℞
[līe′dō-cāne]
AQUEOUS SOLUTIONS FOR ACUTE MANAGEMENT OF CARDIAC ARRHYTHMIAS OR FOR LOCAL ANESTHESIA.

Abboject® Unit of Use Syringe
Ampul
Fliptop Vial
Multiple-dose Fliptop Vial
Pintop Vial
Pressurized Pintop Vial
Universal Additive Syringe

DESCRIPTION

Lidocaine Hydrochloride Injection, USP is a sterile, non-pyrogenic solution of lidocaine hydrochloride in water for injection for parenteral administration in various concentrations with characteristics as follows:

Lidocaine HCl (anhydrous)							
Conc.	0.5%	1%	1.5%	2%	4%	10%*	20%*
mg/mL (anhyd.)	5	10	15	20	40	100	200
pH (approx.)	6.5	6.5	6.5	6.5	6.5	5.7	5.7

*10% and 20% concentrations FOR DILUTION ONLY. **Must not be administered without proper dilution prior to injection.**

Multiple-dose vials contain 0.1% of methylparaben added as preservative. Single-dose vials contain no preservative and unused portions must be discarded after use. May contain sodium hydroxide and hydrochloric acid for pH adjustment. May contain sodium chloride to adjust tonicity.
Lidocaine has cardiac antiarrhythmic properties and is a local anesthetic of the amide type.
Lidocaine Hydrochloride, USP is chemically designated 2-(diethylamino)-2′,6′-acetoxylidide monohydrochloride monohydrate, a white powder freely soluble in water. It has the following structural formula:

$$\text{CH}_3$$
$$-\text{NHCOCH}_2\text{N(C}_2\text{H}_5)_2 \cdot \text{HCl} \cdot \text{H}_2\text{O}$$
$$\text{CH}_3$$

```
FOR CARDIAC
ARRHYTHMIAS
```

CLINICAL PHARMACOLOGY

Mechanism of Action and Electrophysiology:
Studies of the effects of therapeutic concentrations of lidocaine on the electrophysiological properties of mammalian Purkinje fibers have shown that lidocaine attenuates phase 4 diastolic depolarization, decreases automaticity and causes a decrease or no change in excitability and membrane responsiveness. Action potential duration and effective refractory period of Purkinje fibers are decreased while the ratio of effective refractory period to action potential duration is increased. Action potential duration and effective refractory period of ventricular muscle are also decreased. Effective refractory period of the AV node may increase, decrease or remain unchanged and atrial effective refractory period is unchanged. Lidocaine raises the ventricular fibrillation threshold. No significant interactions between lidocaine and the autonomic nervous system have been described and consequently lidocaine has little or no effect on autonomic tone. Clinical electrophysiological studies with lidocaine have demonstrated no change in sinus node recovery time or sino-atrial conduction time, AV nodal conduction time is unchanged or shortened and His-Purkinje conduction time is unchanged.

Hemodynamics:
At therapeutic doses, lidocaine has minimal hemodynamic effects in normal subjects and in patients with heart disease. Lidocaine has been shown to cause no, or minimal decrease in ventricular contractility, cardiac output, arterial pressure or heart rate.

Pharmacokinetics and Metabolism:
Lidocaine is rapidly metabolized by the liver and less than 10% of a dose is excreted unchanged in the urine. Oxidative N-dealkylation, a major pathway of metabolism, results in the metabolites monoethylglycinexylidide and glycinexylidide. The pharmacological/toxicological activities of these metabolites are similar to but less potent than lidocaine. The primary metabolite in urine is a conjugate of 4-hydroxy-2,6-dimethylaniline.
The elimination half-life of lidocaine following an intravenous bolus injection is typically 1.5 to 2.0 hours. There are data that indicate that the half-life may be 3 hours or longer following infusions of greater than 24 hours.
Because of the rapid rate at which lidocaine is metabolized, any condition that alters liver function, including changes in liver blood flow which could result from severe congestive heart failure or shock may alter lidocaine kinetics. The half-life may be two-fold or more greater in patients with liver dysfunction. Renal dysfunction does not affect lidocaine kinetics, but may increase the accumulation of metabolites.
Therapeutic effects of lidocaine are generally associated with plasma levels of 6 to 25 μmole/L (1.5 to 6 μg free base per mL). The blood to plasma distribution ratio is approximately 0.84. Objective adverse manifestations become increasingly apparent with increasing plasma levels above 6.0 μg free base per mL.
The plasma protein binding of lidocaine is dependent on drug concentration and the fraction bound decreases with increasing concentration. At concentrations of 1 to 4 μg free base per mL, 60 to 80 percent of lidocaine is protein bound. In addition to lidocaine concentration, the binding is dependent on the plasma concentration of the α-1-acid glycoprotein.

Lidocaine readily crosses the placental and blood-brain barriers. Dialysis has negligible effects on the kinetics of lidocaine.

INDICATIONS AND USAGE

Lidocaine hydrochloride administered intravenously, is specifically indicated in the acute management of ventricular arrhythmias such as those occurring in relation to acute myocardial infarction, or during cardiac manipulation, such as cardiac surgery.

CONTRAINDICATIONS

Lidocaine hydrochloride is contraindicated in patients with a known history of hypersensitivity to local anesthetics of the amide type. Lidocaine hydrochloride should not be used in patients with Stokes-Adams syndrome, Wolff-Parkinson-White syndrome or with severe degrees of sinoatrial, atrioventricular or intraventricular block in the absence of an artificial pacemaker.

WARNINGS

IN ORDER TO MANAGE POSSIBLE ADVERSE REACTIONS, RESUSCITATIVE EQUIPMENT, OXYGEN AND OTHER RESUSCITATIVE DRUGS SHOULD BE IMMEDIATELY AVAILABLE WHEN LIDOCAINE HYDROCHLORIDE INJECTION IS USED.

THE 10% AND 20% CONCENTRATED SOLUTIONS MUST BE INJECTED UNDILUTED. See DOSAGE AND ADMINISTRATION.

Systemic toxicity may result in manifestations of central nervous system depression (sedation) or irritability (twitching), which may progress to frank convulsions accompanied by respiratory depression and/or arrest. Early recognition of premonitory signs, assurance of adequate oxygenation and, where necessary, establishment of artificial airway with ventilatory support are essential to management of this problem. Should convulsions persist despite ventilatory therapy with oxygen, *small* increments of anticonvulsant drugs may be used intravenously. Examples of such agents include benzodiazepines (e.g., diazepam), ultrashort-acting barbiturates (e.g., thiopental or thiamylal) or a short-acting barbiturate (e.g., pentobarbital or secobarbital). If the patient is under anesthesia, a short-acting muscle relaxant (e.g., succinylcholine) may be used. Longer acting drugs should be used only when recurrent convulsions are evidenced.

Should circulatory depression occur, vasopressors may be used.

Constant electrocardiographic monitoring is essential to the proper administration of lidocaine hydrochloride. Signs of excessive depression of cardiac electrical activity such as sinus node dysfunction, prolongation of the P-R interval and QRS complex or the appearance or aggravation of arrhythmias, should be followed by flow adjustment and, if necessary, prompt cessation of the intravenous infusion of this agent. Occasionally, acceleration of ventricular rate may occur when lidocaine hydrochloride is administered to patients with atrial flutter or fibrillation.

PRECAUTIONS

1. **General:** Caution should be employed in the use of lidocaine hydrochloride in patients with severe liver or kidney disease because accumulation of the drug or metabolites may occur. Lidocaine Hydrochloride Injection, USP should be used with caution in the treatment of patients with hypovolemia, severe congestive heart failure, shock and all forms of heart block. In patients with sinus bradycardia or incomplete heart block, the administration of lidocaine hydrochloride intravenously for the elimination of ventricular ectopic beats without prior acceleration in heart rate (e.g., by atropine, isoproterenol or electric pacing) may promote more frequent and serious ventricular arrhythmias or complete heart block. (See CONTRAINDICATIONS).

Dosage should be reduced for children and for debilitated and/or elderly patients, commensurate with their age and physical status.

The safety of amide local anesthetic agents in patients with genetic predisposition of malignant hyperthermia has not been fully assessed; therefore, lidocaine should be used with caution in such patients.

In hospital environments where drugs known to be triggering agents for malignant hyperthermia (fulminant hyperthermia/hypermetabolism) are administered, it is suggested that a standard protocol for management should be available.

It is not known whether lidocaine may trigger this reaction, however, large doses resulting in significant plasma concentrations, as may be achieved by intravenous infusion, pose potential risk to these individuals. Recognition of early unexplained signs of tachycardia, tachypnea, labile blood pressure and metabolic acidosis may precede temperature elevation. Successful outcome is dependent on early diagnosis, prompt discontinuance of the triggering agent and institution of treatment including oxygen therapy, supportive measures and dantrolene (for details see dantrolene package insert).

2. **Patient Information:** The patient should be advised of the possible occurrence of the experiences listed under ADVERSE REACTIONS.

3. **Laboratory Tests:** None known.

4. **Drug Interactions:** Lidocaine Hydrochloride Injection, USP should be used with caution in patients with digitalis toxicity accompanied by atrioventricular block. Concomitant use of beta-blocking agents may reduce hepatic blood flow and thereby reduce lidocaine clearance.

5. **Carcinogenesis, Mutagenesis, Impairment of Fertility:** Long term studies in animals to evaluate the carcinogenic and mutagenic potential or the effect on fertility of lidocaine HCl have not been conducted.

6. **Pregnancy:**
   Teratogenic Effects: *Pregnancy Category B.* Reproduction studies have been performed in rats at doses up to 6.6 times the maximum human doses and have revealed no significant findings. There are, however, no adequate and well-controlled studies in pregnant women. Because animal reproduction studies are not always predictive of human response, this drug should be used during pregnancy only if clearly needed.

7. **Labor and Delivery:** The effects of lidocaine HCl on the mother and the fetus, when used in the management of cardiac arrhythmias during labor and delivery are not known. Lidocaine readily crosses the placental barrier.

8. **Nursing Mothers:** It is not known whether this drug is excreted in human milk. Because many drugs are excreted in human milk, caution should be exercised when lidocaine is administered to a nursing woman.

9. **Pediatric Use:** Safety and effectiveness in children have not been established by controlled clinical studies. (See DOSAGE AND ADMINISTRATION).

ADVERSE REACTIONS

Adverse experiences following the administration of lidocaine are similar in nature to those observed with other amide local anesthetic agents. Adverse experiences may result from high plasma levels caused by excessive dosage or may result from a hypersensitivity, idiosyncrasy or diminished tolerance on the part of the patient. Serious adverse experiences are generally systemic in nature. The following types are those most commonly reported. The adverse experiences under Central Nervous System and Cardiovascular System are listed in general in a progression from mild to severe.

1. **Central Nervous System**
   CNS reactions are excitatory and/or depressant and may be characterized by light-headedness, nervousness, apprehension, euphoria, confusion, dizziness, drowsiness, tinnitus, blurred or double vision, vomiting, sensations of heat, cold or numbness, twitching, tremors, convulsions, unconsciousness, respiratory depression and arrest. The excitatory reactions may be very brief or may not occur at all, in which case, the first manifestation of toxicity may be drowsiness, merging into unconsciousness and respiratory arrest.

2. **Cardiovascular System**
   Cardiovascular reactions are usually depressant in nature and are characterized by bradycardia, hypotension and cardiovascular collapse, which may lead to cardiac arrest.

3. Allergic reactions as a result of sensitivity to lidocaine are extremely rare and, if they occur, should be managed by conventional means.

DRUG ABUSE AND DEPENDENCE

Although specific studies have not been conducted, lidocaine HCl has been used clinically without evidence of abuse of this drug or of psychological or physical dependence as a result of its use.

OVERDOSAGE

Overdosage of lidocaine HCl usually results in signs of central nervous system or cardiovascular toxicity. See ADVERSE REACTIONS.

Should convulsions or signs of respiratory depression and arrest develop, the patency of the airway and adequacy of ventilation must be assured immediately. Should convulsions persist despite ventilatory therapy with oxygen, small increments of anticonvulsive agents may be given intravenously. Examples of such agents include a benzodiazepine (e.g., diazepam), an ultrashort-acting barbiturate (e.g., thiopental or thiamylal) or a short-acting barbiturate (e.g., pentobarbital or secobarbital). If the patient is under general anesthesia, a short-acting muscle relaxant (e.g., succinylcholine) may be administered.

Should circulatory depression occur, vasopressors may be used.

Dialysis is of negligible value in the treatment of acute overdosage from lidocaine HCl.

DOSAGE AND ADMINISTRATION

Adults

Single Direct Intravenous Injection (bolus): The usual dose is 50 to 100 mg of lidocaine hydrochloride (0.70 to 1.4 mg/kg; 0.32 to 0.63 mg/lb) administered intravenously under ECG monitoring. This dose may be administered at the rate of approximately 25 to 50 mg/min (0.35 to 0.70 mg/kg/min;

0.16 to 0.32 mg/lb/min). Sufficient time should be allowed to enable a slow circulation to carry the drug to the site of action. If the initial injection of 50 to 100 mg does not produce a desired response, a second dose may be injected after five minutes. NO MORE THAN 200 to 300 MG OF LIDOCAINE HYDROCHLORIDE SHOULD BE ADMINISTERED DURING A ONE HOUR PERIOD.

Continuous Intravenous Infusion: Following bolus administration, intravenous infusions of lidocaine hydrochloride may be initiated at the rate of 1 to 4 mg/min of lidocaine hydrochloride (0.014 to 0.057 mg/kg/min; 0.006 to 0.026 mg/lb/min). The rate of intravenous infusions should be reassessed as soon as the patient's basic cardiac rhythm appears to be stable or at the earliest signs of toxicity. It should rarely be necessary to continue intravenous infusions of lidocaine for prolonged periods.

Solutions for intravenous infusion may be prepared by the addition of one gram (or two grams) of lidocaine hydrochloride to one liter of 5% dextrose in water using aseptic technique. Approximately a 0.1% (or 0.2%) solution will result from this procedure; that is, each milliliter will contain approximately 1 (or 2 mg) of lidocaine hydrochloride. In those cases in which fluid restriction is medically appropriate, a more concentrated solution may be prepared.

The 20% concentration of lidocaine hydrochloride should be diluted with a suitable large volume parenteral as follows to achieve the above final concentrations for continuous infusion:

20% (200 mg/mL)	LVP Size	Final Conc.
1 g in 5 mL	1000 mL	0.1%
1 g in 5 mL	500 mL	0.2%
1 g in 5 mL	250 mL	0.4%
2 g in 10 mL	1000 mL	0.2%
2 g in 10 mL	500 mL	0.4%

The 10% concentration of lidocaine hydrochloride should be diluted with a suitable large volume parenteral as follows to achieve the above final concentrations for continuous infusion:

10% (100 mg/mL)	LVP Size	Final Conc.
1 g in 10 mL	1000 mL	0.1%
1 g in 10 mL	500 mL	0.2%
1 g in 10 mL	250 mL	0.4%

Lidocaine Hydrochloride Injection, USP has been found to be chemically stable for 24 hours after dilution in 5% dextrose in water. However, as with all intravenous admixtures, dilution of the solution should be made just prior to its administration.

When administering lidocaine hydrochloride (or any potent medication) by continuous intravenous infusion, it is advisable to use a precision volume control I.V. set.

Pediatric

Although controlled clinical studies to establish pediatric dosing schedules have not been conducted, the American Heart Association's *Standards and Guidelines* recommends a bolus dose of 1 mg/kg followed by an infusion rate of 20 to 50 µg/kg/min.

NOTE

Regarding Prolonged Infusions. There are data that indicate the half-life may be 3 hours or longer following infusions of greater than 24 hours in duration.

Parenteral drug products should be inspected visually for particulate matter and discoloration prior to administration, whenever solution and container permit.

```
FOR LOCAL
ANESTHESIA
```

CLINICAL PHARMACOLOGY

Lidocaine stabilizes the neuronal membrane and prevents the initiation and conduction of nerve impulses, thereby effecting local anesthetic action.

Lidocaine is metabolized mainly in the liver and excreted via the kidneys. Approximately 90% of lidocaine administered is excreted in the form of various metabolites, while less than 10% is excreted unchanged.

INDICATIONS

Lidocaine Hydrochloride Injection, USP is indicated for production of local or regional anesthesia, by infiltration techniques, including percutaneous injection and intravenous regional anesthesia by peripheral nerve block techniques such as brachial plexus and intercostal blocks and by central neural techniques, including epidural and caudal blocks,

Continued on next page

Abbott—Cont.

when the accepted procedures for these techniques as described in standard textbooks are followed.

CONTRAINDICATIONS

Lidocaine hydrochloride is contraindicated in patients with a known history of hypersensitivity either to local anesthetic agents of the amide type or to other components of the injectable formulations.

WARNINGS

1. RESUSCITATIVE EQUIPMENT AND DRUGS, INCLUDING OXYGEN, SHOULD BE IMMEDIATELY AVAILABLE WHEN ANY LOCAL ANESTHETIC AGENT IS USED.
2. **Use in Pregnancy:** Reproductive studies have been performed in rats and rabbits without evidence of harm to the animal fetus. However, the safe use of lidocaine in humans has not been established with respect to possible adverse effects upon fetal development. Careful consideration should be given to this fact before administering this drug to women of childbearing potential, particularly during early pregnancy. This does not exclude the use of the drug at term for obstetrical analgesia. Lidocaine HCl has been used effectively for obstetrical analgesia. Adverse effect on the fetus, course of labor or delivery have rarely been observed when proper dosage and proper technique have been employed.
3. Local anesthetic procedures should be used with caution when there is inflammation and/or sepsis in the region of the proposed injection.
4. Vasopressor agents (administered for the treatment of hypotension related to caudal or other epidural blocks) should be used with caution in the presence of oxytocic drugs, as a severe persistent hypertension and even rupture of a cerebral blood vessel may occur.
5. The solutions which contain a vasoconstrictor should be used with extreme caution for patients whose medical history and physical evaluation suggest the existence of hypertension, arteriosclerotic heart disease, cerebral vascular insufficiency, heart block, thyrotoxicosis or diabetes, etc. The solutions which contain a vasoconstrictor should also be used with extreme caution in patients receiving drugs known to produce blood pressure alterations (e.g., MAO inhibitors, tricyclic antidepressants, phenothiazines, etc.) as either sustained hypotension or hypertension may occur.

PRECAUTIONS

The safety and effectiveness of Lidocaine Hydrochloride Injection, USP depends on proper dosage, correct technique, adequate precautions and readiness for emergencies. Standard textbooks should be consulted for specific techniques and precautions for various regional anesthetic procedures. The lowest dosage that results in effective anesthesia should be used. Injection of repeated doses of lidocaine HCl may cause significant increases in blood levels with each repeated dose due to slow accumulation of lidocaine or its metabolites. Tolerance varies with the status of the patient. Debilitated, elderly patients, acutely ill patients and children should be given reduced doses commensurate with their age and physical status. Lidocaine HCl should also be used with caution in patients with severe shock or heart block.

In using lidocaine HCl for infiltration or regional nerve block anesthesia, injection should always be made slowly and with frequent aspirations. Proper tourniquet technique is essential in the performance of intravenous regional anesthesia. Solutions containing epinephrine or other vasoconstrictors should not be used for this technique.

Epidural anesthesia and caudal anesthesia should be used with extreme caution in persons with the following conditions: Existing neurological disease, spinal deformities, septicemia, severe hypertension and extreme youth.

Fetal bradycardia frequently follows paracervical block and may be associated with fetal acidosis. Fetal heart rate should always be monitored during paracervical anesthesia. Added risk appears to be present in prematurity, postmaturity, toxemia of pregnancy, uteroplacental insufficiency and fetal distress. The physician should weigh the possible advantages against dangers when considering paracervical block in these conditions. When the recommended dose is exceeded, the incidence of fetal bradycardia increases. Short-term neonatal neurobehavioral alterations have been observed in association with some local anesthetics administered during labor and delivery. The short-term and long-term significance of these alterations is not known.

Solutions containing a vasoconstrictor should be used cautiously and in carefully circumscribed quantities in areas of the body supplied by end arteries or having otherwise compromised blood supply (e.g., digits, nose, external ear, penis, etc.). Serious cardiac arrhythmias may occur if preparations containing a vasoconstrictor are employed in patients during or following the administration of chloroform, halothane, cyclopropane, trichloroethylene or other related agents.

Table I
Recommended Dosages of Lidocaine Hydrochloride Injection, USP for Various Anesthetic Procedures in Normal Healthy Adults

Procedure	Conc. (%)	Lidocaine Hydrochloride Injection, USP (without Epinephrine)	
		Vol. (mL)	Total Dose (mg)
Infiltration			
Percutaneous	0.5 or 1.0	1–60	5–300
Intravenous Regional	0.5	10–60	50–300
Peripheral Nerve Blocks, e.g.			
Brachial	1.5	15–20	225–300
Dental	2.0	1–5	20–100
Intercostal	1.0	3	30
Paravertebral	1.0	3–5	30–50
Pudendal (each side)	1.0	10	100
Paracervical			
Obstetrical Analgesia (each side)	1.0	10	100
Sympathetic Nerve Blocks, e.g.			
Cervical (stellate ganglion)	1.0	5	50
Lumbar	1.0	5–10	50–100
Central Neural Blocks			
Epidural*			
Thoracic	1.0	20–30	200–300
Lumbar			
Analgesia	1.0	25–30	250–300
Anesthesia	1.5	15–20	225–300
	2.0	10–15	200–300
Caudal			
Obstetrical Analgesia	1.0	20–30	200–300
Surgical Anesthesia	1.5	15–20	225–300

* Dose determined by number of dermatomes to be anesthetized (2 to 3 mL/dermatome).
THE ABOVE SUGGESTED CONCENTRATIONS AND VOLUMES SERVE ONLY AS A GUIDE. OTHER VOLUMES AND CONCENTRATIONS MAY BE USED PROVIDED THE TOTAL MAXIMUM RECOMMENDED DOSE IS NOT EXCEEDED.

Lidocaine Hydrochloride Injection, USP should be used with caution in persons with known drug sensitivities. Patients allergic to para-aminobenzoic acid derivatives (procaine, tetracaine, benzocaine, etc.) have not shown cross sensitivity to lidocaine.

The safety of amide local anesthetics in patients with malignant hyperthermia has not been assessed, and therefore, these agents should be used with caution in such patients. Drowsiness following an injection of lidocaine HCl is usually an early indication of a high blood level of the drug and may occur following inadvertent intravascular administration or rapid absorption of lidocaine. Local anesthetics react with certain metals and cause the release of their respective ions which, if injected, may cause severe local irritation. Adequate precautions should be taken to avoid this type of interaction. (See STERILIZATION, STORAGE AND TECHNICAL PROCEDURES).

ADVERSE REACTIONS

Reactions to lidocaine HCl are similar in character to those observed with other local anesthetic agents. Adverse reactions may be due to high plasma levels as a result of excessive dosage, rapid absorption or inadvertent intravascular injection. Such reactions are systemic in nature and involve the central nervous system and/or the cardiovascular system. Rarely, reactions may result from hypersensitivity, idiosyncrasy or diminished tolerance on the part of the patient.

CNS reactions are excitatory and/or depressant, and may be characterized by nervousness, dizziness, blurred vision and tremors, followed by drowsiness, convulsions, unconsciousness and, possibly, respiratory arrest. The excitatory reactions may be very brief or may not occur at all, in which case the first manifestations of toxicity may be drowsiness, merging into unconsciousness and respiratory arrest.

Hypotension and bradycardia may occur as normal physiological phenomena following sympathetic block with central neural blocks. Toxic cardiovascular reactions to local anesthetics are usually depressant in nature and are characterized by peripheral vasodilation, hypotension, myocardial depression, bradycardia and, possibly cardiac arrest.

Treatment of a patient with toxic manifestations consists of assuring and maintaining a patent airway, supporting ventilation with oxygen, and assisted or controlled ventilation (respiration) as required. This usually will be sufficient in the management of most reactions.

Should a convulsion persist despite ventilatory therapy with oxygen, small increments of anticonvulsive agents may be given intravenously. Examples of such agents include a benzodiazepine (e.g., diazepam), ultrashort-acting barbiturates (e.g., thiopental or thiamylal) or a short-acting barbiturate (e.g., pentobarbital or secobarbital). Cardiovascular depression may require circulatory assistance with intravenous fluids and/or vasopressors (e.g., ephedrine) as dictated by the clinical situation.

Allergic reactions may occur as a result of sensitivity either to local anesthetics or to the methylparaben used as a preservative in multiple-dose vials. Anaphylactoid type symptomatology and reactions, characterized by cutaneous lesions, urticaria, and edema should be managed by conventional means. The detection of potential sensitivity by skin testing is of limited value.

DOSAGE AND ADMINISTRATION

Table I (Recommended Dosages) summarizes the recommended volumes and concentrations of Lidocaine Hydrochloride Injection, USP for various types of anesthetic procedures. The dosages suggested in this table are for normal healthy adults and refer to the use of epinephrine-free solutions. When larger dosages are required, only solutions containing epinephrine should be used except in those cases where vasopressor drugs may be contraindicated.

These recommended doses serve only as a guide to the amount of anesthetic required for most routine procedures. The actual volume and concentrations to be used depend on a number of factors, such as type and extent of surgical procedure, degree of muscular relaxation required, duration of anesthesia required, the physical state of the patient, etc. In all cases the lowest concentration and smallest dose that will produce the desired result should be given. Dosages should be reduced for children and for elderly and debilitated patients. The onset of anesthesia, the duration of anesthesia and the degree of muscular relaxation are proportional to the volume and concentration of local anesthetic solution used. Thus, an increase in concentration and volume of lidocaine HCl administered will decrease the onset of anesthesia, prolong the duration of anesthesia, provide a greater degree of muscular relaxation and increase the segmental spread of anesthesia. However, increasing the concentration and volume of lidocaine HCl administered may result in a more profound fall in blood pressure when used in epidural anesthesia. Although the incidence of side effects with lidocaine HCl is quite low, caution should be exercised particularly when employing large volumes and concentrations of lidocaine HCl, since the incidence of side effects is directly related to the total dose of local anesthetic agent injected.

It is important that a single-dose container be employed for epidural anesthesia and major peripheral nerve block.

FOR EPIDURAL OR SPINAL ANESTHESIA, USE ONLY SOLUTIONS WITHOUT PRESERVATIVES.

IMPORTANT: *A test dose of 2 to 5 mL should be administered at least 5 minutes prior to injecting the total required volume for central neural blocks (e.g., epidural or caudal anesthesia).*

Maximum Recommended Dosages

For normal healthy adults, the individual dose of lidocaine hydrochloride with epinephrine should be such that the dose of lidocaine hydrochloride is kept below 500 mg and, in any case, should not exceed 7 mg/kg (3.2 mg/lb) of body weight. When used without epinephrine, the amount of Lidocaine Hydrochloride Injection, USP administered should be such that the dose of lidocaine hydrochloride is kept below 300 mg, and in any case, should not exceed 4.5 mg/kg (2.0 mg/lb) of body weight. For continuous epidural or caudal anesthesia, the maximum recommended dosage should not be administered at intervals of less than 90 minutes. For paracervical block for obstetrical analgesia, (including abortion) the maximum recommended dosage (200 mg) should not be administered at intervals of less than 90 minutes. When paracervical block is used for non-obstetrical procedures, more drug may be administered if required to obtain adequate anesthesia. For intravenous regional anesthesia in adults (using lidocaine hydrochloride 0.5% solution without epinephrine), the dose administered should not exceed 4 mg/kg (1.8 mg/lb) of body weight.

Children:
It is difficult to recommend a maximum dose of any drug for children since this varies as a function of age and weight. For children of less than ten years who have a normal lean body mass and normal body development, the maximum dose may be determined by the application of one of the standard pediatric drug formulas (e.g., Clark's rule). For example, in a child of five years weighing 50 lbs, the dose of lidocaine hydrochloride should not exceed 75 to 100 mg when calculated according to Clark's rule. In any case, the maximum dose of lidocaine HCl with epinephrine should not exceed 7 mg/kg (3.2 mg/lb) of body weight. When used without epinephrine, the amount of lidocaine HCl administered should not exceed 4.5 mg/kg (2.0 mg/lb) of body weight. In order to minimize the possibility of toxic reactions, the use of lidocaine HCl 0.5% or 1.0% is recommended for most anesthetic procedures involving pediatric patients. The use of even more dilute solutions (e.g., 0.25% to 0.5%) and total dosages not to exceed 3 mg/kg (1.4 mg/lb) are recommended for induction of intravenous regional anesthesia in children.

Parenteral drug products should be inspected visually for particulate matter and discoloration prior to administration, whenever solution and container permit.
[See table on preceding page].

Sterilization, Storage and Technical Procedures:
Disinfecting agents containing heavy metals, which cause release of respective ions (mercury, zinc, copper, etc.) should not be used for skin or mucous membrane disinfection as they have been related to incidence of swelling and edema. When chemical disinfection of multi-dose vials is desired, either isopropyl alcohol (91%) or 70% ethyl alcohol is recommended. Many commercially available brands of rubbing alcohol, as well as solutions of ethyl alcohol not of USP grade, contain denaturants which are injurious to rubber and, therefore, are not to be used. It is recommended that chemical disinfection be accomplished by wiping the vial or ampul thoroughly with cotton or gauze that has been moistened with the recommended alcohol just prior to use.

HOW SUPPLIED
Lidocaine Hydrochloride Injection, USP is available in a variety of dosage strengths, containers and sizes. Consult Abbott Laboratories, Hospital Products Division for a current listing.
Exposure of pharmaceutical products to heat should be minimized. Avoid excessive heat. Protect from freezing. It is recommended that the product be stored at room temperature (25° C); however, brief exposure up to 40° C does not adversely affect the product.

CAUTION
Federal (USA) law prohibits dispensing without prescription.
06-4067-R17-Rev. Apr., 1987

NEMBUTAL® SODIUM CAPSULES   ℞ Ⓒ
[nêm-bū-tal sō-dī-um]
(pentobarbital sodium capsules, USP)

WARNING: MAY BE HABIT FORMING

DESCRIPTION
The barbiturates are nonselective central nervous system depressants which are primarily used as sedative hypnotics. The barbiturates and their sodium salts are subject to control under the Federal Controlled Substances Act (See "Drug Abuse and Dependence" section).

Barbiturates are substituted pyrimidine derivatives in which the basic structure common to these drugs is barbituric acid, a substance which has no central nervous system (CNS) activity. CNS activity is obtained by substituting alkyl, alkenyl, or aryl groups on the pyrimidine ring. Nembutal (pentobarbital sodium) is chemically represented by sodium 5-ethyl-5-(1-methylbutyl) barbiturate.

The sodium salt of pentobarbital occurs as a white, slightly bitter powder which is freely soluble in water and alcohol but practically insoluble in benzene and ether. Nembutal Sodium capsules for oral administration contain either 50 mg or 100 mg of pentobarbital sodium.

Inactive Ingredients: 50 mg Capsule: FD&C Blue No. 1, FD&C Red No. 3, FD&C Yellow No. 6, gelatin, lactose, magnesium stearate, polacrilin potassium and potassium chloride.
100 mg Capsule: colloidal silicon dioxide, corn starch, FD&C Blue No. 1, FD&C Red No. 3, FD&C Yellow No. 5 (tartrazine), FD&C Yellow No. 6, gelatin, magnesium stearate and potassium chloride.

CLINICAL PHARMACOLOGY
Barbiturates are capable of producing all levels of CNS mood alteration from excitation to mild sedation, to hypnosis, and deep coma. Overdosage can produce death. In high enough therapeutic doses, barbiturates induce anesthesia.
Barbiturates depress the sensory cortex, decrease motor activity, alter cerebellar function, and produce drowsiness, sedation, and hypnosis.
Barbiturate-induced sleep differs from physiological sleep. Sleep laboratory studies have demonstrated that barbiturates reduce the amount of time spent in the rapid eye movement (REM) phase of sleep or dreaming stage. Also, Stages III and IV sleep are decreased. Following abrupt cessation of barbiturates used regularly, patients may experience markedly increased dreaming, nightmares, and/or insomnia. Therefore, withdrawal of a single therapeutic dose over 5 or 6 days has been recommended to lessen the REM rebound and disturbed sleep which contribute to drug withdrawal syndrome (for example, decrease the dose from 3 to 2 doses a day for 1 week).
In studies, secobarbital sodium and pentobarbital sodium have been found to lose most of their effectiveness for both inducing and maintaining sleep by the end of 2 weeks of continued drug administration at fixed doses. The short-, intermediate-, and, to a lesser degree, long-acting barbiturates have been widely prescribed for treating insomnia. Although the clinical literature abounds with claims that the short-acting barbiturates are superior for producing sleep while the intermediate-acting compounds are more effective in maintaining sleep, controlled studies have failed to demonstrate these differential effects. Therefore, as sleep medications, the barbiturates are of limited value beyond short-term use.
Barbiturates have little analgesic action at subanesthetic doses. Rather, in subanesthetic doses these drugs may increase the reaction to painful stimuli. All barbiturates exhibit anticonvulsant activity in anesthetic doses. However, of the drugs in this class, only phenobarbital, mephobarbital, and metharbital have been clinically demonstrated to be effective as oral anticonvulsants in subhypnotic doses.
Barbiturates are respiratory depressants. The degree of respiratory depression is dependent upon dose. With hypnotic doses, respiratory depression produced by barbiturates is similar to that which occurs during physiologic sleep with slight decrease in blood pressure and heart rate.
Studies in laboratory animals have shown that barbiturates cause reduction in the tone and contractility of the uterus, ureters, and urinary bladder. However, concentrations of the drugs required to produce this effect in humans are not reached with sedative-hypnotic doses.
Barbiturates do not impair normal hepatic function, but have been shown to induce liver microsomal enzymes, thus increasing and/or altering the metabolism of barbiturates and other drugs. (See "Precautions—*Drug Interactions*" section).
Pharmacokinetics: Barbiturates are absorbed in varying degrees following oral, rectal, or parenteral administration. The salts are more rapidly absorbed than are the acids. The rate of absorption is increased if the sodium salt is ingested as a dilute solution or taken on an empty stomach.

The onset of action for oral or rectal administration varies from 20 to 60 minutes.
Duration of action, which is related to the rate at which the barbiturates are redistributed throughout the body, varies among persons and in the same person from time to time. In Table 1, the barbiturates are classified according to their duration of action. This classification should not be used to predict the exact duration of effect, but the grouping of drugs should be used as a guide in the selection of barbiturates. No studies have demonstrated that the different routes of administration are equivalent with respect to bioavailability.
[See Table 1 below left]
Barbiturates are weak acids that are absorbed and rapidly distributed to all tissues and fluids with high concentrations in the brain, liver, and kidneys. Lipid solubility of the barbiturates is the dominant factor in their distribution within the body. The more lipid soluble the barbiturate, the more rapidly it penetrates all tissues of the body. Barbiturates are bound to plasma and tissue proteins to a varying degree with the degree of binding increasing directly as a function of lipid solubility. The plasma half-life for pentobarbital in adults is 15 to 50 hours and appears to be dose dependent.
Barbiturates are metabolized primarily by the hepatic microsomal enzyme system, and the metabolic products are excreted in the urine, and less commonly, in the feces. Approximately 25 to 50 percent of a dose of aprobarbital or phenobarbital is eliminated unchanged in the urine, whereas the amount of other barbiturates excreted unchanged in the urine is negligible. The excretion of unmetabolized barbiturate is one feature that distinguishes the long-acting category from those belonging to other categories which are almost entirely metabolized. The inactive metabolites of the barbiturates are excreted as conjugates of glucuronic acid.

INDICATIONS AND USAGE
Oral:
a. Sedatives.
b. Hypnotics, for the short-term treatment of insomnia, since they appear to lose their effectiveness for sleep induction and sleep maintenance after 2 weeks (See "Clinical Pharmacology" section).
c. Preanesthetics.

CONTRAINDICATIONS
Barbiturates are contraindicated in patients with known barbiturate sensitivity. Barbiturates are also contraindicated in patients with a history of manifest or latent porphyria.

WARNINGS
1. *Habit forming:* Barbiturates may be habit forming. Tolerance, psychological and physical dependence may occur with continued use. (See "Drug Abuse and Dependence" and "Pharmacokinetics" sections). Patients who have psychological dependence on barbiturates may increase the dosage or decrease the dosage interval without consulting a physician and may subsequently develop a physical dependence on barbiturates. To minimize the possibility of overdosage or the development of dependence, the prescribing and dispensing of sedative-hypnotic barbiturates should be limited to the amount required for the interval until the next appointment. Abrupt cessation after prolonged use in the dependent person may result in withdrawal symptoms, including delirium, convulsions, and possibly death. Barbiturates should be withdrawn gradually from any patient known to be taking excessive dosage over long periods of time. (See "Drug Abuse and Dependence" section).
2. *Acute or chronic pain:* Caution should be exercised when barbiturates are administered to patients with acute or chronic pain, because paradoxical excitement could be induced or important symptoms could be masked. However, the use of barbiturates as sedatives in the postoperative surgical period and as adjuncts to cancer chemotherapy is well established.
3. *Use in pregnancy:* Barbiturates can cause fetal damage when administered to a pregnant woman. Retrospective, case-controlled studies have suggested a connection between the maternal consumption of barbiturates and a higher than expected incidence of fetal abnormalities. Following oral or parenteral administration, barbiturates readily cross the placental barrier and are distributed throughout fetal tissues with highest concentrations found in the placenta, fetal liver, and brain.

Table 1.—*Classification, Onset, and Duration of Action of Commonly used Barbiturates Taken Orally*

Classification	Onset of action	Duration of action
Long-acting Phenobarbital.	1 hour or longer	10 to 12 hours

Intermediate
  Amobarbital
  Butabarbital.
	¾ to 1 hour	6 to 8 hours

Short-acting
  Pentobarbital
  Secobarbital.
	10 to 15 minutes	3 to 4 hours

Continued on next page

If desired, additional literature on any Abbott Product will be provided upon request to Abbott Laboratories.

Abbott—Cont.

Withdrawal symptoms occur in infants born to mothers who receive barbiturates throughout the last trimester of pregnancy. (See "Drug Abuse and Dependence" section). If this drug is used during pregnancy, or if the patient becomes pregnant while taking this drug, the patient should be apprised of the potential hazard to the fetus.

4. *Synergistic effects:* The concomitant use of alcohol or other CNS depressants may produce additive CNS depressant effects.

PRECAUTIONS

General: Barbiturates may be habit forming. Tolerance and psychological and physical dependence may occur with continuing use. (See "Drug Abuse and Dependence" section). Barbiturates should be administered with caution, if at all, to patients who are mentally depressed, have suicidal tendencies, or a history of drug abuse.

Elderly or debilitated patients may react to barbiturates with marked excitement, depression, and confusion. In some persons, barbiturates repeatedly produce excitement rather than depression.

In patients with hepatic damage, barbiturates should be administered with caution and initially in reduced doses. Barbiturates should not be administered to patients showing the premonitory signs of hepatic coma.

The 100 mg dosage strength of Nembutal Sodium capsules contains FD&C Yellow No. 5 (tartrazine) which may cause allergic-type reactions (including bronchial asthma) in certain susceptible individuals. Although the overall incidence of FD&C Yellow No. 5 (tartrazine) sensitivity in the general population is low, it is frequently seen in patients who also have aspirin hypersensitivity.

Information for the patient: Practitioners should give the following information and instructions to patients receiving barbiturates.

1. The use of barbiturates carries with it an associated risk of psychological and/or physical dependence. The patient should be warned against increasing the dose of the drug without consulting a physician.
2. Barbiturates may impair mental and/or physical abilities required for the performance of potentially hazardous tasks (e.g., driving, operating machinery, etc.).
3. Alcohol should not be consumed while taking barbiturates. Concurrent use of the barbiturates with other CNS depressants (e.g., alcohol, narcotics, tranquilizers, and antihistamines) may result in additional CNS depressant effects.

Laboratory tests: Prolonged therapy with barbiturates should be accompanied by periodic laboratory evaluation of organ systems, including hematopoietic, renal, and hepatic systems. (See "Precautions—*General* " and "Adverse Reactions" sections).

Drug interactions: Most reports of clinically significant drug interactions occurring with the barbiturates have involved phenobarbital. However, the application of these data to other barbiturates appears valid and warrants serial blood level determinations of the relevant drugs when there are multiple therapies.

1. *Anticoagulants:* Phenobarbital lowers the plasma levels of dicumarol (name previously used: bishydroxycoumarin) and causes a decrease in anticoagulant activity as measured by the prothrombin time. Barbiturates can induce hepatic microsomal enzymes resulting in increased metabolism and decreased anticoagulant response of oral anticoagulants (e.g., warfarin, acenocoumarol, dicumarol, and phenprocoumon). Patients stabilized on anticoagulant therapy may require dosage adjustments if barbiturates are added to or withdrawn from their dosage regimen.
2. *Corticosteroids:* Barbiturates appear to enhance the metabolism of exogenous corticosteroids probably through the induction of hepatic microsomal enzymes. Patients stabilized on corticosteroid therapy may require dosage adjustments if barbiturates are added to or withdrawn from their dosage regimen.
3. *Griseofulvin:* Phenobarbital appears to interfere with the absorption of orally administered griseofulvin, thus decreasing its blood level. The effect of the resultant decreased blood levels of griseofulvin on therapeutic response has not been established. However, it would be preferable to avoid concomitant administration of these drugs.
4. *Doxycycline:* Phenobarbital has been shown to shorten the half-life of doxycycline for as long as 2 weeks after barbiturate therapy is discontinued. This mechanism is probably through the induction of hepatic microsomal enzymes that metabolize the antibiotic. If phenobarbital and doxycycline are administered concurrently, the clinical response to doxycycline should be monitored closely.
5. *Phenytoin, sodium valproate, valproic acid:* The effect of barbiturates on the metabolism of phenytoin appears to be variable. Some investigators report an accelerating effect, while others report no effect. Because the effect of barbitu-

rates on the metabolism of phenytoin is not predictable, phenytoin and barbiturate blood levels should be monitored more frequently if these drugs are given concurrently. Sodium valproate and valproic acid appear to decrease barbiturate metabolism; therefore, barbiturate blood levels should be monitored and appropriate dosage adjustments made as indicated.

6. *Central nervous system depressants:* The concomitant use of other central nervous system depressants including other sedatives or hypnotics, antihistamines, tranquilizers, or alcohol, may produce additive depressant effects.
7. *Monoamine oxidase inhibitors (MAOI):* MAOI prolong the effects of barbiturates probably because metabolism of the barbiturate is inhibited.
8. *Estradiol, estrone, progesterone and other steroidal hormones:* Pretreatment with or concurrent administration of phenobarbital may decrease the effect of estradiol by increasing its metabolism. There have been reports of patients treated with antiepileptic drugs (e.g., phenobarbital) who became pregnant while taking oral contraceptives. An alternate contraceptive method might be suggested to women taking phenobarbital.

Carcinogenesis: Adequate data are not available on long-term potential for carcinogenicity in humans or animals for pentobarbital.

Data from one retrospective study of 235 children in which the types of barbiturates are not identified suggested an association between exposure to barbiturates prenatally and an increased incidence of brain tumor. (Gold, E., et al., "Increased Risk of Brain Tumors in Children Exposed to Barbiturates," Journal of National Cancer Institute, 61:1031–1034, 1978).

Pregnancy: 1. *Teratogenic effects.* Pregnancy Category D—See "Warnings—Use in Pregnancy" section.
2. *Nonteratogenic effects.* Reports of infants suffering from long-term barbiturate exposure in utero included the acute withdrawal syndrome of seizures and hyperirritability from birth to a delayed onset of up to 14 days. (See "Drug Abuse and Dependence" section).

Labor and delivery: Hypnotic doses of these barbiturates do not appear to significantly impair uterine activity during labor. Full anesthetic doses of barbiturates decrease the force and frequency of uterine contractions. Administration of sedative-hypnotic barbiturates to the mother during labor may result in respiratory depression in the newborn. Premature infants are particularly susceptible to the depressant effects of barbiturates. If barbiturates are used during labor and delivery, resuscitation equipment should be available. Data are currently not available to evaluate the effect of these barbiturates when forceps delivery or other intervention is necessary. Also, data are not available to determine the effect of these barbiturates on the later growth, development, and functional maturation of the child.

Nursing mothers: Caution should be exercised when a barbiturate is administered to a nursing woman since small amounts of barbiturates are excreted in the milk.

ADVERSE REACTIONS

The following adverse reactions and their incidence were compiled from surveillance of thousands of hospitalized patients. Because such patients may be less aware of certain of the milder adverse effects of barbiturates, the incidence of these reactions may be somewhat higher in fully ambulatory patients.

More than 1 in 100 patients. The most common adverse reaction estimated to occur at a rate of 1 to 3 patients per 100 is:
Nervous System: Somnolence.

Less than 1 in 100 patients. Adverse reactions estimated to occur at a rate of less than 1 in 100 patients listed below, grouped by organ system, and by decreasing order of occurrence are:

Nervous system: Agitation, confusion, hyperkinesia, ataxia, CNS depression, nightmares, nervousness, psychiatric disturbance, hallucinations, insomnia, anxiety, dizziness, thinking abnormality.
Respiratory system: Hypoventilation, apnea.
Cardiovascular system: Bradycardia, hypotension, syncope.
Digestive system: Nausea, vomiting, constipation.
Other reported reactions: Headache, injection site reactions, hypersensitivity reactions (angioedema, skin rashes, exfoliative dermatitis), fever, liver damage, megaloblastic anemia following chronic phenobarbital use.

DRUG ABUSE AND DEPENDENCE

Pentobarbital sodium capsules are subject to control by the Federal Controlled Substances Act under DEA schedule II. Barbiturates may be habit forming. Tolerance, psychological dependence, and physical dependence may occur especially following prolonged use of high doses of barbiturates. Daily administration in excess of 400 mg of pentobarbital or secobarbital for approximately 90 days is likely to produce some degree of physical dependence. A dosage of from 600 to 800 mg taken for at least 35 days is sufficient to produce withdrawal seizures. The average daily dose for the barbiturate addict is usually about 1.5 grams. As tolerance to barbiturates develops, the amount needed to maintain the same

level of intoxication increases; tolerance to a fatal dosage, however, does not increase more than two-fold. As this occurs, the margin between an intoxicating dosage and fatal dosage becomes smaller.

Symptoms of acute intoxication with barbiturates include unsteady gait, slurred speech, and sustained nystagmus. Mental signs of chronic intoxication include confusion, poor judgment, irritability, insomnia, and somatic complaints. Symptoms of barbiturate dependence are similar to those of chronic alcoholism. If an individual appears to be intoxicated with alcohol to a degree that is radically disproportionate to the amount of alcohol in his or her blood the use of barbiturates should be suspected. The lethal dose of a barbiturate is far less if alcohol is also ingested.

The symptoms of barbiturate withdrawal can be severe and may cause death. Minor withdrawal symptoms may appear 8 to 12 hours after the last dose of a barbiturate. These symptoms usually appear in the following order: anxiety, muscle twitching, tremor of hands and fingers, progressive weakness, dizziness, distortion in visual perception, nausea, vomiting, insomnia, and orthostatic hypotension. Major withdrawal symptoms (convulsions and delirium) may occur within 16 hours and last up to 5 days after abrupt cessation of these drugs. Intensity of withdrawal symptoms gradually declines over a period of approximately 15 days. Individuals susceptible to barbiturate abuse and dependence include alcoholics and opiate abusers, as well as other sedative-hypnotic and amphetamine abusers.

Drug dependence to barbiturates arises from repeated administration of a barbiturate or agent with barbiturate-like effect on a continuous basis, generally in amounts exceeding therapeutic dose levels. The characteristics of drug dependence to barbiturates include: (a) a strong desire or need to continue taking the drug; (b) a tendency to increase the dose; (c) a psychic dependence on the effects of the drug related to subjective and individual appreciation of those effects; and (d) a physical dependence on the effects of the drug requiring its presence for maintenance of homeostasis and resulting in a definite, characteristic, and self-limited abstinence syndrome when the drug is withdrawn.

Treatment of barbiturate dependence consists of cautious and gradual withdrawal of the drug. Barbiturate-dependent patients can be withdrawn by using a number of different withdrawal regimens. In all cases withdrawal takes an extended period of time. One method involves substituting a 30 mg dose of phenobarbital for each 100 to 200 mg dose of barbiturate that the patient has been taking. The total daily amount of phenobarbital is then administered in 3 to 4 divided doses, not to exceed 600 mg daily. Should signs of withdrawal occur on the first day of treatment, a loading dose of 100 to 200 mg of phenobarbital may be administered IM in addition to the oral dose. After stabilization on phenobarbital, the total daily dose is decreased by 30 mg a day as long as withdrawal is proceeding smoothly. A modification of this regimen involves initiating treatment at the patient's regular dosage level and decreasing the daily dosage by 10 percent if tolerated by the patient.

Infants physically dependent on barbiturates may be given phenobarbital 3 to 10 mg/kg/day. After withdrawal symptoms (hyperactivity, disturbed sleep, tremors, hyperreflexia) are relieved, the dosage of phenobarbital should be gradually decreased and completely withdrawn over a 2 week period.

OVERDOSAGE

The toxic dose of barbiturates varies considerably. In general, an oral dose of 1 g of most barbiturates produces serious poisoning in an adult. Death commonly occurs after 2 to 10 g of ingested barbiturate. Barbiturate intoxication may be confused with alcoholism, bromide intoxication, and with various neurological disorders.

Acute overdosage with barbiturates is manifested by CNS and respiratory depression which may progress to Cheyne-Stokes respiration, areflexia, constriction of the pupils to a slight degree (though in severe poisoning they may show paralytic dilation), oliguria, tachycardia, hypotension, lowered body temperature, and coma. Typical shock syndrome (apnea, circulatory collapse, respiratory arrest, and death) may occur.

In extreme overdose, all electrical activity in the brain may cease, in which case a "flat" EEG normally equated with clinical death cannot be accepted. This effect is fully reversible unless hypoxic damage occurs. Consideration should be given to the possibility of barbiturate intoxication even in situations that appear to involve trauma.

Complications such as pneumonia, pulmonary edema, cardiac arrhythmias, congestive heart failure, and renal failure may occur. Uremia may increase CNS sensitivity to barbiturates. Differential diagnosis should include hypoglycemia, head trauma, cerebrovascular accidents, convulsive states, and diabetic coma. Blood levels from acute overdosage for some barbiturates are listed in Table 2.
[See table on next page].

Treatment of overdosage is mainly supportive and consists of the following:

1. Maintenance of an adequate airway, with assisted respiration and oxygen administration as necessary.

Table 2.—*Concentration of Barbiturate in the Blood Versus Degree of CNS Depression*
Blood barbiturate level in ppm (μg/ml)

Barbiturate	Onset/ duration	Degree of depression in nontolerant persons*				
		1	2	3	4	5
Pentobarbital	Fast/short	≤ 2	0.5 to 3	10 to 15	12 to 25	15 to 40
Secobarbital	Fast/short	≤ 2	0.5 to 5	10 to 15	15 to 25	15 to 40
Amobarbital	Intermediate/ intermediate	≤ 3	2 to 10	30 to 40	30 to 60	40 to 80
Butabarbital	Intermediate/ intermediate	≤ 5	3 to 25	40 to 60	50 to 80	60 to 100
Phenobarbital	Slow/long	≤ 10	5 to 40	50 to 80	70 to 120	100 to 200

* Categories of degree of depression in nontolerant persons.
1. Under the influence and appreciably impaired for purposes of driving a motor vehicle or performing tasks requiring alertness and unimpaired judgment and reaction time.
2. Sedated, therapeutic range, calm, relaxed, and easily aroused.
3. Comatose, difficult to arose, significant depression of respiration.
4. Compatible with death in aged or ill persons or in presence of obstructed airway, other toxic agents, or exposure to cold.
5. Usual lethal level, the upper end of the range includes those who received some supportive treatment.

2. Monitoring of vital signs and fluid balance.
3. If the patient is conscious and has not lost the gag reflex, emesis may be induced with ipecac. Care should be taken to prevent pulmonary aspiration of vomitus. After completion of vomiting, 30 g activated charcoal in a glass of water may be administered.
4. If emesis is contraindicated, gastric lavage may be performed with a cuffed endotracheal tube in place with the patient in the face down position. Activated charcoal may be left in the emptied stomach and a saline cathartic administered.
5. Fluid therapy and other standard treatment for shock, if needed.
6. If renal function is normal, forced diuresis may aid in the elimination of the barbiturate. Alkalinization of the urine increases renal excretion of some barbiturates, especially phenobarbital, also aprobarbital, and mephobarbital (which is metabolized to phenobarbital).
7. Although not recommended as a routine procedure, hemodialysis may be used in severe barbiturate intoxications or if the patient is anuric or in shock.
8. Patient should be rolled from side to side every 30 minutes.
9. Antibiotics should be given if pneumonia is suspected.
10. Appropriate nursing care to prevent hypostatic pneumonia, decubiti, aspiration, and other complications of patients with altered states of consciousness.

DOSAGE AND ADMINISTRATION

Adults: The usual hypnotic dose consists of 100 mg at bedtime.
Children: The preoperative dose is 2 to 6 mg/kg/24 hours (maximum 100 mg), depending on age, weight, and the desired degree of sedation.
The proper hypnotic dose for children must be judged on the basis of individual age and weight.
Dosages of barbiturates must be individualized with full knowledge of their particular characteristics and recommended rate of administration. Factors of consideration are the patient's age, weight, and condition.
Special patient population: Dosage should be reduced in the elderly or debilitated because these patients may be more sensitive to barbiturates. Dosage should be reduced for patients with impaired renal function or hepatic disease.

HOW SUPPLIED

NEMBUTAL Sodium Capsules (pentobarbital sodium capsules, USP) are supplied as follows:
50 mg transparent and orange-colored capsules in bottles of 100 (**NDC** 0074-3150-11);
100 mg yellow capsules in bottles of 100 (**NDC** 0074-3114-01), 500 (**NDC** 0074-3114-02) and in the Abbo-Pac® unit dose packages of 100 (**NDC** 0074-3114-21).
Abbott Pharmaceuticals, Inc.
North Chicago, IL 60064
Shown in Product Identification Section, page 403

NEMBUTAL® SODIUM SOLUTION   ℞ ©

[nem'-bū-tal]
(pentobarbital sodium injection, USP)
Ampuls—Vials

WARNING: MAY BE HABIT FORMING. DO NOT USE IF MATERIAL HAS PRECIPITATED.

DESCRIPTION

The barbiturates are nonselective central nervous system depressants which are primarily used as sedative hypnotics and also anticonvulsants in subhypnotic doses. The barbiturates and their sodium salts are subject to control under the Federal Controlled Substances Act (See "Drug Abuse and Dependence" section).
The sodium salts of amobarbital, pentobarbital, phenobarbital, and secobarbital are available as sterile parenteral solutions.
Barbiturates are substituted pyrimidine derivatives in which the basic structure common to these drugs is barbituric acid, a substance which has no central nervous system (CNS) activity. CNS activity is obtained by substituting alkyl, alkenyl, or aryl groups on the pyrimidine ring.
NEMBUTAL Sodium Solution (pentobarbital sodium injection) is a sterile solution for intravenous or intramuscular injection. Each ml contains pentobarbital sodium 50 mg, in a vehicle of propylene glycol, 40%, alcohol, 10% and water for injection, to volume. The pH is adjusted to approximately 9.5 with hydrochloric acid and/or sodium hydroxide.
NEMBUTAL Sodium is a short-acting barbiturate, chemically designated as sodium 5-ethyl-5-(1-methylbutyl) barbiturate. The sodium salt occurs as a white, slightly bitter powder which is freely soluble in water and alcohol but practically insoluble in benzene and ether.

CLINICAL PHARMACOLOGY

Barbiturates are capable of producing all levels of CNS mood alteration from excitation to mild sedation, to hypnosis, and deep coma. Overdosage can produce death. In high enough therapeutic doses, barbiturates induce anesthesia.
Barbiturates depress the sensory cortex, decrease motor activity, alter cerebellar function, and produce drowsiness, sedation, and hypnosis.
Barbiturate-induced sleep differs from physiological sleep. Sleep laboratory studies have demonstrated that barbiturates reduce the amount of time spent in the rapid eye movement (REM) phase of sleep or dreaming stage. Also, Stages III and IV sleep are decreased. Following abrupt cessation of barbiturates used regularly, patients may experience markedly increased dreaming, nightmares, and/or insomnia. Therefore, withdrawal of a single therapeutic dose over 5 or 6 days has been recommended to lessen the REM rebound and disturbed sleep which contribute to drug withdrawal syndrome (for example, decrease the dose from 3 to 2 doses a day for 1 week).
In studies, secobarbital sodium and pentobarbital sodium have been found to lose most of their effectiveness for both inducing and maintaining sleep by the end of 2 weeks of continued drug administration at fixed doses. The short-, intermediate-, and, to a lesser degree, long-acting barbiturates have been widely prescribed for treating insomnia. Although the clinical literature abounds with claims that the short-acting barbiturates are superior for producing sleep while the intermediate-acting compounds are more effective in maintaining sleep, controlled studies have failed to demonstrate these differential effects. Therefore, as sleep medications, the barbiturates are of limited value beyond short-term use.
Barbiturates have little analgesic action at subanesthetic doses. Rather, in subanesthetic doses these drugs may increase the reaction to painful stimuli. All barbiturates exhibit anticonvulsant activity in anesthetic doses. However, of the drugs in this class, only phenobarbital, mephobarbital, and metharbital have been clinically demonstrated to be effective as oral anticonvulsants in subhypnotic doses.
Barbiturates are respiratory depressants. The degree of respiratory depression is dependent upon dose. With hypnotic doses, respiratory depression produced by barbiturates is similar to that which occurs during physiologic sleep with slight decrease in blood pressure and heart rate.
Studies in laboratory animals have shown that barbiturates cause reduction in the tone and contractility of the uterus, ureters, and urinary bladder. However, concentration of the drugs required to produce this effect in humans are not reached with sedative-hypnotic doses.

Barbiturates do not impair normal hepatic function, but have been shown to induce liver microsomal enzymes, thus increasing and/or altering the metabolism of barbiturates and other drugs. (See "Precautions—*Drug Interactions*" section).
Pharmacokinetics: Barbiturates are absorbed in varying degrees following oral, rectal, or parenteral administration. The salts are more rapidly absorbed than are the acids.
The onset of action for oral or rectal administration varies from 20 to 60 minutes. For IM administration, the onset of action is slightly faster. Following IV administration, the onset of action ranges from almost immediately for pentobarbital sodium to 5 minutes for phenobarbital sodium. Maximal CNS depression may not occur until 15 minutes or more after IV administration for phenobarbital sodium.
Duration of action, which is related to the rate at which the barbiturates are redistributed throughout the body, varies among persons and in the same person from time to time. No studies have demonstrated that the different routes of administration are equivalent with respect to bioavailability.
Barbiturates are weak acids that are absorbed and rapidly distributed to all tissues and fluids with high concentration in the brain, liver, and kidneys. Lipid solubility of the barbiturates is the dominant factor in their distribution within the body. The more lipid soluble the barbiturate, the more rapidly it penetrates all tissues of the body. Barbiturates are bound to plasma and tissue proteins to a varying degree with the degree of binding increasing directly as a function of lipid solubility. The plasma half-life for pentobarbital in adults is 15 to 50 hours and appears to be dose-dependent.
Barbiturates are metabolized primarily by the hepatic microsomal enzyme system, and the metabolic products are excreted in the urine, and less commonly, in the feces. Approximately 25 to 50 percent of a dose of aprobarbital or phenobarbital is eliminated unchanged in the urine, whereas the amount of other barbiturates excreted unchanged in the urine is negligible. The excretion of unmetabolized barbiturate is one feature that distinguishes the long-acting category from those belonging to other categories which are almost entirely metabolized. The inactive metabolites of the barbiturates are excreted as conjugates of glucuronic acid.

INDICATIONS AND USAGE

Parenteral:
a. Sedatives.
b. Hypnotics, for the short-term treatment of insomnia, since they appear to lose their effectiveness for sleep induction and sleep maintenance after 2 weeks (See "Clinical Pharmacology" section).
c. Preanesthetics.
d. Anticonvulsant, in anesthetic doses, in the emergency control of certain acute convulsive episodes, e.g., those associated with status epilepticus, cholera, eclampsia, meningitis, tetanus, and toxic reactions to strychnine or local anesthetics.

CONTRAINDICATIONS

Barbiturates are contraindicated in patients with known barbiturate sensitivity. Barbiturates are also contraindicated in patients with a history of manifest or latent porphyria.

WARNINGS

1. *Habit forming:* Barbiturates may be habit forming. Tolerance, psychological and physical dependence may occur with continued use. (See "Drug Abuse and Dependence" and "Pharmacokinetics" sections). Patients who have psychological dependence on barbiturates may increase the dosage or decrease the dosage interval without consulting a physician and may subsequently develop a physical dependence on barbiturates. To minimize the possibility of overdosage or the development of dependence, the prescribing and dispensing of sedative-hypnotic barbiturates should be limited to the amount required for the interval until the next appointment. Abrupt cessation after prolonged use in the dependent person may result in withdrawal symptoms, including delirium, convulsions, and possibly death. Barbiturates should be withdrawn gradually from any patient known to be taking excessive dosage over long periods of time. (See "Drug Abuse and Dependence" section).
2. *IV administration:* Too rapid administration may cause respiratory depression, apnea, laryngospasm, or vasodilation with fall in blood pressure.
3. *Acute or chronic pain:* Caution should be exercised when barbiturates are administered to patients with acute or chronic pain, because paradoxical excitement could be induced or important symptoms could be masked. However, the use of barbiturates as sedatives in the postopera-

Continued on next page

Abbott—Cont.

tive surgical period and as adjuncts to cancer chemotherapy is well established.

4. *Use in pregnancy:* Barbiturates can cause fetal damage when administered to a pregnant woman. Retrospective, case-controlled studies have suggested a connection between the maternal consumption of barbiturates and a higher than expected incidence of fetal abnormalities. Following oral or parenteral administration, barbiturates readily cross the placental barrier and are distributed throughout fetal tissues with highest concentrations found in the placenta, fetal liver, and brain. Fetal blood levels approach maternal blood levels following parenteral administration.

Withdrawal symptoms occur in infants born to mothers who receive barbiturates throughout the last trimester of pregnancy. (See "Drug Abuse and Dependence" section). If this drug is used during pregnancy, or if the patient becomes pregnant while taking this drug, the patient should be apprised of the potential hazard to the fetus.

5. *Synergistic effects:* The concomitant use of alcohol or other CNS depressants may produce additive CNS depressant effects.

PRECAUTIONS

General: Barbiturates may be habit forming. Tolerance and psychological and physical dependence may occur with continuing use. (See "Drug Abuse and Dependence" section). Barbiturates should be administered with caution, if at all, to patients who are mentally depressed, have suicidal tendencies, or a history of drug abuse.

Elderly or debilitated patients may react to barbiturates with marked excitement, depression, and confusion. In some persons, barbiturates repeatedly produce excitement rather than depression.

In patients with hepatic damage, barbiturates should be administered with caution and initially in reduced doses. Barbiturates should not be administered to patients showing the premonitory signs of hepatic coma.

Parenteral solutions of barbiturates are highly alkaline. Therefore, extreme care should be taken to avoid perivascular extravasation or intra-arterial injection. Extravascular injection may cause local tissue damage with subsequent necrosis; consequences of intra-arterial injection may vary from transient pain to gangrene of the limb. Any complaint of pain in the limb warrants stopping the injection.

Information for the patient: Practitioners should give the following information and instructions to patients receiving barbiturates.

1. The use of barbiturates carries with it an associated risk of psychological and/or physical dependence. The patient should be warned against increasing the dose of the drug without consulting a physician.

2. Barbiturates may impair mental and/or physical abilities required for the performance of potentially hazardous tasks (e.g., driving, operating machinery, etc.).

3. Alcohol should not be consumed while taking barbiturates. Concurrent use of the barbiturates with other CNS depressants (e.g., alcohol, narcotics, tranquilizers, and antihistamines) may result in additional CNS depressant effects.

Laboratory tests: Prolonged therapy with barbiturates should be accompanied by periodic laboratory evaluation of organ systems, including hematopoietic, renal, and hepatic systems. (See "Precautions-*General*" and "Adverse Reactions" sections).

Drug interactions: Most reports of clinically significant drug interactions occurring with the barbiturates have involved phenobarbital. However, the application of these data to other barbiturates appears valid and warrants serial blood level determinations of the relevant drugs when there are multiple barbiturates.

1. *Anticoagulants:* Phenobarbital lowers the plasma levels of dicumarol (name previously used: bishydroxycoumarin) and causes a decrease in anticoagulant activity as measured by the prothrombin time. Barbiturates can induce hepatic microsomal enzymes resulting in increased metabolism and decreased anticoagulant response of oral anticoagulants (e.g., warfarin, acenocoumarol, dicumarol, and phenprocoumon). Patients stabilized on anticoagulant therapy may require dosage adjustments if barbiturates are added to or withdrawn from their dosage regimen.

2. *Corticosteroids:* Barbiturates appear to enhance the metabolism of exogenous corticosteroids probably through the induction of hepatic microsomol enzymes. Patients stabilized on corticosteroid therapy may require dosage adjustments if barbiturates are added to or withdrawn from their dosage regimen.

3. *Griseofulvin:* Phenobarbital appears to interfere with the absorption of orally administered griseofulvin, thus decreasing its blood level. The effect of the resultant decreased blood levels of griseofulvin on therapeutic response has not been established. However, it would be preferable to avoid concomitant administration of these drugs.

4. *Doxycycline:* Phenobarbital has been shown to shorten the half-life of doxycycline for as long as 2 weeks after barbiturate therapy is discontinued.

This mechanism is probably through the induction of hepatic microsomal enzymes that metabolize the antibiotic. If phenobarbital and doxycycline are administered concurrently, the clinical response to doxycycline should be monitored closely.

5. *Phenytoin, sodium valproate, valproic acid:* The effect of barbiturates on the metabolism of phenytoin appears to be variable. Some investigators report an accelerating effect, while others report no effect. Because the effect of barbiturates on the metabolism of phenytoin is not predictable, phenytoin and barbiturate blood levels should be monitored more frequently if these drugs are given concurrently. Sodium valproate and valproic acid appear to decrease barbiturate metabolism; therefore, barbiturate blood levels should be monitored and appropriate dosage adjustments made as indicated.

6. *Central nervous system depressants:* The concomitant use of other central nervous system depressants, including other sedatives or hypnotics, antihistamines, tranquilizers, or alcohol, may produce additive depressant effects.

7. *Monoamine oxidase inhibitors (MAOI):* MAOI prolong the effects of barbiturates probably because metabolism of the barbiturate is inhibited.

8. *Estradiol, estrone, progesterone and other steroidal hormones:* Pretreatment with or concurrent administration of phenobarbital may decrease the effect of estradiol by increasing its metabolism. There have been reports of patients treated with antiepileptic drugs (e.g., phenobarbital) who became pregnant while taking oral contraceptives. An alternate contraceptive method might be suggested to women taking phenobarbital.

Carcinogenesis: Adequate data are not available on long-term potential for carcinogenicity in humans or animals for pentobarbital.

Data from one retrospective study of 235 children in which the types of barbiturates are not identified suggested an association between exposure to barbiturates prenatally and an increased incidence of brain tumor. (Gold, E., et al., "Increased Risk of Brain Tumors in Children Exposed to Barbiturates," Journal of National Cancer Institute, 61:1031–1034, 1978).

Pregnancy: 1. *Teratogenic effects.* Pregnancy Category D—See "Warnings—Use in Pregnancy" section.

2. *Nonteratogenic effects.* Reports of infants suffering from long-term barbiturate exposure in utero included the acute withdrawal syndrome of seizures and hyperirritability from birth to a delayed onset of up to 14 days. (See "Drug Abuse and Dependence" section).

Labor and delivery: Hypnotic doses of these barbiturates do not appear to significantly impair uterine activity during labor. Full anesthetic doses of barbiturates decrease the force and frequency of uterine contractions. Administration of sedative-hypnotic barbiturates to the mother during labor may result in respiratory depression in the newborn. Premature infants are particularly susceptible to the depressant effects of barbiturates. If barbiturates are used during labor and delivery, resuscitation equipment should be available.

Data are currently not available to evaluate the effect of these barbiturates when forceps delivery or other intervention is necessary. Also, data are not available to determine the effect of these barbiturates on the later growth, development, and functional maturation of the child.

Nursing mothers: Caution should be exercised when a barbiturate is administered to a nursing woman since small amounts of barbiturates are excreted in the milk.

ADVERSE REACTIONS

The following adverse reactions and their incidence were compiled from surveillance of thousands of hospitalized patients. Because such patients may be less aware of certain of the milder adverse effects of barbiturates, the incidence of these reactions may be somewhat higher in fully ambulatory patients.

More than 1 in 100 patients. The most common adverse reaction estimated to occur at a rate of 1 to 3 patients per 100 is: *Nervous System:* Somnolence.

Less than 1 in 100 patients. Adverse reactions estimated to occur at a rate of less than 1 in 100 patients listed below, grouped by organ system, and by decreasing order of occurrence are:

Nervous system: Agitation, confusion, hyperkinesia, ataxia, CNS depression, nightmares, nervousness, psychiatric disturbance, hallucinations, insomnia, anxiety, dizziness, thinking abnormality.

Respiratory system: Hypoventilation, apnea.

Cardiovascular system: Bradycardia, hypotension, syncope.

Digestive system: Nausea, vomiting, constipation.

Other reported reactions: Headache, injection site reactions, hypersensitivity reactions (angioedema, skin rashes, exfoliative dermatitis), fever, liver damage, megaloblastic anemia following chronic phenobarbital use.

DRUG ABUSE AND DEPENDENCE

Pentobarbital sodium injection is subject to control by the Federal Controlled Substances Act under DEA schedule II. Barbiturates may be habit forming. Tolerance, psychological dependence, and physical dependence may occur especially following prolonged use of high doses of barbiturates. Daily administration in excess of 400 mg of pentobarbital or secobarbital for approximately 90 days is likely to produce some degree of physical dependence. A dosage of from 600 to 800 mg taken for at least 35 days is sufficient to produce withdrawal seizures. The average daily dose for the barbiturate addict is usually about 1.5 g. As tolerance to barbiturates develops, the amount needed to maintain the same level of intoxication increases; tolerance to a fatal dosage, however, does not increase more than two-fold. As this occurs, the margin between an intoxicating dosage and fatal dosage becomes smaller.

Symptoms of acute intoxication with barbiturates include unsteady gait, slurred speech, and sustained nystagmus. Mental signs of chronic intoxication include confusion, poor judgment, irritability, insomnia, and somatic complaints. Symptoms of barbiturate dependence are similar to those of chronic alcoholism. If an individual appears to be intoxicated with alcohol to a degree that is radically disproportionate to the amount of alcohol in his or her blood the use of barbiturates should be suspected. The lethal dose of a barbiturate is far less if alcohol is also ingested.

The symptoms of barbiturate withdrawal can be severe and may cause death. Minor withdrawal symptoms may appear 8 to 12 hours after the last dose of a barbiturate. These symptoms usually appear in the following order: anxiety, muscle twitching, tremor of hands and fingers, progressive weakness, dizziness, distortion in visual perception, nausea, vomiting, insomnia, and orthostatic hypotension. Major withdrawal symptoms (convulsions and delirium) may occur within 16 hours and last up to 5 days after abrupt cessation of these drugs. Intensity of withdrawal symptoms gradually declines over a period of approximately 15 days. Individuals susceptible to barbiturate abuse and dependence include alcoholics and opiate abusers, as well as other sedative-hypnotic and amphetamine abusers.

Drug dependence to barbiturates arises from repeated administration of a barbiturate or agent with barbiturate-like effect on a continuous basis, generally in amounts exceeding therapeutic dose levels. The characteristics of drug dependence to barbiturates include: (a) a strong desire or need to continue taking the drug; (b) a tendency to increase the dose; (c) a psychic dependence on the effects of the drug related to subjective and individual appreciation of those effects; and (d) a physical dependence on the effects of the drug requiring its presence for maintenance of homeostasis and resulting in a definite, characteristic, and self-limited abstinence syndrome when the drug is withdrawn.

Treatment of barbiturate dependence consists of cautious and gradual withdrawal of the drug. Barbiturate-dependent patients can be withdrawn by using a number of different withdrawal regimens. In all cases withdrawal takes an extended period of time. One method involves substituting a 30 mg dose of phenobarbital for each 100 to 200 mg dose of barbiturate that the patient has been taking. The total daily amount of phenobarbital is then administered in 3 to 4 divided doses, not to exceed 600 mg daily. Should signs of withdrawal occur on the first day of treatment, a loading dose of 100 to 200 mg of phenobarbital may be administered IM in addition to the oral dose. After stabilization on phenobarbital, the total daily dose is decreased by 30 mg a day as long as withdrawal is proceeding smoothly. A modification of this regimen involves initiating treatment at the patient's regular dosage level and decreasing the daily dosage by 10 percent if tolerated by the patient.

Infants physically dependent on barbiturates may be given phenobarbital 3 to 10 mg/kg/day. After withdrawal symptoms (hyperactivity, disturbed sleep, tremors, hyperreflexia) are relieved, the dosage of phenobarbital should be gradually decreased and completely withdrawn over a 2-week period.

OVERDOSAGE

The toxic dose of barbiturates varies considerably. In general, an oral dose of 1 g of most barbiturates produces serious poisoning in an adult. Death commonly occurs after 2 to 10 g of ingested barbiturate. Barbiturate intoxication may be confused with alcoholism, bromide intoxication, and with various neurological disorders.

Acute overdosage with barbiturates is manifested by CNS and respiratory depression which may progress to Cheyne-Stokes respiration, areflexia, constriction of the pupils to a slight degree (though in severe poisoning they may show paralytic dilation), oliguria, tachycardia, hypotension, lowered body temperature, and coma. Typical shock syndrome (apnea, circulatory collapse, respiratory arrest, and death) may occur.

In extreme overdose, all electrical activity in the brain may cease, in which case a "flat" EEG normally equated with clinical death cannot be accepted. This effect is fully reversible unless hypoxic damage occurs. Consideration should be given to the possibility of barbiturate intoxication even in situations that appear to involve trauma.

Complications such as pneumonia, pulmonary edema, cardiac arrhythmias, congestive heart failure, and renal failure may occur. Uremia may increase CNS sensitivity to barbiturates. Differential diagnosis should include hypoglycemia, head trauma, cerebrovascular accidents, convulsive states, and diabetic coma. Blood levels from acute overdosage for some barbiturates are listed in Table 2. [See Table 2 in Nembutal Capsules prescribing information.]

Treatment of overdosage is mainly supportive and consists of the following:

1. Maintenance of an adequate airway, with assisted respiration and oxygen administration as necessary.
2. Monitoring of vital signs and fluid balance.
3. Fluid therapy and other standard treatment for shock, if needed.
4. If renal function is normal, forced diuresis may aid in the elimination of the barbiturate. Alkalinization of the urine increases renal excretion of some barbiturates, especially phenobarbital, also aprobarbital, and mephobarbital (which is metabolized to phenobarbital).
5. Although not recommended as a routine procedure, hemodialysis may be used in severe barbiturate intoxications or if the patient is anuric or in shock.
6. Patient should be rolled from side to side every 30 minutes.
7. Antibiotics should be given if pneumonia is suspected.
8. Appropriate nursing care to prevent hypostatic pneumonia, decubiti, aspiration, and other complications of patients with altered states of consciousness.

DOSAGE AND ADMINISTRATION

Dosages of barbiturates must be individualized with full knowledge of their particular characteristics and recommended rate of administration. Factors of consideration are the patient's age, weight, and condition. Parenteral routes should be used only when oral administration is impossible or impractical.

Intramuscular Administration: IM injection of the sodium salts of barbiturates should be made deeply into a large muscle, and a volume of 5 ml should not be exceeded at any one site because of possible tissue irritation. After IM injection of a hypnotic dose, the patient's vital signs should be monitored. The usual adult dosage of NEMBUTAL Sodium Solution is 150 to 200 mg as a single IM injection; the recommended pediatric dosage ranges from 2 to 6 mg/kg as a single IM injection not to exceed 100 mg.

Intravenous Administration: IV injection is restricted to conditions in which other routes are not feasible, either because the patient is unconscious (as in cerebral hemorrhage, eclampsia, or status epilepticus, or because the patient resists (as in delirium), or because prompt action is imperative. Slow IV injection is essential and patients should be carefully observed during administration. This requires that blood pressure, respiration, and cardiac function be maintained, vital signs be recorded, and equipment for resuscitation and artificial ventilation be available. The rate of IV injection should not exceed 50 mg/min for pentobarbital sodium.

There is no average intravenous dose of NEMBUTAL Sodium Solution (pentobarbital sodium injection) that can be relied on to produce similar effects in different patients. The possibility of overdose and respiratory depression is remote when the drug is injected slowly in fractional doses.

A commonly used initial dose for the 70 kg adult is 100 mg. Proportional reduction in dosage should be made for pediatric or debilitated patients. At least one minute is necessary to determine the full effect of intravenous pentobarbital. If necessary, additional small increments of the drug may be given up to a total of from 200 to 500 mg for normal adults.

Anticonvulsant use: In convulsive states, dosage of NEMBUTAL Sodium Solution should be kept to a minimum to avoid compounding the depression which may follow convulsions. The injection must be made slowly with due regard to the time required for the drug to penetrate the blood-brain barrier.

Special patient population: Dosage should be reduced in the elderly or debilitated because these patients may be more sensitive to barbiturates. Dosage should be reduced for patients with impaired renal function or hepatic disease.

Inspection: Parenteral drug products should be inspected visually for particulate matter and discoloration prior to administration, whenever solution containers permit. Solutions for injection showing evidence of precipitation should not be used.

HOW SUPPLIED

NEMBUTAL Sodium Solution (pentobarbital sodium injection, USP) is available in the following sizes:
2-ml ampul, 100 mg (1½ gr), in boxes of 25 (**NDC** 0074-6899-04); 20-ml multiple-dose vial, 1 g, in boxes of 5 (**NDC** 0074-3778-04); and 50-ml multiple-dose vial, 2.5 g, in boxes of 5 (**NDC** 0074-3778-05).

Each ml contains:
Pentobarbital Sodium,
derivative of barbituric acid ....50 mg (¾ gr)
Warning—May be habit forming.
Propylene glycol ....40% v/v
Alcohol 10%
Water for Injection ....qs
(pH adjusted to approximately 9.5 with hydrochloric acid and/or sodium hydroxide.)
Exposure of pharmaceutical products to heat should be minimized. Avoid excessive heat. Protect from freezing. It is recommended that the product be stored at room temperature 86°F (30°C), however, brief exposure up to 104°F (40°C) does not adversely affect the product.
Abbott Laboratories
North Chicago, IL 60064
Ref. 07-5165-R3

NEMBUTAL® SODIUM SUPPOSITORIES   ℞ Ⓒ
[nêm-bū'tal]
(pentobarbital sodium suppositories)

WARNING: MAY BE HABIT FORMING

DESCRIPTION

The barbiturates are nonselective central nervous system depressants which are primarily used as sedative hypnotics. The barbiturates and their sodium salts are subject to control under the Federal Controlled Substances Act (See "Drug Abuse and Dependence" section).

Barbiturates are substituted pyrimidine derivatives in which the basic structure common to these drugs is barbituric acid, a substance which has no central nervous system (CNS) activity. CNS activity is obtained by substituting alkyl, alkenyl, or aryl groups on the pyrimidine ring. Nembutal (pentobarbital sodium) is chemically represented by sodium 5-ethyl-5-(1-methylbutyl) barbiturate.

The sodium salt of pentobarbital occurs as a white, slightly bitter powder which is freely soluble in water and alcohol but practically insoluble in benzene and ether. Each rectal suppository contains either 30 mg, 60 mg, 120 mg, or 200 mg of pentobarbital sodium.

Inactive Ingredients: Semi-synthetic glycerides and other ingredients.

CLINICAL PHARMACOLOGY

Barbiturates are capable of producing all levels of CNS mood alteration from excitation to mild sedation, to hypnosis, and deep coma. Overdosage can produce death. In high enough therapeutic doses, barbiturates induce anesthesia.

Barbiturates depress the sensory cortex, decrease motor activity, alter cerebellar function, and produce drowsiness, sedation, and hypnosis.

Barbiturate-induced sleep differs from physiological sleep. Sleep laboratory studies have demonstrated that barbiturates reduce the amount of time spent in the rapid eye movement (REM) phase of sleep or dreaming stage. Also, Stages III and IV sleep are decreased. Following abrupt cessation of barbiturates used regularly, patients may experience markedly increased dreaming, nightmares, and/or insomnia. Therefore, withdrawal of a single therapeutic dose over 5 or 6 days has been recommended to lessen the REM rebound and disturbed sleep which contribute to drug withdrawal syndrome (for example, decrease the dose from 3 to 2 doses a day for 1 week).

In studies, secobarbital sodium and pentobarbital sodium have been found to lose most of their effectiveness for both inducing and maintaining sleep by the end of 2 weeks of continued drug administration at fixed doses. The short-, intermediate-, and, to a lesser degree, long-acting barbiturates have been widely prescribed for treating insomnia. Although the clinical literature abounds with claims that the short-acting barbiturates are superior for producing sleep while the intermediate-acting compounds are more effective in maintaining sleep, controlled studies have failed to demonstrate these differential effects. Therefore, as sleep medications, the barbiturates are of limited value beyond short-term use.

Barbiturates have little analgesic action at subanesthetic doses. Rather, in subanesthetic doses these drugs may increase the reaction to painful stimuli. All barbiturates exhibit anticonvulsant activity in anesthetic doses. However, of the drugs in this class, only phenobarbital, mephobarbital, and metharbital have been clinically demonstrated to be effective as oral anticonvulsants in subhypnotic doses.

Barbiturates are respiratory depressants. The degree of respiratory depression is dependent upon dose. With hypnotic doses, respiratory depression produced by barbiturates is similar to that which occurs during physiologic sleep with slight decrease in blood pressure and heart rate.

Studies in laboratory animals have shown that barbiturates cause reduction in the tone and contractility of the uterus, ureters, and urinary bladder. However, concentrations of the drugs required to produce this effect in humans are not reached with sedative-hypnotic doses.

Barbiturates do not impair normal hepatic function, but have been shown to induce liver microsomal enzymes, thus increasing and/or altering the metabolism of barbiturates and other drugs. (See "Precautions—*Drug Interactions*" section).

Pharmacokinetics: Barbiturates are absorbed in varying degrees following oral, rectal, or parenteral administration. The onset of action for oral or rectal administration varies from 20 to 60 minutes.

Duration of action, which is related to the rate at which the barbiturates are redistributed throughout the body, varies among persons and in the same person from time to time. No studies have demonstrated that the different routes of administration are equivalent with respect to bioavailability.

Barbiturates are weak acids that are absorbed and rapidly distributed to all tissues and fluids with high concentrations in the brain, liver, and kidneys. Lipid solubility of the barbiturates is the dominant factor in their distribution within the body. The more lipid soluble the barbiturate, the more rapidly it penetrates all tissues of the body. Barbiturates are bound to plasma and tissue proteins to a varying degree with the degree of binding increasing directly as a function of lipid solubility. The plasma half-life for pentobarbital in adults is 15 to 50 hours and appears to be dose dependent.

Barbiturates are metabolized primarily by the hepatic microsomal enzyme system, and the metabolic products are excreted in the urine, and less commonly, in the feces. Approximately 25 to 50 percent of a dose of aprobarbital or phenobarbital is eliminated unchanged in the urine, whereas the amount of other barbiturates excreted unchanged in the urine is negligible. The excretion of unmetabolized barbiturate is one feature that distinguishes the long-acting category from those belonging to other categories which are almost entirely metabolized. The inactive metabolites of the barbiturates are excreted as conjugates of glucuronic acid.

INDICATIONS AND USAGE

Rectal: Barbiturates administered rectally are absorbed from the colon and are used when oral or parenteral administration may be undesirable.
1. Sedative.
2. Hypnotic, for the short-term treatment of insomnia, since they appear to lose their effectiveness for sleep induction and sleep maintenance after 2 weeks (See "Clinical Pharmacology" section).

CONTRAINDICATIONS

Barbiturates are contraindicated in patients with known barbiturate sensitivity. Barbiturates are also contraindicated in patients with a history of manifest or latent porphyria.

WARNINGS

1. *Habit forming:* Barbiturates may be habit forming. Tolerance, psychological and physical dependence may occur with continued use. (See "Drug Abuse and Dependence" and "Pharmacokinetics" sections). Patients who have psychological dependence on barbiturates may increase the dosage or decrease the dosage interval without consulting a physician and may subsequently develop a physical dependence on barbiturates. To minimize the possibility of overdosage or the development of dependence, the prescribing and dispensing of sedative-hypnotic barbiturates should be limited to the amount required for the interval until the next appointment. Abrupt cessation after prolonged use in the dependent person may result in withdrawal symptoms, including delirium, convulsions, and possibly death. Barbiturates should be withdrawn gradually from any patient known to be taking excessive dosage over long periods of time. (See "Drug Abuse and Dependence" section).

2. *Acute or chronic pain:* Caution should be exercised when barbiturates are administered to patients with acute or chronic pain, because paradoxical excitement could be induced or important symptoms could be masked. However, the use of barbiturates as sedatives in the postoperative surgical period and as adjuncts to cancer chemotherapy is well established.

3. *Use in pregnancy:* Barbiturates can cause fetal damage when administered to a pregnant woman. Retrospective, case-controlled studies have suggested a connection between the maternal consumption of barbiturates and a higher than expected incidence of fetal abnormalities. Following oral or parenteral administration, barbiturates readily cross the placental barrier and are distributed throughout fetal tissues with highest concentrations found in the placenta, fetal liver, and brain. It is presumed that this effect will also be seen following rectal administration.

Withdrawal symptoms occur in infants born to mothers who receive barbiturates throughout the last trimester of pregnancy. (See "Drug Abuse and Dependence" section). If this

Continued on next page

Abbott—Cont.

drug is used during pregnancy, or if the patient becomes pregnant while taking this drug, the patient should be apprised of the potential hazard to the fetus.

4. *Synergistic effects:* The concomitant use of alcohol or other CNS depressants may produce additive CNS depressant effects.

PRECAUTIONS

General: Barbiturates may be habit forming. Tolerance and psychological and physical dependence may occur with continuing use. (See "Drug Abuse and Dependence" section). Barbiturates should be administered with caution, if at all, to patients who are mentally depressed, have suicidal tendencies, or a history of drug abuse.

Elderly or debilitated patients may react to barbiturates with marked excitement, depression, and confusion. In some persons, barbiturates repeatedly produce excitement rather than depression.

In patients with hepatic damage, barbiturates should be administered with caution and initially in reduced doses. Barbiturates should not be administered to patients showing the premonitory signs of hepatic coma.

Information for the patient: Practitioners should give the following information and instructions to patients receiving barbiturates.

1. The use of barbiturates carries with it an associated risk of psychological and/or physical dependence. The patient should be warned against increasing the dose of the drug without consulting a physician.
2. Barbiturates may impair mental and/or physical abilities required for the performance of potentially hazardous tasks (e.g., driving, operating machinery, etc.)
3. Alcohol should not be consumed while taking barbiturates. Concurrent use of the barbiturates with other CNS depressants (e.g., alcohol, narcotics, tranquilizers, and antihistamines) may result in additional CNS depressant effects.

Laboratory tests: Prolonged therapy with barbiturates should be accompanied by periodic laboratory evaluation of organ systems, including hematopoietic, renal, and hepatic systems. (See "Precautions — *General* " and "Adverse Reactions" sections).

Drug interactions: Most reports of clinically significant drug interactions occurring with the barbiturates have involved phenobarbital. However, the application of these data to other barbiturates appears valid and warrants serial blood level determinations of the relevant drugs when there are multiple therapies.

1. *Anticoagulants:* Phenobarbital lowers the plasma levels of dicumarol (name previously used: bishydroxycoumarin) and causes a decrease in anticoagulant activity as measured by the prothrombin time. Barbiturates can induce hepatic microsomal enzymes resulting in increased metabolism and decreased anticoagulant response of oral anticoagulants (e.g., warfarin, acenocoumarol, dicumarol, and phenprocoumon). Patients stabilized on anticoagulant therapy may require dosage adjustments if barbiturates are added to or withdrawn from their dosage regimen.
2. *Corticosteroids:* Barbiturates appear to enhance the metabolism of exogenous corticosteroids probably through the induction of hepatic microsomal enzymes. Patients stabilized on corticosteroid therapy may require dosage adjustments if barbiturates are added to or withdrawn from their dosage regimen.
3. *Griseofulvin:* Phenobarbital appears to interfere with the absorption of orally administered griseofulvin, thus decreasing its blood level. The effect of the resultant decreased blood levels of griseofulvin on therapeutic response has not been established. However, it would be preferable to avoid concomitant administration of these drugs.
4. *Doxycycline:* Phenobarbital has been shown to shorten the half-life of doxycycline for as long as 2 weeks after barbiturate therapy is discontinued. This mechanism is probably through the induction of hepatic microsomal enzymes that metabolize the antibiotic. If phenobarbital and doxycycline are administered concurrently, the clinical response to doxycycline should be monitored closely.
5. *Phenytoin, sodium valproate, valproic acid:* The effect of barbiturates on the metabolism of phenytoin appears to be variable. Some investigators report an accelerating effect, while others report no effect. Because the effect of barbiturates on the metabolism of phenytoin is not predictable, phenytoin and barbiturate blood levels should be monitored more frequently if these drugs are given concurrently. Sodium valproate and valproic acid appear to decrease barbiturate metabolism; therefore, barbiturate blood levels should be monitored and appropriate dosage adjustments made as indicated.

6. *Central nervous system depressants:* The concomitant use of other central nervous system depressants, including other sedatives or hypnotics, antihistamines, tranquilizers, or alcohol, may produce additive depressant effects.
7. *Monoamine oxidase inhibitors (MAOI):* MAOI prolong the effects of barbiturates probably because metabolism of the barbiturate is inhibited.
8. *Estradiol, estrone, progesterone and other steroidal hormones:* Pretreatment with or concurrent administration of phenobarbital may decrease the effect of estradiol by increasing its metabolism. There have been reports of patients treated with antiepileptic drugs (e.g., phenobarbital) who became pregnant while taking oral contraceptives. An alternate contraceptive method might be suggested to women taking phenobarbital.

Carcinogenesis: Adequate data are not available on long-term potential for carcinogenicity in humans or animals for pentobarbital.

Data from one retrospective study of 235 children in which the types of barbiturates are not identified suggested an association between exposure to barbiturates prenatally and an increased incidence of brain tumor. (Gold, E., et al, "Increased Risk of Brain Tumors in Children Exposed to Barbiturates," Journal of National Cancer Institute, 61:1031–1034, 1978).

Pregnancy: 1. Teratogenic effects. Pregnancy Category D — See "Warnings — Use in Pregnancy" section.

2. *Nonteratogenic effects.* Reports of infants suffering from long-term barbiturate exposure in utero included the acute withdrawal syndrome of seizures and hyperirritability from birth to a delayed onset of up to 14 days. (See "Drug Abuse and Dependence" section).

Labor and delivery: Hypnotic doses of these barbiturates do not appear to significantly impair uterine activity during labor. Full anesthetic doses of barbiturates decrease the force and frequency of uterine contractions. Administration of sedative-hypnotic barbiturates to the mother during labor may result in respiratory depression in the newborn. Premature infants are particularly susceptible to the depressant effects of barbiturates. If barbiturates are used during labor and delivery, resuscitation equipment should be available. Data are currently not available to evaluate the effect of these barbiturates when forceps delivery or other intervention is necessary. Also, data are not available to determine the effect of these barbiturates on the later growth, development, and functional maturation of the child.

Nursing mothers: Caution should be exercised when a barbiturate is administered to a nursing woman since small amounts of barbiturates are excreted in the milk.

ADVERSE REACTIONS

The following adverse reactions and their incidence were compiled from surveillance of thousands of hospitalized patients. Because such patients may be less aware of certain of the milder adverse effects of barbiturates, the incidence of these reactions may be somewhat higher in fully ambulatory patients.

More than 1 in 100 patients. The most common adverse reaction estimated to occur at a rate of 1 to 3 patients per 100 is:

Nervous System: Somnolence.

Less than 1 in 100 patients. Adverse reactions estimated to occur at a rate of less than 1 in 100 patients listed below, grouped by organ system, and by decreasing order of occurrence are:

Nervous system: Agitation, confusion, hyperkinesia, ataxia, CNS depression, nightmares, nervousness, psychiatric disturbance, hallucinations, insomnia, anxiety, dizziness, thinking abnormality.

Respiratory system: Hypoventilation, apnea.

Cardiovascular system: Bradycardia, hypotension, syncope.

Digestive system: Nausea, vomiting, constipation.

Other reported reactions: Headache, injection site reactions, hypersensitivity reactions (angioedema, skin rashes, exfoliative dermatitis), fever, liver damage, megaloblastic anemia following chronic phenobarbital use.

DRUG ABUSE AND DEPENDENCE

Pentobarbital sodium suppositories are subject to control by the Federal Controlled Substances Act under DEA schedule III.

Barbiturates may be habit forming. Tolerance, psychological dependence, and physical dependence may occur especially following prolonged use of high doses of barbiturates. Daily administration in excess of 400 mg of pentobarbital or secobarbital for approximately 90 days is likely to produce some degree of physical dependence. A dosage of from 600 to 800 mg taken for at least 35 days is sufficient to produce withdrawal seizures. The average daily dose for the barbiturate addict is usually about 1.5 grams. As tolerance to barbiturates develops, the amount needed to maintain the same level of intoxication increases; tolerance to a fatal dosage, however, does not increase more than two-fold. As this occurs, the margin between an intoxicating dosage and fatal dosage becomes smaller.

Symptoms of acute intoxication with barbiturates include unsteady gait, slurred speech, and sustained nystagmus. Mental signs of chronic intoxication include confusion, poor judgment, irritability, insomnia, and somatic complaints. Symptoms of barbiturate dependence are similar to those of chronic alcoholism. If an individual appears to be intoxicated with alcohol to a degree that is radically disproportionate to the amount of alcohol in his or her blood the use of barbiturates should be suspected. The lethal dose of a barbiturate is far less if alcohol is also ingested.

The symptoms of barbiturate withdrawal can be severe and may cause death. Minor withdrawal symptoms may appear 8 to 12 hours after the last dose of a barbiturate. These symptoms usually appear in the following order: anxiety, muscle twitching, tremor of hands and fingers, progressive weakness, dizziness, distortion in visual perception, nausea, vomiting, insomnia, and orthostatic hypotension. Major withdrawal symptoms (convulsions and delirium) may occur within 16 hours and last up to 5 days after abrupt cessation of these drugs. Intensity of withdrawal symptoms gradually declines over a period of approximately 15 days. Individuals susceptible to barbiturate abuse and dependence include alcoholics and opiate abusers, as well as other sedative-hypnotic and amphetamine abusers.

Drug dependence to barbiturates arises from repeated administration of a barbiturate or agent with barbiturate-like effect on a continuous basis, generally in amounts exceeding therapeutic dose levels. The characteristics of drug dependence to barbiturates include: (a) a strong desire or need to continue taking the drug; (b) a tendency to increase the dose; (c) a psychic dependence on the effects of the drug related to subjective and individual appreciation of those effects; and (d) a physical dependence on the effects of the drug requiring its presence for maintenance of homeostasis and resulting in a definite, characteristic, and self-limited abstinence syndrome when the drug is withdrawn.

Treatment of barbiturate dependence consists of cautious and gradual withdrawal of the drug. Barbiturate-dependent patients can be withdrawn by using a number of different withdrawal regimens. In all cases withdrawal takes an extended period of time. One method involves substituting a 30 mg dose of phenobarbital for each 100 to 200 mg dose of barbiturate that the patient has been taking. The total daily amount of phenobarbital is then administered in 3 to 4 divided doses, not to exceed 600 mg daily. Should signs of withdrawal occur on the first day of treatment, a loading dose of 100 to 200 mg of phenobarbital may be administered IM in addition to the oral dose. After stabilization on phenobarbital, the total daily dose is decreased by 30 mg a day as long as withdrawal is proceeding smoothly. A modification of this regimen involves initiating treatment at the patient's regular dosage level and decreasing the daily dosage by 10 percent if tolerated by the patient.

Infants physically dependent on barbiturates may be given phenobarbital 3 to 10 mg/kg/day. After withdrawal symptoms (hyperactivity, disturbed sleep, tremors, hyperreflexia) are relieved, the dosage of phenobarbital should be gradually decreased and completely withdrawn over a 2 week period.

OVERDOSAGE

The toxic dose of barbiturates varies considerably. In general, an oral dose of 1 g of most barbiturates produces serious poisoning in an adult. Death commonly occurs after 2 to 10 g of ingested barbiturate. Barbiturate intoxication may be confused with alcoholism, bromide intoxication, and with various neurological disorders.

Acute overdosage with barbiturates is manifested by CNS and respiratory depression which may progress to Cheyne-Stokes respiration, areflexia, constriction of the pupils to a slight degree (though in severe poisoning they may show paralytic dilation), oliguria, tachycardia, hypotension, lowered body temperature, and coma. Typical shock syndrome (apnea, circulatory collapse, respiratory arrest, and death) may occur.

In extreme overdose, all electrical activity in the brain may cease, in which case a "flat" EEG normally equated with clinical death cannot be accepted. This effect is fully reversible unless hypoxic damage occurs. Consideration should be given to the possibility of barbiturate intoxication even in situations that appear to involve trauma.

Complications such as pneumonia, pulmonary edema, cardiac arrhythmias, congestive heart failure, and renal failure may occur. Uremia may increase CNS sensitivity to barbiturates. Differential diagnosis should include hypoglycemia, head trauma, cerebrovascular accidents, convulsive states, and diabetic coma. Blood levels from acute overdosage for some barbiturates are listed in Table 2. [See Table 2 shown in Nembutal Capsules prescribing information.]

Treatment of overdosage is mainly supportive and consists of the following:

1. Maintenance of an adequate airway, with assisted respiration and oxygen administration as necessary.
2. Monitoring of vital signs and fluid balance.
3. Fluid therapy and other standard treatment for shock, if needed.

4. If renal function is normal, forced diuresis may aid in the elimination of the barbiturate. Alkalinization of the urine increases renal excretion of some barbiturates, especially phenobarbital, also aprobarbital, and mephobarbital (which is metabolized to phenobarbital).

5. Although not recommended as a routine procedure, hemodialysis may be used in severe barbiturate intoxications or if the patient is anuric or in shock.

6. Patient should be rolled from side to side every 30 minutes.

7. Antibiotics should be given if pneumonia is suspected.

8. Appropriate nursing care to prevent hypostatic pneumonia, decubiti, aspiration, and other complications of patients with altered states of consciousness.

DOSAGE AND ADMINISTRATION

Typical hypnotic doses for adults and children are given below. These are intended only as a guide, and administration should be adjusted to the individual needs of each patient. For sedation, in children 5–14 years and in adults, reduce dose appropriately.

Adults (average to above average weight)— one 120 mg or one 200 mg suppository.

Children —

12–14 years ....one 60 mg or one (80–110 lbs)	120 mg suppository
5–12 years ....one 60 mg or one (40–80 lbs)	
1–4 years ....one 30 mg or (20–40 lbs)	60 mg suppository
2 months–1 year ....one 30 mg (10–20 lbs)	suppository

Suppositories should not be divided.

Dosages of barbiturates must be individualized with full knowledge of their particular characteristics and recommended rate of administration. Factors of consideration are the patient's age, weight, and condition.

Special patient population: Dosage should be reduced in the elderly or debilitated because these patients may be more sensitive to barbiturates. Dosage should be reduced for patients with impaired renal function or hepatic disease.

HOW SUPPLIED

NEMBUTAL Sodium Suppositories (pentobarbital sodium suppositories) are available as suppositories containing pentobarbital sodium in the amount of 30 mg (½ gr) (NDC 0074-3272-01); 60 mg (1 gr) (NDC 0074-3148-01); 120 mg (2 gr) (NDC 0074-3145-01) and 200 mg (3 gr) (NDC 0074-3164-01). Supplied in boxes of 12 suppositories.

Store in a refrigerator (36°–46°F).

Abbott Laboratories
North Chicago, IL 60064
Ref. 07-5369-R10

NITROPRESS®   ℞

[nī'tro-press]
(Sterile Sodium Nitroprusside, USP)
Univial®
Fliptop Vial

> NITROPRESS is only to be used as an infusion with sterile 5% dextrose injection. Not for direct injection.
> NITROPRESS should be used only when the necessary facilities and equipment for continuous monitoring of blood pressure are available.
> If at infusion rates of up to 10 mcg/kg/minute, an adequate reduction of blood pressure is not obtained within ten minutes, administration of NITROPRESS should be stopped.
> The instructions included herein should be reviewed thoroughly before administration of NITROPRESS.
> As metabolic acidosis is the earliest and most reliable evidence of cyanide toxicity, blood pH and acid base balance should be determined frequently in all patients and, particularly, if there is increased tolerance to the drug.

DESCRIPTION

Sterile Sodium Nitroprusside is an antihypertensive agent for intravenous infusion only, not for direct injection. It contains the equivalent of 50 mg of sodium nitroprusside dihydrate (sodium nitrosylpentacyanoferrate [*III*]) in an amber single use vial.

Chemically, sodium nitroprusside is $Na_2[Fe(CN)_5NO] \cdot 2H_2O$. It is a reddish-brown powder which is soluble in water. In aqueous solutions, it is extremely light sensitive and should be protected from light.

[See Chemical Formula at top of next column].

NITROPRESS (Sterile Sodium Nitroprusside, USP) is available as:

50 mg Unival®—Each 2 mL (when mixed) contains the equivalent of 50 mg sodium nitroprusside dihydrate in sterile water for injection.

Sodium Nitroprusside

50 mg Fliptop Vial—Each 2 mL (when mixed) contains the equivalent of 50 mg sodium nitroprusside dihydrate.

CLINICAL PHARMACOLOGY

NITROPRESS is a potent, immediate acting, intravenous hypotensive agent. This action is probably due to the nitroso (NO) group. Its effect is almost immediate and ends when the IV infusion is stopped. Generally, NITROPRESS is rapidly metabolized to cyanide and subsequently converted to thiocyanate through the mediation of a hepatic enzyme, rhodanase. The rate of conversion from cyanide to thiocyanate is dependent on the availability of sulfur, usually thiosulfate. The hypotensive effect is augmented by ganglionic blocking agents, volatile liquid anesthetics (such as halothane and enflurane), and by most other circulatory depressants.

The hypotensive effects of NITROPRESS are caused by peripheral vasodilation as a result of a direct action on the blood vessels, independent of autonomic innervation. No relaxation is seen in the smooth muscle of the uterus or duodenum *in situ* in animals.

Sodium nitroprusside administered intravenously to hypertensive and normotensive patients produced a marked lowering of the arterial blood pressure, slight increase in heart rate, a mild decrease in cardiac output and a moderate diminution in calculated total peripheral vascular resistance.

The decrease in calculated total peripheral vascular resistance suggests arteriolar vasodilatation. The decreases in cardiac and stroke index noted may be due to the peripheral vascular pooling of blood.

In hypertensive patients, moderate depressor doses induce renal vasodilatation roughly equivalent to the decrease in pressure without an appreciable increase in renal blood flow or a decrease in glomerular filtration.

In normotensive subjects, acute reduction of mean arterial pressure to 60 to 75 mmHg by infusion of sodium nitroprusside caused a significant increase in renin activity of renal venous plasma in correlation with the degree of reduction in pressure. Renal response to reduction in pressure was more striking in renovascular hypertensive patients, with significant increase in renin release occurring from the involved kidney at mean arterial pressures ranging from 90 to 137 mmHg. Furthermore, the magnitude of renin release from the involved kidney was significantly greater when compared with that in normotensive subjects, while in the contralateral, uninvolved kidney, no significant release of renin was detected during the reduction of pressure.

INDICATIONS AND USAGE

NITROPRESS (sterile sodium nitroprusside) is indicated for the immediate reduction of blood pressure of patients in hypertensive crises. Concomitant oral antihypertensive medication should be started while the hypertensive emergency is being brought under control with NITROPRESS.

NITROPRESS is also indicated for producing controlled hypotension during anesthesia in order to reduce bleeding in surgical procedures where surgeon and anesthesiologist deem it appropriate.

CONTRAINDICATIONS

NITROPRESS should not be used in the treatment of compensatory hypertension, *e.g.*, arteriovenous shunt or coarctation of the aorta.

The use of NITROPRESS to produce controlled hypotension during surgery is contraindicated in patients with known inadequate cerebral circulation. NITROPRESS is not intended for use during emergency surgery in moribund patients (A.S.A. Class 5E).

WARNINGS

> If excessive amounts of NITROPRESS are used and/or sulfur—usually thiosulfate—supplies are depleted, cyanide toxicity can occur. (See Overdosage.)
> If sodium nitroprusside infusion is to be extended, particularly if renal impairment is present, close attention should be given to not exceeding the recommended maximum infusion rate of 10 mcg/kg/minute. If in the course of therapy increased tolerance to the drug (as shown by the need for higher infusion rate) develops, it is essential to monitor blood acid-base balance, as metabolic acidosis is the earliest and most reliable evidence of cyanide toxicity. If signs of metabolic acidosis appear, NITROPRESS should be discontinued and an alternate drug administered.
> Serum thiocyanate levels do not reflect cyanide toxicity. However, serum thiocyanate levels should be monitored

---

> daily if treatment is to be extended, especially in patients with renal dysfunction. Thiocyanate accumulation and toxicity may manifest itself as tinnitus, blurred vision, delirium.

Some patients may fail to respond to adequate NITROPRESS administration. Since failure to respond to NITROPRESS may represent associated increase in free cyanide, appearance of increased tolerance to the drug constitutes reason for discontinuing NITROPRESS and promptly instituting alternate therapy.

Prolonged use of sodium nitroprusside may result in excessive thiocyanate formation. Thiocyanate accumulation and toxicity can manifest itself as tinnitus, blurred vision, mental confusion, psychotic behavior, convulsions, delirium, lactic acidosis, bone marrow depression, and hypothyroidism. Plasma thiocyanate concentrations should be monitored daily in any patient receiving therapy for longer than 48 hours, especially in patients with renal or hepatic impairment. Plasma thiocyanate levels above 10 mg/100 mL have been considered toxic and levels of 20 mg/100 mL have been judged fatal.

Since cyanide is converted into thiocyanate through the mediation of a hepatic enzyme, rhodanase, NITROPRESS should be used with caution in patients with hepatic insufficiency.

Since thiocyanate inhibits both the uptake and binding of iodine, caution should be exercised in using NITROPRESS in patients with hypothyroidism or severe renal impairment.

Hypertensive patients are more sensitive to the intravenous effect of sodium nitroprusside than are normotensive subjects. Patients who are receiving concomitant antihypertensive medications are more sensitive to the hypotensive effect of sodium nitroprusside and the dosage of NITROPRESS should be adjusted accordingly.

The following warnings apply to use of NITROPRESS for controlled hypotension during anesthesia:

1. Tolerance to blood loss, anemia and hypovolemia may be diminished. If possible, pre-existing anemia and hypovolemia should be corrected prior to employing controlled hypotension.

2. Hypotensive anesthetic techniques may alter pulmonary ventilation perfusion ratio. Patients intolerant of additional dead air space at ordinary oxygen partial pressure may benefit from higher oxygen partial pressure.

3. Extreme caution should be exercised in patients who are especially poor surgical risks (A.S.A. Class 4 and 4E).

NITROPRESS IS ONLY TO BE USED AS AN INFUSION WITH 5% DEXTROSE INJECTION. NOT FOR DIRECT INJECTION.

Infusion rates greater than 10 mcg/kg/minute are rarely required. If, at this rate, an adequate reduction in blood pressure is not obtained within 10 minutes, administration of NITROPRESS (sterile sodium nitroprusside) should be stopped.

PRECAUTIONS

General: Adequate facilities, equipment and personnel should be available for frequent and vigilant monitoring of blood pressure, since the hypotensive effect of NITROPRESS occurs rapidly.

When the infusion is slowed or stopped, blood pressure usually begins to rise immediately and returns to pretreatment levels within one to ten minutes. It should be used with caution and initially in low doses in elderly patients, since they may be more sensitive to the hypotensive effects of the drug. Young, vigorous males may require somewhat larger than ordinary doses of sodium nitroprusside for hypotensive anesthesia; however, the infusion rate of 10 mcg/kg/minute should not be exceeded. Deepening of anesthesia, if indicated, might permit satisfactory conditions to exist within the recommended dosage range.

Because of the rapid onset of action and potency of NITROPRESS, it should preferably be administered with the use of an infusion pump, micro-drip regulator, or any similar device that would allow precise measurement of the flow rate. Once dissolved in solution. NITROPRESS tends to deteriorate in the presence of light. Therefore, it must be protected from light by covering the container of the prepared solution with the light-protective sleeve supplied with the product, or aluminum foil, or other opaque materials. If properly protected from light, the freshly reconstituted and diluted solution is stable for 24 hours.

NITROPRESS in aqueous solution yields the nitroprusside ion which reacts with even minute quantities of a wide variety of inorganic and organic substances to form usually highly colored reaction products (blue, green or dark red). If this occurs, the infusion should be replaced.

Drug Interactions: The hypotensive effect of sodium nitroprusside is augmented by ganglionic blocking agents. Volatile liquid anesthetics (such as halothane and enflurane) also augment the hypotensive effect. Most other circulatory depressants will augment the hypotensive effect of sodium nitroprusside.

Continued on next page

Abbott—Cont.

Carcinogenesis: No data are available on long-term potential for carcinogenicity in animals or humans for sodium nitroprusside.

Usage During Pregnancy: Pregnancy Category C. Animal reproduction studies have not been conducted with NITROPRESS. It is also not known whether NITROPRESS (sterile sodium nitroprusside) can cause fetal harm when administered to a pregnant woman or can affect reproduction capacity. NITROPRESS should be given to a pregnant woman only if clearly needed.

Nursing Mothers: It is not known whether this drug is excreted in human milk. Because many drugs are excreted in human milk, caution should be exercised when NITROPRESS is administered to a nursing woman.

ADVERSE REACTIONS

Nausea, retching, diaphoresis, apprehension, headache, restlessness, muscle twitching, retrosternal discomfort, palpitations, dizziness and abdominal pain have been noted with too rapid reduction in blood pressure, but these symptoms rapidly disappeared with slowing of the rate of the infusion and did not reappear with continued slower rate of administration. Irritation at the infusion site may occur.

Other adverse reactions reported are:

Cardiovascular:
Bradycardia, electrocardiographic changes, tachycardia.

Dermatologic:
Rash.

Hematologic:
Methemoglobinemia.

Neurologic:
Raised intracranial pressure.

Miscellaneous:
Flushing, venous streaking, irritation at the infusion site. One case of hypothyroidism following prolonged therapy with intravenous sodium nitroprusside has been reported. A patient with severe hypertension with uremia received 3900 mg of sodium nitroprusside intravenously over a period of 21 days. This is one of the longest reported intravenous uses of this agent. There was no tachyphylaxis, but the patient developed evidence of hypothyroidism, together with retention of thiocyanate (9.5 mg/100 mL). With peritoneal dialysis the thiocyanate level diminished and the signs of hypothyroidism subsided.

OVERDOSAGE

The first signs of sodium nitroprusside overdosage are those of profound hypotension. As with instances of depletion of thiosulfate supplies, overdosage may lead to cyanide toxicity. Metabolic acidosis and increasing tolerance to the drug are early indications of overdosage. These may be associated with or followed by dyspnea, headache, vomiting, dizziness, ataxia and loss of consciousness. Sodium nitroprusside should then be immediately discontinued. Other signs of cyanide poisoning are coma, imperceptible pulse, absent reflexes, widely dilated pupils, pink color, distant heart sounds, and shallow breathing. Oxygen alone will not provide relief. Nitrites should be administered to induce methemoglobin formation. Methemoglobin, in turn, combines with cyanide bound to cytochrome oxidase to liberate cytochrome oxidase and form a non-toxic complex, cyanmethemoglobin. Cyanide then gradually dissociates from the latter and is converted by administration of thiosulfate to sodium thiocyanate in the presence of rhodanase.

Treatment: In cases of massive overdosage when signs of cyanide toxicity are present use the following regimen:
1. Discontinue administration of NITROPRESS.
2. Administer amyl nitrite inhalations for 15 to 30 seconds each minute until 3% sodium nitrite solution can be prepared for I.V. administration.
3. Sodium nitrite 3% solution should be injected intravenously at a rate not exceeding 2.5 to 5 mL/minute up to a total dose of 10 to 15 mL with careful monitoring of the blood pressure.
4. Following the above steps, inject sodium thiosulfate intravenously, 12.5 g in 50 mL of 5% dextrose injection over a ten-minute period.
5. Since signs of overdosage may reappear, the patient must be observed for several hours.
6. If signs of overdosage reappear, sodium nitrite and sodium thiosulfate injections are repeated in one-half of the above doses.
7. During the administration of nitrites and later when thiocyanate formation is taking place, blood pressure may drop but can be corrected with vasopressor agents.

The acute toxicity of NITROPRESS is as follows:

Species	Route	LD$_{50}$ ± S.E. (mg/kg)
Mouse	I.V.	8.4 ± 0.3
Rat	I.V.	11.2 ± 1.1
Rabbit	I.V.	2.8 ± 1.1
Dog	I.V.	5

DOSAGE AND ADMINISTRATION

Reconstitution Directions for Univial:
1. Remove protective cap.
   Turn plunger-stopper a quarter turn and press to force sterile water for injection into lower chamber.
2. Shake gently to effect solution.
   Use only a clear solution.
3. Sterilize top of stopper with a suitable germicide.
4. Insert needle through the center of stopper until tip is barely visible. Withdraw dose.

Reconstitution Directions for Fliptop Vial: Dissolve the contents of the Fliptop Vial with 2.3 mL of 5% Dextrose Injection, USP. No other diluent should be used.

Depending on the desired concentration, 2.0 mL (50 mg) of the reconstituted solution should be diluted in 250 to 1000 mL of 5% dextrose injection and promptly covered with light-protective sleeve supplied with the product, or aluminum foil, or other opaque materials to protect from light. *If properly protected from light, the freshly reconstituted and diluted solution is stable for 24 hours.* The freshly prepared solution for infusion has a very faint brownish tint. If it is highly colored, it should be discarded (see PRECAUTIONS). *The infusion fluid used for the administration of NITROPRESS should not be employed as a vehicle for simultaneous administration of any other drug.*

In patients who are not receiving antihypertensive drugs, the average dose of NITROPRESS (sterile sodium nitroprusside) for both adults and children is 3 mcg/kg/minute (range of 0.5 to 10 mcg/kg/minute). Usually, at 3 mcg/kg/minute, blood pressure can be lowered by about 30 to 40% below the pretreatment diastolic levels and maintained. In hypertensive patients receiving concomitant antihypertensive medications, smaller doses are required. In order to avoid excessive levels of thiocyanate and lessen the possibility of a precipitous drop in blood pressure, infusion rates greater than 10 mcg/kg/minute should rarely be used. If, at this rate, an adequate reduction of blood pressure is not obtained within 10 minutes, administration of NITROPRESS should be stopped.

One vial (50 mg) NITROPRESS in 1000 mL of 5% dextrose injection provides a concentration of 50 mcg/mL.
One vial (50 mg) NITROPRESS in 500 mL of 5% dextrose injection provides a concentration of 100 mcg/mL.
One vial (50 mg) NITROPRESS in 250 mL of 5% dextrose injection provides a concentration of 200 mcg/mL.

Dose	mcg/kg/min.
Average	3
Range	0.5 to 10

The intravenous infusion of NITROPRESS should be administered by an infusion pump, micro-drip regulator or any similar device that will allow precise measurement of the flow rate. Care should be taken to avoid extravasation. The rate of administration should be adjusted to maintain the desired antihypertensive or hypotensive effect, as determined by frequent blood pressure determinations. It is recommended that the blood pressure should not be allowed to drop at a too rapid rate and the systolic pressure not be lowered below 60 mmHg. In hypertensive emergencies NITROPRESS infusion may be continued until the patient can safely be treated with oral antihypertensive medications.

Parenteral drug products should be inspected visually for particulate matter and discoloration prior to administration, whenever solution and container permit.

HOW SUPPLIED

NITROPRESS (sterile sodium nitroprusside, USP) is supplied in the following amber-colored, single-dose containers:

List No.	Single-Dose Containers
3019	50 mg/2 mL Univial
3219	50 mg/2 mL Fliptop Vial

Exposure of pharmaceutical products to heat should be minimized. Avoid excessive heat. Protect from freezing. It is recommended that the product be stored at room temperature (25°C); however, brief exposure up to 40°C does not adversely affect the product.
Protect from light—store in carton until use.

Caution: Federal (USA) law prohibits dispensing without prescription.

Univial®—Sterile two-compartment vial, Abbott.

Abbott Laboratories
North Chicago, IL 60064
Ref. 01-2399-R-7 Rev. March, 1987

NORISODRINE® AEROTROL®   ℞
[no-ris 'o-drene air 'ō-trol]
**(isoproterenol hydrochloride inhalation aerosol, USP)
In a Controlled-Dose Nebulizer**

DESCRIPTION

Isoproterenol HCl 0.25% w/w (=2.8 mg/ml) in inert chlorofluorohydrocarbon propellants; alcohol 33%; ascorbic acid 0.1% as preservative; and artificial and natural flavors. Each depression of the valve delivers approximately 0.12 mg to the patient.

ACTIONS

Isoproterenol is a short-acting sympathomimetic drug. It produces pharmacologic response in the cardiovascular system and on the smooth muscles of the bronchial tree. The drug will prevent or overcome histamine-induced asthma in both experimental animals and man, and is effective when used prophylactically. It is one of the most potent bronchodilators known and can be used in patients who do not respond to the bronchodilating action of epinephrine. Isoproterenol has a cardio-accelerating effect, but its vasoconstricting action is less pronounced than that of epinephrine. Therapeutic doses may produce a slight increase in systolic blood pressure, but a slight decrease in diastolic. Larger doses may cause peripheral vasodilatation in the renal, mesenteric and femoral beds and some patients respond with a decrease in diastolic, but no change in systolic pressure. Such effects are usually of very short duration.

INDICATIONS

For the treatment of bronchospasm associated with acute and chronic bronchial asthma, pulmonary emphysema, bronchitis, and bronchiectasis.

CONTRAINDICATIONS

Use of isoproterenol in patients with pre-existing cardiac arrhythmias associated with tachycardia is contraindicated because the cardiac stimulant effects of the drug may aggravate such disorders.

WARNINGS

Excessive use of an adrenergic aerosol should be discouraged, as it may lose its effectiveness. Occasional patients have been reported to develop severe paradoxical airway resistance with repeated excessive use of isoproterenol inhalation preparations. The cause of this refractory state is unknown. It is advisable that in such instances the use of this preparation be discontinued immediately and alternative therapy instituted, since in the reported cases the patients did not respond to other forms of therapy until the drug was withdrawn.

Deaths have been reported following excessive use of isoproterenol inhalation preparations and the exact cause is unknown. Cardiac arrest was noted in several instances.

PRECAUTIONS

Isoproterenol and epinephrine may be used interchangeably if the patient becomes unresponsive to one or the other but should not be used concurrently. If desired, these drugs may be alternated, provided an interval of at least four hours has elapsed.

As with all sympathomimetic drugs, isoproterenol should be used with great caution in the presence of cardiovascular disorders, including coronary insufficiency, hypertension, hyperthyroidism and diabetes, or when there is a sensitivity to sympathomimetic amines.

Although there has been no evidence of teratogenic effects with this drug, use of any drug in pregnancy, lactation, or in women of childbearing age requires that the potential benefit of the drug be weighed against its possible hazard to the mother and child.

ADVERSE REACTIONS

Only a small percentage of patients experience any side effects following oral inhalation of aerosolized isoproterenol. Overdosage may produce tachycardia with resultant coronary insufficiency, palpitations, vertigo, nausea, tremors, headache, insomnia, central excitation, and blood pressure changes. These reactions are similar to those produced by other sympathomimetic agents.

DOSAGE AND ADMINISTRATION

The usual dose for the relief of dyspnea in the acute episode is 1 to 2 inhalations. Start with one inhalation. If no relief is evident after 2 to 5 minutes, a second inhalation may be taken. For daily maintenance, use 1 to 2 inhalations 4 to 6 times daily, or as directed by the physician. The physician should be careful to instruct the patient in the proper technique of administration so that the number of inhalations per treatment and the frequency of treatment may be titrated to the patient's response.

No more than two inhalations should be taken at any one time, or more than 6 inhalations in any hour during a 24-hour period, unless advised by physician.

DIRECTIONS FOR USE

Before each use, remove dust cap and inspect mouthpiece for foreign objects. Assemble.

1. Breathe out fully. Place mouthpiece well into the mouth, aimed at the back of the throat.
2. As you begin to breathe in deeply, press the vial firmly down into the adapter. This releases one dose. Continue to breathe in until your lungs are completely filled.
3. Remove from mouth. Hold your breath for several seconds, then breathe out slowly.
4. Replace dust cap after each use.

WARNING

Do not exceed the dose prescribed by your physician. If difficulty in breathing persists, contact your physician immediately.

HOW SUPPLIED

NORISODRINE AEROTROL (isoproterenol hydrochloride inhalation aerosol, USP), 0.25% w/w, is supplied in a 15 ml controlled-dose nebulizer (**NDC** 0074-6869-03).
Manufactured for
Abbott Laboratories
North Chicago, IL 60064
Ref. 01-2403-R-4

NORISODRINE® WITH CALCIUM IODIDE SYRUP   R

[nō-rĭ 'sō-drēn]
(isoproterenol sulfate and calcium iodide)

HOW SUPPLIED

Each teaspoonful of NORISODRINE WITH CALCIUM IODIDE SYRUP contains 3 mg of isoproterenol sulfate, 150 mg of anhydrous calcium iodide. Norisodrine with Calcium Iodide Syrup is supplied in pint (**NDC** 0074-6953-01) bottles.
Inactive Ingredients: Alcohol 6%, ascorbic acid, caramel coloring, glycerin, liquid glucose, sucrose, water, artificial flavors and other ingredients forming a palatable, aromatic syrup.
Abbott Laboratories
North Chicago, IL 60064
Ref. 07-5699-5/R33

OGEN®   R
(estropipate tablets, USP)
(estropipate vaginal cream, USP)

PRODUCT OVERVIEW

KEY FACTS

OGEN is a natural estrogenic substance prepared from purified crystalline estrone. It is appreciably water soluble and has almost no odor or taste. Ogen is available as tablets for oral administration containing 0.75 mg (OGEN .625), 1.5 mg (OGEN 1.25), 3 mg (OGEN 2.5), and 6 mg (OGEN 5) estropipate. OGEN is also available as OGEN Vaginal Cream containing 1.5 mg estropipate per gram.

MAJOR USES

OGEN tablets are indicated for the treatment of estrogen deficiency associated with moderate to severe vasomotor symptoms of the menopause, atrophic vaginitis, kraurosis vulvae, female hypogonadism, female castration, and primary ovarian failure. OGEN should be administered cyclically, either alone or in conjunction with a progestin. The lowest effective dose that will control symptoms and is appropriate for the specific indication should be prescribed.

SAFETY INFORMATION

Estrogens are contraindicated in women with known or suspected cancer of the breast and known or suspected estrogen-dependant neoplasia and in pregnant women and women who may become pregnant (due to the possibility of harm to the fetus). Other contraindications to estrogen therapy include: undiagnosed abnormal genital bleeding, active thrombophlebitis or thromboembolic disorders or a past history of thrombophlebitis, thrombosis, or thromboembolic disorders associated with previous estrogen use. Because estrogens have been reported to increase the risk of endometrial carcinoma in humans, close clinical surveillance of all women taking estrogens is important.

PRODUCT ILLUSTRATION

625 mg

1.25 mg

2.5 mg

5 mg

PRESCRIBING INFORMATION
OGEN®   R
[ō 'gên]
(estropipate tablets, USP)
(estropipate vaginal cream, USP)

WARNING

1. ESTROGENS HAVE BEEN REPORTED TO INCREASE THE RISK OF ENDOMETRIAL CARCINOMA.
Three independent case control studies have shown an increased risk of endometrial cancer in postmenopausal women exposed to exogenous estrogens for prolonged periods.[1-3] This risk was independent of the other known risk factors for endometrial cancer. These studies are further supported by the finding that incidence rates of endometrial cancer have increased sharply since 1969 in eight different areas of the United States with population-based cancer reporting systems, an increase which may be related to the rapidly expanding use of estrogens during the last decade.[4]
The three case control studies reported that the risk of endometrial cancer in estrogen users was about 4.5 to 13.9 times greater than in nonusers. The risk appears to depend on both duration of treatment[1] and on estrogen dose.[3] In view of these findings, when estrogens are used for the treatment of menopausal symptoms, the lowest dose that will control symptoms should be utilized and medication should be discontinued as soon as possible. When prolonged treatment is medically indicated, the patient should be reassessed on at least a semiannual basis to determine the need for continued therapy. Although the evidence must be considered preliminary, one study suggests that cyclic administration of low doses of estrogen may carry less risk than continuous administration;[3] it therefore appears prudent to utilize such a regimen.
Close clinical surveillance of all women taking estrogens is important. In all cases of undiagnosed persistent or recurring abnormal vaginal bleeding, adequate diagnostic measures should be undertaken to rule out malignancy.
There is no evidence at present that "natural" estrogens are more or less hazardous than "synthetic" estrogens at equiestrogenic doses.
2. OGEN SHOULD NOT BE USED DURING PREGNANCY.
According to some investigators, the use of female sex hormones, both estrogens and progestogens, during early pregnancy may seriously damage the offspring. Studies have reported that females exposed in utero to diethylstilbestrol, a non-steroidal estrogen, have an increased risk of developing in later life a form of vaginal or cervical cancer that is ordinarily extremely rare.[5,6] In one of these studies, this risk was estimated as not greater than 4 per 1000 exposures.[7] Furthermore, there are reports that a high percentage of such exposed women (from 30 to 90 percent) have been found to have vaginal adenosis,[8-12] epithelial changes of the vagina and cervix. Although these reported changes are histologically benign, the investigators have not determined whether they are precursors of adenocarcinoma.
Several reports suggest an association between intrauterine exposure to female sex hormones and congenital anomalies in the offspring, including heart defects and limb reduction defects.[13-16] One case control study[16] estimated a 4.7 fold increased risk of limb reduction defects in infants exposed in utero to sex hormones (oral contraceptives, hormone withdrawal tests for pregnancy, or attempted treatment for threatened abortion). Some of these exposures were very short and involved only a few days of treatment. The data suggest that the risk of limb reduction defects in exposed fetuses is somewhat less than 1 per 1000.
In the past, female sex hormones have been used during pregnancy in an attempt to treat threatened or habitual abortion. OGEN is not intended for these uses nor has it been studied for these uses, and therefore should not be used during pregnancy. There is no evidence from well controlled studies that progestogens are effective for these uses.
If OGEN (estropipate) is used during pregnancy, or if the patient becomes pregnant while taking the tablets or using the vaginal cream, she should be apprised of the potential risks to the fetus, and the question of continuation of the pregnancy should be addressed.

DESCRIPTION

OGEN (estropipate), (formerly piperazine estrone sulfate), is a natural estrogenic substance prepared from purified crystalline estrone, solubilized as the sulfate and stabilized with piperazine. It is appreciably soluble in water and has almost no odor or taste. The amount of piperazine in OGEN is not sufficient to exert a pharmacological action. Its addition ensures solubility, stability, and uniform potency of the estrone sulfate. Chemically estropipate is represented by estra 1,3,5(10) -trien-17-one, 3-(sulfooxy)-, compound with piperazine (1:1).
OGEN is available as tablets for oral administration containing either 0.75 mg (OGEN .625), 1.5 mg (OGEN 1.25), 3 mg (OGEN 2.5) or 6 mg (OGEN 5) estropipate.
Each gram of Ogen Vaginal Cream contains 1.5 mg estropipate.
Inactive Ingredients: OGEN .625 tablet: Corn starch, D&C Yellow No. 10, FD&C Yellow No. 6, hydroxypropyl cellulose, lactose, methylparaben, piperazine, propylparaben, stearic acid and talc.
OGEN 1.25 tablet: Corn starch, FD&C Yellow No. 6, hydroxypropyl cellulose, lactose, methylparaben, piperazine, propylparaben, stearic acid and talc.
OGEN 2.5 tablet: Corn starch, FD&C Blue No. 2, hydroxypropyl cellulose, lactose, methylparaben, piperazine, propylparaben, stearic acid and talc.
OGEN 5 tablet: Corn starch, D&C Yellow No. 10, FD&C Blue No. 2, hydroxypropyl cellulose, lactose, methylparaben, piperazine, propylparaben, stearic acid and talc.
The base of OGEN Vaginal Cream is composed of the following ingredients: glycerin, mineral oil, glyceryl monostearate, polyethylene glycol ether complex of higher fatty alcohols, cetyl alcohol, anhydrous lanolin, sodium biphosphate, cis-N-(3-chloroallyl) hexaminium chloride, propylparaben, methylparaben, piperazine hexahydrate, citric acid and water.

CLINICAL PHARMACOLOGY

Estrogens are important in the development and maintenance of the female reproductive system and secondary sex characteristics. They promote growth and development of the vagina, uterus, and fallopian tubes, and enlargement of the breasts. Indirectly, they contribute to the shaping of the skeleton, maintenance of tone and elasticity of urogenital structures, changes in the epiphyses of the long bones that allow for the pubertal growth spurt and its termination, growth of axillary and pubic hair, and pigmentation of the nipples and genitals. Along with other hormones such as progesterone, estrogens are intricately involved in the process of menstruation. Estrogens also affect the release of pituitary gonadotropins.
OGEN (estropipate) owes its therapeutic action to estrone, one of the three principal estrogenic steroid hormones of man: estradiol, estrone, and estriol. Estradiol is rapidly hydrolyzed in the body to estrone, which in turn may be hydrated to the less active estriol. These transformations occur readily, mainly in the liver, where there is also free interconversion between estrone and estradiol.
A depletion of endogenous estrogens occurs postmenopausally as a result of a decline in ovarian function, and may cause symptomatic vulvovaginal atrophy. The signs and symptoms of these atrophic changes in the vaginal and vulval epithelia may be alleviated by the topical application of an estrogenic hormone such as OGEN.
Gastrointestinal absorption of orally administered estrogens is usually prompt and complete. OGEN Vaginal Cream may be absorbed transmucosally and may produce systemic estrogenic effects. Inactivation of estrogens in the body occurs mainly in the liver. During cyclic passage through the liver, estrogens are degraded to less active estrogenic compounds and conjugated with sulfuric and glucuronic acids. Estrone is 50–80% bound to protein as it circulates in the blood, primarily as a conjugate with sulfate.

INDICATIONS AND USAGE

The cyclic administration (See "DOSAGE AND ADMINISTRATION" section) of OGEN Tablets is indicated for the treatment of estrogen deficiency associated with:
1. Moderate to severe *vasomotor* symptoms of menopause. (There is no evidence that estrogens are effective for nervous symptoms or depression which might occur during menopause, and they should not be used to treat these conditions.)
2. Atrophic vaginitis.
3. Kraurosis vulvae.
4. Female hypogonadism.
5. Female castration.
6. Primary ovarian failure.
The cyclic administration of OGEN Vaginal Cream is indicated for the treatment of atrophic vaginitis or kraurosis vulvae. (See "DOSAGE AND ADMINISTRATION" section.)

Continued on next page

Abbott—Cont.

OGEN (ESTROPIPATE) HAS NOT BEEN TESTED FOR EFFICACY FOR ANY PURPOSE DURING PREGNANCY. SINCE ITS EFFECT UPON THE FETUS IS UNKNOWN, IT CANNOT BE RECOMMENDED FOR ANY CONDITION DURING PREGNANCY (SEE BOXED WARNING).

Concomitant Progestin Use: The lowest effective dose appropriate for the specific indication should be utilized. Studies of the addition of a progestin for seven or more days of a cycle of estrogen administration have reported a lowered incidence of endometrial hyperplasia. Morphological and biochemical studies of endometrium suggest that 10 to 13 days of progestin are needed to provide maximal maturation of the endometrium and to eliminate any hyperplastic changes. Whether this will provide protection from endometrial carcinoma has not been clearly established. There are possible additional risks which may be associated with the inclusion of progestin in estrogen replacement regimens. (See "PRECAUTIONS" section.) The choice of progestin and dosage may be important in minimizing these adverse effects.

CONTRAINDICATIONS

OGEN should not be used in women with any of the following conditions:
1. Known or suspected cancer of the breast.
2. Known or suspected estrogen-dependent neoplasia.
3. OGEN may cause fetal harm when administered to a pregnant woman. OGEN is contraindicated in women who are or may become pregnant (See Boxed Warning).
4. Undiagnosed abnormal genital bleeding.
5. Active thrombophlebitis or thromboembolic disorders.
6. A past history of thrombophlebitis, thrombosis, or thromboembolic disorders associated with previous estrogen use.
OGEN Vaginal Cream is contraindicated in patient's hypersensitive to its ingredients.

WARNINGS

1. *Induction of malignant neoplasms.* Long-term continuous administration of natural and synthetic estrogens in certain animal species has been reported by some investigators to increase the frequency of carcinomas of the breast, cervix, vagina, and liver. There is now evidence that estrogens increase the risk of carcinoma of the endometrium in humans. (See Boxed Warning).

At the present time there is no conclusive evidence that estrogens given to postmenopausal women increase the risk of cancer of the breast.[17,40,41] There are, however, a few retrospective studies which suggest a small but statistically significant increase in the risk factor for breast cancer among these women.[18,42–44] Therefore, caution should be exercised when administering estrogens to women with a strong family history of breast cancer or who have breast nodules, fibrocystic disease, or abnormal mammograms. Careful breast examinations should be performed periodically.

2. *Gallbladder disease.* A recent study has reported a 2 to 3-fold increase in the risk of surgically confirmed gallbladder disease in women receiving postmenopausal estrogens,[17] similar to the 2-fold increase previously noted in users of oral contraceptives.[19,22] In the case of oral contraceptives, the increased risk appeared after two years of use.[22]

3. *Effects similar to those caused by estrogen-progestogen oral contraceptives.* There are several serious adverse effects of oral contraceptives, most of which have not, up to now, been documented as consequences of postmenopausal estrogen therapy. This may reflect the comparatively low doses of estrogen used in postmenopausal women. It would be expected that the larger doses of estrogen used to treat postpartum breast engorgement would be more likely to result in these adverse effects, and, in fact, it has been shown that there is an increased risk of thrombosis in women receiving estrogens for postpartum breast engorgement.[20,21]

a. *Thromboembolic disease.* It is now well established that users of oral contraceptives have an increased risk of various thromboembolic and thrombotic vascular diseases, such as thrombophlebitis, pulmonary embolism, stroke, and myocardial infarction.[22–29] Cases of retinal thrombosis, mesenteric thrombosis, and optic neuritis have been reported in oral contraceptive users. There is evidence that the risk of several of these adverse reactions is related to the dose of the drug.[30,31] An increased risk of post-surgery thromboembolic complications has also been reported in users of oral contraceptives.[32,33] If feasible, estrogen should be discontinued at least 4 weeks before surgery of the type associated with an increased risk of thromboembolism; it should also be discontinued during periods of prolonged immobilization.

While an increased rate of thromboembolic and thrombotic disease in postmenopausal users of estrogens has not been found[17,34] this does not rule out the possibility that such an increase may be present or that subgroups of women who have underlying risk factors or who are receiving relatively large doses of estrogens may have increased risk. Therefore estrogens should not be used in persons with active thrombophlebitis or thromboembolic disorders, and they should not

be used in persons with a history of such disorders in association with estrogen use. They should be used with caution in patients with cerebral vascular or coronary artery disease and only for those in whom estrogens are clearly needed. Large doses of estrogen (5 mg conjugated estrogens per day), comparable to those used to treat cancer of the prostate and breast, have been shown in a large prospective clinical trial in men[35] to increase the risk of nonfatal myocardial infarction, pulmonary embolism and thrombophlebitis. When estrogen doses of this size are used, any of the thromboembolic and thrombotic adverse effects associated with oral contraceptive use should be considered a clear risk.

b. *Hepatic adenoma.* Benign hepatic adenomas appear to be associated with the use of oral contraceptives.[36–38] Although benign, and rare, these may rupture and cause death through intraabdominal hemorrhage. Such lesions have not yet been reported in association with other estrogen or progestogen preparations but should be considered in estrogen users having abdominal pain and tenderness, abdominal mass, or hypovolemic shock. Hepatocellular carcinoma has also been reported in women taking estrogen-containing oral contraceptives.[37] The relationship of this malignancy to these drugs is not known at this time.

c. *Elevated blood pressure.* Increased blood pressure is not uncommon in women using oral contraceptives. There is now a report that this may occur with use of estrogens in the menopause[39] and blood pressure should be monitored with estrogen use, especially if high doses are used.

d. *Glucose tolerance.* A worsening of glucose tolerance has been observed in a significant percentage of patients on estrogen-containing oral contraceptives. For this reason, diabetic patients should be carefully observed while receiving estrogen.

4. *Hypercalcemia.* Administration of estrogens may lead to severe hypercalcemia in patients with breast cancer and bone metastases. If this occurs, the drug should be stopped and appropriate measures taken to reduce the serum calcium level.

PRECAUTIONS

A. General Precautions.

1. A complete medical and family history should be taken prior to the initiation of any estrogen therapy. The pretreatment and periodic physical examinations should include special reference to blood pressure, breasts, abdomen, and pelvic organs, and should include a Papanicolau smear. As a general rule, estrogen should not be prescribed for longer than one year without another physical examination being performed.

2. Diagnostic measures should be taken to rule out gonorrhea or neoplasia before prescribing OGEN Vaginal Cream. Trichomonal, monilial, or bacterial infection should be treated by appropriate anti-microbial therapy.

3. Fluid retention—Estrogens may cause some degree of fluid retention. Therefore, patients with conditions such as epilepsy, migraine, and cardiac or renal dysfunction, which might be influenced by this factor, require careful observation.

4. Certain patients may develop undesirable manifestations of excessive estrogenic stimulation, such as abnormal or excessive uterine bleeding, mastodynia, etc.

5. Oral contraceptives appear to be associated with an increased incidence of mental depression.[22] Although it is not clear whether this is due to the estrogenic or progestogenic component of the contraceptive, patients with a history of depression should be carefully observed.

6. Preexisting uterine leiomyomata may increase in size during estrogen use.

7. The pathologist should be advised of the patient's use of estrogen therapy when relevant specimens are submitted.

8. Patients with a past history of jaundice during pregnancy have an increased risk of recurrence of jaundice while receiving estrogen-containing oral contraceptive therapy. If jaundice develops in any patient receiving estrogen, the medication should be discontinued while the cause is investigated.

9. Estrogens may be poorly metabolized in patients with impaired liver function and they should be administered with caution in such patients.

10. Because estrogens influence the metabolism of calcium and phosphorus, they should be used with caution in patients with metabolic bone diseases that are associated with hypercalcemia or in patients with renal insufficiency.

11. Concomitant Progestin Use: The lowest effective dose appropriate for the specific indication should be utilized. Studies of the addition of a progestin for seven or more days of a cycle of estrogen administration have reported a lowered incidence of endometrial hyperplasia. Morphological and biochemical studies of endometrium suggest that 10 to 13 days of progestin are needed to provide maximal maturation of the endometrium and to eliminate any hyperplastic changes. Whether this will provide protection from endometrial carcinoma has not been clearly established. There are possible additional risks which may be associated with the inclusion of progestin in estrogen replacement regimens. The potential risks may include adverse effects on carbohy-

drate and lipid metabolism. The choice of progestin and dosage may be important in minimizing these adverse effects.

B. Information for the Patient. See text of Patient Package Insert which appears after PHYSICIAN REFERENCES.

C. Drug Interactions. The concomitant use of any drugs which can induce hepatic microsomal enzymes with estrogens may produce estrogen levels which are lower than would be expected from the dose of estrogen administered. The use of *broad spectrum antibiotics* which profoundly effect intestinal flora may influence the oral absorption of steroidal compounds including the estrogens.

Diabetics receiving *insulin* may have increased insulin requirements when receiving estrogens.

Laboratory Test Interference. Certain endocrine and liver function tests may be affected by estrogen-containing oral contraceptives. The following similar changes may be expected with larger doses of estrogen:

a. Increased sulfobromophthalein retention.

b. Increased prothrombin and factors VII, VIII, IX, and X; decreased antithrombin 3; increased norepinephrine-induced platelet aggregability.

c. Increased thyroid binding globulin (TBG) leading to increased circulating total thyroid hormone, as measured by PBI, T4 by column, or T4 by radioimmunoassay. Free T3 resin uptake is decreased, reflecting the elevated TBG; free T4 concentration is unaltered.

d. Abnormal glucose tolerance test results.

e. Decreased pregnanediol excretion.

f. Reduced response to metyrapone test.

g. Reduced serum folate concentration.

h. Increased serum triglyceride and phospholipid concentration.

D. Carcinogenesis. Studies have shown an increased risk of endometrial cancer in postmenopausal women exposed to exogenous estrogens for prolonged periods (see Boxed Warning). At the present time there is no conclusive evidence that estrogens given to postmenopausal women increase the risk of cancer of the breast.[17,40,41] There are, however, a few retrospective studies which suggest a small but statistically significant increase in the risk factor for breast cancer among these women.[18,42–44] (See "WARNINGS" section.)

E. Pregnancy. Pregnancy Category X. See "CONTRAINDICATIONS" section and Boxed Warning.

F. Nursing Mothers. Estrogens have been reported to be excreted in human breast milk. Caution should be excercised when OGEN (estropipate) is administered to a nursing woman.

G. Pediatric Use. Because of the effects of estrogens on epiphyseal closure, they should be used judiciously in young patients in whom bone growth is not complete.

ADVERSE REACTIONS

Hypersensitivity reactions, systemic effects such as breast tenderness, and rarely, withdrawal bleeding, have occurred with the use of topical estrogens. Local irritation (especially when prior inflammation is present) has occurred at initiation of therapy.

(See Warnings regarding reports of possible induction of neoplasia, unknown effects upon the fetus, increased incidence of gallbladder disease, and adverse effects similar to those of oral contraceptives, including thromboembolism.) The following additional adverse reactions in decreasing order of severity within each category have been reported with estrogenic therapy, including oral contraceptives:

1. *Genitourinary system.*
Increase in size of uterine fibromyomata.
Vaginal candidiasis.
Cystitis-like syndrome.
Dysmenorrhea.
Amenorrhea during and after treatment.
Change in cervical eversion and in degree of cervical secretion.
Breakthrough bleeding, spotting, change in menstrual flow.
Premenstrual-like syndrome.
2. *Breast.*
Tenderness, enlargement, secretion.
3. *Gastrointestinal.*
Cholestatic jaundice.
Vomiting, nausea.
Abdominal cramps, bloating.
4. *Skin.*
Hemorrhagic eruption.
Erythema nodosum.
Erythema multiforme.
Hirsutism.
Chloasma or melasma which may persist when drug is discontinued.
Loss of scalp hair.
5. *Eyes.*
Steepening of corneal curvature.
Intolerance to contact lenses.
6. *CNS.*
Chorea.
Mental depression.
Migraine, dizziness, headache.

7. *Miscellaneous.*
Aggravation of porphyria.
Edema.
Reduced carbohydrate tolerance.
Increase or decrease in weight.
Changes in libido.

OVERDOSAGE

Numerous reports of ingestion of large doses of estrogen-containing oral contraceptives by young children indicate that serious ill effects do not occur. Overdosage of estrogen may cause nausea and withdrawal bleeding may occur in females.

DOSAGE AND ADMINISTRATION

OGEN (estropipate) Tablets:
1. *Given cyclically for short-term use:*
For treatment of moderate to severe *vasomotor* symptoms, atrophic vaginitis, or kraurosis vulvae associated with the menopause.
The lowest dose that will control symptoms should be chosen and medication should be discontinued as promptly as possible.
Administration should be cyclic (e.g., 3 weeks on and 1 week off).
Attempts to discontinue or taper medication should be made at 3 to 6 month intervals.
Usual dosage ranges:
Vasomotor symptoms—One OGEN .625 (estropipate) Tablet to one OGEN 5 Tablet per day. The lowest dose that will control symptoms should be chosen. If the patient has not menstruated within the last two months or more, cyclic administration is started arbitrarily. If the patient is menstruating, cyclic administration is started on day 5 of bleeding.
Atrophic vaginitis and kraurosis vulvae—One OGEN .625 Tablet to one OGEN 5 Tablet daily, depending upon the tissue response of the individual patient. The lowest dose that will control symptoms should be chosen. Administer cyclically.
2. *Given cyclically:*
Female hypogonadism; female castration; primary ovarian failure.
Usual dosage ranges:
Female hypogonadism—A daily dose of one OGEN 1.25 Tablet to three OGEN 2.5 Tablets may be given for the first three weeks of a theoretical cycle, followed by a rest period of eight to ten days. The lowest dose that will control symptoms should be chosen. If bleeding does not occur by the end of this period, the same dosage schedule is repeated. The number of courses of estrogen therapy necessary to produce bleeding may vary depending on the responsiveness of the endometrium. If satisfactory withdrawal bleeding does not occur, an oral progestogen may be given in addition to estrogen during the third week of the cycle.
Female castration and primary ovarian failure—A daily dose of one OGEN 1.25 Tablet to three OGEN 2.5 Tablets may be given for the first three weeks of a theoretical cycle, followed by a rest period of eight to ten days. Adjust dosage upward or downward according to severity of symptoms and response of the patient. For maintenance, adjust dosage to lowest level that will provide effective control.
Treated patients with an intact uterus should be monitored closely for signs of endometrial cancer and appropriate diagnostic measures should be taken to rule out malignancy in the event of persistent or recurring abnormal vaginal bleeding.
OGEN (estropipate) Vaginal Cream:
To be administered cyclically for short-term use only:
For treatment of atrophic vaginitis or kraurosis vulvae.
The lowest dose that will control symptoms should be chosen and medication should be discontinued as promptly as possible.
Administration should be cyclic (e.g., three weeks on and one week off).
Attempts to discontinue or taper medication should be made at three to six-month intervals.
Treated patients with an intact uterus should be monitored closely for signs of endometrial cancer and appropriate diagnostic measures should be taken to rule out malignancy in the event of persistent or recurring abnormal vaginal bleeding.
Usual dosage: Intravaginally, 2 to 4 grams of OGEN Vaginal Cream daily, depending upon the severity of the condition. The following instructions for use are intended for the patient and are printed on the carton label for OGEN Vaginal Cream (estropipate).
1. Remove cap from tube.
2. Make sure plunger of applicator is all the way into the barrel.
3. Screw nozzle end of applicator onto the tube.
4. Squeeze tube to force sufficient cream into applicator so that number on plunger indicating prescribed dose is level with top of barrel.
5. Unscrew applicator from tube and replace cap on tube.
6. To deliver medication, insert end of applicator into vagina and push plunger all the way down.
Between uses, pull plunger out of barrel and wash applicator in warm, soapy water. DO NOT PUT APPLICATOR IN HOT OR BOILING WATER.

HOW SUPPLIED

OGEN (estropipate tablets, USP) is supplied as OGEN .625 (0.75 mg estropipate), yellow tablets, **NDC** 0074-3943-04; OGEN 1.25 (1.5 mg estropipate), peach-colored tablets, **NDC** 0074-3946-04; OGEN 2.5 (3 mg estropipate), blue tablets, **NDC** 0074-3951-04; and OGEN 5 (6 mg estropipate), light green tablets, **NDC** 0074-3958-13. Tablets of all four dosage levels are standardized to provide uniform estrone activity and are grooved (Divide-Tab®) to provide dosage flexibility. All tablet sizes of OGEN are available in bottles of 100.
Store tablets below 77°F (25°C).
OGEN (estropipate vaginal cream, USP), 1.5 mg estropipate per gram, is available in packages containing a 1½ oz (42.5 Gm) tube with one plastic applicator calibrated at 1, 2, 3, and 4 Gm levels. (NDC 0074-2467-42).

PHYSICIAN REFERENCES

[1]Ziel, H. K., Finkel, W. D., "Increased Risk of Endometrial Carcinoma Among Users of Conjugated Estrogens", *New England-Journal of Medicine*, 293:1167–1170, 1975.
[2]Smith, D. C., Prentic, R., Thompson, D. J., et al., "Association of Exogenous Estrogen and Endometrial Carcinoma," *New England Journal of Medicine*, 293:1164–1167, 1975.
[3]Mack, T. M., Pike, M. C., Henderson, B. E., et al., "Estrogens and Endometrial Cancer in a Retirement Community," *New England Journal of Medicine*, 294:1262–1267, 1976.
[4]Weiss, N. S., Szekely, D. R., Austin, D. F., "Increasing Incidence of Endometrial Cancer in the United States," *New England Journal of Medicine*, 294:1259–1262, 1976.
[5]Herbst, A. L., Ulfelder, H., Poskanzer, D. C., "Adenocarcinoma of Vagina," *New England Journal of Medicine*, 284:878–881, 1971.
[6]Greenwald, P., Barlow, J., Nasca, P., et al., "Vaginal Cancer after Maternal Treatment with Synthetic Estrogens," *New England Journal of Medicine*, 285:390–392, 1971.
[7]Lanier, A., Noller, K., Decker, D., et al., "Cancer and Stilbestrol. A Follow-up of 1719 Persons Exposed to Estrogens In Utero and Born 1943–1959," *Mayo Clinic Proceedings*, 48:793–799, 1973.
[8]Herbst, A., Kurman, R., Scully, R., "Vaginal and Cervical Abnormalities After Exposure to Stilbestrol In Utero" *Obstetrics and Gynecology*, 40:287–298, 1972.
[9]Herbst, A., Robboy, S., Madonald, G., et al., "The Effects of Local Progesterone on Stilbestrol-Associated Vaginal Adenosis," *American Journal of Obstetrics and Gynecology*, 118:607–615, 1974.
[10]Herbst, A., Poskanzer, D., Robboy, S., et al., "Prenatal Exposure to Stilbestrol, A Prospective Comparison of Exposed Female Offspring with Unexposed Controls," *New England Journal of Medicine*, 292:334–339, 1975.
[11]Stafl, A., Mattingly, R., Foley, D., et al., "Clinical Diagnosis of Vaginal Adenosis," *Obstetrics and Gynecology*, 43:118–128, 1974.
[12]Sherman, A. I., Goldrath, M., Berlin, A., et al., "Cervical-Vaginal Adenosis After In Utero Exposure to Synthetic Estrogens," *Obstetrics and Gynecology*, 44:531–545, 1974.
[13]Gal, I., Kirman, B., Stern, J., "Hormone Pregnancy Tests and Congenital Malformation," *Nature*, 216:83, 1967.
[14]Levy, E. P., Cohen, A., Fraser, F. C., "Hormone Treatment During Pregnancy and Congenital Heart Defects," *Lancet* 1:611, 1973.
[15]Nora, J., Nora, A., "Birth Defects and Oral Contraceptives," *Lancet*, 1:941–942, 1973.
[16]Janerich, D. T., Piper, J. M., Clebatis, D. M., "Oral Contraceptives and Congenital Limb-Reduction Defects," *New England Journal of Medicine*, 291:697–700, 1974.
[17]Boston Collaborative Drug Surveillance Program "Surgically Confirmed Gall Bladder Disease, Venous Thromboembolism and Breast Tumors in Relation to Post-Menopausal Estrogen Therapy," *New England Journal of Medicine*, 290:15–19, 1974.
[18]Brinton, L. A., Hoover, R. N., Szklo, M., et al., "Menopausal Estrogen Use and Risk of Breast Cancer," *Cancer*, 47(10): 2517–2522, 1981.
[19]Boston Collaborative Drug Surveillance Program, "Oral Contraceptives and Venous Thromboembolic Disease, Surgically Confirmed Gall Bladder Disease and Breast Tumors," *Lancet* 1:1399–1404, 1973.
[20]Daniel, D. G., Campbell, H., Turnbull, A. C., "Puerperal Thromboembolism and Suppression of Lactation," *Lancet*, 2:287–289, 1967.
[21]Bailar, J. C., "Thromboembolism and Oestrogen Therapy," *Lancet*, 2:560, 1967.
[22]Royal College of General Practitioners, "Oral Contraception and Thromboembolic Disease," *Journal of the Royal College of General Practitioners*, 13:267–279, 1967.
[23]Inman, W. H. W., Vessey, M. P., "Investigation of Deaths from Pulmonary, Coronary, and Cerebral Thrombosis and Embolism in Women of Child-Bearing Age," *British Medical Journal*, 2:193–199, 1968.
[24]Vessey, M. P., Doll, R., "Investigation of Relation Between Use of Oral Contraceptives and Thromboembolic Disease. A Further Report," *British Medical Journal*, 2:651–657, 1969.
[25]Sartwell, P. E., Masi, A. T., Arthes, F. G., et al., "Thromboembolism and Oral Contraceptives: An Epidemiological Case-Control Study," *American Journal of Epidemiology*, 90:365–380, 1969.
[26]Collaborative Group for the Study of Stroke in Young Women, "Oral Contraception and Increased Risk of Cerebral Ischemia or Thrombosis," *New England Journal of Medicine*, 288:871–878, 1973.
[27]Collaborative Group for the Study of Stroke in Young Women, "Oral Contraceptives and Stroke in Young Women: Associated Risk Factors," *Journal of the American Medical Association*, 231:718–722, 1975.
[28]Mann, J. I., Inman, W. H. W., "Oral Contraceptives and Death from Myocardial Infarction," *British Medical Journal*, 2:245–248, 1975.
[29]Mann, J. I., Vessey, M. P., Thorogood, M., et al., "Myocardial Infarction in Young Women with Special Reference to Oral Contraceptive Practice," *British Medical Journal*, 2:241–245, 1975.
[30]Inman, W. H. W., Vessey, M. P., Westerholm, B., et al., "Thromboembolic Disease and the Steroidal Content of Oral Contraceptives," *British Medical Journal*, 2:203–209, 1970.
[31]Stolley, P. D., Tonascia, J. A., Tockman, M. S., et al., "Thrombosis with Low-Estrogen Oral Contraceptives," *American Journal of Epidemiology*, 102:197–208, 1975.
[32]Vessey, M. P., Doll, R., Fairbairn, A. S., et al., "Post-Operative Thromboembolism and the Use of the Oral Contraceptives," *British Medical Journal*, 3:123–126, 1970.
[33]Greene, G. R., Sartwell, P. E., "Oral Contraceptive Use in Patients with Thromboembolism Following Surgery, Trauma or Infection," *American Journal of Public Health*, 62:680–685, 1972.
[34]Rosenberg, L., Armstrong, M. B., Jick, H., "Myocardial Infarction and Estrogen Therapy in Postmenopausal Women," *New England Journal of Medicine*, 294:1256–1259, 1976.
[35]Coronary Drug Project Research Group, "The Coronary Drug Project: Initial Findings Leading to Modifications of Its Research Protocol," *Journal of the American Medical Association*, 214:1303–1313, 1970.
[36]Baum, J., Holtz, F., Bookstein, J. J., et al., "Possible Association Between Benign Hepatomas and Oral Contraceptives," *Lancet*, 2:926–928, 1973.
[37]Mays, E. T., Christopherson, W. M., Mahr, M. M., et al., "Hepatic Changes in Young Women Ingesting Contraceptive Steroids, Hepatic Hemorrhage and Primary Hepatic Tumors," *Journal of the American Medical Association*, 235:730–732, 1976.
[38]Edmondson, H. A., Henderson, B., Benton, B., "Liver Cell Adenomas Associated with the Use of Oral Contraceptives," *New England Journal of Medicine*, 294:470–472, 1976.
[39]Pfeffer, R. I., Van Den Noort, S., "Estrogen Use and Stroke Risk in Postmenopausal Women," *American Journal of Epidemiology*, 103:445–456, 1976.
[40]Gambrell, R. D., Massey, F. M., Castaneda, T. A., et al., "Estrogen Therapy and Breast Cancer in Postmenopausal Women," *Journal of the American Geriatrics Society*, 28(6): 251–257, 1980.
[41]Kelsey, J. L., Fischer, D. B., Holford, T. R., et al., "Exogenous Estrogens and Other Factors in the Epidemiology of Breast Cancer," *Journal of the National Cancer Institute*, 57(2):327–333, 1981.
[42]Ross, R. K., Paganini-Hill, A., Gerkins, V., et al., "A Case-Control Study of Menopausal Estrogen Therapy and Breast Cancer," *Journal of the American Medical Association*, 243(16):1635–1639, 1980.
[43]Hoover, R., Glass, A., Finkle, W. D., et al., "Conjugated Estrogens and Breast Cancer Risk in Women," *Journal of the National Cancer Institute*, 67(4):815–820, 1981.
[44]Lawson, D. H., Jick, H., Hunter, J. R., et al., "Exogenous Estrogens and Breast Cancer," *American Journal of Epidemiology*, 114(5):710, 1981.

INFORMATION FOR PATIENTS

OGEN®

(estropipate tablets and vaginal cream, USP)
Estrogen cream is used for the local treatment of certain symptoms of estrogen deficiency: the soreness and itching of the vagina and vulva caused by drying and thinning (atrophy) of these tissues.
The discussion that follows is about estrogens that are taken internally for the treatment of symptoms of estrogen deficiency. Some or all of the information below on the systemic use of estrogens may also apply to the estrogen cream.
WHAT YOU SHOULD KNOW ABOUT ESTROGENS: Estrogens are female hormones produced by the ovaries. The ovaries make several different kinds of estrogens. In addition, scientists have been able to make a variety of synthetic estrogens. As far as we know, all these estrogens have similar properties and therefore much the same usefulness, side effects, and risks. This leaflet is intended to help you under-

Continued on next page

Abbott—Cont.

stand what estrogens are used for, the risks involved in their use, and how to use them as safely as possible.

This leaflet includes the most important information about estrogens, but not all the information. If you want to know more, you can ask your doctor or pharmacist to let you read the package insert prepared for the doctor.

Uses of Estrogen: Estrogens are prescribed by doctors for a number of purposes, including:

1. To provide estrogen during a period of adjustment when a woman's ovaries no longer produce it, in order to prevent certain uncomfortable symptoms of estrogen deficiency. (All women normally stop producing estrogens, generally between the ages of 45 and 55; this is called the menopause.)

2. To prevent symptoms of estrogen deficiency when a woman's ovaries have been removed surgically before the natural menopause.

3. To prevent pregnancy. (Estrogens are given along with a progestogen, another female hormone; these combinations are called oral contraceptives or birth control pills. Patient labeling is available to women taking oral contraceptives and they will not be discussed in this leaflet.)

THERE IS NO PROPER USE OF OGEN (ESTROPIPATE) IN A PREGNANT WOMAN.

Estrogens in the Menopause: In the natural course of their lives, all women eventually experience a decrease in estrogen production. This usually occurs between ages 45 and 55 but may occur earlier or later. Sometimes the ovaries may need to be removed before natural menopause by an operation, producing a "surgical menopause."

When the amount of estrogen in the blood begins to decrease, many women may develop typical symptoms: Feelings of warmth in the face, neck, and chest or sudden intense episodes of heat and sweating throughout the body (called "hot flashes" or "hot flushes"). These symptoms are sometimes very uncomfortable. A few women eventually develop changes in the vagina (called "atrophic vaginitis") which cause discomfort, especially during and after intercourse. Estrogens can be prescribed to treat these symptoms of the menopause. It is estimated that considerably more than half of all women undergoing the menopause have only mild symptoms or no symptoms at all and therefore do not need estrogens. Other women may need estrogens for a few months, while their bodies adjust to lower estrogen levels. Sometimes the need will be for periods longer than six months. In an attempt to avoid over-stimulation of the uterus (womb), estrogens are usually given cyclically during each month of use, that is three weeks of pills followed by one week without pills.

Sometimes women experience nervous symptoms or depression during menopause. There is no evidence that estrogens are effective for such symptoms and they should not be used to treat them, although other treatment may be needed.

You may have heard that taking estrogens for long periods (years) after the menopause will keep your skin soft and supple and keep you feeling young. There is no evidence that this is so, however, and such long-term treatment carries important risks.

The Dangers of Estrogens: 1. *Cancer of the uterus.* If estrogens are used in the postmenopausal period for more than a year, there is an increased risk of *endometrial cancer* (cancer of the uterus). Women taking estrogens have roughly 5 to 10 times as great a chance of getting this cancer as women who take no estrogens. To put this another way, while a postmenopausal woman not taking estrogens has 1 chance in 1,000 each year of getting cancer of the uterus, a woman taking estrogens has 5 to 10 chances in 1,000 each year. For this reason *it is important to take estrogens only when you really need them.*

The risk of this cancer is greater the longer estrogens are used and also seems to be greater when larger doses are taken. For this reason *it is important to take the lowest dose of estrogen that will control symptoms and to take it only as long as it is needed.* If estrogens are needed for longer periods of time, your doctor will want to reevaluate your need for estrogens at least every six months.

Women using estrogens should report any irregular vaginal bleeding to their doctors; such bleeding may be of no importance, but it can be an early warning of cancer of the uterus. If you have undiagnosed vaginal bleeding, you should not use estrogens until a diagnosis is made and you are certain there is no cancer of the uterus.

If you have had your uterus completely removed (total hysterectomy), there is no danger of developing cancer of the uterus.

2. *Other possible cancers.* Estrogens can cause development of other tumors in animals, such as tumors of the breast, cervix, vagina, or liver, when given for a long time. At present there is no good evidence that women using estrogen in the menopause have an increased risk of such tumors, but

there is no way yet to be sure they do not; and one study raises the possibility that use of estrogens in the menopause may increase the risk of breast cancer many years later. This is a further reason to use estrogens only when clearly needed. While you are taking estrogens, it is important that you go to your doctor at least once a year for a physical examination. Also, if members of your family have had breast cancer or if you have breast nodules or abnormal mammograms (breast x-rays), your doctor may wish to carry out more frequent examinations of your breasts.

3. *Gallbladder disease.* Women who use estrogens after menopause are more likely to develop gallbladder disease needing surgery than women who do not use estrogens. Birth control pills have a similar effect.

4. *Abnormal blood clotting.* Oral contraceptives increase the risk of blood clotting in various parts of the body. This can result in a stroke (if the clot is in the brain), a heart attack (clot in a blood vessel of the heart), or a pulmonary embolus (a clot which forms in the legs or pelvis, then breaks off and travels to the lungs). Any of these can be fatal.

At this time use of estrogens in the menopause is not known to cause such blood clotting, but this has not been fully studied and there could still prove to be such a risk. It is recommended that if you have had clotting in the legs or lungs or a heart attack or stroke while you were using estrogens or birth control pills, you should not use estrogens. If you have had a stroke or heart attack or if you have angina pectoris, estrogens should be used with great caution and only if clearly needed (for example, if you have severe symptoms of the menopause).

Special Warning About Pregnancy: You should not receive OGEN (estropipate) if you are pregnant. Some scientists have reported that if estrogens are used during pregnancy, there may be a greater than usual chance that the developing baby will be born with a birth defect, although the risk remains small. In addition, other scientists have reported that there is an association between another estrogen-type product (diethylstilbestrol) and appearance of a particular cancer of the vagina or cervix (adenocarcinoma) in young women whose mothers took that drug in pregnancy. Every effort should be made to avoid exposure to OGEN in pregnancy. If exposure occurs, see your doctor.

Other Effects of Estrogens: In addition to the serious known risks of estrogens described above estrogens have the following side effects and potential risks:

1. *Nausea and vomiting.* The most common side effect of estrogen therapy is nausea. Vomiting is less common.

2. *Effects on breasts.* Estrogens may cause breast tenderness or enlargement and may cause the breasts to secrete a liquid. These effects are not dangerous.

3. *Effects on the uterus.* Estrogens may cause benign fibroid tumors of the uterus to get larger.

Some women will have menstrual bleeding when estrogens are stopped. But if the bleeding occurs on days you are still taking estrogens you should report this to your doctor.

4. *Effects on liver.* Women taking oral contraceptives develop on rare occasions a tumor of the liver which can rupture and bleed into the abdomen. So far, these tumors have not been reported in women using estrogens in the menopause, but you should report any swelling or unusual pain or tenderness in the abdomen to your doctor immediately.

Women with a past history of jaundice (yellowing of the skin and white parts of the eyes) may get jaundice again during estrogen use. If this occurs, stop taking estrogens and see your doctor.

5. *Other effects.* Estrogens may cause excess fluid to be retained in the body. This may make some conditions worse, such as epilepsy, migraine, heart disease, or kidney disease.

SUMMARY

Estrogens have important uses, but they have serious risks as well. You must decide, with your doctor, whether the risks are acceptable to you in view of the benefits of treatment. You should not use OGEN (estropipate) if you have cancer of the breast or uterus, are pregnant, have undiagnosed abnormal vaginal bleeding, clotting in the legs or lungs, or have had a stroke, heart attack or angina, or clotting in the legs or lungs in the past while you were taking estrogens.

You can use estrogens as safely as possible by understanding that your doctor will require regular physical examinations while you are taking them and will try to discontinue the drug as soon as possible and use the smallest dose possible. Be alert for signs of trouble including:

1 Abnormal bleeding from the vagina.

2. Pains in the calves or chest or sudden shortness of breath, or coughing blood (indicating possible clots in the legs, heart or lungs).

3. Severe headache, dizziness, faintness, or changes in vision (indicating possible developing clots in the brain or eye).

4. Breast lumps (you should ask your doctor how to examine your own breasts).

5. Jaundice (yellowing of the skin).

6. Mental depression.

Based on his or her assessment of your medical needs, your

doctor has prescribed this drug for you. Do not give the drug to anyone else.

Abbott Laboratories/
Abbott Pharmaceuticals, Inc.
North Chicago, IL 60064
Ref. 03-4358-R13 and 01-2305-R5
Shown in Product Identification Section, page 403

OPTILETS®-500

[ŏp'ti-lets]

High potency multivitamin for use in treatment of multivitamin deficiency.

OPTILETS-M-500®

High potency multivitamin for use in treatment of multivitamin deficiency.
Mineral supplementation added.

(See PDR For Nonprescription Drugs)
Shown in Product Identification Section, page 403

ORETIC®   ℞

[ō-re'tic]

(hydrochlorothiazide tablets, USP)

DESCRIPTION

ORETIC (hydrochlorothiazide) is a member of the benzothiadiazine (thiazide) family of drugs. It is closely related to chlorothiazide. Clinically, ORETIC is an orally active diuretic-antihypertensive agent.

Inactive Ingredients:
25 and 50 mg tablets: corn starch, lactose, magnesium stearate and talc.

ACTIONS

The diuretic and saluretic effects of ORETIC result from a drug-induced inhibition of the renal tubular reabsorption of electrolytes. The excretion of sodium and chloride is greatly enhanced. Potassium excretion is also enhanced to a variable degree, as it is with the other thiazides. Although urinary excretion of bicarbonate is increased slightly, there is usually no significant change in urinary pH. Hydrochlorothiazide has a per mg natriuretic activity approximately 10 times that of the prototype thiazide, chlorothiazide. At maximal therapeutic dosages, all thiazides are approximately equal in their diuretic/natriuretic effects.

There is significant natriuresis and diuresis within two hours after administration of a single oral dose of hydrochlorothiazide. These effects reach a peak in about six hours and persist for about 12 hours following oral administration of a single dose.

Like other benzothiadiazines, ORETIC also has antihypertensive properties, and may be used for this purpose either alone or to enhance the antihypertensive action of other drugs. The mechanism by which the benzothiadiazines, including hydrochlorothiazide, produce a reduction of elevated blood pressure is not known. However, sodium depletion appears to be involved.

ORETIC (hydrochlorothiazide) is readily absorbed from the gastrointestinal tract and is excreted unchanged by the kidneys.

INDICATIONS

ORETIC is indicated in the management of hypertension either as the sole therapeutic agent or to enhance the effect of other antihypertensive drugs in the more severe forms of hypertension.

ORETIC is indicated as adjunctive therapy in edema associated with congestive heart failure, hepatic cirrhosis, and corticosteroid and estrogen therapy.

ORETIC has also been found useful in edema due to various forms of renal dysfunction such as the nephrotic syndrome, acute glomerulonephritis and chronic renal failure.

Usage in Pregnancy: The routine use of diuretics in an otherwise healthy pregnant woman is inappropriate and exposes mother and fetus to unnecessary hazard. Diuretics do not prevent development of toxemia of pregnancy, and there is no satisfactory evidence that they are useful in the treatment of developed toxemia.

Edema during pregnancy may arise from pathological causes or from the physiological and mechanical consequences of pregnancy. Thiazides are indicated in pregnancy when edema is due to pathological causes, just as they are in the absence of pregnancy (however, see Warnings, below). Dependent edema in pregnancy, resulting from restriction of venous return by the expanded uterus, is properly treated through elevation of the lower extremities and use of support hose; use of diuretics to lower intravascular volume in this case is illogical and unnecessary. There is hypervolemia during normal pregnancy which is harmful to neither the fetus nor the mother (in the absence of cardiovascular disease), but which is associated with edema, including generalized edema, in the majority of pregnant women. If this edema produces discomfort, increased recumbency will often provide relief. In rare instances, this edema may cause extreme discomfort which is not relieved by rest. In these cases, a short course of diuretics may provide relief and may be appropriate.

CONTRAINDICATIONS

Renal decompensation.
Hypersensitivity to this or other sulfonamide-derived drugs.

WARNINGS

Hydrochlorothiazide shares with other thiazides the propensity to deplete potassium reserves to an unpredictable degree.

Thiazides should be used with caution in patients with renal disease or significant impairment of renal function, since azotemia may be precipitated and cumulative drug effects may occur.

Thiazides should be used with caution in patients with impaired hepatic function or progressive liver disease, since minor alterations of fluid and electrolyte balance may precipitate hepatic coma.

Thiazides may be additive or potentiative of the action of other antihypertensive drugs. Potentiation occurs with ganglionic or peripheral adrenergic blocking drugs.

Sensitivity reactions may occur in patients with a history of allergy or bronchial asthma.

The possibility of exacerbation or activation of systemic lupus erythematosus has been reported.

Usage in Pregnancy: Thiazides cross the placental barrier and appear in cord blood. The use of thiazides in pregnant women requires that the anticipated benefit be weighed against possible hazards to the fetus. These hazards include fetal or neonatal jaundice, thrombocytopenia, and possible other adverse reactions that have occurred in the adult.

Nursing Mothers: Thiazides appear in breast milk. If use of the drug is deemed essential, the patient should stop nursing.

PRECAUTIONS

Periodic determinations of serum electrolytes should be performed at appropriate intervals for the purpose of detecting possible electrolyte imbalances such as hyponatremia, hypochloremic alkalosis, and hypokalemia. Serum and urine electrolyte determinations are particularly important when a patient is vomiting excessively or receiving parenteral fluids. All patients should be observed for other clinical signs of electrolyte imbalances such as dryness of mouth, thirst, weakness, lethargy, drowsiness, restlessness, muscle pains or cramps, muscular fatigue, hypotension, oliguria, tachycardia, and gastrointestinal disturbances such as nausea and vomiting.

Hypokalemia may develop with thiazides as with any other potent diuretic, especially when brisk diuresis occurs, severe cirrhosis is present, or when corticosteroids or ACTH are given concomitantly. Interference with the adequate oral intake of electrolytes will also contribute to the possible development of hypokalemia. Potassium depletion, even of a mild degree, resulting from thiazide use, may sensitize a patient to the effects of cardiac glycosides such as digitalis. Any chloride deficit is generally mild and usually does not require specific treatment except under extraordinary circumstances (as in liver disease or renal disease). Dilutional hyponatremia may occur in edematous patients in hot weather; appropriate therapy is water restriction rather than administration of salt, except in rare instances when the hyponatremia is life threatening.

In actual salt depletion, appropriate replacement is the therapy of choice.

Hyperuricemia may occur or frank gout may be precipitated in certain patients receiving thiazide therapy.

Insulin requirements in diabetic patients may be increased, decreased, or unchanged. Latent diabetes mellitus may become manifest during thiazide administration.

Thiazide drugs may increase the responsiveness to tubocurarine.

The antihypertensive effects of the drug may be enhanced in the postsympathectomy patient.

Thiazides may decrease arterial responsiveness to norepinephrine. This diminution is not sufficient to preclude effectiveness of the pressor agent for therapeutic use.

If progressive renal impairment becomes evident as indicated by a rising-nonprotein nitrogen or blood urea nitrogen, a careful reappraisal of therapy is necessary with consideration given to withholding or discontinuing diuretic therapy. Thiazides may decrease serum PBI levels without signs of thyroid disturbance.

Thiazides have been reported, on rare occasions, to have elevated serum calcium to hypercalcemic levels. The serum calcium levels have returned to normal when the medication has been stopped. This phenomenon may be related to the ability of the thiazide diuretics to lower the amount of calcium excreted in the urine.

ADVERSE REACTIONS

Gastrointestinal system reactions: Anorexia, gastric irritation, nausea, vomiting, cramping, diarrhea, constipation, jaundice (intrahepatic cholestatic jaundice), pancreatitis. Central nervous system reactions: Dizziness, vertigo, paresthesias, headache, xanthopsia.

Hematologic reactions: Leukopenia, agranulocytosis, thrombocytopenia, aplastic anemia.

Dermatologic — hypersensitivity reactions: Purpura, photosensitivity, rash, urticaria, necrotizing angiitis (vasculitis) (cutaneous vasculitis).

Cardiovascular reaction: Orthostatic hypotension may occur and may be aggravated by alcohol, barbiturates, or narcotics.

Other: Hyperglycemia, glycosuria, hypercalcemia, hyperuricemia, muscle spasm, weakness, restlessness.

There have been isolated reports that certain nonedematous individuals developed severe fluid and electrolyte derangements after only brief exposure to normal doses of thiazide and non-thiazide diuretics. The condition is usually manifested as severe dilutional hyponatremia, hypokalemia, and hypochloremia. It has been reported to be due to inappropriately increased ADH secretion and appears to be idiosyncratic. Potassium replacement is apparently the most important therapy in the treatment of this syndrome along with removal of the offending drug.

Whenever adverse reactions are severe, treatment should be discontinued.

DOSAGE AND ADMINISTRATION

ORETIC (hydrochlorothiazide) is administered orally. Therapy should be individualized according to patient response. This therapy should be titrated to gain maximal therapeutic response as well as the minimal dose possible to maintain that therapeutic response.

For the management of edema the adult dosage ranges from 25 to 200 mg daily and may be given in single or divided doses. Usually 75 to 100 mg will produce the desired diuretic effect.

For the management of hypertension the usual initial adult dosage is 25 to 50 mg two times daily. The dosage may be increased if necessary to a maximum of 100 mg twice daily. When therapy is prolonged or large doses are used, particular attention should be given to the patient's electrolyte status. Supplemental potassium may be required.

In the treatment of hypertension hydrochlorothiazide may be either employed alone or concurrently with other antihypertensive drugs. Combined therapy may provide adequate control of hypertension with lower dosage of the component drugs and fewer or less severe side effects. An enhanced response frequently follows its concurrent administration with Harmonyl® (deserpidine) so that dosage of both drugs may be reduced.

For treatment of moderately severe or severe hypertension, supplemental use of other more potent antihypertensive agents such as Eutonyl® (pargyline hydrochloride) may be indicated.

When other antihypertensive agents are to be added to the regimen, this should be accomplished gradually. Additional potent antihypertensive agents should be given at only half the usual dose since their effect is potentiated by pretreatment with ORETIC.

OVERDOSAGE

Symptoms of overdosage include electrolyte imbalance and signs of potassium deficiency such as confusion, dizziness, muscular weakness, and gastrointestinal disturbances. General supportive measures including replacement of fluids and electrolytes may be indicated in treatment of overdosage.

HOW SUPPLIED

ORETIC (hydrochlorothiazide tablets, USP) is provided in two dosage sizes as white tablets:

   25 mg tablets:
      bottles of 100 (**NDC** 0074-6978-01),
      bottles of 1000 (**NDC** 0074-6978-02),
      Abbo-Pac® unit dose packages, 100 tablets (**NDC** 0074-6978-05).
   50 mg tablets:
      bottles of 100 (**NDC** 0074-6985-01),
      bottles of 1000 (**NDC** 0074-6985-02),
      Abbo-Pac® unit dose packages, 100 tablets (**NDC** 0074-6985-06).

Abbott Laboratories
North Chicago, IL 60064
Ref. 01-4480-R6
   Shown in Product Identification Section, page 403

ORETICYL®   ℞

[ō-re´ti-sill]
(hydrochlorothiazide and
deserpidine tablets)
Oral thiazide-rauwolfia therapy for hypertension.

> **WARNING**
> This fixed combination drug is not indicated for initial therapy of hypertension. Hypertension requires therapy titrated to the individual patient. If the fixed combination represents the dosage so determined, its use may be more convenient in patient management. The treatment of hypertension is not static, but must be reevaluated as conditions in each patient warrant.

DESCRIPTION

ORETICYL is an orally administered combination of Oretic® (hydrochlorothiazide) and Harmonyl® (deserpidine). Hydrochlorothiazide is a diuretic-antihypertensive agent of the benzothiadiazine (thiazide) class. Deserpidine is a purified rauwolfia alkaloid, chemically identified as 11-desmethoxyreserpine, which produces antihypertensive effects.

Inactive Ingredients:
Oreticyl 25 and Oreticyl 50 tablets: corn starch, lactose, magnesium stearate, red ferric oxide, talc and other ingredients. Oreticyl Forte tablets: corn starch, iron oxide, lactose, magnesium stearate, talc and other ingredients.

ACTIONS

The combined antihypertensive actions of hydrochlorothiazide and deserpidine result in a total clinical antihypertensive effect which is greater than can ordinarily be achieved by either drug given individually.

The diuretic and saluretic effects of hydrochlorothiazide result from a drug-induced inhibition of the renal tubular reabsorption of electrolytes. The excretion of sodium and chloride is greatly enhanced. Potassium excretion is also enhanced to a variable degree, as it is with the other thiazides. Although urinary excretion of bicarbonate is increased slightly, there is usually no significant change in urinary pH. Hydrochlorothiazide has a per mg natriuretic activity approximately 10 times that of the prototype thiazide, chlorothiazide. At maximal therapeutic dosages, all thiazides are approximately equal in their diuretic/natriuretic effects. There is significant natriuresis and diuresis within two hours after administration of a single oral dose of hydrochlorothiazide. These effects reach a peak in about six hours and persist for about 12 hours following oral administration of a single dose.

Like other benzothiadiazines, hydrochlorothiazide also has antihypertensive properties, and may be used for this purpose either alone or to enhance the antihypertensive action of other drugs. The mechanism by which the benzothiadiazines, including hydrochlorothiazide, produce a reduction of elevated blood pressure is not known. However, sodium depletion appears to be involved.

Hydrochlorothiazide is readily absorbed from the gastrointestinal tract and is excreted unchanged by the kidneys.

The pharmacologic actions of Harmonyl (deserpidine) are essentially the same as those of other active rauwolfia alkaloids. Deserpidine probably produces its antihypertensive effects through depletion of tissue stores of catecholamines (epinephrine and norepinephrine) from peripheral sites. The antihypertensive effect is often accompanied by bradycardia. There is no significant alteration in cardiac output or renal blood flow. The carotid sinus reflex is inhibited, but postural hypotension is rarely seen with the use of conventional doses of Harmonyl alone.

Deserpidine, like other rauwolfia alkaloids, is characterized by slow onset of action and sustained effect which may persist following withdrawal of the drug.

INDICATIONS

ORETICYL (hydrochlorothiazide and deserpidine) is indicated in the treatment of patients with mild to moderately severe hypertension (see boxed warning). It may be used alone for this purpose or added to other antihypertensive agents for the management of more severe hypertension. When administered with ORETICYL, more potent agents can be given at reduced dosage to minimize undesirable side effects.

CONTRAINDICATIONS

Hydrochlorothiazide is contraindicated in patients with renal decompensation and in those who are hypersensitive to this or other sulfonamide-derived drugs.

Deserpidine is contraindicated in patients with known hypersensitivity, history of mental depression especially with suicidal tendencies, active peptic ulcer, and ulcerative colitis. It is also contraindicated in patients receiving electroconvulsive therapy.

WARNINGS

Hydrochlorothiazide
Hydrochlorothiazide shares with other thiazides the propensity to deplete potassium reserves to an unpredictable degree.

Thiazides should be used with caution in patients with renal disease or significant impairment of renal function, since azotemia may be precipitated and cumulative drug effects may occur.

Thiazides should be used with caution in patients with impaired hepatic function or progressive liver disease, since

Continued on next page

Abbott—Cont.

minor alterations of fluid and electrolyte balance may precipitate hepatic coma.

Thiazides may be additive or potentiative of the action of other antihypertensive drugs. Potentiation occurs with ganglionic or peripheral adrenergic blocking drugs.

Sensitivity reactions may occur in patients with a history of allergy or bronchial asthma.

The possibility of exacerbation or activation of systemic lupus erythematosus has been reported.

Deserpidine

Deserpidine differs slightly in chemical structure from reserpine, however, its actions, indications, cautions and adverse reactions are common to the class of rauwolfia alkaloids. Reserpine may cause mental depression. Recognition of depression may be difficult because this condition may often be disguised by somatic complaints (Masked Depression). The drug should be discontinued at first signs of depression such as despondency, early morning insomnia, loss of appetite, impotence, or self-deprecation. Drug-induced depression may persist for several months after drug withdrawal and may be severe enough to result in suicide.

Usage in Pregnancy and Lactation:

Hydrochlorothiazide

Thiazides cross the placental barrier and appear in cord blood. The use of thiazides in pregnant women requires that the anticipated benefit be weighed against possible hazards to the fetus. These hazards include fetal or neonatal jaundice, thrombocytopenia, and possible other adverse reactions that have occurred in the adult.

Thiazides appear in breast milk. If use of the drug is deemed essential, the patient should stop nursing.

Deserpidine

The safety of deserpidine for use during pregnancy or lactation has not been established; therefore, it should be used in pregnant women or in women of childbearing potential only when in the judgment of the physician its use is deemed essential to the welfare of the patient. Increased respiratory secretions, nasal congestion, cyanosis, and anorexia may occur in infants born to rauwolfia alkaloid-treated mothers, since these preparations are known to cross the placental barrier to enter the fetal circulation and appear in cord blood. They also are secreted by nursing mothers into breast milk.

Reproductive and teratology studies in rats reduced the mating index and neonatal survival indices. The no-effect dosage has not been established.

PRECAUTIONS

Periodic determinations of serum electrolytes should be performed at appropriate intervals for the purpose of detecting possible electrolyte imbalances such as hyponatremia, hypochloremic alkalosis, and hypokalemia. Serum and urine electrolyte determinations are particularly important when a patient is vomiting excessively or receiving parenteral fluids. All patients should be observed for other clinical signs of electrolyte imbalances such as dryness of mouth, thirst, weakness, lethargy, drowsiness, restlessness, muscle pains or cramps, muscular fatigue, hypotension, oliguria, tachycardia, and gastrointestinal disturbances such as nausea and vomiting.

Hypokalemia may develop with thiazides as with any other potent diuretic, especially when brisk diuresis occurs, severe cirrhosis is present, or when corticosteroids or ACTH are given concomitantly. Interference with the adequate oral intake of electrolytes will also contribute to the possible development of hypokalemia. Potassium depletion, even of a mild degree, resulting from thiazide use, may sensitize a patient to the effects of cardiac glycosides such as digitalis. Any chloride deficit is generally mild and usually does not require specific treatment except under extraordinary circumstances (as in liver disease or renal disease). Dilutional hyponatremia may occur in edematous patients in hot weather; appropriate therapy is water restriction rather than administration of salt, except in rare instances when the hyponatremia is life threatening.

In actual salt depletion, appropriate replacement is the therapy of choice.

Hyperuricemia may occur or frank gout may be precipitated in certain patients receiving thiazide therapy.

Insulin requirements in diabetic patients may be increased, decreased, or unchanged. Latent diabetes mellitus may become manifest during thiazide administration.

Thiazide drugs may increase the responsiveness to tubocurarine.

The antihypertensive effects of the drug may be enhanced in the postsympathectomy patient.

Thiazides may decrease arterial responsiveness to norepinephrine. This diminution is not sufficient to preclude effectiveness of the pressor agent for therapeutic use.

If progressive renal impairment becomes evident as indicated by a rising-nonprotein nitrogen or blood urea nitrogen, a careful reappraisal of therapy is necessary with consideration given to withholding or discontinuing diuretic therapy.

Thiazides may decrease serum PBI levels without signs of thyroid disturbance.

Thiazides have been reported, on rare occasions, to have elevated serum calcium to hypercalcemic levels. The serum calcium levels have returned to normal when the medication has been stopped. This phenomenon may be related to the ability of the thiazide diuretics to lower the amount of calcium excreted in the urine.

Because rauwolfia preparations increase gastrointestinal motility and secretion, this drug should be used cautiously in patients with a history of peptic ulcer, ulcerative colitis, or gallstones, where biliary colic may be precipitated.

Caution should be exercised when treating hypertensive patients with renal insufficiency since they adjust poorly to lowered blood pressure levels.

Use deserpidine cautiously with digitalis and quinidine since cardiac arrhythmias have occurred with rauwolfia preparations.

Preoperative withdrawal of deserpidine does not assure that circulatory instability will not occur. It is important that the anesthesiologist be aware of the patient's drug intake and consider this in the overall management, since hypotension has occurred in patients receiving rauwolfia preparations. Anticholinergic and / or adrenergic drugs (metaraminol, norepinephrine) have been employed to treat adverse vagocirculatory effects.

Animal tumorigenicity: There are no studies demonstrating that deserpidine is an animal tumorigen, although it is a prolactin stimulator and structurally related to reserpine. Rodent studies with reserpine, however, have shown that reserpine is an animal tumorigen, causing an increased incidence of mammary fibroadenomas in female mice, malignant tumors of the seminal vesicles in male mice, and malignant adrenal medullary tumors in male rats. These findings arose in 2 year studies in which the drug was administered in the feed at concentrations of 5 and 10 ppm—about 100 to 300 times the usual human dose. The breast neoplasms are thought to be related to reserpine's prolactin-elevating effect. Several other prolactin-elevating drugs have also been associated with an increased incidence of mammary neoplasia in rodents.

The extent to which these findings indicate a risk to humans is uncertain. Tissue culture experiments show that about one-third of human breast tumors are prolactin-dependent *in vitro,* a factor of considerable importance if the use of the drug is contemplated in a patient with previously detected breast cancer. The possibility of an increased risk of breast cancer in reserpine users has been studied extensively; however, no firm conclusion has emerged. Although a few epidemiologic studies have suggested a slightly increased risk (less than twofold in all studies except one) in women who have used reserpine, other studies of generally similar design have not confirmed this. Epidemiologic studies conducted using other drugs (neuroleptic agents) that, like reserpine, increase prolactin levels and, therefore, would be considered rodent mammary carcinogens, have not shown an association between chronic administration of the drug and human mammary tumorigenesis. While long-term clinical observation has not suggested such an association, the available evidence is considered too limited to be conclusive at this time. An association of reserpine intake with pheochromocytoma or tumors of the seminal vesicles has not been explored.

ADVERSE REACTIONS

Hydrochlorothiazide

Gastrointestinal System Reactions: Anorexia, gastric irritation, nausea, vomiting, cramping, diarrhea, constipation, jaundice (intrahepatic cholestatic jaundice), pancreatitis.

Central Nervous System Reactions: Dizziness, vertigo, paresthesias, headache, xanthopsia.

Hematologic Reactions: Leukopenia, agranulocytosis, thrombocytopenia, aplastic anemia.

Dermatologic — Hypersensitivity Reactions: Purpura, photosensitivity, rash, urticaria, necrotizing angitis (vasculitis) (cutaneous vasculitis).

Cardiovascular Reaction: Orthostatic hypotension may occur and may be aggravated by alcohol, barbiturates, or narcotics.

Other: Hyperglycemia, glycosuria, hypercalcemia, hyperuricemia, muscle spasm, weakness, restlessness.

There have been isolated reports that certain nonedematous individuals developed severe fluid and electrolyte derangements after only brief exposure to normal doses of thiazide and non-thiazide diuretics. The condition is usually manifested as severe dilutional hyponatremia, hypokalemia, and hypochloremia. It has been reported to be due to inappropriately increased ADH secretion and appears to be idiosyncratic. Potassium replacement is apparently the most important therapy in the treatment of this syndrome along with the removal of the offending drug.

Whenever adverse reactions are severe, treatment should be discontinued.

Deserpidine

The following adverse reactions have been reported with rauwolfia preparations. These reactions are usually reversible and disappear when the drug is discontinued.

Gastrointestinal: Including hypersecretion, anorexia, diarrhea, nausea, and vomiting.

Cardiovascular: Including angina-like symptoms, arrhythmias (particularly when used concurrently with digitalis or quinidine), and bradycardia.

Central Nervous System: Including drowsiness, depression, nervousness, paradoxical anxiety, nightmares, extrapyramidal tract symptoms, CNS sensitization manifested by dull sensorium, and deafness.

Dermatologic—Hypersensitivity: Including pruritus, rash, and asthma in asthmatic patients.

Ophthalmologic: Including glaucoma, uveitis, optic atrophy, and conjunctival injection.

Hematologic: Thrombocytopenic purpura.

Miscellaneous: Nasal congestion, weight gain, impotence or decreased libido, dysuria, dyspnea, muscular aches, dryness of mouth, dizziness and headache.

DOSAGE AND ADMINISTRATION

Dosage should be determined by individual titration of ingredients (see boxed warning). Dosage of both components should be carefully adjusted to the needs of the individual patient. Since at least ten days to two weeks may elapse before the full effects of the drugs become manifest, the dosage should not be adjusted more frequently.

Three tablet strengths, ORETICYL 25 (hydrochlorothiazide 25 mg, deserpidine 0.125 mg); ORETICYL 50 (hydrochlorothiazide 50 mg, deserpidine 0.125 mg); and ORETICYL FORTE (hydrochlorothiazide 25 mg, deserpidine 0.25 mg), all grooved, are provided to permit considerable latitude in meeting the dosage requirements of individual patients.

The table below will help in determining which dose of ORETICYL 25, ORETICYL 50, or ORETICYL FORTE best represents the equivalent of the titrated dose.

ORETICYL 25	hydro-chlorothiazide	deserpidine
1 tablet bid	25.0 mg bid	0.125 mg bid
1½ tablet bid	37.5 mg bid	0.188 mg bid
2 tablets bid	50.0 mg bid	0.250 mg bid

ORETICYL 50	hydro-chlorothiazide	deserpidine
1 tablet bid	50 mg bid	0.125 mg bid
1½ tablet bid	75 mg bid	0.188 mg bid
2 tablets bid	100 mg bid	0.250 mg bid

ORETICYL FORTE	hydro-chlorothiazide	deserpidine
1 tablet bid	25.0 mg bid	0.250 mg bid
1½ tablet bid	37.5 mg bid	0.375 mg bid
2 tablets bid	50.0 mg bid	0.500 mg bid

The usual adult dosage is one ORETICYL 50 two times daily. When other antihypertensive agents are to be added to the regimen, this should be accomplished gradually. Ganglionic blocking agents should be given at only half the usual dose since their effect is potentiated by pretreatment with ORETICYL (hydrochlorothiazide and deserpidine).

OVERDOSAGE

Symptoms of thiazide overdosage include electrolyte imbalance and signs of potassium deficiency such as confusion, dizziness, muscular weakness, and gastrointestinal disturbances. General supportive measures including replacement of fluids and electrolytes may be indicated in treatment of overdosage.

An overdosage of deserpidine is characterized by flushing of the skin, conjunctival injection, and pupillary constriction. Sedation ranging from drowsiness to coma may occur. Hypotension, hypothermia, central respiratory depression and bradycardia may develop in cases of severe overdosage. Treatment consists of the careful evacuation of stomach contents followed by the usual procedures for the symptomatic management of CNS depressant overdosage. If severe hypotension occurs it should be treated with a direct acting vasopressor such as norepinephrine bitartrate injection.

HOW SUPPLIED

ORETICYL is supplied as grooved tablets in the following dosage sizes:

Rose-colored ORETICYL 25, contains hydrochlorothiazide 25 mg, deserpidine 0.125 mg, in bottles of 100 (**NDC** 0074-6922-01).

Rose-colored ORETICYL 50, contains hydrochlorothiazide 50 mg, deserpidine 0.125 mg, in bottles of 100 (**NDC** 0074-6931-01).

Gray-colored ORETICYL FORTE, contains hydrochlorothiazide 25 mg, deserpidine 0.25 mg, in bottles of 100 (**NDC** 0074-6927-01).

Abbott Laboratories
North Chicago, IL 60064
Ref. 01-2361-R7

PANHEMATIN®   ℞
[pan-hē'ma-tin]
(hemin for injection)
For I.V. Use Only

PANHEMATIN (hemin for injection) should only be used by physicians experienced in the management of porphyrias in hospitals where the recommended clinical and laboratory diagnostic and monitoring techniques are available.
PANHEMATIN therapy should be considered after an appropriate period of alternate therapy (i.e., 400 g glucose/day for 1 to 2 days). (See "WARNINGS", "PRECAUTIONS" and "DOSAGE AND ADMINISTRATION" sections.)

DESCRIPTION

PANHEMATIN (hemin for injection) is an enzyme inhibitor derived from processed red blood cells. Hemin for injection was known previously as hematin. The term hematin has been used to describe the chemical reaction product of hemin and sodium carbonate solution. Hemin is an iron containing metalloporphyrin. Chemically hemin is represented as chloro[7,12-diethenyl-3,8,13,17-tetramethyl-21H,23H-porphine-2,18-dipropanoato (2-)-$N^{21},N^{22}, N^{23}, N^{24}$] iron.
PANHEMATIN is a sterile, lyophilized powder suitable for intravenous administration after reconstitution. Each dispensing vial of PANHEMATIN contains the equivalent of 313 mg hemin, 215 mg sodium carbonate and 300 mg of sorbitol. The pH may have been adjusted with hydrochloric acid; the product contains no preservatives. When mixed as directed with Sterile Water for Injection, USP, each 43 ml provides the equivalent of approximately 301 mg hematin (7 mg/ml).

CLINICAL PHARMACOLOGY

Heme acts to limit the hepatic and/or marrow synthesis of porphyrin. This action is likely due to the inhibition of delta-aminolevulinic acid synthetase, the enzyme which limits the rate of the porphyrin/heme biosynthetic pathway. The exact mechanism by which hematin produces symptomatic improvement in patients with acute episodes of the hepatic porphyrias has not been elucidated.[1,9]
Following intravenous administration of hematin in nonjaundiced human patients, an increase in fecal urobilinogen can be observed which is roughly proportional to the amount of hematin administered. This suggests an enterohepatic pathway as at least one route of elimination. Bilirubin metabolites are also excreted in the urine following hematin injections.[2]
PANHEMATIN (hemin for injection) therapy for the acute porphyrias is not curative. After discontinuation of PANHEMATIN treatment, symptoms generally return although in some cases remission is prolonged. Some neurological symptoms have improved weeks to months after therapy although little or no response was noted at the time of treatment.
Other aspects of human pharmacokinetics have not been defined.

INDICATIONS AND USAGE

PANHEMATIN (hemin for injection) is indicated for the amelioration of recurrent attacks of acute intermittent porphyria temporarily related to the menstrual cycle in susceptible women.
Manifestations such as pain, hypertension, tachycardia, abnormal mental status and mild to progressive neurologic signs may be controlled in selected patients with this disorder.
Similar findings have been reported in other patients with acute intermittent porphyria, porphyria variegata and hereditary coproporphyria. PANHEMATIN is not indicated in porphyria cutanea tarda.

CONTRAINDICATIONS

Hemin for injection is contraindicated in patients with known hypersensitivity to this drug.

WARNINGS

PANHEMATIN (hemin for injection) therapy is intended to limit the rate of porphyria/heme biosynthesis possibly by inhibiting the enzyme delta-aminolevulinic acid synthetase. For this reason, drugs such as estrogens, barbituric acid derivatives and steroid metabolites which increase the activity of delta-aminolevulinic acid synthetase should be avoided.
Also, because PANHEMATIN has exhibited transient, mild anticoagulant effects during clinical studies, concurrent anticoagulant therapy should be avoided.[9] The extent and duration of the hypocoagulable state induced by PANHEMATIN has not been established.

PRECAUTIONS

General:
Clinical benefit from PANHEMATIN depends on prompt administration. Attacks of porphyria may progress to a point where irreversible neuronal damage has occurred. PAN-

HEMATIN therapy is intended to prevent an attack from reaching the critical stage of neuronal degeneration. PANHEMATIN is not effective in repairing neuronal damage.[9]
Recommended dosage guidelines should be strictly followed. Reversible renal shutdown has been observed in a case where an excessive hematin dose (12.2 mg/kg) was administered in a single infusion. Oliguria and increased nitrogen retention occurred although the patient remained asymptomatic.[4] No worsening of renal function has been seen with administration of recommended dosages of hematin.[9]
A large arm vein or a central venous catheter should be utilized for the administration of hemin for injection to avoid the possibility of phlebitis.
Since reconstituted PANHEMATIN is not transparent, any undissolved particulate matter is difficult to see when inspected visually. Therefore, terminal filtration through a sterile 0.45 micron or smaller filter is recommended.
Tests for Diagnosis and Monitoring of Therapy: Before PANHEMATIN therapy is begun, the presence of acute porphyria must be diagnosed using the following criteria:[9]
a.   Presence of clinical symptoms.
b.   Positive Watson-Schwartz or Hoesch test. (A negative Watson-Schwartz or Hoesch test indicates a porphyric attack is highly unlikely. When in doubt quantitative measures of delta-aminolevulinic acid and porphobilinogen in serum or urine may aid in diagnosis.)
Urinary concentrations of the following compounds may be *monitored* during PANHEMATIN therapy. Drug effect will be demonstrated by a decrease in one or more of the following compounds:[3-6] ALA—delta-aminolevulinic acid, UPG —uroporphyrinogen, PBG—porphobilinogen or coproporphyrin.
Carcinogenesis, Mutagenesis, Impairment of Fertility: No data are available on potential for carcinogenicity, mutagenicity or impairment of fertility in animals or humans.
Pregnancy: Teratogenic effects: Pregnancy Category C. Animal reproduction studies have not been conducted with hematin. It is also not known whether hematin can cause fetal harm when administered to a pregnant woman or can affect reproduction capacity. For this reason hemin for injection should not be given to a pregnant woman unless the expected benefits are sufficiently important to the health and welfare of the patient to outweigh the unknown hazard to the fetus.
Nursing Mothers: It is not known whether this drug is excreted in human milk. Because many drugs are excreted in human milk, caution should be exercised when hemin for injection is administered to a nursing woman.
Pediatric Use: Safety and effectiveness in children have not been established.

ADVERSE REACTIONS

Reversible renal shutdown has occurred with administration of excessive doses (See "PRECAUTIONS" section).
Phlebitis with or without leucocytosis and with or without mild pyrexia has occurred after administration of hematin through small arm veins.
There has been one report in the literature[8] of coagulopathy occurring in a patient receiving hematin therapy. This patient exhibited prolonged prothrombin time and partial thromboplastin time, thrombocytopenia, mild hypofibrinogenemia, mild elevation of fibrin split products and a 10% fall in hematocrit.

OVERDOSAGE

Reversible renal shutdown has been observed in a case where an excessive hematin dose (12.2 mg/kg) was administered in a single infusion. Treatment of this case consisted of ethacrynic acid and mannitol.[7]

DOSAGE AND ADMINISTRATION

Before administering hemin for injection, an appropriate period of alternate therapy (i.e., 400 g glucose/day for 1 to 2 days) must be considered. If improvement is unsatisfactory for the treatment of acute attacks of porphyria, an intravenous infusion of PANHEMATIN containing a dose of 1 to 4 mg/kg/day of hematin should be given over a period of 10 to 15 minutes for 3 to 14 days based on the clinical signs. In more severe cases this dose may be repeated no earlier than every 12 hours. No more than 6 mg/kg of hematin should be given in any 24-hour period.
After reconstitution each ml of PANHEMATIN contains the equivalent of approximately 7 mg of hematin. The drug may be administered directly from the vial.

Dosage Calculation Table

1 mg hematin equivalent	= 0.14 ml PANHEMATIN
2 mg hematin equivalent	= 0.28 ml PANHEMATIN
3 mg hematin equivalent	= 0.42 ml PANHEMATIN
4 mg hematin equivalent	= 0.56 ml PANHEMATIN

Since reconstituted PANHEMATIN is not transparent, any undissolved particulate matter is difficult to see when inspected visually. Therefore, terminal filtration through a sterile 0.45 micron or smaller filter is recommended.
Preparation of Solution: Reconstitute PANHEMATIN by aseptically adding 43 ml of Sterile Water for Injection, USP, to the dispensing vial. Immediately after adding diluent, the product should be shaken well for a period of 2 to 3 minutes

to aid dissolution. **NOTE:** Because PANHEMATIN contains no preservative and because PANHEMATIN undergoes rapid chemical decomposition in solution, it should not be reconstituted until immediately before use. After the first withdrawal from the vial, any solution remaining must be discarded.
No drug or chemical agent should be added to a PANHEMATIN fluid admixture unless its effect on the chemical and physical stability has first been determined.

HOW SUPPLIED

PANHEMATIN (hemin for injection) is supplied as a sterile, lyophilized black powder in single dose dispensing vials (**NDC** 0074-2000-43). When mixed as directed with Sterile Water for Injection, USP, each 43 ml provides the equivalent of approximately 301 mg hematin (7 mg/ml). Store lyophilized powder in refrigerator (2–8°C) until time of use.

REFERENCES

1. Bickers, D., Treatment of the Porphyrias: Mechanisms of Action, *J Invest Dermatol* 77(1):107–113, 1981.
2. Watson, C. J., Hematin and Porphyria, editorial, *N Engl J Med* 293(12):605–607, September 18, 1975.
3. Lamon, J. M., Hematin Therapy for Acute Porphyria, *Medicine* 58(3):252–269, 1979.
4. Dhar, G. J., et al., Effects of Hematin in Hepatic Porphyria, *Ann Intern Med* 83:20–30, 1975.
5. Watson, C. J., et al., Use of Hematin in the Acute Attack of the "Inducible" Hepatic Porphyrias, *Adv Intern Med* 23:265–286, 1978.
6. McColl, K. E., et al., Treatment with Haematin in Acute Hepatic Porphyria, *Q J Med*, New Series L (198):161–174, Spring, 1981.
7. Dhar, G. J., et al., Transitory Renal Failure Following Rapid Administration of a Relatively Large Amount of Hematin in a Patient with Acute Intermittent Porphyria in Clinical Remission, *Acta Med Scand* 203:437–443, 1978.
8. Morris, D. L., et al., Coagulopathy Associated with Hematin Treatment for Acute Intermittent Porphyria, *Ann Intern Med* 95:700–701, 1981.
9. Pierach, C. A., Hematin Therapy for the Porphyric Attack, *Semin Liver Dis* 2(2):125–131, May, 1982.

Abbott Laboratories
North Chicago, IL 60064
Ref. 01-2388-R4

PANWARFIN®   ℞
[pan-wăr'fin]
(warfarin sodium tablets, USP)

DESCRIPTION

PANWARFIN (warfarin sodium) is a coumarin anticoagulant, chemically designated as 3-(α-Acetonylbenzyl)-4-hydroxycoumarin sodium salt.
Inactive Ingredients:
2 mg tablets: corn starch, D&C Red No. 30, FD&C Blue No. 1, lactose, magnesium stearate, microcrystalline cellulose, polacrilin potassium and other ingredients.
2.5 mg tablets: corn starch, FD&C Yellow No. 6, lactose, magnesium stearate, microcrystalline cellulose, polacrilin potassium and other ingredients.
5 mg tablets: corn starch, D&C Red No. 30, FD&C Yellow No. 6, lactose, magnesium stearate, microcrystalline cellulose, polacrilin potassium and other ingredients.
7.5 mg tablets: corn starch, FD&C Yellow No. 5 (tartrazine), lactose, magnesium stearate, microcrystalline cellulose, polacrilin potassium and other ingredients.
10 mg tablets: corn starch, lactose, magnesium stearate, microcrystalline cellulose, polacrilin potassium and other ingredients.

ACTIONS

PANWARFIN and other coumarin anticoagulants act by depressing synthesis in the liver of several factors which are known to be active in the coagulation mechanisms in a variety of diseases characterized by thromboembolic phenomena. The resultant **in vivo** effect is a sequential depression of Factors VII, IX, X and II. The degree of depression is dependent upon the dosage administered. Anticoagulants have no direct effect on an established thrombus, nor do they reverse ischemic tissue damage. However, once a thrombosis has occurred, anticoagulant treatment aims to prevent further extension of the formed clot and prevents secondary thromboembolic complications which may result in serious and possible fatal sequelae.
After oral administration, absorption is essentially complete, and maximal plasma concentrations are reached in 1 to 9 hours. Approximately 97% is bound to albumin within the plasma. PANWARFIN usually induces hypoprothrombinemia in 36 to 72 hours, and its duration of action may persist

Continued on next page

Abbott—Cont.

for 4 to 5 days, thus producing a smooth, long lasting response curve. Little is known of the metabolic pathways involved in the biotransformation of oral anticoagulants in man. However, their metabolites appear to be eliminated principally in the urine.

INDICATIONS

PANWARFIN is indicated for the prophylaxis and treatment of venous thrombosis and its extension, the treatment of atrial fibrillation with embolization, the prophylaxis and treatment of pulmonary embolism, and as an adjunct in the treatment of coronary occlusion.

CONTRAINDICATIONS

Anticoagulation is contraindicated in any localized or general physical condition or personal circumstance in which the hazard of hemorrhage might be greater than its potential clinical benefits, such as:

Pregnancy:
PANWARFIN is contraindicated in pregnancy because the drug passes through the placental barrier and may cause fatal hemorrhage to the fetus in utero. Furthermore, there have been reports of birth malformations in children born to mothers who have been treated with warfarin during pregnancy. Women of childbearing potential who are candidates for anticoagulant therapy should be carefully evaluated and the indications critically reviewed with the patient. If the patient becomes pregnant while taking this drug, she should be apprised of the potential risks to the fetus, and the possibility of termination of the pregnancy should be discussed in light of those risks.

Hemorrhagic tendencies or blood dyscrasias.
Recent or contemplated surgery of:
(1) central nervous system; (2) eye; (3) traumatic surgery resulting in large open surfaces.

Bleeding tendencies associated with active ulceration or overt bleeding of:
(1) gastrointestinal, genitourinary or respiratory tracts; (2) cerebrovascular hemorrhage; (3) aneurysms—cerebral, dissecting aorta; (4) pericarditis and pericardial effusions.

Threatened abortion, eclampsia and preeclampsia.

Inadequate laboratory facilities or unsupervised senility, alcoholism, psychosis; or lack of patient cooperation.

Spinal puncture and other diagnostic or therapeutic procedures with potential for uncontrollable bleeding.

Miscellaneous: major regional, lumbar block anesthesia, severe uncontrolled and/or malignant hypertension, subacute bacterial endocarditis, open wounds, visceral carcinoma, vitamin K deficiency, and severe liver or kidney disease.

WARNINGS

The most serious risks associated with anticoagulant therapy with sodium warfarin are hemorrhage in any tissue or organ and, less frequently, necrosis and/or gangrene of skin and other tissues. The risk of hemorrhage is related to the level of intensity and the duration of anticoagulant therapy. Hemorrhage and necrosis have in some cases been reported to result in death or permanent disability. Necrosis appears to be associated with local thrombosis and usually appears within a few days of the start of anticoagulant therapy. In severe cases of necrosis, treatment through debridement or amputation of the affected tissue, limb, breast or penis has been reported. Careful diagnosis is required to determine whether necrosis is caused by an underlying disease. Warfarin therapy should be discontinued when warfarin is suspected to be the cause of developing necrosis and heparin therapy may be considered for anticoagulation. Although various treatments have been attempted, no treatment for necrosis has been considered uniformly effective. See below for information on predisposing conditions. These and other risks associated with anticoagulant therapy must be weighed against the risk of thrombosis or embolization in untreated cases.

Warfarin sodium is a potent drug with a half-life of 2½ days; therefore its effects may become more pronounced as daily maintenance doses overlap. It cannot be emphasized too strongly that treatment of each patient is a highly individualized matter. Dosage should be controlled by periodic determinations of prothrombin time or other suitable coagulation tests. Determinations of whole blood clotting and bleeding times are not effective measures for control of therapy. Heparin prolongs the one-stage prothrombin time. Therefore, to obtain a valid prothrombin time when heparin and PANWARFIN (warfarin sodium) are given together, a period of at least 5 hours should elapse after the last intravenous dose and 24 hours after the last subcutaneous dose of heparin, before blood is drawn.

Caution should be observed when PANWARFIN is administered in any situation or in the presence of any predisposing condition where added risk of hemorrhage or necrosis is present.

Administration of anticoagulants in the following conditions will be based upon clinical judgment in which the risks of

anticoagulant therapy are weighed against the risk of thrombosis or embolization in untreated cases. The following may be associated with these increased risks:

Lactation—Coumarins may pass into the milk of mothers and cause a prothrombinopenic state in the nursing infant.

Mild to moderate hepatic or renal insufficiency.

Infectious diseases or disturbances of intestinal flora—sprue, antibiotic therapy.

Trauma which may result in internal bleeding.

Surgery or trauma resulting in large exposed raw surfaces.

Indwelling catheters and/or drainage tubes in any orifice.

Mild to moderate hypertension.

Known or suspected hereditary, familial or clinical deficiency in protein C—This condition, which should be suspected if there is a history of recurrent episodes of thromboembolic disorders in the patient or in the family, has been associated with an increased risk of developing necrosis following warfarin administration. Skin necrosis may occur in the absence of protein C deficiency. It has been reported that initiation of anticoagulation therapy with heparin for 4 to 5 days before initiation of therapy with PANWARFIN may minimize the incidence of this reaction. Warfarin therapy should be discontinued when warfarin is suspected to be the cause of developing necrosis and heparin therapy may be considered for anticoagulation.

Miscellaneous: polycythemia vera, vasculitis, severe diabetes, severe allergic and anaphylactic disorders, active tuberculosis, history of ulcerative disease of the gastrointestinal tract, and during the postpartum period.

Patients with congestive heart failure may become more sensitive to PANWARFIN, thereby requiring more frequent laboratory monitoring, and reduced doses of PANWARFIN.

Use of anticoagulants with streptokinase or urokinase may be hazardous and caution should be exercised when used concomitantly. (Please note recommendations accompanying these preparations.)

Abrupt cessation of anticoagulant therapy is not generally recommended; taper dose gradually over 3 to 4 weeks.

PRECAUTIONS

Periodic determination of prothrombin time or other suitable coagulation test is essential.

Numerous factors, alone or in combination, including travel, changes in diet, environment, physical state and medication may influence response of the patient to anticoagulants. It is generally good practice to monitor the patient's response with additional prothrombin time determinations in the period immediately after discharge from the hospital, and whenever other medications are initiated, discontinued or taken haphazardly. The following factors are listed for your reference; however, other factors may also affect the prothrombin response.

The following factors alone or in combination, may be responsible for increased prothrombin time response:
ENDOGENOUS FACTORS:
Carcinoma; collagen disease; congestive heart failure; diarrhea; elevated temperature; hepatic disorders—infectious hepatitis, hyperthyroidism, jaundice; poor nutritional state; vitamin K deficiency—steatorrhea.
EXOGENOUS FACTORS:
Alcohol†; allopurinol; aminosalicyclic acid; amiodarone; anabolic steroids; antibiotics; bromelains; chloral hydrate†; chloramphenicol; chlorpropamide; chymotrypsin; cimetidine; cinchophen; clofibrate; PANWARFIN overdosage; dextran; dextrothyroxine; diazoxide; dietary deficiencies; diflunisal; diuretics†; disulfiram; drugs affecting blood elements; ethacrynic acid; fenoprofen; glucagon; hepatotoxic drugs; ibuprofen; indomethacin; influenza virus vaccine; inhalation anesthetics; mefenamic acid; methyldopa; methylphenidate; methylthiouracil; metronidazole; miconazole; monoamine oxidase inhibitors; nalidixic acid; naproxen; nortriptyline; oxolinic acid; oxyphenbutazone; pentoxifylline; phenylbutazone; phenyramidol; phenytoin; prolonged hot weather; prolonged narcotics; propylthiouracil; pyrazolones; quinidine; quinine; ranitidine†; salicylates; sulfinpyrazone; sulfonamides, long acting; sulindac; thyroid drugs; tolbutamide; triclofos sodium; trimethoprim/sulfamethoxazole; unreliable prothrombin time determinations.

The following factors, alone or in combination, may be responsible for decreased prothrombin time response:
ENDOGENOUS FACTORS:
Edema; hereditary resistance to coumarin therapy; hyperlipemia; hyothyroidism.
EXOGENOUS FACTORS:
ACTH; adrenocortical steroids; alochol†; antacids; antihistamines; phenobarbital and other barbiturates; carbamazepine; chloral hydrate†; chlordiazepoxide; cholestyramine; PANWARFIN underdosage; diet high in vitamin K; diuretics†; ethchlorvynol; glutethimide; griseofulvin; haloperidol; meprobamate; oral contraceptives; paraldehyde; primidone; ranitidine†; rifampin; unreliable prothrombin time determinations; vitamin C.
A patient may be exposed to a combination of the above factors, some of which may increase and some decrease his sensitivity to PANWARFIN (warfarin sodium). Because the net effect on his prothrombin time response may be unpredict-

able under these circumstances, more frequent laboratory monitoring is advisable.

Drugs not yet shown to interact or not to interact with coumarins are best regarded with suspicion, and when their administration is started or stopped, the prothrombin time should be determined more often than usual.

Coumarins also affect the action of other drugs. Hypoglycemic agents (chlorpropamide and tolbutamide) and anticonvulsants (phenytoin and phenobarbital) may accumulate in the body as a result of interference with either their metabolism or excretion.

† Increased and decreased prothrombin time responses have been reported.

ADVERSE REACTIONS

Potential adverse reactions to PANWARFIN (warfarin sodium) may include:

Hemorrhage from any tissue or organ. This is a consequence of the anticoagulant effect. The signs and symptoms will vary according to the location and degree or extent of the bleeding. Therefore, the possibility of hemorrhage should be considered in evaluating the condition of any anticoagulated patient with complaints which do not indicate an obvious diagnosis. Bleeding during anticoagulant therapy does not always correlate with prothrombin activity. (See **TREATMENT FOR OVERDOSAGE.**)

Adrenal hemorrhage with resultant acute adrenal insufficiency has occurred during anticoagulant therapy. Anticoagulant therapy should be discontinued in patients who develop signs and symptoms compatible with acute adrenal hemorrhage or insufficiency. Plasma cortisol levels should be measured immediately, and vigorous therapy with intravenous corticosteroids should be instituted promptly. Initiation of therapy should not depend upon laboratory confirmation of the diagnosis, since any delay in an acute situation may result in the patient's death.

Ovarian hemorrhage: Reports indicate that a woman receiving short- or long-term anticoagulant therapy may be at risk of developing ovarian hemorrhage at the time of ovulation.

Paralytic ileus and intestinal obstruction have been reported from submucosal or intramural hemorrhage. Excessive uterine bleeding has occurred but menstrual flow is usually normal.

Bleeding which occurs when the prothrombin time is within the therapeutic range warrants diagnostic investigation since it may unmask a previously unsuspected lesion, e.g. tumor, ulcer, etc.

Necrosis of skin and other tissues. (See **WARNINGS.**)
Other adverse reactions are infrequent and consist of alopecia, urticaria, dermatitis, fever, nausea, diarrhea, abdominal cramping, a syndrome called "purple toes," hypersensitivity reactions, leukopenia, and vomiting.

Priapism has been associated with anticoagulant administration, however, a causal relationship has not been established.

DOSAGE AND LABORATORY CONTROL

The aim of anticoagulant therapy is to impede the coagulation or clotting mechanism to such an extent that thrombosis will not occur, but at the same time avoiding such extensive impairment as might produce spontaneous bleeding. Effective therapeutic levels with minimal complications can best be achieved in cooperative and well-instructed patients, who keep the doctor informed of their status between visits.

The administration and dosage of PANWARFIN must be individualized for each patient according to the particular patient's sensitivity to the drug as indicated by the prothrombin time. The prothrombin time reflects the depression of vitamin K dependent Factors VII, X and II. These factors, in addition to Factor IX, are affected by coumarin anticoagulants. There are several modifications of the Quick one-stage prothrombin time and the physician should become familiar with the specific method used in his laboratory.

Administration of PANWARFIN should be gauged according to prothrombin time determinations by a suitable method. The blood prothrombin time should usually be determined daily after the administration of the initial dose until prothrombin time results stabilize in the therapeutic range. Intervals between subsequent prothrombin time determinations should be based upon the physician's judgment of the patient's reliability and response to warfarin in order to maintain the individual within the therapeutic range. Acceptable intervals for prothrombin time determinations have usually fallen within the range of 1 to 4 weeks. Satisfactory levels for maintenance of therapeutic anticoagulation are 1½ to 2½ times the normal prothrombin time (e.g. 18 to 30 seconds, with a control of 12 seconds).

Induction
Induction may be initiated with 10 to 15 mg daily and thereafter (usually 2 or 3 days) adjusted according to prothrombin time response. The basis for this no-loading dose regimen is that the depression of Factors II, IX, and X is not accelerated by the administration of a loading dose. Avoidance of a large priming dose may minimize the possibility of excessive increases in prothrombin time.

Alternatively, 40 to 60 mg for average adult or 20 to 30 mg for elderly and/or debilitated patients for one dose only administered orally, intravenously, or intramuscularly.

Maintenance

Most patients are satisfactorily maintained at a dose of 2 to 10 mg daily. Flexibility of dosage is provided by breaking scored tablets in half. The individual dose and interval should be gauged by the patient's prothrombin response.

Duration of therapy

The duration of therapy in each patient should be individualized. In general, anticoagulant therapy should be continued until the danger of thrombosis and embolism has passed.

Treatment during dentistry and surgery

The management of patients who undergo dental and surgical procedures requires close liaison between attending physicians, surgeons and dentists. Interruption of anticoagulant therapy may precipitate thromboembolism, and conversely, if anticoagulants are maintained at full doses, some patients may hemorrhage excessively. If it is elected to administer anticoagulants prior to, during, or immediately following dental or surgical procedures, it is recommended that the dosage of PANWARFIN be adjusted to maintain the prothrombin time at approximately $1\frac{1}{2}$ to $2\frac{1}{2}$ times the control level. The operative site should be sufficiently limited to permit the effective use of local procedures for hemostasis including absorbable hemostatic agents, sutures, and pressure dressings if necessary. Under these conditions dental and surgical procedures may be performed without undue risk of hemorrhage.

PANWARFIN WITH HEPARIN

Since a delay intervenes between the administration of the initial dose and the therapeutic prolongation of prothrombin time, it may be advisable in emergency situations to administer sodium heparin initially along with PANWARFIN.

It should be noted that heparin may affect the prothrombin time, and therefore, when patients are receiving both heparin and PANWARFIN, the blood sample for prothrombin time determination should be drawn just prior to the next heparin dosage, at least 5 hours after the last intravenous injection or 24 hours after the last subcutaneous injection.

TREATMENT FOR OVERDOSAGE

Excessive prothrombinopenia, with or without bleeding, is readily controlled by discontinuing PANWARFIN, and if necessary, the oral or parenteral administration of vitamin K_1. The appearance of microscopic hematuria, excessive menstrual bleeding, melena, petechiae or oozing from nicks made while shaving are early manifestations of hypoprothrombinemia beyond a safe and satisfactory level.

In excessive prothrombinopenia with mild or no bleeding, omission of one or more doses of PANWARFIN may suffice; and if necessary, small doses of vitamin K_1 orally, $2\frac{1}{2}$ to 10 mg, will usually correct the problem.

If minor bleeding persists, or progresses to frank bleeding, vitamin K_1 in doses of 5 to 25 mg may be given parenterally. (Please note recommendations accompanying vitamin K preparations prior to use.)

Fresh whole blood transfusions should be considered in cases of severe bleeding or prothrombinopenic states unresponsive to vitamin K_1.

Resumption of PANWARFIN administration reverses the effect of vitamin K_1, and a therapeutic hypoprothrombinemia level can again be obtained. A hypercoagulable state has been reported to occur following rapid reversal of a prolonged prothrombin time, therefore, caution must be used in determining the need for this vitamin.

HOW SUPPLIED

PANWARFIN (warfarin sodium tablets, USP) for oral administration, grooved and bearing dosage strength numerals are available as follows:

2 mg, lavender-colored, in bottles of 100 (NDC 0074-6626-03). Also available in ABBO-PAC® unit dose packages of 100 tablets (NDC 0074-6626-07).

$2\frac{1}{2}$ mg, orange-colored, in bottles of 100 (NDC 0074-7202-01). Also available in ABBO-PAC unit dose packages of 100 tablets (NDC 0074-7202-05).

5 mg, peach-colored, in bottles of 100 (NDC 0074-7210-01) and 500 (NDC 0074-7210-09). Also available in ABBO-PAC unit dose packages of 100 tablets (NDC 0074-7210-05).

$7\frac{1}{2}$ mg, yellow, in bottles of 100 (NDC 0074-6638-03). Also available in ABBO-PAC unit dose packages of 100 tablets (NDC 0074-6638-07).

10 mg, white, in bottles of 100 (NDC 0074-7218-01). Also available in ABBO-PAC unit dose packages of 100 tablets (NDC 0074-7218-05).

Abbott Pharmaceuticals, Inc.
North Chicago, IL 60064
Ref. 03-4306-R5

Shown in Product Identification Section, page 403

PARADIONE®
[pă-ră-dī'own]
(paramethadione)
Capsules and Oral Solution

℞

> BECAUSE OF ITS POTENTIAL TO PRODUCE FETAL MALFORMATIONS AND SERIOUS SIDE EFFECTS, PARADIONE (paramethadione) SHOULD ONLY BE UTILIZED WHEN OTHER LESS TOXIC DRUGS HAVE BEEN FOUND INEFFECTIVE IN CONTROLLING ABSENCE (PETIT MAL) SEIZURES.

DESCRIPTION

PARADIONE (paramethadione) is an antiepileptic agent. An oxazolidinedione compound, it is chemically identified as 5-Ethyl-3,5-dimethyl-2,4-oxazolidinedione. PARADIONE is a synthetic, oily, slightly water-soluble liquid. It is supplied in capsular and liquid forms for oral use only. The capsules are available in two dosage strengths. One strength contains 150 mg the other 300 mg of paramethadione per capsule. Each ml of the liquid contains 300 mg of paramethadione.

Inactive Ingredients: 150 mg capsule: FD&C Yellow No. 6, gelatin, glycerin, methylparaben, olive oil ethyl ester and propylparaben.

300 mg capsule: FD&C Blue No. 1, FD&C Yellow No. 5 (tartrazine), FD&C Yellow No. 6, gelatin, glycerin, methylparaben, olive oil ethyl ester and propylparaben.

Paradione Solution: Alcohol 65% and water.

CLINICAL PHARMACOLOGY

PARADIONE has been shown to prevent pentylenetetrazol-induced and thujone-induced seizures in experimental animals; the drug has a less marked effect on seizures induced by picrotoxin, procaine, cocaine, or strychnine. Unlike the hydantoins and antiepileptic barbiturates, PARADIONE does not modify the maximal seizure pattern in patients undergoing electroconvulsive therapy. PARADIONE has a sedative effect that may increase to the point of ataxia when excessive doses are used. A toxic dose of the drug in animals (approximately 1 g/kg) produced sleep, unconsciousness, and respiratory depression.

Paramethadione is rapidly absorbed from the gastrointestinal tract. It is demethylated by liver microsomes to an active N-demethylated metabolite, and is excreted slowly in this form by the kidney; almost no unmetabolized PARADIONE is excreted.

INDICATIONS AND USAGE

PARADIONE (paramethadione) is indicated for the control of absence (petit mal) seizures that are refractory to treatment with other drugs.

CONTRAINDICATIONS

PARADIONE is contraindicated in patients with a known hypersensitivity to the drug.

WARNINGS

PARADIONE may cause serious side effects. Strict medical supervision of the patient is mandatory, especially during the initial year of therapy.

USAGE DURING PREGNANCY: THERE ARE MULTIPLE REPORTS IN THE CLINICAL LITERATURE WHICH INDICATE THAT THE USE OF ANTIEPILEPTIC DRUGS DURING PREGNANCY RESULTS IN AN INCREASED INCIDENCE OF BIRTH DEFECTS IN THE OFFSPRING. DATA ARE MORE EXTENSIVE WITH RESPECT TO TRIMETHADIONE, PARAMETHADIONE, PHENYTOIN AND PHENOBARBITAL THAN WITH OTHER ANTIEPILEPTIC DRUGS.

THEREFORE, ANTIEPILEPTIC DRUGS SUCH AS PARADIONE (PARAMETHADIONE) SHOULD BE ADMINISTERED TO WOMEN OF CHILDBEARING POTENTIAL ONLY IF THEY ARE CLEARLY SHOWN TO BE ESSENTIAL IN THE MANAGEMENT OF THEIR SEIZURES. EFFECTIVE MEANS OF CONTRACEPTION SHOULD ACCOMPANY THE USE OF PARADIONE IN SUCH PATIENTS. IF A PATIENT BECOMES PREGNANT WHILE TAKING PARADIONE, TERMINATION OF THE PREGNANCY SHOULD BE CONSIDERED. A PATIENT WHO REQUIRES THERAPY WITH PARADIONE AND WHO WISHES TO BECOME PREGNANT SHOULD BE ADVISED OF THE RISKS.

REPORTS HAVE SUGGESTED THAT THE MATERNAL INGESTION OF ANTIEPILEPTIC DRUGS, PARTICULARLY BARBITURATES, IS ASSOCIATED WITH A NEONATAL COAGULATION DEFECT THAT MAY CAUSE BLEEDING DURING THE EARLY (USUALLY WITHIN 24 HOURS OF BIRTH) NEONATAL PERIOD. THE POSSIBILITY OF THE OCCURRENCE OF THIS DEFECT WITH THE USE OF PARADIONE SHOULD BE KEPT IN MIND. THE DEFECT IS CHARACTERIZED BY DECREASED LEVELS OF VITAMIN K-DEPENDENT CLOTTING FACTORS, AND PROLONGATION OF EITHER THE PROTHROMBIN TIME OR THE PARTIAL THROMBOPLASTIN TIME, OR BOTH. IT HAS BEEN SUGGESTED THAT PROPHY-

LACTIC VITAMIN K BE GIVEN TO THE MOTHER ONE MONTH PRIOR TO, AND DURING DELIVERY, AND TO THE INFANT, INTRAVENOUSLY, IMMEDIATELY AFTER BIRTH.

PRECAUTIONS

General: Abrupt discontinuation of PARADIONE may precipitate absence (petit mal) status. PARADIONE (paramethadione) should always be withdrawn gradually unless serious adverse effects dictate otherwise. In the latter case, another antiepileptic may be substituted to protect the patient.

PARADIONE (paramethadione) should be withdrawn promptly if skin rash appears, because of the grave possibility of the occurrence of exfoliative dermatitis or severe forms of erythema multiforme. Even a minor acneiform or morbilliform rash should be allowed to clear completely before treatment with PARADIONE is resumed; reinstitute therapy cautiously. PARADIONE should ordinarily not be used in patients with severe blood dyscrasias.

Hepatitis has been associated rarely with the use of oxazolidinediones. Jaundice or other signs of liver dysfunction are an indication for withdrawal of PARADIONE. PARADIONE should ordinarily not be used in patients with severe hepatic impairment.

Fatal nephrosis has been reported with the use of oxazolidinediones. Persistent or increasing albuminuria, or the development of any other significant renal abnormality, is an indication for withdrawal of the drug. PARADIONE should ordinarily not be used in patients with severe renal dysfunction.

Hemeralopia has occurred with the use of oxazolidinedione compounds; this appears to be an effect of the drugs on the neural layers of the retina, and usually can be reversed by a reduction in dosage. Scotomata are an indication for withdrawal of the drug. Caution should be observed when treating patients who have diseases of the retina or optic nerve.

Manifestations of systemic lupus erythematosus have been associated with the use of the oxazolidinediones, as they have with the use of certain other antiepileptics. Lymphadenopathies simulating malignant lymphoma have also occurred. Lupus-like manifestations or lymph node enlargement are indications for withdrawal of PARADIONE. Signs and symptoms may disappear after discontinuation of therapy, and specific treatment may be unnecessary.

A myasthenia gravis-like syndrome has been associated with the chronic use of the oxazolidinediones. Symptoms suggestive of this condition are indications for withdrawal of PARADIONE.

The 300 mg capsule of PARADIONE contains FD&C Yellow No. 5 (tartrazine) which may cause allergic-type reactions (including bronchial asthma) in certain susceptible individuals. Although the overall incidence of FD&C Yellow No. 5 (tartrazine) sensitivity in the general population is low, it is frequently seen in patients who also have aspirin hypersensitivity.

Information for Patients: Patients should be advised to report immediately such signs and symptoms as sore throat, fever, malaise, easy-bruising, petechiae, or epistaxis, or others that may be indicative of an infection or bleeding tendency.

Laboratory Tests: A complete blood count should be done prior to initiating therapy with PARADIONE, and at monthly intervals thereafter. A marked depression of the blood count is an indication for withdrawal of the drug. If no abnormality appears within 12 months, the interval between blood counts may be extended. A moderate degree of neutropenia with or without a corresponding drop in the leukocyte count is not uncommon. Therapy need not be withdrawn unless the neutrophil count is 2500 or less; more frequent blood examinations should be done when the count is less than 3,000. Other blood dyscrasias, including leukopenia, eosinophilia, thrombocytopenia, pancytopenia, agranulocytosis, hypoplastic anemia, and fatal aplastic anemia, have occurred with the use of oxazolidinediones.

Liver function tests should be done prior to initiating therapy with PARADIONE, and at monthly intervals thereafter. A urinalysis should be done prior to initiating therapy with PARADIONE and at monthly intervals thereafter.

Drug Interactions: Drugs known to cause toxic effects similar to those of the oxazolidinediones should be avoided or used only with extreme caution during therapy with PARADIONE.

Carcinogenesis: No data are available on long-term potential for carcinogenicity in animals or humans.

Pregnancy: Pregnancy Category D. See "Warnings" section.

Nursing Mothers: It is not known whether this drug is excreted in human milk. Because many drugs are excreted in human milk and because of the potential for serious adverse reactions in nursing infants from PARADIONE, a decision

Continued on next page

Abbott—Cont.

should be made whether to discontinue nursing or to discontinue the drug, taking into account the importance of the drug to the mother.

ADVERSE REACTIONS

The following side effects, in decreasing order of severity, have been associated with the use of oxazolidinedione compounds. Although not all of them have been reported with the use of PARADIONE, the possibility of their occurrence should be kept in mind when the drug is prescribed.

Renal: Fatal nephrosis has occurred. Albuminuria.

Hematologic: Fatal aplastic anemia, hypoplastic anemia, pancytopenia, agranulocytosis, leukopenia, neutropenia, thrombocytopenia, eosinophilia, retinal and petechial hemorrhages, vaginal bleeding, epistaxis, and bleeding gums.

Hepatic: Hepatitis has been reported rarely.

Dermatologic: Acneiform or morbilliform skin rash that may progress to severe forms of erythema multiforme or to exfoliative dermatitis. Hair loss.

CNS/Neurologic: A myasthenia gravis-like syndrome has been reported. Precipitation of tonic-clonic (grand mal) seizures, vertigo, personality changes, increased irritability, drowsiness, headache, parasthesias, fatigue, malaise, and insomnia.

Drowsiness usually subsides with continued therapy. If it persists, a reduction in dosage is indicated.

Ophthalmologic: Diplopia, hemeralopia, and photophobia.

Cardiovascular: Changes in blood pressure.

Gastrointestinal: Vomiting, abdominal pain, gastric distress, nausea, anorexia, weight loss, and hiccups.

Other: Lupus erythematosus, and lymphadenopathies simulating malignant lymphoma, have been reported. Pruritus associated with lymphadenopathy and hepatosplenomegaly has occurred in hypersensitive individuals.

OVERDOSAGE

Symptoms of acute PARADIONE overdosage include drowsiness, nausea, dizziness, ataxia, visual disturbances. Coma may follow massive overdosage.

Gastric evacuation, either by induced emesis, or by lavage, or both, should be done immediately. General supportive care, including frequent monitoring of the vital signs and close observation of the patient, are required.

It has been reported that alkalinization of the urine may be expected to increase the excretion of the N-demethylated metabolite of PARADIONE.

A blood count and a careful evaluation of hepatic and renal function should be done following recovery.

DOSAGE AND ADMINISTRATION

PARADIONE is administered orally.

Because PARADIONE Oral Solution contains alcohol 65%, it may be desirable to dilute the preparation with water before administering it to small children.

Usual Adult Dosage: 0.9–2.4 g daily in 3 or 4 equally divided doses (i.e., 300–600 mg 3 or 4 times daily).

Initially, give 0.9 g daily; increase this dose by 300 mg at weekly intervals until therapeutic results are seen or until toxic symptoms appear.

Maintenance dosage should be the least amount of drug required to maintain control.

Children's Dosage: Usually 0.3–0.9 g daily in 3 or 4 equally divided doses.

HOW SUPPLIED

PARADIONE Capsules (paramethadione capsules, USP) are round capsules supplied as 150 mg (orange color) (**NDC** 0074-3976-01), and 300 mg (green color) (**NDC** 0074-3838-01) in bottles of 100.

PARADIONE Solution (paramethadione oral solution, USP), 300 mg per ml, is supplied in 50-ml bottles (**NDC** 0074-3860-01). A dropper is provided with each bottle, which is marked to permit easy measurement of 0.5 ml and 1 ml doses. The solution is clear and colorless.

Abbott Laboratories
North Chicago, IL 60064
01-2349-R7

Shown in Product Identification Section, page 403

PCE®   ℞
(erythromycin particles in tablets)
Dispertab® Tablets

PRODUCT OVERVIEW

KEY FACTS

PCE is an antibacterial product containing specially coated erythromycin base particles. The coating protects the erythromycin from the inactivating effects of gastric acidity and permits efficient absorption of erythromycin in the small intestine. Therapeutic blood levels are achieved when PCE is taken in either the fasting or fed state. Each PCE tablet contains 333 mg erythromycin base for oral administration. The usual adult dose is 333 mg every eight hours. Dosage may be

---

increased up to 4 grams per day depending on the severity of the infection.

MAJOR USES

PCE is indicated for the treatment of upper and lower respiratory tract infections of mild to moderate degree, skin and skin structure infections of mild to moderate degree, and urogenital infections caused by susceptible strains of microorganisms as discussed in further detail in the prescribing information that follows. In penicillin-allergic patients, erythromycin is indicated in the prevention of initial attacks of rheumatic fever and the prevention of bacterial endocarditis. In patients allergic to penicillin and sulfonamides, erythromycin is indicated for the prevention of recurrent attacks of rheumatic fever. Clinical studies suggest that erythromycin is effective in treating Legionnaire's Disease.

SAFETY INFORMATION

PCE is contraindicated in patients with a known hypersensitivity to erythromycin. The most common adverse events associated with erythromycin are gastrointestinal and are dose-related. Caution should be exercised when erythromycin is administered to patients with impaired hepatic function since erythromycin is principally excreted by the liver. Erythromycin has been reported to increase the serum concentrations of theophylline, carbamazepine, and digoxin and to increase the anticoagulant effects of oral anticoagulants. Serum concentrations should be monitored and dose adjustments should be made, if necessary, in patients taking erythromycin in combination with these drugs. Although there is no evidence of teratogenicity associated with erythromycin in animal studies, erythromycin should be used during pregnancy only if clearly needed. Erythromycin has been reported to cross the placental barrier in humans and is excreted in breast milk.

PRODUCT ILLUSTRATION

PRESCRIBING INFORMATION

PCE®   ℞
(erythromycin particles in tablets)
Dispertab® Tablets

DESCRIPTION

PCE (erythromycin particles in tablets) Dispertab tablets are an antibacterial product containing specially coated erythromycin base particles. The coating protects the antibiotic from the inactivating effects of gastric acidity and permits efficient absorption of the antibiotic in the small intestine. Each tablet contains 333 mg of erythromycin base for oral administration.

Inactive ingredients: Cellulosic polymers, citrate ester, colloidal silicon dioxide, D&C Red No. 30, hydrogenated vegetable oil wax, lactose, magnesium stearate, microcrystalline cellulose, povidone, propylene glycol, sodium starch glycolate, stearic acid and vanillin.

Erythromycin is produced by a strain of *Streptomyces erythraeus* and belongs to the macrolide group of antibiotics. It is basic and readily forms salts with acids. Erythromycin is a white to off-white powder, slightly soluble in water, and soluble in alcohol, chloroform, and ether. Erythromycin is known chemically as (3R*, 4S*, 5S*, 6R*, 7R*, 9R*, 11R*, 12R*, 13S*, 14R*)-4-[(2,6-Dideoxy-3-C-methyl-3-0-methyl-α-L-*ribo*-hexopyranosyl)oxy]-14-ethyl-7,12,13-trihydroxy-3, 5, 7, 9, 11, 13-hexamethyl-6-[[3,4,6-trideoxy-3-(dimethylamino)-β-D-*xylo*-hexopyranosyl]oxy]oxacyclotetradecane-2,10-dione.

CLINICAL PHARMACOLOGY

Orally administered erythromycin base and its salts are readily absorbed in the microbiologically active form. Interindividual variations in the absorption of erythromycin are, however, observed, and some patients do not achieve optimal serum levels. Erythromycin is largely bound to plasma proteins. After absorption, erythromycin diffuses readily into most body fluids. In the absence of meningeal inflammation, low concentrations are normally achieved in the spinal fluid but the passage of the drugs across the blood-brain barrier increases in meningitis. Erythromycin crosses the placental barrier and is excreted in breast milk. Erythromycin is not removed by peritoneal dialysis or hemodialysis. In the presence of normal hepatic function, erythromycin is concentrated in the liver and is excreted in the bile; the effect of hepatic dysfunction on biliary excretion of erythromycin is not known. After oral administration, less than 5% of the administered dose can be recovered in the active form in the urine.

The erythromycin particles in PCE (erythromycin particles in tablets) are coated with a polymer whose dissolution is pH dependent. This coating allows for minimal release of erythromycin in acidic environments, e.g. stomach. This delivery

---

system is designed for optimal drug release and absorption in the small intestine. In multiple-dose, steady-state studies, PCE has demonstrated rapid and consistent drug delivery in both fasting and nonfasting conditions. However, optimal blood levels are obtained when PCE is given in the fasting state ($\frac{1}{2}$ hour and preferably 2 hours before meals). Bioavailability data are available from Abbott Laboratories, Dept. 355.

Microbiology:

Erythromycin acts by inhibition of protein synthesis by binding 50 S ribosomal subunits of susceptible organisms. It does not affect nucleic acid synthesis. Antagonism has been demonstrated in vitro between erythromycin and clindamycin, lincomycin, and chloramphenicol.

Many strains of *Haemophilus influenzae* are resistant to erythromycin alone, but are susceptible to erythromycin and sulfonamides together.

Staphylococci resistant to erythromycin may emerge during a course of erythromycin therapy. Culture and susceptibility testing should be performed.

Erythromycin is usually active against the following organisms *in vitro* (prior to use, refer to "Indications and Usage" section):

Gram-positive Bacteria: Staphylococcus aureus (resistant organisms may emerge during treatment), Streptococcus pyogenes (Group A beta-hemolytic streptococci), Alpha-hemolytic streptococci (viridans group), Streptococcus (diplococcus) pneumoniae, Corynebacterium diphtheriae, Corynebacterium minutissimum.

Gram-negative Bacteria: Moraxella (Branhamella) catarrhalis, Neisseria gonorrhoeae, Legionella pneumophila, Bordetella pertussis.

Mycoplasma: Mycoplasma pneumoniae, Ureaplasma urealyticum.

Other Microorganisms: Chlamydia trachomatis, Entamoeba histolytica, Treponema pallidum, Listeria monocytogenes.

Susceptibility Testing:

Quantitative methods that require measurement of zone diameters give the most precise estimates of antibiotic susceptibility. One such standardized single-disc procedure has been recommended for use with discs to test susceptibility to erythromycin.[1] Interpretation involves correlation of the zone diameters obtained in the disc test with minimal inhibitory concentration (MIC) values for erythromycin.

Reports from the laboratory giving results of the standardized single-disc susceptibility test using a 15 mcg erythromycin disc should be interpreted according to the following criteria:

Susceptible organisms produce zones of 18 mm or greater, indicating that the tested organism is likely to respond to therapy.

Resistant organisms produce zones of 13 mm or less, indicating that other therapy should be selected.

Organisms of intermediate susceptibility produce zones of 14 to 17 mm. The "intermediate" category provides a "buffer zone" which should prevent small, uncontrolled technical factors from causing major discrepancies in interpretations; thus, when a zone diameter falls within the "intermediate" range, the results may be considered equivocal. If alternative drugs are not available, confirmation by dilution tests may be indicated.

Standardized procedures require the use of control organisms. The 15 mcg erythromycin disc should give zone diameters between 22 and 30 mm for the *S. aureus* ATCC 25923 control strain.

A bacterial isolate may be considered susceptible if the MIC value[2] for erythromycin is not more than 2 mcg/mL. Organisms are considered resistant if the MIC is 8 mcg/mL or higher. The MIC of erythromycin for *S. aureus* ATCC 29213 control strain should be between 0.12 and 0.5 mcg/mL.

INDICATIONS AND USAGE

PCE (erythromycin particles in tablets) is indicated in the treatment of infections caused by susceptible strains of the designated microorganisms in the diseases listed below:

Upper respiratory tract infections of mild to moderate degree caused by *Streptococcus pyogenes* (Group A beta-hemolytic streptococci); *Streptococcus pneumoniae (Diplococcus pneumoniae)*; *Haemophilus influenzae* (when used concomitantly with adequate doses of sulfonamides, since many strains of *H. influenzae* are not susceptible in the erythromycin concentrations ordinarily achieved). (See appropriate sulfonamide labeling for prescribing information.)

Lower respiratory tract infections of mild to moderate severity caused by *Streptococcus pyogenes* (Group A beta-hemolytic streptococci): *Streptococcus pneumoniae (Diplococcus pneumoniae)*.

Respiratory tract infections due to *Mycoplasma pneumoniae*.

Skin and skin structure infections of mild to moderate severity caused by *Streptococcus pyogenes* and *Staphylococcus aureus* (resistant staphylococci may emerge during treatment).

Pertussis (whooping cough) caused by *Bordetella pertussis*. Erythromycin is effective in eliminating the organism from the nasopharynx of infected individuals, rendering them noninfectious. Some clinical studies suggest that erythromycin may be helpful in the prophylaxis of pertussis in exposed susceptible individuals.

Diphtheria—As an adjunct to antitoxin in infections due to *Corynebacterium diphtheriae*, to prevent establishment of carriers and to eradicate the organism in carriers.

Erythrasma—In the treatment of infections due to *Corynebacterium minutissimum*.

Intestinal amebiasis caused by *Entamoeba histolytica* (oral erythromycins only). Extraenteric amebiasis requires treatment with other agents.

Acute pelvic inflammatory disease caused by *Neisseria gonorrhoeae*: Erythrocin® Lactobionate-I.V. (erythromycin lactobionate for injection, USP) followed by erythromycin base orally, as an alternative drug in treatment of acute pelvic inflammatory disease caused by *N. gonorrhoeae* in female patients with a history of sensitivity to penicillin. Before treatment of gonorrhea, patients who are suspected of also having syphilis should have a microscopic examination for *T. pallidum* (by immunofluorescence or darkfield) before receiving erythromycin and monthly serologic tests for a minimum of 4 months thereafter.

Erythromycins are indicated for treatment of the following infections caused by *Chlamydia trachomatis*: conjunctivitis of the newborn, pneumonia of infancy, and urogenital infections during pregnancy. When tetracyclines are contraindicated or not tolerated, erythromycin is indicated for the treatment of uncomplicated urethral, endocervical, or rectal infections in adults due to *Chlamydia trachomatis*.[3]

When tetracyclines are contraindicated or not tolerated, erythromycin is indicated for the treatment of nongonococcal urethritis caused by *Ureaplasma urealyticum*.[3]

Primary syphilis caused by *Treponema pallidum*. Erythromycin (oral forms only) is an alternative choice of treatment for primary syphilis in patients allergic to the penicillins. In treatment of primary syphilis, spinal fluid should be examined before treatment and as part of the follow-up after therapy.

Legionnaires' Disease caused by *Legionella pneumophila*. Although no controlled clinical efficacy studies have been conducted, *in vitro* and limited preliminary clinical data suggest that erythromycin may be effective in treating Legionnaires' Disease.

Prevention of Initial Attacks of Rheumatic Fever—Penicillin is considered by the American Heart Association to be the drug of choice in the prevention of initial attacks of rheumatic fever (treatment of Group A beta-hemolytic streptococcal infections of the upper respiratory tract e.g., tonsillitis, or pharyngitis).[4] Erythromycin is indicated for the treatment of penicillin-allergic patients. The therapeutic dose should be administered for ten days.

Prevention of Recurrent Attacks of Rheumatic Fever—Penicillin or sulfonamides are considered by the American Heart Association to be the drugs of choice in the prevention of recurrent attacks of rheumatic fever. In patients who are allergic to penicillin and sulfonamides, oral erythromycin is recommended by the American Heart Association in the long-term prophylaxis of streptococcal pharyngitis (for the prevention of recurrent attacks of rheumatic fever).[4]

Prevention of Bacterial Endocarditis—Although no controlled clinical efficacy trials have been conducted, oral erythromycin has been recommended by the American Heart Association for prevention of bacterial endocarditis in penicillin-allergic patients with most congenital cardiac malformations, rheumatic or other acquired valvular dysfunction, idiopathic hypertrophic subaortic stenosis (IHSS), previous history of bacterial endocarditis and mitral valve prolapse with insufficiency when they undergo dental procedures and surgical procedures of the upper respiratory tract.[5]

CONTRAINDICATIONS

Erythromycin is contraindicated in patients with known hypersensitivity to this antibiotic.

WARNINGS

There have been reports of hepatic dysfunction with or without jaundice, occurring in patients receiving oral erythromycin products.

PRECAUTIONS

General: Erythromycin is principally excreted by the liver. Caution should be exercised when erythromycin is administered to patients with impaired hepatic function. (See "Clinical Pharmacology" and "Warnings" sections).

Prolonged or repeated use of erythromycin may result in an overgrowth of nonsusceptible bacteria or fungi. If superinfection occurs, erythromycin should be discontinued and appropriate therapy instituted.

When indicated, incision and drainage or other surgical procedures should be performed in conjunction with antibiotic therapy.

Laboratory Tests: Erythromycin interferes with the fluorometric determination of urinary catecholamines.

Drug Interactions: Erythromycin use in patients who are receiving high doses of theophylline may be associated with an increase of serum theophylline levels and potential theophylline toxicity. Serum theophylline levels should be moni-

tored in patients receiving concomitant erythromycin. The theophylline dose may need to be reduced in some patients. Erythromycin administration in patients receiving carbamazepine has been reported to cause increased serum levels of carbamazepine with subsequent development of signs of carbamazepine toxicity.

Concomitant administration of erythromycin and digoxin has been reported to result in elevated digoxin serum levels. There have been reports of increased anticoagulant effects when erythromycin and oral anticoagulants were used concomitantly.

Carcinogenesis, Mutagenesis, Impairment of Fertility: Long-term (2-year) oral studies conducted in rats with erythromycin base did not provide evidence of tumorigenicity. Mutagenicity studies have not been conducted. There was no apparent effect on male or female fertility in rats fed erythromycin (base) at levels up to 0.25 percent of diet.

Pregnancy: Pregnancy Category B: There is no evidence of teratogenicity or any other adverse effect on reproduction in female rats fed erythromycin base (up to 0.25 percent of diet) prior to and during mating, during gestation, and through weaning of two successive litters. There are, however, no adequate and well-controlled studies in pregnant women. Because animal reproduction studies are not always predictive of human response, this drug should be used during pregnancy only if clearly needed. Erythromycin has been reported to cross the placental barrier in humans, but fetal plasma levels are generally low.

Labor and Delivery: The effect of erythromycin on labor and delivery is unknown.

Nursing Mothers: Erythromycin is excreted in breast milk, therefore, caution should be exercised when erythromycin is administered to a nursing woman.

Pediatric Use: See "Indications and Usage" and "Dosage and Administration" sections.

ADVERSE REACTIONS

The most frequent side effects of oral erythromycin preparations are gastrointestinal and are dose-related. They include nausea, vomiting, abdominal pain, diarrhea and anorexia. Symptoms of hepatic dysfunction and/or abnormal liver function test results may occur (see "Warnings" section). Pseudomembranous colitis has been rarely reported in association with erythromycin therapy.

Allergic reactions ranging from urticaria and mild skin eruptions to anaphylaxis have occurred.

There have been isolated reports of reversible hearing loss occurring chiefly in patients with renal insufficiency and in patients receiving high doses of erythromycin.

OVERDOSAGE

In case of overdosage, erythromycin should be discontinued. Overdosage should be handled with the prompt elimination of unabsorbed drug and all other appropriate measures. Erythromycin is not removed by peritoneal dialysis or hemodialysis.

DOSAGE AND ADMINISTRATION

PCE (erythromycin particles in tablets) is well absorbed and may be given without regard to meals. However, optimal blood levels are obtained when PCE is given in the fasting state ($\frac{1}{2}$ hour and preferably 2 hours before meals).

Adults: The usual dosage is 333 mg every 8 hours. Dosage may be increased up to 4 g per day according to the severity of the infection.

Children: Age, weight, and severity of the infection are important factors in determining the proper dosage. The usual dosage is 30 to 50 mg/kg/day, in equally divided doses. For more severe infections this dosage may be doubled but should not exceed 4 g per day.

In the treatment of Group A beta-hemolytic streptococcal infections of the upper respiratory tract (e.g., tonsillitis or pharyngitis), the therapeutic dosage of erythromycin should be administered for ten days. The American Heart Association suggests a dosage of 250 mg of erythromycin orally, twice a day in long-term prophylaxis of streptococcal upper respiratory tract infections for the prevention of recurring attacks of rheumatic fever in patients allergic to penicillin and sulfonamides.[4]

In prophylaxis against bacterial endocarditis (see "Indications and Usage" section) the oral regimen for penicillin allergic patients is erythromycin 1 gram, 1 hour before the procedure followed by 500 mg six hours later.[5]

Conjunctivitis of the newborn caused by *Chlamydia trachomatis:* Oral erythromycin suspension 50 mg/kg/day in 4 divided doses for at least 2 weeks.[3]

Pneumonia of infancy caused by *Chlamydia trachomatis:* Although the optimal duration of therapy has not been established, the recommended therapy is oral erythromycin suspension 50 mg/kg/day in 4 divided doses for at least 3 weeks.[3]

Urogenital infections during pregnancy due to *Chlamydia trachomatis:* Although the optimal dose and duration of therapy have not been established, the suggested treatment is two erythromycin 333 mg tablets orally every 8 hours or 500 mg of erythromycin by mouth four times a day on an empty stomach for at least 7 days. For women who cannot tolerate

this regimen, a decreased dose of one 333 mg tablet orally every 8 hours or 250 mg by mouth four times a day should be used for at least 14 days.[3,6]

For adults with uncomplicated urethral, endocervical, or rectal infections caused by *Chlamydia trachomatis,* when tetracycline is contraindicated or not tolerated: two 333 mg tablets every 8 hours or 500 mg of erythromycin by mouth four times a day for at least 7 days.[3,6]

For patients with nongonococcal urethritis caused by *Ureaplasma urealyticum* when tetracycline is contraindicated or not tolerated: two 333 mg tablets every 8 hours or 500 mg of erythromycin by mouth four times a day for at least seven days.[3,6]

Primary syphilis: 30 to 40 g given in divided doses over a period of 10 to 15 days.

Acute pelvic inflammatory disease caused by *N. gonorrhoeae*: 500 mg Erythrocin® Lactobionate-I.V. (erythromycin lactobionate for injection, USP) every 6 hours for 3 days, followed by 333 mg of erythromycin base orally every 8 hours for 7 days.

Intestinal amebiasis: Adults: 333 mg every 8 hours or 250 mg every 6 hours for 10 to 14 days. Children: 30 to 50 mg/kg/day in divided doses for 10 to 14 days.

Pertussis: Although optimal dosage and duration have not been established, doses of erythromycin utilized in reported clinical studies were 40 to 50 mg/kg/day, given in divided doses for 5 to 14 days.

Legionnaires' Disease: Although optimal dosage has not been established, doses utilized in reported clinical data were 1 to 4 g daily in divided doses.

HOW SUPPLIED

PCE (erythromycin particles in tablets) Dispertab tablets are supplied as ovaloid, pink-speckled white tablets containing 333 mg of erythromycin in the following sizes: bottles of 60 (NDC 0074-6290-60) and bottles of 500 (NDC 0074-6290-53).

REFERENCES

1. National Committee for Clinical Laboratory Standards, Approved Standard: *Performance Standards for Antimicrobial Disk Susceptibility Tests*, 3rd Edition, Vol. 4(16):M2–A3, Villanova, PA, December 1984.
2. Ericson, H.M., Sherris, J.C., Antibiotic Sensitivity Testing: Report of an International Collaborative Study, *Acta Pathologica et Microbiologica Scandinavica* Section B Suppl. 217:1–90, 1971.
3. CDC Sexually Transmitted Diseases Treatment Guidelines 1985.
4. Committee on Rheumatic Fever and Infective Endocarditis of the Council on Cardiovascular Disease of the Young: Prevention of Rheumatic Fever, *Circulation* 70(6):1118A–1122A, December 1984.
5. Committee on Rheumatic Fever and Infective Endocarditis of the Council on Cardiovascular Disease of the Young: Prevention of Bacterial Endocarditis, *Circulation* 70(6):1123A–1127A, December 1984.
6. Data on file, Abbott Laboratories.

Abbott Health Care Products, Inc.
North Chicago, IL 60064
Ref. 03-4356-R3 Revised: March, 1989
   Shown in Product Identification Section, page 403

PEGANONE®   ℞
[pĕg 'ă-noon]
(ethotoin tablets)

DESCRIPTION

PEGANONE (ethotoin) is an oral antiepileptic of the hydantoin series and is chemically identified as 3-ethyl-5-phenyl-2, 4-imidazolidinedione. PEGANONE tablets are available in two dosage strengths of 250 mg and 500 mg respectively.

Inactive Ingredients: 250 mg and 500 mg tablets: Acacia, lactose, sodium carboxymethylcellulose, stearic acid and talc.

CLINICAL PHARMACOLOGY

PEGANONE (ethotoin) exerts an antiepileptic effect without causing general central nervous system depression. The mechanism of action is probably very similar to that of phenytoin. The latter drug appears to stabilize rather than to raise the normal seizure threshold, and to prevent the spread of seizure activity rather than to abolish the primary focus of seizure discharges.

In laboratory animals, the drug was found effective against electroshock convulsions, and to a lesser extent, against complex partial (psychomotor) and pentylenetetrazol-induced seizures.

In mice, the duration of antiepileptic activity was prolonged by hepatic injury but not by bilateral nephrectomy; the drug is apparently biotransformed by the liver.

Continued on next page

Abbott—Cont.

Ethotoin is fairly rapidly absorbed; the extent of oral absorption is not known. The drug exhibits saturable metabolism with respect to the formation of N-deethyl and p-hydroxyl-ethotoin, the major metabolites. Where plasma concentrations are below about 8 mcg/l, the elimination half-life of ethotoin is in the range of 3 to 9 hours. Above this concentration, the dose-dependent, nonlinear kinetics of the drug preclude definition of any conventional half-life. Experience suggests that therapeutic plasma concentrations fall in the range of 15 to 50 mcg/l; however, this range is not as extensively documented as those quoted for other antiepileptics.

INDICATIONS AND USAGE

PEGANONE (ethotoin) is indicated for the control of tonic-clonic (grand mal) and complex partial (psychomotor) seizures.

CONTRAINDICATIONS

PEGANONE (ethotoin) is contraindicated in patients with hepatic abnormalities or hematologic disorders.

WARNINGS

USAGE DURING PREGNANCY— THERE ARE MULTIPLE REPORTS IN THE CLINICAL LITERATURE WHICH INDICATE THAT THE USE OF ANTIEPILEPTIC DRUGS DURING PREGNANCY RESULTS IN AN INCREASED INCIDENCE OF BIRTH DEFECTS IN THE OFFSPRING. ALTHOUGH DATA ARE MORE EXTENSIVE WITH RESPECT TO TRIMETHADIONE, PARAMETHADIONE, PHENYTOIN, AND PHENOBARBITAL, REPORTS INDICATE A POSSIBLE SIMILAR ASSOCIATION WITH THE USE OF OTHER ANTIEPILEPTIC DRUGS. THEREFORE, ANTIEPILEPTIC DRUGS SHOULD BE ADMINISTERED TO WOMEN OF CHILDBEARING POTENTIAL ONLY IF THEY ARE CLEARLY SHOWN TO BE ESSENTIAL IN THE MANAGEMENT OF THEIR SEIZURES. ANTIEPILEPTIC DRUGS SHOULD NOT BE DISCONTINUED IN PATIENTS IN WHOM THE DRUG IS ADMINISTERED TO PREVENT MAJOR SEIZURES BECAUSE OF THE STRONG POSSIBILITY OF PRECIPITATING STATUS EPILEPTICUS WITH ATTENDANT HYPOXIA AND RISK TO BOTH MOTHER AND THE UNBORN CHILD. CONSIDERATION SHOULD, HOWEVER, BE GIVEN TO DISCONTINUATION OF ANTIEPILEPTICS PRIOR TO AND DURING PREGNANCY WHEN THE NATURE, FREQUENCY AND SEVERITY OF THE SEIZURES DO NOT POSE A SERIOUS THREAT TO THE PATIENT. IT IS NOT, HOWEVER, KNOWN WHETHER EVEN MINOR SEIZURES CONSTITUTE SOME RISK TO THE DEVELOPING EMBRYO OR FETUS. REPORTS HAVE SUGGESTED THAT THE MATERNAL INGESTION OF ANTIEPILEPTIC DRUGS, PARTICULARLY BARBITURATES, IS ASSOCIATED WITH A NEONATAL COAGULATION DEFECT THAT MAY CAUSE BLEEDING DURING THE EARLY (USUALLY WITHIN 24 HOURS OF BIRTH) NEONATAL PERIOD. THE POSSIBILITY OF THE OCCURRENCE OF THIS DEFECT WITH THE USE OF PEGANONE SHOULD BE KEPT IN MIND. THE DEFECT IS CHARACTERIZED BY DECREASED LEVELS OF VITAMIN K-DEPENDENT CLOTTING FACTORS, AND PROLONGATION OF EITHER THE PROTHROMBIN TIME OR THE PARTIAL THROMBOPLASTIN TIME, OR BOTH. IT HAS BEEN SUGGESTED THAT VITAMIN K BE GIVEN PROPHYLACTICALLY TO THE MOTHER ONE MONTH PRIOR TO, AND DURING DELIVERY, AND TO THE INFANT, INTRAVENOUSLY, IMMEDIATELY AFTER BIRTH. THE PHYSICIAN SHOULD WEIGH THESE CONSIDERATIONS IN TREATMENT AND COUNSELING OF EPILEPTIC WOMEN OF CHILDBEARING POTENTIAL.

PRECAUTIONS

General: Blood dyscrasias have been reported in patients receiving PEGANONE. Although the etiologic role of PEGANONE has not been definitely established, physicians should be alert for general malaise, sore throat and other symptoms indicative of possible blood dyscrasia.

There is some evidence suggesting that hydantoin-like compounds may interfere with folic acid metabolism, precipitating a megaloblastic anemia. If this should occur during gestation, folic acid therapy should be considered.

Information for Patients: Patients should be advised to report immediately such signs and symptoms as sore throat, fever, malaise, easy bruising, petechiae, epistaxis, or others that may be indicative of an infection or bleeding tendency.

Laboratory Tests: Liver function tests should be performed if clinical evidence suggests the possibility of hepatic dysfunction. Signs of liver damage are indication for withdrawal of the drug.

It is recommended that blood counts and urinalyses be performed when therapy is begun and at monthly intervals for several months thereafter. As in patients receiving other hydantoin compounds and other antiepileptic drugs, blood dyscrasias have been reported in patients receiving PEGA-

NONE (ethotoin). Marked depression of the blood count is indication for withdrawal of the drug.

Drug Interactions: PEGANONE used in combination with other drugs known to adversely affect the hematopoietic system should be avoided if possible.

Considerable caution should be exercised if PEGANONE is administered concurrently with *Phenurone (phenacemide)* since paranoid symptoms have been reported during therapy with this combination.

A two-way interaction between the hydantoin antiepileptic, *phenytoin,* and the *coumarin anticoagulants* has been suggested. Presumably, phenytoin acts as a stimulator of coumarin metabolism and has been reported to cause decreased serum levels of the coumarin anticoagulants and increased prothrombin-proconvertin concentrations. Conversely, the coumarin anticoagulants have been reported to increase the serum levels and prolong the serum half-life of phenytoin by inhibiting its metabolism. Although there is no documentation of such, a similar interaction between ethotoin and the coumarin anticoagulants may occur. Caution is therefore advised when administering PEGANONE to patients receiving coumarin anticoagulants.

Carcinogenesis: No data are available on long-term potential for carcinogenicity in animals or humans.

Pregnancy: Pregnancy Category C. See "Warnings" section.

Nursing Mothers: Ethotoin is excreted in breast milk. Because of the potential for serious adverse reactions in nursing infants from ethotoin, a decision should be made whether to discontinue nursing or to discontinue the drug, taking into account the importance of the drug to the mother.

ADVERSE REACTIONS

Adverse reactions associated with PEGANONE, in decreasing order of severity, are:

Isolated cases of lymphadenopathy and systemic lupus erythematosus have been reported in patients taking hydantoin compounds, and lymphadenopathy has occurred with PEGANONE. Withdrawal of therapy has resulted in remission of the clinical and pathological findings. Therefore, if a lymphoma-like syndrome develops, the drug should be withdrawn and the patient should be closely observed for regression of signs and symptoms before treatment is resumed.

Ataxia and gum hypertrophy have occurred only rarely—usually only in patients receiving an additional hydantoin derivative. It is of interest to note that ataxia and gum hypertrophy have subsided in patients receiving other hydantoins when PEGANONE was given as a substitute antiepileptic.

Occasionally, vomiting or nausea after ingestion of PEGANONE has been reported, but if the drug is administered after meals, the incidence of gastric distress is reduced. Other side effects have included chest pain, nystagmus, diplopia, fever, dizziness, diarrhea, headache, insomnia, fatigue, numbness and skin rash.

OVERDOSAGE

Symptoms of acute overdosage include drowsiness, visual disturbance, nausea and ataxia. Coma is possible at very high dosage.

Treatment should be begun by inducing emesis; gastric lavage may be considered as an alternative. General supportive measures will be necessary. A careful evaluation of blood-forming organs should be made following recovery.

DOSAGE AND ADMINISTRATION

PEGANONE is administered orally in 4 to 6 divided doses daily. The drug should be taken after food, and doses should be spaced as evenly as practicable. Initial dosage should be conservative. For adults, the initial daily dose should be 1 g or less, with subsequent gradual dosage increases over a period of several days. The optimum dosage must be determined on the basis of individual response. The usual adult maintenance dose is 2 to 3 g daily. Less than 2 g daily has been found ineffective in most adults.

Pediatric dosage depends upon the age and weight of the patient. The initial dose should not exceed 750 mg daily. The usual maintenance dose in children ranges from 500 mg to 1 g daily, although occasionally 2 or (rarely) 3 g daily may be necessary.

If a patient is receiving another antiepileptic drug, it should not be discontinued when PEGANONE therapy is begun. The dosage of the other drug should be reduced gradually as that of PEGANONE is increased. PEGANONE may eventually replace the other drug or the optimal dosage of both antiepileptics may be established.

PEGANONE is compatible with all commonly employed antiepileptic medications with the possible exception of Phenurone® (phenacemide). In tonic-clonic (grand mal) seizures, use of the drug with Gemonil® (metharbital) or phenobarbital may be beneficial. PEGANONE may be used in combination with drugs such as Tridione® (trimethadione) or Paradione® (paramethadione), as an adjunct in those patients with absence (petit mal) associated with tonic-clonic (grand mal).

HOW SUPPLIED

PEGANONE (ethotoin) grooved, white tablets are supplied in two dosage strengths: 250 mg, bottles of 100 (**NDC** 0074-6902-01); 500 mg, bottles of 100 (**NDC** 0074-6905-04).

This product is listed in N.D., a Medicare designated compendium.

Abbott Laboratories
North Chicago, IL 60064
Ref. 01-2360-R6

Shown in Product Identification Section, page 403

PENTHRANE®   ℞
[pen 'thrāne]
(methoxyflurane, USP)

DESCRIPTION

PENTHRANE® (Methoxyflurane, USP), a volatile liquid, is intended only for vaporization at suitable concentrations for administration by inhalation with appropriate anesthesia equipment or devices.

PENTHRANE is an inhalation anesthetic/analgesic which belongs to the fluorinated hydrocarbon group of volatile anesthetics. It is chemically designated 2,2 - dichloro -1, 1 - difluoroethyl methyl ether and has the following structural formula:

$$CH\,Cl_2CF_2 - O - CH_3$$

PENTHRANE has a mildly pungent odor.
Some of the physical constants are:

Molecular weight	164.97
Boiling point at 760 mm Hg	104.6° C
Partition coefficients at 37° C	
Water/gas	4.5
Blood/gas (mean range)	10.20 to 14.06
Oil/gas	825
Vapor Pressure 17.7° C	20 mm Hg
Flash points	
in air	62.8° C
in oxygen (closed system)	32.8° C
in nitrous oxide 50% with 50% oxygen	28.2° C
Lower limits of flammability of vapor concentration	
in air	7.0%
in oxygen	5.4%
in N_2O 50%	4.6%

PENTHRANE (Methoxyflurane, USP) is stable and does not decompose in contact with soda lime. An antioxidant, butylated hydroxytoluene 0.01% w/w is added to insure stability on standing. This slowly oxidizes to a yellow pigment that progressively turns to brown, and which may accumulate on the vaporizer wick. The colored matter may be removed by rinsing the wick with diethyl ether. The wick must be dried after cleaning to avoid introducing diethyl ether into the system.

Polyvinyl chloride plastics are extracted by PENTHRANE, therefore, contact should be avoided. PENTHRANE does not extract polyethylene plastics, polypropylene plastics, fluorinated hydrocarbon plastics or nylon. It is very soluble in rubber and soda lime. Disposable conductive plastic circuits should be discarded after a single use to avoid cross contamination and because PENTHRANE may reduce conductivity of such materials below safe limits for subsequent administration of a flammable anesthetic.

The vapor concentration of PENTHRANE is limited by its vapor pressure at room temperature to a maximum of about 3.5% at 23° C. In practice, this concentration is not easily reached due to the cooling effect of vaporization. PENTHRANE is not flammable except at vapor concentrations well above those recommended for its use. Recommended concentrations are nonflammable and nonexplosive in air, oxygen and nitrous oxide mixtures at ordinary room temperature.

CLINICAL PHARMACOLOGY

PENTHRANE provides anesthesia and/or analgesia.

After surgical anesthesia with PENTHRANE, analgesia and drowsiness may persist after consciousness has returned. This may obviate or reduce the need for narcotics in the immediate postoperative period.

When used alone in safe concentration, PENTHRANE (Methoxyflurane, USP) will not produce appreciable skeletal muscle relaxation. A muscle relaxing agent, e.g., succinylcholine chloride (Quelicin®) or tubocurarine chloride should be used as an adjunct.

Bronchiolar constriction or laryngeal spasm is not ordinarily provoked by PENTHRANE.

During PENTHRANE anesthesia, the cardiac rhythm is usually regular. The myocardium is only minimally sensitized by PENTHRANE to epinephrine. Some decrease in blood pressure often accompanies light planes of anesthesia.

This may be accompanied by bradycardia. The hypotension noted is accompanied by reduced cardiac contractile force and reduced cardiac output.

When used for obstetrical delivery, light planes of PENTHRANE anesthesia have little effect on uterine contractions. There are no known contraindications to the concomitant use of PENTHRANE and oxytocic agents.

Biotransformation of PENTHRANE occurs in man. Approximately 20% of PENTHRANE uptake is recovered in the exhaled air, while urinary excretion of organic fluorine, fluoride and oxalic acid accounts for about 30% of the PENTHRANE uptake.

Studies have shown that higher peak blood fluoride levels are obtained earlier in obese patients than in non-obese.

INDICATIONS AND USAGE

1. PENTHRANE is indicated usually in combination with oxygen and nitrous oxide to provide anesthesia for surgical procedures in which total duration of PENTHRANE administration is anticipated to be 4 hours or less, and in which PENTHRANE is not to be used in concentrations that will provide skeletal muscle relaxation; see WARNINGS regarding time and dose relationships.
2. PENTHRANE (Methoxyflurane, USP) may be used alone with hand held inhalers or in combination with oxygen and nitrous oxide for analgesia in obstetrics and in minor surgical procedures.

CONTRAINDICATIONS

See WARNINGS.

WARNINGS

SEQUENTIAL ANESTHESIA WITH PENTHRANE AND HALOTHANE, OR HALOTHANE AND PENTHRANE, IN EITHER ORDER, HAS BEEN FOLLOWED BY JAUNDICE IN A FEW RARE CASES. WHEN A PREVIOUS EXPOSURE TO PENTHRANE (METHOXYFLURANE, USP) OR HALOTHANE HAS BEEN FOLLOWED BY UNEXPLAINED HEPATIC DYSFUNCTION AND/OR JAUNDICE, CONSIDERATION SHOULD BE GIVEN TO THE USE OF OTHER AGENTS.

THE NEPHROTOXICITY ASSOCIATED WITH PENTHRANE ADMINISTRATION APPEARS TO BE RELATED TO THE TOTAL DOSE (TIME AND CONCENTRATION). SEE PARAGRAPH 5. THE MANIFESTATIONS RANGE IN SEVERITY FROM REVERSIBLE ALTERATIONS IN LABORATORY FINDINGS TO POLYURIC OR OLIGURIC RENAL FAILURE, SOMETIMES FATAL.

POLYURIC RENAL FAILURE IS CHARACTERIZED BY THE DEVELOPMENT, EARLY IN THE POSTOPERATIVE PERIOD, OF THE FOLLOWING:

WEIGHT LOSS

URINE: LOW SPECIFIC GRAVITY, LARGE VOLUME EQUAL TO OR IN EXCESS OF FLUID INTAKE, DECREASED OSMOLALITY.

SERUM/BLOOD: ELEVATION OF SODIUM, CHLORIDE, URIC ACID, BUN, CREATININE.

THIS SYNDROME IS BELIEVED TO BE RELATED TO RELEASE OF THE FLUORIDE ION, A METABOLIC PRODUCT OF PENTHRANE AND TO BE RELATED TO THE TOTAL DOSAGE ADMINISTERED. THEREFORE, THE LOWEST EFFECTIVE DOSAGE SHOULD BE ADMINISTERED, ESPECIALLY IN AGED OR OBESE PATIENTS AND IN SURGICAL PROCEDURES OF LONG DURATION, BEARING IN MIND THAT THE TOTAL DOSE DELIVERED TO THE PATIENT IS A FACTOR OF DURATION OF ADMINISTRATION AND CONCENTRATION OF VAPOR.

OXALATE CRYSTALS AND/OR ACUTE TUBULAR NECROSIS HAVE BEEN NOTED AT AUTOPSY.

The guiding principles in minimizing the possibility of renal injury are:

1. AVOID USING PENTHRANE (METHOXYFLURANE, USP) AS THE SOLE OR PRINCIPLE AGENT TO ACHIEVE MUSCULAR RELAXATION.
2. PATIENTS WITH PRE-EXISTING RENAL DISEASE, IMPAIRMENT OF RENAL FUNCTION, TOXEMIA OF PREGNANCY, AND PATIENTS UNDERGOING VASCULAR SURGERY AT OR NEAR THE RENAL VESSELS SHOULD NOT RECEIVE PENTHRANE UNLESS IN THE JUDGMENT OF THE PHYSICIAN THE BENEFITS OUTWEIGH THE INCREASED RISK OF NEPHROTOXIC EFFECT.
3. URINARY OUTPUT SHOULD BE MONITORED IN ALL PATIENTS IF EXCESSIVE URINE OUTPUT OCCURS, APPROPRIATE LABORATORY STUDIES SHOULD BE DONE TO ASSESS RENAL FUNCTION. IN HIGH RISK PATIENTS (SEE 2, ABOVE) SERIAL TESTS OF RENAL FUNCTION AND MEASUREMENTS OF FLUID AND ELECTROLYTE BALANCE ARE IMPERATIVE. ALL FLUID AND ELECTROLYTE LOSSES SHOULD BE PROMPTLY REPLACED.
4. THE CONCURRENT USE OF TETRACYCLINE AND PENTHRANE HAS BEEN REPORTED TO RESULT IN FATAL RENAL TOXICITY. THE POSSIBILITY EXISTS THAT PENTHRANE MAY ENHANCE THE ADVERSE RENAL EFFECTS OF OTHER DRUGS INCLUDING CERTAIN ANTIBIOTICS OF KNOWN NEPHROTOXIC POTENTIAL SUCH AS GENTAMICIN, KANAMYCIN, COLISTIN, POLYMYXIN B, CEPHALORIDINE AND AMPHOTERICIN B. THIS SHOULD BE CAREFULLY CONSIDERED WHEN PRESCRIBING SUCH DRUGS DURING THE PREOPERATIVE, OPERATIVE AND POSTOPERATIVE PERIODS.
5. BECAUSE OF THE DOSE-RELATED NEPHROTOXICITY POTENTIAL OF PENTHRANE (METHOXYFLURANE, USP), IT IS SUGGESTED THAT THE TOTAL DURATION OF LIGHT ANESTHETIC DEPTH WITH PENTHRANE NOT EXCEED APPROXIMATELY 4 HOURS AT A SINGLE ADMINISTRATION.

PRECAUTIONS

Diabetic patients may have an increased likelihood of developing nephropathy if they have impaired renal function or polyuria, are obese, or are not optimally controlled.

Caution should be exercised in using PENTHRANE in patients under treatment with enzyme inducing drugs (e.g., barbiturates) as such agents may enhance the metabolism of PENTHRANE, resulting in increased fluoride levels.

Ventilation should be assessed carefully and, if depressed, should be augmented to insure adequate oxygenation and carbon dioxide removal. Parenteral anesthetic adjuncts (e.g., barbiturates, narcotics and neuromuscular blocking agents) may also cause depression of respiration requiring assisted or controlled ventilation. A sufficient reduction in respiratory minute volume occurs during deep anesthesia to produce a significant respiratory acidosis if ventilation is not adequately assisted. PENTHRANE causes a slight metabolic acidosis.

PENTHRANE augments the effect of nondepolarizing muscle relaxants so that their usual dosage should be reduced by approximately one-half.

Epinephrine or levarterenol (norepinephrine) should be employed cautiously during PENTHRANE anesthesia.

When PENTHRANE is used under the conditions of dosage and administration shown below, in surgery or obstetrics, inorganic fluoride levels may infrequently reach those at which changes in renal laboratory values have been seen.

General anesthesia, including general anesthesia with PENTHRANE (Methoxyflurane, USP), has been associated in susceptible individuals with the acute onset of fulminant hypermetabolism of skeletal muscle known as *malignant hyperthermic crisis*. This syndrome is characterized by the acute onset of skeletal muscle overactivity and resulting high oxygen demand which usually exceeds supply. TACHYCARDIA and TACHYPNEA are the most important early signs; these may be associated with increased utilization of anesthesia circuit carbon dioxide absorber, arrhythmias, cyanosis, skin mottling, profuse sweating, unstable blood pressure, rapidly rising body temperature (usually appearing sometime after the first signs, when noted) and other indications of markedly increased oxygen demand. Laboratory tests usually confirm the excessive oxygen demand and resulting metabolic acidosis (blood gases); hyperkalemia and myoglobinemia are also frequently noted. Hypoglobinuria and renal failure may develop later. When these signs suggest a diagnosis of malignant hyperthermic crisis, it is important to terminate the anesthetic, cancel the surgery when possible, confirm the diagnosis and initiate management of the condition.

Dantrolene sodium intravenous is indicated, along with supportive measures, in the management of malignant hyperthermic crisis. These necessary supportive measures must be individualized, but will usually involve discontinuance of the suspect triggering agents, attendance to increased oxygen requirements and carbon dioxide production, management of metabolic acidosis, assurance of adequate urinary output, management of electrolyte imbalance and institution of measures to control rising temperature, when indicated. Consult literature references and the prescribing information for dantrolene sodium intravenous for additional information about the management of malignant hyperthermic crisis.

Information for patients:

When appropriate, as in some cases where discharge is anticipated soon after methoxyflurane anesthesia, patients should be cautioned not to drive an automobile, operate hazardous machinery or engage in hazardous sports for 24 hours or more (depending upon total dosage of methoxyflurane, condition of the patient and consideration given to other drugs administered) after anesthesia.

Carcinogenesis, mutagenesis, impairment of fertility:

A 15 month transplacental inhalation study of methoxyflurane at a subanesthetic concentration of 0.13% in the mouse revealed no evidence of anesthetic-related carcinogenesis. This concentration is equivalent to 36 hours of 0.2% methoxyflurane.

Mutagenesis testing of methoxyflurane was negative. Tests included: Ames bacterial assay, mouse sperm morphology assay and sister chromatid exchange in Chinese hamster ovary cells.

Studies of the effect on fertility have not been reported.

Pregnancy Category C: Methoxyflurane has been shown to cause fetal growth retardation in the rat at levels equivalent to 67 hours exposure of 0.2% methoxyflurane. There are no adequate and well-controlled studies in pregnant women. Methoxyflurane should be used during pregnancy only if the potential benefit justifies the potential risk to the fetus.

Nursing Mothers: Caution should be exercised when PENTHRANE (Methoxyflurane, USP) is administered to a nursing mother.

Labor and Delivery: In obstetrics attention should be given to the directions for Dosage and Administration shown below. Fluoride levels in cord blood are usually less than, but may equal those of the mother at delivery. The effect of inorganic fluoride on the infant is not known. However, clinical experience has demonstrated that cases of high output renal failure in either mother or child must be considered unlikely.

Pediatric Use: Safety and effectiveness of PENTHRANE (Methoxyflurane, USP) in children have not been established.

ADVERSE REACTIONS

Renal dysfunction: See WARNINGS.

Hepatic dysfunction, jaundice, and fatal hepatic necrosis have occurred following PENTHRANE anesthesia. Also as with other anesthetics, transient alterations in liver function tests may follow PENTHRANE administration. Hepatic complications rarely have involved reported cross reactions between PENTHRANE and Halothane.

Some patients exhibit pallor during recovery from PENTHRANE anesthesia.

Other adverse reactions which have been reported include cardiac arrest, malignant hyperpyrexia, prolonged postoperative somnolence, respiratory depression laryngospasm, bronchospasm, nausea, vomiting postoperative headache, hypotension and emergence delirium.

OVERDOSAGE

Patients should be closely observed for signs of excessive dosage during administration of PENTHRANE. PENTHRANE overdosage is characterized by decrease in tidal and minute volume; decrease in blood pressure, pallor, cyanosis and muscle relaxation. If the above signs are observed, turn off vaporizer and increase ventilation. If anesthesia exceeds light levels, vapor concentration should be reduced promptly. Prolonged administration (beyond four hours) and/or excessive vapor concentration beyond the equivalent of four hours of 0.25% delivered methoxyflurane may cause nephrotoxic effects attributable to metabolic release of free fluoride ion. See WARNINGS, PRECAUTIONS and DOSAGE AND ADMINISTRATION.

In the event of postoperative excessive urine output, fluid and electrolyte losses should be promptly replaced.

DOSAGE AND ADMINISTRATION

THE LOWEST EFFECTIVE DOSAGE OF PENTHRANE (METHOXYFLURANE, USP) SHOULD BE USED IN ORDER TO MINIMIZE THE POSSIBILITY OF NEPHROPATHY AND TO ALLOW FOR OPTIMAL RECOVERY TIME. IN CASES OF UNUSUALLY HIGH MAINTENANCE REQUIREMENTS, THE USE OF ANESTHETIC ADJUNCTS OR ANOTHER AGENT MAY BE INDICATED. THE ABSENCE OF HYPOTENSION CANNOT BE RELIED UPON AS EVIDENCE THAT DOSAGE HAS NOT BEEN EXCESSIVE DURING MAINTENANCE.

Analgesia

For analgesia, intermittent inhalation of vapor concentrations in the range of 0.3 to 0.8% are recommended. PENTHRANE may be self administered by hand held inhalers (e.g., Analgizer, Cyprane) if the patient is kept under close observation.

For intermittent administration from the hand-held inhaler, dosage for each patient is limited to not more than a single 15 mL charge of liquid PENTHRANE. Such analgesia in labor should not be instituted before relief becomes necessary. Use of the hand-held inhaler does not preclude transfer of the patient to a conventional anesthesia machine for inhalation anesthesia, but concentrations should be kept at the lowest effective dosage. Total time for anesthesia combined with analgesia should be as short as possible, bearing in mind the recommended duration for continuous anesthesia (four hours).

Anesthesia

A light level of anesthesia should be used. The use of deeper levels to achieve muscle relaxation should be avoided.

Apparatus: PENTHRANE should be vaporized by calibrated, temperature compensated, out of circle vaporizers (e.g., Pentec II, Pentomatic) or other methods which provide accurate delivered vapor concentration. Anesthetic uptake by rubber tubing, bags and soda lime which may prolong

Continued on next page

Abbott—Cont.

induction and recovery time can be reduced by the use of nonabsorptive plastic circuit material (not polyvinyl chloride) and fresh moist Baralyme. The fresh gas inlet should be located downstream of the CO_2 absorber in order to avoid excessive anesthetic absorption, and the rebreathing bag and pop-off valve should be located on the expiratory side.

Premedication: The usual preanesthetic medications may be administered prior to PENTHRANE (Methoxyflurane, USP) anesthesia, see PRECAUTIONS.

Induction: Use of a parenteral induction agent (such as an ultra-short acting barbiturate) is recommended unless contraindicated in an individual patient.

Carrier Gases: For general surgery, PENTHRANE should usually be administered with a carrier gas flow consisting of oxygen and at least 50% nitrous oxide in order to minimize the total PENTHRANE dose unless nitrous oxide is contraindicated.

Muscle Relaxation: PENTHRANE should not be administered at levels required to achieve muscle relaxation. Adequate relaxation should be obtained from adjunctive use of a muscle relaxant, e.g., succinylcholine chloride (Quelicin®) or tubocurarine chloride. The usual dosage of nondepolarizing muscle relaxants should be reduced by approximately one-half.

Vapor Concentrations: Initially PENTHRANE concentrations may be increased as tolerated to a maximum of approximately 2.0%. This concentration should only be continued for about two to five minutes, or until patient signs of light anesthesia are evident. The concentration of PENTHRANE should then be reduced by frequent decrements to the lowest possible levels consistent with the maintenance of adequate anesthesia. For example, in a 70 kg patient, the following sequential reduction in the delivered vapor concentration of PENTHRANE (Methoxyflurane, USP) may be appropriate:

Elapsed Minutes				
0 to 5	5 to 20	20 to 60	60 to 120	120 to 240
Vapor Conc.*				
2.0%	0.6%	0.4%	0.2%	0.1%

* Concentrations are approximate and subject to adjustment according to patient signs of anesthesia. Based on 5 liters per minute gas flow and ventilation rate throughout procedure, 50/50 N_2O and oxygen.

Concentration may be increased or decreased according to the requirements of the individual patient. Four hours of 0.25% delivered methoxyflurane should not be exceeded in normal adult patients unless in the opinion of the clinician, the anticipated benefits outweigh the increased risk of dose related nephrotoxicity. The product of these two factors (four hours of 0.25% delivered methoxyflurane) may be used to estimate other combinations of time and dose: Thus two hours of 0.5%, for example, should not ordinarily be exceeded. In sufficiently long cases, PENTHRANE should be discontinued 30 to 40 minutes before the end of surgery. Rapid flushing will not remove PENTHRANE absorbed by rubber circuit components.

Patient signs and levels: The PENTHRANE level of conscious analgesia is suited for pain relief, as in labor and uncomplicated vaginal deliveries. The level of unconscious analgesia is suitable for many minor surgical procedures. The level of light anesthesia is recommended for general surgical use. Deep anesthesia with PENTHRANE (Methoxyflurane, USP) is not recommended.

Appropriate patient signs of PENTHRANE anesthesia should be observed closely as a guide to proper depth. A blood pressure decrease of about 22 mm Hg may be seen during induction. A greater decrease may occur in hypertensive patients. Blood pressure usually recovers as a level of light anesthesia is reached. The absence of hypotension cannot be relied upon as evidence that dosage has not been excessive during maintenance.

HOW SUPPLIED

PENTHRANE (Methoxyflurane, USP) is supplied in 125 ml and 15 ml bottles, List 6864.

Preserve in tight, light-resistant containers and avoid exposure to excessive heat.

Protect from light. Protect from freezing and extreme heat.

Caution: Federal (USA) law prohibits dispensing without prescription.

06-3179-R26-3/82

Marketed by

Abbott Laboratories

PENTOTHAL®

[pen'tōe-thal]

(thiopental sodium

for injection, USP)

WARNING: MAY BE HABIT FORMING.

DESCRIPTION

Pentothal (Thiopental Sodium for Injection, USP) is a thiobarbiturate, the sulfur analogue of sodium pentobarbital. The drug is prepared as a sterile powder and after reconstitution with an appropriate diluent is administered by the intravenous route.

Pentothal is chemically designated sodium 5-ethyl-5-(1-methylbutyl)-2-thiobarbiturate and has the following structural formula:

The drug is a yellowish, hygroscopic powder, stabilized with anhydrous sodium carbonate as a buffer (60 mg/g of thiopental sodium).

CLINICAL PHARMACOLOGY

Pentothal (Thiopental Sodium for Injection, USP) is an ultrashort-acting depressant of the central nervous system which induces hypnosis and anesthesia, but not analgesia. It produces hypnosis within 30 to 40 seconds of intravenous injection. Recovery after a small dose is rapid, with some somnolence and retrograde amnesia. Repeated intravenous doses lead to prolonged anesthesia because fatty tissues act as a reservoir; they accumulate Pentothal in concentrations 6 to 12 times greater than the plasma concentration, and then release the drug slowly to cause prolonged anesthesia. The half-life of the elimination phase after a single intravenous dose is three to eight hours.

The distribution and fate of Pentothal (as with other barbiturates) is influenced chiefly by its lipid solubility (partition coefficient), protein binding and extent of ionization. Pentothal has a partition coefficient of 580.

Approximately 80% of the drug in the blood is bound to plasma protein. Pentothal is largely degraded in the liver and to a smaller extent in other tissues, especially the kidney and brain. It has a pK_a of 7.4.

Concentration in spinal fluid is slightly less than in the plasma.

Biotransformation products of thiopental are pharmacologically inactive and mostly excreted in the urine.

INDICATIONS AND USAGE

Pentothal (Thiopental Sodium for Injection, USP) is indicated (1) as the sole anesthetic agent for brief (15 minute) procedures, (2) for induction of anesthesia prior to administration of other anesthetic agents, (3) to supplement regional anesthesia, (4) to provide hypnosis during balanced anesthesia with other agents for analgesia or muscle relaxation, (5) for the control of convulsive states during or following inhalation anesthesia, local anesthesia, or other causes, (6) in neurosurgical patients with increased intracranial pressure, if adequate ventilation is provided, and (7) for narcoanalysis and narcosynthesis in psychiatric disorders.

CONTRAINDICATIONS

Absolute Contraindications:

(1) Absence of suitable veins for intravenous administration, (2) hypersensitivity (allergy) to barbiturates and (3) variegate porphyria (South African) or acute intermittent porphyria.

Relative Contraindications:

(1) Severe cardiovascular disease, (2) hypotension or shock, (3) conditions in which the hypnotic effect may be prolonged or potentiated — excessive premedication, Addison's disease, hepatic or renal dysfunction, myxedema, increased blood urea, severe anemia, asthma, myasthenia gravis, and (4) status asthmaticus.

WARNINGS

KEEP RESUSCITATIVE AND ENDOTRACHEAL INTUBATION EQUIPMENT AND OXYGEN READILY AVAILABLE. MAINTAIN PATENCY OF THE AIRWAY AT ALL TIMES.

This drug should be administered only by persons qualified in the use of intravenous anesthetics.

Avoid extravasation or intra-arterial injection.

WARNING: MAY BE HABIT FORMING.

PRECAUTIONS

Observe aseptic precautions at all times in preparation and handling of Pentothal (Thiopental Sodium for Injection, USP) solutions.

If used in conditions involving relative contraindications, reduce dosage and administer slowly.

Care should be taken in administering the drug to patients with advanced cardiac disease, increased intracranial pressure, ophthalmoplegia plus, asthma, myasthenia gravis and endocrine insufficiency (pituitary, thyroid, adrenal, pancreas).

Drug Interactions: The following drug interactions have been reported with thiopental:

Drug	Effect
Probenecid	Prolonged action of thiopental
Diazoxide	Hypotension
Zimelidine	Thiopental antagonism
Opioid analgesics	Decreased antinociceptive action
Aminophylline	Thiopental antagonism
Midazolam	Synergism

Nursing Mothers: Thiopental sodium readily crosses the placental barrier and small amounts may appear in the milk of nursing mothers following administration of large doses.

Pregnancy Category C. Animal reproduction studies have not been conducted with Pentothal. It is also not known whether Pentothal can cause fetal harm when administered to a pregnant woman or can affect reproduction capacity. Pentothal should be given to a pregnant woman only if clearly needed.

ADVERSE REACTIONS

Adverse reactions include respiratory depression, myocardial depression, cardiac arrhythmias, prolonged somnolence and recovery, sneezing, coughing, bronchospasm, laryngospasm and shivering.

Anaphylactic and anaphylactoid reactions to Pentothal (Thiopental Sodium for Injection, USP) have been reported. Symptoms, e.g., urticaria, bronchospasm, vasodilation and edema should be managed by conventional means.

Rarely, immune hemolytic anemia with renal failure and radial nerve palsy have been reported.

DRUG ABUSE AND DEPENDENCE

WARNING: MAY BE HABIT FORMING.

Thiopental sodium is classified as a Schedule III controlled substance.

OVERDOSAGE

Overdosage may occur from too rapid or repeated injections. Too rapid injection may be followed by an alarming fall in blood pressure even to shock levels. Apnea, occasional laryngospasm, coughing and other respiratory difficulties with excessive or too rapid injections may occur. In the event of suspected or apparent overdosage, the drug should be discontinued, a patent airway established (intubate if necessary) or maintained, and oxygen should be administered, with assisted ventilation if necessary. The lethal dose of barbiturates varies and cannot be stated with certainty. Lethal blood levels may be as low as 1 mg/100 mL for short-acting barbiturates; less if other depressant drugs or alcohol are also present.

MANAGEMENT OF OVERDOSAGE

It is generally agreed that respiratory depression or arrest due to unusual sensitivity to thiopental sodium or overdosage is easily managed if there is no concomitant respiratory obstruction. If the airway is patent, any method of ventilating the lungs (that prevents hypoxia) should be successful in maintaining other vital functions.

Since depression of respiratory activity is one of the characteristic actions of the drug, it is important to observe respiration closely.

Should laryngeal spasm occur, it may be relieved by one of the usual methods, such as the use of a relaxant drug or positive pressure oxygen. Endotracheal intubation may be indicated in difficult cases.

DOSAGE AND ADMINISTRATION

Pentothal is administered by the intravenous route only. Individual response to the drug is so varied that there can be no fixed dosage. The drug should be titrated against patient requirements as governed by age, sex and body weight. Younger patients require relatively larger doses than middle-aged and elderly persons; the latter metabolize the drug more slowly. Pre-puberty requirements are the same for both sexes, but adult females require less than adult males. Dose is usually proportional to body weight and obese patients require a larger dose than relatively lean persons of the same weight.

Premedication

Premedication usually consists of atropine or scopolamine to suppress vagal reflexes and inhibit secretions. In addition, a barbiturate or an opiate is often given. Sodium pentobarbital injection (Nembutal®) is suggested because it provides a preliminary indication of how the patient will react to barbiturate anesthesia. Ideally, the peak effect of these medications should be reached shortly before the time of induction.

Test Dose

It is advisable to inject a small "test" dose of 25 to 75 mg (1 to 3 mL of a 2.5% solution) of Pentothal (Thiopental Sodium for Injection, USP) to assess tolerance or unusual sensitivity to Pentothal, and pausing to observe patient reaction for at least 60 seconds. If unexpectedly deep anesthesia develops or if respiratory depression occurs, consider these possibilities: (1) the patient may be unusually sensitive to Pentothal, (2) the solution may be more concentrated than had been assumed, or (3) the patient may have received too much premedication.

Use in Anesthesia

Moderately slow induction can usually be accomplished in the "average" adult by injection of 50 to 75 mg (2 to 3 mL of a 2.5% solution) at intervals of 20 to 40 seconds, depending on the reaction of the patient. Once anesthesia is established, additional injections of 25 to 50 mg can be given whenever the patient moves.

Slow injection is recommended to minimize respiratory depression and the possibility of overdosage. The smallest dose consistent with attaining the surgical objective is the desired goal. Momentary apnea following each injection is typical, and progressive decrease in the amplitude of respiration appears with increasing dosage. Pulse remains normal or increases slightly and returns to normal. Blood pressure usually falls slightly but returns toward normal. Muscles usually relax about 30 seconds after unconsciousness is attained, but this may be masked if a skeletal muscle relaxant is used. The tone of jaw muscles is a fairly reliable index. The pupils may dilate but later contract; sensitivity to light is not usually lost until a level of anesthesia deep enough to permit surgery is attained. Nystagmus and divergent strabismus are characteristic during early stages, but at the level of surgical anesthesia, the eyes are central and fixed. Corneal and conjunctival reflexes disappear during surgical anesthesia. When Pentothal (Thiopental Sodium for Injection, USP) is used for induction in balanced anesthesia with a skeletal muscle relaxant and an inhalation agent, the total dose of Pentothal can be estimated and then injected in two to four fractional doses. With this technique, brief periods of apnea may occur which may require assisted or controlled pulmonary ventilation. As an initial dose, 210 to 280 mg (3 to 4 mg/kg) of Pentothal is usually required for rapid induction in the average adult (70 kg).

When Pentothal (Thiopental Sodium for Injection, USP) is used as the sole anesthetic agent, the desired level of anesthesia can be maintained by injection of small repeated doses as needed or by using a continuous intravenous drip in a 0.2% or 0.4% concentration. (Sterile water should not be used as the diluent in these concentrations, since hemolysis will occur.) With continuous drip, the depth of anesthesia is controlled by adjusting the rate of infusion.

Use in Convulsive States

For the control of convulsive states following anesthesia (inhalation or local) or other causes, 75 to 125 mg (3 to 5 mL of a 2.5% solution) should be given as soon as possible after the convulsion begins. Convulsions following the use of a local anesthetic may require 125 to 250 mg of Pentothal given over a ten minute period. If the convulsion is caused by a local anesthetic, the required dose of Pentothal will depend upon the amount of local anesthetic given and its convulsant properties.

Use in Neurosurgical Patients with Increased Intracranial Pressure

In neurosurgical patients, intermittent bolus injections of 1.5 to 3.5 mg/kg of body weight may be given to reduce intraoperative elevations of intracranial pressure, if adequate ventilation is provided.

Use in Psychiatric Disorders

For narcoanalysis and narcosynthesis in psychiatric disorders, premedication with an anticholinergic agent may precede administration of Pentothal. After a test dose, Pentothal (Thiopental Sodium for Injection, USP) is injected at a slow rate of 100 mg/min (4 mL/min of a 2.5% solution) with the patient counting backwards from 100. Shortly after counting becomes confused but before actual sleep is produced, the injection is discontinued. Allow the patient to return to a semidrowsy state where conversation is coherent. Alternatively, Pentothal may be administered by rapid I.V. drip using a 0.2% concentration in 5% dextrose and water. At this concentration, the rate of administration should not exceed 50 mL/min.

MANAGEMENT OF SOME COMPLICATIONS

Respiratory depression (hypoventilation, apnea), which may result from either unusual responsiveness to Pentothal or overdosage, is managed as stated above. Pentothal should be considered to have the same potential for producing respiratory depression as an inhalation agent, and patency of the airway must be protected at all times.

Laryngospasm may occur with light Pentothal narcosis at intubation, or in the absence of intubation if foreign matter or secretions in the respiratory tract create irritation. Laryngeal and bronchial vagal reflexes can be suppressed, and secretions minimized by giving atropine or scopolamine premedication and a barbiturate or opiate. Use of a skeletal muscle relaxant or positive pressure oxygen will usually relieve laryngospasm. Tracheostomy may be indicated in difficult cases.

Myocardial depression, proportional to the amount of drug in direct contact with the heart, can occur and may cause hypotension, particularly in patients with an unhealthy myocardium. Arrhythmias may appear if PCO_2 is elevated, but they are uncommon with adequate ventilation. Management of myocardial depression is the same as for overdosage. Pentothal (Thiopental Sodium for Injection, USP) does not sensitize the heart to epinephrine or other sympathomimetic amines.

Extravascular infiltration should be avoided. Care should be taken to insure that the needle is within the lumen of the vein before injection of Pentothal. Extravascular injection may cause chemical irritation of the tissues varying from slight tenderness to venospasm, extensive necrosis and sloughing. This is due primarily to the high alkaline pH (10 to 11) of clinical concentrations of the drug. If extravasation occurs, the local irritant effects can be reduced by injection of 1% procaine locally to relieve pain and enhance vasodilatation. Local application of heat also may help to increase local circulation and removal of the infiltrate.

Intra-arterial injection can occur inadvertently, especially if an aberrant superficial artery is present at the medial aspect of the antecubital fossa. The area selected for intravenous injection of the drug should be palpated for detection of an underlying pulsating vessel. Accidental intra-arterial injection can cause arteriospasm and severe pain along the course of the artery with blanching of the arm and fingers. Appropriate corrective measures should be instituted promptly to avoid possible development of gangrene. Any patient complaint of pain warrants stopping the injection. Methods suggested for dealing with this complication vary with the severity of symptoms. The following have been suggested:

1. Dilute the injected Pentothal (Thiopental Sodium for Injection, USP) by removing the tourniquet and any restrictive garments.
2. Leave the needle in place, if possible.
3. Inject the artery with a dilute solution of papaverine, 40 to 80 mg, or 10 mL of 1% procaine, to inhibit smooth muscle spasm.
4. If necessary, perform sympathetic block of the brachial plexus and/or stellate ganglion to relieve pain and assist in opening collateral circulation. Papaverine can be injected into the subclavian artery, if desired.
5. Unless otherwise contraindicated, institute immediate heparinization to prevent thrombus formation.
6. Consider local infiltration of an alpha-adrenergic blocking agent such as phentolamine into the vasospastic area.
7. Provide additional symptomatic treatment as required.

Shivering after Pentothal anesthesia, manifested by twitching face muscles and occasional progression to tremors of the arms, head, shoulder and body, is a thermal reaction due to increased sensitivity to cold. Shivering appears if the room environment is cold and if a large ventilatory heat loss has been sustained with balanced inhalation anesthesia employing nitrous oxide. Treatment consists of warming the patient with blankets, maintaining room temperature near 22° C (72° F), and administration of chlorpromazine or methylphenidate.

PREPARATION OF SOLUTIONS

Pentothal (Thiopental Sodium for Injection, USP) is supplied as a yellowish, hygroscopic powder in a variety of different containers. Solutions should be prepared aseptically with one of the three following diluents: Sterile Water for Injection, USP, 0.9% Sodium Chloride Injection, USP or 5% Dextrose Injection, USP. Clinical concentrations used for intermittent intravenous administration vary between 2.0% and 5.0%. A 2.0% or 2.5% solution is most commonly used. A 3.4% concentration in sterile water for injection is isotonic; concentrations less than 2.0% in this diluent are not used because they cause hemolysis. For continuous intravenous drip administration, concentrations of 0.2% or 0.4% are used. Solutions may be prepared by adding Pentothal to 5% Dextrose Injection, USP, 0.9% Sodium Chloride Injection, USP or Normosol®-R pH 7.4.

Since Pentothal contains no added bacteriostatic agent, extreme care in preparation and handling should be exercised at all times to prevent the introduction of microbial contaminants. Solutions should be freshly prepared and used promptly; when reconstituted for administration to several patients, unused portions should be discarded after 24 hours. Sterilization by heating should not be attempted.

WARNING

The 2.5 g and larger sizes contain adequate medication for several patients.

COMPATIBILITY

Any solution of Pentothal (Thiopental Sodium for Injection, USP) with a visible precipitate should not be administered. The stability of Pentothal solutions depends upon several factors, including the diluent, temperature of storage and the amount of carbon dioxide from room air that gains access to the solution. Any factor or condition which tends to lower pH (increase acidity) of Pentothal solutions will increase the likelihood of precipitation of thiopental acid. Such factors include the use of diluents which are too acidic and the absorption of carbon dioxide which can combine with water to form carbonic acid.

Solutions of succinylcholine, tubocurarine or other drugs which have an acid pH should not be mixed with Pentothal solutions. The most stable solutions are those reconstituted in water or isotonic saline, kept under refrigeration and tightly stoppered. The presence or absence of a visible precipitate offers a practical guide to the physical compatibility of prepared solutions of Pentothal.

Calculations for Various Concentrations:

Concentration Desired		Amounts to Use	
Percent	mg/mL	Pentothal g	Diluent mL
0.2	2	1	500
0.4	4	1	250
		2	500
2.0	20	5	250
		10	500
2.5	25	1	40
		5	200
5	50	1	20
		5	100

Reconstituted solutions of Pentothal (Thiopental Sodium for Injection, USP) should be inspected visually for particulate matter and discoloration, whenever solution and container permit.

HOW SUPPLIED

Pentothal is available in a variety of sizes and containers shown at the end of this insert.

Diluents in Pentothal® Kits

READY-TO-MIX SYRINGES AND VIALS
(For preparing solutions of Thiopental Sodium for Injection, USP)

DESCRIPTION

The following diluents in various container, syringe and vial sizes are provided in Pentothal Kits, Pentothal Ready-to-Mix Syringes and Vials for preparing solutions of Pentothal (Thiopental Sodium for Injection, USP) for clinical use:

Sterile Water for Injection, USP is a sterile, nonpyrogenic preparation of water for injection which contains no bacteriostat, antimicrobial agents or added buffers. The pH is 5.7 (5.0 to 7.0).

Sterile Water for Injection, USP is a pharmaceutic aid (solvent) for intravenous administration only after addition of a solute.

Water is chemically designated H_2O.

0.9% Sodium Chloride Injection, USP is a sterile, nonpyrogenic, isotonic solution of sodium chloride and water for injection. Each mL contains sodium chloride 9 mg (308 mOsmol/liter calc). It contains no bacteriostat, antimicrobial agents or added buffers except for pH adjustment. May contain hydrochloric acid and/or sodium hydroxide for pH adjustment. pH is 5.7 (4.5 to 7.0).

0.9% Sodium Chloride Injection, USP is an isotonic vehicle for intravenous administration of another solute.

Sodium chloride is chemically designated NaCl, a white crystalline compound freely soluble in water.

The semi-rigid vial contained in List Nos. 3329, 6418, 6419, 6420 and 6435 is fabricated from a specially formulated polyolefin. It is a copolymer of ethylene and propylene. The safety of the plastic has been confirmed by tests in animals according to USP biological standards for plastic containers. The container requires no vapor barrier to maintain the proper labeled volume.

CLINICAL PHARMACOLOGY

Sterile Water for Injection, USP serves only as a pharmaceutic aid for diluting or dissolving drugs prior to administration.

Water is an essential constituent of all body tissues and accounts for approximately 70% of total body weight. Average normal adult daily requirement ranges from two to three liters (1.0 to 1.5 liters each for insensible water loss by perspiration and urine excretion).

Water balance is maintained by various regulatory mechanisms. Water distribution depends primarily on the concentration of dissociated electrolytes in the body compartments and sodium (Na+) plays a major role in maintaining a physiologic equilibrium between fluid intake and output.

0.9% Sodium Chloride Injection, USP serves only as an isotonic vehicle for drugs prior to administration.

Sodium chloride in water is an electrolyte solution of sodium (Na+) and chloride (Cl−) ions. These ions are normal constituents of the body fluids (principally extracellular) and are essential for maintaining electrolyte balance.

The distribution and excretion of sodium (Na+) and chloride (Cl−) are largely under the control of the kidney which maintains a balance between intake and output of these ions.

The small volumes of fluid and amounts of sodium chloride provided by 0.9% Sodium Chloride Injection in Ready-to-Mix Syringes are unlikely to produce a significant effect on fluid or electrolyte balance.

Continued on next page

Abbott—Cont.

INDICATIONS AND USAGE

These products are indicated only for preparing Pentothal (Thiopental Sodium for Injection, USP) solutions for clinical use.

CONTRAINDICATIONS

Do not use unless the diluent is clear and the bottle or vial seal or syringe package is undamaged.
Diluents in Pentothal Kits, Ready-to-Mix Syringes or Vials should not be used for fluid or sodium chloride replacement.

WARNINGS

Intravenous administration of Sterile Water for Injection, USP without a solute may result in hemolysis.
Use aseptic technique for preparing Pentothal solutions when using Pentothal Kits, Syringes or Vials and during withdrawal from reconstituted single or multiple-use containers.
Administer only clear reconstituted solutions.
Use within 24 hours after reconstitution. Discard unused portions.

PRECAUTIONS

Do not use unless solution is clear and container is undamaged.
Inspect reconstituted (mixed) solutions of Pentothal (Thiopental Sodium for Injection, USP) for clarity and freedom from precipitation or discoloration prior to administration.
Use Transfer Label in each Pentothal Kit and affix to container of reconstituted solution to show concentration and time of preparation.
Pregnancy Category C. Animal reproduction studies have not been conducted with sterile water for injection or sodium chloride injection. It is also not known whether sterile water or sodium chloride injection containing additives can cause fetal harm when administered to a pregnant woman or can affect reproduction capacity. Sterile water for injection or sodium chloride injection with additives should be given to a pregnant woman only if clearly needed.

ADVERSE REACTIONS

Reactions which may occur because of the diluents, technique of preparation or mixing, or administration of reconstituted solutions of Pentothal include febrile response or infection at the site of injection, venous thrombosis or phlebitis extending from the site of injection and extravasation.
If an adverse reaction does occur, discontinue the injection, evaluate the patient, institute appropriate therapeutic countermeasures and save the remainder of unused solution (or the used container or syringe) for examination if deemed necessary.

DRUG ABUSE AND DEPENDENCE

None known.

OVERDOSAGE

Used as diluents for preparing solutions of Pentothal (Thiopental Sodium for Injection, USP) the small volumes of administered fluid (from Sterile Water for Injection in bottles and vials) and amounts of sodium chloride (from 0.9% Sodium Chloride Injection in Ready-to-Mix Syringes) are unlikely to pose a threat of fluid or sodium chloride overload.

DOSAGE AND ADMINISTRATION

Pentothal solutions should be administered only by intravenous injection and by individuals experienced in the conduct of intravenous anesthesia.
The volume and choice of diluent for preparing Pentothal (Thiopental Sodium for Injection, USP) solutions for clinical use depends on the concentration and vehicle desired. Pentothal Kits provide only Sterile Water for Injection as the diluent for individual or multi-patient use; Pentothal Ready-to-

Mix Syringes provide only 0.9% Sodium Chloride Injection, USP as the diluent for individual patient use; vials provide only Sterile Water for Injection, USP as the diluent for individual patient use.
Parenteral drug products should be inspected visually for particulate matter and discoloration prior to administration, whenever solution and container permit. See PRECAUTIONS.

HOW SUPPLIED

The diluent in Pentothal Kits is supplied in various size partial-fill containers with various dosage sizes of Pentothal (Thiopental Sodium for Injection, USP). Kits include all items needed for aseptic transfer of Pentothal powder from a squeeze bottle into the diluent partial-fill container.
The diluent in Pentothal Ready-to-Mix Syringes is supplied in a separate container to permit mixing with the Pentothal in a powder vial to permit immediate intravenous injection of reconstituted solution into a vein or attachment to a standard stopcock assembly.
Vials are supplied in cartons with different dosage sizes of Pentothal for preparing 2.0% or 2.5% concentrations by using a separate syringe (not supplied) for mixing.
See table for list of sizes available.
[See table below].
Store at controlled room temperature 15° to 30° C (59° to 86° F).
Keep reconstituted solution in a cool place.
Caution: Federal (USA) law prohibits dispensing without prescription.
© Abbott 1988
06-4323-R6 Rev. Jan., 1989

PHENURONE®   ℞

[fĕn 'ū-rōne]
(phenacemide tablets, USP)

DESCRIPTION

PHENURONE (phenacemide) is a valuable antiepileptic drug for use in selected patients with epilepsy. Since therapy with PHENURONE involves certain risks, *physicians should thoroughly familiarize themselves with the undesirable side effects which may occur and the precautions to be observed.* PHENURONE (phenacemide) is a substituted acetylurea derivative. Chemically PHENURONE is identified as N-(aminocarbonyl)-benzeneacetamide. PHENURONE tablets contain 500 mg phenacemide for oral administration.
Inactive Ingredients: Corn starch, lactose and talc.

CLINICAL PHARMACOLOGY

In experimental animals, PHENURONE in doses well below those causing neurological signs, elevates the threshold for minimal electroshock convulsions and abolishes the tonic phase of maximal electroshock seizures. The drug prevents or modifies seizures induced by pentylenetetrazol or other convulsants. In comparative tests, PHENURONE was found to be equal or more effective than other commonly used antiepileptics against complex partial (psychomotor) seizures which were induced in mice by low frequency stimulation of the cerebral cortex. Studies in mice have shown that PHENURONE exerts a synergistic antiepileptic effect with mephenytoin, phenobarbital, or trimethadione.
Given orally to laboratory animals, PHENURONE has a low acute toxicity. In mice, slight ataxia appears at 400 mg/kg and light sleep occurs at 800 mg/kg. In high doses the drug causes marked ataxia and coma, the fatal dose being in the range of 3 to 5 g/kg for mice, rats, and cats.
PHENURONE is metabolized by the liver, however, further definition of human pharmacokinetics has not been determined.

INDICATIONS AND USAGE

PHENURONE (phenacemide) is indicated for the control of severe epilepsy, particularly mixed forms of complex partial (psychomotor) seizures, refractory to other drugs.

CONTRAINDICATIONS

PHENURONE should not be administered unless other available antiepileptics have been found to be ineffective in satisfactorily controlling seizures.

WARNINGS

PHENURONE (phenacemide) can produce serious side effects as well as direct organ toxicity. As a consequence its use entails the assumption of certain risks which must be weighed against the benefit to the patient. *Ordinarily* PHENURONE *should not be administered unless other available antiepileptics have been found to be ineffective in controlling seizures.* Death attributable to liver damage during therapy with PHENURONE has been reported. PHENURONE should be used with caution in patients with a history of previous liver dysfunction. If jaundice or other signs of hepatitis appear, the drug should be discontinued.
Aplastic anemia has occurred in association with PHENURONE therapy and death from this condition has been reported. PHENURONE should ordinarily not be used in patients with severe blood dyscrasias. Marked depression of the blood count is an indication for withdrawal of the drug.
Usage During Pregnancy: PHENURONE can cause fetal harm when administered to a pregnant woman. There are multiple reports in the clinical literature which indicate that the use of antiepileptic drugs during pregnancy results in an increased incidence of birth defects in the offspring. Reports have also suggested that the maternal ingestion of antiepileptic drugs, particularly barbiturates, is associated with a neonatal coagulation defect that may cause bleeding during the early (usually within 24 hours of birth) neonatal period. The possibility of the occurrence of this defect with the use of PHENURONE should be kept in mind. The defect is characterized by decreased levels of vitamin K-dependent clotting factors, and prolongation of either the prothrombin time or the partial thromboplastin time, or both. It has been suggested that vitamin K be given prophylactically to the mother one month prior to and during delivery, and to the infant, intravenously, immediately after birth. If this drug is used during pregnancy, or if the patient becomes pregnant while taking this drug, the patient should be apprised of the potential hazard to the fetus.

PRECAUTIONS

General: Extreme caution must be exercised in treating patients who previously have shown personality disorders. It may be advisable to hospitalize such patients during the first week of treatment. Personality changes, including attempts at suicide and the occurrence of psychoses requiring hospitalization, have been reported during therapy with PHENURONE (phenacemide). Severe or exacerbated personality changes are an indication for withdrawal of the drug.
PHENURONE (phenacemide) should be used with caution in patients with a history of previous liver dysfunction.
PHENURONE should be administered with caution to patients with a history of allergy, particularly in association with the administration of other antiepileptics. The drug should be discontinued at the first sign of a skin rash or other allergic manifestation.
Information for Patients: The patient and his family should be aware of the possibility of personality changes so the family can watch for changes in the behavior of the patient such as decreased interest in surroundings, depression, or aggressiveness.
The patient should be told to report immediately any symptoms indicative of a developing blood dyscrasia such as malaise, sore throat, or fever.
Laboratory Tests: Liver function tests should be performed before and during therapy. Death attributable to liver damage during therapy with PHENURONE has been reported. If jaundice or other signs of hepatitis appear, the drug should be discontinued.
Complete blood counts should be made before instituting PHENURONE, and at monthly intervals thereafter. If no abnormality appears within 12 months, the interval between blood counts may be extended. Blood changes have been reported with leukopenia (leukocyte count of 4,000 or less per cubic millimeter of blood) as the most commonly observed effect. However, aplastic anemia has occurred in association with PHENURONE therapy, and death from this condition has been reported. *The total number of each cellular element per cubic millimeter is a better index of possible blood dyscrasia than the percentage of cells.* Marked depression of the blood count is an indication for withdrawal of the drug.
Similarly, as nephritis has occasionally occurred in patients on PHENURONE, the urine should be examined at regular intervals. Abnormal urinary findings are an indication for discontinuance of therapy.
Drug Interactions: Extreme caution is essential if PHENURONE is administered with any other antiepileptic which is known to cause similar toxic effects.

Table: Pentothal® (Thiopental Sodium for Injection, USP) and Diluent in Kits, Ready-to-Mix Syringes and Vials

List No.	Pentothal		Pentothal Container	Diluent (mL)*		Diluent Container	Theoretical Reconstituted Conc.
6259	2.5	g	Squeeze Bottle	W	(125)	PF Bottle	2% (20 mg/mL)
6108	5	g	Squeeze Bottle	W	(250)	PF Bottle	2% (20 mg/mL)
6244	1	g	Squeeze Bottle	W	(40)	PF Bottle	2.5% (25 mg/mL)
6260	2.5	g	Squeeze Bottle	W	(100)	PF Bottle	2.5% (25 mg/mL)
6504	5	g	Squeeze Bottle	W	(200)	Bottle	2.5% (25 mg/mL)
6435	1	g	Vial	W	(50)	Plastic Vial	2% (20 mg/mL)
3329	500	mg	Vial	W	(20)	Plastic Vial	2.5% (25 mg/mL)
6246	400	mg	Syringe	S	(20)	Syringe	2% (20 mg/mL)
6241	250	mg	Syringe	S	(10)	Syringe	2.5% (25 mg/mL)
6243	500	mg	Syringe	S	(20)	Syringe	2.5% (25 mg/mL)
6418	250	mg	Syringe	W	(10)	Plastic Vial	2.5% (25 mg/mL)
6419	400	mg	Syringe	W	(20)	Plastic Vial	2% (20 mg/mL)
6420	500	mg	Syringe	W	(20)	Plastic Vial	2.5% (25 mg/mL)

PF—denotes Partial Fill
W—denotes Sterile Water for Injection, USP
S—denotes 0.9% Sodium Chloride Injection, USP

*Diluent containers are slightly overfilled to assure compliance with USP minimum fill volume requirements.

Considerable caution should be exercised if PHENURONE (phenacemide) is administered concurrently with *Peganone (ethotoin)* since paranoid symptoms have been reported during therapy with this combination.

Carcinogenesis: No data are available on long-term potential for carcinogenicity in animals or humans.

Pregnancy: Pregnancy Category D. See "Warnings" section.

Nursing Mothers: It is not known whether this drug is excreted in human milk. Because many drugs are excreted in human milk and because of the potential for serious adverse reactions in nursing infants from PHENURONE, a decision should be made whether to discontinue nursing or to discontinue the drug, taking into account the importance of the drug to the mother.

Pediatric Use: Safety and effectiveness in children below the age of 5 years have not been established.

ADVERSE REACTIONS

The following adverse effects associated with PHENURONE are listed by decreasing order of frequency based on data from one large clinical study.[1]

Psychiatric: Psychic changes (17 in 100 patients).

Gastrointestinal: Gastrointestinal disturbances (8 in 100 patients), including anorexia (5 in 100 patients) and weight loss (less than 1 in 100 patients).

Dermatologic: Skin rash (5 in 100 patients).

CNS: Drowsiness (4 in 100 patients), headache (2 in 100 patients), insomnia (1 in 100 patients), dizziness and paresthesias (less than 1 in 100 patients).

Hematopoietic: Blood dyscrasias (primarily leukopenia), including fatal aplastic anemia (2 in 100 patients).

Hepatic: Hepatitis, including fatalities (2 in 100 patients).

Renal: Abnormal urinary findings, including a rise in serum creatinine[2], and nephritis (1 in 100 patients or less).

Other: Fatigue, fever, muscle pain and palpitation (less than 1 in 100 patients).

OVERDOSAGE

Symptoms of acute overdosage include excitement or mania, followed by drowsiness, ataxia and coma. In one case of acute overdosage, dizziness was followed by coma which lasted nearly 24 hours. Treatment should be started by inducing emesis; gastric lavage may be considered as an alternative or adjunct. General supportive measures will be necessary. A careful evaluation of liver and kidney function, mental state, and the blood-forming organs should be made following recovery.

DOSAGE AND ADMINISTRATION

PHENURONE is administered orally.

Since PHENURONE may produce serious toxic effects, it is strongly recommended that the dosage be held to the minimum amount necessary to achieve an adequate therapeutic effect.

For adults the usual starting dose is 1.5 g daily, administered in three divided doses of 500 mg each. After the first week, if seizures are not controlled and the drug is well tolerated, an additional 500 mg tablet may be taken upon arising. In the third week, if necessary, the dosage may be further increased by another 500 mg at bedtime. Satisfactory results have been noted in some patients on an initial dose of 250 mg three times per day. The effective total daily dose for adults usually ranges from 2 to 3 g, although some patients have required as much as 5 g daily.

For the pediatric patient from 5 to 10 years of age, approximately one-half the adult dose is recommended. It should be given at the same intervals as for adults.

PHENURONE may be administered alone or in conjunction with other antiepileptics. However, extreme caution must be exercised if other antiepileptics cause toxic effects similar to PHENURONE.

When PHENURONE is to replace other antiepileptic medication, the latter should be withdrawn gradually as the dosage of PHENURONE is increased to maintain seizure control.

HOW SUPPLIED

PHENURONE (Phenacemide Tablets, USP), grooved, white, 500 mg are supplied in bottles of 100 (**NDC** 0074-3971-05).

REFERENCES

1. Tyler, M. W., King, E. Q.: Phenacemide in Treatment of Epilepsy. JAMA 147: 17–21 (1951).
2. Richards, R.K., Bjornsson, T. D., Waterbury, L. D.: Rise in Serum and Urine Creatinine After Phenacemide. Clin. Pharmacol. Ther. 23: 430–437 (1978).

Abbott Laboratories
North Chicago, IL 60064
Ref. 01-2350-R9

PLACIDYL®   ℞ ℂ
[pla'ci-dil]
(ethchlorvynol capsules, USP)
Oral hypnotic

DESCRIPTION

PLACIDYL (ethchlorvynol) is a tertiary carbinol. It is chemically designated as 1-chloro-3-ethyl-1-penten-4-yn-3-ol. Ethchlorvynol occurs as a liquid which is immiscible with water and miscible with most organic solvents. PLACIDYL is an oral hypnotic available in capsule form containing either 200 mg, 500 mg or 750 mg of ethchlorvynol.

Inactive Ingredients: 200 mg capsule: FD&C Red No. 40, gelatin, glycerin, methylparaben, polyethylene glycol, propylparaben, sorbitol, titanium dioxide and other ingredients. 500 mg capsule: FD&C Red No. 40, gelatin, glycerin, iron oxide, methylparaben, polyethylene glycol, propylparaben, sorbitol, titanium dioxide and other ingredients. 750 mg capsule: FD&C Blue No. 1, FD&C Yellow No. 5 (tartrazine), FD&C Yellow No. 6, gelatin, glycerin, iron oxide, methylparaben, polyethylene glycol, propylparaben, sorbitol, titanium dioxide and other ingredients.

CLINICAL PHARMACOLOGY

The usual hypnotic dose of PLACIDYL induces sleep within 15 minutes to one hour. The duration of the hypnotic effect is about five hours. The mechanism of action is unknown.

PLACIDYL is rapidly absorbed from the gastrointestinal tract with peak plasma concentrations usually occurring within two hours after a single oral fasting dose. Plasma concentrations required for hypnotic effects are unknown. The plasma half-life (t½, β) of the parent compound is approximately ten to twenty hours. Studies with ^{14}C-PLACIDYL have demonstrated that within 24 hours, 33% of a single 500 mg dose is excreted in the urine mostly as metabolites. The major plasma and urinary metabolite is the secondary alcohol of PLACIDYL. The free and conjugated forms of this metabolite in the urine account for about 40% of the dose. Other minor metabolites have been identified as the primary alcohol and a secondary alcohol with an altered acetylene group. Studies with ^{14}C-PLACIDYL in animals indicate that the parent compound and its metabolites undergo extensive enterohepatic recirculation.

Distribution studies indicate that there is extensive tissue localization of ethchlorvynol, particularly in adipose tissue. Ethchlorvynol and/or its metabolites have also been detected in liver, kidneys, spleen, brain, bile and cerebrospinal fluid.

INDICATIONS AND USAGE

PLACIDYL is indicated as short-term hypnotic therapy for periods up to one week in duration for the management of insomnia. If retreatment becomes necessary, after drug-free intervals of one or more weeks, it should only be undertaken upon further evaluation of the patient.

CONTRAINDICATIONS

PLACIDYL is contraindicated in patients with known hypersensitivity to the drug and in patients with porphyria.

WARNINGS

PLACIDYL SHOULD BE ADMINISTERED WITH CAUTION TO MENTALLY DEPRESSED PATIENTS WITH OR WITHOUT SUICIDAL TENDENCIES. IT SHOULD ALSO BE ADMINISTERED WITH CAUTION TO THOSE WHO HAVE A PSYCHOLOGICAL POTENTIAL FOR DRUG DEPENDENCE. THE LEAST AMOUNT OF DRUG THAT IS FEASIBLE SHOULD BE PRESCRIBED FOR THESE PATIENTS.

Psychological and Physical Dependence: PROLONGED USE OF PLACIDYL MAY RESULT IN TOLERANCE AND PSYCHOLOGICAL AND PHYSICAL DEPENDENCE. PROLONGED ADMINISTRATION OF THE DRUG IS NOT RECOMMENDED. (See "Drug Abuse and Dependence" section.)

PRECAUTIONS

General: Elderly or debilitated patients should receive the smallest effective amount of PLACIDYL (ethchlorvynol).

Caution should be exercised when treating patients with impaired hepatic or renal function.

Patients who exhibit unpredictable behavior, or paradoxical restlessness or excitement in response to barbiturates or alcohol may react in this manner to PLACIDYL.

PLACIDYL should not be used for the management of insomnia in the presence of pain unless insomnia persists after pain is controlled with analgesics.

The 750 mg dosage strength of PLACIDYL contains FD&C Yellow No. 5 (tartrazine) which may cause allergic-type reactions (including bronchial asthma) in certain susceptible individuals. Although the overall incidence of FD&C Yellow No. 5 (tartrazine) sensitivity in the general population is low, it is frequently seen in patients who also have aspirin hypersensitivity.

Information for Patients: The use of ethchlorvynol carries with it an associated risk of psychological and/or physical dependence. The patient should be warned against increasing the dose of the drug without consulting a physician.

Patients should be advised that, for the duration of the effect of PLACIDYL, mental and/or physical abilities required for the performance of potentially hazardous tasks such as the operation of dangerous machinery including motor vehicles, may be impaired.

Patients should be cautioned to avoid the concomitant use of PLACIDYL with alcohol, barbiturates, other CNS depressants, or MAO inhibitors.

Drug Interactions: The concomitant use of PLACIDYL with alcohol, barbiturates, other CNS depressants, or MAO inhibitors may produce exaggerated depressant effects.

Ethchlorvynol may cause a decreased prothrombin time response to coumarin anticoagulants; therefore, the dosage of these drugs may require adjustment when therapy with ethchlorvynol is initiated and after it is discontinued.

Transient delirium has been reported with the concomitant use of PLACIDYL and amitriptyline; therefore, PLACIDYL should be administered with caution to patients receiving tricyclic antidepressants.

Carcinogenesis: A study in mice receiving oral doses of PLACIDYL up to 7 times the maximum human daily dose for 22 to 24 months produced equivocal results. When compared to controls, a statistically significant increase in total lung tumors was found in female mice given the high dose of PLACIDYL. However, the 48% incidence is not substantially higher than the high value (39%) reported for the historical laboratory controls.

No evidence of carcinogenic potential was observed in rats given PLACIDYL at 5 to 15 times the maximum human daily dose for up to 2 years.

Usage During Pregnancy: 1. Teratogenic—Pregnancy Category C. Ethchlorvynol has been associated with a higher percentage of stillbirths and a lower survival rate of progeny among rats given 40 mg/kg/day. There are no adequate and well-controlled studies in pregnant women. Therefore, ethchlorvynol is not recommended for use during the first and second trimesters of pregnancy. Ethchlorvynol should be used during pregnancy only if the potential benefit justifies the potential risk to the fetus.

2. Non-teratogenic—Clinical experience has indicated that ethchlorvynol taken during the third trimester of pregnancy may produce CNS depression and transient withdrawal symptoms in the newborn. These symptoms resemble congenital narcotic withdrawal symptoms (See "Drug Abuse and Dependence" section).

Nursing Mothers: It is not known whether this drug is excreted in breast milk. Because many drugs are excreted in human milk and because of the potential for serious adverse reactions in nursing infants from PLACIDYL, a decision should be made whether to discontinue nursing or to discontinue the drug, taking into account the importance of the drug to the mother.

Pediatric Use: PLACIDYL is not recommended for use in children since its safety and effectiveness in the pediatric age group has not been determined.

ADVERSE REACTIONS

Adverse effects in decreasing order of severity within each of the following categories are:

Hypersensitivity: cholestatic jaundice, urticaria and rash.

Hematologic: thrombocytopenia—one case of fatal immune thrombocytopenia due to ethchlorvynol has been reported.

Gastrointestinal: vomiting, gastric upset, nausea and aftertaste.

Neurologic: dizziness and facial numbness.

Miscellaneous: blurred vision, hypotension and mild "hangover".

The following idiosyncratic responses have been reported occasionally: syncope without marked hypotension, profound muscular weakness, hysteria, marked excitement, prolonged hypnosis and mild stimulation.

Transient ataxia and giddiness have occurred in patients in whom absorption of the drug is especially rapid. These effects can sometimes be controlled by giving PLACIDYL with food.

(See "Drug Abuse and Dependence" section for the signs and symptoms of chronic intoxication).

DRUG ABUSE AND DEPENDENCE

PLACIDYL is subject to control by the Federal Controlled Substances Act under DEA schedule IV.

Abuse: Pulmonary edema of rapid onset has resulted from the I.V. abuse of PLACIDYL (ethchlorvynol).

Dependence: Signs and symptoms of intoxication have been reported with the prolonged use of doses as low as 1 g/day. Signs and symptoms of chronic intoxication may include incoordination, tremors, ataxia, confusion, slurred speech, hyperreflexia, diplopia, and generalized muscle weakness.

Continued on next page

Abbott—Cont.

Toxic amblyopia, scotoma, nystagmus, and peripheral neuropathy have also been reported with prolonged use of ethchlorvynol; these symptoms are usually reversible.

Severe withdrawal symptoms similar to those seen during barbiturate and alcohol withdrawal have been reported following abrupt discontinuance of prolonged use of PLACIDYL. These symptoms may appear as late as nine days after sudden withdrawal of the drug. Signs and symptoms of PLACIDYL withdrawal may include convulsions, delirium, schizoid reaction, perceptual distortions, memory loss, ataxia, insomnia, slurring of speech, unusual anxiety, irritability, agitation, and tremors. Other signs and symptoms may include anorexia, nausea, vomiting, weakness, dizziness, sweating, muscle twitching, and weight loss.

Management of a patient who manifests withdrawal symptoms from PLACIDYL involves readministration of the drug to approximately the same level of chronic intoxication which existed before the abrupt discontinuance. (Phenobarbital may be substituted for PLACIDYL.) A gradual, stepwise reduction of dosage may then be made over a period of days or weeks. A phenothiazine compound may be used in addition to this regimen for those patients who exhibit psychotic symptoms during the withdrawal period. The patient undergoing withdrawal from PLACIDYL must be hospitalized or closely observed, and given general supportive care as indicated.

In one report an infant born to a mother who received 500 mg PLACIDYL at bedtime daily throughout the third trimester, exhibited withdrawal symptoms on the second day of life. The symptoms included episodic jitteriness, hyperactivity, restlessness, irritability, disturbed sleep and hunger. The neonate responded to a single oral dose of phenobarbital (3 mg/kg). The withdrawal symptoms gradually decreased and completely disappeared by the tenth day of life.

OVERDOSAGE

Acute intoxication is characterized by prolonged deep coma, severe respiratory depression, hypothermia, hypotension, and relative bradycardia. Nystagmus and pancytopenia resulting from acute PLACIDYL overdose have been reported. Although death has occurred following the ingestion of 6 g of PLACIDYL, there have been reports of patients who have survived overdoses of 50 g and more with intensive care. Fatal blood concentrations usually range from 20 to 50 $\mu g/ml$.[1] Because large amounts of ethchlorvynol are taken up by adipose tissue, the blood concentration is an unreliable indicator of the magnitude of overdose.

Management of acute PLACIDYL intoxication is similar to that of acute barbiturate intoxication.[2] Gastric evacuation should be performed immediately. (In the unconscious patient, gastric lavage should be preceded by tracheal intubation with a cuffed tube.) Supportive care (assisted ventilation, frequent and careful monitoring of vital signs, control of blood pressure) is essential. Emphasis should be placed on pulmonary care and monitoring of blood gases. Hemoperfusion utilizing the Amberlite column technique has been reported in the literature to be the most effective method in the management of acute PLACIDYL overdose.[3] In addition, hemodialysis and peritoneal dialysis have each been reported to be of some value. (Aqueous and oil dialysates have been used. Forced diuresis with maintenance of a high urinary output has also been reported of some value.) (See "Drug Abuse and Dependence" section for the signs and symptoms of chronic intoxication.)

DOSAGE AND ADMINISTRATION

The usual adult hypnotic dose of PLACIDYL (ethchlorvynol) is 500 mg taken orally at bedtime. A dose of 750 mg may be required for patients whose sleep response to a 500 mg capsule is inadequate, or for patients being changed from barbiturates or other nonbarbiturate hypnotics. Up to 1000 mg may be given as a single bedtime dose when insomnia is unusually severe. A single supplemental dose of 200 mg may be given to reinstitute sleep in patients who may awaken after the original bedtime dose of 500 or 750 mg.

For patients whose insomnia is characterized only by untimely awakening during the early morning hours, a single dose of 200 mg taken upon awakening may be adequate for relief.

The smallest effective dose of PLACIDYL should be given to elderly or debilitated patients.

PLACIDYL should not be prescribed for periods exceeding one week. (See "Drug Abuse and Dependence" section.)

HOW SUPPLIED

PLACIDYL (ethchlorvynol capsules, USP) is supplied as:
200 mg red capsules:
Bottles of 100 ....(NDC 0074-6661-08).
500 mg red capsules:
Bottles of 100 ....(NDC 0074-6685-15).
Bottles of 500 ....(NDC 0074-6685-02).
ABBO-PAC® unit dose strip packages of 100 ....(NDC 0074-6685-10).

750 mg green capsules:
Bottles of 100 ....(NDC 0074-6630-01).

REFERENCES

1. AMA Dept. of Drugs. *AMA Drug Evaluations*, Massachusetts: Publishing Sciences Group, Inc., 1980.
2. Khantzian, E. J., McKenna, G. J., Acute Toxic and Withdrawal Reactions Associated with Drug Abuse, *Annals of Internal Medicine*, 90:361–372, 1979.
3. Lynn, R.I., et al., Resin Hemoperfusion for Treatment of Ethchlorvynol Overdose, *Annals of Internal Medicine*, 91:549–553, 1979.

Abbott Laboratories
North Chicago, IL 60064
Ref. 01-2363-R7

Shown in Product Identification Section, page 403

QUELIDRINE® SYRUP
[quel 'i-drēen]
(non-narcotic, antihistaminic cough suppressant)

COMPOSITION

Each teaspoonful (5 ml) contains:
Dextromethorphan Hydrobromide ....10 mg
Chlorpheniramine Maleate ....2 mg
Ephedrine Hydrochloride ....5 mg
Phenylephrine Hydrochloride ....5 mg
Ammonium Chloride ....40 mg
Ipecac Fluidextract ....0.005 ml

INACTIVE INGREDIENTS

Alcohol 2%, D&C Red No. 33, glycerin, liquid glucose, magnesium carbonate, methylparaben, propylparaben, sucrose, tolu balsam tincture, water, artificial flavors and other ingredients forming a palatable, aromatic syrup.

ACTION AND INDICATIONS

Quelidrine is designed as an aid in the management of cough associated with acute or subacute simple respiratory infections. Quelidrine provides a wide range of therapeutic action against the cough complex—without the risk of addiction or the production of undue central depression.

WARNINGS

As with any drug, if you are pregnant or nursing a baby, seek the advice of a health professional before using this product. Keep this and all medicines out of the reach of children.

PRECAUTIONS

Quelidrine should be administered with caution to patients with hypertension, serious organic heart disease, angina pectoris, diabetes, thyroid disease, or to persons receiving digitalis. When cough persists or accompanies a high fever, the underlying cause and need for other medication should be reevaluated.

SIDE EFFECTS

Quelidrine is safe for patients of all ages, but professional supervision of dosage for young patients is essential. Side effects are infrequent. Drowsiness, nausea, vomiting, nervousness, palpitation, blurred vision and insomnia may occur in susceptible patients. Constipation is seldom a problem. If side effects are encountered, dosage should be reduced or medication withdrawn.

DOSAGE AND ADMINISTRATION

Adults—1 teaspoonful, one to four times daily. Children 6 years of age or older, ½ teaspoonful, one to four times daily. Children 2 to 6 years old, ¼ teaspoonful one to four times daily. Under 2, as directed by physician. Quelidrine may be diluted with Syrup, NF in order to facilitate pediatric administration.

HOW SUPPLIED

Quelidrine Syrup is supplied in bottles of 4 fluid ounces (NDC 0074-6883-04), with or without a prescription.
Store below 77°F (25°C).
Abbott Laboratories
North Chicago, IL 60064
Ref. 07-5517-4/R21

SELSUN®   ℞
[sel 'sun]
(selenium sulfide lotion, USP)

DESCRIPTION

SELSUN (selenium sulfide lotion) is a liquid antiseborrheic, antifungal preparation for topical application, containing selenium sulfide 2 ½% w/v in aqueous suspension. The product also contains: bentonite, lauric diethanolamide, ethylene glycol monostearate, titanium dioxide, amphoteric-2, sodium lauryl sulfate, sodium phosphate (monobasic), glyceryl monoricinoleate, citric acid, captan, and perfume.

CLINICAL PHARMACOLOGY

Selenium sulfide appears to have a cytostatic effect on cells of the epidermis and follicular epithelium, thus reducing corneocyte production.

INDICATIONS AND USAGE

For the treatment of dandruff and seborrheic dermatitis of the scalp.
For treatment of tinea versicolor.

CONTRAINDICATIONS

SELSUN should not be used by patients allergic to any of its components.

PRECAUTIONS

General: Should not be used when acute inflammation or exudation is present as increased absorption may occur.
Information for Patients: Application to skin or scalp may produce skin irritation or sensitization. If sensitivity reactions occur, use should be discontinued. May be irritating to mucous membranes of the eyes and contact with this area should be avoided. When applied to the body for treatment of tinea versicolor, SELSUN may produce skin irritation especially in the genital area and where skin folds occur. These areas should be thoroughly rinsed after application.
Carcinogenesis: Studies in mice using dermal application of 25% and 50% solutions of 2.5% selenium sulfide lotion over an 88 week period, indicated no carcinogenic effects.
Pregnancy: WHEN USED ON BODY SURFACES FOR THE TREATMENT OF TINEA VERSICOLOR, SELSUN IS CLASSIFIED AS PREGNANCY CATEGORY C. Animal reproduction studies have not been conducted with SELSUN. It is also not known whether SELSUN can cause fetal harm when applied to body surfaces of a pregnant woman or can affect reproduction capacity. Under ordinary circumstances SELSUN should not be used for the treatment of tinea versicolor in pregnant women.
Pediatric Use: Safety and effectiveness in infants have not been established.

ADVERSE REACTIONS

In decreasing order of severity: skin irritation; occasional reports of increase in amount of normal hair loss; discoloration of hair (can be avoided or minimized by thorough rinsing of hair after treatment). As with other shampoos, oiliness or dryness of hair and scalp may occur.

OVERDOSAGE

Accidental Oral Ingestion:
Selsun is intended for external use only. There have been no documented reports of serious toxicity in humans resulting from acute ingestion of SELSUN, however, acute toxicity studies in animals suggest that ingestion of large amounts could result in potential human toxicity. For this reason, evacuation of the stomach contents should be considered in cases of acute oral ingestion.

DOSAGE AND ADMINISTRATION

For treatment of dandruff and seborrheic dermatitis:
1. Massage about 1 or 2 teaspoonfuls of shampoo into wet scalp.
2. Allow product to remain on the scalp for 2 to 3 minutes.
3. Rinse scalp thoroughly.
4. Repeat application and rinse thoroughly.
5. After treatment, wash hands well.
For the usual case, two applications each week for two weeks will afford control. After this, the lotion may be used at less frequent intervals—weekly, every two weeks, or even every 3 or 4 weeks in some cases. The preparation should not be applied more frequently than required to maintain control.
For treatment of tinea versicolor: Apply to affected areas and lather with a small amount of water. Allow product to remain on skin for 10 minutes, rinse the body thoroughly. Repeat this procedure once a day for 7 days. The product may damage jewelry; jewelry should be removed before use.

HOW SUPPLIED

SELSUN (selenium sulfide lotion, USP) is supplied in 4-fluidounce nonbreakable plastic bottles (NDC 0074-2660-04). SELSUN is to be dispensed only on the prescription of a physician.
Abbott Laboratories
North Chicago, IL 60064
Ref. 01-2254-R3

SURBEX®
[sir 'bex]
Vitamin B-Complex
SURBEX® with C
Vitamin B-Complex with Vitamin C

(See PDR For Nonprescription Drugs)

SURBEX-T®
[sir 'bex-t]
High-Potency Vitamin B-Complex with 500 mg of Vitamin C

(See PDR For Nonprescription Drugs)
Shown in Product Identification Section, page 403

SURBEX®–750 with IRON
[*sir'bex ī-ron*]
**High-potency B-complex with iron, vitamin E
and 750 mg vitamin C**

(See PDR For Nonprescription Drugs)
Shown in Product Identification Section, page 403

SURBEX®–750 with ZINC
[*sir'bex zinc*]
**High-potency B-complex with zinc, vitamin E
and 750 mg vitamin C**

(See PDR For Nonprescription Drugs)
Shown in Product Identification Section, page 403

TRANXENE®   ℞ ©
[*tran'zēen*]
(clorazepate dipotassium)
T-TAB™ Tablets
**TRANXENE-SD™
& TRANXENE-SD™ HALF STRENGTH**
(clorazepate dipotassium)
Tablets

PRODUCT OVERVIEW

KEY FACTS
TRANXENE is a long-acting benzodiazepine anxiolytic. TRANXENE T-Tab tablets are uniquely shaped for rapid identification and scored for easy titration. TRANXENE-SD (22.5 mg) and TRANXENE-SD HALF STRENGTH (11.25 mg) tablets are intended for convenient once daily dosing.

MAJOR USES
TRANXENE is approved for use in the short-term management of anxiety, adjunctive therapy in the management of partial seizures, and symptomatic relief of acute alcohol withdrawal.

SAFETY INFORMATION
Contraindicated in patients with hypersensitivity or acute narrow angle glaucoma. Not recommended for use in patients with depressive neurosis, psychotic reactions, or potential for drug dependence. Patients should be cautioned against engaging in hazardous activity (i.e., operating dangerous machinery including motor vehicles).

PRODUCT ILLUSTRATION

3.75 mg

7.5 mg

15 mg

PRESCRIBING INFORMATION

TRANXENE®   ℞ ©
[*tran'zēen*]
(clorazepate dipotassium)
T-TAB™ Tablets
**TRANXENE-SD™
& TRANXENE-SD™ HALF STRENGTH**
(clorazepate dipotassium)
Tablets

DESCRIPTION
Chemically, TRANXENE (clorazepate dipotassium) is a benzodiazepine. The empirical formula is $C_{16}H_{11}ClK_2N_2O_4$; the molecular weight is 408.92.
The compound occurs as a fine, light yellow, practically odorless powder. It is insoluble in the common organic solvents, but very soluble in water. Aqueous solutions are unstable, clear, light yellow, and alkaline.

INACTIVE INGREDIENTS
3.75 mg Tablet: Colloidal silicon dioxide, FD&C Blue No. 2, magnesium oxide, magnesium stearate, microcrystalline cellulose, potassium carbonate, potassium chloride, talc and other ingredients.
7.5 mg Tablet: Colloidal silicon dioxide, FD&C Yellow No. 6, magnesium oxide, magnesium stearate, microcrystalline cellulose, potassium carbonate, potassium chloride, talc and other ingredients.

15 mg Tablet: Colloidal silicon dioxide, FD&C Red No. 3, magnesium oxide, magnesium stearate, microcrystalline cellulose, potassium carbonate, potassium chloride, talc and other ingredients.
Tranxene-SD Tablet, 22.5 mg: Castor oil wax, iron oxide, lactose, magnesium oxide, magnesium stearate, potassium carbonate, potassium chloride, talc and other ingredients.
Tranxene-SD Half Strength Tablet, 11.25 mg: Castor oil wax, FD&C Blue No. 2, lactose, magnesium oxide, magnesium stearate, potassium carbonate, potassium chloride, talc and other ingredients.

ACTIONS
Pharmacologically, clorazepate dipotassium has the characteristics of the benzodiazepines. It has depressant effects on the central nervous system. The primary metabolite, nordiazepam, quickly appears in the blood stream. The serum half-life is about 2 days. The drug is metabolized in the liver and excreted primarily in the urine. (See ANIMAL AND CLINICAL PHARMACOLOGY section).

INDICATIONS
TRANXENE is indicated for the management of anxiety disorders or for the short-term relief of the symptoms of anxiety. Anxiety or tension associated with the stress of everyday life usually does not require treatment with an anxiolytic.
TRANXENE is indicated as adjunctive therapy in the management of partial seizures.
The effectiveness of TRANXENE in long-term management of anxiety, that is, more than 4 months, has not been assessed by systematic clinical studies. Long-term studies in epileptic patients, however, have shown continued therapeutic activity. The physician should reassess periodically the usefulness of the drug for the individual patient.
TRANXENE is indicated for the symptomatic relief of acute alcohol withdrawal.

CONTRAINDICATIONS
TRANXENE is contraindicated in patients with a known hypersensitivity to the drug, and in those with acute narrow angle glaucoma.

WARNINGS
TRANXENE is not recommended for use in depressive neuroses or in psychotic reactions.
Patients on TRANXENE should be cautioned against engaging in hazardous occupations requiring mental alertness, such as operating dangerous machinery including motor vehicles.
Since TRANXENE has a central nervous system depressant effect, patients should be advised against the simultaneous use of other CNS-depressant drugs, and cautioned that the effects of alcohol may be increased.
Because of the lack of sufficient clinical experience, TRANXENE is not recommended for use in patients less than 9 years of age.
Physical and Psychological Dependence: Withdrawal symptoms (similar in character to those noted with barbiturates and alcohol) have occurred following abrupt discontinuance of clorazepate. Symptoms of nervousness, insomnia, irritability, diarrhea, muscle aches and memory impairment have followed abrupt withdrawal after long-term use of high dosage. Withdrawal symptoms have also been reported following abrupt discontinuance of benzodiazepines taken continuously at therapeutic levels for several months.
Caution should be observed in patients who are considered to have a psychological potential for drug dependence.
Evidence of drug dependence has been observed in dogs and rabbits which was characterized by convulsive seizures when the drug was abruptly withdrawn or the dose was reduced; the syndrome in dogs could be abolished by administration of clorazepate.
Usage in Pregnancy: **An increased risk of congenital malformations associated with the use of minor tranquilizers (chlordiazepoxide, diazepam, and meprobamate) during the first trimester of pregnancy has been suggested in several studies. TRANXENE, a benzodiazepine derivative, has not been studied adequately to determine whether it, too, may be associated with an increased risk of fetal abnormality. Because use of these drugs is rarely a matter of urgency, their use during this period should almost always be avoided. The possibility that a woman of childbearing potential may be pregnant at the time of institution of therapy should be considered. Patients should be advised that if they become pregnant during therapy or intend to become pregnant they should communicate with their physician about the desirability of discontinuing the drug.**
Usage during Lactation: TRANXENE should not be given to nursing mothers since it has been reported that nordiazepam is excreted in human breast milk.

PRECAUTIONS
In those patients in which a degree of depression accompanies the anxiety, suicidal tendencies may be present and protective measures may be required. The least amount of drug that is feasible should be available to the patient.
Patients on TRANXENE for prolonged periods should have blood counts and liver function tests periodically. The usual

precautions in treating patients with impaired renal or hepatic function should also be observed.
In elderly or debilitated patients, the initial dose should be small, and increments should be made gradually, in accordance with the response of the patient, to preclude ataxia or excessive sedation.

ADVERSE REACTIONS
The side effect most frequently reported was drowsiness. Less commonly reported (in descending order of occurrence) were: dizziness, various gastrointestinal complaints, nervousness, blurred vision, dry mouth, headache, and mental confusion. Other side effects included insomnia, transient skin rashes, fatigue, ataxia, genitourinary complaints, irritability, diplopia, depression and slurred speech.
There have been reports of abnormal liver and kidney function tests and of decrease in hematocrit.
Decrease in systolic blood pressure has been observed.

DOSAGE AND ADMINISTRATION
For the symptomatic relief of anxiety: TRANXENE (clorazepate dipotassium) T-TAB™ tablets are administered orally in divided doses. The usual daily dose is 30 mg. The dose should be adjusted gradually within the range of 15 to 60 mg daily in accordance with the response of the patient. In elderly or debilitated patients it is advisable to initiate treatment at a daily dose of 7.5 to 15 mg.
TRANXENE may also be administered in a single dose daily at bedtime; the recommended initial dose is 15 mg. After the initial dose, the response of the patient may require adjustment of subsequent dosage. Lower doses may be indicated in the elderly patient. Drowsiness may occur at the initiation of treatment and with dosage increment.
TRANXENE-SD (22.5 mg tablet) may be administered as a single dose every 24 hours. This tablet is intended as an alternate dosage form for the convenience of patients stabilized on a dose of 7.5 mg tablets three times a day. TRANXENE-SD should not be used to initiate therapy.
TRANXENE-SD HALF STRENGTH (11.25 mg tablet) may be administered as a single dose every 24 hours.
For the symptomatic relief of acute alcohol withdrawal:
The following dosage schedule is recommended:

1st 24 hours (Day 1)	30 mg Tranxene, initially; followed by 30 to 60 mg in divided doses
2nd 24 hours (Day 2)	45 to 90 mg in divided doses
3rd 24 hours (Day 3)	22.5 to 45 mg in divided doses
Day 4	15 to 30 mg in divided doses

Thereafter, gradually reduce the daily dose to 7.5 to 15 mg. Discontinue drug therapy as soon as patient's condition is stable.
The maximum recommended total daily dose is 90 mg. Avoid excessive reductions in the total amount of drug administered on successive days.
As an Adjunct to Antiepileptic Drugs:
In order to minimize drowsiness, the recommended initial dosages and dosage increments should not be exceeded.
Adults: The maximum recommended initial dose in patients over 12 years old is 7.5 mg three times a day. Dosage should be increased by no more than 7.5 mg every week and should not exceed 90 mg/day.
Children (9-12 years): The maximum recommended initial dose is 7.5 mg two times a day. Dosage should be increased by no more than 7.5 mg every week and should not exceed 60 mg/day.

DRUG INTERACTIONS
If TRANXENE is to be combined with other drugs acting on the central nervous system, careful consideration should be given to the pharmacology of the agents to be employed. Animal experience indicates that TRANXENE prolongs the sleeping time after hexobarbital or after ethyl alcohol, increases the inhibitory effects of chlorpromazine, but does not exhibit monoamine oxidase inhibition. Clinical studies have shown increased sedation with concurrent hypnotic medications. The actions of the benzodiazepines may be potentiated by barbiturates, narcotics, phenothiazines, monoamine oxidase inhibitors or other antidepressants.
If TRANXENE is used to treat anxiety associated with somatic disease states, careful attention must be paid to possible drug interaction with concomitant medication.

Continued on next page

Abbott—Cont.

In bioavailability studies with normal subjects, the concurrent administration of antacids at therapeutic levels did not significantly influence the bioavailability of TRANXENE.

MANAGEMENT OF OVERDOSAGE

Overdosage is usually manifested by varying degrees of CNS depression ranging from slight sedation to coma. As in the management of overdosage with any drug, it should be borne in mind that multiple agents may have been taken.

There are no specific antidotes for the benzodiazepines. The treatment of overdosage should consist of the general measures employed in the management of overdosage of any CNS depressant. Gastric evacuation either by the induction of emesis, lavage, or both, should be performed immediately. General supportive care, including frequent monitoring of the vital signs and close observation of the patient, is indicated. Hypotension, though rarely reported, may occur with large overdoses. In such cases the use of agents such as Levophed® Bitartrate (norepinephrine bitartrate injection, USP) or Aramine® Injection (metaraminol bitartrate injection, USP) should be considered.

While reports indicate that individuals have survived overdoses of TRANXENE as high as 450 to 675 mg, these doses are not necessarily an accurate indication of the amount of drug absorbed since the time interval between ingestion and the institution of treatment was not always known. Sedation in varying degrees was the most common physiological manifestation of TRANXENE overdosage. Deep coma when it occurred was usually associated with the ingestion of other drugs in addition to TRANXENE.

ANIMAL AND CLINICAL PHARMACOLOGY

Studies in rats and monkeys have shown a substantial difference between doses producing tranquilizing, sedative and toxic effects. In rats, conditioned avoidance response was inhibited at an oral dose of 10 mg/kg; sedation was induced at 32 mg/kg; the LD_{50} was 1320 mg/kg. In monkeys aggressive behavior was reduced at an oral dose of 0.25 mg/kg; sedation (ataxia) was induced at 7.5 mg/kg; the LD_{50} could not be determined because of the emetic effect of large doses, but the LD_{50} exceeds 1600 mg/kg.

Twenty-four dogs were given TRANXENE orally in a 22-month toxicity study; doses up to 75 mg/kg were given. Drug-related changes occurred in the liver; weight was increased and cholestasis with minimal hepatocellular damage was found, but lobular architecture remained well preserved.

Eighteen rhesus monkeys were given oral doses of TRANXENE from 3 to 36 mg/kg daily for 52 weeks. All treated animals remained similar to control animals. Although total leucocyte count remained within normal limits it tended to fall in the female animals on the highest doses.

Examination of all organs revealed no alterations attributable to TRANXENE. There was no damage to liver function or structure.

Reproduction Studies: Standard fertility, reproduction, and teratology studies were conducted in rats and rabbits. Oral doses in rats up to 150 mg/kg and in rabbits up to 15 mg/kg produced no abnormalities in the fetuses. TRANXENE (clorazepate dipotassium) did not alter the fertility indices or reproductive capacity of adult animals. As expected, the sedative effect of high doses interfered with care of the young by their mothers (*see Usage in Pregnancy*).

Clinical Pharmacology: Studies in healthy men have shown that TRANXENE has depressant effects on the central nervous system. Prolonged administration of single daily doses as high as 120 mg was without toxic effects. Abrupt cessation of high doses was followed in some patients by nervousness, insomnia, irritability, diarrhea, muscle aches, or memory impairment.

Absorption —Excretion: After oral administration of TRANXENE , there is essentially no circulating parent drug. Nordiazepam, its primary metabolite, quickly appears in the blood stream. In 2 volunteers given 15 mg (50 μC) of ^{14}C-TRANXENE, about 80% was recovered in the urine and feces within 10 days. Excretion was primarily in the urine with about 1% excreted per day on day 10.

HOW SUPPLIED

TRANXENE (clorazepate dipotassium) is supplied as:
3.75 mg blue-colored, scored T-TAB™ tablets:
Bottles of 100 ....(**NDC** 0074-4389-13).
Bottles of 500 ....(**NDC** 0074-4389-53).
ABBO-PAC® unit dose packages:
100 ....(**NDC** 0074-4389-11).
7.5 mg peach-colored, scored T-TAB™ tablets:
Bottles of 100 ....(**NDC** 0074-4390-13).
Bottles of 500 ....(**NDC** 0074-4390-53).
ABBO-PAC® unit dose packages:
100 ....(**NDC** 0074-4390-11).
15 mg lavender-colored, scored T-TAB™ tablets:
Bottles of 100 ....(**NDC** 0074-4391-13).
Bottles of 500 ....(**NDC** 0074-4391-53).
ABBO-PAC® unit dose packages:
100 ....(**NDC** 0074-4391-11).

PATENT PENDING
TRANXENE-SD™ 22.5 mg tan-colored, single dose tablets:
Bottles of 100 ....(**NDC** 0074-2997-13).
TRANXENE-SD™ HALF STRENGTH 11.25 mg blue-colored, single dose tablets:
Bottles of 100 ....(**NDC** 0074-2699-13).
Abbott Pharmaceuticals, Inc.
North Chicago, IL 60064
Ref. 03-4288-R9
Shown in Product Identification Section, page 403

TRIDIONE®   ℞
[*try'dē-own*]
(trimethadione)
Tablets, Capsules, and Oral Solution

> BECAUSE OF ITS POTENTIAL TO PRODUCE FETAL MALFORMATIONS AND SERIOUS SIDE EFFECTS, TRIDIONE (trimethadione) SHOULD ONLY BE UTILIZED WHEN OTHER LESS TOXIC DRUGS HAVE BEEN FOUND INEFFECTIVE IN CONTROLLING PETIT MAL SEIZURES.

DESCRIPTION

TRIDIONE (trimethadione) is an antiepileptic agent. An oxazolidinedione compound, it is chemically identified as 3,5,5-trimethyloxozolidine-2,4-dione.

TRIDIONE is a synthetic, water-soluble, white, crystalline powder. It is supplied in capsular, tablet, and liquid forms for oral use only.

Inactive Ingredients: 300 mg Capsule: Corn starch, FD&C Blue No. 1, FD&C Red No. 3, FD&C Yellow No. 6, gelatin, titanium dioxide and artificial flavor.

150 mg Dulcet Tablet: Corn starch, lactose, magnesium stearate, magnesium trisilicate, sucrose and natural/synthetic flavor.

Solution: FD&C Yellow No. 6, methylparaben, sucrose, water and natural/synthetic flavors.

CLINICAL PHARMACOLOGY

TRIDIONE has been shown to prevent pentylenetetrazol-induced and thujone-induced seizures in experimental animals; the drug has a less marked effect on seizures induced by picrotoxin, procaine, cocaine, or strychnine. Unlike the hydantoins and antiepileptic barbiturates, TRIDIONE does not modify the maximal seizure pattern in patients undergoing electroconvulsive therapy.

TRIDIONE has a sedative effect that may increase to the point of ataxia when excessive doses are used. A toxic dose of the drug in animals (approximately 2 g/kg) produced sleep, unconsciousness, and respiratory depression.

Trimethadione is rapidly absorbed from the gastrointestinal tract. It is demethylated by liver microsomes to the active metabolite, dimethadione.

Approximately 3% of a daily dose of TRIDIONE is recovered in the urine as unchanged drug. The majority of trimethadione is excreted slowly by the kidney in the form of dimethadione.

INDICATIONS

TRIDIONE (trimethadione) is indicated for the control of petit mal seizures that are refractory to treatment with other drugs.

CONTRAINDICATIONS

TRIDIONE is contraindicated in patients with a known hypersensitivity to the drug.

WARNINGS

TRIDIONE may cause serious side effects. Strict medical supervision of the patient is mandatory, especially during the initial year of therapy.

TRIDIONE (trimethadione) should be withdrawn promptly if skin rash appears, because of the grave possibility of the occurrence of exfoliative dermatitis or severe forms of erythema multiforme. Even a minor acneiform or morbilliform rash should be allowed to clear completely before treatment with TRIDIONE is resumed; reinstitute therapy cautiously.

A complete blood count should be done prior to intiating therapy with TRIDIONE, and at monthly intervals thereafter. A marked depression of the blood count is an indication for withdrawal of the drug. If no abnormality appears within 12 months, the interval between blood counts may be extended. A moderate degree of neutropenia with or without a corresponding drop in the leukocyte count is not uncommon. Therapy need not be withdrawn unless the neutrophil count is 2500 or less; more frequent blood examinations should be done when the count is less than 3,000. Other blood dyscrasias, including leukopenia, eosinophilia, thrombocytopenia, pancytopenia, agranulocytosis, hypoplastic anemia, and fatal aplastic anemia, have occurred. Patients should be advised to report immediately such signs and symptoms as sore throat, fever, malaise, easy bruising, petechiae, or epistaxis, or others that may be indicative of an infection or bleeding tendency. TRIDIONE should ordinarily not be used in patients with severe blood dyscrasias.

Liver function tests should be done prior to initiating therapy with TRIDIONE, and at monthly intervals thereafter. Hepatitis has been reported rarely. Jaundice or other signs of liver dysfunction are an indication for withdrawal of the drug. TRIDIONE should ordinarily not be used in patients with severe hepatic impairment.

A urinalysis should be done prior to initiating therapy with TRIDIONE and at monthly intervals thereafter. Fatal nephrosis has been reported. Persistent or increasing albuminuria, or the development of any other significant renal abnormality, is an indication for withdrawal of the drug. TRIDIONE should ordinarily not be used in patients with severe renal dysfunction.

Hemeralopia has occurred; this appears to be an effect of TRIDIONE on the neural layers of the retina, and usually can be reversed by a reduction in dosage. Scotomata are an indication for withdrawal of the drug. Caution should be observed when treating patients who have diseases of the retina or optic nerve.

Manifestations of systemic lupus erythematosus have been associated with the use of TRIDIONE, as they have with the use of certain other anticonvulsants. Lymphadenopathies simulating malignant lymphoma have occurred. Lupus-like manifestations or lymph node enlargement are indications for withdrawal of the drug. Signs and symptoms may disappear after discontinuation of therapy, and specific treatment may be unnecessary.

A myasthenia gravis-like syndrome has been associated with the chronic use of trimethadione. Symptoms suggestive of this condition are indications for withdrawal of the drug. Drugs known to cause toxic effects similar to those of TRIDIONE should be avoided or used only with extreme caution during therapy with TRIDIONE.

USAGE DURING PREGNANCY AND LACTATION: THERE ARE MULTIPLE REPORTS IN THE CLINICAL LITERATURE WHICH INDICATE THAT THE USE OF ANTICONVULSANT DRUGS DURING PREGNANCY RESULTS IN AN INCREASED INCIDENCE OF BIRTH DEFECTS IN THE OFFSPRING. DATA ARE MORE EXTENSIVE WITH RESPECT TO TRIMETHADIONE, PARAMETHADIONE, PHENYTOIN AND PHENOBARBITAL THAN WITH OTHER ANTICONVULSANT DRUGS. THEREFORE, ANTICONVULSANT DRUGS SUCH AS TRIDIONE (TRIMETHADIONE) SHOULD BE ADMINISTERED TO WOMEN OF CHILDBEARING POTENTIAL ONLY IF THEY ARE CLEARLY SHOWN TO BE ESSENTIAL IN THE MANAGEMENT OF THEIR SEIZURES. EFFECTIVE MEANS OF CONTRACEPTION SHOULD ACCOMPANY THE USE OF TRIDIONE IN SUCH PATIENTS. IF A PATIENT BECOMES PREGNANT WHILE TAKING TRIDIONE, TERMINATION OF THE PREGNANCY SHOULD BE CONSIDERED. A PATIENT WHO REQUIRES THERAPY WITH TRIDIONE AND WHO WISHES TO BECOME PREGNANT SHOULD BE ADVISED OF THE RISKS.

REPORTS HAVE SUGGESTED THAT THE MATERNAL INGESTION OF ANTICONVULSANT DRUGS, PARTICULARLY BARBITURATES, IS ASSOCIATED WITH A NEONATAL COAGULATION DEFECT THAT MAY CAUSE BLEEDING DURING THE EARLY (USUALLY WITHIN 24 HOURS OF BIRTH) NEONATAL PERIOD. THE POSSIBILITY OF THE OCCURRENCE OF THIS DEFECT WITH THE USE OF TRIDIONE SHOULD BE KEPT IN MIND. THE DEFECT IS CHARACTERIZED BY DECREASED LEVELS OF VITAMIN K-DEPENDENT CLOTTING FACTORS, AND PROLONGATION OF EITHER THE PROTHROMBIN TIME OR THE PARTIAL THROMBOPLASTIN TIME, OR BOTH. IT HAS BEEN SUGGESTED THAT PROPHYLACTIC VITAMIN K BE GIVEN TO THE MOTHER ONE MONTH PRIOR TO, AND DURING DELIVERY, AND TO THE INFANT, INTRAVENOUSLY, IMMEDIATELY AFTER BIRTH. THE SAFETY OF TRIDIONE FOR USE DURING LACTATION HAS NOT BEEN ESTABLISHED.

PRECAUTIONS

Abrupt discontinuation of TRIDIONE may precipitate petit mal status. TRIDIONE should always be withdrawn gradually unless serious adverse effects dictate otherwise. In the latter case, another anticonvulsant may be substituted to protect the patient.

Usage during Pregnancy and Lactation:
See WARNINGS.

ADVERSE REACTIONS

The following side effects, some of them serious, have been associated with the use of TRIDIONE.

Gastrointestinal: nausea, vomiting, abdominal pain, gastric distress.

CNS/Neurologic: drowsiness, fatigue, malaise, insomnia, vertigo, headache, paresthesias, precipitation of grand mal seizures, increased irritability, personality changes.

Drowsiness usually subsides with continued therapy. If it persists, a reduction in dosage is indicated.

Hematologic: bleeding gums, epistaxis, retinal and petechial hemorrhages, vaginal bleeding; neutropenia, leukopenia,

eosinophilia, thrombocytopenia, pancytopenia, agranulocytosis, hypoplastic anemia, and fatal aplastic anemia.
Dermatologic: acneiform or morbilliform skin rash that may progress to exfoliative dermatitis or to severe forms of erythema multiforme.
Other: hiccups, anorexia, weight loss, hair loss, changes in blood pressure, albuminuria, hemeralopia, photophobia, diplopia.
Fatal nephrosis has occurred.
Hepatitis has been reported rarely.
Lupus erythematosus, and lymphadenopathies simulating malignant lymphoma, have been reported.
Pruritus associated with lymphadenopathy and hepatosplenomegaly has occurred in hypersensitive individuals.
A myasthenia gravis-like syndrome has been reported.

OVERDOSAGE
Symptoms of acute TRIDIONE overdosage include drowsiness, nausea, dizziness, ataxia, visual disturbances. Coma may follow massive overdosage.
Gastric evacuation, either by induced emesis, or by lavage, or both, should be done immediately. General supportive care, including frequent monitoring of the vital signs and close observation of the patient, are required.
Alkalinization of the urine has been reported to enhance the renal excretion of dimethadione, the active metabolite of TRIDIONE.
A blood count and a careful evaluation of hepatic and renal function should be done following recovery.

DOSAGE AND ADMINISTRATION
TRIDIONE is administered orally.
Usual Adult Dosage: 0.9–2.4 g daily in 3 or 4 equally divided doses (i.e. 300–600 mg 3 or 4 times daily).
Initially, give 0.9 g daily; increase this dose by 300 mg at weekly intervals until therapeutic results are seen or until toxic symptoms appear.
Maintenance dosage should be the least amount of drug required to maintain control.
Children's Dosage: Usually 0.3–0.9 g daily in 3 or 4 equally divided doses.

HOW SUPPLIED
TRIDIONE Capsules (trimethadione capsules, USP), 300 mg (white) are supplied in bottles of 100 (NDC 0074-3709-01).
TRIDIONE Dulcet® Tablets (trimethadione tablets, USP), 150 mg (white) chewable tablets are supplied in bottles of 100 (NDC 0074-3753-01).
TRIDIONE Solution (trimethadione oral solution, USP), 1.2 g per fluidounce (40 mg per ml), is supplied in pint bottles (NDC 0074-3721-01).
Abbott Laboratories/
Abbott Pharmaceuticals, Inc.
North Chicago, IL 60064
®Dulcet—Sweetened tablets, Abbott.
Ref. 01-2368-R5
Shown in Product Identification Section, page 403

TRONOTHANE® HYDROCHLORIDE
[tro 'nō-thāne hy-drō-clō 'rīde]
(pramoxine hydrochloride)
Cream

DESCRIPTION
Tronothane Hydrochloride (pramoxine hydrochloride) is a surface anesthetic agent, chemically unrelated to the benzoate esters of the "caine" type. It is chemically designated as 4-n-butoxyphenyl gammamorpholinopropyl ether hydrochloride.

INDICATIONS
Tronothane Hydrochloride is indicated for temporary relief of pain and itching due to minor burns, sunburn, minor cuts, abrasions, insect bites, minor skin irritations, hemorrhoids and other anorectal disorders.

CONTRAINDICATIONS
Tronothane Hydrochloride is not suitable for and should not be injected into the tissues. It should not be used for bronchoscopy or gastroscopy, or in patients who are hypersensitive to the drug.

WARNINGS
Tronothane Hydrochloride is not intended for prolonged use.
Do not apply to large areas of the body. Do not use in the eyes or nose.
If condition worsens, or persists for 7 days, consult physician.
If bleeding or increased pain occurs when using the product in the rectum, consult physician promptly.
For topical use in children under 2 years or anorectal use in children under 12 years, use only as directed by physician. Keep out of reach of children.

ADVERSE REACTIONS
Local skin reactions, e.g. stinging and burning. Discontinue use if redness, irritation, swelling or pain occur.

DOSAGE AND ADMINISTRATION
Topical—Adults and children 2 years of age or older: Apply to affected area 3 to 4 times daily, or as directed by a physician.
Anorectal—When practical, wash the area with soap and warm water, and rinse off all soap before application. Adults and children 12 years of age or older: Apply up to 5 times daily, especially morning, night and after bowel movements, or as directed by a physician.
External—Apply liberally to affected area.
Intrarectal—Remove cap from tube and attach clean applicator. Squeeze tube to fill and lubricate applicator. Remove cap from applicator. Gently insert applicator into rectum and squeeze tube. Thoroughly cleanse applicator with soap and warm water after use. Replace applicator cap.

HOW SUPPLIED
Tronothane Hydrochloride 1% Cream (pramoxine hydrochloride cream, USP), pramoxine hydrochloride 1% in a water miscible base containing cetyl alcohol, cetyl esters wax, glycerin, sodium lauryl sulfate, methylparaben, and propylparaben, is supplied in a 1-oz tube with rectal applicator (NDC 0074-6645-01).
These products are listed in USP, a Medicare designated compendium.
Abbott Laboratories
North Chicago, IL 60064

If desired, additional literature on any Abbott Product will be provided upon request to Abbott Laboratories.

Adams Laboratories, Inc.
7450 WHITEHALL STREET
FORT WORTH, TX 76118
P.O. DRAWER 487
HURST, TX 76053

ATROHIST® L.A. Tablets   ℞

HOW SUPPLIED
Bottles of 100 tablets (NDC 53014-0021-1).

ATROHIST® SPRINKLE Capsules   ℞

DESCRIPTION
Each ATROHIST® SPRINKLE Capsule provides 2 mg brompheniramine maleate, 25 mg phenyltoloxamine citrate, and 10 mg phenylephrine hydrochloride in a sustained-release formulation intended for oral administration. The microencapsulated contents of a capsule may be sprinkled on a small amount of soft food immediately prior to ingestion, making the product ideal for children and other patients unable to swallow capsules or tablets. Capsules are oversized to facilitate opening but may also be swallowed whole.
ATROHIST® SPRINKLE Capsules have antihistaminic and nasal decongestant effects. The components of ATROHIST® SPRINKLE Capsules have the following chemical names:
Brompheniramine Maleate:
2-[p-bromo-α-[2-(dimethylamino) ethyl] benzyl] pyridine maleate

$C_{16}H_{19}BrN_2 \cdot C_4H_4O_4$ MW = 435.32
Phenyltoloxamine Citrate:
N,N-dimethyl-2(alpha phenyl-ortho-toloxy)-ethylamine

$C_{17}H_{21}NO \cdot C_6H_8O_7$ MW = 447.5
Phenylephrine Hydrochloride:
(R)-3-hydroxy-α-[(methylamino) methyl] benzenemethanol hydrochloride

$C_9H_{13}NO_2 \cdot HCl$ MW = 203.67

CLINICAL PHARMACOLOGY
Brompheniramine maleate and phenyltoloxamine citrate are antihistamines which act on H_1 receptors as antagonists and interfere with the action of histamine, primarily in capillaries surrounding mucous tissues and sensory nerves of nasal and adjacent areas. Both drugs are rapidly and almost completely absorbed from the gastrointestinal tract and distributed throughout the body, including the central nervous system (CNS). Little, if any, of the drugs is excreted unchanged in the urine; most is apparently metabolized by the liver and excreted as degradation products within 24 hours. Alkylamine-type antihistamines such as brompheniramine maleate are among the most potent H_1 blockers and are generally effective in relatively low doses. Although brompheniramine is not so prone as other types of antihistamines to cause drowsiness, a significant proportion of patients do experience this effect. CNS stimulation is more common with alkylamines. Ethanolamine-type antihistamines such as phenyltoloxamine citrate are potent and effective H_1 blockers that possess significant antimuscarinic activity and have a pronounced tendency to induce sedation.
Phenylephrine hydrochloride effects its vasoconstrictor activity by releasing noradrenaline from sympathetic nerve endings, and from direct stimulation of α-adrenoreceptors in blood vessels. Following oral administration, constriction of blood vessels in the nasal mucosa helps relieve nasal congestion. In therapeutic doses the drug causes little, if any, central nervous system stimulation.

INDICATIONS AND USAGE
ATROHIST® SPRINKLE Capsules are indicated for symptomatic relief of seasonal and perennial allergic rhinitis, vasomotor rhinitis, and eustachian tube congestion. The product is particularly suitable for use in children and other patients unable to swallow tablets or capsules.

CONTRAINDICATIONS
This product is contraindicated in patients with hypersensitivity to antihistamines or sympathomimetic amines, and in patients receiving monoamine oxidase (MAO) inhibitor therapy (see **Drug Interactions** section).
Patients known to be hypersensitive to other sympathomimetic amines may exhibit cross sensitivity to phenylephrine. Phenylephrine is contraindicated in patients with severe hypertension or severe coronary artery disease. Patient idiosyncrasy to adrenergic agents may be manifested by insomnia, dizziness, weakness, tremors or arrhythmias.

WARNINGS
Antihistamines should be used with considerable caution in patients with: narrow angle glaucoma; stenosing peptic ulcer; pyloroduodenal obstruction; symptomatic prostatic hypertrophy; bladder neck obstruction.
Sympathomimetic amines should be used with caution in patients with hypertension, ischemic heart disease, diabetes mellitus, increased intraocular pressure, hyperthyroidism, or prostatic hypertropy. Sympathomimetics may produce central nervous system stimulation with convulsions or cardiovascular collapse with accompanying hypotension. Do not exceed recommended dosage.
Hypertensive crises can occur with concurrent use of phenylephrine and monoamine oxidase (MAO) inhibitors, indomethacin or with beta-blockers and methyldopa. If a hypertensive crisis occurs, these drugs should be discontinued immediately and therapy to lower blood pressure should be instituted. Fever should be managed by means of external cooling.

PRECAUTIONS
General: Antihistamines have an atropine-like action and therefore should be used with caution in patients with a history of bronchial asthma, increased intraocular pressure, hyperthyroidism, cardiovascular disease and hypertension. Phenylephrine should be used with caution in patients with diabetes, hypertension, cardiovascular disease and hyperreactivity to ephedrine.
Information for Patients: Antihistamines may impair mental and physical abilities required for the performance of potentially hazardous tasks, such as driving a vehicle or operating machinery. Patients should be warned accordingly. Capsules may be swallowed whole or the entire contents sprinkled on a small amount of soft food (jam etc.) immediately prior to ingestion. Capsule contents should not be subdivided. Capsule contents should not be crushed or chewed.
Pediatric Use: This product is not recommended for use in children under 2 years of age. In infants and children, antihistamines in overdosage may cause hallucinations, convulsions or death. As in adults, antihistamines may diminish mental alertness in children. In the young child particularly, they may produce excitation.
Use in Elderly: The elderly (60 years and older) are more likely to experience adverse reactions to sympathomimetics. Overdosage of sympathomimetics in this age group may

Continued on next page

Adams Laboratories—Cont.

cause hallucinations, convulsions, CNS depression, and death.

Drug Interactions: MAO inhibitors and tricyclic antidepressants may prolong and intensify the anticholinergic (drying) effects of antihistamines. Beta-adrenergic blockers and MAO inhibitors may potentiate the pressor effect of phenylephrine (see **WARNINGS**). Concurrent use of digitalis glycosides may increase the possibility of cardiac arrhythmias. Sympathomimetics may reduce the hypotensive effects of guanethidine, mecamylamine, methyldopa, reserpine and veratrum alkaloids. Concurrent use of tricyclic anticdepressants may antagonize the effects of phenylephrine. Concomitant use of antihistamines with alcohol, tricyclic antidepressants, barbiturates and other CNS depressants may have an additive effect.

Carcinogenesis, Mutagenesis, Impairment of Fertility: No data are available on the long-term potential of the components of this product for carcinogenesis, mutagenesis, or impairment of fertility in animals or humans.

Pregnancy: Category C: Animal reproduction studies have not been conducted with the components of this product. It is also not known whether these drugs can cause fetal harm when administered to a pregnant woman or can effect reproduction capacity. Accordingly, this product should be given to a pregnant woman only if clearly needed.

Nursing Mothers: Use of this product by nursing mothers is not recommended because of the higher than usual risk for infants from sympathomimetic amines.

ADVERSE REACTIONS

Hyper-reactive individuals may display ephedrine-like reactions such as tachycardia, palpitations, headache, dizziness, or nausea. Sympathomimetics have been associated with certain untoward reactions including fear, anxiety, nervousness, restlessness, tremor, weakness, pallor, respiratory difficulty, dysuria, insomnia, hallucinations, convulsions, CNS depression, arrhythmias, and cardiovascular collapse with hypotension.

Possible side effects of antihistamines are drowsiness, dry mouth, anorexia, nausea, vomiting, headache and nervousness, blurring of vision, polyuria, heartburn, dysuria and very rarely, dermatitis.

OVERDOSAGE

Since ATROHIST® SPRINKLE Capsules contain pharmacologically different compounds, treatment of overdosage should be based upon the symptomatology of the patient as it relates to the individual ingredients. A detailed description of the symptoms which are likely to appear after ingestion of an excess of the individual components follows:

Manifestations of antihistamine overdosage may vary from CNS depression (sedation, apnea, cardiovascular collapse) to stimulation (insomnia, hallucinations, tremors or convulsions). Other signs and symptoms may be dizziness, tinnitus, ataxia, blurred vision, and hypotension. Stimulation is particularly likely in children, as are atropine-like signs and symptoms (dry-mouth; fixed, dilated pupils; flushing; hyperthermia and gastrointestinal symptoms).

Overdosage with phenylephrine may manifest itself as excessive CNS stimulation resulting in excitment, tremor, restlessness and insomnia. Other effects may include tachycardia, hypertension, pallor, mydriasis, hyperglycemia and urinary retention. Severe overdosage may cause tachypnea or hyperpnea, hallucination, convulsions or delirium, but in some individuals there may be CNS depression with somnolence, stupor or respiratory depression. Arrhythmias (including ventricular fibrillation) may lead to hypotension and circulatory collapse. Severe hypokalemia can occur, probably due to a compartmental shift rather than a depletion of potassium.

The LD_{50} of phenylephrine (single oral dose) has been reported to be 120 mg/kg in the mouse and 350 mg/kg in the rat. The toxic and lethal concentrations in human biologic fluids are not known. No information is available regarding the LD_{50} of brompheniramine maleate and phenyltoloxamine citrate, and their toxic and lethal concentrations in human biologic fluids are not known. Cases of fatal overdosage with antihistamines have been reported in the literature.

In the event of overdosage, emergency treatment should be started immediately. Since the action of sustained release products may continue for as long as 12 hours, treatment of overdosage should be directed toward reducing further absorption and supporting the patient for at least that length of time. Gastric emptying (Syrup of Ipecac) and/or lavage is recommended as soon as possible after ingestion, even if the patient has vomited spontaneously. Either isotonic or half-isotonic saline may be used for lavage. Administration of an activated charcoal slurry is benefical after lavage and/or emesis if less than 4 hours have passed since ingestion. Saline cathartics, such as Milk of Magnesia, are useful for hastening the evacuation of unreleased medication.

Adrenergic receptor blocking agents are antidotes to phenylephrine. In practice, the most useful is the beta-blocker propranolol which is indicated when there are signs of cardiac toxicity. Theoretically, phenylephrine is dialyzable but procedures have not been clinically established.

In severe cases of overdosage, it is essential to monitor both the heart (by electrocardiograph) and plasma electrolytes, and to give intravenous potassium as indicated. Vasopressors may be used to treat hypotension. Excessive CNS stimulation may be counteracted with parenteral diazepam. Stimulants should not be used. Hyperpyrexia, especially in children, may require treatment with tepid water sponge baths or a hyperthermic blanket. Apnea is treated with ventilatory support.

DOSAGE AND ADMINISTRATION

Adults and children over 12 years of age: Three capsules every 12 hours not to exceed 6 capsules in 24 hours. **Children 6 to 12 years:** One or two capsules every 12 hours not to exceed 4 capsules in 24 hours. **Children 2 to 6 years:** One capsule every 12 hours not to exceed 2 capsules in 24 hours. Capsules may be swallowed whole or the entire contents sprinkled on a small amount of soft food immediately prior to ingestion. **Subdividing the contents of a capsule is not recommended.**

HOW SUPPLIED

Bottles of 100 capsules (NDC 53014-0022-1). White beads in a yellow and clear capsule imprinted with "Adams/0022". Store at controlled room temperature between 15° C and 30° C (59° F and 86° F). Dispense in tight, light-resistant containers.

CAUTION: Federal law prohibits dispensing without prescription.

DECONSAL® II Tablets
PSEUDOEPHEDRINE HCl/GUAIFENESIN

DECONSAL® SPRINKLE Capsules
PHENYLEPHRINE HCl/GUAIFENESIN

DESCRIPTION

DECONSAL® II Tablets: Each scored, dark blue tablet provides 60 mg pseudoephedrine hydrochloride and 600 mg guaifenesin in a sustained-release formulation intended for oral administration.

DECONSAL® SPRINKLE Capsules: Each blue and clear capsule provides 10 mg phenylephrine hydrochloride and 200 mg guaifenesin in a sustained-release formulation intended for oral administration. The microencapsulate contents of a capsule may be sprinkled on a small amount of soft food immediately prior to ingestion, making the product ideal for children and other patients unable to swallow capsules or tablets. Capsules are oversized to facilitate opening but may also be swallowed whole.

Pseudoephedrine hydrochloride and phenylephrine hydrochloride are orally effective nasal decongestants. Chemically, pseudoephedrine hydrochloride is [S-(R*, R*)]-α-[1-(methylamino)ethyl] benzenemethanol hydrochloride. The chemical name for phenylephrine hydrochloride is (R)-3-hydroxy-α-[(methylamino)methyl] benzenemethanol hydrochloride. Guaifenesin is an expectorant. Chemically, it is 3-(2-methoxyphenoxy)-1,2-propanediol.

CLINICAL PHARMACOLOGY

Pseudoephedrine hydrochloride and phenylephrine hydrochloride are orally active sympathomimetic amines which exert a decongestant action on the nasal mucosa.

Pseudoephedrine hydrochloride acts by vasoconstriction which results in reduction of tissue hyperemia, edema, nasal congestion, and an increase in nasal airway patency. The vasoconstriction action of pseudoephedrine is similar to that of ephedrine. In the usual dose it has minimal vasopressor effects. Pseudoephedrine is rapidly and almost completely absorbed from the gastrointestinal tract. It has a plasma half-life of 6 to 8 hours. Acidic urine is associated with faster elimination of the drug. The drug is distributed to body tissues and fluids, including the fetal tissue, breast milk and the central nervous system (CNS). Approximately 50% to 75% of the administered dose is excreted unchanged in the urine; the remainder is apparently metabolized in the liver to inactive compounds by N-demethylation, parahydroxylation, and oxidative deamination.

Phenylephrine hydrochloride effects its vasoconstrictor activity by releasing noradrenaline from sympathetic nerve endings, and from direct stimulation of α-adrenoreceptors in blood vessels. Following oral administration, constriction of blood vessels in the nasal mucosa helps relieve nasal congestion. In therapeutic doses the drug causes little, if any, central nervous system stimulation.

Guaifenesin is an expectorant which increases respiratory tract fluid secretions and helps to loosen phlegm and bronchial secretions. By reducing the viscosity of secretions, guaifenesin increases the efficiency of the cough reflex and of ciliary action in removing accumulated secretions from the trachea and bronchi. Guaifenesin is readily absorbed from

the gastrointestinal tract and is rapidly metabolized and excreted in the urine. Guaifenesin has a plasma half-life of one hour. The major urinary metabolite is β-(2-methoxyphenoxy) lactic acid.

INDICATIONS AND USAGE

DECONSAL® II Tablets and DECONSAL® SPRINKLE Capsules are indicated for the temporary relief of nasal congestion and cough associated with respiratory tract infections and related conditions such as sinusitis, pharyngitis, bronchitis, and asthma, when these conditions are complicated by tenacious mucus and/or mucus plugs and congestion. The products are effective in productive as well as nonproductive cough, but are of particular value in dry, nonproductive cough which tends to injure the mucous membrane of the air passages. DECONSAL® SPRINKLE Capsules are particularly suitable for use in children and other patients unable to swallow tablets or capsules.

CONTRAINDICATIONS

These products are contraindicated in patients with hypersensitivity to guaifenesin or hypersensitivity or idiosyncrasy to sympathomimetic amines which may be manifested by insomnia, dizziness, weakness, tremor, or arrhythmias. Patients known to be hypersensitive to other sympathomimetic amines may exhibit cross sensitivity with phenylephrine or pseudoephedrine. Sympathomimetic amines are contraindicated in patients with severe hypertension, severe coronary artery disease, and patients on monoamine oxidase (MAO) inhibitor therapy (see **Drug Interactions** section).

WARNINGS

Sympathomimetic amines should be used with caution in patients with hypertension, ischemic heart disease, diabetes mellitus, increased intraocular pressure, hyperthyroidism, or prostatic hypertrophy. Sympathomimetics may produce central nervous stimulation with convulsions or cardiovascular collapse with accompanying hypotension. **Do not exceed recommended dosage.**

Hypertensive crises can occur with concurrent use of phenylephrine or pseudoephedrine and monoamine oxidase (MAO) inhibitors, indomethacin, or with beta-blockers and methyldopa. If a hypertensive crisis occurs, these drugs should be discontinued immediately and therapy to lower blood pressure should be instituted. Fever should be managed by means of external cooling.

PRECAUTIONS

General: Use with caution in patients with diabetes, hypertension, cardiovascular disease, or hyperreactivity to ephedrine.

Before prescribing medication to suppress or modify cough, it is important to ascertain that the underlying cause of cough is identified, that modification of cough does not increase the risk of clinical or physiologic complications, and that appropriate therapy for the primary disease is instituted.

Information for Patients: Patients should be instructed to check with physician if symptoms do not improve within 5 days or if fever is present. DECONSAL® SPRINKLE Capsules may be swallowed whole or the entire contents sprinkled on a small amount of soft food (jam, etc.) immediately prior to ingestion. Capsule contents should not be crushed or chewed.

Pediatric Use: These products are not recommended for use in children under 2 years of age.

Use in Elderly: The elderly (60 years and older) are more likely to experience adverse reactions to sympathomimetics. Overdosage of sympathomimetics in this age group may cause hallucinations, convulsions, CNS depression, and death.

Drug Interactions: Beta-adrenergic blockers and MAO inhibitors may potentiate the pressor effects of phenylephrine or pseudoephedrine (see **WARNINGS**). Concurrent use of digitalis glycosides may increase the possibility of cardiac arrhythmias. Sympathomimetics may reduce the hypotensive effects of guanethidine, mecamylamine, methyldopa, reserpine, and veratrum alkaloids. Concurrent use of tricyclic antidepressants may antagonize the effects of phenylephrine and pseudoephedrine.

Drug/Laboratory Test Interactions: Guaifenesin may increase renal clearance for urate and therby lower serum uric acid levels. Guaifenesin may produce an increase in urinary 5-hydroxyindoleacetic acid and may therefore interfere with the interpretation of this test for the diagnosis of carcinoid syndrome. It may also falsely elevate the VMA test for catechols. Administration of this drug should be discontinued 48 hours prior to the collection of urine specimens for such tests.

Carcinogenesis, Mutagenesis, Impairment of Fertility: No data are available on the long-term potential of the components of these products for carcinogenesis, mutagenesis, or impairment of fertility in animals or humans.

Pregnancy: Category C: Animal reproduction studies have not been conducted with the components of these products. It is also not known whether these drugs can cause fetal harm when administered to a pregnant woman or can affect reproduction capacity. Accordingly, these products should be given to a pregnant woman only if clearly needed.

Nursing Mothers: Pseudoephedrine is excreted in breast milk. Use of these products by nursing mothers is not recommended because of the higher than usual risk for infants from sympathomimetic amines.

ADVERSE REACTIONS

Hyperreactive individuals may display ephedrine-like reactions such as tachycardia, palpitations, headache, dizziness, or nausea. Sympathomimetics have been associated with certain untoward reactions including fear, anxiety, nervousness, restlessness, tremor, weakness, pallor, respiratory difficulty, dysuria, insomnia, hallucinations, convulsions, CNS depression, arrhythmias, and cardiovascular collapse with hypotension. No serious side effects have been reported with the use of guaifenesin.

OVERDOSAGE

Since DECONSAL® II Tablets and DECONSAL® SPRINKLE Capsules each contain two pharmacologically different compounds, treatment of overdosage should be based upon the symptomatology of the patient as it relates to the individual ingredients. Treatment of acute overdosage would probably be based upon treating the patient for phenylephrine or pseudoephedrine toxicity which may manifest itself as excessive CNS stimulation resulting in excitement, tremor, restlessness, and insomnia. Other effets may include tachycardia, hypertension, pallor, mydriasis, hyperglycemia and urinary retention. Severe overdosage may cause tachypnea or hyperpnea, hallucinations, convulsions, or delirium, but in some individuals there may be CNS depression. Arrhythmias (including ventricular fibrillation) may lead to hypotension and circulatory collapse. Severe hypokalemia can occur, probably due to a compartmental shift rather than a depletion of potassium. Overdosage with guaifenesin is unlikely to produce toxic effects since its toxicity is much lower than that of phenylephrine or pseudoephedrine.

The LD_{50} of pseudoephedrine (single oral dose) has been reported to be 726 mg/kg in the mouse, 2206 mg/kg in the rat, and 1177 mg/kg in the rabbit. The toxic and lethal concentrations in human biologic fluids are not known. Urinary excretion increases with acidification and decreases with alkalinization of the urine. There are few published reports of toxicity due to pseudoephedrine and no case of fatal overdosage has been reported. The LD_{50} of phenylephrine (single oral dose) has been reported to be 120 mg/kg in the mouse and 350 mg/kg in the rat. The toxic and lethal concentrations in human biologic fluids are not known. Guaifenesin, when administered by stomach tube to test animals in doses up to 5 grams/kg, produced no signs of toxicity.

Since the action of sustained-release products may continue for as long as 12 hours, treatment of overdosage should be directed toward reducing further absorption and supporting the patient for at least that length of time. Gastric emptying (Syrup of Ipecac) and/or lavage is recommended as soon as possible after ingestion, even if the patient has vomited spontaneously. Either isotonic or half-isotonic saline may be used for lavage. Administration of an activated charcoal slurry is beneficial after lavage and/or emesis if less than 4 hours have passed since ingestion. Saline cathartics, such as Milk of Magnesia, are useful for hastening the evacuation of unreleased medication.

Adrenergic receptor blocking agents are antidotes to phenylephrine and pseudoephedrine, in practice, the most useful is the beta-blocker propranolol which is indicated when there are signs of cardiac toxicity. Theoretically, phenylephrine and pseudoephedrine are dialyzable but procedures have not been clinically established.

In severe cases of overdosage, it is essential to monitor both the heart (by electrocardiograph) and plasma electrolytes, and to give intravenous potassium as indicated. Vasopressors may be used to treat hypotension. Excessive CNS stimulation may be counteracted with parenteral diazepam. Stimulants should not be used.

DOSAGE AND ADMINISTRATION

DECONSAL® II Tablets: Adults and children over 12 years of age: One or two tablets every 12 hours not to exceed 4 tablets in 24 hours. **Children 6 to 12 years:** One tablet every 12 hours not to exceed 2 tablets in 24 hours. **Children 2 to 6 years:** ½ tablet every 12 hours not to exceed 1 tablet in 24 hours.

DECONSAL® SPRINKLE Casules: Adults and children over 12 years: Three capsules every 12 hours not to exceed 6 capsules in 24 hours. **Children 6 to 12 years:** One or two capsules every 12 hours not to exceed 4 capsules in 24 hours. **Children 2 to 6 years:** One capsule every 12 hours not to exceed 2 capsules in 24 hours. Capsules may be swallowed whole or the entire contents sprinkled on a small amount of soft food immediately prior to ingestion. **Subdividing the contents of a capsule is not recommended.**

HOW SUPPLIED

DECONSAL® II Tablets: Bottles of 100 tablets (NDC 53014-0017-1). Scored, dark blue tablets are embossed with "Adams/0017".

DECONSAL® SPRINKLE Capsules: Bottles of 100 capsules (NDC 53014-0016-1). White beads in a blue and clear capsule imprinted with "Adams/0016".

Store at controlled room temperature between 15° C and 30° C (59° and 86° F). Dispense in tight containers.

Caution: Federal law prohibits dispensing without prescription.
5/89

DECONSAL® L.A. Tablets   ℞

HOW SUPPLIED

Bottles of 100 tablets (NDC 53014-0015-1).

HUMIBID® L.A. Tablets   ℞
GUAIFENESIN

HUMIBID® SPRINKLE Capsules
GUAIFENESIN

HUMIBID® DM Tablets
GUAIFENESIN/DEXTROMETHORPHAN HYDROBROMIDE

DESCRIPTION

HUMIBID® L.A. Tablets: Each light green, scored, sustained-release tablet provides 600 mg guaifenesin.
HUMIBID® SPRINKLE Capsules: Each green and clear capsule provides 300 mg guaifenesin in a sustained-release formulation intended for oral administration. The microencapsulated contents of a capsule may be sprinkled on a small amount of soft food immediately prior to ingestion, making the product ideal for children and other patients unable to swallow capsules or tablets. Capsules are oversized to facilitate opening but may also be swallowed whole.
HUMIBID® DM Tablets: Each dark green, scored, sustained-release tablet provides 600 mg guaifenesin and 30 mg dextromethorphan hydrobromide.
Chemically, guaifenesin is 3-(2-methoxyphenoxy)-1, 2-propanediol. Dextromethorphan is a salt of the methyl ether of the dextrorotatory isomer of levorphanol, a narcotic analgesic. Chemically, it is 3-methoxy-17-methyl-9α, 13α, 14α-morphinan hydrobromide.

CLINICAL PHARMACOLOGY

Guaifenesin is an expectorant which increases respiratory tract fluid secretions and helps to loosen phlegm and bronchial secretions. By reducing the viscosity of secretions, guaifenesin increases the efficiency of the cough reflex and of ciliary action in removing accumulated secretions from the trachea and bronchi. Guaifenesin is readily absorbed from the gastrointestinal tract and is rapidly metabolized and excreted in the urine. Guaifenesin has a plasma half-life of one hour. The major urinary metabolite is β-(2-methoxyphenoxy) lactic acid.

Dextromethorphan is an antitussive agent which, unlike the isomeric levorphanol, has no analgesic or addictive properties. The drug acts centrally and elevates the threshold for coughing. It is about equal to codeine in depressing the cough reflex. In therapeutic dosage, dextromethorphan does not inhibit ciliary activity. Dextromethorphan is rapidly absorbed from the gastrointestinal tract, metabolized by the liver and excreted primarily in the urine.

INDICATIONS AND USAGE

HUMIBID® L.A. Tablets and HUMIBID® SPRINKLE Capsules are indicated for the temporary relief of coughs associated with respiratory tract infections and related conditions such as sinusitis, pharyngitis and bronchitis, and asthma, when these conditions are complicated by tenacious mucus and/or mucus plugs and congestion.
HUMIBID® DM Tablets are indicated for the temporary relief of coughs associated with upper respiratory tract infections and related conditions such as sinusitis, pharyngitis and bronchitis, particularly when these conditions are complicated by tenacious mucus and/or mucus plugs and congestion.
HUMIBID® L.A. Tablets, HUMIBID® SPRINKLE Capsules, and HUMIBID® DM Tablets are effective in productive as well as non-productive cough, but are of particular value in dry, non-productive cough which tends to injure the mucous membrane of the air passages.

CONTRAINDICATIONS

These products are contraindicated in patients with hypersensitivity to guaifenesin or dextromethorphan.
HUMIBID® DM Tablets should not be used in patients receiving monoamine oxidase (MAO) inhibitor therapy.

PRECAUTIONS

General: Before prescribing medication to suppress or modify cough, it is important that the underlying cause of cough is identified, that modification of cough does not increase the risk of clinical or physiological complications, and that appropriate therapy for the primary disease is instituted.

Dextromethorphan should be used with caution in sedated or debilitated patients, and in patients to be confined to the supine position.

Information for Patients: HUMIBID® SPRINKLE Capsules may be swallowed whole or the entire contents sprinkled on a small amount of soft food (jam, etc.) immediately prior to ingestion. Capsule contents should not be subdivided, nor should they be crushed or chewed.

Drug/Laboratory Test Interactions: Guaifenesin may increase renal clearance for urate and thereby lower serum uric acid levels. Guaifenesin may produce an increase in urinary 5-hydroxyindoleacetic acid and may therefore interfere with the interpretation of this test for the diagnosis of carcinoid syndrome. It may also falsely elevate the VMA test for catechols. Administration of these products should be discontinued 48 hours prior to the collection of urine specimens for such tests.

Carcinogenesis, Mutagenesis, Impairment of Fertility: No data are available on the long-term potential of guaifenesin or of dextromethorphan for carcinogenesis, mutagenesis, or impairment of fertility in animals or humans.

Pregnancy: Category C: Animal reproduction studies have not been conducted with guaifenesin or with dextromethorphan. It is also not known whether these drugs can cause fetal harm when administered to a pregnant woman or can affect reproduction capacity. Therefore, these products should be given to a pregnant woman only if clearly needed.

Nursing Mothers: It is not known whether guaifenesin or dextromethorphan is excreted in human milk. Because many drugs are excreted in human milk, caution should be exercised when these products are administered to a nursing woman and a decision should be made whether to discontinue nursing or to discontinue the drug, taking into account the importance of the drug to the mother.

ADVERSE REACTIONS

No serious side effects from guaifenesin or dextromethorphan have been reported.

OVERDOSAGE

Overdosage with guaifenesin is unlikely to produce toxic effects since its toxicity is low. Guaifenesin, when administered by stomach tube to test animals in doses up to 5 grams/kg, produced no signs of toxicity. In severe cases of overdosage, treatment should be aimed at reducing further absorption of the drug. Gastric emptying (Syrup of Ipecac) and/or lavage is recommended as soon as possible after ingestion.

Overdosage with dextromethorphan may produce central excitement and mental confusion. Very high doses may produce respiratory depression. One case of toxic psychosis (hyperactivity, marked visual and auditory hallucinations) after ingestion of a single 300 mg dose of dextromethorphan has been reported.

DOSAGE AND ADMINISTRATION

HUMIBID® L.A. and HUMIBID® DM Tablets: Adults and children over 12 years of age: One or two tablets every 12 hours not to exceed 4 tablets in 24 hours . **Children 6 to 12 years:** One tablet every 12 hours not to exceed 2 tablets in 24 hours. **Children 2 to 6 years:** ½ tablet every 12 hours not to exceed 1 tablet in 24 hours.
HUMIBID® SPRINKLE Capsules: Adults and children over 12 years of age: Two to four capsules every 12 hours not to exceed 8 capsules in 24 hours. **Children 6 to 12 years:** Two capsules every 12 hours not to exceed 4 capsules in 24 hours. **Children 2 to 6 years:** One capsule every 12 hours not to exceed 2 capsules in 24 hours.

HOW SUPPLIED

HUMIBID® L.A. Tablets: Bottles of 100 tablets (NDC 53014-0012-1) and 500 tablets (NDC 53014-0012-5). Light green, scored tablets are embossed with "Adams/0012".
HUMIBID® SPRINKLE Capsules: Bottles of 100 capsules (NDC 53014-0018-1). White beads in a green and clear capsule imprinted with "Adams/0018".
HUMIBID® DM Tablets: Bottles of 100 tablets (NDC 53014-0030-1). Dark green, scored tablets are embossed with "Adams/0030".
Store at controlled room temperature between 15° C and 30° C (59° F and 86° F). Dispense in tight containers.
CAUTION: Federal law prohibits dispensing without prescription.
5/89

Products are cross-indexed by
generic and chemical names
in the
YELLOW SECTION

Adria Laboratories
Division of Erbamont Inc.
7001 POST ROAD
DUBLIN, OH 43017

PRODUCT IDENTIFICATION CODES

To provide quick and positive identification of Adria Laboratories products, we have imprinted the product identification number on one side of all tablets and capsules. The other side of the tablet displays the name "ADRIA".

In order that you may quickly identify a product by its code number, we have compiled below a numerical list of code numbers of prescription products with their corresponding product names:
[See table below].

ADRIAMYCIN PFS™   ℞
[adrēē'ah-mǐ-cǐn]
(Doxorubicin Hydrochloride, USP)
Injection
FOR INTRAVENOUS USE ONLY

WARNINGS

1. Severe local tissue necrosis will occur if there is extravasation during administration (See Dosage and Administration). ADRIAMYCIN PFS must not be given by the intramuscular or subcutaneous route.
2. Serious irreversible myocardial toxicity with delayed congestive failure often unresponsive to any cardiac supportive therapy may be encountered as total dosage approaches 550 mg/m². This toxicity may occur at lower cumulative doses in patients with prior mediastinal irradiation or on concurrent cyclophosphamide therapy.
3. Dosage should be reduced in patients with impaired hepatic function.
4. Severe myelosuppression may occur.
5. ADRIAMYCIN PFS should be administered only under the supervision of a physician who is experienced in the use of cancer chemotherapeutic agents.

DESCRIPTION

Doxorubicin is a cytotoxic anthracycline antibiotic isolated from cultures of *Streptomyces peucetius* var. *caesius*. Doxorubicin consists of a naphthacenequinone nucleus linked through a glycosidic bond at ring atom 7 to an amino sugar, daunosamine.

Doxorubicin binds to nucleic acids, presumably by specific intercalation of the planar anthracycline nucleus with the DNA double helix. The anthracycline ring is lipophilic but the saturated end of the ring system contains abundant hydroxyl groups adjacent to the amino sugar, producing a hydrophilic center. The molecule is amphoteric, containing acidic functions in the ring phenolic groups and a basic function in the sugar amino group. It binds to cell membranes as well as plasma proteins.

ADRIAMYCIN PFS™ (doxorubicin hydrochloride, USP) Injection is a parenteral, isotonic, preservative-free, single use only solution and is available in 5 mL (10 mg), 10 mL (20 mg), and 25 mL (50 mg) single dose vials and 100 mL (200 mg) multidose vial.

Each mL contains doxorubicin hydrochloride and the following inactive ingredients: sodium chloride 0.9% and water for injection q.s. Hydrochloric acid is used to adjust pH to a target pH of 3.0.

CLINICAL PHARMACOLOGY

Though not completely elucidated, the mechanism of action of doxorubicin is related to its ability to bind DNA and inhibit nucleic acid synthesis. Cell culture studies have demonstrated rapid cell penetration and perinucleolar chromatin binding, rapid inhibition of mitotic activity and nucleic acid synthesis, mutagenesis and chromosomal aberrations. Animal studies have shown activity in a spectrum of experimental tumors, immunosuppression, carcinogenic properties in rodents, induction of a variety of toxic effects, including delayed and progressive cardiac toxicity, myelosuppression in all species and atrophy to testes in rats and dogs.

Pharmacokinetic studies show the intravenous administration of normal or radiolabeled doxorubicin is followed by rapid plasma clearance and significant tissue binding. Urinary excretion, as determined by fluorimetric methods, accounts for approximately 4–5% of the administered dose in five days. Biliary excretion represents the major excretion route, 40–50% of the administered dose being recovered in the bile or the feces in seven days. Impairment of liver function results in slower excretion, and consequently, increased retention and accumulation in plasma and tissues. Doxorubicin does not cross the blood brain barrier.

INDICATIONS AND USAGE

ADRIAMYCIN® (Doxorubicin HCl, USP) for injection has been used successfully to produce regression in disseminated neoplastic conditions such as acute lymphoblastic leukemia, acute myeloblastic leukemia, Wilms' tumor, neuroblastoma, soft tissue and bone sarcomas, breast carcinoma, ovarian carcinoma, transitional cell bladder carcinoma, thyroid carcinoma, lymphomas of both Hodgkin and non-Hodgkin types, bronchogenic carcinoma in which the small cell histologic type is the most responsive compared to other cell types and gastric carcinoma.

A number of other solid tumors have also shown some responsiveness but in numbers too limited to justify specific recommendation. Studies to date have shown malignant melanoma, kidney carcinoma, large bowel carcinoma, brain tumors and metastases to the central nervous system not to be significantly responsive to ADRIAMYCIN therapy.

CONTRAINDICATIONS

ADRIAMYCIN therapy should not be started in patients who have marked myelosuppression induced by previous treatment with other antitumor agents or by radiotherapy. Conclusive data are not available on pre-existing heart disease as a co-factor of increased risk of ADRIAMYCIN induced cardiac toxicity. Preliminary data suggest that in such cases cardiac toxicity may occur at doses lower than the recommended cumulative limit. It is therefore not recommended to start ADRIAMYCIN in such cases. ADRIAMYCIN treatment is contraindicated in patients who received previous treatment with complete cumulative doses of ADRIAMYCIN and/or daunorubicin.

WARNINGS

Special attention must be given to the cardiac toxicity exhibited by ADRIAMYCIN. Although uncommon, acute left ventricular failure has occurred, particularly in patients who have received total dosage of the drug exceeding the currently recommended limit of 550 mg/m². This limit appears to be lower (400 mg/m²) in patients who received radiotherapy to the mediastinal area or concomitant therapy with other potentially cardiotoxic agents such as cyclophosphamide. The total dose of ADRIAMYCIN administered to the individual patient should also take into account a previous or concomitant therapy with related compounds such as daunorubicin. Congestive heart failure and/or cardiomyopathy may be encountered several weeks after discontinuation of ADRIAMYCIN therapy.

Cardiac failure is often not favorably affected by presently known medical or physical therapy for cardiac support. Early clinical diagnosis of drug induced heart failure appears to be essential for successful treatment with digitalis, diuretics, low salt diet and bed rest. Severe cardiac toxicity may occur precipitously without antecedent EKG changes. A baseline EKG and EKGs performed prior to each dose or course after 300 mg/m² cumulative dose has been given is suggested. Transient EKG changes consisting of T-wave flattening, S-T depression and arrhythmias lasting for up to two weeks after a dose or course of ADRIAMYCIN are presently not considered indications for suspension of ADRIAMYCIN therapy. ADRIAMYCIN cardiomyopathy has been reported to be associated with a persistent reduction in the voltage of the QRS wave, a prolongation of the systolic time interval and a reduction of the ejection fraction as determined by echocardiography or radionuclide angiography. None of these tests have yet been confirmed to consistently identify those individual patients that are approaching their maximally tolerated cumulative dose of ADRIAMYCIN. If test results indicate change in cardiac function associated with ADRIAMYCIN the benefit of continued therapy must be carefully evaluated against the risk of producing irreversible cardiac damage.

Acute life-threatening arrhythmias have been reported to occur during or within a few hours after ADRIAMYCIN administration.

There is a high incidence of bone marrow depression, primarily of leukocytes, requiring careful hematologic monitoring. With the recommended dosage schedule, leukopenia is usually transient, reaching its nadir at 10–14 days after treatment with recovery usually occurring by the 21st day. White blood cell counts as low as 1000 mm³ are to be expected during treatment with appropriate doses of ADRIAMYCIN. Red blood cell and platelet levels should also be monitored since they may also be depressed. Hematologic toxicity may require dose reduction or suspension or delay of ADRIAMYCIN therapy. Persistent severe myelosuppression may result in superinfection or hemorrhage.

ADRIAMYCIN may potentiate the toxicity of other anticancer therapies. Exacerbation of cyclophosphamide induced hemorrhagic cystitis and enhancement of the hepatotoxicity of 6-mercaptopurine have been reported. Radiation induced toxicity to the myocardium, mucosae, skin and liver have been reported to be increased by the administration of ADRIAMYCIN.

Toxicity to recommended doses of ADRIAMYCIN is enhanced by hepatic impairment, therefore, prior to the individual dosing, evaluation of hepatic function is recommended using conventional clinical laboratory tests such as SGOT, SGPT, alkaline phosphatase and bilirubin. (See Dosage and Administration).

Necrotizing colitis manifested by typhlitis (cecal inflammation), bloody stools and severe and sometimes fatal infections have been associated with a combination of ADRIAMYCIN given by i.v. push daily for 3 days and cytarabine given by continuous infusion daily for 7 or more days.

On intravenous administration of ADRIAMYCIN extravasation may occur with or without an accompanying stinging or burning sensation and even if blood returns well on aspiration of the infusion needle (See Dosage and Administration). If any signs or symptoms of extravasation have occurred the injection or infusion should be immediately terminated and restarted in another vein.

ADRIAMYCIN and related compounds have also been shown to have mutagenic and carcinogenic properties when tested in experimental models.

Usage in Pregnancy—Safe use of ADRIAMYCIN in pregnancy has not been established. ADRIAMYCIN is embryotoxic and teratogenic in rats and embryotoxic and abortifacient in rabbits. Therefore, the benefits to the pregnant patient should be carefully weighed against the potential toxicity to fetus and embryo. The possible adverse effects on fertility in males and females in humans or experimental animals have not been adequately evaluated.

PRECAUTIONS

Initial treatment with ADRIAMYCIN requires close observation of the patient and extensive laboratory monitoring. It is recommended, therefore, that patients be hospitalized at least during the first phase of the treatment.

Like other cytotoxic drugs, ADRIAMYCIN may induce hyperuricemia secondary to rapid lysis of neoplastic cells. The clinician should monitor the patient's blood uric acid level and be prepared to use such supportive and pharmacologic measures as might be necessary to control this problem.

ADRIAMYCIN imparts a red coloration to the urine for 1–2 days after administration and patients should be advised to expect this during active therapy.

ADRIAMYCIN is not an anti-microbial agent.

ADVERSE REACTIONS

Dose limiting toxicities of therapy are myelosuppression and cardiotoxicity (See Warnings). Other reactions reported are:

Cutaneous—Reversible complete alopecia occurs in most cases. Hyperpigmentation of nailbeds and dermal creases, primarily in children, and onycholysis have been reported in a few cases. Recall of skin reaction due to prior radiotherapy has occurred with ADRIAMYCIN administration.

Gastrointestinal—Acute nausea and vomiting occurs frequently and may be severe. This may be alleviated by antiemetic therapy. Mucositis (stomatitis and esophagitis) may occur 5–10 days after administration. The effect may be severe leading to ulceration and represents a site of origin for severe infections. The dose regimen consisting of administration of ADRIAMYCIN on three successive days results in the greater incidence and severity of mucositis. Ulceration and necrosis of the colon, especially the cecum, may occur leading to bleeding or severe infections which can be fatal. This reaction has been reported in patients with acute non-lymphocytic leukemia treated with a 3-day course of ADRIAMYCIN combined with cytarabine. Anorexia and diarrhea have been occasionally reported.

Vascular—Phlebosclerosis has been reported especially when small veins are used or a single vein is used for re-

---

PRODUCT IDENTIFICATION CODE

peated administration. Facial flushing may occur if the injection is given too rapidly.

Local—Severe cellulitis, vesication and tissue necrosis will occur if ADRIAMYCIN is extravasated during administration. Erythematous streaking along the vein prcximal to the site of the injection has been reported (See Dosage and Administration).

Hypersensitivity—Fever, chills and urticaria have been reported occasionally. Anaphylaxis may occur. A case of apparent cross sensitivity to lincomycin has been reported.

Other—Conjunctivitis and lacrimation occur rarely.

OVERDOSAGE

Acute overdosage with ADRIAMYCIN enhances the toxic effects of mucositis, leukopenia and thrombopenia. Treatment of acute overdosage consists of treatment of the severely myelosuppressed patient with hospitalization, antibiotics, platelet and granulocyte transfusions and symptomatic treatment of mucositis. **The 200 mg vial is packaged as a multiple dose vial and caution should be exercised to prevent inadvertent overdosage.**

Chronic overdosage with cumulative doses exceeding 550 mg/m^2 increases the risk of cardiomyopathy and resultant congestive heart failure. Treatment consists of vigorous management of congestive heart failure with digitalis preparations and diuretics. The use of peripheral vasodilators has been recommended.

DOSAGE AND ADMINISTRATION

Care in the administration of ADRIAMYCIN will reduce the chance of perivenous infiltration. It may also decrease the chance of local reactions such as urticaria and erythematous streaking. On intravenous administration of ADRIAMYCIN, extravasation may occur with or without an accompanying stinging or burning sensation and even if blood returns well on aspiration of the infusion needle. If any signs or symptoms of extravasation have occurred, the injection or infusion should be immediately terminated and restarted in another vein. If it is known or suspected that subcutaneous extravasation has occurred, local infiltration with an injectable corticosteroid and flooding the site with normal saline has been reported to lessen the local reaction. Because of the progressive nature of extravasation reactions, the area of injection should be frequently examined and plastic surgery consultation obtained. If ulceration begins, early wide excision of the involved area should be considered.[1]

The most commonly used dosage schedule is 60–75 mg/m^2 as a single intravenous injection administered at 21-day intervals. The lower dose should be given to patients with inadequate marrow reserves due to old age, or prior therapy, or neoplastic marrow infiltration. An alternative dose schedule is weekly doses of 20 mg/m^2 which has been reported to produce a lower incidence of congestive heart failure. Thirty mg/m^2 on each of three successive days repeated every 4 weeks has also been used. ADRIAMYCIN dosage must be reduced if the bilirubin is elevated as follows: serum bilirubin 1.2–3.0 mg/dL—give ½ normal dose, > 3 mg/dL—give ¼ normal dose.

It is recommended that ADRIAMYCIN PFS be slowly administered into the tubing of a freely running intravenous infusion of Sodium Chloride Injection USP or 5% Dextrose Injection USP. The tubing should be attached to a Butterfly® needle inserted preferably into a large vein. If possible, avoid veins over joints or in extremities with compromised venous or lymphatic drainage. The rate of administration is dependent on the size of the vein and the dosage. However the dose should be administered in not less than 3 to 5 minutes. Local erythematous streaking along the vein as well as facial flushing may be indicative of too rapid an administration. A burning or stinging sensation may be indicative of perivenous infiltration and the infusion should be immediately terminated and restarted in another vein. Perivenous infiltration may occur painlessly.

ADRIAMYCIN should not be mixed with heparin or 5-fluorouracil since it has been reported that these drugs are incompatible to the extent that a precipitate may form. Until specific compatibility data are available, it is not recommended that ADRIAMYCIN PFS be mixed with other drugs. ADRIAMYCIN has been used concurrently with other approved chemotherapeutic agents. Evidence is available that in some types of neoplastic disease combination chemotherapy is superior to single agents. The benefits and risks of such therapy continue to be elucidated.

Handling and Disposal: Skin reactions associated with ADRIAMYCIN have been reported. Caution in the handling of the solution must be exercised and the use of gloves is recommended. If ADRIAMYCIN PFS contacts the skin or mucosae, immediately wash thoroughly with soap and water.

Procedures for proper handling and disposal of anti-cancer drugs should be considered. Several guidelines on this subject have been published.[2–7] There is no general agreement that all of the procedures recommended in the guidelines are necessary or appropriate.

HOW SUPPLIED

ADRIAMYCIN PFS™ (doxorubicin hydrochloride, USP) Injection

Sterile, single use only, contains no preservative
NDC 0013-1136-91 10 mg vial, 2 mg/mL, 5 mL, 10 vial packs.
NDC 0013-1146-94 20 mg vial, 2 mg/mL, 10 mL, 5 vial packs.
NDC 0013-1156-79 50 mg vial, 2 mg/mL, 25 mL, single vial packs.

Store under refrigeration, 2°–8°C (36°–46°F), protect from light and retain in carton until time of use. Discard unused solution.

Sterile, multidose vial, contains no preservative.
NDC 0013-1166-83 200 mg, 2 mg/mL, 100 mL multidose vial, single vial packs.

Store under refrigeration 2°–8°C (36°–46°F), protect from light and retain in carton until time of use.

REFERENCES

1. Rudolph R et al: Skin Ulcers Due to ADRIAMYCIN. Cancer 38: 1087–1094, Sept. 1976.
2. Recommendations for the Safe Handling of Parenteral Antineoplastic Drugs. NIH Publication No. 83-2621. For sale by the Superintendent of Documents, U.S. Government Printing Office, Washington, D.C. 20402.
3. AMA Council Report, Guidelines for Handling Parenteral Antineoplastics. JAMA, March 15, 1985.
4. National Study Commission on Cytotoxic Exposure—Recommendations for Handling Cytotoxic Agents. Available from Louis P. Jeffrey, Sc. D., Director of Pharmacy Services, Rhode Island Hospital, 593 Eddy Street, Providence, Rhode Island 02902.
5. Clinical Oncological Society of Australia: Guidelines and recommendations for safe handling of antineoplastic agents. Med J. Australia 1:426–428, 1983.
6. Jones R., et al. Safe handling of chemotherapeutic agents: A report from the Mount Sinai Medical Center. Ca—A Cancer Journal for Clinicians Sept/Oct, 258–263, 1983.
7. American Society of Hospital Pharmacists technical assistance bulletin on handling cytotoxic drugs in hospitals. Am J Hosp Pharm 42:131–137, 1985.

Manufactured by:
FARMITALIA CARLO ERBA S.p.A.,
MILAN, ITALY
Distributed by:
ADRIA LABORATORIES
Division of Erbamont Inc.
COLUMBUS, OHIO 43215.

ADRIAMYCIN RDF™   ℞
[a'dreeah-mī"sin]
(Doxorubicin Hydrochloride, USP)
For Injection
FOR INTRAVENOUS USE ONLY

PRODUCT OVERVIEW

KEY FACTS

ADRIAMYCIN RDF is a cytotoxic agent active against a variety of hematologic malignancies and solid tumors. The active ingredient, doxorubicin hydrochloride, is an anthracycline antibiotic that selectively kills malignant cells and causes tumor regression. ADRIAMYCIN RDF contains a small amount of methylparaben (to enhance dissolution).

MAJOR USES

ADRIAMYCIN RDF is clinically effective against disseminated neoplastic conditions including acute lymphoblastic and myeloblastic leukemia, Wilm's tumor, neuroblastoma, soft tissue and bone sarcomas, breast carcinoma, ovarian carcinoma, transitional cell bladder carcinoma, thyroid carcinoma, Hodgkin's and non-Hodgkin's lymphoma, bronchogenic carcinoma and gastric carcinoma.

SAFETY INFORMATION

ADRIAMYCIN RDF is intended for intravenous use only. Care must be taken to avoid extravasation. Patients must be carefully monitored and doses adjusted to avoid too severe myelosuppression or mucositis. Too large cumulative doses may cause cardiomyopathy leading to congestive heart failure.

PRESCRIBING INFORMATION

ADRIAMYCIN RDF™   ℞
[a'dreeah-mī"sin]
(Doxorubicin Hydrochloride, USP)
For Injection
FOR INTRAVENOUS USE ONLY

WARNINGS

1. Severe local tissue necrosis will occur if there is extravasation during administration (See Dosage and Administration). ADRIAMYCIN RDF must not be given by the intramuscular or subcutaneous route.
2. Serious irreversible myocardial toxicity with delayed congestive failure often unresponsive to any cardiac

---

supportive therapy may be encountered as total dosage approaches 550 mg/m^2. This toxicity may occur at lower cumulative doses in patients with prior mediastinal irradiation or on concurrent cyclophosphamide therapy.
3. Dosage should be reduced in patients with impaired hepatic function.
4. Severe myelosuppression may occur.
5. ADRIAMYCIN RDF should be administered only under the supervision of a physician who is experienced in the use of cancer chemotherapeutic agents.

DESCRIPTION

Doxorubicin is a cytotoxic anthracycline antibiotic isolated from cultures of *Streptomyces peucetius* var. *caesius*. Doxorubicin consists of a naphthacenequinone nucleus linked through a glycosidic bond at ring atom 7 to an amino sugar, daunosamine.

Doxorubicin binds to nucleic acids, presumably by specific intercalation of the planar anthracycline nucleus with the DNA double helix. The anthracycline ring is lipophilic but the saturated end of the ring system contains abundant hydroxyl groups adjacent to the amino sugar, producing a hydrophilic center. The molecule is amphoteric, containing acidic functions in the ring phenolic groups and a basic function in the sugar amino group. It binds to cell membranes as well as plasma proteins. It is supplied in the hydrochloride form as a freeze-dried powder containing lactose and methylparaben (added to enhance dissolution).

CLINICAL PHARMACOLOGY

Though not completely elucidated, the mechanism of action of doxorubicin is related to its ability to bind to DNA and inhibit nucleic acid synthesis. Cell culture studies have demonstrated rapid cell penetration and perinucleolar chromatin binding, rapid inhibition of mitotic activity and nucleic acid synthesis, mutagenesis and chromosomal aberrations. Animal studies have shown activity in a spectrum of experimental tumors, immunosuppression, carcinogenic properties in rodents, induction of a variety of toxic effects, including delayed and progressive cardiac toxicity, myelosuppression in all species and atrophy to testes in rats and dogs. Pharmacokinetic studies show the intravenous administration of normal or radiolabeled doxorubicin is followed by rapid plasma clearance and significant tissue binding. Urinary excretion, as determined by fluorimetric methods, accounts for approximately 4–5% of the administered dose in five days. Biliary excretion represents the major excretion route, 40–50% of the administered dose being recovered in the bile or the feces in seven days. Impairment of liver function results in slower excretion, and, consequently, increased retention and accumulation in plasma and tissues. Doxorubicin does not cross the blood brain barrier.

INDICATIONS AND USAGE

ADRIAMYCIN® (Doxorubicin HCl, USP) for Injection has been used successfully to produce regression in disseminated neoplastic conditions such as acute lymphoblastic leukemia, acute myeloblastic leukemia, Wilms' tumor, neuroblastoma, soft tissue and bone sarcomas, breast carcinoma, ovarian carcinoma, transitional cell bladder carcinoma, thyroid carcinoma, lymphomas of both Hodgkin and non-Hodgkin types, bronchogenic carcinoma in which the small cell histologic type is the most responsive compared to other cell types and gastric carcinoma.

A number of other solid tumors have also shown some responsiveness but in numbers too limited to justify specific recommendation. Studies to date have shown malignant melanoma, kidney carcinoma, large bowel carcinoma, brain tumors and metastases to the central nervous system not to be significantly responsive to ADRIAMYCIN therapy.

CONTRAINDICATIONS

ADRIAMYCIN therapy should not be started in patients who have marked myelosuppression induced by previous treatment with other antitumor agents or by radiotherapy. Conclusive data are not available on pre-existing heart disease as a co-factor of increased risk of ADRIAMYCIN induced cardiac toxicity. Preliminary data suggest that in such cases cardiac toxicity may occur at doses lower than the recommended cumulative limit. It is therefore not recommended to start ADRIAMYCIN in such cases. ADRIAMYCIN treatment is contraindicated in patients who received previous treatment with complete cumulative doses of ADRIAMYCIN and/or daunorubicin.

WARNINGS

Special attention must be given to the cardiac toxicity exhibited by ADRIAMYCIN. Although uncommon, acute left ventricular failure has occurred, particularly in patients who have received total dosage of the drug exceeding the currently recommended limit of 550 mg/m^2. This limit appears to be lower (400 mg/m^2) in patients who received radiotherapy to the mediastinal area or concomitant therapy with

Continued on next page

Adria—Cont.

other potentially cardiotoxic agents such as cyclophosphamide. The total dose of ADRIAMYCIN administered to the individual patient should also take into account a previous or concomitant therapy with related compounds such as daunorubicin. Congestive heart failure and/or cardiomyopathy may be encountered several weeks after discontinuation of ADRIAMYCIN therapy.

Cardiac failure is often not favorably affected by presently known medical or physical therapy for cardiac support. Early clinical diagnosis of drug induced heart failure appears to be essential for successful treatment with digitalis, diuretics, low salt diet and bed rest. Severe cardiac toxicity may occur precipitously without antecedent EKG changes. A baseline EKG and EKGs performed prior to each dose or course after 300 mg/m^2 cumulative dose has been given is suggested. Transient EKG changes consisting of T-wave flattening. S-T depression and arrhythmias lasting for up to two weeks after a dose or course of ADRIAMYCIN are presently not considered indications for suspension of ADRIAMYCIN therapy. ADRIAMYCIN cardiomyopathy has been reported to be associated with a persistent reduction in the voltage of the QRS wave, a prolongation of the systolic time interval and a reduction of the ejection fraction as determined by echocardiography or radionuclide angiography. None of these tests have yet been confirmed to consistently identify those individual patients that are approaching their maximally tolerated cumulative dose of ADRIAMYCIN. If test results indicate change in cardiac function associated with ADRIAMYCIN the benefit of continued therapy must be carefully evaluated against the risk of producing irreversible cardiac damage.

Acute life-threatening arrhythmias have been reported to occur during or within a few hours after ADRIAMYCIN administration.

There is a high incidence of bone marrow depression, primarily of leukocytes, requiring careful hematologic monitoring. With the recommended dosage schedule, leukopenia is usually transient, reaching its nadir at 10–14 days after treatment with recovery usually occurring by the 21st day. White blood cell counts as low as 1000 mm^3 are to be expected during treatment with appropriate dosages of ADRIAMYCIN. Red blood cell and platelet levels should also be monitored since they may also be depressed. Hematologic toxicity may require dose reduction or suspension or delay of ADRIAMYCIN therapy. Persistent severe myelosuppression may result in superinfection or hemorrhage.

ADRIAMYCIN may potentiate the toxicity of other anticancer therapies. Exacerbation of cyclophosphamide induced hemorrhagic cystitis and enhancement of the hepatotoxicity of 6-mercaptopurine have been reported. Radiation induced toxicity to the myocardium, mucosae, skin and liver have been reported to be increased by the administration of ADRIAMYCIN.

Toxicity to recommended doses of ADRIAMYCIN is enhanced by hepatic impairment, therefore, prior to the individual dosing, evaluation of hepatic function is recommended using conventional clinical laboratory tests, such as SGOT, SGPT, alkaline phosphatase and bilirubin. (See Dosage and Administration).

Necrotizing colitis manifested by typhlitis (cecal inflammation), bloody stools and severe and sometimes fatal infections has been associated with a combination of ADRIAMYCIN given by i.v. push daily for 3 days and cytarabine given by continuous infusion daily for 7 or more days.

On intravenous administration of ADRIAMYCIN extravasation may occur with or without an accompanying stinging or burning sensation and even if blood returns well on aspiration of the infusion needle (See Dosage and Administration). If any signs or symptoms of extravasation have occurred the injection or infusion should be immediately terminated and restarted in another vein.

ADRIAMYCIN and related compounds have also been shown to have mutagenic and carcinogenic properties when tested in experimental models.

Usage in Pregnancy—Safe use of ADRIAMYCIN in pregnancy has not been established. ADRIAMYCIN is embryotoxic and teratogenic in rats and embryotoxic and abortifacient in rabbits. Therefore, the benefits to the pregnant patient should be carefully weighed against the potential toxicity to fetus and embryo. The possible adverse effects on fertility in males and females in humans or experimental animals have not been adequately evaluated.

PRECAUTIONS

Initial treatment with ADRIAMYCIN requires close observation of the patient and extensive laboratory monitoring. It is recommended, therefore, that patients be hospitalized at least during the first phase of the treatment.

Like other cytotoxic drugs, ADRIAMYCIN may induce hyperuricemia secondary to rapid lysis of neoplastic cells. The clinician should monitor the patient's blood uric acid level and be prepared to use such supportive and pharmacologic measures as might be necessary to control this problem.

ADRIAMYCIN imparts a red coloration to the urine for 1-2 days after administration and patients should be advised to expect this during active therapy.

ADRIAMYCIN is not an anti-microbial agent.

ADVERSE REACTIONS

Dose limiting toxicities of therapy are myelosuppression and cardiotoxicity (See Warnings). Other reactions reported are:

Cutaneous—Reversible complete alopecia occurs in most cases. Hyperpigmentation of nailbeds and dermal creases, primarily in children, and onycholysis have been reported in a few cases. Recall of skin reaction due to prior radiotherapy has occurred with ADRIAMYCIN administration.

Gastrointestinal—Acute nausea and vomiting occurs frequently and may be severe. This may be alleviated by antiemetic therapy. Mucositis (stomatitis and esophagitis) may occur 5–10 days after administration. The effect may be severe leading to ulceration and represents a site of origin for severe infections. The dose regimen consisting of administration of ADRIAMYCIN on three successive days results in the greater incidence and severity of mucositis. Ulceration and necrosis of the colon, especially the cecum, may occur leading to bleeding or severe infections which can be fatal. This reaction has been reported in patients with acute non-lymphocytic leukemia treated with a 3-day course of ADRIAMYCIN combined with cytarabine. Anorexia and diarrhea have been occasionally reported.

Vascular—Phlebosclerosis has been reported especially when small veins are used or a single vein is used for repeated administration. Facial flushing may occur if the injection is given too rapidly.

Local—Severe cellulitis, vesication and tissue necrosis will occur if ADRIAMYCIN is extravasated during administration. Erythematous streaking along the vein proximal to the site of the injection has been reported (See Dosage and Administration).

Hypersensitivity—Fever, chills and urticaria have been reported occasionally. Anaphylaxis may occur. A case of apparent cross sensitivity to lincomycin has been reported.

Other—Conjunctivitis and lacrimation occur rarely.

OVERDOSAGE

Acute overdosage with ADRIAMYCIN enhances the toxic effects of mucositis, leukopenia and thrombopenia. Treatment of acute overdosage consists of treatment of the severely myelosuppressed patient with hospitalization, antibiotics, platelet and granulocyte transfusions and symptomatic treatment of mucositis. **The 150 mg is packaged as a multiple dose vial and caution should be exercised to prevent inadvertent overdosage.**

Chronic overdosage with cumulative doses exceeding 550 mg/m^2 increases the risk of cardiomyopathy and resultant congestive heart failure. Treatment consists of vigorous management of congestive heart failure with digitalis preparations and diuretics. The use of peripheral vasodilators has been recommended.

DOSAGE AND ADMINISTRATION

Care in the administration of ADRIAMYCIN will reduce the chance of perivenous infiltration. It may also decrease the chance of local reactions such as urticaria and erythematous streaking. On intravenous administration of ADRIAMYCIN, extravasation may occur with or without accompanying stinging or burning sensation and even if blood returns well on aspiration of the infusion needle. If any signs or symptoms of extravasation have occurred, the injection or infusion should be immediately terminated and restarted in another vein. If it is known or suspected that subcutaneous extravasation has occurred, local infiltration with an injectable corticosteroid and flooding the site with normal saline has been reported to lessen the local reaction. Because of the progressive nature of extravasation reactions, the area of injection should be frequently examined and plastic surgery consultation obtained. If ulceration begins, early wide excision of the involved area should be considered.[1]

The most commonly used dosage schedule is 60–75 mg/m^2 as a single intravenous injection administered at 21-day intervals. The lower dose should be given to patients with inadequate marrow reserves due to old age, or prior therapy, or neoplastic marrow infiltration. An alternative dose schedule is weekly doses of 20 mg/m^2 which has been reported to produce a lower incidence of congestive heart failure. Thirty mg/m^2 on each of three successive days repeated every 4 weeks has also been used. ADRIAMYCIN dosage must be reduced if the bilirubin is elevated as follows: Serum Bilirubin 1.2–3.0 mg/dL-give ½ normal dose, > 3 mg/dL–give ¼ normal dose.

Preparation of Solution: ADRIAMYCIN RDF 10 mg, 20 mg, 50 mg, and 150 mg vials should be reconstituted with 5 mL, 10 mL, 25 mL, and 75 mL respectively, of Sodium Chloride Injection, USP (0.9%) to give a final concentration of 2 mg/mL of doxorubicin hydrochloride. An appropriate volume of air should be withdrawn from the vial during reconstitution to avoid excessive pressure build-up. Bacteriostatic diluents are not recommended.

After adding the diluent, the vial should be shaken and the contents allowed to dissolve. The reconstituted solution is

stable for 7 days at room temperature and under normal room light (100 foot-candles) and 15 days under refrigeration (2°–8°C). It should be protected from exposure to sunlight. Discard any unused solution from the 10 mg, 20 mg and 50 mg single dose vials. Unused solutions of the multiple dose vial remaining beyond the recommended storage times should be discarded.

It is recommended that ADRIAMYCIN be slowly administered into the tubing of a freely running intravenous infusion of Sodium Chloride Injection, USP or 5% Dextrose Injection, USP. The tubing should be attached to a Butterfly® needle inserted preferably into a large vein. If possible, avoid veins over joints or in extremities with compromised venous or lymphatic drainage. The rate of administration is dependent on the size of the vein and the dosage. However, the dose should be administered in not less than 3 to 5 minutes. Local erythematous streaking along the vein as well as facial flushing may be indicative of too rapid an administration. A burning or stinging sensation may be indicative of perivenous infiltration and the infusion should be immediately terminated and restarted in another vein. Perivenous infiltration may occur painlessly.

ADRIAMYCIN should not be mixed with heparin or 5-fluorouracil since it has been reported that these drugs are incompatible to the extent that a precipitate may form. Until specific compatibility data are available, it is not recommended that ADRIAMYCIN be mixed with other drugs.

ADRIAMYCIN has been used concurrently with other approved chemotherapeutic agents. Evidence is available that in some types of neoplastic disease combination chemotherapy is superior to single agents. The benefits and risks of such therapy continue to be elucidated.

Handling and Disposal: Skin reactions associated with ADRIAMYCIN have been reported. Caution in handling and preparation of the powder and solution must be exercised and the use of gloves is recommended. If ADRIAMYCIN powder or solution contacts the skin or mucosae, immediately wash thoroughly with soap and water.

Procedures for proper handling and disposal of anti-cancer drugs should be considered. Several guidelines on this subject have been published.[2-7] There is no general agreement that all of the procedures recommended in the guidelines are necessary or appropriate.

HOW SUPPLIED

ADRIAMYCIN RDF™ (DOXORUBICIN HYDROCHLORIDE, USP) FOR INJECTION is available as follows:

10 mg—Each single dose vial contains 10 mg of doxorubicin HCl, USP, 50 mg of lactose, N.F. and 1 mg of methylparaben, N.F. (added to enhance dissolution) as a sterile red-orange lyophilized powder. Packaged and supplied in 10-vial packs NDC 0013-1086-91.

20 mg—Each single dose vial contains 20 mg of doxorubicin HCl, USP, 100 mg of lactose, N.F. and 2 mg of methylparaben, N.F. (added to enhance dissolution) as a sterile red-orange lyophilized powder. Packaged and supplied in 5-vial packs NDC 0013-1096-94.

50 mg—Each single dose vial contains 50 mg of doxorubicin HCl, USP, 250 mg of lactose, N.F. and 5 mg of methylparaben, N.F. (added to enhance dissolution) as a sterile red-orange lyophilized powder. Packaged and supplied in a single vial pack NDC 0013-1106-79.

Protect from exposure to sunlight and discard any unused solution.

150 mg—Each multi-dose vial contains 150 mg of doxorubicin HCl, USP, 750 mg of lactose, N.F. and 15 mg of methylparaben, N.F. (added to enhance dissolution) as a sterile red-orange lyophilized powder. Packaged and supplied in a single vial pack. NDC 0013-1116-83.

Protect from exposure to sunlight and discard any solution remaining beyond the recommended reconstitution storage times.

REFERENCES

1. Rudolph R et al: Skin Ulcers Due to ADRIAMYCIN. Cancer 38: 1087–1094, Sept. 1976.
2. Recommendations for the Safe Handling of Parenteral Antineoplastic Drugs. NIH Publication No. 83-2621. For sale by the Superintendent of Documents, U.S. Government Printing Office, Washington, D.C. 20402.
3. AMA Council Report. Guidelines for Handling Parenteral Antineoplastics. JAMA, March 15, 1985.
4. National Study Commission on Cytotoxic Exposure—Recommendations for Handling Cytotoxic Agents. Available from Louis P. Jeffrey, Sc. D., Director of Pharmacy Services, Rhode Island Hospital, 593 Eddy Street, Providence, Rhode Island 02902.
5. Clinical Oncological Society of Australia: Guidelines and recommendations for safe handling of antineoplastic agents. Med J Australia 1:426–428 1983.
6. Jones RB, et al. Safe handling of chemotherapeutic agents: A report from the Mount Sinai Medical Center. CA—A Cancer Journal for Clinicians Sept/Oct, 258–263 1983.

7. American Society of Hospital Pharmacists technical assistance bulletin on handling cytotoxic drugs in hospitals. Am J Hosp Pharm 42:131–137, 1985.

Distributed by:
ADRIA LABORATORIES
Division of Erbamont Inc.
COLUMBUS, OHIO 43215.
Manufactured by:
FARMITALIA CARLO ERBA S.p.A.,
MILAN, ITALY

AXOTAL® ℞
[ax 'ō-tall ''']
(Butalbital and Aspirin, Tablets, USP)

WARNING
May be habit forming.

DESCRIPTION
Each AXOTAL tablet for oral administration contains: butalbital, USP, 50 mg (Warning: May be habit forming) and aspirin, USP, 650 mg.
Butalbital, 5-allyl-5-isobutyl barbituric acid, a white odorless crystalline powder, is a short to intermediate-acting barbiturate. Its molecular formula is $C_{11}H_{16}N_2O_3$ and molecular weight 224.26.

ACTIONS
Pharmacologically, AXOTAL combines the analgesic properties of aspirin with the anxiolytic and muscle relaxant properties of butalbital.

INDICATIONS
AXOTAL is indicated for the relief of the symptom complex of tension (or muscle contraction) headaches.

CONTRAINDICATIONS
Hypersensitivity to aspirin or barbiturates. Patients with porphyria.

PRECAUTIONS
General —AXOTAL should be used with caution in patients with certain medical problems, including those with a history of asthma, allergies and nasal polyps. Also, the drug must be prescribed carefully for patients with hemophilia or other bleeding problems, peptic ulcer, renal impairment, or a history of drug abuse or dependence.
Information for patients —AXOTAL may impair the mental and/or physical abilities required for the performance of potentially hazardous tasks, such as driving a car or operating machinery. The patient should be cautioned accordingly.
Drug Interactions —Patients receiving narcotic analgesics, antipsychotics, antianxiety agents, or other CNS depressants (including alcohol) concomitantly with AXOTAL may exhibit additive CNS depressant effects. When combined therapy is contemplated, the dose of one or both agents should be reduced.

Drugs	Effect
Aspirin with anti-inflammatory agents	Increased ulcerogenic effects
Butalbital with coumarin anticoagulants	Decreased effect of anticoagulant because of increased metabolism resulting from enzyme induction.
Butalbital with tricyclic anti-depressants	Decreased blood levels of anti-depressant

Usage in Pregnancy —Adequate studies have not been performed in animals to determine whether this drug affects fertility in males or females, has teratogenic potential or has other adverse effects on the fetus. Although there is no clearly defined risk, experience cannot exclude the possibility of infrequent or subtle damage to the human fetus. AXOTAL should be used in pregnant women only when clearly needed.
Nursing Mothers —The effects of AXOTAL on infants of nursing mothers are not known. Salicylates and barbiturates are excreted in the breast milk of nursing mothers. The serum levels in infants are believed to be insignificant with therapeutic doses.
Pediatric Use —Safety and effectiveness in children below the age of 12 have not been established.

ADVERSE REACTIONS
The most frequent adverse reactions are drowsiness and dizziness. Less frequent adverse reactions are lightheadness and gastrointestinal disturbances including nausea, vomiting and flatulence. Mental confusion or depression can occur due to intolerance or overdosage of butalbital.

DRUG ABUSE AND DEPENDENCE
Prolonged use of barbiturates can produce drug dependence, characterized by psychic dependence, and less frequently, physical dependence, and tolerance. The abuse liability of AXOTAL is similar to that of other barbiturate-containing drug combinations. Caution should be exercised when prescribing medication for patients with a known propensity for taking excessive quantities of drugs which is not uncommon in patients with chronic tension headaches.

OVERDOSAGE
The toxic effects of acute overdosage of AXOTAL are attributable mainly to its barbiturate component and, to a lesser extent, aspirin. Symptoms attributable to acute *barbiturate poisoning* include drowsiness, confusion and coma, respiratory depression, hypertension and shock. Symptoms of *salicylate overdosage* include central nausea and vomiting, tinnitus and deafness, vertigo and headaches, mental dullness and confusion, diaphoresis, rapid pulse and increased respiration leading to respiratory alkalosis. Treatment consists primarily of management of barbiturate intoxication and the correction of acid-base imbalance due to salicylism. Vomiting should be induced mechanically or with emetics, such as ipecac syrup, in the conscious patient. Gastric lavage may be used if the pharyngeal and laryngeal reflexes are present and if less than 4 hours have elapsed since ingestion. A cuffed endotracheal tube should be inserted before gastric lavage of the unconscious patient and when necessary to provide assisted respiration. Gastric lavage followed by activated charcoal is recommended regardless of time since ingestion. Diuresis, alkalinization of the urine, and correction of electrolyte disturbances should be accomplished through administration of intravenous fluids such as 1% sodium bicarbonate in 5% dextrose in water. Meticulous attention should be given to maintaining adequate pulmonary ventilation. Exchange transfusion is most feasible for a small infant while intermittent peritoneal dialysis is useful for cases of moderate severity in adults. Hemodialysis with the artificial kidney is the most effective means of removing salicylate and is indicated for the very severe cases of salicylate intoxication. Hypoprothrombinemia should be treated with intravenous Vitamin K (phytonadione). Methemoglobinemia over 30% should be treated with methylene blue administered slowly intravenously.
In all cases of suspected overdose, immediately call your regional poison center for assistance.

DOSAGE AND ADMINISTRATION
One tablet every four hours as needed. Do not exceed 6 tablets per day.
Medication should be taken with food or a full glass of water or milk to lessen gastric irritation caused by aspirin.

HOW SUPPLIED
Each AXOTAL tablet contains butalbital USP, 50 mg, and aspirin 650 mg.
AXOTAL is available for oral administration as uncoated, white, capsule-shaped tablets coded ADRIA, 130.
Tablets are supplied as follows:
NDC 0013-1301-17 in bottles of 100
NDC 0013-1301-21 in bottles of 500
Store in a tight container below 30°C (86°F). Protect from moisture.

EMETROL®
[ĕm 'ĕ-trŏl]
(Phosphorated Carbohydrate Solution)

For the relief of nausea associated with upset stomach.

DESCRIPTION
EMETROL is an oral solution containing balanced amounts of dextrose (glucose) and levulose (fructose) and phosphoric acid with controlled hydrogen ion concentration. Available in pleasant tasting lemon-mint and cherry flavors.

INGREDIENTS
Each 5 mL teaspoonful contains dextrose (glucose), 1.87 g; levulose (fructose), 1.87 g; and phosphoric acid, 21.5 mg and the following inactive ingredients: D&C yellow No. 10 (lemon mint only) natural color (cherry only), flavors, glycerin, methylparaben and purified water.

ACTION
EMETROL quickly relieves nausea by local action on the wall of the hyperactive G.I. tract. It reduces smooth-muscle contraction in proportion to the amount used. Unlike systemic antinauseants, EMETROL works almost immediately to control nausea.

INDICATIONS
For the relief of nausea associated with upset stomach. For other conditions, take only as directed by your physician.

ADVANTAGES
1. **Fast Action**—works almost immediately by local action on contact with the hyperactive G.I. tract.
2. **Effectiveness**—reduces smooth-muscle contractions in proportion to the amount used—stops nausea.
3. **Safety**—non-toxic—won't mask symptoms of organic pathology.
4. **Convenience**—can be recommended over the phone for any member of the family, even the children—no ℞ required.
5. **Patient Acceptance**—a low cost that patients appreciate—pleasant lemon-mint flavor or cherry flavor that both children and adults like.

USUAL ADULT DOSE
One or two tablespoonsful. Repeat every 15 minutes until distress subsides.

USUAL CHILDREN'S DOSE
One or two teaspoonsful. Repeat dose every 15 minutes until distress subsides. See CAUTION

IMPORTANT
Never dilute EMETROL or drink fluids of any kind immediately before or after taking a dose.

CAUTION
Not to be taken for more than one hour (5 doses) without consulting a physician. If upset stomach continues or recurs frequently, consult a physician promptly as it may be a sign of a serious condition.

WARNINGS
KEEP THIS AND ALL MEDICATIONS OUT OF THE REACH OF CHILDREN. As with any drug, if your are pregnant or nursing a baby, seek the advice of a health professional before using this product.
This product contains fructose and should not be taken by persons with hereditary fructose intolerance (HFI).

> This product contains sugar and should not be taken by diabetics except under the advice and supervision of a physician.

In case of accidental overdose, contact a poison control center, emergency medical facility, or physician immediately for advice.

HOW SUPPLIED
Each 5 mL teaspoonful of EMETROL contains dextrose (glucose), 1.87 g; levulose (fructose), 1.87 g; and phosphoric acid, 21.5 mg in lemon-mint or cherry syrups.
Lemon-Mint
NDC 0013-2113-45 Bottle of 4 fluid ounces (118 mL)
NDC 0013-2113-65 Bottle of 8 fluid ounces (236 mL)
NDC 0013-2113-51 Bottle of 1 pint (473 mL)
Cherry
NDC 0013-2114-45 Bottle of 4 fluid ounces (118 mL)
NDC 0013-2114-65 Bottle of 8 fluid ounces (236 mL)
NDC 0013-2114-51 Bottle of 1 pint (473 mL)
Store at room temperature.

NOTICE
Each bottle is protected by a printed band around the cap. Do not use if band is damaged or missing.
ADRIA LABORATORIES
Division of Erbamont Inc.
COLUMBUS, OHIO 43215
Shown in Product Identification Section, page 404

EVAC-Q-KIT®
[ē-vak 'cue-kit]

DESCRIPTION
Each EVAC-Q-KIT® contains:
1. EVAC-Q-MAG®—10 fl. oz. Sugar-Free. Ingredients: Magnesium citrate, citric acid and potassium citrate in cherry flavored base. Carbonated.
2. EVAC-Q-TABS® — 2 tablets. Ingredients: Each tablet contains 2 grains (130 mg) of phenolphthalein.
3. EVAC-Q-SERT®—2 suppositories. Ingredients: Potassium bitartrate and sodium bicarbonate in polyethylene glycol base.
4. 1 Instruction Sheet (In English and Spanish)

ACTIONS
Bowel Evacuant.

INDICATIONS
EVAC-Q-KIT is indicated for use as a bowel evacuant system in the preparation of the colon for single or multiple radiologic examinations or surgery and endoscopic procedures.

CONTRAINDICATIONS
EVAC-Q-MAG is contraindicated in the presence of severe renal insufficiency.

WARNINGS
Do not use any of these preparations when abdominal pain, nausea, or vomiting are present. Frequent and continued use may cause dependence upon laxatives. Rectal bleeding or failure to respond may indicate a serious condition. Consult physician. As with any drug, if you are pregnant or nursing a

Continued on next page

Adria—Cont.

baby, seek the advice of a health professional before using this product. KEEP OUT OF REACH OF CHILDREN.

PRECAUTIONS
If skin rash appears, do not use this or any other preparation containing phenolphthalein.

DOSAGE AND ADMINISTRATION
Instructions for Patients—early schedule* Your physician is preparing you for an X-ray examination that requires thorough clearing of the intestinal tract. He is using this EVAC-Q-KIT® routine to make this procedure more comfortable for you.
BE SURE TO FOLLOW EACH STEP AND COMPLETE ALL INSTRUCTIONS OR ENTIRE X-RAY EXAMINATION MAY HAVE TO BE REPEATED.

DAY BEFORE EXAMINATION
IMPORTANT: A high fluid intake is essential to the success of this regimen. You MUST take a large glass (8 oz.) of fluid at specified times.

(= 8 oz. fluid.) Drink only black coffee, plain tea, strained fruit juice, soft drinks or water at the times indicated. NO MILK OR CREAM.

☐ **Noon.** Light lunch. Clear soup, two hardboiled eggs, plain Jell-O, fluid.
☐ **12:30 P.M.** (or ½ hr. after lunch) Drink entire contents—EVAC-Q-MAG® (#1 in your kit), over ice.
☐ **1:00 P.M.** +
☐ **3:00 P.M.** Take two (2) EVAC-Q-TABS® laxative tablets (#2 in your kit) with large glass of water.
☐ **4:00 P.M.** +
☐ **5:00 P.M.** Liquid dinner. Clear Soup, plain Jell-O +
☐ **6:00 P.M.** +
☐ **9:00 P.M.** +
☐ **10:00 P.M.** Remove cover from EVAC-Q-SERT® suppository (#3 in your kit). Moisten the suppository in tap water. Insert suppository into rectum. Wait at least 10–15 minutes before evacuating, even if urge is strong.
☐ **BEDTIME:** + .
☐ **DAY OF TEST.** No breakfast.
☐ **6:00 A.M.** (must be at least 2 hours before test). Use remaining EVAC-Q-SERT® suppository (#4 in your kit). Follow same directions as 10:00 P.M. night before.
BE SURE TO DRINK ALL THE FLUID SPECIFIED.
NOTE: This product information is for professional use only.

HOW SUPPLIED
Each EVAC-Q-KIT NDC 0013-2199-76 contains:
1. One 10 fl. oz. EVAC-Q-MAG
2. Two tablets—EVAC-Q-TABS
3. Two suppositories—EVAC-Q-SERT
4. 1 Instruction Sheet
Shipping Unit: 12 EVAC-Q-KIT units per carton.

*Late schedule also available. See Instruction Sheet in EVAC-Q-KIT. (Instruction sheet printed in both English and Spanish.)
EVAC-Q-MAG
Manufactured by:
CumberLand-Swan Inc.
Smyrna, Tennessee 37167
EVAC-Q-KWIK SUPPOSITORY
Manufactured by:
G & W LABORATORIES, INC.
SOUTH PLAINFIELD, NJ 07050
Distributed by:
ADRIA LABORATORIES
Division of Erbamont Inc.
COLUMBUS, OHIO 43215

EVAC-Q-KWIK®
[ē-vak 'cue-kwik]
Bowel Evacuant System

DESCRIPTION
EVAC-Q-KWIK is a bowel evacuant system comprised of three separate products that are intended to be administered sequentially at intervals intended to minimize the overlap of pharmacological activity. These three products are augmented by the sequential administration of liquids in a manner to promote the flushing of the G.I. tract. Together, the products and the liquids comprise the bowel evacuant system.
1. EVAC-Q-MAG®—Each bottle contains 10 fl. oz., magnesium citrate oral solution, USP, in a cherry flavored, sugar-free, carbonated base. It contains sodium 0.84 mEq, potassium 2.1 mEq, magnesium 254 mEq ml/bottle and 66.7 calories.
2. EVAC-Q-TABS®—2 tablets. Each tablet contains phenolphthalein 130 mg.
3. EVAC-Q-KWIK® SUPPOSITORY—bisacodyl 10 mg.
4. Illustrated bilingual instruction sheet.
Magnesium citrate is a saline laxative and has a mild purgative action. It is chemically 2-hydroxy-1,2,3-propanetricarboxylic acid, magnesium salt.
Magnesium citrate occurs as white crystalline powder or granules, slightly soluble in water, soluble in dilute acids. Its molecular weight citrate is 451.12.
Phenolphthalein, a contact laxative, is a diphenylmethane derivative. It is chemically 3,3-bis(4-hydroxyphenyl)-1(3H)-isobenzofuranone.
It occurs as a white, or yellowish-white, crystalline powder and is practically insoluble in water, soluble in alcohol and dilute alkali solutions. Its molecular weight is 318.33.
Bisacodyl, a contact laxative, is also a diphenylmethane derivative. It is chemically 4,4'-(2-pyridylmethylene) diphenol diacetate.
Bisacodyl occurs as a white or off-white crystalline powder, practically insoluble in water, sparingly soluble in alcohol and soluble in chloroform. Its molecular weight is 361.40.

CLINICAL PHARMACOLOGY
Magnesium citrate is a saline laxative. It acts mainly on the small intestine by drawing water into the gut thus increasing intraluminal pressure and intestinal motility, resulting in evacuation of the bowel usually in 3–6 hours or less. Substantial fluid intake is required for this purpose. Approximately 15–30% of the magnesium present in its salts may be absorbed. The magnesium and potassium ions are excreted primarily by the kidney and may accumulate in patients with impaired renal function, in the newborn and in the elderly.
Phenolphthalein, a contact laxative, acts primarily on the large intestine to produce a semifluid stool usually in 4–8 hours. It is dissolved by bile salts and alkaline intestinal secretions and may impart a red color to alkaline feces and urine. Up to 15% of the dose may be absorbed and excreted mainly by the kidney in the conjugated glucuronide form.
Bisacodyl is also a contact laxative which acts on the large intestine to produce brief and strong peristaltic movements resulting in evacuation usually within 15–60 minutes after rectal administration. It is minimally (about 5%) absorbed and excreted mainly in the feces and partly in the urine as the glucuronide.

INDICATIONS AND USAGE
EVAC-Q-KWIK is indicated for use as a bowel evacuant system in the preparation of the colon for single or multiple radiologic examinations or surgery and endoscopic procedures.

CONTRAINDICATIONS
The EVAC-Q-MAG component is contraindicated in patients with severe renal insufficiency.

WARNINGS
Do not use any laxative preparations when abdominal pain, nausea or vomiting are present. Frequent and continued use may cause dependence upon laxatives. Rectal bleeding or failure to respond may indicate a serious underlying condition and require a physician's consultation. KEEP THIS PRODUCT OUT OF REACH OF CHILDREN.
As with any drug, if the patient is pregnant or nursing a baby, she should consult a health professional before using. (See Precautions: Pregnancy, Nursing Mothers.)

PRECAUTIONS
General—If skin rash appears, do not use EVAC-Q-TABS or any other preparation containing phenolphthalein. The EVAC-Q-KWIK SUPPOSITORY should be used with caution in patients with rectal fissures or ulcerated hemorrhoids.
Phenolphthalein, the active ingredient of EVAC-Q-TABS, may color alkaline feces and urine red.
Laboratory Test Interactions—Phenolphthalein in EVAC-Q-TABS may interfere with the ACETEST® and KETOS-TIX® urine tests for ketones to produce a pink color. It may also give false-positive test results for urinary urobilinogen and for estrogens measured by the Kober procedure.
Carcinogenesis, Mutagenesis, Impairment of Fertility—There have been no studies in animals or humans to evaluate the carcinogenesis, mutagenesis or impairment of fertility potential of the EVAC-Q-KWIK.
Pregnancy—Category C. Animal reproduction studies have not been conducted with any of the components of EVAC-Q-KWIK. It is also not known whether the EVAC-Q-KWIK can cause fetal harm when administered to a pregnant woman or can affect reproduction capacity. EVAC-Q-KWIK should be given to a pregnant woman only if clearly needed.
Nursing Mothers—Small amounts of magnesium are excreted in the milk and saliva. Phenolphthalein and bisacodyl are also excreted in human milk. Therefore, caution should be exercised when EVAC-Q-KWIK is administered to a nursing woman.
Pediatric Use—Safety and effectiveness in children below the age of 12 has not been established.

ADVERSE REACTIONS
Excessive bowel activity, usually diarrhea or abdominal discomfort, nausea, vomiting, cramps, weakness, dizziness, palpitations, sweating and fainting may follow the administration of an evacuant. Diarrhea may lead to fluid and electrolyte deficits. Allergic reactions, mainly skin rashes attributed to phenolphthalein, have been reported. Bisacodyl in the EVAC-Q-KWIK SUPPOSITORY may cause irritation or a sensation of burning of the rectal mucosa.

OVERDOSAGE
Accidental or intentional overdosage may lead to severe diarrhea and excessive loss of body fluids and electrolytes, muscle weakness and tremor, gastrointestinal disturbances and fainting. Depressed deep tendon reflexes, sedation, EKG changes or heart block and respiratory paralysis may occur with high plasma magnesium levels.
The excretion of magnesium may be increased by the administration of a diuretic. Only small amounts of phenolphthalein or bisacodyl are absorbed. If ingestion is recent or food is present in the stomach, induction of emesis with ipecac syrup, gastric emptying and lavage and introduction of activated charcoal may be recommended. Fluid and electrolyte administration is also recommended to correct dehydration and electrolyte imbalance.

DOSAGE AND ADMINISTRATION
A high fluid intake and a low residue diet are essential for a successful colon preparation. Recommended liquids are black coffee, plain tea, strained fruit juice, soft drinks or water and use NO MILK OR CREAM. The directions provided in the Instruction Sheet and the following schedule should be adhered to closely.

TIME SCHEDULE
NOON	Light lunch: clear soup, plain gelatin, fluid.
4:00 P.M.	Drink entire contents of EVAC-Q-MAG (#1 in the kit), over ice.
5:00 P.M.	8 oz. of fluid.
6:00 P.M.	Liquid dinner. Clear soup, plain gelatin, 8 oz. of fluid.
7:00 P.M.	Take two (2) EVAC-Q-TABS laxative tablets (#2 in the kit) with a large glass of water.
8:00 P.M.	8 oz. of fluid.
9:00 P.M.	8 oz. of fluid.
10:00 P.M.	Insert one EVAC-Q-KWIK SUPPOSITORY (#3 in the kit) into rectum as far as possible, retain as long as comfort will permit—usually 10–15 minutes—before defecating. Nothing by mouth, after 10:00 P.M. until x-ray examination. Prescription medications can be taken as scheduled with a glass of water.

DRINK ALL THE FLUID SPECIFIED.

ALTERNATE SCHEDULE
(For patients admitted in the afternoon on the day before examination.)
6:00 P.M.	Liquid dinner. Clear soup, plain gelatin, 8 oz. of fluid.
7:00 P.M.	Drink entire contents of EVAC-Q-MAG (#1 in the kit), over ice.
8:00 P.M.	8 oz. of fluid.
9:00 P.M.	8 oz. of fluid.
10:00 P.M.	Take two (2) EVAC-Q-TABS laxative tablets (#2 in the kit) with a large glass of water. Nothing by mouth, after 10:00 p.m. until x-ray examination. Prescription medications can be taken as scheduled with a glass of water.
6:00 A.M.	Insert one EVAC-Q-KWIK SUPPOSITORY (#3 in the kit) into rectum as far as possible, retain as long as comfort will permit—usually 10–15 minutes—before defecating.

DRINK ALL THE FLUID SPECIFIED.
See also: Illustrated Multilingual Instruction Sheet.
NOTE: This product information is for professional use only.

HOW SUPPLIED
Each EVAC-Q-KWIK, NDC 0013-2189-76 contains:
1. One 10 fl. oz. EVAC-Q-MAG
2. Two tablets EVAC-Q-TABS
3. One EVAC-Q-KWIK SUPPOSITORY
4. Instruction Sheet.
Store at controlled room temperature (15–30°C, 59–86°F).
Avoid freezing.

EVAC-Q-MAG
Manufactured by:
CumberLand-Swan Inc.
Smyrna, Tennessee 37167
EVAC-Q-KWIK SUPPOSITORY
Manufactured by:
G & W LABORATORIES, INC.
SOUTH PLAINFIELD, NJ 07050
Distributed by:
ADRIA LABORATORIES
Division of Erbamont Inc.
COLUMBUS, OHIO 43215

ILOPAN® INJECTION   ℞
[ĭ′lō-pan]
(dexpanthenol)
DESCRIPTION
ILOPAN® INJECTION (dexpanthenol) is a derivative of
pantothenic acid, a member of the B complex of vitamins.
ILOPAN INJECTION is a sterile aqueous solution indicated
for use as a gastrointestinal stimulant. The chemical name is
D-(+)-2,   4-dihydroxy-N-(3-hydroxypropyl)-3,3-dimethyl-
butyramide.
Each ml contains dexpanthenol 250 mg in distilled water for
injection.

CLINICAL PHARMACOLOGY
Pantothenic acid is a precursor of coenzyme A, which serves
as a cofactor for a variety of enzyme-catalyzed reactions involving transfer of acetyl groups. The final step in the synthesis of acetylcholine consists of the choline acetylase transfer of an acetyl group from acetylcoenzyme A to choline. Acetylcholine is the neurohumoral transmitter in the parasympathetic system and as such maintains the normal functions
of the intestine. Decrease in acetylcholine content would
result in decreased peristalsis and in extreme cases adynamic ileus. The pharmacological mode of action of the drug
is unknown. Pharmacokinetic data in humans are unavailable.

INDICATIONS AND USAGE
Prophylactic use immediately after major abdominal surgery to minimize the possibility of paralytic ileus. Intestinal
atony causing abdominal distention; postoperative or postpartum retention of flatus, or postoperative delay in resumption of intestinal motility; paralytic ileus.

CONTRAINDICATIONS
There are no known contraindications to the use of ILOPAN
INJECTION.

WARNINGS
There have been rare instances of allergic reactions of unknown cause during the concomitant use of ILOPAN INJEC-
TION with drugs such as antibiotics, narcotics and barbiturates.
Administration of ILOPAN INJECTION directly into the
vein is not advised (See Dosage and Administration).
ILOPAN INJECTION should not be administered within
one hour of succinylcholine.

PRECAUTIONS
General —If any signs of a hypersensitivity reaction appear,
ILOPAN INJECTION should be discontinued. If ileus is a
secondary consequence of mechanical obstruction, primary
attention should be directed to the obstruction.
The management of adynamic ileus includes the correction
of any fluid and electrolyte imbalance (especially hypokalemia), anemia and hypoproteinemia, treatment of infection,
avoidance where possible of drugs which are known to decrease gastrointestinal motility and decompression of the
gastrointestinal tract when considerably distended by
nasogastric suction or use of a long intestinal tube.
Drug Interactions —The effects of succinylcholine appeared
to have been prolonged in a woman administered dexpanthenol.
Carcinogenicity, Mutagenicity, and Impairment of Fertility —
There have been no studies in animals to evaluate the carcinogenic, mutagenic, or impairment of fertility potential of
dexpanthenol.
Pregnancy —Category C. Animal reproduction studies have
not been conducted with ILOPAN INJECTION. It is also not
known whether ILOPAN INJECTION can cause fetal harm
when administered to a pregnant woman or can affect reproduction capacity. ILOPAN INJECTION should be given to a
pregnant woman only if clearly needed.
Nursing Mothers —It is not known whether this drug is excreted in human milk. Because many drugs are excreted in
human milk, caution should be exercised when ILOPAN
INJECTION is administered to a nursing woman.
Pediatric Use —Safety and effectiveness in children have not
been established.

ADVERSE REACTIONS
There have been a few reports of allergic reactions and single
reports of several other adverse events in association with
the administration of dexpanthenol. A causal relationship is

uncertain. One patient experienced itching, tingling, difficulty in breathing. Another patient had red patches of skin.
Two patients had generalized dermatitis and one patient
urticaria.
One patient experienced temporary respiratory difficulty
following administration of ILOPAN INJECTION 5 minutes
after succinylcholine was discontinued.
One patient experienced a noticeable but slight drop in blood
pressure after administration of dexpanthenol while in the
recovery room.
One patient experienced intestinal colic one-half hour after
the drug was administered.
Two patients vomited following administration and two patients had diarrhea 10 days post-surgery and after ILOPAN
INJECTION.
One elderly patient became agitated after administration of
the drug.

DOSAGE AND ADMINISTRATION
Prevention of post-operative adynamic ileus: 250 mg (1 mL)
or 500 mg (2 mL) intramuscularly. Repeat in 2 hours and
then every 6 hours until all danger of adynamic ileus has
passed.
Treatment of adynamic ileus: 500 mg (2 mL) intramuscularly. Repeat in 2 hours and then every 6 hours as needed.
Intravenous administration: ILOPAN INJECTION 2 mL
(500 mg) may be mixed with bulk I.V. solutions such as glucose or Lactated-Ringer's and slowly infused intravenously.
Parenteral drug products should be inspected visually for
particulate matter and discoloration prior to administration,
whenever solution and container permit.

HOW SUPPLIED
Each milliliter of ILOPAN INJECTION contains dexpan-
thenol, 250 mg in Water for Injection. Syringe contains not
more than 0.5% chlorobutanol. ILOPAN INJECTION is
available as follows:
ILOPAN INJECTION
    NDC 0013-2356-95 2 mL Ampuls, Box of 25
ILOPAN INJECTION STAT-PAK® (unit dose)
    NDC 0013-2366-95 Disposable Syringe 2 mL, Box of 25
Mfd. by:
TAYLOR PHARMACAL CO.
DECATUR, ILLINOIS 62525
For:
ADRIA LABORATORIES
Division of Erbamont Inc.
COLUMBUS, OHIO 43215

KAOCHLOR® S–F   ℞
[ka′ō-kloor s-f]
(Potassium Chloride)
10% Liquid
Sugar-Free
KAOCHLOR®   ℞
[ka′ō-kloor]
(Potassium Chloride)
10% Liquid
Contains Sugar
KAON–CL 20%®   ℞
[kā′ŏn-see-el″20%]
(Potassium Chloride)
Sugar-Free

DESCRIPTION
Each 15 ml (tablespoonful) of **KAOCHLOR S-F 10% Liquid**
supplies 20 mEq each of potassium and chloride (as potassium chloride, 1.5g) with saccharin, flavoring, and alcohol
5%. The chemical name of the drug is potassium chloride.
Each 15 ml (tablespoonful) of **KAOCHLOR 10% Liquid**
supplies 20 mEq each of potassium and chloride (as potassium chloride, 1.5 g) with sugar, saccharin, flavoring, and
alcohol 5%. Contains FD&C Yellow No. 5 (tartrazine) as a
color additive. The chemical name of the drug is potassium
chloride.
Each 15 ml (tablespoonful) of **KAON-CL 20%** supplies 40
mEq each of potassium and chloride (as potassium chloride,
3g) with saccharin, flavoring, and alcohol 5%. The chemical
name of the drug is potassium chloride.

CLINICAL PHARMACOLOGY
Potassium ion is the principal intracellular cation of most
body tissues. Potassium ions participate in a number of essential physiological processes including the maintenance of
intracellular tonicity, the transmission of nerve impulses,
the contraction of cardiac, skeletal and smooth muscle and
the maintenance of normal renal function.
Potassium depletion may occur whenever the rate of potassium loss through renal exceretion and/or loss from the gastrointestinal tract exceeds the rate of potassium intake.
Such depletion usually develops slowly as a consequence of
prolonged therapy with oral diuretics, primary or secondary
hyperaldosteronism, diabetic ketoacidosis, or inadequate
replacement of potassium in patients on prolonged parenteral nutrition. Such depletion can develop rapidly with se-

vere diarrhea, especially if associated with vomiting. Potassium depletion due to these causes is usually accompanied by
a concomitant loss of chloride and is manifested by hypokalemia and metabolic alkalosis. Potassium depletion may produce weakness, fatigue, disturbances of cardiac rhythm (primarily ectopic beats), prominent U-waves in the electrocardiogram, and in advanced cases, flaccid paralysis and/or
impaired ability to concentrate urine.
Potassium depletion associated with metabolic alkalosis is
managed by correcting the fundamental cause of the deficiency whenever possible and administering supplemental
potassium chloride, in the form of high potassium food or
potassium chloride solution or tablets.
In rare circumstances (e.g., patients with renal tubular acidosis) potassium depletion may be associated with metabolic
acidosis and hyperchloremia. In such patients potassium
replacement should be accomplished with potassium salts
other than the chloride, such as potassium bicarbonate, potassium citrate, potassium acetate, or potassium gluconate.

INDICATIONS AND USAGE
1. For therapeutic use in patients with hypokalemia with or
   without metabolic alkalosis, in digitalis intoxication and
   in patients with hypokalemic familial periodic paralysis.
2. For the prevention of potassium depletion when the dietary intake is inadequate in the following conditions:
   Patients receiving digitalis and diuretics for congestive
   heart failure, hepatic cirrhosis with ascites, states of aldosterone excess with normal renal function, potassium-
   losing nephropathy, and with certain diarrheal states.
3. The use of potassium salts in patients receiving diuretics
   for uncomplicated essential hypertension is often unnecessary when such patients have a normal dietary pattern.
   Serum potassium should be checked periodically, and if
   hypokalemia occurs, dietary supplementation with potassium-containing foods may be adequate to control milder
   cases. In more severe cases supplementation with potassium salts may be indicated.

CONTRAINDICATIONS
Potassium supplements are contraindicated in patients with
hyperkalemia since a further increase in serum potassium
concentration in such patients can produce cardiac arrest.
Hyperkalemia may complicate any of the following conditions: Chronic renal failure, systemic acidosis such as diabetic acidosis, acute dehydration, extensive tissue breakdown as in severe burns, adrenal insufficiency, or the administration of a potassium-sparing diuretic (e.g., spironolactone, triamterene, amiloride).

WARNINGS
**Do not administer full strength. KAOCHLOR S-F, KAO-
CHLOR 10% LIQUID OR KAON CL 20% will cause gastrointestinal irritation if administered undiluted. For details regarding adequate dilution, see Dosage and Administration.**
Hyperkalemia —In patients with impaired mechanisms for
excreting potassium, the administration of potassium salts
can produce hyperkalemia and cardiac arrest. This occurs
most commonly in patients given potassium by the intravenous route but may also occur in patients given potassium
orally. Potentially fatal hyperkalemia can develop and be
asymptomatic. The use of potassium salts in patients with
chronic renal disease, or any other condition which impairs
potassium excretion, requires particularly careful monitoring of the serum potassium concentration and appropriate
dosage adjustment.
Interaction with Potassium Sparing Diuretics
—Hypokalemia should not be treated by the concomitant
administration of potassium salts and a potassium-sparing
diuretic (e.g., spironolactone, triamterene, amiloride) since
the simultaneous administration of these agents can produce
severe hyperkalemia.
Metabolic Acidosis —Hypokalemia in patients with metabolic acidosis should be treated with an alkalinizing potassium salt such as potassium bicarbonate, potassium citrate,
potassium acetate or potassium gluconate.

PRECAUTIONS
General —The diagnosis of potassium depletion is ordinarily
made by demonstrating hypokalemia in a patient with a
clinical history suggesting some cause for potassium depletion.

KAOCHLOR 10% LIQUID contains FD&C Yellow No. 5
(tartrazine) which may cause allergic-type reactions (including bronchial asthma) in certain susceptible individuals.
Although the overall incidence of FD&C Yellow No. 5 (tartrazine) sensitivity in the general population is low, it is frequently seen in patients who also have aspirin hypersensitivity.
Laboratory Tests —In interpreting the serum potassium
level, the physician should bear in mind that acute alkalosis
per se can produce hypokalemia in the absence of a deficit in
total body potassium while acute acidosis *per se* can increase
the serum potassium concentration into the normal range
even in the presence of a reduced total body potassium. The

Continued on next page

Adria—Cont.

treatment of potassium depletion, particularly in the presence of cardiac disease, renal disease, or acidosis, requires careful attention to acid-base balance and appropriate monitoring of serum electrolytes, the electrocardiogram, and the clinical status of the patient.

It is important to recognize that hyperkalemia is usually asymptomatic and may be manifested only by an increased serum potassium concentration and characteristic electrocardiographic changes (peaking of T-waves, loss of P-wave, depression of S-T segment, and prolongation of the QT interval). (See Contraindications, Warnings and Overdosage.)

The use of potassium salts in patients with chronic renal disease, or any other condition which impairs potassium excretion, requires particularly careful monitoring of the serum potassium concentration and appropriate dosage adjustment.

When blood is drawn for analysis of plasma potassium levels, it is important to recognize that artifactual elevations do occur after repeated fist clenching to make veins more prominent during application of a tourniquet.

Carcinogenesis, Mutagenesis, Impairment of Fertility—There have been no studies in animals or humans to evaluate the carcinogenesis, mutagenesis or impairment of fertility for potassium.

Pregnancy—Category C. Animal reproduction studies have not been conducted with **KAOCHLOR S-F, KAOCHLOR 10% LIQUID OR KAON CL 20%**. It is also not known whether **KAOCHLOR S-F, KAOCHLOR 10% LIQUID OR KAON CL 20%** can cause fetal harm when administered to a pregnant woman or can affect reproduction capacity. **KAOCHLOR S-F, KAOCHLOR 10% LIQUID OR KAON CL 20%** should be given to a pregnant woman only if clearly needed.

Nursing Mothers—It is not known whether this drug is excreted in human milk. Because many drugs are excreted in human milk, caution should be exercised when **KAOCHLOR S-F, KAOCHLOR 10% LIQUID OR KAON CL 20%** is administered to a nursing woman.

Pediatric Use—Safety and effectiveness in children have not been established.

ADVERSE REACTIONS

The most severe adverse effect is hyperkalemia (see Contraindications, Warnings and Overdosage).

The most common adverse reactions to oral potassium salts are nausea, vomiting, abdominal discomfort, and diarrhea. These symptoms are due to irritation of the gastrointestinal tract and are best managed by diluting the preparation further, taking the dose with meals, or reducing the dose.

OVERDOSAGE

The administration of oral potassium to persons with normal excretory mechanisms for potassium rarely causes serious hyperkalemia. However, if excretory mechanisms are impaired or if potassium is administered too rapidly intravenously, potentially fatal hyperkalemia can result (see Contraindications and Warnings). It is important to recognize that hyperkalemia is usually asymptomatic and may be manifested only by an increased serum potassium concentration and characteristic electrocardiographic changes (peaking of T-waves, loss of P-wave, depression of S-T segment, and prolongation of the QT interval). Late manifestations include muscle-paralysis and cardiovascular collapse from cardiac arrest.

Treatment for hyperkalemia includes the following:
1. Elimination of foods and medications containing potassium and potassium-sparing diuretics.
2. Intravenous administration of 300 to 500 ml/hr of 10% dextrose solution containing 10–20 units of crystalline insulin per 1,000 ml.
3. Correction of acidosis, if present, with intravenous sodium bicarbondate.
4. Use of exchange resins, hemodialysis, or peritoneal dialysis.

In treating hyperkalemia, it should be recalled that in patients who have been stabilized on digitalis, too rapid a lowering of the serum potassium concentration can produce digitalis toxicity.

DOSAGE AND ADMINISTRATION

The usual dietary intake of potassium by the average adult is 40 to 80 mEq per day. Potassium depletion sufficient to cause hypokalemia usually requires the loss of 200 or more mEq of potassium from the total body store.

Dosage must be adjusted to the individual needs of each patient but is typically in the range of 20 mEq per day for the prevention of hypokalemia to 40–100 mEq per day or more for the treatment of potassium depletion.

To minimize gastrointestinal irritation, patients must follow directions regarding dilution. Each tablespoonful (15 ml) of **Kaochlor S-F or Kaochlor 10% Liquid** should be diluted with three (3) fluid ounces or more of water or other liquid. Each tablespoonful (15 ml) of **Kaon Cl 20%** should be diluted with six (6) fluid ounces or more of water or other liquid.

One (1) tablespoonful of KAON-CL 20% or two (2) tablespoonsful of **Kaochlor S-F or Kaochlor 10% Liquid** twice daily supplies 40 mEq of potassium. Deviations from this recommendation may be indicated, since no average total daily dose can be defined but must be governed by close observation for clinical effects. However, potassium intoxication may result from any therapeutic dosage. See "Overdosage" and "Precautions".

HOW SUPPLIED

KAOCHLOR S-F 10% LIQUID supplies 20 mEq each of potassium and chloride per tablespoonful (15 ml).
KAOCHLOR S-F 10% LIQUID is supplied in bottles of four (4) fl. oz. (NDC 0013-3093-56), pints (NDC 0013-3093-51).
KAOCHLOR 10% LIQUID supplies 20 mEq each of potassium and chloride per tablespoonful (15 ml).
KAOCHLOR 10% LIQUID is supplied in bottles of pints (NDC 0013-3103-51).
KAON-CL 20% supplies 40 mEq each of potassium and chloride per tablespoonful (15 ml).
NDC 0013-3113-51 Pint
Storage Conditions—Preserve in tight, light resistant containers. Store at room temperature and protect from cold.

KAON® ELIXIR   ℞
[kā'ŏn]
(Potassium Gluconate)
Grape Flavor
Sugar–Free

DESCRIPTION

Each 15 ml (tablespoonful) supplies 20 mEq of potassium (as potassium gluconate, 4.68 g) with saccharin and aromatics and alcohol 5%. The chemical name of the drug is gluconic acid potassium salt.

CLINICAL PHARMACOLOGY

Potassium ion is the principal intracellular cation of most body tissues. Potassium ions participate in a number of essential physiological processes including the maintenance of intracellular tonicity, the transmission of nerve impulses, the contraction of cardiac, skeletal and smooth muscle and the maintenance of normal renal function.

Potassium depletion may occur whenever the rate of potassium loss through renal excretion and/or loss from the gastrointestinal tract exceeds the rate of potassium intake. Potassium depletion sufficient to cause hypokalemia usually requires the loss of 200 or more mEq of potassium from the total body store. Such depletion usually develops slowly as a consequence of prolonged therapy with oral diuretics, primary or secondary hyperaldosteronism, diabetic ketoacidosis, or inadequate replacement of potassium in patients on prolonged parenteral nutrition. Such depletion can develop rapidly with severe diarrhea, especially if associated with vomiting. Potassium depletion may produce weakness, fatigue, disturbances of cardiac rhythm (primarily ectopic beats), prominent U-waves in the electrocardiogram, and in advanced cases, flaccid paralysis and/or impaired ability to concentrate urine.

INDICATIONS AND USAGE

1. For therapeutic use in patients with hypokalemia with or without metabolic alkalosis, in digitalis intoxication and in patients with hypokalemic familial periodic paralysis.
2. For the prevention of potassium depletion when the dietary intake is inadequate in the following conditions: Patients receiving digitalis and diuretics for congestive heart failure; hepatic cirrhosis with ascites, states of aldosterone excess with normal renal function, potassium-losing nephropathy, and with certain diarrheal states.
3. The use of potassium salts in patients receiving diuretics for uncomplicated essential hypertension is often unnecessary when such patients have a normal dietary pattern. Serum potassium should be checked periodically, however, and if hypokalemia occurs, dietary supplementation with potassium-containing foods may be adequate to control milder cases. In more severe cases supplementation with potassium salts may be indicated.
4. Hypokalemia in patients with metabolic acidosis should be treated with an alkalinizing potassium salt such as potassium gluconate.

CONTRAINDICATIONS

Potassium supplements are contraindicated in patients with hyperkalemia since a further increase in serum potassium concentration in such patients can produce cardiac arrest. Hyperkalemia may complicate any of the following conditions: Chronic renal failure, systemic acidosis such as diabetic acidosis, acute dehydration, extensive tissue breakdown as in severe burns, adrenal insufficiency, or the administration of a potassium-sparing diuretic (e.g., spironolactone, triamterene, amiloride).

WARNINGS

Do not administer full strength. KAON ELIXIR may cause gastrointestinal irritation if administered undiluted. For

details regarding adequate dilution, see Dosage and Administration.

Hyperkalemia—In patients with impaired mechanisms for excreting potassium, the administration of potassium salts can produce hyperkalemia and cardiac arrest. This occurs most commonly in patients given potassium by the intravenous route but may also occur in patients given potassium orally. Potentially fatal hyperkalemia can develop rapidly and be asymptomatic. The use of potassium salts in patients with chronic renal disease, or any other condition which impairs potassium excretion, requires particularly careful monitoring of the serum potassium concentration and appropriate dosage adjustment.

Interaction with Potassium Sparing Diuretics—Hypokalemia should not be treated by the concomitant administration of potassium salts and a potassium-sparing diuretic (e.g., spironolactone, triamterene, amiloride) since the simultaneous administration of these agents can produce severe hyperkalemia.

PRECAUTIONS

General—The diagnosis of potassium depletion is ordinarily made by demonstrating hypokalemia in a patient with a clinical history suggesting some cause for potassium depletion.

In hypokalemic states, especially in patients on a low-salt diet, hypochloremic alkalosis is a possibility that may require chloride as well as potassium supplementation. In these circumstances, potassium replacement with potassium chloride may be more advantageous than with other potassium salts.

However, KAON ELIXIR can be supplemented with chloride. Ammonium chloride is an excellent source of chloride ion (18.7 mEq per gram) but it should not be used in patients with hepatic cirrhosis where ammonium salts are contraindicated.

Laboratory Tests—In interpreting the serum potassium level, the physician should bear in mind that acute alkalosis *per se* can produce hypokalemia in the absence of a deficit in total body potassium while acute acidosis *per se* can increase the serum potassium concentration into the normal range even in the presence of a reduced total body potassium. The treatment of potassium depletion, particularly in the presence of cardiac disease, renal disease, or acidosis, requires careful attention to acid-base balance and appropriate monitoring of serum electrolytes, the electrocardiogram, and the clinical status of the patient.

It is important to recognize that hyperkalemia is usually asymptomatic and may be manifested only by an increased serum potassium concentration and characteristic electrocardiographic changes (peaking of T-waves, loss of P-wave, depression of S-T segment, and prolongation of the QT interval). (See Contraindications, Warnings, and Overdosage.)

The use of potassium salts in patients with chronic renal disease, or any other condition which impairs potassium excretion, requires particularly careful monitoring of the serum potassium concentration and appropriate dosage adjustment.

When blood is drawn for analysis of plasma potassium levels, it is important to recognize that artifactual elevations do occur after repeated fist clenching to make veins more prominent during application of a tourniquet.

Carcinogenesis, Mutagenesis, Impairment of Fertility—There have been no studies in animals or humans to evaluate the carcinogenesis, mutagenesis or impairment of fertility for potassium.

Pregnancy—Category C. Animal reproduction studies have not been conducted with KAON ELIXIR. It is also not known whether KAON ELIXIR can cause fetal harm when administered to a pregnant woman or can affect reproduction capacity. KAON ELIXIR should be given to a pregnant woman only if clearly needed.

Nursing Mothers—It is not known whether this drug is excreted in human milk. Because many drugs are excreted in human milk, caution should be exercised when KAON ELIXIR is administered to a nursing woman.

Pediatric Use—Safety and effectiveness in children have not been established.

ADVERSE REACTIONS

The most severe adverse effect is hyperkalemia (see Contraindications, Warnings and Overdosage).

The most common adverse reactions to oral potassium salts are nausea, vomiting, abdominal discomfort, and diarrhea. These symptoms are due to irritation of the gastrointestinal tract and are best managed by diluting the preparation further, taking the dose with meals, or reducing the dose.

OVERDOSAGE

The administration of oral potassium salts to persons with normal excretory mechanisms for potassium rarely causes serious hyperkalemia. However, if excretory mechanisms are impaired or if potassium is administered too rapidly intravenously, potentially fatal hyperkalemia can result (see Contraindications and Warnings). It is important to recognize that hyperkalemia is usually asymptomatic and may be manifested only by an increased serum potassium concentration and characteristic electrocardiographic changes (peaking of T-waves, loss of P-wave, depression of S-T segment, and prolongation of the QT interval). Late manifestations include muscle-paralysis and cardiovascular collapse from cardiac arrest.

Treatment for hyperkalemia includes the following:

1. Elimination of foods and medications containing potassium and potassium-sparing diuretics.
2. Intravenous administration of 300 to 500 ml/hr of 10% dextrose solution containing 10–20 units of crystalline insulin per 1,000 ml.
3. Correction of acidosis, if present, with intravenous sodium bicarbonate.
4. Use of exchange resins, hemodialysis, or peritoneal dialysis.

In treating hyperkalemia, it should be recalled that in patients who have been stabilized on digitalis, too rapid a lowering of the serum potassium concentration can produce digitalis toxicity.

DOSAGE AND ADMINISTRATION

The usual dietary intake of potassium by the average adult is 40 to 80 mEq per day. Potassium depletion sufficient to cause hypokalemia usually requires the loss of 200 or more mEq of potassium from the total body store.

Dosage must be adjusted to the individual needs of each patient but is typically in the range of 20 mEq per day for the prevention of hypokalemia to 40–100 mEq per day or more for the treatment of potassium depletion.

To minimize gastrointestinal irritation, patients must follow directions regarding dilution. Each tablespoonful (15 ml) should be diluted with one fluid ounce or more of water or other liquid.

One tablespoonful twice daily (after morning and evening meals) supplies 40 mEq of potassium. Deviations from this recommendation may be indicated, since no average total daily dose can be defined but must be governed by close observation for clinical effects. However, potassium intoxication may result from any therapeutic dosage. See "Overdosage" and "Precautions".

HOW SUPPLIED

KAON ELIXIR (potassium gluconate), Grape, supplies 20 mEq of potassium (as potassium gluconate, 4.68g) per tablespoonful (15 ml).

NDC 0013-3203-51 Pint
NDC 0013-3203-53 Gallon

Storage Conditions—Preserve in tight, light resistant containers. Store at room temperature and protect from cold.

KAON–CL–10™   ℞

[kā 'ŏn-sēē-ĕl "ten]
(Potassium Chloride)
EXTENDED-RELEASE TABLETS
KAON–CL®   ℞
[kā 'ŏn-sēē-ĕl "]
(Potassium Chloride)
EXTENDED-RELEASE TABLETS

DESCRIPTION

KAON CL-10®is a solid oral dosage form of potassium chloride containing 750 mg of potassium chloride USP equivalent to 10 mEq of potassium in a wax matrix tablet.

KAON CL®is a solid oral dosage form of potassium chloride containing 500 mg of potassium chloride USP equivalent to 6.7 mEq of potassium in a wax matrix tablet.

These formulations are intended to slow the release of potassium so that the likelihood of a high localized concentration of potassium chloride within the gastrointestinal tract is reduced.

KAON CL-10 and KAON-CL are electrolyte replenishers. The chemical name is potassium chloride and the structural formula is KCL. Potassium chloride USP occurs as a white, granular powder or as colorless crystals, It is odorless and has a saline taste. Its solutions are neutral to litmus. It is freely soluble in water and insoluble in alcohol.

Inactive Ingredients: Acacia, Calcium Carbonate, Calcium Stearate, Calcium Sulfate, Carnauba Wax, Microcrystalline Cellulose, Polyethylene Glycol, Purified Water, Shellac, Sodium Benzoate, Stearic Acid, Sucrose, Talc, Titanium Dioxide, Trichloroethylene, White Wax and color additives including FD&C Yellow No. 6 (sunset yellow) aluminum lake (KAON CL-10) and FD&C Yellow No. 5 (tartrazine) aluminum lake (KAON-CL).

CLINICAL PHARMACOLOGY

The potassium ion is the principal intracellular cation of most body tissues. Potassium ions participate in a number of essential physiological processes including the maintenance of intracellular tonicity, the transmission of nerve impulses, the contraction of cardiac, skeletal and smooth muscle and the maintenance of normal renal function.

The intracellular concentration of potassium is approximately 150 to 160 mEq per liter. The normal adult plasma concentration is 3.5 to 5 mEq per liter. An active ion trans-

port system maintains this gradient across the plasma membrane.

Potassium is a normal dietary constituent and under steady state conditions the amount of potassium absorbed from the gastrointestinal tract is equal to the amount excreted in the urine. The usual dietary intake of potassium is 50 to 100 mEq per day.

Potassium depletion will occur whenever the rate of potassium loss through renal excretion and/or loss from the gastrointestinal tract exceeds the rate of potassium intake. Such depletion usually develops as a consequence of therapy with diuretics, primary or secondary hyperaldosteronism, diabetic ketoacidosis, or inadequate replacement of potassium in patients on prolonged parenteral nutrition. Depletion can develop rapidly with severe diarrhea, especially if associated with vomiting. Potassium depletion due to these causes is usually accompanied by a concomitant loss of chloride and is manifested by hypokalemia and metabolic alkalosis. Potassium depletion may produce weakness, fatigue, disturbances of cardiac rhythm (primarily ectopic beats), prominent U-waves in the electrocardiogram, and, in advanced cases, flaccid paralysis and/or impaired ability to concentrate urine.

If potassium depletion associated with metabolic alkalosis cannot be managed by correcting the fundamental cause of the deficiency, e.g., where the patient requires long term diuretic therapy, supplemental potassium in the form of high potassium food or potassium chloride may be able to restore normal potassium levels.

In rare circumstances (e.g., patients with renal tubular acidosis) potassium depletion may be associated with metabolic acidosis and hyperchloremia. In such patients potassium replacement should be accomplished with potassium salts other than chloride, such as potassium bicarbonate, potassium citrate, potassium acetate, or potassium gluconate.

INDICATIONS AND USAGE

BECAUSE OF REPORTS OF INTESTINAL AND GASTRIC ULCERATION AND BLEEDING WITH EXTENDED RELEASE POTASSIUM CHLORIDE PREPARATIONS, THESE DRUGS SHOULD BE RESERVED FOR THOSE PATIENTS WHO CANNOT TOLERATE OR REFUSE TO TAKE LIQUIDS OR EFFERVESCENT POTASSIUM PREPARATIONS OR FOR PATIENTS IN WHOM THERE IS A PROBLEM OF COMPLIANCE WITH THESE PREPARATIONS.

1. For the treatment of patients with hypokalemia, with or without metabolic alkalosis; in digitalis intoxication; and in patients with hypokalemic familial periodic paralysis. If hypokalemia is the result of diuretic therapy, consideration should be given to the use of a lower dose of diuretic, which may be sufficient without leading to hypokalemia.
2. For the prevention of hypokalemia in patients who would be at particular risk if hypokalemia were to develop, e.g., digitalized patients or patients with significant cardiac arrhythmias.

The use of potassium salts in patients receiving diuretics for uncomplicated essential hypertension is often unnecessary when such patients have a normal dietary pattern and when low doses of the diuretic are used. Serum potassium should be checked periodically, however, and if hypokalemia ocurs, dietary supplementation with potassium-containing foods may be adequate to control milder cases. In more severe cases, and if dose adjustment of the diuretic is ineffective or unwarranted, supplementation with potassium salts may be indicated.

CONTRAINDICATIONS

Potassium supplements are contraindicated in patients with hyperkalemia since further increase in serum potassium concentration in such patients can produce cardiac arrest. Hyperkalemia may complicate any of the following conditions: chronic renal failure, systemic acidosis such as diabetic acidosis, acute dehydration, extensive tissue breakdown as in severe burns, adrenal insufficiency, or the administration of a potassium-sparing diuretic (e.g., spironolactone, triamterene, amiloride) (see OVERDOSAGE).

Controlled release formulations of potassium chloride have produced esophageal ulceration in certain cardiac paitents with esophageal compression due to an enlarged left atrium. Potassium supplementation, when indicated in such patients, should be given as a liquid preparation.

All solid oral dosage forms of potassium chloride are contraindicated in any patient in whom there is a structural, pathological (e.g., diabetic gastroparesis) or pharmacologic (use of anticholinergic agents or other agents with anticholinergic properties at sufficient doses to exert anticholinergic effects) cause an arrest or delay in tablet passage through the gastrointestinal tract.

WARNINGS

Hyperkalemia (see OVERDOSAGE)

In patients with impaired mechanisms for excreting potassium, the administration of potassium salts can produce hyperkalemia and cardiac arrest. This occurs most commonly in patients given potassium by the intravenous route but

may also occur in patients given potassium orally. Potentially fatal hyperkalemia can develop rapidly and be asymptomatic. The use of potassium salts in patients with chronic renal disease, or any other condition which impairs potassium excretion, requires particularly careful monitoring of the serum potassium concentration and appropriate dosage adjustment.

Interaction with Potassium Sparing Diuretics

Hypokalemia should not be treated by the concomitant administration of potassium salts and a potassium-sparing diuretic (e.g., spironolactone, triamterene or amiloride) since the simultaneous administration of these agents can produce severe hyperkalemia.

Interaction with Angiotensin Converting Enzyme Inhibitors

Angiotensin converting enzyme (ACE) inhibitors (e.g., captopril, enalapril) will produce some potassium retention by inhibiting aldosterone production. Potassium supplements should be given to patients receiving ACE inhibitors only with close monitoring.

Gastrointestinal Lesions

Solid oral dosage forms of potassium chloride can produce ulcerative and/or stenotic lesions of the gastrointestinal tract. Based on spontaneous adverse reaction reports, enteric coated preparations of potassium chloride are associated with an increased frequency of small bowel lesions (40–50 per 100,000 patient years) compared to sustained release wax matrix formulations (less than one per 100,000 patient years). Because of the lack of extensive marketing experience with microencapsulated products, a comparison between such products and wax matrix or enteric coated products is not available. KAON CL-10 and KAON-CL is a wax matrix tablet formulated to provide a controlled rate of release of potassium chloride and thus to minimize the possibility of a high local concentration of potassium near the gastrointestinal wall.

Prospective trials have been conducted in normal human volunteers in which the upper gastrointestinal tract was evaluated by endoscopic inspection before and after one week of solid oral potassium chloride therapy. The ability of this model to predict events occurring in usual clinical practice is unknown. Trials which approximated usual clinical practice did not reveal any clear differences between the wax matrix and microencapsulated dosage forms. In contrast, there was a higher incidence of gastric and duodenal lesions in subjects receiving a high dose of a wax matrix controlled release formulation under conditions which did not resemble usual or recommended clinical practice (i.e., 96 mEq per day in divided doses of potassium chloride administered to fasted patients, in the presence of an anticholinergic drug to delay gastric emptying; see CONTRAINDICATIONS). The upper gastrointestinal lesions observed by endoscopy were asymptomatic and were not accompanied by evidence of bleeding (Hemoccult® testing). The relevance of these findings to the usual conditions (i.e., non-fasting, no anticholinergic agent, smaller doses) under which controlled release potassium chloride products are used is uncertain; epidemiologic studies have not identified an elevated risk, compared to microencapsulated products, for upper gastrointestinal lesions in patients receiving wax matrix formulations. KAON CL-10 and KAON-CL should be discontinued immediately and the possibility of ulceration, obstruction or perforation considered if severe vomiting, abdominal pain, distention, or gastrointestinal bleeding occurs.

Metabolic Acidosis

Hypokalemia in patients with metabolic acidosis should be treated with an alkalinizing potassium salt such as potassium bicarbonate, potassium citrate, potassium acetate or potassium gluconate.

PRECAUTIONS

General:

The diagnosis of potassium depletion is ordinarily made by demonstrating hypokalemia in a patient with a clinical history suggesting some cause for potassium depletion. In interpreting serum potassium level, the physician should bear in mind that acute alkalosis *per se* can produce hypokalemia in the absence of a deficit in total body potassium while acute acidosis *per se* can increase the serum potassium concentration into the normal range even in the presence of a reduced total body potassium. The treatment of potassium depletion, particularly in the presence of cardiac disease, renal disease, or acidosis requires careful attention to acid-base balance and appropriate monitoring of serum electrolytes, the electrocardiogram, and the clinical status of the patient.

KAON CL-10 contains FD&C Yellow No. 6 (sunset yellow) aluminum lake as a color additive.

KAON-CL contains FD&C Yellow No. 5 (tartrazine) aluminum lake which may cause allergic-type reactions (including bronchial asthma) in certain susceptible persons. Although the overall incidence of FD&C Yellow No. 5 (tartrazine) sensitivity in the general population is low, it is frequently seen in patients who also have aspirin hypersensitivity.

Continued on next page

Adria—Cont.

Information for Patients:
Physicians should consider reminding the patient of the following:
To take each dose with meals and with a full glass of water or other liquid.
To take this medicine following the frequency and amount prescribed by the physician. This is especially important if the patient is also taking diuretics and/or digitalis preparations.
To check with the physician if there is trouble swallowing tablets or if the tablets seem to stick in the throat.
To check with the physician at once if tarry stools or other evidence of gastrointestinal bleeding is noticed.
To take each dose without crushing, chewing or sucking tablets.
Laboratory Tests:
When blood is drawn for analysis of plasma potassium it is important to recognize that artifactual elevations can occur after improper venipuncture technique or as a result of in vitro hemolysis of the sample.
Drug Interactions:
Potassium-sparing diuretics, angiotensin converting enzyme inhibitors: see WARNINGS.
Carcinogenesis, Mutagenesis, Impairment of Fertility:
Carcinogenicity, mutagenicity and fertility studies in animals have not been performed. Potassium is a normal dietary constituent.
Pregnancy Category C:
Animal reproduction studies have not been conducted with KAON CL-10 and KAON CL®. It is unlikely that potassium supplementation that does not lead to hyperkalemia would have an adverse effect on the fetus or would affect reproduction capacity.
Nursing Mothers:
The normal potassium ion content of human milk is about 13 mEq per liter. Since oral potassium becomes part of the body potassium pool, so long as body potassium is not excessive, the contribution of potassium chloride supplementation should have little or no effect on the level of human milk.
Pediatric Use:
Safety and effectiveness on children have not been established.

ADVERSE REACTIONS

One of the most severe adverse effects is hyperkalemia (see CONTRAINDICATIONS, WARNINGS, and OVERDOSAGE). There also have been reports of upper and lower gastrointestinal conditions including obstruction, bleeding, ulceration, and perforation (see CONTRAINDICATIONS and WARNINGS).
The most common adverse reactions to the oral potassium salts are nausea, vomiting, flatulence, abdominal pain/discomfort and diarrhea. These symptoms are due to irritation of the gastrointestinal tract and are best managed by diluting the preparation further, taking the dose with meals, or reducing the amount taken at one time.

OVERDOSAGE

The administration of oral potassium salts to persons with normal excretory mechanisms for potassium rarely causes serious hyperkalemia. However, if excretory mechanisms are impaired, or if potassium is administered too rapidly intravenously, potentially fatal hyperkalemia can result (see CONTRAINDICATIONS and WARNINGS). It is important to recognize that hyperkalemia is usually asymptomatic and may be manifested only by an increased serum potassium concentration (6.5–8.0 mEq/L) and characteristic electrocardiographic changes (peaking of T-waves, loss of P-wave, depression of S-T segment, prolongation of the QT interval). Late manifestations include paralysis and cardiovascular collapse from cardiac arrest (9–12 mEq/L).
Treatment measures for hyperkalemia include the following:
1. Elimination of foods and medications containing potassium and of any agents with potassium-sparing properties;
2. Intravenous administration of 300 to 500 mL/hr of 10% dextrose solution containing 10–20 units of crystalline insulin per 1,000 mL;
3. Correction of acidosis, if present, with intravenous sodium bicarbonate;
4. Use of exchange resins, hemodialysis, or peritoneal dialysis.
In treating hyperkalemia, it should be recalled that in patients who have been stabalized on digitalis, too rapid a lowering of the serum potassium concentration can produce digitalis toxicity.

DOSAGE AND ADMINISTRATION

The usual dietary potassium intake by the average adult is 50 to 100 mEq per day. Potassium depletion sufficient to cause hypokalemia usually requires the loss of 200 or more mEq of potassium from the total body store.

Dosage must be adjusted to the individual needs of each patient. The dose for the prevention of hypokalemia is typically in the range of 20 mEq per day. Doses of 40–100 mEq per day or more are used for the treatment of potassium depletion. Dosage should be divided if more than 20 mEq per day is given such that no more than 20 mEq is given in a single dose.
KAON CL-10 provides 10 mEq of potassium chloride.
KAON-CL provides 6.7 mEq of potassium chloride.
KAON CL-10 and KAON-CL should be taken with meals and with a glass of water or other liquid. This product should not be taken on an empty stomach because of its potential for gastric irritation (see WARNINGS).
Take each dose without crushing, chewing or sucking tablet.

HOW SUPPLIED

Each KAON CL-10® Tablet is a green sugar coated capsule shaped tablet which contains 750 mg of potassium chloride, USP equivalent to 10 mEq of potassium in a wax matrix tablet. Tablets are imprinted with ADRIA/304. They are supplied as follows:

    NDC 0013-3041-17   Bottle of 100
    NDC 0013-3041-21   Bottle of 500
    NDC 0013-3041-23   Bottle of 1000
    NDC 0013-3041-18   STAT-PAK® (unit dose) box of 100

Each KAON-CL Tablet is a yellow round sugar coated tablet which contains 500 mg of potassium chloride USP equivalent to 6.7 mEq of potassium in a wax matrix tablet. Tablets are imprinted with ADRIA/307. They are supplied as follows:

    NDC 0013-3071-17   Bottle of 100
    NDC 0013-3071-19   Bottle of 250
    NDC 0013-3071-23   Bottle of 1000

Store below 30°C (86°F) and protect from moisture.

CAUTION

Federal law prohibits dispensing without a prescription.
ADRIA LABORATORIES
Division of Erbamont, Inc.
COLUMBUS, OHIO 43215
Shown in Product Identification Section, page 404

MAGAN®   ℞
[mā-găn']
(Magnesium Salicylate)

DESCRIPTION

Each MAGAN uncoated, pink, capsule-shaped tablet for oral administration contains 545 mg of magnesium salicylate equivalent to 500 mg of salicylate. Magnesium salicylate is a non-steroidal, antiinflammatory agent with antipyretic and analgesic properties.
Magnesium salicylate is a white, odorless, crystalline powder with a sweet taste. It is soluble in water and alcohol.

CLINICAL PHARMACOLOGY

Salicylic acid is the active moiety released into the plasma by MAGAN (magnesium salicylate). Salicylic acid is enzymatically biotransformed through two pathways to salicyluric acid and salicylphenolic glucuronide and eliminated in the urine.
Oral salicylates are absorbed rapidly, partly from the stomach but mostly from the upper intestine. Salicylic acid is rapidly distributed throughout all body tissues and most transcellular fluids, mainly by pH-dependent passive processes. It can be detected in synovial, spinal and peritoneal fluid, in saliva and in milk. It readily crosses the placental barrier. From 50% to 90% of salicylic acid is bound to plasma proteins, especially albumin.
Following the ingestion of a single dose of 524 mg of magnesium salicylate, a peak concentration of 3.6 mg/dl salicylic acid is reached in 1.5 hours with a T ½ of 2 hours. The major biotransformation paths for the elimination of salicylic acid from the plasma become saturated by low doses of salicylic acid. As a result, repeated doses of MAGAN increase the plasma concentration and markedly prolong the plasma half-time. The plasma concentration of salicylic acid is increased by conditions that reduce the glomerular filtration rate or tubular secretion such as renal disease or the presence of inhibitors that compete for the transport system such as probenecid.
Therapeutic plasma concentrations of salicylic acid for an adequate antiinflammatory effect needed for the treatment of rheumatoid arthritis range between 20–30 mg/dl. Effective analgesia is achieved at lower concentrations. Salicylates relieve pain by both a peripheral and a CNS effect. Salicylates inhibit the synthesis of prostaglandins; the importance of this mechanism in analgesia and antiinflammation has not been fully elucidated. Salicylates have an antipyretic effect in febrile patients but little in subjects with normal temperatures. This appears to be due to the inhibition of the synthesis of prostaglandins which are powerful pyrogens that affect the hypothalamus. Higher therapeutic concentrations cause reversible tinnitus and high tone hearing loss. Full therapeutic doses of salicylates increase oxygen consumption and CO_2 production. They cause an extracellular and intracellular respiratory alkalosis which is rapidly com-

pensated. Salicylates irritate the gastric mucosa and frequently lead to blood loss in the stool; this effect is more pronounced with aspirin than magnesium salicylate. Salicylates in large doses (over 6 g/day) reduce the plasma prothrombin level. In contrast to aspirin, magnesium salicylate does not affect platelets. Salicylic acid increases the urinary excretion of urates at higher doses but may decrease excretion at lower doses.

INDICATIONS AND USAGE

MAGAN is indicated for the relief of the signs and symptoms of rheumatoid arthritis, osteoarthritis, bursitis and other musculoskeletal disorders.

CONTRAINDICATIONS

MAGAN is contraindicated in patients with advanced chronic renal insufficiency. It may counteract the effect of uricosuric agents and should not be prescribed for patients on such drugs.

WARNINGS

As with all salicylates, MAGAN should be avoided or administered with caution to patients with liver damage, pre-existing hypoprothrombinemia, vitamin K deficiency and before surgery.

PRECAUTIONS

General —Appropriate precautions should be taken in prescribing MAGAN for persons known to be sensitive to salicylates and in patients with erosive gastritis or peptic ulcer. If a reaction develops, the drug should be discontinued. MAGAN should be used with caution, if at all, concomitantly with anticoagulants. Appropriate precautions should be taken in administering MAGAN to patients with any impairment of renal function including discontinuing other drugs containing magnesium and monitoring serum magnesium levels if dosage levels of MAGAN are high.
Drug Interactions —Even small doses of MAGAN should not be given with uricosuric agents such as probenecid that decrease tubular reabsorption because it counteracts their effect. Large doses of MAGAN cause hypoprothrombinemia. Lower doses enhance the effects of anticoagulants such as coumadin and must be used with caution in patients receiving anticoagulants that affect the prothrombin time. Caution should also be exercised in patients concurrently treated with a sulfonylurea hypoglycemic agent or methotrexate because of the drug's capability of displacing them from the plasma protein binding sites, resulting in enhanced action of these agents. A similar displacement of barbiturates and diphenylhydantoin may occur; diphenylhydantoin intoxication has been precipitated by the consumption of aspirin. Salicylates inhibit the diuretic action of spironolactone.
Carcinogenesis, Mutagenesis, Impairment of Fertility —There have been no studies in animals or humans to evaluate the carcinogenesis, mutagenesis or impairment of fertility for magnesium salicylate. Aspirin causes testicular atrophy and inhibition of spermatogenesis in animals.
Pregnancy —Category C.
1. *Teratogenic effects* —Aspirin has been shown to be teratogenic in animals and to increase the incidence of still births and neonatal deaths in women. There are no adequate or well-controlled studies of MAGAN in pregnant women. MAGAN should be used during pregnancy only if the potential benefit justifies the potential risk to the fetus.
2. *Non-Teratogenic effects* —Chronic, high dose salicylate therapy of pregnant women increases the length of gestation and the frequency of post maturity and prolongs spontaneous labor. It is recommended MAGAN be taken during the last three months of pregnancy only under the close supervision of a physician.
Nursing Mothers —Since salicylates are excreted in human milk, caution should be exercised when MAGAN is administered to a nursing woman.
Pediatric Use —Safety and effectiveness of MAGAN in children have not been established.

ADVERSE REACTIONS

Magnesium salicylate in large doses has a hypoprothrombinemic effect and should be given with caution in patients receiving anticoagulant drugs, patients with liver damage, pre-existing hypoprothrombinemia, vitamin K deficiency or before surgery.
Salicylates given in overdose produce stimulation (often manifested as tinnitus) followed by depression of the central nervous system. The dosage should be lowered at the onset of tinnitus.
Salicylates may cause gastric mucosal irritation and bleeding. However, fecal blood loss in patients taking MAGAN is significantly less than in those taking aspirin.
MAGAN should not be given to patients with severe renal damage because of the possibility of hypermagnesemia.
In moderate to high doses, salicylates lower the blood glucose in diabetics. Aspirin-induced hypoglycemia has been described in adults undergoing hemodialysis.
Unlike aspirin, magnesium salicylate is not known to affect the platelet adhesiveness involved in the clotting mechanism; and therefore, does not prolong bleeding time. MA-

GAN has not been associated with reactions causing asthmatic attacks in susceptible people.

OVERDOSAGE

Acute overdosage results in salicylate toxicity. Early signs and symptoms from repeated larger doses as well as a large single dose consist of headache, dizziness, tinnitus (which may be absent in children or the elderly), difficulty in hearing, dimness of vision, mental confusion, lassitude, drowsiness, sweating, thirst, hyperventilation, nausea, vomiting and occasionally diarrhea. More severe salicylate poisoning is manifested by CNS disturbances including EEG abnormalities. Hyperventilation occurs producing initial respiratory alkalosis. This is followed by severe metabolic acidosis with dehydration and loss of potassium. Restlessness, garrulity, incoherent speech, apprehension, vertigo, tremor, diplopia, maniacal delirium, hallucinations, generalized convulsions and coma may occur. Toxic symptoms may occur at serum levels greater than 20 mg/dl in patients over 60 years of age. Hyperventilation may occur at plasma salicylate levels over 35 mg/dl. Death may result from salicylate levels between 45–75 mg/dl. As with other salicylates, 10 to 30 g of the drug may be fatal. Renal or hepatic insufficiency and fever and dehydration in children enhance the acute toxicity of salicylate overdoses. Treatment of acute poisoning is a medical emergency and should be undertaken in a hospital. Serum Na, K, Cl, CO_2 levels, pH, BUN, blood glucose and urine pH and specific gravity should be obtained. Emesis should be induced or gastric lavage performed. Activated charcoal may be administered. Hyperthermia should be controlled with tepid water sponging. Dehydration should be treated and acid-base imbalance corrected. A high concentration of salicylic acid in the brain may be fatal. Correction of acidosis shifts salicylate from the brain to the plasma. A bicarbonate solution should be infused to maintain an alkaline diuresis. Care should be taken to avoid pulmonary edema. The blood pH, plasma pCO_2 and plasma glucose level should be monitored frequently. Ketosis and hypoglycemia may be corrected by glucose infusions and hypokalemia by potassium chloride added to the intravenous infusate. Avoid respiratory depressants. Shock may be combatted by plasma infusions. Hemorrhagic phenomena may necessitate whole blood transfusions or vitamin K_1. In severe intoxication, exchange transfusion, peritoneal dialysis, hemodialysis or hemoperfusion should be performed to remove plasma salicylic acid. Dialysis should be seriously considered if the patient's condition is worsening despite appropriate therapy.

DOSAGE AND ADMINISTRATION

The dosage for MAGAN in the treatment of musculoskeletal disorders such as arthritis should be adjusted according to individual patient's needs. The recommended initial regimen is two tablets three times per day. Dosage may be increased, if necessary, to achieve the desired therapeutic effect. In adjusting the dosage, the physician should monitor the dose limiting parameters such as tinnitus and/or serum salicylate over 30 mg/dl.

HOW SUPPLIED

Each MAGAN tablet contains 545 mg of magnesium salicylate equivalent to 500 mg salicylate. MAGAN is available for oral administration as uncoated, pink, capsule-shaped tablets coded Adria 412. They are supplied as follows:
NDC 0013-4121-17 in bottles of 100
NDC 0013-4121-21 in bottles of 500
Store at room temperature and protect from light.

MODANE® SOFT
[mō'dāne soft]
(docusate sodium)
Capsules

DESCRIPTION

Each soft gelatin capsule contains docusate sodium 100 mg. Inactive ingredients include: FD&C Blue No. 1, FD&C Blue No. 2, gelatin, glycerin, methylparaben, polyethylene glycol 400, propylene glycol, propylparaben, sorbitol, and water. Chemically, docusate sodium is butanedioic acid sulfo-1, 4-bis(2-ethylhexyl)ester sodium salt. It is an anionic surfactant.

CLINICAL PHARMACOLOGY

Docusate sodium, an anionic surfactant, allows increased hydration of the stool to produce a softer stool for easier passage usually in 24 to 72 hours. Docusate sodiun is absorbed to some extent in the duodenum and proximal jejunum.

INDICATIONS

For management of functional constipation associated with dry hard stools in adults and children 6 years of age and older. It is especially useful when it is desirable to lessen the strain of defecation (e.g., in persons with painful rectal lesions, hernia or cardiovascular disease).

CONTRAINDICATIONS

Mineral oil administration.

WARNINGS

Do not use any laxative preparation when abdominal pain, nausea or vomiting are present. **KEEP THIS PRODUCT OUT OF REACH OF CHILDREN.** As with any drug, if the patient is pregnant or nursing a baby, she should consult a health professional before using.

PRECAUTIONS

Docusate sodium may increase the intestinal absorption of mineral oil and/or hepatic uptake of other drugs administered concurrently.

ADVERSE REACTIONS

Adverse reactions are uncommon. Diarrhea, nausea, cramping pains and rash have been reported.

OVERDOSAGE

Docusate sodium is relatively nontoxic. Overdosage may be expected to result in anorexia, vomiting, and diarrhea.

DOSAGE AND ADMINISTRATION

Adults: one to three capsules daily, or as directed by a doctor. Children (6 to 12 years): one capsule daily, or as directed by a doctor.

HOW SUPPLIED

Each MODANE SOFT green, soft gelatin capsule contains docusate sodium 100 mg coded 13 503.
NDC 0013-5031-13 Package of 30 Capsules.
Store at controlled room temperature (59°–86°F, 15°–30°C).
Mfd by:
R.P. SCHERER
ST. PETERSBURG, FLORIDA 33702
for: ADRIA LABORATORIES
        Division of Erbamont Inc.
        COLUMBUS, OHIO 43215

MODANE
[mō'dāne]
(phenolphthalein)

DESCRIPTION

MODANE TABLETS (rust red)—Each tablet contains white phenolphthalein 130 mg. Inactive ingredients include acacia, calcium carbonate, calcium sulfate, corn starch, dibasic calcium phosphate, FD&C Red No. 40 aluminum lake, lactose, magnesium stearate, povidone, shellac, sodium benzoate, sucrose, talc, titanium dioxide, water and carnauba wax.
MODANE MILD TABLETS (pink)—Each tablet contains white phenolphthalein 60 mg. Inactive ingredients include acacia, calcium carbonate, calcium sulfate, corn starch, dibasic calcium phosphate, FD&C Red No. 40 aluminum lake, lactose, magnesium stearate, methylparaben, povidone, propylparaben, shellac, sodium benzoate, sucrose, talc, titanium dioxide, water and carnauba wax.

CLINICAL PHARMACOLOGY

Phenolphthalein, a stimulant laxative, acts primarily on the large intestine to produce a semifluid stool usually in 4–8 hours. It is dissolved by bile salts and alkaline intestinal secretions and may impart a red color to alkaline feces and urine.

INDICATIONS

For temporary relief of constipation in adults.

CONTRAINDICATIONS

Sensitivity to phenolphthalein.

WARNINGS

Do not use any laxative preparations when abdominal pain, nausea, or vomiting are present. Frequent and continued use may cause dependence upon laxatives.
KEEP THIS PRODUCT OUT OF REACH OF CHILDREN.
As with any drug, if the patient is pregnant or nursing a baby, she should consult a health professional before using.

PRECAUTIONS

Phenolphthalein may color alkaline feces and urine red. If skin rash appears, do not use this product or any other preparation containing phenolphthalein.

ADVERSE REACTIONS

Excessive bowel activity, usually diarrhea or abdominal discomfort, nausea, vomiting, cramps, weakness, dizziness, palpitations, sweating and fainting may follow the administration of a laxative. Diarrhea may lead to fluid and electrolyte deficits. Allergic reactions, skin rashes attributed to phenolphthalein, have been reported.

OVERDOSAGE

Phenolphthalein is relatively nontoxic. Overdosage may be expected to result in excessive bowel activity. Treatment is symptomatic if the duration of effects is prolonged. Fluid and electrolyte deficits might result from prolonged catharsis.

DOSAGE AND ADMINISTRATION

MODANE Tablet (rust red)—Adults: One tablet daily, or as directed by a doctor. This strength is not recommended for children.
MODANE MILD Tablets (pink)—Adults: One to two tablets daily, or as directed by a doctor. Children (6–12 years): One tablet daily, or as directed by a doctor.
Not recommended for children under 6 years of age.

HOW SUPPLIED

Each MODANE tablet contains white phenolphthalein 130 mg in a rust red, round, sugar coated tablet printed with A on one side and 513 on the other. Store at room temperature. Packages of 10 tablets.
NDC 0013-5131-07
Package of 30 tablets.
NDC 0013-5131-13
Bottle of 100 tablets.
NDC 0013-5131-17
Each MODANE MILD tablet contains white phenolphthalein 60 mg in a pink, round, sugar coated tablet printed with A on one side and 512 on the other. Store at room temperature.
Package of 10 tablets.
NDC 0013-5121-07
Package of 30 tablets.
NDC 0013-5121-13
Bottle of 100 tablets
NDC 0013-5121-17

MODANE PLUS
[mō'dāne plŭs]
(phenolphthalein and docusate sodium)

DESCRIPTION

Each tablet contains white phenolphthalein 65mg and docusate sodium 100mg. Inactive ingredients include acacia, calcium carbonate, calcium sulfate, croscarmellose sodium, FD&C yellow #6 aluminum lake, magnesium stearate, microcrystalline cellulose, povidone, shellac, silica gel, sodium benzoate, sucrose, talc, titanium dioxide, water and carnauba wax.
Phenolphthalein is classified as a stimulant laxative. Chemically phenolphthalein is 3, 3-bis (p-hydroxyphenyl) phthalide.
Chemically, docusate sodium is butanedioic acid, sulfo-1, 4-bis (2-ethylhexyl) ester, sodium salt. It is an anionic surfactant.

CLINICAL PHARMACOLOGY

Phenolphthalein, a stimulant laxative, acts primarily on the large intestine to produce a semifluid stool usually in 4–8 hours. It is dissolved by bile salts and alkaline intestinal secretions and may impart a red color to alkaline feces and urine.
Docusate sodium is classified as a stool softener. It is used in conditions in which it is desirable that the feces be kept soft and straining at the stool be avoided.

INDICATIONS

For temporary relief of constipation in adults.

CONTRAINDICATIONS

Sensitivity to phenolphthalein. Mineral oil administration.

WARNINGS

Do not use any laxative preparations when abdominal pain, nausea or vomiting are present. Frequent and continued use may cause dependence upon laxatives.
KEEP THIS PRODUCT OUT OF REACH OF CHILDREN.
As with any drug, if the patient is pregnant or nursing a baby, she should consult a health professional before using.

PRECAUTIONS

Phenolphthalein may color alkaline feces and urine red.
If skin rash appears, do not use this product or any other preparation containing phenolphthalein.
Docusate sodium may increase the intestinal absorption of mineral oil and/or hepatic uptake of other drugs administered concurrently.

ADVERSE REACTIONS

Excessive bowel activity, usually diarrhea or abdominal discomfort, nausea, vomiting, cramps, weakness, dizziness, palpitations, sweating and fainting may follow the administration of a laxative. Diarrhea may lead to fluid and electrolyte deficits. Allergic reactions, skin rashes attributed to phenolphthalein, have been reported.

OVERDOSAGE

Phenolphthalein is relatively nontoxic. Overdosage may be expected to result in excessive bowel activity. Treatment is symptomatic if the duration of effects is prolonged. Fluid and electrolyte deficits might result from prolonged catharsis.

Continued on next page

Adria—Cont.

DOSAGE AND ADMINISTRATION
Adults: One tablet daily, or as directed by a doctor. This strength is not recommended for children.

HOW SUPPLIED
Each MODANE PLUS tablet contains white phenolphthalein 65 mg and docusate sodium 100 mg in an orange, round, sugar coated tablet printed with A on one side and 514 on the other.
Package of 10 tablets.
NDC 0013-5141-07
Package of 30 tablets.
NDC 0013-5141-13
Bottle of 1u0 tablets.
NDC 0013-5141-17
Store at room temperature.

NEOSAR® FOR INJECTION   ℞
[nē'ō-săr]
(cyclophosphamide USP)

DESCRIPTION
NEOSAR® (Cyclophosphamide for Injection, USP) is supplied as a sterile powder for parenteral use containing 45 mg sodium chloride per 100 mg cyclophosphamide (anhydrous). Cyclophosphamide is a synthetic antineoplastic drug chemically related to the nitrogen mustards. Cyclophosphamide is a white crystalline powder with the molecular formula $C_7H_{15}Cl_2N_2O_2P \cdot H_2O$ and a molecular weight of 279.1. The chemical name for cyclophosphamide is 2-[bis(2-chloroethyl)amino]tetrahydro-2H-1,3,2-oxazaphorine 2-oxide monohydrate. Cyclophosphamide is soluble in water, saline, or ethanol.

CLINICAL PHARMACOLOGY
NEOSAR is biotransformed principally in the liver to active alkylating metabolites by a mixed function microsomal oxidase system. These metabolites interfere with the growth of susceptible rapidly proliferating malignant cells. The mechanism of action is thought to involve cross-linking of tumor cell DNA.
Cyclophosphamide is well absorbed after oral administration with a bioavailability greater than 75%. The unchanged drug has an elimination half-life of 3 to 12 hours. It is eliminated primarily in the form of metabolites, but from 5 to 25% of the dose is excreted in urine as unchanged drug. Several cytotoxic and noncytotoxic metabolites have been identified in urine and in plasma. Concentrations of metabolites reach a maximum in plasma 2 to 3 hours after an intravenous dose. Plasma protein binding of unchanged drug is low but some metabolites are bound to an extent greater than 60%. It has not been demonstrated that any single metabolite is responsible for either the therapeutic or toxic effects of cyclophosphamide. Although elevated levels of metabolites of cyclophosphamide have been observed in patients with renal failure, increased clinical toxicity in such patients has not been demonstrated.

INDICATIONS AND USAGE
NEOSAR, although effective alone in susceptible malignancies, is more frequently used concurrently or sequentially with other antineoplastic drugs. The following malignancies are often susceptible to NEOSAR treatment:
1. Malignant lymphomas (Stages III and IV of the Ann Arbor staging system), Hodgkin's disease, lymphocytic lymphoma (nodular or diffuse), mixed-cell type lymphoma, histiocytic lymphoma, Burkitt's lymphoma.
2. Multiple myeloma.
3. Leukemias: Chronic lymphocytic leukemia, chronic granulocytic leukemia (it is usually ineffective in acute blast crisis), acute myelogenous and monocytic leukemia, acute lymphoblastic (stem cell) leukemia in children (NEOSAR given during remission is effective in prolonging its duration).
4. Cutaneous T-cell lymphoma (Mycosis fungoides-advanced disease).
5. Neuroblastoma (disseminated disease).
6. Adenocarcinoma of the ovary.
7. Retinoblastoma.
8. Carcinoma of the breast.

CONTRAINDICATIONS
Continued use of cyclophosphamide is contraindicated in patients with severely depressed bone marrow function. See WARNINGS and PRECAUTIONS sections.

WARNINGS
Carcinogenesis, Mutagenesis, Impairment of Fertility
Second malignancies have developed in some patients treated with cyclophosphamide used alone or in association with other antineoplastic drugs and/or modalities. Most frequently, they have been urinary bladder, myeloproliferative, or lymphoproliferative malignancies. Second malignan-

cies most frequently were detected in patients treated for primary myeloproliferative or lymphoproliferative malignancies or nonmalignant disease in which immune processes are believed to be involved pathologically. In some cases, the second malignancy developed several years after cyclophosphamide treatment had been discontinued. Urinary bladder malignancies generally have occurred in patients who previously had hemorrhagic cystitis. One case of carcinoma of the renal pelvis was reported in a patient receiving long-term cyclophosphamide therapy for cerebral vasculitis. The possibility of cyclophosphamide-induced malignancy should be considered in any benefit-to-risk assessment for use of the drug.
Cyclophosphamide can cause fetal harm when administered to a pregnant woman and such abnormalities have been reported following cyclophosphamide therapy in pregnant women. Abnormalities were found in two infants and a six-month old fetus born to women treated with cyclophosphamide. Ectrodactylia was found in two of the three cases. Normal infants have also been born to women treated with cyclophosphamide during pregnancy, including the first trimester. If this drug is used during pregnancy, or if the patient becomes pregnant while taking (receiving) this drug, the patient should be apprised of the potential hazard to the fetus. Women of childbearing potential should be advised to avoid becoming pregnant.
Cyclophosphamide interferes with oogenesis and spermatogenesis. It may cause sterility in both sexes. Development of sterility appears to depend on the dose of cyclophosphamide, duration of therapy, and the state of gonadal function at the time of treatment. Cyclophosphamide-induced sterility may be irreversible in some patients.
Amenorrhea associated with decreased estrogen and increased gonadotropin secretion develops in a significant proportion of women treated with cyclophosphamide. Affected patients generally resume regular menses within a few months after cessation of therapy. Girls treated with cyclophosphamide during prepubescence generally develop secondary sexual characteristics normally and have regular menses. Ovarian fibrosis with apparently complete loss of germ cells after prolonged cyclophosphamide treatment in late prepubescence has been reported. Girls treated with cyclophosphamide during prepubescence subsequently have conceived.
Men treated with cyclophosphamide may develop oligospermia or azoospermia associated with increased gonadotropin but normal testosterone secretion. Sexual potency and libido are unimpaired in these patients. Boys treated with cyclophosphamide during prepubescence develop secondary sexual characteristics normally, but may have oligospermia or azoospermia and increased gonadotropin secretion. Some degree of testicular atrophy may occur. Cyclophosphamide-induced azoospermia is reversible in some patients, though the reversibility may not occur for several years after cessation of therapy. Men temporarily rendered sterile by cyclophosphamide have subsequently fathered normal children.
Urinary System
Hemorrhagic cystitis may develop in patients treated with cyclophosphamide. Rarely, this condition can be severe and even fatal. Fibrosis of the urinary bladder, sometimes extensive, also may develop with or without accompanying cystitis. Atypical urinary bladder epithelial cells may appear in the urine. These adverse effects appear to depend on the dose of cyclophosphamide and the duration of therapy. Such bladder injury is thought to be due to cyclophosphamide metabolites excreted in the urine. Forced fluid intake helps to assure an ample output of urine, necessitates frequent voiding, and reduces the time the drug remains in the bladder. This helps to prevent cystitis. Hematuria usually resolves in a few days after cyclophosphamide treatment is stopped, but it may persist. Medical and/or surgical supportive treatment may be required, rarely, to treat protracted cases of severe hemorrhagic cystitis.
Cardiac Toxicity
Although a few instances of cardiac dysfunction have been reported following use of recommended doses of cyclophosphamide, no causal relationship has been established. Cardiotoxicity has been observed in some patients receiving high doses of cyclophosphamide ranging from 120 to 270 mg/kg administered over a period of a few days, usually as a portion of an intensive antineoplastic multi-drug regimen or in conjunction with transplantation procedures. In a few instances with high doses of cyclophosphamide, severe, and sometimes fatal, congestive heart failure has occurred within a few days after the first cyclophosphamide dose. Histopathologic examination has primarily shown hemorrhagic myocarditis. No residual cardiac abnormalities, as evidenced by electrocardiogram or echocardiogram appear to be present in patients surviving episodes of apparent cardiac toxicity associated with high doses of cyclophosphamide.
Cyclophosphamide has been reported to potentiate doxorubicin-induced cardiotoxicity.
Infections
Treatment with cyclophosphamide may cause significant suppression of immune responses. Serious, sometimes fatal, infections may develop in severely immunosuppressed pa-

tients. Cyclophosphamide treatment may not be indicated or should be interrupted or the dose reduced in patients who have or who develop viral, bacterial, fungal, protozoan, or helminthic infections.
Other
Rare instances of anaphylactic reaction including one death have been reported. One instance of possible cross-sensitivity with other alkylating agents has been reported.

PRECAUTIONS
General
Special attention to the possible development of toxicity should be exercised in patients being treated with cyclophosphamide if any of the following conditions are present.
1. Leukopenia
2. Thrombocytopenia
3. Tumor cell infiltration of bone marrow
4. Previous X-ray therapy
5. Previous therapy with other cytotoxic agents
6. Impaired hepatic function
7. Impaired renal function
Laboratory Tests
During treatment, the patient's hematologic profile (particularly neutrophils and platelets) should be monitored regularly to determine the degree of hematopoietic suppression. Urine should also be examined regularly for red cells which may precede hemorrhagic cystitis.
Drug Interactions
The rate of metabolism and the leukopenic activity of cyclophosphamide reportedly are increased by chronic administration of high doses of phenobarbital.
The physician should be alert for possible combined drug actions, desirable or undesirable, involving cyclophosphamide even though cyclophosphamide has been used successfully concurrently with other drugs, including other cytotoxic drugs.
Cyclophosphamide treatment, which causes a marked and persistent inhibition of cholinesterase activity, potentiates the effect of succinylcholine chloride.
If a patient has been treated with cyclophosphamide within 10 days of general anesthesia, the anesthesiologist should be alerted.
Adrenalectomy
Since cyclphosphamide has been reported to be more toxic in adrenalectomized dogs, adjustment of the doses of both replacement steroids and cyclophosphamide may be necessary for the adrenalectomized patient.
Wound Healing
Cyclophosphamide may interfere with normal wound healing.
Carcinogenesis, Mutagenesis, Impairment of Fertility
See WARNINGS section for information on carcinogenesis, mutagenesis, and impairment of fertility.
Pregnancy
Pregnancy Category D—See WARNINGS section.
Nursing Mothers
Cyclophosphamide is excreted in breast milk. Because of the potential for serious adverse reactions and the potential for tumorigenicity shown for cyclophosphamide in humans, a decision should be made whether to discontinue nursing or to discontinue the drug, taking into account the importance of the drug to the mother.

ADVERSE REACTIONS
Information on adverse reactions associated with the use of NEOSAR is arranged according to body system affected or type of reaction. The adverse reactions are listed in order of decreasing incidence. The most serious adverse reactions are described in the WARNINGS section.
Reproductive System
See WARNINGS section for information on impairment of fertility.
Digestive System
Nausea and vomiting commonly occur with cyclophosphamide therapy. Anorexia and, less frequently, abdominal discomfort or pain and diarrhea may occur. There are isolated reports of hemorrhagic colitis, oral mucosal ulceration and jaundice occurring during therapy. These adverse drug effects generally remit when cyclophosphamide treatment is stopped.
Skin and Its Structures
Alopecia occurs commonly in patients treated with cyclophosphamide. The hair can be expected to grow back after treatment with the drug or even during continued drug treatment, though it may be different in texture or color. Skin rash occurs occasionally in patients receiving the drug. Pigmentation of the skin and changes in nails can occur.
Hematopoietic System
Leukopenia occurs in patients treated with cylcophosphamide, is related to the dose of the drug, and can be used as a dosage guide. Leukopenia of less than 2000 cells/mm^3 develops commonly in patients treated with an intial loading dose of the drug, and less frequently in patients maintained on smaller doses. The degree of neutropenia is particularly important because it correlates with a reduction in resistance to infections.

Thrombocytopenia or anemia develop occasionally in patients treated with cyclophosphamide. These hematologic effects usually can be reversed by reducing the drug dose or by interrupting treatment. Recovery from leukopenia usually begins in 7 to 10 days after cessation of therapy.

Urinary System

See WARNINGS section for information on cystitis and urinary bladder fibrosis.

Hemorrhagic ureteritis and renal tubular necrosis have been reported to occur in patients treated with cyclophasphamide. Such lesions usually resolve following cessation of therapy.

Infections

See WARNINGS section for information on reduced host resistance to infections.

Carcinogenesis

See WARNINGS section for information on carcinogenesis.

Respiratory System

Interstitial pulmonary fibrosis has been reported in patients receiving high doses of cyclophosphamide over a prolonged period.

Other

Rare instances of anaphylactic reaction including one death have been reported. One instance of possible cross-sensitivity with other alkylating agents has been reported.

OVERDOSAGE

No specific antidote for cyclophosphamide is known. Overdosage should be managed with supportive measures, including appropriate treatment for any concurrent infection, myelosuppression, or cardiac toxicity should it occur.

DOSAGE AND ADMINISTRATION

Adults and Children

When used as the only oncolytic drug therapy, the initial course of NEOSAR for patients with no hematologic deficiency usually consists of 40 to 50 mg/kg given intravenously in divided doses over a period of 2 to 5 days. Other intravenous regimens include 10 to 15 mg/kg given every 7 to 10 days or 3 to 5 mg/kg twice weekly.

Many other regimens of intravenous NEOSAR have been reported. Dosages must be adjusted in accord with evidence of antitumor activity and/or leukopenia. The total leukocyte count is a good, objective guide for regulating dosage. Transient decreases in the total white blood cell count to 2000 cells/mm^3(following short courses) or more persistent reduction of 300 cells/mm^3(with continuing therapy) are tolerated without serious risk of infection if there is no marked granulocytopenia.

When NEOSAR is included in combined cytotoxic regimens, it may be necessary to reduce the dose of NEOSAR as well as that of the other drugs.

NEOSAR and its metabolites are dialyzable although there are probably quantitative differences depending upon the dialysis system being used. Patients with compromised renal function may show some measurable changes in pharmacokinetic parameters of NEOSAR metabolism, but there is no consistent evidence indicating a need for NEOSAR dosage modification in patients with renal function impairment.

Preparation and Handling of Solutions

Parenteral drug products should be inspected visually for particulate matter and discoloration prior to administration, whenever solution and container permit.

NEOSAR for Injection should be prepared for parenteral use by adding Bacteriostatic Water for Injection, USP, (paraben preserved only) or Sterile Water for Injection, USP to the vial and shaking to dissolve. Use the quantity of diluent shown below to reconstitute the product.

Dosage Strength	Quantity of Diluent
100 mg	5 mL
200 mg	10 mL
500 mg	25 mL
1g	50 mL
2g	100 mL

Solutions of NEOSAR may be injected intravenously, intramuscularly, intraperitoneally, or intrapleurally or they may be infused intravenously in the following:

Dextrose Injection, USP (5% dextrose)
Dextrose and Sodium Chloride Injection, USP (5% dextrose and 0.9% sodium chloride)
5% Dextrose and Ringer's Injection
Lactated Ringer's Injection, USP
Sodium Chloride Injection, USP (0.4% sodium chloride)
Sodium Lactate Injection, USP ($\frac{1}{6}$ molar sodium lactate)
Reconstituted NEOSAR is chemically and physically stable for 24 hours at room temperature or for six days in the refrigerator; it does not contain any antimicrobial preservative and thus care must be taken to assure the sterility of prepared solutions.

NEOSAR prepared by adding Bacteriostatic Water for Injection, USP (paraben preserved only) should be used within 24 hours if stored at room temperature or within 6 days if stored under refrigeration.

If NEOSAR is not prepared by adding Bacteriostatic Water for Injection, USP (paraben preserved only), it is recommended that the solution be used promptly (preferably within six hours).

The osmolarities of solutions of NEOSAR for Injection and normal saline are compared in the following table:

	mOsm/L
NEOSAR	352
Normal saline	287

Extemporaneous liquid preparations of NEOSAR for oral administration may be prepared by dissolving NEOSAR in Aromatic Elixir, N.F. Such preparations should be stored under refrigeration in glass containers and used within 14 days.

Handling and Disposal

Procedures for proper handling and disposal of anticancer drugs should be considered. Several guidelines on this subject have been published.[1-7] There is no general agreement that all the procedures recommended in the guidelines are necessary or appropriate.

HOW SUPPLIED

NEOSAR® (Cyclophosphamide for Injection, USP) contains 45 mg sodium chloride per 100 mg cyclophosphamide (anhydrous) and is available in the following single dose vials:

NDC 0013-5606-93 100 mg vials (yellow cap), cartons of 12
NDC 0013-5616-93 200 mg vials (blue cap), cartons of 12
NDC 0013-5626-93 500 mg vials (red cap), cartons of 12
NDC 0013-5636-70 1 gram vials (gray cap), cartons of 6
NDC 0013-5646-70 2 gram vials (violet cap), cartons of 6

Storage at temperatures not exceeding 25°C (77°F) is recommended. It will withstand brief exposure to temperatures up to 30°C (86°F), but is to be protected from temperatures above 30°C (86°F).

Caution: Federal law prohibits dispensing without prescription.

Manufactured by:

ASTA Pharma AG
BIELEFELD, GERMANY

For:

ADRIA LABORATORIES
Division of Erbamont Inc.
COLUMBUS, OHIO 43215

REFERENCES

1. Recommendations for the Safe Handling of Parenteral Antineoplastic Drugs. NIH Publication No. 83-2621. For sale by the Superintendent of Documents, U.S. Government Printing Office, Washington, D.C. 20402.
2. AMA Council Report. Guidelines for Handling Parenteral Antineoplastics, JAMA, March 15, 1985.
3. National Study Commission on Cytotoxic Exposure—Recommendations for Handling Cytotoxic Agents. Available from Louis P. Jeffrey, ScD., Director of Pharmacy Services, Rhode Island Hospital, 593 Eddy Street, Providence, Rhode Island 02902.
4. Clinical Oncological Society of Australia. Guidelines and recommendations for safe handling of antineoplastic agents. Med J Australia 1:426–428 1983.
5. Jones R.B., et al: Safe handling of chemotherapeutic agents: A report from the Mount Sinai Medical Center, CA-A Cancer Journal for Clinicians Sept./Oct., 258–263 1983.
6. American Society of Hospital Pharmacists technical assistance bulletin on handling cytotoxic drugs in hospitals. Am J Hosp Pharm 42:131–187, 1985.
7. OSHA Work-Practice Guidelines for Personnel Dealing with Cytotoxic (Antineoplastic) Drugs, AM J Hosp Pharm 1986;43:1193–1204.

NITROL® OINTMENT ℞

[nĭ′trŏl]

(2% Nitroglycerin Ointment, USP)

PRODUCT OVERVIEW

KEY FACTS

NITROL Ointment contains 2% nitroglycerin in a controlled release ointment. It is used to relieve pain caused by angina pectoris. It acts by relaxing vascular smooth muscle, producing a vasodilation of both peripheral arteries and veins. This action decreases venous return to the heart and reduces systemic vascular resistance and arterial pressure.

MAJOR USES

NITROL Ointment is used to treat and prevent angina pectoris. A suggested starting dose is $\frac{1}{2}$ inch (7.5 mg) applied to a $2\frac{1}{4} \times 3\frac{1}{2}$ inch area of the skin every 8 hours, covering the area with plastic wrap which can be held in place by adhesive tape. It may also be applied using an Appli-Tape™, a tape surrounded applicator that is applied to the skin.

SAFETY INFORMATION

NITROL Ointment is not to be used for immediate relief of anginal attacks. Severe hypotension especially when upright may occur even with small doses of nitroglycerin. Alcohol may increase the hypotensive effect of nitrates. Symptomatic orthostatic hypotension has been reported with the use of calcium channel blockers and organic nitrates in combination.

PRESCRIBING INFORMATION

NITROL® OINTMENT ℞

[nĭ′trŏl]

(2% Nitroglycerin Ointment)

DESCRIPTION

NITROL® Ointment contains 2% nitroglycerin in a special absorptive base formulated to provide a controlled release of active ingredient. Inactive ingredients: lactose, lanolin, purified water, white petrolatum. Each inch, as squeezed from the tube, contains approximately 15 mg of nitroglycerin.

ACTION

When the ointment is spread on the skin, the active ingredient (nitroglycerin) is continuously absorbed through the skin into the circulation, thus exerting prolonged vasodilator effect. Nitroglycerin ointment is effective in the control of angina pectoris when applied to the trunk or to the proximal parts of extremities.

Nitroglycerin relaxes smooth muscles, principally in the smaller blood vessels and dilates the arterioles and capillaries, especially in the coronary circulation. NITROL Ointment reduces the workload of the heart by virtue of its smooth muscle relaxation. This results predominantly in peripheral venous dilatation which reduces preload, but also to a lesser degree in a peripheral arteriolar dilatation which reduces afterload. These hemodynamic effects have been advanced as explanations for the beneficial actions of nitroglycerin ointment in angina pectoris. Nitroglycerin exerts a favorable influence on myocardial oxygen consumption, resulting in increased myocardial efficiency and significant improvement in left ventricular function. Computerized digital plethysmographic studies have shown the duration of action of NITROL Ointment (2 inches applied to the chest) to be eight hours in comparison to placebo; the onset of action occurred within thirty minutes of administration. Controlled clinical studies have demonstrated that nitroglycerin ointment increased measured exercise tolerance in patients with angina pectoris up to three hours after application (the maximal time interval studied).

INDICATIONS

This drug product has been conditionally approved by the FDA for the prevention and treatment of angina pectoris due to coronary artery disease. The conditional approval reflects a determination that the drug may be marketed pending FDA evaluation of data submitted in support of its effectiveness. A final evaluation of the effectiveness of the product will be announced by the FDA.

CONTRAINDICATIONS

In patients known to be intolerant of the organic nitrate drugs.

WARNINGS

In acute myocardial infarction or congestive heart failure, NITROL Ointment should be used under careful clinical and/or hemodynamic monitoring.

PRECAUTIONS

NITROL Ointment should not be used for treatment of acute anginal attacks. Symptoms of hypotension, particularly when suddenly arising from the recumbent position, are signs of overdosage. When they occur, the dosage should be reduced.

ADVERSE REACTIONS

Transient headaches are the most common side effect, especially at higher dosages. Headaches should be treated with mild analgesics and NITROL Ointment continued. Only with untreatable headaches should the dosage be reduced. Although uncommon, hypotension, an increase in heart rate, faintness, flushing, dizziness, and nausea may occur. These are all attributable to the pharmacologic effects of nitroglycerin on the cardiovascular system, and are symptoms of overdosage. When they occur and persist, the dosage should be reduced. Occasionally, contact dermatitis has been reported with continuous use of topical nitroglycerin. Such incidences may be reduced by changing the site of the application.

MANAGEMENT OF OVERDOSAGE

Severe hypotension may result from overdosage of nitroglycerin ointment. Should hypotension develop, quickly remove the ointment. The patient should be placed in a recumbent position with the legs elevated. In case of persistent hypotension, an IV infusion of 5% dextrose should be started.

Continued on next page

Adria—Cont.

DOSAGE AND ADMINISTRATION

Using Conventional Appli-Rulers™

When applying the ointment, use the Appli-Ruler™ dose determining applicator supplied with the package and squeeze the necessary amount of ointment from the tube on the applicator. Then place the applicator with the ointment side down onto the desired area of the skin, usually the chest (although other areas can be used). Spread the ointment over at least a $2\frac{1}{4} \times 3\frac{1}{2}$ inch area in a thin uniform layer using the applicator. Cover the area with plastic wrap which can be held in place by adhesive tape. The Appli-Ruler allows the patient to measure the necessary amount of ointment and to spread it without being absorbed through the fingers while applying to the skin surface.

Using Appli-Kit™

Measure the desired dosage of NITROL Ointment onto the Tape Surrounded Appli-Tape. Spread the ointment by carefully folding the Appli-Tape™. Be careful not to spread any ointment onto the outer lined border. Bend the Appli-Tape at the star, peel off and discard the outer lined border. Apply the Appli-Tape to the desired body area and press the adhesive border firmly to the skin. To assure proper ointment contact, gently press the entire Appli-Tape.

The usual therapeutic dose is 1 to 2 inches (2.5 to 5.0 cm) applied every eight hours, although some patients may require as much as 4 to 5 inches (10 to 12.5 cm) and/or application every four hours.

Start at $\frac{1}{2}$ inch (1.25 cm) every eight hours and increase the dose by $\frac{1}{2}$ inch (1.25 cm) with each successive application to achieve the desired clinical effects. The optimal dosage should be selected based upon the clinical responses, side effects and effects of therapy upon blood pressure. The greatest attainable decrease in resting blood pressure which is not associated with clinical symptoms of hypotension especially during orthostasis indicates the optimal dosage. To decrease adverse reactions, the dose and frequency of application should be tailored to the individual patient's needs.

The three gram titratable unit dose is a convenient hospital package. The tube has the same orifice as that of larger NITROL tube and any prescribed dose up to four inches may be dispensed from the tube using the instructions described above.

Keep tube tightly closed and store at controlled room temperature 15°–30°C (59°–86°F).

Caution: Federal law prohibits dispensing without prescription.

HOW SUPPLIED

(NDC 0013-5804-55) 30 gram tube
(NDC 0013-5804-56) 60 gram tube
(NDC 0013-5804-57) 30 gram 6 Pack
(NDC 0013-5804-58) 60 gram 6 Pack
(NDC 0013-5804-59) Titratable Unit Dose—50 × 3g Tubes
NITROL Ointment Appli-Kit™
(Packages include a supply of Appli-Tape™ for convenient application)
(NDC 0013-5804-46) 30 gram tube Appli-Kit
(NDC 0013-5804-47) 60 gram tube Appli-Kit
(NDC 0013-5804-48) Titratable Unit Dose—50 × 3g tubes Appli-Kit
Manufactured By:
PACO PHARMACEUTICAL SERVICES, INC.
LAKEWOOD, NJ 08701
For:
ADRIA LABORATORIES
Division of Erbamont Inc.
COLUMBUS, OHIO 43215
Shown in Product Identification Section, page 404

OCTAMIDE PFS™ ℞
(Metoclopramide Injection, USP)

DESCRIPTION

OCTAMIDE PFS™ (metoclopramide injection, USP) is a sterile parenteral, isotonic solution which contains no preservative, and is available in 2 mL (10 mg), 10 mL (50 mg) and 30 mL (150 mg) single dose only vials.

Each mL contains metoclopramide 5 mg (as the hydrochloride), and the following inactive ingredients: sodium chloride 8.5 mg and water for injection q.s. The pH is adjusted to a target pH of 4.0 with sodium hydroxide and/or hydrochloric acid.

Metoclopramide hydrochloride is a white or practically white, crystalline, odorless or practically odorless powder. It is very soluble in water, freely soluble in alcohol, sparingly soluble in chloroform, practically insoluble in ether. Chemically, it is 4-amino-5-chloro-N-[2-(diethylamino)ethyl]-2-methoxy benzamide monohydrochloride monohydrate. Molecular weight: 354.3.

CLINICAL PHARMACOLOGY

Metoclopramide stimulates motility of the upper gastrointestinal tract without stimulating gastric, biliary, or pancreatic secretions. Its mode of action is unclear. It seems to sensitize tissues to the action of acetylcholine. The effect of metoclopramide on motility is not dependent on intact vagal innervation, but it can be abolished by anticholinergic drugs. Metoclopramide increases the tone and amplitude of gastric (especially antral) contractions, relaxes the pyloric sphincter and the duodenal bulb, and increases peristalsis of the duodenum and jejunum resulting in accelerated gastric emptying and intestinal transit. It increases the resting tone of the lower esophageal sphincter. There is little, if any effect on the motility of the colon or gallbladder.

The antiemetic properties of metoclopramide appear to be a result of its antagonism of central and peripheral dopamine receptors. Dopamine produces nausea and vomiting by stimulation of the medullary chemoreceptor trigger zone (CTZ) and metoclopramide blocks stimulation of the CTZ by agents like l-dopa or apomorphine which are known to increase dopamine levels or to possess dopamine-like effects. Metoclopramide also abolishes the slowing of gastric emptying caused by apomorphine.

Like the phenothiazines and related drugs, which are also dopamine antagonists, metoclopramide produces sedation and may produce extrapyramidal reactions, although these are comparatively rare (See WARNINGS). Metoclopramide inhibits the central and peripheral effects of apomorphine, induces release of prolactin and causes a transient increase in circulating aldosterone levels, which may be associated with transient fluid retention.

The onset of pharmacological action of metoclopramide is 1 to 3 minutes following an intravenous dose, 10 to 15 minutes following intramuscular administration, and 30 to 60 minutes following an oral dose; pharmacologic effects persist for 1 to 2 hours.

Pharmcokinetics: It has been shown with an oral preparation that peak concentrations increase linearly with dose; time to peak concentration remains the same; whole body clearance is unchanged; and the elimination rate remains the same. The average elimination half-life in individuals with normal renal function is 5–6 hr. Linear kinetic processes adequately describe the absorption and elimination of metoclopramide.

Approximately 85% of the radioactivity of an orally administered dose appears in the urine within 72 hr. Of the 85% eliminated in the urine, about half is present as free or conjugated metoclopramide.

The drug is not extensively bound to plasma proteins (about 30%). The whole body volume of distribution is high (about 3.5 L/kg) which suggests extensive distribution of drug to the tissues.

Renal impairment affects the clearance of metoclopramide. In a study with patients with varying degrees of renal impairment, a reduction in creatinine clearance was correlated with a reduction in plasma clearance, renal clearance, nonrenal clearance, and increase in elimination half-life. The kinetics of metoclopramide in the presence of renal impairment remained linear however. The reduction in clearance as a result of renal impairment suggests that adjustment downward of maintenance dosage should be done to avoid drug cumulation.

INDICATIONS AND USAGE

Diabetic gastroparesis (diabetic gastric stasis): OCTAMIDE PFS is indicated for relief of symptoms associated with acute and recurrent diabetic gastric stasis. The usual manifestations of delayed gastric emptying (e.g., nausea, vomiting, heartburn, pesistent fullness after meals and anorexia) appear to respond to OCTAMIDE PFS within different time intervals. Significant relief of nausea occurs early and continues to improve over a three-week period. Relief of vomiting and anorexia may precede the relief of abdominal fullness by one week or more.

Prevention of nausea and vomiting associated with emetogenic cancer chemotherapy. OCTAMIDE PFS is indicated for the prophylaxis of vomiting associated with emetogenic cancer chemotherapy.

Small bowel intubation. OCTAMIDE PFS may be used to facilitate small bowel intubation in adults and children in whom the tube does not pass the pylorus with conventional maneuvers.

Radiological examination. OCTAMIDE PFS may be used to stimulate gastric emptying and intestinal transit of barium in cases where delayed emptying interferes with radiological examination of the stomach and/or small intestine.

CONTRAINDICATIONS

Metoclopramide should not be used whenever stimulation of gastrointestinal motility might be dangerous, e.g. in the presence of gastrointestinal hemorrhage, mechanical obstruction, or perforation.

Metoclopramide is contraindicated in patients with pheochromocytoma because the drug may cause a hypertensive crisis, probably due to release of catecholamines from the tumor. Such hypertensive crises may be controlled by phentolamine.

Metoclopramide is contraindicated in patients with known sensitivity or intolerance to the drug.

Metoclopramide should not be used in epileptics or patients receiving other drugs which are likely to cause extrapyramidal reactions, since the frequency and severity of seizures or extrapyramidal reactions may be increased.

WARNINGS

Depression bearing a temporal relationship to metoclopramide administration has been reported.

Extrapyramidal symptoms, manifested primarily as acute dystonic reactions, occur in approximately 1 in 500 patients treated with the usual adult dosages of 30–40 mg/day of metoclopramide. These usually are seen during the first 24–48 hours of treatment with metoclopramide, occur more frequently in children and young adults, and are even more frequent at the higher doses used in prophylaxis of vomiting due to cancer chemotherapy. These symptoms may include involuntary movements of limbs and facial grimacing, torticollis, oculogyric crisis, rhythmic protrusion of tongue, bulbar type of speech, trismus, or dystonic reactions resembling tetanus. Rarely, dystonic reactions may present as stridor and dyspnea, possibly due to laryngospasm. If these symptoms should occur, inject 50 mg diphenhydramine hydrochloride intramuscularly, and they usually will subside. Benztropine mesylate 1 to 2 mg intramuscularly, may also be used to reverse these reactions.

Parkinsonian-like symptoms have occurred, more commonly within the first 6 months after beginning treatment with metoclopramide, but occasionally after long periods. These symptoms generally subside within 2–3 months following discontinuance of metoclopramide.

Tardive Dyskinesia: Tardive dyskinesia, a syndrome consisting of potentially irreversible, involuntary, dyskinetic movements may develop in patients treated with metoclopramide. Although the prevalence of the syndrome appears to be highest among the elderly, especially elderly women, it is impossible to predict which patients are likely to develop the syndrome. Both the risk of developing the syndrome and the likelihood that it will become irreversible are believed to increase with the duration of treatment and the total cumulative dose.

Less commonly, the syndrome can develop after relatively brief treatment periods at low doses; in these cases, symptoms appear more likely to be reversible.

There is no known treatment for established cases of tardive dyskinesia although the syndrome may remit, partially or completely, within several weeks-to-months after metoclopramide is withdrawn. Metoclopramide itself, however, may suppress (or partially suppress) the signs of tardive dyskinesia, thereby masking the underlying disease process. The effect of this symptomatic suppression upon the long-term course of the syndrome is unknown. Therefore, the use of metoclopramide for the symptomatic control of tardive dyskinesia is not recommended.

PRECAUTIONS

General: In one study of hypertensive patients, intravenously administered metoclopramide was shown to release catecholamines: hence, caution should be exercised when metoclopramide is used in patients with hypertension.

Intravenous injections of undiluted metoclopramide should be made slowly allowing 1 to 2 minutes for 10 mg since a transient but intense feeling of anxiety and restlessness, followed by drowsiness, may occur with rapid administration.

Intravenous administration of OCTAMIDE PFS diluted in a parenteral solution should be made slowly over a period of not less than 15 minutes.

Information for patients: Metoclopramide may impair the mental and/or physical abilities required for the performance of hazardous tasks such as operating machinery or driving a motor vehicle. The ambulatory patient should be cautioned accordingly.

Drug Interactions. The effects of metoclopramide on gastrointestinal motility are antagonized by anticholinergic drugs and narcotic analgesics. Additive sedative effects can occur when metoclopramide is given with alcohol, sedatives, hypnotics, narcotics or tranquilizers.

The finding that metoclopramide releases catecholamines in patients with essential hypertension suggests that it should be used cautiously, if at all, in patients receiving monoamine oxidase inhibitors.

Absorption of drugs from the stomach may be diminished (e.g. digoxin) by metoclopramide, whereas absorption of drugs from the small bowel may be accelerated (e.g. acetaminophen, tetracycline, levodopa, ethanol).

Gastroparesis (gastric stasis) may be responsible for poor diabetic control in some patients. Exogenously administered insulin may begin to act before food has left the stomach and lead to hypoglycemia. Because the action of metoclopramide will influence the delivery of food to the intestines and thus the rate of absorption, insulin dosage or timing of dosage may require adjustment.

Carcinogenesis, Mutagenesis, Impairment of Fertility. A 77 week study was conducted in rats with oral doses up to about 40 times the maximum recommended human daily dose. Metoclopramide elevates prolactin levels and the elevation persists during chronic administration. Tissue culture experiments indicate that approximately one-third of human breast cancers are prolactin-dependent *in vitro*, a factor of potential importance if the prescription of metoclopramide is contemplated in a patient with previously detected breast cancer. Although disturbances such as galactorrhea, amenorrhea, gynecomastia, and impotence have been reported with prolactin-elevating drugs, the clinical significance of elevated serum prolactin levels is unknown for most patients. An increase in mammary neoplasms has been found in rodents after chronic administration of prolactin-stimulating neuroleptic drugs and metoclopramide. Neither clinical studies nor epidemiologic studies conducted to date, however, have shown an association between chronic administration of these drugs and mammary tumorigenesis; the available evidence is too limited to be conclusive at this time. An Ames mutagenicity test performed on metoclopramide was negative.

Pregnancy Category B. Reproduction studies performed in rats, mice, and rabbits by the i.v., i.m., s.c. and oral routes at maximum levels ranging from 12 to 250 times the human dose have demonstrated no impairment of fertility or significant harm to the fetus due to metoclopramide. There are, however, no adequate and well-controlled studies in pregnant women. Because animal reproduction studies are not always predictive of human response, this drug should be used during pregnancy only if clearly needed.

Nursing Mothers. Metoclopramide is excreted in human milk. Caution should be exercised when metoclopramide is administered to a nursing mother.

ADVERSE REACTIONS

In general, the incidence of adverse reactions correlates with the dose and duration of metoclopramide administration. The following reactions have been reported, although in most instances, data do not permit an estimate of frequency:

CNS Effects. Restlessness, drowsiness, fatigue and lassitude occur in approximately 10% of patients receiving the most commonly prescribed dosage of 10 mg q.i.d. (see PRECAUTIONS). Insomnia, headache, confusion, dizziness or depression (see WARNINGS) occur less frequently. In cancer chemotherapy patients being treated with 1–2 mg/kg per dose, incidence of drowsiness is about 70%. There are isolated reports of convulsive seizures without clearcut relationship to metoclopramide. Rarely, hallucinations have been reported.

Extrapyramidal Reactions (EPS). Acute dystonic reactions, the most common type of EPS associated with metoclopramide, occur in approximately 0.2% of patients (1 in 500) treated with 30 to 40 mg of metoclopramide per day. In cancer chemotherapy patients receiving 1–2 mg/kg per dose, the incidence is 2% in patients over the age of 30–35, and 25% or higher in children and young adults who have not had prophylactic administration of diphenhydramine. Symptoms include involuntary movements of limbs, facial grimacing, torticollis, oculogyric crisis, rhythmic protusion of the tongue, bulbar type of speech, trismus, opisthotonus (tetanus-like reactions) and rarely, stridor and dyspnea possibly due to laryngospasm; ordinarily these symptoms are readily reversed by diphenhydramine (see WARNINGS).

Parkinsonian-like symptoms may include bradykinesia, tremor, cogwheel rigidity, mask-like facies (see WARNINGS).

Tardive dyskinesia most frequently is characterized by involuntary movements of the tongue, face, mouth or jaw, and sometimes by involuntary movements of the trunk and/or extremities (see WARNINGS).

Motor restlessness (akathisia) may consist of feelings of anxiety, agitation, jitteriness, and insomnia, as well as inability to sit still, pacing, foot-tapping. These symptoms may disappear spontaneously or respond to a reduction in dosage.

Endocrine Disturbances. Galactorrhea, amenorrhea, gynecomastia, impotence secondary to hyperprolactinemia (see PRECAUTIONS). Fluid retention secondary to transient elevation of aldosterone (see CLINICAL PHARMACOLOGY).

Cardiovascular. Hypotension, hypertension and a single instance of supraventricular tachycardia (see CONTRAINDICATIONS and PRECAUTIONS).

Gastrointestinal. Nausea and bowel disturbances, primarily diarrhea.

Hepatic. Rarely, cases of hepatotoxicity, characterized by such findings as jaundice and altered liver function tests, when metroclopramide was administered with other drugs with known hepatotoxic potential.

Renal. Urinary frequency and incontinence.

Hemotologic. A few cases of neutropenia, leukopenia, or agranulocytosis, generally without clearcut relationship to metoclopramide.

Allergic Reactions. A few cases of rash, urticaria, bronchospasm, especially in patients with a history of asthma.

Container	Total Contents*	Concentration	Administration
2 mL single dose vial	10 mg	5 mg/mL	For IV or IM Administration
10 mL single dose vial	50 mg	5mg/mL	For IV Infusion Only; Dilute Before Using
30 mL single dose vial	150 mg	5 mg/mL	For IV Infusion Only; Dilute Before Using

*Metoclopramide (as the hydrochloride)

Rarely, angioneurotic edema, including glossal or laryngeal edema.

Miscellaneous. Visual disturbances. Porphyria. Rare occurences of neuroleptic malignant syndrome (NMS) have been reported. This potentially fatal syndrome is comprised of the symptom complex of hyperthermia, altered consciousness, muscular rigidity and autonomic dysfunction.

Transient flushing of the face and upper body, without alterations in vital signs, following high doses intravenously.

OVERDOSAGE

Symptoms of overdosage may include drowsiness, disorientation and extrapyramidal reactions. Anticholinergic or antiparkinson drugs or antihistamines with anticholinergic properties may be helpful in controlling the extrapyramidal reactions. Symptoms are self-limiting and usually disappear within 24 hours.

Hemodialysis removes relatively little metoclopramide, probably because of the small amount of the drug in blood relative to tissues. Similarly, continuous ambulatory peritoneal dialysis does not remove significant amounts of drug. It is unlikely that dosage would need to be adjusted to compensate for losses through dialysis. Dialysis is not likely to be an effective method of drug removal in overdose situations.

Literature reports describe methemoglobinemia in premature and full term neonates who were given metoclopramide intramuscularly, 1 to 2 mg/kg/day for 3 or more days. Methemoglobinemia has not been reported in similar infants treated with 0.5 mg/kg/day in divided doses. Methemoglobinemia can be reversed by the intravenous administration of methylene blue.

DOSAGE AND ADMINISTRATION

For the relief of symptoms associated with diabetic gastroparesis (diabetic gastric stasis): Administer 10 mg of metoclopramide 30 minutes before each meal and at bedtime for two to eight weeks, depending upon response and the likelihood of continued well-being upon drug discontinuation.

The initial route of administration should be determined by the severity of the presenting symptoms. If only the earliest manifestations of diabetic gastric stasis are present, oral administration of metoclopramide may be initiated. However, if severe symptoms are present, therapy should begin with OCTAMIDE PFS (I.M. or I.V.). Doses of 10 mg may be administered slowly by the intravenous route over a 1 to 2 minute period.

Administration of OCTAMIDE PFS up to 10 days may be required before symptoms subside, at which time oral administration may be instituted. Since diabetic gastric stasis is frequently recurrent, OCTAMIDE PFS therapy should be reinstituted at the earliest manifestation.

For the prevention of nausea and vomiting associated with emetogenic cancer chemotherapy. For doses in excess of 10 mg, OCTAMIDE PFS should be diluted in 50 mL of a parenteral solution.

The preferred parenteral solution is Sodium Chloride Injection (normal saline), which when combined with OCTAMIDE PFS, can be stored frozen for up to 4 weeks. OCTAMIDE PFS is degraded when admixed and frozen with Dextrose-5% in Water. OCTAMIDE PFS diluted in Sodium Chloride Injection, Dextrose-5% in Water, Dextrose-5% in 0.45% Sodium Chloride, Ringer's Injection or Lactated Ringer's Injection may be stored up to 48 hours (without freezing) after preparation if protected from light. All dilutions may be stored unprotected from light under normal light conditions up to 24 hours after preparation.

Intravenous infusions should be made slowly over a period of not less than 15 minutes, 30 minutes before beginning cancer chemotherapy and repeated every 2 hours for two doses, then every 3 hours for three doses.

The initial two doses should be 2 mg/kg if highly emetogenic drugs such as cisplatin or dacarbazine are used alone or in combination. For less emetogenic regimens, 1 mg/kg per dose may be adequate.

If extrapyramidal symptoms should occur, inject diphenhydramine hydrochloride intramuscularly and EPS usually will subside.

To facilitate small bowel intubation. If the tube has not passed the pylorus with conventional maneuvers in 10 minutes, a single dose (undiluted) may be administered slowly by the intravenous route over a 1 to 2 minute period.

The recommended single dose is: Adults—10 mg metoclopramide base (2 mL). Children (6–14 years of age)—2.5 to 5 mg metoclopramide base (0.5 to 1 mL): (under 6 years of age)—0.1 mg metoclopramide base/kg of body weight.

To aid in radiological examinations: In patients where delayed gastric emptying interferes with radiological examination of the stomach and/or small intestine, a single dose may be administered slowly by the intravenous route over a 1 to 2 minute period.

For dosage, see intubation above.

Use in patients with Renal or Hepatic Impairment: Since metoclopramide is excreted principally through the kidneys, in those patients whose creatinine clearance is below 40 mL/min, therapy should be initiated at approximately one-half the recommended dosage. Depending upon clinical efficacy and safety considerations, the dosage may be increased or decreased as appropriate.

See Overdosage Section for information regarding dialysis. Metoclopramide undergoes minimal hepatic metabolism, except for simple conjugation. Its safe use has been described in patients with advanced liver disease whose renal function was normal.

Admixture Compatibilities. OCTAMIDE PFS is compatible for mixing with the following injectable products to the extent indicated below: (Note: specific formulation differences may alter these findings).

Physically and Chemically Compatible up to 48 hours. Cimetidine Hydrochloride (SK&F), Mannitol USP (Abbott), Potassium Acetate, USP (Invenex), Potassium Chloride, USP (ESI), Potassium Phosphate, USP (Invenex).

Physically Compatible up to 48 hours. Ascorbic Acid, USP (Abbott), Benztropine Mesylate, USP (MS&D), Cytarabine, USP (Upjohn), Dexamethasone Sodium Phosphate, USP (ESI, MS&D), Diphenhydramine Hydrochloride, USP (Parke-Davis), Doxorubicin Hydrochloride, USP (Adria), Heparin Sodium, USP (ESI), Hydrocortisone Sodium Phosphate (MS&D), Lidocaine Hydrochloride, USP (ESI), Magnesium Sulfate, USP (ESI), Multi-Vitamin Infusion (must be refrigerated-USV), Vitamin B Complex with Ascorbic Acid (Roche).

Physically Compatible up to 24 hours. (Do not use if precipitation occurs). Aminophylline, USP (ESI), Clindamycin Phosphate, USP (Upjohn), Cyclophosphamide, USP (Mead-Johnson), Insulin, USP (Lilly), Methylprednisolone Sodium Succinate, USP (ESI).

Conditionally Compatible. (Use within one hour after mixing or may be infused into the same running I.V. line). Ampicillin Sodium, USP (Bristol), Calcium Gluconate, USP (ESI), Cisplatin, USP (Bristol), Erythromycin Lactobionate, USP (Abbott), Methotrexate Sodium, USP (Lederle), Penicillin G Potassium, USP (Squibb), Tetracycline Hydrochloride, USP (Lederle).

Incompatible. (Do not mix). Cephalothin Sodium, USP (Lilly), Chloramphenicol Sodium, USP (Parke-Davis), Sodium Bicarbonate, USP (Abbott).

Parenteral drug products should be inspected visually for particulate matter and discoloration prior to administration, whenever solution and container permit.

HOW SUPPLIED

OCTAMIDE PFS™ (metoclopramide injection, USP) Sterile, Isotonic Solution, contains no preservatives

NDC 0013-6106-95, 10 mg vial (mist grey cap), 5 mg per mL, 2 mL, cartons of 25

NDC 0013-6116-95, 50 mg vial (blue cap), 5 mg per mL, 10 mL, cartons of 25

NDC 0013-6126-95, 150 mg vial (red cap), 5 mg per mL, 30 mL, cartons of 25

NDC 0013-6126-70, 150 mg vial (red cap), 5 mg per mL, 30 mL, cartons of 6

[See table above].

Store vials in cartons until time of use. Do not store open vials for later use, as they contain no preservative. **Dilutions may be stored unprotected from light under normal conditions up to 24 hours after preparation.**

STORE PRODUCT AT CONTROLLED ROOM TEMPERATURE, 15°–30°C (59°–86°F).

Manufactured by:
DAVID BULL LABORATORIES, PTY. LTD.
MULGRAVE, VICTORIA 3170 AUSTRALIA
For:
ADRIA LABORATORIES
Division of Erbamont Inc.
COLUMBUS, OHIO 43215

Continued on next page

Adria—Cont.

TYMPAGESIC®   ℞
[tim "pah-jē 'sik]
Otic Solution

Analgesic-Decongestant Ear Drops

DESCRIPTION
TYMPAGESIC Otic Solution, analgesic-decongestant ear drops, contains phenylephrine hydrochloride USP 0.25%, antipyrine USP 5% and benzocaine USP 5% in propylene glycol USP.

Phenylephrine hydrochloride is a sympathomimetic amine with local vasoconstriction or decongestant action. It is chemically (1) Benzenemethanol, 3-hydroxy-α-[(methyl-amino)methyl]-, hydrochloride (R) (2) (—)-*m*-Hydroxy-α-[methylamino)methyl]benzyl alcohol hydrochloride CAS 61-76-7

It occurs as white crystals, has a bitter taste and is freely soluble in water and alcohol.

Antipyrine is an analgesic with local anesthetic action. It is chemically 2,3-dimethyl-1-phenyl-3-pyrazolin-5-one CAS 60-80-0

Antipyrine appears as colorless crystals or white powder, has a slightly bitter taste and is soluble in water and alcohol.

Benzocaine is a local anesthetic. It is chemically ethyl *p*-aminobenzoate CAS 04-09-7

It occurs as white crystals or white crystalline powder and is slightly soluble in water and soluble in organic solvents.

CLINICAL PHARMACOLOGY
Topical application of phenylephrine produces vasoconstriction mainly by a direct effect on α-adrenergic receptors. The effects of phenylephrine are similar to those of epinephrine. However, phenylephrine is considered less CNS and cardiostimulatory than epinephrine. Phenylephrine, after its absorption, is metabolized in the liver and the intestine by the enzyme monoamine oxidase (MAO). The type, route and rate of excretion of metabolites have not been defined.

Like other local anesthetics, benzocaine acts by blocking nerve conduction first in autonomic, then in sensory and finally in motor nerve fibers. Its effect appears to be due to decreased nerve cell membrane permeability to sodium ions or competition with calcium ions for membrane binding sites. A vasoconstrictor, such as phenylephrine, is added to decrease the rate of absorption and prolong the duration of action of the anesthetic. Ester-type anesthetics, which include benzocaine, after absorption are comparatively rapidly degraded by esterases mainly in the liver and excreted in the urine as metabolites and in small amounts as the unchanged drug.

Antipyrine is believed to have analgesic and local anesthetic effects on the nerve endings. After absorption, it is slowly metabolized in the liver by oxidation and conjugation with glucuronic acid and is excreted in the urine mainly in the conjugated form.

INDICATIONS AND USAGE
TYMPAGESIC Otic Solution may be used as a topical anesthetic in the external auditory canal to relieve ear pain.
It may be used concomitantly with systemic antibiotics as in the treatment of acute otitis media.

CONTRAINDICATIONS
TYMPAGESIC 'or any medication for use in the external ear canal is contraindicated in the presence of a perforated tympanic membrane or ear discharge and in individuals with a history of hypersensitivity to any of its ingredients.

WARNINGS
As with all drugs containing a sympathomimetic or an anesthetic, systemic reactions may occur after local application. Phenylephrine may cause blanching and a feeling of coolness in the skin. Allergic and idiosyncratic reactions to local anesthetics have been observed infrequently. Such reactions are unlikely because absorption from the skin of the ear drum or the external ear canal is minimal.
Discontinue promptly if sensitization or irritation occurs.
Cross-sensitivity reactions between members of the *caine* group of local anesthetics have been reported.
Contains *sodium metabisulfite*, a sulfite that may cause allergic-type reactions including anaphylactic symptoms and life-threatening or less severe asthmatic episodes in certain susceptible people. The overall prevalence of sulfite sensitivity in the general population is unknown and probably low. Sulfite sensitivity is seen more frequently in asthmatic than in nonasthmatic people.

PRECAUTIONS
General —Drugs containing a sympathomimetic should be used with caution in the elderly and in patients with hypertension, increased intraocular pressure, diabetes mellitus, ischemic heart disease, hyperthyroidism and prostatic hypertrophy.

High plasma levels of benzocaine and antipyrine may cause CNS stimulation with nausea and vomiting. Such levels, however, are unlikely to be attained following local application in the external ear.
Drug Interactions —MAO inhibitors and β-adrenergic blockers enhance the effects of sympathomimetics. Benzocaine is hydrolyzed in the body to p-aminobenzoic acid which competes with the antibacterial action of sulfonamides. However, these are unlikely to occur because of the limited absorption from the external ear canal.
Carcinogenesis, Mutagenesis, Impairment of Fertility —There have been no studies in animals or humans to evaluate the carcinogenesis, mutagenesis or impairment of fertility for **TYMPAGESIC**.
Pregnancy —Category C. Animal reproduction studies have not been conducted with **TYMPAGESIC**. It is also not known whether **TYMPAGESIC** can cause fetal harm when administered to a pregnant woman or can effect reproduction capacity. **TYMPAGESIC** should be given to a pregnant woman only if clearly needed.
Nursing Mothers —It is not known whether this drug is excreted in human milk. Because many drugs are excreted in human milk, caution should be exercised when **TYMPAGESIC** is administered to a nursing woman.
Pediatric Use —Safety and effectiveness in children below the age of 12 has not been established.

ADVERSE REACTIONS
Following its absorption, phenylephrine may produce a pressor response or cause restlessness, anxiety, nervousness, weakness, pallor, headache and dizziness. Absorption of benzocaine and antipyrine in the plasma may cause chills, nausea, vomiting, tinnitus and agranulocytosis. Such reactions are unlikely following application of **TYMPAGESIC** on the external ear canal.
Benzocaine can cause a hypersensitivity reaction consisting of rash, urticaria and edema. Individuals frequently exposed to ester-type local anesthetics can develop contact dermatitis characterized by erythema and pruritus which may progress to vesiculation and oozing.

OVERDOSAGE
It is more likely to be associated with accidental or deliberate ingestion rather than cutaneous absorption. Phenylephrine present in a bottle (13 mL) of **TYMPAGESIC**, if absorbed, may cause hypertension, headache, vomiting and palpitations. Effects of benzocaine overdosage may include yawning, restlessness, excitement, nausea and vomiting. Antipyrine overdosage may cause giddiness, tremor, sweating and skin eruptions.
Treatment is symptomatic. If ingestion of the contents of a bottle or more of **TYMPAGESIC** is recent or food is present in the stomach, induction of emesis with ipecac syrup, gastric emptying and lavage and introduction of activated charcoal may be recommended.

DOSAGE AND ADMINISTRATION
Using the dropper, instill **TYMPAGESIC** Otic Solution in the external ear canal allowing the solution to run into the canal until filled. Insert a cotton pledget into the meatus after moistening with the otic solution. Repeat every 2 to 4 hours, if necessary, until pain is relieved.
Replace dropper in bottle without rinsing.

HOW SUPPLIED
TYMPAGESIC Otic Solution is supplied in 13 mL amber glass bottle with a dropper.
(NDC 0013-7363-39).
Store at 15°–30°C (59°–86°F).
ADRIA LABORATORIES
Division of Erbamont Inc.
COLUMBUS, OHIO 43215

VANCOR™   ℞
(STERILE VANCOMYCIN HYDROCHLORIDE, USP)
FOR INTRAVENOUS USE

DESCRIPTION
VANCOR™ (Sterile Vancomycin Hydrochloride, USP), intravenous, is a tricyclic glycopeptide antibiotic derived from *Nocardia orientalis* (formerly *Streptomyces orientalis*) and has the chemical formula $C_{66}H_{75}Cl_2N_9O_{24}$. The formula weight is 1449; 500 mg of the base are equivalent to 0.35 mmol.
VANCOR is available in 500 mg and 1 gram strengths, each available as sterile lyophilized powder in vials for single use only.
It is an off-white to buff-colored lyophilized plug. When reconstituted in water, it forms a clear solution with a pH range of 2.5 to 4.5.

CLINICAL PHARMACOLOGY
Vancomycin is poorly absorbed after oral administration; it is given intravenously for therapy of systemic infections. Intramuscular injection is painful.
In subjects with normal kidney function, multiple intravenous dosing of 1 g of vancomycin (15 mg/kg) infused over 60 minutes produces mean plasma concentrations of approximately 63 mg/L immediately at the completion of infusion, mean plasma concentrations of approximately 23 mg/L 2 hours after infusion, and mean plasma concentrations of approximately 8 mg/L 11 hours after the end of the infusion. Multiple dosing of 500 mg infused over 30 minutes produces mean plasma concentrations of about 49 mg/L at the completion of infusion, mean plasma concentrations of about 19 mg/L 2 hours after infusion, and mean plasma concentrations of about 10 mg/L 6 hours after infusion. The plasma concentrations during multiple dosing are similar to those after a single dose.
The mean elimination half-life of vancomycin from plasma is 4 to 6 hours in subjects with normal renal function. In the first 24 hours, about 75% of an administered dose of vancomycin is excreted in urine by glomerular filtration. Mean plasma clearance is about 0.058 L/kg/hr, and mean renal clearance is about 0.048 L/kg/hr. Renal dysfunction slows excretion of vancomycin. In anephric patients, the average half-life of elimination is 7.5 days. The distribution coefficient is from 0.3 to 0.43 L/kg. There is no apparent metabolism of the drug. About 60% of an intraperitoneal dose of vancomycin administered during peritoneal dialysis is absorbed systemically in 6 hours. Serum concentrations of about 10 mg/L are achieved by intraperitoneal injection of 30 mg/kg of vancomycin. Vancomycin is not effectively removed by either hemodialysis or peritoneal dialysis; there have been no reports of vancomycin clearance with hemoperfusion.
Total systemic and renal clearance of vancomycin may be reduced in the elderly.
Vancomycin is approximately 55% serum protein bound as measured by ultrafiltration at vancomycin serum concentrations of 10 to 100 mg/L. After IV administration of vancomycin hydrochloride, inhibitory concentrations are present in pleural, pericardial, ascitic, and synovial fluids; in urine; in peritoneal dialysis fluid; and in atrial appendage tissue. Vancomycin hydrochloride does not readily diffuse across normal meninges into the spinal fluid; but, when the meninges are inflamed, penetration into the spinal fluid occurs.
Microbiology —The bactericidal action of vancomycin results primarily from inhibition of cell-wall biosynthesis. In addition, vancomycin alters bacterial-cell-membrane permeability and RNA synthesis. There is no cross-resistance between vancomycin and other antibiotics. Vancomycin is active against staphylococci, including *Staphylococcus aureus* and *Staphylococcus epidermis* (including heterogeneous methicillin-resistant strains); streptococci, including *Streptococcus pyogenes, Streptococcus pneumoniae* (including penicillin-resistant strains), *Streptococcus agalactiae,* the viridans group, *Streptococcus bovis,* and enterococci (eg, *Streptococcus faecalis*); *Clostridium difficile* (eg, toxigenic strains implicated in pseudomembranous enterocolitis); and diphtheroids. Other organisms that are susceptible to vancomycin in vitro include *Listeria monocytogenes, Lactobacillus* species, *Actinomyces* species, *Clostridium* species, and *Bacillus* species.
Vancomycin is not active in vitro against gram-negative bacilli, mycobacteria, or fungi.
Synergy —The combination of vancomycin and an aminoglycoside acts synergistically in vitro against many strains of *S aureus,* nonenterococcal group D streptococci, enterococci, and *Streptococcus* species (viridans group).
Disc Susceptibility Tests —The standardized method described by the National Committee for Clinical Laboratory Standards has been recommended for use with discs to test susceptibility to vancomycin. Results of standard single-dose susceptibility tests with a 30-μg vancomycin hydrochloride disc should be interpreted according to the following criteria. Susceptible organisms produce zones greater than or equal to 12 mm, indicating that the test organism is likely to respond to therapy. Organisms that produce zones of 10 or 11 mm are considered to be of intermediate susceptibility. Organisms in this category are likely to respond if the infection is confined to tissues or fluids in which high antibiotic concentrations are attained. Resistant organisms produce zones of 9 mm or less, indicating that other therapy should be selected.
With a standardized dilution method, a bacterial isolate may be considered susceptible if the MIC value for vancomycin is 4 mg/L or less. Organisms are considered resistant to vancomycin if the MIC is greater than or equal to 16 mg/L. Organisms having an MIC value of less than 16 mg/L but greater than 4 mg/L are considered to be of intermediate susceptibility.[1–3]
Standardized procedures require the use of laboratory control organisms. The 30-μg vancomycin disc should give zone diameters between 15 and 19 mm for *S aureus* ATCC 25923. As with the standard diffusion methods, dilution procedures require the use of laboratory control organisms. Standard vancomycin powder should give MIC values in the range of 0.5 mg/L to 2.0 mg/L for *S aureus* ATCC 29213. For *S faecalis* ATCC 29212, the MIC range should be 1.0 to 4.0 mg/L.

INDICATIONS AND USAGE

VANCOR is indicated for the treatment of serious or severe infections caused by susceptible strains of methicillin-resistant (β-lactam-resistant) staphylococci. It is indicated for penicillin-allergic patients, for patients who cannot receive or who have failed to respond to other drugs, including the penicillins or cephalosporins, and for infections caused by vancomycin-susceptible organisms that are resistant to other antimicrobial drugs. VANCOR is indicated for initial therapy when methicillin-resistant staphylococci are suspected, but after susceptibility data are available, therapy should be adjusted accordingly.

VANCOR is effective in the treatment of staphylococci endocarditis. Its effectiveness has been documented in other infections due to staphylococci, including septicemia, bone infections, lower respiratory tract infections, and skin and skin-structure infections. When staphylococcal infections are localized and purulent, antibiotics are used as adjuncts to appropriate surgical measures.

VANCOR has been reported to be effective alone or in combination with an aminoglycoside for endocarditis caused by S viridans or S bovis. For endocarditis caused by enterococci (eg, S faecalis), VANCOR has been reported to be effective only in combination with an aminoglycoside.

VANCOR has been reported to be effective for the treatment of diphtheroid endocarditis. VANCOR has been used successfully in combination with rifampin, an aminoglycoside, or both in early-onset prosthetic valve endocarditis caused by S epidermidis or diphtheroids.

Specimens for bacteriologic cultures should be obtained in order to isolate and identify causative organisms and to determine their susceptibility to VANCOR.

The parenteral form of VANCOR may be administered orally for treatment of antibiotic-associated pseudomembranous colitis produced by C difficile. Parenteral administration of VANCOR alone is of unproven benefit for this indication. VANCOR is not effective by the oral route for other types of infection.

Although no controlled clinical efficacy studies have been conducted, intravenous vancomycin has been suggested by the American Heart Association and the American Dental Association for prophylaxis against bacterial endocarditis in patients allergic to penicillin who have congenital heart disease or rheumatic or other acquired valvular heart disease when these patients undergo dental procedures or surgical procedures of the upper respiratory tract.

Note: When selecting antibiotics for the prevention of bacterial endocarditis, the physician or dentist should read the full joint statement of the American Heart Association and the American Dental Association.[4]

CONTRAINDICATIONS

VANCOR is contraindicated in patients with known hypersensitivity to this antibiotic.

WARNINGS

Rapid bolus administration (eg, over several minutes) may be associated with exaggerated hypotension and, rarely, cardiac arrest.

VANCOR should be administered in a dilute solution over a period of not less than 60 minutes to avoid rapid-infusion-related reactions. Stopping the infusion usually results in a prompt cessation of these reactions.

Ototoxicity has occurred in patients receiving vancomycin. It may be transient or permanent. It has been reported mostly in patients who have been given excessive doses, who have an underlying hearing loss, or who are receiving concomitant therapy with another ototoxic agent, such as an aminoglycoside. Vancomycin should be used with caution in patients with renal insufficiency because the risk of toxicity is appreciably increased by high, prolonged blood concentrations.

Dosage of VANCOR must be adjusted for patients with renal dysfunction (see Precautions and Dosage and Administration).

PRECAUTIONS

General —Clinically significant serum concentrations have been reported in some patients being treated for active C difficile-induced pseudomembranous colitis after multiple oral doses of vancomycin.

In order to minimize the risk of nephrotoxicity when treating patients with underlying renal dysfunction or patients receiving concomitant therapy with an aminoglycoside, serial monitoring of renal function should be performed and particular care should be taken in following appropriate dosing schedules (see Dosage and Administration).

Serial tests of auditory function may be helpful in order to minimize the risk of ototoxicity.

Reversible neutropenia has been reported in patients receiving vancomycin hydrochloride (see Adverse Reactions). Patients who will undergo prolonged therapy with VANCOR or those who are receiving concomitant drugs which may cause neutropenia should have periodic monitoring of the leukocyte count.

VANCOR is irritating to tissue and must be given by a secure intravenous route of administration. Pain, tenderness, and necrosis occur with intramuscular injection of VANCOR or with inadvertent extravasation. Thrombophlebitis may occur, the frequency and severity of which can be minimized by administering the drug slowly as a dilute solution (2.5 to 5 g/L) and by rotating the sites of infusion.

There have been reports that the frequency of infusion-related events (including hypotension, flushing, erythema, urticaria, and pruritus) increases with the concomitant administration of anesthetic agents. Infusion-related events may be minimized by the administration of VANCOR as a 60-minute infusion prior to anesthetic induction.

The safety and efficacy of vancomycin administration by the intrathecal (intralumbar or intraventricular) route have not been assessed.

Concurrent and/or sequential systemic or topical use of other potentially neurotoxic and/or nephrotoxic drugs, such as amphotericin B, aminoglycosides, bacitracin, polymyxin B, colistin, viomycin, or cisplatin, requires careful monitoring.

Usage in Pregnancy —Pregnancy Category C —Animal reproduction studies have not been conducted with VANCOR. It is also not known whether VANCOR can cause fetal harm when administered to a pregnant woman or can affect reproduction capacity. VANCOR should be given to a pregnant woman only if clearly needed.

Nursing Mothers —It is not known whether this drug is excreted in human milk. Because many drugs are excreted in human milk, caution should be exercised when VANCOR is administered to a nursing woman. It is unlikely that a nursing infant can absorb a significant amount of vancomycin from the normal gastrointestinal tract.

Usage in Pediatrics —In premature neonates and young infants, it may be appropriate to confirm desired vancomycin serum concentrations. Concomitant administration of vancomycin and anesthetic agents has been associated with erythema and histamine-like flushing in children (see Adverse Reactions).

Geriatrics —The natural decrement of glomerular filtration with increasing age may lead to elevated vancomycin serum concentrations if dosage is not adjusted. Vancomycin dosage schedules should be adjusted in elderly patients (see Dosage and Administration).

ADVERSE REACTIONS

Infusion-Related Events —During or soon after rapid infusion of VANCOR, patients may develop anaphylactoid reactions, including hypotension, wheezing, dyspnea, urticaria, or pruritus. Rapid infusion may also cause flushing of the upper body ("red neck") or pain and muscle spasm of the chest and back. These reactions usually resolve within 20 minutes but may persist for several hours. Such events are infrequent if VANCOR is given by a slow infusion over 60 minutes. In studies of normal volunteers, infusion-related events did not occur when vancomycin hydrochloride was administered at a rate of 10 mg/min or less.

Nephrotoxicity —A few dozen cases of increased serum creatinine or BUN concentrations in patients given vancomycin hydrochloride have been reported. Most of these have occurred in patients who were given aminoglycosides concomitantly or who had preexisting kidney dysfunction. When vancomycin hydrochloride was discontinued, azotemia resolved in most patients.

Ototoxicity —A few dozen cases of hearing loss associated with vancomycin hydrochloride have been reported. Most of these patients had kidney dysfunction, preexisting hearing loss, or concomitant treatment with an ototoxic drug. Vertigo, dizziness, and tinnitus have been reported rarely.

Hematopoietic —Reversible neutropenia, usually starting one week or more after onset of therapy with vancomycin hydrochloride or after a total dose of more than 25 g, has been reported for several dozen patients. Neutropenia appears to be promptly reversible when vancomycin hydrochloride is discontinued. Thrombocytopenia has rarely been reported.

Phlebitis —Inflammation at the injection site has been reported.

Miscellaneous —Infrequently, patients have been reported to have had anaphylaxis, drug fever, chills, and rashes in association with vancomycin hydrochloride.

OVERDOSAGE

Supportive care is advised, with maintenance of glomerular filtration. Vancomycin is poorly removed by dialysis. Hemoperfusion with Amberlite XAD-4 resin has been reported to be of limited benefit.

DOSAGE AND ADMINISTRATION

Patients with Normal Renal Function
Adults —The usual daily intravenous dose is 2 g divided either as 500 mg every 6 hours or 1 g every 12 hours. Each dose should be administered over a period of at least 60 minutes. Other patient factors, such as age or obesity, may call for modification of the usual daily dose.

Children —The total daily intravenous dosage of VANCOR, calculated on the basis of 40 mg/kg of body weight, can be divided and incorporated into the child's 24-hour fluid requirement. Each dose should be administered over a period of at least 60 minutes.

Infants and Neonates —In neonates and young infants, the total daily intravenous dosage may be lower. In both neonates and infants, an initial dose of 15 mg/kg is suggested, followed by 10 mg/kg every 12 hours for neonates in the first week of life and every 8 hours thereafter up to the age of one month. Close monitoring of serum concentrations of vancomycin may be warranted in these patients.

The safety and efficacy of vancomycin administration by the intrathecal (intralumbar or intraventricular) route have not been assessed.

Patients with Impaired Renal Function and Elderly Patients
Dosage adjustment must be made in patients with impaired renal function. In the elderly, dosage reduction may be necessary to a greater extent than expected because of decreasing renal function. Measurement of vancomycin serum concentrations can be helpful in optimizing therapy, especially in seriously ill patients with changing renal function. Vancomycin serum concentrations can be determined by use of microbiologic assay, radioimmunoassay, fluorescence polarization immunoassay, fluorescence immunoassay, or high-pressure liquid chromatography.

If creatinine clearance can be measured or estimated accurately, the dosage for most patients with renal impairment can be calculated by using the following table. The dosage of VANCOR per day in mg is about 15 times the glomerular filtration rate in mL/min:

DOSAGE TABLE FOR VANCOMYCIN IN PATIENTS WITH IMPAIRED RENAL FUNCTION
(Adapted from Moellering et al)[5]

Creatinine Clearance mL/min	Vancomycin Dose mg/24 hr
100	1545
90	1390
80	1235
70	1080
60	925
50	770
40	620
30	465
20	310
10	155

The initial dose should be no less than 15 mg/kg, even in patients with mild to moderate renal insufficiency.

The table is not valid for functionally anephric patients. For such patients, an initial dose of 15 mg/kg of body weight should be given in order to achieve prompt therapeutic serum concentrations. The dose required to maintain stable concentrations is 1.9 mg/kg/24 hr. Since individual maintenance doses of 250 to 1,000 mg are convenient, one dose may be given every several days rather than on a daily basis in patients with marked renal impairment. In anuria, a dose of 1,000 mg every 7 to 10 days has been recommended.

When only serum creatinine concentration is known, the following formula (based on sex, weight, and age of the patient) may be used to calculate creatinine clearance. Calculated creatinine clearances (mL/min) are only estimates. The creatinine clearance should be measured promptly.

Men: $\dfrac{\text{Weight (kg)} \times (140 - \text{age in years})}{72 \times \text{serum creatinine concentration (mg/dL)}}$

Women: $0.85 \times$ above value

The serum creatinine must represent a steady state of renal function. Otherwise, the estimated value for creatinine clearance is not valid. Such a calculated clearance is an overestimate of actual clearance in patients with conditions: (1) characterized by decreasing renal function, such as shock, severe heart failure, or oliguria; (2) in which a normal relationship between muscle mass and total body weight is not present, such as in obese patients or those with liver disease, edema, or ascites; and (3) accompanied by debilitation, malnutrition, or inactivity.

The safety and efficacy of vancomycin administration by the intrathecal (intralumbar or intraventricular) route have not been assessed. Intermittent infusion is the recommended method of administration.

PREPARATION AND STABILITY

At the time of use, reconstitute by adding 10 mL of Sterile Water for Injection to the 500-mg vial or 20 mL of Sterile Water for Injection to the 1 g vial of dry, sterile vancomycin powder. FURTHER DILUTION IS REQUIRED.

After reconstitution, the vials may be stored in a refrigerator for 96 hours without significant loss of potency. Reconstituted solutions containing 500 mg of vancomycin must be diluted with at least 100 mL of diluent. Reconstituted solutions containing 1 g must be diluted with at least 200 mL of diluent. The desired dose diluted in this manner should be administered by intermittent intravenous infusion over a period of at least 60 minutes.

Compatibility with Other Drugs and Intravenous Fluids —The following diluents are physically and chemically compatible (with 4 g/L of VANCOR):

Continued on next page

Adria—Cont.

5% Dextrose Injection, USP
5% Dextrose Injection and 0.9% Sodium Chloride Injection, USP
Lactated Ringer's Injection, USP
Lactated Ringer's and 5% Dextrose Injection
Normosol®-M and 5% Dextrose
0.9% Sodium Chloride Injection, USP
Isolyte® E

These solutions may be stored in a refrigerator for 96 hours. Vancomycin solution has a low pH and may cause physical instability of other compounds. Parenteral drug products should be inspected visually for particulate matter and discoloration prior to administration, whenever solution or container permits.

For Oral Administration —The usual adult total daily dosage for antibiotic-associated pseudomembranous colitis produced by *C difficile* is 500 mg to 2 g given in 3 or 4 divided doses for 7 to 10 days. The total daily dosage in children is 40 mg/kg of body weight in 3 or 4 divided doses. The total daily dosage should not exceed 2 g. The appropriate dose may be diluted in 1 oz. of water and given to the patient to drink. The diluted material may be administered via nasogastric tube. Common flavoring syrups may be added to the solution to improve the taste for oral administration.

HOW SUPPLIED

VANCOR™ (sterile vancomycin hydrochloride, USP)
NDC 0013-7215-86, 500 mg vial (mist grey cap), single pack
NDC 0013-7225-91, 1 g vial (royal blue cap), carton of 10
Store products at controlled room temperature, 15°–30°C (59°–86°F).
CAUTION—Federal law prohibits dispensing without a prescription.
Manufactured by:
THE UPJOHN COMPANY
KALAMAZOO, MICHIGAN 49001
For:
ADRIA LABORATORIES
Division of Erbamont Inc.
COLUMBUS, OHIO 43215

REFERENCES

1. National Committee for Clinical Laboratory Standards, 1984. Performance Standards for Antimicrobial Disk Susceptibility Tests, MZ-A3, NCCLS, Villanova, PA 19805.
2. National Committee for Clinical Laboratory Standards, 1983. Methods for Dilution Antimicrobial Susceptibility Tests for Bacteria that Grow Aerobically, M7-T, NCCLS, Villanova, PA 19805.
3. National Committee for Clinical Laboratory Standards, 1984. Reference Agar Dilution Procedure for Antimicrobial Susceptibility Testing of Anaerobic Bacteria, M11-A, NCCLS, Villanova, PA 19805.
4. Shulman ST, Amren DP, Bisno AL, et al: Prevention of bacterial endocarditis. Circulation, *70* :1123A, 1984.
5. Moellering RC, Krogstad DJ, Greenblatt DJ: Vancomycin therapy in patients with impaired renal function: A nomogram for dosage. Ann Intern Med *94* :343, 1981.

Advanced Nutritional Technology, Inc.
1111 JEFFERSON AVENUE
P.O. BOX 3225
ELIZABETH, NJ 07207-3225

LACTASE ENZYME

DESCRIPTION
Each softgel contains 125 mg. or 260 mg. of lactase enzyme.

HOW SUPPLIED
125 mg. (1750 FCC Units) 100's	NDC #10888-5305-1
125 mg. (1750 FCC Units) 250's	10888-5305-3
260 mg. (3640 FCC Units) 100's	10888-5309-1

LIQUI-CAL®

DESCRIPTION
Two softgels provide 1200 mg. of calcium from calcium carbonate.

HOW SUPPLIED
600 mg. 60's	NDC #10888-5304-6

N'ODOR®

DESCRIPTION
Each softgel contains 50 mg. of chlorophyllin complex effective for urinary & fecal odor control.

HOW SUPPLIED
50 mg. 120's	NDC #10888-1010-5

PHOSCHOL®
[fos 'kol]
Phosphatidylcholine (highly purified lecithin)
Softgels and Concentrate

DESCRIPTION
The active component of PhosChol® is phosphatidylcholine, one of the phospholipids isolated from soya lecithin. Phospholipids are characterized chemically as phosphatides, 1,2-diacyl-SN-glycero-3-phosphoryl derivatives.
PhosChol 900 contains 900 mg of pure phosphatidylcholine in each softgel.
PhosChol 565 contains 565 mg of pure phosphatidylcholine in each softgel.
PhosChol Concentrate contains 3000 mg of pure phosphatidylcholine in each teaspoonful.

ACTION & USES
Choline circulating in the blood after PC ingestion is taken up into all cells of the body. The brain has a unique way of ensuring that its nerve cells will receive adequate supplies of circulating choline.
A special protein molecule within the brain's capillaries traps the circulating choline, and then transports it across the blood-brain barrier, into the brain. Once in the brain, choline is incorporated into the brain's own PC, which is an essential and major part of neuronal membranes. Circulating choline transported into the brain has an additional very important function for a special group of nerve cells that make a biochemical, acetylcholine, which is released into synapses as a neurotransmitter. It provides the essential precursor used to synthesize acetylcholine. Moreover, when nerve cells are active, firing frequently and releasing large quantities of acetylcholine, their ability to make adequate amounts of the neurotransmitter requires that they receive adequate amounts of choline from the blood stream. In the absence of adequate choline, the ability of nerve cells to transmit messages to other cells across synapses is impaired and neuronal cell membranes can be depleted of PC causing cell damage. In contrast, when supplemental choline is provided, these messages can be amplified and membrane structure maintained.
PhosChol® brand of highly purified lecithin has been carefully developed to contain the highest concentration of phosphatidylcholine commercially available and can provide for the highest blood choline levels. By taking 9 g of phosphatidylcholine daily, plasma choline levels will double, thus making available more choline for acetylcholine synthesis.

Figure 1.
LEVELS OF CHOLINE IN HUMAN PLASMA AFTER THE ADMINISTRATION OF 3, 6, 9, AND 18 GRAM DOSES OF LECITHIN AS PHOSCHOL

(One 9-gram dose at baseline, one 9-gram dose at 4 hours)

DOSAGE AND ADMINISTRATION
PhosChol® nutritional supplements may be recommended for two purposes:
To guard against low blood choline levels, and to restore blood choline levels in patients suffering from selected brain disorders. Amounts of PC sufficient to increase blood choline levels would help support normal cellular membrane composition and repair; they would also provide sufficient precursor choline for the maintenance of acetylcholine biosynthesis. Taken according to these schedules, dietary supplements of PC are an aid to good health, and protect against low choline stores.

For optimal results, patients should take 9 g of phosphatidylcholine before noon. With PhosChol® 900, the suggested regimen should be six softgels shortly before breakfast and four softgels shortly before lunch. With PhosChol® 565, nine softgels should be taken before breakfast and seven softgels should be taken before lunch. With PhosChol Concentrate, two teaspoonsful should be taken before breakfast and one teaspoonful before lunch. If ingestion before meals causes intestinal distress, it is recommended that PhosChol be taken either with meals or immediately thereafter.

ADVERSE REACTIONS
No major side effects have been reported in connection with consumption of large quantities of phosphatidylcholine or commercially available (less pure) lecithin.
Minor side effects may be seen such as increased salivation, nausea and upset stomach.

HOW SUPPLIED
Two dosage strengths as clear, amber colored, one-piece sealed softgels.
PhosChol 900 contains 900 mg of pure phosphatidylcholine in each softgel and is available in bottles of 100 and 300 softgels. Ten softgels a day provide 9 grams of phosphatidylcholine.
100's NDC #10888-9000-1
300's NDC #10888-9000-5
PhosChol 565 contains 565 mg of pure phosphatidylcholine and is available in bottles of 100 and 300 softgels. Sixteen softgels a day provide 9 grams of phosphatidylcholine.
100's NDC #10888-5650-1
300's NDC #10888-5650-5
One dosage strength as a liquid concentrate.
PhosChol Concentrate contains 3000 mg of pure phosphatidylcholine in each teaspoonful and is available in 8 oz. and 16 oz. bottles. Three teaspoonsful a day provide 9 grams of phosphatidylcholine.
8 oz. NDC #10888-0121-1
16 oz. NDC #10888-0121-2
Shown in Product Identification Section, page 404

PRECORSIN™

DESCRIPTION
Contains 500 mg. of L-Tryptophan in a liquid centered, easy to swallow softgel.

HOW SUPPLIED
500 mg. 100's	NDC #10888-5308-1
500 mg. 300's	NDC #10888-5308-5

SuperEPA® 1200
Natural source fish oil omega-3 fatty acid concentrate

DESCRIPTION
Each softgel contains
EPA (eicosapentaenoic acid)—360 mg
DHA (docosahexaenoic acid)—240 mg
  Total omega-3 fatty acids—600 mg
No preservatives, sugar, starch or colors added.
Cholesterol-free (less than 1 mg per softgel).

DOSAGE AND ADMINISTRATION
Daily dosage of SuperEPA 1200 is only 1–3 softgels with meals or as advised by the physician.

HOW SUPPLIED
SuperEPA® 1200 is supplied in
Bottles of 60's—NDC #10888-1200-3
Bottles of 90's—NDC #10888-1200-5
Bottles of 180's—NDC #10888-1200-7
Shown in Product Identification Section, page 404

Akorn, Inc.
100 AKORN DRIVE
ABITA SPRINGS, LA 70420

OPHTHALMIC PRODUCTS

For information on Akorn ophthalmic pharmaceutical products, consult the PDR For Ophthalmology. For literature, sample material or service items, please contact Akorn, Inc. directly.

Products are cross-indexed by
generic and chemical names in the
YELLOW SECTION

Alcon Laboratories, Inc.
and its affiliates
CORPORATE HEADQUARTERS:
PO BOX 6600
6201 SOUTH FREEWAY
FORT WORTH, TX 76134

OPHTHALMIC PRODUCTS

For information on Alcon ophthalmic products, consult the PDR for Ophthalmology. See a complete listing of products in the Manufacturer's Index Section of this book. For information, literature, samples or service items contact Alcon Sales Services.

BETOPTIC®
(betaxolol hydrochloride)
0.5% as base
Sterile Ophthalmic Solution

℞

DESCRIPTION

BETOPTIC® Sterile Ophthalmic Solution contains betaxolol hydrochloride, a cardioselective beta-adrenergic receptor blocking agent, in a sterile isotonic solution. Betaxolol hydrochloride is a white, crystalline powder, soluble in water, with a molecular weight of 343.89. The chemical structure is presented below:

$(CH_3)_2CHNHCH_2CHCH_2O$—⬡—$CH_2CH_2OCH_2$—◁ ·HCl
(with OH below)

Empirical Formula:
$C_{18}H_{29}NO_3 \cdot HCl$
Chemical Name
(±)-1-[p-[2-(Cyclopropylmethoxy)ethyl]phenoxy]-3-(isopropylamino)-2-propanol hydrochloride.
Each mL of BETOPTIC Ophthalmic Solution (0.5%) contains: Active: 5.6 mg betaxolol hydrochloride equivalent to betaxolol base 5 mg. Preservative: Benzalkonium Chloride 0.01%. Inactive: Edetate Disodium, Sodium Chloride, Hydrochloric Acid and/or Sodium Hydroxide (to adjust pH), and Purified Water.

CLINICAL PHARMACOLOGY

Betaxolol HCl, a cardioselective (beta-1-adrenergic) receptor blocking agent, does not have significant membrane-stabilizing (local anesthetic) activity and is devoid of intrinsic sympathomimetic action. Orally administered beta-adrenergic blocking agents reduce cardiac output in healthy subjects and patients with heart disease. In patients with severe impairment of myocardial function beta-adrenergic receptor antagonists may inhibit the sympathetic stimulatory effect necessary to maintain adequate cardiac function.
When instilled in the eye, BETOPTIC Ophthalmic Solution has the action of reducing elevated as well as normal intraocular pressure, whether or not accompanied by glaucoma. Ophthalmic betaxolol has minimal effect on pulmonary and cardiovascular parameters.
Ophthalmic betaxolol (one drop in each eye) was compared to timolol and placebo in a three-way crossover study challenging nine patients with reactive airway disease who were selected on the basis of having at least a 15% reduction in the forced expiratory volume in one second (FEV_1) after administration of ophthalmic timolol. Betaxolol HCl had no significant effect on pulmonary function as measured by FEV_1, Forced Vital Capacity (FVC) and FEV_1/VC. Additionally, the action of isoproterenol, a beta stimulant, administered at the end of the study was not inhibited by ophthalmic betaxolol. In contrast, ophthalmic timolol signficantly decreased these pulmonary functions.
[See table above].
No evidence of cardiovascular beta-adrenergic blockade during exercise was observed with betaxolol in a double masked, three-way crossover study in 24 normal subjects comparing ophthalmic betaxolol, timolol and placebo for effect on blood pressure and heart rate. Mean arterial blood pressure was not affected by any treatment; however, ophthalmic timolol produced a significant decrease in the mean heart rate.
[See table below].
Clinical Studies: Optic nerve head damage and visual field loss are the result of a sustained elevated intraocular pressure and poor ocular perfusion. BETOPTIC Ophthalmic Solution has the action of reducing elevated as well as normal intraocular pressure and the mechanism of ocular hypotensive action appears to be a reduction of aqueous production as demonstrated by tonography and aqueous fluorophotometry. The onset of action with BETOPTIC Ophthalmic Solution can generally be noted within 30 minutes and the maximal effect can usually be detected 2 hours after topical administration. A single dose provides a 12-hour reduction in intraocular pressure. Clinical observation of glaucoma patients treated with BETOPTIC Ophthalmic Solution for up to three years shows that the intraocular pressure lowering effect is well maintained.
Clinical studies show that topical BETOPTIC Ophthalmic Solution reduces mean intraocular pressure 25% from baseline. In trials using 22 mmHg as a generally accepted index of intraocular pressure control, BETOPTIC Ophthalmic Solution was effective in more than 94% of the population studied, of which 73% were treated with the beta blocker alone. In controlled, double-masked studies, the magnitude and duration of the ocular hypotensive effect of BETOPTIC Ophthalmic Solution and ophthalmic timolol solution were clinically equivalent.
BETOPTIC Ophthalmic Solution has also been used successfully in glaucoma patients who have undergone a laser trabeculoplasty and have needed additional long-term ocular hypotensive therapy.
BETOPTIC Ophthalmic Solution has been well-tolerated in glaucoma patients wearing hard or soft contact lenses and in aphakic patients.
BETOPTIC Ophthalmic Solution does not produce miosis or accommodative spasm which are frequently seen with miotic agents. The blurred vision and night blindness often associated with standard miotic therapy are not associated with BETOPTIC Ophthalmic Solution. Thus, patients with central lenticular opacities avoid the visual impairment caused by a constricted pupil.

FEV_1 —Percent Change from Baseline[1]

	Betaxolol 1.0%[a]	Timolol 0.5%	Placebo
	Means		
Baseline	1.6	1.4	1.4
60 Minutes	2.3	−25.7*	5.8
120 Minutes	1.6	−27.4*	7.5
240 Minutes	−6.4	−26.9*	6.9
Isoproterenol[b]	36.1	−12.4*	42.8

[1] Schoene, R. B., *et al.* Am. J. Ophthal. 97:86, 1984.
[a] Twice the clinical concentration.
[b] Inhaled at 240 minutes; measurement at 270 minutes.
*Timolol statistically different from betaxolol and placebo (p < 0.05).

INDICATIONS AND USAGE

BETOPTIC® Ophthalmic Solution has been shown to be effective in lowering intraocular pressure and is indicated in the treatment of ocular hypertension and chronic open-angle glaucoma. It may be used alone or in combination with other anti-glaucoma drugs.
In clinical studies BETOPTIC® safely controlled the intraocular pressure of 47 patients with glaucoma and reactive airway disease followed for a mean period of 15 months. However, caution should be used in treating patients with severe reactive airway disease.

CONTRAINDICATIONS

Hypersensitivity to any component of this product.
BETOPTIC Ophthalmic Solution is contraindicated in patients with sinus bradycardia, greater than a first degree atrioventricular block, cardiogenic shock, or patients with overt cardiac failure.

WARNING

Although BETOPTIC Ophthalmic Solution has had little or no effect on heart rate or blood pressure in clinical studies, caution should be observed in treating patients with a history of cardiac failure. Treatment with BETOPTIC Ophthalmic Solution should be discontinued at the first signs of cardiac failure.

PRECAUTIONS

Patients who are receiving a beta-adrenergic blocking agent orally and BETOPTIC Ophthalmic Solution should be observed for a potential additive effect either on the intraocular pressure or on the known systemic effects of beta blockade.
While BETOPTIC Ophthalmic Solution has demonstrated a low potential for systemic effect, it should be used with caution in patients with diabetes (especially labile diabetes) because of possible masking of signs and symptoms of acute hypoglycemia. Beta-adrenergic blocking agents may mask certain signs and symptoms of hyperthyroidism and their abrupt withdrawal might precipitate a thyroid storm.
Consideration should be given to the gradual withdrawal of beta-adrenergic blocking agents prior to general anesthesia because of the reduced ability of the heart to respond to beta-adrenergically mediated sympathetic reflex stimuli.
Pulmonary: Caution should be exercised in the treatment of glaucoma patients with excessive restriction of pulmonary function. Ophthalmic betaxolol has minimal systemic effects and has been used by over 100,000 patients with glaucoma or ocular hypertension and coexisting reactive airway disease. Nonetheless, there have been reports of asthmatic attacks and pulmonary distress during betaxolol treatment. Although rechallenges of such patients with ophthalmic betaxolol have not adversely affected pulmonary function test results, the possibility of adverse pulmonary effects in patients unusually sensitive to beta blockers cannot be ruled out.
Drug Interactions: Although BETOPTIC Ophthalmic Solution used alone has little or no effect on pupil size, mydriasis resulting from concomitant therapy with BETOPTIC Ophthalmic Solution and epinephrine has been reported occasionally. Close observation of the patient is recommended when a beta-blocker is administered to patients receiving catecholamine-depleting drugs such as reserpine, because of possible additive effects and the production of hypotension and/or bradycardia. Caution should be exercised in patients using concomitant adrenergic psychotropic drugs.
Ocular: In patients with angle-closure glaucoma, the immediate treatment objective is to re-open the angle by constriction of the pupil with a miotic agent. Betaxolol has no effect on the pupil; therefore, BETOPTIC Ophthalmic Solution should be used with a miotic to reduce elevated intraocular pressure in angle-closure glaucoma.

Mean Heart Rates[1]

TREATMENT

Bruce Stress Exercise Test

Minutes	Betaxolol 1%[a]	Timolol 0.5%	Placebo
0	79.2	79.3	81.2
2	130.2	126.0	130.4
4	133.4	128.0*	134.3
6	136.4	129.2*	137.9
8	139.8	131.8*	139.4
10	140.8	131.8*	141.3

[1] Atkins, J. M., *et al.* Am. J. Oph. 99:173–175, Feb., 1985.
[a] Twice the clinical concentration
*Mean pulse rate significantly lower for timolol than betaxolol or placebo (p < 0.05).

Continued on next page

Alcon Labs.—Cont.

As with the use of other antiglaucoma drugs, diminished responsiveness to BETOPTIC Ophthalmic Solution after prolonged therapy has been reported in some patients. However in one long-term study in which 250 patients have been followed for a mean period of two years, no significant difference in mean intraocular pressure has been observed after initial stabilization.

ANIMAL STUDIES

No adverse ocular effects were observed following topical ocular administration of BETOPTIC Ophthalmic Solution to rabbits for one year.

CARCINOGENESIS, MUTAGENESIS, IMPAIRMENT OF FERTILITY

Lifetime studies with betaxolol HCl have been completed in mice at oral doses of 6, 20 or 60 mg/kg/day and in rats at 3, 12 or 48 mg/kg/day; betaxolol HCl demonstrated no carcinogenic effect. Higher dose levels were not tested. In a variety of in vitro and in vivo bacterial and mammalian cell assays, betaxolol HCl was nonmutagenic.

Pregnancy Category C: Reproduction, teratology, and peri- and post-natal studies have been conducted with orally administered betaxolol HCl in rats and rabbits. There was evidence of drug related post-implantation loss in rabbits and rats at dose levels above 12 mg/kg and 128 mg/kg, respectively. Betaxolol HCl was not shown to be teratogenic, however, and there were no other adverse effects on reproduction at subtoxic dose levels. There are, however, no adequate and well-controlled studies in pregnant women. Because animal reproductive studies are not always predictive of human response, this drug should be used during pregnancy only if clearly indicated.

Nursing Mothers: It is not known whether BETOPTIC Ophthalmic Solution is excreted in human milk. Because many drugs are excreted in human milk, caution should be exercised when BETOPTIC Ophthalmic Solution is administered to nursing women.

Usage in Children: Clinical studies to establish the safety and efficacy in children have not been performed.

ADVERSE REACTIONS

The following adverse reactions have been reported in clinical trials with BETOPTIC Ophthalmic Solution.

Ocular: BETOPTIC Ophthalmic Solution has been well tolerated. Discomfort of short duration was experienced by one in four patients, but none discontinued therapy; occasional tearing has been reported. Rare instances of decreased corneal sensitivity, erythema, itching sensation, corneal punctate staining, keratitis, anisocoria and photophobia have been reported.

Systemic: Systemic reactions following administration of ophthalmic betaxolol have been reported rarely. These include: insomnia, depression, headache, hives, toxic epidermal necrolysis, bradycardia, asthma, and dyspnea (see Pulmonary Precautions section).

OVERDOSAGE

No information is available on overdosage of humans. The oral LD$_{50}$ of the drug ranged from 350–920 mg/kg in mice and 860–1050 mg/kg in rats. The symptoms which might be expected with an overdose of a systemically administered beta-1-adrenergic receptor blocker agent are bradycardia, hypotension and acute cardiac failure.

A topical overdose of BETOPTIC Ophthalmic Solution may be flushed from the eye(s) with warm tap water.

DOSAGE AND ADMINISTRATION

The usual dose is one drop of BETOPTIC Ophthalmic Solution in the affected eye(s) twice daily. In some patients, the intraocular pressure lowering response to BETOPTIC Ophthalmic Solution may require a few weeks to stabilize. Clinical follow-up should include a determination of the intraocular pressure during the first month of treatment with BETOPTIC Ophthalmic Solution. Thereafter, intraocular pressures should be determined on an individual basis at the judgment of the physician.

When a patient is transferred from a single anti-glaucoma agent, continue the agent already used and add one drop of BETOPTIC Ophthalmic Solution in the affected eye(s) twice a day. On the following day, discontinue the previous anti-glaucoma agent completely and continue with BETOPTIC Ophthalmic Solution.

Because of diurnal variations of intraocular pressure in individual patients, satisfactory response to twice a day therapy is best determined by measuring intraocular pressure at different times during the day. Intraocular pressures ≤ 22 mmHg may not be optimal for control of glaucoma in each patient; therefore, therapy should be individualized.

If the intraocular pressure of the patient is not adequately controlled on this regimen, concomitant therapy with pilocarpine, other miotics, epinephrine or systemically administered carbonic anhydrase inhibitors can be instituted.

When a patient is transferred from several concomitantly administered anti-glaucoma agents, individualization is

required. Adjustment should involve one agent at a time made at intervals of not less than one week. A recommended approach is to continue the agents being used and add one drop of BETOPTIC Ophthalmic Solution in the affected eye(s) twice a day. On the following day, discontinue one of the other anti-glaucoma agents. The remaining anti-glaucoma agents may be decreased or discontinued according to the patient's response to treatment. The physician may be able to discontinue some or all of the other anti-glaucoma agents.

HOW SUPPLIED

BETOPTIC Ophthalmic Solution is a sterile, isotonic, aqueous solution of betaxolol hydrochloride. Supplied as follows: 2.5, 5, 10 and 15 mL in plastic ophthalmic DROP-TAINER® dispensers.

2.5 mL: **NDC** 0065-0245-20
5 mL: **NDC** 0065-0245-05
10 mL: **NDC** 0065-0245-10
15 mL: **NDC** 0065-0245-15

U.S. Patent Nos. 4,252,984; 4,311,708; 4,342,783

STORAGE

Store at room temperature.

NAPHCON-A®   ℞
(naphazoline hydrochloride and pheniramine maleate)
Sterile Ophthalmic Solution

DESCRIPTION

NAPHCON-A® (naphazoline hydrochloride, pheniramine maleate) is a combination of an antihistamine and a decongestant prepared as a sterile topical ophthalmic solution. The active ingredients are represented by the chemical structures:

Established name:
Naphazoline Hydrochloride
Chemical name:
  1H - Imidazole, 4, 5-dihydro- 2-(1- naphthalenylmethyl)- monohydrochloride.

Established name:
  Pheniramine Maleate
Chemical name:
  N,N-Dimethyl -y -phenyl -2- pyridine-propanamine, (Z)-Butenedioic acid.
Each mL contains: Active: Naphazoline Hydrochloride 0.025%, Pheniramine Maleate 0.3%. Preservative: Benzalkonium Chloride 0.01%. Inactive: Boric Acid, Sodium Borate, Edetate Disodium, Sodium Chloride, Sodium Hydroxide and/or Hydrochloric Acid (to adjust pH), and Purified Water.

CLINICAL PHARMACOLOGY

NAPHCON-A® combines the effects of the antihistamine, pheniramine maleate, and the decongestant, naphazoline.

> **INDICATIONS AND USAGE:** Based on a review of a related combination of drugs by the National Academy of Sciences—National Research Council and/or other information, FDA has classified the indications as follows: "Possibly" effective: For relief of ocular irritation and/or congestion or for the treatment of allergic or inflammatory ocular conditions. Final classification of the less-than-effective indication requires further investigation.

CONTRAINDICATIONS

Hypersensitivity to one or more of the components of this preparation.
Do not use in the presence of narrow angle glaucoma or in patients predisposed to narrow angle glaucoma.

WARNINGS

Patients under MAO inhibitors may experience a severe hypertensive crisis if given a sympathomimetic drug such as Naphazoline HCl. Use in infants and children may result in

CNS depression leading to coma and marked reduction in body temperature.

PRECAUTIONS

For topical eye use only—not for injection. This preparation should be used with caution in patients with severe cardiovascular disease including cardiac arrhythmias, patients with poorly controlled hypertension, patients with diabetes, especially those with a tendency toward diabetic ketoacidosis. To prevent contaminating the dropper tip and solution, care should be taken not to touch the eyelids or surrounding area with the dropper tip of the bottle.

ADVERSE REACTIONS

The following adverse reactions may occur: Pupillary dilation, increase in intraocular pressure, systemic effects due to absorption (i.e., hypertension, cardiac irregularities, hyperglycemia).

DOSAGE AND ADMINISTRATION

One or two drops instilled in each eye every 3 to 4 hours or less frequently, as required to relieve symptoms.

HOW SUPPLIED

In 15mL plastic DROP-TAINER® Dispenser.
NDC 0998-0080-15

STORAGE

Store at 36° to 80°F. Keep bottle tightly closed when not in use. Protect from light and excessive heat.

TEARS NATURALE® II Lubricant Eye Drops

DESCRIPTION

TEARS NATURALE II is the only lubricant eye drop preserved with safe, nonsensitizing POLYQUAD 0.001%. In-vitro studies have shown that POLYQUAD substantially avoids the damaging effects of epithelial cell toxicity possible with other tear substitute preservatives, and permits epithelial cell growth. POLYQUAD has been shown to be 99% reaction-free in normal subjects and 97% reaction-free in subjects known to be preservative sensitive.

With its unique mucin-like polymeric formulation and with its neutral pH, low viscosity, and isotonicity, TEARS NATURALE II provides dry eye patients with comfort and prompt long-lasting relief of dry eye symptoms.
Sterile—For Topical Eye Use Only

INGREDIENTS

Each mL contains: **Active:** DUASORB®, a water soluble polymeric system containing Dextran 70 0.1% and Hydroxypropyl Methylcellulose 2910 0.3%. **Preservative:** POLYQUAD®* (Polyquaternium-1) 0.001%. **Inactive:** Edetate Disodium, Potassium Chloride, Sodium Chloride, Purified Water. May contain Hydrochloric Acid and/or Sodium Hydroxide to adjust pH.

INDICATIONS

For the temporary relief of burning and irritation due to dryness of the eye and for use as a protectant against further irritation. For temporary relief of discomfort due to minor irritations of the eye or to exposure to wind or sun.

DIRECTIONS

Instill 1 or 2 drops in the affected eye(s) as needed.

WARNINGS

If you experience eye pain, changes in vision, continued redness or irritation of the eye, or if the condition worsens or persists for more than 72 hours, discontinue use and consult a doctor.
If solution changes color or becomes cloudy, do not use.
To avoid contamination, do not touch tip of container to any surface. Replace cap after using. Keep this and all drugs out of the reach of children. In case of accidental ingestion, seek professional assistance or contact a Poison Control Center immediately.

HOW SUPPLIED

In 15 mL and 30 mL DROP-TAINER® dispensers.
15 mL: NDC 0065-0418-15
30 mL: NDC 0065-0418-30

STORAGE

Store at room temperature.

* U.S. Patent No. 3,931,319 and others.

TOBREX®   ℞
(tobramycin 0.3%)
Ophthalmic Solution and Ointment

DESCRIPTION

TOBREX® (tobramycin* 0.3%) is a sterile topical ophthalmic antibiotic formulation prepared specifically for topical therapy of external infections. This product is supplied in solution and ointment forms. Each mL of TOBREX Ophthalmic solution contains: Active: Tobramycin 0.3% (3 mg). Preservative: Benzalkonium Chloride 0.01%. Inactive: Boric

Acid, Sodium Sulfate, Sodium Chloride, Tyloxapol, Sodium Hydroxide and/or Sulfuric Acid (to adjust pH), and Purified Water.

Each gram of TOBREX Ophthalmic ointment contains: Active: Tobramycin 0.3% (3 mg). Preservative: Chlorobutanol 0.5%. Inactive: Mineral Oil, and White Petrolatum.

The chemical structure of tobramycin is:

Chemical name:
0-{3-amino-3-deoxy-α-D-gluco-pyranosyl-(1→4)}-O-{2, 6-di-amino-2, 3, 6-trideoxy-α-D-ribohexo-pyranosyl-(1→6)}-2-de-oxystreptamine.

Tobramycin is a water-soluble aminoglycoside antibiotic active against a wide variety of gram-negative and gram-positive ophthalmic pathogens.

CLINICAL PHARMACOLOGY

In Vitro Data: *In vitro* studies have demonstrated tobramycin is active against susceptible strains of the following microorganisms:

Staphylococci, including *S. aureus* and *S. epidermidis* (coagulase-positive and coagulase-negative), including penicillin-resistant strains.

Streptococci, including some of the Group A-betahemolytic species, some nonhemolytic species, and some *Streptococcus pneumoniae.*

Pseudomonas aeruginosa, Escherichia coli, Klebsiella pneumoniae, Enterobacter aerogenes, Proteus mirabilis, Morganella morganii, most *Proteus vulgaris* strains, *Haemophilus influenzae* and *H. aegyptius, Moraxella lacunata,* and *Acinetobacter calcoaceticus (Herellea vaginacola)* and some *Neisseria* species. Bacterial susceptibility studies demonstrate that in some cases, microorganisms resistant to gentamicin retain susceptibility to tobramycin. A significant bacterial population resistant to tobramycin has not yet emerged; however, bacterial resistance may develop upon prolonged use.

INDICATIONS AND USAGE

TOBREX® is a topical antibiotic indicated in the treatment of external infections of the eye and its adnexa caused by susceptible bacteria. Appropriate monitoring of bacterial response to topical antibiotic therapy should accompany the use of TOBREX.

Clinical studies have shown tobramycin to be safe and effective for use in children.

CONTRAINDICATIONS

TOBREX Ophthalmic Solution and Ointment are contraindicated in patients with known hypersensitivity to any of their components.

WARNINGS

NOT FOR INJECTION INTO THE EYE. Do not touch tube or dropper tip to any surface, as this may contaminate the contents. Sensitivity to topically applied aminoglycosides may occur in some patients. If a sensitivity reaction to TOBREX® occurs, discontinue use.

PRECAUTIONS

As with other antibiotic preparations, prolonged use may result in overgrowth of nonsusceptible organisms, including fungi. If superinfection occurs, appropriate therapy should be initiated. Ophthalmic ointments may retard corneal wound healing.

Pregnancy Category B. Reproduction studies in three types of animals at doses up to thirty-three times the normal human systemic dose have revealed no evidence of impaired fertility or harm to the fetus due to tobramycin. There are, however, no adequate and well-controlled studies in pregnant women. Because animal studies are not always predictive of human response, this drug should be used during pregnancy only if clearly needed.

Nursing Mothers: Because of the potential for adverse reactions in nursing infants from TOBREX, a decision should be made whether to discontinue nursing the infant or discontinue the drug, taking into account the importance of the drug to the mother.

ADVERSE REACTIONS

The most frequent adverse reactions to TOBREX Ophthalmic Solution and Ointment are localized ocular toxicity and hypersensitivity, including lid itching and swelling, and conjunctival erythema. These reactions occur in less than three of 100 patients treated with TOBREX. Similar reactions may occur with the topical use of other aminoglycoside antibiotics. Other adverse reactions have not been reported from

TOBREX therapy; however, if topical ocular tobramycin is administered concomitantly with systemic aminoglycoside antibiotics, care should be taken to monitor the total serum concentration. In clinical trials, TOBREX Ophthalmic Ointment produced significantly fewer adverse reactions (3.7%) than did GARAMYCIN® Ophthalmic Ointment (10.6%).

OVERDOSAGE

Clinically apparent signs and symptoms of an overdose of TOBREX Ophthalmic Solution or Ointment (punctate keratitis, erythema, increased lacrimation, edema and lid itching) may be similar to adverse reaction effects seen in some patients.

DOSAGE AND ADMINISTRATION

Solution: In mild to moderate disease, instill one or two drops into the affected eye(s) every four hours. In severe infections, instill two drops into the eye(s) hourly until improvement, following which treatment should be reduced prior to discontinuation.

Ointment: In mild to moderate disease, apply a half-inch ribbon into the affected eye(s) two or three times per day. In severe infections, instill a half-inch ribbon into the affected eye(s) every three to four hours until improvement, following which treatment should be reduced prior to discontinuation.

How to Apply TOBREX® Ointment
1. Tilt your head back.
2. Place a finger on your cheek just under your eye and gently pull down until a "V" pocket is formed between your eyeball and your lower lid.
3. Place a small amount (about ½ inch) of TOBREX in the "V" pocket. Do not let the tip of the tube touch your eye.
4. Look downward before closing your eye.

TOBREX Ointment may be used in conjunction with TOBREX Solution.

HOW SUPPLIED

STERILE solution in 5 mL DROP-TAINER® dispenser (NDC 0998-0643-05), containing tobramycin 0.3% (3 mg/mL) and STERILE ointment in 3.5 g ophthalmic tube (NDC 0065-0644-35), containing tobramycin 0.3% (3 mg/g).

STORAGE

Store at 8°–27°C (46°–80°F).
*U.S. Patent No. 3,691,279

Allen & Hanburys
Division of Glaxo Inc.
FIVE MOORE DRIVE
RESEARCH TRIANGLE PARK, NC 27709

BECLOVENT® Inhalation Aerosol ℞
[be′klō-vent″]
(beclomethasone dipropionate, USP)
For Oral Inhalation Only

DESCRIPTION

Beclomethasone dipropionate, USP, the active component of Beclovent® Inhalation Aerosol, is an anti-inflammatory steroid having the chemical name 9-chloro - 11β, 17, 21 - tri-hydroxy - 16β-methylpregna- 1, 4 - diene - 3, 20 - dione 17, 21 - dipropionate.

Beclovent Inhalation Aerosol is a metered-dose aerosol unit containing a microcrystalline suspension of beclomethasone dipropionate-trichloromonofluoromethane clathrate in a mixture of propellants (trichloromonofluoromethane and dichlorodifluoromethane) with oleic acid. Each canister contains beclomethasone dipropionate–trichloromonofluoromethane clathrate having a molecular proportion of beclomethasone dipropionate to trichloromonofluoromethane between 3:1 and 3:2. Each actuation delivers from the mouthpiece a quantity of clathrate equivalent to 42 mcg of beclomethasone dipropionate, USP. The contents of one canister provide at least 200 oral inhalations.

CLINICAL PHARMACOLOGY

Beclomethasone 17, 21-dipropionate is a diester of beclomethasone, a synthetic halogenated corticosteroid. Animal studies show that beclomethasone dipropionate has potent anti-inflammatory activity. When beclomethasone dipropionate was administered systemically to mice, the anti-inflammatory activity was accompanied by other features typical of glucocorticoid action, including thymic involution, liver glycogen deposition, and pituitary-adrenal suppression. However, after systemic administration of beclomethasone dipropionate to rats, the anti-inflammatory action was associated with little or no effect on other tests of glucocorticoid activity.

Beclomethasone dipropionate is sparingly soluble and is poorly mobilized from subcutaneous or intramuscular injection sites. However, systemic absorption occurs after all routes of administration. When given to animals in the form of an aerosolized suspension of the trichloromonofluoromethane clathrate, the drug is deposited in the mouth and nasal passages, the trachea and principal bronchi, and the lung; a

considerable portion of the drug is also swallowed. Absorption occurs rapidly from all respiratory and gastrointestinal tissues, as indicated by the rapid clearance of radioactively labeled drug from local tissues and appearance of tracer in the circulation. There is no evidence of tissue storage of beclomethasone dipropionate or its metabolites. Lung slices can metabolize beclomethasone dipropionate rapidly to beclomethasone 17-monopropionate and more slowly to free beclomethasone (which has very weak anti-inflammatory activity). However, irrespective of the route of administration (injection, oral, or aerosol), the principal route of excretion of the drug and its metabolites is the feces. Less than 10% of the drug and its metabolites is excreted in the urine. In humans, 12% to 15% of an orally administered dose of beclomethasone dipropionate was excreted in the urine as both conjugated and free metabolites of the drug.

The mechanisms responsible for the anti-inflammatory action of beclomethasone dipropionate are unknown. The precise mechanism of the aerosolized drug's action in the lung is also unknown.

INDICATIONS AND USAGE

Beclovent® (beclomethasone dipropionate) Inhalation Aerosol is indicated only for patients who require chronic treatment with corticosteroids for control of the symptoms of bronchial asthma. Such patients would include those already receiving systemic corticosteroids, and selected patients who are inadequately controlled on a nonsteroid regimen and in whom steroid therapy has been withheld because of concern over potential adverse effects.

Beclovent Inhalation Aerosol is NOT indicated:
1. For relief of asthma that can be controlled by bronchodilators and other nonsteroid medications.
2. In patients who require systemic corticosteroid treatment infrequently.
3. In the treatment of nonasthmatic bronchitis.

CONTRAINDICATIONS

Beclovent® (beclomethasone dipropionate) Inhalation Aerosol is contraindicated in the primary treatment of status asthmaticus or other acute episodes of asthma where intensive measures are required.

Hypersensitivity to any of the ingredients of this preparation contraindicates its use.

WARNINGS

Particular care is needed in patients who are transferred from systemically active corticosteroids to Beclovent® (beclomethasone dipropionate) Inhalation Aerosol because deaths due to adrenal insufficiency have occurred in asthmatic patients during and after transfer from systemic corticosteroids to aerosol beclomethasone dipropionate. After withdrawal from systemic corticosteroids, a number of months are required for recovery of hypothalamic-pituitary-adrenal (HPA) function. During this period of HPA suppression, patients may exhibit signs and symptoms of adrenal insufficiency when exposed to trauma, surgery, or infections, particularly gastroenteritis. Although Beclovent Inhalation Aerosol may provide control of asthmatic symptoms during these episodes, it does NOT provide the systemic steroid that is necessary for coping with these emergencies.

During periods of stress or a severe asthmatic attack, patients who have been withdrawn from systemic corticosteroids should be instructed to resume systemic steroids (in large doses) immediately and to contact their physician for further instruction. These patients should also be instructed to carry a warning card indicating that they may need supplementary systemic steroids during periods of stress or a severe asthma attack. To assess the risk of adrenal insufficiency in emergency situations, routine tests of adrenal cortical function, including measurement of early morning resting cortisol levels, should be performed periodically in all patients. An early morning resting cortisol level may be accepted as normal only if it falls at or near the normal mean level.

Localized infections with *Candida albicans* or *Aspergillus niger* have occurred frequently in the mouth and pharynx and occasionally in the larynx. Positive cultures for oral *Candida* may be present in up to 75% of patients. Although the frequency of clinically apparent infection is considerably lower, these infections may require treatment with appropriate antifungal therapy or discontinuation of treatment with Beclovent Inhalation Aerosol.

Beclovent Inhalation Aerosol is not to be regarded as a bronchodilator and is not indicated for rapid relief of bronchospasm.

Patients should be instructed to contact their physician immediately when episodes of asthma that are not responsive to bronchodilators occur during the course of treatment with

Continued on next page

Allen & Hanburys—Cont.

Beclovent Inhalation Aerosol. During such episodes, patients may require therapy with systemic corticosteroids. There is no evidence that control of asthma can be achieved by the administration of Beclovent Inhalation Aerosol in amounts greater than the recommended doses.

Transfer of patients from systemic steroid therapy to Beclovent Inhalation Aerosol may unmask allergic conditions previously suppressed by the systemic steroid therapy, eg, rhinitis, conjunctivitis, and eczema.

PRECAUTIONS

During withdrawal from oral steroids, some patients may experience symptoms of systemically active steroid withdrawal, eg, joint and/or muscular pain, lassitude, and depression, despite maintenance or even improvement of respiratory function (see DOSAGE AND ADMINISTRATION).

In responsive patients, beclomethasone dipropionate may permit control of asthmatic symptoms without suppression of HPA function, as discussed below (see CLINICAL STUDIES). Since beclomethasone dipropionate is absorbed into the circulation and can be systemically active, the beneficial effects of Beclovent® Inhalation Aerosol in minimizing or preventing HPA dysfunction may be expected only when recommended dosages are not exceeded.

The long-term effects of beclomethasone dipropionate in human subjects are still unknown. In particular, the local effects of the agent on developmental or immunologic processes in the mouth, pharynx, trachea, and lung are unknown. There is also no information about the possible long-term systemic effects of the agent.

The potential effects of Beclovent Inhalation Aerosol on acute, recurrent, or chronic pulmonary infections, including active or quiescent tuberculosis, are not known. Similarly, the potential effects of long-term administration of the drug on lung or other tissues are unknown.

Pulmonary infiltrates with eosinophilia may occur in patients on Beclovent Inhalation Aerosol therapy. Although it is possible that in some patients this state may become manifest because of systemic steroid withdrawal when inhalational steroids are administered, a causative role for beclomethasone dipropionate and/or its vehicle cannot be ruled out.

Pregnancy: *Teratogenic Effects:* Glucocorticoids are known teratogens in rodent species and beclomethasone dipropionate is no exception.

Teratology studies were done in rats, mice, and rabbits treated with subcutaneous beclomethasone dipropionate. Beclomethasone dipropionate was found to produce fetal resorption, cleft palate, agnathia, microstomia, absence of tongue, delayed ossification, and partial agenesis of the thymus. Well-controlled trials relating to fetal risk in humans are not available. Glucocorticoids are secreted in human milk. It is not known whether beclomethasone dipropionate would be secreted in human milk, but it is safe to assume that it is likely. The use of beclomethasone dipropionate in pregnant women, nursing mothers, or women of childbearing potential requires that the possible benefits of the drug be weighed against the potential hazards to the mother, embryo, or fetus. Infants born of mothers who have received substantial doses of corticosteroids during pregnancy should be carefully observed for hypoadrenalism.

ADVERSE REACTIONS

Deaths due to adrenal insufficiency have occurred in asthmatic patients during and after transfer from systemic corticosteroids to aerosol beclomethasone dipropionate (see WARNINGS).

Suppression of HPA function (reduction of early morning plasma cortisol levels) has been reported in adult patients who received 1,600-mcg daily doses of Beclovent® (beclomethasone dipropionate) Inhalation Aerosol for one month. A few patients on Beclovent Inhalation Aerosol have complained of hoarseness or dry mouth.

Rare cases of immediate and delayed hypersensitivity reactions, including urticaria, angioedema, rash, and bronchospasm, have been reported after the use of beclomethasone oral or intranasal inhalers.

DOSAGE AND ADMINISTRATION

Adults and Children 12 Years of Age and Older: The usual recommended dosage is two inhalations (84 mcg) given three or four times a day. Alternatively, four inhalations (168 mcg) given twice daily has been shown to be effective in some patients. In patients with severe asthma, it is advisable to start with 12 to 16 inhalations a day and adjust the dosage downward according to the response of the patient. The maximal daily intake should not exceed 20 inhalations, 840 mcg (0.84 mg), in adults.

Children 6 to 12 Years of Age: The usual recommended dosage is one or two inhalations (42 to 84 mcg) given three or four times a day according to the response of the patient. Alternatively, four inhalations (168 mcg) given twice daily has been shown to be effective in some patients. The maximal daily intake should not exceed ten inhalations, 420 mcg

(0.42 mg), in children 6 to 12 years of age. Insufficient clinical data exist with respect to the administration of Beclovent® (beclomethasone dipropionate) Inhalation Aerosol in children below the age of 6.

Rinsing the mouth after inhalation is advised.

Patients receiving bronchodilators by inhalation should be advised to use the bronchodilator before Beclovent Inhalation Aerosol in order to enhance penetration of beclomethasone dipropionate into the bronchial tree. After use of an aerosol bronchodilator, several minutes should elapse before use of the Beclovent Inhalation Aerosol to reduce the potential toxicity from the inhaled fluorocarbon propellants in the two aerosols.

Different considerations must be given to the following groups of patients in order to obtain the full therapeutic benefit of Beclovent Inhalation Aerosol.

Patients Not Receiving Systemic Steroids: The use of Beclovent Inhalation Aerosol is straightforward in patients who are inadequately controlled with nonsteroid medications but in whom systemic steroid therapy has been withheld because of concern over potential adverse reactions. In patients who respond to Beclovent Inhalation Aerosol, an improvement in pulmonary function is usually apparent within one to four weeks after the start of Beclovent Inhalation Aerosol.

Patients Receiving Systemic Steroids: In those patients dependent on systemic steroids, transfer to Beclovent Inhalation Aerosol and subsequent management may be more difficult because recovery from impaired adrenal function is usually slow. Such suppression has been known to last for up to 12 months. Clinical studies, however, have demonstrated that Beclovent Inhalation Aerosol may be effective in the management of these asthmatic patients and may permit replacement or significant reduction in the dosage of systemic corticosteroids.

The patient's asthma should be reasonably stable before treatment with Beclovent Inhalation Aerosol is started. Initially, the aerosol should be used concurrently with the patient's usual maintenance dose of systemic steroid. After approximately one week, gradual withdrawal of the systemic steroid is started by reducing the daily or alternate-daily dose. The next reduction is made after an interval of one or two weeks, depending on the response of the patient. Generally, these decrements should not exceed 2.5 mg of prednisone or its equivalent. A slow rate of withdrawal cannot be overemphasized. During withdrawal some patients may experience symptoms of systemically active steroid withdrawal, eg, joint and/or muscular pain, lassitude, and depression, despite maintenance or even improvement of respiratory function. Such patients should be encouraged to continue with the inhaler but should be watched carefully for objective signs of adrenal insufficiency such as hypotension and weight loss. If evidence of adrenal insufficiency occurs, the systemic steroid dose should be boosted temporarily and thereafter further withdrawal should continue more slowly.

During periods of stress or a severe asthma attack, transfer patients will require supplementary treatment with systemic steroids. Exacerbations of asthma that occur during the course of treatment with Beclovent Inhalation Aerosol should be treated with a short course of systemic steroid that is gradually tapered as these symptoms subside. There is no evidence that control of asthma can be achieved by administration of Beclovent Inhalation Aerosol in amounts greater than the recommended doses.

Directions for Use: Illustrated Patient's Instructions for Use accompany each package of Beclovent Inhalation Aerosol.

CONTENTS UNDER PRESSURE. Do not puncture. Do not use or store near heat or open flame. Exposure to temperatures above 120°F may cause bursting. Never throw container into fire or incinerator. Keep out of reach of children.

HOW SUPPLIED

Beclovent® (beclomethasone dipropionate) Inhalation Aerosol is supplied in a 16.8-g canister containing 200 metered inhalations with oral adapter and patient's instructions (NDC 0173-0312-88). Also available is a 16.8-g refill canister only with patient's instructions (NDC 0173-0360-98).

Store between 2° and 30°C (36° and 86°F). As with most inhaled medications in aerosol canisters, the therapeutic effect of this medication may decrease when the canister is cold. Shake well before using.

ANIMAL PHARMACOLOGY AND TOXICOLOGY

Studies in a number of animal species, including rats, rabbits, and dogs, have shown no unusual toxicity during acute experiments. However, the effects of beclomethasone dipropionate in producing signs of glucocorticoid excess during chronic administration by various routes were dose-related.

CLINICAL STUDIES

The effects of beclomethasone dipropionate on HPA function have been evaluated in adult volunteers. There was no suppression of early morning plasma cortisol concentrations when beclomethasone dipropionate was administered in a dose of 1,000 mcg/day for one month as an aerosol or for

three days by intramuscular injection. However, partial suppression of plasma cortisol concentration was observed when beclomethasone dipropionate was administered in doses of 2,000 mcg/day either intramuscularly or by aerosol. Immediate suppression of plasma cortisol concentrations was observed after single doses of 4,000 mcg of beclomethasone dipropionate.

In one study the effects of beclomethasone dipropionate on HPA function were examined in patients with asthma. There was no change in basal early morning plasma cortisol concentrations or in the cortisol responses to tetracosactrin (ACTH 1:24) stimulation after daily administration of 400, 800, or 1,200 mcg of beclomethasone dipropionate for 28 days. After daily administration of 1,600 mcg each day for 28 days, there was slight reduction in basal cortisol concentrations and a statistically significant (p < .01) reduction in plasma cortisol responses to tetracosactrin stimulation. The effects of a more prolonged period of beclomethasone dipropionate administration on HPA function have not been evaluated. However, a number of investigators have noted that when systemic corticosteroid therapy in asthmatic subjects can be replaced with recommended doses of beclomethasone dipropionate, there is gradual recovery of endogenous cortisol concentrations to the normal range. There is still no documented evidence of recovery from other adverse systemic corticosteroid-induced reactions during prolonged therapy of patients with beclomethasone dipropionate.

Clinical experience has shown that some patients with bronchial asthma who require corticosteroid therapy for control of symptoms can be partially or completely withdrawn from systemic corticosteroids if therapy with beclomethasone dipropionate aerosol is substituted. Beclomethasone dipropionate aerosol is not effective for all patients with bronchial asthma or at all stages of the disease in a given patient.

The early clinical experience has revealed several new problems that may be associated with the use of beclomethasone dipropionate by inhalation for treatment of patients with bronchial asthma.

1. There is a risk of adrenal insufficiency when patients are transferred from systemic corticosteroids to aerosol beclomethasone dipropionate. Although the aerosol may provide adequate control of asthma during the transfer period, it does not provide the systemic steroid that is needed during acute stress situations. Deaths due to adrenal insufficiency have occurred in asthmatic patients during and after transfer from systemic corticosteroids to aerosol beclomethasone dipropionate (see WARNINGS).

2. Transfer of patients from systemic steroid therapy to beclomethasone dipropionate aerosol may unmask allergic conditions that were previously controlled by the systemic steroid therapy, eg, rhinitis, conjunctivitis, and eczema.

3. Localized infections with *C albicans* or *A niger* have occurred frequently in the mouth and pharynx and occasionally in the larynx. It has been reported that up to 75% of the patients who receive prolonged treatment with beclomethasone dipropionate have positive oral cultures for *C albicans*. The incidence of clinically apparent infection is considerably lower but may require therapy with appropriate antifungal agents or discontinuation of treatment with beclomethasone dipropionate aerosol.

The long-term effects of beclomethasone dipropionate in human subjects are still unknown. In particular, the local effects of the agent on developmental or immunologic processes in the mouth, pharynx, trachea, and lung are unknown. There is also no information about the possible long-term systemic effects of the agent. The possible relevance of the data in animal studies to results in human subjects cannot be evaluated.

Shown in Product Identification Section, page 404

BECONASE® Inhalation Aerosol   ℞
[be'kō-nāz"]
(beclomethasone dipropionate, USP)
For Nasal Inhalation Only

BECONASE AQ® Nasal Spray, 0.042%*
[be'kō-nāz"AQ]
(beclomethasone dipropionate, monohydrate)
*Calculated on the dried basis.   **SHAKE WELL**
For Intranasal Use Only   **BEFORE USE.**

DESCRIPTION

Beconase® Inhalation Aerosol:

Beclomethasone dipropionate, USP, the active component of Beconase Inhalation Aerosol, is an anti-inflammatory steroid having the chemical name 9-chloro-11β,17,21-trihydroxy-16β-methylpregna-1, 4-diene-3, 20-dione 17,21-dipropionate.

Beclomethasone dipropionate is a white to creamy-white, odorless powder with a molecular weight of 521.25. It is very slightly soluble in water, very soluble in chloroform, and freely soluble in acetone and in alcohol.

Beconase Inhalation Aerosol is a metered-dose aerosol unit containing a microcrystalline suspension of beclomethasone dipropionate-trichloromonofluoromethane clathrate in a mixture of propellants (trichloromonofluoromethane and dichlorodifluoromethane) with oleic acid. Each canister contains beclomethasone dipropionate-trichloromonofluoromethane clathrate having a molecular proportion of beclomethasone dipropionate to trichloromonofluoromethane between 3:1 and 3:2. Each actuation delivers from the nasal adapter a quantity of clathrate equivalent to 42 mcg of beclomethasone dipropionate, USP. The contents of one canister provide at least 200 metered doses.

Beconase AQ® Nasal Spray:
Beclomethasone dipropionate, monohydrate, the active component of Beconase AQ Nasal Spray, is an anti-inflammatory steroid having the chemical name 9-chloro-11β, 17,21-trihydroxy- 16β-methylpregna-1,4-diene-3,20-dione 17,21-dipropionate.

Beclomethasone dipropionate, monohydrate is a white to creamy-white, odorless powder with a molecular weight of 539.06. It is very slightly soluble in water, very soluble in chloroform, and freely soluble in acetone and in alcohol.

Beconase AQ Nasal Spray is a metered-dose, manual pump spray unit containing a microcrystalline suspension of beclomethasone dipropionate, monohydrate equivalent to 0.042% w/w beclomethasone dipropionate, calculated on the dried basis, in an aqueous medium containing microcrystalline cellulose, carboxymethylcellulose sodium, dextrose, benzalkonium chloride, polysorbate 80, and 0.25% v/w phenylethyl alcohol. Hydrochloric acid may be added to adjust pH. The pH is between 4.5 and 7.0.

After initial priming (three to four actuations), each actuation of the pump delivers from the nasal adapter 100 mg of suspension containing beclomethasone dipropionate, monohydrate equivalent to 42 mcg beclomethasone dipropionate. Each bottle of Beconase AQ Nasal Spray will provide at least 200 metered doses.

CLINICAL PHARMACOLOGY
Beclomethasone 17,21-dipropionate is a diester of beclomethasone, a synthetic halogenated corticosteroid. Animal studies show that beclomethasone dipropionate has potent glucocorticoid and weak mineralocorticoid activity.

The mechanisms for the anti-inflammatory action of beclomethasone dipropionate are unknown. The precise mechanism of the aerosolized drug's action in the nose is also unknown. Biopsies of nasal mucosa obtained during clinical studies showed no histopathologic changes when beclomethasone dipropionate was administered intranasally.

The effects of beclomethasone dipropionate on hypothalamic-pituitary-adrenal (HPA) function have been evaluated in adult volunteers by other routes of administration. Studies with beclomethasone dipropionate by the intranasal route may demonstrate that there is more or that there is less absorption by this route of administration. There was no suppression of early morning plasma cortisol concentrations when beclomethasone dipropionate was administered in a dose of 1,000 mcg/day for one month as an oral aerosol or for three days by intramuscular injection. However, partial suppression of plasma cortisol concentrations was observed when beclomethasone dipropionate was administered in doses of 2,000 mcg/day either by oral aerosol or intramuscular injection. Immediate suppression of plasma cortisol concentrations was observed after single doses of 4,000 mcg of beclomethasone dipropionate. Suppression of HPA function (reduction of early morning plasma cortisol levels) has been reported in adult patients who received 1,600-mcg daily doses of oral beclomethasone dipropionate for one month. In clinical studies using beclomethasone dipropionate aerosol intranasally, there was no evidence of adrenal insufficiency. The effect of Beconase AQ® (beclomethasone dipropionate, monohydrate) Nasal Spray on HPA function was not evaluated but would not be expected to differ from intranasal beclomethasone dipropionate aerosol.

In one study in asthmatic children, the administration of inhaled beclomethasone at recommended daily doses for at least one year was associated with a reduction in nocturnal cortisol secretion. The clinical significance of this finding is not clear. It reinforces other evidence, however, that topical beclomethasone may be absorbed in amounts that can have systemic effects and that physicians should be alert for evidence of systemic effects, especially in chronically treated patients (see PRECAUTIONS).

Beclomethasone dipropionate is sparingly soluble. When given by nasal inhalation in the form of an aqueous or aerosolized suspension, the drug is deposited primarily in the nasal passages. A portion of the drug is swallowed. Absorption occurs rapidly from all respiratory and gastrointestinal tissues. There is no evidence of tissue storage of beclomethasone dipropionate or its metabolites. *In vitro* studies have shown that tissue other than the liver (lung slices) can rapidly metabolize beclomethasone dipropionate to beclomethasone 17-monopropionate and more slowly to free beclomethasone (which has very weak anti-inflammatory activity). However, irrespective of the route of entry, the principal route of excretion of the drug and its metabolites is the feces. In humans, 12% to 15% of an orally administered dose of beclomethasone dipropionate is excreted in the urine as both conjugated and free metabolites of the drug.

Studies have shown that the degree of binding to plasma proteins is 87%.

INDICATIONS AND USAGE
Beconase® (beclomethasone dipropionate) Inhalation Aerosol is indicated for the relief of the symptoms of seasonal or perennial rhinitis in those cases poorly responsive to conventional treatment. **Beconase AQ® (beclomethasone dipropionate, monohydrate) Nasal Spray** is indicated for the relief of the symptoms of seasonal or perennial allergic and nonallergic (vasomotor) rhinitis.

Both preparations are also indicated for the prevention of recurrence of nasal polyps following surgical removal.

Clinical studies with Beconase Inhalation Aerosol in patients with seasonal or perennial rhinitis have shown that improvement is usually apparent within a few days. Results from two clinical trials have shown that significant symptomatic relief was obtained with Beconase AQ Nasal Spray within three days. With either preparation, however, symptomatic relief may not occur in some patients for as long as two weeks. Although systemic effects are minimal at recommended doses, Beconase Inhalation Aerosol and Beconase AQ Nasal Spray should not be continued beyond three weeks in the absence of significant symptomatic improvement. Both preparations should not be used in the presence of untreated localized infection involving the nasal mucosa.

Clinical studies have shown that treatment of the symptoms associated with nasal polyps may have to be continued for several weeks or more before a therapeutic result can be fully assessed. Recurrence of symptoms due to polyps can occur after stopping treatment, depending on the severity of the disease.

CONTRAINDICATIONS
Hypersensitivity to any of the ingredients of either preparation contraindicates its use.

WARNINGS
The replacement of a systemic corticosteroid with Beconase® (beclomethasone dipropionate) Inhalation Aerosol or Beconase AQ® (beclomethasone dipropionate, monohydrate) Nasal Spray can be accompanied by signs of adrenal insufficiency.

Careful attention must be given when patients previously treated for prolonged periods with systemic corticosteroids are transferred to Beconase Inhalation Aerosol or Beconase AQ Nasal Spray. This is particularly important in those patients who have associated asthma or other clinical conditions where too rapid a decrease in systemic corticosteroids may cause a severe exacerbation of their symptoms.

Studies have shown that the combined administration of alternate-day prednisone systemic treatment and orally inhaled beclomethasone increases the likelihood of HPA suppression compared to a therapeutic dose of either one alone. Therefore, Beconase Inhalation Aerosol and Beconase AQ Nasal Spray treatment should be used with caution in patients already on alternate-day prednisone regimens for any disease.

If recommended doses of intranasal beclomethasone are exceeded or if individuals are particularly sensitive or predisposed by virtue of recent systemic steroid therapy, symptoms of hypercorticism may occur, including very rare cases of menstrual irregularities, acneiform lesions, and cushingoid features. If such changes occur, Beconase Inhalation Aerosol and Beconase AQ Nasal Spray should be discontinued slowly consistent with accepted procedures for discontinuing oral steroid therapy.

PRECAUTIONS
General: During withdrawal from oral steroids, some patients may experience symptoms of withdrawal, eg, joint and/or muscular pain, lassitude, and depression.

Rarely, immediate hypersensitivity reactions may occur after the intranasal administration of beclomethasone. Extremely rare instances of wheezing, nasal septum perforation, and increased intraocular pressure have been reported following the intranasal application of aerosolized corticosteroids. Although these have not been observed in clinical trials with Beconase AQ® (beclomethasone dipropionate, monohydrate) Nasal Spray, vigilance should be maintained.

In clinical studies with beclomethasone dipropionate administered intranasally, the development of localized infections of the nose and pharynx with *Candida albicans* has occurred only rarely. When such an infection develops, it may require treatment with appropriate local therapy or discontinuation of treatment with Beconase® (beclomethasone dipropionate) Inhalation Aerosol or Beconase AQ Nasal Spray.

If persistent nasopharyngeal irritation occurs, it may be an indication for stopping Beconase AQ Nasal Spray.

Beclomethasone dipropionate is absorbed into the circulation. Use of excessive doses of Beconase Inhalation Aerosol or Beconase AQ Nasal Spray may suppress HPA function. Beconase Inhalation Aerosol and Beconase AQ Nasal Spray should be used with caution, if at all, in patients with active or quiescent tuberculous infections of the respiratory tract; untreated fungal, bacterial, or systemic viral infections; or ocular herpes simplex.

For either preparation to be effective in the treatment of nasal polyps, the aerosol or spray must be able to enter the nose. Therefore, treatment of nasal polyps with these preparations should be considered adjunctive therapy to surgical removal and/or the use of other medications that will permit effective penetration of these preparations into the nose. Nasal polyps may recur after any form of treatment.

As with any long-term treatment, patients using Beconase Inhalation Aerosol or Beconase AQ Nasal Spray over several months or longer should be examined periodically for possible changes in the nasal mucosa.

Because of the inhibitory effect of corticosteroids on wound healing, patients who have experienced recent nasal septal ulcers, nasal surgery, or trauma should not use a nasal corticosteroid until healing has occurred.

Although systemic effects have been minimal with recommended doses, this potential increases with excessive doses. Therefore, larger than recommended doses of Beconase Inhalation Aerosol and Beconase AQ Nasal Spray should be avoided.

Information for Patients: Patients being treated with Beconase Inhalation Aerosol or Beconase AQ Nasal Spray should receive the following information and instructions. This information is intended to aid in the safe and effective use of medication. It is not a disclosure of all possible adverse or intended effects. Patients should use these preparations at regular intervals since their effectiveness depends on their regular use. The patient should take the medication as directed. It is not acutely effective, and the prescribed dosage should not be increased. Instead, nasal vasoconstrictors or oral antihistamines may be needed until the effects of Beconase Inhalation Aerosol or Beconase AQ Nasal Spray are fully manifested. One to two weeks may pass before full relief is obtained. The patient should contact the doctor if symptoms do not improve, or if the condition worsens, or if sneezing or nasal irritation occurs. For the proper use of either unit and to attain maximum improvement, the patient should read and follow carefully the patient's instructions section of the package insert.

Carcinogenesis, Mutagenesis, Impairment of Fertility: Treatment of rats for a total of 95 weeks, 13 weeks by inhalation and 82 weeks by the oral route, resulted in no evidence of carcinogenic activity. Mutagenic studies have not been performed.

Impairment of fertility, as evidenced by inhibition of the estrous cycle in dogs, was observed following treatment by the oral route. No inhibition of the estrous cycle in dogs was seen following treatment with beclomethasone dipropionate by the inhalation route.

Pregnancy: *Teratogenic Effects: Pregnancy Category C:* Like other corticoids, parenteral (subcutaneous) beclomethasone dipropionate has been shown to be teratogenic and embryocidal in the mouse and rabbit when given in doses approximately ten times the human dose. In these studies, beclomethasone was found to produce fetal resorption, cleft palate, agnathia, microstomia, absence of tongue, delayed ossification, and agenesis of the thymus. No teratogenic or embryocidal effects have been seen in the rat when beclomethasone dipropionate was administered by inhalation at ten times the human dose or orally at 1,000 times the human dose. There are no adequate and well-controlled studies in pregnant women. Beclomethasone dipropionate should be used during pregnancy only if the potential benefit justifies the potential risk to the fetus.

Nonteratogenic Effects: Hypoadrenalism may occur in infants born of mothers receiving corticosteroids during pregnancy. Such infants should be carefully observed.

Nursing Mothers: It is not known whether beclomethasone dipropionate is excreted in human milk. Because other corticosteroids are excreted in human milk, caution should be exercised when Beconase Inhalation Aerosol or Beconase AQ Nasal Spray is administered to a nursing woman.

Pediatric Use: Safety and effectiveness in children below 6 years of age have not been established.

ADVERSE REACTIONS
In general, side effects in clinical studies with both preparations have been primarily associated with irritation of the nasal mucous membranes.

Extremely rare instances of wheezing, nasal septum perforation, and increased intraocular pressure have been reported following the intranasal administration of aerosolized corticosteroids (see PRECAUTIONS).

Rare cases of immediate and delayed hypersensitivity reactions, including urticaria, angioedema, rash, and bronchospasm, have been reported following the oral and intranasal inhalation and administration of beclomethasone.

Beconase® (beclomethasone dipropionate) Inhalation Aerosol: Adverse reactions reported in controlled clinical trials and long-term open studies in patients treated with Beconase Inhalation Aerosol are described below.

Sensations of irritation and burning in the nose (11 per 100 patients) following the use of Beconase Inhalation Aerosol have been reported. Also, occasional sneezing attacks (10 per

Continued on next page

Allen & Hanburys—Cont.

100 adult patients) have occurred immediately following the use of the intranasal inhaler. This symptom may be more common in children. Rhinorrhea may occur occasionally (1 per 100 patients).

Localized infections of the nose and pharynx with *C albicans* have occurred rarely (see PRECAUTIONS).

Transient episodes of epistaxis have been reported in 2 per 100 patients.

Ulceration of the nasal mucosa has been reported rarely. Systemic corticosteroid side effects were not reported during controlled clinical trials with Beconase Inhalation Aerosol. If recommended doses are exceeded, however, or if individuals are particularly sensitive, symptoms of hypercorticism, ie, Cushing's syndrome, could occur.

Beconase AQ® (beclomethasone dipropionate, monohydrate) Nasal Spray: Adverse reactions reported in controlled clinical trials and open studies in patients treated with Beconase AQ Nasal Spray are described below.

Mild nasopharyngeal irritation following the use of beclomethasone aqueous nasal spray has been reported in up to 24% of patients treated, including occasional sneezing attacks (about 4%) occuring immediately following use of the spray. In patients experiencing these symptoms, none had to discontinue treatment. The incidence of transient irritation and sneezing was approximately the same in the group of patients who received placebo in these studies, implying that these complaints may be related to vehicle components of the formulation.

Fewer than 5 per 100 patients reported headache, nausea, or lightheadedness following the use of Beconase AQ Nasal Spray. Fewer than 3 per 100 patients reported nasal stuffiness, nosebleeds, rhinorrhea, or tearing eyes.

OVERDOSAGE

When used at excessive doses, systemic corticosteroid effects such as hypercorticism and adrenal suppression may appear. If such changes occur, the dosage of Beconase® Inhalation Aerosol should be decreased, and Beconase AQ® Nasal Spray should be discontinued slowly consistent with accepted procedures for discontinuing oral steroid therapy. The oral LD_{50} of beclomethasone dipropionate is greater than 1 g/kg in rodents. One canister of Beconase Inhalation Aerosol contains 8.4 mg of beclomethasone dipropionate and one bottle of Beconase AQ Nasal Spray contains beclomethasone dipropionate, monohydrate equivalent to 10.5 mg of beclomethasone dipropionate; therefore, acute overdosage is unlikely.

DOSAGE AND ADMINISTRATION

Beconase® (beclomethasone dipropionate) Inhalation Aerosol: *Adults and Children 12 Years of Age and Older:* The usual dosage is one inhalation (42 mcg) in each nostril two to four times a day (total dose 168 to 336 mcg/day). Patients can often be maintained on a maximum dose of one inhalation in each nostril three times a day (252 mcg/day).

Children 6 to 12 Years of Age: The usual dosage is one inhalation in each nostril three times a day (252 mcg/day). Beconase Inhalation Aerosol is *not* recommended for children below 6 years of age since safety and efficacy studies have not been conducted in this age group.

CONTENTS UNDER PRESSURE. Do not puncture. Do not use or store near heat or open flame. Exposure to temperatures above 120° F may cause bursting. Never throw container into fire or incinerator. Keep out of reach of children.

Beconase AQ® (beclomethasone dipropionate, monohydrate) Nasal Spray: *Adults and Children 6 Years of Age and Older:* The usual dosage is one or two inhalations (42 to 84 mcg) in each nostril twice a day (total dose, 168 to 336 mcg/day).

Beconase AQ Nasal Spray is *not* recommended for children below 6 years of age.

In patients who respond to Beconase Inhalation Aerosol and to Beconase AQ Nasal Spray, an improvement of the symptoms of seasonal or perennial rhinitis usually becomes apparent within a few days after the start of therapy. However, symptomatic relief may not occur in some patients for as long as two weeks. Beconase Inhalation Aerosol and Beconase AQ Nasal Spray should not be continued beyond three weeks in the absence of significant symptomatic improvement.

The therapeutic effects of corticosteroids, unlike those of decongestants, are not immediate. This should be explained to the patient using either preparation in advance in order to ensure cooperation and continuation of treatment with the prescribed dosage regimen.

In the presence of excessive nasal mucus secretion or edema of the nasal mucosa, the drug may fail to reach the site of intended action. In such cases it is advisable to use a nasal vasoconstrictor during the first two to three days of Beconase Inhalation Aerosol or Beconase AQ Nasal Spray therapy.

Directions for Use: Illustrated Patient's Instructions for Use accompany each package of Beconase Inhalation Aerosol and Beconase AQ Nasal Spray.

HOW SUPPLIED

Beconase® (beclomethasone dipropionate) Inhalation Aerosol is supplied in a 16.8-g canister containing 200 metered doses with nasal adapter and patient's instructions (NDC 0173-0336-02). Also available is a 16.8-g refill canister only with patient's instructions (NDC 0173-0360-98).

Store between 2° and 30° C (36° and 86° F). As with most inhaled medications in aerosol canisters, the therapeutic effect of this medication may decrease when the canister is cold. Shake well before using.

Beconase AQ® (beclomethasone dipropionate, monohydrate) Nasal Spray, 0.042%* is supplied in an amber glass bottle fitted with a metering atomizing pump and nasal adapter in a box of one (NDC 0173-0388-79) with patient's instructions for use. Each bottle contains 25 g of suspension.

* Calculated on the dried basis.

Store between 15° and 30° C (59° and 86° F).

Shown in Product Identification Section, page 404

CEFTIN® Tablets   ℞
[*sef'tin*]
(cefuroxime axetil)

DESCRIPTION

Ceftin® (cefuroxime axetil, Glaxo) contains a semisynthetic, broad-spectrum cephalosporin antibiotic for oral administration. Cefuroxime axetil is the 1-(acetyloxy) ethyl ester of cefuroxime (Zinacef®, Glaxo), which in turn is chemically designated as (6R,7R)-3-carbamoyloxymethyl-7- [Z-2-methoxyimino-2- (fur-2-yl) acetamido] ceph-3-em -4-carboxylate. Cefuroxime axetil is in the amorphous form.

Each Ceftin Tablet contains the equivalent of 125, 250, or 500 mg of cefuroxime. Each tablet also contains the inactive ingredients colloidal silicon dioxide, croscarmellose sodium, FD&C Blue No. 1 (250- and 500-mg tablets only), hydrogenated vegetable oil, hydroxypropyl methylcellulose, methylparaben, microcrystalline cellulose, propylene glycol, propylparaben, sodium benzoate (125-mg tablets only), sodium lauryl sulfate, and titanium dioxide.

CLINICAL PHARMACOLOGY

After oral administration, cefuroxime axetil is absorbed from the gastrointestinal tract and rapidly hydrolyzed by nonspecific esterases in the intestinal mucosa and blood to release cefuroxime into the circulation. Cefuroxime is subsequently distributed throughout the extracellular fluids. The axetil moiety is metabolized to acetaldehyde and acetic acid. Cefuroxime is excreted unchanged in the urine.

Serum cefuroxime concentrations and urinary excretion data are shown in the table below.

Bioavailability of Cefuroxime Administered as Cefuroxime Axetil

Dosage* (Cefuroxime Equivalent)	Serum Cefuroxime Concentration+ (mcg/ml)		12-hr Urinary Excretion + (% of dose)
	Peak	6 h	
125 mg	2.1	0.3	52
250 mg	4.1	0.7	51
500 mg	7.0	2.2	48
1,000 mg	13.6	3.4	43

* Administered immediately after a meal.

+ Mean values of 12 normal volunteers. Peak concentrations occurred around two hours after the dose.

While cefuroxime axetil can be taken after food or on an empty stomach, absorption is greater when taken after food (absolute bioavailability of 52% compared with 37%). Peak serum cefuroxime concentrations after a 500-mg dose are also greater when taken with food (mean = 7.0 mcg/ml) compared with the fasting state (mean = 4.9 mcg/ml). Despite this difference in absorption, the clinical and bacteriological responses of patients were independent of food intake at the time of dosing in two studies where this was assessed. Approximately 50% of serum cefuroxime is bound to protein. The half-life of cefuroxime after oral administration of Ceftin® (cefuroxime axetil) is 1.2 hours. Concomitant administration of probenecid increases the area under the serum concentration versus time curve by 50%. Peak serum cefuroxime concentration after a 1.5-g single dose is greater when taken with 1 g of probenecid (mean = 14.8 mcg/ml) than without probenecid (mean = 12.2 mcg/ml). Concomitant probenecid also increases the time for which serum cefuroxime concentrations exceed 0.25 mcg/ml from 10.7 hours to 14.0 hours.

Microbiology: The *in vivo* bactericidal activity of cefuroxime axetil is due to cefuroxime. Cefuroxime has bactericidal activity against a wide range of common pathogens, including many beta-lactamase-producing strains.

Cefuroxime is highly stable to bacterial beta-lactamases, especially plasmid-mediated enzymes that are commonly found in Enterobacteriaceae. The bactericidal action of cefuroxime results from inhibition of cell wall synthesis by binding to essential target proteins.

In vitro, cefuroxime is active against most strains of clinical isolates of the following organisms:

Gram-positive: Staphylococcus aureus (including penicillinase- and non-penicillinase-producing strains), Streptococcus pneumoniae, and Streptococcus pyogenes (group A beta-hemolytic streptococci).

NOTE: Certain strains of enterococci, eg, *Streptococcus faecalis,* are resistant to cefuroxime. Methicillin-resistant staphylococci are resistant to cefuroxime.

Gram-negative: Moraxella (Branhamella) catarrhalis, Escherichia coli, Haemophilus influenzae, Haemophilus parainfluenzae, and Klebsiella pneumoniae.

NOTE: *Pseudomonas* spp and *Campylobacter* spp, *Acinetobacter calcoaceticus,* and most strains of *Serratia* spp and *Proteus vulgaris* are resistant to most first- and second-generation cephalosporins.

Cefuroxime has been shown to be active *in vitro* against the following microorganisms; however, clinical efficacy has not yet been established:

Gram-positive: Staphylococcus epidermidis, Staphylococcus saprophyticus, and Streptococcus agalactiae.

Gram-negative: M catarrhalis (including ampicillin-resistant strains), Citrobacter spp, Enterobacter spp, Klebsiella spp, Morganella morganii, Neisseria gonorrhoeae (including penicillinase- and non-penicillinase-producing strains), Proteus inconstans, Proteus mirabilis, Providencia rettgeri, Salmonella spp, and Shigella spp.

Anaerobes: Bacteroides spp, Clostridium spp, Fusobacterium spp, Peptococcus spp, Peptostreptococcus spp, and Propionibacterium spp.

NOTE: Most strains of *Clostridium difficile* and *Bacteroides fragilis* are resistant to cefuroxime.

Susceptibility Tests: *Diffusion Techniques:* Quantitative methods that require measurement of zone diameters give an estimate of antibiotic susceptibility. One such procedure[1-3] has been recommended for use with disks to test susceptibility to cefuroxime.

Reports from the laboratory giving results of the standard single-disk susceptibility test with a 30-mcg cefuroxime disk should be interpreted according to the following criteria:

Susceptible organisms produce zones of 18 mm or greater, indicating that the test organism is likely to respond to therapy.

Organisms that produce zones of 15 to 17 mm are expected to be susceptible if the infection is confined to tissues and fluids (eg, urine) in which high antibiotic concentrations are attained.

Resistant organisms produce zones of 14 mm or less, indicating that other therapy should be selected.

For gram-positive isolates, the test can be performed with either the cephalosporin-class disk (30 mcg of cephalothin) or the cefuroxime disk (30 mcg of cefuroxime), and a zone of 18 mm or greater indicates a cefuroxime-susceptible organism. Gram-negative organisms should be tested with the cefuroxime disk (using the above criteria), since cefuroxime has been shown by *in vitro* tests to have activity against certain strains of Enterobacteriaceae found resistant when tested with the cephalosporin-class disk. Gram-negative organisms having zones of less than 18 mm around the cephalothin disk are not necessarily of intermediate susceptibility or resistant to cefuroxime.

The cefuroxime disk should not be used for testing susceptibility to other cephalosporins.

Standardized procedures require the use of laboratory control organisms. The 30-mcg cefuroxime disk should give zone diameters between 27 and 35 mm for *S aureus* ATCC 25923. For *E coli* ATCC 25922, the zone diameters should be between 20 and 26 mm.

Dilution Techniques: A bacterial isolate may be considered susceptible if the minimum inhibitory concentration (MIC) value for cefuroxime is less than or equal to 16 mcg/ml. Organisms are considered resistant if the MIC is greater than 32 mcg/ml.

As with standard diffusion methods, dilution procedures require the use of laboratory control organisms. Standard cefuroxime powder should give MIC values in the range of 0.5 and 2 mcg/ml for *S aureus* ATCC 25923. For *E coli* ATCC 25922, the MIC range should be between 2 and 8 mcg/ml.

INDICATIONS AND USAGE

Ceftin® (cefuroxime axetil) is indicated for the treatment of patients with infections caused by susceptible strains of the designated organisms in the following diseases:

1. **Pharyngitis and Tonsillitis** caused by *S pyogenes* (group A beta-hemolytic streptococci). (Penicillin is the usual drug of choice in the treatment and prevention of streptococcal infections, including the prophylaxis of rheumatic fever. Ceftin is generally effective in the eradication of streptococci from the oropharynx. Ceftin is not indicated for the prophylaxis of subsequent rheumatic fever because data to support such use are not yet available.)

2. **Otitis Media** caused by *S pneumoniae, H influenzae* (ampicillin-susceptible and ampicillin-resistant strains), *M catarrhalis* (ampicillin-susceptible strains), and *S pyogenes* (group A beta-hemolytic streptococci).

3. **Lower Respiratory Tract Infections** (bronchitis) caused by *S pneumoniae, H influenzae* (ampicillin-susceptible strains), *H parainfluenzae* (ampicillin-susceptible strains).

4. **Urinary Tract Infections** caused by *E coli* and *K pneumoniae* in the absence of urological complications.

5. **Skin and Skin Structure Infections** caused by *S aureus* and *S pyogenes* (group A beta-hemolytic streptococci).

Bacteriological studies to determine the causative organism and its susceptibility to cefuroxime should be performed. Therapy may be started while awaiting the results of these studies. Once these results become available, antibiotic treatment should be adjusted accordingly.

CONTRAINDICATIONS

Ceftin® (cefuroxime axetil) is contraindicated in patients with known allergy to the cephalosporin group of antibiotics.

WARNINGS

BEFORE THERAPY WITH CEFTIN® (cefuroxime axetil) IS INSTITUTED, CAREFUL INQUIRY SHOULD BE MADE TO DETERMINE WHETHER THE PATIENT HAS HAD PREVIOUS HYPERSENSITIVITY REACTIONS TO CEPHALOSPORINS, PENICILLINS, OR OTHER DRUGS. THIS PRODUCT SHOULD BE GIVEN CAUTIOUSLY TO PENICILLIN-SENSITIVE PATIENTS. ANTIBIOTICS SHOULD BE ADMINISTERED WITH CAUTION TO ANY PATIENT WHO HAS DEMONSTRATED SOME FORM OF ALLERGY, PARTICULARLY TO DRUGS. IF AN ALLERGIC REACTION TO Ceftin OCCURS, DISCONTINUE THE DRUG. SERIOUS ACUTE HYPERSENSITIVITY REACTIONS MAY REQUIRE EPINEPHRINE AND OTHER EMERGENCY MEASURES.

Pseudomembranous colitis has been reported with the use of cephalosporins (and other broad-spectrum antibiotics); therefore, it is important to consider its diagnosis in patients who develop diarrhea in association with antibiotic use.

Treatment with broad-spectrum antibiotics alters normal flora of the colon and may permit overgrowth of clostridia. Studies indicate that a toxin produced by *C difficile* is one primary cause of antibiotic-associated colitis. Cholestyramine and colestipol resins have been shown to bind the toxin *in vitro*.

Mild cases of colitis may respond to drug discontinuation alone. Moderate to severe cases should be managed with fluid, electrolyte, and protein supplementation as indicated. When the colitis is not relieved by drug discontinuation or when it is severe, oral vancomycin is the treatment of choice for antibiotic-associated pseudomembranous colitis produced by *C difficile*. Other causes of colitis should also be considered.

PRECAUTIONS

General: If an allergic reaction to Ceftin® (cefuroxime axetil) occurs, the drug should be discontinued and, if necessary, the patient should be treated with appropriate agents, eg, antihistamines, pressor amines, or corticosteroids.

As with other antibiotics, prolonged use of Ceftin may result in overgrowth of nonsusceptible organisms. If superinfection occurs during therapy, appropriate measures should be taken.

Broad-spectrum antibiotics should be prescribed with caution for individuals with a history of colitis.

Information for Patients: (Pediatric) Ceftin is only available in tablet form. During clinical trials, the tablet was well tolerated by children who could swallow the tablet whole. Children who cannot swallow the tablet whole may have the tablet crushed and mixed with food (eg, applesauce, ice cream). However, it should be noted that the crushed tablet has a strong, persistent, bitter taste. Discontinuation of therapy due to the taste and/or problems of administering this drug occurred in 13% of children (range, 2% to 28% across centers). Thus, the physician and parent should ascertain, preferably while still in the physician's office, that the child can ingest Ceftin reliably. If not, alternative therapy should be considered.

Drug/Laboratory Test Interactions: A false-positive reaction for glucose in the urine may occur with copper reduction tests (Benedict's or Fehling's solution or with Clinitest® tablets), but not with enzyme-based tests for glycosuria (eg, Clinistix®, Tes-Tape®). As a false-negative result may occur in the ferricyanide test, it is recommended that either the glucose oxidase or hexokinase method be used to determine blood plasma glucose levels in patients receiving Ceftin. Cefuroxime does not interfere with the assay of serum and urine creatinine by the alkaline picrate method.

Carcinogenesis, Mutagenesis, Impairment of Fertility: Although no long-term studies in animals have been performed to evaluate carcinogenic potential, no mutagenic potential of cefuroxime was found in standard laboratory tests.

Reproductive studies revealed no impairment of fertility in animals.

Pregnancy: *Pregnancy Category B:* Reproduction studies have been performed in rats and mice at doses up to 50 to 160 times the human dose and have revealed no evidence of impaired fertility or harm to the fetus due to cefuroxime axetil. There are, however, no adequate and well-controlled studies in pregnant women. Because animal reproduction studies are not always predictive of human response, this drug should be used during pregnancy only if clearly needed.

Nursing Mothers: Since cefuroxime is excreted in human milk, consideration should be given to discontinuing nursing temporarily during treatment with Ceftin.

ADVERSE REACTIONS

The adverse reactions to Ceftin® (cefuroxime axetil) are similar to reactions to other orally administered cephalosporins. Ceftin was usually well tolerated in controlled clinical trials.

Pediatric patients taking crushed tablets during clinical trials complained of the bitter taste of Ceftin Tablets (see ADVERSE REACTIONS: Gastrointestinal and PRECAUTIONS: Information for Patients: (Pediatric)). The majority of adverse events were mild, reversible in nature, and did not require discontinuation of the drug. The incidence of gastrointestinal adverse events increased with the higher recommended doses. Twenty-five (25) patients have received Ceftin 500 mg twice a day for one to 2.5 months with no increase in frequency or severity of adverse events.

The following adverse reactions have been reported.

Gastrointestinal: Nausea occurred in 2.4% of patients. Vomiting occurred in 2.0% of patients. Diarrhea occurred in 3.5% of patients. Loose stools occurred in 1.3% of patients. There have been rare reports of pseudomembranous colitis. Crushed tablets have a bitter taste. In pediatric clinical studies conducted with crushed tablets, complaints due to taste ranged from 0/8 (0%) in one center to 47/71 (66%) in another center.

Hypersensitivity: Rash (0.6% of patients), pruritus (0.3% of patients), and urticaria (0.2% of patients) have been observed. One case of severe bronchospasm has been reported among the approximately 1,600 patients treated with Ceftin. Of the patients treated with Ceftin who reported a history of delayed hypersensitivity to a penicillin and not a cephalosporin, 2.9% of patients experienced a delayed hypersensitivity reaction to Ceftin.

Central Nervous System: Headache occurred in less than 0.7% of patients, and dizziness occurred in less than 0.2% of patients.

Other: Vaginitis occurred in 1.9% of female patients.

Clinical Laboratory Tests: Transient elevations in AST (SGOT, 2.0% of patients), ALT (SGPT, 1.6% of patients), and LDH (1.0% of patients) have been observed. Eosinophilia (1.1% of patients) and positive Coombs' test (0.4% of patients) have been reported.

In addition to the adverse reactions listed above that have been observed in patients treated with Ceftin, the following adverse reactions and altered laboratory tests have been reported for cephalosporin class antibiotics.

   Adverse Reactions: Allergic reactions including anaphylaxis, fever, colitis, renal dysfunction, toxic nephropathy, and hepatic dysfunction including cholestasis.

   Several cephalosporins have been implicated in triggering seizures, particularly in patients with renal impairment when the dosage was not reduced. If seizures associated with drug therapy should occur, the drug should be discontinued. Anticonvulsant therapy can be given if clinically indicated.

   Altered Laboratory Tests: Increased prothrombin time, increased BUN, increased creatinine, false-positive test for urinary glucose, increased alkaline phosphatase, neutropenia, thrombocytopenia, and leukopenia.

DOSAGE AND ADMINISTRATION

Ceftin® (cefuroxime axetil) may be given orally without regard to meals. However, absorption is enhanced when Ceftin is administered with food.

Adults and Children 12 Years of Age and Older: The recommended dosage is 250 mg twice a day. For more severe infections or infections caused by less susceptible organisms, the dosage may be increased to 500 mg twice a day.

For uncomplicated urinary tract infections, the usual recommended dosage is 125 mg twice a day. Dosage may be increased to 250 mg twice a day for some patients with urinary tract infections.

Infants and Children Up to 12 Years of Age: The recommended dosage for children is 125 mg twice a day. For children with otitis media, the recommended dosage is 125 mg twice a day for children less than 2 years of age and 250 mg twice a day for children 2 years of age and older.

Ceftin administered as a crushed tablet has a strong, persistent, bitter taste. Alternative therapy should be considered for children who cannot swallow tablets (see PRECAUTIONS: Information for Patients: (Pediatric)).

In the treatment of infections due to *S pyogenes* (group A beta-hemolytic streptococci), a therapeutic dosage of Ceftin should be administered for at least ten days.

HOW SUPPLIED

Ceftin® (cefuroxime axetil) Tablets, 125 mg, are white, capsule-shaped, film-coated tablets engraved with "395" on one side and "GLAXO" on the other in bottles of 20 (NDC 0173-0395-00) and 60 (NDC 0173-0395-01) and unit dose packs of 100 (NDC 0173-0395-02).

Ceftin Tablets, 250 mg, are light blue, capsule-shaped, film-coated tablets engraved with "387" on one side and "GLAXO" on the other in bottles of 20 (NDC 0173-0387-00) and 60 (NDC 0173-0387-42) and unit dose packs of 100 (NDC 0173-0387-01).

Ceftin Tablets, 500 mg, are dark blue, capsule-shaped, film-coated tablets engraved with "394" on one side and "GLAXO" on the other in bottles of 20 (NDC 0173-0394-00) and 60 (NDC 0173-0394-42) and unit dose packs of 50 (NDC 0173-0394-01).

Store between 15° and 30°C (59° and 86°F). Replace cap securely after each opening. Protect unit dose packs from excessive moisture.

REFERENCES

1. Bauer AW, Kirby WMM, Sherris JC, et al: Antibiotic susceptibility testing by a standardized single disc method. *Am J Clin Pathol* 1966;45:493.
2. National Committee for Clinical Laboratory Standards, Approved Standard: Performance Standards for Antimicrobial Disc Susceptibility Tests (M2-A3), December, 1984.
3. Standardized disc susceptibility test. *Federal Register* 1974; 39(May 30):19182–19184.

Shown in Product Identification Section, page 404

CORTICAINE® Cream   ℞
[*kort 'ah-kān"*]
(hydrocortisone acetate)

DESCRIPTION

Corticaine® Cream contains hydrocortisone acetate 0.5% in a washable, nongreasy cream base composed of esters of mixed saturated fatty acids, stearyl alcohol, glycerin, polysorbate 40, menthol, BHA, BHT, disodium EDTA, and purified water with methylparaben and propylparaben as preservatives. Corticaine Cream is an anti-inflammatory and antipruritic cream for topical use.

Chemically, hydrocortisone acetate is 11β, 17-dihydroxy-21-(acetyloxy) pregn-4-ene-3,20-dione.

CLINICAL PHARMACOLOGY

Topical corticosteroids share anti-inflammatory, antipruritic, and vasoconstrictive actions.

The mechanism of anti-inflammatory activity of the topical corticosteroids is unclear. Various laboratory methods, including vasoconstrictor assays, are used to compare and predict potencies and/or clinical efficacies of the topical corticosteroids. There is some evidence to suggest that a recognizable correlation exists between vasoconstrictor potency and therapeutic efficacy in man.

Pharmacokinetics: The extent of percutaneous absorption of topical corticosteroids is determined by many factors, including the vehicle, the integrity of the epidermal barrier, and the use of occlusive dressings.

Topical corticosteroids can be absorbed from normal intact skin. Inflammation and/or other disease processes in the skin increase percutaneous absorption. Occlusive dressings substantially increase the percutaneous absorption of topical corticosteroids. Thus, occlusive dressings may be a valuable therapeutic adjunct for treatment of resistant dermatoses (see DOSAGE AND ADMINISTRATION).

Once absorbed through the skin, topical corticosteroids are handled through pharmacokinetic pathways similar to systemically administered corticosteroids. Corticosteroids are bound to plasma proteins in varying degrees. Corticosteroids are metabolized primarily in the liver and are then excreted by the kidneys. Some of the topical corticosteroids and their metabolites are also excreted into the bile.

INDICATIONS AND USAGE

Corticaine® (hydrocortisone acetate) Cream is indicated for the relief of the inflammatory and pruritic manifestations of corticosteroid-responsive dermatoses and for external anal itching.

CONTRAINDICATIONS

Topical corticosteroids are contraindicated in those patients with a history of hypersensitivity to any of the components of the preparation.

PRECAUTIONS

General: Systemic absorption of topical corticosteroids has produced reversible hypothalamic-pituitary-adrenal (HPA) axis suppression, manifestations of Cushing's syndrome, hyperglycemia, and glucosuria in some patients.

Conditions that augment systemic absorption include the application of the more potent steroids, use over large surface areas, prolonged use, and the addition of occlusive dressings.

Therefore, patients receiving a large dose of a potent topical steroid applied to a large surface area or under an occlusive dressing should be evaluated periodically for evidence of

Continued on next page

Allen & Hanburys—Cont.

HPA axis suppression by using the urinary free cortisol and ACTH stimulation tests. If HPA axis suppression is noted, an attempt should be made to withdraw the drug, to reduce the frequency of application, or to substitute a less potent steroid.

Recovery of HPA axis function is generally prompt and complete upon discontinuation of the drug. Infrequently, signs and symptoms of steroid withdrawal may occur, requiring supplemental systemic corticosteroids.

Children may absorb proportionally larger amounts of topical corticosteroids and thus be more susceptible to systemic toxicity (see PRECAUTIONS: Pediatric Use).

If irritation develops, topical corticosteroids should be discontinued and appropriate therapy instituted.

In the presence of dermatological infections, the use of an appropriate antifungal or antibacterial agent should be instituted. If a favorable response does not occur promptly, the corticosteroid should be discontinued until the infection has been adequately controlled.

Information for the Patient: Patients using topical corticosteroids should receive the following information and instructions:

1. This medication is to be used as directed by the physician. It is for external use only. Avoid contact with the eyes.
2. Patients should be advised not to use this medication for any disorder other than for which it was prescribed.
3. The treated skin area should not be bandaged or otherwise covered or wrapped as to be occlusive unless directed by the physician.
4. Patients should report any signs of local adverse reactions, especially under occlusive dressing.
5. Parents of pediatric patients should be advised not to use tight-fitting diapers or plastic pants on a child being treated in the diaper area, as these garments may constitute occlusive dressings.

Laboratory Tests: The following tests may be helpful in evaluating the HPA axis suppression: Urinary free cortisol test and ACTH stimulation test.

Carcinogenesis, Mutagenesis, Impairment of Fertility: Long-term animal studies have not been performed to evaluate the carcinogenic potential or the effect on fertility of topical corticosteroids.

Studies to determine mutagenicity with prednisolone and hydrocortisone have revealed negative results.

Pregnancy: *Teratogenic Effects: Pregnancy Category C:* Corticosteroids are generally teratogenic in laboratory animals when administered systemically at relatively low dosage levels. The more potent corticosteroids have been shown to be teratogenic after dermal application in laboratory animals. There are no adequate and well-controlled studies in pregnant women on teratogenic effects from topically applied corticosteroids. Therefore, topical corticosteroids should be used during pregnancy only if the potential benefit justifies the potential risk to the fetus. Drugs of this class should not be used extensively on pregnant patients in large amounts or for prolonged periods of time.

Nursing Mothers: It is not known whether topical administration of corticosteroids could result in sufficient systemic absorption to produce detectable quantities in breast milk. Systemically administered corticosteroids are secreted into breast milk in quantities *not* likely to have a deleterious effect on the infant. Nevertheless, caution should be exercised when topical corticosteroids are administered to a nursing woman.

Pediatric Use: *Pediatric patients may demonstrate greater susceptibility to topical corticosteroid-induced HPA axis suppression and Cushing's syndrome than mature patients because of a larger skin surface to body weight ratio.*

HPA axis suppression, Cushing's syndrome, and intracranial hypertension have been reported in children receiving topical corticosteroids. Manifestations of adrenal suppression in children include linear growth retardation, delayed weight gain, low plasma cortisol levels, and absence of response to ACTH stimulation. Manifestations of intracranial hypertension include bulging fontanelles, headaches, and bilateral papilledema.

Administration of topical corticosteroids to children should be limited to the least amount compatible with an effective therapeutic regimen. Chronic corticosteroid therapy may interfere with the growth and development of children.

ADVERSE REACTIONS

The following local adverse reactions are reported infrequently with topical corticosteroids, but may occur more frequently with the use of occlusive dressings. These reactions are listed in an approximate decreasing order of occurrence: burning, itching, irritation, dryness, folliculitis, hypertrichosis, acneiform eruptions, hypopigmentation, perioral dermatitis, allergic contact dermatitis, maceration of the skin, secondary infection, skin atrophy, striae, and miliaria.

OVERDOSAGE

Topically applied corticosteroids can be absorbed in sufficient amounts to produce systemic effects (see PRECAUTIONS).

DOSAGE AND ADMINISTRATION

Topical corticosteroids are generally applied to the affected area as a thin film from one to four times daily depending on the severity of the condition.

Occlusive dressings may be used for the management of psoriasis or recalcitrant conditions.

If an infection develops, the use of occlusive dressings should be discontinued and appropriate antimicrobial therapy instituted.

HOW SUPPLIED

Corticaine® (hydrocortisone acetate) Cream is supplied in a 1-oz tube (NDC 0173-0404-00).

Keep container well closed and store between 15° and 30° C (59° and 86° F).

ETHATAB® Tablets   ℞
[eth ' ah-tab]
(ethaverine hydrochloride)

DESCRIPTION

Each Ethatab® Tablet contains ethaverine hydrochloride 100 mg, D&C Yellow No. 10, FD&C Yellow No. 6, and other ingredients.

ACTION

Ethatab® (ethaverine hydrochloride) acts directly on the smooth muscle cells without involving the autonomic nervous system or its receptors. It produces smooth muscle relaxation, particularly where spasm exists, affecting the larger blood vessels, especially systemic, peripheral, and pulmonary vessels, and smooth muscle of the intestines, biliary tree, and ureters.

INDICATIONS AND USAGE

In peripheral and cerebral vascular insufficiency associated with arterial spasm; also useful as a smooth muscle spasmolytic in spastic conditions of the gastrointestinal and genitourinary tracts.

CONTRAINDICATIONS

The use of Ethatab® (ethaverine hydrochloride) is contraindicated in the presence of complete atrioventricular dissociation.

PRECAUTIONS

As with all vasodilators, Ethatab® (ethaverine hydrochloride) should be administered with caution to patients with glaucoma. The safety of ethaverine hydrochloride during pregnancy or lactation has not been established; therefore, it should not be used in pregnant women or in women of childbearing age unless, in the judgment of the physician, its use is deemed essential to the welfare of the patient.

ADVERSE REACTIONS

Even though the incidence of adverse reactions as reported in the literature is very low, it is possible for a patient to evidence nausea, anorexia, abdominal distress, dryness of the throat, hypotension, malaise, lassitude, drowsiness, flushing, sweating, vertigo, respiratory depression, cardiac depression, cardiac arrhythmia, and headache. If these adverse reactions occur, reduce dosage or discontinue medication.

DOSAGE AND ADMINISTRATION

In mild or moderate disease, the usual dosage for adults is one tablet three times a day. In more difficult cases, dosage may be increased to two tablets three times a day. It is most effective given early in the course of the vascular disorder. Because of the chronic nature of the disease, long-term therapy is required.

HOW SUPPLIED

Ethatab® (ethaverine hydrochloride) Tablets are yellow, oval, scored tablets engraved with "Glaxo" and "281" in bottles of 100 (NDC 0173-0281-43) and unit dose packs of 100 (NDC 0173-0281-47).

THEOBID® and THEOBID® JR. DURACAP®   ℞
[thē 'ō-bid]
(theophylline, anhydrous)
(Sustained-Release)

DESCRIPTION

Theophylline is a bronchodilator structurally classified as a xanthine derivative. It occurs as a white, odorless, crystalline powder having a bitter taste.

Theophylline, anhydrous has the chemical name 1H-Purine-2, 6-dione,3,7-dihydro-1,3-dimethyl.

Each Theobid® or Theobid® Jr. sustained-release capsule for oral administration contains 260 or 130 mg, respectively, of theophylline, anhydrous in a sustained-release bead formulation. Each capsule also contains the inactive ingredi-

ents butylparaben, edetate calcium disodium, FD&C Blue No. 1, FD&C Red No. 3 (Theobid Jr. only), gelatin, methylparaben, pharmaceutical glaze, propylparaben, sodium lauryl sulfate, sodium propionate, corn starch, sucrose, titanium dioxide, and other ingredients.

CLINICAL PHARMACOLOGY

Theophylline directly relaxes the smooth muscle of the bronchial airways and pulmonary blood vessels, thus acting mainly as a bronchodilator and smooth muscle relaxant. It has also been demonstrated that aminophylline has a potent effect on diaphragmatic contractility in normal persons and may then be capable of reducing fatigability and thereby improve contractility in patients with chronic obstructive airway disease. The exact mode of action remains unsettled. Although theophylline does cause inhibition of phosphodiesterase with a resultant increase in intracellular cyclic AMP, other agents similarly inhibit the enzyme, producing a rise of cyclic AMP, but are unassociated with any demonstrable bronchodilation. Other mechanisms proposed include an effect on translocation of intracellular calcium, prostaglandin antagonism, stimulation of catecholamines endogenously, inhibition of cyclic guanosine monophosphate metabolism, and adenosine receptor antagonism. None of these mechanisms has been proved, however.

In vitro, theophylline has been shown to act synergistically with beta-agonists, and data is now available that demonstrates an additive effect in vivo with combined use.

Pharmacokinetics: The half-life of theophylline is influenced by a number of known variables. It may be prolonged in chronic alcoholics, particularly those with liver disease (cirrhosis or alcoholic liver disease), in patients with congestive heart failure, and in those patients taking certain other drugs (see PRECAUTIONS: Drug Interactions). Newborns and neonates have extremely slow clearance rates compared to older infants and children, ie, those over 1 year of age, who have rapid clearance rates. Most nonsmoking adults have clearance rates between these two extremes. In premature neonates the decreased clearance is related to oxidative pathways that have yet to be established.

Theophylline Elimination Characteristics

	Half-life	
	Range	Mean
Children	1–9 h	3.7 h
Adults	3–15 h	7.7 h

In cigarette smokers (one to two packs/day) the mean half-life is four to five hours, much shorter than in nonsmokers. The increase in clearance associated with smoking is presumably due to stimulation of the hepatic metabolic pathway by components of cigarette smoke. The duration of this effect after cessation of smoking is unknown but may require six months to two years before the rate approaches that of the nonsmoker.

In a single-dose study using ten healthy males, with initial fasting of ten hours before dosing and two hours after dosing, Theobid® (theophylline, anhydrous) dosed at 520 mg produced a mean peak theophylline serum level of 10.17 ± 1.01 mcg/ml (mean $\pm$ S.D.) at 5.2 ± 1 hour (mean $\pm$ S.D.) after administration.

In a multiple-dose crossover study of 18 healthy nonsmoking males fasting for ten hours before initial dosing and two hours after dosing. Theobid dosed at 390 mg (mean, 4.8 mg/kg) every 12 hours for five consecutive days produced areas under the curve equivalent to immediate-release aminophylline tablets dosed as 300 mg (mean, 3.2 mg/kg) at eight hours for the same time period.

INDICATIONS AND USAGE

For relief and/or prevention of symptoms from asthma and reversible bronchospasm associated with chronic bronchitis and emphysema.

CONTRAINDICATIONS

This product is contraindicated in individuals who have shown hypersensitivity to its components.

It is also contraindicated in patients with active peptic ulcer disease and in individuals with underlying seizure disorders (unless receiving appropriate anticonvulsant medication).

WARNINGS

Serum levels above 20 mcg/ml are rarely found after appropriate administration of the recommended doses. However, in individuals in whom theophylline plasma clearance is reduced *for any reason*, even conventional doses may result in increased serum levels and potential toxicity. Reduced theophylline clearance has been documented in the following readily identifiable groups: 1) patients with impaired liver function; 2) patients over 55 years of age, particularly males and those with chronic lung disease; 3) those with cardiac failure from any cause; 4) patients with sustained high fever; 5) neonates and infants under 1 year of age; and 6) those patients taking certain drugs (see PRECAUTIONS: Drug Interactions). Such patients frequently have markedly prolonged theophylline serum levels following discontinuation of the drug.

Reduction of dosage and laboratory monitoring is especially appropriate in these individuals.

Serious side effects such as ventricular arrhythmias, convulsions, or even death may appear as the first sign of toxicity without any previous warning. Less serious signs of theophylline toxicity (eg, nausea and restlessness) may occur frequently when initiating therapy, but are usually transient. When such signs are persistent during maintenance therapy, they are often associated with serum concentrations above 20 mcg/ml. Stated differently, *serious toxicity is not reliably preceded by less severe side effects.* A serum concentration measurement is the only reliable method of predicting potentially life-threatening toxicity.

Many patients who require theophylline may exhibit tachycardia due to their underlying disease process; therefore, the cause/effect relationship to elevated serum theophylline concentrations may not be appreciated.

Theophylline products may cause dysrhythmia and/or worsen pre-existing arrhythmias, so any significant change in rate and/or rhythm warrants monitoring and further investigation.

Studies in laboratory animals (minipigs, rodents, and dogs) recorded the occurrence of cardiac arrhythmias and sudden death (with histologic evidence of myocardial necrosis) when beta-agonists and methylxanthines were administered concurrently. The significance of these findings when applied to humans is currently unknown.

PRECAUTIONS

General: On the average theophylline half-life is shorter in cigarette and marijuana smokers than in nonsmokers, but smokers can have half-lives as long as nonsmokers. Theophylline should not be administered concurrently with other xanthines. Use with caution in patients with hypoxemia, hypertension, or those with history of peptic ulcer.

Theophylline may occasionally act as a local irritant to the gastrointestinal tract, although gastrointestinal symptoms are more commonly centrally mediated and associated with serum drug concentrations over 20 mcg/ml.

Information for Patients: The physician should reinforce the importance of taking only the prescribed dose and time interval between doses.

Laboratory Tests: Serum levels should be monitored periodically to determine the theophylline level associated with observed clinical response and to predict toxicity. For such measurements, the serum sample should be obtained at the time of peak concentration, four hours after dosing with Theobid® (theophylline, anhydrous) or Theobid® Jr. (theophylline, anhydrous). It is important that the patient not miss doses or take additional doses during the previous 48 hours and that dosing intervals are reasonably equally spaced. **DOSAGE ADJUSTMENT BASED ON SERUM THEOPHYLLINE MEASUREMENTS WHEN THESE INSTRUCTIONS HAVE NOT BEEN FOLLOWED MAY RESULT IN RECOMMENDATIONS THAT PRESENT RISK OF TOXICITY TO THE PATIENT.**

Drug Interactions: *Drug/Drug:* Toxic synergism with ephedrine has been documented and may occur with some other sympathomimetic bronchodilators. In addition, the following drug interactions have been demonstrated:

Theophylline with:

Allopurinol (high-dose)	Increased serum theophylline levels
Cimetidine	Increased serum theophylline levels
Erythromycin, troleandomycin	Increased serum theophylline levels
Lithium carbonate	Increased renal excretion of lithium
Oral contraceptives	Increased serum theophylline levels
Phenytoin	Decreased theophylline and phenytoin serum levels
Rifampin	Decreased serum theophylline levels

Drug/Food: Theobid and Theobid Jr. have not been adequately studied to determine whether their bioavailability is altered when they are given with food.

Drug/Laboratory Test Interactions: Currently available analytic methods for measuring serum theophylline levels, including high pressure liquid chromatography and immunoassay techniques, are specific. Metabolites and other drugs generally do not affect the results. Other new analytic methods are also now in use. The physician should be aware of the laboratory method used and whether other drugs will interfere with the assay for theophylline.

Carcinogenesis, Mutagenesis, Impairment of Fertility: Long-term carcinogenicity studies have not been performed with theophylline.

Chromosome-breaking activity was detected in human cell cultures at concentrations of theophylline up to 50 times the therapeutic serum concentration in humans. Theophylline was not mutagenic in the dominant lethal assay in male mice given theophylline intraperitoneally in doses up to 30 times the maximum daily human oral dose.

Studies to determine the effect on fertility have not been performed with theophylline.

Serum Theophylline Level		Directions
Within desired range		Maintain dosage if tolerated.
Too high	20 to 25 mcg/ml	Decrease doses by about 10%, and recheck serum theophylline level after three days.
	25 to 30 mcg/ml	Skip the next dose and decrease subsequent doses by about 25%. Recheck serum level after three days.
	Over 30 mcg/ml	Skip next two doses and decrease subsequent doses by 50%. Recheck serum level after three days.
Too low		Increase dosage by 25% at three-day intervals until either the desired serum concentration and/or clinical response is achieved. The total daily dose may need to be administered at more frequent intervals if symptoms occur repeatedly at the end of a dosing interval.

Pregnancy: *Teratogenic Effects: Pregnancy Category C:* Animal reproduction studies have not been conducted with theophylline. It is also not known whether theophylline can cause fetal harm when administered to a pregnant woman or can affect reproduction capacity. Xanthines should be given to a pregnant woman only if clearly needed.

Nursing Mothers: Theophylline is distributed into breast milk and may cause irritability or other signs of toxicity in nursing infants. Because of the potential for serious adverse reactions in nursing infants from theophylline, a decision should be made whether to discontinue nursing or to discontinue the drug, taking into account the importance of the drug to the mother.

Pediatric Use: Safety and effectiveness in children under 6 years of age have not been established for this product.

ADVERSE REACTIONS

The following adverse reactions have been observed, but there has not been enough systematic collection of data to support an estimate of their frequency. The most consistent adverse reactions are usually due to overdosage.

Gastrointestinal: Nausea, vomiting, epigastric pain, hematemesis, diarrhea.

Central Nervous System: Headaches, irritability, restlessness, insomnia, reflex hyperexcitability, muscle twitching, clonic and tonic generalized convulsions.

Cardiovascular: Palpitation, tachycardia, extrasystoles, flushing, hypotension, circulatory failure, ventricular arrhythmias.

Respiratory: Tachypnea.

Renal: Potentiation of diuresis.

Others: Alopecia, hyperglycemia, inappropriate ADH syndrome, rash.

OVERDOSAGE: Management: It is suggested that the management principles outlined below be instituted (consistent with the clinical status of the patient when first seen) and that simultaneous contact with a Regional Poison Control Center be established. In this way both updated information and individualization regarding therapy may be provided.

When Potential Oral Overdose is Established and Seizure Has Not Occurred:

1. If patient is alert and seen within the early hours after ingestion, induction of emesis may be of value. Gastric lavage has been demonstrated to be of no value in influencing outcome in patients who present more than one hour after ingestion.
2. Administer a cathartic. Sorbitol solution is reported to be of value.
3. Administer repeated doses of activated charcoal and monitor theophylline serum levels.
4. Prophylactic administration of phenobarbital has been shown to increase the seizure threshold in laboratory animals, and administration of this drug can be considered.

If Patient Presents with a Seizure:

1. Establish an airway.
2. Administer oxygen.
3. Treat the seizure with intravenous diazepam, 0.1 to 0.3 mg/kg up to 10 mg. If seizures cannot be controlled, the use of general anesthesia should be considered.
4. Monitor vital signs, maintain blood pressure, and provide adequate hydration.

If Post-seizure Coma is Present:

1. Maintain airway and oxygenation.
2. If a result of oral medication, follow above recommendations to prevent absorption of the drug. However, intubation and lavage will have to be performed instead of inducing emesis, and the carthartic and charcoal will need to be introduced via a large bore gastric lavage tube.
3. Continue to provide full supportive care and adequate hydration until the drug is metabolized. In general drug metabolism is sufficiently rapid so as not to warrant dialysis. If repeated oral activated charcoal is ineffective (as noted by stable or rising serum levels) charcoal hemoperfusion may be indicated.

DOSAGE AND ADMINISTRATION

Effective use of theophylline (the concentration of drug in the serum associated with optimal benefit and minimal risk of toxicity) is considered to occur when the theophylline concentration is maintained from 10 to 20 mcg/ml. The early studies from which these levels were derived were carried out in patients immediately or shortly after recovery from acute exacerbations of their disease (some hospitalized with status asthmaticus).

Although the 20-mcg/ml level remains appropriate as a critical value (above which toxicity is more likely to occur), for safety purposes additional data are now available that indicate that the serum theophylline concentrations required to produce maximum physiologic benefit may, in fact, fluctuate with the degree of bronchospasm present and are variable. Therefore, the physician should individualize the range appropriate to the patient's requirements, based on both symptomatic response and improvement in pulmonary function. It should be stressed that serum theophylline concentrations maintained at the upper level of the 10- to 20-mcg/ml range may be associated with potential toxicity when factors known to reduce theophylline clearance are operative (see WARNINGS).

If it is not possible to obtain serum level determinations, restriction of the daily dose (in otherwise healthy adults) to not greater than 13 mg/kg/day, a maximum of 900 mg, in divided doses will result in relatively few patients exceeding serum levels of 20 mcg/ml with the resultant greater risk of toxicity.

Caution should be exercised for younger children who cannot complain of minor side effects. Older adults and those with cor pulmonale, congestive heart failure, and/or liver disease may have unusually low dosage requirements and thus may experience toxicity at the maximal dosage recommended below.

Theophylline does not distribute into fatty tissue. Dosage should be calculated on the basis of lean (ideal) body weight where mg/kg doses are presented.

Frequency of Dosing: When immediate-release products with rapid absorption (such as tablets or liquid) are used, dosing to maintain serum levels generally requires administration every six hours. This is particularly true in children, but dosing intervals as high as eight hours may be satisfactory in adults since they eliminate the drug at a slower rate. Some children, and adults requiring higher than average doses (those having rapid rates of clearance, eg, half-lives of under six hours), may benefit and be more effectively controlled during chronic therapy when given products with sustained-release characteristics, since these provide longer dosing intervals and/or less fluctuation in serum concentration between dosing.

Dosage guidelines are approximations only, and the wide range of theophylline clearance between individuals (particularly those with concomitant disease) makes indiscriminate usage hazardous.

Dosage Guidelines: *Acute Symptoms:* Theobid® (theophylline, anhydrous) and Theobid Jr. (theophylline, anhydrous) are not intended for patients experiencing an acute episode of bronchospasm (associated with asthma, chronic bronchitis, or emphysema). Such patients require *rapid* relief of symptoms and should be treated with an immediate-release or intravenous theophylline preparation (or other bronchodilators) and not with controlled-release products.

Chronic Therapy: Theophylline is a treatment for the management of reversible bronchospasm (asthma, chronic bronchitis, and emphysema) to prevent symptoms and maintain patent airways. It is recommended that the appropriate dosage be established using an immediate-release preparation. A dosage form that allows small, incremental doses is desirable for initiating therapy. A liquid preparation should be considered for children to permit both greater ease and accuracy in adjusting the dosage.

Slow clinical titration is generally preferred to assure acceptance and safety of the medication and to allow the patient to develop tolerance to transient, caffeine-like side effects. Then, if the total 24-hour dose can be given by use of the available strengths of Theobid or Theobid Jr., the patient can usually be switched to the product and given one half of the daily dose at 12-hour intervals. However, certain patients, such as the young, smokers, and some nonsmoking adults, are likely to metabolize theophylline rapidly and require dosing at eight-hour intervals. Such patients can generally be identified as having trough serum concentra-

Continued on next page

Allen & Hanburys—Cont.

tions lower than desired or repeatedly exhibiting symptoms near the end of a dosing interval.

It is important that no patient be maintained on any dosage that is not tolerated. When instructing patients to increase dosage according to the schedule above, they should be told not to take a subsequent dose if apparent side effects occur and to resume therapy at a lower dose once adverse side effects have disappeared.

Maximum Dose of Theophylline Where the Serum Concentration is Not Measured: WARNING: DO NOT ATTEMPT TO MAINTAIN ANY DOSE THAT IS NOT TOLERATED.

Not to exceed the following:

Age <9 years	24 mg/kg/day
Age 9 to 12 years	20 mg/kg/day
Age 12 to 16 years	18 mg/kg/day
Age >16 years	13 mg/kg/day (or 900 mg, whichever is less)

Measurement of Serum Theophylline Concentrations During Chronic Therapy: If the above maximum doses are to be maintained or exceeded, serum theophylline measurement is essential (see PRECAUTIONS: Laboratory Tests).

Final Adjustment of Dosage:
Dosage Adjustment After Serum Theophylline Measurement

[See table on preceding page].

The serum concentration may be rechecked at appropriate intervals, but at least at the end of any adjustment period. When the patient's condition is otherwise clinically stable and none of the recognized factors that alter elimination are present, measurement of serum levels needs to be repeated only every 6 to 12 months.

HOW SUPPLIED

Theobid® (theophylline, anhydrous) Duracap® 260-mg capsules are blue and clear and are imprinted with "Glaxo 268." They are supplied in bottles of 60 (NDC 0173-0268-12) and 500 (NDC 0173-0268-14).

Theobid® Jr. (theophylline, anhydrous) Duracap® 130-mg capsules are two-tone blue and are imprinted with "Glaxo 295." They are supplied in bottles of 60 (NDC 0173-0295-12).

Store between 15° and 30° C (59° and 86°F). Store and dispense in tight containers as defined in USP/NF with child-resistant closures.

Shown in Product Identification Section, page 404

TRANDATE® Injection   ℞
[tran′dāt]
(labetalol hydrochloride)

DESCRIPTION

Trandate® (labetalol HCl) is an adrenergic receptor blocking agent that has both selective alpha$_1$- and nonselective beta-adrenergic receptor blocking actions in a single substance.

Labetalol HCl is 2-hydroxy-5-[1-hydroxy-2-[(1-methyl-3-phenylpropyl)amino]ethyl]benzamide monohydrochloride.

Labetalol HCl has the empirical formula $C_{19}H_{24}N_2O_3 \cdot HCl$ and a molecular weight of 364.9. It has two asymmetric centers and therefore exists as a molecular complex of two diastereoisomeric pairs.

Labetalol HCl is a white or off-white crystalline powder, soluble in water.

Trandate Injection is a clear, colorless to light yellow, aqueous, sterile, isotonic solution for intravenous injection. It has a pH range of 3 to 4. Each ml contains 5 mg labetalol HCl, 45 mg anhydrous dextrose, 0.1 mg edetate disodium; 0.8 mg methylparaben and 0.1 mg propylparaben as preservatives; and citric acid monohydrate and sodium hydroxide, as necessary, to bring the solution into the pH range.

CLINICAL PHARMACOLOGY

Trandate® (labetalol HCl) combines both selective, competitive alpha$_1$-adrenergic blocking and nonselective, competitive beta-adrenergic blocking activity in a single substance. In man, the ratios of alpha- to beta-blockade have been estimated to be approximately 1:3 to 1:7 following oral and intravenous administration, respectively. Beta$_2$-agonist activity has been demonstrated in animals with minimal beta$_1$-agonist (ISA) activity detected. In animals, at doses greater than those required for alpha- or beta-adrenergic blockade, a membrane stabilizing effect has been demonstrated.

Pharmacodynamics: The capacity of labetalol HCl to block alpha receptors in man has been demonstrated by attenuation of the pressor effect of phenylephrine and by a significant reduction of the pressor response caused by immersing the hand in ice-cold water ("cold-pressor test"). Labetalol HCl's beta$_1$-receptor blockade in man was demonstrated by a small decrease in the resting heart rate, attenuation of tachycardia produced by isoproterenol or exercise, and by attenuation of the reflex tachycardia to the hypotension produced by amyl nitrite. Beta$_2$-receptor blockade was dem-

onstrated by inhibition of the isoproterenol-induced fall in diastolic blood pressure. Both the alpha- and beta-blocking actions of orally administered labetalol HCl contribute to a decrease in blood pressure in hypertensive patients. Labetalol HCl consistently, in dose-related fashion, blunted increases in exercise-induced blood pressure and heart rate, and in their double product. The pulmonary circulation during exercise was not affected by labetalol HCl dosing.

Single oral doses of labetalol HCl administered in patients with coronary artery disease had no significant effect on sinus rate, intraventricular conduction, or QRS duration. The atrioventricular (A-V) conduction time was modestly prolonged in two of seven patients. In another study, intravenous labetalol HCl slightly prolonged A-V nodal conduction time and atrial effective refractory period with only small changes in heart rate. The effects on A-V nodal refractoriness were inconsistent.

Labetalol HCl produces dose-related falls in blood pressure without reflex tachycardia and without significant reduction in heart rate, presumably through a mixture of its alpha- and beta-blocking effects. Hemodynamic effects are variable, with small, nonsignificant changes in cardiac output seen in some studies but not others, and small decreases in total peripheral resistance. Elevated plasma renins are reduced. Doses of labetalol HCl that controlled hypertension did not affect renal function in mildly to severely hypertensive patients with normal renal function.

Due to the alpha$_1$-receptor blocking activity of labetalol HCl, blood pressure is lowered more in the standing than in the supine position, and symptoms of postural hypotension can occur. During dosing with intravenous labetalol HCl, the contribution of the postural component should be considered when positioning the patient for treatment, and the patient should not be allowed to move to an erect position unmonitored until his ability to do so is established.

In a clinical pharmacologic study in severe hypertensives, an initial 0.25/kg injection of labetalol HCl administered to patients in the supine position decreased blood pressure by an average of 11/7 mmHg. Additional injections of 0.5 mg/kg at 15-minute intervals up to a total cumulative dose of 1.75 mg/kg of labetalol HCl caused further dose-related decreases in blood pressure. Some patients required cumulative doses of up to 3.25 mg/kg. The maximal effect of each dose level occurred within five minutes. Following discontinuation of intravenous treatment with labetalol HCl, the blood pressure rose gradually and progressively, approaching pretreatment baseline values within an average of 16 to 18 hours in the majority of patients.

Similar results were obtained in the treatment of patients with severe hypertension who required urgent blood pressure reduction with an initial dose of 20 mg (which corresponds to 0.25 mg/kg for an 80-kg patient) followed by additional doses of either 40 or 80 mg at ten-minute intervals to achieve the desired effect, or up to a cumulative dose of 300 mg.

Labetalol HCl administered as a continuous intravenous infusion, with a mean dose of 136 mg (27 to 300 mg) over a period of two to three hours (mean of two hours and 39 minutes), lowered the blood pressure by an average of 60/35 mmHg.

Exacerbation of angina and, in some cases, myocardial infarction and ventricular dysrhythmias have been reported after abrupt discontinuation of therapy with beta-adrenergic blocking agents in patients with coronary artery disease. Abrupt withdrawal of these agents in patients without coronary artery disease has resulted in transient symptoms, including tremulousness, sweating, palpitation, headache, and malaise. Several mechanisms have been proposed to explain these phenomena, among them increased sensitivity to catecholamines because of increased numbers of beta receptors. Although beta-adrenergic receptor blockade is useful in the treatment of angina and hypertension, there are also situations in which sympathetic stimulation is vital. For example, in patients with severely damaged hearts, adequate ventricular function may depend on sympathetic drive. Beta-adrenergic blockade may worsen A-V block by preventing the necessary facilitating effects of sympathetic activity on conduction. Beta$_2$-adrenergic blockade results in passive bronchial constriction by interfering with endogenous adrenergic bronchodilator activity in patients subject to bronchospasm, and it may also interfere with exogenous bronchodilators in such patients.

Pharmacokinetics and Metabolism: Following intravenous infusion of labetalol, the elimination half-life is about 5.5 hours and the total body clearance is approximately 33 ml/min/kg. The plasma half-life of labetalol following oral administration is about six to eight hours. In patients with decreased hepatic or renal function, the elimination half-life of labetalol is not altered; however, the relative bioavailability in hepatically impaired patients is increased due to decreased "first-pass" metabolism.

The metabolism of labetalol is mainly through conjugation to glucuronide metabolites. The metabolites are present in plasma and are excreted in the urine and, via the bile, into the feces. Approximately 55% to 60% of a dose appears in

the urine as conjugates or unchanged labetalol within the first 24 hours of dosing.

Labetalol has also been shown to cross the placental barrier in humans. Only negligible amounts of the drug crossed the blood-brain barrier in animal studies. Labetalol is approximately 50% protein bound. Neither hemodialysis nor peritoneal dialysis removes a significant amount of labetalol HCl from the general circulation (<1%).

INDICATIONS AND USAGE

Trandate® (labetalol HCl) Injection is indicated for control of blood pressure in severe hypertension.

CONTRAINDICATIONS

Trandate® (labetalol HCl) Injection is contraindicated in bronchial asthma, overt cardiac failure, greater-than-first-degree heart block, cardiogenic shock, and severe bradycardia (see WARNINGS).

WARNINGS

Hepatic Injury: Severe hepatocellular injury, confirmed by rechallenge in at least one case, occurs rarely with labetalol therapy. The hepatic injury is usually reversible, but hepatic necrosis and death have been reported. Injury has occurred after both short- and long-term treatment and may be slowly progressive despite minimal symptomatology. Appropriate laboratory testing should be done at the first symptom/sign of liver dysfunction (eg, pruritus, dark urine, persistent anorexia, jaundice, right upper quadrant tenderness, or unexplained "flu-like" symptoms). If the patient has laboratory evidence of liver injury or jaundice, labetalol should be stopped and not restarted.

Cardiac Failure: Sympathetic stimulation is a vital component supporting circulatory function in congestive heart failure. Beta-blockade carries a potential hazard of further depressing myocardial contractility and precipitating more severe failure. Although beta-blockers should be avoided in overt congestive heart failure, if necessary, labetalol HCl can be used with caution in patients with a history of heart failure who are well compensated. Congestive heart failure has been observed in patients receiving labetalol HCl. Labetalol HCl does not abolish the inotropic action of digitalis on heart muscle.

In Patients Without a History of Cardiac Failure: In patients with latent cardiac insufficiency, continued depression of the myocardium with beta-blocking agents over a period of time can, in some cases, lead to cardiac failure. At the first sign or symptom of impending cardiac failure, patients should be fully digitalized and/or be given a diuretic, and the response should be observed closely. If cardiac failure continues despite adequate digitalization and diuretic, Trandate® (labetalol HCl) therapy should be withdrawn (gradually, if possible).

Ischemic Heart Disease: Angina pectoris has not been reported upon labetalol HCl discontinuation. However, following abrupt cessation of therapy with some beta-blocking agents in patients with coronary artery disease, exacerbations of angina pectoris and, in some cases, myocardial infarction have been reported. Therefore, such patients should be cautioned against interruption of therapy without the physician's advice. Even in the absence of overt angina pectoris, when discontinuation of Trandate is planned, the patient should be carefully observed and should be advised to limit physical activity. If angina markedly worsens or acute coronary insufficiency develops, Trandate administration should be reinstituted promptly, at least temporarily, and other measures appropriate for the management of unstable angina should be taken.

Nonallergic Bronchospasm (eg, Chronic Bronchitis and Emphysema): Since Trandate Injection at the usual intravenous therapeutic doses has not been studied in patients with nonallergic bronchospastic disease, it should not be used in such patients.

Pheochromocytoma: Intravenous labetalol HCl has been shown to be effective in lowering blood pressure and relieving symptoms in patients with pheochromocytoma; higher than usual doses may be required. However, paradoxical hypertensive responses have been reported in a few patients with this tumor; therefore, use caution when administering labetalol HCl to patients with pheochromocytoma.

Diabetes Mellitus and Hypoglycemia: Beta-adrenergic blockade may prevent the appearance of premonitory signs and symptoms (eg, tachycardia) of acute hypoglycemia. This is especially important with labile diabetics. Beta-blockade also reduces the release of insulin in response to hyperglycemia; it may therefore be necessary to adjust the dose of antidiabetic drugs.

Major Surgery: The necessity or desirability of withdrawing beta-blocking therapy before major surgery is controversial. Protracted severe hypotension and difficulty in restarting or maintaining a heartbeat have been reported with beta-blockers. The effect of labetalol HCl's alpha-adrenergic activity has not been evaluated in this setting.

A synergism between labetalol HCl and halothane anesthesia has been shown (see PRECAUTIONS: Drug Interactions).

Rapid Decreases of Blood Pressure: Caution must be observed when reducing severely elevated blood pressure. Although such findings have not been reported with intravenous labetalol HCl, a number of adverse reactions, including cerebral infarction, optic nerve infarction, angina, and ischemic changes in the electrocardiogram, have been reported with other agents when severely elevated blood pressure was reduced over time courses of several hours to as long as one or two days. The desired blood pressure lowering should therefore be achieved over as long a period of time as is compatible with the patient's status.

PRECAUTIONS

General: *Impaired Hepatic Function:* Trandate® (labetalol HCl) Injection should be used with caution in patients with impaired hepatic function since metabolism of the drug may be diminished.

Hypotension: Symptomatic postural hypotension (incidence, 58%) is likely to occur if patients are tilted or allowed to assume the upright position within three hours of receiving Trandate Injection. Therefore, the patient's ability to tolerate an upright position should be established before permitting any ambulation.

Jaundice or Hepatic Dysfunction: (see WARNINGS).

Information for Patients: The following information is intended to aid in the safe and effective use of this medication. It is not a disclosure of all possible adverse or intended effects. During and immediately following (for up to three hours) Trandate Injection, the patient should remain supine. Subsequently, the patient should be advised on how to proceed gradually to become ambulatory and should be observed at the time of first ambulation.

When the patient is started on Trandate® (labetalol HCl) Tablets following adequate control of blood pressure with Trandate Injection, appropriate directions for titration of dosage should be provided (see DOSAGE AND ADMINISTRATION).

As with all drugs with beta-blocking activity, certain advice to patients being treated with labetalol HCl is warranted. While no incident of the abrupt withdrawal phenomenon (exacerbation of angina pectoris) has been reported with labetalol HCl, dosing with Trandate Tablets should not be interrupted or discontinued without the physician's advice. Patients being treated with Trandate Tablets should consult a physician at any signs or symptoms of impending cardiac failure or hepatic dysfunction (see WARNINGS). Also, transient scalp tingling may occur, usually when treatment with Trandate Tablets is initiated (see ADVERSE REACTIONS).

Laboratory Tests: Routine laboratory tests are ordinarily not required before or after intravenous labetalol HCl. In patients with concomitant illnesses, such as impaired renal function, appropriate tests should be done to monitor these conditions.

Drug Interactions: Since Trandate Injection may be administered to patients already being treated with other medications, including other antihypertensive agents, careful monitoring of these patients is necessary to detect and treat promptly any undesired effect from concomitant administration.

In one survey, 2.3% of patients taking labetalol HCl orally in combination with tricyclic antidepressants experienced tremor as compared to 0.7% reported to occur with labetalol HCl alone. The contribution of each of the treatments to this adverse reaction is unknown, but the possibility of a drug interaction cannot be excluded.

Drugs possessing beta-blocking properties can blunt the bronchodilator effect of beta-receptor agonist drugs in patients with bronchospasm; therefore, doses greater than the normal antiasthmatic dose of beta-agonist bronchodilator drugs may be required.

Cimetidine has been shown to increase the bioavailability of labetalol HCl administered orally. Since this could be explained either by enhanced absorption or by an alteration of hepatic metabolism of labetalol HCl, special care should be used in establishing the dose required for blood pressure control in such patients.

Synergism has been shown between halothane anesthesia and intravenously administered labetalol HCl. During controlled hypotensive anesthesia using labetalol HCl in association with halothane, high concentrations (3% or above) of halothane should not be used because the degree of hypotension will be increased and because of the possibility of a large reduction in cardiac output and an increase in central venous pressure. The anesthesiologist should be informed when a patient is receiving labetalol HCl.

Labetalol HCl blunts the reflex tachycardia produced by nitroglycerin without preventing its hypotensive effect. If labetalol HCl is used with nitroglycerin in patients with angina pectoris, additional antihypertensive effects may occur.

Drug/Laboratory Test Interactions: The presence of labetalol metabolite in the urine may result in falsely elevated levels of urinary catecholamines, metanephrine, normetanephrine, and vanillylmandelic acid when measured by fluorimetric or photometric methods. In screening patients suspected of having a pheochromocytoma and being treated with labetalol HCl, a specific method, such as a high performance liquid chromatography assay with solid phase extrac-

tion (eg, *J Chromatogr* 385;241,1987) should be employed in determining levels of catecholamines.

Labetalol HCl has also been reported to produce a false-positive test for amphetamine when screening urine for the presence of drugs using the commercially available assay methods Toxi-Lab A® (thin-layer chromatographic assay) and Emit-d.a.u.® (radioenzymatic assay). When patients being treated with labetalol have a positive urine test for amphetamine using these techniques, confirmation should be made by using more specific methods, such as a gas chromatographic-mass spectrometer technique.

Carcinogenesis, Mutagenesis, Impairment of Fertility: Long-term oral dosing studies with labetalol HCl for 18 months in mice and for two years in rats showed no evidence of carcinogenesis. Studies with labetalol HCl using dominant lethal assays in rats and mice and exposing microorganisms according to modified Ames tests showed no evidence of mutagenesis.

Pregnancy: *Teratogenic Effects: Pregnancy Category C:* Teratogenic studies were performed with labetalol in rats and rabbits at oral doses up to approximately six and four times the maximum recommended human dose (MRHD), respectively. No reproducible evidence of fetal malformations was observed. Increased fetal resorptions were seen in both species at doses approximating the MRHD. A teratology study performed with labetalol in rabbits at intravenous doses up to 1.7 times the MRHD revealed no evidence of drug-related harm to the fetus. There are no adequate and well-controlled studies in pregnant women. Labetalol should be used during pregnancy only if the potential benefit justifies the potential risk to the fetus.

Nonteratogenic Effects: Transient hypotension, bradycardia, and hypoglycemia have been rarely observed in infants of mothers who were treated with labetalol HCl for hypertension during pregnancy. Oral administration of labetalol to rats during late gestation through weaning at doses of two to four times the MRHD caused a decrease in neonatal survival.

Labor and Delivery: Labetalol HCl given to pregnant women with hypertension did not appear to affect the usual course of labor and delivery.

Nursing Mothers: Small amounts of labetalol (approximately 0.004% of the maternal dose) are excreted in human milk. Caution should be exercised when Trandate Injection is administered to a nursing woman.

Pediatric Use: Safety and effectiveness in children have not been established.

ADVERSE REACTIONS

Trandate® (labetalol HCl) Injection is usually well tolerated. Most adverse effects have been mild and transient and, in controlled trials involving 92 patients, did not require labetalol HCl withdrawal. Symptomatic postural hypotension (incidence, 58%) is likely to occur if patients are tilted or allowed to assume the upright position within three hours of receiving Trandate Injection. Moderate hypotension occurred in 1 of 100 patients while supine. Increased sweating was noted in 4 of 100 patients, and flushing occurred in 1 of 100 patients.

The following also were reported with Trandate Injection with the incidence per 100 patients as noted:

Cardiovascular System: Ventricular arrhythmia in 1.

Central and Peripheral Nervous Systems: Dizziness in 9, tingling of the scalp/skin in 7, hypoesthesia (numbness) and vertigo in 1 each.

Gastrointestinal System: Nausea in 13, vomiting in 4, dyspepsia and taste distortion in 1 each.

Metabolic Disorders: Transient increases in blood urea nitrogen and serum creatinine levels occurred in 8 of 100 patients; these were associated with drops in blood pressure, generally in patients with prior renal insufficiency.

Psychiatric Disorders: Somnolence/yawning in 3.

Respiratory System: Wheezing in 1.

Skin: Pruritus in 1.

The incidence of adverse reactions depends upon the dose of labetalol HCl. The largest experience is with oral labetalol HCl (see Trandate® (labetalol HCl) Tablets Product Information for details). Certain of the side effects increased with increasing oral dose, as shown in the table above that depicts

the entire US therapeutic trials data base for adverse reactions that are clearly or possibly dose-related.

The oculomucocutaneous syndrome associated with the beta-blocker practolol has not been reported with labetalol HCl during investigational use and extensive foreign marketing experience.

Clinical Laboratory Tests: Among patients dosed with Trandate Tablets, there have been reversible increases of serum transaminases in 4% of patients tested and, more rarely, reversible increases in blood urea.

OVERDOSAGE

Overdosage with Trandate® (labetalol HCl) Injection causes excessive hypotension that is posture sensitive and, sometimes, excessive bradycardia. Patients should be placed supine and their legs raised if necessary to improve the blood supply to the brain. If overdosage with labetalol HCl follows oral ingestion, gastric lavage or pharmacologically induced emesis (using syrup of ipecac) may be useful for removal of the drug shortly after ingestion. The following additional measures should be employed if necessary: **Excessive bradycardia**—administer atropine or epinephrine. **Cardiac failure**—administer a digitalis glycoside and a diuretic. Dopamine or dobutamine may also be useful. **Hypotension**—administer vasopressors, eg, norepinephrine. There is pharmacological evidence that norepinephrine may be the drug of choice. **Bronchospasm**—administer epinephrine and/or an aerosolized beta$_2$-agonist. **Seizures**—administer diazepam.

In severe beta-blocker overdose resulting in hypotension and/or bradycardia, glucagon has been shown to be effective when administered in large doses (5 to 10 mg rapidly over 30 seconds, followed by continuous infusion of 5 mg/h that can be reduced as the patient improves).

Neither hemodialysis nor peritoneal dialysis removes a significant amount of labetalol from the general circulation (<1%).

The oral LD$_{50}$ value of labetalol HCl in the mouse is approximately 600 mg/kg and in the rat is greater than 2 g/kg. The intravenous LD$_{50}$ in these species is 50 to 60 mg/kg.

DOSAGE AND ADMINISTRATION

Trandate® (labetalol HCl) Injection is intended for intravenous use in hospitalized patients. DOSAGE MUST BE INDIVIDUALIZED depending upon the severity of hypertension and the response of the patient during dosing.

Patients should always be kept in a supine position during the period of intravenous drug administration. A substantial fall in blood pressure on standing should be expected in these patients. The patient's ability to tolerate an upright position should be established before permitting any ambulation, such as using toilet facilities.

Either of two methods of administration of Trandate Injection may be used: a) repeated intravenous injection, or b) slow continuous infusion.

Repeated Intravenous Injection: Initially, Trandate Injection should be given in a 20-mg dose (which corresponds to 0.25 mg/kg for an 80-kg patient) by slow intravenous injection over a two-minute period.

Immediately before the injection and at five and ten minutes after injection, supine blood pressure should be measured to evaluate response. Additional injections of 40 or 80 mg can be given at ten-minute intervals until a desired supine blood pressure is achieved or a total of 300 mg of labetalol HCl has been injected. The maximum effect usually occurs within five minutes of each injection.

Slow Continuous Infusion: Trandate Injection is prepared for continuous intravenous infusion by diluting the vial contents with commonly used intravenous fluids (see below). Examples of two methods of preparing the infusion solution are:

Add 40 ml of Trandate Injection to 160 ml of a commonly used intravenous fluid such that the resultant 200 ml of solution contains 200 mg of labetalol HCl, 1 mg/ml. The diluted solution should be administered at a rate of 2 ml/min to deliver 2 mg/min.

Alternatively, add 40 ml of Trandate Injection to 250 ml of a commonly used intravenous fluid. The resultant solution will contain 200 mg of labetalol HCl, approxi-

Continued on next page

Labetalol HCl Daily Dose (mg)	200	300	400	600	800	900	1,200	1,600	2,400
Number of Patients	522	181	606	608	503	117	411	242	175
Dizziness (%)	2	3	3	3	5	1	9	13	16
Fatigue	2	1	4	4	5	3	7	6	10
Nausea	<1	0	1	2	4	0	7	11	19
Vomiting	0	0	<1	<1	<1	0	1	2	3
Dyspepsia	1	0	2	1	1	0	2	2	4
Paresthesia	2	0	2	2	1	1	2	5	5
Nasal Stuffiness	1	1	2	2	2	2	4	5	6
Ejaculation Failure	0	2	1	2	3	0	4	3	5
Impotence	1	1	1	1	2	4	3	4	3
Edema	1	0	1	1	1	0	1	2	2

Allen & Hanburys—Cont.

mately 2 mg/3 ml. The diluted solution should be administered at a rate of 3 ml/min to deliver approximately 2 mg/min.

The rate of infusion of the diluted solution may be adjusted according to the blood pressure response, at the discretion of the physician. To facilitate a desired rate of infusion, the diluted solution can be infused using a controlled administration mechanism, eg, graduated burette or mechanically driven infusion pump.

Since the half-life of labetalol is five to eight hours, steady-state blood levels (in the face of a constant rate of infusion) would not be reached during the usual infusion time period. The infusion should be continued until a satisfactory response is obtained and should then be stopped and oral labetalol HCl started (see below). The effective intravenous dose is usually in the range of 50 to 200 mg. A total dose of up to 300 mg may be required in some patients.

Blood Pressure Monitoring: The blood pressure should be monitored during and after completion of the infusion or intravenous injection. Rapid or excessive falls in either systolic or diastolic blood pressure during intravenous treatment should be avoided. In patients with excessive systolic hypertension, the decrease in systolic pressure should be used as an indicator of effectiveness in addition to the response of the diastolic pressure.

Initiation of Dosing with Trandate® (labetalol HCl) Tablets: Subsequent oral dosing with Trandate Tablets should begin when it has been established that the supine diastolic blood pressure has begun to rise. The recommended initial dose is 200 mg, followed in six to 12 hours by an additional dose of 200 or 400 mg, depending on the blood pressure response. Thereafter, **inpatient titration with Trandate Tablets** may proceed as follows:

Inpatient Titration Instructions

Regimen	Daily Dose*
200 mg bid	400 mg
400 mg bid	800 mg
800 mg bid	1,600 mg
1,200 mg bid	2,400 mg

* If needed, the total daily dose may be given in three divided doses.

The dosage of Trandate Tablets used in the hospital may be increased at one-day intervals to achieve the desired blood pressure reduction.

For subsequent outpatient titration or maintenance dosing, see DOSAGE AND ADMINISTRATION in the Trandate Tablets Product Information for additional recommendations.

Compatibility with Commonly Used Intravenous Fluids: Parenteral drug products should be inspected visually for particulate matter and discoloration prior to administration whenever solution and container permit.

Trandate Injection was tested for compatibility with commonly used intravenous fluids at final concentrations of 1.25 to 3.75 mg of labetalol HCl per ml of the mixture. Trandate Injection was found to be compatible with and stable (for 24 hours refrigerated or at room temperature) in mixtures with the following solutions: Ringer's Injection, USP; Lactated Ringer's Injection, USP; 5% Dextrose and Ringer's Injection; 5% Lactated Ringer's and 5% Dextrose Injection; 5% Dextrose Injection, USP; 0.9% Sodium Chloride Injection, USP; 5% Dextrose and 0.2% Sodium Chloride Injection, USP; 2.5% Dextrose and 0.45% Sodium Chloride Injection, USP; 5% Dextrose and 0.9% Sodium Chloride Injection, USP; and 5% Dextrose and 0.33% Sodium Chloride Injection, USP.

Trandate Injection was NOT compatible with 5% Sodium Bicarbonate Injection, USP.

HOW SUPPLIED

Trandate® (labetalol hydrochloride) Injection, 5 mg/ml, is supplied in 20-ml (100-mg) vials, box of one (NDC 0173-0350-58); 40-ml (200-mg) vials, box of one (NDC 0173-0350-57); 4-ml (20-mg) single-dose, prefilled, disposable syringes, box of one, (NDC 0173-0350-00); and 8-ml (40-mg) single-dose, prefilled, disposable syringes, box of one (NDC 0173-0350-01).

Store between 2° and 30°C (36° and 86°F). Do not freeze. Protect from light.

Note: To insure patient safety, the needle with the prefilled syringes should be handled with care and should be destroyed and discarded if damaged in any manner. If the cannula is bent, no attempt should be made to straighten it. To prevent needle-stick injuries, needles should not be recapped, purposely bent, or broken by hand.

Shown in Product Identification Section, page 404

TRANDATE® Tablets   ℞
[*tran 'dāt*]
(labetalol hydrochloride)

TRANDATE® HCT Tablets   ℞
[*tran 'dāt HCT*]
(labetalol hydrochloride/hydrochlorothiazide)

DESCRIPTION

Trandate® (labetalol HCl) is an adrenergic receptor blocking agent that has both selective alpha$_1$- and nonselective beta-adrenergic receptor blocking actions in a single substance.

Trandate® HCT Tablets for oral administration combine three modes of antihypertensive action: the vasodilating and beta-adrenergic blocking activity of Trandate, plus the known antihypertensive effect of a thiazide diuretic, hydrochlorothiazide.

Labetalol HCl is 2-hydroxy-5-[1-hydroxy-2-[(1-methyl-3-phenylpropyl)amino]ethyl]benzamide monohydrochloride. Labetalol HCl has the empirical formula $C_{19}H_{24}N_2O_3 \cdot HCl$ and a molecular weight of 364.9. It has two asymmetric centers and therefore exists as a molecular complex of two diastereoisomeric pairs.

Labetalol HCl is a white or off-white crystalline powder, soluble in water.

Hydrochlorothiazide is 6-chloro-3,4-dihydro-2H-1,2,4-benzothiadiazine-7-sulfonamide 1,1-dioxide.

Hydrochlorothiazide is a white or practically white crystalline compound, practically insoluble in water but soluble in sodium hydroxide. It has the empirical formula $C_7H_8ClN_3O_4S_2$ and a molecular weight of 297.73.

Trandate Tablets contain 100, 200, or 300 mg of labetalol HCl and are taken orally. The tablets also contain the inactive ingredients corn starch, FD&C Yellow No. 6 (100- and 300-mg tablets only), hydroxypropyl methylcellulose, lactose, magnesium stearate, methylparaben, pregelatinized corn starch, propylparaben, sodium benzoate (200-mg tablet only), talc (100-mg tablet only), and titanium dioxide.

Trandate HCT Tablets are available as 100 mg labetalol HCl/25 mg hydrochlorothiazide; 200 mg labetalol HCl/25 mg hydrochlorothiazide; and 300 mg labetalol HCl/25 mg hydrochlorothiazide.

Each 100/25- and 300/25-mg Trandate HCT tablet also contains the inactive ingredients corn starch, FD&C Yellow No. 6, hydroxypropyl methylcellulose, lactose, magnesium stearate, methylparaben, pregelatinized corn starch, propylparaben, and titanium dioxide.

Each 200/25-mg Trandate HCT tablet also contains the inactive ingredients corn starch, hydroxypropyl methylcellulose, lactose, magnesium stearate, methylparaben, pregelatinized corn starch, propylparaben, and titanium dioxide.

CLINICAL PHARMACOLOGY

Trandate ® HCT (labetalol hydrochloride/hydrochlorothiazide) Tablets: The antihypertensive effects of labetalol and hydrochlorothiazide are additive. Studies have shown that there is no interference with bioavailability when these agents are given together in the single combination tablet. Therefore, this combination provides a convenient formulation for the concomitant administration of these two entities.

Labetalol HCl: Labetalol HCl combines both selective, competitive alpha$_1$-adrenergic blocking and nonselective, competitive beta-adrenergic blocking activity in a single substance. In man, the ratios of alpha- to beta-blockade have been estimated to be approximately 1:3 and 1:7 following oral and intravenous administration, respectively. Beta$_2$-agonist activity has been demonstrated in animals with minimal beta$_1$-agonist (ISA) activity detected. In animals, at doses greater than those required for alpha- or beta-adrenergic blockade, a membrane stabilizing effect has been demonstrated.

Pharmacodynamics: The capacity of labetalol HCl to block alpha receptors in man has been demonstrated by attenuation of the pressor effect of phenylephrine and by a significant reduction of the pressor response caused by immersing the hand in ice-cold water ("cold-pressor test"). Labetalol HCl's beta$_1$-receptor blockade in man was demonstrated by a small decrease in the resting heart rate, attenuation of tachycardia produced by isoproterenol or exercise, and by attenuation of the reflex tachycardia to the hypotension produced by amyl nitrite. Beta$_2$-receptor blockade was demonstrated by inhibition of the isoproterenol-induced fall in diastolic blood pressure. Both the alpha- and beta-blocking actions of orally administered labetalol HCl contribute to a decrease in blood pressure in hypertensive patients. Labetalol HCl consistently, in dose-related fashion, blunted increases in exercise-induced blood pressure and heart rate, and in their double product. The pulmonary circulation during exercise was not affected by labetalol HCl dosing.

Single oral doses of labetalol HCl administered in patients with coronary artery disease had no significant effect on sinus rate, intraventricular conduction, or QRS duration. The atrioventricular (A-V) conduction time was modestly prolonged in two of seven patients. In another study, intravenous labetalol HCl slightly prolonged A-V nodal conduction time and atrial effective refractory period with only small changes in heart rate. The effects on A-V nodal refractoriness were inconsistent.

Labetalol HCl produces dose-related falls in blood pressure without reflex tachycardia and without significant reduction in heart rate, presumably through a mixture of its alpha- and beta-blocking effects. Hemodynamic effects are variable, with small, nonsignificant changes in cardiac output seen in some studies, but not others, and small decreases in total peripheral resistance. Elevated plasma renins are reduced. Doses of labetalol HCl that controlled hypertension did not affect renal function in mildly to severely hypertensive patients with normal renal function.

Due to the alpha$_1$-receptor blocking activity of labetalol HCl, blood pressure is lowered more in the standing than in the supine position, and symptoms of postural hypotension (2%), including rare instances of syncope, can occur. Following oral administration when postural hypotension has occurred, it has been transient and is uncommon when the recommended starting dose and titration increments are closely followed (see DOSAGE AND ADMINISTRATION). Symptomatic postural hypotension is most likely to occur two to four hours after a dose, especially following the use of large initial doses or upon large changes in dose.

The peak effects of single oral doses of labetalol HCl occur within two to four hours. The duration of effect depends upon dose, lasting at least eight hours following single oral doses of 100 mg and more than 12 hours following single oral doses of 300 mg. The maximum, steady-state blood pressure response upon oral, twice-a-day dosing occurs within 24 to 72 hours.

The antihypertensive effect of labetalol has a linear correlation with the logarithm of labetalol plasma concentration, and there is also a linear correlation between the reduction in exercise-induced tachycardia occurring at two hours after oral administration of labetalol HCl and the logarithm of the plasma concentration.

About 70% of the maximum beta-blocking effect is present for five hours after the administration of a single oral dose of 400 mg with suggestion that about 40% remains at eight hours.

The antianginal efficacy of labetalol HCl has not been studied. In 37 patients with hypertension and coronary artery disease, labetalol HCl did not increase the incidence or severity of angina attacks.

Exacerbation of angina and, in some cases, myocardial infarction and ventricular dysrhythmias have been reported after abrupt discontinuation of therapy with beta-adrenergic blocking agents in patients with coronary artery disease. Abrupt withdrawal of these agents in patients without coronary artery disease has resulted in transient symptoms, including tremulousness, sweating, palpitation, headache, and malaise. Several mechanisms have been proposed to explain these phenomena, among them increased sensitivity to catecholamines because of increased numbers of beta receptors. Although beta-adrenergic receptor blockade is useful in the treatment of angina and hypertension, there are also situations in which sympathetic stimulation is vital. For example, in patients with severely damaged hearts, adequate ventricular function may depend on sympathetic drive. Beta-adrenergic blockade may worsen A-V block by preventing the necessary facilitating effects of sympathetic activity on conduction. Beta$_2$-adrenergic blockade results in passive bronchial constriction by interfering with endogenous adrenergic bronchodilator activity in patients subject to bronchospasm and it may also interfere with exogenous bronchodilators in such patients.

Pharmacokinetics and Metabolism: Labetalol HCl is completely absorbed from the gastrointestinal tract with peak plasma levels occurring one to two hours after oral administration. The relative bioavailability of labetalol HCl tablets compared to an oral solution is 100%. The absolute bioavailability (fraction of drug reaching systemic circulation) of labetalol when compared to an intravenous infusion is 25%; this is due to extensive "first-pass" metabolism. Despite "first-pass" metabolism, there is a linear relationship between oral doses of 100 to 3,000 mg and peak plasma levels. The absolute bioavailability of labetalol is increased when administered with food.

The plasma half-life of labetalol following oral administration is about six to eight hours. Steady-state plasma levels of labetalol during repetitive dosing are reached by about the third day of dosing. In patients with decreased hepatic or renal function, the elimination half-life of labetalol is not altered; however, the relative bioavailability in hepatically impaired patients is increased due to decreased "first-pass" metabolism.

The metabolism of labetalol is mainly through conjugation to glucuronide metabolites. These metabolites are present in plasma and are excreted in the urine and, via the bile, into the feces. Approximately 55% to 60% of a dose appears in the urine as conjugates or unchanged labetalol within the first 24 hours of dosing.

Labetalol has been shown to cross the placental barrier in humans. Only negligible amounts of the drug crossed the blood-brain barrier in animal studies. Labetalol is approximately 50% protein bound. Neither hemodialysis nor peritoneal dialysis removes a significant amount of labetalol HCl from the general circulation (<1%).

Hydrochlorothiazide: Hydrochlorothiazide is a diuretic/antihypertensive.

Thiazides affect the renal tubular mechanism of electrolyte reabsorption. At maximal therapeutic dosage, all thiazides are approximately equal in their diuretic potency.

Thiazides increase excretion of sodium and chloride in approximately equivalent amounts. Natriuresis may be accompanied by some loss of potassium and bicarbonate. Following oral administration, the diuretic action of hydrochlorothiazide occurs within two hours, with the peak effect occurring in about four hours. Its action persists for approximately six to twelve hours. Thiazides are eliminated rapidly by the kidney.

Thiazide diuretics have antihypertensive activity per se in hypertensive patients and also may augment the actions of other antihypertensive drugs. The full mechanism of antihypertensive action is not known.

Therapy for hypertension is often initiated with a thiazide diuretic, which induces diuresis, natriuresis, depletion of extracellular fluid, and reduction of cardiac output. Direct arteriolar dilatation may play a role. Thiazides do not affect normal blood pressure.

Plasma renin activity is elevated during thiazide therapy. The aldosterone secretion rate is increased slightly but significantly; this contributes to the hypokalemia caused by thiazides.

INDICATIONS AND USAGE

Trandate® (labetalol HCl) Tablets are indicated in the management of hypertension. Trandate Tablets may be used alone or in combination with other antihypertensive agents, especially thiadize and loop diretics.

Trandate® HCT (labetalol hydrochloride/hydrochlorothiazide) Tablets are indicated in the management of hypertension. THIS FIXED COMBINATION DRUG IS NOT INDICATED FOR INITIAL THERAPY OF HYPERTENSION. IF THE FIXED COMBINATION REPRESENTS THE DOSE TITRATED TO AN INDIVIDUAL PATIENT'S NEEDS, IT MAY BE MORE CONVENIENT THAN THE SEPARATE COMPONENTS.

CONTRAINDICATIONS

Trandate® (labetalol HCl) Tablets and Trandate® HCT (labetalol hydrochloride/hydrochlorothiazide) Tablets are contraindicated in bronchial asthma, overt cardiac failure, greater-than-first-degree heart block, cardiogenic shock, and severe bradycardia (see WARNINGS).

Hydrochlorothiazide is contraindicated in patients with anuria or hypersensitivity to this or other sulfonamide-derived drugs.

WARNINGS

Labetalol HCl: *Hepatic Injury:* Severe hepatocellular injury, confirmed by rechallenge in at least one case, occurs rarely with labetalol therapy. The hepatic injury is usually reversible, but hepatic necrosis and death have been reported. Injury has occurred after both short- and long-term treatment and may be slowly progressive despite minimal symptomatology. Appropriate laboratory testing should be done at the first symptom/sign of liver dysfunction (eg, pruritus, dark urine, persistent anorexia, jaundice, right upper quadrant tenderness, or unexplained "flu-like" symptoms). If the patient has laboratory evidence of liver injury or jaundice, labetalol should be stopped and not restarted.

Cardiac Failure: Sympathetic stimulation is a vital component supporting circulatory function in congestive heart failure. Beta-blockade carries a potential hazard of further depressing myocardial contractility and precipitating more severe failure. Although beta-blockers should be avoided in overt congestive heart failure, if necessary, labetalol HCl can be used with caution in patients with a history of heart failure who are well compensated. Congestive heart failure has been observed in patients receiving labetalol HCl. Labetalol HCl does not abolish the inotropic action of digitalis on heart muscle.

In Patients Without a History of Cardiac Failure: In patients with latent cardiac insufficiency, continued depression of the myocardium with beta-blocking agents over a period of time can, in some cases, lead to cardiac failure. At the first sign or symptom of impending cardiac failure, patients should be fully digitalized and/or be given a diuretic, and the response should be observed closely. If cardiac failure continues despite adequate digitalization and diuretic, Trandate® (labetalol HCl) and Trandate® HCT (labetalol hydrochloride/hydrochlorothiazide) therapy should be withdrawn (gradually, if possible).

Exacerbation of Ischemic Heart Disease Following Abrupt Withdrawal: Angina pectoris has not been reported upon labetalol HCl discontinuation. However, hypersensitivity to catecholamines has been observed in patients withdrawn from beta-blocker therapy; exacerbation of angina and, in some cases, myocardial infarction have occurred after *abrupt* discontinuation of such therapy. When discontinuing chronically administered Trandate or Trandate HCT Tablets, particularly in patients with ischemic heart disease, the dosage should be gradually reduced over a period of one to two weeks and the patient should be carefully monitored. If angina markedly worsens or acute coronary insufficiency develops, labetalol therapy should be reinstituted promptly, at least temporarily, and other measures appropriate for the management of unstable angina should be taken. Patients should be warned against interruption or discontinuation of therapy without the physician's advice. Because coronary artery disease is common and may be unrecognized, it may be prudent not to discontinue Trandate or Trandate HCT therapy abruptly in patients being treated for hypertension.

Bronchospastic Disease: Patients with bronchospastic disease should, in general, not receive antihypertensive drugs possessing beta-blocking properties. Because of labetalol's alpha$_1$-blockade and beta$_2$-agonist actions on airway smooth muscle, however, it may be used with caution in patients who cannot tolerate other antihypertensive treatment. It is nevertheless prudent, if labetalol is used, to use the smallest effective dose, so that inhibition of endogenous or exogenous beta-agonists is minimized.

Pheochromocytoma: Labetalol HCl has been shown to be effective in lowering blood pressure and relieving symptoms in patients with pheochromocytoma. However, paradoxical hypertensive responses have been reported in a few patients with this tumor; therefore, use caution when administering labetalol HCl to patients with pheochromocytoma.

Diabetes Mellitus and Hypoglycemia: Beta-adrenergic blockade may prevent the appearance of premonitory signs and symptoms (eg, tachycardia) of acute hypoglycemia. This is especially important with labile diabetics. Beta-blockade also reduces the release of insulin in response to hyperglycemia; it may therefore be necessary to adjust the dose of antidiabetic drugs.

Major Surgery: The necessity or desirability of withdrawing beta-blocking therapy prior to major surgery is controversial. Protracted severe hypotension and difficulty in restarting or maintaining a heartbeat have been reported with beta-blockers. The effect of labetalol HCl's alpha-adrenergic activity has not been evaluated in this setting.

A synergism between labetalol HCl and halothane anesthesia has been shown (see PRECAUTIONS: Drug Interactions).

Hydrochlorothiazide: Thiazides should be used with caution in severe renal disease. In patients with renal disease, thiazides may precipitate azotemia. Cumulative effects of the drug may develop in patients with impaired renal function.

Thiazides should also be used with caution in patients with impaired hepatic function or progressive liver disease since minor alterations of fluid and electrolyte balance may precipitate hepatic coma.

Thiazides may add to or potentiate the action of other antihypertensive drugs. Potentiation occurs with ganglionic or peripheral adrenergic-blocking drugs.

Sensitivity reactions may occur in patients with a history of allergy or bronchial asthma. The possibility of exacerbation or activation of systemic lupus erythematosus has been reported.

Diabetes mellitus that has been latent may become manifest during thiazide therapy.

PRECAUTIONS

General: *Labetalol HCl: Impaired Hepatic Function:* Labetalol HCl should be used with caution in patients with impaired hepatic function since metabolism of the drug may be diminished.

Jaundice or Hepatic Dysfunction: (see WARNINGS).

Hydrochlorothiazide: Serum and urine electrolyte determinations are particularly important when the patient is vomiting excessively, having diarrhea, or receiving parenteral fluids. Thiazides may cause hyponatremia, hypochloremic alkalosis, hypokalemia, hypomagnesemia, and changes in serum and urine calcium. All patients receiving thiazide therapy should be observed for the clinical warning signs of fluid or electrolyte imbalance, irrespective of cause, which are: dryness of mouth; thirst; weakness; lethargy; drowsiness; restlessness; muscular pains, cramps, or fatigue; hypotension; oliguria, tachycardia; and gastrointestinal disturbances such as nausea and vomiting.

Hypokalemia may develop, especially with brisk diuresis, when severe cirrhosis is present, during concomitant use of corticosteroids or ACTH, or after prolonged therapy. Interference with adequate oral electrolyte intake will also contribute to hypokalemia. Hypokalemia can sensitize or exaggerate the response of the heart to the toxic effects of digitalis (eg, increased ventricular irritability). Hypokalemia may be avoided or treated by use of potassium supplements such as foods with a high potassium content.

Any chloride deficit is generally mild and usually does not require specific treatment except under extraordinary circumstances (as in liver or renal disease). Dilutional hyponatremia may occur in edematous patients in hot weather; appropriate therapy is water restriction, rather than administration of salt, except in rare instances when the hyponatremia is life-threatening. In actual salt depletion, appropriate replacement is the therapy of choice.

Hyperuricemia may occur or acute gout may be precipitated in certain patients receiving thiazides.

The antihypertensive effects of the drug may be enhanced in the postsympathectomy patient.

If progressive renal impairment becomes evident, consider withholding or discontinuing diuretic therapy.

Thiazides may decrease urinary calcium excretion. Thiazides may cause intermittent and slight elevation of serum calcium in the absence of known disorders of calcium metabolism. Marked hypercalcemia may be evidence of hidden hyperparathyroidism.

Information for Patients: As with all drugs with beta-blocking activity, certain advice to patients being treated with labetalol HCl is warranted. This information is intended to aid in the safe and effective use of this medication. It is not a disclosure of all possible adverse or intended effects. While no incidence of the abrupt withdrawal phenomenon (exacerbation of angina pectoris) has been reported with labetalol HCl, dosing with Trandate (labetalol hydrochloride) or Trandate® HCT (labetalol hydrochloride/hydrochlorothiazide) Tablets should not be interrupted or discontinued without a physician's advice. Patients being treated with Trandate or Trandate HCT Tablets should consult a physician at any signs or symptoms of impending cardiac failure or hepatic dysfunction (see WARNINGS). Also, transient scalp tingling may occur, usually when treatment with labetalol HCl is initiated (see ADVERSE REACTIONS).

Laboratory Tests: As with any new drug given over prolonged periods, laboratory parameters should be observed over regular intervals. In patients with concomitant illnesses, such as impaired renal function, appropriate tests should be done to monitor these conditions.

Periodic determination of serum electrolytes to detect possible electrolyte imbalance from the thiazide should be performed at appropriate intervals.

Drug Interactions: *Labetalol HCl:* In one survey, 2.3% of patients taking labetalol HCl in combination with tricyclic antidepressants experienced tremor, as compared to 0.7% reported to occur with labetalol HCl alone. The contribution of each of the treatments to this adverse reaction is unknown, but the possibility of a drug interaction cannot be excluded.

Drugs possessing beta-blocking properties can blunt the bronchodilator effect of beta-receptor agonist drugs in patients with bronchospasm; therefore, doses greater than the normal antiasthmatic dose of beta-agonist bronchodilator drugs may be required.

Cimetidine has been shown to increase the bioavailability of labetalol HCl. Since this could be explained either by enhanced absorption or by an alteration of hepatic metabolism of labetalol HCl, special care should be used in establishing the dose required for blood pressure control in such patients. Synergism has been shown between halothane anesthesia and intravenously administered labetalol HCl. During controlled hypotensive anesthesia using labetalol HCl in association with halothane, high concentrations (3% or above) of halothane should not be used because the degree of hypotension will be increased and because of the possibility of a large reduction in cardiac output and an increase in central venous pressure. The anesthesiologist should be informed when a patient is receiving labetalol HCl.

Labetalol HCl blunts the reflex tachycardia produced by nitroglycerin without preventing its hypotensive effect. If labetalol HCl is used with nitroglycerin in patients with angina pectoris, additional antihypertensive effects may occur.

Hydrochlorothiazide: Insulin requirements in diabetic patients may be increased, decreased, or unchanged.

Thiazide drugs may increase the responsiveness to tubocurarine.

Thiazides may decrease arterial responsiveness to norepinephrine. This diminution is not sufficient to preclude effectiveness of the pressor agent for therapeutic use.

Lithium generally should not be given with diuretics because they reduce its renal clearance and add a high risk of lithium toxicity.

In some patients, the administration of a nonsteroidal anti-inflammatory agent can reduce the diuretic, natriuretic, antihypertensive effects of loop, potassium-sparing, and thiazide diuretics. Therefore, when Trandate HCT and nonsteroidal anti-inflammatory agents are used concomitantly, the patient should be observed closely to determine if the desired effect of the diuretic is obtained.

Drug/Laboratory Test Interactions: *Labetalol HCl:* The presence of labetalol metabolites in the urine may result in falsely elevated levels of urinary catecholamines, metanephrine, normetanephrine, and vanillylmandelic acid when measured by fluorimetric or photometric methods. In screening patients suspected of having a pheochromocytoma and being treated with labetalol HCl, a specific method, such as a high performance liquid chromatographic assay with solid phase extraction (eg, *J Chromatogr* 385:241,1987) should be employed in determining levels of catecholamines.

Continued on next page

Allen & Hanburys—Cont.

Labetalol HCl has also been reported to produce a false-positive test for amphetamine when screening urine for the presence of drugs using the commercially available assay methods Toxi-Lab A® (thin-layer chromatographic assay) and Emit-d.a.u.® (radioenzymatic assay). When patients being treated with labetalol have a positive urine test for amphetamine using these techniques, confirmation should be made by using more specific methods, such as a gas chromatographic-mass spectrometer technique.

Hydrochlorothiazide: Thiazides should be discontinued before carrying out tests for parathyroid function.

Thiazides may decrease serum protein-bound iodine levels without signs of thyroid disturbance.

Carcinogenesis, Mutagenesis, Impairment of Fertility: Labetalol HCl: Long-term oral dosing studies with labetalol HCl for 18 months in mice and for two years in rats showed no evidence of carcinogenesis. Studies with labetalol HCl using dominant lethal assays in rats and mice and exposing microorganisms according to modified Ames tests showed no evidence of mutagenesis. Reproduction studies performed in rats and rabbits dosed orally with labetalol HCl at doses up to ten and eight times the human dose, respectively, revealed no evidence of impaired fertility or harm to the fetus.

Hydrochlorothiazide: Hydrochlorothiazide is presently under study for carcinogenesis in rats and mice in the National Toxicology Research and Testing Program.

Hydrochlorothiazide was not mutagenic in in vitro Ames mutagenicity assays of Salmonella typhimurium strains TA 98, TA 100, TA 1535, TA 1537, and TA 1538 or in in vivo mutagenicity assays of mouse germinal cell chromosomes and Chinese hamster bone marrow cell chromosomes. It was, however, mutagenic in inducing nondisjunction (96% frequency) in diploid strains of Aspergillus nidulans. Hydrochlorothiazide had no adverse effects on fertility in rats at a dose equivalent to the maximum recommended human dose (MRHD) and in mice at a dose equivalent to 25 times the MRHD (4 mg/kg, assumed body weight of 50 kg).

Pregnancy: Teratogenic Effects: Pregnancy Category C: The combination of labetalol HCl and hydrochlorothiazide was not teratogenic in rats and rabbits at oral doses up to approximately 15 and 80 times the MRHD of labetalol (1,200 mg) and hydrochlorothiazide (50 mg), respectively. In rabbits, maternal toxicity was observed with consequent fetotoxicity at the lowest dose tested (3.5 and 20 times the MRHD of labetalol and hydrochlorothiazide, respectively). The combination of labetalol and hydrochlorothiazide appeared to be more toxic in rabbits than was either of the drugs given alone.

Teratogenic studies were performed with labetalol in rats and rabbits at oral doses up to approximately six and four times the MRHD, respectively. No reproducible evidence of fetal malformations was observed. Increased fetal resorptions were seen in both species at doses approximating the MRHD. A teratology study performed with labetalol in rabbits at intravenous doses up to 1.7 times the MRHD revealed no evidence of drug-related harm to the fetus.

Available information indicates that hydrochlorothiazide at doses as high as 330 times the MRHD was not teratogenic in pregnant rats.

There are no adequate and well-controlled studies in pregnant women. Trandate HCT Tablets should be used during pregnancy only if the potential benefit justifies the potential risk to the fetus.

Nonteratogenic Effects: Labetalol HCl: Transient hypotension, bradycardia, and hypoglycemia have been rarely observed in infants of mothers who were treated with labetalol HCl for hypertension during pregnancy. Oral administration of labetalol to rats during late gestation through weaning at doses of two to four times the MRHD caused a decrease in neonatal survival.

Hydrochlorothiazide: Thiazides cross the placental barrier and appear in cord blood. The use of thiazides in pregnant women requires that the anticipated benefit be weighed against possible hazards to the fetus. These hazards include fetal or neonatal jaundice, thrombocytopenia, and possible other adverse reactions that have occurred in the adult.

Labor and Delivery: Labetalol HCl given to pregnant women with hypertension did not appear to affect the usual course of labor and delivery.

Nursing Mothers: Small amounts of labetalol (approximately 0.004% of the maternal dose) are excreted in human milk.

However, thiazides appear in greater amounts in breast milk. Because of the potential for serious adverse reactions in nursing infants from hydrochlorothiazide, a decision should be made whether to discontinue nursing or to discontinue the drug, taking into account the importance of the drug to the mother.

Caution should be exercised when Trandate or Trandate HCT Tablets are administered to a nursing woman.

Pediatric Use: Safety and effectiveness in children have not been established.

ADVERSE REACTIONS

In general, the adverse effects of the combination are the sum of the adverse effects of the two components.

Labetalol HCl: Most adverse effects are mild and transient and occur early in the course of treatment. In controlled clinical trials of three to four months' duration, discontinuation of Trandate® (labetalol hydrochloride) Tablets due to one or more adverse effects was required in 7% of all patients. In these same trials, other agents with solely beta-blocking activity used in the control groups led to discontinuation in 8% to 10% of patients, and a centrally acting alpha-agonist led to discontinuation in 30% of patients.

The incidence rates of adverse reactions listed in the following table were derived from multicenter, controlled clinical trials comparing labetalol HCl, placebo, metoprolol, and propranolol as monotherapy over treatment periods of three and four months. Where the frequency of adverse effects for labetalol HCl and placebo is similar, causal relationship is uncertain. The rates are based on adverse reactions considered probably drug-related by the investigator. If all reports are considered, the rates are somewhat higher (eg, dizziness, 20%; nausea, 14%; fatigue, 11%), but the overall conclusions are unchanged.

[See table below].

The adverse effects were reported spontaneously and are representative of the incidence of adverse effects that may be observed in a properly selected hypertensive patient population, ie, a group excluding patients with bronchospastic disease, overt congestive heart failure, or other contraindications to beta-blocker therapy.

In other studies with labetalol HCl utilizing daily doses up to 2,400 mg, certain of the side effects increased with increasing labetalol dose, including dizziness, fatigue, nausea, paresthesia, nasal stuffiness, ejaculation failure, and impotence.

Labetalol HCl/hydrochlorothiazide: The incidence rates of adverse reactions noted in the following table were derived from multicenter, controlled clinical trials of three months' duration comparing labetalol HCl plus hydrochlorothiazide to labetalol HCl or hydrochlorothiazide alone. The rates are based on adverse reactions considered probably drug-related by the investigators. If all reports are considered, the rates are somewhat higher (eg, dizziness, 16%; headache, 11%; fatigue, 9%), but the overall conclusions are unchanged.

[See table on next page].

In addition, a number of other less common adverse events in patients who were taking labetalol HCl have been reported:

Body as a Whole: Fever

Cardiovascular: Postural hypotension, including, rarely, syncope.

Central and Peripheral Nervous Systems: Paresthesia, most frequently described as scalp tingling. In most cases, it was mild and transient and usually occurred at the beginning of treatment.

Collagen Disorders: Systemic lupus erythematosus and positive antinuclear factor.

Eyes: Dry eyes.

Immunological System: Antimitochondrial antibodies.

Liver and Biliary System: Hepatic necrosis, hepatitis, cholestatic jaundice, elevated liver function tests.

Musculoskeletal System: Muscle cramps, toxic myopathy.

Respiratory System: Bronchospasm.

Skin and Appendages: Rashes of various types, such as generalized maculopapular, lichenoid, urticarial, bullous lichen planus, psoriaform, facial erythema; Peyronie's disease; reversible alopecia.

Urinary System: Difficulty in micturition, including acute urinary bladder retention.

Following approval for marketing in the United Kingdom, a monitored release survey involving approximately 6,800 patients was conducted for further safety and efficacy evaluation of this product. Results of this survey indicate that the type, severity, and incidence of adverse effects were comparable to those cited above.

Potential Adverse Effects: In addition, other adverse effects not listed above have been reported with other beta-adrenergic blocking agents.

Central Nervous System: Reversible mental depression progressing to catatonia, an acute reversible syndrome characterized by disorientation for time and place, short-term memory loss, emotional lability, slightly clouded sensorium, and decreased performance on psychometrics.

Cardiovascular: Intensification of A-V block (see CONTRAINDICATIONS).

Allergic: Fever combined with aching and sore throat, laryngospasm, and respiratory distress.

Hematologic: Agranulocytosis and thrombocytopenic or nonthrombocytopenic purpura.

Gastrointestinal: Mesenteric artery thrombosis and ischemic colitis.

The oculomucocutaneous syndrome associated with the beta-blocker practolol has not been reported with labetalol HCl.

Hydrochlorothiazide: Adverse reactions reported include:

Gastrointestinal System: Anorexia, gastric irritation, nausea, vomiting, cramping, diarrhea, constipation, jaundice (intrahepatic cholestatic jaundice), pancreatitis, sialadenitis.

Central Nervous System: Dizziness, vertigo, paresthesia, headache, and xanthopsia.

Hematologic: Leukopenia, agranulocytosis, thrombocytopenia, aplastic anemia, and hemolytic anemia.

Cardiovascular: Orthostatic hypotension may occur and may be aggravated by alcohol, barbiturates, or narcotics.

Hypersensitivity: Purpura; photosensitivity; rash; urticaria; necrotizing angiitis (vasculitis, cutaneous vasculitis); fever; respiratory distress, including pneumonitis and pulmonary edema; and anaphylactic reactions.

Other: Hyperglycemia, glycosuria, hyperuricemia, muscle spasm, weakness, restlessness, transient blurred vision, severe fluid and electrolyte derangements (rarely).

Whenever adverse reactions are moderate or severe, thiazide dosage should be reduced or therapy withdrawn.

Clinical Laboratory Tests: Labetalol HCl: There have been reversible increases of serum transaminases in 4% of pa-

	Labetalol HCl (N=227) %	Placebo (N=98) %	Propranolol (N=84) %	Metoprolol (N=49) %
Body as a Whole				
fatigue	5	0	12	12
asthenia	1	1	1	0
headache	2	1	1	2
Gastrointestinal				
nausea	6	1	1	2
vomiting	<1	0	0	0
dyspepsia	3	1	1	0
abdominal pain	0	0	1	2
diarrhea	<1	0	2	0
taste distortion	1	0	0	0
Central and Peripheral Nervous Systems				
dizziness	11	3	4	4
paresthesia (usually scalp tingling)	<1	0	0	0
drowsiness	<1	2	2	2
Autonomic Nervous System				
nasal stuffiness	3	0	0	0
ejaculation failure	2	0	0	0
impotence	1	0	1	3
increased sweating	<1	0	0	0
Cardiovascular				
edema	1	0	0	0
postural hypotension	1	0	0	0
bradycardia	0	0	5	12
Respiratory				
dyspnea	2	0	1	2
Skin				
rash	1	0	0	0
Special Senses				
vision abnormality	1	0	0	0
vertigo	2	1	0	0

tients treated with labetalol HCl and tested and, more rarely, reversible increases in blood urea.

OVERDOSAGE

Labetalol HCl: Overdosage with labetalol HCl causes excessive hypotension that is posture sensitive and, sometimes, excessive bradycardia. Patients should be placed supine and their legs raised if necessary to improve the blood supply to the brain. If overdosage with labetalol HCl follows oral ingestion, gastric lavage or pharmacologically induced emesis (using syrup of ipecac) may be useful for removal of the drug shortly after ingestion. The following additional measures should be employed if necessary: *Excessive bradycardia* —administer atropine or epinephrine. *Cardiac failure* —administer a digitalis glycoside and a diuretic. Dopamine or dobutamine may also be useful. *Hypotension* —administer vasopressors, eg, norepinephrine. There is pharmacologic evidence that norepinephrine may be the drug of choice. *Bronchospasm* —administer epinephrine and/or an aerosolized beta₂-agonist. *Seizures* —administer diazepam.

In severe beta-blocker overdose resulting in hypotension and/or bradycardia, glucagon has been shown to be effective when administered in large doses (5 to 10 mg rapidly over 30 seconds, followed by continuous infusion of 5 mg/h that can be reduced as the patient improves).

Neither hemodialysis nor peritoneal dialysis removes a significant amount of labetalol HCl from the general circulation (<1%).

The oral LD_{50} value of labetalol HCl in the mouse is approximately 600 mg/kg and in the rat is greater than 2 g/kg. The intravenous LD_{50} in these species is 50 to 60 mg/kg.

Hydrochlorothiazide: Overdosage symptoms include electrolyte imbalance and signs of potassium deficiency such as confusion, dizziness, muscular weakness, and gastrointestinal disturbances. General supportive measures include replacement of fluids and electrolytes.

DOSAGE AND ADMINISTRATION

Trandate® (labetalol HCl) Tablets: DOSAGE MUST BE INDIVIDUALIZED. The recommended *initial* dosage is 100 mg *twice* daily whether used alone or added to a diuretic regimen. After two or three days, using standing blood pressure as an indicator, dosage may be titrated in increments of 100 mg bid every two or three days. The usual *maintenance* dosage of labetalol HCl is between 200 and 400 mg *twice* daily. Since the full antihypertensive effect of labetalol HCl is usually seen within the first one to three hours of the initial dose or dose increment, the assurance of a lack of an exaggerated hypotensive response can be clinically established in the office setting. The antihypertensive effects of continued dosing can be measured at subsequent visits, approximately 12 hours after a dose, to determine whether further titration is necessary.

Patients with severe hypertension may require from 1,200 to 2,400 mg per day, with or without thiazide diuretics. Should side effects (principally nausea or dizziness) occur with these doses administered bid, the same total daily dose administered tid may improve tolerability and facilitate further titration. Titration increments should not exceed 200 mg bid. When a diuretic is added, an additive antihypertensive effect can be expected. In some cases this may necessitate a labetalol HCl dosage adjustment. As with most antihypertensive drugs, optimal dosages of Trandate® Tablets are usually lower in patients also receiving a diuretic.

When transferring patients from other antihypertensive drugs, Trandate Tablets should be introduced as recommended and the dosage of the existing therapy progressively decreased.

Trandate® HCT Tablets: DOSAGE MUST BE INDIVIDUALIZED. The fixed combination is indicated for patients who, after titration, need the dose of each component present in the combination (see INDICATIONS AND USAGE).

The recommended *initial* dosage of labetalol HCl is 100 mg *twice* daily whether used alone or added to a diuretic regimen. After two or three days, using standing blood pressure as an indicator, dosage may be titrated in increments of 100 mg bid every two or three days. The usual *maintenance* dosage of labetalol HCl is between 200 and 400 mg *twice* daily, although doses up to 1,200 to 2,400 mg have been used. Hydrochlorothiazide is generally started at 25 mg twice daily, although lower doses may be effective in some patients. Most patients do not need dosages greater than 25 mg bid, although dosages of 50 mg bid have been used, and the larger dosages caused increased hypokalemia, hyperuricemia, and hyperglycemia.

The usual dosage of Trandate HCT® Tablets is 200/25 to 300/25 mg twice daily. If doses larger than 600 mg of labetalol are needed, it should be added as the single entity unless there is a specific need and intent to increase the hydrochlorothiazide.

	Labetalol/HCT (N=208) %	HCT (N=95) %	Labetalol (N=106) %
Body as a Whole			
asthenia	1	2	0
leg cramps	1	0	0
fatigue	1	1	2
headache	<1	0	0
malaise	<1	0	0
pain	<1	0	0
rigors	0	0	1
gout	<1	0	0
increased appetite	<1	0	0
creatine phosphokinase	<1	0	0
hypokalemia	1	0	0
Gastrointestinal			
abdominal pain	0	1	0
constipation	<1	0	1
dyspepsia	<1	0	0
flatulence	<1	0	0
gastritis	1	0	0
nausea	2	0	0
Central and Peripheral Nervous Systems			
dizziness	6	2	3
decreased libido	<1	0	0
paresthesia (usually scalp tingling)	<1	0	0
insomnia	0	1	1
paroniria	0	0	1
somnolence	<1	1	0
Cardiovascular			
postural hypotension	<1	0	0
Autonomic Nervous System			
ejaculation failure	<1*	0+	0‡
impotence	1*	1+	0‡
Respiratory System			
bronchospasm	<1	0	0
rhinitis	<1	0	0
Skin and Appendages			
rash	<1	0	0
Urinary System			
micturition frequency	<1	0	0
nocturia	<1	1	0
polyuria	<1	0	0
urinary retention	<1	0	0
Vision			
abnormal vision	<1	0	0

* Based on a male population of 108.
+ Based on a male population of 39.
‡ Based on a male population of 65.

HOW SUPPLIED

Trandate® (labetalol HCl) Tablets, 100 mg, light orange, round, scored, film-coated tablets engraved on one side with "TRANDATE 100 GLAXO," bottles of 100 (NDC 0173-0346-43) and 500 (NDC 0173-0346-44) and unit dose packs of 100 tablets (NDC 0173-0346-47).

Trandate Tablets, 200 mg, white, round, scored, film-coated tablets engraved on one side with "TRANDATE 200 GLAXO," bottles of 100 (NDC 0173-0347-43) and 500 (NDC 0173-0347-44) and unit dose packs of 100 tablets (NDC 0173-0347-47).

Trandate Tablets, 300 mg, peach, round, scored, film-coated tablets engraved on one side with "TRANDATE 300 GLAXO," bottles of 100 (NDC 0173-0348-43) and 500 (NDC 0173-0348-44) and unit dose packs of 100 tablets (NDC 0173-0348-47).

Trandate Tablets should be stored between 2° and 30°C (36° and 86°F). Trandate Tablets in the unit dose boxes should be protected from excessive moisture.

Trandate® HCT Tablets (100 mg labetalol HCl/25 mg hydrochlorothiazide) are pale peach, oval-shaped, film-coated tablets with "371" engraved on one side and "Glaxo" on the other. They are available in bottles of 100 (NDC 0173-0371-00).

Trandate HCT Tablets (200 mg labetalol HCl/25 mg hydrochlorothiazide) are white, oval-shaped, film-coated tablets with "372" engraved on one side and "Glaxo" on the other. They are available in bottles of 100 (NDC 0173-0372-43).

Trandate HCT Tablets (300 mg labetalol HCl/25 mg hydrochlorothiazide) are medium peach, oval-shaped, film-coated tablets with "373" engraved on one side and "Glaxo" on the other. They are available in bottles of 100 (NDC 0173-0373-43).

Trandate HCT Tablets should be stored between 2° and 30°C (36° and 86°F).

Shown in Product Identification Section, page 404

TRINSICON®   ℞
[tren 'sa-kon]
Hematinic Concentrate With Intrinsic Factor
A Highly Potent Oral Antianemia Preparation

TRINSICON® M
Hematinic Concentrate Modified
(Without Folic Acid)

DESCRIPTION

Each Trinsicon® capsule contains:
Special liver-stomach
  concentrate (containing
   intrinsic factor) ....240 mg
Vitamin B₁₂ (activity equivalent) ....15 mcg
Iron, elemental
  (as ferrous fumarate) ....110 mg
Ascorbic acid
  (vitamin C) ....75 mg
Folic acid ....0.5 mg
with other factors of vitamin B complex present in the liver-stomach concentrate.

Each capsule also contains the inactive ingredients FD&C Blue No. 1, FD&C Red No. 3, FD&C Red No. 40, FD&C Yellow No. 6, gelatin, silicone fluid, starch, and titanium dioxide.

Trinsicon® M contains the same ingredients in the same quantities as Trinsicon except folic acid and FD&C Red No. 40.

CLINICAL PHARMACOLOGY

Vitamin B₁₂ with Intrinsic Factor: When secretion of intrinsic factor in gastric juice is inadequate or absent (eg, in Addisonian pernicious anemia or after gastrectomy), vitamin B₁₂ in physiologic doses is absorbed poorly, if at all. The resulting deficiency of vitamin B₁₂ leads to the clinical manifestations of pernicious anemia. Similar megaloblastic anemias may develop in fish tapeworm (*Diphyllobothrium latum*) infec-

Continued on next page

Allen & Hanburys—Cont.

tion or after a surgically created small-bowel blind loop; in these situations, treatment requires freeing the host of the parasites or bacteria that appear to compete for the available vitamin B_{12}. Strict vegetarianism and malabsorption syndromes may also lead to vitamin B_{12} deficiency. In the latter case, parenteral therapy, or oral therapy with so-called massive doses of vitamin B_{12}, may be necessary for adequate treatment of the patient.

Potency of intrinsic factor concentrates is determined physiologically, ie, by their use in patients with pernicious anemia. The liver-stomach concentrate with intrinsic factor and the vitamin B_{12} contained in two Trinsicon® (hematinic concentrate with intrinsic factor) and two Trinsicon® M (hematinic concentrate modified) capsules provide 1½ times the minimum amount of therapeutic agent, which, when given daily in an uncomplicated case of pernicious anemia, will produce a satisfactory reticulocyte response and relief of anemia and symptoms.

Concentrates of intrinsic factor derived from hog gastric, pyloric, and duodenal mucosa have been used successfully in patients who lack intrinsic factor. For example, Fouts et al maintained patients with pernicious anemia in clinical remission with oral therapy (liver extracts or intrinsic factor concentrate with vitamin B_{12}) for as long as 29 years.

After total gastrectomy, Ficarra found multifactor preparations taken orally to be "just as effective in maintaining blood levels as any medication that has to be administered parenterally." His study was based on 24 patients who had survived for five years after total gastrectomy for cancer and who had been taking two Trinsicon capsules daily.

Folic Acid (Trinsicon only): Folic acid deficiency is the immediate cause of most, if not all, cases of nutritional megaloblastic anemia and of the megaloblastic anemias of pregnancy and infancy; usually, it is also at least partially responsible for the megaloblastic anemias of malabsorption syndromes, eg, tropical and nontropical sprue.

It is apparent that in vitamin B_{12} deficiency (eg, pernicious anemia), lack of this vitamin results in impaired utilization of folic acid. There are other evidences of the close folic acid-vitamin B_{12} interrelationship: (1) B_{12} influences the storage, absorption, and utilization of folic acid, and (2) as a deficiency of B_{12} progresses, the requirement for folic acid increases. However, folic acid does not change the requirement for vitamin B_{12}.

Iron: A very common anemia is that due to iron deficiency. In most cases, the response to iron salts is prompt, safe, and predictable. Within limits, the response is quicker and more certain to large doses of iron than to small doses.

Each Trinsicon and each Trinsicon M capsule furnishes 110 mg of elemental iron (as ferrous fumarate) to provide a maximum response.

Ascorbic Acid: Vitamin C plays a role in anemia therapy. It augments the conversion of folic acid to its active form, folinic acid. In addition, ascorbic acid promotes the reduction of ferric iron in food to the more readily absorbed ferrous form. Severe and prolonged vitamin C deficiency is associated with an anemia that is usually hypochromic but occasionally megaloblastic in type.

INDICATIONS AND USAGE

Trinsicon® (hematinic concentrate with intrinsic factor) and Trinsicon® M (hematinic concentrate modified) are multifactor preparations effective in the treatment of anemias that respond to oral hematinics, including pernicious anemia and other megaloblastic anemias and also iron-deficiency anemia. Therapeutic quantities of hematopoietic factors that are known to be important are present in the recommended daily dose.

CONTRAINDICATIONS

Hemochromatosis and hemosiderosis are contraindications to iron therapy.

PRECAUTIONS

General: *Trinsicon® and Trinsicon® M:* Anemia is a manifestation that requires appropriate investigation to determine its cause or causes.

As with all preparations containing intrinsic factor, resistance may develop in some cases of pernicious anemia to the potentiation of absorption of physiologic doses of vitamin B_{12}. If resistance occurs, parenteral therapy or oral therapy with so-called massive doses of vitamin B_{12} may be necessary for adequate treatment of the patient. No single regimen fits all cases, and the status of the patient observed in follow-up is the final criterion for adequacy of therapy. Periodic clinical and laboratory studies are considered essential and are recommended.

Trinsicon®: Folic acid *alone* is unwarranted in the treatment of pure vitamin B_{12} deficiency states, such as pernicious anemia. Folic acid may obscure pernicious anemia in that the blood picture may revert to normal while neurological manifestations remain progressive.

Pregnancy: *Teratogenic Effects: Pregnancy Category C:* Animal reproduction studies have not been conducted

with Trinsicon® (hematinic concentrate with intrinsic factor) or Trinsicon® M (hematinic concentrate modified). It is also not known whether these products can cause fetal harm when administered to a pregnant woman or can affect reproduction capacity. These products should be given to a pregnant woman only if clearly needed.

Nursing Mothers: It is not known whether these drugs are excreted in human milk. Because many drugs are excreted in human milk, caution should be exercised when Trinsicon or Trinsicon M is administered to a nursing woman.

Pediatric Use: Safety and effectiveness in children below the age of 10 have not been established.

ADVERSE REACTIONS

Trinsicon® and Trinsicon® M: Rarely, iron in therapeutic doses produces gastrointestinal reactions, such as diarrhea or constipation. Reducing the dose and administering it with meals will minimize these effects in the iron-sensitive patient.

In extremely rare instances, skin rash suggesting allergy has been noted following the oral administration of liver-stomach material.

Trinsicon: Allergic sensitization has been reported following both oral and parenteral administration of folic acid.

OVERDOSAGE

Symptoms: Those of iron intoxication, which may include pallor and cyanosis, vomiting, hematemesis, diarrhea, melena, shock, drowsiness, and coma.

Treatment: For specific therapy, exchange transfusion and chelating agents. For general management, gastric and rectal lavage with sodium bicarbonate solution or milk, administration of intravenous fluids and electrolytes, and use of oxygen.

DOSAGE AND ADMINISTRATION

One capsule twice a day. (Two capsules daily produce a standard response in the average uncomplicated case of pernicious anemia.)

HOW SUPPLIED

Trinsicon® (hematinic concentrate with intrinsic factor) capsules, dark pink and dark red, are supplied in bottles of 60 (NDC 0173-0364-22) and 500 (NDC 0173-0364-24) and unit dose packs of 100 (NDC 0173-0364-27).

Trinsicon® M (hematinic concentrate modified), pink and red, are supplied in bottles of 16 (NDC 0173-0365-22).

Shown in Product Identification Section, page 404

VENTOLIN® Inhalation Aerosol   ℞
[*vent 'ŏ-lin*]
(albuterol, USP)
Bronchodilator Aerosol
For Oral Inhalation Only

VENTOLIN ROTACAPS®
(albuterol sulfate, USP)
for Inhalation
For Inhalation Only

VENTOLIN® Solution for Inhalation, 0.5%*   ℞
(albuterol sulfate, USP)
*Potency expressed as albuterol.

VENTOLIN® Syrup   ℞
(albuterol sulfate, USP)

VENTOLIN® Tablets   ℞
(albuterol sulfate, USP)

DESCRIPTION

VENTOLIN® Inhalation Aerosol contains albuterol, USP, a relatively selective beta$_2$-adrenergic bronchodilator with the chemical name (α^1-[*tert* -butylamino)methyl]-4-hydroxy-*m* -xylene- α, α' -diol).

Albuterol is the official generic name in the United States. The World Health Organization recommended name for the drug is salbutamol. The molecular weight of albuterol is 239.3, and the empirical formula is $C_{13}H_{21}NO_3$. Albuterol is a white to off-white crystalline solid. It is soluble in ethanol, sparingly soluble in water, and very soluble in chloroform. VENTOLIN Inhalation Aerosol is a metered-dose aerosol unit for oral inhalation. It contains a microcrystalline suspension of albuterol in propellants (trichloromonofluoromethane and dichlorodifluoromethane) with oleic acid. Each actuation delivers from the mouthpiece 90 mcg of albuterol. Each canister provides at least 200 inhalations.

VENTOLIN ROTACAPS® for Inhalation, VENTOLIN® Solution for Inhalation, VENTOLIN® Syrup, and VENTOLIN® Tablets contain albuterol sulfate, USP, a relatively selective beta$_2$-adrenergic bronchodilator with the chemical name α^1-[(*tert* -butylamino]-4-hydroxy-*m* -xylene- α, α' -diol sulfate (2:1)(salt).

The World Health Organization recommended name for albuterol base is salbutamol. Albuterol sulfate has a molecular weight of 576.7, and the empirical formula is $(C_{13}H_{21}NO_3)_2 \cdot H_2SO_4$. Albuterol sulfate is a white crystalline powder, soluble in water and slightly soluble in ethanol.

VENTOLIN ROTACAPS for Inhalation contain a dry powder presentation of albuterol sulfate intended for oral inhalation only. Each light blue and clear, hard gelatin capsule contains a mixture of 200 mcg of microfine albuterol (as the sulfate) with lactose. The contents of each capsule are inhaled using a specially designed plastic device for inhaling powder called the ROTAHALER®. When turned, this device opens the capsule and facilitates dispersion of the albuterol sulfate into the air stream created when the patient inhales through the mouthpiece. VENTOLIN ROTACAPS for Inhalation are an alternative inhalation form of albuterol to the metered-dose pressurized inhaler.

VENTOLIN Solution for Inhalation is in concentrated form. Dilute 0.5 ml of the solution with 2.5 ml of sterile normal saline solution before administration. Each ml of Ventolin Solution for Inhalation contains 5 mg of albuterol (as 6 mg of albuterol sulfate) in an aqueous solution containing benzalkonium chloride; sulfuric acid is used to adjust the pH to between 3 and 5. VENTOLIN Solution for Inhalation contains no sulfiting agents.

VENTOLIN Solution for Inhalation is a clear, colorless to light yellow solution.

VENTOLIN Syrup contains 2 mg of albuterol as 2.4 mg of albuterol sulfate in each teaspoonful (5 ml). VENTOLIN Syrup also contains the inactive ingredients citric acid, FD&C Yellow No. 6, hydroxypropyl methylcellulose, saccharin sodium, sodium benzoate, sodium citrate, artificial strawberry flavor, and purified water.

Each **VENTOLIN Tablet** contains 2 or 4 mg of albuterol as 2.4 or 4.8 mg, respectively, of albuterol sulfate. Each tablet also contains the inactive ingredients corn starch, lactose, and magnesium stearate.

CLINICAL PHARMACOLOGY

In vitro studies and *in vivo* pharmacologic studies have demonstrated that albuterol has a preferential effect on beta$_2$-adrenergic receptors compared with isoproterenol. While it is recognized that beta$_2$-adrenergic receptors are the predominant receptors in bronchial smooth muscle, recent data indicate that there is a population of beta$_2$-receptors in the human heart existing in a concentration between 10% and 50%. The precise function of these, however, is not yet established (see WARNINGS).

The pharmacologic effects of beta-adrenergic agonist drugs, including albuterol, are at least in part attributable to stimulation through beta-adrenergic receptors of intracellular adenyl cyclase, the enzyme that catalyzes the conversion of adenosine triphosphate (ATP) to cyclic-3′,5′-adenosine monophosphate (cyclic AMP). Increased cyclic AMP levels are associated with relaxation of bronchial smooth muscle and inhibition of release of mediators of immediate hypersensitivity from cells, especially from mast cells.

Albuterol has been shown in most controlled clinical trials to have more effect on the respiratory tract, in the form of bronchial smooth muscle relaxation, than isoproterenol at comparable doses while producing fewer cardiovascular effects. Controlled clinical studies and other clinical experience have shown that inhaled albuterol, like other beta-adrenergic agonist drugs, can produce a significant cardiovascular effect in some patients, as measured by pulse rate, blood pressure, symptoms, and/or electrocardiogram changes.

Albuterol is longer acting that isoproterenol in most patients by any route of administration because it is not a substrate for the cellular uptake processes for catecholamines nor for catechol-*O*-methyl transferase.

Because of its gradual absorption from the bronchi, systemic levels of albuterol are low after inhalation of recommended doses. Studies undertaken with four subjects administered tritiated albuterol from a metered-dose aerosol inhaler resulted in maximum plasma concentrations occurring within two to four hours. Due to the sensitivity of the assay method, the metabolic rate and half-life of elimination of albuterol in plasma could not be determined. However, urinary excretion provided data indicating that albuterol has an elimination half-life of 3.8 hours. Approximately 72% of the inhaled dose is excreted within 24 hours in the urine, and consists of 28% as unchanged drug and 44% as metabolite.

Studies is asthmatic patients have shown that less than 20% of a single albuterol dose was absorbed following either intermittent positive-pressure breathing or nebulizer administration; the remaining amount was recovered from the nebulizer and apparatus and expired air. Most of the absorbed dose was recovered in the urine 24 hours after drug administration. Following a 3-mg dose of nebulized albuterol, the maximum albuterol plasma levels at 0.5 hours were 2.1 ng/ml (range, 1.4 to 3.2 ng/ml). There was a significant dose-related response in forced expiratory volume in one second (FEV_1) and peak flow rate. It has been demonstrated that following oral administration of 4 mg of albuterol, the elimination half-life was five to six hours.

Albuterol is rapidly absorbed after oral administration of 10 ml of VENTOLIN® Syrup (4 mg of albuterol) and of 4-mg VENTOLIN® Tablets in normal volunteers. Maximum plasma concentrations of about 18 ng/ml of albuterol are achieved within two hours, and the drug is eliminated with a half-life of about five hours.

In other studies, the analysis of urine samples of patients given 8 mg of tritiated albuterol orally showed that 76% of the dose was excreted over three days, with the majority of the dose being excreted within the first 24 hours. Sixty percent of this radioactivity was shown to be the metabolite. Feces collected over this period contained 4% of the administered dose.

Animal studies show that albuterol does not pass the blood-brain barrier.

Recent studies in laboratory animals (minipigs, rodents, and dogs) recorded the occurrence of cardiac arrhythmias and sudden death (with histologic evidence of myocardial necrosis) when beta-agonists and methylxanthines were administered concurrently. The significance of these findings when applied to humans is currently unknown.

In controlled clinical trials, with VENTOLIN® Inhalation Aerosol, the onset of improvement in pulmonary function was within 15 minutes, as determined by both maximum midexpiratory flow rate (MMEF) and FEV_1. MMEF measurements also showed that near maximum improvement in pulmonary function generally occurs within 60 to 90 minutes following two inhalations of albuterol and that clinically significant improvement generally continues for three to four hours in most patients. In clinical trials, some patients with asthma showed a therapeutic response (defined as maintaining FEV_1 values 15% or more above baseline) that was still apparent at six hours. Continued effectiveness of albuterol was demonstrated over a 13-week period in these same trials.

In clinical studies, two inhalations of albuterol taken approximately 15 minutes before exercise prevented exercise-induced bronchospasm, as demonstrated by the maintenance of FEV_1 within 80% of baseline values in the majority of patients. One of these studies also evaluated the duration of the prophylactic effect to repeated exercise challenges, which was evident at four hours in the majority of patients and at six hours in approximately one third of the patients.

In single, dose-range, crossover trials with VENTOLIN ROTACAPS® for Inhalation, the onset of improvement in pulmonary function was within five minutes, as determined by a 15% increase in FEV_1 following administration of either a 200- or 400-mcg dose. Maximum increases in FEV_1 occurred within 60 minutes following inhalation of either dose. The duration of effect (defined as an increase in FEV_1 of 15% or greater in a single-dose study) was one to two hours after the 200-mcg dose and three to four hours after the 400-mcg dose. In a single-dose study, an increase in forced expiratory flow rate between 25% and 75% of the forced vital capacity of 20% or greater continued for three to four hours after the 200-mcg dose and three to six hours following the 400-mcg dose. A therapeutic response continued for four hours in the majority of patients and six hours in 38% of the patients following the 400-mcg dose. Twenty-two percent of the patients receiving the 200-mcg dose had a duration of effect of eight hours.

In a 12-week, double-blind, comparative evaluation of one 200-mcg VENTOLIN ROTACAPS for Inhalation capsule versus two inhalations of VENTOLIN Inhalation Aerosol, the two dosage regimens were found to be equivalent. Based on a 15% or more increase in FEV_1 determinations, both provided a therapeutic response within 30 minutes that persisted in 50% of patients for two to three hours. Continued effectiveness and safety of VENTOLIN ROTACAPS for Inhalation was demonstrated over the 12-week period.

In controlled clinical trials with VENTOLIN® Solution for Inhalation, most patients exhibited an onset of improvement in pulmonary function within five minutes as determined by FEV_1. FEV_1 measurements also showed that the maximum average improvement in pulmonary function usually occurred at approximately one hour following inhalation of 2.5 mg of albuterol by compressor-nebulizer and remained close to peak for two hours. Clinically significant improvement in pulmonary function (defined as maintenance of a 15% or more increase in FEV_1 over baseline values) continued for three to four hours in most patients, with some patients continuing up to six hours. In repetitive dose studies, continued effectiveness was demonstrated throughout the three-month period of treatment in some patients.

In controlled clinical trials with VENTOLIN Syrup and VENTOLIN Tablets in patients with asthma, the onset of improvement in pulmonary function, as measured by MMEF and FEV_1 and by MMEF, respectively, was within 30 minutes, with peak improvement occurring between two and three hours.

In a controlled clinical trial with VENTOLIN Syrup involving 55 children, clinically significant improvement (defined as maintenance of mean values over baseline of 15% to 20% or more in the FEV_1 and MMEF, respectively) continued to be recorded up to six hours. No decrease in the effectiveness was reported in one uncontrolled study of 32 children who took VENTOLIN Syrup for a three-month period.

In controlled clinical trials with VENTOLIN Tablets in which measurements were conducted for six hours, clinically significant improvement (defined as maintaining a 15% or more increase in FEV_1 and a 20% or more increase in MMEF over baseline values) was observed in 60% of patients at four

hours and in 40% at six hours. In other single-dose, controlled clinical trials, clinically significant improvement was observed in a least 40% of the patients at eight hours. No decrease in the effectiveness of VENTOLIN Tablets has been reported in patients who received long-term treatment with the drug in uncontrolled studies for periods up to six months. The effects of rising doses of albuterol and isoproterenol aerosols were studied in volunteers and asthmatic patients. Results in normal volunteers indicated that albuterol is one half to one quarter as active as isoproterenol in producing increases in heart rate. In asthmatic patients similar cardiovascular differentiation between the two drugs was also seen.

INDICATIONS AND USAGE

VENTOLIN® Inhalation Aerosol is indicated for the prevention and relief of bronchospasm in patients with reversible obstructive airway disease and for the prevention of exercise-induced bronchospasm.

VENTOLIN ROTACAPS® for Inhalation are indicated for the relief of bronchospasm in patients with reversible obstructive airway disease and for the prevention of exercise-induced bronchospasm. This formulation is particularly useful in patients who are unable to properly use the pressurized aerosol form of albuterol or who prefer an alternative formulation. VENTOLIN ROTACAPS for Inhalation can be used with or without concomitant steroid therapy.

VENTOLIN® Solution for Inhalation is indicated for the relief of bronchospasm in patients with reversible obstructive airway disease and acute attacks of bronchospasm.

VENTOLIN® Syrup is indicated for the relief of bronchospasm in adults and children 2 years of age and older with reversible obstructive airway disease.

VENTOLIN® Tablets are indicated for the relief of bronchospasm in patients with reversible obstructive airway disease.

CONTRAINDICATIONS

The VENTOLIN® preparations are contraindicated in patients with a history of hypersensitivity to any of the components.

WARNINGS

As with other inhaled beta-adrenergic agonists, VENTOLIN® Inhalation Aerosol, VENTOLIN ROTACAPS® for Inhalation, and VENTOLIN® Solution for Inhalation can produce paradoxical bronchospasm that can be life-threatening. If it occurs, the preparation should be discontinued immediately and alternative therapy instituted.

Fatalities have been reported in association with excessive use of inhaled sympathomimetic drugs with the home use of nebulizers. The exact cause of death is unknown, but cardiac arrest following the unexpected development of a severe acute asthmatic crisis and subsequent hypoxia is suspected. It is therefore essential that the physician instruct the patient in the need for further evaluation if his/her asthma becomes worse. In individual patients, any beta₂-adrenergic agonist, including albuterol solution for inhalation, may have a clinically significant cardiac effect.

Immediate hypersensitivity reactions may occur after administration of albuterol, as demonstrated by rare cases of urticaria, angioedema, rash, bronchospasm, anaphylaxis, and oropharyngeal edema.

The contents of VENTOLIN Inhalation Aerosol are under pressure. Do not puncture. Do not use or store near heat or open flame. Exposure to temperatures above 120°F may cause bursting. Never throw container into fire or incinerator. Keep out of reach of children.

PRECAUTIONS

General: Although no effect on the cardiovascular system is usually seen after the administration of inhaled albuterol at recommended doses, cardiovascular and central nervous system (CNS) effects seen with all sympathomimetic drugs can occur after use of inhaled albuterol and may require discontinuation of the drug. Albuterol, as with all sympathomimetic amines, should be used with caution in patients with cardiovascular disorders, especially coronary insufficiency, cardiac arrhythmias, and hypertension; in patients with convulsive disorders, hyperthyroidism, or diabetes mellitus; and in patients who are unusually responsive to sympathomimetic amines. Clinically significant changes in systolic and diastolic blood pressure have been seen in individual patients and could be expected to occur in some patients after use of any beta-adrenergic bronchodilator.

Large doses of intravenous albuterol have been reported to aggravate pre-existing diabetes mellitus and ketoacidosis. Additionally, beta-agonists, including albuterol, given intravenously may cause a decrease in serum potassium, possibly through intracellular shunting. The decrease is usually transient, not requiring supplementation. The relevance of these observations to the use of VENTOLIN® products is unknown.

Although there have been no reports concerning the use of VENTOLIN Inhalation Aerosol or VENTOLIN ROTACAPS® for Inhalation during labor and delivery, it has been reported that high doses of albuterol administered intravenously inhibit uterine contractions. Although this effect is

extremely unlikely as a consequence of VENTOLIN Inhalation Aerosol or VENTOLIN ROTACAPS for Inhalation use, it should be kept in mind.

Information for Patients: The action of VENTOLIN Inhalation Aerosol, Solution for Inhalation and Syrup may last up to six hours; the action of VENTOLIN ROTACAPS for Inhalation may last for six hours or longer; and the action of VENTOLIN Tablets may last for eight hours or longer. Therefore they should not be used more frequently than recommended. Do not increase the frequency of doses without medical consultation. If the recommended dosage does not provide relief of symptoms or symptoms become worse, seek immediate medical attention.

While taking VENTOLIN Inhalation Aerosol or VENTOLIN ROTACAPS for Inhalation, other inhaled medicines should not be used unless prescribed. While taking VENTOLIN Solution for Inhalation, other antiasthma medicines should not be used unless prescribed. See package inserts for VENTOLIN Inhalation Aerosol, VENTOLIN ROTACAPS for Inhalation, and VENTOLIN Solution for Inhalation for illustrated Patient's Instructions for Use.

Drug Interactions: Other sympathomimetic aerosol bronchodilators or epinephrine should not be used concomitantly with VENTOLIN Inhalation Aerosol or Solution for Inhalation; other sympathomimetic aerosol bronchodilators should not be used concomitantly with VENTOLIN ROTACAPS for Inhalation becuase they may have additive effects. If additional adrenergic drugs are to be administered by any route to the patient using VENTOLIN Inhalation Aerosol, they should be used with caution to avoid deleterious cardiovascular effects.

In addition, the concomitant use of VENTOLIN Syrup or Tablets and other oral sympathomimetic agents is not recommended since such combined use may lead to deleterious cardiovascular effects. This recommendation does not preclude the judicious use of an aerosol bronchodilator of the adrenergic stimulant type in patients receiving VENTOLIN Syrup or Tablets. Such concomitant use, however, should be individualized and not given on a routine basis. If regular coadministration is required, then alternative therapy should be considered.

Albuterol should be administered with extreme caution to patients being treated with monoamine oxidase inhibitors or tricyclic antidepressants because the action of albuterol on the vascular system may be potentiated.

Beta-receptor blocking agents and albuterol inhibit the effect of each other.

Carcinogenesis, Mutagenesis, Impairment of Fertility: Albuterol sulfate, like other agents in its class, caused a significant dose-related increase in the incidence of benign leiomyomas of the mesovarium in a two-year study in the rat at doses corresponding to 111, 555, and 2,800 times the maximum human aerosol dose; 42, 248, and 1,042 times the maximum human inhalational dose (VENTOLIN ROTACAPS for Inhalation); 10, 50, and 250 times the maximum human nebulizer dose; 2, 9, and 46 times the maximum human (child weighing 21 kg) oral dose (syrup); and 3, 16, and 78 times the maximum human oral dose (tablets). In another study effect was blocked by the coadministration of propranolol. The relevance of these findings to humans is not known. An 18-month study in mice and a lifetime study in hamsters revealed no evidence of tumorigenicity. Studies with albuterol revealed no evidence of mutagenesis. Reproduction studies in rats revealed no evidence of impaired fertility.

Pregnancy: *Teratogenic Effects: Pregnancy Category C:* Albuterol has been shown to be teratogenic in mice when given in doses corresponding to 14 times the human aerosol dose; five times the human inhalational dose (VENTOLIN ROTACAPS for Inhalation); 0.2 times the maximum human (child weighing 21 kg) oral dose (syrup); 0.4 times the maximum human oral dose (tablets); and when given in doses corresponding to the human nebulization dose. There are no adequate and well-controlled studies in pregnant women. Albuterol should be used during pregnancy only if the potential benefit justifies the potential risk to the fetus.

A reproduction study in CD-1 mice given albuterol (0.025, 0.25, and 2.5 mg/kg subcutaneously, corresponding to 1.4, 14, and 140 times the maximum human aerosol dose; 0.5, 5, and 52 times the maximum human inhalational dose (VENTOLIN ROTACAPS for Inhalation); to 0.1, 1, and 12.5 times the maximum human nebulization dose; and 0.5, 5, and 52 times the maximum human oral dose [tablets], respectively) showed cleft palate formation in 5 of 111 (4.5%) fetuses at 0.25 mg/kg and in 10 of 108 (9.3%) fetuses at 2.5 mg/kg. None was observed at 0.025 mg/kg. Cleft palate also occurred in 22 of 72 (30.5%) fetuses treated with 2.5 mg/kg isoproterenol (positive control). A reproduction study in Stride Dutch rabbits revealed cranioschisis in 7 of 19 (37%) fetuses at 50 mg/kg, corresponding to 2,800 times the maximum human inhalational dose, to 250 times the maximum human nebulization dose, to 46 times the maximum human (child weighing 21 kg) oral dose (syrup) of albuterol sulfate,

Continued on next page

Allen & Hanburys—Cont.

and to 78 times the maximum human oral dose (tablets) of albuterol.

Labor and Delivery: Oral albuterol has been shown to delay preterm labor in some reports. There are presently no well-controlled studies that demonstrate that it will stop preterm labor or prevent labor at term. Therefore, cautious use of VENTOLIN ROTACAPS for Inhalation, VENTOLIN Solution for Inhalation, Syrup, or Tablets is required in pregnant patients when given for relief of bronchospasm so as to avoid interference with uterine contractility. Use in such patients should be restricted to those patients in whom the benefits clearly outweigh the risks.

Nursing Mothers: It is not known whether albuterol is excreted in human milk. Because of the potential for tumorigenicity shown for albuterol in some animal studies, a decision should be made whether to discontinue nursing or to discontinue the drug, taking into account the importance of the drug to the mother.

Pediatric Use: Safety and effectiveness have not been established in children below 12 years of age for VENTOLIN ROTACAPS for Inhalation, Inhalation Aerosol, and Solution for Inhalation; in children below 6 years of age for VENTOLIN Tablets; and in children below 2 years of age for VENTOLIN Syrup.

ADVERSE REACTIONS

The adverse reactions to albuterol are similar in nature to reactions to other sympathomimetic agents, although the incidence of certain cardiovascular effects is less with albuterol. Rare cases of urticaria, angioedema, rash, bronchospasm, and oropharyngeal edema have been reported after the use of albuterol. In addition to the reactions given below by specific dosage form, albuterol, like other sympathomimetic agents, can cause adverse reactions such as angina, vomiting, vertigo, CNS stimulation, unusual taste, and drying or irritation of the oropharynx.

VENTOLIN® Inhalation Aerosol: A 13-week double-blind study compared albuterol and isoproterenol aerosols in 147 asthmatic patients. The results of this study showed that the incidence of cardiovascular effects was: palpitations, less than 10 per 100 with albuterol and less than 15 per 100 with isoproterenol; tachycardia, 10 per 100 with both albuterol and isoproterenol; and increased blood pressure, less than 5 per 100 with both albuterol and isoproterenol. In the same study, both drugs caused tremor or nausea in less than 15 patients per 100, and dizziness or heartburn in less than 5 per 100 patients. Nervousness occurred in less than 10 per 100 patients receiving albuterol and in less than 15 per 100 patients receiving isoproterenol.

VENTOLIN ROTACAPS® for Inhalation: The results of clinical trials in 172 patients showed the following side effects:

CNS: Tremors, 6 of 172 patients (3%); nervousness, 5 of 172 patients (3%); headache, 10 of 172 patients (6%); dizziness, 3 of 172 patients (2%); lightheadedness, 4 of 172 patients (2%); insomnia, 1 of 172 patients (<1%); drowsiness, 1 of 172 patients (<1%).

Gastrointestinal: Nausea, burning in stomach, indigestion, each in <1% of patients.

Oropharyngeal: Throat irritation, 3 of 172 patients (2%), dry mouth and voice changes (<1%).

Cardiovascular: 1 of 172 patients (<1%).

Respiratory: Hoarseness, 2 of 172 patients (1%), coughing, 4 of 172 patients (2%).

VENTOLIN® Solution for Inhalation: The results of clinical trials with VENTOLIN Solution for Inhalation in 135 patients showed the following side effects that were considered probably or possibly drug-related:

CNS: Tremor (20%), dizziness (7%), nervousness (4%), headache (3%), insomnia (1%).

Gastrointestinal: Nausea (4%), dyspepsia (1%).

Ear, Nose and Throat: Pharyngitis (<1%), nasal congestion (1%).

Cardiovascular: Tachycardia (1%), hypertension (1%).

Respiratory: Bronchospasm (8%), cough (4%), bronchitis (4%), wheezing (1%).

No clinically relevant laboratory abnormalities related to VENTOLIN Solution for Inhalation administration were determined in these studies.

In comparing the adverse reactions reported for patients treated with VENTOLIN Solution for Inhalation with those of patients treated with isoproterenol during clinical trials of three months, the following moderate to severe reactions, as judged by the investigators, were reported. This table does not include mild reactions.

Percent Incidence of Moderate to Severe Adverse Reactions

Reaction	Albuterol N=65	Isoproterenol N=65
Central Nervous System		
Tremor	10.7%	13.8%
Headache	3.1%	1.5%
Insomnia	3.1%	1.5%
Cardiovascular		
Hypertension	3.1%	3.1%
Arrhythmias	0%	3.0%
Palpitation*	0%	22.0%
Respiratory		
Bronchospasm†	15.4%	18.0%
Cough	3.1%	5.0%
Bronchitis	1.5%	5.0%
Wheezing	1.5%	1.5%
Sputum Increase	1.5%	1.5%
Dyspnea	1.5%	1.5%
Gastrointestinal		
Nausea	3.1%	0%
Dyspepsia	1.5%	0%
Systemic		
Malaise	1.5%	0%

* The finding of no arrhythmias and no palpitations after albuterol administration in this clinical study should not be interpreted as indicating that these adverse effects cannot occur after the administration of inhaled albuterol.

† In most cases of bronchospasm, this term was generally used to describe exacerbations in the underlying pulmonary disease.

VENTOLIN® Syrup: The most frequent adverse reactions to VENTOLIN Syrup in adults and older children were tremor, 10 of 100 patients, and nervousness and shakiness, each in 9 of 100 patients. Other reported adverse reactions were headache, 4 of 100 patients; dizziness and increased appetite, each in 3 of 100 patients; hyperactivity and excitement, each in 2 of 100 patients; and tachycardia, epistaxis, and sleeplessness, each in 1 of 100 patients. The following adverse effects each occurred in less than 1 of 100 patients: muscle spasm, disturbed sleep, epigastric pain, cough, palpitations, stomachache, irritable behavior, dilated pupils, sweating, chest pain, and weakness.

In young children 2 to 6 years of age, some adverse reactions were noted more frequently than in adults and older children. Excitement was noted in approximately 20% of patients and nervousness in 15%. Hyperkinesia occurred in 4% of patients, with insomnia, tachycardia, and gastrointestinal symptoms in 2% each. Anorexia, emotional lability, pallor, fatigue, and conjunctivitis were seen in 1%.

VENTOLIN® Tablets: The most frequent adverse reactions to VENTOLIN Tablets were nervousness and tremor, with each occurring in approximately 20 of 100 patients. Other reported reactions were headache, 7 of 100 patients; tachycardia and palpitations, 5 of 100 patients; muscle cramps, 3 of 100 patients; and insomnia, nausea, weakness, and dizziness, each in 2 of 100 patients. Drowsiness, flushing, restlessness, irritability, chest discomfort, and difficulty in micturition each occurred in less than 1 of 100 patients.

The reactions to VENTOLIN Syrup and Tablets are generally transient in nature, and it is usually not necessary to discontinue treatment. In selected cases, however, dosage may be reduced temporarily; after the reaction has subsided, dosage should be increased in small increments to the optimal dosage.

OVERDOSAGE

Manifestations of overdosage may include anginal pain, hypertension, hypokalemia, and exaggeration of the pharmacologic effects listed in ADVERSE REACTIONS. In these cases, therapy with VENTOLIN® and all beta-adrenergic-stimulating drugs should be stopped, supportive therapy provided, and judicious use of a cardioselective beta-adrenergic blocking agent should be considered, bearing in mind the possibility that such agents can produce profound bronchospasm.

For VENTOLIN® Inhalation Aerosol, as with all sympathomimetic aerosol medications, cardiac arrest and even death may be associated with abuse.

The oral LD$_{50}$ in male and female rats and mice was greater than 2,000 mg/kg. The aerosol LD$_{50}$ could not be determined. Dialysis is not appropriate treatment for overdosage of VENTOLIN® Inhalation Aerosol, VENTOLIN ROTACAPS® for Inhalation, or VENTOLIN® Syrup. The judicious use of a cardioselective beta-receptor blocker, such as metoprolol tartrate, is suggested, bearing in mind the danger of inducing an asthmatic attack. There is insufficient evidence to determine if dialysis is beneficial for overdosage of VENTOLIN® Solution for Inhalation or Tablets.

DOSAGE AND ADMINISTRATION

VENTOLIN® Inhalation Aerosol: For treatment of acute episodes of bronchospasm or prevention of asthmatic symptoms, the usual dosage for adults and children 12 years and older is two inhalations repeated every four to six hours; in some patients, one inhalation every four hours may be sufficient. More frequent administration or a larger number of inhalations is not recommended.

The use of VENTOLIN Inhalation Aerosol can be continued as medically indicated to control recurring bouts of bronchospasm. During this time most patients gain optimal benefit from regular use of the inhaler. Safe usage for periods extending over several years has not been documented.

If a previously effective dosage regimen fails to provide the usual relief, medical advice should be sought immediately as this is often a sign of seriously worsening asthma that would require reassessment of therapy.

Exercise-Induced Bronchospasm Prevention: The usual dosage for adults and children 12 years and older is two inhalations 15 minutes before exercise.

For treatment, see above.

VENTOLIN ROTACAPS® for Inhalation: The usual dosage for adults and children 12 years and older is the contents of one 200-mcg capsule inhaled every four to six hours using a ROTAHALER® inhalation device. In some patients, the contents of two 200-mcg capsules inhaled every four to six hours may be required. Larger doses or more frequent administration is not recommended.

The use of VENTOLIN ROTACAPS for Inhalation can be continued as medically indicated to control recurring bouts of bronchospasm. During this time most patients gain optimal benefit from regular use of the VENTOLIN ROTACAPS for Inhalation formulation.

If a previously effective dosage regimen fails to provide the usual relief, medical advice should be sought immediately as this is often a sign of seriously worsening asthma that would require reassessment of therapy.

VENTOLIN® Solution for Inhalation: The usual dosage for adults and children 12 years and older is 2.5 mg of albuterol administered three to four times daily by nebulization. More frequent administration or higher doses are not recommended. To administer 2.5 mg of albuterol, dilute 0.5 ml of the 0.5% solution for inhalation with 2.5 ml of sterile normal saline solution. The flow rate is regulated to suit the particular nebulizer so that VENTOLIN Solution for Inhalation will be delivered over approximately five to 15 minutes.

The use of VENTOLIN Solution for Inhalation can be continued as medically indicated to control recurring bouts of bronchospasm. During this time most patients gain optimal benefit from regular use of the solution for inhalation.

If a previously effective dosage regimen fails to provide the usual relief, medical advice should be sought immediately as this is often a sign of seriously worsening asthma that would require reassessment of therapy.

VENTOLIN® Syrup: The following dosages of VENTOLIN Syrup are expressed in terms of albuterol base.

Usual Dosage: The usual starting dosage for adults and children over age 14 is 2 mg (1 teaspoonful) or 4 mg (2 teaspoonfuls) three to four times a day.

The usual starting dosage for children 6 to 14 years of age is 2 mg (1 teaspoonful) three or four times a day.

For children 2 to 6 years of age, dosing should be initiated at 0.1 mg/kg of body weight three times a day. This starting dosage should not exceed 2 mg (1 teaspoonful) three times a day.

Dosage Adjustment: For adults and children over age 14, a dosage above 4 mg four times a day should be used *only* when the patient fails to respond. If a favorable response does not occur the dosage may be cautiously increased stepwise, but not to exceed 8 mg four times a day as tolerated.

For children from 6 to 14 years of age who fail to respond to the initial starting dosage of 2 mg four times a day, the dosage may be cautiously increased stepwise, but not to exceed 24 mg per day (given in divided doses).

For children 2 to 6 years of age who do not respond satisfactorily to the initial dosage, the dose may be increased stepwise to 0.2 mg/kg of body weight three times a day, but not to exceed a maximum of 4 mg (2 teaspoonfuls) given three times a day.

Elderly Patients and Those Sensitive to Beta-adrenergic Stimulators: The initial dosage should be restricted to 2 mg three or four times a day and individually adjusted thereafter.

VENTOLIN® Tablets: The following dosages of VENTOLIN Tablets are expressed in terms of albuterol base.

Usual Dosage: The usual starting dosage for adults and children 12 years and older is 2 or 4 mg three or four times a day.

The usual starting dosage for children 6 to 12 years of age is 2 mg three or four times a day.

Dosage Adjustment: For adults and children 12 years and older, a dosage above 4 mg four times a day should be used only when the patient fails to respond. If a favorable response does not occur with the 4-mg initial dosage, it should be cautiously increased stepwise up to a maximum of 8 mg four times a day as tolerated.

For children from 6 to 12 years of age who fail to respond to the initial starting dosage of 2 mg four times a day, the dosage may be cautiously increased stepwise, but not to exceed 24 mg per day (given in divided doses).

Elderly Patients and Those Sensitive to Beta-adrenergic Stimulators: An initial dosage of 2 mg three or four times a day is recommended for elderly patients and for those with a history of unusual sensitivity to beta-adrenergic stimulators. If adequate bronchodilatation is not obtained, dosage may be

increased gradually to as much as 8 mg three or four times a day.
The total daily dosage should not exceed 32 mg in adults and children 12 years and older.

HOW SUPPLIED

VENTOLIN® (albuterol) Inhalation Aerosol is supplied in 17-g canisters containing 200 metered inhalations in boxes of one. Each actuation delivers 90 mcg of albuterol from the mouthpiece. Each canister is supplied with an oral adapter and patient's instructions (NDC 0173-0321-88). Also available, VENTOLIN Inhalation Aerosol Refill 17-g canister only with patient's instructions (NDC 0173-0321-98). **Store between 15° and 30° C (59° and 86° F). As with most inhaled medications in aerosol canisters, the therapeutic effect of this medication may decrease when the canister is cold. Shake well before using.**

VENTOLIN ROTACAPS® (albuterol sulfate) for Inhalation, 200 mcg, are light blue and clear, with "VENTOLIN 200" printed on the blue cap and "GLAXO" printed on the clear body. VENTOLIN ROTACAPS for Inhalation are supplied in a unit dose kit containing one unit dose pack of 96 capsules and one ROTAHALER® inhalation device (NDC 0173-0389-81). **Store between 2° and 30° C (36° and 86° F).**

VENTOLIN® (albuterol sulfate) Solution for Inhalation, 0.5% is supplied in bottles of 20 ml (NDC 0173-0385-58) with accompanying calibrated dropper in boxes of one. **Store between 2° and 30° C (36° and 86°F).**

VENTOLIN® (albuterol sulfate) Syrup, a clear, orange-yellow liquid with a strawberry flavor, contains 2 mg of albuterol as the sulfate per 5 ml in bottles of 16 fluid ounces (one pint) (NDC 0173-0351-54). **Store between 2° and 30°C (36° and 86°F).**

VENTOLIN® (albuterol sulfate) Tablets, 2 mg of albuterol as the sulfate, are white, round, compressed tablets impressed with the product name (VENTOLIN) and the number 2 on one side and scored on the other with "GLAXO" impressed on each side of the score in bottles of 100 (NDC 0173-0341-43) and 500 (NDC 0173-0341-44).

VENTOLIN® (albuterol sulfate) Tablets, 4 mg of albuterol as the sulfate, are white, round, compressed tablets impressed with the product name (VENTOLIN) and the number 4 on one side and scored on the other with "GLAXO" impressed on each side of the score in bottles of 100 (NDC 0173-0342-43) and 500 (NDC 0173-0342-44).

Store between 2° and 30°C (36° and 86°F). Replace cap securely after each opening.

Shown in Product Identification Section, page 404

VICON–C® Capsules
[vī′kon]
(Therapeutic Vitamins and Minerals)

COMPOSITION

Each yellow and orange capsule contains:
Ascorbic acid ....300 mg
Niacinamide ....100 mg
Zinc sulfate, USP* ....80 mg
Magnesium sulfate, USP† ....70 mg
Thiamine mononitrate ....20 mg
d-Calcium pantothenate ....20 mg
Riboflavin ....10 mg
Pyridoxine hydrochloride ....5 mg
* As 50 mg dried zinc sulfate.
† As 50 mg dried magnesium sulfate.
Each capsule also contains D&C Yellow No. 10, FD&C Yellow No. 6, gelatin, microcrystalline cellulose, soybean oil, stearic acid, talc, sodium propionate, and titanium dioxide.

INDICATIONS AND USAGE

Vicon-C® is indicated in the treatment of patients with deficiencies of, or increased requirements for, Vitamin C, B-Complex vitamins, zinc, and/or magnesium. The components of Vicon-C have important roles in nutrition, tissue growth and repair, and the prevention of hemorrhage. Tissue injury resulting from trauma, burns, or surgery may rapidly deplete the body stores of Vitamin C, the B-Complex vitamins, and zinc. Patients maintained on parenteral fluids for extended periods or patients with burns, wounds, or diarrhea often develop deficiencies of Vitamin C, the B-Complex vitamins, and zinc.
Vicon-C is recommended for deficiencies or the prevention of deficiencies of Vitamin C, the B-Complex vitamins, magnesium, and/or zinc in conditions such as febrile diseases, chronic or acute infections, burns, fractures, surgery, toxic conditions, physiologic stress, alcoholism, pregnancy, lactation, geriatrics, gastritis, peptic ulcer, colitis, and in conditions involving special diets and weight-reduction diets. It is also recommended in dentistry for these deficiencies in conditions such as herpetic stomatitis, aphthous stomatitis, cheilosis, herpangina, gingivitis, and states involving oral surgery.

DOSAGE AND ADMINISTRATION

One capsule two or three times daily or as directed by a physician for treatment of deficiencies.

HOW SUPPLIED

Bottles of 60 (NDC 0173-0273-22) and 500 (NDC 0173-0273-24) capsules and unit dose pack of 100 capsules (NDC 0173-0273-27).

Shown in Product Identification Section, page 404

VICON® PLUS Capsules
[vī′kon]
(Therapeutic Vitamins and Minerals)

COMPOSITION

Each red and beige capsule contains:
Vitamin A ....4,000 IU
Vitamin E ....50 IU
Ascorbic acid ....150 mg
Zinc sulfate, USP* ....80 mg
Magnesium sulfate, USP† ....70 mg
Niacinamide ....25 mg
Thiamine mononitrate ....10 mg
d-Calcium pantothenate ....10 mg
Riboflavin ....5 mg
Manganese chloride ....4 mg
Pyridoxine hydrochloride ....2 mg
* As 50 mg dried zinc sulfate.
† As 50 mg dried magnesium sulfate.
Each capsule also contains D&C Yellow No. 10, FD&C Blue No. 1, FD&C Red No. 40, FD&C Yellow No. 6, gelatin, lactose, magnesium stearate, talc, and titanium dioxide.
Vicon® Plus is an extended range vitamin-mineral supplement formulated to aid patient recovery by helping to meet increased nutritional demands.

INDICATIONS AND USAGE

For nutritional supplementation of the patient undergoing physiologic stress due to surgery, burns, trauma, febrile illnesses, or poor nutrition.

DOSAGE AND ADMINISTRATION

One capsule twice daily or as prescribed by a physician for treatment of deficiencies. Dosage should not exceed eight capsules daily due to the possible toxicity of large doses of vitamin A.

HOW SUPPLIED

Bottles of 60 capsules (NDC 0173-0305-22).
Shown in Product Identification Section, page 404

VICON FORTE® Capsules   ℞
[vī′kon for′tā]
(Therapeutic Vitamins-Minerals)

DESCRIPTION

Each black and orange Vicon Forte® capsule for oral administration contains:
Vitamin A ....8,000 IU
Vitamin E ....50 IU
Ascorbic acid ....150 mg
Zinc sulfate, USP* ....80 mg
Magnesium sulfate, USP† ....70 mg
Niacinamide ....25 mg
Thiamine mononitrate ....10 mg
d-Calcium pantothenate ....10 mg
Riboflavin ....5 mg
Manganese chloride ....4 mg
Pyridoxine hydrochloride ....2 mg
Folic acid ....1 mg
Vitamin B$_{12}$ (Cyanocobalamin) ....10 mcg
* As 50 mg dried zinc sulfate.
† As 50 mg dried magnesium sulfate.
Each capsule also contains FD&C Blue No. 1, FD&C Red No. 40, FD&C Yellow No. 6, gelatin, lactose, magnesium stearate, sodium propionate, and titanium dioxide.

INDICATIONS AND USAGE

Vicon Forte® is indicated for the treatment and/or prevention of vitamin and mineral deficiencies associated with restricted diets, improper food intake, alcoholism, and decreased absorption. Vicon Forte is also indicated in patients with increased requirements for vitamins and minerals due to chronic disease, infection, and burns and in persons using alcohol to excess. Preoperative and postoperative use of Vicon Forte can provide the increased amounts of vitamins and minerals necessary for optimal recovery from the stress of surgery.

CONTRAINDICATIONS

None known.

PRECAUTIONS

General: Folic acid in doses above 0.1 mg daily may obscure pernicious anemia in that hematologic remission can occur while neurological manifestations remain progressive.

DOSAGE AND ADMINISTRATION

One capsule daily or as directed by physician.

HOW SUPPLIED

Orange and black capsules imprinted with "Glaxo" and "316" in bottles of 60 (NDC 0173-0316-22) and 500 (NDC 0173-0316-24) and unit dose packs of 100 (NDC 0173-0316-27). Dispense in tight, light-resistant containers as defined in the USP/NF.
Shown in Product Identification Section, page 404

VI–ZAC® Capsules
[vī′zak]
(Therapeutic Vitamin-Mineral)

COMPOSITION

Each orange capsule contains:
Vitamin A ....5,000 IU
Ascorbic acid ....500 mg
Vitamin E ....50 IU
Zinc sulfate, USP* ....80 mg
*As 50 mg dried zinc sulfate.
Each capsule also contains methylcellulose, FD&C Yellow No. 6, FD&C Yellow No. 10, gelatin, lactose, magnesium stearate, and titanium dioxide.

INDICATIONS AND USAGE

Vi-Zac® is indicated in the treatment of patients with deficiencies of, or increased requirements for, Vitamins A, C, and E and zinc. The Vi-Zac formulation is a limited vitamin-mineral formulation designed to meet special needs. It is particularly indicated where there is no requirement for supplemental amounts of the B-Complex vitamins and their attendant appetite stimulation. The formulation is also designed for patients who cannot tolerate magnesium supplements but do need supplemental amounts of zinc.

PRECAUTIONS

Although rarely encountered, vitamin A in large doses daily for several months or longer may cause toxicity.

DOSAGE AND ADMINISTRATION

One or two capsules daily or as directed by the physician for the treatment of deficiencies.

HOW SUPPLIED

Bottles of 60 (NDC 0173-0292-22).
Shown in Product Identification Section, page 404

EDUCATIONAL MATERIAL

Booklets:
"Living With Hypertension"—A patient oriented booklet explains hypertension and is designed to enhance compliance. Free to physicians and pharmacists.
Samples:
Trandate® samples available upon request.

Allergan Optical
Allergan Pharmaceuticals
Divisions of Allergan, Inc.
2525 DUPONT DRIVE
IRVINE, CA 92715

OPHTHALMIC PRODUCTS

For information on Allergan, Inc., prescription, OTC, ophthalmic and contact lens products, consult the Physicians' Desk Reference For Ophthalmology. Allergan OTC artificial tear preparations also appear in the Physicians' Desk Reference For Nonprescription Drugs. For literature, service items or sample material, contact Allergan directly. See a complete listing of products in the Manufacturers' Index section of this book.

Products are
listed alphabetically
in the
PINK SECTION.

Alpha Therapeutic Corporation
5555 VALLEY BOULEVARD
LOS ANGELES, CA 90032

ALBUTEIN® 5% ℞
Albumin (Human), USP, 5% Solution

10 bottles per case.
250mL bottle & IV set	NDC 49669-5211-1
500mL bottle & IV set	NDC 49669-5211-2

ALBUTEIN® 25% ℞
Albumin (Human), USP, 25% Solution

10 bottles per case.
20mL bottle & IV set	NDC 49669-5213-1
50mL bottle & IV set	NDC 49669-5213-2
100mL bottle & IV set	NDC 49669-5213-3

MONOCLATE® ℞
Factor VIII:C, Heat-Treated
Antihemophilic Factor (Human)

Monoclate®, Factor VIII:C, Heat-Treated, Antihemophilic Factor (Human) is supplied in single dose vials (I.U. activity is stated on carton and label of each vial) with sterile diluent, winged infusion set, filter needle, transfer needle and alcohol swabs for reconstitution and administration. Manufactured by Armour Pharmaceutical Company/Kankakee, Illinois 60901 and distributed by Alpha Therapeutic Corporation.

ASSAY Range	NDC CODE
250 (approximate)	49669-9441-1
500 (approximate)	49669-9442-2
1000 (approximate)	49669-9444-3

PLASMATEIN® 5% ℞
Plasma Protein Fraction (Human), USP, 5% Solution

10 bottles per case.
250mL bottle & IV set	NDC 49669-5721-1
500mL bottle & IV set	NDC 49669-5721-2

PROFILATE® HP ℞
Heat-Treated/Solvent Suspension
Antihemophilic Factor (Human), Factor VIII (AHF)

PROFILATE® HP, Heat-Treated/Solvent Suspension, Antihemophilic Factor (Human) is available in 250 and 500 assay ranges with 10 mL diluent; and 750, 1000 and 1100+ assay ranges with 25 mL diluent. For intravenous administration only. Each carton and single dose vial is labeled with AHF dose contained; carton contains sterile diluent, transfer needle, and microaggregate filter. Isoagglutinin titres available upon request. 12 vials per case.
ASSAY RANGE 0–649 AHF Units/vial NDC 49669-4200-1
ASSAY RANGE
    650–2000 AHF Units/vial NDC 49669-4200-2

PROFILATE® SD ℞
Solvent Detergent/Heat-Treated
Antihemophilic Factor (Human), Factor VIII (AHF)

PROFILATE® SD, Solvent Detergent/Heat-Treated, Antihemophilic Factor (Human) is available in 250 and 500 assay ranges with 10 mL diluent; and 750, 1000 and 1100+ assay ranges with 25 mL diluent. For intravenous administration only. Each carton and single dose vial is labeled with AHF dose contained; carton contains sterile diluent, transfer needle, and microaggregate filter. Isoagglutinin titres available upon request. 12 vials per case.
ASSAY RANGE 0–649 AHF Units/vial NDC 49669-4100-1
ASSAY RANGE
    650–2000 AHF Units/vial NDC 49669-4100-2

PROFILNINE® HEAT-TREATED ℞
Wet Method
Factor IX Complex (Human)

PROFILNINE® Heat Treated Wet Method, Factor IX Complex (Human), is available in 250 and 500 assay ranges with 10 mL diluent; and 750, 1000 and 1100+ assay ranges with 25 mL diluent. For intravenous administration only. Each carton and single dose vial is labeled with Factor IX dose contained; carton contains sterile diluent, transfer needle, and microaggregate filter. NAPTT times available upon request. 12 vials per case.
ASSAY RANGE 0–649 AHF Units/vial NDC 49669-3700-1
ASSAY RANGE
    650–2000 AHF Units/vial NDC 49669-3700-2

SOYACAL® 10% ℞
Intravenous Fat Emulsion, 10%

For use with Parenteral Hyperalimentation.
50mL and 100 mL, 20 bottles per case; 250mL and 500 mL, 10 bottles per case.
50mL without IV set	NDC 49669-1310-4
100mL without IV set	NDC 49669-1310-3
250mL without IV set	NDC 49669-1310-2
250mL with IV set	NDC 49669-1310-6
500mL without IV set	NDC 49669-1310-1
500mL with IV set	NDC 49669-1310-5

SOYACAL® 20% ℞
Intravenous Fat Emulsion, 20%

For use with Parenteral Hyperalimentation.
50mL and 100mL, 20 bottles per case; 250mL and 500mL, 10 bottles per case.
50mL without IV set	NDC 49669-1320-4
100mL without IV set	NDC 49669-1320-3
100mL with IV set	NDC 49669-1320-7
250mL without IV set	NDC 49669-1320-2
250mL with IV set	NDC 49669-1320-6
500mL without IV set	NDC 49669-1320-1
500mL with IV set	NDC 49669-1320-5

VENOGLOBULIN®–I ℞
Immune Globulin Intravenous (Human)

Sterile highly purified lyophilized preparation of intact, unmodified immunoglobulin. Supplies broad spectrum of IgG antibodies. Manufacturing process includes cold alcohol fractionation plus purification by PEG fractionation and DEAE Sephadex ion exchange adsorption. For intravenous administration. In 2.5g and 5.0g vials with optional sterile diluent and transfer device. 6 vials per case.
2.5g with reconstitution kit	NDC 49669-1602-1
5.0g with reconstitution kit	NDC 49669-1603-1
2.5g individual vial	NDC 49669-1602-0
5.0g individual vial	NDC 49669-1603-0

EDUCATIONAL MATERIAL

Scientific publications, monographs, product literature, brochures and formulary kits available upon request.

Alra Laboratories, Inc.
3850 CLEARVIEW CT.
GURNEE, IL 60031

ALRAMUCIL INSTANT MIX OTC
Psyllium Hydrophilic Mucilloid For Oral Suspension, USP
Effervescent and Instant mix, Unit dose packets

Each packet provides:
  Psyllium hydrophilic mucilloid .... 3.6 gm.
HOW SUPPLIED
Carton of 30 (NDC 51641-150-03) Regular Flavor
Carton of 30 (NDC 51641-151-03) Orange Flavor

CHOLAC
[ko'lac]
CONSTILAC ℞
[kon'stil-ac]
Lactulose Syrup, USP

Each 15 mL syrup contains:
10 g lactulose (and less than 2.2 g galactose, less than 1.2 g lactose, 1.2 g or less of other sugars); plus water and coloring. Sodium hydroxide used to adjust pH.
HOW SUPPLIED
1 fl. oz. bottle (30 mL) (unit-dose)	NDC #51641-225-61
144 bottles/carton	
8 fl. oz. bottle (240 mL)	NDC #51641-224-68
16 fl oz. bottle (480 mL)	NDC #51641-225-76
32 fl. oz. bottle (960 mL)	NDC #51641-224-82
64 fl. oz. bottle (1920 mL)	NDC #51641-225-94
1 gal. (3785 mL)	NDC #51641-225-97

ERYZOLE Granules for Suspension ℞
erythromycin ethylsuccinate and sulfisoxazole acetyl for oral suspension USP

When reconstituted each 5mL of suspension contains: Erythromycin Ethylsuccinate equivalent to 200mg erythromycin and Sulfisoxazole Acetyl equivalent to 600mg sulfisoxazole.
HOW SUPPLIED
Eryzole suspension is available for teaspoon dosage in bottles of,
100 mL (NDC 51641-111-64)
150 mL (NDC 51641-111-66)
200 mL (NDC 51641-111-68)
in the form of granules to be reconstituted with water.

GELPIRIN TABLETS OTC
Each tablet contains:
Acetaminophen	125 mg.
Aspirin	240 mg.
Caffeine	32 mg.
Along with two buffering agents
HOW SUPPLIED
Bottle of 100 (NDC 51641-711-01)
Bottle of 1000 (NDC 51641-711-10)

GELPIRIN–CCF OTC
Colds, Cough and Fever Tablets

Each tablet contains:
Acetaminophen	325 mg
Guaifensin	25 mg
Phenylpropanolamine HCl	12.5 mg
Chlorpheniramine Maleate	1.0 mg
HOW SUPPLIED
Bottle of 50 (NDC 51641-721-50)

Gen–XENE® ©℞
[jen 'zēn]
Clorazepate Dipotassium Tablets

Gen–XENE Tablets are available in 3.75 mg, 7.5 mg or 15 mg strengths for oral administration.
HOW SUPPLIED
3.75 mg gray, scored tablets debossed with ALRA and GX:
Unit dose packages of 100: NDC 51641-242-11
Bottles of 30 NDC 51641-242-03
Bottles of 100 NDC 51641-242-01
Bottles of 500 NDC 51641-242-05

7.5 mg yellow, scored tablets debossed with ALRA and GT:
Unit dose packages of 100: NDC 51641-243-11
Bottles of 30 NDC 51641-243-03
Bottles of 100 NDC 51641-243-01
Bottles of 500 NDC 51641-243-05

15 mg green, scored tablets debossed with ALRA and GN:
Unit dose packages of 100: NDC 51641-244-11
Bottles of 30 NDC 51641-244-03
Bottles of 100 NDC 51641-244-01
Bottles of 500 NDC 51641-244-05

IBU–TAB
Ibuprofen Tablets, USP

Ibuprofen Tablets are available in 200, 400, 600 and 800 mg strengths for oral administration.
HOW SUPPLIED
Ibuprofen Tablets, 200 mg (orange) film-coated, round tablets. Debossed 'ALRA' on one side and 215 on the other.
Bottles of 30	NDC 51641-215-03
Bottles of 60	NDC 51641-215-60
Bottles of 100	NDC 51641-215-01
Bottles of 250	NDC 51641-215-25
Ibuprofen Tablets, 400 mg (orange) film-coated, round tablets. Debossed 'ALRA' on one side and IF 400 on the other.
Bottles of 100	NDC 51641-214-01
Bottles of 500	NDC 51641-214-05
Bottles of 1000	NDC 51641-214-10
Unit-dose packages of 100	NDC 51641-214-11
Ibuprofen Tablets, 600 mg (orange) film-coated, oval tablets. Debossed 'ALRA' on one side and IF 600 on the other.
Bottles of 100	NDC 51641-213-01
Bottles of 500	NDC 51641-213-05
Bottles of 1000	NDC 51641-213-10
Unit-dose packages of 100	NDC 51641-213-11

Ibuprofen Tablets, 800 mg (light peach) film-coated, oval tablets. Debossed 'ALRA' on one side and IF 800 on the other.

Bottles of 100	NDC 51641-212-01
Bottles of 500	NDC 51641-212-05
Bottles of 1000	NDC 51641-212-10
Unit-dose packages of 100	NDC 51641-212-11

K⁺ 10 ℞
Potassium Chloride Extended-release Tablets, USP

Each K⁺ 10 tablet contains:
Potassium Chloride, USP ....10 mEq (750 mg)
[Equivalent to 10 mEq (390 mg) of potassium and 10 mEq (360 mg) of chloride]

HOW SUPPLIED
Bottle of 100 (NDC #51641-177-01)
Bottle of 500 (NDC #51641-177-05)
Bottle of 1000 (NDC #51641-177-10)
Unit dose packages of 100: NDC 51641-177-11

K⁺ CARE 20 mEq ℞
Potassium Chloride For Oral Solution, USP

Each powder packet provides:
Potassium Chloride .... 20 mEq (1.5 gm.)
[Equivalent to 20 mEq (780 mg) of potassium and 20 mEq (720 mg) of chloride]

HOW SUPPLIED
Carton of 30 (NDC 51641-120-03) Orange flavor
Carton of 30 (NDC 51641-140-03) Fruit flavor
Carton of 100 (NDC 51641-120-01) Orange flavor
Carton of 100 (NDC 51641-140-01) Fruit flavor

K⁺ CARE ET 25 mEq ℞
Potassium Bicarbonate Effervescent Tablets For Oral Solution, USP

Each tablet contains .... 25 mEq of Potassium
(From 2.5 Gm. of Potassium Bicarbonate)

HOW SUPPLIED
Carton of 30 (NDC 51641-135-03) Orange flavor
Carton of 30 (NDC 51641-125-03) Lime flavor
Carton of 100 (NDC 51641-135-01) Orange flavor
Carton of 100 (NDC 51641-125-01) Lime flavor

METHALGEN® OTC
External Analgesic Cream

Methalgen is a combination of Methyl Salicylate, Menthol and Camphor in a water base cream for topical application.

HOW SUPPLIED
Bottle of 2 oz (NDC 51641-301-92)
Jar of 16 oz (NDC 51641-301-96)

Alza Corporation
950 PAGE MILL ROAD
P.O. BOX 10950
PALO ALTO, CA 94303-0802

PROGESTASERT® ℞
[prō-jes-ta-sert]
Intrauterine Progesterone Contraceptive System
Release rated 65 µg/day progesterone for one year

CONTENTS: ONE STERILE SYSTEM
CAUTION: Federal law prohibits dispensing without prescription

NOTICE
You have received Patient Information Leaflets that Federal Regulations (21 CFR 310.502) require you to furnish to each patient who is considering the use of the PROGESTASERT system.
The Patient Information Leaflet contains information on the safety and efficacy of the system. It also contains the Informed Choice Statement. You must not insert the PROGESTASERT system until:
- You have read this physician prescription labeling and are familiar with all the information it contains.
- You and the patient have read and she has initialed each section of the Patient Information Leaflet.
- You have counseled the patient and answered her questions about contraception, the PROGESTASERT system, and the material in the Leaflet.
- You and the patient have reviewed and signed the Informed Choice Statement.
The completely initialed and signed Leaflet, including the signed Informed Choice Statement, should be retained in the patient's records and a second copy of the initialed and signed Leaflet given to the patient for her records.

The Leaflet is also available in Spanish should your practice require it. Address requests to: Customer Service Department, ALZA Corporation, 950 Page Mill Road, P.O. Box 10950, Palo Alto, CA 94303-0802. Telephone (800) 227-9953.

DESCRIPTION
System
The PROGESTASERT system is a white, T-shaped unit constructed of ethylene/vinyl acetate copolymer (EVA) containing titanium dioxide. The 36-mm tubular vertical stem of the T contains a reservoir of 38 mg of progesterone, together with barium sulfate for radiopacity; both are dispersed in medical grade silicone fluid. The 32-mm horizontal cross-arms are solid EVA. Two monofilament blue-black nylon indicator/retrieval threads are fastened to the base of the T stem.

The tip of the shorter indicator thread is 9 cm from the top or leading end of the system and is used to ascertain correct placement at insertion. The long thread extends the length of the inserter, to which it is anchored by a plug that retains the system in the inserter.
Inserter
The inserter is a malleable, curved tube designed to conform to the anatomical configuration of most cervical-uterine cavities. The horizontal arms of the T are positioned outside of the inserter and are folded by an arm-cocker attachment immediately prior to insertion. The inserter does not contain a plunger.
DO NOT REMOVE ANY COMPONENT FROM THE INSERTER BEFORE INSERTION OF THE SYSTEM INTO THE UTERUS.

The PROGESTASERT system inserter permits determination of the depth of uterine placement of the PROGESTASERT system. The curvature of the inserter conforms with the usual orientation of the uterus; however, in cases of extreme flexion, the malleable inserter may need to be gently shaped to the desired curvature prior to insertion.
The PROGESTASERT system is packaged sterile within its inserter. Progesterone is released from the system in situ at an average rate of 65 µg/day for one year by membrane-controlled diffusion from the reservoir. Inert ingredients of the reservoir or membrane—barium sulfate, silicone fluid, titanium dioxide, or EVA—are not released.

CLINICAL PHARMACOLOGY
Available data indicate that the contraceptive effectiveness of the PROGESTASERT system is enhanced by its continuous release of progesterone into the uterine cavity. The mechanism by which progesterone enhances the contraceptive effectiveness of the T is local, not systemic. The concentrations of luteinizing hormone, estradiol, and progesterone in systemic venous plasma follow regular cyclic patterns indicative of ovulation during use of the PROGESTASERT system. Blood chemistry studies related to liver, kidney, and thyroid function also reveal no clinically meaningful changes.
During use of the PROGESTASERT system, the endometrium shows progestational influence. Progesterone released from the system at an average rate of 65 µg/day suppresses endometrial proliferation (an anti-estrogenic effect). Following system removal, the cyclic endometrial pattern rapidly returns to normal. The local mechanism by which continuously released progesterone enhances the contraceptive effectiveness of the T has not been conclusively demonstrated. Two hypotheses have been offered: progesterone-induced inhibition of sperm capacitation or survival; and alteration of the uterine milieu so as to prevent nidation.

INDICATIONS AND USAGE
The PROGESTASERT system is indicated for intrauterine contraception in women who have had at least one child, are in a stable, mutually monogamous relationship, and have no history of pelvic inflammatory disease. The PROGESTASERT system must be replaced every 12 months for continued contraceptive effect.

CONTRAINDICATIONS
The PROGESTASERT system is contraindicated when one or more of the following conditions exist:
1. Pregnancy or suspected pregnancy.
2. History of ectopic pregnancy or a condition that predisposes to ectopic pregnancy (see WARNINGS—Ectopic Pregnancy).

3. Presence of—or a history of—pelvic inflammatory disease (PID) or factors that predispose to PID (See WARNINGS—Pelvic Infection).
4. Patient or her partner has multiple sexual partners.
5. Presence of—or a history of—venereal disease (one or more episodes), including but not limited to gonorrhea or chlamydial infections of the genital tract.
6. Postpartum endometritis or infected abortion.
7. Incomplete involution of the uterus following abortion or childbirth.
8. A previously inserted IUD is still in place.
9. History of pelvic surgery that may be associated with an increased risk of ectopic pregnancy, such as surgery of the fallopian tubes or surgery for pelvic adhesions or endometriosis.
10. Abnormalities of the uterus resulting in distortion of the uterine cavity or uteri that measure less than 6 cm or greater than 10 cm by sounding.
11. Known or suspected uterine or cervical malignancy including an unresolved, abnormal Pap smear.
12. Genital bleeding of unknown etiology.
13. Vaginitis or cervicitis unless and until infection has been completely controlled and has been shown to be non-gonococcal and non-chlamydial.
14. Genital actinomycosis.
15. Conditions or treatments associated with increased susceptibility to infections with microorganisms. Such conditions include, but are not limited to, leukemia, diabetes, certain types of heart disease that are associated with an increased risk of endocarditis, acquired immune deficiency syndrome (AIDS), and conditions requiring chronic corticosteroid therapy.
16. IV drug abuse.

WARNINGS
1. Ectopic Pregnancy
The PROGESTASERT system is contraindicated in patients who, in the physician's judgement, are at special risk of having an ectopic pregnancy. Ectopic pregnancy is potentially fatal and appears to occur more frequently with PROGESTASERT system use than with other IUDs and other contraceptives. Therefore, the possibility of ectopic pregnancy must always be considered in PROGESTASERT system users—including those lacking the specific risk factors described below.
The material that follows is intended to aid the physician in the following:
- Understanding the risks of ectopic pregnancy in PROGESTASERT system users (Section 1a).
- Proper selection of women for PROGESTASERT system use by identifying and excluding those at special risk to ectopic pregnancy (Section 1b).
- Diagnosing and managing ectopic pregnancy in IUD users (Sections 1c and 1d).
- Informing patients of ectopic pregnancy risks (Section 1e).
a. Risks of ectopic pregnancy with PROGESTASERT system use
Should a woman become pregnant while using the PROGESTASERT system, the pregnancy is more likely to be ectopic than pregnancy in a woman using no contraception, ovulation-suppressing oral contraception, or barrier methods.[1,2] This is because the PROGESTASERT system acts in the uterus to prevent uterine pregnancy, but it does not prevent either ovulation or ectopic pregnancy. Thus, each month that the PROGESTASERT system is used, there is protection against uterine pregnancy but not against ectopic pregnancy. In clinical trials of the PROGESTASERT system 1 of 3.6 pregnancies in parous women and 1 of 6.2 pregnancies in nulliparous women were ectopic.
The per-year risk of ectopic pregnancy in PROGESTASERT system users is approximately 5 per 1,000 or 1 ectopic pregnancy in 200 users per year. This risk is approximately the same as in noncontracepting, sexually active women. In contrast, barrier contraceptives, which prevent fertilization, or oral contraceptives that prevent ovulation, reduce the risk of ectopic pregnancy to a few percent of the risk in noncontracepting, sexually active women.
Two clinical studies conducted by the World Health Organization compared the risk of ectopic pregnancies among 2,239 women wearing a progesterone-releasing IUD similar to the PROGESTASERT system with the risk in 3,303 women wearing a copper-releasing IUD. For the first year the risk of ectopic pregnancy was approximately 6 times higher among women using progesterone systems than among women using copper systems. Over the two years that the studies ran, the risk of an ectopic pregnancy with the progesterone-releasing IUD was about 10 times higher than that with copper-releasing IUDs.
b. Women at special risk to ectopic pregnancy
Several factors have been identified as placing a woman at special risk to ectopic pregnancy. The presence of any of these factors contraindicates use of the PROGESTASERT system. Factors indicating high risk to ectopic pregnancy include a history of ectopic pregnancy or a history or pres-

Continued on next page

Alza—Cont.

ence of a condition predisposing to ectopic pregnancy such as PID. A prospective clinical study was conducted over 9.5 years in 415 women who had had verified PID and 100 healthy control subjects. The ratio between ectopic and intrauterine pregnancies after PID was 1/24. In contrast, the ratio in the controls was 1/147. Further analysis of these data suggests that women who have had PID subsequently have an 8- to 10-fold greater risk of ectopic pregnancy than sexually active noncontracepting women who have never had PID.

Factors other than PID may also indicate a high risk to ectopic pregnancy. These factors include multiple sexual partners or a partner with multiple sexual partners, pelvic surgery of certain types, retrograde menstruation, endometritis, and endometriosis.

c. Diagnosis of ectopic pregnancy

The absence of risk factors for ectopic pregnancy described above does not rule out ectopic pregnancy. In every instance of pregnancy occurring in a PROGESTASERT system user it is essential that proper measures be taken to determine if the pregnancy is ectopic.

To determine whether ectopic pregnancy has occurred, special attention should be directed to patients with any of the following symptoms or conditions: unusual, abnormal, or irregular vaginal bleeding; delayed or missed menses; pelvic pain, usually unilateral, which may be associated with fainting or the urge to defecate; unexplained pain in the shoulder; or pain associated with bleeding if not part of the usual menstrual cycle. Ectopic pregnancy should be strongly suspected in patients with a positive pregnancy test or elevated β-HCG values but who lack ultrasonographic or other evidence of intrauterine pregnancy.

d. Management of diagnosed or suspected ectopic pregnancy

When ectopic pregnancy is suspected, diagnostic uncertainty should be resolved as quickly as possible, in view of the life-threatening risk of ruptured ectopic pregnancy. When ectopic pregnancy is diagnosed, immediate surgery is often required because a ruptured ectopic pregnancy may occur at any time.

e. Ectopic pregnancy warning to PROGESTASERT system users

All women who choose the PROGESTASERT system must be informed before insertion that a pregnancy occurring in a PROGESTASERT system user is more likely to be ectopic than one occurring in users of ovulation-preventing oral contraceptives, barrier modes or other IUDs. They should be taught to recognize and report to their physician promptly any symptoms of ectopic pregnancy. Women should also be informed that ectopic pregnancy has been associated with complications leading to loss of fertility.

2. Intrauterine Pregnancy

Intrauterine pregnancy can occur during use of the PROGESTASERT system (see CLINICAL STUDIES section for pregnancy rates).

a. Long-term effects and congenital anomalies

When pregnancy occurs or proceeds with the PROGESTASERT system in place, long-term effects on the offspring are unknown. Congenital anomalies have occurred under such conditions. Their relationship to the PROGESTASERT system has not been established. Systemically administered sex steroids, including progestational agents, have been associated with an increased risk of congenital anomalies. It is not known whether an increased risk of such anomalies exists when pregnancy continues with a PROGESTASERT system in place. The decision to continue or terminate pregnancy should take into account this unknown risk.

b. Septic abortion

Reports have indicated an increased incidence of septic abortion—with septicemia, septic shock, and death—in patients becoming pregnant with an IUD in place. Most of these reports have been associated with the mid-trimester of pregnancy. In some cases, the initial symptoms have been insidi-

ous and not easily recognized. If pregnancy should occur with a PROGESTASERT system *in situ*, the system should be removed if the thread is visible and removal is easily accomplished. Removal or manipulation of the PROGESTASERT system may precipitate abortion. If removal would be or proves to be difficult, or if threads are not visible, termination of the pregnancy should be considered and offered to the patient as an option, bearing in mind that the risks associated with an elective abortion increase with gestational age.

c. Continuation of pregnancy

If the patient chooses to continue the pregnancy with the system in place, she must be warned that this increases the risk of spontaneous abortion and sepsis, which may cause death. In addition, she is at increased risk of premature labor and delivery. As a consequence of premature birth, the fetus is at increased risk of damage. She should be informed more closely than the usual obstetrical patient. She must be advised to report immediately all symptoms such as flu-like syndrome, fever, chills, abdominal cramping and pain, bleeding, or vaginal discharge, because generalized symptoms of septicemia may be insidious.

3. Pelvic Infection (Pelvic Inflammatory Disease)

The PROGESTASERT system is contraindicated in the presence of PID or suspected PID or in women with a history of PID. Use of all IUDs, including the PROGESTASERT system, has been associated with an increased incidence of PID. In hospital-based, case-control study done in the United States in 1976–1978, women using IUD's had a relative risk of PID of 1.6 compared with women using no method.[3] Therefore a decision to use the PROGESTASERT system must include consideration of the risks of PID. The highest rate of PID occurs shortly after insertion and up to four months thereafter. Administration of prophylactic antibiotics may be useful, but the utility of this treatment is still under consideration (see INSERTION PRECAUTIONS). PID can necessitate hysterectomy; can lead to tubo-ovarian abscesses, tubal occlusion and infertility, and tubal damage that predisposes to ectopic pregnancy; can result in peritonitis; and can cause death in infrequent cases. The effect of PID on fertility ie especially important for women who may wish to have children at a later date.

a. Women at special risk to PID

PID is usually a sexually transmitted disease. The risk of PID appears to be greater for women who have multiple sexual partners and also for women whose sexual partner(s) have multiple sexual partners. Women who have ever had PID are at high risk for a recurrence or re-infection.

b. PID warning to PROGESTASERT system users

All women who choose the PROGESTASERT system must be informed prior to insertion that IUD use has been associated with an increased incidence of PID and that PID can necessitate hysterectomy, can cause tubal damage leading to ectopic pregnancy or infertility, or in infrequent cases can cause death. Patients must be taught to recognize and report to their physician promptly any symptoms of pelvic inflammatory disease. These symptoms include development of menstrual disorders (prolonged or heavy bleeding), unusual vaginal discharge, abdominal or pelvic pain or tenderness, dyspareunia, chills, and fever.

c. Asymptomatic PID

PID may be asymptomatic but still result in tubal damage and its sequelae.[4,5]

d. Treatment of PID

Following diagnosis of PID, or suspected PID, bacteriologic specimens should be obtained and antibiotic therapy should be initiated promptly. Removal of the PROGESTASERT system soon after initiation of antibiotic therapy is required. Guidelines for PID treatment are available from the Center for Disease Control (CDC), Atlanta, Georgia. A copy of the printed guidelines has been provided to you by ALZA Corporation. The guidelines were established after deliberation by a group of experts and staff of the CDC but they should not be construed as rules suitable for use in all patients. Adequate PID treatment requires the application of current standards of therapy prevailing at the time of occurrence of the infec-

tion with reference to the specific antibiotic's prescription labeling.

Genital actinomycosis has been associated primarily with long-term IUD use. If it occurs, promptly institute appropriate antibiotic therapy and remove the PROGESTASERT system.

4. Embedment

Partial penetration or embedment of the PROGESTASERT system in the endometrium or myometrium may decrease contraceptive effectiveness and can result in difficult removals. In some cases, this can result in fragmentation of the IUD, necessitating surgical removal.

5. Fragmentation

If fragmentation of the PROGESTASERT system occurs, all pieces should be removed if possible. Verification of removal should take into account that the horizontal crossarms are not radiopaque.

6. Perforation

Partial or total perforation of the uterine wall or cervix may occur with the use of the PROGESTASERT system. The possibility of perforation must be kept in mind during insertion and at the time of any subsequent examination. It is recommended that the PROGESTASERT system insertion be postponed postpartum or post abortion until involution of the uterus is complete since the incidence of perforation and expulsion is greater if involution is not complete. Involution may be delayed in nursing mothers; there is an increased risk of perforation in women who are lactating. If perforation occurs, the PROGESTASERT system should be removed. A surgical procedure may be required. Adhesions, foreign body reactions, peritonitis, cystic masses in the pelvis, intestinal penetrations, intestinal obstruction and local inflammatory reaction with abscess formation and erosion of adjacent viscera may result if an IUD is left in the peritoneal cavity.

7. Risks of Mortality

The available data from a variety of sources have been analyzed to estimate the risk of death associated with various methods of contraception. The estimates of risk of death include the combined risk of the contraceptive method plus the risk of pregnancy or abortion in the event of method failure. The findings of the analysis are shown in Table I.[6]
[See table below left].

PRECAUTIONS

1. Patient Counseling

a. Patients must be informed of the availability, effectiveness, and risks of the PROGESTASERT system and other forms of contraception. They should also be informed of the health risks associated with pregnancy resulting from failure to use any contraception.

b. Prior to insertion of the PROGESTASERT system, the physician, nurse, or other trained health professional must provide the patient with the Patient Information Leaflet. The patient must read the leaflet in its entirety and discuss fully any questions she has concerning the PROGESTASERT system and other methods of contraception. She must then initial and sign the leaflet, including the Informed Choice Statement, where indicated.

2. Patient Evaluation and Clinical Considerations

a. A complete medical history should be obtained to determine conditions that might influence the selection of the PROGESTASERT system or contraindicate its use (see CONTRAINDICATIONS). Physical examination should include a pelvic examination, Pap smear, N. gonorrhea and Chlamydia culture (or other specific tests for these organisms) and, if indicated, appropriate tests for other forms of venereal disease. **Special attention must be given to ascertaining whether the woman is at a risk of ectopic pregnancy or PID. The PROGESTASERT system is contraindicated in these women.**

b. The PROGESTASERT system is not intended for immediate postabortion or postpartum insertion. It should not be inserted until involution of the uterus is complete. (Involution may be delayed in nursing mothers.) The incidence of perforation and expulsion is greater if involution is not completed. Data also suggests there may be an increased risk of perforation and expulsion if the woman is lactating.[7,8]

c. **The physician should determine that the patient is not pregnant.** The possibility of insertion in the presence of an existing undetermined pregnancy is reduced if insertion is performed during or shortly following a menstrual period.

d. Patients with certain types of valvular heart disease and surgically constructed systemic-pulmonary shunts have an increased risk of infective endocarditis. Use of a PROGESTASERT system in these patients may represent a potential source of septic emboli and is contraindicated. Other conditions predisposing to infection (see CONTRAINDICATIONS) are also contraindications to PROGESTASERT system insertion.

e. IUDs should be used with caution in those patients who have an anemia or a history of menorrhagia or hypermenorrhea. Patients experiencing menorrhagia and/or metrorrhagia following IUD insertion may be at risk for the development of hypochromic microcytic anemia. Also,

TABLE I—Annual Number of Birth-Related or Method-Related Deaths Associated with Control of Fertility per 100,000 Nonsterile Women, by Fertility Control Method According to Age

Method of control and outcome	15–19	20–24	25–29	30–34	35–39	40–44
No fertility control methods*	7.0	7.4	9.1	14.8	25.7	28.2
Oral contraceptives non-smokers**	0.3	0.5	0.9	1.9	13.8	31.6
Oral contraceptives smokers**	2.2	3.4	6.6	13.5	51.1	117.2
IUD**	0.8	0.8	1.0	1.0	1.4	1.4
Condom*	1.1	1.6	0.7	0.2	0.3	0.4
Diaphragm/spermicide*	1.9	1.2	1.2	1.3	2.2	2.8
Periodic abstinence*	2.5	1.6	1.6	1.7	2.9	3.6

* Deaths are birth related

** Deaths are method related

IUDs should be used with caution in patients who have a coagulopathy or are receiving anticoagulants.

f. Use of the PROGESTASERT system in patients with vaginitis or cervicitis should be postponed until proper treatment has cleared up the infection and until the cervicitis has been shown not to be due to gonorrhea or chlamydia (see CONTRAINDICATIONS).

3. Insertion Precautions

a. Because the presence of organisms capable of establishing PID cannot be determined by appearance, and because IUD insertion may be associated with introduction of vaginal bacteria into the uterus, administration of prophylactic antibiotics may be considered, but the utility of this treatment is still under evaluation. Regimens include doxycycline 200 mg orally 1 hour before insertion or erythromycin 500 mg orally 1 hours before insertion and 500 mg orally 6 hours after insertion. The use of antibiotics in nursing mothers is not recommended. Before prescribing the above mentioned antibiotics, refer to their prescription drug labeling, and make certain that the patient is a suitable candidate for the drug.

b. The uterus should be carefully sounded prior to insertion to determine the degree of patency of the endocervical canal and the internal os, and the direction and depth of the uterine cavity. In occasional cases, severe cervical stenosis may be encountered. Do not use excessive force to overcome this resistance.

c. The uterus should sound to a depth of 6 to 10 centimeters (cm). Insertion of the PROGESTASERT system into a uterine cavity measuring less than 6.5 cm by sounding may increase the incidence of expulsion, bleeding, and pain.

d. Syncope, bradycardia, or other neurovascular episodes may occur during insertion or removal of the PROGESTASERT system, especially in patients with a previous disposition to these conditions or cervical stenosis. If decreased pulse, perspiration, or pallor are observed, the patient should remain supine until these signs have disappeared.

e. The patient should be told that some bleeding and/or cramps may occur during the first few weeks after insertion. If her symptoms continue or are severe she should report them to her physician. She should also be given instructions on what other symptoms require her to call her physician. She should be instructed on how to check after her menstrual period to make certain that the thread still protrudes from the cervix and cautioned not to pull on the thread and displace the PROGESTASERT system. She should be informed that there is no contraceptive protection if the PROGESTASERT system is displaced or expelled. If a partial expulsion occurs, removal is indicated.

f. **The patient must be told to return within 3 months for a checkup and at 12 months after insertion for removal of the PROGESTASERT system. Patient reminder cards must be properly completed and given to the patient.**

4. Requirements for Continuation and Removal

a. The PROGESTASERT system must be replaced every 12 months. There is no evidence of decreasing contraceptive efficacy with time before 12 months, but contraceptive effectiveness after 12 months decreases; therefore, the patient should be informed of the known duration of contraceptive efficacy and be advised to return in 12 months for removal and possible insertion of a new PROGESTASERT system.

b. The PROGESTASERT system should be removed for the following medical reasons: menorrhagia- and/or metrorrhagia-producing anemia; pelvic infection; endometritis; genital actinomycosis; intractable pelvic pain; dyspareunia; pregnancy; endometrial or cervical malignancy; uterine or cervical perforation; increase in length of the threads extending from the cervix, or any other indication of partial expulsion.

c. If the retrieval threads are not visible, they may have retracted into the uterus or have been broken, or the PROGESTASERT system may have been broken, perforated the uterus, or have been expelled. Location may be determined by feeling with a probe, X-ray, or sonography.

5. Continuing Care of patients Using the PROGESTASERT System

a. Any inquiries regarding pain, odorous discharge, bleeding, fever, genital lesions or sores, or a missed period should be promptly responded to and prompt examination recommended.

b. If examination during visits subsequent to insertion reveals that the length of the threads has visibly or palpably changed from the length at time of insertion, the system should be considered displaced and should be removed. A new system may be inserted at that time or during the next menses if it is certain that conception has not occurred. When the thread cannot be seen by the physician, further investigation is necessary.

c. Since the PROGESTASERT system may be expelled or displaced, patients should be reexamined and evaluated shortly after the first postinsertion menses, but definitely within 3 months after insertion. **The PROGESTASERT** system must be removed every 12 months because of diminished contraceptive effectiveness thereafter. At the time of reinsertion, appropriate medical and laboratory examinations should be carried out.

d. In the event a pregnancy is confirmed during PROGESTASERT system use, the following steps should be taken:

• Determine whether pregnancy is ectopic and take appropriate measures if it is.

• Inform patient of the risks of leaving an IUD *in situ* or removing it during pregnancy and of the lack of data on the PROGESTASERT system's long-term effects on the offspring of women who had it *in utero* during conception or gestation (see WARNINGS).

• If possible the PROGESTASERT system should be removed after the patient has been warned of the risks of removal. If removal is difficult, the patient should be counseled about and offered pregnancy termination.

• If the PROGESTASERT system is left in place, the patient's course should be followed closely.

ADVERSE REACTIONS

These adverse reactions are not listed in any order of frequency or severity.

Reported adverse reactions with intrauterine contraceptives include: endometritis; spontaneous abortion; septic abortion; septicemia; perforation of the uterus and cervix; embedment; fragmentation of the IUD; pelvic infection; tubo-ovarian abscess; tubal damage; vaginitis; leukorrhea; cervical erosion; pregnancy; ectopic pregnancy; fetal damage and congenital anomalies; difficult removal; complete or partial expulsion of the IUD; intermenstrual spotting; prolongation of menstrual flow; anemia; amenorrhea or delayed menses; pain and cramping; dysmenorrhea; backaches; dyspareunia; neurovascular episodes, including bradycardia and syncope secondary to insertion. Uterine perforation and IUD displacement into the abdomen have been followed by peritonitis, abdominal adhesions, intestinal penetration, intestinal obstruction, local inflammatory reaction with abscess formation and erosion of adjacent viscera, and cystic masses in the pelvis. Certain of these adverse reactions can lead to loss of fertility, partial or total removal of reproductive organs, hormonal imbalance, or death.

DIRECTIONS FOR USE

A single PROGESTASERT system is to be inserted into the uterine cavity (see PRECAUTIONS). The system must be removed 12 months after insertion and replaced for continued contraceptive effectiveness. See INSERTION AND REMOVAL INSTRUCTIONS.

CLINICAL STUDIES

Different event rates have been reported with the use of different IUDs. Inasmuch as these rates are usually derived from separate studies conducted by different investigators in several population groups, they cannot be compared with precision. Clinical trials of the PROGESTASERT system were conducted by ALZA and the World Health Organization from 1970 to 1981; use-effectiveness was determined from combined data as tabulated by the life table method. (Rates are expressed as events per 100 women through 12 months of use.) This experience is based on 5104 women who completed 12 months of use.

	12 Months	
	Parous*	Nulliparous*
Pregnancy		
Intrauterine	1.3	2.1
Extrauterine (ectopic)	0.5	0.4
Total	1.8	2.5
Expulsion	2.7	7.6
Medical Removals	9.3	12.0
Continuation Rate	81.2	73.4

* Columns do not total 100 because rates are not included for the following: scheduled removals, removals for planned pregnancy, release from studies, and lost-to-follow-up.

The lowest expected and typical failure rates during the first year of continuous use of all contraceptive methods are listed in Table 2.[9]

TABLE 2—Percentage of Women Experiencing an Accidental Pregnancy in the First Year of Continuous Use

Method	Lowest Expected*	Typical**
No Contraception	89	89
Oral Contraceptives		3.0
combined	0.1	N/A***
progestin only	0.5	N/A***
Diaphragm with spermicidal cream or jelly	3.0	18.0
Spermicides alone (foam, creams, jellies, and vaginal suppositories)	3.0	21.0
Vaginal Sponge		
nulliparous	5.0	18.0
multiparous	>8.0	>28.0
IUD (medicated)	1.0	6.0†
Condom		
without spermicides	3.0	12.0
Periodic abstinence (all methods)	2.0–8.0	20.0
Female sterilization	0.3	0.4
Male sterilization	0.1	0.15

* The authors' best guess of the percentage of women expected to experience an accidental pregnancy among couples who initiate a method (not necessarily for the first time) and who use it consistently and correctly during the first year if they do not stop for any other reason.

** This term represents "typical" couples who initiate use of a method (not necessarily for the first time), who experience an accidental pregnancy during the first year if they do not stop use for any other reason.

*** N/A—Data not available.

† Combined typical rate for both medicated and non-medicated IUD. The rate for the medicated IUD alone is not available.

HOW SUPPLIED

Available in cartons containing six packages, each with a sterile system and sterile inserter in a Tyvek polyethylene pouch.

INSERTION AND REMOVAL INSTRUCTIONS

NOTE: Physicians are cautioned to become thoroughly familiar with the insertion instructions in their entirety before attempting placement of the PROGESTASERT system. There is debate as to how many IUD insertions constitute adequate training for a clinician. It is probably wise to have done 15–25 insertions under supervision prior to inserting an IUD unsupervised. A practitioner with only 4–6 insertions would probably not have had adequate experience with difficult insertions.

The insertion technique is different in several respects from that used with other intrauterine contraceptives and the physician should pay particular attention to the drawings and commentary accompanying these instructions.

The usual time of insertion is during the latter part of the menstrual period, or one or two days thereafter.

The PROGESTASERT system retains its efficacy for 12 months. Therefore, it must be removed and a new one inserted no more than 12 months after insertion for continued contraceptive efficacy.

PRELIMINARY PREPARATION

1. Before insertion, the patient must read and initial each section of the Patient Information Leaflet; the medical and social history and counseling of the patient must be completed; and the Informed Choice Statement must be signed by the patient and by the doctor.

2. Refer to CONTRAINDICATIONS, WARNINGS, and PRECAUTIONS.

3. Prior to insertion of the PROGESTASERT system, a cervical Pap smear, N. gonorrhea and Chlamydia cultures (or specific tests for these organisms), and pelvic examination are to be performed.

4. If used, commence antibiotic prophylaxis one hour before insertion.

5. Use of aseptic technique during insertion is essential.

6. The endocervix should be cleansed with an antiseptic solution and a tenaculum applied to the cervix with downward traction for correction of the angulation of the cervix and stabilization of the cervix.

7. Prior to insertion, determine by uterine sounding the depth and position of the uterus and the patency of the cervical canal. Insertion into a uterus that sounds less than 6 cm or more than 10 cm is contraindicated.

8. THE PROGESTASERT SYSTEM MUST BE USED ONLY WITH ITS SPECIALLY DESIGNED INSERTER. This inserter will facilitate fundal placement and is designed to decrease the possibility of uterine perforation. No component should be removed from the inserter before insertion of the system into the uterus.

NOTE: Any intrauterine procedure can result in severe pain, bradycardia, and syncope.

SYSTEM INSERTION

1. Place the pouch on a hard, flat surface. Peel the clear cover back completely. Inspect the inserter to make sure the thread-retaining plug is secure at the end of the inserter with 2.5–5.0 cm of the long "retainer" thread protruding. Do not insert the system if the plug cannot be easily secured.

Continued on next page

Alza—Cont.

Remove the system and inserter by grasping the inserter at a point between two sets of graduations. DO NOT CONTAMINATE THE END CONTAINING THE SYSTEM.

2. IMMEDIATELY PRIOR TO INSERTION, cock the arms of the PROGESTASERT system by holding the inserter vertically with arm cocker flat on the sterile interior of the pouch. Press down firmly to cock the arms. This will cause the arms to fold against the sides of the inserter.

NOTE: To avoid alteration of system shape, do not leave the system cocked for more than five minutes.

3. Examine the curvature of the inserter. Make any necessary adjustments to the curvature of the inserter to fit the flexion of the uterus, maintaining aseptic technique. For an anteverted uterus, the black numbers on the inserter should face up; they should face down for a retroverted uterus. Be certain that the thread-retaining plug is still secure in the end of the inserter, then introduce the inserter into the cervical canal. The feet of the arm-cocker will rest centered on the cervical os as you push the inserter gently but steadily through the cervical canal.

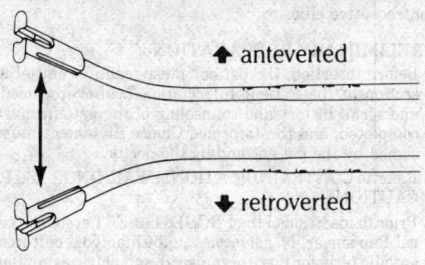

↑ anteverted

↓ retroverted

4. When the fundus is reached, the number on the inserter at the base of the arm-cocker should equal the previously sounded uterine depth.

5. DO NOT PULL BACK ON THE ARMCOCKER OR INSERTER. Release the PROGESTASERT system by squeezing the wings of the thread-retaining plug and removing it.

6. Slowly withdraw the inserter. The PROGESTASERT system remains in the uterus as the inserter is withdrawn. After insertion is complete, check to make certain that **no** components of the inserter are in the uterus. Dispose of the inserter shaft with attached armcocker, as well as the thread-retaining plug.

CORRECT FUNDAL PLACEMENT

To be fully effective, the PROGESTASERT system must be placed at the fundus. To confirm the correct position of the PROGESTASERT system. measure the length of the short "indicator" thread against the graduations on the thread-retaining end of the inserter. The length of this short thread should be the difference between 9 cm and the uterine depth.

2 cm

For example, if the uterus was sounded to 7 cm, the short "indicator" thread should extend out of the cervix 9 cm — 7 cm = 2 cm.

Cut the long "retainer" thread to a standard length of your choice—at least 3 cm from the cervix. This can be used for future reference in determining if fundal placement is being maintained. (If pregnancy, displacement, or perforation occurs, the thread may be drawn up through the cervix.) Record uterine depth and length of cut "retainer" thread in the patient's chart.

3 cm

SYSTEM REMOVAL

To remove the PROGESTASERT system, pull gently on the exposed threads. The arms of the system will fold upward as it is withdrawn from the uterus. Even if removal proves difficult, the system should not remain in the uterus after one year.

CAUTION: Federal law prohibits dispensing without prescription.

© ALZA Corporation, 1989

REFERENCES
1. World Health Organization's Special Programme of Research, Development and Research Training in Human Reproduction: A multi-national case-control study of ectopic pregnancy. "Clin Reprod Fertil." 1985; 3: 131–143.
2. Ory H.W., Women's Health Study: Ectopic pregnancy and intrauterine contraceptive devices: New perspectives. "Obstet. Gynecol." 1981; 57: 137–144.
3. Lee, N.C., Rubin, G.L., and Borucki, R. The Intrauterine Device and Pelvic Inflammatory Disease Revisited: New Results From the Women's Health Study. "Obstet. Gynecol." 1988; 72: 1–6.
4. Cramer D.W. et al: Tubal infertility and the intrauterine device. "N. Engl. J. Med." 1985; 312: 941–947.
5. Daling J.R. et al: Primary tubal infertility in relation to the use of an intrauterine device. "N. Engl. J. Med." 1985; 312: 937–941.
6. Ory H.W.: Mortality associated with fertility and fertility control. "Family Planning Perspective" 1983; 15: 57–63.
7. Heartwell S.F., Schlesselman S.: Risk of uterine perforation among users of intrauterine devices. "Obstet. Gynecol." 1983; 61: 31–36.
8. Chi I.C., Kelly E.: Is lactation a risk factor of IUD and sterilisation-related uterine perforations? A hypothesis. "Int. J. Gynaecol. Obstet." 1984; 22: 315–317.
9. Trussell J., Kost K.: Contraceptive failure in the United States: A critical review of the literature. "Studies in Family Planning" 1987; 18: 237–283.

PROGESTASERT®   ℞

Intrauterine Progesterone Conntraceptive System

PATIENT INFORMATION

INTRODUCTION

ALZA's intrauterine device, the PROGESTASERT® system, is the only hormone-releasing IUD and has been available in the United States since 1976. It was tested in more than 5000 women and over a million units have been used since its introduction. However, as with all methods of contraception, its use is associated with some risks. The purpose of this brochure is to explain those risks to you.

IMPORTANT NOTICE

To understand the risks and benefits of the PROGESTASERT system you will need to read and understand this entire leaflet and discuss it with your doctor. It contains information vital to your health. A more technical leaflet is available, which is written for the medical professional. If you would like to read that leaflet, ask your doctor for a copy. You may need the doctor's help to understand some of the information.

If you have difficulty understanding any of the technical terms in this brochure, check the glossary on page 7 and ask your doctor for clarification.

Intrauterine devices (IUDs) have been the subject of many personal injury lawsuits. Several IUD manufacturers have discontinued U.S. sales of their IUDs. Nevertheless, many doctors consider IUDs to be the best contraceptive choice for certain women. The PROGESTASERT system is most appropriately used in women who have had at least one child and are in a stable, mutually monogamous relationship, and have no history of pelvic inflammatory disease (PID). In addition to reading this leaflet, you should also learn about sterilization and other birth control methods. One of these methods may be more suitable or safer for you than the PROGESTASERT system. To make the appropriate decision, you must discuss your questions about the PROGESTASERT and other kinds of birth control with your doctor. Also, have the doctor explain to your satisfaction anything you do not understand in this leaflet.

Under certain conditions you should not have the PROGESTASERT system inserted; the risks to your health or your ability to bear children may be too great. Such conditions are described under SPECIAL RISK FACTORS and WHAT YOU SHOULD DISCUSS WITH YOUR DOCTOR. Even if none of these conditions applies to you, you may still experience serious problems while using the PROGESTASERT system. These problems require immediate medical attention. They can cause damage to your reproductive organs and the ability to bear children or in infrequent cases can cause death. You may have to undergo major surgery, and you may become temporarily or permanently sterile (see SPECIAL RISK FACTORS). Prompt medical treatment, though absolutely necessary, may not always be effective.

To become familiar with the danger signs of IUD use read ADVERSE REACTIONS, SIDE EFFECTS, AND WARNINGS. Then discuss these sections of the leaflet with your doctor.

I have read this notice, and I understand it; I must initial all sections of the leaflet where indicated and will discuss its contents with my doctor. I will not use the PROGESTASERT system without fully understanding this information. I also understand that I am free to choose not to use the PROGESTASERT system.

_____
Signature

_____
Date

DESCRIPTION

The PROGESTASERT system is a type of IUD that contains progesterone and is inserted into the uterus (womb) to prevent pregnancy. Like all other contraceptives, it is not 100%

effective. (See USE EFFECTIVENESS for pregnancy rates during its use.)

The PROGESTASERT system is small, flexible, and T-shaped, with a hollow stem containing the hormone progesterone. The T itself measures 1.26 inches across the arms and 1.42 inches in length and is made of a flexible material (ethylene/vinyl acetate copolymer). This material permits the continuous release of progesterone into the uterus for 12 months. **The PROGESTASERT system must be replaced every 12 months to maintain its contraceptive effect.** Two blue-black threads extend from the base of the T. They will extend into your vagina, indicate the presence of the system, and aid in its removal.

THE PROGESTERONE IN THE PROGESTASERT SYSTEM

The PROGESTASERT system is the only intrauterine contraceptive to use progesterone, a hormone chemically identical to a hormone that your ovaries make. In 12 months the PROGESTASERT system releases only a little more progesterone than your body produces in one day during the latter part of a normal menstrual cycle.

Other contraceptive methods rely on different principles and materials to help prevent pregnancy. For instance, birth control pills rely on substances (progestins and estrogens) that differ from those made by your body.

The PROGESTASERT system is also unique in another way. The hormone it delivers does not travel through the bloodstream. Instead, the progesterone acts locally, directly on the lining of your uterus.

HOW THE PROGESTASERT SYSTEM ACTS AS A CONTRACEPTIVE

How IUDs act as contraceptives is not competely understood. Several theories have been suggested. IUDs seem to interfere in some manner with fertilization, or they may prevent the fertilized egg from remaining in the uterus. IUDs do not prevent ovulation (release of an egg by the ovary).

The PROGESTASERT system acts only within the uterus. Thus, it does not always prevent ectopic pregnancy (pregnancy outside the uterus). Ectopic pregnancy can require surgery and can make you unable to bear children; in infrequent cases it can cause death. (See SPECIAL RISK FACTORS—Ectopic Pregnancy.)

I have read this section and understand it or will discuss it with my doctor.

_____ Initials

USE-EFFECTIVNESS

In clinical trials the incidence of unplanned pregnancies in women who used the PROGESTASERT system was 2 to 3 per 100 woman-years, or 2 to 3 women out of 100 became pregnant in a year while using the PROGESTASERT intrauterine progesterone contraceptive system. The number of pregnancies includes both uterine and ectopic (outside the uterus).

In these studies 3 to 8 women out of 100 expelled the system during the first year. Nine to 12 women per year had an adverse reaction requiring system removal. Some of these adverse reactions were pelvic inflammatory disease (PID), an infection of the reproduction organs. The number of women in the studies who used the system continously for one year was 73 to 81 out of 100.

The typical failure rates for all methods of birth control during the first year are listed below in Table 1.[1] The failure rate tabulated below for IUDs includes all IUDs combined.

Table 1—Typical Failure Rates for All Methods	
Method	Rate
Oral Contraceptives	3%
IUD	6%
Diaphragm with Spermicides	18%
Vaginal Sponge	
among women who have never been pregnant	18%
among women who have been pregnant	> 28%
Condom alone	12%
Periodic abstinence	20%
No method	89%

[1]Trussel J. Kost K: Contraceptive failure in the United States. A critical review of the literature. *Studies in Family Planning* 1987: 18:237–283

I have read this section and understand it or will discuss it with my doctor.

_____ Initials

LOSS OF CONTRACEPTIVE EFFECT AFTER PROGESTASERT SYSTEM REMOVAL

After discontinuation of PROGESTASERT system use, its contraceptive effect on the uterus is reversed. Usually, but not always, a woman is able to become pregnant. In a study of 154 women seeking pregnancy, 76% became pregnant within a year following discontinuation.

I have read this section and understand it or will discuss it with my doctor.

_____ Initials

SPECIAL RISK FACTORS

The conditions discussed below can significantly increase your chances of developing serious complications while using an IUD. Some of these conditions can necessitate surgery, can make you unable to have children, or can cause death. Therefore it is important that you have access to emergency care if it becomes necessary. Read the information carefully and discuss it with your doctor.

Special Risk Factors for Ectopic Pregnancy

Ectopic pregnancy is a dangerous type of pregnancy that develops outside the uterus. The PROGESTASERT system—unlike some other contraceptives—does not prevent ectopic pregnancy. Studies indicate that PROGESTASERT system users have approximately the same risk of ectopic pregnancy as sexually active women using no contraception. But among women in the clinical studies who became pregnant while using the PROGESTASERT system, 1 out of 3 to 4 pregnancies among women who had borne one or more children was ectopic; among women who had not had children, 1 out of 6 pregnancies was ectopic.

PROGESTASERT system users are also more apt to have an ectopic pregnancy than users of other IUDs. Two clinical studies conducted by the World Health Organization compared the risk of ectopic pregnancies among women wearing a progesterone-releasing IUD similar to the PROGESTASERT system with the risk in women wearing a copper-releasing IUD. From the combined data of the two studies, the risk of an ectopic pregnancy in the first year was approximately 6 times higher among women using progesterone systems than among women using copper IUDs. Over the two years that the studies ran, the risk of an ectopic pregnancy with the progesterone IUD was about 10 times higher than that with copper-releasing IUDs.

If you have ever had an ectopic pregnancy, you have an increased risk of having another one. You also have an increased risk of an ectopic pregnancy if you have ever had certain infections. These infections include pelvic inflammatory disease (PID) or any venereal disease (VD) caused by gonorrhea or chlamydia. **If you have ever had an ectopic pregnancy or these kinds of infections, you must not use the PROGESTASERT system.** Other contraceptive methods may be more suitable for you. Discuss this matter with your doctor.

If you are using the PROGESTASERT system, you should immediately call your doctor if you develop any of the following symptoms, which may indicate ectopic pregnancy:

- A missed period, or delayed period followed by spotting or scanty or irregular bleeding
- Cramping, tenderness, or sharp pain in your pelvis or lower abdomen
- Fainting associated with pelvic or lower abdominal pain or with an urge to have a bowel movement
- Pelvic or lower abdominal pain radiating down your legs
- Pain in your shoulder
- Pain associated with vaginal bleeding
- Any unusual or abnormal vaginal bleeding

Failure to seek and receive prompt and adequate treatment could greatly increase the changes of sterility or the need for surgery or could result in death.

Special Risk Factors for Pelvic Infection (Pelvic Inflammatory Disease).

Evidence indicates that IUD users are more likely than other women to suffer a serious infection called pelvic inflammatory disease (PID), particularly in women with multiple sexual partners. PID is the medical term for infection in the upper pelvic area. This area includes the uterus (womb), fallopian tubes, ovaries, and surrounding tissues. (Vaginitis, a local infection of the vagina, is not PID.) Studies indicate that the highest rate of PID occurs shortly after insertion and up to 4 months thereafter. PID can cause permanent blockage of the tubes and sterility, ectopic pregnancy, or, in infrequent cases, death. **If you have or have ever had PID, you must not use the PROGESTASERT system.**

PID is an infection caused by gonorrhea, chlamydia, or other bacteria. PID is usually a sexually transmitted disease, and your chances of getting PID increase greatly if you have more than one sexual partner. Your risk of getting PID also increases if you have a sexual partner who has sexual intercourse with others. **If you have an increased risk of getting PID, you must not use the PROGESTASERT system.** You should consider using a barrier method which may provide partial protection against sexually transmitted diseases. Treatment of PID may require surgical removal of your uterus (hysterectomy), tubes, and ovaries. Removing the ovaries may result in lifelong need for hormonal treatments. Such surgery may have to be done on an emergency basis and may result in death.

Symptoms of PID include pelvic or lower abdominal pain, chills, fever, abnormal vaginal discharge, abnormal menstrual bleeding, or painful sexual intercourse. PID and damage to your tubes can occur even without these symptoms. If you are using the PROGESTASERT system and develop any of these symptoms, see your doctor as soon as possible. If you have PID, you should receive appropriate antibiotic therapy, and the PROGESTASERT system should be removed. **Failure to seek and receive prompt and adequate treatment will greatly increase the chances that you will become sterile, require surgery, or have life-threatening or fatal PID.** Even prompt and adequate treatment cannot guarantee that these events will not occur.

Other Conditions That Increase Risk of Infection

Some conditions make you susceptible to infection during IUD use or following IUD insertion. These conditions include diabetes, leukemia, acquired immune deficiency syndrome (AIDS). IV drug abuse, and long-term steroid therapy. In addition, certain defects or diseases of the heart valves, such as rheumatic heart disease, may make you more likely than other IUD users to develop heart inflammation or infection. If you have any of these conditions you should not use the PROGESTASERT system.

I have read this section and understand it or will discuss it with my doctor.

_____ Initials

SIDE EFFECTS

The following may occur while the PROGESTASERT system is being inserted or afterwards.

1. Pain, usually uterine cramps or low backache, occur at the time of insertion and may persist. (Pain and cramping may also occur at removal.) If pain is severe, becomes worse, or persists, contact your doctor.
2. Fainting may occur at the time of insertion or removal of an IUD.
3. Some bleeding occurs following insertion in most women.
4. Partial or total perforation of the uterus may occur at the time of or after PROGESTASERT system insertion. If you think the system may be displaced, check with your doctor (see WARNINGS—Tail or thread disappearance). Perforation could result in abdominal adhesions, (scars), intestinal obstruction or penetration, inflammation, serious infection, and loss of contraceptive protection. Perforation and its complications may require surgery and in infrequent cases may result in death.
5. Bleeding between menstrual periods may occur during the first 2 or 3 months after insertion. The first few menstrual periods after insertion may be heavier and longer than usual. If these conditions continue for longer than 2 or 3 months, consult your doctor.
6. Occasionally you may miss a menstrual period while using the PROGESTASERT system. It is important to determine if you are pregnant; report this without delay to your doctor.
7. The PROGESTASERT system may come out of your uterus through the cervical opening. This is called expulsion, and is most likely to occur during the first 2 or 3 menstrual cycles following insertion. Expulsion leaves you unprotected against pregnancy. Refer to the section called DIRECTIONS FOR USE for information on how to check to see if your system is properly postioned. If you think the IUD has come out or has been displaced, use another birth control method, such as contraceptive vaginal foam, cream, or jelly, or condoms (rubbers), until you can be checked by your doctor. (These alternative methods are not as effective in preventing uterine pregnancy as the PROGESTASERT system.) Call your doctor for an examination.

I have read this section and understand it or will discuss it with my doctor.

_____ Initials

WHAT YOU SHOULD DISCUSS WITH YOUR DOCTOR

Before you have the PROGESTASERT system inserted, you should discuss with your doctor your plans for having children. Also indicate below if you have ever had—or suspect you have ever had—any of the conditions listed below. **Some of these conditions, especially those highlighted, might make the PROGESTASERT system an unsuitable contraceptive for you:**
[See table on bottom next page].

I have read this section and understand it or will discuss it with my doctor.

_____ Initials

ADVERSE REACTIONS

The following adverse reactions have been reported and may be caused by the PROGESTASERT system:

Continued on next page

Alza—Cont.

- Abdominal infection or adhesions (scar tissue)
- Anemia
- Backache
- Birth Defects
- Blood poisoning (septicemia)
- Bowel obstruction
- Cervical infection or erosion
- Cysts on ovaries and tubes
- Delayed menstruation
- Difficult removal
- Ectopic pregnancy
- Embedment (IUD surrounded by uterine tissue)
- Expulsion (IUD comes completely or partially out of the uterus)
- Fainting and pain at the time of insertion or removal
- Fetal damage
- Fragmentation (break-up) of the IUD
- Infertility
- Intermenstrual spotting
- Miscarriage (spontaneous abortion)
- Pain and cramps
- Painful intercourse
- Pelvic infection (PID), which may result in surgical removal of your reproductive organs (hysterectomy)
- Perforation of the uterus (womb) or cervix (IUD passes through uterine tissue)
- Pregnancy
- Premature birth
- Prolonged or heavy menstrual flow
- Septic abortion (infected miscarriage) followed in some cases by blood poisoning (septicemia), which can lead to death
- Vaginal discharge and infection

I have read this section and understand it or will discuss it with my doctor.

———————————— Initials ————————————

WARNINGS

If you have a PROGESTASERT system inserted, call your doctor immediately for any of the following reasons:

1. **A missed period.** This may mean you are pregnant and the IUD should be removed.
2. **Unexplained or abnormal vaginal bleeding or discharge.** This could indicate a serious complication such as an infection or ectopic pregnancy.
3. **A delayed period followed by scanty or irregular bleeding.** This could indicate an ectopic pregnancy.
4. **Pelvic or lower abdominal pain or cramps or unexplained fever.** Such symptoms could mean an ectopic pregnancy or infection has developed requiring immediate treatment.

Table 2—Annual Number of Birth-Related or Method-Related Deaths Associated with Control of Fertility per 100,000 Nonsterile Women, by Fertility Control Method According to Age

Method of control and outcome	15–19	20–24	25–29	30–34	35–39	40–44
No fertility control methods*	7.0	7.4	9.1	14.8	25.7	28.2
Oral contraceptives/nonsmokers**	0.3	0.5	0.9	1.9	13.8	31.6
Oral contraceptives/smokers**	2.2	3.4	6.6	13.5	51.1	117.2
IUD**	0.8	0.8	1.0	1.0	1.4	1.4
Condom*	1.1	1.6	0.7	0.2	0.3	0.4
Diaphragm/spermicide*	1.9	1.2	1.2	1.3	2.2	2.8
Periodic abstinence*	2.5	1.6	1.6	1.7	2.9	3.6

  * Deaths are birth related
 ** Deaths are method related

5. **Exposure to venereal disease (VD), also called sexually transmitted disease (STD).** The use of the PROGESTASERT system does not prevent venereal disease. If exposure to venereal disease is suspected, report for examination and treatment promptly. Failure to do so could result in serious pelvic infection.
6. **Genital sores or lesions, or fever with vaginal discharge.** These may indicate an infection.
7. **Severe or prolonged menstrual bleeding.** If the flow is heavier and lasts much longer than your usual menstrual flow, you may need to have the PROGESTASERT system removed to prevent anemia.
8. **Thread disappearance or pain during sex.** If you cannot feel the tail or thread coming through the cervix or have pain during sex, the PROGESTASERT system may have been expelled or displaced or may have perforated the uterus. If any of these has occurred, you are no longer protected from pregnancy. Use another birth control method, such as contraceptive vaginal foam, cream, or jelly, or condoms (rubbers) until you can be checked. (These alternative methods are not as effective against uterine pregnancy as the PROGESTASERT system.) If perforation has occurred, removal of the PROGESTASERT system is necessary, usually by surgery.
9. **Risk of death.** Available data from a variety of sources have been analyzed to estimate the risk of death associated with various methods of contraception. The estimates of risk of death include the combined risk of the contraceptive method plus the risk of pregnancy or abortion in the event of method failure. The findings of the analysis are shown in Table 2.[2]

I have read this section and understand it or will discuss it with my doctor.

———————————— Initials ————————————

[See table above].

[2] Ory, HW: Mortality associated with fertility and fertility control *Family Planning Perspectives* 1983; 15:57–63

I have read this section and understand it or will discuss it with my doctor.

———————————— Initials ————————————

SPECIAL WARNING ABOUT UTERINE PREGNANCY WITH A PROGESTASERT SYSTEM IN PLACE

Some women become pregnant while using the PROGESTASERT system. If you miss your menstrual period, or if you suspect you are pregnant, see your doctor right away. When a pregnancy continues with the IUD in place, serious complications may occur: sepsis (severe blood infection); spontaneous miscarriage (abortion); septic abortion (infected miscarriage); and death. These may occur at any time during the pregnancy, but most of these serious complications have been reported in the middle three months of pregnancy.

When the PROGESTASERT system remains in the uterus during conception or pregnancy, the long-term effects on the child (or fetus) are not known. Under such conditions some birth defects have occurred. Although it has been suggested, their relationship to the PROGESTASERT system has not been established. You should discuss all your questions about this with your doctor.

If your doctor confirms that you are pregnant, the PROGESTASERT system should be removed. Removal of the system may cause a miscarriage. However, successful IUD removal in pregnancy decreases the likelihood of subsequent complications, including miscarriage.

In some cases removal of the PROGESTASERT system may prove to be difficult. If so, you and your doctor should discuss at that time the question of continuing the pregnancy in view of the serious complications (described above) that may occur. In reaching a decision about termination of pregnancy, you should be aware that the risks associated with abortion increase with the length of time you have been pregnant.

If you continue your pregnancy with the PROGESTASERT system in place, you will need your physician to follow your course more closely than usual throughout your pregnancy. Be sure to report immediately to the doctor if you have any of the following symptoms or signs:

- Bleeding from the vagina
- Pelvic or lower abdominal pain or cramping
- Flu-like symptoms such as chills or fever
- Unusual vaginal discharge
- Ruptured membranes
- Any other signs or symptoms which gives you concern

Any of these symptoms could indicate that you are having a miscarriage that is complicated by an infection or that you are beginning, or about to begin, premature labor. Such an infection can cause infertility or death. Premature labor may lead to delivery of a premature infant. Premature infants have a higher chance of dying, mental retardation, cerebral palsy, or other serious medical problems. Therefore, report any symptoms without delay to your doctor, so that you can obtain immediate treatment.

I have read this section and understand it or will discuss it with my doctor.

———————————— Initials ————————————

GLOSSARY OF TERMS

Anemia—condition in which the blood does not have enough red blood cells.

Cervix—the narrow lower end of the uterus which opens into the vagina.

Chlamydia—a type of infection in the vagina and uterus, spread by sexual contact.

Contraceptive—a drug or device that prevents ovulation, fertilization, or implantation of the fertilized egg in the uterus.

Ectopic Pregnancy—development of the fertilized egg outside the uterus.

Expulsion—condition in which the IUD is forced out of the uterus.

Fertilization—process in which the sperm penetrates the egg of the female.

Please Check Appropriate Box

	Yes	No	Don't know—will discuss with my doctor
- Abnormalities of the uterus (womb)	☐	☐	☐
- Acquired immune deficiency syndrome (AIDS)	☐	☐	☐
- Anemia or blood clotting problems	☐	☐	☐
- Bleeding between periods	☐	☐	☐
- Cancer of the uterus (womb) or cervix	☐	☐	☐
- History of other types of cancer	☐	☐	☐
- Corticosteroid therapy	☐	☐	☐
- Current suspected or possible pregnancy	☐	☐	☐
- Diabetes	☐	☐	☐
- Ectopic pregnancy (pregnancy outside of the uterus)	☐	☐	☐
- Fainting attacks	☐	☐	☐
- Genital sores or lesions	☐	☐	☐
- Heart disease	☐	☐	☐
- Heart murmur	☐	☐	☐
- Heavy menstrual flow	☐	☐	☐
- Hepatitis or severe liver disease	☐	☐	☐
- Infection of the uterus (womb) or cervix	☐	☐	☐
- IUD in place now	☐	☐	☐
- IV drug abuse	☐	☐	☐
- Leukemia	☐	☐	☐
- Multiple sexual partners	☐	☐	☐
- A sexual partner who has multiple sexual partners	☐	☐	☐
- Pelvic infection (including pus in fallopian tubes)	☐	☐	☐
- Prior IUD use	☐	☐	☐
- Recent abortion or miscarriage	☐	☐	☐
- Recent pregnancy	☐	☐	☐
- Severe menstrual cramps	☐	☐	☐
- Sexually transmitted disease (venereal disease), such as gonorrhea, chlamydia	☐	☐	☐
- Suspicious or abnormal Pap smear	☐	☐	☐
- Unexplained genital bleeding	☐	☐	☐
- Uterine or pelvic surgery	☐	☐	☐
- Vaginal discharge or infection	☐	☐	☐

Gonorrhea—a contagious infection of the genital area, spread by sexual contact.

Hysterectomy—surgical procedure in which the uterus is removed.

Monogamous—having only one sexual partner.

Ovulation—release of an egg from the ovary into the fallopian tube.

Perforation—tearing of the wall of the uterus when the IUD is pushed through accidentally.

Sepsis—infection of the bloodstream usually resulting from the spread of bacteria from a localized infection.

Septic Abortion—miscarriage or abortion caused by an infection of the uterus; may cause sepsis.

Sterilization—procedure to make a man or woman unable to reproduce.

Progestasert®
Intrauterine Progesterone Contraceptive System

PATIENT INFORMATION

INFORMED CHOICE STATEMENT

I have read this leaflet in its entirety and discussed its contents with my doctor. My doctor has answered all my questions and has advised me of the risks and benefits associated with the use of the PROGESTASERT system, with other forms of contraception, and with no form of contraception. I understand that while using the PROGESTASERT system I may experience serious medical problems thay may not be caused by any defect in the PROGESTASERT system or inadequacy of medical care. These problems could lead to surgery, sterility, permanent hormonal imbalance, or death. I have considered all factors and voluntarily choose to have the PROGESTASERT system inserted by

Dr._____on date_____

_____
Patient Signature

The patient has signed this leaflet in my presence after I counseled her and answered all her questions.

_____ _____
Doctor   Date

This system is scheduled for removal on _____
                                    Date

I have chosen not to use the PROGESTASERT system.

_____
Patient Signature

© ALZA Corporation
Edition Date March 1989
Shown in Product Identification Section, page 404

EDUCATIONAL MATERIAL

Booklets - Brochures
A. Patient Information Leaflet
    (free to patients)
B. Spanish Patient Information Leaflet
    (free to patients)
C. Demonstration Kit (free)

Films - Slides - Videos
A. Progestasert® System Insertion Technique Videocassette
    (free)
B. Patient Audiocassette Tape
    (free)
C. Tape Player/Recorder ($20.00)

American Dermal Corporation
BEDMINSTER INDUSTRIAL PARK
PO BOX 900
PLUMSTEADVILLE, PA 18949

DRITHOCREME®   ℞
(anthralin) 0.1%, 0.25%, 0.5%, 1.0% (HP)

DESCRIPTION

Drithocreme is a pale yellow topical cream containing 0.1%, 0.25%, 0.5% or 1.0% (HP) anthralin USP in a base of white petrolatum, sodium lauryl sulfate, cetostearyl alcohol, ascorbic acid, salicylic acid, chlorocresol and purified water. The chemical name of anthralin is 1,8,dihydroxy-9-anthrone or 1,8,9-trihydroxyanthracene.

CLINICAL PHARMACOLOGY

Although the precise mechanism of anthralin's anti-psoriatic action is not fully understood, in vitro evidence suggests that its antimitotic effect results from inhibition of DNA synthesis. Additionally, the chemically reducing properties of anthralin may upset oxidative metabolic processes, providing a further slowing down of epidermal mitosis. Absorption in man has not been finally determined, but in a limited clinical study of Drithocreme, no traces of anthraquinone metabolites were detected in the urine of subjects treated. However, caution is advised in patients with renal disease.

INDICATIONS AND USAGE

An aid in the topical treatment of quiescent or chronic psoriasis. Treatment should be continued until the skin is entirely clear i.e. when there is nothing to feel with the fingers and the texture is normal.

CONTRAINDICATIONS

In patients with acute or actively inflamed psoriatic eruptions, or a history of hypersensitivity to any of the ingredients.

WARNINGS

Avoid contact with the eyes or mucous membranes. Exercise care when applying Drithocreme to the face or intertriginous skin areas and do not use high strengths in these sites. Discontinue use if a sensitivity reaction occurs or if excessive irritation develops on uninvolved skin areas.

PRECAUTIONS

For external use only. Keep out of the reach of children. To prevent the possibility of staining clothing or bed linen while gaining experience in using Drithocreme, it may be advisable to use protective dressings. To prevent the possibility of discoloration particularly where Drithocreme HP (1.0%) has been used, always rinse the bath/shower with hot water immediately after washing/showering and then use a suitable cleanser to remove any deposit on the surface of the bath or shower. Contact with fabrics, plastics and other materials may cause staining and should be avoided. Always wash hands thoroughly after use. Long-term studies in animals have not been performed to evaluate the carcinogenic potential of the drug. Although anthralin has been found to have tumor-promoting properties on mouse skin, there have been no reports to suggest carcinogenic effects in humans after many years of clinical use.

PREGNANCY

Pregnancy Category C. Animal reproduction studies have not been conducted with Drithocreme. It is also not known whether Drithocreme can cause fetal harm when administered to a pregnant woman or can affect reproduction capacity. Drithocreme should be given to a pregnant woman only if clearly needed.

NURSING MOTHERS

It is not known whether this drug is excreted in human milk. Because many drugs are excreted in milk and because of the potential for tumorigenicity shown for anthralin in animal studies, a decision should be made whether to discontinue nursing or to discontinue the drug, taking into account the importance of the drug to the mother.

PEDIATRIC USE

Safety and effectiveness in children have not been specifically established.

ADVERSE REACTIONS

Very few instances of contact allergic reactions to anthralin have been reported. However, transient primary irritation of normal skin or uninvolved skin surrounding the treated lesions is more frequently seen. If the initial treatment produces excessive soreness or if the lesions spread, reduce frequency of application and, in extreme cases, discontinue use and consult physician. Some temporary discoloration of hair and fingernails may arise during the period of treatment but should be minimized by careful application. Drithocreme may stain skin, hair or fabrics. Staining of fabrics may be permanent, so contact should be avoided.

DOSAGE AND ADMINISTRATION

Generally, it is recommended that Drithocreme be applied once a day. Anthralin is known to be a potential skin irritant.The irritant potential of anthralin is directly related to the strength being used and each patient's individual tolerance. Therefore, where the response to anthralin treatment has not previously been established, always commence treatment for at least one week using 0.1% Drithocreme. Increase to the 0.25%, 0.5% or 1.0% (HP) strengths if appropriate. To open the tube, unscrew the cap and invert to pierce membrane.

Drithocreme should normally be applied once daily and removed by washing or showering. The optimal period of contact will vary according to the strength used and the patient's response to treatment.

For The Skin: Apply sparingly only to the psoriatic lesions and rub gently and carefully into the skin until absorbed. It is most important to avoid applying an excessive quantity which may cause unnecessary soiling and staining of the clothing and/or bed linen. At the end of each period of treatment, a bath or shower should be taken to remove any surplus cream which may have become red/brown in color. The margins of the lesions may gradually become stained purple/brown as treatment progresses, but this will disappear after cessation of treatment.

For The Scalp: Comb the hair to remove scalar debris and, after suitably parting, rub the cream well into the lesions. Keep Drithocreme away from the eyes. Care should be taken to avoid application of the cream to uninvolved scalp margins. Remove any unintended residue which may be deposited behind the ears. At the end of each period of contact, wash the hair and scalp to remove any surplus cream (which may have become red/brown in color). Keep tightly capped when not in use. Store in a cool place (46°–59°F)

HOW SUPPLIED

50g tubes
Drithocreme 0.1%   NDC 51201-0029-1
Drithocreme 0.25%   NDC 51201-0028-1
Drithocreme 0.5%   NDC 51201-0027-1
Drithocreme HP 1.0%   NDC 51201-0026-1

CAUTION

Federal law prohibits dispensing without prescription.
Revised 6/89
AMERICAN DERMAL CORPORATION
Plumsteadville, PA 18949

DRITHO-SCALP®   ℞
(anthralin) 0.25%, 0.5%

CONTAINS

0.25% or 0.5% anthralin USP in a base of white petrolatum, mineral oil, sodium lauryl sulfate, cetostearyl alcohol, ascorbic acid, salicylic acid, chlorocresol and purified water. The chemical name of anthralin is 1,8,dihydroxy-9-anthrone.

HOW SUPPLIED

50g tube with special applicator
Dritho-Scalp 0.25% NDC 51202-0024-1
Dritho-Scalp 0.5% NDC 51201-0023-1

VIRANOL® GEL   ℞
12.0% Salicylic Acid USP,
in a collodion gel containing lactic acid,
camphor, pyroxylin, ethyl alcohol and
ethyl acetate

DESCRIPTION

Viranol Gel is a gel formulation for topical application containing 12.0% Salicylic Acid USP in an evaporative gel containing lactic acid, camphor, pyroxylin, ethyl alcohol and ethyl acetate.

ACTION

The active ingredient, Salicylic Acid, is believed to exert a keratolytic action which effects the removal of wart epidermal cells infected by deoxyribonucleic acid viruses.

INDICATIONS

Viranol Gel is indicated as an aid in the treatment and removal of plantar warts and other common warts.

CONTRAINDICATIONS

Viranol Gel should not be used by diabetics, individuals with impaired blood circulation or by patients who are sensitive to any of the ingredients.

WARNINGS

Viranol Gel should not be applied to moles, birthmarks, unusual warts with protruding hair, genital warts, or warts on the face.

PRECAUTIONS

Viranol Gel is for external use only.
Discontinue use if excessive irritation occurs on normal skin areas. Avoid contact with eyes and mucous membranes. If contact with eyes or mucous membranes should occur, flush with water to remove collodion film, continue rinsing for an additional 15 minutes and consult physician. Viranol Gel is highly flammable and should not be used or stored near fire or flame. Avoid inhaling vapors. Avoid contact with clothing, fabrics, plastics, wood, metal and other materials, which may cause damage.

ADVERSE REACTIONS

Viranol Gel may cause local irritation on normal skin. Care should be used to avoid contact with normal surrounding skin areas while applying Viranol Gel directly to wart.

DOSAGE AND ADMINISTRATION

Before initial use, the tube membrane should be pierced by inverting the standard cap, which should then be discarded. The accompanying special applicator should then be screwed firmly onto the tube. This special applicator includes its own cap which should always be replaced between treatments.

Continued on next page

American Dermal—Cont.

Once daily application.

1. Every night, soak the affected site in warm water for 2–3 minutes. 2. Dry thoroughly with your own towel. 3. Remove applicator cap, locate tip of applicator precisely at site of lesion and gently squeeze the tube. Apply one or two drops of the gel carefully to the lesion and allow to dry over its surface. Take care to avoid spreading on to surrounding normal skin. No adhesive bandage is necessary. Always recap the applicator after use. 4. The following evening, carefully remove and discard the elastic film formed from the previous application, and re-apply the gel. 5. Once a week, gently rub away the treated surface using an emery board or pumice stone before re-applying the gel. 6. Some mild transient irritation may be expected, but treatment should be discontinued in case of more severe irritation. If you are in any doubt about your treatment, consult your doctor or nurse.

HOW SUPPLIED

8g tube.
NDC 51201-5007-1.
Keep tube tightly capped and stored at controlled room temperature.
Keep out of the reach of children.

CAUTION

Federal law prohibits dispensing without prescription.
Revised 12/87
Viranol is a registered trademark.
American Dermal Corporation
U.S.A.: Plumsteadville, PA 18949
UK: Hitchin, Herts. Made in UK.   WA4/7/2

VIRANOL®   ℞

DESCRIPTION

Viranol® is a solution for topical application containing 16.7% Salicylic Acid U.S.P., and 16.7% Lactic Acid U.S.P. in a vehicle of Flexible Collodion U.S.P.

HOW SUPPLIED

10 ml bottle with applicator, NDC 51201-5006-1 Keep bottle tightly capped and store in an upright position at controlled room temperature. Keep out of reach of Children.

Amgen Inc.
1900 OAK TERRACE LANE
THOUSAND OAKS, CA 91320

EPOGEN®   ℞
EPOETIN ALFA
For Injection

DESCRIPTION

Erythropoietin is a glycoprotein which stimulates red blood cell production. It is produced in the kidney and stimulates the division and differentiation of committed erythroid progenitors in the bone marrow. EPOGEN® is the Amgen Inc. trademark for Epoetin alfa which has been selected as the proper name for recombinant human erythropoietin. EPOGEN® (Epoetin alfa), a 165 amino acid glycoprotein manufactured by recombinant DNA technology, has the same biological effects as endogenous erythropoietin.[1] It has a molecular weight of 30,400 daltons and is produced by mammalian cells into which the human erythropoietin gene has been introduced. The product contains the identical amino acid sequence of isolated natural erythropoietin.
EPOGEN® is formulated as a sterile, colorless, preservative-free liquid for intravenous or subcutaneous administration. Each single-use vial contains 2,000, 4,000, or 10,000 units of EPOGEN® formulated in an isotonic sodium chloride/sodium citrate buffered solution (pH 6.9 ± 0.3) containing Albumin (Human) (2.5 mg), sodium citrate (5.8 mg), sodium chloride (5.8 mg), and citric acid (0.06 mg) in Water for Injection, USP. Filling and packaging operations for EPOGEN® are performed by an outside FDA-approved contractor.

CLINICAL PHARMACOLOGY

Erythropoietin is a glycoprotein which stimulates red blood cell production. Endogenous production of erythropoietin is normally regulated by the level of tissue oxygenation. Hypoxia and anemia generally increase the production of erythropoietin, which in turn stimulates erythropoiesis.[2] In normal subjects, plasma erythropoietin levels range from 0.01 to 0.03 U/mL,[2,3] and increase up to 100- to 1000-fold during hypoxia or anemia.[2,3] In contrast, in patients with chronic renal failure (CRF), production of erythropoietin is impaired, and this erythropoietin deficiency is the primary cause of their anemia.[3,4]

Chronic renal failure is the clinical situation in which there is a progressive and usually irreversible decline in kidney function. Such patients may manifest the sequelae of renal dysfunction, including anemia, but do not necessarily require regular dialysis. Patients with end-stage renal disease (ESRD) are those patients with CRF who require regular dialysis or kidney transplantation for survival.
EPOGEN® has been shown to stimulate erythropoiesis in anemic patients with CRF, including both patients on dialysis and those who do not require regular dialysis.[4–13] The first evidence of a response to the three times weekly (T.I.W.) administration of EPOGEN® is an increase in the reticulocyte count within 10 days, followed by increases in the red cell count, hemoglobin, and hematocrit, usually within 2–6 weeks.[4,5] Because of the length of time required for erythropoiesis—several days for erythroid progenitors to mature and be released into the circulation—a clinically significant increase in hematocrit is usually not observed in less than 2 weeks and may require up to 6 weeks in some patients. Once the hematocrit reaches the target range (30–33%), that level can be sustained by EPOGEN® (Epoetin alfa) therapy in the absence of iron deficiency and concurrent illnesses.
The rate of hematocrit increase varies between patients and is dependent upon the dose of EPOGEN®, within a therapeutic range of approximately 50–300 U/kg T.I.W.;[4] a greater biologic response is not observed at doses exceeding 300 U/kg T.I.W.[6] Other factors affecting the rate and extent of response include availability of iron stores, the baseline hematocrit, and the presence of concurrent medical problems.

PHARMACOKINETICS

Intravenously administered EPOGEN® is eliminated at a rate consistent with first order kinetics with a circulating half-life ranging from approximately 4 to 13 hours in patients with CRF. Within the therapeutic dose range, detectable levels of plasma erythropoietin are maintained for at least 24 hours.[7] After subcutaneous administration of EPOGEN® to patients with CRF, peak serum levels are achieved within 5–24 hours after administration and decline slowly thereafter. There is no apparent difference in half-life between patients not on dialysis whose serum creatinine levels were greater than 3, and patients maintained on dialysis.

INDICATIONS AND USAGE

EPOGEN® is indicated in the treatment of anemia associated with chronic renal failure, including patients on dialysis (end-stage renal disease) and patients not on dialysis. EPOGEN® is indicated to elevate or maintain the red blood cell level (as manifested by the hematocrit or hemoglobin determinations) and to decrease the need for transfusions in these patients.
EPOGEN® is not intended for patients who require immediate correction of severe anemia.
EPOGEN® may obviate the need for maintenance transfusions but is not a substitute for emergency transfusion.
Prior to initiation of therapy, the patient's iron stores, including transferrin saturation and serum ferritin, should be evaluated. Transferrin saturation should be at least 20% and ferritin at least 100 ng/mL. Blood pressure should be adequately controlled prior to initiation of EPOGEN® therapy, and must be closely monitored and controlled during therapy. Non-dialysis patients with symptomatic anemia considered for therapy should have a hematocrit less than 30%. All patients on EPOGEN® therapy should be regularly monitored (see "Laboratory Monitoring" and "Precautions").
EPOGEN® should be administered under the guidance of a qualified physician (see "Dosage and Administration").

CLINICAL EXPERIENCE: RESPONSE TO EPOGEN®

Response to EPOGEN® was consistent across all studies. In the presence of adequate iron stores (see "Pre-Therapy Iron Evaluation"), the time to reach the target hematocrit is a function of the baseline hematocrit and the rate of hematocrit rise.
The rate of increase in hematocrit is dependent upon the dose of EPOGEN® administered and individual patient variation. In clinical trials at starting doses of 50–150 U/kg T.I.W., patients responded with an average rate of hematocrit rise of:

HEMATOCRIT INCREASE		
Starting Dose (T.I.W., IV)	Hematocrit Points/Day	Hematocrit Points/2 Weeks
50 U/kg	0.11	1.5
100 U/kg	0.18	2.5
150 U/kg	0.25	3.5

Over this dose range, approximately 95% of all patients responded with a clinically significant increase in hematocrit, and by the end of approximately two months of therapy virtually all patients were transfusion-independent. Once the target hematocrit was achieved, the maintenance dose was individualized for each patient.

Clinical Experience in Patients on Dialysis

Thirteen clinical studies were conducted, involving intravenous administration to a total of 1010 anemic patients on dialysis for 986 patient-years of EPOGEN® (Epoetin alfa) therapy. In the three largest of these clinical trials, the median maintenance dose necessary to maintain the hematocrit between 30–36% was approximately 75 U/kg (T.I.W.). In the U.S. multicenter Phase III study, approximately 65% of the patients required doses of 100 U/kg T.I.W., or less, to maintain their hematocrit at approximately 35%. Almost 10% of patients required a dose of 25 U/kg, or less, and approximately 10% required a dose of more than 200 U/kg T.I.W. to maintain their hematocrit at this level.

Clinical Experience in Patients with CRF Not Requiring Dialysis

Four clinical trials were conducted in patients with CRF not on dialysis involving 181 EPOGEN®-treated patients for approximately 67 patient-years of experience. These patients responded to EPOGEN® therapy in a manner similar to that observed in patients on dialysis. Patients with CRF not on dialysis demonstrated a dose-dependent and sustained increase in hematocrit when EPOGEN® was administered by either an intravenous (IV) or subcutaneous (SC) route, with similar rates of rise of hematocrit when EPOGEN® was administered by either route. Moreover, EPOGEN® doses of 75–150 U/kg per week have been shown to maintain hematocrits of 36–38% for up to six months.

CONTRAINDICATIONS

EPOGEN® is contraindicated in patients with:
1) Uncontrolled hypertension
2) Known hypersensitivity to mammalian cell-derived products
3) Known hypersensitivity to Albumin (Human).

WARNINGS

Hypertension: Patients with uncontrolled hypertension should not be treated with EPOGEN®; blood pressure should be controlled adequately before initiation of therapy. Blood pressure may rise during EPOGEN® therapy, often during the early phase of treatment when the hematocrit is increasing.
For patients who respond to EPOGEN® with a rapid increase in hematocrit (e.g., more than 4 points in any two-week period), the dose of EPOGEN® should be reduced because of the possible association of excessive rate of rise of hematocrit with an exacerbation of hypertension.
Seizures: Seizures have occurred in patients with CRF participating in EPOGEN® clinical trials.
In patients on dialysis, there was a higher incidence of seizures during the first 90 days of therapy (occurring in approximately 2.5% of patients), as compared with later timepoints.
Given the potential for an increased risk of seizures during the first 90 days of therapy, blood pressure and the presence of premonitory neurologic symptoms should be monitored closely. Patients should be cautioned to avoid potentially hazardous activities such as driving or operating heavy machinery during this period.
Thrombotic Events: During hemodialysis, patients treated with EPOGEN® (Epoetin alfa) may require increased anticoagulation with heparin to prevent clotting of the artificial kidney. Clotting of the vascular access (A-V shunt) has occurred at an annualized rate of about 0.25 events per patient-year on EPOGEN® therapy.
Overall, for patients with CRF (whether on dialysis or not), other thrombotic events (e.g., myocardial infarction, cerebrovascular accident, transient ischemic attack) have occurred at an annualized rate of less than 0.04 events per patient-year of EPOGEN® therapy. Patients with pre-existing vascular disease should be monitored closely.

PRECAUTIONS

General: The parenteral administration of any biologic product should be attended by appropriate precautions in case allergic or other untoward reactions occur (see "Contraindications"). While transient rashes have occasionally been observed concurrently with EPOGEN® therapy, no serious allergic or anaphylactic reactions have been reported.
The safety and efficacy of EPOGEN® therapy have not been established in patients with a known history of a seizure disorder or underlying hematologic disease (e.g., sickle cell anemia, myelodysplastic syndromes, or hypercoagulable disorders).
In some female patients, menses have resumed following EPOGEN® therapy; the possibility of potential pregnancy should be discussed and the need for contraception evaluated.
Patients with CRF Not Requiring Dialysis: Blood pressure and hematocrit should be monitored no less frequently than for patients maintained on dialysis. Renal function and fluid and electrolyte balance should be closely monitored, as an improved sense of well-being may obscure the need to initiate dialysis in some patients.
Hematology: In order to avoid reaching the target hematocrit too rapidly, or exceeding the target range (hematocrit of 30–33%), the guidelines for dose and frequency of dose ad-

justments (see "Dosage and Administration") should be followed.

For patients who respond to EPOGEN® with a rapid increase in hematocrit (e.g., more than 4 points in any two-week period), the dose of EPOGEN® should be reduced because of the possible association of excessive rate of rise of hematocrit with an exacerbation of hypertension.

The elevated bleeding time characteristic of CRF decreases toward normal after correction of anemia in EPOGEN®-treated patients. Reduction of bleeding time also occurs after correction of anemia by transfusion.

Sufficient time should be allowed to determine a patient's responsiveness to a dosage of EPOGEN® before adjusting the dose. Because of the time required for erythropoiesis and the red cell half-life, an interval of 2–6 weeks may occur between the time of a dose adjustment (initiation, increase, decrease, or discontinuation) and a significant change in hematocrit.

Exacerbation of porphyria has been observed rarely in patients with CRF treated with EPOGEN®. However, EPOGEN® has not caused urinary excretion of porphyrin metabolites in normal volunteers, even in the presence of a rapid erythropoietic response. Nevertheless, EPOGEN® should be used with caution in patients with known porphyria.

In pre-clinical studies in dogs and rats, but not in monkeys, EPOGEN® therapy was associated with subclinical bone marrow fibrosis. Bone marrow fibrosis is a known complication of CRF in humans and may be related to secondary hyperparathyroidism or unknown factors. The incidence of bone marrow fibrosis was not increased in a study of patients on dialysis who were treated with EPOGEN® (Epoetin alfa) for 12–19 months, compared to the incidence of bone marrow fibrosis in a matched group of patients who had not been treated with EPOGEN®.

Delayed or Diminished Response: If the patient fails to respond or to maintain a response, the following etiologies should be considered and evaluated:

1) Iron deficiency: functional iron deficiency may develop with normal ferritin levels but low transferrin saturation (less than 20%), presumably due to the inability to mobilize iron stores rapidly enough to support increased erythropoiesis. Virtually all patients will eventually require supplemental iron therapy.
2) Underlying infectious, inflammatory, or malignant processes.
3) Occult blood loss.
4) Underlying hematoligic diseases (i.e., thalassemia, refractory anemia, or other myelodysplastic disorders).
5) Vitamin deficiencies: folic acid or vitamin B_{12}.
6) Hemolysis.
7) Aluminum intoxication.
8) Osteitis fibrosa cystica.

Laboratory Monitoring: The hematocrit should be determined twice a week until it has stabilized in the target range and the maintenance dose has been established. After any dose adjustment, the hematocrit should also be determined twice weekly for at least 2–6 weeks until it has been determined that the hematocrit has stabilized in response to the dose change. The hematocrit should then be monitored at regular intervals.

A complete blood count with differential and platelet count should be performed regularly. During clinical trials, modest increases were seen in platelets and white blood cell counts. While these changes were statistically significant, they were not clinically significant and the values remained within normal ranges.

In patients with CRF, serum chemistry values [including blood urea nitrogen (BUN), uric acid, creatinine, phosphorus, and potassium] should be monitored regularly. During clinical trials in patients on dialysis, modest increases were seen in BUN, creatinine, phosphorus, and potassium. In some patients with CRF not on dialysis treated with EPOGEN®, modest increases in serum uric acid and phosphorus were observed. While changes were statistically significant, the values remained within the ranges normally seen in patients with CRF.

Iron Evaluation: Prior to and during EPOGEN® (Epoetin alfa) therapy, the patient's iron stores, including transferrin saturation (serum iron divided by iron binding capacity) and serum ferritin, should be evaluated. Transferrin saturation should be at least 20%, and ferritin should be at least 100 ng/mL. Supplemental iron may be required to increase and maintain transferrin saturation to levels that will adequately support EPOGEN®-stimulated erythropoiesis.

Hypertension: Patients with uncontrolled hypertension should not be treated with EPOGEN®; blood pressure should be adequately controlled before initiation of therapy. Blood pressure may rise and episodes of hypertension may increase during EPOGEN® therapy in all CRF patients, whether or not they require dialysis, often during the early phase of treatment when the hematocrit is increasing. To prevent hypertension and its sequelae, particular care needs to be taken in patients treated with EPOGEN® to monitor and aggressively control blood pressure. During the period when the hematocrit is increasing, approximately 25% of

patients on dialysis may require initiation of, or increases in, antihypertensive therapy. Patients should be advised as to the importance of compliance with antihypertensive therapy and dietary restrictions. For patients who respond to EPOGEN® with a rapid increase in hematocrit (e.g., more than 4 points in any two-week period), the dose of EPOGEN® should be reduced because of the possible association of excessive rate of rise of hematocrit with an exacerbation of hypertension. If blood pressure is difficult to control, the dose of EPOGEN® should be reduced; if clinically indicated, EPOGEN® may be withheld until blood pressure control is re-established.

Seizures: Seizures have occurred in patients with CRF participating in EPOGEN® clinical trials. In patients on dialysis, there was a higher incidence of seizures during the first 90 days of therapy (occurring in approximately 2.5% of patients), as compared with later timepoints.

Given the potential for an increased risk of seizures during the first 90 days of therapy, blood pressure and the presence of premonitory neurologic symptoms should be monitored closely. Patients should be cautioned to avoid potentially hazardous activities such as driving or operating heavy machinery during this period.

Thrombotic Events: During hemodialysis, patients treated with EPOGEN® may require increased anticoagulation with heparin to prevent clotting of the artificial kidney. Clotting of the vascular access has occurred at an annualized rate of about 0.25 events per patient-year on EPOGEN® therapy.

A relationship has not been established with statistical certainty between a rise in hematocrit and the rate of thrombotic events [including thrombosis of vascular access (A-V shunt)] in EPOGEN®-treated patients. Overall, in patients with CRF (whether on dialysis or not), other thrombotic events (e.g., myocardial infarction, cerebrovascular accident, transient ischemic attack) have occurred at an annualized rate of less than 0.04 events per patient-year of EPOGEN® therapy. Patients with pre-existing vascular disease should be monitored closely.

Diet: As the hematocrit increases and patients experience an improved sense of well-being and quality of life, the importance of compliance with dietary and dialysis prescriptions should be reinforced. In particular, hyperkalemia is not uncommon in patients with CRF. In U.S. studies in patients on dialysis, hyperkalemia has occurred at an annualized rate of approximately 0.11 episodes per patient-year of EPOGEN® therapy, often in association with poor compliance to medication, dietary and/or dialysis prescriptions.

Dialysis Management: Therapy with EPOGEN® (Epoetin alfa) results in an increase in hematocrit and a decrease in plasma volume which could affect dialysis efficiency. In studies to date, the resulting increase in hematocrit did not appear to adversely affect dialyzer function[9,10] or the efficiency of high flux hemodialysis.[11] During hemodialysis, patients treated with EPOGEN® may require increased anticoagulation with heparin to prevent clotting of the artificial kidney. Patients who are marginally dialyzed may require adjustments in their dialysis prescription. As with all patients on dialysis, the serum chemistry values [including blood urea nitrogen (BUN), creatinine, phosphorus, and potassium] in EPOGEN®-treated patients should be monitored regularly to assure the adequacy of the dialysis prescription.

Renal Function

In patients with CRF not on dialysis, renal function and fluid and electrolyte balance should be closely monitored, as an improved sense of well-being may obscure the need to initiate dialysis in some patients. In patients with CRF not on dialysis, placebo-controlled studies of progression of renal dysfunction over periods of greater than one year have not been completed. In shorter-term trials in patients with CRF not on dialysis, changes in creatinine and creatinine clear-

ance were not significantly different in patients treated with EPOGEN® (Epoetin alfa), compared with placebo-treated patients. Analysis of the slope of 1/serum creatinine vs. time plots in these patients indicates no significant change in the slope after the initiation of EPOGEN® therapy.

Drug Interaction: No evidence of interaction of EPOGEN® with other drugs was observed in the course of clinical trials.

Carcinogenesis, Mutagenesis, and Impairment of Fertility: Carcinogenic potential of EPOGEN® has not been evaluated. EPOGEN® does not induce bacterial gene mutation (Ames Test), chromosomal aberrations in mammalian cells, micronuclei in mice, or gene mutation at the HGPRT locus. In male and female rats treated intravenously with EPOGEN®, there was a trend for slightly increased fetal wastage at doses of 100 and 500 U/kg; this trend was not statistically significant.

Pregnancy Category C: EPOGEN® has been shown to have adverse effects in rats when given in doses five times the human dose. There are no adequate and well-controlled studies in pregnant women. EPOGEN® should be used during pregnancy only if potential benefit justifies the potential risk to the fetus.

In studies in female rats, there were decreases in body weight gain, delays in appearance of abdominal hair, delayed eyelid opening, delayed ossification, and decreases in the number of caudal vertebrae in the F1 fetuses of the 500 U/kg group. In female rats treated intravenously, there was a trend for slightly increased fetal wastage at doses of 100 and 500 U/kg; this trend was not statistically significant. EPOGEN® has not shown any adverse effect at doses as high as 500 U/kg in pregnant rabbits (from day 6 to 18 of gestation).

Nursing Mothers: Postnatal observations of the live offspring (F1 generation) of female rats treated with EPOGEN® during gestation and lactation revealed no effect of EPOGEN® at doses of up to 500 U/kg. There were, however, decreases in body weight gain, delays in appearance of abdominal hair, eyelid opening, and decreases in the number of caudal vertebrae in the F1 fetuses of the 500 U/kg group. There were no EPOGEN®-related effects on the F2 generation fetuses.

It is not known whether EPOGEN® is excreted in human milk. Because many drugs are excreted in human milk, caution should be exercised when EPOGEN® is administered to a nursing woman.

Pediatric Use: The safety and effectiveness of EPOGEN® in children have not been established.

ADVERSE REACTIONS

Studies analyzed to date indicate that EPOGEN® (Epoetin alfa) is generally well tolerated. The adverse events reported are frequent sequelae of CRF and are not necessarily attributable to EPOGEN® therapy. In double-blind, placebo-controlled studies involving over 300 patients with CRF, the events reported in greater than 5% of EPOGEN®-treated patients during the blinded phase were:

[See table above].

In the U.S. EPOGEN® studies in patients on dialysis (over 567 patients) the incidence (number of events per patient-year) of the most frequently reported adverse events were: hypertension (0.75), headache (0.40), tachycardia (0.31), nausea/vomiting (0.26), clotted vascular access (0.25), shortness of breath (0.14), hyperkalemia (0.11), and diarrhea (0.11). Other reported events occurred at a rate of less than 0.10 events per patient per year.

Events reported to have occurred within several hours of administration of EPOGEN® were rare, mild and transient, and included flu-like symptoms such as arthralgias and myalgias.

Event	Percent of Patients Reporting Event	
	EPOGEN®-Treated Patients (n = 200)	Placebo-Treated Patients (n = 135)
Hypertension	24.0%	18.5%
Headache	16.0%	11.9%
Arthralgias	11.0%	5.9%
Nausea	10.5%	8.9%
Edema	9.0%	10.4%
Fatigue	9.0%	14.1%
Diarrhea	8.5%	5.9%
Vomiting	8.0%	5.2%
Chest Pain	7.0%	8.8%
Skin Reaction (Administration Site)	7.0%	11.9%
Asthenia	7.0%	11.9%
Dizziness	7.0%	12.6%
Clotted Access	6.8%	2.3%

Significant adverse events of concern in patients with CRF treated in double-blinded, placebo-controlled trials occurred in the following percent of patients during the blinded phase of the studies:

Event	EPOGEN®-Treated	Placebo-Treated
Seizure	1.1%	1.1%
CVA/TIA	0.4%	0.6%
MI	0.4%	1.1%
Death	0	1.7%

Continued on next page

Amgen—Cont.

In all studies analyzed to date, EPOGEN® administration was generally well tolerated, irrespective of the route of administration.

Allergic Reactions: There have been no reports of serious allergic reactions or anaphylaxis associated with EPOGEN® administration. Skin rashes and urticaria have been observed rarely and when reported have been mild and transient in nature. There has been no evidence for development of antibodies to erythropoietin in patients tested to date, including those receiving intravenous EPOGEN® for over two years. Nevertheless, if an anaphylactoid reaction occurs, EPOGEN® should be immediately discontinued and appropriate therapy initiated.

Seizures: The relationship, if any, of EPOGEN® therapy to seizures is uncertain. The baseline incidence of seizures in the untreated dialysis population is difficult to determine; it appears to be in the range of 5–10 per patient-year.[14–16] There have been 47 seizures in 1010 patients on dialysis treated with EPOGEN® with an exposure of 986 patient-years for a rate of approximately 0.048 events per patient-year. However, there appeared to be a higher rate of seizures during the first 90 days of therapy (occurring in approximately 2.5% of patients), when compared to subsequent 90-day time periods. While the relationship between seizures and the rate of rise of hematocrit is uncertain, it is recommended that the dose of EPOGEN® be decreased if the hematocrit increase exceeds 4 points in any two-week period.

Hypertension: Up to 80% of patients with CRF have a history of hypertension.[17] Blood pressure may rise during EPOGEN® therapy in CRF patients whether or not maintained on dialysis; during the early phase of treatment when hematocrit is increasing, approximately 25% of patients on dialysis may require initiation or increases in antihypertensive therapy. Hypertensive encephalopathy and seizures have been observed in patients with CRF treated with EPOGEN® (Epoetin alfa). Increases in blood pressure may be associated with the rate of increase in hematocrit. It is recommended that the dose of EPOGEN® be decreased if the hematocrit increase exceeds 4 points in any two-week period.

Increases in blood pressure have been reported in clinical trials, often during the first 90 days of therapy. When data from all patients in the U.S. Phase III multicenter trial were analyzed, there was an apparent trend of more reports of hypertensive adverse events in patients on dialysis with a faster rate of rise of hematocrit (greater than 4 hematocrit points in any two-week period). However, in a double-blind, placebo-controlled trial, hypertensive adverse events were not reported at an increased rate in the EPOGEN®-treated group (150 U/kg T.I.W.) relative to the placebo group. There do not appear to be any direct pressor effects of EPOGEN®. Special care should be taken to closely monitor and control blood pressure in EPOGEN®-treated patients.

Thrombotic Events: During hemodialysis, patients treated with EPOGEN® may require increased anticoagulation with heparin to prevent clotting of the artificial kidney. Clotting of the vascular access has occurred at an annualized rate of about 0.25 events per patient-year on EPOGEN® therapy.

A relationship has not been established with statistical certainty between a rise in hematocrit and the rate of thrombotic events [including thrombosis of vascular access (A-V shunt)] in EPOGEN®-treated patients. Overall, for patients with CRF (whether on dialysis or not), other thrombotic events (e.g., myocardial infarction, cerebrovascular accident, transient ischemic attack) have occurred at an annualized rate of less than 0.04 events per patient-year of EPOGEN® therapy.

Patients with pre-existing vascular disease should be monitored closely.

OVERDOSAGE

The maximum amount of EPOGEN® (Epoetin alfa) that can be safely administered in single or multiple doses has not been determined. Doses of up to 1500 U/kg T.I.W. for three to four weeks have been administered without any direct toxic effects of EPOGEN® itself.[6]

Therapy with EPOGEN® can result in polycythemia if the hematocrit is not carefully monitored and the dose appropriately adjusted. If the target range is exceeded, EPOGEN® may be temporarily withheld until the hematocrit returns to the target range; EPOGEN® therapy may then be resumed using a lower dose (see "Dosage and Administration"). If polycythemia is of concern, phlebotomy may be indicated to decrease the hematocrit to within acceptable ranges.

DOSAGE AND ADMINISTRATION

Starting doses of EPOGEN® over the range of 50–100 U/kg three times weekly (T.I.W.) have been shown to be safe and effective in increasing hematocrit and eliminating transfusion dependency in patients with CRF (see Clinical Experience). The dose of EPOGEN® should be reduced when the hematocrit reaches the target range of 30–33% or increases by more than 4 points in any two-week period. The dosage of

EPOGEN® must be individualized to maintain the hematocrit within the target range. Dose changes should generally be in the range of 25 U/kg, T.I.W. The table below provides general therapeutic guidelines.

Starting Dose	50–100 U/kg T.I.W.; IV: Dialysis Patients; IV or SC: Non-dialysis CRF Patients.
Reduce Dose When:	1) Target range is reached, or 2) Hematocrit increases >4 points in any two-week period.
Increase Dose If:	Hematocrit does not increase by 5–6 points after 8 weeks of therapy, and hematocrit is below target range.
Maintenance Dose	Individually titrate.
Target Hematocrit Range	30–33% (max: 36%)

In patients on dialysis, EPOGEN® usually has been administered as an IV bolus T.I.W. While the administration of EPOGEN® is independent of the dialysis procedure, EPOGEN® may be administered into the venous line at the end of the dialysis procedure to obviate the need for additional venous access. In patients with CRF not on dialysis, EPOGEN® may be given either as an intravenous or subcutaneous injection.

During therapy, hematological parameters should be monitored regularly (see "Laboratory Monitoring").

Pre-Therapy Iron Evaluation: Prior to and during EPOGEN® therapy, the patient's iron stores, including transferrin saturation (serum iron divided by iron binding capacity) and serum ferritin, should be evaluated. Transferrin saturation should be at least 20%, and ferritin should be at least 100 ng/mL. Supplemental iron may be required to increase and maintain transferrin saturation to levels that will adequately support EPOGEN®-stimulated erythropoiesis.

Dose Adjustment

- When the hematocrit reaches 30–33%, the dosage should be decreased by approximately 25 U/kg T.I.W., to avoid exceeding the target range. Once the hematocrit is within the target range, the maintenance dose must be individualized for each patient (see "Maintenance Dose").
- At any time, if the hematocrit increases by more than 4 points in a two-week period, the dose should be immediately decreased. After the dose reduction, the hematocrit should be monitored twice weekly for 2–6 weeks, and further dose adjustments should be made as outlined in "Maintenance Dose."
- As the hematocrit approaches, or if it exceeds 36%, EPOGEN® should be temporarily withheld until the hematocrit decreases to the target range of 30–33%; the dose should be reduced by approximately 25 U/kg T.I.W. upon re-initiation of therapy.
- If a hematocrit increase of 5–6 points is not achieved after an eight-week period and iron stores are adequate (see "Delayed or Diminished Response"), the dose of EPOGEN® may be increased in increments of 25 U/kg T.I.W. Further increases of 25 U/kg T.I.W. may be made at 4–6 week intervals until the desired response is attained.

Maintenance Dose

The maintenance dose must be individualized for each patient. As the hematocrit approaches, or if it exceeds 36%, EPOGEN® should be temporarily withheld until the hematocrit is 33% or less. Upon re-initiation of therapy, the dose should be reduced by approximately 25 U/kg T.I.W., or doses omitted, and an appropriate time interval (i.e., 2–6 weeks) allowed for stabilization of response.

If the hematocrit remains below, or falls below the target range, iron stores should be re-evaluated. If the transferrin saturation is less than 20%, supplemental iron should be administered. If the transferrin saturation is greater than 20%, the dose of EPOGEN® may be increased by 25 U/kg T.I.W. Such dose increases should not be made more frequently than once a month, unless clinically indicated, as the response time of the hematocrit to a dose increase can be 2–6 weeks. Hematocrit should be measured twice weekly for 2–6 weeks following dose increases. In the U.S. Phase III multicenter trial in patients on hemodialysis, the median maintenance dose was 75 U/kg T.I.W., with approximately 65% of the patients requiring doses of 100 U/kg T.I.W., or less, to maintain their hematocrit within the range of 32–38% (maintenance doses ranged from 12.5 to 525 U/kg T.I.W.). Almost 10% of the patients required a dose of 25 U/kg, or less, and approximately 10% of the patients required more than 200 U/kg T.I.W. to maintain their hematocrit in this range.

In patients with CRF not on dialysis, the maintenance dose must also be individualized. EPOGEN® (Epoetin alfa) doses of 75–150 U/kg per week have been shown to maintain hematocrits of 36–38% for up to six months.

Delayed or Diminished Response

Over 95% of patients with CRF responded with clinically significant increases in hematocrit, and virtually all patients were transfusion-independent within approximately two months of initiation of EPOGEN® therapy.

If a patient fails to respond or maintain a response, other etiologies should be considered and evaluated as clinically

indicated. See "Precautions" section for discussion of delayed or diminished response.

PREPARATION AND ADMINISTRATION OF EPOGEN®

1. DO NOT SHAKE. Shaking may denature the glycoprotein, rendering it biologically inactive.
2. Parenteral drug products should be inspected visually for particulate matter and discoloration prior to administration. Do not use any vials exhibiting particulate matter or discoloration.
3. Using aseptic techniques, attach a sterile needle to a sterile syringe. Remove the flip top from the vial containing EPOGEN®, and wipe the septum with a disinfectant. Insert the needle into the vial, and withdraw into the syringe an appropriate volume of solution.
4. Use only one dose per vial; do not re-enter the vial. Discard unused portions. Contains no preservative.
5. Do not administer in conjunction with other drug solutions.

HOW SUPPLIED

EPOGEN® is available in vials containing 2,000 (NDC 5551-3126-10), 4,000 (NDC 5551-3148-10), or 10,000 (NDC 5551-3144-10) units of Epoetin alfa in 1.0 mL of a sterile, preservative-free solution. Each dosage form is supplied in boxes containing 10 single-use vials.

STORAGE

Store at 2° to 8°C (36° to 46°F). Do not freeze or shake.

REFERENCES

1. Egrie JC, Strickland TW, Lane J, et al., (1986). "Characterization and Biological Effects of Recombinant Human Erythropoietin." *Immunobiol.* 72: 213–224.
2. Graber SE, and Krantz SB, (1978). "Erythropoietin and the Control of Red Cell Production." *Ann. Rev. Med.* 29: 51–66.
3. Eschbach JW, and Adamson JW, (1985). "Anemia of End-Stage Renal Disease (ESRD)." *Kidney Intl.* 28: 1–5.
4. Eschbach JW, Egrie JC, Downing MR, Browne JK, and Adamson JW, (1987). "Correction of the Anemia of End-Stage Renal Disease with Recombinant Human Erythropoietin." *NEJM* 316: 73–78.
5. Eschbach JW, Adamson JW, and Cooperative Multicenter r-HuEPO Trial Group, (1988). "Correction of the Anemia of Hemodialysis (HD) Patients with Recombinant Human Erythropoietin (r-HuEPO): Results of a Multicenter Study." *Kidney Intl.* 33: 189.
6. Eschbach JW, Egrie JC, Downing MR, Browne JK, Adamson JW, (1989). "The Use of Recombinant Human Erythropoietin (r-HuEPO): Effect in End-Stage Renal Disease (ESRD)," *Prevention of Chronic Uremia*, (Friedman, Beyer, DeSanto, Giordano, eds.), Field and Wood Inc., Philadelphia, PA, pp 148–155.
7. Egrie JC, Eschbach JW, McGuire T, and Adamson JW, (1988). "Pharmacokinetics of Recombinant Human Erythropoietin (r-HuEPO) Administered to Hemodialysis (HD) Patients." *Kidney Intl.* 33: 262.
8. Lundin AP, Delano BG, Stein R, Quinn RM, and Friedman EA, (1988). "Recombinant Human Erythropoietin (r-HuEPO) Treatment Enhances Exercise Tolerance in Hemodialysis Patients." *Kidney Intl.* 33: 200.
9. Paganini E, Garcia J, Ellis P, Bodnar D, and Magnussen M, (1988). "Clinical Sequelae of Correction of Anemia with Recombinant Human Erythropoietin (r-HuEPO); Urea Kinetics, Dialyzer Function and Reuse." *Am. J. Kid. Dis.* 11: 16.
10. Delano BG, Lundin AP, Golansky R, Quinn RM, Rao TKS, and Friedman EA, (1988). "Dialyzer Urea and Creatinine Clearances Not Significantly Changed in r-HuEPO Treated Maintenance Hemodialysis (MD) Patients." *Kidney Intl.* 33: 219.
11. Stivelman J, Van Wyck D, and Ogden D, (1988). "Use of Recombinant Erythropoietin (r-HuEPO) with High Flux Dialysis (HFD) Does Not Worsen Azotemia or Shorten Access Survival." *Kidney Intl.* 33: 239.
12. Lim VS, DeGowin RL, Zavala D, Kirchner PT, Abels R, Perry P, and Fangman J, (1989). "Recombinant Human Erythropoietin Treatment in Pre-Dialysis Patients: A Double-Blind Placebo-Controlled Trial." *Ann. Int. Med.* 110: 108–114.
13. Stone WJ, Graber SE, Krantz SB, et al., (1988). "Treatment of the Anemia of Pre-Dialysis Patients with Recombinant Human Erythropoietin: A Randomized, Placebo-Controlled Trial." *Am. J. Med. Sci.* 296: 171–179.
14. Raskin NH, and Fishman RA, (1976). "Neurologic Disorders in Renal Failure (First of Two Parts)." *NEJM* 294: 143–148.
15. Raskin NH, and Fishman RA, (1976). "Neurologic Disorders in Renal Failure (Second of Two Parts)." *NEJM* 294: 204–210.
16. Messing RO, and Simon RP, (1986). "Seizures as a Manifestation of Systemic Disease." *Neurologic Clinics* 4: 563–584.
17. Kerr DN, (1979), "Chronic Renal Failure," *Cecil Textbook of Medicine*, (Beeson PB, McDermott W, Wyng-

aarden JB, eds.), W.B. Saunders, Philadelphia, PA, pp 1351–1367.
Manufactured by:
AMGEN Inc.
1900 Oak Terrace Lane
Thousand Oaks, CA 91320   Issue Date: 06/15/89
       0126G201
Shown in Product Identification Section, page 405

Anaquest
2005 WEST BELTLINE HIGHWAY
MADISON WI 53713-2318

ENLON®   ℞
[ĕn'lon]
(edrophonium chloride injection, USP)

DESCRIPTION
ENLON (edrophonium chloride injection, USP) is a rapid acting cholinergic (cholinesterase inhibitor). Chemically edrophonium chloride is ethyl (m-hydroxyphenyl) dimethylammonium chloride and its structural formula is:

ENLON contains in each mL of sterile solution:
10 mg edrophonium chloride compounded with 0.45% phenol and 0.2% sodium sulfite as preservative, buffered with sodium citrate and citric acid. Its pH is adjusted to approximately 5.4.

CLINICAL PHARMACOLOGY
ENLON (edrophonium chloride injection, USP) activates neuromuscular transmission primarily by inhibiting or inactivating acetylcholinesterase. By inactivating the acetylcholinesterase enzyme, acetylcholine is not hydrolyzed by acetylcholinesterase and is thereby allowed to accumulate. The accumulation of acetylcholine at the sites of cholinergic transmission facilitates transmission of impulses across the myoneural junction.

INDICATIONS AND USAGE
ENLON (edrophonium chloride injection, USP) is recommended as a reversal agent or antagonist of nondepolarizing muscle relaxants such as tubocurarine, metocurine, atracurium, vecuronium, or pancuronium. It is not effective against depolarizing relaxants such as succinylcholine and decamethonium. It is also useful if used adjunctively in the treatment of respiratory depression caused by curare overdosage.
ENLON is recommended for use in the differential diagnosis of myasthenia gravis. It may also be used as an adjunct to evaluate treatment requirements of the disease, and for evaluating emergency treatment in myasthenic crisis. It is not recommended for maintenance therapy in myasthenia gravis.

CONTRAINDICATIONS
ENLON (edrophonium chloride injection, USP) is not to be used in patients with known hypersensitivity to anticholinesterase agents, or in patients having urinary obstructions of mechanical type.

WARNINGS
Contains sodium sulfite, a sulfite that may cause allergic-type reactions including anaphylactic symptoms and life-threatening or less severe asthmatic episodes in certain susceptible people. The overall prevalence of sulfite sensitivity in the general population is unknown and probably low. Sulfite sensitivity is seen more frequently in asthmatic than in nonasthmatic people.
It is recommended that 1 mg atropine sulfate should be made available for immediate use, to counteract any severe cholinergic reaction. ENLON (edrophonium chloride injection, USP) should be used with caution in patients with bronchial asthma or cardiac dysrhythmias. Transient bradycardia may occur and be relieved by atropine sulfate. Isolated instances of cardiac and respiratory arrest following administration of edrophonium chloride have been reported. It is postulated that these are vagotonic effects.

PRECAUTIONS
General: As with any antagonist of nondepolarizing muscle relaxants, adequate recovery of voluntary respiration and neuromuscular transmission must be obtained prior to discontinuation of respiratory assistance. Should a patient develop "anticholinesterase insensitivity" for brief or prolonged periods, the patient should be carefully monitored and the dosage of anticholinesterase drugs reduced or withheld until the patient again becomes sensitive to them.
Drug Interactions: The drug should not be administered prior to the administration of any nondepolarizing muscle relaxants. The drug should be administered with caution to patients with symptoms of myasthenic weakness who are also on anticholinesterase drugs. Anticholinesterase overdosage (cholinergic crisis) symptoms may mimic underdosage (myasthenic weakness) so the use of this drug may worsen the condition of these patients (see OVERDOSAGE section for treatment).
Pregnancy Category C: It is not known whether ENLON (edrophonium chloride injection, USP) can cause fetal harm when administered to a pregnant woman or can affect reproduction capacity, since there have been no adequate and well controlled studies in humans.
Labor and Delivery: The effect of ENLON on the mother and fetus, on the duration of labor or delivery, on the possibility that forceps delivery or other intervention or resuscitation of the newborn will be necessary is not known. The effect of the drug on the later growth, development and functional maturation of the child is also unknown.
Nursing Mothers: The safety of ENLON during lactation in humans has not been established.

ADVERSE REACTIONS
A patient in myasthenic crisis, being treated with ENLON (edrophonium chloride injection, USP) should be observed for bradycardia or cardiac standstill and cholinergic reactions if an overdosage is given. Reactions common to anticholinesterase agents such as edrophonium chloride are:
Cardiovascular: arrhythmias (especially bradycardia), fall in output leading to hypotension;
Respiratory: increased tracheobronchial secretions, laryngospasm, bronchiolar constriction and respiratory muscle paralysis;
Neurologic: convulsion, dysarthria, dysphonia, and dysphagia;
Gastrointestinal: nausea, vomiting, increased peristalsis, increased gastric and intestinal secretions, diarrhea, abdominal cramps;
Musculoskeletal: weakness and fasciculations;
Miscellaneous: increased urinary frequency, diaphoresis, increased lacrimation, pupillary constriction, diplopia, and conjunctival hyperemia.

OVERDOSAGE
Muscarine-like symptoms (nausea, vomiting, diarrhea, sweating, increased bronchial and salivary secretions and bradycardia) may appear with overdosage (cholinergic crisis) of ENLON (edrophonium chloride injection, USP) but may be managed by the use of atropine. Obstruction of the airway by bronchial secretions can arise and may be managed with suction (especially if tracheostomy has been performed) and by the use of atropine. Signs of atropine overdosage such as dry mouth, flush and tachycardia should be avoided as tenacious secretions and bronchial plugs may form. Should edrophonium chloride overdosage occur:
1. Maintain respiratory exchange.
2. Monitor cardiac function.
Appropriate measures should be taken if convulsions or shock are present.

DOSAGE AND ADMINISTRATION
The recommended adult intravenous injection for antagonism of neuromuscular block:
Administer 1 mL (10 mg) slowly within a period of 30 to 45 seconds, the dosage may be repeated to a maximum total dose of 4 mL (40 mg). Its onset of action is manifest within 30 to 60 seconds after injection. Response should be monitored carefully and assisted ventilation should always be employed. When given to counteract muscle relaxant overdosage, the dose effect on respiration should be observed prior to repeat dosages and assisted ventilation should be employed.
ENLON (edrophonium chloride injection, USP) Test in Differential Diagnosis of Myasthenia Gravis:
Adults:
Intravenous Dosage: Prepare a tuberculin syringe with 1 mL (10 mg) of ENLON and an intravenous needle; intravenously inject 0.2 mL (2 mg) within 15 to 30 seconds. The needle should be left in situ. If a cholinergic reaction (muscarinic side effects, skeletal muscle fasciculations and increased muscle weakness) occurs, discontinue test and intravenously administer 0.4 mg to 0.5 mg atropine sulfate. Inject the remaining 0.8 mL (8 mg) only if no reaction occurs after 45 seconds. The test may be repeated after one-half hour.
Intramuscular Dosage: Intramuscularly inject 1 mL (10 mg) of ENLON. If hyperreactivity (cholinergic reaction) is demonstrated, retest the patient after one-half hour with another intramuscular injection of 0.2 mL (2 mg) ENLON. This will eliminate the possibility of false-negative reactions.
Children:
Intravenous dose in children weighing up to 75 pounds: Intravenously inject 0.1 mL (1 mg) ENLON. If there is no response within 45 seconds, incremental doses of 0.1 mg (1 mg) given every 30 to 45 seconds may be administered to a maximum total dose of 0.5 mL (5 mg). The recommended dose in infants is 0.05 mL (0.5 mg).
Intravenous dose in children weighing above 75 pounds: Intravenously inject 0.2 mL (2 mg) ENLON. If there is no response within 45 seconds, incremental doses of 0.1 mL (1 mg) given every 30 to 45 seconds may be administered to a maximum total dose of 1 mL (10 mg).
Intramuscular Dose: Intramuscularly inject 0.2 mL (2 mg) ENLON in children weighing up to 75 pounds; above this weight, the dose is 0.5 mL (5 mg). All signs of hyperreactivity (cholinergic reaction) noted in the intravenous test will be demonstrated in the intramuscular test; however, there is a two to ten minute delay before reaction.
ENLON (edrophonium chloride injection, USP) Test to Evaluate Treatment Requirements in Myasthenia Gravis: The test dose of ENLON should follow one hour after oral intake of the drug being used to treat the disease. The recommended dose is 0.1 mL to 0.2 mL (1 mg to 2 mg) administered intravenously. Response to ENLON test dose in treated myasthenic patients is summarized as follows:
Undertreated patient: Myasthenic response; characterized by increased muscle strength (ptosis, diplopia, dysphonia, dysphagia, dysarthria, respiration, limb strength). This indicates inadequate treatment of the myasthenic condition.
Controlled patient: Adequate response; characterized by no change in muscle strength with minimal side reactions (lacrimation, diaphoresis, salivation, abdominal cramps, nausea, vomiting, diarrhea). Fasciculations (orbicularis oculi, facial muscles, limb muscles) may or may not occur. This response indicates that therapy is stabilized.
Overtreated patient: Cholinergic response; characterized by decreased muscle strength and severe side reactions. Fasciculations may be observed. This response occurs in myasthenics who have been overtreated with anticholinesterase drugs.
ENLON (edrophonium chloride injection, USP) Test in Crisis: Crisis in the myasthenic patient is characterized as a state of severe respiratory distress with inadequate ventilatory exchange, and unpredictable response to medication. If the patient is apneic, achieve ventilatory exchange immediately to avoid cardiac arrest and irreversible central nervous system damage.
The ENLON Test should not be conducted until respiratory exchange is maintained. The cholinergic patient will exhibit further weakness in the muscles of respiration and will have increased oropharyngeal secretions if ENLON is administered. Whereas, upon administration of ENLON the myasthenic patient will demonstrate improved respiration and can be given additional medication. To perform the test prepare a syringe with 0.2 mL (2 mg) ENLON and intravenously inject 0.1 mL (1 mg). The patient's cardiac and respiratory actions should be observed for change. The remaining 0.1 mL (1 mg) may be injected after one minute if no response is noted. If, after the entire 0.2 mL (2 mg) dose has been injected, no improvement in respiration occurs, discontinue all anticholinesterase drugs. Controlled ventilation can be achieved by tracheostomy with assisted respiration.

HOW SUPPLIED
ENLON (edrophonium chloride injection, USP):
NDC 10019-873-15   15 mL multidose vials.
Mfd. for: Anaquest, Madison, Wisconsin 53713
By: Taylor Pharmacal Co., Decatur, Illinois 62525
                       A-0389 Rev 1-87
Shown in Product Identification Section, page 405

ETHRANE®   ℞
[ē'thrān]
(enflurane, USP)
Liquid For Inhalation

CAUTION: Federal Law Prohibits Dispensing without Prescription.

DESCRIPTION
ETHRANE (enflurane, USP), a nonflammable liquid administered by vaporizing, is a general inhalation anesthetic drug. It is 2-chloro-1,1,2-trifluoroethyl difluoroethyl ether (CHF_2OCF_2CHFCl). The boiling point is 56.5°C at 760 mm Hg, and the vapor pressure (in mm Hg) is 175 at 20°C, 218 at 25°C, and 345 at 36°C. Vapor pressures can be calculated using the equation:
$$\log_{10}P_{vap} = A + \frac{B}{T}$$
$$A = 7.967$$
$$B = -1678.4$$
$$T = °C + 273.16 \text{ (Kelvin)}$$
The specific gravity (25°/25°C) is 1.517. The refractive index at 20°C is 1.3026–1.3030. The blood/gas coefficient is 1.91 at 37°C and the oil/gas coefficient is 98.5 at 37°C.
Enflurane is a clear, colorless, stable liquid whose purity exceeds 99.9% (area percent by gas chromatography). No stabilizers are added as these have been found, through controlled laboratory tests, to be unnecessary even in the presence of ultraviolet light. Enflurane is stable to strong base and does not decompose in contact with soda lime and does

Continued on next page

Anaquest—Cont.

not react with aluminum, tin, brass, iron or copper. The partition coefficients of enflurane at 25°C are 74 in conductive rubber and 120 in polyvinyl chloride.

CLINICAL PHARMACOLOGY

ĖTHRANE (enflurane, USP) is an inhalation anesthetic. The MAC (minimum alveolar concentration) in man is 1.68% in pure oxygen, 0.57 in 70% nitrous oxide-30% oxygen, and 1.17 in 30% nitrous oxide-70% oxygen.

Induction of and recovery from anesthesia with enflurane are rapid. Enflurane has a mild, sweet odor. Enflurane may provide a mild stimulus to salivation or tracheobronchial secretions. Pharyngeal and laryngeal reflexes are readily obtunded. The level of anesthesia can be changed rapidly by changing the inspired enflurane concentration. Enflurane reduces ventilation as depth of anesthesia increases. High $PaCO_2$ levels can be obtained at deeper levels of anesthesia if ventilation is not supported. Enflurane provokes a sigh response reminiscent of that seen with diethyl ether.

There is a decrease in blood pressure with induction of anesthesia, followed by a return to near normal with surgical stimulation. Progressive increases in depth of anesthesia produce corresponding increases in hypotension. Heart rate remains relatively constant without significant bradycardia. Electrocardiographic monitoring or recordings indicate that cardiac rhythm remains stable. Elevation of the carbon dioxide level in arterial blood does not alter cardiac rhythm. Studies in man indicate a considerable margin of safety in the administration of epinephrine-containing solutions during enflurane anesthesia. Enflurane anesthesia has been used in excision of pheochromocytoma in man without ventricular arrhythmias. On the basis of studies in patients anesthetized with enflurane and injected with epinephrine-containing solutions to achieve hemostasis in a highly vascular area (transsphenoidal surgery), up to 2 micrograms per kilogram (2 μg/kg) of epinephrine may be injected subcutaneously over a 10 minute period in patients judged to have ordinary tolerance to epinephrine administration. This would represent up to 14 mL of 1:100,000 epinephrine-containing solution (10 μg/mL), or the equivalent quantity, in a 70 kilogram patient. This may be repeated up to 3 times per hour (total 42 mL per hour). The concomitant administration of lidocaine enhances the safety of the use of epinephrine during enflurane anesthesia. This effect of lidocaine is dose related. All customary precautions in the use of vasoconstrictor substances should be observed.

Muscle relaxation may be adequate for intra-abdominal operations at normal levels of anesthesia. Muscle relaxants may be used to achieve greater relaxation and all commonly used muscle relaxants are compatible with enflurane. THE NONDEPOLARIZING MUSCLE RELAXANTS ARE POTENTIATED. In the normal 70 kg adult, 6 to 9 mg of d-tubocurarine or 1.0 to 1.5 mg of pancuronium will produce a 90% or greater depression of twitch height. Neostigmine does not reverse the direct effect of enflurane.

Enflurane 0.25 to 1.0% (average 0.5%) provides analgesia equal to that produced by 30 to 60% (average 40%) nitrous oxide for vaginal delivery. With either agent, patients remain awake, cooperative and oriented. Maternal blood losses are comparable. These clinical approaches produce normal Apgar scores. Serial neurobehavioral testing of the newborn during the first 24 hours of life reveals that neither enflurane nor nitrous oxide analgesia is associated with obvious neurobehavioral alterations. Neither enflurane nor nitrous oxide when used for obstetrical analgesia alters BUN, creatinine, uric acid or osmolality. The only difference in the use of these two agents for obstetrical analgesia appears to be higher inspired oxygen concentration that may be used with enflurane.

Analgetic doses of enflurane, up to approximately 1.0%, do not significantly depress the rate or force of uterine contraction during labor and delivery. A slowing of the rate of uterine contraction and a diminution of the force of uterine contraction is noted between the administration of 1.0 and 2.0% delivered enflurane; concentrations somewhere between 2.0 and 3.0% delivered enflurane may abolish uterine contractions. Enflurane displaces the myometrial response curve to oxytocin so that at lower concentrations of enflurane oxytocin will restore uterine contractions; however, as the dose of enflurane progresses (somewhere between 1.5 and 3.0% delivered enflurane) the response to oxytocin is diminished and then abolished. Uterine bleeding may be increased when enflurane is used in higher concentrations for vaginal delivery or to facilitate delivery by Cesarean section; however, this has not been demonstrated within the recommended dosage range (see DOSAGE AND ADMINISTRATION section). Mean estimated blood loss in patients anesthetized for therapeutic termination of pregnancy with 1.0% enflurane in 70% nitrous oxide with oxygen is approximately twice that noted following therapeutic termination of pregnancy performed with the use of a local anesthetic technique (40 mL versus 20 mL).

Pharmacokinetics: Biotransformation of enflurane in man results in low peak levels of serum fluoride averaging 15 μmol/L. These levels are well below the 50 μmol/L threshold level which can produce minimal renal damage in normal subjects. However, patients chronically ingesting isoniazid or other hydrazine-containing compounds may metabolize greater amounts of enflurane. Although no significant renal dysfunction has been found thus far in such patients, peak serum fluoride levels can exceed 50 μmol/L, particularly when anesthesia goes beyond 2 MAC hours. Depression of lymphocyte transformation does not follow prolonged enflurane anesthesia in man in the absence of surgery. Thus enflurane does not depress this aspect of the immune response.

INDICATIONS AND USAGE

ĖTHRANE (enflurane, USP) may be used for induction and maintenance of general anesthesia. Enflurane may be used to provide analgesia for vaginal delivery. Low concentrations of enflurane (see DOSAGE AND ADMINISTRATION) may also be used to supplement other general anesthetic agents during delivery by Cesarean section. Higher concentrations of enflurane may produce uterine relaxation and an increase in uterine bleeding.

CONTRAINDICATIONS

Seizure disorders (see WARNINGS).
Known sensitivity to ĖTHRANE (enflurane, USP) or other halogenated anesthetics.
Known or suspected genetic susceptibility to malignant hyperthermia.

WARNINGS

Increasing depth of anesthesia with ĖTHRANE (enflurane, USP) may produce a change in the electroencephalogram characterized by high voltage, fast frequency, progressing through spike-dome complexes alternating with periods of electrical silence to frank seizure activity. The latter may or may not be associated with motor movement. Motor activity, when encountered, generally consists of twitching or "jerks" of various muscle groups; it is self-limiting and can be terminated by lowering the anesthetic concentration. This electroencephalographic pattern associated with deep anesthesia is exacerbated by low arterial carbon dioxide tension. A reduction in ventilation and anesthetic concentrations usually suffices to eliminate seizure activity. Cerebral blood flow and metabolism studies in normal volunteers immediately following seizure activity show no evidence of cerebral hypoxia. Mental function testing does not reveal any impairment of performance following prolonged enflurane anesthesia associated with or not associated with seizure activity.

Since onset of anesthesia may be altered easily and rapidly, only vaporizers producing predictable concentrations should be used. Hypotension and respiratory exchange can serve as a guide to depth of anesthesia. Deep levels of anesthesia may produce marked hypotension and respiratory depression.

When previous exposure to a halogenated anesthetic is known to have been followed by evidence of unexplained hepatic dysfunction, consideration should be given to use of an agent other than enflurane.

PRECAUTIONS

General: ĖTHRANE (enflurane, USP) should be used with caution in patients who by virtue of medical or drug history could be considered more susceptible to cortical stimulation produced by this drug.

Information to Patients: Enflurane, as well as other general anesthetics, may cause a slight decrease in intellectual function for 2 to 3 days following anesthesia. As with other anesthetics, small changes in moods and symptoms may persist for several days following anesthesia.

Laboratory Tests: Bromsulfalein (BSP) retention is mildly elevated postoperatively in some cases. This may relate to the effect of surgery since prolonged anesthesia (5 to 7 hours) in human volunteers does not result in BSP elevation. There is some elevation of glucose and white blood count intraoperatively. Glucose elevation should be considered in diabetic patients.

Drug Interactions: The action of nondepolarizing relaxants is augmented by enflurane. Less than the usual amounts of these drugs should be used. If the usual amounts of nondepolarizing relaxants are given, the time for recovery from neuromuscular blockade will be longer in the presence of enflurane than when halothane or nitrous oxide with a balanced technique are used.

Carcinogenesis/Mutagenesis: Swiss ICR mice were given enflurane to determine whether such exposure might induce neoplasia. Enflurane was given at $\frac{1}{2}$, $\frac{1}{8}$ and $\frac{1}{32}$ MAC for four in-utero exposures and for 24 exposures to the pups during the first nine weeks of life. The mice were killed at 15 months of age. The incidence of tumors in these mice was the same as in untreated control mice who were given the same background gases, but not the anesthetic.

Exposure of mice to 20 hours of 1.2% enflurane causes a small (about $\frac{1}{2}$ of 1.0%) but statistically significant increase in sperm abnormalities. In contrast to these results, in vitro approaches to the study of mutagenesis (Ames test, sister

chromatid exchange test, and the 8-azaguanine system) have not shown a mutagenic effect of enflurane.

Pregnancy Category B: Reproduction studies have been performed in rats and rabbits at doses up to four times the human dose and have revealed no evidence of impaired fertility or harm to the fetus due to enflurane. There are, however, no adequate and well controlled studies in pregnant women. Because animal reproduction studies are not always predictive of human response, this drug should be used during pregnancy only if clearly needed.

Nursing Mothers: It is not known whether this drug is excreted in human milk. Because many drugs are excreted in human milk, caution should be exercised when enflurane is administered to a nursing woman.

Malignant Hyperthermia: In susceptible individuals, enflurane anesthesia may trigger a skeletal muscle hypermetabolic state leading to high oxygen demand and the clinical syndrome known as malignant hyperthermia. The syndrome includes nonspecific features such as muscle rigidity, tachycardia, tachypnea, cyanosis, arrhythmias and unstable blood pressure. (It should also be noted that many of these nonspecific signs may appear with light anesthesia, acute hypoxia, etc. The syndrome of malignant hyperthermia secondary to enflurane appears to be rare; by March 1980, 35 cases had been reported in North America for an approximate incidence of 1:725,000 enflurane anesthetics.) An increase in overall metabolism may be reflected in an elevated temperature (which may rise rapidly early or late in the case, but usually is not the first sign of augmented metabolism) and an increased usage of the CO_2 absorption system (hot canister). PaO_2 and pH may decrease, and hyperkalemia and a base deficit may appear. Treatment includes discontinuance of triggering agents (e.g., enflurane), administration of intravenous dantrolene sodium, and applications of supportive therapy. Such therapy includes vigorous efforts to restore body temperature to normal, respiratory and circulatory support as indicated, and management of electrolyte-fluid-acid-base derangement. (Consult prescribing information for dantrolene sodium intravenous for additional information on patient management.) Renal failure may appear later, and urine flow should be sustained if possible.

ADVERSE REACTIONS

1. Malignant hyperthermia (see PRECAUTIONS).
2. Motor activity exemplified by movements of various muscle groups and/or seizures may be encountered with deep levels of ĖTHRANE (enflurane, USP) anesthesia, or light levels with hypocapnia.
3. Hypotension and respiratory depression have been reported.
4. Arrhythmias, shivering, nausea and vomiting have been reported.
5. Elevation of the white blood count has been observed.
6. Unexplained mild, moderate and severe liver injury may rarely follow anesthesia with enflurane. Serum transaminases may be increased and histologic evidence of injury may be found. The histologic changes are neither unique nor consistent. In several of these cases, it has not been possible to exclude enflurane as the cause or as a contributing cause of liver injury. The incidence of unexplained hepatotoxicity following the administration of enflurane is unknown, but it appears to be rare and not dose related.

OVERDOSAGE

In the event of overdosage, or what may appear to be overdosage, the following action should be taken.
Stop drug administration, establish a clear airway and initiate assisted or controlled ventilation with pure oxygen.

DOSAGE AND ADMINISTRATION

The concentration of ĖTHRANE (enflurane, USP) being delivered from a vaporizer during anesthesia should be known. This may be accomplished by using:
a) vaporizers calibrated specifically for enflurane;
b) vaporizers from which delivered flows can easily and readily be calculated.

Preanesthetic Medication: Preanesthetic medication should be selected according to the need of the individual patient, taking into account that secretions are weakly stimulated by enflurane and that enflurane does not alter heart rate. The use of anticholinergic drugs is a matter of choice.

Surgical Anesthesia: Induction may be achieved using enflurane alone with oxygen or in combination with oxygen-nitrous oxide mixtures. Under these conditions some excitement may be encountered. If excitement is to be avoided, a hypnotic dose of a short-acting barbiturate should be used to induce unconsciousness, followed by the enflurane mixture. In general, inspired concentrations of 2.0 to 4.5% enflurane produce surgical anesthesia in 7 to 10 minutes.

Maintenance: Surgical levels of anesthesia may be maintained with 0.5 to 3.0% enflurane. Maintenance concentrations should not exceed 3.0%. If added relaxation is required, supplemental doses of muscle relaxants may be used. Ventilation to maintain the tension of carbon dioxide in arterial blood in the 35 to 45 mm Hg range is preferred. Hyperventilation should be avoided in order to minimize possible CNS excitation.

The level of blood pressure during maintenance is an inverse function of enflurane concentration in the absence of other complicating problems. Excessive decreases (unless related to hypovolemia) may be due to depth of anesthesia and in such instances should be corrected by lightening the level of anesthesia.

Analgesia: Enflurane 0.25 to 1.0% provides analgesia for vaginal delivery equal to that produced by 30 to 60% nitrous oxide. These concentrations normally do not produce amnesia. See also the information on the effects of enflurane on uterine contraction contained in the CLINICAL PHARMACOLOGY section.

Cesarean Section: Enflurane should ordinarily be administered in the concentration range of 0.5 to 1.0% to supplement other general anesthetics. See also the information on the effects of enflurane on uterine contraction contained in the CLINICAL PHARMACOLOGY section.

HOW SUPPLIED

ETHRANE (enflurane, USP) is packaged in 125 and 250 mL amber-colored bottles.

125 mL—NDC 10019-350-50
250 mL—NDC 10019-350-60

Storage: Store at room temperature 15–30°C (59–86°F). Enflurane contains no additives and has been demonstrated to be stable at room temperature for periods in excess of five years.

A-0408 Rev 5-87

Shown in Product Identification Section, page 405

FORANE®   ℞
[for ´an]
(isoflurane, USP)
Liquid for Inhalation

CAUTION: Federal Law Prohibits Dispensing without Prescription.

DESCRIPTION

FORANE (isoflurane, USP) a nonflammable liquid administered by vaporizing, is a general inhalation anesthetic drug. It is 1-chloro-2,2,2-trifluoroethyl difluoromethyl ether, and its structural formula is:

```
      F   H        F
      |   |        |
  F — C — C — O — C — H
      |   |        |
      F   Cl       F
```

Some physical constants are:

Molecular weight	184.5
Boiling point at 760 mm Hg	48.5°C (uncorr.)
Refractive index $n^{20}D$	1.2990–1.3005
Specific gravity 25°/25°C	1.496
Vapor pressure in mm Hg** 20°C	238
25°C	295
30°C	367
35°C	450

** Equation for vapor pressure calculation:

$$\log_{10}P_{vap} = A + \frac{B}{T} \text{ where: } A = 8.056$$
$$B = -1664.58$$
$$T = °C + 273.16 \text{ (Kelvin)}$$

Partition coefficients at 37°C

Water/gas	0.61
Blood/gas	1.43
Oil/gas	90.8

Partition coefficients at 25°C—rubber and plastic

Conductive rubber/gas	62.0
Butyl rubber/gas	75.0
Polyvinyl chloride/gas	110.0
Polyethylene/gas	~2.0
Polyurethane/gas	~1.4
Polyolefin/gas	~1.1
Butyl acetate/gas	~2.5
Purity by gas chromatography	>99.9%

Lower limit of flammability in oxygen or nitrous oxide at 9 joules/sec. and 23°C   None

Lower limit of flammability in oxygen or nitrous oxide at 900 joules/sec. and 23°C   Greater than useful concentration in anesthesia.

Isoflurane is a clear, colorless, stable liquid containing no additives or chemical stabilizers. Isoflurane has a mildly pungent, musty, ethereal odor. Samples stored in indirect sunlight in clear, colorless glass for five years, as well as samples directly exposed for 30 hours to a 2 amp, 115 volt, 60 cycle long wave U.V. light were unchanged in composition as determined by gas chromatography. Isoflurane in one normal sodium methoxide-methanol solution, a strong base, for over six months consumed essentially no alkali, indicative of strong base stability. Isoflurane does not decompose in the presence of soda lime, and does not attack aluminum, tin, brass, iron or copper.

CLINICAL PHARMACOLOGY

FORANE (isoflurane, USP) is an inhalation anesthetic. The MAC (minimum alveolar concentration) in man is as follows:

Age	100% Oxygen	70% N₂O
26 ± 4	1.28	0.56
44 ± 7	1.15	0.50
64 ± 5	1.05	0.37

Induction of and recovery from isoflurane anesthesia are rapid. Isoflurane has a mild pungency which limits the rate of induction, although excessive salivation or tracheobronchial secretions do not appear to be stimulated. Pharyngeal and laryngeal reflexes are readily obtunded. The level of anesthesia may be changed rapidly with isoflurane. Isoflurane is a profound respiratory depressant. RESPIRATION MUST BE MONITORED CLOSELY AND SUPPORTED WHEN NECESSARY. As anesthetic dose is increased, tidal volume decreases and respiratory rate is unchanged. This depression is partially reversed by surgical stimulation, even at deeper levels of anesthesia. Isoflurane evokes a sigh response reminiscent of that seen with diethyl ether and enflurane, although the frequency is less than with enflurane. Blood pressure decreases with induction of anesthesia but returns toward normal with surgical stimulation. Progressive increases in depth of anesthesia produce corresponding decreases in blood pressure. Nitrous oxide diminishes the inspiratory concentration of isoflurane required to reach a desired level of anesthesia and may reduce the arterial hypotension seen with isoflurane alone. Heart rhythm is remarkably stable. With controlled ventilation and normal PaCO₂, cardiac output is maintained despite increasing depth of anesthesia primarily through an increase in heart rate which compensates for a reduction in stroke volume. The hypercapnia which attends spontaneous ventilation during isoflurane anesthesia further increases heart rate and raises cardiac output above awake levels. Isoflurane does not sensitize the myocardium to exogenously administered epinephrine in the dog. Limited data indicate that subcutaneous injection of 0.25 mg of epinephrine (50 mL of 1:200,000 solution) does not produce an increase in ventricular arrhythmias in patients anesthetized with isoflurane. Muscle relaxation is often adequate for intra-abdominal operations at normal levels of anesthesia. Complete muscle paralysis can be attained with small doses of muscle relaxants. ALL COMMONLY USED MUSCLE RELAXANTS ARE MARKEDLY POTENTIATED WITH ISOFLURANE, THE EFFECT BEING MOST PROFOUND WITH THE NONDEPOLARIZING TYPE. Neostigmine reverses the effect of nondepolarizing muscle relaxants in the presence of isoflurane. All commonly used muscle relaxants are compatible with isoflurane.

Pharmacokinetics: Isoflurane undergoes minimal biotransformation in man. In the postanesthesia period, only 0.17% of the isoflurane taken up can be recovered as urinary metabolites.

INDICATIONS AND USAGE

FORANE (isoflurane, USP) may be used for induction and maintenance of general anesthesia. Adequate data have not been developed to establish its application in obstetrical anesthesia.

CONTRAINDICATIONS

Known sensitivity to FORANE (isoflurane, USP) or to other halogenated agents.
Known or suspected genetic susceptibility to malignant hyperthermia.

WARNINGS

Since levels of anesthesia may be altered easily and rapidly, only vaporizers producing predictable concentrations should be used. Hypotension and respiratory depression increase as anesthesia is deepened.
Increased blood loss comparable to that seen with halothane has been observed in patients undergoing abortions.
FORANE (isoflurane, USP) markedly increases cerebral blood flow at deeper levels of anesthesia. There may be a transient rise in cerebral spinal fluid pressure which is fully reversible with hyperventilation.

PRECAUTIONS

General: As with any potent general anesthetic, FORANE (isoflurane, USP) should only be administered in an adequately equipped anesthetizing environment by those who are familiar with the pharmacology of the drug and qualified by training and experience to manage the anesthetized patient.
Information to Patients: Isoflurane, as well as other general anesthetics, may cause a slight decrease in intellectual function for 2 or 3 days following anesthesia. As with other anesthetics, small changes in moods and symptoms may persist for up to 6 days after administration.
Laboratory Tests: Transient increases in BSP retention, blood glucose and serum creatinine with decrease in BUN, serum cholesterol and alkaline phosphatase have been observed.

Drug Interactions: Isoflurane potentiates the muscle relaxant effect of all muscle relaxants, most notably nondepolarizing muscle relaxants, and MAC (minimum alveolar concentration) is reduced by concomitant administration of N₂O. See CLINICAL PHARMACOLOGY.

Carcinogenesis: Swiss ICR mice were given isoflurane to determine whether such exposure might induce neoplasia. Isoflurane was given at ½, ⅛ and 1/32 MAC for four in-utero exposures and for 24 exposures to the pups during the first nine weeks of life. The mice were killed at 15 months of age. The incidence of tumors in these mice was the same as in untreated control mice which were given the same background gases, but not the anesthetic.

Pregnancy Category C: Isoflurane has been shown to have a possible anesthetic-related fetotoxic effect in mice when given in doses 6 times the human dose. There are no adequate and well-controlled studies in pregnant women. Isoflurane should be used during pregnancy only if the potential benefit justifies the potential risk to the fetus.

Nursing Mothers: It is not known whether this drug is excreted in human milk. Because many drugs are excreted in human milk, caution should be exercised when isoflurane is administered to a nursing woman.

Malignant Hyperthermia: In susceptible individuals, isoflurane anesthesia may trigger a skeletal muscle hypermetabolic state leading to high oxygen demand and the clinical syndrome known as malignant hyperthermia. The syndrome includes nonspecific features such as muscle rigidity, tachycardia, tachypnea, cyanosis, arrhythmias, and unstable blood pressure. (It should also be noted that many of these nonspecific signs may appear with light anesthesia, acute hypoxia, etc.) An increase in overall metabolism may be reflected in an elevated temperature (which may rise rapidly early or late in the case, but usually is not the first sign of augmented metabolism) and an increased usage of the CO₂ absorption system (hot canister). PaO₂ and pH may decrease, and hyperkalemia and a base deficit may appear. Treatment includes discontinuance of triggering agents (e.g., isoflurane), administration of intravenous dantrolene sodium, and application of supportive therapy. Such therapy includes vigorous efforts to restore body temperature to normal, respiratory and circulatory support as indicated, and management of electrolyte-fluid-acid-base derangements. (Consult prescribing information for dantrolene sodium intravenous for additional information on patient management.) Renal failure may appear later, and urine flow should be sustained if possible.

ADVERSE REACTION

Adverse reactions encountered in the administration of FORANE (isoflurane, USP) are in general dose dependent extensions of pharmacophysiologic effects and include respiratory depression, hypotension and arrhythmias.
Shivering, nausea, vomiting and ileus have been observed in the postoperative period.
As with all other general anesthetics, transient elevations in white blood count have been observed even in the absence of surgical stress.
See PRECAUTIONS for information regarding malignant hyperthermia.

OVERDOSAGE

In the event of overdosage, or what may appear to be overdosage, the following action should be taken:
Stop drug administration, establish a clear airway and initiate assisted or controlled ventilation with pure oxygen.

DOSAGE AND ADMINISTRATION

Premedication: Premedication should be selected according to the need of the individual patient, taking into account that secretions are weakly stimulated by FORANE (isoflurane, USP) and the heart rate tends to be increased. The use of anticholinergic drugs is a matter of choice.
Inspired Concentration: The concentration of isoflurane being delivered from a vaporizer during anesthesia should be known. This may be accomplished by using:
a) vaporizers calibrated specifically for isoflurane;
b) vaporizers from which delivered flows can be calculated, such as vaporizers delivering a saturated vapor which is then diluted. The delivered concentration from such a vaporizer may be calculated using the formula:

$$\% \text{ isoflurane} = \frac{100\, P_V F_V}{F_T (P_A - P_V)}$$

where:
     P_A = Pressure of atmosphere
     P_V = Vapor pressure of isoflurane
     F_V = Flow of gas through vaporizer (mL/min)
     F_T = Total gas flow (mL/min)

Isoflurane contains no stabilizer. Nothing in the agent alters calibration or operation of these vaporizers.
Induction: Induction with isoflurane in oxygen or in combination with oxygen-nitrous oxide mixtures may produce coughing, breath holding, or laryngospasm. These difficulties may be avoided by the use of a hypnotic dose of an ultrashort-acting barbiturate. Inspired concentrations of 1.5 to

Continued on next page

Anaquest—Cont.

3.0% isoflurane usually produce surgical anesthesia in 7 to 10 minutes.

Maintenance: Surgical levels of anesthesia may be sustained with a 1.0 to 2.5% concentration when nitrous oxide is used concomitantly. An additional 0.5 to 1.0% may be required when isoflurane is given using oxygen alone. If added relaxation is required, supplemental doses of muscle relaxants may be used.

The level of blood pressure during maintenance is an inverse function of isoflurane concentration in the absence of other complicating problems. Excessive decreases may be due to depth of anesthesia and in such instances may be corrected by lightening anesthesia.

HOW SUPPLIED

FORANE (isoflurane, USP), NDC 10019-360-40, is packaged in 100 mL amber-colored bottles.

Storage: Store at room temperature 15–30°C (59–86°F). Isoflurane contains no additives and has been demonstrated to be stable at room temperature for periods in excess of five years.

A-0409 Rev 5-87

Shown in Product Identification Section, page 405

> ### EDUCATIONAL MATERIAL

Educational Resources

Anaquest offers a wide range of educational materials free of charge to physicians, nurse-anesthetists and hospital pharmacists. They are available from Anaquest representatives, by writing to: Anaquest, 2005 West Beltline Highway, Madison, WI 53713-2318, or by calling "(800) ANA-DRUG".

- Audio-visual library—films, slides, and audiocassettes available from Anaquest representatives
- Product compendiums and monographs
- Speakers bureau
- Continuing education—AANA-accredited home-study program for nurse-anesthetists and hospital pharmacists (ACPE-approved provider); AMA-accredited computerized case simulations for physicians
- Computerized drug information—available through Anaquest representatives

---

Arco Pharmaceuticals, Inc.
105 ORVILLE DRIVE
BOHEMIA, NY 11716

ARCO-LASE®
(broad pH spectrum digestant)

COMPOSITION

Each soft, mint flavored tablet contains Trizyme*, 38 mg., and Lipase, 25 mg.
*Contains the following standardized enzymes: amylolytic 30 mg.; proteolytic 6 mg.; cellulolytic 2 mg.

ACTION AND USES

Indicated for most gastrointestinal disorders due to poor digestion. Flatulence, gas and bloating, dyspepsia, distention, fullness, heartburn, or in any condition where normal digestion is impaired by digestive insufficiencies. Arcolase provides the highest standardized enzymatic activity, plus the protective action of the widest pH range. Thus it is effective throughout the entire G.I. tract. Requiring no enteric coating, there is assurance of a positive breakdown of its factors. This is advantageous, because quite often patients with digestive disorders cannot digest their food properly, let alone hard, or enteric coated capsules or tablets.

SIDE EFFECTS
None.

ADMINISTRATION AND DOSAGE

One tablet with or immediately following meals. Tablet may be swallowed or chewed.

SUPPLIED
Bottles of 50's. NDC 275-4040.

ARCO-LASE® PLUS   ℞

COMPOSITION

Same as Arco-Lase, plus the addition of Hyoscyamine sulfate 0.10 mg., atropine sulfate 0.02 mg. and phenobarbital ⅛ gr. (Warning: may be habit forming.)

ACTION AND USES

Gastrointestinal disturbances, such as cramps, bloating, spasms, diarrhea, nausea, vomiting and peptic ulcer. The enzymes correct the digestive insufficiencies.

The antispasmodic and phenobarbital contribute to the symptomatic relief of hypermotility and nervous tension, which usually accompanies functional disturbances of the bowel.

ADMINISTRATION AND DOSAGE
One tablet following meals.

SIDE EFFECTS

May cause rapid pulse, dryness of mouth and blurred vision.

CONTRAINDICATIONS

This product is contraindicated in the presence of glaucoma or prostatic hypertrophy.

SUPPLIED
Bottles of 50's. NDC 275-45-45.

LITERATURE AVAILABLE
Yes.

MEGA-B®
(super potency vitamin B complex, sugar & starch free)

COMPOSITION

Each Mega-B Tablet contains the following Mega Vitamins:

B_1 (Thiamine Mononitrate)	100 mg.
B_2 (Riboflavin)	100 mg.
B_6 (Pyridoxine Hydrochloride)	100 mg.
B_{12} (Cyanocobalamin)	100 mcg.
Choline Bitartrate	100 mg.
Inositol	100 mg.
Niacinamide	100 mg.
Folic Acid	100 mcg.
Pantothenic Acid	100 mg.
d-Biotin	100 mcg.
Para-Aminobenzoic Acid (PABA)	100 mg.

In a base of yeast to provide the identified and unidentified B-Complex Factors.

ADVANTAGES

Each Mega-B capsule-shaped tablet provides the highest vitamin B complex available in a single dose.

Mega-B was designed for those patients who require truly Mega vitamin potencies with the convenience of minimum dosage.

INDICATIONS

Mega-B is indicated in conditions characterized by depletions or increased demand of the water-soluble B-complex vitamins. It may be useful in the nutritional management of patients during prolonged convalescence associated with major surgery. It is also indicated for stress conditions, as an adjunct to antibiotics and diuretic therapy, pre and post operative cases, liver conditions, gastrointestinal disorders interfering with intake or absorption of water-soluble vitamins, prolonged or wasting diseases, diabetes, burns, fractures, severe infections, and some psychological disorders.

WARNING

NOT INTENDED FOR TREATMENT OF PERNICIOUS ANEMIA, OR OTHER PRIMARY OR SECONDARY ANEMIAS.

DOSAGE

Usual dosage is one Mega-B tablet daily, or varied, depending on clinical needs.

SUPPLIED

Yellow capsule shaped tablets in bottles of 30, 100 and 500.

MEGADOSE™
(multiple mega-vitamin formula with minerals, sugar and starch free)

COMPOSITION

Vitamin A	25,000 USP Units
Vitamin D	1,000 USP Units
Vitamin C w/Rose Hips	250 mg.
Vitamin E	100 IU
Folic Acid	400 mcg.
Vitamin B_1	80 mg.
Vitamin B_2	80 mg.
Niacinamide	80 mg.
Vitamin B_6	80 mg.
Vitamin B_{12}	80 mcg.
Biotin	80 mcg.
Pantothenic Acid	80 mg.
Choline Bitartrate	80 mg.
Inositol	80 mg.
Para-Aminobenzoic Acid	80 mg.
Rutin	30 mg.
Citrus Bioflavonoids	30 mg.
Betaine Hydrochloride	30 mg.
Glutamic Acid	30 mg.
Hesperidin Complex	5 mg.
Iodine (from Kelp)	0.15 mg.
Calcium Gluconate*	50 mg.
Zinc Gluconate*	25 mg.
Potassium Gluconate*	10 mg.
Ferrous Gluconate*	10 mg.
Magnesium Gluconate*	7 mg.
Manganese Gluconate*	6 mg.
Copper Gluconate*	0.5 mg.

*Natural mineral chelates in a base containing natural ingredients.

DOSAGE
One tablet daily.

SUPPLIED
Capsule shaped tablets in bottles of 30, 100 and 250.

Armour Pharmaceutical Company
SUITE 200
920A HARVEST DRIVE
BLUE BELL, PA 19422

PLASMA DERIVATIVE PRODUCTS

ALBUMINAR®-5   ℞
[al-byōō′mĭn-är]
Albumin
(Human) U.S.P. 5%

ALBUMINAR®-5 Albumin (Human) is supplied as a 5% solution in:
- 50 mL bottles containing 2.5 grams of albumin
- 250 mL bottles containing 12.5 grams of albumin
- 500 mL bottles containing 25.0 grams of albumin
- 1000 mL bottles containing 50 grams of albumin

For use with intravenous administration set. See directions on set supplied.

ALBUMINAR®-25   ℞
[ăl-byōō′mĭn-är″]
Albumin
(Human) U.S.P. 25%

ALBUMINAR®-25 Albumin (Human), is supplied as a 25% solution in:
- 20 mL vials containing 5.0 grams of albumin
- 50 mL vials containing 12.5 grams of albumin
- 100 mL vials containing 25.0 grams of albumin

For use with intravenous administration set. See directions on set supplied.

GAMMAR®   ℞
[găm′är]
Immune Globulin
(Human) U.S.P.

GAMMAR® Immune Globulin (Human) U.S.P. is supplied in 2 mL and 10 mL vials.

GAMULIN® Rh   ℞
[găm′yōō-lĭn″]
Rh₀ (D) Immune Globulin (Human)

A sterile Immune Globulin Solution containing Rh_o (D) antibodies. Supplied in individual package containing a single dose vial of Gamulin Rh, patient identification card, directions for use, and patient information brochure and cartons containing 25 single dose vials of Gamulin Rh, 25 patient identification cards, 10 sets of directions for use, and 25 patient information brochures and plastic cases containing 6 single dose syringes of Gamulin Rh, 6 patient identification cards, directions for use, 6 patient information brochures, and 6 laboratory control forms.

HUMATE-P™   ℞
[hyōō′māt]
Antihemophilic Factor (Human), Pasteurized

Humate-P™, Antihemophilic Factor (Human), Pasteurized, is supplied in single dose vials (I.U. activity is stated on label of each vial) with sterile diluent and needles for reconstitution and withdrawal. Manufactured by Behringwerke AG, Marburg/Lahn West Germany and distributed by Armour Pharmaceutical Company.

MINI–GAMULIN™ Rh   ℞
[mĭ-nē "găm 'yoo-lĭn]
Rh₀ (D) Immune Globulin (Human)

A sterile Immune Globulin Solution containing Rh₀ (D) antibodies. Mini-Gamulin Rh contains one-sixth the quantity of Rh₀ (D) antibody contained in a standard dose of Rh₀ (D) Immune Globulin (Human). Mini-Gamulin is supplied in individual packages of single dose vials and cartons of 25 single dose vials and plastic cases containing 6 single dose syringes of Mini-Gamulin Rh, 6 patient identification cards, directions for use, 6 patient information brochures, and 6 laboratory control forms.

MONOCLATE® Factor VIII:C, Heat-Treated   ℞
[mŏn 'ō-clāte "]
Antihemophilic Factor (Human)

MONOCLATE®, Factor VIII:C, Heat-Treated, Antihemophilic Factor (Human) is supplied in single dose vials (I.U. activity is stated on carton and label of each vial) with sterile diluent, winged administration set, filter needle, transfer needle and alcohol swabs for reconstitution and administration.

PLASMA–PLEX®   ℞
[plăz 'ma-plĕks]
Plasma Protein Fraction (Human) U.S.P.

As a 5% Solution in:
50 mL bottles containing 2.5 g of selected plasma proteins
250 mL bottles containing 12.5 g of selected plasma proteins
500 mL bottles containing 25.0 g of selected plasma proteins.
For use with intravenous administration set. See directions on set supplied.

EDUCATIONAL MATERIAL

Albuminar
"The Clinical Uses of Normal Serum Albumin (human)"
(CME—Rutgers) cassette and accompanying brochure.
—Management in Shock
Available to physicians and pharmacists—contact Armour Corporate Headquarters.

Gamulin
"Confidence Factor" booklets
—in Rh negative women
—in a matter of choice
—in antepartum prophylaxis
—in prenatal diagnostic testing
The above literature is available to physicians, pharmacists and patients.
Monograph Series—"The Prevention of Rh Isoimmunization"
#1— Amniocentesis and Rh Isoimmunization
#2— Antenatal Rh Immune Globulin Use in an Uneventful Pregnancy
#3— Management of the High-Risk Pregnancy
#4— Massive Transplacental Hemorrhage, the Laboratory and the Blood Bank
Film—"Hemolytic disease of the newborn"
The Monograph Series and film are available to physicians and pharmacists—contact Armour Corporate Headquarters.

Monoclate® Factor VIII:C
Question and Answer Booklet
Monoclonal Antibody Technology
Summary of Pre-clinical and Clinical Data
Available to physicians and pharmacists—contact Armour Corporate Headquarters.

Products are cross-indexed
by product classifications
in the
BLUE SECTION

Arther, Inc.
P.O. BOX 1455
W. CALDWELL, NJ 07007-1455

TRYPTACIN®
[trĭp 'tă-sĭn]
(brand of l-tryptophan)

DESCRIPTION
TRYPTACIN - Chemically, aminoindole-3-propionic acid is white to slightly yellowish white crystals or crystalline powder, taste slightly bitter. Contains not less than 98.5% and not more than 100.5% of l-tryptophan($C_{11}H_{12}N_2O_2$).

ACTION AND USES
Dietary supplement. L-tryptophan is a precursor of the neurotransmitter, serotonin (5-hydroxytryptamine).

ADMINISTRATION AND DOSAGE
2 to 4 500 mg. tablets or 1 to 2 1000 mg tablets one half hour before bedtime.

HOW SUPPLIED
500 mg. Capsule shaped, scored white tablets.
Bottle of 100's—NDC 48558-001-10
Bottle of 250's—NDC 48558-001-25
Box of 100's—NDC 48558-001-01 (Unit Dose)
1000 mg. Capsule shaped, white tablets.
Bottle of 100's—NDC 48558-010-10

REFERENCES
Age of Alcoholism Onset: Relationship to Serotonin Precursor Availability
Arch. Gen. Psychiatry, Vol. 46, March 1989: 231-236

Dietary Tryptophan Reverses Alcohol-induced Impairment of Facial Recognition but not Verbal Recall
Alcoholism: Clinical and Experimental Research, Vol. 12, 1988, 531–33

The Effect of Altered Tryptophan Levels on Mood and Behavior in Normal Human Males
Clinical Neuropharmacology, Vol. 11, Suppl. 1, 1988: S207-S215

Clomipramine, Tryptophan and Lithium in Combination for Resistant Endogenous Depression: Seven Case Studies
British Jrl of Psychiatry, 1987, 151:213–217

Use of L-Tryptophan as a Sleep Aid in the Elderly
The Psychiatric Forum, Vol. 13, No. 2, 1985–86: 82–85

Trazodone/Tryptophan for Aggressive Behavior
Lancet: Apr. 18, 1987, 929–30

L-Tryptophan Administered to Chronic Sleep-Onset Insomnias: Late appearing reduction of Sleep latency
Psychopharmacology (1986) 90: 151–155

The Use of Tryptophan in Normal-Weight Bulimia Can. J of Psych., Nov., Vol. 31 (8) 755–6, 1986

Monoamine Precursors in The Affective Disorders.
Advances in Human Psychopharmacology, 3:251–285, 1984

B.F. Ascher & Company, Inc.
15501 WEST 109TH STREET
LENEXA, KS 66219

ADIPOST™ Capusles   ⓒ ℞
[ad-uh-post]

Phendimetrazine tartrate slow-release
  capsules ....105 mg

HOW SUPPLIED
White/clear capsules with NDC 225/470 printed in red on each capsule half. Contains white slow-release beads.
Bottles of 100—NDC 0225-0470-15

ALLENT® Capsules   ℞
[all 'ent]

Brompheniramine maleate, U.S.P. .... 12 mg
Pseudoephedrine hydrochloride, U.S.P. ....120 mg

HOW SUPPLIED
Clear capsules containing white, slow-release beads with the NDC number 225-480 printed in black iron oxide to insure product is dye-free.
Bottles of 100—NDC 0225-2480-15

ANASPAZ® Tablets   ℞
[an 'ah-spāz]

(l-hyoscyamine sulfate) ....0.125 mg

HOW SUPPLIED
Light yellow, compressed, scored tablets with the Ascher logo on one side and the NDC 225/295 on the other.
Bottles of 100—NDC 0225-0295-15
Bottles of 500—NDC 0225-0295-20

AYR® Saline Nasal Mist and Drops

(See PDR For Nonprescription Drugs)

DRIZE® Capsules   ℞
[driz]

Chlorpheniramine maleate ....12 mg.
Phenylpropanolamine HCl ....75 mg.

HOW SUPPLIED
Clear capsules with white extended-release beads with the NDC 225-405 imprinted in iron oxide black to insure the product is dye-free.
Bottles of 100—NDC 0225-0405-15

HY-PHEN® Tablets   ⓒ ℞
formerly Hycodaphen
[hi-fen]
hydrocodone bitartrate 5 mg
  (WARNING: May be habit forming.)
acetaminophen 500 mg

HOW SUPPLIED
HY-PHEN is available as a compressed, white, capsule shaped, bisected tablet impressed with two Ascher logos in juxtaposition with the score on one side and 225-450 on the other in bottles of 100 tablets (NDC 0225-0450-15) and 500 tablets (NDC 0225-0450-20) and Hospital Unit Dose Package of 100 Tablets (NDC 0225-0450-21).

KWELCOF® Liquid   ⓒ ℞
[kwel 'cof]

Each teaspoonful (5 ml) contains:
Hydrocodone bitartrate ....5 mg
    (WARNING: May be habit-forming)
Guaifenesin ....100 mg

HOW SUPPLIED
Clear, fruit-flavored liquid which is alcohol-free, dye-free, sugar-free and corn products-free.
1 pint bottles—NDC 0225-0420-45
Unit Dose: 10 × 5 ml cups—NDC 0225-0420-75
Unit Dose: 100 × 5 ml cups—NDC 0225-0420-15

MOBIGESIC® Analgesic Tablets

(See PDR For Nonprescription Drugs)

MOBISYL® Analgesic Creme

(See PDR For Nonprescription Drugs)

PEN●KERA® Creme

(See PDR For Nonprescription Drugs)

TOLFRINIC® Tablets   ℞
[tol-fren-ic]

Each tablet contains:
Ferrous fumarate ....600 mg
    (Provides elemental iron 200 mg)
Vitamin B₁₂ (cyanocobalamin) ....25 mcg
                            (anhydrous)
Ascorbic acid ....100 mg

HOW SUPPLIED
Dark brown, film-coated tablet with 225/105 on one side.
Bottles of 100—NDC 0225-0105-15

UNILAX® Softgel Capsules

(See PDR For Nonprescription Drugs)

Astra Pharmaceutical Products, Inc.
50 OTIS STREET
WESTBORO, MA 01581-4428

ASTRAMORPH™ PF   ℞
[ås'-trå-mörf"]
(morphine sulfate injection, USP) Preservative-Free

DESCRIPTION
Morphine is the most important alkaloid of opium and is a phenanthrene derivative . It is available as the sulfate, having the following structural formula:

7,8-Didehydro-4,5-epoxy-17-methyl-(5α,6α)-morphinan-3,6-diol sulfate (2:1)(salt), pentahydrate

Preservative-free ASTRAMORPH PF (Morphine Sulfate Injection, USP) is a sterile, pyrogen-free, isobaric solution free of antioxidants, preservatives or other potentially neurotoxic additives, and is intended for intravenous, epidural or intrathecal administration as a narcotic analgesic. Each milliliter contains morphine sulfate 0.5 mg or 1 mg (Warning: May Be Habit Forming) and sodium chloride 9 mg in Water for Injection. pH may be adjusted with hydrochloric acid to 2.5–6.0. Containers are sealed under nitrogen. Each container is intended for SINGLE USE ONLY. Discard any unused portion. DO NOT AUTOCLAVE.

CLINICAL PHARMACOLOGY
Morphine exerts its primary effects on the central nervous system and organs containing smooth muscle. Pharmacologic effects include analgesia, drowsiness, alteration in mood (euphoria), reduction in body temperature (at low doses), dose-related depression of respiration, interference with adrenocortical response to stress (at high doses), reduction in peripheral resistance with little or no effect on cardiac index and miosis.

Morphine, as other opioids, acts as an agonist interacting with stereo-specific and saturable binding sites/receptors in the brain, spinal cord and other tissues. These sites have been classified as μ receptors and are widely distributed throughout the central nervous system being present in highest concentration in the limbic system (frontal and temporal cortex, amygdala and hippocampus), thalamus, striatum, hypothalamus, midbrain and laminae I, II, IV and V of the dorsal horn in the spinal cord. It has been postulated that exogenously administered morphine exerts its analgesic effect, in part, by altering the central release of neurotransmitter from afferent nerves sensitive to noxious stimuli. Peripheral threshold or responsiveness to noxious stimuli is unaffected leaving monosynaptic reflexes such as the patellar or the Achilles tendon reflex intact.

Autonomic reflexes are not affected by epidural or intrathecal morphine, however morphine exerts spasmogenic effects on the gastrointestinal tract that result in decreased peristaltic activity.

Central nervous system effects of intravenously administered morphine sulfate are influenced by ability to cross the blood-brain barrier. The delay in the onset of analgesia following epidural or intrathecal injection may be attributed to its relatively poor lipid solubility (i.e., an oil/water partition coefficient of 1.42), and its slow access to the receptor sites. The hydrophilic character of morphine may also explain its retention in the CNS and its slow release into the systemic circulation, resulting in a prolonged effect.

Nausea and vomiting may be prominent and are thought to be the result of central stimulation of the chemoreceptor trigger zone. Histamine release is common; allergic manifestations of urticaria and, rarely, anaphylaxis may occur. Bronchoconstriction may occur either as an idiosyncratic reaction or from large dosages.

Approximately one-third of intravenous morphine is bound to plasma proteins. Free morphine is rapidly redistributed in parenchymatous tissues. The major metabolic pathway is through conjugation with glucuronic acid in the liver. Elimination half-life is approximately 1.5 to 2 hours in healthy volunteers. For intravenously administered morphine, 90% is excreted in the urine within 24 hours and traces are detectable in urine up to 48 hours. About 7–10% of administered morphine eventually appears in the feces as conjugated morphine.

Peak serum levels following epidural or intrathecal administration of ASTRAMORPH-PF are reached within 30 minutes in most subjects and decline to very low levels during the next 2 to 4 hours. The onset of action occurs in 15 to 60 minutes following epidural administration or intrathecal administration; analgesia may last up to 24 hours. Due to this extended duration of action, sustained pain relief can be provided with lower daily doses (by these two routes) than are usually required with intravenous or intramuscular morphine administration.

INDICATIONS AND USAGE
Preservative-free ASTRAMORPH PF is a systemic narcotic analgesic for administration by the intravenous, epidural or intrathecal routes. It is used for the management of pain not responsive to non-narcotic analgesics. Morphine sulfate, administered epidurally or intrathecally, provides pain relief for extended periods without attendant loss of motor, sensory or sympathetic function.

CONTRAINDICATIONS
ASTRAMORPH PF is contraindicated in those medical conditions which would preclude the administration of opioids by the intravenous route—allergy to morphine or other opiates, acute bronchial asthma, upper airway obstruction. Administration of morphine by the epidural or intrathecal route is contraindicated in the presence of infection at the injection site, anticoagulant therapy, bleeding diathesis, parenterally administered corticosteroids within a two week period or other concomitant drug therapy or medical condition which would contraindicate the technique of epidural or intrathecal analgesia.

WARNINGS
ASTRAMORPH PF administration should be limited to use by those familiar with the management of respiratory depression, and in the case of epidural or intrathecal administration, familiar with the techniques and patient management problems associated with epidural or intrathecal drug administration. Because epidural administration has been associated with lessened potential for immediate or late adverse effects than intrathecal administration, the epidural route should be used whenever possible. Rapid intravenous administration may result in chest wall rigidity.

FACILITES WHERE ASTRAMORPH PF IS ADMINISTERED MUST BE EQUIPPED WITH RESUSCITATIVE EQUIPMENT, OXYGEN, NALOXONE INJECTION, AND OTHER RESUSCITATIVE DRUGS. WHEN THE EPIDURAL OR INTRATHECAL ROUTE OF ADMINISTRATION IS EMPLOYED, PATIENTS MUST BE OBSERVED IN A FULLY EQUIPPED AND STAFFED ENVIRONMENT FOR AT LEAST 24 HOURS. SEVERE RESPIRATORY DEPRESSION UP TO 24 HOURS FOLLOWING EPIDURAL OR INTRATHECAL ADMINISTRATION HAS BEEN REPORTED.

Morphine sulfate may be habit forming. (See Drug Abuse and Dependence section).

PRECAUTIONS
General
Preservative-free ASTRAMORPH PF (Morphine Sulfate Injection, USP) should be administered with extreme caution in aged or debilitated patients, in the presence of increased intracranial/intraocular pressure and in patients with head injury. Pupillary changes (miosis) may obscure the course of intracranial pathology. Care is urged in patients who have a decreased respiratory reserve (e.g., emphysema, severe obesity, kyphoscoliosis).

Seizures may result from high doses. Patients with known seizure disorders should be carefully observed for evidence of morphine-induced seizure activity.

It is recommended that administration of ASTRAMORPH PF by the epidural or intrathecal routes be limited to the lumbar area. Intrathecal use has been associated with a higher incidence of respiratory depression than epidural use. Smooth muscle hypertonicity may result in biliary colic, difficulty in urination and possible urinary retention requiring catheterization. Consideration should be given to risks inherent in urethral catheterization, e.g., sepsis, when epidural or intrathecal administration is considered, especially in the perioperative period.

Elimination half-life may be prolonged in patients with reduced metabolic rates and with hepatic or renal dysfunction. Hence, care should be exercised in administering morphine in these conditions, particularly with repeated dosing.

Patients with reduced circulating blood volume, impaired myocardial function or on sympatholytic drugs should be observed carefully for orthostatic hypotension, particularly in transport.

Patients with chronic obstructive pulmonary disease and patients with acute asthmatic attack may develop acute respiratory failure with administration of morphine. Use in these patients should be reserved for those whose conditions require endotracheal intubation and respiratory support or control of ventilation.

Drug Interactions
Depressant effects of morphine are potentiated by either concomitant administration or in the presence of other CNS depressants such as alcohol, sedatives, antihistaminics or psychotropic drugs (e.g., MAO inhibitors, phenothiazines, butyrophenones and tricyclic antidepressants). Premedication or intra-anesthetic use of neuroleptics with morphine may increase the risk of respiratory depression.

Carcinogenesis, Mutagenesis, Impairment of Fertility
Studies of morphine sulfate in animals to evaluate the carcinogenic and mutagenic potential or the effect on fertility have not been conducted.

Pregnancy
Teratogenic effects—Pregnancy Category C
Animal reproduction studies have not been conducted with morphine sulfate. It is also not known whether morphine sulfate can cause fetal harm when administered to a pregnant woman or can affect reproduction capacity. Morphine sulfate should be given to a pregnant woman only if clearly needed.

Nonteratogenic effects
Infants born from mothers who have been taking morphine chronically may exhibit withdrawal symptoms.

Labor and Delivery
Intravenous morphine readily passes into the fetal circulation and may result in respiratory depression in the neonate. Naloxone and resuscitative equipment should be available for reversal of narcotic-induced respiratory depression in the neonate. In addition, intravenous morphine may reduce the strength, duration and frequency of uterine contraction resulting in prolonged labor.

Epidurally and intrathecally administered morphine readily passes into the fetal circulation and may result in respiratory depression of the neonate. Controlled clinical studies have shown that *epidural* administration has little or no effect on the relief of labor pain.

However, studies have suggested that in most cases 0.2 to 1 mg of morphine *intrathecally* provides adequate pain relief with little effect on the duration of first stage labor. The second stage labor, though, may be prolonged if the parturient is not encouraged to bear down. A continuous intravenous infusion of naloxone, 0.6 mg/hr. for 24 hours after intrathecal injection may be employed to reduce the incidence of potential side effects.

Nursing Mothers
Morphine is excreted in maternal milk. Effect on the nursing infant is not known.

Pediatric Use
Safety and effectiveness in children have not been established.

ADVERSE REACTIONS
The most serious side effect is respiratory depression. Because of delay in maximum CNS effect with intravenously administered drug (30 min), rapid administration may result in overdosing. Bolus administration by the epidural or intrathecal route may result in early respiratory depression due to direct venous redistribution of morphine to the respiratory centers in the brain. Late (up to 24 hours) onset of acute respiratory depression has been reported with administration by the epidural or intrathecal route and is believed to be the result of rostral spread. Reports of respiratory depression following intrathecal administration have been more frequent, but the dosage used in most of these cases has been considerably higher than that recommended. This depression may be severe and could require intervention (see Warnings and Overdosage sections). Even without clinical evidence of ventilatory inadequacy, a diminished CO_2 ventilation response may be noted for up to 22 hours following epidural or intrathecal administration.

While low doses of intravenously administered morphine have little effect on cardiovascular stability, high doses are excitatory, resulting from sympathetic hyperactivity and increase in circulating catecholamines. Excitation of the central nervous system resulting in convulsions may accompany high doses of morphine given intravenously. Dysphoric reactions may occur and toxic psychoses have been reported. Epidural or intrathecal administration is accompanied by a high incidence of pruritus which is dose related but not confined to site of administration. Nausea and vomiting are frequently seen in patients following morphine administration. Urinary retention which may persist for 10–20 hours following single epidural or intrathecal administration has been reported in approximately 90% of males. Incidence is somewhat lower in females. Patients may require catheterization (see Precautions). Pruritus, nausea/vomiting and urinary retention frequently can be alleviated by the intravenous administration of low doses of naloxone (0.2 mg). Tolerance and dependence to chronically administered morphine, by whatever route, is known to occur (see Drug Abuse and Dependence section).

Miscellaneous side effects include constipation, headache, anxiety, depression of cough reflex, interference with thermal regulation and oliguria. Evidence of histamine release such as urticaria, wheals and/or local tissue irritation may occur.

In general, side effects are amenable to reversal by narcotic antagonists. NALOXONE INJECTION AND RESUSCITATIVE EQUIPMENT SHOULD BE IMMEDIATELY AVAILABLE FOR ADMINISTRATION IN CASE OF LIFE THREATENING OR INTOLERABLE SIDE EFFECTS.

DRUG ABUSE AND DEPENDENCE
Controlled Substance
Morphine sulfate is a Schedule II substance under the Drug Enforcement Administration classification.
Abuse
Morphine has recognized abuse and dependence potential.
Dependence
Cerebral and spinal receptors may develop tolerance/dependence independently, as a function of local dosage. Care must be taken to avert withdrawal in those patients who have been maintained on parenteral/oral narcotics when epidural or intrathecal administration is considered. Withdrawal may occur following chronic epidural or intrathecal administration, as well as the development of tolerance to morphine by these routes. (**See nonteratogenic effects under Pregnancy**).

OVERDOSAGE
Overdosage is characterized by respiratory depression with or without concomitant CNS depression. Since respiratory arrest may result either through direct depression of the respiratory center or as the result of hypoxia, primary attention should be given to the establishment of adequate respiratory exchange through provision of a patent airway and institution of assisted or controlled ventilation. The narcotic antagonist, naloxone hydrochloride, is a specific antidote. Naloxone hydrochloride (see package insert for full prescribing information) should be administered intravenously, simultaneously with respiratory resuscitation. *As the duration of effect of naloxone is considerably shorter than that of epidural or intrathecal morphine, repeated administration may be necessary.* Patients should be closely observed for evidence of renarcotization.
Note: *Respiratory depression may be delayed in onset up to 24 hours* following epidural or intrathecal administration. In painful conditions, reversal of narcotic effect may result in acute onset of pain and release of catecholamines. Careful administration of naloxone may permit reversal of side effects without affecting analgesia. Parenteral administration of narcotics in patients receiving epidural or intrathecal morphine may result in overdosage.

DOSAGE AND ADMINISTRATION
Preservative-free ASTRAMORPH PF (Morphine Sulfate Injection, USP) is intended for intravenous, epidural or intrathecal administration.
Intravenous Administration
Dosage
The initial dose of morphine should be 2 mg to 10 mg/70 kg of body weight. Patients under the age of 18; no information available.
Epidural Administration
ASTRAMORPH PF SHOULD BE ADMINISTERED EPIDURALLY ONLY BY PHYSICIANS EXPERIENCED IN THE TECHNIQUES OF EPIDURAL ADMINISTRATION AND WHO ARE THOROUGHLY FAMILIAR WITH THE LABELING. IT SHOULD BE ADMINISTERED ONLY IN SETTINGS WHERE ADEQUATE PATIENT MONITORING IS POSSIBLE. RESUSCITATIVE EQUIPMENT AND A SPECIFIC ANTAGONIST (NALOXONE HYDROCHLORIDE INJECTION) SHOULD BE IMMEDIATELY AVAILABLE FOR THE MANAGEMENT OF RESPIRATORY DEPRESSION AS WELL AS COMPLICATIONS WHICH MIGHT RESULT FROM INADVERTENT INTRATHECAL OR INTRAVASCULAR INJECTION. (NOTE: INTRATHECAL DOSAGE IS USUALLY 1/10 OF EPIDURAL DOSAGE). PATIENT MONITORING SHOULD BE CONTINUED FOR AT LEAST 24 HOURS AFTER EACH DOSE, SINCE DELAYED RESPIRATORY DEPRESSION MAY OCCUR.
Proper placement of a needle or catheter in the epidural space should be verified before ASTRAMORPH PF is injected. Acceptable techniques for verifying proper placement include: a) aspiration to check for absence of blood or cerebrospinal fluid, or b) administration of 5 mL (3 mL in obstetric patients) of 1.5% UNPRESERVED Lidocaine and Epinephrine (1:200,000) Injection and then observe the patient for lack of tachycardia (this indicates that vascular injection has *not* been made) and lack of sudden onset of segmental anesthesia (this indicates that intrathecal injection has *not* been made).
Epidural Adult Dosage
Initial injection of 5 mg in the lumbar region may provide satisfactory pain relief for up to 24 hours. If adequate pain relief is not achieved within one hour, careful administration of incremental doses of 1 to 2 mg at intervals sufficient to assess effectiveness may be given. No more than 10 mg/24 hr should be administered.
Thoracic administration has been shown to dramatically increase the incidence of early and late respiratory depression even at doses of 1 to 2 mg.
For continuous infusion an initial dose of 2 to 4 mg/24 hours is recommended. Further doses of 1 to 2 mg may be given if pain relief is not achieved initially.
Aged or debilitated patients-Administer with extreme caution (**see Precautions section**). Doses of less than 5 mg may provide satisfactory pain relief for up to 24 hours.

Epidural Pediatric Use
No information on use in pediatric patients is available.
Intrathecal Administration

> NOTE: INTRATHECAL DOSAGE IS USUALLY 1/10 THAT OF EPIDURAL DOSAGE

ASTRAMORPH PF SHOULD BE ADMINISTERED INTRATHECALLY ONLY BY PHYSICIANS EXPERIENCED IN THE TECHNIQUES OF INTRATHECAL ADMINISTRATION AND WHO ARE THOROUGHLY FAMILIAR WITH THE LABELING. IT SHOULD BE ADMINISTERED ONLY IN SETTINGS WHERE ADEQUATE PATIENT MONITORING IS POSSIBLE. RESUSCITATIVE EQUIPMENT AND A SPECIFIC ANTAGONIST (NALOXONE HYDROCHLORIDE INJECTION) SHOULD BE IMMEDIATELY AVAILABLE FOR THE MANAGEMENT OF RESPIRATORY DEPRESSION AS WELL AS COMPLICATIONS WHICH MIGHT RESULT FROM INADVERTENT INTRAVASCULAR INJECTION. PATIENT MONITORING SHOULD BE CONTINUED FOR AT LEAST 24 HOURS AFTER EACH DOSE, SINCE DELAYED RESPIRATORY DEPRESSION MAY OCCUR. RESPIRATORY DEPRESSION (BOTH EARLY AND LATE ONSET) HAS OCCURRED MORE FREQUENTLY FOLLOWING INTRATHECAL ADMINISTRATION.
Intrathecal Adult Dosage
A single injection of 0.2 to 1 mg may provide satisfactory pain relief for up to 24 hours. (**CAUTION: THIS IS ONLY 0.4 TO 2 ML OF THE 0.5 MG/ML POTENCY OR 0.2 to 1 ML OF THE 1 MG/ML POTENCY OF ASTRAMORPH PF). DO NOT INJECT INTRATHECALLY MORE THAN 2 ML OF THE 0.5 MG/ML POTENCY OR 1 ML OF THE 1 MG/ML POTENCY. USE IN THE LUMBAR AREA ONLY IS RECOMMENDED.** Repeated intrathecal injections of ASTRAMORPH PF are not recommended. A constant intravenous infusion of naloxone hydrochloride, 0.6 mg/hr, for 24 hours after intrathecal injection may be used to reduce the incidence of potential side effects.
Aged or debilitated patients-Administer with extreme caution (**see Precautions section**). A lower dosage is usually satisfactory.
Repeat Dosage
If pain recurs, alternative routes of administraion should be considered, since experience with repeated doses of morphine by the intrathecal route is limited.
Intrathecal Pediatric Use
No information on use in pediatric patients is available. Parenteral drug products should be inspected for particulate matter and discoloration prior to administration, whenever solution and container permit.

HOW SUPPLIED
The following strengths and container types of ASTRAMORPH PF are available:
(.05 mg/mL)
NDC 0186-1159-03 — 2 mL (1 mg) Ampule, Boxes of 10
NDC 0186-1150-02 — 10 mL (5 mg) Ampule, Boxes of 5
NDC 0186-1152-12 — 10 mL (5 mg) Single Dose Vial, Astra E-Z OFF™ vial closure Boxes of 5
(1 mg/mL)
NDC 0186-1160-03 — 2 mL (2 mg) Ampule, Boxes of 10
NDC 0186-1151-02 — 10 mL (10 mg) Ampule, Boxes of 5
NDC 0186-1153-12 — 10 mL (10 mg) Single Dose Vial, Astra E-Z OFF™ vial closure Boxes of 5
Storage
Protect from light. Store in carton at controlled room temperature, 15° to 30° C (59°F to 86°F) until ready to use. ASTRAMORPH PF contains no preservative. **DISCARD ANY UNUSED PORTION. DO NOT AUTOCLAVE.** Do not use the Injection if darker than pale yellow or if discolored in any other way, or if it contains a precipitate.
Caution: Federal law prohibits dispensing without prescription.
021865R02 — Rev. 11/88(2)

ATROPINE SULFATE ℞
[ā'trow-peen]
Injection, USP
0.1 mg/ml
Adult Strength

(For details of indications, dosage and administration, precautions, and adverse reactions, see circular in package.)

HOW SUPPLIED
Prefilled syringes equipped with 21 g 15/16″ needle:
5 ml (0.5 mg) NDC 0186-0648-01
10 ml (1 mg) NDC 0186-0649-01
Solution should be stored at controlled room temperature 15°–30°C (59°–86°F)
021880R00 — Iss. 1/87

BRETYLIUM TOSYLATE INJECTION ℞
For Intramuscular or Intravenous Use

For details of indications, dosage and administration, precautions, and adverse reactions, see circular in package.

HOW SUPPLIED
NDC 0186-1131-04 10 mL single dose vial
NDC 0186-0663-01 10 mL syringe
Each unit contains 500 mg bretylium tosylate in Water for Injection, USP. The pH is adjusted, when necessary with dilute hydrochloric acid and/or sodium hydroxide. Sterile, non-pyrogenic.
021864R02 — 5/87(2)

10% CALCIUM CHLORIDE ℞
[cal'cium chlor'ide]
Injection, USP
1 gram (100 mg/ml)
27.3 mg (1.4 mEq) Ca++/ml
2.04 mOsm/ml (calc.)
A Hypertonic Solution for Intravenous Injection

Caution: This solution must not be injected intramuscularly or subcutaneously.

(For details of indications, dosage and administration, precautions, and adverse reactions, see circular in package.)

HOW SUPPLIED
10% Calcium Chloride Injection, USP is supplied as follows:
NDC 0186-1166-04 10 ml single dose vials in packages of 25.
NDC 0186-0651-01 10 ml prefilled syringes with 21 g 15/16″ needle.
The solution should be stored at controlled room temperature 15°–30°C (59°–86°F).
021882R00 — Iss. 1/87

10% CALCIUM GLUCONATE ℞
[cal'cium glu'con-ate]
Injection, USP
0.465 mEq/mL
0.7 mOsm/mL (calculated)
For Intravenous Use Only

(For details of indications, dosage and administration, precautions, and adverse reactions, see circular in package.)

HOW SUPPLIED
Calcium Gluconate USP, 10% is supplied in the following forms:
NDC 0186-1172-04 10 mL Single Dose Vial in packages of 25
NDC 0186-0655-01 10 mL Syringe in packages of 10
Store at controlled room temperature 15°–30°C (59°–86°F).
Note: Supersaturated solutions are prone to supersaturation. See PRECAUTIONS for instructions for dissolving crystals.
021706R00 — Rev. 7/88

CLINDAMYCIN PHOSPHATE INJECTION, USP ℞
[klin"dah-mī'sin]
Sterile Solution
For Intramuscular and Intravenous Use

> **WARNING**
> Clindamycin therapy has been associated with severe colitis which may end fatally. Therefore, it should be reserved for serious infections where less toxic antimicrobial agents are inappropriate, as described in the Indications Section. It should not be used in patients with nonbacterial infections, such as most upper respiratory tract infections. Studies indicate a toxin(s) produced by *Clostridia* is one primary cause of antibiotic associated colitis. Cholestyramine and colestipol resins have been shown to bind the toxin *in vitro*. See WARNINGS section. The colitis is usually characterized by severe, persistent diarrhea and severe abdominal cramps and may be associated with the passage of blood and mucus. Endoscopic examination may reveal pseudomembranous colitis. Stool culture for *Clostridium difficile* and stool assay for *C. difficile* toxin may be helpful diagnostically.
> When significant diarrhea occurs, the drug should be discontinued or, if necessary, continued only with close observation of the patient. Large bowel endoscopy has been recommended.
> Antiperistaltic agents such as opiates and diphenoxylate with atropine may prolong and/or worsen the condition. Vancomycin has been found to be effective in the treatment of antibiotic associated pseudomembranous colitis produced by *Clostridium difficile*. The usual adult

Continued on next page

Astra—Cont.

dose is 500 milligrams to 2 grams of vancomycin orally per day in three to four divided doses administered for 7 to 10 days. Cholestyramine or colestipol resins bind vancomycin *in vitro*. If both a resin and vancomycin are to be administered concurrently, it may be advisable to separate the time of administration of each drug. Diarrhea, colitis, and pseudomembranous colitis have been observed to begin up to several weeks following cessation of therapy with clindamycin.

(For details of indications, dosage and administration, precautions, and adverse reactions, see circular in package.)

HOW SUPPLIED

Each mL of Clindamycin Phosphate Injection, USP contains clindamycin phosphate equivalent to 150 mg clindamycin; 0.5 mg disodium edetate; 9.45 mg benzyl alcohol added as preservative. When necessary, pH is adjusted with sodium hydroxide and/or hydrochloric acid. Clindamycin Phosphate Injection, USP is available in the following packages:

2 mL vials	NDC 0186-1450-04 Boxes of 25
4 mL vials	NDC 0186-1451-04 Boxes of 25
6 mL vials	NDC 0186-1452-04 Boxes of 25
60 mL Pharmacy Bulk Package	NDC 0186-1453-01 Box of 1

Store at controlled room temperature 15°–30°C(59°–86°F).
Caution: Federal law prohibits dispensing without prescription.
021898R00   Iss. 6/88

50% DEXTROSE   ℞

[dex'trose]
Injection, USP
Concentrated Dextrose
For Intravenous
Administration

NOTE: This solution is hypertonic—see Warnings and Precautions

(For details of indications, dosage and administration, precautions, and adverse reactions, see circular in package.)

HOW SUPPLIED

Dextrose Injection USP, 50% is supplied as follows:
50 ml Prefilled Syringe with 19 g $^{15}/_{16}$″ needle, NDC 0186-0654-01
The solution should be stored at controlled room temperature 15°–30° (59°–86°F).
021857R01   Rev. 7/88

DOPAMINE HCl Injection, USP   ℞

[dó-pa-mean]

(For details of indications, dosage and administration, precautions, and adverse reactions, see circular in package.)

HOW SUPPLIED

Dopamine HCl 200 mg is supplied in the following forms:
  Ampule—5 ml (40 mg/ml) NDC 0186-1050-03
  Single Dose Vial—5 ml (40 mg/ml) NDC 0186-1010-13
  Additive Syringe—5 ml (40 mg/ml) NDC 0186-0638-01
Dopamine HCl 400 mg is supplied in the following forms:
  Ampule   —5 ml (80 mg/ml) NDC 0186-1051-03
          —10 ml (40 mg/ml) NDC 0186-1055-03
  Single Dose Vial—5 ml (80 mg/ml) NDC 0186-1012-13
  Additive Syringe—5 ml (80 mg/ml) NDC 0186-0641-01
          —10 ml (40 mg/ml) NDC 0186-0639-01
Dopamine HCl 800 mg is supplied in the following forms:
  Ampule—5 ml (160 mg/ml) NDC 0186-1052-03
  Single Dose Vial—5 ml (160 mg/ml) NDC 0186-1014-13
  Additive Syringe—5 ml (160 mg/ml) NDC 0186-0642-01
Packages are color coded according to the total dosage content; 200 mg coded blue/white, 400 mg coded green/white and 800 mg coded yellow/white.

Store at controlled room temperature 15°–30°C (59°–86°F). Protect from light.
Avoid contact with alkalies (including sodium bicarbonate), oxidizing agents, or iron salts.
NOTE: Do not use the Injection if it is darker than slightly yellow or discolored in any other way.
021861R03   Rev. 4/86 (3)

DROPERIDOL INJECTION, USP   ℞
FOR INTRAVENOUS OR INTRAMUSCULAR USE ONLY

(For details of indications, dosage and administration, precautions, and adverse reactions, see circular in package.)

HOW SUPPLIED

Droperidol injection is available as:
Ampules, 2.5 mg/mL
2 mL, (5 mg/2 mL),   box of 10   NDC 0186-1220-03
5 mL, (12.5 mg/5 mL),   box of 10   NDC 0186-1221-03
Single Dose Vials, 2.5 mg/mL
2 mL, (5 mg/2 mL),   box of 10   NDC 0186-1226-13
5 mL, (12.5 mg/5 mL),   box of 10   NDC 0186-1227-13
Multiple Dose Vials, 2.5 mg/mL
10 mL,   box of 1   NDC 0186-1224-12
PROTECT FROM LIGHT, STORE AT CONTROLLED ROOM TEMPERATURE 15°–30°C (59°–86°F).
021879R02   9/88(2)

DURANEST®   ℞
[dur'a-nest]
(etidocaine hydrochloride)
Injections for infiltration and nerve block

DESCRIPTION

Duranest (etidocaine HCl) Injections are sterile aqueous solutions that contain a local anesthetic agent and are administered parenterally by injection. See INDICATIONS AND USAGE for specific uses. The specific quantitative composition of each available solution is shown in Table 1. Duranest Injections contain etidocaine HCl, which is chemically designated as butanamide, N-(2,6-dimethylphenyl)-2-(ethylpropylamino)-, monohydrochloride and has the following structural formula:

Epinephrine is (-)-3, 4-Dihydroxy-α-[(methylamino) methyl] benzyl alcohol and has the following structural formula:

The pKa of etidocaine (7.74) is similar to that of lidocaine (7.86). However, etidocaine possesses a greater degree of lipid solubility and protein binding capacity than does lidocaine. Duranest Injections are sterile and, except for the 1.5% concentration, are available with or without epinephrine 1:200,000. Single dose containers of Duranest Injection without epinephrine may be reautoclaved if necessary.
See Table 1 below. Composition of available solutions.

CLINICAL PHARMACOLOGY

Mechanism of action: Etidocaine stabilizes the neuronal membrane by inhibiting the ionic fluxes required for the initiation and conduction of impulses, thereby effecting local anesthetic action.
Onset and duration of action: In vivo animal studies have shown that etidocaine has a rapid onset (3–5 minutes) and a prolonged duration of action (5–10 hours). Based on compara-

tive clinical studies of lidocaine and etidocaine, the anesthetic properties of etidocaine in man may be characterized as follows: Initial onset of sensory analgesia and motor blockade is rapid (usually 3–5 minutes) and similar to that produced by lidocaine. Duration of sensory analgesia is 1.5 to 2 times longer than that of lidocaine by the peridural route. The difference in analgesic duration between etidocaine and lidocaine may be even greater following peripheral nerve blockade than following central neural block. Duration of analgesia in excess of 9 hours is not infrequent when etidocaine is used for peripheral nerve blocks such as brachial plexus blockade. Etidocaine produces a profound degree of motor blockade and abdominal muscle relaxation when used for peridural analgesia.
Hemodynamics: Excessive blood levels may cause changes in cardiac output, total peripheral resistance and mean arterial pressure. With central neural blockade these changes may be attributable to block of autonomic fibers, a direct depressant effect on the local anesthetic agent on various components of the cardiovascular system, and/or the beta-adrenergic receptor stimulating action of epinephrine when present. The net effect is normally a modest hypotension when the recommended dosages are not exceeded.
Pharmacokinetics and metabolism: Information derived from diverse formulations, concentrations and usages reveals that etidocaine is completely absorbed following parenteral administration, its rate of absorption depending, for example, upon such factors as the site of administration and the presence or absence of a vasoconstrictor agent. Except for intravenous administration, the highest blood levels are obtained following intercostal nerve block and the lowest after subcutaneous administration.
The plasma binding of etidocaine is dependent on drug concentration, and the fraction bound decreases with increasing concentration. At 0.5–1.0 μL, 95% is bound to plasma protein.
Etidocaine crosses the blood-brain barrier and placental barriers, presumably by passive diffusion.
Etidocaine is metabolized rapidly by the liver, and metabolites and unchanged drug are excreted by the kidney. Biotransformation includes oxidative N-dealkylation, ring hydroxylation, cleavage of the amide linkage, and conjugation. To date, approximately 20 metabolites of etidocaine have been found in the urine. The percent of dose excreted as unchanged drug is less than 10%.
The mean elimination half-life of etidocaine following a bolus intravenous injection is about 2.5 hours. Because of the rapid rate at which etidocaine is metabolized, any condition that affects liver function may alter etidocaine kinetics. Renal dysfunction may not affect etidocaine kinetics but may increase the accumulation of metabolites.
Factors such as acidosis and the concomitant use of CNS stimulants and depressants affect the CNS levels of etidocaine required to produce overt systemic effects. In the rhesus monkey arterial blood levels of 4.5 μg/mL have been shown to be threshold for convulsive activity.

INDICATIONS AND USAGE

Duranest (etidocaine HCl) Solutions are indicated for infiltration anesthesia, peripheral nerve blocks (e.g., brachial plexus, intercostal, retrobulbar, ulnar, inferior alveolar), and central neural block (i.e., lumbar or caudal epidural blocks).

CONTRAINDICATIONS

Etidocaine is contraindicated in patients with a known history of hypersensitivity to local anesthetics of the amide type.

WARNINGS

DURANEST INJECTIONS FOR INFILTRATION AND NERVE BLOCK SHOULD BE EMPLOYED ONLY BY CLINICIANS WHO ARE WELL VERSED IN DIAGNOSIS AND MANAGEMENT OF DOSE-RELATED TOXICITY AND OTHER ACUTE EMERGENCIES THAT MIGHT ARISE FROM THE BLOCK TO BE EMPLOYED AND THEN ONLY AFTER ENSURING THE *IMMEDIATE* AVAILABILITY OF OXYGEN, OTHER RESUSCITATIVE DRUGS, CARDIOPULMONARY EQUIPMENT, AND THE PERSONNEL NEEDED FOR PROPER MANAGEMENT OF TOXIC REACTIONS AND RELATED EMERGENCIES (See also ADVERSE REACTIONS and PRECAUTIONS). DELAY IN PROPER MANAGEMENT OF DOSE-RELATED TOXICITY, UNDERVENTILATION FROM ANY CAUSE AND/OR ALTERED SENSITIVITY MAY LEAD TO THE DEVELOPMENT OF ACIDOSIS, CARDIAC ARREST AND, POSSIBLY, DEATH.
To avoid intravascular injection, aspiration should be performed before the local anesthetic solution is injected. The needle must be repositioned until no return of blood can be elicited by aspiration. Note, however, that the absence of blood in the syringe does not guarantee that intravascular injection has been avoided.
Local anesthetic solutions containing antimicrobial preservatives (e.g., methylparaben) should not be used for epidural anesthesia because the safety of these agents has not been

Table 1. Composition of Available Solutions

Product Identification			Formula			
Duranest (etidocaine HCl) Concentration %	Epinephrine Dilution (as the bitartrate)	pH	Sodium chloride (mg/mL)	Single Dose Vials/ Dental Cartridge Sodium metabisulfite (mg/mL)	Citric acid (mg/mL)	
1.0	None	4.0–5.0	7.1	None	—	
1.0	1:200,000	3.0–4.5	7.1	0.5	0.2	
1.5	1:200,000	3.0–4.5	6.2	0.5	0.2	

NOTE: pH of all solutions adjusted with sodium hydroxide or hydrochloric acid. Duranest dental cartridges are only available as 1.5% solution with epinephrine 1:200,000 established with regard to intrathecal injection, either intentional or accidental.

Vasopressor agents administered for the treatment of hypotension related to caudal or other epidural blocks should not be used in the presence of ergot-type oxytocic drugs, since severe persistent hypertension and even rupture of cerebral blood vessels may occur.

Duranest with epinephrine solutions contain sodium metabisulfite, a sulfite that may cause allergic-type reactions including anaphylactic symptoms and life-threatening or less severe asthmatic episodes in certain susceptible people. The overall prevalence of sulfite sensitivity in the general population is unknown and probably low. Sulfite sensitivity is seen more frequently in asthmatic than in nonasthmatic people.

PRECAUTIONS

General: The safety and effectiveness of etidocaine depend on proper dosage, correct technique, adequate precautions, and readiness for emergencies. Standard textbooks should be consulted for specific techniques and precautions for various regional anesthetic procedures. Resuscitative equipment, oxygen, and other resuscitative drugs should be available for immediate use (See WARNINGS and ADVERSE REACTIONS.) The lowest dosage that results in effective anesthesia should be used to avoid high plasma levels and serious adverse effects. Syringe aspirations should also be performed before and during each supplemental injection when using indwelling catheter techniques. During the administration of epidural anesthesia, it is recommended that a test dose be administered initially and that the patient be monitored for central nervous system toxicity and cardiovascular toxicity, as well as for signs of unintended intrathecal administration, before proceeding. When clinical conditions permit, consideration should be given to employing local anesthetic solutions that contain epinephrine for the test dose because circulatory changes compatible with epinephrine may also serve as a warning sign of unintended intravascular injection. An intravascular injection is still possible even if aspirations for blood are negative. Repeated doses of etidocaine may cause significant increases in blood levels with each repeated dose because of slow accumulation of the drug or its metabolites. Tolerance to elevated blood levels varies with the status of the patient. Debilitated, elderly patients, acutely ill patients, and children should be given reduced doses commensurate with their age and physical condition. Etidocaine should also be used with caution in patients with severe shock or heart block.

Lumbar and caudal epidural anesthesia should be used with extreme caution in persons with the following conditions: existing neurological disease, spinal deformities, septicemia and severe hypertension.

Local anesthetic solutions containing a vasoconstrictor should be used cautiously and in carefully circumscribed quantities in areas of the body supplied by end arteries or having otherwise compromised blood supply. Patients with peripheral vascular disease and those with hypertensive vascular disease may exhibit exaggerated vasoconstrictor response. Ischemic injury or necrosis may result. Preparations containing a vasoconstrictor should be used with caution in patients during or following the administration of potent general anesthetic agents, since cardiac arrhythmias may occur under such conditions.

Careful and constant monitoring of cardiovascular and respiratory (adequacy of ventilation) vital signs and the patient's state of consciousness should be accomplished after each local anesthetic injection. It should be kept in mind at such times that restlessness, anxiety, tinnitus, dizziness, blurred vision, tremors, depression or drowsiness may be early warning signs of central nervous system toxicity.

Since amide-type local anesthetics are metabolized by the liver, Duranest Injections should be used with caution in patients with hepatic disease.

Patients with severe hepatic disease, because of their inability to metabolize local anesthetics normally, are a greater risk of developing toxic plasma concentrations. Duranest Injection should also be used with caution in patients with impaired cardiovascular function since they may be less able to compensate for functional changes associated with the prolongation of A-V conduction produced by these drugs.

Many drugs used during the conduct of anesthesia are considered potential triggering agents for familial malignant hyperthermia. Since it is not known whether amide-type local anesthetics may trigger this reaction and since the need for supplemental general anesthesia cannot be predicted in advance, it is suggested that a standard protocol for the management of malignant hyperthermia should be available. Early unexplained signs of tachycardia, tachypnea, labile blood pressure and metabolic acidosis may precede temperature elevation. Successful outcome is dependent on early diagnosis, prompt discontinuance of the suspect triggering agent(s) and institution of treatment, including oxygen therapy, indicated supportive measures and dantrolene (consult dantrolene sodium intravenous package insert before using).

Etidocaine should be used with caution in persons with known drug sensitivities. Patients allergic to para-aminobenzoic acid derivatives (procaine, tetracaine, benzocaine, etc.) have not shown cross sensitivity to etidocaine.

Use in the Head and Neck Area: Small doses of local anesthetics injected into the head and neck area, including retrobulbar, dental and stellate ganglion blocks, may produce adverse reactions similar to systemic toxicity seen with unintentional intravascular injections of larger doses. The injection procedures require the utmost care. Confusion, convulsions, respiratory depression and/or respiratory arrest, and cardiovascular stimulation or depression have been reported. These reactions may be due to intra-arterial injection of the local anesthetic with retrograde flow to the cerebral circulation. They may also be due to puncture of the dural sheath of the optic nerve during retrobulbar block with diffusion of any local anesthetic along the subdural space to the midbrain. Patients receiving these blocks should have their circulation and respiration monitored and be constantly observed. Resuscitative equipment and personnel for treating adverse reactions should be immediately available. Dosage recommendations should not be exceeded. (See DOSAGE AND ADMINISTRATION.)

Use in Ophthalmic Surgery: When local anesthetic solutions are employed for retrobulbar block, lack of corneal sensation should not be relied upon to determine whether or not the patient is ready for surgery since corneal sensation usually precedes clinically acceptable external ocular muscle akinesia.

Use in Dentistry: Because of the long duration of anesthesia, when Duranest 1.5% with epinephrine is used for dental injections, patients should be cautioned about the possibility of inadvertent trauma to tongue, lips and buccal mucosa and advised not to chew solid foods or test the anesthetized area by biting or probing.

Information for Patients: When appropriate, patients should be informed in advance that they may experience temporary loss of sensation and motor activity, usually in the lower half of the body, following proper administration of epidural anesthesia.

Clinically significant drug interactions: The administration of local anesthetic solutions containing epinephrine or norepinephrine to patients receiving monoamine oxidase inhibitors, tricyclic antidepressants or phenothiazines may produce severe, prolonged hypotension or hypertension. Concurrent use of these agents should generally be avoided. In situations when concurrent therapy is necessary, careful patient monitoring is essential.

Concurrent administration of vasopressor drugs (for the treatment of hypotension related to epidural blocks) and ergot-type oxytocic drugs may cause severe, persistent hypertension or cerebrovascular accidents.

Drug Laboratory test interactions: The intramuscular injection of etidocaine may result in an increase in creatine phosphokinase levels. Thus, the use of this enzyme determination, without isoenzyme separation, as a diagnostic test for the presence of acute myocardial infarction may be compromised by the intramuscular injection of etidocaine.

Carcinogenesis, mutagenesis, impairment of fertility: Studies of etidocaine in animals to evaluate the carcinogenic and mutagenic potential have not been conducted. Studies in rats at 1.7 times the maximum recommended human dose have revealed no impairment of fertility.

Use in Pregnancy: Teratogenic Effects. Pregnancy Category B. Reproduction studies have been performed in rats and rabbits at doses up to 1.7 times the human dose and have revealed no evidence of harm to the fetus caused by etidocaine. There are, however, no adequate and well-controlled studies in pregnant women. Animal reproduction studies are not always predictive of human response. General consideration should be given to this fact before administering etidocaine to women of childbearing potential, especially during early pregnancy when maximum organogenesis takes place.

Labor and delivery: Local anesthetics rapidly cross the placenta and when used for epidural, paracervical, pudendal or caudal block anesthesia, can cause varying degrees of maternal, fetal and neonatal toxicity. (See CLINICAL PHARMACOLOGY—Pharmacokinetics). The incidence and degree of toxicity depend upon the procedure performed, the type and amount of drug used, and the technique of drug administration. Adverse reactions in the parturient, fetus and neonate involve alterations of the central nervous system, peripheral vascular tone and cardiac function.

Maternal hypotension has resulted from regional anesthesia. Local anesthetics produce vasodilation by blocking sympathetic nerves. Elevating the patient's legs and positioning her on her left side will help prevent decreases in blood pressure. The fetal heart rate also should be monitored continuously and electronic fetal monitoring is highly advisable.

Epidural anesthesia may alter the forces of parturition through changes in uterine contractility or maternal expulsive efforts. Because Duranest Injection may produce profound motor block, it is not recommended for epidural anesthesia in normal delivery. Duranest Injection is, however, recommended for epidural anesthesia when caesarian section is to be performed.

The use of some local anesthetic drug products during labor and delivery may be followed by diminished muscle strength and tone for the first day or two of life. The long-term significance of these observations is unknown.

Fetal bradycardia may occur in 20 to 30 percent of patients receiving paracervical nerve block anesthesia with the amide-type local anesthetics and may be associated with fetal acidosis. Fetal heart rate should always be monitored during paracervical anesthesia. The physician should weigh the possible advantages against risks when considering paracervical block in prematurity, toxemia of pregnancy, and fetal distress. Careful adherence to recommended dosage is of the utmost importance in obstetrical paracervical block. Failure to achieve adequate analgesia with recommended doses should arouse suspicion of intravascular or fetal intracranial injection. Cases compatible with unintended fetal intracranial injection of local anesthetic solution have been reported following intended paracervical or pudendal block or both. Babies so affected present with unexplained neonatal depression at birth, which correlates with high local anesthetic serum levels, and often manifest seizures within six hours. Prompt use of supportive measures combined with forced urinary excretion of the local anesthetic has been used successfully to manage this complication. Case reports of maternal convulsions and cardiovascular collapse following use of some local anesthetics for paracervical block in early pregnancy (as anesthesia for elective abortion) suggest that systemic absorption under these circumstances may be rapid. There are inadequate data in support of safe and effective use of etidocaine for obstetrical or non-obstetrical paracervical block, therefore, such use is not recommended.

Nursing mothers: It is not known whether this drug is excreted in human milk. Because many drugs are excreted in human milk, caution should be exercised when etidocaine is administered to a nursing woman.

Pediatric use: No information is currently available on appropriate pediatric doses.

ADVERSE REACTIONS

Systemic: Adverse experiences following the administration of etidocaine are similar in nature to those observed with other amide local anesthetic agents. These adverse experiences are, in general, dose-related and may result from high plasma levels caused by excessive dosage, rapid absorption or unintended intravascular injection, or may result from a hypersensitivity, idiosyncrasy or diminished tolerance on the part of the patient. Serious adverse experiences are generally systemic in nature. The following types are those most commonly reported:

Central nervous system: CNS manifestations are excitatory and/or depressant and may be characterized by lightheadedness, nervousness, apprehension, euphoria, confusion, dizziness, drowsiness, tinnitus, blurred or double vision, vomiting, sensations of heat, cold or numbness, twitching, tremors, convulsions, unconsciousness, respiratory depression and arrest. The excitatory manifestations may be very brief or may not occur at all, in which case the first manifestation of toxicity may be drowsiness merging into unconsciousness and respiratory arrest.

Drowsiness following the administration of etidocaine is usually an early sign of a high blood level of the drug and may occur as a consequence of rapid absorption.

Cardiovascular system: Cardiovascular manifestations are usually depressant and are characterized by bradycardia, hypotension, and cardiovascular collapse, which may lead to cardiac arrest.

Allergic: Allergic reactions are characterized by cutaneous lesions, urticaria, edema or anaphylactoid reactions. Allergic reactions may occur as a result of sensitivity either to local anesthetic agents or to the methylparaben used as a preservative in multiple dose vials. The detection of sensitivity by skin testing is of doubtful value.

Neurologic: The incidences of adverse reactions associated with the use of local anesthetics may be related to the total dose of local anesthetic administered and are also dependent upon the particular drug used, the route of administration and the physical status of the patient.

In the practice of caudal or lumbar epidural block, occasional unintentional penetration of the subarachnoid space by the catheter may occur. Subsequent adverse effects may depend partially on the amount of drug administered subdurally. These may include spinal block of varying magnitude (including total spinal block), hypotension secondary to spinal block, loss of bladder and bowel control, and loss of perineal sensation and sexual function. Persistent motor, sensory and/or autonomic (sphincter control) deficit of some lower spinal segments with slow recovery (several months) or incomplete recovery have been reported in rare instances when caudal or lumbar epidural block has been attempted. Backache and headache have also been noted following use of these anesthetic procedures.

Continued on next page

Astra—Cont.

Dosage Form and Volume	Duranest Injection Concentration	Epinephrine Dilution (as the bitartrate)	pH	NDC Number
Single Dose Vials 30 mL	1.0%	None	4.0–5.0	0186-0820-01
	1.0%	1:200,000	3.0–4.5	0186-0825-01
20 mL	1.5%	1:200,000	3.0–4.5	0186-0836-03
Dental Cartridge 1.8 mL	1.5%	1:200,000	3.0–4.5	0186-0840-14

OVERDOSAGE

Acute emergencies from local anesthetics are generally related to high plasma levels encountered during therapeutic use of local anesthetics or to unintended subarachnoid injection of local anesthetic solution (see ADVERSE REACTIONS, WARNINGS, and PRECAUTIONS).

Management of local anesthetic emergencies: The first consideration is prevention, best accomplished by careful and constant monitoring of cardiovascular and respiratory vital signs and the patient's state of consciousness after each local anesthetic injection. At the first sign of change, oxygen should be administered.

The first step in the management of convulsions, as well as underventilation or apnea due to unintentional subarachnoid injection of drug solution, consists of immediate attention to the maintenance of a patent airway and assisted or controlled ventilation with oxygen and a delivery system capable of permitting immediate positive airway pressure by mask. Immediately after the institution of these ventilatory measures, the adequacy of the circulation should be evaluated, keeping in mind that drugs used to treat convulsions sometimes depress the circulation when administered intravenously. Should convulsions persist despite adequate respiratory support, and if the status of the circulation permits, small increments of an ultra-short acting barbiturate (such as thiopental or thiamylal) or a benzodiazepine (such as diazepam) may be administered intravenously. The clinician should be familiar, prior to use of local anesthetics, with these anticonvulsant drugs. Supportive treatment of circulatory depression may require administration of intravenous fluids and, when appropriate, a vasopressor as directed by the clinical situation (e.g., ephedrine).

If not treated immediately, both convulsions and cardiovascular depression can result in hypoxia, acidosis, bradycardia, arrhythmias and cardiac arrest. Underventilation or apnea due to unintentional subarachnoid injection of local anesthetic solution may produce these same signs and also lead to cardiac arrest if ventilatory support is not instituted. If cardiac arrest should occur, standard cardiopulmonary resuscitative measures should be instituted.

Endotracheal intubation, employing drugs and techniques familiar to the clinician, may be indicated, after initial administration of oxygen by mask, if difficulty is encountered in the maintenance of a patent airway or if prolonged ventilatory support (assisted or controlled) is indicated.

Dialysis is of negligible value in the treatment of acute overdosage with etidocaine.

The intravenous LD_{50} of etidocaine HCl in female mice is 7.6 (6.6–8.5) mg/kg and the subcutaneous LD_{50} is 112 (96–166) mg/kg.

DOSAGE AND ADMINISTRATION

As with all local anesthetic agents, the dose of Duranest (etidocaine HCl) Injection to be employed will depend upon the area to be anesthetized, the vascularity of the tissues, the number of neuronal segments to be blocked, the type of regional anesthetic technique, and the physical condition and tolerance of the individual patient.

The maximum dose to be employed as a single injection should be determined on the basis of the status of the patient and the type of regional anesthetic technique to be performed. Although single injections of 450 mg have been employed for regional anesthesia without adverse effects, at present it is strongly recommended that the maximal dose as a single injection should not exceed 400 mg (approximately 8.0 mg/kg or 3.6 mg/lb based on a 50 kg person) with epinephrine 1:200,000 and 300 mg (approximately 6 mg/kg and 2.7 mg/lb based on a 50 kg person) without epinephrine. Because etidocaine has been shown to disappear quite rapidly from blood, toxicity is influenced by rapidity of administration, and therefore slow injection in vascular areas is highly recommended. Incremental doses of Duranest Injection may be repeated at 2–3 hour intervals.

Caudal and lumbar epidural block: As a precaution against the adverse experiences sometimes observed following unintentional penetration of the subarachnoid space, a test dose of 2–5 mL should be administered at least 5 minutes prior to injecting the total volume required for a lumbar or caudal epidural block. The test dose should be repeated if the patient is moved in a manner that may have displaced the catheter. Epinephrine, if contained in the test dose (10–15μg have been suggested), may serve as a warning of unintentional intravascular injection. If injected into a blood vessel this amount of epinephrine is likely to produce a transient "epinephrine response" within 45 seconds, consisting of an increase in heart rate and systolic blood pressure, circumoral pallor, palpitations and nervousness in the unsedated patient. The sedated patient may exhibit only a pulse rate increase of 20 or more beats per minute for 15 or more seconds. Patients on beta-blockers may not manifest changes in heart rate, but blood pressure monitoring can detect an evanescent rise in systolic blood pressure. Adequate time should be allowed for onset of anesthesia after administration of each test dose. The rapid injection of a large volume of Duranest Injection through the catheter should be avoided, and when feasible fractional doses should be administered.

In the event of the known injection of a large volume of local anesthetic solution into the subarachnoid space after suitable resuscitation and if the catheter is in place, consider attempting the recovery of drug by draining a moderate amount of cerebrospinal fluid (such as 10 mL) through the epidural catheter.

Use in Dentistry: When used for local anesthesia in dental procedures the dosage of Duranest (etidocaine HCl) Injection depends on the physical status of the patient, the area of the oral cavity to be anesthetized, the vascularity of the oral tissues, and the technique of anesthesia. The least volume of solution that results in effective local anesthesia should be administered. For specific techniques and procedures of local anesthesia in the oral cavity, refer to standard textbooks.

Dosage requirements should be determined on an individual basis. In maxillary infiltration and/or inferior alveolar nerve block, initial dosages of 1.0–5.0 mL (½–2½ cartridges) of Duranest Injection 1.5% with epinephrine 1:200,000 are usually effective.

Aspiration is recommended since it reduces the possibility of intravascular injection, thereby keeping the incidence of side effects and anesthetic failures to a minimum.

The following dosage recommendations are intended as guides for the use of Duranest Injection in the average adult patient. As indicated previously, the dosage should be reduced for elderly or debilitated patients or patients with severe renal disease.

NOTE:

Parenteral drug products should be inspected visually for particulate matter and discoloration prior to administration whenever the solution and container permit. Solutions that are discolored and/or contain particulate matter should not be used.

[See table below left].

HOW SUPPLIED

[See table above].

Store at controlled room temperature 15°–30°C (59°–86°F).

021842R03   Rev.1/87(3)

DYCLONE® 0.5% and 1%   ℞

[*dié-clone*]

(dyclonine HCl)

Topical Solutions, U.S.P.

DESCRIPTION

Dyclone (dyclonine HCl) 0.5% and 1% Topical Solutions contain a local anesthetic agent and are administered topically. See INDICATIONS for specific uses.

Dyclone 0.5% and 1% Topical Solutions contain dyclonine HCl, which is chemically designated as 4'-butoxy-3-piperidinopropiophenone HCl. Dyclonine HCl is a white crystalline powder that is sparingly soluble in water and has the following structural formula:

COMPOSITIONS OF DYCLONE 0.5% AND 1% TOPICAL SOLUTIONS

Each ml of Dyclone 0.5% Solution contains dyclonine HCl, 5 mg.

Each ml of Dyclone 1% Solution contains dyclonine HCl, 10 mg.

Both solutions also contain chlorbutanol hydrous and sodium chloride, and the pH is adjusted to 3.5–5.0 by means of hydrochloric acid and/or sodium hydroxide.

CLINICAL PHARMACOLOGY

Dyclone Topical Solutions effect surface anesthesia when applied topically to mucous membranes. Effective anesthesia varies with different patients, but usually occurs from 2 to 10 minutes after application and persists for approximately 30 minutes.

INDICATIONS AND USAGE

Dyclone Topical Solutions are indicated for anesthetizing accessible mucous membranes (e.g., the mouth, pharynx, larynx, trachea, esophagus, and urethra) prior to various endoscopic procedures.

Dyclone 0.5% Topical Solution may also be used to block the gag reflex, to relieve the pain of oral ulcers or stomatitis and to relieve pain associated with ano-genital lesions.

CONTRAINDICATIONS

Dyclonine is contraindicated in patients known to be hypersensitive (allergic) to the local anesthetic or to other components of Dyclone Topical Solutions.

WARNINGS

IN ORDER TO MANAGE POSSIBLE ADVERSE REACTIONS, RESUSCITATIVE EQUIPMENT, OXYGEN AND OTHER RESUSCITATIVE DRUGS SHOULD BE IMMEDIATELY AVAILABLE WHENEVER LOCAL ANESTHETIC AGENTS, SUCH AS DYCLONINE, ARE ADMINISTERED TO MUCOUS MEMBRANES.

Dyclone Topical Solutions should not be injected into tissue or used in the eyes because of highly irritant properties.

Dyclone Topical Solutions should be used with extreme caution in the presence of sepsis or severely traumatized mucosa in the area of application since under such conditions there is the potential for rapid systemic absorption.

PRECAUTIONS

General: The safety and effectiveness of dyclonine depend on proper dosage, correct technique, adequate precautions, and readiness for emergencies (See WARNINGS and ADVERSE REACTIONS). The lowest dosage that results in effective anesthesia should be used to avoid high plasma levels and serious adverse effects. Repeated doses of dyclonine may cause significant increases in blood levels with each repeated dose because of slow accumulation of the drug or its metabolites. Tolerance to elevated blood levels varies with the status of the patient. Debilitated, elderly patients, acutely ill patients, and children should be given reduced

Table 2. Dosage Recommendations

PROCEDURE	Duranest HCl with epinephrine 1:200,000			PROCEDURE	Duranest HCl with epinephrine 1:200,000		
	Conc. (%)	Vol. (mL)	Total Dose (mg)		Conc. (%)	Vol. (mL)	Total Dose (mg)
Peripheral Nerve Block	1.0	5–40	50–400	Caudal	1.0	10–30	100–300
				Retrobulbar	1.0 or 1.5	2–4	20–60
Central Neural Block Lumbar Peridural				Maxillary Infiltration and/or Inferior Alveolar Nerve Block	1.5	1–5	15–75
Intraabdominal or Pelvic Surgery Lower Limb Surgery	1.0 or	10–30	100–300				
Caesarean Section	1.5	10–20	150–300				

doses commensurate with their age, weight and physical condition. Dyclonine should also be used with caution in patients with severe shock or heart block.

Dyclone Topical Solutions should be used with caution in persons with known drug sensitivities.

Information for Patients: When topical anesthetics are used in the mouth or throat, the patient should be aware that the production of topical anesthesia may impair swallowing and thus enhance the danger of aspiration. For this reason, food should not be ingested for 60 minutes following use of local anesthetic preparations in the mouth or throat area. This is particularly important in children because of their frequency of eating.

Numbness of the tongue or buccal mucosa may increase the danger of biting trauma. When Dyclone 0.5% Topical Solution is used to relieve the pain of oral ulcers or stomatitis which interferes with eating, patients should be warned about the risk of biting trauma before they accept this treatment; caution should be exercised in selecting food and eating. Following other uses in the mouth and throat area, food and/or chewing gum should not be used while the area is anesthetized.

Drug/Laboratory Test Interactions: Dyclone Topical Solutions should not be used in cystoscopic procedures following intravenous pyelography because an iodine precipitate occurs which interferes with visualization.

Carcinogenesis, mutagenesis, impairment of fertility: Studies of dyclonine in animals to evaluate the carcinogenic and mutagenic potential or the effect on fertility have not been conducted.

Use in Pregnancy: Teratogenic Effects:
Pregnancy Category C. Animal reproduction studies have not been conducted with dyclonine. It is also not known whether dyclonine can cause fetal harm when administered to a pregnant woman or can affect reproduction capacity. General consideration should be given to this fact before administering dyclonine to women of childbearing potential, especially during early pregnancy when maximum organogenesis takes place.

Nursing Mothers: It is not known whether this drug is excreted in human milk. Because many drugs are excreted in human milk, caution should be exercised when dyclonine is administered to a nursing woman.

Pediatric Use: Safety and effectiveness in children under the age of 12 have not been established.

ADVERSE REACTIONS

Adverse experiences following the administration of dyclonine are similar in nature to those observed with other local anesthetic agents. These adverse experiences are, in general, dose-related and may result from high plasma levels caused by excessive dosage or rapid absorption, or may result from a hypersensitivity, idiosyncrasy or diminished tolerance on the part of the patient. Serious adverse experiences are generally systemic in nature. The following types are those most commonly reported:

Central nervous system: CNS manifestations are excitatory and/or depressant and may be characterized by lightheadedness, nervousness, apprehension, euphoria, confusion, dizziness, drowsiness, tinnitus, blurred or double vision, vomiting, sensations of heat, cold or numbness, twitching, tremors, convulsions, unconsciousness, repiratory depression and arrest. The excitatory manifestations may be very brief or may not occur at all, in which case the first manifestation of toxicity may be drowsiness merging into unconsciousness and respiratory arrest.

Drowsiness following the administration of dyclonine is usually an early sign of a high blood level of the drug and may occur as a consequence of rapid absorption.

Cardiovascular system: Cardiovascular manifestations are usually depressant and are characterized by bradycardia, hypotension, and cardiovascular collapse, which may lead to cardiac arrest.

Allergic: Allergic reactions are characterized by cutaneous lesions, urticaria, edema or anaphylactoid reactions. Allergic reactions may occur as a result of sensitivity either to the local anesthetic agent or to the other ingredients used in this formulation. Allergic reactions, if they occur, should be managed by conventional means. The detection of sensitivity by skin testing is of doubtful value. Local reactions include irritation, stinging, urethritis with and without bleeding.

OVERDOSAGE

Acute emergencies from local anesthetics are generally related to high plasma levels encountered during therapeutic use of local anesthetics. (See ADVERSE REACTIONS, WARNINGS, and PRECAUTIONS.)

Management of local anesthetic emergencies: The first consideration is prevention, best accomplished by careful and constant monitoring of cardiovascular and respiratory vital signs and the patient's state of consciousness after each local anesthetic administration.

The first step in the management of convulsions consists of immediate attention to the maintenance of a patent airway and assisted or controlled ventilation with oxygen and a delivery system capable of permitting immediate positive air-

way pressure by mask. Immediately after the institution of these ventilatory measures, the adequacy of the circulation should be evaluated, keeping in mind that drugs used to treat convulsions sometimes depress the circulation when administered intravenously. Should convulsions persist despite adequate respiratory support, and if the status of the circulation permits, small increments of an ultra-short acting barbiturate (such as thiopental or thiamylal) or a benzodiazepine (such as diazepam) may be administered intravenously. The clinician should be familiar, prior to use of local anesthetics, with these anticonvulsant drugs. Supportive treatment of circulatory depression may require administration of intravenous fluids and, when appropriate, a vasopressor as directed by the clinical situation (e.g., ephedrine).

If not treated immediately, both convulsions and cardiovascular depression can result in hypoxia, acidosis, bradycardia, arrhythmias and cardiac arrest. If cardiac arrest should occur, standard cardiopulmonary resuscitative measures should be instituted.

The mean lethal dose (LD$_{50}$) of dyclonine HCl administered orally to female rats is 176 mg/kg and 90 mg/kg in female mice. Intraperitoneally the LD$_{50}$ in female rats is 31 mg/kg and 43 mg/kg in female mice.

DOSAGE AND ADMINISTRATION

As with all local anesthetics, the dosage varies and depends upon the area to be anesthetized, vascularity of the tissues, individual tolerance and the technique of anesthesia. The lowest dosage needed to provide effective anesthesia should be administered.

A maximum dose of 30 ml of 1% Dyclone Topical Solution (300 mg of dyclonine HCl) may be used, although satisfactory anesthesia is usually produced within the range of 4 to 20 ml. For specific techniques and procedures refer to standard textbooks.

Although as much as 300 mg of dyclonine HCl (as a 1% solution) have been tolerated, this dosage as a 0.5% solution has not been administered primarily because satisfactory anesthesia in endoscopic procedures can usually be produced by lesser amounts. For specific techniques for endoscopic procedures refer to standard textbooks.

PROCTOLOGY
Apply pledgets of cotton or sponges moistened with the Dyclone 0.5% Solution to postoperative wounds for the relief of discomfort and pain.

GYNECOLOGY
Apply Dyclone 0.5% Solution as wet compresses or as a spray to relieve the discomfort of episiotomy or perineorrhaphy wounds.

ONCOLOGY-RADIOLOGY
Apply Dyclone 0.5% Solution as a rinse or swab to inflamed or ulcerated mucous membrane of the mouth caused by antineoplastic chemotherapy or radiation therapy. In lesions of the esophagus, 5–15 ml of the anesthetic may be swallowed to relieve pain and allow more comfortable deglutition.

OTORHINOLARYNGOLOGY
To suppress the gag reflex and to facilitate examination of the posterior pharynx or larynx, apply Dyclone 0.5% Solution as a spray or gargle.

Dyclone 0.5% Solution may be applied as a rinse or swab to relieve the discomfort of aphthous stomatitis, herpetic stomatitis, or other painful oral lesions.

DENTISTRY
Dyclone 0.5% Topical Solution is useful to suppress the gag reflex in the positioning of x-ray films, making prosthetic impressions, and doing surgical procedures in the molar areas. It is also useful as a preinjection mucous membrane anesthetic or applied to the gums prior to scaling (prophylaxis). The anesthetic can be applied as a mouthwash or gargle and the excess spit out.

HOW SUPPLIED
Sterile, in one fluid ounce bottles, DYCLONE 0.5% TOPICAL SOLUTION (NDC 0186-3001-01) and DYCLONE 1% TOPICAL SOLUTION (NDC 0186-3002-01). Keep tightly closed. Store at controlled room temperature: 15°–30°C (59°–86°F). Avoid excessive heat (temperatures above 40°C (104°F). Subject to damage by freezing.
021859R01   Rev. 6/86

EPINEPHRINE   ℞
[ep-ē-nef'-rin]
Injection, USP
1:10,000 (0.1 mg/ml)
Adult Strength

(For details of indications, dosage and administration, precautions, and adverse reactions, see circular in package.)

HOW SUPPLIED
Epinephrine Injection USP, 1:10,000, is supplied in 10 mL prefilled syringes with a 21 g $^{15}/_{16}$" needle. (NDC 0186-0653-01). The solution should be stored at controlled room temper-

ature 15°–30°C (59°–86°F) and should be protected from light by storage in the original carton until use.
021883R00   Rev. 1/87

FENTANYL CITRATE* and DROPERIDOL   ℂ ℞
INJECTION
*WARNING (May be habit forming)
For INTRAVENOUS OR INTRAMUSCULAR USE ONLY

> The two components of Fentanyl Citrate and Droperidol Injection, fentanyl citrate and droperidol, have different pharmacologic actions. Before administering Fentanyl Citrate and Droperidol Injection, the user should become familiar with the special properties of each drug, particularly the widely differing durations of action.

(For details of indication, dosage and administration, precautions, and adverse reactions, see circular in package.)

HOW SUPPLIED
Each mL of Fentanyl Citrate and Droperidol Injection contains fentanyl citrate (WARNING: May be habit forming) equivalent to 0.05 mg (50 mcg) of fentanyl base, droperidol 2.5 mg and lactic acid to adjust pH and is available in the following dosage forms:
Ampules
NDC 0186-1230-03, 2 mL ampule in packages of 10
NDC 0186-1231-03, 5 mL ampule in packages of 10
Vials
NDC 0186-1232-13, 2 mL single dose vial in packages of 10
NDC 0186-1233-13, 5 mL single dose vial in packages of 10
(FOR INTRAVENOUS USE BY HOSPITAL PERSONNEL SPECIFICALLY TRAINED IN THE USE OF OPIOID ANALGESICS.)
PROTECT FROM LIGHT. STORE AT CONTROLLED ROOM TEMPERATURE 15°–30°C (59°–86°F).
021881R01   5/89(1)

FUROSEMIDE INJECTION, USP   ℞
[fū "rŏ'sĕ-mīde]
10 mg/mL

PROTECT FROM LIGHT ● DO NOT USE IF THE SOLUTION IS DISCOLORED ● STORE AT CONTROLLED ROOM TEMPERATURE

> WARNING: Furosemide is a potent diuretic which if given in excessive amounts can lead to a profound diuresis with water and electrolyte depletion. Therefore, careful medical supervision is required, and the individual dose and the dosage schedule have to be adjusted to each patient's needs.
> (See under "DOSAGE AND ADMINISTRATION")

(For details of indications, dosage, and administration, precautions, and adverse reactions, see circular in package.)

HOW SUPPLIED
Furosemide injection, USP, 10 mg/mL is supplied in the following forms:
Single Dose Vials:
2 mL (20 mg), 25 per package, NDC 0186-1114-13
4 mL (40 mg), 25 per package, NDC 0186-1115-13
8 mL (80 mg), 25 per package, NDC 0186-1116-12
10 mL (100 mg), 25 per package, NDC 0186-1117-12
Prefilled Syringes:
4 mL (40 mg), NDC 0186-0635-01
10 mL (100 mg), NDC 0186-0636-01
Syringes supplied with 21 gauge × $^{15}/_{16}$" needle.
All solutions should be stored at controlled room temperature 15°–30°C (59°–86°F) and should be protected from light. Do not use if the solution is discolored.
021877R01   4/88(1)

Continued on next page

Astra—Cont.

HEMOPAD®   ℞
[hē'mō-păd]
Absorbable Collagen Hemostat

DESCRIPTION
HEMOPAD® Absorbable Collagen Hemostat is a purified bovine collagen. The material, prepared as a textured pad, is sterile, nonpyrogenic, and absorbable. Hemostatic activity, which is an inherent property of collagen, is largely dependent on the basic helical structure of this protein. The helical structure of native collagen is preserved during the manufacture of HEMOPAD Hemostat. When collagen comes into contact with blood, platelets aggregate on the collagen and release coagulation factors which, together with plasma factors result in the formation of fibrin, and finally in the formation of a clot.

INDICATIONS
HEMOPAD is indicated in surgical procedures (other than in neurological, urological and ophthalmological surgery) for use as an adjunct to hemostasis when control of bleeding by ligature or other conventional methods is ineffective or impractical.

CONTRAINDICATIONS
HEMOPAD is contraindicated in the closure of skin incisions as it may interfere with the healing of skin edges. This interference is due to simple mechanical interposition of dry collagen and not due to any intrinsic interference with wound healing.
HEMOPAD is contraindicated on bone surfaces to which prosthetic materials are to be attached with methylmethacrylate adhesives. It has been reported with another absorbable collagen hemostat, that by filling porosities of cancellous bone, collagen may reduce the bonding strength of methylmethacrylate.

WARNINGS
HEMOPAD is inactivated by autoclaving. It should not be resterilized. As with any foreign substance, use in contaminated wounds may enhance infection.
HEMOPAD should not be used in instances of pumping arterial hemorrhage.
HEMOPAD should not be used where blood or other fluids have pooled or in cases where the point of hemorrhage is submerged. HEMOPAD will not act as a tampon or plug in a bleeding site nor will it close off an area of blood collecting behind a tampon.
Only the amount of HEMOPAD necessary to provide hemostasis should be used. The long-term effects of leaving HEMOPAD *in situ* are unknown. Opened, unused HEMOPAD should be discarded because it cannot be resterilized.

PRECAUTIONS
As with other hemostatic agents, it is not recommended that HEMOPAD be left in an infected nor contaminated space, nor is it recommended for use in persons known to be sensitive to material of bovine origin. When placed into cavities or closed spaces, care should be exercised to avoid overpacking HEMOPAD as it may absorb fluid and expand and press against neighboring structures.
Safety of this product has not been established in children and pregnant women: therefore, HEMOPAD should only be used when benefit to risk clearly warrants its use.
HEMOPAD is not intended to be used to treat systemic coagulation disorders.

ADVERSE REACTIONS
HEMOPAD is a collagen product. Although several types of post-operative complications were observed in HEMOPAD treated patients, none were attributed to HEMOPAD by the investigator. Adverse reactions reported for other collagen hemostats include hematoma, potentiation of infection, wound dehiscence, inflammation and edema. Other reported adverse reactions that may be related to the use of collagen hemostats include adhesion formation, allergic reaction, foreign body reaction and subgaleal seroma (in a single case). The use of microfibrillar collagen in dental extraction sockets has been reported to increase the incidence of alveolalgia. The possibility that all of the above reactions may occur with HEMOPAD cannot be excluded.

ADMINISTRATION
HEMOPAD is applied directly to the bleeding surface with pressure. HEMOPAD can be cut to size. The amount needed and the period of time necessary to apply pressure will vary with the type and amount of bleeding to be controlled. Hemostasis time depends upon the type of surgery and degree of pretreatment bleeding. It usually occurred between 2 to 6 minutes with HEMOPAD.
HEMOPAD maintains its integrity in the presence of blood and is not dispersed when wet. It is easily removed from the site following hemostatsis. It is most effective when used dry. HEMOPAD may be left *in situ* whenever necessary. However, the surgeon, at his discretion, should remove any excess of HEMOPAD prior to wound closure. Animal implant studies have demonstrated that absorption and tissue reaction to HEMOPAD are similar to those observed with another absorbable collagen hemostatic agent.

CLINICAL STUDIES
The safety, effectiveness and handling characteristics of HEMOPAD Collagen Absorbable Hemostat were evaluated in a variety of surgical procedures. The average time to hemostasis for HEMOPAD was 4.4 minutes. Passive Hemagglutination Assay (PHA) and Enzyme-Linked Immunoabsorbent Assay (ELISA) methods have been used to evaluate the immunological potential for HEMOPAD to produce antibodies in animals. These assays revealed little if any elevation of antibody titers in HEMOPAD treated animals while in animals treated with a collagen control hemostat, mild elevation of antibodies occurred. The handling properties of HEMOPAD were judged superior to those of the collagen control hemostat.

HOW SUPPLIED
HEMOPAD is supplied in a nonwoven form in peelable plastic pouches in the following sizes:
2.5cm × 5cm IN BOXES OF 10
            PRODUCT No. 0166-2001-00
5cm × 8cm IN BOXES OF 10
            PRODUCT No. 0186-2002-00
8cm × 10cm IN BOXES OF 10
            PRODUCT No. 0186-2003-00
The sterility of the product is guaranteed unless the individual envelope is damaged or opened.
CAUTION: Federal (U.S.A.) law restricts this device to sale, distribution, and use by or on the order of a physician.
HEMOPAD is manufactured by DATASCOPE CORP.
021873 R00   *Rev. 12/87*

HYDROMORPHONE HCL INJECTION   ℂ
(For details of indications, dosages and administration, precautions, and adverse reactions, see circular in package.)
HOW SUPPLIED
2 mg/mL—20 mL multiple dose vials—NDC 0186-1309-01
Storage: Store at 59°–86°F (15°–30°C). Protect from light.
021888R00   Iss. 12/87

MAGNESIUM SULFATE INJECTION, USP   ℞
(For details of indications, dosages and administration, precautions, and adverse reactions, see circular in package.)
[See table below left].
No preservative added. Unused portion of container should be discarded. Use only if solution is clear, and seal intact.
021874R01   2/88

MANNITOL Injection, USP, 25%   ℞
[man-ĭ-tall]
For Intravenous Injection; or
Urologic Irrigation

For details of indications, dosage and administration, precautions, and adverse reactions, see circular in package.

HOW SUPPLIED
Mannitol Injection USP, 25% is a sterile solution supplied in single dose containers as follows:
NDC 0186-1168-04: 50 ml vials, 25 vials per package
NDC 0186-0652-01: 50 ml syringes, 10 syringes per package
CAUTION: Federal law prohibits dispensing without prescription.
Store at controlled room temperature 15°–30°C (59°–86°F).
Note: Crystals may form in mannitol solutions especially if solutions are chilled. See PRECAUTIONS to dissolve the crystals.
021855R01   Rev. 5/86(1)

MEPERIDINE HCl INJECTION, USP   ℂ ℞
(For details of indications, dosage and administration, precautions, and adverse reactions, see circular in package.)
HOW SUPPLIED
Meperidine Hydrochloride Injection, USP is available as:
Multiple Dose Vials
NDC 0186-1283-01   100 mg/mL,   20 mL vial, box of 1
NDC 0186-1284-01   50 mg/mL,   30 mL vial, box of 1
Store at controlled room temperature 15°–30°C (59°–86°F).
021889R02   Iss. 2/89(2)

METHOTREXATE SODIUM INJECTION, USP   ℞
NOTE
See Box "WARNINGS".
(For details of indications, dosages and administration, precautions, and adverse reactions, see circular in package.)

HOW SUPPLIED
Methotrexate Sodium Injection Preservative-Free Solution 25 mg/mL. Single use vials only.
NDC 0186-1420-13   2 mL (50 mg)
NDC 0186-1421-13   4 mL (100 mg)
NDC 0186-1422-12   10 mL (250 mg)
NDC 0186-1423-04   10 mL (250 mg)
Manufactured by Pharmachemie BV Haarlem, Holland
021894R01   8/88

MORPHINE SULFATE INJECTION, USP   ℂ
(morphine sulfate injection, USP)

(For details of indications, dosage and administration, precautions, and adverse reactions, see circular in package.)
HOW SUPPLIED
Morphine Sulfate Injection, USP, is available in the following dosage strengths:
8 mg (⅛ gr.)/mL, 2 mL (1 mL fill); Ampule
            NDC 0186-1155-03, Boxes of 25
10 mg (⅙ gr.)/mL, 2 mL (1 mL fill); Ampule
            NDC 0186-1156-03, Boxes of 25
15 mg (¼ gr.)/mL, 2 mL (1 mL fill); Ampule
            NDC 0186-1157-03, Boxes of 25
8 mg (⅛ gr.)/mL, 2 mL (1 mL fill); Vial
            NDC 0186-1138-13, Boxes of 25
10 mg (⅙ gr.)/mL, 2 mL (1 mL fill); Vial
            NDC 0186-1139-13, Boxes of 25
15 mg (¼ gr.)/mL, 2 mL (1 mL fill); Vial
            NDC 0186-1140-13, Boxes of 25
15 mg (¼ gr.)/mL, 20 mL Multiple dose vial;
            NDC 0186-1158-02, Boxes of 5
Protect from light. Store at controlled room temperature 15°–30°C (59°–86°F).
021869R03   Iss. Rev. 11/87 (3)

NDC No. 0186-	Magnesium Sulfate Heptahydrate Concentration	Container Type	Fill Volume	Magnesium per mL	Sulfate per mL
1203-04	10%	Vial	20 mL	9.9 mg	38.9 mg
1204-04	10%	Vial	50 mL	9.9 mg	38.9 mg
1209-04	50%	Vial	2 mL	49.3 mg	194.7 mg
1210-04	50%	Vial	10 mL	49.3 mg	194.7 mg
1211-04	50%	Vial	20 mL	49.3 mg	194.7 mg
0684-01	50%	Additive Syringe	5 mL	49.3 mg	194.7 mg
0685-01	50%	Additive Syringe	10 mL	49.3 mg	194.7 mg

NALBUPHINE HCl INJECTION ℞

(For details of indications, dosage and administration, precautions, and adverse reactions, see circular in package.)

HOW SUPPLIED

Nalbuphine HCl Injection for intramuscular, subcutaneous or intravenous use is available in the following dosage forms:

Vials
10 mg/mL, 10 mL vial (box of 1)   NDC 0186-1262-12
20 mg/mL, 10 mL vial (box of 1)   NDC 0186-1266-12
Store at controlled room temperature 15°–30°C (59°–86°F).
Protect from light.
021886R03   Iss. 10/88(3)

NALOXONE HCl INJECTION, USP ℞
Narcotic Antagonist

(For details of indications, dosage and administration, precautions, and adverse reactions, see circular in package.)

HOW SUPPLIED

Naloxone HCl Injection for intravenous, intramuscular and subcutaneous administration is available as:
0.02 mg/mL
2 mL vial,   box of 10   NDC 0186-1252-13
0.4 mg/mL
1 mL vial,   box of 10   NDC 0186-1250-13
10 mL vial,   box of 1   NDC 0186-1254-12
1 mg/mL
1 mL vial,   box of 10   NDC 0186-1251-13
5 mL vial,   box of 1   NDC 0186-1253-13
10 mL vial,   box of 1   NDC 0186-1255-12
Store at controlled room temperature 15°–30°C (59°–86°F).
021885R03   5/89(3)

NESACAINE® ℞
[nes 'a-caine]
(Chloroprocaine HCl) Injection
NESACAINE®MPF
(Chloroprocaine HCl) Injection
for Infiltration and Nerve Block

DESCRIPTION

Nesacaine and Nesacaine-MPF Injections are sterile non-pyrogenic local anesthetics. The active ingredient in Nesacaine and Nesacaine-MPF Injections is chloroprocaine HCl (benzoic acid, 4-amino-2-chloro-2-(diethylamino)ethyl ester, monohydrochloride), which is represented by the following structural formula:

$$NH_2-\bigcirc-COOCH_2CH_2N(C_2H_5)_2 \cdot HCl$$

Cl

Table 1. Composition of Available Solutions
[See table above right].
The solutions are adjusted to pH 2.7–4.0 by means of sodium hydroxide and/or hydrochloric acid.
Nesacaine and Nesacaine-MPF injections should not be re-sterilized by autoclaving.

CLINICAL PHARMACOLOGY

Chloroprocaine, like other local anesthetics, blocks the generation and the conduction of nerve impulses, presumably by increasing the threshold for electrical excitation in the nerve, by slowing the propagation of the nerve impulse and by reducing the rate of rise of the action potential. In general, the progression of anesthesia is related to the diameter, myelination and conduction velocity of affected nerve fibers. Clinically, the order of loss of nerve function is as follows: (1) pain, (2) temperature, (3) touch, (4) proprioception, and (5) skeletal muscle tone.
Systemic absorption of local anesthetics produces effects on the cardiovascular and central nervous systems. At blood concentrations achieved with normal therapeutic doses, changes in cardiac conduction, excitability, refractoriness, contractility, and peripheral vascular resistance are minimal. However, toxic blood concentrations depress cardiac conduction and excitability, which may lead to atrioventricular block and ultimately to cardiac arrest. In addition, with toxic blood concentration myocardial contractility may be depressed and peripheral vasodilation may occur, leading to decreased cardiac output and arterial blood pressure.
Following systemic absorption, toxic blood concentrations of local anesthetics can produce central nervous system stimulation, depression, or both. Apparent central stimulation may be manifested as restlessness, tremors and shivering, which may progress to convulsions. Depression and coma may occur, possibly progressing ultimately to respiratory arrest.
However, the local anesthetics have a primary depressant effect on the medulla and on higher centers. The depressed

Product Identification	Chloroprocaine HCl	Formula (mg/mL)			
		Sodium Chloride	Disodium EDTA dihydrate	Methylparaben	
Nesacaine 1%	10	6.7	0.111	1.0	
Nesacaine 2%	20	4.7	0.111	1.0	
Nesacaine-MPF 2%	20	4.7	0.111	—	
Nesacaine-MPF 3%	30	3.3	0.111	—	

stage may occur without a prior stage of central nervous system stimulation.

PHARMACOKINETICS

The rate of systemic absorption of local anesthetic drugs is dependent upon the total dose and concentration of drug administered, the route of administration, the vascularity of the administration site, and the presence or absence of epinephrine in the anesthetic solution. Epinephrine usually reduces the rate of absorption and plasma concentration of local anesthetics and is sometimes added to local anesthetic solutions in order to prolong the duration of action.
The onset of action with chloroprocaine is rapid (usually within 6 to 12 minutes), and the duration of anesthesia, depending upon the amount used and the route of administration, may be up to 60 minutes.
Local anesthetics appear to cross the placenta by passive diffusion. However, the rate and degree of diffusion varies considerably among the different drugs as governed by: (1) the degree of plasma protein binding, (2) the degree of ionization, and (3) the degree of lipid solubility. Fetal/maternal ratios of local anesthetics appear to be inversely related to the degree of plasma protein binding, since only the free, unbound drug is available for placental transfer. Thus, drugs with the highest protein binding capacity may have the lowest fetal/maternal ratios. The extent of placental transfer is also determined by the degree of ionization and lipid solubility of the drug. Lipid soluble, nonionized drugs readily enter the fetal blood from the maternal circulation.
Depending upon the route of administration, local anesthetics are distributed to some extent to all body tissues, with high concentrations found in highly perfused organs such as the liver, lungs, heart and brain.
Various pharmacokinetic parameters of the local anesthetics can be significantly altered by the presence of hepatic or renal disease, addition of epinephrine, factors affecting urinary pH, renal blood flow, the route of administration, and the age of the patient. The in vitro plasma half-life of chloroprocaine in adults is 21 ± 2 seconds for males and 25 ± 1 seconds for females. The in vitro plasma half-life in neonates is 43 ± 2 seconds.
Chloroprocaine is rapidly metabolized in plasma by hydrolysis of the ester linkage by pseudocholinesterase. The hydrolysis of chloroprocaine results in the production of β-diethylaminoethanol and 2-chloro-4-aminobenzoic acid, which inhibits the action of the sulfonamides (SEE PRECAUTIONS). The kidney is the main excretory organ for most local anesthetics and their metabolites. Urinary excretion is affected by urinary perfusion and factors affecting urinary pH.

INDICATIONS AND USAGE

Nesacaine 1% and 2% Injections, in multidose vials with methylparaben as preservative, are indicated for the production of local anesthesia by infiltration and peripheral nerve block. They are not to be used for lumbar or caudal epidural anesthesia.
Nesacaine-MPF 2% and 3% Injections, in single-dose vials without preservative, are indicated for the production of local anesthesia by infiltration, peripheral and central nerve block, including lumbar and caudal epidural blocks.
Nesacaine and Nesacaine-MPF Injections, are not to be used for subarachnoid administration.

CONTRAINDICATIONS

Nesacaine and Nesacaine-MPF Injections are contraindicated in patients hypersensitive (allergic) to drugs of the PABA ester group.
Lumbar and caudal epidural anesthesia should be used with extreme caution in persons with the following conditions; existing neurological disease, spinal deformities, septicemia and severe hypertension.

WARNINGS

LOCAL ANESTHETICS SHOULD ONLY BE EMPLOYED BY CLINICIANS WHO ARE WELL VERSED IN DIAGNOSIS AND MANAGEMENT OF DOSE RELATED TOXICITY AND OTHER ACUTE EMERGENCIES WHICH MIGHT ARISE FROM THE BLOCK TO BE EMPLOYED, AND THEN ONLY AFTER ENSURING THE *IMMEDIATE* AVAILABILITY OF OXYGEN, OTHER RESUSCITATIVE DRUGS, CARDIOPULMONARY RESUSCITATIVE EQUIPMENT, AND THE PERSONNEL RESOURCES NEEDED FOR PROPER MANAGEMENT OF TOXIC REACTIONS AND RELATED EMERGENCIES (See also *ADVERSE REACTIONS and PRECAUTIONS*.) DELAY IN PROPER MANAGEMENT OF DOSE RELATED TOXICITY, UNDERVENTILATION FROM ANY CAUSE AND/

OR ALTERED SENSITIVITY MAY LEAD TO THE DEVELOPMENT OF ACIDOSIS, CARDIAC ARREST AND, POSSIBLY, DEATH. NESACAINE (chloroprocaine HCl) INJECTION contains methylparaben and should not be used for lumbar or caudal epidural anesthesia because safety of this antimicrobial preservative has not been established with regard to intrathecal injection, either intentional or unintended. NESACAINE-MPF Injection contains no preservative; discard unused solution remaining in vial after initial use.
Vasopressors should not be used in the presence of ergot-type oxytocic drugs, since a severe persistent hypertension may occur.
To avoid intravascular injection, aspiration should be performed before the anesthetic solution is injected. The needle must be repositioned until no blood return can be elicited. However, the absence of blood in the syringe does not guarantee that intravascular injection has been avoided.
Mixtures of local anesthetics are sometimes employed to compensate for the slower onset of one drug and the shorter duration of action of the second drug. Experiments in primates suggest that toxicity is probably additive when mixtures of local anesthetics are employed, but some experiments in rodents suggest synergism. Caution regarding toxic equivalence should be exercised when mixtures of local anesthetics are employed.

PRECAUTIONS

General: The safety and effective use of chloroprocaine depend on proper dosage, correct technique, adequate precautions and readiness for emergencies. Resuscitative equipment, oxygen and other resuscitative drugs should be available for immediate use. (See WARNINGS and ADVERSE REACTIONS). The lowest dosage that results in effective anesthesia should be used to avoid high plasma levels and serious adverse effects. Injections should be made slowly, with frequent aspirations before and during the injection to avoid intravascular injection. Syringe aspirations should also be performed before and during each supplemental injection in continuous (intermittent) catheter techniques. During the administration of epidural anesthesia, it is recommended that a test dose be administered (3 mL of 3% or 5 mL of 2% Nesacaine-MPF Injection) initially and that the patient be monitored for central nervous system toxicity and cardiovascular toxicity, as well as for signs of unintended intrathecal administration, before proceeding. When clinical conditions permit, consideration should be given to employing a chloroprocaine solution that contains epinephrine for the test dose because circulatory changes characteristic of epinephrine may also serve as a warning sign of unintended intravascular injection. An intravascular injection is still possible even if aspirations for blood are negative. With the use of continuous catheter techniques, it is recommended that a fraction of each supplemental dose be administered as a test dose in order to verify proper location of the catheter.
Injection of repeated doses of local anesthetics may cause significant increases in plasma levels with each repeated dose due to slow accumulation of the drug or its metabolites. Tolerance to elevated blood levels varies with the physical condition of the patient. Debilitated, elderly patients, acutely ill patients, and children should be given reduced doses commensurate with their age and physical status. Local anesthetics should also be used with caution in patients with hypotension or heart block.
Careful and constant monitoring of cardiovascular and respiratory (adequacy of ventilation) vital signs and the patient's state of consciousness should be accomplished after each local anesthetic injection. It should be kept in mind at such times that restlessness, anxiety, tinnitus, dizziness, blurred vision, tremors, depression or drowsiness may be early warning signs of central nervous system toxicity.
Local anesthetic solutions containing a vasoconstrictor should be used cautiously and in carefully circumscribed quantities in areas of the body supplied by end arteries or having otherwise compromised blood supply. Patients with peripheral vascular disease and those with hypertensive vascular disease may exhibit exaggerated vasoconstrictor response. Ischemic injury or necrosis may result.
Since ester-type local anesthetics are hydrolyzed by plasma cholinesterase produced by the liver, chloroprocaine should be used cautiously in patients with hepatic disease.
Local anesthetics should also be used with caution in patients with impaired cardiovascular function since they may

Continued on next page

Astra—Cont.

be less able to compensate for functional changes associated with the prolongation of A-V conduction produced by these drugs.

Use in Ophthalmic Surgery: When local anesthetic solutions are employed for retrobulbar block, lack of corneal sensation should not be relied upon to determine whether or not the patient is ready for surgery. This is because complete lack of corneal sensation usually precedes clinically acceptable external ocular muscle akinesia.

INFORMATION FOR PATIENTS

When appropriate, patients should be informed in advance that they may experience temporary loss of sensation and motor activity, usually in the lower half of the body, following proper administration of epidural anesthesia.

Clinically Significant Drug Interactions: The administration of local anesthetic solutions containing epinephrine or norepinephrine to patients receiving monoamine oxidase inhibitors, tricyclic antidepressants or phenothiazines may produce severe, prolonged hypotension or hypertension. Concurrent use of these agents should generally be avoided. In situations when concurrent therapy is necessary, careful patient monitoring is essential.

Concurrent administration of vasopressor drugs (for the treatment of hypotension related to obstetric blocks) and ergot-type oxytocic drugs may cause severe, presistent hypertension or cerebrovascular accidents.

The para-aminobenzoic acid metabolite of chloroprocaine inhibits the action of sulfonamides. Therefore, chloroprocaine should not be used in any condition in which a sulfonamide drug is being administered.

Carcinogenesis, Mutagenesis, and Impairment of Fertility: Long-term studies in animals to evaluate carcinogenic potential and reproduction studies to evaluate mutagenesis or impairment of fertility have not been conducted with chloroprocaine.

Pregnancy Category C: Animal reproduction studies have not been conducted with chloroprocaine. It is also not known whether chloroprocaine can cause fetal harm when administered to a pregnant woman or can affect reproduction capacity. Chloroprocaine should be given to a pregnant woman only if clearly needed. This does not preclude the use of chloroprocaine at term for the production of obstetrical anesthesia.

Labor and Delivery: Local anesthetics rapidly cross the placenta, and when used for epidural, paracervical, pudendal or caudal block anesthesia, can cause varying degrees of maternal, fetal and neonatal toxicity.

(See CLINICAL PHARMACOLOGY—Pharmacokinetics) The incidence and degree of toxicity depend upon the procedure performed, the type and amount of drug used, and the technique of drug administration. Adverse reactions in the parturient, fetus and neonate involve alterations of the central nervous system, peripheral vascular tone and cardiac function.

Maternal hypotension has resulted from regional anesthesia. Local anesthetics produce vasodilation by blocking sympathetic nerves. Elevating the patient's legs and positioning her on her left side will help prevent decreases in blood pressure. The fetal heart rate also should be monitored continuously, and electronic fetal monitoring is highly advisable.

Epidural, paracervical, or pudendal anesthesia may alter the forces of parturition through changes in uterine contractility or maternal expulsive efforts. In one study, paracervical block anesthesia was associated with a decrease in the mean duration of first stage labor and facilitation of cervical dilation. However, epidural anesthesia has also been reported to prolong the second stage of labor by removing the parturient's reflex urge to bear down or by interfering with motor function. The use of obstetrical anesthesia may increase the need for forceps assistance.

The use of some local anesthetic drug products during labor and delivery may be followed by diminished muscle strength and tone for the first day or two of life. The long-term significance of these observations is unknown.

Careful adherence to recommended dosage is of the utmost importance in obstetrical paracervical block. Failure to achieve adequate analgesia with recommended doses should arouse suspicion of intravascular or fetal intracranial injection. Cases compatible with unintended fetal intracranial injection of local anesthetic solution have been reported following intended paracervical or pudendal block or both. Babies so affected present with unexplained neonatal depression at birth which correlates with high local anesthetic serum levels and usually manifest seizures within six hours. Prompt use of supportive measures combined with forced urinary excretion of the local anesthetic has been used successfully to manage this complication.

Case reports of maternal convulsions and cardiovascular collapse following use of some local anesthetics for paracervical block in early pregnancy (as anesthesia for elective abortion) suggest that systemic absorption under these circumstances may be rapid. The recommended maximum dose of each drug should not be exceeded. Injection should be made slowly and with frequent aspiration. Allow a 5-minute interval between sides.

There are no data concerning use of chloroprocaine for obstetrical paracervical block when toxemia of pregnancy is present or when fetal distress or prematurity is anticipated in advance of the block; such use is, therefore, not recommended.

The following information should be considered by clinicians who select chloroprocaine for obstetrical paracervical block anesthesia: 1) Fetal bradycardia (generally a heart rate of less than 120 per minute for more than 2 minutes) has been noted by electronic monitoring in about 5 to 10 percent of the cases (various studies) where initial total doses of 120 mg to 400 mg of chloroprocaine were employed. The incidence of bradycardia, within this dose range, might not be dose related. 2) Fetal acidosis has not been demonstrated by blood gas monitoring around the time of bradycardia or afterwards. These data are limited and generally restricted to nontoxemic cases where fetal distress or prematurity was not anticipated in advance of the block. 3) No intact chloroprocaine and only trace quantities of a hydrolysis product, 2-chloro-4-aminobenzoic acid, have been demonstrated in umbilical cord arterial or venous plasma following properly administered paracervical block with chloroprocaine. 4) The role of drug factors and non-drug factors associated with fetal bradycardia following paracervical block are unexplained at this time.

Nursing Mothers: It is not known whether this drug is excreted in human milk. Because many drugs are excreted in human milk, caution should be exercised when chloroprocaine is administered to a nursing woman.

Pediatric Use: Guidlines for the administration of Nesacaine and Nesacaine-MPF Injections to children are presented in DOSAGE AND ADMINISTRATION.

ADVERSE REACTIONS

Systemic: The most commonly encountered acute adverse experiences that demand immediate countermeasures are related to the central nervous system and the cardiovascular system. These adverse experiences are generally dose related and may result from rapid absorption from the injection site, diminished tolerance, or from unintentional intravascular injection of the local anesthetic solution. In addition to systemic dose-related toxicity, unintentional subarachnoid injection of drug during the intended performance of caudal or lumbar epidural block or nerve blocks near the vertebral column (especially in the head and neck region) may result in underventilation or apnea ("Total Spinal"). Factors influencing plasma protein binding, such as acidosis, systemic diseases that alter protein production, or competition of other drugs for protein binding sites, may diminish individual tolerance. Plasma cholinesterase deficiency may also account for diminished tolerance to ester type local anesthetics.

Central Nervous System Reactions: These are characterized by excitation and/or depression. Restlessness, anxiety, dizziness, tinnitus, blurred vision or tremors may occur, possibly proceeding to convulsions. However, excitement may be transient or absent, with depression being the first manifestation of an adverse reaction. This may quickly be followed by drowsiness merging into unconsciousness and respiratory arrest.

The incidence of convulsions associated with the use of local anesthetics varies with the procedure used and the total dose administered. In a survey of studies of epidural anesthesia, overt toxicity progressing to convulsions occurred in approximately 0.1 percent of local anesthetic administrations.

Cardiovascular System Reactions: High doses, or unintended intravascular injection, may lead to high plasma levels and related depression of the myocardium, hypotension, bradycardia, ventricular arrhythmias and, possibly, cardiac arrest.

Allergic: Allergic type reactions are rare and may occur as a result of sensitivity to the local anesthetic or to other formulation ingredients, such as the antimicrobial preservative methylparaben, contained in multiple dose vials. These reactions are characterized by signs such as urticaria, pruritis, erythema, angioneurotic edema (including laryngeal edema), tachycardia, sneezing, nausea, vomiting, dizziness, syncope, excessive sweating, elevated temperature, and possibly, anaphylactoid type symptomatology (including severe hypotension). Cross sensitivity among members of the ester-type local anesthetic group has been reported. The usefulness of screening for sensitivity has not been definitely established.

Neurologic: In the practice of caudal or lumbar epidural block, occasional unintentional penetration of the subarachnoid space by the catheter may occur (see PRECAUTIONS). Subsequent adverse observations may depend partially on the amount of drug administered intrathecally. These observations may include spinal block of varying magnitude (including total spinal block), hypotension secondary to spinal block, loss of bladder, and bowel control, and loss of perineal sensation and sexual function. Arachnoiditis, persistent motor, sensory and/or autonomic (sphincter control) deficit of some lower spinal segments with slow recovery (several months) or incomplete recovery have been reported in rare instances. (See DOSAGE AND ADMINISTRATION discussion of Caudal and Lumbar Epidural Block). Backache and headache have also been noted following lumbar epidural or caudal block.

OVERDOSAGE

Acute emergencies from local anesthetics are generally related to high plasma levels encountered during therapeutic use of local anesthetics or to unintended subarachnoid injection of local anesthetic solution (see ADVERSE REACTIONS, WARNINGS, and PRECAUTIONS).

In mice, the intravenous LD_{50} of chloroprocaine HCl is 97 mg/kg and the subcutaneous LD_{50} of chloroprocaine HCl is 950 mg/kg.

Management of Local Anesthetic Emergencies: The first consideration is prevention, best accomplished by careful and constant monitoring of cardiovascular and respiratory vital signs and the patient's state of consciousness after each local anesthetic injection. At the first sign of change, oxygen should be administered.

The first step is the management of convulsions, as well as underventilation or apnea due to unintentional subarachnoid injection of drug solution, consists of immediate attention to the maintenance of a patent airway and assisted or controlled ventilation with oxygen and a delivery system capable of permitting immediate positive airway pressure by mask. Immediately after the institution of these ventilatory measures, the adequacy of the circulation should be evaluated, keeping in mind that drugs used to treat convulsions sometimes depress the circulation when administered intravenously. Should convulsions persist despite adequate respiratory support, and if the status of the circulation permits, small increments of an ultra-short acting barbiturate (such as thiopental or thiamylal) or a benzodiazepine (such as diazepam) may be administered intravenously; the clinician should be familiar, prior to use of local anesthetics, with these anticonvulsant drugs. Supportive treatment of circulatory depression may require administration of intravenous fluids and, when appropriate, a vasopressor dictated by the clinical situation (such as ephedrine to enhance myocardial contractile force).

If not treated immediately, both convulsions and cardiovascular depression can result in hypoxia, acidosis, bradycardia, arrhythmias and cardiac arrest. Underventilation or apnea due to unintentional subarachnoid injection of local anesthetic solution may produce these same signs and also lead to cardiac arrest if ventilatory support is not instituted. If cardiac arrest should occur, standard cardiopulmonary resuscitative measures should be instituted. Recovery has been reported after prolonged resuscitative efforts.

Endotracheal intubation, employing drugs and techniques familiar to the clinician, may be indicated, after initial administration of oxygen by mask, if difficulty is encountered in the maintenance of a patent airway or if prolonged ventilatory support (assisted or controlled) is indicated.

DOSAGE AND ADMINISTRATION

Chloroprocaine may be administered as a single injection or continuously through an indwelling catheter. As with all local anesthetics, the dose administered varies with the anesthetic procedure, the vascularity of the tissues, the depth of anesthesia and degree of muscle relaxation required, the duration of anesthesia desired, and the physical condition of the patient. The smallest dose and concentration required to produce the desired result should be used. Dosage should be reduced for children, elderly and debilitated patients and patients with cardiac and/or liver disease. The maximum single recommended doses of chloroprocaine in adults are: without epinephrine, 11 mg/kg, not to exceed a maximum total dose of 800 mg; with epinephrine (1:200,000), 14 mg/kg, not to exceed a maximum total dose of 1000 mg. For specific techniques and procedures, refer to standard textbooks.

Caudal and Lumbar Epidural Block: In order to guard against adverse experiences sometimes noted following unintended penetration of the subarachnoid space, the following procedure modifications are recommended: 1. Use an adequate test dose (3 mL of Nesacaine-MPF 3% Injection or 5 mL of Nesacaine-MPF 2% Injection) prior to induction of complete block. This test dose should be repeated if the patient is moved in such a fashion as to have displaced the epidural catheter. Allow adequate time for onset of anesthesia following administration of each test dose. 2. Avoid the rapid injection of a large volume of local anesthetic solution through the catheter. Consider fractional doses, when feasible. 3. In the event of the known injection of a large volume of local anesthetic solution into the subarachnoid space, after suitable resuscitation and if the catheter is in place, consider attempting the recovery of drug by draining a moderate amount of cerebrospinal fluid (such as 10 mL) through the epidural catheter.

As a guide for some routine procedures, suggested doses are given below:

1. Infiltration and Peripheral Nerve Block: NESACAINE or NESACAINE-MPF (Chloroprocaine HCl) INJECTION [See table right].
2. Caudal and Lumbar Epidural Block: NESACAINE-MPF INJECTION. For caudal anesthesia, the initial dose is 15 to 25 mL of a 2% or 3% solution. Repeated doses may be given at 40 to 60 minutes intervals.

For lumbar epidural anesthesia, 2.0 to 2.5 mL per segment of a 2% or 3% solution can be used. The usual total volume of Nesacaine-MPF Injection is from 15 to 25 mL. Repeated doses 2 to 6 mL less than the original dose may be given at 40 to 50 minutes intervals.

The above dosages are recommended as a guide for use in the average adult. Maximum dosages of all local anesthetics must be individualized after evaluating the size and physical condition of the patient and the rate of systemic absorption from a particular injection site.

Pediatric Dosage: It is difficult to recommend a maximum dose of any drug for children, since this varies as a function of age and weight. For children over 3 years of age who have a normal lean body mass and normal body development, the maximum dose is determined by the child's age and weight and should not exceed 11 mg/kg (5 mg/lb). For example, in a child of 5 years weighing 50 lbs (23 kg), the dose of chloroprocaine HCl without epinephrine would be 250 mg. Concentrations of 0.5–1.0% are suggested for infiltration and 1.0–1.5% for nerve block. In order to guard against systemic toxicity, the lowest effective concentration and lowest effective dose should be used at all times. Some of the lower concentrations for use in infants and smaller children are not available in pre-packaged containers; it will be necessary to dilute available concentrations with the amount of 0.9% sodium chloride injection necessary to obtain the required final concentration of chloroprocaine solution.

Preparation of Epinephrine Solutions—To prepare a 1:200,000 epinephrine-chloroprocaine HCl solution, add 0.15 mL of a 1 to 1000 Epinephrine Injection U.S.P. to 30 mL of Nesacaine-MPF Injection.

Chloroprocaine is incompatible with caustic alkalis and their carbonates, soaps, silver salts, iodine and iodides.

Parenteral drug products should be inspected visually for particulate matter and discoloration prior to administration, whenever solution and container permit. As with other anesthetics having a free aromatic amino group, Nesacaine and Nesacaine-MPF Injections are slightly photosensitive and may become discolored after prolonged exposure to light. It is recommended that these vials be stored in the original outer containers, protected from direct sunlight. Discolored solution should not be administered. If exposed to low temperature, Nesacaine and Nesacaine-MPF Injections may deposit crystals of chloroprocaine HCl which will redissolve with shaking when returned to room temperature. The product should not be used if it contains undissolved (e.g., particulate) material.

HOW SUPPLIED

NESACAINE (Chloroprocaine HCl) INJECTION with preservatives is supplied as follows:

   1% solution (NDC 0186-0971-66) in 30 mL multiple dose vials.

   2% solution (NDC 0186-0972-66) in 30 mL multiple dose vials.

NESACAINE-MPF (Chloroprocaine HCl) INJECTION without preservatives is supplied as follows:

   2% solution (NDC 0186-0993-66) in 30 mL single dose vials.

   3% solution (NDC 0186-0994-66) in 30 mL single dose vials.

Keep from freezing. Protect from light. Store at controlled room temperature: 15°–30°C (59°–86°F).

021849R05   Rev. 5/87(5)

PANCURONIUM BROMIDE INJECTION   ℞

> THIS DRUG SHOULD BE ADMINISTERED BY ADEQUATELY TRAINED INDIVIDUALS FAMILIAR WITH ITS ACTIONS, CHARACTERISTICS, AND HAZARDS.

HOW SUPPLIED

Pancuronium Bromide Injection is packaged in the following forms:

Vials, 1 mg/mL
NDC 0186-1322-12, 10 mL size—boxes of 5, Flip-Off vial closure

Vials, 2 mg/mL
NDC 0186-1331-13, 2 mL size—boxes of 10, Astra E-Z OFF™ vial closure
NDC 0186-1334-03, 2 mL size—boxes of 10, Flip-Off vial closure
NDC 0186-1332-13, 5 mL size—boxes of 10, Astra E-Z OFF™ vial closure
NDC 0186-1335-03, 5 mL size—boxes of 10, Flip-off vial closure

Anesthetic Procedure	Solution Concentration %	Volume (mL)	Total Dose (mg)
Mandibular	2	2–3	40–60
Infraorbital	2	0.5–1	10–20
Brachial plexus	2	30–40	600–800
Digital (without epinephrine)	1	3–4	30–40
Pudendal	2	10 each side	400
Paracervical (see also PRECAUTIONS)	1	3 per each of 4 sites	up to 120

Syringes, 2 mg/mL
NDC 0186-1333-23, 2 mL size—boxes of 10, 22G, 1¼″ needle
NDC 0186-1336-23, 2 mL size—boxes of 10, Luer Hub Only
NDC 0186-0676-01, 5 mL size—box of 1, 21G, ¹⁵/₁₆″ needle
NDC 0186-0692-01, 5 mL size—box of 1, Luer Hub Only

STORAGE

Both concentrations of Pancuronium Bromide Injection will maintain full clinical potency for six months if kept at a room temperature of 18° to 22°C (65° to 72°F), or for 18 months when refrigerated at 2° to 8°C (36° to 46°F).

021887R04   12/88 (4)

POLOCAINE®   ℞
[pō′-lō-caine ″]
(mepivacaine hydrochloride Injection, USP)
THESE SOLUTIONS ARE NOT INTENDED FOR SPINAL ANESTHESIA OR DENTAL USE

(For details of indications, dosages and administration, precautions, and adverse reactions, see circular in package.)

HOW SUPPLIED

1% Single Dose Vial	30 mL	(NDC 0186-0412-01)
1% Multiple Dose Vial	50 mL	(NDC 0186-0410-01)
1.5% Single Dose Vial	30 mL	(NDC 0186-0418-01)
2% Single Dose Vial	20 mL	(NDC 0186-0422-01)
2% Multiple Dose Vial	50 mL	(NDC 0186-0420-01)

Unused portions of solutions not containing preservatives should be discarded.

021863R00   Issue 11/85

SENSORCAINE®   ℞
[sén-sor-caine]
(Bupivacaine HCl Injection, USP)
SENSORCAINE® with Epinephrine 1:200,000 (as bitartrate) (Bupivacaine and Epinephrine Injection, USP)

DESCRIPTION

Sensorcaine® (bupivacaine HCl) injections are sterile isotonic solutions that contain a local anesthetic agent with and without epinephrine (as bitartrate) 1:200,000 and are administered parenterally by injection. See INDICATIONS AND USAGE for specific uses. Solutions of bupivacaine HCl may be autoclaved if they do not contain epinephrine.

Sensorcaine® Injections contain bupivacaine HCl which is chemically designated as 2-piperidinecarboxamide, 1-butyl-N-(2,6-dimethylphenyl)-monohydrochloride, monohydrate and has the following structure:

Epinephrine is (-)-3,4-Dihydroxy-α-[(methylamino)methyl] benzyl alcohol. It has the following structural formula:

The pKa of bupivacaine (8.1) is similar to that of lidocaine (7.86). However, bupivacaine possesses a greater degree of lipid solubility and is protein bound to a greater extent than lidocaine.

Bupivacaine is related chemically and pharmacologically to the aminoacyl local anesthetics. It is a homologue of mepivacaine and is chemically related to lidocaine. All three of these anesthetics contain an amide linkage between the aromatic nucleus and the amino or piperidine group. They differ in this respect from the procaine-type local anesthetics, which have an ester linkage.

Sensorcaine is a sterile isotonic solution containing sodium chloride. In multiple dose vials each mL also contains 1 mg methylparaben as antiseptic preservative. The pH of these solutions is adjusted to between 4.5 and 6.5 with sodium hydroxide and/or hydrochloric acid.

Sensorcaine with Epinephrine 1:200,000 (as bitartrate) is a sterile isotonic solution containing sodium chloride. Each mL contains bupivacaine hydrochloride and 0.005 mg epinephrine, with 0.5 mg sodium metabisulfite as an antioxidant and 0.2 mg citric acid (anhydrous) as stabilizer. In multiple dose vials, each mL also contains 1 mg methylparaben as antiseptic preservative. The pH of these solutions is adjusted to between 3.3 and 5.5 with sodium hydroxide and/or hydrochloric acid.

CLINICAL PHARMACOLOGY

Local anesthetics block the generation and the conduction of nerve impulses, presumably by increasing the threshold for electrical excitation in the nerve, by slowing the propagation of the nerve impulse, and by reducing the rate of rise of the action potential. In general, the progression of anesthesia is related to the diameter, myelination and conduction velocity of affected nerve fibers. Clinically, the order of loss of nerve function is as follows: (1) pain, (2) temperature, (3) touch, (4) proprioception, and (5) skeletal muscle tone.

Systemic absorption of local anesthetics produces effects on the cardiovascular and central nervous systems. At blood concentrations achieved with therapeutic doses, changes in cardiac conduction, excitability, refractoriness, contractility, and peripheral vascular resistance are minimal. However, toxic blood concentrations depress cardiac conduction and excitability, which may lead to atrioventricular block, ventricular arrhythmias and to cardiac arrest, sometimes resulting in fatalities. In addition, myocardial contractility is depressed and peripheral vasodilation occurs, leading to decreased cardiac output and arterial blood pressure.

Recent clinical reports and animal research suggest that these cardiovascular changes are more likely to occur after unintended intravascular injection of bupivacaine. Therefore incremental dosing is necessary.

Following systemic absorption, local anesthetics can produce central nervous system stimulation, depression or both. Apparent central stimulation is usually manifested as restlessness, tremors and shivering, progressing to convulsions, followed by depression and coma, progressing ultimately to respiratory arrest. However, the local anesthetics have a primary depressant effect on the medulla and on higher centers. The depressed stage may occur without a prior excited stage.

Pharmacokinetics: The rate of systemic absorption of local anesthetics is dependent upon the total dose and concentration of drug administered, the route of administration, the vascularity of the administration site, and the presence or absence of epinephrine in the anesthetic solution. A dilute concentration of epinephrine (1:200,000 or 5 μg/mL) usually reduces the rate of absorption and peak plasma concentration of bupivacaine, permitting the use of moderately larger total doses and sometimes prolonging the duration of action. The onset of action with bupivacaine is rapid and anesthesia is long-lasting. The duration of anesthesia is significantly longer with bupivacaine than with any other commonly used local anesthetic. It has also been noted that there is a period of analgesia that persists after the return of sensation, during which time the need for potent analgesics is reduced.

Local anesthetics are bound to plasma proteins in varying degrees. Generally, the lower the plasma concentration of drug, the higher the percentage of drug bound to plasma proteins.

Local anesthetics appear to cross the placenta by passive diffusion. The rate and degree of diffusion is governed by: (1) the degree of plasma protein binding, (2) the degree of ionization, and (3) the degree of lipid solubility. Fetal/maternal ratios of local anesthetics appear to be inversely related to the degree of plasma protein binding, because only the free, unbound drug is available for placental transfer. Bupivacaine, with a high protein binding capacity (95%), has a low fetal/maternal ratio (0.2-0.4). The extent of placental transfer is also determined by the degree of ionization and lipid solubility of the drug. Lipid soluble, nonionized drugs readily enter the fetal blood from the maternal circulation.

Depending upon the route of administration, local anesthetics are distributed to some extent to all body tissues, with high concentrations found in highly perfused organs such as the liver, lungs, heart and brain.

Continued on next page

Astra—Cont.

Pharmacokinetic studies on the plasma profile of bupivacaine after direct intravenous injection suggest a three-compartment open model. The first compartment is represented by the rapid intravascular distribution of the drug. The second compartment represents the equilibration of the drug throughout the highly perfused organs such as the brain, myocardium, lungs, kidneys and liver. The third compartment represents an equilibration of the drug, with poorly perfused tissues, such as muscle and fat. The elimination of drug from tissue depends largely upon the ability of binding sites in the circulation to carry it to the liver where it is metabolized.

After injection of Sensorcaine (bupivacaine HCl) injection for caudal, epidural or peripheral nerve block in man, peak levels of bupivacaine in the blood are reached in 30 to 45 minutes, followed by a decline to insignificant levels during the next 3 to 6 hours.

Various pharmacokinetic parameters of the local anesthetics can be significantly altered by the presence of hepatic or renal disease, addition of epinephrine, factors affecting urinary pH, renal blood flow, the route of drug administration, and the age of the patient. The half-life of bupivacaine in adults is 3.5 ± 2.0 hours and in neonates 8.1 hours.

Amide-type local anesthetics such as bupivacaine are metabolized primarily in the liver via conjugation with glucuronic acid.

Patients with hepatic disease, especially those with severe hepatic disease, may be more susceptible to the potential toxicities of the amide-type local anesthetics. The major metabolite of bupivacaine is 2,6-pipecoloxylidine.

The kidney is the main excretory organ for most local anesthetics and their metabolites. Urinary excretion is affected by renal perfusion and factors affecting urinary pH. Only 5% of bupivacaine is excreted unchanged in the urine.

When administered in recommended doses and concentrations, Sensorcaine (bupivacaine HCl) injection does not ordinarily produce irritation or tissue damage and does not cause methemoglobinemia.

INDICATIONS AND USAGE

Sensorcaine (bupivacaine HCl) injection is indicated for the production of local or regional anesthesia or analgesia for surgery, for oral surgery procedures, for diagnostic and therapeutic procedures and for obstetrical procedures. Only the 0.25% and 0.5% concentrations are indicated for obstetrical anesthesia. (See WARNINGS.)

Experience with non-obstetrical surgical procedures in pregnant patients is not sufficient to recommend use of the 0.75% concentration in these patients. Sensorcaine (bupivacaine HCl) injection is not recommended for intravenous regional anesthesia (Bier Block). See WARNINGS.

The routes of administration and indicated Sensorcaine (bupivacaine HCl) concentrations are:

local infiltration	0.25%
peripheral nerve block	0.25%, 0.5%
retrobulbar block	0.75%
sympathetic block	0.25%
lumbar epidural	0.25%, 0.5% and 0.75% (non-obstetrical)
caudal	0.25%, 0.5%

epidural test dose (see PRECAUTIONS)
(See DOSAGE AND ADMINISTRATION for additional information.) Standard textbooks should be consulted to determine the accepted procedures and techniques for the administration of Sensorcaine (bupivacaine HCl).

CONTRAINDICATIONS

Sensorcaine (bupivacaine HCl) injection is contraindicated in obstetrical paracervical block anesthesia. Its use by this technique has resulted in fetal bradycardia and death.
Sensorcaine (bupivacaine HCl) is contraindicated in patients with a known hypersensitivity to it or to any local anesthetic agent of the amide type or to other components of bupivacaine solutions.

WARNINGS

THE 0.75% CONCENTRATION OF SENSORCAINE (BUPIVACAINE HYDROCHLORIDE) INJECTION IS NOT RECOMMENDED FOR OBSTETRICAL ANESTHESIA. THERE HAVE BEEN REPORTS OF CARDIAC ARREST WITH DIFFICULT RESUSCITATION OR DEATH DURING USE OF BUPIVACAINE FOR EPIDURAL ANESTHESIA IN OBSTETRICAL PATIENTS. IN MOST CASES, THIS HAS FOLLOWED USE OF THE 0.75% CONCENTRATION. RESUSCITATION HAS BEEN DIFFICULT OR IMPOSSIBLE DESPITE APPARENTLY ADEQUATE PREPARATION AND APPROPRIATE MANAGEMENT. CARDIAC ARREST HAS OCCURRED AFTER CONVULSIONS RESULTING FROM SYSTEMIC TOXICITY, PRESUMABLY FOLLOWING UNINTENTIONAL INTRAVASCULAR INJECTION. THE 0.75% CONCENTRA-

TION SHOULD BE RESERVED FOR SURGICAL PROCEDURES WHERE A HIGH DEGREE OF MUSCLE RELAXATION AND PROLONGED EFFECT ARE NECESSARY.

LOCAL ANESTHETICS SHOULD ONLY BE EMPLOYED BY CLINICIANS WHO ARE WELL VERSED IN DIAGNOSIS AND MANAGEMENT OF DOSE-RELATED TOXICITY AND OTHER ACUTE EMERGENCIES WHICH MIGHT ARISE FROM THE BLOCK TO BE EMPLOYED, AND THEN ONLY AFTER ENSURING THE *IMMEDIATE* AVAILABILITY OF OXYGEN, OTHER RESUSCITATIVE DRUGS, CARDIOPULMONARY RESUSCITATIVE EQUIPMENT, AND THE PERSONNEL RESOURCES NEEDED FOR PROPER MANAGEMENT OF TOXIC REACTIONS AND RELATED EMERGENCIES. (See also ADVERSE REACTIONS, PRECAUTIONS, and OVERDOSAGE.) DELAY IN PROPER MANAGEMENT OF DOSE-RELATED TOXICITY, UNDERVENTILATION FROM ANY CAUSE AND/OR ALTERED SENSITIVITY MAY LEAD TO THE DEVELOPMENT OF ACIDOSIS, CARDIAC ARREST AND, POSSIBLY, DEATH.

Local anesthetic solutions containing antimicrobial preservatives, i.e. those supplied in multiple dose vials, should not be used for epidural or caudal anesthesia because safety has not been established with regard to intrathecal injection, either intentional or unintentional, of such preservatives.
It is essential that aspiration for blood or cerebrospinal fluid (where applicable) be done prior to injecting any local anesthetic, both the original dose and all subsequent doses, to avoid intravascular or subarachnoid injection. However, a negative aspiration does *not* ensure against an intravascular or subarachnoid injection.
Bupivacaine and Epinephrine Injection or other vasopressors should not be used concomitantly with ergot-type oxytocic drugs, because a severe persistent hypertension may occur. Likewise, solutions of bupivacaine containing a vasoconstrictor, such as epinephrine, should be used with extreme caution in patients receiving monoamine oxidase (MAO) inhibitors or antidepressants of the triptyline or imipramine types, because severe prolonged hypertension may result.
Until further experience is gained in children younger than 12 years, administration of bupivacaine in this age group is not recommended.
Reports of cardiac arrest and death have occurred with the use of bupivacaine for intravenous regional anesthesia (Bier Block). Information on safe dosages or techniques of administration of this product are lacking; therefore bupivacaine is not recommended for use by this technique.
Prior use of chloroprocaine may interfere with subsequent use of bupivacaine. Because of this, and because safety of intercurrent use of bupivacaine and chloroprocaine has not been established, such use is not recommended.
Sensorcaine with epinephrine solutions contain sodium metabisulfite, a sulfite that may cause allergic-type reactions including anaphylactic symptoms and life-threatening or less severe asthmatic episodes in certain susceptible people. The overall prevalence of sulfite sensitivity in the general population is unknown and probably low. Sulfite sensitivity is seen more frequently in asthmatic than in nonasthmatic people.

PRECAUTIONS

General: The safety and effectiveness of local anesthetics depend on proper dosage, correct technique, adequate precautions and readiness for emergencies. Resuscitative equipment, oxygen and other resuscitative drugs should be available for immediate use. (See WARNINGS, ADVERSE REACTIONS, and OVERDOSAGE.) During major regional nerve blocks, the patient should have I.V. fluids running via an indwelling catheter to assure a functioning intravenous pathway. The lowest dosage of local anesthetic that results in effective anesthesia should be used to avoid high plasma levels and serious adverse effects. The rapid injection of a large volume of local anesthetic solution should be avoided and fractional (incremental) doses should be used when feasible.
Epidural Anesthesia: During epidural administration of bupivacaine, concentrated solutions (0.5–0.75%) should be administered in incremental doses of 3 to 5 mL with sufficient time between doses to detect toxic manifestations of unintentional intravascular or intrathecal injection. Syringe aspirations should also be performed before and during each supplemental injection in continuous (intermittent) catheter techniques. An intravascular injection is still possible even if aspirations for blood are negative.
During the administration of epidural anesthethesia, it is recommended that a test dose be administered initially and the effects monitored before the full dose is given. When using a "continuous" catheter technique, test doses should be given prior to both the original and all reinforcing doses, because plastic tubing in the epidural space can migrate into a blood vessel or through the dura. When clinical conditions permit, the test dose should contain epinephrine (10 to 15 μg have been suggested) to serve as a warning of unintentional intravascular injection. If injected into a blood vessel, this

amount of epinephrine is likely to produce a transient "epinephrine response" within 45 seconds, consisting of an increase in heart rate and systolic blood pressure, circumoral pallor, palpitations and nervousness in the unsedated patient. The sedated patient may exhibit only a pulse rate increase of 20 or more beats per minute for 15 or more seconds. Therefore, following the test dose, the heart rate should be monitored for a heart rate increase. Patients on beta-blockers may not manifest changes in heart rate, but blood pressure monitoring can detect an evanescent rise in systolic blood pressure. The test dose should also contain 10 to 15 mg of Sensorcaine (bupivacaine HCl) injection or an equivalent dose of a short-acting amide anesthetic such as 30 to 40 mg of lidocaine, to detect an unintentional intrathecal administration. This will be manifested within a few minutes by signs of spinal block (e.g. decreased sensation of the buttocks, paresis of the legs, or, in the sedated patient, absent knee jerk). An intravascular or subarachnoid injection is still possible even if results of the test dose are negative. The test dose itself may produce a systemic toxic reaction, high spinal or epinephrine-induced cardiovascular effects.

Injection of repeated doses of local anesthetics may cause significant increases in plasma levels with each repeated dose due to slow accumulation of the drug or its metabolites or to slow metabolic degradation. Tolerance to elevated blood levels varies with the physical condition of the patient. Debilitated, elderly patients, acutely ill patients and children should be given reduced doses commensurate with their age and physical condition. Local anesthetics should also be used with caution in patients with hypotension or heart block.
Careful and constant monitoring of cardiovascular and respiratory vital signs (adequacy of ventilation) and the patient's state of consciousness should be performed after each local anesthetic injection. It should be kept in mind at such times that restlessness, anxiety, incoherent speech, light-headedness, numbness and tingling of the mouth and lips, metallic taste, tinnitus, dizziness, blurred vision, tremors, twitching, depression, or drowsiness may be early warning signs of central nervous system toxicity.
Local anesthetic solutions containing a vasoconstrictor should be used cautiously and in carefully restricted quantities in areas of the body supplied by end arteries or having otherwise compromised blood supply such as digits, nose, external ear, penis, etc. Patients with hypertensive vascular disease may exhibit exaggerated vasoconstrictor response. Ischemic injury or necrosis may result.
Because amide-type local anesthetics such as bupivacaine are metabolized by the liver, these drugs, especially repeat doses, should be used cautiously in patients with hepatic disease. Patients with severe hepatic disease, because of their inability to metabolize local anesthetics normally, are at a greater risk of developing toxic plasma concentrations. Local anesthetics should also be used with caution in patients with impaired cardiovascular function because they may be less able to compensate for functional changes associated with the prolongation of A-V conduction produced by these drugs.
Serious dose-related cardiac arrythmias may occur if preparations containing a vasoconstrictor such as epinephrine are employed in patients during or following the administration of potent inhalation anesthetics. In deciding whether to use these products concurrently in the same patient, the combined action of both agents upon the myocardium, the concentration and volume of vasoconstrictor used, and the time since injection, when applicable, should be taken into account.
Many drugs used during the conduct of anesthesia are considered potential triggering agents for familial malignant hyperthermia. Because it is not known whether amide-type local anesthetics may trigger this reaction and because the need for supplemental general anesthesia cannot be predicted in advance, it is suggested that a standard protocol for management should be available. Early unexplained signs of tachycardia, tachypnea, labile blood pressure and metabolic acidosis may precede temperature elevation. Successful outcome is dependent on early diagnosis, prompt discontinuance of the suspect triggering agent(s) and prompt treatment, including oxygen therapy, dantrolene (consult dantrolene sodium intravenous package insert before using) and other supportive measures.
Use in Head and Neck Area: Small doses of local anesthetics injected into the head and neck area, including retrobulbar, dental and stellate ganglion blocks, may produce adverse reactions similar to systemic toxicity seen with unintentional intravascular injections of larger doses. The injection procedures require the utmost care. Confusion, convulsions, respiratory depression and/or respiratory arrest, and cardiovascular stimulation or depression have been reported. These reactions may be due to intraarterial injection of the local anesthetic with retrograde flow to the cerebral circulation. They also may be due to puncture of the dural sheath of the optic nerve during retrobulbar block with diffusion of any local anesthetic along the subdural space to the midbrain. Patients receiving these blocks should have their circulation and respiration monitored and be constantly observed. Resuscitative equipment and personnel for treating

adverse reactions should be immediately available. Dosage recommendations should not be exceeded. (See DOSAGE AND ADMINISTRATION.)

Use in Ophthalmic Surgery: Clinicians who perform retrobulbar blocks should be aware that there have been reports of respiratory arrest following local anesthetic injection. Prior to retrobulbar block, as with all other regional procedures the immediate availability of equipment, drugs, and personnel to manage respiratory arrest or depression, convulsions, and cardiac stimulation or depression should be assured (see also WARNINGS and USE IN HEAD AND NECK AREA, above). As with other anesthetic procedures, patients should be constantly monitored following ophthalmic blocks for signs of these adverse reactions, which may occur following relatively low total doses. A concentration of 0.75% bupvacaine is indicated for retrobulbar block, however this concentration is not indicated for any other peripheral nerve block, including the facial nerve and not indicated for local infiltration, including the conjunctiva (See INDICATIONS and PRECAUTIONS, General). Mixing Sensorcaine with other local anesthetics is not recommended because of insufficient data on the clinical use of such mixtures. When Sensorcaine 0.75% is used for retrobulbar block, complete corneal anesthesia usually precedes onset of clinically acceptable external ocular muscle akinesia. Therefore, the presence of akinesia rather than anesthesia alone should determine readiness of the patient for surgery.

Information for Patients: When appropriate, patients should be informed in advance that they may experience temporary loss of sensation and motor activity, usually in the lower half of the body following proper administration of caudal or lumbar epidural anesthesia. Also, when appropriate, the physician should discuss other information including adverse reactions in the Sensorcaine (bupivacaine HCl) package insert.

Clinically Significant Drug Interactions: The administration of local anesthetic solutions containing epinephrine or norepinephrine to patients receiving monoamine oxidase inhibitors or tricyclic antidepressants may produce severe, prolonged hypertension. Concurrent use of these agents should generally be avoided. In situations in which concurrent therapy is necessary, careful patient monitoring is essential.

Concurrent administration of vasopressor drugs and of ergot-type oxytocic drugs may cause severe, persistent hypertension or cerebrovascular accidents.

Phenothiazines and butyrophenones may reduce or reverse the pressor effect of epinephrine.

Carcinogenesis, Mutagenesis, and Impairment of Fertility: - Long-term studies in animals of most local anesthetics, including bupivacaine, to evaluate the carcinogenic potential have not been conducted. Mutagenic potential or the effect on fertility have not been determined. There is no evidence from human data that bupivacaine may be carcinogenic or mutagenic or that it impairs fertility.

Pregnancy Category C: Decreased pup survival in rats and embryocidal effect in rabbits have been observed when bupivacaine HCl was administered to these species in doses comparable to nine and five times, respectively, the maximum recommended daily human dose (400 mg). There are no adequate and well-controlled studies in pregnant women of the effect of bupivacaine on the developing fetus. Sensorcaine (bupivacaine HCl) injection should be used during pregnancy only if the potential benefit justifies the potential risk to the fetus. This does not exclude the use of Sensorcaine (bupivacaine HCl) injection (0.25% and 0.5% concentrations) at term for obstetrical anesthesia or analgesia. (See LABOR AND DELIVERY.)

Labor and Delivery: See Box WARNING regarding obstetrical use of 0.75% concentration.

Sensorcaine (bupivacaine HCl) injection is contraindicated in obstetrical paracervical block anesthesia.

Local anesthetics rapidly cross the placenta, and when used for epidural, caudal or pudendal block anesthesia, can cause varying degrees of maternal, fetal and neonatal toxicity. (See Pharmacokinetics in CLINICAL PHARMACOLOGY.) The incidence and degree of toxicity depend upon the procedure performed, the type and amount of drug used, and the technique of drug administration. Adverse reactions in the parturient, fetus and neonate involve alterations of the central nervous system, peripheral vascular tone and cardiac function.

Maternal hypotension has resulted from regional anesthesia. Local anesthetics produce vasodilation by blocking sympathetic nerves. Elevating the patient's legs and positioning her on her left side will help prevent decreases in blood pressure. The fetal heart rate also should be monitored continuously, and electronic fetal monitoring is highly advisable. Epidural, caudal, or pudendal anesthesia may alter the forces of parturition through changes in uterine contractility or maternal expulsive efforts. Epidural anesthesia has been reported to prolong the second stage of labor by removing the parturient's reflex urge to bear down or by interfering with motor function. The use of obstetrical anesthesia may increase the need for forceps assistance.

The use of some local anesthetic drug products during labor and delivery may be followed by diminished muscle strength and tone for the first day or two of life. This has not been reported with Sensorcaine (bupivacaine HCl) injection.

It is extremely important to avoid aortocaval compression by the gravid uterus during administration of regional block to parturients. To do this, the patient must be maintained in the left lateral decubitus position or a blanket roll or sandbag may be placed beneath the right hip and the gravid uterus displaced to the left.

Nursing Mothers: It is not known whether local anesthetic drugs are excreted in human milk. Because many drugs are excreted in human milk, caution should be exercised when local anesthetics are administered to a nursing mother.

Pediatric Use: Until further experience is gained in children younger than 12 years, administration of Sensorcaine (bupivacaine HCl) injection in this age group is not recommended.

ADVERSE REACTIONS

Reactions to bupivacaine are characteristic of those associated with other amide-type local anesthetics. A major cause of adverse reactions to this group of drugs may be associated with its excessive plasma levels, which may be due to overdosage, unintentional intravascular injection or slow metabolic degradation.

Systemic: The most commonly encountered acute adverse experiences that demand immediate countermeasures are related to the central nervous system and the cardiovascular system. These adverse experiences are generally dose related and due to high plasma levels which may result from overdosage, rapid absorption from the injection site, diminished tolerance or from unintentional intravascular injection of the local anesthetic solution. In addition to systemic dose-related toxicity, unintentional subarachnoid injection of drug during the intended performance of caudal or lumbar epidural block or nerve blocks near the vertebral column (especially in the head and neck region) may result in underventilation or apnea ("Total or High Spinal"). Also, hypotension due to loss of sympathetic tone and respiratory paralysis or underventilation due to cephalad extension of the motor level of anesthesia may occur. This may lead to secondary cardiac arrest if untreated. Factors influencing plasma protein binding, such as acidosis, systemic diseases that alter protein production or competition with other drugs for protein binding sites, may diminish individual tolerance.

Central Nervous System Reactions: These are characterized by excitation and/or depression. Restlessness, anxiety, dizziness, tinnitus, blurred vision or tremors may occur, possibly proceeding to convulsions. However, excitement may be transient or absent, with depression being the first manifestation of an adverse reaction. This may quickly be followed by drowsiness merging into unconsciousness and respiratory arrest. Other central nervous system effects may be nausea, vomiting, chills, and constriction of the pupils.

The incidence of convulsions associated with the use of local anesthetics varies with the procedure used and the total dose administered. In a survey of studies of epidural anesthesia, overt toxicity progressing to convulsions occurred in approximately 0.1 percent of local anesthetic administrations.

Cardiovascular System Reactions: High doses or unintentional intravascular injection may lead to high plasma levels and related depression of the myocardium, decreased cardiac output, heart block, hypotension, bradycardia, ventricular arrhythmias, including ventricular tachycardia and ventricular fibrillation, and cardiac arrest. (See WARNINGS, PRECAUTIONS, and OVERDOSAGE sections).

Allergic: Allergic type reactions are rare and may occur as a result of sensitivity to the local anesthetic or to other formulation ingredients, such as the antimicrobial preservative methylparaben contained in multiple dose vials or sulfites in epinephrine-containing solutions (see WARNINGS). These reactions are characterized by signs such as urticaria, pruritis, erythema, angioneurotic edema (including laryngeal edema), tachycardia, sneezing, nausea, vomiting, dizziness, syncope, excessive sweating, elevated temperature, and possibly, anaphylactoid symptomatology (including severe hypotension). Cross sensitivity among members of the amide-type local anesthetic group has been reported. The usefulness of screening for sensitivity has not been definitely established.

Neurologic: The incidence of adverse neurologic reactions associated with the use of local anesthetics may be related to the total dose of local anesthetic administered and are also dependent upon the particular drug used, the route of administraion and the physical status of the patient. Many of these effects may be related to local anesthetic techniques, with or without a contribution from the drug.

In the practice of caudal or lumbar epidural block, occasional unintentional penetration of the subarachnoid space by the catheter or needle may occur. Subsequent adverse effects may depend partially on the amount of drug administered intrathecally and the physiological and physical effects of a dural puncture. A high spinal is characterized by paralysis of the legs, loss of consciousness, respiratory paralysis and bradycardia.

Neurologic effects following unintentional subarachnoid administration during epidural or caudal anesthesia may include spinal block by varying magnitude (including high or total spinal block); hypotension secondary to spinal block; urinary retention; fecal and urinary incontinence; loss of perineal sensation and sexual function; persistent anesthesia, paresthesia, weakness, paralysis of the lower extremities and loss of sphincter control, all of which may have slow, incomplete or no recovery; headache; backache; septic meningitis; meningismus; slowing of labor; increased incidence of forceps delivery; or cranial nerve palsies due to traction on nerves from loss of cerebrospinal fluid.

OVERDOSAGE

Acute emergencies from local anesthetics are generally related to high plasma levels encountered during therapeutic use of local anesthetics or to unintended subarachnoid injection of local anesthetic solution. (See ADVERSE REACTIONS, WARNINGS, and PRECAUTIONS.)

Management of Local Anesthetic Emergencies: The first consideration is prevention, best accomplished by careful and constant monitoring of cardiovascular and respiratory vital signs and the patient's state of consciousness after each local anesthetic injection . At the first sign of change, oxygen should be administered.

The first step in the management of systemic toxic reactions, as well as underventilation or apnea due to unintentional subarachnoid injection of drug solution, consists of immediate attention to the establishment and maintenance of a patent airway and effective assisted or controlled ventilation with 100% oxygen with a delivery system capable of permitting immediate positive airway pressure by mask. This may prevent convulsions if they have not already occurred.

If necessary, use drugs to control the convulsions. A 50 to 100 mg bolus I.V. injection of succinylcholine will paralyze the patient without depressing the central nervous or cardiovascular systems and facilitate ventilation. A bolus I.V. dose of 5 to 10 mg of diazepam or 50 to 100 mg of thiopental will permit ventilation and counteract central nervous system stimulation, but these drugs also depress the central nervous system, respiratory and cardiac function, add to postictal depression, and may result in apnea. Intravenous barbiturates, anticonsulsant agents, or muscle relaxants should only be administered by those familiar with their use. Immediately after the institution of these ventilatory measures, the adequacy of the circulation should be evaluated. Supportive treatment of circulatory depression may require administration of intravenous fluids, and, when appropriate, a vasopressor dictated by the clinical situation (such as ephedrine or epinephrine to enhance myocardial contractile force).

If difficulty is encountered in the maintenance of a patent airway or if prolonged ventilatory support (assisted or controlled) is indicated, endotracheal intubation, employing drugs and techniques familiar to the clinician, may be indicated after initial administration of oxygen by mask.

Recent clinical data from patients experiencing local anesthetic induced convulsions demonstrated rapid development of hypoxia, hypercarbia and acidosis wih bupivacaine within a minute of the onset of convulsions. These observations suggest the oxygen consumption and carbon dioxide production are greatly increased during local anesthetic convulsions and emphasize the importance of immediate and effective ventilation with oxygen which may avoid cardiac arrest.

If not treated immediately, convulsions with simultaneous hypoxia, hypercarbia and acidosis, plus myocardial depression from the direct effects of the local anesthetic may result in cardiac arrhythmias, bradycardia, asystole, ventricular fibrillation, or cardiac arrest. Respiratory abnormalities, including apnea, may occur. Underventilation or apnea due to unintentional subarachnoid injection of local anesthetic solution may produce these same signs and also lead to cardiac arrest if ventilatory support is not instituted. If cardiac arrest should occur, a successful outcome may require prolonged resuscitative efforts.

The supine position is dangerous in pregnant women at term because of aortocaval compression by the gravid uterus. Therefore, during treatment of systemic toxicity, maternal hypotension or fetal bradycardia following regional block, the parturient should be maintained in the left lateral decubitus position if possible, or manual displacement of the uterus off the great vessels be accomplished.

The mean seizure dosage of bupivacaine in rhesus monkeys was found to be 4.4 mg/kg with mean arterial plasma concentration of 4.5 mcg/mL. The intravenous and subcutaneous LD_{50} in mice is 6 to 8mg/kg and 38 to 54mg/kg respectively.

DOSAGE AND ADMINISTRATION

The dosage of any local anesthetic administered varies with the anesthetic procedure, the area to be anesthetized, the vascularity of the tissues, the number of neuronal segments to be blocked, the depth of anesthesia and degree of muscle relaxation required, the duration of anesthesia desired, indi-

Continued on next page

Astra—Cont.

vidual tolerance, and the physical condition of the patient. The smallest dose and concentration required to produce the desired result should be administered. Dosage of SENSOR-CAINE should be reduced for young, elderly and debilitated patients and patients with cardiac and/or liver disease. The rapid injection of a large volume of local anesthetic solution should be avoided and fractional (incremental) doses should be used when feasible. For specific techniques and procedures, refer to standard textbooks.

In recommended doses, SENSORCAINE produces complete sensory block, but the effect on motor function differs among the three concentrations.

0.25%—when used for caudal, epidural, or peripheral nerve block, produces incomplete motor block. Should be used for operations in which muscle relaxation is not important, or when another means of providing muscle relaxation is used concurrently. Onset of action may be slower than with the 0.5% or 0.75% solutions.

0.5%—provides motor blockade for caudal, epidural, or nerve block, but muscle relaxation may be inadequate for operations in which complete muscle relaxation is essential.

0.75%—produces complete motor block. Most useful for epidural block in abdominal operations requiring complete muscle relaxation, and for retrobulbar anesthesia. Not for obstetrical anesthesia.

The duration of anesthesia with SENSORCAINE is such that for most indications, a single dose is sufficient.

Maximum dosage limit must be individualized in each case after evaluating the size and physical status of the patient, as well as the usual rate of systemic absorption from a particular injection site. Most experience to date is with single doses of SENSORCAINE up to 225 mg with epinephrine 1:200,000 and 175 mg without epinephrine, more or less drug may be used depending on individualization of each case. These doses may be repeated up to once every three hours. In clinical studies to date, total daily doses up to 400 mg have been reported. Until further experience is gained, this dose should not be exceeded in 24 hours. The duration of anesthetic effect may be prolonged by the addition of epinephrine.

The dosages in Table 1 have generally proved satisfactory and are recommended as a guide for use in the average adult. These dosages should be reduced for young, elderly or debilitated patients. Until further experience is gained, SENSORCAINE is not recommended for children younger than 12 years. SENSORCAINE is contraindicated in obstetrical paracervical blocks and is not recommended for intravenous regional anesthesia (Bier Block).

Use in Epidural Anesthesia: During epidural administration of SENSORCAINE, 0.5% and 0.75% solutions should be administered in incremental doses of 3 mL to 5 mL, with sufficient time between doses to detect toxic manifestations of unintentional intravascular or intrathecal injection . In obstetrics, only the 0.5% and 0.25% concentrations should be used; incremental doses of 3 mL to 5 mL of the 0.5% solution, not exceeding 50 mg to 100 mg at any dosing interval, are recommended. Repeat doses should be preceded by a test dose containing epinephrine if not contraindicated.

Use only the single-dose ampules and single-dose vials for caudal or epidural anesthesia, the multiple-dose vials contain a preservative and therefore should not be used for these procedures.

Test dose for Caudal and Lumbar Epidural Blocks: See PRECAUTIONS.

HOW SUPPLIED
Sensorcaine (bupivacaine HCl) injections

Dosage Form	Concentrate	Astra Sterile-Pak®
Single Dose Vials, 10 mL	0.25%, 0.5% and 0.75% without epinephrine 0.25%, 0.5%, 0.75% with epinephrine 1:200,000	
Single Dose Vials, 30 mL	0.25%, 0.5% and 0.75% without epinephrine 0.25%, 0.5% and 0.75% with epinephrine 1:200,000	x (not 0.75%) x (not 0.25%)
Multiple dose Vials, 50 mL	0.25% and 0.5% without epinephrine 0.25% and 0.5% with epinephrine 1:200,000	
Single Dose Ampules, 30 mL	0.25%, 0.5%, 0.75% without epinephrine 0.5% and 0.75% with epinephrine 1:200,000	x x
Single Dose Ampules, 5 mL	0.5% with epinephrine 1:200,000	

x–Package forms—also available in Astra Sterile-Pak® Pre-sterilized vials or ampules in a Convenient Dispenser Carton.

Unused portions of solutions in single dose containers should be discarded, since this product form contains no preservatives.
[See table below].
NOTE: Parenteral drug products should be inspected visually for particulate matter and discoloration prior to administration whenever the solution and container permit. Solutions that are discolored and/or contain particulate matter should not be used.

HOW SUPPLIED
SOLUTIONS OF SENSORCAINE(BUPIVACAINE HYDROCHLORIDE) SHOULD NOT BE USED FOR THE PRODUCTION OF SPINAL ANESTHESIA (SUBARACHNOID BLOCK) BECAUSE OF INSUFFICIENT DATA TO SUPPORT SUCH USE.
[See table above].
Disinfecting agents containing heavy metals, which cause release of respective ions (mercury, zinc, copper, etc.), should not be used for skin or mucous membrane disinfection since they have been related to incidents of swelling and edema. When chemical disinfection of the container surface is desired, either isopropyl alcohol (91%) or ethyl alcohol (70%) is recommended. It is recommended that chemical disinfection be accomplished by wiping the ampule or vial stopper thoroughly with cotton or gauze that has been moistened with the recommended alcohol just prior to use.
Solutions should be stored at controlled room temperature 15° to 30° C (59°–86°F).
Solutions containing epinephrine should be protected from light.

021851R11   Rev. 9/87(11)

SENSORCAINE® SPINAL   ℞
[sén-sor-caine]
(Bupivacaine in Dextrose Injection USP)
Bupivacaine HCl 0.75% in Dextrose 8.25% Injection
Sterile Hyperbaric Solution for Spinal Anesthesia

(For details of indications, dosages and administration, precautions, and adverse reactions, see circular in package.)

DOSAGE AND ADMINISTRATION
The dose of any local anesthetic administered varies with the anesthetic procedure, the area to be anesthetized, the vascularity of the tissues, the number of neuronal segments to be blocked, the depth of anesthesia and degree of muscle relaxation required, the duration of anesthesia desired, individual tolerance, and the physical condition of the patient. The smallest dose and concentration required to produce the desired result should be administered. Dosages of Sensorcaine Spinal (Bupivacaine in Dextrose Injection USP) should be reduced for elderly and debilitated patients and patients with cardiac and/or liver disease.

For specific techniques and procedures, refer to standard textbooks.

The extent and degree of spinal anesthesia depend upon several factors including dosage, specific gravity of the anesthetic solution, volume of solution used, force of injection, level of puncture, and position of the patient during and immediately after injection.

Seven and one-half mg (7.5 mg or 1.0 mL) Sensorcaine Spinal has generally proven satisfactory for spinal anesthesia for lower extremity and perineal procedures including TURP and vaginal hysterectomy. Twelve mg (12 mg or 1.6 mL) has been used for lower abdominal procedures such as abdominal hysterectomy, tubal ligation, and appendectomy. These doses are recommended as a guide for use in the average adult and may be reduced for the elderly or debilitated patients. Because experience with Sensorcaine Spinal is limited in patients below the age of 18 years, dosage recommendations in this age group cannot be made.

Obstetrical Use
Doses as low as 6 mg of bupivacaine hydrochloride have been used for vaginal delivery under spinal anesthesia. The dose range of 7.5 mg to 10.5 mg (1 mL to 1.4 mL) bupivacaine hydrochloride has been used for Cesarean section under spinal anesthesia.

In recommended doses, Sensorcaine Spinal produces complete motor and sensory block.

Unused portions of solutions should be discarded following initial use.

Sensorcaine Spinal should be inspected visually for discoloration and particulate matter prior to administration; solutions which are discolored or which contain particulate matter should not be used.

Sensorcaine Spinal solution may be autoclaved once at 15 pound pressure, 121° C (250° F) for 15 minutes. Do not administer any solution which is discolored or contains particulate matter.

HOW SUPPLIED
NDC 0186-1026-03 2 mL ampule (15 mg bupivacaine HCl with 165 mg dextrose), boxes of 10.
Store at controlled room temperature, between 15° C and 30° C (59° F and 86° F).
021868R00   Iss. 12/86

SODIUM BICARBONATE   ℞
[so '-dēum by-car '-bōw-nāte]
Injection, USP

FOR CORRECTION OF METABOLIC ACIDOSIS AND OTHER CONDITIONS REQUIRING SYSTEMIC ALKALINIZATION
(For details of indications, dosage and administration, precautions, and adverse reactions, see circular in package.)

HOW SUPPLIED
Sodium Bicarbonate Injection, USP is supplied in the following dosage forms:
[See table on top next page].
Solutions should be stored at controlled room temperature 15°–30°C (59°–86–86°F).
021852R00   Rev. 7/88

TABLE 1. DOSAGE RECOMMENDATIONS—SENSORCAINE (bupivacaine HCl) INJECTIONS

Type of Block	conc.(%)	Each Dose (mL.)	Each Dose (mg.)	Motor Block[1]
Local infiltration	0.25[4]	up to max.	up to max.	—
Epidural	0.75[2,4]	10–20	75–150	Complete
	0.50[4]	10–20	50–100	Moderate to complete
	0.25[4]	10–20	25–50	Partial to moderate
Caudal	0.50[4]	15–30	75–150	Moderate to complete
	0.25[4]	15–30	37.5–75	Moderate
Peripheral	0.50[4]	5 to max.	25 to max.	Moderate to complete
	0.25[4]	5 to max.	12.5 to max.	Moderate to complete
Retrobulbar[3]	0.75[4]	2–4	15–30	Complete
Sympathetic[3]	0.25	20–50	50–125	—
Epidural Test Dose	0.5 w/epi.	2–3	10–15 (see PRECAUTIONS)	—

[1]With continuous (intermittent) techniques, repeat doses increase the degree of motor block. The first repeat dose of 0.5% may produce complete motor block. Intercostal nerve block with 0.25% may also produce complete motor block for intra-abdominal surgery.
[2]For single dose; not for intermittent (catheter) epidural technique. Not for obstetrical anesthesia.
[3]See PRECAUTIONS.
[4]Solutions with or without epinephrine.

NDC No. 0186-	Dosage Form	Conc. %	mg/mL (NaHCO₃)	mEq/mL; (Na+)	mEq/mL (HCO₃)	mEq/Container size (mL)	mOsm
0650-01	Syringe	8.4	84	1.0	1.0	50/50	2/mL
0656-01	Syringe (Pediatric)	8.4	84	1.0	1.0	10/10	2/mL
0647-01	Syringe	7.5	75	0.9	0.9	44.6/50	1.79/mL
0646-01	Syringe (Infant)	4.2	42	0.5	0.5	5/10	1/mL
0645-01	Syringe (Infant)	4.2	42	0.5	0.5	2.5/5	1/mL

XYLOCAINE® (lidocaine hydrochloride)   ℞

[zī'lo-caine]

INJECTIONS
Local anesthetic for
infiltration and nerve block

DESCRIPTION

Xylocaine (lidocaine HCl) Injections are sterile non-pyrogenic aqueous solutions that contain a local anesthetic agent and are administered parenterally by injection. See INDICATIONS for specific uses. The specific quantitative composition for each available solution is shown in Table 1.

Xylocaine solutions contain lidocaine HCl, which is chemically designated as acetamide 2-(diethylamino)-N-(2,6-dimethylphenyl)-monohydrochloride and has the molecular wt. 270.8.

Epinephrine is (−)-3.4-Dihydroxy-α-[(methylamino) methyl] benzyl alcohol and has the molecular wt. 183.21. [See table below].

CLINICAL PHARMACOLOGY

Mechanism of action: Lidocaine stabilizes the neuronal membrane by inhibiting the ionic fluxes required for the initiation and conduction of impulses, thereby effecting local anesthetic action.

Hemodynamics: Excessive blood levels may cause changes in cardiac output, total peripheral resistance, and mean arterial pressure. With central neural blockade these changes may be attributable to block of autonomic fibers, a direct depressant effect of the local anesthetic agent on various components of the cardiovascular system and/or the beta-adrenergic receptor stimulating action of epinephrine when present. The net effect is normally a modest hypotension when the recommended dosages are not exceeded.

Pharmacokinetics and metabolism: Information derived from diverse formulations, concentrations and usages reveals that lidocaine is completely absorbed following parenteral administration, its rate of absorption depending, for example, upon various factors such as the site of administration and the presence or absence of a vasoconstrictor agent. Except for intravascular administration, the highest blood levels are obtained following intercoastal nerve block and the lowest after subcutaneous administration.

The plasma binding of lidocaine is dependent on drug concentration, and the fraction bound decreases with increasing concentration. At concentrations of 1 to 4 μg of free base per mL 60 to 80 percent of lidocaine is protein bound. Binding is also dependent on the plasma concentration of the alpha-1-acid glycoprotein.

Lidocaine crosses the blood-brain and placental barriers, presumably by passive diffusion.

Lidocaine is metabolized rapidly by the liver, and metabolites and unchanged drug are excreted by the kidneys. Biotransformation includes oxidative N-dealkylation, ring hydroxylation, cleavage of the amide linkage, and conjugation. N-dealkylation, a major pathway of biotransformation, yields the metabolites monoethylglycinexylidide and glycinexylidide. The pharmacological/toxicological actions of these metabolites are similar to, but less potent than, those of lidocaine. Approximately 90% of lidocaine administered is excreted in the form of various metabolites, and less than 10% is excreted unchanged. The primary metabolite in urine is a conjugate of 4-hyroxy-2, 6-dimethylaniline.

The elimination half-life of lidocaine following an intravenous bolus injection is typically 1.5 to 2.0 hours. Because of the rapid rate at which lidocaine is metabolized, any condition that affects liver function may alter lidocaine kinetics. The half-life may be prolonged two-fold or more in patients with liver dysfunction. Renal dysfunction does not affect lidocaine kinetics but may increase the accumulation of metabolites.

Factors such as acidosis and the use of CNS stimulants and depressants affect the CNS levels of lidocaine required to produce overt systemic effects. Objective adverse manifestations become increasingly apparent with increasing venous plasma levels above 6.0 μg free base per mL. In the rhesus monkey arterial blood levels of 18–21 μg/mL have been shown to be threshold for convulsive activity.

INDICATIONS AND USAGE

Xylocaine (lidocaine HCl) Injections are indicated for production of local or regional anesthesia by infiltration techniques such as percutaneous injection and intravenous regional anesthesia by peripheral nerve block techniques such as brachial plexus and intercostal and by central neural techniques such as lumbar and caudal epidural blocks, when the accepted procedures for these techniques as described in standard textbooks are observed.

CONTRAINDICATIONS

Lidocaine is contraindicated in patients with a known history of hypersensitivity to local anesthetics of the amide type.

WARNINGS

XYLOCAINE INJECTIONS FOR INFILTRATION AND NERVE BLOCK SHOULD BE EMPLOYED ONLY BY CLINICIANS WHO ARE WELL VERSED IN DIAGNOSIS AND MANAGEMENT OF DOSE-RELATED TOXICITY AND OTHER ACUTE EMERGENCIES THAT MIGHT ARISE FROM THE BLOCK TO BE EMPLOYED AND THEN ONLY AFTER ENSURING THE *IMMEDIATE* AVAILABILITY OF OXYGEN, OTHER RESUSCITATIVE DRUGS, CARDIOPULMONARY EQUIPMENT, AND THE PERSONNEL NEEDED FOR PROPER MANAGEMENT OF TOXIC REACTIONS AND RELATED EMERGENCIES (See also ADVERSE REACTIONS and PRECAUTIONS). DELAY IN PROPER MANAGEMENT OF DOSE-RELATED TOXICITY, UNDERVENTILATION FROM ANY CAUSE AND/OR ALTERED SENSITIVITY MAY LEAD TO THE DEVELOPMENT OF ACIDOSIS, CARDIAC ARREST AND, POSSIBLY, DEATH.

To avoid intravascular injection, aspiration should be performed before the local anesthetic solution is injected. The needle must be repositioned until no return of blood can be elicited by aspiration. Note, however, that the absence of blood in the syringe does not guarantee that intravascular injection has been avoided.

Local anesthetic solutions containing antimicrobial preservatives (e.g., methylparaben) should not be used for epidural or spinal anesthesia because the safety of these agents has not been established with regard to intrathecal injection, either intentional or accidental.

Xylocaine with epinephrine solutions contain sodium metabisulfite, a sulfite that may cause allergic-type reactions including anaphylactic symptoms and life-threatening or less severe asthmatic episodes in certain susceptible people. The overall prevalence of sulfite sensitivity in the general population is unknown and probably low. Sulfite sensitivity is seen more frequently in asthmatic than in nonasthmatic people.

PRECAUTIONS

General: The safety and effectivness of lidocaine depend on proper dosage, correct technique, adequate precautions, and readiness for emergencies. Standard textbooks should be consulted for specific techniques and precautions for various regional anesthetic procedures.

Resuscitative equipment, oxygen, and other resuscitative drugs should be available for immediate use. (See WARNINGS and ADVERSE REACTIONS). The lowest dosage that results in effective anesthesia should be used to avoid high plasma levels and serious adverse effects. Syringe aspirations should also be performed before and during each supplemental injection when using indwelling catheter techniques. During the administration of epidural anesthesia, it is recommended that a test dose be administered initially and that the patient be monitored for central nervous system toxicity and cardiovascular toxicity, as well as for signs of unintended intrathecal administration before proceeding. When clinical conditions permit, consideration should be given to employing local anesthetic solutions that contain epinephrine for the test dose because circulatory changes compatible with epinephrine may also serve as a warning sign of unintended intravascular injection. An intravascular injection is still possible even if aspirations for blood are negative. Repeated doses of lidocaine may cause significant increases in blood levels with each repeated dose because of slow accumulation of the drug or its metabolites. Tolerance to elevated blood levels varies with the status of the patient. Debilitated, elderly patients, acutely ill patients and children should be given reduced doses commensurate with their age and physical condition. Lidocaine should also be used with caution in patients with severe shock or heart block. Lumbar and caudal epidural anesthesia should be used with extreme caution in persons with the following conditions: existing neurological disease, spinal deformities, septicemia and severe hypertension.

Local anesthetic solutions containing a vasoconstrictor should be used cautiously and in carefully circumscribed quantities in areas of the body supplied by end arteries or having otherwise compromised blood supply. Patients with peripheral vascular disease and those with hypertensive vascular disease may exhibit exaggerated vasoconstrictor response. Ischemic injury or necrosis may result. Preparations containing a vasoconstrictor should be used with caution in patients during or following the administration of potent general anesthetic agents, since cardiac arrhythmias may occur under such conditions.

Careful and constant monitoring of cardiovascular and respiratory (adequacy of ventilation) vital signs and the patient's state of consciousness should be accomplished after each local anesthetic injection. It should be kept in mind at such times that restlessness, anxiety, tinnitus, dizziness, blurred vision,

Continued on next page

TABLE I COMPOSITION OF AVAILABLE SOLUTIONS

PRODUCT IDENTIFICATION		FORMULA						
		SINGLE DOSE VIALS AND AMPULES			MULTIPLE DOSE VIALS			
Xylocaine (lidocaine HCl) Injection (Percent)	Epinephrine (dilution)	Sodium Chloride (mg/mL)	Sodium Metabisulfite (mg/mL)	Citric Acid (mg/mL)	Sodium Chloride (mg/mL)	Sodium Metabisulfite (mg/mL)	Citric Acid (mg/mL)	Methyl-Paraben (mg/mL)
0.5	None	8.0	None	None	8.0	None	None	1.0
0.5	1:200,000	N.S.	N.S.	N.S.	8.0	0.5	0.2	1.0
1.0	None	7.0	None	None	7.0	None	None	1.0
1.0	1:200,000	7.0	0.5	0.2	N.S.	N.S.	N.S.	N.S.
1.0	1:100,000	N.S.	N.S.	N.S.	7.0	0.5	0.2	1.0
1.5	None	6.5	None	None	N.S.	N.S.	N.S.	N.S.
1.5	1:200,000	6.5	0.5	0.2	N.S.	N.S.	N.S.	N.S.
2.0	None	6.0	None	None	6.0	None	None	1.0
2.0	1:200,000	6.0	0.5	0.2	N.S.	N.S.	N.S.	N.S.
2.0	1:100,000	N.S.	N.S.	N.S.	6.0	0.5	0.2	1.0

N.S. Not Supplied

NOTE: pH of all solutions adjusted to USP limits with sodium hydroxide and/or hydrochloric acid.

Astra—Cont.

tremors, depression or drowsiness may be early warning signs of central nervous system toxicity.

Since amide-type local anesthetics are metabolized by the liver, Xylocaine Injection should be used with caution in patients with hepatic disease. Patients with severe hepatic disease because of their inability to metabolize local anesthetics normally, are at greater risk of developing toxic plasma concentrations. Xylocaine Injection should also be used with caution in patients with impaired cardiovascular function since they may be less able to compensate for functional changes associated with the prolongation of A-V conduction produced by these drugs.

Many drugs used during the conduct of anesthesia are considered potential triggering agents for familial malignant hyperthermia. Since it is not known whether amide-type local anesthetics may trigger this reaction and since the need for supplemental general anesthesia cannot be predicted in advance, it is suggested that a standard protocol for the management of malignant hyperthermia should be available. Early unexplained signs of tachycardia, tachypnea, labile blood pressure and metabolic acidosis may precede temperature elevation. Successful outcome is dependent on early diagnosis, prompt discontinuance of the suspect triggering agent(s) and institution of treatment, including oxygen therapy, indicated supportive measures and dantrolene (consult dantrolene sodium intravenous package insert before using).

Proper tourniquet technique, as described in publications and standard textbooks, is essential in the performance of intravenous regional anesthesia. Solutions containing epinephrine or other vasoconstrictors should not be used for this technique.

Lidocaine should be used with caution in persons with known drug sensitivities. Patients allergic to para-aminobenzoic acid derivatives (procaine, tetracaine, benzocaine, etc.) have not shown cross sensitivity to lidocaine.

Use in the Head and Neck Area: Small doses of local anesthetics injected into the head and neck area, including retrobulbar, dental and stellate ganglion blocks, may produce adverse reactions similar to systemic toxicity seen with unintentional intravascular injections of larger doses. Confusion, convulsions, respiratory depression and/or respiratory arrest, and cardiovascular stimulation or depression have been reported. These reactions may be due to intra-arterial injection of the local anesthetic with retrograde flow to the cerebral circulation. Patients receiving these blocks should have their circulation and respiration monitored and be constantly observed. Resuscitative equipment and personnel for treating adverse reactions should be immediately available. Dosage recommendations should not be exceeded. (See DOSAGE and ADMINISTRATION).

Information for Patients: When appropriate, patients should be informed in advance that they may experience temporary loss of sensation and motor activity, usually in the lower half of the body, following proper administration of epidural anesthesia.

Clinically significant drug interactions: The administration of local anesthetic solutions containing epinephrine or norepinephrine to patients receiving monamine oxidase inhibitors or tricyclic antidepressants may produce severe, prolonged hypertension.

Phenothiazines and butyrophenones may reduce or reverse the pressor effect of epinephrine.

Concurrent use of these agents should generally be avoided. In situations when concurrent therapy is necessary, careful patient monitoring is essential.

Concurrent administration of vasopressor drugs (for the treatment of hypotension related to obstetric blocks) and ergot-type oxytocic drugs may cause severe, persistent hypertension or cerebrovascular accidents.

Drug Laboratory test interactions: The intramuscular injection of lidocaine may result in an increase in creatine phosphokinase levels. Thus, the use of this enzyme determination without isoenzyme separation, as a diagnostic test for the presence of acute myocardial infarction may be compromised by the intramuscular injection of lidocaine.

Carcinogenesis, mutagenesis, impairment of fertility: Studies of lidocaine in animals to evaluate the carcinogenic and mutagenic potential or the effect on fertility have not been conducted.

Pregnancy: Teratogenic Effects. Pregnancy Category B. Reproduction studies have been performed in rats at doses up to 6.6 times the human dose and have revealed no evidence of harm to the fetus caused by lidocaine. There are, however, no adequate and well-controlled studies in pregnant women. Animal reproduction studies are not always predictive of human response. General consideration should be given to this fact before administering lidocaine to women of childbearing potential, especially during early pregnancy when maximum organogenesis takes place.

Labor and delivery: Local anesthetics rapidly cross the placenta and when used for epidural, paracervical, pudendal or caudal block anesthesia, can cause varying degrees of maternal, fetal and neonatal toxicity (See CLINICAL PHARMACOLOGY—Pharmacokinetics). The potential for toxicity depends upon the procedure performed, the type and amount of drug used, and the technique of drug administration. Adverse reactions in the parturient, fetus and neonate involve alterations of the central nervous system peripheral vascular tone and cardiac function.

Maternal hypotension has resulted from regional anesthesia. Local anesthetics produce vasodilation by blocking sympathetic nerves. Elevating the patient's legs and positioning her on her left side will help prevent decreases in blood pressure. The fetal heart rate also should be monitored continuously, and electronic fetal monitoring is highly advisable.

Epidural, spinal, paracervical, or pudendal anesthesia may alter the forces of parturition through changes in uterine contractility or maternal expulsive efforts. In one study paracervical block anesthesia was associated with a decrease in the mean duration of first stage labor and facilitation of cervical dilation. However, spinal and epidural anesthesia have also been reported to prolong the second stage of labor by removing the parturient's reflex urge to bear down or by interfering with motor function. The use of obstetrical anesthesia may increase the need for forceps assistance.

The use of some local anesthetic drug products during labor and delivery may be followed by diminished muscle strength and tone for the first day or two of life. The long term significance of these observations is unknown. Fetal bradycardia may occur in 20 to 30 percent of patients receiving paracervical nerve block anesthesia with the amide-type local anesthetics and may be associated with fetal acidosis. Fetal heart rate should always be monitored during paracervical anesthesia. The physician should weigh the possible advantages against risks when considering paracervical block in prematurity, toxemia of pregnancy, and fetal distress. Careful adherence to recommended dosage is of the utmost importance in obstetrical paracervical block. Failure to achieve adequate analgesia with recommended doses should arouse suspicion of intravascular or fetal intracranial injection. Cases compatible with unintended fetal intracranial injection of local anesthetic solution have been reported following intended paracervical or pudendal block or both. Babies so affected present with unexplained neonatal depression at birth, which correlates with high local anesthetic serum levels, and often manifest seizures within six hours. Prompt use of supportive measures combined with forced urinary excretion of the local anesthetic has been used successfully to manage this complication.

Case reports of maternal convulsions and cardiovascular collapse following use of some local anesthetics for paracervical block in early pregnancy (as anesthesia for elective abortion) suggest that systemic absorption under these circumstances may be rapid. The recommended maximum dose of each drug should not be exceeded. Injection should be made slowly and with frequent aspiration. Allow a 5-minute interval between sides.

Nursing mothers: It is not known whether this drug is excreted in human milk. Because many drugs are excreted in human milk, caution should be exercised when lidocaine is administered to a nursing woman.

Pediatric use: Dosages in children should be reduced, commensurate with age, body weight and physical condition. See DOSAGE AND ADMINISTRATION.

ADVERSE REACTIONS

Systemic: Adverse experiences following the administration of lidocaine are similar in nature to those observed with other amide local anesthetic agents. These adverse experiences are, in general, dose-related and may result from high plasma levels caused by excessive dosage, rapid absorption or inadvertent intravascular injection, or may result from a hypersensitivity, idiosyncrasy or diminished tolerance on the part of the patient. Serious adverse experiences are generally systemic in nature. The following types are those most commonly reported:

Central nervous system: CNS manifestations are excitatory and/or depressant and may be characterized by lightheadedness, nervousness, apprehension, euphoria, confusion, dizziness, drowsiness, tinnitus, blurred or double vision, vomiting, sensations of heat, cold or numbness, twitching, tremors, convulsions, unconsciusness, respiratory depression and arrest. The excitatory manifestations may be very brief or may not occur at all, in which case the first manifestation of toxicity may be drowsiness merging into unconsciousness and respiratory arrest.

Drowsiness following the administration of lidocaine is usually an early sign of a high blood level of the drug and may occur as a consequence of rapid absorption.

Cardiovascular system: Cardiovascular manifestations are usually depressant and are characterized by bradycardia, hypotension, and cardiovascular collapse, which may lead to cardiac arrest.

Allergic: Allergic reactions are characterized by cutaneous lesions, urticaria, edema or anaphylactoid reactions. Allergic reactions may occur as a result of sensitivity either to local anesthetic agents or to the methylparaben used as a preservative in multiple dose vials. Allergic reactions as a result of sensitivity to lidocaine are extremely rare and, if they occur, should be managed by conventional means. The detection of sensitivity by skin testing is of doubtful value.

Neurologic: The incidences of adverse reactions associated with the use of local anesthetics may be related to the total dose of local anesthetic administered and are also dependent upon the particular drug used, the route of administration and the physical status of the patient. In a prospective review of 10,440 patients who received lidocaine for spinal anesthesia, the incidences of adverse reactions were reported to be about 3 percent each for positional headaches, hypotension and backache; 2 percent for shivering; and less than 1 percent each for peripheral nerve symptoms, nausea, respiratory inadequacy and double vision. Many of these observations may be related to local anesthetic techniques, with or without a contribution from the local anesthetic.

In the practice of caudal or lumbar epidural block, occasional unintentional penetration of the subarachnoid space by the catheter may occur. Subsequent adverse effects may depend partially on the amount of drug administered subdurally. These may include spinal block of varying magnitude (including total spinal block), hypotension secondary to spinal block, loss of bladder and bowel control, and loss of perineal sensation and sexual function. Persistent motor, sensory and/or autonomic (sphincter control) deficit of some lower spinal segments with slow recovery (several months) or incomplete recovery have been reported in rare instances when caudal or lumbar epidural block has been attempted. Backache and headache have also been noted following use of these anesthetic procedures.

OVERDOSAGE

Acute emergencies from local anesthetics are generally related to high plasma levels encountered during therapeutic use of local anesthetics or to unintended subarachnoid injection of local anesthetic solution (see ADVERSE REACTIONS, WARNINGS and PRECAUTIONS).

Management of local anesthetic emergencies: The first consideration is prevention, best accomplished by careful and constant monitoring of cardiovascular and respiratory vital signs and the patient's state of consciousness after each local anesthetic injection. At the first sign of change, oxygen should be administered.

The first step in the management of convulsions, as well as underventilation or apnea due to unintended subarachnoid injection of drug solution, consists of immediate attention to the maintenance of a patent airway and assisted or controlled ventilation with oxygen and a delivery system capable of permitting immediate positive airway pressure by mask. Immediately after the institution of these ventilatory measures, the adequacy of the circulation should be evaluated, keeping in mind that drugs used to treat convulsions sometimes depress the circulation when administered intravenously. Should convulsions persist despite adequate respiratory support, and if the status of the circulation permits, small increments of an ultra-short acting barbiturate (such as thiopental or thiamylal) or a benzodiazepine (such as diazepam) may be administered intravenously. The clinician should be familiar, prior to use of local anesthetics, with these anticonvulsant drugs. Supportive treatment of circulatory depression may require administration of intravenous fluids and, when appropriate, a vasopressor as directed by the clinical situation (e.g. ephedrine).

If not treated immediately, both convulsions and cardiovascular depression can result in hypoxia, acidosis, bradycardia, arrhythmias and cardiac arrest. Underventilation or apenea due to unintentional subarachnoid injection of local anesthetic solution may produce these same signs and also lead to cardiac arrest if ventilatory support is not instituted. If cardiac arrest should occur standard cardiopulmonary resuscitative measures should be instituted.

Endotracheal intubation, employing drugs and techniques familiar to the clinician, may be indicated, after initial administration of oxygen by mask, if difficulty is encountered in the maintenance of a patent airway or if prolonged ventilatory support (assisted or controlled) is indicated.

Dialysis is of negligible value in the treatment of acute overdosage with lidocaine.

The oral LD_{50} of lidocaine HCl in non-fasted female rats is 459 (346–773) mg/kg (as the salt) and 214 (159–324) mg/kg (as the salt) in fasted female rats.

DOSAGE AND ADMINISTRATION

Table II (Recommended Dosages) summarizes the recommended volumes and concentrations of Xylocaine Injection for various types of anesthetic procedures. The dosages suggested in this table are for normal healthy adults and refer to the use of epinephrine-free solutions. When larger volumes are required only solutions containing epinephrine should be used, except in those cases where vasopressor drugs may be contraindicated.

These recommended doses serve only as a guide to the amount of anesthetic required for most routine procedures. The actual volumes and concentrations to be used depend on a number of factors such as type and extent of surgical procedure, depth of anesthesia and degree of muscular relaxation required, duration of anesthesia required, and the physical condition of the patient. In all cases the lowest concentration and smallest dose that will produce the desired result should be given. Dosages should be reduced for children and for elderly and debilitated patients and patients with cardiac and/or liver disease.

The onset of anesthesia, the duration of anesthesia and the degree of muscular relaxation are proportional to the volume and concentration (i.e. total dose) of local anesthetic used. Thus, an increase in volume and concentration of Xylocaine Injection will decrease the onset of anesthesia, prolong the duration of anesthesia, provide a greater degree of muscular relaxation and increase the segmental spread of anesthesia. However, increasing the volume and concentration of Xylocaine Injection may result in a more profound fall in blood pressure when used in epidural anesthesia. Although the incidence of side effects with lidocaine is quite low, caution should be exercised when employing large volumes and concentrations, since the incidence of side effects is directly proportional to the total dose of local anesthetic agent injected.

For intravenous regional anesthesia, only the 50 mL single dose vial containing Xylocaine (lidocaine HCl) 0.5% Injection should be used.

Epidural Anesthesia
For epidural anesthesia, only the following dosage forms of Xylocaine Injection are recommended:
1% without epinephrine .... 30 mL ampules
                                     30 mL single dose vials
1% with epinephrine 1:200,000 .... 30 mL ampules
                                     30 mL single dose vials
1.5% without epinephrine .... 20 mL ampules
                                     20 mL single dose vials
1.5% with epinephrine 1:200,000 .... 30 mL ampules
                                     30 mL single dose vials
2% without epinephrine .... 10 mL ampules
                                     10 mL single dose vials
2% with epinephrine 1:200,000 .... 20 mL ampules
                                     20 mL single dose vials
Although these solutions are intended specifically for epidural anesthesia, they may also be used for infiltration and peripheral nerve block, provided they are employed as single dose units. These solutions contain no bacteriostatic agent. In epidural anesthesia, the dosage varies with the number of dermatomes to be anesthetized (generally 2-3 mL of the indicated concentration per dermatome).

Caudal and lumbar epidural block: As a precaution against the adverse experience sometimes observed following unintentional penetration of the subarachnoid space, a test dose such as 2-3 mL of 1.5% lidocaine should be administered at least 5 minutes prior to injecting the total volume required for a lumbar or caudal epidural block. The test dose should be repeated if the patient is moved in a manner that may have displaced the catheter. Epinephrine, if contained in the test dose (10-15 µg have been suggested), may serve as a warning of unintentional intravascular injection. If injected into a blood vessel, this amount of epinephrine is likely to produce a transient "epinephrine response" within 45 seconds, consisting of an increase in heart rate and systolic blood pressure, circumoral pallor, palpitations and nervousness in the unsedated patient. The sedated patient may exhibit only a pulse rate increase of 20 or more beats per minutes for 15 or more seconds. Patients on beta-blockers may not manifest changes in heart rate, but blood pressure monitoring can detect an evanescent rise in systolic blood pressure. Adequate time should be allowed for onset of anesthesia after administration of each test dose. The rapid injection of a large volume of Xylocaine Injection through the catheter should be avoided, and, when feasible, fractional doses should be administered.

In the event of the known injection of a large volume of local anesthetic solution into the subarachnoid space, after suitable resuscitation and if the catheter is in place, consider attempting the recovery of drug by draining a moderate amount of cerebrospinal fluid (such as 10 mL) through the epidural catheter.

MAXIMUM RECOMMENDED DOSAGES

Adults: For normal healthy adults, the individual maximum recommended dose of lidocaine HCl with epinephrine should not exceed 7 mg/kg (3.5 mg/lb) of body weight and in general it is recommended that the maximum total dose not exceed 500 mg. When used without epinephrine, the maximum individual dose should not exceed 4.5 mg/kg (2 mg per lb) of body weight, and in general it is recommended that the maximum total dose does not exceed 300 mg. For continuous epidural or caudal anesthesia, the maximum recommended dosage should not be administered at intervals of less than 90 minutes. When continuous lumbar or caudal epidural anesthesia is used for non-obstetrical procedures, more drug may be administered if required to produce adequate anesthesia.

The maximum recommended dose per 90 minute period of lidocaine hydrochloride for paracervical block in obstetrical patients and non-obstetrical patients is 200 mg total. One

HOW SUPPLIED

Xylocaine (lidocaine HCl) Concentration	/Epinephrine Dilution (if present)	Ampules (mL)					Single Dose Vials (mL)						Multiple Dose Vials (mL)		
		2	5	10	20	30	2*	5	10	20	30	50	10	20	50
0.5%							X	X	X			X	X		X
0.5%	/1:200,000												X		
1%		X	X			X	X	X	X		X		X	X	X
1%	/1:100,000												X	X	X
1%	/1:200,000					X		X	X	X					
1.5%				X					X	X					
1.5%	/1:200,000		X			X		X	X						
2%		X	X				X	X	X				X	X	X
2%	/1:100,000												X	X	X
2%	/1:200,000			X				X	X	X					

All solutions should be stored at controlled room temperatures 15°–30°C (59°–86°F).   * = 3 mL vial with 2 mL fill

half of the total dose is usually administered to each side. Inject slowly five minutes between sides. (See also discussion of paracervical block in PRECAUTIONS.)

For intravenous regional anesthesia, the dose administered should not exceed 4 mg/kg in adults.

Children: It is difficult to recommend a maximum dose of any drug for children, since this varies as a function of age and weight. For children over 3 years of age who have a normal lean body mass and normal body development, the maximum dose is determined by the child's age and weight. For example, in a child of 5 years weighing 50 lbs., the dose of lidocaine HCl should not exceed 75–100 mg (1.5–2 mg/lb). The use of even more dilute solutions (i.e., 0.25–0.5%) and total dosages not to exceed 3 mg/kg (1.4 mg/lb) are recommended for induction of intravenous regional anesthesia in children.

In order to guard against systemic toxicity, the lowest effective concentration and lowest effective dose should be used at all times. In some cases it will be necessary to dilute available concentrations with 0.9% sodium chloride injection in order to obtain the required final concentration.

NOTE: Parenteral drug products should be inspected visually for particulate matter and discoloration prior to administration whenever the solution and container permit. Solutions that are discolored, cloudy and/or contain particulate matter should not be used.

TABLE II   Recommended Dosages

PROCEDURE	Xylocaine (lidocaine hydrochloride) Injection (without epinephrine)		
	Conc (%)	Vol (mL)	Total Dose (mg)
Infiltration			
Percutaneous	0.5 or 1	1–60	5–300
Intravenous regional	0.5	10–60	50–300
Peripheral Nerve Blocks, e.g.			
Brachial	1.5	15–20	225–300
Dental	2	1–5	20–100
Intercostal	1	3	30
Paravertebral	1	3–5	30–50
Pudendal (each side)	1	10	100
Paracervical			
Obstetrical analgesia (each side)			
	1	10	100
Sympathetic Nerve Blocks, e.g.			
Cervical (stellate ganglion)	1	5	50
Lumbar	1	5–10	50–100
Central Neural Blocks			
Epidural*			
Thoracic	1	20–30	200–300
Lumbar			
Analgesia	1	25–30	250–300
Anesthesia	1.5	15–20	225–300
	2	10–15	200–300
Caudal			
Obstetrical analgesia	1	20–30	200–300
Surgical anesthesia	1.5	15–20	225–300

* Dose determined by number of dermatomes to be anesthetized (2–3 mL/dermatome).
THE ABOVE SUGGESTED CONCENTRATIONS AND VOLUMES SERVE ONLY AS A GUIDE. OTHER VOLUMES AND CONCENTRATIONS MAY BE USED PROVIDED THE TOTAL MAXIMUM RECOMMENDED DOSE IS NOT EXCEEDED.

Sterilization, Storage and Technical Procedures: Disinfecting agents containing heavy metals, which cause release of respective ions (mercury, zinc, copper, etc.) should not be used for skin or mucous membrane disinfection as they have been related to incidents of swelling and edema. When chemical disinfection of multi-dose vials is desired, either isopropyl alcohol (91%) or ethyl alcohol (70%) is recommended. Many commercially available brands of rubbing alcohol as well as solutions of ethyl alcohol not of U.S.P. grade, contain denaturants which are injurious to rubber and therefore are not to be used.

HOW SUPPLIED
[See table above].
Protect from light.
021850R09   Rev. 11/88(9)

XYLOCAINE® INJECTION   ℞
[zī'lo-caine]
(lidocaine hydrochloride)
FOR VENTRICULAR ARRHYTHMIAS

DESCRIPTION
Xylocaine (lidocaine hydrochloride) Injection is a sterile and non-pyrogenic solution of an antiarrhythmic agent administered intravenously by either direct injection or continuous infusion or intramuscularly by injection. The specific quantitative for each available solution appears in Table 1.
See Table 1 on next page
Xylocaine Injections are composed of aqueous solutions of lidocaine hydrochloride. Lidocaine hydrochloride ($C_{14}H_{22}N_2O \cdot HCl$) is chemically designated acetamide, 2-(diethylamino)-N-(2, 6 dimethylphenyl)-, monohydrochloride and is represented by the following structural formula:

CLINICAL PHARMACOLOGY
Mechanism of action and electrophysiology:
Studies of the effects of therapeutic concentrations of lidocaine on the electrophysiological properties of mammalian Purkinje fibers have shown that lidocaine attenuates phase 4 diastolic depolarization, decreases automaticity, and causes a decrease or no change in excitability and membrane responsiveness. Action potential duration and effective refractory period of Purkinje fibers are decreased, while the ratio of effective refractory period to action potential duration is increased. Action potential duration and effective refractory period of ventricular muscle are also decreased. Effective refractory period of the AV node may increase, decrease or remain unchanged, and atrial effective refractory period is unchanged. Lidocaine raises the ventricular fibrillation threshold. No significant interactions between lidocaine and the automatic nervous shstem have been described and consequently, lidocaine has little or no effect on autonomic tone.
Clinical electrophysiological studies with lidocaine have demonstrated no change in sinus node recovery time or sino-

Continued on next page

Astra—Cont.

atrial conduction time. AV nodal conduction time is unchanged or shortened, and His-Purkinje conduction time is unchanged.

Hemodynamics:
At therapeutic doses, lidocaine has minimal hemodynamic effects in normal subjects and in patients with heart disease. Lidocaine has been shown to cause no, or minimal, decrease in ventricular contractility, cardiac output, arterial pressure or heart rate.

Pharmacokinetics and metabolism:
Lidocaine is rapidly metabolized by the liver, and less than 10% of a dose is excreted unchanged in the urine. Oxidative N-dealkylation, a major pathway of metabolism, results in the metabolites monoethylglycinexylidide and glycinexylidide. The pharmacological/toxicological activities of these metabolites are similar to, but less potent than, lidocaine. The primary metabolite in urine is a conjugate of 4-hydroxy-2,6-dimethylaniline.

The elimination half-life of lidocaine following an intravenous bolus injection is typically 1.5 to 2.0 hours. There are data that indicate that the half-life may be 3 hours or longer following infusions of greater than 24 hours.

Because of the rapid rate at which lidocaine is metabolized, any condition that alters liver function, including changes in liver blood flow, which could result from severe congestive heart failure or shock, may alter lidocaine kinetics. The half-life may be two-fold or more greater in patients with liver dysfunction. Renal dysfunction does not affect lidocaine kinetics, but may increase the accumulation of metabolites. Therapeutic effects of lidocaine are generally associated with plasma levels of 6 to 25 μmole/L (1.5 to 6μg free base per mL). The blood to plasma distribution ratio is approximately 0.84. Objective adverse manifestations become increasingly apparent with increasing plasma levels above 6.0 μg free base per mL.

The plasma protein binding of lidocaine is dependent on drug concentration, and the fraction bound decreases with increasing concentration. At concentrations of 1 to 4 μg free base per mL, 60 to 80 percent of lidocaine is protein bound. In addition to lidocaine concentration, the binding is dependent on the plasma concentration of the α-1-acid glycoprotein.

Lidocaine readily crosses the placental and blood-brain barriers. Dialysis has negligible effects on the kinetics of lidocaine.

When an appropriate dose of Xylocaine Injection is administered intramuscularly into the deltoid muscle, effective antiarrhythmic blood levels are usually obtained within 5 to 15 minutes and usually persist for 60 to 90 minutes. Absorption from other intramuscular sites such as the vastus lateralis and gluteus maximus is slower, resulting in significantly lower blood levels during the first hour.

INDICATIONS AND USAGE
Xylocaine Injection, administered intravenously or intramuscularly, is specifically indicated in the acute management of ventricular arrhythmias such as those occurring in relation to acute myocardial infarction, or during cardiac manipulation, such as cardiac surgery.

CONTRAINDICATIONS
Xylocaine Injection is contraindicated in patients with a known history of hypersensitivity to local anesthetics of the amide type. Xylocaine Injection should not be used in patients with Stokes-Adams syndrome, Wolff-Parkinson-White syndrome, or with severe degrees of sinoatrial, atrioventricular, or intraventicular block in the absence of an artificial pacemaker.

WARNINGS
IN ORDER TO MANAGE POSSIBLE ADVERSE REACTIONS, RESUSCITATIVE EQUIPMENT, OXYGEN AND OTHER RESUSCITATIVE DRUGS SHOULD BE IMMEDIATELY AVAILABLE WHEN XYLOCAINE (LIDOCAINE HYDROCHLORIDE) INJECTION IS USED.

Systemic toxicity may result in manifestations of central nervous sytem depression (sedation) or irritability (twitching), which may progress to frank convulsions accompanied by respiratory depression and/or arrest. Early recognition of premonitory signs, assurance of adequate oxygenation and, where necessary, establishment of artificial airway with ventilatory support are essential to management of this problem. Should convulsions persist despite ventilatory therapy with oxygen, *small* increments of anticonvulsant drugs may be used intravenously. Examples of such agents include benzodiazepines (e.g., diazepam), ultra short-acting barbiturates (e.g., thiopental or thiamylal), or a short-acting barbiturate (e.g., pentobarbital or secobarbital). If the patient is under anesthesia, a short-acting muscle relaxant (e.g., succinylcholine) may be used. Longer acting drugs should be used only when recurrent convulsions are evidenced.

Should circulatory depression occur, vasopressors may be used.

Constant electrocardiographic monitoring is essential to the proper administration of Xylocaine Injections. Signs of excessive depression of cardiac electrical activity such as sinus node dysfunction, prolongation of the P-R interval and QRS complex or the appearance or aggravation of arrhythmias, should be followed by flow adjustment and, if necessary, prompt cessation of the intravenous infusion of this agent. Occasionally, acceleration of ventricular rate may occur when Xylocaine Injection is administered to patients with atrial flutter or fibrillation.

PRECAUTIONS
1. **General:** Caution should be employed in the use of Xylocaine Injection in patients with severe liver or kidney disease because accumulation of the drug or metabolites may occur.

Xylocaine Injection should be used with caution in the treatment of patients with hypovolemia, severe congestive heart failure, shock, and all forms of heart block. In patients with sinus bradycardia or incomplete heart block, the administration of Xylocaine Injection intravenously for the elimination of ventricular ectopic beats, without prior acceleration in heart rate (e.g., by atropine, isoproterenol or electric pacing), may promote more frequent and serious ventricular arrhythmias or complete heart block (see CONTRAINDICATIONS).

Dosage should be reduced for children and for debilitated and/or elderly patients, commensurate with their age and physical status.

The safety of amide local anesthetic agents in patients with genetic predispositon to malignant hyperthermia has not been fully assessed; therefore, lidocaine should be used with caution in such patients.

In hospital environments where drugs known to be triggering agents for malignant hyperthermia (fulminant hypermetabolism) are administered, it is suggested that a standard protocol for management should be available. It is not known whether lidocaine may trigger this reaction; however, large doses resulting in significant plasma concentrations, as may be achieved by intravenous infusion, pose potential risk to these individuals. Recognition of early unexplained signs of tachycardia, tachypnea, labile blood pressure and metabolic acidosis may precede temperature elevation. Successful outcome is dependent on early diagnosis, prompt discontinuance of the triggering agent and institution of treatment including oxygen

therapy, supportive measures and dantrolene (for details see dantrolene package insert).

2. **Patient information:** The patient should be advised of the possible occurrence of the experiences listed under ADVERSE REACTIONS.
3. **Laboratory tests:** None known.
4. a. **Drug interactions:** Xylocaine Injections should be used with caution in patients with digitalis toxicity accompanied by atrioventricular block. Concomitant use of beta-blocking agents or cimetidine may reduce hepatic blood flow and thereby reduce lidocaine clearance.

    Lidocaine and tocainide are pharmacodynamically similar. The concomitant use of these two agents may cause an increased incidence of adverse reactions, including central nervous system adverse reactions such as seizure.
   b. **Drug/Laboratory test interactions:** The intramuscular use of Xylocaine Injection may result in an increase in creatine phosphokinase levels. Thus, the use of this enzyme determination, without isoenzyme separation, as a diagnostic test for the presence of acute myocardial infarction may be compromised by the use of intramuscular Xylocaine Injection.
5. **Carcinogenesis, mutagenesis, impairment of fertility:** Long term studies in animals to evaluate the carcinogenic and mutagenic potential or the effect on fertility of Xylocaine Injection have not been conducted.
6. **Pregnancy:**
   a. **Teratogenic effects:** Pregnancy Category B. Reproduction studies have been performed in rats at doses up to 6.6 times the maximum human doses and have revealed no significant findings. There are, however, no adequate and well-controlled studies in pregnant women. Because animal reproduction studies are not always predictive of human response, this drug should be used during pregnancy only if clearly needed.
7. **Labor and delivery:** The effects of Xylocaine Injection on the mother and the fetus, when used in the management of cardiac arrhythmias during labor and delivery, are not known. Lidocaine readily crosses the placental barrier.
8. **Nursing mothers:** It is not known whether this drug is excreted in human milk. Because many drugs are excreted in human milk, caution should be exercised when lidocaine is administered to a nursing woman.
9. **Pediatric use:** Safety and effectiveness in children have not been established by controlled clinical studies. (See DOSAGE AND ADMINISTRATION).

ADVERSE REACTIONS
Adverse experiences following the administration of lidocaine are similar in nature to those observed with other amide local anesthetic agents. Adverse experiences may result from high plasma levels caused by excessive dosage or may result from a hypersensitivity, idiosyncrasy or diminished tolerance on the part of the patient. Serious adverse experiences are generally systemic in nature. The following types are those most commonly reported. The adverse experiences under Central Nervous System and Cardiovascular System are listed, in general, in a progression from mild to severe.

1. **Central Nervous System:**
   CNS reactions are excitatory and/or depressant, and may be characterized by light-headedness, nervousness, apprehension, euphoria, confusion, dizziness, drowsiness, tinnitus, blurred or double vision, vomiting, sensations of heat, cold or numbness, twitching, tremors, convulsions, unconsciousness, respiratory depression and arrest. The excitatory reactions may be very brief or may not occur at all, in which case, the first manifestation of toxicity may be drowsiness, merging into unconsciousness and respiratory arrest.
2. **Cardiovascular System:**
   Cardiovascular reactions are usually depressant in nature and are characterized by bradycardia, hypotension, and cardiovascular collapse, which may lead to cardiac arrest.
3. Allergic reactions as a result of sensitivity to lidocaine are extremely rare and, if they occur, should be managed by conventional means.

DRUG ABUSE AND DEPENDENCE
Although specific studies have not been conducted, Xylocaine Injection has been used clinically without evidence of abuse of this drug or of psychological or physical dependence as a result of its use.

OVERDOSAGE
Overdosage of Xylocaine (lidocaine hydrochloride) Injection usually results in signs of central nervous system or cardiovascular toxicity. See ADVERSE REACTIONS.

Should convulsions or signs of respiratory depression and arrest develop, the patency of the airway and adequacy of ventilation must be assured immediately. Should convulsions persist despite ventilatory therapy with oxygen, small increments of anticonvulsive agents may be given intravenously. Examples of such agents include a benzodiazepine

TABLE 1 Composition of available solutions:

		Composition*	
	Dosage Form	lidocaine hydrochloride (mg per mL)	sodium chloride (mg per mL)
For Direct Intravenous Injection	5 mL (50 mg) prefilled syringe	10	7
	5 mL (100 mg) prefilled syringe	20	6
	5 mL (100 mg) ampule	20	6
For Preparation of Intravenous Infusion Injections	25 mL (One Gram) single use vial	40	None
	50 mL (Two Grams) single use vial	40	None
	5 mL (One Gram) additive syringe	200	None
	10 mL (Two Grams) additive syringe	200	None
For Intramuscular Injection	5 mL (500 mg) ampule	100	None

*pH of all solutions adjusted to 5.0-7.0 with sodium hydroxide and/or hydrochloric acid.
All containers are for single use: solutions do not contain preservatives.

(e.g., diazepam), an ultrashort-acting barbiturate (e.g., thiopental or thiamylal), or a short-acting barbiturate (e.g., pentobarbital or secobarbital). If the patient is under general anesthesia, a short-acting muscle relaxant (e.g., succinylcholine) may be administered.

Should circulatory depression occur, vasopressors may be used. Should cardiac arrest occur, standard CPR procedures should be instituted.

Dialysis is of negligible value in the treatment of acute overdosage from Xylocaine Injection.

DOSAGE AND ADMINISTRATION

Adults

Single Direct Intravenous Injection (bolus):
ONLY THE 5 ML, 50 MG OR 100 MG DOSAGE SIZES should be used for direct intravenous injection. The usual dose is 50 to 100 mg of lidocaine hydrochloride (0.70 to 1.4 mg/kg: 0.32 to 0.63 mg/lb) administered intravenously under ECG monitoring. This dose may be administered at the rate of approximately 25 to 50 mg/min (0.35 to 0.70 mg/kg/min; 0.16 to 0.32 mg/lb/min). Sufficient time should be allowed to enable a slow circulation to carry the drug to the site of action. If the initial injection of 50 to 100 mg does not produce a desired response, a second dose may be injected after 5 minutes. The syringe should be activated immediately prior to the injection. (See illustrated instructions for use on produce package.) NO MORE THAN 200 TO 300 MG OF LIDOCAINE HYDROCHLORIDE SHOULD BE ADMINISTERED DURING A ONE HOUR PERIOD.

Continuous Intravenous Infusion:
Following bolus administration, intravenous infusions of Xylocaine Injection may be initiated at the rate of 1 to 4 mg/min of lidocaine hydrochloride (0.014 to 0.057 mg/kg/min; 0.006 to 0.026 mg/lb/min). The rate of intravenous infusions should be reassessed as soon as the patient's basic cardiac rhythm appears to be stable or at the earliest signs of toxicity. It should rarely be necessary to continue intravenous infusions of lidocaine for prolonged periods. Solutions for intravenous infusion may be prepared by the addition of one gram (or two grams) of lidocaine hydrochloride to one liter of 5% dextrose in water using aseptic technique. Approximately a 0.1% (or 0.2%) solution will result from this procedure; that is, each milliliter will contain approximately 1 (or 2 mg) of lidocaine hydrochloride. In those cases in which fluid restriction is medically appropriate, a more concentrated solution may be prepared.

Xylocaine Injection has been found to be chemically stable for 24 hours after dilution in 5% dextrose in water. However, as with all intravenous admixtures, dilution of the solution should be made just prior to its administration.

Parenteral drug products should be inspected visually for particulate matter and discoloration prior to administration whenever the solution and container permit. Do not use if solution is discolored or cloudy.

Intramuscular Injection:
The recommended dose of lidocaine hydrochloride by the intramuscular route is 300 mg (approximately 4.3 mg/kg or 2.0 mg/lb). The deltoid muscle is recommended as the preferred site of injection, since therapeutic blood levels of lidocaine occur faster and the peak blood level is significantly higher following deltoid administration as compared to injections into the lateral thigh or gluteus. Injections should be made with frequent aspiration to avoid possible inadvertent intravascular injection.

As soon as possible, and when indicated, patients should be changed to an intravenous infusion of Xylocaine Injection. However, if necessary, an additional intramuscular injection may be made after an interval of 60-90 minutes.

Pediatric

Although controlled clinical studies to establish pediatric dosing schedules have not been conducted, the American Heart Association's *Standards and Guidelines* recommends a bolus dose of 1 mg/kg followed by an infusion rate of 30 µg/kg/min.

Note regarding prolonged infusions: There are data that indicate the half-life may be 3 hours or longer following infusions of greater than 24 hours in duration.

HOW SUPPLIED

For direct intravenous injection, Xylocaine (lidocaine hydrochloride) Injection without preservatives is supplied in 5 mL, 50 mg and 100 mg prefilled syringes and in 5 mL, 100 mg ampules.

For intramuscular injection, Xylocaine Injection without preservatives is supplied in 5 mL, 500 mg ampules (100 mg/mL).

For preparing solutions for intravenous infusions, Xylocaine Injection without sodium chloride or preservatives is supplied in one and two gram additive syringes and in one and two gram single use vials. Vials are available with or without pre-sterilized transfer unit manufactured by the West Company.

Injections should be stored at controlled room temperature 15°-30°C (59°-86°F).

021834R04   Rev. 2/88(4)

XYLOCAINE® (lidocaine HCl)   ℞
[zī'lo-caine]
4% STERILE SOLUTION
For transtracheal use,
retrobulbar injection,
and for topical application

DESCRIPTION

Xylocaine (lidocaine HCl) 4% Sterile Solution contains a local anesthetic agent and is administered topically or by injection. See INDICATIONS for specific uses.

Xylocaine 4% Sterile Solution contains lidocaine HCl, which is chemically designated as acetamide, 2-(diethylamino)-N-(2,6-dimethylphenyl)-monohydrochloride.

Xylocaine 4% Sterile Solution is 5 ml ampules may be autoclaved repeatedly if necessary.

Composition of Xylocaine 4% Sterile Solution
Each ml contains lidocaine HCl, 40.0 mg, and sodium hydroxide and/or hydrochloric acid to adjust pH to 5.0–7.0. A sterile, aqueous solution.

CLINICAL PHARMACOLOGY

Mechanism of action: Lidocaine stabilizes the neuronal membrane by inhibiting the ionic fluxes required for the initiation and conduction of impulses, thereby effecting local anesthetic action.

Oneset and duration of anesthesia: The onset of action is rapid. For retrobulbar injection, 4 ml of Xylocaine 4% Sterile Solution provides an average duration of action of 1 to 1 1/2 hours. This duration may be extended for ophthalmic surgery by the addition of epinephrine, the usual recommended dilution being 1:50,000 to 1:100,000.

Hemodynamics: Excessive blood levels may cause changes in cardiac output, total peripheral resistance, and mean arterial pressure. These changes may be attributable to a direct depressant effect of the local anesthetic agent on various components of the cardiovascular system. The net effect is normally a modest hypotension when the recommended dosages are not exceeded.

Pharmacokinetics and metabolism: Information derived from other formulations, concentrations and usages reveals that lidocaine is completely absorbed following parenteral administration, its rate of absorption depending, for example, upon such factors as the site of administration and the presence or absence of a vasoconstrictor agent. Lidocaine may be absorbed following topical administration to mucous membranes, its rate and extent of absorption depending upon concentration and total dose administered, the specific site of application and duration of exposure. In general, the rate of absorption of local anesthetic agents following topical application occurs most rapidly after intratracheal administration. Lidocaine is also well absorbed from the gastrointestinal tract, but little intact drug appears in the circulation because of biotransformation by the liver.

Lidocaine is metabolized rapidly by the liver, and metabolites and unchanged drug are excreted by the kidneys. Biotransformation includes oxidative N-dealkylation, ring hydroxylation, cleavage of the amide linkage, and conjugation. N-dealkylation, a major pathway of biotransformation, yields the metabolites monoethylglycinexylidide and glycinexylidide. The pharmacological/toxicological actions of these metabolites are similar to, but less potent than, those of lidocaine. Approximately 90% of lidocaine administered is excreted in the form of various metabolites, and less than 10% is excreted unchanged. The primary metabolite in urine is a conjugate of 4-hydroxy-2,6-dimethylaniline.

Studies have shown that peak blood levels of lidocaine may occur as early as 5 and as late as 30 minutes after endotracheal administration of a 4% lidocaine HCl solution.

The plasma binding of lidocaine is dependent on drug concentration, and the fraction bound decreases with increasing concentration. At concentrations of 1 to 4 µg of free base per ml, 60 to 80 percent of lidocaine is protein bound. Binding is also dependent on the plasma concentration of the alpha-1-acid glycoprotein.

Lidocaine crosses the blood-brain and placental barriers, presumably by passive diffusion.

Studies of lidocaine metabolism following intravenous bolus injections have shown that the elimination half-life of this agent is typically 1.5 to 2.0 hours. Because of the rapid rate at which lidocaine is metabolized, any condition that affects liver function may alter lidocaine kinetics. The half-life may be prolonged two-fold or more in patients with liver dysfunction. Renal dysfunction does not affect lidocaine kinetics but may increase the accumulation of metabolites.

Factors such as acidosis and the use of CNS stimulants and depressants affect the CNS levels of lidocaine required to produce overt systemic effects. Objective adverse manifestations become increasingly apparent with increasing venous plasma levels above 6.0 µg free base per ml. In the rhesus monkey arterial blood levels of 18–21 µg/ml have been shown to be threshold for convulsive activity.

INDICATIONS AND USAGE

Xylocaine (lidocaine HCl) 4% Sterile Solution is indicated for the production of topical anesthesia of the mucous membranes of the respiratory tract or the genito-urinary tract. It may be injected trans-tracheally to anesthetize the larynx and trachea, and it may be administered by retrobulbar injection to provide anesthesia for ophthalmic surgery.

CONTRAINDICATIONS

Lidocaine is contraindicated in patients with a known history of hypersensitivity to local anesthetics of the amide type.

WARNINGS

XYLOCAINE 4% STERILE SOLUTION SHOULD BE EMPLOYED ONLY BY CLINICIANS WHO ARE WELL VERSED IN DIAGNOSIS AND MANAGEMENT OF DOSE-RELATED TOXICITY AND OTHER ACUTE EMERGENCIES THAT MIGHT ARISE AND THEN ONLY AFTER ENSURING THE *IMMEDIATE* AVAILABILITY OF OXYGEN, OTHER RESUSCITATIVE DRUGS, CARDIOPULMONARY EQUIPMENT, AND THE PERSONNEL NEEDED FOR PROPER MANAGEMENT OF TOXIC REACTIONS AND RELATED EMERGENCIES (See also ADVERSE REACTIONS and PRECAUTIONS.) DELAY IN PROPER MANAGEMENT OF DOSE-RELATED TOXICITY, UNDERVENTILATION FROM ANY CAUSE AND/OR ALTERED SENSITIVITY MAY LEAD TO THE DEVELOPMENT OF ACIDOSIS, CARDIAC ARREST AND, POSSIBLY, DEATH.

To avoid intravascular injection, aspiration should be performed before the local anesthetic solution is injected. The needle must be repositioned until no return of blood can be elicited by aspiration. Note, however, that the absence of blood in the syringe does not guarantee that intravascular injection has been avoided.

Xylocaine 4% Sterile Solution should be used with extreme caution if there is sepsis or severely traumatized mucosa in the area of application, since under such conditions there is the potential for rapid systemic absorption.

PRECAUTIONS

General: The safety and effectiveness of lidocaine depend on proper dosage, correct technique, adequate precautions, and readiness for emergencies. Resuscitative equipment, oxygen and other resuscitative drugs should be available for immediate use. (See WARNINGS and ADVERSE REACTIONS.) The lowest dosage that results in effective anesthesia should be used to avoid high plasma levels and serious adverse effects. Repeated doses of lidocaine may cause significant increases in blood levels with each repeated dose, because of slow accumulation of the drug or its metabolites. Tolerance to elevated blood levels varies with the status of the patient. Debilitated, elderly patients, acutely ill patients, and children should be given reduced doses commensurate with their age and physical status. Lidocaine should also be used with caution in patients with severe shock or heart block.

Local anesthetic solutions containing a vasoconstrictor should be used cautiously and in carefully circumscribed quantities in areas of the body supplied by end arteries or having otherwise compromised blood supply. Patients with peripheral vascular disease and those with hypertensive vascular disease may exhibit exaggerated vasoconstrictor response. Ischemic injury or necrosis may result. Preparations containing a vasoconstrictor should be used with caution in patients during or following the administration of potent general anesthetic agents, since cardiac arrhythmias may occur under such conditions.

Careful and constant monitoring of cardiovascular and respiratory (adequacy of ventilation) vital signs and the patient's state of consciousness should be accomplished after each local anesthetic injection. It should be kept in mind at such times that restlessness, anxiety, tinnitus, dizziness, blurred vision, tremors, depression or drowsiness may be early warning signs of central nervous system toxicity.

Since amide-type local anesthetics are metabolized by the liver, Xylocaine 4% Sterile Solution should be used with caution in patients with hepatic disease.

Patients with severe hepatic disease, because of their inability to metabolize local anesthetic normally, are a greater risk of developing toxic plasma concentrations. Xylocaine 4% Sterile Solution should also be used with caution in patients with impaired cardiovascular function since they may be less able to compensate for functional changes associated with the prolongation of A-V conduction produced by these drugs.

Use in Ophthalmic Surgery: When local anesthetic solutions are employed for retrobulbar block, lack of corneal sensation should not be relied upon to determine whether or not the patient is ready for surgery since corneal sensation usually precedes clinically acceptable external ocular muscle akinesia.

Many drugs used during the conduct of anesthesia are considered potential triggering agents for familial malignant hyperthermia. Since it is not known whether amide-type local anesthetics may trigger this reaction and since the need for supplemental general anesthesia cannot be predicted in advance, it is suggested that a standard protocol for

Continued on next page

Astra—Cont.

management should be available. Early unexplained signs of tachycardia, tachypnea, labile blood pressure and metabolic acidosis may precede temperature elevation. Successful outcome is dependent on early diagnosis, prompt discontinuance of the suspect triggering agent(s) and institution of treatment, including oxygen theray, indicated supportive measures and dantrolene (consult dantrolene sodium intravenous package insert before using).

Lidocaine should be used with caution in persons with known drug sensitivities. Patients allergic to para-aminobenzoic acid derivatives (procaine, tetracaine, benzocaine, etc.) have not shown cross sensitivity to lidocaine.

Use in the Head and Neck Area: Small doses of local anesthetics injected into the head and neck area, including retrobulbar, dental and stellate ganglion blocks, may produce adverse reactions similar to systemic toxicity seen with unintentional intravascular injections of larger doses. Confusion, convulsions, respiratory depression and/or respiratory arrest, and cardiovascular stimulation or depression have been reported. These reactions may be due to intra-arterial injection of the local anesthetic with retrograde flow to the cerebral circulation. Patients receiving these blocks should have their circulation and respiration monitored and be constantly observed. Resuscitative equipment and personnel for treating adverse reactions should be immediately available. Dosage recommendations should not be exceeded. (See DOSAGE AND ADMINISTRATION.)

Information for Patients: When topical anesthetics are used in the mouth, the patient should be aware that the production of topical anesthesia may impair swallowing and thus enhance the danger of aspiration. For this reason, food should not be ingested for 60 minutes following use of local anesthetic preparations in the mouth or throat area. This is particularly important in children because of their frequency of eating.

Numbness of the tongue or buccal mucosa may enhance the danger of unintentional biting trauma. Food and chewing gum should not be taken while the mouth or throat area is anesthetized.

Clinically significant drug interactions: The administration of local anesthetic solutions containing epinephrine or norepinephrine to patients receiving monoamine oxidase inhibitors, tricyclic antidepressants or phenothiazines may produce severe, prolonged hypotension or hypertension. Concurrent use of these agents should generally be avoided. In situations when concurrent therapy is necessary, careful patient monitoring is essential.

Drug/Laboratory test interactions: The intramuscular injection of lidocaine may result in an increase in creatine phosphokinase levels. Thus, the use of this enzyme determination, without isoenzyme separation, as a diagnostic test for the presence of acute myocardial infarction may be compromised by the intramuscular injection of lidocaine.

Carcinogenesis, mutagenesis, impairment of fertility: Studies of lidocaine in animals to evaluate the carcinogenic and mutagenic potential or the effect on fertility have not been conducted.

Use in Pregnancy: Teratogenic Effects. Pregnancy Category B. Reproduction studies have been performed in rats at doses up to 6.6 times the human dose and have revealed no evidence of harm to the fetus caused by lidocaine. There are, however, no adequate and well-controlled studied in pregnant women. Animal reproduction studies are not always predictive of human response. General consideration should be given to this fact before administering lidocaine to women of childbearing potential, especially during early pregnancy when maximum organogenesis takes place.

Labor and delivery: Lidocaine is not contraindicated in labor and delivery. Should Xylocaine 4% Sterile Solution be used concomitantly with other products containing lidocaine, the total dose contributed by all formulations must be kept in mind.

Nursing mothers: It is not known whether this drug is excreted in human milk. Because many drugs are excreted in human milk, caution should be exercised when lidocaine is administered to a nursing woman.

Pediatric use: Dosages in children should be reduced, commensurate with age and body weight. See DOSAGE AND ADMINISTRATION.

ADVERSE REACTIONS

Adverse experiences following the administration of lidocaine are similar in nature to those observed with other amide local anesthetic agents. These adverse experiences are, in general, dose-related and may result from high plasma levels caused by excessive dosage, rapid absorption or inadvertent intravascular injection, or may result from a hypersensitivity, idiosyncrasy or diminished tolerance on the part of the patient. Serious adverse experiences are generally systemic in nature. The following types are those most commonly reported:

Central nervous system: CNS manifestations are excitatory and/or depressant and may be characterized by lightheaded-

ness, nervousness, apprehension, euphoria, confusion, dizziness, drowsiness, tinnitus, blurred or double vision, vomiting, sensations of heat, cold or numbness, twitching, tremors, convulsions, unconsciousness, respiratory depression and arrest. The excitatory manifestations may be very brief or may not occur at all, in which case the first manifestation of toxicity may be drowsiness merging into unconsciousness and respiratory arrest.

Drowsiness following the administration of lidocaine is usually an early sign of a high blood level of the drug and may occur as a consequence of rapid absorption.

Cardiovascular system: Cardiovascular manifestations are usually depressant and are characterized by bradycardia, hypotension, and cardiovascular collapse, which may lead to cardiac arrest.

Allergic: Allergic reactions are characterized by cutaneous lesions, urticaria, edema or anaphylactoid reactions. Allergic reactions as a result of sensitivity to lidocaine are extremely rare and, if they occur, should be managed by conventional means. The detection of sensitivity by skin testing is of doubtful value.

Neurologic: The incidences of adverse reactions associated with the use of local anesthetics may be related to the total dose of local anesthetic administered and are also dependent upon the particular drug used, the route of administration and the physical status of the patient.

OVERDOSAGE

Acute emergencies from local anesthetics are generally related to high plasma levels encountered during therapeutic use of local anesthetics or to unintended subarachnoid injection of local anesthetic solution (see ADVERSE REACTIONS, WARNINGS, and PRECAUTIONS).

Management of local anesthetic emergencies: The first consideration is prevention, best accomplished by careful and constant monitoring of cardiovascular and respiratory vital signs and the patient's state of consciousness after each local anesthetic injection. At the first sign of change, oxygen should be administered.

The first step in the management of convulsions consists of immediate attention to the maintenance of a patent airway and assisted or controlled ventilation with oxygen and a delivery system capable of permitting immediate positive airway pressure by mask. Immediately after the institution of these ventilatory measures, the adequacy of the circulation should be evaluated, keeping in mind that drugs used to treat convulsions sometimes depress the circulation when administered intravenously. Should convulsions persist despite adequate respiratory support, and if the status of the circulation permits, small increments of an ultra-short acting barbiturate (such as thiopental or thiamylal) or a benzodiazepine (such as diazepam) may be administered intravenously. The clinician should be familiar, prior to use of local anesthetics, with these anticonvulsant drugs. Supportive treatment of circulatory depression may require administration of intravenous fluids and, when appropriate, a vasopressor as directed by the clinical situation (e.g., ephedrine).

If not treated immediately, both convulsions and cardiovascular depression can result in hypoxia, acidosis, bradycardia, arrhythmias and cardiac arrest. If cardiac arrest should occur, standard cardiopulmonary resuscitative measures should be instituted.

Endotracheal intubation, employing drugs and techniques familiar to the clinician, may be indicated, after initial administration of oxygen by mask, if difficulty is encountered in the maintenance of a patent airway or if prolonged ventilatory support (assisted or controlled) is indicated.

Dialysis is of negligible value in the treatment of acute overdosage with lidocaine.

The intravenous LD_{50} of lidocaine HCl in female mice is 26 (21–31) mg/kg and the subcutaneous LD_{50} is 264 (203–304) mg/kg.

DOSAGE AND ADMINISTRATION

When Xylocaine 4% Sterile Solution is used concomitantly with other products containing lidocaine, the total dose contributed by all formulations must be kept in mind.

The dosage varies and depends upon the area to be anesthetized, vascularity of the tissues, individual tolerance and the technique of anesthesia. The lowest dosage needed to provide effective anesthesia should be administered. Dosages should be reduced for children and for elderly and debilitated patients.

Although the incidence of adverse effects with Xylocaine 4% Sterile Solution is quite low, caution should be exercised, particularly when employing large volumes and concentrations of Xylocaine 4% Sterile Solution since the incidence of adverse effects is directly proportional to the total dose of local anesthetic agent administered. For specific techniques and procedures refer to standard textbooks.

The dosages below are for normal, healthy adults.

RETROBULBAR INJECTION: The suggested dose for a 70 kg person is 3–5 ml (120–200 mg of lidocaine HCl), i.e., 1.7–3 mg/kg or 0.9–1.5 mg/lb body weight. A portion of this is injected retrobulbarly and the rest may be used to block the facial nerve.

TRANSTRACHEAL INJECTION: For local anesthesia by the transtracheal route 2–3 ml should be injected through a large enough needle so that the injection can be made rapidly. By injecting during inspiration some of the drug will be carried into the bronchi and the resulting cough will distribute the rest of the drug over the vocal cords and the epiglottis.

Occasionally it may be necessary to spray the pharynx by oropharyngeal spray to achieve complete analgesia. For the combination of the injection and spray, it should rarely be necessary to utilize more than 5 ml (200 mg of lidocaine HCl), i.e., 3 mg/kg or 1.5 mg/lb body weight.

TOPICAL APPLICATION: For laryngoscopy, bronchoscopy and endotracheal intubation, the pharynx may be sprayed with 1–5 ml (40–200 mg of lidocaine HCl), i.e., 0.6–3 mg/kg or 0.3–1.5 mg/lb body weight.

MAXIMUM RECOMMENDED DOSAGES

Normal Healthy Adults: The maximum recommended dose of Xylocaine 4% Sterile Solution should be such that the dose of lidocaine HCl is kept below 300 mg and in any case should not exceed 4.5 mg/kg (2 mg/lb) body weight.

Children:

It is difficult to recommend a maximum dose of any drug for children since this varies as a function of age and weight. For children of less than ten years who have a normal lean body mass and normal body development, the maximum dose may be determined by the application of one of the standard pediatric drug formulas (e.g. Clark's rule). For example, in a child of five years weighing 50 lbs., the dose of lidocaine hydrochloride should not exceed 75–100 mg when calculated according to Clark's rule. In any case, the maximum dose of Xylocaine Solution with epinephrine should not exceed 7 mg/kg (3.2 mg/lb.) of body weight. When used without epinephrine, the amount of Xylocaine Solution administered should be such that the dose of lidocaine is kept below 300 mg and in any case should not exceed 4.5 mg/kg (2.0 mg/lb) of body weight. NOTE: Parenteral drug products should be inspected visually for particulate matter and discoloration prior to administration whenever the solution and container permit. Solutions that are discolored and/or contain particulate matter should not be used.

HOW SUPPLIED

Xylocaine (lidocaine HCl) 4% Sterile Solution, 5 ml ampule (NDC 0186-0235-03) and 5 ml prefilled sterile disposable syringe packaged in a presterilized kit containing a laryngotracheal cannula (NDC 0186-0235-72).

Store at controlled room temperature: 15°C–30°C (59°–86°F).
021562R05   Rev. 3/86(5)

XYLOCAINE® (lidocaine hydrochloride) ℞
[zī'lo-caine]
4% TOPICAL SOLUTION
For topical application

DESCRIPTION

Xylocaine (lidocaine HCl) 4% Topical Solution contains a local anesthetic agent and is administered topically. See INDICATIONS for specific uses.

Xylocaine 4% Topical Solution contains lidocaine HCL, which is chemically designated as acetamide, 2-(diethylamino)-N-(2,6-dimethylphenyl)-, monohydrochloride.

The 50ml screw-cap bottle should not be autoclaved, because the closure employed cannot withstand autoclaving temperatures and pressures. Composition of Xylocaine (lidocaine HCl) 4% Topical Solution: Each ml contains lidocaine HCl, 40mg, methylparaben, and sodium hydroxide and/or hydrochloric acid to adjust pH to 6.0–7.0.

An aqueous solution. NOT FOR INJECTION

HOW SUPPLIED

Xylocaine (lidocaine HCl) 4% Topical Solution 50ml screw-cap bottle, cartoned (NDC 0186-0320-01). NOT FOR INJECTION.

Store at controlled room temperature: 15°-30°C (59°-86°F).
021802R01   7/84

XYLOCAINE® (lidocaine) ℞
[zī'lo-caine]
HYDROCHLORIDE 1.5% WITH
DEXTROSE 7.5%
    Sterile Hyperbaric Solution Only
    for Spinal Anesthesia
    in Obstetrics

(For details of indications, dosage and administration, precautions, and adverse reactions, see circular in package.)

HOW SUPPLIED

Xylocaine® (lidocaine HCl) 1.5% Solution with Dextrose 7.5% (NDC 0186-0212-03) is supplied in 2 ml ampules in packages of 10. Store at controlled room temperature 15°-30°C (59°-86°F).
021836R04   3/84

XYLOCAINE® (lidocaine hydrochloride) ℞
[zī'lo-cain]

5% SOLUTION WITH GLUCOSE 7.5%
Sterile Hyperbaric Solution
for Spinal Anesthesia

(For details of indications, dosage and administration, precautions, and adverse reactions, see circular in package.)

HOW SUPPLIED
Xylocaine® (lidocaine HCl) 5% solution with Glucose 7.5% (NDC 0186-0225-03) is supplied in 2 mL ampules in packages of 10.
Store at controlled room temperatures 15°–30°C (59°–86°F).
021564R09   1/88(9)

XYLOCAINE® 2% (lidocaine hydrochloride) ℞
[zī'lo-caine]

JELLY
A Topical Anesthetic
for Urological Procedures
and Lubrication
of Endotracheal Tubes

DESCRIPTION
Xylocaine (lidocaine HCl) 2% Jelly is a sterile aqueous product that contains a local anesthetic agent and is administered topically. See INDICATIONS for specific uses.
Xylocaine 2% Jelly contains lidocaine HCl which is chemically designated as acetamide, 2-(diethylamino)-N-(2,6-dimethylphenyl)-, monohydrochloride and has the following structural formula:

$$CH_3, C_2H_5, NH\text{-}CO\text{-}CH_2\text{-}N \cdot HCl, CH_3, C_2H_5$$

Xylocaine 2% Jelly also contains hydroxypropylmethylcellulose, and the resulting mixture maintains contact with mucosa and provides lubrication for instrumentation.
The unused portion should be discarded after initial use.
Composition of Xylocaine 2% Jelly:
Each ml contains 20 mg of lidocaine HYCl. The formulation also contains methylparaben, propylparaben, hydroxypropylmethylcellulose, and sodium hydroxide and/or hydrochloric acid to adjust pH to 6.0–7.0

CLINICAL PHARMACOLOGY
Mechanism of action: Lidocaine stabilizes the neuronal membrane by inhibiting the ionic fluxes required for the initiation and conduction of impulses, thereby effecting local anesthetic action.
Onset of action: The onset of action is 3–5 minutes. It is ineffective when applied to intact skin.
Hemodynamics: Excessive blood levels may cause changes in cardiac output, total peripheral resistance, and mean arterial pressure. These changes may be attributable to a direct depressant effect of the local anesthetic agent on various components of the cardiovascular system.
Pharmacokinetics and metabolism: Lidocaine may be absorbed following topical administration to mucous membranes, its rate and extent of absorption depending upon concentration and total dose administered, the specific site of application and duration of exposure. In general, the rate of absorption of local anesthetic agents following topical application occurs most rapidly after intratracheal administration. Lidocaine is also well-absorbed from the gastrointestinal tract, but little intact drug may appear in the circulation because of biotransformation in the liver.
Lidocaine is metabolized rapidly by the liver, and metabolites and unchanged drug are excreted by the kidneys. Biotransformation includes oxidative N-dealkylation, ring hydroxylation, cleavage of the amide linkage, and conjugation. N-dealkylation, a major pathway of biotransformation, yields the metabolites monoethylglycinexylidide and glycinexylidide. The pharacological/toxicological actions of these metabolites are similar to, but less potent than, those of lidocaine. Approximately 90% of lidocaine administered is excreted in the form of various metabolites, and less than 10% is excreted unchanged. The primary metabolite in urine is a conjugate of 4-hydroxy-2,6-dimethylaniline.
The plasma binding of lidocaine is dependent on drug concentration, and the fraction bound decreases with increasing concentration. At concentrations of 1 to 4 µg of free base per ml, 60 to 80 percent of lidocaine is protein bound. Binding is also dependent on the plasma concentration of the alpha-1-acid glycoprotein.
Lidocaine crosses the blood-brain and placental barriers, presumably by passive diffusion.
Studies of lidocaine metabolism following intravenous bolus injections have shown that the elimination half-life of this agent is typically 1.5 to 2.0 hours. Because of the rapid rate at which lidocaine is metabolized, any condition that affects liver function may alter lidocaine kinetics. The half-life may be prolonged two-fold or more in patients with liver dysfunction. Renal dysfunction does not affect lidocaine kinetics but may increase the accumulation of metabolites.
Factors such as acidosis and the use of CNS stimulants and depressants affect the CNS levels of lidocaine required to produce overt systemic effects. Objective adverse manifestations become increasingly apparent with increasing venous plasma levels above 6.0 µg free base per ml. In the rhesus monkey arterial blood levels of 18–21 µg/ml have been shown to be threshold for convulsive activity.

INDICATIONS AND USAGE
Xylocaine (lidocaine HCl) 2% Jelly is indicated for prevention and control of pain in procedures involving the male and female urethra, for topical treatment of painful urethritis, and as an anesthetic lubricant for endotracheal intubation (oral and nasal).

CONTRAINDICATIONS
Lidocaine is contraindicated in patients with a known history of hypersensitivity to local anesthetics of the amide type or to other components of Xylocaine 2% Jelly.

WARNINGS
EXCESSIVE DOSAGE, OR SHORT INTERVALS BETWEEN DOSES, CAN RESULT IN HIGH PLASMA LEVELS AND SERIOUS ADVERSE EFFECTS. PATIENTS SHOULD BE INSTRUCTED TO STRICTLY ADHERE TO THE RECOMMENDED DOSAGE AND ADMINISTRATION GUIDELINES AS SET FORTH IN THIS PACKAGE INSERT.
THE MANAGEMENT OF SERIOUS ADVERSE REACTIONS MAY REQUIRE THE USE OF RESUSCITATIVE EQUIPMENT, OXYGEN, AND OTHER RESUSCITATIVE DRUGS.
Xylocaine 2% Jelly should be used with extreme caution in the presence of sepsis or severely traumatized mucosa in the area of application, since under such conditions there is the potential for rapid systemic absorption.
When used for endotracheal tube lubrication care should be taken to avoid introducing the product into the lumen of the tube. Do not use the jelly to lubricate the endotracheal stylettes. If allowed into the inner lumen, the jelly may dry on the inner surface leaving a residue which tends to clump with flexion, narrowing the lumen. There have been rare reports in which this residue has caused the lumen to occlude. See also ADVERSE REACTION and DOSAGE & ADMINISTRATION.

PRECAUTIONS
General: The safety and effectiveness of lidocaine depend on proper dosage, correct technique, adequate precautions, and readiness for emergencies. (See WARNINGS and ADVERSE REACTIONS.) The lowest dosage that results in effective anesthesia should be used to avoid high plasma levels and serious adverse effects. Repeated doses of lidocaine may cause significant increases in blood levels with each repeated dose because of slow accumulation of the drug or its metabolites. Tolerance to elevated blood levels varies with the status of the patient. Debilitated, elderly patients, acutely ill patients, and children should be given reduced doses commensurate with their age and physical status. Lidocaine should also be used with caution in patients with severe shock or heart block.
Xylocaine 2% Jelly should be used with caution in patients with known drug sensitivities. Patients allergic to para-aminobenzoic acid derivatives (procaine, tetracaine, benzocaine, etc.) have not shown cross sensitivity to lidocaine.
Many drugs used during the conduct of anesthesia are considered potential triggering agents for familial malignant hyperthermia. Since it is not known whether amide-type local anesthetics may trigger this reaction and since the need for supplemental general anesthesia cannot be predicted in advance, it is suggested that a standard protocol for management should be available. Early unexplained signs of tachycardia, tachypnea, labile blood pressure and metabolic acidosis may precede temperature elevation. Successful outcome is dependent on early diagnosis, prompt discontinuance of the suspect triggering agent(s) and institution of treatment, including oxygen therapy, indicated supportive measures and dantrolene (consult dantrolene sodium intravenous package insert before using).
Information for Patients: When topical anesthetics are used in the mouth, the patient should be aware that the production of topical anesthesia may impair swallowing and thus enhance the danger of aspiration. For this reason, food should not be ingested for 60 minutes following use of local anesthetic preparations in the mouth or throat area. This is particularly important in children because of their frequency of eating.
Numbness of the tongue or buccal mucosa may enhance the danger of unintentional biting trauma. Food and chewing gum should not be taken while the mouth or throat area is anesthetized.

Carcinogenesis, mutagenesis, impairment of fertility: Studies of lidocaine in animals to evaluate the carcinogenic and mutagenic potential or the effect on fertility have not been conducted.
Use in Pregnancy: Teratogenic Effects. Pregnancy Category B. Reproduction studies have been performed in rats at doses up to 6.6 times the human dose and have revealed no evidence of harm to the fetus caused by lidocaine. There are, however, no adequate and well-controlled studies in pregnant women. Animal reproduction studies are not always predictive of human response. General consideration should be given to this fact before administering lidocaine to women of childbearing potential, especially during early pregnancy when maximum organogenesis takes place.
Labor and Delivery: Lidocaine is not contraindicated in labor and delivery. Should Xylocaine 2% Jelly be used concomitantly with other products containing lidocaine, the total dose contributed by all formulations must be kept in mind.
Nursing mothers: It is not known whether this drug is excreted in human milk. Because many drugs are excreted in human milk, caution should be exercised when lidocaine is administered to a nursing woman.
Pediatric use: Dosages in children should be reduced, commensurate with age, body weight and physical condition. See DOSAGE AND ADMINISTRATION.

ADVERSE REACTIONS
Adverse experiences following the administration of lidocaine are similar in nature to those observed with other amide local anesthetic agents. These adverse experiences are, in general, dose-related and may result from high plasma levels caused by excessive dosage or rapid absorption, or may result from a hypersensitivity, idiosyncrasy or diminished tolerance on the part of the patient. Serious adverse experiences are generally systemic in nature. The following types are those most commonly reported:
There have been rare reports of endotracheal tube occlusion associated with the presence of dried jelly residue in the inner lumen of the tube. See also WARNINGS and DOSAGE & ADMINISTRATION.
Central nervous system. CNS manifestations are excitatory and/or depressant and may be characterized by lightheadedness, nervousness, apprehension, euphoria, confusion, dizziness, drowsiness, tinnitus, blurred or double vision, vomiting, sensations of heat, cold or numbness, twitching, tremors, convulsions, unconsciousness, respiratory depression and arrest. The excitatory manifestations may be very brief or may not occur at all, in which case the first manifestation of toxicity may be drowsiness merging into unconsciousness and respiratory arrest.
Drowsiness following the administration of lidocaine is usually an early sign of a high blood level of the drug and may occur as a consequence of rapid absorption.
Cardiovascular system: Cardiovascular manifestations are usually depressant and are characterized by bradycardia, hypotension, and cardiovascular collapse, which may lead to cardiac arrest.
Allergic: Allergic reactions are characterized by cutaneous lesions, urticaria, edema or anaphylactoid reactions. Allergic reactions may occur as a result of sensitivity either to the local anesthetic agent or to other components in the formulation. Allergic reactions as a result of sensitivity to lidocaine are extremely rare and, if they occur, should be managed by conventional means. The detection of sensitivity by skin testing is of doubtful value.

OVERDOSAGE
Acute emergencies from local anesthetics are generally related to high plasma levels encountered during therapeutic use of local anesthetics. (See ADVERSE REACTIONS, WARNINGS, and PRECAUTIONS.)
Management of local anesthetic emergencies: The first consideration is prevention, best accomplished by careful and constant monitoring of cardiovascular and respiratory vital signs and the patient's state of consciousness after each local anesthetic administration. At the first sign of change, oxygen should be administered.
The first step in the management of convulsions consists of immediate attention to the maintenance of a patent airway and assisted or controlled ventilation with oxygen and a delivery system capable of permitting immediate positive airway pressure by mask. Immediately after the institution of these ventilatory measures, the adequacy of the circulation should be evaluated, keeping in mind that drugs used to treat convulsions sometimes depress the circulation when administered intravenously. Should convulsions persist despite adequate respiratory support, and if the status of the circulation permits, small increments of an ultra-short acting barbiturate (such as thiopental or thiamylal) or a benzodiazepine (such as diazepam) may be administered intravenously. The clinician should be familiar, prior to use of local anesthetics, with these anticonvulsant drugs. Supportive treatment or circulatory depression may require administra-

Continued on next page

Astra—Cont.

tion of intravenous fluids and, when appropriate, a vasopressor as directed by the clinical situation (e.g. ephedrine).
If not treated immediately, both convulsions and cardiovascular depression can result in hypoxia, acidosis, bradycardia, arrhythmias and cardiac arrest. If cardiac arrest should occur, standard cardiopulmonary resuscitative measures should be instituted.
Dialysis is of negligible value in the treatment of acute overdosage with lidocaine.
The oral LD_{50} of lidocaine HCl in non-fasted female rats is 459 (346–773) mg/kg (as the salt) and 214 (159–324) mg/kg (as the salt) in fasted female rats.

DOSAGE AND ADMINISTRATION

When Xylocaine 2% Jelly is used concomitantly with other products containing lidocaine, the total dose contributed by all formulations must be kept in mind.
The dosage varies and depends upon the area to be anesthetized, vascularity of the tissues, individual tolerance, and the technique of anesthesia. The lowest dosage needed to provide effective anesthesia should be administered. Dosages should be reduced for children and for elderly and debilitated patients. Although the incidence of adverse effects with Xylocaine 2% Jelly is quite low, caution should be exercised, particularly when employing large amounts, since the incidence of adverse effects is directly proportional to the total dose of local anesthetic agent administered.
For surface anesthesia of the male adult urethra: The plastic cone is sterilized for 5 minutes in boiling water, cooled, and attached to the tube. The cone may be gas sterilized or cold sterilized, as preferred. The jelly is instilled slowly into the urethra by gently expressing the contents of the tube until the patient has a feeling of tension or until almost half the tube (15 ml; *i.e.*, 300 mg of lidocaine HCl) is emptied. A penile clamp is then applied for several minutes at the corona and then the remaining contents of the tube are instilled.
Prior to sounding or cystoscopy, a penile clamp should be applied for 5 to 10 minutes to obtain adequate anesthesia. The contents of one tube (30 ml, *i.e.*, 600 mg) are usually required to fill and dilate the male urethra.
Prior to catheterization, smaller volumes (5–10 ml, *i.e.*, 100–200 mg) are usually adequate for lubrication.
For surface anesthesia of the female adult urethra: The plastic cone is sterilized for 5 minutes in boiling water, cooled, and attached to the tube. The cone may be gas sterilized or cold sterilized, as preferred. Three to five ml of the jelly is instilled slowly into the urethra by gently expressing approximately 10–20% of the contents of the tube. If desired, some jelly may be deposited on a cotton swab and introduced into the urethra. In order to obtain adequate anesthesia, several minutes should be allowed prior to performing urological procedures.
Lubrication for endotracheal intubation: Apply a moderate amount of jelly to the external surface of the endotracheal tube shortly before use. Care should be taken to avoid introducing the product into the lumen of the tube. Do not use the jelly to lubricate endotracheal stylettes. See WARNINGS and ADVERSE REACTIONS concerning rare reports of inner lumen occlusion. It is also recommended that use of endotracheal tubes with dried jelly on the external surface be avoided for lack of lubricating effect.
MAXIMUM DOSAGE: No more than one tube (600 mg of lidocaine HCl) should be given in any 12 hour period.
Children: It is difficult to recommend a maximum dose of any drug for children since this varies as a function of age and weight. For children less than ten years who have a normal lean body mass and a normal lean body development, the maximum dose may be determined by the application of one of the standard pediatric drug formulas (e.g., Clark's rule). For example, in a child of five years weighing 50 lbs., the dose of lidocaine hydrochloriide should not exceed 75–100 mg when calculated according to Clark's rule. In any case, the maximum amount of Xylocaine administered should not exceed 4.5 mg/kg (2.0 mg/lb) of body weight.

HOW SUPPLIED

Xylocaine (lidocaine HCl) 2% Jelly (NDC 0186-0330-01) is supplied in collapsible tubes that deliver 30 ml. A detachable applicator cone and a key for expressing the contents are included in each package.
Store at controlled room temperature 15°–30°C (59°–86°F).
021838R11   Rev. 6/86(11)

5% XYLOCAINE (lidocaine)   ℞
[zī'lo-caine]
Ointment
A Water-Soluble Topical Anesthetic Ointment

DESCRIPTION

Xylocaine (lidocaine) 5% Ointment contains a local anesthetic agent and is administered topically. See INDICATIONS for specific uses.

Xylocaine 5% Ointment contains lidocaine, which is chemically designated as acetamide, 2-(diethylamino)-N-(2,6-dimethylphenyl)-, and has the following structural formula:

Composition of Xylocaine 5% Ointment
Each gram of the plain and flavored ointments contains lidocaine, 50 mg, polyethylene glycol 1500, polyethylene glycol 4000, propylene gylcol and sodium saccharin. The flavored ointment contains peppermint oil and spearmint oil.

CLINICAL PHARMACOLOGY

Mechanism of action:
Lidocaine stabilizes the nueronal membrane by inhibiting the ionic fluxes required for the initiation and conduction of impulses, thereby effecting local anesthetic action.
Onset of anesthesia:
Xylocaine (lidocaine) 5% Ointment effects local, topical anesthesia. The onset of action is 3–5 minutes. It is ineffective when applied to intact skin.
Hemodynamics:
Excessive blood levels may cause changes in cardiac output, total peripheral resistance, and mean arterial pressure. These changes may be attributable to a direct depressant effect of the local anesthetic agent on various components of the cardiovascular system.
Pharmacokinetics and metabolism:
Lidocaine may be absorbed following topical administration to mucous membranes, its rate and extent of absorption depending upon the specific site of application, duration of exposure, concentration, and total dosage. In general, the rate of absorption of local anesthetic agents following topical application occurs most rapidly after intratracheal administration. Lidocaine is also well-absorbed from the gastrointestinal tract, but little intact drug appears in the circulation because of biotransformation in the liver.
Lidocaine is metabolized by the liver, and metabolites and unchanged drug are excreted by the kidneys. Biotransformation includes oxidative N-dealkylation, ring hydroxylation, cleavage of the amide linkage, and conjugation. N-dealkylatgion, a major pathway of biotransformation, yields the metabolites monoethylglycinexylidide and glycinexylidide. The pharmacological/toxicological actions of these metabolites are similar to, but less potent than, those of lidocaine. Approximately 90% of lidocaine administered is excreted in the form of various metabolites, and less than 10% is excreted unchanged. The primary metabolite in urine is a conjugate of 4-hydroxy-2, 6-dimethylaniline.
The plasma binding of lidocaine is dependent on drug concentration, and the fraction bound decreases with increasing concentration. At concentrations of 1 to 4 μg of free base per ml, 60 to 80 percent of lidocaine is protein bound. Binding is also dependent on the plasma concentration of the alpha-1-acid glycoprotein.
Lidocaine crosses the blood-brain and placental barriers, presumably by passive diffusion.
Studies of lidocaine metabolism following intravenous bolus injections have shown that the elimination half-life of this agent is typically 1.5 to 2.0 hours. Because of the rapid rate at which lidocaine is metabolized, any condition that affects liver function may alter lidocaine kinetics. The half-life may be prolonged two-fold or more in patients with liver dysfunction. Renal dysfunction does not affect lidocaine kinetics but may increase the accumulation of metabolites.
Factors such as acidosis and the use of CNS stimulants and depressants affect the CNS levels of lidocaine required to produce overt systemic effects. Objective adverse manifestations become increasingly apparent with increasing venous plasma levels above 6.0 μg free base per mL. In the rhesus monkey arterial blood levels of 18–21 μg/mL have been shown to be threshold for convulsive activity.

INDICATIONS AND USAGE

Xylocaine (lidocaine) 5% Ointment is indicated for production of anesthesia of accessible mucous membranes of the oropharynx.
It is also useful as an anesthetic lubricant for intubation and for the temporary relief of pain associated with minor burns, including sunburn, abrasions of the skin, and insect bites.

CONTRAINDICATIONS

Lidocaine is contraindicated in patients with a known history of hyersensitivity to local anesthetics of the amide type or to other components of Xylocaine 5% Ointment.

WARNINGS

EXCESSIVE DOSAGE, OR SHORT INTERVALS BETWEEN DOSES, CAN RESULT IN HIGH PLASMA LEVELS AND SERIOUS ADVERSE EFFECTS, PATIENTS SHOULD BE INSTRUCTED TO STRICTLY ADHERE TO THE RECOMMENDED DOSAGE AND ADMINISTRA-

TION GUIDELINES AS SET FORTH IN THIS PACKAGE INSERT.
THE MANAGEMENT OF SERIOUS ADVERSE REACTIONS MAY REQUIRE THE USE OF RESUSCITATIVE EQUIPMENT, OXYGEN, AND OTHER RESUSCITATIVE DRUGS.
Xylocaine 5% Ointment should be used with extreme caution in the presence of sepsis or severely traumatized mucosa in the area of application, since under such conditions there is the potential for rapid systemic absorption.

PRECAUTIONS

General:
The safety and effectiveness of lidocaine depend on proper dosage, correct technique, adequate precautions, and readiness for emergencies. (See WARNINGS and ADVERSE REACTIONS). The lowest dosage that results in effective anesthesia should be used to avoid high plasma levels and serious adverse effects. Repeated doses of lidocaine may cause significant increases in blood levels with each repeated dose because of slow accumulation of the drug and/or its metabolites. Tolerance to elevated blood levels varies with the status of the patient. Debilitated, elderly patients, acutely ill patients, and children should be given reduced doses commensurate with their age and physical condition. Lidocaine should also be used with caution in patients with severe shock or heart block.
Xylocaine 5% Ointment should be used with caution in patients with known drug sensitivities. Patients allergic to paraaminobenzoic acid derivatives (procaine, tetracaine, benzocaine, etc.) have not shown cross sensitivity to lidocaine. Many drugs used during the conduct of anesthesia are considered potential triggering agents for familial malignant hyperthermia. Since it is not known whether amide-type local anesthetics may trigger this reaction and since the need for supplemental general anesthesia cannot be predicted in advance, it is suggested that a standard protocol for the management of malignant hyperthermia should be available. Early unexplained signs of tachycardia, tachypnea, labile blood pressure and metabolic acidosis may precede temperature elevation. Successful outcome is dependent on early diagnosis, prompt discontinuance of the suspect triggering agent(s) and institution of treatment, including oxygen therapy, indicated supportive measures and dantrolene (consult dantrolene sodium intravenous package insert before using).
Information for Patients:
When topical anesthetics are used in the mouth, the patient should be aware that the production of topical anesthesia may impair swallowing and thus enhance the danger of aspiration. For this reason, food should not be ingested for 60 minutes following the use of local anesthetic preparations in the mouth or throat area. This is particularly important in children because of their frequency of eating.
Numbness of the tongue or buccal mucosa may enhance the danger of unintentional biting trauma. Food and chewing gum should not be taken while the mouth or throat area is anesthetized.
Carcinogenesis, mutagenesis, impairment of fertility:
Studies of lidocaine in animals to evaluate the carcinogenic and mutagenic potential or the effect on fertility have not been conducted.
Use in Pregnancy:
Teratogenic Effects. Pregnancy Category B. Reproduction studies have been performed in rats at doses up to 6.6 times the human dose and have revealed no evidence of harm to the fetus caused by lidocaine. There are, however, no adequate and well-controlled studies in pregnant women. Animal reproduction studies are not always predictive of human response. General consideration should be given to this fact before administering lidocaine to women of childbearing potential, especially during early pregnancy when maximum organogenesis takes place.
Labor and Delivery:
Lidocaine is not contraindicated in labor and delivery. Should Xylocaine 5% Ointment be used concomitantly with other products containing lidocaine, the total dose contributed by all formulations must be kept in mind.
Nursing Mothers:
It is not known whether this drug is excreted in human milk. Because many drugs are excreted in human milk, caution should be exercised when lidocaine is administered to a nursing woman.
Pediatric use:
Dosage in children should be reduced, commensurate with age, body weight and physical condition. Caution must be taken to avoid overdosage when applying Xylocaine 5% Ointment to large areas of injured or abraded skin, since the systemic absorption of lidocaine may be increased under such conditions. See DOSAGE and ADMINISTRATION.

ADVERSE REACTIONS

Adverse experiences following the administration of lidocaine are similar in nature to those observed with other amide local anesthetic agents. These adverse experiences are, in general, dose-related and may result from high plasma levels caused by excessive dosage or rapid absorption, or may result from a hypersensitivity, idiosyncrasy or diminished tolerance on the part of the patient. Serious adverse experiences are generally systemic in nature. The following types are those most commonly reported:

Central nervous system:

CNS manifestations are excitatory and/or depressant and may be characterized by lightheadedness, nervousness, apprehension, euphoria, confusion, dizziness, drowsiness, tinnitus, blurred or double vision, vomiting, sensations of heat, cold or numbness, twitching, tremors, convulsions, unconsciousness, respiratory depression and arrest. The excitatory manifestations may be very brief or may not occur at all, in which case the first manifestation of toxicity may be drowsiness merging into unconsciousness and respiratory arrest. Drowsiness following the administration of lidocaine is usually an early sign of a high blood level of the drug and may occur as a consequence of rapid absorption.

Cardiovascular system:

Cardiovascular manifestations are usually depressant and are characterized by bradycardia, hypotension, and cardiovascular collapse, which may lead to cardiac arrest.

Allergic:

Allergic reactions are characterized by cutaneous lesions, urticaria, edema or anaphylactoid reactions. Allergic reactions may occur as a result of sensitivity either to the local anesthetic agent or to other components in the formulation. Allergic reactions as a result of sensitivity to lidocaine are extremely rare and, if they occur, should be managed by conventional means. The detection of sensitivity by skin testing is of doubtful value.

OVERDOSAGE

Acute emergencies from local anesthetics are generally related to high plasma levels encountered during therapeutic use of local anesthetics. (see ADVERSE REACTIONS, WARNINGS, and PRECAUTIONS).

Management of local anesthetic emergencies:

The first consideration is prevention, best accomplished by careful and constant monitoring of cardiovascular and respiratory vital signs and the patient's state of consciousness after each local anethetic administration. At the first sign of change, oxygen should be administered.

The first step in the management of convulsions consists of immediate attention to the maintenance of a patent airway and assisted or controlled ventilation with oxygen and a delivery system capable of permitting immediate positive airway pressure by mask. Immediately after the institution of these ventilatory measures, the adequacy of the circulation should be evaluated, keeping in mind that drugs used to treat convulsions sometimes depress the circulation when administered intravenously. Should convulsions persist despite adequate respiratory support, and if the status of the circulation permits, small increments of an ultra-short acting barbiturate (such as thiopental or thiamylal) or a benzodiazepine (such as diazepam) may be administered intravenously. The clinician should be familiar, prior to use of local anesthetics, with these anticonvulsant drugs. Supportive treatment of circulatory depression may require administration of intravenous fluids and, when appropriate, a vasopressor as directed by the clinical situation (e.g., ephedrine).

If not treated immediately, both convulsions and cardiovascular depression can result in hypoxia, acidosis, bradycardia, arrhythmias and cardiac arrest. If cardiac arrest should occur, standard cardiopulmonary resuscitative measures should be instituted.

Dialysis is of negligible value in the treatment of acute overdosage with lidocaine.

The oral LD_{50} of lidocaine HCl in non-fasted female rats is 459 (346-773) mg/kg (as the salt) and 214 (159-324) mg/kg (as the salt) in fasted female rats.

DOSAGE AND ADMINISTRATION

When Xylocaine 5% Ointment is used concomitantly with other products containing lidocaine, the total dose contributed by all formulations must be kept in mind.

Adult

A single application should not exceed 5 gm of Xylocaine 5% Ointment, containing 250 mg of Xylocaine base (equivalent chemically to approximately 300 mg of Xylocaine hydrochloride). This is roughly equivalent to squeezing a six (6) inch length of ointment from the tube. In a 70 kg adult this dose equals 3.6 mg/kg (1.6 mg/lb) lidocaine base. No more than one-half tube, approximately 17–20 gm of ointment or 850–1000 mg Xylocaine base, should be administered in any one day.

Although the incidence of adverse effects with Xylocaine 5% Ointment is quite low, caution should be exercised, particularly when employing large amounts, since the incidence of adverse effects is directly proportional to the total dose of local anesthetic agent administered.

Dosage for children

It is difficult to recommend a maximum dose of any drug for children since this varies as a function of age and weight. For children less than ten years who have a normal lean body mass and a normal lean body development, the maximum dose may be determined by the application of one of the standard pediatric drug formulas (e.g., Clark's rule). For example, in a child of five years weighing 50 lbs., the dose of lidocaine should not exceed 75–100 mg when calculated according to Clark's rule. In any case, the maximum amount of Xylocaine administered should not exceed 4.5 mg/kg (2.0 mg/lb) of body weight.

Administration

For medical use, apply topically for adequate control of symptoms. The use of a sterile gauze pad is suggested for application to broken skin tissue. Apply to the tube prior to intubation.

In dentistry, apply to previously dried oral mucosa. Subsequent removal of excess saliva with cotton rolls or saliva ejector minimizes dilution of the ointment, permits maximum penetration, and minimizes the possibility of swallowing the topical ointment.

For use in connection with the insertion of new dentures, apply to all denture surfaces contacting mucosa.

IMPORTANT: Patients should consult a dentist at intervals not exceeding 48 hours throughout the fitting period.

HOW SUPPLIED

Xylocaine (lidocaine) 5% Ointment (NDC 0186-0315-21) is available in 35 gm tubes.

Xylocaine (lidocaine) 5% Ointment Flavored for application within the oral cavity, is dispensed in 3.5 gram tubes, 10 tubes per carton (NDC 0186-0350-03), and in 35-gram jars (NDC 0186-0350-01).

KEEP CONTAINER TIGHTLY CLOSED AT ALL TIMES WHEN NOT IN USE.

Store at controlled room temperature 15°C–30°C (59°–86°F).

021709R11   Rev. 12/86 (11)

XYLOCAINE ® (lidocaine)
[zi'lo-cain]
2.5% OINTMENT

(See PDR For Nonprescription Drugs)

XYLOCAINE® (lidocaine)   ℞
[zi'lo-caine]
10% Oral Spray
     Flavored Topical Anesthetic Aerosol
     For Use In The Oral Cavity

WARNING—CONTENTS UNDER PRESSURE.

DESCRIPTION

Xylocaine (lidocaine) 10% Oral Spray contains a local anesthetic agent and is administered topically in the oral cavity. See INDICATIONS for specific uses.

Xylocaine 10% Oral Spray contains lidocaine, which is chemically designated as acetamide,2-(diethylamino)-N-(2,6-dimethylphenyl)-, and has the following structural formula:

Composition of Xylocaine (lidocaine) 10% Oral Spray
Each actuation of the metered dose valve delivers 0.1ml of solution containing lidocaine, 10mg, cetylpyridinium chloride, absolute alcohol, saccharin, flavor, and polyethylene glycol.

And as propellants: trichlorofluoromethane/dichlorodifluoromethane (65%/35%).

CLINICAL PHARMACOLOGY

Mechanism of action: Lidocaine stabilizes the neuronal membrane by inhibiting the ionic fluxes required for the initiation and conduction of impulses, thereby effecting local anesthetic action.

Onset and duration of action: Xylocaine (lidocaine) 10% Oral Spray acts on intact mucous membranes to produce local anesthesia. Anesthesia occurs usually within 1–2 minutes and persists for approximately 10–15 minutes.

Hemodynamics: Excessive blood levels may cause changes in cardiac output, total peripheral resistance, and mean arterial pressure. These changes may be attributable to a direct depressant effect of the local anesthetic agent on various components of the cardiovascular system.

Pharmacokinetics and metabolism: Lidocaine may be absorbed following topical administration to mucous membranes, its rate of absorption and percent of dose absorbed depending upon concentration and total dose administered, the specific site of application and duration of exposure. In general, the rate of absorption of local anesthetic agents following topical application occurs most rapidly after intratracheal administration. Lidocaine is well-absorbed from the gastrointestinal tract, but little intact drug appears in the circulation because of biotransformation in the liver.

Lidocaine is metabolized rapidly by the liver, and metabolites and unchanged drug are excreted by the kidney. Biotransformation includes oxidative N-dealkylation, ring hydroxylation, cleavage of the amide linkage, and conjugation. N-dealkylation, a major pathway of biotransformation, yields the metabolites monoethylglycinexylidide and glycinexylidide. The pharmacological/toxicological actions of these metabolites are similar to, but less potent than, those of lidocaine. Approximately 90% of lidocaine administered is excreted in the form of various metabolites, and less than 10% is excreted unchanged. The primary metabolite in urine is a conjugate of 4-hydroxy-2, 6-dimethylaniline.

The plasma binding of lidocaine is dependent on drug concentration, and the fraction bound decreases with increasing concentration. At concentrations of 1 to 4 μg of free base per ml, 60 to 80 percent of lidocaine is protein bound. Binding is also dependent on the plasma concentration of the alpha-1-acid glycoprotein.

Lidocaine crosses the blood-brain and placental barriers, presumably by passive diffusion.

Studies of lidocaine metabolism following intravenous bolus injections have shown that the elimination half-life of this agent is typically 1.5 to 2.0 hours. Because of the rapid rate at which lidocaine is metabolized, any condition that affects liver function may alter lidocaine kinetics. The half-life may be prolonged two-fold or more in patients with liver dysfunction. Renal dysfunction does not affect lidocaine kinetics but may increase the accumulation of metabolites.

Factors such as acidosis and the use of CNS stimulants and depressants affect the CNS levels of lidocaine required to produce overt systemic effects. Objective adverse manifestations become increasingly apparent with increasing venous plasma levels above 6.0 μg free base per mL. In the rhesus monkey arterial blood levels of 18–21 μg/ mL have been shown to be threshold for convulsive activity.

INDICATIONS AND USAGE

Xylocaine (lidocaine) 10% Oral Spray is indicated for the production of topical anesthesia of the accessible mucous membranes of the mouth and oropharynx.

CONTRAINDICATIONS

Lidocaine is contraindicated in patients with a known history of hypersensitivity to local anesthetics of the amide type or to other components of Xylocaine 10% Oral Spray.

WARNINGS

IN ORDER TO MANAGE POSSIBLE ADVERSE REACTIONS, RESUSCITATIVE EQUIPMENT, OXYGEN AND OTHER RESUSCITATIVE DRUGS MUST BE IMMEDIATELY AVAILABLE WHEN LOCAL ANESTHETIC AGENTS, SUCH AS LIDOCAINE, ARE ADMINISTERED TO MUCOUS MEMBRANES.

Xylocaine 10% Oral Spray should be used with extreme caution if there is sepsis or extremely traumatized mucosa in the area of application, since under such conditions there is the potential for rapid systemic absorption.

PRECAUTIONS

General: The safety and effectiveness of lidocaine depend on proper dosage, correct technique, adequate precautions, and readiness for emergencies. Resuscitative equipment, oxygen, and other resuscitative drugs should be available for immediate use. (See WARNINGS and ADVERSE REACTIONS). The lowest dosage that results in effective anesthesia should be used to avoid high plasma levels and serious adverse effects. Repeated doses of lidocaine may cause significant increases in blood levels with each repeated dose because of slow accumulation of the drug or its metabolites. Tolerance varies with the status of the patient. Debilitated, elderly patients, acutely ill patients, and children should be given reduced doses commensurate with their age and physical status. Lidocaine should also be used with caution in patients with severe shock or heart block.

Xylocaine 10% Oral Spray should be used with caution in patients with known drug sensitivities. Patients allergic to para-aminobenzoic acid derivatives (procaine, tetracaine, benzocaine, etc.) have not shown cross sensitivity to lidocaine.

Many drugs used during the conduct of anesthesia are considered potential triggering agents for familial malignant hyperthermia. Since it is not known whether amide-type local anesthetics may trigger this reaction and since the need for supplemental general anesthesia cannot be predicted in advance, it is suggested that a standard protocol for management should be available. Early unexplained signs of tachycardia, tachypnea, labile blood pressure and metabolic acidosis may precede temperature elevation. Successful outcome is dependent on early diagnosis, prompt discontinuance of the suspect triggering agent(s) and institution of treatment, including oxygen therapy, indicated supportive measures and dantrolene (consult dantrolene sodium intravenous package insert before using).

Continued on next page

Astra—Cont.

Information for Patients: When topical anesthetics are used in the mouth, the patient should be aware that the production of topical anesthesia may impair swallowing and thus enhance the danger of aspiration. For this reason, food should not be ingested for 60 minutes following use of local anesthetic preprations in the mouth or throat area. This is particularly important in children because of their frequency of eating.

Numbness of the tongue or buccal mucosa may enhance the danger of unintentional biting trauma. Food and chewing gum should not be taken while the mouth or throat area is anesthetized.

Carcinogenesis, mutagenesis, impairment of fertility: Studies of lidocaine in animals to evaluate the carcinogenic and mutagenic potential or the effect on fertility have not been conducted.

Use in Pregnancy: Teratogenic Effects. Pregnancy Category B. Reproduction studies have been performed in rats at doses up to 6.6 times the human dose and have revealed no evidence of harm to the fetus caused by lidocaine. There are, however, no adequate and well-controlled studies in pregnant women. Animal reproduction studies are not always predictive of human response. General consideration should be given to this fact before administering lidocaine to women of childbearing potential, especially during early pregnancy when maximum organogenesis takes place.

Labor and Delivery: Lidocaine is not contraindicated in labor and delivery. Should Xylocaine 10% Oral Spray be used concomitantly with other products containing lidocaine, the total dose contributed by all formulations must be kept in mind.

Nursing mothers: It is not known whether this drug is excreted in human milk. Because many drugs are excreted in human milk, caution should be exercised when lidocaine is administered to a nursing woman.

Pediatric use: Safety and effectiveness in children below the age of 12 years have not been established.

ADVERSE REACTIONS

Adverse experiences following the administration of lidocaine are similar in nature to those observed with other amide local anesthetic agents. These adverse experiences are, in general, dose-related and may result from high plasma levels caused by excessive dosage or rapid absorption, or may result from a hypersensitivity, idiosyncrasy or diminished tolerance on the part of the patient. Serious adverse experiences are generally systemic in nature. The following types are those most commonly reported:

Central nervous system: CNS manifestations are excitatory and/or depressant and may be characterized by lightheadedness, nervousness, apprehension, euphoria, confusion, dizziness, drowsiness, tinnitus, blurred or double vision, vomiting, sensations of heat, cold or numbness, twitching, tremors, convulsions, unconsciousness, respiratory depression and arrest. The excitatory manifestations may be very brief or may not occur at all, in which case the first manifestation of toxicity may be drowsiness merging into unconsciousness and respiratory arrest.

Drowsiness following the administration of lidocaine is usually an early sign of a high blood level of the drug and may occur as a consequence of rapid absorption.

Cardiovascular system: Cardiovascular manifestations are usually depressant and are characterized by bradycardia, hypotension, and cardiovascular collapse, which may lead to cardiac arrest.

Allergic: Allergic reactions are characterized by cutaneous lesions, urticaria, edema or anaphylactoid reactions. Allergic reactions may occur as a result of sensitivity either to the local anesthetic agent or to other ingredients in the formulation. Allergic reactions as a result of sensitivity to lidocaine are extremely rare and, if they occur, should be managed by conventional means. The detection of sensitivity by skin testing is of doubtful value.

OVERDOSAGE

Acute emergencies from local anesthetics are generally related to high plasma levels encountered during therapeutic use of local anesthetics. (see ADVERSE REACTIONS, WARNINGS, and PRECAUTIONS).

Management of local anesthetic emergencies: The first consideration is prevention, best accomplished by careful and constant monitoring of cardiovascular and respiratory vital signs and the patient's state of consciousness after each local anesthetic administration. At the first sign of change, oxygen should be administered.

The first step in the management of convulsions consists of immediate attention to the maintenance of a patent airway and assisted or controlled ventilation with oxygen and a delivery system capable of permitting immediate positive airway pressure by mask. Immediately after the institution of these ventilatory measures, the adequacy of the circulation should be evaluated, keeping in mind that drugs used to treat convulsions sometimes depress the circulation when administered intravenously. Should convulsions persist despite adequate respiratory support, and if the status of the circulation permits, small increments of an ultra-short acting barbiturate (such as thiopental or thiamylal) or a benzodiazepine (such as diazepam) may be administered intravenously. The clinician should be familiar, prior to use of local anesthetics, with these anticonvulsant drugs. Supportive treatment of circulatory depression may require administration of intravenous fluids and, when appropriate, a vasopressor as directed by the clinical situation (e.g., ephedrine).

If not treated immediately, both convulsions and cardiovascular depression can result in hypoxia, acidosis, bradycardia, arrhythmias and cardiac arrest. If cardiac arrest should occur, standard cardiopulmonary resuscitative measures should be instituted.

Dialysis is of negligible value in the treatment of acute overdosage with lidocaine.

The intravenous LD_{50} of lidocaine HCl in female mice is 26(21–31) mg/kg and the subcutaneous LD_{50} is 264(203–304) mg/kg.

DOSAGE AND ADMINISTRATION

When Xylocaine 10% Oral Spray is used concomitantly with other products containing lidocaine, the total dose contributed by all formulations must be kept in mind.

Two metered doses per quadrant are recommended as the upper limit and, *under no circumstances* should one exceed three metered doses per quadrant of oral mucosa over a one-half hour period to produce the desired anesthetic effect. Experience in children is inadequate to recommend a pediatric dose at this time.

HOW SUPPLIED

NDC 0186-0356-01. A 26.8 mL aerosol container provides a total amount of 3.3 g (w/w) of the active ingredient lidocaine. Each actuation of the metered dose valve delivers 10mg of lidocaine.

Contents under pressure. Do not puncture or incinerate container. Do not expose to heat or store at temperatures above 120°F. Avoid contact with the eyes. Inhalation and swallowing should be avoided.

Keep out of the reach of children.

Use only as directed; intentional misuse by deliberately concentrating and inhaling the contents can be harmful or fatal.

STORE AT CONTROLLED ROOM TEMPERATURE 15°–30°C (59°–86°F).

Manufactured by Armstrong Laboratories, Inc., West Roxbury, MA 02132

021731R06   Rev. 3/89(6)

XYLOCAINE® 2% (lidocaine hydrochloride) VISCOUS SOLUTION   ℞
[zī'lo-caine]
A Topical Anesthetic for the Mucous Membranes of the Mouth and Pharynx

DESCRIPTION

Xylocaine (lidocaine HCl) 2% Viscous Solution contains a local anesthetic agent and is administered topically. Xylocaine 2% Viscous Solution contains lidocaine HCl, which is chemically designated as acetamidine, 2-(diethylamino)-N-(2,6-dimethylphenyl)-, monohydrochloride.

The molecular formula of lidocaine is $C_{14}H_{22}N_2O$. The molecular weight is 234.34.

COMPOSITION OF SOLUTION

Each ml contains 20 mg of lidocaine HCl, flavoring, sodium saccharin, methylparaben, propylparaben and sodium carboxymethylcellulose in purified water. The pH is adjusted to 6.0–7.0 by means of sodium hydroxide and/or hydrochloric acid.

CLINICAL PHARMACOLOGY

Mechanism of action: Lidocaine stabilizes the neuronal membrane by inhibiting the ionic fluxes required for the initiation and conduction of impulses, thereby effecting local anesthetic action.

Hemodynamics: Excessive blood levels may cause changes in cardiac output, total peripheral resistance, and mean arterial pressure. These changes may be attributable to a direct depressant effect of the local anesthetic agent on various components of the cardiovascular system. The net effect is normally a modest hypotension when the recommended dosages are not exceeded.

Pharmacokinetics and metabolism: Lidocaine is absorbed following topical administration to mucous membranes, its rate and extent of absorption being dependent upon concentration and total dose administered, the specific site of application, and duration of exposure. In general, the rate of absorption of local anesthetic agents following topical application occurs most rapidly after intratracheal administration. Lidocaine is also well-absorbed from the gastrointestinal tract, but little intact drug appears in the circulation because of biotransformation in the liver.

The plasma binding of lidocaine is dependent on drug concentration, and the fraction bound decreases with increasing concentration. At concentrations of 1 to 4 μg of free base per ml, 60 to 80 percent of lidocaine is protein bound. Binding is also dependent on the plasma concentration of the alpha-1-acid glycoprotein.

Lidocaine crosses the blood-brain and placental barriers, presumably by passive diffusion.

Lidocaine is metabolized rapidly by the liver, and metabolites and unchanged drug are excreted by the kidneys. Biotransformation includes oxidative N-dealkylation, ring hydroxylation, cleavage of the amide linkage, and conjugation. N-dealkylation, a major pathway of biotransformation, yields the metabolites monoethylglycinexylidide and glycinexylidide. The pharmacological/toxicological actions of these metabolites are similar to, but less potent than, those of lidocaine. Approximately 90% of lidocaine administered is excreted in the form of various metabolites, and less than 10% is excreted unchanged. The primary metabolite in urine is a conjugate of 4-hydroxy-2, 6-dimethylaniline.

The elimination half-life of lidocaine following an intravenous bolus injection is typically 1.5 to 2.0 hours. Because of the rapid rate at which lidocaine is metabolized, any condition that affects liver function may alter lidocaine kinetics. The half-life may be prolonged two-fold or more in patients with liver dysfunction. Renal dysfunction does not affect lidocaine kinetics but may increase the accumulation of metabolites.

Factors such as acidosis and the use of CNS stimulants and depressants affect the CNS levels of lidocaine required to produce overt systemic effects. Objective adverse manifestations become increasingly apparent with increasing venous plasma levels above 6.0 ug free base per ml. In the rhesus monkey arterial blood levels of 28–21 μg/ml have been shown to be threshold for convulsive activity.

INDICATIONS AND USAGE

Xylocaine (lidocaine HCl) 2% Viscous Solution is indicated for the production of topical anesthesia of irritated or inflamed mucous membranes of the mouth and pharynx. It is also useful for reducing gagging during the taking of X-ray pictures and dental impressions.

CONTRAINDICATIONS

Lidocaine is contraindicated in patients with a known history of hypersensitivity to local anesthetics of the amide type, or to other components of the solution.

WARNINGS

EXCESSIVE DOSAGE, OR SHORT INTERVALS BETWEEN DOSES, CAN RESULT IN HIGH PLASMA LEVELS AND SERIOUS ADVERSE EFFECTS. PATIENTS SHOULD BE INSTRUCTED TO STRICTLY ADHERE TO THE RECOMMENDED DOSAGE AND ADMINISTRATION GUIDELINES AS SET FORTH IN THIS PACKAGE INSERT.

THE MANAGEMENT OF SERIOUS ADVERSE REACTIONS MAY REQUIRE THE USE OF RESUSCITATIVE EQUIPMENT, OXYGEN, AND OTHER RESUSCITATIVE DRUGS.

Xylocaine 2% Viscous Solution should be used with extreme caution if the mucosa in the area of application has been traumatized, since under such conditions there is the potential for rapid systemic absorption.

PRECAUTIONS

General: The safety and effectiveness of lidocaine depend on proper dosage, correct technique, adequate precautions, and readiness for emergencies (See WARNINGS and ADVERSE REACTIONS). The lowest dosage that results in effective anesthesia should be used to avoid high plasma levels and serious adverse effects. Repeated doses of lidocaine may cause significant increases in blood levels with each repeated dose because of slow accumulation of the drug and/or its metabolites. Tolerance varies with the status of the patient. Debilitated, elderly patients, acutely ill patients, and children should be given reduced doses commensurate with their age, weight and physical condition. Lidocaine should also be used with caution in patients with severe shock or heart block.

Xylocaine 2% Viscous Solution should be used with caution in persons with known drug sensitivities. Patients allergic to para-aminobenzoic acid derivatives (procaine, tetracaine, benzocaine, etc.) have not shown cross sensitivity to lidocaine.

Information for Patients: When topical anesthetics are used in the mouth or throat, the patient should be aware that the production of topical anesthesia may impair swallowing and thus enhance the danger of aspiration. For this reason, food should not be ingested for 60 minutes following use of local anesthetic preparations in the mouth or throat area. This is particularly important in children because of their frequency of eating.

Numbness of the tongue or buccal mucosa may increase the danger of biting trauma. For this reason food and/or chewing gum should not be used while the mouth or throat area is anesthetized.

PATIENTS SHOULD BE INSTRUCTED TO STRICTLY ADHERE TO DOSING INSTRUCTIONS, AND TO KEEP THE SUPPLY OF MEDICATION OUT OF THE REACH OF CHILDREN.

Carcinogenesis, mutagenesis, impairment of fertility: Studies of lidocaine in animals to evaluate the carcinogenic and mutagenic potential or the effect on fertility have not been conducted.

Pregnancy: Teratogenic Effects. Pregnancy Category B. Reproduction studies have been performed in rats at doses up to 6.6 times the human dose and have revealed no evidence of harm to the fetus caused by lidocaine. There are, however, no adequate and well-controlled studies in pregnant women. Because animal reproduction studies are not always predictive of human response, this drug should be used in pregnancy only if clearly needed.

Nursing mothers: It is not known whether this drug is excreted in human milk. Because many drugs are excreted in human milk, caution should be exercised when lidocaine is administered to nursing women.

Pediatric use: Dosages in children should be reduced, commensurate with age, body weight and physical condition. See DOSAGE AND ADMINISTRATION.

ADVERSE REACTIONS

Adverse experiences following the adminstration of lidocaine are similar in nature to those observed with other amide local anesthetic agents. These adverse experiences are, in general, dose-related and may result from high plasma levels caused by excessive dosage or rapid absorption, or may result from a hypersensitivity, idiosyncrasy or diminished tolerance on the part of the patient. Serious adverse experiences are generally systemic in nature. The following types are those most commonly reported:

Central nervous system: CNS manifestations are excitatory and/or depressant and may be characterized by lightheadedness, nervousness, apprehension, euphoria, confusion, dizziness, drowsiness, tinnitus, blurred or double vision, vomiting, sensations of heat, cold or numbness, twitching, tremors, convulsions, unconsciousness, respiratory depression and arrest. The excitatory manifestations may be very brief or may not occur at all, in which case the first manifestation of toxicity may be drowsiness merging into unconsciousness and respiratory arrest.

Drowsiness following the administration of lidocaine is usually an early sign of a high blood level of the drug and may occur as a consequence of rapid absorption.

Cardiovascular system: Cardiovascular manifestations are usually depressant and are characterized by bradycardia, hypotension, and cardiovascular collapse, which may lead to cardiac arrest.

Allergic: Allergic reactions are characterized by cutaneous lesions, urticaria, edema or anaphylactoid reactions. Allergic reactions may occur as a result of sensitivity either to the local anesthetic agent or to the methylparaben and/or propylparaben used in this formulation. Allergic reactions as a result of sensitivity to lidocaine are extremely rare and, if they occur, should be managed by conventional means. The detection of sensitivity by skin testing is of doubtful value.

OVERDOSAGE

Acute emergencies from local anesthetics are generally related to high plasma levels encountered during therapeutic use of local anesthetics (see ADVERSE REACTIONS, WARNINGS, and PRECAUTIONS).

Management of local anesthetic emergencies: The first consideration is prevention, best accomplished by careful and constant monitoring of cardiovascular and respiratory vital signs and the patient's state of consciousness after each local anesthetic administration.

The first step in the management of convulsions consists of immediate attention to the maintenance of a patent airway and assisted or controlled ventilation with oxygen. In situations where trained personnel are readily available, ventilation should be maintained and oxygen should be delivered by a delivery system capable of permitting immediate positive airway pressure by mask. Immediately after the institution of these ventilatory measures, the adequacy of the circulation should be evaluated, keeping in mind that drugs used to treat convulsions sometimes depress the circulation when administered intravenously. Should convulsions persist despite adequate respiratory support, and if the status of the circulation permits, small increments of an ultra-short acting barbiturate (such as thiopental or thiamylal) or a benzodiazepine (such as diazepam) may be administered intravenously. The clinician should be familiar, prior to use of local anesthetics, with these anticonvulsant drugs. Supportive treatment of circulatory depression may require administration of intravenous fluids and, when appropriate, a vasopressor as indicated by the clinical situation (e.g., ephedrine).

If not treated immediately, both convulsions and cardiovascular depression can result in hypoxia, acidosis, bradycardia, arrhythmias and cardiac arrest. If cardiac arrest should occur, standard cardiopulmonary resuscitative measures should be instituted.

Dialysis is of negligible value in the treatment of acute overdosage with lidocaine.

The oral LD_{50} of lidocaine in non-fasted female rats is 459 (346–773) mg/kg (as the salt) and 214 (159–324) mg/kg (as the salt) in fasted female rats.

DOSAGE AND ADMINISTRATION

Adult

The maximum recommended single dose of Xylocaine (lidocaine HCl) 2% Viscous Solution for healthy adults should be such that the dose of lidocaine HCl does not exceed 4.5 mg/kg or 2 mg/lb body weight and does not in any case exceed a total of 300 mg.

For symptomatic treatment of irritated or inflamed mucous membranes of the mouth and pharynx, the usual adult dose is one 15 mL tablespoonful undiluted. For use in the mouth, the solution should be swished around in the mouth and spit out. For use on the pharynx, the undiluted solution should be gargled and may be swallowed. This dose should not be administered at intervals of less than three hours, and not more than eight doses should be given in a 24-hour period. The dosage should be adjusted commensurate with the patient's age, weight and physical condition (see PRECAUTIONS).

Pediatric

It is difficult to recommend a maximum dose of any drug for children since this varies as function of age and weight. For children over 3 years of age who have a normal lean body mass and normal body development, the maximum dose is determined by the child's weight or age. For example: in a child of 5 years weighing 50 lbs., the dose of lidocaine hydrochloride should not exceed 75–100 mg (¾ to 1 teaspoonful). For infants and in children under 3 years of age, ¼ teaspoon of the solution should be accurately measured and applied to the immediate area with a cotton-tipped applicator. This dose should not be administered at intervals of less than three hours. Not more than four doses should be given in a 12-hour period.

HOW SUPPLIED

Xylocaine 2% (lidocaine HCl) Viscous Solution is available in 100 mL (NDC 0186-0360-01) and 450 mL (NDC 0186-0360-11) polyethylene squeeze bottles and in unit of use (adult dose) packages of 25 (20 mL) polyethylene bottles (NDC 0186-0361-78).

The solutions should be stored at controlled room temperature 15°–30°C (59°–86°F).

021899R00   Iss. 1/88

YUTOPAR®   ℞

[yoū 'tow-par]
(ritodrine hydrochloride)
Sterile Solution and Tablets

CAUTION: Federal law prohibits dispensing without prescription.

DESCRIPTION

Yutopar, which contains the betamimetic (beta sympathomimetic amine) ritodrine hydrochloride, is available in two dosage forms. Yutopar for parenteral (intravenous) use is a clear, colorless, sterile, aqueous solution; each milliliter contains either 10 mg. or 15 mg. of ritodrine hydrochloride, 0.44% (w/v) of acetic acid, 0.24% (w/v) sodium hydroxide, 0.1% (w/v) of sodium metabisulfite, and 0.29% (w/v) of sodium chloride in water for injection USP. Hydrochloric acid or additional sodium hydroxide is used to adjust pH. **FOR INTRAVENOUS USE ONLY. MUST BE DILUTED BEFORE USE. FOR DOSAGE AND ADMINISTRATION INSTRUCTIONS, SEE PRODUCT INFORMATION BELOW. DO NOT USE IF SOLUTION IS DISCOLORED OR CONTAINS A PRECIPITATE.**

Each Yutopar tablet contains 10 mg. of ritodrine hydrochloride and the following inactive ingredients (in alphabetical order): corn starch, iron oxide yellow synthetic, lactose, magnesium stearate, povidone, and talc.

Ritodrine hydrochloride is a white, odorless crystalline powder, freely soluble in water, with a melting point between 196° and 205°C. The chemical name of ritodrine hydrochloride is erythro-p-hydroxy-α-[1[(p-hydroxyphenethyl)amino]ethyl]benzyl alcohol hydrochloride and has the chemical structure:

CLINICAL PHARMACOLOGY

Yutopar (ritodrine hydrochloride) is a beta-receptor agonist, which has been shown by *in vitro* and *in vivo* pharmacologic studies in animals to exert a preferential effect on the β_2 adrenergic receptors such as those in the uterine smooth muscle. Stimulation of the β_2 receptors inhibits contractility of the uterine smooth muscle.

In humans, intravenous infusions of 0.05 to 0.30 mg/min. or single oral doses of 10 to 20 mg. decreased the intensity and

frequency of uterine contractions. These effects were antagonized by beta-blocking compounds. Intravenous administration induced an immediate dose-related elevation of heart rate with maximum mean increases between 19 and 40 beats per minute. Widening of the pulse pressure was also observed; the average increase in systolic blood pressure was 4.0 mm. Hg, and the average decrease in diastolic pressure was 12.3 mm. Hg. With oran intake, the increase in heart rate was mild and delayed.

During intravenous infusion in humans, transient elevations of blood glucose, insulin, and free fatty acids have been observed. Decreased serum potassium has also been found, but effects on other electrolytes have not been reported.

Serum kinetics in humans (non-pregnant females) of an intravenous infusion of 60 minutes duration were determined by measuring serum ritodrine levels by a radioimmunoassay technique. The distribution half-life was found to be 6 to 9 minutes, and the effective half-life 1.7 to 2.6 hours. In a study of serum kinetics after oral ingestion (male subjects), the decline of serum drug levels could be described in terms of a two-phase decay with an initial half-life of 1.3 hours and a final half-life of 12 hours. With either route of administration, 90% of the excretion was completed within 24 hours after the dose.

Comparison of ritodrine serum levels after intravenous administration with those after oral dosage indicates the oral bioavailability is about 30%. Intravenous infusion at a rate of 0.15 mg./min. for 1 hour yielded maximum serum levels ranging between 32 and 52 ng./mL in a group of 6 non-pregnant female volunteers; maximum serum levels following single and repeated (4 × 10 mg./24 hr.) 10 mg. oral doses ranged between 5 and 15 ng./mL and were obtained within 30 to 60 minutes after ingestion.

Placental transfer was confirmed by measurement of drug concentrations in cord blood showing that ritodrine and its conjugates reach the fetal circulation.

INDICATIONS AND USAGE

Yutopar is indicated for the management of preterm labor in suitable patients.

Administered intravenously, the drug will decrease uterine activity and thus prolong gestation in the majority of such patients. After intravenous Yutopar has arrested the acute episode, oral administration may help to avert relapse. Additional acute episodes may be treated by repeating the intravenous infusion. The incidence of neonatal mortality and respiratory distress syndrome increases when the normal gestation period is shortened.

Since successful inhibition of labor is more likely with early treatment, therapy with Yutopar should be instituted as soon as the diagnosis of preterm labor is established and contraindications ruled out in pregnancies of 20 or more weeks' gestation. The efficacy and safety of Yutopar in advanced labor, that is, when cervical dilatation is more than 4 cm. or effacement is more than 80%, have not been established.

CONTRAINDICATIONS

Yutopar is contraindicated before the 20th week of pregnancy.

Yutopar is also contraindicated in those conditions of the mother or fetus in which continuation of pregnancy is hazardous; specific contraindications include:

1. Antepartum hemorrhage which demands immediate delivery
2. Eclampsia and severe preeclampsia
3. Intrauterine fetal death
4. Chorioamnionitis
5. Maternal cardiac disease
6. Pulmonary hypertension
7. Maternal hyperthyroidism
8. Uncontrolled maternal diabetes mellitus (See PRECAUTIONS.)
9. Pre-existing maternal medical conditions that would be seriously affected by the known pharmacologic properties of a betamimetic drug; such as: hypovolemia, cardiac arrhythmias associated with tachycardia or digitalis intoxication, uncontrolled hypertension, pheochromocytoma, bronchial asthma already treated by betamimetics and/or steroids
10. Known hypersensitivity to any component of the product

WARNINGS

Maternal pulmonary edema has been reported in patients treated with Yutopar, sometimes after delivery. It has occurred more often when patients were treated concomitantly with corticosteroids. Maternal death from this condition has been reported with or without corticosteroids given concomitantly with drugs of this class.

Patients so treated must be closely monitored in the hospital. The patient's state of hydration should be carefully monitored; fluid overload must be avoided. (See

Continued on next page

Astra—Cont.

DOSAGE AND ADMINISTRATION.) Intravenous fluid loading may be aggravated by the use of betamimetics with or without corticosteroids and may turn into manifest circulatory overloading with subsequent pulmonary edema. If pulmonary edema develops during administration, the drug should be discontinued. Edema should be managed by conventional means.

Intravenous administration of Yutopar should be supervised by persons having knowledge of the pharmacology of the drug and who are qualified to identify and manage complications of drug administration and pregnancy. Beta-adrenergic drugs increase cardiac output, and even in a normal healthy heart this added myocardial oxygen demand can sometimes lead to myocardial ischemia. Complications may include: myocardial necrosis, which may result in death; arrhythmias, including premature atrial and ventricular contractions, ventricular tachycardia, and bundle branch block; anginal pain, with or without ECG changes. *Because cardiovascular responses are common and more pronounced during intravenous administration of Yutopar, cardiovascular effects, including maternal pulse rate and blood pressure and fetal heart rate, should be closely monitored. Care should be exercised for maternal signs and symptoms of pulmonary edema. A persistent high tachycardia (over 140 beats per minute) may be one of the signs of impending pulmonary edema with drugs of this class. Occult cardiac disease may be unmasked with the use of Yutopar. If the patient complains of chest pain or tightness of chest, the drug should be temporarily discontinued and an ECG should be done as soon as possible.* The drug should not be administered to patients with mild to moderate preeclampsia, hypertension, or diabetes unless the attending physician considers that the benefits clearly outweigh the risks.

Yutopar Solution contains sodium metabisulfite, a sulfite that may cause serious allergic-type reactions including anaphylactic symptoms and life-threatening or less severe asthmatic episodes in certain susceptible people. The overall prevalence of sulfite sensitivity in the general population is unknown and probably low. Sulfite sensitivity is seen more frequently in asthmatic than in nonasthmatic people.

PRECAUTIONS

When Yutopar is used for the management of preterm labor in a patient with premature rupture of the membranes, the benefits of delaying delivery should be balanced against the potential risks of development of chorioamnionitis.

Among low birth weight infants, approximately 9% may be growth retarded for gestational age. Therefore, Intra-Uterine Growth Retardation (IUGR) should be considered in the differential diagnosis of preterm labor; this is especially important when the gestational age is in doubt. The decision to continue or reinitiate the administration of Yutopar will depend on an assessment of fetal maturity. In addition to clinical parameters, other studies, such as sonography or amniocentesis, may be helpful in establishing the state of fetal maturity if it is in doubt.

Baseline EKG
This should be done to rule out occult maternal heart disease.

Laboratory Tests
Because intravenous administration of Yutopar has been shown to elevate plasma insulin and glucose and to decrease plasma potassium concentrations, monitoring of glucose and electrolyte levels is recommended during protracted infusions. Decrease of plasma potassium concentrations is usually transient, returning to normal within 24 hours. Special attention should be paid to biochemical variables when treating diabetic patients or those receiving potassium-depleting diuretics.
Serial hemograms may be helpful as an index of state of hydration.

Drug Interactions
Corticosteroids used concomitantly may lead to pulmonary edema. (See Warnings.)
Cardiovascular effects of Yutopar solution (especially cardiac arrhythmia or hypotension) may be potentiated by concomitant use of the following drugs.
1. magnesium sulfate
2. diazoxide
3. meperidine
4. potent general anesthetic agents
Systemic hypertension may be exaggerated in the presence of parasympatholytic agents such as atropine.
The effects of other sympathomimetic amines may be potentiated when concurrently administered and these effects may be additive. A sufficient time interval should elapse prior to administration of another sympathomimetic drug. With either oral or intravenous administration, 90% of the excretion of Yutopar is completed within 24 hours after the dose.

(See CLINICAL PHARMACOLOGY.)
Beta-adrenergic blocking drugs inhibit the action of Yutopar; coadministration of these drugs should, therefore, be avoided.
With anesthetics used in surgery, the possibility that hypotensive effects may be potentiated should be considered.
Migraine Headache
Transient cerebral ischemia associated with beta sympathomimetic therapy has been reported in two patients with migraine headache.
Carcinogenesis, Mutagenesis, Impairment of Fertility
In rats given oral doses of 1, 10 and 150 mg./kg./day of ritodrine hydrochloride for 82 weeks, benign and malignant tumors were found in the various dosage groups. Since there were no important differences between untreated controls and treated groups and no dose-related trends, it was concluded that there was no evidence of tumorigenicity. The incidence (2–4%) of tumors of the type found in this study is not unusual in this species.
Reproduction studies in rats and rabbits have revealed no evidence of impaired fertility due to ritodrine hydrochloride.
Pregnancy
Teratogenic Effects
(Pregnancy Category B)
Reproduction studies were performed in rats and rabbits. The doses employed intravenously were $\frac{1}{9}$ (1 mg./kg.), $\frac{1}{3}$ (3 mg./kg.), and 1 (9 mg./kg.) times the maximum human daily intravenous dose (but given to the animals as a bolus rather than by infusion). The oral doses, 10 and 100 mg./kg. represented 5 and 50 times the maximum human daily oral maintenance dose. The results of these studies have revealed no evidence of impaired fertility or harm to the fetus due to ritodrine hydrochloride.
No adverse fetal effects were encountered when single intravenous doses of 1, 3, and 9 mg./kg./day or oral doses of 10 and 100 mg./kg./day were given to rats and rabbits on Days 6 through 15 and 6 through 18 of gestation, respectively. Intravenous doses of 1 and 8 mg./kg./day or oral doses of 10 and 100 mg./kg./day administered to the mother from Day 15 of pregnancy to Day 21 postpartum did not affect perinatal or postnatal development in rats. A slight increase in fetal weight in the rat was observed. Oral administration to both sexes did not impair fertility or reproductive performance. Lethal doses to pregnant rats did not cause immediate fetal demise. There are no adequate and well-controlled studies of Yutopar effects in pregnant women before 20 weeks' gestation; *therefore, this drug should not be used before the 20th week of pregnancy.* Studies of Yutopar administered to pregnant women from the 20th week of gestation have not shown increased risk of fetal abnormalities. Follow-up of selected variables in a small number of children for up to 2 years has not revealed harmful effects on growth, developmental or functional maturation. Nonetheless, although clinical studies did not demonstrate a risk of permanent adverse fetal effects from Yutopar, the possibility cannot be excluded; therefore, Yutopar should be used only when clearly indicated.
Some studies indicate that infants born before 36 weeks' gestation make up less than 10% of all births but account for as many as 75% of perinatal deaths and one-half of all neurologically handicapped infants. There are data available indicating that infants born at any time prior to full term may manifest a higher incidence of neurologic or other handicaps than occurs in the total population of infants born at or after full term. In delaying or preventing preterm labor, the use of Yutopar should result in an overall increase in neonatal survival. Handicapped infants who might not have otherwise survived may survive.

ADVERSE REACTIONS

The unwanted effects of Yutopar are related to its betamimetic activity and usually are controlled by suitable dosage adjustment.
Effects Associated with Intravenous Administration
Usual effects (80–100% of patients)
Intravenous infusion of Yutopar leads almost invariably to dose-related alterations in maternal and fetal heart rates and in maternal blood pressure. During clinical studies in which the maximum infusion rate was limited to 0.35 mg./min. (one patient received 0.40 mg./min.), the maximum maternal and fetal heart rates averaged, respectively, 130 (range 60 to 180) and 164 (range 130 to 200) beats per minute. The maximum maternal systolic blood pressures averaged 128 mm. Hg (range 96 to 162 mm. Hg), an average increase of 12 mm. Hg from pretreatment levels. The minimum maternal diastolic blood pressures averaged 48 mm. Hg (range 0 to 76 mm. Hg), an average decrease of 23 mm. Hg from pretreatment levels. While the more severe effects were usually managed effectively by dosage adjustments, in less than 1% of patients, persistent maternal tachycardia or decreased diastolic blood pressure required withdrawal of the drug. A persistent high tachycardia (over 140 beats per minute) may be one of the signs of impending pulmonary edema. (See WARNINGS.)
Yutopar infusion is associated with transient elevation of blood glucose and insulin, which decreases toward normal

values after 48 to 72 hours despite continued infusion. Elevation of free fatty acids and cAMP has been reported. Reduction of potassium levels should be expected; other biochemical effects have not been reported.
Frequent effects (10–50% of patients)
Intravenous Yutopar, in about one-third of the patients, was associated with palpitation. Tremor, nausea, vomiting, headache, or erythema was observed in 10 to 15% of patients.
Occasional effects (5–10% of patients)
Nervousness, jitteriness, restlessness, emotional upset, or anxiety was reported in 5 to 6% of patients and malaise in similar numbers.
Infrequent effects (1–3% of patients)
Cardiac symptoms including chest pain or tightness (rarely associated with abnormalities of ECG) and arrhythmia were reported in 1 to 2% of patients. (See Warnings.)
Other infrequently reported maternal effects included: anaphylactic shock, rash, heart murmur, epigastric distress, ileus, bloating, constipation, diarrhea, dyspnea, hyperventilation, hemolytic icterus, glycosuria, lactic acidosis, sweating, chills, drowsiness, and weakness. Impaired liver function (i.e., increased transaminase levels and hepatitis) have also been reported infrequently (less than 1%) with the use of ritodrine and other beta sympathomimetics.
Neonatal Effects
Infrequently reported neonatal symptoms include hypoglycemia and ileus. In addition, hypocalcemia and hypotension have been reported in neonates whose mothers were treated with other betamimetic agents.
Effects Associated with Oral Administration
Frequent effects (< 50% of patients)
Oral ritodrine in clinical studies was often associated with small increases in maternal heart rate, but little or no effect upon either maternal systolic or diastolic blood pressure or upon fetal heart rate was found.
Oral ritodrine in 10 to 15% of patients was associated with palpitation or tremor. Nausea and jitterness were less frequent (5 to 8%), while rash was observed in some patients (3 to 4%), and arrhythmia was infrequent (about 1%). Impaired liver function (i.e., increased transaminase levels and hepatitis) have also been reported infrequently (less than 1%) with the use of ritodrine and other beta sympathomimetics.

OVERDOSAGE

The symptoms of overdosage are those of excessive beta-adrenergic stimulation including exaggeration of the known pharmacologic effects, the most prominent being tachycardia (maternal and fetal), palpitation, cardiac arrhythmia, hypotension, dyspnea, nervousness, tremor, nausea, and vomiting. If an excess of ritodrine tablets is ingested, gastric lavage or induction of emesis should be carried out followed by administration of activated charcoal. When symptoms of overdose occur as a result of intravenous administration, ritodrine should be discontinued; an appropriate beta-blocking agent may be used as an antidote. Ritodrine hydrochloride is dialyzable.
Acute intravenous toxicity was studied in rats and rabbits and acute oral toxicity in mice, rats, guinea pigs, and dogs. The LD50 values in the most sensitive of the species used were 64 mg./kg. intravenously in the nonpregnant rabbit and 540 mg./kg. orally in the nonpregnant mouse. The intravenous LD50 value in the pregnant rat was 85 mg./kg. The amount of drug required to produce symptoms of overdose in humans is individually variable. No reports of human mortality due to overdose have been received.

DOSAGE AND ADMINISTRATION

In the management of preterm labor, the initial intravenous treatment should usually be followed by oral administration. The optimum dose of Yutopar is determined by a clinical balance of uterine response and unwanted effects.
Intravenous Therapy
Do not use intravenous Yutopar if the solution is discolored or contains any precipitate or particulate matter. Yutopar solution should be used promptly after preparation, but in no case after 48 hours of preparation.
Method of Administration: To minimize the risks of hypotension, the patient should be maintained in the left lateral position throughout infusion and careful attention given to her state of hydration, but fluid overload must be avoided. For appropriate control and dose titration, a controlled infusion device is recommended to adjust the rate of flow in drops/minute. An i.v. microdrip chamber (60 drops/mL) can provide a convenient range of infusion rates within the recommended dose range for Yutopar.
Recommended Dilution: 150 mg. ritodrine hydrochloride in 500 mL fluid yielding a final concentration of 0.3 mg/mL*. Ritodrine for intravenous infusion should be diluted with 5% w/v dextrose solution. Because of the increased probability of pulmonary edema, saline diluents such as:
—0.9% w/v sodium chloride solution,
—compound sodium chloride solution (Ringer's solution)
—and Hartmann's solution, should be reserved for cases where dextrose solution is medically undesirable e.g. diabetes mellitus.

* In those cases where fluid restriction is medically desirable, a more concentrated solution may be prepared.

Intravenous therapy should be started as soon as possible after diagnosis. The usual initial dose is 0.1 mg./minute (0.33 mL/min., 20 drops/min. using a microdrip chamber at the recommended dilution), to be gradually increased according to the results by 0.05 mg./minute (0.17 mL/min., 10 drops/min. using a microdrip chamber at the recommended dilution) every 10 minutes until the desired result is attained. The effective dosage usually lies between 0.15 and 0.35 mg./minute (0.50 to 1.17 mL/min., 30–70 drops/min. using a microdrip chamber at the recommended dilution). Frequent monitoring of maternal uterine contractions, heart rate, and blood pressure, and of fetal heart rate is required, with dosage individually titrated according to response. If other drugs need to be given intravenously, the use of "piggyback" or other site of intravenous administration permits the continued independent control of the rate of infusion of the Yutopar.

The infusion should generally be continued for at least 12 hours after uterine contractions cease. With the recommended dilution, the maximum volume of fluid that might be administered after 12 hours at the highest dose (0.35 mg./min.) will be approximately 840 mL.

The amount of i.v. fluids administered and the rate of administration should be monitored to avoid circulatory fluid overload (over-hydration). (See PRECAUTIONS, Laboratory Tests.)

Oral Maintenance
One tablet (10 mg.) may be given approximately 30 minutes before the termination of intravenous therapy. The usual dosage schedule for the first 24 hours of oral administration is 1 tablet (10 mg.) every two hours. Thereafter, the usual maintenance is 1 or 2 tablets (10 to 20 mg.) every four to six hours, the dose depending on uterine activity and unwanted effects. The total daily dose of oral ritodrine should not exceed 120 mg. The treatment may be continued as long as the physician considers it desirable to prolong pregnancy.

Recurrence of unwanted preterm labor may be treated with repeated infusion of Yutopar.

HOW SUPPLIED
NDC 0186-0569-13: 5 mL vial in boxes of 10. Each vial contains 50 mg (10 mg/mL) of ritodrine hydrochloride.
NDC 0186-0599-03: 5 mL ampuls in boxes of 10. Each ampul contains 50 mg (10 mg/mL) of ritodrine hydrochloride.
NDC 0186-0597-12: 10 mL vial in boxes of 6. Each vial contains 150 mg (15 mg/mL) of ritodrine hydrochloride.
NDC 0186-0595-60: 10 mg tablets in bottles of 60. Each round, yellow tablet contains 10 mg ritodrine hydrochloride and is inscribed YUTOPAR on one side and scored on the other.
NDC 0186-0595-78: 10 mg unit dose tablets in boxes of 100. Each round, yellow tablet contains 10 mg ritodrine hydrochloride and is inscribed YUTOPAR on one side and scored on the other.
NDC 0186-0644-01: 10 mL syringe in boxes of 10. Each syringe contains 150 mg (15 mg/mL) of ritodrine hydrochloride.

Both the tablet and intravenous dosage forms should be stored at room temperature, preferably below 86°F. (30°C). Protect from excessive heat.

Oral dosage form manufactured by DUPHAR B.V., Amsterdam, Holland for
ASTRA®
Astra Pharmaceuticals Products, Inc.
Westborough MA 01581
Yutopar® licensed by Duphar B. V. Amsterdam, Holland
021843R06   Rev. 7/87(6)

For information on Astra products, write to:
Professional Information Dept.
Astra Pharmaceutical Products, Inc.
50 Otis Street
Westborough Massachusetts 01581-4428

IDENTIFICATION PROBLEM?
Consult PDR's
Product Identification Section
where you'll find over 1700
products pictured actual size
and in full color.

Ayerst Laboratories
Division of American Home
Products Corporation
685 THIRD AVE.
NEW YORK, NY 10017-4071

As a result of a merger of Wyeth Laboratories and Ayerst Laboratories, all prescription products of both companies and all nonprescription products of Wyeth are now products of Wyeth-Ayerst Laboratories.

All of Ayerst's consumer products are now products of Whitehall Laboratories.

Baker Cummins
Pharmaceuticals, Inc.
8800 N. W. 36TH STREET
MIAMI, FL 33178

DORAL™   ℂ
brand of quazepam
Tablets

DESCRIPTION
DORAL (brand of quazepam) Tablets contain quazepam, a trifluoroethyl benzodiazepine hypnotic agent, having the chemical name 7-chloro-5-(o-fluorophenyl)-1,3-dihydro-1-(2,2,2-trifluoroethyl)-2H -1,4-benzodiazepine-2-thione and the following structural formula:

Quazepam has the empirical formula $C_{17}H_{11}ClF_4N_2S$, and a molecular weight of 386.8. It is a white crystalline compound, soluble in ethanol and insoluble in water.

Each DORAL Tablet contains either 7.5 or 15 mg of quazepam.

The inactive ingredients for DORAL Tablets 7.5 or 15 mg include cellulose, corn starch, FD&C Yellow No. 6 A1 Lake, lactose, magnesium stearate, silicon dioxide, and sodium lauryl sulfate.

CLINICAL PHARMACOLOGY
Central nervous system agents of the 1,4-benzodiazepine class presumably exert their effects by binding to stereospecific receptors at several sites within the central nervous system (CNS). Their exact mechanism of action is unknown.

In a sleep laboratory study, DORAL Tablets significantly decreased sleep latency and total wake time, and significantly increased total sleep time and percent sleep time, for one or more nights. Quazepam 15 mg was effective on the first night of administration. Sleep latency, total wake time and wake time after sleep onset were still decreased and percent sleep time was still increased for several nights after the drug was discontinued. Percent slow wave sleep was decreased, and REM sleep was essentially unchanged. No transient sleep disturbance, such as "rebound insomnia", was observed after withdrawal of the drug in sleep laboratory studies in 12 patients using 15 mg doses.

In outpatient studies, DORAL Tablets improved all subjective measures of sleep including sleep induction time, duration of sleep, number of nocturnal awakenings, occurrences of early morning awakening, and sleep quality. Some effects were evident on the first night of administration of DORAL Tablets (sleep induction time, number of nocturnal awakenings, and duration of sleep). Residual medication effects ("hangover") were minimal.

Quazepam is rapidly (absorption half-life of about 30 minutes) and well absorbed from the gastrointestinal tract. The peak plasma concentration of quazepam is approximately 20 ng/ml after a 15 mg dose and is obtained at about 2 hours. Quazepam, the active parent compound, is extensively metabolized in the liver; two of the plasma metabolites are 2-oxoquazepam and N-desalkyl-2-oxoquazepam. All three compounds show pharmacological central nervous system activity in animals.

Following administration of ^{14}C-quazepam, approximately 31% of the dose appears in the urine and 23% in the feces over a five-day period; only trace amounts of unchanged drug are present in the urine.

The mean elimination half-life of quazepam and 2-oxoquazepam is 39 hours and that of N-desalkyl-2-oxoquazepam is 73 hours. Steady-state levels of quazepam and 2-oxoquazepam are attained by the seventh daily dose

and that of N-desalkyl-2-oxoquazepam by the thirteenth daily dose.

The pharmacokinetics of quazepam and 2-oxoquazepam in geriatric subjects are comparable to those seen in young adults; as with desalkyl metabolites of other benzodiazepines, the elimination half-life of N-desalkyl-2-oxoquazepam in geriatric patients is about twice that of young adults.

The degree of plasma protein binding for quazepam and its two major metabolites is greater than 95%. The absorption, distribution, metabolism, and excretion of benzodiazepines may be altered in various disease states including alcoholism, impaired hepatic function, and impaired renal function.

The type and duration of hypnotic effects and the profile of unwanted effects during administration of benzodiazepine drugs may be influenced by the biologic half-life of administered drug and any active metabolites formed. When half-lives are long, drug or metabolites may accumulate during periods of nightly administration and be associated with impairments of cognitive and or motor performance during waking hours; the possibility of interaction with other psychoactive drugs or alcohol will be enhanced. In contrast, if half-lives are short, drug and metabolites will be cleared before the next dose is ingested, and carryover effects related to excessive sedation or CNS depression should be minimal or absent. However, during nightly use for an extended period, pharmacodynamic tolerance or adaptation to some effects of benzodiazepine hypnotics may develop. If the drug has a short half-life of elimination, it is possible that a relative deficiency of the drug or its active metabolites (i.e., in relationship to the receptor site) may occur at some point in the interval between each night's use. This sequence of events may account for two clinical findings reported to occur after several weeks of nightly use of rapidly eliminated benzodiazepine hypnotics, namely, increased wakefulness during the last third of the night, and the appearance of increased signs of daytime anxiety in selected patients.

Quazepam crosses the placental barrier of mice. Quazepam, 2-oxoquazepam and N-desalkyl-2-oxoquazepam are present in breast milk of lactating women, but the total amount found in the milk represents only about 0.1% of the administered dose.

INDICATIONS AND USAGE
DORAL Tablets are indicated for the treatment of insomnia characterized by difficulty in falling asleep, frequent nocturnal awakenings, and/or early morning awakenings. The effectiveness of DORAL has been established in placebo-controlled clinical studies of 5 nights duration in acute and chronic insomnia. The sustained effectiveness of DORAL has been established in chronic insomnia in a sleep lab (polysomnographic) study of 28 nights duration.

Because insomnia is often transient and intermittent, the prolonged administration of DORAL Tablets is generally not necessary or recommended. Since insomnia may be a symptom of several other disorders, the possibility that the complaint may be related to a condition for which there is a more specific treatment should be considered.

CONTRAINDICATIONS
DORAL Tablets are contraindicated in patients with known hypersensitivity to this drug or other benzodiazepines, and in patients with established or suspected sleep apnea.

Usage in Pregnancy: Benzodiazepines may cause fetal damage when administered during pregnancy. An increased risk of congenital malformations associated with the use of diazepam and chlordiazepoxide during the first trimester of pregnancy has been suggested in several studies. Transplacental distribution has resulted in neonatal CNS depression following ingestion of therapeutic doses of a benzodiazepine hypnotic during the last weeks of pregnancy.

DORAL Tablets are contraindicated in pregnancy because the potential risks outweigh the possible advantages of their use during this period. If there is a likelihood of the patient becoming pregnant while receiving DORAL she should be warned of the potential risk to the fetus. Patients should be instructed to discontinue the drug prior to becoming pregnant. The possibility that a woman of childbearing potential may be pregnant at the time of institution of therapy should be considered (See **Teratogenic Effects: Pregnancy Category X.**)

WARNINGS
Patients receiving benzodiazepines should be cautioned about possible combined effects with alcohol and other CNS depressants. Also, caution patients that an additive effect may occur if alcoholic beverages are consumed during the day following the use of benzodiazepines for nighttime sedation. The potential for this interaction continues for several days following their discontinuance until serum levels of psychoactive metabolites have declined.

Patients should also be cautioned about engaging in hazardous occupations requiring complete mental alertness such as operating machinery or driving a motor vehicle, after ingesting benzodiazepines, including potential impairment of the

Continued on next page

Baker Cummins—Cont.

performance of such activities which may occur the day following ingestion.

Withdrawal symptoms of the type associated with sedatives/hypnotics (e.g., barbiturates, bromides, etc.) and alcohol have been reported after the discontinuation of benzodiazepines. While these symptoms have been more frequently reported after the discontinuation of excessive benzodiazepine doses, there have also been controlled studies demonstrating the occurrence of such symptoms after discontinuation of therapeutic doses of benzodiazepines, generally following prolonged use (but in some instances after periods as brief as six weeks). It is generally believed that the gradual reduction of dosage will diminish the occurrence of such symptoms (see **Drug Abuse and Dependence**).

PRECAUTIONS

General: Impaired motor and/or cognitive performance attributable to the accumulation of benzodiazepines and their active metabolites following several days of repeated use at their recommended doses is a concern in certain vulnerable patients (e.g., those especially sensitive to the effects of benzodiazepines or those with reduced capacity to metabolize and eliminte them). Consequently, elderly or debilitated patients and those with impaired renal or hepatic function should be cautioned about the risk and advised to monitor themselves for signs of excessive sedation or impaired coordination.

The possibility of respiratory depression in patients with chronic pulmonary insufficiency should be considered.

When benzodiazepines are administered to depressed patients, there is a risk that the signs or symptoms of depression may be intensified. Consequently, appropriate precautions (e.g., limiting the total prescription size and increased monitoring for suicidal ideation) should be considered.

Information for Patients It is suggested that physicians discuss the following information with patients. This information is intended to aid in the safe and effective use of this medication. It is not a disclosure of all possible adverse or intended effects.

1. Inform your physician about any alcohol consumption and medicine your are taking now, including drugs you may buy without a prescription. Alcohol should generally not be used during treatment with hypnotics.
2. Inform your physician if you are planning to become pregnant, if you are pregnant, or if you become pregnant while you are taking this medicine.
3. Inform your physician if you are nursing.
4. Until you experience how this medicine affects you, do not drive a car or operate potentially dangerous machinery, etc.
5. Benzodiazepines may cause daytime sedation, which may persist for several days following drug discontinuation.
6. Patients should be told not to increase the dose on their own and should inform their physician if they believe the drug "does not work anymore".
7. If benzodiazepines are taken on a prolonged and regular basis (even for periods as brief as six weeks), patients should be advised not to stop taking them abruptly or to decrease the dose without consulting their physician, because withdrawal symptoms may occur.

Laboratory Tests: Laboratory tests are not ordinarily required in otherwise healthy patients when quazepam is used as recommended.

Drug Interactions: The benzodiazepines, including DORAL Tablets, produce additive CNS depressant effects when coadministered with psychotropic medications, anticonvulsants, antihistamines, ethanol, and other drugs which produce CNS depression.

Carcinogenesis, Mutagenesis, Impairment of Fertility: Quazepam showed no evidence of carcinogenicity or other significant pathology in oral oncogenicity studies in mice and hamsters.

Quazepam was tested for mutagenicity using the L5178Y TK+, —Mouse Lymphoma Mutagenesis Assay and Ames Test. The L5178Y TK+,—Assay was equivocal and the Ames Test did not show mutagenic activity.

Reproduction studies in mice conducted with quazepam at doses equal to 60 and 180 times the human dose of 15 mg, and with diazepam at 67 times the human dose, produced slight reductions in the pregnancy rate. Similar reduction in pregnancy rates have been reported in mice dosed with other benzodiazepines, and is believed to be related to the sedative effects of these drugs at high doses.

Teratogenic Effects: Pregnancy Category X (See CONTRA-INDICATIONS, Usage in Pregnancy section.) Reproduction studies of quazepam in mice at doses up to 400 times the human dose revealed no major drug-related malformations. Minor developmental variations that occurred were delayed ossification of the sternum, vertebrae, distal phalanges and supraoccipital bones, at doses of 66 and 400 times the human dose. Studies with diazepam at 200 times the human dose showed a similar or greater incidence than quazepam. A reproduction study of quazepam in New Zealand rabbits at doses up to 134 times the human dose demonstrated no effect on fetal morphology or development of offspring.

Nonteratogenic Effects: The child born of a mother who is taking benzodiazepines may be at some risk of withdrawal symptoms from the drug during the postnatal period. Neonatal flaccidity has been reported in children born of mothers who had been receiving benzodiazepines.

Labor and Delivery: DORAL Tablets have no established use in labor or delivery.

Nursing Mothers: Quazepam and its metabolites are excreted in the milk of lactating women. Therefore, administration of DORAL Tablets to nursing women is not recommended.

Pediatric Use: Safety and effectiveness in children below the age of 18 years have not been established.

ADVERSE REACTIONS

Adverse events most frequently encountered in patients treated with quazepam are drowsiness and headache.

Accurate estimates of the incidence of adverse events asociated with the use of any drug are difficult to obtain. Estimates are influenced by drug dose, detection technique, setting, physician judgments, etc. Consequently, the table below is presented solely to indicate the relative frequency of adverse events reported in representative controlled clinical studies conducted to evaluate the safety and efficacy of quazepam. The figures cited cannot be used to predict precisely the incidence of such events in the course of usual medical practice. These figures, also, cannot be compared with those obtained from other clinical studies involving related drug products and placebo.

The figures cited below are estimates of untoward clinical event incidences of 1% or greater among subjects who participated in the relatively short duration placebo-controlled clinical trials of quazepam.

	DORAL (15 mg)	PLACEBO
NUMBER OF PATIENTS TREATED	267	268
% OF PATIENTS REPORTING		
Central Nervous System		
Daytime Drowsiness	12.0%	3.3%
Headache	4.5%	2.2%
Fatigue	1.9%	0
Dizziness	1.5%	<1%
Autonomic Nervous System		
Dry Mouth	1.5%	<1%
Gastrointestinal System		
Dyspepsia	1.1%	<1%

The following incidences of laboratory abnormalities occurred at a rate of 1% or greater in patients receiving quazepam and the corresponding placebo group. None of these changes were considered to be of physiological significance.

	DORAL		PLACEBO	
NUMBER OF PATIENTS	234		244	
% of Patients Reporting	Low	High	Low	High
Hematology				
Hemoglobin	1.4	0	1.2	0
Hematocrit	1.5	0	1.7	0
Lymphocyte	1.3	1.6	1.2	1.9
Eosinophil	*	1.5	*	1.3
SEG	1.1	*	1.6	*
Monocyte	*	1.1	*	*
Blood Chemistry				
Glucose	*	*	*	1.2
SGOT	*	1.3	*	1.1
Urinalysis				
Specific Gravity	*	*	*	1.1
WBC	0	2.6	0	3.0
RBC	0	*	0	1.1
Epithelial Cells	0	2.5	0	3.2
Crystals	0	*	0	1.0

* These laboratory abnormalities occurred in less than 1% of patients. In addition, abnormalities in the following laboratory tests were observed in less than 1% of the patients evaluated; WBC count, platelet count, total protein, albumin, BUN, creatinine, total bilirubin, alkaline phosphatase, and SGPT.

The following additional events occurred among individuals receiving quazepam at doses equivalent to or greater than those recommended during its clinical testing and development. There is no way to estabish whether or not the administration of DORAL caused these events.

Hypokinesia, ataxia, confusion, incoordination, hyperkinesia, speech disorder, and tremor were reported.

Also, depression, nervousness, agitation, amnesia, anorexia, anxiety, apathy, euphoria, impotence, decreased libido, paranoid reaction, nightmares, abnormal thinking, abnormal taste perception, abnormal vision, and cataract were reported.

Also reported were urinary incontinence, palpitations, nausea, constipation, diarrhea, abdominal pain, pruritus, rash, asthenia, and malaise.

The following list provides an overview of adverse experiences that have been reported and are considered to be reasonably related to the administration of benzodiazepines; incontinence, slurred speech, urinary retention, jaundice, dysarthria, dystonia, changes in libido, irritability, and menstrual irregularities.

As with all benzodiazepines, paradoxical reactions such as stimulation, agitation, increased muscle spasticity, sleep disturbances, hallucinations, and other adverse behavioral effects may occur in rare instances and in a random fashion. Should these occur,use of the drug should be discontinued.

There have been reports of withdrawal signs and symptoms of the type associated with withdrawal from CNS depressant drugs following the rapid decrease or the abrupt discontinuation of benzodiazepines (see **Drug Abuse and Dependence** section).

DRUG ABUSE AND DEPENDENCE

Withdrawal symptoms similar in character to those noted with sedatives/hypnotics and alcohol have occurred following the abrupt discontinuation of drugs in the benzodiazepine class. The symptoms can range from mild dysphoria and insomnia to a major syndrome which may include abdominal and muscle cramps, vomiting, sweating, tremors, and convulsions.

Although withdrawal symptoms are more commonly noted after the discontinuation of higher than therapeutic doses of benzodiazepines, a proportion of patients taking benzodiazepines chronically at therapeutic doses may become physically dependent upon them. Available data, however, cannot provide a reliable estimate of the incidence of dependency or the relationship of the dependency to dose and duration of treatment. Evidence of physical dependency has been obtained in controlled studies that rely upon the finding that some patients exhibit signs and symptoms upon drug discontinuation that cannot be attributed to the return of the psychopathology for which the benzodiazepine was initially prescribed. There is some evidence to suggest that gradual reduction of dosage will attenuate or eliminate these withdrawal phenomena. In most instances, the withdrawal phenomena have been relatively mild and transient; however, life-threatening events (e.g., seizures, delirium, etc.) have been reported.

Gradual withdrawal is the preferred course for any patient taking benzodiazepines for a prolonged period. Patients with a history of seizures, regardless of their concomitant anti-seizure drug therapy, should not be withdrawn abruptly from benzodiazepines.

Individuals with a history of addition to, or abuse of, drugs or alcohol should be under careful surveillance when receiving benzodiazepines because of the risk to such patients of habituation and dependence.

Controlled Substance Class: DORAL is a controlled substance under the Controlled Substance Act and has been assigned by the Drug Enforcement Administration to Schedule IV.

OVERDOSAGE

Overdosage of DORAL Tablets has not been reported. Manifestations of overdosage seen with other benzodiazepines include somnolence, confusion, and coma. In the event that an overdose occurs, the following is the recommended treatment. Respiration, pulse, and blood pressure should be monitored, as in all cases of drug overdosage. General supportive measures should be employed, along with immediate gastric lavage. Intravenous fluids should be administered and an adequate airway maintained. Hypotension may be treated with the use of Levophed® (levarterenol) or Aramine® (metaraminol). Dialysis is of limited value. Animal experiments suggest that forced diuresis of hemodialysis are probably of little value in treating overdosage. As with the management of intentional overdosing with any drug, it should be borne in mind that multiple agents may have been ingested.

The oral LD_{50} in mice was greater than 5,000 mg/kg.

DOSAGE AND ADMINISTRATION

Adults: Initate therapy at 15 mg until individual responses are determined. In some patients, the dose may then be reduced to 7.5 mg.

Elderly and debilitated patients: Because the elderly and debilitated may be more sensitive to benzodiazepines, attempts to reduce the nightly dosage after the first one or two nights of therapy are suggested.

HOW SUPPLIED

DORAL Tablets, 7.5 mg, capsule-shaped, light orange, slightly white speckled tablets, impressed with the product identification number 7.5 on one side of the tablet, and the product name (DORAL) on the other; bottles of 100 (NDC 0575-9000-01).

DORAL Tablets, 15 mg, capsule-shaped, light orange, slightly white speckled tablets, scored and impressed with the product identification number 15 on one side of the tab-

let, and the product name (DORAL) on the other; bottles of 100 (NDC 0575-9001-01).
Store DORAL Tablets between 2° and 30°C (36° and 86°F).

Manufactured by
Schering Corporation
for
Baker Cummins Pharmaceuticals, Inc.
Miami, FL 33178 USA

7/89   I-000152
Copyright © 1989

Barr Laboratories, Inc.
2 QUAKER ROAD
P.O. BOX D-2900
POMONA, NY 10970

Barr Product Listing
Barr manufactures all of its own products so you can be assured of product identification, consistency in color and size batch-to-batch, day-to-day, year-to-year.
Our broad product line includes the analgesics, antibiotics, antidiabetics, antihypertensives, anti-infectives, cardiovasculars, psychotherapeutics, steroids and others. The following is a selective representation of Barr products. For a full product listing and further information, please call **1-800-222-4043** or **1-800-222-0190**.

NDC # 0555	PRODUCT	
0198	Acetaminophen w/ Codeine Tablets 300 mg/30 mg	℃
0229	Acetaminophen w/ Codeine Tablets 300 mg/60 mg	℃
0294	Aspirin w/ Codeine Tablets 325 mg/15 mg	℃
0264	Aspirin w/ Codeine Tablets 325 mg/30 mg	℃
0280	Aspirin w/ Codeine Tablets 325 mg/60 mg	℃
0514	Cephalexin Capsules 250 mg	℞
0515	Cephalexin Capsules 500 mg	℞
0525	Cephalexin for Oral Suspension 125 mg/5 ml	℞
0526	Cephalexin for Oral Suspension 250 mg/5 ml	℞
0545	Cephalexin Tablets 250 mg	℞
0546	Cephalexin Tablets 500 mg	℞
0550	Cephradine Capsules 250 mg	℞
0551	Cephradine Capsules 500 mg	℞
0553	Cephradine for Oral Suspension 125 mg/5 ml	℞
0552	Cephradine for Oral Suspension 250 mg/5 ml	℞
0585	Chlorzoxazone Tablets 500 mg	℞
0163	Diazepam Tablets 2 mg	℃
0363	Diazepam Tablets 5 mg	℃
0164	Diazepam Tablets 10 mg	℃
0252	Dipyridamole Tablets 25 mg	℞
0285	Dipyridamole Tablets 50 mg	℞
0286	Dipyridamole Tablets 75 mg	℞
0296	Doxycycline Capsules 50 mg (DOXY-CAPS™)	℞
0297	Doxycycline Capsules 100 mg (DOXY-CAPS™)	℞
0295	Doxycycline Tablets 100 mg (DOXY-TABS™)	℞
0533	Erythromycin Delayed-Release Tablets 500 mg (E-BASE®)	℞
0584	Erthromycin Delayed-Release Capsules 250 mg	℞
0230	Erythromycin Estolate Capsules 250 mg	℞
0215	Erythromycin Ethylsuccinate for Oral Suspension 200 mg/5 ml.	℞
0259	Erythromycin Ethylsuccinate Tablets 400 mg	℞
0445	Erythromycin Ethylsuccinate and Sulfisoxazole Acetyl for Oral Suspension 200 mg/600 mg/5 ml (E.S.P.™)	℞
0013	Erythromycin Stearate Tablets 250 mg	℞

0377	Flurazepam Capsules 15 mg	℃
0378	Flurazepam Capsules 30 mg	℃
0325	Hydrocodone Bitartrate w/ Acetaminophen Tablets 5 mg/500 mg	℃
0419	Ibuprofen Tablets 400 mg	℞
0420	Ibuprofen Tablets 600 mg	℞
0499	Ibuprofen Tablets 800 mg	℞
0336	Indomethacin Tablets 25 mg	℞
0337	Indomethacin Capsules 50 mg	℞
0066	Isoniazid Tablets 100 mg	℞
0071	Isoniazid Tablets 300 mg	℞
0484	Leucovorin Ca Tablets 5mg	℞
0485	Leucovorin Ca Tablets 25 mg	℞
0370	Lorazepam Tablets 0.5 mg	℃
0371	Lorazepam Tablets 1.0 mg	℃
0372	Lorazepam Tablets 2.0 mg	℃
0381	Meperidine HCl Tablets 50 mg	℃
0382	Meperidine HCl Tablets 100 mg	℃
0291	Metronidazole Tablets 250 mg	℞
0292	Metronidazole Tablets 500 mg	℞
0374	Oxazepam Capsules 10 mg	℃
0375	Oxazepam Capsules 15 mg	℃
0376	Oxazepam Capsules 30 mg	℃
0373	Oxazepam Tablets 15 mg	℃
0278	Oxycodone w/ Acetaminophen Tablets 5 mg/325 mg	℃
0293	Oxycodone w/ Aspirin Tablets 4.5 mg/325 mg	℃
0395	Phenylbutazone Tablets 100 mg	℞
0396	Phenylbutazone Capsules 100 mg	℞
0317	Propoxyphene Napsylate and Acetaminophen Tablets 50 mg/325 mg	℃
0318	Propoxyphene Napsylate and Acetaminophen Tablets 100 mg/650 mg White	℃
0470	Propoxyphene Napsylate and Acetaminophen Tablets 100 mg/650 mg Pink	℃
0321	Sulfamethoxazole w/ Trimethoprim Tablets 400 mg/80 mg	℞
0322	Sulfamethoxazole w/ Trimethoprim Tablets 800 mg/160 mg	℞
0487	Temazepam Capsules 15 mg	℃
0488	Temazepam Capsules 30 mg	℃
0011	Tetracycline Capsules 250 mg	℞
0010	Tetracycline Capsules 500 mg	℞
0489	Trazodone HCl Tablets 50 mg	℞
0490	Trazodone HCl Tablets 100 mg	℞
0444	Triamterene w/Hydrochlorothiazide Tablets 75 mg/50 mg	℞
0429	Trimethoprim Tablets 100 mg	℞
0425	Verapamil HCl Tablets 80 mg	℞
0455	Verapamil HCl Tablets 120 mg	℞

Barry Laboratories
2100 PARK CENTRAL BLVD. NORTH
SUITE 500
POMPANO BEACH, FL 33064

ALLERGENIC EXTRACTS, DIAGNOSIS AND/OR IMMUNOTHERAPY   ℞

COMPOSITION
Fluid allergens are available from the following categories: pollens, foods, dusts, epidermals, insects, fungi (molds & smuts), yeasts, and others.

ACTION AND USES
For diagnosis and immunotherapy.

PRECAUTIONS
Usual precautions used in testing or treating hypersensitive individuals. See product information circulars accompanying each product.

HOW SUPPLIED
Diagnostic materials are available for cutaneous or intracutaneous testing.
Diagnostic Test Sets include a comprehensive selection of perennial and seasonal allergens for each of five botanical zones.
Diagnostic Test Sets available: Multi-Test® , 50 Plus, Food and Intradermal.

Immunorex®—Prescription Allergy Treatment Sets— Individualized, four vial treatment sets are prepared from the physician's instructions, based on the patient's skin test reactions and history. RAST based prescriptions and refills of any dilutions are also available.

LITERATURE AVAILABLE
Send for free descriptive literature, report and case history forms.

Beach Pharmaceuticals
Division of BEACH PRODUCTS, INC.
5220 SOUTH MANHATTAN AVE.
TAMPA, FL 33611

BEELITH Tablets   OTC
Magnesium/Vitamin B$_6$ Supplement

DESCRIPTION
Each tablet contains magnesium oxide 600 mg and pyridoxine hydrochloride (Vitamin B$_6$) 25 mg equivalent to B$_6$ 20 mg. **Inactive Ingredients:** Castor oil, hydroxypropyl methylcellulose, magnesium stearate, microcrystalline cellulose, pharmaceutical glaze, povidone and sodium starch glycolate. May contain hydroxypropyl cellulose, polyethylene glycol and propylene glycol. Also, FD&C Blue #2, D&C Yellow #10, FD&C Yellow #6 (Sunset Yellow), and titanium dioxide.

WARNINGS
Keep this and all drugs out of the reach of children. In case of accidental overdose seek professional assistance or contact a Poison Control Center immediately. As with any drug, if you are pregnant or nursing a baby, seek the advise of a health professional before using this product.

ACTIONS AND USES
BEELITH is a dietary supplement for patients deficient in magnesium and/or pyridoxine. Each tablet yeilds approximately 362 mg of elemental magnesium and supplies 1000% of the Adult U.S. Recommended Daily Allowance (RDA) for Vitamin B$_6$ and 90% of the Adult RDA for magnesium.

DOSAGE
The usual adult dose is one or two tablets daily.

PRECAUTION
Excessive dosage might cause laxation.

CAUTION
Use only under the supervision of a physician. Use with caution in renal insufficiency.

DRUG INTERACTION PRECAUTIONS
Do not take this product if you are presently taking a prescription antibiotic drug containing any form of tetracycline.

HOW SUPPLIED
Golden yellow film coated tablet with the name **BEACH** and the number **1132** printed on each tablet. Bottle of 100 (NDC 0486-1132-01) tablets.
Shown in Product Identification Section, page 405

Continued on next page

Beach—Cont.

CITROLITH TABLETS   ℞

DESCRIPTION
Each white, capsule shaped tablet contains potassium citrate, anhydrous 50 mg and sodium citrate, anhydrous 950 mg.

K-PHOS® M.F.   ℞
K-PHOS® No.2   ℞
Phosphate Urinary Acidifiers

DESCRIPTION
K-PHOS® M.F.: Each tablet contains potassium acid phosphate 155 mg and sodium acid phosphate, anhydrous 350 mg. Each tablet yields approximately 125.6 mg of phosphorus, 44.5 mg of potassium or 1.1 mEq and 67 mg of sodium or 2.9 mEq. **K-PHOS® No.2:** Each tablet contains potassium acid phosphate 305 mg and sodium acid phosphate, anhydrous, 700 mg. Each tablet yields approximately 250 mg of phosphorus, 88 mg of potassium or 2.3 mEq and 134 mg of sodium or 5.8 mEq.

ACTIONS
These products are highly effective urinary acidifiers.

INDICATIONS
For use in patients with elevated urinary pH. These products help keep calcium soluble and reduce odor and rash caused by ammoniacal urine. Also, by acidifying the urine they increase the antibacterial activity of methenamine mandelate and methenamine hippurate.

CONTRAINDICATIONS
These products are contraindicated in patients with infected phosphate stones; in patients with severely impaired renal function (less than 30% of normal) and in the presence of hyperphosphatemia.

PRECAUTIONS
Drug Interactions: Use of antacids containing magnesium, aluminum or calcium in conjunction with phosphate preparations may bind the phosphate and prevent its absorption. Concurrent use of antihypertensives, especially diazoxide, guanethidine, hydralazine, methyldopa or rauwolfia alkaloids; or corticosteroids, especially mineralocorticoids or corticotropin, with sodium phosphate may result in hypernatremia. Potassium-containing medications or potassium-sparing diuretics may cause hyperkalemia when used with potassium phosphates. Patients should have serum potassium level determinations at periodic intervals. Plasma levels of salicylates may be increased since salicylate excretion is decreased in acidified urine; administration of monobasic phosphates to patients stabilized on salicylates may lead to toxic salicylate levels.
General: Contains potassium and sodium and should be used with caution if regulation of these elements is desired. Occasionally, some individuals may experience a mild laxative effect during the first few days of phosphate therapy. If laxation persists to an unpleasant degree, reduce the daily dosage until this effect subsides or, if necessary, discontinue the use of this product. Use of this medication should be carefully considered when the following medical problems exist: Cardiac disease (particularly in digitalized patients), Addison's disease, acute dehydration, extensive tissue breakdown, myotonia congenita, cardiac failure, cirrhosis of the liver or severe hepatic disease, peripheral and pulmonary edema, hypernatremia, hypertension, toxemia of pregnancy, hypoparathyroidism, and acute pancreatitis. Rickets may benefit from phosphate therapy but caution should be observed. High serum phosphate levels increase the risk of extraskeletal calcification.
Information for Patients: Patients with kidney stones may pass old stones when phosphate therapy is started and should be warned of this possibility. Patients should be advised to avoid the use of antacids containing aluminum, magnesium or calcium which may prevent the absorption of phosphate.
Laboratory Tests: Careful monitoring of renal function and serum electrolytes (calcium, phosphorus, potassium, sodium) may be required at periodic intervals. Other tests may be warranted in some patients, depending on conditions.
Carcinogenesis, mutagenesis, impairment of fertility: Long term animal studies to evaluate the carcinogenic, mutagenic, or teratogenic potential of these products have not been performed.
Pregnancy: Pregnancy Category C. Animal reproduction studies have not been conducted with these products. It is also not known whether these products can cause fetal harm when administered to a pregnant woman or can affect reproduction capacity. These products should be given to a pregnant woman only if clearly needed.
Nursing Mothers: It is not known whether these drugs are excreted in human milk. Because many drugs are excreted in human milk, caution should be exercised when these products are administered to a nursing woman.

ADVERSE REACTIONS
Gastrointestinal upset (diarrhea, nausea, stomach pain and vomiting) may occur with phosphate therapy. Also, bone and joint pain (possible phosphate-induced osteomalacia) could occur. The following adverse effects may be observed (primarily from sodium or potassium): headaches; dizziness; mental confusion; seizures; weakness or heaviness of legs; unusual tiredness or weakness; muscle cramps; numbness, tingling, pain, or weakness of hands or feet; numbness or tingling around lips; fast or irregular heartbeat; shortness of breath or troubled breathing; swelling of feet or lower legs; unusual weight gain; low urine output unusual thirst.

DIRECTIONS
K-PHOS® M.F.: Two tablets four times daily with a full glass of water.
K-PHOS® No.2: One tablet four times daily with a full glass of water. When the urine is difficult to acidify administer one tablet every two hours not to exceed eight tablets in a 24 hour period.

HOW SUPPLIED
K-PHOS® M.F.: White scored tablet with the name **BEACH** and the number **1135** embossed on each tablet. Bottles of 100 (NDC 0486-1135-01) and bottles of 500 (NDC 0486-1135-05) tablets. **K-PHOS® No.2:** Brown capsule shaped tablet with the name **BEACH** and the number **1134** embossed on each tablet. Bottles of 100 (NDC 0486-1134-01) and bottles of 500 (NDC 0486-1134-05) tablets.

CAUTION
Federal law prohibits dispensing without prescription.
Shown in Product Identification Section, page 405

K-PHOS® NEUTRAL   ℞
Supplies 250 mg of phosphorus per tablet.

DESCRIPTION
Each tablet contains 852 mg dibasic sodium phosphate anhydrous, 155 mg monobasic potassium phosphate, and 130 mg monobasic sodium phosphate monohydrate. Each tablet yields approximately 250 mg of phosphorus, 298 mg of sodium (13.0 mEq) and 45 mg of potassium (1.1 mEq).

INDICATIONS
K-PHOS® NEUTRAL increases urinary phosphate and pyrophosphate. As a phosphorous supplement, each tablet supplies 25% of the U.S. Recommended Daily Allowance (U.S.RDA) of phosphorus for adults.

CONTRAINDICATIONS
This product is contraindicated in patients with infected phosphate stones, in patients with severely impaired renal function (less than 30% of normal) and in the presence of hyperphosphatemia.

PRECAUTIONS
General: This product contains potassium and sodium and should be used with caution if regulation of these elements is desired. Occasionally, some individuals may experience a mild laxative effect during the first few days of phosphate therapy. If laxation persists to an unpleasant degree, reduce the daily dosage until this effect subsides or, if necessary, discontinue the use of this product.
Caution should be exercised when prescribing this product in the following conditions: Cardiac disease (particularly in digitalized patients); severe adrenal insufficiency (Addison's disease); acute dehydration; severe renal insufficiency; renal function impairment or chronic renal disease; extensive tissue breakdown (such as severe burns); myotonia congenita; cardiac failure; cirrhosis of the liver or severe hepatic disease; peripheral or pulmonary edema; hypernatremia; hypertension; toxemia of pregnancy; hypoparathyroidism; and acute pancreatitis. Rickets may benefit from phosphate therapy, but caution should be exercised. High serum phosphate may increase the incidence of extra-skeletal calcification.
Information for Patients: Patients with kidney stones may pass old stones when phosphate therapy is started and should be warned of this possibility. Patients should be advised to avoid the use of antacids containing aluminum, magnesium or calcium which may prevent the absorption of phosphate.
Laboratory Tests: Careful monitoring of renal function and serum electrolytes (calcium, phosphorus, potassium, sodium) may be required at periodic intervals during phosphate therapy. Other tests may be warranted in some patients, depending on conditions.
Drug Interactions: The use of antacids containing magnesium, aluminum or calcium in conjunction with phosphate preparations may bind the phosphate and prevent its absorption. Concurrent use of antihypertensives, especially diazoxide, guanethidine, hydralazine, methyldopa, or rauwolfia alkaloids; or corticosteroids, especially mineralocorticoids or corticotropin, with sodium phosphate may result in hypernatremia. Calcium-containing preparations and/or vitamin D may antagonize the effects of phosphates in the treatment of hypercalcemia. Potassium-containing medications or potassium-sparing diuretics may cause hyperkalemia. Patients should have serum potassium level determinations at periodic intervals.
Carcinogenesis, Mutagenesis, Impairment of Fertility: There have been no studies in animals or humans to evaluate the carcinogenesis, mutagenesis, or impairment of fertility for this product.
Pregnancy: Pregnancy Category C. Animal reproduction studies have not been conducted with this product. It is also not known whether this product can cause fetal harm when administered to a pregnant woman or can affect reproduction capacity. This product should be given to a pregnant woman only if clearly needed.
Nursing Mothers: It is not known whether this drug is excreted in human milk. Because many drugs are excreted in human milk, caution should be exercised when this product is administered to a nursing woman.

ADVERSE REACTIONS
Gastrointestinal upset (diarrhea, nausea, stomach pain, and vomiting) may occur with phosphate therapy. Also, bone and joint pain (possible phosphate-induced osteomalacia) could occur. The following adverse effects may be observed (primarily from sodium or potassium): headaches; dizziness; mental confusion; seizures; weakness or heaviness of legs; unusual tiredness or weakness; muscle cramps; numbness, tingling, pain, or weakness of hands or feet; numbness or tingling around lips; fast or irregular heartbeat; shortness of breath or troubled breathing; swelling of feet or lower legs; unusual weight gain; low urine output; unusual thirst.

DIRECTIONS
Adults: One or two tablets four times a day with a full glass of water.

HOW SUPPLIED
White, film coated, capsule-shaped tablet with the name **BEACH** and number **1125** embossed on each tablet. Bottles of 100 (NDC 0486-1125-01) and 500 (NDC 0486-1125-05) tablets.

CAUTION
Federal law prohibits dispensing without a prescription.
Shown in Product Identification Section, page 405

K-PHOS® ORIGINAL (Sodium Free)   ℞
(Potassium Acid Phosphate)
Urinary Acidifier
Supplies 114 mg of phosphorus per tablet.

DESCRIPTION
Each tablet contains potassium acid phosphate 500 mg. Each tablet yields approximately 114 mg of phosphorus and 144 mg of potassium or 3.7 mEq.

ACTIONS
K-PHOS® ORIGINAL (Sodium Free) is a highly effective urinary acidifier.

INDICATIONS
For use in patients with elevated urinary pH. Helps keep calcium soluble and reduces odor and rash caused by ammoniacal urine. Also, by acidifying the urine, it increases the antibacterial activity of methenamine mandelate and methenamine hippurate.

CONTRAINDICATIONS
This product is contraindicated in patients with infected phosphate stones; in patients with severely impaired renal function (less than 30% of normal) and in the presence of hyperphosphatemia and hyperkalemia.

PRECAUTIONS
General: This product contains potassium and should be used with caution if regulation of this element is desired. Occasionally, some individuals may experience a mild laxative effect during the first few days of phosphate therapy. If laxation persists to an unpleasant degree, reduce the daily dosage until this effect subsides or, if necessary, discontinue the use of this product.
Caution should be exercised when prescribing this product in the following conditions: Cardiac disease (particularly in digitalized patients); severe adrenal insufficiency (Addison's disease); acute dehydration; severe renal insufficieny or chronic renal disease; extensive tissue breakdown (such as severe burns); myotonia congenita; hypoparathyroidism; and acute pancreatitis. Rickets may benefit from phosphate therapy, but caution should be exercised. High serum phosphate levels may increase the incidence of extraskeletal calcification.
Information for Patients: Patients with kidney stones may pass old stones when phosphate therapy is started and should be warned of this possibility. Patients should be advised to avoid the use of antacids containing aluminum, calcium, or magnesium which may prevent the absorption of

phosphate. To assure against gastrointestinal injury associated with oral ingestion of concentrated potassium salt preparations, patients should be instructed to dissolve tablets completely in an appropriate amount of water before taking.

Laboratory Tests: Careful monitoring of renal function and serum electrolytes (calcium, phosphorous, potassium) may be required at periodic intervals during phosphate therapy. Other tests may be warranted in some patients, depending on conditions.

Drug Interactions: The use of antacids containing magnesium, calcium, or aluminum in conjunction with phosphate preparations may bind the phosphate and prevent its absorption. Potassium-containing medications or potassium-sparing diuretics may cause hyperkalemia when used concurrently with potassium salts. Patients should have serum potassium level determinations at periodic intervals. Concurrent use of salicylates may lead to increased serum salicylate levels since excretion of salicylates is reduced in acidified urine. Serum salicylate levels should be closely monitored to avoid toxicity.

Carcincogenesis, Mutagenesis, Impairment of Fertility: There have been no studies in animals or humans to evaluate the carcinogenesis, mutagenesis, or impairment of fertility for this product.

Pregnancy: Pregnancy Category C. Animal reproduction studies have not been conducted with this product. It is also not known whether this product can cause fetal harm when administered to a pregnant woman or can affect reproduction capacity. This product should be given to a pregnant woman only if clearly needed.

Nursing Mothers: It is not known whether this drug is excreted in human milk. Because many drugs are excreted in human milk, caution should be exercised when this product is administered to a nursing woman.

ADVERSE REACTIONS

Gastrointestinal upset (diarrhea, nausea, stomach pain, and vomiting) may occur with the use of potassium phosphates. Also, bone and joint pain (possible phosphate-induced osteomalacia) could occur. The following adverse effects may be observed with potassium administration: irregular heartbeat; dizziness; mental confusion; weakness or heaviness of legs; unusual tiredness; muscle cramps; numbness, tingling, pain, or weakness in hands or feet; numbness or tingling around lips; shortness of breath or troubled breathing.

DIRECTIONS

Two tablets dissolved in 6–8 oz. of water 4 times daily with meals and at bedtime. For best results, let the tablets soak in water for 2 to 5 minutes, or more if necessary, and stir. If any tablet particles remain undissolved, they may be crushed and stirred vigorously to speed dissolution.

HOW SUPPLIED

White scored tablet with the name **BEACH** and the number **1111** embossed on each tablet. Bottles of 100 (NDC 0486-1111-01) and bottles of 500 (NDC 0486-1111-05) tablets.

CAUTION

Federal law prohibits dispensing without prescription.
Shown in Product Identification Section, page 405

THIACIDE TABLETS ℞
[thī-ă-sīd]
SODIUM FREE

DESCRIPTION

Each tablet contains methenamine mandelate 500 mg. and potassium acid phosphate 250 mg.
Shown in Product Identification Section, page 405

UROQID–Acid® Tablets ℞
UROQID–Acid®No. 2 Tablets ℞

DESCRIPTION

Each **UROQID-Acid®** tablet contains methenamine mandelate 350 mg and sodium acid phosphate, monohydrate 200 mg. Each **UROQID-Acid®No. 2** tablet contains methenamine mandelate 500 mg and sodium acid phosphate, monohydrate 500 mg.

CLINICAL PHARMACOLOGY

Methenamine mandelate is rapidly absorbed and excreted in the urine. Formaldehyde is released by acid hydrolysis from methenamine with bactericidal levels rapidly reached at pH 5.0–5.5. Proportionally less formaldehyde is released as urinary pH approaches 6.0 and insufficient quantities are released above this level for therapeutic response. In acid urine, mandelic acid exerts its antibacterial action and also contributes to the acidification of the urine. Mandelic acid is excreted by both glomerular filtration and tubular excretion. In acid urine, there is equally effective antibacterial activity against both gram-positive and gram-negative organisms, since the antibacterial action of mandelic acid and formaldehyde is nonspecific. With Proteus vulgaris and urea splitting strains of Pseudomonas and Aerobacter, results

may be discouraging and particular attention is required in monitoring urinary pH and overall management.

INDICATIONS AND USAGE

For the suppression or elimination of bacteriuria associated with chronic and recurrent infections of the urinary tract, including pyelitis, pyelonephritis, cystitis, and infected residual urine accompanying neurogenic bladder. When used as recommended, **UROQUID-Acid®** and **UROQUID- Acid® No. 2** are particularly suitable for long-term therapy because of their relative safety and because resistance to the nonspecific bactericidal action of formaldehyde does not develop. Pathogens resistant to other antibacterial agents may respond because of the nonspecific effect of formaldehyde formed in an acid urine.

Prophylactic Use Rationale: Urine is a good culture medium for many urinary pathogens. Inoculation by a few organisms (relapse or reinfection) may lead to bacteriuria in susceptible individuals. Thus, the rationale of management in recurring urinary tract infection (bacteriuria) is to change the urine from a growth-supporting to a growth-inhibiting medium. There is a growing body of evidence that long-term administration of methenamine can prevent recurrence of bacteriuria in patients with chronic pyelonephritis.

Therapeutic Use Rationale: Helps to sterilize the urine and, in some situations in which underlying pathologic conditions prevent sterilization by any means, they can help to suppress bacteriuria. As part of the overall management of the urinary tract infection, a thorough diagnostic evaluation should accompany the use of these products.

CONTRAINDICATIONS

UROQID-Acid® and **UROQID-Acid®No. 2** are contraindicated in patients with renal insufficiency, severe hepatic disease, severe dehydration, hyperphosphatemia, and in patients who have exhibited hypersensitivity to any components of these products.

PRECAUTIONS

General: These products should not be used as the sole therapeutic agent in acute parenchymal infections causing systemic symptoms such as chills anf fever.

UROQID-Acid® and **UROQID-Acid®No. 2** contain approximately 33 mg and 83 mg of sodium per tablet, respectively, and should be used with caution in patients on a sodium-restricted diet.

Sodium phosphates should be used with caution in the following conditions: cardiac failure; peripheral or pulmonary edema; hypernatremia; hypertension; toxemia of pregnancy; hypoparathyroidism; and acute pancreatitis. High serum phosphate levels increase the incidence of extraskeletal calcification.

Large doses of methenamine (8 grams daily for 3 to 4 weeks) have caused bladder irritation, painful and frequent micturation, albuminuria and gross hematuria. Dysuria may occur, although usually at higher than recommended doses, and can be controlled by reducing the dosage. These products contain a urinary acidifier and can cause metabolic acidosis. Care should be taken to maintain an acid urinary pH (below 5.5), especially when treating infections due to urea-splitting organisms such as Proteus and strains of Pseudomonas. Drugs and/or foods which produce an alkaline urine should be restricted. Frequent urine pH tests are essential. If acidification of the urine is contraindicated or unattainable, use of these products should be discontinued.

Information for Patients: To assure an acidic pH, patients should be instructed to restrict or avoid most fruits, milk and milk products, and antacids containing sodium carbonate or bicarbonate.

Laboratory Tests: As with all urinary tract infections, the efficacy of therapy should be monitored by repeated urine cultures. During long-term therapy, careful monitoring of renal function, serum phosphorus and sodium may be required at periodic intervals.

Drug Interactions: Formaldehyde and sulfonamides form an insoluble precipitate in acid urine and increase the risk of crystalliuria; therefore, these products should not be used concurrently. Thiazide diuretics, carbonic anhydrase inhibitors, antacids, or urinary alkalinizing agents should not be used concurrently since they may cause the urine to become alkaline and reduce the effectiveness of methenamine by inhibiting its conversion to formaldehyde. Concurrent use of antihypertensives, especially diazoxide, guanethidine, hydralazine, methyldopa, or rauwolfia alkaloids; or corticosteroids, especially mineralocorticoids or corticotropin, with sodium phosphates may result in hypernatremia. Concurrent use of salicylates may lead to increased serum salicylate levels since excretion of salicylates is reduced in acidified urine. Serum salicylate levels should be closely monitored to avoid toxicity.

Laboratory Test Interactions: Formaldehyde interferes with fluorometric procedures for determination of urinary catecholamines and vanilmandelic acid (VMA) causing erroneously high results. Formaldehyde also causes falsely decreased urine estriol levels by reacting with estriol when acid hydrolysis techniques are used; estriol determinations which use enzymatic hydrolysis are unaffected by folmalde-

hyde. Formaldehyde causes falsely elevated 17-hydroxycorticosteroid levels when the Porter-Silber method is used and falsely decreased 5-hydroxyindoleacetic acid (5HIAA) levels by inhibiting color development when nitrosonaphthol methods are used.

Carcinogenesis, Mutagenesis, Impairment of Fertility: Long-term animal studies to evaluate the carcinogenic, mutagenic, or impairment of fertility potential of these products have not been performed.

Pregnancy: Pregnancy Category C. Animal reproduction studies have not been conducted with these products. It is also not known whether these products can cause fetal harm when administered to a pregnant woman or can affect reproduction capacity. Since methenamine is known to cross the placental barrier, these products should be given to a pregnant woman only if clearly needed.

Nursing Mothers: Methenamine is excreted in breast milk. Caution should be exercised when these products are administered to a nursing woman.

ADVERSE REACTIONS

Gastrointestinal disturbances (nausea, stomach upset), generalized skin rash, dysuria, painful or difficult urination may occur occasionally with the use of methenamine preparations. Microscopic and rarely, gross hematuria have also been reported.

Gastrointestinal upsets (diarrhea, nausea, stomach pain, and vomiting) may occur with the use of sodium phosphates. Also, bone or joint pain (possible phosphate induced osteomalacia) could occur. The following adverse effects may be observed (primarily from sodium or potassium): headaches; dizziness; mental confusion; seizures; weakness or heaviness of legs; unusual tiredness or weakness; muscle cramps; numbness, tingling, pain or weakness of hands or feet; numbness or tingling around lips; fast or irregular heartbeat; shortness of breath or troubled breathing; swelling of feet or lower legs; unusual weight gain; low urine output; unusual thirst.

DIRECTIONS

UROQID-Acid®: Initially, 3 tablets 4 times daily. For maintenance, 1 or 2 tablets 4 times daily. **UROQID-Acid® No. 2:** Initially, 2 tablets 4 times daily. For maintenance, 2 to 4 tablets daily, in divided doses. Give these products with a full glass of water.

HOW SUPPLIED

UROQID-Acid® is a yellow, sugar coated, tablet with the name **BEACH** and the number **1112** printed on each tablet. Packaged in bottles of 100 (NDC 0486-1112-01) and 500 (NDC 0486-1112-05) tablets. **UROQID-Acid®No. 2** is a yellow, film coated, capsule shaped tablet with the name **BEACH** and the number **1114** embossed on each tablet. Packaged in bottles of 100 (NDC 0486-1114-01) and 500 (NDC 0486-1114-05) tablets.

CAUTION

Federal law prohibits dispensing without prescription.
Shown in Product Identification Section, page 405

Beecham Products USA
DIVISION OF BEECHAM INC.
POST OFFICE BOX 1467
PITTSBURGH, PA 15230

A-200™ Pediculicide Shampoo, Gel

A-200™ Shampoo

DESCRIPTION

Active ingredients: Pyrethrins 0.33%, piperonyl butoxide technical 4% (equivalent to 3.2% (butylcarbityl) (6-propylpiperonyl) ether and .8% related compounds).
Inert ingredients: Benzyl alcohol, butyl stearate, fragrance, octoxynol-9, oleic acid, oleoresin parsley seed, petroleum distillate, water.

A-200™ Gel

DESCRIPTION

Active ingredients: pyrethrins 0.33%, piperonyl butoxide technical 4% (equivalent to 3.2% (butylcarbityl) (6-propylpiperonyl) ether and 0.8% related compounds).
Inert ingredients: benzyl alcohol, butyl stearate, carbomer 940, fragrance, octoxynol-9, oleic acid, oleoresin parsley seed, petroleum distillate, triisopropanolamine, water.

ACTIONS

A-200 is an effective pediculicide for control of head lice (Pediculus humanus capitis), pubic lice (Phthirus pubis) and body lice (Pediculus humanus corporis), and their nits.

INDICATIONS

A-200 Shampoo and Gel are indicated for the treatment of human pediculosis—head lice, body lice and pubic lice, and their eggs. A-200 Gel is specially formulated for pubic lice

Continued on next page

Beecham Products—Cont.

and head lice in children, where control of application is desirable.

CONTRAINDICATIONS

A-200 is contraindicated in individuals hypersensitive to any of its ingredients or allergic to ragweed.

PRECAUTIONS

A-200 is for external use only. It is harmful if swallowed or inhaled. It may be irritating to the eyes and mucous membranes. In case of accidental contact with eyes, they should be immediately flushed with water. In order to prevent reinfestation with lice, all clothing and bedding must be sterilized or treated concurrent with the application of this preparation. If skin irritation or signs of infection are present, a physician should be consulted.

ADMINISTRATION AND DOSAGE

Apply A-200 to **dry** hair and scalp or other infested areas. Use enough to completely wet area being treated. Massage in. (For head lice, avoid getting product into eyes. Helpful hint: When shampooing a child's head, place towel across forehead.) Allow product to remain for 10 minutes, but no longer. Add small quantities of water, and work rich lather into hair and scalp. Rinse thoroughly with warm water. Towel dry. Comb hair with special A-200 precision comb to remove dead lice and eggs. Repeat treatment in 7-10 days or earlier if reinfestation has occurred. Do not use more than 2 applications of A-200 in 24 hours. When used on children, adult supervision is recommended.

HOW SUPPLIED

A-200 Shampoo in 2 and 4 fl. oz. unbreakable plastic bottles with special comb. A-200 Gel in 1 oz. tubes.

LITERATURE AVAILABLE

Patient literature available upon request.
Shown in Product Identification Section, page 405

ESOTÉRICA® MEDICATED FADE CREAM
Regular
Facial
Fortified with Sunscreen Scented
Fortified with Sunscreen Unscented

(See PDR For Nonprescription Drugs)

LIQUIPRIN® Drops and Elixir
(acetaminophen)

(See PDR For Nonprescription Drugs)

MASSENGILL® Douches
[mas 'sen-gil]

PRODUCT OVERVIEW
KEY FACTS

Massengill is the brand name for a line of douches which are recommended for routine cleansing and for temporary relief of vaginal itching and irritation. Massengill Disposable douches are available in two Vinegar & Water formulas (Extra Mild and Extra Cleansing), a Baking Soda formula, three Cosmetic solutions (Country Flowers, Belle-Mai, and Mountain Herbs) an Unscented solution, and a Medicated formula (with povidone-iodine). Massengill also is available in a Medicated liquid concentrate (povidone-iodine) and a Non-Medicated liquid concentrate and powder form.

MAJOR USES

Massengill's Vinegar & Water, Baking Soda & Water, Unscented, and Cosmetic douches are recommended for routine douching, or for cleansing following menstruation or the prescribed use of vaginal medication or contraceptives. Massengill Medicated is recommended in a seven day regimen for the symptomatic relief of minor itching and irritation associated with vaginitis due to Candida albicans, Trichomonas vaginalis and Gardnerella vaginalis.

SAFETY INFORMATION

Do not douche during pregnancy unless directed by a physician.
Massengill Vinegar & Water, Baking Soda & Water, Unscented, and Cosmetic Douches—If irritation occurs, discontinue use.
Massengill Medicated — Women with iodine-sensitivity should not use this product. If symptoms persist after seven days, or if redness, swelling or pain develop, consult a physician. Do not use while nursing unless directed by a physician.

PRODUCT INFORMATION
MASSENGILL®
[mas 'sen-gil]
Disposable Douches

MASSENGILL®
Liquid Concentrate
MASSENGILL® Powder
INGREDIENTS

DISPOSABLES: Extra Mild Vinegar and Water—Water and Vinegar.
Extra Cleansing Vinegar and Water—Water, Vinegar, Puraclean™ (Cetylpyridinium Chloride), Diazolidinyl Urea, Disodium EDTA.
Baking Soda and Water—Sanitized Water, Sodium Bicarbonate (Baking Soda).
Belle-Mai—Water, SD Alcohol 40, Lactic Acid, Sodium Lactate, Octoxynol-9, Cetylpyridinium Chloride, Propylene Glycol (and) Diazolidinyl Urea (and) Methyl Paraben (and) Propyl Paraben, Disodium EDTA, Fragrance, FD&C Blue #1.
Country Flowers—Water, SD Alcohol 40, Lactic Acid, Sodium Lactate, Octoxynol-9, Cetylpyridinium Chloride, Propylene Glycol (and) Diazolidinyl Urea (and), Methyl Paraben (and) Propyl Paraben, Disodium EDTA, Fragrance, D&C Red #28, FD&C Blue #1.
Mountain Herbs—Water, SD Alcohol 40, Lactic Acid, Sodium Lactate, Octoxynol-9, Cetylpyridinium Chloride, Propylene Glycol (and) Diazolidinyl Urea (and) Methyl Paraben (and) Propyl Paraben, Disodium EDTA, Fragrance, D&C Yellow #10, FD&C Blue #1.
Unscented—Water, SD Alcohol 40, Lactic Acid, Sodium Lactate, Octoxynol-9, Cetylpyridinium Chloride, Propylene Glycol (and) Diazolidinyl Urea (and) Methyl Paraben (and) Propyl Paraben, Disodium EDTA.
LIQUID CONCENTRATE: Water, SD Alcohol 40, Lactic Acid, Sodium Bicarbonate, Octoxynol-9, Fragrance, D&C Yellow #10, FD&C Yellow #6 (Sunset Yellow).
POWDER: Sodium Chloride, Ammonium alum, PEG-8, Phenol, Methyl Salicylate, Eucalyptus Oil, Menthol, Thymol, D&C Yellow #10, FD&C Yellow #6 (Sunset Yellow).
FLORAL POWDER: Sodium Chloride, Ammonium alum, Octoxynol-9, SD Alcohol 23-A, Fragrance, and FD&C Yellow #6 (Sunset Yellow).

INDICATIONS

Recommended for routine cleansing at the end of menstruation, after use of contraceptive creams or jellies (check the contraceptive package instructions first) or to rinse out the residue of prescribed vaginal medication (as directed by physician).

ACTIONS

The buffered acid solutions of Massengill Douches are valuable adjuncts to specific vaginal therapy following the prescribed use of vaginal medication or contraceptives and in feminine hygiene.

DIRECTIONS

DISPOSABLES: Twist off flat, wing-shaped tab from bottle containing premixed solution, attach nozzle supplied and use. The unit is completely disposable.
LIQUID CONCENTRATE: Fill cap ¾ full, to measuring line, and pour contents into douche bag containing 1 quart of warm water. Mix thoroughly.
POWDER: Dissolve two rounded teaspoonfuls in a douche bag containing 1 quart of warm water. Mix thoroughly.

WARNING

Vaginal cleansing douches should not be used more than twice weekly except on the advice of a physician. If irritation occurs, discontinue use. Keep out of reach of children. In case of accidental ingestion, seek professional assistance by contacting your physician, the local poison control center, or the Rocky Mt. Poison Control Center at 303-592-1710 (Collect), 24 hours a day.

HOW SUPPLIED

Disposable—6 oz. disposable plastic bottle.
Liquid Concentrate—4 oz., 8 oz., plastic bottles.
Powder—4 oz., 8 oz., 16 oz., Packettes—10's, 12's.

MASSENGILL® Medicated
[mas 'sen-gil]
Disposable Douche
MASSENGILL® Medicated
Liquid Concentrate

ACTIVE INGREDIENT

DISPOSABLE: Cepticin™ (povidone-iodine)
LIQUID CONCENTRATE: Cepticin™ (povidone-iodine)

INDICATIONS

For symptomatic relief of minor irritation and itching associated with vaginitis due to Candida albicans, Trichomonas vaginalis, and Gardnerella vaginalis.

ACTION

Povidone-iodine is widely recognized as an effective broad spectrum microbicide against both gram negative and gram positive bacteria, fungi, yeasts and protozoa. While remaining active in the presence of blood, serum or bodily secretions, it possesses virtually none of the irritating properties of iodine.

WARNINGS

If symptoms persist after seven days of use, or if redness, swelling or pain develop during treatment, consult a physician. Women with iodine-sensitivity should not use this product. Women may douche during menstruation if they douche gently. Do not douche during pregnancy or while nursing unless directed by a physician. Douching does not prevent pregnancy. Keep out of reach of children. In case of accidental ingestion, seek professional assistance by contacting your physician, the local poison control center, or the Rocky Mt. Poison Control Center at 303-592-1710 (Collect), 24 hours a day.

DOSAGE AND ADMINISTRATION

DISPOSABLE: Dosage is provided as a single unit concentrate to be added to 6 oz. of sanitized water supplied in a disposable bottle. A specially designed nozzle is provided. After use, the unit is discarded. Use one bottle a day. Although symptoms may be relieved earlier, for maximum relief, use for seven days.
LIQUID CONCENTRATE: Pour one capful into douche bag containing one quart of water. Mix thoroughly. Use once daily. Although symptoms may be relieved earlier, for maximum relief, use for seven days.

HOW SUPPLIED

Disposable—6 oz. bottle of sanitized water with 0.17 oz. vial of povidone-iodine and nozzle.
Liquid Concentrate—4 oz., 8 oz. plastic bottles.

MASSENGILL® Medicated
[mas 'sen-gil]
Soft Cloth Towelette

ACTIVE INGREDIENT
Hydrocortisone (0.5%)

INDICATIONS

For soothing relief of minor external feminine itching or other itching associated with minor skin irritations, inflammation, and rashes.

ACTION

Massengill Medicated Soft Cloth Towelettes contain hydrocortisone, a proven anti-inflammatory, anti-pruritic ingredient. The towelette delivery system makes the application soothing, soft, and gentle.

WARNING

For external use only. Avoid contact with eyes, If condition worsens, symptoms persist for more than seven days, or symptoms recur within a few days, discontinue use and consult a physician. If experiencing a vaginal discharge, see a physician.
Keep this and all drugs out of the reach of children. As with any drug, if pregnant or nursing a baby, seek the advice of a health professional before using this product. In case of accidental ingestion, seek professional assistance or contact a Poison Control Center immediately.

DIRECTIONS

Adults and Children two years of age and older—apply to the affected area not more than three to four times daily. Children under two years of age—consult a physician before using. Remove towelette from foil packet, gently wipe, and discard. Throw away towelette after it has been used once.

HOW SUPPLIED

Ten individually wrapped, disposable towelettes per carton.

MASSENGILL®
[mas 'sen-gil]
Unscented Soft Cloth Towelette

INACTIVE INGREDIENTS

Water, Octoxynol-9, Lactic Acid, Sodium Lactate, Potassium Sorbate, Disodium EDTA, and Cetylpyridinium Chloride.

INDICATIONS

For cleansing and refreshing the external vaginal area.

ACTIONS

Massengill Unscented Soft Cloth Towelettes safely cleanse the external vaginal area and do not contain fragrance. The towelette delivery system makes the application soft and gentle.

WARNINGS

For external use only. Avoid contact with eyes.

DIRECTIONS

Remove towelette from foil packet, unfold, and gently wipe. Throw away towelette after it has been used once.

HOW SUPPLIED

Sixteen individually wrapped, disposable towelettes per carton.

NATURE'S REMEDY® Laxative

(See PDR For Nonprescription Drugs)

NoSalt®

Salt Alternative
Regular and Seasoned

(See PDR For Nonprescription Drugs)

OXY CLEAN®

Medicated Cleanser
Medicated Soap
Lathering Facial Scrub

(See PDR For Nonprescription Drugs)

OXY CLEAN® MEDICATED PADS

Regular Strength, Sensitive Skin, and Maximum Strength Formulas

(See PDR For Nonprescription Drugs)

OXY–5® Vanishing & Tinted
OXY–10® Vanishing & Tinted

Benzoyl Peroxide Lotion 5% and 10%

(See PDR For Nonprescription Drugs)

OXY-10® DAILY FACE WASH

Antibacterial Skin Wash

(See PDR for Nonprescription Drugs)

OXY NIGHT WATCH™

Nighttime Acne Medication
Maximum Strength and Sensitive Skin Formulas

(See PDR for Nonprescription Drugs)

TUMS® Antacid Tablets, Regular and Extra Strength
TUMS® Liquid Extra Strength Antacid
TUMS® Liquid Extra Strength Antacid with Simethicone

(See PDR For Nonprescription Drugs)

EDUCATIONAL MATERIAL

Booklet:
"A Personal Guide to Feminine Freshness"
A 16 page illustrated booklet on vaginal infections, feminine hygiene and douching. Free to physicians, pharmacists and patients in limited quantities by writing Beecham or calling 800-BEECHAM. (PA residents 800-242-1718)
Film, Video:
"Feminine Hygiene and You"
This 14 minute color film begins with a simple explanation of how a woman's body works (reproductive system, menstrual cycle, and vaginal secretions) then explains douching. Free loan to physicians, pharmacists and clinics. Available in 16mm, and VHS by writing Beecham or calling 800-BEE-CHAM. (PA residents 800-242-1718)

Important Notice
Before prescribing or administering
any product described in
PHYSICIANS' DESK REFERENCE
always consult the PDR Supplement for
possible new or revised information

Beecham Laboratories
DIV. OF BEECHAM INC.
501 FIFTH STREET
BRISTOL, TN 37620

PRODUCT IDENTIFICATION CODES

To provide quick and positive identification of Beecham Laboratories' products, we have imprinted a code number or brand name on tablet and capsule products. In order that you may identify a product by its code and number, we have compiled below a numerical list of code numbers with their corresponding product names. The code number as it appears on tablets and capsules bears the letters BMP plus the numerical code. Amoxil®, Fastin®, Nucofed® and Tigan® Capsules and Amoxil® Chewable Tablets bear the brand name only. Augmentin® swallow tablets have the name scored on one side and the strength on the other side.

BMP Code No.	Product
112	DASIN® Capsules
121	LIVITAMIN® Capsules
122	LIVITAMIN® w/INTRINSIC FACTOR Capsules
123	LIVITAMIN® CHEWABLE Tablets
125	MENEST™ (Esterified Estrogens, U.S.P.) Tablets 0.3 mg.
126	MENEST™ (Esterified Estrogens, U.S.P.) Tablets 0.625 mg.
127	MENEST™ (Esterified Estrogens, U.S.P.) Tablets 1.25 mg.
128	MENEST™ (Esterified Estrogens, U.S.P.) Tablets 2.5 mg.
140	TOTACILLIN® (Ampicillin) Capsules 250 mg.
141	TOTACILLIN® (Ampicillin) Capsules 500 mg.
143	BACTOCILL® (Oxacillin Sodium) Capsules 250 mg.
144	BACTOCILL® (Oxacillin Sodium) Capsules 500 mg.
145	DARICON® (Oxyphencyclimine HCl) Tablets 10 mg.
156	TIGAN® (Trimethobenzamide HCl) Capsules 100 mg.
157	TIGAN® (Trimethobenzamide HCl) Capsules 250 mg.
165	DYCILL® (Dicloxacillin Sodium) Capsules 250 mg.
166	DYCILL® (Dicloxacillin Sodium) Capsules 500 mg.
169	CLOXAPEN® (Cloxacillin Sodium) Capsules 250 mg.
170	CLOXAPEN® (Cloxacillin Sodium) Capsules 500 mg.
182	NUCOFED® Capsules
185	BEEPEN–VK® (Penicillin V Potassium) Tablets 250 mg.
186	BEEPEN–VK® (Penicillin V Potassium) Tablets 500 mg.
188	ANEXSIA® 7.5 Tablets
189	AUGMENTIN® (Amoxicillin/Clavulanate Potassium) '125' Chewable Tablets
190	AUGMENTIN® (Amoxicillin/Clavulanate Potassium) '250' Chewable Tablets
192	MAXOLON® (Metoclopramide Hydrochloride) 10 mg Tablets
207	ANEXSIA® Tablets
210	CONAR®-A Tablets
211	LAROTID® (Amoxicillin) 250 mg Capsules
212	LAROTID® (Amoxicillin) 500 mg Capsules

AMOXIL®   ℞

[ā-mŏx'ĭl]
(amoxicillin)
capsules, powder for oral suspension
and chewable tablets

DESCRIPTION

AMOXIL (amoxicillin) is a semisynthetic antibiotic, an analog of ampicillin, with a broad spectrum of bactericidal activity against many Gram-positive and Gram-negative microorganisms. Chemically it is D-(-)-α-amino-p-hydroxybenzyl penicillin trihydrate. **Inactive Ingredients:** Capsules—Magnesium Stearate, and Magnesium Sulfate. Chewable Tablets—Citric Acid, Corn Starch, F D & C Red 3, Flavorings, Glycine, Mannitol, Magnesium Stearate, Saccharin Sodium, Silica Gel and Sucrose. Oral Suspension—F D & C Red 3, Flavorings, Silica Gel, Sodium Benzoate, Sodium Citrate, Sucrose, and Xanthan Gum.

ACTIONS

PHARMACOLOGY

Amoxicillin is stable in the presence of gastric acid and may be given without regard to meals. It is rapidly absorbed after oral administration. It diffuses readily into most body tissues and fluids, with the exception of brain and spinal fluid, except when meninges are inflamed. The half-life of amoxicillin is 61.3 minutes. Most of the amoxicillin is excreted unchanged in the urine; its excretion can be delayed by concurrent administration of probenecid. Amoxicillin is not highly protein-bound. In blood serum, amoxicillin is approximately 20% protein-bound as compared to 60% for penicillin G. Orally administered doses of 250 mg and 500 mg amoxicillin capsules result in average peak blood levels one to two hours after administration in the range of 3.5 mcg/mL to 5.0 mcg/mL and 5.5 mcg/mL to 7.5 mcg/mL respectively. Orally administered doses of amoxicillin suspension 125 mg/5 mL and 250 mg/5 mL result in average peak blood levels one to two hours after administration in the range of 1.5 mcg/mL to 3.0 mcg/mL and 3.5 mcg/mL to 5.0 mcg/mL respectively. Amoxicillin chewable tablets, 125 mg and 250 mg, produced blood levels similar to those achieved with the corresponding doses of amoxicillin oral suspensions.

Detectable serum levels are observed up to 8 hours after an orally administered dose of amoxicillin. Following a 1 g dose and utilizing a special skin window technique to determine levels of the antibiotic, it was noted that therapeutic levels were found in the interstitial fluid. Approximately 60 percent of an orally administered dose of amoxicillin is excreted in the urine within six to eight hours.

MICROBIOLOGY:

AMOXIL (amoxicillin) is similar to ampicillin in its bactericidal action against susceptible organisms during the stage of active multiplication. It acts through the inhibition of biosynthesis of cell wall mucopeptide. *In vitro* studies have demonstrated the susceptibility of most strains of the following Gram-positive bacteria: alpha- and beta-hemolytic streptococci, *Diplococcus pneumoniae*, nonpenicillinase-producing staphylococci, and *Streptococcus faecalis*. It is active *in vitro* against many strains of *Haemophilus influenzae*, *Neisseria gonorrhoeae*, *Escherichia coli* and *Proteus mirabilis*. Because it does not resist destruction by penicillinase, it is not effective against penicillinase-producing bacteria, particularly resistant staphylococci. All strains of Pseudomonas and most strains of Klebsiella and Enterobacter are resistant.

DISC SUSCEPTIBILITY TESTS: Quantitative methods that require measurement of zone diameters give the most precise estimates of antibiotic susceptibility. One such procedure* has been recommended for use with discs for testing susceptibility to ampicillin-class antibiotics. Interpretations correlate diameters of the disc test with MIC values for amoxicillin. With this procedure, a report from the laboratory of "susceptible" indicates that the infecting organism is likely to respond to therapy. A report of "resistant" indicates that the infecting organism is not likely to respond to therapy. A report of "intermediate susceptibility" suggests that the organism would be susceptible if high dosage is used, or if the infection is confined to tissues and fluids (e.g., urine), in which high antibiotic levels are attained.

*Bauer, A. W., Kirby, W. M. M., Sherris, J. C., and Turck, M.: Antibiotic Testing by a Standardized Single Disc Method, Am. J. Clin. Pathol., 45:493, 1966. Standardized Disc Susceptibility Test, FEDERAL REGISTER 37:20527–29, 1972.

Continued on next page

Beecham Laboratories—Cont.

INDICATIONS

AMOXIL (amoxicillin) is indicated in the treatment of infections due to susceptible strains of the following:

Gram-negative organisms—*H. influenzae, E. coli, P. mirabilis* and *N. gonorrhoeae.*

Gram-positive organisms—Streptococci (including *Streptococcus faecalis*), *D. pneumoniae* and nonpenicillinase-producing staphylococci.

Therapy may be instituted prior to obtaining results from bacteriological and susceptibility studies to determine the causative organisms and their susceptibility to amoxicillin. Indicated surgical procedures should be performed.

CONTRAINDICATIONS

A history of allergic reaction to any of the penicillins is a contraindication.

WARNINGS

SERIOUS AND OCCASIONALLY FATAL HYPERSENSITIVITY (ANAPHYLACTOID) REACTIONS HAVE BEEN REPORTED IN PATIENTS ON PENICILLIN THERAPY. ALTHOUGH ANAPHYLAXIS IS MORE FREQUENT FOLLOWING PARENTERAL THERAPY, IT HAS OCCURRED IN PATIENTS ON ORAL PENICILLINS. THESE REACTIONS ARE MORE LIKELY TO OCCUR IN INDIVIDUALS WITH A HISTORY OF SENSITIVITY TO MULTIPLE ALLERGENS. THERE HAVE BEEN REPORTS OF INDIVIDUALS WITH A HISTORY OF PENICILLIN HYPERSENSITIVITY WHO HAVE EXPERIENCED SEVERE REACTIONS WHEN TREATED WITH CEPHALOSPORINS. BEFORE THERAPY WITH ANY PENICILLIN, CAREFUL INQUIRY SHOULD BE MADE CONCERNING PREVIOUS HYPERSENSITIVITY REACTIONS TO PENICILLINS, CEPHALOSPORINS, OR OTHER ALLERGENS. IF AN ALLERGIC REACTION OCCURS, APPROPRIATE THERAPY SHOULD BE INSTITUTED AND DISCONTINUANCE OF AMOXICILLIN THERAPY CONSIDERED. SERIOUS ANAPHYLACTOID REACTIONS REQUIRE IMMEDIATE EMERGENCY TREATMENT WITH EPINEPHRINE, OXYGEN, INTRAVENOUS STEROIDS, AND AIRWAY MANAGEMENT, INCLUDING INTUBATION, SHOULD ALSO BE ADMINISTERED AS INDICATED.

USAGE IN PREGNANCY

Safety for use in pregnancy has not been established.

PRECAUTIONS

As with any potent drug, periodic assessment of renal, hepatic and hematopoietic function should be made during prolonged therapy.

The possibility of superinfections with mycotic or bacterial pathogens should be kept in mind during therapy. If superinfections occur (usually involving Enterobacter, Pseudomonas or Candida), the drug should be discontinued and/or appropriate therapy instituted.

ADVERSE REACTIONS

As with other penicillins, it may be expected that untoward reactions will be essentially limited to sensitivity phenomena. They are more likely to occur in individuals who have previously demonstrated hypersensitivity to penicillins and in those with a history of allergy, asthma, hay fever or urticaria. The following adverse reactions have been reported as associated with the use of the penicillins:

Gastrointestinal: Nausea, vomiting and diarrhea.

Hypersensitivity Reactions: Erythematous maculopapular rashes and urticaria have been reported.

NOTE: Urticaria, other skin rashes and serum sickness-like reactions may be controlled with antihistamines and, if necessary, systemic corticosteroids. Whenever such reactions occur, amoxicillin should be discontinued unless, in the opinion of the physician, the condition being treated is life-threatening and amenable only to amoxicillin therapy.

Liver: A moderate rise in serum glutamic oxaloacetic transaminase (SGOT) has been noted, but the significance of this finding is unknown.

Hemic and Lymphatic Systems: Anemia, thrombocytopenia, thrombocytopenic purpura, eosinophilia, leukopenia and agranulocytosis have been reported during therapy with the penicillins. These reactions are usually reversible on discontinuation of therapy and are believed to be hypersensitivity phenomena.

Central Nervous System: Reversible hyperactivity, agitation, anxiety, insomnia, confusion, behavioral changes, and/or dizziness have been reported rarely.

DOSAGE AND ADMINISTRATION

Infections of the ear, nose and throat due to streptococci, pneumococci, nonpenicillinase-producing staphylococci and *H. influenzae;*

Infections of the genitourinary tract due to *E. coli, Proteus mirabilis* and *Streptococcus faecalis;*

Infections of the skin and soft-tissues due to streptococci, susceptible staphylococci and *E. coli.*

USUAL DOSAGE:

Adults: 250 mg every 8 hours.

Children: 20 mg/kg/day in divided doses every 8 hours.

Children weighing 20 kg or more should be dosed according to the adult recommendations.

In severe infections or those caused by less susceptible organisms:

500 mg every 8 hours for adults and 40 mg/kg/day in divided doses every 8 hours for children may be needed.

Infections of the lower respiratory tract due to streptococci, pneumococci, nonpenicillinase-producing staphylococci and *H. influenzae:*

USUAL DOSAGE:

Adults: 500 mg every 8 hours.

Children: 40 mg/kg/day in divided doses every 8 hours.

Children weighing 20 kg or more should be dosed according to the adult recommendations.

Gonorrhea, acute uncomplicated ano-genital and urethral infections due to *N. gonorrhoeae* (males and females):

USUAL DOSAGE:

Adults: 3 grams as a single oral dose.

Prepubertal children: 50 mg/kg amoxicillin combined with 25 mg/kg probenecid as a single dose.

NOTE: SINCE PROBENECID IS CONTRAINDICATED IN CHILDREN UNDER 2 YEARS, THIS REGIMEN SHOULD NOT BE USED IN THESE CASES.

Cases of gonorrhea with a suspected lesion of syphilis should have dark-field examinations before receiving amoxicillin, and monthly serological tests for a minimum of four months. Larger doses may be required for stubborn or severe infections.

The children's dosage is intended for individuals whose weight will not cause a dosage to be calculated greater than that recommended for adults.

It should be recognized that in the treatment of chronic urinary tract infections, frequent bacteriological and clinical appraisals are necessary. Smaller doses than those recommended above should not be used. Even higher doses may be needed at times. In stubborn infections, therapy may be required for several weeks. It may be necessary to continue clinical and/or bacteriological follow-up for several months after cessation of therapy. Except for gonorrhea, treatment should be continued for a minimum of 48 to 72 hours beyond the time that the patient becomes asymptomatic or evidence of bacterial eradication has been obtained. It is recommended that there be at least 10 days' treatment for any infection caused by hemolytic streptococci to prevent the occurrence of acute rheumatic fever or glomerulonephritis.

DOSAGE AND ADMINISTRATION OF PEDIATRIC DROPS

Usual dosage for all indications except infections of the lower respiratory tract:

Under 6 kg (13 lbs): 0.75 mL every 8 hours.

6–7 kg (13–15 lbs): 1.0 mL every 8 hours.

8 kg (16–18 lbs): 1.25 mL every 8 hours.

Infections of the lower respiratory tract:

Under 6 kg (13 lbs): 1.25 mL every 8 hours.

6–7 kg (13–15 lbs): 1.75 mL every 8 hours.

8 kg (16–18 lbs): 2.25 mL every 8 hours.

Children weighing more than 8 kg (18 lbs) should receive the appropriate dose of the Oral Suspension 125 mg or 250 mg/5 mL.

After reconstitution, the required amount of suspension should be placed directly onto the child's tongue for swallowing. Alternate means of administration are to add the required amount of suspension to formula, milk, fruit juice, water, ginger ale or cold drinks. These preparations should then be taken immediately. To be certain the child is receiving full dosage, such preparations should be consumed in entirety.

DIRECTIONS FOR MIXING ORAL SUSPENSION

Prepare suspension at time of dispensing as follows: Tap bottle until all powder flows freely. Add approximately ⅓ of the total amount of water for reconstitution (see table below) and shake vigorously to wet powder. Add remainder of the water and again shake vigorously.

125 mg per 5 mL

Bottle Size	Amount of Water Required for Reconstitution
80 mL	62 mL
100 mL	78 mL
150 mL	116 mL

Each teaspoonful (5 mL) will contain 125 mg amoxicillin.

125 mg unit dose   5 mL

250 mg per 5 mL

Bottle Size	Amount of Water Required for Reconstitution
80 mL	59 mL
100 mL	74 mL
150 mL	111 mL

Each teaspoonful (5 mL) will contain 250 mg amoxicillin.

250 mg unit dose   5 mL

DIRECTIONS FOR MIXING PEDIATRIC DROPS

Prepare pediatric drops at time of dispensing as follows: Add the required amount of water (see table below) to the bottle and shake vigorously. Each mL of suspension will then contain amoxicillin trihydrate equivalent to 50 mg amoxicillin.

Bottle Size	Amount of Water Required for Reconstitution
15 mL	12 mL
30 mL	23 mL

NOTE: SHAKE BOTH ORAL SUSPENSION AND PEDIATRIC DROPS WELL BEFORE USING. Keep bottle tightly closed. Any unused portion of the reconstituted suspension must be discarded after 14 days. Refrigeration preferable, but not required.

HOW SUPPLIED

AMOXIL (amoxicillin) **Capsules.** Each capsule contains 250 mg or 500 mg amoxicillin as the trihydrate.

250 mg/Capsule

NDC 0029-6006-30 ....bottles of 100
NDC 0029-6006-32 ....bottles of 500
NDC 0029-6006-31 ....unit dose carton of 100

500 mg/Capsule

NDC 0029-6007-30 ....bottles of 100
NDC 0029-6007-32 ....bottles of 500
NDC 0029-6007-31 ....unit dose cartons of 100

AMOXIL (amoxicillin) **Chewable Tablets.** Each tablet contains 125 mg or 250 mg amoxicillin as the trihydrate.

125 mg/Tablet

NDC 0029-6004-39 ....bottles of 60

250 mg/Tablet

NDC 0029-6005-30 ....bottles of 100

AMOXIL (amoxicillin) **for Oral Suspension.**

125 mg/5 mL

NDC 0029-6008-21 ....80 mL bottle
NDC 0029-6008-23 ....100 mL bottle
NDC 0029-6008-22 ....150 mL bottle

250 mg/5 mL

NDC 0029-6009-21 ....80 mL bottle
NDC 0029-6009-23 ....100 mL bottle
NDC 0029-6009-22 ....150 mL bottle

Each 5 mL of reconstituted suspension contains 125 mg or 250 mg amoxicillin as the trihydrate.

NDC 0029-6008-18 ....125 mg unit dose bottle
NDC 0029-6009-18 ....250 mg unit dose bottle

AMOXIL (amoxicillin) **Pediatric Drops for Oral Suspension.** Each mL of reconstituted suspension contains 50 mg amoxicillin as the trihydrate.

NDC 0029-6035-20 ....15 mL bottle
NDC 0029-6038-39 ....30 mL bottle

Rev. February, 1989

9416642

Shown in Product Identification Section, page 405

ANEXSIA® 5/500   Ⓒ
Hydrocodone Bitartrate and Acetaminophen Tablets

DESCRIPTION

Each tablet contains: hydrocodone bitartrate, 5 mg (**Warning:** May be habit forming); and acetaminophen, 500 mg. **Inactive Ingredients:** Magnesium Stearate, Pregelatinized Starch, Starch (corn), and Stearic Acid.

Hydrocodone bitartrate is an opioid analgesic and antitussive and occurs as fine, white crystals or as a crystalline powder. It is affected by light. The chemical name is: 4,5α-epoxy-3-methoxy-17-methylmorphinan-6-one tartrate (1:1) hydrate (2:5). Its structure is as follows:

$C_{18}H_{21}NO_3 \cdot C_4H_6O_6 \cdot 2\frac{1}{2}H_2O$ M.W. 494.50

Acetaminophen, 4'-hydroxyacetanilide, is a non-opiate, non-salicylate analgesic and antipyretic which occurs as a white, odorless crystalline powder possessing a slightly bitter taste. Its structure is as follows:

$C_8H_9NO_2$ M.W. 151.16

CLINICAL PHARMACOLOGY

Hydrocodone is a semisynthetic narcotic analgesic and antitussive with multiple actions qualitatively similar to those of codeine. Most of these involve the central nervous system and smooth muscle. The precise mechanism of action of hydrocodone and other opiates is not known, although it is believed to relate to the existence of opiate receptors in the central nervous system. In addition to analgesia, narcotics may produce drowsiness, changes in mood and mental clouding.

Radioimmunoassay techniques have recently been developed for the analysis of hydrocodone in human plasma. After a 10 mg oral dose of hydrocodone bitartrate, a mean peak serum drug level of 23.6 ng/mL and an elimination half-life of 3.8 hours were found.

The analgesic action of acetaminophen involves peripheral and central influences, but the specific mechanism is as yet undetermined. Antipyretic activity is mediated through hypothalamic heat regulating centers. Acetaminophen inhibits prostaglandin synthetase. Therapeutic doses of acetaminophen have negligible effects on the cardiovascular or respiratory systems; however, toxic doses may cause circulatory failure and rapid, shallow breathing. Acetaminophen is rapidly and almost completely absorbed from the gastrointestinal tract, producing maximum serum concentrations within 30 minutes to one hour. The plasma half-life in adults and children ranges from 0.90 hours to 3.25 hours with an average of approximately 2 hours. The drug distributes uniformly in most body fluids and is approximately 25% protein bound. Acetaminophen is conjugated in the liver, with less than 3% of the dose excreted unchanged in 24 hours. The primary metabolic pathway is conjugation to sulfate and glucuronide by-products. A minor oxidative pathway forms cysteine and mercapturic acid. These compounds are subsequently excreted by the kidneys into the urine.

INDICATIONS AND USAGE

For the relief of moderate to moderately severe pain.

CONTRAINDICATIONS

Hypersensitivity to acetaminophen or hydrocodone.

WARNINGS

Respiratory Depression: At high doses or in sensitive patients, hydrocodone may produce dose-related respiratory depression by acting directly on the brain stem respiratory center. Hydrocodone also affects the center that controls respiratory rhythm, and may produce irregular and periodic breathing.

Head Injury and Increased Intracranial Pressure: The respiratory depressant effects of narcotics and their capacity to elevate cerebrospinal fluid pressure may be markedly exaggerated in the presence of head injury, other intracranial lesions or a pre-existing increase in intracranial pressure. Furthermore, narcotics produce adverse reactions which may obscure the clinical course of patients with head injuries.

Acute Abdominal Conditions: The administration of narcotics may obscure the diagnosis or clinical course of patients with acute abdominal conditions.

PRECAUTIONS

Special Risk Patients: As with any narcotic analgesic agent, Hydrocodone Bitartrate and Acetaminophen Tablets should be used with caution in elderly or debilitated patients and those with severe impairment of hepatic or renal function, hypothyroidism, Addison's disease, prostatic hypertrophy or urethral stricture. The usual precautions should be observed and the possibility of respiratory depression should be kept in mind.

Information for Patients: Hydrocodone Bitartrate and Acetaminophen Tablets, like all narcotics, may impair the mental and/or physical abilities required for the performance of potentially hazardous tasks such as driving a car or operating machinery; patients should be cautioned accordingly.

Cough Reflex: Hydrocodone suppresses the cough reflex; as with all narcotics, caution should be exercised when Hydrocodone Bitartrate and Acetaminophen Tablets are used postoperatively and in patients with pulmonary disease.

Drug Interactions: Patients receiving other narcotic analgesics, antipsychotics, antianxiety agents, or other CNS depressants (including alcohol) concomitantly with hydrocodone and acetaminophen tablets may exhibit an additive CNS depression. When combined therapy is contemplated, the dose of one or both agents should be reduced.

The use of MAO inhibitors or tricyclic antidepressants with hydrocodone preparations may increase the effect of either the antidepressant or hydrocodone.

The concurrent use of anticholinergics with hydrocodone may produce paralytic ileus.

Usage in Pregnancy:

Teratogenic Effects: Pregnancy Category C. Hydrocodone has been shown to be teratogenic in hamsters when given in doses 700 times the human dose. There are no adequate and well-controlled studies in pregnant women. Hydrocodone Bitartrate and Acetaminophen Tablets should be used during pregnancy only if the potential benefit justifies the potential risk to the fetus.

Nonteratogenic Effects: Babies born to mothers who have been taking opioids regularly prior to delivery will be physically dependent. The withdrawal signs include irritability and excessive crying, tremors, hyperactive reflexes, increased respiratory rate, increased stools, sneezing, yawning, vomiting, and fever. The intensity of the syndrome does not always correlate with the duration of maternal opioid use or dose. There is no consensus on the best method of managing withdrawal. Chlorpromazine 0.7 to 1 mg/kg q6h, and paregoric 2 to 4 drops/kg q4h, have been used to treat with-

drawal symptoms in infants. The duration of therapy is 4 to 28 days, with the dosage decreased as tolerated.

Labor and Delivery: As with all narcotics, administration of Hydrocodone Bitartrate and Acetaminophen Tablets to the mother shortly before delivery may result in some degree of respiratory depression in the newborn, especially if higher doses are used.

Nursing Mothers: It is not known whether this drug is excreted in human milk. Because many drugs are excreted in human milk and because of the potential for serious adverse reactions in nursing infants from Hydrocodone Bitartrate and Acetaminophen Tablets, a decision should be made whether to discontinue nursing or to discontinue the drug, taking into account the importance of the drug to the mother.

Pediatric Use: Safety and effectiveness in children have not been established.

ADVERSE REACTIONS

The most frequently observed adverse reactions include lightheadedness, dizziness, sedation, nausea and vomiting. These effects seem to be more prominent in ambulatory than in nonambulatory patients and some of these adverse reactions may be alleviated if the patient lies down.

Other adverse reactions include:

Central Nervous System: Drowsiness, mental clouding, lethargy, impairment of mental and physical performance, anxiety, fear, dysphoria, psychic dependence, mood changes.

Gastrointestinal System: The antiemetic phenothiazines are useful in suppressing the nausea and vomiting which may occur (see above); however, some phenothiazine derivatives seem to be antianalgesic and to increase the amount of narcotic required to produce pain relief, while other phenothiazines reduce the amount of narcotic required to produce a given level of analgesia. Prolonged administration of Hydrocodone Bitartrate and Acetaminophen Tablets may produce constipation.

Genitourinary System: Ureteral spasm, spasm of vesical sphincters and urinary retention have been reported.

Respiratory Depression: Hydrocodone bitartrate may produce dose-related respiratory depression by acting directly on the brain stem respiratory center. Hydrocodone also affects the center that controls respiratory rhythm, and may produce irregular and periodic breathing. If significant respiratory depression occurs, it may be antagonized by the use of naloxone hydrochloride. Apply other supportive measures when indicated.

DRUG ABUSE AND DEPENDENCE

Hydrocodone Bitartrate and Acetaminophen Tablets are subject to the Federal Controlled Substance Act (Schedule III).

Psychic dependence, physical dependence, and tolerance may develop upon repeated administration of narcotics; therefore, Hydrocodone Bitartrate and Acetaminophen Tablets should be prescribed and administered with caution. However, psychic dependence is unlikely to develop when Hydrocodone Bitartrate and Acetaminophen Tablets are used for a short time for the treatment of pain.

Physical dependence, the condition in which continued administration of the drug is required to prevent the appearance of a withdrawal syndrome, assumes clinically significant proportions only after several weeks of continued narcotic use, although some mild degree of physical dependence may develop after a few days of narcotic therapy. Tolerance, in which increasingly large doses are required in order to produce the same degree of analgesia, is manifested initially by a shortened duration of analgesic effect, and subsequently by decreases in the intensity of analgesia. The rate of development of tolerance varies among patients.

OVERDOSAGE

Acetaminophen

Signs and Symptoms: In acute acetaminophen overdosage, dose-dependent, potentially fatal hepatic necrosis is the most serious adverse effect. Renal tubular necrosis, hypoglycemic coma, and thrombocytopenia may also occur.

In adults, hepatic toxicity has rarely been reported with acute overdoses of less than 10 grams and fatalities with less than 15 grams. Importantly, young children seem to be more resistant than adults to the hepatotoxic effect of an acetaminophen overdose. Despite this, the measures outlined below should be initiated in any adult or child suspected of having ingested an acetaminophen overdose.

Early symptoms following a potentially hepatotoxic overdose may include: nausea, vomiting, diaphoresis and general malaise. Clinical and laboratory evidence of hepatic toxicity may not be apparent until 48 to 72 hours post-ingestion.

Treatment: The stomach should be emptied promptly by lavage or by induction of emesis with syrup of ipecac. Patients' estimates of the quantity of a drug ingested are notoriously unreliable. Therefore, if an acetaminophen overdose is suspected, a serum acetaminophen assay should be obtained as early as possible, but no sooner than four hours following ingestion. Liver function studies should be obtained initially and repeated at 24-hour intervals.

The antidote, N-acetylcysteine, should be administered as early as possible, preferably within 16 hours of the overdose ingestion for optimal results, but in any case, within 24 hours. Following recovery, there are no residual, structural or functional hepatic abnormalities.

Hydrocodone

Signs and Symptoms: Serious overdose with hydrocodone is characterized by respiratory depression (a decrease in respiratory rate and/or tidal volume, Cheyne-Stokes respiration, cyanosis), extreme somnolence progressing to stupor or coma, skeletal muscle flaccidity, cold and clammy skin, and sometimes bradycardia and hypotension. In severe overdose, apnea, circulatory collapse, cardiac arrest and death may occur.

Treatment: Primary attention should be given to the re-establishment of adequate respiratory exchange through provision of a patent airway and the institution of assisted or controlled ventilation. The narcotic antagonist naloxone is a specific antidote against respiratory depression which may result from overdosage or unusual sensitivity to narcotics, including hydrocodone. Therefore, an appropriate dose of naloxone hydrochloride (see package insert) should be administered, preferably by the intravenous route, and simultaneously with efforts at respiratory resuscitation. Since the duration of action of hydrocodone may exceed that of the antagonist, the patient should be kept under continued surveillance and repeated doses of the antagonist should be administered as needed to maintain adequate respiration.

An antagonist should not be administered in the absence of clinically significant respiratory or cardiovascular depression. Oxygen, intravenous fluids, vasopressors and other supportive measures should be employed as indicated.

Gastric emptying may be useful in removing unabsorbed drug.

DOSAGE AND ADMINISTRATION

Dosage should be adjusted according to the severity of pain and the response of the patient. However, it should be kept in mind that tolerance to hydrocodone can develop with continued use and that the incidence of untoward effects is dose related.

The usual adult dosage is one or two tablets every four to six hours as needed for pain. The total 24 hour dose should not exceed 8 tablets.

HOW SUPPLIED

Hydrocodone Bitartrate and Acetaminophen Tablets
Each tablet contains: hydrocodone bitartrate 5 mg and acetaminophen 500 mg.
They are available as white, round bisected tablets debossed with a logo identified as BMP 207.
Bottles of 100 ....NDC 0029-1365-30
Storage: Store at controlled room temperature 15°–30°C. (59°–86°F.).
A Schedule III Narcotic.
0938010   Revised February, 1988
Shown in Product Identification Section, page 405

ANEXSIA® 7.5/650   (III)
Hydrocodone Bitartrate and Acetaminophen Tablets

DESCRIPTION

Each tablet contains: hydrocodone bitartrate, 7.5 mg (**Warning:** May be habit forming); and acetaminophen, 650 mg.
Inactive Ingredients: Magnesium Stearate, Pregelatinized Starch, Starch (corn), Stearic Acid, and FD&C Yellow No. 6.
Hydrocodone bitartrate is an opioid analgesic and antitussive and occurs as fine, white crystals or as a crystalline powder. It is affected by light. The chemical name is: 4,5α-epoxy-3-methoxy-17-methylmorphinan-6-one tartrate (1:1) hydrate (2:5). Its structure is as follows:

$C_{18}H_{21}NO_3 \cdot C_4H_6O_6 \cdot 2\frac{1}{2}H_2O$ M.W. 494.50

Acetaminophen, 4'-hydroxyacetanilide, is a nonopiate, non-salicylate analgesic and antipyretic which occurs as a white, odorless crystalline powder possessing a slightly bitter taste. Its structure is as follows:

$C_8H_9NO_2$ M.W. 151.16

Continued on next page

Beecham Laboratories—Cont.

CLINICAL PHARMACOLOGY

Hydrocodone is a semisynthetic narcotic analgesic and antitussive with multiple actions qualitatively similar to those of codeine. Most of these involve the central nervous system and smooth muscle. The precise mechanism of action of hydrocodone and other opiates is not known, although it is believed to relate to the existence of opiate receptors in the central nervous system. In addition to analgesia, narcotics may produce drowsiness, changes in mood and mental clouding.

Radioimmunoassay techniques have recently been developed for the analysis of hydrocodone in human plasma. After a 10 mg oral dose of hydrocodone bitartrate, a mean peak serum drug level of 23.6 ng/mL and an elimination half-life of 3.8 hours were found.

The analgesic action of acetaminophen involves peripheral and central influences, but the specific mechanism is as yet undetermined. Antipyretic activity is mediated through hypothalamic heat regulating centers. Acetaminophen inhibits prostaglandin synthetase. Therapeutic doses of acetaminophen have negligible effects on the cardiovascular or respiratory systems; however, toxic doses may cause circulatory failure and rapid, shallow breathing. Acetaminophen is rapidly and almost completely absorbed from the gastrointestinal tract, producing maximum serum concentrations within 30 minutes to one hour. The plasma half-life in adults and children ranges from 0.90 hours to 3.25 hours with an average of approximately 2 hours. The drug distributes uniformly in most body fluids and is approximately 25% protein bound. Acetaminophen is conjugated in the liver, with less than 3% of the dose excreted unchanged in 24 hours. The primary metabolic pathway is conjugation to sulfate and glucuronide by-products. A minor oxidative pathway forms cysteine and mercapturic acid. These compounds are subsequently excreted by the kidneys into the urine.

INDICATIONS AND USAGE

For the relief of moderate to moderately severe pain.

CONTRAINDICATIONS

Hypersensitivity to acetaminophen or hydrocodone.

WARNINGS

Respiratory Depression: At high doses or in sensitive patients, hydrocodone may produce dose-related respiratory depression by acting directly on brain stem respiratory centers. Hydrocodone also affects centers that control respiratory rhythm, and may produce irregular and periodic breathing.

Head Injury and Increased Intracranial Pressure: The respiratory depressant effects of narcotics and their capacity to elevate cerebrospinal fluid pressure may be markedly exaggerated in the presence of head injury, other intracranial lesions or a pre-existing increase in intracranial pressure. Furthermore, narcotics produce adverse reactions which may obscure the clinical course of patients with head injuries.

Acute Abdominal Conditions: The administration of narcotics may obscure the diagnosis or clinical course of patients with acute abdominal conditions.

PRECAUTIONS

Special Risk Patients: As with any narcotic analgesic agent, Hydrocodone Bitartrate and Acetaminophen Tablets should be used with caution in elderly or debilitated patients and those with severe impairment of hepatic or renal function, hypothyroidism, Addison's disease, prostatic hypertrophy or urethral stricture. The usual precautions should be observed and the possibility of respiratory depression should be kept in mind.

Information for Patients: Hydrocodone Bitartrate and Acetaminophen Tablets like all narcotics, may impair the mental and/or physical abilities required for the performance of potentially hazardous tasks such as driving a car or operating machinery; patients should be cautioned accordingly.

Cough Reflex: Hydrocodone suppresses the cough reflex; as with all narcotics, caution should be exercised when Hydrocodone Bitartrate and Acetaminophen Tablets are used postoperatively and in patients with pulmonary disease.

Drug Interactions: Patients receiving other narcotic analgesics, antipsychotics, antianxiety agents, or other CNS depressants (including alcohol) concomitantly with Hydrocodone Bitartrate and Acetaminophen tablets may exhibit an additive CNS depression. When combined therapy is contemplated, the dose of one or both agents should be reduced.

The use of MAO inhibitors or tricyclic antidepressants with hydrocodone preparations may increase the effect of either the antidepressant or hydrocodone.

The concurrent use of anticholinergics with hydrocodone may produce paralytic ileus.

Usage in Pregnancy:

Teratogenic Effects: Pregnancy Category C. Hydrocodone has been shown to be teratogenic in hamsters when given in doses 700 times the human dose. There are no adequate and well-controlled studies in pregnant women. Hydrocodone Bitartrate and Acetaminophen Tablets should be used during pregnancy only if the potential benefit justifies the potential risk to the fetus.

Nonteratogenic Effects: Babies born to mothers who have been taking opioids regularly prior to delivery will be physically dependent. The withdrawal signs include irritability and excessive crying, tremors, hyperactive reflexes, increased respiratory rate, increased stools, sneezing, yawning, vomiting, and fever. The intensity of the syndrome does not always correlate with the duration of maternal opioid use or dose. There is no consensus on the best method of managing withdrawal. Chlorpromazine 0.7 to 1 mg/kg q6h, and paregoric 2 to 4 drops/kg q4h, have been used to treat withdrawal symptoms in infants. The duration of therapy is 4 to 28 days, with the dosage decreased as tolerated.

Labor and Delivery: As with all narcotics, administration of Hydrocodone Bitartrate and Acetaminophen Tablets to the mother shortly before delivery may result in some degree of respiratory depression in the newborn, especially if higher doses are used.

Nursing Mothers: It is not known whether this drug is excreted in human milk. Because many drugs are excreted in human milk and because of the potential for serious adverse reactions in nursing infants from Hydrocodone Bitartrate and Acetaminophen Tablets, a decision should be made whether to discontinue nursing or to discontinue the drug, taking into account the importance of the drug to the mother.

Pediatric Use: Safety and effectiveness in children have not been established.

ADVERSE REACTIONS

The most frequently observed adverse reactions include lightheadedness, dizziness, sedation, nausea and vomiting. These effects seem to be more prominent in ambulatory than in nonambulatory patients and some of these adverse reactions may be alleviated if the patient lies down.

Other adverse reactions include:

Central Nervous System: Drowsiness, mental clouding, lethargy, impairment of mental and physical performance, anxiety, fear, dysphoria, dizziness, psychic dependence, mood changes.

Gastrointestinal System: The antiemetic phenothiazines are useful in suppressing the nausea and vomiting which may occur (see above); however, some phenothiazine derivatives seem to be antianalgesic and to increase the amount of narcotic required to produce pain relief, while other phenothiazines reduce the amount of narcotic required to produce a given level of analgesia. Prolonged administration of Hydrocodone Bitartrate and Acetaminophen Tablets may produce constipation.

Genitourinary System: Ureteral spasm, spasm of vesical sphincters and urinary retention have been reported.

Respiratory Depression: Hydrocodone bitartrate may produce dose-related respiratory depression by acting directly on the brain stem respiratory center. Hydrocodone also affects centers that control respiratory rhythm, and may produce irregular and periodic breathing. If significant respiratory depression occurs, it may be antagonized by the use of naloxone hydrochloride. Apply other supportive measures when indicated.

DRUG ABUSE AND DEPENDENCE

Hydrocodone Bitartrate and Acetaminophen Tablets are subject to the Federal Controlled Substance Act (Schedule III). Psychic dependence, physical dependence, and tolerance may develop upon repeated administration of narcotics; therefore, Hydrocodone Bitartrate and Acetaminophen Tablets should be prescribed and administered with caution. However, psychic dependence is unlikely to develop when Hydrocodone Bitartrate and Acetaminophen Tablets are used for a short time for the treatment of pain.

Physical dependence, the condition in which continued administration of the drug is required to prevent the appearance of a withdrawal syndrome, assumes clinically significant proportions only after several weeks of continued narcotic use, although some mild degree of physical dependence may develop after a few days of narcotic therapy. Tolerance, in which increasingly large doses are required in order to produce the same degree of analgesia, is manifested initially by a shortened duration of analgesic effect, and subsequently by decreases in the intensity of analgesia. The rate of development of tolerance varies among patients.

OVERDOSAGE

Acetaminophen

Signs and Symptoms: In acute acetaminophen overdosage, dose-dependent, potentially fatal hepatic necrosis is the most serious adverse effects. Renal tubular necrosis, hypoglycemic coma, and thrombocytopenia may also occur.

In adults, hepatic toxicity has rarely been reported with acute overdoses of less than 10 grams and fatalities with less than 15 grams. Importantly, young children seem to be more resistant than adults to the hepatotoxic effect of an acetaminophen overdose. Despite this, the measures outlined below should be initiated in any adult or child suspected of having ingested an acetaminophen overdose.

Early symptoms following a potentially hepatotoxic overdose may include: nausea, vomiting, diaphoresis and general malaise. Clinical and laboratory evidence of hepatic toxicity may not be apparent until 48 to 72 hours post-ingestion.

Treatment: The stomach should be emptied promptly by lavage or by induction of emesis with syrup of ipecac. Patients' estimates of the quantity of a drug ingested are notoriously unreliable. Therefore, if an acetaminophen overdose is suspected, a serum acetaminophen assay should be obtained as early as possible, but no sooner than four hours following ingestion. Liver function studies should be obtained initially and repeated at 24-hour intervals.

The antidote, N-acetylcysteine, should be administered as early as possible, preferably within 16 hours of the overdose ingestion for optimal results, but in any case, within 24 hours. Following recovery, there are no residual, structural or functional hepatic abnormalities.

Hydrocodone

Signs and Symptoms: Serious overdose with hydrocodone is characterized by respiratory depression (a decrease in respiratory rate and/or tidal volume, Cheyne-Stokes respiration, cyanosis), extreme somnolence progressing to stupor or coma, skeletal muscle flaccidity, cold and clammy skin, and sometimes bradycardia and hypotension. In severe overdose, apnea, circulatory collapse, cardiac arrest and death may occur.

Treatment: Primary attention should be given to the reestablishment of adequate respiratory exchange through provision of a patent airway and the institution of assisted or controlled ventilation. The narcotic antagonist naloxone is a specific antidote against respiratory depression which may result from overdosage or unusual sensitivity to narcotics, including hydrocodone. Therefore, an appropriate dose of naloxone hydrochloride (see package insert) should be administered, preferably by the intravenous route, and simultaneously with efforts at respiratory resuscitation. Since the duration of action of hydrocodone may exceed that of the antagonist, the patient should be kept under continued surveillance and repeated doses of the antagonist should be administered as needed to maintain adequate respiration.

An antagonist should not be administered in the absence of clinically significant respiratory or cardiovascular depression. Oxygen, intravenous fluids, vasopressors and other supportive measures should be employed as indicated.

Gastric emptying may be useful in removing unabsorbed drug.

DOSAGE AND ADMINISTRATION

Dosage should be adjusted according to the severity of pain and the response of the patient. However, it should be kept in mind that tolerance to hydrocodone can develop with continued use and that the incidence of untoward effects is dose related.

The usual adult dosage is one tablet every four to six hours as needed for pain. The total 24 hour dose should not exceed 6 tablets.

HOW SUPPLIED

Hydrocodone Bitartrate and Acetaminophen Tablets
Each tablet contains: hydrocodone bitartrate 7.5 mg and acetaminophen 650 mg.
They are available as peach colored, capsule shaped tablets with a bisecting line and debossed with a BMP 188 identification number.
Bottles of 100 ....*NDC* 0029-1362-30
Storage: Store at controlled room temperature 15°–30°C. (59°–86°F.)
A Schedule III Narcotic.
0938000   Revised January, 1988

Shown in Product Identification Section, page 405

AUGMENTIN®   ℞
(amoxicillin/clavulanate potassium)
Tablets, Powder for Oral Suspension
and Chewable Tablets

DESCRIPTION

AUGMENTIN is an oral antibacterial combination consisting of the semisynthetic antibiotic amoxicillin and the β-lactamase inhibitor, clavulanate potassium (the potassium salt of clavulanic acid). Amoxicillin is an analog of ampicillin, derived from the basic penicillin nucleus, 6-aminopenicillanic acid. Chemically, amoxicillin is D-(-)-α-amino-p-hydroxybenzyl-penicillin trihydrate and may be represented structurally as:

Clavulanic acid is produced by the fermentation of *Streptomyces clavuligerus*. It is a β-lactam structurally related to the penicillins and possesses the ability to inactivate a wide variety of β-lactamases by blocking the active sites of these enzymes. Clavulanic acid is particularly active against the clinically important plasmid mediated β-lactamases frequently responsible for transferred drug resistance to penicillins and cephalosporins. Chemically clavulanate potassium is potassium Z-(3R, 5R)-2-(β-hydroxyethylidene) clavam-3-carboxylate and may be represented structurally as:

Inactive Ingredients: Tablets—Colloidal Silicon Dioxide, Ethyl Cellulose, Hydroxypropyl Cellulose, Hydroxypropyl Methylcellulose, Magnesium Stearate, Microcrystalline Cellulose, Sodium Starch Glycolate and Titanium Dioxide. Powder for Oral Suspension—Colloidal Silicon Dioxide, Flavorings, Mannitol, Silica Gel, Sodium Saccharin, Succinic Acid and Xanthan Gum. Chewable Tablets—Colloidal Silcon Dioxide, D & C Yellow No. 10, Glycine, Magnesium Stearate and Mannitol.

AUGMENTIN is available in '250' and '500' white film-coated tablets and '125' and '250' chewable tablets, and '125' banana flavored and '250' orange flavored oral suspensions. Each AUGMENTIN '250' and '500' tablet contains 250 mg and 500 mg amoxicillin as the trihydrate, respectively, together with 125 mg clavulanic acid as the potassium salt. Each '125' chewable tablet and each teaspoonful (5 mL) of reconstituted AUGMENTIN '125' oral suspension contain 125 mg amoxicillin and 31.25 mg clavulanic acid as the potassium salt while each '250' chewable tablet and each 5 mL of reconstituted AUGMENTIN '250' oral suspension contain 250 mg amoxicillin and 62.5 mg clavulanic acid as the potassium salt.

Each AUGMENTIN tablet contains 0.63 mEq potassium. Each '125' chewable tablet and each 5 mL of reconstituted AUGMENTIN '125' oral suspension contain 0.16 mEq potassium. Each '250' chewable tablet and each 5 mL of reconstituted AUGMENTIN '250' oral suspension contain 0.32 mEq potassium.

CLINICAL PHARMACOLOGY

Amoxicillin and clavulanate potassium are well absorbed from the gastrointestinal tract after oral administration of AUGMENTIN. AUGMENTIN is stable in the presence of gastric acid and may be given without regard to meals.

Oral administration of one AUGMENTIN '250' or AUGMENTIN '500' tablet provides average peak serum concentrations one to two hours after dosing of 4.4 mcg/mL and 7.6 mcg/mL, respectively, for amoxicillin and 2.3 mcg/mL for clavulanic acid. The areas under the serum concentration curves obtained during the first 6 hours after dosing were 11.4 mcg/mL.hr and 20.2 mcg/mL.hr for amoxicillin, respectively, when one AUGMENTIN '250' or '500' tablet was administered to adult volunteers. The corresponding area under the serum concentration curve for clavulanic acid was 5 mcg/mL.hr. Oral administration of 5 mL of AUGMENTIN '250' suspension or equivalent dose of 10 mL of AUGMENTIN '125' suspension provides average peak serum concentrations approximately one hour after dosing of 6.9 mcg/mL for amoxicillin and 1.6 mcg/mL for clavulanic acid. The areas under the serum concentration curves obtained during the first 6 hours after dosing were 12.6 mcg/mL.hr for amoxicillin and 2.9 mcg/mL.hr for clavulanic acid when 5 mL of AUGMENTIN '250' suspension or equivalent dose of 10 mL of AUGMENTIN '125' suspension was administered to adult volunteers. One AUGMENTIN '250' chewable tablet or two AUGMENTIN '125' chewable tablets are equivalent to 5 mL of AUGMENTIN '250' suspension and provide similar serum levels of amoxicillin and clavulanic acid.

Amoxicillin serum concentrations achieved with AUGMENTIN are similar to those produced by the oral administration of equivalent doses of amoxicillin alone. The half life of amoxicillin after the oral administration of AUGMENTIN is 1.3 hours and that of clavulanic acid is 1.0 hour.

Approximately 50–70% of the amoxicillin and approximately 25–40% of the clavulanic acid are excreted unchanged in urine during the first six hours after administration of a single AUGMENTIN '250' or '500' tablet or 10 mL of AUGMENTIN '250' suspension.

Concurrent administration of probenecid delays amoxicillin excretion but does not delay renal excretion of clavulanic acid.

Neither component in AUGMENTIN is highly protein-bound; clavulanic acid has been found to be approximately 30% bound to human serum and amoxicillin approximately 20% bound.

Amoxicillin diffuses readily into most body tissues and fluids with the exception of the brain and spinal fluids. The results of experiments involving the administration of clavulanic acid to animals suggest that this compound, like amoxicillin, is well distributed in body tissues.

Two hours after oral administration of a single 35 mg/kg dose of AUGMENTIN suspension to fasting children, average concentrations of 3.0 mcg/mL of amoxicillin and 0.5 mcg/mL of clavulanic acid were detected in middle ear effusions.

Recommended AUGMENTIN Susceptibility Ranges[1,2]

ORGANISMS	RESISTANT	INTERMEDIATE	SUSCEPTIBLE	MIC[3] CORRELATES mcg/mL	
				R	S
Gram Negative Enteric Bacteria	≤13 mm	14–17 mm	≥18 mm	≥32/16	≤8/4
Staphylococcus[4] and Hemophilus spp	≤19 mm	—	≥20 mm		≤4/2 ≤4/2

Microbiology: Amoxicillin is a semisynthetic antibiotic with a broad spectrum of bactericidal activity against many Gram-positive and Gram-negative microorganisms. Amoxicillin is, however, susceptible to degradation by β-lactamases and therefore the spectrum of activity does not include organisms which produce these enzymes.

Clavulanic acid is a β-lactam, structurally related to the penicillins, which possesses the ability to inactivate a wide range of β-lactamase enzymes commonly found in microorganisms resistant to penicillins and cephalosporins. In particular, it has good activity against the clinically important plasmid mediated β-lactamases frequently responsible for transferred drug resistance.

The formulation of amoxicillin with clavulanic acid in AUGMENTIN protects amoxicillin from degradation by β-lactamase enzymes and effectively extends the antibiotic spectrum of amoxicillin to include many bacteria normally resistant to amoxicillin and other β-lactam antibiotics. Thus AUGMENTIN possesses the distinctive properties of a broad spectrum antibiotic and a β-lactamase inhibitor.

While *in vitro* studies have demonstrated the susceptibility of most strains of the following organisms, clinical efficacy for infections other than those included in the Indications and Usage section has not been documented.

GRAM-POSITIVE BACTERIA: *Staphylococcus aureus* (β-lactamase and non-β-lactamase producing), *Staphylococcus epidermidis* (β-lactamase and non-β-lactamase producing), *Staphylococcus saprophyticus* (β-lactamase and non-β-lactamase producing), *Streptococcus faecalis** (Enterococcus), *Streptococcus pneumoniae** (D. pneumoniae), *Streptococcus pyogenes**, *Streptococcus viridans**

ANAEROBES: *Clostridium* species*, *Peptococcus* species*, *Peptostreptococcus* species*

* These are non-β-lactamase producing strains and therefore are susceptible to amoxicillin alone.

GRAM-NEGATIVE BACTERIA: *Hemophilus influenzae* (β-lactamase and non-β-lactamase producing), *Branhamella catarrhalis* (*Neisseria catarrhalis*) (β-lactamase and non-β-lactamase producing); *Escherichia coli* (β-lactamase and non-β-lactamase producing), *Klebsiella* species (All known strains are β-lactamase producing), *Enterobacter* species (Although most strains of *Enterobacter* species are resistant *in vitro*, clinical efficacy has been demonstrated with AUGMENTIN in urinary tract infections caused by these organisms.), *Proteus mirabilis* (β-lactamase and non-β-lactamase producing), *Proteus vulgaris* (β-lactamase and non-β-lactamase producing), *Neisseria gonorrhoeae* (β-lactamase and non-β-lactamase producing), *Legionella* species (β-lactamase and non-β-lactamase producing).

ANAEROBES: *Bacteroides* species, including *B. fragilis* (β-lactamase and non-β-lactamase producing).

SUSCEPTIBILITY TESTING

Diffusion Technique: For Kirby-Bauer method of susceptibility testing, a 30 mcg AUGMENTIN (20 mcg amoxicillin + 10 mcg clavulanic acid) diffusion disk should be used. With this procedure, a report from the laboratory of "Susceptible" indicates that the infecting organism is likely to respond to AUGMENTIN therapy and a report of "Resistant" indicates that the infecting organism is not likely to respond to therapy. An "intermediate susceptibility" report suggests that the infecting organism would be susceptible to AUGMENTIN if the higher dosage is used or if the infection is confined to tissues or fluids (e.g. urine) in which high antibiotic levels are attained.

Dilution Techniques: Broth or agar dilution methods may be used to determine the minimal inhibitory concentration (MIC) value for susceptibility of bacterial isolates to AUGMENTIN. Tubes should be inoculated to contain 10^4 to 10^5 organisms/mL or plates "spotted" with 10^3 to 10^4 organisms. The recommended dilution method employs a constant amoxicillin/clavulanic acid ratio of 2 to 1 in all tubes with increasing concentrations of amoxicillin. MIC's are reported in terms of amoxicillin concentration in the presence of clavulanic acid at a constant 2 parts amoxicillin to 1 part clavulanic acid.

[See table above].

[1] The non-β-lactamase-producing organisms which are normally susceptible to ampicillin, such as *Streptococci*, will have similar zone sizes as for ampicillin disks.

[2] The quality control cultures should have the following assigned daily ranges for AUGMENTIN:

		Disks	MIC Range (mcg/mL)
E. coli	(ATCC 25922)	19–25 mm	2/1–8/4
S. aureus	(ATCC 25923)	28–36 mm	0.25/0.12–0.5/0.25
E. coli	(ATCC 35218)	18–22 mm	4/2–16/8

[3] Expressed as concentration of amoxicillin/clavulanic acid

[4] Organisms which show susceptibility to AUGMENTIN but are resistant to methicillin/oxacillin should be considered resistant.

INDICATIONS AND USAGE

AUGMENTIN is indicated in the treatment of infections caused by susceptible strains of the designated organisms in the conditions listed below:

Lower Respiratory Infections—caused by β-lactamase producing strains of *Hemophilus influenzae* and *Branhamella catarrhalis*.

Otitis Media—caused by β-lactamase producing strains of *Hemophilus influenzae* and *Branhamella catarrhalis*.

Sinusitis—caused by β-lactamase producing strains of *Hemophilus influenzae* and *Branhamella catarrhalis*.

Skin and Skin Structure Infections—caused by β-lactamase producing strains of *Staphylococcus aureus*, *Escherichia coli*, and *Klebsiella* spp.

Urinary Tract Infections—caused by β-lactamase producing strains of *Escherichia coli*, *Klebsiella* spp. and *Enterobacter* spp.

While AUGMENTIN is indicated only for the conditions listed above, infections caused by ampicillin susceptible organisms are also amenable to AUGMENTIN treatment due to its amoxicillin content. Therefore, mixed infections caused by ampicillin susceptible organisms and β-lactamase producing organisms susceptible to AUGMENTIN should not require the addition of another antibiotic.

Bacteriological studies, to determine the causative organisms and their susceptibility to AUGMENTIN, should be performed together with any indicated surgical procedures. Therapy may be instituted prior to obtaining the results from bacteriological and susceptibility studies to determine the causative organisms and their susceptibility to AUGMENTIN when there is reason to believe the infection may involve any of the β-lactamase producing organisms listed above. Once the results are known, therapy should be adjusted, if appropriate.

CONTRAINDICATIONS

A history of allergic reactions to any penicillin is a contraindication.

WARNINGS

SERIOUS AND OCCASIONALLY FATAL HYPERSENSITIVITY (ANAPHYLACTOID) REACTIONS HAVE BEEN REPORTED IN PATIENTS ON PENICILLIN THERAPY. ALTHOUGH ANAPHYLAXIS IS MORE FREQUENT FOLLOWING PARENTERAL THERAPY, IT HAS OCCURRED IN PATIENTS ON ORAL PENICILLINS. THESE REACTIONS ARE MORE LIKELY TO OCCUR IN INDIVIDUALS WITH A HISTORY OF PENICILLIN HYPERSENSITIVITY AND/OR A HISTORY OF SENSITIVITY TO MULTIPLE ALLERGENS. THERE HAVE BEEN REPORTS OF INDIVIDUALS WITH A HISTORY OF PENICILLIN HYPERSENSITIVITY WHO HAVE EXPERIENCED SEVERE REACTIONS WHEN TREATED WITH CEPHALOSPORINS. BEFORE INITIATING THERAPY WITH ANY PENICILLIN, CAREFUL INQUIRY SHOULD BE MADE CONCERNING PREVIOUS HYPERSENSITIVITY REACTIONS TO PENICILLINS, CEPHALOSPORINS, OR OTHER ALLERGENS. IF AN ALLERGIC REACTION OCCURS, AUGMENTIN SHOULD BE DISCONTINUED AND THE APPROPRIATE THERAPY INSTITUTED. **SERIOUS ANAPHYLACTOID REACTIONS REQUIRE IMMEDIATE EMERGENCY**

Continued on next page

Beecham Laboratories—Cont.

TREATMENT WITH EPINEPHRINE. OXYGEN, INTRAVE-NOUS STEROIDS, AND AIRWAY MANAGEMENT, IN-CLUDING INTUBATION, SHOULD ALSO BE ADMINIS-TERED AS INDICATED.

PRECAUTIONS

General: While AUGMENTIN possesses the characteristic low toxicity of the penicillin group of antibiotics, periodic assessment of organ system functions, including renal, hepatic and hematopoietic function is advisable during prolonged therapy.

A high percentage of patients with mononucleosis who receive ampicillin develop a skin rash. Thus, ampicillin class antibiotics should not be administered to patients with mononucleosis.

The possibility of superinfections with mycotic or bacterial pathogens should be kept in mind during therapy. If superinfections occur (usually involving *Pseudomonas* or *Candida*), the drug should be discontinued and/or appropriate therapy instituted.

Drug Interactions: Probenecid decreases the renal tubular secretion of amoxicillin. Concurrent use with AUGMENTIN may result in increased and prolonged blood levels of amoxicillin.

The concurrent administration of allopurinol and ampicillin increases substantially the incidence of rashes in patients receiving both drugs as compared to patients receiving ampicillin alone. It is not known whether this potentiation of ampicillin rashes is due to allopurinol or the hyperuricemia present in these patients. There are no data with AUGMENTIN and allopurinol administered concurrently.

AUGMENTIN should not be co-administered with ANTA-BUSE® (disulfiram).

Drug/Laboratory Test Interactions: Oral administraion of AUGMENTIN will result in high urine concentrations of amoxicillin. High urine concentrations of ampicillin may result in false positive reactions when testing for the presence of glucose in urine using Clinitest™, Benedict's Solution or Fehling's Solution. Since this effect may also occur with amoxicillin and therefore AUGMENTIN, it is recommended that glucose tests based on enzymatic glucose oxidase reactions (such as Clinistix™ or Testape™) be used. Following administration of ampicillin to pregnant women a transient decrease in plasma concentration of total conjugated estriol, estriol-glucuronide, conjugated estrone and estradiol has been noted. This effect may also occur with amoxicillin and therefore AUGMENTIN.

Carcinogenesis, Mutagenesis, Impairment of Fertility: Longterm studies in animals have not been performed to evaluate carcinogenic or mutagenic potential.

Pregnancy (Category B): Reproduction studies have been performed in mice and rats at doses up to ten (10) times the human dose and have revealed no evidence of impaired fertility or harm to the fetus due to AUGMENTIN. There are, however, no adequate and well-controlled studies in pregnant women. Because animal reproduction studies are not always predictive of human response, this drug should be used during pregnancy only if clearly needed.

Labor and Delivery: Oral ampicillin class antibiotics are generally poorly absorbed during labor. Studies in guinea pigs have been shown that intravenous administration of ampicillin decreased the uterine tone, frequency of contractions, height of contractions and duration of contractions. However, it is not known whether the use of AUGMENTIN in humans during labor or delivery has immediate or delayed adverse effects on the fetus, prolongs the duration of labor or increases the likelihood that forceps delivery or other obstetrical intervention or resuscitation of the newborn will be necessary.

Nursing Mothers: Ampicillin class antibiotics are excreted in the milk; therefore, caution should be exercised when AUGMENTIN is administered to a nursing woman.

ADVERSE REACTIONS

AUGMENTIN is generally well tolerated. The majority of side effects observed in clinical trials were of a mild and transient nature and less than 3% of patients discontinued therapy because of drug related side effects. The most frequently reported adverse effects were diarrhea/loose stools (9%), nausea (3%), skin rashes and urticaria (3%), vomiting (1%), and vaginitis (1%). The overall incidence of side effects, and in particular diarrhea, increased with the higher recommended dose. Other less frequently reported reactions include: abdominal discomfort, flatulence and headache.

The following adverse reactions have been reported for ampicillin class antibiotics:

Gastrointestinal: Diarrhea, nausea, vomiting, indigestion, gastritis, stomatitis, glossitis, black "hairy" tongue, enterocolitis and pseudomembraneous colitis.

Hypersensitivity reactions: Skin rashes, urticaria, angioedema, serum sickness-like reactions (urticaria or skin rash accompanied by arthritis, arthralgia, myalgia, and frequently fever), erythema multiforme (rarely Stevens-John-

son Syndrome), and an occasional case of exfoliative dermatitis have been reported. These reactions may be controlled with antihistamines and, if necessary, systemic corticosteroids. Whenever such reactions occur, the drug should be discontinued, unless the opinion of the physician dictates otherwise. Serious and occasional fatal hypersensitivity (anaphylactic) reactions can occur with oral penicillin (See Warnings).

Liver: A moderate rise in SGOT and/or SGPT has been noted in patients treated with ampicillin class antibiotics as well as with AUGMENTIN, but the significance of these findings is unknown. As with some other penicillins, and some cephalosporins, transient hepatitis and cholestatic jaundice have been reported rarely.

Hemic and Lymphatic Systems: Anemia, thrombocytopenia, thrombocytopenic purpura, eosinophilia, leukopenia and agranulocytosis have been reported during therapy with penicillins. These reactions are usually reversible on discontinuation of therapy and are believed to be hypersensitivity phenomena. A slight thrombocytosis was noted in less than 1% of the patients treated with AUGMENTIN.

Central Nervous System: Reversible hyperactivity, agitation, anxiety, insomnia, confusion, behaviorial changes, and/or dizziness have been reported rarely.

OVERDOSAGE

Amoxicillin may be removed from circulation by hemodialysis.

The molecular weight, degree of protein binding and pharmacokinetic profile of clavulanic acid together with information from a single patient with renal insufficiency all suggest that this compound may also be removed by hemodialysis.

DOSAGE AND ADMINISTRATION

Dosage:

Adults: The usual adult dose is one AUGMENTIN '250' tablet every eight hours. For more severe infections and infections of the respiratory tract, the dose should be one AUGMENTIN '500' tablet every eight hours.

Since both the AUGMENTIN '250' and '500' tablets contain the same amount of clavulanic acid (125 mg, as the potassium salt), two AUGMENTIN '250' tablets are not equivalent to one AUGMENTIN '500' tablet. Therefore, two AUGMENTIN '250' tablets should not be substituted for one AUGMENTIN '500' tablet for treatment of more severe infections.

Children: The usual dose is 20 mg/kg/day, based on amoxicillin component, in divided doses every eight hours. For otitis media, sinusitis and lower respiratory infections, the dose should be 40 mg/kg/day, based on the amoxicillin component, in divided doses every eight hours. Severe infections should be treated with the higher recommended dose.

Children weighing 40 kg and more should be dosed according to the adult recommendations.

DIRECTIONS FOR MIXING ORAL SUSPENSION

Prepare a suspension at time of dispensing as follows: Tap bottle until all the powder flows freely. Add approximately 2/3 of the total amount of water for reconstitution (see table below) and shake vigorously to suspend powder. Add remainder of the water and again shake vigorously.

AUGMENTIN '125' Suspension

Bottle Size	Amount of Water Required for Reconstitution
75 mL	67 mL
150 mL	134 mL

Each teaspoonful (5 mL) will contain 125 mg amoxicillin and 31.25 mg of clavulanic acid as the potassium salt.

AUGMENTIN '250' Suspension

Bottle Size	Amount of Water Required for Reconstitution
75 mL	65 mL
150 mL	130 mL

Each teaspoonful (5 mL) will contain 250 mg amoxicillin and 62.5 mg of clavulanic acid as the potassium salt.

Note: SHAKE ORAL SUSPENSION WELL BEFORE USING.

Reconstituted suspension must be stored under refrigeration and discarded after 10 days.

Administration: The absorption of AUGMENTIN is unaffected by food. Therefore, AUGMENTIN may be administered without regard to meals.

HOW SUPPLIED

AUGMENTIN '250' TABLETS: Each white oval filmcoated tablet, debossed with AUGMENTIN on one side and 250/125 on the other side, contains 250 mg amoxicillin as the trihydrate and 125 mg clavulanic acid as the potassium salt.

NDC 0029-6075-27 .... bottles of 30
NDC 0029-6075-31 ....Unit Dose (10×10) 100 tablets

AUGMENTIN '500' TABLETS: Each white oval filmcoated tablet, debossed with AUGMENTIN on one side and 500/125 on the other side, contains 500 mg amoxicillin as the trihydrate and 125 mg clavulanic acid as the potassium salt.

NDC 0029-6080-27 .... bottles of 30
NDC 0029-6080-31 ....Unit Dose (10×10) 100 tablets

AUGMENTIN '125' FOR ORAL SUSPENSION: Each 5 mL of reconstituted banana flavored suspension contains 125 mg amoxicillin and 31.25 mg clavulanic acid as the potassium salt.

NDC 0029-6085-39 .... 75 mL bottle
NDC 0029-6085-22 .... 150 mL bottle

AUGMENTIN '250' FOR ORAL SUSPENSION: Each 5 mL of reconstituted orange flavored suspension contains 250 mg amoxicillin and 62.5 mg clavulanic acid as the potassium salt.

NDC 0029-6090-39 .... 75 mL bottle
NDC 0029-6090-22 .... 150 mL bottle

AUGMENTIN '125' CHEWABLE TABLETS: Each yellow mottled round tablet, debossed with BMP 189, contains 125 mg amoxicillin as the trihydrate and 31.25 mg clavulanic acid as the potassium salt.

NDC 0029-6073-47 ....carton of 30 (5×6) tablets

AUGMENTIN '250' CHEWABLE TABLETS: Each yellow mottled round tablet, debossed with BMP 190, contains 250 mg amoxicillin as the trihydrate and 62.5 mg clavulanic acid as the potassium salt.

NDC 0029-6074-47 ....carton of 30 (5×6) tablets

REVISED DECEMBER, 1988
9417094

Shown in Product Identification Section, page 405

BACTROBAN®   ℞
(mupirocin)
Ointment 2%
For Dermatologic Use

DESCRIPTION

Each gram of BACTROBAN® Ointment 2% contains 20 mg mupirocin in a bland water miscible ointment base consisting of polyethylene glycol 400 and polyethylene glycol 3350 (polyethylene glycol ointment, N.F.). Mupirocin is a naturally-occurring antibiotic. The chemical name is 9-4-[5S-(2S,3S-epoxy-5S-hydroxy-4S-methylhexyl)-3R, 4R-dihydroxytetrahydropyran-2S-yl]-3-methylbut-2(E)-enoyloxy-nonanoic acid. The chemical structure is:

mupirocin

CLINICAL PHARMACOLOGY

Mupirocin is produced by fermentation of the organism *Pseudomonas fluorescens*. Mupirocin inhibits bacterial protein synthesis by reversibly and specifically binding to bacterial isoleucyl transfer-RNA synthetase. Due to this mode of action, mupirocin shows no cross resistance with chloramphenicol, erythromycin, fusidic acid, gentamicin, lincomycin, methicillin, neomycin, novobiocin, penicillin, streptomycin, and tetracycline.

Application of ^{14}C-labeled mupirocin ointment to the lower arm of normal male subjects followed by occlusion for 24 hours showed no measurable systemic absorption, (<1.1 nanogram mupirocin per milliliter of whole blood). Measurable radioactivity was present in the stratum corneum of these subjects 72 hours after application.

Microbiology: The following bacteria are susceptible to the action of mupirocin *in vitro:* the aerobic isolates of *Staphylococcus aureus* (including methicillin-resistant and β-lactamase producing strains), *Staphylococcus epidermidis, Staphylococcus saprophyticus,* and *Streptococcus pyogenes.*

Only the organisms listed in the **INDICATIONS AND USAGE** section have been shown to be clinically susceptible to mupirocin.

INDICATIONS AND USAGE

BACTROBAN® (mupirocin) Ointment is indicated for the topical treatment of impetigo due to: *Staphylococcus aureus,* beta hemolytic Streptococcus*, and *Streptococcus pyogenes.*

* Efficacy for this organism in this organ system was studied in fewer than ten infections.

CONTRAINDICATIONS

This drug is contraindicated in individuals with a history of sensitivity reactions to any of its components.

WARNINGS

BACTROBAN® Ointment is not for ophthalmic use.

PRECAUTIONS

If a reaction suggesting sensitivity or chemical irritation should occur with the use of BACTROBAN® Ointment, treatment should be discontinued and appropriate alternative therapy for the infection instituted.

As with other antibacterial products prolonged use may result in overgrowth of nonsusceptible organisms, including fungi.

Pregnancy category B: Reproduction studies have been performed in rats and rabbits at systemic doses, i.e., orally, subcutaneously, and intramuscularly, up to 100 times the human topical dose and have revealed no evidence of impaired fertility or harm to the fetus due to mupirocin. There are, however, no adequate and well-controlled studies in pregnant women. Because animal studies are not always predictive of human response, this drug should be used during pregnancy only if clearly needed.

Nursing mothers: It is not known whether BACTROBAN® is present in breast milk. Nursing should be temporarily discontinued while using BACTROBAN®.

ADVERSE REACTIONS

The following local adverse reactions have been reported in connection with the use of BACTROBAN® Ointment: burning, stinging, or pain in 1.5% of patients; itching in 1% of patients; rash, nausea, erythema, dry skin, tenderness, swelling, contact dermatitis, and increased exudate in less than 1% of patients.

DOSAGE AND ADMINISTRATION

A small amount of BACTROBAN® Ointment should be applied to the affected area three times daily. The area treated may be covered with a gauze dressing if desired. Patients not showing a clinical response within 3 to 5 days should be re-evaluated.

HOW SUPPLIED

BACTROBAN® (mupirocin) Ointment 2% is supplied in 15 gram tubes.
(NDC # 0029-1525-22)
Store between 15° and 30°C (59° and 86°F).
REVISED FEB., 1988
0938020

Shown in Product Identification Section, page 405

FASTIN® Capsules
[fǎs 'tĭn]
(phentermine hydrochloride)

DESCRIPTION

Each FASTIN (phentermine hydrochloride) capsule contains phentermine hydrochloride, 30 mg (equivalent to 24 mg Phentermine).

Phentermine hydrochloride is a white crystalline powder, very soluble in water and alcohol. Chemically, the product is phenyl-tertiary-butylamine hydrochloride. *Inactive Ingredients:* FD&C Blue 1, Methylcellulose, Polyethylene Glycol, Starch, Titanium Dioxide, Sucrose and Invert Sugar. The branding ink used on the gelatin capsules contains: Ethyl Alcohol, F D & C Blue 1 Aluminum Lake, Isopropyl Alcohol, n-Butyl Alcohol, Propylene Glycol, Pharmaceutical Shellac (modified) or Refined Shellac (Food Grade).

ACTIONS

FASTIN is a sympathomimetic amine with pharmacologic activity similar to the prototype drugs of this class used in obesity, the amphetamines. Actions include central nervous system stimulation and elevation of blood pressure. Tachyphylaxis and tolerance have been demonstrated with all drugs of this class in which these phenomena have been looked for.

Drugs of this class used in obesity are commonly known as "anorectics" or "anorexigenics." It has not been established that the action of such drugs in treating obesity is primarily one of appetite suppression. Other central nervous system actions, or metabolic effects may be involved, for example. Adult obese subjects instructed in dietary management and treated with "anorectic" drugs, lose more weight on the average than those treated with placebo and diet, as determined in relatively short-term clinical trials.

The magnitude of increased weight loss of drug-treated patients over placebo-treated patients is only a fraction of a pound a week. The rate of weight loss is greatest in the first weeks of therapy for both drug and placebo subjects and tends to decrease in succeeding weeks. The possible origins of the increased weight loss due to the various drug effects are not established. The amount of weight loss associated with the use of an "anorectic" drug varies from trial to trial, and the increased weight loss appears to be related in part to variables other than the drugs prescribed, such as the physician-investigator, the population treated, and the diet prescribed. Studies do not permit conclusions as to the relative importance of the drug and nondrug factors on weight loss.

The natural history of obesity is measured in years, whereas the studies cited are restricted to a few weeks duration; thus, the total impact of drug-induced weight loss over that of diet alone must be considered clinically limited.

INDICATION

FASTIN is indicated in the management of exogenous obesity as a short term (a few weeks) adjunct in a regimen of weight reduction based on caloric restriction. The limited usefulness of agents of this class (see ACTIONS) should be measured against possible risk factors inherent in their use such as those described below.

CONTRAINDICATIONS

Advanced arteriosclerosis, symptomatic cardiovascular disease, moderate to severe hypertension, hyperthyroidism, known hypersensitivity, or idiosyncrasy to the sympathomimetic amines, glaucoma.
Agitated states.
Patients with a history of drug abuse.
During or within 14 days following the administration of monoamine oxidase inhibitors (hypertensive crises may result).

WARNINGS

Tolerance to the anorectic effect usually develops within a few weeks. When this occurs, the recommended dose should not be exceeded in an attempt to increase the effect; rather, the drug should be discontinued.

FASTIN may impair the ability of the patient to engage in potentially hazardous activities such as operating machinery or driving a motor vehicle; the patient should therefore be cautioned accordingly.

Drug Dependence: FASTIN is related chemically and pharmacologically to the amphetamines. Amphetamines and related stimulant drugs have been extensively abused, and the possibility of abuse of FASTIN should be kept in mind when evaluating the desirability of including a drug as part of a weight reduction program. Abuse of amphetamines and related drugs may be associated with intense psychological dependence and severe social dysfunction. There are reports of patients who have increased the dosage to many times that recommended. Abrupt cessation following prolonged high dosage administration results in extreme fatigue and mental depression; changes are also noted on the sleep EEG. Manifestations of chronic intoxication with anorectic drugs include severe dermatoses, marked insomnia, irritability, hyperactivity, and personality changes. The most severe manifestation of chronic intoxications is psychosis, often clinically indistinguishable from schizophrenia.

Usage in Pregnancy: Safe use in pregnancy has not been established. Use of FASTIN by women who are or who may become pregnant, and those in the first trimester of pregnancy, requires that the potential benefit be weighed against the possible hazard to mother and infant.

Usage in Children: FASTIN is not recommended for use in children under 12 years of age.

Usage with Alcohol: Concomitant use of alcohol with FASTIN may result in an adverse drug interaction.

PRECAUTIONS

Caution is to be exercised in prescribing FASTIN for patients with even mild hypertension.

Insulin requirements in diabetes mellitus may be altered in association with the use of FASTIN and the concomitant dietary regimen.

FASTIN may decrease the hypotensive effect of guanethidine.

The least amount feasible should be prescribed or dispensed at one time in order to minimize the possibility of overdosage.

ADVERSE REACTIONS

Cardiovascular: Palpitation, tachycardia, elevation of blood pressure.
Central Nervous System: Overstimulation, restlessness, dizziness, insomnia, euphoria, dysphoria, tremor, headache; rarely psychotic episodes at recommended doses.
Gastrointestinal: Dryness of the mouth, unpleasant taste, diarrhea, constipation, other gastrointestinal disturbances.
Allergic: Urticaria.
Endocrine: Impotence, changes in libido.

DOSAGE AND ADMINISTRATION

Exogenous Obesity: One capsule at approximately 2 hours after breakfast for appetite control. Late evening medication should be avoided because of the possibility of resulting insomnia.

Administration of one capsule (30 mg) daily has been found to be adequate in depression of the appetite for twelve to fourteen hours.

FASTIN is not recommended for use in children under 12 years of age.

OVERDOSAGE

Manifestations of acute overdosage with phentermine include restlessness, tremor, hyperreflexia, rapid respiration, confusion, assaultiveness, hallucinations, panic states. Fatigue and depression usually follow the central stimulation.

Cardiovascular effects include arrhythmias, hypertension or hypotension, and circulatory collapse. Gastrointestinal symptoms include nausea, vomiting, diarrhea, and abdominal cramps. Fatal poisoning usually terminates in convulsions and coma.

Management of acute phentermine intoxication is largely symptomatic and includes lavage and sedation with a barbiturate. Experience with hemodialysis or peritoneal dialysis is inadequate to permit recommendations in this regard. Acidification of the urine increases phentermine excretion. Intravenous phentolamine (REGITINE) has been suggested for possible acute, severe hypertension, if this complicates phentermine overdosage.

CAUTION

Federal law prohibits dispensing without prescription.

HOW SUPPLIED

Blue and clear capsules with blue and white beads containing 30 mg phentermine hydrochloride (equivalent to 24 mg phentermine).
NDC 0029-2205-30 ....bottles of 100
NDC 0029-2205-39 ....bottles of 450
NDC 0029-2205-31 ....pack of 30
DGB-0047/10-87   Revised October, 1987

Shown in Product Identification Section, page 405

NUCOFED®
[nū 'cō-fĕd]
Syrup and Capsules

DESCRIPTION

Nucofed Syrup and Capsules is an antitussive-decongestant containing in each 5 mL (teaspoonful) and each capsule: codeine phosphate, 20 mg (Warning: May Be Habit Forming); pseudoephedrine hydrochloride, 60 mg. Nucofed Syrup contains no alcohol and contains 2.25 g of sucrose per 5 mL (teaspoonful). Codeine phosphate and pseudoephedrine hydrochloride may be represented by the following chemical names and structural formulas:

Codeine Phosphate

7,8-didehydro-4,5α-epoxy-3-methoxy-17-methylmorphinan-6α-ol Phosphate (1:1) salt hemihydrate

Pseudoephedrine HCl

[S-(R*,R*)]-α-[1-(methylamino) ethyl]benzene methanol hydrochloride.

Inactive Ingredients, Syrup: Citric Acid, Flavorings, Glycerin, Propylene Glycol, Sodium Benzoate, Sorbitol, Sucrose, D&C Yellow 10, and FD&C Blue 1. **Capsules:** Starch, Lactose, Magnesium Stearate, FD&C Yellow No. 6, FD&C Blue No. 1, and D&C Yellow No. 10.

CLINICAL PHARMACOLOGY

Nucofed Syrup and Capsules
The clinical pharmacology of this formulated product is thought to be due to the action of its ingredients, codeine phosphate and pseudoephedrine hydrochloride.

Codeine Phosphate. Codeine causes suppression of the cough reflex by a direct effect on the cough center in the medulla and appears to exert a drying effect on respiratory tract mucosa and to increase viscosity of bronchial secretions.

Codeine is well absorbed from the gastrointestinal tract. Following oral administration, peak antitussive effects usually can be expected to occur within 1–2 hours and may persist for a period of four hours. Codeine is metabolized in the liver. The drug undergoes O-demethylation, N-demethylation, and partial conjugation with glucuronic acid, and is excreted mainly in the urine as norcodeine and morphine in the free and conjugated forms.

Codeine appears in breast milk of nursing mothers and has been reported to cross the placental barrier.

Pseudoephedrine Hydrochloride. Pseudoephedrine is a physiologically active stereoisomer of ephedrine which acts directly on *alpha*, and, to a lesser degree, *beta* -adrenergic receptors. The *alpha* -adrenergic effects are believed to result from the reduced production of cyclic adenosine-3',5'

Continued on next page

Beecham Laboratories—Cont.

monophosphate (cyclic 3′,5′-AMP) by inhibition of the enzyme adenyl cyclase, where *beta*-adrenergic effects appear to be caused by the stimulation of adenyl cyclase activity. Pseudoephedrine acts directly on *alpha*-adrenergic receptors in the respiratory tract mucosa producing vasoconstriction resulting in shrinkage of swollen nasal mucous membranes, reduction of tissue hyperemia, edema, and nasal congestion, and an increase in nasal airway patency. Drainage of sinus secretions is increased and obstructed eustachian ostia may be opened. Relaxation of bronchial smooth muscle by stimulation of *beta*₂ adrenergic receptors may also occur. Following oral administration significant bronchodilation has not been demonstrated consistently.

Nasal decongestion usually occurs within 30 minutes and persists for 4–6 hours after oral administration of 60 mg of pseudoephedrine hydrochloride.

Although specific information is not available, pseudoephedrine is presumed to cross the placenta and to enter cerebrospinal fluid. It is incompletely metabolized in the liver by N-demethylation to an inactive metabolite. Both are excreted in the urine with 55%–75% of a dose being unchanged.

INDICATIONS AND USAGE
NUCOFED is indicated for symptomatic relief when both coughing and congestion are associated with upper respiratory infections and related conditions such as common cold, bronchitis, influenza, and sinusitis.

CONTRAINDICATIONS
Hypersensitivity to product's active ingredients.

WARNINGS
Persons with persistent cough such as occurs with smoking, asthma, emphysema, or where cough is accompanied by excessive secretions should not take this product except under the advice and supervision of a physician.

May cause or aggravate constipation.

Do not give this product to children taking other drugs except under the advice and supervision of a physician.

Persons with a chronic pulmonary disease or shortness of breath, high blood pressure, heart disease, diabetes or thyroid disease should not take this product except under the advice and supervision of a physician.

Do not exceed recommended dosage because at higher doses nervousness, dizziness, or sleeplessness may occur.

If symptoms do not improve within 7 days or are accompanied by high fever, consult a physician before continuing use.

PRECAUTIONS
General
Inasmuch as the active ingredients of Nucofed Syrup and Capsules consist of codeine phosphate and pseudoephedrine hydrochloride, this medication should be used with caution in the presence of the following:
- Cardiovascular disease (of any etiology)
- Diabetes mellitus
- Hypertension (of any severity)
- Abnormal thyroid function
- Prostatic hypertrophy
- Addison's disease
- Chronic ulcerative colitis
- History of drug abuse or dependence
- Chronic respiratory disease or impairment
- Functional impairment of the liver or kidney

Patients taking Nucofed Syrup and Capsules should be cautioned when driving or doing jobs requiring alertness and to get up slowly from a lying or sitting position, or to lie down if nausea occurs.

Possible Drug Interactions
Because of the potential for drug interactions, persons currently taking any of the following medications should take Nucofed Syrup and Capsules on the advice and under the supervision of a physician.
- Beta adrenergic blockers—concurrent use may increase the pressor effect of pseudoephedrine.
- Digitalis glycosides—concurrent use with pseudoephedrine may increase the possibility of cardiac arrhythmias.
- Antihypertensive agents including Veratrum alkaloids—hypotensive effects may be decreased by the concurrent use of pseudoephedrine.
- Monoamine oxidase (MAO) inhibitors— these agents may potentiate the pressor effect of pseudoephedrine and may result in a hypertensive crisis; pseudoephedrine should not be administered during or within 14 days of MAO inhibitors.
- Sympathomimetics, other — sympathomimetics used concurrently may increase the effects either of these agents or of pseudoephedrine, thereby increasing the potential for side effects.
- Tricyclic antidepressants—the concurrent use of tricyclic antidepressants may antagonize the effects of pseudoephedrine and may increase the effects either of the antidepressants themselves or of the codeine component.
- CNS depressants

- Alcohol
- General anesthetics
- Anticholinergics—concurrent use may result in paralytic ileus.

Drug/Laboratory Test Interactions
- Codeine may cause an elevation in serum amylase levels due to the spasm producing potential of narcotic analgesics on the sphincter of Oddi.

Pregnancy: Category C
Animal reproduction studies of the components of Nucofed Syrup and Capsules (codeine, pseudoephedrine) have not been conducted. Thus, it is not known whether these agents can cause fetal harm when administered to pregnant women or whether they affect reproductive capacity. Accordingly, Nucofed Syrup and Capsules should be given to pregnant women only where clearly needed.

Nursing Mothers
Codeine and pseudoephedrine are excreted in breast milk; therefore, caution should be exercised when this medication is prescribed for a nursing mother.

Pediatric Use
Do not give Nucofed Syrup and Capsules to children under two years of age except on the advice and under the supervision of a physician.

ADVERSE REACTIONS
Based on the composition of Nucofed Syrup and Capsules the following side effects may occur: nervousness, restlessness, trouble in sleeping, drowsiness, difficult or painful urination, dizziness or lightheadedness, headache, nausea and vomiting, constipation, trembling, troubled breathing, increase in sweating, unusual paleness, weakness, changes in heart rate.

DRUG ABUSE AND DEPENDENCE
NUCOFED is placed in Schedule III of the Controlled Substances Act.

OVERDOSAGE
Nucofed Syrup and Capsules contain codeine phosphate and pseudoephedrine hydrochloride. Overdosage as a result of this product should be treated based upon the symptomatology of the patient as it relates to the individual ingredient. Treatment of acute overdosage would probably be based upon treating the patient for codeine toxicity which may be manifested as:
- Gradual drowsiness, dizziness, heaviness of the head, weariness, diminution of sensibility, loss of pain and other modalities of sensation.
- Nausea and vomiting.
- A transient excitement stage, characterized by extreme restlessness, delirium, and rarely epileptiform convulsions, is sometimes seen in children and rarely in adult women.
- Bilateral miosis, progressing to pinpoint pupils, which do not react to light or accommodation. The pupils may dilate during terminal asphyxia.
- Itching of the skin and nose, sometimes with skin rashes and urticaria.
- Coma, with muscular relaxation and depressed or absent superficial and deep reflexes. A Babinski toe sign may appear.
- Marked slowing of the respiratory rate with inadequate pulmonary ventilation and consequent cyanosis. Breathing becomes stertorous and irregular (Cheyne-Stokes or Biot).
- The pulse is slow and the blood pressure gradually falls to shock levels. Urine formation ceases or is reduced to a very low rate.

The lethal dose of codeine for an adult is about 0.5–1.0 g. Treatment is as recommended for narcotics.

DOSAGE AND ADMINISTRATION
RECOMMENDED DOSAGE: CAPSULE
Adults: 1 capsule every 6 hours, not to exceed 4 capsules in 24 hours.
RECOMMENDED DOSAGE: SYRUP
Adults: 1 teaspoonful every 6 hours, not to exceed 4 teaspoonfuls in 24 hours.
Children:
    6 to under 12 years: ½ teaspoonful every 6 hours, not to exceed 2 teaspoonfuls in 24 hours.
    2 to under 6 years: ¼ teaspoonful every 6 hours, not to exceed 1 teaspoonful in 24 hours.
Do not give this product to children under 2 years, except under the advice and supervision of a physician.

HOW SUPPLIED
Nucofed Syrup, Green, Mint Flavored
    NDC 0029-3135-34   Pints
Nucofed Capsules, Green Top, Clear Bottom
    NDC 0029-3138-39   Bottles of 60

CAUTION
Federal law prohibits dispensing without prescription.
DGB—0491/1-88
Revised January, 1988
    Shown in Product Identification Section, page 405

NUCOFED® EXPECTORANT   ℞
[nū ′cō-fĕd]
SYRUP

DESCRIPTION
Nucofed Expectorant is an antitussive-decongestant-expectorant syrup for oral administration containing in each 5 mL (teaspoonful): codeine phosphate, 20 mg (Warning: May Be Habit Forming); pseudoephedrine HCl, 60 mg; guaifenesin, 200 mg; alcohol, 12.5%.

Codeine phosphate, pseudoephedrine hydrochloride and guaifenesin may be represented by the following chemical names and structural formulas:

Codeine Phosphate

$H_2PO_4^- \cdot \frac{1}{2}H_2O$

7,8-didehydro-4,5α-epoxy-3-methoxy-17-methylmorphinan-6α-ol Phosphate (1:1) salt hemihydrate

Pseudoephedrine HCl

[S-(R*,R*)]-α-[1-(methylamino) ethyl]benzene methanol hydrochloride

Guaifenesin

$OCH_2CH(OH)CH_2OH$
OCH_3

3-(0-methoxyphenoxy)-1,2-propanediol

Inactive Ingredients: D & C Yellow 10, F D & C Red 40, Flavoring, Glycerin, Saccharin Sodium, Sodium Chloride and Sucrose.

CLINICAL PHARMACOLOGY
Nucofed Expectorant
The clinical pharmacology of this formulated product is thought to be due to the action of its ingredients, codeine phosphate, pseudoephedrine hydrochloride and guaifenesin.

Codeine Phosphate. Codeine causes suppression of the cough reflex by a direct effect on the cough center in the medulla and appears to exert a drying effect on respiratory tract mucosa and to increase viscosity of bronchial secretions.

Codeine is well absorbed from the gastrointestinal tract. Following oral administration, peak antitussive effects can be expected to occur within one to two hours and may persist for a period of four hours. Codeine is metabolized in the liver. The drug undergoes O-demethylation, N-demethylation, and partial conjugation with glucuronic acid, and is excreted mainly in the urine as norcodeine and morphine in the free and conjugated forms.

Codeine appears in breast milk of nursing mothers and has been reported to cross the placental barrier.

Pseudoephedrine Hydrochloride. Pseudoephedrine is a physiologically active stereoisomer of ephedrine which acts directly on *alpha,* and to a lesser degree, *beta*-adrenergic receptors. The *alpha*-adrenergic effects are believed to result from the reduced production of cyclic adenosine-3′,5′ monophosphate (cyclic 3′,5′-AMP) by inhibition of the enzyme adenyl cyclase, whereas *beta*-adrenergic effects appear to be caused by the stimulation of adenyl cyclase activity.

Pseudoephedrine acts directly on *alpha*-adrenergic receptors in the respiratory tract mucosa producing vasoconstriction resulting in shrinkage of swollen nasal mucous membranes, reduction of tissue hyperemia, edema, and nasal congestion, and an increase in nasal airway patency. Drainage of sinus secretions is increased and obstructed eustachian ostia may be opened. Relaxation of bronchial smooth muscle by stimulation of *beta*₂ adrenergic receptors may also occur. Following oral administration significant bronchodilation has not been demonstrated consistently.

Nasal decongestion usually occurs within 30 minutes and persists for 4–6 hours after oral administration of 60 mg of pseudoephedrine hydrochloride.

Although specific information is not available, pseudoephedrine is presumed to cross the placenta and to enter cerebrospinal fluid. It is incompletely metabolized in the liver by

N-demethylation to an inactive metabolite. Both are excreted in the urine with 55%–75% of a dose being unchanged.

Guaifenesin. Guaifenesin, by increasing respiratory tract fluid, reduces the viscosity of tenacious secretions and acts as an expectorant.

Guaifenesin is excreted in the urine mainly as glucuronates and sulfonates.

INDICATIONS AND USAGE

NUCOFED EXPECTORANT is indicated for symptomatic relief when both coughing and congestion are associated with upper respiratory infections and related conditions such as common colds, bronchitis, influenza, and sinusitis.

CONTRAINDICATIONS

Hypersensitivity to product's active ingredients.

WARNINGS

Persons with persistent cough such as occurs with smoking, asthma, emphysema, or where cough is accompanied by excessive secretions should not take this product except under the advice and supervision of a physician.

Do not give this product to children taking other drugs except under the advice and supervision of a physician.

Persons with a chronic pulmonary disease or shortness of breath, high blood pressure, heart disease, diabetes or thyroid disease should not take this product except under the advice and supervision of a physician.

Do not exceed recommended dosage because at higher doses nervousness, dizziness, or sleeplessness may occur.

If symptoms do not improve within 7 days or are accompanied by high fever, consult a physician before continuing use.

PRECAUTIONS

General. Inasmuch as the active ingredient of Nucofed Expectorant consist of codeine phosphate, pseudoephedrine hydrochloride and guaifenesin, this medication should be used with caution in the presence of the following:
- Cardiovascular disease (of any etiology)
- Diabetes mellitus
- Hypertension (of any severity)
- Abnormal thyroid function
- Prostatic hypertrophy
- Addison's disease
- Chronic ulcerative colitis
- History of drug abuse or dependence
- Chronic respiratory disease or impairment
- Functional impairment of the liver or kidney

Patients taking Nucofed Expectorant should be cautioned when driving or doing jobs requiring alertness and to get up slowly from a lying or sitting position, or to lie down if nausea occurs.

Possible Drug Interactions. Because of the potential for drug interactions, persons currently taking any of the following medications should take Nucofed Expectorant only on the advice and under the supervision of a physician.
- Beta adrenergic blockers—concurrent use may increase the pressor effect of pseudoephedrine.
- Digitalis glycosides—concurrent use with pseudoephedrine may increase the possibility of cardiac arrhythmias.
- Antihypertensive agents including Veratrum alkaloids—hypotensive effects may be decreased by the concurrent use of pseudoephedrine.
- Monoamine oxidase (MAO) inhibitors—these agents may potentiate the pressor effect of pseudoephedrine and may result in a hypertensive crisis; pseudoephedrine should not be administered during or within 14 days of MAO inhibitors.
- Sympathomimetics, other—sympathomimetics used concurrently may increase the effects either of these agents or of pseudoephedrine, thereby increasing the potential for side effects.
- Tricyclic antidepressants—the concurrent use of tricyclic antidepressants may antagonize the effects of pseudoephedrine and may increase the effects either of the antidepressants themselves or of the codeine component.
- CNS depressants
- Alcohol
- General anesthetics
- Anticholinergics—concurrent use may result in paralytic ileus.

Drug/Laboratory Test Interactions
- Codeine may cause an elevation in serum amylase levels due to the spasm producing potential of narcotic analgesics on the sphincter of Oddi.
- Guaifenesin is known to interfere with the colorimetric determination of 5-hydroxy-indole-acetic acid (5-HIAA) and vanilmandelic acid (VMA).

Pregnancy: Category C
Animal reproduction studies of the components of Nucofed Expectorant (codeine, pseudoephedrine and guaifenesin) have not been conducted. Thus, it is not known whether these agents can cause fetal harm when administered to pregnant women or whether they affect reproductive capacity. Accordingly, Nucofed Expectorant should be given to pregnant women only where clearly needed.

Nursing Mothers
Codeine and pseudoephedrine, two of the ingredients in Nucofed Expectorant, are excreted in breast milk; therefore, caution should be exercised when this medication is prescribed for a nursing mother.

Pediatric Use
Do not give Nucofed Expectorant to children under two years of age except on the advice and under the supervision of a physician.

ADVERSE REACTIONS

Based on the composition of Nucofed Expectorant the following side effects may occur: nervousness, restlessness, trouble in sleeping, drowsiness, difficult or painful urination, dizziness or lightheadedness, headache, nausea or vomiting, constipation, trembling, troubled breathing, increase in sweating, unusual paleness, weakness, changes in heart rate.

DRUG ABUSE AND DEPENDENCE

Nucofed Expectorant has been placed in Schedule III of the Controlled Substances Act.

OVERDOSAGE

Nucofed Expectorant contains codeine phosphate, pseudoephedrine hydrochloride and guaifenesin. Overdosage as a result of this product should be treated based upon the symptomatology of the patient as it relates to the individual ingredient. Treatment of acute overdosage would probably be based upon treating the patient for codeine toxicity which may be manifested as:
- Gradual drowsiness, dizziness, heaviness of the head, weariness, diminution of sensibility, loss of pain and other modalities of sensation.
- Nausea and vomiting.
- A transient excitement stage, characterized by extreme restlessness, delirium, and rarely epileptiform convulsions, is sometimes seen in children and rarely in adult women.
- Bilateral miosis, progressing to pinpoint pupils, which do not react to light or accommodation. The pupils may dilate during terminal asphyxia.
- Itching of the skin and nose, sometimes with skin rashes and urticaria.
- Coma, with muscular relaxation and depressed or absent superficial and deep reflexes. A Babinski toe sign may appear.
- Marked slowing of the respiratory rate with inadequate pulmonary ventilation and consequent cyanosis. Breathing becomes stertorous and irregular (Cheyne-Stokes or Biot).
- The pulse is slow and the blood pressure gradually falls to shock levels. Urine formation ceases or is reduced to a very low rate.

The lethal dose of codeine for an adult is about 0.5–1.0 g. Treatment is as recommended for narcotics.

DOSAGE AND ADMINISTRATION

RECOMMENDED DOSAGE:

Adults: 1 teaspoonful every 6 hours, not to exceed 4 teaspoonfuls in 24 hours.

Children:
    6 to under 12 years: ½ teaspoonful every 6 hours, not to exceed 2 teaspoonfuls in 24 hours.
    2 to under 6 years: ¼ teaspoonful every 6 hours, not to exceed 1 teaspoonful in 24 hours.
Do not give this product to children under 2 years, except under the advice and supervision of a physician.

HOW SUPPLIED

Red, Wintergreen Flavored Syrup
    NDC 0029-3142-34   Pints

CAUTION

Federal law prohibits dispensing without prescription.
DGB—1266/2-88
Revised February, 1988

NUCOFED®   © ℞

[nū ′cō-fĕd]
PEDIATRIC EXPECTORANT
SYRUP

DESCRIPTION

Nucofed Pediatric Expectorant is an antitussive-decongestant-expectorant syrup for oral administration containing in each 5 mL (teaspoonful): codeine phosphate, 10 mg (Warning: May Be Habit Forming); pseudoephedrine HCl, 30 mg; guaifenesin, 100 mg; alcohol, 6%

Codeine phosphate, pseudoephedrine hydrochloride and guaifenesin may be represented by the following chemical names and structural formulas:

[See Chemical Formula at top of next column].

Codeine Phosphate

7,8-didehydro-4,5α-epoxy-3-methoxy-17-methylmorphinan-6α-ol Phosphate (1:1) salt hemihydrate

Pseudoephedrine HCl

[S-(R*,R*)]-α-[1-(methylamino) ethyl]benzene methanol hydrochloride

Guaifenesin

OCH₂CH(OH)CH₂OH

3-(0-methoxyphenoxy)-1,2-propanediol

Inactive Ingredients: Edetate Disodium, F D & C Red 40, Flavorings, Glycerin, Potassium Sorbate, Saccharin Sodium, Sodium Chloride and Sucrose.

CLINICAL PHARMACOLOGY

Nucofed Pediatric Expectorant
The clinical pharmacology of this formulated product is thought to be due to the action of its ingredients, codeine phosphate, pseudoephedrine hydrochloride and guaifenesin.

Codeine Phosphate. Codeine causes suppression of the cough reflex by a direct effect on the cough center in the medulla and appears to exert a drying effect on respiratory tract mucosa and to increase viscosity of bronchial secretions.

Codeine is well absorbed from the gastrointestinal tract. Following oral administration, peak antitussive effect usually can be expected to occur within one to two hours and may persist for a period of four hours. Codeine is metabolized in the liver. The drug undergoes O-demethylation, N-demethylation, and partial conjugation with glucuronic acid, and is excreted mainly in the urine as norcodeine and morphine in the free and conjugated forms.

Codeine appears in breast milk of nursing mothers and has been reported to cross the placental barrier.

Pseudoephedrine Hydrochloride. Pseudoephedrine is a physiologically active stereoisomer of ephedrine which acts directly on *alpha*, and to a lesser degree, *beta* -adrenergic receptors. The *alpha* -adrenergic effects are believed to result from the reduced production of cyclic adenosine-3′,5′ monophosphate (cyclic 3′,5′-AMP) by inhibition of the enzyme adenyl cyclase, whereas *beta* -adrenergic effects appear to be caused by the stimulation of adenyl cyclase activity.

Pseudoephedrine acts directly on *alpha* -adrenergic receptors in the respiratory tract mucosa producing vasoconstriction resulting in shrinkage of swollen nasal mucous membranes, reduction of tissue hyperemia, edema, and nasal congestion, and an increase in nasal airway patency. Drainage of sinus secretions is increased and obstructed eustachian ostia may be opened. Relaxation of bronchial smooth muscle by stimulation of $beta_2$ adrenergic receptors may also occur. Following oral administration significant bronchodilation has not been demonstrated consistently.

Nasal decongestion usually occurs within 30 minutes and persists for 4–6 hours after oral administration of 30 mg of pseudoephedrine hydrochloride.

Although specific information is not available, pseudoephedrine is presumed to cross the placenta and to enter cerebrospinal fluid. It is incompletely metabolized in the liver by N-demethylation to an inactive metabolite. Both are excreted in the urine with 55%–75% of a dose being unchanged.

Guaifenesin. Guaifenesin, by increasing respiratory tract fluid, reduces the viscosity of tenacious secretions and acts as an expectorant.

Guaifenesin is excreted in the urine mainly as glucuronates and sulfonates.

INDICATIONS AND USAGE

NUCOFED PEDIATRIC EXPECTORANT is indicated for symptomatic relief when both coughing and congestion are associated with upper respiratory infections and related conditions such as common cold, bronchitis, influenza, and sinusitis.

CONTRAINDICATIONS

Hypersensitivity to product's active ingredients.

WARNINGS

Persons with persistent cough such as occurs with smoking, asthma, emphysema, or where cough is accompanied by ex-

Continued on next page

Beecham Laboratories—Cont.

cessive secretions should not take this product except under the advice and supervision of a physician.

Do not give this product to children taking other drugs except under the advice and supervision of a physician.

Persons with a chronic pulmonary disease or shortness of breath, high blood pressure, heart disease, diabetes or thyroid disease should not take this product except under the advice and supervision of a physician.

Do not exceed recommended dosage because at higher doses nervousness, dizziness, or sleeplessness may occur.

If symptoms do not improve within 7 days or are accompanied by high fever, consult a physician before continuing use.

PRECAUTIONS

General. Inasmuch as the active ingredients of Nucofed Pediatric Expectorant consist of codeine phosphate, pseudoephedrine hydrochloride and guaifenesin, this medication should be used with caution in the presence of the following:
- Cardiovascular disease (of any etiology)
- Diabetes mellitus
- Hypertension (of any severity)
- Abnormal thyroid function
- Prostatic hypertrophy
- Addison's disease
- Chronic ulcerative colitis
- History of drug abuse or dependence
- Chronic respiratory disease or impairment
- Functional impairment of the liver or kidney

Patients taking Nucofed Pediatric Expectorant should be cautioned when driving or doing jobs requiring alertness and to get up slowly from a lying or sitting position, or to lie down if nausea occurs.

Possible Drug Interactions. Because of the potential for drug interactions, persons currently taking any of the following medications should take Nucofed Pediatric Expectorant only on the advice and under the supervision of a physician.
- Beta adrenergic blockers—concurrent use may increase the pressor effect of pseudoephedrine.
- Digitalis glycosides—concurrent use with pseudoephedrine may increase the possibility of cardiac arrhythmias.
- Antihypertensive agents including Veratrum alkaloids—hypotensive effects may be decreased by the concurrent use of pseudoephedrine.
- Monoamine oxidase (MAO) inhibitors—these agents may potentiate the pressor effect of pseudophedrine and may result in a hypertensive crisis; pseudoephedrine should not be administered during or within 14 days of MAO inhibitors.
- Sympathomimetics, other—sympathomimetics used concurrently may increase the effects either of these agents or of pseudoephedrine, thereby increasing the potential for side effects.
- Tricyclic antidepressants—the concurrent use of tricyclic antidepressants may antagonize the effects of pseudoephedrine and may increase the effects either of the antidepressants themselves or of the codeine component.
- CNS depressants
- Alcohol
- General anesthetics
- Anticholinergics—concurrent use may result in paralytic ileus.

Drug/Laboratory Test Interactions
- Codeine may cause an elevation in serum amylase levels due to the spasm producing potential of narcotic analgesics on the sphincter of Oddi.
- Guaifenesin is known to interfere with the colorimetric determination of 5-hydroxyindole-acetic acid (5-HIAA) and vanilmandelic acid (VMA).

Pregnancy: Category C
Animal reproduction studies of the components of Nucofed Pediatric Expectorant (codeine, pseudoephedrine and guaifensin) have not been conducted. Thus, it is not known whether these agents can cause fetal harm when administered to pregnant women or whether they affect reproductive capacity. Accordingly, Nucofed Pediatric Expectorant should be given to pregnant women only where clearly needed.

Nursing Mothers
Codeine and pseudoephedrine, two of the ingredients in Nucofed Pediatric Expectorant, are excreted in breast milk; therefore, caution should be exercised when this medication is prescribed for a nursing mother.

Pediatric Use
Do not give Nucofed Pediatric Expectorant to children under two years of age except on the advice and under the supervision of a physician.

ADVERSE REACTIONS

Based on the composition of Nucofed Pediatric Expectorant the following side effects may occur: nervousness, restlessness, trouble in sleeping, drowsiness, difficult or painful urination, dizziness or lightheadedness, headache, nausea or vomiting, constipation, trembling, troubled breathing, in-

crease in sweating, unusual paleness, weakness, changes in heart rate.

DRUG ABUSE AND DEPENDENCE

Nucofed Pediatric Expectorant has been placed in Schedule V of the Controlled Substances Act.

OVERDOSAGE

Nucofed Pediatric Expectorant contains codeine phosphate, pseudoephedrine hydrochloride and guaifenesin. Overdosage as a result of this product should be treated based upon the symptomatology of the patient as it relates to the individual ingredient. Treatment of acute overdosage would probably be based upon treating the patient for codeine toxicity which may be manifested as:
- Gradual drowsiness, dizziness, heaviness of the head, weariness, diminution of sensibility, loss of pain and other modalities of sensation.
- Nausea and vomiting.
- A transient excitement stage, characterized by extreme restlessness, delirium, and rarely epileptiform convulsions, is sometimes seen in children and rarely in adult women.
- Bilateral miosis, progressing to pinpoint pupils, which do not react to light or accommodation. The pupils may dilate during terminal asphyxia.
- Itching of the skin and nose, sometimes with skin rashes and urticaria.
- Coma, with muscular relaxation and depressed or absent superficial and deep reflexes. A Babinski toe sign may appear.
- Marked slowing of the respiratory rate with inadequate pulmonary ventilation and consequent cyanosis. Breathing becomes stertorous and irregular (Cheyne-Stokes or Biot).
- The pulse is slow and the blood pressure gradually falls to shock levels. Urine formation ceases or is reduced to a very low rate.

The lethal dose of codeine for an adult is approximately 0.5–1.0 g. Reliable information regarding the lethal dose in children is not available. Treatment is as recommended for narcotics.

DOSAGE AND ADMINISTRATION
RECOMMENDED DOSAGE:

Adults and Children 12 years of age and over: 2 teaspoonfuls every 6 hours, not to exceed 8 teaspoonfuls in 24 hours.

Children:
  6 to under 12 years: 1 teaspoonful every 6 hours, not to exceed 4 teaspoonfuls in 24 hours.
  2 to under 6 years: $\frac{1}{2}$ teaspoonful every 6 hours, not to exceed 2 teaspoonfuls in 24 hours.

Do not give this product to children under 2 years, except under the advice and supervision of a physician.

HOW SUPPLIED
Red, Strawberry Flavored Syrup
NDC 0029-3130-39   Pints

CAUTION
Federal law prohibits dispensing without prescription.
DGB—2010/5-88
Revised May, 1988

TICAR®   ℞
[tĭ'kar]
sterile ticarcillin disodium
for Intramuscular or Intravenous Administration

DESCRIPTION

TICAR (ticarcillin disodium) is a semisynthetic injectable penicillin derived from the penicillin nucleus, 6-aminopenicillanic acid. Chemically, it is 6-[(Carboxy-3-thienylacetyl)amino]3, 3-dimethyl-7-oxo-4-thia-1-azabicyclo [3.2.0]heptane-2-carboxylic acid disodium salt.

[See Chemical Formula at top of next column].

It is supplied as a white to pale yellow powder for reconstitution. The reconstituted solution is clear, colorless or pale yellow, having a pH of 6.0–8.0. Ticarcillin is very soluble in water, its solubility is greater than 600 mg/ml.

ACTIONS
PHARMACOLOGY

Ticarcillin is not absorbed orally, therefore, it must be given intravenously or intramuscularly. Following intramuscular administration, peak serum concentrations occur within $\frac{1}{2}$–1 hour. Somewhat higher and more prolonged serum levels can be achieved with the concurrent administration of probenecid.

The minimum inhibitory concentrations (MIC) for many strains of *Pseudomonas* are relatively high by usual standards; serum levels of 60 mcg/ml or greater are required. However, the low degree of toxicity of ticarcillin permits the use of doses large enough to achieve inhibitory levels for these strains in serum or tissues. Other susceptible organisms usually require serum levels in the 10–25 mcg/ml range.
[See table below].

As with other penicillins, ticarcillin is eliminated by glomerular filtration and tubular secretion. It is not highly bound to serum protein (approximately 45%) and is excreted unchanged in high concentrations in the urine. After the administration of a 1–2 Gm I.M. dose, a urine concentration of 2000–4000 mcg/ml may be obtained in patients with normal renal function. The serum half-life of ticarcillin in normal individuals is approximately 70 minutes.

An inverse relationship exists between serum half-life and creatinine clearance, but the dosage of TICAR need only be adjusted in cases of severe renal impairment (see DOSAGE AND ADMINISTRATION). The administered ticarcillin may be removed from patients undergoing dialysis; the actual amount removed depends on the duration and type of dialysis.

Ticarcillin can be detected in tissues and interstitial fluid following parenteral administration. Penetration into the cerebrospinal fluid, bile and pleural fluid has been demonstrated.

MICROBIOLOGY
Ticarcillin is bactericidal and demonstrates substantial *in vitro* activity against both Gram-positive and Gram-negative organisms. Many strains of the following organisms were found to be susceptible to ticarcillin *in vitro*:
Pseudomonas aeruginosa (and other species)
Escherichia coli
Proteus mirabilis
Morganella morganii (formerly *Proteus morganii*)
Providencia rettgeri (formerly *Proteus rettgeri*)
Proteus vulgaris
Enterobacter species
Haemophilus influenzae
Neisseria species
Salmonella species
Staphylococcus aureus (non-penicillinase producing)
Staphylococcus epidermidis
Beta-hemolytic streptococci (Group A)
Streptococcus faecalis (Enterococcus)
Streptococcus pneumoniae
Anaerobic bacteria, including:
Bacteroides species including *B. fragilis*
Fusobacterium species
Veillonella species
Clostridium species
Eubacterium species
Peptococcus species
Peptostreptococcus species
In vitro synergism between ticarcillin and gentamicin sulfate, tobramycin sulfate or amikacin sulfate against certain strains of *Pseudomonas aeruginosa* has been demonstrated.

TICARCILLIN SERUM LEVELS
mcg/ml

Dosage	Route	$\frac{1}{4}$ hr.	$\frac{1}{2}$ hr.	1 hr.	2 hr.	3 hr.	4 hr.	6 hr.
Adults:								
500 mg	IM	—	7.7	8.6	6.0	4.0	—	2.9
1 Gm	IM	—	31.0	18.7	15.7	9.7	—	3.4
2 Gm	IM	—	63.6	39.7	32.3	18.9	—	3.4
3 Gm	IV	190.0	140.0	107.0	52.2	31.3	13.8	4.2
5 Gm	IV	327.0	280.0	175.0	106.0	63.0	28.5	9.6
3 Gm +	IV	223.0	166.0	123.0	78.0	54.0	35.4	17.1
1 Gm	Oral							
Probenecid								

Neonates:		$\frac{1}{2}$ hr.	1 hr.	$1\frac{1}{2}$ hr.	2 hr.	4 hr.	8 hr.	
50 mg/kg	IM	64.0	70.7	63.7	60.1	33.2	11.6	

Some strains of such microorganisms as *Mima-Herellea (Acinetobacter)*, *Citrobacter* and *Serratia* have shown susceptibility.

Ticarcillin is not stable in the presence of penicillinase.

Some strains of *Pseudomonas* have developed resistance fairly rapidly.

DISK SUSCEPTIBILITY TESTS

Susceptibility Tests: Ticarcillin disks or powders should be used for testing susceptibility to ticarcillin. However, organisms reportedly susceptible to carbenicillin are susceptible to ticarcillin.

Diffusion Techniques: For the disk diffusion method of susceptibility testing a 75 mcg TICAR DISK should be used. The method for this test is the one outlined in NCCLS publication M2-A3* with the following interpretative criteria:

[See table above right].

Dilution Techniques: Dilution techniques for determining the MIC (minimum inhibitory concentration) are published by NCCLS for the broth and agar dilution procedures. The MIC data should be interpreted in light of the concentrations present in serum, tissue, and body fluids. Organisms with MIC ≤ 64 are considered susceptible when they are in tissue but organisms with MIC ≤ 128 would be susceptible in urine where the TICAR concentrations are much greater. At present, only dilution methods can be recommended for testing antibiotic susceptibility of obligate anaerobes.

Susceptibility testing methods require the use of control organisms. The 75 mcg ticarcillin disk should give zone diameters between 22 and 28 mm for *P. aeruginosa* ATCC 27853 and 24 and 30 mm for *E. Coli* ATCC 25922. Reference strains are available for dilution testing of ticarcillin. 95% of the MIC's should fall within the following MIC ranges and the majority of MIC's should be at values close to the center of the pertinent range. (Reference NCCLS publication M7-A**) *S. aureus* ATCC 29213, 2.0–8.0 mcg/ml; *S. faecalis* ATCC 29212, 16–64 mcg/ml; *E. coli* ATCC 25922, 2.0–8.0 mcg/ml; *P. aeruginosa* ATCC 27853, 8.0–32 mcg/ml.

*Performance standards for Antimicrobial Disk Susceptibility Tests, National Committee for Clinical Laboratory Standards, Vol. 4, No. 16, pp. 369–402, 1984.

**Methods for Dilution Antimicrobial Susceptibility Tests for Bacteria That Grow Aerobically, Vol. 5, No. 22, pp. 579–618. 1985.

INDICATIONS

TICAR (ticarcillin disodium) is indicated for the treatment of the following infections:

Bacterial septicemia (†)

Skin and soft-tissue infections (†)

Acute and chronic respiratory tract infections (†)(‡)

  (†) caused by susceptible strains of *Pseudomonas aeruginosa, Proteus* species (both indole-positive and indole-negative) and *Escherichia coli.*

  (‡) (Though clinical improvement has been shown, bacteriological cures cannot be expected in patients with chronic respiratory disease or cystic fibrosis.)

Genitourinary tract infections (complicated and uncomplicated) due to susceptible strains of *Pseudomonas aeruginosa, Proteus* species (both indole-positive and indole-negative), *Escherichia coli, Enterobacter* and *Streptococcus faecalis* (enterococcus).

Ticarcillin is also indicated in the treatment of the following infections due to susceptible anaerobic bacteria:
1. Bacterial septicemia.
2. Lower respiratory tract infections such as empyema, anaerobic pneumonitis and lung abscess.
3. Intra-abdominal infections such as peritonitis and intra-abdominal abscess (typically resulting from anaerobic organisms resident in the normal gastrointestinal tract).
4. Infections of the female pelvis and genital tract, such as endometritis, pelvic inflammatory disease, pelvic abscess and salpingitis.
5. Skin and soft-tissue infections.

Culture	Susceptible	Intermediate	Resistant
P. aeruginosa and *Enterobacteriaceae*	≥ 15 mm	12–14 mm	≤ 11 mm

The MIC correlates are:

Resistant > 128 mcg/ml
Susceptible ≤ 64 mcg/ml

DOSAGE AND ADMINISTRATION

Clinical experience indicates that in serious urinary tract and systemic infections, intravenous therapy in the higher doses should be used. Intramuscular injections should not exceed 2 grams per injection.

Adults:

Bacterial Septicemia Respiratory Tract Infections Skin and Soft-Tissue Infections Intra-Abdominal Infections Infections of the Female Pelvis and Genital Tract	200–300 mg/kg/day by I.V. infusion in divided doses every 4 or 6 hours. [The usual dose is 3 gm given every 4 hours (18 gm/day) or 4 gm given every 6 hours (16 gm/day) depending on weight and the severity of the infection.]
Urinary Tract Infections Complicated:	150–200 mg/kg/day by I.V. infusion in divided doses every 4 or 6 hours. [Usual recommended dosage for average (70 kg) adults: 3 grams q.i.d.]
Uncomplicated:	1 gram I.M. or direct I.V. every 6 hours.

Infections complicated by renal insufficiency: (1)

Initial loading dose of 3 grams I.V. followed by I.V. doses, based on creatinine clearance and type of dialysis, as indicated below:

Creatinine clearance ml/min.:	
over 60	3 grams every 4 hours
30–60	2 grams every 4 hours
10–30	2 grams every 8 hours
less than 10	2 grams every 12 hours (or 1 gram I.M. every 6 hours)
less than 10 with hepatic dysfunction	2 grams every 24 hours (or 1 gram I.M. every 12 hours)
patients on peritoneal dialysis	3 grams every 12 hours
patients on hemodialysis	2 grams every 12 hours supplemented with 3 grams after each dialysis

To calculate creatinine clearance* from a serum creatinine value use the following formula:

$$C_{cr} = \frac{(140-\text{Age})\ (\text{wt in kg})}{72 \times S_{cr}(\text{mg}/100\ \text{ml})}$$

This is the calculated creatinine clearance for adult males; for females it is 15% less.

* Cockcroft, D.W., et al, "Prediction of Creatinine Clearance from Serum Creatinine" Nephron 16:31–41 (1976).

(1) The half-life of ticarcillin in patients with renal failure is approximately 13 hours.

Children: Under 40 kg (88 lbs)

The daily dose for children should not exceed the adult dosage.

Bacterial Septicemia Respiratory Tract Infections Skin and Soft-Tissue Infections Intra-Abdominal Infections Infections of the Female Pelvis and Genital Tract	200–300 mg/kg/day by I.V. infusion in divided doses every 4 or 6 hours.
Urinary Tract Infections Complicated:	150–200 mg/kg/day by I.V. infusion in divided doses every 4 or 6 hours.
Uncomplicated:	50–100 mg/kg/day I.M. or direct I.V. in divided doses every 6 or 8 hours.

Infections complicated by renal insufficiency:

Clinical data is insufficient to recommend an optimum dose.

Children weighing more than 40 kg (88 lbs) should receive adult dosages.

Neonates: In the neonate, for severe infections (sepsis) due to susceptible strains of *Pseudomonas, Proteus,* and *E. coli,* the following ticarcillin dosages may be given I.M. or by 10–20 minutes I.V. infusion:

Infants under 2000 grams body weight:		Infants over 2000 grams body weight:	
Aged 0–7 days	75 mg/kg/12 hours (150 mg/kg/day)	Ages 0–7 days	75 mg/kg/8 hours (225 mg/kg/day)
Aged over 7 days	75 mg/kg/8 hours (225 mg/kg/day)	Aged over 7 days	100 mg/kg/8 hours (300 mg/kg/day)

This dosage schedule is intended to produce peak serum concentrations of 125–150 mcg/ml one hour after a dose of ticarcillin and trough concentrations of 25–50 mcg/ml immediately before the next dose.

NOTE: Gentamicin, tobramycin or amikacin may be used concurrently with ticarcillin for initial therapy until results of culture and susceptibility studies are known. **Seriously ill patients should receive the higher doses. TICAR has proved to be useful in infections in which protective mechanisms are impaired, such as in acute leukemia and during therapy with immunosuppressive or oncolytic drugs.**

Continued on next page

Beecham Laboratories—Cont.

STABILITY PERIOD

Intravenous Solution (concentration of 10 mg/ml to 100 mg/ml)	Room Temperature (70°–75°F).	Refrigeration (40°F)
Sodium Chloride Injection, U.S.P.	72 hours	14 days
Dextrose Injection 5%	72 hours	14 days
Lactated Ringer's Injection	48 hours	14 days

Although ticarcillin is primarily indicated in Gram-negative infections, its *in vitro* activity against Gram-positive organisms should be considered in treating infections caused by both Gram-negative and Gram-positive organisms (see MICROBIOLOGY).

Based on the *in vitro* synergism between ticarcillin and gentamicin sulfate, tobramycin sulfate or amikacin sulfate against certain strains of *Pseudomonas aeruginosa*, combined therapy has been successful, using full therapeutic dosages. (For additional prescribing information, see the gentamicin sulfate, tobramycin sulfate and amikacin sulfate package inserts.)

NOTE: Culturing and susceptibilty testing should be performed initially and during treatment to monitor the effectiveness of therapy and the susceptibility of the bacteria.

CONTRAINDICATIONS

A history of allergic reaction to any of the penicillins is a contraindication.

WARNINGS

Serious and occasionally fatal hypersensitivity (anaphylactoid) reactions have been reported in patients receiving penicillin. These reactions are more likely to occur in persons with a history of sensitivity to multiple allergens.

There are reports of patients with a history of penicillin hypersensitivity reactions who experience severe hypersensitivity reactions when treated with a cephalosporin. Before therapy with a penicillin, careful inquiry should be made about previous hypersensitivity reactions to penicillins, cephalosporins, and other allergens. If a reaction occurs, the drug should be discontinued unless, in the opinion of the physician, the condition being treated is life-threatening and amenable only to ticarcillin therapy. **Serious anaphylactoid reactions require immediate emergency treatment with epinephrine. Oxygen, intravenous steroids, airway management, including intubation, should also be administered as indicated.**

Some patients receiving high doses of ticarcillin may develop hemorrhagic manifestations associated with abnormalities of coagulation tests, such as bleeding time and platelet aggregation. On withdrawal of the drug, the bleeding should cease and coagulation abnormalities revert to normal. Other causes of abnormal bleeding should also be considered. Patients with renal impairment, in whom excretion of ticarcillin is delayed, should be observed for bleeding manifestations. Such patients should be dosed strictly according to recommendations (see DOSAGE AND ADMINISTRATION). If bleeding manifestations appear, ticarcillin treatment should be discontinued and appropriate therapy instituted.

PRECAUTIONS

Although TICAR (ticarcillin disodium) exhibits the characteristic low toxicity of the penicillins, as with any other potent agent, it is advisable to check periodically for organ system dysfunction (including renal, hepatic and hematopoietic) during prolonged treatment. If overgrowth of resistant organisms occurs, the appropriate therapy should be initiated.

Since the theoretical sodium content is 5.2 milliequivalents (120 mg) per gram of ticarcillin, and the actual vial content can be as high as 6.5 mEq/Gm, electrolyte and cardiac status should be monitored carefully.

In a few patients receiving intravenous ticarcillin, hypokalemia has been reported. Serum potassium should be measured periodically, and, if necessary, corrective therapy should be implemented.

As with any penicillin, the possibility of an allergic response, including anaphylaxis, exists, particularly in hypersensitive patients.

USAGE DURING PREGNANCY

Reproduction studies have been performed in mice and rats and have revealed no evidence of impaired fertility or harm to the fetus due to ticarcillin. There are no well-controlled studies in pregnant women, but investigational experience does not include any positive evidence of adverse effects on the fetus. Although there is no clearly defined risk, such experience cannot exclude the possibility of infrequent or subtle damage to the fetus. Ticarcillin should be used in pregnant women only when clearly needed.

ADVERSE REACTIONS

The following adverse reactions may occur:

Hypersensitivity Reactions: Skin rashes, pruritus, urticaria, drug fever.

Gastrointestinal Disturbances: Nausea and vomiting.

Hemic and Lymphatic Systems: As with other penicillins, anemia, thrombocytopenia, leukopenia, neutropenia and eosinophilia.

Abnormalities of Blood, Hepatic and Renal Laboratory Studies: As with other semisynthetic penicillins, SGOT and SGPT elevations have been reported. To date, clinical manifestations of hepatic or renal disorders have not been observed which could be ascribed solely to ticarcillin.

CNS: Patients, especially those with impaired renal function, may experience convulsions or neuromuscular excitability when very high doses of the drug are administered.

Other: Local reactions such as pain (rarely accompanied by induration) at the site of the injection have been reported.

Vein irritation and phlebitis can occur, particularly when undiluted solution is directly injected into the vein.

[See table on bottom preceding page]

DIRECTIONS FOR USE

—1 Gm, 3 Gm and 6 Gm Standard Vials—

INTRAMUSCULAR USE: (Concentration of approximately 385 mg/ml).

For initial reconstitution use Sterile Water for Injection, U.S.P., Sodium Chloride Injection, U.S.P. or 1% Lidocaine Hydrochloride solution* (without epinephrine).

Each gram of ticarcillin should be reconstituted with 2 ml of Sterile Water for Injection, U.S.P., Sodium Chloride Injection, U.S.P. or 1% Lidocaine Hydrochloride solution* (without epinephrine) and used promptly. Each 2.6 ml of the resulting solution will then contain 1 Gm of ticarcillin.

*[For full product information, refer to manufacturer's package insert for Lidocaine Hydrochloride.]

As with all intramuscular preparations, TICAR (ticarcillin disodium) should be injected well within the body of a relatively large muscle, using usual techniques and precautions.

INTRAVENOUS ADMINISTRATION: (Concentration of approximately 200 mg/ml).

For initial reconstitution use Sodium Chloride Injection, U.S.P., Dextrose Injection 5% or Lactated Ringer's Injection.

Reconstitute each gram of ticarcillin with 4 ml of the appropriate diluent. After the addition of 4 ml of diluent per gram of ticarcillin each 1.0 ml of the resulting solution will have an approximate concentration of 200 mg. Once dissolved, further dilute if desired.

DIRECT INTRAVENOUS INJECTION: In order to avoid vein irritation, administer solution as slowly as possible.

INTRAVENOUS INFUSION: Administer by continuous or intermittent intravenous drip. Intermittent infusion should be administered over a 30 minute to 2 hour period in equally divided doses. **—3 Gm Piggyback Bottles—**

DIRECT INTRAVENOUS INJECTION: (Concentrations of approximately 29 mg/ml to 100 mg/ml).

The 3 gram bottle should be reconstituted with a minimum of 30 ml of the desired intravenous solution listed below.

Amount of Diluent	Concentration of Solution
100 ml	1 Gm/34 ml (~29 mg/ml)
60 ml	1 Gm/20 ml (50 mg/ml)
30 ml	1 Gm/10 ml (100 mg/ml)

In order to avoid vein irritation, the solution should be administered as slowly as possible. A dilution of approximately 50 mg/ml or more will further reduce the incidence of vein irritation.

INTRAVENOUS INFUSION: Stability studies in the intravenous solutions listed below indicate that ticarcillin disodium will provide sufficient activity at room temperature (70°–75°F) within the stated time periods at concentrations between 10 mg/ml and 50 mg/ml—see Stability Period section below. After reconstitution and prior to administration Ticar as with other parenteral drugs should be inspected visually for particulate matter and discoloration.

[See table above].

Refrigerated solutions stored longer than 72 hours should not be used for multidose purposes.

After reconstitution and dilution to a concentration of 10 mg/ml to 100 mg/ml, this solution can be frozen (0°F) and stored for up to 30 days. The thawed solution must be used within 24 hours. Unused solutions should be discarded after the time periods mentioned above.

It is recommended that TICAR and gentamicin sulfate, tobramycin sulfate or amikacin sulfate not be mixed together in the same I.V. solution due to the gradual inactivation of gentamicin sulfate, tobramycin sulfate or amikacin sulfate under these circumstances. The therapeutic effect of TICAR and these aminoglycoside drugs remains unimpaired when administered separately.

HOW SUPPLIED

TICAR (sterile ticarcillin disodium). Each vial contains ticarcillin disodium equivalent to 1 Gm, 3 Gm, 6 Gm, ticarcillin.

NDC 0029-6550-22 ....1 Gm Vial
NDC 0029-6552-26 ....3 Gm Vial
NDC 0029-6555-26 ....6 Gm Vial
NDC 0029-6552-21 ....3 Gm Piggyback Bottle

Ticar is also supplied as:

NDC 0029-6558-21 ....20 Gm Pharmacy Bulk Package
NDC 0029-6559-21 ....30 Gm Pharmacy Bulk Package
NDC 0029-6552-40 ......3 Gm ADD-Vantage® ANTIBIOTIC VIAL

TICAR (sterile ticarcillin disodium). Each vial contains ticarcillin disodium equivalent to 20 Gm, 30 Gm, 3 Gm ticarcillin.

STORE DRY POWDER AT ROOM TEMPERATURE or BELOW.

June, 1988
7182/C

TIGAN®   ℞

[tī'găn]
(trimethobenzamide HCl)

DESCRIPTION

Chemically, trimethobenzamide HCl is N-[p-[2-(dimethylamino) -ethoxy] benzyl]-3,4,5-trimethoxybenzamide hydrochloride. It has a molecular weight of 424.93 and the following structural formula:

$$(CH_3)_2N-CH_2CH_2O-\!\!\!\!\bigcirc\!\!\!\!-CH_2NHC\overset{O}{\underset{\parallel}{}}-\!\!\!\!\bigcirc\!\!\!\!\begin{smallmatrix}OCH_3\\OCH_3\\OCH_3\end{smallmatrix} \cdot HCl$$

Capsules: Blue, each containing 250 mg trimethobenzamide hydrochloride; blue and white, each containing 100 mg trimethobenzamide hydrochloride.

Inactive Ingredients: Lactose, Magnesium Stearate and Starch.

Suppositories, (200 mg): Each suppository contains 200 mg trimethobenzamide hydrochloride and 2% benzocaine in a base compounded with polysorbate 80, white beeswax and propylene glycol monostearate.

Suppositories, Pediatric (100 mg): Each suppository contains 100 mg trimethobenzamide hydrochloride and 2% benzocaine in a base compounded with polysorbate 80, white beeswax and propylene glycol monostearate.

Ampuls: Each 2-mL ampul contains 200 mg trimethobenzamide hydrochloride compounded with 0.2% parabens (methyl and propyl) as preservatives, 1 mg sodium citrate and 0.4 mg citric acid as buffers and pH adjusted to approximately 5.0 with sodium hydroxide.

Multiple Dose Vials: Each mL contains 100 mg trimethobenzamide hydrochloride compounded with 0.45% phenol as preservative, 0.5 mg sodium citrate and 0.2 mg citric acid as buffers and pH adjusted to approximately 5.0 with sodium hydroxide.

Thera-Ject® (Disposable Syringes): Each 2 mL contains 200 mg trimethobenzamide hydrochloride compounded with 0.45% phenol as preservative, 1 mg sodium citrate and 0.4 mg citric acid as buffers, 0.2 mg disodium edetate as stabilizer and pH adjusted to approximately 5.0 with sodium hydroxide.

ACTIONS

The mechanism of action of Tigan as determined in animals is obscure, but may be the chemoreceptor trigger zone (CTZ), an area in the medulla oblongata through which emetic impulses are conveyed to the vomiting center; direct impulses to the vomiting center apparently are not similarly inhibited. In dogs pretreated with trimethobenzamide HCl, the emetic response to apomorphine is inhibited, while little or no protection is afforded against emesis induced by intragastric copper sulfate.

INDICATIONS

Tigan is indicated for the control of nausea and vomiting.

CONTRAINDICATIONS

The injectable form of Tigan in children, the suppositories in premature or newborn infants, and use in patients with known hypersensitivity to trimethobenzamide are contraindicated. Since the suppositories contain benzocaine they should not be used in patients known to be sensitive to this or similar local anesthetics.

WARNINGS

Caution should be exercised when administering Tigan to children for the treatment of vomiting. Antiemetics are not recommended for treatment of uncomplicated vomiting in children and their use should be limited to prolonged vomiting of known etiology. There are three principal reasons for caution:

1. There has been some suspicion that centrally acting antiemetics may contribute, in combination with viral illnesses (a possible cause of vomiting in children), to development of Reye's syndrome, a potentially fatal acute childhood encephalopathy with visceral fatty degeneration, especially involving the liver. Although there is no confirmation of this suspicion, caution is nevertheless recommended.

2. The extrapyramidal symptoms which can occur secondary to Tigan may be confused with the central nervous system signs of an undiagnosed primary disease responsible for the vomiting, e.g., Reye's syndrome or other encephalopathy.

3. It has been suspected that drugs with hepatotoxic potential, such as Tigan, may unfavorably alter the course of Reye's syndrome. Such drugs should therefore be avoided in children whose signs and symptoms (vomiting) could represent Reye's syndrome. It should also be noted that salicylates and acetaminophen are hepatotoxic at large doses. Although it is not known that at usual doses they would represent a hazard in patients with the underlying hepatic disorder of Reye's syndrome, these drugs, too, should be avoided in children whose signs and symptoms could represent Reye's syndrome, unless alternative methods of controlling fever are not successful.

Tigan may produce drowsiness. Patients should not operate motor vehicles or other dangerous machinery until their individual responses have been determined. Reye's syndrome has been associated with the use of TIGAN and other drugs, including antiemetics, although their contribution, if any, to the cause and course of the disease hasn't been established. This syndrome is characterized by an abrupt onset shortly following a nonspecific febrile illness, with persistent, severe vomiting, lethargy, irrational behavior, progressive encephalopathy leading to coma, convulsions and death.

Usage in Pregnancy: Trimethobenzamide hydrochloride was studied in reproduction experiments in rats and rabbits and no teratogenicity was suggested. The only effects observed were an increased percentage of embryonic resorptions or stillborn pups in rats administered 20 mg and 100 mg/kg and increased resorptions in rabbits receiving 100 mg/kg. In each study these adverse effects were attributed to one or two dams. The relevance to humans is not known. Since there is no adequate experience in pregnant or lactating women who have received this drug, safety in pregnancy or in nursing mothers has not been established.

Usage with Alcohol: Concomitant use of alcohol with Tigan may result in an adverse drug interaction.

PRECAUTIONS

During the course of acute febrile illness, encephalitides, gastroenteritis, dehydration and electrolyte imbalance, especially in children and the elderly or debilitated, CNS reactions such as opisthotonos, convulsions, coma and extrapyramidal symptoms have been reported with and without use of Tigan or other antiemetic agents. In such disorders caution should be exercised in administering Tigan, particularly to patients who have recently received other CNS-acting agents (phenothiazines, barbiturates, belladonna derivatives). It is recommended that severe emesis should not be treated with an antiemetic drug alone; where possible the cause of vomiting should be established. Primary emphasis should be directed toward the restoration of body fluids and electrolyte balance, the relief of fever and relief of the causative disease process. Overhydration should be avoided since it may result in cerebral edema.

The antiemetic effects of Tigan may render diagnosis more difficult in such conditions as appendicitis and obscure signs of toxicity due to overdosage of other drugs.

ADVERSE REACTIONS

There have been reports of hypersensitivity reactions and Parkinson-like symptoms. There have been instances of hypotension reported following parenteral administration to surgical patients. There have been reports of blood dyscrasias, blurring of vision, coma, convulsions, depression of mood, diarrhea, disorientation, dizziness, drowsiness, headache, jaundice, muscle cramps and opisthotonos. If these occur, the administration of the drug should be discontinued. Allergic-type skin reactions have been observed; therefore, the drug should be discontinued at the first sign of sensitization. While these symptoms will usually disappear spontaneously, symptomatic treatment may be indicated in some cases.

SERUM LEVELS IN ADULTS
AFTER A 30-MINUTE IV INFUSION OF TIMENTIN

TICARCILLIN SERUM LEVELS (mcg/ml)							
Dose	0	15 min.	30 min.	1 hr.	1.5 hr.	3.5 hr.	5.5 hr.
3.1 Gm	324 (293–388)	223 (184–293)	176 (135–235)	131 (102–195)	90 (65–119)	27 (19–37)	6 (5–7)
3.2 Gm	336 (301–386)	214 (180–258)	186 (160–218)	122 (108–136)	78 (33–113)	29 (19–44)	10 (5–15)

CLAVULANIC ACID SERUM LEVELS (mcg/ml)							
Dose	0	15 min.	30 min.	1 hr.	1.5 hr.	3.5 hr.	5.5 hr.
3.1 Gm	8.0 (5.3–10.3)	4.6 (3.0–7.6)	2.6 (1.8–3.4)	1.8 (1.6–2.2)	1.2 (0.8–1.6)	0.3 (0.2–0.3)	0
3.2 Gm	15.8 (11.7–21.0)	8.3 (6.4–10.0)	5.2 (3.5–6.3)	3.4 (1.9–4.0)	2.5 (1.3–3.4)	0.5 (0.2–0.8)	0

DOSAGE AND ADMINISTRATION
(See WARNINGS and PRECAUTIONS.)
Dosage should be adjusted according to the indication for therapy, severity of symptoms and the response of the patient.
CAPSULES, 250 mg and 100 mg
Usual Adult Dosage
  One 250-mg capsule t.i.d. or q.i.d.
Usual Children's Dosage
  30 to 90 lbs: One or two 100-mg capsules t.i.d. or q.i.d.
SUPPOSITORIES, 200 mg (Not to be used in premature or newborn infants.)
Usual Adult Dosage
  One suppository (200 mg) t.i.d. or q.i.d.
Usual Children's Dosage
  Under 30 lbs: One-half suppository (100 mg) t.i.d. or q.i.d.
  30 to 90 lbs: One-half to one suppository (100 to 200 mg) t.i.d. or q.i.d.
SUPPOSITORIES, PEDIATRIC, 100 mg (Not to be used in premature or newborn infants).
Usual Children's Dosage
  Under 30 lbs; One suppository (100 mg) t.i.d. or q.i.d.
  30 to 90 lbs; One to two suppositories (100 to 200 mg) t.i.d. or q.i.d.
INJECTABLE, 100 mg/mL (Not recommended for use in children.)
Usual Adult Dosage:
  2 mL (200 mg) t.i.d. or q.i.d. intramuscularly.
Intramuscular administration may cause pain, stinging, burning, redness and swelling at the site of injection. Such effects may be minimized by deep injection into the upper outer quadrant of the gluteal region, and by avoiding the escape of solution along the route.
Note: The injectable form is intended for intramuscular administration only; it is not recommended for intravenous use.

CAUTION
Federal law prohibits dispensing without prescription.

HOW SUPPLIED
Capsules, 250 mg trimethobenzamide hydrochloride each, bottles of 100 and 500; 100 mg trimethobenzamide hydrochloride each, bottles of 100.
Suppositories, 200 mg, boxes of 10 and 50
Suppositories, Pediatric, 100 mg, boxes of 10
Ampuls, 2 mL, boxes of 10
Multiple Dose Vials, 20 mL
Thera-Ject® (Disposable Syringes), 2 mL, boxes of 25
DGB—0059/1-87   Revised January, 1987
Shown in Product Identification Section, page 405

TIMENTIN®   ℞
[tĭ′mĕn-tĭn]
sterile ticarcillin disodium
and clavulanate potassium
for Intravenous Administration

DESCRIPTION
TIMENTIN is an injectable antibacterial combination consisting of the semisynthetic antibiotic, ticarcillin disodium and the β-lactamase inhibitor, clavulanate potassium (the potassium salt of clavulanic acid) for intravenous administration. Ticarcillin is derived from the basic penicillin nucleus, 6-amino-penicillanic acid. Chemically, it is 6-[(carboxy-3-thienylacetyl)amino]-3,3-dimethyl-7-oxo-4-thia-1-azabicyclo[3.2.0]heptane-2-carboxylic acid disodium salt and may be represented as:

Clavulanic acid is produced by the fermentation of *Streptomyces clavuligerus*. It is a β-lactam structurally re-

lated to the penicillins and possesses the ability to inactivate a wide variety of β-lactamases by blocking the active sites of these enzymes. Clavulanic acid is particularly active against the clinically important plasmid mediated β-lactamases frequently responsible for transferred drug resistance to penicillins and cephalosporins.

Chemically, clavulanate potassium is potassium Z-(3R,5R)-2-(β-hydroxyethylidene) clavam-3-carboxylate and may be represented structurally as:

TIMENTIN is supplied as a white to pale yellow powder for reconstitution. TIMENTIN is very soluble in water; its solubility being greater than 600 mg/ml. The reconstituted solution is clear, colorless or pale yellow, having a pH of 5.5 to 7.5. For the TIMENTIN 3.1 Gm and 3.2 Gm vials, the theoretical sodium content is 4.75 mEq (109 mg) per gram of TIMENTIN. The theoretical potassium content is 0.15 mEq (6 mg) and 0.3 mEq (11.9 mg) per gram of TIMENTIN for the 3.1 Gm vial and 3.2 Gm vial, respectively.

CLINICAL PHARMACOLOGY
After an intravenous infusion (30 min.) of 3.1 Gm or 3.2 Gm TIMENTIN, peak serum concentrations of both ticarcillin and clavulanic acid are attained immediately after completion of infusion. Ticarcillin serum levels are similar to those produced by the administration of equivalent amounts of ticarcillin alone with a mean peak serum level of 330 mcg/ml for the 3.1 Gm and 3.2 Gm formulations. The corresponding mean peak serum levels for clavulanic acid were 8 mcg/ml and 16 mcg/ml for the 3.1 Gm and 3.2 Gm formulations, respectively.
[See table above].
The mean area under the serum concentration curves for ticarcillin was 485 mcg/ml.hr for the TIMENTIN 3.1 Gm and 3.2 Gm formulations. The corresponding areas under the serum concentration curves for clavulanic acid were 8.2 mcg/ml.hr and 15.6 mcg/ml.hr for the TIMENTIN 3.1 Gm and 3.2 Gm formulations, respectively.
The mean serum half-lives of ticarcillin and clavulanic acid in healthy volunteers were 68 minutes and 64 minutes, respectively, following administration of 3.1 Gm or 3.2 Gm of TIMENTIN.
Approximately 60–70% of ticarcillin and approximately 35–45% of clavulanic acid are excreted unchanged in urine during the first 6 hours after administration of a single dose of TIMENTIN to normal volunteers with normal renal function. Two hours after an intravenous injection of 3.1 Gm or 3.2 Gm TIMENTIN, concentrations of ticarcillin in urine generally exceed 1500 mcg/ml. The corresponding concentrations of clavulanic acid in urine generally exceed 40 mcg/ml and 70 mcg/ml following administration of the 3.1 Gm and 3.2 Gm doses, respectively. By 4-6 hours after injection, the urine concentrations of ticarcillin and clavulanic acid usually decline to approximately 190 mcg/ml and 2 mcg/ml, respectively, for both doses.
Neither component of TIMENTIN is highly protein bound; ticarcillin has been found to be approximately 45% bound to human serum protein and clavulanic acid approximately 9% bound.
Somewhat higher and more prolonged serum levels of ticarcillin can be achieved with the concurrent administration of probenecid; however, probenecid does not enhance the serum levels of clavulanic acid.
Ticarcillin can be detected in tissues and interstitial fluid following parenteral administration.
Penetration of ticarcillin into the bile, pleural fluid and cerebrospinal fluid with inflamed meninges has been demonstrated. The results of experiments involving the administration of clavulanic acid to animals suggest that this compound, like ticarcillin, is well distributed in body tissues.
An inverse relationship exists between the serum half-life of ticarcillin and creatinine clearance. The dosage of TIMEN-

Continued on next page

Beecham Laboratories—Cont.

TIN need only be adjusted in cases of severe renal impairment (see Dosage and Administration).
Ticarcillin may be removed from patients undergoing dialysis; the actual amount removed depends on the duration and type of dialysis.
MICROBIOLOGY: Ticarcillin is a semisynthetic antibiotic with a broad spectrum of bactericidal activity against many Gram-positive and Gram-negative aerobic and anaerobic bacteria.
Ticarcillin is, however, susceptible to degradation by β-lactamases and therefore the spectrum of activity does not normally include organisms which produce these enzymes.
Clavulanic acid is a β-lactam, structurally related to the penicillins, which possesses the ability to inactivate a wide range of β-lactamase enzymes commonly found in microorganisms resistant to penicillins and cephalosporins. In particular, it has good activity against the clinically important plasmid mediated β-lactamases frequently responsible for transferred drug resistance.
The formulation of ticarcillin with clavulanic acid in TIMENTIN protects ticarcillin from degradation by β-lactamase enzymes and effectively extends the antibiotic spectrum of ticarcillin to include many bacteria normally resistant to ticarcillin and other β-lactam antibiotics. Thus TIMENTIN possesses the distinctive properties of a broad spectrum antibiotic and a β-lactamase inhibitor.
While *in vitro* studies have demonstrated the susceptibility of most strains of the following organisms, clinical efficacy for infections other than those included in the Indications section has not been documented.
GRAM-NEGATIVE BACTERIA: *Pseudomonas aeruginosa* (β-lactamase and non-β-lactamase producing), *Pseudomonas* species including *P. maltophilia* (β-lactamase and non-β-lactamase producing), *Escherichia coli* (β-lactamase and non-β-lactamase producing), *Proteus mirabilis* (β-lactamase and non-β-lactamase producing), *Proteus vulgaris* (β-lactamase and non-β-lactamase producing), *Providencia rettgeri* (formerly *Proteus rettgeri*) (β-lactamase and non-β-lactamase producing), *Providencia stuartii* (β-lactamase and non-β-lactamase producing), *Morganella morganii* (formerly *Proteus morganii*) (β-lactamase and non-β-lactamase producing), *Enterobacter* species (Although most strains of *Enterobacter* species are resistant *in vitro*, clinical efficacy has been demonstrated with TIMENTIN in urinary tract infections caused by these organisms). *Acinetobacter* species (β-lactamase and non-β-lactamase producing), *Hemophilus influenzae* (β-lactamase and non-β-lactamase producing), *Branhamella catarrhalis* (β-lactamase and non-β-lactamase producing), *Serratia* species including *S. marcescens* (β-lactamase and non-β-lactamase producing), *Neisseria gonorrhoeae* (β-lactamase and non-β-lactamase producing), *Neisseria meningitidis**, *Salmonella* species (β-lactamase and non-β-lactamase producing), *Klebsiella* species including *K. pneumoniae* (β-lactamase and non-β-lactamase producing), *Citrobacter* species including *C. freundii, C. diversus* and *C. amalonaticus* (β-lactamase and non-β-lactamase producing).
GRAM-POSITIVE BACTERIA: *Staphylococcus aureus* (β-lactamase and non-β-lactamase producing), *Staphylococcus saprophyticus, Staphylococcus epidermidis* (coagulase negative *Staphylococci*) (β-lactamase and non-β-lactamase producing), *Streptococcus pneumoniae** (*D. pneumoniae*), *Streptococcus bovis *, Streptococcus agalactiae ** (Group B), *Streptococcus faecalis ** (Enterococcus), *Streptococcus pyogenes ** (Group A, β-hemolytic), Viridans group *Streptococci **.
ANAEROBIC BACTERIA: *Bacteroides* species, including *B. fragilis* group (*B. fragilis, B. vulgatus*) (β-lactamase and non-β-lactamase producing), Non-*B. fragilis* (*B. melaninogenicus*) (β-lactamase and non-β-lactamase producing), *B. thetaiotaomicron, B. ovatus, B. distasonis,* (β-lactamase and non-β-lactamase producing), *Clostridium* species including *C. perfringens, C. difficile, C. sporogenes, C. ramosum* and *C. bifermentans *, Eubacterium* species, *Fusobacterium* species including *F. nucleatum* and *F. necrophorum *, Peptococcus* species*, *Peptostreptococcus* species*, *Veillonella* species.
* These are non-β-lactamase producing strains and therefore are susceptible to ticarcillin alone. Some of the β-lactamase producing strains are also susceptible to ticarcillin alone.
In vitro synergism between TIMENTIN and gentamicin, tobramycin or amikacin against multi-resistant strains of *Pseudomonas aeruginosa* has been demonstrated.
SUSCEPTIBILITY TESTING:
Diffusion Technique: An 85 mcg TIMENTIN (75 mcg ticarcillin plus 10 mcg clavulanic acid) diffusion disk is available for use with the Kirby-Bauer method. Based on the zone sizes given below, a report of "Susceptible" indicates that the infecting organism is likely to respond to TIMENTIN therapy, while a report of "Resistant" indicates that the organism is not likely to respond to therapy with this antibiotic. A report of "Intermediate" susceptibility indicates that the organism would be susceptible to TIMENTIN at a higher dosage or if

the infection is confined to tissues or fluids (e.g., urine) in which high antibiotic levels are attained.
Dilution Technique: Broth or agar dilution methods may be used to determine the minimal inhibitory concentration (MIC) values for bacterial isolates to TIMENTIN. Tubes should be inoculated with the test culture containing 10^4 to 10^5 CFU/ml or plates spotted with a test solution containing 10^3 to 10^4 CFU/ml.
The recommended dilution pattern utilizes a constant level of clavulanic acid, 2 mcg/ml, in all tubes together with varying amounts of ticarcillin. MIC's are expressed in terms of the ticarcillin concentration in the presence of 2 mcg/ml clavulanic acid.
RECOMMENDED RANGES FOR TIMENTIN SUSCEPTIBILITY TESTING[1,2,3]

Diffusion Method
Disk Zone Size, mm

Res. ≤11	Inter. 12–14	Susc. ≥15

Dilution Method
MIC Correlates[4], mcg/ml

Res. ≥128	Susc. ≤64

[1] The non-β-lactamase producing organisms which are normally susceptible to ticarcillin will have similar zone sizes as for ticarcillin.
[2] Staphylococci which are susceptible to TIMENTIN but resistant to methicillin, oxacillin or nafcillin must be considered as resistant.
[3] The quality control cultures should have the following assigned daily ranges for TIMENTIN:

		Disks	MIC Range (mcg/ml)
E. coli	(ATCC 25922)	24–30 mm	2/2–8/2
S. aureus	(ATCC 25923)	32–40 mm	
Ps. aeruginosa	(ATCC 27853)	20–28 mm	8/2–32/2
E. coli	(ATCC 35218)	21–25 mm	4/2–16/2
S. aureus	(ATCC 29213)	—	0.5/2–2/2

[4] Expressed as concentration of ticarcillin in the presence of a constant 2.0 mcg/ml concentration of clavulanic acid.

INDICATIONS AND USAGE

TIMENTIN is indicated in the treatment of infections caused by susceptible strains of the designated organisms in the conditions listed below:
Septicemia: including bacteremia, caused by β-lactamase producing strains of *Klebsiella* spp.*, *E. coli*, Staphylococcus aureus** and *Pseudomonas aeruginosa** (and other *Pseudomonas* species*).
Lower Respiratory Infections: caused by β-lactamase producing strains of *Staphylococcus aureus, Hemophilus influenzae** and *Klebsiella* spp.*
Bone and Joint Infections: caused by β-lactamase producing strains of *Staphylococcus aureus.*
Skin and Skin Structure Infections: caused by β-lactamase producing strains of *Staphylococcus aureus, Klebsiella* spp.* and *E. coli*.*
Urinary Tract Infections (complicated and uncomplicated): caused by β-lactamase producing strains of *E. coli, Klebsiella* spp., *Pseudomonas aeruginosa** (and other *Pseudomonas* spp.*), *Citrobacter* spp.*, *Enterobacter cloacae*, Serratia marcescens** and *Staphylococcus aureus*.*
Gynecologic Infections: Endometritis caused by B-lactamase producing strains of *B. melaninogenicus*, Enterobacter* spp. (including *E. cloacae**), *Escherichia coli, Klebsiella pneumoniae*, Staphlococcus aureus* and *Staphylococcus epidermidis.*
*Efficacy for this organism in this organ system was studied in fewer than 10 infections.
While TIMENTIN is indicated only for the conditions listed above, infections caused by ticarcillin susceptible organisms are also amenable to TIMENTIN treatment due to its ticarcillin content. Therefore, mixed infections caused by ticarcillin susceptible organisms and β-lactamase producing organisms susceptible to TIMENTIN should not require the addition of another antibiotic.
Appropriate culture and susceptibility tests should be performed before treatment in order to isolate and identify organisms causing infection and to determine their susceptibility to TIMENTIN. Because of its broad spectrum of bactericidal activity against Gram-positive and Gram-negative bacteria, TIMENTIN is particularly useful for the treatment of mixed infections and for presumptive therapy prior to the identification of the causative organisms. TIMENTIN has been shown to be effective as single drug therapy in the treatment of some serious infections where normally combination antibiotic therapy might be employed. Therapy with TIMENTIN may be initiated before results of such tests are known when there is reason to believe the infection may involve any of the β-lactamase producing organisms listed above; however, once these results become available, appropriate therapy should be continued.
Based on the *in vitro* synergism between TIMENTIN and aminoglycosides against certain strains of *Pseudomonas aeruginosa*, combined therapy has been successful, especially in patients with impaired host defenses. Both drugs should be

used in full therapeutic doses. As soon as results of culture and susceptibility tests become available, antimicrobial therapy should be adjusted as indicated.

CONTRAINDICATIONS

TIMENTIN is contraindicated in patients with a history of hypersensitivity reactions to any of the penicillins.

WARNINGS

SERIOUS AND OCCASIONALLY FATAL HYPERSENSITIVITY (ANAPHYLACTOID) REACTIONS HAVE BEEN REPORTED IN PATIENTS ON PENICILLIN THERAPY. THESE REACTIONS ARE MORE LIKELY TO OCCUR IN INDIVIDUALS WITH A HISTORY OF PENICILLIN HYPERSENSITIVITY AND/OR A HISTORY OF SENSITIVITY TO MULTIPLE ALLERGENS. THERE HAVE BEEN REPORTS OF INDIVIDUALS WITH A HISTORY OF PENICILLIN HYPERSENSITIVITY WHO HAVE EXPERIENCED SEVERE REACTIONS WHEN TREATED WITH CEPHALOSPORINS. BEFORE INITIATING THERAPY WITH TIMENTIN, CAREFUL INQUIRY SHOULD BE MADE CONCERNING PREVIOUS HYPERSENSITIVITY REACTIONS TO PENICILLINS, CEPHALOSPORINS, OR OTHER DRUGS. IF AN ALLERGIC REACTION OCCURS, TIMENTIN SHOULD BE DISCONTINUED AND THE APPROPRIATE THERAPY INSTITUTED. SERIOUS ANAPHYLACTOID REACTIONS REQUIRE IMMEDIATE EMERGENCY TREATMENT WITH EPINEPHRINE, OXYGEN, INTRAVENOUS STEROIDS, AND AIRWAY MANAGEMENT, INCLUDING INTUBATION, SHOULD ALSO BE PROVIDED AS INDICATED.

PRECAUTIONS

General: While TIMENTIN possesses the characteristic low toxicity of the penicillin group of antibiotics, periodic assessment of organ system functions, including renal, hepatic and hematopoietic function is advisable during prolonged therapy.
Bleeding manifestations have occurred in some patients receiving beta-lactam antibiotics. These reactions have been associated with abnormalities of coagulation tests such as clotting time, platelet aggregation and prothrombin time and are more likely to occur in patients with renal impairment. If bleeding manifestations appear, TIMENTIN treatment should be discontinued and appropriate therapy instituted.
TIMENTIN has only rarely been reported to cause hypokalemia; however, the possibility of this occurring should be kept in mind particularly when treating patients with fluid and electrolyte imbalance. Periodic monitoring of serum potassium may be advisable in patients receiving prolonged therapy.
The theoretical sodium content is 4.75 mEq (109 mg) per gram of TIMENTIN. This should be considered when treating patients requiring restricted salt intake.
As with any penicillin, an allergic reaction, including anaphylaxis, may occur during TIMENTIN administration, particularly in a hypersensitive individual.
The possibility of superinfections with mycotic or bacterial pathogens should be kept in mind, particularly during prolonged treatment. If superinfections occur, appropriate measures should be taken.
Drug/Laboratory Test Interactions: As with other penicillins, the mixing of TIMENTIN with an aminoglycoside in solutions for parenteral administration can result in substantial inactivation of the aminoglycoside.
Probenecid interferes with the renal tubular secretion of ticarcillin, thereby increasing serum concentrations and prolonging serum half-life of the antibiotic.
High urine concentrations of ticarcillin may produce false positive protein reactions (pseudoproteinuria) with the following methods: sulfosalicylic acid and boiling test, acetic acid test, biuret reaction, and nitric acid test. The bromphenol blue (Multi-stix®) reagent strip test has been reported to be reliable.
The presence of clavulanic acid in TIMENTIN may cause a non-specific binding of IgG and albumin by red cell membranes leading to a false positive Coombs test.
Carcinogenesis, Mutagenesis, Impairment of Fertility: Long-term studies in animals have not been performed to evaluate carcinogenic or mutagenic potential.
Pregnancy (Category B): Reproduction studies have been performed in rats given doses up to 1050 mg/kg/day and have revealed no evidence of impaired fertility or harm to the fetus due to TIMENTIN. There are, however, no adequate and well-controlled studies in pregnant women. Because animal reproduction studies are not always predictive of human response, this drug should be used during pregnancy only if clearly needed.
Nursing Mothers: Caution should be exercised when TIMENTIN is administered to a nursing woman.
Pediatric Use: The efficacy and safety of TIMENTIN have not been established in infants and children under the age of 12.
Drug Abuse and Dependence: Neither TIMENTIN abuse nor TIMENTIN dependence has been reported.

ADVERSE REACTIONS

As with other penicillins, the following adverse reactions may occur:

Hypersensitivity reactions: skin rash, pruritus, urticaria, arthralgia, myalgia, drug fever, chills, chest discomfort, and anaphylactic reactions.

Central nervous system: headache, giddiness, neuromuscular hyperirritability or convulsive seizures.

Gastro-intestinal disturbances: disturbances of taste and smell, stomatitis, flatulence, nausea, vomiting and diarrhea, epigastric pain.

Hemic and Lymphatic systems: thrombocytopenia, leukopenia, neutropenia, eosinophilia and reduction of hemoglobin or hematocrit. Prolongation of prothrombin time and bleeding time.

Abnormalities of hepatic and renal function tests: elevation of serum aspartate aminotransferase (SGOT), serum alanine aminotransferase (SGPT), serum alkaline phosphatase, serum LDH, serum bilirubin. Rarely, transient hepatitis and cholestatic jaundice—as with some other penicillins and some cephalosporins. Elevation of serum creatinine and/or BUN, hypernatremia. Reduction in serum potassium and uric acid.

Local reactions: pain, burning, swelling and induration at the injection site and thrombophlebitis with intravenous administration.

Overdosage: As with other penicillins, TIMENTIN in overdosage has the potential to cause neuromuscular hyperirritability or convulsive seizures. Ticarcillin may be removed from circulation by hemodialysis. The molecular weight, degree of protein binding and pharmacokinetic profile of clavulanic acid together with information from a single patient with renal insufficiency all suggest that this compound may also be removed by hemodialysis.

DOSAGE AND ADMINISTRATION

TIMENTIN should be administered by intravenous infusion (30 min.).

Adults: The usual recommended dosage for systemic and urinary tract infections for average (60 kg) adults is 3.1 Gm TIMENTIN (3.1 Gm vial containing 3 Gm ticarcillin and 100 mg clavulanic acid) given every 4 to 6 hours. For Gynecologic infections, TIMENTIN should be adminstered as follows: Moderate infections 200 mg/kg/day in divided doses every 6 hours and for severe infections 300 mg/kg/day in divided doses every 4 hours. For patients weighing less than 60 kg, the recommended dosage is 200–300 mg/kg/day, based on ticarcillin content, given in divided doses every 4 to 6 hours. In urinary tract infections, a dosage of 3.2 Gm TIMENTIN (3.2 Gm vial containing 3 Gm ticarcillin and 200 mg clavulanic acid) given every 8 hours is adequate.

For infections complicated by renal insufficiency[1], an initial loading dose of 3.1 Gm should be followed by doses based on creatinine clearance and type of dialysis as indicated below:

Creatinine clearance ml/min.	Dosage
over 60	3.1 Gm every 4 hrs
30–60	2 Gm every 4 hrs
10–30	2 Gm every 8 hrs
less than 10	2 Gm every 12 hrs
Less than 10 with hepatic dysfunction	2 Gm every 24 hrs
patients on peritoneal dialysis	3.1 Gm every 12 hrs
patients on hemodialysis	2 Gm every 12 hrs supplemented with 3.1 Gm after each dialysis

To calculate creatinine clearance* from a serum creatinine value use the following formula:

$$C_{cr} = \frac{(140\text{-Age}) \ (\text{wt in kg})}{72 \times S_{cr}(\text{mg}/100 \ \text{ml})}$$

This is the calculated creatinine clearance for adult males, for females it is 15% less.

* Cockcroft, D. W., et al, "Prediction of Creatinine Clearance from Serum Creatinine", Nephron 16:31-41 (1976).

[1] The half-life of Ticarcillin in patients with renal failure is approximately 13 hours.

Dosage for any individual patient must take into consideration the site and severity of infection, the susceptibility of the organisms causing infection, and the status of the patient's host defense mechanisms.

The duration of therapy depends upon the severity of infection. Generally, TIMENTIN should be continued for at least 2 days after the signs and symptoms of infection have disappeared. The usual duration is 10 to 14 days; however, in difficult and complicated infections, more prolonged therapy may be required.

Frequent bacteriologic and clinical appraisal is necessary during therapy of chronic urinary tract infection and may be required for several months after therapy has been completed; persistent infections may require treatment for several weeks and doses smaller than those indicated above should not be used.

In certain infections, involving abscess formation, appropriate surgical drainage should be performed in conjunction with antimicrobial therapy.

INTRAVENOUS ADMINISTRATION

DIRECTIONS FOR USE

3.1 Gm and 3.2 Gm Vials and Piggyback Bottles

The 3.1 Gm or 3.2 Gm vial should be reconstituted by adding approximately 13 ml of Sterile Water for Injection, U.S.P. or Sodium Chloride Injection, U.S.P.; and shaking well. When dissolved, the concentration of ticarcillin will be approximately 200 mg/ml with corresponding concentrations of 6.7 mg/ml and 13.4 mg/ml clavulanic acid for the 3.1 Gm and 3.2 Gm respective doses. Conversely, each 5.0 ml of the 3.1 Gm dose reconstituted with approximately 13 ml of diluent will contain approximately 1 Gm of ticarcillin and 33 mg of clavulanic acid. For the 3.2 Gm dose reconstituted with 13 ml of diluent, each 5.0 ml will contain 1 Gm of ticarcillin and 66 mg of clavulanic acid.

INTRAVENOUS INFUSION: The dissolved drug should be further diluted to desired volume using the recommended solution listed in the **Compatibility and Stability Section (Stability Period)** to a concentration between 10 mg/ml to 100 mg/ml. The solution of reconstituted drug may then be administered over a period of 30 minutes by direct infusion or through a Y-type intravenous infusion set. If this method or the "piggyback" method of administration is used, it is advisable to discontinue temporarily the administration of any other solutions during the infusion of TIMENTIN.

Stability—For I.V. solutions, see **Stability Period** below.

When TIMENTIN is given in combination with another antimicrobial, such as an aminoglycoside, each drug should be given separately in accordance with the recommended dosage and routes of administration for each drug.

After reconstitution and prior to administration, TIMENTIN, as with other parenteral drugs, should be inspected visually for particulate matter. If this condition is evident, the solution should be discarded. The color of reconstituted solutions of TIMENTIN normally ranges from light to dark yellow depending on concentration, duration and temperature of storage while maintaining label claim characteristics.

COMPATIBILITY AND STABILITY

3.1 Gm and 3.2 Gm Vials and Piggyback Bottles

(Dilutions derived from a stock solution of 200 mg/ml)

The concentrated stock solution at 200 mg/ml is stable for up to 6 hours at room temperature (70°–75°F) or up to 72 hours under refrigeration (40°F).

If the concentrated stock solution (200 mg/ml) is held for up to 6 hours at room temperature (70°–75°F) or up to 72 hours under refrigeration (40°F) and further diluted to a concentration between 10 mg/ml and 100 mg/ml with any of the diluents listed below, then the following stability periods apply.

STABILITY PERIOD
(3.1 Gm and 3.2 Gm Vials and Piggyback Bottles)

Intravenous Solution (Ticarcillin Concentrations of 10 mg/ml to 100 ml)	Room Temperature (70°–75°F)	Refrigerated (40°F)
Dextrose Injection 5%, U.S.P.	24 hours	3 days
Sodium Chloride Injection, U.S.P.	24 hours	7 days
Lactated Ringer's Injection, U.S.P.	24 hours	7 days

If the concentrated stock solution (200 mg/ml) is stored for up to 6 hours at room temperature and then further diluted to a concentration between 10 mg/ml and 100 mg/ml, solutions of Sodium Chloride Injection, U.S.P., and Lactated Ringer's Injection, U.S.P. may be stored frozen (0°F) for up to 30 days. Solutions prepared with Dextrose Injection 5%. U.S.P. may be stored frozen (0°F) for up to 7 days. All thawed solutions should be used within 8 hours or discarded. Once thawed, solutions should not be refrozen.

NOTE: TIMENTIN is incompatible with Sodium Bicarbonate. Unused solutions must be discarded after the time periods listed above.

HOW SUPPLIED

TIMENTIN (Sterile Ticarcillin Disodium and Clavulanate Potassium).

Each 3.1 Gm vial contains sterile ticarcillin disodium equivalent to 3 Gm ticarcillin and sterile clavulanate potassium equivalent to 0.1 Gm clavulanic acid.

NDC 0029-6571-26 .... 3.1 Gm Vial
NDC 0029-6571-21 .... 3.1 Gm Piggyback Bottle

Each 3.2 Gm vial contains sterile ticarcillin disodium equivalent to 3 Gm ticarcillin and sterile clavulanate potassium equivalent to 0.2 Gm clavulanic acid.

NDC 0029-6572-26 .... 3.2 Gm Vial
NDC 0029-6572-21 .... 3.2 Gm Piggyback Bottle

TIMENTIN is also supplied as:

NDC 0029-6571-40 ....3.1 Gm ADD-Vantage®
Antibiotic Vial

NDC 0029-6579-21 ....31 Gm Pharmacy Bulk Package

Each 31 Gm vial contains sterile ticarcillin disodium equivalent to 30 Gm ticarcillin and sterile clavulanate potassium equivalent to 1 Gm clavulanic acid.

TIMENTIN vials should be stored at room temperature or below.

Rev. January, 1989

7548/H

Shown in Product Identification Section, page 405

Beiersdorf Inc
P.O. BOX 5529
NORWALK, CT 06856-5529

AQUAPHOR®

Ointment

NDC Numbers– 10356-020-01
10356-020-02
10356-020-03
10356-020-06
10356-020-07

COMPOSITION

Petrolatum, mineral oil, mineral wax, wool wax alcohol.

ACTIONS AND USES

Aquaphor is a stable, neutral, odorless, anhydrous ointment base. Miscible with water or aqueous solutions, Aquaphor will absorb several times its own weight, forming smooth, creamy water-in-oil emulsions. In its pure form, Aquaphor is recommended for use as a topical preparation to help soothe, protect and heal minor cuts and burns. Helps prevent and protect chapped, cracked and extremely dry skin and lips.

ADMINISTRATION AND DOSAGES

Use Aquaphor alone or in compounding virtually any ointment using aqueous solutions alone or in combination with other oil-based substances, and all common topical medications. Apply Aquaphor liberally to affected area. In the case of wounds, clean area prior to application.

PRECAUTIONS

For external use only. Avoid contact with eyes. Not be applied over third degree burns, deep or puncture wounds, infections or lacerations. If condition worsens or does not improve within 7 days, patient should consult a doctor.

HOW SUPPLIED

1.75 oz. tube—List No. 45583
3.25 oz. jar—List No. 45584
16 oz. jar—List No. 45585
5 lb. jar—List. No. 45586
45 lb. drum—List No. 45587

EUCERIN® Cleansing Bar

[ū'sir-in]

Unscented Moisturizing Formula

ACTIVE INGREDIENT

Eucerite®

ACTIONS AND USES

Eucerin® Cleansing Bar has been specially formulated for use on sensitive skin. The formulation contains Eucerite®, a special blend of ingredients that closely resemble the natural oils of the skin, thus providing excellent moisturizing properties. This formulation is unscented and non-comedogenic. Additionally, the ph value of Eucerin Cleansing Bar is maintained at 5.5 in order to match the skin's normal acid mantle.

DIRECTIONS

Use during shower, bath, or regular cleansing, or as directed by physician

HOW SUPPLIED

3 ounce bar.
List number 3852

EUCERIN® Creme

[ū'sir-in]

Unscented Moisturizing Formula

NDC Numbers–10356-090-01
10356-090-05
10356-090-04

COMPOSITION

Water, petrolatum, mineral oil, mineral wax, wool wax alcohol, methylchoroisothiazolinone-methylisothiazolinone.

Continued on next page

Beiersdorf—Cont.

ACTIONS AND USES

A gentle, non-comedogenic, unscented water-in-oil emulsion, Eucerin helps alleviate excessively dry skin and may be helpful in conditions such as chapped or chafed skin, sunburn, windburn, and itching associated with dryness.

ADMINISTRATION AND DOSAGES

Apply freely to affected areas of the skin as often as necessary or as directed by physician.

PRECAUTIONS

For external use only.

HOW SUPPLIED

16 oz. jar—List Number 0090
8 oz. jar—List Number 3774
4 oz. jar—List Number 3797

EUCERIN® Lotion
[ū 'sir-in]
Unscented Moisturizing Formula
NDC Numbers–10356-793-01
          10356-793-04
          10356-793-06

COMPOSITION

Water, Mineral Oil, Isopropyl Myristate, PEG-40 Sorbitan Peroleate, Lanolin Acid Glycerin Ester, Sorbitol, Propylene Glycol, Cetyl Palmitate, Magnesium Sulfate, Aluminum Stearate, Lanolin Alcohol, BHT, Methylchloroisothiazolinone · Methylisothiazolinone.

ACTIONS AND USES

Eucerin Lotion is a non-comedogenic, unscented, unique water-in-oil formulation that will help to alleviate and soothe excessively dry skin, and provide long-lasting moisturization.

ADMINISTRATION AND DOSAGE

Apply Eucerin Lotion all over body—hands, arms, legs, and feet—to help moisturize, smooth and soothe rough, dry skin.

PRECAUTIONS

For external use only.

HOW SUPPLIED

4 fluid oz. plastic bottle—List Number 3771
8 fluid oz. plastic bottle—List Number 3793
16 fluid oz. plastic bottle—List number 3794

Berlex Laboratories, Inc.
300 FAIRFIELD ROAD
WAYNE, NJ 07470

DECONAMINE® Tablets   ℞
[dē "con 'uh-mēēn]
DECONAMINE® SR Capsules   ℞
DECONAMINE® Syrup   ℞
(chlorpheniramine maleate; d-pseudoephedrine hydrochloride)

DESCRIPTION
Tablets
Each scored, white tablet contains:
  chlorpheniramine maleate ....4 mg
  d-pseudoephedrine hydrochloride ....60 mg
Each DECONAMINE® Tablet also contains the following inactive ingredients: dibasic calcium phosphate, magnesium stearate, microcrystalline cellulose, pregelatinized starch, silica gel, starch (corn), and stearic acid.
SR Capsules
Each sustained-release blue and yellow capsule contains:
  chlorpheniramine maleate ....8 mg
  d-pseudoephedrine hydrochloride ....120 mg
Each DECONAMINE® SR Capsule also contains the following inactive ingredients: coloring agents, gelatin, starch, and sucrose.
Each DECONAMINE® SR Capsule contains FD&C Yellow No. 6 as a color additive.
Each DECONAMINE® SR Capsule may also contain one or more of the following inactive ingredients: butyl paraben, methyl paraben, propyl paraben, titanium dioxide and other ingredient(s).
  The capsules are designed to provide prolonged release of medication.
Syrup—No alcohol, no dye
Each 5 mL (teaspoonful) clear, colorless to slightly yellow liquid contains:
  chlorpheniramine maleate ....2 mg
  d-pseudoephedrine hydrochloride ....30 mg
in a grape-flavored, aromatic vehicle

DECONAMINE® Syrup also contains the following inactive ingredients: citric acid, flavoring agent, glycerin, sodium benzoate, sodium chloride, sorbitol, sucrose, and water.

CLINICAL PHARMACOLOGY

Chlorpheniramine maleate antagonizes the physiological action of histamine by acting as an H_1 receptor blocking agent.
Pseudoephedrine is an orally active sympathomimetic amine and exerts a decongestant action on the nasal mucosa. It does this by vasoconstriction, which results in reduction of tissue hyperemia, edema, nasal congestion and an increase in nasal airway patency. The vasoconstrictive action of pseudoephedrine is similar to that of ephedrine. In the usual dose it has minimal vasopressor effects.

INDICATIONS

For relief of nasal congestion associated with the common cold, hay fever and other allergies, sinusitis, eustachian tube blockage, and vasomotor and allergic rhinitis.

CONTRAINDICATIONS

Patients with severe hypertension, severe coronary artery disease and patients on MAO inhibitor therapy.
DECONAMINE® medications are also contraindicated in patients sensitive to antihistamines or sympathomimetic agents.

WARNINGS

Chlorpheniramine maleate should be used with extreme caution in patients with narrow angle glaucoma; stenosing peptic ulcer; pyloroduodenal obstruction; symptomatic prostatic hypertrophy; or bladder neck obstruction. Due to its mild atropine-like action, chlorpheniramine maleate should be used cautiously in patients with bronchial asthma.
Sympathomimetic amines should be used with caution in patients with hypertension, ischemic heart disease, diabetes mellitus, increased intraocular pressure, hyperthyroidism and prostatic hypertrophy. Sympathomimetics may produce central nervous system stimulation with convulsions or cardiovascular collapse with accompanying hypotension.

PRECAUTIONS

Information for patients:
Antihistamines may impair mental and physical abilities required for the performance of potentially hazardous tasks, such as driving a vehicle or operating machinery. Patients should also be warned about possible additive effects with alcohol and other central nervous system depressants (hypnotics, sedatives, tranquilizers).
Drug interactions:
Pseudoephedrine-containing drugs should not be given to patients treated with monoamine oxidase (MAO) inhibitors because of the possibility of precipitating a hypertensive crisis. MAO inhibitors also prolong and intensify the anticholinergic effects of antihistamines. Sympathomimetics may reduce the antihypertensive effect of methyldopa, reserpine, veratrum alkaloids and mecamylamine.
Alcohol and other sedative drugs will potentiate the sedative effects of chlorpheniramine.
Care should be taken in administering DECONAMINE® medications concomitantly with other sympathomimetic amines, since their combined effects on the cardiovascular system may be harmful to the patient.
Pregnancy:
Pregnancy Category C: Animal reproduction studies have not been conducted with DECONAMINE® medications. It is also not known whether DECONAMINE® medications can cause fetal harm when administered to a pregnant woman or can affect reproduction capacity. DECONAMINE® medications should be given to a pregnant woman only if clearly needed.
Nursing Mothers: Due to the possible passage of pseudoephedrine and chlorpheniramine into breast milk, and, because of the higher than usual risk for infants from sympathomimetic amines and antihistamines, the benefit to the mother vs. the potential risk should be considered and a decision should be made whether to discontinue nursing or to discontinue the drug.
Pediatric Use: DECONAMINE® Capsules or Tablets should not be given to children under 12 years of age.

ADVERSE REACTIONS
Chlorpheniramine maleate
Slight to moderate drowsiness may occur and is the most frequent side effect. Other possible side effects of antihistamines in general include:
General: urticaria, drug rash, anaphylactic shock, photosensitivity, excessive perspiration, chills, dryness of mouth, nose and throat;
Cardiovascular: hypotension, headache, palpitation, tachycardia, extrasystoles;
Hematological: hemolytic anemia, thrombocytopenia, agranulocytosis;

CNS: sedation, dizziness, disturbed coordination, fatigue, confusion, restlessness, excitation, nervousness, tremor, irritability, insomnia, euphoria, paresthesia, blurred vision, diplopia, vertigo, tinnitus, hysteria, neuritis, convulsion;
Gastrointestinal: epigastric distress, anorexia, nausea, vomiting, diarrhea, constipation;
Genitourinary: urinary frequency, difficult urination, urinary retention, early menses;
Respiratory: thickening of bronchial secretions, tightness of chest, wheezing and nasal stuffiness.
Pseudoephedrine hydrochloride
Pseudoephedrine may cause mild central nervous system stimulation, especially in those patients who are hypersensitive to sympathomimetic drugs. Nervousness, excitability, restlessness, dizziness, weakness and insomnia may also occur. Headache and drowsiness have also been reported. Large doses may cause lightheadedness, nausea and/or vomiting. Sympathomimetic drugs have also been associated with certain untoward reactions including fear, anxiety, tenseness, restlessness, tremor, weakness, pallor, respiratory difficulty, dysuria, insomnia, hallucination, convulsion, CNS depression, arrhythmias and cardiovascular collapse with hypotension.

OVERDOSAGE

Acute overdosage may produce clinical signs of CNS stimulation and variable cardiovascular effects. Pressor amines should be used with great caution in the presence of pseudoephedrine. Patients with signs of stimulation should be treated conservatively.

DOSAGE AND ADMINISTRATION
Tablets
Adults and children over 12 years, 1 tablet three or four times daily.
Children under 12 years, DECONAMINE® Syrup is recommended.
Syrup
Adults and children over 12 years, 1 to 2 teaspoonfuls (5 to 10 mL) three or four times daily.
Children 6 to 12 years, ½ to 1 teaspoonful (2.5 to 5 mL) three or four times daily, not to exceed 4 teaspoonfuls in 24 hours.
Children 2 to 6 years, ½ teaspoonful (2.5 mL) three or four times daily, not to exceed 2 teaspoonfuls in 24 hours.
Children under two years, as directed by physician.
SR Capsules
Adults and children over 12 years, 1 capsule every 12 hours.
Children under 12 years, DECONAMINE® Syrup is recommended.

HOW SUPPLIED
In bottles of:
Tablets
  100 ....NDC 50419-184-10
SR Capsules
  100 ....NDC 50419-181-10
  500 ....NDC 50419-181-50
Syrup
  473 mL ....NDC 50419-185-16
Store at controlled room temperature.
Manufactured by or for
BERLEX Laboratories, Inc.
Wayne, NJ 07470
Rev. 1/88   60565-2
Shown in Product Identification Section, page 405

QUINAGLUTE®   ℞
[kwĭn 'uh-glōōt "]
(quinidine gluconate)
DURA–TABS®
(sustained-release tablets)

DESCRIPTION

Each QUINAGLUTE® (brand of quinidine gluconate) DURA-TABS® (brand of sustained-release tablets) Tablet contains 324 mg quinidine gluconate (equivalent to 202 mg quinidine base) in a tablet matrix specially designed for the sustained-release (8 to 12 hours) of the drug in the gastrointestinal tract. QUINAGLUTE® DURA-TABS® Tablets are to be administered orally.
Quinidine gluconate is the gluconate salt of quinidine [6-methoxy-α-(5-vinyl-2-quinuclidinyl)-4-quinoline-methanol], a dextrorotatory isomer of quinine. Quinidine gluconate is represented by the following structural formula:

Quinidine gluconate contains 62.3% of the anhydrous quinidine alkaloid, whereas quinidine sulfate contains 82.86%. In prescribing QUINAGLUTE® DURA-TABS® Tablets, this factor should be considered.

Therapeutic category: Type I antiarrhythmic.

Each QUINAGLUTE® DURA-TABS® Tablet also contains the following inactive ingredients: confectioner's sugar, magnesium stearate, starch (corn), and other ingredient(s).

CLINICAL PHARMACOLOGY

The antiarrhythmic activity consists of the following basic actions:

1. In arrhythmias due to enhanced automaticity, quinidine decreases the rate of rise of slow diastolic (Phase 4) depolarization, thereby depressing automaticity, particularly in ectopic foci.
2. In addition to the above, quinidine slows depolarization, repolarization and amplitude of the action potential, thus increasing its duration leading to an increase in the refractoriness of atrial and ventricular tissue. Prolongation of the effective refractory period and an increase in conduction time may prevent the reentry phenomenon.
3. Quinidine exerts an indirect anticholinergic effect through blockade of vagal innervation. This anticholinergic effect may facilitate conduction in the atrioventricular junction.

Quinidine absorption from QUINAGLUTE® DURA-TABS® Tablets proceeds at a slower rate than the immediate-release products. In a single-dose pharmacokinetic study conducted in normal volunteers, the time of peak quinidine serum concentration was 1.6 hours for quinidine sulfate tablets and 3.6 hours for QUINAGLUTE® DURA-TABS® Tablets.

The apparent elimination half-life of quinidine ranges from 4 to 10 hours in healthy persons with a usual mean value of 6 to 7 hours. The half-life may be prolonged in elderly persons. From 60% to 80% of the dose is metabolized by the liver. Renal excretion of the intact drug comprises the remainder of the total clearance. Quinidine is approximately 75% bound to serum proteins.

In the past, plasma levels of 1.5 to 5 μg/mL have been reported as therapeutic,[1] based on non-specific assay methodology that quantitates quinidine metabolites as well as intact quinidine. The therapeutic plasma level range using newer, more specific assays has not been definitively established; however, effective reduction of premature ventricular contractions has been reported with blood levels less than 1.0 μg/mL.[2] In general, plasma quinidine levels are lower using specific assays. Clinicians requesting serum quinidine determinations should therefore also ask that the method of analysis be specified.

Due to the wide individual variation in response to quinidine therapy, the usefulness of serum quinidine levels in the planning of optimal quinidine therapy has not been clearly established. A serum quinidine concentration within the reported therapeutic range may not necessarily be the optimal concentration for some patients. In the absence of toxicity, such patients may warrant an increase in dose to achieve the desired therapeutic effect. However, for those patients in whom a high blood level has been achieved without significant therapeutic response, increasing the dose to potentially toxic levels is not warranted and consideration should be given to combination or alternate therapy. In all cases, the physician should carefully consider the patient response and evidence of toxicity along with blood levels in determining optimal quinidine therapy.

[1] Koch-Weser, Arch. Int. Med. 1972, 129:763-772.
[2] Carliner et al, Am. Heart Journ. 1980, 100:483-489.

INDICATIONS AND USAGE

QUINAGLUTE® DURA-TABS® Tablets are indicated in the prevention and/or treatment of:

1. Ventricular arrhythmias
   Premature ventricular contractions
   Ventricular tachycardia (when not associated with complete heartblock)
2. Junctional (nodal) arrhythmias
   AV junctional premature complexes
   Paroxysmal junctional tachycardia
3. Supraventricular (atrial) arrhythmias
   Premature atrial contractions
   Paroxysmal atrial tachycardia
   Atrial flutter
   Atrial fibrillation (chronic and paroxysmal)

CONTRAINDICATIONS

1. Idiosyncrasy or hypersensitivity to quinidine.
2. Complete AV block.
3. Complete bundle branch block or other severe intraventricular conduction defects, especially those exhibiting a marked grade of QRS widening.
4. Digitalis intoxication manifested by AV conduction disorders.
5. Myasthenia gravis.
6. Aberrant impulses and abnormal rhythms due to escape mechanisms.

WARNINGS

1. In the treatment of atrial flutter, reversion to sinus rhythm may be preceded by a progressive reduction in the degree of AV block to a 1:1 ratio resulting in an extremely rapid ventricular rate. This possible hazard may be reduced by digitalization prior to administration of quinidine.
2. Recent reports indicate that plasma concentrations of digoxin increase and may even double when quinidine is administered concurrently. Patients on concomitant therapy should be carefully monitored. Reduction of digoxin dosage may have to be considered.
3. Manifestations of quinidine cardiotoxicity such as excessive prolongation of the QT interval, widening of the QRS complex and ventricular tachyarrhythmias mandate immediate discontinuation of the drug and/or close clinical and electrocardiographic monitoring.
4. In susceptible individuals, such as those with marginally compensated cardiovascular disease, quinidine may produce clinically important depression of cardiac function such as hypotension, bradycardia, or heartblock. Quinidine therapy should be carefully monitored in such individuals.
5. Quinidine should be used with extreme caution in patients with incomplete AV block since complete block and asystole may be produced. Quinidine may cause abnormalities of cardiac rhythm in digitalized patients and therefore should be used with caution in the presence of digitalis intoxication.
6. Quinidine should be used with caution in patients exhibiting renal, cardiac or hepatic insufficiency because of potential accumulation of quinidine in plasma leading to toxicity.
7. Patients taking quinidine occasionally have syncopal episodes, usually resulting from ventricular tachycardia or fibrillation. This syndrome has not been shown to be related to dose or plasma levels. Syncopal episodes frequently terminate spontaneously or in response to treatment, but sometimes are fatal.
8. A few cases of hepatotoxicity, including granulomatous hepatitis, due to quinidine hypersensitivity have been reported in patients taking quinidine. Unexplained fever and/or elevation of hepatic enzymes, particularly in the early stages of therapy, warrant consideration of possible hepatotoxicity. Monitoring liver function during the first 4 to 8 weeks should be considered. Cessation of quinidine in these cases usually results in the disappearance of toxicity.

PRECAUTIONS

General: The precautions to be observed include all those applicable to quinidine. A preliminary test dose of a single tablet of quinidine sulfate may be administered to determine if the patient has an idiosyncrasy to quinidine. Hypersensitivity to quinidine, although rare, should constantly be considered, especially during the first weeks of therapy. Hospitalization for close clinical observation, electrocardiographic monitoring, and possible determination of plasma quinidine levels is indicated when large doses are used, or with patients who present an increased risk.

Information for Patients: As with all solid oral dosage medications, QUINAGLUTE® DURA-TABS® Tablets should be taken with an adequate amount of fluid, preferably in an upright position, to facilitate swallowing.

Drug Interactions:

Drug	Effect
Quinidine with anticholinergic drugs	Additive vagolytic effect
Quinidine with cholinergic drugs	Antagonism of cholinergic effects
Quinidine with carbonic anhydrase inhibitors, sodium bicarbonate, thiazide diuretics	Alkalinization of urine resulting in decreased excretion of quinidine
Quinidine with coumarin anticoagulants	Reduction of clotting factor concentrations
Quinidine with tubocurare, succinylcholine and decamethonium	Potentiation of neuromuscular blockade
Quinidine with phenothiazines and reserpine	Additive cardiac depressive effects
Quinidine with hepatic enzyme-inducing drugs (phenobarbital, phenytoin, rifampin)	Potential for reduction of quinidine plasma levels
Quinidine with cimetidine	Potential for elevation of quinidine plasma levels
Quinidine with digoxin	Increased plasma concentrations of digoxin (See WARNINGS)

Carcinogenesis, Mutagenesis and Impairment of Fertility: Long-term studies in animals have not been performed to evaluate the carcinogenic potential of quinidine. There is currently no evidence of quinidine-induced mutagenesis or impairment of fertility.

Pregnancy: Teratogenic Effects: Pregnancy Category C. Animal reproduction studies have not been conducted with quinidine. There are no adequate and well-controlled studies in pregnant women. QUINAGLUTE® DURA-TABS® Tablets should be administered to a pregnant woman only if clearly indicated.

Nonteratogenic Effects: Like quinine, quinidine has been reported to have oxytocic properties. The significance of this property in the clinical setting has not been established.

Nursing Mothers: Because of passage of the drug into breast milk, caution should be exercised when QUINAGLUTE® DURA-TABS® Tablets are administered to a nursing woman.

Pediatric Use: There are no adequate and well-controlled studies establishing the safety and effectiveness of QUINAGLUTE® DURA-TABS® Tablets in children.

ADVERSE REACTIONS

Symptoms of cinchonism, ringing in ears, headache, nausea, and/or disturbed vision may appear in sensitive patients after a single dose of the drug.

The most frequently encountered side effects to quinidine are gastrointestinal in nature. These gastrointestinal effects include nausea, vomiting, abdominal pain, diarrhea, and rarely, esophagitis.

Less frequently encountered adverse reactions:

Cardiovascular: Widening of QRS complex, cardiac asystole, ventricular ectopic beats, idioventricular rhythms including ventricular tachycardia and fibrillation, paradoxical tachycardia, arterial embolism and hypotension.

Hematologic: Acute hemolytic anemia, hypoprothrombinemia, thrombocytopenia (purpura), agranulocytosis.

Central Nervous System: Headache, fever, vertigo, apprehension, excitement, confusion, delirium and syncope, disturbed hearing (tinnitus, decreased auditory acuity), disturbed vision (mydriasis, blurred vision, disturbed color perception, reduced vision field, photophobia, diplopia, night blindness, scotomata), optic neuritis.

Dermatologic: Rash, cutaneous flushing with intense pruritus, urticaria. Photosensitivity has also been reported.

Hypersensitivity Reactions: Angioedema, acute asthmatic episode, vascular collapse, respiratory arrest, hepatotoxicity including granulomatous hepatitis (See WARNINGS).

Although rare, there have been reports of lupus erythematosus in patients taking quinidine.

OVERDOSAGE

If ingestion of quinidine is recent, gastric lavage, emesis and/or administration of activated charcoal may reduce absorption. Management of overdosage includes symptomatic treatment, ECG and blood pressure monitoring, cardiac pacing if indicated, and acidification of the urine. Artificial respiration and other supportive measures may be required. IV infusion of $\frac{1}{6}$ molar sodium lactate reportedly reduces the cardiotoxic effects of quinidine. Since marked CNS depression may occur even in the presence of convulsions, CNS depressants should not be administered. Hypotension may be treated, if necessary, with metaraminol or norepinephrine after adequate fluid volume replacement. Hemodialysis has been reported to be effective in the treatment of quinidine overdosage in adults and children, but is rarely warranted.

DOSAGE AND ADMINISTRATION

The dosage varies considerably depending upon the general condition and cardiovascular state of the patient. The quantity and frequency of administration of QUINAGLUTE® DURA-TABS® Tablets that will achieve the desired clinical results must be determined for each patient.

The ideal dosage is the minimum amount of total dose and frequency of daily administration that will prevent premature contractions, paroxysmal tachycardias and maintain normal sinus rhythm.

Prevention of premature atrial, nodal or ventricular contractions:
1 to 2 tablets every 8 or 12 hours.

Maintenance of normal sinus rhythm following conversion of paroxysmal tachycardias:
2 tablets every 12 hours or 1 $\frac{1}{2}$ to 2 tablets every 8 hours are usually required.

Continued on next page

Information on the Berlex products appearing here is based on the labeling in effect on June 1, 1989. Further information for these and other products may be obtained from the Professional Services Department, Berlex Laboratories, Inc., 300 Fairfield Road, Wayne, New Jersey 07470 (201) 292-3007.

Berlex—Cont.

Although most patients may be maintained in normal rhythm on a dosage of 1 QUINAGLUTE® DURA-TABS® Tablet every 8 or 12 hours, other patients may require larger doses or more frequent administration (ie every 6 hours) than the usually recommended schedule. Such increased dosage should be instituted only after careful clinical and laboratory evaluation of the patient, including monitoring of plasma quinidine levels and, if possible, serial electrocardiograms.

QUINAGLUTE® DURA-TABS® Tablets are generally well tolerated. Gastrointestinal disturbances, if they occur, may be minimized by administering the drug with food.

It is frequently desirable to determine if a patient can tolerate maintenance quinidine therapy prior to electrical conversion. Therefore, maintenance therapy may be initiated 2 to 3 days before electrical conversion is attempted.

QUINAGLUTE® DURA-TABS® Tablets are well suited for such a program and can be administered at a maintenance dose felt necessary for a given patient as indicated above.

Note: Dosage may be titrated by breaking the tablet in half. Do not crush or chew since sustained-release properties will be lost.

HOW SUPPLIED

White to off-white round tablet imprinted with:

In bottles of:

100 Tablets	NDC 50419-101-10
250 Tablets	NDC 50419-101-25
	NSN 6505-00-728-2009
500 Tablets	NDC 50419-101-50
Unit Dose Boxes of 100	NDC 50419-101-11

Store at controlled room temperature, between 15° and 30°C (59° and 86°F).

* Tablet designs are registered trademarks of Berlex Laboratories, Inc.

Revised 12/86   60536-6

Shown in Product Identification Section, page 405

TRI-LEVLEN® 21   ℞
[*trī-lĕv́lĕn*]
Tablets
(levonorgestrel and ethinyl estradiol tablets—triphasic regimen)

TRI-LEVLEN® 28   ℞
[*trī-lĕv́lĕn*]
Tablets
(levonorgestrel and ethinyl estradiol tablets—triphasic regimen)

LEVLEN® 21   ℞
[*lĕv́lĕn*]
Tablets
(levonorgestrel and ethinyl estradiol tablets)

LEVLEN® 28   ℞
Tablets
(levonorgestrel and ethinyl estradiol tablets)

DESCRIPTION

TRI-LEVLEN® 21 tablets
Each cycle of TRI-LEVLEN® 21 (Levonorgestrel and Ethinyl Estradiol Tablets—Triphasic Regimen) tablets consists of three different drug phases as follows: Phase 1 comprised of 6 brown tablets, each containing 0.050 mg of levonorgestrel (d(-)-13 beta-ethyl-17-alpha-ethinyl-17-beta-hydroxygon-4-en-3-one), a totally synthetic progestogen, and 0.030 mg of ethinyl estradiol (19-nor-17α-pregna-1,3,5(10)-trien-20-yne-3,17-diol); phase 2 comprised of 5 white tablets, each containing 0.075 mg levonorgestrel and 0.040 mg ethinyl estradiol; and, phase 3 comprised of 10 light-yellow tablets, each containing 0.125 mg levonorgestrel and 0.030 mg ethinyl estradiol. The inactive ingredients present are calcium carbonate, glycerin, iron oxides, lactose, magnesium stearate, methylparaben, polyethylene glycol, povidone, propylparaben, sodium benzoate, starch, sucrose, talc, and titanium dioxide.

TRI-LEVLEN® 28 tablets
Each cycle of TRI-LEVLEN® 28 (Levonorgestrel and Ethinyl Estradiol Tablets—Triphasic Regimen) tablets consists of three different drug phases as follows: Phase 1 comprised of 6 brown tablets, each containing 0.050 mg of levonorgestrel (d(-)-13 beta-ethyl-17-alpha-ethinyl-17-beta-hydroxygon-4-en-3-one), a totally synthetic progestogen, and 0.030 mg of ethinyl estradiol (19-nor-17 α-pregna-1,3,5(10)-trien-20-yne-3, 17-diol); phase 2 comprised of 5 white tablets, each containing 0.075 mg levonorgestrel and 0.040 mg ethinyl estradiol; and phase 3 comprised of 10 light-yellow tablets, each con-

taining 0.125 mg levonorgestrel and 0.030 mg ethinyl estradiol; then followed by 7 light-green inert tablets. The inactive ingredients present are calcium carbonate, cellulose, FD&C Blue 1, glycerin, iron oxides, lactose, magnesium stearate, methylparaben, polyethylene glycol, povidone, propylparaben, sodium benzoate, starch, sucrose, talc, and titanium dioxide.

LEVLEN® 21 tablets:
Each LEVLEN® 21 tablet contains 0.15 mg of levonorgestrel (d(-)-13 beta-ethyl-17-alpha-ethinyl-17-beta-hydroxygon-4-en-3-one), a totally synthetic progestogen, and 0.03 mg of ethinyl estradiol (19-nor-17 α-pregna-1,3,5(10)-trien-20-yne-3, 17-diol). The inactive ingredients present are cellulose, FD&C Yellow 6, lactose, magnesium stearate, and polacrillin potassium.

LEVLEN® 28 tablets:
21 light-orange LEVLEN® tablets, each containing 0.15 mg of levonorgestrel (d(-)-13 beta-ethyl-17-alpha-ethinyl-17-beta-hydroxygon-4-en-3-one), a totally synthetic progestogen, and 0.03 mg of ethinyl estradiol (19-nor-17 α-pregna-1,3,5(10)-trien-20-yne-3, 17-diol), and 7 pink inert tablets. The inactive ingredients present are cellulose, FD&C Red 3, FD&C Yellow 6, lactose, magnesium stearate, and polacrillin potassium.

Levonorgestrel   Ethinyl Estradiol

CLINICAL PHARMACOLOGY

Combination oral contraceptives act primarily through the mechanism of gonadotropin suppression due to the estrogenic and progestational activity of the ingredients. Although the primary mechanism of action is inhibition of ovulation, alterations in the genital tract, including changes in the cervical mucus (which increase the difficulty of sperm penetration) and the endometrium (which reduce the likelihood of implantation), may also contribute to contraceptive effectiveness.

INDICATIONS AND USAGE

TRI-LEVLEN® tablets and LEVLEN® tablets are indicated for the prevention of pregnancy in women who elect to use oral contraceptives as a method of contraception. Oral contraceptives are highly effective. The pregnancy rate in women using conventional combination oral contraceptives (containing 35 mcg or more of ethinyl estradiol or 50 mcg or more of mestranol) is generally reported as less than one pregnancy per 100 woman-years of use. Slightly higher rates (somewhat more than 1 pregnancy per 100 woman-years of use) are reported for some combination products containing 35 mcg or less of ethinyl estradiol, and rates on the order of 3 pregnancies per 100 woman-years are reported for the progestogen-only oral contraceptives.

These rates are derived from separate studies conducted by different investigators in several population groups and cannot be compared precisely. Furthermore, pregnancy rates tend to be lower as clinical studies are continued, possibly due to selective retention in the longer studies of those patients who accept the treatment regimen and do not discontinue as a result of adverse reactions, pregnancy, or other reasons.

In clinical trials with TRI-LEVLEN® tablets, 3,546 patients completed 35,036 cycles, and a total of nine pregnancies were reported. This represents a pregnancy rate of 0.33 per 100 woman-years. When used as directed, two pregnancies resulted for a corrected pregnancy rate of 0.07 per 100 woman-years.

In clincal trials with LEVLEN® tablets, 1,084 patients completed 8.186 cycles, and a total of three pregnancies were reported. This represents a pregnancy rate of 0.48 per 100 woman-years.

Table 1 gives ranges of pregnancy rates reported in the literature[1] for other means of contraception. The efficacy of these means of contraception (except the IUD) depends upon the degree of adherence to the method.

TABLE 1
PREGNANCIES PER 100 WOMAN-YEARS
IUD, less than 1–6; Diaphragm with spermicidal products (creams or jellies), 2–20; Condom, 3–36; Aerosol foams, 2–29; Jellies and creams, 4–36; Periodic abstinence (rhythm) all types, less than 1–47:

1. Calendar method, 14–47;
2. Temperature method, 1–20;
3. Temperature method—intercourse only in postovulatory phase, less than 1–7;
4. Mucus method, 1–25;

No contraception, 60–80.

Dose-Related Risk of Thromboembolism from Oral Contraceptives: Two studies have shown a positive association between the dose of estrogens in oral contraceptives

and the risk of thromboembolism.[2,3] For this reason, it is prudent and in keeping with good principles of therapeutics to minimize exposure to estrogen. The oral-contraceptive product prescribed for any given patient should be that product which contains the least amount of estrogen that is compatible with an acceptable pregnancy rate and patient acceptance. It is recommended that new acceptors of oral contraceptives be started on preparations containing 0.05 mg or less of estrogen.

CONTRAINDICATIONS

Oral contraceptives should not be used in women with any of the following conditions:

1. Thrombophlebitis or thromboembolic disorders.
2. A past history of deep-vein thrombophlebitis or thromboembolic disorders.
3. Cerebral-vascular or coronary-artery disease.
4. Known or suspected carcinoma of the breast.
5. Known or suspected estrogen-dependent neoplasia.
6. Undiagnosed abnormal genital bleeding.
7. Known or suspected pregnancy (see Warning No. 5).
8. Benign or malignant liver tumor which developed during the use of oral contraceptives or other estrogen-containing products.

WARNINGS

> Cigarette smoking increases the risk of serious cardio-vascular side effects from oral-contraceptive use. This risk increases with age and with heavy smoking (15 or more cigarettes per day) and is quite marked in women over 35 years of age. Women who use oral contraceptives should be strongly advised not to smoke.
>
> The use of oral contraceptives is associated with increased risk of several serious conditions, including thromboembolism, stroke, myocardial infarction, hepatic adenoma, gallbladder disease, hypertension. Practitioners prescribing oral contraceptives should be familiar with the following information relating to these risks.

1. *Thromboembolic Disorders and Other Vascular Problems:* An increased risk of thromboembolic and thrombotic disease associated with the use of oral contraceptives is well-established. Three principal studies in Great Britain[4-6] and three in the United States[7-10] have demonstrated an increased risk of fatal and nonfatal venous thromboembolism and stroke, both hemorrhagic and thrombotic. These studies estimate that users of oral contraceptives are 4 to 11 times more likely than nonusers to develop these diseases without evident cause (Table 2).

CEREBROVASCULAR DISORDERS
In a collaborative American study[9,10] of cerebrovascular disorders in women with and without predisposing causes, it was estimated that the risk of hemorrhagic stroke was 2.0 times greater in users than nonusers and the risk of thrombotic stroke was 4 to 9.5 times greater in users than in nonusers (Table 2).

TABLE 2
SUMMARY OF RELATIVE RISK OF THROMBOEMBOLIC DISORDERS AND OTHER VASCULAR PROBLEMS IN ORAL-CONTRACEPTIVE USERS COMPARED TO NONUSERS

	Relative risk, times greater
Idiopathic thromboembolic disease	4–11
Postsurgery thromboembolic complications	4–6
Thrombotic stroke	4–9.5
Hemorrhagic stroke	2
Myocardial infarction	2–12

MYOCARDIAL INFARCTION
An increased risk of myocardial infarction associated with the use of oral contraceptives has been reported,[11-13] confirming a previously suspected association. These studies, conducted in the United Kingdom, found, as expected, that the greater the number of underlying risk factors for coronary-artery disease (cigarette smoking, hypertension, hypercholesterolemia, obesity, diabetes, history of preeclamptic toxemia) the higher the risk of developing myocardial infarction, regardless of whether the patient was an oral-contraceptive user or not. Oral contraceptives, however, were found to be a clear additional risk factor.

In terms of relative risk, it has been estimated[52] that oral-contraceptive users who do not smoke (smoking is considered a major predisposing condition to myocardial infarction) are about twice as likely to have a fatal myocardial infarction as nonusers who do not smoke. Oral-contraceptive users who are also smokers have about a 5-fold increased risk of fatal infarction compared to users who do not smoke, but about a 10- to 12-fold increased risk compared to nonusers who do not smoke. Furthermore, the amount of smoking is also an important factor. In determining the importance of these relative risks, however, the baseline rates for various age groups, as shown in Table 3, must be given serious consideration. The importance of other predisposing conditions mentioned above in determining relative and absolute risks has not as yet been quantified; it is quite likely that the same synergistic action exists, but perhaps to a lesser extent.

TABLE 3

Estimated annual mortality rate per 100,000 women from myocardial infarction by use of oral contraceptives, smoking habits, and age (in years):

	Myocardial infarction			
	Women aged 30–39		Women aged 40–44	
Smoking habits	Users	Non-users	Users	Non-users
All smokers	10.2	2.6	62.0	15.9
Heavy*	13.0	5.1	78.7	31.3
Light	4.7	0.9	28.6	5.7
Nonsmokers	1.8	1.2	10.7	7.4
Smokers and nonsmokers	5.4	1.9	32.8	11.7

*Heavy smoker: 15 or more cigarettes per day.
From JAIN, A.K., *Studies in Family Planning*, 8 :50, 1977.

RISK OF DOSE

In an analysis of data derived from several national adverse-reaction reporting systems,[2] British investigators concluded that the risk of thromboembolism, including coronary thrombosis, is directly related to the dose of estrogen used in oral contraceptives. Preparations containing 100 mcg or more of estrogen were associated with a higher risk of thromboembolism than those containing 50–80 mcg of estrogen. Their analysis did suggest, however, that the quantity of estrogen may not be the sole factor involved. This finding has been confirmed in the United States.[3] Careful epidemiological studies to determine the degree of thromboembolic risk associated with progestogen-only oral contraceptives have not been performed. Cases of thromboembolic disease have been reported in women using these products, and they should not be presumed to be free of excess risk.

ESTIMATE OF EXCESS MORTALITY FROM CIRCULATORY DISEASES

A large prospective study[53] carried out in the U.K. estimated the mortality rate per 100,000 women per year from diseases of the circulatory system for users and nonusers of oral contraceptives according to age, smoking habits, and duration of use. The overall excess death rate annually from circulatory diseases for oral-contraceptive users was estimated to be 20 per 100,000 (ages 15–34—5/100,000; ages 35–44—33/100,000; ages 45–49—140/100,000), the risk being concentrated in older women, in those with a long duration of use, and in cigarette smokers. It was not possible, however, to examine the interrelationships of age, smoking, and duration of use, nor to compare the effects of continuous vs. intermittent use. Although the study showed a 10-fold increase in death due to circulatory diseases in users for 5 or more years, all of these deaths occurred in women 35 or older. Until larger numbers of women under 35 with continuous use for 5 or more years are available, it is not possible to assess the magnitude of the relative risk for this younger age group. The available data from a variety of sources have been analyzed[14] to estimate the risk of death associated with various methods of contraception. The estimates of risk of death for each method include the combined risk of the contraceptive method (e.g., thromboembolic and thrombotic disease in the case of oral contraceptives) plus the risk attributable to pregnancy or abortion in the event of method failure. This latter risk varies with the effectiveness of the contraceptive method. The findings of this analysis are shown in the bar graph (Figure 1).[14] The study concluded that the mortality associated with all methods of birth control is low and below that associated with childbirth, with the exception of oral contraceptives in women over 40 who smoke. (The rates given for Pill only/smokers for each age group are for smokers as a class. For "heavy" smokers [more than 15 cigarettes a day], the rates given would be about double; for "light" smokers [less than 15 cigarettes a day], about 50 percent.) The lowest mortality is associated with the condom or diaphragm backed up by early abortion. The risk of thromboembolic and thrombotic disease associated with oral contraceptives increases with age after approximately age 30 and, for myocardial infarction, is further increased by hypertension, hypercholesterolemia, obesity, diabetes, or history of pre-eclamptic toxemia and, especially, by cigarette smoking. Based on the data currently available, the following chart gives a gross estimate of the risk of death from circulatory disorders associated with the use of oral contraceptives:

SMOKING HABITS AND OTHER PREDISPOSING CONDITIONS—RISK ASSOCIATED WITH USE OF ORAL CONTRACEPTIVES

Age	Below 30	30–39	40+
Heavy smokers	C	B	A
Light smokers	D	C	B
Nonsmokers (no predisposing conditions)	D	C, D	C
Nonsmokers (other predisposing conditions)	C	C, B	B, A

A—Use associated with very high risk.
B—Use associated with high risk.
C—Use associated with moderate risk.
D—Use associated with low risk.

The physician and the patient should be alert to the earliest manifestations of thromboembolic and thrombotic disorders (e.g., thrombophlebitis, pulmonary embolism, cerebrovascular insufficiency, coronary occlusion, retinal thrombosis, and mesenteric thrombosis). Should any of these occur or be suspected, the drug should be discontinued immediately.

A four- to six-fold increased risk of postsurgery thromboembolic complications has been reported in oral-contraceptive users.[15,16] If feasible, oral contraceptives should be discontinued at least 4 weeks before surgery of a type associated with an increased risk of thromboembolism or prolonged immobilization.

Figure 1. Estimated annual number of deaths associated with control of fertility and no control per 100,000 non-sterile women, by regimen of control and age of women.

Regimen of control

□ No method ▦ Abortion only ▨ Pill only/nonsmokers ☐ Pill only/smokers

▦ IUDs only ▨ Traditional contraception only (diaphragm or condom) ■ Traditional contraception and abortion

PERSISTENCE OF RISK OF VASCULAR DISORDERS

Findings from one study in Great Britain involving cerebrovascular disease[54] and another study in the United States concerning myocardial infarction[55] suggest that an increased risk of these conditions in users of oral contraceptives persists after discontinuation of the oral contraceptive. In the British study, the risk of cerebrovascular disease remained elevated in former oral-contraceptive users for at least six years after discontinuation. In the U.S. study, an increased risk of myocardial infarction persisted for at least 9 years in women 40- to 49-years-old who had used oral contraceptives for five or more years. The findings in both these studies require confirmation since they are inconsistent with other published information.[9,11,13,56–60]

2. *Ocular Lesions:*

There have been reports of neuro-ocular lesions such as optic neuritis or retinal thrombosis associated with the use of oral contraceptives. Discontinue oral-contraceptive medication if there is unexplained, sudden or gradual, partial or complete loss of vision; onset of proptosis or diplopia; papilledema; or retinal-vascular lesions, and institute appropriate diagnostic and therapeutic measures.

3. *Carcinoma:*

Long-term continuous administration of either natural or synthetic estrogen in certain animal species increases the frequency of carcinoma of the breast, cervix, vagina, and liver. Certain synthetic progestogens, none currently contained in oral contraceptives, have been noted to increase the incidence of mammary nodules, benign and malignant, in dogs.

In humans, three case-control studies have reported an increased risk of endometrial carcinoma associated with the prolonged use of exogenous estrogen in postmenopausal women.[17–19] One publication[20] reported on the first 21 cases submitted by physicians to a registry of cases of adenocarcinoma of the endometrium in women under 40 on oral contraceptives. Of the cases found in women without predisposing risk factors for adenocarcinoma of the endometrium (e.g., irregular bleeding at the time oral contraceptives were first given, polycystic ovaries), nearly all occurred in women who had used a sequential oral contraceptive. These products are no longer marketed. No evidence has been reported suggesting an increased risk of endometrial cancer in users of conventional combination or progestogen-only oral contraceptives.

Several studies[8,21–24] have found no increase in breast cancer in women taking oral contraceptives or estrogens. One study,[25] however, while also noting no overall increased risk of breast cancer in women treated with oral contraceptives, found an excess risk in the subgroups of oral-contraceptive users with documented benign breast disease. A reduced occurrence of benign breast tumors in users of oral contraceptives has been well-documented.[8,21,25–27]

In summary, there is at present no confirmed evidence from human studies of an increased risk of cancer associated with oral contraceptives. Close clinical surveillance of all women taking oral contraceptives is, nevertheless, essential. In all cases of undiagnosed persistent or recurrent abnormal vaginal bleeding, appropriate diagnostic measures should be taken to rule out malignancy. Women with a strong family history of breast cancer or who have breast nodules, fibrocystic disease, or abnormal mammograms should be monitored with particular care if they elect to use oral contraceptives instead of other methods of contraception.

4. *Hepatic Tumors:*

Benign hepatic adenomas have been found to be associated with the use of oral contraceptives.[28–30,46] One study[46] showed that oral contraceptive formulations with high hormonal potency were associated with a higher risk than lower potency formulations. Although benign, hepatic adenomas may rupture and may cause death through intra-abdominal hemorrhage. This has been reported in short-term as well as long-term users of oral contraceptives. Two studies relate risk with duration of use of the contraceptive, the risk being much greater after 4 or more years of oral-contraceptive use.[30,46] While hepatic adenoma is a rare lesion, it should be considered in women presenting abdominal pain and tenderness, abdominal mass or shock. A few cases of hepatocellular carcinoma have been reported in women taking oral contraceptives. The relationship of these drugs to this type of malignancy is not known at this time.

5. *Use in or Immediately Preceding Pregnancy, Birth Defects in Offspring, and Malignancy in Female Offspring:*

The use of female sex hormones—both estrogenic and progestational agents—during early pregnancy may seriously damage the offspring. It has been shown that females exposed in utero to diethylstilbestrol, a non-steroidal estrogen, have an increased risk of developing in later life a form of vaginal or cervical cancer that is ordinarily extremely rare.[31,32] This risk has been estimated to be of the order of 1 in 1,000 exposures or less.[33,47] Although there is no evidence at the present time that oral contraceptives further enhance the risk of developing this type of malignancy, such patients should be monitored with particular care if they elect to use oral contraceptives instead of other methods of contraception. Furthermore, a high percentage of such exposed women (from 30 to 90%) have been found to have epithelial changes of the vagina and cervix.[34–38] Although these changes are histologically benign, it is not known whether this condition is a precursor of vaginal malignancy. Male children so exposed may develop abnormalities of the urogenital tract.[48–50] Although similar data are not available with the use of other estrogens, it cannot be presumed that they would not induce similar changes. An increased risk of congenital anomalies, including heart defects and limb defects, has been reported with the use of sex hormones, including oral contraceptives, in pregnancy.[39–42,51] One case-control study[42] has estimated a 4.7-fold increase in risk of limb-reduction defects in infants exposed in utero to sex hormones (oral contraceptives, hormonal withdrawal tests for pregnancy, or attempted treatment for threatened abortion).

Continued on next page

Information on the Berlex products appearing here is based on the labeling in effect on June 1, 1989. Further information for these and other products may be obtained from the Professional Services Department, Berlex Laboratories, Inc., 300 Fairfield Road, Wayne, New Jersey 07470 (201) 292-3007.

Berlex—Cont.

Some of these exposures were very short and involved only a few days of treatment. The data suggest that the risk of limb-reduction defects in exposed fetuses is somewhat less than one in 1,000 live births.

In the past, female sex hormones have been used during pregnancy in an attempt to treat threatened or habitual abortion. There is considerable evidence that estrogens are ineffective for these indications, and there is no evidence from well-controlled studies that progestogens are effective for these uses.

There is some evidence that triploidy and possibly other types of polyploidy are increased among abortuses from women who become pregnant soon after ceasing oral contraceptives.[43] Embryos with these anomalies are virtually always aborted spontaneously. Whether there is an overall increase in spontaneous abortion of pregnancies conceived soon after stopping oral contraceptives is unknown. It is recommended that, for any patient who has missed two consecutive periods, pregnancy should be ruled out before continuing the contraceptive regimen. If the patient has not adhered to the prescribed schedule, the possibility of pregnancy should be considered at the time of the first missed period (or after 45 days from the last menstrual period if the progestogen-only oral contraceptives are used), and further use of oral contraceptives should be withheld until pregnancy has been ruled out. If pregnancy is confirmed, the patient should be apprised of the potential risks to the fetus, and the advisability of continuation of the pregnancy should be discussed in the light of these risks.

It is also recommended that women who discontinue oral contraceptives with the intent of becoming pregnant use an alternate form of contraception for a period of time before attempting to conceive. Many clinicians recommend 3 months, although no precise information is available on which to base this recommendation. The administration of progestogen-only or progestogen-estrogen combinations to induce withdrawal bleeding should not be used as a test of pregnancy.

6. *Gallbladder Disease:*
Studies[8,23,26] report an increased risk of surgically confirmed gallbladder disease in users of oral contraceptives and estrogens. In one study, an increased risk appeared after 2 years of use and doubled after 4 or 5 years of use. In one of the other studies, an increased risk was apparent between 6 and 12 months of use.

7. *Carbohydrate and Lipid Metabolic Effects:*
A decrease in glucose tolerance has been observed in a significant percentage of patients on oral contraceptives. For this reason, prediabetic and diabetic patients should be carefully observed while receiving oral contraceptives.

An increase in triglycerides and total phospholipids has been observed in patients receiving oral contraceptives.[44] Three studies[61-63] have been performed with the TRI-LEVLEN® tablets formulation and no significant alterations in lipid metabolism were noted with the exception of a slight increase in triglyceride levels in one study.[62] The clinical significance of these findings remains to be defined.

8. *Elevated Blood Pressure:*
An increase in blood pressure has been reported in patients receiving oral contraceptives.[26] In some women, hypertension may occur within a few months of beginning oral-contraceptive use. In the first year of use, the prevalence of women with hypertension is low in users and may be no higher than that of a comparable group of nonusers. The prevalence in users increases, however, with longer exposure, and in the fifth year of use is two-and-a-half to three times the reported prevalence in the first year. Age is also strongly correlated with the development of hypertension in oral-contraceptive users. Women who previously have had hypertension during pregnancy may be more likely to develop elevation of blood pressure when given oral contraceptives. Hypertension that develops as a result of taking oral contraceptives usually returns to normal after discontinuing the drug.

9. *Headache:*
The onset or exacerbation of migraine or development of headache of a new pattern which is recurrent, persistent, or severe, requires discontinuation of oral contraceptives and evaluation of the cause.

10. *Bleeding Irregularities:*
Breakthrough bleeding, spotting, and amenorrhea are frequent reasons for patients discontinuing oral contraceptives. In breakthrough bleeding, as in all cases of irregular bleeding from the vagina, nonfunctional causes should be borne in mind. In undiagnosed persistent or recurrent abnormal bleeding from the vagina, adequate diagnostic measures are indicated to rule out pregnancy or malignancy. If pathology has been excluded, time or a change to another formulation may solve the problem. Changing to an oral contraceptive with a higher estrogen content, while potentially useful in minimizing menstrual irregularity, should be done only if

necessary, since this may increase the risk of thromboembolic disease.

Women with a past history of oligomenorrhea or secondary amenorrhea or young women without regular cycles may have a tendency to remain anovulatory or to become amenorrheic after discontinuation of oral contraceptives. Women with these preexisting problems should be advised of this possibility and encouraged to use other contraceptive methods. Post-use anovulation, possibly prolonged, may also occur in women without previous irregularities.

11. *Ectopic Pregnancy:*
Ectopic as well as intrauterine pregnancy may occur in contraceptive failures. However, in progestogen-only oral contraceptive failures, the ratio of ectopic to intrauterine pregnancies is higher than in women who are not receiving oral contraceptives, since the drugs are more effective in preventing intrauterine than ectopic pregnancies.

12. *Breast-feeding:*
Oral contraceptives given in the postpartum period may interfere with lactation. There may be a decrease in the quantity and quality of the breast milk. Furthermore, a small fraction of the hormonal agents in oral contraceptives has been identified in the milk of mothers receiving these drugs.[45,64,65] The effects, if any, on the breast-fed child have not been determined. If feasible, the use of oral contraceptives should be deferred until the infant has been weaned.

PRECAUTIONS
GENERAL
1. A complete medical and family history should be taken prior to initiation of oral contraceptives. The pretreatment and periodic physical examinations should include special reference to blood pressure, breasts, abdomen and pelvic organs, including Papanicolaou smear and relevant laboratory tests. As a general rule, oral contraceptives should not be prescribed for longer than 1 year without another physical examination and PAP smear being performed.
2. Under the influence of estrogen-progestogen preparations, preexisting uterine leiomyomata may increase in size.
3. Patients with a history of psychic depression should be carefully observed and the drug discontinued if depression recurs to a serious degree. Patients becoming significantly depressed while taking oral contraceptives should stop the medication and use an alternate method of contraception in an attempt to determine whether the symptom is drug-related.
4. Oral contraceptives may cause some degree of fluid retention. They should be prescribed with caution, and only with careful monitoring, in patients with conditions which might be aggravated by fluid retention, such as convulsive disorders, migraine syndrome, asthma, or cardiac or renal insufficiency.
5. Patients with a past history of jaundice during pregnancy have an increased risk of recurrence of jaundice while receiving oral-contraceptive therapy. If jaundice develops in any patient receiving such drugs, the medication should be discontinued.
6. Steroid hormones may be poorly metabolized in patients with impaired liver function and should be administered with caution in such patients.
7. Oral-contraceptive users may have disturbances in normal tryptophan metabolism which may result in a relative pyridoxine deficiency. The clinical significance of this is yet to be determined.
8. Serum folate levels may be depressed by oral-contraceptive therapy. Since the pregnant woman is predisposed to the development of folate deficiency and the incidence of folate deficiency increases with increasing gestation, it is possible that if a woman becomes pregnant shortly after stopping oral contraceptives, she may have a greater chance of developing folate deficiency and complications attributed to this deficiency.
9. The pathologist should be advised of oral-contraceptive therapy when relevant specimens are submitted.
10. Certain endocrine- and liver-function tests and blood components may be affected by estrogen-containing oral contraceptives:
a. Increased sulfobromophthalein retention.
b. Increased prothrombin and factors VII, VIII, IX, and X; decreased antithrombin 3; increased norepinephrine-induced platelet aggregability.
c. Increased thyroid-binding globulin (TBG) leading to increased circulating total-thyroid hormone, as measured by protein-bound iodine (PBI), T4 by column, or T4 by radioimmunoassay. Free T3 resin uptake is decreased, reflecting the elevated TBG; free T4 concentration is unaltered.
d. Decreased pregnanediol excretion.
e. Reduced response to metyrapone test.

INFORMATION FOR THE PATIENT
(See patient labeling which follows.)

DRUG INTERACTIONS
Reduced efficacy and increased incidence of breakthrough bleeding have been associated with concomitant use of rifampin. A similar association has been suggested with barbitu-

rates, phenylbutazone, phenytoin sodium, ampicillin, and tetracycline.

CARCINOGENESIS, MUTAGENESIS, IMPAIRMENT OF FERTILITY
See "Warnings" section #3,4 and 5, for information on the carcinogenesis, mutagenesis, and impairment of fertility.

PREGNANCY
Pregnancy Cagtegory X. See "Contraindications" and "Warnings."

NURSING MOTHERS
See "Warnings." Because of the potential for adverse reactions in nursing infants from oral-contraceptive tablets, a decision should be made whether to discontinue the drug, taking into account the importance of the drug to the mother.

ADVERSE REACTIONS
An increased risk of the following serious adverse reactions has been associated with the use of oral contraceptives (see "Warnings"):

Thrombophlebitis.	Hypertension.
Pulmonary embolism.	Gallbladder disease.
Coronary thrombosis.	Benign hepatomas.
Cerebral thrombosis.	Congenital anomalies.
Cerebral hemorrhage.	

There is evidence of an association between the following conditions and the use of oral contraceptives, although additional confirmatory studies are needed:
Mesenteric thrombosis.
Neuro-ocular lesions, e.g., retinal thrombosis and optic neuritis.
The following adverse reactions have been reported in patients receiving oral contraceptives and are believed to be drug-related:
Nausea and/or vomiting, usually the most common adverse reactions, occur in approximately 10 percent or less of patients during the first cycle. Other reactions, as a general rule, are seen much less frequently or only occasionally.
Gastrointestinal symptoms (such as abdominal cramps and bloating).
Breakthrough bleeding.
Spotting.
Change in menstrual flow.
Dysmenorrhea.
Amenorrhea during and after treatment.
Temporary infertility after discontinuance of treatment.
Edema.
Chloasma or melasma which may persist.
Breast changes: tenderness, enlargement, and secretion.
Change in weight (increase or decrease).
Change in cervical erosion and cervical secretion.
Possible diminution in lactation when given immediately postpartum.
Cholestatic jaundice.
Migraine.
Increase in size of uterine leiomyomata.
Rash (allergic).
Mental depression.
Reduced tolerance to carbohydrates.
Vaginal candidiasis.
Change in corneal curvature (steepening).
Intolerance to contact lenses.
The following adverse reactions have been reported in users of oral contraceptives, and the association has been neither confirmed nor refuted:

Premenstrual-like syndrome.	Hirsutism.
Cataracts.	Loss of scalp hair.
Changes in libido.	Erythema multiforme.
Chorea.	Erythema nodosum.
Changes in appetite.	Hemorrhagic eruption.
Cystitis-like syndrome.	Vaginitis.
Headache.	Porphyria.
Nervousness.	Hemolytic uremic
Dizziness.	syndrome.

ACUTE OVERDOSE
Serious ill effects have not been reported following acute ingestion of large doses of oral contraceptives by young children. Overdosage may cause nausea, and withdrawal bleeding may occur in females.

DOSAGE AND ADMINISTRATION
TRI-LEVLEN® tablets
To achieve maximum contraceptive effectiveness, TRI-LEVLEN® tablets (Levonorgestrel and Ethinyl Estradiol Tablets—Triphasic Regimen) must be taken exactly as directed and at intervals not exceeding 24 hours.
TRI-LEVLEN® 21 TABLETS (LEVONORGESTREL AND ETHINYL ESTRADIOL TABLETS—TRIPHASIC REGIMEN)
TRI-LEVLEN® 21 tablets are a three-phase preparation. The dosage of TRI-LEVLEN® 21 tablets is **one tablet daily** for 21 consecutive days per menstrual cycle in the following order: 6 brown tablets (phase 1), followed by 5 white tablets

(phase 2), and then followed by the last 10 light-yellow tablets (phase 3), according to the prescribed schedule. Tablets are then discontinued for 7 days (three weeks on, one week off).

It is recommended that TRI-LEVLEN® 21 tablets be taken at the same time each day, preferably after the evening meal or at bedtime. During the first cycle of medication, the patient should be instructed to take one TRI-LEVLEN® 21 tablet daily in the order of 6 brown, 5 white and, finally, 10 light-yellow tablets for twenty-one (21) consecutive days, beginning on day one (1) of her menstrual cycle. (The first day of menstruation is day one.) The tablets are then discontinued for one week (7 days). Withdrawal bleeding usually occurs within 3 days following discontinuation of TRI-LEVLEN® 21 Tablets. (If TRI-LEVLEN® 21 tablets are first taken later than the first day of the first menstrual cycle of medication or postpartum, contraceptive reliance should not be placed on TRI-LEVLEN® 21 tablets until after the first 7 consecutive days of administration. The possibility of ovulation and conception prior to initiation of medication should be considered.)

When switching from another oral contraceptive, TRI-LEVLEN® 21 tablets should be started on the first day of bleeding following the last tablet taken of the previous oral contraceptive.

The patient begins her next and all subsequent 21-day courses of TRI-LEVLEN® 21 tablets on the same day of the week that she began her first course, following the same schedule: 21 days on—7 days off. She begins taking her brown tablets on the 8th day after discontinuance regardless of whether or not a menstrual period has occurred or is still in progress. Any time the next cycle of TRI-LEVLEN® 21 tablets are started later than the 8th day, the patient should be protected by another means of contraception until she has taken a tablet daily for seven consecutive days.

If spotting or breakthrough bleeding occurs, the patient is instructed to continue on the same regimen. This type of bleeding is usually transient and without significance; however, if the bleeding is persistent or prolonged, the patient is advised to consult her physician. Although the occurrence of pregnancy is highly unlikely if TRI-LEVLEN® 21 tablets are taken according to directions, if withdrawal bleeding does not occur, the possibility of pregnancy must be considered. If the patient has not adhered to the prescribed schedule (missed one or more tablets or started taking them on a day later than she should have), the probability of pregnancy should be considered at the time of the first missed period and appropriate diagnostic measures taken before the medication is resumed. If the patient has adhered to the prescribed regimen and misses two consecutive periods, pregnancy should be ruled out before continuing the contraceptive regimen.

The patient should be instructed to take a missed tablet as soon as it is remembered. If two consecutive tablets are missed they should both be taken as soon as remembered. The next tablet should be taken at the usual time.

Any time the patient misses one or two tablets she should also use another method of contraception until she has taken a tablet daily for seven consecutive days. If breakthrough bleeding occurs following missed tablets it will usually be transient and of no consequence. While there is little likelihood of ovulation occurring if only one or two tablets are missed, the possibility of ovulation increases with each successive day that scheduled tablets are missed. If three consecutive tablets are missed, all medication should be discontinued and the remainder of the package discarded. A new package of TRI-LEVLEN® 21 tablets should be started on the first day of the patient's next bleed after the last tablet was taken. An alternate means of contraception should be prescribed during the days without tablets and continued until the patient has taken a tablet daily for seven consecutive days. In the nonlactating mother, TRI-LEVLEN® 21 tablets may be prescribed in the postpartum period either immediately or at the first postpartum examination whether or not menstruation has resumed.

TRI-LEVLEN® 28 TABLETS (LEVONORGESTREL AND ETHINYL ESTRADIOL TABLETS—TRIPHASIC REGIMEN)

TRI-LEVLEN® 28 tablets are a three-phase preparation plus 7 inert tablets. The dosage of TRI-LEVLEN® 28 tablets is **one tablet daily** for 28 consecutive days per menstrual cycle in the following order: 6 brown tablets (phase 1), followed by 5 white tablets (phase 2), followed by 10 light-yellow tablets (phase 3), plus 7 light-green inert tablets according to the prescribed schedule.

It is recommended that TRI-LEVLEN® 28 tablets be taken at the same time each day, preferably after the evening meal or at bedtime. During the first cycle of medication, the patient should be instructed to take one TRI-LEVLEN® 28 tablet daily in the order of 6 brown, 5 white, 10 light-yellow tablets, and then 7 light-green inert tablets for twenty-eight (28) consecutive days, beginning on day one (1) of her menstrual cycle. (The first day of menstruation is day one). Withdrawal bleeding usually occurs within 3 days following the last light-yellow tablet. (If TRI-LEVLEN® 28 tablets are first taken later than the first day of the first menstual cycle

of medication or postpartum, contraceptive reliance should not be placed on TRI-LEVLEN® 28 tablets until after the first 7 consecutive days of administration. The possibility of ovulation and conception prior to initiation of medication should be considered.)

When switching from another oral contraceptive, TRI-LEVLEN® 28 tablets should be started on the first day of bleeding following the last tablet taken on the previous oral contraceptive.

The patient begins her next and all subsequent 28-day courses of TRI-LEVLEN® 28 tablets on the same day of the week that she began her first course, following the same schedule. She begins taking her brown tablets on the next day after ingestion of the last light-green tablet, regardless of whether or not a menstrual period has occurred or is still in progress. Any time a subsequent cycle of TRI-LEVLEN® 28 tablets is started later than the next day, the patient should be protected by another means of contraception until she has taken a tablet daily for seven consecutive days.

If spotting or breakthrough bleeding occurs, the patient is instructed to continue on the same regimen. This type of bleeding is usually transient and without significance, however, if the bleeding is persistent or prolonged, the patient is advised to consult her physician. Although the occurrence of pregnancy is highly unlikely if TRI-LEVLEN® 28 tablets are taken according to directions, if withdrawal bleeding does not occur, the possibility of pregnancy must be considered. If the patient has not adhered to the prescribed schedule (missed one or more tablets or started taking them on a day later than she should have), the probability of pregnancy should be considered at the time of the first missed period and appropriate diagnostic measures taken before the medication is resumed. If the patient has adhered to the prescribed regimen and misses two consecutive periods, pregnancy should be ruled out before continuing the contraceptive regimen.

The patient should be instructed to take a missed brown, white, or light-yellow tablet as soon as it is remembered. If two consecutive brown, white or light-yellow tablets are missed, they should both be taken as soon as remembered. The next tablet should be taken at the usual time.

Any time the patient misses one or two brown, white, or light-yellow tablets, she should also use another method of contraception until she has taken a brown, white, or light-yellow tablet for seven consecutive days. If the patient misses one or more light-green tablets, she is still protected against pregnancy provided she begins taking brown tablets again on the proper day. If breakthrough bleeding occurs following missed brown, white, or light-yellow tablets, it will usually be transient and of no consequence. While there is little likelihood of ovulation occurring if only one or two brown, white or light-yellow tablets are missed, the possibility of ovulation increases with each successive day that scheduled tablets are missed. If three consecutive brown, white, or light-yellow tablets are missed, all medication should be discontinued and the remainder of the package discarded. A new package of TRI-LEVLEN® 28 tablets should be started on the first day of the patient's next bleed after the last tablet was taken. An alternate means of contraception should be prescribed during the days without tablets and continued until the patient has taken a tablet daily for seven consecutive days. In the nonlactating mother, TRI-LEVLEN® 28 tablets may be prescribed in the postpartum period either immediately or at the first postpartum examination whether or not menstruation has resumed.

LEVLEN® tablets

To achieve maximum contraceptive effectiveness, LEVLEN® 21 tablets and LEVLEN® 28 tablets must be taken exactly as directed and at intervals not exceeding 24 hours.

LEVLEN® 21 TABLETS (LEVONORGESTREL AND ETHINYL ESTRADIOL TABLETS)

The dosage of LEVLEN® 21 is one tablet daily for 21 consecutive days per menstrual cycle according to prescribed schedule. Tablets are then discontinued for 7 days (three weeks on, one week off).

It is recommended that LEVLEN® 21 tablets be taken at the same time each day, preferably after the evening meal or at bedtime.

During the first cycle of medication, the patient is instructed to take one LEVLEN® 21 tablet daily for twenty-one consecutive days beginning on day five of her menstrual cycle. (The first day of menstruation is day one.) The tablets are then discontinued for one week (7 days). Withdrawal bleeding should usually occur within three days following discontinuation of LEVLEN® 21 tablets.

(If LEVLEN® 21 tablets are first taken later than the fifth day of the first menstrual cycle of medication or postpartum, contraceptive reliance should not be placed on LEVLEN® 21 tablets until after the first seven consecutive days of administration. The possibility of ovulation and conception prior to initiation of medication should be considered.)

The patient begins her next and all subsequent 21-day courses of LEVLEN® 21 tablets on the same day of the week

that she began her first course, following the same schedule: 21 days on—7 days off. She begins taking her tablets on the 8th day after discontinuance regardless of whether or not a menstrual period has occurred or is still in progress. Any time a new cycle of LEVLEN® 21 tablets is started later than the 8th day the patient should be protected by another means of contraception until she has taken a tablet daily for seven consecutive days.

If spotting or breakthrough bleeding occurs, the patient is instructed to continue on the same regimen. This type of bleeding is usually transient and without significance; however, if the bleeding is persistent or prolonged, the patient is advised to consult her physician. Although the occurrence of pregnancy is highly unlikely if LEVLEN® 21 tablets are taken according to directions, if withdrawal bleeding does not occur, the possiblity of pregnancy must be considered. If the patient has not adhered to the prescribed schedule (missed one or more tablets or started taking them on a day later than she should have), the probability of pregnancy should be considered at the time of the first missed period and appropriate diagnostic measures taken before the medication is resumed. If the patient has adhered to the prescribed regimen and misses two consecutive periods, pregnancy should be ruled out before continuing the contraceptive regimen.

The patient should be instructed to take a missed tablet as soon as it is remembered. If two consecutive tablets are missed, they should both be taken as soon as remembered. The next tablet should be taken at the usual time.

Any time the patient misses one or two tablets, she should also use another method of contraception until she has taken a tablet daily for seven consecutive days. If breakthrough bleeding occurs following missed tablets, it will usually be transient and of no consequence. While there is little likelihood of ovulation occurring if only one or two tablets are missed, the possibility of ovulation increases with each successive day that scheduled tablets are missed. If three consecutive tablets are missed, all medication should be discontinued and the remainder of the package discarded. A new tablet cycle should be started on the 8th day after the last tablet was taken, and an alternated means of contraception should be prescribed during the seven days without tablets and until the patient has taken a tablet daily for seven consecutive days. In the nonlactating mother, LEVLEN® tablets may be prescribed in the postpartum period either immediately or at the first postpartum examination whether or not menstruation has resumed.

LEVLEN® 28 TABLETS (LEVONORGESTREL AND ETHINYL ESTRADIOL TABLETS)

The dosage of LEVLEN® 28 tablets is one light-orange tablet daily for 21 consecutive days, followed by one pink inert tablet daily for 7 consecutive days, according to prescribed schedule. It is recommended that tablets be taken at the same time each day, preferably after the evening meal or at bedtime. During the first cycle of medication, the patient is instructed to begin taking LEVLEN® 28 tablets on the first Sunday after the onset of menstruation. If menstruation begins on a Sunday, the first tablet (light-orange) is taken that day. One light-orange tablet should be taken daily for 21 consecutive days, followed by one pink inert tablet daily for 7 consecutive days. Withdrawal bleeding should usually occur within three days following discontinuation of light-orange tablets.

During the first cycle, contraceptive reliance should not be placed on LEVLEN® 28 tablets until a light-orange tablet has been taken daily for 7 consecutive days. The possibility of ovulation and conception prior to initiation of medication should be considered.

The patient begins her next and all subsequent 28-day courses of tablets on the same day of the week (Sunday) on which she began her first course, following the same schedule: 21 days on light-orange tablets—7 days on pink inert tablets. If in any cycle the patient starts tablets later than the proper day, she should protect herself by using another method of birth control until she has taken a light-orange tablet daily for 7 consecutive days.

If spotting or breakthrough bleeding occurs, the patient is instructed to continue on the same regimen. This type of bleeding is usually transient and without significance; however, if the bleeding is persistent or prolonged, the patient is advised to consult her physician. Although the occurrence of pregnancy is highly unlikely if LEVLEN® 28 tablets are taken according to directions, if withdrawal bleeding does not occur, the possiblilty of pregnancy must be considered. If the patient has not adhered to the prescribed schedule (missed one or more tablets or started taking them on a day

Continued on next page

Information on the Berlex products appearing here is based on the labeling in effect on June 1, 1989. Further information for these and other products may be obtained from the Professional Services Department, Berlex Laboratories, Inc., 300 Fairfield Road, Wayne, New Jersey 07470 (201) 292-3007.

Berlex—Cont.

later than she should have), the probability of pregnancy should be considered at the time of the first missed period and appropriate diagnostic measures taken before the medication is resumed. If the patient has adhered to the prescribed regimen and misses two consecutive periods, pregnancy should be ruled out before continuing the contraceptive regimen.

The patient should be instructed to take a missed light-orange tablet as soon as it is remembered. If two consecutive light-orange tablets are missed, they should both be taken as soon as remembered. The next tablet should be taken at the usual time.

Any time the patient misses one or two light-orange tablets, she should also use another method of contraception until she has taken a light-orange tablet daily for seven consecutive days. If the patient misses one or more pink tablets, she is still protected against pregnancy *provided* she begins taking light-orange tablets again on the proper day.

If breakthrough bleeding occurs following missed light-orange tablets, it will usually be transient and of no consequence. While there is little likelihood of ovulation occurring if only one or two light-orange tablets are missed, the possibility of ovulation increases with each successive day that scheduled light-orange tablets are missed. (If three consecutive light-orange LEVLEN® tablets are missed, all medication should be discontinued and the remainder of the 28-day package discarded. A new tablet cycle should be started on the first Sunday following the last missed tablet, and an alternate means of contraception should be prescribed during the days without tablets and until the patient has taken a light-orange tablet daily for 7 consecutive days.) In the non-lactating mother, LEVLEN® tablets may be prescribed in the postpartum period either immediately or at the first postpartum examination whether or not menstruation has resumed.

HOW SUPPLIED

TRI-LEVLEN® tablets

TRI-LEVLEN® 21 tablets (Levonorgestrel and Ethinyl Estradiol Tablets—Triphasic Regimen), Berlex, NDC 50419-430-21, are available in packages of 3 SLIDECASE™ dispensers. Each cycle contains 21 round, coated tablets as follows:
NDC 50419-095, six brown tablets marked "B" on one side and "95" on the other side, each containing 0.050 mg levonorgestrel and 0.030 mg ethinyl estradiol;
NDC 50419-096, five white to off-white tablets marked "B" on one side and "96" on the other side, each containing 0.075 mg levonorgestrel and 0.040 mg ethinyl estradiol; and
NDC 50419-097, ten light-yellow tablets marked "B" on one side and "97" on the other side, each containing 0.125 mg levonorgestrel and 0.030 mg ethinyl estradiol.
TRI-LEVLEN® 28 tablets (Levonorgestrel and Ethinyl Estradiol Tablets—Triphasic Regimen), Berlex, NDC 50419-431-28, are available in packages of 3 SLIDECASE™ dispensers. Each cycle contains 28 round, coated tablets as follows:
NDC 50419-095, six brown tablets marked "B" on one side and "95" on the other side, each containing 0.050 mg levonorgestrel and 0.030 mg ethinyl estradiol; NDC 50419-096, five white to off-white tablets marked "B" on one side and "96" on the other side, each containing 0.075 mg levonorgestrel and 0.040 mg ethinyl estradiol;
NDC 50419-097, ten light-yellow tablets marked "B" on one side and "97" on the other side, each containing 0.125 mg levonorgestrel and 0.030 mg ethinyl estradiol; and
NDC 50419-011, seven light-green inert tablets marked "B" on one side and "11" on the other side.
LEVLEN® tablets
LEVLEN® 21 tablets (0.15 mg levonorgestrel and 0.03 mg ethinyl estradiol), Berlex, are available in packages of 3 SLIDECASE™ dispensers of 21 tablets each as follows:
NDC 50419-021, light orange, round tablet marked "B" on one side and "21" on the other side.
LEVLEN® 28 tablets (0.15 mg levonorgestrel and 0.03 mg ethinyl estradiol). Berlex, are available in packages of 3 SLIDECASE™ dispensers, each containing 28 tablets as follows:
21 active tablets, NDC 50419-021, light-orange, round tablet marked "B" on one side and "21" on the other side.
7 inert tablets, NDC 50419-028, pink, round tablet marked "B" on one side and "28" on the other side.

REFERENCES

1. *"Population Reports,"* Series H, Number 2, May 1974; Series I, Number 1, June 1974; Series B, Number 2, January 1975; Series H, Number 3, 1975; Series H, Number 4, January 1976 (published by the Population Information Program, The George Washington University Medical Center, 2001 S St. NW., Washington, D.C.).
2. Inman, W. H. W., Vessey, M. P., Westerholm, B., and Engelund, A., "Thromboembolic disease and the steroidal con-

tent of oral contraceptives. A report to the Committee on Safety of Drugs," Brit Med J 2 :203–209, 1970.
3. Stolley, P. D., Tonascia, J. A., Tockman, M. S., Sartwell, P. E., Rutledge, A. H., and Jacobs, M. P., "Thrombosis with low-estrogen oral contraceptives," Am J Epidemiol 102 :197–208, 1975.
4. Royal College of General Practitioners, "Oral contraception and thromboembolic disease," J Coll Gen Pract 13 :267–279, 1967.
5. Inman, W. H. W., and Vessey, M. P., "Investigation of deaths from pulmonary, coronary and cerebral thrombosis and embolism in women of childbearing age," Brit Med J 2 :193–199, 1968.
6. Vessey, M. P., and Doll, R., "Investigation of relation between use of oral contraceptives and thromboembolic disease. A further report," Brit Med J 2 :651–657, 1969.
7. Sartwell, P. E., Masi, A. T., Arthes, F. G., Greene, G. R., and Smith, H. E., "Thromboembolism and oral contraceptives: an epidemiological case control study," Am J Epidemiol 90 :365–380, 1969.
8. Boston Collaborative Drug Surveillance Program, "Oral contraceptives and venous thromboembolic disease, surgically confirmed gallbladder disease and breast tumors," Lancet 1 :1399–1404, 1973.
9. Collaborative Group for the Study of Stroke in Young Women, "Oral contraception and increased risk of cerebral ischemia or thrombosis," N Engl J Med 288 :871–878, 1973.
10. Collaborative Group for the Study of Stroke in Young Women, "Oral contraceptives and stroke in young women: associated risk factors," JAMA 231 :718–722, 1975.
11. Mann, J. I., and Inman, W. H. W., "Oral contraceptives and death from myocardial infarction," Brit Med J 2 :245–248, 1975.
12. Mann, J. I., Inman, W. H. W., and Thorogood, M., "Oral contraceptive use in older women and fatal myocardial infarction," Brit Med J 2 :445–447, 1976.
13. Mann, J. I., Vessey, M. P., Thorogood, M., and Doll, R., "Myocardial infarction in young women with special reference to oral contraceptive practice," Brit Med J 2 :241–245, 1975.
14. Tietze, C., "New Estimates of Mortality Associated with Fertility Control," Family Planning Perspectives, 9 :74–76, 1977.
15. Vessey, M. P., Doll, R., Fairbairn, A. S., and Glober, G., "Post-operative thromboembolism and the use of oral contraceptives," Brit Med J 3 :123–126, 1970.
16. Greene, G. R., and Sartwell, P. E., "Oral contraceptive use in patients with thromboembolism following surgery, trauma, or infection," Am J Pub Health 62 :680–685, 1972.
17. Smith, D. C., Prentice, R., Thompson, D. J., and Herrmann, W. L., "Association of exogenous estrogen and endometrial carcinoma," N Engl J Med 293 :1164–1167, 1975.
18. Ziel, H. K., and Finkle, W. D., "Increased risk of endometrial carcinoma among users of conjugated estrogens," N Engl J Med 293 :1167–1170, 1975.
19. Mack, T. N., Pike, M. C., Henderson, B. E., Pfeffer, R. I., Gerkins, V. R., Arthur, M., and Brown, S. E., "Estrogens and endometrial cancer in a retirement community," N Engl J Med 294 :1262–1267, 1976.
20. Silverberg, S. G., and Makowski, E. L., "Endometrial carcinoma in young women taking oral contraceptive agents," Obstet Gynecol 46 :503–506, 1975.
21. Vessey, M. P., Doll, R., and Sutton, P. M., "Oral contraceptives and breast neoplasia: a retrospective study," Brit Med J 3 :719–724, 1972.
22. Vessey, M. P., Doll, R., and Jones K., "Oral contraceptives and breast cancer. Progress report of an epidemiological study," Lancet 1 :941–943, 1975.
23. Boston Collaborative Drug Surveillance Program, "Surgically confirmed gallbladder disease, venous thromboembolism and breast tumors in relation to postmenopausal estrogen therapy," N Engl J Med 290 :15–19, 1974.
24. Arthes, F. G., Sartwell, P. E., and Lewison, E. F., "The pill, estrogens, and the breast. Epidemiologic aspects," Cancer 28 :1391–1394, 1971.
25. Fasal, E., and Paffenbarger, R. S., "Oral contraceptives as related to cancer and benign lesions of the breast," J Natl Cancer Inst 55 :767–773, 1975.
26. Royal College of General Practitioners, "Oral Contraceptives and Health," London, Pitman, 1974.
27. Ory, H., Cole P., MacMahon, B., and Hoover, R., "Oral contraceptives and reduced risk of benign breast diseases," N Engl J Med 294 :419–422, 1976.
28. Baum, J., Holtz, F., Bookstein, J. J., and Klein, E. W., "Possible association between benign hepatomas and oral contraceptives," Lancet 2 :926–928, 1973.
29. Mays, E. T., Christopherson, W. M., Mahr, M. M., and Williams, H. C., "Hepatic changes in young women ingesting contraceptive steroids. Hepatic hemorrhage and primary hepatic tumors," JAMA 235 :730–732, 1976.
30. Edmondson, H. A., Henderson, B., and Benton, B., "Liver-cell adenomas associated with use of oral contraceptives," N Engl J Med 294 :470–472, 1976.
31. Herbst, A. L., Ulfedler, H., and Poskanzer, D. C., "Adenocarcinoma of the vagina," N Engl J Med 284 :878–881, 1971.

32. Greenwald, P., Barlow, J. J., Nasca, P. C., and Burnett, W., "Vaginal cancer after maternal treatment with synthetic estrogens," N Engl J Med 285 :390–392, 1971.
33. Lanier, A. P., Noller, K. L., Decker, D. G., Elveback, L., and Kurland, L. T., "Cancer and stilbestrol. A follow-up of 1719 persons exposed to estrogens in utero and born 1943–1959," Mayo Clin Pro 48 :793–799, 1973.
34. Herbst, A. L., Kurman, R. J., and Scully, R. E., "Vaginal and cervical abnormalities after exposure to stilbestrol in utero," Obstet Gynecol 40 :287–298, 1972.
35. Herbst, A. L., Robboy, S. J., Macdonald, G. J., and Scully, R. E., "The effects of local progesterone on stilbestrol-associated vaginal adenosis," Am J Obstet Gynecol 118 :607–615, 1974.
36. Herbst, A. L., Poskanzer, D. C., Robboy, S. J., Friedlander, L., and Scully, R. E., "Prenatal exposure to stilbestrol: a prospective comparison of exposed female offspring with unexposed controls," N Engl J Med 292 :334–339, 1975.
37. Stafl, A., Mattingly, R. F., Foley, D. V., Fetherston, W., "Clinical diagnosis of vaginal adenosis," Obstet Gynecol 43 :118–128, 1974.
38. Sherman, A. I., Goldrath, M., Berlin, A., Vakhariya, V., Banooni, F., Michaels, W., Goodman, P., and Brown, S., "Cervical-vaginal adenosis after in utero exposure to synthetic estrogens," Obstet Gynecol 44 :531–545, 1974.
39. Gal, I., Kirman, B., and Stern, J., "Hormone pregnancy tests and congenital malformation," Nature 216 :83, 1967.
40. Levy, E. P., Cohen, A., and Fraser, F. C., "Hormone treatment during pregnancy and congenital heart defects," Lancet 1 :611, 1973.
41. Nora, J. J., and Nora, A. H., "Birth defects and oral contraceptives," Lancet 1 :941–942, 1973.
42. Janerich, D. T., Piper, J. M., and Glebatis, D. M., "Oral contraceptives and congenital limb-reduction defects," N Engl J Med 291 :697–700, 1974.
43. Carr, D. H., "Chromosome studies in selected spontaneous abortions: I. Conception after oral contraceptives," Canad Med Assoc J 103 :343–348, 1970.
44. Wynn, V., Doar, J. W. H., and Mills, G. L., "Some effects of oral contraceptives on serum-lipid and lipoprotein levels," Lancet 2 :720–723, 1966.
45. Laumas, K. R., Malkani, P. K., Bhatnagar, S., and Laumas, V., "Radioactivity in the breast milk of lactating women after oral administration of 3 H-norethynodrel," Am J Obstet Gynecol 98 :411–413, 1967.
46. Center for Disease Control, "Increased Risk of Hepatocellular Adenoma in Women with Long-term use of Oral Contraceptives," Morbidity and Mortality Weekly Report, 26 :293–294, 1977.
47. Herbst, A. L., Cole, P., Colton, T., Robboy, S. J., and Scully, R. E., "Age-incidence and Risk of Diethylstilbestrol-related Clear Cell Adenocarcinoma of the Vagina and Cervix," Am J Obstet Gynecol 128 :43–50, 1977.
48. Bibbo, M., Al-Naqeeb, M., Baccarini, I., Gill, W., Newton, M., Sleeper, K. M., Sonek, M., and Wied, G. L., "Follow-up Study of Male and Female Offspring of DES-treated Mothers. A Preliminary Report," J of Repro Med 15 :29–32, 1975.
49. Gill, W. B., Schumacher, G. F. B., and Bibbo, M., "Structural and Functional Abnormalities in the Sex Organs of Male Offspring of Mothers Treated with Diethylstilbestrol (DES)," J of Repro Med 16 :147–153, 1976.
50. Henderson, B. E., Senton, B., Cosgrove, M., Baptista, J., Aldrich, J., Townsend, D., Hart, W., and Mack, T., "Urogenital Tract Abnormalities in Sons of Women Treated with Diethylstilbestrol," Pediatrics, 58 :505–507, 1976.
51. Heinonen, O. P., Slone, D., Nonson, R. R., Hook, E. B., and Shapiro, S., "Cardiovascular Birth Defects and Antenatal Exposure to Female Sex Hormones," N Engl J Med 296 :67–70, 1977.
52. Jain, A. K., "Mortality Risk Associated with the Use of Oral Contraceptives," Studies in Family Planning, 8 :50–54, 1977.
53. Beral, V., "Mortality Among Oral Contraceptive Users," Lancet, 2 :727–731, 1977.
54. Royal College of General Practitioners' Oral contraception study, "Incidence of arterial disease among oral contraceptive users," J Royal Col Gen Pract 33 :75–82, 1983.
55. Slone, D., Shapiro, S., Kaufman, D. W., Rosenberg, L., Miettinen, O., and Stolley, P., "Risk of myocardial infarction in relation to current and discontinued use of oral contraceptives," N Engl J Med 305 :420–424, 1981.
56. Inman, W.H.W., "Oral contraceptives and fatal subarachnoid haemorrhage," Brit Med J 2 :1468–1470, 1979.
57. Petitti, D. B., and Wingerd, J., "Use of oral contraceptives, cigarette smoking and risk of subarachnoid haemorrhage," Lancet 2 :234–236, 1978.
58. Thorogood, M., Adam, S. A., and Mann, J. I., "Fatal subarachnoid haemorrhage in young women: role of oral contraceptives," Brit Med J 283 :762, 1981.
59. Rosenberg, L., Hennekens, C.H., Rosner, B., Belanger, C., Rothman, K. J., and Speizer, F. E., "Oral contraceptive use in relation to nonfatal myocardial infarction," Am J Epidemiol 111 :59–66, 1980.
60. Adam, S. A., Thorogood, M., and Mann, J. I., "Oral contraception and myocardial infarction revisited: the effects of

new preparations and prescribing patterns," Brit J Obstet Gynaecol 88:838–845, 1981.

61. Data on file.
62. Briggs, M. H., "Implications and assessment of metabolic effects of oral contraceptives." New considerations in oral contraception. Proceedings of an international symposium, Catholic University-Leuven, Leuven, Belgium. September, 1981 Ed. I. Brosens.
63. Vermeulen, A., and Thiery, M., "Metabolic effects of the triphasic oral contraceptive Trigynon®." Contraception 26:505–513, 1982.
64. Nilsson, S., Nygren, K., and Johansson, E., "Ethinyl Estradiol in Human Milk and Plasma after Oral Administration." Contraception 17:131–139, 1978.
65. Nilsson, S., Nygren, K., and Johansson, E., "d-Norgestrel Concentrations in Maternal Plasma, Milk, and Child Plasma During Administration of Oral Contraceptives to Nursing Women." Am J Obstet Gynecol 129:178, 1977.

The patient labeling for oral-contraceptive drug products is set forth below:

Brief Summary Patient Package Insert

> Cigarette smoking increases the risk of serious adverse effects on the heart and blood vessels from oral-contraceptive use. This risk increases with age and with heavy smoking (15 or more cigarettes per day) and is quite marked in women over 35 years of age. Women who use oral contraceptives should not smoke.

Oral contraceptives taken as directed are about 99% effective in preventing pregnancy. (The mini-pill, however, is somewhat less effective.) Forgetting to take your pills increases the chance of pregnancy. Women who have or have had clotting disorders, cancer of the breast or sex organs, unexplained vaginal bleeding, a stroke, heart attack, angina pectoris, or who suspect they may be pregnant should not use oral contraceptives. Various drugs, such as some antibiotics, may also decrease the effectiveness of oral contraceptives.

Most side effects of the pill are not serious. The most common side effects are nausea, vomiting, bleeding between menstrual periods, weight gain, and breast tenderness. However, proper use of oral contraceptives requires that they be taken under your doctor's continuous supervision, because they can be associated with serious side effects which may be fatal. Fortunately, these occur very infrequently.
The serious side effects are:
1. Blood clots in the legs, lungs, brain, heart, or other organs, and hemorrhage into the brain due to bursting of a blood vessel. Certain of these effects may occur after pill use has been stopped.
2. Liver tumors, which may rupture and cause severe bleeding.
3. Birth defects if the pill is taken while you are pregnant.
4. High blood pressure.
5. Gallbladder disease.
The symptoms associated with these serious side effects are discussed in the detailed leaflet given you with your supply of pills. Notify your doctor if you notice any unusual physical disturbance while taking the pill.

The estrogen in oral contraceptives has been found to cause breast cancer and other cancers in certain animals. These findings suggest that oral contraceptives may also cause cancer in humans. However, studies to date in women taking currently marketed oral contraceptives have not confirmed that oral contraceptives cause cancer in humans.
The detailed leaflet describes more completely the benefits and risks of oral contraceptives. It also provides information on other forms of contraception. Read it carefully. If you have any questions, consult your doctor.

CAUTION: Oral contraceptives are of no value in the prevention or treatment of venereal disease.
DETAILED PATIENT LABELING
WHAT YOU SHOULD KNOW ABOUT ORAL CONTRACEPTIVES
Oral contraceptives ("the pill") are the most effective way (except for sterilization) to prevent pregnancy. They are also convenient and, for most women, free of serious or unpleasant side effects. Oral contraceptives must always be taken under the continuous supervision of a physician.
It is important that any woman who considers using an oral contraceptive understand the risks involved. Although the oral contraceptives have important advantages over other methods of contraception, they have certain risks that no other method has. Only you can decide whether the advantages are worth these risks. This leaflet will tell you about the most important risks. It will explain how you can help your doctor prescribe the pill as safely as possible by telling him about yourself and being alert for the earliest signs of trouble. And it will tell you how to use the pill properly, so that it will be as effective as possible. There is more detailed information available in the leaflet prepared for doctors. Your pharmacist can show you a copy; you may need your doctor's help in understanding parts of it.

WHO SHOULD NOT USE ORAL CONTRACEPTIVES
A. If you have any of the following conditions, you should not use the pill:
1. Clots in the legs or lungs.
2. Angina pectoris.
3. Known or suspected cancer of the breast or sex organs.
4. Unusual vaginal bleeding that has not yet been diagnosed.
5. Known or suspected pregnancy.
B. If you have had any of the following conditions, you should not use the pill:
1. Heart attack or stroke.
2. Clots in the legs or lungs.

> C. Cigarette smoking increases the risk of serious adverse effects on the heart and blood vessels from oral-contraceptive use. This risk increases with age and with heavy smoking (15 or more cigarettes per day) and is quite marked in women over 35 years of age. Women who use oral contraceptives should not smoke.

D. If you have scanty or irregular periods or are a young woman without a regular cycle, you should use another method of contraception because, if you use the pill, you may have difficulty becoming pregnant or may fail to have menstrual periods after discontinuing the pill.
DECIDING TO USE ORAL CONTRACEPTIVES
If you do not have any of the conditions listed above and are thinking about using oral contraceptives, to help you decide, you need information about the advantages and risks of oral contraceptives and of other contraceptive methods as well. This leaflet describes the advantages and risks of oral contraceptives. Except for sterilization, the IUD, and abortion, which have their own inherent risks, the only risks of other methods of contraception are those due to pregnancy should the method fail. Your doctor can answer questions you have with respect to other methods of contraception. He can also answer any questions you may have after reading this leaflet on oral contraceptives.
1. What Oral Contraceptives Are and How They Work. Oral contraceptives are of two types. The most common, often simply called "the pill," is a combination of an estrogen and a progestogen, the two kinds of female hormones. The amount of estrogen and progestogen can vary, but the amount of estrogen is most important because both the effectiveness and some of the dangers of oral contraceptives are related to the amount of estrogen. This kind of oral contraceptive works principally by preventing release of an egg from the ovary. When the amount of estrogen is 50 micrograms or more, and the pill is taken as directed, oral contraceptives are more than 99% effective (i.e., there would be less than 1 pregnancy if 100 women used the pill for 1 year). Pills that contain 20 to 35 micrograms of estrogen vary slightly in effectiveness, ranging from 98% to more than 99% effective.
The second type of oral contraceptive, often called the "mini-pill," contains only a progestogen. It works in part by preventing release of an egg from the ovary but also by keeping sperm from reaching the egg and by making the uterus (womb) less receptive to any fertilized egg that reaches it. The mini-pill is less effective than the combination oral contraceptive, about 97% effective. In addition, the progestogen-only pill has a tendency to cause irregular bleeding which may be quite inconvenient, or cessation of bleeding entirely. The progestogen-only pill is used despite its lower effectiveness in the hope that it will prove not to have some of the serious side effects of the estrogen-containing pill (see below), but it is not yet certain that the mini-pill does in fact have fewer serious side effects. The discussion below, while based mainly on information about the combination pills, should be considered to apply as well to the mini-pill.
2. Other Nonsurgical Ways to Prevent Pregnancy. As this leaflet will explain, oral contraceptives have several serious risks. Other methods of contraception have lesser risks or none at all. They are also less effective than oral contraceptives, but, used properly, may be effective enough for many women.
The following table gives reported pregnancy rates (the number of women out of 100 who would become pregnant in 1 year) for these methods.
PREGNANCIES PER 100 WOMEN PER YEAR
Intrauterine device (IUD), less than 1–6; Diaphragm with spermicidal products (creams or jellies), 2–20; Condom (rubber), 3–36; Aerosol foams, 2–29; Jellies and creams, 4–36; Periodic abstinence (rhythm) all types, less than 1–47:
1. Calendar method, 14–47;
2. Temperature method, 1–20;
3. Temperature method—intercourse only in postovulatory phase, less than 1–7;
4. Mucus method, 1–25;
No contraception, 60–80.
The figures (except for the IUD) vary widely because people differ in how well they use each method. Very faithful users of the various methods obtain very good results, except for users of the calendar method of periodic abstinence (rhythm). Except for the IUD, effective use of these methods

requires somewhat more effort than simply taking a single pill every day, but it is an effort that many couples undertake successfully. Your doctor can tell you a great deal more about these methods of contraception.
3. The Dangers of Oral Contraceptives.
a. *Circulatory disorders (abnormal blood clotting and stroke due to hemorrhage).* Blood clots (in various blood vessels of the body) are the most common of the serious side effects of oral contraceptives. A clot can result in a stroke (if the clot is in the brain), a heart attack (if the clot is in a blood vessel of the heart), or a pulmonary embolus (a clot which forms in the legs or pelvis, then breaks off and travels to the lungs). Any of these can be fatal. Clots also occur rarely in the blood vessels of the eye, resulting in blindness or impairment of vision in that eye. There is evidence that the risk of clotting increases with higher estrogen doses. It is therefore important to keep the dose of estrogen as low as possible, so long as the oral contraceptive used has an acceptable pregnancy rate and doesn't cause unacceptable changes in the menstrual pattern. Furthermore, cigarette smoking by oral-contraceptive users increases the risk of serious adverse effects on the heart and blood vessels. This risk increases with age and with heavy smoking (15 or more cigarettes per day) and begins to become quite marked in women over 35 years of age. For this reason, women who use oral contraceptives should not smoke.
The risk of abnormal clotting increases with age in both users and nonusers of oral contraceptives, but the increased risk from the contraceptive appears to be present at all ages. For oral-contraceptive users in general, it has been estimated that in women between the ages of 15 and 34 the risk of death due to a circulatory disorder is about 1 in 12,000 per year, whereas for nonusers the rate is about 1 in 50,000 per year. In the age group 35 to 44, the risk is estimated to be about 1 in 2,500 per year for oral-contraceptive users and about 1 in 10,000 per year for nonusers.
Even without the pill, the risk of having a heart attack increases with age and is also increased by such heart attack risk factors as high blood pressure, high cholesterol, obesity, diabetes, and cigarette smoking. Without any risk factors present, the use of oral contraceptives alone may double the risk of heart attack. However, the combination of cigarette smoking, especially heavy smoking, and oral contraceptive use greatly increases the risk of heart attack. Oral-contraceptive users who smoke are about 5 times more likely to have a heart attack than users who do not smoke and about 10 times more likely to have a heart attack than nonusers who do not smoke. It has been estimated that users between the ages of 30 and 39 who smoke have about a 1 in 10,000 chance each year of having a fatal heart attack compared to about a 1 in 50,000 chance in users who do not smoke, and about a 1 in 100,000 chance in nonusers who do not smoke. In the age group 40 to 44, the risk is about 1 in 1,700 per year for users who smoke compared to about 1 in 10,000 for users who do not smoke and to about 1 in 14,000 per year for nonusers who do not smoke. Heavy smoking (about 15 cigarettes or more a day) further increases the risk. If you do not smoke and have none of the other heart attack risk factors described above, you will have a smaller risk than listed. If you have several heart attack risk factors, the risk may be considerably greater than listed. In addition to blood-clotting disorders, it has been estimated that women taking oral contraceptives are twice as likely as nonusers to have a stroke due to rupture of a blood vessel in the brain. There is evidence that patients who stop taking oral contraceptives after using them continuously for five or more years may continue to have an increased risk of stroke or heart attack for at least six to nine years after discontinuation.
b. *Formation of tumors.* Studies have found that when certain animals are given the female sex hormone, estrogen, which is an ingredient of oral contraceptives, continuously for long periods, cancers may develop in the breast, cervix, vagina, and liver.
These findings suggest that oral contraceptives may cause cancer in humans. However, studies to date in women taking currently marketed oral contraceptives have not confirmed that oral contraceptives cause cancer in humans. Several studies have found no increase in breast cancer in users, although one study suggested oral contraceptives might cause an increase in breast cancer in women who already have benign breast disease (e.g., cysts).
Women with a strong family history of breast cancer or who have breast nodules, fibrocystic disease, or abnormal mammograms or who were exposed to DES (diethylstilbestrol), an estrogen, during their mother's pregnancy must be followed

Continued on next page

Information on the Berlex products appearing here is based on the labeling in effect on June 1, 1989. Further information for these and other products may be obtained from the Professional Services Department, Berlex Laboratories, Inc., 300 Fairfield Road, Wayne, New Jersey 07470 (201) 292-3007.

Berlex—Cont.

very closely by their doctors if they choose to use oral contraceptives instead of another method of contraception. Many studies have shown that women taking oral contraceptives have less risk of getting benign breast disease than those who have not used oral contraceptives. Recently, strong evidence has emerged that estrogens (one component of oral contraceptives), when given for periods of more than one year to women after the menopause, increase the risk of cancer of the uterus (womb). There is also some evidence that a kind of oral contraceptive which is no longer marketed, the sequential oral contraceptive, may increase the risk of cancer of the uterus. There remains no evidence, however, that the oral contraceptives now available increase the risk of this cancer. Oral contraceptives do cause, although rarely, a benign (nonmalignant) tumor of the liver. These tumors do not spread, but they may rupture and cause internal bleeding, which may be fatal. A few cases of cancer of the liver have been reported in women using oral contraceptives, but it is not yet known whether the drug caused them.

c. *Dangers to a developing child if oral contraceptives are used in or immediately preceding pregnancy.* Oral contraceptives should not be taken by pregnant women because they may damage the developing child. An increased risk of birth defects, including heart defects and limb defects, has been associated with the use of sex hormones, including oral contraceptives, in pregnancy. In addition, the developing female child whose mother has received DES (diethylstilbestrol), an estrogen, during pregnancy has a risk of getting cancer of the vagina or cervix in her teens or young adulthood. This risk is estimated to be about 1 in 1,000 exposures or less. Abnormalities of the urinary and sex organs have been reported in male offspring so exposed. It is possible that other estrogens, such as the estrogens in oral contraceptives, could have the same effect in the child if the mother takes them during pregnancy.

If you stop taking oral contraceptives to become pregnant, your doctor may recommend that you use another method of contraception for a short while. The reason for this is that there is evidence from studies in women who have had "miscarriages" soon after stopping the pill, that the lost fetuses are more likely to be abnormal. Whether there is an overall increase in "miscarriage" in women who become pregnant soon after stopping the pill as compared with women who do not use the pill is not known, but it is possible that there may be. If, however, you do become pregnant soon after stopping oral contraceptives, and do not have a miscarriage, there is no evidence that the baby has an increased risk of being abnormal.

d. *Gallbladder disease.* Women who use oral contraceptives have a greater risk than nonusers of having gallbladder disease requiring surgery. The increased risk may first appear within 1 year of use and may double after 4 or 5 years of use.

e. *Other side effects of oral contraceptives.* Some women using oral contraceptives experience unpleasant side effects that are not dangerous and are not likely to damage their health. Some of these may be temporary. Your breasts may feel tender, nausea and vomiting may occur, you may gain or lose weight, and your ankles may swell. A spotty darkening of the skin, particularly of the face, is possible and may persist. You may notice unexpected vaginal bleeding or changes in your menstrual period. Irregular bleeding is frequently seen when using the mini-pill or combination oral contraceptives containing less than 50 micrograms of estrogen. More serious side effects include worsening of migraine, asthma, epilepsy, and kidney or heart disease because of a tendency for water to be retained in the body when oral contraceptives are used.

Other side effects are growth of preexisting fibroid tumors of the uterus; mental depression, and liver problems with jaundice (yellowing of the skin). Your doctor may find that levels of sugar and fatty substances in your blood are elevated; the long-term effects of these changes are not known. Some women develop high blood pressure while taking oral contraceptives, which ordinarily returns to the original levels when the oral contraceptive is stopped.

Other reactions, although not proved to be caused by oral contraceptives, are occasionally reported. These include more frequent urination and some discomfort when urinating, blood-cell breakdown with kidney failure, nervousness, dizziness, some loss of scalp hair, an increase in body hair, an increase or decrease in sex drive, appetite changes, cataracts, and a need for a change in contact lens prescription, or inability to use contact lenses. After you stop using oral contraceptives, there may be a delay before you are able to become pregnant or before you resume having menstrual periods. This is especially true of women who had irregular menstrual cycles prior to the use of oral contraceptives. As discussed previously, your doctor may recommend that you wait a short while after stopping the pill before you try to become pregnant. During this time, use another form of contraception. You should consult your physician before resuming use of oral contraceptives after childbirth, especially if

you plan to nurse your baby. Drugs in oral contraceptives are known to appear in the milk, and the long-range effect on infants is not known at this time. Furthermore, oral contraceptives may cause a decrease in your milk supply as well as in the quality of the milk.

4. Comparison of the Risks of Oral Contraceptives and Other Contraceptive Methods. The many studies on the risks and effectiveness of oral contraceptives and other methods of contraception have been analyzed to estimate the risk of death associated with various methods of contraception. This risk has two parts: (a) the risk of the method itself (e.g., the risk that oral contraceptives will cause death due to abnormal clotting), and (b) the risk of death due to pregnancy or abortion in the event the method fails. The results of this analysis are shown in the bar graph (Figure 1). The height of the bars is the number of deaths per 100,000 women each year. There are six sets of bars, each set referring to a specific age group of women. Within each set of bars, there is a single bar for each of the different contraceptive methods. For oral contraceptives, there are two bars—one for smokers and the other for nonsmokers. The analysis is based on present knowledge, and new information could, of course, alter it. The analysis shows that the risk of death from all methods of birth control is low and below that associated with childbirth, except for oral contraceptives in women over 40 who smoke. It shows that the lowest risk of death is associated with the condom or diaphragm (traditional contraception) backed up by early abortion in case of failure of the condom or diaphragm to prevent pregnancy. Also, at any age the risk of death (due to unexpected pregnancy) from the use of traditional contraception, even without a backup of abortion, is generally the same as or less than that from use of oral contraceptives.

Figure 1. Estimated annual number of deaths associated with control of fertility and no control per 100,000 nonsterile women, by regimen of control and age of women.

Regimen of control

☐ No method   ▨ Abortion only   ▧ Pill only/ nonsmokers   ☐ Pill only/ smokers

▨ IUDs only   ▧ Traditional contraception only (diaphragm or condom)   ■ Traditional contraception and abortion

HOW TO USE ORAL CONTRACEPTIVES AS SAFELY AND EFFECTIVELY AS POSSIBLE, ONCE YOU HAVE DECIDED TO USE THEM

1. What to tell your Doctor.

You can make use of the pill as safely as possible by telling your doctor if you have any of the following:

a. Conditions that mean you should not use oral contraceptives:

Clots in the legs or lungs.
Clots in the legs or lungs in the past.
A stroke, heart attack, or angina pectoris.
Known or suspected cancer of the breast or sex organs.

Unusual vaginal bleeding that has not yet been diagnosed.
Known or suspected pregnancy.

b. Conditions that your doctor will want to watch closely or which might cause him to suggest another method of contraception:

A family history of breast cancer.
Breast nodules, fibrocystic disease of the breast, or an abnormal mammogram.

Diabetes.	Heart or kidney disease.
High blood pressure.	Epilepsy.
High cholesterol.	Mental depression.
Cigarette smoking.	Fibroid tumors of the uterus.
Migraine headaches.	Gallbladder disease.

c. Once you are using oral contraceptives, you should be alert for signs of a serious adverse effect and call your doctor if they occur.

Sharp pain in the chest, coughing blood, or sudden shortness of breath (indicating possible clots in the lungs).
Pain in the calf (possible clot in the leg).
Crushing chest pain or heaviness (indicating possible heart attack).
Sudden severe headache or vomiting, dizziness or fainting, disturbance of vision or speech, or weakness or numbness in an arm or leg (indicating a possible stroke).
Sudden partial or complete loss of vision (indicating a possible clot in the eye).
Breast lumps (you should ask your doctor to show you how to examine your own breasts).
Severe pain in the abdomen (indicating a possible ruptured tumor of the liver).
Severe depression.
Yellowing of the skin (jaundice).

2. How to Take the Pill So That It is Most Effective.

Reduced effectiveness and an increased incidence of breakthrough bleeding have been associated with the use of oral contraceptives with antibiotics such as rifampin, ampicillin, and tetracycline or with certain other drugs such as barbiturates, phenylbutazone or phenytoin sodium. You should use an additional means of contraception during any cycle in which any of these drugs are taken.

To achieve maximum contraceptive effectiveness, oral contraceptives must be taken exactly as directed and at intervals not exceeding 24 hours. It is recommended that tablets be taken at the same time each day, preferably after the evening meal or at bedtime. Taking them on a definite schedule will decrease the chance of forgetting a tablet and also help keep the proper amount of medication in your system. See detailed instructions below for TRI-LEVLEN® 21 tablets (Levonorgestrel and Ethinyl Estradiol Tablets—Triphasic Regimen), TRI-LEVLEN® 28 tablets (Levonorgestrel and Ethinyl Estradiol Tablets—Triphasic Regimen), LEVLEN® 21 and LEVLEN® 28 tablets.

For specific instructions on **how to use your particular package**, refer to the Brief Summary Patient Package insert provided with your pill package.

TRI-LEVLEN® 21 TABLETS (LEVONORGESTREL AND ETHINYL ESTRADIOL TABLETS—TRIPHASIC REGIMEN)

TRI-LEVLEN® is a three-phased contraceptive, different from the usual same-dose-every-day combination oral contraceptive.

TRI-LEVLEN® 21 tablets contain 21 active pills divided among 6 brown pills, 5 white pills, and 10 light-yellow pills in each package.

The dosage of TRI-LEVLEN® 21 tablets is **one pill daily** for 21 days in a row in your menstrual cycle beginning with the first brown pill, continuing through the white pills and finishing the cycle with the light-yellow pills, **in that order.** Pills are then discontinued for 7 days. The basic schedule is 21 days on—7 days off. In the first month, you should begin taking TRI-LEVLEN® 21 tablets on day one (1) of your menstrual cycle, which is the first day of your menstruation regardless of the amount of bleeding or spotting. (Day 1 is the first day of menstruation, even if it is almost midnight when you start.) Note: During the first month on TRI-LEVLEN® 21 tablets, if you start taking pills later than day 1 of your menstrual cycle, you should protect yourself by also using another method of birth control until you have taken a pill daily for seven days in a row (6 brown pills followed by 1 white pill). Thereafter, if you follow directions carefully you will obtain the full contraceptive benefit. If you begin taking pills later than the proper day, the possibility of ovulation and pregnancy occurring before or during the taking of the brown pills should be considered.

Take one pill every day until you finish all 21 pills. No pills are then taken for one week (7 days). Your period will usually begin about three days after you take the last light-yellow pill. Don't be alarmed if the amount of bleeding is not the same as before. On the 8th day, start with a brown pill from a new package, even if you still have your period. If, for example, you took TRI-LEVLEN® 21 tablets for the first time on a Tuesday, the 8th day will also be a Tuesday. **If you have taken the pills as directed,** you will begin the next cycle on the same day of the week. If you start taking pills later than the 8th day, you should protect yourself by also using another method of birth control until you have taken a pill daily for seven days in a row.

When switching from another oral contraceptive, TRI-LEVLEN® 21 tablets should be started on the first day of bleeding following the last pill taken of the previous oral contraceptive.

TRI-LEVLEN® 28 TABLETS (LEVONORGESTREL AND ETHINYL ESTRADIOL TABLETS—TRIPHASIC REGIMEN)

TRI-LEVLEN® is a three-phased contraceptive, different from the usual same-dose-every-day combination oral contraceptive.

TRI-LEVLEN® 28 tablets contain active pills divided among 6 brown pills, 5 white pills, and 10 light-yellow pills plus 7 light-green inactive pills per package. The dosage of TRI-LEVLEN® 28 tablets is one active pill daily for 21 days in a row beginning with the 6 brown pills, followed by the 5 white pills, followed by the 10 light-yellow pills, and then one of the 7 light-green inactive pills daily for the next 7 days, **in that order**, for a total of 28 days or 4 weeks. The basic schedule is 21 days on active pills (brown, white, and light-yellow)—7 days on light-green inactive pills. Always take all of the 21 active pills (brown, white, and light-yellow) in each package before taking the light-green pills.

When you start your **first** cycle of TRI-LEVLEN® 28 tablets, you should begin taking your pills on the **first** day of your next menstrual period, regardless of the day of the week or the amount of the bleeding or spotting. Note: During the first month on TRI-LEVLEN® 28 tablets, if you start taking pills later than day 1 of your menstrual cycle, you should protect yourself by also using another method of birth control until you have taken a pill daily for seven days in a row (6 brown pills followed by 1 white pill). Thereafter, if you follow directions carefully you will obtain the full contraceptive benefit. If you begin taking pills later than the proper day, the possibility of ovulation and pregnancy occurring before or during the taking of the brown pills should be considered. Take one pill every day until you finish all 6 brown, 5 white, and 10 light-yellow pills in a package followed by all 7 light-green pills. Your period will usually begin about three days after you take the last light-green pill, which will be during the time you are taking the light-green pills. Don't be alarmed if the amount of bleeding is not the same as before.

The day after you have taken your last light-green pill, begin a new package of pills (first taking the 6 brown, then the 5 white, and then the 10 light-yellow pills one a day just as you did before) so that you will take a pill every day without interruption. **If you have taken the pills as directed,** the starting day for each new package will always be the same day as in the previous cycle. When switching from another oral contraceptive, TRI-LEVLEN® 28 tablets should be started on the first day of bleeding following the last pill taken of the previous oral contraceptive.

Spotting or Breakthrough Bleeding:

Spotting is slight staining between menstrual periods which may not even require a pad. Breakthrough bleeding is a flow much like a regular period, requiring sanitary protection. Spotting is more common than breakthrough bleeding, and both occur more often in the first few cycles than in later cycles. These types of bleeding are usually temporary and without significance. It is important to continue taking your pills on schedule. If the bleeding persists for more than a few days, consult your doctor.

MISSED PILLS

There is a chance of becoming pregnant if you miss one brown, white, or light-yellow pill, and that chance increases with each additional brown, white, or light-yellow pill missed. If you miss any one of these pills, it is important it be taken as soon as remembered. If you miss any two of these pills consecutively, it is important both be taken as soon as remembered. The next pill should then be taken at the usual time. Any time you miss one or two brown, white, or light-yellow pills, **or begin a new package later than directed,** you should also use another method of birth control until you have taken a brown, white, or light-yellow pill daily for seven consecutive days. If you miss one or more light-yellow inactive pills (TRI-LEVLEN® 28 tablets only), you are still protected against pregnancy **provided** you begin taking your next brown pill on the proper day. If breakthrough bleeding occurs following missed pills, it will usually be temporary and of no consequence.

If you forget to take brown, white, or light-yellow pills three days in a row, do not take them when you remember but stop the medication and discard the package. Begin a new package, as directed above, on the first day of bleeding of your next period. During the days without pills, and until you have taken 6 brown and a white pill daily for seven consecutive days, you should protect yourself from pregnancy by also using another method of birth control.

LEVLEN® 21 TABLETS (LEVONORGESTTREL AND ETHINYL ESTRADIOL TABLETS)

The dosage of LEVLEN® 21 tablets is one tablet daily for 21 days in a row per menstrual cycle. Tablets are then discontinued for 7 days. The basic schedule is 21 days on—7 days off.

During the first month, you should begin taking LEVLEN® 21 tablets on Day 5 of your menstrual cycle whether or not you still have your period. (Day 1 is the first day of menstruation, even if it is almost midnight when you start.) Note: During your first month on LEVLEN® 21 tablets if you start taking tablets later than Day 5 of your menstrual cycle, you should protect yourself by also using another method of birth control until you have taken a tablet daily for seven consecutive days. Thereafter, if you follow directions carefully you will obtain the full contraceptive benefit. If you begin taking tablets later than the proper day, the possibility of ovulation and pregnancy occurring before beginning medication should be considered. Take one tablet every day until you finish all 21 tablets. No tablets are then taken for one week (7 days). Your period will usually begin about three days after you take the last tablet. Don't be alarmed if the amount of bleeding is not the same as before. On the 8th day, start a new SLIDECASE™ dispenser even if you still have your period. If, for example, you took LEVLEN® 21 tablets for the first time on a Tuesday, the 8th day will also be a Tuesday. Thus, you will always begin a new cycle on the same day of the week as long as you do not interrupt your original schedule. If you start taking tablets later than the 8th day, you should protect yourself by also using another method of birth control until you have taken a tablet daily for seven days in a row.

LEVLEN® 28 (LEVONORGESTREL AND ETHINYL ESTRADIOL TABLETS)

The dosage of LEVLEN® 28 tablets is one light-orange active tablet daily for 21 consecutive days followed by one pink inactive tablet daily for 7 consecutive days. The basic schedule is 21 days on light-orange active tablets—7 days on pink inactive tablets. Always take all 21 light-orange tablets in each SLIDECASE™ dispenser before taking the pink tablets.

You should begin taking LEVLEN® 28 tablets on the first Sunday after your menstrual period begins, whether or not you are still bleeding. If your period begins on a Sunday, take your first tablet that very same day. Your first light-orange tablet is marked with the word "Start". Note: During the first month on LEVLEN® 28 tablets, you should protect yourself by also using another method of birth control until you have taken a light-orange tablet daily for seven consecutive days. Thereafter, if you follow directions carefully, you will obtain the full contraceptive benefit. If you begin taking tablets later than the proper day, the possibility of ovulation and pregnancy occuring before beginning medication should be considered. Take one tablet every day until you finish all 21 light-orange tablets in a SLIDECASE™ dispenser, followed by all seven pink tablets. Your period will usually begin about three days after you take the last light-orange tablet, which will be during the time you are taking the pink tablets. Don't be alarmed if the amount of bleeding is not the same as before. The day after you have taken your last pink tablet, begin a new SLIDECASE™ despenser of tablets (taking all 21 light-orange tablets first, just as you did before) so that you will take a tablet every day without interruption. The starting day for each new SLIDECASE™ dispenser will always be Sunday. If in any cycle you start tablets later than the proper day, you should also use another method of birth control until you have taken a light-orange tablet daily for 7 days in a row.

Spotting or Breakthrough Bleeding:

Spotting is slight staining between menstrual periods which may not even require a pad. Breakthrough bleeding is a flow much like a regular period, requiring sanitary protection. Spotting is more common than breakthrough bleeding, and both occur more often in the first few cycles than in later cycles. These types of bleeding are usually temporary and without significance. It is important to continue taking your pills on schedule. If the bleeding persists for more than a few days, consult your doctor.

Forgotten Pills:

LEVLEN® 21 tablets contain 21 active light-orange tablets per SLIDECASE™ dispenser. LEVLEN® 28 tablets contain 21 active light-orange tablets plus 7 pink inactive tablets per SLIDECASE™ dispenser.

The chance of becoming pregnant is probably quite small if you miss only one light-orange tablet in a cycle. Of course, with each additional one you skip, the chance increases. If you miss one or more pink tablets (LEVLEN® 28 tablets), you are still protected against pregnancy as long as you begin taking your next light-orange tablet on the proper day. It is important to take a missed light-orange tablet as soon as it is remembered. If two consecutive light-orange tablets are missed they should both be taken as soon as remembered. The next tablet should then be taken at the usual time. Any time you miss one or two light-orange tablets, or begin a new SLIDECASE™ dispenser after the proper starting day, you should also use another method of birth control until you have taken a light-orange tablet daily for seven consecutive days. If breakthrough bleeding occurs following missed tablets, it will usually be temporary and of no consequence. While there is little likelihood of pregnancy occuring if only one or two light-orange tablets are missed, the possibility of

pregnancy increases with each successive day that scheduled light-orange tablets are missed.

If you are taking LEVLEN® 21 tablets and forget to take three light-orange tablets in a row, do not take them when you remember. Wait four more days—which makes a whole week without tablets. Then begin a new SLIDECASE™ dispenser on the 8th day after the last tablet was taken. During the seven days without tablets, and until you have taken a light-orange tablet daily for seven consecutive days, you should protect yourself from pregnancy by also using another method of birth control.

If you are taking LEVLEN® 28 tablets and forget to take three light-orange tablets in a row, do not take them when you remember. Stop taking all medication until the first Sunday following the last missed tablet. Then, whether or not you have had your period, and even if you are still bleeding, start a new SLIDECASE™ dispenser. During the days without tablets, and until you have taken a light-orange tablet daily for seven consecutive days, you should protect yourself from pregnancy by also using another method of birth control.

———

At times there may be no menstrual period after a cycle of pills. Therefore, if you miss one menstrual period but have taken the pills **exactly as you were supposed to,** continue as usual into the next cycle. If you have not taken the pills correctly and miss a menstrual period, you may be pregnant and should stop taking oral contraceptives until your doctor determines whether or not you are pregnant. Until you can get to your doctor, use another form of contraception. If two consecutive menstrual periods are missed, you should stop taking pills until it is determined whether you are pregnant. If you do become pregnant while using oral contraceptives, you should discuss the risks to the developing child with your doctor.

3. Periodic Examination.

Your doctor will take a complete medical and family history before prescribing oral contraceptives. At that time and about once a year thereafter, he will generally examine your blood pressure, breasts, abdomen, and pelvic organs (including a Papanicolaou smear, i.e., test for cancer).

SUMMARY

Oral contraceptives are the most effective method, except sterilization, for preventing pregnancy. Other methods when used conscientiously, are also very effective and have fewer risks. The serious risks of oral contraceptives are uncommon, and the "pill" is a very convenient method of preventing pregnancy. If you have certain conditions or have had these conditions in the past, you should not use oral contraceptives, because the risk is too great. These conditions are listed in the leaflet. If you do not have these conditions, and decide to use the "pill", please read the leaflet carefully so that you can use the "pill" most safely and effectively. Based on his or her assessment of your medical needs, your doctor has prescribed this drug for you. Do not give the drug to anyone else.

Manufactured for
BERLEX Laboratories, Inc., Wayne, NJ 07470

Issued May 1986   60611-1
                                                                60612-0

Shown in Product Identification Section, page 405

———

Beutlich, Inc.
7149 N. AUSTIN AVENUE
NILES, IL 60648

CEO–TWO® SUPPOSITORIES

COMPOSITION

Each adult rectal suppository contains sodium bicarbonate and potassium bitartrate in a water soluble polyethylene glycol base.

ACTIONS AND USES

CEO-TWO® is successfully used as a bowel evacuant, and for bowel retraining programs. The gentle pressure of the released CO_2 in the rectum stimulates peristalsis, and defecation usually results in 10 to 20 minutes. CEO-TWO® is especially helpful for spinal cord injury patients. It is gentle as well as safe. Unlike many other rectal suppositories, CEO-TWO® is not an irritant. It is, however, effective and predictable and will not cause an embarrassment at some later inconvenient time and place. Also used pre and post partum, pre and post operatively, or whenever the last 25cm of the lower bowel must be emptied.

ADMINISTRATION AND DOSAGE

One or two suppositories can be used as needed. Moisten CEO-TWO® with warm water before inserting. Patient should retain as long as possible. Dosage can be repeated in 4-6 hours if necessary.

Continued on next page

Beutlich—Cont.

CONTRAINDICATIONS
As with other enemas or laxatives.

HOW SUPPLIED
In packages of 10, white opaque suppositories. Keep in cool, dry place.
DO NOT REFRIGERATE

HURRICAINE® TOPICAL
ANESTHETIC
LIQUID AND GEL

COMPOSITION
HURRICAINE® (20% Benzocaine)

ACTION AND INDICATION
HURRICAINE® is quick, 15 to 30 seconds, effective and safe topical anesthetic that controls pain on any accessible mucous membrane, as well as to suppress the gag reflex, and it tastes good.

ADVANTAGES
Anesthesia is of short duration (12–15 minutes) with virtually no systemic absorption. True allergic reactions are rare. HURRICAINE® is also used in many dental and medical procedures with excellent patient acceptance.
PATIENTS WITH A KNOWN HYPERSENSITIVITY TO BENZOCAINE SHOULD NOT USE HURRICAINE®.
DO NOT USE IN EYES.
NOT FOR INJECTION.
KEEP OUT OF REACH OF CHILDREN.

HOW SUPPLIED
LIQUID or GEL in 1 oz. bottles & 1/8 oz. individual patient unit dose tubes.
FLAVORS—ORIGINAL CHERRY AND PINA COLADA.

HURRICAINE® TOPICAL
ANESTHETIC
AEROSOL SPRAY

COMPOSITION
20% Benzocaine

ACTION AND INDICATION
HURRICAINE® SPRAY is a good tasting topical anesthetic for oral and mucousal application, will help to control pain as well as to suppress the gag reflex during certain endoscopic procedures.

ADVANTAGES
HURRICAINE® is probably the agent of choice in endoscopy because of its safety, effectiveness, and patients' acceptance. HURRICAINE® provides you with rapid onset of action (15–30 seconds) and short duration (12–15 minutes) with virtually no systemic absorption. True allergic reactions are rare.
PATIENTS WITH A KNOWN HYPERSENSITIVITY TO BENZOCAINE SHOULD NOT USE.
DO NOT USE IN EYES.
NOT FOR INJECTION.
KEEP OUT OF REACH OF CHILDREN.

HOW SUPPLIED
Aerosol SPRAY 2 oz. can

HURRICAINE® TOPICAL
ANESTHETIC
SPRAY KIT

COMPOSITION
HURRICAINE® SPRAY 2 oz. aerosol can 20% benzocaine with 200 disposable extension tubes.

ADVANTAGES
The use of disposable extention tubes will minimize the risk of infection thru cross contamination. Clean, quick and easy to attach.
PATIENTS WITH A KNOWN HYPERSENSITIVITY TO BENZOCAINE SHOULD NOT USE HURRICAINE®.
DO NOT USE IN EYES.
NOT FOR INJECTION.
KEEP OUT OF REACH OF CHILDREN.

HOW SUPPLIED
2 oz. Aerosol with 200 disposable extension tubes

MEVANIN-C CAPSULES

COMPOSITION
Each capsule contains: Ascorbic Acid 200 mg., Hesperidin Complex 30 mg., Calcium Lactate 300 mg., Cyanocobalamin

---

1 mcg., Ferrous Sulfate 65 mg., Folic Acid 0.1 mg., Vitamin A 3000 USP units, Vitamin D 300 USP units, Thiamine HCl 2 mg., Riboflavin 2 mg., Pyridoxine HCl 0.5 mg., Niacin 5 mg., plus trace amounts of copper, zinc, manganese, magnesium, potassium and iodine.

ADMINISTRATION AND DOSAGE
One capsule daily.

HOW SUPPLIED
In bottles of 90 and 450 red and white capsules.

PERIDIN-C®

COMPOSITION
Each tablet contains Hesperidin Methyl Chalcone 50 mg., Hesperidin Complex 150 mg., Ascorbic Acid 200 mg.

DOSAGE
1 tablet daily.

HOW SUPPLIED
In bottles of 100 and 500 orange tablets.

Biocraft Laboratories, Inc.
92 ROUTE 46
ELMWOOD PARK, NJ 07407

NDC 0332	PRODUCT	PROD. ID. NO.
	ALBUTEROL SULFATE TABLETS ℞	
2226	2 mg	130
2228	4 mg	131
	AMILORIDE HYDROCHLORIDE AND HYDROCHLOROTHIAZIDE TABLETS ℞	
2205	5 mg/50 mg	52
	AMITRIPTYLINE HCL TABLETS ℞	
2120	10 mg	22
2122	25 mg	23
2124	50 mg	24
2126	75 mg	25
2128	100 mg	26
	AMOXICILLIN CAPSULES ℞	
3107	250 mg	01
3109	500 mg	03
	AMOXICILLIN SUSPENSION ℞	
4150	125 mg/5 mL	
4155	250 mg/5 mL	
	AMPICILLIN CAPSULES ℞	
3111	250 mg	05
3113	500 mg	06
	AMPICILLIN SUSPENSION ℞	
4129	125 mg/5 mL	
4131	250 mg/5 mL	
	AMPICILLIN-PROBENECID SUSPENSION ℞	
4140	1 gm Probenecid; 3.5 gm Amp	
	CEFADROXIL CAPSULES ℞	
3159	500 mg	114
	CEFADROXIL SUSPENSION ℞	
4169	125 mg/5 mL	
4171	250 mg/5 mL	
4173	500 mg/5 mL	
	CEPHALEXIN CAPSULES ℞	
3145	250 mg	115
3147	500 mg	117
	CEPHALEXIN SUSPENSION ℞	
4175	125 mg/5 mL	
4177	250 mg/5 mL	
	CEPHALEXIN TABLETS ℞	
2238	250 mg	136
2240	500 mg	137
	CEPHRADINE CAPSULES ℞	
3153	250 mg	112
3155	500 mg	113
	CEPHRADINE SUSPENSION ℞	
4165	125 mg/5 mL	
4167	250 mg/5 mL	
	CHLOROQUINE PHOSPHATE TABLETS ℞	
2160	250 mg	38
	CLOXACILLIN CAPSULES ℞	
3119	250 mg	28
3121	500 mg	30
	CLOXACILLIN SOLUTION ℞	
4159	125 mg/5 mL	
	CYCLACILLIN TABLETS ℞	
2207	250 mg	94
2208	500 mg	95
	DICLOXACILLIN CAPSULES ℞	
3123	250 mg	02
3125	500 mg	04
	DISOPYRAMIDE PHOSPHATE CAPSULES ℞	
3127	100 mg	40
3129	150 mg	41

	HYDROCORTISONE TOPICAL CREAM	
5125	1%	
	IMIPRAMINE HCL TABLETS ℞	
2111	10 mg	19
2113	25 mg	20
2117	50 mg	21
	METOCLOPRAMIDE SYRUP ℞	
6105	5 mg/5 mL	
	METOCLOPRAMIDE TABLETS ℞	
2203	10 mg	93
	NEOMYCIN SULFATE TABLETS ℞	
1177	500 mg	18
	NYSTATIN SUSPENSION ℞	
6109	100,000 units/mL	
	OXACILLIN CAPSULES ℞	
3115	250 mg	12
3117	500 mg	14
	OXACILLIN SOLUTION ℞	
4157	250 mg/5 mL	
	PENICILLIN G POTASSIUM TABLETS ℞	
1117	200,000 Units	07
1121	250,000 Units	09
1123	400,000 Units	10
	PENICILLIN V POTASSIUM SOLUTION ℞	
4125	125 mg/5 mL	
4127	250 mg/5 mL	
	PENICILLIN V POTASSIUM TABLETS ℞	
1171	250 mg ROUND	15
1172	250 mg OVAL	16
1173	500 mg ROUND	17
1174	500 mg OVAL	49
	SULFAMETHOXAZOLE AND TRIMETHOPRIM PEDIATRIC SUSPENSION ℞	
6100	200 mg/40 mg per 5 mL	
	SULFAMETHOXAZOLE AND TRIMETHOPRIM TABLETS ℞	
2130	400 mg/80 mg (Single Strength)	32
2132	800 mg/160 mg (Double Strength)	33
	TRIMETHOPRIM TABLETS ℞	
2158	100 mg	34
2159	200 mg	35

Bio-Tech Pharmacal, Inc.
P.O. BOX 1992
FAYETTEVILLE, AR 72702

B-12 RESIN (Sublingual)
Each tablet contains 1,000mcg Vit B-12 on ion Exchange Resin.

BIO-STATIN   ℞
POWDER
Pure Nystatin pre-packaged in bottles of 150,000MM Units (30 gm; approx. 300 doses).
CAPSULES
500,000 or 1,000,000 Units Pure Nystatin per capsule.

BROMASE
(Proteolytic Enzyme)
(Bromelain)

ACTIVE INGREDIENTS
Each BROMASE capsule contains 500 mg of Bromelain (2400mcu/gm), 15 mg Ascorbic Acid.

INDICATIONS
Due to its action as a prostaglandin modulator, BROMASE is useful as a supplement for inflammatory conditions resulting from prostaglandin metabolism, surgical procedures, sports activities, and other trauma.

PRECAUTION AND DRUG INTERACTION
Virtually non-toxic; no LD50 up to 10g/kg. Chronic use well-tolerated. Concomitant use with Coumadin or in hemophillacs and others with bleeding tendencies inadvisable. Safe use during pregnancy not established.

DOSAGE AND ADMINISTRATION
One or more capsules BID or TID; between meals preferably.

HOW SUPPLIED
Bottles of 60s. NDC #53191-151-06.

C-MAX
Each gradual release tablet contains Vit C (from ascorbic acid; Mg, Zn, K, Mn Ascorbate) 1,000mg; Mg (Ascorbate) 40 mg; Zn (Ascorbate) 5mg; K (Ascorbate) 10mg; Mn (Ascorbate) 1 mg; Pectin 10mg.

MAG-L

Each enteric-coated tablet contains Mg Cl 535mg.

OB-20-℞Pre- and Peri-Natal (YEAST FREE)   ℞

Each 3 tablets contain Beta Carotene 8000 USP Units; Vit D3 400 USP Units; Vit E (d-Alpha Tocopherol) 30 USP Units; Vit C (Ascorbic Acid, Mn, Zn Ascorbate) 120mg; Folic Acid 1.0mg; Vit B1 1.7mg; Vit B2 2mg; Vit B3 20mg; Vit B6 10mg; Vit B12 (Resin Adsorbate) 8mcg; Biotin 150mcg; Pantothenic Acid 10mg; Ca (Citrate) 500mg; Iron (Fe Gluconate) 50mg; Mg (Cl) 150mg; Zn (Ascorbate) 25mg; Mn (Ascorbate 5mg; Cr (Chelate) Non Yeast 25mcg; Se (Chelate) 25 mcg.

PROS-TECH

Each capsule contains Glutamic Acid, Alanine, Glycine.

Blaine Company, Inc.
2700 DIXIE HIGHWAY
FT. MITCHELL, KY 41017

MAG-OX 400   OTC

DESCRIPTION
Each tablet contains Magnesium Oxide 400 mg. U.S.P. (Heavy), or 241.3 mg. Elemental Magnesium (19.86 mEq.)

INDICATIONS AND USAGE
Hypomagnesemia, magnesium deficiencies and/or magnesium depletion resulting from malnutrition, restricted diet, alcoholism or magnesium depleting drugs. An antacid. For increasing urinary magnesium excretion.

WARNINGS
Do not take more than 2 tablets in a 24 hour period, or use this maximum dosage for more than 2 weeks, except under the advice and supervision of a physician. Do not use this product except under the advice and supervision of a physician if you have a kidney disease. May have laxative effect. As with any drug, if you are pregnant or nursing a baby, seek professional advice before using this product. Keep this and all medicines out of children's reach.

DOSAGE
Adult dose 1 or 2 tablets daily or as directed by a physician.

HOW SUPPLIED
Bottles of 100 and 1000.

URO-MAG   OTC

DESCRIPTION
Each capsule contains Magnesium Oxide 140 mg. U.S.P. (Heavy), or 84.5 mg. Elemental Magnesium (6.93 mEq.)

INDICATIONS AND USAGE
Hypomagnesemia, magnesium deficiencies and/or magnesium depletion resulting from malnutrition, restricted diet, alcoholism or magnesium depleting drugs. An antacid. For increasing urinary magnesium excretion.

WARNINGS
Do not take more than 4 capsules in a 24 hour period, or use this maximum dosage for more than 2 weeks, except under the advice and supervision of a physician. Do not use this product except under the advice and supervision of a physician if you have a kidney disease. May have laxative effect. As with any drug, if you are pregnant or nursing a baby, seek professional advice before using this product. Keep this and all medicines out of children's reach.

DOSAGE
Adult dose 3–4 capsules daily or as directed by a physician.

HOW SUPPLIED
Bottles of 100 and 1000.

EDUCATIONAL MATERIAL

Samples and literature available to physicians upon request.

Products are cross-indexed by
generic and chemical names in the
YELLOW SECTION

Bock Pharmacal Company
P.O. BOX 8519
ST. LOUIS, MO 63126-0519

BRONCHOLATE CS   ℂ

Each 5 ml cherry flavored red syrup contains:
Codeine Phosphate	10.00 mg
(Warning: May be habit forming)	
Ephedrine HCl	6.25 mg
Guaifenesin	100.00 mg

HOW SUPPLIED
Bottles of 16 oz.

BRONCHOLATE SOFTGELS   ℞

Each orange football shaped softgel contains:
Ephedrine HCl	12.5 mg
Guaifenesin	200.0 mg

HOW SUPPLIED
Bottles of 100

BRONCHOLATE SYRUP   ℞

Each 5 ml orange flavored syrup contains:
Ephedrine HCl	6.25 mg
Guaifenesin	100.00 mg

HOW SUPPLIED
Bottles of 16 oz.

DOLPRN #3 TABLETS   ℞ ℂ

Each green layered tablet embossed BOCK contains:
Codeine Phosphate	30.0 mg
(Warning: May be habit forming)	
Acetaminophen	400.0 mg
Aspirin	250.0 mg
Magnesium Hydroxide	60.0 mg
Dried Aluminum Hydroxide Gel USP	60.0 mg

HOW SUPPLIED
Bottles of 100.

HEMASPAN TABLETS

Each round beige tablet embossed BOCK 330 contains:
*Iron, Elemental (as Ferrous Fumarate)	110.0 mg
Vitamin C	200.0 mg
Docusate Sodium	20.0 mg

*In a special base to provide delayed therapeutic action.

HOW SUPPLIED
Bottles of 100

HISTUSSIN HC   ℞ ℂ

Each 5 ml orange/pineapple flavored syrup contains:
Hydrocodone Bitartrate	2.5 mg
(Warning: May be habit forming.)	
Phenylephrine Hydrochloride	5.0 mg
Chlorpheniramine Maleate	2.0 mg

HOW SUPPLIED
Bottles of 16 oz.

POLY-HISTINE CS   ℞ ℂ

Each 5 ml cherry flavored red syrup contains:
Codeine Phosphate	10.0 mg
(Warning: May be habit forming.)	
Phenylpropanolamine HCl	12.5 mg
Brompheniramine Maleate	2.0 mg

HOW SUPPLIED
Bottles of 16 oz.

POLY-HISTINE ELIXIR   ℞

Each 5 ml lemon-lime flavored green elixir contains:
Phenyltoloxamine Citrate	4.0 mg
Pyrilamine Maleate	4.0 mg
Pheniramine Maleate	4.0 mg
Alcohol	4%

HOW SUPPLIED
Bottles of 16 oz.

POLY-HISTINE
EXPECTORANT

Each 5 ml cherry flavored red syrup contains:
Phenylpropanolamine HCl	12.5 mg
Guaifenesin	100.0 mg

HOW SUPPLIED
Bottles of 16 oz.

POLY-HISTINE-D CAPSULES   ℞

Each red-clear timed release capsule* imprinted BOCK contains:
Phenylpropanolamine HCl	50.0 mg
Phenyltoloxamine Citrate	16.0 mg
Pyrilamine Maleate	16.0 mg
Pheniramine Maleate	16.0 mg

*In a special base to provide prolonged therapeutic action.

HOW SUPPLIED
Bottles of 100.

POLY-HISTINE-D ELIXIR   ℞

Each 5 ml wild cherry flavored red elixir contains:
Phenylpropanolamine HCl	12.5 mg
Phenyltoloxamine Citrate	4.0 mg
Pyrilamine Maleate	4.0 mg
Pheniramine Maleate	4.0 mg
Alcohol	4%

HOW SUPPLIED
Bottles of 16 oz.

POLY-HISTINE-D PED CAPS   ℞

Each clear timed release capsule* imprinted BOCK contains:
Phenylpropanolamine HCl	25.0 mg
Phenyltoloxamine Citrate	8.0 mg
Pyrilamine Maleate	8.0 mg
Pheniramine Maleate	8.0 mg

*In a special base to provide prolonged therapeutic action.

HOW SUPPLIED
Bottles of 100.

POLY-HISTINE DM SYRUP   ℞

Each 5 ml black-raspberry flavored purple syrup contains:
Dextromethorphan HBr	10.0 mg
Phenylpropanolamine HCl	12.5 mg
Brompheniramine Maleate	2.0 mg

HOW SUPPLIED
Bottles of 16 oz.

PRENATE 90®   ℞
Vitamin-Mineral Supplement

Each white film coated tablet embossed BOCK contains:
*Iron (Ferrous Fumarate)	90.0 mg*
Iodine (Potassium Iodide)	0.15 mg
Calcium (Calcium Carbonate)	250.0 mg
Copper (Cupric Oxide)	2.0 mg
Zinc (Zinc Oxide)	25.0 mg
Folic Acid	1.0 mg
Vitamin A (Acetate)	4000.0 I.U.
Vitamin D (Ergocalciferol)	400.0 I.U.
Vitamin E (Acetate)	30.0 I.U.
Vitamin C (Ascorbic Acid)	120.0 mg
Vitamin B_1 (Thiamine Mononitrate)	3.0 mg
Vitamin B_2 (Riboflavin)	3.4 mg
Vitamin B_6 (Pyridoxine HCl)	20.0 mg
Vitamin B_{12} (Cyanocobalamin)	12.0 mcg
Niacinamide	20.0 mg
Docusate Sodium	50.0 mg

*MICRO IRON (A special base to provide delayed therapeutic action)

HOW SUPPLIED
Bottles of 100.

THEON SYRUP   ℞

Each 5 ml dye-free syrup contains:
Theophylline (Anhydrous)	50.0 mg
Alcohol	1%

HOW SUPPLIED
Bottles of 16 oz.

Continued on next page

Bock—Cont.

ZEPHREX TABLETS   ℞

Each blue film coated tablet embossed BOCK contains:
Pseudoephedrine HCl ....60.0 mg
Guaifenesin ....400.0 mg

HOW SUPPLIED
Bottles of 100.

ZEPHREX–LA TABLETS   ℞

Each orange timed release tablet* embossed BOCK contains:
Pseudoephedrine HCl ....120.0 mg
Guaifenesin ....600.0 mg
*In a special base to provide prolonged therapeutic action.

HOW SUPPLIED
Bottles of 100.

Boehringer Ingelheim Pharmaceuticals, Inc.

A subsidiary of Boehringer Ingelheim Corporation
90 EAST RIDGE
POST OFFICE BOX 368
RIDGEFIELD, CT 06877

ALUPENT®   ℞
[al'u-pent]
(metaproterenol sulfate, USP)
Bronchodilator

Tablets 10 mg	BI-CODE 74
Tablets 20 mg	BI-CODE 72
Inhalation Aerosol 10 ml	BI-CODE 70
Syrup 10 mg/5 ml	BI-CODE 73
Inhalation Solution 5%	BI-CODE 71
Inhalation Solution	BI-CODE 69
Unit-dose Vials 0.4% and 0.6%	

DESCRIPTION

Alupent® (metaproterenol sulfate USP) Inhalation Aerosol is administered by oral inhalation. Each canister of Inhalation Aerosol contains 150 mg of metaproterenol sulfate as a micronized powder. This is sufficient medication for 200 inhalations. Each metered dose delivers through the mouthpiece 0.65 mg of metaproterenol sulfate (each ml contains 15 mg). The inert ingredients are dichlorodifluoromethane, dichlorotetrafluoroethane and trichloromonofluoromethane as propellants, and soya lecithin.

Alupent Inhalation Solution is administered by oral inhalation with the aid of a hand-bulb nebulizer or an intermittent positive pressure breathing apparatus (IPPB). It contains Alupent 5% in a pH-adjusted aqueous solution containing benzalkonium chloride and edetate disodium as preservatives.

Alupent Inhalation Solution Unit-dose Vial is administered by oral inhalation with the aid of an IPPB. It contains Alupent 0.4% or 0.6% in a sterile pH-adjusted aqueous solution with edetate disodium and sodium chloride.

Alupent Syrup is administered orally. Each teaspoonful (5 ml) of syrup contains metaproterenol sulfate 10 mg. The inactive ingredients are edetate disodium, FD&C Red No. 40, hydroxyethylcellulose, imitation black cherry flavor, methylparaben, propylparaben, saccharin, sorbitol solution.

Alupent Tablets are administered orally. Each tablet contains metaproterenol sulfate 10 mg or 20 mg. The inactive ingredients are colloidal silicon dioxide, corn starch, dibasic calcium phosphate, lactose, magnesium stearate.

Chemically, Alupent is 1-(3,5 dihydroxyphenyl)-2-isopropylaminoethanol sulfate, a white crystalline, racemic mixture of two optically active isomers. It differs from isoproterenol hydrochloride by having two hydroxyl groups attached at the meta positions on the benzene ring rather than one at the meta and one at the para position.

metaproterenol sulfate (Alupent)
[See Chemical Formula at top of next column].

isoproterenol hydrochloride

CLINICAL PHARMACOLOGY

Alupent (metaproterenol sulfate USP) is a potent beta-adrenergic stimulator. Alupent Inhalation Aerosol and Inhalation Solution have a rapid onset of action. It is postulated that beta-adrenergic stimulants produce many of their pharmacological effects by activation of adenyl cyclase, the enzyme that catalyzes the conversion of adenosine triphosphate to cyclic adenosine monophosphate.

Pharmacokinetics: Absorption, biotransformation and excretion studies in humans following administration by inhalation have shown that approximately 3 percent of the actuated dose is absorbed intact through the lungs.

Following oral administration in humans, an average of 40% of the drug is absorbed; it is not metabolized by catechol-O-methyltransferase or sulfatase enzymes in the gut, but is excreted primarily as glucuronic acid conjugates.

When administered orally or by inhalation, Alupent decreases reversible bronchospasm. Pulmonary function tests performed concomitantly usually show improvement following aerosol Alupent administration, e.g., an increase in the one-second forced expiratory volume (FEV_1), an increase in maximum expiratory flow rate, an increase in peak expiratory flow rate, an increase in forced vital capacity, and/or a decrease in airway resistance. The resultant decrease in airway obstruction may relieve the dyspnea associated with bronchospasm.

Controlled single- and multiple-dose studies have been performed with pulmonary function monitoring. The duration of effect of a *single dose* of Alupent Tablets 20 mg or Alupent Syrup (that is, the period of time during which there is a 15% or greater increase in FEV_1) was up to 4 hours. Four controlled multiple-dose 60-day studies, comparing the effectiveness of Alupent Tablets with ephedrine tablets, have been performed. Because of difficulties in study design, only one study was available which could be analyzed in depth. This study showed a loss of efficacy with time for both Alupent and ephedrine. Therefore, the physician should take this phenomenon into account in evaluating the individual patient's overall management. Further studies are in progress to adequately explain these results.

Controlled single- and multiple-dose studies have been performed with pulmonary function monitoring. The duration of effect of a *single dose* of two to three inhalations of Alupent Inhalation Aerosol (that is, the period of time during which there is a 20% or greater increase in FEV_1) has varied from 1 to 5 hours.

In repetitive-dosing studies (up to q.i.d.) the duration of effect for a similar dose of Alupent Inhalation Aerosol has ranged from about 1 to 2.5 hours. Present studies are inadequate to explain the divergence in duration of the FEV_1 effect between single- and repetitive-dosing studies, respectively.

Following controlled single dose studies with Alupent Inhalation Solution by an intermittent positive pressure breathing apparatus (IPPB) and by hand-bulb nebulizers, significant improvement (15% or greater increase in FEV_1) occurred within 5 to 30 minutes and persisted for periods varying from 2 to 6 hours.

In these studies, the longer duration of effect occurred in the studies in which the drug was administered by IPPB, i.e., 6 hours, versus 2 to 3 hours when administered by hand-bulb nebulizer. In these studies the doses used were 0.3 ml by IPPB and 10 inhalations by hand-bulb nebulizer.

In controlled repetitive-dosing studies with Alupent Inhalation Solution by IPPB and by hand-bulb nebulizer the onset of effect occurred within 5 to 30 minutes and duration ranged from 4 to 6 hours. In these studies the doses used were 0.3 ml b.i.d. or t.i.d. when given by IPPB, and 10 inhalations q.i.d. (no more often than q4h) when given by hand-bulb nebulizer. As in the single dose studies, effectiveness was measured as a sustained increase in FEV_1 of 15% or greater. In these repetitive-dosing studies there was no apparent difference in duration between the two methods of delivery.

Clinical studies were conducted in which the effectiveness of Alupent Inhalation Solution was evaluated by comparison with that of isoproterenol hydrochloride over periods of two to three months. Both drugs continued to produce significant improvement in pulmonary function throughout this period of treatment.

Recent studies in laboratory animals (minipigs, rodents and dogs) recorded the occurrence of cardiac arrhythmias and sudden death (with histologic evidence of myocardial necrosis) when beta agonists and methylxanthines were administered concurrently. The significance of these findings when applied to humans is currently unknown.

INDICATIONS AND USAGE

Alupent® (metaproterenol sulfate USP) is indicated as a bronchodilator for bronchial asthma and for reversible bronchospasm which may occur in association with bronchitis and emphysema.

CONTRAINDICATIONS

Use in patients with cardiac arrhythmias associated with tachycardia is contraindicated.

Although rare, immediate hypersensitivity reactions can occur. Therefore, Alupent® (metaproterenol sulfate USP) is contraindicated in patients with a history of hypersensitivity to any of its components.

WARNINGS

Excessive use of adrenergic aerosols is potentially dangerous. Fatalities have been reported following excessive use of Alupent® (metaproterenol sulfate USP) as with other sympathomimetic inhalation preparations, and the exact cause is unknown. Cardiac arrest was noted in several cases.

Alupent, like other beta adrenergic agonists, can produce a significant cardiovascular effect in some patients, as measured by pulse rate, blood pressure, symptoms and/or ECG changes. As with other beta adrenergic aerosols, Alupent can produce paradoxical bronchospasm (which can be life threatening). If it occurs, the preparation should be discontinued immediately and alternative therapy instituted. Alupent® (metaproterenol sulfate USP) should not be used more often than prescribed. Patients should be advised to contact their physician in the event that they do not respond to their usual dose of sympathomimetic amine aerosol.

PRECAUTIONS

General: Extreme care must be exercised with respect to the administration of additional sympathomimetic agents. Since metaproterenol is a sympathomimetic amine it should be used with caution in patients with cardiovascular disorders, including ischemic heart disease, hypertension or cardiac arrhythmias, in patients with hyperthyroidism or diabetes mellitus, and in patients who are unusually responsive to sympathomimetic amines or who have convulsive disorders. Significant changes in systolic and diastolic blood pressure could be expected to occur in some patients after use of any beta adrenergic bronchodilator.

Information for Patients: Extreme care must be exercised with respect to the administration of additional sympathomimetic agents. A sufficient interval of time should elapse prior to administration of another sympathomimetic agent.

Drug Interactions: Other beta adrenergic aerosol bronchodilators should not be used concomitantly with Alupent because they may have additive effects. Beta adrenergic agonists should be administered with caution to patients being treated with monoamine oxidase inhibitors or tricyclic antidepressants, since the action of beta adrenergic agonists on the vascular system may be potentiated.

Carcinogenesis/Mutagenesis/Impairment of Fertility: In an 18-month study in mice, Alupent produced an increase in benign ovarian tumors in females at doses corresponding to 320 and 640 times the maximum recommended dose (based on a 50 kg individual). In a two-year study in rats, a non-significant incidence of benign leiomyomata of the mesovarium was noted at 640 times the maximum recommended dose. The relevance of these findings to man is not known. Mutagenic studies with Alupent have not been conducted. Reproduction studies in rats revealed no evidence of impaired fertility.

Pregnancy: *Teratogenic Effects: Pregnancy Category C.* Alupent has been shown to be teratogenic and embryotoxic in rabbits when given orally in doses 620 times the human inhalation dose and 62 times the human oral dose. There are no adequate and well-controlled studies in pregnant women. Alupent should be used during pregnancy only if the potential benefit justifies the potential risk to the fetus.

Oral reproduction studies in mice, rats and rabbits showed no teratogenic or embryocidal effects at 50 mg/kg corresponding to 310 times the human inhalation dose and 31 times the human oral dose. Teratogenic effects in the rabbit included skeletal abnormalities and hydrocephalus with bone separation.

Nursing Mothers: It is not known whether this drug is excreted in human milk. Because many drugs are excreted in human milk, caution should be exercised when Alupent is administered to a nursing woman.

Pediatric Use: See **DOSAGE AND ADMINISTRATION.**

ADVERSE REACTIONS

Adverse reactions are similar to those noted with other sympathomimetic agents. Adverse reactions such as tachycardia, hypertension, palpitations, nervousness, tremor, nausea and vomiting have been reported.

The most frequent adverse reaction to Alupent® (metaproterenol sulfate USP) administered by metered-dose inhaler among 251 patients in 90-day controlled clinical trials was nervousness. This was reported in 6.8% of patients. Less frequent adverse experiences, occurring in 1–4% of patients were headache, dizziness, palpitations, gastrointestinal distress, tremor, throat irritation, nausea, vomiting, cough and asthma exacerbation. Tachycardia occurred in less than 1% of patients.

OVERDOSAGE

The expected symptoms with overdosage are those of excessive beta-adrenergic stimulation and/or any of the symptoms listed under adverse reactions, e.g. angina, hypertension or hypotension, arrhythmias, nervousness, headache, tremor, dry mouth, palpitation, nausea, dizziness, fatigue, malaise and insomnia.

Treatment consists of discontinuation of metaproterenol together with appropriate symptomatic therapy.

DOSAGE AND ADMINISTRATION

If Alupent® (metaproterenol sulfate USP) is administered before or after other sympathomimetic bronchodilators, caution should be exercised with respect to possible potentiation of adrenergic effects.

Inhalation Aerosol: The usual single dose is two to three inhalations. With repetitive dosing, inhalation should usually not be repeated more often than about every three to four hours. Total dosage per day should not exceed 12 inhalations. Alupent Inhalation Aerosol is not recommended for use in children under 12 years of age.

Inhalation Solution: Usually treatment need not be repeated more often than every four hours to relieve acute attacks of bronchospasm. As part of a total treatment program in chronic bronchospastic pulmonary diseases, Alupent Inhalation Solution may be administered three to four times a day.

As with all medications, the physician should begin therapy with the lowest effective dose and then titrate the dosage according to the individual patient's requirements. Alupent Inhalation Solution is not recommended for use in children under 12 years of age.

Inhalation Solution 5%: Alupent Inhalation Solution is administered by oral inhalation with the aid of a hand bulb nebulizer or an intermittent positive pressure breathing apparatus (IPPB).

Method of Administration	Usual Single Dose	Range	Dilution
Hand-bulb nebulizer	10 inhalations	5–15 inhalations	No dilution
IPPB	0.3 ml	0.2–0.3 ml	Diluted in approx. 2.5 ml of saline solution or other diluent

Inhalation Solution 0.4% and 0.6% Unit-dose Vials: Alupent Inhalation Solution Unit-dose Vial is administered by oral inhalation using an IPPB device. The usual adult dose is one vial per nebulization treatment. Each vial of Alupent Inhalation Solution 0.4% is equivalent to 0.2 ml Alupent Inhalation Solution 5% diluted to 2.5 ml with normal saline; each vial of Alupent Inhalation Solution 0.6% is equivalent to 0.3 ml Alupent Inhalation Solution 5% diluted to 2.5 ml with normal saline.

Syrup: Children aged six to nine years or weight under 60 lbs—one teaspoonful three or four times a day. Children over nine years or weight over 60 lbs—two teaspoonfuls three or four times a day. Experience in children under the age of six is limited to 78 children. Of this number, 40 were treated with Alupent syrup for at least one month. In this group daily doses of approximately 1.3 to 2.6 mg/kg were well tolerated. Adults—two teaspoonfuls three or four times a day.

Tablets: *Adults:* The usual dose is 20 mg three or four times a day. *Children:* Aged six to nine years or weight under 60 lbs—10 mg three or four times a day. Over nine years or weight over 60 lbs—20 mg three or four times a day. Alupent tablets are not recommended for use in children under six years at this time.

HOW SUPPLIED

Inhalation Aerosol: Each Alupent® Inhalation Aerosol contains 150 mg of metaproterenol sulfate as a micronized powder in inert propellants. Each metered dose delivers through the mouthpiece 0.65 mg metaproterenol sulfate (each ml contains 15 mg). Alupent Inhalation Aerosol with Mouthpiece (NDC 0597-0070-17), net contents 14g (10 ml), equipped with blue protective cap. Alupent Inhalation Aerosol Refill (NDC 0597-0070-18), net contents 14g (10 ml). Store between 59°F (15°C) and 77°F (25°C). Avoid excessive humidity.

Inhalation Solution: Alupent Inhalation Solution is supplied as a 5% solution in bottles of 10 ml or 30 ml with accompanying calibrated dropper. Store below 77°F (25°C). Protect from light. Do not use the solution if it is brown or has a precipitate.

Alupent Inhalation Solution Unit-dose Vial is supplied as a 0.4% or 0.6% clear colorless or nearly colorless solution containing 2.5 ml with 25 vials per box. Store below 77°F (25°C). Protect from light. Do not use the solution if it is brown or has a precipitate.

Syrup: Alupent is available as a cherry-flavored syrup, 10 mg per teaspoonful (5 ml) in 16 fl. oz. bottles. Store below 86°F (30°C). Protect from light.

Tablets: Alupent is supplied in two dosage strengths as scored round white tablets in bottles of 100. Tablets of 10 mg coded BI/74. Tablets of 20 mg coded BI/72. Storage for bottles: Store below 86°F (30°C). Protect from light. Storage for blister samples: Store below 77°F (25°C). Protect from light.

CAUTION

Federal law prohibits dispensing without prescription.

AL-PI-12/88

Shown in Product Identification Section, page 405

ATROVENT® ℞
[ă'trō"věnt]
(ipratropium bromide)
Inhalation Aerosol
Bronchodilator

PRODUCT OVERVIEW

KEY FACTS

The active ingredient in Atrovent® (ipratropium bromide) Inhalation Aerosol is ipratropium bromide. It is an anticholinergic bronchodilator classified as a synthetic quaternary ammonium compound. The bronchodilating effect of Atrovent is primarily local and site specific. It is not well absorbed systemically, resulting in a low potential for toxicity.

MAJOR USES

Atrovent Inhalation Aerosol has proved to be clinically effective for maintenance treatment of bronchospasm associated with chronic obstructive pulmonary disease, including chronic bronchitis and emphysema.

SAFETY INFORMATION

Atrovent Inhalation Aerosol is contraindicated for patients with a hypersensitivity to atropine or its derivatives. It is not intended for treatment of acute episodes of bronchospasm where rapid response is required.

Before prescribing, please consult full prescribing information below.

PRESCRIBING INFORMATION

ATROVENT® ℞
[ă'trō"věnt]
(ipratropium bromide)
Inhalation Aerosol
Bronchodilator

DESCRIPTION

The active ingredient in Atrovent® (ipratropium bromide) Inhalation Aerosol is ipratropium bromide. It is an anticholinergic bronchodilator chemically described as 8-azoniabicyclo[3.2.1]-octane, 3-(3-hydroxy-1-oxo-2-phenylpropoxy)-8-methyl-8-(1-methylethyl)-, bromide, monohydrate (endo, syn)-, (±)-; a synthetic quaternary ammonium compound, chemically related to atropine. It has the following structural formula:

Ipratropium bromide is a white crystalline substance, freely soluble in water and lower alcohols but insoluble in lipophilic solvents such as ether, chloroform, and fluorocarbons. Atrovent Inhalation Aerosol is an inhalation aerosol for oral administration. The net weight is 14 grams; it yields 200 inhalations. Each actuation of the valve delivers 18 mcg of ipratropium bromide from the mouthpiece. The inert ingredients are dichlorodifluoromethane, dichlorotetrafluoroethane, and trichloromonofluoromethane as propellants and soya lecithin.

CLINICAL PHARMACOLOGY

Atrovent® (ipratropium bromide) is an anticholinergic (parasympatholytic) agent which, based on animal studies, appears to inhibit vagally mediated reflexes by antagonizing the action of acetylcholine, the transmitter agent released from the vagus nerve. Anticholinergics prevent the increases in intracellular concentration of cyclic guanosine monophosphate (cyclic GMP) which are caused by interaction of acetylcholine with the muscarinic receptor on bronchial smooth muscle.

The bronchodilation following inhalation of Atrovent is primarily a local, site-specific effect, not a systemic one. Much of an inhaled dose is swallowed as shown by fecal excretion studies. Atrovent is not readily absorbed into the systemic circulation either from the surface of the lung or from the gastrointestinal tract as confirmed by blood level and renal excretion studies.

The half-life of elimination is about 2 hours after inhalation or intravenous administration. Autoradiographic studies in rats have shown that Atrovent does not penetrate the blood-brain barrier.

In controlled 90-day studies in patients with bronchospasm associated with chronic obstructive pulmonary disease (chronic bronchitis and emphysema) significant improvements in pulmonary function (FEV_1 and $FEF_{25-75}\%$ increases of 15% or more) occurred within 15 minutes, reached a peak in 1–2 hours, and persisted for periods of 3 to 4 hours in the majority of patients and up to 6 hours in some patients. In addition, significant increases in Forced Vital Capacity (FVC) have been demonstrated.

Controlled clinical studies have demonstrated that Atrovent (ipratropium bromide) does not alter either mucociliary clearance or the volume or viscosity of respiratory secretions. In studies without a positive control Atrovent did not alter pupil size, accommodation or visual acuity (See ADVERSE REACTIONS).

Ventilation/perfusion studies have shown no clinically significant effects on pulmonary gas exchange or arterial oxygen tension. Atrovent does not produce clinically significant changes in pulse rate or blood pressure.

INDICATIONS AND USAGE

Atrovent® (ipratropium bromide) is indicated as a bronchodilator for maintenance treatment of bronchospasm associated with chronic obstructive pulmonary disease, including chronic bronchitis and emphysema.

CONTRAINDICATIONS

Hypersensitivity to atropine or its derivatives.

WARNINGS

Atrovent® (ipratropium bromide) is not indicated for the initial treatment of acute episodes of bronchospasm where rapid response is required.

PRECAUTIONS

General: Atrovent® (ipratropium bromide) should be used with caution in patients with narrow-angle glaucoma, prostatic hypertrophy or bladder-neck obstruction.

Information for Patients: Patients should be advised that temporary blurring of vision may result if the aerosol is sprayed into the eyes.

Patients should be reminded that Atrovent is not intended for occasional use, but rather, in order to be maximally effective, must be used consistently as prescribed throughout the course of therapy.

Drug Interactions: Atrovent has been used concomitantly with other drugs, including sympathomimetic bronchodilators, methylxanthines, steroids and cromolyn sodium, commonly used in the treatment of chronic obstructive pulmonary disease, without adverse drug reactions. There are no formal studies fully evaluating the interactive effects of Atrovent and these drugs with respect to effectiveness.

Carcinogenesis, Mutagenesis, Impairment of Fertility: Two-year oral carcinogenicity studies in rats and mice have revealed no carcinogenic potential at doses up to 1,250 times the maximum recommended human daily dose for Atrovent. Results of various mutagenicity studies were negative. Fertility of male or female rats at oral doses up to approximately 10,000 times the maximum recommended human daily dose was unaffected by Atrovent administration. At doses above 18,000 times the maximum recommended human daily dose, increased resorption and decreased conception rates were observed.

Pregnancy: *TERATOGENIC EFFECTS Pregnancy Category B.* Oral reproduction studies performed in mice, rats and rabbits (at doses approximately 2,000, 200,000 and 26,000 times the maximum recommended human daily dose, respectively) and inhalation reproduction studies in rats and rabbits (at doses approximately 312 and 375 times the maximum recommended human daily dose, respectively) have demonstrated no evidence of teratogenic effects as a result of Atrovent. However, no adequate or well controlled studies have been conducted in pregnant women. Because animal reproduction studies are not always predictive of human response, Atrovent® (ipratropium bromide) should be used during pregnancy only if clearly needed.

Nursing Mothers: It is not known whether Atrovent is excreted in human milk. Although lipid-insoluble quaternary bases pass into breast milk, it is unlikely that Atrovent would reach the infant to an important extent, especially when taken by aerosol. However, because many drugs are excreted in human milk, caution should be exercised when Atrovent is administered to a nursing woman.

Pediatric Use: Safety and effectiveness in children below the age of 12 have not been established.

ADVERSE REACTIONS

Adverse reaction information concerning Atrovent® (ipratropium bromide) is derived from 90 day controlled clinical trials (N = 254), other controlled clinical trials using recom-

Continued on next page

Boehringer Ingelheim—Cont.

mended doses of Atrovent (N = 377) and an uncontrolled study (N = 1924). Additional information is derived from the foreign post-marketing experience and the published literature.

Adverse reactions occurring in greater than one percent of patients in the 90 day controlled clinical trials appear in the following table:

Reaction	Percent of Patients	
	Ipratropium bromide N = 254	Metaproterenol sulfate N = 249
Cardiovascular		
Palpitations	1.8	1.6
Central Nervous System		
Nervousness	3.1	6.8
Dizziness	2.4	2.8
Headache	2.4	2.0
Dermatological		
Rash	1.2	0.4
Gastrointestinal		
Nausea	2.8	1.2
Gastrointestinal distress	2.4	2.8
Vomiting	0	1.2
Musculoskeletal		
Tremor	0	2.4
Ophthalmological		
Blurred vision	1.2	0.8
Oro-Otolaryngeal		
Dry mouth	2.4	0.8
Irritation from aerosol	1.6	1.6
Respiratory		
Cough	5.9	1.2
Exacerbation of symptoms	2.4	3.6

Additional adverse reactions reported in less than one percent of the patients considered possibly due to Atrovent include urinary difficulty, fatigue, insomnia and hoarseness. The large uncontrolled, open-label study included seriously ill patients. About 7% of patients treated discontinued the program because of adverse events.

Of the 2301 patients treated in the large uncontrolled study and in clinical trials other than the 90-day studies, the most common adverse reactions reported were: dryness of the oropharynx, about 5 in 100; cough, exacerbation of symptoms and irritation from aerosol, each about 3 in 100; headache, about 2 in 100; nausea, dizziness, blurred vision/difficulty in accommodation, and drying of secretions, each about 1 in 100. Less frequently reported adverse reactions that were possibly due to Atrovent® (ipratropium bromide) include tachycardia, paresthesias, drowsiness, coordination difficulty, itching, hives, flushing, alopecia, constipation, tremor, mucosal ulcers.

Cases of precipitation or worsening of narrow-angle glaucoma, acute eye pain and hypotension have been reported. A case of giant urticaria with positive rechallenge has been reported from the foreign marketing experience. (See CONTRAINDICATIONS).

OVERDOSAGE

Acute overdosage by inhalation is unlikely since Atrovent® (ipratropium bromide) is not well absorbed systemically after aerosol or oral administration. The oral LD_{50} of Atrovent ranged between 1001 and 2010 mg/kg in mice; between 1667 and more than 4000 mg/kg in rats; and between 400 and 1300 mg/kg in dogs.

DOSAGE AND ADMINISTRATION

The usual starting dose of Atrovent® (ipratropium bromide) is two inhalations (36 mcg) four times a day. Patients may take additional inhalations as required; however, the total number of inhalations should not exceed 12 in 24 hours.

HOW SUPPLIED

Atrovent® (ipratropium bromide) Inhalation Aerosol is supplied as a metered dose inhaler with mouthpiece. Each 14 gram vial provides sufficient medication for 200 inhalations. NDC 0597-0082-14. Each actuation delivers 18 mcg of ipratropium bromide from the mouthpiece.
Store below 30°C (86°F); avoid excessive humidity.

CAUTION

Federal law prohibits dispensing without prescription.

AT-PI-8/88

Shown in Product Identification Section, page 405

CATAPRES®   ℞
[kah 'tah-pres]
(clonidine hydrochloride USP)
Oral Antihypertensive

Tablets, 0.1 mg ....BI-CODE 06
Tablets, 0.2 mg ....BI-CODE 07
Tablets, 0.3 mg ....BI-CODE 11

DESCRIPTION

Catapres® (clonidine hydrochloride USP) is a centrally acting antihypertensive agent available as tablets for oral administration in three dosage strengths: 0.1 mg, 0.2 mg and 0.3 mg. The 0.1 mg tablet is equivalent to 0.087 mg of the free base.

The inactive ingredients are colloidal silicon dioxide, corn starch, dibasic calcium phosphate, FD&C Yellow No. 6, gelatin, glycerin, lactose, magnesium stearate, methyl paraben, propylparaben. The Catapres 0.1 mg tablet also contains FD&C Blue No. 1 and FD&C Red No. 3.

Clonidine hydrochloride is an imidazoline derivative and exists as a mesomeric compound. The chemical name is 2-(2,6-dichlorophenylamino)-2-imidazoline hydrochloride. The following is the structural formula:

$C_9H_9Cl_2N_3 \cdot HCl$ Mol. Wt. 266.56

Clonidine hydrochloride is an odorless, bitter, white crystalline substance soluble in water and alcohol.

CLINICAL PHARMACOLOGY

Catapres® (clonidine hydrochloride USP) acts relatively rapidly. The patient's blood pressure declines within 30 to 60 minutes after an oral dose, the maximum decrease occurring within 2 to 4 hours. The plasma level of Catapres peaks in approximately 3 to 5 hours and the plasma half-life ranges from 12 to 16 hours. The half-life increases up to 41 hours in patients with severe impairment of renal function. Following oral administration about 40-60% of the absorbed dose is recovered in the urine as unchanged drug in 24 hours. About 50% of the absorbed dose is metabolized in the liver.

Clonidine stimulates alpha-adrenoreceptors in the brain stem, resulting in reduced sympathetic outflow from the central nervous system and a decrease in peripheral resistance, renal vascular resistance, heart rate, and blood pressure. Renal blood flow and glomerular filtration rate remain essentially unchanged. Normal postural reflexes are intact and therefore orthostatic symptoms are mild and infrequent.

Acute studies with clonidine hydrochloride in humans have demonstrated a moderate reduction (15% to 20%) of cardiac output in the supine position with no change in the peripheral resistance; at a 45° tilt there is a smaller reduction in cardiac output and a decrease of peripheral resistance. During long-term therapy, cardiac output tends to return to control values, while peripheral resistance remains decreased. Slowing of the pulse rate has been observed in most patients given clonidine, but the drug does not alter normal hemodynamic response to exercise.

Other studies in patients have provided evidence of a reduction in plasma renin activity and in the excretion of aldosterone and catecholamines, but the exact relationship of these pharmacologic actions to the antihypertensive effect has not been fully elucidated.

Clonidine acutely stimulates growth hormone release in both children and adults, but does not produce a chronic elevation of growth hormone with long-term use.

Tolerance may develop in some patients, necessitating a reevaluation of therapy.

INDICATIONS AND USAGE

Catapres® (clonidine hydrochloride USP) is indicated in the treatment of hypertension. Catapres may be employed alone or concomitantly with other antihypertensive agents.

CONTRAINDICATIONS

None known.

PRECAUTIONS

General In patients who have developed localized contact sensitization to Catapres-TTS® (clonidine), substitution of oral clonidine hydrochloride therapy may be associated with the development of a generalized skin rash.

In patients who develop an allergic reaction from Catapres-TTS® (clonidine) that extends beyond the local patch site (such as generalized skin rash, urticaria, or angioedema), oral clonidine hydrochloride substitution may elicit a similar reaction.

As with all antihypertensive therapy, Catapres® (clonidine hydrochloride USP) should be used with caution in patients with severe coronary insufficiency, recent myocardial infarction, cerebrovascular disease or chronic renal failure.

Withdrawal Patients should be instructed not to discontinue therapy without consulting their physician. Sudden cessation of clonidine treatment has resulted in subjective symptoms such as nervousness, agitation and headache, accompanied or followed by a rapid rise in blood pressure and elevated catecholamine concentrations in the plasma, but such occurrences have usually been associated with previous administration of high oral doses (exceeding 1.2 mg/day) and/or with continuation of concomitant beta-blocker therapy. Rare instances of hypertensive encephalopathy and death have been reported. When discontinuing therapy with Catapres, the physician should reduce the dose gradually over 2 to 4 days to avoid withdrawal symptomatology.

An excessive rise in blood pressure following Catapres discontinuance can be reversed by administration of oral clonidine or by intravenous phentolamine. If therapy is to be discontinued in patients receiving beta-blockers and clonidine concurrently, beta-blockers should be discontinued several days before the gradual withdrawal of Catapres.

Perioperative Use Administration of Catapres should be continued to within four hours of surgery and resumed as soon as possible thereafter. The blood pressure should be carefully monitored and appropriate measures instituted to control it as necessary.

Information for Patients Patients who engage in potentially hazardous activities, such as operating machinery or driving, should be advised of a potential sedative effect of clonidine. Patients should be cautioned against interruption of Catapres therapy without a physician's advice.

Drug Interactions If a patient receiving clonidine hydrochloride is also taking tricyclic antidepressants, the effect of clonidine may be reduced, thus necessitating an increase in dosage. Clonidine hydrochloride may enhance the CNS-depressive effects of alcohol, barbiturates or other sedatives. Amitriptyline in combination with clonidine enhances the manifestation of corneal lesions in rats (see Toxicology).

Carcinogenesis, Mutagenesis, Impairment of Fertility In a 132-week (fixed concentration) dietary administration study in rats, clonidine hydrochloride administered at 32 to 46 times the maximum recommended daily human dose was unassociated with evidence of carcinogenic potential. Fertility of male or female rats was unaffected by clonidine hydrochloride doses as high as 150 mcg/kg or about 3 times the maximum recommended daily human dose (MRDHD). Fertility of female rats did, however, appear to be affected (in another experiment) at dose levels of 500 to 2000 mcg/kg or 10 to 40 times the MRDHD.

Usage in Pregnancy *TERATOGENIC EFFECTS Pregnancy Category C* Reproduction studies performed in rabbits at doses up to approximately 3 times the maximum recommended daily human dose (MRDHD) of clonidine hydrochloride have revealed no evidence of teratogenic or embryotoxic potential in rabbits. In rats, however, doses as low as 1/3 the MRDHD were associated with increased resorptions in a study in which dams were treated continuously from 2 months prior to mating. Increased resorptions were not associated with treatment at the same or at higher dose levels (up to 3 times the MRDHD) when dams were treated days 6–15 of gestation. Increased resorptions were observed at much higher levels (40 times the MRDHD) in rats and mice treated days 1–14 of gestation (lowest dose employed in that study was 500 mcg/kg). There are, however, no adequate and well-controlled studies in pregnant women. Because animal reproduction studies are not always predictive of human response, this drug should be used during pregnancy only if clearly needed.

Nursing Mothers As clonidine hydrochloride is excreted in human milk, caution should be exercised when Catapres® (clonidine hydrochloride USP) is administered to a nursing woman.

Pediatric Use Safety and effectiveness in children have not been established.

ADVERSE REACTIONS

Most adverse effects are mild and tend to diminish with continued therapy. The most frequent (which appear to be dose-related) are dry mouth, occurring in about 40 of 100 patients; drowsiness, about 33 in 100; dizziness, about 16 in 100; constipation and sedation, each about 10 in 100.

The following less frequent adverse experiences have also been reported in patients receiving Catapres® (clonidine hydrochloride USP), but in many cases patients were receiving concomitant medication and a causal relationship has not been established.

Gastrointestinal Nausea and vomiting, about 5 in 100 patients; anorexia and malaise, each about 1 in 100; mild transient abnormalities in liver function tests, about 1 in 100; rare reports of hepatitis; parotitis, rarely.

Metabolic Weight gain, about 1 in 100 patients; gynecomastia, about 1 in 1000; transient elevation of blood glucose or serum creatine phosphokinase, rarely.

Central Nervous System Nervousness and agitation, about 3 in 100 patients; mental depression, about 1 in 100; headache, about 1 in 100; insomnia, about 5 in 1000. Vivid dreams or nightmares, other behavioral changes, restlessness, anxiety, visual and auditory hallucinations and delirium have been reported.

Cardiovascular Orthostatic symptoms, about 3 in 100 patients; palpitations and tachycardia, bradycardia, each about 5 in 1000. Raynaud's phenomenon, congestive heart failure, and electrocardiographic abnormalities i.e. conduction disturbances and arrhythmias have been reported rarely. Rare cases of sinus bradycardia and atrioventricular block have been reported, both with and without the use of concomitant digitalis.

Dermatological Rash, about 1 in 100 patients; pruritus, about 7 in 1000; hives, angioneurotic edema and urticaria, about 5 in 1000; alopecia, about 2 in 1000.

Genitourinary Decreased sexual activity, impotence and loss of libido, about 3 in 100 patients; nocturia, about 1 in 100; difficulty in micturition, about 2 in 1000; urinary retention, about 1 in 1000.

Other Weakness, about 10 in 100 patients; fatigue, about 4 in 100; discontinuation syndrome, about 1 in 100; muscle or joint pain, about 6 in 1000 and cramps of the lower limbs, about 3 in 1000. Dryness, burning of the eyes, blurred vision, dryness of the nasal mucosa, pallor, weakly positive Coombs' test, increased sensitivity to alcohol and fever have been reported.

OVERDOSAGE

The signs and symptoms of clonidine hydrochloride overdosage include hypotension, bradycardia, lethargy, irritability, weakness, somnolence, diminished or absent reflexes, miosis, vomiting and hypoventilation. With large overdoses, reversible cardiac conduction defects or arrhythmias, apnea, seizures and transient hypertension have been reported. The oral LD_{50} of clonidine in rats was 465 mg/kg, and in mice 206 mg/kg.

The general treatment of Catapres® (clonidine hydrochloride USP) overdosage may include intravenous fluids as indicated. Bradycardia can be treated with intravenous atropine sulfate and hypotension with dopamine infusion in addition to intravenous fluids. Hypertension, associated with overdosage, has been treated with intravenous furosemide or diazoxide or alpha-blocking agents such as phentolamine. Tolazoline, an alpha-blocker, in intravenous doses of 10 mg at 30-minute intervals, may reverse clonidine's effects if other efforts fail. Routine hemodialysis is of limited benefit, since a maximum of 5% of circulating clonidine is removed.

In a patient who ingested 100 mg clonidine hydrochloride, plasma clonidine levels were 60 ng/ml (one hour), 190 ng/ml (1.5 hours), 370 ng/ml (two hours) and 120 ng/ml (5.5 and 6.5 hours). This patient developed hypertension followed by hypotension, bradycardia, apnea, hallucinations, semicoma, and premature ventricular contractions. The patient fully recovered after intensive treatment.

DOSAGE AND ADMINISTRATION

Adults: The dose of Catapres® (clonidine hydrochloride USP) must be adjusted according to the patient's individual blood pressure response. The following is a general guide to its administration.

Initial Dose 0.1 mg tablet twice daily (morning and bedtime). Elderly patients may benefit from a lower initial dose.

Maintenance Dose Further increments of 0.1 mg per day may be made if necessary until the desired response is achieved. Taking the larger portion of the total daily dose at bedtime may minimize transient adjustment effects of dry mouth and drowsiness. The therapeutic doses most commonly employed have ranged from 0.2 mg to 0.6 mg per day given in divided doses. Studies have indicated that 2.4 mg is the maximum effective daily dose, but doses as high as this have rarely been employed.

Renal Impairment Dosage must be adjusted according to the degree of impairment, and patients should be carefully monitored. Since only a minimal amount of clonidine is removed during routine hemodialysis, there is no need to give supplemental clonidine following dialysis.

HOW SUPPLIED

Catapres® (clonidine hydrochloride USP) is supplied in tablets containing 0.1 mg, 0.2 mg or 0.3 mg of clonidine hydrochloride.

Catapres® 0.1 mg tablets are tan, oval shaped and single scored with the marking BI 6. Available in bottles of 100 (NDC 0597-0006-01) and 1000 (NDC 0597-0006-10) and unit-dose packages of 100 (NDC 0597-0006-61).

Catapres® 0.2 mg tablets are orange, oval shaped and single scored with the marking BI 7. Available in bottles of 100 (NDC 0597-0007-01) and 1000 (NDC 0597-0007-10) and unit-dose packages of 100 (NDC 0597-0007-61).

Catapres® 0.3 mg tablets are peach, oval shaped and single scored with the marking BI 11. Available in bottles of 100 (NDC 0597-0011-01).

Store below 86°F (30°C).

Dispense in tight, light-resistant container.

Caution Federal law prohibits dispensing without prescription.

TOXICOLOGY

In several studies, oral clonidine hydrochloride produced a dose-dependent increase in the incidence and severity of spontaneously occurring retinal degeneration in albino rats treated for 6 months or longer. Tissue distribution studies in dogs and monkeys revealed that clonidine hydrochloride was concentrated in the choroid of the eye. In view of the retinal degeneration observed in rats, eye examinations were performed in 908 patients prior to the start of clonidine hydrochloride therapy, who were then examined periodically thereafter. In 353 of these 908 patients, examinations were performed for periods of 24 months or longer. Except for some dryness of the eyes, no drug-related abnormal ophthalmologic findings were recorded and clonidine hydrochloride did not alter retinal function as shown by specialized tests such as the electroretinogram and macular dazzle. In rats, clonidine hydrochloride in combination with amitriptyline produced corneal lesions within 5 days.

CA-PI-4/88

Shown in Product Identification Section, page 406

CATAPRES–TTS® ℞

(clonidine)   Catapres-TTS®-1
Transdermal Therapeutic   Catapres-TTS®-2
System   Catapres-TTS®-3
                          (clonidine)
Programmed delivery *in vivo* of 0.1, 0.2 or 0.3 mg clonidine per day, for one week

PRODUCT OVERVIEW

KEY FACTS

Catapres-TTS® (clonidine) delivers a therapeutic dose of the antihypertensive clonidine through an adhesive patch applied to the skin. Each patch delivers clonidine at a constant rate for 7 days, permitting once-a-week dosing.

MAJOR USES

Catapres-TTS has been proven effective in the treatment of hypertension in controlled clinical trials. It may be used alone or with other antihypertensives.

SAFETY INFORMATION

Catapres-TTS is contraindicated in patients with known hypersensitivity to clonidine or any other component of the adhesive layer therapeutic system. As with other antihypertensive medications, patients should be instructed not to discontinue therapy without consulting their physician. Before prescribing, please consult full prescribing information below.

PRESCRIBING INFORMATION

CATAPRES–TTS® ℞

(clonidine)   Catapres-TTS®-1
Transdermal Therapeutic   Catapres-TTS®-2
System   Catapres-TTS®-3
                          (clonidine)
Programmed delivery *in vivo* of 0.1, 0.2 or 0.3 mg clonidine per day, for one week

DESCRIPTION

Catapres-TTS® (clonidine) is a transdermal system providing continuous systemic delivery of clonidine for 7 days at an approximately constant rate. Clonidine is a centrally acting alpha agonist and is an antihypertensive agent. It is an imidazoline derivative whose chemical name is 2, 6-dichloro-N-2-imidazolidinylidenebenzenamine and has the following chemical structure:

(clonidine)

System Structure and Components Catapres-TTS is a multilayered film, 0.2 mm thick, containing clonidine as the active agent. System area is 3.5, 7.0, or 10.5 cm² and the amount of drug released is directly proportional to area. (See Release Rate Concept.) The composition per unit area of all three dosages is identical.

Proceeding from the visible surface towards the surface attached to the skin, are four layers: 1) a backing layer of pigmented polyester film; 2) a drug reservoir of clonidine, mineral oil, polyisobutylene, and colloidal silicon dioxide; 3) a microporous polypropylene membrane that controls the rate of delivery of clonidine from the system to the skin surface; 4) an adhesive formulation of clonidine, mineral oil, polyisobutylene, and colloidal silicon dioxide. Prior to use, a protective peel strip of polyester that covers layer 4 is removed.

Release Rate Concept Catapres-TTS is programmed to release clonidine at an approximately constant rate for 7 days. The energy source for drug release derives from the concentration gradient existing between a saturated solu-

tion of drug in the system and the much lower concentration prevailing in the skin. Clonidine flows in the direction of the lower concentration at a constant rate, limited by the rate-controlling membrane, so long as a saturated solution is maintained in the drug reservoir.

Following system application to intact skin, clonidine in the adhesive layer saturates the skin sites below the system. Clonidine from the drug reservoir then begins to flow through the rate-controlling membrane and the adhesive layer of the system into the systemic circulation via the capillaries beneath the skin. Therapeutic plasma clonidine levels are achieved 2 to 3 days after initial application of Catapres-TTS.

The 3.5, 7.0, and 10.5 cm² systems respectively deliver 0.1, 0.2, and 0.3 mg clonidine per day. To ensure constant release of drug over 7 days, the total drug content of the system is greater than the total amount of drug delivered. Application of a new system to a fresh skin site at weekly intervals continuously maintains therapeutic plasma concentrations of clonidine. If the Catapres-TTS is removed and not replaced with a new system, therapeutic plasma clonidine levels will persist for about 8 hours and then decline slowly over several days. Over this time period, blood pressure returns gradually to pretreatment levels. If the patient experiences localized skin irritation before completing 7 days of use, the system may be removed and replaced with a new one applied on a fresh skin site.

CLINICAL PHARMACOLOGY

The plasma half-life of clonidine is 12.7 ± 7 hours. Following oral administration, about 40–60% of the absorbed dose is recovered in the urine as unchanged drug in 24 hours. About 50% of the absorbed dose is metabolized in the liver.

Clonidine stimulates alpha-adrenoreceptors in the brain stem, resulting in reduced sympathetic outflow from the central nervous system and a decrease in peripheral resistance, renal vascular resistance, heart rate, and blood pressure. Renal blood flow and glomerular filtration rate remain essentially unchanged. Normal postural reflexes are intact, and therefore orthostatic symptoms are mild and infrequent. Acute studies with clonidine hydrochloride in humans have demonstrated a moderate reduction (15% to 20%) of cardiac output in the supine position with no change in the peripheral resistance; at a 45° tilt there is a smaller reduction in cardiac output and a decrease of peripheral resistance. During long-term therapy, cardiac output tends to return to control values, while peripheral resistance remains decreased. Slowing of the pulse rate has been observed in most patients given clonidine, but the drug does not alter normal hemodynamic response to exercise.

Other studies in patients have provided evidence of a reduction in plasma renin activity and in the excretion of aldosterone and catecholamines, but the exact relationship of these pharmacologic actions to the antihypertensive effect has not been fully elucidated.

Clonidine acutely stimulates growth hormone release in both children and adults, but does not produce a chronic elevation of growth hormone with long-term use.

Tolerance may develop in some patients, necessitating a reevaluation of therapy.

INDICATIONS FOR USE

Catapres-TTS® (clonidine) is indicated in the treatment of hypertension. It may be employed alone or concomitantly with other antihypertensive agents.

CONTRAINDICATIONS

Catapres-TTS® (clonidine) should not be used in patients with known hypersensitivity to clonidine or to any other component of the adhesive layer of the therapeutic system.

PRECAUTIONS

General In patients who have developed localized contact sensitization to Catapres-TTS® (clonidine), substitution of oral clonidine hydrochloride therapy may be associated with development of a generalized skin rash.

In patients who develop an allergic reaction to Catapres-TTS that extends beyond the local patch site (such as generalized skin rash, urticaria, or angioedema) oral clonidine hydrochloride substitution may elicit a similar reaction.

As with all antihypertensive therapy, Catapres-TTS should be used with caution in patients with severe coronary insufficiency, recent myocardial infarction, cerebrovascular disease, or chronic renal failure.

Transdermal clonidine systems should be removed before attempting defibrillation or cardioversion because of the potential for altered electrical conductivity which may enhance the possibility of arcing, a phenomenon associated with the use of defibrillators.

Withdrawal Patients should be instructed not to discontinue therapy without consulting their physician. Sudden cessation of clonidine treatment has resulted in subjective symptoms such as nervousness, agitation and headache, accompanied or followed by a rapid rise in blood pressure and elevated catecholamine concentrations in the plasma,

Continued on next page

Boehringer Ingelheim—Cont.

but such occurrences have usually been associated with previous administration of high oral doses (exceeding 1.2 mg/day) and/or with continuation of concomitant beta-blocker therapy. Rare instances of hypertensive encephalopathy and death have been reported.

An excessive rise in blood pressure following Catapres-TTS discontinuance can be reversed by administration of oral clonidine or by intravenous phentolamine. If therapy is to be discontinued in patients receiving beta-blockers and clonidine concurrently, beta-blockers should be discontinued several days before cessation of Catapres-TTS administration.

Perioperative Use As with oral clonidine therapy, Catapres-TTS therapy should not be interrupted during the surgical period. Blood pressure should be carefully monitored during surgery and additional measures to control blood pressure should be available if required. Physicians considering starting Catapres-TTS therapy during the perioperative period must be aware that therapeutic plasma clonidine levels are not achieved until 2 to 3 days after initial application of Catapres-TTS (See DOSAGE AND ADMINISTRATION).

Information for Patients Patients who engage in potentially hazardous activities, such as operating machinery or driving, should be advised of a potential sedative effect of clonidine. Patients should be cautioned against interruption of Catapres-TTS therapy without a physician's advice. Patients should be advised that if the system begins to loosen from the skin after application, the adhesive overlay should be applied directly over the system to ensure good adhesion over its 7-day lifetime. Instructions for using the system are provided. Patients who develop moderate or severe erythema and/or localized vesicle formation at the site of application, or a generalized skin rash, should consult their physician promptly about the possible need to remove the patch.

Drug Interactions If a patient receiving clonidine is also taking tricyclic antidepressants, the effect of clonidine may be reduced, thus necessitating an increase in dosage. Clonidine may enhance the CNS-depressive effects of alcohol, barbiturates or other sedatives. Amitriptyline in combination with clonidine enhances the manifestation of corneal lesions in rats. (See TOXICOLOGY section.)

Carcinogenesis, Mutagenesis, Impairment of Fertility In a 132-week (fixed concentration) dietary administration study in rats, Catapres® (clonidine HCl) administered at 32 to 46 times the oral maximum recommended daily human dose (MRDHD) was unassociated with evidence of carcinogenic potential. Results from the Ames test with clonidine hydrochloride revealed no evidence of mutagenesis. Fertility of male or female rats was unaffected by clonidine doses as high as 150 mcg/kg or about 3 times the oral MRDHD. Fertility of female rats did, however, appear to be affected (in another experiment) at the dose levels of 500 to 2000 mcg/kg or 10 to 40 times the oral MRDHD.

Pregnancy *TERATOGENIC EFFECTS Pregnancy Category C* Reproduction studies performed in rabbits at doses up to approximately 3 times the oral maximum recommended daily human dose (MRDHD) of Catapres® (clonidine HCl) have revealed no evidence of teratogenic or embryotoxic potential in rabbits. In rats, however, doses as low as ⅓ the oral MRDHD of clonidine were associated with increased resorptions in a study in which dams were treated continuously from 2 months prior to mating. Increased resorptions were not associated with treatment at the same or at higher dose levels (up to 3 times the oral MRDHD) when dams were treated days 6–15 of gestation. Increased resorptions were observed at much higher levels (40 times the oral MRDHD) in rats and mice treated days 1–14 of gestation (lowest dose employed in the study was 500 mcg/kg). There are, however, no adequate and well-controlled studies in pregnant women. Because animal reproduction studies are not always predictive of human response, this drug should be used during pregnancy only if clearly needed.

Nursing Mothers As clonidine is excreted in human milk, caution should be exercised when Catapres-TTS is administered to a nursing woman.

Pediatric Use Safety and effectiveness in children below the age of twelve have not been established.

ADVERSE REACTIONS

Most systemic adverse effects during therapy with Catapres-TTS® (clonidine) have been mild and have tended to diminish with continued therapy. In a 3-month, multiclinic trial of Catapres-TTS in 101 hypertensive patients, the most frequent systemic reactions were dry mouth (25 patients) and drowsiness (12 patients).

Transient localized skin reactions, primarily localized pruritus, occurred in 51 patients. Twenty-six patients experienced localized erythema. This erythema and pruritus were more common in patients utilizing an adhesive overlay for the entire 7-day treatment period. Allergic contact sensitization to Catapres-TTS was observed in 5 patients.

In additional clinical experience contact dermatitis resulting in treatment discontinuation was observed in 128 of 673 patients (about 19 in 100) after a mean duration of treatment of 37 weeks. The incidence in white females was about 34 in 100; in white males about 18 in 100; in black females about 14 in 100; and in black males about 8 in 100.

The following less frequent adverse experiences were also reported in patients involved in this multiclinic trial with Catapres-TTS.

Gastrointestinal Constipation (1 patient); nausea (1); and change in taste (1).

Central Nervous System Fatigue (6 patients); headache (5); lethargy (3); sedation (3); insomnia (2); dizziness (2); and nervousness (1).

Genitourinary Impotence/sexual dysfunction (2 patients).

Dermatological Localized vesiculation (7 patients); hyperpigmentation (5); edema (3); excoriation (3); burning (3); papules (1); throbbing (1); blanching (1); and generalized macular rash (1).

In additional clinical experience involving 3539 patients, less common dermatologic reactions have occurred, where a causal relationship to Catapres-TTS was not established: maculopapular skin rash (10 cases); urticaria (2 cases); angioedema involving the face (2 cases), one of which also involved the tongue.

Oro-otolaryngeal Dry throat (2 patients).

In long experience with oral Catapres, the most common adverse reactions have been dry mouth (about 40%), drowsiness (about 35%) and sedation (about 8%). In addition, the following adverse reactions have been reported less frequently:

Gastrointestinal Nausea and vomiting, about 5 in 100 patients; anorexia and malaise, each about 1 in 100; mild transient abnormalities in liver function tests, about 1 in 100; rare reports of hepatitis; parotitis, rarely.

Metabolic Weight gain, about 1 in 100 patients; gynecomastia, about 1 in 1000; transient elevation of blood glucose or serum creatine phosphokinase, rarely.

Central Nervous System Nervousness and agitation, about 3 in 100 patients; mental depression, about 1 in 100 and insomnia, about 5 in 1000. Vivid dreams or nightmares, other behavioral changes, restlessness, anxiety, visual and auditory hallucinations and delirium have been reported.

Cardiovascular Orthostatic symptoms, about 3 in 100 patients; palpitations and tachycardia, and bradycardia, each about 5 in 1000. Raynaud's phenomenon, congestive heart failure, and electrocardiographic abnormalities (i.e. conduction disturbances and arrythmias) have been reported rarely. Rare cases of sinus bradycardia and atrioventricular block have been reported, both with and without the use of concomitant digitalis.

Dermatological Rash, about 1 in 100 patients; pruritus, about 7 in 1000; hives, angioneurotic edema and urticaria, about 5 in 1000; alopecia, about 2 in 1000.

Genitourinary Decreased sexual activity, impotence and loss of libido, about 3 in 100 patients; nocturia, about 1 in 100; difficulty in micturition, about 2 in 1000; urinary retention, about 1 in 1000.

Other Weakness, about 10 in 100 patients; fatigue, about 4 in 100; headache, and discontinuation syndrome, each about 1 in 100; muscle or joint pain, about 6 in 1000 and cramps of the lower limbs, about 3 in 1000. Dryness, burning of the eyes, blurred vision, dryness of the nasal mucosa, pallor, weakly positive Coombs' test, increased sensitivity to alcohol and fever have been reported.

OVERDOSAGE

If symptoms of overdosage occur, remove all Catapres-TTS® (clonidine) systems. The signs and symptoms of clonidine overdosage include hypotension, bradycardia, lethargy, irritability, weakness, somnolence, diminished or absent reflexes, miosis, vomiting and hypoventilation. With large overdoses, reversible cardiac conduction defects or arrhythmias, apnea, seizures and transient hypertension have been reported. The oral LD$_{50}$ of clonidine in rats was 465 mg/kg, and in mice 206 mg/kg.

The general treatment of Catapres-TTS overdosage may include intravenous fluids as indicated. Bradycardia can be treated with intravenous atropine sulfate and hypotension with dopamine infusion in addition to intravenous fluids. Hypertension associated with overdosage has been treated with intravenous furosemide or diazoxide or alpha-blocking

agents such as phentolamine. Tolazoline, an alpha-blocker, in intravenous doses of 10 mg at 30-minute intervals, may reverse clonidine's effects if other efforts fail. Routine hemodialysis is of limited benefit, since a maximum of 5% of circulating clonidine is removed.

In a patient who ingested 100 mg clonidine hydrochloride, plasma clonidine levels were 60 ng/ml (1 hour), 190 ng/ml (1.5 hours), 370 ng/ml (2 hours) and 120 ng/ml (5.5 and 6.5 hours). This patient developed hypertension followed by hypotension, bradycardia, apnea, hallucinations, semicoma, and premature ventricular contractions. The patient fully recovered after intensive treatment.

DOSAGE AND ADMINISTRATION

Apply Catapres-TTS® (clonidine) to a hairless area of intact skin on the upper arm or torso, once every 7 days. Each new application of Catapres-TTS should be on a different skin site from the previous location. If the system loosens during 7-day wearing, the adhesive overlay should be applied directly over the system to ensure good adhesion.

To initiate therapy, Catapres-TTS dosage should be titrated according to individual therapeutic requirements, starting with Catapres-TTS-1. If after one or two weeks the desired reduction in blood pressure is not achieved, increase the dosage by adding an additional Catapres-TTS-1 or changing to a larger system. An increase in dosage above two Catapres-TTS-3 is usually not associated with additional efficacy.

When substituting Catapres-TTS in patients on prior antihypertensive therapy, physicians should be aware that the antihypertensive effect of Catapres-TTS may not commence until 2 to 3 days after initial application. Therefore, gradual reduction of prior drug dosage is advised. Some or all previous antihypertensive treatment may have to be continued, particularly in patients with more severe forms of hypertension.

HOW SUPPLIED

Catapres-TTS®-1 (clonidine) and Catapres-TTS-2 are supplied as 4 pouched systems and 4 adhesive overlays per carton, 3 cartons per shipper (NDC 0597-0031-12 and 0597-0032-12, respectively). Catapres-TTS-3 is supplied as 4 pouched systems and 4 adhesive overlays per carton (NDC 0597-0033-34).

See chart below left.

Storage and Handling: Store below 86°F (30°C).

Caution: Federal law prohibits dispensing without prescription.

TOXICOLOGY

In several studies, oral clonidine hydrochloride produced a dose-dependent increase in the incidence and severity of spontaneously occurring retinal degeneration in albino rats treated for six months or longer. Tissue distribution studies in dogs and monkeys revealed that clonidine hydrochloride was concentrated in the choroid of the eye. In view of the retinal degeneration observed in rats, eye examinations were performed in 908 patients prior to the start of clonidine hydrochloride therapy, who were then examined periodically thereafter. In 353 of these 908 patients, examinations were performed for periods of 24 months or longer. Except for some dryness of the eyes, no drug-related abnormal ophthalmologic findings were recorded and clonidine hydrochloride did not alter retinal function as shown by specialized tests such as the electroretinogram and macular dazzle.

In rats, clonidine hydrochloride in combination with amitriptyline produced corneal lesions within 5 days.

CT-PI-7/88

Shown in Product Identification Section, page 406

COMBIPRES®   ℞

[kom 'be-pres]

Each tablet contains:
clonidine hydrochloride USP,
0.1 mg or 0.2 mg or 0.3 mg
and chlorthalidone USP, 15 mg
Oral Antihypertensive

Tablets 0.1	**BI-CODE 08**
Tablets 0.2	**BI-CODE 09**
Tablets 0.3	**BI-CODE 10**

WARNING

This fixed combination drug is not indicated for initial therapy of hypertension. Hypertension requires therapy titrated to the individual patient. If the fixed combination represents the dosage so determined, its use may be more convenient in patient management. The treatment of hypertension is not static, but must be reevaluated as conditions in each patient warrant.

DESCRIPTION

Combipres® is a combination of clonidine hydrochloride and chlorthalidone. Clonidine hydrochloride, an antihypertensive agent, is an imidazoline derivative and exists as a

	Programmed Delivery Clonidine *in vivo* Per Day Over 1 Week	Clonidine Content	Size	Code
Catapres-TTS®-1 (clonidine)	0.1 mg	2.5 mg	3.5 cm^2	BI-31
Catapres-TTS®-2 (clonidine)	0.2 mg	5.0 mg	7.0 cm^2	BI-32
Catapres-TTS®-3 (clonidine)	0.3 mg	7.5 mg	10.5 cm^2	BI-33

mesomeric compound. The chemical name for clonidine hydrochloride is 2-(2,6-dichlorophenylamino)-2-imidazoline hydrochloride, and its structural formula is:

clonidine hydrochloride

It is an odorless, bitter, white crystalline substance soluble in water and alcohol, with a molecular weight of 266.57. The 0.1 mg tablet is equivalent to 0.087 mg of the free base. Chlorthalidone is 2-chloro-5-(1-hydroxy-3-oxo-1-isoindolinyl) benzenesulfonamide, and has the following structural formula:

chlorthalidone

Chlorthalidone is an oral diuretic agent indicated for the treatment of edema and hypertension. The drug has a prolonged action. It differs from other sulfonamide diuretics in that a double ring system is incorporated in its chemical structure.

ACTIONS

Combipres®:

Combipres produces a more pronounced antihypertensive response than occurs after either clonidine hydrochloride or chlorthalidone alone in equivalent doses.

Clonidine hydrochloride:

Clonidine hydrochloride is an antihypertensive agent whose mechanism of action appears to be central alpha-adrenergic stimulation as demonstrated in animal studies. This results in the inhibition of bulbar sympathetic cardioaccelerator and sympathetic vasoconstrictor centers, thereby causing a decrease in sympathetic outflow from the brain. Initially, clonidine hydrochloride stimulates peripheral alpha-adrenergic receptors producing transient vasoconstriction.

Clonidine hydrochloride acts relatively rapidly. The patient's blood pressure declines within 30 to 60 minutes after an oral dose, the maximum decrease occurring within 2 to 4 hours. The antihypertensive effect in humans lasts approximately 6 to 8 hours. The peak plasma level of clonidine hydrochloride occurs in approximately 3 to 5 hours with a plasma half-life of 12 to 16 hours. Clonidine hydrochloride and its metabolites are excreted mainly in the urine. When labeled drug was administered, unchanged drug appearing in the urine accounted for about 32 percent of administered radioactivity.

Orthostatic effects are mild and infrequent since supine pressure is reduced to essentially the same extent as standing pressure. Clonidine hydrochloride does not alter normal hemodynamic responses to exercise. Acute studies with clonidine hydrochloride in humans have demonstrated a moderate reduction (15 to 20%) of cardiac output in the supine position with no change in the peripheral resistance, while at a 45° tilt there is a smaller reduction in cardiac output and a decrease of peripheral resistance. Renal blood flow and the glomerular filtration rate remain essentially unchanged. During long-term therapy, cardiac output tends to return to control values while peripheral resistance remains decreased. Slowing of the pulse rate has been observed in most patients given clonidine hydrochloride.

Other studies in humans have provided evidence of a reduction in plasma renin activity and in the excretion of aldosterone and catecholamines in patients treated with clonidine hydrochloride.

The exact relationship between these pharmacologic actions of clonidine hydrochloride in humans and its antihypertensive effect in individual patients has not been fully elucidated at this time.

Clonidine hydrochloride has been administered together with hydralazine, guanethidine, methyldopa, reserpine, spironolactone, furosemide, chlorthalidone and thiazide diuretics without drug-to-drug interactions.

Chlorthalidone:

The diuretic action of chlorthalidone is thought to be due to inhibition of sodium and chloride reabsorption in the proximal tubule. It has been suggested that the initial antihypertensive action of the drug is due to a reduction of plasma volume.

INDICATION

Combipres® is indicated in the treatment of hypertension (see box warning).

CONTRAINDICATIONS

Combipres® is contraindicated in patients with known hypersensitivity to chlorthalidone and in patients with severe renal or hepatic diseases.

WARNINGS

Tolerance may develop in some patients treated with Combipres.® When this occurs therapy should be reevaluated.

USE IN PREGNANCY

No teratogenic changes have been observed following concomitant administration of chlorthalidone and clonidine hydrochloride to pregnant rats in doses up to 0.128 mg/kg of clonidine hydrochloride and 32 mg/kg of chlorthalidone. However, when animals were given clonidine hydrochloride alone in doses as low as 0.015 mg/kg (one-third the maximum recommended dose) some embryotoxicity was evident. In view of these findings and since information on possible adverse effects in pregnant women is limited to uncontrolled clinical data, Combipres is not recommended in women who are or may become pregnant, unless the potential benefit outweighs the potential risk to mother and infant.

USE IN CHILDREN

No clinical experience is available with the use of Combipres® in children. Studies are being performed with clonidine hydrochloride to evaluate its use in the treatment of hypertension in children.

PRECAUTIONS

General:

In patients who have developed localized contact sensitization to Catapres-TTS® (clonidine), substitution of oral clonidine hydrochloride therapy may be associated with development of a generalized skin rash.

In patients who develop an allergic reaction to Catapres-TTS that extends beyond the local patch site (such as generalized skin rash, urticaria, or angioedema), oral clonidine hydrochloride substitution may elicit a similar reaction.

Clonidine hydrochloride:

WITHDRAWAL

Patients should be instructed not to discontinue therapy without consulting their physician. Sudden cessation of clonidine treatment has resulted in subjective symptoms such as nervousness, agitation and headache, accompanied or followed by a rapid rise in blood pressure and elevated catecholamine concentrations in the plasma, but such occurrences have usually been associated with previous administration of high oral doses (exceeding 1.2 mg/day) and/or with continuation of concomitant beta-blocker therapy. Rare instances of hypertensive encephalopathy and death have been reported. When discontinuing therapy with oral clonidine, the physician should reduce the dose gradually over 2 to 4 days to avoid withdrawal symptomatology.

An excessive rise in blood pressure following oral clonidine discontinuation can be reversed by administration of oral clonidine or by intravenous phentolamine. If therapy is to be discontinued in patients receiving beta-blockers and clonidine concurrently, beta-blockers should be discontinued several days before the gradual withdrawal of oral clonidine. Patients who engage in potentially hazardous activities, such as operating machinery or driving, should be advised of the sedative effect of the clonidine hydrochloride component. Like any other antihypertensive agent, Combipres should be used with caution in patients with severe coronary insufficiency, recent myocardial infarction, cerebrovascular disease or chronic renal failure.

As an integral part of their overall long-term care, patients treated with Combipres should receive periodic eye examinations (see Toxicology).

DRUG INTERACTIONS

If a patient receiving clonidine hydrochloride is also taking tricyclic antidepressants, the effect of clonidine may be reduced, thus necessitating an increase in dosage. Clonidine hydrochloride may enhance the CNS-depressive effects of alcohol, barbiturates or other sedatives. Amitriptyline in combination with clonidine enhances the manifestation of corneal lesions in rats (see Toxicology).

Chlorthalidone:

Patients predisposed toward or affected by diabetes should be tested periodically while receiving Combipres, because of the hyperglycemic effect of chlorthalidone.

Because of the possibility of progression of renal failure, periodic determination of the BUN is indicated. If, in the physician's opinion, a rising BUN is significant, the drug should be stopped.

The chlorthalidone component of Combipres may lead to sodium and/or potassium depletion. Muscular weakness, muscle cramps, anorexia, nausea, vomiting, constipation, lethargy or mental confusion may occur. Severe dietary salt restriction is not recommended in patients receiving Combipres.

Periodic determinations of the serum potassium level will aid the physician in the detection of hypokalemia. Extra care should be given to detection of hypokalemia in patients receiving adrenal corticosteroids, ACTH or digitalis. Hypochlo-

remic alkalosis often precedes other evidences of severe potassium deficiency. Frequently, therefore, more sensitive indicators than the potassium serum level are the serum bicarbonate and chloride concentrations. Also indicative of potassium depletion can be electrocardiographic alterations such as changes in conduction time, reduction in amplitude of the T wave, ST segment depression, prominent U wave. These abnormalities may appear with potassium depletion before the serum level of potassium decreases. To lessen the possibility of potassium deficiency, the diet, in addition to meat and vegetables, should include potassium-rich foods, such as citrus fruits and bananas. If significant potassium depletion should occur during therapy, oral potassium supplements in the form of potassium chloride (3 to 4.5 g/day), fruit juice and bananas should be given.

ADVERSE REACTIONS

Combipres® is generally well tolerated. The most common reactions associated with Combipres are dry mouth (about 40%), drowsiness (about 35%), and sedation (about 8%). Constipation, dizziness, headache and fatigue have been reported. Generally, these effects tend to diminish with continued therapy.

In addition to the reactions listed above, certain adverse reactions associated with the component drugs of Combipres are shown below.

Clonidine hydrochloride:

Gastrointestinal: Anorexia, malaise, nausea, vomiting, parotid pain, mild transient abnormalities in liver function tests. One case of possible drug-induced hepatitis without icterus or hyperbilirubinemia has been reported in a patient receiving clonidine hydrochloride, chlorthalidone and papaverine hydrochloride.

Metabolic: Weight gain, transient elevation of blood glucose or serum creatine phosphokinase, gynecomastia.

Cardiovascular: Congestive heart failure, Raynaud's phenomenon, and electrocardiographic abnormalities manifested as Wenckebach period or ventricular trigeminy. Rare cases of sinus bradycardia and atrioventricular block have been reported, both with and without the use of concomitant digitalis.

Central Nervous System: Vivid dreams or nightmares, insomnia, other behavioral changes, nervousness, restlessness, anxiety, mental depression.

Dermatologic: Rash, angioneurotic edema, hives, urticaria, thinning of the hair, pruritus not associated with a rash.

Genitourinary: Impotence, urinary retention.

Other: Increased sensitivity to alcohol, dryness, itching or burning of the eyes, dryness of the nasal mucosa, pallor or weakly positive Coombs' test.

Chlorthalidone:

Symptoms such as nausea, gastric irritation, anorexia, constipation and cramping, weakness, dizziness, transient myopia and restlessness are occasionally observed. Headache and impotence or dysuria may occur rarely. Orthostatic hypotension has been reported and may be potentiated when chlorthalidone is combined with alcohol, barbiturates or narcotics. Skin rashes, urticaria and purpura have been reported in a few instances.

A decreased glucose tolerance evidenced by hyperglycemia and glycosuria may develop inconsistently. This condition, usually reversible on discontinuation of therapy, responds to control with antidiabetic treatment. Diabetics and those predisposed should be checked regularly.

As with other diuretic agents, hypokalemia may occur (see Precautions). Hyperuricemia may be observed on occasion and acute attacks of gout have been precipitated. In cases where prolonged and significant elevation of blood uric acid concentration is considered potentially deleterious, concomitant use of a uricosuric agent is effective in reversing hyperuricemia without loss of diuretic and/or antihypertensive activity.

Idiosyncratic drug reactions such as aplastic anemia, thrombocytopenia, leukopenia, agranulocytosis and necrotizing angiitis have occurred, but are rare.

The remote possibility of pancreatitis should be considered when epigastric pain or unexplained gastrointestinal symptoms develop after prolonged administration.

Other adverse reactions which have been reported with this general class of compounds include: jaundice, xanthopsia, paresthesia and photosensitization.

DOSAGE AND ADMINISTRATION

DOSAGE: As determined by individual titration of clonidine hydrochloride and chlorthalidone (see box warning).

The following is a general guide to the administration of the individual components of Combipres®:

Clonidine hydrochloride:

Initial dose: One 0.1 mg tablet twice daily. *Maintenance dose:* Further increments of 0.1 mg or 0.2 mg per day may be made until the desired response is achieved. The therapeutic doses most commonly employed have ranged from 0.2 to 0.8 mg per day, given in divided doses. Studies have indi-

Continued on next page

Boehringer Ingelheim—Cont.

cated that 2.4 mg is the maximum effective daily dose but doses as high as this have rarely been employed.

Chlorthalidone:
The usual initial dose is 50 mg daily, which may be given in divided doses.
If the individual doses of clonidine hydrochloride and chlorthalidone determined by titration represent the dose contained in Combipres, for convenience the patient may then be given Combipres.

OVERDOSAGE

Clonidine hydrochloride:
Profound hypotension, weakness, somnolence, diminished or absent reflexes and vomiting followed the accidental ingestion of clonidine hydrochloride by several children from 19 months to 5 years of age. Gastric lavage and administration of an analeptic and vasopressor led to complete recovery within 24 hours. Tolazoline in intravenous doses of 10 mg at 30-minute intervals usually abolishes all effects of clonidine hydrochloride overdosage.

Chlorthalidone:
Symptoms of overdosage include nausea, weakness, dizziness, and disturbances of electrolyte balance. There is no specific antidote, but gastric lavage is recommended, followed by supportive treatment. Where necessary, this may include intravenous dextrose and saline with potassium, administered with caution.

TOXICOLOGY

In several studies, clonidine hydrochloride produced a dose-dependent increase in the incidence and severity of spontaneously occurring retinal degeneration in albino rats treated for 6 months or longer. Tissue distribution studies in dogs and monkeys revealed that clonidine hydrochloride was concentrated in the choroid of the eye. In view of the retinal degeneration observed in rats, eye examinations were performed in 908 patients prior to the start of clonidine hydrochloride therapy, who were then examined periodically thereafter. In 353 of these 908 patients, examinations were performed for periods of 24 months or longer. Except for some dryness of the eyes, no drug-related abnormal ophthalmologic findings were recorded and clonidine hydrochloride did not alter retinal function as shown by specialized tests such as the electroretinogram and macular dazzle.
In rats, clonidine hydrochloride in combination with amitriptyline produced corneal lesions within 5 days.

HOW SUPPLIED

Combipres® 0.1 (each tablet contains clonidine hydrochloride, 0.1 mg +chlorthalidone, 15 mg). It is available as pink, oval, single-scored compressed tablets in bottles of 100 and 1000.
Combipres® 0.2 (each tablet contains clonidine hydrochloride, 0.2 mg +chlorthalidone, 15 mg). It is available as blue, oval, single-scored compressed tablets in bottles of 100 and 1000.
Combipres® 0.3 (each tablet contains clonidine hydrochloride, 0.3 mg +chlorthalidone, 15 mg). It is available as white, oval, single-scored compressed tablets in bottles of 100.
The inactive ingredients are colloidal silicon dioxide, corn starch, dibasic calcium phosphate, gelatin, glycerin, lactose, magnesium stearate, methyl paraben, propyl paraben. Combipres 0.1 and Combipres 0.2 also contain FD&C Red No. 3 and FD&C Blue No. 1, respectively.
Store below 86°F (30°C). Avoid excessive humidity.

CAUTION

Federal law prohibits dispensing without prescription.

CM-PI-3/88

Shown in Product Identification Section, page 406

DULCOLAX®

[dul'co-lax]
(bisacodyl USP)

Tablets of 5 mg...BI-CODE 12
Suppositories of 10 mg ....BI-CODE 52

Laxative

DESCRIPTION

Dulcolax® (bisacodyl) is a contact laxative acting directly on the colonic mucosa to produce normal peristalsis throughout the large intestine. Its unique mode of action permits either oral or rectal administration, according to the requirements of the patient. Because of its gentleness and reliability of action, Dulcolax may be used whenever constipation is a problem. In preparation for surgery, proctoscopy, or radiologic examination, Dulcolax provides satisfactory cleansing of the bowel, obviating the need for an enema.
The active ingredient in Dulcolax, bisacodyl, is a colorless, tasteless compound that is practically insoluble in water and alkaline solution. It is designated chemically bis(p-acetoxyphenyl)-2-pyridyl-methane.

Tablet: Active Ingredient: bisacodyl USP 5 mg per tablet.
Also Contains: acacia, acetylated monoglyceride, carnauba wax, cellulose acetate phthalate, corn starch, D&C Red No. 30 aluminum lake, D&C Yellow No. 10 aluminum lake, dibutyl phthalate, docusate sodium, gelatin, glycerin, iron oxides, kaolin, lactose, magnesium stearate, methylparaben, pharmaceutical glaze, polyethylene glycol, povidone, propylparaben, sodium benzoate, sorbitan monooleate, sucrose, talc, titanium dioxide, white wax.
Suppository: Active Ingredient: bisacodyl USP 10 mg per suppository. **Also Contains:** hydrogenated vegetable oil.

ACTIONS

Dulcolax® (bisacodyl) differs markedly from other laxatives in its mode of action: it is virtually nontoxic, and its laxative effect occurs on contact with the colonic mucosa, where it stimulates sensory nerve endings to produce parasympathetic reflexes resulting in increased peristaltic contractions of the colon. Administered orally, Dulcolax is absorbed to a variable degree from the small bowel but such absorption is not related to the mode of action of the compound. Dulcolax administered rectally in the form of suppositories is negligibly absorbed. The contact action of the drug is restricted to the colon, and motility of the small intestine is not appreciably influenced. Local axon reflexes, as well as segmental reflexes, are initiated in the region of contact and contribute to the widespread peristaltic activity producing evacuation. For this reason, Dulcolax may often be employed satisfactorily in patients with ganglionic blockage or spinal cord damage (paraplegia, poliomyelitis, etc.).

INDICATIONS

Acute Constipation: Taken at bedtime, Dulcolax® (bisacodyl) tablets are almost invariably effective the following morning. When taken before breakfast, they usually produce an effect within six hours. For a prompter response and to replace enemas, the suppositories, which are usually effective in 15 minutes to one hour, can be used.
Chronic Constipation and Bowel Retraining: Dulcolax is extremely effective in the management of chronic constipation, particularly in older patients. By gradually lengthening the interval between doses as colonic tone improves, the drug has been found to be effective in redeveloping proper bowel hygiene. There is no tendency to "rebound."
Preparation for Radiography: Dulcolax tablets are excellent in eliminating fecal and gas shadows from x-rays taken of the abdominal area. For barium enemas, no food should be given following the administration of the tablets, to prevent reaccumulation of material in the cecum, and a suppository should be given one to two hours prior to examination.
Preoperative Preparation: Dulcolax tablets have been shown to be an ideal laxative in emptying the G.I. tract prior to abdominal surgery or to other surgery under general anesthesia. They may be supplemented by suppositories to replace the usual enema preparation. Dulcolax will not replace the colonic irrigations usually given patients before intracolonic surgery, but is useful in the preliminary emptying of the colon prior to these procedures.
Postoperative Care: Suppositories can be used to replace enemas, or tablets given as an oral laxative, to restore normal bowel hygiene after surgery.
Antepartum Care: Either tablets or suppositories can be used for constipation in pregnancy without danger of stimulating the uterus.
Preparation for Delivery: Suppositories can be used to replace enemas in the first stage of labor provided that they are given at least two hours before the onset of the second stage.
Postpartum Care: The same indications apply as in postoperative care, with no contraindication in nursing mothers.
Preparation for Sigmoidoscopy or Proctoscopy: For unscheduled office examinations, adequate preparation is usually obtained with a single suppository. For sigmoidoscopy scheduled in advance, however, administration of tablets the night before in addition will result in adequate preparation almost invariably.
Colostomies: Tablets the night before or a suppository inserted into the colostomy opening in the morning will frequently make irrigations unnecessary, and in other cases will expedite the procedure.

CONTRAINDICATION

There is no contraindication to the use of Dulcolax® (bisacodyl), other than an acute surgical abdomen.

PRECAUTION

Caution for Patients: Do not use laxative products when abdominal pain, nausea, or vomiting are present unless directed by a doctor. As with all medicines, keep these tablets/suppositories out of reach of children. Frequent or continued use of this preparation may result in dependence on laxatives.

ADVERSE REACTIONS

As with any laxative, abdominal cramps are occasionally noted, particularly in severely constipated individuals.

DOSAGE

Tablets
Tablets must be swallowed whole, not chewed or crushed, and should not be taken within one hour of antacids or milk.
Adults: Two or three (usually two) tablets suffice when an ordinary laxative effect is desired. This usually results in one or two soft, formed stools.
Up to six tablets may be safely given in preparation for special procedures when greater assurance of complete evacuation of the colon is desired. In producing such thorough emptying, these higher doses may result in several loose, unformed stools.
Children: One or two tablets, depending on age and severity of constipation, administered as above. Tablets should not be given to a child too young to swallow them whole.
Suppositories
Adults: One suppository at the time a bowel movement is required. Usually effective in 15 minutes to one hour.
Children: Half a suppository is generally effective for infants and children under two years of age. Above this age, a whole suppository is usually advisable.
Combined
In preparation for surgery, radiography and sigmoidoscopy, a combination of tablets the night before and a suppository in the morning is recommended (see Indications).

HOW SUPPLIED

Dulcolax® (bisacodyl): Yellow, enteric-coated tablets of 5 mg in boxes of 24, bottles of 100, 1000 and unit-strip packages of 100; Suppositories of 10 mg in boxes of 2, 4, 8, 50 and 500.

NOTE

Dulcolax® (bisacodyl) suppositories and tablets should be stored at temperatures below 77°F (25°C) and excessive humidity should be avoided.

CLINICAL APPLICATIONS

Dulcolax® (bisacodyl) can be used in virtually any patient in whom a laxative or enema is indicated. It has no effect on the blood picture, erythrocyte sedimentation rate, urinary findings, or hepatic or renal function. It may be safely given to infants and the aged, pregnant or nursing women, debilitated patients, and may be prescribed in the presence of such conditions as cardiovascular, renal, or hepatic diseases.

ALSO AVAILABLE

Dulcolax® (bisacodyl) Bowel Prep Kit. Each kit contains:
1 Dulcolax suppository of 10 mg bisacodyl;
4 Dulcolax tablets of 5 mg bisacodyl;
Complete patient instructions.

DU-PI-4/87

Shown in Product Identification Section, page 406

MEXITIL® ℞
(mexiletine hydrochloride)
Oral Antiarrhythmic
Capsules of 150 mg, 200 mg and 250 mg

PRODUCT OVERVIEW

KEY FACTS

Mexitil® (mexiletine hydrochloride) is an orally active Class 1B antiarrhythmic agent that is structurally similar to lidocaine. It has no significant negative inotropic effects, nor does it affect QRS or QT intervals.

MAJOR USES

Mexitil has proven to be effective in the suppression of symptomatic ventricular arrhythmias (ventricular tachycardia, couplets and PVCs) in controlled clinical trials and in long-term use.

SAFETY INFORMATION

Mexitil is contraindicated in the presence of cardiogenic shock or pre-existing second- or third-degree AV block (if no pacemaker is present). It is important to optimize response and tolerance for each patient by careful dosage titration. Although serious adverse events have occasionally been reported, the most common adverse reactions to Mexitil are reversible upper GI and CNS effects, which can often be avoided by administration with food and careful dosage titration.
Before prescribing, please consult full prescribing information below.

PRESCRIBING INFORMATION

MEXITIL® ℞
(mexiletine hydrochloride)
Oral Antiarrhythmic
Capsules of 150 mg, 200 mg and 250 mg

DESCRIPTION

Mexitil® (mexiletine hydrochloride) is an orally active antiarrhythmic agent available as 150 mg, 200 mg and 250 mg capsules. 100 mg of mexiletine hydrochloride is equivalent to 83.31 mg of mexiletine base. It is a white to off-white crystalline powder with a slightly bitter taste, freely soluble in water and in alcohol. Mexitil has a pKa of 9.2.

Chemically, Mexitil is 1-methyl-2-(2,6-xylyloxy)-ethylamine hydrochloride and has the following structural formula:
$C_{11}H_{17}NO \cdot HCl$ Mol. Wt. 215.73

mexiletine hydrochloride (Mexitil)

Mexitil Capsules contain the following inactive ingredients: colloidal silicon dioxide, corn starch, magnesium stearate, titanium dioxide, gelatin, FD&C Red No. 40 and FD&C Blue No. 1; the Mexitil 150 mg capsule also contains FD&C Yellow No. 6 and FD&C Red No. 3; the Mexitil 250 mg capsule also contains D&C Yellow No. 10 and D&C Red No. 28. Mexitil capsules may contain one or more of the following components: sodium lauryl sulfate, sodium propionate, edetate calcium disodium, benzyl alcohol, carboxymethylcellulose sodium, glycerin, butyl paraben, propyl paraben, methyl paraben, pharmaceutical glaze, ethylene glycol monoethyl ether, soya lecithin, dimethylpolysiloxane, refined shellac (food grade) and other inactive ingredients.

CLINICAL PHARMACOLOGY

Mechanism of Action Mexitil® (mexiletine hydrochloride) is a local anesthetic, antiarrhythmic agent, structurally similar to lidocaine, but orally active. In animal studies, Mexitil has been shown to be effective in the suppression of induced ventricular arrhythmias, including those induced by glycoside toxicity and coronary artery ligation. Mexitil, like lidocaine, inhibits the inward sodium current, thus reducing the rate of rise of the action potential, Phase 0. Mexitil decreased the effective refractory period (ERP) in Purkinje fibers. The decrease in ERP was of lesser magnitude than the decrease in action potential duration (APD), with a resulting increase in the ERP/APD ratio.

Electrophysiology in Man Mexiletine is a Class 1B antiarrhythmic compound with electrophysiologic properties in man similar to those of lidocaine, but dissimilar from quinidine, procainamide, and disopyramide.

In patients with normal conduction systems, Mexitil has a minimal effect on cardiac impulse generation and propagation. In clinical trials, no development of second-degree or third-degree AV block was observed. Mexitil did not prolong ventricular depolarization (QRS duration) or repolarization (QT intervals) as measured by electrocardiography. Theoretically, therefore, Mexitil may be useful in the treatment of ventricular arrhythmias associated with a prolonged QT interval.

In patients with pre-existing conduction defects, depression of the sinus rate, prolongation of sinus node recovery time, decreased conduction velocity and increased effective refractory period of the intraventricular conduction system have occasionally been observed.

The antiarrhythmic effect of Mexitil has been established in controlled comparative trials against placebo, quinidine, procainamide and disopyramide. Mexitil, at doses of 200–400 mg q8h, produced a significant reduction of ventricular premature beats, paired beats, and episodes of non-sustained ventricular tachycardia compared to placebo and was similar in effectiveness to the active agents. Among all patients entered into the studies, about 30% in each treatment group had a 70% or greater reduction in PVC count and about 40% failed to complete the three-month studies because of adverse effects. Follow-up of patients from the controlled trials has demonstrated continued effectiveness of Mexitil in long-term use.

Hemodynamics Hemodynamic studies in a limited number of patients, with normal or abnormal myocardial function, following oral administration of Mexitil, have shown small, usually not statistically significant, decreases in cardiac output and increases in systemic vascular resistance, but no significant negative inotropic effect. Blood pressure and pulse rate remain essentially unchanged. Mild depression of myocardial function, similar to that produced by lidocaine, has occasionally been observed following intravenous Mexitil therapy in patients with cardiac disease.

Pharmacokinetics Mexitil is well absorbed (~90%) from the gastrointestinal tract. Unlike lidocaine, its first-pass metabolism is low. Peak blood levels are reached in two to three hours. In normal subjects, the plasma elimination half-life of Mexitil is approximately 10–12 hours. It is 50–60% bound to plasma protein, with a volume of distribution of 5–7 liters/kg. Mexitil is metabolized in the liver. Approximately 10% is excreted unchanged by the kidney. While urinary pH does not normally have much influence on elimination, marked changes in urinary pH influence the rate of excretion: acidification accelerates excretion, while alkalinization retards it.

Several metabolites of mexiletine have shown minimal antiarrhythmic activity in animal models. The most active is the minor metabolite N-methylmexiletine, which is less than

20% as potent as mexiletine. The urinary excretion of N-methylmexiletine in man is less than 0.5%. Thus the therapeutic activity of Mexitil is due to the parent compound. Hepatic impairment prolongs the elimination half-life of Mexitil. In eight patients with moderate to severe liver disease, the mean half-life was approximately 25 hours. Consistent with the limited renal elimination of Mexitil, little change in the half-life has been detected in patients with reduced renal function. In eight patients with creatinine clearance less than 10 ml/min, the mean plasma elimination half-life was 15.7 hours; in seven patients with creatinine clearance between 11–40 ml/min, the mean half-life was 13.4 hours.

The absorption rate of Mexitil is reduced in clinical situations such as acute myocardial infarction in which gastric emptying time is increased. Narcotics, atropine and magnesium-aluminum hydroxide have also been reported to slow the absorption of Mexitil. Metoclopramide has been reported to accelerate absorption.

Mexiletine plasma levels of at least 0.5 mcg/ml are generally required for therapeutic response. An increase in the frequency of central nervous system adverse effects has been observed when plasma levels exceed 2.0 mcg/ml. Thus the therapeutic range is approximately 0.5 to 2.0 mcg/ml. Plasma levels within the therapeutic range can be attained with either three times daily or twice daily dosing but peak to trough differences are greater with the latter regimen, creating the possibility of adverse effects at peak and arrhythmic escape at trough. Nevertheless, some patients may be transferred successfully to the twice daily regimen (See DOSAGE AND ADMINISTRATION).

INDICATIONS

Mexitil® (mexiletine hydrochloride) is indicated for the suppression of symptomatic ventricular arrhythmias, including frequent premature ventricular contractions, unifocal or multifocal, couplets and ventricular tachycardia.

Like other antiarrhythmics, mexiletine has not been shown to prevent sudden death in patients with serious ventricular ectopic activity, and also, like other antiarrhythmics, it has potentially serious adverse effects, including the ability to worsen arrhythmias. It is therefore essential that each patient given mexiletine be evaluated electrocardiographically and clinically prior to and during mexiletine therapy to determine whether the response to mexiletine supports continued treatment.

CONTRAINDICATIONS

Mexitil® (mexiletine hydrochloride) is contraindicated in the presence of cardiogenic shock or pre-existing second- or third-degree AV block (if no pacemaker is present).

PRECAUTIONS

General If a ventricular pacemaker is operative, patients with second or third degree heart block may be treated with Mexitil® (mexiletine hydrochloride) if continuously monitored. A limited number of patients (45 of 475 in controlled clinical trials) with pre-existing first degree AV block were treated with Mexitil; none of these patients developed second or third degree AV block. Caution should be exercised when it is used in such patients or in patients with pre-existing sinus node dysfunction or intraventricular conduction abnormalities.

Like other antiarrhythmics Mexitil® (mexiletine hydrochloride) can cause worsening of arrhythmias. This has been uncommon in patients with less serious arrhythmias (frequent premature beats or non-sustained ventricular tachycardia: see ADVERSE REACTIONS), but is of greater concern in patients with life-threatening arrhythmias such as sustained ventricular tachycardia. In patients with such arrhythmias subjected to programmed electrical stimulation or to exercise provocation, 10–15% of patients had exacerbation of the arrhythmia, a rate not greater than that of other agents.

Mexitil should be used with caution in patients with hypotension and severe congestive heart failure.

Since Mexitil is metabolized in the liver, and hepatic impairment has been reported to prolong the elimination half-life of Mexitil, patients with liver disease should be followed carefully while receiving Mexitil. The same caution should be observed in patients with hepatic dysfunction secondary to congestive heart failure.

Concurrent drug therapy or dietary regimens which may markedly alter urinary pH should be avoided during Mexitil therapy. The minor fluctuations in urinary pH associated with normal diet do not affect the excretion of Mexitil.

SGOT Elevation and Liver Injury In three-month controlled trials, elevations of SGOT greater than three times the upper limit of normal occurred in about 1% of both mexiletine-treated and control patients. Approximately 2% of patients in the mexiletine compassionate use program had elevations of SGOT greater than or equal to three times the upper limit of normal. These elevations frequently occurred in association with identifiable clinical events and therapeutic measures such as congestive heart failure, acute myocardial infarction, blood transfusions and other medications. These elevations were often asymptomatic and transient, usually

not associated with elevated bilirubin levels and usually did not require discontinuation of therapy. Marked elevations of SGOT (> 1000 U/L) were seen before death in four patients with end-stage cardiac disease (severe congestive heart failure, cardiogenic shock).

In foreign marketing experience rare instances of severe liver injury, including hepatic necrosis, have been reported in association with Mexitil treatment. It is recommended that patients in whom an abnormal liver test has occurred, or who have signs or symptoms suggesting liver dysfunction, be carefully evaluated. If persistent or worsening elevation of hepatic enzymes is detected, consideration should be given to discontinuing therapy.

Blood Dyscrasias Blood dyscrasias were not seen in the controlled trials. Among 10,867 patients treated with mexiletine in the compassionate use program, marked leukopenia (neutrophils less than 1000/mm^3) or agranulocytosis were seen in 0.06%, and milder depressions of leukocytes were seen in 0.08%, and thrombocytopenia was observed in 0.16%. Many of these patients were seriously ill and receiving concomitant medications with known hematologic adverse effects. Rechallenge with mexiletine in several cases was negative. Marked leukopenia or agranulocytosis did not occur in any patient receiving Mexitil alone; five of the six cases of agranulocytosis were associated with procainamide (sustained release preparations in four) and one with vinblastine. If significant hematologic changes are observed, the patient should be carefully evaluated, and, if warranted, Mexitil should be discontinued. Blood counts usually return to normal within one month of discontinuation. (See ADVERSE REACTIONS.)

Convulsions (seizures) did not occur in Mexitil controlled clinical trials. In the compassionate use program, convulsions were reported in about 2 of 1000 patients. Twenty-eight percent of these patients discontinued therapy. Convulsions were reported in patients with and without a prior history of seizures. Mexiletine should be used with caution in patients with known seizure disorder.

Drug Interactions In a large compassionate use program Mexitil has been used concurrently with commonly employed antianginal, antihypertensive, and anticoagulant drugs without observed interactions. A variety of antiarrhythmics such as quinidine or propranolol were also added, sometimes with improved control of ventricular ectopy. When phenytoin or other hepatic enzyme inducers such as rifampin and phenobarbital have been taken concurrently with Mexitil, lowered Mexitil plasma levels have been reported. Monitoring of Mexitil plasma levels is recommended during such concurrent use to avoid ineffective therapy.

In a formal study, benzodiazepines were shown not to affect Mexitil plasma concentrations. ECG intervals (PR, QRS and QT) were not affected by concurrent Mexitil and digoxin, diuretics, or propranolol.

Concurrent administration of cimetidine and Mexitil has been reported to increase, decrease, or leave unchanged Mexitil plasma levels; therefore patients should be followed carefully during concurrent therapy.

Mexitil does not alter serum digoxin levels, but magnesium-aluminum hydroxide, when used to treat gastrointestinal symptoms due to Mexitil, has been reported to lower serum digoxin levels.

There have been isolated reports of increased plasma theophylline levels following concomitant administration of Mexitil.

Carcinogenesis, Mutagenesis and Impairment of Fertility Studies of carcinogenesis in rats (24 months) and mice (18 months) did not demonstrate any tumorigenic potential. Mexitil was found to be non-mutagenic in the Ames test. Mexitil did not impair fertility in the rat.

Pregnancy/Teratogenic Effects
PREGNANCY CATEGORY C
Reproduction studies performed with Mexitil® in rats, mice and rabbits at doses up to four times the maximum human oral dose (20 mg/kg in a 50 kg patient) revealed no evidence of teratogenicity or impaired fertility but did show an increase in fetal resorption. There are no adequate and well-controlled studies in pregnant women; this drug should be used in pregnancy only if the potential benefit justifies the potential risk to the fetus.

Nursing Mothers Mexitil appears in human milk in concentrations similar to those observed in plasma. Therefore, if the use of Mexitil is deemed essential, an alternative method of infant feeding should be considered.

Pediatric Use Safety and effectiveness in children have not been established.

ADVERSE REACTIONS

Mexitil® (mexiletine hydrochloride) commonly produces reversible gastrointestinal and nervous system adverse reactions but is otherwise well tolerated. Mexitil has been evaluated in 483 patients in one-month and three-month controlled studies and in over 10,000 patients in a large compassionate use program. Dosages in the controlled studies ranged from 600–1200 mg/day; some patients (8%) in the

Continued on next page

Boehringer Ingelheim—Cont.

compassionate use program were treated with higher daily doses (1600–3200 mg/day). In the three-month controlled trials comparing Mexitil to quinidine, procainamide and disopyramide, the most frequent adverse reactions were upper gastrointestinal distress (41%), lightheadedness (10.5%), tremor (12.6%) and coordination difficulties (10.2%). Similar frequency and incidence were observed in the one-month placebo-controlled trial. Although these reactions were generally not serious, and were dose-related and reversible with a reduction in dosage, by taking the drug with food or antacid or by therapy discontinuation, they led to therapy discontinuation in 40% of patients in the controlled trials. A tabulation of the adverse events reported in the one-month placebo-controlled trial follows:

COMPARATIVE INCIDENCE (%) OF ADVERSE EVENTS AMONG PATIENTS TREATED WITH MEXILETINE AND PLACEBO IN THE 4-WEEK, DOUBLE-BLIND CROSSOVER TRIAL

	Mexiletine N = 53	Placebo N = 49
Cardiovascular		
Palpitations	7.5	10.2
Chest Pain	7.5	4.1
Increased Ventricular Arrhythmias/PVC's	1.9	—
Digestive		
Nausea/Vomiting/Heartburn	39.6	6.1
Central Nervous System		
Dizziness/Lightheadedness	26.4	14.3
Tremor	13.2	—
Nervousness	11.3	6.1
Coordination Difficulties	9.4	—
Changes in Sleep Habits	7.5	16.3
Paresthesias/Numbness	3.8	2.0
Weakness	1.9	4.1
Fatigue	1.9	2.0
Tinnitus	1.9	4.1
Confusion/Clouded Sensorium	1.9	2.0
Other		
Headache	7.5	6.1
Blurred Vision/Visual Disturbances	7.5	2.0
Dyspnea/Respiratory	5.7	10.2
Rash	3.8	2.0
Non-specific Edema	3.8	—

A tabulation of adverse reactions occurring in one percent or more of patients in the three-month controlled studies follows:

[See table below].

Less than 1%: Syncope, edema, hot flashes, hypertension, short-term memory loss, loss of consciousness, other psychological changes, diaphoresis, urinary hesitancy/retention, malaise, impotence/decreased libido, pharyngitis.

In postmarketing experience, there have been isolated, spontaneous reports of pulmonary changes including pulmonary fibrosis during Mexitil therapy in association with other drugs or diseases that are known to produce pulmonary toxicity.

A causal relationship to Mexitil therapy has not been established.

An additional group of over 10,000 patients has been treated in a program allowing administration of Mexitil® (mexiletine hydrochloride) under compassionate use circumstances. These patients were seriously ill with the large majority on multiple drug therapy. Twenty-four percent of the patients continued in the program for one year or longer. Adverse reactions leading to therapy discontinuation occurred in 15 percent of patients (usually upper gastrointestinal system or nervous system effects). In general, the more common adverse reactions were similar to those in the controlled trials. Less common adverse events possibly related to Mexitil use include:

Cardiovascular System: Syncope and hypotension, each about 6 in 1000; bradycardia, about 4 in 1000; angina/angina-like pain, about 3 in 1000; edema, atrioventricular block/conduction disturbances and hot flashes, each about 2 in 1000; atrial arrhythmias, hypertension and cardiogenic shock, each about 1 in 1000.

Central Nervous System: Short-term memory loss, about 9 in 1000 patients; hallucinations and other psychological changes, each about 3 in 1000; psychosis and convulsions/seizures, each about 2 in 1000; loss of consciousness, about 6 in 10,000.

Digestive: Dysphagia, about 2 in 1000; peptic ulcer, about 8 in 10,000; upper gastrointestinal bleeding, about 7 in 10,000; esophageal ulceration, about 1 in 10,000.

Laboratory: Abnormal liver function tests, about 5 in 1000 patients; positive ANA and thrombocytopenia, each about 2 in 1000; leukopenia (including neutropenia and agranulocytosis), about 1 in 1000; myelofibrosis, about 2 in 10,000 patients.

Other: Diaphoresis, about 6 in 1000; altered taste, about 5 in 1000; salivary changes, hair loss and impotence/decreased libido, each about 4 in 1000; malaise, about 3 in 1000; urinary hesitancy/retention, each about 2 in 1000; hiccups, dry skin, laryngeal and pharyngeal changes and changes in oral mucous membranes, each about 1 in 1000; SLE syndrome, about 4 in 10,000.

Hematology: Blood dyscrasias were not seen in the controlled trials but did occur among the 10,867 patients treated with mexiletine in the compassionate use program (see PRECAUTIONS).

Myelofibrosis was reported in two patients in the compassionate use program: one was receiving long-term thiotepa therapy and the other had pretreatment myeloid abnormalities.

OVERDOSAGE

Nine cases of Mexitil® (mexiletine hydrochloride) overdosage have been reported; two were fatal. In one fatality, 4400 mg of the drug was ingested. In the other death, the dose ingested was unknown. There has been a report of non-fatal ingestion of 8000 mg. Symptoms associated with overdosage include nausea, hypotension, sinus bradycardia, paresthesia seizures, intermittent left bundle branch block and temporary asystole.

There is no specific antidote for Mexitil. Acidification of the urine, which will accelerate the excretion of mexiletine, may be useful. Treatment of overdosage should be supportive, and may include the administration of atropine if hypotension or bradycardia occurs.

DOSAGE AND ADMINISTRATION

The dosage of Mexitil® (mexiletine hydrochloride) must be individualized on the basis of response and tolerance, both of which are dose-related. Administration with food or antacid is recommended. Initiate Mexitil therapy with 200 mg every eight hours when rapid control of arrhythmia is not essential. A minimum of two to three days between dose adjustments is recommended. Dose may be adjusted in 50 or 100 mg increments up or down.

As with any antiarrhythmic drug, clinical and electrocardiographic evaluation (including Holter monitoring if necessary for evaluation) are needed to determine whether the desired antiarrhythmic effect has been obtained and to guide titration and dose adjustment.

Satisfactory control can be achieved in most patients by 200 to 300 mg given every eight hours with food or antacid. If satisfactory response has not been achieved at 300 mg q8h, and the patient tolerates Mexitil well, a dose of 400 mg q8h may be tried. As the severity of CNS side effects increases with total daily dose, the dose should not exceed 1200 mg/day.

In general, patients with renal failure will require the usual doses of Mexitil. Patients with severe liver disease, however, may require lower doses and must be monitored closely. Similarly, marked right-sided congestive heart failure can reduce hepatic metabolism and reduce the needed dose. Plasma level may also be affected by certain concomitant drugs (see PRECAUTIONS: Drug Interactions).

Loading Dose: When rapid control of ventricular arrhythmia is essential, an initial loading dose of 400 mg of Mexitil may be administered, followed by a 200 mg dose in eight hours. Onset of therapeutic effect is usually observed within 30 minutes to two hours.

Q12H Dosage Schedule: Some patients responding to Mexitil may be transferred to a 12-hour dosage schedule to improve convenience and compliance. If adequate suppression is achieved on a Mexitil dose of 300 mg or less every eight hours, the same total daily dose may be given in divided doses every 12 hours while carefully monitoring the degree of suppression of ventricular ectopy. This dose may be adjusted up to a maximum of 450 mg every 12 hours to achieve the desired response.

Transferring to Mexitil: The following dosage schedule, based on theoretical considerations rather than experimental data, is suggested for transferring patients from other Class I oral antiarrhythmic agents to Mexitil: Mexitil treatment may be initiated with a 200 mg dose, and titrated to response as described above, 6–12 hours after the last dose of quinidine sulfate, 3–6 hours after the last dose of procainamide, 6–12 hours after the last dose of disopyramide or 8–12 hours after the last dose of tocainide.

In patients in whom withdrawal of the previous antiarrhythmic agent is likely to produce life-threatening arrhythmias, hospitalization of the patient is recommended.

When transferring from lidocaine to Mexitil, the lidocaine infusion should be stopped when the first oral dose of Mexitil is administered. The infusion line should be left open until suppression of the arrhythmia appears to be satisfactorily maintained. Consideration should be given to the similarity of the adverse effects of lidocaine and Mexitil and the possibility that they may be additive.

HOW SUPPLIED

Mexitil® (mexiletine hydrochloride) is supplied in hard gelatin capsules containing 150 mg, 200 mg or 250 mg of mexiletine hydrochloride:

Mexitil® 150 mg capsules are red and caramel with the marking BI 66. Available in bottles of 100 (NDC 0597-0066-01) and individually blister-sealed unit-dose cartons of 100 (NDC 0597-0066-61).

COMPARATIVE INCIDENCE (%) OF ADVERSE EVENTS AMONG PATIENTS TREATED WITH MEXILETINE OR CONTROL DRUGS IN THE 12-WEEK DOUBLE-BLIND TRIALS

	Mexiletine N = 430	Quinidine N = 262	Procainamide N = 78	Disopyramide N = 69
Cardiovascular				
Palpitations	4.3	4.6	1.3	5.8
Chest Pain	2.6	3.4	1.3	2.9
Angina/Angina-like Pain	1.7	1.9	2.6	2.9
Increased Ventricular Arrhythmias/PVC's	1.0	2.7	2.6	—
Digestive				
Nausea/Vomiting/Heartburn	39.3	21.4	33.3	14.5
Diarrhea	5.2	33.2	2.6	8.7
Constipation	4.0	—	6.4	11.6
Changes in Appetite	2.6	1.9	—	—
Abdominal Pain/Cramps/Discomfort	1.2	1.5	—	1.4
Central Nervous System				
Dizziness/Lightheadedness	18.9	14.1	14.1	2.9
Tremor	13.2	2.3	3.8	1.4
Coordination Difficulties	9.7	1.1	1.3	—
Changes in Sleep Habits	7.1	2.7	11.5	8.7
Weakness	5.0	5.3	7.7	2.9
Nervousness	5.0	1.9	6.4	5.8
Fatigue	3.8	5.7	5.1	1.4
Speech Difficulties	2.6	0.4	—	—
Confusion/Clouded Sensorium	2.6	—	3.8	—
Paresthesias/Numbness	2.4	2.3	2.6	—
Tinnitus	2.4	1.5	—	—
Depression	2.4	1.1	1.3	1.4
Other				
Blurred Vision/Visual Disturbances	5.7	3.1	5.1	7.2
Headache	5.7	6.9	7.7	4.3
Rash	4.2	3.8	10.3	1.4
Dyspnea/Respiratory	3.3	3.1	5.1	2.9
Dry Mouth	2.8	1.9	5.1	14.5
Arthralgia	1.7	2.3	5.1	1.4
Fever	1.2	3.1	2.6	—

Mexitil® 200 mg capsules are red with the marking BI 67. Available in bottles of 100 (NDC 0597-0067-01) and individually blister-sealed unit-dose cartons of 100 (NDC 0597-0067-61).

Mexitil® 250 mg capsules are red and aqua green with the marking BI 68. Available in bottles of 100 (NDC 0597-0068-01) and individually blister-sealed unit-dose cartons of 100 (NDC 0597-0068-61).

Store below 86°F (30°C).

Caution: Federal law prohibits dispensing without prescription.

ME-PI-10/88

Shown in Product Indentification Section, page 406

PERSANTINE®   ℞

[per-san 'tēn]
(dipyridamole USP)

Tablets of 25 mg	BI-CODE 17
Tablets of 50 mg	BI-CODE 18
Tablets of 75 mg	BI-CODE 19

DESCRIPTION

Persantine® (dipyridamole USP) is a platelet inhibitor chemically described as 2,6-bis(diethanol-amino)-4,8-dipiperidino-pyrimido-(5,4-d) pyrimidine. It has the following structural formula:

$C_{24}H_{40}N_8O_4$ Mol. Wt. 504.63

Dipyridamole is an odorless yellow crystalline powder, having a bitter taste. It is soluble in dilute acids, methanol and chloroform, and practically insoluble in water.

Persantine tablets for oral administration contain:

Active Ingredient: *TABLETS 25, 50 and 75 mg:* dipyridamole USP 25, 50 and 75 mg respectively.

Inactive Ingredients: *TABLET 25 mg:* acacia, carnauba wax, corn starch, FD&C blue No. 1 aluminum lake, FD&C red No. 3 aluminum lake, FD&C yellow No. 6 aluminum lake, lactose, magnesium stearate, polyethylene glycol, povidone, shellac, sodium benzoate, sucrose, talc, titanium dioxide, white wax.

TABLETS 50 and 75 mg: acacia, carnauba wax, corn starch, FD&C blue No. 1 aluminum lake, FD&C yellow No. 6, lactose, magnesium stearate, polyethylene glycol, povidone, shellac, sucrose, talc, titanium dioxide, white wax.

CLINICAL PHARMACOLOGY

It is believed that platelet reactivity and interaction with prosthetic cardiac valve surfaces, resulting in abnormally shortened platelet survival time, is a significant factor in thromboembolic complications occurring in connection with prosthetic heart valve replacement.

Persantine® (dipyridamole USP) has been found to lengthen abnormally shortened platelet survival time in a dose-dependent manner.

In three randomized controlled clinical trials involving 854 patients who had undergone surgical placement of a prosthetic heart valve, Persantine, in combination with warfarin, decreased the incidence of postoperative thromboembolic events by 62% to 91% compared to warfarin treatment alone. The incidence of thromboembolic events in patients receiving the combination of Persantine and warfarin ranged from 1.2% to 1.8%. In three additional studies involving 392 patients taking Persantine and coumarin-like anticoagulants, the incidence of thromboembolic events ranged from 2.3% to 6.9%.

In these trials, the coumarin anticoagulant was begun between 24 hours and 4 days postoperatively, and the Persantine was begun between 24 hours and 10 days postoperatively. The length of follow-up in these trials varied from 1 to 2 years.

Persantine does not influence prothrombin time or activity measurements when administered with warfarin.

Mechanism of Action: Persantine is a platelet adhesion inhibitor, although the mechanism of action has not been fully elucidated. The mechanism may relate to inhibition of red blood cell uptake of adenosine, itself an inhibitor of platelet reactivity, phosphodiesterase inhibition leading to increased cyclic-3', 5'-adenosine monophosphate within platelets, and inhibition of thromboxane A_2 formation, which is a potent stimulator of platelet activation.

Hemodynamics: In dogs intraduodenal doses of Persantine of 0.5 to 4.0 mg/kg produced dose-related decreases in systemic and coronary vascular resistance leading to decreases in systemic blood pressure and increases in coronary blood flow. Onset of action was in about 24 minutes and effects persisted for about 3 hours.

Similar effects were observed following IV Persantine in doses ranging from 0.025 to 2.0 mg/kg.

In man the same qualitative hemodynamic effects have been observed. However, acute intravenous administration of Persantine may worsen regional myocardial perfusion distal to partial occlusion of coronary arteries.

Pharmacokinetics and Metabolism: Following an oral dose of Persantine, the average time to peak concentration is about 75 minutes. The decline in plasma concentration following a dose of Persantine fits a two-compartment model. The alpha half-life (the initial decline following peak concentration) is approximately 40 minutes. The beta half-life (the terminal decline in plasma concentration) is approximately 10 hours. Persantine is highly bound to plasma proteins. It is metabolized in the liver where it is conjugated as a glucuronide and excreted with the bile.

INDICATIONS AND USAGE

Persantine® (dipyridamole USP) is indicated as an adjunct to coumarin anticoagulants in the prevention of postoperative thromboembolic complications of cardiac valve replacement.

CONTRAINDICATIONS

None known.

PRECAUTIONS

General: Persantine® (dipyridamole USP) should be used with caution in patients with hypotension since it can produce peripheral vasodilation.

Carcinogenesis, Mutagenesis, Impairment of Fertility: In a 111 week oral study in mice and in a 128-142 week oral study in rats, Persantine produced no significant carcinogenic effects at doses of 8, 25 and 75 mg/kg (1, 3.1 and 9.4 times the maximum recommended daily human dose). Mutagenicity testing with Persantine was negative. Reproduction studies with Persantine revealed no evidence of impaired fertility in rats at doses up to 60 times the maximum recommended human dose. A significant reduction in number of corpora lutea with consequent reduction in implantations and live fetuses was, however, observed at 155 times the maximum recommended human dose.

Teratogenic Effects: *PREGNANCY CATEGORY B* Reproduction studies have been performed in mice and rats at doses up to 125 mg/kg (15.6 times the maximum recommended daily human dose) and rabbits at doses up to 20 mg/kg and have revealed no evidence of harm to the fetus due to Persantine. There are, however, no adequate and well-controlled studies in pregnant women. Because animal reproduction studies are not always predictive of human response, this drug should be used during pregnancy only if clearly needed.

Nursing Mothers: As dipyridamole is excreted in human milk, caution should be exercised when Persantine is administered to a nursing woman.

Pediatric Use: Safety and effectiveness in children below the age of 12 years has not been established.

ADVERSE REACTIONS

Adverse reactions at therapeutic doses are usually minimal and transient. On long-term use of Persantine® (dipyridamole USP) initial side effects usually disappear. The following reactions were reported in two heart valve replacement trials comparing Persantine and warfarin therapy to either warfarin alone or warfarin and placebo:

	Persantine/ Warfarin (N=147)	Placebo/ Warfarin (N=170)
Dizziness	13.6%	8.2%
Abdominal distress	6.1%	3.5%
Headache	2.3%	0.0
Rash	2.3%	1.1%

Other reactions from uncontrolled studies include diarrhea, vomiting, flushing and pruritus. In addition, angina pectoris has been reported rarely. On those uncommon occasions when adverse reactions have been persistent or intolerable, they have ceased on withdrawal of the medication.

When Persantine was administered concomitantly with warfarin, bleeding was no greater in frequency or severity than that observed when warfarin was administered alone.

OVERDOSAGE

Hypotension, if it occurs, is likely to be of short duration, but a vasopressor drug may be used if necessary. The oral LD_{50} in rats is greater than 6,000 mg/kg while in the dogs, the oral LD_{50} is approximately 400 mg/kg. Since Persantine® (dipyridamole USP) is highly protein bound, dialysis is not likely to be of benefit.

DOSAGE AND ADMINISTRATION

Adjunctive Use in Prophylaxis of Thromboembolism after Cardiac Valve Replacement The recommended dose is 75–100 mg four times daily as an adjunct to the usual warfarin therapy. Please note that aspirin is not to be administered concomitantly with coumarin anticoagulants.

HOW SUPPLIED

Persantine® (dipyridamole USP) is available as round, orange, sugar-coated tablets of 25 mg, 50 mg and 75 mg coded BI/17, BI/18 and BI/19 respectively.

They are available in the following package sizes:

25 mg Tablets	
Bottles of 100	(NDC 0597-0017-01)
Bottles of 1000	(NDC 0597-0017-10)
Unit Dose Packages of 100	(NDC 0597-0017-61)
50 mg Tablets	
Bottles of 100	(NDC 0597-0018-01)
Bottles of 1000	(NDC 0597-0018-10)
Unit Dose Packages of 100	(NDC 0597-0018-61)
75 mg Tablets	
Bottles of 100	(NDC 0597-0019-01)
Bottles of 500	(NDC 0597-0019-05)
Unit Dose Packages of 100	(NDC 0597-0019-61)

Store below 86°F (30°C).

Caution: Federal law prohibits dispensing without prescription.

PE-PI-5/88

Shown in Product Identification Section, page 406

PRELUDIN®   C℞

[pra-lu 'din]
(phenmetrazine hydrochloride USP)
Endurets® (prolonged-action

tablets), 75 mg ....BI-CODE 62

DESCRIPTION

Preludin® (phenmetrazine hydrochloride USP) belongs to the oxazine group of compounds and is designated chemically as 2-phenyl-3-methyltetrahydro-1,4-oxazine hydrochloride.

Phenmetrazine hydrochloride is a white, water-soluble, crystalline powder.

Active Ingredient: Each prolonged-action tablet contains phenmetrazine hydrochloride 75 mg.

Inactive Ingredients: Aluminum tristearate, confectioner's sugar, corn starch, FD&C Blue No. 2, FD&C Red No. 3, FD&C Yellow No. 5 (tartrazine), FD&C Yellow No. 6, gelatin, magnesium stearate, silica gel, stearic acid, talc and other ingredients.

ACTIONS

Preludin (phenmetrazine hydrochloride USP) is a sympathomimetic amine with pharmacologic activity similar to the prototype drugs of this class used in obesity, the amphetamines. Actions include central nervous system stimulation and elevation of blood pressure. Tachyphylaxis and tolerance have been demonstrated with all drugs of this class in which these phenomena have been looked for.

Drugs of this class used in obesity are commonly known as "anorectics" or "anorexigenics." It has not been established, however, that the action of such drugs in treating obesity is primarily one of appetite suppression. Other central nervous system actions, or metabolic effects, may be involved, for example.

Adult obese subjects instructed in dietary management and treated with "anorectic" drugs lose more weight on the average than those treated with placebo and diet, as determined in relatively short-term clinical trials.

The magnitude of increased weight loss of drug-treated patients over placebo-treated patients is only a fraction of a pound a week. The rate of weight loss is greatest in the first weeks of therapy for both drug and placebo subjects and tends to decrease in succeeding weeks. The possible origins of the increased weight loss due to the various drug effects are not established. The amount of weight loss associated with the use of an "anorectic" drug varies from trial to trial, and the increased weight loss appears to be related in part to variables other than the drug prescribed, such as the physician-investigator, the population treated, and the diet prescribed. Studies do not permit conclusions as to the relative importance of the drug and non-drug factors on weight loss. The natural history of obesity is measured in years, whereas the studies cited are restricted to a few weeks' duration; thus, the total impact of drug-induced weight loss over that of diet alone must be considered clinically limited.

Preludin Endurets are formulated to release the active drug substance *in vivo* in a more gradual fashion than the stan-

Continued on next page

Boehringer Ingelheim—Cont.

dard formulation, as demonstrated by blood levels. The formulation has not been shown superior in effectiveness with respect to weight loss over the same dosage of the standard, noncontrolled-release formulations.

INDICATION

Preludin (phenmetrazine hydrochloride USP) is indicated in the management of exogenous obesity as a short-term (a few weeks) adjunct in a regimen of weight reduction based on caloric restriction. The limited usefulness of agents of this class (see Actions) should be measured against possible risk factors inherent to their use such as those described below.

CONTRAINDICATIONS

Advanced arteriosclerosis, symptomatic cardiovascular disease, moderate to severe hypertension, hyperthyroidism, known hypersensitivity or idiosyncrasy to sympathomimetic amines, glaucoma. Agitated states. Patients with a history of drug abuse. Concomitant use of CNS stimulants. During or within 14 days following the administration of monoamine oxidase inhibitors (hypertensive crises may result).

WARNINGS

Tolerance usually develops within a few weeks. When this occurs, the recommended dose should not be exceeded in an attempt to increase anorectic effect; rather, the drug should be discontinued.

Preludin (phenmetrazine hydrochloride USP) may impair the ability of the patient to engage in potentially hazardous activities such as operating machinery or driving a motor vehicle; the patient should therefore be cautioned accordingly.

Drug Dependence Preludin (phenmetrazine hydrochloride USP) is related chemically and pharmacologically to the amphetamines. Amphetamines and related stimulant drugs have been extensively abused, and the possibility of abuse of Preludin (phenmetrazine hydrochloride USP) should be kept in mind when evaluating the desirability of including a drug as part of a weight reduction program. Abuse of amphetamines and related drugs may be associated with intense psychological dependence and severe social dysfunction. There are reports of patients who have increased the dosage to many times that recommended. Abrupt cessation following prolonged high dosage administration results in extreme fatigue and mental depression; changes are also noted on the sleep EEG. Manifestations of chronic intoxication with anorectic drugs include severe dermatoses, marked insomnia, irritability, hyperactivity, and personality changes. The most severe manifestation of chronic intoxication is psychosis, often clinically indistinguishable from schizophrenia.

Usage in Pregnancy Safe use in pregnancy has not been established. Animal reproductive studies demonstrated no teratogenic effects. However, the conception rate was adversely affected, as well as survival and body weight of pups at weaning. There have been clinical reports of congenital malformation associated with the use of this compound but a causal relationship has not been proved. Until more information is available, Preludin (phenmetrazine hydrochloride USP) should not be used by women who are or may become pregnant, particularly in the first trimester, unless in the opinion of the prescribing physician the potential benefits outweigh the possible risks.

Usage in Children Preludin (phenmetrazine hydrochloride USP) is not recommended for use in children under 12 years of age.

PRECAUTIONS

Caution should be exercised in prescribing Preludin (phenmetrazine hydrochloride USP) for patients with even mild hypertension. Insulin requirements in diabetes mellitus may be altered in association with the use of Preludin (phenmetrazine hydrochloride USP) and the concomitant dietary regimen. Preludin (phenmetrazine hydrochloride USP) may decrease the hypotensive effect of guanethidine. The least amount feasible should be prescribed or dispensed at one time in order to minimize the possibility of overdosage. Preludin Endurets, 75 mg, contain FD&C Yellow No. 5 (tartrazine) which may cause allergic-type reactions (including bronchial asthma) in certain susceptible individuals. Although the overall incidence of FD&C Yellow No. 5 (tartrazine) sensitivity in the general population is low, it is frequently seen in patients who also have aspirin hypersensitivity.

ADVERSE REACTIONS

Cardiovascular Palpitation, tachycardia, elevation of blood pressure.

Central Nervous System Overstimulation, restlessness, dizziness, insomnia, euphoria, dysphoria, tremor, headache; rarely psychotic episodes at recommended doses.

Gastrointestinal Dryness of the mouth, unpleasant taste, diarrhea, constipation, other gastrointestinal disturbances.

Allergic Urticaria.

Endocrine Impotence, changes in libido.

DOSAGE AND ADMINISTRATION

Preludin (phenmetrazine hydrochloride USP) is not recommended for use in children under 12 years of age.

The maximum adult dosage is one 75 mg Endurets prolonged-action tablet taken daily. Since an Endurets tablet provides appetite suppression for approximately 12 hours, the time of administration should be determined by the period of the day over which the anorectic effect is desired.

OVERDOSAGE

Manifestations of acute overdosage with phenmetrazine hydrochloride include restlessness, tremor, hyperreflexia, rapid respiration, confusion, assaultiveness, hallucinations, panic states. Fatigue and depression usually follow the central stimulation.

Cardiovascular effects include arrhythmias, hypertension, or hypotension and circulatory collapse. Gastrointestinal symptoms include nausea, vomiting, diarrhea and abdominal cramps. Poisoning may result in convulsions, coma, and death.

Management of acute phenmetrazine hydrochloride intoxication is largely symptomatic and includes lavage and sedation with a barbiturate. Experience with hemodialysis or peritoneal dialysis is inadequate to permit recommendation in this regard. As with the amphetamines, acidification of the urine should increase phenmetrazine hydrochloride excretion. Intravenous phentolamine has been suggested for possible acute, severe hypertension if this complicates phenmetrazine overdosage.

HOW SUPPLIED

Preludin (phenmetrazine hydrochloride USP) is available as pink, round Endurets prolonged-action tablets of 75 mg for once-a-day administration. Bottles of 100. NDC 0597-0062-01.

PR-PI-6/85

Shown in Product Identification Section, page 406

PRELU-2®   Ⓒ Ⓡ
[pra 'lu (2)]
(phendimetrazine tartrate)
Timed Release Capsules   **BI-CODE 64**
    105 mg

DESCRIPTION

Chemical name: phendimetrazine tartrate (+) 3, 4 dimethyl-2-phenylmorpholine tartrate. Phendimetrazine tartrate is a white, odorless powder with a bitter taste. It is soluble in water, methanol and ethanol. It has a molecular weight of 341, and has the following molecular structure:

d-3, 4-dimethyl-2-phenylmorpholine tartrate

The capsule is manufactured in a special base which is designed for prolonged release.

Active Ingredient: Each timed-release capsule contains phendimetrazine tartrate 105 mg.

Inactive Ingredients: D&C Red No. 33, D&C Yellow No. 10, FD&C Blue No. 1, FD&C Yellow No. 6, gelatin, povidone, shellac, silica gel, starch, sucrose, talc, titanium dioxide.

CLINICAL PHARMACOLOGY

Phendimetrazine tartrate is a sympathomimetic amine with pharmacologic activity similar to the prototype of drugs of this class used in obesity, the amphetamines. Actions include central nervous system stimulation and elevation of blood pressure. Tachyphylaxis and tolerance have been demonstrated with all drugs of this class in which these phenomena have been looked for.

Drugs of this class used in obesity are commonly known as 'anorectics' or 'anorexigenics.' It has not been established, however, that the action of such drugs in treating obesity is primarily one of appetite suppression. Other central nervous system actions, or metabolic effects, may be involved, for example.

Adult obese subjects instructed in dietary management and treated with 'anorectic' drugs lose more weight on the average than those treated with placebo and diet, as determined in relatively short-term clinical trials.

The magnitude of increased weight loss of drug-treated patients over placebo-treated patients is only a fraction of a pound a week. The rate of weight loss is greatest in the first weeks of therapy for both drug and placebo subjects and tends to decrease in succeeding weeks. The possible origins of the increased weight loss due to the various drug effects are not established. The amount of weight loss associated with the use of an 'anorectic' drug varies from trial to trial, and the increased weight loss appears to be related in part to

variables other than the drug prescribed, such as the physician-investigator, the population treated, and the diet prescribed. Studies do not permit conclusions as to the relative importance of the drug and non-drug factors on weight loss. The natural history of obesity is measured in years, whereas the studies cited are restricted to a few weeks duration; thus, the total impact of drug-induced weight loss over that of diet alone must be considered clinically limited.

The active drug, 105 mg of phendimetrazine tartrate in each capsule of this special timed release dosage form, approximates the action of three 35 mg non-timed doses taken at four-hour intervals.

The major route of elimination is via the kidneys where most of the drug and metabolites are excreted. Some of the drug is metabolized to phenmetrazine and also phendimetrazine-N-oxide.

The average half-life of elimination when studied under controlled conditions is about 3.7 hours for both the timed and non-timed forms. The absorption half-life of the drug from conventional non-timed 35 mg phendimetrazine tablets is appreciably more rapid than the absorption rate of the drug from the timed release formulation.

INDICATIONS AND USAGE

Phendimetrazine tartrate is indicated in the management of exogenous obesity as a short-term adjunct (a few weeks) in a regimen of weight reduction based on caloric restriction. The limited usefulness of agents of this class (see Clinical Pharmacology) should be measured against possible risk factors inherent in their use such as those described below.

CONTRAINDICATIONS

Advanced arteriosclerosis, symptomatic cardiovascular disease, moderate to severe hypertension, hyperthyroidism, known hypersensitivity, or idiosyncrasy to the sympathomimetic amines, glaucoma.
Agitated states.
Patients with a history of drug abuse.
During or within 14 days following the administration of monoamine oxidase inhibitors (hypertensive crises may result).

WARNINGS

Tolerance to the anorectic effect usually develops within a few weeks. When this occurs, the recommended dose should not be exceeded in an attempt to increase the effect; rather, the drug should be discontinued.

Phendimetrazine tartrate may impair the ability of the patient to engage in potentially hazardous activities such as operating machinery or driving a motor vehicle; the patient should therefore be cautioned accordingly.

DRUG DEPENDENCE

Phendimetrazine tartrate is related chemically and pharmacologically to the amphetamines. Amphetamines and related stimulant drugs have been extensively abused, and the possibility of abuse of phendimetrazine tartrate should be kept in mind when evaluating the desirability of including a drug as part of a weight reduction program. Abuse of amphetamines and related drugs may be associated with intense psychological dependence and severe social dysfunction. There are reports of patients who have increased the dosage to many times that recommended. Abrupt cessation following prolonged high dosage administration results in extreme fatigue and mental depression; changes are also noted on the sleep EEG. Manifestations of chronic intoxication with anorectic drugs include severe dermatoses, marked insomnia, irritability, hyperactivity, and personality changes. The most severe manifestation of chronic intoxication is psychosis, often clinically indistinguishable from schizophrenia.

Usage in Pregnancy: The safety of phendimetrazine tartrate in pregnancy and lactation has not been established. Therefore phendimetrazine tartrate should not be taken by women who are or may become pregnant.

Usage in Children: Phendimetrazine tartrate is not recommended for use in children under 12 years of age.

PRECAUTIONS

Caution is to be exercised in prescribing phendimetrazine tartrate for patients with even mild hypertension.

Insulin requirements in diabetes mellitus may be altered in association with the use of phendimetrazine tartrate and the concomitant dietary regimen.

Phendimetrazine tartrate may decrease the hypotensive effect of guanethidine.

The least amount feasible should be prescribed or dispensed at one time in order to minimize the possibility of overdosage.

ADVERSE REACTIONS

Cardiovascular: Palpitation, tachycardia, elevation of blood pressure.

Central Nervous System: Overstimulation, restlessness, dizziness, insomnia, euphoria, dysphoria, tremor, headache; rarely psychotic episodes at recommended doses.

Gastrointestinal: Dryness of the mouth, unpleasant taste, diarrhea, constipation, other gastrointestinal disturbances.

Allergic: Urticaria.
Endocrine: Impotence, changes in libido.

OVERDOSAGE

Manifestations of acute overdosage with phendimetrazine tartrate include restlessness, tremor, hyperreflexia, rapid respiration, confusion, assaultiveness, hallucinations, panic states.

Fatigue and depression usually follow the central stimulation.

Cardiovascular effects include arrhythmias, hypertension or hypotension and circulatory collapse. Gastrointestinal symptoms include nausea, vomiting, diarrhea, and abdominal cramps. Fatal poisoning usually terminates in convulsions and coma. Management of acute phendimetrazine tartrate intoxication is largely symptomatic and includes lavage and sedation with a barbiturate. Experience with hemodialysis or peritoneal dialysis is inadequate to permit recommendation in this regard. Acidification of the urine increases phendimetrazine tartrate excretion. Intravenous phentolamine (Regitine) has been suggested for possible acute, severe hypertension, if this complicates phendimetrazine tartrate overdosage.

DOSAGE AND ADMINISTRATION

Since this product is a timed release dosage form, limit to one timed release capsule (105 mg phendimetrazine tartrate) in the morning.

Phendimetrazine tartrate is not recommended for use in children under 12 years of age.

HOW SUPPLIED

105 mg capsules (celery and green) in bottles of 100.
Federal law prohibits dispensing without a prescription.
P2-PI-9/85
Shown in Product Identification Section, page 406

RESPBID® ℞

[resp'bid]
(anhydrous theophylline)
Sustained release
Tablets of 250 mg and 500 mg
Oral Bronchodilator

Prescribing Information

DESCRIPTION

Theophylline is a bronchodilator structurally classified as a xanthine derivative. It occurs as a white, odorless, crystalline powder having a bitter taste. Theophylline anhydrous has the chemical name, 1H-Purine-2, 6-dione, 3,7-dihydro-1,3-dimethyl-, and is represented by the following structural formula:

$C_7H_8N_4O_2$ Molecular Weight 180.17
Respbid® (anhydrous theophylline) Tablets contain 250 or 500 mg theophylline anhydrous, in a sustained-release formulation for oral administration. Respbid Tablets also contain: cellulose acetate phthalate, lactose, magnesium stearate.

CLINICAL PHARMACOLOGY

Theophylline directly relaxes the smooth muscle of the bronchial airways and pulmonary blood vessels, thus acting mainly as a bronchodilator and smooth muscle relaxant. It has also been demonstrated that aminophylline has a potent effect on diaphragmatic contractility in normal persons and may then be capable of reducing fatigability and thereby improve contractility in patients with chronic obstructive airways disease. The exact mode of action remains unsettled. Although theophylline does cause inhibition of phosphodiesterase with a resultant increase in intracellular cyclic AMP, other agents similarly inhibit the enzyme producing a rise of cyclic AMP but are unassociated with any demonstrable bronchodilation. Other mechanisms proposed include an effect on translocation of intracellular calcium; prostaglandin antagonism; stimulation of catecholamines endogenously; inhibition of cyclic guanosine monophosphate metabolism and adenosine receptor antagonism. None of these mechanisms has been proved, however.

In vitro, theophylline has been shown to act synergistically with beta agonists and there are now available data which do demonstrate an additive effect *in vivo* with combined use.

Pharmacokinetics: The half-life of theophylline is influenced by a number of known variables. It may be prolonged in chronic alcoholics, particularly those with liver disease (cirrhosis or alcoholic liver disease), in patients with congestive heart failure, and in those patients taking certain other drugs (see PRECAUTIONS, Drug Interactions). Newborns and neonates have extremely slow clearance rates compared to older infants and children, i.e., those over 1 year. Older children have rapid clearance rates while most non-smoking adults have clearance rates between these two extremes. In premature neonates the decreased clearance is related to oxidative pathways that have yet to be established.

Theophylline Elimination Characteristics

	Half-Life (in Hours)	
	Range	Mean
Children	1–9	3.7
Adults	3–15	7.7

In cigarette smokers (1–2 packs/day) the mean half-life is 4–5 hours, much shorter than in non-smokers. The increase in clearance associated with smoking is presumably due to stimulation of the hepatic metabolic pathway by components of cigarette smoke. The duration of this effect after cessation of smoking is unknown but may require 6 months to 2 years before the rate approaches that of the non-smoker.

A single 500 mg dose of Respbid® (anhydrous theophylline) in 8 healthy male subjects fasted for 10 hours predose (overnight) through 4 hours postdose resulted in mean peak theophylline plasma levels of 9.1 ± 3.8 (SD) mcg/ml occurring at 5.0 ± 1.5 hours following dose administration. The extent of theophylline absorption from Respbid® (anhydrous theophylline) was complete in these subjects when compared with that from an immediate-release tablet. In another single dose study, comparable rates and extents of theophylline absorption were seen for the 250 mg Respbid Tablets in 18 healthy male subjects, fasted as above.

In a five-day multiple-dose study, 18 healthy male subjects received 250 mg Respbid Tablets in doses ranging from 375 mg to 625 mg twice dailiy (mean dose of 11 mg/kg per day). Subjects were allowed to take drug with milk and were permitted their normal daily meals except for fasting from 10 hours before through 4 hours after the morning dose on day 5. Following that dose, mean minimum and maximum plasma theophylline levels were 7.3 ± 2.3 mcg/ml and 10.8 ± 3.1 mcg/ml, respectively. The average percent fluctuation $[(C_{max} - C_{min}/C_{min}) \times 100]$ was 48%. The extent of theophylline absorption from Respbid averaged $94 \pm 19\%$ of that from an immediate-release liquid given four times daily.

In other studies: A single 500 mg dose of Respbid was administered to 35 healthy volunteers in both a fasting state and with a high-fat content breakfast. The resultant pharmacokinetic values recorded a delay in the rate of absorption (but not the extent) for the fed group.

In a multiple-dose study involving 12 adolescent patients, the rate and extent of absorption was similar whether the drug was taken immediately after, or two hours after, a low-fat content breakfast (see PRECAUTIONS, Drug/Food Interactions).

INDICATIONS AND USAGE

For relief and/or prevention of symptoms from asthma and reversible bronchospasm associated with chronic bronchitis and emphysema.

CONTRAINDICATIONS

Respbid® (anhydrous theophylline) Tablets are contraindicated in individuals who are hypersensitive to theophylline or any of the tablet components. It is also contraindicated in patients with active peptic ulcer disease, and in individuals with underlying seizure disorders (unless receiving appropriate anti-convulsant therapy).

WARNINGS

Serum levels above 20 mcg/ml are rarely found after appropriate administration of the recommended doses. However, in individuals in whom theophylline plasma clearance is reduced for any reason, even conventional doses may result in increased serum levels and potential toxicity. Reduced theophylline clearance has been documented in the following readily identifiable groups: 1) patients with impaired liver function; 2) patients over 55 years of age, particularly males and those with chronic lung disease; 3) those with cardiac failure from any cause; 4) those with sustained high fever; 5) neonates and infants under 1 year of age; and 6) those patients taking certain drugs (see PRECAUTIONS, Drug Interactions). Frequently, such patients have markedly prolonged theophylline serum levels following discontinuation of the drug.

Reduction of dosage and laboratory monitoring is especially appropriate in the above individuals.

Serious side effects such as ventricular arrhythmias, convulsions or even death may appear as the first sign of toxicity without any previous warning. Less serious signs of theophylline toxicity (i.e., nausea and restlessness) may occur frequently when initiating therapy, but are usually transient; when such signs are persistent during maintenance therapy; they are often associated with serum concentrations above 20 mcg/ml. Stated differently: serious toxicity is not reliably preceded by less severe side effects. A serum concentration measurement is the only reliable method of predicting potentially life-threatening toxicity.

Many patients who require theophylline exhibit tachycardia due to their underlying disease process so that the cause/effect relationship to elevated serum theophylline concentrations may not be appreciated.

Theophylline products may cause dysrhythmia and/or worsen pre-existing arrhythmias and any significant change in rate and/or rhythm warrants monitoring and further investigation.

Studies in laboratory animals (minipigs, rodents, and dogs) recorded the occurrence of cardiac arrhythmias and sudden death (with histologic evidence of myocardial necrosis) when beta-agonists and methylxanthines were administered concurrently. The significance of these findings when applied to humans is currently unknown.

PRECAUTIONS

General: On the average, theophylline half-life is shorter in cigarette and marijuana smokers than in non-smokers, but smokers can have half-lives as long as non-smokers. Theophylline should not be administered concurrently with other xanthines. Use with caution in patients with hypoxemia, hypertension, or those with history of peptic ulcer. Theophylline may occasionally act as a local irritant to G.I. tract although gastrointestinal symptoms are more commonly centrally mediated and associated with serum drug concentrations over 20 mcg/ml.

Information for Patients: If nausea, vomiting, restlessness, irregular heartbeat, or convulsions occur, contact a physician immediately.

Take only the amount of drug that has been prescribed. Do not take a larger dose, or take the drug more often, or for a longer time than recommended.

Take this drug consistently with respect to food: either with meals, or fasted (at least two hours pre- or 2 hours post-meals).

Do not take other medicines, especially those for pulmonary disorders, except on the advice of a physician.

Contact your physician if pulmonary symptoms occur repeatedly, especially at the end of a dosing interval.

Avoid drinking large amounts of caffeine-containing beverages, such as coffee, tea, cocoa, or cola, or eating large quantities of chocolate while taking this medicine, since these foods increase the side effects of theophylline.

Respbid® (anhydrous theophylline) Tablets should not be chewed or crushed.

Laboratory Tests: Serum levels should be monitored periodically to determine the theophylline level associated with observed clinical response and as the method of predicting toxicity. For such measurements, the serum sample should be obtained four to six hours after administration of Respbid Tablets. It is important that the patient will not have missed or taken additional doses during the previous 48 hours and that dosing intervals will have been reasonably equally spaced. DOSAGE ADJUSTMENT BASED ON SERUM THEOPHYLLINE MEASUREMENTS WHEN THESE INSTRUCTIONS HAVE NOT BEEN FOLLOWED MAY RESULT IN RECOMMENDATIONS THAT PRESENT RISK OF TOXICITY TO THE PATIENT.

Drug Interactions: *Drug/Drug*—Toxic synergism with ephedrine has been documented and may occur with other sympathomimetic bronchodilators. In addition, the following drug interactions have been demonstrated:
Theophylline with:

Allopurinol (high-dose)	Increased serum theophylline levels
Cimetidine	Increased serum theophylline levels
Erythromycin, Troleandomycin	Increased serum theophylline levels
Lithium carbonate	Increased renal excretion of lithium
Oral Contraceptives	Increased serum theophylline levels
Phenytoin	Decreased theophylline and phenytoin serum levels
Rifampin	Decreased serum theophylline levels

Drug/Food —Administration of a single dose of Respbid immediately after a high-fat content breakfast (8 ounces of whole milk, 2 fried eggs, 2 bacon strips, 2 ounces of hash browns and 2 slices of buttered toast, which equates to approximately 71 grams of fat and 985 calories) to 35 healthy volunteers resulted in plasma concentration levels (for the first 8 hours) of 40–60% of those noted during the fasted state and a delay in the time to peak plasma level (T-max) of 17.1 hours in contrast to the 5.1 hours observed during the fasted state.

However, when Respbid was administered on an every 12 hour schedule for 5 days, no consequential effect on absorption was noted following similar high-fat content breakfast, and the time to peak concentration averaged 5.4 hours. The rate and extent of absorption seen was similar when the drug was taken immediately after, and two hours after, a low-fat content breakfast.

The effect of other types and amounts of food, and the pharmacokinetic profile following an evening meal is not presently known.

Continued on next page

Boehringer Ingelheim—Cont.

Drug-Laboratory Test Interactions: Currently available analytical methods, including high pressure liquid chromatography and immunoassay techniques, for measuring serum theophylline levels are specific. Metabolites and other drugs generally do not affect the results. Other new analytic methods are also now in use. The physician should be aware of the laboratory method used and whether other drugs will interfere with the assay for theophylline.

Carcinogenesis, Mutagenesis, and Impairment of Fertility: Long-term carcinogenicity studies have not been performed with theophylline.

Chromosome-breaking activity was detected in human cell cultures at concentrations of theophylline up to 50 times the therapeutic serum concentration in humans. Theophylline was not mutagenic in the dominant lethal assay in male mice given theophylline intraperitoneally in doses up to 30 times the maximum daily human oral dose.

Studies to determine the effect on fertility have not been performed with theophylline.

Pregnancy: Category C—Animal reproduction studies have not been conducted with theophylline. It is also not known whether theophylline can cause fetal harm when administered to a pregnant woman or can affect reproduction capacity. Xanthines should be given to a pregnant woman only if clearly needed.

Nursing Mothers: Theophylline is distributed into breast milk and may cause irritability or other signs of toxicity in nursing infants. Because of the potential for serious adverse reactions in nursing infants from theophylline, a decision should be made whether to discontinue nursing or to discontinue the drug, taking into account the importance of the drug to the mother.

Pediatric Use: Respbid® (anhydrous theophylline) Tablets are not recommended for administration to children less than six years of age.

ADVERSE REACTIONS

The following adverse reactions have been observed, but there has not been enough systematic collection of data to support an estimate of their frequency. The most consistent adverse reactions are usually due to overdosage.

1. *Gastrointestinal:* nausea, vomiting, epigastric pain, hematemesis, diarrhea.
2. *Central nervous system:* headaches, irritability, restlessness, insomnia, reflex hyperexcitability, muscle twitching, clonic and tonic generalized convulsions.
3. *Cardiovascular:* palpitation, tachycardia, extrasystoles, flushing, hypotension, circulatory failure, ventricular arrhythmias.
4. *Respiratory:* tachypnea.
5. *Renal:* potentiation of diuresis.
6. *Others:* alopecia, hyperglycemia, inappropriate ADH syndrome, rash.

OVERDOSAGE

Management: It is suggested that the management principles (consistent with the clinical status of the patient when first seen) outlined below be instituted and that simultaneous contact with a Regional Poison Control Center be established. In this way both updated information and individualization regarding required therapy may be provided.

1. When potential oral overdose is established and seizure has not occurred:
a) If patient is alert and seen within the early hours after ingestion, induction of emesis may be of value. Gastric lavage has been demonstrated to be of no value in influencing outcome in patients who present more than 1 hour after ingestion.
b) Administer a cathartic. Sorbitol solution is reported to be of value.
c) Administer repeated doses of activated charcoal and monitor theophylline serum levels.
d) Prophylactic administration of phenobarbital has been shown to increase the seizure threshold in laboratory

animals, and administration of this drug can be considered.

2. If patient presents with a seizure:
a) Establish an airway.
b) Administer oxygen.
c) Treat the seizure with intravenous diazepam, 0.1 to 0.3 mg/kg up to 10 mg. If seizures cannot be controlled, the use of general anesthesia should be considered.
d) Monitor vital signs, maintain blood pressure and provide adequate hydration.

3. If post-seizure coma is present:
a) Maintain airway and oxygenation.
b) If a result of oral medication, follow above recommendations to prevent absorption of the drug, but intubation and lavage will have to be performed instead of inducing emesis, and the cathartic and charcoal will need to be introduced via a large bore gastric lavage tube.
c) Continue to provide full supportive care and adequate hydration until the drug is metabolized. In general, drug metabolism is sufficiently rapid so as not to warrant dialysis. If repeated oral activated charcoal is ineffective (as noted by stable or rising serum levels) charcoal hemoperfusion may be indicated.

DOSAGE AND ADMINISTRATION

Effective use of theophylline (i.e., the concentration of drug in the serum associated with optimal benefit and minimal risk of toxicity) is considered to occur when the theophylline concentration is maintained from 10 to 20 mcg/ml. The early studies from which these levels were derived were carried out in patients immediately or shortly after recovery from acute exacerbations of their disease (some hospitalized with status asthmaticus).

Although the 20 mcg/ml level remains appropriate as a critical value (above which toxicity is more likely to occur) for safety purposes, additional data are now available which indicate that the serum theophylline concentrations required to produce maximum physiologic benefit may, in fact, fluctuate with the degree of bronchospasm present and are variable. Therefore, the physician should individualize the range appropriate to the patient's requirements, based on both symptomatic response and improvement in pulmonary function. It should be stressed that serum theophylline concentrations maintained at the upper level of the 10 to 20 mcg/ml range may be associated with potential toxicity when factors known to reduce theophylline clearance are operative (see WARNINGS).

If it is not possible to obtain serum level determinations, restriction of the daily dose (in otherwise healthy adults) to not greater than 13 mg/kg/day, to a maximum of 900 mg, in divided doses, will result in relatively few patients exceeding serum levels of 20 mcg/ml and the resultant greater risk of toxicity.

Caution should be exercised for younger children who cannot complain of minor side effects. Older adults, those with cor pulmonale, congestive heart failure, and/or liver diseases may have unusually low dosage requirements and thus may experience toxicity at the maximal dosage recommended below.

Theophylline does not distribute into fatty tissue. Dosage should be calculated on the basis of lean (ideal) body weight where mg/kg doses are presented.

Dosage guidelines are approximations only and the wide range of theophylline clearance between individuals (particularly those with concomitant disease) makes indiscriminate usage hazardous.

Respbid® (anhydrous theophylline) Tablets Should Not Be Chewed or Crushed.

Dosage Guidelines: There is information which shows that taking Respbid consistently after both high-fat and low-fat content breakfasts does not result in a decrease in peak concentration or delay in time to peak concentration that are seen when a single dose of Respbid is taken immediately after a high-fat content breakfast. Therefore, Respbid® (anhydrous theophylline) should be administered consistently with respect to food; either with meals, or fasted (at least 2 hours pre- or 2 hours post-meals). (See PRECAUTIONS, Drug/Food Interactions.)

Status asthmaticus should be considered a medical emergency and is defined as that degree of bronchospasm which is not rapidly responsive to usual doses of conventional bronchodilators. Optimal therapy for such patients frequently requires both <u>additional medication</u>, parenterally administered, and <u>close monitoring</u>, preferably in an intensive care setting.

Acute Symptoms—Respbid Tablets are not intended for patients experiencing an acute episode of bronchospasm (associated with asthma, chronic bronchitis, or emphysema). Such patients require <u>rapid</u> relief of symptoms and should be treated with an immediate release theophylline preparation, an intravenous theophylline preparation or other bronchodilators, and not with controlled-release products.

Chronic Symptoms—Theophylline administration is a treatment for the management of reversible bronchospasm (asthma, chronic bronchitis and emphysema) to prevent symptoms and maintain patent airways. The appropriate dosage of theophylline can be established using an immediate-release preparation. Slow clinical titration is preferred to help assure acceptance and safety of the medication. When appropriate theophylline serum levels have been attained and clinical improvement has been maintained, the patient can usually be switched to Respbid Tablets by dividing the total daily dose of immediate-release theophylline by two and administering the appropriate Respbid Tablet every 12 hours (see conversion chart below). However, certain patients, such as the young, smokers, or some non-smoking adults are likely to metabolize theophylline rapidly and require the total daily dose administered as three equal doses at eight-hour intervals. Such patients can generally be identified as having trough serum levels lower than desired or repeatedly exhibited symptoms near the end of a dosing interval.

If the established daily dose is:	The q 12 hr regimen is: no. tablets:	strength:
500 mg	1	Respbid 250 mg
1000 mg	1	Respbid 500 mg

Alternatively, therapy can be initiated with Respbid since it is available in dosage strengths which permit titration and adjustment of dosage as noted above. A liquid preparation should be considered for children to permit both greater ease of and more accurate dosage adjustment.

Recommended Doses for Initiating Therapy with Respbid:
Initial Dose—As an initial dose, 16 mg/kg per 24 hours or 400 mg per 24 hours (whichever is less) of Respbid® (anhydrous theophylline) Tablets in divided doses at 8- or 12-hour intervals, as appropriate (see DOSAGE AND ADMINISTRATION).

Increasing Dose—The above dosage may be increased in approximately 25% increments at three-day intervals so long as the drug is tolerated, until clinical response is satisfactory or the maximum dose as indicated in the following section is reached. The serum concentration may be checked at these intervals, but at a minimum, should be determined at the end of this adjustment period.

IT IS IMPORTANT THAT NO PATIENT BE MAINTAINED ON ANY DOSAGE THAT IS NOT TOLERATED. In instructing patients to increase dosage, they should be instructed not to take a subsequent dose if side effects occur and to resume therapy at a lower dose once adverse effects have disappeared.

Maximum Dose Where the Serum Concentration Is Not Measured:
WARNING: DO NOT ATTEMPT TO MAINTAIN ANY DOSE THAT IS NOT TOLERATED.
Do not exceed the following (or 900 mg, whichever is less):

Age	Dose
Age 6–9 years	24 mg/kg/day
Age 9–12 years	20 mg/kg/day
Age 12–16 years	18 mg/kg/day
Age 16 years and older	13 mg/kg/day

Measurement of Serum Theophylline Concentrations During Chronic Therapy: If the above maximum doses are to be maintained or exceeded, serum theophylline measurement is essential (see PRECAUTIONS, Laboratory Tests, for guidance).

Dosage Adjustment After Serum Theophylline Measurement:
[See table left].

HOW SUPPLIED

Respbid® brand anhydrous theophylline is supplied as 250 mg white, round, scored sustained release tablets imprinted with "BI 48" (NDC 0597-0048-01) and 500 mg white, capsule-shaped, scored sustained release tablets imprinted with "BI 49" (NDC 0597-0049-01) in bottles of 100.
STORE AT CONTROLLED ROOM TEMPERATURE 15°–30°C (59°–86°F).
Caution: Federal law prohibits dispensing without prescription.

RE-PI- 10/87
Shown in Product Identification Section, page 406

If serum theophylline is:		Directions:
Within desired range		Maintain dosage if tolerated. Recheck serum theophylline concentration at 6- to 12-month intervals.*
Too high	20 to 25 mcg/ml	Decrease doses by about 10% and recheck serum level after 3 days.
	25 to 30 mcg/ml	Skip the next dose and decrease subsequent doses by about 25%. Recheck serum level after 3 days.
	Over 30 mcg/ml	Skip next two doses and decrease subsequent doses by 50%. Recheck serum level after 3 days.
Too low		Increase dosage by 25% at 3 day intervals until either the desired serum concentration and/or clinical response is achieved.* The total daily dose may need to be administered at more frequent intervals if symptoms occur repeatedly at the end of a dosing interval.

The serum concentration may be rechecked at appropriate intervals, but at least at the end of any adjustment period. When the patient's condition is otherwise clinically stable, and none of the recognized factors which alter elimination are present, measurement of serum levels need be repeated only every 6 to 12 months.

*Finer adjustments in dosage may be needed for some patients.

SERENTIL® ℞

[seh-ren'til]

(mesoridazine USP) besylate

Tablets, 10 mg	BI-CODE 20
Tablets, 25 mg	BI-CODE 21
Tablets, 50 mg	BI-CODE 22
Tablets, 100 mg	BI-CODE 23
Concentrate of 25 mg/ml	BI-CODE 25
Ampuls of 1 ml (25 mg)	BI-CODE 27

DESCRIPTION

Serentil® (mesoridazine USP), the besylate salt of a metabolite of thioridazine, is a phenothiazine tranquilizer that is effective in the treatment of schizophrenia, organic brain disorders, alcoholism and psychoneuroses.

Serentil is 10-[2(1-methyl-2-piperidyl) ethyl]-2- (methyl-sulfinyl)-phenothiazine [as the besylate].

Tablet, 10 mg, for oral administration—Active Ingredient: mesoridazine (as the besylate), 10 mg. Inactive Ingredients: acacia, carnauba wax, colloidal silicon dioxide, FD&C Red No. 40 aluminum lake, lactose, microcrystalline cellulose, povidone, sodium benzoate, starch, stearic acid, sucrose, talc, titanium dioxide, and other ingredients.

Tablet, 25 mg, for oral administration—Active Ingredient: mesoridazine (as the besylate), 25 mg. Inactive Ingredients: acacia, carnauba wax, colloidal silicon dioxide, FD&C Red No. 40 aluminum lake, lactose, microcrystalline cellulose, povidone, sodium benzoate, stearic acid, sucrose, talc, titanium dioxide, and other ingredients.

Tablet, 50 mg, for oral administration—Active Ingredient: mesoridazine (as the besylate), 50 mg. Inactive Ingredients: acacia, carnauba wax, colloidal silicon dioxide, FD&C Red No. 40 aluminum lake, gelatin, lactose, microcrystalline cellulose, povidone, sodium benzoate, starch, stearic acid, sucrose, talc, titanium dioxide, and other ingredients.

Tablet, 100 mg, for oral administration—Active Ingredient: mesoridazine (as the besylate), 100 mg. Inactive Ingredients: acacia, carnauba wax, colloidal silicon dioxide, FD&C Red No. 40 aluminum lake, gelatin, lactose, microcrystalline cellulose, povidone, sodium benzoate, starch, stearic acid, sucrose, talc, titanium dioxide, and other ingredients.

Ampuls, 1 ml, for intramuscular administration—Active Ingredient: mesoridazine (as the besylate), 25 mg. Inactive Ingredients: edetate disodium USP, 0.5 mg; sodium chloride USP, 7.2 mg; carbon dioxide gas (bone dry) q.s., water for injection USP, q.s. to 1 ml.

Concentrate, for oral administration—Active Ingredient: mesoridazine (as the besylate), 25 mg per ml. Inactive Ingredients: alcohol, 0.61% by volume; citric acid; FD&C Red No. 40; flavors; methylparaben; propylparaben; purified water; sodium citrate, sorbitol.

ACTIONS

Based upon animal studies Serentil® (mesoridazine USP), like other phenothiazines, acts indirectly on reticular formation, whereby neuronal activity into reticular formation is reduced without affecting its intrinsic ability to activate the cerebral cortex. In addition, the phenothiazines exhibit at least part of their activities through depression of hypothalamic centers. Neurochemically, the phenothiazines are thought to exert their effects by a central adrenergic blocking action.

INDICATIONS

In clinical studies Serentil® (mesoridazine USP) has been found useful in the following disease states:

Schizophrenia: Serentil is effective in the treatment of schizophrenia. It substantially reduces the severity of emotional withdrawal, conceptual disorganization, anxiety, tension, hallucinatory behavior, suspiciousness and blunted affect in schizophrenic patients. As with other phenothiazines, patients refractory to previous medication may respond to Serentil.

Behavioral Problems in Mental Deficiency and Chronic Brain Syndrome: The effect of Serentil was found to be excellent or good in the management of hyperactivity and uncooperativeness associated with mental deficiency and chronic brain syndrome.

Alcoholism—Acute and Chronic: Serentil ameliorates anxiety, tension, depression, nausea and vomiting in both acute and chronic alcoholics without producing hepatic dysfunction or hindering the functional recovery of the impaired liver.

Psychoneurotic Manifestations: Serentil reduces the symptoms of anxiety and tension, prevalent symptoms often asso-ciated with neurotic components of many disorders, and benefits personality disorders in general.

CONTRAINDICATIONS

As with other phenothiazines, Serentil® (mesoridazine USP) is contraindicated in severe central nervous system depression or comatose states from any cause. Serentil is contraindicated in individuals who have previously shown hypersensitivity to the drug.

WARNINGS

Tardive Dyskinesia: Tardive dyskinesia, a syndrome consisting of potentially irreversible, involuntary, dyskinetic movements may develop in patients treated with neuroleptic (antipsychotic) drugs. Although the prevalence of the syndrome appears to be highest among the elderly, especially elderly women, it is impossible to rely upon prevalence estimates to predict, at the inception of neuroleptic treatment, which patients are likely to develop the syndrome. Whether neuroleptic drug products differ in their potential to cause tardive dyskinesia is unknown.

Both the risk of developing the syndrome and the likelihood that it will become irreversible are believed to increase as the duration of treatment and the total cumulative dose of neuroleptic drugs administered to the patient increase. However, the syndrome can develop, although much less commonly, after relatively brief treatment periods at low doses.

There is no known treatment for established cases of tardive dyskinesia, although the syndrome may remit, partially or completely, if neuroleptic treatment is withdrawn. Neuroleptic treatment, itself, however, may suppress (or partially suppress) the signs and symptoms of the syndrome and thereby may possibly mask the underlying disease process. The effect that symptomatic suppression has upon the long-term course of the syndrome is unknown.

Given these considerations, neuroleptics should be prescribed in a manner that is most likely to minimize the occurrence of tardive dyskinesia. Chronic neuroleptic treatment should generally be reserved for patients who suffer from a chronic illness 1) that is known to respond to neuroleptic drugs, and 2) for which alternative, equally effective but potentially less harmful treatments are *not* available or appropriate. In patients who do require chronic treatment, the smallest dose and the shortest duration of treatment producing a satisfactory clinical response should be sought. The need for continued treatment should be reassessed periodically.

If signs and symptoms of tardive dyskinesia appear in a patient on neuroleptics, drug discontinuation should be considered. However, some patients may require treatment despite the presence of the syndrome.

(For further information about the description of tardive dyskinesia and its clinical detection, please refer to the sections on Information for Patients and Adverse Reactions.)

Neuroleptic Malignant Syndrome (NMS) A potentially fatal symptom complex sometimes referred to as Neuroleptic Malignant Syndrome (NMS) has been reported in association with antipsychotic drugs. Clinical manifestations of NMS are hyperpyrexia, muscle rigidity, altered mental status and evidence of autonomic instability (irregular pulse or blood pressure, tachycardia, diaphoresis, and cardiac dysrhythmias).

The diagnostic evaluation of patients with this syndrome is complicated. In arriving at a diagnosis, it is important to identify cases where the clinical presentation includes both serious medical illness (e.g., pneumonia, systemic infection, etc.) and untreated or inadequately treated extrapyramidal signs and symptoms (EPS). Other important considerations in the differential diagnosis include central anticholinergic toxicity, heat stroke, drug fever and primary central nervous system (CNS) pathology.

The management of NMS should include 1) immediate discontinuation of antipsychotic drugs and other drugs not essential to concurrent therapy, 2) intensive symptomatic treatment and medical monitoring, and 3) treatment of any concomitant serious medical problems for which specific treatments are available. There is no general agreement about specific pharmacological treatment regimens for uncomplicated NMS. If a patient requires antipsychotic drug treatment after recovery from NMS, the potential reintroduction of drug therapy should be carefully considered. The patient should be carefully monitored, since recurrences of NMS have been reported.

Where patients are participating in activities requiring complete mental alertness (e.g., driving), it is advisable to administer the phenothiazines cautiously and to increase the dosage gradually.

Usage in Pregnancy: The safety of this drug in pregnancy has not been established; hence, it should be given only when the anticipated benefits to be derived from treatment exceed the possible risks to mother and fetus.

Usage in Children: The use of Serentil® (mesoridazine USP) in children under 12 years of age is not recommended, because safe conditions for its use have not been established. Attention should be paid to the fact that phenothiazines are capable of potentiating central nervous system depressants (e.g., anesthetics, opiates, alcohol, etc.) as well as atropine and phosphorus insecticides.

PRECAUTIONS

While ocular changes have not to date been related to Serentil® (mesoridazine USP), one should be aware that such changes have been seen with other drugs of this class.

Because of possible hypotensive effects, reserve parenteral administration for bedfast patients or for acute ambulatory cases, and keep patient lying down for at least one-half hour after injection.

Leukopenia and/or agranulocytosis have been attributed to phenothiazine therapy. A single case of transient granulocytopenia has been associated with Serentil. Since convulsive seizures have been reported, patients receiving anticonvulsant medication should be maintained on that regimen while receiving Serentil.

Neuroleptic drugs elevate prolactin levels; the elevation persists during chronic administration. Tissue culture experiments indicate that approximately one-third of human breast cancers are prolactin dependent in vitro, a factor of potential importance if the prescription of these drugs is contemplated in a patient with a previously detected breast cancer. Although disturbances such as galactorrhea, amenorrhea, gynecomastia, and impotence have been reported, the clinical significance of elevated serum prolactin levels is unknown for most patients. An increase in mammary neoplasms has been found in rodents after chronic administration of neuroleptic drugs. Neither clinical studies nor epidemiologic studies conducted to date, however, have shown an association between chronic administration of these drugs and mammary tumorigenesis; the available evidence is considered too limited to be conclusive at this time.

Information for Patients: Given the likelihood that some patients exposed chronically to neuroleptics will develop tardive dyskinesia, it is advised that all patients in whom chronic use is contemplated be given, if possible, full information about this risk.

ADVERSE REACTIONS

Drowsiness and hypotension were the most prevalent side effects encountered. Side effects tended to reach their maximum level of severity early with the exception of a few (rigidity and motoric effects) which occurred later in therapy.

With the exceptions of tremor and rigidity, adverse reactions were generally found among those patients who received relatively high doses early in treatment. Clinical data showed no tendency for the investigators to terminate treatment because of side effects.

Serentil® (mesoridazine USP) has demonstrated a remarkably low incidence of adverse reactions when compared with other phenothiazine compounds.

Central Nervous System: Drowsiness, Parkinson's syndrome, dizziness, weakness, tremor, restlessness, ataxia, dystonia, rigidity, slurring, akathisia, motoric reactions (opisthotonos) have been reported.

Autonomic Nervous System: Dry mouth, nausea and vomiting, fainting, stuffy nose, photophobia, constipation and blurred vision have occurred in some instances.

Genitourinary System: Inhibition of ejaculation, impotence, enuresis, incontinence have been reported.

Skin: Itching, rash, hypertrophic papillae of the tongue and angioneurotic edema have been reported.

Cardiovascular System: Hypotension and tachycardia have been reported. EKG changes have occurred in some instances (see Phenothiazine Derivatives: Cardiovascular Effects).

Phenothiazine Derivatives: It should be noted that efficacy, indications and untoward effects have varied with the different phenothiazines. The physician should be aware that the following have occurred with one or more phenothiazines and should be considered whenever one of these drugs is used:

Autonomic Reactions: Miosis, obstipation, anorexia, paralytic ileus.

Cutaneous Reactions: Erythema, exfoliative dermatitis, contact dermatitis.

Blood Dyscrasias: Agranulocytosis, leukopenia, eosinophilia, thrombocytopenia, anemia, aplastic anemia, pancytopenia.

Allergic Reactions: Fever, laryngeal edema, angioneurotic edema, asthma.

Hepatotoxicity: Jaundice, biliary stasis.

Cardiovascular Effects: Changes in the terminal portion of the electrocardiogram, including prolongation of the Q-T interval, lowering and inversion of the T wave and appearance of a wave tentatively identified as a bifid T or a U wave have been observed in some patients receiving the phenothiazine tranquilizers, including Serentil. To date, these appear to be due to altered repolarization and not related to myocardial damage. They appear to be reversible. While there is no evidence at present that these changes are in any way precursors of any significant disturbance of cardiac rhythm, it should be noted that sudden and unexpected deaths appar-

Continued on next page

Boehringer Ingelheim—Cont.

ently due to cardiac arrest have occurred in patients previously showing characteristic electrocardiographic changes while taking the drug. The use of periodic electrocardiograms has been proposed but would appear to be of questionable value as a predictive device.

Hypotension, rarely resulting in cardiac arrest, has been noted.

Extrapyramidal Symptoms: Akathisia, agitation, motor restlessness, dystonic reactions, trismus, torticollis, opisthotonos, oculogyric crises, tremor, muscular rigidity, akinesia.

Tardive dyskinesia: Chronic use of neuroleptics may be associated with the development of tardive dyskinesia. The salient features of this syndrome are described in the **Warnings** section and below.

The syndrome is characterized by involuntary choreoathetoid movements which variously involve the tongue, face, mouth, lips, or jaw (e.g., protrusion of the tongue, puffing of cheeks, puckering of the mouth, chewing movements), trunk and extremities. The severity of the syndrome and the degree of impairment produced vary widely.

The syndrome may become clinically recognizable either during treatment, upon dosage reduction, or upon withdrawal of treatment. Movements may decrease in intensity and may disappear altogether if further treatment with neuroleptics is withheld. It is generally believed that reversibility is more likely after short- rather than long-term neuroleptic exposure. Consequently, early detection of tardive dyskinesia is important. To increase the likelihood of detecting the syndrome at the earliest possible time, the dosage of neuroleptic drug should be reduced periodically (if clinically possible) and the patient observed for signs of the disorder. This maneuver is critical, for neuroleptic drugs may mask the signs of the syndrome.

Endocrine Disturbances: Menstrual irregularities, altered libido, gynecomastia, lactation, weight gain, edema. False positive pregnancy tests have been reported.

Urinary Disturbances: Retention, incontinence.

Others: Hyperpyrexia. Behavioral effects suggestive of a paradoxical reaction have been reported. These include excitement, bizarre dreams, aggravation of psychoses and toxic confusional states. More recently, a peculiar skin-eye syndrome has been recognized as a side effect following longterm treatment with phenothiazines. This reaction is marked by progressive pigmentation of areas of the skin or conjunctiva and/or accompanied by discoloration of the exposed sclera and cornea. Opacities of the anterior lens and cornea described as irregular or stellate in shape have also been reported. Systemic lupus erythematosus-like syndrome.

DOSAGE AND ADMINISTRATION

The dosage of Serentil® (mesoridazine USP), as with most medications, should be adjusted to the needs of the individual. The lowest effective dosage should always be used. When maximum response is achieved, dosage may be reduced gradually to a maintenance level.

Schizophrenia: For most patients, regardless of symptom severity, a starting dose of 50 mg t.i.d. is recommended. The usual optimum total daily dose range is 100-400 mg per day.

Behavioral Problems in Mental Deficiency and Chronic Brain Syndrome: For most patients a starting dose of 25 mg t.i.d. is recommended. The usual optimum total daily dose range is 75-300 mg per day.

Alcoholism: For most patients the usual starting dose is 25 mg b.i.d. The usual optimum total daily dose range is 50-200 mg per day.

Psychoneurotic Manifestations: For most patients the usual starting dose is 10 mg t.i.d. The usual optimum total daily dose range is 30-150 mg per day.

Injectable Form: In those situations in which an intramuscular form of medication is indicated, Serentil® (mesoridazine USP) injectable is available. For most patients a starting dose of 25 mg is recommended. The dose may be repeated in 30 to 60 minutes, if necessary. The usual optimum total daily dose range is 25-200 mg per day.

HOW SUPPLIED

Tablets: 10 mg, 25 mg, 50 mg, and 100 mg mesoridazine (as the besylate). Bottles of 100.

Ampuls: 1 ml [25 mg mesoridazine (as the besylate)]. Boxes of 20.

Concentrate: Contains 25 mg mesoridazine (as the besylate) per ml; alcohol, USP, 0.61% by volume. Immediate containers: Amber glass bottles of 4 fl oz (118 ml) packaged in cartons of 12 bottles, with an accompanying dropper graduated to deliver 10 mg, 25 mg and 50 mg of mesoridazine (as the besylate).

STORAGE

Tablets: Below 86°F. Injection: Below 86°F; protect from light. Oral Solution:
Below 77°F. Protect from light. Dispense in amber glass bottles only.

The concentrate may be diluted with distilled water, acidified tap water, orange juice or grape juice.

Each dose should be diluted just prior to administration. Preparation and storage of bulk dilutions is not recommended.

Additional information available to physicians.

PHARMACOLOGY

Pharmacological studies in laboratory animals have established that Serentil® (mesoridazine USP) has a spectrum of pharmacodynamic actions typical of a major tranquilizer. In common with other tranquilizers it inhibits spontaneous motor activity in mice, prolongs thiopental and hexobarbital sleeping time in mice and produces spindles and block of arousal reaction in the EEG of rabbits. It is effective in blocking spinal reflexes in the cat and antagonizes d-amphetamine excitation and toxicity in grouped mice. It shows a moderate adrenergic blocking activity in vitro and in vivo and antagonizes 5-hydroxytryptamine in vivo. Intravenously administered, it lowers the blood pressure of anesthetized dogs. It has a weak antiacetylcholine effect in vitro.

The most outstanding activity of Serentil is seen in tests developed to investigate antiemotive activity of drugs. Such tests are those in which the rat reacts to acute or chronic stress by increased defecation (emotogenic defecation) or tests in which "emotional mydriasis" is elicited in the mouse by an electric shock. In both of these tests Serentil is effective in reducing emotive reactions. Its ED$_{50}$ in inhibiting emotogenic defecation in the rat is 0.053 mg/kg (subcutaneous administration). Serentil has a potent antiemetic action. The intravenous ED$_{50}$ against apomorphine-induced emesis in the dog is 0.64 mg/kg. Serentil, in common with other phenothiazines, demonstrates antiarrhythmic activity in anesthetized dogs.

Metabolic studies in the dog and rabbit with tritium labeled mesoridazine demonstrate that the compound is well absorbed from the gastrointestinal tract. The biological half-life of Serentil in these studies appears to be somewhere between 24 and 48 hours. Although significant urinary excretion was observed following the administration of Serentil, these studies also suggest that biliary excretion is an important excretion route for mesoridazine and/or its metabolites.

Toxicity Studies
Acute LD$_{50}$ (mg/kg):

Route	Mouse	Rat	Rabbit	Dog
Oral	560±62.5	644±48	MLD=800	MLD=800
I.M.	—	509M 584 F	405	—
I.V.	26±0.08	—	—	—

Chronic toxicity studies were conducted in rats and dogs. Rats were administered Serentil, orally seven days per week for a period of 17 months in doses up to 160 mg/kg per day. Dogs were administered Serentil orally seven days per week for a period of 13 months. The daily dosage of the drug was increased during the period of this test such that the "topdose" group received a daily dose of 120 mg/kg of mesoridazine for the last month of the study.

Untoward effects that occurred upon chronic administration of high dose levels included:

Rats: Reduction of food intake, slowed weight gain, morphological changes in pituitary-supported endocrine organs, and melanin-like pigment deposition in renal tissues.

Dogs: Emesis, muscle tremors, decreased food intake and death associated with aspiration of oral-gastric contents into the respiratory system.

Increased intrauterine resorptions were seen with Serentil in rats at 70 mg/kg and in rabbits at 125 mg/kg but not at 60 and 100 mg/kg, respectively. No drug-related teratology was suggested by these reproductive studies.

Local irritation from the intramuscular injection of Serentil was of the same order of magnitude as with other phenothiazines.

Caution: Federal law prohibits dispensing without prescription.

SE-PI-10/87

Shown in Product Identification Section, page 406

THALITONE®   ℞
[*thal'ih-tŏn*]
(chlorthalidone USP)
Tablets of 15 or 25 mg

Prescribing Information

DESCRIPTION

Thalitone® (chlorthalidone USP) is an antihypertensive/diuretic supplied as 15 or 25 mg tablets for oral use. It is a monosulfamyl diuretic that differs chemically from thiazide diuretics in that a double ring system is incorporated in its structure. It is racemic mixture of 2-chloro- 5-(1-hydroxy-

---

3-oxo-1-isoindolinyl) benzenesulfonamide with the following structural formula:

$$C_{14}H_{11}ClN_2O_4S \qquad\qquad 338.76$$

Chlorthalidone is practically insoluble in water, in ether and in chloroform; soluble in methanol, slightly soluble in alcohol.

The inactive ingredients are colloidal silicon dioxide, lactose, magnesium stearate, microcrystalline cellulose, povidone, sodium starch glycolate.

CLINICAL PHARMACOLOGY

Chlorthalidone is a long-acting oral diuretic with antihypertensive activity. Its diuretic action commences a mean of 2.6 hours after dosing and continues for up to 72 hours. The drug produces diuresis with increased excretion of sodium and chloride. The diuretic effects of chlorthalidone and the benzothiadiazine (thiazide) diuretics appear to arise from similar mechanisms and the maximal effect of chlorthalidone and the thiazides appears to be similar. The site of action appears to be the distal convoluted tubule of the nephron. The diuretic effects of chlorthalidone lead to decreased extracellular fluid volume, plasma volume, cardiac output, total exchangeable sodium, glomerular filtration rate, and renal plasma flow. Although the mechanism of action of chlorthalidone and related drugs is not wholly clear, sodium and water depletion appear to provide a basis for its antihypertensive effect. Like the thiazide diuretics, chlorthalidone produces dose-related reductions in serum potassium levels, elevations in serum uric acid and blood glucose, and it can lead to decreased sodium and chloride levels.

The mean plasma half-life of chlorthalidone is about 40 to 60 hours. It is eliminated primarily as unchanged drug in the urine. Non-renal routes of elimination have yet to be clarified. In the blood, approximately 75% of the drug is bound to plasma proteins.

INDICATIONS AND USAGE

Thalitone® (chlorthalidone) is indicated in the management of hypertension, either alone or in combination with other antihypertensive drugs.

Chlorthalidone is indicated as adjunctive therapy in edema associated with congestive heart failure, hepatic cirrhosis and corticosteroid and estrogen therapy.

Chlorthalidone has also been found useful in edema due to various forms of renal dysfunction such as nephrotic syndrome, acute glomerulonephritis, and chronic renal failure.

Usage in Pregnancy: The routine use of diuretics in an otherwise healthy woman is inappropriate and exposes mother and fetus to unnecessary hazard. Diuretics do not prevent development of toxemia of pregnancy and there is no satisfactory evidence that they are useful in the treatment of developed toxemia.

Edema during pregnancy may arise from pathological causes or from the physiologic and mechanical consequences of pregnancy. Chlorthalidone is indicated in pregnancy when edema is due to pathologic causes just as it is in the absence of pregnancy (however, see **WARNINGS** below). Dependent edema in pregnancy resulting from restriction of venous return by the expanded uterus is properly treated through elevation of the lower extremities and use of support hose; use of diuretics to lower intravascular volume in this case is illogical and unnecessary. There is hypervolemia during normal pregnancy that is harmful to neither the fetus nor the mother (in the absence of cardiovascular disease) but that is associated with edema, including generalized edema, in the majority of pregnant women. If this edema produces discomfort, increased recumbency will often provide relief. In rare instances, this edema may cause extreme discomfort that is not relieved by rest. In these cases, a short course of diuretics may provide relief and may be appropriate.

CONTRAINDICATIONS

Anuria
Known hypersensitivity to chlorthalidone or other sulfonamide-derived drugs.

WARNINGS

Thalitone® (chlorthalidone USP) should be used with caution in severe renal disease. In patients with renal disease, chlorthalidone or related drugs may precipitate azotemia. Cumulative effects of the drug may develop in patients with impaired renal function.

Chlorthalidone should be used with caution in patients with impaired hepatic function or progressive liver disease, because minor alterations of fluid and electrolyte balance may precipitate hepatic coma.

Sensitivity reactions may occur in patients with a history of allergy or bronchial asthma.

The possibility of exacerbation or activation of systemic lupus erythematosus has been reported with thiazide diuretics which are structurally related to chlorthalidone. However, systemic lupus erythematosus has not been reported following chlorthalidone administration.

PRECAUTIONS

General: Hypokalemia and other electrolyte abnormalities, including hyponatremia and hypochloremic alkalosis, are common in patients receiving chlorthalidone. These abnormalities are dose-related but may occur even at the lowest marketed doses of chlorthalidone. Serum electrolytes should be determined before initiating therapy and at periodic intervals during therapy. Serum and urine electrolyte determinations are particularly important when the patient is vomiting excessively or receiving parenteral fluids. All patients taking chlorthalidone should be observed for clinical signs of electrolyte imbalance, including dryness of mouth, thirst, weakness, lethargy, drowsiness, restlessness, muscle pains or cramps, muscular fatigue, hypotension, oliguria, tachycardia, palpitations and gastrointestinal disturbances, such as nausea and vomiting. Digitalis therapy may exaggerate metabolic effects of hypokalemia especially with reference to myocardial activity.

Any chloride deficit is generally mild and usually does not require specific treatment except under extraordinary circumstances (as in liver disease or renal disease). Dilutional hyponatremia may occur in edematous patients in hot weather; appropriate therapy is water restriction, rather than administration of salt, except in rare instances when the hyponatremia is life-threatening. In cases of actual salt depletion, appropriate replacement is the therapy of choice.

Uric Acid: Hyperuricemia may occur or frank gout may be precipitated in certain patients receiving chlorthalidone.

Other: Increases in serum glucose may occur and latent diabetes mellitus may become manifest during chlorthalidone therapy (see **PRECAUTIONS** Drug Interactions). Chlorthalidone and related drugs may decrease serum PBI levels without signs of thyroid disturbance.

Information For Patients: Patients should inform their doctor if they have: 1) had an allergic reaction to chlorthalidone or other diuretics or have asthma 2) kidney disease 3) liver disease 4) gout 5) systemic lupus erythematosus, or 6) been taking other drugs such as cortisone, digitalis, lithium carbonate, or drugs for diabetes.

Patients should be cautioned to contact their physician if they experience any of the following symptoms of potassium loss: excess thirst, tiredness, drowsiness, restlessness, muscle pains or cramps, nausea, vomiting or increased heart rate or pulse.

Patients should also be cautioned that taking alcohol can increase the chance of dizziness occurring.

Laboratory Tests: Periodic determination of serum electrolytes to detect possible electrolyte imbalance should be performed at appropriate intervals.

All patients receiving chlorthalidone should be observed for clinical signs of fluid or electrolyte imbalance: namely, hyponatremia, hypochloremic alkalosis and hypokalemia. Serum and urine electrolyte determinations are particularly important when the patient is vomiting excessively or receiving parenteral fluids.

Drug Interactions: Chlorthalidone may add to or potentiate the action of other antihypertensive drugs.

Insulin requirements in diabetic patients may be increased, decreased or unchanged. Higher dosage of oral hypoglycemic agents may be required.

Chlorthalidone and related drugs may increase the responsiveness to tubocurarine.

Chlorthalidone and related drugs may decrease arterial responsiveness to norepinephrine. This diminution is not sufficient to preclude effectiveness of the pressor agent for therapeutic use.

Lithium renal clearance is reduced by chlorthalidone, increasing the risk of lithium toxicity.

Drug/Laboratory Test Interactions: Chlorthalidone and related drugs may decrease serum PBI levels without signs of thyroid disturbance.

Carcinogenesis, Mutagenesis, Impairment of Fertility: No information is available.

Pregnancy/Teratogenic Effects: *PREGNANCY CATEGORY B:* Reproduction studies have been performed in the rat and the rabbit at doses up to 420 times the human dose and have revealed no evidence of impaired fertility or harm to the fetus due to chlorthalidone. There are, however, no adequate and well-controlled studies in pregnant women. Because animal reproduction studies are not always predictive of human response, this drug should be used during pregnancy only if clearly needed.

Pregnancy/Non-Teratogenic Effects: Thiazides cross the placental barrier and appear in cord blood. The use of chlorthalidone and related drugs in pregnant women requires that the anticipated benefits of the drug be weighed against possible hazards to the fetus. These hazards include fetal or neonatal jaundice, thrombocytopenia, and possibly other adverse reactions that have occurred in the adult.

Nursing Mothers: Thiazides are excreted in human milk. Because of the potential for serious adverse reactions in nursing infants from chlorthalidone, a decision should be made whether to discontinue nursing or to discontinue the drug, taking into account the importance of the drug to the mother.

Pediatric Use: Safety and effectiveness in children have not been established.

ADVERSE REACTIONS

The following adverse reactions have been observed but there is not enough systematic collection of data to support an estimate of their frequency.

Gastrointestinal System Reactions: anorexia, gastric irritation, nausea, vomiting, cramping, diarrhea, constipation, jaundice (intrahepatic cholestatic jaundice), pancreatitis.

Central Nervous System Reactions: dizziness, vertigo, paresthesias, headache, xanthopsia.

Hematologic Reactions: leukopenia, agranulocytosis, thrombocytopenia, aplastic anemia.

Dermatologic-Hypersensitivity Reactions: purpura, photosensitivity, rash, urticaria, necrotizing angiitis (vasculitis) (cutaneous vasculitis), Lyell's syndrome (toxic epidermal necrolysis).

Cardiovascular Reaction: Orthostatic hypotension may occur and may be aggravated by alcohol, barbiturates or narcotics.

Other Adverse Reactions: hyperglycemia, glycosuria, hyperuricemia, muscle spasm, weakness, restlessness, impotence. Whenever adverse reactions are moderate or severe, chlorthalidone dosage should be reduced or therapy withdrawn.

OVERDOSAGE

Symptoms of acute overdosage include nausea, weakness, dizziness and disturbances of electrolyte balance. The oral LD_{50} of the drug in the mouse and the rat is more than 25,000 mg/kg body weight. The minimum lethal dose (MLD) in humans has not been established. There is no specific antidote but gastric lavage is recommended, followed by supportive treatment. Where necessary, this may include intravenous dextrose-saline with potassium administered with caution.

DOSAGE AND ADMINISTRATION

Therapy should be initiated with the lowest possible dose, then titrated according to individual patient response. A single dose given in the morning with food is recommended; divided doses are not necessary.

Hypertension: Therapy in most patients should be initiated with a single daily dose of 15 mg. If the response is insufficient after a suitable trial, the dosage may be increased to 30 mg and then to a single daily dose of 45–50 mg. If additional control is required, the addition of a second antihypertensive drug is recommended. Increases in serum uric acid and decreases in serum potassium are dose-related over the 15–50 mg/day range and beyond.

Edema *INITIATION:* Adults, initially 50 to 100 mg daily or 100 mg on alternate days. Some patients may require 150 to 200 mg at these intervals or up to 200 mg daily. Dosages above this level, however, do not usually produce a greater response.

MAINTENANCE: Maintenance doses may often be lower than initial doses and should be adjusted according to the individual patient. Effectiveness is well sustained during continued use.

HOW SUPPLIED

White, kidney-shaped compressed tablets, coded BI/77 containing 15 mg of chlorthalidone in bottles of 100 (NDC 0597-0077-01) and coded BI/76 containing 25 mg of chlorthalidone in bottles of 100 (NDC 0597-0076-01).

Store below 30° C (86° F).

Caution: Federal law prohibits dispensing without prescription.

Th- PI- 11/88

Shown in Product Identification Section, page 406

Bolar Pharmaceutical Co., Inc.
33 RALPH AVENUE
COPIAGUE, NY 11726

CARISOPRODOL COMPOUND TABLETS ℞
(Carisoprodol and Aspirin Tablets, USP)

DESCRIPTION

Carisoprodol compound is a combination product containing carisoprodol, a centrally-acting muscle relaxant, plus aspirin, an analgesic with antipyretic and anti-inflammatory properties. It is available as a two-layered, white and lavender, round tablet for oral administration. Each tablet contains carisoprodol 200 mg and aspirin 325 mg. Chemically, carisoprodol is N-isopropyl-2-methyl-2-propyl-1, 3-propanediol dicarbamate. Its chemical formula is $C_{12}H_{24}N_2O_4$, with a molecular weight of 260.33.

Chemically, aspirin is Benzoic acid, 2-(acetyloxy)-, its chemical formula is $C_9H_8O_4$, with a molecular weight of 180.16.

The chemical structural formulas for carisoprodol and aspirin are as follows:

[See Chemical Formula at top of next column].

ASPIRIN

CARISOPRODOL

Carisoprodol Compound tablets contain: Dibasic Calcium Phosphate, Povidone, Sodium Lauryl Sulfate, Sodium Starch Glycolate, Stearic Acid, FD&C Blue #1 Aluminum Lake, and FD&C Red #3 Aluminum Lake.

CLINICAL PHARMACOLOGY

Carisoprodol: Carisoprodol is a centrally-acting muscle relaxant that does not directly relax tense skeletal muscles in man. The mode of action of carisoprodol in relieving acute muscle spasm of local origin has not been clearly identified, but may be related to its sedative properties. In animals, carisoprodol has been shown to produce muscle relaxation by blocking interneuronal activity and depressing transmission of polysynaptic neurons in the spinal cord and in the descending reticular formation of the brain. The onset of action is rapid and lasts four to six hours.

Carisoprodol is metabolized in the liver and is excreted by the kidneys. It is dialyzable by peritoneal and hemodialysis.

Aspirin: Aspirin is a non-narcotic analgesic with anti-inflammatory and antipyretic activity. Inhibition of prostaglandin biosynthesis appears to account for most of its anti-inflammatory and for at least part of its analgesic and antipyretic properties.

Aspirin is rapidly absorbed and almost totally hydrolyzed to salicylic acid following oral administration. Although aspirin has a half-life of only about 15 minutes, the apparent biologic half-life of salicylic acid in the therapeutic plasma concentration range is between 6 and 12 hours. Salicylic acid is eliminated by renal excretion and by biotransformation to inactive metabolites. Clearance of salicylic acid in the high-dose range is sensitive to urinary pH (see **Drug Interactions**) and is reduced by renal dysfunction.

INDICATIONS AND USAGE

As an adjunct to rest, physical therapy and other measures for the relief of discomfort associated with acute, painful musculoskeletal conditions. The mode of action of carisoprodol has not been clearly identified, but may be related to its sedative properties. Carisoprodol does not directly relax skeletal muscles in man.

CONTRAINDICATIONS

Acute intermittent porphyria; bleeding disorders, allergic or idiosyncratic reactions to carisoprodol, aspirin or related compounds.

WARNINGS

On very rare occasions, the first dose of carisoprodol has been followed by an idiosyncratic reaction with symptoms appearing within minutes or hours. These may include extreme weakness, transient quadriplegia, dizziness, ataxia, temporary loss of vision, diplopia, mydriasis, dysarthia, agitation, euphoria, confusion and disorientation. Although symptoms usually subside over the course of the next several hours, discontinue carisoprodol compound and initiate appropriate supportive and symptomatic therapy, which may include epinephrine and/or antihistamines. In severe cases, corticosteroids may be necessary. Severe reactions have been manifested by asthmatic episodes, fever, weakness, dizziness, angioneurotic edema, smarting eyes, hypotension and anaphylactoid shock.

The effects of carisoprodol with agents such as alcohol, other CNS depressants, or psychotropic drugs may be additive. Appropriate caution should be exercised with patients who may take one or more of these agents simultaneously with carisoprodol compound.

PRECAUTIONS

General: To avoid excessive accumulation of carisoprodol, aspirin, or their metabolites, use carisoprodol compound with caution in patients with compromised liver or kidney function, or in elderly or debilitated patients (see **CLINICAL PHARMACOLOGY**).

Use with caution in patients with history of gastritis or peptic ulcer, in patients on anticoagulant therapy and in addiction-prone individuals.

Information for Patients: Caution patients that this drug may impair the mental and/or physical abilities required for the performance of potentially hazardous tasks such as driving a motor vehicle or operating machinery.

Caution patients with a predisposition for gastrointestinal bleeding that concomitant use of aspirin and alcohol may have an additive effect in this regard.

Continued on next page

Bolar—Cont.

Caution patients that dosage of medications used for gout, arthritis, or diabetes may have to be adjusted when aspirin is administered or discontinued (see **Drug Interactions**).

Drug Interactions: Clinically important interactions may occur when certain drugs are administered concomitantly with aspirin or aspirin-containing drugs.

1. Oral Anticoagulants—By interfering with platelet function or decreasing plasma prothrombin concentration, aspirin enhances the potential for bleeding in patients on anticoagulants.
2. Methotrexate—Aspirin enhances the toxic effects of this drug.
3. Probenecid and Sulfinpyrazone—Large doses of aspirin reduce the uricosuric effect of both drugs. Renal excretion of salicylate may also be reduced.
4. Oral Antidiabetic Drug—Enhancement of hypoglycemia may occur.
5. Antacids—To the extent that they raise urinary pH, antacids may substantially decrease plasma salicylate concentrations: conversely, their withdrawal can result in a substantial increase.
6. Ammonium Chloride—This and other drugs that acidify a relatively alkaline urine can elevate plasma salicylate concentrations.
7. Ethyl Alcohol—Enhanced aspirin-induced fecal blood loss has been reported.
8. Corticosteroids—Salicylate plasma levels may be decreased when adrenal corticosteroids are given, and may be increased substantially when they are discontinued.

Carcinogenesis, Mutagenesis, Impairment of Fertility: No long-term studies have been done with carisoprodol compound.

Pregnancy-Teratogenic Effects: Pregnancy Category C. Adequate animal reproduction studies have not been conducted with carisoprodol compound. It is also not known whether carisoprodol compound can cause fetal harm when administered to a pregnant woman or can affect reproduction capacity. Carisoprodol compound should be given to a pregnant woman only if clearly needed.

Studies in rodents have shown salicylates to be teratogenic when given in early gestation, and embryocidal when given in later gestation in doses considerably greater than usual therapeutic dose in humans. Studies in women who took aspirin during pregnancy have not demonstrated an increased incidence of congenital abnormalities in the offspring.

Labor and Delivery: Ingestion of aspirin near term or prior to delivery may prolong delivery or lead to bleeding in mother, fetus or neonate.

Nursing Mothers: Carisoprodol is excreted in human milk in concentrations two-to-four times that in maternal plasma. Aspirin is excreted in human milk in moderate amounts and can produce a bleeding tendency in nursing infants. Because of the potential for serious adverse reactions in nursing infants, a decision should be made whether to discontinue nursing or the drug, taking into account the importance of the drug to the mother.

Pediatric Use: Safety and effectiveness in children below the age of twelve have not been established.

ADVERSE REACTIONS

If severe reactions occur, discontinue carisoprodol compound and initiate appropriate symptomatic and supportive therapy.

The following side effects which have occurred with the administration of the individual ingredients alone may also occur with the combination.

Carisoprodol:

Central Nervous System: Drowsiness is the most frequent complaint and along with other CNS effects may require dosage reduction. Observed less frequently are dizziness, vertigo and ataxia. Tremor, agitation, irritability, headache, depressive reactions, syncope and insomnia have been infrequent or rare.

Idiosyncratic: Idiosyncratic reactions are very rare. They are usually seen within the period of the first to fourth dose in patients having had no previous contact with the drug (see **WARNINGS**).

Allergic: Skin rash, erythema multiforme, pruritus, eosinophilia and fixed drug eruptions with cross-reaction to meprobamate have been reported. If allergic reactions occur, discontinue carisoprodol compound and treat symptomatically. In evaluating possible allergic reactions, also consider allergy to excipients (information on excipients is available to physicians on request).

Cardiovascular: Tachycardia, postural hypotension and facial flushing.

Gastrointestinal: Nausea, vomiting, epigastric distress and hiccup.

Hematologic: No serious blood dyscrasias have been attributed to carisoprodol alone. Leukopenia and pancytopenia have been reported, very rarely, in situations in which other drugs or viral infections may have been responsible.

Aspirin: The most common adverse reactions associated with the use of aspirin have been gastrointestinal, including nausea, vomiting, gastritis, occult bleeding, constipation and diarrhea. Gastric erosion, angioedema, asthma, rash, pruritus and urticaria have been reported less commonly. Tinnitus is a sign of high serum salicylate levels (see **OVERDOSAGE**).

Aspirin Intolerance: Allergic type reactions in aspirin-sensitive individuals may involve the respiratory tract or the skin. Symptoms of the former range from rhinorrhea and shortness of breath to severe asthma, and the latter may consist of urticaria, edema, rash or angioedema (giant hives). These may occur independently or in combination.

DRUG ABUSE AND DEPENDENCE

Abuse: In clinical use, abuse has been rare.

Dependence: In clinical use, dependence with carisoprodol compound has been rare and there have been no reports of significant abstinence signs. Nevertheless, the following information on the individual ingredients should be kept in mind.

Carisoprodol: In dogs, no withdrawal symptoms occurred after abrupt cessation of carisoprodol from dosages as high as 1 gm/kg/day. In a study in man, abrupt cessation of 100 mg/kg/day (about five times the recommended daily adult dosage) was followed in some subjects by mild withdrawal symptoms such as abdominal cramps, insomnia, chills, headache and nausea. Delirium and convulsions did not occur (see **PRECAUTIONS**).

OVERDOSAGE

Signs and Symptoms: Any of the following which have been reported with the individual ingredients may occur and may be modified to a varying degree by the effects of the other ingredients present in carisoprodol compound.

Carisoprodol: Stupor, coma, shock, respiratory depression and very rarely, death. Overdosage with carisoprodol in combination with alcohol, other CNS depressants, or psychotropic agents can have additive effects, even when one of the agents has been taken in the usually recommended dosage.

Aspirin: Headache, tinnitus, hearing difficulty, dim vision, dizziness, lassitude, hyperpnea, rapid breathing, thirst, nausea, vomiting, sweating and occasionally diarrhea are characteristic of mild to moderate salicylate poisoning. Salicylate poisoning should be considered in children with symptoms of vomiting, hyperpnea, and hyperthermia. Hyperpnea is an early sign of salicylate poisoning, but dyspnea supervenes at plasma levels above 50 mg/dl. These respiratory changes eventually lead to serious acid-base disturbances. Metabolic acidosis is a constant finding in infants but occurs in older children only with severe poisoning; adults usually exhibit respiratory alkalosis initially and acidosis terminally.

Other symptoms of severe salicylate poisoning include hyperthermia, dehydration, delirium and mental disturbances. Skin eruptions, GI hemorrhage, or pulmonary edema are less common. Early CNS stimulation is replaced by increasing depression, stupor and coma. Death is usually due to respiratory failure or cardiovascular collapse.

Treatment-General: Provide symptomatic and supportive treatment, as indicated. Any drug remaining in the stomach should be removed using appropriate procedures and caution to protect the airway and prevent aspiration, especially in the stuporous or comatose patient. Incomplete gastric emptying with delayed absorption of carisoprodol has been reported as a cause for relapse. Should respiration or blood pressure become compromised, respiratory assistance, central nervous system stimulants and pressor agents should be administered cautiously, as indicated.

Carisoprodol: The following have been used successfully in overdosage with the related drug meprobamate: diuretics, osmotic (mannitol) diuresis, peritoneal dialysis, and hemodialysis (see **CLINICAL PHARMACOLOGY**). Careful monitoring of urinary output is necessary and caution should be taken to avoid overhydration. Carisoprodol can be measured in biological fluid by gas chromatography (Douglas, J.F., et al: J Pharm Sci 58:145, 1969).

Aspirin: Since there are no specific antidotes for salicylate poisoning, the aim of treatment is to enhance elimination of salicylate and prevent or reduce further absorption; to correct any fluid electrolyte or metabolic imbalance; and to provide general and cardiorespiratory support. If acidosis is present, intravenous sodium bicarbonate must be given, along with adequate hydration, until salicylate levels decrease to within the therapeutic range. To enhance elimination, forced diuresis and alkalinization of the urine may be beneficial. The need for hemoperfusion or hemodialysis is rare and should be used only when other measures have failed.

DOSAGE AND ADMINISTRATION

Usual Adult Dosage: 1 or 2 tablets, four times daily. Not recommended for use in children under age twelve (see **PRECAUTIONS**).

HOW SUPPLIED

—Tablets containing 200 mg of Carisoprodol and 325 mg of Aspirin.

—White and lavender colored, double layered, round shape, unscored tablet debossed with Bolar logo on one side and product identification number 144 on the other side of tablet

—Bottles of 100, 500 and 1000

- 100 NDC # 0725-0144-01
   500 NDC # 0725-0144-05
 1000 NDC # 0725-0144-10

STORE AT CONTROLLED ROOM TEMPERATURE 15°–30°C (59°–86°F)

CAUTION

Federal law prohibits dispensing without prescription.
PROTECT FROM MOISTURE
REVISION DATE: FEBRUARY 1989
MANUFACTURED BY: Bolar Pharmaceutical Co., Inc., Copiague, New York 11726   9B
Shown in Product Identification Section, page 406

DISOPYRAMIDE PHOSPHATE   ℞ CONTROLLED-RELEASE CAPSULES

DESCRIPTION

Disopyramide phosphate is an antiarrhythmic drug available for oral administration in controlled-release capsules equivalent to 100 mg and 150 mg of disopyramide base. The base content of the phosphate salt is 77.66%. The structural formula of disopyramide phosphate is:

$[(CH_3)_2CH]_2NCH_2\,CH_2CCONH_2 \cdot H_3PO_4$

α-[2-(Diisopropylamino)ethyl]-α-phenyl-2-pyridineacetamide phosphate (1:1) 22059-60-5
Disopyramide phosphate is freely soluble in water, and the free base (pKa 10.4) has an aqueous solubility of 1mg/ml. The chloroform water partition coefficient of the base is 3.1 at pH 7.2.

Disopyramide phosphate is a racemic mixture of d-and l-isomers. This drug is not chemically related to other antiarrhythmic drugs.

Disopyramide Phosphate Controlled-Release Capsules are designed to afford a gradual and consistent release of disopyramide. Thus, for maintenance therapy, Disopyramide Phosphate Controlled-Release Capsules provide the benefit of less frequent dosing (every 12 hours) as compared with the every-6-hour dosage schedule of immediate-release capsules.

Disopyramide Phosphate Controlled-Release Capsules contain corn starch, cellulose derivatives, dye (FD&C Blue #1, FD&C Red #40, D&C Red #28, D&C Yellow #10), gelatin, pharmaceutical glaze, povidone, sucrose, titanium dioxide, and other ingredients.

CLINICAL PHARMACOLOGY

Mechanisms of Action:
Disopyramide phosphate is a Type 1 antiarrhythmic drug (i.e., similar to procainamide and quinidine). **In animal studies**, disopyramide phosphate decreases the rate of diastolic depolarization (phase 4) in cells with augmented automaticity, decreases the upstroke velocity (phase 0) and increases the action potential duration of normal cardiac cells, decreases the disparity in refractoriness between infarcted and adjacent normally perfused myocardium and has no effect on alpha- or beta-adrenergic receptors.

Electrophysiology:
In man, disopyramide at therapeutic plasma levels shorten the sinus node recovery time, lengthens the effective refractory period of the atrium, and has a minimal effect on the effective refractory period of the AV node. Little effect has been shown on AV-nodal and His-Purkinje conduction times or QRS duration. However, prolongation of conduction in accessory pathways occur.

Hemodynamics:
At recommended oral doses, disopyramide phosphate rarely produces significant alterations of blood pressure in patients without congestive heart failure (See WARNINGS). With intravenous disopyramide phosphate, either increases in systolic/diastolic or decreases in systolic blood pressure have been reported, depending on the infusion rate and the patient population. Intravenous disopyramide phosphate may cause cardiac depression with an approximate mean 10% reduction of cardiac output, which is more pronounced in patients with cardiac dysfunction.

Anticholinergic Activity
The **in vitro** anticholinergic activity of disopyramide is approximately 0.06% that of atropine, however, the usual dose for disopyramide is 150 mg every 6 hours and for Disopyra-

mide Phosphate Controlled-Release 300 mg every 12 hours compared to 0.4–0.6 mg for atropine (see WARNINGS and ADVERSE REACTIONS for anticholinergic side effects).

Pharmacokinetics:
The usual therapeutic plasma levels of disopyramide base are 2–4 mcg/ml and at these concentrations protein binding varies from 50–65%. Because of concentration-dependent protein binding, it is difficult to predict the concentration of the free drug when total drug is measured.

The mean plasma half-life of disopyramide in healthy humans is 6.7 hours (range of 4 to 10 hours). In patients with impaired renal function (creatinine clearance less than 40 ml/min), disopyramide half-life values were 8 to 18 hours. After the administration of 200 mg of immediate-release disopyramide to 10 cardiac patients with borderline to moderate heart failure, the time to peak serum concentration was increased to 2.3 ($\pm$1.5) hours from 2.0 hours. The mean peak serum concentration was increased to 4.8 ($\pm$1.6) mcg/ml from the 2-4 mcg/ml range found in normal healthy volunteers. After intravenous administration in these same patients, the mean elimination half-life was 9.7 ($\pm$4.2) hours, compared to a range in healthy volunteers of 4.4 to 7.8 hours. In a second study of the oral administration of disopyramide in patients with heart disease, including left ventricular dysfunction, the mean plasma half-life was slightly prolonged to 7.8 ($\pm$1.9) hours, with a range of 5.0 to 9.5 hours. In healthy men, about 50% of a given dose of disopyramide is excreted in the urine as the unchanged drug, about 20% as the mono-N-dealkylated metabolite and 10% as the other metabolites. The plasma concentration of the major metabolite is approximately one tenth that of disopyramide. Altering the urinary pH in man does not affect the plasma half-life of disopyramide.

In a single-dose crossover study in 12 healthy subjects, the mean peak serum concentration of disopyramide following a single 150 mg oral dose of KV's Disopyramide Phosphate Controlled-Release Capsules was 2.39 ($\pm$0.89) mcg/ml, achieved at 5.58 ($\pm$1.44) hours. Following multiple doses (300 mg every 12 hours), of KV's Disopyramide Phosphate Controlled-Release Capsules, steady-state plasma levels of between 2 and 4 mcg/ml were attained. Total bioavailability was shown to be similar to an immediate-release product.

INDICATIONS AND USAGE
Disopyramide Phosphate Controlled-Release Capsules should be prescribed only after appropriate electrocardiographic assessment.

Disopyramide Phosphate Controlled-Release Capsules are indicated for suppression and prevention of recurrence of the following cardiac arrhythmias when they occur singly or in combination:
1. Unifocal premature (ectopic) ventricular contractions.
2. Premature (ectopic) ventricular contractions of multifocal origin.
3. Paired premature ventricular contractions (couplets).
4. Episodes of ventricular tachycardia (persistent ventricular tachycardia is ordinarily treated with D.C. cardioversion).

In controlled trials of ambulatory patients, 150 mg of disopyramide every 6 hours was as effective as 325 mg of quinidine every 6 hours in reducing the frequency of ventricular ectopic activity. Disopyramide phosphate was equally effective in digitalized and nondigitalized patients. Disopyramide phosphate is also equally effective in the treatment of primary cardiac arrhythmias and those which occur in association with organic heart disease including coronary artery disease.

Oral disopyramide phosphate has not been adequately studied in patients with acute myocardial infarction or in patients with persistent ventricular tachycardia or atrial arrhythmias.

Disopyramide Phosphate Controlled-Release Capsules should not be used initially if rapid establishment of disopyramide plasma levels are desired.

Type 1 antiarrhythmic drugs are usually not effective in treating arrhythmias secondary to digitalis intoxication and therefore, Disopyramide Phosphate Controlled-Release Capsules are not indicated for such cases.

The value of antiarrhythmic drugs in preventing sudden death in patients with serious ventricular ectopic activity has not been established.

CONTRAINDICATIONS
Disopyramide Phosphate Controlled-Release Capsules are contraindicated in the presence of cardiogenic shock, preexisting second- or third-degree AV block (if no pacemaker is present), congenital Q-T prolongation, or known hypersensitivity to the drug.

WARNINGS
Negative Inotropic Properties:
Heart Failure/Hypotension
Disopyramide may cause or worsen congestive heart failure or produce severe hypotension as a consequence of its negative inotropic properties. Hypotension has been observed primarily in patients with primary cardiomyopathy or inadequately compensated congestive heart failure. Disopyra-

mide phosphate should not be used in patients with uncompensated or marginally compensated congestive heart failure or hypotension unless the congestive heart failure or hypotension is secondary to cardiac arrhythmia. Patients with a history of heart failure may be treated with disopyramide but careful attention must be given to the maintenance of cardiac function, including optimal digitalization. If hypotension occurs or congestive heart failure worsens, disopyramide should be discontinued and, if necessary, restarted at a lower dosage only after adequate cardiac compensation has been established.

QRS Widening:
Although it is unusual, significant widening (greater than 25%) of QRS complex may occur during disopyramide administration; in such cases disopyramide phosphate should be discontinued.

Q-T Prolongation:
As with other Type 1 antiarrhythmic drugs, prolongation of the Q-T interval (corrected) and worsening of the arrhythmia, including ventricular tachycardia and ventricular fibrillation may occur. Patients who have evidenced prolongation of the Q-T interval in response to quinidine may be at particular risk. If a Q-T prolongation of greater than 25% is observed and if ectopy continues, the patient should be monitored closely, and consideration be given to discontinuing disopyramide phosphate.

Hypoglycemia:
In rare instances significant lowering of blood glucose values has been reported during disopyramide phosphate administration. The physician should be alert to this possibility, especially in patients with congestive heart failure, chronic malnutrition, hepatic, renal or other diseases or drugs (e.g., beta adrenoceptor blockers, alcohol) which could compromise preservation of the normal glucoregulatory mechanisms in the absence of food. In these patients the blood glucose levels should be carefully followed.

Concomitant Antiarrhythmic Therapy:
The concomitant use of disopyramide phosphate with other Type 1 antiarrhythmic agents (such as quinidine or procainamide) and/or propranolol should be reserved for patients with life-threatening arrhythmias who are demonstrably unresponsive to single-agent antiarrhythmic therapy. Such use may produce serious negative inotropic effects, or may excessively prolong conduction. This should be considered particularly in patients with any degree of cardiac decompensation or those with a prior history thereof. Patients receiving more than one antiarrhythmic drug must be carefully monitored.

Heart Block:
If first-degree heart block develops in a patient receiving disopyramide phosphate, the dosage should be reduced. If the block persists despite reduction of dosage, continuation of the drug must depend upon weighing the benefit being obtained against the risk of higher degrees of heart block. Development of second- or third-degree AV block or unifascicular, bifascicular or trifascicular block requires discontinuation of disopyramide phosphate therapy, unless the ventricular rate is adequately controlled by a temporary or implanted ventricular pacemaker.

Anticholinergic Activity:
Because of its anticholinergic activity, disopyramide phosphate should not be used in patients with glaucoma, myasthenia gravis or urinary retention unless adequate overriding measures are taken; these consist of the topical application of potent miotics (e.g., pilocarpine) for patients with glaucoma, and catheter drainage or operative relief for patients with urinary retention. Urinary retention may occur in patients of either sex as a consequence of disopyramide phosphate administration, but males with benign prostatic hypertrophy are at particular risk. In patients with a family history of glaucoma, intraocular pressure should be measured before initiating therapy. Disopyramide phosphate should be used with special care in patients with myasthenia gravis since its anticholinergic properties could precipitate a myasthenic crisis in such patients.

PRECAUTIONS
General
Atrial Tachyarrhythmias:
Patients with atrial flutter or fibrillation should be digitalized prior to disopyramide administration to ensure that drug-induced enhancement of AV conduction does not result in an increase of ventricular rate beyond physiologically acceptable limits.

Conduction Abnormalities:
Care should be taken when prescribing disopyramide phosphate for patients with sick sinus syndrome (bradycardia-tachycardia syndrome). Wolff-Parkinson-White syndrome (WPW), or bundle branch block. The effect of disopyramide in these conditions is uncertain at present.

Cardiomyopathy:
Patients with myocarditis or other cardiomyopathy may develop significant hypotension in response to the usual dosage of disopyramide, probably due to cardiodepressant mechanisms. Therefore, a loading dose of disopyramide phosphate should not be given to such patients and initial dosage and

subsequent dosage adjustments should be made under close supervision (see DOSAGE AND ADMINISTRATION).
Renal Impairment:
More than 50% of disopyramide is excreted in the urine unchanged. Therefore, dosage should be reduced in patients with impaired renal function (see DOSAGE AND ADMINISTRATION). The electrocardiogram should be carefully monitored for prolongation of PR interval, evidence of QRS widening or other signs of overdosage (see OVERDOSAGE). Disopyramide phosphate is not recommended for patients with severe renal insufficiency (creatinine clearance 40 ml/min. or less).

Hepatic Impairment:
Hepatic impairment also causes an increase in the plasma half-life of disopyramide. Dosage should be reduced for patients with such impairment. The electrocardiogram should be carefully monitored for signs of overdosage (see OVERDOSAGE).
Patients with cardiac dysfunction have a higher potential for hepatic impairment; this should be considered when administering disopyramide phosphate.

Potassium Imbalance:
Antiarrhythmic drugs may be ineffective in patients with hypokalemia, and their toxic effects may be enhanced in patients with hyperkalemia. Therefore, potassium abnormalities should be corrected before starting disopyramide phosphate therapy.

Drug Interactions:
If phenytoin or other hepatic enzyme inducers are taken concurrently with disopyramide phosphate lower plasma levels of disopyramide may occur. Monitoring of disopyramide plasma levels is recommended in such concurrent use to avoid ineffective therapy. Other antiarrhythmic drugs (e.g., quinidine, procainamide, lidocaine, propranolol) have occasionally been used concurrently with disopyramide phosphate. Excessive widening of the QRS complex and/or prolongation of the Q-T interval may occur in these situations (see WARNINGS). In healthy subjects, no significant drug-drug interaction was observed when disopyramide phosphate was coadministered with either propranolol or diazepam. Concomitant administration of disopyramide phosphate and quinidine resulted in slight increases in plasma disopyramide levels and slight decreases in plasma quinidine levels. Disopyramide does not increase serum digoxin levels.

Carcinogenesis, Mutagenesis, Impairment Of Fertility:
Eighteen months of disopyramide phosphate administration to rats, at oral doses of up to 400 mg/kg/day of disopyramide (about 30 times the usual daily human dose of 600 mg/day, assuming a patient weight of at least 50 kg), revealed no evidence of carcinogenic potential. An evaluation of mutagenic potential by Ames test was negative. Disopyramide at doses up to 250 mg/kg/day, did not adversely affect fertility of rats.

Pregnancy:
Teratogenic effects: Pregnancy Category C. Disopyramide was associated with decreased numbers of implantation sites and decreased growth and survival of pups when administered to pregnant rats at 250 mg/kg/day (20 or more times the usual daily human dose of 12 mg/kg, assuming a patient weight of at least 50 kg), a level at which weight gain and food consumption of dams were also reduced. Increased resorption rates were reported in rabbits at 60 mg/kg/day (5 or more times the usual daily human dose). Effects on implantation, pup growth, and survival were not evaluated in rabbits. There are no adequate and well-controlled studies in pregnant women. Disopyramide Phosphate Controlled-Release Capsules should be used during pregnancy only if the potential benefit justifies the potential risk to the fetus.
Nonteratogenic Effects: Disopyramide has been reported to stimulate contractions of the pregnant uterus. Disopyramide has been found in human fetal blood.

Labor And Delivery:
It is not known whether the use of disopyramide phosphate during labor or delivery has immediate or delayed adverse effects on the fetus or whether it prolongs the duration of labor or increases the need for forceps delivery or other obstetric intervention.

Nursing Mothers:
Studies in rats have shown that the concentration of disopyramide and its metabolites is between one and three times greater in milk than it is in plasma. Following oral administration disopyramide has been detected in human milk at a concentration not exceeding that in plasma. Because of the potential for serious adverse reactions in nursing infants from Disopyramide Phosphate Controlled-Release Capsules a decision should be made whether to discontinue nursing or to discontinue the drug, taking into account the importance of the drug to the mother.

ADVERSE REACTIONS
The adverse reactions which were reported in disopyramide phosphate clinical trials encompass observations in 1,500 patients, including 90 patients studied for at least 4 years.

Continued on next page

Bolar—Cont.

The most serious adverse reactions are hypotension and congestive heart failure. The most common adverse reactions which are dose dependent are associated with the anticholinergic properties of the drug. These may be transitory but may be persistent or can be severe. Urinary retention is the most serious anticholinergic effect.

The following reactions were reported in 10–40% of patients:
Anticholinergic: dry mouth (32%), urinary hesitancy (14%), constipation (11%)

The following reactions were reported in 3–9% of patients:
Anticholinergic: blurred vision, dry nose/eyes/throat.
Genitourinary: urinary retention, urinary frequency and urgency.
Gastrointestinal: nausea, pain/bloating/gas.
General: dizziness, general fatigue/muscle weakness, headache, malaise, aches/pains.

The following reactions were reported in 1–3% of patients:
Genitourinary: impotence.
Cardiovascular: hypotension with or without congestive heart failure, increased congestive heart failure (see WARNINGS), cardiac conduction disturbances (see WARNINGS), edema/weight gain, shortness of breath, syncope, chest pain.
Gastrointestinal: anorexia, diarrhea, vomiting.
Dermatologic: generalized rash/dermatoses, itching.
Central nervous system: nervousness.
Other: hypokalemia, elevated cholesterol/triglycerides.

The following reactions were reported in less than 1%:
Depression, insomnia, dysuria, numbness/tingling, elevated liver enzymes, AV block, elevated BUN, elevated creatinine, decreased hemoglobin/hematocrit.
Hypoglycemia has been reported in association with disopyramide phosphate administration (see WARNINGS).

Infrequent occurrences of reversible cholestatic jaundice, fever, and respiratory difficulty have been reported in association with disopyramide therapy as have rare instances of thrombocytopenia, reversible agranulocytosis and gynecomastia. Some cases of LE (lupus erythematosus) symptoms have been reported; most cases occurred in patients who had been switched to disopyramide from procainamide following the development of LE symptoms. Rarely, acute psychosis has been reported following disopyramide phosphate therapy, with prompt return to normal mental status when therapy was stopped. The physician should be aware of these possible reactions and should discontinue disopyramde phosphate therapy promptly if they occur.

OVERDOSAGE

Symptoms
Deliberate or accidental overdose of oral disopyramide may be followed by apnea, loss of consciousness, cardiac arrhythmias and loss of spontaneous respiration. Death has occurred following overdose.
Toxic plasma levels of disopyramide produce excessive widening of the QRS complex and Q-T interval, worsening of congestive heart failure, hypotension, varying kinds and degrees of conduction disturbance, bradycardia, and finally asystole. Obvious anticholinergic effects are also observed. The approximate oral LD_{50} disopyramide phosphate is 580 and 700 mg/kg for rats and mice, respectively.

Treatment
Experience indicates that prompt and vigorous treatment of overdosage is necessary, even in the absence of symptoms. Such treatment may be lifesaving. No specific antidote for disopyramide phosphate has been identified. Treatment should be symptomatic and may include induction of emesis or gastric lavage, administration of a cathartic followed by activated charcoal by mouth or stomach tube, intravenous administration of isoproterenol and dopamine, insertion of an intra-aortic balloon for counterpulsation, and mechanically assisted ventilation. Hemodialysis or, preferably, hemoperfusion with charcoal may be employed to lower serum concentration of the drug.
The electrocardiogram should be monitored, and supportive therapy with cardiac glycosides and diuretics should be given as required.
If progressive AV block should develop, endocardial pacing should be implemented. In case of any impaired renal function, measures to increase the glomerular filtration rate may reduce the toxicity (disopyramide is excreted primarily by the kidney).
The anticholinergic effects can be reversed with neostigmine at the discretion of the physician.
Altering the urinary pH in humans does not affect the plasma half-life or the amount of disopyramide excreted in the urine.

DOSAGE AND ADMINISTRATION

The dosage of disopyramide (as the phosphate) must be individualized for each patient on the basis of response and tolerance. The usual adult dosage of disopyramide is 400 to 800 mg per day given in divided doses. The recommended dosage

---

for most adults is 600 mg/day given in divided doses. For patients whose body weight is less than 110 pounds (50 kg), the recommended dosage is 400 mg/day given in divided doses.

For patients with cardiomyopathy or possible cardiac decompensation, a loading dose should not be given, initial dosage should be limited to 100 mg of immediate-release disopyramide every 6–8 hours. Subsequent dosage adjustments should be made gradually, with close monitoring for the possible development of hypotension and/or congestive heart failure (see WARNINGS).

For patients with moderate renal insufficiency (creatinine clearance greater than 40 ml/min) or hepatic insufficiency, the recommended dosage is 400 mg/day given in divided doses.

Disopyramide Phosphate Controlled-Release Capsules are not recommended for patients with severe renal insufficiency.

Disopyramide Phosphate Controlled-Release Capsules should not be used initially if rapid establishment of disopyramide plasma levels is desired.

Transferring to Disopyramide Phosphate Controlled-Release Capsules:
The following dosage schedule based on theoretical considerations rather than experimental data is suggested for transferring patients with normal renal function from either quinidine sulfate or procainamide therapy (Type 1 antiarrhythmic agents) to Disopyramide Phosphate Controlled-Release Capsules therapy.
Disopyramide Phosphate Controlled-Release Capsules should be started using the regular maintenance schedule **without a loading dose** 6–12 hours after the last dose of quinidine sulfate or 3–6 hours after the last dose of procainamide. In patients where withdrawal of quinidine sulfate or procainamide is likely to produce life-threatening arrhythmias, the physician should consider hospitalization of the patient. When transferring a patient from immediate-release disopyramide to Disopyramide Controlled-Release, the maintenance schedule of Disopyramide Phosphate Controlled-Release Capsules may be started 6 hours after the last dose of immediate-release disopyramide phosphate capsules.

Pediatric Dosage:
Controlled clinical studies have not been conducted in pediatric patients.

HOW SUPPLIED

100 mg
—Capsules containing 100 mg of disopyramide (as the phosphate) in controlled-release beads.
—Purple and yellow capsule printed BOLAR/KV and DISO-$^{12}/_{100}$ on the capsule.
—Bottles of 100, 500, and 1000.

150 mg
—Capsules containing 150 mg of disopyramide (as the phosphate) in controlled-release beads.
—Purple and orange capsule printed BOLAR/KV and DISO-$^{12}/_{150}$ on the capsule.
—Bottles of 100, 500 and 1,000
Store at controlled room temperature 15°–30°C (59°–86°F).

CAUTION
Federal Law Prohibits Dispensing Without Prescription
REVISION DATE: August 1988

Manufactured For:
Bolar Pharmaceutical Co., Inc.
Copiague, NY 11726
Manufactured By:
KV Pharmaceutical Company
St. Louis, Missouri 63144   8H
Shown in Product Identification Section, page 406

NITROFURANTOIN CAPSULES   ℞
(Macrocrystalline)

DESCRIPTION
Macrocrystalline nitrofurantoin is a synthetic chemical of controlled crystal size. It is a stable, yellow crystalline compound. Nitrofurantoin is an antibacterial agent for specific urinary tract infections. It is available in 50 mg and 100 mg capsules for oral administration. Its chemical formula is $C_8H_6N_4O_5$ and is designated chemically as 1-[(5-Nitrofurfurylidene)amino]hydantoin. It has the following chemical structure:

Inactive Ingredients: Gelatin, Magnesium Stearate, Pregelatinized Starch, Talc, Titanium Dioxide, D&C Yellow #10 and FD&C Yellow #6.

CLINICAL PHARMACOLOGY
Macrocrystalline nitrofurantoin is a larger crystal form of nitrofurantoin. The absorption of macrocrystalline nitrofurantoin is slower and its excretion somewhat less when compared to microcrystalline nitrofurantoin. Blood concentrations at therapeutic dosage are usually low. Many patients who cannot tolerate microcrystalline nitrofurantoin are able to take nitrofurantoin macrocrystalline capsules without nausea. It is highly soluble in urine, to which it may impart a brown color.
Unlike many drugs, the presence of food or agents delaying gastric emptying can increase the bioavailability of macrocrystalline nitrofurantoin, presumably by allowing better dissolution in gastric juices.
Microbiology: Nitrofurantoin, *in vitro*, is bacteriostatic in low concentrations (5–10 mcg/mL) and is considered to be bactericidal in higher concentrations. Its mode of action is presumed to be interference with several bacterial enzyme systems. Bacteria develop only a limited resistance to furan derivatives.
While *in vitro* studies have demonstrated the susceptibility of most strains of the following organisms, clinically efficacy for infections other than those included in the INDICATIONS AND USAGE section has not been documented.
Escherichia coli, enterococci (e.g., *Streptococcus faecalis*), *Staphylococcus aureus, Staphylococcus epidermidis.*
NOTE: Some strains of *Enterobacter* species and *Klebsiella* species, are resistant to nitrofurantoin. It is not active against most strains of *Proteus* and *Serratia* species. It has no activity against *Pseudomonas* species.
Antagonism has been demonstrated between nitrofurantoin and both nalidixic acid and oxolinic acid *in vitro*.
Susceptibility Tests—Quantitative methods that require measurement of zone diameters give the most precise estimates of antimicrobial susceptibility. One recommended procedure (NCCLS, ASM-2)*, uses a disc containing 300 micrograms for testing susceptibility; interpretations correlate zone diameters of this disc test with MIC values for nitrofurantoin. Reports from the laboratory should be interpreted according to the following criteria:
Susceptible organisms produce zones of 17 mm or greater, indicating that the tested organism is likely to respond to therapy.
Organisms of intermediate susceptibility produce zones of 15 to 16 mm, indicating that the tested organism would be susceptible if high dosage is used.
Resistant organisms produce zones of 14 mm or less, indicating that other therapy should be selected.
A bacterial isolate may be considered susceptible if the MIC value for nitrofurantoin is 25 micrograms per mL or less. Organisms are considered resistant if the MIC is 100 micrograms per mL or more.
NOTE: Specimens for culture and susceptibility testing should be obtained prior to and during drug administration.

INDICATIONS AND USAGE
Nitrofurantoin capsules (macrocrystalline) are specifically indicated for the treatment of urinary tract infections when due to susceptible strains of *E. coli*, enterococci, *S. aureus* (it is not indicated for the treatment of associated renal cortical or perinephric abscesses), and certain susceptible strains of *Klebsiella, Enterobacter* and *Proteus* species.

CONTRAINDICATIONS
Anuria, oliguria, or significant impairment of renal function (creatinine clearance under 40 mL per minute) are contraindications. Treatment of this type of patient carries an increased risk of toxicity because of impaired excretion of the drug.
The drug is contraindicated in pregnant patients at term (during labor and delivery) as well as in infants under one month of age because of the possibility of hemolytic anemia in the fetus or in the newborn infant due to immature enzyme systems (glutathione instability).
The drug is also contraindicated in those patients with known hypersensitivity to nitrofurantoin.

WARNINGS
**ACUTE, SUBACUTE, OR CHRONIC PULMONARY REACTIONS HAVE BEEN OBSERVED IN PATIENTS TREATED WITH NITROFURANTOIN. IF THESE REACTIONS OCCUR, NITROFURANTOIN SHOULD BE DISCONTINUED AND APPROPRIATE MEASURES TAKEN. REPORTS HAVE CITED PULMONARY REACTIONS AS A CONTRIBUTING CAUSE OF DEATH.
CHRONIC PULMONARY REACTIONS (DIFFUSE INTERSTITIAL PNEUMONITIS OR PULMONARY FIBROSIS, OR BOTH) CAN DEVELOP INSIDIOUSLY. THESE REACTIONS OCCUR RARELY AND GENERALLY IN PATIENTS RECEIVING THERAPY FOR SIX MONTHS OR LONGER. CLOSE MONITORING OF THE PULMONARY CONDITION OF PATIENTS RECEIVING LONG-TERM THERAPY IS WARRANTED AND REQUIRES THAT THE BENEFITS OF THERAPY BE WEIGHED AGAINST POTENTIAL RISKS (SEE RESPIRATORY REACTIONS).**

Hepatitis, including chronic hepatitis, occurs rarely. Fatalities have been reported. The onset of chronic active hepatitis may be insidious, and patients receiving long-term therapy should be monitored periodically for changes in liver function. If hepatitis occurs, the drug should be withdrawn immediately and appropriate measures should be taken.

Peripheral neuropathy which may become severe or irreversible has occurred. Fatalities have been reported. Conditions such as renal impairment (creatinine clearance under 40 mL per minute), anemia, diabetes mellitus, electrolyte imbalance, vitamin B deficiency, and debilitating disease may enhance such occurrence of peripheral neuropathy.

Cases of hemolytic anemia of the primaquine sensitivity type have been induced by nitrofurantoin. Hemolysis appears to be linked to a glucose-6-phosphate dehydrogenase deficiency in the red blood cells of the affected patients. This deficiency is found in 10 percent of blacks and a small percentage of ethnic groups of Mediterranean and Near-Eastern origin. Hemolysis is an indication to discontinuing nitrofurantoin. Hemolysis ceases when the drug is withdrawn.

PRECAUTIONS

Drug Interactions: Magnesium trisilicate, when administered concomitantly with nitrofurantoin, reduces both the rate and extent of absorption. The mechanism for this interaction probably is adsorption of drug onto the surface of magnesium trisilicate.

Uricosuric drugs such as probenecid and sulfinpyrazone may inhibit renal tubular secretion of nitrofurantoin. The resulting increase in serum levels may increase toxicity and the decreased urinary levels could lessen its efficacy as a urinary tract antibacterial.

Carcinogenesis, Mutagenesis: Nitrofurantoin, when fed to female Holtzman rats at levels of 0.3% in commercial diet for up to 44.5 weeks, was not carcinogenic. Nitrofurantoin was not carcinogenic when female Sprague-Dawley rats were fed a commercial diet with nitrofurantoin levels at 0.1% to 0.187% (total cumulative, 9.25 g) for 75 weeks. Further studies of the effects of chronic administration to rodents are in progress.

Results of microbial *in vitro* tests using *Escherichia coli, Salmonella typhimurium,* and *Aspergillis nidulans* suggest that nitrofurantoin is a weak mutagen. Results of a dominant lethal assay in the mouse were negative.

Impairment of Fertility: The administration of high doses of nitrofurantoin to rats causes temporary spermatogenic arrest; this is reversible on discontinuing the drug. Doses of 10 mg/kg or greater in healthy human males may, in certain unpredictable instances, produce slight to moderate spermatogenic arrest with a decrease in sperm count.

Pregnancy: The safety of nitrofurantoin during pregnancy and lactation has not been established. Use of this drug in women of childbearing potential requires that the anticipated benefit be weighed against the possible risks.

Labor and Delivery: See CONTRINDICATIONS.

Nursing Mothers: Nitrofurantoin has been detected in breast milk, in trace amounts. Caution should be exercised when nitrofurantoin is administered to a nursing mother, especially if the infant is known or suspected to have a glucose-6-phosphate dehydrogenase deficiency.

Pediatric Use: Contraindicated in infants under one month of age. (See CONTRAINDICATIONS.)

ADVERSE REACTIONS

Respiratory:
CHRONIC, SUBACUTE, OR ACUTE PULMONARY HYPERSENSITIVITY REACTIONS MAY OCCUR.
CHRONIC PULMONARY REACTIONS OCCUR GENERALLY IN PATIENTS WHO HAVE RECEIVED CONTINUOUS TREATMENT FOR SIX MONTHS OR LONGER. MALAISE, DYSPNEA ON EXERTION, COUGH, AND ALTERED PULMONARY FUNCTION ARE COMMON MANIFESTATIONS WHICH CAN OCCUR INSIDIOUSLY. RADIOLOGIC AND HISTOLOGIC FINDINGS OF DIFFUSE INTERSTITIAL PNEUMONITIS OR FIBROSIS, OR BOTH, ARE ALSO COMMON MANIFESTATIONS OF THE CHRONIC PULMONARY REACTION. FEVER IS RARELY PROMINENT.
THE SEVERITY OF CHRONIC PULMONARY REACTIONS AND THEIR DEGREE OF RESOLUTION APPEAR TO BE RELATED TO THE DURATION OF THERAPY AFTER THE FIRST CLINICAL SIGNS APPEAR. PULMONARY FUNCTION MAY BE IMPAIRED PERMANENTLY, EVEN AFTER CESSATION OF THERAPY. THE RISK IS GREATER WHEN CHRONIC PULMONARY REACTIONS ARE NOT RECOGNIZED EARLY.
In subacute pulmonary reactions, fever and eosinophilia occur less often than in the acute form. Upon cessation of therapy, recovery may require several months. If the symptoms are not recognized as being drug-related and nitrofurantoin therapy is not stopped, the symptoms may become more severe.
Acute pulmonary reactions are commonly manifested by fever, chills, cough, chest pain, dyspnea, pulmonary infiltration with consolidation or pleural effusion on X-ray, and eosinophilia. Acute reactions usually occur within the first

week of treatment and are reversible with cessation of therapy. Resolution often is dramatic. (See WARNINGS.)
Gastrointestinal: Hepatitis, including chronic active hepatitis and cholestatic jaundice occur rarely.
Nausea, emesis and anorexia occur most often. Abdominal pain and diarrhea are less common gastrointestinal reactions. These dose-related reactions can be minimized by reduction of dosage.
Neurologic: Peripheral neuropathy, which may become severe or irreversible has occured. Fatalities have been reported. Conditions such as renal impairment (creatinine clearance under 40 mL per minute), anemia, diabetes mellitus, electrolyte imbalance, vitamin B deficiency, and debilitating diseases may increase the possibility of peripheral neuropathy.
Less frequent reactions of unknown causal relationship are nystagmus, vertigo, dizziness, asthenia, headache, and drowsiness.
Dermatologic: Exfoliative dermatitis and erythema multiforme (including Stevens-Johnson Syndrome) has been reported rarely. Transient alopecia has been reported.
Allergic Reactions: Lupus-like syndrome associated with pulmonary reaction to nitrofurantoin has been reported. Also angioedema, maculopapular, erythematous or eczematous eruptions, urticaria, rash and pruritus have occurred. Anaphylaxis, sialadenitis, pancreatitis, arthralgia, myalgia, drug fever, and chills or chills and fever have been reported.
Hematologic: Agranulocytosis, leukopenia, granulocytopenia, hemolytic anemia, thrombocytopenia, glucose-6-phosphate dehydrogenase deficiency anemia, megaloblastic anemia, and eosinophilia have occured. Cessation of therapy has returned the blood picture to normal. Aplastic anemia has been reported rarely.
Miscellaneous: As with other antimicrobial agents, superinfections by resistant organisms, e.g., Pseudomonas, may occur. However, these are limited to the genitourinary tract because suppression of normal bacterial flora does not occur elsewhere in the body.

OVERDOSAGE

Occasional incidents of acute overdosage of nitrofurantoin have not resulted in any specific symptoms other than vomiting. In case vomiting does not occur soon after an excessive dose, induction of emesis is recommended. There is no specific antidote, but a high fluid intake should be maintained to promote urinary excretion of the drug. It is dialyzable.

DOSAGE AND ADMINISTRATION

Nitrofurantoin capsules (macrocrystalline) should be given with food to improve drug absorption and, in some patients tolerance.
Adults: 50–100 mg four times a day—the lower dosage level is recommended for uncomplicated urinary tract infections.
Children: 5–7 mg/kg of body weight per 24 hours given in four divided doses (contraindicated under one month of age). Therapy should be continued for one week or for at least 3 days after sterility of the urine is obtained. Continued infection indicates the need for reevaluation.
For long-term suppressive therapy in adults, a reduction of dosage to 50–100 mg at bedtime may be adequate. For long-term suppressive therapy in children, doses as low as 1 mg/kg per 24 hours, given in a single or in two divided doses, may be adequate. **See WARNINGS SECTION REGARDING RISKS ASSOCIATED WITH LONG-TERM THERAPY.**

HOW SUPPLIED

50 mg
—Capsules containing 50 mg of nitrofurantoin macrocrystals
—Opaque white/opaque yellow capsules printed in red with **NITROFURANTOIN MACROCRYSTALS** on cap and **BOLAR 1016** on body.
—Bottles of 100, 500 and 1000
100 mg
—Capsules containing 100 mg of nitrofurantoin macrocrystals
—Opaque yellow capsules printed in red with **NITROFURANTOIN MACROCRYSTALS** on cap and **BOLAR 1015** on body.
—Bottles of 100, 500 and 1000
CAUTION:
Federal law prohibits dispensing without prescription.
STORE AT CONTROLLED ROOM TEMPERATURE 15°–30°C (59°–86°F)
REVISION DATE: FEBRUARY 1989
MANUFACTURED BY:
BOLAR PHARMACEUTICAL CO., INC.
COPIAGUE, NEW YORK 11726
*National Committee for Clinical Laboratory Standards. Approved Standard: ASM-2. Performance Standards for Antimicrobial Disc Susceptibility Tests July, 1975.
9B
Shown in Product Identification Section, page 406

NITROGLYCERIN TRANSDERMAL SYSTEM   ℞

DESCRIPTION

The Nitroglycerin Transdermal System contains nitroglycerin in a laminated matrix composed of polyvinyl chloride/polyvinyl acetate copolymer, di-(2-ethylhexyl) phthalate, isopropyl palmitate, colloidal silicon dioxide, aluminum foil laminate, polyethylene foam and acrylic adhesive to provide a continuous source of the active ingredient. Nitroglycerin Transdermal System is available in dosage strengths which deliver 5 mg/24 hrs (10 cm^2), 10 mg/24 hrs (20 cm^2), and 15 mg/24 hrs (30 cm^2) containing 62.5 mg, 125.0 mg, and 187.5 mg of nitroglycerin, respectively, thereby providing a range of dosing levels of nitroglycerin. The excess nitroglycerin remains in the system and serves as the reservoir to facilitate release of the drug. The rate of release of the drug is dependent upon the area of the system: approximately 0.5 mg nitroglycerin is released for every cm^2 of system size per 24 hours.
Each unit is sealed in polyester-foil-polyethylene laminate. The bandage portion consists of a medical grade acrylic based adhesive backed with polyethylene foam.

CLINICAL PHARMACOLOGY

When the Nitroglycerin Transdermal System is applied to the skin, nitroglycerin is absorbed continuously through the skin into the systemic circulation. This results in active drug reaching the target organs (heart, extremities) before deactivation by the liver. Nitroglycerin is a smooth muscle relaxant with vascular effects manifested predominantly by venous dilation and pooling. The major beneficial effect of nitroglycerin in angina pectoris is a reduction in myocardial oxygen consumption secondary to vascular smooth muscle relaxation with resultant reduction in cardiac preload and afterload. In recent years there has been an increasing recognition of a direct vasodilator effect of nitroglycerin on the coronary vessels.
In a bioavailability study using healthy volunteers, transdermal absorption of nitroglycerin from the Nitroglycerin Transdermal System achieved steady state venous plasma levels, and maintained these levels for 24 hours. Detectable plasma levels were attained within a ½ hour after application of the system, and were still detectable ½ hour after removal of the system. Precise definition of "therapeutic plasma level" is not known at this time.
The amount of nitroglycerin released (5 mg, 10 mg or 15 mg per 24 hours) represents the mean release rate of nitroglycerin from the system as determined from healthy volunteers, and hence, the amount potentially available for absorption through the skin. Absorption will vary among individuals.

INDICATIONS AND USAGE
This drug product has been conditionally approved by the FDA for the prevention and treatment of angina pectoris due to coronary artery disease. The conditional approval reflects a determination that the drug may be marketed while further investigation of its effectiveness is undertaken. A final evaluation of the effectiveness of the product will be announced by the FDA.

CONTRAINDICATIONS

Intolerance of organic nitrate drugs, marked anemia.

WARNINGS

The Nitroglycerin Transdermal System should be used under careful clinical and/or hemodynamic monitoring in patients with acute myocardial infarction or congestive heart failure.
In terminating treatment of anginal patients, both the dosage and frequency of application must be gradually reduced over a period of 4 to 6 weeks in order to prevent sudden withdrawal reactions, which are characteristic of all vasodilators in the nitroglycerin class.

PRECAUTIONS

Symptoms of hypotension, such as faintness, weakness or dizziness, particularly orthostatic hypotension, may be due to overdosage. If during the course of treatment these symptoms occur, the dosage should be reduced or use of the product discontinued.
Nitroglycerin Transdermal System is not intended for use in treatment of acute anginal attacks. For this purpose, occasional use of sublingual nitroglycerin may be necessary.
Pregnancy:
Pregnancy Category C. Animal reproduction studies have not been conducted with Nitroglycerin Transdermal System. It is also not known whether nitroglycerin can cause fetal harm when administered to a pregnant woman or can affect reproduction capacity. Nitroglycerin should be given to a pregnant woman only if clearly needed.

Continued on next page

Bolar—Cont.

Nursing Mothers:
It is not known whether nitroglycerin is excreted in human milk. Because many drugs are excreted in human milk, caution should be exercised when Nitroglycerin Transdermal System is administered to a nursing woman.

ADVERSE REACTIONS

Transient headache is the most common side effect, especially when higher doses of the drug are administered. Headaches should be treated with mild analgesics while continuing Nitroglycerin Transdermal System therapy. If headache persists, the Nitroglycerin Transdermal System dosage should be reduced or use of the product discontinued.
Adverse reactions reported less frequently include hypotension, increased heart rate, faintness, flushing, dizziness, nausea, vomiting and dermatitis. Except for dermatitis, these symptoms are attributed to the pharmacologic effects of nitroglycerin. However, they may be symptoms of overdosage. When they persist, the Nitroglycerin Transdermal System dosage should be reduced or use of the product discontinued.

DOSAGE AND ADMINISTRATION

To apply the Nitroglycerin Transdermal System, tear away the printed foil surface, using the tear notch provided. Apply the Nitroglycerin Transdermal System firmly to the skin surface. The initial starting dose is usually 5 mg/24 hrs (10 cm^2 system). To achieve optimum therapeutic effect in some patients, it may be necessary to titrate to a higher dosage strength. Dosage should be titrated while monitoring clinical response, i.e., blood pressure, episodes of angina and subsequent use of sublingual nitroglycerin. The Nitroglycerin Transdermal System, may remain in place for periods up to 24 hours as required to provide continuous levels of nitroglycerin.
The Nitroglycerin Transdermal System may be applied to any convenient skin area; a recommended site of application is the arm or chest. A suitable area may be shaved if necessary. Do not apply the Nitroglycerin Transdermal System to the distal part of the extremities.

STORAGE CONDITIONS

Store at controlled room temperature 15°–30°C (59°–86°F). **Do not refrigerate.**

HOW SUPPLIED

Nitroglycerin Transdermal System.
5 mg/24 hrs (10 cm^2)
10 mg/24 hrs (20 cm^2)
15 mg/24 hrs (30 cm^2)
Available in packages of 30 Units.

CAUTION

Federal law prohibits dispensing without prescription.
PATIENT INSTRUCTIONS FOR APPLICATION:
Patient Instructions are furnished with each carton.
REVISION DATE: MAY 1988
MANUFACTURED FOR BOLAR PHARMACEUTICAL CO., INC., COPIAGUE, NY 11726
BY HERCON LABORATORIES CORPORATION, HEALTH-CHEM, SOUTH PLAINFIELD, NEW JERSEY 07080

8E

PATIENT PACKAGE INSERT
Instructions For The Patient
NTS™
(nitroglycerin transdermal system)
Once-a-Day Therapy for Angina Pectoris

HOW NTS WORKS

NTS is a sustained-release nitroglycerin product. Nitroglycerin or related medications are available in several forms. Sublingual tablets, which are to be placed under the tongue, act quickly, but they have an effect for only a short period of time. Long-acting products such as capsules or tablets that are swallowed or ointments that are applied to the skin, are available. These are normally used several times a day.
NTS is designed to provide you with a continuous, uniform amount of preventative medication in a once-a-day dosage form. When **NTS** is applied to the skin, the nitroglycerin is absorbed slowly through the skin and into the blood stream. The circulatory system takes the nitroglycerin directly to the heart and to other parts of the body.

SOME SPECIAL ADVICE

NTS (nitroglycerin) is to be used for preventing attacks of angina. It is **not** meant to be used for stopping an attack that has already started.
Perspiration does not interfere with the action of **NTS** as long as it stays **tightly attached** to the skin.
Some people get headaches when they first start using nitroglycerin. These headaches usually become less severe or even disappear as treatment continues. If you develop headaches, your doctor may adjust your dosage and/or recommend that you also take headache medication.

Although uncommon, faintness, flushing, weakness, dizziness may occur, especially when suddenly arising from a lying, sitting, or bending position. Nausea, vomiting, and skin rash are other uncommon side effects. If any of these persist, you should notify your physician.
If your angina attacks change for the worse —if they become more severe, occur more frequently, last longer, or change in any way —notify your physician promptly.

Directions for Use of NTS

1. **REMOVE THE PROTECTIVE ALUMINUM FOIL LAYER BY HOLDING THE PRE-NOTCHED TAB BETWEEN THUMB AND FOREFINGER. GENTLY PULL THE TAB IN THE DIRECTION OF THE ARROW, AS SHOWN, TO BREAK THE TWO NOTCHES THAT HOLD THE TAB IN PLACE. THEN GENTLY PEEL THE FOIL LAYER AWAY FROM THE ADHESIVE FOAM PAD. FINALLY, REMOVE THE CORNER TAB FROM THE ADHESIVE FOAM PAD. IF ANY TRACES OF PAPER STICK TO THE ADHESIVE SURFACE, JUST PEEL OFF BEFORE USE.**

2. • Before applying, make sure the "medicated square" is attached to the adhesive foam pad, as shown.

• If the "medicated square" is attached to the protective aluminum foil, remove it with clean hands and place it on the foam adhesive pad. Wash hands.
• Should the "medicated square" be dropped, please discard and apply a new **NTS** (nitroglycerin).

3. For sensitive skin, reduce adhesion strength by touching the adhesive lightly with a dry, lint-free cloth. **Be careful not to remove too much adhesive.**

4. Place **NTS** (nitroglycerin) firmly on site free of hair on chest or on inner side of upper arm. Change application site each time to avoid skin irritation.

5. • To remove, just peel from skin. Apply a new **NTS** every 24 hours to a different site.
• If the **NTS** falls off or loosens apply a new **NTS**.

NOTE: Store between 59°–86°F (15°–30°C). **Do not refrigerate.** Avoid extremes of temperature and/or humidity during storage.

Shown in Product Identification Section, page 406

EXTENDED PHENYTOIN SODIUM CAPSULES, USP   ℞

DESCRIPTION

Phenytoin Sodium is an antiepileptic drug. Phenytoin sodium is related to the barbiturates in chemical structure, but has a five-membered ring. The chemical name for phenytoin sodium is 2,4-Imidazotidinedione, 5,5-diphenyl-, monosodium salt. The structural formula of phenytoin is:

Each Extended Phenytoin Sodium Capsule contains 100 mg of phenytoin sodium. Product *in vivo* performance is characterized by a slow and extended rate of absorption with peak blood concentrations expected in 4 to 12 hours as contrasted to Prompt Phenytoin Sodium Capsules USP with a rapid rate of absorption with peak blood concentration expected in $1\frac{1}{2}$ to 3 hours.
Phenytoin sodium extended capsules contain confectioner's sugar, gelatin, lactose hydrous, magnesium stearate, talc, and other ingredients.

CLINICAL PHARMACOLOGY

Phenytoin is an antiepileptic drug which can be useful in the treatment of epilepsy. The primary site of action appears to be *the motor cortex* where spread of seizure activity is inhibited. Possibly by promoting sodium efflux from neurons, phenytoin tends to *stabilize* the threshold against hyperexcitability caused by excessive stimulation or environmental changes capable of reducing membrane sodium gradient. This includes the reduction of post-tetanic potentiation at synapses. Loss of post-tetanic potentiation prevents cortical seizure foci from detonating adjacent cortical areas. Phenytoin reduces the maximal activity of brain stem centers responsible for the tonic phase of tonic-clonic (grand mal) seizures.
The plasma half-life in man after oral administration of phenytoin averages 22 hours, with a range of 7 to 42 hours. Steady-state therapeutic levels are achieved 7 to 10 days after initiation of therapy with recommended doses of 300 mg/day.
When serum level determinations are necessary, they should be obtained at least 5–7 half-lives after treatment initiation, dosage change, or addition or subtraction of another drug to the regimen so that equilibrium or steady-state will have been achieved. Trough levels provide information about clinically effective serum level range and confirm patient compliance and are obtained just prior to the patient's next scheduled dose. Peak levels indicate an individual's threshold for emergence of dose-related side effects and are obtained at the time of expected peak concentration. For Extended Phenytoin Sodium Capsules, peak serum levels occur 4–12 hours after administration.

Optimum control without clinical signs of toxicity occurs more often with serum levels between 10 and 20 mcg/ml, although some mild cases of tonic-clonic (grand mal) epilepsy may be controlled with lower-serum levels of phenytoin.

In most patients maintained at a steady dosage, stable phenytoin serum levels are achieved. There may be wide inter-patient variability in phenytoin serum levels with equivalent dosages. Patients with unusually low levels may be non-compliant or hypermetabolizers of phenytoin. Unusually high levels result from liver disease, congenital enzyme deficiency or drug interactions which result in metabolic interference. The patient with large variations in phenytoin plasma levels, despite standard doses, presents a difficult clinical problem. Serum level determinations in such patients may be particularly helpful.

Most of the drug is excreted in the bile as inactive metabolites which are then reabsorbed from the intestinal tract and excreted in the urine. Urinary excretion of phenytoin and its metabolites occurs partly with glomerular filtration but more importantly, by tubular secretion. Because phenytoin is hydroxylated in the liver by an enzyme system which is saturable, small incremental doses may produce very substantial increases in serum levels, when these are in the upper range. The steady-state level may be disproportionately increased, with resultant intoxication, from an increase in dosage of 10% or more.

INDICATIONS AND USAGE

Extended phenytoin sodium capsules are indicated for the control of tonic-clonic and psychomotor (grand mal and temporal lobe) seizures and prevention and treatment of seizures occurring during or following neurosurgery.

Phenytoin serum level determinations may be necessary for optimal dosage adjustment (see DOSAGE AND ADMINISTRATION).

CONTRAINDICATIONS

Phenytoin is contraindicated in those patients who are hypersensitive to phenytoin or other hydantoins.

WARNINGS

Abrupt withdrawal of phenytoin in epileptic patients may precipitate status epilepticus. When, in the judgement of the clinician, the need for dosage reduction, discontinuation, or substitution of alternative antiepileptic medication arises, this should be done gradually. However, in the event of an allergic or hypersensitivity reaction, rapid substitution of alternative therapy may be necessary. In this case, alternative therapy should be an antiepileptic drug not belonging to the hydantoin chemical class.

There have been a number of reports suggesting a relationship between phenytoin and the development of lymphadenopathy (local or generalized) including benign lymph node hyperplasia, pseudolymphoma, lymphoma and Hodgkin's Disease.

Although a cause and effect relationship has not been established, the occurrence of lymphadenopathy indicates the need to differentiate such a condition from other types of lymph node pathology. Lymph node involvement may occur with or without symptoms and signs resembling serum sickness eg, fever, rash and liver involvement.

In all cases of lymphadenopathy, follow-up observation for an extended period is indicated and every effort should be made to achieve seizure control using alternative antiepileptic drugs.

Acute alcoholic intake may increase phenytoin serum levels while chronic alcoholic use may decrease serum levels.

Use in Pregnancy: A number of reports suggest an association between the use of antiepileptic drugs by women with epilepsy and a higher incidence of birth defects in children born to these women. Data are more extensive with respect to phenytoin and phenobarbital, but these are also the most commonly prescribed antiepileptic drugs; less systematic or anecdotal reports suggest a possible similar association with the use of all known antiepileptic drugs.

The reports suggesting a higher incidence of birth defects in children of drug-treated epileptic women cannot be regarded as adequate to prove a definite cause and effect relationship. There are intrinsic methodologic problems in obtaining adequate data on drug teratogenicity in humans; genetic factors or the epileptic condition itself may be more important than drug therapy in leading to birth defects. The great majority of the mothers on antiepileptic medication deliver normal infants. It is important to note that antiepileptic drugs should not be discontinued in patients in whom the drug is administered to prevent major seizures, because of the strong possibility of precipitating status epilepticus with attendant hypoxia and threat to life. In individual cases where the severity and frequency of the seizure disorder are such that the removal of medication does not pose a serious threat to the patient, discontinuation of the drug may be considered prior to and during pregnancy, although it cannot be said with any confidence that even minor seizures do not pose some hazards to the developing embryo or fetus. The prescribing physician will wish to weigh these considerations in treating and counseling epileptic women of childbearing potential.

In addition to the reports of increased incidence of congenital malformation, such as cleft lip/palate and heart malformations in children of women receiving phenytoin and other antiepileptic drugs, there have more recently been reports of a fetal hydantoin syndrome. This consists of prenatal growth deficiency, microcephaly and mental deficiency in children born to mothers who have received phenytoin, barbiturates, alcohol, or trimethadione. However, these features are all interrelated and are frequently associated with intrauterine growth retardation from other causes.

There have been isolated reports of malignancies, including neuroblastoma, in children whose mothers received phenytoin during pregnancy.

An increase in seizure frequency during pregnancy occurs in a high proportion of patients because of altered phenytoin absorption or metabolism. Periodic measurement of serum phenytoin levels is particularly valuable in the management of a pregnant epileptic patient as a guide to an appropriate adjustment of dosage. However, postpartum restoration of the original dosage will probably be indicated.

Neonatal coagulation defects have been reported within the first 24 hours in babies born to the epileptic mothers receiving phenobarbital and/or phenytoin. Vitamin K_1 has been shown to prevent or correct this defect and has been recommended to be given to the mother before delivery and the neonate after birth.

PRECAUTIONS

General: The liver is the chief site of biotransformation of phenytoin; patients with impaired liver function, elderly patients, or those who are gravely ill may show early signs of toxicity. A small percentage of individuals who have been treated with phenytoin have been shown to metabolize the drug slowly. Slow metabolism may be due to limited enzyme availability and lack of induction; it appears to be genetically determined.

Phenytoin should be discontinued if a skin rash appears (see WARNINGS section regarding drug discontinuation). If the rash is exfoliative, purpuric, or bullous or if lupus erythematosus or Stevens-Johnson syndrome is suspected, use of the drug should not be resumed. (See ADVERSE REACTIONS.) If the rash is of a milder type (measles-like or scarlatiniform), therapy may be resumed after the rash has completely disappeared. If the rash recurs upon reinstitution of therapy, further phenytoin medication is contraindicated.

Hyperglycemia, resulting from the drug's inhibitory effects on insulin release, has been reported. Phenytoin may also raise the serum glucose level in diabetic patients.

Osteomalacia has been associated with phenytoin therapy and is considered to be due to phenytoin's interference with Vitamin D metabolism.

Phenytoin is not indicated for seizures due to hypoglycemic or other causes. Appropriate diagnostic procedures should be performed as indicated.

Phenytoin is not effective for absence (petit mal) seizures. If tonic-clonic (grand mal) and absence (petit mal) seizures are present, combined drug therapy is needed.

Serum levels of phenytoin sustained above the optimal range may produce confusional states referred to as "delirium", "psychosis", or "encephalopathy", or rarely irreversible cerebellar dysfunction. Accordingly, at the first sign of acute toxicity, plasma levels are recommended. Dose reduction of phenytoin therapy is indicated if plasma levels are excessive, if symptoms persist, termination is recommended. (See WARNINGS).

Information for Patients: Patients taking phenytoin should be advised of the importance of adhering strictly to the prescribed dosage regimen and of informing the physician of any clinical condition in which it is not possible to take the drug orally as prescribed, eg, surgery, etc.

Patients should also be cautioned on the use of other drugs or alcoholic beverages without first seeking the physician's advice.

The importance of good dental hygiene should be stressed in order to minimize the development of gingival hyperplasia and its complications.

Patients should be instructed to call their physician if skin rash develops.

Laboratory Tests: Phenytoin serum level determinations may be necessary to achieve optimal dosage adjustments.

Drug Interactions:

There are many drugs which may increase or decrease phenytoin levels or which phenytoin may affect. The most commonly occurring drug interactions are listed below:

1. Drug which may increase phenytoin serum levels include: chloramphenicol, dicumarol, disulfiram, tolbutamide, isoniazid, phenylbutazone, acute alcohol intake, salicylates, chlordiazepoxide, phenothiazines, diazepam, estrogens, ethosuximide, halothane, methylphenidate, sulfonamides, cimetidine, trazodone.

2. Drugs which may decrease phenytoin serum levels include: carbamazepine, chronic alcohol abuse, reserpine. Molindone Hydrochloride contains calcium ions which interfere with the absorption of phenytoin. Ingestion times, of phenytoin and antacid preparations containing

calcium should be staggered in patients with low serum phenytoin levels to prevent absorption problems.

3. Drugs which may either increase or decrease phenytoin serum levels include: phenobarbital, valproic acid and sodium valproate. Similarly, the effect of phenytoin on phenobarbital, valproic acid and sodium valproate serum levels is unpredictable.

4. Although not a true drug interaction, trycyclic antidepressants may precipitate seizures in susceptible patients and phenytoin dosage may need to be adjusted.

5. Drugs whose efficacy is impaired by phenytoin include: corticosteroids, coumarin anticoagulants, oral contraceptives, quinidine and vitamin D, digitoxin, rifampin, doxycycline, estrogens, furosemide.

Serum level determinations are especially helpful when possible drug interactions are suspected.

Drug/Laboratory Test Interactions: Phenytoin may cause decreased serum levels of protein-bound iodine (PBI). It may also produce lower than normal values for dexamethasone or metyrapone tests. Phenytoin may cause raised serum levels of glucose, alkaline phosphatase and gamma glutamyl transpeptidase (GGT).

Carcinogenesis: See WARNINGS section for information on carcinogenesis.

Pregnancy: See WARNINGS.

Nursing Mothers: Infant breast feeding is not recommended for women taking this drug because phenytoin appears to be secreted in low concentrations in human milk.

ADVERSE REACTIONS

Central Nervous System: The most common manifestations encountered with phenytoin therapy are referable to this system and are usually dose-related. These include nystagmus, ataxia, slurred speech and mental confusion. Dizziness, insomnia, transient nervousness, motor twitchings and headaches have also been observed.

There have also been rare reports of phenytoin induced dyskinesias including chorea, dystonia, tremor and asterixis, similar to those induced by phenothiazine and other neuroleptic drugs.

A predominantly sensory peripheral polyneuropathy has been observed in patients receiving long-term phenytoin therapy.

Gastrointestinal System: Nausea, vomiting and constipation.

Integumentary System: Dermatological manifestations sometimes accompanied by fever have included scarlatiniform or morbilliform rashes. A morbilliform rash (measles-like) is the most common; other types of dermatitis are seen more rarely. Other more serious forms which may be fatal have included bullous, exfoliative or purpuric dermatitis, lupus erythematosus, and Stevens-Johnson syndrome (see PRECAUTIONS).

Hemopoietic System: Hemopoietic complications, some fatal, have occasionally been reported in association with administration of phenytoin. These have included thrombocytopenia, leukopenia, granulocytopenia, agranulocytosis and pancytopenia. While macrocytosis and megaloblastic anemia have occurred, these conditions usually respond to folic acid therapy. Lymphadenopathy including benign lymph node hyperplasia, pseudolymphoma, lymphoma and Hodgkin's Disease have been reported (see WARNINGS).

Connective Tissue System: Coarsening of the facial features, enlargement of the lips, gingival hyperplasia, hirsutism and Peyronie's Disease.

Other: Systemic lupus erythematosus, periarteritis nodosa, toxic hepatitis, liver damage, and immuno-globulin abnormalities may occur.

OVERDOSAGE

The lethal dose in children is not known. The lethal dose in adults is estimated to be 2 to 5 grams. The initial symptoms are nystagmus, ataxia and dysarthria. Other signs are tremor, hyperflexia, lethargy, slurred speech, nausea, vomiting. The patient may become comatose and hypertensive. Death is due to respiratory and circulatory depression.

There are marked variations among individuals with respect to phenytoin plasma levels where toxicity may occur. Nystagmus, on lateral gaze, usually appears at 20 mcg/ml, ataxia at 30 mcg/ml, dysarthria and lethargy appear when the plasma concentration is over 40 mcg/ml, but as high a concentration as 50 mcg/ml has been reported without evidence of toxicity. As much as 25 times the therapeutic dose has been taken to result in a serum concentration over 100 mcg/ml with complete recovery.

Treatment: Treatment is nonspecific since there is no known antidote.

The adequacy of the respiratory and circulatory systems should be carefully observed and appropriate supportive measures employed. Hemodialysis can be considered since phenytoin is not completely bound to plasma proteins. Total exchange transfusion has been used in the treatment of severe intoxication in children.

Continued on next page

Bolar—Cont.

In acute overdosage the possibility of other CNS depressants, including alcohol, should be borne in mind.

DOSAGE AND ADMINISTRATION

Serum concentrations should be monitored in changing from Extended Phenytoin Sodium Capsules USP to Prompt Phenytoin Sodium Capsules USP, and from the sodium salt to the free acid form. Because there is approximately an 8% increase in drug content with the free acid form than the sodium salt, dosage adjustments and serum level monitoring may be necessary when switching from a product formulated with the free acid to a product formulated with the sodium salt and vice versa.

General: Dosage should be individualized to provide maximum benefit. In some cases serum blood level determinations may be necessary for optimal dosage adjustments—the clinically effective serum level is usually 10–20 mcg/ml. With recommended dosage, a period of seven to ten days may be required to achieve steady-state blood levels with phenytoin and changes in dosage (increase or decrease) should not be carried out at intervals shorter than seven to ten days.

Adult Dosage: Divided Daily Dosage: Patients who have received no previous treatment may be started on one 100 mg Extended Phenytoin Sodium Capsule three times daily and the dosage then adjusted to suit individual requirements. For most adults, the satisfactory maintenance dosage will be one capsule three to four times a day. An increase up to two capsules three times a day may be made if necessary.

Once-a-Day Dosage: In adults, if seizure control is established with divided doses of three 100 mg Extended Phenytoin Sodium Capsules daily, once-a-day dosage with 300 mg of extended phenytoin sodium capsules may be considered. Studies comparing divided doses of 300 mg with a single dose of this quantity indicated absorption, peak plasma levels, biologic half-life, difference between peak and minimum values and urinary recovery were equivalent. Once-a-day dosage offers a convenience to the individual patient or to nursing personnel for institutionalized patients and is intended to be used only for patients requiring this amount of drug daily. A major problem in motivating noncompliant patients may also be lessened when the patient can take this drug once a day. However, patients should be cautioned not to miss a dose, inadvertently.

Only extended phenytoin sodium capsules are recommended for once-a-day dosing, Inherent differences in dissolution characteristics and resultant absorption rates of phenytoin due to different manufacturing procedures and/or dosage forms preclude such recommendation for other phenytoin products. When a change in the dosage form or brand is prescribed, careful monitoring of phenytoin serum levels should be carried out.

Loading Dose: Some authorities have advocated use of an oral loading dose of phenytoin in adults who require rapid steady state serum levels and where intravenous administration is not desirable. This dosing regimen should be reserved for patients in a clinic or hospital setting where phenytoin serum levels can be closely monitored. Patients with a history of renal or liver disease should not receive the oral loading regimen.

Initially, one gram of phenytoin capsules is divided into 3 doses (400 mg, 300 mg, 300 mg) and administered at two-hourly intervals. Normal maintenance dosage is then instituted 24 hours after the loading dose, with frequent serum level determinations.

Pediatric Dosage: Initially, 5 mg/kg/day in two or three equally divided doses, with subsequent dosage individualized to a maximum of 300 mg daily. A recommended daily maintenance dosage is usually 4 to 8 mg/kg. Children over 6 years old may require the minimum adult dose (300 mg/day).

HOW SUPPLIED

—Capsules containing 100 mg of phenytoin sodium
—Clear capsules imprinted in black with "Bolar" on the cap and product identification number 0084 on the body
—Bottles of 100, 500 and 1000
Store at Controlled Room Temperature 15 °–30 °C (59 °–86 °F)

CAUTION

Federal law prohibits dispensing without prescription.
REVISION DATE: April 1989
MANUFACTURED BY: Bolar Pharmaceutical Co., Inc.
Copiague, New York 11726   9D
Shown in Product Identification Section, page 406

QUINIDINE GLUCONATE EXTENDED-RELEASE TABLETS   ℞

DESCRIPTION

Quinidine gluconate occurs as a white powder. It is odorless and has a very bitter taste. It is freely soluble in water and slightly soluble in alcohol.

Quinidine gluconate is the gluconate salt of quinidine (cinchonan-9-ol,6'-methoxy-,(9s)-,mono-D-gluconate) a diastereomer of quinine.
The structural formula is as follows:

$C_{20}H_{24}N_2O_2 \cdot C_6H_{12}O_7$ M.W. 520.58

Each extended-release tablet for oral administration contains 324 mg of quinidine gluconate (equivalent to 202 mg of quinidine alkaloid), in a tablet matrix specially designed for the prolonged (8 to 12 hours) release of the drug in the gastrointestinal tract.

Inactive ingredients: DiBasic Calcium Phosphate, Magnesium Stearate, Microcrystalline Cellulose, Povidone, Stearic Acid, Silica Gel and other ingredients.

CLINICAL PHARMACOLOGY

The action of quinidine in preventing aberrant cardiac rhythms of atrial and ventricular origin resides in its ability to (a) depress excitability of cardiac muscle, (b) slow the rate of spontaneous rhythm, (c) decrease vagal tone, and (d) prolong conduction and effective refractory period. Besides these direct effects, quinidine exerts some indirect activity on the heart through an anticholinergic action. Large oral doses may reduce the arterial pressure by means of peripheral vasodilation. Hypotension of a serious degree is more likely with the parenteral use of the drug.

Quinidine absorption from Quinidine Gluconate Extended-Release Tablets proceeds at a slower rate than the immediate-release products. Peak plasma concentrations of quinidine from immediate-release quinidine gluconate occurs in approximately 60 to 90 minutes. In a two-way multiple dose crossover bioavailability study conducted in normal volunteers, the time of peak quinidine serum concentration was 4 hours for Bolar's Quinidine Gluconate Extended-Release Tablets.

The apparent elimination half-life of quinidine ranges from 4 to 10 hours in healthy persons with a usual mean value of 6 to 7 hours. The half-life may be prolonged in elderly persons. From 60% to 80% of the dose is metabolized by the liver. Renal excretion of the intact drug comprises the remainder of the total clearance. Quinidine is approximately 75% bound to serum proteins.

Serum levels of quinidine can be measured. Values vary according to the assay employed. Traditionally, plasma concentrations for effective use of quinidine have been reported to range from 2–7 mcg/mL, and levels of 8 mcg/mL or greater are associated with toxicity. This information is based upon less specific analytic methods which quantitate metabolites as well as intact quinidine. However, plasma quinidine concentrations will be lower using more specific assays. Therefore, clinicians requesting serum quinidine determinations should be aware of the method of analysis. There is a wide individual variation in response to quinidine therapy. In all cases, the physician should carefully consider patient response and evidence of toxicity along with blood levels in determining optimal quinidine therapy.

INDICATIONS AND USAGE

Quinidine Gluconate is indicated in the treatment of:
1. Premature atrial and ventricular contractions.
2. Paroxysmal atrial tachycardia.
3. Paroxysmal atrioventricular (AV) junctional rhythm.
4. Atrial flutter.
5. Paroxysmal atrial fibrillation.
6. Established atrial fibrillation when therapy is appropriate.
7. Paroxysmal ventricular tachycardia when not associated with complete heart block.
8. Maintenance therapy after electrical conversion of atrial fibrillation and/or flutter.

CONTRAINDICATIONS

Hypersensitivity or idiosyncrasy to the drug, digitalis intoxication manifested by AV conduction disorders, complete AV block with an AV nodal or idioventricula pacemaker, left bundle block or other severe intraventricular conduction defects with marked QRS widening. Ectopic impulses and abnormal rhythms due to escape mechanisms. Also, myasthenia gravis.

WARNINGS

In the treatment of atrial flutter, reversion to sinus rhythm may be preceded by a progressive reduction in the degree of AV block to a 1:1 ratio, which results in extremely rapid ventricular rate. This possible hazard may be reduced by digitalization prior to administration of quinidine.

In susceptible individuals, such as those with marginally compensated cardiovascular disease, quinidine may produce clinically important depression of cardiac function manifested by hypotension, bradycardia, or heartblock. Quinidine therapy should be carefully monitored in such individuals. Evidence of quinidine cardiotoxicity, (excessive prolongation of Q-T interval, widening of QRS complex, and ventricular tachyarrhythmias) mandates immediate discontinuation of the drug and subsequent close clinical and electrocardiographic monitoring of the patient.

Quinidine should be used with extreme caution where there is incomplete AV block, since complete block and asystole may result. This drug may cause unpredictable abnormalities of rhythm in digitalized hearts, and it should be used with special caution in the presence of digitalis intoxication. The cardiotoxic effect of quinidine is increased by hyperkalemia and decreased by hypokalemia.

Patients taking quinidine occasionally have syncopal episodes which usually result from ventricular tachycardia or fibrillation. This syndrome has not been shown to be related to dose or serum levels. Syncopal episodes frequently terminate spontaneously or in response to treatment, but sometimes are fatal.

Recent reports have described increased, potentially toxic, digoxin serum levels when quinidine is administered concurrently. When concurrent use is necessary, reduction of digoxin dosage may have to be considered, its serum concentration should be monitored and the patient observed closely for digitalis intoxication.

Caution should be used when quinidine is administered concurrently with coumarin anticoagulants. This combination may reduce prothrombin levels and cause bleeding.

Quinidine should be used with caution in patients exhibiting renal, cardiac or hepatic insufficiency because of potential accumulation of quinidine in serum leading to toxicity.

Cases of hepatotoxicity, including granulomatous hepatitis, due to quinidine hypersensitivity have been reported. Unexplained fever and/or elevation of hepatic enzymes, particularly in the early stages of therapy, warrant consideration of possible hepatotoxicity. Monitoring liver function during the first 4–8 weeks should be considered. Cessation of quinidine in these cases usually results in the disappearance of toxicity.

PRECAUTIONS

General: A preliminary test dose of a single tablet of quinidine gluconate may be administered to determine if the patient has an idiosyncrasy to quinidine. Hypersensitivity to quinidine, although rare, should constantly be considered, especially during the first weeks of therapy. Hospitalization for close clinical observation, electrocardiographic monitoring and possible determination of serum quinidine levels is indicated when large doses are used, or with patients who present an increased risk.

Information for Patients: As with all solid oral dosage medication, quinidine gluconate should be taken with an adequate amount of fluid, preferably in an upright position, to facilitate swallowing.

Drug Interactions:

Drug	Effect
Quinidine with:	
Anticholinergics	Additive vagolytic effect
Cholinergics	Antagonism of cholinergic effects
Carbonic anhydrase inhibitors, Sodium bicarbonate, thiazide diuretcs	Alkalinization of urine resulting in decreased excretion of quinidine
Coumarin anticoagulants	Reduction of clotting factor concentrations (see WARNINGS)
Tubocuraine, succinylcholine decamethonium and pancuronium	Potentiation of neuromuscular blockade
Phenothiazines and reserpine	Additive cardiac depressive effects
Hepatic enzyme-inducing drugs (phenobarbital, phenytoin, rifampin)	Decreased plasma half-life of quinidine
Digoxin	Increased serum concentrations of digoxin (See WARNINGS)
Amiodarone	Increased serum concentration of quinidine
Cimetidine	Prolonged quinidine half-life and increased in serum quinidine level
Ranitidine	Premature ventricular contractions and/or bigeminy
Verapamil	Increased quinidine half-life and an increase in serum quinidine level; potential hypotensive reactions
Nifedipine	Decreased serum concentrations of quinidine

Laboratory Tests: Continuous electrocardiographic monitoring and determination of serum quinidine levels are indicated when large doses are used.

Periodic blood counts and liver and kidney function tests should be performed during long-term therapy; the drug should be discontinued if blood dyscrasias or evidence of hepatic or renal dysfunction occurs.

Carcinogenesis, Mutagenesis and Impairment of Fertility: Studies in animals have not been performed to evaluate the carcinogenic potential of quinidine.

Usage in Pregnancy:

Teratogenic Effects: Pregnancy Category C. Animal reproduction studies have not been conducted with quinidine. There are no adequate and well-controlled studies in pregnant women. Quinidine should be given to a pregnant woman only if clearly needed.

Nonteratogenic Effects: Like quinine, quinidine has been reported to have oxytocic properties. The significance of this property in the clinical setting has not been established.

Labor and Delivery: There is no known use of quinidine gluconate in labor and delivery. However, quinidine has been reported to have oxytocic properties. The significance of this property in the clinical setting has not been established.

Nursing Mothers: Caution should be exercised when quinidine is administered to a nursing mother due to passage of the drug into breast milk.

Pediatric Use: There are no adequate and well-controlled studies establishing the safety and effectiveness of quinidine gluconate in children.

ADVERSE REACTIONS

Symptoms of cinchonism, such as ringing in ears, loss of hearing, dizziness, lightheadedness, headache, nausea and/or disturbed vision may appear in sensitive patients after a single dose of the drug. The most frequently encountered side effects to quinidine are gastrointestinal.

Gastrointestinal: Nausea, vomiting, abdominal pain, diarrhea, anorexia, granulomatous hepatitis (which may be preceded by fever), esophagitis.

Cardiovascular: Ventricular extrasystoles occuring at a rate of one or more every 6 normal beats; widening of the QRS complex and prolonged QT interval; complete AV block; ventricular tachycardia and fibrillation; ventricular flutter, torsade de pointes; arterial embolism; hypotension, syncope.

Central Nervous System: Headache, vertigo, apprehension, excitement, confusion, delirium, dementia, ataxia, depression.

Ophthalmologic and Otologic: Disturbed hearing (tinnitus, decreased auditory acuity), disturbed vision (mydriasis, blurred-vision, disturbed color perception, photophobia, diplopia, night blindness, scotomata), optic neuritis, reduced visual field.

Dermatologic: Cutaneous flushing with intense pruritus, photosensitivity, urticaria, rash, eczema, exfoliative eruptions, psoriasis, abnormalities of pigmentation.

Hypersensitivity: Angioedema, acute asthmatic episode, vascular collapse, respiratory arrest, hepatotoxicity, granulomatous hepatitis (see WARNINGS), purpura vasculitis.

Hematologic: Thrombocytopenia, thrombocytopenic purpura, agranulocytosis, acute hemolytic anemia, hypoprothrombinemia, leukocytosis, shift to left in WBC differential, neutropenia.

Immunologic: Systemic lupus erythematosus, lupus nephritis.

Miscellaneous: Fever, increase in serum skeletal muscle creatine phosphokinase, arthralgia, myalgia.

OVERDOSAGE

Symptoms: Overdosage of quinidine can lead to accelerated idioventricular rhythm, morphologic appearance of QRS complexes, prolonged QT intervals, intermittent sinus capture beats, paroxysms of tachycardia, ventricular arrhythmias, hypotension, oliguria, respiratory depression, pulmonary edema, acidosis, seizures, and coma.

Treatment: Early treatment to empty the stomach using syrup of ipecac and/or gastric lavage is recommended. Administration of activated charcoal may reduce absorption. Other general supportive measures should be employed as indicated by patient response in severe cases, circulation should be stabilized and measurements of pulmonary capillary wedge pressure should be performed to assure adequate left ventricular filling pressure. Electrolyte and blood gas abnormalities should be corrected. In quinidine-induced vasodilation, catecholamines and other alpha-adrenergic agonists may be tried. Arrhythmias may be treated with lidocaine, pacing, and cardioversion. Administration of sodium lactate reportedly reduces the cardiotoxicity of quinidine, however sodium lactate is contraindicated in the presence of alkalosis as increased urinary pH can lead to an increase in the renal tubular absorption of quinidine. Acidification of the urine may enhance the urinary excretion of quinidine.

DOSAGE AND ADMINISTRATION

The dosage varies considerably depending upon the general condition and cardiovascular state of the patient. The quantity and frequency of administration of quinidine gluconate extended-release tablets that will achieve the desired clinical results, must be determined for each patient.

The ideal dosage is the minimum amount of total dose and frequency of daily administration that will prevent premature contractions, paroxysmal tachycardias and maintain normal sinus rhythm.

Prevention of premature atrial, nodal or ventricular contractions: 1 to 2 tablets every 8 to 12 hours.

Maintenance of normal sinus rhythm following conversion of paroxysmal tachycardias: 2 tablets every 12 hours or 1½ to 2 tablets every 8 hours usually are required.

Although most patients may be maintained in normal rhythm on a dosage of one quinidine gluconate extended-release tablet every 8 to 12 hours, other patients may require larger doses or more frequent administration (i.e., every 6 hours) than the usually recommended schedule. Such increased dosage should be instituted only after careful clinical and laboratory evaluation of the patient, including monitoring of plasma quinidine levels and, if possible, serial electrocardiograms.

It is frequently desirable to determine if a patient can tolerate maintenance quinidine therapy prior to electrical conversion. Therefore, maintenance therapy may be initiated 2 to 3 days before electrical conversion is attempted. Quinidine Gluconate Extended-Release tablets are well suited for such a program and can be administered at a maintenance dose felt necessary for a given patient as indicated above.

Note: Do not crush or chew since extended-release properties will be lost.

HOW SUPPLIED

—Each extended-release tablet contains 324 mg of quinidine gluconate.

—White, round shaped, scored tablet debossed with Bolar logo on one side and product identification number 3000 on the other side of tablet.

—Bottles of 100, 250 and 500.

STORE AT CONTROLLED ROOM TEMPERATURE 15°–30°C (59°–86°F).

CAUTION

FEDERAL LAW PROHIBITS DISPENSING WITHOUT PRESCRIPTION.

REVISION DATE: October 1988

MANUFACTURED BY:
Bolar Pharmaceutical Co., Inc.
Copiague, New York 11726   8J
Shown in Product Identification Section, page 406

TRIAMTERENE AND   ℞
HYDROCHLOROTHIAZIDE CAPSULES

DESCRIPTION

Each triamterene and hydrochlorothiazide capsule for oral use, contains hydrochlorothiazide 25 mg and triamterene 50 mg. Hydroclorothiazide is a diuretic/antihypertensive agent and triamterene is an antikaliuretic agent.

Hydrochlorothiazide is slightly soluble in water. It is soluble in dilute ammonia, dilute aqueous sodium hydroxide and dimethylformamide. It is sparingly soluble in methanol.

Hydrochlorothiazide is 6-chloro-3,4-dihydro-2H-1,2,4-benzothiadiazine-7-sulfonamide 1,1-dioxide and its structural formula is:

At 50°C, triamterene is practically insoluble in water (less than 0.1%). It is soluble in formic acid, sparingly soluble in methoxyethanol and very slightly soluble in alcohol.

Triamterene is 2,4,7-triamino-6-phenylpteridine and its structural formula is:

Inactive Ingredients: Gelatin, Lactose Anhydrous, Magnesium Stearate, Titanium Dioxide, FD&C Red #40, and other ingredients.

CLINICAL PHARMACOLOGY

Triamterene and Hydrochlorothiazide Capsules are a diuretic antihypertensive drug product that combines natriuretic and antikaliuretic effects. Each component complements the action of the other. The hydrochlorothiazide component blocks the reabsorption of sodium and chloride ions, and thereby increases the quantity of sodium traversing the distal tubule and the volume of water excreted. A portion of the additional sodium presented to the distal tubule is ex-

changed there for potassium and hydrogen ions. With continued use of hydrochlorothiazide and depletion of sodium, compensatory mechanisms tend to increase this exchange and may produce excessive loss of potassium, hydrogen and chloride ions. Hydrochlorothiazide also decreases the excretion of calcium and uric acid, may increase the excretion of iodide and may reduce glomerular filtration rate. The exact mechanism of the antihypertensive effect of hydrochlorothiazide is not known.

The triamterene component exerts its diuretic effect on the distal renal tubule to inhibit the reabsorption of sodium in exchange for potassium and hydrogen ions. Its natriuretic activity is limited by the amount of sodium reaching this site of action. Although it blocks the increase in this exchange that is stimulated by mineralocorticoids (chiefly aldosterone) it is not a competitive antagonist of aldosterone and its activity can be demonstrated in adrenalectomized rats and patients with Addison's disease. As a result, the dose of triamterene required is not proportionally related to the level of mineralocorticoid activity, but is dictated by the response of the individual patients, and the kaliuretic effect of concomitantly administered drugs. By inhibiting the distal tubular exchange mechanism, triamterene maintains or increases the sodium excretion and reduces the excess loss of potassium, hydrogen, and chloride ions induced by hydrochlorothiazide. As with hydrochlorothiazide, triamterene may reduce glomerular filtration and renal plasma flow. Via this mechanism it may reduce uric acid excretion although it has no tubular effect on uric acid reabsorption or secretion. Triamterene does not affect calcium excretion. No predictable antihypertensive effect has been demonstrated for triamterene.

Duration of diuretic activity and effective dosage range of the hydrochlorothiazide and triamterene components are similar. Onset of diuresis with Triamterene and Hydrochlorothiazide Capsules takes place within one hour, peaks at two to three hours and tapers off during the subsequent seven to nine hours.

The bioavailability of the hydrochlorothiazide and the triamterene components of this product are, in each case, about 50% of that observed with an aqueous suspension of the components. (See PRECAUTIONS, Bioavailability.)

INDICATIONS AND USAGE

This fixed combination drug is not indicated for the initial therapy of edema or hypertension except in individuals in whom the development of hypokalemia cannot be risked. Triamterene and Hydrochlorothiazide Capsules are indicated for the treatment of hypertension or edema in patients who develop hypokalemia on hydrochlorothiazide alone.

Triamterene and hydrochlorothiazide is also indicated for those patients who require a thiazide diuretic and in whom the development of hypokalemia cannot be risked.

Triamterene and hydrochlorothiazide may be used alone or as an adjunct to other antihypertensive drugs, such as beta-blockers. Since triamterene and hydrochlorothiazide may enhance the action of these agents, dosage adjustments may be necessary.

Usage in Pregnancy: The routine use of diuretics in an otherwise healthy woman is inappropriate and exposes mother and fetus to unnecessary hazard. Diuretics do not prevent development of toxemia of pregnancy, and there is no satisfactory evidence that they are useful in the treatment of developed toxemia.

Edema during pregnancy may arise from pathological causes or from the physiologic and mechanical consequences of pregnancy. Diuretics are indicated in pregnancy when edema is due to pathologic causes, just as they are in the absence of pregnancy. Dependent edema in pregnancy resulting from restriction of venous return by the expanded uterus is properly treated through elevation of the lower extremities and use of support hose; use of diuretics to lower intravascular volume in this case is illogical and unnecessary. There is hypervolemia during normal pregnancy which is harmful to neither the fetus nor the mother (in the absence of cardiovascular disease), but which is associated with edema, including generalized edema in the majority of pregnant women. If this edema produces discomfort, increased recumbency will often provide relief. In rare instances this edema may cause extreme discomfort which is not relieved by rest. In these cases a short course of diuretics may provide relief and may be appropriate.

CONTRAINDICATIONS

Antikaliuretic Therapy and Potassium Supplementation: Triamterene and hydrochlorothiazide should not be given to patients receiving other potassium-conserving agents such as spironolactone, amiloride or other formulations containing triamterene. Concomitant potassium-containing salt substitutes should also not be used.

Potassium supplementation should not be used with triamterene and hydrochlorothiazide except in severe cases of hypokalemia. Such concomitant therapy can be associated with rapid increases in serum potassium level. If potassium sup-

Continued on next page

Bolar—Cont.

plementation is used, careful monitoring of the serum potassium level is necessary.

Impaired Renal Function: Triamterene and hydrochlorothiazide is contraindicated in patients with anuria, acute and chronic renal insufficiency of significant renal impairment.

Hypersensitivity: Hypersensitivity to either drug in the preparation or to other sulfonamide derived drugs is a contraindication.

Hyperkalemia: Triamterene and hydrochlorothiazide should not be used in patients with preexisting elevated serum potassium.

WARNINGS
Hyperkalemia:

> Abnormal elevation of serum potassium levels (greater than or equal to 5.5. mEq/liter) can occur with all potassium-conserving diuretic combinations, including triamterene and hydrochlorothiazide. Hyperkalemia is more likely to occur in patients with renal impairment, diabetes (even without evidence of renal impairment), elderly or severely ill patients. Since uncorrected hyperkalemia may be fatal, serum potassium levels must be monitored at frequent intervals especially in patients first receiving triamterene and hydrochlorothiazide when dosages are changed or with any illness that may influence renal function.

If hyperkalemia is suspected (warning signs include paresthesias, muscular weakness, fatigue, flaccid paralysis of the extremities, bradycardia and shock), an electrocardiogram (ECG) should be obtained. However, it is important to monitor serum potassium levels because hyperkalemia may not be associated with ECG changes.

If hyperkalemia is present, triamterene and hydrochlorothiazide should be discontinued immediately and a thiazide alone should be substituted. If the serum potassium exceeds 6.5 mEq/liter, more vigorous therapy is required. The clinical situation dictates the procedures to be employed. These include the intravenous administration of calcium chloride injection, sodium bicarbonate injection and/or the oral or parenteral administration of glucose with a rapid-acting insulin preparation. Cationic exchange resins such as sodium polystyrene sulfonate may be orally or rectally administered. Persistent hyperkalemia may require dialysis.

The development of hyperkalemia associated with potassium-sparing diuretics is accentuated in the presence of renal impairment (see CONTRAINDICATIONS section). Patients with mild renal functional impairment should not receive this drug without frequent and continuing monitoring of serum electrolytes. Cumulative drug effects may be observed in patients with impaired renal function. The renal clearances of hydrochlorothiazide and the pharmacologically active metabolite of triamterene, the sulfate ester of hydroxytriamterene have been shown to be reduced and the plasma levels increased following triamterene and hydrochlorothiazide administration to elderly patients and patients with impaired renal function.

Hyperkalemia has been reported in diabetic patients with the use of potassium-conserving agents even in the absence of apparent renal impairment. Accordingly, serum electrolytes must be frequently monitored if triamterene and hydrochlorothiazide is used in diabetic patients.

Metabolic or Respiratory Acidosis: Potassium-conserving therapy should also be avoided in severely ill patients in whom respiratory or metabolic acidosis may occur. Acidosis may be associated with rapid elevations in serum potassium levels. If triamterene and hydrochlorothiazide is employed, frequent evaluations of acid/base balance and serum electrolytes are necessary.

PRECAUTIONS

General: Bioavailability: The bioavailability of the hydrochlorothiazide and triamterene components in this formulation of Triamterene and Hydrochlorothiazide Capsule is about 50% of the maximum obtainable with oral therapy. Theoretically, a patient transferred from therapy with hydrochlorothiazide with or without triamterene might show an increase in blood pressure, fluid retention, or change in serum potassium. Extensive clinical experience with triamterene and hydrochlorothiazide, however, suggests that these conditions have not been commonly observed in clinical practice. (See CLINICAL PHARMACOLOGY.)

Impaired Hepatic Function: Thiazides should be used with caution in patients with impaired hepatic function. They can precipitate hepatic coma in patients with severe liver disease. Potassium depletion induced by the thiazide may be important in this connection. Administer triamterene and hydrochlorothiazide cautiously and be alert for such early signs of impending coma as confusion, drowsiness and tremor; if mental confusion increases discontinue triamterene and hydrochlorothiazide for a few days. Attention must be given to other factors that may precipitate hepatic coma,

such as blood in the gastrointestinal tract or preexisting potassium depletion.

Hypokalemia: Hypokalemia is uncommon with triamterene and hydrochlorothiazide, but, should it develop, corrective measures should be taken such as potassium supplementation or increased intake of potassium-rich foods. Institute such measures cautiously with frequent determinations of serum potassium levels, especially in patients receiving digitalis or with a history of cardiac arrhythmias. If serious hypokalemia (serum potassium less than 3.0 mEq/L) is demonstrated by repeat serum potassium determinations, triamterene and hydrochlorothiazide should be discontinued and potassium chloride supplementation initiated. Less serious hypokalemia should be evaluated with regard to other coexisting conditions and treated accordingly.

Electrolyte Imbalance: Electrolyte imbalance, often encountered in such conditions as heart failure, renal disease or cirrhosis of the liver, may also be aggravated by diuretics and should be considered during triamterene and hydrochlorothiazide therapy when using high doses for prolonged periods or in patients on a salt-restricted diet. Serum determinations of electrolytes should be performed, and are particularly important if the patient is vomiting excessively or receiving fluids parenterally. Possible fluid and electrolyte imbalance may be indicated by such warning signs as: dry mouth, thirst, weakness, lethargy, drowsiness, restlessness, muscle pain or cramps, muscular fatigue, hypotension, oliguria, tachycardia and gastrointestinal symptoms.

Hypochloremia: Although any chloride deficit is generally mild and usually does not require specific treatment except under extraordinary circumstances (as in liver disease or renal disease), chloride replacement may be required in the treatment of metabolic alkalosis. Dilutional hyponatremia may occur in edematous patients in hot weather; appropriate therapy is water restriction, rather than administration of salt, except in rare instances when the hyponatremia is life threatening. In actual salt depletion, appropriate replacement is the therapy of choice.

Renal Stones: Triamterene has been found in renal stones in association with the other usual calculus components. Triamterene and hydrochlorothiazide should be used with caution in patients with a history of renal stones.

Laboratory Tests: *Serum Potassium:* The normal adult range of serum potassium is 3.5 to 5.0 mEq per liter with 4.5 mEq often being used for a reference point. If hypokalemia should develop, corrective measures should be taken such as potassium supplementation or increased dietary intake of potassium-rich foods.

Institute such measures cautiously with frequent determinations of serum potassium levels. Potassium levels persistently above 6 mEq per liter require careful observation and treatment. Serum potassium levels do not necessarily indicate true body potassium concentration. A rise in plasma pH may cause a decrease in plasma potassium concentration and an increase in the intracellular potassium concentration. Discontinue corrective measures for hypokalemia immediately if laboratory determinations reveal an abnormal elevation of serum potassium. Discontinue triamterene and hydrochlorothiazide and substitute a thiazide diuretic alone until potassium levels return to normal.

Serum Creatinine and BUN: Triamterene and hydrochlorothiazide may produce an elevated blood urea nitrogen level, creatinine level or both. This apparently is secondary to a reversible reduction of glomerular filtration rate or a depletion of intravascular fluid volume (prerenal azotemia) rather than renal toxicity; levels usually return to normal when triamterene and hydrochlorothiazide is discontinued. If azotemia increases, discontinue triamterene and hydrochlorothiazide. Periodic BUN or serum creatinine determinations should be made, especially in elderly patients and in patients with suspected or confirmed renal insufficiency.

Serum PBI: Thiazide may decrease serum PBI levels without sign of thyroid disturbance.

Parathyroid Function: Thiazides should be discontinued before carrying out tests for parathyroid function. Calcium excretion is decreased by thiazides. Pathologic changes in the parathyroid glands with hypercalcemia and hypophosphatemia have been observed in a few patients on prolonged thiazide therapy. The common complications of hyperparathyroidism such as bone resorption and peptic ulceration have not been seen.

Drug Interactions: *Angiotensin-converting enzyme inhibitors:* Potassium-sparing agents should be used with caution in conjunction with angiotensin-converting enzyme (ACE) inhibitors due to an increased risk of hyperkalemia. *Oral hypoglycemic drugs:* Concurrent use with chlorpropamide may increase the risk of severe hyponatremia. *Nonsteroidal anti-inflammatory drugs:* A possible interaction resulting in acute renal failure has been reported in a few patients on triamterene and hydrochlorothiazide when treated with indomethacin, a nonsteroidal anti-inflammatory agent. Caution is advised in administering nonsteroidal anti-inflammatory agents with triamterene and hydrochlorothiazide.

Lithium: Lithium generally should not be given with diuretics because they reduce its renal clearance and increase

the risk of lithium toxicity. Read circulars for lithium preparations before use of such concomitant therapy with triamterene and hydrochlorothiazide.

Surgical considerations: Thiazides have been shown to decrease arterial responsiveness to norepinephrine (an effect attributed to loss of sodium). This diminution is not sufficient to preclude effectiveness of the pressor agent for therapeutic use. Thiazides have also been shown to increase the paralyzing effect of nondepolarizing muscle relaxants such as tubocurarine (an effect attributed to potassium loss); consequently caution should be observed in patients undergoing surgery.

Other Considerations: Concurrent use of hydrochlorothiazide with amphotericin B or corticosteroids or corticotropin (ACTH) may intensify electrolyte imbalance, particularly hypokalemia, although the presence of triamterene minimizes the hypokalemic effect.

Thiazides may add to or potentiate the action of other antihypertensive drugs. See INDICATIONS AND USAGE for concomitant use with other antihypertensive drugs.

The effect of oral anticoagulants may be decreased when used concurrently with hydrochlorothiazide; dosage adjustments may be necessary.

Triamterene and hydrochlorothiazide may raise the level of blood uric acid; dosage adjustment of antigout medication may be necessary to control hyperuricemia and gout.

The following agents given together with triamterene may promote serum potassium accumulation and possibly result in hyperkalemia because of the potassium-sparing nature of triamterene, especially in patients with renal insufficiency; blood from blood bank (may contain up to 30 mEq of potassium per liter of plasma or up to 65 mEq per liter of whole blood when stored for more than 10 days); low-salt milk (may contain up to 60 mEq of potassium per liter); potassium-containing medications (such as parenteral penicillin G potassium); salt substitutes (most contain substantial amounts of potassium).

Exchange resins, such as sodium polystyrene sulfonate, whether administered orally or rectally, reduce serum potassium levels by sodium replacement of the potassium; fluid retention may occur in some patients because of the increased sodium intake.

Chronic or overuse of laxatives may reduce serum potassium levels by promoting excessive potassium loss from the intestinal tract; laxatives may interfere with the potassium-retaining effects of triamterene.

The effectiveness of methenamine may be decreased when used concurrently with hydrochlorothiazide because of alkalinization of the urine.

Drug/Laboratory Test Interactions: Triamterene and quinidine have similar fluorescence spectra; thus, triamterene and hydrochlorothiazide will interfere with the fluorescent measurements of quinidine.

Pregnancy: Category C: *Teratogenic Effects*—The safe use of triamterene and hydrochlorothiazide in pregnancy has not been established. Animal reproduction studies have not been conducted with triamterene and hydrochlorothiazide. It is also not known if triamterene and hydrochlorothiazide can cause fetal harm when administered to a pregnant woman or can affect reproductive capacity. Triamterene and hydrochlorothiazide should be given to a pregnant woman only if clearly needed.

Nonteratogenic Effects—Thiazides cross the placental barrier and appear in cord blood. The use of thiazides in pregnant women requires that the anticipated benefit be weighed against possible hazards to the fetus. These hazards include fetal or neonatal jaundice, thrombocytopenia, and possible other adverse reactions which have occurred in the adult. Triamterene has been shown to cross the placental barrier and appear in the cord blood of animals. The use of triamterene in pregnant women requires that the anticipated benefit be weighed against possible hazards to the fetus. These possible hazards include adverse reactions which have occurred in the adult.

Nursing Mothers—Thiazides appear and triamterene may appear in breast milk. If use of the drug product is deemed essential, the patient should stop nursing.

Pediatric Use—Safety and effectiveness in children have not been established.

ADVERSE REACTIONS

Adverse effects are listed in decreasing order of frequency, however, the most serious adverse effects are listed first regardless of frequency. The serious adverse effects associated with triamterene and hydrochlorothiazide have commonly occurred in less than 0.1% of patients treated with this product.

Hypersensitivity: anaphylaxis, rash, urticaria, photosensitivity.

Cardiovascular: arrhythmia, postural hypotension.

Metabolic: diabetes mellitus, hyperkalemia, hyperglycemia, glycosuria, hyperuricemia, hypokalemia, hyponatremia, acidosis, hypochloremia.

Gastrointestinal: jaundice and/or liver enzyme abnormalities, pancreatitis, nausea and vomiting, diarrhea, constipation, abdominal pain.

Renal: acute renal failure, interstitial nephritis, renal stones composed primarily of triamterene, elevated BUN and serum creatinine, abnormal urinary sediment.
Hematologic: leukopenia, thrombocytopenia and purpura, megaloblastic anemia.
Musculoskeletal: Muscle cramps.
Central Nervous System: weakness, fatigue, dizziness, headache, dry mouth.
Miscellaneous: impotence, sialadenitis.
Thiazides alone have been shown to cause the following additional adverse reactions:
Central Nervous System: paresthesias, vertigo.
Ophthalmic: xanthopsia, transient blurred vision.
Respiratory: allergic pneumonitis, pulmonary edema, respiratory distress.
Other: necrotizing vasculitis, exacerbation of lupus.
Hematologic: aplastic anemia, agranulocytosis, hemolytic anemia.
Neonate and infancy: thrombocytopenia and pancreatitis-rarely, in newborns whose mothers have received thiazides during pregnancy.

DOSAGE AND ADMINISTRATION
The usual dosage of Triamterene and Hydrochlorothiazide Capsules, 50 mg/25 mg, is one or two capsules given once daily, with appropriate monitoring of serum potassium and of the clinical effect. [See WARNINGS, Hyperkalemia and PRECAUTIONS, Bioavailability.)

OVERDOSAGE
Electrolyte imbalance is the major concern (see WARNINGS section). Symptoms reported include: polyuria, nausea, vomiting, weakness, lassitude, fever, flushed face, and hyperactive deep tendon reflexes. If hypotension occurs, it may be treated with pressor agents such as levarterenol to maintain blood pressure. Carefully evaluate the electrolyte pattern and fluid balance. Induce immediate evacuation of the stomach through emesis or gastric lavage. There is no specific antidote.
Reversible acute renal failure following ingestion of 50 tablets of a product containing a combination of 50 mg triamterene and 25 mg hydrochlorothiazide has been reported. Although triamterene is largely protein-bound (approximately 67%), there may be some benefit to dialysis in cases of overdosage.

HOW SUPPLIED
—Capsules containing 50 mg of triamterene and 25 mg of hydrochlorothiazide
—Opaque red capsule printed with BOLAR and product identification number 227
—Bottles of 100, 250, 500 and 1000
STORE AT CONTROLLED ROOM TEMPERATURE 15°-30°C (59°-86°F)
CAUTION: FEDERAL LAW PROHIBITS DISPENSING WITHOUT PRESCRIPTION.
REVISION DATE: JULY 1988
MANUFACTURED BY:
BOLAR PHARMACEUTICAL CO., INC.
COPIAGUE, NEW YORK 11726   8G
Shown in Product Identification Section, page 406

Boots Pharmaceuticals, Inc.
A subsidiary of The Boots Company (USA) Inc.
8800 ELLERBE ROAD
SHREVEPORT, LA 71106 U.S.A.

PRODUCT INFORMATION WAS PREPARED IN MAY, 1989. FOR FURTHER INFORMATION ON THESE AND OTHER BOOTS PRODUCTS CONTACT YOUR BOOTS REPRESENTATIVE OR WRITE BOOTS PHARMACEUTICALS, INC., P. O. BOX 6750, SHREVEPORT, LA 71136.

E-MYCIN®   ℞
(erythromycin delayed-release)
Tablets, USP
250 mg/333 mg

Each E-MYCIN tablet contains erythromycin as the base.

DESCRIPTION
Erythromycin is produced by a strain of *Streptomyces erythreus* and belongs to the macrolide group of antibiotics. It is basic and readily forms salts with acids. The base is white to off-white crystals or powder slightly soluble in water, soluble in alcohol, in chloroform, and in ether. The chemical name for erythromycin is (3R*, 4S*, 5S*, 6R*, 7R*, 9R*, 11R*, 12R*, 13S*, 14R*)-4-[2,6-Dideoxy-3-C-methyl-3-O-methyl-α-L-ribo-hexopyranosyl)-oxy]-14-ethyl-7, 12, 13-trihydroxy-3,5,7,9,11,13-hexamethyl-6-[[3, 4, 6 -trideoxy -3 -(dimethylamino) β-D-$xylo$-yexopyranosyl]oxy]oxacyclotetra-

decane - 2,10-dione and the molecular weight is 733.94. The structural formula is represented below:

E-MYCIN® (erythromycin delayed-release) Tablets, USP available in 250 mg and 333 mg strengths, are specially coated to protect the contents from the inactivating effects of gastric acidity and to permit efficient absorption of the antibiotic in the small intestine.
Inactive Ingredients: carboxymethylcellulose calcium, carnauba wax, cellulose acetate phthalate, corn starch, hydroxypropyl cellulose, lactose, magnesium stearate, mineral oil, propylene glycol, sorbic acid, sorbitan monooleate, sucrose, talc, titanium dioxide. The 250 mg tablet also contains erythrosine sodium and FD&C Yellow No. 6 (sunset yellow) as a color additive.

CLINICAL PHARMACOLOGY
The mode of action of erythromycin is inhibition of protein synthesis without affecting nucleic acid synthesis. Resistance to erythromycin of some strains of *Haemophilus influenzae* and staphylococci has been demonstrated. Culture and susceptibility testing should be done. If the Kirby-Bauer method of disk susceptibility is used, a 15 mcg erythromycin disk should give a zone diameter of at least 18 mm when tested against an erythromycin susceptible organism.
Bioavailability data are available from The Boots Company (USA) Inc.
E-MYCIN Tablets are well absorbed and may be given without regard to meals.
After absorption, erythromycin diffuses readily into most body fluids. Low concentrations are normally achieved in the spinal fluid but passage of the drug across the blood-brain barrier increases in meningitis. In the presence of normal hepatic function, erythromycin is concentrated in the liver and excreted in the bile; the effect of hepatic dysfunction on excretion of erythromycin by the liver into the bile is not known. After oral administration, less than 5 percent of the activity of the administered dose can be recovered in the urine.
Erythromycin crosses the placental barrier but fetal plasma levels are low.
Antagonism in antibacterial activity has been demonstrated between clindamycin and erythromycin *in vitro.*

INDICATIONS AND USAGE
Streptococcus pyogenes (Group A beta hemolytic streptococcus): For upper and lower respiratory tract, skin, and soft tissue infections of mild to moderate severity.
Injectable benzathine penicillin G is considered by the American Heart Association to be the drug of choice in the treatment and prevention of streptococcal pharyngitis and in long-term prophylaxis of rheumatic fever.
When oral medication is preferred for treatment of the above conditions, penicillin G, V, or erythromycin are alternate drugs of choice.
When oral medication is given, the importance of strict adherence by the patient to the prescribed dosage regimen must be stressed. A therapeutic dose should be administered for at least 10 days.
Alpha-hemolytic streptococci (viridans group): Although no controlled clinical efficacy trials have been conducted, oral erythromycin has been suggested by the American Heart Association and American Dental Association for use in the prophylaxis against bacterial endocarditis in patients hypersensitive to penicillin who have congenital heart disease or rheumatic or other acquired valvular heart disease when they undergo dental procedures and surgical procedures of the upper respiratory tract.[1] Erythromycin is not suitable prior to genitourinary or gastrointestinal tract surgery except as described under **DOSAGE AND ADMINISTRATION.**
NOTE: When selecting antibiotics for the prevention of bacterial endocarditis the physician or dentist should read the full joint statement of the American Heart Association and the American Dental Association.[1]
Staphylococcus aureus: For acute infections of skin and soft tissue of mild to moderate severity. Resistant organisms may emerge during treatment.
Streptococcus pneumoniae (Diplococcus pneumoniae): For upper respiratory tract infections (eg, otitis media, pharyngitis) and lower respiratory tract infections (eg, pneumonia) of mild to moderate degree.
Mycoplasma pneumoniae (Eaton agent, PPLO): For respiratory infections due to those organism.

Hemophilus infuenzae: For upper respiratory tract infections of mild to moderate severity when used concomitantly with adequate doses of sulfonamides. Not all strains of this organism are susceptible at the erythromycin concentrations ordinarily achieved (see appropriate sulfonamide labeling for prescribing information).
Treponema pallidum: Erythromycin is an alternate choice of treatment for primary syphillis in patients allergic to the penicillins. In treatment of primary syphilis, spinal fluid examinations should be done before treatment and as part of follow-up after therapy.
Corynebacterium diphtheriae and C. minutissimum: As an adjunct to antitoxin, to prevent establishment of carriers, and to eradicate the organism in carriers.
In the treatment of erythrasma.
Entamoeba histolytica: In the treatment of intestinal amebiasis only. Extraenteric amebiasis requires treatment with other agents.
Listeria monocytogenes: Infections due to this organism.
Neisseria gonorrhoeae: Erythromycin lactobionate for injection in conjunction with erythromycin base orally, as an alternative drug in treatment of acute pelvic inflammatory disease caused by *N. gonorrhoeae* in female patients with a history of sensitivity to penicillin. Before treatment of gonorrhea, patients who are suspected of also having syphillis should have a microscopic examination for *T. pallidum* (by immunofluorescence or dark-field) before receiving erythromycin, and monthly serologic tests for a minimum of 4 months.
Chlamydia trachomatis: Erythromycins are indicated for treatment of the following infections caused by *Chlamydia trachomatis:* conjunctivitis of the newborn, pneumonia of infancy, urogenital infections during pregnancy. When tetracyclines are contraindicated or not tolerated, erythromycin is indicated for the treatment of uncomplicated urethral, endocervical, or rectal infections in adults due to *Chlamydia trachomatis.*[2]
Bordetella pertussis: Erythromycin is effective in eliminating the organism from the nasopharynx of infected individuals, rendering them noninfectious. Some clinical studies suggest that erythromycin may be helpful in the prophylaxis of pertussis in exposed susceptible individuals.
Legionnaires Disease: Although no controlled clinical efficacy studies have been conducted, *in vitro* and limited preliminary clinical data suggest that erythromycin can be effective in treating Legionnaires Disease.

CONTRAINDICATIONS
Erythromycin is contraindicated in patients with known hypersensitivity to this antibiotic.

WARNING
Usage in pregnancy: Safety for use in pregnancy has not been established.

PRECAUTIONS
General: Erythromycin is principally excreted by the liver. Caution should be exercised in administering the antibiotic to patients with impaired hepatic function.
There have been reports of hepatic dysfunction, with or without jaundice, occurring in patients receiving oral erythromycin products. Nevertheless a thorough evaluation of the jaundice should be performed.
Drug interactions: Recent data from studies of erythromycin reveal that its use in patients who are receiving high doses of theophylline may be associated with an increase of serum theophylline levels and potential theophylline toxicity. In cases of theophylline toxicity and/or elevated serum theophylline levels, the dose of theophylline should be reduced while the patient is receiving concomitant erythromycin therapy.
Erythromycin administration in children receiving carbamazepine has been reported to cause increased blood levels of carbamazepine with subsequent development of signs of carbamazepine toxicity (ataxia, dizziness, vomiting).
Erythromycin may decrease the clearance of warfarin and thus potentiate the hypoprothrombinemic effect of warfarin.
Erythromycin has been reported to decrease the clearance of triazolam and thus may increase the pharmacologic effect of triazolam.
Erythromycin has been reported to decrease the clearance of cyclosporine causing elevated cyclosporine levels and associated increased serum creatinine. Renal function as well as serum concentration of cyclosporine should be closely monitored when both drugs are administered concomitantly.
An interaction between erythromycin and ergotamine has been reported to increase the vasospasm associated with ergotamine.

ADVERSE REACTIONS
The most frequent side effects of erythromycin preparations are gastrointestinal, such as abdominal cramping and discomfort, and are dose related. Nausea, vomiting, and diarrhea occur infrequently with usual oral doses.

Continued on next page

Boots Pharm.—Cont.

During prolonged or repeated therapy, there is a possibility of overgrowth of nonsusceptible bacteria or fungi. If such infections occur, the drug should be discontinued and appropriate therapy instituted.

Mild allergic reactions such as urticaria and other skin rashes have occurred. Serious allergic reactions, including anaphylaxis, have been reported.

There have been isolated reports of reversible hearing loss occurring chiefly in patients with renal insufficiency and in patients receiving high doses of erythromycin.

DOSAGE AND ADMINISTRATION

E-MYCIN® (erythromycin delayed-release) Tablets, USP are well absorbed and may be given without regard to meals.

Adults: The usual dose is 250 mg four times daily or 333 mg every 8 hours.

If twice a day dosage is desired, the recommended dose is 500 mg every 12 hours.

Dosage may be increased up to 4 or more grams per day according to the severity of the infection. Twice-a-day dosing is not recommended when doses larger than 1 gram daily are administered.

Children: Age, weight, and severity of the infection are important factors in determining the proper dosage. 30 to 50 mg/kg/day, in divided doses, is the usual dose. For more severe infections, this dose may be doubled.

In the treatment of streptococcal infections, a therapeutic dosage of erythromycin should be administered for at least 10 days. In continuous prophylaxis of streptococcal infections in persons with a history of rheumatic heart disease, the dose is 250 mg twice a day.

For prophylaxis against bacterial endocarditis[1] in patients with congenital heart disease or rheumatic, or other acquired valvular heart disease when undergoing dental procedures or surgical procedures of the upper respiratory tract, give 1.0 gram (20 mg/kg for children) orally 1½–2 hours before the procedure and then 500 mg (10 mg/kg for children) orally every 6 hours for 8 doses.

For treatment of primary syphilis: 30 to 40 grams given in divided doses over a period of 10 to 15 days.

For treatment of acute pelvic inflammatory disease caused by *N. gonorrhoeae*: After initial treatment with erythromycin lactobionate for injection (500 mg every 6 hours for 3 days), the oral dosage recommendation is 250 mg every 6 hours for 7 days or 333 mg every 8 hours for 7 days.

Urogenital infections during pregnancy due to *Chlamydia trachomatis*: Although the optimal dose and duration of therapy have not been established, the suggested treatment is erythromycin 500 mg, by mouth, four times a day or two 333 mg tablets every eight hours for at least seven days. For women who cannot tolerate this regimen, a decreased dose of 250 mg, by mouth, four times a day or one 333 mg tablet every eight hours should be used for at least 14 days.[2]

For adults with uncomplicated urethral, endocervical or rectal infections caused by *Chlamydia trachomatis* in whom tetracyclines are contraindicated or not tolerated: 500 mg, by mouth, four times a day or two 333 mg tablets every eight hours for at least seven days.[2]

For dysenteric amebiasis: 250 mg four times daily or 333 mg every 8 hours for 10 to 14 days, for adults; 30 to 50 mg/kg/day in divided doses for 10 to 14 days for children.

For use in pertussis: Although optimal dosage and duration have not been established, doses of erythromycin utilized in reported clinical studies were 40 to 50 mg/kg/day, given in divided doses for 5 to 14 days.

For treatment of Legionnaires Disease: Although optimal doses have not been established, doses utilized in reported clinical data were those recommended above (1 to 4 grams erythromycin base daily in divided doses).

Preoperative Prophylaxis for Elective Colorectal Surgery: Listed below is an example of a recommended bowel preparation regimen. A proposed surgery time of 8:00 a.m. has been used.

Pre-op Day 3: Minimum residue or clear liquid diet. Bisacodyl, 1 tablet orally at 6:00 p.m.

Pre-op Day 2: Minimum residue or clear liquid diet. Magnesium sulfate, 30 mL, 50% solution (15g) orally at 10:00 a.m., 2:00 p.m. and 6:00 p.m. Enema at 7:00 p.m. and 8:00 p.m.

Pre-op Day 1: Clear liquid diet Supplemental (IV) fluids as needed. Magnesium sulfate, 30 mL, 50% solution (15g) orally at 10:00 a.m. and 2:00 p.m. Neomycin sulfate (1.0g) and erythromycin base (three 333 mg tablets or four 250 mg tablets) orally at 1:00 p.m., 2:00 p.m. and 11:00 p.m. No enema.

Day of operation: Patient evacuates rectum at 6:30 a.m. for scheduled operation at 8:00 a.m.

TREATMENT OF OVERDOSAGE

Allergic reactions associated with acute overdosage should be handled in the usual manner—that is, by the administration of adrenalin, corticosteroids, and antihistamines as indicated and the prompt elimination of unabsorbed drug, in addition to all needed supportive measures.

HOW SUPPLIED

E-MYCIN Tablets 250 mg: round, convex, light peach, enteric-coated, tablet with "E-MYCIN 250 mg" printed in black on one face.

Bottles of 40	NDC 0524-0207-99
Bottles of 100	NDC 0524-0207-01
Unit Dose Pkg of 100	NDC 0524-0207-21
Bottles of 500	NDC 0524-0207-05

E-MYCIN Tabits 333 mg: round, convex, white, enteric-coated tablet with "E-MYCIN 333 mg" printed in orange on one face.

Bottles of 30	NDC 0524-0208-30
Bottles of 100	NDC 0524-0208-01
Unit Dose Pkg of 100	NDC 0524-0208-21
Bottles of 500	NDC 0524-0208-05

Store at controlled room temperature, 15°–30°C (59°–86° F).

CAUTION

Federal (USA) law prohibits dispensing without prescription.

[1] American Heart Association 1977. Prevention of bacterial endocarditis. Circulation 56: 139A–143A.

[2] CDC Sexually Transmitted Diseases Treatment Guidelines 1982.

Manufactured For:
Boots Pharmaceuticals, Inc.
Shreveport, Louisiana 71106 USA
a subsidiary of
The Boots Company (USA) Inc.
By:
The Upjohn Company
Kalamazoo, Michigan 49001 USA

Revised 5/8/89

Shown in Product Identification Section, page 406

RUFEN®
[*roo-fin*]
(ibuprofen)   ℞

DESCRIPTION

RUFEN (ibuprofen) is ($\pm$)-2-(p-isobutylphenyl) propionic acid. It is a white powder with a melting point of 74–77°C and is very slightly soluble in water (<1 mg/mL) and readily soluble in organic solvents such as ethanol and acetone. Its structural formula is:

RUFEN is a nonsteroidal anti-inflammatory agent. It is available in 400, 600 and 800 mg tablets for oral administration.

CLINICAL PHARMACOLOGY

RUFEN is a nonsteroidal anti-inflammatory agent that possesses analgesic and antipyretic activities. Its mode of action, like that of other nonsteroidal anti-inflammatory agents, is not completely understood, but may be related to prostaglandin synthetase inhibition.

In clinical studies in patients with rheumatoid arthritis and osteoarthritis, RUFEN has been shown to be comparable to aspirin in controlling pain and inflammation and to be associated with a statistically significant reduction in the milder gastrointestinal side effects (see **ADVERSE REACTIONS**). RUFEN may be well tolerated in some patients who have had gastrointestinal side effects with aspirin, but these patients when treated with RUFEN should be carefully followed for signs and symptoms of gastrointestinal ulceration and bleeding.

Although it is not definitely known whether ibuprofen causes less peptic ulceration than aspirin, in one study involving 885 patients with rheumatoid arthritis treated for up to one year, there were no reports of gastric ulceration with ibuprofen whereas frank ulceration was reported in 13 patients in the aspirin group (statistically significant $p < .001$). Gastroscopic studies at varying doses show an increased tendency toward gastric irritation at higher doses. However, at comparable doses gastric irritation is approximately half that seen with aspirin. Studies using ^{51}Cr-tagged red cells indicate that fecal blood loss associated with ibuprofen in doses up to 2400 mg daily did not exceed the normal range, and was significantly less than that seen in aspirin-treated patients.

In clinical studies in patients with rheumatoid arthritis, ibuprofen has been shown to be comparable to indomethacin in controlling aforementioned signs and symptoms of disease activity and to be associated with a statistically significant reduction of the milder gastrointestinal (see **ADVERSE REACTIONS**) and CNS side effects.

RUFEN may be used in combination with gold salts and/or corticosteroids.

Controlled studies have demonstrated that ibuprofen is a more effective analgesic than propoxyphene for the relief of episiotomy pain, pain following dental extraction procedures, and for the relief of the symptoms of primary dysmenorrhea.

In patients with primary dysmenorrhea, ibuprofen has been shown to reduce elevated levels of prostaglandin activity in the menstrual fluid and to reduce resting and active intrauterine pressure, as well as the frequency of uterine contractions. The probable mechanism of action is to inhibit prostaglandin synthesis rather than simply to provide analgesia.

Pharmacokinetics: RUFEN is rapidly absorbed when administered orally. Peak serum ibuprofen levels are generally attained one to two hours after administration. With single doses up to 800 mg, linear relationship exists between amount of drug administered and the integrated area under the serum drug concentration vs time curve. Above 800 mg, however, the area under the curve increases less than proportional to increases in dose. There is no evidence of drug accumulation or enzyme induction.

The administration of RUFEN tablets either under fasting conditions or immediately before meals yields quite similar serum ibuprofen concentration-time profiles. When RUFEN is administered immediately after a meal, there is a reduction in the rate of absorption but no appreciable decrease in the extent of absorption. The bioavailability of RUFEN is minimally altered by the presence of food.

A bioavailability study has shown that there was no interference with the absorption of ibuprofen when given in conjunction with an antacid containing both aluminum hydroxide and magnesium hydroxide.

Ibuprofen is rapidly metabolized and eliminated in the urine. The excretion of ibuprofen is virtually complete 24 hours after the last dose. The serum half-life is 1.8 to 2.0 hours.

Studies have shown that following ingestion of the drug 45% to 79% of the dose was recovered in the urine within 24 hours as metabolite A (25%), (+)-2-4'-(2 hydroxy-2-methylpropyl)-phenyl propionic acid and metabolite B (37%), (+)-2-4'-(2 carboxypropyl) phenyl propionic acid, the percentages of free and conjugated ibuprofen were approximately 1% and 14%, respectively.

INDICATIONS AND USAGE

RUFEN is indicated for relief of the signs and symptoms of rheumatoid arthritis and osteoarthritis.

RUFEN is indicated for the relief of mild to moderate pain.

RUFEN is also indicated for the treatment of primary dysmenorrhea.

Since there have been no controlled trials to demonstrate whether there is any beneficial effect or harmful interaction with the use of RUFEN in conjunction with aspirin, the combination cannot be recommended (see **Drug Interactions**). Controlled clinical trials to establish the safety and effectiveness of RUFEN in children have not been conducted.

CONTRAINDICATIONS

RUFEN tablets should not be used in patients who have previously exhibited hypersensitivity to it, or in individuals with all or part of the syndrome of nasal polyps, angioedema and bronchospastic reactivity to aspirin, or other nonsteroidal anti-inflammatory agents. Anaphylactoid reactions have occurred in such patients.

WARNINGS

Risk of GI Ulceration, Bleeding and Perforation with NSAID Therapy. Serious gastrointestinal toxicity such as bleeding, ulceration, and perforation, can occur at any time, with or without warning symptoms, in patients treated chronically with NSAID therapy. Although minor upper gastrointestinal problems, such as dyspepsia, are common, usually developing early in therapy, physicians should remain alert for ulceration and bleeding in patients treated chronically with NSAIDs even in the absence of previous GI trace symptoms. In patients observed in clinical trials of several months to two years duration, symptomatic upper GI ulcers, gross bleeding or perforation appear to occur in approximately 1% of patients treated for 3–6 months, and in about 2–4% of patients treated for one year. Physicians should inform patients about the signs and/or symptoms of serious GI toxicity and what steps to take if they occur.

Studies to date have not identified any subset of patients not at risk of developing peptic ulceration and bleeding. Except for a prior history of serious GI events and other risk factors known to be associated with peptic ulcer disease, such as alcoholism, smoking, etc., no risk factors (e.g., age, sex) have been associated with increased risk. Elderly or debilitated patients seem to tolerate ulceration or bleeding less well than other individuals and most spontaneous reports of fatal GI events are in this population. Studies to date are inconclusive concerning the relative risk of various NSAIDs in causing such reactions. High doses of any NSAID probably carry a greater risk of these reactions, although controlled clinical trials showing this do not exist in most cases. In considering the use of relatively large doses (within the recommended dosage range), sufficient benefit should be anticipated to offset the potential increased risk of GI toxicity.

PRECAUTIONS

General: Blurred and/or diminished vision, scotomata, and/or changes in color vision have been reported. If a patient develops such complaints while receiving RUFEN the drug should be discontinued and the patient should have an ophthalmologic examination which includes central visual fields and color vision testing.

Fluid retention and edema have been reported in association with RUFEN, therefore, the drug should be used with caution in patients with a history of cardiac decompensation or hypertension.

RUFEN, like other nonsteroidal anti-inflammatory agents, can inhibit platelet aggregation but the effect is quantitatively less and of shorter duration than that seen with aspirin. Ibuprofen has been shown to prolong bleeding time (but within the normal range), in normal subjects. Because this prolonged bleeding effect may be exaggerated in patients with underlying hemostatic defects, RUFEN should be used with caution in persons with intrinsic coagulation defects and those on anticoagulant therapy.

Patients on RUFEN should report to their physicians signs or symptoms of gastrointestinal ulceration or bleeding, blurred vision or other eye symptoms, skin rash, weight gain, or edema.

In order to avoid exacerbation of disease or adrenal insufficiency, patients who have been on prolonged corticosteroid therapy should have their therapy tapered slowly rather than discontinued abruptly when RUFEN is added to the treatment program.

The antipyretic and anti-inflammatory activity of ibuprofen may reduce fever and inflammation, thus diminishing their utility as diagnostic signs in detecting complications of presumed noninfectious, noninflammatory painful conditions.

Liver Effects: As with other nonsteroidal anti-inflammatory drugs, borderline elevations of one or more liver tests may occur in up to 15% of patients. These abnormalities may progress, may remain essentially unchanged, or may be transient with continued therapy. The SGPT (ALT) test is probably the most sensitive indicator of liver dysfunction. Meaningful (3 times the upper limit of normal), elevations of SGPT or SGOT (AST) occurred in controlled clinical trials in less than 1% of patients. A patient with symptoms and/or signs suggesting liver dysfunction, or in whom an abnormal liver test has occurred, should be evaluated for evidence of the development of more severe hepatic reactions while on therapy with ibuprofen. Severe hepatic reactions, including jaundice and cases of fatal hepatitis, have been reported with ibuprofen as with other nonsteroidal anti-inflammatory drugs. Although such reactions are rare, if abnormal liver tests persist or worsen, if clinical signs and symptoms consistent with liver disease develop, or if systemic manifestations occur (e.g., eosinophilia, rash, etc.) RUFEN should be discontinued.

Hemoglobin Levels: In cross-study comparisons with doses ranging from 1200 mg to 3200 mg daily for several weeks, a slight dose-response decrease in hemoglobin/hematocrit was noted. This has been observed with other nonsteroidal anti-inflammatory drugs; the mechanism is unknown. However, even with daily doses of 3200 mg, the total decrease in hemoglobin usually does not exceed 1 gram; if there are no signs of bleeding, it is probably not clinically important.

In two postmarketing clinical studies the incidence of a decreased hemoglobin level was greater than previously reported. Decrease in hemoglobin of 1 gram or more was observed in 17.1% of 193 patients on 1600 mg ibuprofen daily (osteoarthritis), and in 22.8% of 189 patients taking 2400 mg of ibuprofen daily (rheumatoid arthritis). Positive stool occult blood tests and elevated serum creatinine levels were also observed in these studies.

Aseptic Meningitis: Aseptic meningitis with fever and coma has been observed on rare occasions in patients on ibuprofen therapy. Although it is probably more likely to occur in patients with systemic lupus erythematosus and related connective tissue diseases, it has been reported in patients who do not have an underlying chronic disease. If signs or symptoms of meningitis develop in a patient on RUFEN, the possibility of its being related to ibuprofen should be considered.

Renal Effects: As with other nonsteroidal anti-inflammatory drugs, long term administration of ibuprofen to animals has resulted in renal papillary necrosis and other abnormal renal pathology. In humans, there have been reports of acute interstitial nephritis with hematuria, proteinuria, and occasionally nephrotic syndrome.

A second form of renal toxicity has been seen in patients with prerenal conditions leading to a reduction in renal blood flow or blood volume, where the renal prostaglandins have a supportive role in the maintenance of renal perfusion. In these patients administration of a nonsteroidal anti-inflammatory drug may cause a dose dependent reduction in prostaglandin formation and may precipitate overt renal decompensation. Patients at greatest risk of this reaction are those with impaired renal function, heart failure, liver dysfunction, those taking diuretics and the elderly. Discontinua-

tion of nonsteroidal anti-inflammatory drug therapy is typically followed by recovery to the pretreatment state.

Those patients at high risk who chronically take RUFEN should have renal function monitored if they have signs or symptoms which may be consistent with mild azotemia, such as malaise, fatigue, loss of appetite, etc. Occasional patients may develop some elevation of serum creatinine and BUN levels without signs or symptoms.

Since ibuprofen is eliminated primarily by the kidneys, patients with significantly impaired renal function should be closely monitored and a reduction in dosage should be anticipated to avoid drug accumulation. Prospective studies on the safety of ibuprofen in patients with chronic renal failure have not been conducted.

Information for Patients: Ibuprofen, like other drugs of its class, is not free of side effects. The side effects of these drugs can cause discomfort and rarely, there are more serious side effects, such as gastrointestinal bleeding, which may result in hospitalization and even fatal outcomes.

NSAIDs (Nonsteroidal Anti-Inflammatory Drugs) are often essential agents in the management of arthritis and have a major role in the treatment of pain, but they also may be commonly employed for conditions which are less serious. Physicians may wish to discuss with their patients the potential risks (see **WARNINGS, PRECAUTIONS,** and **ADVERSE REACTIONS** sections) and likely benefits of NSAID treatment, particularly when the drugs are used for less serious conditions where treatment without NSAIDS may represent an acceptable alternative to both the patient and physician.

Laboratory Tests: Because serious GI tract ulceration and bleeding can occur without warning symptoms, physicians should follow chronically treated patients for the signs and symptoms of ulceration and bleeding and should inform them of the importance of this follow-up (see **WARNINGS**).

Drug Interactions: *Coumarin-type anticoagulants.* Several short-term controlled studies failed to show that ibuprofen significantly affected prothrombin times or a variety of other clotting factors when administered to individuals on coumarin-type anticoagulants. However, because bleeding has been reported when RUFEN® (ibuprofen) and other nonsteroidal anti-inflammatory agents have been administered to patients on coumarin-type anticoagulants, the physician should be cautious when administering RUFEN to patients on anticoagulants.

Aspirin: Animal studies show that aspirin given with nonsteroidal anti-inflammatory agents, including ibuprofen, yields a net decrease in anti-inflammatory activity with lowered blood levels of the non-aspirin drug. Single dose bioavailability studies in normal volunteers have failed to show an effect of aspirin on ibuprofen blood levels. Correlative clinical studies have not been done.

Methotrexate: Ibuprofen, as well as other nonsteroidal anti-inflammatory drugs, has been reported to competitively inhibit methotrexate accumulation in rabbit kidney slices. This may indicate that ibuprofen could enhance the toxicity of methotrexate. Caution should be used if RUFEN is administered concomitantly with methotrexate.

H-2 Antagonists: In studies with human volunteers, coadministration of cimetidine or ranitidine with ibuprofen had no substantive effect on ibuprofen serum concentrations.

Furosemide: Clinical studies, as well as random observations, have shown that ibuprofen can reduce the natriuretic effect of furosemide and thiazides in some patients. This response has been attributed to inhibition of renal prostaglandin synthesis. During concomitant therapy with ibuprofen, the patient should be observed closely for signs of renal failure (see **PRECAUTIONS. Renal Effects**), as well as to assure diuretic efficacy.

Lithium: Ibuprofen produced an elevation of plasma lithium levels and a reduction in renal lithium clearance in a study of eleven normal volunteers. The mean minimum lithium concentration increased 15% and the renal clearance of lithium was decreased by 19% during this period of concomitant drug administration.

This effect has been attributed to inhibition of renal prostaglandin synthesis by ibuprofen. Thus, when ibuprofen and lithium are administered concurrently, subjects should be observed carefully for signs of lithium toxicity. (Read circulars for lithium preparation before use of such concurrent therapy.)

Pregnancy. Reproductive studies conducted in rats and rabbits at doses somewhat less than the maximal clinical dose did not demonstrate evidence of developmental abnormalities. However, animal reproduction studies are not always predictive of human response. As there are no adequate and well-controlled studies in pregnant women, this drug should be used during pregnancy only if clearly needed. Because of the known effects of nonsteroidal anti-inflammatory drugs on the fetal cardiovascular system (closure of ductus arteriosus) use during late pregnancy should be avoided. As with other drugs known to inhibit prostaglandin synthesis, an increased incidence of dystocia and delayed parturition occurred in rats. Administration of RUFEN is not recommended during pregnancy.

Nursing Mothers: In limited studies, an assay capable of detecting 1 mcg/mL did not demonstrate ibuprofen in the milk of lactating mothers. However, because of the limited nature of the studies and the possible adverse effects of prostaglandin inhibiting drugs on neonates, RUFEN is not recommended for use in nursing mothers.

ADVERSE REACTIONS

The most frequent type of adverse reaction occurring with ibuprofen is gastrointestinal. In controlled clinical trials, the percentage of patients reporting one or more gastrointestinal complaints ranged from 4% to 16%.

In controlled studies when ibuprofen was compared to aspirin and indomethacin in equally effective doses, the overall incidence of gastrointestinal complaints was about half that seen in either the aspirin-or indomethacin-treated patients. Adverse reactions observed during controlled clinical trials at an incidence greater than 1% are listed in the following paragraphs. Those reactions listed under the heading, Incidence Greater Than 1% (but less than 3%) Probable Causal Relationship, encompass observations in approximately 3,000 patients. More than 500 of these patients were treated for periods of at least 54 weeks.

Still other reactions occurring less frequently than 1 in 100 were reported in controlled clinical trials and from marketing experience. These reactions have been divided into two categories: Precise Incidence Unknown (but less than 1%) Probable Causal Relationship, lists reactions with ibuprofen therapy where the probability of a causal relationship exists; Precise Incidence Unknown (but less than 1%) Causal Relationship Unknown, lists reactions with ibuprofen therapy where a causal relationship has not been established.

Reported side effects were higher at doses of 3200 mg/day than at doses of 2400 mg or less per day in clinical trials of patients with rheumatoid arthritis. The increases in incidence were slight and still within the ranges reported in the following paragraphs.

Incidence greater than 1% (but less than 3%)
Probable Causal Relationship

Gastrointestinal: Nausea*, epigastric pain*, heartburn*, diarrhea, abdominal distress, nausea and vomiting, indigestion, constipation, abdominal cramps or pain, fullness of the GI tract (bloating and flatulence).

Central Nervous System: Dizziness*, headache, nervousness.

Dermatologic: Rash* (including maculopapular type), pruritus.

Special Senses: Tinnitus.

Metabolic/Endocrine: Decreased appetite.

Cardiovascular: Edema, fluid retention (generally responds promptly to drug discontinuation) (see **PRECAUTIONS**).

Precise Incidence Unknown (but less than 1%)
Probable Causal Relationship**

Gastrointestinal: Gastric or duodenal ulcer with bleeding and/or perforation, gastrointestinal hemorrhage, pancreatitis, melena, gastritis, hepatitis, jaundice, abnormal liver function tests.

Central Nervous System: Depression, insomnia, confusion, emotional lability, somnolence, aseptic meningitis with fever and coma. (See **PRECAUTIONS**.)

Dermatologic: Vesiculobullous eruptions, urticaria, erythema multiforme, Stevens-Johnson syndrome and alopecia.

Special Senses: Hearing loss, amblyopia (blurred and/or diminished vision, scotomata and/or changes in color vision). (see **PRECAUTIONS**).

Hematologic: Neutropenia, agranulocytosis, aplastic anemia, hemolytic anemia (sometimes Coombs positive), thrombocytopenia with or without purpura, eosinophilia, decrease in hemoglobin and hematocrit (see **PRECAUTIONS**).

Cardiovascular: Congestive heart failure in patients with marginal cardiac function, elevated blood pressure, palpitations.

Allergic: Syndrome of abdominal pain, fever, chills, nausea and vomiting, anaphylaxis, bronchospasm (see **CONTRAINDICATIONS**).

Renal: Acute renal failure in patients with pre-existing significantly impaired renal function (see **PRECAUTIONS**), decreased creatinine clearance, polyuria, azotemia, cystitis, hematuria.

Miscellaneous: Dry eyes and mouth, gingival ulcer, rhinitis.

Precise Incidence Unknown (but less than 1%)
Causal Relationship Unknown**

Central Nervous System: Paresthesias, hallucinations, dream abnormalities, pseudotumor cerebri.

Dermatologic: Toxic epidermal necrolysis, photoallergic skin reactions.

Special Senses: Conjunctivitis, diplopia, optic neuritis, cataracts.

Continued on next page

Boots Pharm.—Cont.

Hematologic: Bleeding episodes (e.g., epistaxis, menorrhagia).

Metabolic/Endocrine: Gynecomastia, hypoglycemic reactions, acidosis.

Cardiovascular: Arrhythmias (sinus tachycardia, sinus bradycardia).

Allergic: Serum sickness, lupus erythematosus syndrome, Henoch-Schonlein vasculitis, angioedema.

Renal: Renal papillary necrosis.

* Reactions occurring in 3% to 9% of patients treated with ibuprofen. (Those reactions occurring in less than 3% of the patients are unmarked).

** Reactions are classified under "Probable Causal Relationship (PCR)", if there has been one positive rechallenge or if three or more cases occur which might be casually related. Reactions are classified under "Causal Relationship Unknown", if seven or more events have been reported but the criteria for PCR have not been met.

OVERDOSAGE

Approximately 1½ hours after the reported ingestion of from 7 to 10 ibuprofen tablets (400 mg), a 19-month old child weighing 12 kg was seen in the hospital emergency room, apneic and cyanotic, responding only to painful stimuli. This type of stimulus, however, was sufficient to induce respiration. Oxygen and parenteral fluids were given; a greenish-yellow fluid was aspirated from the stomach with no evidence to indicate the presence of ibuprofen. Two hours after ingestion the child's condition seemed stable, she still responded only to painful stimuli and continued to have periods of apnea lasting from 5 to 10 seconds. She was admitted to intensive care and sodium bicarbonate was administered as well as infusions of dextrose and normal saline. By four hours post-ingestion she could be aroused easily, sit by herself and respond to spoken commands. Blood level of ibuprofen was 102.9 mcg/mL approximately 8½ hours after accidental ingestion. At 12 hours she appeared to be completely recovered.

In two other reported cases where children (each weighing approximately 10 kg) accidentally, acutely ingested approximately 120 mg/kg, there were no signs of acute intoxication or late sequelae. Blood level in one child 90 minutes after ingestion was 700 mcg/mL, about 10 times the peak levels seen in absorption-excretion studies.

A 19-year old male who had taken 8,000 mg of ibuprofen over a period of a few hours complained of dizziness, and nystagmus was noted. After hospitalization, parenteral hydration and three days bed rest, he recovered with no reported sequelae.

In cases of acute overdosage, the stomach should be emptied by vomiting or lavage, though little drug will likely be recovered if more than an hour has elapsed since ingestion. Because the drug is acidic and is excreted in the urine, it is theoretically beneficial to administer alkali and induce diuresis. In addition to supportive measures, the use of oral activated charcoal may help reduce the absorption and reabsorption of ibuprofen.

DOSAGE AND ADMINISTRATION

Do not exceed 3200 mg total daily dose. If gastrointestinal complaints occur, administer RUFEN with meals or milk.

Rheumatoid arthritis and osteoarthritis, including flareups of chronic disease: *Suggested Dosage:* 1200–3200 mg daily (300 mg q.i.d., or 400 mg, 600 mg or 800 t.i.d. or q.i.d.). Individual patients may show a better response to 3200 mg daily, as compared with 2400 mg, although in well-controlled clinical trials patients on 3200 mg did not show a better mean response in terms of efficacy. Therefore, when treating patients with 3200 mg/day, the physician should observe sufficient increased clinical benefits to offset potential increased risk.

The dose of ibuprofen should be tailored to each patient, and may be lowered or raised from the suggested doses depending on the severity of symptoms either at time of initiating drug therapy or as the patient responds or fails to respond.

In general, patients with rheumatoid arthritis seem to require higher doses of ibuprofen than do patients with osteoarthritis.

The smallest dose of RUFEN that yields acceptable control should be employed. A linear blood level dose-response relationship exists with single doses up to 800 mg (see **CLINICAL PHARMACOLOGY, Pharmacokinetcs** for effects of food on rate of absorption).

In chronic conditions, a therapeutic response to RUFEN therapy is sometimes seen in a few days to a week but most often is observed by two weeks. After a satisfactory response has been achieved, the patient's dose should be reviewed and adjusted as required.

Mild to moderate pain: 400 mg every 4 to 6 hours as necessary for the relief of pain.

In controlled analgesic clinical trials, doses of ibuprofen greater than 400 mg were no more effective than the 400 mg dose.

Dysmenorrhea: For the treatment of dysmenorrhea, beginning with the earliest onset of such pain, RUFEN should be given in a dose of 400 mg every 4 hours as necessary for the relief of pain.

HOW SUPPLIED

RUFEN Tablets 400 mg: round, magenta, sugar-coated tablets, printed RUFEN 400.

Bottles of 100	NDC 0524-0039-01
Bottles of 500	NDC 0524-0039-05
Unit Dose Cartons of 100	NDC 0524-0039-21

Manufactured for:
Boots Pharmaceuticals, Inc.
Shreveport, Louisiana 71106 USA
By:
The Boots Company PLC
Nottingham, England

RUFEN Tablets USP 600 mg: white, film-coated, elongated tablets printed RUFEN 6.

Bottles of 100	NDC 0524-0062-01
Bottles of 500	NDC 0524-0062-05
Unit Dose Cartons of 100	NDC 0524-0062-21

RUFEN Tablets 800 mg: white, film-coated, elongated tablets, printed RUFEN 8:

Bottles of 100	NDC 0524-0073-01
Bottles of 500	NDC 0524-0073-05
Unit Dose Cartons of 100	NDC 0524-0073-21

Manufactured and Distributed by:
Boots Pharmaceuticals, Inc.
Shreveport, Louisiana 71106, USA
a subsidiary of
The Boots Company (USA) Inc.

Caution: Federal (USA) law prohibits dispensing without prescription.

Rev. 2/10/89   26225-03

Shown in Product Identification Section, page 406

Boots-Flint, Inc.
A subsidiary of The Boots Company (USA) Inc.
300 TRI-STATE INTERNATIONAL CENTER
SUITE 200
LINCOLNSHIRE, IL 60069

CHOLOXIN® Tablets   ℞
[kō "lŏcks 'ĭn]
(Dextrothyroxine Sodium Tablets, USP)

DESCRIPTION

Dextrothyroxine Sodium, USP is the sodium salt of the dextrorotatory isomer of thyroxine useful in the treatment of hyperlipidemia. It is chemically described as D-3,5,3′,5′-tetraiodothyronine sodium salt.

CHOLOXIN (Dextrothyroxine Sodium) Tablets, USP are available for oral use containing 1, 2, 4, or 6 mg of dextrothyroxine sodium.

CHOLOXIN Tablets contain the following inactive ingredients: Acacia, confectioners' sugar, gelatin, lactose, magnesium stearate, polysorbate 80 (1, 2, and 6 mg tablets only), povidone and talc. The following are the color additives per tablet strength:

Strength (mg)	Color Additive(s)
1 mg	FD&C Yellow No. 6 (Sunset Yellow)
2 mg	FD&C Yellow No. 5 (tartrazine)
4 mg	None
6 mg	FD&C Yellow No. 5, (tartrazine) FD&C Blue No. 1

CLINICAL PHARMACOLOGY

The predominant effect of CHOLOXIN is the reduction of elevated serum cholesterol levels. Beta lipoprotein and triglyceride fractions may also be reduced from previously elevated levels.

Available evidence indicates that CHOLOXIN stimulates the liver to inrease catabolism and excretion of cholesterol and its degradation products via the biliary route into the feces. Cholesterol synthesis is not inhibited and abnormal metabolic end products do not accumulate in the blood.

INDICATION AND USAGE

CHOLOXIN may be indicated as an adjunct to diet for the reduction of elevated low density lipoprotein (LDL) cholesterol in patients with primary hypercholesterolemia (Types IIa and IIb) with no known or suspected heart disease, whose response to diet and other nonpharmacologic measures has been inadequate.

This is not an innocuous drug. Strict attention be paid to the indications nad contraindications.

After establishing that the elevation in serum cholesterol represents a primary disorder not due to secondary conditions such as poorly controlled diabetes mellitus, hypothyroidism, the nephrotic syndrome, liver disease, or dys-

proteinemias, it should be determined that a patient for whom treatment with CHOLOXIN is being considered has a pesistently elevated LDL cholesterol as the cause of an elevated total serum cholesterol. This may be particularly relevant for patients with elevated total triglycerides or with markedly elevated HDL-C values, where non-LDL lipoprotein fractions may contribute significantly to total cholesterol levels without apparent increase in cardiovascular risk. In most patients, LDL-C may be estimated according to the following equation:

$$LDL\text{-}C = \text{total cholesterol} - [(0.16 \times \text{triglycerides}) + HDL\text{-}C].$$

When total triglycerides are greater than 400 mg/dL this equation is less accurate. In such patients, LDL-Cholesterol may be obtained by ultracentrifugation.

It has not been clearly established whether dextrothyroxine induced lowering of serum cholesterol or lipid levels has a detrimental, beneficial, or no effect on the morbidity or mortality due to atherosclerosis of coronary heart disease. CHOLOXIN may have a detrimental effect on morbidity and mortality in patients with established coronary heart disease (see CONTRAINDICATIONS).

CONTRAINDICATIONS

The administration of CHOLOXIN to euthyroid patients with one or more of the following conditions is contraindicated.

1. Known or suspected organic heart disease, especially coronary artery disease, including angina pectoris; history of myocardial infarction; cardiac arrhythmia or tachycardia, either active or in patients with demonstrated propensity for arrhythmias; rheumatic heart disease; history of congestive heart failure; and decompensated or borderline compensated cardiac status. In a large study, involving men who had had a myocardial infarction, use of the drug was discontinued because of a trend to increased mortality in dextrothyroxine-treated subjects compared with placebo-treated patients.
2. Hypertension (other than mild, labile systolic hypertension.)
3. Pregnancy.
4. Nursing mothers.
5. History of iodism.
6. Safety and effectiveness in children have not been established.
7. In patients with advanced liver or kidney diseases.

WARNINGS

> Drugs with thyroid hormone activity, alone or together with other therapeutic agents, have been used for the treatment of obesity. In euthyroid patients, doses within the range of daily hormonal requirements are ineffective for weight reduction. Larger doses may produce serious or even life threatening manifestations of toxicity, particularly when given in association with sympathomimetic amines such as those used for their anorectic effects.
>
> In a large study, in men who have had a myocardial infarction, use of the drug was discontinued because of a trend to increased mortality in dextrothyroxine-treated subjects compared with placebo-treated patients. Even in subjects without known or suspected coronary disease, the potential benefits and risks of using CHOLOXIN should be carefully considered in patients presenting increased risk of coronary disease because of age, sex, obesity, history of smoking, hypertension and/or other factors increasing the risk of coronary artery disease, such as positive family history of premature coronary artery disease.

CHOLOXIN may potentiate the effects of anticoagulants on prothrombin time.
Reductions of anticoagulant by as much as 30% have been required in some patients.
Consequently, the dosage of anticoagulants should be reduced by one third upon initiation of CHOLOXIN therapy and the dosage subsequently readjusted on the basis of prothrombin time. The prothrombin time of patients receiving anticoagulant therapy concomitantly with CHOLOXIN therapy should be observed as frequently as necessary, at least weekly during the first few weeks of treatment.

In the surgical patient, it is wise to consider withdrawal of the drug two weeks prior to surgery if the use of anticoagulants during surgery is contemplated.

CHOLOXIN should not be used with thyroid replacement drugs.

Since the possibility of precipitating cardiac arrhythmias during surgery may be greater in patients treated with thyroid hormones, it may be wise to discontinue CHOLOXIN in euthyroid patients at least two weeks prior to an elective operation. Thus during emergency surgery in euthyroid patients, the patients should be carefully observed.

There are reports that dextrothyroxine sodium in diabetic patients is capable of increasing blood sugar levels with a resultant increase in requirements of insulin or oral hypoglycemic agents. Special attention should be paid to parameters necessary for good control of the diabetic state in dextrothyroxine sodium-treated subjects and to dosage requirements of insulin or other antidiabetic drugs. If dextrothyroxine sodium is later withdrawn from patients who had required a dosage increase of insulin or oral hypoglycemic agents during its administration, the dosage of antidiabetic drugs should be reduced and adjusted to maintain good control of the diabetic state.

When impaired liver and/or kidney function are present, the advantages of CHOLOXIN therapy must be weighed against the possibility of deleterious results (see CONTRAINDICATIONS).

PRECAUTIONS

General: It is expected that patients on CHOLOXIN therapy will show increased serum thyroxine levels. These increased serum thyroxine values are evidence of absorption and transport of the drug, and should NOT be interpreted as evidence of hypermetabolism; therefore, they may not be used to determine the effective dose of dextrothyroxine sodium. Thyroxine values in the range of 10 to 25 mcg% in dextrothyroxine sodium-treated patients are common.

If signs or symptoms of iodism develop during dextrothyroxine sodium therapy, the drug should be discontinued.

The 2 mg and 6 mg CHOLOXIN tablets contain FD&C Yellow No. 5 (tartrazine) which may cause allergic-type reactions (including bronchial asthma) in certain susceptible individuals. Although the overall incidence of FD&C Yellow No. 5 (tartrazine) sensitivity in the general population is low, it is frequently seen in patients who also have aspirin hypersensitivity.

Information for patients: Patients should receive instruction in appropriate dietary and other nonpharmacologic measures designed to reduce serum cholesterol levels. These include restriction of intake of cholesterol, total calories, and saturated fatty acids, and increasing the ratio of polyunsaturated to saturated fats.

Patients should be instructed to notify physician if any of the following occur: Palpitations, chest pain, diarrhea, excessive sweating, rash or acne, insomnia, headache, increasing nervousness, or visual disturbances.

Drug interactions: Dextrothyroxine sodium potentiates the effect of anticoagulants on prothrombin time, thus indicating a decrease in the dosage requirements of the anticoagulants. On the other hand, dosage requirements of antidiabetic drugs have been reported to be increased during dextrothyroxine sodium therapy (see **WARNINGS.**)

Carcinogenesis, mutagenesis, impairment of fertility: Long term studies in animals to evaluate carcinogenic potential have not been performed.

Pregnancy: Teratogenic effects—Pregnancy Category B. Reproduction studies have been performed in rabbits and rats at doses up to 100 times (mg/kg) the expected maximum daily dose for humans and have revealed no evidence of impaired fertility or harm to the fetus due to CHOLOXIN. There are, however, no adequate and well-controlled studies in pregnant women. Because animal reproduction studies are not always predictive of human response, this drug should be used during pregnancy only if clearly needed.

Women of childbearing age who require drug therapy for hypercholesterolemia should consider use of a bile acid sequestering resin. Since pregnancy may occur despite the use of birth control procedures, administration of CHOLOXIN to women of this age group should be undertaken only after weighing the possible risk to the fetus against the possible benefits to the mother.

Nursing mothers: It is not known whether dextrothyroxine sodium is excreted in human milk. Because many drugs are excreted in human milk, caution should be exercised when CHOLOXIN is administered to a nursing woman (see **CONTRAINDICATIONS**).

PEDIATRIC USE

Safety and effectiveness in children have not been established (see **CONTRAINDICATIONS**).

ADVERSE REACTIONS

The side effects attributed to CHOLOXIN therapy are, for the most part, due to increased metabolism, and may be minimized by following the recommended dosage schedule. Adverse effects are least commonly seen in euthyroid patients with no signs or symptoms of organic heart disease.

In the absence of known organic heart disease, some cardiac changes may be precipitated during dextrothyroxine sodium therapy. Angina pectoris, extrasystoles, ectopic beats, supraventricular tachycardia, ECG evidence of ischemic myocardial changes and increase in heart size have all been observed. Myocardial infarctions, both fatal and nonfatal, have occurred, but theses are not unexpected in untreated patients in the age groups studied. It is not known whether any of these infarcts were drug related.

However, should any of these signs or symptoms develop, or other evidence of cardiac disease appear, CHOLOXIN is contraindicated and should be discontinued.

Changes in clinical status that may be related to the metabolic action of the drug include the development of insomnia,

nervousness, palpitations, tremors, loss of weight, lid lag, sweating, flushing, hyperthermia, hair loss, diuresis, and menstrual irregularities. Gastrointestinal complaints during therapy have included dyspepsia, nausea and vomiting, constipation, diarrhea, and decrease in appetite.

Other side effects reported to be associated with dextrothyroxine sodium therapy include the development of headache, changes in libido (increase or decrease), hoarseness, tinnitus, dizziness, peripheral edema, malaise, tiredness, visual disturbances, psychological changes, paresthesia, muscle pain, and various bizarre subjective complaints. Skin rashes, including a few which appeared to be due to iodism, and itching have been attributed to dextrothyroxine sodium by some investigators. Gallstones have been discovered in occasional dextrothyroxine sodium-treated patients and cholestatic jaundice has occurred in one patient, although its relationship to dextrothyroxine sodium therapy was not established.

In several instances, the previously existing conditions of the patient appeared to continue or progress during the administration of dextrothyroxine sodium. A worsening of peripheral vascular disease, altered sensorium, exophthalmos and retinopathy have been reported.

OVERDOSAGE

Overdosage with CHOLOXIN may result in signs and symptoms of thyrotoxicosis. The dosage at which such symptoms may appear will depend on the previous thyroid status of the patient, and their individual sensitivity to the drug. CHOLOXIN is somewhat protein-bound and would not be expected to be appreciably dialyzable. Treatment of overdosage is similar to that of thyrotoxic storm and may include hydration, sedation, and use of beta-adrenergic blocking agents.

DOSAGE AND ADMINISTRATION

For adult euthroid hypercholesterolemic patients, the recommended maintenance dose of CHOLOXIN is 4 to 8 mg per day. The initial dose should be 1 to 2 mg daily, to be increased in 1 to 2 mg increments at intervals of not less that one month to a maximal level of 4 to 8 mg daily.

If signs and symptoms of cardiac disease develop during the treatment period, the drug should be withdrawn.

HOW SUPPLIED

CHOLOXIN® (Dextrothyroxine Sodium), USP Tablets are supplied as scored, color-coded tablets in 4 strengths as shown below:

Strength and Color	Tablets per Container	Code	NDC
1 mg Orange	100	3P1413	0048-1230-03
2 mg Yellow	100	3P1423	0048-1250-03
4 mg White	100	3P1433	0048-1270-03
6 mg Green	100	3P1463	0048-1290-03

TABLE 1
NUMBER OF SENSITIVE BURN ISOLATED STRAINS/
TOTAL BURN ISOLATED STRAINS TESTED

Genus & Species	CONCENTRATION OF SILVER SULFADIAZINE 62.5 mcg/ml	125 mcg/ml
Pseudomonas aeruginosa	46/54	50/54
Pseudomonas cepacia	2/3	2/3
Pseudomonas species	2/3	2/3
Enterobacter cloacae	6/14	6/14
Enterobacter aerogenes	4/6	4/6
Enterobacter agglomerans	1/1	1/1
Klebsiella pneumoniae	4/4	4/4
Klebsiella species	1/3	1/3
Escherichia coli	11/15	11/15
Serratia liquifaciens	3/3	3/3
Serratia marcescens	6/6	6/6
Serratia rubidae	2/2	2/2
Serratia species	0/1	1/1
Proteus mirabilis	8/8	8/8
Proteus morganii	8/9	8/9
Proteus rettgeri	1/1	1/1
Proteus vulgaris	3/4	4/4
Providencia species	3/3	3/3
Citrobacter diversus	0/2	0/2
Shigella species	1/2	1/2
Acinetobacter anitratum	2/2	2/2
Aeromonas hydrophilia	3/3	3/3
Arizona hinshawii	1/1	1/1
Alcaligenes faecalis	2/2	2/2
Staphylococcus aureus	7/7	7/7
Streptococcus Group D (including *Enterococcus*)	17/18	18/18
Bacillus species	0/1	1/1
Candida albicans	1/3	3/3
Candida species	0/1	1/1

Store at controlled room temperature, 15°–30° C (59°–86° F).
Caution: Federal (USA) law prohibits dispensing without a prescription.
Manufactured by:
Boots Puerto Rico, Inc.
Jayuya, Puerto Rico 00664-0795
For
Boots-Flint, Inc.
Lincolnshire, IL 60069 USA
a subsidiary of
The Boots Company (USA) Inc.
1230-02
Rev. 04/89
Shown in Product Identification Section, page 406

FLINT SSD™   ℞
(1% Silver Sulfadiazine Cream)

DESCRIPTION

Flint SSD™ (1% Silver Sulfadiazine Cream) is a topical antibacterial preparation which has as its active antimicrobial ingredient silver sulfadiazine. The active moiety is contained within an opaque, white, water-miscible cream base.

Each 1000 grams of FLINT SSD™ Cream contains 10 grams of silver sulfadiazine. The cream base contains White Petrolatum, USP; Polyoxyl 40 Stearate, NF; Cetyl Alcohol, NF; Stearyl Alcohol, NF; Propylene Glycol, USP; Isopropyl Myristate, NF; Sorbitan Monooleate, NF; Sodium Hydroxide, Purified Water, USP; with 0.3% Methylparaben, NF, as a preservative.

Silver sulfadiazine has an empirical formula of $C_{10}H_9AgN_4O_2S$, molecular weight of 357.14, and structural formula as shown:

CLINICAL PHARMACOLOGY

Flint SSD™ Cream has demonstrated *in vitro* antimicrobial activity against actual clinical burn wound isolates. Representative organisms included numerous strains of gramnegative and gram-positive bacteria and yeasts. *In vitro* test results evaluating the antimicrobial effectiveness of silver sulfadiazine are summarized in Table 1. All microorganisms analyzed for susceptibility are isolates from burn patients obtained nationwide.
[See table above].
Flint SSD™ (1% Silver Sulfadiazine Cream) exerts its principal antimicrobial effect at the level of the cell membrane and cell wall. The mechanism and site of action differ from sodium sulfadiazine and silver nitrate. *In vitro* analysis has

Continued on next page

Boots-Flint—Cont.

demonstrated that the bactericidal activity exerted by Flint SSD™ (1% Silver Sulfadiazine Cream) is superior to sulfadiazine alone.

Flint SSD™ Cream may be especially applicable to the treatment of pediatric burn patients, because it is not a carbonic anhydrase inhibitor. There have been no reports of acidosis attributable to treatment with Flint SSD™ Cream.

INDICATIONS AND USAGE

Flint SSD™ Cream is a topical antibacterial preparation which is indicated as an adjunct to currently accepted principles of burn wound care, for the prevention and treatment of burn wound sepsis in patients with partial and full thickness burns.

CONTRAINDICATIONS

Since sulfonamide derivatives are known to increase the possibility of kernicterus[1], Flint SSD™ Cream should not be used in pregnant women approaching or at term, premature infants, or neonates less than two months of age.

WARNINGS

Flint SSD™ Cream should be administered with caution to patients with a history of hypersensitivity to silver sulfadiazine. It is not known whether prior sensitivity to other sulfonamides will precipitate an allergic response to Flint SSD™ Cream.

Should manifestation of allergic response to Flint SSD™ Cream be observed, continuation of therapy must be weighed against the potential hazards of the particular allergic reaction.

While Flint SSD™ Cream is exerting a bacteriostatic effect on the burn wound, fungal proliferation in and below the eschar may occur. However, the incidence of clinically reported fungal superinfection is low.

Flint SSD™ Cream should be used with caution in patients with a history of glucose-6-phosphate dehydrogenase deficiency, as hemolysis may occur.

When treatment with Flint SSD™ Cream involves prolonged administration and/or large burn surfaces, considerable amounts of silver sulfadiazine are absorbed. Serum sulfa concentrations may approach adult therapeutic levels (8-12 mg%).

In extensively burned patients, serum sulfa concentrations and renal function should be closely monitored, and urine should be analyzed for presence of sulfa crystals.

PRECAUTIONS

Following administration of Flint SSD™ (1% Silver Sulfadiazine Cream), absorption of sulfadiazine has been reported. In addition, small amounts of silver are absorbed over the course of repeated application of Flint SSD™ Cream. Impairment of hepatic and renal functions which results in diminished excretion of drug constituents may lead to accumulation of silver and sulfadiazine moieties. In the presence of hepatic and/or renal dysfunction, the therapeutic benefits of continued silver sulfadiazine administration must be assessed in light of the possibility of accumulation of by-products.

When utilizing topical enzymatic preparations for debridement of partial and full thickness burn wounds, concomitant or alternating topical antimicrobial therapy must be employed.

Pregnancy: Teratogenic effects

Pregnancy Category C: Animal reproduction studies have not been conducted with Flint SSD™ Cream. It is also not known whether Flint SSD™ Cream can cause fetal harm when administered to a pregnant woman or can affect reproduction capacity. Flint SSD™ Cream should be given to a pregnant woman only if clearly needed.

There are no reports in the medical literature which associate Flint SSD™ Cream therapy with adverse effects on the fetus or reproductive capacity.

Flint SSD™ Cream should be administered to pregnant women only when the physician decides that the potentially life-saving benefits of silver sulfadiazine therapy in the larger burn (extent greater than 20% body surface area) outweigh possible hazard to the fetus.

Nursing mothers: There is no evidence that topical application of Flint SSD™ Cream results in excretion of any of its constituents in human milk. However, since all sulfonamide derivatives are known to increase the possibility of kernicterus, caution should be exercised when Flint SSD™ Cream is administered to nursing women.

ADVERSE REACTIONS

Several cases of transient leukopenia have been reported in patients receiving silver sulfadiazine therapy. Leukopenia associated with silver sulfadiazine administration is primarily characterized by decreased neutrophil count. Maximal white blood cell depression occurs within two to four days of initiation of therapy. Rebound to normal leukocyte levels follows onset within two to three days. Recovery is not influenced by continuation of silver sulfadiazine therapy. The incidence of leukopenia in various reports averages about

20%, although an incidence as high as 55% has been noted (Caffee and Bingham, 1982). An even higher incidence has been seen in patients simultaneously treated with cimetidine.

A low incidence of other adverse reactions has been reported. These include burning sensation, rashes and pruritus, and rarely, interstitial nephritis.

It is often difficult to differentiate topical reactions which are precipitated by Flint SSD™ (1% Silver Sulfadiazine Cream) from those resulting from routine burn wound effects, or caused by hypersensitivity to other therapeutic agents being administered concurrently to the patient.

During the treatment of burns over large body surfaces (greater than 20% body surface area), significant amounts of silver sulfadiazine are systemically absorbed. Therefore, it is possible that any adverse reactions associated with sulfonamides may occur.

DOSAGE AND ADMINISTRATION

In the patient with a major burn, evaluation of airway and fluid replacement needs should precede treatment of the burn wound. After appropriate resuscitative measures are instituted, the burn wound is evaluated for extent and depth, and an appropriate treatment regimen is instituted.

Flinit SSD™ Cream should be applied to a thickness of at least 1/16 inch, to selected burned surfaces once or twice daily.

It is recommended that a protocol for management of the burn wound using accepted principles and techniques of debridement be followed. Flint SSD™ Cream should be applied with sterile gloves.

Flint SSD™ Cream will provide antimicrobial protection when used with either open treatment or occlusive dressing regimens. When treating patients utilizing the open method, care must be taken to promptly reapply Flint SSD™ Cream whenever it is removed by patient movement.

Daily hydrotherapy facilitates debridement of loosened eschar and removal of accumulated debris. Flint SSD™ Cream should be reapplied immediately after hydrotherapy.

Treatment of burns with topical antimicrobial agents has been reported to allow spontaneous healing of deep partial thickness burn wounds, by preventing bacterial proliferation which could otherwise cause conversion to full thickness loss. However, delayed separation of eschar associated with the use of topical antimicrobial agents such as Flint SSD™ Cream may require definitive surgical treatment of the eschar.

Flint SSD™ Cream should be applied continually until either spontaneous healing or grafting of the burn wound is achieved.

In order to avoid the possibility of infection, Flint SSD™ Cream should not be withdrawn from the therapeutic regimen until definitive wound closure is accomplished, unless there is a significant adverse reaction to the drug.

HOW SUPPLIED

FLINT SSD Cream (1% Silver Sulfadiazine Cream) is supplied as follows:

3P4000 NDC 0048-2100-71	50 gram jar
3P4007 NDC 0048-2100-70	400 gram jar
3P4009 NDC 0048-2100-73	1000 gram jar

Store at controlled room temperatures 15°–30° C (59°–86° F).

CAUTION

Federal law prohibits dispensing without prescription.

REFERENCES

1. American Medical Association, eds. 1980. Sulfonamides and related compounds, in: **AMA Drug Evaluations**, ed. 4., chap. 77, 1305.
2. Caffee H. Bingham H. 1982. Leukopenia and Silver Sulfadiazine **J. Trauma** 22: No. 7 586-587.
3. Delaveau P, Friedrich-Noue P. 1977. Cutaneous absorption and urinary elimination of silver sulfadiazine compounds used in the treatment of burns. **Therapie** 32:563-572. (Fr)
4. Dimick AR. 1977. Experience with the use of proteolytic enzyme (Travase®) in burn patients. **J Trauma** 17:948-955.
5. Fox CL Jr. 1968. Silver Sulfadiazine—A new topical therapy for Pseudomonas in burns. Therapy of Pseudomonas infection in burns. **Arch Surg** 96:184-188.
6. Fox CL Jr. Modak SM, 1974. Mechanism of silver sulfadiazine action of burn wound infections. **Antimicrob Agents for Chemother** 5:582-588.
7. Harrison HN. 1979. Pharmacology of sulfadiazine silver. Its attachment to burned human and rat skin and studies of gastrointestinal absorption and extension. **Arch Surg** 114-:281-285.
8. Jarret F. et al. 1978. Acute leukopenia during topical burn therapy with silver sulfadiazine. **Amer J Surg** 135:818-819.
9. Kiker RG. et al. 1977. A controlled study of the effects of silver sulfadiazine on white blood cell counts in burned children. **J Trauma** 17:835-835.
10. Krizek TJ. et al. 1975. Emergency nonsurgical escharotomy in the burned extremity. **Orthop Rev** (July), 53-55.
11. Pennisi VR. et al. 1976. The combined efficacy of Travase and silver sulfadiazine in the acute burn. **Burns** 2:169-172.
12. Rodeheaver G, et al. 1975. Proteolytic enzymes as adjuncts to antimicrobial prophylaxis of contaminated wounds. **Am J Surg** 129:537-544.

Manufactured for
Boots-Flint, Inc.
Lincolnshire, Illinois 60069 USA
a subsidiary of The Boots Company (USA) Inc.
By Paco Laboratories, Inc.
Lakewood, NJ 08701, USA

12/87

Shown in Product Indentification Section, page 406

RU-TUSS® TABLETS   ℞
[roo-tŭs]

DESCRIPTION

Each prolonged action tablet contains:

Phenylephrine Hydrochloride	25 mg
Phenylpropanolamine Hydrochloride	50 mg
Chlorpheniramine Maleate	8 mg
Hyoscyamine Sulfate	0.19 mg
Atropine Sulfate	0.04 mg
Scopolamine Hydrobromide	0.01 mg

RU-TUSS Tablets act continuously for 10 to 12 hours.

RU-TUSS Tablets are an oral antihistaminic, nasal decongestant and anti-secretory preparation.

INDICATIONS AND USAGE

RU-TUSS Tablets provide relief of the symptoms resulting from irritation of sinus, nasal and upper respiratory tract tissues. Phenylephrine and phenylpropanolamine combine to exert a vasoconstrictive and decongestive action while chlorpheniramine maleate decreases the symptoms of watering eyes, post nasal drip and sneezing which may be associated with an allergic-like response. The belladonna alkaloids, hyoscyamine, atropine and scopolamine further augment the anti-secretory activity of RU-TUSS Tablets.

CONTRAINDICATIONS

Hypersensitivity to antihistamines or sympathomimetics. RU-TUSS Tablets are contraindicated in children under 12 years of age and in patients with glaucoma, bronchial asthma and women who are pregnant. Concomitant use of MAO inhibitors is contraindicated.

WARNINGS

RU-TUSS Tablets may cause drowsiness. Patients should be warned of the possible additive effects caused by taking antihistamines with alcohol, hypnotics, sedatives or tranquilizers.

PRECAUTIONS

RU-TUSS Tablets contain belladonna alkaloids, and must be administered with care to those patients with urinary bladder neck obstruction. Caution should be exercised when RU-TUSS Tablets are given to patients with hypertension, cardiac or peripheral vascular disease or hyperthyroidism. Patients should avoid driving a motor vehicle or operating dangerous machinery (See **WARNINGS**).

OVERDOSAGE

Since the action of sustained release products may continue for as long as 12 hours, treatment of overdoses directed at reversing the effects of the drug and supporting the patient should be maintained for at least that length of time. Saline cathartics are useful for hastening evacuation of unreleased medication. In children and infants, antihistamine overdosage may produce convulsions and death.

ADVERSE REACTIONS

Hypersensitivity reactions such as rash, urticaria, leukopenia, agranulocytosis, and thrombocytopenia may occur. Other adverse reactions to RU-TUSS Tablets may be drowsiness, lassitude, giddiness, dryness of the mucous membranes, tightness of the chest, thickening of bronchial secretions, urinary frequency and dysuria, palpitation, tachycardia, hypotension/hypertension, faintness, dizziness, tinnitus, headache, incoordination, visual disturbances, mydriasis, xerostomia, blurred vision, anorexia, nausea, vomiting, diarrhea, constipation, epigastric distress, hyperirritability, nervousness, and insomnia. Large overdoses may cause tachypnea, delirium, fever, stupor, coma and respiratory failure.

DOSAGE AND ADMINISTRATION

Adults and children over 12 years of age, one tablet morning and evening. Not recommended for children under 12 years of age. Tablets are to be swallowed whole.

HOW SUPPLIED

Bottles of 100 Tablets	NDC 0048-0058-01
Bottles of 500 Tablets	NDC 0048-0058-05

Federal law prohibits dispensing without prescription.

Manufactured by:
Vitarine Company, Inc.
Springfield Gardens, New York, 11413 USA
For
Boots-Flint Inc.
Lincolnshire, Illinois 60069 USA
a subsidiary of
The Boots Company (USA) Inc.
Rev. 10/87   0058-04
Shown in Product Identification Section, page 406

RU–TUSS® II CAPSULES   ℞
[*roo-tŭs*]
Phenylpropanolamine Hydrochloride 75 mg
Chlorpheniramine Maleate 12 mg

DESCRIPTION
Each slow-release capsule contains 12 mg of chlorpheniramine maleate and 75 mg of phenylpropanolamine hydrochloride so prepared that an initial dose is released promptly (approximately one-third of the contents) and the remaining medication is released gradually over a prolonged period. White beads are DYE-FREE.
Chlorpheniramine maleate is 2-[p-chloro-α[2-(dimethylamino) ethyl] benzyl] pyridine maleate(1:1), an antihistamine, phenylpropanolamine hydrochloride is benzenemethanol, α-(1-aminoethyl)-hydrochloride, (R*, S*)-, (±), an adrenergic agent.
The structural formulas are as follows:

Chlorpheniramine Maleate
M.W.390.87

Phenylpropanolamine HCl
M.W. 187.67

CLINICAL PHARMACOLOGY
Chlorpheniramine Maleate: An antihistamine with anticholinergic (drying) and sedative side effects. Antihistamines appear to compete with histamine for cell receptor sites on effector cells. Chlorpheniramine maleate is a member of the alkylamine class of antihistamines which are among the least sedating antihistamines.
Phenylpropanolamine Hydrochloride: The drug may directly stimulate adrenergic receptors but probably indirectly stimulates both alpha (*a*) and beta (*b*) adrenergic receptors by releasing norepinephrine from its storage sites. Phenylpropanolamine increases heart rate, force of contraction and cardiac output, and excitability. It acts on alpha receptors in the mucosa of the respiratory tract, producing vasoconstriction which results in shrinkage of swollen mucous membranes, reduction of tissue, hyeremia, edema and nasal congestion, and an increase in nasal airway patency. Phenylpropanolamine causes CNS stimulation and reportedly has an anorexigenic effect.
Pharmacokinetics: The active drugs, 12 mg of chlorpheniramine maleate and 75 mg of phenylpropanolamine hydrochloride, in each capsule of this special slow-release dosage form approximate the serum levels of two liquid doses containing 6 mg of chlorpheniramine maleate and 37.5 mg of phenylpropanolamine hydrochloride taken at six hour intervals. The absorption half-life of the drugs from a non-timed liquid is appreciably more rapid than from the slow-release formulation.
When studied under controlled conditions, the peak chlorpheniramine serum level occurs about 5.5 hours after administration and the peak phenylpropanolamine level occurs after about 3.5 hours. The average half-life of elimination is about 17.5 hours for chlorpheniramine and 5.0 hours for phenylpropanolamine.

INDICATIONS AND USAGE
For the treatment of the symptoms of seasonal and perennial allergic rhinitis and vasomotor rhinitis, including nasal obstruction (congestion).

CONTRAINDICATIONS
Hypersensitivity to either ingredient; severe hypertension; coronary artery disease; stenosing peptic ulcer; pyloroduodenal or bladder neck obstruction.
These capsules should NOT be used to treat lower respiratory tract conditions, including asthma.
As with any product containing a sympathomimetic, capsules should NOT be used in patients taking MAO inhibitors. Because of the higher risk of antihistamine side effects in infants generally, and for newborns and premature in partic-

ular, antihistamine therapy is contraindicated in nursing mothers. Capsules should NOT be used in newborns or premature infants.

WARNINGS
Caution patients about activities requiring alertness (e.g. operating vehicles or machinery). Patients should also be warned about the possible additive effects of alcohol and other CNS depressants (hypnotics, sedatives, tranquilizers, etc.).

PRECAUTIONS
General: Capsules should be used with considerable caution in patients with narrow angle glaucoma, stenosing peptic ulcer, pyloroduodenal obstruction, symptomatic prostatic hypertrophy, bladder neck obstruction, hypertension, thyroid disease, diabetes and heart disease. The risk of antihistamine induced dizziness, sedation and hypotension is greater in elderly patients (over 60 years)
Drug Interactions: These capsules should not be used in patients taking MAO inhibitors. Antihistamines have additive effects with alcohol and other CNS depressants (hypnotics, sedatives, tranquilizers, etc.).
Usage in Pregnancy: Pregnancy Category C. Animal reproduction studies have not been conducted. It is also not known whether this product can cause fetal harm when administered to a pregnant woman or can affect reproduction capacity. Capsules should be given to pregnant women only if clearly needed.
Nursing Mothers: It is not known whether this drug is excreted in human milk. Because many drugs are excreted in human milk, caution should be exercised when this product is administered to a nursing mother.
Pediatric Use: Safety and effectiveness in children below the age of 12 have not been established.

ADVERSE REACTIONS
General: Urticaria, drug rash, anaphylactic shock, photosensitivity, excessive perspiration, chills, dryness of the mouth, nose and throat.
Cardiovascular System: Hypotension, hypertension, headache palpitations, tachycardia, extrasystoles and angina pain.
Hematologic System: Hemolytic anemia, thrombocytopenia, agranulocytosis.
Nervous System: Sedation, dizziness, disturbed coordination, fatigue, confusion, restlessness, excitation, nervousness, tremor, irritability, insomnia, euphoria, paresthesias, blurred vision, diplopia, vertigo, tinnitus, acute labyrinthitis, hysteria, neuritis and convulsions.
Gastrointestinal System: Epigastric distress, anorexia, nausea, vomiting, diarrhea, constipation.
Genitourinary System: Urinary frequency, difficult urination, urinary retention, early menses.
Respiratory System: Thickening of bronchial secretions, tightness of chest and wheezing, nasal stuffiness.

OVERDOSAGE
Symptoms: Overdosage symptoms may vary from central nervous system depression to stimulation. Peripheral atropine-like signs and symptoms as well as gastrointestinal symptoms may occur. Marked cerebral irritation resulting in jerking of muscles and possible convulsions may be followed by deep stupor and respiratory failure. Acute hypertension or cardiovascular collapse with accompanying hypotension may occur.
Treatment: If spontaneous vomiting has not occurred, immediate evacuation of the stomach should be induced by emesis or gastric lavage. Saline cathartics, such as milk of magnesia, draw water into the bowel by osmosis, and therefore, are valuable for their action in rapid dilution of bowel content. Respiratory depression should be treated promptly with oxygen. Do not treat CNS depression with analeptics which might precipitate convulsion. If convulsions or marked CNS excitement occur, use only short-acting depressants.

DOSAGE AND ADMINISTRATION
Adults and children over 12 years of age—one capsule every 12 hours. Should not be used in children under 12.

HOW SUPPLIED
Available for oral administration in green/clear, slow-release capsules, printed "Ru-Tuss II" over "31" on body and "Boots" over "31" on cap in gold ink.
100 Capsule Bottle NDC 0048-0031-01
Storage Conditions: Protect from light. Store in dry place 59°–86°F.
CAUTION: Federal law prohibits dispensing without prescription.

Manufactured by
KV Pharmaceutical Company
St. Louis, Missouri 63144
For
Boots-Flint, Inc.
Lincolnshire, Illinois 60069 USA
a subsidiary of
The Boots Company (USA) Inc.
Rev. 10/87   0031-05
Shown in Product Identification Section, page 406

RU–TUSS®   Ⓒ
With Hydrocodone
[*roo-tŭs*]

DESCRIPTION
Each fluid ounce of RU-TUSS® with Hydrocodone contains:
Hydrocodone Bitartrate .... 10 mg
(WARNING: MAY BE HABIT FORMING)
Phenylephrine Hydrochloride .... 30 mg
Phenylpropanolamine Hydrochloride .... 20 mg
Pheniramine Maleate .... 20 mg
Pyrilamine Maleate .... 20 mg
Alcohol 5%
Contains FD&C Yellow No. 6 (Sunset Yellow) as a color additive.
RU-TUSS with Hydrocodone is an oral antitussive, antihistaminic and nasal decongestant preparation.

INDICATIONS AND USAGE
RU-TUSS with Hydrocodone is indicated for the temporary relief of symptoms associated with hay fever, allergies, nasal congestion and cough due to the common cold.

CONTRAINDICATIONS
Hypersensitivity to antihistamines. Concomitant use of antihypertensive or antidepressant drugs containing a monoamine oxidase inhibitor is contraindicated.
RU-TUSS with Hydrocodone is contraindicated in patients with glaucoma, bronchial asthma and in women who are pregnant.

WARNINGS
Patients should be warned of the potential that RU-TUSS with Hydrocodone may be habit forming.
RU-TUSS with Hydrocodone may cause drowsiness.
Patients should be warned of the possible additive effects caused by taking antihistamines with alcohol, hypnotics, sedatives and tranquilizers.

PRECAUTIONS
Patients taking RU-TUSS with Hydrocodone should avoid driving a motor vehicle or operating dangerous machinery (See **WARNINGS**).
Caution should be taken with patients having hypertension and cardiovascular disease.

ADVERSE REACTIONS
RU-TUSS with Hydrocodone may cause drowsiness, lassitude, giddiness, dryness of mucous membranes, tightness of the chest, thickening of bronchial secretions, urinary frequency and dysuria, palpitation, tachycardia, hypotension/hypertension, faintness, dizziness, tinnitus, headache, incoordination, visual disturbances, mydriasis, xerostomia, blurred vision, anorexia, nausea, vomiting, diarrhea, constipation, epigastric distress, hyperirritability, nervousness and insomnia.
Overdoses may cause restlessness, excitation, delirium, tremors, euphoria, stupor, tachycardia and even convulsions.

DOSAGE AND ADMINISTRATION
Adults: 2 teaspoonfuls, orally, every 4 to 6 hours.
Children 6 to 12 years of age: 1 teaspoonful every 4 to 6 hours.
Children 2 to 6 years of age: ½ to 1 teaspoonful every 4 to 6 hours, according to age. Doses for children should not be repeated more than 4 times in any 24 hour period.

HOW SUPPLIED
Pint Bottles (16 fl. oz.)   NDC 0048-1007-16
Caution: Federal law prohibits dispensing without prescription.

Manufactured by
Boots Pharmaceuticals, Inc.
Shreveport, Louisiana 71106 USA
For
Boots-Flint, Inc.
Lincolnshire, Illinois 60069 USA
a subsidiary of
The Boots Company (USA) Inc.
Rev. 10/87   20725-01

Continued on next page

Boots-Flint—Cont.

SYNTHROID®   ℞

[sĭn 'throid]
(Levothyroxine Sodium, USP)
Synthroid Tablets—for oral administration
Synthroid Injection—for parenteral
administration after reconstitution

DESCRIPTION

SYNTHROID (Levothyroxine Sodium, USP) **Tablets** and **Injection** contain synthetic crystalline L-3,3',5,5'-tetraiodothyronine sodium salt (levothyroxine (T_4) sodium). Synthetic T_4 is similar to that produced in the human thyroid gland. T_4 contains four iodine atoms and is formed by the coupling of two molecules of diiodotyrosine (DIT).
Levothyroxine (T_4) Sodium has an empirical formula of $C_{15}H_{10}I_4NNaO_4xH_2O$, molecular weight of 798.86 (anhydrous), and structural formula as shown:

LEVOTHYROXINE SODIUM

SYNTHROID **Tablets** contain the following inactive ingredients: Acacia, gelatin (50 mcg strength only), lactose, magnesium stearate, povidone, confectioners' sugar, and talc. The following are the color additives per tablet strength:

Strength (mcg)	Color Additive(s)
25	FD&C Yellow No. 6 (Sunset Yellow)
50	None
75	FD&C Red No. 40, FD&C Blue No. 2
100	FD&C Yellow No. 5 (tartrazine)
112	FD&C Red No. 3, FD&C Blue No. 2.
125	FD&C Yellow No. 6 (Sunset Yellow), FD&C Red No. 40, FD&C Blue No. 1
150	FD&C Blue No. 2
175	FD&C Blue No. 1, D&C Red No. 27 & 30
200	FD&C Red No. 40
300	FD&C Blue No. 1, FD&C Yellow No. 5 (tartrazine)

CLINICAL PHARMACOLOGY

The steps in the synthesis of thyroid hormones are controlled by thyrotropin (Thyroid Stimulating Hormone, TSH) secreted by the anterior pituitary. This hormone's secretion is in turn controlled by a feedback mechanism effected by the thyroid hormones themselves and by thyrotropin releasing hormone (TRH), a tripeptide of hypothalamic origin. Endogenous thyroid hormone secretion is suppressed when exogenous thyroid hormones are administered to euthyroid individuals in excess of the normal gland's secretion.
The mechanisms by which thyroid hormones exert their physiologic action are not well understood. These hormones enhance oxygen consumption by most tissues of the body and increase the basal metabolic rate and the metabolism of carbohydrates, lipids, and proteins. Thus they exert a profound influence on every organ system in the body and are of particular importance in the development of the central nervous system.
The normal thyroid gland contains approximately 200 mcg of levothyroxine (T_4) per gram of gland, and 15 mcg of triiodothyronine (T_3) per gram. The ratio of these two hormones in the circulation does not represent the ratio in the thyroid gland, since about 80 percent of peripheral triiodothyronine comes from monodeiodination of levothyroxine at the 5 position (outer ring). Peripheral levothyroxine at the 5 position (inner ring) results in the formation of reverse triiodothyronine (rT_3), which is calorigenically inactive. These facts would seem to advocate levothyroxine as the treatment of choice for the hypothyroid patient and to militate against the administration of hormone combinations which, while normalizing thyroxine levels may produce triiodothyronine levels in the thyrotoxic range.
Triiodothyronine (T_3) level is low in the fetus and newborn, in old age, in chronic caloric deprivation, hepatic cirrhosis, renal failure, surgical stress, and chronic illnesses representing what has been called the "low triiodothyronine syndrome."

PHARMACOKINETICS

Animal studies have shown that T_4 is only partially absorbed from the gastrointestinal tract. The degree of absorption is dependent on the vehicle used for its administration and by the character of the intestinal contents, the intestinal flora, including plasma protein, soluble dietary factors, all of which bind thyroid and thereby make it unavailable for diffusion.

Depending on other factors, absorption has varied from 48 to 79 percent of the administered dose. Fasting increases absorption. Malabsorption syndromes, as well as dietary factors, (children's soybean formula, concomitant use of anionic exchange resins such as cholestyramine) cause excessive fecal loss.
More than 99 percent of circulating hormones are bound to serum proteins, including thyroxine-binding globulin (TBG), thyroxine-binding prealbumin (TBPA), and albumin (TBa), whose capacities and affinities vary for the hormones. The higher affinity of levothyroxine (T_4) for both TBG and TBPA as compared to triiodothyronine (T_3) partially explains the higher serum levels and longer half-life of the former hormone. Both protein-bound hormones exist in equilibrium with minute amounts of free hormone, the latter accounting for the metabolic activity.
Deiodination of levothyroxine (T_4) occurs at a number of sites, including liver, kidney, and other tissues. The conjugated hormone, in the form of glucuronide or sulfate, is found in the bile and gut where it may complete an enterohepatic circulation. Eight-five percent of levothyroxine (T_4) metabolized daily is deiodinated.

INDICATIONS AND USAGE

SYNTHROID (Levothyroxine Sodium, USP) is indicated:
1. As replacement or supplemental therapy in patients with hypothyroidism of any etiology, except transient hypothyroidism during the recovery phase of subacute thyroiditis. This category includes cretinism, myxedema, and ordinary hypothyroidism in patients of any age (children, adults, the elderly), or state (including pregnancy); primary hypothyroidism resulting from functional deficiency, primary atrophy, partial or total absence of thyroid gland, or the effects of surgery, radiation, or drugs, with or without the presence of goiter; and secondary (pituitary), or tertiary (hypothalamic) hypothyroidism (See **CONTRAINDICATIONS** and **PRECAUTIONS**). SYNTHROID **Injection** can be used intravenously whenever a rapid onset of effect is critical and either intravenously or intramuscularly in hypothyroid patients whenever the oral route is precluded for long periods of time.
2. As a pituitary TSH suppressant, in the treatment or prevention of various types of euthyroid goiters, including thyroid nodules, subacute or chronic lymphocytic thyroiditis (Hashimoto's), multinodular goiter, and in the management of thyroid cancer.
3. As a diagnostic agent in suppression tests to aid in the diagnosis of suspected mild hyperthyroidism or thyroid gland autonomy.

CONTRAINDICATIONS

Thyroid hormone preparations are generally contraindicated in patients with diagnosed but as yet uncorrected adrenal cortical insufficiency, untreated thyrotoxicosis, and apparent hypersensitivity to any of their active or extraneous constituents. There is no well documented evidence from the literature, however, of true allergic or idiosyncratic reactions to thyroid hormone.

WARNINGS

Drugs with thyroid hormone activity, alone or together with other therapeutic agents, have been used for the treatment of obesity. In euthyroid patients, doses within the range of daily hormonal requirements are ineffective for weight reduction. Larger doses may produce serious or even life threatening manifestations of toxicity, particularly when given in association with sympathomimetic amines such as those used for their anorectic effects.

The use of thyroid hormones in the therapy of obesity, alone or combined with other drugs, is unjustified and has been shown to be ineffective. Neither is their use justified for the treatment of male or female infertility unless this condition is accompanied by hypothyroidism.

PRECAUTIONS

General. Thyroid hormones should be used with great caution in a number of circumstances where the integrity of the cardiovascular system, particularly the coronary arteries, is suspected. These include patients with angina pectoris or the elderly, who have a greater likelihood of occult cardiac disease. In these patients, therapy should be initiated with low doses, i.e., 25–50 mcg levothyroxine (T_4). When, in such patients, a euthyroid state can only be reached at the expense of an aggravation of the cardiovascular disease, thyroid hormone dosage should be reduced.
Thyroid hormone therapy in patients with concomitant diabetes mellitus or insipidus or adrenal cortical insufficiency aggravates the intensity of their symptoms. Appropriate adjustments of the various therapeutic measures directed at these concomitant endocrine diseases are required. The therapy of myxedema coma may require simultaneous administration of glucocorticoids (See **DOSAGE AND ADMINISTRATION**).

Hypothyroidism decreases and hyperthyroidism increases the sensitivity to oral anticoagulants. Prothrombin time should be closely monitored in thyroid treated patients on oral anticoagulants and dosage of the latter agents adjusted on the basis of frequent prothrombin time determinations. In infants, excessive doses of thyroid hormone preparations may produce craniosynostosis.
The 100 mcg (0.1 mg) and 300 mcg (0.3 mg) tablets of SYNTHROID (Levothyroxine Sodium, USP) contain FD&C Yellow No. 5 (tartrazine) which may cause allergic-type reactions (including bronchial asthma) in certain susceptible individuals. Although the overall incidence of FD&C Yellow No. 5 (tartrazine) sensitivity in the general population is low, it is frequently seen in patients who also have aspirin hypersensitivity.
Information for the Patient. Patients on thyroid hormone preparations and parents of children on thyroid therapy should be informed that:
1. Replacement therapy is to be taken essentially for life, with the exception of cases of transient hypothyroidism, usually associated with thyroiditis, and in those patients receiving a therapeutic trial of the drug.
2. They should immediately report during the course of therapy any signs or symptoms of thyroid hormone toxicity, e.g., chest pain, increased pulse rate, palpitations, excessive sweating, heat intolerance, nervousness, or any other unusual event.
3. In case of concomitant diabetes mellitus, the daily dosage of antidiabetic medication may need readjustment as thyroid hormone replacement is achieved. If thyroid medication is stopped, a downward readjustment of the dosage of insulin or oral hypoglycemic agent may be necessary to avoid hypoglycemia. At all times, close monitoring of blood or urinary glucose levels is mandatory in such patients.
4. In case of concomitant oral anticoagulant therapy, the prothrombin time should be measured frequently to determine if the dosage of oral anticoagulants is to be readjusted.
5. Partial loss of hair may be experienced by children in the first few months of thyroid therapy, but this is usually a transient phenomenon and later recovery is usually the rule.
Laboratory Tests. Treatment of patients with thyroid hormones requires the periodic assessment of thyroid status by means of appropriate laboratory tests, by full clinical evaluation, or both. The TSH suppression test can be used to test the effectiveness of any thyroid preparation bearing in mind the relative insensitivity of the infant pituitary to the negative feedback effect of thyroid hormones. Serum T_4 levels can be used to test the effectiveness of levothyroxine sodium. When the total serum T_4 is low by TSH is normal, a test specific to assess unbound (free) T_4 levels is warranted. Specific measurements of T_4 and T_3 by competitive protein binding or radioimmunoassay are not influenced by blood levels of organic or inorganic iodine and have essentially replaced older tests of thyroid hormone measurements, i.e., PBI, BEI, and T_4 by column.
Drug Interactions: *Oral Anticoagulants*—Thyroid hormones appear to increase catabolism of vitamin K-dependent clotting factors. If oral anticoagulants are also being given, compensatory increases in clotting factor synthesis are impaired. Patients stabilized on oral anticoagulants who are found to require thyroid replacement therapy should be watched very closely when thyroid is started. If a patient is truly hypothyroid, it is likely that a reduction in anticoagulant dosage will be required. No special precautions appear to be necessary when oral anticoagulant therapy is begun in a patient already stabilized on maintenance thyroid replacement therapy.
Insulin or Oral Hypoglycemics—Initiating thyroid replacement therapy may cause increases in insulin or oral hypoglycemic requirements. The effects seen are poorly understood and depend upon a variety of factors such as dose and type of thyroid preparations and endocrine status of the patient. Patients receiving insulin or oral hypoglycemics should be closely watched during initiation of thyroid replacement therapy.
Cholestyramine—Cholestyramine binds both T_4 and T_3 in the intestine, thus impairing absorption of these thyroid hormones. *In vitro* studies indicate that the binding is not easily reversed. Therefore, four to five hours should elapse between administration of cholestyramine and thyroid hormones.
Estrogen, Oral Contraceptives—Estrogens tend to increase serum thyroxine-binding globulin (TBG). In a patient with a nonfunctioning thyroid gland who is receiving thyroid replacement therapy, free levothyroxine may be decreased when estrogens are started thus increasing thyroid requirements. However, if the patient's thyroid gland has sufficient function, the decreased free thyroxine will result in a compensatory increase in thyroxine output by the thyroid. Therefore, patients without a functioning thyroid gland who are on thyroid replacement therapy may need to increase their thyroid dose if estrogens or estrogen-containing oral contraceptives are given.

Drug/Laboratory Test Interactions. The following drugs or moieties are known to interfere with some laboratory tests performed in patients on thyroid hormone therapy: Androgens, corticosteroids, estrogens, oral contraceptives containing estrogens, iodine-containing preparations, and the numerous preparations containing salicylates.

1. Changes in TBG concentration should be taken into consideration in the interpretation of T_4 and T_3 values. Pregnancy, estrogens, and estrogen-containing oral contraceptives increase TBG concentrations. TBG may also be increased during infectious hepatitis. Decreases in TBG concentrations are observed in nephrosis, acromegaly, and after androgen or corticosteroid therapy. Familial hyper- or hypo-thyroxine-binding-globulinemias have been described. The incidence of TBG deficiency approximates 1 in 9000. The binding of thyroxine by TBPA is inhibited by salicylates. In such cases, the unbound (free) hormone should be measured. Alternatively, an indirect measure of free thyroxine, such as the Free Thyroxine Index (FTI) may be used.

2. Medicinal or dietary iodine interferes with all *in vivo* tests of radioiodine uptake, producing low uptakes which may not indicate a true decrease in hormone synthesis.

3. The persistence of clinical and laboratory evidence of hypothyroidism in spite of adequate dosage replacement indicates either poor patient compliance, poor absorption, or inactivity of the preparation. Intracellular resistance to thyroid hormone is quite rare, and is suggested by clinical signs and symptoms of hypothyroidism in the presence of high serum T_4 levels.

Carcinogenesis, Mutagenesis, and Impairment of Fertility. A reported association between prolonged thyroid therapy and breast cancer has not been confirmed and patients on thyroid for established indications should not discontinue therapy. No confirmatory long-term studies in animals have been performed to evaluate carcinogenic potential, mutagenicity, or impairment of fertility in either males or females.

Pregnancy—Category A. Thyroid hormones do not readily cross the placental barrier. The clinical experience to date does not indicate any adverse effect on fetuses when thyroid hormones are administered to pregnant women. On the basis of current knowledge, thyroid replacement therapy to hypothyroid women should not be discontinued during pregnancy.

Nursing Mothers. Minimal amounts of thyroid hormones are excreted in human milk. Thyroid is not associated with serious adverse reactions and does not have known tumorigenic potential. While caution should be exercised when thyroid is administered to a nursing woman, adequate replacement doses of levothyroxine are generally needed to maintain normal lactation.

Pediatric Use. Pregnant mothers provide little or no thyroid hormone to the fetus. The incidence of congenital hypothyroidism is relatively high (1 in 4,000) and the hypothyroid fetus would not derive any benefit from the small amounts of hormone crossing the placental barrier. Routine determinations of serum T_4 and/or TSH is strongly advised in neonates in view of the deleterious effects of thyroid deficiency on growth and development.

Treatment should be initiated immediately upon diagnosis, and maintained for life, unless transient hypothyroidism is suspected; in which case, therapy may be interrupted for 2 to 8 weeks after the age of 3 years to reassess the condition. Cessation of therapy is justified in patients who have maintained a normal TSH during those 2 to 8 weeks.

ADVERSE REACTIONS

Adverse reactions other than those indicative of hyperthyroidism because of therapeutic overdosage, either initially or during the maintenance periods, are rare (See **OVERDOSAGE**).

OVERDOSAGE

Signs and Symptoms. Excessive doses of thyroid result in hypermetabolic state resembling in every respect the condition of endogenous origin. The condition may be self-induced.

Treatment of Overdosage. Dosage should be reduced or therapy temporarily discontinued if signs and symptoms of overdosage appear. Treatment may be reinstated at a lower dosage. In normal individuals, normal hypothalamic-pituitary-thyroid axis function is restored in 6 to 8 weeks after thyroid suppression.

Treatment of acute massive thyroid hormone overdosage is aimed at reducing gastrointestinal absorption of the drugs and counteracting central and peripheral effects, mainly those of increased sympathetic activity. Vomiting may be induced initially if further gastrointestinal absorption can reasonably be prevented and barring contraindications such as coma, convulsions, or loss of the gagging reflex. Treatment is symptomatic and supportive. Oxygen may be administered and ventilation maintained. Cardiac glycosides may be indicated if congestive heart failure develops. Measures to control fever, hypoglycemia, or fluid loss should be instituted if needed. Antiadrenergic agents, particularly propranolol, have been used advantageously in the treatment of in-

creased sympathetic activity. Propranolol may be administered intravenously at a dosage of 1 to 3 mg over a 10 minute period or orally, 80 to 160 mg/day, especially when no contraindications exist for its use. Other adjunctive measures may include administration of cholestyramine to interfere with thyroxine absorption, and glucocorticoids to inhibit conversion of T_4 to T_3.

DOSAGE AND ADMINISTRATION

The dosage and rate of administration of SYNTHROID® (Levothyroxine Sodium, USP) is determined by the indication and must in every case be individualized according to patient response and laboratory findings.

Hypothyroidism. SYNTHROID **Tablets** are usually instituted using low doses, with increments which depend on the cardiovascular status of the patient. The usual starting dose is 50 mcg, with increments of 25 mcg every 2 to 3 weeks. A lower starting dosage, 25 mcg/day or less, is recommended in patients with long standing hypothyroidism, particularly if cardiovascular impairment is suspected, in which case extreme caution is recommended. The appearance of angina is an indication for a reduction in dosage. Most patients require not more than 200 mcg/day. Failure to respond to doses of 300 mcg suggests lack of compliance or malabsorption. Adequate therapy usually results in normal TSH and T_4 levels after 2 to 3 weeks of the maintenance dose.

Readjustment of SYNTHROID **Tablets** dosage should be made within the first four weeks of therapy, after proper clinical and laboratory evaluations.

SYNTHROID **Injection** by intravenous or intramuscular routes can be substituted for the oral dosage form when ingestion of SYNTHROID **Tablets** is precluded for long periods of time. The initial parenteral dosage should be approximately one half of the previously established oral dosage of levothyroxine sodium tablets. Close observation of the patient, with individual adjustment of the dosage as needed, is recommended.

Myxedema Coma. Myxedema coma is usually precipitated in the hypothyroid patient by intercurrent illness or drugs such as sedatives and anesthetics and should be considered a medical emergency. Therapy should be directed at the correction of electrolyte disturbances and possible infection besides the administration of thyroid hormones. Corticosteroids should be administered routinely. T_4 may be administered via a nasogastric tube but the preferred route of administration is intravenous. Sodium levothyroxine (T_4) is given at a starting dose of 400 mcg (100 mcg/mL) given rapidly, and is usually well tolerated, even in the elderly. In the presence of concomitant heart disease, the sudden administration of such large doses of L-thyroxine intravenously is clearly not without its cardiovascular risks. Under such circumstances, intravenous therapy should not be undertaken without weighing the alternative risks of the myxedema coma and the cardiovascular disease. Clinical judgement in this situation may dictate smaller intravenous doses of SYNTHROID **Injection**. The initial dose is followed by daily supplements of 100 to 200 mcg given intravenously. Normal T_4 levels are achieved in 24 hours followed in 3 days by three-fold evaluation of T_3. Continued daily administration of lesser amounts parenterally should be maintained until the patient is fully capable of accepting a daily oral dose. A daily maintenance dose of 50 to 100 mcg parenterally should suffice to maintain the euthyroid state, once established. Oral therapy would be resumed as soon as the clinical situation has been stabilized and the patient is able to take oral medication.

TSH Suppression in Thyroid Cancer, Nodules, and Euthyroid Goiters. Exogenous thyroid hormone may produce regression of metastases from follicular and papillary carcinoma of the thyroid and is used as ancillary therapy of these conditions following surgery or radioactive iodine. Medullary carcinoma of the thyroid is usually unresponsive to this therapy. TSH should be suppressed to low or undetectable levels. Therefore, larger amounts of thyroid hormone than those used for replacement therapy are frequently required. This therapy is also used in treating nontoxic solitary nodules and multinodular goiters, and to prevent thyroid enlargement in chronic (Hashimoto's) thyroiditis.

Thyroid Suppression Therapy. Administration of thyroid hormone in doses higher than those produced physiologically by the gland results in suppression of the production of endogenous hormone. This is the basis for the thyroid suppression test and is used as an aid in the diagnosis of patients with signs of mild hyperthyroidism in whom base line laboratory tests appear normal, or to demonstrate thyroid gland autonomy in patients with Graves' ophthalmopathy. [131]I uptake is determined before and after the administration of the exogenous hormone. A fifty percent or greater suppression of uptake indicates a normal thyroid-pituitary axis and thus rules out thyroid gland autonomy.

For adults, the average suppressive dose of levothyroxine (T_4) is 2.6 mcg/kg of body weight per day given for 7 to 10 days. These doses usually yield normal serum T_4 and T_3 levels and lack of response to TSH.

Levothyroxine sodium should be administered cautiously to patients in whom there is a strong suspicion of thyroid gland

autonomy, in view of the fact that the exogenous hormone effects will be additive to the endogenous source.

Pediatric Dosage. Pediatric dosage should follow the recommendations summarized in Table I. In infants with congenital hypothyroidism, therapy with full doses should be instituted as soon as the diagnosis has been made. SYNTHROID **Tablets** may be given to infants and children who cannot swallow intact tablets by crushing the proper dose tablet and suspending the **freshly crushed** tablet in a small amount of water or formula. The suspension can be given by spoon or dropper. DO NOT STORE THE SUSPENSION FOR ANY PERIOD OF TIME. The crushed tablet may also be sprinkled over a small amount of food, such as cooked cereal or apple sauce.

Table I
**Recommended Pediatric Dosage
For Congenital Hypothyroidism***

	SYNTHROID (Levothyroxine Sodium Tablets, USP)	
Age	Dose per day	Daily dose per kg of body weight
0– 6 mos	25– 50 mcg	8–10 mcg
6–12 mos	50– 75 mcg	6– 8 mcg
1– 5 yrs	75–100 mcg	5– 6 mcg
6–12 yrs	100–150 mcg	4– 5 mcg

*To be adjusted on the basis of clinical response and laboratory tests (See **Laboratory Tests**).

HOW SUPPLIED

SYNTHROID **Tablets** (Levothyroxine Sodium Tablets, USP) are supplied as scored, color coded potency-marked tablets as follows:

25 mcg, orange
Bottles of 100, Code 3P1023   NDC 0048-1020-03
Bottles of 1000, Code 3P1025   NDC 0048-1020-05
50 mcg, white
Bottles of 100, Code 3P1043   NDC 0048-1040-03
Bottles of 1000, Code 3P1045   NDC 0048-1040-05
Unit Dose Cartons of 100, Code 3P1033 NDC 0048-1040-13
75 mcg, violet
Bottles of 100, Code 3P1053   NDC 0048-1050-03
Bottles of 1000, Code 3P1055   NDC 0048-1050-05
Unit Dose Cartons of 100, Code 3P1003 NDC 0048-1050-13
100 mcg, yellow
Bottles of 100, Code 3P1073   NDC 0048-1070-03
Bottles of 1000, Code 3P1075   NDC 0048-1070-05
Unit Dose Cartons of 100, Code 3P1063 NDC 0048-1070-13
112 mcg, rose
Bottles of 100, Code 3P1183   NDC 0048-1080-03
Bottles of 1000, Code 3P1185   NDC 0048-1080-05
Unit Dose Cartons of 100, Code 3P1193 NDC 0048-1080-13
125 mcg, brown
Bottles of 100, Code 3P1103   NDC 0048-1130-03
Bottles of 1000, Code 3P1105   NDC 0048-1130-05
Unit Dose Cartons of 100, Code 3P1113 NDC 0048-1130-13
150 mcg, blue
Bottles of 100, Code 3P1093   NDC 0048-1090-03
Bottles of 1000, Code 3P1095   NDC 0048-1090-05
Unit Dose Cartons of 100, Code 3P1083 NDC 0048-1090-13
175 mcg, lilac
Bottles of 100, Code 3P1153   NDC 0048-1100-03
200 mcg, pink
Bottles of 100, Code 3P1143   NDC 0048-1140-03
Bottles of 1000, Code 3P1145   NDC 0048-1140-05
Unit Dose Cartons of 100, Code 3P1133 NDC 0048-1140-13
300 mcg, green
Bottles of 100, Code 3P1173   NDC 0048-1170-03
Bottles of 1000, Code 3P1175   NDC 0048-1170-05
Unit Dose Cartons of 100, Code 3P1163 NDC 0048-1170-13
Store at controlled room temperature 15°–30° C (59°–86° F).
SYNTHROID (Levothyroxine Sodium, USP) **Injection** is lyophilized with 10 mg Mannitol, USP and 0.7 mg tribasic sodium phosphate anhydrous in 10 mL vials. The pH may be adjusted with sodium hydroxide. It is supplied in color coded vials as follows:
200 mcg, gray
10 mL One Dose Vial, Code 3P1312   NDC 0048-1014-99
500 mcg, yellow
10 mL One Dose Vial, Code 3P1302   NDC 0048-1012-99
Store at controlled room temperature 15°–30° C (59°–86° F).

DIRECTIONS FOR RECONSTITUTION

Reconstitute the lyophilized levothyroxine sodium by aseptically adding 5 mL of 0.9% Sodium Chloride Injection, USP or Bacteriostatic Sodium Chloride Injection, USP with Benzyl Alcohol, only. Shake vial to insure complete mixing. Use immediately after reconstitution. Do not add to other intravenous fluids. Discard any unused portion.

Continued on next page

Boots-Flint—Cont.

Reference articles are available on request.
Caution: Federal law prohibits dispensing without a prescription.
Tablets
Manufactured by
Boots Puerto Rico, Inc.
Jayuya, Puerto Rico 00664-0795
Injection
Manufactured by
Baxter Healthcare Corporation
Cleveland, Mississippi 38732
             For
Boots-Flint, Inc.
Lincolnshire, Illinois 60069 USA
a subsidiary of The Boots Company (USA) Inc.
1020-04
8/88
Shown in Product Identification Section, page 406

TRAVASE® OINTMENT   ℞

[*trăv 'āz*]
(Sutilains Ointment USP)

DESCRIPTION

TRAVASE® Ointment (Sutilains Ointment, USP) is a sterile topical preparation in one-half ounce tubes. It contains proteolytic enzymes, elaborated by *Bacillus subtilis*, in a hydrophobic ointment base consisting of 95% mineral oil and 5% polyethylene. One gram of ointment contains approximately 82,000 USP Casein Units* of proteolytic activity.
*One USP Casein Unit of proteolytic activity is contained in the amount of sutilains which, when incubated with 35 mg of denatured casein at 37°C, produces in one minute a hydrolysate whose absorbance at 275 nm is equal to that of a tyrosine solution containing 1.5 micrograms of USP Tyrosine Reference Standard per mL.

CLINICAL PHARMACOLOGY

TRAVASE Ointment selectively digests necrotic soft tissues by proteolytic action. It dissolves and facilitates the removal of necrotic tissue and purulent exudates that otherwise impair formation of granulation tissue and delay wound healing.
At body temperatures these proteolytic enzymes have optimal activity in the pH range from 6.0 to 6.8.

INDICATIONS AND USAGE

For wound debridement—TRAVASE Ointment is indicated as an adjunct to establishing methods of wound care for biochemical debridement of the following lesions:
    Second and third degree burns,
    Decubitus ulcers,
    Incisional, traumatic, and pyogenic wounds,
    Ulcers secondary to peripheral vascular disease.

CONTRAINDICATIONS

Application of TRAVASE® Ointment (Sutilains Ointment, USP) is contraindicated in the following conditions:
    Wounds communicating with major body cavities,
    Wounds containing exposed major nerves or nervous tissue,
    Fungating neoplastic ulcers.

WARNING

Do not permit TRAVASE Ointment to come into contact with the eyes. In treatment of burns or lesions about the head or neck, should the ointment inadvertently come in contact with the eyes, the eyes should be immediately rinsed with copious amounts of water, preferably sterile.

PRECAUTIONS

A moist environment is essential to optimal activity of the enzyme. Enzyme activity may be impaired by certain agents. *In vitro*, several detergents and antiseptics (benzalkonium chloride, hexachlorophene, iodine, and nitrofurazone) may render the substrate indifferent to the action of the enzyme. Compounds such as thimerosal, containing metallic ions, interfere directly with enzyme activity to a slight degree, whereas neomycin, sulfamylon, streptomycin, and penicillin do not affect enzyme activity. In cases where adjunctive topical therapy has been used and no dissolution of slough occurs after treatment with TRAVASE Ointment for 24 to 48 hours, further application, because of interference by the adjunctive agents, is unlikely to be rewarding.
In cases where there is existent or threatening invasive infection, appropriate systemic antibiotic therapy should be instituted concurrently.
Although there have been no reports of systemic allergic reaction to TRAVASE Ointment in humans, studies have shown that there may be an antibody response in humans to absorbed enzyme material.

Pregnancy: Teratogenic Effects
Pregnancy Category B. Reproduction studies have been performed in rabbits at doses up to two times the maximum human dose and have revealed no evidence of impaired fertility or harm to fetus due to TRAVASE Ointment. There are, however, no adequate and well controlled studies in women. Because animal reproductive studies are not always predicative of human response, this drug should be used during pregnancy only if clearly needed.
Pediatric Use
Safety and effectiveness in children have not been established.

ADVERSE REACTIONS

Adverse reactions consist of mild, transient pain, paresthesias, bleeding and transient dermatitis. Pain usually can be controlled by administration of mild analgesics. Side effects severe enough to warrant discontinuation of therapy occasionally have occurred.
If bleeding or dermatitis occurs as a result of the application of TRAVASE® Ointment (Sutilains Ointment, USP) therapy should be discontinued. No systemic toxicity has been observed as a result of the topical application of TRAVASE Ointment.

DOSAGE AND ADMINISTRATION

STRICT ADHERENCE TO THE FOLLOWING IS REQUIRED FOR EFFECTIVE RESULTS OF TREATMENT:
1. Thoroughly cleanse and irrigate wound area with sodium chloride solution or water. Wounds **MUST** be cleansed of antiseptics or heavy-metal antibacterials which may denature enzyme or alter substrate characteristics (e.g., hexachlorophene, silver nitrate, benzalkonium chloride, nitrofurazone).
2. Thoroughly moisten wound area either through tubbing, showering, or wet soaks (e.g. sodium chloride solution or water).
3. Apply TRAVASE Ointment in a thin layer assuring intimate contact with necrotic tissue and complete wound coverage extending to ¼ to ½ inch beyond the area to be debrided
4. Apply loose, moist dressings.
5. Repeat entire procedure 3 to 4 times per day for best results.

HOW SUPPLIED

TRAVASE Ointment (Sutilains Ointment, USP) is supplied as follows:
3P3002 NDC 0048-1500-52 one-half ounce (14.2 g) tube.
Refrigerate at 2° to 8°C (36°–46°F).
Manufactured for
Boots-Flint, Inc.
Lincolnshire, Illinois 60069 USA
a subsidiary of
The Boots Company (USA) Inc.
by Smith Kline & French Laboratories
Philadelphia, PA 19101 USA
Printed in USA
27201-01
5/88
Shown in Product Identification Section, page 406

ZORprin®   ℞

(aspirin 800 mg)
Zero-Order Release

DESCRIPTION

Each capsule-shaped ZORprin® (aspirin) tablet contains 800 mg of aspirin in a special matrix formulated to control the release of aspirin after oral administration. The tablet matrix is designed to release aspirin in a linear, pH dependent fashion thereby reducing the potential for gastrointestinal irritation and providing a more convenient dosage regimen. *In vitro* studies have shown that aspirin release from the ZORprin matrix approximates a zero-order mode. The tablet contains Cellulose Acetate Phthalate, NF and Starch, NF (Corn Starch) as inactive ingredients.
The structural formula of aspirin is:

CLINICAL PHARMACOLOGY

Aspirin, as contained in ZORprin, has demonstrated anti-inflammatory and analgesic activity. Its mode of action as an anti-inflammatory and analgesic agent primarily involves inhibition of prostaglandin synthesis.
The ZORprin matrix releases aspirin in a linear, pH dependent manner. In an acid environment such as the stomach, ZORprin releases little aspirin whereas in an alkaline environment such as the lower duodenum, aspirin is released in a linear fashion. It is the pH dependence of aspirin release from ZORprin that reduces direct contact between aspirin

and the gastric mucosa, resulting in a reduction in the potential for direct irritation.
Bioavailability data for ZORprin demonstrate that detectable levels of salicylate, the active circulating form of aspirin, are present twenty-four hours following a single oral dose, indicative of the prolonged release kinetics of ZORprin. This dose of ZORprin produced a reduction in circulating prostaglandin levels up to 14 hours after administration, compared to six hours for an equivalent dose of immediate release aspirin. Multiple doses bioavailability studies showed similar steady-state salicylate levels of ZORprin as for immediate release aspirin using the same total daily dose. In addition, clinical studies demonstrate that comparable therapeutic blood levels can be maintained by patients whether receiving ZORprin twice daily or aspirin four times daily. Long-term monitoring of ZORprin therapy showed no signs of salicylate accumulation once steady-state salicylate levels were reached (4–6 days). These studies substantiate a twice daily dosage regimen.
Studies in humans indicate that salicylates are excreted in the urine as free salicylic acid (10%); salicyluric acid (75%); salicylic phenolic (10%); and acyl glucuronides (5%) and gentisic acid (<1%).

INDICATIONS AND USAGE

ZORprin is indicated for the treatment of rheumatoid arthritis and osteoarthritis. The safety and efficacy of ZORprin have not been established in patients who are designated by the American Rheumatism Association as Functional Class IV.
In patients treated with ZORprin for rheumatoid arthritis and osteoarthritis, the efficacy of ZORprin has been shown by reduction in pain, morning stiffness and disease activity as assessed by both investigators and patients. The pain relief and improvement in clinical symptoms observed in patients taking ZORprin were comparable to immediate release aspirin, but ZORprin was associated with a statistically significant reduction in the milder gastrointestinal side effects (see **ADVERSE REACTIONS**). ZORprin may be well tolerated in some patients who have had gastrointestinal side effects with immediate release aspirin, but these patients when treated with ZORprin should be carefully followed for signs and symptoms of gastrointestinal bleeding and ulceration.
ZORprin use concurrently with other nonsteroidal anti-inflammatory agents cannot be recommended because the appropriate studies have not been performed (see **Drug Interactions**).
Sustained release aspirin products, such as ZORprin, are not recommended for antipyresis or for short-term analgesia.

CONTRAINDICATIONS

ZORprin should not be used in patients known to be hypersensitive to salicylates or in individuals with nasal polyps, angioedema, bronchospastic reactivity to aspirin, renal or hepatic insufficiency, hypoprothrombinemia or other bleeding disorders. ZORprin is contraindicated in all children with fever.

WARNINGS

ZORprin should be used with caution when anticoagulants are prescribed concurrently, since aspirin may depress platelet aggregation and increase bleeding time. Salicylates may have a hypoglycemic action. They may also potentiate the effect of oral hypoglycemics and the concomitant use of these agents is not recommended. However, if such use is necessary, reduced dosage of the hypoglycemic agent may be necessary. The hypoglycemic action of salicylates may also necessitate adjustment of the insulin dose of diabetics.
While salicylates in large doses have a uricosuric effect, smaller amounts may reduce urate excretion and increase serum uric acid. Therefore, patients with gout should avoid the use of salicylates.

WARNINGS

Children and teenagers should not use this medicine for chicken pox or flu symptoms before a doctor is consulted about Reye's Syndrome, a rare but serious illness reported to be associated with aspirin.

USE IN PREGNANCY

ZORprin can cause fetal harm when administered to pregnant women. Aspirin has produced teratogenic effects and increases the incidence of stillbirths and neonatal deaths in animals. If this drug is used in pregnancy, or if the patient becomes pregnant while taking this drug, the patient should be apprised of the potential hazard to the fetus.
Aspirin interferes with maternal and infant hemostasis and may lengthen the duration of pregnancy and parturition. Aspirin should not be taken during the last 3 months of pregnancy.

PRECAUTIONS

General: Particular care should be used when prescribing this medication to patients with erosive gastritis, peptic ulcer, mild diabetes or gout. As with all salicylate drugs, caution should be exercised in prescribing ZORprin for those patients with bleeding tendencies or those on anticoagulants.

Patients receiving aspirin may develop mild salicylate intoxication (salicylism) that may be reversed by dosage reduction.

Salicylates can produce changes in thyroid function tests. Salicylates should be used with caution in patients with severe hepatic damage, preexisting hypoprothrombinemia, Vitamin K deficiency and in those undergoing surgery.

Since aspirin release from ZORprin® (aspirin) is pH dependent it may change in those conditions where gastric pH has been increased as a result of antacids, gastric secretion inhibitors or surgical procedures.

Drug Interactions: (see **WARNINGS**) Aspirin may interfere with some anticoagulant and hypoglycemic drugs. Drugs which lower serum uric acid excretion may be antagonized by the concomitant use of aspirin, particularly in doses less than 2.0 grams/day. Nonsteroidal anti-inflammatory drugs may be competitively displaced from their albumin binding sites by aspirin. This interaction may alter the clinical efficacy of both drugs. Concomitant administration of other anti-inflammatory drugs may increase the risk of gastrointestinal ulceration. Also, the combination of alcohol and aspirin may increase the risk of gastrointestinal bleeding.

Aspirin may enhance the activity of methotrexate and increase its toxicity.

Sodium excretion produced by spironolactone and perhaps other diuretics may be decreased in the presence of salicylates. Urinary alkalinizers may decrease the serum concentration of salicylates by increasing the rate of renal salicylate excretion. Phenobarbital may also decrease the serum concentration of salicylates via enzyme induction.

Pregnancy Category D: See **WARNINGS** Section.

Nursing Mothers: Salicylates have been detected in the breast milk of nursing mothers. Because of the potential for serious adverse reactions in nursing infants from aspirin, a decision should be made whether to discontinue nursing or discontinue the drug, taking into account the benefit of the drug to the mother.

ADVERSE REACTIONS

Hematologic: Aspirin interferes with hemostasis and those patients with a history of blood coagulation defects or receiving anticoagulant drugs or with severe anemia should not take ZORprin. The chronic use of aspirin may cause persistent iron deficiency anemia (see **Gastrointestinal**).

Gastrointestinal: Aspirin may potentiate peptic ulcer, and cause stomach distress or heartburn. Aspirin can cause an increase in occult bleeding and in some patients massive gastrointestinal bleeding. However, the greatest release of active drug from ZORprin is designed to occur in the small intestine in a linear fashion. This has resulted in fewer symptomatic gastrointestinal side effects.

Allergic: Allergic and anaphylactic reactions have been noted when hypersensitive individuals have taken aspirin. Fatal anaphylactic shock, while not common, has been reported.

Respiratory: Aspirin sensitivity, manifested by exacerbations of bronchospasm and rhinitis, may occur in patients with a history of nasal polyps, asthma or rhinitis.

Dermatologic: Hives, rashes, and angioedema may occur, especially in patients suffering from chronic urticaria.

Central Nervous System: Taken in overdoses, aspirin may cause tinnitus. Depression of the central nervous system may also be noted, following initial stimulation.

Renal: Aspirin may aggravate chronic kidney disease.

Hepatic: High doses of aspirin have been reported to produce reversible hepatic dysfunction.

OVERDOSAGE

Overdosage may result in the usual symptoms of salicylism: tinnitus, vertigo, headache, confusion, drowsiness, sweating, hyperventilation, vomiting or diarrhea. Plasma salicylate levels in adults may range from 50 to 80 mg/dl in the mildly intoxicated patient to 110 to 160 mg/dl in the severely intoxicated patient. Aspirin intoxication can cause metabolic acidosis in young children, and an initial respiratory alkalosis followed by metabolic acidosis in adults. Treatment for mild intoxication should include emptying the stomach with an emetic, gastric lavage or administration of activated charcoal. In addition to these measures, individuals suffering from severe intoxication should have forced alkaline diuresis. In extreme cases, hemodialysis or peritoneal dialysis may be required.

The clearance of salicylate in children is much slower than adults and this should receive due consideration when aspirin overdosages occur in children; salicylate half-lives of 30 hours have been reported in infants 4–8 months old.

DOSAGE AND ADMINISTRATION

In order to achieve a zero-order release, the tablets of ZORprin should be swallowed intact. ZORprin should also be taken with ample fluids (8 oz or more).

Breaking the tablets or disrupting the structure will alter the release profile of the drug.

Adult Dosage: The recommended initial dose of ZORprin is two 800 mg tablets twice a day. However, the anti-inflammatory dose range of aspirin therapy extends to 6000 mg per day. Incremental adjustment of the dosage should be determined by the physician, based upon the patient's response and needs and serum salicylate concentrations. Maximum anti-inflammatory effects are often not realized at serum salicylate levels below 20–25 mg/dl. Since it will take 4–6 days to reach steady-state levels of salicylic acid with ZORprin, it is recommended that dosages be given for at least one week before further adjustment. In general, patients with rheumatoid arthritis seem to require higher doses of ZORprin than do patients with osteoarthritis.

ZORprin is not recommended for children below the age of 12.

HOW SUPPLIED

ZORprin® (aspirin) Zero-Order Release tablets are supplied as 800 mg; plain, white elongated tablets with debossed stylized Boots "B" and "57".

Bottles of 100   NDC 0048-0057-01

Store at controlled room temperature 15°–30°C (59°–86°F).

Caution: Federal (USA) law prohibits dispensing without a prescription.

U.S. Patent No. 4,308,251

Manufactured by:
Boots Pharmaceuticals, Inc.
Shreveport, Louisiana 71106 USA
For:
Boots-Flint, Inc.
Lincolnshire, Illinois 60069 USA
a subsidiary of
The Boots Company (USA) Inc.
Rev. 9/28/88   25725-02
© Copyright 1988
All rights reserved by Boots Pharmaceuticals, Inc.
Shown in Product Identification Section, page 406

EDUCATIONAL MATERIAL

Booklet-Pamphlet

"Thyroid Today" various authors, publication issued 4 times per year. Publication provides information written by physicians for physicians concerning thyroid disease diagnosis and treatment. Free to Physicians and Pharmacists.

"A Closer Look at Your Thyroid" patient publication on hypothyroidism. Free to Physicians and Pharmacists.

Samples

Provide physicians with professional supply of SYN-THROID® (Levothyroxine Sodium, USP) for personal use;-mast written prescription is included. (Allow 8 wks. delivery.) Strengths include 0.025 mg., 0.05 mg., 0.075 mg., 0.1 mg., 0.112 mg, 0.125 mg, 0.150 mg, 0.175 mg, 0.2 mg, 0.3 mg in unit size of 100 tablets per bottle. Only 2 samples per order.

Educational Programs

BOOTS-FLINT offers a modular series of educational programs on thyroid disease free to registered pharmacists, physicians.

Braintree Laboratories, Inc.
P.O. BOX 361
BRAINTREE, MA 02184

GoLYTELY®   ℞
[go-līt´lē]
PEG-3350 and Electrolytes For Oral Solution

DESCRIPTION

A white powder for reconstitution containing 236 g polyethylene glycol 3350, 22.74 g sodium sulfate, 6.74 g sodium bicarbonate, 5.86 g sodium chloride, and 2.97 g potassium chloride. When dissolved in water to a volume of 4 liters, GoLYTELY is an isosmotic solution having a mildly salty taste. GoLYTELY is administered orally or via nasogastric tube.

CLINICAL PHARMACOLOGY

GoLYTELY induces a diarrhea which rapidly cleanses the bowel, usually within four hours. The osmotic activity of polyethylene glycol 3350 and the electrolyte concentration result in virtually no net absorption or excretion of ions or water. Accordingly, large volumes may be administered without significant changes in fluid or electrolyte balance.

INDICATIONS AND USAGE

GoLYTELY is indicated for bowel cleansing prior to colonoscopy and barium enema x-ray examination.

CONTRAINDICATIONS

GoLYTELY is contraindicated in patients with gastrointestinal obstruction, gastric retention, bowel perforation, toxic colitis, toxic megacolon or ileus.

WARNINGS

No additional ingredients, e.g. flavorings, should be added to the solution. GoLYTELY should be used with caution in patients with severe ulcerative colitis.

PRECAUTIONS

General: Patients with impaired gag reflex, unconscious or semiconscious patients, and patients prone to regurgitation or aspiration, should be observed during the administration of GoLYTELY, especially if it is administered via nasogastric tube. If a patient experiences severe bloating, distention or abdominal pain, administration should be slowed or temporarily discontinued until the symptoms abate. If gastrointestinal obstruction or perforation is suspected, appropriate studies should be performed to rule out these conditions before administration of GoLYTELY.

Information for patients: GoLYTELY produces a watery stool which cleanses the bowel before examination. Prepare the solution according to the instructions on the bottle. It is more palatable if chilled. For best results, no solid food should be consumed during the 3 to 4 hour period before drinking the solution, but in no case should solid foods be eaten within 2 hours of taking GoLYTELY.

Drink 240 ml (8 oz.) every 10 minutes. Rapid drinking of each portion is better than drinking small amounts continuously. The first bowel movement should occur approximately one hour after the start of GoLYTELY administration. You may experience some abdominal bloating and distention before the bowels start to move. If severe discomfort or distention occur, stop drinking temporarily or drink each portion at longer intervals until these symptoms disappear. Continue drinking until the watery stool is clear and free of solid matter. This usually requires at least 3 liters and it is best to drink all of the solution. Any unused portion should be discarded.

Drug Interactions: Oral medication administered within one hour of the start of administration of GoLYTELY may be flushed from the gastrointestinal tract and not absorbed.

Carcinogenesis, Mutagenesis, Impairment of Fertility: Carcinogenic and reproductive studies with animals have not been performed.

Pregnancy: Category C. Animal reproduction studies have not been conducted with GoLYTELY. It is also not known whether GoLYTELY can cause fetal harm when administered to a pregnant woman or can affect reproductive capacity. GoLYTELY should be given to a pregnant woman only if clearly needed.

Pediatric Use: Safety and effectiveness in children have not been established.

ADVERSE REACTIONS

Nausea, abdominal fullness and bloating are the most common adverse reactions (occurring in up to 50% of patients) to administration of GoLYTELY. Abdominal cramps, vomiting and anal irritation occur less frequently. These adverse reactions are transient and subside rapidly. Isolated cases of urticaria, rhinorrhea and dermatitis have been reported which may represent allergic reactions.

DOSAGE AND ADMINISTRATION

The recommended dose for adults is 4 liters of GoLYTELY solution prior to gastrointestinal examination, as ingestion of this dose produces a satisfactory preparation in over 95% of patients. Ideally the patient should fast for approximately three or four hours prior to GoLYTELY administration, but in no case should solid food be given for at least two hours before the solution is given.

GoLYTELY is usually administered orally, but may be given via nasogastric tube to patients who are unwilling or unable to drink the solution. **Oral administration** is at a rate of 240 ml (8 oz.) every 10 minutes, until 4 liters are consumed or the rectal effluent is clear. Rapid drinking of each portion is preferred to drinking small amounts continuously. **Nasogastric tube administration** is at the rate of 20–30 ml per minute (1.2–1.8 liters per hour). The first bowel movement should occur approximately one hour after the start of GoLYTELY administration.

Various regimens have been used. One method is to schedule patients for examination in midmorning or later, allowing the patients three hours for drinking and an additional one hour period for complete bowel evacuation. Another method is to administer GoLYTELY on the evening before the examination, particularly if the patient is to have a barium enema.

Preparation of the solution: GoLYTELY solution is prepared by filling the container to the 4 liter mark with water and shaking vigorously several times to insure that the ingredients are dissolved. Dissolution is facilitated by using lukewarm water. The solution is more palatable if chilled before administration. The reconstituted solution should be refrigerated and used within 48 hours. Discard any unused portion.

Continued on next page

Braintree—Cont.

HOW SUPPLIED

In powdered form, for oral administration as a solution following reconstitution. Each disposable jug contains, in powdered form: polyethylene glycol 3350 236 g, sodium sulfate 22.74 g, sodium bicarbonate 6.74 g, sodium chloride 5.86 g, potassium chloride 2.97 g. When made up to 4 liters volume with water, the solution contains PEG 3350 17.6 mmol/L, sodium 125 mmol/L, sulfate 40 mmol/L, chloride 35 mmol/L, bicarbonate 20 mmol/L and potassium 10 mmol/L.

CAUTION

Federal law prohibits dispensing without prescription.

STORAGE

Store in sealed container at 59°–86°F. When reconstituted, keep solution refrigerated. Use within 48 hours. Discard unused portion.

NDC 52268-0100-01

Revised 7/1/87

Made by Lyne Laboratories, Stoughton, MA 02072 for BRAINTREE LABORATORIES, INC., Box 361, Braintree, MA 02184

Shown in Product Identification Section, page 406

EDUCATIONAL MATERIAL

Booklets

A complimentary patient booklet is available: "Bowel Preparation Before Your Colonoscopy."

Bristol Laboratories
A Bristol-Myers Company
EVANSVILLE, IN 47721

AMIKIN®   ℞
[ah-mi'kin]
(amikacin sulfate) Injectable, 500 mg vial NSN 6505-01-033-0058 (M & VA)
Injectable, 1 g vial NSN 6505-01-056-1950 (M & VA)

WARNINGS

Patients treated with parenteral aminoglycosides should be under close clinical observation because of the potential ototoxicity and nephrotoxicity associated with their use. Safety for treatment periods which are longer than 14 days has not been established.

Neurotoxicity, manifested as vestibular and permanent bilateral auditory ototoxicity, can occur in patients with preexisting renal damage and in patients with normal renal function treated at higher doses and/or for periods longer than those recommended. The risk of aminoglycoside-induced ototoxicity is greater in patients with renal damage. High frequency deafness usually occurs first and can be detected only by audiometric testing. Vertigo may occur and may be evidence of vestibular injury. Other manifestations of neurotoxicity may include numbness, skin tingling, muscle twitching and convulsions. The risk of hearing loss due to aminoglycosides increases with the degree of exposure to either high peak or high trough serum concentrations. Patients developing cochlear damage may not have symptoms during therapy to warn them of developing eighth-nerve toxicity, and total or partial irreversible bilateral deafness may occur after the drug has been discontinued. Aminoglycoside-induced ototoxicity is usually irreversible.

Aminoglycosides are potentially nephrotoxic. The risk of nephrotoxicity is greater in patients with impaired renal function and in those who receive high doses or prolonged therapy.

Neuromuscular blockade and respiratory paralysis have been reported following parenteral injection, topical instillation (as in orthopedic and abdominal irrigation or in local treatment of empyema), and following oral use of aminoglycosides. The possibility of these phenomena should be considered if aminoglycosides are administered by any route, especially in patients receiving anesthetics, neuromuscular blocking agents such as tubocurarine, succinylcholine, decamethonium, or in patients receiving massive transfusions of citrate-anticoagulated blood. If blockage occurs, calcium salts may reverse these phenomena, but mechanical respiratory assistance may be necessary.

Renal and eighth-nerve function should be closely monitored especially in patients with known or suspected renal impairment at the onset of therapy and also in

those whose renal function is initially normal but who develop signs of renal dysfunction during therapy. Serum concentrations of amikacin should be monitored when feasible to assure adequate levels and to avoid potentially toxic levels and prolonged peak concentrations above 35 μg per mL. Urine should be examined for decreased specific gravity, increased excretion of proteins, and the presence of cells or casts. Blood urea nitrogen, serum creatinine, or creatinine clearance should be measured periodically. Serial audiograms should be obtained where feasible in patients old enough to be tested, particularly high risk patients. Evidence of ototoxicity (dizziness, vertigo, tinnitus, roaring in the ears, and hearing loss) or nephrotoxicity requires discontinuation of the drug or dosage adjustment.

Concurrent and/or sequential systemic, oral or topical use of other neurotoxic or nephrotoxic products, particularly bacitracin, cisplatin, amphotericin B, cephaloridine, paromomycin, viomycin, polymyxin B, colistin, vancomycin, or other aminoglycosides should be avoided. Other factors that may increase risk of toxicity are advanced age and dehydration.

The concurrent use of AMIKIN with potent diuretics (ethacrynic acid, or furosemide) should be avoided since diuretics by themselves may cause ototoxicity. In addition, when administered, intravenously, diuretics may enhance aminoglycoside toxicity by altering antibiotic concentrations in serum and tissue.

DESCRIPTION

Amikacin sulfate is a semi-synthetic aminoglycoside antibiotic derived from kanamycin. It is $C_{22}H_{43}N_5O_{13} \cdot 2H_2SO_4$. D-Streptamine, 0-3-amino-3-deoxy-α-D-glucopyranosyl-(1 → 6)-0-[6-amino-6-deoxy-α-D-glucopyranosyl-(1 → 4)]-N1-(4-amino-2-hydroxyl-1-oxobutyl)-2-deoxy-, (S)-, sulfate (1:2) (salt).

The dosage form is supplied as a sterile, colorless to light straw colored solution. The 100 mg per 2 mL vial contains, in addition to amikacin sulfate, 0.13% sodium bisulfite and 0.5% sodium citrate with pH adjusted to 4.5 with sulfuric acid. The 500 mg per 2 mL vial and the 1 gram per 4 mL vial contain 0.66% sodium bisulfite and 2.5% sodium citrate with pH adjusted to 4.5 with sulfuric acid.

CLINICAL PHARMACOLOGY

Intramuscular Administration—AMIKIN is rapidly absorbed after intramuscular administration. In normal adult volunteers, average peak serum concentrations of about 12, 16, and 21 μg/mL are obtained 1 hour after intramuscular administration of 250-mg (3.7mg/kg), 375-mg (5 mg/kg), 500-mg (7.5 mg/kg), single doses, respectively. At 10 hours, serum levels are about 0.3 μg/mL, 1.2 μg/mL, and 2.1 μg/mL, respectively.

Tolerance studies in normal volunteers reveal that amikacin is well tolerated locally following repeated intramuscular dosing, and when given at maximally recommended doses, no ototoxicity or nephrotoxicity has been reported. There is no evidence of drug accumulation with repeated dosing for 10 days when administered according to recommended doses.

With normal renal function, about 91.9% of an intramuscular dose is excreted unchanged in the urine in the first 8 hours, and 98.2% within 24 hours. Mean urine concentrations for 6 hours are 563 μg/mL following a 250-mg dose, 697 μg/mL following a 375-mg dose, and 832 μg/mL following a 500-mg dose.

Preliminary intramuscular studies in newborns of different weights (less than 1.5 kg, 1.5 to 2.0 kg, over 2.0 kg) at a dose of 7.5 mg/kg revealed that, like other aminoglycosides, serum half-life values were correlated inversely with postnatal age and renal clearances of amikacin. The volume of distribution indicates that amikacin, like other aminoglycosides, remains primarily in the extracellular fluid space of neonates. Repeated dosing every 12 hours in all the above groups did not demonstrate accumulation after 5 days.

Intravenous Administration—Single doses of 500 mg (7.5 mg/kg) administered to normal adults as an infusion over a period of 30 minutes produced a mean peak serum concentration of 38 μg/mL at the end of the infusion, and levels of 24 μg/mL, 18 μg/mL, and 0.75 μg/mL at 30 minutes, 1 hour and 10 hours postinfusion, respectively. Eighty-four percent of the administered dose was excreted in the urine in 9 hours and about 94% within 24 hours.

Repeat infusions of 7.5 mg/kg every 12 hours in normal adults were well tolerated and caused no drug accumulation. **General**—Pharmacokinetic studies in normal adult subjects reveal the mean serum half-life to be slightly over 2 hours with a mean total apparent volume of distribution of 24 liters (28% of the body weight). By the ultrafiltration technique, reports of serum protein binding range from 0% to 11%. The mean serum clearance rate is about 100 mL/min and the renal clearance rate is 94 mL/min in subjects with normal renal function.

Amikacin is excreted primarily by glomerular filtration. Patients with impaired renal function or diminished glomerular filtration pressure excrete the drug much more slowly (effectively prolonging the serum half-life). Therefore, renal function should be monitored carefully and dosage adjusted accordingly (see suggested dosage schedule under "Dosage and Administration").

Following administration at the recommended dose, therapeutic levels are found in bone, heart, gallbladder, and lung tissue in addition to significant concentrations in urine, bile, sputum, bronchial secretions, interstitial, pleural and synovial fluids.

Spinal fluid levels in normal infants are approximately 10% to 20% of the serum concentrations and may reach 50% when the meninges are inflamed. AMIKIN has been demonstrated to cross the placental barrier and yield significant concentrations in amniotic fluid. The peak fetal serum concentration is about 16% of the peak maternal serum concentration and maternal and fetal serum half-life values are about 2 and 3.7 hours, respectively.

Microbiology

Gram-negative—Amikacin is active **in vitro** against **Pseudomonas** species, **Escherichia coli, Proteus** species (indole-positive and indole-negative), **Providencia** species, **Klebsiella-Enterobacter-Serratia** species, **Acinetobacter** (formerly **Mima-Herellea**) species, and **Citrobacter freundii.**

When strains of the above organisms are found to be resistant to other aminoglycosides, including gentamicin, tobramycin and kanamycin, many are susceptible to amikacin **in vitro.**

Gram-positive—Amikacin is active **in vitro** against penicillinase and nonpenicillinase-producing **Staphylococcus** species including methicillin-resistant strains. However, aminoglycosides in general have a low order of activity against other Gram-positive organisms; viz, **Streptococcus pyogenes,** enterococci, and **Streptococcus pneumoniae** (formerly **Diplococcus pneumoniae**).

Amikacin resists degradation by most aminoglycoside inactivating enzymes known to affect gentamicin, tobramycin, and kanamycin.

In vitro studies have shown that AMIKIN combined with a beta-lactam antibiotic acts synergistically against many clinically significant gram-negative organisms.

Disc Susceptibility Tests—Quantitative methods that require measurement of zone diameters give the most precise estimates of antibiotic susceptibility. One such procedure* has been recommended for use with discs to test susceptibility to amikacin. Interpretation involves correlation of the diameters obtained in the disc test with MIC values for amikacin. When the causative organism is tested by the Kirby-Bauer method of disc susceptibility, a 30-μg amikacin disc should give a zone of 17 mm or greater to indicate susceptibility. Zone sizes of 14 mm or less indicate resistance. Zone sizes of 15 to 16 mm indicate intermediate susceptibility. With this procedure, a report from the laboratory of "susceptible" indicates that the infecting organism is likely to respond to therapy. A report of "resistant" indicates that the infecting organism is not likely to respond to therapy. A report of "intermediate susceptibility" suggests that the organism would be susceptible if the infection is confined to tissues and fluids (eg, urine) in which high antibiotic levels are attained.

INDICATIONS AND USAGE

AMIKIN is indicated in the short-term treatment of serious infections due to susceptible strains of Gram-negative bacteria, including **Pseudomonas** species, **Escherichia coli,** species of indole-positive and indole-negative **Proteus, Providencia** species, **Klebsiella-Enterobacter-Serratia** species, and **Acinetobacter (Mima-Herellea)** species.

Clinical studies have shown AMIKIN to be effective in bacterial septicemia (including neonatal sepsis); in serious infections of the respiratory tract, bones and joints, central nervous system (including meningitis) and skin and soft tissue; intra-abdominal infections (including peritonitis); and in burns and postoperative infections (including postvascular surgery). Clinical studies have shown AMIKIN also to be effective in serious complicated and recurrent urinary tract infections due to these organisms. Aminoglycosides, including AMIKIN injectable, are not indicated in uncomplicated initial episodes of urinary tract infections unless the causative organisms are not susceptible to antibiotics having less potential toxicity.

Bacteriologic studies should be performed to identify causative organisms and their susceptibilities to amikacin. AMIKIN may be considered as initial therapy in suspected Gram-negative infections and therapy may be instituted before obtaining the results of susceptibility testing. Clinical trials demonstrated that AMIKIN was effective in infections caused by gentamicin and/or tobramycin-resistant strains of Gram-negative organisms, particularly **Proteus rettgeri, Providencia stuartii, Serratia marcescens,** and **Pseudomonas aeruginosa.** The decision to continue therapy with the drug should be based on results of the susceptibility tests, the severity of the infection, the response of the patient and the important additional considerations contained in the "Warnings" box above.

AMIKIN has also been shown to be effective in staphylococcal infections and may be considered as initial therapy under certain conditions in the treatment of known or suspected staphylococcal disease such as, severe infections where the causative organism may be either a Gram-negative bacterium or a staphylococcus, infections due to susceptible strains of staphylococci in patients allergic to other antibiotics, and in mixed staphylococcal/Gram-negative infections. In certain severe infections such as neonatal sepsis, concomitant therapy with a penicillin-type drug may be indicated because of the possibility of infections due to Gram-positive organisms such as streptococci or pneumococci.

CONTRAINDICATIONS

A history of hypersensitivity to amikacin is a contraindication for its use. A history of hypersensitivity or serious toxic reactions to aminoglycosides may contraindicate the use of any other aminoglycoside because of the known cross-sensitivities of patients to drugs in this class.

WARNINGS

See "Warnings" box above.

Aminoglycosides can cause fetal harm when administered to a pregnant woman. Aminoglycosides cross the placenta and there have been several reports of total irreversible, bilateral congenital deafness in children whose mothers received streptomycin during pregnancy. Although serious side effects to the fetus or newborns have not been reported in the treatment of pregnant women with other aminoglycosides, the potential for harm exists. Reproduction studies of amikacin have been performed in rats and mice and revealed no evidence of impaired fertility or harm to the fetus due to amikacin. There are no well controlled studies in pregnant women, but investigational experience does not include any positive evidence of adverse effects to the fetus. If this drug is used during pregnancy, or if the patient becomes pregnant while taking this drug, the patient should be apprised of the potential hazard to the fetus.

Contains sodium bisulfite, a sulfite that may cause allergic-type reactions including anaphylactic symptoms and life-threatening or less severe asthmatic episodes in certain susceptible people. The overall prevalence of sulfite sensitivity in the general population is unknown and probably low. Sulfite sensitivity is seen more frequently in asthmatic than nonasthmatic people.

PRECAUTIONS

Aminoglycosides are quickly and almost totally absorbed when they are applied topically, except to the urinary bladder, in association with surgical procedures. Irreversible deafness, renal failure, and death due to neuromuscular blockade have been reported following irrigation of both small and large surgical fields with an aminoglycoside preparation.

AMIKIN is potentially nephrotoxic, ototoxic and neurotoxic. The concurrent or serial use of other ototoxic or nephrotoxic agents should be avoided either systemically or topically because of the potential for additive effects. Increased nephrotoxicity has been reported following concomitant parenteral administration of aminoglycoside antibiotics and cephalosporins. Concomitant cephalosporins may spuriously elevate creatinine determinations.

Since AMIKIN is present in high concentrations in the renal excretory system, patients should be well hydrated to minimize chemical irritation of the renal tubules. Kidney function should be assessed by the usual methods prior to starting therapy and daily during the course of treatment.

If signs of renal irritation appear (casts, white or red cells, or albumin), hydration should be increased. A reduction in dosage (see "Dosage and Administration") may be desirable if other evidence of renal dysfunction occurs such as decreased creatinine clearance; decreased urine specific gravity; increased BUN, creatinine, or oliguria. If azotemia increases or if a progressive decrease in urinary output occurs, treatment should be stopped.

Note: When patients are well hydrated and kidney function is normal the risk of nephrotoxic reactions with amikacin is low if the dosage recomendations (see "Dosage and Administration") are not exceeded.

Elderly patients may have reduced renal function which may not be evident in routine screening tests such as BUN or serum creatinine. A creatinine clearance determination may be more useful. Monitoring of renal function during treatment with aminoglycosides is particularly important.

Aminoglycosides should be used with caution in patients with muscular disorders such as myasthenia gravis or parkinsonism since these drugs may aggravate muscle weakness because of their potential curare-like effect on the neuromuscular junction.

In vitro mixing of aminoglycosides with beta-lactam antibiotics (penicillin or cephalosporins) may result in a significant mutual inactivation. A reduction in serum half-life or serum level may occur when an aminoglycoside or penicillin-type drug is administered by separate routes. Inactivation of the aminoglycoside is clinically significant only in patients with severely impaired renal function. Inactivation may continue in specimens of body fluids collected for assay, resulting in inaccurate aminoglycoside readings. Such specimens should be properly handled (assayed promptly, frozen, or treated with beta-lactamase).

Cross-allergenicity among aminoglycosides has been demonstrated.

As with other antibiotics, the use of amikacin may result in overgrowth of nonsusceptible organisms. If this occurs, appropriate therapy should be instituted.

Aminoglycosides should not be given concurrently with potent diuretics (See "Warnings" box).

Carcinogenesis, Mutagenesis, Impairment of Fertility—Studies in humans have not been performed with the aminoglycosides to determine their effect on carcinogenesis, mutagenesis, or impairment of fertility.

Pregnancy—Category D (See "Warnings" section).

Nursing Mothers—It is not known whether this drug is excreted in human milk. As a general rule, nursing should not be undertaken while a patient is on a drug since many drugs are excreted in human milk.

PEDIATRIC USE—Aminoglycosides should be used with caution in premature and neonatal infants because of the renal immaturity of these patients and the resulting prolongation of serum half-life of these drugs.

ADVERSE REACTIONS

All aminoglycosides have the potential to induce auditory, vestibular, and renal toxicity and neuromuscular blockade (see "Warnings" box). They occur more frequently in patients with present or past history of renal impairment, of treatment with other ototoxic or nephrotoxic drugs, and in patients treated for longer periods and/or with higher doses than recommended.

Neurotoxicity-Ototoxicity—Toxic effects on the eighth cranial nerve can result in hearing loss, loss of balance, or both. Amikacin primarily affects auditory function. Cochlear damage includes high frequency deafness and usually occurs before clinical hearing loss can be detected.

Neurotoxicity-Neuromuscular Blockage—Acute muscular paralysis and apnea can occur following treatment with aminoglycoside drugs.

Nephrotoxicity—Elevation of serum creatinine, albuminuria, presence of red and white cells, casts, azotemia, and oliguria have been reported. Renal function changes are usually reversible when the drug is discontinued.

Other—In addition to those described above, other adverse reactions which have been reported on rare occasions are skin rash, drug fever, headache, paresthesia, tremor, nausea and vomiting, eosinophilia, arthralgia, anemia, and hypotension.

Overdosage—In the event of overdosage or toxic reaction, peritoneal dialysis or hemodialysis will aid in the removal of amikacin from the blood. In the newborn infant, exchange transfusion may also be considered.

DOSAGE AND ADMINISTRATION

The patient's pretreatment body weight should be obtained for calculation of correct dosage. AMIKIN may be given intramuscularly or intravenously.

The status of renal function should be estimated by measurement of the serum creatinine concentration or calculation of the endogenous creatinine clearance rate. The blood urea nitrogen (BUN) is much less reliable for this purpose. Reassessment of renal function should be made periodically during therapy.

Whenever possible, amikacin concentrations in serum should be measured to assure adequate but not excessive levels. It is desirable to measure both peak and trough serum concentrations intermittently during therapy. Peak concentrations (30–90 minutes after injection) above 35 μg per mL and trough concentrations (just prior to the next dose) above 10 μg per mL should be avoided. Dosage should be adjusted as indicated.

Intramuscular Administration for Patients with Normal Renal Function—The recommended dosage for adults, children and older infants (see "Warnings" box) with normal renal function is 15 mg/kg/day divided into 2 or 3 equal doses administered at equally-divided intervals, ie, 7.5 mg/kg q.12h or 5 mg/kg q.8h. Treatment of patients in the heavier weight classes should not exceed 1.5 gram/day.

When amikacin is indicated in newborns (see "Warnings" box), it is recommended that a loading dose of 10 mg/kg be administered initially to be followed with 7.5 mg/kg every 12 hours.

The usual duration of treatment is 7 to 10 days. It is desirable to limit the duration of treatment to short term whenever feasible. The total daily dose by all routes of administration should not exceed 15 mg/kg/day. In difficult and complicated infections where treatment beyond 10 days is considered, the use of AMIKIN should be reevaluated. If continued, amikacin serum levels, and renal, auditory, and vestibular functions should be monitored. At the recommended dosage level, uncomplicated infections due to amikacin-sensitive organisms should respond in 24 to 48 hours. If definite clinical response does not occur within 3 to 5 days, therapy should be stopped and the antibiotic susceptibility pattern of the invading organism should be rechecked. Failure of the infection to respond may be due to resistance of the organism or to the presence of septic foci requiring surgical drainage.

When AMIKIN is indicated in uncomplicated urinary tract infections, a dose of 250 mg twice daily may be used. [See table above].

Intramuscular Administration for Patients with Impaired Renal Function—Whenever possible, serum amikacin concentrations should be monitored by appropriate assay procedures. Doses may be adjusted in patients with impaired renal function either by administering normal doses at prolonged intervals or by administering reduced doses at a fixed interval.

Both methods are based on the patient's creatinine clearance or serum creatinine values since these have been found to correlate with aminoglycoside half-lives in patients with diminished renal function. These dosage schedules must be used in conjunction with careful clinical and laboratory observations of the patient and should be modified as necessary. Neither method should be used when dialysis is being performed.

Normal Dosage at Prolonged Intervals—If the creatinine clearance rate is not available and the patient's condition is stable, a dosage interval in hours for the normal dose can be calculated by multiplying the patient's serum creatinine by 9, eg, if the serum creatinine concentration is 2 mg/100 mL, the recommended single dose (7.5 mg/kg) should be administered every 18 hours.

Reduced Dosage at Fixed Time Intervals—When renal function is impaired and it is desirable to administer AMIKIN at a fixed time interval, dosage must be reduced. In these patients, serum AMIKIN concentrations should be measured to assure accurate administration of AMIKIN and to avoid concentrations above 35 μg/mL. If serum assay determinations are not available and the patient's condition is stable,

Continued on next page

DOSAGE GUIDELINES

ADULTS AND CHILDREN WITH NORMAL RENAL FUNCTION

Patient Weight		Dosage		
lbs.	kg	7.5 mg/kg q. 12h	OR	5mg/kg q. 8h
99	45	337.5 mg		225 mg
110	50	375 mg		250 mg
121	55	412.5 mg		275 mg
132	60	450 mg		300 mg
143	65	487.5 mg		325 mg
154	70	525 mg		350 mg
165	75	562.6 mg		375 mg
176	80	600 mg		400 mg
187	85	637.5 mg		425 mg
198	90	675 mg		450 mg
209	95	712.5 mg		475 mg
220	100	750 mg		500 mg

Available as: 100 mg/2 mL vial, 500 mg/2 mL vial, 1g/4 mL vial, 500 mg/2 mL Disposable Syringe

Bristol Labs.—Cont.

serum creatinine and creatinine clearance values are the most readily available indicators of the degree of renal impairment to use as a guide for dosage.

First, initiate therapy by administering a normal dose, 7.5 mg/kg, as a loading dose. This loading dose is the same as the normally recommended dose which would be calculated for a patient with a normal renal function as described above.

To determine the size of maintenance doses administered every 12 hours, the loading dose should be reduced in proportion to the reduction in the patient's creatinine clearance rate:

$$\text{Maintenance Dose Every 12 hours} = \frac{\text{observed CC in mL/min}}{\text{normal CC in mL/min}} \times \text{calculated loading dose in mg}$$

(CC—creatinine clearance rate)

An alternate rough guide for determining reduced dosage at 12-hour intervals (for patients whose steady state serum creatinine values are known) is to divide the normally recommended dose by the patient's serum creatinine.

The above dosage schedules are not intended to be rigid recommendations but are provided as guides to dosage when the measurement of amikacin serum levels is not feasible.

Intravenous Administration—The individual dose, the total daily dose, and the total cumulative dose of AMIKIN are identical to the dose recommended for intramuscular administration. The solution for intravenous use is prepared by adding the contents of a 0.5 gram vial to 100–200 mL of sterile diluent such as Normal Saline or 5% Dextrose in Water or any other compatible solution.

The solution is administered to adults over a 30 to 60 minute period. The total daily dose should not exceed 15 mg/kg/day and may be divided into either 2 or 3 equally-divided doses at equally-divided intervals.

In pediatric patients the amount of fluid used will depend on the amount ordered for the patient. It should be a sufficient amount to infuse the amikacin over a 30 to 60 minute period. Infants should receive a 1 to 2 hour infusion.

Amikacin should not be physically premixed with other drugs but should be administered separately according to the recommended dose and route.

Stability in IV Fluids—AMIKIN is stable for 24 hours at room temperature at concentrations of 0.25 and 5.0 mg/mL in the following solutions:

5% Dextrose Injection, USP
5% Dextrose and 0.2% Sodium Chloride Injection, USP
5% Dextrose and 0.45% Sodium Chloride Injection, USP
0.9% Sodium Chloride Injection, USP
Lactated Ringer's Injection, USP
Normosol®M in 5% Dextrose Injection, USP (or Plasma-Lyte 56 Injection in 5% Dextrose in Water)
Normosol®R in 5% Dextrose Injection, USP (or Plasma-Lyte 148 Injection in 5% Dextrose in Water)

In the above solutions with AMIKIN concentrations of 0.25 and 5.0 mg/mL, solutions aged for 60 days at 4°C and then stored at 25°C had utility times of 24 hours.

At the same concentrations, solutions frozen and aged for 30 days at −15°C, thawed, and stored at 25°C had utility times of 24 hours.

Parenteral drug products should be inspected visually for particulate matter and discoloration prior to administration whenever the solution and container permit.

Aminoglycosides administered by any of the above routes should not be physically premixed with other drugs but should be administered separately.

Because of the potential toxicity of aminoglycosides, "fixed dosage" recommendations which are not based upon body weight are not advised. Rather, it is essential to calculate the dosage to fit the needs of each patient.

SUPPLY

AMIKIN is supplied as a colorless solution which requires no refrigeration. It is stable at room temperature for at least two years. At times the solution may become a very pale yellow; this does not indicate a decrease in potency.

AMIKIN (amikacin sulfate injection)
NDC 0015-3015-20—100 mg per 2 mL
NDC 0015-3020-20—500 mg per 2 mL
NDC 0015-3020-21—Disposable Syringe (500 mg per 2 mL)
NDC 0015-3023-20—1 gram per 4 mL
U.S. Patent Nos. 3,781,268, 4,424,343

*Bauer, A. W., Kirby, W. M. M., Sherris, J. C., and Turck, M.: Antibiotic Testing by a Standardized Single Disc Method, Am. J. Clin. Pathol. 45:493, 1966; Standardized Disc Susceptibility Test, FEDERAL REGISTER, 37:20527–29, 1972.

ENKAID®   ℞
[ĕn´-kād]
(encainide HCl)

DESCRIPTION

ENKAID®, encainide hydrochloride, is an antiarrhythmic drug supplied as 25, 35, and 50 mg capsules for oral administration. The chemical name of ENKAID is (±)-4-methoxy-N-[2-[2-(1-methyl-2-piperidinyl)ethyl]phenyl]benzamide hydrochloride. Its molecular weight is 388.94 and the structural formula is represented as follows:

Encainide hydrochloride is a white solid which is freely soluble in water, slightly soluble in ethanol, and insoluble in heptane. The pH of a 1% aqueous solution is 5.8. In addition to the hard gelatin capsule shell, the other inactive ingredients are lactose, magnesium stearate and sodium starch glycolate.

CLINICAL PHARMACOLOGY

Mechanism of Action

The mechanisms of the antiarrhythmic effects of ENKAID are unknown but probably are the result of its ability to slow conduction, reduce membrane responsiveness, inhibit automaticity, and increase the ratio of the effective refractory period to action potential duration. ENKAID produces a differentially greater effect on the ischemic zone as compared with normal cells in the myocardium. This could result in the elimination of the disparity in the electrophysiologic properties between these two zones and eliminate pathways of abnormal impulse conduction, development of boundary currents and/or sites of abnormal impulse generation.

Electrophysiology

ENKAID is a Class IC antiarrhythmic agent, ie, is a blocker of the sodium channel of Purkinje fibers and the myocardium.

In isolated Purkinje and myocardial cells its electrophysiologic profile is characterized by a dose-related slowing of phase O depolarization and little effect on either the action potential duration or repolarization. This profile differs from that of Class IA drugs (eg, quinidine, disopyramide, procainamide) that slow phase O depolarization and prolong action potential duration or Class IB agents (eg, lidocaine, tocainide and mexiletine) that slow phase O depolarization only slightly and shorten the action potential duration.

In the intact animal and man, the electrophysiologic effects of encainide are a result not only of encainide but of two metabolites as well, each of which is present in most patients (over 90%) at therapeutically active levels. Encainide and its metabolites produce a dose-related decrease in intracardiac conduction in all parts of the heart, with slowing of conduction in the His-Purkinje system and AV node and an increase in the refractoriness of the atrium and ventricle. (See **WARNINGS: Electrocardiographic Changes**).

Each variable studied in normal and ischemic tissues is altered in the same manner in both, but more markedly in ischemic tissues.

ENKAID has also been shown to slow conduction and increase refractoriness in accessory atrioventricular pathways and in the AV node.

HEMODYNAMICS

In oral studies of hemodynamic effects, using invasive and noninvasive measurements of cardiac function, ENKAID had no effects on measurements of cardiac performance such as cardiac or stroke volume index, pulmonary capillary wedge pressure or peripheral blood pressure either at rest or during exercise. In noninvasive studies that included both geriatric patients and younger patients with impaired left ventricular function (New York Heart Association Class III & IV) there were no detrimental effects on ejection fractions acutely or after more than 12 months of therapy in some cases. Doses of 75–300 mg/day of ENKAID, which reduced the incidence of premature ventricular complexes by at least 80%, did not adversely affect exercise tolerance, and were well tolerated clinically by patients with markedly impaired left ventricular function. In a few instances, however, apparent new or worsened congestive heart failure has developed during treatment with ENKAID (See **WARNINGS**).

CLINICAL ACTIONS

Although ENKAID should not be used for the treatment of nonlife-treatening arrhythmias, in premarketing, placebo-controlled trials ENKAID caused a dose-related reduction in the occurrence of single, repetitive, and multiform premature ventricular complexes. ENKAID has been shown to reduce the incidence of nonsustained ventricular tachycar-

dia. Doses of 75–150 mg per day were needed in most patients to attain 75% or greater suppression. In programmed electrical stimulation studies, ENKAID has prevented the induction of ventricular tachycardia in about 20% to 30% of the patients. ENKAID has also been shown to reduce the recurrence of sustained ventricular tachycardia in patients with a history of malignant arrhythmias.

ENKAID is effective in treating ventricular arrhythmias in patients with and without organic heart disease and has frequently been effective in patients who were unresponsive to, or intolerant of, one or more other antiarrhythmic agents. When ENKAID therapy was discontinued, such as during placebo phases in the premarketing clinical trials, ventricular ectopy returned to rates that did not differ significantly from the baseline values. That is, no clinical evidence of arrhythmia exacerbation or "rebound" has been noted following discontinuation.

PHARMACOKINETICS

The absorption of ENKAID after oral administration is nearly complete with peak plasma levels present 30 to 90 minutes after dosing.

There are two major genetically determined patterns of encainide metabolism. In over 90% of patients the drug is rapidly and extensively metabolized with an elimination half-life of 1 to 2 hours. These patients convert encainide to two active metabolites, O-demethylencainide (ODE) and 3-methoxy-O-demethylencainide (MODE), that are more active (on a per mg basis) than encainide itself. These metabolites are eliminated more slowly than encainide, with half-lives of 3 to 4 hours for ODE and 6 to 12 hours for MODE. A radiolabeled dose of encainide is excreted in approximately equal amounts in the urine and feces. A major urinary metabolite is ODE, with lesser amounts of encainide and MODE present.

In less than 10% of patients, metabolism of encainide is slower and the estimated encainide elimination half-life is 6 to 11 hours. Slow metabolism of encainide is associated with a diminished ability to metabolize debrisoquin. In these patients the renal excretion of encainide is a major route of elimination and little if any MODE and only small amounts of ODE are present in their plasma.

Despite the differences in pharmacogenetics, in all patients 3 to 5 days of dosing are required to achieve steady state conditions. Based on clinical experience and pharmacokinetic considerations, the recommended dosage regimen (see **DOSAGE AND ADMINISTRATION**) is appropriate for all patients regardless of their genetically determined capacity to metabolize encainide.

Encainide, ODE, and MODE follow a nonlinear pharmacokinetic disposition, although ODE and MODE differ from linearity only to a small extent. The absorption of ENKAID is retarded by food, but the overall bioavailability is not altered. The pharmacokinetics of ENKAID do not change with increasing age over 21, and are not different between men and women.

The clearance of encainide and conversion to active metabolites is reduced in patients with hepatic disease, but serum concentrations of ODE and MODE are similar to those in normal patients. There is insufficient experience to be certain about the need for alteration in the normal dose and/or dosing interval when ENKAID is administered to patients with hepatic disease, but it is prudent to increase doses cautiously.

The clearance of encainide is reduced, and plasma levels of the active metabolites ODE and MODE are increased in patients with significant renal impairment and the dosage should be reduced in these patients (see **PRECAUTIONS.**). Encainide and ODE are bound to a moderate extent to plasma proteins (75%–85%) while the binding of MODE, at about 92%, is somewhat greater.

For information on potential drug interactions see **PRECAUTIONS: Drug Interactions.**

INDICATIONS AND USAGE

ENKAID is indicated for the treatment of documented ventricular arrhythmias, such as sustained ventricular tachycardia that, in the judgement of the physician, are life-threatening. Because of the proarrhythmic effects of ENKAID, its use should be reserved for patients in whom, in the opinion of the physician, the benefits of treatment outweigh the risks. ENKAID should not be used in patients with less severe ventricular arrhythmias, even if the patients are symptomatic.

Treatment with ENKAID should be initiated in a hospital. Patients should also be hospitalized at the time of a dose increase to 200 mg per day or above (see DOSAGE AND ADMINISTRATION).

The effects of ENKAID in patients with supraventricular arrhythmias and patients with recent myocardial infarction (except as described in the WARNINGS section) have not been adequately studied.

As is the case for other antiarrhythmic agents, there is no evidence from controlled trials that the use of ENKAID favorably affects survival or the incidence of sudden death.

CONTRAINDICATIONS

ENKAID is contraindicated in patients with preexisting second- or third-degree AV block, or with right bundle branch block when associated with a left hemiblock (bifascicular block), unless a pacemaker is present to sustain the cardiac rhythm should complete heart block occur. ENKAID is also contraindicated in the presence of cardiogenic shock or known hypersensitivity to the drug.

WARNINGS

Mortality

ENKAID was included in the National Heart Lung and Blood Institute's Cardiac Arrhythmia Suppression Trial (CAST), a long-term, multicenter, randomized, double-blind study in patients with asymptomatic nonlife-threatening arrhythmias who had a myocardial infarction more than 6 days, but less than 2 years previously. An excessive mortality or nonfatal cardiac arrest rate was seen in patients treated with ENKAID compared with that seen in a carefully matched placebo-treated group. This rate was 40/415 (9.6%) for ENKAID and 15/416 (3.6%) for its matched placebo. The average duration of treatment with ENKAID in this study was 10 months.

The applicability of the CAST results to other populations (eg, those without recent myocardial infarction) is uncertain, but at present it is prudent to consider the risks of class IC agents, coupled with the lack of any evidence of improved survival, unacceptable in patients without life-threatening ventricular arrhythmias, even if the patients are experiencing unpleasant, but not life-threatening, symptoms or signs.

Proarrhythmia

ENKAID, like other antiarrhythmic agents, can cause new or worsened arrhythmias. Such proarrhythmic effects range from an increase in frequency of PVCs to the development of more severe ventricular tachycardia; eg, tachycardia that is more sustained or more resistant to conversion to sinus rhythm, with potentially fatal consequences.

In patients with malignant arrhythmias, it is often difficult to distinguish a spontaneous variation in the patient's underlying rhythm disorder from drug induced worsening, so the following occurrence rates must be considered approximations.

Overall, in premarketing clinical trials with ENKAID about 10% of all patients had proarrhythmic events, about 6% of them representing new or worsened ventricular tachycardia. Provocation or aggravation occurred most frequently in patients who had a history of sustained ventricular tachycardia (12% of such patients), cardiomyopathy (16%), congestive heart failure (12%), or sustained ventricular tachycardia with cardiomyopathy or congestive heart failure (17%). The incidence of proarrhythmic events in patients without ventricular tachycardia or overt manifestations of clinical heart disease ranged from 3% to 4%. Proarrhythmia occurred least frequently in patients with no known structural heart disease. Age, sex, baseline ECG intervals, or ECG changes caused by ENKAID were not predictive of the occurrence of proarrhythmia.

A review of deaths in premarketing clinical trials indicates that about 1% of patients might have died of a possible proarrhythmic effect of ENKAID, virtually all of them patients with a history of ventricular tachycardia. In most cases, patients had a history of sustained ventricular tachycardia or ventricular fibrillation.

Proarrhythmic events in premarketing clinical trials occurred most commonly during the first week of therapy and were much more common when doses exceeded 200 mg/day. Initiating therapy at 75 mg/day combined with gradual dose adjustment reduced the risk of proarrhythmia (see DOSAGE AND ADMINISTRATION).

Congestive Heart Failure

New or worsened congestive heart failure (CHF) attributed to ENKAID occurred infrequently (< 1%); nevertheless, ENKAID should be used cautiously in patients with CHF or congestive cardiomyopathy.

Electrolyte Disturbances

Hypokalemia or hyperkalemia may alter the effects of Class I antiarrhythmic drugs. Preexisting hypokalemia or hyperkalemia should be corrected before administration of ENKAID.

Sick Sinus Syndrome—(Bradycardia-Tachycardia Syndrome)

ENKAID should be used only with extreme caution in patients with sick sinus syndrome because it may cause sinus bradycardia, sinus pause, or sinus arrest.

Electrocardiographic Changes

ENKAID slows conduction and consequently produces dose-related changes in the PR and QRS intervals. The intervals increase in a linear manner at doses from 30 to 225 mg/day. There is no consistent change in JT. The QTc interval is increased, but only to the extent of the increase in QRS interval.

Changes in ECG Intervals*

| | Total Daily Dose (mg) | | | | | |
| | 75 | | 150 | | 200 | |
Interval	sec	(%)	sec	(%)	sec	(%)
PR	0.02	(12)	0.04	(21)	0.04	(24)
QRS	0.01	(12)	0.02	(23)	0.02	(26)

* Percent change based on mean baseline values of PR = 0.169 and QRS = 0.088 from a group of 504 patients treated for ventricular arrhythmias.

Unlike the changes in the PR, QRS, and QTc intervals observed with the Class 1A drugs, the ECG changes induced by ENKAID are not in themselves indications of effectiveness, toxicity or overdosage nor can they routinely be used to predict efficacy.

Clinically significant changes in cardiac conduction have been observed. Sinus bradycardia, sinus pause, or sinus arrest occurred in 1% of the patients and prolongation of QRS interval to greater than/or equal to 0.20 sec developed in about 7% of the patients. The incidence of second- or third-degree AV block was less, 0.5% and 0.2% respectively.

Effects on Pacemaker Thresholds

The safety of ENKAID in patients with permanently implanted programmable pacemakers has been established in a small (10 patient) study which evaluated the effects of increasing doses on pacemaker thresholds. ENKAID has a limited potential for increasing pacemaker thresholds. Only one subject had a clinically significant change that would require pacemaker reprogramming and that occurred only at the highest dose tested (75 mg t.i.d.). These effects were reversed when the drug was discontinued. It is advisable to establish pacemaker threshold prior to encainide administration and at regular intervals during therapy. Reprogramming of multiprogrammable pacemakers may be required to increase voltage or pulse width. ENKAID should not be administered to patients with existing poor thresholds or nonprogrammable pacemakers unless suitable pacing rescue is available. In addition to possible rise in pacing threshold, ENKAID may suppress ventricular escape rhythms.

PRECAUTIONS

Drug Interactions

In prospective studies single and multiple doses of ENKAID have had no significant effect on serum digoxin levels. Likewise, combined digoxin/ENKAID therapy has been administered without adverse effects.

Experience has indicated no obvious problems with the combined use of ENKAID and other antiarrhythmic agents, diuretics, beta blockers or calcium channel blockers. However, because of possible additive pharmacologic effects, caution is indicated when ENKAID is used with another antiarrhythmic agent or any other drug that affects cardiac conduction. Cimetidine (300 mg q.i.d.) increases plasma concentrations of encainide and its active metabolites. Although no clinically significant consequences have been reported, caution should be utilized when the two drugs are administered simultaneously. ENKAID dosage should be reduced if cimetidine is to be given to a patient taking ENKAID.

In vitro binding studies with several drugs that may be administered concomitantly have not revealed any significant alteration in the protein binding of encainide, ODE, or MODE; nor did high concentrations of encainide and its metabolites alter the binding of the other medications including such highly protein bound drugs as warfarin.

Hepatic Impairment

Patients with hepatic impairment have a significantly reduced rate of elimination of encainide, probably as a consequence of decreased metabolism to ODE and MODE; serum concentrations of ODE and MODE, however, are little altered. There is insufficient experience to be certain about the need for alterations in the dose and/or dosing interval of ENKAID in patients with hepatic disease, but it is prudent to increase doses cautiously.

Renal Impairment

Limited data suggest that reduction in the elimination of encainide and its active metabolites ODE and MODE in patients with severe renal impairment (serum creatinine > 3.5 mg/dL or creatinine clearance of less than 20 mL/min) results in significant accumulation of metabolites and, to a lesser degree, encainide. In such patients, therapy with ENKAID should be initiated with a single daily dose of 25 mg. If needed the dose may be increased to 25 mg b.i.d. after at least 7 days, and again to 25 mg t.i.d. after an additional 7 days if necessary. Doses above 150 mg per day are not recommended. Consideration should be given to reducing ENKAID dosage if renal function deteriorates significantly.

Carcinogenesis, Mutagenesis, Impairment of Fertility

Carcinogenicity studies have been performed by the oral route in rats and mice at doses up to 30 mg/kg/day and 135 mg/kg/day, respectively. No drug-related increase in tumor incidence was observed. Bacterial and mammalian mutagenicity tests with encainide have been negative. No reduction in fertility occurred in rats at oral doses up to 14 mg/kg/day. Fertility was reduced when both male and female rats received oral doses of 28 mg/kg/day (approximately 13 times the average human dose) prior to mating; there was no reduction with treatment of each sex separately at the same dose.

Pregnancy Category B

Reproduction studies have been performed in rats and rabbits at doses up to 13 and 9 times the average human dose, respectively, and have revealed no evidence of harm to the fetus due to encainide. There are, however, no adequate and well-controlled studies in pregnant women. Because animal reproduction studies are not always predictive of human response, this drug should be used during pregnancy only if clearly needed.

Nursing Mothers

Encainide is excreted in the milk of laboratory animals and has been reported to be present in human milk. Although no overt postnatal effects were observed in the postnatal phase of the rodent reproduction studies, other than decreased weight at the highest dose of 28 mg/kg/day (13 times human dose), the potential for serious adverse reactions in nursing infants from ENKAID is unknown. A decision should be made whether to discontinue nursing or to discontinue the drug, taking into account the importance of the drug to the mother.

Pediatric Use

The safety and effectiveness of ENKAID in children less than 18 years of age have not been established.

ADVERSE REACTIONS

In the National Heart Lung and Blood Institute's Cardiac Arrhythmia Suppression Trial (CAST), the incidence of total mortality and nonfatal cardiac arrest in the ENKAID group was 40/415 (9.6%), and that in the placebo group was 15/416 (3.6%). (See boxed **WARNINGS**).

The most serious adverse reactions reported for ENKAID in premarketing clinical trials were the provocation or aggravation of ventricular arrhythmias (See **WARNINGS**). These occurred during the course of the clinical research program in about 10% of the patients who received a wide range of doses under a variety of circumstances. In some cases this resulted in the development of sustained ventricular tachycardia or ventricular fibrillation.

Only 0.4% of patients discontinued ENKAID therapy due to congestive heart failure or related causes. Second- or third-degree AV block developed in 0.5% and 0.2% of the patients respectively. Sinus bradycardia, sinus pause or sinus arrest occurred in 1% of the patients. There have been rare reports of elevated serum liver enzymes (alkaline phosphatase, serum transaminases), hepatitis, and jaundice, in which a relation to encainide is possible and there has been one instance of a rechallenge-confirmed elevation of transaminases. There have also been rare reports of elevated blood glucose levels or of increased insulin requirements in diabetic patients. Although no cause and effect relationship has been established, caution is advised in patients who develop unexplained jaundice or signs of hepatic dysfunction or hyperglycemia and consideration should be given to discontinuing therapy.

In premarketing evaluations 2400 subjects were exposed to ENKAID, of whom more than 500 were maintained on drug for two years or longer. Adverse events were sufficiently troublesome to cause discontinuation in about 7% of the patients participating in premarketing clinical trials. The most frequently reported adverse events were dizziness, blurred or abnormal vision, and headache.

The following table lists the most common adverse events that occurred in two multi-center premarketing clinical trials, one of which compared encainide to placebo, the other to quinidine. This table lists all such adverse events reported by at least 3% of the patients and thus may include symptoms of the underlying disease, intercurrent illness or adverse reactions to drug therapy.

[See table on bottom next page].

The following table gives the incidence of the most common adverse events at selected doses of ENKAID that were used during the premarketing clinical trials which involved a total of 749 patients with ventricular arrhythmias. The incidence figures in the "0 mg" column are based on events that occurred while patients were on placebo or in drug-free wash out periods.

[See table on top next page].

Other adverse events occurring in less than 1% of the patients receiving ENKAID include: malaise, decreased or increased blood pressure, confusion, ataxia, abnormal gait, abnormal sensation, abnormal dreams, diplopia, photophobia and periorbital edema.

POSTINTRODUCTION CLINICAL EXPERIENCE

Other than the clinical experience in the CAST study described above (see boxed **WARNINGS** and **ADVERSE REACTIONS**), postmarketing experience has shown an adverse experience profile similar to that described for the premarketing clinical trials. Voluntary reports since introduction include rare reports (less than one report per 10,000 patients) of arthralgia, fever, leukopenia, positive ANA test,

Continued on next page

Bristol Labs.—Cont.

and thrombocytopenia. Because of the uncontrolled nature of these voluntary reports, and because most of the patients were receiving concomitant medications, any causal relationship to ENKAID treatment is difficult to establish.

OVERDOSAGE

Intentional or accidental overdosages with ENKAID have resulted in death.

Signs, Symptoms, and Laboratory Findings Associated with an Overdosage of the Drug

Overdosage with ENKAID may produce excessive widening of the QRS complex and QT interval and AV dissociation. Hypotension, bradycardia and finally asystole may develop. A variety of conduction disturbances may be observed. Convulsions have occurred in one case of intentional overdosage.

Oral LD$_{50}$ of the Drug in Animals

The acute, oral LD$_{50}$ values for encainide are estimated to be 80 mg/kg in the mouse and 59 mg/kg in the rat.

Recommended General Treatment Procedures

In the event of overdosage with ENKAID, patients should be hospitalized and provided with cardiac monitoring and advanced life support systems. No specific antidote for EN-KAID has been identified; however, one report has suggested hypertonic sodium bicarbonate may be useful in managing the cardiac toxicity associated with an ENKAID overdosage. Acute overdosages should be treated by gastric lavage followed by activated charcoal. Treatment of overdosage should be supportive.

DOSAGE AND ADMINISTRATION

As with other antiarrhythmic agents, ENKAID therapy in patients with sustained ventricular tachycardia should be initiated in a hospital setting with facilities for cardiac rhythm monitoring. Hospitalization is also recommended for patients with sinus node dysfunction or cardiomyopathy and/or congestive heart failure even if there is no history of sustained ventricular tachycardia, and at the time of a dose increase to 200 mg per day or above.

ENKAID should be administered only after appropriate clinical assessment and the dosage of ENKAID must be individualized for each patient on the basis of therapeutic response and tolerance.

The recommended initial dosing schedule for adults is one 25 mg ENKAID capsule t.i.d. at approximately 8-hour intervals. After a period of 3 to 5 days, the dosage may be increased to 35 mg t.i.d. if necessary. If the desired therapeutic response is not achieved after an additional 3 to 5 days, the dose may again be adjusted to 50 mg t.i.d. Rapid dose escalation should be avoided.

Patients with hepatic disease or severe renal impairment may require dose and/or dosing interval adjustment (See **PRECAUTIONS**).

Incidence (%) of the Most Common Adverse Events at Various Doses.
(Includes all adverse events regardless of relationship to drug therapy.)

Body Systems	0 mg (N=479)	75 mg (N=298)	150 mg (N=260)	>200 mg (N=208)
Body as a Whole				
abdominal pain	1	2	2	3
asthenia	4	4	5	9
chest pain	3	5	2	6
headache	6	3	5	12
lower extremity pain	3	<1	1	3
upper extremity pain	1	<1	<1	2
pain	<1	<1	<1	<1
paresthesia	<1	1	<1	2
Cardiovascular				
congestive heart failure	<1	<1	1	2
palpitations	5	4	3	8
premature ventricular contraction	<1	<1	<1	3
QRS interval prolonged ≥0.20	<1	<1	3	4
syncope	<1	<1	1	5
ventricular tachycardia	<1	3	3	8
Digestive				
constipation	1	<1	<1	2
diarrhea	2	<1	<1	2
dyspepsia	1	<1	<1	3
nausea	2	2	2	6
Nervous				
dizziness	7	6	10	18
tremor	<1	<1	<1	2
Respiratory				
dyspnea	2	2	5	4
increased cough	<1	<1	1	2
Skin and Appendages				
rash	2	<1	<1	4
Special Senses				
abnormal/blurred vision	5	4	8	26
taste perversion	<1	1	2	1

Dosages of ENKAID should be adjusted gradually allowing 3 to 5 days between dosing increments.

This will allow all patients, (even the minority that metabolize the drug very slowly) to achieve "steady state" blood levels of encainide and its active metabolites before increasing the dose. Gradual dose adjustments will help prevent the usage of doses which are higher than necessary to control the arrhythmia and which may increase the risk of proarrhythmic events.

In an occasional patient, the dosage may have to be increased to 50 mg q.i.d. to achieve the desired therapeutic response. Higher doses are not normally recommended. However, after the careful dose titration as described above has failed,

patients with documented life-threatening arrhythmias may be treated with up to 75 mg q.i.d. Patients should be hospitalized at the time of these dose increases to 200 mg per day or above. Once the desired therapeutic response is achieved, many patients can be adequately maintained on chronic therapy at doses lower than the maximum achieved during titration.

Patients with malignant arrhythmias who exhibit a beneficial response as judged by objective criteria (Holter monitoring, programmed electrical stimulation, exercise testing, etc.) can be maintained on chronic ENKAID therapy.

Some patients whose arrhythmias are well controlled by dosages of 50 mg t.i.d. or less may be transferred to a 12-hour dosage regimen if necessary to increase convenience and help assure compliance. Only those patients who have had an adequate response to 50 mg t.i.d. or less should be transferred to a 12-hour dosage regimen. The total daily dose may be given in two equally divided doses at approximately 12-hour intervals and the patient should be carefully monitored to ensure that an adequate suppression of ventricular ectopy is maintained. The maximum single dose that should be utilized is 75 mg.

Use of higher initial doses and more rapid dosage adjustments have resulted in an increased incidence of proarrhythmic events particularly during the first few days of dosing, therefore, a loading dose is not recommended.

Although limited experience with the concomitant use of ENKAID and intravenous lidocaine has revealed no adverse effects, there are no formal studies to demonstrate the utility of such combined therapy. Clinical experience on transferring patients to ENKAID from another antiarrhythmic drug is also limited. As a general principle, antiarrhythmic therapy should be withdrawn for two to four plasma half-lives before ENKAID is started. If withdrawing antiarrhythmic therapy is potentially life-threatening, consideration should be given to hospitalization.

Facilities for determining plasma levels of encainide and its metabolites are not readily available and the utility of such measurements in guiding the care of patients has not been demonstrated.

HOW SUPPLIED

Capsules, 25 mg, green and yellow hard gelatin capsule imprinted with ENKAID, 25 mg, Bristol and 732.
NDC 0087-0732-41 Bottles of 100.
NDC 0087-0732-42 Cartons of 100 Unit Dose.
NDC 0087-0732-43 Bottles of 500
Capsules, 35 mg, green and orange hard gelatin capsule imprinted with ENKAID, 35 mg, Bristol and 734.
NDC 0087-0734-41 Bottles of 100.
NDC 0087-0734-42 Cartons of 100 Unit Dose.
NDC 0087-0734-43 Bottles of 500
Capsules, 50 mg, green and brown hard gelatin capsule imprinted with ENKAID, 50 mg, Bristol and 735.

Incidence (%) of Adverse Events

	Encainide/Placebo Trial		Encainide/Quinidine Trial	
Body System	Encainide (N=88)	Placebo (N=37)	Encainide (N=153)	Quinidine (N=154)
Body as a whole				
abdominal pain	2.3	0	1.3	3.9
asthenia	14.8	16.2	6.5	13.6
chest pains	10.2	8.1	8.5	8.4
death	3.4	0	1.3	0
fever	—	—	0	7.8
headache	5.7	5.4	8.5	15.6
lower extremity pain	5.7	0	4.6	5.2
malaise	—	—	0	3.9
upper extremity pain	4.5	5.4	2.0	3.9
Cardiovascular				
palpitations	12.5	18.9	7.2	5.8
peripheral edema	2.3	0	1.3	3.2
proarrhythmia	3.4	0	0.7	0.6
Digestive				
constipation	2.2	0	4.6	2.6
diarrhea	0	8.1	9.2	39.0
dry mouth	—	—	3.9	2.6
dyspepsia	5.7	5.4	4.6	9.7
nausea	2.3	2.7	8.5	10.4
vomiting	2.3	0	0.7	3.2
Nervous				
anorexia	1.1	0	2.0	3.2
dizziness	15.9	10.8	15.7	14.9
insomnia	3.4	0	2.0	1.3
nervousness	1.1	0	2.0	3.2
somnolence	-	-	3.9	1.9
Respiratory				
dyspnea	8.0	10.8	3.9	8.4
Skin and Appendages				
rash	1.1	0	2.0	4.5
Special Senses				
abnormal/blurred vision	3.4	2.7	11.1	5.8
tinnitus	—	—	3.9	3.9

NDC 0087-0735-41 Bottles of 100.
NDC 0087-0735-42 Cartons of 100 Unit Dose.
Store at room temperature—Protect from temperatures
greater than 86°F (30°C).
U.S. Pat. No. 3,931,195
U.S. Patent No. Re. 30,811
Shown in Product Identification Section, page 406

K–LYTE®   ℞
[*k ' līt*]
Effervescent Tablets
Lime, box of 30 NSN 6505-00-934-3477 (M & VA)

Each tablet in solution provides 25 mEq (978 mg) potassium
as bicarbonate and citrate.

K–LYTE® DS   ℞
Effervescent Tablets
Each tablet in solution provides 50 mEq (1955 mg) potassium
as bicarbonate and citrate.

K–LYTE/CL®   ℞
Effervescent Tablets
Each tablet in solution provides the equivalent of 25 mEq
(1865 mg) potassium chloride.

K–LYTE/CL® 50   ℞
Effervescent Tablets
Each tablet in solution provides the equivalent of 50 mEq
(3730 mg) potassium chloride.

DESCRIPTION
[See table above right].
Inactive Ingredients: All of the K-LYTE line of effervescent
tablets contain docusate sodium, natural and/or artificial
flavors, light mineral oil, saccharin and talc.
K-LYTE® and K-LYTE® DS lime tablets, and
K-LYTE/Cl® and K-LYTE/Cl® 50 citrus tablets have D&C
Yellow No. 10. K-LYTE® and K-LYTE® DS orange tablets
and K-LYTE/Cl® and K-LYTE/Cl® 50 fruit punch tablets
have FD&C Yellow No. 6. K-LYTE orange and lime tablets
have dextrose, and K-LYTE DS orange and lime tablets have
lactose.
Note: This listing of inactive ingredients is a voluntary
action of Pharmaceutical Manufacturers Association members.

CLINICAL PHARMACOLOGY
Potassium ion is the principal intracellular cation of most
body tissues and participates in a number of essential physiological processes. These include numerous enzymatic reactions in intermediary metabolism, the maintenance of intracellular tonicity, the transmission of nerve impulses, and the
function of cardiac, skeletal, and smooth muscle. Disturbances in potassium metabolism may, therefore, elicit a broad
range of clinical disorders. The normal serum potassium
level is maintained principally by close renal regulation of
potassium balance.
Potassium depletion may occur whenever potassium loss
through renal excretion and/or loss from the gastrointestinal tract exceeds the potassium intake. Such depletion usually develops slowly as a consequence of prolonged therapy
with oral diuretics, primary or secondary hyperaldosteronism, diabetic ketoacidosis, severe vomiting and diarrhea, or
inadequate replacement of potassium in patients on prolonged parenteral nutrition. Potassium depletion may be
accompanied by hypokalemia as well as hypochloremia and
metabolic alkalosis.
Potassium deficiency may be manifested by generalized
weakness, drowsiness, anorexia, and nausea; oliguria,
edema, and chronic ileus with distention; shallow and infrequent respirations; low blood pressure, altered cardiac
rhythms, and systolic murmurs; hypokalemia and such ECG
changes as prominent U wave, lengthening of the Q-T interval, depression of the S-T segment, and depression or inversion of the T wave.

INDICATIONS AND USAGE
All K-LYTE® products are used for therapy or prophylaxis
of potassium deficiency. They are useful when thiazide diuretics, corticosteroids, or vomiting and diarrhea cause excessive potassium loss; and when dietary potassium is low.
These products may also be useful when potassium therapy
is indicated in digitalis intoxication. K-LYTE/Cl and
K-LYTE/Cl 50 are recommended in the management of hypokalemia accompanied by metabolic alkalosis and hypochloremia, eg, as induced by vomiting.

CONTRAINDICATIONS
Potassium supplements are contraindicated in patients with
hyperkalemia since a further increase in serum potassium
concentration in such patients can produce cardiac arrest.
Hyperkalemia may complicate any of the following conditions: chronic renal impairment, metabolic acidosis such as
diabetic acidosis, acute dehydration, extensive tissue breakdown as in severe burns or adrenal insufficiency. Hypokalemia should not be treated by the concomitant administration
of potassium salts and a potassium-sparing diuretic (eg,

	K-LYTE	K-LYTE DS	K-LYTE/CL	K-LYTE/CL 50
Potassium Chloride	—	—	1.5 g	2.24 g
Potassium Bicarbonate	2.5 g	2.5 g	0.5 g	2.0 g
Potassium Citrate	—	2.7 g	—	—
L-lysine Monohydro-chloride	—	—	0.91 g	3.65 g
Citric Acid	2.1 g	2.1 g	0.55 g	1.0 g

spironolactone or triamterene), since the simultaneous administration of these agents can produce severe hyperkalemia.

WARNINGS
In patients with impaired mechanisms for excreting potassium, the administration of potassium salts can produce hyperkalemia and cardiac arrest. This occurs most commonly
in patients given potassium by the intravenous route but
may also occur in patients given potassium orally. Potentially fatal hyperkalemia can develop rapidly and may be
asymptomatic. The use of potassium salts in patients with
chronic renal disease, or any other condition which impairs
potassium excretion, requires particularly careful monitoring of the serum potassium concentration and appropriate
dosage adjustment.

PRECAUTIONS
General precautions—The diagnosis of potassium depletion
is ordinarily made by demonstrating hypokalemia in a patient with a clinical history suggesting some cause for potassium depletion. When interpreting the serum potassium
level, the physician should bear in mind that acute alkalosis
per se can produce hypokalemia in the absence of a deficit in
total body potassium, while acute acidosis *per se* can increase
the serum potassium concentration into the normal range
even in the presence of a reduced total body potassium.
Therefore, the treatment of potassium depletion requires
careful attention to acid-base balance and appropriate monitoring of serum electrolytes, the ECG, and the clinical status
of the patient.
Information for patients—To minimize the possibility of
gastrointestinal irritation associated with the oral ingestion
of concentrated potassium salt preparations, patients should
be carefully directed to dissolve each dose completely in the
stated amount of water.
Laboratory tests—Frequent clinical evaluation of the patient should include ECG and serum potassium determinations.
Drug interactions—The simultaneous administration of
potassium supplements and a potassium-sparing diuretic
can produce severe hyperkalemia (see Contraindications).
Potassium supplements should be used cautiously in patients who are using salt substitutes because most of the latter contain substantial amounts of potassium. Such concomitant use could result in hyperkalemia.
Usage in Pregnancy—Pregnancy Category C —Animal reproduction studies have not been conducted with any of the
K-LYTE products. It is also not known whether these products can cause fetal harm when administered to a pregnant
woman or can affect reproduction capacity. They should be
given to a pregnant woman only if clearly needed.
Nursing Mothers—Many drugs are excreted in human milk
and because of the potential for serious adverse reactions in
nursing infants from oral potassium supplements, a decision
should be made whether to discontinue nursing or discontinue the drug, taking into account the importance of the
drug to the mother.
Usage in Children—Safety and effectiveness in children have
not been established.

ADVERSE REACTIONS
The most common adverse reactions to oral potassium supplements are nausea, vomiting, diarrhea and abdominal
discomfort. These side effects occur more frequently when
the medication is not taken with food or is not diluted properly or dissolved completely.
Hyperkalemia occurs only rarely in patients with normal
renal function receiving potassium supplements orally.
Signs and symptoms of hyperkalemia are cardiac arrhythmias, mental confusion, unexplained anxiety, numbness or tingling in hands, feet or lips, shortness of breath or
difficult breathing, unusual tiredness or weakness and weakness or heaviness of legs (see Contraindications, Warnings
and Overdosage).

OVERDOSAGE
The administration of oral potassium salts to persons with
normal renal function rarely causes serious hyperkalemia.
However, in patients with chronic renal disease, or any other
condition which impairs potassium excretion or if potassium
is administered too rapidly intravenously, potentially fatal
hyperkalemia can result (see Contraindications and Warnings). The earliest clinical manifestations of this condition
may be only increased serum potassium levels and characteristic ECG changes such as peaking of T-waves, loss of P-
wave, depression of S-T segment and prolongation of the QT
interval. These changes in the ECG usually appear when
serum potassium concentration reaches 7 to 8 mEq per liter.
Other clinical manifestations occurring at a concentration of
9 to 10 mEq per liter may include muscle paralysis and death
from cardiac arrest.
The treatment of severe hyperkalemia should focus on reducing the serum potassium concentration by promoting the
transfer of potassium from the extracellular to the intracellular space. The measures taken may include the following:
a) intravenous administration of 1 liter of a 10 percent glucose solution containing 30-40 units of insulin; b) in the acidotic patient, intravenous administration of 150 mEq to 300
mEq of sodium bicarbonate. Other measures should include
the elimination of potassium-containing medications and
potassium-sparing diuretics and frequently the oral administration of a cation exchange resin (such as sodium polystyrene sulfonate) to remove gastrointestinal potassium. To
assure rapid movement of the resin through the gastrointestinal tract, a nonabsorbable polyhydric alcohol (eg, sorbitol)
should be given in quantities sufficient to induce a soft to
semiliquid bowel movement every few hours.
Hemodialysis is an effective alternative means of removing
excess potassium.

DOSAGE AND ADMINISTRATION
Adults—One (1) K-LYTE/Cl 50 tablet (50 mEq potassium
and chloride) or one (1) K-LYTE DS tablet (50 mEq potassium) completely dissolved in 6 to 8 ounces of cold or ice water, 1 to 2 times daily, depending on the requirements of the
patient. One (1) K-LYTE/Cl tablet (25 mEq potassium and
chloride) or one (1) K-LYTE tablet (25 mEq potassium) completely dissolved in 3 to 4 ounces of cold or ice water, 2 to 4
times daily, depending on the requirements of the patient.
Note: It is suggested that all K-LYTE products be taken with
meals and sipped slowly over a 5 to 10 minute period.

HOW SUPPLIED
K-LYTE® Effervescent Tablets. Each tablet in solution pro-
vides 25 mEq (978 mg) potassium.
  NDC 0087-0760-01 Lime flavor, Boxes of 30
  NDC 0087-0760-43 Lime flavor, Boxes of 100
  NDC 0087-0760-02 Lime flavor, Boxes of 250
  NDC 0087-0761-01 Orange flavor, Boxes of 30
  NDC 0087-0761-43 Orange flavor, Boxes of 100
  NDC 0087-0761-02 Orange flavor, Boxes of 250
K-LYTE® DS Effervescent Tablets. Each tablet provides 50
mEq (1955 mg) potassium.
  NDC 0087-0772-41 Lime flavor, Boxes of 30
  NDC 0087-0772-42 Lime flavor, Boxes of 100
  NDC 0087-0771-41 Orange flavor, Boxes of 30
  NDC 0087-0771-42 Orange flavor, Boxes of 100
K-LYTE/CL® Effervescent Tablets. Each tablet in solution
provides the equivalent of 25 mEq (1865 mg) potassium chlo-
ride.
  NDC 0087-0766-41 Citrus flavor, Boxes of 30
  NDC 0087-0766-43 Citrus flavor, Boxes of 100
  NDC 0087-0766-42 Citrus flavor, Boxes of 250
  NDC 0087-0767-41 Fruit Punch flavor, Boxes of 30
  NDC 0087-0767-43 Fruit Punch flavor, Boxes of 100
  NDC 0087-0767-42 Fruit Punch flavor, Boxes of 250

Continued on next page

Bristol Labs.—Cont.

K-LYTE/CL® 50 mEq Effervescent Tablets. Each tablet in solution provides the equivalent of 50 mEq (3730 mg) potassium chloride.

NDC 0087-0757-41 Fruit Punch flavor, Boxes of 30
NDC 0087-0757-42 Fruit Punch flavor, Boxes of 100
NDC 0087-0758-41 Citrus flavor, Boxes of 30
NDC 0087-0758-42 Citrus flavor, Boxes of 100
Store Below 86°F (30°C).
U.S. Patent No. 3,970,750
Shown in Product Identification Section, page 406

NALDECON®

[nal'dĕ-côn]
**Tablets, Syrup, Pediatric Drops
and Pediatric Syrup
For Oral Use Only**
Pediatric Syrup, 16 oz bottle NSN 6505-01-094-1974 (M)

DESCRIPTION
NALDECON is a preparation containing:
(1) phenylpropanolamine hydrochloride

Benzenemethanol, α-(1-aminoethyl)- hydrochloride
(2) phenylephrine hydrochloride

1-m-hydroxy-α-[(methylamino)methyl]benzyl alcohol hydrochloride
(3) phenyltoloxamine citrate

N, N-dimethyl-2(alpha phenyl-ortho-toloxy)-ethylamine citrate
(4) chlorpheniramine maleate

2-[p-chloro-α-[2-(dimethylamino)ethyl]benzyl]pyridine maleate
Inactive ingredients in NALDECON tablets are: acacia, FD&C Red No. 3, gelatin, lactose, magnesium stearate, polyethylene glycol 8000, starch, sucrose, carnauba wax, and white wax.

Inactive ingredients in NALDECON syrup, pediatric syrup, and pediatric drops are D&C Red No. 33, D&C Yellow No. 10, natural and artificial flavorings, glycerin, povidone, purified water, sodium benzoate and sorbitol.
[See table below].

CLINICAL PHARMACOLOGY
Phenylpropanolamine Hydrochloride
The drug may directly stimulate adrenergic receptors but probably indirectly stimulates both alpha (α) and beta (β) adrenergic receptors by releasing norepinephrine from its storage sites. Phenylpropanolamine increases heart rate, force of contraction and cardiac output, and excitability. It acts on α receptors in the mucosa of the respiratory tract, producing vasoconstriction which results in shrinkage of swollen mucous membranes, reduction of tissue, hyperemia, edema and nasal congestion, and an increase in nasal airway patency. Phenylpropanolamine causes CNS stimulation and reportedly has an anorexigenic effect.
Phenylephrine Hydrochloride
Phenylephrine acts predominantly by a direct action on alpha (α) adrenergic receptors. In therapeutic doses, the drug has no significant stimulant effect on the beta (β) adrenergic receptors of the heart. Following oral administration, constriction of blood vessels in the nasal mucosa may relieve nasal congestion. In therapeutic doses the drug causes little, if any, central nervous system stimulation.
Phenyltoloxamine Citrate
Phenyltoloxamine is an H_1 blocking agent which interferes with the action of histamine primarily in capillaries surrounding mucous tissues and sensory nerves of nasal and adjacent areas. It has the ability to interfere with certain actions of acetylcholine-inhibiting secretions in the nose, mouth and pharynx. It commonly causes CNS depression.
Chlorpheniramine Maleate
Chlorpheniramine competitively antagonizes most of the smooth muscle stimulating actions of histamine on the H_1 receptors of the GI tract, uterus, large blood vessels and bronchial muscle. It also antagonizes the action of histamine that results in increased capillary permeability and the formation of edema.

INDICATIONS AND USAGE
For the relief of nasal congestion and eustachian tube congestion associated with the common cold, sinusitis and acute upper respiratory infections. Also indicated for symptomatic relief of perennial and seasonal allergic rhinitis, vasomotor rhinitis.

Decongestants in combination with antihistamines have been used to relieve eustachian tube congestion associated with acute eustachian salpingitis, aerotitis and serous otitis media.

CONTRAINDICATIONS
Patients with severe hypertension, severe coronary artery disease, patients on MAO inhibitor therapy; patients with narrow angle glaucoma, urinary retention, peptic ulcer and during an asthmatic attack. Also contraindicated in patients with hypersensitivity or idiosyncrasy to sympathomimetic amines or antihistamines.

WARNINGS
Sympathomimetic amines should be used judiciously and sparingly in patients with hypertension, diabetes mellitus, ischemic heart disease, increased intraocular pressure, hyperthyroidism or prostatic hypertrophy. See, however, CONTRAINDICATIONS. Sympathomimetics may produce central nervous system stimulation with convulsions or cardiovascular collapse with accompanying hypotension.
Antihistamines may impair mental and physical abilities required for the performance of potentially hazardous tasks, such as driving a vehicle or operating machinery, and may impair mental alertness in children. Chlorpheniramine

and phenyltoloxamine have an atropine-like action and should be used with caution in patients with increased intraocular pressure, cardiovascular disease, hypertension or in patients with a history of bronchial asthma. See, however, CONTRAINDICATIONS.
Do not exceed recommended dosage.

PRECAUTIONS
Patients with diabetes, hypertension, cardiovascular disease and hyperreactivity to ephedrine. The antihistaminics may cause drowsiness and ambulatory patients who operate machinery or motor vehicles should be cautioned accordingly.

DRUG INTERACTIONS
MAO inhibitors and beta adrenergic blockers increase the effect of sympathomimetics. Sympathomimetics may reduce the antihypertensive effects of methyldopa, mecamylamine, reserpine and veratrum alkaloids. Concomitant use of antihistamines with alcohol, tricyclic antidepressants, barbiturates and other CNS depressants may have an additive effect.

PREGNANCY CATEGORY C
Animal reproduction studies have not been conducted with NALDECON. It is also not known whether NALDECON can cause fetal harm when administered to a pregnant woman or can affect reproductive capacity. NALDECON should be given to a pregnant woman only if clearly needed.

NURSING MOTHERS
Caution should be exercised when this drug is given to nursing mothers due to the higher than usual risk of the sympathomimetic amines in infants.

ADVERSE REACTIONS
Hyperreactive individuals may display ephedrine-like reactions such as tachycardia, palpitations, headache, dizziness or nausea. Patients sensitive to antihistamines may experience mild sedation. Sympathomimetics have been associated with certain untoward reactions including restlessness, tremor, weakness, pallor, respiratory difficulty, dysuria, insomnia, hallucinations, convulsions, CNS depression, arrhythmias and cardiovascular collapse with hypotension. Possible side effects of antihistamines are drowsiness, restlessness, dizziness, weakness, dry mouth, anorexia, nausea, vomiting, headache, nervousness, blurring of vision, polyuria, heartburn, dysuria and, very rarely, dermatitis.

OVERDOSAGE
In the event of overdosage, emergency treatment should be started immediately.
Symptoms: Overdosage symptoms may vary from central nervous system depression to stimulation. Symptoms may include: nervousness, dry mouth, possible convulsions, respiratory failure, acute hypertension. In both children and adults, coma and cardiovascular collapse may occur.
Management: It is suggested that the management principles (consistent with the clinical status of the patient when first seen) outlined below be instituted and that simultaneous contact with a Regional Poison Control Center be established. In this way both updated information and individualization regarding required therapy may be provided.
Induction of emesis and gastric lavage may be performed if the patient is alert and seen within early hours after ingestion. Drug remaining in the stomach may be adsorbed by the administration of activated charcoal.
Respiratory distress should be treated promptly. *Stimulants* (analeptic agents) should *not* be used because they may precipitate convulsions. Use of a short-acting barbiturate is recommended if convulsions or marked CNS excitement occur.

DOSAGE AND ADMINISTRATION
This chart represents single dosages for the products listed below. Usual dosage schedule for NALDECON Pediatric Drops, NALDECON Pediatric Syrup and NALDECON Syrup is every 3 to 4 hours, not to exceed four doses in a 24-hour period. For sustained-action NALDECON Tablets, doses should be administered on arising, in midafternoon, and at bedtime.
[See table on next page].

HOW SUPPLIED
NDC 0015-5600—NALDECON Tablets
NDC 0015-5601—NALDECON Syrup
NDC 0015-5615—NALDECON Pediatric Drops
NDC 0015-5616—NALDECON Pediatric Syrup
For information on package sizes available, refer to the current price schedule.
BRISTOL, NALDECON and the distinctive speckled tablets are trademarks.
Shown in Product Identification Section, page 406

	For immediate action	For delayed action	Total contents
Each sustained-action tablet contains:			
Phenylpropanolamine hydrochloride	20.0 mg	20.0 mg	40.0 mg
Phenylephrine hydrochloride	5.0 mg	5.0 mg	10.0 mg
Phenyltoloxamine citrate	7.5 mg	7.5 mg	15.0 mg
Chlorpheniramine maleate	2.5 mg	2.5 mg	5.0 mg
Each teaspoonful (5 mL) of syrup contains:			
Phenylpropanolamine hydrochloride			20.0 mg
Phenylephrine hydrochloride			5.0 mg
Phenyltoloxamine citrate			7.5 mg
Chlorpheniramine maleate			2.5 mg

	Pediatric Syrup each 5 mL contains:	Pediatric Drops each 1 mL contains:
Each pediatric formulation contains the following ingredients:		
Phenylpropanolamine hydrochloride	5.0 mg	5.0 mg
Phenylephrine hydrochloride	1.25 mg	1.25 mg
Phenyltoloxamine citrate	2.0 mg	2.0 mg
Chlorpheniramine maleate	0.5 mg	0.5 mg

Single Dosage for ...	NALDECON Pediatric Drops	NALDECON Pediatric Syrup	NALDECON Syrup	NALDECON Tablets
3 to 6 months (12–17 lbs)	¼ mL			
6 to 12 months (17–24 lbs)	½ mL	½ teaspoonful		
1 to 6 years (24–50 lbs)	1 mL	1 teaspoonful		
6 to 12 years (over 50 lbs)		2 teaspoonfuls	½ teaspoonful	½ tablet
over 12 years			1 teaspoonful	1 tablet

NALDECON CX® ADULT LIQUID   Ⓒ

[nal 'dĕ-côn]

Nasal Decongestant/Expectorant/Cough Suppressant

DESCRIPTION

Each teaspoonful (5 mL) of NALDECON CX Adult Liquid contains:

Phenylpropanolamine hydrochloride .... 12.5 mg
Guaifenesin (glyceryl guaiacolate) .... 200 mg
Codeine Phosphate .... 10 mg
   (Warning: May be Habit Forming)

This combination product is antihistamine-free, alcohol-free and sugar-free.

INACTIVE INGREDIENTS

Citric Acid, FD&C Blue No. 1, FD&C Red No. 40, Hydrogenated Glucose Syrup, Natural & Artificial Flavor, Polyethylene Glycol, Purified Water, Sodium Benzoate, Sodium Citrate, Sodium Saccharin.

INDICATIONS

For the temporary relief of nasal congestion due to the common cold (cold), hay fever or other respiratory allergies (allergic rhinitis), or associated with sinusitis. Helps loosen phlegm (sputum) and thin bronchial secretions to rid the bronchial passageways of bothersome mucus. Temporarily quiets cough due to minor throat and bronchial irritation as may occur with a cold or inhaled irritants.

CONTRAINDICATIONS

Do not take if hypersensitive to guaifenesin, codeine or sympathomimetic amines.

WARNINGS

As with any drug, if you are pregnant or nursing a baby, seek the advice of a health professional before using this product. Do not give this product to children under 12 years of age unless directed by a physician. Do not exceed recommended dosage because at higher doses nervousness, dizziness, or sleeplessness may occur. Do not take this product for more than 7 days. If symptoms do not improve or are accompanied by fever, consult a physician. Do not take this product if you have heart disease, high blood pressure, thyroid disease, diabetes, or difficulty in urination due to enlargement of the prostate gland unless directed by a physician. *Drug Interaction Precaution:* Do not take this product if you are presently taking a prescription drug for high blood pressure or depression, without first consulting your physician. A persistent cough may be a sign of a serious condition. If cough persists for more than 1 week, tends to recur, or is accompanied by fever, rash, or persistent headache, consult a physician. Do not take this product for persistent or chronic cough such as occurs with smoking, asthma, chronic bronchitis, or emphysema, or if cough is accompanied by excessive phlegm (sputum) unless directed by a physician. Do not take this product if you have a chronic pulmonary disease or shortness of breath unless directed by a physician. May cause or aggravate constipation. Keep this and all drugs out of the reach of children. In case of accidental overdose, seek professional assistance or contact a Poison Control Center immediately.

DOSAGE AND ADMINISTRATION

Adults and children 12 years of age and over: Oral dosage is 2 teaspoonsful every 4 hours, not to exceed 6 doses in 24 hours, or as directed by a physician.

HOW SUPPLIED

NALDECON CX Adult Liquid—4oz. and pint bottles.
Store at room temperature. Avoid excessive heat.
Also Described in PDR For Nonprescription Drugs

NALDECON DX® ADULT LIQUID   OTC

[nal 'dĕ-côn Dx]

Nasal Decongestant/Expectorant/Cough Suppressant

DESCRIPTION

Each teaspoonful (5 mL) of NALDECON DX Adult Liquid contains:

Phenylpropanolamine hydrochloride .... 12.5 mg
Guaifenesin (glyceryl guaiacolate) .... 200 mg
Dextromethorphan hydrobromide .... 10 mg

This combination product is antihistamine-free, sugar-free and alcohol-free.

INACTIVE INGREDIENTS

Citric Acid, FD&C Yellow No. 6, Nat. & Art. Flavor, Polyethylene Glycol, Purified Water, Sodium Benzoate, Sodium Citrate, Sodium Saccharin and Sorbitol.

INDICATIONS

For the temporary relief of nasal congestion due to the common cold (cold), hay fever or other respiratory allergies (allergic rhinitis), or associated with sinusitis. Helps loosen phlegm (sputum) and thin bronchial secretions to rid the bronchial passageways of bothersome mucus. Temporarily quiets cough due to minor throat and bronchial irritation as may occur with a cold or inhaled irritants.

CONTRAINDICATIONS

Do not take if hypersensitive to guaifenesin, dextromethorphan or sympathomimetic amines.

WARNINGS

As with any drug, if you are pregnant or nursing a baby, seek the advice of a health professional before using this product. Do not give this product to children under 12 years of age unless directed by a physician. Do not exceed recommended dosage because at higher doses nervousness, dizziness or sleeplessness may occur. Do not take this product for more than 7 days. If symptoms do not improve or are accompanied by fever, consult a physician. Do not take this product if you have heart disease, high blood pressure, thyroid disease, diabetes, or difficulty in urination due to enlargement of the prostate gland unless directed by a physician. *Drug Interaction Precaution:* Do not take this product if you are presently taking a prescription drug for high blood pressure or depression, without first consulting your physician. A persistent cough may be a sign of a serious condition. If cough persists for more than one week, tends to recur, or is accompanied by fever, rash, or persistent headache, consult a physician. Do not take this product for persistent or chronic cough such as occurs with smoking, asthma, chronic bronchitis, or emphysema, or if cough is accompanied by excessive phlegm (sputum) unless directed by a physician. Keep this and all drugs out of the reach of children. In case of accidental overdose, seek professional assistance or contact a poison control center immediately.

DOSAGE AND ADMINISTRATION

Adults and children 12 years of age and over: Oral dosage is 2 teaspoonsful every 4 hours, not to exceed 6 doses in 24 hours, or as directed by a physician.

HOW SUPPLIED

NALDECON DX Adult Liquid—4 oz. and pint bottles.
Store at room temperature. Avoid excessive heat.
Also Described in PDR For Nonprescription Drugs

NALDECON DX® PEDIATRIC DROPS   OTC

[nal 'dĕ-côn Dx]

Nasal Decongestant/Expectorant/Cough Suppressant

DESCRIPTION

Each 1 mL of NALDECON DX Pediatric Drops contains:

Phenylpropanolamine hydrochloride .... 6.25 mg
Guaifenesin (glyceryl guaiacolate) .... 30 mg
Dextromethorphan hydrobromide .... 5 mg
Alcohol .... 0.6% V/V

This combination product is antihistamine-free and sugar-free.

INACTIVE INGREDIENTS

Alcohol (0.6% V/V), Citric Acid, FD&C Yellow No. 6, Nat. & Art. Flavors, Propylene Glycol, Purified Water, Sodium Benzoate, Sodium Saccharin and Sorbitol

INDICATIONS

For the temporary relief of nasal congestion due to the common cold (cold), hay fever or other respiratory allergies (allergic rhinitis), or associated with sinusitis. Helps loosen phlegm (sputum) and thin bronchial secretions to rid the bronchial passageways of bothersome mucus. Temporarily quiets cough due to minor throat and bronchial irritation as may occur with a cold or inhaled irritants.

CONTRAINDICATIONS

Do not take if hypersensitive to guaifenesin, dextromethorphan, or sympathomimetic amines.

WARNINGS

Take by mouth only. Do not exceed recommended dosage because at higher doses nervousness, dizziness or sleeplessness may occur. Do not give this product to children for more than 7 days. If symptoms do not improve or are accompanied by fever, consult a physician. Do not give this product to children who have heart disease, high blood pressure, thyroid disease, or diabetes, unless directed by a physician. *Drug Interaction Precaution:* Do not give this product to a child who is taking a prescription drug for high blood pressure or depression, without first consulting the child's physician. A persistent cough may be a sign of a serious condition. If cough persists for more than 1 week, tends to recur, or is accompanied by fever, rash, or persistent headache, consult a physician. Do not give this product for persistent or chronic cough such as occurs with smoking, asthma, chronic bronchitis, or emphysema, or if cough is accompanied by excessive phlegm (sputum) unless directed by a physician. Keep this and all drugs out of the reach of children. In case of accidental overdose, seek professional assistance or contact a poison control center immediately.

DOSAGE AND ADMINISTRATION

Children 2 to under 6 years of age: Oral dosage is 1 mL every 4 hours, not to exceed 6 doses in 24 hours, or as directed by a physician. Children under 2 years of age: Consult a physician.

HOW SUPPLIED

NALDECON DX Pediatric Drops—30mL bottle with calibrated dropper.
Store at room temperature. Protect from freezing.
Also Described in PDR For Nonprescription Drugs

NALDECON DX®   OTC

[nal 'dĕ-côn Dx]

CHILDREN'S SYRUP

Nasal Decongestant/Expectorant/Cough Suppressant

DESCRIPTION

Each teaspoonful (5 mL) of NALDECON DX Children's Syrup contains:

Phenylpropanolamine hydrochloride .... 6.25 mg
Guaifenesin (glyceryl guaiacolate) .... 100 mg
Dextromethorphan hydrobromide .... 5 mg

This combination product is antihistamine-free.

INACTIVE INGREDIENTS

Alcohol (5% V/V), FD&C Yellow No. 6, Fructose, Glycerin, Nat. & Art. Flavors, Purified Water, Sodium Benzoate, Sucrose and Tartaric Acid.

INDICATIONS

For the temporary relief of nasal congestion due to the common cold (cold), hay fever or other respiratory allergies (allergic rhinitis), or associated with sinusitis. Helps loosen phlegm (sputum) and thin bronchial secretions to rid the bronchial passageways of bothersome mucus. Temporarily quiets cough due to minor throat and bronchial irritation as may occur with a cold or inhaled irritants.

CONTRAINDICATIONS

Do not take if hypersensitive to guaifenesin, dextromethorphan, or sympathomimetic amines.

WARNINGS

Do not exceed recommended dosage because at higher doses nervousness, dizziness, or sleeplessness may occur. Do not give this product to children for more than 7 days. If symptoms do not improve or are accompanied by fever, consult a physician. Do not give this product to children who have heart disease, high blood pressure, thyroid disease, or diabetes, unless directed by a physician. *Drug Interaction Precaution:* Do not give this product to a child who is taking a prescription drug for high blood pressure or depression, without first consulting the child's physician. A persistent cough may be a sign of a serious condition. If cough persists for more than 1 week, tends to recur, or is accompanied by fever, rash, or persistent headache, consult a physician. Do not give this product for persistent or chronic cough such as occurs with smoking, asthma, chronic bronchitis, or emphysema, or if cough is accompanied by excessive phlegm (sputum) unless directed by a physician. Keep this and all drugs out of the

Continued on next page

Bristol Labs.—Cont.

reach of children. In case of accidental overdose, seek professional assistance or contact a poison control center immediately.

DOSAGE AND ADMINISTRATION

Children 6 to under 12 years of age: Oral dosage is 2 teaspoonsful every 4 hours, not to exceed 6 doses in 24 hours, or as directed by a physician. Children 2 to under 6 years of age: Oral dosage is 1 teaspoonful every 4 hours, not to exceed 6 doses in 24 hours, or as directed by a physician. Children under 2 years of age: Consult a physician.

HOW SUPPLIED

NALDECON DX Children's Syrup—4 oz. and pint bottles. Store at room temprature. Protect from excessive heat and freezing.

Also Described in PDR For Nonprescription Drugs

NALDECON EX® PEDIATRIC DROPS　　　　OTC
[nal'dĕ-côn Ex]
Nasal Decongestant/Expectorant

DESCRIPTION

Each 1 mL of NALDECON EX Pediatric Drops contains:
Phenylpropanolamine hydrochloride .... 6.25 mg
Guaifenesin (glyceryl guaiacolate) .... 30 mg
This combination product is antihistamine-free.

INACTIVE INGREDIENTS

Alcohol (0.6% V/V), Citric Acid, D&C Yellow No. 10, Nat. & Art. Flavors, Propylene Glycol, Purified Water, Sodium Benzoate, and Sucrose
Store at room temperature. Protect from excessive heat and freezing.

INDICATIONS

For the temporary relief of nasal congestion due to the common cold (cold), hay fever or other respiratory allergies (allergic rhinitis), or associated with sinusitis. Helps loosen phlegm (sputum) and thin bronchial secretions to rid the bronchial passageways of bothersome mucus.

CONTRAINDICATIONS

Do not take if hypersensitive to guaifenesin or sympathomimetic amines.

WARNINGS

Take by mouth only. Do not exceed recommended dosage because at higher doses nervousness, dizziness or sleeplessness may occur. Do not give this product to children for more than 7 days. If symptoms do not improve or are accompanied by fever, consult a physician. Do not give this product to children who have heart disease, high blood pressure, thyroid disease, or diabetes, unless directed by a physician. *Drug Interaction Precaution:* Do not give this product to a child who is taking a prescription drug for high blood pressure or depression, without first consulting the child's physician. A persistent cough may be a sign of a serious condition. If cough persists for more than 1 week, tends to recur, or is accompanied by fever, rash, or persistent headache, consult a physician. Do not give this product for persistent or chronic cough such as occurs with smoking, asthma, chronic bronchitis, or emphysema, or if cough is accompanied by excessive phlegm (sputum) unless directed by a physician. Keep this and all drugs out of the reach of children. In case of accidental overdose, seek professional assistance or contact a poison control center immediately. Your physician or pharmacist is the best source of information on this medication.

DOSAGE AND ADMINISTRATION

Children 2 to under 6 years of age: Oral dosage is 1 mL every 4 hours, not to exceed 6 doses in 24 hours, or as directed by a physician. Children under 2 years of age: Consult a physician.

HOW SUPPLIED

NALDECON EX Pediatric Drops—30 mL bottle with calibrated dropper.
Store at room temperature. Protect from excessive heat and freezing.

Also Described in PDR For Nonprescription Drugs

NALDECON EX® CHILDREN'S SYRUP　　　　OTC
[nal'dĕ-côn Ex]
Nasal Decongestant/Expectorant

DESCRIPTION

Each teaspoonful (5 mL) of NALDECON EX Children's Syrup contains:
Phenylpropanolamine hydrochloride .... 6.25 mg
Guaifenesin (glyceryl guaiacolate) .... 100 mg
Alcohol .... 5% V/V
This combination product is antihistamine-free and sugar-free.

INACTIVE INGREDIENTS

Alcohol (5% V/V), D&C Yellow No. 10, Glycerin, Nat. & Art. Flavor, Propylene Glycol, Purified Water, Sodium Benzoate, Sodium Saccharin, Sorbitol and Tartaric Acid.

INDICATIONS

For the temporary relief of nasal congestion due to the common cold (cold), hay fever or other respiratory allergies (allergic rhinitis), or associated with sinusitis. Helps loosen phlegm (sputum) and thin bronchial secretions to rid the bronchial passageways of bothersome mucus.

CONTRAINDICATIONS

Do not take if hypersensitive to guaifenesin or sympathomimetic amines.

WARNINGS

Do not exceed recommended dosage because at higher doses nervousness, dizziness or sleeplessness may occur. Do not give this product to children for more than 7 days. If symptoms do not improve or are accompanied by fever, consult a physician. Do not give this product to children who have heart disease, high blood pressure, thyroid disease, or diabetes, unless directed by a physician. *Drug Interaction Precaution:* Do not give this product to a child who is taking a prescription drug for high blood pressure or depression, without first consulting the child's physician. A persistent cough may be a sign of a serious condition. If cough persists for more than 1 week, tends to recur, or is accompanied by fever, rash, or persistent headache, consult a physician. Do not give this product for persistent or chronic cough such as occurs with smoking, asthma, chronic bronchitis, or emphysema, or if cough is accompanied by excessive phlegm (sputum) unless directed by a physician. Keep this and all drugs out of the reach of children. In case of accidental overdose, seek professional assistance or contact a poison control center immediately. Your physician or pharmacist is the best source of information on this medication.

DOSAGE AND ADMINISTRATION

Children 6 to under 12 years of age: Oral dosage is 2 teaspoonsful every 4 hours not to exceed 6 doses in 24 hours, or as directed by a physician. Children 2 to under 6 years of age: Oral dosage is 1 teaspoonful every 4 hours, not to exceed 6 doses in 24 hours, or as directed by a physician. Children under 2 years of age: consult a physician.

HOW SUPPLIED

NALDECON EX Children's Syrup—4 oz. and pint bottles. Store at room temperature. Protect from excessive heat and freezing.

Also Described in PDR For Nonprescription Drugs

NALDECON SENIOR DX®　　　　OTC
[nal'dĕ-côn]
Expectorant/Cough Suppressant
Cough/Cold Liquid
for Adults 50 and Over

DESCRIPTION

Each teaspoonful (5 mL) of Naldecon Senior DX Cough/Cold Liquid contains:
Guaifenesin ....200 mg
Dextromethorphan hydrobromide ....15 mg

INACTIVE INGREDIENTS

Citric acid, FD&C Blue No. 1, FD&C Red No. 40, natural & artificial flavorings, polyethylene glycol, purified water, sodium benzoate, sodium citrate, sodium saccharin, sorbitol.

INDICATIONS

Non-narcotic cough suppressant for the temporary relief of coughing. Helps loosen phlegm (sputum) and bronchial secretions and rid the bronchial passageways of bothersome mucus.

CONTRAINDICATIONS

Do not take if hypersensitive to guaifenesin or dextromethorphan.

WARNINGS

A persistent cough may be a sign of a serious condition. If cough persists for more than 1 week, tends to recur, or is accompanied by fever, rash, or persistent headache, consult a physician. Do not take this product for persistent or chronic cough such as occurs with smoking, asthma, emphysema, or if cough is accompanied by excessive phlegm (mucus) unless directed by a physician. Do not exceed recommended dose or give this product to children under 12 years of age unless directed by a physician. As with any drug, if you are pregnant or nursing a baby, seek the advice of a health professional before using this product. Keep this and all drugs out of the reach of children. In case of accidental overdose, seek professional assistance or contact a Poison Control Center immediately.

DOSAGE AND ADMINISTRATION

Adults: Oral dosage is 2 teaspoonsful every 6 to 8 hours, not to exceed 4 doses in 24 hours, or as directed by a physician. Children under 12 years of age: consult a physician.

HOW SUPPLIED

Naldecon Senior DX Cough/Cold Liquid—4 oz and pint bottles.
Store at room temperature.
Also described in PDR for Nonprescription Drugs.

NALDECON SENIOR EX®　　　　OTC
[nal'dĕ-côn]
(guaifenesin)
Expectorant
Cough/Cold Liquid
for Adults 50 and Over

DESCRIPTION

Each teaspoonful (5 mL) of Naldecon Senior EX Cough/Cold Liquid contains:
Guaifenesin ....200 mg

INACTIVE INGREDIENTS

Citric acid, FD&C Blue No. 1, FD&C Red No. 40, natural & artificial flavorings, polyethylene glycol, purified water, sodium benzoate, sodium citrate, sodium saccharin, sorbitol.

INDICATIONS

Helps loosen phlegm (sputum) and bronchial secretions and rid the bronchial passageways of bothersome mucus.

CONTRAINDICATIONS

Do not take if hypersensitive to guaifenesin.

WARNINGS

A persistent cough may be a sign of a serious condition. If cough persists for more than 1 week, tends to recur, or is accompanied by fever, rash, or persistent headache, consult a physician. Do not take this product for persistent or chronic cough such as occurs with smoking, asthma, emphysema, or if cough is accompanied by excessive phlegm (mucus) unless directed by a physician. Do not exceed recommended dose or give this product to children under 12 years of age unless directed by a physician. As with any drug, if you are pregnant or nursing a baby, seek the advice of a health professional before using this product. Keep this and all drugs out of the reach of children. In case of accidental overdose, seek professional assistance or contact a Poison Control Center immediately.

DOSAGE AND ADMINISTRATION

Adults: Oral dosage is 2 teaspoonful every 4 hours, not to exceed 6 doses in 24 hours, or as directed by a physician. Children under 12 years of age: consult a physician.

HOW SUPPLIED

Naldecon Senior EX Cough/Cold Liquid—4 oz and pint bottles.
Store at room temperature.
Also described in PDR for Nonprescription Drugs.

QUESTRAN® POWDER　　　　℞
[kwest'răn]
(Cholestyramine for Oral Suspension)
Box of 60, 4 g packets NSN 6505-00-105-0372 (M&VA)
Can, 378 g NSN 6505-01-274-2720 (M)

DESCRIPTION

QUESTRAN Powder, the chloride salt of a basic anion exchange resin, a cholesterol lowering agent, is intended for oral administration. Cholestyramine resin is quite hydrophilic, but insoluble in water. The cholestyramine resin in QUESTRAN is not absorbed from the digestive tract. Nine grams of QUESTRAN Powder contain 4 grams of anhydrous cholestyramine resin. It is represented by the following structural formula:

Representation of structure of main polymeric groups
This product contains the following inactive ingredients: acacia, citric acid, D&C Yellow No. 10, FD&C Yellow No. 6, flavor (natural and artificial), polysorbate 80, propylene glycol alginate, and sucrose.

CLINICAL PHARMACOLOGY

Cholesterol is probably the sole precursor of bile acids. During normal digestion, bile acids are secreted into the intestines. A major portion of the bile acids is absorbed from the intestinal tract and returned to the liver via the enterohepatic circulation. Only very small amounts of bile acids are found in normal serum.

QUESTRAN resin adsorbs and combines with the bile acids in the intestine to form an insoluble complex which is excreted in the feces. This results in a partial removal of bile acids from the enterohepatic circulation by preventing their absorption.

The increased fecal loss of bile acids due to QUESTRAN administration leads to an increased oxidation of cholesterol to bile acids, a decrease in beta lipoprotein or low density lipoprotein plasma levels and a decrease in serum cholesterol levels. Although in man, QUESTRAN produces an increase in hepatic synthesis of cholesterol, plasma cholesterol levels fall.

In patients with partial biliary obstruction, the reduction of serum bile acid levels by QUESTRAN reduces excess bile acids deposited in the dermal tissue with resultant decrease in pruritus.

INDICATIONS AND USAGE

1) QUESTRAN is indicated as adjunctive therapy to diet for the reduction of elevated serum cholesterol in patients with primary hypercholesterolemia (elevated low density lipoprotein [LDL] cholesterol) who do not respond adequately to diet. QUESTRAN may be useful to lower LDL cholesterol in patients who also have hypertriglyceridemia, but it is not indicated where hypertriglyceridemia is the abnormality of most concern.

In a large, placebo-controlled, multi-clinic study, the LRC-CPPT[a], hypercholesterolemic subjects treated with QUESTRAN had significant reductions in total and low-density lipoprotein cholesterol (LDL-C). Over the seven-year study period the QUESTRAN group experienced a 19% reduction in the combined rate of coronary heart disease death plus nonfatal myocardial infarction (cumulative incidences of 7% Questran and 8.6% placebo). The subjects included in the study were middle-aged men (age 35–59) with serum cholesterol levels above 265 mg/dL and no previous history of heart disease. It is not clear to what extent these findings can be extrapolated to other segments of the hypercholesterolemic population not studied.

Dietary therapy specific for the type of hyperlipoproteinemia is the initial treatment of choice. Excess body weight may be an important factor and caloric restriction for weight normalization should be addressed prior to drug therapy in the overweight. The use of drugs should be considered only when reasonable attempts have been made to obtain satisfactory results with nondrug methods. If the decision ultimately is to use drugs, the patient should be instructed that this does not reduce the importance of adhering to diet.

2) QUESTRAN is indicated for the relief of pruritus associated with partial biliary obstruction. QUESTRAN has been shown to have a variable effect on serum cholesterol in these patients. Patients with primary biliary cirrhosis may exhibit an elevated cholesterol as part of their disease.

CONTRAINDICATIONS

QUESTRAN is contraindicated in patients with complete biliary obstruction where bile is not secreted into the intestine and in those individuals who have shown hypersensitivity to any of its components.

PRECAUTIONS

General: Before instituting therapy with QUESTRAN, diseases contributing to increased blood cholesterol such as hypothyroidism, diabetes mellitus, nephrotic syndrome, dysproteinemias and obstructive liver disease should be looked for and specifically treated. A favorable trend in cholesterol reduction should occur during the first month of QUESTRAN therapy. The therapy should be continued to sustain cholesterol reduction. If adequate cholesterol reduction is not attained, QUESTRAN therapy should be discontinued.

Chronic use of QUESTRAN may be associated with increased bleeding tendency due to hypoprothrombinemia associated with Vitamin K deficiency. This will usually respond promptly to parenteral Vitamin K_1 and recurrences can be prevented by oral administration of Vitamin K_1. Reduction of serum or red cell folate has been reported over long term administration of QUESTRAN. Supplementation with folic acid should be considered in these cases.

There is a possibility that prolonged use of QUESTRAN, since it is a chloride form of anion exchange resin, may produce hyperchloremic acidosis. This would especially be true in younger and smaller patients where the relative dosage may be higher.

QUESTRAN may produce or worsen pre-existing constipation. Dosage should be reduced or discontinued in such cases. Fecal impaction and aggravation of hemorrhoids may occur. Every effort should be made to avert severe constipation and its inherent problems in those patients with clinically symptomatic coronary artery disease.

Information for Patients: Inform your physician if you are pregnant or plan to become pregnant or are breast-feeding. Drink plenty of fluids and mix each 9-gram dose of QUESTRAN Powder in at least 2 to 6 ounces of fluid before taking.

Laboratory Tests: Serum cholesterol levels should be determined frequently during the first few months of therapy and periodically thereafter. Serum triglyceride levels should be measured periodically to detect whether significant changes have occurred.

The LRC-CPPT showed a dose-related increase in serum triglycerides of 10.7%–17.1% in the cholestyramine-treated group, compared with an increase of 7.9%–11.7% in the placebo group. Based on the mean values and adjusting for the placebo group, the cholestyramine-treated group showed an increase of 5% over pre-entry levels the first year of the study and an increase of 4.3% the seventh year.

Drug Interactions: QUESTRAN may delay or reduce the absorption of concomitant oral medication such as phenylbutazone, warfarin, chlorothiazide (acidic) or propranolol (basic), as well as tetracycline, penicillin G, phenobarbital, thyroid and thyroxine preparations, and digitalis. The discontinuance of QUESTRAN could pose a hazard to health if a potentially toxic drug such as digitalis has been titrated to a maintenance level while the patient was taking QUESTRAN.

Because cholestyramine binds bile acids, QUESTRAN may interfere with normal fat digestion and absorption and thus may prevent absorption of fat soluble vitamins such as A, D and K. When QUESTRAN is given for long periods of time, concomitant supplementation with water-miscible (or parenteral) form of vitamins A and D should be considered.

SINCE **QUESTRAN** MAY BIND OTHER DRUGS GIVEN CONCURRENTLY, PATIENTS SHOULD TAKE OTHER DRUGS AT LEAST ONE HOUR BEFORE OR 4–6 HOURS AFTER **QUESTRAN** (OR AT AS GREAT AN INTERVAL AS POSSIBLE) TO AVOID IMPEDING THEIR ABSORPTION.

Carcinogenesis, Mutagenesis and Impairment of Fertility: In studies conducted in rats in which cholestyramine resin was used as a tool to investigate the role of various intestinal factors, such as fat, bile salts and microbial flora, in the development of intestinal tumors induced by potent carcinogens, the incidence of such tumors was observed to be greater in cholestyramine resin-treated rats than in control rats.

The relevance of this laboratory observation from studies in rats to the clinical use of QUESTRAN is not known. In the LRC-CPPT study referred to above, the total incidence of fatal and nonfatal neoplasms was similar in both treatment groups. When the many different categories of tumors are examined, various alimentary system cancers were somewhat more prevalent in the cholestyramine group. The small numbers and the multiple categories prevent conclusions from being drawn. However, in view of the fact that cholestyramine resin is confined to the GI tract and not absorbed, and in light of the animal experiments referred to above, further follow-up of the LRC-CPPT participants is planned for cause-specific mortality and cancer morbidity.

Pregnancy: Since QUESTRAN is not absorbed systemically, it is not expected to cause fetal harm when administered during pregnancy in recommended dosages. There are, however, no adequate and well controlled studies in pregnant women, and the known interference with absorption of fat-soluble vitamins may be detrimental even in the presence of supplementation.

Nursing Mothers: Caution should be exercised when QUESTRAN is administered to a nursing mother. The possible lack of proper vitamin absorption described in the "Pregnancy" section may have an effect on nursing infants.

Pediatric Use: As experience in infants and children is limited, a practical dosage schedule has not been established. In calculating pediatric dosages, 44.4 mg of anhydrous cholestyramine resin are contained in 100 mg of QUESTRAN. The effects of long-term drug administration, as well as its effect in maintaining lowered cholesterol levels in pediatric patients, are unknown.

ADVERSE REACTIONS

The most common adverse reaction is constipation. When used as a cholesterol-lowering agent predisposing factors for most complaints of constipation are high dose and increased age (more than 60 years old). Most instances of constipation are mild, transient, and controlled with conventional therapy. Some patients require a temporary decrease in dosage or discontinuation of therapy.

Less Frequent Adverse Reactions: Abdominal discomfort, flatulence, nausea, vomiting, diarrhea, heartburn, anorexia, indigestive feeling and steatorrhea, bleeding tendencies due to hypoprothrombinemia (Vitamin K deficiency) as well as Vitamin A (one case of night blindness reported) and D deficiencies, hyperchloremic acidosis in children, osteoporosis, rash and irritation of the skin, tongue and perianal area. One ten-month-old baby with biliary atresia had an impaction presumed to be due to QUESTRAN after three days administration of 9 grams daily. She developed acute intestinal sepsis and died.

Occasional calcified material has been observed in the biliary tree, including calcification of the gallbladder, in patients to whom cholestyramine resin has been given. However, this may be a manifestation of the liver disease and not drug related.

One patient experienced biliary colic on each of three occasions on which he took QUESTRAN. One patient diagnosed as acute abdominal symptom complex was found to have a "pasty mass" in the transverse colon on x-ray.

Other events (not necessarily drug related) reported in patients taking QUESTRAN include:

Gastrointestinal—GI-rectal bleeding, black stools, hemorrhoidal bleeding, bleeding from known duodenal ulcer, dysphagia, hiccups, ulcer attack, sour taste, pancreatitis, rectal pain, diverticulitis.

Hematologic—Prolonged prothrombin time, ecchymosis, anemia.

Hypersensitivity—Urticaria, asthma, wheezing, shortness of breath.

Musculoskeletal—Backache, muscle and joint pains, arthritis.

Neurologic—Headache, anxiety, vertigo, dizziness, fatigue, tinnitus, syncope, drowsiness, femoral nerve pain, paresthesia.

Eye—Uveitis.

Renal—Hematuria, dysuria, burnt odor to urine, diuresis.

Miscellaneous—Weight loss, weight gain, increased libido, swollen glands, edema, dental bleeding.

OVERDOSAGE

Overdosage of QUESTRAN has not been reported. Should overdosage occur, however, the chief potential harm would be obstruction of the gastrointestinal tract. The location of such potential obstruction, the degree of obstruction, and the presence or absence of normal gut motility would determine treatment.

DOSAGE AND ADMINISTRATION

The recommended adult dose is one packet or one level scoopful (9 grams of QUESTRAN Powder contain 4 grams of anhydrous cholestyramine resin) one to six times daily. Dosage may be adjusted as required to meet the patient's needs. **QUESTRAN Powder should not be taken in its dry form. Always mix QUESTRAN Powder with water or other fluids before ingesting. See Preparation Instructions.**

PREPARATION

The color of QUESTRAN may vary somewhat from batch to batch, but this variation does not affect the performance of the product. Place the contents of one packet or one level scoopful of QUESTRAN in a glass or cup. Add at least 2–6 ounces of water or the beverage of your choice. Stir to a uniform consistency.

QUESTRAN may also be mixed with highly fluid soups or pulpy fruits with a high moisture content such as applesauce or crushed pineapple.

HOW SUPPLIED

QUESTRAN is available in cartons of sixty 9-gram packets and in cans containing 378 grams. Nine grams of QUESTRAN Powder contain 4 grams of anhydrous cholestyramine resin.

NDC 0087-0580-11 Cartons of 60 packets
NDC 0087-0580-05 Cans, 378 g

CLINICAL STUDIES

The NIH has concluded a 10-year randomized double-blind placebo-controlled study[a] in 12 lipid research clinics on the effect of lowering plasma cholesterol on coronary heart disease (CHD) risk (the risk of either coronary death or nonfatal myocardial infarction). Plasma cholesterol was lowered by a combination of a modest cholesterol-lowering diet and QUESTRAN. The dose response relationship between the amount of QUESTRAN ingested daily, the lowering of total plasma cholesterol, and the reduction in CHD risk is summarized below:

RELATION OF REDUCTION IN CHOLESTEROL TO REDUCTION IN CORONARY HEART DISEASE RISK

Packet Count	No.	Total Cholesterol Lowering	Reduction in CHD Risk
0–2	439	4.4%	10.9%
2–5	496	11.5%	26.1%
5–6	965	19.0%	39.3%

REFERENCE

[a]Anon: The Lipid Research Clinics Coronary Primary Prevention Trial Results: (I) Reduction in Incidence of Coronary Heart Disease; (II) The Relationship of Reduction in Incidence of Coronary Heart Disease to Cholesterol Lowering. JAMA 1984; 251:351–374.

Continued on next page

Bristol Labs.—Cont.

QUESTRAN® LIGHT   ℞
[kwest′rän līt]
(Cholestyramine for Oral Suspension)

DESCRIPTION

QUESTRAN LIGHT (cholestyramine for oral suspension), the chloride salt of a basic anion exchange resin, a cholesterol-lowering agent, is intended for oral administration. Cholestyramine resin is quite hydrophilic, but insoluble in water. The cholestyramine resin in QUESTRAN LIGHT is not absorbed from the digestive tract. Five grams of QUESTRAN LIGHT contain 4 grams of anhydrous cholestyramine resin. It is represented by the following structural formula:

Representation of structure of main polymeric groups
This product contains the following inactive ingredients: aspartame, citric acid, D&C Yellow No. 10, FD&C Red No. 40, flavor (natural and artificial), propylene glycol alginate, colloidal silicon dioxide, sucrose, and xanthan gum.

CLINICAL PHARMACOLOGY

Cholesterol is probably the sole precursor of bile acids. During normal digestion, bile acids are secreted into the intestines. A major portion of the bile acids is absorbed from the intestinal tract and returned to the liver via the enterohepatic circulation. Only very small amounts of bile acids are found in normal serum.

Cholestyramine resin adsorbs and combines with the bile acids in the intestine to form an insoluble complex which is excreted in the feces. This results in a partial removal of bile acids from the enterohepatic circulation by preventing their absorption.

The increased fecal loss of bile acids due to cholestyramine resin administration leads to an increased oxidation of cholesterol to bile acids, a decrease in beta lipoprotein or low density lipoprotein plasma levels and a decrease in serum cholesterol levels. Although in man cholestyramine resin produces an increase in hepatic synthesis of cholesterol, plasma cholesterol levels fall.

In patients with partial biliary obstruction, the reduction of serum bile acid levels by cholestyramine resin reduces excess bile acids deposited in the dermal tissue with resultant decrease in pruritus.

INDICATIONS AND USAGE

1. QUESTRAN LIGHT is indicated as adjunctive therapy to diet for the reduction of elevated serum cholesterol in patients with primary hypercholesterolemia (elevated low density lipoprotein [LDL] cholesterol) who do not respond adequately to diet. Cholestyramine resin may be useful to lower LDL cholesterol in patients who also have hypertriglyceridemia, but it is not indicated where hypertriglyceridemia is the abnormality of most concern.

In a large, placebo-controlled, multi-clinic study, the LRC-CPPT,[a] hypercholesterolemic subjects treated with cholestyramine resin had significant reductions in total and low-density lipoprotein cholesterol (LDL-C). Over the seven-year study period the cholestyramine resin group experienced a 19% reduction in the combined rate of coronary heart disease death plus nonfatal myocardial infarction (cumulative incidences of 7% cholestyramine resin and 8.6% placebo). The subjects included in the study were middle-aged men (age 35-59) with serum cholesterol levels above 265 mg/dL and no previous history of heart disease. It is not clear to what extent these findings can be extrapolated to other segments of the hypercholesterolemic population not studied.

Dietary therapy specific for the type of hyperlipoproteinemia is the initial treatment of choice. Excess body weight may be an important factor and caloric restriction for weight normalization should be addressed prior to drug therapy in the overweight. The use of drugs should be considered only when reasonable attempts have been made to obtain satisfactory results with nondrug methods. If the decision ultimately is to use drugs, the patient should be instructed that this does not reduce the importance of adhering to diet.

2. QUESTRAN LIGHT is indicated for the relief of pruritus associated with partial biliary obstruction. Cholestyramine resin has been shown to have a variable effect on serum cholesterol in these patients. Patients with primary biliary cirrhosis may exhibit an elevated cholesterol as part of their disease.

CONTRAINDICATIONS

Cholestyramine resin is contraindicated in patients with complete biliary obstruction where bile is not secreted into the intestine and in those individuals who have shown hypersensitivity to any of its components.

WARNING

PHENYLKETONURICS: QUESTRAN LIGHT CONTAINS 16.8 mg PHENYLALANINE PER 5-GRAM DOSE.

PRECAUTIONS

General

Before instituting therapy with cholestyramine resin, diseases contributing to increased blood cholesterol such as hypothyroidism, diabetes mellitus, nephrotic syndrome, dysproteinemias and obstructive liver disease should be looked for and specifically treated. A favorable trend in cholesterol reduction should occur during the first month of cholestyramine resin therapy. The therapy should be continued to sustain cholesterol reduction. If adequate cholesterol reduction is not attained, cholestyramine resin therapy should be discontinued.

Chronic use of cholestyramine resin may be associated with increased bleeding tendency due to hypoprothrombinemia associated with Vitamin K deficiency. This will usually respond promptly to parenteral Vitamin K_1 and recurrences can be prevented by oral administration of Vitamin K_1. Reduction of serum or red cell folate has been reported over long term administration of cholestyramine resin. Supplementation with folic acid should be considered in these cases. There is a possibility that prolonged use of QUESTRAN LIGHT, since it is a chloride form of anion exchange resin, may produce hyperchloremic acidosis. This would especially be true in younger and smaller patients where the relative dosage may be higher.

Cholestyramine resin may produce or worsen pre-existing constipation. Dosage should be reduced or discontinued in such cases. Fecal impaction and aggravation of hemorrhoids may occur. Every effort should be made to avert severe constipation and its inherent problems in those patients with clinically symptomatic coronary artery disease.

Information for Patients

Inform your physician if you are pregnant or plan to become pregnant or are breast feeding. Drink plenty of fluids and mix each 5-gram dose of QUESTRAN LIGHT in at least 2–3 ounces of fluid before taking.

Laboratory Tests

Serum cholesterol levels should be determined frequently during the first few months of therapy and periodically thereafter. Serum triglyceride levels should be measured periodically to detect whether significant changes have occurred.

The LRC-CPPT showed a dose-related increase in serum triglycerides of 10.7%–17.1% in the cholestyramine-treated group, compared with an increase of 7.9%–11.7% in the placebo group. Based on the mean values and adjusting for the placebo group, the cholestyramine-treated group showed an increase of 5% over pre-entry levels the first year of the study and an increase of 4.3% the seventh year.

Drug Interactions

Cholestyramine resin may delay or reduce the absorption of concomitant oral medication such as phenylbutazone, warfarin, chlorothiazide (acidic), or propranolol (basic), as well as tetracycline, penicillin G, phenobarbital, thyroid and thyroxine preparations, and digitalis. The discontinuance of cholestyramine resin could pose a hazard to health if a potentially toxic drug such as digitalis has been titrated to a maintenance level while the patient was taking cholestyramine resin.

Because cholestyramine binds bile acids, cholestyramine resin may interfere with normal fat digestion and absorption and thus may prevent absorption of fat soluble vitamins such as A, D and K. When cholestyramine resin is given for long periods of time, concomitant supplementation with water-miscible (or parenteral) form of vitamins A and D should be considered.

SINCE CHOLESTYRAMINE RESIN MAY BIND OTHER DRUGS GIVEN CONCURRENTLY, PATIENTS SHOULD TAKE OTHER DRUGS AT LEAST ONE HOUR BEFORE OR 4 TO 6 HOURS AFTER CHOLESTYRAMINE RESIN (OR AT AS GREAT AN INTERVAL AS POSSIBLE) TO AVOID IMPEDING THEIR ABSORPTION.

Carcinogenesis, Mutagenesis and Impairment of Fertility

In studies conducted in rats in which cholestyramine resin was used as a tool to investigate the role of various intestinal factors, such as fat, bile salts and microbial flora, in the development of intestinal tumors induced by potent carcinogens, the incidence of such tumors was observed to be greater in cholestyramine resin treated rats than in control rats. The relevance of this laboratory observation from studies in rats to the clinical use of cholestyramine resin is not known. In the LRC-CPPT study referred to above, the total incidence of fatal and nonfatal neoplasms was similar in both treatment groups. When the many different categories of tumors are examined, various alimentary system cancers were somewhat more prevalent in the cholestyramine group. The small numbers and the multiple categories prevent conclusions from being drawn. However, in view of the fact that cholestyramine resin is confined to the GI tract and not absorbed, and in light of the animal experiments referred to above, further follow-up of the LRC-CPPT participants is planned for cause-specific mortality and cancer morbidity.

Pregnancy

Since cholestyramine resin is not absorbed systemically, it is not expected to cause fetal harm when administered during pregnancy in recommended dosages. There are, however, no adequate and well controlled studies in pregnant women, and the known interference with absorption of fat soluble vitamins may be detrimental even in the presence of supplementation.

Nursing Mothers

Caution should be exercised when cholestyramine resin is administered to a nursing mother. The possible lack of proper vitamin absorption described in the "Pregnancy" section may have an effect on nursing infants.

Pediatric Use

As experience in infants and children is limited, a practical dosage schedule has not been established.

In calculating pediatric dosages, 80 mg of anhydrous cholestyramine resin are contained in 100 mg of QUESTRAN LIGHT.

The effects of long-term drug administration, as well as its effect in maintaining lowered cholesterol levels in pediatric patients, are unknown.

ADVERSE REACTIONS

The most common adverse reaction is constipation. When used as a cholesterol-lowering agent, predisposing factors for most complaints of constipation are high dose and increased age (more than 60 years old). Most instances of constipation are mild, transient, and controlled with conventional therapy. Some patients require a temporary decrease in dosage or discontinuation of therapy.

Less Frequent Adverse Reactions: Abdominal discomfort, flatulence, nausea, vomiting, diarrhea, heartburn, anorexia, indigestive feeling and steatorrhea, bleeding tendencies due to hypoprothrombinemia (Vitamin K deficiency) as well as Vitamin A (one case of night blindness reported) and D deficiencies, hyperchloremic acidosis in children, osteoporosis, rash and irritation of the skin, tongue and perianal area. One ten-month-old baby with biliary atresia had an impaction presumed to be due to cholestyramine resin after three days administration of 9 grams daily. She developed acute intestinal sepsis and died.

Occasional calcified material has been observed in the biliary tree, including calcification of the gallbladder, in patients to whom cholestyramine resin has been given. However, this may be a manifestation of the liver disease and not drug related.

One patient experienced biliary colic on each of three occasions on which he took cholestyramine resin. One patient diagnosed as acute abdominal symptom complex was found to have a "pasty mass" in the transverse colon on x-ray.

Other events (not necessarily drug related) reported in patients taking cholestyramine resin include:

Gastrointestinal—GI-rectal bleeding, black stools, hemorrhoidal bleeding, bleeding from known duodenal ulcer, dysphagia, hiccups, ulcer attack, sour taste, pancreatitis, rectal pain, diverticulitis.

Hematologic—Prolonged prothrombin time, ecchymosis, anemia.

Hypersensitivity—Urticaria, asthma, wheezing, shortness of breath.

Musculoskeletal—Backache, muscle and joint pains, arthritis.

Neurologic—Headache, anxiety, vertigo, dizziness, fatigue, tinnitus, syncope, drowsiness, femoral nerve pain, paresthesia.

Eye—Uveitis.

Renal—Hematuria, dysuria, burnt odor to urine, diuresis.

Miscellaneous—Weight loss, weight gain, increased libido, swollen glands, edema, dental bleeding.

OVERDOSAGE

Overdosage of cholestyramine resin has not been reported. Should overdosage occur, however, the chief potential harm would be obstruction of the gastrointestinal tract. The location of such potential obstruction, the degree of obstruction, and the presence or absence of normal gut motility would determine treatment.

DOSAGE AND ADMINISTRATION

The recommended adult dose is one single dose packet or one level scoopful (5 grams of QUESTRAN LIGHT contain 4 grams of anhydrous cholestyramine resin) one to six times daily. Dosage may be adjusted as required to meet the patient's needs.

QUESTRAN LIGHT should not be taken in its dry form. Always mix QUESTRAN LIGHT with water or other fluids before ingesting. See Preparation instructions.

PREPARATION

The color of QUESTRAN LIGHT may vary somewhat from batch to batch but this variation does not affect the performance of the product. Place the contents of one single-dose packet or one level scoopful of cholestyramine resin in a glass or cup. Add at least 2–3 ounces of water or the beverage of your choice. Stir to a uniform consistency.

QUESTRAN LIGHT may also be mixed with highly fluid soups or pulpy fruits with a high moisture content such as applesauce or crushed pineapple.

HOW SUPPLIED

QUESTRAN LIGHT is available in cartons of sixty 5-gram packets and in cans containing 210 grams. Five grams of QUESTRAN LIGHT contain 4 grams of anhydrous cholestyramine resin.

NDC 0087-0589-01   210 g cans, 42 doses
NDC 0087-0589-03   Cartons of 60, 5 g packets
Store at room temperature.

CLINICAL STUDIES

The NIH has concluded a 10-year randomized double-blind placebo-controlled study[a] in 12 lipid research clinics on the effect of lowering plasma cholesterol on coronary heart disease (CHD) risk (the risk of either coronary death or nonfatal myocardial infarction). Plasma cholesterol was lowered by a combination of a modest cholesterol-lowering diet and cholestyramine resin. The dose response relationship between the amount of cholestyramine resin ingested daily, the lowering of total plasma cholesterol, and the reduction of CHD risk is summarized below:

RELATION OF REDUCTION IN CHOLESTEROL TO REDUCTION IN CORONARY HEART DISEASE RISK

No. of Doses* Per Day	No.	Total Cholesterol Lowering	Reduction in CHD Risk
0–2	439	4.4%	10.9%
2–5	496	11.5%	26.1%
5–6	965	19.0%	39.3%

*One dose contains 4 g cholestyramine resin.

REFERENCES

a. Anon: The Lipid Research Clinics Coronary Primary Prevention Trial Results: (I) Reduction in Incidence of Coronary Heart Disease; (II) The Relationship of Reduction in Incidence of Coronary Heart Disease to Cholesterol Lowering. JAMA 1984; 251:351–374.

QUIBRON®   ℞
[kwĭ'bron]
(Theophylline-Guaifenesin)
Capsules, 1000s   NSN 6505-00-764-3366(M)

DESCRIPTION

Each QUIBRON® soft gelatin capsule or tablespoon (15 mL) of liquid contains 150 mg of theophylline (anhydrous) and 90 mg of guaifenesin, as an oral bronchodilator-expectorant. QUIBRON Liquid contains no alcohol and is dye-free.

QUIBRON®-300   ℞
(Theophylline-Guaifenesin)

DESCRIPTION

Each QUIBRON®-300 soft gelatin capsule contains 300 mg of theophylline (anhydrous) and 180 mg of guaifenesin, as an oral bronchodilator-expectorant. The structural formula for the active ingredients of QUIBRON and QUIBRON-300 are presented below:

Theophylline
[1,3 Dimethylxanthine]

Guaifenesin
[3-(o-Methoxyphenoxy)-1,2-propanediol]

Theophylline, a xanthine compound, is a white, odorless crystalline powder, having a bitter taste.
Guaifenesin, a guaiacol compound, is a white to slightly yellow crystalline powder with a bitter, aromatic taste.

INACTIVE INGREDIENTS

QUIBRON and QUIBRON-300 Capsules contain: D&C Yellow No. 10, non-porcine gelatin, glycerin, edible ink, polyethylene glycol, and titanium dioxide.
QUIBRON Liquid contains: flavors, propylene glycol, sodium hydroxide, sorbitol solution, sucrose, and purified water.

CLINICAL PHARMACOLOGY
THEOPHYLLINE
Mode of Action

Theophylline acts as a bronchodilator by direct relaxation of bronchial smooth muscle. Theophylline is a competitive inhibitor of cyclic nucleotide phosphodiesterase resulting in increased intracellular levels of cAMP which mediates smooth muscle relaxation. Like some other xanthines, theophylline acts as a coronary vasodilator, cardiac stimulant, skeletal muscle stimulant, central nervous system stimulant and diuretic.

Pharmacokinetics

As theophylline is released from the formulation it is, under usual conditions, absorbed completely and fairly rapidly. Excretion, principally as inactive metabolites, occurs primarily via the kidney. The half-life of theophylline varies among individuals with a wide range having been documented. Theophylline half-life is shortened in cigarette smokers. Half-life is prolonged in alcoholism, reduced hepatic or renal function, congestive heart failure and patients receiving antibiotics such as troleandomycin or erythromycin. High fever for prolonged periods may decrease theophylline elimination. The theophylline half-life is generally shorter in children.

Representative Theophylline Serum Half-lives

	Half-life (hours)	
	Mean	Range
Adults		
non-smokers	8.7	6.1–12.8
smokers	5.5	4.0– 7.7
congestive heart failure	22.9	3.1–82.0
Children (6–16 yrs)	3.7	1.4– 7.9

Therapeutic serum theophylline levels are usually 10–20 µg/mL.

Binding to plasma proteins is not extensive and theophylline is not preferentially taken up by any particular organ.
Theophylline-containing products may increase the plasma levels of free fatty acids and the urinary levels of epinephrine and norepinephrine.
Apparently no development of tolerance occurs with chronic use of theophylline.

CLINICAL PHARMACOLOGY
GUAIFENESIN
Mode of Action

Guaifenesin increases respiratory tract secretions, possibly by stimulating the goblet cells.

Pharmacokinetics

Guaifenesin appears to be well absorbed, but its pharmacokinetics has not been well studied.

INDICATIONS AND USAGE

QUIBRON and QUIBRON-300 are indicated for the symptomatic treatment of bronchospasm associated with such conditions as bronchial asthma, chronic bronchitis and pulmonary emphysema.

CONTRAINDICATIONS

QUIBRON products are contraindicated in individuals who have shown hypersensitivity to any of their components or xanthine derivatives.

WARNINGS

Excessive theophylline doses may be associated with toxicity; thus serum theophylline levels should be monitored to assure maximal benefit without excessive risk.
Serum levels of theophylline above the accepted therapeutic range (10–20 µg/mL) are associated with an increased incidence of toxicity. Such levels may be reached with customary doses in individuals who metabolize the drug slowly, especially patients (1) with lowered body plasma clearance, (2) with liver dysfunction or chronic obstructive pulmonary disease or (3) older than 55 years of age, particularly males. Serious toxicity, such as a seizure or ventricular arrhythmias, is not necessarily preceded by less serious side-effects such as nausea, irritability or restlessness.
Many patients who have higher (greater than 20 µg/mL) theophylline serum levels exhibit tachycardia. Theophylline products may exacerbate pre-existing arrhythmias.

PRECAUTIONS
General

Use with caution in patients with severe cardiac disease, hypertension, acute myocardial injury, congestive heart failure, cor pulmonale, severe hypoxemia, hyperthyroidism, hepatic impairment, history of peptic ulcer, alcoholism and in the elderly. Concurrent administration with certain antibiotics (see DRUG INTERACTIONS section) may result in increased serum theophylline levels.
A decrease in serum half-life is seen in smokers (see CLINICAL PHARMACOLOGY/Pharmacokinetics).
Particular caution should be used in administering theophylline to patients in congestive heart failure. Reduced theophylline clearance in these patients may cause theophylline blood levels to persist long after discontinuing the drug.

Theophylline should not be administered concurrently with other xanthine medications.

Usage in Pregnancy

Teratogenic effects: Pregnancy Category C. Animal reproduction studies have not been conducted with QUIBRON products. It is also not known whether QUIBRON products can cause fetal harm when administered to a pregnant woman or can affect reproduction capacity. QUIBRON products should be given to a pregnant woman only if clearly indicated.

Nonteratogenic effects: It is not known whether use of this drug during labor or delivery has immediate or delayed adverse effects on the fetus, or whether it prolongs the duration of labor or increases the possibility of forceps delivery or other obstetrical intervention.

Nursing Mothers

Theophylline has been reported to be excreted in human milk and to have caused irritability in a nursing infant. Because of the potential for serious adverse reactions, a decision should be made whether to discontinue nursing or to discontinue QUIBRON or QUIBRON-300, taking into account the importance of this drug to the mother.

Pediatric Use

Sufficient numbers of infants under the age of 1 year have not been studied in clinical trials to support the use of theophylline in this age group; however, there is evidence recorded that the use of dosage recommendations for older infants and young children (16 mg/kg/24 hours) may result in the development of toxic serum levels. Such findings very probably reflect differences in the metabolic handling of theophylline related to absent or underdeveloped enzyme systems. Consequently, the use of theophylline in this age group should carefully consider the associated benefits and risks. If used, the maintenance dose must be conservative and in accord with the following guidelines:

Initial Maintenance Dosage:

Premature Infants:
Up to 24 days postnatal age—1.0 mg/kg q.12h

Beyond 24 days postnatal age—1.5 mg/kg q.12h

Infants 6 to 52 Weeks:
$[(0.2 \times \text{age in weeks}) + 5.0] \times \text{kg body wt} = 24$ hour dose in mg.

Up to 26 weeks, divide into q.8h dosing intervals.
From 26–52 weeks, divide into q.6h dosing intervals.

Final dosage should be guided by serum concentration after a steady state (no further accumulation of drug) has been achieved.

Drug Interactions

Drug	Effect
Theophylline with lithium carbonate	Increased renal excretion of lithium
Theophylline with propranolol	Mutual antagonism of therapeutic effects
Theophylline with furosemide	Increased diuresis
Theophylline with reserpine	Tachycardia
Theophylline with chlordiazepoxide	Fatty acid mobilization
Theophylline with troleandomycin or erythromycin	Increased theophylline plasma levels

Drug/Laboratory Test Interactions

Theophylline may interfere with the assay of uric acid, especially the phosphotungstate method. Thus, serum uric acid levels may be overestimated. Metabolites of guaifenesin may contribute to increased 5–hydroxyindoleacetic acid readings when determined with nitrosonaphthol reagent.

ADVERSE REACTIONS

The frequency of adverse reactions is related to serum theophylline levels and is usually not a problem at levels below 20 µg/mL. The most consistent adverse reactions are usually due to overdosage and, while all have not been reported with QUIBRON or QUIBRON-300, the following reactions may be considered when theophylline is administered. Central nervous system: clonic and tonic generalized convulsions, muscle twitching, reflex hyperexcitability, headaches, insomnia, restlessness, and irritability. Cardiovascular: circulatory failure, ventricular arrhythmias, hypotension, extrasystoles, tachycardia, palpitation, and flushing. Gastrointestinal: hematemesis, vomiting, diarrhea, epigastric pain, and nausea. Renal: increased excretion of renal tubular cells and red blood cells, albuminuria, and diuresis. Respiratory: tachypnea. Others: hyperglycemia and inappropriate ADH syndrome.

OVERDOSAGE
Symptoms

Nervousness, agitation, headache, insomnia, vomiting, tachycardia, extrasystoles, hyperreflexia, fasciculations and

Continued on next page

Bristol Labs.—Cont.

clonic and tonic convulsions. Children may be particularly prone to restlessness and hyperactivity that can proceed to convulsions.

Management

If potential oral overdose is established and seizure has **not** occurred:

1. Induce vomiting.
2. Administer a cathartic (this is particularly important if sustained release preparations have been taken).
3. Administer activated charcoal.
4. Monitor vital signs, maintain blood pressure and provide adequate hydration.

If patient is having seizure:

1. Establish an airway.
2. Administer O_2.
3. Treat the seizure with intravenous diazepam 0.1 to 0.3 mg/kg up to 10 mg.
4. Monitor vital signs, maintain blood pressure and provide adequate hydration.

Post-Seizure Coma

1. Maintain airway and oxygenation.
2. If a result of oral medication, follow above recommendations to prevent absorption of drug, but intubation and lavage will have to be performed instead of inducing emesis and the cathartic and charcoal will need to be introduced via a large bore gastric lavage tube.
3. Continue to provide full supportive care and adequate hydration while waiting for drug to be metabolized. In general, the drug is metabolized rapidly enough so as to not warrant consideration of dialysis.

General

The oral LD_{50} of theophylline in mice is 350 mg/kg. The oral LD_{50} of guaifenesin in mice is 1725 mg/kg. In humans, adverse reactions often occur when serum theophylline levels exceed 20 μg/mL. Information on physiological variables which influence excretion of theophylline can be found under the heading "Clinical Pharmacology."

DOSAGE AND ADMINISTRATION

General

Therapeutic serum levels associated with optimal likelihood for benefit and minimal risk of toxicity are considered to be between 10 and 20 μg/mL, although levels of 5-10 μg/mL are reported to be effective for some patients. Levels above 20 μg/mL may produce toxic effects. There is great variation from patient to patient and dosage must be individualized because there is a relatively narrow range between therapeutic and toxic levels of theophylline. Monitoring of serum theophylline levels is highly recommended. Since theophylline does not distribute into fatty tissue, dosage should be calculated on the basis of ideal body weight.

Giving theophylline with food may prevent the rare case of stomach irritation and, although absorption may be slower, it is still complete.

QUIBRON

Treatment should be initiated at 150 mg theophylline every 6 hours for adults and 4 mg/kg every 6 hours for children. The usual recommended dosages are—Adults: 1–2 capsules or 1–2 tablespoons (15 mL) liquid every 6–8 hours. Children 9 to 12: 4–5 mg theophylline/kg body weight every 6–8 hours. Children 1 to 9: 4 mg theophylline/kg body weight every 6–8 hours. For children under 1 year see **PRECAUTIONS** section. Approximate mg/kg dosage by TEASPOON (5 mL) of QUIBRON Liquid may be determined from the following table:

AVERAGE DOSAGE IN TEASPOONS (5 mL) TO PROVIDE THE FOLLOWING MG OF THEOPHYLLINE/KG BODY WEIGHT/DOSE

BODY WEIGHT		4 mg/kg	5 mg/kg	6 mg/kg
Lbs	kgs			
20	9	$\frac{3}{4}$	1	1
30	14	1	$1\frac{1}{2}$	$1\frac{3}{4}$
40	18	$1\frac{1}{2}$	2	$2\frac{1}{4}$
50	23	$1\frac{3}{4}$	$2\frac{1}{4}$	$2\frac{3}{4}$
60	27	2	$2\frac{3}{4}$	$3\frac{1}{4}$
70	32	$2\frac{1}{2}$	3	$3\frac{3}{4}$
80	36	3	$3\frac{1}{2}$	$4\frac{1}{4}$
90	41	$3\frac{1}{4}$	4	5
100	46	$3\frac{1}{2}$	$4\frac{1}{2}$	$5\frac{1}{2}$

If the desired response is not achieved with the recommended initial dose, and there are no adverse reactions, the dose may be cautiously adjusted upward in increments of no more than 25 percent at 2–3 day intervals until the following MAXIMUM DOSE WITHOUT MEASUREMENT OF SERUM CONCENTRATION or a maximum of 900 mg in any 24 hour period (whichever is less) is attained:

MAXIMUM DAILY DOSE WITHOUT MEASUREMENT OF SERUM CONCENTRATION

	mg per kg Body Weight*
Children (under 9)	24
Children (9–12)	20
Adolescents (12–16)	18
Adults	13

*Use ideal body weight for obese patients

Do not attempt to maintain any dose that is not tolerated. If doses higher than those contained in the above MAXIMUM DOSE WITHOUT MEASUREMENT OF SERUM CONCENTRATION are necessary, it is recommended that serum theophylline levels be monitored. For therapeutic levels, draw blood sample just before next dose is due; for toxic levels, draw blood sample when last dose peaks ($\simeq$2 hours after dosing). It is important that the patient has missed no doses during the previous 72 hours and that dosing intervals have been reasonably typical with no added doses during that period of time. DOSAGE ADJUSTMENT BASED ON SERUM THEOPHYLLINE MEASUREMENTS WHEN THESE INSTRUCTIONS HAVE **NOT** BEEN FOLLOWED, MAY RESULT IN RECOMMENDATIONS THAT PRESENT RISK OF TOXICITY TO THE PATIENT.

QUIBRON-300 Capsules

QUIBRON-300 is appropriate therapy when higher theophylline dosages are required. The usual recommended dosages for QUIBRON-300 are—**Adults:** 1 capsule every 6–8 hours for patients whose dosage has been adjusted upward to achieve therapeutic serum levels.

HOW SUPPLIED

QUIBRON® Capsules (yellow) in bottles of 100 (NDC 0087-0516-01); and 1000 (NDC 0087-0516-02); Unit Dose 100s (NDC 0087-0516-03).

QUIBRON® Liquid in 1 pint (NDC 0087-0510-03) and 1 gallon (NDC 0087-0510-01).

QUIBRON-300 Capsules (yellow and white) in bottles of 100 (NDC 0087-0515-41).

Store at controlled room temperature of 59°–86°F (15°–30°C).

Shown in Product Identification Section, page 406

QUIBRON®-T   ℞

[kwĭ'bran]
(theophylline tablets, USP)
DIVIDOSE® TABLETS
IMMEDIATE RELEASE BRONCHODILATOR

DESCRIPTION

Theophylline is a bronchodilator structurally classified as a xanthine derivative. It occurs as a white, odorless, crystalline powder having a bitter taste. Theophylline anhydrous has the chemical name, 1H-purine-2,6-dione, 3,7-dihydro-1,3-dimethyl-, and is represented by the following structural formula:

QUIBRON®-T tablets provide 300 mg of anhydrous theophylline as an oral bronchodilator in an immediate release formulation combined with the convenience of the unique DIVIDOSE® tablet design. With functional trisects and bisects, QUIBRON-T can be conveniently and accurately divided into 100, 150, and 200 mg segments to provide a variety of dosing increments, as required.

QUIBRON-T tablets

One-third tablet	= 100 mg
One-half tablet	= 150 mg
Two-thirds tablet	= 200 mg
One tablet	= 300 mg

This product contains the following inactive ingredients: microcrystalline cellulose, yellow ferric oxide, hydroxypropyl methylcellulose 2910, lactose, magnesium stearate, colloidal silicon dioxide, and sodium starch glycolate.

CLINICAL PHARMACOLOGY

Mode of Action

Theophylline directly relaxes the smooth muscle of the bronchial airways and pulmonary blood vessels, thus acting mainly as a bronchodilator and smooth muscle relaxant. It has also been demonstrated that aminophylline has a potent effect on diaphragmatic contractility in normal persons and may then be capable of reducing fatigability and thereby improve contractility in patients with chronic obstructive airways disease. The exact mode of action remains unsettled.

Although theophylline does cause inhibition of phosphodiesterase with a resultant increase in intracellular cyclic AMP, other agents similarly inhibit the enzyme producing a rise of cyclic AMP but are unassociated with any demonstrable bronchodilation. Other mechanisms proposed include an effect on translocation of intracellular calcium; prostaglandin antagonism; stimulation of catecholamines endogenously; inhibition of cyclic guanosine monophosphate metabolism and adenosine receptor antagonism. None of these mechanisms has been proved, however.

In vitro, theophylline has been shown to act synergistically with *beta*-agonists and there are now available data which do demonstrate an additive effect *in vivo* with combined use.

Pharmacokinetics

The half-life of theophylline is influenced by a number of known variables. It may be prolonged in chronic alcoholics, particularly those with liver disease (cirrhosis or alcoholic liver disease), in patients with congestive heart failure, and in those patients taking certain other drugs (see PRECAUTIONS, Drug Interactions). Newborns and neonates have extremely slow clearance rates compared to older infants and children, ie, those over 1 year. Older children have rapid clearance rates while most nonsmoking adults have clearance rates between these two extremes. In premature neonates the decreased clearance is related to oxidative pathways that have yet to be established.

Theophylline Elimination Characteristics

	Half-life (in hours)	
	Range	Mean
Children	1–9	3.7
Adults	3–15	7.7

In cigarette smokers (1 to 2 packs/day) the mean half-life is 4 to 5 hours, much shorter than in nonsmokers. The increase in clearance associated with smoking is presumably due to stimulation of the hepatic metabolic pathway by components of cigarette smoke. The duration of this effect after cessation of smoking is unknown but may require 6 months to 2 years before the rate approaches that of the nonsmoker.

INDICATIONS AND USAGE

QUIBRON-T tablets are indicated for relief and/or prevention of symptoms from asthma and reversible bronchospasm associated with chronic bronchitis and emphysema.

CONTRAINDICATIONS

QUIBRON-T tablets are contraindicated in individuals who have shown hypersensitivity to its components. It is also contraindicated in patients with active peptic ulcer disease, and in individuals with underlying seizure disorders (unless receiving appropriate anticonvulsant medication).

WARNINGS

Excessive doses may be associated with toxicity, although increasing the dose of theophylline may enhance response. The likelihood of serious toxicity increases substantially when the serum theophylline concentration exceeds 20 μg/mL. Therefore, determination of serum theophylline levels is recommended to assure maximal benefit without excessive risk.

Serum levels above 20 μg/mL are rarely found after appropriate administration of the recommended doses. However, in individuals in whom theophylline plasma clearance is reduced *for any reason*, even conventional doses may result in increased serum levels and potential toxicity. Reduced theophylline clearance has been documented in the following readily identifiable groups: 1) patients with impaired liver function; 2) patients over 55 years of age, particularly males and those with chronic lung disease; 3) those with cardiac failure from any cause; 4) patients with sustained high fever; 5) neonates and infants under 1 year of age; and 6) those patients taking certain drugs (see PRECAUTIONS, Drug Interactions). Frequently, such patients have markedly prolonged theophylline serum levels following discontinuation of the drug. Reduction of dosage and laboratory monitoring is especially appropriate in the above individuals.

Serious side effects such as ventricular arrhythmias, convulsions or even death may appear as the first sign of toxicity without any previous warning. Less serious signs of theophylline toxicity (ie, nausea and restlessness) may occur frequently when initiating therapy, but are usually transient; when such signs are persistent during maintenance therapy, they are often associated with serum concentrations above 20 μg/mL. Stated differently; *serious toxicity is not reliably preceded by less severe side effects.* A serum concentration measurement is the only reliable method of predicting potentially life-threatening toxicity.

Many patients who require theophylline exhibit tachycardia due to their underlying disease process so that the cause/effect relationship to elevated serum theophylline concentrations may not be appreciated.

Theophylline products may cause dysrhythmia and/or worsen pre-existing arrhythmias and any significant change in rate and/or rhythm warrants monitoring and further investigation.

Studies in laboratory animals (minipigs, rodents, and dogs) recorded the occurrence of cardiac arrhythmias and sudden death (with histologic evidence of myocardial necrosis) when *beta*-agonists and methylxanthines were administered concurrently. The significance of these findings when applied to humans is currently unknown.

PRECAUTIONS

General
On the average, theophylline half-life is shorter in cigarette and marijuana smokers than in nonsmokers, but smokers can have half-lives as long as nonsmokers. Theophylline should not be administered concurrently with other xanthines. Use with caution in patients with hypoxemia, hypertension, or those with history of peptic ulcer. Theophylline may occasionally act as a local irritant to G.I. tract although gastrointestinal symptoms are more commonly centrally mediated and associated with serum drug concentrations over 20 $\mu g/mL$.

Information for Patients
The importance of taking only the prescribed dose and time interval between doses should be reinforced.

Laboratory Tests
Serum levels should be monitored periodically to determine the theophylline level associated with observed clinical response and as the method of predicting toxicity. For such measurements, the serum sample should be obtained at the time of peak concentration, 1 to 2 hours after administration for immediate release products. It is important that the patient will not have missed or taken additional doses during the previous 48 hours and that dosing intervals will have been reasonably equally spaced. DOSAGE ADJUSTMENT BASED ON SERUM THEOPHYLLINE MEASUREMENTS WHEN THESE INSTRUCTIONS HAVE NOT BEEN FOLLOWED MAY RESULT IN RECOMMENDATIONS THAT PRESENT RISK OF TOXICITY TO THE PATIENT.

Drug Interactions
Toxic synergism with ephedrine has been documented and may occur with other sympathomimetic bronchodilators. In addition, the following drug interactions have been demonstrated:

Theophylline with:

Allopurinol (high dose)	Increased serum theophylline levels
Cimetidine	Increased serum theophylline levels
Erythromycin, Troleandomycin	Increased serum theophylline levels
Lithium Carbonate	Increased renal excretion of lithium
Oral Contraceptives	Increased serum theophylline levels
Phenytoin	Decreased theophylline and phenytoin serum levels
Rifampin	Decreased serum theophylline levels

Drug/Laboratory Test Interactions
Currently available analytical methods, including high pressure liquid chromatography and immunoassay techniques, for measuring serum theophylline levels are specific. Metabolites and other drugs generally do not affect the results. Other new analytic methods are also now in use. The physician should be aware of the laboratory method used and whether other drugs will interfere with the assay for theophylline.

Carcinogenesis, Mutagenesis, and Impairment of Fertility
Long-term carcinogenicity studies have not been performed with theophylline.

Chromosome-breaking activity was detected in human cell cultures at concentrations of theophylline up to 50 times the therapeutic serum concentration in humans. Theophylline was not mutagenic in the dominant lethal assay in male mice given theophylline intraperitoneally in doses up to 30 times the maximum daily human oral dose.

Studies to determine the effect on fertility have not been performed with theophylline.

Pregnancy
Category C—Animal reproduction studies have not been conducted with theophylline. It is also not known whether theophylline can cause fetal harm when administered to a pregnant woman or can affect reproduction capacity. Xanthines should be given to a pregnant woman only if clearly needed.

Nursing Mothers
Theophylline is distributed into breast milk and may cause irritability or other signs of toxicity in nursing infants. Because of the potential for serious adverse reactions in nursing infants from theophylline, a decision should be made whether to discontinue nursing or to discontinue the drug, taking into account the importance of the drug to the mother.

Pediatric Use
Safety and effectiveness of theophylline immediate-release products in children under 1 year of age have not been established. Because of the potential difficulty of drug administration (eg, tablet swallowability) and the inability to provide small and precise incremental doses, it is recommended that a liquid theophylline preparation be used for children under 6 years of age.

ADVERSE REACTIONS
The following adverse reactions have been observed, but there has not been enough systematic collection of data to support an estimate of their frequency. The most consistent adverse reactions are usually due to overdosage.
1. **Gastrointestinal:** nausea, vomiting, epigastric pain, hematemesis, diarrhea.
2. **Central nervous system:** headaches, irritability, restlessness, insomnia, reflex hyperexcitability, muscle twitching, clonic and tonic generalized convulsions.
3. **Cardiovascular:** palpitation, tachycardia, extrasystoles, flushing, hypotension, circulatory failure, ventricular arrhythmias.
4. **Respiratory:** tachypnea.
5. **Renal:** potentiation of diuresis.
6. **Others:** alopecia, hyperglycemia, inappropriate ADH syndrome, rash.

OVERDOSAGE

Management
It is suggested that the management principles (consistent with the clinical status of the patient when first seen) outlined below be instituted and that simultaneous contact with a Regional Poison Control Center be established. In this way both updated information and individualization regarding required therapy may be provided.
1. When potential oral overdose is established and seizure has not occurred:
   a) If patient is alert and seen within the early hours after ingestion, induction of emesis may be of value. Gastric lavage has been demonstrated to be of no value in influencing outcome in patients who present more than 1 hour after ingestion.
   b) Administer a cathartic. Sorbitol solution is reported to be of value.
   c) Administer repeated doses of activated charcoal and monitor theophylline serum levels.
   d) Prophylactic administration of phenobarbital has been shown to increase the seizure threshold in laboratory animals, and administration of this drug can be considered.
2. If patient presents with a seizure:
   a) Establish an airway.
   b) Administer oxygen.
   c) Treat the seizure with intravenous diazepam, 0.1 to 0.3 mg/kg, up to 10 mg. If seizures cannot be controlled, the use of general anesthesia should be considered.
   d) Monitor vital signs, maintain blood pressure, and provide adequate hydration.
3. If postseizure coma is present:
   a) Maintain airway and oxygenation.
   b) If a result of oral medication, follow above recommendations to prevent absorption of the drug, but intubation and lavage will have to be performed instead of inducing emesis, and the cathartic and charcoal will need to be introduced via a large bore gastric lavage tube.
   c) Continue to provide full supportive care and adequate hydration until the drug is metabolized. In general, drug metabolism is sufficiently rapid so as not to warrant dialysis. If repeated oral activated charcoal is ineffective (as noted by stable or rising serum levels) charcoal hemoperfusion may be indicated.

DOSAGE AND ADMINISTRATION
Effective use of theophylline, (ie, the concentration of drug in the serum associated with optimal benefit and minimal risk of toxicity) is considered to occur when the theophylline concentration is maintained from 10 to 20 $\mu g/mL$. The early studies from which these levels were derived were carried out in patients immediately or shortly after recovery from acute exacerbations of their disease (some hospitalized with status asthmaticus).

Although the 20 $\mu g/mL$ level remains appropriate as a critical value (above which toxicity is more likely to occur) for safety purposes, additional data are now available which indicate that the serum theophylline concentrations required to produce maximum physiologic benefit may, in fact, fluctuate with the degree of bronchospasm present and are variable. Therefore, the physician should individualize the range appropriate to the patient's requirements, based on both symptomatic response and improvement in pulmonary function. It should be stressed that serum theophylline concentrations maintained at the upper level of the 10 to 20 $\mu g/mL$ range may be associated with potential toxicity when factors known to reduce theophylline clearance are operative. (See WARNINGS.)

If it is not possible to obtain serum level determinations, restriction of the daily dose (in otherwise healthy adults) to not greater than 13 mg/kg/day, to a maximum of 900 mg, in divided doses will result in relatively few patients exceeding serum levels of 20 $\mu g/mL$ and the resultant greater risk of toxicity.

Caution should be exercised for younger children who cannot complain of minor side effects. Older adults, those with cor pulmonale, congestive heart failure, and/or liver disease may have unusually low dosage requirements and thus may experience toxicity at the maximal dosage recommended below.

Theophylline does not distribute into fatty tissue. Dosage should be calculated on the basis of lean (ideal) body weight where mg/kg doses are presented.

Frequency of Dosing: When immediate-release products with rapid absorption are used, dosing to maintain serum levels generally requires administration every 6 hours. This is particularly true in children, but dosing intervals up to 8 hours may be satisfactory in adults since they eliminate the drug at a slower rate. Some children, and adults requiring higher-than-average doses (those having rapid rates of clearance, eg, half-lives of under 6 hours), may benefit and be more effectively controlled during chronic therapy when given products with sustained-release characteristics since these provide longer dosing intervals and/or less fluctuation in serum concentration between dosing.

Dosage guidelines are approximations only and the wide range of theophylline clearance between individuals (particularly those with concomitant disease) makes indiscriminate usage hazardous.

Dosage Guidelines
I. Acute symptoms of bronchospasm requiring rapid attainment of theophylline serum levels for bronchodilation.

   NOTE: Status asthmaticus should be considered a medical emergency and is defined as that degree of bronchospasm which is not rapidly responsive to usual doses of conventional bronchodilators. Optimal therapy for such patients frequently requires both *additional medication,* parenterally administered, and *close monitoring,* preferably in an intensive care setting.

   A. Patients not currently receiving theophylline products.

	Theophylline Dosage Oral	
	Loading	Maintenance:
Children age: 6 to 9 years	5 mg/kg	4 mg/kg q.6 hours
Children age: 9 to 16 years and smokers	5 mg/kg	3 mg/kg q.6 hours
Otherwise healthy nonsmoking adults	5 mg/kg	3 mg/kg q.8 hours
Older patients and patients with cor pulmonale	5 mg/kg	2 mg/kg q.8 hours
Patients with congestive heart failure	5 mg/kg	1–2 mg/kg q.12 hours

   B. Patients currently receiving theophylline products: Determine, where possible, the time, amount, dosage form, and route of administration of the last dose the patient received.

   The loading dose for theophylline is based on the principle that each 0.5 mg/kg of theophylline administered as a loading dose will result in a 1.0 $\mu g/mL$ increase in serum theophylline concentration. Ideally, the loading dose should be deferred if a serum theophylline concentration can be obtained rapidly.

   If this is not possible, the clinician must exercise judgment in selecting a dose based on the potential for benefit and risk. When there is sufficient respiratory distress to warrant a small risk, then 2.5 mg/kg of theophylline administered in rapidly-absorbed form is likely to increase serum concentration by approximately 5 $\mu g/mL$. If the patient is not experiencing theophylline toxicity, this is unlikely to result in dangerous adverse effects.

   Subsequent to the decision regarding use of a loading dose for this group of patients, the maintenance dosage recommendations are the same as those described above.

II. Chronic Therapy
   Theophylline is a treatment for the management of reversible bronchospasm (asthma, chronic bronchitis and emphysema) to prevent symptoms and maintain patent airways. A dosage form which allows small incremental doses is desirable for initiating therapy. A liquid preparation should be considered for children to permit greater ease of and more accurate dosage adjustment. Slow clinical titration is generally preferred to assure acceptance and safety of the medication, and to allow the patient to develop tolerance to transient caffeine-like side effects.

Initial Dose:
16 mg/kg/24 hours or 400 mg/24 hours (whichever is less) of theophylline in divided doses at 6- or 8-hour intervals.

Increasing Dose:
The above dosage may be increased in approximately 25% increments at 3-day intervals so long as the drug is tolerated; until clinical response is satisfactory or the maximum dose as indicated in Section III (below) is reached. The serum concentration may be checked at

Continued on next page

Bristol Labs.—Cont.

these intervals, but at a minimum, should be determined at the end of this adjustment period.

It is important that no patient be maintained on any dosage that is not tolerated. When instructing patients to increase dosage according to the schedule above, they should be told not to take a subsequent dose if apparent side effects occur and to resume therapy at a lower dose once adverse effects have disappeared.

III. Maximum Dose of Theophylline Where the Serum Concentration is Not Measured

WARNING: DO NOT ATTEMPT TO MAINTAIN ANY DOSE THAT IS NOT TOLERATED.

Not to exceed the following: (or 900 mg, whichever is less)

Age 6–9 years	24 mg/kg/day
Age 9–12 years	20 mg/kg/day
Age 12–16 years	18 mg/kg/day
Age 16 years and older	13 mg/kg/day

IV. Measurement of Serum Theophylline Concentrations During Chronic Therapy:

If the above maximum doses are to be maintained or exceeded, serum theophylline measurement is essential. (See PRECAUTIONS, Laboratory Tests, for guidance).

V. Final Adjustment of Dosage:

Dosage adjustment after serum theophylline measurement

[See table below].

The serum concentration may be rechecked at appropriate intervals, but at least at the end of any adjustment period. When the patient's condition is otherwise clinically stable and none of the recognized factors which alter elimination are present, measurement of serum levels need be repeated only every 6 to 12 months.

DOSAGE OF THEOPHYLLINE TO PROVIDE mg ANHYDROUS THEOPHYLLINE/kg BODY WEIGHT*/DOSE

Body Weight*		Approximate Dose in mg		
Lbs.	kg	3 mg/kg	4 mg/kg	5 mg/kg
40	18	54	72	90
60	27	81	108	135
70	32	96	128	160
80	36	108	144	180
90	41	123	164	205
100	45	135	180	225
120	55	165	220	275
140	64	192		320
160	73	219		365
180	82	246		410
200	91	273		455
220	100	300		500

* For obese patients, use lean (ie, ideal) body weight.

HOW SUPPLIED

QUIBRON-T Tablets: Ivory, in the Dividose® tablet design with debossed "BL" logo and "512" on one side containing 300 mg anhydrous theophylline.

NDC 0087-0512-41	Bottles of 100
NDC 0087-0512-44	Bottles of 500

Store below 86°F (30°C).

Shown in Product Identification Section, page 406

QUIBRON®–T/SR   ℞

[kwi'bran]
(Theophylline Anhydrous)
DIVIDOSE® TABLETS
SUSTAINED RELEASE BRONCHODILATOR

DESCRIPTION

QUIBRON-T/SR tablets provide 300 mg of anhydrous theophylline as an oral bronchodilator in a sustained release formulation combined with the convenience of the unique Dividose® tablet design. With functional trisects and bisects, QUIBRON-T/SR tablets can be conveniently and accurately divided into 100, 150, and 200 mg segments to provide a variety of dosing increments, as required.

QUIBRON-T/SR tablets	
One-third tablet	= 100 mg
One-half tablet	= 150 mg
Two-thirds tablet	= 200 mg
One tablet	= 300 mg

If serum theophylline is:		Directions:
Within desired range		Maintain dosage if tolerated.
Too high	20 to 25 µg/mL	Decrease doses by about 10% and recheck serum level after 3 days.
	25 to 30 µg/mL	Skip the next dose and decrease subsequent doses by about 25%. Recheck serum level after 3 days.
	Over 30 µg/mL	Skip next 2 doses and decrease subsequent doses by 50%. Recheck serum level after 3 days.
Too low		Increase dosage by 25% at 3-day intervals until either the desired serum concentration and/or clinical response is achieved. The total daily dose may need to be administered at more frequent intervals if symptoms occur repeatedly at the end of a dosing interval.

Theophylline is a white odorless crystalline powder which has a bitter taste. It is chemically related to caffeine and its structure is shown below:

Theophylline
(1*H*-Purine-2,6-dione,3,7-dihydro-1,3-dimethyl-)

This product contains the following inactive ingredient: magnesium stearate.

CLINICAL PHARMACOLOGY

Mode of Action

Theophylline acts as a bronchodilator by direct relaxation of bronchial smooth muscle. Theophylline is a competitive inhibitor of cyclic nucleotide phosphodiesterase resulting in increased intracellular levels of cAMP which mediates smooth muscle relaxation. Like some other xanthines, theophylline acts as a coronary vasodilator, cardiac stimulant, skeletal muscle stimulant, cerebral stimulant and diuretic. *In vitro*, theophylline has been shown to act synergistically with beta agonists that increase intracellular cyclic AMP through the stimulation of adenyl cyclase, but synergism has not been demonstrated in patient studies. More data are needed to determine if theophylline and beta agonists have a clinically important additive effect *in vivo*. Apparently, no development of tolerance occurs with chronic use of theophylline.

Pharmacokinetics

Theophylline excretion, principally as inactive metabolites, occurs primarily via the kidney. The half-life of theophylline varies among individuals with a wide range having been documented. Theophylline half-life is shorter in cigarette smokers. Half-life is prolonged in alcoholism, reduced hepatic or renal function, congestive heart failure and in patients receiving macrolide antibiotics (troleandomycin and erythromycin) or cimetidine. High fever for prolonged periods may decrease theophylline elimination. Older adults (over age 55) and patients with chronic obstructive pulmonary disease, with or without cor pulmonale, may have much slower clearance rates. For such patients, the theophylline half-life may exceed 24 hours. The theophylline half-life is generally shorter in children.

It appears that between three months and two years of cessation of smoking may be necessary for elimination of the effect of smoking on theophylline pharmacokinetics.

Representative Theophylline Serum Half-lives

	Half-life (hours)	
	Mean	Range
Adults		
non-smokers	8.7	6.1–12.8
smokers	5.5	4.0–7.7
congestive heart failure	22.9	3.1–82.0
Children (6–16 years)	3.7	1.4–7.9

Therapeutic serum theophylline levels are usually 10–20 µg/mL.

Binding to plasma proteins is not extensive and theophylline is not preferentially taken up by any particular organ.

Theophylline-containing products may increase the plasma levels of free fatty acids and the urinary levels of epinephrine and norepinephrine.

Apparently no development of tolerance occurs with chronic use of theophylline.

In a single-dose study of QUIBRON-T/SR, a 300 mg dose in 12 fasted normal male subjects gave a mean peak plasma level of 5.26 ± 1.04 (S.D.) µg/mL at 6.25 ± 1.10 (S.D.) hours. In a multi-dose, steady state study of 16 adult patients with a mean age of 39.0 years, the patients were dose-titrated to a therapeutically effective level without toxicity. Doses were administered once every 12 hours and ranged from 7.8 mg/kg/24 hours to 18.6 mg/kg/24 hours with a mean dose of 10.0 ± 2.8 (S.D.) mg/kg/24 hours. No food-fasting conditions

---

were imposed in the study. A mean C_{max} of 13.9 ± 3.2 (S.D.) µg/mL, a mean C_{min} of 7.7 ± 2.0 (S.D.) µg/mL, and a mean percent fluctuation of 87.1 ± 49.6 (S.D.) resulted from the study.

In a multi-dose, steady state study of 15 patients with a mean age of 14.4 years, the patients were dose-titrated to a therapeutically effective level without toxicity. Doses were administered once every 12 hours and ranged from 9.1 mg/kg/24 hours to 22.6 mg/kg/24 hours with a mean dose of 13.3 ± 3.9 (S.D.) mg/kg/24 hours. No food-fasting conditions were imposed in the study. A mean C_{max} of 13.8 ± 3.9 (S.D.) µg/mL, a mean C_{min} of 8.0 ± 2.5 (S.D.) µg/mL, and a mean percent fluctuation of 85.4 ± 57.7 (S.D.) resulted from the study.

INDICATIONS AND USAGE

QUIBRON-T/SR tablets are indicated for relief and/or prevention of symptoms from asthma and reversible bronchospasm associated with chronic bronchitis and emphysema.

CONTRAINDICATIONS

QUIBRON-T/SR tablets are contraindicated in individuals who have shown hypersensitivity to any of its components or xanthine derivatives.

WARNINGS

Excessive theophylline doses may be associated with toxicity; thus serum theophylline levels should be monitored to assure maximal benefit without excessive risk.

Status asthmaticus should be considered a medical emergency and is defined as that degree of bronchospasm which is not rapidly responsive to usual doses of conventional bronchodilators. Optimal therapy for such patients frequently requires both *additional medication*, parenterally administered, and *close monitoring*, preferably in an intensive care setting.

Although increasing the dose of theophylline may bring about relief, such treatment may be associated with toxicity. The likelihood of the development of such toxicity increases significantly when the serum theophylline concentration exceeds 20 µg/mL. Therefore, determination of serum theophylline levels is recommended to assure maximal benefit without excessive risk.

Serum levels above 20 µg/mL are rarely found after appropriate administration of the recommended doses. However, in individuals in whom theophylline plasma clearance is reduced for any reason, even conventional doses may result in increased serum levels and potential toxicity. Reduced theophylline clearance has been documented in the following readily identifiable groups: 1) patients with impaired renal or liver function; 2) patients over 55 years of age, particularly males and those with chronic lung disease; 3) those with cardiac failure from any cause; 4) neonates; and 5) those patients taking certain drugs (macrolide antibiotics and cimetidine). Decreased clearance of theophylline may be associated with either influenza immunization or active influenza infection. Reduction in dosage and laboratory monitoring are especially appropriate in the above individuals. Serious toxic side effects, such as seizure, ventricular arrhythmia, or even death, are not necessarily preceded by less serious side effects such as nausea, irritability, or restlessness. Many patients who have higher (> 20 µg/mL) theophylline serum levels exhibit tachycardia. Theophylline products may cause dysrhythmia and/or worsen pre-existing arrhythmias. Any significant change in heart rate and/or rhythm warrants monitoring and further investigation.

PRECAUTIONS

General

QUIBRON-T/SR tablets should not be chewed or crushed. Use with caution in neonates, the elderly (especially males), and in patients with severe cardiac disease, hypertension, acute myocardial injury, congestive heart failure, cor pulmonale, severe hypoxemia, hyperthyroidism, hepatic impairment, history of peptic ulcer or alcoholism.

Concurrent administration with certain antibiotics (see DRUG INTERACTIONS section) may result in increased serum theophylline levels.

A decrease in serum half-life is seen in smokers (see Clinical Pharmacology/Pharmacokinetics).

Particular caution should be used in administering theophylline to patients in congestive heart failure. Reduced theophylline clearance in these patients may cause theophylline blood levels to persist long after discontinuing the drug.

Theophylline should not be administered concurrently with other xanthine medications.

Use theophylline cautiously in patients with a history of peptic ulcer. Theophylline may occasionally act as a local irritant to the GI tract, although gastrointestinal symptoms are more commonly centrally mediated and associated with serum drug concentrations over 20 µg/mL.

Sustained release theophylline is not useful in status asthmaticus.

Information for Patients

Patients should be instructed carefully on how to divide QUIBRON-T/SR tablets along the appropriate tablet score.

The physician should reinforce the importance of taking only the prescribed dose and observing the correct time interval between doses.

The patient should alert the physician if symptoms occur repeatedly, especially near the end of a dosing interval.

Drug Interactions

Drug—Drug: Toxic synergism with ephedrine has been documented and may occur with some other sympathomimetic bronchodilators. In addition, the following drug interactions have been demonstrated:

Drug	Effect
Theophylline with lithium carbonate	Increased renal excretion of lithium
Theophylline with propranolol	Mutual antagonism of therapeutic effects
Theophylline with cimetidine	Increased serum theophylline levels
Theophylline with troleandomycin or erythromycin	Increased serum theophylline levels

Drug—Food: QUIBRON-T/SR has not been adequately studied to determine whether its bioavailability is altered when it is given with food.

Available data suggests that drug administration at the time of food ingestion may influence the absorption characteristics of some or all theophylline controlled-release products, resulting in serum values different from those found after administration in the fasting state.

A drug-food effect, if any, would likely have its greatest clinical significance when high theophylline serum levels are being maintained and/or when large single doses (>13 mg/kg or 900 mg) of a controlled-release theophylline product are given. The influence of type and amount of food on performance of controlled-release theophylline products is under study at this time.

Drug-Laboratory Test Interactions:
Spectrophotometric determination of theophylline is affected by coffee, tea, cola beverages, chocolate, and acetaminophen, which contribute to falsely high values.

Carcinogenesis, Mutagenesis, and Impairment of Fertility

Long-term animal studies have not been performed to evaluate the carcinogenic potential, mutagenic potential, or the effect on fertility of xanthine compounds.

Usage in Pregnancy

Teratogenic Effects
Pregnancy Category C. Animal reproduction studies have not been conducted with QUIBRON-T/SR. It is also not known whether QUIBRON-T/SR tablets can cause fetal harm when administered to a pregnant woman or can affect reproduction capacity. QUIBRON-T/SR tablets should be given to a pregnant woman only if clearly indicated.

Nonteratogenic Effects
It is not known whether use of this drug during labor or delivery has immediate or delayed adverse effects on the fetus, or whether it prolongs the duration of labor or increases the possibility of forceps delivery or other obstetrical intervention.

Nursing Mothers

Theophylline has been reported to be excreted in human milk and to have caused irritability in a nursing infant. Because of the potential for serious adverse reactions, a decision should be made whether to discontinue nursing or to discontinue QUIBRON-T/SR tablets, taking into account the importance of this drug to the mother.

Pediatric Use

Safety and effectiveness in children under 6 years of age have not been established with this product.

ADVERSE REACTIONS

The frequency of adverse reactions is related to serum theophylline levels and is usually not a problem at levels below 20 μg/mL. The most consistent adverse reactions are usually due to overdosage and, while not all have not been reported with QUIBRON-T and/or with QUIBRON-T/SR tablets, the following reactions may be considered when theophylline is administered. Central nervous system: clonic and tonic generalized convulsions, muscle twitching, reflex hyperexcitability, headaches, insomnia, restlessness, and irritability. Cardiovascular: circulatory failure, ventricular arrhythmias, hypotension, extrasystoles, tachycardia, palpitation, and flushing. Gastrointestinal: hematemesis, vomiting, diarrhea, epigastric pain, and nausea. Renal: increased excretion of renal tubular cells and red blood cells, albuminuria, and diuresis. Respiratory: tachypnea. Others: hyperglycemia and inappropriate ADH syndrome, and rash.

OVERDOSAGE

Symptoms

Nervousness, agitation, headache, insomnia, nausea, vomiting, tachycardia, extrasystoles, hyperreflexia, fasciculations and clonic and tonic convulsions. Children may be particularly prone to restlessness and hyperactivity that can proceed to convulsions.

If serum theophylline level is:		Directions:
Within normal limits	10 to 20 μg/mL	Maintain dosage if tolerated. Recheck serum theophylline concentration at 6- to 12-month intervals.*
Too high	20 to 25 μg/mL	Decrease doses by about 10%. Recheck serum theophylline concentration at 6- to 12-month intervals.*
	25 to 30 μg/mL	Skip next dose and decrease subsequent doses by about 25%.
	Over 30 μg/mL	Skip next 2 doses and decrease subsequent doses by 50%. Recheck serum theophylline.
Too low	7.5 to 10 μg/mL	Increase dose by about 25%. Recheck serum theophylline concentration at 6- to 12-month intervals.**
	5 to 7.5 μg/mL	Increase dose by about 25% to the nearest dose increment and recheck serum theophylline for guidance in further dosage adjustment (another increase will probably be needed, but this provides a safety check).

* Finer adjustments may be needed for some patients.
** Dividing the daily dosage into 3 doses administered at 8 hour intervals may be indicated if symptoms occur repeatedly at the end of a dosing interval.
From the Journal of Respiratory Diseases 2(7): 16, 1981.

Management

If potential oral overdose is established and seizure has *not* occurred:
1. Induce vomiting.
2. Administer a cathartic (this is particularly important if a sustained release preparation has been taken).
3. Administer activated charcoal.
4. Monitor vital signs, maintain blood pressure and provide adequate hydration.

If patient is having a seizure:
1. Establish an airway.
2. Administer O₂.
3. Treat the seizure with intravenous diazepam 0.1 to 0.3 mg/kg up to a total dose of 10 mg.
4. Monitor vital signs, maintain blood pressure and provide adequate hydration.

Post-seizure Coma:
1. Maintain airway and oxygenation.
2. If the reaction occurs after oral medication, follow above recommendations to prevent absorption of drug, but intubation and lavage will have to be performed instead of inducing emesis and the cathartic and charcoal will need to be introduced via a large bore gastric lavage tube.
3. Continue to provide full supportive care and adequate hydration while waiting for drug to be metabolized. In general, the drug is metabolized sufficiently rapidly enough so as to not warrant consideration of dialysis, however, if serum levels exceed 50 μg/mL, charcoal hemoperfusion may be indicated.

General

The oral LD₅₀ of theophylline in mice is 350 mg/kg. In humans, adverse reactions often occur when serum theophylline levels exceed 20 μg/mL. Information on physiological variables which influence excretion of theophylline can be found under the heading "Clinical Pharmacology."

DOSAGE AND ADMINISTRATION

General

QUIBRON-T/SR has not been adequately studied for its bioavailability when administered with food (see PRECAUTIONS, DRUG-FOOD INTERACTIONS).

Therapeutic serum levels associated with optimal likelihood for benefit and minimal risk of toxicity are considered to be between 10 μg/mL and 20 μg/mL. Levels above 20 μg/mL may produce toxic effects and, in a small number of patients, toxicity may even be seen with serum levels between 15–20 μg/mL, particularly during initiation of therapy. Because of the variable rates of theophylline elimination among patients, the dose necessary to achieve the desired serum level of 10–20 μg theophylline per mL varies from patient to patient. Therefore, it is essential that not only must dosage be individualized, but titration and monitoring of serum levels be utilized where available.

When serum concentrations cannot be obtained, restriction of dosage to amounts and intervals recommended in the guidelines listed below becomes essential.

Since theophylline does not distribute into fatty tissue, dosage should be calculated on the basis of ideal body weight.

Acute Symptoms

QUIBRON-T/SR is not intended for use in status asthmaticus or with patients experiencing an acute episode of bronchospasm (associated with asthma, chronic bronchitis, or emphysema). Such patients require rapid relief of symptoms and should be treated with an immediate-release or intravenous theophylline preparation (or other bronchodilators) and not with controlled-release products.

Chronic therapy

It is recommended that the appropriate dosage be established using an immediate-release preparation. Slow clinical titration is generally preferred to help assure acceptance and safety of the medication, and to allow the patient to develop tolerance to transient caffeine-like side effects. For children under 25 kg, proper dosage should be established with a liquid preparation to permit titration in small increments. Then, the patient can usually be switched to

QUIBRON-T/SR, giving one-half of the daily dose at 12-hour intervals. However, certain patients, such as the young, smokers, and some non-smoking adults, are likely to metabolize theophylline rapidly and require dosing at eight-hour intervals. Such patients can generally be identified as having trough serum concentrations lower than desired or repeatedly exhibiting symptoms near the end of the dosage interval.

The average initial adult and children's (over 25 kg) dose is two-thirds (200 mg) of a QUIBRON-T/SR tablet q.12 h

If the desired response is not achieved with the recommended initial dose, and there are no adverse reactions, the dose may be cautiously adjusted upward in increments of no more than 25 percent at 3 day intervals until the following MAXIMUM DOSE WITHOUT MEASUREMENT OF SERUM CONCENTRATION or, in the case of adults, a maximum of 900 mg in any 24 hour period (whichever is less) is attained.

Following each adjustment, if the clinical response is satisfactory, that dosage level should be maintained.

MAXIMUM DOSE WITHOUT MEASUREMENT OF SERUM CONCENTRATION

	mg per kg Body Weight* per day
Children (under 9)	24
Children (9–12)	20
Adolescents (12–16)	18
Adults	13 (or 900 mg, whichever is less)

*Use ideal body weight for obese patients.

Do not attempt to maintain any dose that is not tolerated. If doses higher than those contained in the above MAXIMUM DOSE WITHOUT MEASUREMENT OF SERUM CONCENTRATION are necessary, it is recommended that serum theophylline levels be monitored. For therapeutic levels, draw blood sample when last dose peaks (4–5 hours after dosing). It is important that the patient has missed no doses during the previous 72 hours and that dosing intervals have been reasonably typical with no doses added during that period of time. DOSE ADJUSTMENT BASED ON SERUM THEOPHYLLINE MEASUREMENTS MADE WHEN THESE INSTRUCTIONS HAVE **NOT** BEEN FOLLOWED, MAY RESULT IN RECOMMENDATIONS THAT PRESENT RISK OF TOXICITY TO THE PATIENT.

[See table above].

Caution should be exercised for younger children who cannot complain of minor side effects. Older adults, those with cor pulmonale, congestive heart failure, and/or liver disease may have unusually low dosage requirements and thus may experience toxicity at the maximal dosage recommended above.

It is important that no patient be maintained on any dosage that is not tolerated. In instructing patients to increase dosage according to the schedule above, they should be instructed not to take a subsequent dose if apparent side effects occur and to resume therapy at a lower dose once adverse effects have disappeared.

HOW SUPPLIED

QUIBRON-T/SR tablets (white, in the Dividose® tablet design) containing 300 mg anhydrous theophylline.

NDC-0087-0519-41	Bottles of 100
NDC 0087-0519-44	Bottles of 500

Store below 86°F (30°C).
Patent Nos. 4,465,660, 4,547,358, 4,215,104

Shown in Product Identification Section, page 407

Continued on next page

Bristol Labs.—Cont.

SALURON® ℞
[săl-ū-rŏn]
(hydroflumethiazide)

DESCRIPTION
SALURON (hydroflumethiazide) is a potent oral diuretic-antihypertensive agent of low toxicity. Each tablet contains 50 mg hydroflumethiazide.
SALURON is 3,4-hydro-7-sulfamyl-6-trifluoromethyl-1,2,4-benzothiadiazine 1,1-dioxide. Hydroflumethiazide is very slightly soluble in water, soluble in methanol and freely soluble in acetone. Inactive ingredients in SALURON tablets are: cellulose microcrystalline, lactose, magnesium stearate, silicon dioxide colloidal and sodium starch glycolate. It has the following structural formula:

CLINICAL PHARMACOLOGY
Hydroflumethiazide is incompletely but fairly rapidly absorbed from the gastrointestinal tract. It appears to have a biphasic biological half-life with an estimated alpha-phase of about 2 hours and an estimated beta-phase of about 17 hours; it has a metabolite with a longer half-life, which is extensively bound to the red blood cells. Hydroflumethiazide is excreted in the urine; its metabolite has also been detected in the urine.
The mechanism of action results in an interference with the renal tubular mechanism of electrolyte reabsorption. At maximal therapeutic dosage all thiazides are approximately equal in their diuretic potency. The mechanism whereby thiazides function in the control of hypertension is unknown.

INDICATIONS AND USAGE
SALURON is indicated as adjunctive therapy in edema associated with congestive heart failure, hepatic cirrhosis, and corticosteroid and estrogen therapy.
SALURON has also been found useful in edema due to various forms of renal dysfunction such as nephrotic syndrome, acute glomerulonephritis, and chronic renal failure.
SALURON is indicated in the management of hypertension either as the sole therapeutic agent or to enhance the effectiveness of other antihypertensive drugs in the more severe forms of hypertension.
Usage in Pregnancy—The routine use of diuretics in an otherwise healthy woman is inappropriate and exposes mother and fetus to unnecessary hazard. Diuretics do not prevent development of toxemia of pregnancy, and there is no satisfactory evidence that they are useful in the treatment of developed toxemia.
Edema during pregnancy may arise from pathological causes or from the physiologic and mechanical consequences of pregnancy. Thiazides are indicated in pregnancy when edema is due to pathologic causes, just as they are in the absence of pregnancy (however, see **Precautions,** Pregnancy below). Dependent edema in pregnancy, resulting from restriction of venous return by the expanded uterus, is properly treated through elevation of the lower extremities and use of support hose; use of diuretics to lower intravascular volume in this case is illogical and unnecessary. There is hypervolemia during normal pregnancy which is harmful to neither the fetus nor the mother (in the absence of cardiovascular disease), but which is associated with edema, including generalized edema, in the majority of pregnant women. If this edema produces discomfort, increased recumbency will often provide relief. In rare instances, this edema may cause extreme discomfort which is not relieved by rest. In these cases, a short course of diuretics may provide relief and may be appropriate.

CONTRAINDICATIONS
SALURON is contraindicated in patients with anuria or hypersensitivity to this or other sulfonamide derived drugs.

WARNINGS
SALURON should be used with caution in severe renal disease. In patients with renal disease, thiazide may precipitate azotemia. Cumulative effects of the drug may develop in patients with impaired renal function.
Thiazides should be used with caution in patients with impaired hepatic function or progressive liver disease, since minor alterations of fluid and electrolyte balance may precipitate hepatic coma.
Thiazides may be additive or potentiative of the action of other antihypertensive drugs. Potentiation occurs with ganglionic or peripheral adrenergic blocking drugs.
Sensitivity reactions may occur in patients with a history of allergy or bronchial asthma.
The possibility of exacerbation or activation of systemic lupus erythematosus has been reported.

PRECAUTIONS
General—All patients receiving thiazide therapy should be observed for clinical signs of fluid or electrolyte imbalance; namely, hyponatremia, hypochloremic alkalosis, and hypokalemia. Serum and urine electrolyte determinations are particularly important when the patient is vomiting excessively or receiving parenteral fluids. Medication such as digitalis may also influence serum electrolytes. Warning signs, irrespective of cause, are: dryness of mouth, thirst, weakness, lethargy, drowsiness, restlessness, muscle pains or cramps, muscular fatigue, hypotension, oliguria, tachycardia, and gastrointestinal disurbances such as nausea and vomiting.
Hypokalemia may develop with thiazides as with any other potent diuretic, especially with brisk diuresis, when severe cirrhosis is present, or during concomitant use of corticosteroids or ACTH.
Interference with adequate oral electrolyte intake will also contribute to hypokalemia. Digitalis therapy may exaggerate metabolic effects of hypokalemia especially with reference to myocardial activity.
Any chloride deficit is generally mild and usually does not require specific treatment except under extraordinary circumstances (as in liver disease or renal disease). Dilutional hyponatremia may occur in edematous patients in hot weather; appropriate therapy is water restriction, rather than administration of salt except in rare instances when the hyponatremia is life-threatening. In actual salt depletion, appropriate replacement is the therapy of choice.
Hyperuricemia may occur or frank gout may be precipitated in certain patients receiving thiazide therapy.
Insulin requirements in diabetic patients may be increased, decreased, or unchanged. Latent diabetes mellitus may become manifested during thiazide administration.
The antihypertensive effects of the drug may be enhanced in the postsympathectomy patient.
If progressive renal impairment becomes evident, as indicated by a rising creatinine or blood urea nitrogen, a careful reappraisal of therapy is necessary with consideration given to withholding or discontinuing diuretic therapy.
Thiazides may decrease serum PBI levels without signs of thyroid disturbance.
Lithium generally should not be given with diuretics because they reduce its renal clearance and increase the risk of lithium toxicity. Read circulars for lithium preparations before use of such concomitant therapy with "SALURON."
Thiazides have been shown to increase the urinary excretion of magnesium; this may result in hypomagnesemia.
Calcium excretion is decreased by thiazides. Pathological changes in the parathyroid gland with hypercalcemia and hypophosphatemia have been observed in a few patients on prolonged thiazide therapy. The common complications of hyperparathyroidism such as renal lithiasis, bone resorption and peptic ulceration have not been seen.
Information for Patients—This medicine may cause a loss of potassium from your body. To help prevent this, your doctor may want you to:
- eat or drink foods that have a high potassium content (for example, orange or other citrus fruit juices), or
- take a potassium supplement, or
- take another medicine to help prevent the loss of the potassium in the first place.
It is very important to follow these directions. Also, it is important not to change your diet on your own. This is more important if you are already on a special diet (as for diabetes), or if you are taking a potassium supplement or a medicine to reduce potassium loss. Extra potassium may not be necessary and, in some cases, too much potassium could be harmful.
Check with your doctor if you become sick and have severe or continuing vomiting or diarrhea. These problems may cause you to lose additional water and potassium.

Caution: Diabetics—Thiazide diuretics may raise blood sugar levels. While you are using this medicine, be especially careful in testing for sugar in your urine. If you have any questions about this, check with your doctor.
A few people who take this medicine may become more sensitive to sunlight than they are normally. When you begin to take this medicine, avoid too much sun or use of a sunlamp until you see how you react, especially if you tend to burn easily. If you have a severe reaction, check with your doctor.
For patients taking this medicine for high blood pressure:
- **Do not take other medicines unless they have been discussed with your doctor.** This especially includes over-the-counter (nonprescription) medicines for appetite control, asthma, colds, cough, hay fever, or sinus.

Abstracted from USP DI "Advice for the Patient"
©1984 USP Convention: permission granted.

Laboratory Tests—Periodic determination of serum electrolytes to detect possible electrolyte imbalance should be performed at appropriate intervals.

Drug Interactions—Anticoagulants, oral
(effects may be decreased when used concurrently with thiazide diuretics; dosage adjustments may be necessary)
Antigout medications
(thiazide diuretics may raise the level of blood uric acid; dosage adjustment of antigout medications may be necessary to control hyperuricemia and gout)
Antihypertensive medications, other, especially diazoxide, or Preanesthetic and anesthetic agents used in surgery or Skeletal muscle relaxants, nondepolarizing, used in surgery
(effects may be potentiated when used concurrently with thiazide diuretics; dosage adjustments may be necessary)
Amphotericin B or Corticosteroids or Corticotropin (ACTH)
(concurrent use with thiazide diuretics may intensify electrolyte imbalance, particularly hypokalemia)
Cardiac glycosides
(concurrent use with thiazide diuretics may enhance the possibility of digitalis toxicity associated with hypokalemia)
Colestipol
(may inhibit gastrointestinal absorption of the thiazide diuretics; administration 1 hour before or 4 hours after colestipol is recommended)
Hypoglycemics
(thiazide diuretics may raise blood glucose levels; for adult-onset diabetics, dosage adjustment of hypoglycemic medications may be necessary during and after thiazide diuretic therapy; insulin requirements may be increased, decreased, or unchanged)
Lithium salts
(concurrent use with thiazide diuretics is not recommended, as they may provoke lithium toxicity because of reduced renal clearance)
Methenamine
(effectiveness may be decreased when used concurrently with thiazide diuretics because of alkalinization of the urine)
Nonsteroidal anti-inflammatory agents (in some patients, the steroidal anti-inflammatory agent can reduce the diuretic, natriuretic, and antihypertensive effects of loop, potassium sparing and thiazide diuretics. Therefore, when hydroflumethiazide and nonsteroidal anti-inflammatory agents are used concomitantly, the patient should be observed closely to determine if the desired effect of the diuretic is obtained.)
Norepinephrine (thiazides may decrease arterial responsiveness to norepinephrine. This diminution is not sufficient to preclude effectiveness of the pressor agent for therapeutic use.)
Tubocurarine (thiazide drugs may increase the responsiveness to tubocurarine.)
Diagnostic Interference—With expected physiologic effects
Blood and urine glucose levels (usually only in patients with a predisposition to glucose intolerance) and
Serum bilirubin levels (by displacement from albumin binding) and
Serum calcium levels (thiazide diuretics should be discontinued before parathyroid function tests are carried out) and
Serum uric acid levels (may be increased)
Serum magnesium, potassium, and sodium levels (may be decreased; serum magnesium levels may increase in uremic patients)
Serum protein-bound iodine (PBI) levels (may be decreased). Thiazides should be discontinued before carrying out tests for parathyroid function (see PRECAUTIONS, General, calcium excretion).
Carcinogenesis, Mutagenesis, Impairment of Fertility—No studies have been performed to evaluate carcinogenic or mutagenic potential of SALURON or the potential of SALURON to impair fertility.
Pregnancy:—*Teratogenic Effects—Pregnancy Category C.* Animal reproduction studies have not been conducted with SALURON. It is also not known whether SALURON can cause fetal harm when administered to a pregnant woman or can affect reproduction capacity. SALURON should be given to a pregnant woman only if clearly needed. *Nonteratogenic Effects*— Fetal or neonatal jaundice, thrombocytopenia and possibly other adverse reactions which have occurred in the adult.
Nursing Mothers—Thiazides appear in breast milk. If use of the drug is deemed essential, the patient may consider stopping nursing.
Pediatric Use—Safety and effectiveness in children have not been established.

ADVERSE REACTIONS
The following adverse reactions have been observed, but there is not enough systematic collection of data to support an estimate of their frequency.
A. Gastrointestinal system reactions: Anorexia, gastric irritation, nausea, vomiting, cramping, diarrhea, constipation, jaundice (intrahepatic cholestatic jaundice), pancreatitis.

B. Central nervous system reactions: Dizziness, vertigo, parathesias, headache, xanthopsia.

C. Hematologic reactions: Leukopenia, agranulocytosis, thrombocytopenia, aplastic anemia.

D. Dermatologic-Hypersensitivity reactions: Purpura, photosensitivity, rash, urticaria, necrotizing angiitis (vasculitis) (cutaneous vasculitis).

E. Cardiovascular reaction: Orthostatic hypotension may occur and may be aggravated by alcohol, barbiturates, or narcotics.

F. Other: Hyperglycemia; glycosuria, hyperuricemia, muscle spasm, weakness, restlessness.

Whenever adverse reactions are moderate or severe, thiazide dosage should be reduced or therapy withdrawn.

OVERDOSAGE

Signs and Symptoms—Diuresis, lethargy progressing to coma, with minimal cardiorespiratory depression and with or without significant serum electrolyte changes or dehydration; GI irritation; hypermotility; transient elevation in BUN level.

Treatment—Empty stomach by gastric lavage, taking care to avoid aspiration. Monitor serum electrolyte levels and renal function, and institute supportive measures, as required to maintain hydration, electrolyte balance, respiration, and cardiovascular and renal function. Treat GI effects symptomatically.

DOSAGE AND ADMINISTRATION

The average adult diuretic dose is 25 to 200 mg per day. The average adult antihypertensive dose is 50 to 100 mg per day. Therapy should be individualized according to patient response. This therapy should be titrated to gain maximal therapeutic response as well as the minimal dose possible to maintain that therapeutic response.

HOW SUPPLIED

NDC 0015-5410—SALURON Tablets, scored, 50 mg.
Store at room temperature (approximately 25°C).
For information on package sizes available, refer to the current price schedule.

PHYSICIAN REFERENCES

1. USP DI ©1984 USP Convention.
Shown in Product Identification Section, page 407

SALUTENSIN®   ℞
SALUTENSIN–DEMI®
[săl-ū-těn 'sĭn]
(Hydroflumethiazide, Reserpine Antihypertensive Formulation)

> **WARNING**
>
> This fixed combination drug is not indicated for initial therapy of hypertension. Hypertension requires therapy titrated to the individual patient. If the fixed combination represents the dosage so determined, its use may be more convenient in patient management. The treatment of hypertension is not static, but must be reevaluated as conditions in each patient warrant.

DESCRIPTION

Salutensin tablets for oral administration combine two antihypertensive agents: Saluron® (hydroflumethiazide) and reserpine. The chemical name for hydroflumethiazide is 3,4-dihydro-7-sulfamyl-6-trifluoromethyl-2H-1,2,4-benzothiadiazine-1,1-dioxide. Hydroflumethiazide is very slightly soluble in water, soluble in methanol and freely soluble in acetone. It has the following structural formula:

Hydroflumethiazide

Reserpine (3,4,5-trimethoxybenzoyl methyl reserpate) is a crystalline alkaloid derived from Rauwolfia serpentina. It is very slightly soluble in water, slightly soluble in acetone, methanol and ethanol and freely soluble in chloroform and methylene chloride. It has the following structural formula:

Reserpine

Each Salutensin tablet contains:

Saluron (hydroflumethiazide)	50 mg.
Reserpine	0.125 mg.

Each Salutensin-Demi tablet contains:

Saluron (hydroflumethiazide)	25 mg.
Reserpine	0.125 mg.

Inactive ingredients in Salutensin tablets are: D&C Yellow No. 10 Lake, FD&C Blue 1 Lake 12%, lactose, magnesium stearate, povidone, starch and sucrose.

Inactive ingredients in Salutensin-Demi tablets are: D&C Red No. 30 Lake, D&C Yellow No. 10 Lake, lactose, magnesium stearate, povidone, starch and sucrose.

CLINICAL PHARMACOLOGY

Hydroflumethiazide is incompletely but fairly rapidly absorbed from the gastrointestinal tract. It appears to have a biphasic biological half-life with an estimated alpha-phase of about 2 hours and an estimated beta-phase of about 17 hours; it has a metabolite with a longer half-life, which is extensively bound to the red blood cells. Hydroflumethiazide is excreted in the urine; its metabolite has also been detected in the urine.

Hydroflumethiazide is an oral diuretic-antihypertensive agent. It exerts its effect by inhibiting renal tubular reabsorption, including increased excretion of sodium and chloride and water with variable concomitant loss of potassium and bicarbonate as well. When used alone as an antihypertensive agent, hydroflumethiazide usually induces a gradual but sustained decrease in abnormally elevated blood-pressure—both systolic and diastolic. Hypertensive patients who have been maintained on chlorothiazide or hydrochlorothiazide may also be maintained on hydroflumethiazide.

Reserpine is absorbed from the gastrointestinal tract. About 6% has been reported to be excreted in the urine in the first 24 hours and about 8% in the first 4 days, mainly as the metabolite trimethoxybenzoic acid. Over 60% is excreted in the faeces in the first 4 days, mainly unchanged. Reserpine crosses the placental barrier and also appears in breast milk. The component, reserpine, probably produces its antihypertensive effects through depletion of tissue stores of catecholamines (epinephrine and norepinephrine) from peripheral sites. By contrast, its sedative and tranquilizing properties are thought to be related to depletion of 5-hydroxytryptamine from the brain.

Reserpine is characterized by slow onset of action and sustained effect. Both its cardiovascular and central nervous system effects may persist following withdrawal of the drug. Careful observation for changes in blood pressure must be made when Salutensin is used with other antihypertensive drugs.

INDICATIONS AND USAGE

Hypertension (see box warning).

CONTRAINDICATIONS

Salutensin is contraindicated in patients with a history of mental depression because of the possibility that it will potentiate depression and increase the possibility of suicide or in patients who have previously demonstrated hypersensitivity to its components. Patients with anuria or oliguria should not be given this medication. The presence of an active peptic ulcer, ulcerative colitis or depression contraindicates the use of reserpine. If electroshock therapy is necessary, treatment with Salutensin should be discontinued at least seven (7) days prior to this therapy.

WARNINGS

Azotemia may be precipitated or increased by hydroflumethiazide. Special caution is necessary in patients with impaired renal function to avoid cumulative or toxic effects. Since in hepatic cirrhosis, minor alterations of fluid and electrolyte balance may precipitate coma, hydroflumethiazide should be given with caution.

The possibility of sensitivity reactions should be considered in patients with a history of allergy or bronchial asthma. Hydroflumethiazide potentiates the action of other antihypertensive drugs. Therefore, the dosage of these agents, especially the ganglion blockers, must be reduced by at least 50 percent as soon as hydroflumethiazide is added to the regimen.

The possibility of exacerbation or activation of systemic lupus erythematosus has been reported for sulfonamide derivatives (including thiazides) and reserpine.

Reserpine may cause mental depression. Recognition of depression may be difficult because depression may often be disguised by somatic complaints (Masked Depression). The drug should be discontinued at first signs of depression such as despondency, early morning insomnia, loss of appetite, impotence, or self-deprecation. Drug-induced depression may persist for several months after drug withdrawal and may be severe enough to result in suicide.

PRECAUTIONS

General—Salutensin is a combination product containing hydroflumethiazide and reserpine. Precautions to be observed are associated with the individual components and are listed below.

Hydroflumethiazide—Careful check should be kept for signs of fluid and electrolyte imbalance. Serum and urine electrolyte determinations are particularly important when the patient is vomiting excessively or receiving parenteral fluids. Warning signs, irrespective of cause, are: dryness of mouth, thirst, weakness, lethargy, drowsiness, restlessness, muscle pains or cramps, muscular fatigue, hypotension, oliguria, tachycardia, and gastrointestinal disturbances.

Potassium excretion is usually minimal. However, hypokalemia may develop with hydroflumethiazide as with any other potent diuretic, especially with brisk diuresis, when severe cirrhosis is present, or during concomitant use of steroids or ACTH. Interference with adequate electrolyte intake will contribute to hypokalemia. Digitalis therapy may exaggerate metabolic effects of hypokalemia especially with reference to myocardial activity. If dietary salt is unduly restricted, especially during hot weather, in severely edematous patients with congestive failure or renal disease, a low salt syndrome may complicate therapy with thiazides.

Hypokalemia may be avoided or treated by use of potassium chloride or giving foods with a high potassium content. Any chloride deficit may similarly be corrected by use of ammonium chloride (excepting patients with hepatic disease) and largely prevented by a near normal salt intake.

Thiazide drugs may increase the responsiveness to tubocurarine. The antihypertensive effect of the drug may be enhanced in the post-sympathectomy patient. Hydroflumethiazide decreases arterial responsiveness to norepinephrine, as do other thiazides, necessitating due care in surgical patients. It is recommended that thiazides be discontinued 48 hours before elective surgery. Orthostatic hypotension may occur and may be potentiated by alcohol, barbiturates, or narcotics.

Pathological changes in the parathyroid glands with hypercalcemia and hypophosphatemia have been observed in a few patients on prolonged thiazide therapy. The common complications of hyperparathyroidism such as renal lithiasis, bone resorption, and peptic ulceration have not been seen. The effect of discontinuance of thiazide therapy on serum calcium and phosphorus levels may be helpful in assessing the need for parathyroid surgery in such patients. Parathyroidectomy has been followed by subjective clinical improvement in most patients, but is without effect on the hypertension. Following surgery, thiazide therapy may be resumed.

Caution is necessary in patients with hyperuricemia or a history of gout, since gout may be precipitated. Insulin requirements in diabetic patients may be increased, decreased, or unchanged. In latent diabetics, hydroflumethiazide, in common with other benzothiadiazines, may cause hyperglycemia and glycosuria.

Reserpine—Since reserpine may increase gastric secretion and motility, it should be used cautiously in patients with a history of peptic ulcer, ulcerative colitis, or other gastrointestinal disorders. This compound may precipitate biliary colic in patients with gallstones, or bronchial asthma in susceptible persons.

Reserpine may cause hypotension including orthostatic hypotension. In hypertensive patients on reserpine therapy significant hypotension and bradycardia may develop during surgical anesthesia. Therefore, the drug should be discontinued two weeks before giving anesthesia. For emergency surgical procedures, it may be necessary to give vagal blocking agents parenterally to prevent or reverse hypotension and/or bradycardia.

Anxiety or depression, as well as psychosis, may develop during reserpine therapy. If depression is present when therapy is begun, it may be aggravated. Mental depression is unusual with reserpine doses of 0.25 mg daily or less. In any case, Salutensin should be discontinued at the first sign of depression.

As with most antihypertensive therapy, caution should be exercised when treating hypertensive patients with renal insufficiency, since they adjust poorly to lowered blood pressure levels. Use reserpine cautiously with digitalis and quinidine; cardiac arrhythmias have occurred with reserpine preparations. Thiazides may decrease serum P.B.I. levels without signs of thyroid disturbance.

Information for Patients—If you miss a dose of this medicine, take it as soon as possible. If it is almost time for your next dose, do not take the missed dose at all and do not double the next one. Instead, go back to your regular dosing schedule. If you have any questions about this, check with your doctor.

This medicine may cause a loss of potassium from your body. To help prevent this, your doctor may want you to:

- eat or drink foods that have a high potassium content (for example, orange or other citrus fruit juices,) or
- take a potassium supplement, or
- take another medicine to help prevent the loss of the potassium in the first place.

Continued on next page

Bristol Labs.—Cont.

It is very important to follow these directions. Also, it is important not to change your diet on your own. This is more important if you are already on a special diet (as for diabetes), or if you are taking a potassium supplement or a medicine to reduce potassium loss. Extra potassium may not be necessary and, in some cases, too much potassium could be harmful.

Check with your doctor if you become sick and have severe or continuing vomiting or diarrhea. These problems may cause you to lose additional water and potassium.

Caution: Diabetics—This medicine may raise blood sugar levels. While you are using this medicine, be especially careful in testing for sugar in your urine. If you have any questions about this, check with your doctor.

A few people who take this medicine may become more sensitive to sunlight than they are normally. When you begin to take this medicine, avoid too much sun or use of a sunlamp until you see how you react, especially if you tend to burn easily. If you have a severe reaction, check with your doctor.

This medicine may cause some people to become drowsy or less alert than they are normally. This is more likely to happen when you begin to take it or when you increase the amount of medicine you are taking. **Make sure you know how you react to this medicine before you drive, use machines, or do other jobs that require you to be alert.**

Dizziness, lightheadedness, or fainting may occur, especially when you get up from a lying or sitting position. Getting up slowly may help but if the problem continues or gets worse, check with your doctor.

In some patients, this medicine may cause mental depression. **Tell your doctor right away:**
- if you or anyone else notices unusual changes in your moods.
- if you start having early-morning sleeplessness or unusually vivid dreams or nightmares.

This medicine will add to the effects of alcohol and other medicines (CNS depressants) that slow down the nervous system. Some examples of CNS depressants are antihistamines or medicine for hay fever, other allergies, or colds; sedatives, tranquilizers, or sleeping medicine; prescription pain medicine or narcotics; barbiturates; medicine for seizures; tricyclic antidepressants (medicine for depression); or anesthetics, including dental anesthetics. **Check with your doctor before taking any of the above while you are taking this medicine.**

Before having any kind of surgery (including dental surgery), or emergency treatment, **make sure the doctor or dentist in charge knows that you are taking this medicine.**

This medicine may cause stuffiness in the nose. However, do not use nasal decongestant medicines without first checking with your doctor or pharmacist.

Do not take other medicines unless they have been discussed with your doctor. This especially includes over-the-counter (nonprescription) medicines for appetite control, asthma, colds, cough, hay fever, or sinus, since they may tend to increase your blood pressure.

Your mouth, nose, and throat may feel very dry while you are taking this medicine. To help relieve mouth dryness, chew sugarless gum or dissolve bits of ice in your mouth.
Abstracted from USP DI "Advice for the Patient" ©1984 USP Convention; permission granted.

Laboratory Tests—Determination of serum electrolytes to detect possible electrolyte imbalance should be performed at appropriate intervals.

DRUG INTERACTIONS

Reserpine
Alcohol or
CNS depressants
(concurrent use may enhance the CNS depressant effects of either these medications or rauwolfia alkaloids)
Antihypertensives, other, or
Diuretics
(antihypertensive effects may be potentiated when used concurrently with rauwolfia alkaloids; although some combinations are frequently used for therapeutic advantage, when used concurrently dosage adjustments may be necessary)
Beta-blockers
(concurrent administration with beta-blockers may result in additive and possible excessive beta-adrenergic blockage. Although this effect is largely theoretical, close observation is recommended)
Digitalis glycosides or
Quinidine
(concurrent use may result in cardiac arrhythmias; although this interaction is controversial and does not appear to be significant with usual doses, caution is recommended, especially when large doses of rauwolfia alkaloids are used in digitalized patients)

Levodopa
(since rauwolfia alkaloids may cause dopamine depletion and parkinsonism effects, concurrent use is not recommended)
Methotrimeprazine
(concurrent use may result in additive hypotension)
Monoamine oxidase (MAO) inhibitors
(concurrent use with rauwolfia alkaloids may result in moderate to sudden and severe hypertension and hyperpyrexia which can reach crisis levels)
Sympathomimetics
Indirect-acting amines such as amphetamines, ephedrine, methylphenidate, phenylpropanolamine, pseudoephedrine, tryamine
(rauwolfia alkaloids inhibit the action of indirect-acting sympathomimetics by depleting catecholamine stores)
Direct-acting amines such as epinephrine, isoproterenol, and norepinephrine (levarterenol). Included are metaraminol and phenylephrine which are thought to act both directly and indirectly
(rauwolfia alkaloids may theoretically prolong the action of direct-acting sympathomimetics by preventing uptake into storage granules; a "denervation supersensitivity" response is also possible, although concurrent use with rauwolfia alkaloids is not known to produce severe adverse effects, a significant increase in blood pressure has been documented when phenylephrine ophthalmic drops have been administered to patients taking reserpine, and caution and close observation are recommended)
Tricyclic antidepressants
(concurrent use may decrease the hypotensive effects of rauwolfia alkaloids and interfere with the antidepressant effects of these medications)
Hydroflumethiazide
Antihypertensive medications, other, especially diazoxide, or
Preanesthetic and anesthetic agents used in surgery or
Skeletal muscle relaxants, nondepolarizing, used in surgery
(effects may be potentiated when used concurrently with thiazide diuretics, dosage adjustments may be necessary)
Amphotericin B or
Corticosteroids or
Corticotropin (ACTH)
(concurrent use with thiazide diuretics may intensify electrolyte imbalance, particularly hypokalemia)
Cardiac glycosides
(concurrent use with thiazide diuretics may enhance the possibility of digitalis toxicity associated with hypokalemia)
Colestipol
(may inhibit gastrointestinal absorption of the thiazide diuretics; administration 1 hour before or 4 hours after colestipol is recommended)
Hypoglycemics
(thiazide diuretics may raise blood glucose levels, for adult-onset diabetics, dosage adjustment of hypoglycemic medications may be necessary during and after thiazide diuretic therapy; insulin requirements may be increased, decreased, or unchanged)
Lithium salts
(concurrent use with thiazide diuretics is not recommended, as they may provoke lithium toxicity because of reduced renal clearance)
Methenamine
(effectiveness may be decreased when used concurrently with thiazide diuretics because of alkalinization of the urine)
Nonsteroidal anti-inflammatories (In some patients, the administration of a nonsteroidal anti-inflammatory agent can reduce the diuretic, natriuretic and antihypertensive effects of loop, potassium-sparing and thiazide diuretics. Therefore, when Salutensin/Salutensin-Demi and nonsteroidal anti-inflammatory agents are used concomitantly, the patient should be observed closely to determine if the desired effect of the diuretic is obtained.)
Diagnostic Interference
Reserpine
With diagnostic test results
Urinary steroid colorimetric determinations by modified Glenn-Nelson technique or Holtorff-Koch modification of Zimmerman reaction (falsely low because rauwolfia alkaloids slightly decrease absorbance)
With expected physiologic effects
Serum prolactin levels (may be increased)
Urinary catecholamine excretion (large parenteral doses of reserpine may cause an initial increase, although an overall decrease is usually noted with chronic administration of rauwolfia alkaloids)
Urinary vanilmandelic acid (VMA) excretion (intramuscular administration of reserpine causes an initial increase of about 40%, followed by a decrease by the end of the second day, chronic or parenteral administration of rauwolfia alkaloids results in an overall decrease)

Hydroflumethiazide
With expected physiologic effects
Blood and urine glucose levels (usually only in patients with a predisposition to glucose intolerance) and
Serum bilirubin levels (by displacement from albumin binding) and
Serum calcium levels (thiazide diuretics should be discontinued before parathyroid function tests are carried out) and
Serum uric acid levels (may be increased)
Serum magnesium, potassium, and sodium levels (may be decreased; serum magnesium levels may increase in uremic patients)
Serum protein bound iodine (PBI) levels (may be decreased)
Animal Tumorigenicity—Rodent studies have shown that reserpine is an animal tumorigen, causing an increased incidence of mammary fibroadenomas in female mice, malignant tumors of the seminal vesicals in male mice, and malignant adrenal medullary tumors in male rats. These findings arose in 2 year studies in which the drug was administered in the feed at concentrations of 5 and 10 ppm—about 100 to 300 times the usual human dose. The breast neoplasms are thought to be related to reserpine's prolactin-elevating effect. Several other prolactin-elevating drugs have also been associated with an increased incidence of mammary neoplasia in rodents.

The extent to which these findings indicate a risk to humans is uncertain. Tissue culture experiments show that about one-third of human breast tumors are prolactin-dependent in vitro, a factor of considerable importance if the use of the drug is contemplated in a patient with previously detected breast cancer. The possibility of an increased risk of breast cancer in reserpine users has been studied extensively; however, no firm conclusion has emerged. Although a few epidemiologic studies have suggested a slightly increased risk (less than two-fold in all studies except one) in women who have used reserpine, other studies of generally similar design have not confirmed this. Epidemiologic studies conducted using other drugs (neuroleptic agents) that, like reserpine, increase prolactin levels and therefore would be considered rodent mammary carcinogens, have not shown an association between chronic administration of the drug and human mammary tumorigenesis. While long-term clinical observation has not suggested such an association, the available evidence is considered too limited to be conclusive at this time. An association of reserpine intake with pheochromocytoma or tumors of the seminal vesicles has not been explored.

Pregnancy: Teratogenic Effects—Pregnancy Category C—Animal reproduction studies have not been conducted with Salutensin. It is also not known whether Salutensin can cause fetal harm when administered to a pregnant woman or can affect reproduction capacity. Salutensin should be given to a pregnant woman only if clearly indicated.
Nonteratogenic Effects—There is some evidence that side effects such as nasal congestion, lethargy, depressed Moro reflex, and bradycardia may appear in infants born of reserpine-treated mothers. Thiazides cross the placental barrier and appear in cord blood. When Salutensin is used in women of childbearing age, the potential benefits of the drug should be weighed against the possible hazards to the fetus. These hazards included fetal or neonatal jaundice, thrombocytopenia, and possibly other adverse reactions which have occurred in the adult.
Nursing Mothers—Thiazides and reserpine appear in breast milk. If use of the drug is deemed essential, the mother may consider stopping nursing.
Pediatric Use—Safety and effectiveness in children have not been established.

ADVERSE REACTIONS

The following adverse reactions have been observed, but there is not enough systematic collection of data to support an estimate of their frequency.
Hydroflumethiazide
A. Gastrointestinal System Reactions: anorexia, gastric irritation, nausea, vomiting, cramping, diarrhea, constipation, jaundice (intrahepatic cholestatic jaundice), pancreatitis, hyperglycemia, and glycosuria.
B. Central Nervous System Reactions: dizziness, vertigo paresthesias, headache and xanthopsia.
C. Hematologic Reactions: leukopenia, thrombocytopenia, agranulocytosis, and aplastic anemia.
D. Dermatologic Hypersensitivity Reactions: purpura, photosensitivity, rash, urticaria, and necrotizing angiitis (vasculitis) (cutaneous vasculitis).
E. Cardiovascular Reaction: orthostatic hypotension may occur and may be aggravated by alcohol, barbiturates or narcotics.
F. Miscellaneous: muscle spasm, weakness, restlessness, fever, respiratory distress including pneumonitis, pulmonary edema and anaphylactic reactions.
Whenever adverse reactions are moderate or severe, thiazide dosage should be reduced or therapy withdrawn.
Reserpine
A. Gastrointestinal System Reactions: anorexia, nausea, increased intestinal motility, diarrhea, dryness of the mouth, increased salivation, vomiting.

B. Central Nervous System Reactions: excessive sedation, nightmares, headaches, dizziness, blurred vision, syncope, impotence or decreased libido, mental depression, nervousness, paradoxical anxiety, dull sensorium, deafness, glaucoma, uveitis, optic atrophy, Parkinsonian-like syndrome.

C. Hematologic Reactions: epistaxis, purpura due to thrombocytopenia.

D. Dermatological Reactions: conjunctival injection, flushing of the skin, pruritus, rash.

E. Cardiovascular Reactions: bradycardia dyspnea, angina pectoris and other direct cardiac effects (eg, premature ventricular contractions, fluid retention, congestive failure).

F. Miscellaneous: nasal congestion, weight gain, muscular aches, enhanced susceptibility to colds, dysuria, non-puerperal lactation.

OVERDOSAGE

Signs and Symptoms—Hydroflumethiazide-related effects: diuresis, lethargy progressing to coma with minimal cardiorespiratory depression, GI irritation, hypermotility, elevated BUN, serum electrolyte changes.

Reserpine-related effects: impairment of consciousness ranging from drowsiness to coma, flushing, conjunctival injection, miosis, hypotension, hypothermia, respiratory depression, bradycardia, diarrhea.

Treatment—Induce emesis or use gastric lavage, followed by activated charcoal, to empty stomach. Treat hypotension by volume expansion, if possible. If a vasopressor is needed, use phenylephrine, levarterenol, or metaminol. Treat significant bradycardia with vagal blocking agents, along with other appropriate measures. Monitor serum electrolytes and renal function and institute supportive measures, as required. Treat GI effects symptomatically. Observe patient for at least 72 hours.

Dialyzability

There is no information available on the dialyzability of reserpine and hydroflumethiazide.

DOSAGE AND ADMINISTRATION

As determined by individual titration (see box warning). The usual adult dose of Salutensin is one tablet once or twice daily. If a smaller amount of thiazide diuretic is desired, Salutensin-Demi, one tablet once or twice daily, can be given. Most patients will respond to this dosage level. In cases where a patient has been previously titrated to a higher dose of reserpine than that contained in 1 or 2 tablets of Salutensin, reserpine should be added as the single entity alone. Doses of hydroflumethiazide greater than 100 mg a day can significantly increase the incidence of hypokalemia and other adverse effects without any evidence that such doses increase the antihypertensive efficacy of the combination.

HOW SUPPLIED

Salutensin tablets, which are round and green, contain 50 mg Saluron (hydroflumethiazide) and 0.125 mg reserpine.
NDC 0015-5436-60 Bottles of 100
NDC 0015-5436-90 Bottles of 1000
Store below 86°F (30°C).
Salutensin-Demi tablets, which are round and pale yellow, contain 25 mg Saluron (hydroflumethiazide) and 0.125 mg reserpine.
NDC 0015-5455-60 Bottles of 100
Store below 86°F (30°C).

PHYSICIAN REFERENCES

1. USP DI ©1984 USP Convention.
For information on package sizes available, refer to the current price schedule.
Shown in Product Identification Section, page 407

STADOL®   ℞

[stā'dŏl]
(butorphanol tartrate)

DESCRIPTION

Stadol (butorphanol tartrate), sterile, parenteral, narcotic analgesic agent with agonist-antagonist activity, is a member of the phenanthrene series. The chemical name is levo-N-cyclobutylmethyl-6, 10aβ-dihydroxy-1,2,3,9,10, 10a-hexahydro- (4H) - 10, 4a-iminoethanophenanthrene tartrate. It is a white crystalline substance soluble in aqueous solution. The dose is expressed as the salt. One milligram of tartrate salt is equivalent to 0.68 milligram of base. In addition to Stadol (butorphanol tartrate), each mL contains 3.3 mg citric acid, 6.4 mg sodium citrate and 6.4 mg sodium chloride. The structural formula is:

The molecular weight is 477.56 and the molecular formula is $C_{21}H_{29}NO_2 \cdot C_4H_6O_6$

CLINICAL PHARMACOLOGY

Stadol is a potent analgesic. The duration of analgesia is generally 3 to 4 hours and is approximately equivalent to that of morphine. The onset time for analgesia is within 10 minutes following intramuscular injection and very rapidly following intravenous administration. Peak analgesic activity is obtained at 30 to 60 minutes following intramuscular injection and more rapidly following intravenous injection.

Narcotic Antagonist Activity

Stadol has narcotic antagonist activity which is approximately equivalent to that of nalorphine, 30 times that of pentazocine and 1/40 that of naloxone (Narcan®) as measured by the antagonism of morphine analgesia in the rat tail flick test.

Mechanism of Analgesic Action

The exact mechanism of action of Stadol is unknown. It is felt that the class of narcotic agonist-antagonist analgesics exert their analgesic effect via a central nervous system mechanism. Currently, it is believed the site of action of centrally acting analgesics is subcortical, possibly in the limbic system.

Effect on Respiration

At the analgesic dose of 2 mg, Stadol depresses respiration to a degree equal to 10 mg morphine. The magnitude of respiratory depression with Stadol is not appreciably increased at doses of 4 mg. In contrast to the magnitude of respiratory depression, the duration of respiratory depression with Stadol is dose related. Any respiratory depression produced by Stadol is reversible by naloxone which is a specific antagonist.

Cardiovascular Effects

The hemodynamic changes after the intravenous administration of Stadol are similar to the reported hemodynamic changes after pentazocine. The changes include increased pulmonary artery pressure, pulmonary wedge pressure, left ventricular end diastolic pressure, systemic arterial pressure, and pulmonary vascular resistance. Although smaller than those following pentazocine, these changes are nevertheless in a direction which increases the work of the heart, especially in the pulmonary circuit.

INDICATIONS AND USAGE

Stadol is recommended for the relief of moderate to severe pain. Stadol can also be used for preoperative or preanesthetic medication, as a supplement to balanced anesthesia, and for the relief of prepartum pain.

CONTRAINDICATIONS

Stadol should not be administered to patients who have been shown to be hypersensitive to it.

WARNINGS

Patients Physically Dependent on Narcotics

Because of its antagonist properties, Stadol is not recommended for patients physically dependent on narcotics. Detoxification in such patients is required prior to use.
Due to the difficulty in assessing addiction in patients who have recently received substantial amounts of narcotic medication, caution should be used in the administration of Stadol. Detoxification of such patients prior to usage should be carefully considered.

Use During Balanced Anesthesia

Since the combined respiratory depressant effect of all intravenous medication used during conduct of general anesthesia may lead to under-ventilation or apnea, butorphanol should be administered during balanced anesthesia only by persons specifically trained in the use of intravenous anesthetics and adjuncts, the maintenance of a patent airway and management of respiratory effects of all intravenous medication administered.
An opioid antagonist, resuscitative and intubation equipment and oxygen should be readily available.

Drug Dependence

Special care should be exercised in administering Stadol to emotionally unstable patients and to those with a history of drug misuse. When long term therapy is contemplated, such patients should be closely supervised. Even though Stadol has a low physical dependence liability, care should be taken that individuals who may be prone to drug abuse are closely supervised. It is important to avoid increases in dose and frequency of injections by the patient and to prevent the use of the drug in anticipation of pain rather than for the relief of pain.

Head Injury and Increased Intracranial Pressure

Although there is no clinical experience in patients with head injury, it can be assumed that Stadol, like other potent analgesics, elevates cerebrospinal fluid pressure. Therefore the use of Stadol in cases of head injury can produce effects (e.g., miosis) which may obscure the clinical course of patients with head injuries. In such patients Stadol must be used with extreme caution and only if its use is deemed essential.

Cardiovascular Effects

Because Stadol increases the work of the heart, especially the pulmonary circuit, (see Clinical Pharmacology), the use of this drug in acute myocardial infarction or in cardiac patients with ventricular dysfunction or coronary insufficiency should be limited to those who are hypersensitive to morphine sulfate or meperidine.

PRECAUTIONS

Certain Respiratory Conditions

Because Stadol causes some respiratory depression, it should be administered only with caution and low dosage to patients with respiratory depression (e.g., from other medication, uremia, or severe infection), severely limited respiratory reserve, bronchial asthma, obstructive respiratory conditions, or cyanosis.

Impaired Renal or Hepatic Function

Although laboratory tests have not indicated that Stadol causes or increases renal or hepatic impairment, the drug should be administered with caution to patients with such impairment. Extensive liver disease may predispose to greater side effects and greater activity from the usual clinical dose, possibly the result of decreased metabolism of the drug by the liver.

Biliary Surgery

Clinical studies have not been done to establish the safety of Stadol administration to patients about to undergo surgery of the biliary tract.

Usage as a Preoperative or Preanesthetic Medication

Slight increases in systolic blood pressure may occur, therefore caution should be employed when Stadol is used in the hypertensive patient.

Usage in Pregnancy

The safety of Stadol for use in pregnancy prior to the labor period has not been established; therefore, this drug should be used in pregnant patients only when in the judgment of the physician its use is deemed essential to the welfare of the patient.
Reproduction studies have been performed in rats, mice, and rabbits and have revealed no evidence of impaired fertility or harm to the fetus due to Stadol at about 2.5 to 5 times the human dose.

Usage in Labor and Delivery

In general, the safety to the mother and fetus following the administration of Stadol during labor has been established, however, there have been a few reports of infant respiratory distress/apnea occurring after delivery (less than 1%; see Adverse Reactions). Patients receiving Stadol during labor have experienced no adverse effects other than those observed with commonly used analgesics. Stadol should be used with caution in women delivering premature infants.

Usage in Nursing Mothers

The use of Stadol in lactating mothers who are nursing their infants is not recommended, since it is not known whether this drug is excreted in milk. Stadol has been used safely for labor pain in mothers who subsequently nursed their infants.

Usage in Children

Safety and efficacy in children below age 18 years have not been established at present.

ADVERSE REACTIONS

The most frequent adverse reactions in 1250 patients treated with Stadol are: sedation (503, 40%), nausea (82, 6%), clammy/sweating (76, 6%).
Less frequent reactions are: headache (35, 3%), vertigo (33, 3%), floating feeling (33, 3%), dizziness (23, 2%), lethargy (19, 2%), confusion (15, 1%), lightheadedness (12, 1%).
Other adverse reactions which may occur (reported incidence of less than 1%) are:
CNS: nervousness, unusual dreams, agitation, euphoria, hallucinations, seizures
Autonomic: flushing and warmth, dry mouth, sensitivity to cold
Cardiovascular: palpitation, increase or decrease of blood pressure
Gastrointestinal: vomiting
Respiratory: slowing of respiration, shallow breathing, apnea
Dermatological: rash or hives
Eye: diplopia or blurred vision

OVERDOSAGE

Manifestations

Although there have been no experiences of overdosage with Stadol during clinical trials, this may occur due to accidental or intentional misuse as well as therapeutic use. Based on the pharmacology of Stadol, overdosage could produce some degree of respiratory depression and variable cardiovascular and central nervous system effects.

Treatment

The immediate treatment of suspected Stadol overdosage is intravenous naloxone. The respiratory and cardiac status of the patient should be evaluated constantly and appropriate

Continued on next page

Bristol Labs.—Cont.

supportive measures instituted, such as oxygen, intravenous fluids, vasopressors, and assisted or controlled respiration.

DOSAGE AND ADMINISTRATION
USE FOR PAIN
Adults:

Intramuscular—The usual recommended single dose for I.M. administration is 2 mg. This may be repeated every three to four hours, as necessary. The effective dosage range, depending on the severity of pain, is 1 to 4 mg repeated every three to four hours. At this time, there is insufficient clinical data to recommend single doses beyond 4 mg.

Intravenous—The usual recommended single dose for I.V. administration is 1 mg repeated every three to four hours as necessary. The effective dosage range, depending on the severity of pain, is 0.5 to 2 mg repeated every three to four hours.

Children:

Since there is no clinical experience in children under 18 years, Stadol is not recommended in this age group.

Concomitant Use with Tranquilizers

According to accepted procedure, the dose of Stadol should be reduced when administered concomitantly with phenothiazines and other tranquilizers which may potentiate the action of Stadol.

USE IN ANESTHESIA

For analgesic action during the anesthetic periods, premedication, and maintenance. Some of the factors to be considered in determining the dose are age, body weight, physical status, underlying pathological condition, use of other drugs, type of anesthesia to be used and surgical procedure involved.

Premedication: Preoperative medication dosage of butorphanol should be individualized. The usual adult dose is 2 mg IM, administered 60–90 minutes before surgery. This is approximately equivalent in sedative effect to 10 mg morphine or 80 mg meperidine.

Maintenance: Incremental use of intravenous butorphanol during maintenance in balanced anesthesia must be individualized. The usual incremental dose of butorphanol is 0.5 to 1.0 mg intravenously. The incremental dose may be higher, up to 0.06 mg/kg (4 mg/70 kg), depending on previous sedative, analgesic and hypnotic drugs administered. Butorphanol should not be relied upon as the only intravenous drug to supplement nitrous oxide because it may fail to provide adequate analgesia. A failure to achieve successful analgesia during balanced anesthesia is commonly reflected by increases in general sympathetic tone. Consequently, if blood pressure continues to rise after repeated doses of butorphanol, consideration should be given to adding a potent volatile liquid inhalational anesthetic or another intravenous medication (such as a thiobarbiturate or benzodiazepine). The total dose of butorphanol will vary, however, patients seldom require less than 4 mg or more than 12.5 mg (approximately 0.06 to 0.18 mg/kg).

Storage Conditions

Store at room temperature.

Parenteral drug products should be inspected visually for particulate matter and discoloration prior to administration, whenever solution and container permit.

SUPPLY

Stadol (butorphanol tartrate) Injection for I.M. or I.V. use is available as follows:

NDC 0015-5644-20—2 mg per mL, 2-mL vial
NDC 0015-5645-20—1 mg per mL, 1-mL vial
NDC 0015-5646-20—2 mg per mL, 1-mL vial
NDC 0015-5648-20—2 mg per mL, 10-mL multi-dose vial
U.S. Patent Nos. 3,819,635, 4,139,534

For information on package sizes available, refer to the current price schedule.

ULTRACEF®   ℞
[ul-trah-sef]
cefadroxil monohydrate
CAPSULES, TABLETS AND ORAL SUSPENSION

DESCRIPTION

ULTRACEF (cefadroxil monohydrate) is a semisynthetic cephalosporin antibiotic intended for oral administration. It is a white to yellowish-white crystalline powder. It is soluble in water and it is acid-stable. It is chemically designated as 7-[[D-2-amino-2-(4-hydroxyphenyl) acetyl]amino]-3- methyl-8-oxo-5-thia-1-azabicyclo [4.2.0]oct-2-ene-2- carboxylic acid monohydrate.

Inactive ingredient in ULTRACEF capsules is: magnesium stearate.

Inactive ingredients in ULTRACEF tablets are: cellulose microcrystalline and magnesium stearate.

Inactive ingredients in ULTRACEF for oral suspension are: Avicel, FD& C Red No. 40, natural & artificial flavorings, Polysorbate 80, sodium benzoate, sucrose and tragacanth. It has the following structural formula.

CLINICAL PHARMACOLOGY

ULTRACEF is rapidly absorbed after oral administration. Following single doses of 500 and 1000 mg, average peak serum concentrations were approximately 16 and 28 μg/mL, respectively. Measurable levels were present 12 hours after administration. Over 90 percent of the drug is excreted unchanged in the urine within 24 hours. Peak urine concentrations are approximately 1800 μg/mL during the period following a single 500-mg dose. Increases in dosage generally produce a proportionate increase in ULTRACEF urinary concentration. The urine antibiotic concentration, following a 1-gram dose, was maintained well above the MIC of susceptible urinary pathogens for 20 to 22 hours.

MICROBIOLOGY

In vitro tests demonstrate that the cephalosporins are bactericidal because of their inhibition of cell-wall synthesis. ULTRACEF is active against the following organisms **in vitro:**
> Beta-hemolytic streptococci
> Staphylococci, including coagulase-positive, coagulasenegative, and penicillinase-producing strains
> **Streptococcus (Diplococcus) pneumoniae**
> **Escherichia coli**
> **Proteus mirabilis**
> **Klebsiella** species
> **Moraxella (Branhamella) catarrhalis**

Note: Most strains of Enterococci (**Streptococcus faecalis** and **S. faecium**) are resistant to ULTRACEF. It is not active against most strains of **Enterobacter** species. **P. Morganii**, and **P. vulgaris**. It has no activity against **Pseudomonas** species and **Acinetobacter calcoaceticus** (formerly **Mima** and **Herellea** species).

Disc Susceptibility Tests—Quantitative methods that require measurement of zone diameters give the most precise estimates of antibiotic susceptibility. One recommended procedure (CFR Section 460.1) uses a cephalosporin-class disc for testing susceptibility; interpretations correlate zone diameters of this disc test with MIC values for ULTRACEF. With this procedure, a report from the laboratory of "resistant" indicates that the infecting organism is not likely to respond to therapy. A report of "intermediate susceptibility" suggests that the organism would be susceptible if the infection is confined to the urinary tract, as ULTRACEF produces high antibiotic levels in the urine.

INDICATIONS AND USAGE

ULTRACEF is indicated for the treatment of the following infections when caused by susceptible strains of the designated microorganisms:

Urinary tract infections caused by **E. coli, P. mirabilis,** and **Klebsiella** species.

Skin and skin structure infections caused by staphylococci and/or streptococci.

Pharyngitis and tonsillitis caused by Group A beta-hemolytic streptococci. (Penicillin is the usual drug of choice in the treatment and prevention of streptococcal infections, including the prophylaxis of rheumatic fever. ULTRACEF is generally effective in the eradication of streptococci from the nasopharynx; however substantial data establishing the efficacy of ULTRACEF in the subsequent prevention of rheumatic fever are not available at present.)

Note: Culture and susceptibility tests should be initiated prior to and during therapy. Renal function studies should be performed when indicated.

CONTRAINDICATIONS

ULTRACEF is contraindicated in patients with known allergy to the cephalosporin group of antibiotics.

WARNING

IN PENICILLIN-ALLERGIC PATIENTS, CEPHALOSPORIN ANTIBIOTICS SHOULD BE USED WITH GREAT CAUTION. THERE IS CLINICAL AND LABORATORY EVIDENCE OF PARTIAL CROSS-ALLERGENICITY OF THE PENICILLINS AND THE CEPHALOSPORINS, AND THERE ARE INSTANCES OF PATIENTS WHO HAVE HAD REACTIONS TO BOTH DRUGS (INCLUDING FATAL ANAPHYLAXIS AFTER PARENTERAL USE).

Any patient who has demonstrated a history of some form of allergy, particularly to drugs, should receive antibiotics cautiously and then only when absolutely necessary. No exception should be made with regard to ULTRACEF.

Pseudomembranous colitis has been reported with the use of cephalosporins (and other broad spectrum antibiotics); therefore, it is important to consider its diagnosis in patients who develop diarrhea in association with antibiotic use.

Treatment with broad spectrum antibiotics alters normal flora of the colon and may permit overgrowth of clostridia. Studies indicate a toxin produced by **Clostridium difficile** is one primary cause of antibiotic-associated colitis. Cholestyramine and colestipol resins have been shown to bind the toxin **in vitro.**

Mild cases of colitis may respond to drug discontinuance alone.

Moderate to severe cases should be managed with fluid, electrolyte and protein supplementation as indicated.

When the colitis is not relieved by drug discontinuance or when it is severe, oral vancomycin is the treatment of choice for antibiotic-associated pseudomembranous colitis produced by **C. difficile.** Other causes of colitis should also be considered.

PRECAUTIONS

General: Patients should be followed carefully so that any side effects or unusual manifestations of drug idiosyncrasy may be detected. If a hypersensitivity reaction occurs, the drug should be discontinued and the patient treated with the usual agents (eg, epinephrine or other pressor amines, antihistamines, or corticosteroids).

ULTRACEF should be used with caution in the presence of markedly impaired renal function (creatinine clearance rate of less than 50 mL/min/1.73M²). (See DOSAGE AND ADMINISTRATION.) In patients with known or suspected renal impairment, careful clinical observation and appropriate laboratory studies should be made prior to and during therapy.

Prolonged use of ULTRACEF may result in the overgrowth of nonsusceptible organisms. Careful observation of the patient is essential. If superinfection occurs during therapy, appropriate measures should be taken.

Positive direct Coombs' tests have been reported during treatment with the cephalosporin antibiotics. In hematologic studies or in transfusion cross-matching procedures when antiglobulin tests are performed on the minor side or in Coombs' testing of newborns whose mothers have received cephalosporin antibiotics before parturition, it should be recognized that a positive Coombs' test may be due to the drug.

ULTRACEF should be prescribed with caution in individuals with a history of gastrointestinal disease, particularly colitis.

Carcinogenesis, Mutagenesis and Impairment of Fertility: No long-term studies have been performed to determine carcinogenic potential. No genetic toxicity tests have been performed.

USAGE IN PREGNANCY

Pregnancy Category B: Reproduction studies have been performed in mice and rats at doses up to 11 times the human dose and have revealed no evidence of impaired fertility or harm to the fetus due to cefadroxil monohydrate. There are, however, no adequate and well-controlled studies in pregnant women. Because animal reproduction studies are not always predictive of human response, this drug should be used during pregnancy only if clearly needed.

Nursing Mothers: Caution should be exercised when cefadroxil monohydrate is administered to a nursing mother.

ADVERSE REACTIONS

Gastrointestinal — Symptoms of pseudomembranous colitis can appear during antibiotic treatment. Nausea and vomiting have been reported rarely. Diarrhea and dysuria have also occurred.

Hypersensitivity — Allergies (in the form of rash, urticaria, and angioedema) have been observed. These reactions usually subsided upon discontinuation of the drug.

Other reactions have included genital pruritus, genital moniliasis, vaginitis, and moderate transient neutropenia.

DOSAGE AND ADMINISTRATION

ULTRACEF is acid stable and may be administered orally without regard to meals. Administration with food may be helpful in diminishing potential gastrointestinal complaints occasionally associated with oral cephalosporin therapy.

Adults

Urinary Tract Infections — For uncomplicated lower urinary tract infections (ie, cystitis) the usual dosage is 1 or 2 grams per day in single (q.d.) or divided doses (b.i.d.).

For all other urinary tract infections the usual dosage is 2 grams per day in divided doses (b.i.d.).

Skin and Skin Structure Infections — For skin and skin structure infections the usual dosage is 1 gram per day in single (q.d.) or divided doses (b.i.d.).

Pharyngitis and Tonsillitis — Treatment of Group A beta-hemolytic streptococcal pharyngitis and tonsillitis — 1 gram per day in single (q.d.) or divided doses (b.i.d.) for 10 days.

Children — For urinary tract infections and for skin and skin structure infections, the recommended daily dosage for children is 30 mg/kg/day in divided doses every 12 hours. For pharyngitis and tonsillitis, the recommended daily dosage

for children is 30 mg/kg/day in single (q.d.) or divided doses (b.i.d.). In the treatment of beta-hemolytic streptococcal infections, a therapeutic dosage of ULTRACEF should be administered for at least 10 days.
See chart for total daily dosage for children.

DAILY DOSAGE OF ULTRACEF SUSPENSION

Child's Weight

lbs	kg	125 mg/5 mL	250 mg/5 mL
10	4.5	1 tsp	—
20	9.1	2 tsp	1 tsp
30	13.6	3 tsp	1 ½ tsp
40	18.2	4 tsp	2 tsp
50	22.7	5 tsp	2 ½ tsp
60	27.3	6 tsp	3 tsp
70 & above	31.8+	—	4 tsp

In patients with renal impairment, the dosage of cefadroxil monohydrate should be adjusted according to creatinine clearance rates to prevent drug accumulation. The following schedule is suggested. In adults, the initial dose is 1000 mg of ULTRACEF and the maintenance dose (based on the creatinine clearance rate mL/min/1.73m^2) is 500 mg at the time intervals listed below.

Creatinine Clearances	Dosage Interval
0-10 mL/min	36 hours
10-25 mL/min	24 hours
25-50 mL/min	12 hours

Patients with creatinine clearance rates over 50 mL/min may be treated as if they were patients having normal renal function.

HOW SUPPLIED

ULTRACEF (cefadroxil monohydrate) tablets. Each tablet contains cefadroxil monohydrate equivalent to 1 gram cefadroxil.
NDC 0015-7286—1 gram
ULTRACEF (cefadroxil monohydrate) capsules. Each capsule contains cefadroxil monohydrate equivalent to 500 mg cefadroxil.
NDC 0015-7271—500 mg
ULTRACEF (cefadroxil monohydrate) for oral suspension. Each 5 mL of reconstituted suspension contains cefadroxil monohydrate equivalent to 125 mg or 250 mg cefadroxil.
NDC 0015-7283—125 mg
NDC 0015-7284—250 mg
U.S. Patent Nos. 4,160,863, 4,504,657
Directions for mixing are included on the label. Shake well before using. Keep container tightly closed.
Store reconstituted suspension in refrigerator, discard unused portion after 14 days.
For information on package sizes available, refer to the current price schedule.

Bristol-Myers Institutional Products
A Bristol-Myers Company
2400 W. LLOYD EXPRESSWAY
EVANSVILLE, IN 47721-0001

BRISTOL-MYERS INSTITUTIONAL PRODUCTS

COMPLETE LISTING OF BRISTOL-MYERS INSTITUTIONAL PRODUCTS

NDC	Product
	BETAPEN®-VK (penicillin V potassium)
0015-7506-40	Betapen-VK O/Sol 125 mg/5 mL, 100 mL
0015-7506-64	Betapen-VK O/Sol 125 mg/5 mL, 200 mL
0015-7507-40	Betapen-VK O/Sol 250 mg/5 mL, 100 mL
0015-7507-64	Betapen-VK O/Sol 250 mg/5 mL, 200 mL
0015-7508-60	Betapen-VK Tabs 250 mg, 100s
0015-7508-90	Betapen-VK Tabs 250 mg, 1,000s
0015-7509-60	Betapen-VK Tabs 500 mg, 100s
0015-7509-80	Betapen-VK Tabs 500 mg, 500s
	CEFADYL® (sterile cephapirin sodium)
0015-7613-20	Cefadyl for Inj 20 g (Bulk vial), 100 mL
0015-7627-28	Cefadyl for Inj 0.5 g/15 mL vial
0015-7628-22	Cefadyl for Inj 1 g/Piggyback 100 mL vial
0015-7628-20	Cefadyl for Inj 1 g/15 mL vial
0015-7629-30	Cefadyl for Inj 2 g/15 mL vial
0015-7629-28	Cefadyl for Inj 2 g/Piggyback 100 mL vial
0015-7630-20	Cefadyl for Inj 4 g/Piggyback 100 mL vial
0015-7628-18	Cefadyl 1 g in ADD-Vantage® vial
0015-7629-18	Cefadyl 2 g in ADD-Vantage vial

	DYNAPEN® (dicloxacillin sodium)
0015-7658-50	Dynapen Caps 500 mg, 50s
0015-7856-35	Dynapen O/Susp 62.5 mg/5 mL, 80 mL
0015-7856-40	Dynapen O/Susp 62.5 mg/5 mL, 100 mL
0015-7856-64	Dynapen O/Susp 62.5 mg/5 mL, 200 mL
0015-7892-30	Dynapen Caps 125 mg, 24s
0015-7892-60	Dynapen Caps 125 mg, 100s
0015-7893-30	Dynapen Caps 250 mg, 24s
0015-7893-60	Dynapen Caps 250 mg, 100s
0015-7893-66	Dynapen Caps 250 mg, DOSA-TROL® 100s
	KANTREX® (kanamycin sulfate)
0015-3502-20	Kantrex Inj* 500 mg/2 mL vial
0015-3503-20	Kantrex Inj* 1 g/3 mL vial
0015-3506-25	Kantrex Caps 500 mg, 20s
0015-3506-60	Kantrex Caps 500 mg, 100s
0015-3512-20	Kantrex Ped Inj* 75 mg/2 mL vial
	*(see full prescribing information at end of listing)
	MUCOMYST® (acetylcysteine)
	Mucomyst 20% acetylcysteine solution 200 mg/mL
0087-0570-03	three 10 mL vials, 1 dropper
0087-0570-09	three 30 mL vials
0087-0570-07	twelve 4 mL vials
	Mucomyst-10 10% acetylcysteine solution 100 mg/mL
0087-0572-01	three 10 mL vials, 1 dropper
0087-0572-02	three 30 mL vials
0087-0572-03	twelve 4 mL vials
	NAFCIL™ (nafcillin sodium for injection)
0015-7101-28	Nafcil Inj 10 g (Bulk vial), 100 mL
0015-7224-20	Nafcil Inj Buf 500 mg, vial
0015-7225-28	Nafcil Inj 1 g/Piggyback 100 mL vial
0015-7225-20	Nafcil Inj Buf l g, vial
0015-7226-28	Nafcil Inj 2 g/Piggyback 100 mL vial
0015-7226-20	Nafcil Inj Buf 2 g, vial
0015-7225-18	Nafcil 1 g in ADD-Vantage® Vial
0015-7226-18	Nafcil 2 g in ADD-Vantage Vial
	POLYCILLIN-N® (ampicillin sodium for injection)
0015-7100-28	Polycillin-N Inj 10 g (Bulk vial), 100 mL
0015-7401-20	Polycillin-N Inj 125 mg, vial
0015-7402-20	Polycillin-N Inj 250 mg, vial
0015-7403-31	Polycillin-N Inj 500 mg/Piggyback 100 mL vial
0015-7403-20	Polycillin-N Inj 500 mg, vial
0015-7404-36	Polycillin-N Inj 1 g/Piggyback 100 mL vial
0015-7404-20	Polycillin-N Inj 1 g, vial
0015-7405-28	Polycillin-N Inj 2 g/Piggyback 100 mL vial
0015-7405-20	Polycillin-N Inj 2 g, vial
0015-7404-18	Polycillin-N 1 g in ADD-Vantage Vial
0015-7405-18	Polycillin-N 2 g in ADD-Vantage Vial
	POLYCILLIN® (oral ampicillin)
0015-7884-20	Polycillin Ped Drops, 100 mg/mL, 20 mL
0015-7884-40	Polycillin O/Sus 500 mg/5 mL, 100 mL
0015-7884-77	Polycillin O/Sus 500 mg/bottle, DOSA-TROL®, 5 mL, 25 pk
0015-7988-40	Polycillin O/Sus 125 mg/5 mL, 100 mL
0015-7988-50	Polycillin O/Sus 125 mg/5 mL, 150 mL
0015-7988-64	Polycillin O/Sus 125 mg/5 mL, 200 mL
0015-7988-77	Polycillin O/Sus 125 mg/bottle, DOSA-TROL®, 5 mL, 25 pk
0015-7992-60	Polycillin Caps 250 mg, 100s
0015-7992-66	Polycillin Caps 250 mg, DOSA-TROL®, 100s
0015-7992-80	Polycillin Caps 250 mg, 500s
0015-7992-90	Polycillin Caps 250 mg, 1000s
0015-7993-60	Polycillin Caps 500 mg, 100s
0015-7993-66	Polycillin Caps 500 mg, DOSA-TROL, 100s
0015-7993-80	Polycillin Caps 500 mg, 500s
0015-7998-40	Polycillin O/Sus 250 mg/5 mL, 100 mL
0015-7998-50	Polycillin O/Sus 250 mg/5 mL, 150 mL
0015-7998-64	Polycillin O/Sus 250 mg/5 mL, 200 mL
0015-7998-77	Polycillin O/Sus 250 mg/bottle, DOSA-TROL, 5 mL, 25 pk
	POLYCILLIN-PRB® (ampicillin-probenecid)
0015-7607-27	Polycillin-PRB O/Sus 3.5 g
	POLYMOX® (amoxicillin)
0015-7276-35	Polymox O/Sus 125 mg/5 mL, 80 mL
0015-7276-41	Polymox O/Sus 125 mg/5 mL, 100 mL
0015-7276-50	Polymox O/Sus 125 mg/5 mL, 150 mL
0015-7276-77	Polymox O/Sus 125 mg/btl, DOSA-TROL 5 mL, 25 pk
0015-7277-16	Polymox Ped Drops 50 mg/mL, 15 mL
0015-7277-35	Polymox O/Sus 250 mg/5 mL, 80 mL
0015-7277-41	Polymox O/Sus 250 mg/5 mL, 100 mL
0015-7277-50	Polymox O/Sus 250 mg/5 mL, 150 mL
0015-7277-77	Polymox O/Sus 250 mg/btl, DOSA-TROL 5 mL, 25 pk
0015-7278-60	Polymox Caps 250 mg, 100s
0015-7278-66	Polymox Caps 250 mg, DOSA-TROL, 100s
0015-7278-80	Polymox Caps 250 mg, 500s
0015-7279-50	Polymox Caps 500 mg, 50s
0015-7279-60	Polymox Caps 500 mg, 100s
0015-7279-66	Polymox Caps 500 mg, DOSA-TROL, 100s
0015-7279-80	Polymox Caps 500 mg, 500s

	PROSTAPHLIN® (oxacillin sodium)
0015-7103-28	Prostaphlin Inj 10 g (Bulk vial), 100 mL
0015-7300-29	Prostaphlin Inj 4 g/Piggyback 100 mL vial
0015-7970-28	Prostaphlin Inj 2 g/Piggyback 100 mL vial
0015-7970-20	Prostaphlin Inj 2 g, vial
0015-7977-45	Prostaphlin Caps 250 mg, 48s
0015-7977-58	Prostaphlin Caps 250 mg, 100s
0015-7977-66	Prostaphlin Caps 250 mg, DOSA-TROL®, 100s
0015-7978-20	Prostaphlin Inj 250 mg, vial
0015-7979-20	Prostaphlin Inj 500 mg, vial
0015-7981-28	Prostaphlin Inj 1 g/Piggyback 100 mL vial
0015-7981-20	Prostaphlin Inj 1 g, vial
0015-7982-45	Prostaphlin Caps 500 mg, 48s
0015-7982-58	Prostaphlin Caps 500 mg, 100s
0015-7982-66	Prostaphlin Caps 500 mg, DOSA-TROL, 100s
0015-7985-40	Prostaphlin O/S 250 mg/5 mL, 100 mL
0015-7981-18	Prostaphlin 1 g in ADD-Vantage® Vial
0015-7970-18	Prostaphlin 2 g in ADD-Vantage Vial
	STAPHCILLIN® (methicillin sodium for injection)
0015-7102-28	Staphcillin Inj 10 g (Bulk vial), 100 mL
0015-7961-28	Staphcillin Inj 1 g/Piggyback 100 mL vial
0015-7961-20	Staphcillin Inj Buf, 1 g, vial
0015-7964-20	Staphcillin Inj Buf, 4 g, vial
0015-7965-20	Staphcillin Inj Buf, 6 g, vial
	TEGOPEN® (cloxacillin sodium)
0015-7496-60	Tegopen Caps 500 mg, 100s
0015-7935-60	Tegopen Caps 250 mg, 100s
0015-7941-40	Tegopen O/Sus 125 mg/5 mL, 100 mL
0015-7941-64	Tegopen O/Sus 125 mg/5 mL, 200 mL
	ZOLICEF™ (sterile cefazolin sodium, USP)
0015-7338-12	Zolicef Inj 500 mg, vial
0015-7339-12	Zolicef Inj 1 g, vial

Bristol-Myers Institutional Products in ADD-Vantage®

KANTREX® ℞
INJECTION
Kanamycin Sulfate Injection
500 mg per 2 mL; 1 g per 3 mL
KANTREX® ℞
PEDIATRIC INJECTION
Kanamycin Sulfate Injection
75 mg per 2 mL

WARNING
Patients treated with aminoglycosides by any route should be under close clinical observation because of the potential toxicity associated with their use. As with other aminoglycosides, the major toxic effects of kanamycin sulfate are its action on the auditory and vestibular branches of the eighth nerve and the renal tubules. Neurotoxicity is manifested by bilateral auditory toxicity which often is permanent and, sometimes, by vestibular ototoxicity. Loss of high frequency perception usually occurs before there is noticeable clinical hearing loss and can be detected by audiometric testing. There may not be clinical symptoms to warn of developing cochlear damage. Vertigo may occur and may be evidence of vestibular injury. Other manifestations of neurotoxicity may include numbness, skin tingling, muscle twitching, and convulsions. The risk of hearing loss increases with the degree of exposure to either high peak or high trough serum concentrations and continues to progress after drug withdrawal.
Renal impairment may be characterized by decreased creatinine clearance, the presence of cells or casts, oliguria, proteinuria, decreased urine specific gravity, or evidence of increasing nitrogen retention (increasing BUN, NPN or serum creatinine).
The risks of severe ototoxic and nephrotoxic reactions are sharply increased in patients with impaired renal function and in those with normal renal function who receive high doses or prolonged therapy.
Renal and eighth nerve function should be closely monitored, especially in patients with known or suspected reduced renal function at the onset of therapy, and also in those whose renal function is initially normal but who develop signs of renal dysfunction during therapy. Serum concentrations of parenterally administered aminoglycosides should be monitored when feasible to assure adequate levels and to avoid potentially toxic levels. Urine should be examined for decreased specific gravity, increased excretion of protein and the presence of cells or casts. Blood urea nitrogen, serum creatinine, or creatinine clearance should be measured periodically. Serial audiograms should be obtained when feasible in patients old enough to be tested, particularly high risk patients. Evidence of ototoxicity (dizziness, vertigo, tinnitus, roaring in the ears, and hearing loss) or nephrotoxicity requires dosage adjustment or discontinuance of the drug.

Continued on next page

Bristol-Myers Institutional—Cont.

Neuromuscular blockade with respiratory paralysis may occur when kanamycin sulfate is instilled intraperitonealy concomitantly with anesthesia and muscle-relaxing drugs. Neuromuscular blockade has been reported following parenteral injection and the oral use of aminoglycosides. The possibility of the occurrence of neuromuscular blockade and respiratory paralysis should be considered if aminoglycosides are administered by any route, especially in patients receiving anesthetics, neuromuscular-blocking agents such as tubocurarine, succinylcholine, decamethonium, or in patients receiving massive transfusions of citrate-anticoagulated blood. If blockage occurs, calcium salts may reduce these phenomena but mechanical respiratory assistance may be necessary.

The concurrent and/or sequential systemic, oral, or topical use of kanamycin and other potentially nephrotoxic, and/or neurotoxic drugs, particularly polymyxin B, bacitracin, colistin, amphotericin B, cisplatin, vancomycin and all other aminoglycosides (including paromomycin) should be avoided because the toxicity may be additive. Other factors which may increase patient risk of toxicity are advanced age and dehydration.

Kanamycin sulfate should not be given concurrently with potent diuretics (ethacrynic acid, furosemide, meralluride sodium, sodium mercaptomerin, or mannitol). Some diuretics themselves cause ototoxicity, and intravenously administered diuretics may enhance aminoglycoside toxicity by altering antibiotic concentrations in serum and tissue.

DESCRIPTION

Kanamycin sulfate is an aminoglycoside antibiotic produced by **Streptomyces kanamyceticus.** It is $C_{18}H_{36}N_4O_{11} \cdot 2H_2SO_4 \cdot$ D-Streptamine, 0-3-amino-3-deoxy-α-D-glucopyranosyl—(1→6)-0-[6-amino-6-deoxy-α-D-glucopyranosyl-(1→4)]-2-deoxy, sulfate 1:2 (salt). It consists of two amino sugars glycosidically linked to deoxystreptamine.

Kanamycin sulfate injection, sterile solution for parenteral administration, contains respectively: kanamycin sulfate 75 mg, 500 mg, and 1.0 g; sodium bisulfite, an antioxidant, 0.099%, 0.66%, and 0.45%; and sodium citrate, 0.33%, 2.2%, and 2.2% with pH of each dosage form adjusted to 4.5 with sulfuric acid.

CLINICAL PHARMACOLOGY

The drug is rapidly absorbed after intramuscular injection and peak serum levels are generally reached within approximately one hour. Doses of 7.5 mg/kg give mean peak levels of 22 µg/mL. At 8 hours following a 7.5 mg/kg dose, mean serum levels are 3.2 µg/mL. The serum half-life is 2½ hours. Intravenous administration of kanamycin over a period of one hour resulted in serum concentrations similar to those obtained by intramuscular administration.

Kanamycin diffuses rapidly into most body fluids including synovial and peritoneal fluids and bile. Significant levels of the drug appear in cord blood and amniotic fluid following intramuscular administration to pregnant patients. Spinal fluid concentrations in normal infants are approximately 10 to 20 percent of serum levels and may reach 50 percent when the meninges are inflamed.

Studies in normal adult patients have shown only trace levels of kanamycin in spinal fluid. No data are available on adults with meningitis.

The drug is excreted almost entirely by glomerular filtration and is not reabsorbed by the renal tubules. Hence, high concentrations are attained in the nephron, and the urine may contain levels 10 to 20 times higher than those in serum. Little, if any, metabolic transformation occurs. Renal excretion is extremely rapid. In patients with normal renal function, approximately one-half of the administered dose is cleared within 4 hours and excretion is complete within 24 to 48 hours. Patients with impaired renal function or with diminished glomerular filtration pressure excrete kanamycin more slowly. Such patients may build up excessively high blood levels which greatly increase the risk of ototoxic reactions. In severely burned patients the half-life may be significantly decreased and resulting serum concentrations may be lower than anticipated from the mg per kg dose.

Microbiology

Kanamycin sulfate is a bactericidal antibiotic which acts by inhibiting the synthesis of protein in susceptible microorganisms. Kanamycin sulfate is active **in vitro** against many strains of **Staphylococcus aureus** (including penicillinase and nonpenicillinase-producing strains), **Staphylococcus epidermidis, N. gonorrhoeae, H. influenzae, E. coli, Enterobacter aerogenes, Shigella** and **Salmonella** species, **K. pneumoniae, Serratia marcescens, Providencia** species, **Acinetobacter** species and **Citrobacter freundii** and **Citrobacter species,** and many strains of both indole-positive and indole-negative **Proteus** strains that are frequently resistant to other antibiotics.

Aminoglycosides have a low order of activity against most gram-positive organisms including **Streptococcus pyogenes, Streptococcus pneumoniae** and **enterococci. In vitro** studies have demonstrated that an aminoglycoside combined with an antibiotic which interferes with cell wall synthesis (ie, Penicillin G or ampicillin affects some Group D streptococcal strains synergistically. Bacteriological testing and tests for antibiotic synergism are necessary.

Enzymatic inactivation of deoxystreptamine is the principal mechanism of resistance.

Susceptibility Testing: Quantitative methods for susceptibility testing that require measurement of zone diameters give the most precise estimates of antibiotic susceptibility. One such procedure has been recommended for use with discs to test susceptibility to kanamycin. Interpretation involves correlation of the diameters obtained in the disc test with minimal inhibitory concentration (MIC) values for kanamycin.

Reports from the laboratory give results of the standardized single disc susceptibility test (Bauer, et al, Am J Clin Path 1966; 45:493 and Federal Register 37:20525-20529, 1972), using a 30-µg kanamycin disc should be interpreted according to the following criteria:

Organisms producing zones of 18 mm or greater, or MICs of 16 µg or less are considered susceptible, indicating that the test organism is likely to respond to therapy.

Resistant organisms produce zones of 14 mm or less or MICs of 16 µg or greater. A report of "resistant" from the laboratory indicates that the infecting organism is not likely to respond to therapy.

Zones greater than 14 mm and less than 18 mm, or MICs of greater than 16 µg and less than 65 µg, indicate intermediate susceptibility. A report of "intermediate" susceptibility suggests that the organism would be susceptible if the infection is confined to tissues and fluids (eg, urine), in which high antibiotic levels are attained.

Control organisms are recommended for susceptibility testing. Each time the test is performed one or more of the following organisms should be included: **Escherichia coli** ATCC 15922, **Staphylococcus aureus** ATCC 25923 and **Pseudomonas aeruginosa** ATCC 27853. The control organisms should produce zones of inhibition within the following ranges:

Escherichia coli (ATCC 15922)	22–30 mm
Staphylococcus aureus (ATCC 25923)	22–31 mm
Pseudomonas aeruginosa (ATCC 27853)	17–23 mm

INDICATIONS AND USAGE

Kanamycin is indicated in the short-term treatment of serious infections caused by susceptible strains of the designated microorganisms below. Bacteriological studies to identify the causative organisms and to determine their susceptibility to kanamycin should be performed. Therapy may be instituted prior to obtaining the results of susceptibility testing. Kanamycin may be considered as initial therapy in the treatment of infections where one or more of the following are the known or suspected pathogens: **E. coli, Proteus** species (both indole-positive and indole-negative), **Enterobacter aerogenes, Klebsiella pneumoniae, Serratia marcescens, Acinetobacter** species. The decision to continue therapy with the drug should be based on results of the susceptibility tests, the response of the infection to therapy, and the important additional concepts contained in the "Warning" box above.

In serious infections when the causative organisms are unknown, Kantrex may be administered as initial therapy in conjunction with a penicillin- or cephalosporin-type drug before obtaining results of susceptibility testing. If anerobic organisms are suspected, consideration should be given to using other suitable antimicrobial therapy in conjunction with kanamycin.

Although kanamycin is not the drug of choice for staphylococcal infections, it may be indicated under certain conditions for the treatment of known or suspected staphylococcal disease. These situations include the initial therapy of severe infections where the organism is thought to be either a Gram-negative bacterium or a staphylococcus, infections due to susceptible strains of staphylococci in patients allergic to other antibiotics, and mixed staphylococcal/Gram-negative infections.

CONTRAINDICATIONS

A history of hypersensitivity or toxic reaction to one aminoglycoside may also contraindicate the use of any other

aminoglycoside, because of the known cross-sensitivity and cumulative effects of drugs in this category.

THIS DRUG IS **NOT** INDICATED IN LONG-TERM THERAPY (eg, Tuberculosis) BECAUSE OF THE TOXIC HAZARD ASSOCIATED WITH EXTENDED ADMINISTRATION.

WARNING

See "Warning" box above.

Aminoglycosides can cause fetal harm when administered to pregnant women. Aminoglycoside antibiotics cross the placenta and there have been several reports of total, irreversible, bilateral congenital deafness in children whose mothers received streptomycin during pregnancy. Although serious side effects to fetus or newborn have not been reported in treatment of pregnant women with other aminoglycosides, the potential for harm exists.

Reproductive studies have been performed in rats and rabbits and have revealed no evidence of impaired fertility or teratogenic effects. Dosages of 200 mg/kg/day in pregnant rats and pregnant guinea pigs led to hearing impairment in the offspring. There are no well-controlled studies in pregnant women but clinical experience does not include any positive evidence of adverse effects on the fetus. However, if the drug is used during pregnancy, or if the patient becomes pregnant while taking this drug, the patient should be apprised of the potential hazard on the fetus.

Contains sodium bisulfite, a sulfite that may cause allergic-type reactions including anaphylactic symptoms and life-threatening or less severe asthmatic episodes in certain susceptible people. The overall prevalence of sulfite sensitivity in the general population is unknown and probably low. Sulfite sensitivity is seen more frequently in asthmatic than in nonasthmatic people.

PRECAUTIONS

General

Neurotoxic and nephrotoxic antibiotics may be almost completely absorbed from body surfaces (except the urinary bladder) after local irrigation and after topical application during surgical procedures. The potential toxic effects of antibiotics administered in this fashion (oto- and nephrotoxicity, neuromuscular blockade, respiratory paralysis) should be considered. (See "Warning" box).

Increased nephrotoxicity has been reported following concomitant administration of aminoglycoside antibiotics with some cephalosporins.

Aminoglycosides should be used with caution in patients with neuromuscular disorders such as myasthenia gravis, Parkinsonism, or infant botulism, since these drugs may aggravate muscle weakness because of their potential curare-like effect on neuromuscular junction.

Elderly patients may have a decrease in renal function which may not be evident in the results of routine screening tests, such as BUN or serum creatinine levels. Measurement of creatinine clearance or an estimate based on published nomograms or equations may be more useful. Monitoring of renal function during treatment with kanamycin as with other aminoglycosides, is particularly important in such patients.

Because of high concentrations of kanamycin sulfate in the urinary excretory system, patients should be well hydrated before treatment to prevent irritation of the renal tubules.

NOTE: The risk of toxic reactions is low in well-hydrated patients with normal kidney function, who receive a total dose of 15 g of kanamycin or less.

Treatment with kanamycin may result in overgrowth of nonsusceptible organisms. If this occurs kanamycin should be discontinued and appropriate therapy initiated.

Laboratory Tests

Tests of eighth cranial nerve functions: Serial audiometric tests are suggested, particularly when renal function is impaired and/or prolonged aminoglycoside therapy is required; such tests should also be repeated periodically after treatment if there is evidence of a hearing deficit or vestibular abnormalities before or during therapy, or when consecutive or concomitant use of other potentially ototoxic drug is unavoidable.

Test of renal function: It should be emphasized that since renal function may alter appreciably during therapy, renal function should be tested daily or more frequently. Urine should be examined for increased excretion of protein and for presence of cells and casts, keeping in mind the effects of the primary illness on these tests. One or more of the following laboratory measurements should be obtained at the onset of therapy, frequently during therapy, and at, or shortly after, the end of therapy:

Creatinine clearance rate (either carefully measured or estimated from published nomograms or equations based on patient's age, sex, body weight, and serial creatinine concentrations) (preferred over BUN).

Serum creatinine concentration (preferred over BUN).

Blood urea nitrogen (BUN).

More frequent testing is desirable if renal function is changing. If signs of renal irritation appear, such as casts, white or red cells, and albumin, hydration should be increased and a reduction in dosage may be desirable (see "Dosage and Administration"). These signs usually disappear when treatment is completed. However, if azotemia or a progressive decrease of urine output occurs, treatment should be stopped.

Drug Interactions: In vitro mixing of an aminoglycoside with beta-lactam-type antibiotics (penicillins or cephalosporins) may result in a significant mutual inactivation. Even when an aminoglycoside and a penicillin-type drug are administered separately by different routes, a reduction in aminoglycoside serum half-life or serum levels has been reported in patients with impaired renal function and in some patients with normal renal function. Usually, such inactivation of the aminoglycoside is clinically significant only in patients with severely impaired renal function. (See also "Laboratory test interactions"). See "Warnings" box regarding concurrent use of potent diuretics, concurrent and/or sequential use of other neurotoxic and/or nephrotoxic antibiotics, and for other essential information.

Laboratory Test Interactions: Concomitant cephalosporin therapy may spuriously elevate creatinine determinations. The inactivation between aminoglycosides and beta-lactam antibiotics described in "Drug Interactions" may continue in specimens of body fluids collected for assay, resulting in inaccurate, false low aminoglycoside readings. Such specimens should be properly handled, ie assayed promptly, frozen, or treated with beta-lactamase.

Carcinogenesis, mutagenesis, impairment of fertility: Studies have not been performed with kanamycin to determine its effect in carcinogenesis, mutagenesis or impairment of fertility.

Pregnancy Category D: (See "Warnings" Section.)

Nursing mothers: Kanamycin sulfate is excreted in minute amounts in human milk. Because of the potential for serious adverse reactions from aminoglycosides in nursing infants, a decision should be made whether to discontinue nursing or to discontinue the drug taking into account the importance of the drug to the mother.

Pediatric Use: Aminoglycosides should be used with caution in prematures and neonates because of the renal immaturity of these patients and the resulting prolongation of serum half-life of these drugs.

ADVERSE REACTIONS

Kanamycin has the potential to induce auditory and sometimes vestibular toxicity, renal toxicity, and neuromuscular blockade. The risks are higher for patients with a present or past history of renal impairment (especially if hemodialysis is required), for those receiving concomitant or sequential treatment with other ototoxic or nephrotoxic drugs or rapid acting diuretic agents given intravenously (ethacrynic acid, furosemide, and mannitol), and for patients treated for longer periods and/or with higher doses than recommended.

Ototoxicity: Toxic effects of kanamycin on the eighth cranial nerve can result in partially reversible or irreversible bilateral loss of hearing, loss of balance, or both. Tinnitus or vertigo may or may not be experienced. Cochlear damage is usually manifested initially by small changes in audiometric test results at the high frequencies and may not be associated with subjective hearing loss. Vestibular dysfunction is usually manifested by nystagmus, vertigo, nausea, vomiting, or acute Meniere's syndrome.

Nephrotoxicity: Albuminuria, presence of red and white cells, and granular casts; azotemia and oliguria have been reported. Renal function changes are usually reversible when the drug is discontinued. Renal impairment may be characterized by a rise in serum creatinine and may be accompanied by oliguria, presence of casts, cells, and protein in the urine, by rising levels of BUN or by decrease in creatinine clearance.

Neuromuscular blockade: Acute muscular paralysis and apnea can occur following treatment with aminoglycoside antibiotics. Neurotoxicity can occur after intrapleural and interperitoneal instillation of large doses of an aminoglycoside; however, the reaction has followed intravenous, intramuscular, and even the oral administration of these agents.

Other: Some local irritation or pain may follow the intramuscular injection of kanamycin. Other adverse reactions of the drug reported on rare occasions are skin rash, drug fever, headache, paresthesia, nausea, vomiting, and diarrhea. The "malabsorption syndrome" characterized by an increase in fecal fat, decrease in serum carotene and fall in xylose absorption, reportedly has occurred with prolonged therapy.

OVERDOSAGE

In the event of overdosage or toxic reaction, hemodialysis or peritoneal dialysis will aid in the removal of kanamycin from the blood. In the newborn infant, exchange transfusions may also be considered.

DOSAGE AND ADMINISTRATION

Kanamycin injection may be given intramuscularly or intravenously. The patient's pretreatment body weight should be obtained for calculation of the correct dosage. The dosage of an aminoglycoside in obese patients should be based on an estimate of the lean body mass. The status of renal function should be determined by measurement of serum creatinine

concentration or calculation of the endogenous creatinine clearance rate. The blood urea nitrogen (BUN) level is much less reliable for this purpose. Renal function should be reassessed frequently during therapy.

It is desirable to measure both peak and trough serum concentrations intermittently during therapy since both concentrations are used to determine the adequacy and safety of the dose and to adjust the dosage during treatment. Peak serum concentrations (30 to 90 minutes after injection) above 35 μg per mL and trough concentrations (just prior to the next dose) above 10 μg per mL should be avoided.

Intramuscular Route: Inject deeply into the upper outer quadrant of the gluteal muscle. The recommended dose for adults or children is 15 mg/kg/day in two equally divided dosages administered at equally divided intervals, ie, 7.5 mg/kg q12h. If continuously high blood levels are desired, the daily dose of 15 mg/kg may be given in equally divided doses every 6 or 8 hours. Treatment of patients in the heavier weight classes, ie, 100 kg, should not exceed 1.5 g/day.

In patients with impaired renal function, it is desirable to follow therapy by appropriate serum assays. If this is not feasible, a suggested method is to reduce the frequency of administration in patients with renal dysfunction. The interval between doses may be calculated with the following formula:

Serum creatinine (mg/100 mL) × 9 = Dosage Interval (in hours); eg, if the serum creatinine is 2 mg, the recommended dose (7.5 mg/kg) should be administered every 18 hours. Changes in creatinine concentration during therapy would, of course, necessitate changes in the dosage frequency.

It is desirable to limit the duration of treatment with kanamycin to short term. The usual duration of treatment is 7 to 10 days. Total daily dose by all routes of administration should not exceed 1.5 g/day. If longer therapy is required, measurement of kanamycin peak and trough serum concentrations is particularly important as a basis for determining the adequacy and safety of the dose. These patients should be carefully monitored for changes in renal, auditory, and vestibular function. Dosage should be adjusted as needed. The risks of toxicity multiply as the length of treatment increases.

At the recommended dosage level, uncomplicated infections due to kanamycin-susceptible organisms should respond to therapy in 24 to 48 hours. If definite clinical response does not occur within 3 to 5 days, therapy should be stopped and the antibiotic susceptibility pattern of the invading organism should be rechecked. Failure of the infection to respond may be due to resistance of the organism or to the presence of septic foci requiring surgical drainage.

Intravenous Administration: The dose should not exceed 15 mg/kg per day and must be administered slowly. The solution for intravenous use is prepared by adding the contents of a 500-mg vial to 100 to 200 mL of sterile diluent such as Normal Saline or 5% Dextrose in Water, or the contents of a 1.0-g vial to 200 to 400 mL of sterile diluent. The appropriate dose is administered over a 30- to 60-minute period. The total daily dose should be divided into 2 or 3 equally divided doses. In pediatric patients the amount of diluent used should be sufficient to infuse the kanamycin sulfate over a 30- to 60-minute period.

Kanamycin sulfate injection should not be physically mixed with other antibacterial agents but each should be administered separately in accordance with its recommended route of administration and dosage schedule.

Intraperitoneal Use: (following exploration for established peritonitis or after peritoneal contamination due to fecal spill during surgery.)

Adults: 500 mg diluted in 20 mL sterile distilled water may be instilled through a polyethylene catheter sutured into the wound at closure. If possible, instillation should be postponed until the patient has fully recovered from the effects of anesthesia and muscle-relaxing drugs (see duration of treatment statement above and "Warning" box). Serum levels should be carefully monitored during treatment.

Aerosol Treatment: 250 mg 2 to 4 times a day. Withdraw 250 mg (1.0 mL) from a 500-mg vial and dilute it with 3 mL Physiological Saline and nebulize. Serum levels should be carefully monitored during treatment.

Other Routes of Administration: Kantrex Injection in concentrations of 0.25 percent (2.5 mg/mL) has been used as an irrigating solution in abscess cavities, pleural space, peritoneal and ventricular cavities. Possible absorption of Kantrex by such routes must be taken into account and dosage adjustments should be arranged so that a maximum total dose of 1.5 g/day by all routes of administration is not exceeded. Serum levels should be carefully monitored during treatment.

PEDIATRIC DOSAGE GUIDE FOR
KANTREX PEDIATRIC INJECTION,
75 mg/2 mL—
AMOUNT PER 24 HOURS
TO BE GIVEN IN DIVIDED DOSES

Weight in Pounds	Weight in Kilograms	Daily Dosage in Milligrams	Daily Dosage in Milliliters
2.2	1.00	15.0	0.4
2.8	1.25	18.8	0.5
3.3	1.50	22.5	0.6
3.9	1.75	26.2	0.7
4.4	2.00	30.0	0.8
5.0	2.25	33.8	0.9
5.5	2.50	37.5	1.0
6.0	2.75	41.2	1.1
6.6	3.00	45.0	1.2
7.7	3.50	52.5	1.4
8.8	4.00	60.0	1.6
9.9	4.50	67.5	1.8
11.0	5.00	75.0	2.0

STABILITY

Occasionally, some vials may darken during the shelf life of the product, but this does not indicate a loss of potency. Parenteral drug products should be inspected visually for particulate matter and discoloration prior to administration, whenever container and solution permit.

HOW SUPPLIED

KANTREX INJECTION (kanamycin sulfate injection)
    NDC 0015-3502-20—500 mg per 2 mL
    NDC 0015-3502-24—Disposable Syringe (500 mg per 2 mL)
    NDC 0015-3503-20—1 g per 3 mL
KANTREX PEDIATRIC INJECTION (kanamycin sulfate injection)
    NDC 0015-3512-20—75 mg per 2 mL
    (activity assayed as kanamycin base)
For information on package sizes available, refer to the current price schedule.

Bristol-Myers Oncology Division
(A Bristol-Myers Company)
2404 W. PENNSYLVANIA STREET
EVANSVILLE, IN 47721

BiCNU®   ℞
[bĭk′nū]
(sterile carmustine [BCNU])

> **WARNINGS**
> BiCNU (sterile carmustine [BCNU]) should be administered under the supervision of a qualified physician experienced in the use of cancer chemotherapeutic agents.
> Bone marrow suppression, notably thrombocytopenia and leukopenia, which may contribute to bleeding and overwhelming infections in an already compromised patient, is the most common and severe of the toxic effects of BiCNU (see "WARNINGS" and "ADVERSE REACTIONS").
> Since the major toxicity is delayed bone marrow suppression, blood counts should be monitored weekly for at least six weeks after a dose (see "ADVERSE REACTIONS"). At the recommended dosage, courses of BiCNU should not be given more frequently than every six weeks.
> The bone marrow toxicity of BiCNU is cumulative and therefore dosage adjustment must be considered on the basis of nadir blood counts from prior dose (see "Dosage Adjustment Table" under "DOSAGE AND ADMINISTRATION").
> Pulmonary toxicity from BiCNU appears to be dose related. Patients receiving greater than 1400 mg/m^2 cumulative dose are at significantly higher risk than those receiving less.

DESCRIPTION

BiCNU (sterile carmustine [BCNU]) is one of the nitrosoureas used in the treatment of certain neoplastic diseases. It is 1,3-bis (2-chloroethyl)-1-nitrosourea. It is lyophilized pale yellow flakes or congealed mass with a molecular weight of 214.06. It is highly soluble in alcohol and lipids, and poorly soluble in water. BiCNU is administered by intravenous infusion after reconstitution as recommended.

Continued on next page

Bristol-Myers Oncology—Cont.

The structural formula is:

$$Cl-CH_2-CH_2-N-C-NH-CH_2-CH_2-Cl$$
$$\underset{NO}{|} \qquad \overset{O}{\overset{||}{}}$$

Sterile BiCNU is available in 100 mg single dose vials of lyophilized material.

CLINICAL PHARMACOLOGY

Although it is generally agreed that BiCNU alkylates DNA and RNA, it is not cross resistant with other alkylators. As with other nitrosoureas, it may also inhibit several key enzymatic processes by carbamoylation of amino acids in proteins.

Intravenously-administered BiCNU is rapidly degraded, with no intact drug detectable after 15 minutes. However, in studies with C–14 labeled drug, prolonged levels of the isotope were detected in the plasma and tissue, probably representing radioactive fragments of the parent compound.

It is thought that the antineoplastic and toxic activities of BiCNU may be due to metabolites. Approximately 60 to 70% of a total dose is excreted in the urine in 96 hours and about 10% as respiratory CO_2. The fate of the remainder is undetermined.

Because of the high lipid solubility and the relative lack of ionization at physiological pH, BiCNU crosses the blood-brain barrier quite effectively. Levels of radioactivity in the CSF are $\geq$ 50% of those measured concurrently in plasma.

INDICATIONS AND USAGE

BiCNU is indicated as palliative therapy as a single agent or in established combination therapy with other approved chemotherapeutic agents in the following:

1. Brain tumors—glioblastoma, brainstem glioma, medulloblastoma, astrocytoma, ependymoma, and metastatic brain tumors.
2. Multiple myeloma—in combination with prednisone.
3. Hodgkin's Disease—as secondary therapy in combination with other approved drugs in patients who relapse while being treated with primary therapy, or who fail to respond to primary therapy.
4. Non-Hodgkin's lymphomas—as secondary therapy in combination with other approved drugs for patients who relapse while being treated with primary therapy, or who fail to respond to primary therapy.

CONTRAINDICATIONS

BiCNU should not be given to individuals who have demonstrated a previous hypersensitivity to it.

WARNINGS

Since the major toxicity is delayed bone marrow suppression, blood counts should be monitored weekly for at least six weeks after a dose (see "ADVERSE REACTIONS"). At the recommended dosage, courses of BiCNU should not be given more frequently than every six weeks.

The bone marrow toxicity of BiCNU is cumulative and therefore dosage adjustment must be considered on the basis of nadir blood counts from prior dose (see "Dosage Adjustment Table" under "DOSAGE AND ADMINISTRATION").

Pulmonary toxicity from BiCNU appears to be dose related. Patients receiving greater than 1400 mg/m^2 cumulative dose are at significantly higher risk than those receiving less (see "ADVERSE REACTIONS").

Long term use of nitrosoureas has been reported to be associated with the development of secondary malignancies.

Liver and renal function tests should be monitored periodically (see "ADVERSE REACTIONS").

BiCNU may cause fetal harm when administered to a pregnant woman. BiCNU has been shown to be embryotoxic in rats and rabbits and teratogenic in rats when given in doses equivalent to the human dose. There are no adequate and well-controlled studies in pregnant women. If this drug is used during pregnancy, or if the patient becomes pregnant while taking (receiving) this drug, the patient should be apprised of the potential hazard to the fetus. Women of childbearing potential should be advised to avoid becoming pregnant.

BiCNU has been administered through an intra-arterial intracarotid route; this procedure is investigational and has been associated with ocular toxicity.

PRECAUTIONS

General: In all instances where the use of BiCNU is considered for chemotherapy, the physician must evaluate the need and usefulness of the drug against the risks of toxic effects or adverse reactions. Most such adverse reactions are reversible if detected early. When such effects or reactions do occur, the drug should be reduced in dosage or discontinued and appropriate corrective measures should be taken according to the clinical judgment of the physician. Reinstitution of BiCNU therapy should be carried out with caution, and with adequate consideration of the further need for the drug and alertness as to possible recurrence of toxicity.

Laboratory Tests: Due to delayed bone marrow suppression, blood counts should be monitored weekly for at least six weeks after a dose.

Baseline pulmonary function studies should be conducted along with frequent pulmonary function tests during treatment. Patients with a baseline below 70% of the predicted Forced Vital Capacity (FVC) or Carbon Monoxide Diffusing Capacity (DL$_{CO}$) are particularly at risk.

Since BiCNU may cause liver dysfunction, it is recommended that liver function tests be monitored.

Renal function tests should also be monitored periodically.

Carcinogenesis, Mutagenesis, Impairment of Fertility: BiCNU is carcinogenic in rats and mice, producing a marked increase in tumor incidence in doses approximating those employed clinically. Nitrosourea therapy does have carcinogenic potential in humans (see "ADVERSE REACTIONS"). BiCNU also affects fertility in male rats at doses somewhat higher than the human dose.

Pregnancy: Pregnancy "Category D," see "WARNINGS."

Nursing Mothers: It is not known whether this drug is excreted in human milk. Because many drugs are excreted in human milk and because of the potential for serious adverse reactions in nursing infants from BiCNU, a decision should be made whether to discontinue nursing or to discontinue the drug, taking into account the importance of the drug to the mother.

Pediatric Use: Safety and effectiveness in children have not been established.

ADVERSE REACTIONS

Hematologic Toxicity: The most frequent and most serious toxicity of BiCNU is delayed myelosuppression. It usually occurs four to six weeks after drug administration and is dose related. Thrombocytopenia occurs at about four weeks postadministration and persists for one to two weeks. Leukopenia occurs at five to six weeks after a dose of BiCNU and persists for one to two weeks. Thrombocytopenia is generally more severe than leukopenia. However, both may be dose-limiting toxicities.

BiCNU may produce cumulative myelosuppression, manifested by more depressed indices or longer duration of suppression after repeated doses.

The occurrence of acute leukemia and bone marrow dysplasias have been reported in patients following long term nitrosourea therapy.

Anemia also occurs, but is less frequent and less severe than thrombocytopenia or leukopenia.

Pulmonary Toxicity: Pulmonary toxicity characterized by pulmonary infiltrates and/or fibrosis has been reported with BiCNU and related nitrosoureas. Most of these patients were receiving prolonged therapy with total doses of BiCNU greater than 1400 mg/m^2. However, there have been reports of pulmonary fibrosis in patients receiving lower total doses. Other risk factors include past history of lung disease and duration of treatment. Cases of fatal pulmonary toxicity with BiCNU have been reported.

Gastrointestinal Toxicity: Nausea and vomiting after IV administration of BiCNU are noted frequently. This toxicity appears within two hours of dosing, usually lasting four to six hours, and is dose related. Prior administration of antiemetics is effective in diminishing and sometimes preventing this side effect.

Hepatotoxicity: A reversible type of hepatic toxicity, manifested by increased transaminase, alkaline phosphatase and bilirubin levels, has been reported in a small percentage of patients receiving BiCNU.

Nephrotoxicity: Renal abnormalities consisting of progressive azotemia, decrease in kidney size and renal failure have been reported in patients who received large cumulative doses after prolonged therapy with BiCNU and related nitrosoureas. Kidney damage has also been reported occasionally in patients receiving lower total doses.

Other Toxicities: Accidental contact of reconstituted BiCNU with skin has caused burning and hyperpigmentation of the affected areas.

Rapid IV infusion of BiCNU may produce intensive flushing of the skin and suffusion of the conjunctiva within two hours, lasting about four hours. It is also associated with burning at the site of injection although true thrombosis is rare.

Neuroretinitis has been reported.

OVERDOSAGE

No proven antidotes have been established for BiCNU overdosage.

DOSAGE AND ADMINISTRATION

The recommended dose of BiCNU as a single agent in previously untreated patients is 150 to 200 mg/m^2 intravenously every six weeks. This may be given as a single dose or divided into daily injections such as 75 to 100 mg/m^2 on two successive days. When BiCNU is used in combination with other myelosuppressive drugs or in patients in whom bone marrow reserve is depleted, the doses should be adjusted accordingly. Doses subsequent to the initial dose should be adjusted according to the hematologic response of the patient to the preceding dose. The following schedule is suggested as a guide to dosage adjustment:

Nadir After Prior Dose		Percentage of Prior Dose to be Given
Leukocytes/mm^3	Platelets/mm^3	
> 4000	> 100,000	100%
3000–3999	75,000–99,999	100%
2000–2999	25,000–74,999	70%
< 2000	< 25,000	50%

A repeat course of BiCNU should not be given until circulating blood elements have returned to acceptable levels (platelets above 100,000/mm^3, leukocytes above 4,000/mm^3), and this is usually in six weeks. Adequate number of neutrophils should be present on a peripheral blood smear. Blood counts should be monitored weekly and repeat courses should not be given before six weeks because the hematologic toxicity is delayed and cumulative.

Administration Precautions: As with other potentially toxic compounds, caution should be exercised in handling BiCNU and preparing the solution of BiCNU. Accidental contact of reconstituted BiCNU with the skin has caused transient hyperpigmentation of the affected areas. The use of gloves is recommended. If BiCNU lyophilized material or solution contacts the skin or mucosa, immediately wash the skin or mucosa thoroughly with soap and water.

The reconstituted solution should be used intravenously only and should be administered by IV drip. Injection of BiCNU over shorter periods of time than one to two hours may produce intense pain and burning at the site of injection.

Preparation of Intravenous Solutions: First, dissolve BiCNU with 3 mL of the supplied sterile diluent (Dehydrated Alcohol Injection, USP). Second, aseptically add 27 mL Sterile Water for Injection, USP. Each mL of resulting solution contains 3.3 mg of BiCNU in 10% ethanol, pH 5.6 to 6.0. Reconstitution as recommended results in a clear, colorless to yellowish solution which may be further diluted with 0.9% Sodium Chloride Injection, USP, or 5% Dextrose Injection, USP. Parenteral drug products should be inspected visually for particulate matter and discoloration prior to administration, whenever solution and container permit.

Important Note: The lyophilized dosage formulation contains no preservatives and is not intended as a multiple dose vial.

Stability: Unopened vials of the dry drug must be stored in a refrigerator (2°C to 8°C). The recommended storage of unopened vials provides a stable product for two years. After reconstitution as recommended, BiCNU is stable for eight hours at room temperature (25°C) or 24 hours under refrigeration (4°C).

Vials reconstituted as directed and further diluted to a concentration of 0.2 mg/mL in 5% Dextrose Injection, USP, or 0.9% Sodium Chloride Injection, USP, are stable for 48 hours under refrigeration (4°C) and an additional 8 hours at room temperature (25°C) under normal room fluorescent light.

Glass containers were used for the stability data provided in this section. Only use glass containers for BiCNU administration.

Important Note: BiCNU has a low melting point (30.5° to 32.0°C or 86.9° to 89.6°F). Exposure of the drug to this temperature or above will cause the drug to liquefy and appear as an oil film on the vials. This is a sign of decomposition and vials should be discarded. If there is a question of adequate refrigeration upon receipt of this product, immediately inspect the larger vial in each individual carton. Hold the vial to a bright light for inspection. The BiCNU will appear as a very small amount of dry flakes or dry congealed mass. If this is evident, the BiCNU is suitable for use and should be refrigerated immediately.

Procedures for proper handling and disposal of anticancer drugs should be considered. Several guidelines on this subject have been published.[1-7] There is no general agreement that all of the procedures recommended in the guidelines are necessary or appropriate.

REFERENCES

1. Recommendations for the Safe Handling of Parenteral Antineoplastic Drugs, NIH Publication No. 83–2621. For sale by the Superintendent of Documents, US Government Printing Office, Washington, DC 20402.
2. AMA Council Report, Guidelines for Handling Parenteral Antineoplastics. JAMA 1985 March 15.
3. National Study Commission on Cytotoxic Exposure—Recommendations for Handling Cytotoxic Agents. Available from Louis P. Jeffrey, ScD., Chairman, National Study Commission on Cytotoxic Exposure, Massachusetts College of Pharmacy and Allied Health Sciences, 179 Longwood Avenue, Boston, Massachusetts 02115.
4. Clinical Oncological Society of Australia. Guidelines and Recommendations for Safe Handling of Antineoplastic Agents. Med J Australia 1983; 1:426–428.

5. Jones RB, et al: Safe handling of chemotherapeutic agents: a report from the Mount Sinai Medical Center, CA—A Cancer Journal for Clinicians 1983; (Sept/Oct) 258–263.
6. American Society of Hospital Pharmacists Technical Assistance Bulletin on Handling Cytotoxic Drugs in Hospitals. Am J Hosp Pharm 1985; 42:131–137.
7. OSHA Work-Practice Guidelines for Personnel Dealing with Cytotoxic (Antineoplastic) Drugs. Am J Hosp Pharm 1986; 43:1193–1204.

SUPPLY

BiCNU (sterile carmustine [BCNU]). Each package contains a vial containing 100 mg carmustine and a vial containing 3 mL sterile diluent.
NDC 0015-3012
Store dry powder in refrigerator (2° to 8°C).
For information on package sizes available refer to the current price schedule.
Manufactured by Ben Venue Laboratories, Inc., Bedford, Ohio 44146

BLENOXANE®   ℞
[blĕ-nŏk'sān]
(sterile bleomycin sulfate, USP)
vial, 15 units NSN 6505-01-060-4278(m)

WARNING

It is recommended that Blenoxane be administered under the supervision of a qualified physician experienced in the use of cancer chemotherapeutic agents.

Appropriate management of therapy and complications is possible only when adequate diagnostic and treatment facilities are readily available.

Pulmonary fibrosis is the most severe toxicity associated with Blenoxane. The most frequent presentation is pneumonitis occasionally progressing to pulmonary fibrosis. Its occurrence is higher in elderly patients and in those receiving greater than 400 units total dose, but pulmonary toxicity has been observed in young patients and those treated with low doses.

A severe idiosyncratic reaction consisting of hypotension, mental confusion, fever, chills, and wheezing has been reported in approximately 1% of lymphoma patients treated with Blenoxane.

DESCRIPTION

Blenoxane (sterile bleomycin sulfate, USP) is a mixture of cytotoxic glycopeptide antibiotics isolated from a strain of **Streptomyces verticillus**. It is freely soluble in water.
Note: A unit of bleomycin is equal to the formerly used milligram activity. The term milligram activity is a misnomer and was changed to units to be more precise.

ACTION

Although the exact mechanism of action of Blenoxane is unknown, available evidence would seem to indicate that the main mode of action is the inhibition of DNA synthesis with some evidence of lesser inhibition of RNA and protein synthesis.

In mice, high concentrations of Blenoxane are found in the skin, lungs, kidneys, peritoneum, and lymphatics. Tumor cells of the skin and lungs have been found to have high concentrations of Blenoxane in contrast to the low concentrations found in hematopoietic tissue. The low concentrations of Blenoxane found in bone marrow may be related to high levels of Blenoxane degradative enzymes found in that tissue.

In patients with a creatinine clearance of > 35 mL per minute, the serum or plasma terminal elimination half-life of bleomycin is approximately 115 minutes. In patients with a creatinine clearance of < 35 mL per minute, the plasma or serum terminal elimination half-life increases exponentially as the creatinine clearance decreases. In humans, 60% to 70% of an administered dose is recovered in the urine as active bleomycin.

INDICATIONS

Blenoxane should be considered a palliative treatment. It has been shown to be useful in the management of the following neoplasms either as a single agent or in proven combinations with other approved chemotherapeutic agents:
Squamous Cell Carcinoma—Head and neck (including mouth, tongue, tonsil, nasopharynx, oropharynx, sinus, palate, lip, buccal mucosa, gingiva, epiglottis, larynx), skin, penis, cervix, and vulva. The response to Blenoxane is poorer in patients with head and neck cancer previously irradiated.
Lymphomas—Hodgkin's, reticulum cell sarcoma, lymphosarcoma.
Testicular Carcinoma—Embryonal cell, choriocarcinoma, and teratocarcinoma.

CONTRAINDICATIONS

Blenoxane is contraindicated in patients who have demonstrated a hypersensitive or an idiosyncratic reaction to it.

WARNINGS

Patients receiving Blenoxane must be observed carefully and frequently during and after therapy. It should be used with extreme caution in patients with significant impairment of renal function or compromised pulmonary function.
Pulmonary toxicities occur in 10% of treated patients. In approximately 1%, the nonspecific pneumonitis induced by Blenoxane progresses to pulmonary fibrosis, and death. Although this is age and dose related, the toxicity is unpredictable. Frequent roentgenograms are recommended.
Idiosyncratic reactions similar to anaphylaxis have been reported in 1% of lymphoma patients treated with Blenoxane. Since these usually occur after the first or second dose, careful monitoring is essential after these doses.
Renal or hepatic toxicity, beginning as a deterioration in renal or liver function tests, have been reported infrequently. These toxicities may occur, however, at any time after initiation of therapy.
Usage in Pregnancy: Safe use of Blenoxane in pregnant women has not been established.

ADVERSE REACTIONS

Pulmonary—This is potentially the most serious side effect, occurring in approximately 10% of treated patients. The most frequent presentation is pneumonitis occasionally progressing to pulmonary fibrosis. Approximately 1% of patients treated have died of pulmonary fibrosis. Pulmonary toxicity is both dose and age related, being more common in patients over 70 years of age and in those receiving over 400 units total dose. This toxicity, however, is unpredictable and has been seen occasionally in young patients receiving low doses.
Because of lack of specificity of the clinical syndrome, the identification of patients with pulmonary toxicity due to Blenoxane has been extremely difficult. The earliest symptom associated with Blenoxane pulmonary toxicity is dyspnea. The earliest sign is fine rales.
Radiographically, Blenoxane-induced pneumonitis produces nonspecific patchy opacities, usually of the lower lung fields. The most common changes in pulmonary function tests are a decrease in total lung volume and a decrease in vital capacity. However, these changes are not predictive of the development of pulmonary fibrosis.
The microscopic tissue changes due to Blenoxane toxicity include bronchiolar squamous metaplasia, reactive macrophages, atypical alveolar epithelial cells, fibrinous edema, and interstitial fibrosis. The acute stage may involve capillary changes and subsequent fibrinous exudation into alveoli producing a change similar to hyaline membrane formation and progressing to a diffuse interstitial fibrosis resembling the Hamman-Rich syndrome. These microscopic findings are nonspecific, e.g., similar changes are seen in radiation pneumonitis, pneumocystic pneumonitis.
To monitor the onset of pulmonary toxicity, roentgenograms of the chest should be taken every 1 to 2 weeks. If pulmonary changes are noted, treatment should be discontinued until it can be determined if they are drug related. Recent studies have suggested that sequential measurement of the pulmonary diffusion capacity for carbon monoxide (DL_{co}) during treatment with Blenoxane may be an indicator of subclinical pulmonary toxicity. It is recommended that the DL_{co} be monitored monthly if it is to be employed to detect pulmonary toxicities, and thus the drug should be discontinued when the DL_{co} falls below 30% to 35% of the pretreatment value.
Because of bleomycin's sensitization of lung tissue, patients who have received bleomycin are at greater risk of developing pulmonary toxicity when oxygen is administered in surgery. While long exposure to very high oxygen concentrations is a known cause of lung damage, after bleomycin administration, lung damage can occur at lower concentrations than usually would be considered safe. Suggestive preventive measures are:
(1) Maintain Fl O_2 at concentrations approximating that of room air (25%) during surgery and the postoperative period.
(2) Monitor carefully fluid replacement, focusing more on colloid administration rather than crystalloid.
Sudden onset of an acute chest pain syndrome suggestive of pleuropericarditis has been rarely reported during Blenoxane infusions. Although each patient must be individually evaluated, further courses of Blenoxane do not appear to be contraindicated.
Idiosyncratic Reactions—In approximately 1% of the lymphoma patients treated with Blenoxane an idiosyncratic reaction, similar to anaphylaxis clinically, has been reported. The reaction may be immediate or delayed for several hours, and usually occurs after the first or second dose. It consists of hypotension, mental confusion, fever, chills, and wheezing. Treatment is symptomatic including volume expansion, pressor agents, antihistamines, and corticosteroids.
Integument and Mucous Membranes—These are the most frequent side effects being reported in approximately 50% of treated patients. These consist of erythema, rash, striae, vesiculation, hyperpigmentation, and tenderness of the skin.

Hyperkeratosis, nail changes, alopecia, pruritus, and stomatitis have also been reported. It was necessary to discontinue Blenoxane therapy in 2% of treated patients because of these toxicities.
Skin toxicity is a relatively late manifestation usually developing in the 2nd and 3rd week of treatment after 150 to 200 units of Blenoxane have been administered and appears to be related to the cumulative dose.
Other—Vascular toxicities coincident with the use of Blenoxane in combination with other antineoplastic agents have been reported rarely. The events are clinically heterogeneous and may include myocardial infarction, cerebrovascular accident, thrombotic microangiopathy (HUS) or cerebral arteritis. Various mechanisms have been proposed for these vascular complications. There are also reports of Raynaud's phenomenon occurring in patients treated with Blenoxane in combination with vinblastine with or without cisplatin or, in a few cases, with Blenoxane as a single agent. It is currently unknown if the cause of Raynaud's phenomenon in these cases is the disease, underlying vascular compromise, Blenoxane, vinblastine, hypomagnesemia, or a combination of any of these factors.
Fever, chills, and vomiting were frequently reported side effects. Anorexia and weight loss are common and may persist long after termination of this medication. Pain at tumor site, phlebitis, and other local reactions were reported infrequently.

DOSAGE

Because of the possibility of an anaphylactoid reaction, lymphoma patients should be treated with two units or less for the first two doses. If no acute reaction occurs, then the regular dosage schedule may be followed.
The following dose schedule is recommended: **Squamous cell carcinoma, lymphosarcoma, reticulum cell sarcoma, testicular carcinoma**—0.25 to 0.50 units/kg (10 to 20 units/m^2) given intravenously, intramuscularly, or subcutaneously weekly or twice weekly.
Hodgkin's Disease—0.25 to 0.50 units/kg (10 to 20 units/m^2) given intravenously, intramuscularly, or subcutaneously weekly or twice weekly. After a 50% response, a maintenance dose of one unit daily or five units weekly intravenously or intramuscularly should be given.
Pulmonary toxicity of Blenoxane appears to be dose related with a striking increase when the total dose is over 400 units. Total doses over 400 units should be given with great caution.
NOTE: When Blenoxane is used in combination with other antineoplastic agents, pulmonary toxicities may occur at lower doses.
Improvement of Hodgkin's Disease and testicular tumors is prompt and noted within 2 weeks. If no improvement is seen by this time, improvement is unlikely. Squamous cell cancers respond more slowly, sometimes requiring as long as 3 weeks before any improvement is noted.

ADMINISTRATION

Blenoxane may be given by the intramuscular, intravenous, or subcutaneous routes.
Intramuscular or Subcutaneous—Dissolve the contents of a Blenoxane vial in 1 to 5 mL of Sterile Water for Injection, U.S.P., Sodium Chloride for Injection, U.S.P., 5% Dextrose Injection, U.S.P., or Bacteriostatic Water for Injection, U.S.P.
Intravenous—Dissolve the contents of the vial in 5 mL or more of a solution suitable for injection, e.g., physiologic saline or glucose, and administer slowly over a period of 10 minutes.

STABILITY

The sterile powder is stable under refrigeration (2°–8°C) and should not be used after the expiration date is reached.
Blenoxane is stable for 24 hours at room temperature in Sodium Chloride or 5% Dextrose Solution.
Blenoxane is stable for 24 hours in 5% Dextrose containing heparin 100 units per mL or 1000 units per mL.
Procedures for proper handling and disposal of anticancer drugs should be considered. Several guidelines on this subject have been published.[1-7] There is no general agreement that all of the procedures recommended in the guidelines are necessary or appropriate.

REFERENCES

1. Recommendations for the Safe Handling of Parenteral Antineoplastic Drugs. NIH Publication No. 83-2621. For sale by the Superintendent of Documents, US Government Printing Office, Washington, D.C. 20402.
2. AMA Council Report. Guidelines for Handling Parenteral Antineoplastics, JAMA 1985 March 15.
3. National Study Commission on Cytotoxic Exposure—Recommendations for Handling Cytotoxic Agents. Available from Louis P. Jeffrey, Sc.D., Chairman, National Study Commission on Cytotoxic Exposure, Massachusetts College of Pharmacy and Allied Health Sciences, 179 Longwood Avenue, Boston, Massachusetts 02115.

Continued on next page

Bristol-Myers Oncology—Cont.

4. Clinical Oncological Society of Australia. Guidelines and Recommendations for Safe Handling of Antineoplastic Agents. Med J Australia 1983; 1:426-428.
5. Jones, RB, et. al. Safe handling of chemotherapeutic agents: A Report from the Mount Sinai Medical Center, CA—A Cancer Journal for Clinicians 1983; (Sept/Oct) 258-263.
6. American Society of Hospital Pharmacists Technical Assistance Bulletin on Handling Cytotoxic Drugs in Hospitals. Am J Hosp Pharm 1985; 42:131-137.
7. OSHA Work-Practice Guidelines for Personnel Dealing with Cytotoxic (Antineoplasic) Drugs, Am J Hosp Pharm 1986; 43:1193-1204.

SUPPLY

Each vial contains 15 units of Blenoxane as sterile bleomycin sulfate USP.
NDC 0015-3010-20
Manufactured by Nippon Kayaku Co., Ltd.
Tokyo, Japan
For information on package sizes available, refer to the current price sheet.

CeeNU®   R

[cē'nū]
(lomustine [CCNU]) capsules

WARNINGS

CeeNU (lomustine) should be administered under the supervision of a qualified physician experienced in the use of cancer chemotherapeutic agents.

Bone marrow suppression, notably thrombocytopenia and leukopenia, which may contribute to bleeding and overwhelming infections in an already compromised patient, is the most common and severe of the toxic effects of CeeNU (see "WARNINGS" and "ADVERSE REACTIONS").

Since the major toxicity is delayed bone marrow suppression, blood counts should be monitored weekly for at least six weeks after a dose (see "ADVERSE REACTIONS"). At the recommended dosage, courses of CeeNU should not be given more frequently than every six weeks.

The bone marrow toxicity of CeeNU is cumulative and therefore dosage adjustment must be considered on the basis of nadir blood counts from prior dose (see Dosage Adjustment Table under "DOSAGE AND ADMINISTRATION").

DESCRIPTION

CeeNU (lomustine) (CCNU) is one of the nitrosoureas used in the treatment of certain neoplastic diseases. It is 1-(2-chloroethyl)-3-cyclohexyl-1-nitrosourea. It is a yellow powder with the empirical formula of $C_9H_{16}ClN_3O_2$ and a molecular weight of 233.71. CeeNU is soluble in 10% ethanol (0.05 mg per mL) and in absolute alcohol (70 mg per mL). CeeNU is relatively insoluble in water (< 0.05 mg per mL).
It is relatively unionized at a physiological pH.
Inactive ingredients in CeeNU capsules are: magnesium stearate and mannitol.
The structural formula is:

CeeNU is available in 10 mg, 40 mg and 100 mg capsules for oral administration.

CLINICAL PHARMACOLOY

Although it is generally agreed that CeeNU alkylates DNA and RNA, it is not cross resistant with other alkylators. As with other nitrosoureas, it may also inhibit several key enzymatic processes by carbamoylation of amino acids in proteins.
CeeNU may be given orally. Following oral administration of radioactive CeeNU at doses ranging from 30 mg/m^2 to 100 mg/m^2, about half of the radioactivity given was excreted in the form of degradation products within 24 hours.
The serum half-life of the metabolites ranges from 16 hours to two days. Tissue levels are comparable to plasma levels at 15 minutes after intravenous administration.
Because of the high lipid solubility and the relative lack of ionization at a physiological pH, CeeNU crosses the blood-brain barrier quite effectively. Levels of radioactivity in the CSF are 50% or greater than those measured concurrently in plasma.

INDICATIONS AND USAGE

CeeNU has been shown to be useful as a single agent in addition to other treatment modalities, or in established combination therapy with other approved chemotherapeutic agents in the following:
Brain tumors—both primary and metastatic, in patients who have already received appropriate surgical and/or radiotherapeutic procedures.
Hodgkin's Disease—secondary therapy in combination with other approved drugs in patients who relapse while being treated with primary therapy, or who fail to respond to primary therapy.

CONTRAINDICATIONS

CeeNU should not be given to individuals who have demonstrated a previous hypersensitivity to it.

WARNINGS

Since the major toxicity is delayed bone marrow suppression, blood counts should be monitored weekly for at least six weeks after a dose (see "ADVERSE REACTIONS"). At the recommended dosage, courses of CeeNU should not be given more frequently than every six weeks.
The bone marrow toxicity of CeeNU is cumulative and therefore dosage adjustment must be considered on the basis of nadir blood counts from prior dose (see Dosage Adjustment Table under "DOSAGE AND ADMINISTRATION").
Pulmonary toxicity from CeeNU appears to be dose related (see "ADVERSE REACTIONS").
Long term use in nitrosoureas has been reported to be possibly associated with the development of secondary malignancies.
Liver and renal function tests should be monitored periodically (see "ADVERSE REACTIONS").
Pregnancy Category D: CeeNU can cause fetal harm when administered to a pregnant woman. CeeNU is embryotoxic and teratogenic in rats and embryotoxic in rabbits at dose levels equivalent to the human dose. There are no adequate and well controlled studies in pregnant women. If this drug is used during pregnancy, or if the patient becomes pregnant while taking (receiving) this drug, the patient should be apprised of the potential hazard to the fetus. Women of childbearing potential should be advised to avoid becoming pregnant.

PRECAUTIONS

General: In all instances where the use of CeeNU is considered for chemotherapy, the physician must evaluate the need and usefulness of the drug against the risks of toxic effects or adverse reactions. Most such adverse reactions are reversible if detected early. When such effects or reactions do occur, the drug should be reduced in dosage or discontinued and appropriate corrective measures should be taken according to the clinical judgment of the physician. Reinstitution of CeeNU therapy should be carried out with caution and with adequate consideration of the further need for the drug and alertness as to possible recurrence of toxicity.
Laboratory Tests: Due to delayed bone marrow suppression, blood counts should be monitored weekly for at least six weeks after a dose.
Baseline pulmonary function studies should be conducted along with frequent pulmonary function tests during treatment. Patients with a baseline below 70% of the predicted Forced Vital Capacity (FVC) or Carbon Monoxide Diffusing Capacity (DL_{co}) are particularly at risk.
Since CeeNU may cause liver dysfunction, it is recommended that liver function tests be monitored periodically. Renal function tests should also be monitored periodically.
Carcinogenesis, Mutagenesis, Impairment of Fertility: CeeNU is carcinogenic in rats and mice, producing a marked increase in tumor incidence in doses approximating those employed clinically. Nitrosourea therapy does have carcinogenic potential in humans (see "ADVERSE REACTIONS"). CeeNU also affects fertility in male rats at doses somewhat higher than the human dose.
Pregnancy: Pregnancy "Category D"—See "WARNINGS" section.
Nursing Mothers: It is not known whether this drug is excreted in human milk. Because many drugs are excreted in human milk and because of the potential for serious adverse reactions in nursing infants from CeeNU, a decision should be made whether to discontinue nursing or to discontinue the drug, taking into account the importance of the drug to the mother.
Information for the Patient: Patients receiving CeeNU should be given the following information and instructions by the physician:
1. Patients should be told that CeeNU is an anticancer drug and belongs to the group of medicines known as alkylating agents.
2. In order to provide the proper dose of CeeNU, patients should be aware that there may be two or more different types and colors of capsules in the container dispensed by the pharmacist.
3. Patients should be told that CeeNU is given as a single oral dose and will not be repeated for at least 6 weeks.
4. Patients should be told that nausea and vomiting usually last less than 24 hours, although loss of appetite may last for several days.
5. If any of the following reactions occur, notify the physician: fever, chills, sore throat, unusual bleeding or bruising, shortness of breath, dry cough, swelling of feet or lower legs, mental confusion or yellowing of eyes and skin.

ADVERSE REACTIONS

Hematologic Toxicity: The most frequent and most serious toxicity of CeeNU is delayed myelosuppression. It usually occurs four to six weeks after drug administration and is dose related. Thrombocytopenia occurs at about four weeks postadministration and persists for one to two weeks. Leukopenia occurs at five to six weeks after a dose of CeeNU and persists for one to two weeks. Approximately 65% of patients receiving 130 mg/m^2 develop white blood counts below 5000 wbc/mm^3. Thirty-six percent developed white blood counts below 3000 wbc/mm^3. Thrombocytopenia is generally more severe than leukopenia. However, both may be dose-limiting toxicities.
CeeNU may produce cumulative myelosuppression, manifested by more depressed indices or longer duration of suppression after repeated doses.
The occurrence of acute leukemia and bone marrow dysplasias have been reported in patients following long term nitrosourea therapy.
Anemia also occurs, but is less frequent and less severe than thrombocytopenia or leukopenia.
Pulmonary Toxicity: Pulmonary toxicity characterized by pulmonary infiltrates and/or fibrosis has been reported rarely with CeeNU. Onset of toxicity has occurred after an interval of six months or longer from the start of therapy with cumulative doses of CeeNU usually greater than 1100 mg/m^2. There is one report of pulmonary toxicity at a cumulative dose of only 600 mg.
Gastrointestinal Toxicity: Nausea and vomiting may occur three to six hours after an oral dose and usually lasts less than 24 hours. Prior administration of antiemetics is effective in diminishing and sometimes preventing this side effect. Nausea and vomiting can also be reduced if CeeNU is administered to fasting patients.
Hepatotoxicity: A reversible type of hepatic toxicity, manifested by increased transaminase, alkaline phosphatase and bilirubin levels, has been reported in a small percentage of patients receiving CeeNU.
Nephrotoxicity: Renal abnormalities consisting of progressive azotemia, decrease in kidney size and renal failure have been reported in patients who received large cumulative doses after prolonged therapy with CeeNU. Kidney damage has also been reported occasionally in patients receiving lower total doses.
Other Toxicities: Stomatitis and alopecia have been reported infrequently.
Neurological reactions such as disorientation, lethargy, ataxia, and dysarthria have been noted in some patients receiving CeeNU. However, the relationship to medication in these patients is unclear.

OVERDOSAGE

No proven antidotes have been established for CeeNU overdosage.

DOSAGE AND ADMINISTRATION

The recommended dose of CeeNU in adults and children as a single agent in previously untreated patients is 130 mg/m^2 as a single oral dose every six weeks. In individuals with compromised bone marrow function, the dose should be reduced to 100 mg/m^2 every 6 weeks. When CeeNU is used in combination with other myelosuppressive drugs, the doses should be adjusted accordingly.
Doses subsequent to the initial dose should be adjusted according to the hematologic response of the patient to the preceding dose. The following schedule is suggested as a guide to dosage adjustment:

Nadir After Prior Dose		Percentage of Prior Dose to be Given
Leukocytes	Platelets	
>4000	>100,000	100%
3000–3999	75,000–99,999	100%
2000–2999	25,000–74,999	70%
<2000	<25,000	50%

A repeat course of CeeNU should not be given until circulating blood elements have returned to acceptable levels (platelets above 100,000/mm^3; leukocytes above 4,000/mm^3) and this is usually in 6 weeks. Adequate number of neutrophils should be present on a peripheral blood smear. Blood counts should be monitored weekly and repeat courses should not be given before 6 weeks because the hematologic toxicity is delayed and cumulative.

HOW SUPPLIED

The dose pack of CeeNU (lomustine, CCNU) **NDC** 0015-3034-10 Capsules contains;

2—100 mg capsules (Green/Green)
2—40 mg capsules (White/Green)
2—10 mg capsules (White/White)

Stability: CeeNU Capsules are stable for the lot life indicated on package labeling when stored at room temperature in well closed containers. Avoid excessive heat (over 40°C).

Directions to the Pharmacist: The dose pack contains a total of 300 mg and will provide enough medication for titration of a single dose. The total dose prescribed by the physician can be obtained (to within 10 mg) by determining the appropriate combination of the enclosed capsule strengths. The appropriate number of capsules of each size should be placed in a single vial to which the patient information label (gummed label provided) explaining the differences in the appearance of the capsules is affixed. Each color-coded capsule is imprinted with the dose in milligrams.

A patient information sticker, to be placed on dispensing container, is enclosed.

Also available: Individual bottles of 20 capsules each.

NDC 0015-3032-20—100 mg capsules (Green/Green)
NDC 0015-3031-20—40 mg capsules (White/Green)
NDC 0015-3030-20—10 mg capsules (White/White)

Procedures for proper handling and disposal of anticancer drugs should be considered. Several guidelines on this subject have been published.[1-7] There is no general agreement that all of the procedures recommended in the guidelines are necessary or appropriate.

REFERENCES

1. Recommendations for the Safe Handling of Parenteral Antineoplastic Drugs. NIH Publication No. 83-2621. For sale by the Superintendent of Documents, U.S. Government Printing Office, Washington, D.C. 20402.
2. AMA Council Report. Guidelines for Handling Parenteral Antineoplastics. JAMA, 1985; March 15.
3. National Study Commission on Cytotoxic Exposure—Recommendations for Handling Cytotoxic Agents. Available from Louis P. Jeffrey, Sc.D., Chairman, National Study Commission on Cytotoxic Exposure, Massachusetts College of Pharmacy and Allied Health Sciences, 179 Longwood Avenue, Boston, Massachusetts 02115.
4. Clinical Oncological Society of Australia: Guidelines and Recommendations for Safe Handling of Antineoplastic Agents. Med. J. Australia 1983; 1:426-428.
5. Jones, R. B., et. al. Safe Handling of Chemotherapeutic Agents: A report from the Mount Sinai Medical Center, Ca—A Cancer Journal for Clinicians 1983; Sept./Oct., 258-263.
6. American Society of Hospital Pharmacists Technical Assistance Bulletin on Handling Cytotoxic Drugs in Hospitals. Am. J. Hosp. Pharm. 1985; 42:131-137.
7. OSHA Work-Practice Guidelines for Personnel Dealing with Cytotoxic (Antineoplastic) Drugs. Am. J. Hosp. Pharm. 1986; 43:1193-1204.

Shown in Product Identification Section, page 407

CYTOXAN®   ℞

[sī-taks'an]
(Cyclophosphamide, USP)
Lyophilized Cytoxan
Injectable, 2.0 g vials (6)   NSN 6505-01-219-3900(m)

DESCRIPTION

CYTOXAN (cyclophosphamide) is supplied as a sterile powder for parenteral use containing 45 mg sodium chloride per 100 mg cyclophosphamide (anhydrous), a sterile lyophilizate for parenteral use containing 75 mg mannitol per 100 mg cyclophosphamide (anhydrous), a tablet for oral use containing 25 mg cyclophosphamide (anhydrous), and a tablet for oral use containing 50 mg cyclophosphamide (anhydrous). Inactive ingredients in CYTOXAN tablets are: acacia, FD&C Blue No. 1, D&C Yellow No. 10 Aluminum Lake, lactose, magnesium stearate, starch, stearic acid and talc. Cyclophosphamide is a synthetic antineoplastic drug chemically related to the nitrogen mustards. Cyclophosphamide is a white crystalline powder with the molecular formula of $C_7H_{15}Cl_2N_2O_2P \cdot H_2O$ and a molecular weight of 279.1. The chemical name for cyclophosphamide is 2-[bis(2-chloroethyl)amino]tetrahydro-2H-1,3,2-oxazaphosphorine 2-oxide monohydrate. Cyclophosphamide is soluble in water, saline, or ethanol and has the following structural formula:

CLINICAL PHARMACOLOGY

CYTOXAN (cyclophosphamide) is biotransformed principally in the liver to active alkylating metabolites by a mixed function microsomal oxidase system. These metabolites interfere with the growth of susceptible rapidly proliferating malignant cells. The mechanism of action is thought to involve cross-linking of tumor cell DNA.

CYTOXAN is well absorbed after oral administration with a bioavailability greater than 75%. The unchanged drug has an elimination half-life of 3 to 12 hours. It is eliminated primarily in the form of metabolites, but from 5% to 25% of the dose is excreted in urine as unchanged drug. Several cytotoxic and noncytotoxic metabolites have been identified in urine and in plasma. Concentrations of metabolites reach a maximum in plasma 2 to 3 hours after an intravenous dose. Plasma protein binding of unchanged drug is low but some metabolites are bound to an extent greater than 60%. It has not been demonstrated that any single metabolite is responsible for either the therapeutic or toxic effects of cyclophosphamide. Although elevated levels of metabolites of cyclophosphamide have been observed in patients with renal failure, increased clinical toxicity in such patients has not been demonstrated.

INDICATION AND USAGE

Malignant Diseases—CYTOXAN, although effective alone in susceptible malignancies, is more frequently used concurrently or sequentially with other antineoplastic drugs.

The following malignancies are often susceptible to CYTOXAN treatment:

1. Malignant lymphomas (Stages III and IV of the Ann Arbor staging system), Hodgkin's disease, lymphocytic lymphoma (nodular or diffuse), mixed-cell type lymphoma, histiocytic lymphoma, Burkitt's lymphoma. 2. Multiple myeloma. 3. Leukemias: Chronic lymphocytic leukemia, chronic granulocytic leukemia (it is usually ineffective in acute blastic crisis), acute myelogenous and monocytic leukemia, acute lymphoblastic (stem-cell) leukemia in children (CYTOXAN given during remission is effective in prolonging its duration). 4. Mycosis fungoides (advanced disease), 5. Neuroblastoma (disseminated disease). 6. Adenocarcinoma of the ovary. 7. Retinoblastoma. 8. Carcinoma of the breast.

Nonmalignant Disease: Biopsy Proven "Minimal Change" Nephrotic Syndrome in Children—CYTOXAN is useful in carefully selected cases of biopsy proven "minimal change" nephrotic syndrome in children but should not be used as primary therapy. In children whose disease fails to respond adequately to appropriate adrenocorticosteroid therapy or in whom the adrenocorticosteroid therapy produces or threatens to produce intolerable side effects. CYTOXAN may induce a remission. CYTOXAN is not indicated for the nephrotic syndrome in adults or for any other renal disease.

CONTRAINDICATIONS

Continued use of cyclophosphamide is contraindicated in patients with severely depressed bone marrow function. Cyclophosphamide is contraindicated in patients who have demonstrated a previous hypersensitivity to it. See WARNINGS and PRECAUTIONS sections.

WARNINGS

Carcinogenesis, Mutagenesis, Impairment of Fertility—Second malignancies have developed in some patients treated with cyclophosphamide used alone or in association with other antineoplastic drugs and/or modalities. Most frequently, they have been urinary bladder, myeloproliferative, or lymphoproliferative malignancies. Second malignancies most frequently were detected in patients treated for primary myeloproliferative or lymphoproliferative malignancies or nonmalignant disease in which immune processes are believed to be involved pathologically. In some cases, the second malignancy developed several years after cyclophosphamide treatment had been discontinued. Urinary bladder malignancies generally have occurred in patients who previously had hemorrhagic cystitis. One case of carcinoma of the renal pelvis was reported in a patient receiving long-term cyclophosphamide therapy for cerebral vasculitis. The possibility of cyclophosphamide-induced malignancy should be considered in any benefit-to-risk assessment for use of the drug.

Cyclophosphamide can cause fetal harm when administered to a pregnant woman and such abnormalities have been reported following cyclophosphamide therapy in pregnant women. Abnormalities were found in two infants and a six-month old fetus born to women treated with cyclophosphamide. Ectrodactylia was found in two of the three cases. Normal infants have also been born to women treated with cyclophosphamide during pregnancy, including the first trimester. If this drug is used during pregnancy, or if the patient becomes pregnant while taking (receiving) this drug, the patient should be apprised of the potential hazard to the fetus. Women of childbearing potential should be advised to avoid becoming pregnant.

Cyclophosphamide interferes with oogenesis and spermatogenesis. It may cause sterility in both sexes. Development of sterility appears to depend on the dose of cyclophosphamide, duration of therapy, and the state of gonadal function at the time of treatment. Cyclophosphamide-induced sterility may be irreversible in some patients.

Amenorrhea associated with decreased estrogen and increased gonadotropin secretion develops in a significant proportion of women treated with cyclophosphamide. Affected patients generally resume regular menses within a few months after cessation of therapy. Girls treated with cyclophosphamide during prepubescence generally develop secondary sexual characteristics normally and have regular menses. Ovarian fibrosis with apparently complete loss of germ cells after prolonged cyclophosphamide treatment in late prepubescence has been reported. Girls treated with cyclophosphamide during prepubescence subsequently have conceived.

Men treated with cyclophosphamide may develop oligospermia or azoospermia associated with increased gonadotropin but normal testosterone secretion. Sexual potency and libido are unimpaired in these patients. Boys treated with cyclophosphamide during prepubescence develop secondary sexual characteristics normally, but may have oligospermia or azoospermia and increased gonadotropin secretion. Some degree of testicular atrophy may occur. Cyclophosphamide-induced azoospermia is reversible in some patients, though the reversibility may not occur for several years after cessation of therapy. Men temporarily rendered sterile by cyclophosphamide have subsequently fathered normal children.

Urinary System—Hemorrhagic cystitis may develop in patients treated with cyclophosphamide. Rarely, this condition can be severe and even fatal. Fibrosis of the urinary bladder, sometimes extensive, also may develop with or without accompanying cystitis. Atypical urinary bladder epithelial cells may appear in the urine. These adverse effects appear to depend on the dose of cyclophosphamide and the duration of therapy. Such bladder injury is thought to be due to cyclophosphamide metabolites excreted in the urine. Forced fluid intake helps to assure an ample output of urine, necessitates frequent voiding, and reduces the time the drug remains in the bladder. This helps to prevent cystitis. Hematuria usually resolves in a few days after cyclophosphamide treatment is stopped, but it may persist. Medical and/or surgical supportive treatment may be required, rarely, to treat protracted cases of severe hemorrhagic cystitis. It is usually necessary to discontinue cyclophosphamide therapy in instances of severe hemorrhagic cystitis.

Cardiac Toxicity—Although a few instances of cardiac dysfunction have been reported following use of recommended doses of cyclophosphamide, no causal relationship has been established. Cardiotoxicity has been observed in some patients receiving high doses of cyclophosphamide ranging from 120 to 270 mg/kg administered over a period of a few days, usually as a portion of an intensive antineoplastic multidrug regimen or in conjunction with transplantation procedures. In a few instances with high doses of cyclophosphamide, severe, and sometimes fatal, congestive heart failure has occurred within a few days after the first cyclophosphamide dose. Histopathologic examination has primarily shown hemorrhagic myocarditis.

No residual cardiac abnormalities, as evidenced by electrocardiogram or echocardiogram appear to be present in patients surviving episodes of apparent cardiac toxicity associated with high doses of cyclophosphamide.

Cyclophosphamide has been reported to potentiate doxorubicin-induced cardiotoxicity.

Infections—Treatment with cyclophosphamide may cause significant suppression of immune responses. Serious, sometimes fatal, infections may develop in severely immunosuppressed patients. Cyclophosphamide treatment may not be indicated or should be interrupted or the dose reduced in patients who have or who develop viral, bacterial, fungal, protozoan, or helminthic infections.

Other—Rare instances of anaphylactic reaction including one death have been reported. One instance of possible cross-sensitivity with other alkylating agents has been reported.

PRECAUTIONS

General—Special attention to the possible development of toxicity should be exercised in patients being treated with cyclophosphamide if any of the following conditions are present.

1. Leukopenia. 2. Thrombocytopenia. 3. Tumor cell infiltration of bone marrow. 4. Previous X-ray therapy. 5. Previous therapy with other cytotoxic agents. 6. Impaired hepatic function. 7. Impaired renal function.

Laboratory Tests—During treatment, the patient's hematologic profile (particularly neutrophils and platelets) should be monitored regularly to determine the degree of hematopoietic suppression. Urine should also be examined regularly for red cells which may precede hemorrhagic cystitis.

Drug Interactions—The rate of metabolism and the leukopenic activity of cyclophosphamide reportedly are increased by chronic administration of high doses of phenobarbital.

The physician should be alert for possible combined drug actions, desirable or undesirable, involving cyclophosphamide even though cyclophosphamide has been used successfully concurrently with other drugs, including other cytotoxic drugs.

Continued on next page

Bristol-Myers Oncology—Cont.

Cyclophosphamide treatment, which causes a marked and persistent inhibition of cholinesterase activity, potentiates the effect of succinylcholine chloride.

If a patient has been treated with cyclophosphamide within 10 days of general anesthesia, the anesthesiologist should be alerted.

Adrenalectomy—Since cyclophosphamide has been reported to be more toxic in adrenalectomized dogs, adjustment of the doses of both replacement steroids and cyclophosphamide may be necessary for the adrenalectomized patient.

Wound Healing—Cyclophosphamide may interfere with normal wound healing.

Carcinogenesis, Mutagenesis, Impairment of Fertility—See WARNINGS section for information on carcinogenesis, mutagenesis, and impairment of fertility.

Pregnancy—Pregnancy Category D. See WARNINGS section.

Nursing Mothers—Cyclophosphamide is excreted in breast milk. Because of the potential for serious adverse reactions and the potential for tumorigenicity shown for cyclophosphamide in humans, a decision should be made whether to discontinue nursing or to discontinue the drug, taking into account the importance of the drug to the mother.

ADVERSE REACTIONS

Information on adverse reactions associated with the use of CYTOXAN is arranged according to body system affected or type of reaction. The adverse reactions are listed in order of decreasing incidence. The most serious adverse reactions are described in the WARNINGS section.

Reproductive System—See WARNINGS section for information on impairment of fertility.

Digestive System—Nausea and vomiting commonly occur with cyclophosphamide therapy. Anorexia and, less frequently, abdominal discomfort or pain and diarrhea may occur. There are isolated reports of hemorrhagic colitis, oral mucosal ulceration and jaundice occurring during therapy. These adverse drug effects generally remit when cyclophosphamide treatment is stopped.

Skin and Its Structures—Alopecia occurs commonly in patients treated with cyclophosphamide. The hair can be expected to grow back after treatment with the drug or even during continued drug treatment, though it may be different in texture or color. Skin rash occurs occasionally in patients receiving the drug. Pigmentation of the skin and changes in nails can occur.

Hematopoietic System—Leukopenia occurs in patients treated with cyclophosphamide, is related to the dose of the drug, and can be used as a dosage guide. Leukopenia of less than 2000 cells/mm^3 develops commonly in patients treated with an initial loading dose of the drug, and less frequently in patients maintained on smaller doses. The degree of neutropenia is particularly important because it correlates with a reduction in resistance to infections. Thrombocytopenia or anemia develop occasionally in patients treated with CYTOXAN. These hematologic effects usually can be reversed by reducing the drug dose or by interrupting treatment. Recovery from leukopenia usually begins in 7 to 10 days after cessation of therapy.

Urinary System—See WARNINGS section for information on cystitis and urinary bladder fibrosis.

Hemorrhagic ureteritis and renal tubular necrosis have been reported to occur in patients treated with cyclophosphamide. Such lesions usually resolve following cessation of therapy.

Infections—See WARNINGS section for information on reduced host resistance to infections.

Carcinogenesis—See WARNINGS section for information on carcinogenesis.

Respiratory System—Interstitial pulmonary fibrosis has been reported in patients receiving high doses of cyclophosphamide over a prolonged period.

Other—Rare instances of anaphylactic reaction including one death have been reported. One instance of possible cross-sensitivity with other alkylating agents has been reported.

OVERDOSAGE

No specific antidote for cyclophosphamide is known. Overdosage should be managed with supportive measures, including appropriate treatment for any concurrent infection, myelosuppression, or cardiac toxicity should it occur.

DOSAGE AND ADMINISTRATION

Treatment of Malignant Diseases: Adults and Children—When used as the only oncolytic drug therapy, the initial course of CYTOXAN for patients with no hematologic deficiency usually consists of 40 to 50 mg/kg given intravenously in divided doses over a period of 2 to 5 days. Other intravenous regimens include 10 to 15 mg/kg given every 7 to 10 days or 3 to 5 mg/kg twice weekly.

Oral CYTOXAN dosing is usually in the range of 1 to 5 mg/kg/day for both initial and maintenance dosing.

Many other regimens of intravenous and oral CYTOXAN have been reported. Dosages must be adjusted in accord with

evidence of antitumor activity and/or leukopenia. The total leukocyte count is a good, objective guide for regulating dosage. Transient decreases in the total white blood cell count to 2000 cells/mm^3 (following short courses) or more persistent reduction to 3000 cells/mm^3 (with continuing therapy) are tolerated without serious risk of infection if there is no marked granulocytopenia.

When CYTOXAN is included in combined cytotoxic regimens, it may be necessary to reduce the dose of CYTOXAN as well as that of the other drugs.

CYTOXAN and its metabolites are dialyzable although there are probably quantitative differences depending upon the dialysis system being used. Patients with compromised renal function may show some measurable changes in pharmacokinetic parameters of CYTOXAN metabolism, but there is no consistent evidence indicating a need for CYTOXAN dosage modification in patients with renal function impairment.

Treatment of Nonmalignant Diseases: Biopsy Proven "Minimal Change" Nephrotic Syndrome in Children—An oral dose of 2.5 to 3 mg/kg daily for a period of 60 to 90 days is recommended. In males, the incidence of oligospermia and azoospermia increases if the duration of Cytoxan treatment exceeds 60 days. Treatment beyond 90 days increases the probability of sterility. Adrenocorticosteroid therapy may be tapered and discontinued during the course of CYTOXAN therapy. See PRECAUTIONS section concerning hematologic monitoring.

Preparation and Handling of Solutions—Parenteral drug products should be inspected visually for particulate matter and discoloration prior to administration, whenever solution and container permit.

CYTOXAN for Injection and Lyophilized CYTOXAN for Injection should be prepared for parenteral use by adding Bacteriostatic Water for Injection, U.S.P., (paraben preserved only) or Sterile Water for Injection, U.S.P., to the vial and shaking to dissolve. Use the quantity of diluent shown below to reconstitute the product.

Dosage Strength	Cytoxan for Injection Quantity of Diluent	Lyophilized Cytoxan for Injection Quantity of Diluent
100 mg	5 mL	5 mL
200 mg	10 mL	10 mL
500 mg	25 mL	20–25 mL
1 g	50 mL	50 mL
2 g	100 mL	80–100 mL

Solutions of CYTOXAN for Injection and Lyophilized CYTOXAN for Injection may be injected intravenously, intramuscularly, intraperitoneally, or intrapleurally or they may be infused intravenously in the following:

Dextrose Injection, U.S.P. (5% dextrose)

Dextrose and Sodium Chloride Injection, U.S.P. (5% dextrose and 0.9% sodium chloride)

5% Dextrose and Ringer's Injection

Lactated Ringer's Injection, U.S.P.

Sodium Chloride Injection, U.S.P. (0.45% sodium chloride)

Sodium Lactate Injection, U.S.P. (1/6 molar sodium lactate)

Reconstituted CYTOXAN for Injection and Lyophilized CYTOXAN for Injection are chemically and physically stable for 24 hours at room temperature or for 6 days in the refrigerator; it does not contain any antimicrobial preservative and thus care must be taken to assure the sterility of prepared solutions.

CYTOXAN for Injection and Lyophilized CYTOXAN for Injection prepared by adding Bacteriostatic Water for Injection U.S.P. (paraben preserved only) should be used within 24 hours if stored at room temperature or within 6 days if stored under refrigeration.

If CYTOXAN for Injection or Lyophilized CYTOXAN for Injection is not prepared by adding Bacteriostatic Water for Injection U.S.P. (paraben preserved only), it is recommended that the solution be used promptly (preferably within 6 hours).

The osmolarities of solutions of CYTOXAN for Injection, Lyophilized CYTOXAN for Injection, and normal saline are compared in the following table:

	mOsm/L
Lyophilized CYTOXAN for Injection 4 mL diluent per 100 mg cyclophosphamide	219
5 mL diluent per 100 mg cyclophosphamide	172
CYTOXAN for Injection	352
Normal saline	287

Lyophilized CYTOXAN for Injection is slightly hypotonic with respect to normal saline.

Extemporaneous liquid preparations of CYTOXAN for oral administration may be prepared by dissolving CYTOXAN for Injection or Lyophilized CYTOXAN for Injection in Aromatic Elixir, N.F. Such preparations should be stored under refrigeration in glass containers and used within 14 days.

HOW SUPPLIED

CYTOXAN for Injection contains 45 mg of sodium chloride per 100 mg of cyclophosphamide (anhydrous) and is supplied in vials for single dose use.

CYTOXAN for Injection (cyclophosphamide for injection, USP).

NDC 0015-0500-41   100 mg vials, carton of 12, case of 1 carton

NDC 0015-0501-41   200 mg vials, carton of 12, case of 1 carton

NDC 0015-0502-41   500 mg vials, carton of 12, case of 1 carton

NDC 0015-0505-41   1.0 g vials, carton of 6

NDC 0015-0506-41   2.0 g vials, carton of 6

Lyophilized CYTOXAN for Injection contains 75 mg mannitol per 100 mg cyclophosphamide (anhydrous) and is supplied in vials for single-dose use.

Lyophilized CYTOXAN for Injection (cyclophosphamide for injection, USP)

U.S. Patent No. 4,537,883

NDC 0015-0539-41   100 mg vials, carton of 12, case of 1 carton

NDC 0015-0546-41   200 mg vials, carton of 12, case of 1 carton

NDC 0015-0547-41   500 mg vials, carton of 12, case of 1 carton

NDC 0015-0548-41   1.0 g vials, carton of 6

NDC 0015-0549-41   2.0 g vials, carton of 6

CYTOXAN Tablets, 25 mg, and CYTOXAN Tablets, 50 mg, are white tablets with blue flecks containing 25 mg and 50 mg cyclophosphamide (anhydrous), respectively.

CYTOXAN Tablets (cyclophosphamide tablets, USP)

NDC 0015-0503-01   50 mg, bottles of 100

NDC 0015-0503-02   50 mg, bottles of 1000

NDC 0015-0503-03   50 mg, Unit Dose, cartons of 100

NDC 0015-0503-48   50 mg, Compliance Pack, cartons of 28

NDC 0015-0504-01   25 mg, bottles of 100

Storage at or below 77°F (25°C) is recommended; this product will withstand brief exposure to temperatures up to 86°F (30°C) but should be protected from temperatures above 86°F (30°C).

Procedures for proper handling and disposal of anticancer drugs should be considered. Several guidelines on this subject have been published.[1-7] There is no general agreement that all of the procedures recommended in the guidelines are necessary or appropriate.

REFERENCES

1. Recommendations for the Safe Handling of Parenteral Antineoplastic Drugs. NIH Publication No. 83-2621. For sale by the Superintendent of Documents, US Government Printing Office, Washington, DC 20402.
2. AMA Council Report, Guidelines for Handling Parenteral Antineoplastics, JAMA 1985 March 15.
3. National Study Commission on Cytotoxic Exposure—Recommendations for Handling Cytotoxic Agents. Available from Louis P. Jeffrey, Sc.D., Chairman, National Study Commission on Cytotoxic Exposure, Massachusetts College of Pharmacy and Allied Health Sciences, 179 Longwood Avenue, Boston, Massachusetts 02115.
4. Clinical Oncological Society of Australia. Guidelines and Recommendations for Safe Handling of Antineoplastic Agents. Med J Australia 1983; 1:426-428.
5. Jones RB, et al: Safe handling of chemotherapeutic agents: A report from the Mount Sinai Medical Center. CA—A Cancer Journal for Clinicians 1983; (Sept/Oct) 258-263.
6. American Society of Hospital Pharmacists Technical Assistance Bulletin on Handling Cytotoxic Drugs in Hospitals. Am J Hosp Pharm 1985; 42:131-137.
7. OSHA Work-Practice Guidelines for Personnel Dealing with Cytotoxic (Antineoplastic) Drugs. Am J Hosp Pharm 1986; 43:1193-1204.

Shown in Product Identification Section, page 407

IFEX®   ℞

[*i-fĕx*]

(sterile ifosfamide)

WARNING

IFEX should be administered under the supervision of a qualified physician experienced in the use of cancer chemotherapeutic agents. Urotoxic side effects, especially hemorrhagic cystitis, as well as CNS toxicities such as confusion and coma have been assoicated with the use of IFEX. When they occur, they may require cessation of IFEX therapy. Severe myelosuppression has been reported. (See "Adverse Reactions" section.)

DESCRIPTION

IFEX (sterile ifosfamide) single-dose vials for constitution and administration by intravenous infusion each contain 1 gram of sterile ifosfamide. Ifosfamide is a chemotherapeutic agent chemically related to the nitrogen mustards and a synthetic analog of cyclophosphamide. Ifosfamide is 3-(2-chloroethyl)-2-[(2-chloroethyl) amino] tetrahydro-2H-1,3,2-oxazaphosphorine 2-oxide. The molecular formula is $C_7H_{15}Cl_2N_2O_2P$ and its molecular weight is 261.1. Its structural formula is:

Ifosfamide is a white crystalline powder that is soluble in water.

CLINICAL PHARMACOLOGY

Ifosfamide has been shown to require metabolic activation by microsomal liver enzymes to produce biologically active metabolites. Activation occurs by hydroxylation at the ring carbon atom 4 to form the unstable intermediate 4-hydroxyifosfamide. This metabolite rapidly degrades to the stable urinary metabolite 4-ketoifosfamide. Opening of the ring results in formation of the stable urinary metabolite, 4-carboxyifosfamide. These urinary metabolites have not been found to be cytotoxic. N, N-bis (2-chloroethyl)-phosphoric acid diamide (ifosphoramide) and acrolein are also found. Enzymatic oxidation of the chloroethyl side chains and subsequent dealkylation produces the major urinary metabolites, dechloroethyl ifosfamide and dechloroethyl cyclophosphamide. The alkylated metabolites of ifosfamide have been shown to interact with DNA.

In vitro incubation of DNA with activated ifosfamide has produced phosphotriesters. The treatment of intact cell nuclei may also result in the formation of DNA-DNA crosslinks. DNA repair most likely occurs in G-1 and G-2 stage cells.

Pharmacokinetics

Ifosfamide exhibits dose-dependent pharmacokinetics in humans. At single doses of 3.8–5.0 g/m², the plasma concentrations decay biphasically and the mean terminal elimination half-life is about 15 hours. At doses of 1.6–2.4 g/m²/day, the plasma decay is monoexponential and the terminal elimination half-life is about seven hours. Ifosfamide is extensively metabolized in humans and the metabolic pathways appear to be saturated at high doses.

After administration of doses of 5 g/m² of ¹⁴C-labeled ifosfamide, from 70% to 86% of the dosed radioactivity was recovered in the urine, with about 61% of the dose excreted as parent compound. At doses of 1.6–2.4 g/m² only 12% to 18% of the dose was excreted in the urine as unchanged drug within 72 hours.

Two different dechloroethylated derivatives of ifosfamide, 4-carboxyifosfamide, thiodiacetic acid and cysteine conjugates of chloroacetic acid have been identified as the major urinary metabolites of ifosfamide in humans and only small amounts of 4-hydroxyifosfamide and acrolein are present. Small quantities (nmole/mL) of ifosfamide mustard and 4-hydroxyifosfamide are detectable in human plasma. Metabolism of ifosfamide is required for the generation of the biologically active species and while metabolism is extensive, it is also quite variable among patients.

In a study at Indiana University, 50 fully evaluable patients with germ cell testicular cancer were treated with IFEX in combination with cisplatin and either vinblastine or etoposide after failing (47 of 50 patients) at least two prior chemotherapy regimens consisting of cisplatin/vinblastine/ bleomycin, (PVB), cisplatin/vinblastine/actinomycin D/bleomycin/cyclophosphamide, (VAB6), or the combination of cisplatin and etoposide. Patients were selected for remaining cisplatin sensitivity because they had previously responded to a cisplatin containing regimen and had not progressed while on the cisplatin containing regimen or within 3 weeks of stopping it. Patients served as their own control based on the premise that long term complete responses could not be achieved by retreatment with a regimen to which they had previously responded and subsequently relapsed.

Ten of 50 fully evaluable patients were still alive 2 to 5 years after treatment. Four of the 10 long term survivors were rendered free of cancer by surgical resection after treatment with the ifosfamide regimen; median survival for the entire group of 50 fully evaluable patients was 53 weeks.

INDICATION AND USAGE

IFEX, used in combination with certain other approved antineoplastic agents, is indicated for third line chemotherapy of germ cell testicular cancer. It should ordinarily be used in combination with a prophylactic agent for hemorrhagic cystitis, such as mesna.

CONTRAINDICATIONS

Continued use of IFEX is contraindicated in patients with severely depressed bone marrow function (See WARNINGS and PRECAUTIONS sections). IFEX is also contraindicated in patients who have demonstrated a previous hypersensitivity to it.

WARNINGS

Urinary System

Urotoxic side effects, especially hemorrhagic cystitis, have been frequently associated with the use of IFEX. It is recommended that a urinalysis should be obtained prior to each dose of IFEX. If microscopic hematuria (greater than 10 RBCs per high power field), is present, then subsequent administration should be withheld until complete resolution. Further administration of IFEX should be given with vigorous oral or parenteral hydration.

Hematopoietic System

When IFEX is given in combination with other chemotherapeutic agents, severe myelosuppression is frequently observed. Close hematologic monitoring is recommended. White blood cell (WBC) count, platelet count and hemoglobin should be obtained prior to each administration and at appropriate intervals. Unless clinically essential, IFEX should not be given to patients with a WBC count below 2000/μL and/or a platelet count below 50,000/μL.

Central Nervous System

Neurologic manifestations consisting of somnolence, confusion, hallucinations and in some instances, coma, have been reported following IFEX therapy. The occurrence of these symptoms requires discontinuing IFEX therapy. The symptoms have usually been reversible and supportive therapy should be maintained until their complete resolution.

Pregnancy

Animal studies indicate that the drug is capable of causing gene mutations and chromosomal damage in vivo. Embryotoxic and teratogenic effects have been observed in mice, rats and rabbits at doses 0.05–0.075 times the human dose. Ifosfamide can cause fetal damage when administered to a pregnant woman. If IFEX is used during pregnancy, or if the patient becomes pregnant while taking this drug, the patient should be apprised of the potential hazard to the fetus.

PRECAUTIONS

General

IFEX should be given cautiously to patients with impaired renal function as well as to those with compromised bone marrow reserve, as indicated by: leukopenia, granulocytopenia, extensive bone marrow metastases, prior radiation therapy, or prior therapy with other cytotoxic agents.

Laboratory Tests

During treatment, the patient's hematologic profile (particularly neutrophils and platelets) should be monitored regularly to determine the degree of hematopoietic suppression. Urine should also be examined regularly for red cells which may precede hemorrhagic cystitis.

Drug Interactions

The physician should be alert for possible combined drug actions, desirable or undesirable, involving ifosfamide even though ifosfamide has been used successfully concurrently with other drugs, including other cytotoxic drugs.

Wound Healing

Ifosfamide may interfere with normal wound healing.

Pregnancy

Pregnancy "Category D." See WARNINGS section.

Nursing Mothers

Ifosfamide is excreted in breast milk. Because of the potential for serious adverse events and the tumorigenicity shown for ifosfamide in animal studies, a decision should be made whether to discontinue nursing or to discontinue the drug, taking into account the importance of the drug to the mother.

Carcinogenesis, Mutagenesis, Impairment of Fertility.

Ifosfamide has been shown to be carcinogenic in rats, with female rats showing a significant incidence of leiomyosarcomas and mammary fibroadenomas.

The mutagenic potential of ifosfamide has been documented in bacterial systems in vitro and mammalian cells in vivo. In vivo, ifosfamide has induced mutagenic effects in mice and Drosophila melanogaster germ cells, and has induced a significant increase in dominant lethal mutations in male mice as well as recessive sex-linked lethal mutations in Drosophila. In pregnant mice, resorptions increased and anomalies were present at day 19 after 30 mg/m² dose of ifosfamide was administered on day 11 of gestation. Embryolethal effects were observed in rats following the administration of 54 mg/m² doses of ifosfamide from the sixth through the fifteenth day of gestation and embryotoxic effects were apparent after dams received 18 mg/m² doses over the same dosing period. Ifosfamide is embryotoxic to rabbits receiving 88 mg/m²/day doses from the sixth through the eighteenth day after mating. The number of anomalies was also significantly increased over the control group.

Pediatric Use

Safety and effectiveness in children have not been established.

ADVERSE REACTIONS

In patients receiving IFEX as a single agent, the dose-limiting toxicities are myelosuppression and urotoxicity. Dose fractionation, vigorous hydration, and a protector such as mesna can significantly reduce the incidence of hematuria, especially gross hematuria, associated with hemorrhagic cystitis. At a dose of 1.2 g/m² daily for five consecutive days, leukopenia, when it occurs, is usually mild to moderate. Other significant side effects include alopecia, nausea, vomiting, and central nervous system toxicities.

Adverse Reaction	*Incidence %
Alopecia	83
Nausea-Vomiting	58
Hematuria	46
Gross Hematuria	12
CNS Toxicity	12
Infection	8
Renal Impairment	6
Liver Dysfunction	3
Phlebitis	2
Fever	1
Allergic Reaction	<1
Anorexia	<1
Cardiotoxicity	<1
Coagulopathy	<1
Constipation	<1
Dermatitis	<1
Diarrhea	<1
Fatigue	<1
Hypertension	<1
Hypotension	<1
Malaise	<1
Polyneuropathy	<1
Pulmonary Symptoms	<1
Salivation	<1
Stomatitis	<1

* Based upon 2,070 patients from the published literature in 30 single agent studies.

Hematologic Toxicity

Myelosuppression was dose related and dose limiting. It consisted mainly of leukopenia and, to a lesser extent, thrombocytopenia. A WBC count <3000/μL is expected in 50% of the patients treated with IFEX single agent at doses of 1.2 g/m² per day for five consecutive days. At this dose level, thrombocytopenia (platelets < 100,000/μL) occurred in about 20% of the patients. At higher dosages, leukopenia was almost universal, at total dosages of 10–12 g/m²/cycle, one-half of the patients had a WBC count below 1000/μL and 8% of patients had platelet counts less than 50,000/μL. Myelosuppression was usually reversible and treatment can be given every 3 to 4 weeks. When IFEX is used in combination with other myelosuppressive agents, adjustments in dosing may be necessary. Patients who experience severe myelosuppression are potentially at increased risk for infection.

Digestive System

Nausea and vomiting occurred in 58% of the patients who received IFEX. They were usually controlled by standard antiemetic therapy. Other gastrointestinal side effects include anorexia, diarrhea, and in some cases, constipation.

Urinary System

Urotoxicity consisted of hemorrhagic cystitis, dysuria, urinary frequency and other symptoms of bladder irritation. Hematuria occurred in 6% to 92% of patients treated with IFEX. The incidence and severity of hematuria can be significantly reduced by using vigorous hydration, a fractionated dose schedule and a protector such as mesna. At daily doses of 1.2 g/m² for five consecutive days without a protector, microscopic hematuria is expected in about one-half of the patients and gross hematuria in about 8% of patients. Renal toxicity occurred in 6% of the patients treated with ifosfamide as a single agent. Clinical signs, such as elevation in BUN or serum creatinine or decrease in creatinine clearance, were usually transient. They were most likely to be related to tubular damage. One episode of renal tubular acidosis which progressed into chronic renal failure was reported. Proteinuria and acidosis also occurred in rare instances. Metabolic acidosis was reported in 31% of patients in one study when IFEX was administered at doses of 2.0–2.5 g/m²/day for four days.

Central Nervous System

CNS side effects were observed in 12% of patients treated with IFEX. Those most commonly seen were somnolence, confusion, depressive psychosis, and hallucinations. Other less frequent symptoms include dizziness, disorientation, and cranial nerve dysfunction. Seizures and coma were occasionally reported. The incidence of CNS toxicity may be higher in patients with altered renal function.

Other

Alopecia occurred in approximately 83% of the patients treated with IFEX as a single agent. In combination, this incidence may be as high as 100%, depending on the other agents included in the chemotherapy regimen. Increases in liver enzymes and/or bilirubin were noted in 3% of the patients. Other less frequent side effects included phlebitis,

Continued on next page

Bristol-Myers Oncology—Cont.

pulmonary symptoms, fever of unknown origin, allergic reactions, stomatitis, cardiotoxicity, and polyneuropathy.

OVERDOSAGE

No specific antidote for IFEX is known. Management of overdosage would include general supportive measures to sustain the patient through any period of toxicity that might occur.

DOSAGE AND ADMINISTRATION

IFEX should be administered intravenously at a dose of 1.2 g/m^2 per day for five consecutive days. Treatment is repeated every 3 weeks or after recovery from hematologic toxicity (Platelets $\geq 100,000/\mu L$, WBC $\geq 4,000/\mu L$). In order to prevent bladder toxicity, IFEX should be given with extensive hydration consisting of at least two liters of oral or intravenous fluid per day. A protector, such as mesna, should also be used to prevent hemorrhagic cystitis. IFEX should be administered as a slow intravenous infusion lasting a minimum of 30 minutes. Although IFEX has been administered to a small number of patients with compromised hepatic and/or renal function, studies to establish optimal dose schedules of IFEX in such patients have not been conducted.

Preparation for Intravenous Administration/Stability

Injections are prepared for parenteral use by adding *Sterile Water for Injection USP or Bacteriostatic Water for Injection USP* (benzyl alcohol or parabens preserved) to the vial and shaking to dissolve. Use the quantity of diluent shown below to reconstitute the product:

Dosage Strength	Quantity of Diluent	Final Concentration
1 gram	20 mL	50 mg/mL

Reconstituted solutions are chemically and physically stable for one week at 30°C or three weeks at 5°C.
Solutions of ifosfamide may be diluted further to achieve concentrations of 0.6 to 20 mg/mL in the following fluids:

  5% Dextrose Injection, USP
  0.9% Sodium Chloride Injection, USP
  Lactated Ringer's Injection, USP
  Sterile Water for Injection, USP

Such admixtures, when stored in large volume parenteral glass bottles, Viaflex bags, or PAB™ bags, are physically and chemically stable for at least one week at 30°C or six weeks at 5°C.
Because essentially identical stability results were obtained for Sterile Water admixtures as for the other admixtures (5% Dextrose Injection, 0.9% Sodium Chloride Injection, and Lactated Ringer's Injection), the use of large volume parenteral glass bottles, Viaflex bags or PAB™ bags that contain intermediate concentrations or mixtures of excipients (eg, 2.5% Dextrose Injection, 0.45% Sodium Chloride Injection, or 5% Dextrose and 0.9% Sodium Chloride Injection) is also acceptable.
The microbiological qualities of the constituted products or prepared admixtures should be considered, particularly where unpreserved vehicles are used.
Dilutions of IFEX not prepared by constitution with Bacteriostatic Water for Injection, USP, (benzyl alcohol or parabens preserved), should be refrigerated and used within six hours.
Parenteral drug products should be inspected visually for particulate matter and discoloration prior to administration.

HOW SUPPLIED

IFLEX (sterile ifosfamide) is only available in a combination package with the uroprotective agent Mesnex (mesna) injection.
IFEX (sterile ifosfamide) Mesnex™ (mesna) injection.
NDC 0015-3558-41—1 gram Single Dose Vial, carton of 5
   —200 mg Single Dose Ampule, carton of 15
The dry powder may be stored at room temperature. Storage above 104°F (40°C) should be avoided.
Procedures for proper handling and disposal of anticancer drugs should be considered. Skin reactions associated with accidental exposure to IFEX may occur. The use of gloves is recommended. If IFEX solution contacts the skin or mucosa, immediately wash the skin thoroughly with soap and water or rinse the mucosa with copious amounts of water. Several guidelines on this subject have been published.[1-7] There is no general agreement that all of the procedures recommended in the guidelines are necessary or appropriate.

REFERENCES

1. Recommendations for the Safe Handling of Parenteral Antineoplastic Drugs. NIH Publication No. 83-2621. For sale by the Superintendent of Documents, U.S. Government Printing Office, Washington, DC 20402.
2. AMA Council Report, Guidelines for Handling Parenteral Antineoplastics, JAMA 1985; March 15.
3. National Study Commission on Cytotoxic Exposure—Recommendations for Handling Cytotoxic Agents. Available from Louis P. Jeffrey, Sc.D., Chairman, National Study Commission on Cytotoxic Exposure, Massachusetts College of Pharmacy and Allied Health Sciences, 179 Longwood Avenue, Boston Massachusetts 02115.
4. Clinical Oncological Society of Australia: Guidelines and Recommendations for Safe Handling of Antineoplastic Agents. Med J Australia 1983; 1:426–428.
5. Jones, RB, *et al:* Safe Handling of Chemotherapuetic Agents: A Report from the Mount Sinai Medical Center, CA-A Cancer Journal for Clinicians 1983; Sept/Oct. 258–263.
6. American Society of Hospital Pharmacists Technical Assistance Bulletin on Handling Cytotoxic Drugs in Hospitals, Am J Hosp Pharm 1985; 42:131–137.
7. OSHA Work-Practice Guidelines for Personnel Dealing with Cytotoxic (Antineoplastic) Drugs. Am J Hosp Pharm 1986; 43:1193–1204.

LYSODREN®   ℞
[li 'sō-drĕn "]
(mitotane
tablets, USP)

WARNINGS

Lysodren (mitotane) should be administered under the supervision of a qualified physician experienced in the uses of cancer chemotherapeutic agents. Lysodren should be temporarily discontinued immediately following shock or severe trauma since adrenal suppression is its prime action. Exogenous steroids should be administered in such circumstances, since the depressed adrenal may not immediately start to secrete steroids.

DESCRIPTION

Lysodren (mitotane) is an oral chemotherapeutic agent. It is best known by its trivial name, o,p'-DDD, and is chemically, 1.1-dichloro-2-(o-chlorophenyl) -2- (p-chlorophenyl) ethane. The chemical structure is shown below.

Lysodren is a white granular solid composed of clear colorless crystals. It is tasteless and has a slight pleasant aromatic odor. It is soluble in ethanol, isoctane and carbon tetrachloride. It has a molecular weight of 320.05.
Inactive ingredients in Lysodren tablets are: avicel, polyethylene glycol 3350, silicon dioxide, and starch.
Lysodren is available as 500 mg scored tablets for oral administration.

CLINICAL PHARMACOLOGY

Lysodren can best be described as an adrenal cytotoxic agent, although it can cause adrenal inhibition, apparently without cellular destruction. Its biochemical mechanism of action is unknown. Data are available to suggest that the drug modifies the peripheral metabolism of steroids as well as directly suppressing the adrenal cortex. The administration of Lysodren alters the extra-adrenal metabolism of cortisol in man, leading to a reduction in measurable 17-hydroxy corticosteroids, even though plasma levels of corticosteroids do not fall. The drug apparently causes increased formation of 6-β-hydroxyl cortisol.
Data in adrenal carcinoma patients indicate that about 40% of oral Lysodren is absorbed and approximately 10% of administered dose is recovered in the urine as a water-soluble metabolite. A variable amount of metabolite (1 to 17%) is excreted in the bile and the balance is apparently stored in the tissues.
Following discontinuation of Lysodren, the plasma terminal half life has ranged from 18 to 159 days. In most patients blood levels become undetectable after six to nine weeks. Autopsy data have provided evidence that Lysodren is found in most tissues of the body; however, fat tissues are the primary site of storage. Lysodren is converted to a water-soluble metabolite.
No unchanged Lysodren has been found in urine or bile.

INDICATIONS AND USAGE

Lysodren is indicated in the treatment of inoperable adrenal cortical carcinoma of both functional and nonfunctional types.

CONTRAINDICATIONS

Lysodren should not be given to individuals who have demonstrated a previous hypersensitivity to it.

WARNINGS

Lysodren should be temporarily discontinued immediately following shock or severe trauma, since adrenal suppression is its prime action. Exogenous steroids should be administered in such circumstances, since the depressed adrenal may not immediately start to secrete steroids.
Lysodren should be administered with care to patients with liver disease other than metastatic lesions from the adrenal cortex, since the metabolism of Lysodren may be interfered with and the drug may accumulate.
All possible tumor tissues should be surgically removed from large metastatic masses before Lysodren administration is instituted. This is necessary to minimize the possibility of infarction and hemorrhage in the tumor due to a rapid cytotoxic effect of the drug.
Long-term continuous administration of high doses of Lysodren may lead to brain damage and impairment of function. Behavioral and neurological assessments should be made at regular intervals when continuous Lysodren treatment exceeds two years.
A substantial percentage of the patients treated show signs of adrenal insufficiency. It therefore appears necessary to watch for and institute steroid replacement in those patients. However, some investigators have recommended that steroid replacement therapy be administered concomitantly with Lysodren. It has been shown that the metabolism of exogenous steroids is modified and consequently somewhat higher doses than normal replacement therapy may be required.

PRECAUTIONS

General: Adrenal insufficiency may develop in patients treated with Lysodren, and adrenal steroid replacement should be considered for these patients.
Since sedation, lethargy, vertigo, and other CNS side effects can occur, ambulatory patients should be cautioned about driving, operating machinery, and other hazardous pursuits requiring mental and physical alertness.
Drug Interactions: Lysodren has been reported to accelerate the metabolism of warfarin by the mechanism of hepatic microsomal enzyme induction, leading to an increase in dosage requirements for warfarin. Therefore, physicians should closely monitor patients for a change in anticoagulant dosage requirements when administering Lysodren to patients on coumarin-type anticoagulants. In addition, Lysodren should be given with caution to patients receiving other drugs susceptible to the influence of hepatic enzyme induction.
Carcinogenesis, Mutagenesis, Impairment of Fertility: The carcinogenic and mutagenic potentials of Lysodren are unknown. However, the mechanism of action of this compound suggests that it probably has less carcinogenic potential than other cytotoxic chemotherapeutic drugs.
Pregnancy: Pregnancy "Category C." Animal reproduction studies have not been conducted with Lysodren. It is also not known whether Lysodren can cause fetal harm when administered to a pregnant woman or can affect reproduction capacity. Lysodren should be given to a pregnant woman only if clearly needed.
Nursing Mothers: It is not known whether this drug is excreted in human milk. Because many drugs are excreted in human milk and because of the potential for adverse reactions in nursing infants from mitotane, a decision should be made whether to discontinue nursing or to discontinue the drug, taking into account the importance of the drug to the mother.

ADVERSE REACTIONS

A very high percentage of patients treated with Lysodren has shown at least one type of side effect. The main types of adverse reactions consist of the following:
1. Gastrointestinal disturbances, which consist of anorexia, nausea or vomiting, and in some cases diarrhea, occur in about 80% of the patients.
2. Central nervous system side effects occur in 40% of the patients. These consist primarily of depression as manifested by lethargy and somnolence (25%), and dizziness or vertigo (15%).
3. Skin toxicity has been observed in about 15% of the cases. These skin changes consist primarily of transient skin rashes which do not seem to be dose related. In some instances, this side effect subsided while the patients were maintained on the drug without a change of dose.
Infrequently occurring side effects involve the eye (visual blurring, diplopia, lens opacity, toxic retinopathy); the genitourinary system (hematuria, hemorrhagic cystitis, and albuminuria); cardiovascular system (hypertension, orthostatic hypotension, and flushing); and some miscellaneous effects including generalized aching, hyperpyrexia, and lowered protein bound iodine (PBI).

OVERDOSAGE

No proven antidotes have been established for Lysodren overdosage.

DOSAGE AND ADMINISTRATION

The recommended treatment schedule is to start the patient at 2 to 6 g of Lysodren per day in divided doses, either three or four times a day. Doses are usually increased incrementally to 9 to 10 g per day. If severe side effects appear, the dose should be reduced until the maximum tolerated dose is achieved. If the patient can tolerate higher doses and improved clinical response appears possible, the dose should be increased until adverse reactions interfere. Experience has shown that the maximum tolerated dose (MTD) will vary from 2 to 16 g per day, but has usually been 9 to 10 g per day. The highest doses used in the studies to date were 18 to 19 g per day.

Treatment should be instituted in the hospital until a stable dosage regimen is achieved.

Treatment should be continued as long as clinical benefits are observed. Maintenance of clinical status or slowing of growth of metastatic lesions can be considered clinical benefits if they can clearly be shown to have occurred.

If no clinical benefits are observed after three months at the maximum tolerated dose, the case would generally be considered a clinical failure. However, 10% of the patients who showed a measurable response required more than three months at the MTD. Early diagnosis and prompt institution of treatment improve the probability of a positive clinical response. Clinical effectiveness can be shown by reduction in tumor mass; reduction in pain, weakness or anorexia; and reduction of symptoms and signs due to excessive steroid production.

A number of patients have been treated intermittently with treatment being restarted when severe symptoms have reappeared. Patients often do not respond after the third or fourth such course. Experience accumulated to date suggests that continuous treatment with the maximum possible dosage of Lysodren is the best approach.

Procedures for proper handling and disposal of anticancer drugs should be considered. Several guidelines on this subject have been published.[1-7] There is no general agreement that all of the procedures recommended in the guidelines are necessary or appropriate.

REFERENCES

1. Recommendations for the Safe Handling of Parenteral Antineoplastic Drugs. NIH Publication No. 83-2621. For sale by the Superintendent of Documents, U.S. Government Printing Office, Washington, D.C. 20402.
2. AMA Council Report. Guidelines for Handling Parenteral Antineoplastics. JAMA, 1985; March 15.
3. National Study Commission on Cytotoxic Exposure—Recommendations for Handling Cytotoxic Agents. Available from Louis P. Jeffrey, Sc.D., Chairman, National Study Commission on Cytotoxic Exposure, Massachusetts College of Pharmacy and Allied Health Sciences, 179 Longwood Avenue, Boston, Massachusetts 02115.
4. Clinical Oncological Society of Australia: Guidelines and Recommendations for Safe Handling of Antineoplastic Agents. Med. J. Australia 1983; 1:426–428.
5. Jones, R. B., et. al. Safe Handling of Chemotherapeutic Agents: A Report from the Mount Sinai Medical Center, CA—A Cancer Journal for Clinicians 1983; Sept./Oct., 258–263.
6 American Society of Hospital Pharmacists Technical Assistance Bulletin on Handling Cytotoxic Drugs in Hospitals. Am. J. Hosp. Pharm. 1985; 42:131–137.
7. OSHA Work-Practice Guidelines for Personnel Dealing with Cytotoxic (Antineoplastic) Drugs. Am. J. Hosp. Pharm. 1986; 43:1193–1204.

HOW SUPPLIED

Lysodren (mitotane) Tablets, USP
NDC 0015-3080-60—500 mg Tablets, bottle of 100
Tablets may be stored at room temperature.
Shown in Product Identification Section, page 407

MEGACE® ℞

[mĕg 'ace]
(megestrol acetate tablets, USP)
40 mg tablets, bottle of 100s NSN 6505-01-070-1493(M)

THE USE OF MEGACE DURING THE FIRST 4 MONTHS OF PREGNANCY IS NOT RECOMMENDED
Progestational agents have been used beginning with the first trimester of pregnancy in an attempt to prevent habitual abortion. There is no adequate evidence that such use is effective when such drugs are given during the first 4 months of pregnancy. Furthermore, in the vast majority of women, the cause of abortion is a defective ovum, which progestational agents could not be expected to influence. In addition, the use of progestational agents, with their uterine-relaxant properties, in patients with fertilized defective ova may cause a delay in spontaneous abortion. Therefore, the use of such drugs during the first 4 months of pregnancy is not recommended.
Several reports suggest an association between intrauterine exposure to progestational drugs in the first trimester of pregnancy and genital abnormalities in male and female fetuses. The risk of hypospadias, 5 to 8 per 1,000 male births in the general population, may be approximately doubled with exposure to these drugs. There are insufficient data to quantify the risk to exposed female fetuses, but insofar as some of these drugs induce mild virilization of the external genitalia of the

---

female fetus, and because of the increased association of hypospadias in the male fetus, it is prudent to avoid the use of these drugs during the first trimester of pregnancy.
If the patient is exposed to Megace during the first 4 months of pregnancy or if she becomes pregnant while taking this drug, she should be apprised of the potential risks to the fetus.

DESCRIPTION

Megestrol acetate is a white, crystalline solid chemically described as 17α-acetoxy-6-methylpregna-4, 6-diene-3, 20-dione. Its molecular weight is 384.5. Inactive ingredients in Megace tablets are: acacia, calcium phosphate, FD&C Blue No. 1, Aluminum Lake, lactose, magnesium stearate, silicon dioxide colloidal and starch. The empirical formula is $C_{24}H_{32}O_4$ and the structural formula is:

MEGESTROL ACETATE

ACTIONS

While the precise mechanism by which Megace (megestrol acetate) produces its antineoplastic effects against endometrial carcinoma is unknown at the present time, an antiluteinizing effect mediated via the pituitary has been postulated. There is also evidence to suggest a local effect as a result of the marked changes brought about by the direct instillation of progestational agents into the endometrial cavity. Likewise, the antineoplastic action of Megace (megestrol acetate) on carcinoma of the breast is unclear.

INDICATIONS

Megace (megestrol acetate) is indicated for the palliative treatment of advanced carcinoma of the breast or endometrium (ie, recurrent, inoperable, or metastatic disease). It should not be used in lieu of currently accepted procedures such as surgery, radiation, or chemotherapy.

CONTRAINDICATIONS

As a diagnostic test for pregnancy.

WARNINGS

Administration for up to 7 years of megestrol acetate to female dogs is associated with an increased incidence of both benign and malignant tumors of the breast. Comparable studies in rats and studies in monkeys are not associated with an increased incidence of tumors. The relationship of the dog tumors to humans is unknown but should be considered in assessing the benefit-to-risk ratio when prescribing Megace and in surveillance of patients on therapy.
The use of Megace (megestrol acetate) in other types of neoplastic disease is not recommended.

PRECAUTIONS

There are no specific precautions identified for the use of Megace (megestrol acetate) when used as recommended. Close, customary surveillance is indicated for any patient being treated for recurrent or metastatic cancer. Use with caution in patients with a history of thrombophlebitis.

ADVERSE REACTIONS

Weight Gain: Weight gain is a frequent side effect of Megace. This gain has been associated with increased appetite and is not necessarily associated with fluid retention.
Thromboembolic Phenomena: Thromboembolic phenomena including thrombophlebitis and pulmonary embolism have been rarely reported.
Other Adverse Reactions: Nausea and vomiting, edema, breakthrough bleeding, dyspnea, tumor flare (with or without hypercalcemia), hyperglycemia, alopecia, carpal tunnel syndrome, and rash.

OVERDOSAGE

No serious side effects have resulted from studies involving Megace (megestrol acetate) administered in dosages as high as 800 mg/day.

DOSAGE AND ADMINISTRATION

Breast cancer: 160 mg/day (40 q.i.d.)
Endometrial carcinoma: 40—320 mg/day in divided doses. At least two months of continuous treatment is considered an adequate period for determining the efficacy of Megace (megestrol acetate).

HOW SUPPLIED

Megace® is available as light blue, scored tablets containing 20 mg or 40 mg megestrol acetate.

NDC 0015-0595-01, Bottles of 100 20 mg tablet
NDC 0015-0596-41, Bottles of 100 40 mg tablet
NDC 0015-0596-45, Bottles of 500 40 mg tablet
NDC 0015-0596-46 Bottles of 250 40 mg tablet
Shown in Product Identification Section, page 407

MESNEX™ ℞

[mĕs-nĕx]
(Mesna) Injection

DESCRIPTION

Mesnex Injection is a detoxifying agent to inhibit the hemorrhagic cystitis induced by ifosfamide (Ifex®). The active ingredient mesna is a synthetic sulfhydryl compound designated as sodium 2-mercaptoethanesulfonate with a molecular formula of $C_2H_5NaO_3S_2$ and a molecular weight of 164.18. Its structural formula is as follows:

$$HS\text{-}CH_2\text{-}CH_2SO_3\text{-}Na^+$$

Mesnex Injection is a sterile preservative-free aqueous solution of clear and colorless appearance in clear glass ampules for intravenous administration. Mesnex Injection contains 100 mg/mL mesna, 0.25 mg/mL edetate disodium and sodium hydroxide for pH adjustment. The solution has a pH range of 6.5–8.5.

CLINICAL PHARMACOLOGY

Mesnex was developed as a prophylactic agent to prevent the hemorrhagic cystitis induced by ifosfamide.

Analogous to the physiological cysteine-cystine system, following intravenous administration mesna is rapidly oxidized to its only metabolite, mesna disulfide (dimesna). Mesna disulfide remains in the intravascular compartment and is rapidly eliminated by the kidneys.

In the kidney, the mesna disulfide is reduced to the free thiol compound, mesna, which reacts chemically with the urotoxic ifosfamide metabolites (acrolein and 4-hydroxy-ifosfamide) resulting in their detoxification. The first step in the detoxification process is the binding of mesna to 4-hydroxy-ifosfamide forming a non-urotoxic 4-sulfoethylthioifosfamide. Mesna also binds to the double bonds of acrolein and other urotoxic metabolites.

After administration of an 800 mg dose the half-lives of mesna and dimesna in the blood are 0.36 hours and 1.17 hours, respectively. Approximately 32% and 33% of the administered dose was eliminated in the urine in 24 hours as mesna and dimesna, respectively. The majority of the dose recovered was eliminated within 4 hours. Mesna has a volume of distribution of 0.652 l/kg and a plasma clearance of 1.23 l/kg/hour.

Ifosfamide has been shown to have dose dependent pharmacokinetics in humans. At doses of 2–4 g, its terminal elimination half-life is about 7 hours. As a result, in order to maintain adequate levels of mesna in the urinary bladder during the course of elimination of the urotoxic ifosfamide metabolites, repeated doses of Mesnex are required.

Based on the pharmacokinetic profiles of mesna and ifosfamide as discussed above, Mesnex was given as bolus doses prior to ifosfamide and at 4 and 8 hours after ifosfamide administration. The hemorrhagic cystitis produced by ifosfamide is dose dependent. At a dose of 1.2 g/m² ifosfamide administered daily for 5 days, 16%–26% of the patients who received conventional uroprophylaxis (high fluid intake, alkalinization of the urine and the administration of diuretics) developed hematuria (> 50 rbc/hpf or macrohematuria). In contrast none of the patients who received Mesnex together with this dose of ifosfamide developed hematuria. Higher doses of ifosfamide from 2–4 g/m² administered for 3 to 5 days, produced hematuria in 31%–100% of the patients. When Mesnex was administered together with these doses of ifosfamide the incidence of hematuria was less than 7%.

INDICATIONS AND USAGE

Mesnex has been shown to be effective as a prophylactic agent in reducing the incidence of ifosfamide induced hemorrhagic cystitis.

CONTRAINDICATIONS

Mesnex is contraindicated in patients known to be hypersensitive to mesna or other thiol compounds.

WARNINGS

Mesnex has been developed as an agent to prevent ifosfamide induced hemorrhagic cystitis. It will not prevent or alleviate any of the other adverse reactions or toxicities associated with ifosfamide therapy.

Mesnex does not prevent hemorrhagic cystitis in all patients. Up to 6% of patients treated with mesna have developed hematuria (> 50 rbc/hpf or WHO grade 2 and above). As a result, a morning specimen of urine should be examined for the presence of hematuria (red blood cells) each day prior to ifosfamide therapy. If hematuria develops when Mesnex is given with ifosfamide according to the recommended dosage schedule, depending on the severity of the hematuria, dosage

Continued on next page

Bristol-Myers Oncology—Cont.

reductions or discontinuation of ifosfamide therapy may be initiated.

In order to obtain adequate protection, Mesnex must be administered with each dose of ifosfamide as outlined in the Dosage and Administration section. Mesnex is not effective in preventing hematuria due to other pathological conditions such as thrombocytopenia.

PRECAUTIONS

Laboratory Tests

A false positive test for urinary ketones may arise in patients treated with Mesnex. In this test, a red-violet color develops which, with the addition of glacial acetic acid, will return to violet.

Drug Interactions

In vitro and in vivo animal tumor models have shown that mesna dose not have any effect on the antitumor efficacy of concomitantly administered cytotoxic agents.

Carcinogenesis, Mutagenesis and Impairment of Fertility

No long term animal studies have been performed to evaluate the carcinogenic potential of mesna. The Ames **Salmonella typhimurium** test, mouse micronucleus assay and frequency of sister chromatid exchange and chromosomal aberrations in PHA stimulated lymphocytes in vitro assays revealed no mutagenic activity.

Pregnancy

Pregnancy Category B. Reproduction studies in rats and rabbits with oral doses up to 1000 mg/kg have revealed no harm to the fetus due to mesna. It is not known whether Mesnex can cause fetal harm when administered to a pregnant woman or can affect reproductive capacity. Mesnex should be given to a pregnant woman only if the benefits clearly outweigh any possible risks.

Teratology studies in rats and rabbits have shown no effects.

Nursing Mothers

It is not known whether mesna or dimesna is excreted in human milk. Because many drugs are excreted in human milk and because of the potential for adverse reactions in nursing infants, a decision should be made whether to discontinue nursing or discontinue the drug, taking into account the importance of the drug to the mother.

ADVERSE REACTIONS

Because Mesnex is used in combination with ifosfamide and other chemotherapeutic agents with documented toxicities, it is difficult to distinguish the adverse reactions which may be due to Mesnex from those caused by the concomitantly administered cytostatic agents. As a result, the adverse reaction profile of Mesnex was determined in three Phase I studies (16 subjects) utilizing intravenous and oral administration and two controlled studies in which ifosfamide and Mesnex were compared to ifosfamide and standard prophylaxis.

In Phase I studies in which i.v. bolus doses of 0.8–1.6 g/m^2 Mesnex were administered as single or three repeated doses to a total of 10 patients, a bad taste in the mouth (100%) and soft stools (70%) were reported. At intravenous and oral bolus doses of 2.4 g/m^2 which are approximately 10 times the recommended clinical doses (0.24 g/m^2) headache (50%), fatigue (33%), nausea (33%), diarrhea (83%), limb pain (50%), hypotension (17%) and allergy (17%) have also been reported in the six patients who participated in this study.

In controlled clinical studies, adverse reactions which can be reasonably associated with Mesnex were vomiting, diarrhea and nausea.

OVERDOSAGE

There is no known antidote for Mesnex.

DOSAGE AND ADMINISTRATION

For the prophylaxis of ifosfamide induced hemorrhagic cystitis, Mesnex may be given on a fractionated dosing schedule of bolus intravenous injections as outlined below.

Mesnex is given as intravenous bolus injections in a dosage equal to 20% of the ifosfamide dosage (w/w) at the time of ifosfamide administration and 4 and 8 hours after each dose of ifosfamide. The total daily dose of Mesnex is 60% of the ifosfamide dose.

The recommended dosing schedule is outlined below:

	0 Hours	4 Hours	8 Hours
Ifosfamide	1.2 g/m^2	—	—
Mesnex	240 mg/m^2	240 mg/m^2	240 mg/m^2

In order to maintain adequate protection, this dosing schedule should be repeated on each day that ifosfamide is administered. When the dosage of ifosfamide is adjusted (either increased or decreased), the dose of Mesnex should be modified accordingly. When exposed to oxygen, mesna is oxidized to the disulfide, dimesna. As a result, any unused drug remaining in the ampules after dosing should be discarded and new ampules used for each administration.

Preparation of Intravenous Solutions/Stability

For i.v. administration the drug can be diluted by adding the contents of a Mesnex ampule to any of the following fluids

obtaining final concentrations of 20 mg mesna/mL fluid:
  5% Dextrose Injection, USP
  5% Dextrose and Sodium Chloride Injection, USP
  0.9% Sodium Chloride Injection, USP
  Lactated Ringer's Injection, USP
For example:
One ampule of Mesnex Injection 200 mg/2 mL may be added to 8 mL, or one ampule of Mesnex Injection 400 mg/4 mL may be added to 16 mL of any of the solutions listed above to create a final concentration of 20 mg mesna/mL fluid. Diluted solutions are chemically and physically stable for 24 hours at 25°C (77°F).

It is recommended that solutions of Mesnex be refrigerated and used within 6 hours.

Mesna is not compatible with cisplatin.

Parenteral drug products should be inspected visually for particulate matter and discoloration prior to administration.

HOW SUPPLIED

Mesnex™(Mesna) Injection 100 mg/mL
NDC 0015-3560-41 200 mg Single Dose Ampule,
  Box of 15 Ampules of 2 mL (color-ring coding: turquoise/yellow)
NDC 0015-3561-41 400 mg Single Dose Ampule,
  Box of 15 Ampules of 4 mL (color-ring coding: blue/green)
NDC 0015-3562-41 1 g Single Dose Ampule,
  Box of 10 Ampules of 10 mL (color-ring coding: blue/green)
Store at room temperature.

MUTAMYCIN®   ℞

[mū''-tĕ-mī'-sĭn]
(mitomycin for injection)

WARNING

Mutamycin should be administered under the supervision of a qualified physician experienced in the use of cancer chemotherapeutic agents. Appropriate management of therapy and complications is possible only when adequate diagnostic and treatment facilities are readily available.

Bone marrow suppression, notably thrombocytopenia and leukopenia, which may contribute to overwhelming infections in an already compromised patient, is the most common and severe of the toxic effects of Mutamycin (see "Warnings" and "Adverse Reactions" sections). Hemolytic Uremic Syndrome (HUS) a serious complication of chemotherapy, consisting primarily of microangiopathic hemolytic anemia, thrombocytopenia, and irreversible renal failure, has been reported in patients receiving systemic Mutamycin. The syndrome may occur at any time during systemic therapy with Mutamycin as a single agent or in combination with other cytotoxic drugs, however, most cases occur at doses ≥ 60 mg of Mutamycin. Blood product transfusion may exacerbate the symptoms associated with this syndrome. The incidence of the syndrome has not been defined.

DESCRIPTION

Mutamycin (also known as mitomycin and/or mitomycin-C) is an antibiotic isolated from the broth of **Streptomyces caespitosus** which has been shown to have antitumor activity. The compound is heat stable, has a high melting point, and is freely soluble in organic solvents.

ACTION

Mutamycin selectively inhibits the synthesis of deoxyribonucleic acid (DNA). The guanine and cytosine content correlates with the degree of Mutamycin-induced cross-linking. At high concentrations of the drug, cellular RNA and protein synthesis are also suppressed.

In humans, Mutamycin is rapidly cleared from the serum after intravenous administration. Time required to reduce the serum concentration by 50% after a 30 mg. bolus injection is 17 minutes. After injection of 30 mg., 20 mg., or 10 mg. I.V., the maximal serum concentrations were 2.4 μg./mL, 1.7 μg./mL, and 0.52 μg./mL, respectively. Clearance is effected primarily by metabolism in the liver, but metabolism occurs in other tissues as well. The rate of clearance is inversely proportional to the maximal serum concentration because, it is thought, of saturation of the degradative pathways.

Approximately 10% of a dose of Mutamycin is excreted unchanged in the urine. Since metabolic pathways are saturated at relatively low doses, the percent of a dose excreted in urine increases with increasing dose. In children, excretion of intravenously administered Mutamycin is similar.

Animal Toxicology—Mutamycin has been found to be carcinogenic in rats and mice. At doses approximating the recommended clinical dose in man, it produces a greater than 100 percent increase in tumor incidence in male Sprague-Dawley rats, and a greater than 50 percent increase in tumor incidence in female Swiss mice.

INDICATIONS

Mutamycin is not recommended as single-agent, primary therapy. It has been shown to be useful in the therapy of dis-

seminated adenocarcinoma of the stomach or pancreas in proven combinations with other approved chemotherapeutic agents and as palliative treatment when other modalities have failed. Mutamycin is not recommended to replace appropriate surgery and /or radiotherapy.

CONTRAINDICATIONS

Mutamycin is contraindicated in patients who have demonstrated a hypersensitive or idiosyncratic reaction to it in the past.

Mutamycin is contraindicated in patients with thrombocytopenia, coagulation disorder, or an increase in bleeding tendency due to other causes.

WARNINGS

Patients being treated with Mutamycin must be observed carefully and frequently during and after therapy.

The use of Mutamycin results in a high incidence of bone marrow suppression, particularly thrombocytopenia and leukopenia. Therefore, the following studies should be obtained repeatedly during therapy and for at least 8 weeks following therapy: platelet count, white blood cell count, differential, and hemoglobin. The occurrence of a platelet count below 100,000/mm^3 or a WBC below 4,000/mm^3 or a progressive decline in either is an indication to withhold further therapy until blood counts have recovered above these levels.

Patients should be advised of the potential toxicity of this drug, particularly bone marrow suppression. Deaths have been reported due to septicemia as a result of leukopenia due to the drug.

Patients receiving Mutamycin should be observed for evidence of renal toxicity. Mutamycin should not be given to patients with a serum creatinine greater than 1.7 mg. percent.

Usage in Pregnancy—Safe use of Mutamycin in pregnant women has not been established. Teratological changes have been noted in animal studies. The effect of Mutamycin on fertility is unknown.

PRECAUTIONS

Acute shortness of breath and severe bronchospasm have been reported following the administration of vinca alkaloids in patients who had previously or simultaneously received Mutamycin. The onset of this acute respiratory distress occurred within minutes to hours after the vinca alkaloid injection. The total number of doses for each drug has varied considerably. Bronchodilators, steroids and/or oxygen have produced symptomatic relief.

A few cases of adult respiratory distress syndrome have been reported in patients receiving Mutamycin in combination with other chemotherapy and maintained at F10$_2$ concentrations greater than 50% perioperatively. Therefore, caution should be exercised using only enough oxygen to provide adequate arterial saturation since oxygen itself is toxic to the lungs. Careful attention should be paid to fluid balance and overhydration should be avoided.

ADVERSE REACTIONS

Bone Marrow Toxicity— This was the most common and most serious toxicity, occurring in 605 of 937 patients (64.4%). Thrombocytopenia and/or leukopenia may occur anytime within 8 weeks after onset of therapy with an average time of 4 weeks. Recovery after cessation of therapy was within 10 weeks. About 25% of the leukopenic or thrombocytopenic episodes did not recover. Mutamycin produces cumulative myelosuppression.

Integument and Mucous Membrane Toxicity— This has occurred in approximately 4% of patients treated with Mutamycin. Cellulitis at the injection site has been reported and is occasionally severe. Stomatitis and alopecia also occur frequently. Rashes are rarely reported. The most important dermatological problem with this drug, however, is the necrosis and consequent sloughing of tissue which results if the drug is extravasated during injection. Extravasation may occur with or without an accompanying stinging or burning sensation and even if there is adequate blood return when the injection needle is aspirated. There have been reports of delayed erythema and/or ulceration occurring either at or distant from the injection site, weeks to months after Mutamycin, even when no obvious evidence of extravasation was observed during administration. Skin grafting has been required in some cases.

Renal Toxicity—2% of 1,281 patients demonstrated a statistically significant rise in creatinine. There appeared to be no correlation between total dose administered or duration of therapy and the degree of renal impairment.

Pulmonary Toxicity—This has occurred infrequently but can be severe and may be life threatening. Dyspnea with a nonproductive cough and radiographic evidence of pulmonary infiltrates may be indicative of Mutamycin-induced pulmonary toxicity. If other etiologies are eliminated, Mutamycin therapy should be discontinued. Steroids have been employed as treatment of this toxicity, but the therapeutic value has not been determined.

A few cases of adult respiratory distress syndrome have been reported in patients receiving Mutamycin in combination with other chemotherapy and maintained at FIO_2 concentrations greater than 50% perioperatively.

Hemolytic Uremic Syndrome (HUS)—This serious complication of chemotherapy, consisting primarily of microangiopathic hemolytic anemia (hematocrit $\leq 25\%$), thrombocytopenia ($\leq 100,000/mm^3$), and irreversible renal failure (serum creatinine ≥ 1.6 mg/dl) has been reported in patients receiving systemic Mutamycin. Microangiopathic hemolysis with fragmented red blood cells on peripheral blood smears has occurred in 98% of patients with the syndrome. Other less frequent complications of the syndrome may include pulmonary edema (65%), neurologic abnormalities (16%), and hypertension. Exacerbation of the symptoms associated with HUS has been reported in some patients receiving blood product transfusions. A high mortality rate (52%) has been associated with this syndrome.

The syndrome may occur at any time during systemic therapy with Mutamycin as a single agent or in combination with other cytotoxic drugs. Less frequently, HUS has also been reported in patients receiving combinations of cytotoxic drugs not including Mutamycin. Of 83 patients studied, 72 developed the syndrome at total doses exceeding 60 mg of Mutamycin. Consequently, patients receiving ≥ 60 mg of Mutamycin should be monitored closely for unexplained anemia with fragmented cells on peripheral blood smear, thrombocytopenia, and decreased renal function.

The incidence of the syndrome has not been defined. Therapy for the syndrome is investigational.

Acute Side Effects Due to Mutamycin were fever, anorexia, nausea, and vomiting. They occurred in about 14% of 1,281 patients.

Other Undesirable Side Effects that have been reported during Mutamycin therapy have been headache, blurring of vision, confusion, drowsiness, syncope, fatigue, edema, thrombophlebitis, hematemesis, diarrhea, and pain. These did not appear to be dose related and were not unequivocally drug related. They may have been due to the primary or metastatic disease processes.

DOSAGE AND ADMINISTRATION

Mutamycin should be given intravenously only, using care to avoid extravasation of the compound. If extravasation occurs, cellulitis, ulceration, and slough may result.

Each vial contains either mitomycin 5 mg and mannitol 10 mg, mitomycin 20 mg and mannitol 40 mg, or mitomycin 40 mg and mannitol 80 mg. To administer, add Sterile Water for Injection, 10 mL, 40 mL or 80 mL, respectively. Shake to dissolve. If product does not dissolve immediately, allow to stand at room temperature until solution is obtained.

After full hematological recovery (see guide to dosage adjustment) from any previous chemotherapy, the following dosage schedule may be used at 6 to 8 week intervals:

  20 mg/m² intravenously as a single dose via a functioning intravenous catheter.

Because of cumulative myelosuppression, patients should be fully reevaluated after each course of Mutamycin, and the dose reduced if the patient has experienced any toxicities. Doses greater than 20 mg/m² have not been shown to be more effective, and are more toxic than lower doses.

The following schedule is suggested as a guide to dosage adjustment:

Nadir After Prior Dose

Leukocytes/mm³	Platelets/mm³	Percentage of Prior Dose To be Given
>4000	>100,000	100%
3000–3999	75,000–99,999	100%
2000–2999	25,000–74,999	70%
<2000	<25,000	50%

No repeat dosage should be given until leukocyte count has returned to 4000/mm³ and platelet count to 100,000/mm³. When Mutamycin is used in combination with other myelosuppressive agents, the doses should be adjusted accordingly. If the disease continues to progress after two courses of Mutamycin, the drug should be stopped since chances of response are minimal.

STABILITY

1. **Unreconstituted** Mutamycin stored at room temperature is stable for the lot life indicated on the package. Avoid excessive heat (over 40°C).
2. **Reconstituted** with Sterile Water for Injection to a concentration of 0.5 mg. per mL, Mutamycin is stable for 14 days refrigerated or 7 days at room temperature.
3. **Diluted** in various IV fluids at room temperature, to a concentration of 20 to 40 micrograms per mL:

IV Fluid	Stability
5% Dextrose Injection	3 hours
0.9% Sodium Chloride Injection	12 hours
Sodium Lactate Injection	24 hours

4. **The combination** of Mutamycin (5 mg. to 15 mg.) and heparin (1,000 units to 10,000 units) in 30 mL of 0.9% Sodium Chloride Injection is stable for 48 hours at room temperature.

Procedures for proper handling and disposal of anticancer drugs should be considered. Several guidelines on this subject have been published.[1-7] There is no general agreement that all of the procedures recommended in the guidelines are necessary or appropriate.

REFERENCES

1. Recommendations for the Safe Handling of Parenteral Antineoplastic Drugs. NIH Publication No. 83-2621. For sale by the Superintendent of Documents, U.S. Government Printing Office, Washington, D.C. 20402.
2. AMA Council Report. Guidelines for Handling Parenteral Antineoplastics, JAMA, 1985; March 15.
3. National Study Commission on Cytotoxic Exposure—Recommendations for Handling Cytotoxic Agents. Available from Louis P. Jeffrey, Sc.D., Chairman, National Study Commission on Cytotoxic Exposure, Massachusetts College of Pharmacy and Allied Health Sciences, 179 Longwood Avenue, Boston, Massachusetts 02115.
4. Clinical Oncological Society of Australia: Guidelines and Recommendations for Safe Handling of Antineoplastic Agents. Med. J. Australia 1983; 1:426–428.
5. Jones, R. B., et. al. Safe Handling of Chemotherapeutic Agents: A Report from the Mount Sinai Medical Center, Ca—A Cancer Journal for Clinicians 1983; Sept./Oct., 258–263.
6. American Society of Hospital Pharmacists Technical Assistance Bulletin on Handling Cytotoxic Drugs in Hospitals, Am. J. Hosp. Pharm. 1985; 42:131–137.
7. OSHA Work-Practice Guidelines for Personnel Dealing with Cytotoxic (antineoplastic) Drugs. Am. J. Hosp. Pharm. 1986; 43:1193–1204.

SUPPLY

Mutamycin (mitomycin for Injection).
NDC 0015-3001-20—Each vial contains 5 mg. mitomycin.
NDC 0015-3002-20—Each vial contains 20 mg. mitomycin.
NDC 0015-3059-20—Each vial contains 40 mg mitomycin.
Shown in Product Identification Section, page 407

PARAPLATIN®   ℞
[păr-a-plătin]
(Carboplatin for Injection)

WARNING

PARAPLATIN® (carboplatin for injection) should be administered under the supervision of a qualified physician experienced in the use of cancer chemotherapeutic agents. Appropriate management of therapy and complications is possible only when adequate treatment facilities are readily available.

Bone marrow suppression is dose related and may be severe, resulting in infection and/or bleeding. Anemia may be cumulative and may require transfusion support. Vomiting is another frequent drug-related side effect.

Anaphylactic-like reactions to PARAPLATIN have been reported and may occur within minutes of PARAPLATIN administration. Epinephrine, corticosteroids, and antihistamines have been employed to alleviate symptoms.

DESCRIPTION

PARAPLATIN® (carboplatin for injection) is supplied as a sterile lyophilized powder available in single-dose vials containing 50 mg, 150 mg, and 450 mg of carboplatin for administration by intravenous infusion. Each vial contains equal parts by weight of carboplatin and mannitol.

Carboplatin is a platinum coordination compound that is used as a cancer chemotherapeutic agent. The chemical name for carboplatin is platinum, diammine [1,1-cyclobutane-dicarboxylato(2-)-0,0']-, (SP-4-2), and has the following structural formula:

Carboplatin is a white to off-white crystalline powder with the molecular formula of $C_6H_{12}N_2O_4Pt$ and a molecular weight of 371.25. It is soluble in water at a rate of approximately 14 mg/mL, and the pH of a 1% solution is 5–7. It is virtually insoluble in ethanol, acetone, and dimethylacetamide.

CLINICAL PHARMACOLOGY

Carboplatin, like cisplatin, produces predominantly interstrand DNA cross-links rather than DNA-protein cross-links. This effect is apparently cell-cycle nonspecific. The aquation of carboplatin, which is thought to produce the active species, occurs at a slower rate than in the case of cisplatin. Despite this difference, it appears that both carboplatin and cisplatin induce equal numbers of drug-DNA cross-links, causing equal lesions and biological effects. The differences in potencies for carboplatin and cisplatin appear to be directly related to the difference in aquation rates.

In patients with creatinine clearances of about 60 mL/min or greater, plasma levels of intact carboplatin decay in a biphasic manner after a 30-minute intravenous infusion of 300 to 500 mg/m² of PARAPLATIN. The initial plasma half-life (alpha) was found to be 1.1 to 2.0 hours (N=6), and the postdistribution plasma half-life (beta) was found to be 2.6 to 5.9 hours (N=6). The total body clearance, apparent volume of distribution and mean residence time for carboplatin are 4.4 L/hour, 16 L and 3.5 hours, respectively. The Cmax values and areas under the plasma concentration vs time curves from 0 to infinity (AUC inf) increase linearly with dose, although the increase was slightly more than dose proportional. Carboplatin, therefore, exhibits linear pharmacokinetics over the dosing range studied (300 to 500 mg/m²).

Carboplatin is not bound to plasma proteins. No significant quantities of protein-free, ultrafilterable platinum-containing species other than carboplatin are present in plasma. However, platinum from carboplatin becomes irreversibly bound to plasma proteins and is slowly eliminated with a minimum half-life of 5 days.

The major route of elimination of carboplatin is renal excretion. Patients with creatinine clearances of approximately 60 mL/min or greater excrete 65% of the dose in the urine within 12 hours and 71% of the dose within 24 hours. All of the platinum in the 24-hour urine is present as carboplatin. Only 3% to 5% of the administered platinum is excreted in the urine between 24 and 96 hours. There are insufficient data to determine whether biliary excretion occurs.

In patients with creatinine clearances below 60 mL/min the total body and renal clearances of carboplatin decrease as the creatinine clearance decreases. PARAPLATIN dosages should therefore be reduced in these patients (see "DOSAGE AND ADMINISTRATION").

In two randomized controlled studies in patients with advanced ovarian cancer previously treated with chemotherapy, PARAPLATIN achieved six clinical complete responses in 47 patients. The duration of these responses ranged from 45 to 71+ weeks.

INDICATIONS

PARAPLATIN is indicated for the palliative treatment of patients with ovarian carcinoma recurrent after prior chemotherapy, including patients who have been previously treated with cisplatin.

Within the group of patients previously treated with cisplatin, those who have developed progressive disease while receiving cisplatin therapy may have a decreased response rate.

CONTRAINDICATIONS

PARAPLATIN is contraindicated in patients with a history of severe allergic reactions to cisplatin or other platinum-containing compounds, or mannitol.

PARAPLATIN should not be employed in patients with severe bone marrow depression or significant bleeding.

WARNINGS

Bone marrow suppression (leukopenia, neutropenia, and thrombocytopenia) is dose dependent and is also the dose-limiting toxicity. Peripheral blood counts should be frequently monitored during PARAPLATIN treatment and, when appropriate, until recovery is achieved. Median nadir occurs at day 21 in patients receiving single-agent PARAPLATIN. In general, single intermittent courses of PARAPLATIN should not be repeated until leukocyte, neutrophil, and platelet counts have recovered.

Since anemia is cumulative, transfusions may be needed during treatment with PARAPLATIN, particularly in patients receiving prolonged therapy.

Bone marrow suppression is increased in patients who have received prior therapy, especially regimens including cisplatin. Marrow suppression is also increased in patients with impaired kidney function. Initial PARAPLATIN dosages in these patients should be appropriately reduced (see "DOSAGE AND ADMINISTRATION") and blood counts should be carefully monitored between courses. The use of PARAPLATIN in combination with other bone marrow suppressing therapies must be carefully managed with respect to dosage and timing in order to minimize additive effects. PARAPLATIN has limited nephrotoxic potential, but concomitant treatment with aminoglycosides has resulted in increased renal and/or audiologic toxicity, and caution must be exercised when a patient receives both drugs.

Continued on next page

Bristol-Myers Oncology—Cont.

PARAPLATIN can induce emesis, which can be more severe in patients previously receiving emetogenic therapy. The incidence and intensity of emesis have been reduced by using premedication with antiemetics. Although no conclusive efficacy data exist with the following schedules of PARAPLATIN, lengthening the duration of single intravenous administration to 24 hours or dividing the total dose over five consecutive daily pulse doses has resulted in reduced emesis.

Although peripheral neurotoxicity is infrequent, its incidence is increased in patients older than 65 years and in patients previously treated with cisplatin. Pre-existing cisplatin-induced neurotoxicity does not worsen in about 70% of the patients receiving PARAPLATIN as secondary treatment.

As in the case of other platinum coordination compounds, allergic reactions to PARAPLATIN have been reported. These may occur within minutes of administration and should be managed with appropriate supportive therapy. High dosages of PARAPLATIN (more than four times the recommended dose) have resulted in severe abnormalities of liver function tests.

PARAPLATIN may cause fetal harm when administered to a pregnant woman. PARAPLATIN has been shown to be embryotoxic and teratogenic in rats. There are no adequate and well-controlled studies in pregnant women. If this drug is used during pregnancy, or if the patient becomes pregnant while receiving this drug, the patient should be apprised of the potential hazard to the fetus. Women of childbearing potential should be advised to avoid becoming pregnant.

PRECAUTIONS

General: Needles or intravenous administration sets containing aluminum parts that may come in contact with PARAPLATIN should not be used for the preparation or administration of the drug. Aluminum can react with carboplatin causing precipitate formation and loss of potency.

Drug Interactions: The renal effects of nephrotoxic compounds may be potentiated by PARAPLATIN.

Carcinogenesis, mutagenesis, impairment of fertility: The carcinogenic potential of carboplatin has not been studied, but compounds with similar mechanisms of action and mutagenicity profiles have been reported to be carcinogenic. Carboplatin has been shown to be mutagenic both in vitro and in vivo. It has also been shown to be embryotoxic and teratogenic in rats receiving the drug during organogenesis.

Pregnancy: Pregnancy "category D": (see "Warnings").

Nursing mothers: It is not known whether carboplatin is excreted in human milk. Because there is a possibility of toxicity in nursing infants secondary to PARAPLATIN treatment of the mother, it is recommended that breast-feeding be discontinued if the mother is treated with PARAPLATIN.

ADVERSE REACTIONS

Data in the following table are based on the experience of 553 patients with previously treated ovarian carcinoma who received single-agent PARAPLATIN.

ADVERSE EXPERIENCES IN 553 PREVIOUSLY TREATED OVARIAN CANCER PATIENTS RECEIVING SINGLE-AGENT PARAPLATIN

Bone Marrow		Percent
Thrombocytopenia,	$<100,000/mm^3$	62
	$<50,000/mm^3$	35
Neutropenia,	$<2,000$ cells/mm^3	67
	$<1,000$ cells/mm^3	21
Leukopenia,	$<4,000$ cells/mm^3	85
	$<2,000$ cells/mm^3	26
Anemia,	<11 g/dL	90
	<8 g/dL	21
Infections		5
Bleeding		5
Transfusions		44
Gastrointestinal		
Nausea and vomiting		92
Vomiting		81
Other GI side effects		21
Neurologic		
Peripheral neuropathies		6
Ototoxicity		1
Other sensory side effects		1
Central neurotoxicity		5
Renal		
Serum creatinine elevations		10
Blood urea elevations		22
Hepatic		
Bilirubin elevations		5
SGOT elevations		19
Alkaline phosphatase elevations		37

Electrolytes Loss	
Sodium	47
Potassium	28
Calcium	31
Magnesium	43
Other Side Effects	
Pain	23
Asthenia	11
Cardiovascular	6
Respiratory	6
Allergic	2
Genitourinary	2
Alopecia	2
Mucositis	1

In the narrative section that follows, the incidences of adverse events are based on data from 1893 patients with various types of tumors who received PARAPLATIN as single-agent therapy.

Hematologic toxicity: Bone marrow suppression is the dose-limiting toxicity of PARAPLATIN. Thrombocytopenia with platelet counts below 50,000/mm^3 occurs in 25% of the patients (35% of pretreated ovarian cancer patients); neutropenia with granulocyte counts below 1,000/mm^3 occurs in 16% of the patients (21% of pretreated ovarian cancer patients); leukopenia with WBC counts below 2,000/mm^3 occurs in 15% of the patients (26% of pretreated ovarian cancer patients). The nadir usually occurs about day 21 in patients receiving single-agent therapy. By day 28, 90% of patients have platelet counts above 100,000/mm^3; 74% have neutrophil counts above 2,000/mm^3; 67% have leukocyte counts above 4,000/mm^3.

Marrow suppression is usually more severe in patients with impaired kidney function. Patients with poor performance status have also experienced a higher incidence of severe leukopenia and thrombocytopenia.

The hematologic effects, although usually reversible, have resulted in infectious or hemorrhagic complications in 5% of the patients treated with PARAPLATIN, with drug-related death occurring in less than 1% of the patients.

Anemia with hemoglobin less than 11 g/dL has been observed in 71% of the patients who started therapy with a baseline above that value. The incidence of anemia increases with increasing exposure to PARAPLATIN. Transfusions have been administered to 26% of the patients treated with PARAPLATIN (44% of previously treated ovarian cancer patients).

Bone marrow depression may be more severe when PARAPLATIN is combined with other bone marrow suppressing drugs or with radiotherapy.

Gastrointestinal toxicity: Vomiting occurs in 65% of the patients (81% of previously treated ovarian cancer patients) and in about one-third of these patients it is severe. Carboplatin, as a single agent or in combination, is significantly less emetogenic than cisplatin; however, patients previously treated with emetogenic agents, especially cisplatin, appear to be more prone to vomiting. Nausea alone occurs in an additional 10% to 15% of patients. Both nausea and vomiting usually cease within 24 hours of treatment and are often responsive to antiemetic measures. Although no conclusive efficacy data exist with the following schedules, prolonged administration of PARAPLATIN, either by continuous 24-hour infusion or by daily pulse doses given for 5 consecutive days, was associated with less severe vomiting than the single dose intermittent schedule. Emesis was increased when PARAPLATIN was used in combination with other emetogenic compounds. Other gastrointestinal effects observed frequently were pain, in 17% of the patients; diarrhea, in 6%; and constipation, also in 6%.

Neurologic toxicity: Peripheral neuropathies have been observed in 4% of the patients receiving PARAPLATIN (6% of pretreated ovarian cancer patients) with mild paresthesias occurring most frequently. Carboplatin therapy produces significantly fewer and less severe neurologic side effects than dose therapy with cisplatin. However, patients older than 65 years and/or previously treated with cisplatin appear to have an increased risk (10%) for peripheral neuropathies. In 70% of the patients with pre-existing cisplatin-induced peripheral neurotoxicity, there was no worsening of symptoms during therapy with PARAPLATIN. Clinical ototoxicity and other sensory abnormalities such as visual disturbances and change in taste have been reported in only 1% of the patients. Central nervous system symptoms have been reported in 5% of the patients and appear to be most often related to the use of antiemetics.

Although the overall incidence of peripheral neurologic side effects induced by PARAPLATIN is low, prolonged treatment, particularly in cisplatin pretreated patients, may result in cumulative neurotoxicity.

Nephrotoxicity: Development of abnormal renal function test results is uncommon, despite the fact that carboplatin, unlike cisplatin, has usually been administered without high-volume fluid hydration and/or forced diuresis. The incidences of abnormal renal function tests reported are 6% for serum creatinine and 14% for blood urea nitrogen (10% and 22%, respectively, in pretreated ovarian cancer pa-

tients). Most of these reported abnormalities have been mild and about one-half of them were reversible.

Creatinine clearance has proven to be the most sensitive measure of kidney function in patients receiving PARAPLATIN, and it appears to be the most useful test for correlating drug clearance and bone marrow suppression. Twenty-seven percent of the patients who had a baseline value of 60 mL/min or more demonstrated a reduction below this value during PARAPLATIN therapy.

Hepatic toxicity: The incidences of abnormal liver function tests in patients with normal baseline values were reported as follows: total bilirubin, 5%; SGOT, 15%; and alkaline phosphatase, 24%; (5%, 19%, and 37%, respectively, in pretreated ovarian cancer patients). These abnormalities have generally been mild and reversible in about one half of the cases, although the role of metastatic tumor in the liver may complicate the assessment in many patients. In a limited series of patients receiving very high dosages of PARAPLATIN and autologous bone marrow transplantation, severe abnormalities of liver function tests were reported.

Electrolyte changes: The incidences of abnormally decreased serum electrolyte values reported were as follows: sodium, 29%; potassium, 20%; calcium, 22%; and magnesium, 29%; (47%, 28%, 31%, and 43%, respectively, in pretreated ovarian cancer patients). Electrolyte supplementation was not routinely administered concomitantly with PARAPLATIN, and these electrolyte abnormalities were rarely associated with symptoms.

Allergic reactions: Hypersensitivity to PARAPLATIN has been reported in 2% of the patients. These allergic reactions have been similar in nature and severity to those reported with other platinum-containing compounds, ie, rash, urticaria, erythema, pruritus, and rarely bronchospasm and hypotension. These reactions have been successfully managed with standard epinephrine, corticosteroid, and antihistamine therapy.

Other events: Pain and asthenia were the most frequently reported miscellaneous adverse effects; their relationship to the tumor and to anemia was likely. Alopecia was reported (3%). Cardiovascular, respiratory, genitourinary, and mucosal side effects have occurred in 6% or less of the patients. Cardiovascular events (cardiac failure, embolism, cerebrovascular accidents) were fatal in less than 1% of the patients and did not appear to be related to chemotherapy.

OVERDOSAGE

There is no known antidote for PARAPLATIN overdosage. The anticipated complications of overdosage would be secondary to bone marrow suppression and/or hepatic toxicity.

DOSAGE AND ADMINISTRATION

NOTE: Aluminum reacts with carboplatin causing precipitate formation and loss of potency, therefore, needles or intravenous sets containing aluminum parts that may come in contact with the drug must not be used for the preparation or administration of PARAPLATIN.

PARAPLATIN, as a single agent, has been shown to be effective in patients with recurrent ovarian carcinoma at a dosage of 360 mg/m^2 I.V. on day 1 every 4 weeks. In general, however, single intermittent courses of PARAPLATIN should not be repeated until the neutrophil count is at least 2000 and the platelet count is at least 100,000.

The dose adjustments shown in the table below are modified from a controlled trial in previously treated patients with ovarian carcinoma. Blood counts were done weekly, and the recommendations are based on the lowest posttreatment platelet or neutrophil value.

Platelets	Neutrophils	Adjusted Dose (From Prior Course)
$>100,000$	$>2,000$	125%
50–100,000	500–2,000	No Adjustment
$<50,000$	<500	75%

Only one escalation should be made. Doses greater than 125% of the starting dose are not recommended.

PARAPLATIN is usually administered by an infusion lasting 15 minutes or longer. No pretreatment or posttreatment hydration or forced diuresis is required.

Patients with impaired kidney function: Patients with creatinine clearance values below 60 mL/min are at increased risk of severe bone marrow suppression. In renally-impaired patients who received single agent PARAPLATIN therapy, the incidence of severe leukopenia, neutropenia, or thrombocytopenia has been about 25% when the dosage modifications in the table below have been used.

Baseline Creatinine Clearance	Recommended Dose on Day 1
41–59 mL/min	250 mg/m^2
16–40 mL/min	200 mg/m^2

The data available for patients with severely impaired kidney function (creatinine clearance below 15 mL/min) are too limited to permit a recommendation for treatment.[1,2] These dosing recommendations apply to the initial course of treatment. Subsequent dosages should be adjusted according to the patient's tolerance based on the degree of bone marrow suppression.

PREPARATION OF INTRAVENOUS SOLUTIONS

Immediately before use, the content of each vial must be reconstituted with either Sterile Water for Injection, USP, 5% Dextrose in Water, or 0.9% Sodium Chloride Injection, USP, according to the following schedule:

Vial Strength	Diluent Volume
50 mg	5 mL
150 mg	15 mL
450 mg	45 mL

These dilutions all produce a carboplatin concentration of 10 mg/mL.

PARAPLATIN can be further diluted to concentrations as low as 0.5 mg/mL with 5% Dextrose in Water (D₅W) or 0.9% Sodium Chloride Injection, USP (NS).

STABILITY

Unopened vials of PARAPLATIN for Injection are stable for the life indicated on the package when stored at controlled room temperature 15°–30°C (59°–86°F), and protected from light.

When prepared as directed, PARAPLATIN solutions are stable for 8 hours at room temperature (25°C). Since no antibacterial preservative is contained in the formulation, it is recommended that PARAPLATIN solutions be discarded 8 hours after dilution.

Parenteral drug products should be inspected visually for particulate matter and discoloration prior to administration.

HOW SUPPLIED

NDC 0015-3213-30   50 mg vials, individually cartoned, shelf packs of 10 cartons, 10 shelf packs per case. (Yellow flip-off seals)

NDC 0015-3214-30   150 mg vials, individually cartoned, shelf packs of 10 cartons, 10 shelf packs per case. (Violet flip-off seals)

NDC 0015-3215-30   450 mg vials, individually cartoned, shelf packs of 6 cartons, 10 shelf packs per case. (Blue flip-off seals)

STORAGE

Store the unopened vials at controlled room temperature 15°–30°C (59°–86°F). Protect from light. Solutions for infusion should be discarded 8 hours after preparation.

HANDLING AND DISPOSAL

Procedures for proper handling and disposal of anticancer drugs should be considered. Several guidelines on this subject have been published.[3–9] There is no general agreement that all of the procedures recommended in the guidelines are necessary or appropriate.

REFERENCES

1. Egorin, MJ, et al: Pharmacokinetics and dosage reduction of cis-diammine (1,1-cyclobutanedicarboxylato) platinum in patients with impaired renal function. Cancer Res 1984;44:5432–5438.
2. Carboplatin, Etoposide, and Bleomycin for Treatment of Stage IIC Seminoma Complicated by Acute Renal Failure. Cancer Treatment Reports, Vol. 71, No. 11, pp 1123–1124, November 1987.
3. Recommendations for the Safe Handling of Parenteral Antineoplastic Drugs. NIH Publication No. 83–2621. For sale by the Superintendent of Documents, US Government Printing Office, Washington, DC 20402.
4. AMA Council Report. Guidelines for Handling Parenteral Antineoplastics. JAMA 1985 March 15.
5. National Study Commission Cytotoxic Exposure—Recommendations for Handling Cytotoxic Agents. Available from Louis P. Jeffrey, Chairman, National Study Commission on Cytotoxic Exposure, Massachusetts College of Pharmacy and Allied Health Sciences, 179 Longwood Avenue, Boston, Massachusetts, 02115.
6. Clinical Oncological Society of Australia. Guidelines and Recommendations for Safe Handling of Antineoplastic Agents. Med J Australia 1983; 1:426–428.
7. Jones RB, et al: Safe handling of chemotherapeutic agents: A report from the Mount Sinai Medical Center. CA—A Cancer Journal for Clinicians 1983; (Sept/Oct) 258–263.
8. American Society of Hospital Pharmacists Technical Assistance Bulletin on Handling Cytotoxic Drugs in Hospitals. Am J Hosp Pharm 1985; 42:131–137.
9. OSHA Work-Practice Guidelines for Personnel Dealing with Cytotoxic (Antineoplastic) Drugs. Am J Hosp Pharm 1986; 43:1193–1204.

U.S. Patent Nos. 4,140,707
4,657,927

PLATINOL®   ℞

[plă′tĭ-nŏl″]
(cisplatin for injection, USP)

Injectable, 10 mg vial

       NSN 6505-01-074-7590 (M&VA)

Injectable, 50 mg vial

       NSN 6505-01-097-2935 (M&VA)

WARNING

Platinol (cisplatin) should be administered under the supervision of a qualified physician experienced in the use of cancer chemotherapeutic agents. Appropriate management of therapy and complications is possible only when adequate diagnostic and treatment facilities are readily available.

Cumulative renal toxicity associated with Platinol is severe. Other major dose-related toxicities are myelosuppression, nausea and vomiting.

Ototoxicity, which may be more pronounced in children, and is manifested by tinnitus, and/or loss of high frequency hearing and occasionally deafness, is significant.

Anaphylactic-like reactions to Platinol have been reported. Facial edema, bronchoconstriction, tachycardia, and hypotension may occur within minutes of Platinol administration. Epinephrine, corticosteroids, and antihistamines have been effectively employed to alleviate symptoms (see "Warnings" and "Adverse Reactions" sections).

DESCRIPTION

Platinol (cisplatin) (cis-diamminedichloroplatinum) is a heavy metal complex containing a central atom of platinum surrounded by two chloride atoms and two ammonia molecules in the cis position. It is a white lyophilized powder with the molecular formula Pt $Cl_2H_6N_2$, and a molecular weight of 300.1. It is soluble in water or saline at 1 mg/mL and in dimethylformamide at 24 mg/mL. It has a melting point of 207°C.

ACTION

Platinol has biochemical properties similar to that of bifunctional alkylating agents, producing interstrand and intrastrand cross-links in DNA. It is apparently cell-cycle nonspecific. Following a single I.V. dose, Platinol concentrates in liver, kidneys and large and small intestines in animals and humans. Platinol apparently has poor penetration into the CNS.

Plasma levels of radioactivity decay in a biphasic manner after an I.V. bolus dose of radioactive Platinol to patients. The initial plasma half-life is 25 to 49 minutes, and the postdistribution plasma half-life is 58 to 73 hours. During the postdistribution phase, greater than 90% of the radioactivity in the blood is protein bound. Platinol is excreted primarily in the urine. However, urinary excretion is incomplete with only 27% to 43% of the radioactivity being excreted within the first 5 days post-dose in human beings. There are insufficient data to determine whether biliary or intestinal excretion occurs.

INDICATIONS

Platinol is indicated as palliative therapy to be employed as follows:

Metastatic Testicular Tumors—in established combination therapy with other approved chemotherapeutic agents in patients with metastatic testicular tumors who have already received appropriate surgical and/or radiotherapeutic procedures. An established combination therapy consists of Platinol, Blenoxane (bleomycin sulfate) and Velban (vinblastine sulfate).

Metastatic Ovarian Tumors—in established combination therapy with other approved chemotherapeutic agents in patients with metastatic ovarian tumors who have already received appropriate surgical and/or radiotherapeutic procedures. An established combination consists of Platinol and Adriamycin (doxorubicin hydrochloride). Platinol, as a single agent, is indicated as secondary therapy in patients with metastatic ovarian tumors refractory to standard chemotherapy who have not previously received Platinol therapy.

Advanced Bladder Cancer—Platinol is indicated as a single agent for patients with transitional cell bladder cancer which is no longer amenable to local treatments such as surgery and/or radiotherapy.

CONTRAINDICATIONS

Platinol is contraindicated in patients with preexisting renal impairment. Platinol should not be employed in myelosuppressed patients, or patients with hearing impairment.

Platinol is contraindicated in patients with a history of allergic reactions to Platinol or other platinum-containing compounds.

WARNINGS

Platinol produces cumulative nephrotoxicity which is potentiated by aminoglycoside antibiotics. The serum creatinine, BUN, creatinine clearance and magnesium, potassium and calcium levels should be measured prior to initiating therapy, and prior to each subsequent course. At the recommended dosage, Platinol should not be given more frequently than once every 3 to 4 weeks (see "Adverse Reactions").

There are reports of severe neuropathies in patients in whom regimens are employed using higher doses of Platinol or greater dose frequencies than those recommended. These neuropathies may be irreversible and are seen as paresthesias in a stocking-glove distribution, areflexia, and loss of proprioception and vibratory sensation. Loss of motor function has also been reported.

Anaphylactic-like reactions to Platinol have been reported. These reactions have occurred within minutes of administration to patients with prior exposure to Platinol, and have been alleviated by administration of epinephrine, corticosteroids and antihistamines.

Since ototoxicity of Platinol is cumulative, audiometric testing should be performed prior to initiating therapy and prior to each subsequent dose of drug (see "Adverse Reactions").

Safe use in human pregnancy has not been established. Platinol is mutagenic in bacteria and produces chromosome aberrations in animal cells in tissue culture. In mice Platinol is teratogenic and embryotoxic.

Platinol has not been studied for its carcinogenic potential but compounds with similar mechanisms of action and mutagenicity have been reported to be carcinogenic.

PRECAUTIONS

Peripheral blood counts should be monitored weekly. Liver function should be monitored periodically. Neurologic examination should also be performed regularly (see "Adverse Reactions").

ADVERSE REACTIONS

Nephrotoxicity—Dose-related and cumulative renal insufficiency is the major dose-limiting toxicity. Renal toxicity has been noted in 28% to 36% of patients treated with a single dose of 50 mg/m². It is first noted during the second week after a dose and is manifested by elevations in BUN and creatinine, serum uric acid and/or a decrease in creatinine clearance. **Renal toxicity becomes more prolonged and severe with repeated courses of the drug. Renal function must return to normal before another dose of Platinol can be given.**

Impairment of renal function has been associated with renal tubular damage. The administration of Platinol using a 6- to 8-hour infusion with intravenous hydration, and mannitol has been used to reduce nephrotoxicity. However, renal toxicity still can occur after utilization of these procedures.

Ototoxicity—Ototoxicity has been observed in up to 31% of patients treated with a single dose of Platinol 50 mg/m², and is manifested by tinnitus and/or hearing loss in the high frequency range (4,000 to 8,000 Hz). Decreased ability to hear normal conversational tones may occur occasionally. Ototoxic effects may be more severe in children receiving Platinol. Hearing loss can be unilateral or bilateral and tends to become more frequent and severe with repeated doses. It is unclear whether Platinol-induced ototoxicity is reversible. Careful monitoring of audiometry should be performed prior to initiation of therapy and prior to subsequent doses of Platinol.

Vestibular toxicity has also been reported.

Hematologic—Myelosuppression occurs in 25% to 30% of patients treated with Platinol. The nadirs in circulating platelets and leukocytes occur between days 18 to 23 (range 7.5 to 45) with most patients recovering by day 39 (range 13 to 62). Leukopenia and thrombocytopenia are more pronounced at higher doses (> 50 mg/m²). Anemia (decrease of 2 g hemoglobin/100 mL) occurs at approximately the same frequency and with the same timing as leukopenia and thrombocytopenia.

In addition to anemia secondary to myelosuppression, a Coombs' positive hemolytic anemia has been reported. In the presence of cisplatin hemolytic anemia, a further course of treatment may be accompanied by increased hemolysis and this risk should be weighed by the treating physician.

Gastrointestinal—Marked nausea and vomiting occur in almost all patients treated with Platinol, and are occasionally so severe that the drug must be discontinued. Nausea and vomiting usually begin within one to four hours after treatment and last up to 24 hours. Various degrees of nausea and anorexia may persist for up to one week after treatment.

OTHER TOXICITIES

Vascular toxicities coincident with the use of Platinol in combination with other antineoplastic agents have been reported rarely. The events are clinically heterogeneous and

Continued on next page

Bristol-Myers Oncology—Cont.

may include myocardial infarction, cerebrovascular accident, thrombotic microangiopathy (HUS) or cerebral arteritis. Various mechanisms have been proposed for these vascular complications. There are also reports of Raynaud's phenomenon occurring in patients treated with the combination of bleomycin, vinblastine with or without Platinol. It has been suggested that hypomagnesemia developing coincident with the use of Platinol may be an added, although not essential, factor associated with this event. However, it is currently unknown if the cause of Raynaud's phenomenon in these cases is the disease, underlying vascular compromise, bleomycin, vinblastine, hypomagnesemia, or a combination of any of these factors.

Serum Electrolyte Disturbances—Hypomagnesemia, hypocalcemia, hyponatremia, hypokalemia and hypophosphatemia have been reported to occur in patients treated with Platinol and are probably related to renal tubular damage. Tetany has occasionally been reported in those patients with hypocalcemia and hypomagnesemia. Generally, normal serum electrolyte levels are restored by administering supplemental electrolytes and discontinuing Platinol. Inappropriate antidiuretic hormone syndrome has also been reported.

Hyperuricemia—Hyperuricemia has been reported to occur at approximately the same frequency as the increases in BUN and serum creatinine.
It is more pronounced after doses greater than 50 mg/m², and peak levels of uric acid generally occur between 3 to 5 days after the dose. Allopurinol therapy for hyperuricemia effectively reduces uric acid levels.

Neurotoxicity (see "Warnings" section)—Neurotoxicity, usually characterized by peripheral neuropathies, has been reported. The neuropathies usually occur after prolonged therapy (4 to 7 months): however, neurologic symptoms have been reported to occur after a single dose. Platinol therapy should be discontinued when the symptoms are first observed. Preliminary evidence suggests peripheral neuropathy may be irreversible in some patients.
Lhermitte's sign and autonomic neuropathy have also been reported.
Loss of taste and seizures have also been reported.

Ocular Toxicity—Optic neuritis, papilledema and cerebral blindness have been reported infrequently in patients receiving standard recommended doses of Platinol. Improvement and/or total recovery usually occurs after discontinuing Platinol. Steroids with or without mannitol have been used, however, efficacy has not been established.
Blurred vision and altered color perception have been reported after the use of regimens with higher doses of Platinol or greater dose frequencies than those recommended in the package insert. The altered color perception manifests as a loss of color discrimination, particularly in the blue-yellow axis. The only finding on fundoscopic exam is irregular retinal pigmentation of the macular area.

Anaphylactic-like Reactions—Anaphylactic-like reactions have been occasionally reported in patients previously exposed to Platinol. The reactions consist of facial edema, wheezing, tachycardia and hypotension within a few minutes of drug administration. Reactions may be controlled by intravenous epinephrine, corticosteroids or antihistamines. Patients receiving Platinol should be observed carefully for possible anaphylactic-like reactions and supportive equipment and medication should be available to treat such a complication.
Other toxicities reported to occur infrequently are cardiac abnormalities, anorexia elevated SGOT and rash.

DOSAGE AND ADMINISTRATION

Note: Needles or intravenous sets containing aluminum parts that may come in contact with Platinol should not be used for preparation or administration. Aluminum reacts with Platinol, causing precipitate formation and a loss of potency.

Metastatic Testicular Tumors—An effective combination for the treatment of patients with metastatic testicular carcinomas includes Platinol, Blenoxane (bleomycin sulfate) and Velban (vinblastine sulfate). Remission induction therapy consists of Platinol, Blenoxane (bleomycin sulfate) and Velban (vinblastine sulfate) in the following doses:
     PLATINOL—20 mg/m² I.V. daily for 5 days (days 1 to 5) every 3 weeks for three courses.
     BLENOXANE®—(bleomycin sulfate)—30 units I.V. weekly (day 2 of each week) for 12 consecutive doses.
     VELBAN®—(vinblastine sulfate)—0.15 to 0.2 mg/kg I.V. twice weekly (days 1 and 2) every 3 weeks for four courses (a total of eight doses).
Maintenance therapy for patients who respond to the above regimen consists of Velban (vinblastine sulfate) 0.3 mg/kg I.V. every 4 weeks for a total of 2 years.
For directions for the administration of Blenoxane (bleomycin sulfate) and Velban (vinblastine sulfate), refer to their respective package insert.

Metastatic Ovarian Tumors—An effective combination for the treatment of patients with metastatic ovarian tumors includes Platinol and Adriamycin (doxorubicin hydrochloride) in the following doses:
     PLATINOL—50 mg/m² I.V. once every 3 weeks (day 1).
     ADRIAMYCIN™ (doxorubicin hydrochloride)—50 mg/m² I.V. once every 3 weeks (day 1).
For directions for the administration of Adriamycin (doxorubicin hydrochloride), refer to the Adriamycin (doxorubicin hydrochloride) package insert.
In combination therapy, Platinol and Adriamycin (doxorubicin hydrochloride) are administered sequentially.
As a single agent, Platinol should be administered at a dose of 100 mg/m² I.V. once every 4 weeks.

Advanced Bladder Cancer—Platinol should be administered as a single agent at a dose of 50–70 mg/m² I.V. once every 3 to 4 weeks depending on the extent of prior exposure to radiation therapy and/or prior chemotherapy. For heavily pretreated patients an initial dose of 50 mg/m² repeated every 4 weeks is recommended.
Pretreatment hydration with 1 to 2 liters of fluid infused for 8 to 12 hours prior to a Platinol dose is recommended. The drug is then diluted in 2 liters of 5% Dextrose in ½ or ⅓N Saline containing 37.5 g of mannitol, and infused over a 6- to 8-hour period. Adequate hydration and urinary output must be maintained during the following 24 hours.
A repeat course of Platinol should not be given until the serum creatinine is below 1.5 mg/100 mL, and/or the BUN is below 25 mg/100 mL. A repeat course should not be given until circulating blood elements are at an acceptable level (platelets $\geq$ 100,000/mm³, WBC $\geq$ 4,000/mm³). Subsequent doses of Platinol should not be given until an audiometric analysis indicates that auditory acuity is within normal limits.
As with other potentially toxic compounds, caution should be exercised in handling the powder and preparing the solution of cisplatin. Skin reactions associated with accidental exposure to cisplatin may occur. The use of gloves is recommended. If cisplatin powder or solution contacts the skin or mucosae, immediately wash the skin or mucosae thoroughly with soap and water.

PREPARATION OF INTRAVENOUS SOLUTIONS

The 10 mg and 50 mg vials should be reconstituted with 10 mL or 50 mL of Sterile Water for Injection, USP, respectively. Each mL of the resulting solution will contain 1 mg of Platinol.
Reconstitution as recommended results in a clear, colorless solution.
The reconstituted solution should be used intravenously only and should be administered by I.V. infusion over a 6- to 8-hour period. (See "Dosage and Administration".)

STABILITY

Unopened vials of dry powder are stable for the lot life indicated on the package when stored at room temperature (27℃).
The reconstituted solution is stable for 20 hours at room temperature (27℃).
Important Note: Once reconstituted, the solution should be kept at room temperature (27℃). If the reconstituted solution is refrigerated a precipitate will form.
Procedures for proper handling and disposal of anticancer drugs should be considered. Several guidelines on this subject have been published.[1–7] There is no general agreement that all of the procedures recommended in the guidelines are necessary or appropriate.

References:

1. Recommendations for the Safe Handling of Parenteral Antineoplastic Drugs. NIH Publication No. 83-2621. For sale by the Superintendent of Documents, U.S. Government Printing Office, Washington, D.C. 20402.
2. AMA Council Report. Guidelines for Handling Parenteral Antineoplastics. JAMA, 1985; March 15.
3. National Study Commission on Cytotoxic Exposure—Recommendations for Handling Cytotoxic Agents. Available from Louis P. Jeffrey, Sc.D., Chairman, National Study Commission on Cytotoxic Exposure, Massachusetts College of Pharmacy and Allied Health Sciences, 179 Longwood Avenue, Boston, Massachusetts 02115.
4. Clinical Oncological Society of Australia: Guidelines and Recommendations for Safe Handling of Antineoplastic Agents. Med. J. Australia 1983; 1:426–428.
5. Jones, R. B., et. al. Safe Handling of Chemotherapeutic Agents: A Report from the Mount Sinai Medical Center. Ca—A Cancer Journal for Clinicians 1983; Sept./Oct., 258–263.
6. American Society of Hospital Pharmacists Technical Assistance Bulletin on Handling Cytotoxic Drugs in Hospitals. Am. J. Hosp. Pharm. 1985; 42:131–137.
7. OSHA Work-Practice Guidelines for Personnel Dealing with Cytotoxic (Antineoplastic) Drugs. Am. J. Hosp. Pharm. 1986; 43:1193–1204.

HOW SUPPLIED

Platinol (cisplatin for Injection)
     NDC 0015-3070-20—Each amber vial contains 10 mg of cisplatin.
     NDC 0015-3072-20—Each amber vial contains 50 mg of cisplatin.
U.S. Patent No. 4,177,263
     Shown in Product Identification Section, page 407

PLATINOL®-AQ   ℞
[pla-ti-nol -AQ]
cisplatin injection

WARNING

Platinol (cisplatin) should be administered under the supervision of a qualified physician experienced in the use of cancer chemotherapeutic agents. Appropriate management of therapy and complications is possible only when adequate diagnostic and treatment facilities are readily available.
Cumulative renal toxicity associated with Platinol is severe. Other major dose-related toxicities are myelosuppression, nausea and vomiting.
Ototoxicity, which may be more pronounced in children, and is manifested by tinnitus, and/or loss of high frequency hearing and occasionally deafness, is significant.
Anaphylactic-like reactions to Platinol have been reported. Facial edema, bronchoconstriction, tachycardia, and hypotension may occur within minutes of Platinol administration. Epinephrine, corticosteroids, and antihistamines have been effectively employed to alleviate symptoms (see "Warnings" and "Adverse Reactions" sections).

DESCRIPTION

Cisplatin (cis-diamminedichloroplatinum) is a heavy metal complex containing a central atom of platinum surrounded by two chloride atoms and two ammonia molecules in the cis position. It is a white powder with the molecular formula Pt $Cl_2H_6N_2$, and a molecular weight of 300.1. It is soluble in water or saline at 1 mg/mL and in dimethylformamide at 24 mg/mL. It has a melting point of 207℃. Platinol-AQ is a sterile aqueous solution, each mL containing 1.0 mg cisplatin and 9 mg sodium chloride. HCl and/or sodium hydroxide added to adjust pH.

ACTION

Platinol has biochemical properties similar to that of bifunctional alkylating agents, producing interstrand and intrastrand cross-links in DNA. It is apparently cell-cycle nonspecific. Following a single I.V. dose, Platinol concentrates in liver, kidneys and large and small intestines in animals and humans. Platinol apparently has poor penetration into the CNS.
Plasma levels of radioactivity decay in a biphasic manner after an I.V. bolus dose of radioactive Platinol to patients. The initial plasma half-life is 25 to 49 minutes, and the postdistribution plasma half-life is 58 to 73 hours. During the postdistribution phase, greater than 90% of the radioactivity in the blood is protein bound. Platinol is excreted primarily in the urine. However, urinary excretion is incomplete with only 27% to 43% of the radioactivity being excreted within the first 5 days post-dose in human beings. There are insufficient data to determine whether biliary or intestinal excretion occurs.

INDICATIONS

Platinol is indicated as palliative therapy to be employed as follows:
Metastatic Testicular Tumors—In established combination therapy with other approved chemotherapeutic agents in patients with metastatic testicular tumors who have already received appropriate surgical and/or radiotherapeutic procedures. An established combination therapy consists of Platinol, Blenoxane (bleomycin sulfate) and Velban (vinblastine sulfate).
Metastatic Ovarian Tumors—In established combination therapy with other approved chemotherapeutic agents in patients with metastatic ovarian tumors who have already received appropriate surgical and/or radiotherapeutic procedures. An established combination consists of Platinol and Adriamycin™ (doxorubicin hydrochloride). Platinol, as a single agent, is indicated as secondary therapy in patients with metastatic ovarian tumors refractory to standard chemotherapy who have not previously received Platinol therapy.

Advanced Bladder Cancer—Platinol is indicated as a single agent for patients with transitional cell bladder cancer which is no longer amenable to local treatments such as surgery and/or radiotherapy.

CONTRAINDICATIONS

Platinol is contraindicated in patients with preexisting renal impairment. Platinol should not be employed in myelosuppressed patients, or patients with hearing impairment. Platinol is contraindicated in patients with a history of allergic reactions to Platinol or other platinum-containing compounds.

WARNINGS

Platinol produces cumulative nephrotoxicity which is potentiated by aminoglycoside antibiotics. The serum creatinine, BUN, creatinine clearance and magnesium, potassium and calcium levels should be measured prior to initiating therapy, and prior to each subsequent course. At the recommended dosage, Platinol should not be given more frequently than once every 3 to 4 weeks (see "Adverse Reactions"). There are reports of severe neuropathies in patients in whom regimens are employed using higher doses of Platinol or greater dose frequencies than those recommended. These neuropathies may be irreversible and are seen as paresthesias in a stocking-glove distribution, areflexia, and loss of proprioception and vibratory sensation.
Loss of motor function has also been reported.
Anaphylactic-like reactions to Platinol have been reported. These reactions have occurred within minutes of administration to patients with prior exposure to Platinol, and have been alleviated by administration of epinephrine, corticosteroids and antihistamines.
Since ototoxicity of Platinol is cumulative, audiometric testing should be performed prior to initiating therapy and prior to each subsequent dose of drug (see "Adverse Reactions").
Safe use in human pregnancy has not been established. Platinol is mutagenic in bacteria and produces chromosome aberrations in animal cells in tissue culture. In mice Platinol is teratogenic and embryotoxic.
Platinol has not been studied for its carcinogenic potential but compounds with similar mechanisms of action and mutagenicity have been reported to be carcinogenic.

PRECAUTIONS

Peripheral blood counts should be monitored weekly. Liver function should be monitored periodically. Neurologic examination should also be performed regularly (see "Adverse Reactions").
Drug Interactions—Plasma levels of anticonvulsant agents may become subtherapeutic during cisplatin therapy.

ADVERSE REACTIONS

Nephrotoxicity—Dose-related and cumulative renal insufficiency is the major dose-limiting toxicity of Platinol. Renal toxicity has been noted in 28% to 36% of patients treated with a single dose of 50 mg/m². It is first noted during the second week after a dose and is manifested by elevations in BUN and creatinine, serum uric acid and/or a decrease in creatinine clearance. **Renal toxicity becomes more prolonged and severe with repeated courses of the drug. Renal function must return to normal before another dose of Platinol can be given.**
Impairment of renal function has been associated with renal tubular damage. The administration of Platinol using a 6- to 8-hour infusion with intravenous hydration, and mannitol has been used to reduce nephrotoxicity. However, renal toxicity still can occur after utilization of these procedures.
Ototoxicity—Ototoxicity has been observed in up to 31% of patients treated with a single dose of Platinol 50 mg/m², and is manifested by tinnitus and/or hearing loss in the high frequency range (4,000 to 8,000 Hz). Decreased ability to hear normal conversational tones may occur occasionally. Ototoxic effects may be more severe in children receiving Platinol. Hearing loss can be unilateral or bilateral and tends to become more frequent and severe with repeated doses. Ototoxicity may be enhanced with prior or simultaneous cranial irradiation. It is unclear whether Platinol-induced ototoxicity is reversible. Careful monitoring of audiometry should be performed prior to initiation of therapy and prior to subsequent doses of Platinol.
Vestibular toxicity has also been reported.
Hematologic—Myelosuppression occurs in 25% to 30% of patients treated with Platinol. The nadirs in circulating platelets and leukocytes occur between days 18 to 23 (range 7.5 to 45) with most patients recovering by day 39 (range 13 to 62). Leukopenia and thrombocytopenia are more pronounced at higher doses (> 50 mg/m²). Anemia (decrease of 2 g hemoglobin/100 mL) occurs at approximately the same frequency and with the same timing as leukopenia and thrombocytopenia.
In addition to anemia secondary to myelosuppression, a Coombs' positive hemolytic anemia has been reported. In the presence of cisplatin hemolytic anemia, a further course of treatment may be accompanied by increased hemolysis and this risk should be weighed by the treating physician.

Gastrointestinal—Marked nausea and vomiting occur in almost all patients treated with Platinol, and are occasionally so severe that the drug must be discontinued. Nausea and vomiting usually begin within 1 to 4 hours after treatment and last up to 24 hours. Various degrees of nausea and anorexia may persist for up to 1 week after treatment.

OTHER TOXICITIES

Vascular toxicities coincident with the use of Platinol in combination with other antineoplastic agents have been reported rarely. The events are clinically heterogeneous and may include myocardial infarction, cerebrovascular accident, thrombotic microangiopathy (HUS) or cerebral arteritis. Various mechanisms have been proposed for these vascular complications. There are also reports of Raynaud's phenomenon occurring in patients treated with the combination of bleomycin, vinblastine with or without Platinol. It has been suggested that hypomagnesemia developing coincident with the use of Platinol may be an added, although not essential, factor associated with this event. However, it is currently unknown if the cause of Raynaud's phenomenon in these cases is the disease, underlying vascular compromise, bleomycin, vinblastine, hypomagnesemia, or a combination of any of these factors.
Serum Electrolyte Disturbances—Hypomagnesemia, hypocalcemia, hyponatremia, hypokalemia and hypophosphatemia have been reported to occur in patients treated with Platinol and are probably related to renal tubular damage. Tetany has occasionally been reported in those patients with hypocalcemia and hypomagnesemia. Generally, normal serum electrolyte levels are restored by administering supplemental electrolytes and discontinuing Platinol.
Inappropriate antidiuretic hormone syndrome has also been reported.
Hyperuricemia—Hyperuricemia has been reported to occur at approximately the same frequency as the increases in BUN and serum creatinine.
It is more pronounced after doses greater than 50 mg/m², and peak levels of uric acid generally occur between 3 to 5 days after the dose. Allopurinol therapy for hyperuricemia effectively reduces uric acid levels.
Neurotoxicity (see "Warnings" section)—Neurotoxicity, usually characterized by peripheral neuropathies, has been reported. The neuropathies usually occur after prolonged therapy (4 to 7 months): however, neurologic symptoms have been reported to occur after a single dose. Platinol therapy should be discontinued when the symptoms are first observed. Preliminary evidence suggests peripheral neuropathy may be irreversible in some patients.
Lhermitte's sign and autonomic neuropathy have also been reported.
Loss of taste and seizures have also been reported.
Ocular Toxicity—Optic neuritis, papilledema and cerebral blindness have been reported infrequently in patients receiving standard recommended doses of Platinol. Improvement and/or total recovery usually occurs after discontinuing Platinol. Steroids with or without mannitol have been used, however, efficacy has not been established.
Blurred vision and altered color perception have been reported after the use of regimens with higher doses of Platinol or greater dose frequencies than those recommended in the package insert. The altered color perception manifests as a loss of color discrimination, particularly in the blue-yellow axis. The only finding on funduscopic exam is irregular retinal pigmentation of the macular area.
Anaphylactic-like Reactions—Anaphylactic-like reactions have been occasionally reported in patients previously exposed to Platinol. The reactions consist of facial edema, wheezing, tachycardia and hypotension within a few minutes of drug administration. Reactions may be controlled by intravenous epinephrine, corticosteroids or antihistamines. Patients receiving Platinol should be observed carefully for possible anaphylactic-like reactions and supportive equipment and medication should be available to treat such a complication.
Other toxicities reported to occur infrequently are cardiac abnormalities, anorexia, elevated SGOT and rash. Alopecia has also been reported.

DOSAGE AND ADMINISTRATION

Note: Needles or intravenous sets containing aluminum parts that may come in contact with Platinol should not be used for preparation or administration. Aluminum reacts with Platinol, causing precipitate formation and a loss of potency.
Metastatic Testicular Tumors—An effective combination for the treatment of patients with metastatic testicular carcinomas includes Platinol, Blenoxane (bleomycin sulfate) and Velban (vinblastine sulfate). Remission induction therapy consists of Platinol, Blenoxane (bleomycin sulfate) and Velban (vinblastine sulfate) in the following doses:
PLATINOL—20 mg/m² I.V. daily for 5 days (days 1 to 5) every 3 weeks for three courses.
BLENOXANE®—(bleomycin sulfate)—30 units I.V. weekly (day 2 of each week) for 12 consecutive doses.

VELBAN®—(vinblastine sulfate)—0.15 to 0.2 mg/kg I.V. twice weekly (days 1 and 2) every 3 weeks for four courses (a total of eight doses).
Maintenance therapy for patients who respond to the above regimen consists of Velban (vinblastine sulfate) 0.3 mg/kg I.V. every 4 weeks for a total of 2 years.
For directions for the administration of Blenoxane (bleomycin sulfate) and Velban (vinblastine sulfate), refer to their respective package insert.
Metastatic Ovarian Tumors—An effective combination for the treatment of patients with metastatic ovarian tumors includes Platinol and Adriamycin (doxorubicin hydrochloride) in the following doses:
PLATINOL—50 mg/m² I.V. once every 3 weeks (day 1).
ADRIAMYCIN™ (doxorubicin hydrochloride)—50 mg/m² I.V. once every 3 weeks (day 1).
For directions for the administration of Adriamycin (doxorubicin hydrochloride), refer to the Adriamycin (doxorubicin hydrochloride) package insert.
In combination therapy, Platinol and Adriamycin (doxorubicin hydrochloride) are administered sequentially.
As a single agent, Platinol should be administered at a dose of 100 mg/m² I.V. once every 4 weeks.
Advanced Bladder Cancer—Platinol should be administered as a single agent at a dose of 50–70 mg/m² I.V. once every 3 to 4 weeks depending on the extent of prior exposure to radiation therapy and/or prior chemotherapy. For heavily pretreated patients an initial dose of 50 mg/m² repeated every 4 weeks is recommended.
Pretreatment hydration with 1 to 2 liters of fluid infused for 8 to 12 hours prior to a Platinol dose is recommended. The drug is then diluted in 2 liters of 5% Dextrose in ½ or ⅓N Saline containing 37.5 g of mannitol, and infused over a 6- to 8-hour period. Do not dilute Platinol-AQ in just 5% Dextrose Injection. Adequate hydration and urinary output must be maintained during the following 24 hours.
A repeat course of Platinol should not be given until the serum creatinine is below 1.5 mg/100 mL, and/or the BUN is below 25 mg/100 mL. A repeat course should not be given until circulating blood elements are at an acceptable level (platelets ≥ 100,000/mm³, WBC ≥ 4,000/mm³). Subsequent doses of Platinol should not be given until an audiometric analysis indicates that auditory acuity is within normal limits.
As with other potentially toxic compounds, caution should be exercised in handling aqueous solution. Skin reactions associated with accidental exposure to cisplatin may occur. The use of gloves is recommended. If cisplatin solution contacts the skin or mucosae, immediately wash the skin or mucosae thoroughly with soap and water.
The aqueous solution should be used intravenously only and should be administered by I.V. infusion over a 6- to 8-hour period.

STABILITY

Store at 15°C–25°C. Do not refrigerate. Protect from light.
Procedures for proper handling and disposal of anticancer drugs should be considered. Several guidelines on this subject have been published.[1-7] There is no general agreement that all of the procedures recommended in the guidelines are necessary or appropriate.

REFERENCES

1. Recommendations for the Safe Handling of Parenteral Antineoplastic Drugs. NIH Publication No. 83-2621. For sale by the Superintendent of Documents, US Government Printing Office, Washington, D.C. 20402.
2. AMA Council Report. Guidelines for Handling Parenteral Antineoplastics. JAMA 1985 March 15.
3. National Study Commission on Cytotoxic Exposure—Recommendations for Handling Cytotoxic Agents. Available from Louis P. Jeffrey, Sc.D., Chairman, National Study Commission on Cytotoxic Exposure, Massachusetts College of Pharmacy and Allied Health Sciences, 179 Longwood Avenue, Boston, Massachusetts 02115.
4. Clinical Oncological Society of Australia: Guidelines and Recommendations for Safe Handling of Antineoplastic Agents. Med J Australia 1983; 1:426–428.
5. Jones, RB, et. al. Safe Handling of Chemotherapeutic Agents: A Report from the Mount Sinai Medical Center. Ca—A Cancer Journal for Clinicians 1983; (Sept/Oct) 258–263.
6. American Society of Hospital Pharmacists Technical Assistance Bulletin on Handling Cytotoxic Drugs in Hospitals. Am J Hosp Pharm 1985; 42:131–137.
7. OSHA Work-Practice Guidelines for Personnel Dealing with Cytotoxic (Antineoplastic) Drugs. Am J Hosp Pharm 1986; 43:1193–1204.

HOW SUPPLIED

Platinol-AQ (cisplatin) injection.
NDC 0015-3220-22—Each single dose vial contains 50 mg of cisplatin
NDC 0015-3221-22—Each single dose vial contains 100 mg of cisplatin
U.S. Patent No. 4,177,263
Shown in Product Identification Section, page 407

Continued on next page

Bristol-Myers Oncology—Cont.

RUBEX™   ℞

[ru'bĕx]
(doxorubicin hydrochloride
for injection, USP)
FOR INTRAVENOUS USE ONLY

WARNINGS

1. Severe local tissue necrosis will occur if there is extravasation during administration (See **DOSAGE AND ADMINISTRATION**). Doxorubicin must not be given by the intramuscular or subcutaneous route.
2. Serious irreversible myocardial toxicity with delayed congestive failure often unresponsive to any cardiac supportive therapy may be encountered as total dosage approaches 550 mg/m². This toxicity may occur at lower cumulative doses in patients with prior mediastinal irradiation or on concurrent cyclophosphamide therapy.
3. Dosage should be reduced in patients with impaired hepatic function.
4. Severe myelosuppression may occur.
5. Doxorubicin should be administered only under the supervision of a physician who is experienced in the use of cancer chemotherapeutic agents.

DESCRIPTION

Doxorubicin is a cytotoxic anthracycline antibiotic isolated from cultures of **Streptomyces peucetius** var. **caesius**. Doxorubicin consists of a naphthacenequinone nucleus linked through a glycosidic bond at ring atom 7 to an amino sugar, daunosamine. The structural formula is as follows:

$C_{27}H_{29}NO_{11}HCl$ Formula Weight —579.99

Doxorubicin binds to nucleic acids, presumably by specific intercalation of the planar anthracycline nucleus with the DNA double helix. The anthracycline ring is lipophilic but the saturated end of the ring system contains abundant hydroxyl groups adjacent to the amino sugar, producing a hydrophilic center. The molecule is amphoteric, containing acidic functions in the ring phenolic groups and a basic function in the sugar amino group. It binds to cell membranes as well as plasma proteins. Rubex (doxorubicin hydrochloride for injection, USP) is for intravenous use only. It is available in 50 mg and 100 mg single dose vials as a lyophilized, sterile powder with added lactose (anhydrous), 250 mg and 500 mg respectively.

CLINICAL PHARMACOLOGY

Though not completely elucidated, the mechanism of action of doxorubicin is related to its ability to bind to DNA and inhibit nucleic acid synthesis. Cell culture studies have demonstrated rapid cell penetration and perinucleolar chromatin binding, rapid inhibition of mitotic activity and nucleic acid synthesis, mutagenesis and chromosomal aberrations. Animal studies have shown activity in a spectrum of experimental tumors, immunosuppression, carcinogenic properties in rodents, induction of a variety of toxic effects, including delayed and progressive cardiac toxicity, myelosuppression in all species and atrophy to testes in rats and dogs.
Pharmacokinetic studies show the intravenous administration of normal or radiolabeled doxorubicin is followed by rapid plasma clearance and significant tissue binding. Urinary excretion, as determined by fluorimetric methods, accounts for approximately 4%-5% of the administered dose in 5 days. Biliary excretion represents the major excretion route, 40%-50% of the administered dose being recovered in the bile or the feces in 7 days. Impairment of liver function results in slower excretion, and, consequently, increased retention and accumulation in plasma and tissues. Doxorubicin does not cross the blood brain barrier.

INDICATIONS AND USAGE

Doxorubicin hydrochloride for injection has been used successfully to produce regression in disseminated neoplastic conditions such as acute lymphoblastic leukemia, acute myeloblastic leukemia, Wilms' tumor, neuroblastoma, soft tissue and bone sarcomas, breast carcinoma, ovarian carcinoma, transitional cell bladder carcinoma, thyroid carcinoma, lymphomas of both Hodgkin and non-Hodgkin types, bronchogenic carcinoma in which the small cell histologic type is the most responsive compared to other cell types and gastric carcinoma.
A number of other solid tumors have also shown some responsiveness but in numbers too limited to justify specific recommendation. Studies to date have shown malignant melanoma, kidney carcinoma, large bowel carcinoma, brain tumors and metastases to the central nervous system not to be significantly responsive to doxorubicin therapy.

CONTRAINDICATIONS

Doxorubicin therapy should not be started in patients who have marked myelosuppression induced by previous treatment with other antitumor agents or by radiotherapy. Conclusive data are not available on pre-existing heart disease as a co-factor of increased risk of doxorubicin induced cardiac toxicity. Preliminary data suggest that in such cases cardiac toxicity may occur at doses lower than the recommended cumulative limit. It is therefore not recommended to start doxorubicin in such cases. Doxorubicin treatment is contraindicated in patients who received previous treatment with complete cumulative doses of doxorubicin and/or daunorubicin.

WARNINGS

Special attention must be given to the cardiac toxicity exhibited by doxorubicin. Although uncommon, acute left ventricular failure has occurred, particularly in patients who have received total dosage of the drug exceeding the currently recommended limit of 550 mg/m². This limit appears to be lower (400 mg/m²) in patients who received radiotherapy to the mediastinal area or concomitant therapy with other potentially cardiotoxic agents such as cyclophosphamide. The total dose of doxorubicin administered to the individual patient should also take into account previous or concomitant therapy with related compounds such as daunorubicin. Congestive heart failure and/or cardiomyopathy may be encountered several weeks after discontinuation of doxorubicin therapy.
Cardiac failure is often not favorably affected by presently known medical or physical therapy for cardiac support. Early clinical diagnosis of drug induced heart failure appears to be essential for successful treatment with digitalis, diuretics, low salt diet and bed rest. Severe cardiac toxicity may occur precipitously without antecedent EKG changes. A baseline EKG and EKGs performed prior to each dose or course after 300 mg/m² cumulative dose has been given is suggested. Transient EKG changes consisting of T-wave flattening, S-T depression and arrhythmias lasting for up to 2 weeks after a dose or course of doxorubicin are presently not considered indications for suspension of doxorubicin therapy. Doxorubicin cardiomyopathy has been reported to be associated with a persistent reduction in the voltage of the QRS wave, a prolongation of the systolic time interval and a reduction of the ejection fraction as determined by echocardiography or radionuclide angiography. None of these tests have yet been confirmed to consistently identify those individual patients that are approaching their maximally tolerated cumulative dose of doxorubicin. If test results indicate change in cardiac function associated with doxorubicin the benefit of continued therapy must be carefully evaluated against the risk of producing irreversible cardiac damage. Acute life-threatening arrhythmias have been reported to occur during or within a few hours after doxorubicin hydrochloride administration.
There is a high incidence of bone marrow depression, primarily of leukocytes, requiring careful hematologic monitoring. With the recommended dosage schedule, leukopenia is usually transient, reaching its nadir at 10 to 14 days after treatment with recovery usually occurring by the 21st day. White blood cell counts as low as 1000/mm³ are to be expected during treatment with appropriate doses of doxorubicin. Red blood cell and platelet levels should also be monitored since they may also be depressed. Hematologic toxicity may require dose reduction or suspension or delay of doxorubicin therapy. Persistent severe myelosuppression may result in superinfection or hemorrhage.
Doxorubicin may potentiate the toxicity of other anticancer therapies. Exacerbation of cyclophosphamide induced hemorrhagic cystitis and enhancement of the hepatotoxicity of 6-mercaptopurine have been reported. Radiation induced toxicity to the myocardium, mucosae, skin and liver have been reported to be increased by the administration of doxorubicin.
Toxicity to recommended doses of doxorubicin hydrochloride is enhanced by hepatic impairment, therefore, prior to the individual dosing, evaluation of hepatic function is recommended using conventional clinical laboratory tests such as

SGOT, SGPT, alkaline phosphatase and bilirubin. (See **DOSAGE AND ADMINISTRATION**).
Necrotizing colitis manifested by typhlitis (cecal inflammation), bloody stools and severe and sometimes fatal infections have been associated with a combination of doxorubicin hydrochloride given by I.V. push daily for 3 days and cytarabine given by continuous infusion daily for 7 or more days.
On intravenous administration of doxorubicin extravasation may occur with or without an accompanying stinging or burning sensation and even if blood returns well on aspiration of the infusion needle (See **DOSAGE AND ADMINISTRATION**). If any signs or symptoms of extravasation have occurred the injection or infusion should be immediately terminated and restarted in another vein.
Doxorubicin and related compounds have also been shown to have mutagenic and carcinogenic properties when tested in experimental models.
Usage in Pregnancy—Safe use of doxorubicin in pregnancy has not been established. Doxorubicin is embryotoxic and teratogenic in rats and embryotoxic and abortifacient in rabbits. Therefore, the benefits to the pregnant patient should be carefully weighed against the potential toxicity to fetus and embryo. The possible adverse effects on fertility in males and females in humans or experimental animals have not been adequately evaluated.

PRECAUTIONS

Initial treatment with doxorubicin requires close observation of the patient and extensive laboratory monitoring. It is recommended, therefore, that patients be hospitalized at least during the first phase of the treatment.
Like other cytotoxic drugs, doxorubicin may induce hyperuricemia secondary to rapid lysis of neoplastic cells. The clinician should monitor the patient's blood uric acid level and be prepared to use such supportive and pharmacologic measures as might be necessary to control this problem.
Doxorubicin imparts a red coloration to the urine for 1 to 2 days after administration and patients should be advised to expect this during active therapy.
Doxorubicin is not an antimicrobial agent.

ADVERSE REACTIONS

Dose limiting toxicities of therapy are myelosuppression and cardiotoxicity (See **WARNINGS**). Other reactions reported are:
Cutaneous—Reversible complete alopecia occurs in most cases. Hyperpigmentation of nailbeds and dermal creases, primarily in children, and onycholysis have been reported in a few cases. Recall of skin reaction due to prior radiotherapy has occurred with doxorubicin administration.
Gastrointestinal—Acute nausea and vomiting occurs frequently and may be severe. This may be alleviated by antiemetic therapy. Mucositis (stomatitis and esophagitis) may occur 5 to 10 days after administration. The effect may be severe leading to ulceration and represents a site of origin for severe infections. The dosage regimen consisting of administration of doxorubicin on 3 successive days results in the greater incidence and severity of mucositis. Ulceration and necrosis of the colon, especially the cecum, may occur leading to bleeding or severe infections which can be fatal. This reaction has been reported in patients with acute nonlymphocytic leukemia treated with a 3-day course of doxorubicin combined with cytarabine. Anorexia and diarrhea have been occasionally reported.
Vascular—Phlebosclerosis has been reported especially when small veins are used or a single vein is used for repeated administration. Facial flushing may occur if the injection is given too rapidly.
Local—Severe cellulitis, vesication and tissue necrosis will occur if doxorubicin is extravasated during administration. Erythematous streaking along the vein proximal to the site of the injection has been reported (See **DOSAGE AND ADMINISTRATION**).
Hypersensitivity—Fever, chills and urticaria have been reported occasionally. Anaphylaxis may occur. A case of apparent cross sensitivity to lincomycin has been reported.
Other—Conjunctivitis and lacrimation occur rarely.

OVERDOSAGE

Acute overdosage with doxorubicin enhances the toxic effects of mucositis, leukopenia and thrombopenia. Treatment of acute overdosage consists of treatment of the severely myelosuppressed patient with hospitalization, antibiotics, platelet and granulocyte transfusions and symptomatic treatment of mucositis.
Chronic overdosage with cumulative doses exceeding 550 mg/m² increases the risk of cardiomyopathy and resultant congestive heart failure. Treatment consists of vigorous management of congestive heart failure with digitalis preparations and diuretics. The use of peripheral vasodilators has been recommended.

DOSAGE AND ADMINISTRATION

Care in the administration of doxorubicin hydrochloride will reduce the chance or perivenous infiltration. It may also decrease the chance of local reactions such as urticaria and erythematous streaking. On intravenous administration of doxorubicin, extravasation may occur with or without an accompanying stinging or burning sensation and even if blood returns well on aspiration of the infusion needle. If any signs or symptoms of extravasation have occurred, the injection or infusion should be immediately terminated and restarted in another vein. If it is known or suspected that subcutaneous extravasation has occurred, local infiltration with an injectable corticosteroid and flooding the site with normal saline have been reported to lessen the local reaction. Because of the progressive nature of extravasation reactions, the area of injection should be frequently examined and plastic surgery consultation obtained. If ulceration begins, early wide excision of the involved area should be considered[1].

The most commonly used dosage schedule is 60–75 mg/m^2 as a single intravenous injection administered at 21-day intervals. The lower dose should be given to patients with inadequate marrow reserves due to old age, or prior therapy, or neoplastic marrow infiltration. An alternative dosage schedule is weekly doses of 20 mg/m^2 which has been reported to produce a lower incidence of congestive heart failure. Thirty (30) mg/m^2 on each of 3 successive days repeated every 4 weeks has also been used. Doxorubicin dosage must be reduced if the bilirubin is elevated as follows: Serum Bilirubin 1.2–3.0 mg/dL—give $\frac{1}{2}$ normal dose, >3 mg/dL—give $\frac{1}{4}$ normal dose.

Preparation of solution—Doxorubicin hydrochloride for injection, USP, 50 mg and 100 mg vials should be reconstituted with 25 mL and 50 mL respectively of Sodium Chloride Injection, USP (0.9%) to give a final concentration of 2 mg/mL of doxorubicin hydrochloride. An appropriate volume of air should be withdrawn from the vial during reconstitution to avoid excessive pressure build-up. Bacteriostatic diluents are not recommended.

After adding the diluent, the vial should be shaken and the contents allowed to dissolve. The reconstituted solution is stable for 24 hours at room temperature and 48 hours under refrigeration 2°–8°C (36°–46°F). It should be protected from exposure to sunlight and any unused solution should be discarded.

It is recommended that doxorubicin be slowly administered into the tubing of a freely running intravenous infusion of Sodium Chloride Injection, USP, or 5% Dextrose Injection, USP. The tubing should be attached to a Butterfly® needle inserted preferably into a large vein. If possible, avoid veins over joints or in extremities with compromised venous or lymphatic drainage. The rate of administration is dependent on the size of the vein and the dosage. However, the dose should be administered in not less than 3 to 5 minutes. Local erythematous streaking along the vein as well as facial flushing may be indicative of too rapid an administration. A burning or stinging sensation may be indicative of perivenous infiltration and the infusion should be immediately terminated and restarted in another vein. Perivenous infiltration may occur painlessly.

Doxorubicin should not be mixed with heparin or fluorouracil since it has been reported that these drugs are incompatible to the extent that a precipitate may form. Until specific compatibility data are available, it is not recommended that doxorubicin be mixed with other drugs.

Doxorubicin has been used concurrently with other approved chemotherapeutic agents. Evidence is available that in some types of neoplastic disease combination chemotherapy is superior to single agents. The benefits and risks of such therapy continue to be elucidated.

Parenteral drug products should be inspected visually for particulate matter and discoloration prior to administration, whenever solution and container permit.

Handling and Disposal—Skin reactions associated with doxorubicin have been reported. Caution in the handling and preparation of the powder and solution must be exercised and the use of gloves is recommended. If doxorubicin powder or solution contacts the skin or mucosae, immediately wash thoroughly with soap and water.

Procedures for proper handling and disposal of anticancer drugs should be considered. Several guidelines on this subject have been published[2–8]. There is no general agreement that all of the procedures recommended in the guidelines are necessary or appropriate.

HOW SUPPLIED

Doxorubincin hydrochloride for injection, USP, is available as follows:

50 mg—Each single-dose vial contains 50 mg of doxorubicin HCl, USP, as a sterile red-orange lyophilized powder, NDC 0015-3352-22. Available as one individually cartoned vial.

100 mg—Each single-dose vial contains 100 mg of doxorubicin HCl, USP, as a sterile red-orange lyophilized powder, NDC 0015-3353-22. Available as one individually cartoned vial.

Store dry powder at controlled room temperature 15°–30°C (59°–86°F).

The reconstituted solution is stable for 24 hours at room temperature or 48 hours under refrigeration 2°–8°C (36°–46°F). Protect from exposure to sunlight. Retain in carton until time of use.

REFERENCES

1. Rudolph R, et al: Skin Ulcers Due to ADRIAMYCIN. Cancer 38;1087–1094, Sept. 1976.
2. Recommendations for the Safe Handling of Parenteral Antineoplastic Drugs. NIH Publication No. 83-2621. For sale by the Superintendent of Documents, US Government Printing Office, Washington, DC 20402.
3. AMA Council Report. Guidelines for Handling Parenteral Antineoplastics. JAMA 1985 March 15.
4. National Study Commission on Cytotoxic Exposure—Recommendations for Handling Cytotoxic Agents. Available from Louis P. Jeffrey, Sc.D., Chairman, National Study Commission of Cytotoxic Exposure, Massachusetts College of Pharmacy and Allied Health Sciences, 179 Longwood Avenue, Boston, Massachusetts 02115.
5. Clinical Oncological Society of Australia. Guidelines and Recommendations for Safe Handling of Antineoplastic Agents. Med J Australia 1983; 1:426–428.
6. Jones RB, et al: Safe Handling of Chemotherapeutic Agents: A Report from the Mount Sinai Medical Center. CA—A Cancer Journal of Clinicians 1983; (Sept/Oct) 258–263.
7. American Society of Hospital Pharmacists Technical Assistance Bulletin on Handling Cytotoxic Drugs in Hospitals. Am J Hosp Pharm 1985; 42:131–137.
8. OSHA Work-Practice Guidelines for Personnel Dealing with Cytotoxic (Antineoplastic) Drugs. Am J Hosp Pharm 1986; 43:1193–1204.

VEPESID®   ℞
(etoposide)
INJECTION AND CAPSULES

WARNINGS

VePesid (etoposide) should be administered under the supervision of a qualified physician experienced in the use of cancer chemotherapeutic agents. Severe myelosuppression with resulting infection or bleeding may occur.

DESCRIPTION

VePesid (etoposide) (also commonly known as VP-16) is a semisynthetic derivative of podophyllotoxin used in the treatment of certain neoplastic diseases. It is 4'-demethylepipodophyllotoxin 9-[4,6-0-(R)-ethylidene-β-D-glucopyranoside]. It is very soluble in methanol and chloroform, slightly soluble in ethanol and sparingly soluble in water and ether. It is made more miscible with water by means of organic solvents. It has a molecular weight of 588.58 and a molecular formula of $C_{29}H_{32}O_{13}$.

VePesid may be administered either intravenously or orally. VePesid injection is available in 100 mg (5 mL) sterile, multiple dose vials. The pH of the clear yellow solution is 3 to 4. Each mL contains 20 mg etoposide, 2 mg citric acid, 30 mg benzyl alcohol, 80 mg polysorbate 80/tween 80, 650 mg polyethylene glycol 300, and 30.5% (v/v) alcohol.

VePesid is also available as 50 mg pink capsules. Each liquid filled, soft gelatin capsule contains 50 mg of etoposide in a vehicle consisting of citric acid, glycerin, purified water and polyethylene glycol 400. The soft gelatin capsules contain gelatin, glycerin, sorbitol, purified water and parabens (ethyl and propyl) with the following dye system: iron oxide (red) and titanium dioxide; the capsules are printed with edible ink.

The structural formula is:

CLINICAL PHARMACOLOGY

VePesid has been shown to cause metaphase arrest in chick fibroblasts. Its main effect, however, appears to be at the G_2 portion of the cell cycle in mammalian cells. Two different dose-dependent responses are seen. At high concentrations (10 μg/mL or more), lysis of cells entering mitosis is observed. At low concentrations (0.3 to 10 μg/mL), cells are inhibited from entering prophase. It does not interfere with microtubular assembly. The predominant macromolecular effect of VePesid appears to be DNA synthesis inhibition.

Pharmacokinetics: On intravenous administration, the disposition of etoposide is best described as a biphasic process with a distribution half-life of about 1.5 hours and terminal elimination half-life ranging from 4 to 11 hours. Total body clearance values range from 33 to 48 mL/min or 16 to 36 mL/min/m^2 and, like the terminal elimination half-life, are independent of dose over a range 100 to 600 mg/m^2. Over the same dose range, the areas under the plasma concentration vs. time curves (AUC) and the maximum plasma concentration (Cmax) values increase linearly with dose. Etoposide does not accumulate in the plasma following daily administration of 100 mg/m^2 for 4 to 5 days.

The mean volumes of distribution at steady state fall in the range of 18 to 29 liters or 7 to 17 L/m^2. Etoposide enters the CSF poorly. Although it is detectable in CSF and intracerebral tumors, the concentrations are lower than in extracerebral tumors and in plasma. Etoposide concentrations are higher in normal lung than in lung metastases and are similar in primary tumors and normal tissues of the myometrium. **In vitro**, etoposide is highly protein bound (97%) to human plasma proteins. An inverse relationship between plasma albumin levels and etoposide renal clearance is found in children. The effect of other highly bound drugs or of disease states on the protein binding of etoposide is not known.

After intravenous administration of ^{3}H-etoposide (70 to 290 mg/m^2), mean recoveries of radioactivity in the urine range from 42% to 67%, and fecal recoveries range from 0% to 16% of the dose. Less than 50% of an intravenous dose is excreted in the urine as etoposide with mean recoveries of 8% to 35% within 24 hours.

In children, approximately 55% of the dose is excreted in the urine as etoposide in 24 hours. The mean renal clearance of etoposide is 7 to 10 mL/min/m^2 or about 35% of the total body clearance over a dose range of 80 to 600 mg/m^2. Etoposide, therefore, is cleared by both renal and nonrenal processes, i.e., metabolism and biliary excretion. The effect of renal disease on plasma etoposide clearance is not known. Biliary excretion appears to be a minor route of etoposide elimination. Only 6% or less of an intravenous dose is recovered in the bile as etoposide. Metabolism accounts for most of the nonrenal clearance of etoposide. The major urinary metabolite of etoposide in adults and children is the hydroxy acid [4'-demethylepipodophyllic acid-9-(4, 6-0-(R)-ethylidene-β-D-glucopyranoside)], formed by opening of the lactone ring. It is also present in human plasma, presumably as the **trans** isomer. Glucuronide and/or sulfate conjugates of etoposide are excreted in human urine and represent 5% to 22% of the dose.

After either intravenous infusion or oral capsule administration, the Cmax and AUC values exhibit marked intrasubject and intersubject variability. This results in variability in the estimates of the absolute oral bioavailability of etoposide oral capsules.

Cmax and AUC values for orally administered etoposide capsules consistently fall in the same range as the Cmax and AUC values for an intravenous dose of one half the size of the oral dose. The overall mean value of oral capsule bioavailability is approximately 50% (range 25%–75%). Dose proportionality in absorption following oral capsule administration has not been established.

There is no evidence of a first-pass effect for etoposide. For example, no correlation exists between the absolute oral bioavailability of etoposide capsules and nonrenal clearance. No evidence exists for any other differences in etoposide metabolism and excretion after administration of oral capsules as compared to intravenous infusion.

In adults, the total body clearance of etoposide is correlated with creatinine clearance, serum albumin concentration, and nonrenal clearance. In children, elevated serum SGPT levels are associated with reduced drug total body clearance. Prior use of cisplatin may also result in a decrease of etoposide total body clearance in children.

INDICATION AND USAGE

VePesid is indicated in the management of the following neoplasms:

Refractory Testicular Tumors—VePesid Injection in combination therapy with other approved chemotherapeutic agents in patients with refractory testicular tumors who have already received appropriate surgical, chemotherapeutic and radiotherapeutic therapy.

Adequate data on the use of VePesid Capsules in the treatment of testicular cancer are not available.

Small cell lung cancer—VePesid Injection and/or Capsules in combination with other approved chemotherapeutic agents as first line treatment in patients with small cell lung cancer.

CONTRAINDICATIONS

VePesid is contraindicated in patients who have demonstrated a previous hypersensitivity to it.

Continued on next page

Bristol-Myers Oncology—Cont.

WARNINGS

Patients being treated with VePesid must be frequently observed for myelosuppression both during and after therapy. Dose-limiting bone marrow suppression is the most significant toxicity associated with VePesid therapy. Therefore, the following studies should be obtained at the start of therapy and prior to each subsequent dose of VePesid: platelet count, hemoglobin, white blood cell count and differential. The occurrence of a platelet count below 50,000/mm³ or an absolute neutrophil count below 500/mm³ is an indication to withhold further therapy until the blood counts have sufficiently recovered.

Physicians should be aware of the possible occurrence of an anaphylactic reaction manifested by chills, fever, tachycardia, bronchospasm, dyspnea and hypotension. (See "ADVERSE REACTIONS" section.) Treatment is symptomatic. The infusion should be terminated immediately, followed by the administration of pressor agents, corticosteroids, antihistamines, or volume expanders at the discretion of the physician.

For parenteral administration, VePesid should be given only by slow intravenous infusion (usually over a 30- to 60-minute period) since hypotension has been reported as a possible side effect of rapid intravenous injection.

Pregnancy: Pregnancy "Category D." VePesid can cause fetal harm when administered to a pregnant woman. VePesid has been shown to be teratogenic in mice and rats. There are no adequate and well-controlled studies in pregnant women. If this drug is used during pregnancy, or if the patient becomes pregnant while receiving this drug, the patient should be apprised of the potential hazard to the fetus. Women of childbearing potential should be advised to avoid becoming pregnant.

VePesid is teratogenic and embryocidal in rats and mice at doses of 1% to 3% of the recommended clinical dose based on body surface area.

In a teratology study in SPF rats, VePesid was administered intravenously at doses of 0.13, 0.4, 1.2 and 3.6 mg/kg/day on days 6 to 15 of gestation. VePesid caused dose-related maternal toxicity, embryotoxicity, and teratogenicity at dose levels of 0.4 mg/kg/day and higher. Embryonic resorptions were 90% and 100% at the two highest dosages. At 0.4 and 1.2 mg/kg, fetal weights were decreased and fetal abnormalities including decreased weight, major skeletal abnormalities, exencephaly, encephalocele and anophthalmia occurred. Even at the lowest dose tested, 0.13 mg/kg, a significant increase in retarded ossification was observed.

VePesid administered as a single intraperitoneal injection in Swiss-Albino mice at dosages of 1, 1.5 and 2 mg/kg on days 6, 7 or 8 of gestation caused dose-related embryotoxicity, cranial abnormalities and major skeletal malformations.

PRECAUTIONS

General: In all instances where the use of VePesid is considered for chemotherapy, the physician must evaluate the need and usefulness of the drug against the risk of adverse reactions. Most such adverse reactions are reversible if detected early. If severe reactions occur, the drug should be reduced in dosage or discontinued and appropriate corrective measures should be taken according to the clinical judgment of the physician. Reinstitution of VePesid therapy should be carried out with caution, and with adequate consideration of the further need for the drug and alertness as to possible recurrence of toxicity.

Laboratory Tests: Periodic complete blood counts should be done during the course of VePesid treatment. They should be performed prior to therapy and at appropriate intervals during and after therapy. At least one determination should be done prior to each dose of VePesid.

Carcinogenesis, Mutagenesis, Impairment of Fertility: Carcinogenicity tests with VePesid have not been conducted in laboratory animals. VePesid should be considered a potential carcinogen in humans (see "ADVERSE REACTIONS" section).

The mutagenic and genotoxic potential of VePesid has been established in mammalian cells. VePesid caused aberrations in chromosome number and structure in embryonic murine cells and human hematopoietic cells; gene mutations in Chinese hamster ovary cells; and DNA damage by strand breakage and DNA-protein cross-links in mouse leukemia cells. VePesid also caused a dose-related increase in sister chromatid exchanges in Chinese hamster ovary cells.

Treatment of Swiss-Albino mice with 1.5 mg/kg IP of VePesid on day 7 of gestation increased the incidence of intrauterine death and fetal malformations as well as significantly decreased the average fetal body weight. Maternal weight gain was not affected.

Treatment of pregnant SPF rats with 1.2 mg/kg/day IV of VePesid for 10 days led to a prenatal mortality of 92%, and 50% of the implanting fetuses were abnormal.

Pregnancy: Pregnancy "Category D." (See "WARNINGS" section.)

Nursing Mothers: It is not known whether this drug is excreted in human milk. Because many drugs are excreted in human milk and because of the potential for serious adverse reactions in nursing infants from VePesid, a decision should be made whether to discontinue nursing or to discontinue the drug, taking into account the importance of the drug to the mother.

Pediatric Use: Safety and effectiveness in children have not been established.

VePesid injection contains polysorbate 80. In premature infants, a life-threatening syndrome consisting of liver and renal failure, pulmonary deterioration, thrombocytopenia and ascites has been associated with an injectable vitamin E product containing polysorbate 80.

ADVERSE REACTIONS

The following data on adverse reactions are based on both oral and intravenous administration of VePesid as a single agent, using several different dose schedules for treatment of a wide variety of malignancies.

Hematologic Toxicity: Myelosuppression is dose related and dose limiting with granulocyte nadirs occurring 7 to 14 days after drug administration and platelet nadirs occurring 9 to 16 days after drug administration. Bone marrow recovery is usually complete by day 20, and no cumulative toxicity has been reported.

The occurrence of acute leukemia with or without a preleukemic phase has been reported rarely in patients treated with VePesid in association with other antineoplastic agents.

Gastrointestinal Toxicity: Nausea and vomiting are the major gastrointestinal toxicities. The severity of such nausea and vomiting is generally mild to moderate with treatment discontinuation required in 1% of patients. Nausea and vomiting can usually be controlled with standard antiemetic therapy. Gastrointestinal toxicities are slightly more frequent after oral administration than after intravenous infusion.

Hypotension: Transient hypotension following rapid intravenous administration has been reported in 1% to 2% of patients. It has not been associated with cardiac toxicity or electrocardiographic changes. No delayed hypotension has been noted. To prevent this rare occurrence, it is recommended that VePesid be administered by slow intravenous infusion over a 30- to 60-minute period. If hypotension occurs, it usually responds to cessation of the infusion and administration of fluids or other supportive therapy as appropriate. When restarting the infusion, a slower administration rate should be used.

Allergic Reactions: Anaphylactic-like reactions characterized by chills, fever, tachycardia, bronchospasm, dyspnea and hypotension have been reported to occur in 0.7% to 2% of patients receiving intravenous VePesid and in less than 1% of the patients treated with the oral capsules. These reactions have usually responded promptly to the cessation of the infusion and administration of pressor agents, corticosteroids, antihistamines or volume expanders as appropriate. One fatal acute reaction associated with bronchospasm has been reported. Hypertension and flushing have also been reported. Blood pressure usually normalizes within a few hours after cessation of the infusion.

Alopecia: Reversible alopecia, sometimes progressing to total baldness was observed in up to 66% of patients.

Other Toxicities: The following adverse reactions have been infrequently reported: aftertaste, rash, fever, pigmentation, pruritus, abdominal pain, constipation, dysphagia, transient cortical blindness and a single report of radiation recall dermatitis.

The incidences of adverse reactions in the table that follows are derived from multiple data bases from studies in 2,081 patients when VePesid was used either orally or by injection as a single agent.

ADVERSE DRUG EFFECT	PERCENT RANGE OF REPORTED INCIDENCE
Hematologic toxicity	
Leukopenia (less than 1,000 WBC/mm³)	3–17
Leukopenia (less than 4,000 WBC/mm³)	60–91
Thrombocytopenia (less than 50,000 platelets/mm³)	1–20
Thrombocytopenia (less than 100,000 platelets/mm³)	22–41
Anemia	0–33
Gastrointestinal toxicity	
Nausea and vomiting	31–43
Abdominal pain	0–2
Anorexia	10–13
Diarrhea	1–13
Stomatitis	1–6
Hepatic	0–3
Alopecia	8–66
Peripheral neurotoxicity	1–2
Hypotension	1–2
Allergic reaction	1–2

OVERDOSAGE

No proven antidotes have been established for VePesid overdosage.

DOSAGE AND ADMINISTRATION

Note: Plastic devices made of acrylic or ABS (a polymer composed of acrylonitrile, butadiene and styrene) have been reported to crack and leak when used with undiluted VePesid Injection. This effect has not been reported with diluted VePesid.

VePesid Injection: The usual dose of VePesid Injection in testicular cancer in combination with other approved chemotherapeutic agents ranges from 50 to 100 mg/m²/day on days 1 through 5 to 100 mg/m²/day on days 1, 3 and 5.

In small cell lung cancer, the VePesid Injection dose in combination with other approved chemotherapeutic drugs ranges from 35 mg/m²/day for 4 days to 50 mg/m²/day for 5 days.

Chemotherapy courses are repeated at 3- to 4-week intervals after adequate recovery from any toxicity.

VePesid Capsules: In small cell lung cancer, the recommended dose of VePesid Capsules is two times the IV dose rounded to the nearest 50 mg.

The dosage, by either route, should be modified to take into account the myelosuppressive effects of other drugs in the combination or the effects of prior x-ray therapy or chemotherapy which may have compromised bone marrow reserve.

Administration Precautions: As with other potentially toxic compounds, caution should be exercised in handling and preparing the solution of VePesid. Skin reactions associated with accidental exposure to VePesid may occur. The use of gloves is recommended. If VePesid solution contacts the skin or mucosa, immediately wash the skin or mucosa thoroughly with soap and water.

Preparation for Intravenous Administration: VePesid Injection must be diluted prior to use with either 5% Dextrose Injection, USP, or 0.9% Sodium Chloride Injection, USP, to give a final concentration of 0.2 or 0.4 mg/mL. If solutions are prepared at concentrations above 0.4 mg/mL, precipitation may occur. Hypotension following rapid intravenous administration has been reported, hence, it is recommended that the VePesid solution be administered over a 30- to 60-minute period or longer. **VePesid should not be given by rapid intravenous injection.**

Parenteral drug products should be inspected visually for particulate matter and discoloration (see "DESCRIPTION" section) prior to administration whenever solution and container permit.

Stability: Unopened vials of VePesid Injection are stable for 24 months at room temperature (25℃). Vials diluted as recommended to a concentration of 0.2 or 0.4 mg/mL are stable for 96 and 48 hours, respectively, at room temperature (25℃) under normal room fluorescent light in both glass and plastic containers.

VePesid Capsules must be stored under refrigeration 2°–8℃ (36°–46°F). The capsules are stable for 24 months under such refrigerated conditions.

Procedures for proper handling and disposal of anticancer drugs should be considered. Several guidelines on this subject have been published.[1-7] There is no general agreement that all of the procedures recommended in the guidelines are necessary or appropriate.

References
1. Recommendations for the Safe Handling of Parenteral Antineoplastic Drugs. NIH Publication No. 83-2621. For sale by the Superintendent of Documents, U.S. Government Printing Office, Washington, D.C. 20402.
2. AMA Council Report. Guidelines for Handling Parenteral Antineoplastics. JAMA, 1985; March 15.
3. National Study Commission on Cytotoxic Exposure—Recommendations for Handling Cytotoxic Agents. Available from Louis P. Jeffrey, Sc.D., Chairman, National Study Commission on Cytotoxic Exposure, Massachusetts College of Pharmacy and Allied Health Sciences, 179 Longwood Avenue, Boston, Massachusetts 02115.
4. Clinical Oncological Society of Australia: Guidelines and Recommendations for Safe Handling of Antineoplastic Agents. Med. J. Australia 1983; 1:426–428.
5. Jones, R. B., et. al. Safe Handling of Chemotherapeutic Agents: A Report from the Mount Sinai Medical Center. Ca—A Cancer Journal for Clinicians 1983; Sept./Oct., 258–263.
6. American Society of Hospital Pharmacists Technical Assistance Bulletin on Handling Cytotoxic Drugs in Hospitals Am. J. Hosp. Pharm. 1985; 42:131–137.
7. OSHA Work-Practice Guidelines for Personnel Dealing with Cytotoxic (Antineoplastic) Drugs. Am. J. Hosp. Pharm. 1986; 43:1193–1204.

HOW SUPPLIED

VePesid (etoposide) Injection

NDC 0015-3095-20—100 mg/5 mL Sterile Multiple Dose Vial, 10's

VePesid (etoposide) Capsules

NDC 0015-3091-45—50 mg pink capsules with "BRISTOL 3091" printed in black in blisterpacks of 20 individually labeled blisters, each containing one capsule.

Capsules are to be stored under refrigeration 2°–8°C (36°–46°F).

DO NOT FREEZE.

Dispense in child-resistant containers.

For information on package sizes available, refer to the current price schedule.

Shown in Product Identification Section, page 407

Bristol-Myers Products
(Div. of Bristol-Myers Co.)
345 PARK AVENUE
NEW YORK, NY 10154

Tri-Buffered BUFFERIN®
[bŭf'fĕr-ĭn]
Analgesic

COMPOSITION

Active Ingredient: Each coated tablet or caplet contains Aspirin 325 mg in a formulation buffered with Calcium Carbonate, Magnesium Oxide and Magnesium Carbonate.

Other Ingredients: Benzoic Acid, Carnauba Wax, Citric Acid, Corn Starch, FD&C Blue No. 1, Hydroxypropyl Methylcellulose, Mineral Oil, Polysorbate 20, Povidone, Propylene Glycol, Simethicone Emulsion, Sodium Phosphate, Sorbitan Monolaurate, Titanium Dioxide. May also contain: Glyceryl Behenate, Magnesium Stearate, Sodium Lauryl Sulfate, Sodium Stearyl Fumarate, Stearic Acid, Zinc Stearate.

ACTION AND USES

For effective relief from headaches, pain and fever of colds and flu, muscle aches, temporary relief of minor arthritis pain and inflammation, mentrual pain and toothaches. Buffered formulation helps prevent the stomach upset that plain aspirin can cause. Coated tablets for easy swallowing.

CONTRAINDICATIONS

Hypersensitivity to salicylates.

CAUTION

If pain persists for more than 10 days or redness is present, or in arthritic or rheumatic conditions affecting children under 12, consult a physician immediately. Do not take without consulting a physician if under medical care. Consult a dentist for toothache promptly.

WARNING

Children and teenagers should not use this medicine for chicken pox or flu symptoms before a doctor is consulted about Reye syndrome, a rare but serious illness reported to be associated with aspirin. KEEP THIS AND ALL MEDICINES OUT OF CHILDREN'S REACH. IN CASE OF ACCIDENTAL OVERDOSE, CONTACT A PHYSICIAN OR POISON CONTROL CENTER IMMEDIATELY. If dizziness, impaired hearing or ringing in the ears occurs, discontinue use. As with any drug, if you are pregnant or nursing a baby, seek the advice of a health professional before using this product.

ADMINISTRATION AND DOSAGE

Adults: 2 tablets or caplets with water every 4 hours as needed. Do not exceed 12 tablets or caplets in 24 hours, unless directed by physician. For children 6 to under 12, one-half adult dose. Under 6, consult physician.

OVERDOSE

(Symptoms and treatment) Typical of aspirin.

HOW SUPPLIED

Tri-Buffered BUFFERIN is supplied as:
Coated circular white tablet with letter "B" debossed on one surface.
NDC 19810-0073-2 Bottle of 12's
NDC 19810-0073-3 Bottle of 36's
NDC 19810-0073-4 Bottle of 60's
NDC 19810-0073-5 Bottle of 100's
NDC 19810-0073-6 Bottle of 200's
NDC 19810-0093-2 Bottle of 275's
NDC 19810-0073-7 Bottle of 1000's for hospital and clinical use.
NDC 19810-0073-9 Boxed 200 × 2 tablet foil pack for hospital and clinical use.
Coated scored white caplet with letter "B" debossed on each side of scoring.
NDC 19810-0072-1 Bottle of 36's
NDC 19810-0072-2 Bottle of 60's
NDC 19810-0072-3 Bottle of 100's
All consumer sizes have child resistant closures except 100's for tablets and 60's for caplets which are sizes recommended for households without young children. Store at room temperature.

Professional samples available on request.
Also described in PDR for Nonprescription Drugs.

PROFESSIONAL LABELING

1. Tri-Buffered BUFFERIN® FOR RECURRENT TRANSIENT ISCHEMIC ATTACKS

INDICATION

For reducing the risk of recurrent transient ischemic attacks (TIA's) or stroke in men who have had transient ischemia of the brain due to fibrin platelet emboli. There is inadequate evidence that aspirin or buffered aspirin is effective in reducing TIA's in women at the recommended dosage. There is no evidence that aspirin or buffered aspirin is of benefit in the treatment of completed strokes in men or women.

CLINICAL TRIALS

The indication is supported by the results of a Canadian study (1) in which 585 patients with threatened stroke were followed in a randomized clinical trial for an average of 26 months to determine whether aspirin or sulfinpyrazone, singly or in combination, was superior to placebo in preventing transient ischemic attacks, stroke, or death. The study showed that, although sulfinpyrazone had no statistically significant effect, aspirin reduced the risk of continuing transient ischemic attacks, stroke, or death by 19 percent and reduced the risk of stroke or death by 31 percent. Another aspirin study carried out in the United States with 178 patients, showed a statistically significant number of "favorable outcomes," including reduced transient ischemic attacks, storke, and death (2).

PRECAUTIONS

Patients presenting with signs and symptoms of TIA's should have a complete medical and neurologic evaluation. Consideration should be given to other disorders that resemble TIA's. Attention should be given to risk factors: it is important to evaluate and treat, if appropriate, other diseases associated with TIA's and stroke, such as hypertension and diabetes.

Concurrent administration of absorbable antacids at therapeutic doses may increase the clearance of salicylates in some individuals. The concurrent administration of nonabsorbable antacids may alter the rate of absorption of aspirin, thereby resulting in a decreased acetylsalicylic acid/salicylate ratio in plasma. The clinical significance of these decreases in available aspirin is unknown.

Aspirin at dosages of 1,000 milligrams per day has been associated with small increases in blood pressure, blood urea nitrogen, and serum uric acid levels. It is recommended that patients placed on long-term aspirin treatment be seen at regular intervals to assess changes in these measurements.

ADVERSE REACTIONS

At dosages of 1,000 milligrams or higher of aspirin per day, gastrointestinal side effects include stomach pain, heartburn, nausea and/or vomiting, as well as increased rates of gross gastrointestinal bleeding.

DOSAGE AND ADMINISTRATION

Adult oral dosage for men is 1,300 milligrams a day, in divided doses of 650 milligrams twice a day or 325 milligrams four times a day.

REFERENCES

(1) The Canadian Cooperative Study Group. "A Randomized Trial of Aspirin and Sulfinpyrazone in Threatened Stroke," *New England Journal of Medicine,* 299:53–59, 1978.

(2) Fields, W.S., et al., "Controlled Trial of Aspirin in Cerebral Ischemia," *Stroke* 8:301–316, 1977.

2. Tri-Buffered BUFFERIN® FOR MYOCARDIAL INFARCTION

INDICATION

Aspirin is indicated to reduce the risk of death and/or nonfatal myocardial infarction in patients with a previous infarction or unstable angina pectoris.

CLINICAL TRIALS

The indication is supported by the results of six, large, randomized multicenter, placebo-controlled studies[1–7] involving 10,816, predominantly male, post-myocardial infarction (MI) patients and one randomized placebo-controlled study of 1,266 men with unstable angina. Therapy with aspirin was begun at intervals after the onset of acute MI varying from less than 3 days to more than 5 years and continued for periods of from less than one year to four years. In the unstable angina study, treatment was started within 1 month after the onset of unstable angina and continued for 12 weeks and complicating conditions such as congestive heart failure were not included in the study.

Aspirin therapy in MI patients was associated with about a 20 percent reduction in the risk of subsequent death and/or nonfatal reinfarction, a median absolute decrease of 3 percent from the 12 to 22 percent event rates in the placebo groups. In the aspirin-treated unstable angina patients the reduction in risk was about 50 percent, a reduction in the

event rate of 5% from the 10% rate in the placebo group over the 12 weeks of the study.

Daily dosage of aspirin in the post-myocardial infarction studies was 300 mg. in one study and 900 and 1500 mg. in five studies. A dose of 325 mg. was used in the study of unstable angina.

ADVERSE REACTIONS

Gastrointestinal Reactions: Doses of 1000 mg. per day of aspirin caused gastrointestinal symptoms and bleeding that in some cases were clinically significant. In the largest post-infarction study (The Aspirin Myocardial Infaraction Study (AMIS) with 4,500 people), the percentage incidences of gastrointestinal symptoms for the aspirin (1000 mg. of a standard, solid-tablet formulation) and placebo-treated subjects, respectively, were: stomach pain (14.5%; 4.4%); heartburn (11.9%; 4.8%); nausea and/or vomiting (7.6%; 2.1%); hospitalization for gastrointestinal disorder (4.8%; 3.5%). In the AMIS and other trials, aspirin treated patients had increased rates of gross gastrointestinal bleeding. Symptoms and signs of gastrointestinal irritation were not significantly increased in subjects treated for unstable angina with buffered aspirin in solution.

Cardiovascular and Biochemical:
In the AMIS trial, the dosage of 1000 mg. per day of aspirin was associated with small increases in systolic blood pressure (BP) (average 1.5 to 2.1 mm) and diastolic BP (0.5 to 0.6 mm), depending upon whether maximal or last available readings were used. Blood urea nitrogen and uric acid levels were also increased, but by less than 1.0 mg%.

Subjects with marked hypertension or renal insufficiency had been excluded from the trial so that the clinical importance of these observations for such subjects or for any subjects treated over more prolonged periods is not known. It is recommended that patients placed on long-term aspirin treatment, even at doses of 300 mg. per day, be seen at regular intervals to asess changes in these measurements.

REFERENCES

1. Elwood P.C., et al., "A Randomized Controlled Trial of Acetylsalicylic Acid in the Secondary Prevention of Mortality from Myocardial Infarction," British Medical Journal, 1:436–440, 1974. 2. The Coronary Drug Project Reserach Group, "Aspirin in Coronary Heart Disease," Journal of Chronic Disease, 29:625–642, 1976. 3. Breddin K, et al., "Secondary Prevention of Myocardial Infarction; Comparison of Acetylsalicylic Acid Phenprocoumon and Placebo," Thromb. Haemost., 41:225–236, 1979. 4. Aspirin Myocardial Infarction Study Research Group, "A Randomized, Controlled Trial of Aspirin in Persons Recovered from Myocardial Infarction," Journal American Medical Association, 243:661–669, 1980. 5. Elwood P.C., and Sweetnam, P.M., "Aspirin and Secondary Mortality after Myocardial Infarction," Lancet, pp. 1313–1315, December 22–29, 1979. 6. The Persantine-Aspirin Reinfarction Study Research Group. "Persantine and Aspirin in Coronary Heart Disease," Circulation 62;449–460, 1980. 7. Lewis H.D., et al., "Protective Effects of Aspirin Against Acute Myocardial Infarction and Death in Men with Unstable Angina, Results of a Veterans Administration Cooperative Study," New England Journal of Medicine, 309;396–403, 1983.

ADMINISTRATION AND DOSAGE

Although most of the studies used dosages exceeding 300 mg., two trials used only 300 mg. and pharmacologic data indicate that this dose inhibits platelet function fully. Therefore, 300 mg. or a conventional 325 mg. aspirin dose is a reasonable, routine dose that would minimize gastrointestinal adverse reactions.

Shown in Product Identification Section, page 407

Arthritis Strength Tri-Buffered BUFFERIN®
[bŭf'fĕr-ĭn]
Analgesic

COMPOSITION

Active Ingredients: Aspirin (500 mg) in a formulation buffered with Calcium Carbonate, Magnesium Oxide and Magnesium Carbonate.

Other Ingredients: Benzoic Acid, Carnauba Wax, Citric Acid, Corn Starch, FD&C Blue No. 1, Hydroxpropyl Methylcellulose, Mineral Oil, Polysorbate 20, Povidone, Propylene Glycol, Simethicone Emulsion, Sodium Phosphate, Sorbitan Monolaurate, Titanium Dioxide. May also contain: Glyceryl Behenate, Magnesium Stearate, Sodium Lauryl Sulfate, Sodium Stearyl Fumarate, Stearic Acid, Zinc Stearate.

ACTION AND USES

For temporary relief from the minor aches and pains, stiffness, swelling and inflammation of arthritis. Buffered formulation helps prevent the stomach upset that plain aspirin can cause. Coated caplets for easy swallowing.

Continued on next page

Bristol-Myers Products—Cont.

CONTRAINDICATIONS

Hypersensitivity to salicylates.

CAUTION

If pain persists for more than 10 days or redness is present or in arthritic or rheumatic conditions affecting children under 12 consult physician immediately. Do not take without consulting physician if under medical care.

WARNING

Children and teenagers should not use this medicine for chicken pox or flu symptoms before a doctor is consulted about Reye syndrome, a rare but serious illness reported to be associated with aspirin. KEEP THIS AND ALL MEDICINES OUT OF CHILDREN'S REACH. IN CASE OF ACCIDENTAL OVERDOSE, CONTACT A PHYSICIAN OR POISON CONTROL CENTER IMMEDIATELY. If dizziness, impaired hearing or ringing in the ears occurs, discontinue use. As with any drug, if you are pregnant or nursing a baby, seek the advice of a health professional before using this product.

ADMINISTRATION AND DOSAGE

Adults: Two caplets with water every 4 hours as needed. Do not exceed 8 caplets in 24 hours, or give to children under 12 unless directed by a physician.

OVERDOSE

(Symptoms and treatment) Typical of aspirin.

HOW SUPPLIED

Arthritis Strength Tri-Buffered BUFFERIN® is supplied as:
Plain white coated caplet "ABS" debossed on one side.
NDC 19810-0051-1 Bottle of 40's
NDC 19810-0051-2 Bottle of 100's
The 40 caplet size does not have a child resistant closure and is recommended for households without young children.
Store at room temperature.
Also described in PDR For Nonprescription Drugs.
Shown in Product Identification Section, page 407

Extra Strength Tri-Buffered BUFFERIN®
[bŭf'fĕr-ĭn]
Analgesic

COMPOSITION

Active Ingredients: Aspirin (500 mg) in a formulation buffered with Calcium Carbonate, Magnesium Oxide and Magnesium Carbonate.
Other Ingredients: Benzoic Acid, Carnuaba Wax, Citric Acid, Corn Starch, FD&C Blue No. 1, Hydroxypropyl Methylcellulose, Mineral Oil, Polyorbate 20, Povidone, Propylene Glycol, Simethicone Emulsion, Sodium Phosphate, Sorbitan Monolaurate, Titanium Dioxide. May also contain: Glyceryl Behenate, Magnesium Stearate, Sodium Lauryl Sulfate, Sodium Stearyl Fumarate, Stearic Acid, Zinc Stearate.

ACTION AND USES

Contains aspirin for relief from headaches, pain and fever of colds and flu, muscle aches, temporary relief of minor arthritis pain and inflammation, menstrual pain and toothaches. Buffered formulation which helps prevent the stomach upset that plain aspirin can cause. Each tablet is coated for easy swallowing.

CONTRAINDICATIONS

Hypersensitivity to salicylates.

CAUTION

If pain persists for more than 10 days, or redness is present, or in arthritic or rheumatic conditions affecting children under 12, consult a physician immediately. Do not take without consulting a physician if under medical care. Consult a dentist for toothache promptly.

WARNING

Children and teenagers should not use this medicine for chicken pox or flu symptoms before a doctor is consulted about Reye syndrome, a rare but serious illness reported to be associated with aspirin. KEEP THIS AND ALL MEDICINES OUT OF CHILDREN'S REACH. IN CASE OF ACCIDENTAL OVERDOSE, CONTACT A PHYSICIAN OR POISON CONTROL CENTER IMMEDIATELY. If dizziness, impaired hearing or ringing in the ears occurs, discontinue use. As with any drug, if you are pregnant or nursing a baby, seek the advice of a health professional before using this product.

ADMINISTRATION AND DOSAGE

Adults: Two tablets with water every 4 hours as needed. Do not exceed 8 tablets in 24 hours, or give to children under 12 unless directed by a physician.

OVERDOSE

(Symptoms and treatment) Typical of aspirin.

HOW SUPPLIED

Extra Strength Tri-Buffered BUFFERIN® is supplied as: White elongated coated tablet with "ESB" debossed on one side.
NDC 19810-0074-1 Bottle of 30's
NDC 19810-0074-2 Bottle of 60's
NDC 19810-0074-3 Bottle of 100's
All sizes have child resistant closures except 60's which is recommended for households without young children.
Store at room temperature.
Also described in PDR For Nonprescription Drugs.
Shown in Product Identification Section, page 407

COMTREX®
[cŏm'trĕx]
Multi-Symptom Cold Reliever

COMPOSITION

Each tablet, caplet, liqui-gel and fluid ounce (30 ml.) contains:
[See table below].

ACTIONS AND USES

COMTREX® tablets, caplets, liqui-gels, and liquid contain four important ingredients for safe and effective relief. A **decongestant**-pseudoephedrine HCl-(Phenylpropanolamine HCl in Liqui-Gels) to relieve nasal and sinus congestion. An **antihistamine**-chlorpheniramine maleate-to dry up runny nose. A **cough suppressant**-dextromethorphan HBr-to quiet cough. A **non-aspirin analgesic**-acetaminophen-to relieve body aches and pain.

CONTRAINDICATIONS

Hypersensitivity to acetaminophen or antihistamines.

WARNING

KEEP THIS AND ALL OTHER MEDICATIONS OUT OF THE REACH OF CHILDREN. IN CASE OF ACCIDENTAL OVERDOSE, SEEK PROFESSIONAL ASSISTANCE OR CONTACT A POISON CONTROL CENTER IMMEDIATELY. PROMPT MEDICAL ATTENTION IS CRITICAL FOR ADULTS AS WELL AS CHILDREN EVEN IF YOU DO NOT NOTICE ANY SYMPTOMS. As with any drug, if you are pregnant or nursing a baby, seek the advice of a health professional before using this product. Do not take this product for more than 7 days (for adults) or 5 days (for children), or for fever for more than 3 days unless directed by a doctor. Do not exceed recommended dosage because at higher doses nervousness, dizziness or sleeplessness may occur. May cause excitablility especially in children. A persistent cough may be a sign of a serious condition. If cough persists for more than 7 days, tends to recur, or is accompanied by rash, persistent headache, fever that lasts for more than 3 days or if new symptoms occur, consult a doctor. Do not take this product for persistent or chronic cough such as occurs with smoking, asthma or emphysema, or if cough is accompanied by excessive phlegm (mucus) unless directed by a doctor. If sore throat is severe, persists for more than 2 days, is accompanied or followed by a fever, headache, rash, nausea or vomiting, consult a doctor promptly. This product should not be taken by persons who have asthma, glaucoma, emphysema, chronic pulmonary disease, high blood pressure, heart disease, thyroid disease, diabetes, shortness of breath, difficulty in breathing or difficulty in urination due to enlargement of the prostate gland unless directed by a doctor. May cause marked drowsiness. Use caution when driving a motor vehicle or operating machinery. Avoid alcoholic beverages and do not take this product if you are taking sedatives or tranquilizers without first consulting your doctor.

DRUG INTERACTION PRECAUTION

This product should not be taken by any adult or child who is taking a prescription medication for high blood pressure or depression without first consulting a doctor.

ADMINISTRATION AND DOSAGE

Tablets or Caplets: **Adults,** 2 tablets or caplets every 4 hours as needed not to exceed 8 tablets or caplets in 24 hours. **Children** 6 to under 12 years: one tablet every 4 hours as needed, not to exceed 4 tablets or caplets in 24 hours. Under 6, consult a doctor.
Liqui-Gel: **Adults,** two liqui-gels every 4 hours as needed, not to exceed 12 liqui-gels in 24 hours. **Children** 6 to under 12 years; 1 liqui-gel every 4 hours as needed, not to exceed 6 liqui-gels in 24 hours. Under 6 consult a doctor.
Liquid: **Adults,** 1 fluid ounce (30 ml.) every 4 hours as needed, not to exceed 4 fluid ounces (120 ml.) in 24 hours. **Children** 6–12 years: ½ the adult dose. Under 6, consult a physician.

OVERDOSE

For overdose treatment information, consult a regional poison control center. (Also see Allergy-Sinus COMTREX®, Cough Formula COMPTREX®)

HOW SUPPLIED

COMTREX® is supplied as:
Yellow tablet with letter "C" debossed on one surface.
NDC 19810-0790-1 Blister packages of 24's
NDC 19810-0790-2 Bottles of 50's
Coated yellow caplet with "Comtrex" printed in red on one side.
NDC 19810-0792-3 Blister packages of 24's
NDC 19810-0792-4 Bottles of 50's
Yellow Liqui-gel with "Comtrex" printed in red on one side.
NDC 19810-0561-1 Blister packages of 24's
NDC 19810-0561-2 Blister packages of 50's
Clear orange liquid:
NDC 19810-0791-1 6 oz. plastic bottles
NDC 19810-0791-2 10 oz. plastic bottles
All sizes packaged in child resistant closures except for 24's for tablets, caplets and liqui-gels and 6 oz. liquid which are sizes recommended for households without young children. Store caplets, tablets and liquid at room temperature. Store liqui-gels below 86° F. (30° C.). Keep from freezing.
Also described in PDR For Nonprescription Drugs.
Shown in Product Identification Section, page 407

ALLERGY–SINUS COMTREX
[cŏm'trĕx]
Multi-Symptom Allergy/Sinus Formula

COMPOSITION

ACTIVE INGREDIENTS
Each coated tablet or caplet contains 500 mg acetaminophen, 30 mg pseudoephedrine HCl, 2 mg chlorpheniramine maleate.
OTHER INGREDIENTS
Benzoic acid, carnauba wax, corn starch, D&C yellow no. 10 lake, FD&C blue no. 1 lake, FD&C Red No. 40 lake, hydroxypropyl methylcellulose, mineral oil, polysorbate 20, povidone, propylene glycol, simethicone emulsion, sodium citrate, sorbitan monolaurate, stearic acid, titanium dioxide. May also contain: crospovidone, D&C yellow no. 10, erythorbic acid, FD&C blue No. 1, magnesium stearate, methylparaben, microcrystalline cellulose, polysorbate 80, propylparaben, silicon dioxide, wood cellulose.

	COMTREX Per Tablet or Caplet	COMTREX Liquid-Gel per Liqui-Gel	COMTREX Liquid Per Fl. Ounce
Acetaminophen:	325 mg.	325 mg.	650 mg.
Pseudoephedrine HCl:	30 mg.	—	60 mg.
Phenylpropanolamine HCl:	—	12.5 mg.	—
Chlorpheniramine Maleate:	2 mg.	2 mg.	4 mg.
Dextromethorphan HBr:	10 mg.	10 mg.	20 mg.

Other Ingredients:

Tablet	Caplet	Liqui-Gels	Liquid
Corn Starch	Benzoic Acid	D&C Yellow No. 10	Alcohol (20% by volume)
D&C Yellow No. 10 Lake	Carnauba Wax	FD&C Red No. 40	Citric Acid
FD&C Red No. 40 Lake	Corn Starch	Gelatin	D&C Yellow No. 10
Magnesium Stearate	D&C Yellow No. 10 Lake	Glycerin	FD&C Red No. 40
Methylparaben	FD&C Red No. 40 Lake	Polyethylene Glycol	Flavors
Propylparaben	Hydroxypropylmethylcellulose	Povidone	Polyethylene Glycol
Stearic Acid	Magnesium Stearate	Propylene Glycol	Povidone
	Methylparaben	Silicon Dioxide	Sodium Citrate
	Mineral Oil	Sorbitol	Sucrose
	Polysorbate 20	Titanium Dioxide	Water
	Povidone	Water	
	Propylene Glycol		
	Propylparaben		
	Simethicone Emulsion		
	Sorbitan Monolaurate		
	Stearic Acid		
	Titanium Dioxide		

INDICATIONS

ALLERGY-SINUS COMTREX provides temporary relief of these upper respiratory allergy, hay fever, and sinusitis symptoms: sneezing, itchy, watery eyes, runny nose, headache, nasal and sinus pressure and congestion.

PRODUCT INFORMATION

ALLERGY-SINUS COMTREX tablets and camplets contain three important ingredients for safe and effective relief. A maximum dose of **non-aspirin analgesic**-acetaminophen-to relief sinus headache pain. A **decongestant**-pseudoephedrine HCl-to relieve nasal and sinus congestion. A **antihistamine**-chlorpheniramine maleate-to relieve sneezing, runny nose, and itchy eyes.

CONTRAINDICATIONS

Hypersitivity to acetaminophen, pseudoephedrine or antihistamines.

WARNINGS

KEEP THIS AND ALL MEDICINE OUT OF CHILDREN'S REACH. In case of accidental overdose, contact a physician or Poison Control Center immediately. Do not give to children under 12 or exceed recommended dosage. Reduce dosage if nervousness, restlessness or sleeplessness occurs. Do not use for more than 10 days unless directed by a physician. Do not take without consulting a physician if under medical care. Individuals with high blood pressure, diabetes, heart or thyroid disease, asthma, glaucoma, or difficulty in urination due to enlargement of the prostate gland should not take this preparation unless directed by a physician. As with any drug, if you are pregnant or nursing a baby, seek the advice of a health professional before using this product. Do not drive or operate machinery while taking this medicine as it may cause drowsiness.

ADMINISTRATION AND DOSAGE

Adults, two tablets or caplets every 6 hours, as needed, not to exceed 8 tablets or caplets in 24 hours.

OVERDOSE

For overdose treatment information, consult a regional poison control center. (See also Comtrex Tablets, Caplets and Liquid, Cough Formula Comtrex).

HOW SUPPLIED

Allergy-Sinus COMTREX® is supplied as:
Coated green tablets with "Comtrex A/S" printed in black on one side.
NDC 19810-0774-1 Blister packages of 24's
NDC 19810-0774-2 Bottles of 50's
Coated green caplets with "A/S" debossed on one surface.
NDC 19810-0081-4 Blister packages of 24's
NDC 19810-0081-5 Bottles of 50's
All sizes packaged in child resistant closures except 24's for tablets and caplets which are sizes recommended for households without young children.
Store at room temperature.
Also described in PDR For Nonprescription Drugs.
Shown in Product Identification Section, page 407

Cough Formula COMTREX®

[cŏm'trĕx]
Multi-Symptom Cough Formula

COMPOSITION

ACTIVE INGREDIENTS

Each 4 teaspoonfuls (⅔ fl. oz.) contains:
—EXPECTORANT—200 mg Guaifenesin
—COUGH SUPPRESSANT—30 mg Dextromethorphan HBr
—ANALGESIC—500 mg Acetaminophen
—DECONGESTANT—60 MG Pseudoephedrine HCl

OTHER INGREDIENTS

Alcohol (20% by volume), Citric Acid, FD&C Red No. 40, Flavor, Menthol, Povidone, Saccharin Sodium, Sodium Citrate, Sucrose, Water.

INDICATIONS AND USES

For temporary relief of coughs, nasal and upper chest congestion fever and pain due to a chest cold.

BENEFITS OF COUGH FORMULA COMTREX

—Relieves upper chest congestion by loosening phlegm and mucus.
—Relieves your cough for up to 8 hours.
—Relieves muscle pain due to excessive coughing.
—Soothes irritated sore throat.
—Helps clear nasal passages to relieve congestion.

CONTRAINDICATIONS

Hypersitivity to Acetaminophen or Pseudoephedrine

WARNING

KEEP THIS AND ALL OTHER MEDICATIONS OUT OF THE REACH OF CHILDREN. IN CASE OF ACCIDENTAL OVERDOSE, SEEK PROFESSIONAL ASSISTANCE OR CONTACT A POISON CONTROL CENTER IMMEDIATELY. PROMPT MEDICAL ATTENTION IS CRITICAL

FOR ADULTS AS WELL AS FOR CHILDREN EVEN IF YOU DO NOT NOTICE ANY SYMPTOMS. As with any drug, if you are pregnant or nursing a baby, seek the advice of a health professional before using this product. Do not take this product for more than 7 days (for adults) or 5 days (for children) or for fever for more than 3 days unless directed by a doctor. Do not exceed recommended dosage because at higher doses nervousness, dizziness or sleeplessness may occur. A persistent cough may be a sign of a serious condition. If cough persists for more than 7 days, tends to recur or is accompanied by rash, persistent headache, fever that lasts for more than 3 days, or if new symptoms occur, consult a doctor. Do not take this product for persistent or chronic cough such as occurs with smoking, asthma, chronic bronchitis or emphysema or if cough is accompanied by excessive phlegm (mucus) unless directed by a doctor. If sore throat is severe, persists for more than 2 days, is accompanied or followed by a fever, headache, rash, nausea or vomiting, consult a doctor promptly. This product should not be taken by persons who have asthma, glaucoma, emphysema, chronic pulmonary disease, high blood pressure, thyroid disease, diabetes, shortness of breath, difficulty in breathing or difficulty in urination due to enlargement of the prostate gland unless directed by a doctor.

PRECAUTION

This product should not be taken by any adult or child who is taking a prescription medication for high blood pressure or depression without first consulting a doctor.

ADMINISTRATION AND DOSAGE

Adult Dose: (12 years and over):
Take ⅔ fl. oz. in dosage cup or four teaspoonfuls. Repeat every 6 hours as needed. No more than 4 doses in a 24-hour period.
Child Dose: (6 to under 12 years):
Take ⅓ fl. oz. in dosage cup or two teaspoonfuls. Repeat every 6 hours as needed. No more than 4 doses in a 24-hour period.
DO NOT ADMINISTER TO CHILDREN UNDER 6 YEARS OF AGE.

OVERDOSE

For overdose treatment information consult a regional poison control center.

HOW SUPPLIED

Cough Formula COMTREX® is supplied as a clear red raspberry flavored liquid:
NDC 19810-0781-1 4 oz. plastic bottle
NDC 19810-0781-3 8 oz. plastic bottle
The 4 oz. size is not child resistant and is recommended for households without young children.
Store at room temperature.
Also described in PDR For Nonprescription Drugs.
Shown in Product Identification Section, page 407

CONGESPIRIN® for Children Aspirin Free Chewable Cold Tablets

[cŏn"gĕs'pir-in]

COMPOSITION

Each tablet contains acetaminophen 81 mg. (1¼ grains), phenylephrine hydrochloride 1¼ mg. Also Contains: Calcium Stearate, D&C Red No. 30 Aluminum Lake, D&C Yellow No. 10 Aluminum Lake, Ethyl Cellulose, Flavor, Mannitol, Microcrystalline Cellulose, Polyethylene, Saccharin, Calcium, Sucrose.

ACTION AND USES

A non-aspirin analgesic/nasal decongestant that temporarily reduces fever and relieves aches, pains and nasal congestion associated with colds and "flu."

WARNINGS

KEEP THIS AND ALL MEDICINES OUT OF CHILDREN'S REACH. IN CASE OF ACCIDENTAL OVERDOSE, CONTACT A PHYSICIAN IMMEDIATELY.

CAUTION

If child is under medical care, do not administer without consulting physician. Do not exceed recommended dosage. Consult your physician if symptoms persist or if high blood pressure, heart disease, diabetes or thyroid disease is present. Do not administer for more than 10 days unless directed by physician.

DOSAGE AND ADMINISTRATION

Under 2, consult your physician.

2–3 years	2 tablets
4–5 years	3 tablets
6–8 years	4 tablets
9–10 years	5 tablets
11–12 years	6 tablets
over 12 years	8 tablets

Repeat dose in four hours if necessary. Do not give more than four doses per day unless prescribed by your physician.

OVERDOSE

For overdose treatment information consult a regional poison control center. See also: Congespirin for Children Aspirin Free Liquid Cold Medicine and Congespirin for Children Cough Syrup.

HOW SUPPLIED

CONGESPIRIN Aspirin Free Chewable Cold Tablets are supplied as scored orange tablets with "C" on one side.
NDC 19810-0748-1 Bottles of 24's.
Bottles are child resistant.
Store at room temperature.
Also described in PDR for Nonprescription Drugs.

Extra-Strength DATRIL®

[dā'trĭl]
Analgesic

COMPOSITION

Each tablet or caplet contains acetaminophen, 500 mg. Other Ingredients: (Tablets) Corn Starch, Stearic Acid. Tablets may also contain: Croscamellose Sodium, Crospovidone, Erythorbic Acid, Methylparaben, Povidone, Propylparaben, Silicon Dioxide, Sodium Lauryl Sulfate, Wood Cellulose. Caplets also contain: Carnauba Wax, Corn Starch, FD&C Blue No. 1, Hydroxypropyl Methylcellulose, Mineral Oil, Polysorbate 20, Povidone, Propylene Glycol, Simethicone Emulsion, Sorbitan Monolaurate, Stearic Acid, Titanium Dioxide. May also contain: Benzoic Acid, Croscarmellose Sodium, Crospovidone, Erythorbic Acid, Methylparaben, Propylparaben, Silicon Dioxide, Sodium Lauryl Sulfate, Wood Cellulose.

ACTIONS AND USES

Extra-Strength DATRIL contains non-aspirin acetaminophen which is less likely to irritate the stomach than plain aspirin. Extra-Strength DATRIL is intended for the temporary relief of minor aches, pains, headaches and fever. For most persons with peptic ulcer Extra-Strength DATRIL may be used when taken as directed for recommended conditions.

CONTRAINDICATIONS

There have been rare reports of skin rash or glossitis attributed to acetaminophen. Discontinue use if a sensitivity reaction occurs. However, acetaminophen is usually well tolerated by aspirin-sensitive patients.

CAUTION

Severe or recurrent pain, high or continued fever may be indicative of serious illness. Under these conditions consult a physician. **If pain persists for more than 10 days or redness is present, or in arthritic conditions affecting children under 12, consult a physician immediately.** Do not take without consulting a physician if under medical care.

WARNINGS

Keep this and all medicines out of the reach of children. In case of accidental overdose, contact a physician or Poison Control Center immediately. Do not give to children 12 and under or use for more than 10 days unless directed by a physician. As with any drug, if you are pregnant or nursing a baby, seek the advice of a health professional before using this product.

DOSAGE

Adults: Two tablets or caplets. May be repeated in 4 hours if needed. Do not exceed 8 tablets or caplets in any 24 hour period.

OVERDOSE

MUCOMYST (acetylcysteine) As An Antidote For Acetaminophen Overdose)
Acetaminophen is rapidly absorbed from the upper gastrointestinal tract with peak plasma levels occurring between 30 and 60 minutes after therapeutic doses and usually within 4 hours following an overdose. The parent compound, which is nontoxic, is extensively metabolized in the liver to form principally the sulfate and glucuronide conjugates which are also nontoxic and are rapidly excreted in the urine. A small fraction of an ingested dose is metabolized in the liver by the cytochrome P-450 mixed function oxidase enzyme system to form a reactive, potentially toxic, intermediate metabolite which preferentially conjugates with hepatic glutathione to form the nontoxic cysteine and mercapturic acid derivatives which are then excreted by the kidney. Therapeutic doses of acetaminophen do not saturate the glucuronide and sulfate conjugation pathways and do not result in the formation of sufficient reactive metabolite to deplete glutathione stores. However, following ingestion of a large overdose (150 mg/kg or greater) the glucuronide and sulfate conjugation pathways are saturated resulting in a larger fraction of the drug being metabolized via the P-450 pathway. The increased formation of reactive metabolite may deplete the hepatic stores of glutathione with subsequent binding of the metabolite to protein molecules within the hepatocyte resulting in

Continued on next page

Bristol-Myers Products—Cont.

cellular necrosis. Acetylcysteine has been shown to reduce the extent of liver injury following acetaminophen overdose. Early symptoms following a potentially hepatotoxic overdose may include: nausea, vomiting, diaphoresis and general malaise. Clinical and laboratory evidence of hepatic toxicity may not be apparent until 48 to 72 hours postingestion. In adults and adolescents, regardless of the quantity of acetaminophen reported to have been ingested, administer MUCOMYST® acetylcysteine immediately. MUCOMYST acetylcysteine therapy should be initiated and continued for a full course of therapy. Its effectiveness depends on early administration, with benefit seen principally in patients treated within 16 hours of the overdose.

If acetaminophen plasma assay capability is not available, and the estimated acetaminophen ingestion exceeds 150 mg/kg, MUCOMYST acetylcysteine therapy should be initiated and continued for a full course of therapy.

For full prescribing information, refer to the MUCOMYST package insert. Do not await the results of assays for acetaminophen level before initiating treatment with MUCOMYST acetylcysteine. The following additional procedures are recommended: The stomach should be emptied promptly by lavage or by induction of emesis with syrup of ipecac. A serum acetaminophen assay should be obtained as early as possible, but no sooner than four hours following ingestion. Liver function studies should be obtained initially and repeated at 24-hour intervals.

For additional emergency information call your regional poison center or toll-free (1-800-525-6115) to the Rocky Mountain Poison Center for assistance in diagnosis and for directions in the use of MUCOMYST acetylcysteine as an antidote.

HOW SUPPLIED

Extra Strength DATRIL® is supplied as:
White circular tablets with "DATRIL" debossed on one surface.
NDC 19810-0705-1 Bottles of 30's
NDC 19810-0705-2 Bottles of 60's
NDC 19810-0705-3 Bottles of 100's
Coated white caplet with "Datril" debossed on one side.
NDC 19810-0799-1 Bottles of 24's
NDC 19810-0799-2 Bottles of 50's
All sizes packaged in child resistant closures except 50's for caplets and 60's for tablets which are sizes recommended for households without young children.
Store at room temperature.
Also described in PDR For Nonprescription Drugs.
Shown in Product Identification Section, page 407

EXCEDRIN® Extra-Strength
Analgesic
[ĕx "cĕd 'rĭn]

COMPOSITION

Each tablet or caplet contains Acetaminophen 250 mg.; Aspirin 250 mg.; and Caffeine 65 mg.
OTHER INGREDIENTS: (Tablets) Microcrystalline Cellulose, Stearic Acid. Tablets may also contain: Hydroxypropylcellulose. **(Caplets)** Carnauba Wax, FD&C Blue No. 1, Hydroxypropyl Methylcellulose, Microcrystalline Cellulose, Mineral Oil, Polysorbate 20, Povidone, Propylene Glycol, Simethicone Emulsion, Sorbitan Monolaurate, Stearic Acid, Titanium Dioxide. Caplets may also contain: Benzoic Acid, Hydroxypropylcellulose.

ACTION AND USES

Extra-Strength EXCEDRIN is intended for the relief of pain from: headache, sinusitis, colds or 'flu', muscular aches and menstrual discomfort. Also recommended for temporary relief of toothaches and minor arthritic pains.

CONTRAINDICATIONS

Hypersensitivity to salicylates or acetaminophen.

CAUTION

If pain persists for more than 10 days, or redness is present, or in arthritic conditions affecting children under 12, consult physician immediately. Consult dentist for toothache promptly. Do not take without consulting physician if under medical care. Store at room temperature.

WARNING

Children and teenagers should not use this medicine for chicken pox or flu symptoms before a doctor is consulted about Reye syndrome, a rare but serious illness reported to be associated with aspirin. Do not exceed 8 tablets or caplets in 24 hours or use for more than 10 days unless directed by physician, or give to children under 12. KEEP THIS AND ALL MEDICINES OUT OF CHILDREN'S REACH. IN CASE OF ACCIDENTAL OVERDOSE, CONTACT A PHYSICIAN IMMEDIATELY. As with any drug, if you are pregnant or nursing a baby, seek the advice of a health professional before using this product.

ADMINISTRATION AND DOSAGE

Tablets or Caplets—Individuals 12 and over, take 2 tablets or caplets every 4 hours as needed.

OVERDOSE

For overdose treatment information, consult a regional poison control center.

HOW SUPPLIED

Extra Strength EXCEDRIN® is supplied as:
White circular tablet with letter "E" debossed on one side.
NDC 19810-0700-2 Bottles of 12's
NDC 19810-0772-9 Bottles of 30's
NDC 19810-0700-4 Bottles of 60's
NDC 19810-0700-5 Bottles of 100's
NDC 19810-0700-6 Bottles of 165's
NDC 19810-0700-7 Bottles of 225's
NDC 19810-0782-2 Bottles of 275's
NDC 19810-0700-1 A metal tin of 12's
Coated while caplets with "Excedrin" printed in red on one side.
NDC 19810-0002-1 Bottles of 24's
NDC 19810-0002-2 Bottles of 50's
NDC 19810-0002-3 Bottles of 80's
All sizes packaged in child resistant closures except 100's for tablets, 80's for caplets which are sizes recommended for households without young children.
Store at room temperature.
Also described in PDR For Nonprescription Drugs.
Shown in Product Identification Section, page 407

EXCEDRIN P.M.®
[ĕx "cĕd 'rĭn]
Analgesic Sleeping Aid

COMPOSITION

Each tablet or caplet contains Acetaminophen 500 mg. and Diphenhydramine citrate 38 mg. Tablets also Contain: Corn Starch Pregelatinized, D&C Yellow No. 10, D&C Yellow No. 10 Aluminum Lake, FD&C Blue No. 1, FD&C Blue No. 1 Aluminum Lake, Magnesium Stearate, Methylparaben, Propylparaben, Stearic Acid. May Also Contain: Microcrystalline Cellulose, Povidone.
Caplets also Contain: Benzoic Acid; Carauba Wax; Corn Starch; D&C Yellow No. 10; D&C Yellow No. 10 Aluminum Lake; FD&C Blue No. 1; FD&C Blue No. 1 Aluminum Lake; Hydroxypropyl Methylcellulose; Methylparaben; Magnesium Stearate; Propylene Glycol; Propylparaben; Simethicone Emulsion; Stearic Acid; Titanium Dioxide.

ACTION AND USES

For the temporary relief of occasional headaches and minor aches and pains with accompanying sleeplessness.

CONTRAINDICATIONS

Hypersensitivity to acetaminophen or antihistamines.

CAUTION

Do not drive a car or operate machinery while taking this medication. Do not take without consulting physician if under medical care.

WARNING

KEEP THIS AND ALL MEDICINES OUT OF CHILDREN'S REACH. IN CASE OF ACCIDENTAL OVERDOSE, CONTACT A PHYSICIAN IMMEDIATELY. Do not give to children under 12 years of age or use for more than 10 days unless directed by a physician. Consult your physician if symptoms persist or new ones occur or if fever persists more than 3 days (72 hours) or recurs, or if sleeplessness persists continuously for more than two weeks. Insomnia may be a symptom of serious underlying medical illness. Take this product with caution if alcohol is being consumed. DO NOT TAKE THIS PRODUCT IF YOU HAVE ASTHMA, GLAUCOMA OR ENLARGEMENT OF THE PROSTATE GLAND EXCEPT UNDER THE ADVICE AND SUPERVISION OF A PHYSICIAN. As with any drug, if you are pregnant or nursing a baby, seek the advice of a health professional before using this product.

ADMINISTRATION AND DOSAGE

Adults take two tablets at bedtime or as directed by a physician. Do not exceed recommended dosage.

OVERDOSE

For overdose treatment information, consult a regional poison control center.

HOW SUPPLIED

EXCEDRIN P.M.® is supplied as:
Light blue circular tablets with "PM" debossed on one side.
NDC 19810-0763-6 Bottles of 10's
NDC 19810-0763-3 Bottles of 30's
NDC 19810-0763-4 Bottles of 50's
NDC 19810-0763-5 Bottles of 80's
Light blue coated caplet with "Exedrin P.M." imprinted on one side.

NDC 19810-0032-2 Bottles of 30's
NDC 19810-0032-3 Bottles of 50's
All sizes packaged in child resistant closures except 50's which is recommended for households without young children.
Store at room temperature.
Also described in PDR For Nonprescription Drugs.

Sinus EXCEDRIN®
[ex "cĕd 'rĭn]
Analgesic, Decongestant

COMPOSITION

Each coated tablet or caplet contains 500 mg Acetaminophen and 30 mg Pseudoephedrine HCl.

OTHER INGREDIENTS

Corn Starch, D&C Yellow No. 10 Lake, FD&C Red No. 40 Lake, Hydroxypropylcellulose, Hydroxypropyl Methylcellulose, Mineral Oil, Polysorbate 20, Povidone, Propylene Glycol, Simethicone Emulsion, Sorbitan Monolaurate, Stearic Acid, Titanium Dioxide. May also contain: Benzoic Acid, Carnauba Wax.

ACTION AND USES

Sinus EXCEDRIN is intended for the temporary relief of headache and sinus pain and for the relief of sinus pressure due to sinusitis or the common cold.

CONTRAINDICATIONS

Hypersensitivity to acetaminophen or pseudoephedrine.

WARNINGS

KEEP THIS AND ALL MEDICINES OUT OF CHILDREN'S REACH. In case of accidental overdose, contact a physician or Poison Control Center immediately. Do not exceed recommended dosage. Reduce dosage if nervousness, dizziness or sleeplessness occurs. Do not take this product for more than 7 days. If symptoms do not improve or are accompanied by a fever, consult a doctor. If you have heart disease, diabetes, high blood pressure, thyroid disease or difficulty in urination due to enlargement of the prostrate gland, or are presently taking a prescription drug for high blood pressure or depression, do not take this medicine unless directed by a physician. As with any drug, if you are pregnant or nursing a baby, seek the advice of a health professional before using this product.

ADMINISTRATION AND DOSAGE

Adults and Children over 12: two tablets or caplets every 6 hours as needed, not to exceed 8 tablets or caplets in 24 hours. Children 12 and under should use only as directed by a doctor.

HOW SUPPLIED

Sinus EXCEDRIN® is supplied as:
Coated circular orange tablets with "Sinus Excedrin" imprinted in green on one side.
NDC 19810-0080-1 Blister packages of 24's
NDC 19810-0080-2 Bottles of 50's
Coated orange caplets with "Sinus Excedrin" imprinted in green on one side.
NDC 19810-0077-1 Blister packages of 24's
NDC 19810-0077-2 Bottles of 50's
All sizes have child resistant closures except 24's for tablets and caplets which are recommended for households without young children.
Store at room temperature.
Also described in PDR For Nonprescription Drugs.

4—WAY® Cold Tablets

COMPOSITION

"New Aspirin-Free Formula"
Each tablet contains acetaminophen 325 mg., phenylpropanolamine HCl 12.5 mg., and chlorpheniramine maleate 2 mg.
Other Ingredients: Corn Starch, Corn Starch Pregelatinized, Microcrystalline Cellulose, Sodium Starch Glycolate, Stearic Acid, Sucrose.

ACTIONS AND USES

For temporary relief of 1) nasal congestion, 2) runny nose, 3) fever, and 4) minor aches and pains as may occur in the common cold.

DOSAGE AND ADMINISTRATION

Adults—2 tablets every 4 hours, as needed. Do not exceed 12 tablets in 24 hours. Children 6 to under 12 years—one half the adult dosage.

CAUTION

Do not drive or operate machinery while taking this medication as it may cause drowsiness.

WARNING

Keep this and all medicines out of children's reach. In case of accidental overdose, contact a physician or poison control center immediately. Do not exceed the recommended dosage.

Do not give to children under 6 or use for more than 10 days (for adults) or 5 days (for children) unless directed by a physician. If symptoms do not improve or are accompanied by fever that lasts for mroe than 3 days or if new symptoms occur, consult a doctor. Persons with high blood pressure, diabetes, heart or thyroid disease, asthma, glaucoma, or difficulty in urination due to enlargement of the prostate gland or persons under a doctor's care should not use this preparation unless directed by a physician. May cause excitablity in children. Reduce dosage if nervousness, restlessness, or sleeplessness occurs. As with any drug, if you are pregnant or nursing a baby, seek the advice of a health professional before using this product. Do not drive a car or operate machinery while taking this medicine as it may cause drowsiness.

DRUG INTERACTION PRECAUTION

Do not take this product if you are presently taking a prescription drug for high blood pressure or depression without first consulting your doctor.

HOW SUPPLIED

4-WAY Cold Tablets are supplied as a white tablet with the number "4" debossed on one surface.
NDC 19810-0040-1 Bottle of 36's
NDC 19810-0040-2 Bottle of 60's
All sizes packaged in child resistant bottle closures.
Store at room temperature.
Also described in PDR For Nonprescription Drugs.

4-WAY® Fast Acting Nasal Spray

COMPOSITION

Phenylephrine hydrochloride 0.5%, naphazoline hydrochloride 0.05%, pyrilamine maleate 0.2%, in a buffered isotonic aqueous solution with thimerosal 0.005% added as a preservative. Also Contains: Benzalkonium Chloride, Poloxamer 188, Potassium Phosphate, Sodium Chloride, Sodium Phosphate, Water. Also available in a mentholated formula containing Phenylephrine hydrochloride 0.5%, naphazoline hydrochloride 0.05%, pyrilamine maleate 0.2%, in a buffered isotonic aqueous solution with thimerosal 0.005% added as a preservative. Also Contains: Benzalkonium Chloride, Camphor, Eucalyptol, Menthol, Poloxamer 188, Polysorbate 80, Potassium Phosphate, Sodium Chloride, Sodium Phosphate, Water.

ACTION AND USES

For prompt, temporary relief of nasal congestion due to the common cold, sinusitis, hay fever or other upper respiratory allegeries.

DOSAGE AND ADMINISTRATION

DOSAGE: Adults: Spray twice into each nostril. Repeat every 6 hours if needed. Do not give to children under 12 years of age unless directed by physician. **DIRECTIONS:** Remove protective cap. Hold bottle with thumb at base and nozzle between first and second fingers. With head upright, insert metered pump spray nozzle into nostril. Depress pump twice, all the way down, with a firm even stroke. Do not tilt head backward while spraying. Wipe tip clean after each use.

WARNING

Do not exceed recommended dosage because symptoms may occur such as burning, stinging, sneezing or increase of nasal discharge. Overdosage in young children may cause marked sedation. Follow directions carefully. Do not use this product for more than 3 days. If symptoms persist, consult a physician. The use of this dispenser by more than one person may spread infection. Store at room temperature. Keep this and all medicines out of children's reach. In case of accidental ingestion, contact a physician or Poison Control Center immediately.

OVERDOSAGE

For overdose treatment information, contact a regional poison control center.

HOW SUPPLIED

4-WAY® Fast Acting Nasal Spray is supplied as:
Regular formula:
NDC 19810-0001-1 Atomizer of ½ fluid ounce.
NDC 19810-0001-2 Atomizer of 1 fluid ounce.
NDC 19810-0001-3 Metered pump of ½ fluid ounce.
Mentholated formula:
NDC 19810-0003-1 Atomizer of ½ fluid ounce.
NDC 19810-0003-2 Atomizer of 1 fluid ounce.
Store at room temperature.
Also described in the PDR for Nonprescription Drugs.

4-WAY® Long Lasting Nasal Spray

COMPOSITION

Oxymetazoline Hydrochloride 0.05% in a buffered isotonic aqueous solution. Phenylmercuric Acetate 0.002% added as a preservative. Also Contains: Benzalkonium Chloride, Glycine, Sorbitol, Water.

ACTION AND USES

Provides temporary relief of nasal congestion due to the common cold, sinusitis, hayfever or other upper respiratory allergies.

DOSAGE AND ADMINISTRATION

DOSAGE: Adults—and children 6 years of age and older (with adult supervision): Spray 2 or 3 times into each nostril twice daily—once in the morning and once in the evening. Not recommended for children under 6. **DIRECTIONS:** Remove protective cap. Hold bottle with thumb at base and nozzle between first and second fingers. With head upright, insert metered pump spray nozzle into nostril. Depress pump 2 or 3 times, all the way down, with a firm even stroke and sniff deeply. Repeat in other nostril. Do not tilt head backward while spraying. Wipe tip clean after each use.

WARNING

Do not give this product to children under 6 years of age except under the advice and supervision of a physician. Do not exceed recommended dosage because symptoms may occur such as burning, stinging, sneezing or increase of nasal discharge. Do not use this product for more than 3 days. If symptoms persist, consult a physician. The use of this dispenser by more than one person may spread infection. Store at room temperature. Keep this and all medicines out of children's reach. In case of accidental ingestion, contact a physician or Poison Control Center immediately.

OVERDOSAGE

For overdose treatment information, contact a regional poison control center.

HOW SUPPLIED

4-WAY Long Lasting Nasal Spray is supplied as:
Atomizers and a metered pump:
NDC 19810-0728-1 Atomizers of ½ fluid ounce.
NDC 19810-0728-3 Metered pump of ½ fluid ounce.
Store at room temperature.
Also described in the PDR for Nonprescription Drugs.

NO DOZ® Tablets
[nō'dōz]

COMPOSITION

Each tablet contains 100 mg. Caffeine. Other Ingredients: Cornstarch, Flavors, Mannitol, Microcrystalline Cellulose, Stearic Acid, Sucrose.

INDICATIONS

Helps restore mental alertness or wakefulness when experiencing fatigue or drowsiness.

DOSAGE AND ADMINISTRATION

Adults and children 12 years of age and over: One or two tablets not more often than every 3 to 4 hours.

CAUTION

Do not take without consulting physician if under medical care. No stimulant should be substituted for normal sleep in activities requiring physical alertness.

WARNING

For occasional use only. Not intended for use as a substitute for sleep. If fatigue or drowsiness persists or continues to recur, consult a doctor. The recommended dose of this product contains about as much caffeine as a cup of coffee. Limit the use of caffeine-containing medications, foods, or beverages while taking this product because too much caffeine may cause nervousness, irritability, sleeplessness and, occasionally, rapid heart beat. Do not give to children under 12 years of age. **KEEP THIS AND ALL MEDICINES OUT OF THE REACH OF CHILDREN. IN CASE OF ACCIDENTAL OVERDOSE, SEEK PROFESSIONAL ASSISTANCE OR CONTACT A POISON CONTROL CENTER IMMEDIATELY.** As with any drug, if you are pregnant or nursing a baby, seek the advice of a health professional before using this product.

OVERDOSE

Typical of caffeine.

HOW SUPPLIED

NO DOZ® is supplied as:
A circular white tablet with "NoDoz" debossed on one side.
NDC 19810-0063-2 Blister pack of 16's
NDC 19810-0063-3 Blister pack of 36's
NDC 19810-0062-5 Bottle of 60's
Store at room temperature.
Also described in the PDR for Nonprescription Drugs.

NUPRIN®
(ibuprofen)
Analgesic

WARNING

ASPIRIN SENSITIVE PATIENTS should not take this product if they have had a severe allergic reaction to aspirin, e.g.—asthma, swelling, shock or hives, because even though this product contains no aspirin or salicylates, cross-reactions may occur in patients allergic to aspirin.

COMPOSITION

Each tablet or caplet contains ibuprofen USP, 200 mg. **Other Ingredients:** Carnauba wax, cornstarch, D&C Yellow No. 10, FD&C Yellow No. 6, hydroxypropyl methylcellulose, propylene glycol, silicon dioxide, stearic acid, titanium dioxide.

ACTION AND USES

For the temporary relief of minor aches and pains associated with the common cold, headache, toothache, muscular aches, backache, for the minor pain of arthritis, for the pain of menstrual cramps and for reduction of fever.

WARNINGS

The following warnings are stated on the Nuprin label: Do not take for pain for more than 10 days or for fever for more than 3 days unless directed by a doctor. If pain or fever persists or gets worse, if new symptoms occur, or if the painful area is red or swollen, consult a doctor. These could be signs of serious illness. If you are under a doctor's care for any serious condition, consult a doctor before taking this product. As with aspirin and acetaminophen, if you have any condition which requires you to take prescription drugs or if you have had any problems or serious side effects from taking any non-prescription pain reliever, do not take NUPRIN without first discussing it with your doctor. If you experience any symptoms which are unusual or seem unrelated to the condition for which you took ibuprofen, consult a doctor before taking any more of it. Although ibuprofen is indicated for the same conditions as aspirin and acetaminophen, it should not be taken with them except under a doctor's direction. Do not combine this product with any other ibuprofen-containing product. As with any drug, if you are pregnant or nursing a baby, seek the advice of a health professional before using this product. IT IS ESPECIALLY IMPORTANT NOT TO USE IBUPROFEN DURING THE LAST 3 MONTHS OF PREGNANCY UNLESS SPECIFICALLY DIRECTED TO DO SO BY A DOCTOR BECAUSE IT MAY CAUSE PROBLEMS IN THE UNBORN CHILD OR COMPLICATIONS DURING DELIVERY. Keep this and all drugs out of the reach of children. In case of accidental overdose, seek professional assistance or contact a poison control center immediately.

CAUTION

Store at room temperature. Avoid excessive heat 40°C (104°F).

ADMINISTRATION AND DOSAGE

Directions. Adults: Take 1 tablet or caplet every 4 to 6 hours while symptoms persist. If pain or fever does not respond to 1 tablet or caplet, 2 tablets or caplets may be used but do not exceed 6 tablets or caplets in 24 hours, unless directed by a doctor. The smallest effective dose should be used. Take with food or milk if occasional and mild heartburn, upset stomach, or stomach pain occurs with use. Consult a doctor if these symptoms are more than mild or if they persist. Children: Do not give this product to children under 12 except under the advice and supervision of a doctor.

OVERDOSAGE

For overdose treatment information, consult a regional poison control center.

HOW SUPPLIED

NUPRIN® is supplied as:
Golden yellow round tablets with "NUPRIN" printed in black on one side.
NDC 19810-0767-5 Blister card of 8's
NDC 19810-0767-2 Bottles of 24's
NDC 19810-0767-3 Bottles of 50's
NDC 19810-0767-4 Bottles of 100's
NDC 19810-0767-7 Bottles of 150's
NDC 19810-0767-8 Bottles of 225's
Golden yellow caplets with "NUPRIN" printed in black on one side.
NDC 19810-0796-1 Bottles of 24's
NDC 19810-0796-2 Bottles of 50's
NDC 19810-0796-3 Bottles of 100's
All sizes packaged in child resistant closures except 24's for tablets and 24's for caplets, which are sizes recommended for households without young children.
Store at room temperature. Avoid excessive heat 40°C. (104°F.).
Distributed by Bristol-Myers Company
Also described in the PDR For Nonprescription Drugs.
Shown in Product Identification Section, page 407

PAZO® Hemorrhoid
Ointment/Suppositories

COMPOSITION

Ointment: Triolyte®, [Bristol-Myers brand of the combination of benzocaine (0.8%) and ephedrine sulphate (0.2%)];

Continued on next page

Bristol-Myers Products—Cont.

zinc oxide (4.0%); camphor (2.18%). Also Contains: Lanolin, Petrolatum.

Suppositories (per suppository): Triolyte® [Bristol-Myers brand of the combination of benzocaine (15.44 mg) and ephedrine sulfate(3.86 mg)]; zinc oxide (77.2 mg); camphor (42.07 mg). Also Contains: Hydrogenated Vegetable Oil.

ACTION AND USES
Pazo helps shrink swelling of inflamed hemorrhoid tissue. Provides prompt, temporary relief of burning itch and pain in many cases.

ADMINISTRATION
Ointment—Apply Pazo well up in rectum night and morning, and after each bowel movement. Repeat as often during the day as may be necessary to maintain comfort. Continue for one week after symptoms subside. When applicator is used, lubricate applicator first with Pazo. Insert slowly, then simply press tube.
Suppositories—Remove foil and insert one Pazo suppository night and morning, and after each bowel movement. Repeat as often during the day as may be necessary to maintain comfort. Continue for one week after symptoms subside.

WARNING
If the underlying condition persists or recurs frequently, despite treatment, or if any bleeding or hard irreducible swelling is present, consult your physician.
Keep out of children's reach. Keep in a cool place.

HOW SUPPLIED
PAZO® ointment is supplied with a plastic applicator as:
NDC 19810-0768-1 One ounce tubes
NDC 19810-0768-2 Two ounce tubes
PAZO® suppositories are silver foil wrapped and supplied as:
NDC 19810-0703-1 Box of 12's
NDC 19810-0703-2 Box of 24's
Keep in a cool place.
Also described in the PDR For Nonprescription Drugs.

THERAPEUTIC MINERAL ICE

ACTIVE INGREDIENT
Menthol.
The cool blue Therapeutic Mineral Ice gel base is specially formulated to dry quickly with no grease or lingering unpleasant odor.

INDICATIONS
An external pain relieving coolant gel for the temporary relief of minor aches and pains of muscles and joints associated with arthritis, simple backache, strains, bruises, sprains and sports injuries. **USE ONLY AS DIRECTED. Read all warnings before use.**

WARNING
KEEP OUT OF THE REACH OF CHILDREN. For external use only. Not for internal use. Avoid contact with eyes and mucous membranes. Do not use with other ointments, creams, sprays, or liniments. **Do not use with Heating Pads or Heating Devices.** If condition worsens, or if symptoms persist for more than 7 days, or clear up and occur again within a few days, discontinue use of this product and consult your doctor. Do not apply to wounds or damaged skin. Do not bandage tightly. If you have sensitive skin, consult doctor **before** use. If skin irritation develops, discontinue use and consult your doctor. As with any drug, if you are pregnant or nursing a baby, seek the advice of a health professional **before** using this product. Store in a cool place. Keep lid tightly closed. Do not use, pour, spill or store near heat or open flame. **Note:** you can always use Mineral Ice as directed, but its use is never intended to replace your doctor's advice.

DIRECTIONS
Adults and children 2 years of age and older: Clean skin of all other ointments, creams, sprays, or liniments. Apply to affected areas not more than 3 to 4 times daily. May be used with wet or dry bandages or with ice packs. Not greasy. No protective cover needed.
Children: Do not use on children under 2 years of age, except under the advice and supervision of a doctor.

HOW SUPPLIED
Available in 3.5 oz., 8 oz., and 16 oz. containers.
Shown in Product Identification Section, page 407

The Brown Pharmaceutical Company, Inc.
See ICN PHARMACEUTICALS, INC.

Burroughs Wellcome Co.
**3030 CORNWALLIS ROAD
RESEARCH TRIANGLE PARK,
NC 27709**

LITERATURE AVAILABLE: Folders, packaging inserts, file cards, films, slides, lecture guides, monographs, cassettes, videos and continuing education material.

ACTIDIL® Tablets and Syrup
[ăk ′tuh-dĭl]
Antihistamine

(See PDR For Nonprescription Drugs)
Tablets shown in Product Identification Section, page 407

ACTIFED® Tablets, Syrup, Capsules and 12-Hour Capsules
[ăk ′tĭ-fĕd]
Antihistamine/Nasal Decongestant

(See PDR For Nonprescription Drugs)
Tablets, Capsules and 12-Hour Capsules shown in Product Identification Section, page 407

ACTIFED® with CODEINE　　　　　　℞ ℂ
[ăk ′tĭ-fed]
Cough Syrup

DESCRIPTION
Each 5 ml (1 teaspoonful) contains: codeine phosphate 10 mg (Warning—may be habit-forming), Actidil® (triprolidine hydrochloride) 1.25 mg, Sudafed® (pseudoephedrine hydrochloride) 30 mg and the inactive ingredients: alcohol 4.3%, sodium benzoate 0.1% and methylparaben 0.1% (added as preservatives), flavors, glycerin, and sorbitol. This medication is intended for oral administration.
Actifed with Codeine Cough Syrup has antitussive, antihistaminic and nasal decongestant effects. The components of Actifed with Codeine Cough Syrup have the following chemical names.
Codeine Phosphate, U.S.P.:
7,8-didehydro-4,5α-epoxy-3-methoxy-17-methyl-morphinan-6α-ol phosphate (1:1) (salt) hemihydrate
Triprolidine Hydrochloride Monohydrate:
(E)-2-[3-(1-pyrrolidinyl)-1-(p-tolyl)propenyl]pyridine monohydrochloride monohydrate
Pseudoephedrine Hydrochloride:
[S-(R *,R *)]-α-[1-(methylamino)ethyl]benzenemethanol hydrochloride

CLINICAL PHARMACOLOGY
Codeine: Codeine probably exerts its antitussive activity by depressing the medullary (brain) cough center, thereby raising its threshold for incoming cough impulses.
Codeine is readily absorbed from the gastrointestinal tract, with a therapeutic dose reaching peak antitussive effectiveness in about 2 hours and persisting for 4 to 6 hours. Codeine is rapidly distributed from blood to body tissues and taken up preferentially by parenchymatous organs such as liver, spleen and kidney. It passes the blood brain barrier and is found in fetal tissue and breast milk.
The drug is not bound by plasma proteins nor is it accumulated in body tissues. Codeine is metabolized in the liver to morphine and norcodeine, each representing about 10 percent of the administered codeine dose. About 90 percent of the dose is excreted within 24 hours, primarily through the kidneys. Urinary excretion products are free and glucuronide-conjugated codeine (about 70%), free and conjugated norcodeine (about 10%), free and conjugated morphine (about 10%), normorphine (under 4%) and hydrocodone (< 1%). The remainder of the dose appears in the feces.
Triprolidine: Antihistamines such as triprolidine hydrochloride act as antagonists of the H₁ histamine receptor. Consequently, they prevent histamine from eliciting typical immediate hypersensitivity responses in the nose, eyes, lungs and skin.

Animal distribution studies have shown localization of triprolidine in lung, spleen and kidney tissue. Liver microsome studies have revealed the presence of several metabolites with an oxidized product of the toluene methyl group predominating.
Pseudoephedrine: Pseudoephedrine acts as an indirect sympathomimetic agent by stimulating sympathetic (adrenergic) nerve endings to release norepinephrine. Norepinephrine in turn stimulates alpha and beta receptors throughout the body. The action of pseudoephedrine hydrochloride is apparently more specific for the blood vessels of the upper respiratory tract and less specific for the blood vessels of the systemic circulation. The vasoconstriction elicited at these sites results in the shrinkage of swollen tissues in the sinuses and nasal passages.
Pseudoephedrine is rapidly and almost completely absorbed from the gastrointestinal tract. Considerable variation in half-life has been observed (from about 4½ to 10 hours), which is attributed to individual differences in absorption and excretion. Excretion rates are also altered by urine pH, increasing with acidification and decreasing with alkalinization. As a result, mean half-life falls to about 4 hours at pH 5 and increases to 12 to 13 hours at pH 8.
After administration of a 60 mg tablet, 87 to 96% of the pseudoephedrine is cleared from the body within 24 hours. The drug is distributed to body tissues and fluids, including fetal tissue, breast milk and the central nervous system (CNS). About 55 to 75% of an administered dose is excreted unchanged in the urine; the remainder is apparently metabolized in the liver to inactive compounds by N-demethylation, parahydroxylation and oxidative deamination.
The pharmacokinetic properties of codeine, triprolidine and pseudoephedrine from 10 ml of Actifed with Codeine Cough Syrup were investigated compared to a reference preparation of equal component doses in 18 healthy adults. The results of this study showed that Actifed with Codeine Cough Syrup and the reference preparation were bioequivalent.
Pharmacokinetic parameters for Actifed with Codeine Cough Syrup are as follows:
[See table below].

INDICATIONS AND USAGE
Actifed with Codeine Cough Syrup is indicated for temporary relief of coughs and upper respiratory symptoms, including nasal congestion, associated with allergy or the common cold.

CONTRAINDICATIONS
Actifed with Codeine Cough Syrup is contraindicated under the following conditions:
Use in Newborn or Premature Infants: This drug should *not* be used in newborn or premature infants.
Use in Lower Respiratory Disease: Antihistamines should *not* be used to treat lower respiratory tract symptoms, including asthma.
Hypersensitivity to: 1) codeine phosphate or other narcotics; 2) triprolidine hydrochloride or other antihistamines of similar chemical structure; or 3) sympathomimetic amines, including pseudoephedrine.
Sympathomimetic amines are contraindicated in patients with severe hypertension, severe coronary artery disease and in patients on monoamine oxidase (MAO) inhibitor therapy (see Drug Interaction Section).

WARNINGS
Actifed with Codeine Cough Syrup should be used with considerable caution in patients with increased intraocular pressure (narrow angle glaucoma), stenosing peptic ulcer, pyloroduodenal obstruction, symptomatic prostatic hypertrophy, bladder neck obstruction, hypertension, diabetes mellitus, ischemic heart disease, and hyperthyroidism.
In the presence of head injury or other intracranial lesions, the respiratory depressant effects of codeine and other narcotics may be markedly enhanced, as well as their capacity for elevating cerebrospinal fluid pressue.
Narcotics also produce other CNS depressant effects, such as drowsiness, that may further obscure the clinical course of patients with head injuries.
Codeine or other narcotics may obscure signs on which to judge the diagnosis or clinical course of patients with acute abdominal conditions.

Parameter	Codeine*	Triprolidine†	Pseudoephedrine‡
Elimination Half Life (hr)	2.7 ± 0.4§	4.0 ± 2.2	5.5 ± 0.9
Time to Maximum Concentration (hr)	1.2 ± 0.5	1.8 ± 0.7	2.6 ± 1.0
Maximum Plasma Concentration (ng/ml)	44.8 ± 11.7	4.9 ± 1.8	189 ± 44
Area Under Plasma Curve from t = 0 to t = ∞ (ng/ml·hr)	226 ± 41	42.5 ± 34.0	1938 ± 440

* 20 mg Codeine Phosphate hemihydrate (equivalent to 14.7 mg free base)
† 2.5 mg Triprolidine HCl monohydrate (equivalent to 2.1 mg free base)
‡ 60 mg Pseudoephedrine HCl (equivalent to 49.1 mg free base)
§ Means ± S.D.

PRECAUTIONS

General: Actifed with Codeine Cough Syrup should be prescribed with caution for certain special-risk patients, such as the eldery or debilitated, and for those with severe impairment of renal or hepatic function, gallbladder disease or gallstones, respiratory impairment, cardiac arrhythmias, history of bronchial asthma, prostatic hypertrophy or urethral stricture, and in patients known to be taking other antitussive, antihistamine or decongestant medications. Patients' self-medication habits should be investigated to determine their use of such medications. Actifed with Codeine Cough Syrup is intended for short-term use only.

Information for Patients:

1. Patients should be warned about engaging in activities requiring mental alertness such as driving a car, operating dangerous machinery or hazardous appliances.
2. Patients with a history of glaucoma, peptic ulcer, urinary retention or pregnancy should be cautioned before starting Actifed.
3. Patients should be told not to take alcohol, sleeping pills, sedatives or tranquilizers while taking Actifed.
4. Antihistamines as in Actifed, may cause dizziness, drowsiness, dry mouth, blurred vision, weakness, nausea, headache or nervousness in some patients.
5. Patients should be told to store this medicine in a tightly closed container in a dry, cool place away from heat or direct sunlight and out of the reach of children.
6. **Nursing Mothers** refer to following section titled "Nursing Mothers."

Actifed with Codeine Cough Syrup should not be used by persons intolerant to sympathomimetics used for the relief of nasal or sinus congestion. Such drugs include ephedrine, epinephrine, phenylpropanolamine, and phenylephrine. Symptoms of intolerance include drowsiness, dizziness, weakness, difficulty in breathing, tenseness, muscle tremors or palpitations.

Codeine may be habit-forming when used over long periods or in high doses. Patients should take the drug only for as long, in the amounts, and as frequently as prescribed.

Drug Interactions: Actifed with Codeine Cough Syrup may **enhance** the effects of:

1. monoamine oxidase (MAO) inhibitors;
2. other narcotic analgesics, alcohol, general anesthetics, tranquilizers, sedative-hypnotics, surgical skeletal muscle relaxants, or other CNS depressants, by causing increased CNS depression.

Actifed with Codeine Cough Syrup may **diminish:**
the antihypertensive effects of guanethidine, bethanidine, methyldopa, and reserpine.

Drug/Laboratory Test Interactions:
Codeine: Narcotic administration may increase serum amylase levels.

Carcinogenesis, Mutagenesis, Impairment of Fertility: No adequate studies have been conducted in animals to determine whether the components of Actifed with Codeine Cough Syrup have a potential for carcinogenesis, mutagenesis or impairment of fertility.

Pregnancy: *Teratogenic Effects:* Pregnancy Category C. Animal reproduction studies have not been conducted with Actifed with Codeine Cough Syrup. It is also not known whether Actifed with Codeine Cough Syrup can cause fetal harm when administered to a pregnant woman or can affect reproduction capacity. Actifed with Codeine Cough Syrup should be given to a pregnant woman only if clearly needed. Teratology studies have been conducted with three ingredients of Actifed with Codeine Cough Syrup. Pseudoephedrine studies were conducted in rats at doses up to 150 times the human dose; triprolidine was studied in rats and rabbits at doses up to 125 times the human dose, and codeine studies were conducted in rats and rabbits at doses up to 150 times the human dose. No evidence of teratogenic harm to the fetus was revealed in any of these studies. However, overt signs of toxicity were observed in the dams which received pseudoephedrine. This was reflected in reduced average weight and length and rate of skeletal ossification in their fetuses.

Nursing Mothers: The components of Actifed with Codeine Cough Syrup are excreted in breast milk in small amounts, but the significance of their effects on nursing infants is not known. Because of the potential for serious adverse reactions in nursing infants from maternal ingestion of Actifed with Codeine Cough Syrup, a decision should be made whether to discontinue nursing or to discontinue the drug, taking into account the importance of the drug to the mother.

Pediatric Use: As in adults, the combination of an antihistamine, sympathomimetic amine and codeine can elicit either mild stimulation or mild sedation in children. In infants and children particularly, the ingredients in this drug product **in overdosage** may produce hallucinations, convulsions and death. Symptoms of toxicity in children may include fixed dilated pupils, flushed face, dry mouth, fever, excitation, hallucinations, ataxia, incoordination, athetosis, tonic clonic convulsions and postictal depression, (see CONTRAINDICATIONS and OVERDOSAGE sections).

Use in Elderly (approximately 60 years or older): The ingredients in Actifed with Codeine Cough Syrup are more likely to cause adverse reactions in elderly patients.

ADVERSE REACTIONS

(The most frequent adverse reactions are underlined.)

General: Dryness of mouth, dryness of nose, dryness of throat, urticaria, drug rash, anaphylactic shock, photosensitivity, excessive perspiration and chills.
Cardiovascular System: Hypotension, headache, palpitations, tachycardia, extrasystoles.
Hematologic System: Hemolytic anemia, thrombocytopenia, agranulocytosis.
Nervous System: Sedation, sleepiness, dizziness, disturbed coordination, fatigue, confusion, restlessness, excitation, anxiety, nervousness, tremor, irritability, insomnia, euphoria, paresthesias, blurred vision, diplopia, vertigo, tinnitus, acute labyrinthitis, hysteria, neuritis, convulsions, CNS depression, hallucination.
G.I. System: Epigastric distress, anorexia, nausea, vomiting, diarrhea, constipation.
G.U. System: Urinary frequency, difficult urination, urinary retention, early menses.
Respiratory System: Thickening of bronchial secretions, tightness of chest and wheezing, nasal stuffiness, respiratory depression.

DRUG ABUSE AND DEPENDENCE

Like other medications containing a narcotic, Actifed with Codeine Cough Syrup is controlled by the Drug Enforcement Administration. It is classified under Schedule V.

Actifed with Codeine Cough Syrup can produce drug dependence of the morphine type, and therefore it has a potential for being abused. Psychic dependence, physical dependence and tolerance may develop on repeated administration.

The dependence liability of codeine has been found to be too small to permit a full definition of its characteristics. Studies indicate that addiction to codeine is extremely uncommon and requires very high parenteral doses.

When dependence on codeine occurs at therapeutic doses, it appears to require from one to two months to develop, and withdrawal symptoms are mild. Most patients on long-term oral codeine therapy show no signs of physical dependence upon abrupt withdrawal.

OVERDOSAGE

Since Actifed with Codeine Cough Syrup is comprised of three pharmacologically different compounds, it is difficult to predict the exact manifestation of symptoms in a given individual. Reaction to an overdosage of Actifed with Codeine Cough Syrup may vary from CNS depression to stimulation. A detailed description of symptoms which are likely to appear after ingestion of an excess of the individual components follows:

Overdosage with codeine can cause transient euphoria, drowsiness, dizziness, weariness, diminution of sensibility, loss of sensation, vomiting, transient excitement in children and occasionally in adult women, miosis progressing to nonreactive pinpoint pupils, itching sometimes with skin rashes and urticaria, and clammy skin with mottled cyanosis. In more severe cases, muscular relaxation with depressed or absent superficial and deep reflexes and a positive Babinski sign may appear. Marked slowing of the respiratory rate with inadequate pulmonary ventilation and consequent cyanosis may occur. Terminal signs include shock, pulmonary edema, hypostatic or aspiration pneumonia and respiratory arrest, with death occurring within 6–12 hours following ingestion.

Overdoses of antihistamines may cause hallucinations, convulsions, or possibly death, especially in infants and children. Antihistamines are more likely to cause dizziness, sedation, and hypotension in elderly patients.

Overdosage with triprolidine may produce reactions varying from depression to stimulation of the Central Nervous System (CNS); the latter is particularly likely in children. Atropine-like signs and symptoms (dry mouth, fixed dilated pupils, flushing, tachycardia, hallucinations, convulsions, urinary retention, cardiac arrthymias and coma) may occur.

Overdosage with pseudoephedrine can cause excessive CNS stimulation resulting in excitement, nervousness, anxiety, tremor, restlessness and insomnia. Other effects include tachycardia, hypertension, pallor, mydriasis, hyperglycemia and urinary retention. Severe overdosage may cause tachypnea or hyperpnea, hallucinations, convulsions, or delirium, but in some individuals there may be CNS depression with somnolence, stupor or respiratory depression. Arrhythmias (including ventricular fibrillation) may lead to hypotension and circulatory collapse. Severe hypokalemia can occur, probably due to compartmental shift rather than depletion of potassium. No organ damage or significant metabolic derangement is associated with pseudoephedrine overdosage.

The toxic plasma concentration of codeine is not known with certainty. Experimental production of mild to moderate CNS depression in healthy, nontolerant subjects occurs at plasma concentrations of 0.5–1.9 µg/ml when codeine is given by

intravenous infusion. The single lethal dose of codeine in adults is estimated to be from 0.5 to 1.0 gram. It is also estimated that 5 mg/kg could be fatal in children.

The LD_{50} (single, oral dose) of triprolidine is 163 to 308 mg/kg in the mouse (depending upon strain) and 840 mg/kg in the rat.

Insufficient data are available to estimate the toxic and lethal doses of triprolidine in humans. No reports of acute poisoning with triprolidine have appeared.

The LD_{50} (single, oral dose) of pseudoephedrine is 726 mg/kg in the mouse, 2206 mg/kg in the rat and 1177 mg/kg in the rabbit. The toxic and lethal concentrations in human biologic fluids are not known. Excretion rates increase with urine acidification and decrease with alkalinization. Few reports of toxicity due to pseudoephedrine have been published and no case of fatal overdosage is known.

Therapy, if instituted within 4 hours of overdosage, is aimed at reducing further absorption of the drug. In the conscious patient, vomiting should be induced even though it may have occurred spontaneously. If vomiting cannot be induced, gastric lavage is indicated. Adequate precautions must be taken to protect against aspiration, especially in infants and children. Charcoal slurry or other suitable agents should be instilled into the stomach after vomiting or lavage. Saline cathartics or milk of magnesia may be of additional benefit. In the unconscious patient, the airway should be secured with a cuffed endotracheal tube before attempting to evacuate the gastric contents. Intensive supportive and nursing care is indicated, as for any comatose patient.

If breathing is significantly impaired, maintenance of adequate airway and mechanical support of respiration is the most effective means of providing adequate oxygenation. Hypotension is an early sign of impending cardiovascular collapse and should be treated vigorously. Do not use CNS stimulants. Convulsions should be controlled by careful administration of diazepam or short-acting barbiturate, repeated as necessary. Physostigmine may be also considered for use in controlling centrally mediated convulsions.

Ice packs and cooling sponge baths, not alcohol, can aid in reducing the fever commonly seen in children.

For codeine, continuous stimulation that arouses, but does not exhaust, the patient is useful in preventing coma. Continuous or intermittent oxygen therapy is usually indicated, while Naloxone is useful as a codeine antidote. Close nursing care is essential.

Saline cathartics, such as Milk of Magnesia, help to dilute the concentration of the drugs in the bowel by drawing water into the gut, thereby hastening drug elimination.

Adrenergic receptor blocking agents are antidotes to pseudoephedrine. In practice, the most useful is the beta-blocker propranolol, which is indicated when there are signs of cardiac toxicity.

There are no specific antidotes to triprolidine. Histamine should not be given.

Pseudoephedrine and codeine are theoretically dialyzable, but the procedures have not been clinically established.

In severe cases of overdosage, it is essential to monitor both the heart (by electrocardiograph) and plasma electrolytes and to give intravenous potassium as indicated by these continuous controls. Vasopressors may be used to treat hypotension, and excessive CNS stimulation may be counteracted with parenteral diazepam. Stimulants should not be used.

DOSAGE AND ADMINISTRATION

DOSAGE SHOULD BE INDIVIDUALIZED ACCORDING TO THE NEEDS AND RESPONSE OF THE PATIENT.
Usual Dose:

	Teaspoonfuls (5 ml)	
Adults and children 12 years and older	2	every 4–6 hours not to exceed 4 doses in a 24-hour period
Children 6 to under 12 years	1	
Children 2 to under 6 years	½	

HOW SUPPLIED

Bottle of one pint (NDC-0081-0025-96).
Store at 15°–30°C (59°–86°F) and protect from light.

ACTIFED® PLUS Tablets and Caplets
[ăk´tĭ-fĕd]
Anagelsic/Antihistamine/Nasal Decongestant

(See PDR For Nonprescription Drugs)
Tablets and Caplets shown in Product Identification Section, page 407

Continued on next page

Burroughs Wellcome—Cont.

ALKERAN® ℞
[al-kur'an]
(Melphalan)
2 mg Scored Tablets

> **WARNING:** Melphalan is leukemogenic in humans. Melphalan produces chromosomal aberrations *in vitro* and *in vivo* and therefore should be considered potentially mutagenic in humans. Melphalan produces amenorrhea.

DESCRIPTION

Alkeran (melphalan), also known as L-phenylalanine mustard, phenylalanine mustard, L-PAM, or L-sarcolysin, is a phenylalanine derivative of nitrogen mustard. Alkeran is a bifunctional alkylating agent which is active against selective human neoplastic diseases. It is known chemically as 4-[bis(2-chloroethyl)amino]-*L* - phenylalanine.

Melphalan is the active L-isomer of the compound and was first synthesized in 1953 by Bergel and Stock; the D-isomer, known as medphalan, is less active against certain animal tumors, and the dose needed to produce effects on chromosomes is larger than that required with the L-isomer. The racemic (DL–) form is known as merphalan or sarcolysin. Melphalan is insoluble in water and has a pKa_1 of ~ 2.1. Alkeran (melphalan) is available in tablet form for oral administration. Each scored tablet contains 2 mg melphalan and the inactive ingredients lactose, magnesium stearate, potato starch, povidone, and sucrose.

CLINICAL PHARMACOLOGY

Alberts *et al* [1] found that plasma melphalan levels are highly variable after oral dosing, both with respect to the time of the first appearance of melphalan in plasma (range 0 to 336 minutes) and to the peak plasma concentration (range 0.166 to 3.741 μg/ml) achieved.[2] These results may be due to incomplete intestinal absorption, a variable "first pass" hepatic metabolism, or to rapid hydrolysis. Five patients were studied after both oral and intravenous dosing with 0.6 mg/kg as a single bolus dose by each route. The areas under the plasma concentration-time curves after oral administration averaged 61 ± 26% (± standard deviation; range 25 to 89%) of those following intravenous administration. In 18 patients given a single oral dose of 0.6 mg/kg of melphalan, the terminal plasma half-disappearance time of parent drug was 89.5 ± 50 minutes. The 24-hour urinary excretion of parent drug in these patients was 10 ± 4.5%, suggesting that renal clearance is not a major route of elimination of parent drug. Tattersall *et al*,[3] using universally labeled ^{14}C-melphalan, found substantially less radioactivity in the urine of patients given the drug by mouth (30% of administered dose in nine days) than in the urine of those given it intravenously (35 to 65% in seven days). Following either oral or intravenous administration, the pattern of label recovery was similar, with the majority being recovered in the first 24 hours. Following oral administration, peak radioactivity occurred in plasma at two hours and then disappeared with a half-life of approximately 160 hours. In one patient where parent drug (rather than just radiolabel) was determined, the melphalan half-disappearance time was 67 minutes.[3]

INDICATIONS AND USAGE

Alkeran (melphalan) is indicated for the palliative treatment of multiple myeloma and for the palliation of non-resectable epithelial carcinoma of the ovary.

CONTRAINDICATIONS

Melphalan should not be used in patients whose disease has demonstrated a prior resistance to this agent. Patients who have demonstrated hypersensitivity to melphalan should not be given the drug.

WARNINGS

As with other nitrogen mustard drugs, excessive dosage will produce marked bone marrow depression. Frequent blood counts are essential to determine optimal dosage and to avoid toxicity. The drug should be discontinued or the dosage reduced upon evidence of depression of the bone marrow. There are many reports of patients with multiple myeloma who have developed acute, nonlymphocytic leukemia or myeloproliferative syndrome following therapy with alkylating agents (including melphalan). Evaluation of published reports strongly suggests that melphalan is leukemogenic (see PRECAUTIONS: Carcinogenesis). The potential benefits from the drug and potential risk of carcinogenesis must be evaluated on an individual basis.

Pregnancy: "Pregnancy Category D." Melphalan may cause fetal harm when administered to a pregnant woman. Animal reproduction studies have not been conducted with melphalan. There are no adequate and well-controlled studies in pregnant women. If this drug is used during preg-

nancy, or if the patient becomes pregnant while taking this drug, the patient should be apprised of the potential hazard to the fetus. Women of childbearing potential should be advised to avoid becoming pregnant.

PRECAUTIONS

General: Melphalan should be used with extreme caution in patients whose bone marrow reserve may have been compromised by prior irradiation or chemotherapy, or whose marrow function is recovering from previous cytotoxic therapy. If the leukocyte count falls below 3,000/μl, or the platelet count below 100,000 μl, the drug should be discontinued until the peripheral blood cell counts have recovered.

A recommendation as to whether or not dosage reduction should be made routinely in patients with impaired creatinine clearance cannot be made because:

(a) There is considerable inherent patient-to-patient variability in the systemic availability of melphalan in patients with normal renal function.

(b) There is only a small amount of the administered dose that appears as parent drug in the urine of patients with normal renal function.

Patients with azotemia should be closely observed, however, in order to make dosage reductions, if required, at the earliest possible time.

Information for Patients: Patients should be informed that the major toxicities of melphalan are related to myelosuppression, hypersensitivity, gastrointestinal toxicity, pulmonary toxicity, infertility, and nonlymphocytic leukemia and myeloproliferative syndrome. Patients should never be allowed to take the drug without close medical supervision and should be advised to consult their physician if they experience skin rash, vasculitis, bleeding, fever, persistent cough, nausea, vomiting, amenorrhea, weight loss, or unusual lumps/masses. Women of childbearing potential should be advised to avoid becoming pregnant.

Laboratory Tests: Weekly examination of the blood should be made to determine hemoglobin levels, total and differential leukocyte counts, and platelet enumeration. Patients may develop symptoms of anemia if the hemoglobin falls below 9–10 gm/dl, and are at risk of severe infection if the absolute neutrophil count is below 1,000/mm³, and may bleed if the platelet count falls below 50,000/mm³.

Drug Interactions: There are no known drug/drug interactions with melphalan.

Carcinogenesis, Mutagenesis, Impairment of Fertility: In an animal study to evaluate carcinogenesis, rats were given melphalan i.p. 3 times weekly for six months in doses ten to twenty times greater than the recommended dose in man. Fifty percent (50%) of the animals developed peritoneal sarcomas. Males and females developed lung tumors in excess of controls.[4] In a 39-week test melphalan produced a dose-related increase in lung tumors in mice.[5]

Acute nonlymphocytic leukemia and myeloproliferative syndrome have been reported in patients with cancer treated with alkylating agents (including melphalan).[6,7,8] Some patients also received other chemotherapeutic agents or radiation therapy. Precise quantitation of the risk of acute leukemia, myeloproliferative syndrome or carcinoma is not possible. Published reports of leukemia in patients who have received melphalan (and other alkylating agents) suggest that the risk of leukemogenesis increases with chronicity of treatment and with cumulative dose. Two studies[7,8] showed that the 10 year cumulative risk of developing acute leukemia or myeloproliferative syndrome after melphalan therapy was less than 2% for cumulative doses under 600 mg. This does not mean that there is a cumulative dose below which there is no risk of the induction of secondary malignancy. The potential benefits from melphalan therapy must be weighed on an individual basis against the possible risk of the induction of a second malignancy.

Melphalan has been shown to cause chromatid or chromosome damage in man.[9] Melphalan causes suppression of ovarian function in pre-menopausal women, resulting in amenorrhea in a significant number of patients.[10,11]

Pregnancy: *Teratogenic Effects:* Pregnancy Category D: See WARNINGS section.

Nursing Mothers: It is not known whether this drug is excreted in human milk. Because many drugs are excreted in human milk and because of the potential for serious adverse reactions in nursing infants from melphalan, a decision should be made whether to discontinue nursing or to discontinue the drug, taking into account the importance of the drug to the mother.

Pediatric Use: The safety and effectiveness in children have not been established.

ADVERSE REACTIONS

Hematologic Effects: The most common side effect is bone marrow suppression.[12] Although bone marrow suppression frequently occurs, it is usually reversible if melphalan is withdrawn early enough. However, irreversible bone marrow failure has been reported.[13,14]

Gastrointestinal: Gastrointestinal disturbances such as nausea and vomiting, diarrhea and oral ulceration occur infrequently.

Miscellaneous: Other reported adverse reactions include: pulmonary fibrosis[15,16] and interstitial pneumonitis, skin hypersensitivity, vasculitis, alopecia, hemolytic anemia, and allergic reaction.

OVERDOSAGE

Immediate effects are likely to be vomiting, ulceration of the mouth, diarrhea and hemorrhage of the gastrointestinal tract. The main toxic effect is on the bone marrow, and there is no known antidote. The blood picture should be closely followed for three to six weeks. General supportive measures, together with appropriate blood transfusions and antibiotics, should be instituted if necessary. This drug is not removed from plasma to any significant degree by hemodialysis.[17]

The oral LD_{50} dose in mice is 21 mg/kg.

DOSAGE AND ADMINISTRATION

Multiple Myeloma: The usual oral dose is 6 mg (3 tablets) daily. The entire daily dose may be given at one time. It is adjusted, as required, on the basis of blood counts done at approximately weekly intervals. After two to three weeks of treatment, the drug should be discontinued for up to four weeks during which time the blood count should be followed carefully. When the white blood cell and platelet counts are rising, a maintenance dose of 2 mg daily may be instituted. Because of the patient-to-patient variation in melphalan plasma levels following oral administration of the drug, several investigators have recommended that melphalan dosage be cautiously escalated until some myelosuppression is observed, in order to assure that potentially therapeutic levels of the drug have been reached.[1,3]

Other dosage regimens have been used by various investigators. Osserman and Takatsuki have used an initial course of 10 mg/day for seven to ten days.[18,19] They report that maximal suppression of the leukocyte and platelet counts occurs within three to five weeks and recovery within four to eight weeks. Continuous maintenance therapy with 2 mg/day is instituted when the white blood cell count is greater than 4,000 and the platelet count is greater than 100,000. Dosage is adjusted to between 1 and 3 mg/day depending upon the hematological response. It is desirable to try to maintain a significant degree of bone marrow depression so as to keep the leukocyte count in the range of 3,000 to 3,500 cells/μl. Hoogstraten *et al* have started treatment with 0.15 mg/kg/day for seven days.[20] This is followed by a rest period of at least 14 days, but it may be as long as five to six weeks. Maintenance therapy is started when the white blood cell and platelet counts are rising. The maintenance dose is 0.05 mg/kg per day or less and is adjusted according to the blood count.

Available evidence suggests that about one third to one half of the patients with multiple myeloma show a favorable response to oral administration of the drug.

One study by Alexanian *et al* has shown that the use of melphalan in combination with prednisone significantly improves the percentage of patients with multiple myeloma who achieve palliation.[21] One regimen has been to administer courses of melphalan at 0.25 mg/kg/day for four consecutive days (or, 0.20 mg/kg/day for five consecutive days) for a total dose of 1 mg/kg per course. These four- to five-day courses are then repeated every four to six weeks if the granulocyte count and the platelet count have returned to normal levels.

It is to be emphasized that response may be very gradual over many months; it is important that repeated courses or continuous therapy be given since improvement may continue slowly over many months, and the maximum benefit may be missed if treatment is abandoned too soon.

In patients with moderate to severe renal impairment, currently available pharmacokinetic data does not justify an absolute recommendation on dosage reduction to those patients, but it may be prudent to use a reduced dose initially.[22,23]

Epithelial Ovarian Cancer: One commonly employed regimen for the treatment of ovarian carcinoma has been to administer melphalan at a dose of 0.2 mg/kg daily for five days as a single course. Courses are repeated every four to five weeks depending upon hematologic tolerance.[24,25]

Procedures for proper handling and disposal of anti-cancer drugs should be considered. Several guidelines on this subject have been published.[26-32]

There is no general agreement that all of the procedures recommended in the guidelines are necessary or appropriate.

HOW SUPPLIED

White, scored tablets containing 2 mg melphalan, imprinted with "ALKERAN" and "A2A"; in bottle of 50 (NDC-0081-0045-35).

Store at 15°–25°C (59°–77°F) in a dry place, protect from light, and dispense in glass.

REFERENCES

1. Alberts DS *et al:* Oral melphalan kinetics. *Clin Pharmacol Ther*, 1979; 26(6):737-745.

2. Alberts DS *et al*: Unpublished data on file with Burroughs Wellcome Co., 1981.

3. Tattersall MHN *et al*: Pharmacokinetics of melphalan following oral or intravenous administration in patients with malignant disease. *Europ J Cancer* 1977; *11*: 507–513.

4. Weisburger JH *et al*: The Carcinogenic properties of some of the principal drugs used in clinical cancer chemotherapy. *Recent Results Cancer Res* 1975; *52*: 1–17.

5. Shimkin MB *et al*: Bioassay of 29 alkylating chemicals by the pulmonary-tumor response in strain A mice. *J Natl Cancer Inst* 1966; *36*: 915–935.

6. Einhorn N *et al*: Acute leukemia after chemotherapy (melphalan). *Cancer* 1978; *41*: 444–447.

7. Fisher B *et al*: Leukemia in breast cancer patients following adjuvant chemotherapy or postoperative radiation: the NSABP experience. *J Clin Oncol* 1985; 3:1640-1658.

8. Greene MH *et al*: Melphalan may be a more potent leukemogen than cyclophosphamide. *Ann Int Med* 1986; 105:360-367.

9. Sharpe HB: Observations on the effect of therapy with nitrogen mustard or a derivative on chromosomes of human peripheral blood lymphocytes. *Cell Tissue Kinet* 1971; *4*: 501–504.

10. Rose DP, David TE: Ovarian function in patients receiving adjuvant chemotherapy for breast cancer. *Lancet* 1977; *1*: 1174–1176.

11. Ahmann DL *et al*: Repeated adjuvant chemotherapy with phenylalanine mustard or 5-fluorouracil, cyclophosphamide and prednisone with or without radiation, after mastectomy for breast cancer. *Lancet* 1978; *1*:893–896.

12. Speed DE *et al*: Melphalan in the treatment of myelomatosis. *Br Med J*, 1964; *1*: 1664–1669.

13. Smith JP, Rutledge F: Chemotherapy in the treatment of cancer of the ovary. *Am J Obstet Gynecol* 1970; *107*: 691–703.

14. Bergsagel DE *et al*: The treatment of plasma cell myeloma. *Adv Cancer Research* 1967; *10*: 311–359.

15. Taetle R, Dickman PS, Feldman PS. Pulmonary histopathologic changes associated with melphalan therapy. *Cancer* 1978; *42*: 1239–1245.

16. Westerfield BT *et al*: Reversible melphalan-induced lung damage. *Am J Med* 1980; *68*: 767–771.

17. Pallante SL *et al*: Quantitation by gas chromatography-chemical ionization-mass spectrometry of phenylalanine mustard in plasma of patients. *Cancer Res* 1980; *40*: 2268–2272.

18. Osserman EF: Therapy of plasma cell myeloma with melphalan. *Proc Am Assoc Cancer Res* 1963; *4*: 50.

19. Osserman EF and Takatsuki K: Plasma cell myeloma: gamma globulin synthesis and structure. *Medicine* 1963; *42*: 357–384.

20. Hoogstraten B *et al*: Melphalan in multiple myeloma. *Blood* 1967; *30(1)*: 74–83.

21. Alexanian R *et al*: Treatment for multiple myeloma. *JAMA* 1969; *208(9)*: 1680–1685.

22. Alberts DS *et al*: Comparative pharmokinetics of chlorambucil and melphalan in man. *Recent Results Cancer Res* 1980; *74*: 124–131.

23. Alberts DS *et al*: Effect of renal dysfunction in dogs on the disposition and marrow toxicity of melphalan. *Brit J Cancer* 1981; *43*: 330–334.

24. Smith JP and Rutledge FN: Chemotherapy in advanced ovarian cancer. *Natl Cancer Inst Monogr* 1975; *42*: 141–143.

25. Young RC *et al*: Advanced ovarian adenocarcinoma. *N Engl J Med* 1978; *299(23)*: 1261–1266.

26. Recommendations for the safe handling of parenteral antineoplastic drugs. NIH Publications No. 83-2621. For sale by the Superintendent of Documents, U.S. Government Printing Office, Washington, D.C. 20402.

27. AMA Council Report. Guidelines for handling parenteral antineoplastics. *JAMA*, March 15, 1985.

28. National Study Commission on Cytotoxic Exposure—Recommendations for handling cytotoxic agents. Available from Louis P. Jeffrey, Sc.D., Director of Pharmacy Services, Rhode Island Hospital, 593 Eddy Street, Providence, Rhode Island 02902.

29. Clinical Oncological Society of Australia: Guidelines and recommendations for safe handling of antineoplastic agents. *Med J Australia* 1983; 1:426–428.

30. Jones RB *et al*: Safe handling of chemotherapeutic agents: A report from the Mount Sinai Medical Center. *Ca—A Cancer Journal for Clinicians* 1983; Sept/Oct: 258–263.

31. American Society of Hospital Pharmacists technical assistance bulletin on handling cytotoxic drugs in hospitals. *Am J Hosp Pharm* 1985; 42:131–137.

32. Yodaiken RE, Bennett D: OSHA work-practice guidelines for personnel dealing with cytotoxic (antineoplastic) drugs. *Am J Hosp Pharm* 1986; 43:1193–1204.

Shown in Product Identification Section, page 407

ALLERACT™ DECONGESTANT Tablets and Caplets
[ˈal-ər-ˈakt]
Antihistamine/Nasal Decongestant

(See PDR For Nonprescription Drugs)
Tablets and Caplets shown in Product Identification Section, page 407

ALLERACT™ Tablets
[ˈal-ər-ˈakt]
Antihistamine

(See PDR For Nonprescription Drugs)
Shown in Product Identification Section, page 407

ANECTINE®   ℞
[ă-nĕk ˈtēn]
(Succinylcholine Chloride)
Injection, USP

ANECTINE®   ℞
(Succinylcholine Chloride)
Sterile Powder Flo-Pack®

> This drug should be used only by individuals familiar with its actions, characteristics and hazards.

DESCRIPTION

Anectine (succinylcholine chloride) is an ultra short-acting depolarizing-type, skeletal muscle relaxant for intravenous administration.

Succinylcholine chloride is a white, odorless, slightly bitter powder and very soluble in water. The drug is unstable in alkaline solutions but relatively stable in acid solutions, depending upon the concentration of the solution and the storage temperature. Solutions of succinylcholine chloride should be stored under refrigeration to preserve potency. Anectine Injection is a sterile non-pyrogenic solution for intravenous injection, containing 20 mg succinylcholine chloride in each ml and made isotonic with sodium chloride. The pH is adjusted to 3.5 with hydrochloric acid. Methylparaben (0.1%) is added as a preservative. Anectine Flo-Pack is a sterile powder, containing either 500 mg or 1000 mg of succinylcholine chloride in each vial.

The chemical name for succinylcholine chloride is 2,2′-[(1,4-dioxo-1,4-butanediyl)bis(oxy)]bis[N,N,N trimethylethanaminium] dichloride.

CLINICAL PHARMACOLOGY

Succinylcholine is a depolarizing skeletal muscle relaxant. As does acetylcholine, it combines with the cholinergic receptors of the motor end plate to produce depolarization. This depolarization may be observed as fasciculations. Subsequent neuromuscular transmission is inhibited so long as adequate concentration of succinylcholine remains at the receptor site. Onset of flaccid paralysis is rapid (less than one minute after intravenous administration), and with single administration lasts approximately 4–6 minutes.

Succinylcholine is rapidly hydrolyzed by plasma pseudocholinesterase to succinylmonocholine (which possesses nondepolarizing muscle relaxant properties) and then more slowly to succinic acid and choline. About 10% of the drug is excreted unchanged in the urine. The paralysis following administration of succinylcholine is selective, initially involving consecutively the levator muscles of the face, muscles of the glottis and finally the intercostals and the diaphragm and all other skeletal muscles.

Succinylcholine has no direct action on the uterus or other smooth muscle structures. Because it is highly ionized and has low fat solubility, it does not readily cross the placenta. Tachyphylaxis occurs with repeated administration.

When succinylcholine is given over a prolonged period of time, the characteristic depolarizing neuromuscular block (Phase I block) may change to a block with characteristics superficially resembling a non-depolarizing block (Phase II block). This may be associated with prolonged respiratory depression or apnea in patients who manifest the transition to Phase II block. When this diagnosis is confirmed by peripheral nerve stimulation, it may be reversed with anticholinesterase drugs such as neostigmine (See Precautions).

While succinylcholine has no direct effect on the myocardium, changes in rhythm may result from vagal stimulation, such as may result from surgical procedures (particularly in children) or from potassium-mediated alterations in electrical conductivity. These effects are enhanced by cyclopropane and halogenated anesthetics.

Succinylcholine causes a slight, transient increase in intraocular pressure immediately after its injection and during the fasciculation phase, and slight increases may persist after onset of complete paralysis. This suggests that the drug should not be used in the presence of open eye injuries.

As with other neuromuscular blockers, the potential for releasing histamine is present following succinylcholine administration. Serious histamine-mediated flushing, hypotension and bronchoconstriction are, however, uncommon in normal clinical usage.

Succinylcholine has no effect on consciousness, pain threshold or cerebration. It should be used only with adequate anesthesia.

INDICATIONS AND USAGE

Succinylcholine chloride is indicated as an adjunct to general anesthesia, to facilitate endotracheal intubation, and to provide skeletal muscle relaxation during surgery or mechanical ventilation.

CONTRAINDICATIONS

Succinylcholine is contraindicated for persons with genetically determined disorders of plasma pseudocholinesterase, personal or familial history of malignant hyperthermia, myopathies associated with elevated creatine phosphokinase (CPK) values, known hypersensitivity to the drug, acute narrow angle glaucoma, and penetrating eye injuries.

WARNINGS

Succinylcholine should be used only by those skilled in the management of artificial respiration and only when facilities are instantly available for endotracheal intubation and for providing adequate ventilation of the patient, including the administration of oxygen under positive pressure and the elimination of carbon dioxide. The clinician must be prepared to assist or control respiration.

Succinylcholine should not be mixed with short-acting barbiturates in the same syringe or administered simultaneously during intravenous infusion through the same needle. Solutions of succinylcholine have an acid pH, whereas those of barbiturates are alkaline. Depending upon the resultant pH of a mixture of solutions of these drugs, either free barbituric acid may be precipitated or succinylcholine hydrolyzed.

Succinylcholine administration has been associated with acute onset of fulminant hypermetabolism of skeletal muscle known as malignant hyperthermic crisis. This frequently presents as intractable spasm of the jaw muscles which may progress to generalized rigidity, increased oxygen demand, tachycardia, tachypnea and profound hyperpyrexia. Successful outcome depends on recognition of early signs, such as jaw muscle spasm, lack of laryngeal relaxation or generalized rigidity to initial administration of succinylcholine for endotracheal intubation, or failure of tachycardia to respond to deepening anesthesia. Skin mottling, rising temperature and coagulopathies occur late in the course of the hypermetabolic process. Recognition of the syndrome is a signal for discontinuation of anesthesia, attention to increased oxygen consumption, correction of metabolic acidosis, support of circulation, assurance of adequate urinary output and institution of measures to control rising temperature. Dantrolene sodium, intravenously, is recommended as an adjunct to supportive measures in the management of this problem. Consult literature references or the dantrolene prescribing information for additional information about the management of malignant hyperthermic crisis. Routine, continuous monitoring of temperature is recommended as an aid to early recognition of malignant hyperthermia.

PRECAUTIONS

General: Low levels or abnormal variants of pseudocholinesterase may be associated with prolonged respiratory depression or apnea following the use of succinylcholine. Low levels of pseudocholinesterase may occur in patients with the following conditions: burns, severe liver disease or cirrhosis, cancer, severe anemia, pregnancy, malnutrition, severe dehydration, collagen diseases, myxedema, and abnormal body temperature. Also, exposure to neurotoxic insecticides, antimalarial or anti-cancer drugs, monoamine oxidase inhibitors, contraceptive pills, pancuronium, chlorpromazine, ecothiopate iodide, or neostigmine may result in low levels of pseudocholinesterase. Succinylcholine should be administered with extreme care to such patients. If low pseudocholinesterase activity is suspected, a small test dose of from 5 to 10 mg of succinylcholine may be administered, or relaxation may be produced by the cautious administration of a 0.1% solution of the drug by intravenous drip. Apnea or prolonged muscle paralysis should be treated with controlled respiration.

Succinylcholine should be administered with great caution to patients recovering from severe trauma, those suffering from electrolyte imbalance, those receiving quinidine, and those who have been digitalized recently or who may have digitalis toxicity, because in these circumstances it may induce serious cardiac arrhythmias or cardiac arrest. Great caution should be observed also in patients with pre-existing hyperkalemia, those who are paraplegic, or have suffered extensive or severe burns, extensive denervation of skeletal muscle due to disease or injury of the central nervous system, or have degenerative or dystrophic neuromuscular disease, because such patients tend to become severely hyperkalemic when given succinylcholine.

Continued on next page

Burroughs Wellcome—Cont.

When succinylcholine is given over a prolonged period of time, the characteristic depolarization block of the myoneural junction (Phase I block) may change to a block with characteristics superficially resembling a non-depolarizing block (Phase II block). Prolonged respiratory depression or apnea may be observed in patients manifesting this transition to Phase II block. The transition from Phase I to Phase II block has been reported in 7 of 7 patients studied under halothane anesthesia after an accumulated dose of 2 to 4 mg/kg succinylcholine (administered in repeated, divided doses). The onset of Phase II block coincided with the onset of tachyphylaxis and prolongation of spontaneous recovery. In another study, using balanced anesthesia (N_2O/O_2/narcotic-thiopental) and succinylcholine infusion, the transition was less abrupt, with great individual variability in the dose of succinylcholine required to produce Phase II block. Of 32 patients studied, 24 developed Phase II block. Tachyphylaxis was not associated with the transition to Phase II block, and 50% of the patients who developed Phase II block experienced prolonged recovery.

When Phase II block is suspected in cases of prolonged neuromuscular blockade, positive diagnosis should be made by peripheral nerve stimulation, prior to administration of any anticholinesterase drug. Reversal of Phase II block is a medical decision which must be made upon the basis of the individual clinical pharmacology and the experience and judgment of the physician. The presence of Phase II block is indicated by fade of responses to successive stimuli (preferably "train of four"). The use of anticholinesterase drugs to reverse Phase II block should be accompanied by appropriate doses of atropine to prevent disturbances of cardiac rhythm. After adequate reversal of Phase II block with an anticholinesterase agent, the patient should be continually observed for at least 1 hour for signs of return of muscle relaxation. Reversal should not be attempted unless: (1) a peripheral nerve stimulator is used to determine the presence of Phase II block (since anticholinesterase agents will potentiate succinylcholine-induced Phase I block), and (2) spontaneous recovery of muscle twitch has been observed for at least 20 minutes and has reached a plateau with further recovery proceeding slowly; this delay is to ensure complete hydrolysis of succinylcholine by pseudocholinesterase prior to administration of the anticholinesterase agent. Should the type of block be misdiagnosed, depolarization of the type initially induced by succinylcholine, that is depolarizing block, will be prolonged by an anticholinesterase agent.

Succinylcholine should be used with caution, if at all, during ocular surgery and in patients with glaucoma. The drug should be employed with caution in patients with fractures or muscle spasm because the initial muscle fasciculations may cause additional trauma.

Succinylcholine may increase intragastric pressure, which could result in regurgitation and possible aspiration of stomach contents.

Neuromuscular blockade may be prolonged in patients with hypokalemia or hypocalcemia.

Drug Interactions: Drugs which may enhance the neuromuscular blocking action of succinylcholine include: phenelzine, promazine, oxytocin, aprotinin, certain nonpenicillin antibiotics, quinidine, β-adrenergic blockers, procainamide, lidocaine, trimethaphan, lithium carbonate, magnesium salts, quinine, chloroquine, propanidid, diethylether, and isoflurane.

If other relaxants are to be used during the same procedure, the possibility of a synergistic or antagonistic effect should be considered.

Pregnancy: *Teratogenic Effects:* Pregnancy Category C. Animal reproduction studies have not been conducted with succinylcholine chloride. It is also not known whether succinylcholine can cause fetal harm when administered to a pregnant woman or can affect reproduction capacity. Succinylcholine should be given to a pregnant woman only if clearly needed.

Nonteratogenic Effects: Pseudocholinesterase levels are decreased by approximately 24% during pregnancy and for several days postpartum. Therefore, a higher proportion of patients may be expected to show sensitivity (prolonged apnea) to succinylcholine when pregnant than when nonpregnant.

Labor and Delivery: Succinylcholine is commonly used to provide muscle relaxation during delivery by caesarean section. While small amounts of succinylcholine are known to cross the placental barrier, under normal conditions the quantity of drug that enters fetal circulation after a single dose of 1 mg/kg to the mother will not endanger the fetus. However, since the amount of drug that crosses the placental barrier is dependent on the concentration gradient between the maternal and fetal circulations, residual neuromuscular blockade (apnea and flaccidity) may occur in the neonate after repeated high doses to, or in the presence of atypical pseudocholinesterase in, the mother.

ADVERSE REACTIONS

Adverse reactions consist primarily of an extension of the drug's pharmacological actions. It causes profound muscle relaxation resulting in respiratory depression to the point of apnea; this effect may be prolonged. Hypersensitivity to the drug may exist in rare instances. The following additional adverse reactions have been reported: cardiac arrest, malignant hyperthermia, arrhythmias, bradycardia, tachycardia, hypertension, hypotension, hyperkalemia, prolonged respiratory depression or apnea, increased intraocular pressure, muscle fasciculation, postoperative muscle pain, rhabdomyolysis with possible myoglobinuric acute renal failure, excessive salivation, and rash.

DOSAGE AND ADMINISTRATION

The dosage of succinylcholine is essentially individualized and its administration should always be determined by the clinician after careful assessment of the patient. To avoid distress to the patient, succinylcholine should not be administered before unconsciousness has been induced. Succinylcholine should not be mixed with short-acting barbiturates in the same syringe or administered simultaneously during intravenous infusion through the same needle.

For Short Surgical Procedures: The average dose for relaxation of short duration is 0.6 mg/kg (~2.0 ml) Anectine (succinylcholine chloride) Injection given intravenously. The optimum dose will vary among individuals and may be from 0.3 to 1.1 mg/kg for adults (1.0 to 4.0 ml). Following administration of doses in this range, relaxation develops in about 1 minute; maximum muscular paralysis may persist for about 2 minutes, after which recovery takes place within 4 to 6 minutes. However, very large doses may result in more prolonged apnea. An initial test dose of 0.1 mg/kg (~0.5 ml) may be used to determine the sensitivity of the patient and the individual recovery time.

For Long Surgical Procedures: The dosage of succinylcholine administered by infusion depends upon the duration of the surgical procedure and the need for muscle relaxation. The average rate for an adult ranges between 2.5 and 4.3 mg per minute.

Solutions containing from 0.1% to 0.2% (1 to 2 mg per ml) succinylcholine have commonly been used for continuous intravenous drip. Solutions of 0.1% or 0.2% may conveniently be prepared by adding 1 g succinylcholine (the contents of one Anectine Sterile Powder Flo-Pack unit containing 1 g succinylcholine chloride) respectively to 1,000 or 500 ml of sterile solution, such as sterile 5% dextrose solution or sterile isotonic saline solution. The more dilute solution (0.1% or 1 mg per ml) is probably preferable from the standpoint of ease of control of the rate of administration of the drug and, hence, of relaxation. This intravenous drip solution containing 1 mg per ml may be administered at a rate of 0.5 mg (0.5 ml) to 10 mg (10 ml) per minute to obtain the required amount of relaxation. The amount required per minute will depend upon the individual response as well as the degree of relaxation required. The 0.2% solution may be especially useful in those cases where it is desired to avoid overburdening the circulation with a large volume of fluid. It is recommended that neuromuscular function be carefully monitored with a peripheral nerve stimulator when using succinylcholine by infusion in order to avoid overdose, detect development of Phase II block, follow its rate of recovery, and assess the effects of reversing agents.

Solutions of succinylcholine must be used within 24 hours after preparation. Discard unused solutions.

Intermittent intravenous injections of succinylcholine may also be used to provide muscle relaxation for long procedures. An intravenous injection of 0.3 to 1.1 mg/kg may be given initially, followed, at appropriate intervals, by further injections of 0.04 to 0.07 mg/kg to maintain the degree of relaxation required.

Pediatric Use: For endotracheal intubation, the intravenous dose of succinylcholine is 2 mg/kg for infants and small children; for older children and adolescents the dose is 1 mg/kg.

Intravenous bolus administration of succinylcholine in infants or children may result in profound bradycardia or, rarely, asystole. As in adults, the incidence of bradycardia in children is higher following a second dose of succinylcholine. The occurrence of bradyarrhythmias may be reduced by pretreatment with atropine.

Intramuscular Use: If necessary, succinylcholine may be given intramuscularly to infants, older children or adults when a suitable vein is inaccessible. A dose of up to 3 to 4 mg/kg may be given, but not more than 150 mg total dose should be administered by this route. The onset of effect of succinylcholine given intramuscularly is usually observed in about 2 to 3 minutes.

Parenteral drug products should be inspected visually for particulate matter and discoloration prior to administration whenever solution and container permit.

HOW SUPPLIED

For immediate injection of single doses for short procedures: Anectine® Injection, 20 mg succinylcholine chloride in each ml.

Multiple-dose vials of 10 ml.
Box of 12 vials (NDC-0081-0071-95).
Store in refrigerator at 2° to 8°C (36° to 46°F). The multi-dose vials are stable for up to 14 days at room temperature without significant loss of potency.
For preparation of intravenous drip solutions only:
Anectine® Flo-Pack®, 500 mg sterile succinylcholine chloride powder.
Box of 12 vials (NDC-0081-0085-15).
Anectine® Flo-Pack®, 1000 mg sterile succinylcholine chloride powder.
Box of 12 vials (NDC-0081-0086-15).
Anectine Flo-Pack does not require refrigeration. Store at 15° to 30°C (59° to 86°F). Solutions of succinylcholine must be used within 24 hours after preparation. Discard unused solutions.

CARDILATE® TABLETS   ℞
[kar 'dĭ-lāt]
(Erythrityl Tetranitrate)

DESCRIPTION

Cardilate (erythrityl tetranitrate) is an antianginal drug that belongs to the organic nitrate class of pharmaceutical agents. Erythrityl tetranitrate is soluble in alcohol, ether and glycerol, but insoluble in water. It has the empirical formula $C_4H_6N_4O_{12}$, molecular weight of 302.12 and melting point of 61°C.

Erythrityl tetranitrate is known chemically as $(R*S*)$-1,2,3,4-butanetetrol tetranitrate.

In the pure state, erythrityl tetranitrate will explode upon percussion, but properly diluted with lactose, as in Cardilate tablets, it is nonexplosive. Since it is a low melting solid, erythrityl tetranitrate does not evaporate from the Cardilate tablets.

Cardilate Oral/Sublingual Tablets contain 10 mg erythrityl tetranitrate and the inactive ingredients lactose, magnesium stearate and potato starch, with disintegration characteristics that permit sublingual or oral (swallowed) administration.

CLINICAL PHARMACOLOGY

Cardilate exerts its effects by relaxation of vascular smooth muscle.[1] The action is maximal on the post-capillary vessels, including the large veins. Venodilatation results in peripheral blood pooling, which decreases venous return to the heart, central venous pressure and pulmonary capillary wedge pressure (preload reduction).[2] Pulmonary arteriolar dilatation causes a reduction in pulmonary vascular resistance.[2] A decrease in systemic arterial pressure (afterload reduction) can also occur, but is usually less pronounced. Augmentation of cardiac output generally occurs in those patients with increased filling pressures and high resting systemic vascular resistance.[2]

Mechanism of Action: The inadequate myocardial oxygenation that precipitates angina can be corrected by: (1) increasing the supply of oxygen to ischemic myocardium through direct dilatation of the large coronary conductance vessels or (2) decreasing the myocardial oxygen demand secondary to a reduction of cardiac work (preload and afterload reduction).[3] The beneficial effect of Cardilate probably involves both mechanisms.

Pharmacokinetics and Metabolism: Cardilate is readily absorbed from the sublingual, buccal and gastrointestinal mucosae. The peak effect from a swallowed dose is diminished but of longer duration when compared to the sublingual route.[4] The biotransformation of Cardilate is thought to occur by reductive hydrolysis catalyzed by the hepatic enzyme glutathione-organic nitrate reductase.[3] Differences in response among various nitrates may relate to both intrinsic potency at cardiovascular sites, as well as factors related to pharmacokinetics and biotransformation.[5]

Time to onset of effect is approximately 5 minutes for the sublingual route and 15 to 30 minutes for swallowed tablets, with peak effect in 15 minutes and 60 minutes, respectively. Duration of action will vary, but vasodilatory effects have been demonstrated for up to 3 hours after sublingual administration[4,6] and for 6 hours after the oral (swallowed) route.[4]

INDICATIONS AND USAGE

Cardilate (erythrityl tetranitrate) is intended for the prophylaxis and long-term treatment of patients with frequent or recurrent anginal pain and reduced exercise tolerance associated with angina pectoris, rather than for the treatment of the acute attack of angina pectoris, since its onset is somewhat slower than that of nitroglycerin.

CONTRAINDICATIONS

Cardilate should not be administered to individuals with a known hypersensitivity or idiosyncratic reaction to organic nitrates.

WARNINGS

The use of nitrates in acute myocardial infarction or congestive heart failure should be undertaken only under close clinical observation and/or in conjunction with hemodynamic monitoring.

PRECAUTIONS

General: Cardilate should be used with caution in patients with severe liver or renal disease. Development of tolerance and cross-tolerance to the effects of erythrityl tetranitrate and other organic nitrates may occur. However, recent studies in patients with chronic heart failure[1] indicate that nitrates produce sustained beneficial hemodynamic effects.

Carcinogenesis, Mutagenesis, Impairment of Fertility: No long-term studies in animals have been performed.

Pregnancy: *Teratogenic Effects.* Pregnancy Category C. Animal reproduction studies have not been conducted with Cardilate. It is also not known whether Cardilate can cause fetal harm when administered to a pregnant woman or can affect reproduction capacity. Cardilate should be given to a pregnant woman only if clearly needed.

Nursing Mothers: It is not known whether this drug is excreted in human milk. Because many drugs are excreted in human milk, caution should be exercised when Cardilate is administered to a nursing woman.

Pediatric Use: Safety and effectiveness in children have not been established.

ADVERSE REACTIONS

The most frequent adverse reaction in patients treated with Cardilate is headache. Lowering the dose and the use of analgesics will help control headaches, which usually diminish or disappear as therapy is continued. Other adverse reactions occurring are the following: cutaneous vasodilatation with flushing, and transient episodes of dizziness and weakness, plus other signs of cerebral ischemia associated with postural hypotension. Occasional individuals exhibit marked sensitivity to the hypotensive effects of organic nitrates, and severe responses (eg, nausea, vomiting, weakness, restlessness, pallor, perspiration and collapse) can occur even with the usual therapeutic dose. Alcohol may enhance this effect. Drug rash and/or exfoliative dermatitis may occasionally occur.

OVERDOSAGE

Accidental overdosage of Cardilate may result in severe hypotension and reflex tachycardia, which can be treated by laying the patient down and elevating the legs. If further treatment is required, the administration of intravenous fluids or other means of treating hypotension should be considered.

DOSAGE AND ADMINISTRATION

The Cardilate Oral/ Sublingual Tablet can be placed under the tongue or swallowed. Sublingual therapy may be initiated with a dose of 5 to 10 mg prior to each anticipated physical or emotional stress, and at bedtime for patients subject to nocturnal attacks of angina. The dose may be increased as needed.

If the patient is to swallow the tablet, therapy may be initiated with 10 mg before each meal, as well as mid-morning and mid-afternoon if needed, and at bedtime for patients subject to nocturnal attacks. The dose may be increased or decreased as needed.

Dosage titration up to 100 mg daily has been well tolerated, but temporary headache is more apt to occur with increasing doses. When headache occurs, the dose should be reduced for a few days. If headache is troublesome during adjustment of dosage, it may be effectively relieved with an analgesic.

HOW SUPPLIED

Square, white, scored tablets containing 10 mg erythrityl tetranitrate, imprinted with "CARDILATE" and "X7A" on each tablet; bottle of 100 (NDC 0081-0168-55).

Store at 15°–25°C (59°– 77°F) in a dry place and dispense in glass.

REFERENCES

1. Chatterjee K, Parmley WW: Vasodilator therapy for chronic heart failure. *Ann Rev Pharmacol Toxicol*, 1980;20:475–512.
2. Goldberg S. Mann T, Grossman W: Nitrate therapy of heart failure in valvular heart disease. *Am J Med* 1978;65:161–166.
3. Needleman P, Johnson EM: Vasodilators and the treatment of angina. in Gilman AG, Goodman LS, Gilman A, (eds): *The Pharmacological Basis of Therapeutics*, ed 6. New York, Macmillan Publishing Co Inc, 1980, pp 819–833.
4. Hanneman RE, Erb RJ, Stoltman WP, et al: Digital plethysmography for assessing erythrityl tetranitrate bioavailability. *Clin Pharmacol Ther* 1981;29:35–39.
5. Wastila WB, Namm DH, Maxwell RA: Comparison of the vascular effects of several organic nitrates in anesthetized rats and dogs after intravenous and intraportal administration, in *Second International Symposium on Vascular Neuroeffector Mechanisms, Odense, 1975.* Basel, Karger 1976, pp 216–225.
6. Haffty GB, Nakamura Y, Spodick DH, et al: Bioavailability of organic nitrates: A comparison of methods for evalu-
ating plethysmographic responses. *J Clin Pharmacol*, 1982;22:117–124.

Shown in Product Identification Section, page 407

CORTISPORIN® CREAM   ℞
[kor'tĭ-spor''ĭn krēm]
(Polymyxin B Sulfate-Neomycin Sulfate-Hydrocortisone Acetate)

DESCRIPTION

Cortisporin® Cream (polymyxin B sulfate-neomycin sulfate-hydrocortisone acetate) is a topical antibacterial cream. Each gram contains: Aerosporin® (polymyxin B sulfate) 10,000 units; neomycin sulfate equivalent to 3.5 mg neomycin base; and hydrocortisone acetate 5 mg (0.5%). The inactive ingredients are liquid petrolatum, white petrolatum, propylene glycol, polyoxyethylene polyoxypropylene compound, emulsifying wax, purified water, and 0.25% methylparaben added as a preservative. Sodium hydroxide or sulfuric acid may be added to adjust pH.

Polymyxin B sulfate is the sulfate salt of polymyxin B_1 and B_2, which are produced by the growth of *Bacillus polymyxa* (Prazmowski) Migula (Fam. Bacillaceae). It has a potency of not less than 6,000 polymyxin B units per mg, calculated on an anhydrous basis.

Neomycin sulfate is the sulfate salt of neomycin B and C, which are produced by the growth of *Streptomyces fradiae* Waksman (Fam. Streptomycetaceae). It has a potency equivalent of not less than 600 µg of neomycin standard per mg, calculated on an anhydrous basis.

Hydrocortisone acetate is the acetate ester of hydrocortisone, an anti-inflammatory hormone. Its chemical name is 21-(acetyloxy)-11β,17-dihydroxypregn-4-ene-3,20-dione.

The base is a smooth vanishing cream with a pH of approximately 5.0.

CLINICAL PHARMACOLOGY

Corticoids suppress the inflammatory response to a variety of agents and they may delay healing. Since corticoids may inhibit the body's defense mechanism against infection, a concomitant antimicrobial drug may be used when this inhibition is considered to be clinically significant in a particular case.

The anti-infective components in the combination are included to provide action against specific organisms susceptible to them. Polymyxin B sulfate and neomycin sulfate together are considered active against the following microorganisms: *Staphylococcus aureus, Escherichia coli, Haemophilus influenzae, Klebsiella-Enterobacter* species, *Neisseria* species and *Pseudomonas aeruginosa*. The product does not provide adequate coverage against *Serratia marcescens* and streptococci, including *Streptococcus pneumoniae*.

The relative potency of corticosteroids depends on the molecular structure, concentration and release from the vehicle. The acid pH helps restore normal cutaneous acidity. Owing to its excellent spreading and penetrating properties, the cream facilitates treatment of hairy and intertriginous areas. It may also be of value in selective cases where the lesions are moist.

INDICATIONS AND USAGE

For the treatment of corticosteroid-responsive dermatoses with secondary infection. It has not been demonstrated that this steroid-antibiotic combination provides greater benefit than the steroid component alone after 7 days of treatment (see WARNINGS section).

CONTRAINDICATIONS

Not for use in the eyes or in the external ear canal if the eardrum is perforated. This product is contraindicated in tuberculous, fungal or viral lesions of the skin (herpes simplex, vaccinia and varicella). This product is contraindicated in those individuals who have shown hypersensitivity to any of its components.

WARNINGS

Because of the concern of nephrotoxicity and ototoxicity associated with neomycin, this combination should not be used over a wide area or for extended periods of time.

PRECAUTIONS

General: As with any antibacterial preparation, prolonged use may result in overgrowth of nonsusceptible organisms, including fungi. Appropriate measures should be taken if this occurs. Use of steroids on infected areas should be supervised with care as anti-inflammatory steroids may encourage spread of infection. If this occurs, steroid therapy should be stopped and appropriate antibacterial drugs used. Generalized dermatological conditions may require systemic corticosteroid therapy.

Signs and symptoms of exogenous hyperadrenocorticism can occur with the use of topical corticosteroids, including adrenal suppression. Systemic absorption of topically applied steroids will be increased if extensive body surface areas are treated or if occlusive dressings are used. Under these circumstances, suitable precautions should be taken when long-term use is anticipated.

Information for Patients: If redness, irritation, swelling or pain persists or increases, discontinue use and notify physician. Do not use in the eyes.

Laboratory Tests: Systemic effects of excessive levels of hydrocortisone may include a reduction in the number of circulating eosinophils and a decrease in urinary excretion of 17-hydroxycorticosteroids.

Carcinogenesis, Mutagenesis, Impairment of Fertility: Long-term studies in animals (rats, rabbits, mice) showed no evidence of carcinogenicity attributable to oral administration of corticosteroids.

Pregnancy: *Teratogenic Effects:* Pregnancy Category C. Corticosteroids have been shown to be teratogenic in rabbits when applied topically at concentrations of 0.5% on days 6–18 of gestation and in mice when applied topically at a concentration of 15% on days 10–13 of gestation. There are no adequate and well controlled studies in pregnant women. Corticosteroids should be used during pregnancy only if the potential benefit justifies the potential risk to the fetus.

Nursing Mothers: Hydrocortisone acetate appears in human milk following oral administration of the drug. Since systemic absorption of hydrocortisone may occur when applied topically, caution should be exercised when Cortisporin Cream is used by a nursing woman.

Pediatric Use: Sufficient percutaneous absorption of hydrocortisone can occur in infants and children during prolonged use to cause cessation of growth, as well as other systemic signs and symptoms of hyperadrenocorticism.

ADVERSE REACTIONS

Neomycin occasionally causes skin sensitization. Ototoxicity and nephrotoxicity have also been reported (see WARNINGS section). Adverse reactions have occurred with topical use of antibiotic combinations including neomycin and polymyxin B. Exact incidence figures are not available since no denominator of treated patients is available. The reaction occurring most often is allergic sensitization. In one clinical study using a 20% neomycin patch, neomycin-induced allergic skin reactions occurred in two of 2,175 (0.09%) individuals in the general population.[1] In another study, the incidence was found to be approximately 1%.[2]

The following local adverse reactions have been reported with topical corticosteroids, especially under occlusive dressings: burning, itching, irritation, dryness, folliculitis, hypertrichosis, acneiform eruptions, hypopigmentation, perioral dermatitis, allergic contact dermatitis, maceration of the skin, secondary infection, skin atrophy, striae, and miliaria. When steroid preparations are used for long periods of time in intertriginous areas or over extensive body areas, with or without occlusive non-permeable dressings, striae may occur; also there exists the possibility of systemic side effects when steroid preparations are used over large areas or for a long period of time.

DOSAGE AND ADMINISTRATION

A small quantity of the cream should be applied 2 to 4 times daily, as required. The cream should, if conditions permit, be gently rubbed into the affected areas.

HOW SUPPLIED

Tube of 7.5 g (NDC-0081-0185-98).
Store at 15°–25°C (59°–77°F).

REFERENCES

1. Leyden JJ, Kligman AM: Contact dermatitis to neomycin sulfate. *JAMA* 1979;242(12):1276–1278.
2. Prystowsky SD, Allen AM, Smith RW, *et al:* Allergic contact hypersensitivity to nickel, neomycin, ethylenediamine, and benzocaine. *Arch Dermatol* 1979;115:959–962.

CORTISPORIN® OINTMENT   ℞
[kor'tĭ-spor''ĭn]
(Polymyxin B Sulfate-Bacitracin Zinc-Neomycin Sulfate-Hydrocortisone)

DESCRIPTION

Cortisporin® Ointment (polymyxin B sulfate-bacitracin zinc-neomycin sulfate-hydrocortisone) is a topical antibacterial ointment. Each gram contains: Aerosporin® (polymyxin B sulfate) 5,000 units, bacitracin zinc 400 units, neomycin sulfate equivalent to 3.5 mg neomycin base, hydrocortisone 10 mg (1%), and special white petrolatum qs.

Polymyxin B sulfate is the sulfate salt of polymyxin B_1 and B_2, which are produced by the growth of *Bacillus polymyxa* (Prazmowski) Migula (Fam. Bacillaceae). It has a potency of not less than 6,000 polymyxin B units per mg, calculated on an anhydrous basis.

Bacitracin zinc is the zinc salt of bacitracin, a mixture of related cyclic polypeptides (mainly bacitracin A) produced by the growth of an organism of the *licheniformis* group of *Bacillis subtilis* (Fam. Bacillaceae). It has a potency of not less than 40 bacitracin units per mg.

Neomycin sulfate is the sulfate salt of neomycin B and C, which are produced by the growth of *Streptomyces fradiae*

Continued on next page

Burroughs Wellcome—Cont.

Waksman (Fam. Streptocmycetaceae). It has a potency equivalent of not less than 600 µg of neomycin standard per mg, calculated on an anhydrous basis.

Hydrocortisone, 11β, 17, 21-trihydroxypregn-4-ene-3, 20-dione, is an anti-inflammatory hormone.

CLINICAL PHARMACOLOGY

Corticoids suppress the inflammatory response to a variety of agents and they may delay healing. Since corticoids may inhibit the body's defense mechanism against infection, a concomitant antimicrobial drug may be used when this inhibition is considered to be clinically significant in a particular case.

The anti-infective components in the combination are included to provide action against specific organisms susceptible to them. Polymyxin B sulfate, bacitracin zinc and neomycin sulfate together are considered active against the following microorganisms: *Staphylococcus aureus*, streptococci, including *Streptococcus pneumoniae*, *Escherichia coli*, *Haemophilus influenzae*, *Klebsiella-Enterobacter* species, *Neisseria* species and *Pseudomonas aeruginosa*.

The product does not provide adequate coverage against *Serratia marcescens*.

The relative potency of corticosteroids depends on the molecular structure, concentration and release from the vehicle.

INDICATIONS AND USAGE

For the treatment of corticosteroid-responsive dermatoses with secondary infection. It has not been demonstrated that this steroid-antibiotic combination provides greater benefit than the steroid component alone after 7 days of treatment (see WARNINGS section).

CONTRAINDICATIONS

Not for use in the eyes or in the external ear canal if the eardrum is perforated. This product is contraindicated in tuberculous, fungal or viral lesions of the skin (herpes simplex, vaccinia and varicella). This product is contraindicated in those individuals who have shown hypersensitivity to any of its components.

WARNINGS

Because of the concern of nephrotoxicity and ototoxicity associated with neomycin, this combination should not be used over a wide area or for extended periods of time.

PRECAUTIONS

General: As with any antibiotic preparation, prolonged use may result in the overgrowth of nonsusceptible organisms, including fungi. Appropriate measures should be taken if this occurs. Use of steroids on infected areas should be supervised with care as anti-inflammatory steroids may encourage spread of infection. If this occurs, steroid therapy should be stopped and appropriate antibacterial drugs used. Generalized dermatological conditions may require systemic corticosteroid therapy.

Signs and symptoms of exogenous hyperadrenocorticism can occur with the use of topical corticosteroids, including adrenal suppression. Systemic absorption of topically applied steroids will be increased if extensive body surface areas are treated or if occlusive dressings are used. Under these circumstances, suitable precautions should be taken when long-term use is anticipated.

Information for Patients: If redness, irritation, swelling or pain persists or increases, discontinue use and notify physician. Do not use in the eyes.

Laboratory Tests: Systemic effects of excessive levels of hydrocortisone may include a reduction in the number of circulating eosinophils and a decrease in urinary excretion of 17-hydroxycorticosteroids.

Carcinogenesis, Mutagenesis, Impairment of Fertility: Long-term studies in animals (rats, rabbits, mice) showed no evidence of carcinogenicity attributable to oral administration of corticosteroids.

Pregnancy: *Teratogenic Effects:* Pregnancy Category C. Corticosteroids have been shown to be teratogenic in rabbits when applied topically at concentrations of 0.5% on days 6–18 of gestation and in mice when applied topically at a concentration of 15% on days 10–13 of gestation. There are no adequate and well-controlled studies in pregnant women. Corticosteroids should be used during pregnancy only if the potential benefit justifies the potential risk to the fetus.

Nursing Mothers: Hydrocortisone appears in human milk following oral administration of the drug. Since systemic absorption of hydrocortisone may occur when applied topically, caution should be exercised when Cortisporin Ointment is used by a nursing woman.

Pediatric Use: Sufficient percutaneous absorption of hydrocortisone can occur in infants and children during prolonged use to cause cessation of growth, as well as other systemic signs and symptoms of hyperadrenocorticism.

ADVERSE REACTIONS

Neomycin occasionally causes skin sensitization. Ototoxicity and nephrotoxicity have also been reported (see WARN-

INGS section). Adverse reactions have occurred with topical use of antibiotic combinations including neomycin, bacitracin and polymyxin B. Exact incidence figures are not available since no denominator of treated patients is available. The reaction occurring most often is allergic sensitization. In one clinical study, using a 20% neomycin patch, neomycin-induced allergic skin reactions occurred in two of 2,175 (0.09%) individuals in the general population.[1] In another study, the incidence was found to be approximately 1%.[2]

The following local adverse reactions have been reported with topical corticosteroids, especially under occlusive dressings: burning, itching, irritation, dryness, folliculitis, hypertrichosis, acneiform eruptions, hypopigmentation, perioral dermatitis, allergic contact dermatitis, maceration of the skin, secondary infection, skin atrophy, striae and miliaria. When steroid preparations are used for long periods of time in intertriginous areas or over extensive body areas, with or without occlusive non-permeable dressings, striae may occur; also there exists the possibility of systemic side effects when steroid preparations are used over larger areas or for a long period of time.

DOSAGE AND ADMINISTRATION

A thin film is applied 2 to 4 times daily to the affected area.

HOW SUPPLIED

Tube of ½ oz with applicator tip (NDC 0081-0196-88). Store at 15°–25°C (59°–77°F).

REFERENCES

1. Leyden JJ, Kligman AM: Contact dermatitis to neomycin sulfate. *JAMA* 1979;242:1276–1278.
2. Prystowsky SD, Allen AM, Smith RW, et al: Allergic contact hypersensitivity to nickel, neomycin, ethylenediamine, and benzocaine. *Arch Dermatol* 1979;115:959–962.

CORTISPORIN® OPHTHALMIC   ℞
[kor'tĭ-spor"ĭn]
OINTMENT Sterile
(Polymyxin B Sulfate-Bacitracin Zinc-Neomycin Sulfate-Hydrocortisone)

DESCRIPTION

Cortisporin® Ophthalmic Ointment (polymyxin B sulfate-bacitracin zinc-neomycin sulfate-hydrocortisone) is a sterile antimicrobial and anti-inflammatory ointment for ophthalmic use. Each gram contains: Aerosporin® (polymyxin B sulfate) 10,000 units, bacitracin zinc 400 units, neomycin sulfate equivalent to 3.5 mg neomycin base, hydrocortisone 10 mg (1%) and special white petrolatum, qs.

Polymyxin B sulfate is the sulfate salt of polymyxin B_1 and B_2, which are produced by the growth of *Bacillus polymyxa* (Prazmowski) Migula (Fam. Bacillaceae). It has a potency of not less than 6,000 polymyxin B units per mg, calculated on an anhydrous basis.

Bacitracin zinc is the zinc salt of bacitracin, a mixture of related cyclic polypeptides (mainly bacitracin A) produced by the growth of an organism of the *licheniformis* group of *Bacillus subtilis* (Fam. Bacillaceae). It has a potency of not less than 40 bacitracin units per mg.

Neomycin sulfate is the sulfate salt of neomycin B and C, which are produced by the growth of *Streptomyces fradiae* Waksman (Fam. Streptomycetaceae). It has a potency equivalent of not less than 600 µg of neomycin standard per mg, calculated on an anhydrous basis.

Hydrocortisone, 11β, 17, 21-trihydroxypregn-4-ene-3, 20-dione, is an anti-inflammatory hormone.

CLINICAL PHARMACOLOGY

Corticoids suppress the inflammatory response to a variety of agents and they may delay healing. Since corticoids may inhibit the body's defense mechanism against infection, a concomitant antimicrobial drug may be used when this inhibition is considered to be clinically significant in a particular case.

The anti-infective components in the combination are included to provide action against specific organisms susceptible to them.

Polymyxin B sulfate, bacitracin zinc and neomycin sulfate together are considered active against the following microorganisms: *Staphylococcus aureus*, streptococci, including *Streptococcus pneumoniae*, *Escherichia coli*, *Haemophilus influenzae*, *Klebsiella-Enterobacter* species, *Neisseria* species and *Pseudomonas aeruginosa*.

When used topically, polymyxin B, bacitracin and neomycin are rarely irritating, and absorption from the intact skin or mucous membrane is insignificant. The incidence of skin sensitization to this combination has been shown to be low on normal skin.[1,2] Since these antibiotics are seldom used systemically, the patient is spared sensitization to those antibiotics which might later be required systemically.

When a decision to administer both a corticoid and antimicrobials is made, the administration of such drugs in combination has the advantage of greater patient compliance and convenience, with the added assurance that the intended dosage of both drugs is administered, plus assured compati-

bility of ingredients when both types of drug are in the same formulation and particularly that the intended volume of each drug is delivered simultaneously, thereby avoiding dilution of either medication by successive applications.

The relative potency of corticosteroids depends on the molecular structure, concentration and release from the vehicle.

INDICATIONS AND USAGE

For steroid-responsive inflammatory ocular conditions for which a corticosteroid is indicated and where bacterial infection or a risk of bacterial ocular infection exists.

Ocular steroids are indicated in inflammatory conditions of the palpebral and bulbar conjunctiva, cornea and anterior segment of the globe where the inherent risk of steroid use in certain infective conjunctivitides is accepted to obtain a diminution in edema and inflammation. They are also indicated in chronic anterior uveitis and corneal injury from chemical, radiation, or thermal burns, or penetration of foreign bodies. The use of a combination drug with an anti-infective component is indicated where the risk of infection is high or where there is an expectation that potentially dangerous numbers of bacteria will be present in the eye.

The particular anti-infective drugs in this product are active against the following common bacterial eye pathogens: *Staphylococcus aureus*, streptococci, including *Streptococcus pneumoniae*, *Escherichia coli*, *Haemophilus influenzae*, *Klebsiella-Enterobacter* species, *Neisseria* species, and *Pseudomonas aeruginosa*.

The product does not provide adequate coverage against *Serratia marcescens*.

CONTRAINDICATIONS

Epithelial herpes simplex keratitis (dendritic keratitis), vaccinia, varicella, and many other viral diseases of the cornea and conjunctiva. Mycobacterial infection of the eye. Fungal diseases of ocular structures. Hypersensitivity to a component of the medication. (Hypersensitivity to the antibiotic component occurs at a higher rate than for other components.)

The use of these combinations is always contraindicated after uncomplicated removal of a corneal foreign body.

WARNINGS

Prolonged use may result in glaucoma, with damage to the optic nerve, defects in visual acuity and fields of vision, and posterior subcapsular cataract formation. Prolonged use may suppress the host response and thus increase the hazard of secondary ocular infections. In those diseases causing thinning of the cornea or sclera, perforations have been known to occur with the use of topical steroids. In acute purulent conditions of the eye, steroids may mask infection or enhance existing infection. If these products are used for 10 days or longer, intraocular pressure should be routinely monitored even though it may be difficult in children and uncooperative patients.

Employment of steroid medication in the treatment of herpes simplex requires great caution.

Neomycin sulfate may cause cutaneous sensitization. A precise incidence of hypersensitivity reactions (primarily skin rash) due to topical neomycin is not known.

The manifestations of sensitization to neomycin are usually itching, reddening and edema of the conjunctiva and eyelid. It may be manifest simply as a failure to heal. During long-term use of neomycin-containing products, periodic examination for such signs is advisable, and the patient should be told to discontinue the product if they are observed. These symptoms subside quickly on withdrawing the medication. Neomycin-containing applications should be avoided for the patient thereafter.

PRECAUTIONS

General: The initial prescription and renewal of the medication order beyond 8 grams should be made by a physician only after examination of the patient with the aid of magnification, such as slit lamp biomicroscopy and, where appropriate, fluorescein staining.

The possibility of persistent fungal infections of the cornea should be considered after prolonged steroid dosing.

Allergic cross-reactions may occur which could prevent the use of any or all of the following antibiotics for the treatment of future infections: kanamycin, paromomycin, streptomycin, and possibly gentamicin.

Carcinogenesis, Mutagenesis, Impairment of Fertility: Long-term studies in animals (rats, rabbits, mice) showed no evidence of carcinogenicity attributable to oral administration of corticosteroids.

Pregnancy: *Teratogenic Effects:* Pregnancy Category C. Corticosteroids have been shown to be teratogenic in rabbits when applied topically at concentrations of 0.5% on days 6-18 of gestation and in mice when applied topically at a concentration of 15% on days 10-13 of gestation. There are no adequate and well-controlled studies in pregnant women. Corticosteroids should be used during pregnancy only if the potential benefit justifies the potential risk to the fetus.

Nursing Mothers: Hydrocortisone appears in human milk following oral administration of the drug. Since systemic absorption of hydrocortisone may occur when applied topically, caution should be exercised when Cortisporin Ophthalmic Ointment is used by a nursing woman.

ADVERSE REACTIONS

Adverse reactions have occurred with steroid/anti-infective combination drugs which can be attributed to the steroid component, the anti-infective component, or the combination. Reactions occurring most often from the presence of the anti-infective ingredient are localized hypersensitivity, including itching, swelling and conjunctival erythema. Local irritation on instillation has also been reported. Exact incidence figures are not available since no denominator of treated patients is available.

The reactions due to the steroid component in decreasing order of frequency are: elevation of intraocular pressure (IOP) with possible development of glaucoma, and infrequent optic nerve damage; posterior subcapsular cataract formation; and delayed wound healing.

Secondary Infection: The development of secondary infection has occurred after use of combinations containing steroids and antimicrobials. Fungal infections of the cornea are particularly prone to develop coincidentally with long-term applications of steroid. The possibility of fungal invasion must be considered in any persistent corneal ulceration where steroid treatment has been used.

Secondary bacterial ocular infection following suppression of host responses also occurs.

DOSAGE AND ADMINISTRATION

Apply the ointment in the affected eye every 3 or 4 hours, depending on the severity of the condition.

Not more than 8 grams should be prescribed initially and the prescription should not be refilled without further evaluation as outlined in PRECAUTIONS above.

HOW SUPPLIED

Tube of 1/8 oz with ophthalmic tip (NDC-0081-0197-86). Store at 15°–25°C (59°–77°F).

REFERENCES:

1. Leyden JJ and Kligman AM. Contact Dermatitis to Neomycin Sulfate. JAMA 242 (12):1276-1278, 1979.
2. Prystowsky SD, Allen AM, Smith RW, Nonomura JH, Odom RB and Akers WA. Allergic Contact Hypersensitivity to Nickel, Neomycin, Ethylenediamine, and Benzocaine. Arch Dermatol 115 :959-962, 1979.
DoD NSN 6505-01-102-4303

CORTISPORIN® ℞
[kor'ti-spor"in]
OPHTHALMIC SUSPENSION Sterile
(Polymyxin B Sulfate-Neomycin Sulfate-Hydrocortisone)

DESCRIPTION

Cortisporin® Ophthalmic Suspension (polymyxin B sulfate-neomycin sulfate-hydrocortisone) is a sterile antimicrobial and anti-inflammatory suspension for ophthalmic use. Each ml contains: Aerosporin® (polymyxin B sulfate) 10,000 units, neomycin sulfate equivalent to 3.5 mg neomycin base and hydrocortisone 10 mg (1%). The vehicle contains thimerosal 0.001% (added as a preservative) and the inactive ingredients cetyl alcohol, glyceryl monosterate, mineral oil, polyoxyl 40 stearate, propylene gylcol and water for injection. Sulfuric acid may be added to adjust pH.

Polymyxin B sulfate is the sulfate salt of polymyxin B_1 and B_2, which are produced by the growth of *Bacillus polymyxa* (Prazmowski) Migula (Fam. Bacillaceae). It has a potency of not less than 6,000 polymyxin B units per mg, calculated on an anhydrous basis.

Neomycin sulfate is the sulfate salt of neomycin B and C, which are produced by the growth of *Streptomyces fradiae* Waksman (Fam. Streptomycetaceae). It has a potency equivalent of not less than 600 μg of neomycin standard per mg, calculated on an anhydrous basis.

Hydrocortisone, 11β, 17, 21-trihydroxypregn-4-ene-3,20-dione, is an anti-inflammatory hormone.

CLINICAL PHARMACOLOGY

Corticoids suppress the inflammatory response to a variety of agents and they may delay healing. Since corticoids may inhibit the body's defense mechanism against infection, a concomitant antimicrobial drug may be used when this inhibition is considered to be clinically significant in a particular case.

The anti-infective components in the combination are included to provide action against specific organisms susceptible to them. Polymyxin B sulfate and neomycin sulfate together are considered active against the following microorganisms: *Staphylococcus aureus, Escherichia coli, Haemophilus influenzae, Klebsiella-Enterobacter* species, *Neisseria* species and *Pseudomonas aeruginosa.*

When used topically, polymyxin B and neomycin are rarely irritating, and absorption from the intact skin or mucous membrane is insignificant. The incidence of skin sensitization to this combination has been shown to be low on normal skin.[1,2] Since these antibiotics are seldom used systemically,

the patient is spared sensitization to those antibiotics which might later be required systemically.

When a decision to administer both a corticoid and antimicrobials is made, the administration of such drugs in combination has the advantage of greater patient compliance and convenience, with the added assurance that the intended dosage of both drugs is administered, plus assured compatibility of ingredients when both types of drug are in the same formulation and, particularly that the intended volume of each drug is delivered simultaneously, thereby avoiding dilution of either medication by successive instillations.

The relative potency of corticosteroids depends on the molecular structure, concentration, and release from the vehicle.

INDICATIONS AND USAGE

For steroid-responsive inflammatory ocular conditions for which a corticosteroid is indicated and where bacterial infection or a risk of bacterial ocular infection exists.

Ocular steroids are indicated in inflammatory conditions of the palpebral and bulbar conjunctiva, cornea and anterior segment of the globe where the inherent risk of steroid use in certain infective conjunctivities is accepted to obtain a diminution in edema and inflammation. They are also indicated in chronic anterior uveitis and corneal injury from chemical, radiation, or thermal burns, or penetration of foreign bodies.

The use of a combination drug with an anti-infective component is indicated where the risk of infection is high or where there is an expectation that potentially dangerous numbers of bacteria will be present in the eye.

The particular anti-infective drugs in this product are active against the following common bacterial eye pathogens: *Staphylococcus aureus, Escherichia coli, Haemophilus influenzae, Klebsiella-Enterobacter* species, *Neisseria* species, and *Pseudomonas aeruginosa.*

The product does not provide adequate coverage against *Serratia marcescens* and streptococci, including *Streptococcus pneumoniae.*

CONTRAINDICATIONS

Epithelial herpes simplex keratitis (dendritic keratitis), vaccinia, varicella, and many other viral diseases of the cornea and conjunctiva. Mycobacterial infection of the eye. Fungal diseases of ocular structures. Hypersensitivity to a component of the medication. (Hypersensitivity to the antibiotic component occurs at a higher rate than for other components.)

The use of these combinations is always contraindicated after uncomplicated removal of a corneal foreign body.

WARNINGS

Prolonged use may result in glaucoma, with damage to the optic nerve, defects in visual acuity and fields of vision, and posterior subcapsular cataract formation. Prolonged use may suppress the host response and thus increase the hazard of secondary ocular infections. In those diseases causing thinning of the cornea or sclera, perforations have been known to occur with the use of topical steroids. In acute purulent conditions of the eye, steroids may mask infection or enhance existing infection. If these products are used for 10 days or longer, intraocular pressure should be routinely monitored even though it may be difficult in children and uncooperative patients.

Employment of steroid medication in the treatment of herpes simplex requires great caution.

Neomycin sulfate may cause cutaneous sensitization. A precise incidence of hypersensitivity reactions (primarily skin rash) due to topical neomycin is not known.

The manifestations of sensitization to neomycin are usually itching, reddening and edema of the conjunctiva and eyelid. It may be manifest simply as a failure to heal. During long-term use of neomycin-containing products, periodic examination for such signs is advisable, and the patient should be told to discontinue the product if they are observed. These symptoms subside quickly on withdrawing the medication. Neomycin-containing applications should be avoided for the patient thereafter.

PRECAUTIONS

General: The initial prescription and renewal of the medication order beyond 20 milliliters should be made by a physician only after examination of the patient with the aid of magnification, such as slit lamp biomicroscopy and, where appropriate, fluorescein staining.

The possibility of persistent fungal infections of the cornea should be considered after prolonged steroid dosing.

Allergic cross-reactions may occur which could prevent the use of any or all of the following antibiotics for the treatment of future infections: kanamycin, paromomycin, streptomycin, and possibly gentamicin.

Carcinogenesis, Mutagenesis, Impairment of Fertility: Long-term studies in animals (rats, rabbits, mice) showed no evidence of carcinogenicity attributable to oral administration of corticosteroids.

Pregnancy: *Teratogenic Effects:* Pregnancy Category C. Corticosteroids have been shown to be teratogenic in rabbits when applied topically at concentrations of 0.5% on days 6–18 of gestation and in mice when applied topically at a

concentration of 15% on days 10–13 of gestation. There are no adequate and well-controlled studies in pregnant women. Corticosteroids should be used during pregnancy only if the potential benefit justifies the potential risk to the fetus.

Nursing Mothers: Hydrocortisone appears in human milk following oral administration of the drug. Since systemic absorption of hydrocortisone may occur when applied topically, caution should be exercised when Cortisporin Ophthalmic Suspension is used by a nursing woman.

ADVERSE REACTIONS

Adverse reactions have occurred with steroid/anti-infective combination drugs which can be attributed to the steroid component, the anti-infective component, or the combination. Reactions occurring most often from the presence of the anti-infective ingredient are localized hypersensitivity, including itching, swelling and conjunctival erythema. Local irritation on instillation has also been reported. Exact incidence figures are not available since no denominator of treated patients is available.

The reactions due to the steroid component in decreasing order of frequency are: elevation of intraocular pressure (IOP) with possible development of glaucoma, and infrequent optic nerve damage; posterior subcapsular cataract formation; and delayed wound healing.

Secondary Infection: The development of secondary infection has occurred after use of combinations containing steroids and antimicrobials. Fungal infections of the cornea are particularly prone to develop coincidentally with long-term applications of steroid. The possibility of fungal invasion must be considered in any persistent corneal ulceration where steroid treatment has been used.

Secondary bacterial ocular infection following suppression of host responses also occurs.

DOSAGE AND ADMINISTRATION

One or two drops in the affected eye every 3 or 4 hours, depending on the severity of the condition. The suspension may be used more frequently if necessary.

Not more than 20 milliliters should be prescribed initially and the prescription should not be refilled without further evaluation as outlined in PRECAUTIONS above.

SHAKE WELL BEFORE USING.

HOW SUPPLIED

Plastic DROP DOSE® dispenser bottle of 7.5 ml (NDC-0081-0193-02). Store at 15°–25°C (59°–77°F).

REFERENCES

1. Leyden JJ and Kligman AM. Contact Dermatitis to Neomycin Sulfate. JAMA 242 (12): 1276–1278, 1979.
2. Prystowsky SD, Allen AM, Smith RW, Nonomura JH, Odom RB and Akers WA. Allergic Contact Hypersensitivity to Nickel, Neomycin, Ethylenediamine, and Benzocaine. Arch Dermatol 115 :959–962, 1979.
DOD NSN 6505-00-764-9042

CORTISPORIN® OTIC SOLUTION Sterile ℞
[kor'ti-spor"in ō-tik]
(Polymyxin B Sulfate-Neomycin Sulfate-Hydrocortisone)

DESCRIPTION

Cortisporin Otic Solution (polymyxin B sulfate-neomycin sulfate-hydrocortisone) is a sterile antibacterial and anti-inflammatory solution for otic use. Each ml contains: Aerosporin® (polymyxin B sulfate) 10,000 units, neomycin sulfate equivalent to 3.5 mg neomycin base, and hydrocortisone 10 mg (1%). The vehicle contains potassium metabisulfite 0.1% (added as a preservative) and the inactive ingredients cupric sulfate, glycerin, hydrochloric acid, propylene glycol, and Water for Injection.

Polymyxin B sulfate is the sulfate salt of polymyxin B_1 and B_2, which are produced by the growth of *Bacillus polymyxa* (Prazmowski) Migula (Fam. Bacillaceae). It has a potency of not less than 6,000 polymyxin B units per mg, calculated on an anhydrous basis.

Neomycin sulfate is the sulfate salt of neomycin B and C, which are produced by the growth of *Streptomyces fradiae* Waksman (Fam. Streptomycetaceae). It has a potency equivalent of not less than 600 μg of neomycin standard per mg, calculated on an anhydrous basis.

Hydrocortisone, 11β, 17, 21-trihydroxypregn-4-ene-3, 20-dione, is an anti-inflammatory hormone.

CLINICAL PHARMACOLOGY

Corticoids suppress the inflammatory response to a variety of agents and they may delay healing. Since corticoids may inhibit the body's defense mechanism against infection, a concomitant antimicrobial drug may be used when this inhibition is considered to be clinically significant in a particular case.

The anti-infective components in the combination are included to provide action against specific organisms susceptible to them. Polymyxin B sulfate and neomycin sulfate to-

Continued on next page

Burroughs Wellcome—Cont.

gether are considered active against the following microorganisms: *Staphylococcus aureus, Escherichia coli, Haemophilus influenzae, Klebsiella-Enterobacter* species, *Neisseria* species, and *Pseudomonas aeruginosa*. This product does not provide adequate coverage against *Serratia marcescens* and streptococci, including *Streptococcus pneumonia*.

The relative potency of corticosteroids depends on the molecular structure, concentration, and release from the vehicle.

INDICATIONS AND USAGE

For the treatment of superficial bacterial infections of the external auditory canal caused by organisms susceptible to the action of the antibiotics.

CONTRAINDICATIONS

This product is contraindicated in those individuals who have shown hypersensitivity to any of its components, and in herpes simplex, vaccinia and varicella infections.

WARNINGS

This product should be used with care when the integrity of the tympanic membrane is in question because of the possibility of ototoxicity, and because stinging and burning may occur when this product gains access to the middle ear.

Neomycin sulfate may cause cutaneous sensitization. A precise incidence of hypersensitivity reactions (primarily skin rash) due to topical neomycin is not known.

When using neomycin-containing products to control secondary infection in the chronic dermatoses, such as chronic otitis externa or stasis dermatitis, it should be borne in mind that the skin in these conditions is more liable than is normal skin to become sensitized to many substances, including neomycin. The manifestation of sensitization to neomycin is usually a low-grade reddening with swelling, dry scaling and itching; it may be manifest simply as a failure to heal. Periodic examination for such signs is advisable, and the patient should be told to discontinue the product if they are observed. These symptoms regress quickly on withdrawing the medication. Neomycin-containing applications should be avoided for the patient thereafter.

Contains potassium metabisulfite, a sulfite that may cause allergic-type reactions including anaphylactic symptoms and life-threatening or less severe asthmatic episodes in certain susceptible people. The overall prevalence of sulfite sensitivity in the general population is unknown and probably low. Sulfite sensitivity is seen more frequently in asthmatic than in nonasthmatic people.

PRECAUTIONS

General: As with other antibiotic preparations, prolonged use may result in overgrowth of nonsusceptible organisms, including fungi.

If the infection is not improved after one week, cultures and susceptibility tests should be repeated to verify the identity of the organism and to determine whether therapy should be changed.

Treatment should not be continued for longer than ten days. Allergic cross-reactions may occur which could prevent the use of any or all of the following antibiotics for the treatment of future infections: kanamycin, paromomycin, streptomycin, and possibly gentamicin.

Information for Patients: Avoid contaminating the dropper with material from the ear, fingers, or other source. This caution is necessary if the sterility of the drops is to be preserved.

If sensitization or irritation occurs, discontinue use immediately and contact your physician.

Do not use in the eyes.

Laboratory Tests: Systemic effects of excessive levels of hydrocortisone may include a reduction in the number of circulating eosinophils and a decrease in urinary excretion of 17-hydroxycorticosteroids.

Carcinogenesis, Mutagenesis, Impairment of Fertility: Long-term studies in animals (rats, rabbits, mice) showed no evidence of carcinogenicity attributable to oral administration of corticosteroids.

Pregnancy: Teratogenic effects: Pregnancy Category C. Corticosteroids have been shown to be teratogenic in rabbits when applied topically at concentrations of 0.5% on days 6 to 18 of gestation and in mice when applied topically at a concentration of 15% on days 10 to 13 of gestation. There are no adequate and well-controlled studies in pregnant women. Corticosteroids should be used during pregnancy only if the potential benefit justifies the potential risk to the fetus.

Nursing Mothers: Hydrocortisone appears in human milk following oral administration of the drug. Since systemic absorption of hydrocortisone may occur when applied topically, caution should be exercised when Cortisporin Otic Solution is used by a nursing woman.

Pediatric Use: See **DOSAGE AND ADMINISTRATION**.

ADVERSE REACTIONS

Neomycin occasionally causes skin sensitization. Ototoxicity and nephrotoxicity have also been reported (See **WARNINGS** section). Adverse reactions have occurred with topical use of antibiotic combinations including neomycin and polymyxin B. Exact incidence figures are not available since no denominator of treated patients is available. The reaction occurring most often is allergic sensitization. In one clinical study, using a 20% neomycin patch, neomycin-induced allergic skin reactions occurred in two of 2,175 (0.9%) individuals in the general population.[1] In another study, the incidence was found to be approximately 1%.[2]

The following local adverse reactions have been reported with topical corticosteroids, especially under occlusive dressings: burning, itching, irritation, dryness, folliculitis, hypertrichosis, acneiform eruptions, hypopigmentation, perioral dermatitis, allergic contact dermatitis, maceration of the skin, secondary infection, skin atrophy, striae, and miliaria. Stinging and burning have been reported when this product has gained access to the middle ear.

DOSAGE AND ADMINISTRATION

The external auditory canal should be thoroughly cleansed and dried with a sterile cotton applicator.

For adults, 4 drops of the solution should be instilled into the affected ear 3 or 4 times daily. For infants and children, 3 drops are suggested because of the smaller capacity of the ear canal.

The patient should lie with the affected ear upward and then the drops should be instilled. This position should be maintained for 5 minutes to facilitate penetration of the drops into the ear canal.

Repeat, if necessary, for the opposite ear.

If preferred, a cotton wick may be inserted into the canal and then the cotton may be saturated with the solution. This wick should be kept moist by adding further solution every four hours. The wick should be replaced at least once every 24 hours.

HOW SUPPLIED

Bottle of 10 ml with sterilized dropper. (NDC 0081-0199-92). Store at 15° to 25°C (59° to 77°F).

Also Available: Cortisporin Otic Suspension bottle of 10 ml with sterilized dropper.

Pediotic™ Suspension bottle of 7.5 ml with sterilized dropper.

REFERENCES

1. Leyden JJ, Kligman AM. Contact dermatitis to neomycin sulfate, *JAMA* 1979;242(12):1276–1278.
2. Prystowsky SD, Allen AM, Smith RW, et al: Allergic contact hypersensitivity to nickel, neomycin, ethylenediamine, and benzocaine. *Arch Dermatol* 1979; 115:959–962.

CORTISPORIN® OTIC SUSPENSION   ℞

[kor 'tĭ-spor "ĭn ŏ-tĭk]
Sterile
(Polymyxin B Sulfate-Neomycin Sulfate-Hydrocortisone)

DESCRIPTION

Cortisporin Otic Suspension (polymyxin B sulfate-neomycin sulfate-hydrocortisone) is a sterile antibacterial and anti-inflammatory suspension for otic use. Each ml contains: Aerosporin® (polymyxin B sulfate) 10,000 units, neomycin sulfate equivalent to 3.5 mg neomycin base, and hydrocortisone 10 mg (1%). The vehicle contains thimerosal 0.01% (added as a preservative) and the inactive ingredients cetyl alcohol, propylene glycol, polysorbate 80, and Water for Injection. Sulfuric acid may be added to adjust pH.

Polymyxin B sulfate is the sulfate salt of polymyxin B_1 and B_2, which are produced by the growth of *Bacillus polymyxa* (Prazmowski) Migula (Fam. Bacillaceae). It has a potency of not less than 6,000 polymyxin B units per mg, calculated on an anhydrous basis.

Neomycin sulfate is the sulfate salt of neomycin B and C, which are produced by the growth of *Streptomyces fradiae* Waksman (Fam. Streptomycetaceae). It has a potency equivalent of not less than 600 μg of neomycin standard per mg, calculated on an anhydrous basis.

Hydrocortisone, 11β, 17, 21-trihydroxypregn-4-ene-3, 20-dione, is an anti-inflammatory hormone.

CLINICAL PHARMACOLOGY

Corticoids suppress the inflammatory response to a variety of agents and they may delay healing. Since corticoids may inhibit the body's defense mechanism against infection, a concomitant antimicrobial drug may be used when this inhibition is considered to be clinically significant in a particular case.

The anti-infective components in the combination are included to provide action against specific organisms susceptible to them. Polymyxin B sulfate and neomycin sulfate together are considered active against the following microorganisms: *Staphylococcus aureus, Escherichia coli, Haemophilus influenzae, Klebsiella-Enterobacter* species, *Neisseria* species, and *Pseudomonas aeruginosa*. This product does not provide adequate coverage against *Serratia marcescens* and streptococci, including *Streptococcus pneumonia*.

The relative potency of corticosteroids depends on the molecular structure, concentration, and release from the vehicle.

INDICATIONS AND USAGE

For the treatment of superficial bacterial infections of the external auditory canal caused by organisms susceptible to the action of the antibiotics, and for the treatment of infections of mastoidectomy and fenestration cavities caused by organisms susceptible to the antibiotics.

CONTRAINDICATIONS

This product is contraindicated in those individuals who have shown hypersensitivity to any of its components, and in herpes simplex, vaccinia and varicella infections.

WARNINGS

This product should be used with care in cases of perforated eardrum and in long-standing cases of chronic otitis media because of the possibility of ototoxicity.

Neomycin sulfate may cause cutaneous sensitization. A precise incidence of hypersensitivity reactions (primarily skin rash) due to topical neomycin is not known.

When using neomycin-containing products to control secondary infection in the chronic dermatoses, such as chronic otitis externa or stasis dermatitis, it should be borne in mind that the skin in these conditions is more liable than is normal skin to become sensitized to many substances, including neomycin. The manifestation of sensitization to neomycin is usually a low-grade reddening with swelling, dry scaling and itching; it may be manifest simply as a failure to heal. Periodic examination for such signs is advisable, and the patient should be told to discontinue the product if they are observed. These symptoms regress quickly on withdrawing the medication. Neomycin-containing applications should be avoided for the patient thereafter.

PRECAUTIONS

General: As with other antibiotic preparations, prolonged use may result in overgrowth of nonsusceptible organisms, including fungi.

If the infection is not improved after one week, cultures and susceptibility tests should be repeated to verify the identity of the organism and to determine whether therapy should be changed.

Treatment should not be continued for longer than ten days. Allergic cross-reactions may occur which could prevent the use of any or all of the following antibiotics for the treatment of future infections: kanamycin, paromomycin, streptomycin, and possibly gentamicin.

Information for Patients: Avoid contaminating the dropper with material from the ear, fingers, or other source. This caution is necessary if the sterility of the drops is to be preserved.

If sensitization or irritation occurs, discontinue use immediately and contact your physician.

Do not use in the eyes.

SHAKE WELL BEFORE USING.

Laboratory Tests: Systemic effects of excessive levels of hydrocortisone may include a reduction in the number of circulating eosinophils and a decrease in urinary excretion of 17-hydroxycorticosteroids.

Carcinogenesis, Mutagenesis, Impairment of Fertility: Long-term studies in animals (rats, rabbits, mice) showed no evidence of carcinogenicity attributable to oral administration of corticosteroids.

Pregnancy: Teratogenic effects: Pregnancy Category C. Corticosteroids have been shown to be teratogenic in rabbits when applied topically at concentrations of 0.5% on days 6 to 18 of gestation and in mice when applied topically at a concentration of 15% on days 10 to 13 of gestation. There are no adequate and well-controlled studies in pregnant women. Corticosteroids should be used during pregnancy only if the potential benefit justifies the potential risk to the fetus.

Nursing Mothers: Hydrocortisone appears in human milk following oral administration of the drug. Since systemic absorption of hydrocortisone may occur when applied topically, caution should be exercised when Cortisporin Otic Suspension is used by a nursing woman.

Pediatric Use: See DOSAGE AND ADMINISTRATION.

ADVERSE REACTIONS

Neomycin occasionally causes skin sensitization. Ototoxicity and nephrotoxicity have also been reported (See WARNINGS section). Adverse reactions have occurred with topical use of antibiotic combinations including neomycin and polymyxin B. Exact incidence figures are not available since no denominator of treated patients is available. The reaction occurring most often is allergic sensitization. In one clinical study, using a 20% neomycin patch, neomycin-induced allergic skin reactions occurred in two of 2,175 (0.09%) individuals in the general population.[1] In another study, the incidence was found to be approximately 1%.[2]

The following local adverse reactions have been reported with topical corticosteroids, especially under occlusive dressings: burning, itching, irritation, dryness, folliculitis, hypertrichosis, acneiform eruptions, hypopigmentation, perioral dermatitis, allergic contact dermatitis, maceration of the skin, secondary infection, skin atrophy, striae and miliaria. Stinging and burning have been reported rarely when this drug has gained access to the middle ear.

DOSAGE AND ADMINISTRATION

The external auditory canal should be thoroughly cleansed and dried with a sterile cotton applicator.

For adults, 4 drops of the suspension should be instilled into the affected ear 3 or 4 times daily.

For infants and children, 3 drops are suggested because of the smaller capacity of the ear canal.

The patient should lie with the affected ear upward and then the drops should be instilled. This position should be maintained for 5 minutes to facilitate penetration of the drops into the ear canal.

Repeat, if necessary, for the opposite ear.

If preferred, a cotton wick may be inserted into the canal and then the cotton may be saturated with the suspension. This wick should be kept moist by adding further suspension every four hours. The wick should be replaced at least once every 24 hours.

SHAKE WELL BEFORE USING.

HOW SUPPLIED

Bottle of 10 ml with sterilized dropper. (NDC 0081-0198-92). Store at 15° to 25°C (59° to 77°F).

Also Available: Cortisporin Otic Solution bottle of 10 ml with sterilized dropper.

Pediotic™ Suspension bottle of 7.5 ml with sterilized dropper.

REFERENCES

1. Leyden JJ, Kligman AM. Contact dermatitis to neomycin sulfate. *JAMA* 1979;242(12):1276-1278.
2. Prystowsky SD, Allen AM, Smith RW, et al: Allergic contact hypersensitivity to nickel, neomycin, ethylenediamine, and benzocaine. *Arch Dermatol* 1979;115:959-962.

DARAPRIM®
[dair'ah-prïm '']   ℞
(Pyrimethamine)
25 mg Scored Tablets

DESCRIPTION

Daraprim (pyrimethamine) is an antiparasitic available in tablet form for oral administration. Each scored tablet contains 25 mg pyrimethamine and the inactive ingredients corn and potato starch, lactose, and magnesium stearate. Pyrimethamine is known chemically as 2,4-diamino-5-(p-chlorophenyl)-6-ethylpyrimidine.

CLINICAL PHARMACOLOGY

Pyrimethamine is well absorbed, with peak levels occurring between 2 to 6 hours following administration. It is eliminated slowly and has a plasma half-life of approximately 96 hours. Pyrimethamine is 87% bound to human plasma proteins.

Microbiology: Pyrimethamine is a folic acid antagonist and the rationale for its therapeutic action is based on the differential requirement between host and parasite for nucleic acid precursors involved in growth. This activity is highly selective against plasmodia and *Toxoplasma gondii*.

Pyrimethamine possesses blood schizonticidal and some tissue schizonticidal activity against malaria parasites of man. However, its blood schizonticidal activity may be slower than that of 4-aminoquinoline compounds. It does not destroy gametocytes, but arrests sporogony in the mosquito. The action of Daraprim against *Toxoplasma gondii* is greatly enhanced when used in conjunction with sulfonamides. This was demonstrated by Eyles and Coleman[1] in the treatment of experimental toxoplasmosis in the mouse. Jacobs et al [2] demonstrated that combination of the two drugs effectively prevented the development of severe uveitis in most rabbits following the inoculation of the anterior chamber of the eye with toxoplasma.

INDICATIONS AND USAGE

Daraprim (Pyrimethamine) is indicated for the chemoprophylaxis of malaria due to susceptible strains of plasmodia. It should not be used alone to treat an acute attack of malaria. Fast-acting schizonticides such as chloroquine or quinine are indicated and preferable for the treatment of acute attacks. However, conjoint use of Daraprim will initiate *transmission control* and *suppressive cure* for susceptible strains of plasmodia.

Daraprim is also indicated for the treatment of toxoplasmosis. For this purpose the drug should be used conjointly with a sulfonamide since synergism exists with this combination.

CONTRAINDICATIONS

Use of Daraprim is contraindicated in patients with known hypersensitivity to pyrimethamine. Use of the drug is also contraindicated in patients with documented megaloblastic anemia due to folate deficiency.

WARNINGS

The dosage of pyrimethamine required for the treatment of toxoplasmosis is 10 to 20 times the recommended antimalaria dosage and approaches the toxic level. If signs of folate deficiency develop (see ADVERSE REACTIONS) reduce the dosage or discontinue the drug according to the response of the patient. Folinic acid (leucovorin) should be administered in a dosage of 5 to 15 mg daily (orally, I.V. or I.M.) until normal hematopoiesis is restored.

Daraprim should be kept out of the reach of children as children and infants are extremely susceptible to adverse effects from an overdose. Deaths in children have been reported after accidental ingestion.

PRECAUTIONS

General: The recommended dosage for chemoprophylaxis of malaria should not be exceeded. A small "starting" dose for toxoplasmosis is recommended in patients with convulsive disorders to avoid the potential nervous system toxicity of pyrimethamine. Daraprim should be used with caution in patients with impaired renal or hepatic function or in patients with possible folate deficiency, such as individuals with malabsorption syndrome, alcoholism or pregnancy, and those receiving therapy, such as phenytoin, affecting folate levels (see "Pregnancy" subsection).

Information for Patients: Patients should be warned that at the first appearance of a skin rash they should stop use of Daraprim and seek medical attention immediately. Patients should also be warned that the appearance of sore throat, pallor, purpura or glossitis may be early indications of serious disorders which require prophylactic treatment to be stopped, and medical treatment to be sought. Patients should be warned to keep Daraprim out of the reach of children. Patients should be warned that if anorexia and vomiting occur, they may be minimized by taking the drug with meals.

Laboratory Tests: In patients receiving high dosage, as for the treatment of toxoplasmosis, semiweekly blood counts, including platelet counts, should be done.

Drug Interactions: Pyrimethamine may be used with sulfonamides, quinine and other antimalarials, and with other antibiotics. However, the concomitant use of other antifolic drugs, such as sulfonamides or trimethoprim-sulfamethoxazole combinations, while the patient is receiving pyrimethamine for antimalarial prophylaxis, may increase the risk of bone marrow suppression. If signs of folate deficiency develop, pyrimethamine should be discontinued. Folinic acid (leucovorin) should be administered until normal hematopoiesis is restored (see WARNINGS). Mild hepatotoxicity has been reported in some patients when lorazepam and pyrimethamine were administered concomitantly.

Carcinogenesis, Mutagenesis, Impairment of Fertility:
Carcinogenesis: Pyrimethamine has been reported to produce a significant increase in the number of lung tumors per mouse when given intraperitoneally at high doses (0.025 g/kg).[3] There have been two reports of cancer associated with pyrimethamine administration: a 51-year-old female who developed chronic granulocytic leukemia after taking pyrimethamine for two years for toxoplasmosis,[4] and a 56-year-old patient who developed reticulum cell sarcoma after 14 months of pyrimethamine for toxoplasmosis.[5]

Mutagenesis: Pyrimethamine has been shown to be nonmutagenic in the following *in vitro* assays: the Ames point mutation assay, the Rec assay and the *E. coli* WP2 assay. It was positive in the L5178Y/TK +/− mouse lymphoma assay in the absence of exogenous metabolic activation.[6] Human blood lymphocytes cultured *in vitro* had structural chromosome aberrations induced by pyrimethamine.

In vivo, chromosomes analyzed from the bone marrow of rats dosed with pyrimethamine showed an increased number of structural and numerical aberrations.

Impairment of Fertility: The effects of pyrimethamine on rat pregnancy seem to indicate that the fertility index of rats treated with pyrimethamine is lowered only when the higher dosage is used, suggesting a possible toxic effect upon the whole organism and/or the conceptuses.[7]

Pregnancy: *Teratogenic Effects:* Pregnancy Category C. Pyrimethamine has been shown to be teratogenic in rats, hamsters and Goettingen miniature pigs. There are no adequate and well-controlled studies in pregnant women. Daraprim should be used during pregnancy only if the potential benefit justifies the potential risk to the fetus. Concurrent administration of folinic acid is strongly recommended when used for the treatment of toxoplasmosis during pregnancy. Thiersch[8] reported that when rats were given an oral dose of pyrimethamine of 12.5 mg/kg from day 7 to 9 of the gestation period, there was 66.2% resorption and 32.8% of the live fetuses were stunted. When lower doses of 1 mg/kg and 0.5 mg/kg were given for 10 days, days 4 to 13 of gestation, there was 15% and 8.5% resorption, respectively, and 16.6% and 6.9% of the live fetuses were stunted. A daily oral dose as low as 0.3 mg/kg given for days 7 to 16 of gestation still resulted in 2.7% of the fetuses being stunted.

Sullivan and Takacs[9] found that less than 10% of hamster fetuses died or were malformed following single doses of 20 mg to the mother, which on a mg/kg basis was eight to nine times greater than that given to rats.

Hayama and Kokue[10] reported on the administration of pyrimethamine to pregnant female Goettingen miniature pigs. Sows given 0.9 mg/kg/day, during days 11 to 35 of pregnancy, i.e. the period of organogenesis in the pig, delivered normal offspring. Sows administered a high dose 3.6 mg/kg/day during the same gestational period delivered offspring with a high incidence of malformations including cleft palate, club foot, and micrognathia.

Nursing Mothers: Pyrimethamine is excreted in human milk. Milk samples obtained from lactating mothers after treatment with pyrimethamine were found to have measurable concentrations of the drug, with peak concentration at 6 hours postadministration. It is estimated that after a single 75 mg dose of oral pyrimethamine, approximately 3 to 4 mg of the drug would be passed on to the feeding child over a 48-hour period.

Because of the potential for serious adverse reactions in nursing infants from Daraprim, a decision should be made whether to discontinue nursing or to discontinue the drug, taking into account the importance of the drug to the mother. (See "Carcinogenesis, Mutagenesis, Impairment of Fertility" and "Pregnancy" subsections.)

Pediatric Use: See DOSAGE AND ADMINISTRATION

ADVERSE REACTIONS

Hypersensitivity reactions, occasionally severe, can occur at any dose, particularly when pyrimethamine is administered concomitantly with a sulfonamide. With large doses of pyrimethamine, anorexia and vomiting may occur. Vomiting may be minimized by giving the medication with meals: it usually disappears promptly upon reduction of dosage. Doses used in toxoplasmosis may produce megaloblastic anemia, leukopenia, thrombocytopenia, pancytopenia, atrophic glossitis, hematuria and disorders of cardiac rhythm. Hematologic effects, however, may also occur at low doses in certain individuals (see PRECAUTIONS—General).

Insomnia, diarrhea, headache, light-headedness, dryness of the mouth or throat, fever, malaise, dermatitis, abnormal skin pigmentation, depression, seizures, pulmonary eosinophilia, and hyperphenylalaninemia have been reported rarely.

OVERDOSAGE

Acute intoxication may follow the ingestion of an excessive amount of pyrimethamine. Gastrointestinal and/or central nervous system signs may be present, including convulsions. The initial symptoms are usually gastrointestinal and may include abdominal pain, nausea, severe and repeated vomiting, possibly including hematemesis. Central nervous system toxicity may be manifest by initial excitability, generalized and prolonged convulsions which may be followed by respiratory depression, circulatory collapse and death within a few hours. Neurological symptoms appear rapidly (30 minutes to 2 hours after drug ingestion), suggesting that in gross overdosage pyrimethamine has a direct toxic effect on the central nervous system.

The fatal dose is variable, with the smallest reported fatal single dose being 250 mg to 300 mg. There are, however, reports of children who have recovered after taking 375 mg to 625 mg.

There is no specific antidote to acute pyrimethamine poisoning. Gastric lavage is recommended and is effective if carried out very soon after drug ingestion. A parenteral barbiturate may be indicated to control convulsions. Folinic acid may also be given to counteract effects on the hematopoietic system (see WARNINGS).

DOSAGE AND ADMINISTRATION

For Chemoprophylaxis of Malaria:
Adults and children over 10 years—25 mg (1 tablet) once weekly

Children 4 through 10 years—12.5 mg (½ tablet) once weekly

Infants and children under 4 years—6.25 mg (¼ tablet) once weekly

Regimens planned to include *suppressive cure* should be extended through any characteristic periods of early recrudescence and late relapse for at least 10 weeks in each case.

For Treatment of Acute Attacks: Daraprim is recommended in areas where only susceptible plasmodia exist. This drug is not recommended alone in the treatment of acute attacks of malaria in nonimmune persons. Fast-acting schizonticides such as chloroquine or quinine are indicated for treatment of acute attacks. However, conjoint Daraprim dosage of 25 mg daily for 2 days will initiate *transmission control* and *suppressive cure*. Should circumstances arise wherein Daraprim must be used alone in semi-immune persons, the adult dosage for an acute attack is 50 mg for 2 days; children 4 through 10 years old may be given 25 mg daily for 2 days. In any event, clinical cure should be followed by the once-weekly regimen described above.

For Toxoplasmosis: The dosage of Daraprim for the treatment of toxoplasmosis must be carefully adjusted so as to provide maximum therapeutic effect and a minimum of side effects. At the high dosage required, there is a marked variation in the tolerance to the drug. Young patients may tolerate higher doses than older individuals.

The adult *starting* dose is 50 to 75 mg of the drug daily, together with 1 to 4 g daily of a sulfonamide of the sulfapyrimidine type, e.g., sulfadiazine. This dosage is ordinarily continued for 1 to 3 weeks, depending on the response of the patient

Continued on next page

Burroughs Wellcome—Cont.

and his tolerance of the therapy. The dosage may then be reduced to about one-half that previously given for each drug and continued for an additional 4 to 5 weeks.

The pediatric dosage of Daraprim is 1 mg/kg per day divided into 2 equal daily doses; after 2 to 4 days this dose may be reduced to one-half and continued for approximately one month. The usual pediatric sulfonamide dosage is used in conjunction with Daraprim.

HOW SUPPLIED

White, scored tablets containing 25 mg pyrimethamine, imprinted with "DARAPRIM" and "A3A" in bottles of 100 (NDC 0081-0201-55). Store at 15° to 25°C (59° to 77°F) in a dry place and protect from light.

REFERENCES

1. Eyles DE, Coleman N: Synergistic effect of sulfadiazine and Daraprim against experimental toxoplasmosis in the mouse. *Antibiot Chemother* 1953;3:483-490.
2. Jacobs L, Melton ML, Kaufman HE: Treatment of experimental ocular toxoplasmosis, *Arch Ophthalmol* 1964;71:111-118.
3. Bahna L; Pyrimethamine. *LARC Monogr Eval Carcinog Risk Chem* 1977; 13:233-242.
4. Jim RTS, Elizaga FV: Development of chronic granulocytic leukemia in a patient treated with pyrimethamine. *Hawaii Med J* 1977;36(6):173-176.
5. Sadoff L: Antimalarial drugs and Burkitt's lymphoma. *Lancet* 1973; 2(7840):1262-1263.
6. Clive D, Johnson KO, Spector JKS et al.: Validation and characterization of the L5178Y/TK +/− mouse lymphoma mutagen assay system. *Mut Res* 1979;59:61-108.
7. Andrade ATL, Guerra MO, Silva NOG et al.: Antifertility effects of pyrimethamine. *Excerpta Med Int Cong Ser* 1976;370:317-321.
8. Thiersch JB: Effects of certain 2,4-diaminopyrimidine antagonists of folic acid on pregnancy and rat fetus. *Proc Soc Exp Biol Med* 1954;87:571-577.
9. Sullivan GE, Takacs E: Comparative teratogenicity of pyrimethamine in rats and hamsters. *Teratology* 1971;4:205-210.
10. Hayama T, Kokue E: Use of Goettingen miniature pigs for studying pyrimethamine teratogenesis, *CRC Crit Rev Toxicol* 1985;14(4):403-421.

Shown in Product Identification Section, page 407

DIGIBIND®   B̶
[di'gi-bind]
Digoxin Immune Fab (Ovine)

DESCRIPTION

Digibind, Digoxin Immune Fab (Ovine), is a sterile lyophilized powder of antigen binding fragments (Fab) derived from specific antidigoxin antibodies raised in sheep. Production of antibodies specific for digoxin involves conjugation of digoxin as a hapten to human albumin. Sheep are immunized with this material to produce antibodies specific for the antigenic determinants of the digoxin molecule. The antibody is then papain digested and digoxin-specific Fab fragments of the antibody are isolated and purified by affinity chromatography. These antibody fragments have a molecular weight of approximately 50,000.

Each vial which will bind approximately 0.6 mg of digoxin (or digitoxin) contains 40 mg of digoxin-specific Fab fragments derived from sheep plus 75 mg of sorbitol as a stabilizer and 28 mg of sodium chloride. It contains no preservatives.

Digibind is administered by intravenous injection after reconstitution with Sterile Water for Injection (4 ml per vial).

CLINICAL PHARMACOLOGY

After intravenous injection of Digoxin Immune Fab (Ovine) in the baboon, digoxin-specific Fab fragments are excreted in the urine with a biological half-life of about 9 to 13 hours.[1] In humans with normal renal function the half-life appears to be 15 to 20 hours.[2] Experimental studies in animals indicate that these antibody fragments have a large volume of distribution in the extracellular space, unlike whole antibody which distributes in a space only about twice the plasma volume.[1] Ordinarily, following administration of Digibind, improvement in signs and symptoms of digitalis intoxication begins within one-half hour or less.[2,3,4,5]

The affinity of Digibind for digoxin is in the range of 10^9 to 10^{10} M^{-1}, which is greater than the affinity of digoxin for (sodium, potassium) ATPase, the presumed receptor for its toxic effects. The affinity of Digibind for digitoxin is about 10^8 to 10^9 M^{-1}.[6]

Digibind binds molecules of digoxin, making them unavailable for binding at their site of action on cells in the body. The Fab fragment-digoxin complex accumulates in the blood, from which it is excreted by the kidney. The net effect is to shift the equilibrium away from binding of digoxin to its receptors in the body, thereby reversing its effects.

INDICATIONS AND USAGE

Digibind, Digoxin Immune Fab (Ovine), is indicated for treatment of potentially life-threatening digoxin intoxication.[3] Although designed specifically to treat life-threatening digoxin overdose, it has also been used successfully to treat life-threatening digitoxin overdose.[3] Since human experience is limited and the consequences of repeated exposures are unknown, Digibind is not indicated for milder cases of digitalis toxicity.

Manifestations of life-threatening toxicity include severe ventricular arrhythmias such as ventricular tachycardia or ventricular fibrillation, or progressive bradyarrhythmias such as severe sinus bradycardia or second or third degree heart block not responsive to atropine.

Ingestion of more than 10 mg of digoxin in previously healthy adults or 4 mg of digoxin in previously healthy children, or ingestion causing steady-state serum concentrations greater than 10 ng/ml, often results in cardiac arrest. Digitalis-induced progressive elevation of the serum potassium concentration also suggests imminent cardiac arrest. If the potassium concentration exceeds 5 mEq/L in the setting of severe digitalis intoxication, Digibind therapy is indicated.

CONTRAINDICATIONS

There are no known contraindications to the use of Digibind.

WARNINGS

Suicidal ingestion often involves more than one drug; thus toxicity from other drugs should not be overlooked.

One should consider the possibility of anaphylactic, hypersensitivity or febrile reactions. If an anaphylactoid reaction occurs, the drug infusion should be discontinued and appropriate therapy initiated using aminophylline, oxygen, volume expansion, diphenhydramine, corticosteroids and airway management as indicated. The need for epinephrine should be balanced against its potential risk in the setting of digitalis toxicity.

Since the Fab fragment of the antibody lacks the antigenic determinants of the Fc fragment, it should pose less of an immunogenic threat to patients than does an intact immunoglobulin molecule. Patients with known allergies would be particularly at risk, as would individuals who have previously received antibodies or Fab fragments raised in sheep. Skin testing for allergy was performed during the clinical investigation of Digibind. Only one patient developed erythema at the site of skin testing, with no accompanying wheal reaction; this individual had no adverse reaction to systemic treatment with Digibind. Since allergy testing can delay urgently needed therapy, it is not routinely required before treatment of life-threatening digitalis toxicity with Digibind.

Skin testing may be appropriate for high risk individuals, especially patients with known allergies or those previously treated with Digoxin Immune Fab (Ovine). The intradermal skin test can be performed by: 1. Diluting 0.1 ml of reconstituted Digibind (10 mg/ml) in 9.9 ml sterile isotonic saline (1:100 dilution, 100 μg/ml). 2. Inject 0.1 ml of the 1:100 dilution (10μg) intradermally and observe for an urticarial wheal surrounded by a zone of erythema. The test should be read at 20 minutes.

The scratch test procedure is performed by placing one drop of a 1:100 dilution of Digibind on the skin and then making a ¼-inch scratch through the drop with a sterile needle. The scratch site is inspected at 20 minutes for an urticarial wheal surrounded by erythema.

If skin testing causes a systemic reaction, a tourniquet should be applied above the site of testing and measures to treat anaphylaxis should be instituted. Further administration of Digibind should be avoided unless its use is absolutely essential, in which case the patient should be pretreated with corticosteroids and diphenhydramine, and preparations made for treating anaphylaxis.

PRECAUTIONS

General: Digoxin Immune Fab (Ovine) has been used on only a limited scale in man and its safety has therefore not yet been completely defined.

Standard therapy for digitalis intoxication includes withdrawal of the drug and correction of factors that may contribute to toxicity, such as electrolyte disturbances, hypoxia, acid-base disturbances and agents such as catecholamines. Also, treatment of arrhythmias may include judicious potassium supplements, lidocaine, phenytoin, procainamide and /or propranolol; treatment of sinus bradycardia or atrioventricular block may involve atropine or pacemaker insertion. Massive digitalis intoxication can cause hyperkalemia; administration of potassium supplements in the setting of massive intoxication may be hazardous (see Laboratory Tests). After treatment with Digibind, the serum potassium concentration may drop rapidly[2] and must be monitored frequently, especially over the first several hours after Digibind is given (see Laboratory Tests).

The elimination half-life in the setting of renal failure has not been clearly defined. Several patients with mild to moderate renal dysfunction have been successfully treated with Digibind.[4] There is no evidence to suggest the time course of

therapeutic effect is any different in these patients than in patients with normal renal function, but excretion of the Fab fragment-digoxin complex from the body is probably delayed. In patients who are functionally anephric, one would anticipate failure to clear the Fab fragment-digoxin complex from the blood by glomerular filtration and renal excretion. In this setting the reticuloendothelial system might eliminate the complex. Whether this would lead to detoxification or to reintoxication following release of newly unbound digoxin into the blood is uncertain. Such patients should be monitored for a prolonged period for possible recurrence of digitalis toxicity.

Patients with intrinsically poor cardiac function may deteriorate from withdrawal of the inotropic action of digoxin. Studies in animals have shown that the reversal of inotropic effect is relatively gradual, occurring over hours. When needed, additional support can be provided by use of intravenous inotropes, such as dopamine or dobutamine, or vasodilators. One must be careful in using catecholamines not to aggravate digitalis toxic rhythm disturbances. Clearly, other types of digitalis glycosides should not be used in this setting. Redigitalization should be postponed, if possible, until the Fab fragments have been eliminated from the body, which may require several days. Patients with impaired renal function may require a week or longer.

Laboratory Tests: Serum digoxin or digitoxin concentration should be obtained before Digibind administration if at all possible. These measurements may be difficult to interpret if drawn soon after the last digitalis dose, since at least 6 to 8 hours are required for equilibration of digoxin between serum and tissue. Patients should be closely monitored, including temperature, blood pressure, electrocardiogram and potassium concentration, during and after administration of Digibind. The total serum digoxin concentration may rise precipitously following administration of Digibind but this will be almost entirely bound to the Fab fragment and therefore not able to react with receptors in the body. Digibind will interfere with digitalis immunoassay measurements.[7] Thus, the standard serum digoxin concentration measurement can be clinically misleading until the Fab fragment is eliminated from the body, which may require several days. Patients with impaired renal function may require a week or longer before the standard serum digoxin concentration assay will give reliable results.

Potassium concentrations should be followed carefully. Severe digitalis intoxication can cause life-threatening elevation in serum potassium concentration by shifting potassium from inside to outside the cell. The elevation in serum potassium concentration can lead to increased renal excretion of potassium. Thus, these patients may have hyperkalemia with a total body deficit of potassium. When the effect of digitalis is reversed by Digibind, potassium shifts back inside the cell, with a resulting decline in serum potassium concentration.[4] Hypokalemia may thus develop rapidly. For these reasons, serum potassium concentration should be monitored repeatedly, especially over the first several hours after Digibind is given, and cautiously treated when necessary.

Carcinogenesis, Mutagenesis, Impairment of Fertility: There have been no long-term studies performed in animals to evaluate carcinogenic potential.

Pregnancy: Pregnancy Category C. Animal reproduction studies have not been conducted with Digibind. It is also not known whether Digibind can cause fetal harm when administered to a pregnant woman or can affect reproduction capacity. Digibind should be given to a pregnant woman only if clearly needed.

Nursing Mothers: It is not known whether this drug is excreted in human milk. Because many drugs are excreted in human milk, caution should be exercised when Digibind is administered to a nursing woman.

Pediatric Use: Digibind has been successfully used in infants with no apparent adverse sequelae. As in all other circumstances, use of this drug in infants should be based on careful consideration of the benefits of the drug balanced against the potential risk involved.

ADVERSE REACTIONS

Allergic reactions to Digibind have been reported rarely. Atopic patients appear to be at particular risk. In a few instances, low cardiac output states and congestive heart failure could have been exacerbated by withdrawal of the inotropic effects of digitalis. Hypokalemia may occur from reactivation of (sodium, potassium) ATPase (see Laboratory Tests). Patients with atrial fibrillation may develop a rapid ventricular response from withdrawal of the effects of digitalis on the atrioventricular node.[4]

DOSAGE AND ADMINISTRATION

Digibind, Digoxin Immune Fab (Ovine), is administered by the intravenous route over 30 minutes. It is recommended that it be infused through a 0.22 μm membrane filter. If cardiac arrest is imminent, it can be given as a bolus injection. The dosage of Digibind varies according to the amount of digoxin to be neutralized. The average dose used during clinical testing was 10 vials. Dosing guidelines are given below. If after several hours toxicity has not adequately reversed or appears to recur, readministration of Digibind at a dose guided by clinical judgment may be required. If a patient presents with digitalis toxicity from an acute ingestion, and neither a serum digitalis concentration nor an estimated ingestion amount is available, 20 vials (800 mg) of Digibind can be administered. This amount will be adequate to treat most life-threatening ingestions in both adults and children. However, in small children it is important to monitor for volume overload. Failure to respond to Digibind raises the possibility that the clinical problem is not caused by digitalis intoxication. If there is no response to an adequate dose of Digibind, the diagnosis of digitalis toxicity should be questioned.

Dosage Estimates: The dose administered need not be exactly equimolar, especially since digoxin body load calculations are only approximate. In general, a large Digibind dose has a faster onset of effect but may enhance the possibility of a febrile reaction. The following tables give approximate Digibind doses rounded off and expressed as number of vials to administer or, for infants, number of milligrams. More accurate calculations to estimate Digibind requirements are given below.

Table 1 gives dosage estimates of Digibind for adults and children who have ingested a large single dose of digoxin.

TABLE 1: Approximate Digibind dose for Reversal of a Single Ingestion Digoxin Overdose

NUMBER OF DIGOXIN TABLETS OR CAPSULES INGESTED*	DIGIBIND DOSE	
	mg	# of Vials
25	340	8.5
50	680	17
75	1000	25
100	1360	34
150	2000	50
200	2680	67

*0.25 mg tablets with 80% bioavailability or 0.2 mg Lanoxicaps® Capsules

Table 2 gives dosage estimates of Digibind **for adults**, derived from the steady state serum digoxin concentration. The dose is expressed in number of vials.
[See table above].

Table 3 gives dosage estimates of Digibind **for infants and children**, derived from the steady state serum digoxin concentration. Since infants can have much smaller dosage requirements, it is recommended that the 40 mg vial be reconstituted as directed and administered with a tuberculin syringe. For very small doses, a reconstituted vial can be diluted with 36 ml of sterile isotonic saline to achieve a concentration of 1 mg/ml.
[See table below].

Exact Dosage Calculation: The equimolar dose of Digibind required is calculated from the total amount of digoxin (or digitoxin) in the patient's body. An estimate of total body load is based either on the known acutely ingested dose or is estimated by using a steady state serum concentration. For toxicity from an acute ingestion, the total body load of digoxin in mg will be approximately equal to the dose ingested in mg ($\times$ 0.80 to correct for incomplete absorption of tablets). The total body load of digitoxin in mg is equal to the dose ingested in mg.

To estimate total load from the steady-state serum concentration, the patient's serum digoxin concentration in ng/ml is multiplied by the mean volume of distribution of digoxin in the body (5.6 L/kg times patient weight in kg) to give total body load in μg. This is divided by 1000 to obtain the estimated amount of digoxin in the body in mg.

For digoxin: Body load in mg = (serum digoxin concentration)(5.6)(weight in kg) $\div$ 1000

For patients toxic from digitoxin, total body load can be estimated by using the 0.56 L/kg volume of distribution in place of the 5.6 L/kg for digoxin.

For digitoxin: Body load in mg = (serum digitoxin concentration)(0.56)(weight in kg) $\div$ 1000

Each vial of Digibind contains 40 mg of purified digoxin-specific Fab fragments which will bind approximately 0.6 mg of digoxin (or digitoxin). Thus, one can calculate the total number of vials required by dividing the total body load in mg by 0.6 mg/vial.

TABLE 2: Adult Dose Estimate of Digibind (in # of Vials) From Serum Digoxin Concentration

		SERUM DIGOXIN CONCENTRATION (ng/ml)						
		1	2	4	8	12	16	20
PATIENT	40	0.5 v	1 v	2 v	3 v	5 v	6 v	8 v
WEIGHT	60	0.5 v	1 v	2 v	5 v	7 v	9 v	11 v
	70	1 v	2 v	3 v	5 v	8 v	11 v	13 v
(kg)	80	1 v	2 v	3 v	6 v	9 v	12 v	15 v
	100	1 v	2 v	4 v	8 v	11 v	15 v	19 v

v = vials

$$\text{Dose (in \# of vials)} = \frac{\text{Body load (mg)}}{0.6 \text{ (mg/vial)}}$$

The above calculations can be rounded off and simplified as:
Dose (in # of vials) = (serum digoxin concentration)(weight in kg) $\div$ 100
or (serum digitoxin concentration)(weight in kg) $\div$ 1000

If the calculation based on ingested dose differs substantially from the calculation based on serum digoxin or digitoxin concentration, it may be preferable to administer an amount based on the higher calculation. Erroneous calculations may result from inaccurate estimates of the amount ingested or absorbed or from non-steady state serum digoxin or digitoxin concentrations. Inaccurate serum digoxin concentration measurements are a possible source of error; this is especially so for very high values, since most assay kits are not designed to measure values above 5 ng/ml.

The volume of distribution at steady state of 5.6 L/kg for digoxin and 0.56 L/kg for digitoxin are population averages. Individual patients may vary from this average value. Thus, further dosing may be required guided by clinical judgment.

Reconstitution: The contents in each vial to be used should be dissolved with 4 ml of Sterile Water for Injection, by gentle mixing, to give an approximately isosmotic solution with a protein concentration of 10 mg/ml. Reconstituted product should be used promptly. If it is not used immediately, it may be stored under refrigeration at 2 to 8°C (36 to 46°F) for up to 4 hours. The reconstituted product may be diluted if desired with sterile isotonic saline to a convenient volume. Parenteral drug products should be inspected visually for particulate matter and discoloration prior to administration, whenever solution and container permit.

HOW SUPPLIED
Vials containing 40 mg of purified lyophilized digoxin-specific Fab fragments. Box of 1. (NDC-0081-0230-44).

STORAGE
Refrigerate at 2 to 8°C (36 to 46°F).

REFERENCES
1. Smith TW, Lloyd BL, Spicer N, Haber E. Immunogenicity and kinetics of distribution and elimination of sheep digoxin-specific IgG and Fab fragments in the rabbit and baboon. *Clin Exp Immunol* 1979; 36:384–396.
2. Smith TW, Haber E, Yeatman L, Butler VP Jr. Reversal of advanced digoxin intoxication with Fab fragments of digoxin-specific antibodies. *N Engl J Med* 1976; 294:797–800.
3. Smith TW, Butler VP Jr, Haber E, Fozzard H, Marcus Fl, Bremner WF, Schulman IC, Phillips A. Treatment of life-threatening digitalis intoxication with digoxin-specific Fab antibody fragments: Experience in 26 cases. *N Engl J Med* 1982; 307:1357–1362.
4. Wenger TL, Butler VP Jr, Haber E, Smith TW. Treatment of 63 severely digitalis-toxic patients with digoxin-specific antibody fragments. *J Am Coll Cardiol* 1985; 5:118A–123A.
5. Spiegel A, Marchlinski FE. Time course for reversal of digoxin toxicity with digoxin-specific antibody fragments. *Am Heart J* 1985; 109 :1397–1399.
6. Smith TW, Butler VP, Haber E. Characterization of antibodies of high affinity and specificity for the digitalis glycoside digoxin. *Biochemistry* 1970; 9:331–337.
7. Gibb I, Adams PC, Parnham AJ, Jennings K. Plasma digoxin: Assay anomalies in Fab-treated patients. *Br J Clin Pharmacol* 1983; 16:445–447.

EMPIRIN® Tablets
[ĭm'per-ĭn]
Analgesic

(See PDR For Nonprescription Drugs)
Shown in Product Identification Section, page 407

EMPIRIN® with Codeine Tablets   ℞©
[ĭm'per-ĭn with kō'dēn]

DESCRIPTION
Empirin with Codeine is supplied in tablet form for oral administration. Each tablet contains aspirin (acetylsalicylic acid) 325 mg, codeine phosphate in one of the following strengths: No. 2, 15 mg; No. 3, 30 mg and No. 4, 60 mg (Warning—may be habit-forming), and the inactive ingredients colloidal silicon dioxide, microcrystalline cellulose, potato starch, and stearic acid.
Empirin with Codeine has analgesic, antipyretic and anti-inflammatory effects.
The components of Empirin with Codeine have the following chemical names:
a. Aspirin (acetylsalicylic acid): 2-(acetyloxy)benzoic acid
b. Codeine phosphate U.S.P.: 7,8-didehydro-4, 5α-epoxy-3-methoxy-17-methylmorphinan-6α-ol phosphate (1:1) (salt) hemihydrate

CLINICAL PHARMACOLOGY
Aspirin: The analgesic, anti-inflammatory and antipyretic effects of aspirin are believed to result from inhibition of the synthesis of certain prostaglandins. Aspirin interferes with clotting mechanisms primarily by diminishing platelet aggregation; at high doses prothrombin synthesis can be inhibited.
Aspirin in solution is rapidly absorbed from the stomach and from the upper small intestine. About 50 percent of an oral dose is absorbed in 30 minutes and peak plasma concentrations are reached in about 40 minutes. Higher than normal stomach pH or the presence of food slightly delays absorption.
Once absorbed, aspirin is mainly hydrolyzed to salicylic acid and distributed to all body tissues and fluids, including fetal tissue, breast milk and the central nervous system (CNS). Highest concentrations are found in plasma, liver, renal cortex, heart and lung.
From 50 to 80 percent of the salicylic acid and its metabolites in plasma are loosely bound to proteins. The plasma half-life of total salicylate is about 3.0 hours, with a 650 mg dose. Higher doses of aspirin cause increases in plasma salicylate half-life. Metabolism occurs primarily in the hepatocytes. The major metabolites are salicyluric acid (75%), the phenolic and acyl glucuronides of salicylate (15%), and gentisic and gentisuric acid (<1%).
Almost all of a therapeutic dose of aspirin is excreted through the kidneys, either as salicylic acid or the above-mentioned metabolic products. Renal clearance of salicylates is greatly augmented by an alkaline urine, as is produced by concurrent administration of sodium bicarbonate or potassium citrate.
Toxic salicylate blood levels are usually above 30 mg/100 ml. The single lethal dose of aspirin in normal adults is approximately 25–30 g, but patients have recovered from much larger doses with appropriate treatment.
Codeine: Codeine probably exerts its analgesic effect through actions on opiate receptors in the CNS.
Codeine is readily absorbed from the gastrointestinal tract, and a therapeutic dose reaches peak analgesic effectiveness in about 2 hours and persists for 4 to 6 hours. Oral codeine (60 mg) given to healthy males has been shown to achieve peak blood levels of 0.016 mg/100 ml at approximately one hour post-dose. The codeine plasma half-life for a 60 mg oral dose is about 2.9 hours. Blood levels causing CNS depression begin at 0.05–0.19 mg/100 ml. The single lethal dose of codeine in adults is estimated to be approximately 0.5–1.0 g. Codeine is rapidly distributed from blood to body tissues and taken up preferentially by parenchymatous organs such as liver, spleen and kidney. It passes the blood-brain barrier and is found in fetal tissue and breast milk.

TABLE 3: Infants and Children Dose Estimates of Digibind (in mg) From Serum Digoxin Concentration

		SERUM DIGOXIN CONCENTRATION (ng/ml)						
		1	2	4	8	12	16	20
PATIENT	1	0.5* mg	1* mg	1.5* mg	3 mg	5 mg	6 mg	8 mg
WEIGHT	3	1* mg	2* mg	5 mg	9 mg	13 mg	18 mg	22 mg
(kg)	5	2* mg	4 mg	8 mg	15 mg	22 mg	30 mg	40 mg
	10	4 mg	8 mg	15 mg	30 mg	40 mg	60 mg	80 mg
	20	8 mg	15 mg	30 mg	60 mg	80 mg	120 mg	160 mg

*Dilution of reconstituted vial of 1 mg/ml may be desirable

Continued on next page

Burroughs Wellcome—Cont.

The drug is not bound by plasma proteins nor is it accumulated in body tissues. Codeine is metabolized in liver to morphine and norcodeine, each representing about 10 percent of the administered dose of codeine. About 90 percent of the dose is excreted within 24 hours, primarily through the kidneys. Urinary excretion products are free and glucuronide-conjugated codeine (about 70%), free and conjugated norcodeine (about 10%), free and conjugated morphine (about 10%), normorphine (under 4%) and hydrocodone (<1%). The remainder of the dose appears in the feces.

INDICATIONS AND USAGE

Empirin with Codeine is indicated for the relief of mild, moderate, and moderate to severe pain.

CONTRAINDICATIONS

Empirin with Codeine is contraindicated under the following conditions:

(1) hypersensitivity or intolerance to aspirin or codeine,
(2) severe bleeding, disorders of coagulation or primary hemostasis, including hemophilia, hypoprothrombinemia, von Willebrand's disease, the thrombocytopenias, thrombasthenia and other ill-defined hereditary platelet dysfunctions, as well as such associated conditions as severe vitamin K deficiency and severe liver damage,
(3) anticoagulant therapy, and
(4) peptic ulcer, or other serious gastrointestinal lesions.

WARNINGS

Therapeutic doses of aspirin can cause anaphylactic shock and other severe allergic reactions. A history of allergy is often lacking.

Significant bleeding can result from aspirin therapy in patients with peptic ulcer or other gastrointestinal lesions, and in patients with bleeding disorders. Aspirin administered pre-operatively may prolong the bleeding time.

In the presence of head injury or other intracranial lesions, the respiratory depressant effects of codeine and other narcotics may be markedly enhanced, as well as their capacity for elevating cerebrospinal fluid pressure. Narcotics also produce other CNS depressant effects, such as drowsiness, that may further obscure the clinical course of patients with head injuries.

Codeine or other narcotics may obscure signs on which to judge the diagnosis or clinical course of patients with acute abdominal conditions.

Results from pilot epidemiologic studies suggest an association between aspirin and Reye Syndrome. Caution should be used in administering this product to children, including teenagers, with chicken pox or flu.

PRECAUTIONS

General: Empirin with Codeine should be prescribed with caution for certain special-risk patients such as the elderly or debilitated, and those with severe impairment of renal or hepatic function, gallbladder disease or gallstones, respiratory impairment, cardiac arrhythmias, inflammatory disorders of the gastrointestinal tract, hypothyroidism, Addison's disease, prostatic hypertrophy or urethral stricture, coagulation disorders, head injuries, or acute abdominal conditions. Empirin with Codeine should not be prescribed for long-term therapy unless specifically indicated.

Precautions should be taken when administering salicylates to persons with known allergies. Hypersensitivity to aspirin is particularly likely in patients with nasal polyps, and relatively common in those with asthma.

Information for Patients: Empirin with Codeine may impair the mental and/or physical abilities required for the performance of potentially hazardous tasks such as driving a car or operating machinery. Such tasks should be avoided while taking Empirin with Codeine.

Alcohol and other CNS depressants may produce an additive CNS depression when taken with Empirin with Codeine, and should be avoided.

Codeine may be habit-forming when used over long periods or in high doses. Patients should take the drug only for as long as it is prescribed, in the amounts prescribed, and no more frequently than prescribed.

Laboratory Tests: Hypersensitivity to aspirin cannot be detected by skin testing or radioimmunoassay procedures. The primary screening tests for detecting a bleeding tendency are platelet count, bleeding time, activated partial thromboplastin time and prothrombin time.

In patients with severe hepatic or renal disease, effects of therapy should be monitored with serial liver and/or renal function tests.

Drug Interactions: Empirin with Codeine may *enhance* the effects of:

(1) monoamine oxidase (MAO) inhibitors,
(2) oral anticoagulants, causing bleeding by inhibiting prothrombin formation in the liver and displacing anticoagulants from plasma protein binding sites,
(3) oral antidiabetic agents and insulin, causing hypoglycemia by contributing an additive effect, and by displacing the oral antidiabetic agents from secondary binding sites,
(4) 6-mercaptopurine and methotrexate, causing bone marrow toxicity and blood dyscrasias by displacing these drugs from secondary binding sites,
(5) penicillins and sulfonamides, increasing their blood levels by displacing these drugs from protein binding sites,
(6) non-steroidal anti-inflammatory agents, increasing the risk of peptic ulceration and bleeding by contributing additive effects,
(7) other narcotic analgesics, alcohol, general anesthetics, tranquilizers such as chlordiazepoxide, sedative-hypnotics, or other CNS depressants, causing increased CNS depression,
(8) corticosteroids, potentiating steroid anti-inflammatory effects by displacing steroids from protein binding sites. Aspirin intoxication may occur with corticosteroid withdrawal because steroids promote renal clearance of salicylates.

Empirin with Codeine may *diminish* the effects of:

(1) uricosuric agents such as probenecid and sulfinpyrazone, reducing their effectiveness in the treatment of gout. Aspirin competes with these agents for protein binding sites.

Aspirin and its metabolites may be caused to accumulate in the body, perhaps to toxic levels, by para-aminosalicylic acid, furosemide, and vitamin C.

Drug/Laboratory Test Interactions:

Aspirin: Aspirin may interfere with the following laboratory determinations in blood: serum amylase, fasting blood glucose, carbon dioxide, cholesterol, protein, protein bound iodine, uric acid, prothrombin time, bleeding time, and spectrophotometric detection of barbiturates. Aspirin may interfere with the following laboratory determinations in urine: glucose, 5-hydroxyindoleacetic acid, Gerhardt ketone, vanillylmandelic acid (VMA), protein, uric acid, and diacetic acid.

Codeine: Codeine may increase serum amylase levels.

Carcinogenesis, Mutagenesis, Impairment of Fertility: No adequate long-term studies have been conducted in animals to determine whether codeine has a potential for carcinogenesis, mutagenesis, or impairment of fertility.

Adequate long-term studies have been conducted in mice and rats with aspirin, alone or in combination with other drugs, in which no evidence of carcinogenesis was seen. No adequate studies have been conducted in animals to determine whether aspirin has a potential for mutagenesis or impairment of fertility.

Pregnancy: *Teratogenic Effects:* Pregnancy Category C. Animal reproduction studies have not been conducted with Empirin with Codeine. It is also not known whether Empirin with Codeine can cause fetal harm when administered to a pregnant woman or can affect reproduction capacity. Empirin with Codeine should be given to a pregnant woman only if clearly needed.

Reproductive studies in rats and mice have shown aspirin to be teratogenic and embryocidal at four to six times the human therapeutic dose. Studies in pregnant women, however, have not shown that aspirin increases the risk of abnormalities when administered during the first trimester of pregnancy. In controlled studies involving 41,337 pregnant women and their offspring, there was no evidence that aspirin taken during pregnancy caused stillbirth, neonatal death or reduced birthweight. In controlled studies of 50,282 pregnant women and their offspring, aspirin administration in moderate and heavy doses during the first four lunar months of pregnancy showed no teratogenic effect.

Reproduction studies have been performed in rabbits and rats at doses up to 150 times the human dose and have revealed no evidence of impaired fertility or harm to the fetus due to codeine.

Nonteratogenic Effects: Therapeutic doses of aspirin in pregnant women close to term may cause bleeding in mother, fetus, or neonate. During the last six months of pregnancy, regular use of aspirin in high doses may prolong pregnancy and delivery.

Labor and Delivery: Ingestion of aspirin prior to delivery may prolong delivery or lead to bleeding in the mother or neonate. Use of codeine during labor may lead to respiratory depression in the neonate.

Nursing Mothers: Aspirin and codeine are excreted in breast milk in small amounts, but the significance of their effects on nursing infants is not known. Because of the potential for serious adverse reactions in nursing infants from Empirin with Codeine, a decision should be made whether to discontinue nursing or to discontinue the drug, taking into account the importance of the drug to the mother.

ADVERSE REACTIONS

Codeine: The most frequently observed adverse reactions to codeine include light-headedness, dizziness, drowsiness, nausea, vomiting, constipation and depression of respiration. Less common reactions to codeine include euphoria, dysphoria, pruritus and skin rashes.

Aspirin: Mild aspirin intoxication (salicylism) can occur in response to chronic use of large doses. Manifestations include nausea, vomiting, hearing impairment, tinnitus, diminished vision, headache, dizziness, drowsiness, mental confusion, hyperpnea, hyperventilation, tachycardia, sweating and thirst.

Therapeutic doses of aspirin can induce mild or severe allergic reactions manifested by skin rashes, urticaria, angioedema, rhinorrhea, asthma, abdominal pain, nausea, vomiting, or anaphylactic shock. A history of allergy is often lacking, and allergic reactions may occur even in patients who have previously taken aspirin without any ill effects. Allergic reactions to aspirin are most likely to occur in patients with a history of allergic disease, especially in patients with nasal polyps or asthma.

Some patients are unable to take aspirin or other salicylates without developing nausea or vomiting. Occasional patients respond to aspirin (usually in large doses) with dyspepsia or heartburn, which may be accompanied by occult bleeding. Excessive bruising or bleeding is sometimes seen in patients with mild disorders of primary hemostasis who regularly use low doses of aspirin.

Prolonged use of aspirin can cause painless erosion of gastric mucosa, occult bleeding and, infrequently, iron-deficiency anemia. High doses of aspirin can exacerbate symptoms of peptic ulcer and, occasionally, cause extensive bleeding. Excessive bleeding can follow injury or surgery in patients with or without known bleeding disorders who have taken therapeutic doses of aspirin within the preceding 10 days. Hepatotoxicity has been reported in association with prolonged use of large doses of aspirin in patients with lupus erythematosus, rheumatoid arthritis and rheumatic disease. Bone marrow depression, manifested by weakness, fatigue, or abnormal bruising or bleeding, has occasionally been reported.

In patients with glucose-6-phosphate dehydrogenase deficiency, aspirin can cause a mild degree of hemolytic anemia. In hyperuricemic persons, low doses of aspirin may reduce the effectiveness of uricosuric therapy or precipitate an attack of gout.

DRUG ABUSE AND DEPENDENCE

Like other medications containing a narcotic analgesic, Empirin with Codeine is controlled by the Drug Enforcement Administration and is classified under Schedule III.

Empirin with Codeine can produce drug dependence of the morphine type, therefore, it has a potential for being abused. Psychic dependence, physical dependence and tolerance may develop on repeated administration.

The dependence liability of codeine has been found to be too small to permit a full definition of its characteristics. Studies indicate that addiction to codeine is extremely uncommon and requires very high parenteral doses.

When dependence on codeine occurs at therapeutic doses, it appears to require from one to two months to develop, and withdrawal symptoms are mild. Most patients on long-term oral codeine therapy show no signs of physical dependence upon abrupt withdrawal.

OVERDOSAGE

Severe intoxication, caused by overdose of Empirin with Codeine may produce: skin eruptions, dyspnea, vertigo, double vision, delusions, hallucinations, garbled speech, excitability, restlessness, delirium, constricted pupils, a positive Babinski sign, respiratory depression (slow and shallow breathing; Cheyne-Stokes respiration), cyanosis, clammy skin, muscle flaccidity, circulatory collapse, stupor and coma. In children, difficulty in hearing, tinnitus, dim vision, headache, dizziness, drowsiness, confusion, rapid breathing, sweating, thirst, nausea, vomiting, hyperpyrexia, dehydration and convulsions are prominent signs. The most severe manifestations from aspirin result from cardiovascular and respiratory insufficiency secondary to acid-base and electrolyte disturbances, complicated by hyperthermia and dehydration. The most severe manifestations from codeine are associated with respiratory depression.

Respiratory alkalosis is characteristic of the early phase of intoxication with aspirin while hyperventilation is occurring, but is quickly followed by metabolic acidosis in most people with severe intoxication. This occurs more readily in children. Hypoglycemia may occur in children who have taken large overdoses. Other laboratory findings associated with aspirin intoxication include ketonuria, hyponatremia, hypokalemia, and occasionally proteinuria. A slight rise in lactic dehydrogenase and hydroxybutyric dehydrogenase may occur.

Concentrations of aspirin in plasma above 30 mg/100 ml are associated with toxicity. (See Clinical Pharmacology section for information on factors influencing aspirin blood levels.) The single lethal dose of aspirin in adults is probably about 25–30 g, but is not known with certainty.

The toxic plasma concentration of codeine is not known with certainty. Experimental production of mild to moderate CNS depression in healthy, nontolerant subjects occurred at plasma concentrations of 0.05–0.19 mg/100 ml when codeine was given by intravenous infusion. The single lethal dose of codeine in adults is estimated to be from 0.5–1.0 g. It is also estimated that 5 mg/kg could be fatal in children. Hemodialysis and peritoneal dialysis can be performed to reduce the body aspirin content. Codeine is theoretically dialyzable but the procedure has not been clinically established.

Treatment of overdosage consists primarily of support of vital functions, management of codeine-induced respiratory depression, increasing salicylate elimination, and correcting the acid-base imbalance due primarily to salicylism.

In a comatose patient, primary attention should be given to establishment of adequate respiratory exchange through provisions of a patent airway and the institution of assisted or controlled ventilation. The narcotic antagonist naloxone is a specific antidote for respiratory depression which may result from overdose or unusual sensitivity to narcotics. Therefore, an appropriate dose of an antagonist should be administered, preferably by the intravenous route, simultaneously with efforts at respiratory resuscitation. Since the duration of action of Empirin with Codeine may exceed that of the antagonist, the patient should be kept under continued surveillance and repeated doses of the antagonist should be administered as needed to maintain adequate respiration. A narcotic antagonist should not be administered in the absence of clinically significant respiratory or cardiovascular depression.

Gastric emptying (Syrup of Ipecac) and/or lavage is recommended as soon as possible after ingestion, even if the patient has vomited spontaneously. (Apomorphine should not be used as an emetic for Empirin with Codeine, since it may potentiate hypotension and respiratory depression.) Administration of activated charcoal as a slurry is beneficial after lavage and/or emesis, if less than three hours have passed since ingestion. Charcoal adsorption should *not* be employed prior to emesis or lavage.

Severity of aspirin intoxication is determined by measuring the blood salicylate level. Acid-base status should be closely followed with serial blood gas and serum pH measurements. Fluid and electrolyte balance should also be regularly monitored.

A serum salicylate level of 30 mg/100 ml or higher indicates a need for enhanced salicylate excretion that can be achieved through body-fluid supplementation and urine alkalinization if renal function is normal. In mild intoxication, urine flow can be increased by forcing oral fluids and giving potassium citrate capsules.

(DO NOT GIVE BICARBONATE BY MOUTH SINCE IT INCREASES THE RATE OF SALICYLATE ABSORPTION.) In severe cases, hyperthermia and hypovolemia, as well as respiratory depression are the major immediate threats to life. Children should be sponged with tepid water. Replacement fluid should be administered intravenously and augmented with sufficient bicarbonate to correct acidosis, with monitoring of plasma electrolytes and pH, to promote alkaline diuresis of salicylate if renal function is normal. Complete control may also require infusion of glucose to control hypoglycemia.

Potassium deficiency may also be corrected through the infusion, once adequate urinary output is assured. Plasma or plasma expanders may be needed if fluid replacement is insufficient to maintain normal blood pressure or adequate urinary output.

In patients with renal insufficiency or in cases of life-threatening intoxication, dialysis is usually required. Peritoneal dialysis or exchange transfusion is indicated in infants and young children, and hemodialysis in older patients.

Oxygen, intravenous fluids, vasopressors and other supportive measures should be employed as needed.

DOSAGE AND ADMINISTRATION

Dosage is adjusted according to the severity of pain and the response of the patient. It may occasionally be necessary to exceed the usual dosage recommended below when pain is severe or the patient has become tolerant to the analgesic effect of codeine. Empirin with Codeine is given orally. The usual adult dose for Empirin with Codeine No. 2 and No. 3 is one or two tablets every four hours as required. The usual adult dose for Empirin with Codeine No. 4 is one tablet every four hours as required.

Empirin with Codeine should be taken with food or a full glass of milk or water to lessen gastric irritation.

HOW SUPPLIED

Empirin with Codeine No. 2, 15 mg: (white tablet imprinted with "EMPIRIN" and "2")

Bottle of 100	NDC 0081-0215-55
Bottle of 1000	NDC 0081-0215-75

Empirin with Codeine No. 3, 30 mg: (white tablet imprinted with "EMPIRIN" and "3")

Bottle of 100	NDC 0081-0220-55
	VA NSN 6505-00-959-4431
Bottle of 500	NDC 0081-0220-70
Bottle of 1000	NDC 0081-0220-75
	DoD NSN 6505-00-149-0116
Dispenserpak® of 25	NDC 0081-0220-25
	DoD NSN 6505-06-118-2347

Empirin with Codeine No. 4, 60 mg: (white tablet imprinted with "EMPIRIN" and "4")

Bottle of 100	NDC 0081-0225-55
Bottle of 500	NDC 0081-0225-70
Dispenserpak® of 25	NDC 0081-0225-25

Store at 15°–30°C (59°–86°F) in a dry place and protect from light.

Shown in Product Identification Section, page 407

IMURAN®   ℞
[ĭm′ū-ran″]
(Azathioprine)
50 mg Scored Tablets
20 mg vial (as the sodium salt) for I.V. injection, equivalent to 100 mg Azathioprine sterile lyophilized material.

> **WARNING**
> Chronic immunosuppression with this purine antimetabolite increases *risk of neoplasia* in humans. Physicians using this drug should be very familiar with this risk as well as with the mutagenic potential to both men and women and with possible hematologic toxicities. See below under WARNINGS.

DESCRIPTION

Imuran (Azathioprine), an immunosuppressive antimetabolite, is available in tablet form for oral administration and 100 mg vials for intravenous injection. Each scored tablet contains 50 mg azathioprine and the inactive ingredients lactose, magnesium stearate, potato starch, povidone, and stearic acid. Each 100 mg vial contains azathioprine, as the sodium salt, equivalent to 100 mg azathioprine sterile lyophilized material and sodium hydroxide to adjust pH.

Azathioprine is chemically 6-[(1-methyl-4-nitroimidazol-5-yl)thio] purine. It is an imidazolyl derivative of 6-mercaptopurine (Purinethol®) and many of its biological effects are similar to those of the parent compound.

Azathioprine is insoluble in water, but may be dissolved with addition of one molar equivalent of alkali. The sodium salt of azathioprine is sufficiently soluble to make a 10 mg/ml water solution which is stable for 24 hours at 59° to 77°F (15° to 25°C). Azathioprine is stable in solution at neutral or acid pH but hydrolysis to mercaptopurine occurs in excess sodium hydroxide (0.1N), especially on warming. Conversion to mercaptopurine also occurs in the presence of sulfhydryl compounds such as cysteine, glutathione and hydrogen sulfide.

CLINICAL PHARMACOLOGY AND ACTIONS

Metabolism[1]: Azathioprine is well absorbed following oral administration. Maximum serum radioactivity occurs at one to two hours after oral ^{35}S-azathioprine and decays with a half-life of five hours. This is not an estimate of the half-life of azathioprine itself but is the decay rate for all ^{35}S-containing metabolites of the drug. Because of extensive metabolism, only a fraction of the radioactivity is present as azathioprine. Usual doses produce blood levels of azathioprine, and of mercaptopurine derived from it, which are low (<1 mcg/ml). Blood levels are of little predictive value for therapy since the magnitude and duration of clinical effects correlate with thiopurine nucleotide levels in tissues rather than with plasma drug levels. Azathioprine and mercaptopurine are moderately bound to serum proteins (30%) and are partially dialyzable.

Azathioprine is cleaved *in vivo* to mercaptopurine. Both compounds are rapidly eliminated from blood and are oxidized or methylated in erythrocytes and liver; no azathioprine or mercaptopurine is detectable in urine after eight hours. Conversion to inactive 6-thiouric acid by xanthine oxidase is an important degradative pathway, and the inhibition of this pathway in patients receiving allopurinol (Zyloprim®) is the basis for the azathioprine dosage reduction required in these patients (see DOSAGE AND ADMINISTRATION). Proportions of metabolites are different in individual patients, and this presumably accounts for variable magnitude and duration of drug effects. Renal clearance is probably not important in predicting biological effectiveness or toxicities, although dose reduction is practiced in patients with poor renal function.

Homograft Survival[1,2]: Summary information from transplant centers and registries indicates relatively universal use of Imuran with or without other immunosuppressive agents.[3,4,5] Although the use of azathioprine for inhibition of renal homograft rejection is well established, the mechanism(s) for this action are somewhat obscure. The drug suppresses hypersensitivities of the cell-mediated type and causes variable alterations in antibody production. Suppression of T-cell effects, including ablation of T-cell suppression, is dependent on the temporal relationship to antigenic stimulus or engraftment. This agent has little effect on established graft rejections or secondary responses.

Alterations in specific immune responses or immunologic functions in transplant recipients are difficult to relate specifically to immunosuppression by azathioprine. These patients have subnormal responses to vaccines, low numbers of

T-cells, and abnormal phagocytosis by peripheral blood cells, but their mitogenic responses, serum immunoglobulins and secondary antibody responses are usually normal. Transplant recipients on azathioprine also receive corticosteroids and may be given antilymphocyte globulin; there are no known hazards or toxicities due to interactions of these agents.

Immunoinflammatory Response: Azathioprine suppresses disease manifestations as well as underlying pathology in animal models of auto-immune disease. For example, the severity of adjuvant arthritis is reduced by azathioprine. The mechanisms whereby azathioprine affects auto-immune diseases are not known. Azathioprine is immunosuppressive, delayed hypersensitivity and cellular cytotoxicity tests being suppressed to a greater degree than are antibody responses. In the rat model of adjuvant arthritis, azathioprine has been shown to inhibit the lymph node hyperplasia which precedes the onset of the signs of the disease. Both the immunosuppressive and therapeutic effects in animal models are dose-related. Azathioprine is considered a slow-acting drug and effects may persist after the drug has been discontinued.

INDICATIONS AND USAGE

Imuran is indicated as an adjunct for the prevention of rejection in renal homotransplantation. It is also indicated for the management of severe, active rheumatoid arthritis unresponsive to rest, aspirin or other nonsteroidal anti-inflammatory drugs, or to agents in the class of which gold is an example.

Renal Homotransplantation: Imuran is indicated as an adjunct for the prevention of rejection in renal homotransplantation. Experience with over 16,000 transplants shows a five-year patient survival of 35% to 55%, but this is dependent on donor, match for HLA antigens, anti-donor or anti B-cell alloantigen antibody and other variables. The effect of Imuran on these variables has not been tested in controlled trials.

Rheumatoid Arthritis[6,7]: Imuran is indicated only in adult patients meeting criteria for classic or definite rheumatoid arthritis as specified by the American Rheumatism Association.[8] Imuran should be restricted to patients with severe, active and erosive disease not responsive to conventional management including rest, aspirin or other non-steroidal drugs or to agents in the class of which gold is an example. Rest, physiotherapy and salicylates should be continued while Imuran is given, but it may be possible to reduce the dose of corticosteroids in patients on Imuran. The combined use of Imuran with gold, antimalarials or penicillamine has not been studied for either added benefit or unexpected adverse effects. The use of Imuran with these agents cannot be recommended.

CONTRAINDICATIONS

Imuran should not be given to patients who have shown hypersensitivity to the drug.

Imuran should not be used for treating rheumatoid arthritis in pregnant women.

Patients with rheumatoid arthritis previously treated with alkylating agents (cyclophosphamide, chlorambucil, melphalan or others) may have a prohibitive risk of neoplasia if treated with Imuran.

WARNINGS

Severe *leukopenia and/or thrombocytopenia* may occur in patients on Imuran. Macrocytic anemia and severe bone marrow depression may also occur. Hematologic toxicities are dose related and may be more severe in renal transplant patients whose homograft is undergoing rejection. It is suggested that patients on Imuran have complete blood counts, including platelet counts, weekly during the first month, twice monthly for the second and third months of treatment, then monthly or more frequently if dosage alterations or other therapy changes are necessary. Delayed hematologic suppression may occur. Prompt reduction in dosage or temporary withdrawal of the drug may be necessary if there is a rapid fall in, or persistently low leukocyte count or other evidence of bone marrow depression. Leukopenia does not correlate with therapeutic effect; therefore the dose should not be increased intentionally to lower the white blood cell count.

Serious infections are a constant hazard for patients on chronic immunosuppression, especially for homograft recipients. Fungal, viral, bacterial and protozoal infections may be fatal and should be treated vigorously. Reduction of azathioprine dosage and/or use of other drugs should be considered. Imuran® is mutagenic in animals and humans, carcinogenic in animals, and may increase the patient's *risk of neoplasia*. Renal transplant patients are known to have an increased risk of malignancy, predominantly skin cancer and reticulum cell or lymphomatous tumors.[9] Information is available on the spontaneous neoplasia risk in Rheumatoid Arthritis,[11] and on neoplasia following immunosuppressive therapy of other autoimmune diseases.[12] It has not been possible to define the precise risk of neoplasia due to Imuran,[10] but the risk is lower for patients with rheumatoid arthritis

Continued on next page

Burroughs Wellcome—Cont.

than for transplant recipients. However, acute myelogenous leukemia as well as solid tumors have been reported in patients with rheumatoid arthritis who have received azathioprine. Data on neoplasia in patients receiving Imuran can be found under Adverse Reactions.

Pregnancy Warning[13]: Imuran should not be given during pregnancy without careful weighing of risk versus benefit. Whenever possible, use of Imuran in pregnant patients should be avoided.

Imuran has been shown to be mutagenic in both male and female animals. Chromosomal abnormalities have also been documented in patients; however, the abnormalities in humans were reversed upon discontinuance of the drug.[14] Imuran is teratogenic in rodents. Transplacental transmission of azathioprine and its metabolites has been reported in man.[15] Limited immunologic and other abnormalities have occurred in some infants born of renal homograft recipients on Imuran. Benefit versus risk must be weighed carefully before use of Imuran in patients of reproductive potential. This drug should not be used for treating rheumatoid arthritis in pregnant women.

PRECAUTIONS

Patient Information: Patients being started on Imuran should be informed of the necessity of periodic blood counts while they are receiving the drug and should be encouraged to report any unusual bleeding or bruising to their physician. They should be advised of the danger of infection while receiving Imuran and encouraged to report signs and symptoms of infection to their physician. Careful dosage instructions should be given to the patient, especially when Imuran is being administered in the presence of impaired renal function or concomitantly with allopurinol (see DOSAGE AND ADMINISTRATION). Patients should be advised of the potential risks of the use of Imuran during pregnancy and during the nursing period. The increased risk of neoplasia following Imuran therapy should be explained to the patient.

ADVERSE REACTIONS

The principal and potentially serious toxic effects of Imuran are hematologic and gastrointestinal. The risks of secondary infection and neoplasia are also important. The frequency and severity of adverse reactions depend on the dose and duration of Imuran as well as on the patient's underlying disease or concomitant therapies. The incidence of hematologic toxicities and neoplasia encountered in groups of renal homograft recipients is significantly higher than that in studies employing Imuran for rheumatoid arthritis. The relative incidences in clinical studies are summarized below:

Toxicity	Renal Homograft	Rheumatoid Arthritis
Leukopenia		
Any Degree	>50%	28%
<2500/mm^3	16%	5.3%
Neoplasia		
Lymphoma	0.5%	
Others	2.8%	*

*18 reported cases; denominator unknown.

Hematologic: Leukopenia and/or thrombocytopenia are dose dependent and may occur late in the course of Imuran therapy. Dose reduction or temporary withdrawal allows reversal of these toxicities. Infection may occur as a secondary manifestation of bone marrow suppression or leukopenia, but the incidence of infection in renal homotransplantation is 30 to 60 times that in rheumatoid arthritis. Macrocytic anemia and/or bleeding have been reported in two patients on Imuran.

Gastrointestinal: Nausea and vomiting may occur within the first few months of Imuran therapy, and occurred in approximately 12% of 676 rheumatoid arthritis patients. The frequency of gastric disturbance can be reduced by administration of the drug in divided doses and/or after meals. Vomiting with abdominal pain may occur rarely with a hypersensitivity pancreatitis. Hepatotoxicity manifest by elevation of serum alkaline phosphatase, bilirubin and/or serum transaminases is known to occur following azathioprine use, primarily in allograft recipients. Hepatotoxicity has been uncommon (less than 1%) in rheumatoid arthritis patients. Hepatotoxicity following transplantation most often occurs within 6 months of transplantation and is generally reversible after interruption of Imuran. A rare, but life-threatening hepatic veno-occlusive disease associated with chronic administration of azathioprine has been described in transplant patients and in one patient receiving Imuran for panuveitis.[16,17,18] Periodic measurement of serum transaminases, alkaline phosphatase and bilirubin is indicated for early detection of hepatotoxicity. If hepatic veno-occlusive disease is clinically suspected, Imuran should be permanently withdrawn.

Others: Additional side effects of low frequency have been reported. These include skin rashes (approximately 2%), alopecia, fever, arthralgias, diarrhea, steatorrhea and negative nitrogen balance (all less than 1%).

DOSAGE AND ADMINISTRATION

Renal Homotransplantation: The dose of Imuran required to prevent rejection and minimize toxicity will vary with individual patients; this necessitates careful management. Initial dose is usually 3 to 5 mg/kg daily, beginning at the time of transplant. Imuran is usually given as a single daily dose on the day of, and in a minority of cases one to three days before, transplantation. Imuran is often initiated with the intravenous administration of the sodium salt, with subsequent use of tablets (at the same dose level) after the postoperative period. Intravenous administration of the sodium salt is indicated only in patients unable to tolerate oral medications. Dose reduction to maintenance levels of 1 to 3 mg/kg daily is usually possible. The dose of Imuran should not be increased to toxic levels because of threatened rejection. Discontinuation may be necessary for severe hematologic or other toxicity, even if rejection of the homograft may be a consequence of drug withdrawal.

Rheumatoid Arthritis: Imuran is usually given on a daily basis. The initial dose should be approximately 1.0 mg/kg (50 to 100 mg) given as a single dose or on a twice daily schedule. The dose may be increased, beginning at six to eight weeks and thereafter by steps at four-week intervals, if there are no serious toxicities and if initial response is unsatisfactory. Dose increments should be 0.5 mg/kg daily, up to a maximum dose of 2.5 mg/kg/day. Therapeutic response occurs after several weeks of treatment, usually six to eight; an adequate trial should be a minimum of 12 weeks. Patients not improved after twelve weeks can be considered refractory. Imuran may be continued long-term in patients with clinical response, but patients should be monitored carefully, and gradual dosage reduction should be attempted to reduce risk of toxicities.

Maintenance therapy should be at the lowest effective dose, and the dose given can be lowered decrementally with changes of 0.5 mg/kg or approximately 25 mg daily every four weeks while other therapy is kept constant. The optimum duration of maintenance Imuran has not been determined. Imuran can be discontinued abruptly, but delayed effects are possible.

Use in Renal Dysfunction: Relatively oliguric patients, especially those with tubular necrosis in the immediate postcadaveric transplant period, may have delayed clearance of Imuran or its metabolites, may be particularly sensitive to this drug and may require lower doses.

Use with Allopurinol (Zyloprim®): The principal pathway for detoxification of Imuran is inhibited by allopurinol (Zyloprim). Patients receiving Imuran and Zyloprim concomitantly should have a dose reduction of Imuran, to approximately $\frac{1}{3}$ to $\frac{1}{4}$ the usual dose.

Parenteral Administration: Add 10 ml of Sterile Water for Injection, and swirl until a clear solution results. This solution is for intravenous use only; it has a pH of approximately 9.6, and it should be used within twenty-four hours. Further dilution into sterile saline or dextrose is usually made for infusion; the final volume depends on time for the infusion, usually 30-60 minutes but as short as 5 minutes and as long as 8 hours for the daily dose.

HOW SUPPLIED

50 mg overlapping circle-shape, yellow to off-white, scored tablets imprinted with "IMURAN" and "50" on each tablet; bottle of 100 (NDC 0081-0597-55) and unit dose pack of 100 (NDC 0081-0597-56). Store at 15° to 25°C (59° to 77°F) in a dry place and protect from light. **DoD & VA NSN 6505-00-119-9317**

20 ml vial (NDC 0081-0598-71) containing the equivalent of 100 mg azathioprine (as the sodium salt). Store at 15° to 25°C (59° to 77°F) and protect from light. The sterile, lyophilized sodium salt is yellow, and should be dissolved in Sterile Water for Injection (see Parenteral Administration under DOSAGE AND ADMINISTRATION).

REFERENCES

1. Elion, G.B. and G.H. Hitchings, "Azathioprine" in *Handbook of Experimental Pharmacology*, Vol. 38, ed. by Sartorelli and Johns, Springer Verlag, New York, 1975.
2. McIntosh, J., P. Hansen *et al.*, "Defective Immune and Phagocytic Functions in Uremia and Renal Transplantation," *Int. Arch. Allergy Appl. Immunol.*, 51:544–559, 1976.
3. Advisory Committee, Renal Transplant Registry, "The 12th Report of the Human Renal Transplant Registry," *JAMA*, 233:787–796, 1975.
4. McGeown, M., "Immunosuppression for Kidney Transplantation," *Lancet*, ii:310–312, 1973.
5. Simmons, R.L., E.J. Thompson *et al.*, "115 Patients with First Cadaver Kidney Transplants Followed Two to Seven and a Half Years," *Am. J. Med.*, 62:234–242, 1977.
6. Fye, K. and N. Talal, "Cytotoxic Drugs in the Treatment of Rheumatoid Arthritis," *Ration. Drug Ther. 9* (4): 1–5, 1975.
7. Davis, J.D., H.B. Muss, and R.A. Turner, "Cytotoxic Agents in the Treatment of Rheumatoid Arthritis," *South. Med. J.*, 71 (1): 58–64, 1978.
8. McEwen, C., "The Diagnosis and Differential Diagnosis of Rheumatoid Arthritis," *Arthritis and Allied Conditions*, Philadelphia, Lea and Febiger, pp. 403–418, 1972.
9. Hoover, R. and J.F. Fraumeni, "Risk of Cancer in Renal Transplant Recipients," *Lancet*, 2:55–57, 1973.
10. Sieber, S.M. and R.H. Adamson, "Toxicity of Antineoplastic Agents in Man," *Adv. Cancer Res.*, 22:57–155, 1975.
11. Lewis, R.B., C.W. Castor, R.E. Knisley, and G.C. Bole, "Frequency of Neoplasia in Systemic Lupus Erythematosus and Rheumatoid Arthritis," *Arthritis Rheum.*, 19 (6): 1256–1260, 1976.
12. Louie, S. and R.S. Schwartz, "Immunodeficiency and the Pathogenesis of Lymphoma and Leukemia," *Semin. Hematol.*, 15 (2): 117–138, 1978.
13. Tagatz, G.E. and R.L. Simmons, "Pregnancy After Renal Transplantation," *Ann. Intern. Med.*, 82:113–114, 1975 (Editorial).
14. Hunter, T., M.B. Urowitz, D.A. Gordon, H.A. Smythe and M.A. Ogryzlo, Azathioprine in Rheumatoid Arthritis. A Long-Term Follow-Up Study, Arthritis Rheum., 18 (1): 15–20, 1975.
15. Saarikoski, S. and M. Sepalla, Immunosuppression During Pregnancy: Transmission of Azathioprine and its Metabolites from the Mother to the Fetus, Am. J. Obstet. Gynecol., 115 (8): 1100–1106, 1973.
16. Read AE, Wiesner RH, LaBrecque DR, et al: Hepatic veno-occlusive disease associated with renal transplantation and azathioprine therapy. Ann Intern Med 1986;104:651–655.
17. Katzka DA, Saul SH, Jorkasky D, et al: Azathioprine and hepatic venocclusive disease in renal transplant patients. Gastroenterology 1986;90:446–454.
18. Weitz H, Gokel JM, Loeschke K, et al: Veno-occlusive disease of the liver in patients receiving immunosuppressive therapy. Virchows Arch [A] 1982;395:245–256.
Shown in Product Identification Section, page 407

KEMADRIN®   ℞

[kĕm'ah-drĭn]
(Procyclidine Hydrochloride)
5 mg Scored Tablets

DESCRIPTION

Kemadrin (Procyclidine Hydrochloride) is a synthetic antispasmodic compound of relatively low toxicity. It has been shown to be useful for the symptomatic treatment of parkinsonism (paralysis agitans) and extrapyramidal dysfunction caused by tranquilizer therapy. Procyclidine hydrochloride was developed at The Wellcome Research Laboratories as the most promising of a series of antiparkinsonism compounds produced by chemical modification of antihistamines. Procyclidine hydrochloride is a white crystalline substance which is soluble in water and almost tasteless. It is known chemically as α-cyclohexyl-α-phenyl-1-pyrrolidinepropanol hydrochloride.

Kemadrin® (Procyclidine Hydrochloride) is available in tablet form for oral administration. Each scored tablet contains 5 mg procyclidine hydrochloride and the inactive ingredients corn and potato starch, lactose, and magnesium stearate.

CLINICAL PHARMACOLOGY

Pharmacologic tests have shown that procyclidine hydrochloride has an atropine-like action and exerts an antispasmodic effect on smooth muscle. It is a potent mydriatic and inhibits salivation. It has no sympathetic ganglion blocking activity in doses as high as 4 mg/kg, as measured by the lack of inhibition of the response of the nictitating membrane to preganglionic electrical stimulation.

The intravenous LD$_{50}$ in mice was about 60 mg/kg. Subcutaneously, doses of 300 mg/kg were not toxic. In dogs the intraperitoneal administration of procyclidine hydrochloride in doses of 5 mg/kg caused maximal dilation of the pupil and inhibition of salivation, but had no toxic action. When the dose was increased to 20 mg/kg the same symptoms occurred, and in addition there were tremors and ataxia lasting 4 to 5 hours. In one animal convulsions occurred which were controlled by pentobarbital. In all animals behavior returned to normal within 24 hours.

Chronic toxicity tests in rats showed that the compound caused only a very slight retardation in growth, and no change in the erythrocyte count or the histological appearance of the lungs, liver, spleen and kidney when as much as 10 mg/kg body weight was given subcutaneously daily for 9 weeks.

INDICATIONS

Kemadrin (Procyclidine Hydrochloride) is indicated in the treatment of parkinsonism including the postencephalitic, arteriosclerotic and idiopathic types. Partial control of the parkinsonism symptoms is the usual therapeutic accomplishment. Procyclidine hydrochloride is usually more efficacious in the relief of rigidity than tremor; but tremor, fatigue, weakness and sluggishness are frequently beneficially

PRODUCT	BIOAVAILABILITY	EQUIVALENT DOSES (IN MG)*		
Lanoxin® Tablet	60–80%	0.125	0.25	0.5
Lanoxin Elixir	70–85%	0.125	0.25	0.5
Lanoxin Injection/IM	70–85%	0.125	0.25	0.5
Lanoxin Injection/IV	100%	0.1	0.2	0.4
Lanoxicaps Capsules	90–100%	0.1	0.2	0.4

*1 mg = 1000 µg

influenced. It can be substituted for all the previous medications in mild and moderate cases. For the control of more severe cases other drugs may be added to procyclidine therapy as indications warrant.

Clinical reports indicate that procyclidine often successfully relieves the symptoms of extrapyramidal dysfunction (dystonia, dyskinesia, akathisia and parkinsonism) which accompany the therapy of mental disorders with phenothiazine and rauwolfia compounds. In addition to minimizing the symptoms induced by tranquilizing drugs, the drug effectively controls sialorrhea resulting from neuroleptic medication. At the same time freedom from the side effects induced by tranquilizer drugs, as provided by the administration of procyclidine, permits a more sustained treatment of the patient's mental disorder.

Clinical results in the treatment of parkinsonism indicate that most patients experience subjective improvement characterized by a feeling of well-being and increased alertness, together with diminished salivation and a marked improvement in muscular coordination as demonstrated by objective tests of manual dexterity and by increased ability to carry out ordinary self-care activities. While the drug exerts a mild atropine-like action and therefore causes mydriasis, this may be kept minimal by careful adjustment of the daily dosage.

CONTRAINDICATIONS

Procyclidine hydrochloride should not be used in angle-closure glaucoma although simple type glaucomas do not appear to be adversely affected.

WARNINGS: Use in Children:

Safety and efficacy have not been established in the pediatric age group; therefore, the use of procyclidine hydrochloride in this age group requires that the potential benefits be weighed against the possible hazards to the child.

Pregnancy Warning: The safe use of this drug in pregnancy has not been established; therefore, the use of procyclidine hydrochloride in pregnancy, lactation or in women of childbearing age requires that the potential benefits be weighed against the possible hazards to the mother and child.

PRECAUTIONS

Conditions in which inhibition of the parasympathetic nervous system is undesirable such as tachycardia and urinary retention (such as may occur with marked prostatic hypertrophy) require special care in the administration of the drug. Hypotensive patients who receive the drug should be observed closely. Occasionally, particularly in older patients, mental confusion and disorientation may occur with the development of agitation, hallucinations and psychotic-like symptoms.

Patients with mental disorders occasionally experience a precipitation of a psychotic episode when the dosage of antiparkinsonism drugs is increased to treat the extrapyramidal side effects of phenothiazine and rauwolfia derivatives.

ADVERSE REACTIONS

Anticholinergic effects can be produced by therapeutic doses although these can frequently be minimized or eliminated by careful dosage. They include: dryness of the mouth, mydriasis, blurring of vision, giddiness, lightheadedness and gastrointestinal disturbances such as nausea, vomiting, epigastric distress and constipation. Occasionally an allergic reaction such as a skin rash may be encountered. Feelings of muscular weakness may occur. Acute suppurative parotitis as a complication of dry mouth has been reported.

DOSAGE AND ADMINISTRATION

For Parkinsonism: The dosage of the drug for the treatment of parkinsonism depends upon the age of the patient, the etiology of the disease, and individual responsiveness. Therefore, the dosage must remain flexible to permit adjustment to the individual tolerance and requirements of each patient. In general, younger and postencephalitic patients require and tolerate a somewhat higher dosage than older patients and those with arteriosclerosis.

For Patients Who Have Received No Other Therapy: The usual dose of procyclidine hydrochloride for initial treatment is 2.5 mg administered three times daily after meals. If well tolerated, this dose may be gradually increased to 5 mg three times a day and occasionally 5 mg given before retiring. In some cases smaller doses may be employed with good therapeutic results.

Occasionally a patient is encountered who cannot tolerate a bedtime dose of the drug. In such cases it may be desirable to adjust dosage so that the bedtime dose is omitted and the total daily requirement is administered in three equal daytime doses. It is best administered during or after meals to minimize the development of side reactions.

To Transfer Patients to Kemadrin (Procyclidine Hydrochloride) from Other Therapy: Patients who have been receiving other drugs may be transferred to procyclidine hydrochloride. This is accomplished gradually by substituting 2.5 mg three times a day for all or part of the original drug. The dose of procyclidine is then increased as required while that of the other drug is correspondingly omitted or decreased

until complete replacement is achieved. The total daily dosage may then be adjusted to the level which produces maximum benefit.

For Drug-Induced Extrapyramidal Symptoms: For treatment of symptoms of extrapyramidal dysfunction induced by tranquilizer drugs during the therapy of mental disorders, the dosage of procyclidine hydrochloride will depend on the severity of side effects associated with tranquilizer administration. In general the larger the dosage of the tranquilizer the more severe will be the associated symptoms, including rigidity and tremors. Accordingly, the drug dosage should be adjusted to suit the needs of the individual patient and to provide maximum relief of the induced symptoms. A convenient method to establish the daily dosage of procyclidine is to begin with the administration of 2.5 mg three times daily. This may be increased by 2.5 mg daily increments until the patient obtains relief of symptoms. In most cases excellent results will be obtained with 10 to 20 mg daily.

HOW SUPPLIED

White, scored tablets containing 5 mg procyclidine hydrochloride imprinted with "KEMADRIN" and "S3A" in bottles of 100 (NDC 0081-0604-55).

Store at 15°–30°C (59°–86°F) in a dry place.

Shown in Product Identification Section, page 407

LANOXICAPS®   ℞
[lă-nŏx 'ĭ-kăps"]
(Digoxin Solution in Capsules)
 50 µg (0.05 mg) I.D. Imprint A2C (red)
 100 µg (0.1 mg) I.D. Imprint B2C (yellow)
 200 µg (0.2 mg) I.D. Imprint C2C (green)

DESCRIPTION

Digoxin is one of the cardiac (or digitalis) glycosides, a closely related group of drugs having in common specific effects on the myocardium. These drugs are found in a number of plants. Digoxin is extracted from the leaves of *Digitalis lanata*. The term "digitalis" is used to designate the whole group. The glycosides are composed of two portions: a sugar and a cardenolide (hence "glycosides").

Digoxin has the molecular formula $C_{41}H_{64}O_{14}$, a molecular weight of 780.95 and melting and decomposition points above 235°C. The drug is practically insoluble in water and in ether; slightly soluble in diluted (50%) alcohol and in chloroform; and freely soluble in pyridine. Digoxin powder is composed of odorless white crystals.

Digoxin has the chemical name: 3β-[(O -2, 6-dideoxy- β -D-ribo -hexopyranosyl- (1→4) -O-2, 6-dideoxy- β -D-ribo -hexopyranosyl -(1→4)- 2,6-dideoxy-β-D-ribo -hexopyranosyl) oxy]-12β, 14-dihydroxy-5β-card-20(22)-enolide.

Lanoxicaps is a stable solution of digoxin enclosed within a soft gelatin capsule for oral use. Each capsule contains the labeled amount of digoxin USP dissolved in a solvent comprised of polyethylene glycol 400 USP, 8 percent ethyl alcohol, propylene glycol USP and purified water USP. Inactive ingredients in the capsule shell include FD&C Red No. 40 (0.05 mg Capsule), D&C Yellow No. 10 (0.1 mg and 0.2 mg Capsules), FD&C Blue No. 1 (0.2 mg Capsule), gelatin, glycerin, methylparaben and propylparaben (added as preservatives), purified water, and sorbitol. Capsules printed with edible ink.

CLINICAL PHARMACOLOGY

Mechanism of Action: The influence of digitalis glycosides on the myocardium is dose-related, and involves both a direct action on cardiac muscle and the specialized conduction system, and indirect actions on the cardiovascular system mediated by the autonomic nervous system. The indirect actions mediated by the autonomic nervous system involve a vagomimetic action, which is responsible for the effects of digitalis on the sino-atrial (SA) and atrioventricular (AV) nodes; and also a baroreceptor sensitization which results in increased carotid sinus nerve activity and enhanced sympathetic withdrawal for any given increment in mean arterial pressure. The pharmacologic consequences of these direct and indirect effects are: 1) an increase in the force and velocity of myocardial systolic contraction (positive inotropic action); 2) a slowing of heart rate (negative chronotropic effect); and 3) decreased conduction velocity through the AV node. In higher doses, digitalis increases sympathetic outflow from the central nervous system (CNS) to both cardiac and peripheral sympathetic nerves. This increase in sympathetic activity may be an important factor in digitalis cardiac toxicity.

Most of the extracardiac manifestations of digitalis toxicity are also mediated by the CNS.

Pharmacokinetics:

Absorption—Gastrointestinal absorption of digoxin is a passive process. Absorption of digoxin from Lanoxicaps capsules has been demonstrated to be 90 to 100% complete compared to an identical intravenous dose of digoxin. Conventional digoxin tablets are absorbed 60 to 80%. The enhanced absorption from Lanoxicaps compared to digoxin tablets and elixir is associated with reduced between-patient and within-patient variability in steady-state serum concentrations. The peak serum concentrations are higher than those observed after tablets. When digoxin tablets or capsules are taken after meals, the rate of absorption is slowed, but the total amount of digoxin absorbed is usually unchanged. When taken with meals high in bran fiber, however, the amount absorbed from an oral dose may be reduced. Comparisons of the systemic availability and equivalent doses for digoxin preparations are shown in the following table:

[See table above].

In some patients, orally administered digoxin is converted to cardioinactive reduction products (e.g., dihydrodigoxin) by colonic bacteria in the gut. Data suggest that one in ten patients treated with digoxin tablets will degrade 40% or more of the ingested dose. This phenomenon is minimized with Lanoxicaps because they are rapidly absorbed in the upper gastrointestinal tract.

Distribution—Following drug administration, a 6 to 8 hour distribution phase is observed. This is followed by a much more gradual serum concentration decline, which is dependent on digoxin elimination from the body. The peak height and slope of the early portion (absorption/distribution phases) of the serum concentration-time curve are dependent upon the route of administration and the absorption characteristics of the formulation. Clinical evidence indicates that the early high serum concentrations (particularly high for digoxin capsules) do not reflect the concentration of digoxin at its site of action, but that with chronic use, the steady-state post-distribution serum levels are in equilibrium with tissue levels and correlate with pharmacologic effects. In individual patients, these post-distribution serum concentrations are linearly related to maintenance dosage and may be useful in evaluating therapeutic and toxic effects (see Serum Digoxin Concentrations in DOSAGE AND ADMINISTRATION section).

Digoxin is concentrated in tissues and therefore has a large apparent volume of distribution. Digoxin crosses both the blood-brain barrier and the placenta. At delivery, serum digoxin concentration in the newborn is similar to the serum level in the mother. Approximately 20 to 25% of plasma digoxin is bound to protein. Serum digoxin concentrations are not significantly altered by large changes in fat tissue weight, so that its distribution space correlates best with lean (ideal) body weight, not total body weight.

Pharmacologic Response—The approximate times to onset of effect and to peak effect of all the Lanoxin and Lanoxicaps preparations are given in the following table:

[See table on next page].

Excretion—Elimination of digoxin follows first-order kinetics (that is, the quantity of digoxin eliminated at any time is proportional to the total body content). Following intravenous administration to normal subjects, 50 to 70% of a digoxin dose is excreted unchanged in the urine. Renal excretion of digoxin is proportional to glomerular filtration rate and is largely independent of urine flow. In subjects with normal renal function, digoxin has a half-life of 1.5 to 2.0 days. The half-life in anuric patients is prolonged to 4 to 6 days. Digoxin is not effectively removed from the body by dialysis, exchange transfusion or during cardiopulmonary by-pass because most of the drug is in tissue rather than circulating in the blood.

INDICATIONS AND USAGE

Heart Failure: The increased cardiac output resulting from the inotropic action of digoxin ameliorates the disturbances characteristic of heart failure (venous congestion, edema, dyspnea, orthopnea and cardiac asthma).

Digoxin is more effective in "low output" (pump) failure than in "high output" heart failure secondary to arteriovenous fistula, anemia, infection or hyperthyroidism.

Digoxin is usually continued after failure is controlled, unless some known precipitating factor is corrected. Studies have shown, however, that even though hemodynamic ef-

Continued on next page

Burroughs Wellcome—Cont.

fects can be demonstrated in almost all patients, corresponding improvement in the signs and symptoms of heart failure is not necessarily apparent. Therefore, in patients in whom digoxin may be difficult to regulate, or in whom the risk of toxicity may be great (e.g., patients with unstable renal function or whose potassium levels tend to fluctuate) a cautious withdrawal of digoxin may be considered. If digoxin is discontinued, the patient should be regularly monitored for clinical evidence of recurrent heart failure.

Atrial Fibrillation: Digoxin reduces ventricular rate and thereby improves hemodynamics. Palpitation, precordial distress or weakness are relieved and concomitant congestive failure ameliorated. Digoxin should be continued in doses necessary to maintain the desired ventricular rate.

Atrial Flutter: Digoxin slows the heart and regular sinus rhythm may appear. Frequently the flutter is converted to atrial fibrillation with a controlled ventricular response. Digoxin treatment should be maintained if atrial fibrillation persists. (Electrical cardioversion is often the treatment of choice for atrial flutter. See discussion of cardioversion in PRECAUTIONS section.)

Paroxysmal Atrial Tachycardia (PAT): Digoxin may convert PAT to sinus rhythm by slowing conduction through the AV node. If heart failure has ensued or paroxysms recur frequently, digoxin should be continued. In infants, digoxin is usually continued for 3 to 6 months after a single episode of PAT to prevent recurrence.

CONTRAINDICATIONS

Digitalis glycosides are contraindicated in ventricular fibrillation.

In a given patient, an untoward effect requiring permanent discontinuation of other digitalis preparations usually constitutes a contraindication to digoxin. Hypersensitivity to digoxin itself is a contraindication to its use. Allergy to digoxin, though rare, does occur. It may not extend to all such preparations, and another digitalis glycoside may be tried with caution.

WARNINGS

Digitalis alone or with other drugs has been used in the treatment of obesity. This use of digoxin or other digitalis glycosides is unwarranted. Moreover, since they may cause potentially fatal arrhythmias or other adverse effects, the use of these drugs solely for the treatment of obesity is dangerous. It is recommended that digoxin in soft capsules be administered in divided daily doses to minimize any potential adverse reactions, since peak serum digoxin concentrations resulting from the capsules are approximately twice those after bioequivalent tablet doses (400 µg of Lanoxicaps are bioequivalent to 500 µg of tablets). Studies are underway to determine if there are any increased risks associated with the higher peaks that occur with single daily dosing of soft gelatin capsules.

Anorexia, nausea, vomiting and arrhythmias may accompany heart failure or may be indications of digitalis intoxication. Clinical evaluation of the cause of these symptoms should be attempted before further digitalis administration. In such circumstances determination of the serum digoxin concentration may be an aid in deciding whether or not digitalis toxicity is likely to be present. If the possibility of digitalis intoxication cannot be excluded, cardiac glycosides should be temporarily withheld, if permitted by the clinical situation.

Patients with renal insufficiency require smaller than usual maintenance doses of digoxin (see DOSAGE AND ADMINISTRATION section).

Heart failure accompanying acute glomerulonephritis requires extreme care in digitalization. Relatively low loading and maintenance doses and concomitant use of antihypertensive drugs may be necessary and careful monitoring is essential. Digoxin should be discontinued as soon as possible.

Patients with severe carditis, such as carditis associated with rheumatic fever or viral myocarditis, are especially sensitive to digoxin-induced disturbances of rhythm.

Newborn infants display considerable variability in their tolerance to digoxin. Premature and immature infants are particularly sensitive, and dosage must not only be reduced but must be individualized according to their degree of maturity.

Note: Digitalis glycosides are an important cause of accidental poisoning in children.

PRECAUTIONS

General: Digoxin toxicity develops more frequently and lasts longer in patients with renal impairment because of the decreased excretion of digoxin. Therefore, it should be anticipated that dosage requirements will be decreased in patients with moderate to severe renal disease (see DOSAGE AND ADMINISTRATION section). Because of the prolonged half-life, a longer period of time is required to achieve an initial or new steady-state concentration in patients with renal impairment than in patients with normal renal function.

In patients with hypokalemia, toxicity may occur despite serum digoxin concentrations within the "normal range", because potassium depletion sensitizes the myocardium to digoxin. Therefore, it is desirable to maintain normal serum potassium levels in patients being treated with digoxin. Hypokalemia may result from diuretic, amphotericin B or corticosteroid therapy, and from dialysis or mechanical suction of gastrointestinal secretions. It may also accompany malnutrition, diarrhea, prolonged vomiting, old age and long-standing heart failure. In general, rapid changes in serum potassium or other electrolytes should be avoided, and intravenous treatment with potassium should be reserved for special circumstances as described below (see TREATMENT OF ARRHYTHMIAS PRODUCED BY OVERDOSAGE section).

Calcium, particularly when administered rapidly by the intravenous route, may produce serious arrhythmias in digitalized patients. Hypercalcemia from any cause predisposes the patient to digitalis toxicity. On the other hand, hypocalcemia can nullify the effects of digoxin in man; thus, digoxin may be ineffective until serum calcium is restored to normal. These interactions are related to the fact that calcium affects contractility and excitability of the heart in a manner similar to digoxin.

Hypomagnesemia may predispose to digitalis toxicity. If low magnesium levels are detected in a patient on digoxin, replacement therapy should be instituted.

Quinidine, verapamil, and amiodarone cause a rise in serum digoxin concentration, with the implication that digitalis intoxication may result. This rise appears to be proportional to the dose. The effect is mediated by a reduction in the digoxin clearance and, in the case of quinidine, decreased volume of distribution as well.

Certain antibiotics may increase digoxin absorption in patients who convert digoxin to inactive metabolites in the gut (see Pharmacokinetics portion of the CLINICAL PHARMACOLOGY section). Recent studies have shown that specific colonic bacteria in the lower gastrointestinal tract convert digoxin to cardioinactive reduction products, thereby reducing its bioavailability. Although inactivation of these bacteria by antibiotics is rapid, the serum digoxin concentration will rise at a rate consistent with the elimination half-life of digoxin. The magnitude of rise in serum digoxin concentration relates to the extent of bacterial inactivation, and may be as much as two-fold in some cases. This interaction is significantly reduced if digoxin is given as Lanoxicaps.

Patients with acute myocardial infarction or severe pulmonary disease may be unusually sensitive to digoxin-induced disturbances of rhythm.

Atrial arrhythmias associated with hypermetabolic states (e.g. hyperthyroidism) are particularly resistant to digoxin treatment. Large doses of digoxin are not recommended as the only treatment of these arrhythmias and care must be taken to avoid toxicity if large doses of digoxin are required. In hypothyroidism, the digoxin requirements are reduced. Digoxin responses in patients with compensated thyroid disease are normal.

Reduction of digoxin dosage may be desirable prior to electrical cardioversion to avoid induction of ventricular arrhythmias, but the physician must consider the consequences of rapid increase in ventricular response to atrial fibrillation if digoxin is withheld 1 to 2 days prior to cardioversion. If there is a suspicion that digitalis toxicity exists, elective cardioversion should be delayed. If it is not prudent to delay cardioversion, the energy level selected should be minimal at first and carefully increased in an attempt to avoid precipitating ventricular arrhythmias.

Incomplete AV block, especially in patients with Stokes-Adams attacks, may progress to advanced or complete heart block if digoxin is given.

In some patients with sinus node disease (i.e. Sick Sinus Syndrome), digoxin may worsen sinus bradycardia or sino-atrial block.

In patients with Wolff-Parkinson-White Syndrome and atrial fibrillation, digoxin can enhance transmission of impulses through the accessory pathway. This effect may result in extremely rapid ventricular rates and even ventricular fibrillation.

Digoxin may worsen the outflow obstruction in patients with idiopathic hypertrophic subaortic stenosis (IHSS). Unless cardiac failure is severe, it is doubtful whether digoxin should be employed.

Patients with chronic constrictive pericarditis may fail to respond to digoxin. In addition, slowing of the heart rate by digoxin in some patients may further decrease cardiac output.

Patients with heart failure from amyloid heart disease or constrictive cardiomyopathies respond poorly to treatment with digoxin.

Digoxin is not indicated for the treatment of sinus tachycardia unless it is associated with heart failure.

Digoxin may produce false positive ST-T changes in the electrocardiogram during exercise testing.

Intramuscular injection of digoxin is extremely painful and offers no advantages unless other routes of administration are contraindicated.

Laboratory Tests: Patients receiving digoxin should have their serum electrolytes and renal function (BUN and/or serum creatinine) assessed periodically; the frequency of assessments will depend on the clinical setting. For discussion of serum digoxin concentrations, see DOSAGE AND ADMINISTRATION section.

Drug Interactions: Potassium-depleting *corticosteroids* and *diuretics* may be major contributing factors to digitalis toxicity. *Calcium*, particularly if administered rapidly by the intravenous route, may produce serious arrhythmias in digitalized patients. *Quinidine, verapamil*, and *amiodarone* cause a rise in serum digoxin concentration, with the implication that digitalis intoxication may result. Certain *antibiotics* increase digoxin absorption in patients who inactivate digoxin by bacterial metabolism in the lower intestine, so that digitalis intoxication may result. *Propantheline* and *diphenoxylate*, by decreasing gut motility, may increase digoxin absorption. *Antacids, kaolin-pectin, sulfasalazine, neomycin, cholestyramine* and certain *anticancer drugs* may interfere with intestinal digoxin absorption, resulting in unexpectedly low serum concentrations. There have been inconsistent reports regarding the effects of other drugs on the serum digoxin concentration. *Thyroid* administration to a digitalized, hypothyroid patient may increase the dose requirement of digoxin. Concomitant use of digoxin and *sympathomimetics* increases the risk of cardiac arrhythmias, because both enhance ectopic pacemaker activity. *Succinylcholine* may cause a sudden extrusion of potassium from muscle cells, and may thereby cause arrhythmias in digitalized patients. Although β adrenergic blockers or calcium channel blockers and digoxin may be useful in combination to control atrial fibrillation, their additive effects on AV node conduction can result in complete heart block.

Due to the considerable variability of these interactions, digoxin dosage should be carefully individualized when patients receive coadministered medications. Furthermore, caution should be exercised when combining digoxin with any drug that may cause a significant deterioration in renal function, since this may impair the excretion of digoxin.

Carcinogenesis, Mutagenesis, Impairment of Fertility: There have been no long-term studies performed in animals to evaluate carcinogenic potential.

Pregnancy: *Teratogenic Effects:* Pregnancy Category C. Animal reproduction studies have not been conducted with digoxin. It is also not known whether digoxin can cause fetal harm when administered to a pregnant woman or can affect reproduction capacity. Digoxin should be given to a pregnant woman only if clearly needed.

Nursing Mothers: Studies have shown that digoxin concentrations in the mother's serum and milk are similar. However, the estimated daily dose to a nursing infant will be far below the usual infant maintenance dose. Therefore, this amount should have no pharmacologic effect upon the infant. Nevertheless, caution should be exercised when digoxin is administered to a nursing woman.

ADVERSE REACTIONS

The frequency and severity of adverse reactions to digoxin depend on the dose and route of administration, as well as on the patient's underlying disease or concomitant therapies (see PRECAUTIONS section and Serum Digoxin Concentrations subsection of DOSAGE AND ADMINISTRATION). The overall incidence of adverse reactions has been reported as 5 to 20%, with 15 to 20% of them being considered serious (one to four percent of patients receiving digoxin). Evidence suggests that the incidence of toxicity has decreased since the introduction of the serum digoxin assay and improved standardization of digoxin tablets. Cardiac toxicity accounts for about one-half, gastrointestinal disturbances for about

PRODUCT	TIME TO ONSET OF EFFECT*	TIME TO PEAK EFFECT*
Lanoxin® Tablet	0.5–2 hours	2–6 hours
Lanoxin Elixir	0.5–2 hours	2–6 hours
Lanoxin Injection/IM	0.5–2 hours	2–6 hours
Lanoxin Injection/IV	5–30 minutes†	1–4 hours
Lanoxicaps Capsules	0.5–2 hours	2–6 hours

*Documented for ventricular response rate in atrial fibrillation, inotropic effect and electrocardiographic changes.
†Depending upon rate of infusion.

one-fourth, and CNS and other toxicity for about one-fourth of these adverse reactions.

Adults:

Cardiac—Unifocal or multiform ventricular premature contractions, especially in bigeminal or trigeminal patterns, are the most common arrhythmias associated with digoxin toxicity in adults with heart disease. Ventricular tachycardia may result from digitalis toxicity. Atrioventricular (AV) dissociation, accelerated junctional (nodal) rhythm and atrial tachycardia with block are also common arrhythmias caused by digoxin overdosage.

Excessive slowing of the pulse is a clinical sign of digoxin overdosage. AV block (Wenckebach) of increasing degree may proceed to complete heart block.

Note: The electrocardiogram is fundamental in determining the presence and nature of these cardiac disturbances. Digoxin may also induce other changes in the ECG (e.g. PR prolongation, ST depression), which represent digoxin effect and may or may not be associated with digitalis toxicity.

Gastrointestinal—Anorexia, nausea, vomiting and, less commonly, diarrhea are common early symptoms of overdosage. However, uncontrolled heart failure may also produce such symptoms. Digitalis toxicity very rarely may cause abdominal pain and hemorrhagic necrosis of the intestines.

CNS—Visual disturbances (blurred or yellow vision), headache, weakness, dizziness, apathy and psychosis can occur.

Other—Gynecomastia is occasionally observed. Maculopapular rash or other skin reactions are rarely observed.

Infants and Children: Toxicity differs from the adult in a number of respects. Anorexia, nausea, vomiting, diarrhea and CNS disturbances may be present but are rare as initial symptoms in infants. Cardiac arrhythmias are more reliable signs of toxicity. Digoxin in children may produce any arrhythmia. The most commonly encountered are conduction disturbances or supraventricular tachyarrhythmias, such as atrial tachycardia with or without block, and junctional (nodal) tachycardia. Ventricular arrhythmias are less common. Sinus bradycardia may also be a sign of impending digoxin intoxication, especially in infants, even in the absence of first degree heart block. Any arrhythmia or alteration in cardiac conduction that develops in a child taking digoxin should initially be assumed to be a consequence of digoxin intoxication.

OVERDOSAGE:

Treatment of Arrhythmias Produced by Overdosage:

Adults: Digoxin should be discontinued until all signs of toxicity are gone. Discontinuation may be all that is necessary if toxic manifestations are not severe and appear only near the expected time for maximum effect of the drug. Correction of factors that may contribute to toxicity such as electrolyte disturbances, hypoxia, acid-base disturbances and removal of aggravating agents such as catecholamines, should also be considered. Potassium salts may be indicated, particularly if hypokalemia in present. Potassium administration may be dangerous in the setting of massive digitalis overdosage (see Massive Digitalis Overdosage subsection below). Potassium chloride in divided oral doses totaling 3 to 6 grams of the salt (40 to 80 mEq K +) for adults may be given provided renal function is adequate (see below for potassium recommendations in Infants and Children).

When correction of the arrhythmia is urgent and the serum potassium concentration is low or normal, potassium should be administered intravenously in 5% dextrose injection. For adults, a total of 40 to 80 mEq (diluted to a concentration of 40 mEq per 500 ml) may be given at a rate not exceeding 20 mEq per hour, or slower if limited by pain due to local irritation. Additional amounts may be given if the arrhythmia is uncontrolled and potassium well-tolerated. ECG monitoring should be performed to watch for any evidence of potassium toxicity (e.g. peaking of T waves) and to observe the effect on the arrhythmia. The infusion may be stopped when the desired effect is achieved.

Note: Potassium should not be used and may be dangerous in heart block due to digoxin, unless primarily related to supraventricular tachycardia.

Other agents that have been used for the treatment of digoxin intoxication include lidocaine, procainamide, propranolol and phenytoin, although use of the latter must be considered experimental. In advanced heart block, atropine and/or temporary ventricular pacing may be beneficial. Digibind®, Digoxin Immune Fab (Ovine), can be used to reverse potentially life-threatening digoxin (or digitoxin) intoxication. Improvement in signs and symptoms of digitalis toxicity usually begins within ½ hour of Digibind administration. Each 40 mg vial of Digibind will neutralize 0.6 mg of digoxin (which is a usual body store of an adequately digitalized 70 kg patient).

Infants and Children: See Adult section for general recommendations for the treatment of arrhythmias produced by overdosage and for cautions regarding the use of potassium. If a potassium preparation is used to treat toxicity, it may be given orally in divided doses totaling 1 to 1.5 mEq K + per kilogram (kg) body weight (1 gram of potassium chloride contains 13.4 mEq K +).

When correction of the arrhythmia with potassium is urgent, approximately 0.5 mEq/kg of potassium per hour may be given intravenously, with careful ECG monitoring. The intravenous solution of potassium should be dilute enough to avoid local irritation; however, especially in infants, care must be taken to avoid intravenous fluid overload.

MASSIVE DIGITALIS OVERDOSAGE

Manifestations of life-threatening toxicity include severe ventricular arrhythmias such as ventricular tachycardia or ventricular fibrillation, or progressive bradyarrhythmias such as severe sinus bradycardia or second or third degree heart block not responsive to atropine. An overdosage of more than 10 mg of digoxin in previously healthy adults or 4 mg in previously healthy children or overdosage resulting in steady-state serum concentrations greater than 10 ng/ml, often results in cardiac arrest. Severe digitalis intoxication can cause life-threatening elevation in serum potassium concentration by shifting potassium from inside to outside the cell resulting in hyperkalemia. Administration of potassium supplements in the setting of massive intoxication may be hazardous.

Digibind®, Digoxin Immune Fab (Ovine), may be used at a dose equimolar to digoxin in the body to reverse the effects of ingestion of a massive overdose. The decision to administer Digibind before the onset of toxic manifestations will depend on the likelihood that life-threatening toxicity will occur (see above).

Patients with massive digitalis ingestion should receive large doses of activated charcoal to prevent absorption and bind digoxin in the gut during enteroenteric recirculation. Emesis or gastric lavage may be indicated especially if ingestion has occurred within 30 minutes of the patient's presentation at the hospital. Emesis should not be induced in patients who are obtunded. If a patient presents more than 2 hours after ingestion or already has toxic manifestations, it may be unsafe to induce vomiting or attempt passage of a gastric tube, because such maneuvers may induce an acute vagal episode that can worsen digitalis-toxic arrhythmias.

DOSAGE AND ADMINISTRATION

Recommended dosages are average values that may require considerable modification because of individual sensitivity or associated conditions. Diminished renal function is the most important factor requiring modification of recommended doses.

Due to the more complete absorption of digoxin from soft capsules, recommended oral doses are only 80 percent of those for Tablets, Elixir and I.M. Injection.

Because the significance of the higher peak serum concentrations associated with once daily capsules is not established, divided daily dosing is presently recommended for:

1. Infants and children under 10 years of age;
2. Patients requiring a daily dose of 300 μg (0.3 mg) or greater;
3. Patients with a previous history of digitalis toxicity;
4. Patients considered likely to become toxic;
5. Patients in whom compliance is not a problem.

Where compliance is considered a problem, single daily dosing may be appropriate.

In deciding the dose of digoxin, several factors must be considered:

1. The disease being treated. Atrial arrhythmias may require larger doses than heart failure.
2. The body weight of the patient. Doses should be calculated based upon lean or ideal body weight.
3. The patient's renal function, preferably evaluated on the basis of creatinine clearance.
4. Age is an important factor in infants and children.
5. Concomitant disease states, drugs or other factors likely to alter the expected clinical response to digoxin (see PRECAUTIONS and Drug Interactions sections).

Digitalization may be accomplished by either of two general approaches that vary in dosage and frequency of administration, but reach the same endpoint in terms of total amount of digoxin accumulated in the body.

1. Rapid digitalization may be achieved by administering a loading dose based upon projected peak body digoxin stores, then calculating the maintenance dose as a percentage of the loading dose.
2. More gradual digitalization may be obtained by beginning an appropriate maintenance dose, thus allowing digoxin body stores to accumulate slowly. Steady-state serum digoxin concentrations will be achieved in approximately 5 half-lives of the drug for the individual patient. Depending upon the patient's renal function, this will take between one and three weeks.

Adults:

Adults—Rapid Digitalization with a Loading Dose: Peak body digoxin stores of 8 to 12 μg/kg should provide therapeutic effect with minimum risk of toxicity in most patients with

$$\text{Maintenance Dose} = \text{Peak Body Stores (i.e. Loading Dose)} \times \frac{\% \text{ Daily Loss}}{100}$$

Where: % Daily Loss = 14 + Ccr/5

heart failure and normal sinus rhythm. Larger stores (10 to 15 μg/kg) are often required for adequate control of ventricular rate in patients with atrial flutter or fibrillation. Because of altered digoxin distribution and elimination, projected peak body stores for patients with renal insufficiency should be conservative (i.e. 6 to 10 μg/kg) [see PRECAUTIONS section].

The loading dose should be based on the projected peak body stores and administered in several portions, with roughly half the total given as the first dose. Additional fractions of this planned total dose may be given at 6 to 8 hour intervals, **with careful assessment of clinical response before each additional dose.**

If the patient's clinical response necessitates a change from the calculated dose of digoxin, then calculation of the maintenance dose should be based upon the amount actually given.

In previously undigitalized patients, a single initial Lanoxicaps dose of 400 to 600 μg (0.4 to 0.6 mg) usually produces a detectable effect in 0.5 to 2 hours that becomes maximal in 2 to 6 hours. Additional doses of 100 to 300 μg (0.1 to 0.3 mg) may be given cautiously at 6 to 8 hour intervals until clinical evidence of an adequate effect is noted. The usual amount of Lanoxicaps that a 70 kg patient requires to achieve 8 to 15 μg/kg peak body stores is 600 to 1000 μg (0.6 to 1.0 mg).

Although peak body stores are mathematically related to loading doses and are utilized to calculate maintenance doses, they do not correlate with measured serum concentrations. This discrepancy is caused by digoxin distribution within the body during the first 6 to 8 hours following a dose. Serum concentrations drawn during this time are usually not interpretable.

The maintenance dose should be based upon the percentage of the peak body stores lost each day through elimination. The following formula has had wide clinical use:

[See table above.]

Ccr is creatinine clearance, corrected to 70 kg body weight or 1.73 m² body surface area. **For adults,** if only serum creatinine concentrations (Scr) are available, a Ccr (corrected to 70 kg body weight) may be estimated in men as (140 − Age)/Scr. For women, this result should be multiplied by 0.85.

Note: This equation cannot be used for estimating creatinine clearance in infants or children.

A common practice involves the use of Lanoxin® Injection to achieve rapid digitalization, with conversion to Lanoxicaps or Lanoxin Tablets for maintenance therapy. If patients are switched from IV to oral digoxin formulations, allowances must be made for differences in bioavailability when calculating maintenance dosages (see table, CLINICAL PHARMACOLOGY section).

Adults—Gradual Digitalization with a Maintenance Dose: The following table provides average Lanoxicaps daily maintenance dose requirements for patients with heart failure based upon lean body weight and renal function:

[See table on bottom next page.]

Example—based on the above table, a patient in heart failure with an estimated lean body weight of 70 kg and a Ccr of 60 ml/min, should be given 200 μg (0.2 mg) of Lanoxicaps per day, usually taken as a 100 μg (0.1 mg) capsule after the morning and evening meals. Steady-state serum concentrations should not be anticipated before 11 days.

Infants and Children: Digitalization must be individualized. Divided daily dosing is recommended for infants and young children. In these patients, where dosage adjustment is frequent and outside the fixed dosages available, Lanoxicaps may not be the formulation of choice. Children over 10 years of age require adult dosages in proportion to their body weight.

In the newborn period, renal clearance of digoxin is diminished and suitable dosage adjustments must be observed. This is especially pronounced in the premature infant. Beyond the immediate newborn period, children generally require proportionally larger doses than adults on the basis of body weight or body surface area.

Lanoxin® Injection Pediatric can be used to achieve rapid digitalization, with conversion to an oral Lanoxin formulation for maintenance therapy. If patients are switched from IV to oral digoxin tablets or elixir, allowances must be made for differences in bioavailability when calculating maintenance dosages (see bioavailability table in CLINICAL PHARMACOLOGY section and dosing table below).

Intramuscular injection of digoxin is extremely painful and offers no advantages unless other routes of administration are contraindicated.

Digitalizing and daily maintenance doses for each age group are given below and should provide therapeutic effect with

Continued on next page

Burroughs Wellcome—Cont.

minimum risk of toxicity in most patients with heart failure and normal sinus rhythm. Larger doses are often required for adequate control of ventricular rate in patients with atrial flutter or fibrillation.

The loading dose should be administered in several portions, with roughly half the total given as the first dose. Additional fractions of this planned total dose may be given at 6 to 8 hour intervals, **with careful assessment of clinical response before each additional dose**. If the patient's clinical response necessitates a change from the calculated dose of digoxin, then calculation of the maintenance dose should be based upon the amount actually given.

[See table right].

More gradual digitalization can also be accomplished by beginning an appropriate maintenance dose. The range of percentages provided above can be used in calculating this dose for patients with normal renal function. In children with renal disease, digoxin dosing must be carefully titrated based upon desired clinical response.

Long-term use of digoxin is indicated in many children who have been digitalized for acute heart failure, unless the cause is transient. Children with severe congenital heart disease, even after surgery, may require digoxin for prolonged periods.

It cannot be overemphasized that both the adult and pediatric dosage guidelines provided are based upon average patient response and substantial individual variation can be expected. Accordingly, ultimate dosage selection must be based upon clinical assessment of the patient.

Serum Digoxin Concentrations: Measurement of serum digoxin concentrations can be helpful to the clinician in determining the state of digitalization and in assigning certain probabilities to the likelihood of digoxin intoxication. Studies in adults considered adequately digitalized (without evidence of toxicity) show that about two-thirds of such patients have serum digoxin levels ranging from 0.8 to 2.0 ng/ml. Patients with atrial fibrillation or atrial flutter require and appear to tolerate higher levels than do patients with other indications. On the other hand, in adult patients with clinical evidence of digoxin toxicity, about two-thirds will have serum digoxin levels greater than 2.0 ng/ml. Thus, whereas levels less than 0.8 ng/ml are infrequently associated with toxicity, levels greater than 2.0 ng/ml are often associated with toxicity. Values in between are not very helpful in deciding whether a certain sign or symptom is more likely caused by digoxin toxicity or by something else. There are rare patients who are unable to tolerate digoxin even at serum concentrations below 0.8 ng/ml. Some researchers suggest that infants and young children tolerate slightly higher serum concentrations than do adults.

To allow adequate time for equilibration of digoxin between serum and tissue, **sampling of serum concentrations for clinical use should be at least 6 to 8 hours after the last dose**, regardless of the route of administration or formulation used. On a twice daily dosing schedule, there will be only minor differences in serum digoxin concentrations whether sampling is done at 8 or 12 hours after a dose. After a single daily dose, the concentration will be 10 to 25% lower when sampled at 24 versus 8 hours, depending upon the patient's renal function. Ideally, sampling for assessment of steady-state concentrations should be done just before the next dose.

If a discrepancy exists between the reported serum concentration and the observed clinical response, the clinician should consider the following possibilities:

1. Analytical problems in the assay procedure.
2. Inappropriate serum sampling time.
3. Administration of a digitalis glycoside other than digoxin.
4. Conditions (described in WARNINGS and PRECAUTIONS sections) causing an alteration in the sensitivity of the patient to digoxin.
5. The patient falls outside the norm in his response to or handling of digoxin. This decision should only be

Usual Digitalizing and Maintenance Dosages for Lanoxicaps in Children with **Normal Renal Function Based on Lean Body Weight**

Age	Digitalizing* Dose (µg/kg)	Daily † Maintenance Dose (µg/kg)
2–5 Years	25–35	25–35% of the oral or IV loading dose ‡
5–10 Years	15–30	
Over 10 years	8–12	

*IV digitalizing doses are the same as Lanoxicaps digitalizing doses.
†Divided daily dosing is recommended for children under 10 years of age.
‡Projected or actual digitalizing dose providing desired clinical response.

reached after exclusion of the other possibilities and generally should be confirmed by additional correlations of clinical observations with serum digoxin concentrations.

The serum concentration data should always be interpreted in the overall clinical context and an isolated serum concentration value should not be used alone as a basis for increasing or decreasing digoxin dosage.

Adjustment of Maintenance Dose in Previously Digitalized Patients: Lanoxicaps maintenance doses in individual patients on steady-state digoxin can be adjusted upward or downward in proportion to the ratio of the desired versus the measured serum concentration. For example, a patient at steady-state on 100 µg (0.1 mg) of Lanoxicaps per day with a measured serum concentration of 0.7 ng/ml, should have the dose increased to 200 µg (0.2 mg) per day to achieve a steady-state serum concentration of 1.4 ng/ml, **assuming the serum digoxin concentration measurement is correct, renal function remains stable during this time and the needed adjustment is not the result of a problem with compliance.**

Dosage Adjustment When Changing Preparations: The absolute bioavailability of the capsule formulation is greater than that of the standard tablets and very near that of the intravenous dosage form. As a result the doses recommended for Lanoxicaps capsules are the same as those for Lanoxin® Injection (see CLINICAL PHARMACOLOGY section). Adjustments in dosage will seldom be necessary when converting a patient from intravenous to Lanoxicaps formulation. The differences in bioavailability between injectable Lanoxin or Lanoxicaps, and Lanoxin Elixir Pediatric or Lanoxin Tablets must be considered when changing patients from one dosage form to another.

Lanoxin Injection and Lanoxicaps doses of 100 µg (0.1 mg) and 200 µg (0.2 mg) are approximately equivalent to 125 µg (0.125 mg) and 250 µg (0.25 mg) doses of Lanoxin Tablets and Elixir Pediatric (see table in CLINICAL PHARMACOLOGY section). Intramuscular injection of digoxin is extremely painful and offers no advantages unless other routes of administration are contraindicated.

HOW SUPPLIED

LANOXICAPS (DIGOXIN SOLUTION IN CAPSULES), 50 µg (0.05 mg): bottles of 100 (NDC-0081-0270-55). Imprint A2C (red).
LANOXICAPS (DIGOXIN SOLUTION IN CAPSULES), 100 µg (0.1 mg)* bottles of 100 (NDC-0081-0272-55); Unit Dose Pack of 100 (NDC-0081-0272-56); Unit of Use bottles of 30 (NDC-0081-0272-30). Imprint B2C (yellow).
LANOXICAPS (DIGOXIN SOLUTION IN CAPSULES), 200 µg (0.2 mg)* bottles of 100 (NDC-0081-0274-55); Unit Dose Pack of 100 (NDC-0081-0274-56); Unit of Use bottles of 30 (NDC-0081-0274-30). Imprint C2C (green).
Store at 15°–30°C (59°–86°F) in a dry place and protect from light.
Also Available:
LANOXIN® (DIGOXIN) TABLETS, Scored 125 µg (0.125 mg): Bottles of 100 and 1000; Unit Dose Pack of 100; Unit of Use bottles of 30.
LANOXIN (DIGOXIN) TABLETS, Scored 250 µg (0.25 mg): Bottles of 100, 1000 and 5000; Unit Dose Pack of 100; Unit of Use bottles of 30.
LANOXIN (DIGOXIN) TABLETS Scored 500 µg (0.5 mg): Bottles of 100.

LANOXIN (DIGOXIN) ELIXIR PEDIATRIC, 50 µg (0.05 mg) per ml; bottle of 60 ml with calibrated dropper.
LANOXIN (DIGOXIN) INJECTION, 500 µg (0.5 mg) in 2 ml (250 µg [0.25 mg] per ml); boxes of 10 and 50 ampuls.
LANOXIN (DIGOXIN) INJECTION PEDIATRIC, 100 µg (0.1 mg) in 1 ml; box of 10 ampuls.
*U.S. Patent No. 4088750
Shown in Product Identification Section, page 407

LANOXIN®   ℞
[lă-nŏx 'ĭn ʺ]
(Digoxin)
Tablets/Injections/Elixir Pediatric

DESCRIPTION

Digoxin is one of the cardiac (or digitalis) glycosides, a closely related group of drugs having in common specific effects on the myocardium. These drugs are found in a number of plants. Digoxin is extracted from the leaves of *Digitalis lanata*. The term "digitalis" is used to designate the whole group. The glycosides are composed of two portions: a sugar and a cardenolide (hence "glycosides").

Digoxin has the molecular formula $C_{41}H_{64}O_{14}$, a molecular weight of 780.95 and melting and decomposition points above 235°C. The drug is practically insoluble in water and in ether; slightly soluble in diluted (50%) alcohol and in chloroform; and freely soluble in pyridine. Digoxin powder is composed of odorless white crystals.

Digoxin has the chemical name: 3β-[(O-2,6- dideoxy- β -D-ribo -hexopyranosyl -(1→4)- O -2,6- dideoxy- β -D-ribo-hexopyranosyl - (1→4)- 2,6-dideoxy -β-D-ribo -hexopyranosyl) oxy]-12β, 14-dihydroxy-5β-card-20(22)-enolide.

Lanoxin Tablets with 125 µg (0.125 mg), 250 µg (0.25 mg) or 500 µg (0.5 mg) digoxin USP are intended for oral use. Each tablet contains the labeled amount of digoxin USP and the inactive ingredients: 0.125 mg tablet—corn and potato starch, D&C Yellow No. 10, FD&C Yellow No. 6, lactose, and magnesium stearate; 0.25 mg tablet—corn and potato starch, lactose, magnesium stearate, and stearic acid; 0.5 mg tablet—corn and potato starch, D&C Green No. 5 and Yellow No. 10, FD&C Red No. 40, lactose, magnesium stearate, and stearic acid.

Lanoxin (Digoxin) Injection and Injection Pediatric are sterile solutions of digoxin for intravenous or intramuscular injection. The vehicle contains 40% propylene glycol and 10% alcohol. The injection is buffered to a pH of 6.8 to 7.2 with 0.3 percent sodium phosphate and 0.08 percent anhydrous citric acid. Each 2 ml ampul of Lanoxin Injection contains 500 µg (0.5 mg) digoxin [250 µg (0.25 mg) per ml]. Each 1 ml ampul of Lanoxin Injection Pediatric contains 100 µg (0.1 mg) digoxin. Dilution is not required.

Lanoxin Elixir Pediatric is a stable solution of digoxin specially formulated for oral use in infants and children. Each ml contains 50 µg (0.05 mg) digoxin USP. The lime-flavored elixir contains 10% alcohol and methylparaben 0.1% (added as a preservative), citric acid, D&C Green No. 5 and Yellow No. 10, flavor, propylene glycol, sodium phosphate, and sucrose. Each package is supplied with a specially calibrated dropper to facilitate the administration of accurate dosage even in premature infants. Starting at 0.2 ml, this 1 ml dropper is marked in divisions of 0.1 ml, each corresponding to 5 µg (0.005 mg) digoxin.

CLINICAL PHARMACOLOGY
Mechanism of Action:

The influence of digitalis glycosides on the myocardium is dose-related, and involves both a direct action on cardiac muscle and the specialized conduction system, and indirect actions on the cardiovascular system mediated by the autonomic nervous system. The indirect actions mediated by the autonomic nervous system involve a vagomimetic action, which is responsible for the effects of digitalis on the sinoatrial (SA) and atrioventricular (AV) nodes; and also a baroreceptor sensitization which results in increased carotid sinus nerve activity and enhanced sympathetic withdrawal for any given increment in mean arterial pressure. The pharmacologic consequences of these direct and indirect effects are: 1) an increase in the force and velocity of myocardial systolic contraction (positive inotropic action); 2) a slowing of heart rate (negative chronotropic effect); and 3) decreased conduction velocity through the AV node. In higher doses,

Usual Lanoxicaps Daily Maintenance Dose Requirements (µg) for Estimated Peak Body Stores of 10 µg/kg

		50/110	60/132	70/154	80/176	90/198	100/220		
				Lean Body Weight (kg/lbs)					
	0	50	100	100	100	150	150	22	
	10	100	100	100	150	150	150	19	
	20	100	100	150	150	150	200	16	
Corrected	30	100	150	150	150	200	200	14	Number of
Ccr	40	100	150	150	200	200	250	13	Days
(ml/min	50	150	150	200	200	250	250	12	Before
per 70 kg)	60	150	150	200	200	250	300	11	Steady-State
	70	150	200	200	250	250	300	10	Achieved
	80	150	200	200	250	300	300	9	
	90	150	200	250	250	300	350	8	
	100	200	200	250	300	300	350	7	

digitalis increases sympathetic outflow from the central nervous system (CNS) to both cardiac and peripheral sympathetic nerves. This increase in sympathetic activity may be an important factor in digitalis cardiac toxicity. Most of the extracardiac manifestations of digitalis toxicity are also mediated by the CNS.

Pharmacokinetics:

Note: The following data are from studies performed in adults, unless otherwise stated.

Absorption —Gastrointestinal absorption of digoxin is a passive process. Absorption of digoxin from the Lanoxin® tablet formulation has been demonstrated to be 60 to 80% complete and absorption of digoxin from the Lanoxin® Elixir Pediatric formulation 70 to 85% complete compared to an identical intravenous dose of digoxin (absolute bioavailability). When digoxin elixir or tablets are taken after meals, the rate of absorption is slowed, but the total amount of digoxin absorbed is usually unchanged. When taken with meals high in bran fiber, however, the amount absorbed from an oral dose may be reduced. Comparison of the systemic availability and equivalent doses for digoxin preparations are shown in the following table.

[See table above right].

In some patients, orally administered digoxin is converted to cardioinactive reduction products (e.g., dihydrodigoxin) by colonic bacteria in the gut. Data suggest that one in ten patients treated with digoxin tablets will degrade 40% or more of the ingested dose.

Distribution —Following drug administration, a 6 to 8 hour distribution phase is observed. This is followed by a much more gradual serum concentration decline, which is dependent on digoxin elimination from the body. The peak height and slope of the early portion (absorption/distribution phases) of the serum concentration-time curve are dependent upon the route of administration and the absorption characteristics of the formulation. Clinical evidence indicates that the early high serum concentrations do not reflect the concentration of digoxin at its site of action, but that with chronic use, the steady-state post-distribution serum levels are in equilibrium with tissue levels and correlate with pharmacologic effects. In individual patients, these post-distribution serum concentrations are linearly related to maintenance dosage and may be useful in evaluating therapeutic and toxic effects (see Serum Digoxin Concentrations in DOSAGE AND ADMINISTRATION section).

Digoxin is concentrated in tissues and therefore has a large apparent volume of distribution. Digoxin crosses both the blood-brain barrier and the placenta. At delivery, serum digoxin concentration in the newborn is similar to the serum level in the mother. Approximately 20 to 25% of plasma digoxin is bound to protein. Serum digoxin concentrations are not significantly altered by large changes in fat tissue weight, so that its distribution space correlates best with lean (ideal) body weight, not total body weight.

Pharmacologic Response —The approximate times to onset of effect and to peak effect of all the Lanoxin® preparations are given in the following table:

[See table below].

Excretion —Elimination of digoxin follows first-order kinetics (that is, the quantity of digoxin eliminated at any time is proportional to the total body content). Following intravenous administration to normal subjects, 50 to 70% of a digoxin dose is excreted unchanged in the urine. Renal excretion of digoxin is proportional to glomerular filtration rate and is largely independent of urine flow. In subjects with normal renal function, digoxin has a half-life of 1.5 to 2.0 days. The half-life in anuric patients is prolonged to 4 to 6 days. Digoxin is not effectively removed from the body by dialysis, exchange transfusion or during cardiopulmonary by-pass because most of the drug is in tissue rather than circulating in the blood.

INDICATIONS AND USAGE

Heart Failure:

The increased cardiac output resulting from the inotropic action of digoxin ameliorates the disturbances characteristic of heart failure (venous congestion, edema, dyspnea, orthopnea and cardiac asthma).

Digoxin is more effective in "low output" (pump) failure than in "high output" heart failure secondary to arteriovenous fistula, anemia, infection or hyperthyroidism.

Digoxin is usually continued after failure is controlled, unless some known precipitating factor is corrected. Studies

PRODUCT	ABSOLUTE BIOAVAILABILITY	EQUIVALENT DOSES (IN MG*)		
Lanoxin Tablet	60–80%	0.125	0.25	0.5
Lanoxin Elixir	70–85%	0.125	0.25	0.5
Lanoxin Injection/IM	70–85%	0.125	0.25	0.5
Lanoxin Injection/IV	100%	0.1	0.2	0.4
Lanoxicaps Capsules	90–100%	0.1	0.2	0.4

*1 mg = 1000 μg

have shown, however, that even though hemodynamic effects can be demonstrated in almost all patients, corresponding improvement in the signs and symptoms of heart failure is not necessarily apparent. Therefore, in patients in whom digoxin may be difficult to regulate, or in whom the risk of toxicity may be great (e.g., patients with unstable renal function or whose potassium levels tend to fluctuate) a cautious withdrawal of digoxin may be considered. If digoxin is discontinued, the patient should be regularly monitored for clinical evidence of recurrent heart failure.

Atrial Fibrillation:

Digoxin reduces ventricular rate and thereby improves hemodynamics. Palpitation, precordial distress or weakness are relieved and concomitant congestive failure ameliorated. Digoxin should be continued in doses necessary to maintain the desired ventricular rate.

Atrial Flutter:

Digoxin slows the heart and regular sinus rhythm may appear. Frequently the flutter is converted to atrial fibrillation with a controlled ventricular response. Digoxin treatment should be maintained if atrial fibrillation persists. (Electrical cardioversion is often the treatment of choice for atrial flutter. See discussion of cardioversion in PRECAUTIONS section.)

Paroxysmal Atrial Tachycardia (PAT):

Digoxin may convert PAT to sinus rhythm by slowing conduction through the AV node. If heart failure has ensued or paroxysms recur frequently, digoxin should be continued. In infants, digoxin is usually continued for 3 to 6 months after a single episode of PAT to prevent recurrence.

CONTRAINDICATIONS

Digitalis glycosides are contraindicated in ventricular fibrillation.

In a given patient, an untoward effect requiring permanent discontinuation of other digitalis preparations usually constitutes a contraindication to digoxin. Hypersensitivity to digoxin itself is a contraindication to its use. Allergy to digoxin, though rare, does occur. It may not extend to all such preparations, and another digitalis glycoside may be tried with caution.

WARNINGS

Digitalis alone or with other drugs has been used in the treatment of obesity. This use of digoxin or other digitalis glycosides is unwarranted. Moreover, since they may cause potentially fatal arrhythmias or other adverse effects, the use of these drugs solely for the treatment of obesity is dangerous. Anorexia, nausea, vomiting and arrhythmias may accompany heart failure or may be indications of digitalis intoxication. Clinical evaluation of the cause of these symptoms should be attempted before further digitalis administration. In such circumstances determination of the serum digoxin concentration may be an aid in deciding whether or not digitalis toxicity is likely to be present. If the possibility of digitalis intoxication cannot be excluded, cardiac glycosides should be temporarily withheld, if permitted by the clinical situation.

Patients with renal insufficiency require smaller than usual maintenance doses of digoxin (see DOSAGE AND ADMINISTRATION section).

Heart failure accompanying acute glomerulonephritis requires extreme care in digitalization. Relatively low loading and maintenance doses and concomitant use of antihypertensive drugs may be necessary and careful monitoring is essential. Digoxin should be discontinued as soon as possible. Patients with severe carditis, such as carditis associated with rheumatic fever or viral myocarditis, are especially sensitive to digoxin-induced disturbances of rhythm.

Newborn infants display considerable variability in their tolerance to digoxin. Premature and immature infants are

particularly sensitive, and dosage must not only be reduced but must be individualized according to their degree of maturity.

Note: Digitalis glycosides are an important cause of accidental poisoning in children.

PRECAUTIONS

General:

Digoxin toxicity develops more frequently and lasts longer in patients with renal impairment because of the decreased excretion of digoxin. Therefore, it should be anticipated that dosage requirements will be decreased in patients with moderate to severe renal disease (see DOSAGE AND ADMINISTRATION section). Because of the prolonged half-life, a longer period of time is required to achieve an initial or new steady-state concentration in patients with renal impairment than in patients with normal renal function.

In patients with hypokalemia, toxicity may occur despite serum digoxin concentrations within the "normal range", because potassium depletion sensitizes the myocardium to digoxin. Therefore, it is desirable to maintain normal serum potassium levels in patients being treated with digoxin. Hypokalemia may result from diuretic, amphotericin B or corticosteroid therapy, and from dialysis or mechanical suction of gastrointestinal secretions. It may also accompany malnutrition, diarrhea, prolonged vomiting, old age and long-standing heart failure. In general, rapid changes in serum potassium or other electrolytes should be avoided, and intravenous treatment with potassium should be reserved for special circumstances as described below (see TREATMENT OF ARRHYTHMIAS PRODUCED BY OVERDOSAGE section). Calcium, particularly when administered rapidly by the intravenous route, may produce serious arrhythmias in digitalized patients. Hypercalcemia from any cause predisposes the patient to digitalis toxicity. On the other hand, hypocalcemia can nullify the effects of digoxin in man; thus, digoxin may be ineffective until serum calcium is restored to normal. These interactions are related to the fact that calcium affects contractility and excitability of the heart in a manner similar to digoxin.

Hypomagnesemia may predispose to digitalis toxicity. If low magnesium levels are detected in a patient on digoxin, replacement therapy should be instituted.

Quinidine, verapamil, and amoidarone cause a rise in serum digoxin concentration, with the implication that digitalis intoxication may result. This rise appears to be proportional to the dose. The effect is mediated by a reduction in the digoxin clearance and, in the case of quinidine, decreased volume of distribution as well.

Certain antibiotics may increase digoxin absorption in patients who convert digoxin to inactive metabolites in the gut (see Pharmacokinetics portion of the CLINICAL PHARMACOLOGY section). Recent studies have shown that specific colonic bacteria in the lower gastrointestinal tract convert digoxin to cardioinactive reduction products, thereby reducing its bioavailability. Although inactivation of these bacteria by antibiotics is rapid, the serum digoxin concentration will rise at a rate consistent with the elimination half-life of digoxin. The magnitude of rise in serum digoxin concentration relates to the extent of bacterial inactivation, and may be as much as two-fold in some cases.

Patients with acute myocardial infarction or severe pulmonary disease may be unusually sensitive to digoxin-induced disturbances of rhythm.

Atrial arrhythmias associated with hypermetabolic states (e.g. hyperthyroidism) are particularly resistant to digoxin treatment. Large doses of digoxin are not recommended as the only treatment of these arrhythmias and care must be taken to avoid toxicity if large doses of digoxin are required. In hypothyroidism, the digoxin requirements are reduced. Digoxin responses in patients with compensated thyroid disease are normal.

Reduction of digoxin dosage may be desirable prior to electrical cardioversion to avoid induction of ventricular arrhythmias, but the physician must consider the consequences of rapid increase in ventricular response to atrial fibrillation if digoxin is withheld 1 to 2 days prior to cardioversion. If there is a suspicion that digitalis toxicity exists, elective cardioversion should be delayed. If it is not prudent to delay cardioversion, the energy level selected should be minimal at first and carefully increased in an attempt to avoid precipitating ventricular arrhythmias.

PRODUCT	TIME TO ONSET OF EFFECT*	TIME TO PEAK EFFECT*
Lanoxin Tablet	0.5–2 hours	2–6 hours
Lanoxin Elixir	0.5–2 hours	2–6 hours
Lanoxin Injection/IM	0.5–2 hours	2–6 hours
Lanoxin Injection/IV	5–30 minutes†	1–4 hours
Lanoxicaps Capsules	0.5–2 hours	2–6 hours

*Documented for ventricular response rate in atrial fibrillation, inotropic effect and electrocardiographic changes.
†Depending upon rate of infusion.

Continued on next page

Burroughs Wellcome—Cont.

Incomplete AV block, especially in patients with Stokes-Adams attacks, may progress to advanced or complete heart block if digoxin is given.

In some patients with sinus node disease (i.e. Sick Sinus Syndrome), digoxin may worsen sinus bradycardia or sino-atrial block.

In patients with Wolff-Parkinson-White Syndrome and atrial fibrillation, digoxin can enhance transmission of impulses through the accessory pathway. This effect may result in extremely rapid ventricular rates and even ventricular fibrillation.

Digoxin may worsen the outflow obstruction in patients with idiopathic hypertrophic subaortic stenosis (IHSS). Unless cardiac failure is severe, it is doubtful whether digoxin should be employed.

Patients with chronic constrictive pericarditis may fail to respond to digoxin. In addition, slowing of the heart rate by digoxin in some patients may further decrease cardiac output.

Patients with heart failure from amyloid heart disease or constrictive cardiomyopathies respond poorly to treatment with digoxin.

Digoxin is not indicated for the treatment of sinus tachycardia unless it is associated with heart failure.

Digoxin may produce false positive ST-T changes in the electrocardiogram during exercise testing.

Intramuscular injection of digoxin is extremely painful and offers no advantages unless other routes of administration are contraindicated.

Laboratory Tests:

Patients receiving digoxin should have their serum electrolytes and renal function (BUN and/or serum creatinine) assessed periodically; the frequency of assessments will depend on the clinical setting. For discussion of serum digoxin concentrations, see DOSAGE AND ADMINISTRATION section.

Drug Interactions:

Potassium-depleting *corticosteroids* and *diuretics* may be major contributing factors to digitalis toxicity. *Calcium*, particularly if administered rapidly by the intravenous route, may produce serious arrhythmias in digitalized patients. *Quinidine, verapamil,* and *amiodarone* cause a rise in serum digoxin concentration, with the implication that digitalis intoxication may result. Certain *antibiotics* increase digoxin absorption in patients who inactivate digoxin by bacterial metabolism in the lower intestine, so that digitalis intoxication may result. *Propantheline* and *diphenoxylate*, by decreasing gut motility, may increase digoxin absorption. *Antacids, kaolin-pectin, sulfasalazine, neomycin, cholestyramine* and certain *anticancer drugs* may interfere with intestinal digoxin absorption, resulting in unexpectedly low serum concentrations. There have been inconsistent reports regarding the effects of other drugs on the serum digoxin concentration. *Thyroid* administration to a digitalized, hypothyroid patient may increase the dose requirement of digoxin. Concomitant use of digoxin and *sympathomimetics* increases the risk of cardiac arrhythmias because both enhance ectopic pacemaker activity. *Succinylcholine* may cause a sudden extrusion of potassium from muscle cells, and may thereby cause arrhythmias in digitalized patients. Although β adrenergic blockers or calcium channel blockers and digoxin may be useful in combination to control atrial fibrillation, their additive effects on AV node conduction can result in complete heart block.

Due to the considerable variability of these interactions, digoxin dosage should be carefully individualized when patients receive coadministered medications.

Furthermore, caution should be exercised when combining digoxin with any drug that may cause a significant deterioration in renal function, since this may impair the excretion of digoxin.

Carcinogenesis, Mutagenesis, Impairment of Fertility:

There have been no long-term studies performed in animals to evaluate carcinogenic potential.

Pregnancy: *Teratogenic Effects:* Pregnancy Category C.

Animal reproduction studies have not been conducted with digoxin. It is also not known whether digoxin can cause fetal harm when administered to a pregnant woman or can affect reproduction capacity. Digoxin should be given to a pregnant woman only if clearly needed.

Nursing Mothers:

Studies have shown that digoxin concentrations in the mother's serum and milk are similar. However, the estimated daily dose to a nursing infant will be far below the usual infant maintenance dose. Therefore, this amount should have no pharmacologic effect upon the infant. Nevertheless, caution should be exercised when digoxin is administered to a nursing woman.

ADVERSE REACTIONS

The frequency and severity of adverse reactions to digoxin depend on the dose and route of administration, as well as on the patient's underlying disease or concomitant therapies

(see PRECAUTIONS section and Serum Digoxin Concentrations subsection of DOSAGE AND ADMINISTRATION). The overall incidence of adverse reactions has been reported as 5 to 20%, with 15 to 20% of them being considered serious (one to four percent of patients receiving digoxin). Evidence suggests that the incidence of toxicity has decreased since the introduction of the serum digoxin assay and improved standardization of digoxin tablets. Cardiac toxicity accounts for about one-half, gastrointestinal disturbances for about one-fourth, and CNS and other toxicity for about one-fourth of these adverse reactions.

Adults:

Cardiac—Unifocal or multiform ventricular premature contractions, especially in bigeminal or trigeminal patterns, are the most common arrhythmias associated with digoxin toxicity in adults with heart disease.

Ventricular tachycardia may result from digitalis toxicity. Atrioventricular (AV) dissociation, accelerated junctional (nodal) rhythm and atrial tachycardia with block are also common arrhythmias caused by digoxin overdosage.

Excessive slowing of the pulse is a clinical sign of digoxin overdosage. AV block (Wenckebach) of increasing degree may proceed to complete heart block.

Note: The electrocardiogram is fundamental in determining the presence and nature of these cardiac disturbances. Digoxin may also induce other changes in the ECG (e.g. PR prolongation, ST depression), which represent digoxin effect and may or may not be associated with digitalis toxicity.

Gastrointestinal—Anorexia, nausea, vomiting and less commonly diarrhea are common early symptoms of overdosage. However, uncontrolled heart failure may also produce such symptoms. Digitalis toxicity very rarely may cause abdominal pain and hemorrhagic necrosis of the intestines.

CNS—Visual disturbances (blurred or yellow vision), headache, weakness, dizziness, apathy and psychosis can occur.

Other—Gynecomastia is occasionally observed. Maculopapular rash or other skin reactions are rarely observed.

Infants and Children:

Toxicity differs from the adult in a number of respects. Anorexia, nausea, vomiting, diarrhea and CNS disturbances may be present but are rare as initial symptoms in infants. Cardiac arrhythmias are more reliable signs of toxicity. Digoxin in children may produce any arrhythmia.

Cardiac—Conduction disturbances or supraventricular tachyarrhythmias, such as atrioventricular (AV) block (Wenckebach), atrial tachycardia with or without block and junctional (nodal) tachycardia are the most common arrhythmias associated with digoxin toxicity in children. Ventricular arrhythmias, such as unifocal or multiform ventricular premature contractions, especially in bigeminal or trigeminal patterns, are less common. Ventricular tachycardia may result from digitalis toxicity. Sinus bradycardia may also be a sign of impending digoxin intoxication, especially in infants, even in the absence of first degree heart block. Any arrhythmias or alteration in cardiac conduction that develops in a child taking digoxin should initially be assumed to be a consequence of digoxin intoxication.

Note: The electrocardiogram is fundamental in determining the presence and nature of these cardiac disturbances. Digoxin may also induce other changes in the ECG (e.g. PR prolongation, ST depression), which represent digoxin effect and may or may not be associated with digitalis toxicity.

Gastrointestinal—Anorexia, nausea, vomiting and diarrhea may be early symptoms of overdosage. However, uncontrolled heart failure may also produce such symptoms. Digitalis toxicity very rarely may cause abdominal pain and hemorrhagic necrosis of the intestines.

CNS—Visual disturbances (blurred or yellow vision), headache, weakness, dizziness, apathy and psychosis can occur. These may be difficult to recognize in infants and children.

Other—Gynecomastia is occasionally observed. Maculopapular rash or other skin reactions are rarely observed.

OVERDOSAGE

Treatment of Arrhythmias Produced by Overdosage:

Adults:

Digoxin should be discontinued until all signs of toxicity are gone. Discontinuation may be all that is necessary if toxic manifestations are not severe and appear only near the expected time for maximum effect of the drug.

Correction of factors that may contribute to toxicity such as electrolyte disturbances, hypoxia, acid-base disturbances and removal of aggravating agents such as catecholamines, should also be considered. Potassium salts may be indicated, particularly if hypokalemia is present. Potassium administration may be dangerous in the setting of massive digitalis overdosage (see Massive Digitalis Overdosage subsection below). Potassium chloride in divided oral doses totaling 3 to 6 grams of the salt (40 to 80 mEq K+) for adults may be given provided renal function is adequate (see below for potassium recommendations in Infants and Children).

When correction of the arrhythmia is urgent and the serum potassium concentration is low or normal, potassium should be administered intravenously in 5% dextrose injection. For

adults, a total of 40 to 80 mEq (diluted to a concentration of 40 mEq per 500 ml) may be given at a rate not exceeding 20 mEq per hour, or slower if limited by pain due to local irritation. Additional amounts may be given if the arrhythmia is uncontrolled and potassium well-tolerated. ECG monitoring should be performed to watch for any evidence of potassium toxicity (e.g. peaking of T waves) and to observe the effect on the arrhythmia. The infusion may be stopped when the desired effect is achieved.

Note: Potassium should not be used and may be dangerous in heart block due to digoxin, unless primarily related to supraventricular tachycardia.

Other agents that have been used for the treatment of digoxin intoxication include lidocaine, procainamide, propranolol and phenytoin, although use of the latter must be considered experimental. In advanced heart block, atropine and/or temporary ventricular pacing may be beneficial. Digibind®, Digoxin Immune Fab (Ovine), can be used to reverse potentially life-threatening digoxin (or digitoxin) intoxication. Improvement in signs and symptoms of digitalis toxicity usually begins within ½ hour of Digibind administration. Each 40 mg vial of Digibind will neutralize 0.6 mg of digoxin (which is a usual body store of an adequately digitalized 70 kg patient).

Infants and Children:

See Adult section for general recommendations for the treatment of arrhythmias produced by overdosage and for cautions regarding the use of potassium.

If a potassium preparation is used to treat toxicity, it may be given orally in divided doses totaling 1 to 1.5 mEq K+ per kilogram (kg) body weight (1 gram of potassium chloride contains 13.4 mEq K+).

When correction of the arrhythmia with potassium is urgent, approximately 0.5 mEq/kg of potassium per hour may be given intravenously, with careful ECG monitoring. The intravenous solution of potassium should be dilute enough to avoid local irritation; however, especially in infants, care must be taken to avoid intravenous fluid overload.

Massive Digitalis Overdosage

Manifestations of life-threatening toxicity include severe ventricular arrhythmias much as ventricular tachycardia or ventricular fibrillation, or progressive bradyarrhythmias much as severe sinus bradycardia or second or third degree heart block not responsive to atropine. An overdosage of more than 10 mg of digoxin in previously healthy adults or 4 mg in previously healthy children or overdosage resulting in steady-state serum concentrations greater than 10 ng/ml, often results in cardiac arrest.

Severe digitalis intoxication can cause life-threatening elevation in serum potassium concentration by shifting potassium from inside to outside the cell resulting in hyperkalemia. Administration of potassium supplements in the setting of massive intoxication may be hazardous.

Digibind®, Digoxin Immune Fab (Ovine), may be used at a dose equimolar to digoxin in the body to reverse the effects of ingestion of a massive overdose. The decision to administer Digibind before the onset of toxic manifestations will depend on the likelihood that life-threatening toxicity will occur (see above).

Patients with massive digitalis ingestion should receive large doses of activated charcoal to prevent absorption and bind digoxin in the gut during enteroenteric recirculation. Emesis of gastric lavage may be indicated especially if ingestion has occurred within 30 minutes of the patient's presentation at the hospital. Emesis should not be induced in patients who are obtunded. If a patient presents more than 2 hours after ingestion or already has toxic manifestations, it may be unsafe to induce vomiting or attempt passage of a gastric tube, because such maneuvers may induce an acute vagal episode that can worsen digitalis-toxic arrhythmias.

DOSAGE AND ADMINISTRATION

Recommended dosages are average values that may require considerable modification because of individual sensitivity or associated conditions. Diminished renal function is the most important factor requiring modification of recommended doses.

Parenteral administration of digoxin should be used only when the need for rapid digitalization is urgent or when the drug cannot be taken orally. Intramuscular injection can lead to severe pain at the injection site, thus intravenous administration is preferred. If the drug must be administered by the intramuscular route, it should be injected deep into the muscle followed by massage. No more than 500 μg (2 ml) of Lanoxin Injection or 200 μg (2 ml) of Lanoxin Injection Pediatric should be injected into a single site.

Lanoxin® Injection and Injection Pediatric can be administered undiluted or diluted with a 4-fold or greater volume of sterile water for injection, 0.9% sodium chloride injection or 5% dextrose injection. The use of less than a 4-fold volume of diluent could lead to precipitation of the digoxin. Immediate use of the diluted product is recommended.

If tuberculin syringes are used to measure very small doses, one must be aware of the problem of inadvertent overadministration of digoxin. The syringe should *not* be flushed with the parenteral solution after its contents are expelled into an indwelling vascular catheter.

Slow infusion of Lanoxin® Injection or Injection Pediatric is preferable to bolus administration. Rapid infusion of digitalis glycosides has been shown to cause systemic and coronary arteriolar constriction, which may be clinically undesirable. Caution is thus advised and Lanoxin Injection or Injection Pediatric should probably be administered over a period of 5 minutes or longer. Mixing of Lanoxin Injections with other drugs in the same container or simultaneous administration in the same intravenous line is not recommended.

In deciding the dose of digoxin, several factors must be considered:

1. The disease being treated. Atrial arrhythmias may require larger doses than heart failure.
2. The body weight of the patient. Doses should be calculated based upon lean or ideal body weight.
3. The patient's renal function, preferably evaluated on the basis of creatinine clearance.
4. Age is an important factor in infants and children.
5. Concomitant disease states, drugs or other factors likely to alter the expected clinical response to digoxin (see PRECAUTIONS and Drug Interactions sections).

Digitalization may be accomplished by either of two general approaches that vary in dosage and frequency of administration, but reach the same endpoint in terms of total amount of digoxin accumulated in the body.

1. Rapid digitalization may be achieved by administering a loading dose based upon projected peak body digoxin stores, then calculating the maintenance dose as a percentage of the loading dose.
2. More gradual digitalization may be obtained by beginning an appropriate maintenance dose, thus allowing digoxin body stores to accumulate slowly. Steady-state serum digoxin concentrations will be achieved in approximately 5 half-lives of the drug for the individual patient. Depending upon the patient's renal function, this will take between one and three weeks.

Adults:

Adults—Rapid Digitalization with a Loading Dose. Peak body digoxin stores of 8 to 12 µg/kg should provide therapeutic effect with minimum risk of toxicity in most patients with heart failure and normal sinus rhythm. Larger stores (10 to 15 µg/kg) are often required for adequate control of ventricular rate in patients with atrial flutter or fibrillation. Because of altered digoxin distribution and elimination, projected peak body stores for patients with renal insufficiency should be conservative (i.e. 6 to 10 µg/kg) [see PRECAUTIONS section].

The loading dose should be based on the projected peak body stores and administered in several portions, with roughly half the total given as the first dose. Additional fractions of this planned total dose may be given at 4 to 8 hour intervals IV or 6 to 8 hour intervals orally, with **careful assessment of clinical response before each additional dose.**

If the patient's clinical response necessitates a change from the calculated dose of digoxin, then calculation of the maintenance dose should be based upon the amount actually given.

In previously undigitalized patients, a single initial intravenous Lanoxin® Injection dose of 400 to 600 µg (0.4 to 0.6 mg) usually produces a detectable effect in 5 to 30 minutes that becomes maximal in 1 to 4 hours. Additional doses of 100 to 300 µg (0.1 to 0.3 mg) may be given cautiously at 4 to 8 hour intervals until clinical evidence of an adequate effect is noted. The usual amount of Lanoxin Injection that a 70 kg patient requires to achieve 8 to 15 µg/kg peak body stores is 600 to 1000 µg (0.6 to 1.0 mg).

In previously undigitalized patients, a single initial Lanoxin® Tablet or Elixir Pediatric dose of 500 to 750 µg (0.5 to 0.75 mg) usually produces a detectable effect in 0.5 to 2 hours that becomes maximal in 2 to 6 hours. Additional doses of 125 to 375 µg (0.125 to 0.375 mg) may be given cautiously at 6 to 8 hour intervals until clinical evidence of an adequate effect is noted. The usual amount of Lanoxin Tablets or Elixir that a 70 kg patient requires to achieve 8 to 15 µg/kg peak body stores is 750 to 1250 µg (0.75 to 1.25 mg).

Although peak body stores are mathematically related to loading doses and are utilized to calculate maintenance doses, they do not correlate with measured serum concentrations. This discrepancy is caused by digoxin distribution within the body during the first 6 to 8 hours following a dose. Serum concentrations drawn during this time are usually not interpretable.

The maintenance dose should be based upon the percentage of the peak body stores lost each day through elimination. The following formula has had wide clinical use:
[See table above.]

Ccr is creatinine clearance, corrected to 70 kg body weight or 1.73 m² body surface area. *For adults,* if only serum creatinine concentrations (Scr) are available, a Ccr (corrected to 70 kg body weight) may be estimated in men as $(140 - Age)/Scr$. For women, this result should be multiplied by 0.85.

Note: This equation cannot be used for estimating creatinine clearance in infants or children.

A common practice involves the use of Lanoxin® Injection to achieve rapid digitalization, with conversion to Lanoxin Tablets or Lanoxicaps for maintenance therapy. If patients are switched from IV to oral digoxin formulations, allowances must be made for differences in bioavailability when calculating maintenance dosages (see table, CLINICAL PHARMACOLOGY section).

Adults—Gradual Digitalization with a Maintenance Dose: The following table provides average Lanoxin Tablet daily maintenance dose requirements for patients with heart failure based upon lean body weight and renal function:
[See table below].

Infants and Children:

Digitalization must be individualized. Divided daily dosing is recommended for infants and young children. Children over 10 years of age require adult dosages in proportion to their body weight.

In the newborn period, renal clearance of digoxin is diminished and suitable dosage adjustments must be observed. This is especially pronounced in the premature infant. Beyond the immediate newborn period, children generally require proportionally larger doses than adults on the basis of body weight or body surface area.

Infants and Children— Rapid Digitalization with a Loading Dose: Lanoxin Injection Pediatric can be used to achieve rapid digitalization, with conversion to an oral Lanoxin formulation for maintenance therapy. If patients are switched from IV to oral digoxin tablets or elixir, allowances must be made for differences in bioavailability when calculating maintenance dosages (see bioavailability table in CLINICAL PHARMACOLOGY section and dosing tables below).

Intramuscular injection of digoxin is extremely painful and offers no advantages unless other routes of administration are contraindicated.

Digitalizing and daily maintenance doses for each age group are given below and should provide therapeutic effect with minimum risk of toxicity in most patients with heart failure and normal sinus rhythm. Larger doses are often required

for adequate control of ventricular rate in patients with atrial flutter or fibrillation.

The loading dose should be administered in several portions, with roughly half the total given as the first dose. Additional fractions of this planned total dose may be given at 6 to 8 hour intervals with Lanoxin Tablets or Elixir or at 4 to 8 hour intervals with Lanoxin Injection or Injection Pediatric **with careful assessment of clinical response before each additional dose.** If the patient's clinical response necessitates a change from the calculated dose of digoxin, then calculation of the maintenance dose should be based upon the amount actually given.
[See table on next page].

Infants and Children—Gradual Digitalization With A Maintenance Dose: More gradual digitalization can also be accomplished by beginning an appropriate maintenance dose. The range of percentages provided above can be used in calculating this dose for patients with normal renal function. In children with renal disease, digoxin dosing must be carefully titrated based upon clinical response.

Long-term use of digoxin is indicated in many children who have been digitalized for acute heart failure, unless the cause is transient. Children with severe congenital heart disease, even after surgery, may require digoxin for prolonged periods.

It cannot be overemphasized that both the adult and pediatric dosage guidelines provided are based upon average patient response and substantial individual variation can be expected. Accordingly, ultimate dosage selection must be based upon clinical assessment of the patient.

Serum Digoxin Concentrations:

Measurement of serum digoxin concentrations can be helpful to the clinician in determining the state of digitalization and in assigning certain probabilities to the likelihood of digoxin intoxication. Studies in adults considered adequately digitalized (without evidence of toxicity) show that about two-thirds of such patients have serum digoxin levels ranging from 0.8 to 2.0 ng/ml. Patients with atrial fibrillation or atrial flutter require and appear to tolerate higher levels than do patients with other indications. On the other hand, in adult patients with clinical evidence of digoxin toxicity, about two-thirds will have serum digoxin levels greater than 2.0 ng/ml. Thus, whereas levels less than 0.8 ng/ml are infrequently associated with toxicity, levels greater than 2.0 ng/ml are often associated with toxicity. Values in between are not very helpful in deciding whether a certain sign or symptom is more likely caused by digoxin toxicity or by something else. There are rare patients who are unable to tolerate digoxin even at serum concentrations below 0.8 ng/ml. Some researchers suggest that infants and young children tolerate slightly higher serum concentrations than do adults.

To allow adequate time for equilibration of digoxin between serum and tissue, **sampling of serum concentrations for clinical use should be at least 6 to 8 hours after the last dose,** regardless of the route of administration or formulation used. On a twice daily dosing schedule, there will be only minor differences in serum digoxin concentrations whether sampling is done at 8 or 12 hours after a dose. After a single daily dose, the concentration will be 10 to 25% lower when sampled at 24 versus 8 hours, depending upon the patient's renal function. Ideally, sampling for assessment of steady-state concentrations should be done just before the next dose.

If a discrepancy exists between the reported serum concentration and the observed clinical response, the clinician should consider the following possibilities:

1. Analytical problems in the assay procedure.
2. Inappropriate serum sampling time.
3. Administration of a digitalis glycoside other than digoxin.
4. Conditions (described in WARNINGS and PRECAUTIONS sections) causing an alteration in the sensitivity of the patient to digoxin.
5. The patient falls outside the norm in his response to or handling of digoxin. This decision should only be reached after exclusion of the other possibilities and generally should be confirmed by additional correlations of clinical observations with serum digoxin concentrations.

The serum concentration data should always be interpreted in the overall clinical context and an isolated serum concentration value should not be used alone as a basis for increasing or decreasing digoxin dosage.

Adjustment of Maintenance Dose in Previously Digitalized Patients:

Maintenance doses in individual patients on steady-state digoxin can be adjusted upward or downward in proportion

---

Lanoxin

$$Maintenance\ Dose = Peak\ Body\ Stores\ (i.e.\ Loading\ Dose)\ x\ \frac{\%\ Daily\ Loss}{100}$$

$$Where:\ \%\ Daily\ Loss = 14 + Ccr/5$$

Usual Lanoxin Daily Maintenance Dose Requirements (µg)
For Estimated Peak Body Stores of 10 µg/kg

		Lean Body Weight (kg/lbs)							
		50/110	60/132	70/154	80/176	90/198	100/220		
	0	63*†	125	125	125	188††	188	22	
	10	125	125	125	188	188	188	19	
	20	125	125	188	188	188	250	16	
Corrected	30	125	188	188	188	250	250	14	Number of
Ccr	40	125	188	188	250	250	250	13	Days
(ml/min	50	188	188	250	250	250	250	12	Before
per 70 kg)	60	188	188	250	250	250	375	11	Steady-State
	70	188	250	250	250	250	375	10	Achieved
	80	188	250	250	250	375	375	9	
	90	188	250	250	250	375	500	8	
	100	250	250	250	375	375	500	7	

* 63 µg = 0.063 mg
† ½ of 125 µg tablet or 125 µg every other day
†† 1½ of 125 µg tablet.

Example —based on the above table, a patient in heart failure with an estimated lean body weight of 70 kg and a Ccr of 60 ml/min, should be given a 250 µg (0.25 mg) Lanoxin® Tablet each day, usually taken after the morning meal. Steady-state serum concentrations should not be anticipated before 11 days.

Continued on next page

Burroughs Wellcome—Cont.

to the ratio of the desired versus the measured serum concentration. For example, a patient at steady-state on 125 μg (0.125 mg) of Lanoxin Tablets per day with a measured serum concentration of 0.7 ng/ml, should have the dose increased to 250 μg (0.25 mg) per day to achieve a steady-state serum concentration of 1.4 ng/ml, **assuming the serum digoxin concentration measurement is correct, renal function remains stable during this time and the needed adjustment is not the result of a problem with compliance.**

Dosage Adjustment When Changing Preparations:
The difference in bioavailability between injectable Lanoxin or Lanoxicaps and Lanoxin Elixir Pediatric or Lanoxin Tablets must be considered when changing patients from one dosage form to another.

Lanoxin Injection and Lanoxicaps doses of 100 μg (0.1 mg) and 200 μg (0.2 mg) are approximately equivalent to 125 μg (0.125 mg) and 250 μg (0.25 mg) doses of Lanoxin Tablets and Elixir Pediatric (see table in CLINICAL PHARMACOLOGY section). Intramuscular injection of digoxin is extremely painful and offers no advantages unless other routes of administration are contraindicated.

HOW SUPPLIED

LANOXIN® (DIGOXIN) TABLETS, Scored 125 μg (0.125 mg): Bottles of 100 (NDC-0081-0242-55) and 1000 (NDC-0081-0242-75); Unit dose pack of 100 (NDC 0081-0242-56); Unit of Use bottles of 30 (NDC-0081-0242-30) **VA NSN** 6505-01-049-6807. Imprinted with LANOXIN and Y3B (yellow). Store at 15°–30°C (59°–86°F) in a dry place and protect from light.

LANOXIN (DIGOXIN) TABLETS, Scored 250 μg (0.25 mg): Bottles of 100 (NDC-0081-0249-55) **DoD DSN** 6505-00-116-7750. 1000 (NDC-0081-0249-75) **VA NSN** 6505-00-611-7898 and 5000 (NDC-0081-0249-80); Unit dose pack of 100 (10 x 10) (NDC-0081-0249-56) **DoD NSN** 6505-00-117-5689; Unit of Use bottles of 30 (NDC-0081-0249-30) **VA NSN** 6505-01-035-2104. Imprinted with LANOXIN and X3A (white). Store at 15°–30°C (59°–86°F) in a dry place.

LANOXIN (DIGOXIN) TABLETS, Scored 500 μg (0.5 mg): Bottles of 100 (NDC-0081-0253-55). Imprinted with LANOXIN and T9A (green). Store at 15°–30°C (59°–86°F) in a dry place and protect from light.

LANOXIN (DIGOXIN) INJECTION, 500 μg (0.5 mg) in 2 ml (250 μg [0.25 mg] per ml); boxes of 10 (NDC-0081-0260-10) **DoD NSN** 6505-00-531-7761 and 50 ampuls (NDC-0081-0260-35). Store at 15°–30°C (59°–86°F) and protect from light.

LANOXIN (DIGOXIN) INJECTION PEDIATRIC, 100 μg (0.1 mg) in 1 ml; box of 10 ampuls (NDC-0081-0262-10). Store at 15°–30°C (59°– 86°F) and protect from light.

LANOXIN (DIGOXIN) ELIXIR PEDIATRIC, 50 μg (0.05 mg) per ml; bottle of 60 ml with calibrated dropper (NDC-0081-0264-27) **DoD NSN** 6505-00-890-1726. Store at 15°–25°C (59°–77°F) and protect from light.

ALSO AVAILABLE

LANOXICAPS (DIGOXIN SOLUTION IN CAPSULES), 50 μg (0.05 mg) bottles of 100; 100 μg (0.1 mg) bottles of 100, Unit dose pack of 100, Unit of use bottles of 30; 200 μg (0.2 mg) bottles of 100, Unit dose pack of 100, Unit of use bottles of 30.

Tablets Shown in Product Identification Section, page 407

LEUCOVORIN CALCIUM FOR INJECTION   ℞
WELLCOVORIN® brand STERILE POWDER
25, 50 or 100 mg per vial

DESCRIPTION

Wellcovorin brand Leucovorin Calcium For Injection Sterile Powder is a sterile preparation containing leucovorin present as the calcium salt pentahydrate of N-[4-[[(2-amino-5-formyl-1, 4, 5, 6, 7, 8-hexahydro-4-oxo-6-pteridinyl)methyl] amino]benzoyl]-L-glutamic acid. Each 5 mg of leucovorin is equivalent to 5.40 mg of anhydrous leucovorin calcium. Leucovorin is a water soluble vitamin in the folate group; it is useful as an antidote to drugs which act as folic acid antagonists.

Each 25 mg, 50 mg or 100 mg vial of Wellcovorin brand Leucovorin Calcium For Injection Sterile Powder, when reconstituted with 2.5 mL, 5 mL or 10 mL, respectively, of sterile diluent, contains leucovorin (as the calcium salt) 10 mg/mL. The inactive ingredients are sodium chloride 20 mg, 40 mg or 80 mg per vial, respectively, and sodium hydroxide and/or hydrochloric acid added to adjust the pH to approximately 8.1. The dry product contains no preservative. Dilute with Bacteriostatic Water for Injection USP, which contains benzyl alcohol (see WARNINGS section), or with Sterile Water for Injection, USP.

Wellcovorin brand Leucovorin Calcium For Injection Sterile Powder, when reconstituted as directed, is suitable for IM or IV administration.

There is 0.004 mEq of calcium per mg leucovorin.

CLINICAL PHARMACOLOGY

Leucovorin is a mixture of the diastereoisomers of the 5-formyl derivative of tetrahydrofolic acid. The biologically active compound of the mixture is the (-)-L-isomer, known as Citrovorum factor or (-)-folinic acid. Leucovorin does not require reduction by the enzyme dihydrofolate reductase in order to participate in reactions utilizing folates as a source of "one-carbon" moieties. After intravenous administration of 25 mg calcium leucovorin, total reduced folate (as measured by *Lactobacillus casei* assay) reached a mean peak of 1259 ng/mL (range 897–1625).

The mean time to peak was 10 minutes. This initial rise in total reduced folate was primarily due to the parent compound 5-formyl THF (measured by S. *faecalis* assay) which rose to 1206 ng/mL at 10 minutes. A sharp drop in parent compound follows and coincides with the appearance of the metabolite (also active) 5-CH$_3$-THF which becomes the predominant circulating form of the drug. The mean peak of 5-CH$_3$-THF was 258 ng/mL occurring at 1.3 hours. The t½ was 6.2 hours for total reduced folates. After intramuscular injection of 25 mg the mean peak total THF was 436 ng/mL (range 240–725) which occurred at a mean time of 52 minutes. Similar to IV administration, the initial sharp rise was due to the parent compound (5-CHO-THF) 360 ng/mL at 28 minutes and the level of the metabolite 5-CH$_3$-THF increased subsequently over time until at 1.5 hours it represented 50% of the circulating total folate. The mean peak of 5-CH$_3$-THF was 226 ng/mL at 2.8 hours. The t½ of total reduced folate was 6.2 hours. There was no difference of statistical significance between IM and IV administration in the AUC for the total THF, 5-CHO-THF or 5-CH$_3$-THF.

INDICATIONS AND USAGE

Wellcovorin brand Leucovorin Calcium For Injection Sterile Powder is indicated (a) to diminish the toxicity and counteract the effect of inadvertently administered overdosages of folic acid antagonists and (b) in the treatment of the megaloblastic anemias due to sprue, nutritional deficiency, pregnancy, and infancy when oral therapy is not feasible.

CONTRAINDICATIONS

Leucovorin is improper therapy for pernicious anemia and other megaloblastic anemias secondary to the lack of vitamin B$_{12}$. A hematologic remission may occur while neurologic manifestations remain progressive.

WARNINGS

In the treatment of accidental overdosage of folic acid antagonists, leucovorin should be administered as promptly as possible. As the time interval between antifolate administration (e.g., methotrexate [MTX]) and leucovorin rescue increases, leucovorin's effectiveness in counteracting hematologic toxicity diminishes.

Monitoring of serum MTX concentration is essential in determining the optimal dose and duration of treatment with leucovorin which should be such that the resulting levels of tetrahydrofolate are equal to or greater than that of MTX. In determining the dose and duration of leucovorin therapy, it should be remembered that there may be a delay of MTX excretion in the presence of a third space (i.e., ascites, pleural effusion) or if renal insufficiency or inadequate hydration exists. Under such circumstances, high doses of leucovorin are recommended. These doses are higher than those recommended for oral use and must be given intravenously.

If MTX is administered intrathecally as local therapy and leucovorin is administered concurrently, the presence of tetrahydrofolate which diffuses readily into the cerebrospinal fluid may negate the antineoplastic effect of MTX.

Because of the preservative contained in Bacteriostatic Water for Injection, USP (benzyl alcohol preserved), doses greater than 10 mg/m^2 with this diluent are not recommended. If greater doses are required (see DOSAGE AND ADMINISTRATION) the desiccated powder should be reconstituted with Sterile Water for Injection, USP, and used immediately.

PRECAUTIONS

General: Following chemotherapy with folic acid antagonists, parenteral administration of leucovorin is preferable to oral dosing if there is a possibility that the patient may vomit and not absorb the leucovorin. In the presence of pernicious anemia, a hematologic remission may occur while neurologic manifestations remain progressive. Leucovorin has no effect on other established toxicities of MTX such as the nephrotoxicity resulting from drug precipitation in the kidney.

Drug Interactions: Folic acid in large amounts may counteract the antiepileptic effect of phenobarbital, phenytoin and primidone, and increase the frequency of seizures in susceptible children.

Leucovorin may enhance the toxicity of fluorouracil.

Pregnancy: Teratogenic Effects: Pregnancy Category C. Animal reproduction studies have not been conducted with leucovorin. It is also not known whether leucovorin can cause fetal harm when administered to a pregnant woman or can affect reproduction capacity. Leucovorin should be given to a pregnant woman only if clearly needed.

Nursing Mothers: It is not known whether this drug is excreted in human milk. Because many drugs are excreted in human milk, caution should be exercised when leucovorin is administered to a nursing mother.

Pediatric Use: See "Drug Interactions."

ADVERSE REACTIONS

Allergic sensitization has been reported following both oral and parenteral administration of folic acid.

OVERDOSAGE

Excessive amounts of leucovorin may nullify the chemotherapeutic effect of folic acid antagonists.

DOSAGE AND ADMINISTRATION

Inadvertent Overdosage of Antifol: As soon as possible after an inadvertent overdosage of the antifol, MTX, leucovorin should be given in a dosage regimen of 10 mg/m^2 every 6 hours IV or IM until the serum MTX levels are below 10^{-8} M. If there is adequate gastrointestinal function, doses subsequent to the initial dose may be given orally (see labeling of oral product). Concomitant hydration (3L/d) and urinary alkalinization with sodium bicarbonate should be employed. The bicarbonate dose should be adjusted to maintain a urinary pH at 7 or greater.

Serum samples should be assayed for creatinine levels and MTX levels at 24-hour intervals. If the 24-hour serum creatinine level has increased 50% over baseline or if the 24-hour MTX level is > 5 × 10^{-6} M or the 48-hour MTX level is > 9

Usual Digitalizing and Maintenance Dosages for Lanoxin® Tablets or Lanoxin® Elixir Pediatric in Children with Normal Renal Function Based on Lean Body Weight

Age	Digitalizing* Dose (μg/kg)	Daily † Oral Maintenance Dose (μg/kg)
Premature	20–30	20–30% of *oral* loading dose††
Full-Term	25–35	
1–24 Months	35–60	
2–5 Years	30–40	25–35% of *oral* loading dose††
5–10 Years	20–35	
Over 10 years	10–15	

Usual Digitalizing and Maintenance Dosages for Lanoxin® Injection or Lanoxin® Injection Pediatric in Children with Normal Renal Function Based on Lean Body Weight

Age	Digitalizing* Dose (μg/kg)	Daily † IV Maintenance Dose (μg/kg)
Premature	15–25	20–30% of the IV loading dose††
Full-Term	20–30	
1–24 Months	30–50	
2–5 Years	25–35	25–35% of the IV loading dose††
5–10 Years	15–30	
Over 10 Years	8–12	

*   IV digitalizing doses are 80% of oral digitalizing doses.
†   Divided daily dosing is recommended for children under 10 years of age.
††   Projected or actual digitalizing dose providing clinical response.

$\times 10^{-7}$ M, the doses of leucovorin should be increased to 100 mg/m^2 q 3 hours IV until the MTX level is $<10^{-8}$ M. When such doses are administered, a non-preserved diluent should be used (see WARNINGS). The rate of injection of leucovorin calcium should not exceed 17.5 mL (175 mg leucovorin) per minute.

Megaloblastic Anemia: No more than or up to 1 mg daily. There is no evidence that doses > 1 mg daily have greater efficacy than those of 1 mg; additionally, loss of folate in urine becomes roughly logarithmic as the amount administered exceeds 1 mg.

Instructions for Reconstitution: Read WARNINGS for considerations in choice of diluent. The contents of each vial should be reconstituted with Bacteriostatic Water for Injection, USP (benzyl alcohol preserved) or with Sterile Water for Injection, USP as follows:

Contents of Vial	Amount of Diluent
25 mg	2.5 mL
50 mg	5 mL
100 mg	10 mL

The resulting solution in each case contains 10 mg leucovorin per mL.

When reconstituted with Bacteriostatic Water for Injection, the resulting solution must be used within 7 days. If reconstituted with Sterile Water for Injection, use immediately and discard any unused portion.

Parenteral drug products should be inspected visually for particulate matter and discoloration prior to administration, whenever solution and container permit.

HOW SUPPLIED

25 mg/vial, Box of 1 (NDC 0081-0636-93); 50 mg/vial, Box of 1 (NDC 0081-0637-93); 100 mg/vial, Box of 1 (NDC 0081-0638-93).

Store dry powder and reconstituted solution at controlled room temperature 15° to 30°C (59° to 86°F). Protect from light.

LEUKERAN®   ℞

[lū́'kŭh-răn]
(Chlorambucil)
2 mg Sugar-coated Tablets

WARNING: Leukeran (chlorambucil) can severely suppress bone marrow function. Chlorambucil is a carcinogen in humans. Chlorambucil is probably mutagenic and teratogenic in humans. Chlorambucil produces human infertility. See "WARNINGS" and "PRECAUTIONS" sections.

DESCRIPTION

Leukeran (chlorambucil) was first synthesized by Everett et al.[1] It is a bifunctional alkylating agent of the nitrogen mustard type that has been found active against selected human neoplastic diseases. Chlorambucil is known chemically as 4-[bis(2-chlorethyl)amino]benzenebutanoic acid.

Chlorambucil hydrolyzes in water and has a pKa of 5.8.

Leukeran (chlorambucil) is available in tablet form for oral administration. Each sugar-coated tablet contains 2 mg chlorambucil and the inactive ingredients corn and wheat starch, gum acacia, lactose, magnesium stearate, polysorbate 60, sucrose, and talc.

CLINICAL PHARMACOLOGY

Chlorambucil is rapidly and completely absorbed from the gastrointestinal tract. After single oral doses of 0.6-1.2 mg/kg, peak plasma chlorambucil levels are reached within one hour and the terminal half-life of the parent drug is estimated at 1.5 hours. Chlorambucil undergoes rapid metabolism to phenylacetic acid mustard, the major metabolite, and the combined chlorambucil and phenylacetic acid mustard urinary excretion is extremely low—less than 1% in 24 hours. The peak plasma levels of chlorambucil and phenylacetic acid mustard are similar, approximating 1 μg/ml; however, the metabolite's half-life is 1.6 times greater than the parent drug.[2,3]

Chlorambucil and its metabolites are extensively bound to plasma and tissue proteins. In vitro, chlorambucil is 99% bound to plasma proteins, specifically albumin.[4] Cerebrospinal fluid levels of chlorambucil have not been determined. Evidence of human teratogenicity suggests that the drug crosses the placenta.[5,6]

Chlorambucil is extensively metabolized in the liver primarily to phenylacetic acid mustard which has antineoplastic activity.[2,3] Chlorambucil and its major metabolite spontaneously degrade in vivo forming monohydroxy and dihydroxy derivatives.[2] After a single dose of radiolabeled chlorambucil (^{14}C) approximately 15% to 60% of the radioactivity appears in the urine after 24 hours. Again, less than 1% of the urinary radioactivity is in the form of chlorambucil or phenylacetic acid mustard.[2] In summary, the pharmacokinetic data suggest that oral chlorambucil undergoes rapid gastrointestinal absorption and plasma clearance and that it is almost completely metabolized, having extremely low urinary excretion.

INDICATIONS AND USAGE

Leukeran (chlorambucil) is indicated in the treatment of chronic lymphatic (lymphocytic) leukemia, malignant lymphomas including lymphosarcoma, giant follicular lymphoma and Hodgkin's disease. It is not curative in any of these disorders but may produce clinically useful palliation.

CONTRAINDICATIONS

Chlorambucil should not be used in patients whose disease has demonstrated a prior resistance to the agent. Patients who have demonstrated hypersensitivity to chlorambucil should not be given the drug.[7] There may be cross-hypersensitivity (skin rash) between chlorambucil and other alkylating agents.[8]

WARNINGS

Because of its carcinogenic properties, chlorambucil should not be given to patients with conditions other than chronic lymphatic leukemia or malignant lymphomas. Convulsions,[9] infertility,[10] leukemia[11,12] and secondary malignancies[13] have been observed when chlorambucil was employed in the therapy of malignant and non-malignant diseases.

There are many reports of acute leukemia arising in patients with both malignant[15] and non-malignant[16] diseases following chlorambucil treatment. In many instances, these patients also received other chemotherapeutic agents or some form of radiation therapy. The quantitation of the risk of chlorambucil-induction of leukemia or carcinoma in humans is not possible. Evaluation of published reports of leukemia developing in patients who have received chlorambucil (and other alkylating agents) suggests that the risk of leukemogenesis increases with both chronicity of treatment and large cumulative doses. However, it has proved impossible to define a cumulative dose below which there is no risk of the induction of secondary malignancy. The potential benefits from chlorambucil therapy must be weighed on an individual basis against the possible risk of the induction of a secondary malignancy.

Chlorambucil has been shown to cause chromatid or chromosome damage in man.[17,18] Both reversible and permanent sterility have been observed in both sexes receiving chlorambucil.

A high incidence of sterility has been documented when chlorambucil is administered to prepubertal and pubertal males.[19] Prolonged or permanent azoospermia has also been observed in adult males.[20] While most reports of gonadal dysfunction secondary to chlorambucil have related to males, the induction of amenorrhea in females with alkylating agents is well documented and chlorambucil is capable of producing amenorrhea. Autopsy studies of the ovaries from women with malignant lymphoma treated with combination chemotherapy including chlorambucil have shown varying degrees of fibrosis, vasculitis, and depletion of primordial follicles.[21,22]

Pregnancy: "Pregnancy Category D": Chlorambucil can cause fetal harm when administered to a pregnant woman. Unilateral renal agenesis has been observed in two offspring whose mothers received chlorambucil during the first trimester.[5,6] Urogenital malformations including absence of a kidney were found in fetuses of rats given chlorambucil.[14] There are no adequate and well-controlled studies in pregnant women. If this drug is used during pregnancy, or if the patient becomes pregnant while taking this drug, the patient should be apprised of the potential hazard to the fetus. Women of childbearing potential should be advised to avoid becoming pregnant.

PRECAUTIONS

General: Many patients develop a slowly progressive lymphopenia during treatment. The lymphocyte count usually rapidly returns to normal levels upon completion of drug therapy. Most patients have some neutropenia after the third week of treatment and this may continue for up to ten days after the last dose. Subsequently, the neutrophil count usually rapidly returns to normal. Severe neutropenia appears to be related to dosage and usually occurs only in patients who have received a total dosage of 6.5 mg/kg or more in one course of therapy with continuous dosing. About one-quarter of all patients receiving the continuous-dose schedule, and one-third of those receiving this dosage in eight weeks or less may be expected to develop severe neutropenia.[23]

While it is not necessary to discontinue chlorambucil at the first evidence of a fall in neutrophil count, it must be remembered that the fall may continue for ten days after the last dose and that as the total dose approaches 6.5 mg/kg there is a risk of causing irreversible bone marrow damage. The dose of chlorambucil should be decreased if leukocyte or platelet counts fall below normal values and should be discontinued for more severe depression.

Chlorambucil should **not** be given at full dosages before four weeks after a full course of radiation therapy or chemotherapy because of the vulnerability of the bone marrow to damage under these conditions. If the pretherapy leukocyte or platelet counts are depressed from bone marrow disease process prior to institution of therapy, the treatment should be instituted at a reduced dosage.

Persistently low neutrophil and platelet counts or peripheral lymphocytosis suggest bone marrow infiltration. If confirmed by bone marrow examination, the daily dosage of chlorambucil should not exceed 0.1 mg/kg. Chlorambucil appears to be relatively free from gastrointestinal side effects or other evidence of toxicity apart from the bone marrow depressant action. In humans, single oral doses of 20 mg or more may produce nausea and vomiting.

Children with nephrotic syndrome[9] and patients receiving high pulse doses of chlorambucil[24] may have an increased risk of seizures. As with any potentially epileptogenic drug, caution should be exercised when administering chlorambucil to patients with a history of seizure disorder, head trauma or receiving other potentially epileptogenic drugs.

Information for Patients: Patients should be informed that the major toxicities of chlorambucil are related to hypersensitivity, drug fever, myelosuppression, hepatotoxicity, infertility, seizures, gastrointestinal toxicity, and secondary malignancies. Patients should never be allowed to take the drug without medical supervision and should consult their physician if they experience skin rash, bleeding, fever, jaundice, persistent cough, seizures, nausea, vomiting, amenorrhea, or unusual lumps/masses. Women of childbearing potential should be advised to avoid becoming pregnant.

Laboratory Tests: Patients must be followed carefully to avoid life-endangering damage to the bone marrow during treatment. Weekly examination of the blood should be made to determine hemoglobin levels, total and differential leukocyte counts, and quantitative platelet counts. Also, during the first 3 to 6 weeks of therapy, it is recommended that white blood cell counts be made 3 or 4 days after each of the weekly complete blood counts. Galton et al[23] have suggested that in following patients it is helpful to plot the blood counts on a chart at the same time that body weight, temperature, spleen size, etc., are recorded. It is considered dangerous to allow a patient to go more than two weeks without hematological and clinical examination during treatment.

Drug Interactions: There are no known drug/drug interactions with chlorambucil.

Carcinogenesis, Mutagenesis, Impairment of Fertility: See WARNINGS section for information on carcinogenesis, mutagenesis and impairment of fertility.

Pregnancy: Teratogenic Effects: Pregnancy Category D: See WARNINGS section.

Nursing Mothers: It is not known whether this drug is excreted in human milk. Because many drugs are excreted in human milk and because of the potential for serious adverse reactions in nursing infants from chlorambucil, a decision should be made whether to discontinue nursing or to discontinue the drug, taking into account the importance of the drug to the mother.

Pediatric Use: The safety and effectiveness in children have not been established.

ADVERSE REACTIONS

Hematologic: The most common side effect is bone marrow suppression.[25] Although bone marrow suppression frequently occurs, it is usually reversible if the chlorambucil is withdrawn early enough. However, irreversible bone marrow failure has been reported.[26,27]

Gastrointestinal: Gastrointestinal disturbances such as nausea and vomiting, diarrhea and oral ulceration occur infrequently.

CNS: Tremors, muscular twitching, confusion, agitation, ataxia, flaccid paresis and hallucinations have been reported as rare adverse experiences to chlorambucil which resolve upon discontinuation of drug. Rare, focal and/or generalized seizures have been reported to occur in both children[9,28,29] and adults[24,30–33] at both therapeutic daily doses, pulse dosing regimens and in acute overdose (see PRECAUTIONS-General).

Miscellaneous: Other reported adverse reactions include: pulmonary fibrosis, hepatotoxicity and jaundice, drug fever, skin hypersensitivity, peripheral neuropathy, interstitial pneumonia, sterile cystitis, infertility, leukemia and secondary malignancies (see WARNINGS).

OVERDOSAGE

Reversible pancytopenia was the main finding of inadvertent overdoses of chlorambucil.[34,35] Neurological toxicity ranging from agitated behavior and ataxia to multiple grand mal seizures has also occurred.[28,34] As there is no known antidote, the blood picture should be closely monitored and general supportive measures should be instituted, together with appropriate blood transfusions if necessary. Chlorambucil is not dialyzable.

Continued on next page

Burroughs Wellcome—Cont.

Oral LD_{50} single doses in mice are 123 mg/kg. In rats, a single intraperitoneal dose of 12.5 mg/kg of chlorambucil produces typical nitrogen-mustard effects; these include atrophy of the intestinal mucous membrane and lymphoid tissues, severe lymphopenia becoming maximal in four days, anemia and thrombocytopenia. After this dose, the animals begin to recover within three days and appear normal in about a week although the bone marrow may not become completely normal for about three weeks. An intraperitoneal dose of 18.5 mg/kg kills about 50% of the rats with development of convulsions. As much as 50 mg/kg has been given orally to rats as a single dose, with recovery. Such a dose causes bradycardia, excessive salivation, hematuria, convulsions, and respiratory dysfunction.

DOSAGE AND ADMINISTRATION

The usual oral dosage is 0.1 to 0.2 mg/kg body weight daily for three to six weeks as required. This usually amounts to 4 to 10 mg a day for the average patient. The entire daily dose may be given at one time. These dosages are for initiation of therapy or for short courses of treatment. The dosage must be carefully adjusted according to the response of the patient and must be reduced as soon as there is an abrupt fall in the white blood cell count. Patients with Hodgkin's disease usually require 0.2 mg/kg daily whereas patients with other lymphomas or chronic lymphocytic leukemia usually require only 0.1 mg/kg daily. When lymphocytic infiltration of the bone marrow is present, or when the bone marrow is hypoplastic, the daily dose should not exceed 0.1 mg/kg (about 6 mg for the average patient).

Alternate schedules for the treatment of chronic lymphocytic leukemia employing intermittent, bi-weekly or once monthly pulse doses of chlorambucil have been reported.[36,37] Intermittent schedules of chlorambucil begin with an initial single dose of 0.4 mg/kg. Doses are generally increased by 0.1 mg/kg until control of lymphocytosis or toxicity is observed. Subsequent doses are modified to produce mild hematologic toxicity. It is felt that the response rate of chronic lymphocytic leukemia to the bi-weekly or once monthly schedule of chlorambucil administration is similar or better to that previously reported with daily administration and that hematologic toxicity was less than or equal to that encountered in studies using daily chlorambucil.

Radiation and cytotoxic drugs render the bone marrow more vulnerable to damage and chlorambucil should be used with particular caution within four weeks of a full course of radiation therapy or chemotherapy. However, small doses of palliative radiation over isolated foci remote from the bone marrow will not usually depress the neutrophil and platelet count. In these cases chlorambucil may be given in the customary dosage.

It is presently felt that short courses of treatment are safer than continuous maintenance therapy although both methods have been effective. It must be recognized that continuous therapy may give the appearance of "maintenance" in patients who are actually in remission and have no immediate need for further drug. If maintenance dosage is used, it should not exceed 0.1 mg/kg daily and may well be as low as 0.03 mg/kg daily. A typical maintenance dose is 2 mg to 4 mg daily, or less, depending on the status of the blood counts. It may, therefore, be desirable to withdraw the drug after maximal control has been achieved since intermittent therapy reinstituted at time of relapse may be as effective as continuous treatment.

Procedures for proper handling and disposal of anti-cancer drugs should be considered. Several guidelines on this subject have been published.[38-44] There is no general agreement that all of the procedures recommended in the guidelines are necessary or appropriate.

HOW SUPPLIED

White sugar-coated tablet containing 2 mg chlorambucil; bottle of 50 (NDC-0081-0635-35).

Store at 15°–25°C (59°–77°F) in a dry place.

REFERENCES

1. Everett JL, Roberts JJ, Ross WCJ: Aryl-2-halogenoalkylamines. Part XII. Some carboxylic derivatives of NN-Di-2-chloroethylaniline. J Chem Soc 1953, 3:2386–2392.
2. Alberts DS, Chang SY, Chen H-SG, et al: Pharmacokinetics and metabolism of chlorambucil in man: A preliminary report. Cancer Treat Rev, 1979;6 (suppl):9–17.
3. McLean A, Woods RL, Catovsky D, et al: Pharmacokinetics and metabolism of chlorambucil in patients with malignant disease. Cancer Treat Rev, 1979;6(suppl):33–42.
4. Ehrsson H, Lönroth U, Wallin I, et al: Degradation of chlorambucil in aqueous solution: Influence of human albumin binding. J Pharm Pharmacol, 1981;33:313–315.
5. Shotton D, Monie IW: Possible teratogenic effect of chlorambucil on a human fetus. JAMA 1963;186:74–75.
6. Steege JF, Caldwell DS: Renal agenesis after first trimester exposure to chlorambucil. South Med J 1980;73:1414–1415.
7. Knisley RE, Settipane GA, Albala MM: Unusual reaction to chlorambucil in a patient with chronic lymphocytic leukemia. Arch Dermatol 1971;104:77–79.
8. Weiss RB, Bruno S: Hypersensitivity reactions to cancer chemotherapeutic agents. Ann Intern Med 1981; 94:66–72.
9. Williams SA, Makker SP, Grupe WE: Seizures: A significant side effect of chlorambucil therapy in children. J Pediatr 1978;93:516–518.
10. Freckman HA, Fry HL, Mendez FL, et al: Chlorambucil-prednisolone therapy for disseminated breast carcinoma. JAMA 1964;189:23–26.
11. Aymard JP, Frustin J, Witz F, et al: Acute leukemia after prolonged chlorambucil treatment for non-malignant disease: A report of a new case and literature survey. Acta Haematol 1980;63:283–285.
12. Berk PD, Goldberg JD, Silverstein MN, et al: Increased incidence of acute leukemia in polycythemia vera associated with chlorambucil therapy. N Engl J Med, 1981;304:441–447.
13. Lerner HJ: Acute myelogenous leukemia in patients receiving chlorambucil as long-term adjuvant chemotherapy for stage II breast cancer. Cancer Treat Rep 1978;62:1135–1138.
14. Monie IW: Chlorambucil-induced abnormalities of the urogenital system of rat fetuses. Anat Rec 1961;139:145–153.
15. Zarrabi MH, Grüwald HW, Rosner F: Chronic lymphocytic leukemia terminating in acute leukemia. Arch Intern Med 1977;137:1059–1064.
16. Cameron S: Chlorambucil and leukemia. N Eng J Med 1977; 296:1065.
17. Lawler SD, Lele KP: Chromosomal damage induced by chlorambucil in chronic lymphocytic leukemia. Scand J Haematol 1972;9:603–612.
18. Stevenson AC, Patel C: Effects of chlorambucil on human chromosomes. Mutat Res 1973;18:333–351.
19. Guesry P, Lenoir G, Broyer M: Gonadal effects of chlorambucil given to prepubertal and pubertal boys for nephrotic syndrome. J Pediatr 1978;92:299–303.
20. Richter P, Calamera JC, Morgenfeld MC, et al: Effect of chlorambucil on spermatogenesis in the human with malignant lymphoma. Cancer 1970;25:1026–1030.
21. Morgenfeld MC, Goldberg V, Parisier H, et al: Ovarian lesions due to cytostatic agents during the treatment of Hodgkin's disease. Surg Gynecol Obstet 1972; 134:826–828.
22. Sobrinho LG, Levine RA, DeConti RC: Amenorrhea in patients with Hodgkin's disease treated with antineoplastic agents. Am J Obstet Gynecol 1971;109:135–139.
23. Galton DAG, Israels LG, Nabarro JDN, et al: Clinical trials of p-(Di-2-chloroethylamino)-phenylbutyric acid (CB 1348) in malignant lymphoma. Br Med J 1955;2:1172–1176.
24. Ciobanu N, Runowicz C, Gucalp R, et al: Reversible central nervous system toxicity associated with high-dose chlorambucil in autologous bone marrow transplantation for ovarian cancer. Cancer Treat Rep 1987;71:1324–1325.
25. Moore GE, Bross IDJ, Ausman R, et al: Effects of chlorambucil (NSC-3088) in 374 Patients with advanced cancer. Cancer Chemother Rep 1968;52(pt 1):661–666.
26. Galton DAG, Wiltshaw E, Szur L, et al: The use of chlorambucil and steroids in the treatment of chronic lymphocytic leukemia. Br J Haematol 1961;7:73–98.
27. Rudd P, Fries JF, Epstein WV: Irreversible bone marrow failure with chlorambucil. J Rheumatol 1975;2:421–429.
28. Wolfson S, Olney MB: Accidental ingestion of a toxic dose of chlorambucil: Report of a case in a child. JAMA 1957;165:239–240.
29. Bryne TN, Moseley TAE, Finer MA: Myoclonic seizures following chlorambucil overdose. Ann Neurol 1981;9:191–194.
30. LaDelfa I, Myers BR, Hoffstein V: Chlorambucil induced myoclonic seizures in an adult. J Clin Oncol 1985;3:1691–1692.
31. Naysmith A, Robson RH: Focal fits during chlorambucil therapy. Postgrad Med J 1979;55:806–807.
32. Blank DW, Nanji AA, Schreiber DH, et al: Acute renal failure and seizures associated with chlorambucil overdose. J. Toxicol Clin Toxicol 1983;20:361–365.
33. Ammenti A, Reitter B, Muller-Wiefel DE: Chlorambucil neurotoxicity: Report of two cases. Helv Paediatr Acta 1980;35:281–287.
34. Green AA, Naiman JL: Chlorambucil poisoning. Am J Dis Child 1968;116:190–191.
35. Enck RE, Bennett JM: Inadvertent chlorambucil overdose in adults. NY State J Med 1977;77:1480–1481.
36. Knospe WH, Loeb V Jr, Huguley CM: Bi-weekly chlorambucil treatment of chronic lymphocytic leukemia. Cancer 1974;33:555–562.
37. Sawitsky A, Rai KR, Glidewell O, et al: Comparison of daily versus intermittent chlorambucil and prednisone therapy in the treatment of patients with chronic lymphocytic leukemia. Blood 1977;50:1049–1059.
38. Recommendations for the safe handling of parenteral antineoplastic drugs. US Dept of Health and Human Services publications No. (NIH) 83-2621. Government Printing Office, 1983.
39. Council on Scientific Affairs: Guidelines for handling parenteral antineoplastic drugs. AMA COUNCIL REPORT. JAMA 1985;253:1590–1592.
40. National Study Commission on Cytotoxic Exposure: Recommendations for Handling Cytotoxic Agents. (Available from L.P. Jeffrey, Director of Pharmacy Services, Rhode Island Hospital, 593 Eddy St, Providence, RI 02902.)
41. Clinical Oncological Society of Australia: Guidelines and recommendations for safe handling of antineoplastic agents. Med J Australia 1983;1:426–428.
42. Jones RB, Frank R, Mass T: Safe handling of chemotherapeutic agents: A report from the Mount Sinai Medical Center. CA-A Cancer J for Clin 1983;33:258–263.
43. American Society of Hospital Pharmacists technical assistance bulletin on handling cytotoxic drugs in hospitals. Am J Hosp Pharm 1985;42:131–137.
44. Yodaiken RE, Bennett D: OSHA work-practice guidelines for personnel dealing with cytotoxic (antineoplastic) drugs. AM J Hosp Pharm 1986;43:1193–1204.
Shown in Product Identification Section, page 407

MANTADIL® CREAM   ℞
[măn′tah-dĭl″]

DESCRIPTION

Mantadil® Cream contains the antihistamine chlorcyclizine hydrochloride 2% and the corticosteroid hydrocortisone acetate 0.5%, with methylparaben 0.25% (added as a preservative) in a vanishing cream base. The inactive ingredients are liquid and white petrolatum, emulsifying wax and purified water.

Mantadil Cream is an ANTIPRURITIC-ANTI-INFLAMMATORY-ANESTHETIC for topical administration.

Chlorcyclizine hydrochloride is known chemically as 1-[(4-chlorophenyl)phenylmethyl]-4-methylpiperazine monohydrochloride.

Hydrocortisone acetate is the acetate ester of cortisol, known chemically as 21-(acetyloxy)-11β,17-dihydroxypregn-4-ene-3,20-dione.

The pH of this product is approximately 4.5.

CLINICAL PHARMACOLOGY

Chlorcyclizine hydrochloride is an H_1 histamine-receptor antagonist that will occupy receptor sites in effector cells to the exclusion of histamine. It blocks most of the effects of histamine mediated by H_1 receptors, including contraction of smooth muscle and increased capillary permeability. Absorption of chlorcyclizine hydrochloride into the skin is rapid following topical application, whereas systemic absorption from the skin is minimal. Chlorcyclizine hydrochloride prevents local edema and provides local anesthetic and antipruritic action in the skin.

Hydrocortisone acetate administered topically suppresses most inflammatory and allergic responses in the skin. Following topical application, it is absorbed rapidly into the skin, where it reduces local heat, redness, swelling, and tenderness. A small part of the dose applied to broken skin is absorbed systemically and metabolized by the liver.

INDICATIONS AND USAGE

Mantadil Cream is indicated for the treatment of pruritic skin eruptions and other dermatoses including: eczema (allergic, nuchal and nummular); dermatitis (atopic, lichenoid and seborrheic); contact dermatitis including poison ivy, poison oak and poison sumac; localized neurodermatitis; insect bites; sunburn; intertrigo; and anogenital pruritus.

CONTRAINDICATIONS

This preparation is contraindicated in patients who are hypersensitive to any of its components; in tuberculosis of the skin, vaccinia, varicella, and herpes simplex. As with other topical products containing hydrocortisone, the cream should not be used in bacterial infections of the skin unless antibacterial therapy is concomitant.

Not for ophthalmic use.

WARNINGS

Oral chlorcyclizine is teratogenic in animals. Long-term reproduction studies of topical chlorcyclizine have not been conducted in humans.

PRECAUTIONS

General: If signs of irritation develop with use of this cream, treatment should be discontinued and appropriate therapy instituted.

Any of the side effects reported following systemic use of corticosteroids, including adrenal suppression, may also occur following their topical use, especially in infants and children. Systemic absorption of topically applied steroids will be increased if extensive body surface areas are treated or if the occlusive technique is used. Under these circumstances, suitable precautions should be taken when long-term use is anticipated, particularly in infants and children.

Carcinogenesis, Mutagenesis, Impairment of Fertility:
Oral chlorcyclizine is teratogenic in animals. Long-term reproduction studies of topical chlorcyclizine have not been conducted. It is poorly absorbed percutaneously.

Pregnancy: *Teratogenic Effects:* Pregnancy Category C. Animal reproduction studies have not been conducted with Mantadil Cream. It is also not known whether Mantadil Cream can cause fetal harm when administered to a pregnant woman or can affect reproduction capacity. Mantadil Cream should be given to a pregnant woman only if clearly needed.

Nursing Mothers: Hydrocortisone acetate appears in human milk following oral administration of the drug. Caution should be exercised when hydrocortisone acetate is administered to a nursing woman.
It is not known whether chlorcyclizine hydrochloride is excreted in human milk. Because many drugs are excreted in human milk, caution should be exercised when chlorcyclizine hydrochloride is administered to a nursing woman.

ADVERSE REACTIONS
Allergic contact dermatitis may occur with topical application of chlorcyclizine hydrochloride. Systemic side effects have been reported after topical application of antihistamines to large areas of skin.
The following local adverse reactions have been reported with topical corticosteroids, especially under occlusive dressings: irritation, folliculitis, hypertrichosis, acneiform eruptions, hypopigmentation, allergic contact dermatitis, secondary infection, skin atrophy, striae and miliaria.

OVERDOSAGE
With continued application of topical corticosteroid on large areas of damaged skin and under occlusion, there is a remote possibility that sufficient absorption could occur to produce Cushing's syndrome. This is more likely in children.
Systemic toxicity following topical application of chlorcyclizine has never been reported.
The oral LD_{50} of chlorcyclizine hydrochloride in the mouse is 300 mg/kg.
The intraperitoneal LD_{50} of hydrocortisone acetate in the mouse is 2300 mg/kg.

DOSAGE AND ADMINISTRATION
Apply to the skin two to five times daily. If the condition of the skin will permit, the cream should be well rubbed in.

HOW SUPPLIED
Mantadil Cream (Chlorcyclizine hydrochloride 2% and hydrocortisone acetate 0.5%) is available in 15 gram tubes (NDC-0081-0650-94).
Store at 15°-25°C (59°-77°F).

MAREZINE®   ℞
[mair'uh-zēn'']
(Cyclizine Lactate)
Injection
50 mg in 1 ml

DESCRIPTION
Chemically, cyclizine is N-benzhydryl-N'-methylpiperazine, and has a molecular weight of 266.4.
It is a white crystalline solid having a bitter taste, and is soluble in water and isotonic saline.
Marezine (Cyclizine Lactate) Injection is a sterile solution for INTRAMUSCULAR INJECTION ONLY.

ACTION
Marezine (Cyclizine Lactate) has antiemetic, anticholinergic and antihistaminic properties. It also reduces the sensitivity of the labyrinthine apparatus. The exact mechanism of action is unknown. In dogs the drug prevents emesis from intravenous threshold doses of apomorphine, but it is much less effective in blocking emesis from orally administered copper sulfate. These data suggest that the action is mediated through the chemoreceptive trigger zone.

INDICATIONS
For the treatment of nausea and vomiting of motion sickness when the oral route cannot be used.

CONTRAINDICATIONS
Marezine is contraindicated in individuals who have shown a previous hypersensitivity to the drug.

WARNINGS
Patients may become drowsy while taking Marezine and should be cautioned against engaging in activities requiring mental alertness, e.g., driving a car or operating heavy machinery or appliances.
Use in Children: Clinical studies establishing safety and efficacy in children have not been done; therefore, usage in this age group and nursing mothers cannot be recommended.

COMPATIBILITY TABLE
Marezine (Cyclizine Lactate) Injection

Forms a clear solution with: (i.e., can be mixed with)	Is not compatible with: (requires separate injection)
Atropine sulfate	Oxytetracycline hydrochloride
Meperidine hydrochloride (Demerol)	Chlortetracycline hydrochloride
Morphine sulfate	Penicillin
Tetracycline hydrochloride	Any solution with pH of 6.8
Streptomycin sulfate	or higher (this includes
Pyridoxine hydrochloride*	Pentothal sodium and other
Codeine phosphate and sulfate	soluble barbiturates)
Alphaprodine HCl (Nisentil)	
Scopolamine hydrobromide*	
Pantopon (Hydrochlorides of opium alkaloids)*	
Hydromorphone (Dilaudid)*	*Administer within 4–10 minutes

Use with CNS Depressants: May have additive effects with alcohol and other CNS depressants (hypnotics, sedatives, tranquilizers, antianxiety agents, etc.).

PRECAUTIONS
Because of its anticholinergic action, Marezine should be used with caution and appropriate monitoring in patients with glaucoma, obstructive disease of the gastrointestinal or genitourinary tract, and in elderly males with possible prostatic hypertrophy. Incipient glaucoma may be precipitated by anticholinergic drugs such as Marezine. The drug may have a hypotensive action. This may be confusing or dangerous in postoperative patients and should influence the decision on using the drug postoperatively.

ADVERSE REACTIONS
Urticaria, drug rash, dryness of mouth, nose and throat, drowsiness, restlessness, excitation, nervousness, insomnia, euphoria, anorexia, nausea, vomiting, diarrhea, constipation, hypotension, blurred vision, diplopia, vertigo, tinnitus, palpitation, tachycardia, urinary frequency, difficult urination, urinary retention, auditory and visual hallucinations have been reported, particularly when dosage recommendations are exceeded. Cholestatic jaundice has occurred in association with the use of Marezine. Following oral administration, a case of reversible agranulocytosis has been reported.

DOSAGE AND ADMINISTRATION
Marezine (Cyclizine Lactate) Injection is administered INTRAMUSCULARLY. The usual dose is 1 ml (50 mg) every 4 to 6 hours as necessary.

OVERDOSAGE
Symptoms of Overdosage: Moderate overdosage may cause hyperexcitability alternating with drowsiness. Massive overdosage may cause convulsions; hallucinations; respiratory paralysis.
Treatment: Appropriate supportive and symptomatic treatment. Consider dialysis.
Caution: Do not use morphine or other respiratory depressants.
[See table above].

HOW SUPPLIED
MAREZINE® (CYCLIZINE LACTATE) INJECTION
50 mg in 1 ml
Boxes of 10 ampuls (NDC-0081-0663-10)
The injection should be stored in a cold place. It may develop a slight yellow tint if stored at room temperature for several months; however, it retains full potency.
Also Available:
MAREZINE® (CYCLIZINE HYDROCHLORIDE)
50 mg Scored TABLETS
Boxes of 12
Bottles of 100

MAREZINE® Tablets
[mâr'uh-zēn'']
Antiemetic

(See PDR For Nonprescription Drugs)
Shown in Product Identification Section, page 407

MYLERAN®   ℞
[mī'lah-răn'']
(Busulfan)
2 mg Scored Tablets

WARNING
Myleran® (busulfan) is a potent drug. It should not be used unless a diagnosis of chronic myelogenous leukemia has been adequately established and the responsible physician is knowledgeable in assessing response to chemotherapy.
Myleran (busulfan) can induce severe bone marrow hypoplasia. Reduce or discontinue the dosage immediately at the first sign of any unusual depression of bone marrow function as reflected by an abnormal decrease in any of the formed elements of the blood. A bone marrow examination should be performed if the bone marrow status is uncertain.
SEE "WARNINGS" SECTION FOR INFORMATION REGARDING BUSULFAN-INDUCED LEUKEMOGENESIS IN HUMANS.

DESCRIPTION
Myleran (busulfan) is a bifunctional alkylating agent. Busulfan is known chemically as 1,4-butanediol dimethanesulfonate and has the following structural formula:
$$CH_3SO_2O(CH_2)_4OSO_2CH_3$$
Busulfan is *not* a structural analog of the nitrogen mustards. Myleran (busulfan) is available in tablet form for oral administration. Each scored tablet contains 2 mg busulfan and the inactive ingredients magnesium stearate and sodium chloride.
The activity of busulfan in chronic myelogenous leukemia was first reported by D.A.G. Galton in 1953.[1]

CLINICAL PHARMACOLOGY
No analytical method has been found which permits the quantitation of non-radiolabeled busulfan or its metabolites in biological tissues or plasma. All studies of the pharmacokinetics of busulfan in humans have employed radiolabeled drug using either sulfur-35 (labeling the "carrier" portion of the molecule) or carbon-14 or tritium in the alkane portion of the 4-carbon chain (labels in the "alkylating" portion of the molecule).
Studies with ^{35}S-busulfan.[2] Following the intravenous administration of a single therapeutic dose of ^{35}S-busulfan, there was rapid disappearance of radioactivity from the blood; 90 to 95% of the ^{35}S-label disappeared within three to five minutes after injection. Thereafter, a constant, low level of radioactivity (1 to 3% of the injected dose) was maintained during the subsequent forty-eight hour period of observation. Following the oral administration of ^{35}S-busulfan, there was a lag period of one-half to two hours prior to the detection of radioactivity in the blood. However, at four hours the (low) level of circulating radioactivity was comparable to that obtained following intravenous administration. After either oral or intravenous administration of ^{35}S-busulfan to humans, 45 to 60% of the radioactivity was recovered in the urine in the forty-eight hours after administration; the majority of the total urinary excretion occurred in the first twenty-four hours. In man, over 95% of the urinary sulfur-35 occurs as ^{35}S-methanesulfonic acid.
The fact that urinary recovery of sulfur-35 was equivalent, irrespective of whether the drug was given intravenously or orally, suggests virtually complete absorption by the oral route.
Studies with ^{14}C-busulfan.[2] Oral and intravenous administration of 1,4-^{14}C-busulfan showed the same rapid initial disappearance of plasma radioactivity with a subsequent low-level plateau as observed following the administration of ^{35}S-labeled drug. Cumulative radioactivity in the urine after forty-eight hours was 25 to 30% of the administered dose (contrasting with 45 to 60% for ^{35}S-busulfan) and suggests a slower excretion of the alkylating portion of the molecule and its metabolites than for the sulfonoxymethyl moieties. Regardless of the route of administration, 1,4-^{14}C-busulfan yielded a complex mixture of at least 12 radiolabeled metabolites in urine; the main metabolite being 3-hydroxy-tetrahydrothiophene-1, 1-dioxide.
Studies with ^{3}H-busulfan.[3] Human pharmacokinetic studies have been conducted employing busulfan labeled with

Continued on next page

Burroughs Wellcome—Cont.

tritium on the tetramethylene chain. These experiments confirmed a rapid initial clearance of the radioactivity from plasma, irrespective of whether the drug was given orally or intravenously, and showed a gradual accumulation of radioactivity in the plasma after repeated doses. Urinary excretion of less than 50% of the total dose given suggested a slow elimination of the metabolic products from the body.

There is no experience with the use of dialysis in an attempt to modify the clinical toxicity of busulfan. One technical difficulty would derive from the extremely poor water solubility of busulfan. Additionally, all studies of the metabolism of busulfan employing radiolabeled materials indicate rapid chemical reactivity of the parent compound with prolonged retention of some of the metabolites (particularly the metabolites arising from the "alkylating" portion of the molecule). The effectiveness of dialysis at removing significant quantities of unreacted drug would be expected to be minimal in such a situation.

No information is available regarding the penetration of busulfan into brain or cerebrospinal fluid.

Biochemical Pharmacology: In aqueous media, busulfan undergoes a wide range of nucleophilic substitution reactions. While this chemical reactivity is relatively non-specific, alkylation of the DNA is felt to be an important biological mechanism for its cytotoxic effect.[4] Coliphage T7 exposed to busulfan was found to have the DNA crosslinked by intrastrand crosslinkages, but no interstrand linkages were found.

The metabolic fate of busulfan has been studied in rats and humans using ^{14}C- and ^{35}S-labeled materials.[2,5,6] In man,[2] as in the rat,[6] almost all of the radioactivity in ^{35}S-labeled busulfan is excreted in the urine in the form of ^{35}S-methanesulfonic acid. No unchanged drug was found in human urine,[2] although a small amount has been reported in rat urine.[6] Roberts and Warwick demonstrated that the formation of methanesulfonic acid *in vivo* in the rat is not due to a simple hydrolysis of busulfan to 1,4-butanediol, since only about 4% of 2,3-^{14}C-busulfan was excreted as carbon dioxide whereas 2,3-^{14}C-1,4-butanediol was converted almost exclusively to carbon dioxide.[5] The predominant reaction of busulfan in the rat is the alkylation of sulfhydryl groups (particularly cysteine and cysteine-containing compounds) to produce a cyclic sulfonium compound which is the precursor of the major urinary metabolite of the 4-carbon portion of the molecule, 3-hydroxytetrahydrothiophene-1, 1-dioxide.[5] This has been termed a "sulfur-stripping" action of busulfan and it may modify the function of certain sulfur-containing amino acids, polypeptides, and proteins; whether this action makes an important contribution to the cytotoxicity of busulfan is unknown.

The biochemical basis for acquired resistance to busulfan is largely a matter of speculation. Although altered transport of busulfan into the cell is one possibility, increased intracellular inactivation of the drug before it reaches the DNA is also possible. Experiments with other alkylating agents have shown that resistance to this class of compounds may reflect an acquired ability of the resistant cell to repair alkylation damage more effectively.[4]

INDICATIONS AND USAGE

Myleran® (busulfan) is indicated for the palliative treatment of chronic myelogenous (myeloid, myelocytic, granulocytic) leukemia. Although not curative, busulfan reduces the total granulocyte mass, relieves symptoms of the disease, and improves the clinical state of the patient. Approximately 90% of adults with previously untreated chronic myelogenous leukemia will obtain hematologic remission with regression or stabilization of organomegaly following the use of busulfan. It has been shown to be superior to splenic irradiation with respect to survival times and maintenance of hemoglobin levels, and to be equivalent to irradiation at controlling splenomegaly.[7]

It is not clear whether busulfan unequivocally prolongs the survival of responding patients beyond the 31 months experienced by an untreated group of historical controls.[8] Median survival figures of 31–42 months have been reported for several groups of patients treated with busulfan, but concurrent control groups of comparable, untreated patients are not available.[7,9,10,11] The median survival figures reported from different studies will be influenced by the percentage of "poor risk" patients initially entered into the particular study. Patients who are alive two years following the diagnosis of chronic myelogenous leukemia, and who have been treated during that period with busulfan, are estimated to have a mean annual mortality rate during the second to fifth year which is approximately two-thirds that of patients who received either no treatment, conventional x-ray or ^{32}P-irradiation, or chemotherapy with minimally active drugs.[12]

Busulfan is clearly less effective in patients with chronic myelogenous leukemia who lack the Philadelphia (Ph[1]) chromosome.[13] Also, the so-called "juvenile" type of chronic myelogenous leukemia, typically occurring in young children and associated with the absence of a Philadelphia chromo-

some, responds poorly to busulfan.[14] The drug is of no benefit in patients whose chronic myelogenous leukemia has entered a "blastic" phase.

CONTRAINDICATIONS

Myleran® (busulfan) should not be used unless a diagnosis of chronic myelogenous leukemia has been adequately established and the responsible physician is knowledgeable in assessing response to chemotherapy.

Myleran should not be used in patients whose chronic myelogenous leukemia has demonstrated prior resistance to this drug.

Myleran is of no value in chronic lymphocytic leukemia, acute leukemia, or in the "blastic crisis" of chronic myelogenous leukemia.

WARNINGS

The most frequent, serious side effect of treatment with busulfan is the induction of bone marrow failure (which may or may not be anatomically hypoplastic) resulting in severe pancytopenia. The pancytopenia caused by busulfan may be more prolonged than that induced with other alkylating agents. It is generally felt that the usual cause of busulfan-induced pancytopenia is the failure to stop administration of the drug soon enough; individual idiosyncrasy to the drug does not seem to be an important factor. *Myleran should be used with extreme caution and exceptional vigilance in patients whose bone marrow reserve may have been compromised by prior irradiation or chemotherapy, or whose marrow function is recovering from previous cytotoxic therapy.* Although recovery from busulfan-induced pancytopenia may take from one month to two years, this complication is potentially reversible and the patient should be vigorously supported through any period of severe pancytopenia.[15]

A rare, important complication of busulfan therapy is the development of bronchopulmonary dysplasia with pulmonary fibrosis.[16] Symptoms have been reported to occur within eight months to ten years after initiation of therapy—the average duration of therapy being four years. The histologic findings associated with "busulfan lung" mimic those seen following pulmonary irradiation. Clinically, patients have reported the insidious onset of cough, dyspnea, and low-grade fever. Pulmonary function studies have revealed diminished diffusion capacity and decreased pulmonary compliance. It is important to exclude more common conditions (such as opportunistic infections or leukemic infiltration of the lungs) with appropriate diagnostic techniques. If measures such as sputum cultures, virologic studies, and exfoliative cytology fail to establish an etiology for the pulmonary infiltrates, lung biopsy may be necessary to establish the diagnosis. Treatment of established busulfan-induced pulmonary fibrosis is unsatisfactory; in most cases the patients have died within six months after the diagnosis was established. There is no specific therapy for this complication other than the immediate discontinuation of busulfan. The administration of corticosteroids has been suggested, but the results have not been impressive or uniformly successful.

Busulfan may cause cellular dysplasia in many organs in addition to the lung. Cytologic abnormalities characterized by giant, hyperchromatic nuclei have been reported in lymph nodes, pancreas, thyroid, adrenal glands, liver, and bone marrow. This cytologic dysplasia may be severe enough to cause difficulty in interpretation of exfoliative cytologic examinations from the lung, bladder, breast, and the uterine cervix.

In addition to the widespread epithelial dysplasia that has been observed during busulfan therapy, chromosome aberrations have been reported in cells from patients receiving busulfan.

Busulfan is mutagenic in mice and, possibly, in man.

A number of malignant tumors have been reported in patients on busulfan therapy and this drug may be a human carcinogen. Four cases of acute leukemia occurred among 243 patients treated with busulfan as adjuvant chemotherapy following surgical resection of bronchogenic carcinoma. All four cases were from a subgroup of 19 of these 243 patients who developed pancytopenia while taking busulfan five to eight years before leukemia became clinically apparent. These findings suggest that busulfan is leukemogenic, although its mode of action is uncertain.[17]

Ovarian suppression and amenorrhea with menopausal symptoms commonly occur during busulfan therapy in premenopausal patients. Busulfan interferes with spermatogenesis in experimental animals, and there have been clinical reports of sterility, azoospermia and testicular atrophy in male patients.

Pregnancy: "Pregnancy Category D." Busulfan may cause fetal harm when administered to a pregnant woman. Although there have been a number of cases reported where apparently normal children have been born after busulfan treatment during pregnancy,[18] one case has been cited where a malformed baby was delivered by a mother treated with busulfan. During the pregnancy that resulted in the malformed infant, the mother received x-ray therapy early in the first trimester, mercaptopurine until the third month,

then busulfan until delivery.[19] In pregnant rats, busulfan produces sterility in both male and female offspring due to the absence of germinal cells in testes and ovaries.[20] Germinal cell aplasia or sterility in offspring of mothers receiving busulfan during pregnancy has not been reported in humans. There are no adequate and well-controlled studies in pregnant women. If this drug is used during pregnancy, or if the patient becomes pregnant while taking this drug, the patient should be apprised of the potential hazard to the fetus. Women of childbearing potential should be advised to avoid becoming pregnant.

PRECAUTIONS

General: The most consistent, dose-related toxicity is bone marrow suppression. This may be manifest by anemia, leukopenia, thrombocytopenia, or any combination of these. It is imperative that patients be instructed to report promptly the development of fever, sore throat, signs of local infection, bleeding from any site, or symptoms suggestive of anemia. Any one of these findings may indicate busulfan toxicity; however, they may also indicate transformation of the disease to an acute "blastic" form. Since busulfan may have a delayed effect, it is important to withdraw the medication temporarily at the first sign of an abnormally large or exceptionally rapid fall in any of the formed elements of the blood. *Patients should never be allowed to take the drug without close medical supervision.*

Information for Patients: Patients beginning therapy with busulfan should be informed of the importance of having periodic blood counts and to immediately report any unusual fever or bleeding. Aside from the major toxicity of myelosuppression, patients should be instructed to report any difficulty in breathing, persistent cough or congestion. They should be told that diffuse pulmonary fibrosis is an infrequent but serious and potentially life-threatening complication of long-term bulsulfan therapy. Patients should be alerted to report any signs of abrupt weakness, unusual fatigue, anorexia, weight loss, nausea and vomiting, and melanoderma that could be associated with a syndrome resembling adrenal insufficiency. Patients should never be allowed to take the drug without medical supervision and they should be informed that other encountered toxicities to busulfan include infertility, amenorrhea, skin hyperpigmentation, drug hypersensitivity, dryness of the mucous membranes and rarely cataract formation. Women of childbearing potential should be advised to avoid becoming pregnant. The increased risk of a second malignancy should be explained to the patient.

Laboratory Tests: It is recommended that evaluation of the hemoglobin or hematocrit, total white blood cell count and differential count, and quantitative platelet count be obtained weekly while the patient is on busulfan therapy. In cases where the cause of fluctuation in the formed elements of the peripheral blood is obscure, bone marrow examination may be useful for evaluation of marrow status. A decision to increase, decrease, continue, or discontinue a given dose of busulfan must be based not only on the absolute hematologic values, but also on the rapidity with which changes are occurring. The dosage of busulfan may need to be reduced if this agent is combined with other drugs whose primary toxicity is myelosuppression. Occasional patients may be unusually sensitive to busulfan administered at standard dosage and suffer neutropenia or thrombocytopenia after a relatively short exposure to the drug. Busulfan should not be used where facilities for complete blood counts, including quantitative platelet counts, are not available at weekly (or more frequent) intervals.

Drug Interactions: There are no known drug/drug interactions with busulfan other than additive myelosuppression with other myelosuppressive drugs.

Carcinogenesis, Mutagenesis, Impairment of Fertility: See WARNINGS section.

Pregnancy: *Teratogenic effects:* Pregnancy Category D. See WARNINGS section.

Non-Teratogenic effects: There have been reports in the literature of small infants being born after the mothers received busulfan during pregnancy, in particular, during the third trimester.[21] One case was reported where an infant had mild anemia and neutropenia at birth after busulfan was administered to the mother from the eighth week of pregnancy to term.[18]

Nursing Mothers: It is not known whether this drug is excreted in human milk. Because of the potential for tumorigenicity shown for busulfan in animal and human studies, a decision should be made whether to discontinue nursing or to discontinue the drug, taking into account the importance of the drug to the mother.

ADVERSE REACTIONS

Hematological Effects: The most frequent, serious, toxic effect of busulfan is myelosuppression resulting in leukopenia, thrombocytopenia, and anemia. Myelosuppression is most frequently the result of a failure to discontinue dosage in the face of an undetected decrease in leukocyte or platelet counts.[15]

Pulmonary: Interstitial pulmonary fibrosis has been reported rarely, but it is a clinically significant adverse effect when observed and calls for immediate discontinuation of further administration of the drug. The role of corticosteroids in arresting or reversing the fibrosis has been reported to be beneficial in some cases and without effect in others.[16]

Cardiac: One case of endocardial fibrosis has been reported in a 79-year-old woman who received a total dose of 7,200 mg of busulfan over a period of nine years for the management of chronic myelogenous leukemia.[22] At autopsy, she was found to have endocardial fibrosis of the left ventricle in addition to interstitial pulmonary fibrosis.

Ocular: Busulfan is capable of inducing cataracts in rats and there have been several reports indicating that this is a rare complication in humans. In the few cases reported in humans, cataracts have occurred only after prolonged administration of busulfan.[23]

Dermatologic: Hyperpigmentation is the most common adverse skin reaction and occurs in 5–10% of patients, particularly those with a dark complexion.

Metabolic: In a few cases, a clinical syndrome closely resembling adrenal insufficiency and characterized by weakness, severe fatigue, anorexia, weight loss, nausea and vomiting, and melanoderma has developed after prolonged busulfan therapy. The symptoms have sometimes been reversible when busulfan was withdrawn. Adrenal responsiveness to exogenously administered ACTH has usually been normal. However, pituitary function testing with metyrapone revealed a blunted urinary 17-hydroxycorticosteroid excretion in two patients.[24] Following the discontinuation of busulfan (which was associated with clinical improvement), rechallenge with metyrapone revealed normal pituitary-adrenal function.

Hyperuricemia and/or hyperuricosuria are not uncommon in patients with chronic myelogenous leukemia. Additional rapid destruction of granulocytes may accompany the initiation of chemotherapy and increase the urate pool. Adverse effects can be minimized by increased hydration, urine alkalinization, and the prophylactic administration of a xanthine oxidase inhibitor such as Zyloprim® (allopurinol).

Miscellaneous: Other reported adverse reactions include: urticaria, erythema multiforme, erythema nodosum, alopecia, porphyria cutanea tarda, excessive dryness and fragility of the skin with anhidrosis, dryness of the oral mucous membranes and cheilosis, gynecomastia, cholestatic jaundice, and myasthenia gravis. Most of these are single case reports, and in many a clear cause and effect relationship with busulfan has not been demonstrated.

OVERDOSAGE

There is no known antidote to busulfan. The principal toxic effect is on the bone marrow. Survival after a single 140 mg dose has been reported in an 18 kg, 4-year-old child,[25] but hematologic toxicity is likely to be more profound with chronic overdosage. The hematologic status should be closely monitored and vigorous supportive measures instituted if necessary. Induction of vomiting or gastric lavage followed by administration of charcoal may be indicated if ingestion were recent. It is not known whether busulfan is dialyzable (see CLINICAL PHARMACOLOGY).

Oral LD_{50} single doses in mice are 120 mg/kg. Two distinct types of toxic responses are seen at median lethal doses given intraperitoneally. Within a matter of hours there are signs of stimulation of the central nervous system with convulsions and death on the first day. Mice are more sensitive to this effect than are rats. With doses at the LD_{50} there is also delayed death due to damage to the bone marrow. At three times the LD_{50}, atrophy of the mucosa of the large intestine is found after a week, whereas that of the small intestine is little affected.[26] After doses in the order of 10 times those used therapeutically were added to the diet of rats, irreversible cataracts were produced after several weeks. Small doses had no such effect.[27]

DOSAGE AND ADMINISTRATION

Busulfan is administered orally. The usual adult dose range for *remission induction* is four to eight mg, total dose, daily. Dosing on a weight basis is the same for both children and adults, approximately 60 μg per kg of body weight or 1.8 mg per square meter of body surface, daily. Since the rate of fall of the leukocyte count is dose related, daily doses exceeding four mg per day should be reserved for patients with the most compelling symptoms; the greater the total daily dose, the greater is the possibility of inducing bone marrow aplasia.

A decrease in the leukocyte count is not usually seen during the first ten to fifteen days of treatment; the leukocyte count may actually increase during this period and it should not be interpreted as resistance to the drug, nor should the dose be increased.[28] Since the leukocyte count may continue to fall for more than one month after discontinuing the drug, it is important that busulfan be discontinued *prior* to the total leukocyte count falling into the normal range. When the total leukocyte count has declined to approximately 15,000/μl, the drug should be withheld.

With a constant dose of busulfan, the total leukocyte count declines exponentially; a weekly plot of the leukocyte count on semi-logarithmic graph paper aids in predicting the time when therapy should be discontinued.[29] With the recommended dose of busulfan, a normal leukocyte count is usually achieved in twelve to twenty weeks.

During remission, the patient is examined at monthly intervals and treatment resumed with the induction dosage when the total leukocyte count reaches approximately 50,000/μl. When remission is shorter than three months, maintenance therapy of 1 to 3 mg daily may be advisable in order to keep the hematological status under control and prevent rapid relapse.

Procedures for proper handling and disposal of anti-cancer drugs should be considered. Several guidelines on this subject have been published.[30–35]

There is no general agreement that all of the procedures recommended in the guidelines are necessary or appropriate.

HOW SUPPLIED

White, scored tablets containing 2 mg busulfan, imprinted with "MYLERAN" and "K2A" on each tablet; bottle of 25 (NDC-0081-0713-25). Store at 15°–30°C (59°–86°F) in a dry place.

REFERENCES

1. Galton DAG: Myleran in chronic myeloid leukaemia. *Lancet* 1953; 1:208–213.
2. Nadkarni MV, Trams EG, Smith PK: Preliminary studies on the distribution and fate of TEM, TEPA, and Myleran in the human. *Cancer Res* 1959;19:713–718.
3. Vodopick H, Hamilton HE, Jackson HL, et al: Metabolic fate of tritiated Busulfan in man. *J Lab Clin Med* 1969;73:266–276.
4. Fox BW: Mechanism of action of methanesulfonates in Sartorelli AC, Johns DG (eds): *Antineoplastic and Immunosuppressive Agents*, Part II. Berlin, Springer-Verlag, 1975, pp 34–46.
5. Roberts JJ, Warwick GP: The mode of action of alkylating agents—III. The formation of 3-hydroxytetrahydrothiophene-1:1-dioxide from 1:4-dimethanesulphonyloxybutane (Myleran), S-β-L-alanyltetrahydrothiophenium mesylate, tetrahydrothiophene and tetrahydrothiophene-1:1-dioxide in the rat, rabbit and mouse. *Biochem Pharmacol* 1961;6:217–227.
6. Peng CT: Distribution and metabolic fate of S-35 labeled Myleran (Busulfan) in normal and tumor bearing rats. *J Pharmacol Exp Ther* 1957;120:229–238.
7. Medical research council's working party for therapeutic trials in leukaemia: Chronic granulocytic leukaemia: Comparison of radiotherapy and busulphan therapy. *Br Med J* 1968;1:201–208.
8. Minot GR, Buckman TE, Isaacs R: Chronic myelogenous leukemia: Age incidence, duration, and benefit derived from irradiation. *JAMA* 1924;82:1489–1494.
9. Haut A, Abbott WS, Wintrobe MM, et al: Busulfan in the treatment of chronic myelocytic leukemia. The effect of long term intermittent therapy. *Blood* 1961;17:1–19.
10. Monfardini S, Gee T, Fried J, et al: Survival in chronic myelogenous leukemia: Influence of treatment and extent of disease at diagnosis. *Cancer* 1973;31:492–501.
11. Conrad FG: Survival in chronic granulocytic leukemia. *Arch Intern Med* 1973;131:684–685.
12. Sokal JE: Evaluation of survival data for chronic myelocytic leukemia. *Am J Med* 1976;1:493–500.
13. Ezdinli EZ, Sokal JE, Crosswhite L, et al: Philadelphia-Chromosome-Positive and -Negative chronic myelocytic leukemia. *Ann Intern Med* 1970;72:175–182.
14. Smith KL, Johnson W: Classification of chronic myelocytic leukemia in children. *Cancer* 1974; 34:670–679.
15. Stuart JJ, Crocker DL, Roberts HR: Treatment of Busulfan-induced pancytopenia. *Arch Intern Med* 1977; 136:1181–1183.
16. Sostman HD, Matthay RA, Putman CE: Cytotoxic drug-induced lung disease. *Am J Med* 1977;62:608–615.
17. Stott H, Fox W, Girling DJ, et al: Acute leukaemia after Busulphan. *Br Med J* 1977;2:1513–1517.
18. Dugdale M, Fort AT: Busulfan treatment of leukemia during pregnancy. Case report and review of the literature. *JAMA* 1967;199:131–133.
19. Diamond I, Anderson MM, McCreadie SR: Transplacental transmission of busulfan (Myleran®) in a mother with leukemia. *Pediatrics* 1960;25:85–90.
20. Bollag W: Cytostatica in der Schwangerschaft. *Schweiz Med Wochenschr* 1954;84:393–395.
21. Boros SJ, Reynolds JW: Intrauterine growth retardation following third-trimester exposure to Busulfan. *Am J Obstet Gynecol* 1977;129:111–112.
22. Weinberger A, Pinkhas J, Sandbank U, et al: Endocardial fibrosis following Busulfan treatment. *JAMA* 1975;231:495.
23. Ravindranathan MP, Paul VJ, Kuriakose ET: Cataract after Busulphan treatment. *Br Med J* 1972;1:218–219.
24. Vivacqua RJ, Haurani FI, Erslev AJ: "Selective" pituitary insufficiency secondary to Busulfan. *Ann Intern Med* 1967;67:380–387.
25. De Oliveira HP, Cruz E, Fonseca A de S, et al: Accidental ingestion of a toxic dose of Myleran by a child. *Acta Haemat* (Basel) 1963;29:249–255.
26. Sternberg SS, Phillips FS, Scholler J: Pharmacological and pathological effects of alkylating agents. *Ann NY Acad Sci* 1958;68:811–825.
27. Solomon C, Light AE, de Beers EJ: Cataracts produced in rats by 1,4-dimethanesulfonoxybutane (Myleran). *AMA Arch Ophthal* 1955;54:850–852.
28. Stryckmans PA: Current concepts in chronic myelogenous leukemia. *Semin Hematol* 1974; 11:101–139.
29. Galton DAG: Chemotherapy of chronic myelocytic leukaemia. *Semin Hematol* 1969;6:323–343.
30. Recommendations for the Safe Handling of Parenteral Antineoplastic Drugs. NIH Publications No. 83-2621. For sale by the Superintendent of Documents, U.S. Government Printing Office, Washington, D.C. 20402.
31. AMA Council Report. Guidelines for Handling Parenteral Antineoplastics. *JAMA*, March 15, 1985.
32. National Study Commission on Cytotoxic Exposure-Recommendations for Handling Cytotoxic Agents. Available from Louis P. Jeffrey, Sc.D., Director of Pharmacy Services, Rhode Island Hospital, 593 Eddy Street, Providence, Rhode Island 02902.
33. Clinical Oncological Society of Australia. Guidelines and recommendations for safe handling of antineoplastic agents. *Med J Australia* 1:426–428, 1983.
34. Jones R.B., et al. Safe handling of chemotherapeutic agents: A Report from the Mount Sinai Medical Center. *Ca—A Cancer Journal for Clinicians* Sept/Oct, 258–263, 1983.
35. American Society of Hospital Pharmacists technical assistance bulletin on handling cytotoxic drugs in hospitals. *Am J Hosp Pharm* 42:131–137, 1985.
Shown in Product Identification Section, page 407

Professional Labeling
NEOSPORIN® CREAM   OTC
[ne″o-spor′in]
(Polymyxin B Sulfate-Neomycin Sulfate)

DESCRIPTION
Neosporin Cream (polymyxin B sulfate-neomycin sulfate) is a topical first aid antibiotic cream. Each gram contains: Aerosporin® (polymyxin B sulfate) 10,000 units and neomycin 3.5 mg.

The vehicle contains the inactive ingredients: methylparaben 0.25% (added as a preservative); emulsifying wax, mineral oil, polyoxyethylene polyoxypropylene compound, propylene glycol, purified water and white petrolatum.

INDICATIONS
First aid to help prevent infection in minor cuts, scrapes and burns.

CONTRAINDICATIONS
Not for use in the eyes or in the external ear canal if the eardrum is perforated. This product is contraindicated in those individuals who have shown hypersensitivity to any of its components.

WARNINGS
Because of the concern of nephrotoxicity and ototoxicity associated with neomycin, this combination should not be used over a wide area or for extended periods of time.

PRECAUTIONS
General: As with other antibacterial preparations, prolonged use may result in overgrowth of non-susceptible organisms, including fungi. Appropriate measures should be taken if this occurs.

Information for Patients: For external use only. Do not use in the eyes or apply over large areas of the body. In case of deep or puncture wounds, animal bites or serious burns, consult a physician. Stop use and consult a physician if the condition persists or gets worse. Do not use longer than 1 week unless directed by a physician.

ADVERSE REACTIONS
Neomycin occasionally causes skin sensitization. Ototoxicity and nephrotoxicity have also been reported (see WARNINGS section). Adverse reactions have occurred with topical use of antibiotic combinations including neomycin and polymyxin B. Exact incidence figures are not available since no denominator of treated patients is available. The reaction occurring most often is allergic sensitization. In one clinical study, using a 20% neomycin patch, neomycin-induced allergic skin reactions occurred in two of 2,175 (0.09%) individuals in the general population.[1] In another study the incidence was found to be approximately 1%.[2]

Continued on next page

Burroughs Wellcome—Cont.

DOSAGE AND ADMINISTRATION
Clean the affected area. Apply a small amount of this product (an amount equal to the surface area of the tip of a finger) on the area 1 to 3 times daily. May be covered with a sterile bandage.

HOW SUPPLIED
Tube of ½ oz; ¹⁄₃₂ oz (approx.) foil packets packed 144 per carton.
Store at 15° to 25°C (59° to 77°F).

REFERENCES
1. Leyden JJ, Kligman AM: Contact dermatitis to neomycin sulfate. *JAMA* 1979; 242:1276–1278.
2. Prystowsky SD, Allen AM, Smith RW et al: Allergic contract hypersensitivity to nickle, neomycin, ethylenediamine, and benzocaine. *Arch Dermatol* 1979; 115:959–962.
PL 2

NEOSPORIN® G.U. IRRIGANT   ℞
[ne"o-spor'in]
Sterile
(Neomycin Sulfate-Polymyxin B Sulfate
Solution for Irrigation)
NOT FOR INJECTION

DESCRIPTION
Neosporin G.U. Irrigant is a concentrated sterile antibiotic solution to be diluted for urinary bladder irrigation. Each ml contains neomycin sulfate equivalent to 40 mg neomycin base, 200,000 units polymyxin B sulfate and water for injection. The 20-ml multiple-dose vial contains, in addition to the above, 1 mg methylparaben (0.1%) added as a preservative. Neomycin sulfate, an antibiotic of the aminoglycoside group, is the sulfate salt of neomycin B and C produced by *Streptomyces fradiae*. It has a potency equivalent to not less than 600 µg of neomycin per mg.
Polymyxin B sulfate, a polypeptide antibiotic, is the sulfate salt of polymyxin B₁ and B₂ produced by the growth of *Bacillus polymyxa*. It has a potency of not less than 6,000 polymyxin B units per mg.

CLINICAL PHARMACOLOGY
After prophylactic irrigation of the intact urinary bladder, neomycin and polymyxin B are absorbed in clinically insignificant quantities. A neomycin serum level of 0.1 µg/ml was observed in three of 33 patients receiving the rinse solution. This level is well below that which has been associated with neomycin-induced toxicity.
When used topically, polymyxin B sulfate and neomycin are rarely irritating.
Microbiology: The prepared Neosporin G.U. Irrigant Sterile solution is bactericidal. The aminoglycosides act by inhibiting normal protein synthesis in susceptible microorganisms. Polymyxins increase the permeability of bacterial cell wall membranes. The solution is active *in vitro* against
Escherichia coli
Staphylococcus aureus
Haemophilus influenzae
Klebsiella and *Enterobacter* species
Neisseria species, and
Pseudomonas aeruginosa
It is not active *in vitro* against *Serratia marcescens* and streptococci.
Bacterial resistance may develop following the use of the antibiotics in the catheter-rinse solution.

INDICATIONS AND USAGE
Neosporin G.U. Irrigant is indicated for short-term use (up to 10 days) as a continuous irrigant or rinse in the urinary bladder of abacteriuric patients to help prevent bacteriuria and gram-negative rod septicemia associated with the use of indwelling catheters.
Since organisms gain entrance to the bladder by way of, through, and around the catheter, significant bacteriuria is induced by bacterial multiplication in the bladder urine, in the mucoid film often present between catheter and urethra, and in other sites. Urinary tract infection may result from the repeated presence in the urine of large numbers of pathogenic bacteria. The use of closed systems with indwelling catheters has been shown to reduce the risk of infection. A three-way closed catheter system with constant neomycin-polymyxin B bladder rinse is indicated to prevent the development of infection while using indwelling catheters.
If uropathogens are isolated, they should be identified and tested for susceptibility so that appropriate antimicrobial therapy for systemic use can be initiated.

CONTRAINDICATIONS
Hypersensitivity to neomycin, the polymyxins, or any ingredient in the solution is a contraindication to its use. A history of hypersensitivity or serious toxic reaction to an aminoglycoside may also contraindicate the use of any other

aminoglycoside because of the known cross-sensitivity of patients to drugs of this class.

WARNINGS
PROPHYLACTIC BLADDER CARE WITH NEOSPORIN G.U. IRRIGANT STERILE SHOULD NOT BE GIVEN WHERE THERE IS A POSSIBILITY OF SYSTEMIC ABSORPTION. NEOSPORIN G.U. IRRIGANT STERILE SHOULD NOT BE USED FOR IRRIGATION OTHER THAN FOR THE URINARY BLADDER. Systemic absorption after topical application of neomycin to open wounds, burns, and granulating surfaces is significant and serum concentrations comparable to and often higher than those attained following oral and parenteral therapy have been reported. Absorption of neomycin from the denuded bladder surface has been reported.
However, the likelihood of toxicity following topical irrigation of the intact urinary bladder with Neosporin G.U. Irrigant Sterile is low since no appreciable amounts of these antibiotics enter the systemic circulation by this route if irrigation does not exceed ten days.
Neosporin G.U. Irrigant is intended for continuous prophylactic irrigation of the lumen of the intact urinary bladder of patients with indwelling catheters. Patients should be under constant supervision by a physician. Irrigation should be avoided in patients with defects in the bladder mucosa or bladder wall, such as vesical rupture, or in association with operative procedures on the bladder wall, because of the risk of toxicity due to systemic absorption following diffusion into absorptive tissues and spaces. When absorbed, neomycin and polymyxin B are nephrotoxic antibiotics, and the nephrotoxic potentials are additive. In addition, both antibiotics, when absorbed, are neurotoxins: neomycin can destroy fibers of the acoustic nerve causing permanent bilateral deafness; neomycin and polymyxin B are additive in their neuromuscular blocking effects, not only in terms of potency and duration but also in terms of characteristics of the blocks produced.
Aminoglycosides, when absorbed, can cause fetal harm when administered to a pregnant woman. Aminoglycoside antibiotics cross the placenta and there have been reports of total, irreversible, bilateral, congenital deafness in children whose mothers received streptomycin during pregnancy. Although serious side effects have not been reported in the treatment of pregnant women with other aminoglycosides, the potential for harm exists. If Neosporin G.U. Irrigant Sterile is used during pregnancy, the patient should be apprised of the potential hazard to the fetus (See PRECAUTIONS).

PRECAUTIONS
General: Ototoxicity, nephrotoxicity, and neuromuscular blockade may occur if Neosporin G.U. Irrigant ingredients are systemically absorbed (See WARNINGS). Absorption of neomycin from the denuded bladder surface has been reported. Patients with impaired renal function, infants, dehydrated patients, elderly patients, and patients receiving high doses of prolonged treatment are especially at risk for the development of toxicity.
Irrigation of the bladder with Neosporin G.U. Irrigant may result in overgrowth of nonsusceptible organisms, including fungi. Appropriate measures should be taken if this occurs. The safety and effectiveness of the preparation for use in the care of patients with recent lower urinary tract surgery have not been established.
Urine specimens should be collected during prophylactic bladder care for urinalysis, culture, and susceptibility testing. Positive cultures suggest the presence of organisms which are resistant to the bladder rinse antibiotics.
Pregnancy: *Teratogenic Effects:* Pregnancy Category D. (See WARNINGS section).

ADVERSE REACTIONS
Neomycin occasionally causes skin sensitization when applied topically; however, topical application to mucus membranes rarely results in local or systemic hypersensitivity reactions.
Irritation of the urinary bladder mucosa has been reported.
Signs of ototoxicity and nephrotoxicity have been reported following parenteral use of these drugs and following the oral and topical use of neomycin (See WARNINGS).

DOSAGE AND ADMINISTRATION
This preparation is specifically designed for use with "three-way" catheters or with other catheter systems permitting **continuous** irrigation of the urinary bladder. The usual irrigation dose is one 1-ml ampul a day for up to ten days.
Using strict aseptic techniques, the contents of one 1-ml ampul of Neosporin G.U. Irrigant Sterile (Neomycin Sulfate-Polymyxin B Sulfate Solution for Irrigation) should be added to a 1,000-ml container of isotonic saline solution. This container should then be connected to the inflow lumen of the "three-way" catheter which has been inserted with full aseptic precautions; use of a sterile lubricant is recommended during insertion of the catheter. The outflow lumen should be connected, via a sterile disposable plastic tube, to a disposable plastic collection bag. Stringent procedures, such as taping the inflow and outflow junction at the catheter,

should be observed when necessary to insure the junctional integrity of the system.
For most patients, the inflow rate of the 1,000-ml saline solution of neomycin and polymyxin B should be adjusted to a slow drip to deliver about 1,000 ml every twenty-four hours. If the patient's urine output exceeds 2 liters per day, it is recommended that the inflow rate be adjusted to deliver 2,000 ml of the solution in a twenty-four hour period.
It is important that the rinse of the bladder be **continuous**; the inflow or rinse solution should not be interrupted for more than a few minutes.
Preparation of the irrigation solution should be performed with strict aseptic techniques. The prepared solution should be stored at 4°C, and should be used within 48 hours following preparation to reduce the risk of contamination with resistant microorganisms.

HOW SUPPLIED
1-ml ampuls, boxes of 10 (NDC-0081-0748-10) and 50 ampuls (NDC-0081-0748-35); 20-ml multi-dose vial (NDC-0081-0748-93).
Store at 2° to 8°C (36° to 46°F).

Professional Labeling
NEOSPORIN® OINTMENT   OTC
MAXIMUM STRENGTH NEOSPORIN® OINTMENT
[ne"ō-spor'in]
(Polymyxin B Sulfate-Bacitracin Zinc-Neomycin Sulfate)

DESCRIPTION
Neosporin Ointment (polymyxin B sulfate-bacitracin zinc-neomycin sulfate) is a topical first aid antibiotic ointment. Each gram of Neosporin Ointment contains: polymyxin B sulfate 5,000 units, bacitracin zinc 400 units and neomycin 3.5 mg in a special white petrolatum base.
Each gram of Maximum Strength Neosporin Ointment contains: polymyxin B sulfate 10,000 units, bacitracin zinc 500 units and neomycin 3.5 mg in a special white petrolatum base.

INDICATIONS
First aid to help prevent infection in minor cuts, scrapes and burns.

CONTRAINDICATIONS
Not for use in the eyes or in the external ear canal if the eardrum is perforated. This product is contraindicated in those individuals who have shown hypersensitivity to any of its components.

WARNINGS
Because of the concern of nephrotoxicity and ototoxicity associated with neomycin, this combination should not be used over a wide area or for extended periods of time.

PRECAUTIONS
General: As with other antibacterial preparations, prolonged use may result in overgrowth of non-susceptible organisms, including fungi. Appropriate measures should be taken if this occurs.
Information for Patients: For external use only. Do not use in the eyes or apply over large areas of the body. In case of deep or puncture wounds, animal bites, or serious burns, consult a physician. Stop use and consult a physician if the condition persists or gets worse. Do not use longer than 1 week unless directed by a physician.

ADVERSE REACTIONS
Neomycin occasionally causes skin sensitization. Ototoxicity and nephrotoxicity have also been reported (see WARNINGS section). Adverse reactions have occurred with topical use of antibiotic combinations including neomycin and polymyxin B. Exact incidence figures are not available since no denominator of treated patients is available. The reaction occurring most often is allergic sensitization. In one clinical study, using a 20% neomycin patch, neomycin-induced allergic skin reactions occurred in two of 2,175 (0.09%) individuals in the general population.[1] In another study the incidence was found to be approximately 1%.[2]

DOSAGE AND ADMINISTRATION
Clean the affected area. Apply a small amount of this product (an amount equal to the surface area of the tip of a finger) on the area 1 to 3 times daily. May be covered with a sterile bandage.

HOW SUPPLIED
Neosporin Ointment:
Tubes of ½ oz and 1 oz; ¹⁄₃₂ oz (approx.) foil packets packed 144 per carton.
Maximum Strength Neosporin Ointment:
Tube of ½ oz.
Store at 15° to 25°C (59° to 77°F).

REFERENCES
1. Leyden JJ, Kligman AM: Contact dermatitis to neomycin sulfate. *JAMA* 1979; 242:1276–1278.

2. Prystowsky SD, Allen AM, Smith RW, et al: Allergic contact hypersensitivity to nickle, neomycin, ethylenediamine, and benzocaine. *Arch Dermatol* 1979; 115:959–962.
PL 3

NEOSPORIN® ℞
[nē″ō-spor′in]
OPHTHALMIC OINTMENT Sterile
(Polymyxin B Sulfate-Bacitracin Zinc-Neomycin Sulfate)

DESCRIPTION

Neosporin Ophthalmic Ointment (polymyxin B sulfate-bacitracin zinc-neomycin sulfate) is a sterile antimicrobial ointment for ophthalmic use. Each gram contains: Aerosporin® (polymyxin B sulfate) 10,000 units, bacitracin zinc 400 units, neomycin sulfate equivalent to 3.5 mg neomycin base and special white petrolatum, qs.

Polymyxin B sulfate is the sulfate salt of polymyxin B_1 and B_2 which are produced by the growth of *Bacillus polymyxa* (Prazmowski) Migula (Fam. Bacillaceae). It has a potency of not less than 6,000 polymyxin B units per mg, calculated on an anhydrous basis.

Bacitracin zinc is the zinc salt of bacitracin, a mixture of related cyclic polypeptides (mainly bacitracin A) produced by the growth of an organism of the *licheniformis* group of *Bacillus subtilis* (Fam. Bacillaceae). It has a potency of not less than 40 bacitracin units per mg. The precise formula is not known.

Neomycin sulfate is the sulfate salt of neomycin B and C, which are produced by the growth of *Streptomyces fradiae* Waksman (Fam. Streptomycetaceae). It has a potency equivalent of not less than 600 μg of neomycin standard per mg, calculated on an anhydrous basis.

CLINICAL PHARMACOLOGY

A wide range of antibacterial action is provided by the overlapping spectra of polymyxin B sulfate, bacitracin and neomycin. The spectrum of action encompasses most bacterial pathogens capable of causing external infections of the eye and its adnexa.

Polymyxin B is bactericidal for a variety of gram-negative organisms. It increases the permeability of the bacterial cell membrane by interacting with the phospholipid components of the membrane.

Bacitracin is bactericidal for a variety of gram-positive and gram-negative organisms. It interferes with bacterial cell wall synthesis by inhibition of the regeneration of phospholipid receptors involved in peptidoglycan synthesis.

Neomycin is bactericidal for many gram-positive and gram-negative organisms. It is an aminoglycoside antibiotic which inhibits protein synthesis by binding with ribosomal RNA and causing misreading of the bacterial genetic code.

When used topically, polymyxin B, bacitracin and neomycin are rarely irritating, and absorption from the intact skin or mucous membrane is insignificant. The incidence of skin sensitization to this combination has been shown to be low on normal skin.[1,2] Since these antibiotics are seldom used systemically, the patient is spared sensitization to those antibiotics which might later be required systemically.

Microbiology: Polymyxin B sulfate, bacitracin zinc and neomycin sulfate together are considered active against the following microorganisms: *Staphylococcus aureus*, streptococci, including *Streptococcus pneumoniae*, *Escherichia coli*, *Haemophilus influenzae*, *Klebsiella-Enterobacter* species, *Neisseria* species and *Pseudomonas aeruginosa*. The product does not provide adequate coverage against *Serratia marcescens*.

INDICATIONS AND USAGE

Neosporin Ophthalmic Ointment is indicated in the short-term treatment of superficial external ocular infections caused by organisms susceptible to one or more of the antibiotics contained therein.

CONTRAINDICATIONS

This product is contraindicated in those individuals who have shown hypersensitivity to any of its components.

WARNINGS

The manifestations of sensitization to neomycin are usually itching, reddening and edema of the conjunctiva and eyelid. It may be manifest simply as a failure to heal. During long-term use of neomycin-containing products, periodic examination for such signs is advisable, and the patient should be told to discontinue the product if they are observed. These symptoms subside quickly on withdrawing the medication. Neomycin-containing applications should be avoided for the patient thereafter.

PRECAUTIONS

General: As with other antibiotic preparations, prolonged use may result in overgrowth of nonsusceptible organisms including fungi. Appropriate measures should be taken if this occurs.

Allergic cross-reactions may occur which could prevent the use of any or all of the following antibiotics for the treatment of future infections: kanamycin, paromomycin, streptomycin, and possibly gentamicin.

Information for Patients: If redness, irritation, swelling or pain persists or increases, discontinue use and contact your physician.

Avoid contaminating the applicator tip with material from the eye, fingers, or other source. This caution is necessary if the sterility of the ointment is to be preserved.

ADVERSE REACTIONS

Neomycin Sulfate may cause cutaneous and conjunctival sensitization. A precise incidence of hypersensitivity reactions (primarily skin rash) due to topical neomycin is not known.

DOSAGE AND ADMINISTRATION

Apply the ointment every 3 or 4 hours for 7 to 10 days, depending on the severity of the infection.

HOW SUPPLIED

Tube of $\frac{1}{8}$ oz with ophthalmic tip. (NDC 0081-0732-86)
Store at 15°–25°C (59°–77°F).
$\frac{1}{8}$ oz. × 12—DoD   NSN 6505-01-143-4644

REFERENCES

1. Leyden JJ, and Kligman AM. Contact Dermatitis to Neomycin Sulfate, *JAMA* 242 (12): 1276–1278, 1979.
2. Prystowsky SD, Allen AM, Smith RW, Nonomura JH, Odom RB, and Akers WA. Allergic Contact Hypersensitivity to Nickle, Neomycin, Ethylenediamine, and Benzocaine. *Arch Dermatol* 115: 959–962, 1979.

NEOSPORIN® OPHTHALMIC ℞
SOLUTION Sterile
[nē′ō-spor′in]
(Polymyxin B Sulfate-Neomycin Sulfate-Gramicidin)

DESCRIPTION

Neosporin Ophthalmic Solution (polymyxin B sulfate-neomycin sulfate-gramicidin) is a sterile antimicrobial solution for ophthalmic use. Each ml contains: Aerosporin® (polymyxin B sulfate) 10,000 units, neomycin sulfate equivalent to 1.75 mg neomycin base and gramicidin 0.025 mg. The vehicle contains alcohol 0.5%, thimerosal 0.001% (added as a preservative) and the inactive ingredients propylene glycol, polyoxyethylene polyoxypropylene compound, sodium chloride and water for injection.

Polymyxin B sulfate is the sulfate salt of polymyxin B_1 and B_2 which are produced by the growth of *Bacillus polymyxa* (Prazmowski) Migula (Fam. Bacillaceae). It has a potency of not less than 6,000 polymyxin B units per mg, calculated on an anhydrous basis.

Neomycin sulfate is the sulfate salt of neomycin B and C, which are produced by the growth of *Streptomyces fradiae* Waksman (Fam. Streptomycetaceae). It has a potency equivalent of not less than 600 μg of neomycin standard per mg, calculated on an anhydrous basis.

Gramicidin (also called Gramicidin D) is a mixture of three pairs of antibacterial substances (Gramicidin A, B and C) produced by the growth of *Bacillus brevis* Dubos (Fam. Bacillaceae). It has a potency of not less than 900 μg of standard gramicidin per mg.

CLINICAL PHARMACOLOGY

A wide range of antibacterial action is provided by the overlapping spectra of polymyxin B sulfate, neomycin and gramicidin. The spectrum of action encompasses most bacterial pathogens capable of causing external infections of the eye and its adnexa.

Polymyxin B is bactericidal for a variety of gram-negative organisms. It increases the permeability of the bacterial cell membrane by interacting with the phospholipid components of the membrane.

Neomycin is bactericidal for many gram-positive and gram-negative organisms. It is an aminoglycoside antibiotic which inhibits protein synthesis by binding with ribosomal RNA and causing misreading of the bacterial genetic code.

Gramicidin is bactericidal for a variety of gram-positive organisms. It increases the permeability of the bacterial cell membrane to inorganic cations by forming a network of channels through the normal lipid bilayer of the membrane.

When used topically, polymyxin B, neomycin and gramicidin are rarely irritating, and absorption from the intact skin or mucous membrane is insignificant. The incidence of skin sensitization to this combination has been shown to be low on normal skin.[1,2] Since these antibiotics are seldom used systemically, the patient is spared sensitization to those antibiotics which might later be required systemically.

Microbiology: Polymyxin B sulfate, neomycin sulfate and gramicidin together are considered active against the following microorganisms: *Staphylococcus aureus*, streptococci, including *Streptococcus pneumoniae*, *Escherichia coli*, *Haemophilus influenzae*, *Klebsiella-Enterobacter* species, *Neisseria* species and *Pseudomonas aeruginosa*. The product does not provide adequate coverage against *Serratia marcescens*.

INDICATIONS AND USAGE

Neosporin Ophthalmic Solution is indicated in the short-term treatment of superficial external ocular infections caused by organisms susceptible to one or more of the antibiotics contained therein.

CONTRAINDICATIONS

This product is contraindicated in those individuals who have shown hypersensitivity to any of its components.

WARNINGS

The manifestations of sensitization to neomycin are usually itching, reddening and edema of the conjunctiva and eyelid. It may be manifest simply as a failure to heal. During long-term use of neomycin-containing products, periodic examination for such signs is advisable, and the patient should be told to discontinue the product if they are observed. These symptoms subside quickly on withdrawing the medication. Neomycin-containing applications should be avoided for the patient thereafter.

PRECAUTIONS

General: As with other antibiotic preparations, prolonged use may result in overgrowth of nonsusceptible organisms including fungi. Appropriate measures should be taken if this occurs.

Allergic cross-reactions may occur which could prevent the use of any or all of the following antibiotics for the treatment of future infections: kanamycin, paromomycin, streptomycin, and possibly gentamicin.

Information for Patients: If redness, irritation, swelling or pain persists or increases, discontinue use and contact your physician.

Avoid contaminating the applicator tip with material from the eye, fingers, or other source. This caution is necessary if the sterility of the drops is to be preserved.

ADVERSE REACTIONS

Neomycin Sulfate may cause cutaneous and conjunctival sensitization. A precise incidence of hypersensitivity reactions (primarily skin rash) due to topical neomycin is not known.

DOSAGE AND ADMINISTRATION

The suggested dosage is one or two drops in the affected eye two to four times daily, or more frequently as required, for 7 to 10 days. In acute infections, initiate therapy with one or two drops every 15 to 30 minutes, reducing the frequency of instillation gradually as the infection is controlled.

HOW SUPPLIED

Drop Dose® of 10 ml (plastic dispenser bottle). (NDC-0081-0728-69)
Store at 15°–25°C (59°–77°F) and protect from light.
10 ml-DoD & VA   NSN 6505-01-143-4643

REFERENCES

1. Leyden JJ, and Kligman AM. Contact Dermatitis to Neomycin Sulfate. *JAMA* 242 (12): 1276–1278, 1979.
2. Prystowsky SD, Allen AM, Smith RW, Nonomura JH, Odom RB and Akers WA, Allergic Contact Hypersensitivity to Nickel, Neomycin, Ethylenediamine, and Benzocaine. *Arch Dermatol* 115: 959–962, 1979.

NIX™ ℞
[niks]
(Permethrin) 1%
Creme Rinse

DESCRIPTION

Nix™ (Permethrin) 1% Creme Rinse is a topical pediculicide and ovicide for the treatment of infestation with *Pediculus humanus* var. *capitis* (the head louse) and its nits (eggs). The product is a creme rinse, each gram containing Permethrin 10 mg (1%). Inactive ingredients are: stearalkonium chloride, hydrolyzed animal protein, cetyl alcohol, polyoxyethylene 10 cetyl ether, hydroxyethylcellulose, balsam canada, fragrance, citric acid, propylene glycol and FD&C Yellow No. 6. Also contains isopropyl alcohol 200 mg (20%) and added as preservatives, methylparaben 2 mg (0.2%), propylparaben 0.8 mg (0.08%) and imidazolidinyl urea 2 mg (0.2%). Permethrin is a mixture of the *cis* and *trans* isomers of the synthetic pyrethroid ($\pm$)-3-phenoxybenzyl 3-(2,2-dichlorovinyl)-2,2-dimethylcyclopropanecarboxylate (*cis: trans*/25:75). It is a yellow to light orange-brown low melting solid or viscous liquid. The molecular weight is 391.29.

CLINICAL PHARMACOLOGY

Permethrin is a synthetic pyrethroid, active against lice, ticks, mites, and fleas. It acts on the nerve cell membrane to disrupt the sodium channel current by which the polarization of the membrane is regulated. Delayed repolarization and paralysis of the pests are the consequences of this disturbance.

Permethrin is rapidly metabolized by ester hydrolysis to inactive metabolites which are excreted primarily in the

Continued on next page

Burroughs Wellcome—Cont.

urine. Although the amount of permethrin absorbed after a single application of the 1% Creme Rinse has not been determined precisely, preliminary data suggest it is less than 2% of the amount applied. Residual persistence of Nix is detectable on the hair for at least 10 days following a single application.

PEDICULICIDAL/OVICIDAL ACTIVITIES

In vitro data indicate that permethrin has pediculicidal and ovicidal activity against *Pediculus humanus* var. *capitis*. The high cure rate (97–99%) of Nix in patients with head lice demonstrated at 14 days following a single application is attributable to a combination of its pediculicidal and ovicidal activities and its residual persistence on the hair which may also prevent reinfestation.

INDICATIONS AND USAGE

Nix is indicated for the single-application treatment of infestation with *Pediculus humanus* var. *capitis* (the head louse) and its nits (eggs). Retreatment for recurrences is required in less than 1% of patients since the ovicidal activity may be supplemented by residual persistence in the hair. If live lice are observed after at least seven days following the initial application, a second application can be given.

CONTRAINDICATIONS

Nix is contraindicated in patients with known hypersensitivity to any of its components, to any synthetic pyrethroid or pyrethrin, or to chrysanthemums.

WARNING

If hypersensitivity to Nix occurs, discontinue use.

PRECAUTIONS

General: Head lice infestation is often accompanied by pruritus, erythema, and edema. Treatment with Nix may temporarily exacerbate these conditions.

Information for Patients: Patients with head lice should be advised that itching, redness, or swelling of the scalp may occur after application of Nix. If irritation persists, they should consult their physician. Nix is not irritating to the eyes; however, patients should be advised to avoid contact with eyes during application and to flush with water immediately if Nix gets in the eyes. In order to prevent accidental ingestion by children, the remaining contents of Nix should be discarded after use.

Removal of nits (eggs) is recommended for reasons of personal hygiene and compliance with school 'no nit' policies. The nits can be combed from the hair treated with Nix after drying.

Carcinogenesis, Mutagenesis, Impairment of Fertility: Six carcinogenicity bioassays were evaluated with permethrin, three each in rats and mice. No tumorigenicity was seen in the rat studies. However, species-specific increases in pulmonary adenomas, a common benign tumor of mice of high spontaneous background incidence, were seen in the three mouse studies. In one of these studies there was an increased incidence of pulmonary alveolar-cell carcinomas and benign liver adenomas only in female mice when permethrin was given in their food at a concentration of 5000 ppm. Mutagenicity assays, which give useful correlative data for interpreting results from carcinogenicity bioassays in rodents, were negative. Permethrin showed no evidence of mutagenic potential in a battery of *in vitro* and *in vivo* genetic toxicity studies.

Permethrin did not have any adverse effect on reproductive function at a dose of 180 mg/kg/day orally in a three-generation rat study.

Pregnancy: *Teratogenic Effects:* Pregnancy Category B: Reproduction studies have been performed in mice, rats, and rabbits (200–400 mg/kg/day orally) and have revealed no evidence of impaired fertility or harm to the fetus due to permethrin. There are, however, no adequate and well controlled studies in pregnant women. Because animal reproduction studies are not always predictive of human response, this drug should be used during pregnancy only if clearly needed.

Nursing Mothers: It is not known whether this drug is excreted in human milk. Because many drugs are excreted in human milk and because of the evidence for tumorigenic potential of permethrin in animal studies, consideration should be given to discontinuing nursing temporarily or withholding the drug while the mother is nursing.

Pediatric Use: Nix is safe and effective in children two years of age and older. Safety and effectiveness in children less than two years of age have not been established.

ADVERSE REACTIONS

The most frequent adverse reaction to Nix is pruritus. This is usually a consequence of head lice infestation itself, but may be temporarily aggravated following treatment with Nix. 5.9% of patients in clinical studies experienced mild temporary itching; 3.4% experienced mild transient burning/ stinging, tingling, numbness, or scalp discomfort; and 2.1%

experienced mild transient erythema, edema, or rash of the scalp.

OVERDOSAGE

No instance of accidental ingestion of Nix has been reported. If ingested, gastric lavage and general supportive measures should be employed.

DOSAGE AND ADMINISTRATION

Adults and Children: Nix is intended for use after the hair has been washed with shampoo, rinsed with water and towel dried. Apply a sufficient volume of Nix to saturate the hair and scalp (especially behind the ears and on nape of the neck). Nix should remain on the hair for 10 minutes before being rinsed off with water. A single treatment is sufficient to eliminate head lice infestation. Removal of nits (eggs) is recommended for reasons of personal hygiene and compliance with school 'no nit' policies. A nit comb is provided.

SHAKE WELL BEFORE USING.

HOW SUPPLIED

Nix (Permethrin) 1% (wt./wt.) Creme Rinse is supplied in plastic squeeze bottles that contain 2 fl oz weighing 56 g. (NDC 0081-0780-81)

Store at 15°–25°C (59°–77°F).

PEDIOTIC® SUSPENSION Sterile   ℞
['pēd-ē- 'ōt-ik]
(Polymyxin B Sulfate-Neomycin Sulfate-Hydrocortisone Otic Suspension)

DESCRIPTION

Pediotic (polymyxin B sulfate-neomycin sulfate-hydrocortisone Otic Suspension) is a sterile antibacterial and anti-inflammatory suspension for otic use. Each ml contains: Aerosporin® (polymyxin B sulfate) 10,000 units, neomycin sulfate equivalent to 3.5 mg neomycin base, and hydrocortisone 10 mg (1%). The vehicle contains thimerosal 0.001% (added as a preservative) and the inactive ingredients cetyl alcohol, glyceryl monostearate, mineral oil, polyoxyl 40 stearate, propylene glycol, and Water for Injection. Sulfuric acid may be added to adjust pH. Pediotic Suspension has a minimum pH of 4.1, which is less acidic than the minimum pH of 3.0 for Cortisporin® Otic Suspension.

Polymyxin B sulfate is the sulfate salt of polymyxin B_1 and B_2, which are produced by the growth of *Bacillus polymyxa* (Prazmowski) Migula (Fam. Bacillaceae). It has a potency of not less than 6,000 polymyxin B units per mg, calculated on an anhydrous basis.

Neomycin sulfate is the sulfate salt of neomycin B and C, which are produced by the growth of *Streptomyces fradiae* Waksman (Fam. Streptomycetaceae). It has a potency equivalent of not less than 600 μg of neomycin standard per mg, calculated on an anhydrous basis.

Hydrocortisone, 11B, 17, 21-trihydroxypregn-4-ene-3,20-dione, is an anti-inflammatory hormone.

CLINICAL PHARMACOLOGY

Corticoids suppress the inflammatory response to a variety of agents and they may delay healing. Since corticoids may inhibit the body's defense mechanism against infection, a concomitant antimicrobial drug may be used when this inhibition is considered to be clinically significant in a particular case.

The anti-infective components in the combination are included to provide action against specific organisms susceptible to them. Polymyxin B sulfate and neomycin sulfate together are considered active against the following microorganisms: *Staphylococcus aureus*, *Escherichia coli*, *Haemophilus influenzae*, *Klebsiella-Enterobacter* species, *Neisseria* species, and *Pseudomonas aeruginosa*. This product does not provide adequate coverage against *Serratia marcescens* and streptococci, including *Streptococcus pneumonia*.

The relative potency of corticosteroids depends on the molecular structure, concentration, and release from the vehicle.

INDICATIONS AND USAGE

For the treatment of superficial bacterial infections of the external auditory canal caused by organisms susceptible to the action of the antibiotics, and for the treatment of infections of mastoidectomy and fenestration cavities caused by organisms susceptible to the antibiotics.

CONTRAINDICATIONS

This product is contraindicated in those individuals who have shown hypersensitivity to any of its components, and in herpes simplex, vaccinia, and varicella infections.

WARNINGS

This product should be used with care in cases of perforated eardrum and in long-standing cases of chronic otitis media because of the possibility of ototoxicity.

Neomycin sulfate may cause cutaneous sensitization. A precise incidence of hypersensitivity reactions (primarily skin rash) due to topical neomycin is not known.

When using neomycin-containing products to control secondary infection in the chronic dermatoses, such as chronic otitis externa or stasis dermatitis, it should be borne in mind

that the skin in these conditions is more liable than is normal skin to become sensitized to many substances, including neomycin. The manifestation of sensitization to neomycin is usually a low-grade reddening with swelling, dry scaling and itching; it may be manifest simply as a failure to heal. Periodic examination for such signs is advisable, and the patient should be told to discontinue the product if they are observed. These symptoms regress quickly on withdrawing the medication. Neomycin-containing applications should be avoided for the patient thereafter.

PRECAUTIONS

General: As with other antibacterial preparations, prolonged use may result in overgrowth of non-susceptible organisms, including fungi.

If the infection is not improved after one week, cultures and susceptibility tests should be repeated to verify the identity of the organism and to determine whether therapy should be changed.

Treatment should not be continued for longer than ten days. Allergic cross-reactions may occur which could prevent the use of any or all of the following antibiotics for the treatment of future infections: kanamycin, paromomycin, streptomycin, and possibly gentamicin.

Information for Patients: Avoid contaminating the dropper with material from the ear, fingers, or other source. This caution is necessary if the sterility of the drops is to be preserved. If sensitization or irritation occurs, discontinue use immediately and contact your physician. Do not use in the eyes.

SHAKE WELL BEFORE USING.

Laboratory Tests: Systemic effects of excessive levels of hydrocortisone may include a reduction in the number of circulating eosinophils and a decrease in urinary excretion of 17-hydroxycorticosteroids.

Carcinogenesis, Mutagenesis, Impairment of Fertility: Long-term studies in animals (rats, rabbits, mice) showed no evidence of carcinogenicity attributable to oral administration of corticosteroids.

Pregnancy: *Teratogenic Effects:* Pregnancy Category C. Corticosteroids have been shown to be teratogenic in rabbits when applied topically at concentrations of 0.5% on days 6–18 of gestation and in mice when applied topically at a concentration of 15% on days 10–13 of gestation. There are no adequate and well-controlled studies in pregnant women. Corticosteroids should be used during pregnancy only if the potential benefit justifies the potential risk to the fetus.

Nursing Mothers: Hydrocortisone appears in human milk following oral administration of the drug. Since systemic absorption of hydrocortisone may occur when applied topically, caution should be exercised when Pediotic is used by a nursing woman.

Pediatric Use: See DOSAGE AND ADMINISTRATION.

ADVERSE REACTIONS

Neomycin occasionally causes skin sensitization. Ototoxicity and nephrotoxicity have also been reported (see WARNINGS section). Adverse reactions have occurred with topical use of antibiotic combinations including neomycin and polymyxin B. Exact incidence figures are not available since no denominator of treated patients is available. The reaction occurring most often is allergic sensitization. In one clinical study, using a 20% neomycin patch, neomycin-induced allergic skin reactions occurred in two of 2,175 (0.09%) individuals in the general population.[1] In another study, the incidence was found to be approximately 1%.[2]

The following local adverse reactions have been reported with topical corticosteroids, especially under occlusive dressings: burning, itching, irritation, dryness, folliculitis, hypertrichosis, acneiform eruptions, hypopigmentation, perioral dermatitis, allergic contact dermatitis, maceration of the skin, secondary infection, skin atrophy, striae, and miliaria. Stinging and burning have been reported rarely when this drug has gained access to the middle ear.

DOSAGE AND ADMINISTRATION

The external auditory canal should be thoroughly cleansed and dried with a sterile cotton applicator.

For adults, 4 drops of the suspension should be instilled into the affected ear 3 or 4 times daily. For infants and children, 3 drops are suggested because of the smaller capacity of the ear canal.

The patient should lie with the affected ear upward and then the drops should be instilled. This position should be maintained for 5 minutes to facilitate penetration of the drops into the ear canal. Repeat, if necessary, for the opposite ear. If preferred, a cotton wick may be inserted into the canal and then the cotton may be saturated with the suspension. This wick should be kept moist by adding further suspension every four hours. The wick should be replaced at least once every 24 hours.

SHAKE WELL BEFORE USING.

HOW SUPPLIED

Bottle of 7.5 ml with sterilized dropper. NDC 0081-0910-02.
Store at 15° to 25°C (59° to 77°F).

REFERENCES

1. Leyden JJ, Kligman AM: Contact dermatitis to neomycin sulfate. *JAMA* 1979;242:1276–1278.
2. Prystowsky SD, Allen AM, Smith RW, et al: Allergic contact hypersensitivity to nickel, neomycin, ethylenediamine, and benzocaine. *Arch Dermatol* 1979;115:959–962.

POLYMYXIN B SULFATE   ℞
AEROSPORIN® brand
Sterile Powder
Polymyxin B Sulfate for Parenteral and/or
Ophthalmic Administration

WARNING

CAUTION: WHEN THIS DRUG IS GIVEN INTRAMUSCULARLY AND/OR INTRATHECALLY, IT SHOULD BE GIVEN ONLY TO HOSPITALIZED PATIENTS, SO AS TO PROVIDE CONSTANT SUPERVISION BY A PHYSICIAN.
RENAL FUNCTION SHOULD BE CAREFULLY DETERMINED AND PATIENTS WITH RENAL DAMAGE AND NITROGEN RETENTION SHOULD HAVE REDUCED DOSAGE. PATIENTS WITH NEPHROTOXICITY DUE TO POLYMYXIN B SULFATE USUALLY SHOW ALBUMINURIA, CELLULAR CASTS, AND AZOTEMIA. DIMINISHING URINE OUTPUT AND A RISING BUN ARE INDICATIONS FOR DISCONTINUING THERAPY WITH THIS DRUG.
NEUROTOXIC REACTIONS MAY BE MANIFESTED BY IRRITABILITY, WEAKNESS, DROWSINESS, ATAXIA, PERIORAL PARESTHESIA, NUMBNESS OF THE EXTREMITIES, AND BLURRING OF VISION. THESE ARE USUALLY ASSOCIATED WITH HIGH SERUM LEVELS FOUND IN PATIENTS WITH IMPAIRED RENAL FUNCTION AND/OR NEPHROTOXICITY. THE CONCURRENT USE OF OTHER NEPHROTOXIC AND NEUROTOXIC DRUGS, PARTICULARLY KANAMYCIN, STREPTOMYCIN, CEPHALORIDINE, PAROMOMYCIN, TOBRAMYCIN, POLYMYXIN E (COLISTIN), NEOMYCIN, GENTAMICIN, AND VIOMYCIN, SHOULD BE AVOIDED.
THE NEUROTOXICITY OF POLYMYXIN B SULFATE CAN RESULT IN RESPIRATORY PARALYSIS FROM NEUROMUSCULAR BLOCKADE, ESPECIALLY WHEN THE DRUG IS GIVEN SOON AFTER ANESTHESIA AND/OR MUSCLE RELAXANTS.
USAGE IN PREGNANCY: THE SAFETY OF THIS DRUG IN HUMAN PREGNANCY HAS NOT BEEN ESTABLISHED.

DESCRIPTION

Polymyxin B sulfate is one of a group of basic polypeptide antibiotics derived from *B polymyxa* (*B aerosporous*). Aerosporin brand Polymyxin B Sulfate is in powder form suitable for preparation of sterile solutions for intramuscular, intravenous drip, intrathecal, or ophthalmic use.
In the medical literature, dosages have frequently been given in terms of equivalent weight of pure polymyxin B base. Each milligram of pure polymyxin B base is equivalent to 10,000 units of polymyxin B and each microgram of pure polymyxin B base is equivalent to 10 units of polymyxin B. Aqueous solutions of Aerosporin brand Polymyxin B Sulfate may be stored up to 12 months without significant loss of potency if kept under refrigeration. In the interest of safety, solutions for parenteral use should be stored under refrigeration and any unused portion should be discarded after 72 hours. Polymyxin B sulfate should not be stored in alkaline solutions since they are less stable.

ACTIONS

Polymyxin B sulfate has a bactericidal action against almost all gram-negative bacilli except the Proteus group. Polymyxins increase the permeability of bacterial cell wall membranes. All gram-positive bacteria, fungi, and the gram-negative cocci, *N gonorrhoeae* and *N meningitidis*, are resistant. Susceptibility plate testing: If the Kirby-Bauer method of disc susceptibility testing is used, a 300-unit polymyxin B disc should give a zone of over 11 mm when tested against a polymyxin B-susceptible bacterial strain.
Polymyxin B sulfate is not absorbed from the normal alimentary tract. Since the drug loses 50 percent of its activity in the presence of serum, active blood levels are low. Repeated injections may give a cumulative effect. Levels tend to be higher in infants and children. The drug is excreted slowly by the kidneys. Tissue diffusion is poor and the drug does not pass the blood brain barrier into the cerebrospinal fluid. In therapeutic dosage, polymyxin B sulfate causes some nephrotoxicity with tubule damage to a slight degree.

INDICATIONS

Acute Infections Caused by Susceptible Strains of *Pseudomonas aeruginosa*. Polymyxin B sulfate is a drug of choice in the treatment of infections of the urinary tract, meninges, and bloodstream caused by susceptible strains of *Ps aeruginosa*. It may also be used topically and subconjunctivally in the treatment of infections of the eye caused by susceptible strains of *Ps aeruginosa*.
It may be indicated in serious infections caused by susceptible strains of the following organisms, when less potentially toxic drugs are ineffective or contraindicated:
H influenzae, specifically meningeal infections.
Escherichia coli, specifically urinary tract infections.
Aerobacter aerogenes, specifically bacteremia.
Klebsiella pneumoniae, specifically bacteremia.
Note: In Meningeal Infections, Polymyxin B Sulfate Should Be Administered Only by the Intrathecal Route.

CONTRAINDICATIONS

This drug is contraindicated in persons with a prior history of hypersensitivity reactions to the polymyxins.

PRECAUTIONS

See "Warning" box.
Baseline renal function should be done prior to therapy, with frequent monitoring of renal function and blood levels of the drug during parenteral therapy.
Avoid concurrent use of a curariform muscle relaxant and other neurotoxic drugs (ether, tubocurarine, succinylcholine, gallamine, decamethonium and sodium citrate) which may precipitate respiratory depression. If signs of respiratory paralysis appear, respiration should be assisted as required, and the drug discontinued.
As with other antibiotics, use of this drug may result in overgrowth of nonsusceptible organisms, including fungi. If superinfection occurs, appropriate therapy should be instituted.

ADVERSE REACTIONS

See "Warning" box.
Nephrotoxic reactions: Albuminuria, cylinduria, azotemia, and rising blood levels without any increase in dosage.
Neurotoxic reactions: Facial flushing, dizziness progressing to ataxia, drowsiness, peripheral paresthesias (circumoral and stocking glove), apnea due to concurrent use of curariform muscle relaxants and other neurotoxic drugs or inadvertent overdosage, and signs of meningeal irritation with intrathecal administration, e.g., fever, headache, stiff neck and increased cell count and protein cerebrospinal fluid.
Other reactions occasionally reported: Drug fever, urticarial rash, pain (severe) at intramuscular injection sites, and thrombophlebitis at intravenous injection sites.

DOSAGE AND ADMINISTRATION

PARENTERAL:
Intravenous. Dissolve 500,000 units polymyxin B sulfate in 300-500 cc of 5 percent dextrose in water for continuous intravenous drip.
Adults and children. 15,000-25,000 units/kg body weight/day in individuals with normal kidney function. This amount should be reduced from 15,000 units/kg downward for individuals with kidney impairment. Infusions may be given every 12 hours; however, the total daily dose must not exceed 25,000 units/kg/day.
Infants. Infants with normal kidney function may receive up to 40,000 units/kg/day without adverse effects.
Intramuscular. Not recommended routinely because of severe pain at injection sites, particularly in infants and children. Dissolve 500,000 units polymyxin B sulfate in 2 cc sterile distilled water. (Water for Injection, U.S.P.) or sterile physiologic saline (Sodium Chloride Injection, U.S.P.) or 1 percent procaine hydrochloride solution.
Adults and children. 25,000-30,000 units/kg/day. This should be reduced in the presence of renal impairment. The dosage may be divided and given at either 4- or 6-hour intervals.
Infants. Infants with normal kidney function may receive up to 40,000 units/kg/day without adverse effects.
Note: Doses as high as 45,000 units/kg/day have been used in limited clinical studies in treating prematures and newborn infants for sepsis caused by *Ps aeruginosa*.
Intrathecal. A treatment of choice for *Ps aeruginosa* meningitis. Dissolve 500,000 units polymyxin B sulfate in 10 cc of sterile physiologic saline (Sodium Chloride Injection, U.S.P.) for 50,000 units per ml dosage unit.
Adults and children over 2 years of age. Dosage is 50,000 units once daily intrathecally for 3-4 days, then 50,000 units once every other day for at least 2 weeks after cultures of the cerebrospinal fluid are negative and sugar content has returned to normal.
Children under 2 years of age. 20,000 units once daily, intrathecally for 3-4 days or 25,000 units once every other day. Continue with a dose of 25,000 units once every other day for at least 2 weeks after cultures of the cerebrospinal fluid are negative and sugar content has returned to normal.
IN THE INTEREST OF SAFETY, SOLUTIONS FOR PARENTERAL USE SHOULD BE STORED UNDER REFRIGERATION, AND ANY UNUSED PORTIONS SHOULD BE DISCARDED AFTER 72 HOURS.

TOPICAL:
Ophthalmic. Dissolve 500,000 units polymyxin B sulfate in 20-50 cc sterile distilled water (Water for Injection, U.S.P.) or sterile physiologic saline (Sodium Chloride Injection, U.S.P.) for a 10,000-25,000 units per cc concentration.
For the treatment of *Ps aeruginosa* infections of the eye, a concentration of 0.1 percent to 0.25 percent (10,000 units to 25,000 units per cc) is administered 1-3 drops every hour, increasing the intervals as response indicates.
Subconjunctival injection of up to 10,000 units/day may be used for the treatment of *Ps aeruginosa* infections of the cornea and conjunctiva.
Note: Avoid total systemic and ophthalmic instillation over 25,000 units/kg/day.

HOW SUPPLIED

POLYMYXIN B SULFATE STERILE POWDER, AEROSPORIN brand, 500,000 units per vial
500,000 units per vial
Rubber-stoppered glass vial with flip-off cap, box of 1 (NDC 0081-0035-93) and tray of 10 (NDC 0081-0035-10).
Store at 15° to 30°C (59° to 86°F).
Vial—VA NSN 6505-00-913-3124

POLYSPORIN® OINTMENT
[pah "lĕ-spor 'ĭn]
First Aid Antibiotic

(See PDR For Nonprescription Drugs)

POLYSPORIN® OPHTHALMIC
[pah "lĕ-spor 'ĭn]
OINTMENT Sterile   ℞
(Polymyxin B-Bacitracin)

DESCRIPTION
Each gram contains Aerosporin® (Polymyxin B Sulfate) 10,000 units, bacitracin zinc 500 units, special white petrolatum qs.

ACTIONS
Polymyxin B attacks gram-negative bacilli, including virtually all strains of *Pseudomonas aeruginosa* and *H influenzae* species.
Bacitracin is active against most gram-positive bacilli and cocci, including hemolytic streptococci.

INDICATIONS
For the treatment of superficial ocular infections involving the conjunctiva and/or cornea caused by organisms susceptible to polymyxin B sulfate and bacitracin zinc.

CONTRAINDICATIONS
This product is contraindicated in those individuals who have shown hypersensitivity to any of its components.

WARNINGS
Ophthalmic ointments may retard corneal healing.

PRECAUTIONS
As with other antibiotic preparations, prolonged use may result in overgrowth of nonsusceptible organisms, including fungi. Appropriate measures should be taken if this occurs.

DOSAGE AND ADMINISTRATION
Apply the ointment every 3 or 4 hours, depending on the severity of the infection.

HOW SUPPLIED
Tube of 1/8 oz with ophthalmic tip. (NDC 0081-0797-86)

POLYSPORIN® POWDER
[pah "lĕ-spor 'ĭn]
First Aid Antibiotic

(See PDR For Nonprescription Drugs)

POLYSPORIN® SPRAY
[pah "lĕ-spor 'ĭn]
First Aid Antibiotic

(See PDR For Nonprescription Drugs)

PROLOPRIM®   ℞
[prō 'lah-prĭm "]
(Trimethoprim)
100 mg and 200 mg Scored Tablets

DESCRIPTION
Proloprim® (trimethoprim)* is a synthetic antibacterial, available in tablet form for oral administration. Each scored white tablet contains 100 mg trimethoprim and the inactive ingredients corn starch, lactose, magnesium stearate, and

Continued on next page

Burroughs Wellcome—Cont.

sodium starch glycolate. Each scored yellow tablet contains 200 mg trimethoprim and the inactive ingredients corn starch, D&C Yellow No. 10, magnesium stearate, and sodium starch glycolate.

Trimethoprim is 2, 4-diamino-5-(3,4,5,-trimethoxybenzyl)-pyrimidine. It is a white to light yellow, odorless, bitter compound with a molecular weight of 290.3 and the molecular formula $C_{14}H_{18}N_4O_3$.

CLINICAL PHARMACOLOGY

Trimethoprim is rapidly absorbed following oral administration. It exists in the blood as unbound, protein-bound and metabolized forms. Ten to twenty percent of trimethoprim is metabolized, primarily in the liver; the remainder is excreted unchanged in the urine. The principal metabolites of trimethoprim are the 1- and 3-oxides and the 3'- and 4'-hydroxy derivatives. The free form is considered to be the therapeutically active form. Approximately 44% of trimethoprim is bound to plasma proteins.

Mean peak plasma concentrations of approximately 1.0 mcg/ml occur 1 to 4 hours after oral administration of a single 100 mg dose. A single 200 mg dose will result in serum levels approximately twice as high. The half-life of trimethoprim ranges from 8 to 10 hours. However, patients with severely impaired renal function exhibit an increase in the half-life of trimethoprim, which requires either dosage regimen adjustment or not using the drug in such patients (see DOSAGE AND ADMINISTRATION section). During a 13-week study of trimethoprim administrered at a daily dosage of 200 mg (50 mg *q.i.d.*), the mean minimum steady-state concentration of the drug was 1.1 mcg/ml. Steady-state concentrations were achieved within two to three days of chronic administration and were maintained throughout the experimental period.

Excretion of trimethoprim is primarily by the kidneys through glomerular filtration and tubular secretion. Urine concentrations of trimethoprim are considerably higher than are the concentrations in the blood. After a single oral dose of 100 mg, urine concentrations of trimethoprim ranged from 30 to 160 mcg/ml during the 0 to 4 hour period and declined to approximately 18 to 91 mcg/ml during the 8 to 24 hour period. A 200 mg single oral dose will result in trimethoprim urine levels approximately twice as high. After oral administration, 50% to 60% of trimethoprim is excreted in the urine within 24 hours, approximately 80% of this being unmetabolized trimethoprim.

Since normal vaginal and fecal flora are the source of most pathogens causing urinary tract infections, it is relevant to consider the distribution of trimethoprim into these sites. Concentrations of trimethoprim in vaginal secretions are consistently greater than those found simultaneously in serum, being typically 1.6 times the concentrations of simultaneously obtained serum samples. Sufficient trimethoprim is excreted in the feces to markedly reduce or eliminate trimethoprim-susceptible organisms from the fecal flora. Trimethoprim also passes the placental barrier and is excreted in human milk.

Microbiology: Proloprim blocks the production of tetrahydrofolic acid from dihydrofolic acid by binding to and reversibly inhibiting the required enzyme dihydrofolate reductase. This binding is very much stronger for the bacterial enzyme than for the corresponding mammalian enzyme. Thus, Proloprim selectively interferes with bacterial biosynthesis of nucleic acids and proteins.

In vitro serial dilution tests have shown that the spectrum of antibacterial activity of Proloprim includes the common urinary tract pathogens with the exception of *Pseudomonas aeruginosa*.

The dominant non-*Enterobacteriaceae* fecal organisms, *Bacteroides* spp. and *Lactobacillus* spp., are not susceptible to trimethoprim concentrations obtained with the recommended dosage.

REPRESENTATIVE MINIMUM INHIBITORY CONCENTRATIONS FOR TRIMETHOPRIM-SUSCEPTIBLE ORGANISMS

Bacteria	Trimethoprim MIC— mcg/ml (Range)
Escherichia coli	0.05–1.5
Proteus mirabilis	0.5 –1.5
Klebsiella pneumoniae	0.5 –5.0
Enterobacter species	0.5 –5.0
Staphylococcus species, coagulase-negative	0.15–5.0

Susceptibility Testing: The recommended quantitative disc susceptibility method[1,2] may be used for estimating the susceptibility of bacteria to Proloprim. With this procedure, reports from the laboratory giving results using the 5 mcg trimethoprim disc should be interpreted according to the following criteria: Organisms producing zones of 16 mm or greater are classified as susceptible, whereas those producing zones of 11 to 15 mm are classified as having intermediate susceptibility. A report from the laboratory of "Susceptible to trimethoprim" or "Intermediate susceptibility to trimethoprim" indicates that the infection is likely to respond when, as in uncomplicated urinary tract infections, effective therapy is dependent upon the urine concentration of trimethoprim. Organisms producing zones of 10 mm or less are reported as resistant, indicating that other therapy should be selected.

Dilution methods for determining susceptibility are also used, and results are reported as the minimum drug concentration inhibiting microbial growth (MIC).[3] If the MIC is 8 mcg per ml or less, the microorganism is considered "susceptible." If the MIC is 16 mcg per ml or greater, the microorganism is considered "resistant."

INDICATIONS AND USAGE

For the treatment of initial episodes of uncomplicated urinary tract infections due to susceptible strains of the following organisms: *Escherichia coli*, *Proteus mirabilis*, *Klebsiella pneumoniae* and *Enterobacter* species and coagulase-negative *Staphylococcus* species, including *S. saprophyticus*.

Cultures and susceptibility tests should be performed to determine the susceptibility of the bacteria to trimethoprim. Therapy may be initiated prior to obtaining the results of these tests.

CONTRAINDICATIONS

Proloprim is contraindicated in individuals hypersensitive to trimethoprim and in those with documented megaloblastic anemia due to folate deficiency.

WARNINGS

Serious hypersensitivity reactions have been reported rarely in patients on trimethoprim therapy. Trimethoprim has been reported rarely to interfere with hematopoiesis, especially when administered in large doses and/or for prolonged periods.

The presence of clinical signs such as sore throat, fever, pallor or purpura may be early indications of serious blood disorders (see Chronic Overdosage).

Complete blood counts should be obtained if any of these signs are noted in a patient receiving trimethoprim and the drug discontinued if a significant reduction in the count of any formed blood element is found.

PRECAUTIONS

General: Trimethoprim should be given with caution to patients with possible folate deficiency. Folates may be administered concomitantly without interfering with the antibacterial action of trimethoprim. Trimethoprim should also be given with caution to patients with impaired renal or hepatic function (see CLINICAL PHARMACOLOGY and DOSAGE AND ADMINISTRATION).

Drug Interactions: Proloprim may inhibit the hepatic metabolism of phenytoin. Trimethoprim, given at a common clinical dosage, increased the phenytoin half-life by 51% and decreased the phenytoin metabolic clearance rate by 30%. When administering these drugs concurrently, one should be alert for possible excessive phenytoin effect.

Drug/Laboratory Test Interactions: Trimethoprim can interfere with a serum methotrexate assay as determined by the competitive binding protein technique (CBPA) when a bacterial dihydrofolate reductase is used as the binding protein. No interference occurs, however, if methotrexate is measured by a radioimmunoassay (RIA).

The presence of trimethoprim may also interfere with the Jaffé alkaline picrate reaction assay for creatinine resulting in overestimations of about 10% in the range of normal values.

Carcinogenesis, Mutagenesis, Impairment of Fertility:

Carcinogenesis: Long-term studies in animals to evaluate carcinogenic potential have not been conducted with trimethoprim.

Mutagenesis: Trimethoprim was demonstrated to be non-mutagenic in the Ames assay. In studies at two laboratories no chromosomal damage was detected in cultured Chinese hamster ovary cells at concentrations approximately 500 times human plasma levels; at concentrations approximately 1000 times human plasma levels in these same cells a low level of chromosomal damage was induced at one of the laboratories. No chromosomal abnormalities were observed in cultured human leukocytes at concentrations of trimethoprim up to 20 times human steady state plasma levels. No chromosomal effects were detected in peripheral lymphocytes of human subjects receiving 320 mg of trimethoprim in combination with up to 1600 mg of sulfamethoxazole per day for as long as 112 weeks.

Impairment of Fertility: No adverse effects on fertility or general reproductive performance were observed in rats given trimethoprim in oral dosages as high as 70 mg/kg/day for males and 14 mg/kg/day for females.

Pregnancy: *Teratogenic Effects:* Pregnancy Category C. Trimethoprim has been shown to be teratogenic in the rat when given in doses 40 times the human dose. In some rabbit studies, an overall increase in fetal loss (dead and resorbed and malformed conceptuses) was associated with doses 6 times the human therapeutic dose.

While there are no large well-controlled studies on the use of trimethoprim in pregnant women, Brumfitt and Pursell,[4] in a retrospective study, reported the outcome of 186 pregnancies during which the mother received either placebo or trimethoprim in combination with sulfamethoxazole. The incidence of congenital abnormalities was 4.5% (3 of 66) in those who received placebo and 3.3% (4 of 120) in those receiving trimethoprim and sulfamethoxazole. There were no abnormalities in the 10 children whose mothers received the drug during the first trimester. In a separate survey, Brumfitt and Pursell also found no congenital abnormalities in 35 children whose mothers had received trimethoprim and sulfamethoxazole at the time of conception or shortly thereafter.

Because trimethoprim may interfere with folic acid metabolism, Proloprim should be used during pregnancy only if the potential benefit justifies the potential risk to the fetus.

Nonteratogenic Effects: The oral administration of trimethoprim to rats at a dose of 70 mg/kg/day commencing with the last third of gestation and continuing through parturition and lactation caused no deleterious effects on gestation or pup growth and survival.

Nursing Mothers: Trimethoprim is excreted in human milk. Because trimethoprim may interfere with folic acid metabolism, caution should be exercised when Proloprim is administered to a nursing mother.

Pediatric Use: The safety of trimethoprim in infants under two months has not been demonstrated. The effectiveness of trimethoprim as a single agent has not been established in children under 12 years of age.

ADVERSE REACTIONS

The adverse effects encountered most often with trimethoprim were rash and pruritus.

Dermatologic: Rash, pruritus and phototoxic skin eruptions. At the recommended dosage regimens of 100 mg *b.i.d.*, or 200 mg *q.d.*, each for 10 days, the incidence of rash is 2.9% to 6.7%. In clinical studies which employed high doses of Proloprim, an elevated incidence of rash was noted. These rashes were maculopapular, morbilliform, pruritic and generally mild to moderate, appearing 7 to 14 days after the initiation of therapy.

Hypersensitivity: Rare reports of exfoliative dermatitis, erythema multiforme, Stevens-Johnson syndrome, Lyell syndrome and anaphylaxis have been received.

Gastrointestinal: Epigastric distress, nausea, vomiting, and glossitis. Elevation of serum transminase and bilirubin has been noted, but the significance of this finding is unknown. Cholestatic jaundice has been rarely reported.

Hematologic: Thrombocytopenia, leukopenia, neutropenia, megaloblastic anemia, and methemoglobinemia.

Miscellaneous: Fever, and increases in BUN and serum creatinine levels.

OVERDOSAGE

Acute: Signs of acute overdosage with trimethoprim may appear following ingestion of 1 gram or more of the drug and include nausea, vomiting, dizziness, headaches, mental depression, confusion and bone marrow depression (see Chronic Overdosage).

Treatment consists of gastric lavage and general supportive measures. Acidification of the urine will increase renal elimination of trimethoprim. Peritoneal dialysis is not effective and hemodialysis only moderately effective in eliminating the drug.

Chronic: Use of trimethoprim at high doses and/or for extended periods of time may cause bone marrow depression manifested as thrombocytopenia, leukopenia and/or megaloblastic anemia. If signs of bone marrow depression occur, trimethoprim should be discontinued and the patient should be given leucovorin; 5 to 15 mg leucovorin daily has been recommended by some investigatiors.

DOSAGE AND ADMINISTRATION

The usual oral adult dosage is 100 mg of Proloprim every 12 hours or 200 mg Proloprim every 24 hours, each for 10 days. The use of trimethoprim in patients with a creatinine clearance of less than 15 ml/min is not recommended. For patients with a creatinine clearance of 15 to 30 ml/min, the dose should be 50 mg every 12 hours.

The effectiveness of trimethoprim has not been established in children under 12 years of age.

HOW SUPPLIED

100 mg Tablets (white, scored, round-shaped), containing 100 mg trimethoprim—bottle of 100 (NDC 0081-0820-55). Imprint on tablets "PROLOPRIM 09A." Store at 15°-30°C (59°-86°F) in a dry place. 200 mg Tablets (yellow, scored, round-shaped), containing 200 mg trimethoprim—bottle of 100 (NDC 0081-0825-55). Imprint on tablets "PROLOPRIM 200." Store at 15°-30°C (59°-86°F) in a dry place and protect from light.

REFERENCES

1. Bauer AW, Kirby WMM, Sherris JC, Turck M: Antibiotic Susceptibility Testing by Standardized Single Disk Method. *Am J Clin Path* 45: 493–496, 1966.

2. Approved Standard ASM-2 Performance Standards for Antimicrobial Disc Susceptibility Test: National Committee for Clinical Laboratory Standards, 771 East Lancaster Avenue, Villanova, Pennsylvania 19085.

3. Ericsson HM and Sherris JC: Antibiotic Sensitivity Testing. Report of an International Collaborative Study. *Acta Pathol Microbiol Scand* [B] (Suppl. 217): 1–90, 1971.

4. Brumfitt W and Pursell R: Trimethoprim/Sulfamethoxazole in the Treatment of Bacteriuria in Women. *J Infect Dis* 128 (Suppl): S657–S663, November 1973.

*Mfd. under U.S. Pat. #3,956,327.

Shown in Product Identification Section, page 407

PURINETHOL®   ℞

[*pur'in-thawl'*]
(Mercaptopurine)
50 mg Scored Tablets

Caution: Purinethol (mercaptopurine) is a potent drug. It should not be used unless a diagnosis of acute lymphatic leukemia has been adequately established and the responsible physician is knowledgeable in assessing response to chemotherapy.

DESCRIPTION

Purinethol (mercaptopurine) was synthesized and developed by Hitchings, Elion, and associates at the Wellcome Research Laboratories.[1] It is one of a large series of purine analogues which interfere with nucleic acid biosynthesis and has been found active against human leukemias.

Mercaptopurine, known chemically as 1,7-dihydro-6H-purine-6-thione monohydrate, is an analogue of the purine bases adenine and hypoxanthine.

Purinethol (mercaptopurine) is available in tablet form for oral administration. Each scored tablet contains 50 mg mercaptopurine and the inactive ingredients corn and potato starch, lactose, magnesium stearate, and stearic acid.

CLINICAL PHARMACOLOGY

Clinical studies have shown that the absorption of an oral dose of mercaptopurine in man is incomplete and variable, averaging approximately 50% of the administered dose.[2] The factors influencing absorption are unknown. Intravenous administration of an investigational preparation of mercaptopurine revealed a plasma half-disappearance time of 21 minutes in children and 47 minutes in adults. The volume of distribution usually exceeded that of the total body water.[2]

Following the oral administration of ^{35}S-6-mercaptopurine in one subject, a total of 46% of the dose could be accounted for in the urine (as parent drug and metabolites) in the first 24 hours. Metabolites of mercaptopurine were found in urine within the first 2 hours after administration. Radioactivity (in the form of sulfate) could be found in the urine for weeks afterwards.[3]

There is negligible entry of mercaptopurine into cerebrospinal fluid.

Plasma protein binding averages 19% over the concentration range 10 to 50 micrograms per milliliter (a concentration only achieved by intravenous administration of mercaptopurine at doses exceeding 5 to 10 mg/kg).[2]

Monitoring of plasma levels of mercaptopurine during therapy is of questionable value.[3] There is technical difficulty in determining plasma concentrations which are seldom greater than 1 to 2 micrograms per ml after a therapeutic oral dose. More significantly, mercaptopurine enters rapidly into the anabolic and catabolic pathways for purines, and the active intracellular metabolites have appreciably longer half-lives than the parent drug. The biochemical effects of a single dose of mercaptopurine are evident long after the parent drug has disappeared from plasma. Because of this rapid metabolism of mercaptopurine to active intracellular derivatives, hemodialysis would not be expected to appreciably reduce toxicity of the drug. There is no known pharmacologic antagonist to the biochemical actions of mercaptopurine *in vivo*.

Mercaptopurine competes with hypoxanthine and guanine for the enzyme hypoxanthine-guanine phosphoribosyltransferase (HGPRTase) and is itself converted to thioinosinic acid (TIMP). This intracellular nucleotide inhibits several reactions involving inosinic acid (IMP), including the conversion of IMP to xanthylic acid (XMP) and the conversion of IMP to adenylic acid (AMP) via adenylosuccinate (SAMP). In addition, 6-methylthioinosinate (MTIMP) is formed by the methylation of TIMP. Both TIMP and MTIMP have been reported to inhibit glutamine-5-phosphoribosylpyrophosphate amidotransferase, the first enzyme unique to the *de novo* pathway for purine ribonucleotide synthesis.[3]

Experiments indicate that radiolabeled mercaptopurine may be recovered from the DNA in the form of deoxythioguanosine.[4] Some mercaptopurine is converted to nucleotide derivatives of 6-thioguanine (6-TG) by the sequential actions of inosinate (IMP) dehydrogenase and xanthylate (XMP) aminase, converting TIMP to thioguanylic acid (TGMP).

Animal tumors that are resistant to mercaptopurine often have lost the ability to convert mercaptopurine to TIMP. However, it is clear that resistance to mercaptopurine may be acquired by other means as well, particularly in human leukemias.

It is not known exactly which of any one or more of the biochemical effects of mercaptopurine and its metabolites are directly or predominantly responsible for cell death.[5]

The catabolism of mercaptopurine and its metabolites is complex. In man, after oral administration of ^{35}S-6-mercaptopurine, urine contains intact mercaptopurine, thiouric acid (formed by direct oxidation by xanthine oxidase, probably via 6-mercapto-8-hydroxypurine), and a number of 6-methylated thiopurines. The methylthiopurines yield appreciable amounts of inorganic sulfate.[3] The importance of the metabolism by xanthine oxidase relates to the fact that Zyloprim® (allopurinol) inhibits this enzyme and retards the catabolism of mercaptopurine and its active metabolites. A significant reduction in mercaptopurine dosage is mandatory if a potent xanthine oxidase inhibitor and Purinethol (mercaptopurine) are used simultaneously in a patient (see "PRECAUTIONS").

INDICATIONS AND USAGE

Purinethol (mercaptopurine) is indicated for remission induction and maintenance therapy of acute lymphatic leukemia. The response to this agent depends upon the particular subclassification of acute lymphatic leukemia and the age of the patient (child or adult).

Acute Lymphatic (Lymphocytic, Lymphoblastic) Leukemia: Given as a single agent for remission induction, mercaptopurine induces complete remission in approximately 25% of children and 10% of adults. However, reliance upon mercaptopurine alone is not justified for initial remission induction of acute lymphatic leukemia since combination chemotherapy with vincristine, prednisone, and L-asparaginase results in more frequent complete remission induction than with mercaptopurine alone or in combination. The duration of complete remission induced in acute lymphatic leukemia is so brief without the use of maintenance therapy that some form of drug therapy is considered essential. Mercaptopurine, as a single agent, is capable of significantly prolonging complete remission duration; however, combination therapy has produced remission duration longer than that achieved with mercaptopurine alone.

Acute Myelogenous (and Acute Myelomonocytic) Leukemia: As a single agent, mercaptopurine will induce complete remission in approximately 10% of children and adults with acute myelogenous leukemia or its subclassifications. These results are inferior to those achieved with combination chemotherapy employing optimum treatment schedules.

Central Nervous System Leukemia: Mercaptopurine is not effective for prophylaxis or treatment of central nervous system leukemia.

Other Neoplasms: Purinethol (mercaptopurine) is not effective in chronic lymphatic leukemia, the lymphomas (including Hodgkin's Disease), or solid tumors.

CONTRAINDICATIONS

Purinethol (mercaptopurine) should not be used unless a diagnosis of acute lymphatic leukemia has been adequately established and the responsible physician is knowledgeable in assessing response to chemotherapy.

Mercaptopurine should not be used in patients whose disease has demonstrated prior resistance to this drug. In animals and man, there is usually complete cross-resistance between Purinethol (mercaptopurine) and Tabloid® brand thioguanine.

WARNINGS

SINCE DRUGS USED IN CANCER CHEMOTHERAPY ARE POTENTIALLY HAZARDOUS, IT IS RECOMMENDED THAT ONLY PHYSICIANS EXPERIENCED WITH THE RISKS OF MERCAPTOPURINE AND KNOWLEDGEABLE IN THE NATURAL HISTORY OF ACUTE LEUKEMIAS ADMINISTER THIS DRUG.

Bone Marrow Toxicity: The most consistent, dose-related toxicity is bone marrow suppression. This may be manifest by anemia, leukopenia, thrombocytopenia, or any combination of these. Any of these findings may also reflect progression of the underlying disease. Since mercaptopurine may have a delayed effect, it is important to withdraw the medication temporarily at the first sign of an abnormally large fall in any of the formed elements of the blood.

Hepatotoxicity: Purinethol (mercaptopurine) is hepatotoxic in animals and man. A small number of deaths have been reported which may have been attributed to hepatic necrosis due to administration of mercaptopurine. Hepatic injury can occur with any dosage, but seems to occur with more frequency when doses of 2.5 mg/kg/day are exceeded.

The histologic pattern of mercaptopurine hepatotoxicity includes features of both intrahepatic cholestasis and parenchymal cell necrosis, either of which may predominate. It is not clear how much of the hepatic damage is due to direct toxicity from the drug and how much may be due to a hypersensitivity reaction. In some patients jaundice has cleared following withdrawal of mercaptopurine and reappeared with its reintroduction.[6]

Published reports have cited widely varying incidences of overt hepatotoxicity. In a large series of patients with various neoplastic diseases, mercaptopurine was administered orally in doses ranging from 2.5 mg/kg to 5.0 mg/kg without any evidence of hepatotoxicity. It was noted by the authors that no definite clinical evidence of liver damage could be ascribed to the drug, although an occasional case of serum hepatitis did occur in patients receiving 6-MP who previously had transfusions.[6] In reports of smaller cohorts of adult and pediatric leukemic patients, the incidence of hepatotoxicity ranged from 0 to 6%.[7,8,9] In an isolated report by Einhorn and Davidsohn, jaundice was observed more frequently (40%), especially when doses exceeded 2.5 mg/kg.[10] Usually, clinically detectable jaundice appears early in the course of treatment (one to two months). However, jaundice has been reported as early as one week and as late as eight years after the start of treatment with mercaptopurine.[11] Monitoring of serum transaminase levels, alkaline phosphatase, and bilirubin levels may allow early detection of hepatotoxicity. It is advisable to monitor these liver function tests at weekly intervals when first beginning therapy and at monthly intervals thereafter. Liver function tests may be advisable more frequently in patients who are receiving mercaptopurine with other hepatotoxic drugs or with known pre-existing liver disease.

The concomitant administration of mercaptopurine with other hepatotoxic agents requires especially careful clinical and biochemical monitoring of hepatic function. Combination therapy involving mercaptopurine with other drugs not felt to be hepatotoxic should nevertheless be approached with caution. The combination of mercaptopurine with doxorubicin (Adriamycin) was reported to be hepatotoxic in 19 of 20 patients undergoing remission-induction therapy for leukemia resistant to previous therapy.[12]

The hepatotoxicity has been associated in some cases with anorexia, diarrhea, jaundice, and ascites. Hepatic encephalopathy has occurred.

The onset of clinical jaundice, hepatomegaly, or anorexia with tenderness in the right hypochondrium are immediate indications for withholding mercaptopurine until the exact etiology can be identified. Likewise, any evidence of deterioration in liver function studies, toxic hepatitis, or biliary stasis should prompt discontinuation of the drug and a search for an etiology of the hepatotoxicity.

Immunosuppression: Mercaptopurine recipients may manifest decreased cellular hypersensitivities and impaired allograft rejection. Induction of immunity to infectious agents or vaccines will be subnormal in these patients; the degree of immunosuppression will depend on antigen dose and temporal relationship to drug. This immunosuppressive effect should be carefully considered with regard to intercurrent infections and risk of subsequent neoplasia.

Pregnancy: "Pregnancy Category D." Mercaptopurine can cause fetal harm when administered to a pregnant woman. Women receiving mercaptopurine in the first trimester of pregnancy have an increased incidence of abortion; the risk of malformation in offspring surviving first trimester exposure is not accurately known.[13] In a series of twenty-eight women receiving mercaptopurine after the first trimester of pregnancy, three mothers died undelivered, one delivered a stillborn child, and one aborted; there were no cases of macroscopically abnormal fetuses.[14] Since such experience cannot exclude the possibility of fetal damage, mercaptopurine should be used during pregnancy only if the benefit clearly justifies the possible risk to the fetus, and particular caution should be given to the use of mercaptopurine in the first trimester of pregnancy.

There are no adequate and well controlled studies in pregnant women. If this drug is used during pregnancy or if the patient becomes pregnant while taking the drug, the patient should be apprised of the potential hazard to the fetus. Women of childbearing potential should be advised to avoid becoming pregnant.

PRECAUTIONS

General: The safe and effective use of Purinethol demands a thorough knowledge of the natural history of the condition being treated. After selection of an initial dosage schedule, therapy will frequently need to be modified depending upon the patient's response and manifestations of toxicity.

The most frequent, serious, toxic effect of mercaptopurine is myelosuppression resulting in leukopenia, thrombocytopenia, and anemia. These toxic effects are often unavoidable during the induction phase of adult acute leukemia if remission induction is to be successful. Whether or not these manifestations demand modification or cessation of dosage de-

Continued on next page

Burroughs Wellcome—Cont.

pends both upon the response of the underlying disease and a careful consideration of supportive facilities (granulocyte and platelet transfusions) which may be available. Life-threatening infections and bleeding have been observed as a consequence of mercaptopurine-induced granulocytopenia and thrombocytopenia. Severe hematologic toxicity may require supportive therapy with platelet transfusions for bleeding, and antibiotics and granulocyte transfusions if sepsis is documented.

If it is not the intent to deliberately induce bone marrow hypoplasia, it is important to discontinue the drug temporarily at the first evidence of an abnormally large fall in white blood cell count, platelet count, or hemoglobin concentration. In many patients with severe depression of the formed elements of the blood due to mercaptopurine, the bone marrow appears hypoplastic on aspiration or biopsy, whereas in other cases it may appear normocellular. The qualitative changes in the erythroid elements toward the megaloblastic series, characteristically seen with the folic acid antagonists and some other antimetabolites, are not seen with this drug. It is probably advisable to start with smaller dosages in patients with impaired renal function, since the latent might result in slower elimination of the drug and metabolites and a greater cumulative effect.

Information for Patients: Patients should be informed that the major toxicities of mercaptopurine are related to myelo-suppression, hepatotoxicity and gastrointestinal toxicity. Patients should never be allowed to take the drug without medical supervision and should be advised to consult their physician if they experience fever, sore throat, jaundice, nausea, vomiting, signs of local infection, bleeding from any site, or symptoms suggestive of anemia. Women of childbearing potential should be advised to avoid becoming pregnant.

Laboratory Tests: It is recommended that evaluation of the hemoglobin or hematocrit, total white blood cell count and differential count, and quantitative platelet count be obtained weekly while the patient is on mercaptopurine therapy. In cases where the cause of fluctuations in the formed elements in the peripheral blood is obscure, bone marrow examination may be useful for the evaluation of marrow status. The decision to increase, decrease, continue, or discontinue a given dosage of mercaptopurine must be based not only on the absolute hematologic values, but also upon the rapidity with which changes are occurring. In many instances, particularly during the induction phase of acute leukemia, complete blood counts will need to be done more frequently than once weekly in order to evaluate the effect of the therapy.

Drug Interactions:

Interaction with allopurinol: When allopurinol and mercaptopurine are administered concomitantly, it is imperative that the dose of mercaptopurine be reduced to one-third to one-quarter of the usual dose. Failure to observe this dosage reduction will result in a delayed catabolism of mercaptopurine and the strong likelihood of inducing severe toxicity.

There is usually complete cross-resistance between Purinethol® (mercaptopurine) and Tabloid® brand thioguanine.

The dosage of mercaptopurine may need to be reduced when this agent is combined with other drugs whose primary or secondary toxicity is myelosuppression. Enhanced marrow suppression has been noted in some patients also receiving trimethoprim-sulfamethoxazole.[15,16]

Carcinogenesis, Mutagenesis, Impairment of Fertility: Purinethol (mercaptopurine) causes chromosomal aberrations in animals and man and induces dominant-lethal mutations in male mice. In mice, surviving female offspring of mothers who received chronic low doses of mercaptopurine during pregnancy were found sterile or if they became pregnant had smaller litters and more dead fetuses as compared to control animals.[17] Carcinogenic potential exists in man, but the extent of the risk is unknown.

The effect of mercaptopurine on human fertility is unknown for either males or females.

Pregnancy: *Teratogenic Effects:* Pregnancy Category D. See WARNINGS section.

Nursing Mothers: It is not known whether this drug is excreted in human milk. Because many drugs are excreted in human milk, and because of the potential for serious adverse reactions in nursing infants from mercaptopurine, a decision should be made whether to discontinue nursing or to discontinue the drug, taking into account the importance of the drug to the mother.

ADVERSE REACTIONS

The principal and potentially serious toxic effects of Purinethol are bone marrow toxicity and hepatotoxicity (see WARNINGS).

Hematologic Effects: The most frequent adverse reaction to mercaptopurine is myelosuppression. The induction of complete remission of acute lymphatic leukemia frequently is associated with marrow hypoplasia. Maintenance of remission generally involves multiple drug regimens whose component agents cause myelosuppression. Anemia, leukopenia, and thrombocytopenia are frequently observed. Dosages and schedules are adjusted to prevent life-threatening cytopenias.

Renal: Hyperuricemia may occur in patients receiving mercaptopurine as a consequence of rapid cell lysis accompanying the antineoplastic effect. Adverse effects can be minimized by increased hydration, urine alkalinization, and the prophylactic administration of a xanthine oxidase inhibitor such as allopurinol. The dosage of mercaptopurine should be reduced to one-third to one-quarter of the usual dose if allopurinol is given concurrently.

Gastrointestinal: Intestinal ulceration has been reported.[18] Nausea, vomiting and anorexia are uncommon during initial administration. Mild diarrhea and sprue-like symptoms have been noted occasionally, but it is difficult at present to attribute these to the medication. Oral lesions are rarely seen, and when they occur they resemble thrush rather than antifolic ulcerations.

An increased risk of pancreatitis may be associated with the investigational use of Purinethol in inflammatory bowel disease.[19,20,21]

Miscellaneous: While dermatologic reactions can occur as a consequence of disease, the administration of Purinethol has been associated with skin rashes and hyperpigmentation.[22] Drug fever has been very rarely reported with mercaptopurine. Before attributing fever to mercaptopurine, every attempt should be made to exclude more common causes of pyrexia, such as sepsis, in patients with acute leukemia.

OVERDOSAGE

Signs and symptoms of overdosage may be immediate such as anorexia, nausea, vomiting and diarrhea; or delayed such as myelosuppression, liver dysfunction and gastroenteritis. Dialysis cannot be expected to clear mercaptopurine. Hemodialysis is thought to be of marginal use due to the rapid intracellular incorporation of mercaptopurine into active metabolites with long persistence. The oral LD_{50} of mercaptopurine was determined to be 480 mg/kg in the mouse and 425 mg/kg in the rat.[23]

There is no known pharmacologic antagonist of mercaptopurine. The drug should be discontinued immediately if unintended toxicity occurs during treatment. If a patient is seen immediately following an accidental overdosage of the drug, it may be useful to induce emesis.

DOSAGE AND ADMINISTRATION

Induction Therapy: Purinethol (mercaptopurine) is administered orally. The dosage which will be tolerated and be effective varies from patient to patient, and therefore careful titration is necessary to obtain the optimum therapeutic effect without incurring excessive, unintended toxicity. The usual initial dosage for children and adults is 2.5 mg/kg of body weight per day (100 to 200 mg in the average adult and 50 mg in an average 5-year-old child). Children with acute leukemia have tolerated this dose without difficulty in most cases; it may be continued daily for several weeks or more in some patients. If, after four weeks at this dosage, there is no clinical improvement and no definite evidence of leukocyte or platelet depression, the dosage may be increased up to 5 mg/kg daily. About 2.5 mg/kg per day may result in a rapid fall in leukocyte count within 1 to 2 weeks in some adults with acute lymphatic leukemia and high total leukocyte counts.

The total daily dosage may be given at one time. It is calculated to the nearest multiple of 25 mg. The dosage of mercaptopurine should be reduced to one-third to one-quarter of the usual dose if allopurinol is given concurrently. Because the drug may have a delayed action, it should be discontinued at the first sign of an abnormally large or rapid fall in the leukocyte or platelet count. If subsequently the leukocyte count or platelet count remains constant for two or three days, or rises, treatment may be resumed.

Maintenance Therapy: Once a complete hematologic remission is obtained, maintenance therapy is considered essential. Maintenance doses will vary from patient to patient. A usual daily maintenance dose of mercaptopurine is 1.5 to 2.5 mg/kg/day as a single dose. It is to be emphasized that in children with acute lymphatic leukemia in remission, superior results have been obtained when mercaptopurine has been combined with other agents (most frequently with methotrexate) for remission maintenance. Mercaptopurine should rarely be relied upon as a single agent for the maintenance of remissions induced in acute leukemia.

Procedures for proper handling and disposal of anti-cancer drugs should be considered. Several guidelines on this subject have been published.[18–23]

There is no general agreement that all of the procedures recommended in the guidelines are necessary or appropriate.

HOW SUPPLIED

Off-white, scored tablets containing 50 mg mercaptopurine, imprinted with "PURINETHOL" and "04A"; bottles of 25 (NDC 0081-0807-25) and 250 (NDC 0081-0807-65). Store at 15°–25°C (59°–77°F) in a dry place.

REFERENCES

1. Hitchings GH, Elion GB: The chemistry and biochemistry of purine analogs. *Ann NY Acad Sci* 1954; 60:195–199.
2. Loo TL, Luce JK, Sullivan MP, et al: Clinical pharmacologic observations on 6-mercaptopurine and 6-methylthiopurine ribonucleoside. *Clin Pharmacol Ther* 1968; 9:180–194.
3. Elion GB: Biochemistry and pharmacology of purine analogs. *Fed Proc* 1967; 26:898–904.
4. Scannell JP, Hitchings GH: Thioguanine in deoxyribonucleic acid from tumors of 6-mercaptopurine-treated mice. *Proc Soc Exp Biol Med* 1966; 122:627–629.
5. Paterson ARP, Tidd DM: 6-thiopurines, in Sartorelli AC, Johns DG (eds): *Antineoplastic and Immunosuppressive Agents*, Part II. Berlin, Springer-Verlag, 1975, pp 384–403.
6. Burchenal JH, Ellison RR, Murphy ML, et al: Clinical studies on 6-mercaptopurine. *Ann NY Acad Sci* 1954; 60:359–368.
7. Farber S: Summary of experience with 6-mercaptopurine. *Ann NY Acad Sci* 1954; 60:412–414.
8. Fountain JR: Clinical observations of the treatment of leukemia and allied disorders with 6-mercaptopurine. *Ann NY Acad Sci* 1954; 60:439–446.
9. Hyman GA, Gellhorn A, Wolff JA: The therapeutic effect of mercaptopurine in a variety of human neoplastic diseases. *Ann NY Acad Sci* 1954; 60:430–435.
10. Einhorn M, Davidsohn I: Hepatotoxicity of mercaptopurine. *JAMA* 1964; 188:802–806.
11. Schein PS, Winokur SH: Immunosuppressive and cytotoxic chemotherapy: long-term complications. *Ann Intern Med* 1975; 82:84–95.
12. Stern MH, Minow RA, Casey JH, et al: Hepatotoxicity in patients treated with adriamycin and 6-mercaptopurine for refractory leukemia. *Am J Clin Pathol* 1975; 63:758–759.
13. Blatt J, Mulvihill JJ, Ziegler JL, et al: Pregnancy outcome following cancer chemotherapy. *Am J Med* 1980; 69:828–832.
14. Nicholson HO: Cytotoxic drugs in pregnancy. *J Obstet Gynaec Brit Cwlth* 1968; 75:307–312.
15. Woods WG, Daigle AE, Hutchinson RJ, et al: Myelosuppression associated with co-trimoxazole as a prophylactic antibiotic in the maintenance phase of childhood acute lymphocytic leukemia. *J Pediatr* 1984; 105:639–644.
16. Rees CA, Lennard L, Lilleyman JS, et al: Disturbance of 6-mercaptopurine metabolism by cotrimoxazole in childhood lymphoblastic leukaemia. *Cancer Chemother Pharmacol* 1984; 12:87–89.
17. Reimers TJ, Sluss PM: 6-mercaptopurine treatment of pregnant mice: effects on second and third generations. *Science* 1978; 201:65–67.
18. Clark PA, Hsia YE, Huntsman RG: Toxic complications of treatment with 6-mercaptopurine. *Br Med J* 1960; 1:393–395.
19. Present DH, Meltzer SJ, Wolke A, et al: Short and long term toxicity to 6-mercaptopurine in the management of inflammatory bowel disease. *Gastroenterology* 1985; 88:1545.
20. Bank L, Wright JP: 6-mercaptopurine-related pancreatitis in 2 patients with inflammatory bowel disease, abstract. *Dig Dis Sci* 1984; 29:357–359.
21. Singleton JW, Law DH, Kelley Jr ML, et al: National Cooperative Crohn's Disease Study: Adverse reactions to study drugs. *Gastroenterology* 1979; 77:870–882.
22. Dreizen S, Bodey GP, Rodriguez V, et al: Cutaneous complications of cancer chemotherapy. *Postgrad Med* 1975; 58:150–158.
23. Unpublished data on file with Burroughs Wellcome Co.
24. Recommendations for the Safe Handling of Parenteral Antineoplastic Drugs. NIH Publications No. 83–2321. For sale by the Superintendent of Documents, U.S. Government Printing Office, Washington, D.C. 20402.
25. AMA Council Report. Guidelines for Handling Parenteral Antineoplastics, *JAMA*, March 15, 1985.
26. National Study Commission on Cytotoxic Exposure—Recommendations for Handling Cytotoxic Agents. Available from Louis P. Jeffrey, Sc.D., Director of Pharmacy Services, Rhode Island Hospital, 593 Eddy Street, Providence, Rhode Island 02902.
27. Clinical Oncological Society of Australia: Guidelines and recommendations for safe handling of antineoplastic agents. *Med J Australia* 1983; 1:426–428.
28. Jones RB, et al: Safe handling of chemotherapeutic agents: A report from the Mount Sinai Medical Center. *Ca—A Cancer Journal for Clinicians* 1983; Sept/Oct:258–263.
29. American Society of Hospital Pharmacists technical assistance bulletin on handling cytotoxic drugs in hospitals. *Am J Hosp Pharm* 1985; 42:131–137.

Shown in Product Identification Section, page 407

RETROVIR® Capsules   ℞
[rĕt-rō-vēr']
(Zidovudine)

WARNING

THERAPY WITH RETROVIR (ZIDOVUDINE) IS OFTEN ASSOCIATED WITH HEMATOLOGIC TOXICITY INCLUDING GRANULOCYTOPENIA AND SEVERE ANEMIA REQUIRING TRANSFUSIONS (SEE WARNINGS). IN ADDITION, PATIENTS TREATED WITH ZIDOVUDINE MAY CONTINUE TO DEVELOP OPPORTUNISTIC INFECTIONS (OI'S) AND OTHER COMPLICATIONS OF THE ACQUIRED IMMUNODEFICIENCY SYNDROME (AIDS) AND AIDS RELATED COMPLEX (ARC) CAUSED BY THE HUMAN IMMUNODEFICIENCY VIRUS (HIV). THEREFORE, PATIENTS ON ZIDOVUDINE SHOULD BE UNDER CLOSE CLINICAL OBSERVATION BY PHYSICIANS EXPERIENCED IN THE TREATMENT OF PATIENTS WITH DISEASES ASSOCIATED WITH HIV. THE SAFETY AND EFFICACY OF ZIDOVUDINE HAVE BEEN ESTABLISHED ONLY FOR CERTAIN ADULT AIDS AND ADVANCED ARC PATIENTS (SEE "INDICATIONS AND USAGE").

DESCRIPTION

Retrovir is the brand name for zidovudine [formerly called azidothymidine (AZT)], an antiretroviral drug active against human immunodeficiency virus (HIV). Retrovir Capsules are for oral administration. Each capsule contains 100 mg of zidovudine and the inactive ingredients corn starch, magnesium stearate, microcrystalline cellulose, and sodium starch glycolate. The 100 mg empty hard gelatin capsule, printed with edible black ink, consists of gelatin and titanium dioxide. The blue band around the capsule consists of gelatin and FD&C Blue No. 2.

The chemical name of zidovudine is 3'-azido-3'-deoxythymidine.

Zidovudine is a white to off-white, odorless, crystalline solid with a molecular weight of 267.24 daltons and the molecular formula $C_{10}H_{13}N_5O_4$.

CLINICAL PHARMACOLOGY

Zidovudine is an inhibitor of the *in vitro* replication of some retroviruses including HIV (also known as HTLV III, LAV, or ARV). This drug is a thymidine analogue in which the 3'-hydroxyl (-OH) group is replaced by an azido (-N₃) group. Cellular thymidine kinase converts zidovudine into zidovudine monophosphate. The monophosphate is further converted into the diphosphate by cellular thymidylate kinase and to the triphosphate derivative by other cellular enzymes. Zidovudine triphosphate interferes with the HIV viral RNA dependent DNA polymerase (reverse transcriptase) and thus, inhibits viral replication. Zidovudine triphosphate also inhibits cellular α-DNA polymerase, but at concentrations 100-fold higher than those required to inhibit reverse transcriptase. *In vitro*, zidovudine triphosphate has been shown to be incorporated into growing chains of DNA by viral reverse transcriptase. When incorporation by the viral enzyme occurs, the DNA chain is terminated. Studies in cell culture suggest that zidovudine incorporation by cellular α-DNA polymerase may occur, but only to a very small extent and not in all test systems. Chain termination has not been demonstrated with cellular α-DNA polymerase.

Microbiology: The relationship between *in vitro* susceptibility of HIV to zidovudine and the inhibition of HIV replication in man or clinical response to therapy has not been established. *In vitro* sensitivity results vary greatly depending upon the time between virus infection and zidovudine treatment, the particular assay used, the cell type employed, and the laboratory performing the test. In addition, the methods currently used to establish virologic responses in clinical trials may be relatively insensitive in detecting changes in the quantities of actively replicating HIV or reactivation of these viruses.

Zidovudine blocked 90% of detectable HIV replication *in vitro* at concentrations of ≤ 0.13 μg/ml (ID₉₀) when added shortly after laboratory infection of susceptible cells. This level of antiviral effect was observed in experiments measuring reverse transcriptase activity in H9 cells, PHA stimulated peripheral blood lymphocytes, and unstimulated peripheral blood lymphocytes. The concentration of drug required to produce a 50% decrease in supernatant reverse transcriptase was 0.013 μg/ml (ID₅₀) in both H9 cells and peripheral blood lymphocytes. Zidovudine at concentrations of 0.13 μg/ml also provided > 90% protection from a strain of HIV (HTLV IIIB) induced cytopathic effects in two tetanus-specific T4 cell lines. p24 gag protein expression was also undetectable at the same concentration in these cells. Partial inhibition of viral activity in cells with chronic HIV infection (presumed to carry integrated HIV DNA) required concentrations of zidovudine (8.8 μg/ml in one laboratory to 13.3 μg/ml in another) which are approximately 100 times

as high as those necessary to block HIV replication in acutely infected cells. Because a limited number of virus isolates have been tested for sensitivity to zidovudine, these results may not reflect the susceptibility of all HIV strains causing disease in the general population.

Although limited testing has demonstrated no HIV isolates resistant to zidovudine, the development of resistance to zidovudine has not been adequately studied and the frequency of zidovudine-resistant isolates existing in the general population is unknown.

The major metabolite of zidovudine, 3'-azido-3'-deoxy-5'-O-β-D-glucopyranuronosylthymidine (GAZT), does not inhibit HIV replication *in vitro*. GAZT does not antagonize the antiviral effect of zidovudine *in vitro* nor does GAZT compete with zidovudine triphosphate as an inhibitor of HIV reverse transcriptase.

The cytotoxicity of zidovudine for various cell lines was determined using a cell growth assay. ID₅₀ values for several human cell lines showed little growth inhibition by zidovudine except at concentrations > 50 μg/ml. However, one human T-lymphocyte cell line was sensitive to the cytotoxic effect of zidovudine with an ID₅₀ of 5 μg/ml. Moreover, in a colony-forming unit assay designed to assess the toxicity of zidovudine for human bone marrow, an ID₅₀ value of < 1.25 μg/ml was estimated. Two of ten human lymphocyte cultures tested were found to be sensitive to zidovudine at 5 μg/ml or less.

Zidovudine has antiviral activity against some mammalian retroviruses in addition to HIV. No significant inhibitory activity was exhibited against a variety of other human and animal viruses, except an ID₅₀ of 1.4 to 2.7 μg/ml against the Epstein-Barr virus, the clinical significance of which is not known at this time.

The following microbiological activities of zidovudine have been observed *in vitro* but the clinical significance is unknown. Many *Enterobacteriaceae*, including strains of *Shigella, Salmonella, Klebsiella, Enterobacter, Citrobacter,* and *Escherichia coli* are inhibited *in vitro* by low concentrations of zidovudine (0.005 to 0.5 μg/ml). Synergy of zidovudine with trimethoprim has been observed against some of these bacteria *in vitro*. Limited data suggest that bacterial resistance to zidovudine develops rapidly. Zidovudine has no activity against gram positive organisms, anaerobes, mycobacteria, or fungal pathogens including *Candida albicans* and *Cryptococcus neoformans*. Although *Giardia lamblia* is inhibited by 1.9 μg/ml of zidovudine, no activity was observed against other protozoal pathogens.

Pharmacokinetics: The pharmacokinetics of zidovudine has been evaluated in 22 adult HIV-infected patients in a Phase I dose-escalation study. Cohorts of 3 to 7 patients received 1 hour intravenous infusions of an investigational formulation of zidovudine ranging from 1 to 2.5 mg/kg every 8 hours to 2.5 to 7.5 mg/kg every 4 hours (3 to 45 mg/day) for 14 to 28 days followed by oral dosing ranging from 2 to 5 mg/kg every 8 hours to 5 to 10 mg/kg every 4 hours (6 to 60 mg/kg/day) for an additional 32 days. After oral dosing, zidovudine was rapidly absorbed from the gastrointestinal tract with peak serum concentrations occurring within 0.5 to 1.5 hours. Dose-independent kinetics was observed over the range of 2 mg/kg every 8 hours to 10 mg/kg every 4 hours. The mean zidovudine half-life was approximately 1 hour and ranged from 0.78 to 1.93 hours following oral dosing.

Steady-state serum concentrations of zidovudine following chronic oral administration of 250 mg every 4 hours (3.0 to 5.4 mg/kg) were determined in 21 patients (body weight ranged from 46.0 to 83.6 kg) in a Phase II trial. Mean steady-state predose and 1.5 hours postdose zidovudine concentrations were 0.16 μg/ml (range 0 to 0.84 μg/ml) and 0.62 μg/ml (range 0.05 to 1.46 μg/ml), respectively.

Zidovudine is rapidly metabolized to 3'-azido-3'-deoxy-5'-O-β-D-glucopyranuronosylthymidine (GAZT) which has an apparent elimination half-life of 1 hour (range 0.61 to 1.73 hours). Following oral administration, urinary recoveries of zidovudine and GAZT accounted for 14 and 74% of the dose, respectively, and the total urinary recovery averaged 90% (range 63 to 95%), indicating a high degree of absorption. However, as a result of first-pass metabolism, the average oral capsule bioavailability of zidovudine is 65% (range 52 to 75%).

Additional pharmacokinetic data following intravenous dosing indicated dose-independent kinetics over the range of 1 to 5 mg/kg with a mean zidovudine half-life of 1.1 hours (range 0.48 to 2.86 hours). Total body clearance averaged 1900 ml/min/70 kg and the apparent volume of distribution was 1.6 L/kg. Renal clearance is estimated to be 400 ml/min/70 kg, indicating glomerular filtration and active tubular secretion by the kidneys. Zidovudine plasma protein binding is 34 to 38%, indicating that drug interactions involving binding site displacement are not anticipated.

The zidovudine cerebrospinal fluid (CSF)/plasma concentration ratio measured 1.8 hours following oral dosing at 2 mg/kg was 0.15 (n = 1). The ratios measured at 2 to 4 hours following intravenous dosing of 2.5 mg/kg and 5.0 mg/kg were 0.20 (n = 1) and 0.64 (n = 3), respectively.

INDICATIONS AND USAGE

Retrovir Capsules are indicated for the management of certain adult patients with symptomatic HIV infection (AIDS and advanced ARC) who have a history of cytologically confirmed *Pneumocystis carinii* pneumonia (PCP) or an absolute CD4 (T4 helper/inducer) lymphocyte count of less than 200/mm³ in the peripheral blood before therapy is begun. This indication is based primarily on the results of a randomized, double-blind, placebo-controlled trial conducted at 12 medical centers in the United States in which 281 patients with AIDS or advanced ARC were studied for an average of four and a half months. Additional data have been collected on approximately 80% of these patients who have received zidovudine in an open-label extension of this trial for an average of five more months.

The patient population of the controlled trial consisted of 160 AIDS patients (85 Retrovir and 75 placebo) who had recovered from their first episode of PCP diagnosed within the previous four months and 121 ARC patients (59 Retrovir and 62 placebo) with multiple signs and symptoms of HIV infection, including mucocutaneous candidiasis and/or unexplained weight loss (≥ 15 lbs or > 10% of prior body weight). All patients had evidence of impaired cellular immunity with an absence of delayed cutaneous hypersensitivity and a decreased number of CD4 (T4) lymphocytes in the peripheral circulation. Two hundred twenty-one (79% of all patients) had fewer than 200 T4 cells/mm³ at entry (95% of AIDS patients and 57% of ARC patients). All patients began therapy at a dose of 250 mg every 4 hours around the clock. This dosage was reduced or temporarily or permanently discontinued if serious marrow toxicity occurred. The trial was stopped because of a significant reduction in mortality before all patients had completed the planned 24 weeks of treatment. There were 19 deaths in the placebo group and 1 in the Retrovir group (p < .001). All deaths were apparently due to opportunistic infections (OI) or other complications of HIV infection. Treatment duration ranged from 12 weeks to 26 weeks, with a mean and median duration of 17 and 18 weeks, respectively.

Retrovir also significantly reduced the risk of acquiring an AIDS-defining OI in patients after 6 weeks of treatment (p < .001). In addition, patients who received Retrovir generally did better than the placebo group in terms of several other measures of efficacy including performance level, neuropsychiatric function, maintenance of body weight and the number and severity of symptoms associated with HIV infection. A modest increase in mean CD4 (T4) counts was seen in the zidovudine group but the significance of this finding is unclear as the CD4 (T4) counts declined again in some patients.

The most significant adverse reaction noted in the study was a depression of formed elements in the peripheral blood, which necessitated dose reduction or drug discontinuation in 49 of the 144 (34%) participants. Of those participants whose baseline CD4 (T4) lymphocyte counts were ≤ 200, 47% of those receiving Retrovir and 10% of those receiving placebo developed a granulocyte count of < 750/mm³. Similarly, 45% of Retrovir recipients and only 14% of placebo recipients had a > 25% reduction in hemoglobin (see ADVERSE REACTIONS). Transfusions were administered to some patients with anemia. 47 of 114 (41%) Retrovir recipients and 17 of 107 (16%) placebo recipients with < 200 CD4 lymphocytes at entry were transfused. Only one of 30 Retrovir recipients and none of 30 placebo recipients with > 200 CD4 lymphocytes required transfusion.

Although mean platelet counts in Retrovir recipients were statistically increased compared to mean baseline values, thrombocytopenia did occur in some patients. Twelve percent (12%) of Retrovir recipients compared to 5% of placebo recipients had > 50% decreases from baseline platelet count. At the conclusion of the placebo-controlled trial, 127 Retrovir recipients and 102 placebo recipients elected to enroll in an uncontrolled extension protocol in which all patients received Retrovir at a dose of 200 mg every four hours. This dose was chosen because of concern about cumulative hematologic toxicity and to allow for greater flexibility in dosing. Over the subsequent five months, opportunistic infections continued to occur and additional patients died in both groups. Sixteen patients from the original placebo cohort died after the conclusion of the controlled trial. Four of these 16 never received Retrovir and seven expired during the first month of therapy. Ten additional deaths occurred among the original Retrovir recipients. With respect to these data, termination of the controlled trial precludes direct comparisons of mortality and morbidity between the original placebo and drug recipients. Long-term follow-up of these patients, however, will allow for examination of the natural history of prolonged zidovudine therapy.

CONTRAINDICATIONS

Retrovir Capsules are contraindicated for patients who have potentially life-threatening allergic reactions to any of the components of the formulation.

Continued on next page

Burroughs Wellcome—Cont.

		Pretreatment CD4 (T4) Levels			
		≤200/mm³		>200/mm³	
Abnormality	% Decrease from Baseline	Zidovudine (n=113)	Placebo (n=105)	Zidovudine (n=30)	Placebo (n=30)
Granulocytopenia	>50%	55%	19%	40%	13%
Anemia	>25%	45%	14%	10%	10%

WARNINGS

Zidovudine has been carefully studied in limited numbers of seriously ill HIV-infected patients treated for a limited period of time. Therefore, the full safety and efficacy profile of zidovudine has not been completely defined, particularly in regard to prolonged use, and especially in HIV-infected individuals who have less advanced disease.

Zidovudine should be used with extreme caution in patients who have bone marrow compromise evidenced by granulocyte count <1000/mm³ or hemoglobin <9.5 g/dl. In the placebo-controlled study, anemia and granulocytopenia were the most significant adverse events observed (see ADVERSE REACTIONS). There have been reports of pancytopenia associated with the use of zidovudine, which was reversible in most instances after discontinuance of the drug. Significant anemia most commonly occurred after 4 to 6 weeks of therapy and in many cases required dose adjustment, discontinuation of zidovudine, and/or blood transfusions. Frequent (at least every 2 weeks) blood counts are strongly recommended in patients taking zidovudine. If anemia or granulocytopenia develops, dosage adjustments may be necessary (see DOSAGE AND ADMINISTRATION). Coadministration of zidovudine with other drugs metabolized by glucuronidation should be avoided because the toxicity of either drug may be potentiated (see Drug Interactions under PRECAUTIONS). Zidovudine recipients who used acetaminophen during the controlled trial had an increased incidence of granulocytopenia which appeared to be correlated with the duration of acetaminophen use.

PRECAUTIONS

General: Zidovudine is eliminated from the body primarily by renal excretion following metabolism in the liver (glucuronidation). There are currently no data available concerning the use of zidovudine in patients with impaired renal or hepatic function, and such patients may be at a greater risk of toxicity from zidovudine.

Information for Patients: Zidovudine is not a cure for HIV infections, and patients may continue to acquire illnesses associated with AIDS or ARC, including opportunistic infections. Therefore, patients should be advised to seek medical care for any significant change in their health status.

Patients should be informed that the major toxicities of zidovudine are granulocytopenia and/or anemia. They should be told that they may require transfusions or dose modifications including possible discontinuation if toxicity develops. They should be told of the extreme importance of having their blood counts followed closely while on therapy. They should be cautioned about the use of other medications such as acetaminophen that may exacerbate the toxicity of zidovudine.

Retrovir Capsules are for oral ingestion only. Patients should be told of the importance of taking zidovudine exactly as prescribed, and that administration every 4 hours includes dosing around the clock, even though it may interrupt their normal sleep. They should be told not to share medication and not to exceed the recommended dose. They should be told that the long-term effects of zidovudine are unknown at this time.

Patients should be advised that zidovudine therapy has not been shown to reduce the risk of transmission of HIV to others through sexual contact or blood contamination.

Drug Interactions: The interaction of other drugs with zidovudine has not been studied in a systematic manner. Coadministration of zidovudine with drugs that are nephrotoxic, cytotoxic, or which interfere with RBC/WBC number or function (e.g., dapsone, pentamidine, amphotericin B, flucytosine, vincristine, vinblastine, adriamycin, or interferon) may increase the risk of toxicity. Limited data suggest that probenecid may inhibit glucuronidation and/or reduce renal excretion of zidovudine. In addition, other drugs (e.g., acetaminophen, aspirin, or indomethacin) may competitively inhibit glucuronidation (see WARNINGS). Phenytoin levels have been reported to be low in some patients receiving zidovudine, while in one case a high level was documented. These observations suggest that phenytoin levels should be carefully monitored in patients receiving zidovudine since many patients with advance HIV injections have CNS conditions which may predispose to seizure activity.

Some experimental nucleoside analogues which are being evaluated in AIDS and ARC patients may affect RBC/WBC number or function and may increase the potential for hematologic toxicity of zidovudine. Some experimental nucleoside analogues affecting DNA replication antagonize the in vitro antiviral activity of zidovudine against HIV and thus, concomitant use of such drugs should be avoided.

Some drugs such as trimethoprim-sulfamethoxazole, pyrimethamine, and acyclovir may be necessary for the management or prevention of opportunistic infections. In the controlled trial, increased toxicity was not detected for limited exposure to these drugs. However, there is one published report of neurotoxicity (profound lethargy) associated with concomitant use of zidovudine and acyclovir.

Carcinogenesis, Mutagenesis, Impairment of Fertility: Long-term carcinogenicity studies of zidovudine in animals have not been completed. However, in an in vitro mammalian cell transformation assay, zidovudine was positive at concentrations of 0.5 µg/ml and higher.

No evidence of mutagenicity (with or without metabolic activation) was observed in the Ames Salmonella mutagenicity assay. In a mutagenicity assay conducted in L5178Y/TK$^{+/-}$ mouse lymphoma cells, zidovudine was weakly mutagenic in the absence of metabolic activation only at the highest concentrations tested (4000 and 5000 µg/ml). In the presence of metabolic activation, the drug was weakly mutagenic at concentrations of 1000 µg/ml and higher. In an in vitro cytogenetic study performed in cultured human lymphocytes, zidovudine induced dose-related structural chromosomal abnormalities at concentrations of 3 µg/ml and higher. No such effects were noted at the two lowest concentrations tested, 0.3 and 1 µg/ml. In an in vivo cytogenetic study in rats given a single intravenous injection of zidovudine at doses of 37.5 to 300 mg/kg, there were no treatment-related structural or numerical chromosomal alterations in spite of plasma levels that were as high as 453 µg/ml five minutes after dosing.

Effects of zidovudine on fertility have not been studied.

Pregnancy: Pregnancy Category C. An oral teratology study in pregnant rats using doses up to 20 times the human dose has revealed no evidence of harm to the fetus due to zidovudine. Other teratology and reproduction/fertility tests in animals have not been completed. It is not known whether zidovudine can cause fetal harm when administered to a pregnant woman or can affect reproductive capacity. Zidovudine should be given to a pregnant woman only if clearly needed.

Nursing Mothers: It is not known whether zidovudine is excreted in human milk. Because many drugs are excreted in human milk and because of the potential for serious adverse reactions from zidovudine in nursing infants, mothers should be instructed to discontinue nursing if they are receiving zidovudine.

Pediatric Use: Safety and effectiveness in children have not been established.

ADVERSE REACTIONS

The most frequent adverse events and abnormal laboratory values reported in the placebo-controlled clinical trial of oral zidovudine administration in 281 patients (144 patients zidovudine; 137 patients placebo) were granulocytopenia and anemia. The occurrence of these hematologic toxicities was inversely related to CD4 (T4) lymphocyte number, hemoglobin, and granulocyte count at study entry, and directly related to dose and duration of therapy. The frequency of granulocytopenia and anemia according to the patients' CD4 (T4) levels is shown in the following table:

[See table below.]

Because many patients were anemic and/or granulocytopenic before starting therapy with zidovudine, examining the degree of change when compared to baseline, as shown in the table below, may be more informative.

[See table above.]

The anemia appeared to be the result of impaired erythrocyte maturation as evidenced by increasing macrocytosis (MCV) while on drug.

The 281 patients treated in this controlled trial had serious underlying disease with multiple baseline symptoms and clinical abnormalities. The following table summarizes those reported clinical adverse events which occurred in at least 5% of all patients treated with zidovudine. Severe headache, nausea, insomnia and myalgia were reported at a significantly greater rate in zidovudine recipients.

[See table on top next page].

Clinical adverse events which occurred in less than 5% of all patients treated with zidovudine are listed below. Since many of these adverse events were seen in placebo-treated patients as well as zidovudine recipients, they may not be attributable to the drug.

Body as a whole: body odor, chills, edema of the lip, flu syndrome, hyperalgesia, back pain, chest pain, lymphadenopathy.
Cardiovascular: vasodilation.
Gastrointestinal: constipation, dysphagia, edema of the tongue, eructation, flatulence, bleeding gums, rectal hemorrhage, mouth ulcer.
Musculoskeletal: arthralgia, muscle spasm, tremor, twitch.
Nervous: anxiety, confusion, depression, emotional lability, nervousness, syncope, loss of mental acuity, vertigo.
Respiratory: cough, epistaxis, pharyngitis, rhinitis, sinusitis, hoarseness.
Skin: acne, pruritus, urticaria.
Special senses: amblyopia, hearing loss, photophobia.
Urogenital: dysuria, polyuria, urinary frequency, urinary hesitancy.

The following events have been reported in patients treated with zidovudine. They may also occur as part of the underlying disease process. As such, the relationship between these events and the use of zidovudine is uncertain: seizures, myopathy, nail pigmentation.

OVERDOSAGE

One patient who ingested 10 to 20 grams (~110 to 220 mg/kg) of zidovudine as part of an intentional multidrug overdose (which also included triazolam and barbiturates) experienced mild ataxia acutely but exhibited no hematologic abnormalities on extended follow-up. If overdosage occurs, intensive observation for marrow suppression with transfusions and protective measures for granulocytopenia may be needed until marrow function returns. Although other nucleoside analogues have been partially removed by peritoneal dialysis or hemodialysis, it is not known whether zidovudine can be removed in this manner.

DOSAGE AND ADMINISTRATION

The recommended starting dose of Retrovir is 200 mg (two 100 mg capsules) administered orally every four hours around the clock. In a 70 kg patient this dose corresponds to 2.9 mg/kg every four hours. The dose administered in the placebo-controlled clinical trial was 250 mg (2.3 to 5.9 mg/kg depending on body weight) every four hours (see INDICATIONS AND USAGE).

Hematologic toxicities appear to be related to pretreatment bone marrow reserve and to dose and duration of therapy. Careful monitoring of hematologic indices every two weeks is recommended to detect serious anemia or granulocytopenia. In patients with hematologic toxicity, reduction in hemoglobin may occur as early as 2 to 4 weeks, and granulocytopenia usually occurs after 6 to 8 weeks.

Dose Adjustment: Significant anemia (hemoglobin of <7.5 g/dl or reduction of >25% of baseline) and/or significant granulocytopenia (granulocyte count of <750/mm³ or reduction of >50% from baseline) may require a dose interruption until some evidence of marrow recovery is observed. For less severe anemia or granulocytopenia, a reduction in daily dose may be adequate. In patients who develop significant anemia, dose modification does not necessarily eliminate the need for transfusion. If marrow recovery occurs following dose modification, gradual increases in dose may be appropriate depending on hematologic indices and patient tolerance.

	Pretreatment CD4 (T4) Levels			
	≤200/mm³		>200/mm³	
Abnormality	Zidovudine (n=113)	Placebo (n=105)	Zidovudine (n=30)	Placebo (n=30)
Granulocytopenia (<750/mm³)	47%	10%	10%	3%
Anemia (Hgb <7.5 g/dl)	30%	6%	3%	0%

Percentage (%) of Patients with Clinical Events

Adverse Event	Zidovudine (n=144) %	Placebo (n=137) %	Adverse Event	Zidovudine (n=144) %	Placebo (n=137) %
BODY AS A WHOLE			MUSCULOSKELETAL		
Asthenia	19	18	Myalgia	8	2
Diaphoresis	5	4	NERVOUS		
Fever	16	12	Dizziness	6	4
Headache	42	37	Insomnia	5	1
Malaise	8	7	Paresthesia	6	3
GASTROINTESTINAL			Somnolence	8	9
Anorexia	11	8	RESPIRATORY		
Diarrhea	12	18	Dyspnea	5	3
Dyspepsia	5	4	SKIN		
GI Pain	20	19	Rash	17	15
Nausea	46	18	SPECIAL SENSES		
Vomiting	6	3	Taste Perversion	5	8

HOW SUPPLIED

Retrovir Capsules 100 mg (white, opaque cap and body with a dark blue band) containing 100 mg zidovudine and printed with "Wellcome" and unicorn logo on cap and "Y9C" and "100" on body. Bottles of 100 (NDC 0081-0108-55).

Store at 15° to 25°C (59° to 77°F) and protect from light and moisture.

U.S. Patent No. 4724232 (Use Patent) Other Pats. Pending
Shown in Product Identification Section, page 407

SEPTRA® I.V. INFUSION   ℞
[sĕp'trah]
(Trimethoprim and Sulfamethoxazole)

DESCRIPTION

Septra I.V. Infusion (Trimethoprim and Sulfamethoxazole), a sterile solution for intravenous infusion only, is a synthetic antibacterial combination product. Each ml contains 16 mg trimethoprim* and 80 mg sulfamethoxazole compounded with 40% propylene glycol, 10% ethyl alcohol and 0.3% diethanolamine; 1% benzyl alcohol and 0.1% sodium metabisulfite added as preservatives, water for injection, and pH adjusted to approximately 10 with sodium hydroxide.

Trimethoprim is 2,4-diamino-5-(3,4,5-trimethoxybenzyl)-pyrimidine. It is a white to light yellow, odorless, bitter compound with a molecular weight of 290.3 and the molecular formula $C_{14}H_{18}N_4O_3$.

Sulfamethoxazole is N^1-(5-methyl-3-isoxazolyl)sulfanilamide. It is an almost white, odorless, tasteless compound with a molecular weight of 253.28 and the molecular formula $C_{10}H_{11}N_3O_3S$.

CLINICAL PHARMACOLOGY

Following a one-hour intravenous infusion of a single dose of 160 mg trimethoprim and 800 mg sulfamethoxazole to 11 patients whose weight ranged from 105 lbs. to 165 lbs. (mean, 143 lbs.), the mean peak plasma concentrations of trimethoprim and sulfamethoxazole were 3.4 ± 0.3 µg/ml and 46.3 ± 2.7 µg/ml, respectively. Following repeated intravenous administration of the same dose at eight-hour intervals, the mean plasma concentrations just prior to and immediately after each infusion at steady state were 5.6 ± 0.6 µg/ml and 8.8 ± 0.9 µg/ml for trimethoprim and 70.6 ± 7.3 µg/ml and 105.6 ± 10.9 µg/ml for sulfamethoxazole. The mean plasma half-life was 11.3 ± 0.7 hours for trimethoprim and 12.8 ± 1.8 hours for sulfamethoxazole. All of these 11 patients had normal renal function and their ages ranged from 17 to 78 years (median, 60 years)[1].

Pharmacokinetic studies in children and adults suggest an age-dependent half-life of trimethoprim as indicated in the following table.[2]

Age (yrs.)	No. of Patients	Mean TMP Half-life (hours)
<1	2	7.67
1–10	9	5.49
10–20	5	8.19
20–63	6	12.82

Patients with severely impaired renal function exhibit an increase in the half-lives of both components, requiring dosage regimen adjustment (see DOSAGE AND ADMINISTRATION section).

Both trimethoprim and sulfamethoxazole exist in the blood as unbound, protein-bound and metabolized forms; sulfamethoxazole also exists as the conjugated form. The metabolism of sulfamethoxazole occurs predominately by N_4-acetylation, although the glucuronide conjugate has been identified. The principal metabolites of trimethoprim are the 1- and 3- oxides and the 3'- and 4'-hydroxy derivatives. The free forms of trimethoprim and sulfamethoxazole are considered to be the therapeutically active forms. Approximately 44% of trimethoprim and 70% of sulfamethoxazole are bound to plasma proteins. The presence of 10 mg percent sulfamethoxazole in plasma decreases the protein binding of trimethoprim by an insignificant degree; trimethoprim does not influence the protein binding of sulfamethoxazole.

Excretion of trimethoprim and sulfamethoxazole is primarily by the kidneys through both glomerular filtration and tubular secretion. Urine concentrations of both trimethoprim and sulfamethoxazole are considerably higher than are the concentrations in the blood. The percent of dose excreted in urine over a 12-hour period following the intravenous administration of the first dose of 240 mg of trimethoprim and 1200 mg of sulfamethoxazole on day 1 ranged from 17% to 42.4% as free trimethoprim; 7% to 12.7% as free sulfamethoxazole; and 36.7% to 56% as total (free plus the N_4-acetylated metabolite) sulfamethoxazole. When administered together as Septra, neither trimethoprim nor sulfamethoxazole affects the urinary excretion pattern of the other.

Both trimethoprim and sulfamethoxazole distribute to sputum and vaginal fluid; trimethoprim also distributes to bronchial secretions and both pass the placental barrier and are excreted in human milk.

Microbiology: Sulfamethoxazole inhibits bacterial synthesis of dihydrofolic acid by competing with *para*-aminobenzoic acid (PABA). Trimethoprim blocks the production of tetrahydrofolic acid from dihydrofolic acid by binding to and reversibly inhibiting the required enzyme, dihydrofolate reductase. Thus, Septra blocks two consecutive steps in the biosynthesis of nucleic acids and proteins essential to many bacteria.

In vitro studies have shown that bacterial resistance develops more slowly with Septra than with trimethoprim or sulfamethoxazole alone.

In vitro serial dilution tests have shown that the spectrum of antibacterial activity of Septra includes common bacterial pathogens with the exception of *Pseudomonas aeruginosa*. The following organisms are usually susceptible: *Escherichia coli, Klebsiella* species, *Enterobacter* species, *Morganella morganii, Proteus mirabilis*, indole-positive *Proteus* species, including *Proteus vulgaris, Haemophilus influenzae* (including ampicillin-resistant strains), *Streptococcus pneumoniae, Shigella flexneri* and *Shigella sonnei*. It should be noted, however, that there are little clinical data on the use of Septra I.V. Infusion in serious systemic infections due to *Haemophilus influenzae* and *Streptococcus pneumoniae*.
[See table below].

Susceptibility Testing: The recommended quantitative disc susceptibility method may be used for estimating the susceptibility of bacteria to Septra.[3,4] With this procedure, a report from the laboratory of "Susceptible to trimethoprim and sulfamethoxazole" indicates that the infection is likely to respond to therapy with Septra. If the infection is confined to the urine, a report of "Intermediate susceptibility to trimethoprim and sulfamethoxazole" also indicates that the infection is likely to respond. A report of "Resistant to trimethoprim and sulfamethoxazole" indicates that the infection is unlikely to respond to therapy with Septra.

INDICATIONS AND USAGE

PNEUMOCYSTIS CARINII PNEUMONIA: Septra I.V. Infusion is indicated in the treatment of *Pneumocystis carinii* pneumonia in children and adults.

SHIGELLOSIS: Septra I.V. Infusion is indicated in the treatment of enteritis caused by susceptible strains of *Shigella flexneri* and *Shigella sonnei* in children and adults.

URINARY TRACT INFECTIONS: Septra I.V. Infusion is indicated in the treatment of severe or complicated urinary tract infections due to susceptible strains of *Escherichia coli, Klebsiella* species, *Enterobacter* species, *Morganella morganii*, and *Proteus* species when oral administration of Septra is not feasible and when the organism is not susceptible to single agent antibacterials effective in the urinary tract.

Although appropriate culture and susceptibility studies should be performed, therapy may be started while awaiting the results of these studies.

CONTRAINDICATIONS

Hypersensitivity to trimethoprim or sulfonamides. Patients with documented megaloblastic anemia due to folate deficiency. Pregnancy at term and during the nursing period, because sulfonamides pass the placenta and are excreted in the milk and may cause kernicterus. Infants less than two months of age.

WARNINGS

FATALITIES ASSOCIATED WITH THE ADMINISTRATION OF SULFONAMIDES, ALTHOUGH RARE, HAVE OCCURRED DUE TO SEVERE REACTIONS, INCLUDING STEVENS-JOHNSON SYNDROME, TOXIC EPIDERMAL NECROLYSIS, FULMINANT HEPATIC NECROSIS, AGRANULOCYTOSIS, APLASTIC ANEMIA, OTHER BLOOD DYSCRASIAS AND HYPERSENSITIVITY OF THE RESPIRATORY TRACT.

SEPTRA SHOULD BE DISCONTINUED AT THE FIRST APPEARANCE OF SKIN RASH OR ANY SIGN OF ADVERSE REACTION. Clinical signs, such as rash, sore throat, fever, arthralgia, cough, shortness of breath, pallor, purpura or jaundice may be early indications of serious reactions. In rare instances, a skin rash may be followed by more severe reactions, such as Stevens-Johnson syndrome, toxic epidermal necrolysis, hepatic necrosis or serious blood disorder. Complete blood counts should be done frequently in patients receiving sulfonamides.

SEPTRA SHOULD NOT BE USED IN THE TREATMENT OF STREPTOCOCCAL PHARYNGITIS. Clinical studies have documented that patients with group A β-hemolytic streptococcal tonsillopharyngitis have a greater incidence of bacteriologic failure when treated with Septra than do those patients treated with penicillin, as evidenced by failure to eradicate this organism from the tonsillopharyngeal area.

Contains sodium metabisulfite, a sulfite that may cause allergic-type reactions including anaphylactic symptoms and life-threatening or less severe asthmatic episodes in certain susceptible people. The overall prevalence of sulfite sensitivity in the general population is unknown and probably low. Sulfite sensitivity is seen more frequently in asthmatic than in nonasthmatic people.

PRECAUTIONS

General: Septra should be given with caution to patients with impaired renal or hepatic function, to those with possi-

---

REPRESENTATIVE MINIMUM INHIBITORY CONCENTRATION VALUES FOR SEPTRA SUSCEPTIBLE ORGANISMS (MIC-µg/ml)

Bacteria	TMP Alone	SMX Alone	TMP/SMX (1:19) TMP	TMP/SMX (1:19) SMX
Escherichia coli	0.05–1.5	1.0–245	0.05–0.5	0.95–9.5
Proteus species (indole positive)	0.5–5.0	7.35–300	0.05–1.5	0.95–28.5
Morganella morganii	0.5–5.0	7.35–300	0.05–1.5	0.95–28.5
Proteus mirabilis	0.5–1.5	7.35–30	0.05–0.15	0.95–2.85
Klebsiella species	0.15–5.0	2.45–245	0.05–1.5	0.95–28.5
Enterobacter species	0.15–5.0	2.45–245	0.05–1.5	0.95–28.5
Haemophilus influenzae	0.15–1.5	2.85–95	0.015–0.15	0.285–2.85
Streptococcus pneumoniae	0.15–1.5	7.35–24.5	0.05–0.15	0.95–2.85
Shigella flexneri †	<0.01–0.04	<0.16–>320	<0.002–0.03	0.04–0.625
Shigella sonnei †	0.02–0.08	0.625–>320	0.004–0.06	0.08–1.25

TMP = Trimethoprim   SMX = Sulfamethoxazole
†Rudoy RC, Nelson JD, Haltalin KC. *Antimicrobial Agents and Chemotherapy* 5:439-43, 1974.

Continued on next page

Burroughs Wellcome—Cont.

ble folate deficiency (e.g., the elderly, chronic alcoholics, patients receiving anticonvulsant therapy, patients with malabsorption syndrome, and patients in malnutrition states) and to those with severe allergy or bronchial asthma. In glucose-6-phosphate dehydrogenase-deficient individuals, hemolysis may occur. This reaction is frequently dose-related. Adequate fluid intake must be maintained in order to prevent crystalluria and stone formation. (See CLINICAL PHARMACOLOGY and DOSAGE AND ADMINISTRATION.)

Local irritation and inflammation due to extravascular infiltration of the infusion has been observed with Septra I.V. Infusion. If these occur the infusion should be discontinued and restarted at another site.

Use in the Elderly: There may be an increased risk of severe adverse reactions in elderly patients, particularly when complicating conditions exist, e.g., impaired kidney and/or liver function, or concomitant use of other drugs. Severe skin reactions, or generalized bone marrow suppression (see WARNINGS and ADVERSE REACTIONS sections) or a specific decrease in platelets (with or without purpura) are the most frequently reported severe adverse reactions in elderly patients. In those concurrently receiving certain diuretics, primarily thiazides, an increased incidence of thrombocytopenia with purpura has been reported. Appropriate dosage adjustments should be made for patients with impaired kidney function (see DOSAGE AND ADMINISTRATION section).

Use in the Treatment of *Pneumocystis carinii* Pneumonia in Patients with Acquired Immunodeficiency Syndrome (AIDS): The incidence of side effects, particularly rash, fever, leukopenia, and elevated aminotransferase (transaminase) values with Septra therapy in AIDS patients who are being treated for *Pneumocystis carinii* pneumonia has been reported to be greatly increased compared with the incidence normally associated with the use of Septra in non-AIDS patients.

Laboratory Tests: Appropriate culture and susceptibility studies should be performed before and throughout treatment. Complete blood counts should be done frequently in patients receiving Septra; if a significant reduction in the count of any formed blood element is noted, Septra should be discontinued. Urinalyses with careful microscopic examination and renal function tests should be performed during therapy, particularly for those patients with impaired renal function.

Drug Interactions: In elderly patients concurrently receiving certain diuretics, primarily thiazides, an increased incidence of thrombocytopenia with purpura has been reported.

It has been reported that Septra may prolong the prothrombin time in patients who are receiving the anticoagulant warfarin. This interaction should be kept in mind when Septra is given to patients already on anticoagulant therapy, and the coagulation time should be reassessed.

Septra may inhibit the hepatic metabolism of phenytoin. Septra, given at a common clinical dosage, increased the phenytoin half-life by 39% and decreased the phenytoin metabolic clearance rate by 27%. When administering these drugs concurrently, one should be alert for possible excessive phenytoin effect.

Sulfonamides can also displace methotrexate from plasma protein binding sites, thus increasing free methotrexate concentrations.

Drug/Laboratory Test Interactions: Septra, specifically the trimethoprim component, can interfere with a serum methotrexate assay as determined by the competitive binding protein technique (CBPA) when a bacterial dihydrofolate reductase is used as the binding protein. No interference occurs, however, if methotrexate is measured by a radioimmunoassay (RIA).

The presence of trimethoprim and sulfamethoxazole may also interfere with the Jaffé alkaline picrate reaction assay for creatinine resulting in over-estimations of about 10% in the range of normal values.

Carcinogenesis, Mutagenesis, Impairment of Fertility:
Carcinogenesis: Long-term studies in animals to evaluate carcinogenic potential have not been conducted with Septra I.V. Infusion.

Mutagenesis: Bacterial mutagenic studies have not been performed with sulfamethoxazole and trimethoprim in combination. Trimethoprim was demonstrated to be non-mutagenic in the Ames assay. In studies at two laboratories no chromosomal damage was detected in cultured Chinese hamster ovary cells at concentrations approximately 500 times human plasma levels; at concentrations approximately 1000 times human plasma levels in these same cells a low level of chromosomal damage was induced at one of the laboratories. No chromosomal abnormalities were observed in cultured human leukocytes at concentrations of trimethoprim up to 20 times human steady state plasma levels. No chromosomal effects were detected in peripheral lymphocytes of human subjects receiving 320 mg of trimethoprim in combination

with up to 1600 mg of sulfamethoxazole per day for as long as 112 weeks.

Impairment of Fertility: Septra I.V. Infusion has not been studied in animals for evidence of impairment of fertility. However, studies in rats at oral dosages as high as 70 mg/kg trimethoprim plus 350 mg/kg sulfamethoxazole daily showed no adverse effects on fertility or general reproductive performance.

Pregnancy: *Teratogenic Effects:* Pregnancy Category C. In rats, oral doses of 533 mg/kg sulfamethoxazole or 200 mg/kg trimethoprim produced teratological effects manifested mainly as cleft palates. The highest dose which did not cause cleft palates in rats was 512 mg/kg sulfamethoxazole or 192 mg/kg trimethoprim when administered separately. In two studies in rats, no teratology was observed when 512 mg/kg of sulfamethoxazole was used in combination with 128 mg/kg of trimethoprim. In one study, however, cleft palates were observed in one litter out of 9 when 355 mg/kg of sulfamethoxazole was used in combination with 88 mg/kg of trimethoprim.

In some rabbit studies, an overall increase in fetal loss (dead and resorbed and malformed conceptuses) was associated with doses of trimethoprim 6 times the human therapeutic dose.

While there are no large, well-controlled studies on the use of trimethoprim and sulfamethoxazole in pregnant women, Brumfitt and Pursell[5], in a retrospective study, reported the outcome of 186 pregnancies during which the mother received either placebo or oral trimethoprim and sulfamethoxazole. The incidence of congenital abnormalities was 4.5% (3 of 66) in those who received placebo and 3.3% (4 of 120) in those receiving trimethoprim and sulfamethoxazole. There were no abnormalities in the 10 children whose mothers received the drug during the first trimester. In a separate survey, Brumfitt and Pursell also found no congenital abnormalities in 35 children whose mothers had received oral trimethoprim and sulfamethoxazole at the time of conception or shortly thereafter.

Because trimethoprim and sulfamethoxazole may interfere with folic acid metabolism, Septra I.V. Infusion should be used during pregnancy only if the potential benefit justifies the potential risk to the fetus.

Nonteratogenic Effects: See CONTRAINDICATIONS section.

Nursing Mothers: See CONTRAINDICATIONS section.

Pediatric Use: Septra I.V. Infusion is not recommended for infants younger than two months of age (see CONTRAINDICATIONS section).

ADVERSE REACTIONS

The most common adverse effects are gastrointestinal disturbances (nausea, vomiting, anorexia) and allergic skin reactions (such as rash and urticaria). **FATALITIES ASSOCIATED WITH THE ADMINISTRATION OF SULFONAMIDES, ALTHOUGH RARE, HAVE OCCURRED DUE TO SEVERE REACTIONS, INCLUDING STEVENS-JOHNSON SYNDROME, TOXIC EPIDERMAL NECROLYSIS, FULMINANT HEPATIC NECROSIS, AGRANULOCYTOSIS, APLASTIC ANEMIA, OTHER BLOOD DYSCRASIAS AND HYPERSENSITIVITY OF THE RESPIRATORY TRACT (SEE WARNINGS SECTION).** Local reaction, pain and slight irritation on I.V. administration are infrequent. Thrombophlebitis has rarely been observed.

Hematologic: Agranulocytosis, aplastic anemia, thrombocytopenia, leukopenia, neutropenia, hemolytic anemia, megaloblastic anemia, hypoprothrombinemia, methemoglobinemia, eosinophilia.

Allergic Reactions: Stevens-Johnson syndrome, toxic epidermal necrolysis, anaphylaxis, allergic myocarditis, erythema multiforme, exfoliative dermatitis, angioedema, drug fever, chills, Henoch-Schoenlein purpura, serum sickness-like syndrome, generalized allergic reactions, generalized skin eruptions, conjunctival and scleral injection, photosensitivity, pruritus, urticaria and rash. In addition, periarteritis nodosa and systemic lupus erythematosus have been reported.

Gastrointestinal: Hepatitis including cholestatic jaundice and hepatic necrosis, elevation of serum transaminase and bilirubin, pseudomembranous enterocolitis, pancreatitis, stomatitis, glossitis, nausea, emesis, abdominal pain, diarrhea, anorexia.

Genitourinary: Renal failure, interstitial nephritis, BUN and serum creatinine elevation, toxic nephrosis with oliguria and anuria, and crystalluria.

Neurologic: Aseptic meningitis, convulsions, peripheral neuritis, ataxia, vertigo, tinnitus, headache.

Psychiatric: Hallucinations, depression, apathy, nervousness.

Endocrine: The sulfonamides bear certain chemical similarities to some goitrogens, diuretics (acetazolamide and the thiazides) and oral hypoglycemic agents. Cross-sensitivity may exist with these agents. Diuresis and hypoglycemia have occurred rarely in patients receiving sulfonamides.

Musculoskeletal: Arthralgia and myalgia.

Respiratory System: Pulmonary infiltrates, cough, shortness of breath.

Miscellaneous: Weakness, fatigue, insomnia.

OVERDOSAGE

Acute: Since there has been no extensive experience in humans with single doses of Septra I.V. Infusion in excess of 25 ml (400 mg trimethoprim and 2000 mg sulfamethoxazole), the maximum tolerated dose in humans is unknown. Signs and symptoms of overdosage reported with sulfonamides include anorexia, colic, nausea, vomiting, dizziness, headache, drowsiness and unconsciousness. Pyrexia, hematuria and crystalluria may be noted. Blood dyscrasias and jaundice are potential late manifestations of overdosage. Signs of acute overdosage with trimethoprim include nausea, vomiting, dizziness, headache, mental depression, confusion and bone marrow depression.

General principles of treatment include the administration of intravenous fluids if urine output is low and renal function is normal. Acidification of the urine will increase renal elimination of trimethoprim. The patient should be monitored with blood counts and appropriate blood chemistries, including electrolytes. If a significant blood dyscrasia or jaundice occurs, specific therapy should be instituted for these complications. Peritoneal dialysis is not effective and hemodialysis is only moderately effective in eliminating trimethoprim and sulfamethoxazole.

Chronic: Use of Septra I.V. Infusion at high doses and/or for extended periods of time may cause bone marrow depression manifested as thrombocytopenia, leukopenia, and/or megaloblastic anemia. If signs of bone marrow depression occur, the patient should be given leucovorin; 5 to 15 mg leucovorin daily has been recommended by some investigators.

Animal Toxicity: The LD_{50} of Septra I.V. Infusion in mice is 700 mg/kg or 7.3 ml/kg; in rats and rabbits the LD_{50} is > 500 mg/kg or > 5.2 ml/kg. The vehicle produced the same LD_{50} in each of these species as the active drug.

The signs and symptoms noted in mice, rats and rabbits with Septra I.V. Infusion or its vehicle at the high I.V. doses used in acute toxicity studies included ataxia, decreased motor activity, loss of righting reflex, tremors or convulsions, and/or respiratory depression.

DOSAGE AND ADMINISTRATION

CONTRAINDICATED IN INFANTS LESS THAN TWO MONTHS OF AGE. CAUTION—SEPTRA I.V. INFUSION MUST BE DILUTED IN 5% DEXTROSE IN WATER SOLUTION PRIOR TO ADMINISTRATION. DO NOT MIX SEPTRA I.V. INFUSION WITH OTHER DRUGS OR SOLUTIONS. RAPID INFUSION OR BOLUS INJECTION MUST BE AVOIDED.

DOSAGE

Children and Adults:
PNEUMOCYSTIS CARINII PNEUMONIA: Total daily dose is 15 to 20 mg/kg (based on the trimethoprim component) given in three to four equally divided doses every 6 or 8 hours for up to 14 days. One investigator noted that a total daily dose of 10 to 15 mg/kg was sufficient in 10 adult patients with normal renal function.[6]
SEVERE URINARY TRACT INFECTIONS AND SHIGELLOSIS: Total daily dose is 8 to 10 mg/kg (based on the trimethoprim component) given in two to four equally divided doses every 6, 8 or 12 hours for up to 14 days for severe urinary tract infections and 5 days for shigellosis. The maximum recommended daily dose is 60 ml per day.

For Patients with Impaired Renal Function: When renal function is impaired, a reduced dosage should be employed using the following table:

Creatinine Clearance (ml/min)	Recommended Dosage Regimen
Above 30	Use Standard Regimen
15–30	½ the Usual Regimen
Below 15	Use Not Recommended

Method of Preparation: Septra I.V. Infusion must be diluted. EACH 5 ML SHOULD BE ADDED TO 125 ML OF 5% DEXTROSE IN WATER. After diluting with 5% dextrose in water the solution should not be refrigerated and should be used within 6 hours. If a dilution of 5 ml per 100 ml of 5% dextrose in water is desired, it should be used within 4 hours. If upon visual inspection there is cloudiness or evidence of crystallization after mixing, the solution should be discarded and a fresh solution prepared.

Multiple Dose Vial: After initial entry into the vial, the remaining contents must be used within 48 hours.

The following infusion systems have been tested and found satisfactory: unit-dose glass containers; unit-dose polyvinyl chloride and polyolefin containers. No other systems have been tested and therefore no others can be recommended.

Dilution: EACH 5 ML OF SEPTRA I.V. INFUSION SHOULD BE ADDED TO 125 ML OF 5% DEXTROSE IN WATER.

NOTE: In those instances where fluid restriction is desirable, each 5 ml may be added to 75 ml of 5% dextrose in water. Under these circumstances the solution should be mixed just prior to use and should be administered within two (2) hours. If upon visual inspection there is cloudiness or evidence of crystallization after mixing, the solution should be discarded and a fresh solution prepared.

DO NOT MIX SEPTRA I.V. INFUSION-5% DEXTROSE IN WATER WITH DRUGS OR SOLUTIONS IN THE SAME CONTAINER.

ADMINISTRATION

The solution should be given by intravenous infusion over a period of 60 to 90 minutes. Rapid infusion or bolus injections must be avoided. Septra I.V. Infusion should not be given intramuscularly.

HOW SUPPLIED

5 ml ampuls, containing 80 mg trimethoprim (16 mg/ml) and 400 mg sulfamethoxazole (80 mg/ml) for infusion with 5% dextrose in water. Box of 10 (NDC-0081-0856-10).

5 ml vials, containing 80 mg trimethoprim (16 mg/ml) and 400 mg sulfamethoxazole (80 mg/ml) for infusion with 5% dextrose in water. Tray of 10 (NDC-0081-0856-44).

10 ml multiple dose vials, containing 160 mg trimethoprim (16 mg/ml) and 800 mg sulfamethoxazole (80 mg/ml) for infusion with 5% dextrose in water. Tray of 10 (NDC-0081-0856-95).

20 ml multiple dose vial, containing 320 mg trimethoprim (16 mg/ml) and 1600 mg sulfamethoxazole (80 mg/ml) for infusion with 5% dextrose in water. Box of 1 (NDC-0081-0856-93).

50 ml multiple dose vial, containing 800 mg trimethoprim (16 mg/ml) and 4000 mg sulfamethoxazole (80 mg/ml) for infusion with 5% dextrose in water. Box of 1 (NDC-0081-0856-02).

STORE AT 15°-25°C (59°-77°F). DO NOT REFRIGERATE. Also available in tablets containing 80 mg trimethoprim and 400 mg sulfamethoxazole (bottles of 100 and 500; unit dose pack of 100); DS (double strength) tablets containing 160 mg trimethoprim and 800 mg sulfamethoxazole (bottles of 100 and 250; unit dose pack of 100, unit of use bottle of 20 with child-resistant cap); and oral suspension containing 40 mg trimethoprim and 200 mg sulfamethoxazole in each 5 ml (pink, cherry flavored: bottle of 1 pint [473 ml]; unit of use bottles of 20 ml—tray of 12, 100 ml—box of 1, 150 ml—tray of 6 and 200 ml—tray of 6 with child-resistant caps; and purple, grape flavored: bottle of 1 pint [473 ml]).

REFERENCES

1. Grose WE, Bodey GP, Loo TL: Clinical Pharmacology of Intravenously Administered Trimethoprim-Sulfamethoxazole. *Antimicrob Agents Chemother* 15: 447–451, March 1979.
2. Siber GR, Gorham C, Durbin W, Lesko L, Levin MJ: Pharmacology of Intravenous Trimethoprim-Sulfamethoxazole in Children and Adults. Current Chemotherapy and Infectious Diseases, American Society for Microbiology, Washington, D.C., 1980, Vol. 1, pp. 691–692.
3. Bauer AW, Kirby WMM, Sherris JC, Turck M: Antibiotic Susceptibility Testing by Standardized Single Disk Method. *Am J Clin Path* 45: 493–496, April 1966.
4. Approved Standard ASM-2 Performance Standards for Antimicrobial Disc Susceptibility Test: National Committee for Clinical Laboratory Standards, 771 East Lancaster Avenue, Villanova, Pennsylvania 19085.
5. Brumfitt W and Pursell R: Trimethoprim/Sulfamethoxazole in the Treatment of Bacteriuria in Women. *J Infect Dis* 128 (Suppl): S657–S663, Nov. 1973.
6. Winston DJ, Lau WK, Gale RP, Young LS: Trimethoprim-Sulfamethoxazole for the Treatment of *Pneumocystis carinii* pneumonia. *Ann Int Med* 92: 762–769, June 1980.
* Mfd. under U.S. Patent No. 3,956,327

SEPTRA® I.V. INFUSION ℞
[sĕp'trah]
ADD-Vantage® Vials
(Trimethoprim and Sulfamethoxazole)

DESCRIPTION

Septra I.V. Infusion (Trimethoprim and Sulfamethoxazole), a sterile solution for intravenous infusion only, is a synthetic antibacterial combination product. Each ml contains 16 mg trimethoprim* and 80 mg sulfamethoxazole compounded with 40% propylene glycol, 10% ethyl alcohol and 0.3% diethanolamine; 1% benzyl alcohol and 0.1% sodium metabisulfite added as preservatives, water for injection, and pH adjusted to approximately 10 with sodium hydroxide.
Trimethoprim is 2,4-diamino-5-(3,4,5-trimethoxybenzyl) pyrimidine. It is a white to light yellow, odorless, bitter compound with a molecular weight of 290.3 and the molecular formula $C_{14}H_{18}N_4O_3$.
Sulfamethoxazole is N^1-(5-methyl-3-isoxazolyl) sulfanilamide. It is an almost white, odorless, tasteless compound with a molecular weight of 253.28 and the molecular formula $C_{10}H_{11}N_3O_3S$.

CLINICAL PHARMACOLOGY

Following a one-hour intravenous infusion of a single dose of 160 mg trimethoprim and 800 mg sulfamethoxazole to 11 patients whose weight ranged from 105 lbs. to 165 lbs. (mean, 143 lbs.), the mean peak plasma concentrations of trimethoprim and sulfamethoxazole were 3.4 ± 0.3 μg/ml and $46.3 \pm$

REPRESENTATIVE MINIMUM INHIBITORY CONCENTRATION VALUES FOR SEPTRA SUSCEPTIBLE ORGANISMS (MIC-μg/ml)

Bacteria	Trimethoprim Alone	Sulfamethoxazole Alone	Trimethoprim/Sulfamethoxazole (1:19) Trimethoprim	Sulfamethoxazole
Escherichia coli	0.05–1.5	1.0–245	0.05–0.5	0.95–9.5
Proteus species (indole positive)	0.5–5.0	7.35–300	0.05–1.5	0.95–28.5
Morganella morganii	0.5–5.0	7.35–300	0.05–1.5	0.95–28.5
Proteus mirabilis	0.5–1.5	7.35–30	0.05–0.15	0.95–2.85
Klebsiella species	0.15–5.0	2.45–245	0.05–1.5	0.95–28.5
Enterobacter species	0.15–5.0	2.45–245	0.05–1.5	0.95–28.5
Haemophilus influenzae	0.15–1.5	2.85–95	0.015–0.15	0.285–2.85
Streptococcus pneumoniae	0.15–1.5	7.35–24.5	0.05–0.15	0.95–2.85
Shigella flexneri †	<0.01–0.04	<0.16–>320	<0.002–0.03	0.04–0.625
Shigella sonnei †	0.02–0.08	0.625–>320	0.004–0.06	0.08–1.25

† Rudoy RC, Nelson JD, Haltalin KC. *Antimicrobial Agents and Chemotherapy* 5:439–43, 1974.

2.7 μg/ml, respectively. Following repeated intravenous administration of the same dose at eight-hour intervals, the mean plasma concentrations just prior to and immediately after each infusion at steady state were 5.6 ± 0.6 μg/ml and 8.8 ± 0.9 μg/ml for trimethoprim and 70.6 ± 7.3 μg/ml and 105.6 ± 10.9 μg/ml for sulfamethoxazole. The mean plasma half-life was 11.3 ± 0.7 hours for trimethoprim and 12.8 ± 1.8 hours for sulfamethoxazole. All of these 11 patients had normal renal function and their ages ranged from 17 to 78 years (median, 60 years)[1].
Pharmacokinetic studies in children and adults suggest an age-dependent half-life of trimethoprim as indicated in the following table.[2]

Age (yrs.)	No. of Patients	Mean Trimethoprim Half-life (hours)
<1	2	7.67
1–10	9	5.49
10–20	5	8.19
20–63	6	12.82

Patients with severely impaired renal function exhibit an increase in the half-lives of both components, requiring dosage regimen adjustment (see DOSAGE AND ADMINISTRATION section).
Both trimethoprim and sulfamethoxazole exist in the blood as unbound, protein-bound and metabolized forms; sulfamethoxazole also exists as the conjugated form. The metabolism of sulfamethoxazole occurs predominately by N_4-acetylation, although the glucuronide conjugate has been identified. The principal metabolites of trimethoprim are the 1- and 3- oxides and the 3'- and 4'-hydroxy derivatives. The free forms of trimethoprim and sulfamethoxazole are considered to be the therapeutically active forms. Approximately 44% of trimethoprim and 70% of sulfamethoxazole are bound to plasma proteins. The presence of 10 mg percent sulfamethoxazole in plasma decreases the protein binding of trimethoprim by an insignificant degree; trimethoprim does not influence the protein binding of sulfamethoxazole.
Excretion of trimethoprim and sulfamethoxazole is primarily by the kidneys through both glomerular filtration and tubular secretion. Urine concentrations of both trimethoprim and sulfamethoxazole are considerably higher than are the concentrations in the blood. The percent of dose excreted in urine over a 12-hour period following the intravenous administration of the first dose of 240 mg of trimethoprim and 1200 mg of sulfamethoxazole on day 1 ranged from 17% to 42.4% as free trimethoprim; 7% to 12.7% as free sulfamethoxazole; and 36.7% to 56% as total (free plus the N_4-acetylated metabolite) sulfamethoxazole. When administered together as Septra, neither trimethoprim nor sulfamethoxazole affects the urinary excretion pattern of the other.
Both trimethoprim and sulfamethoxazole distribute to sputum and vaginal fluid; trimethoprim also distributes to bronchial secretions and both pass the placental barrier and are excreted in breast milk.
Microbiology: Sulfamethoxazole inhibits bacterial synthesis of dihydrofolic acid by competing with *para*-aminobenzoic acid (PABA). Trimethoprim blocks the production of tetrahydrofolic acid from dihydrofolic acid by binding to and reversibly inhibiting the required enzyme, dihydrofolate reductase. Thus, Septra blocks two consecutive steps in the biosynthesis of nucleic acids and proteins essential to many bacteria.
In vitro studies have shown that bacterial resistance develops more slowly with Septra than with trimethoprim or sulfamethoxazole alone.
In vitro serial dilution tests have shown that the spectrum of antibacterial activity of Septra includes common bacterial pathogens with the exception of *Pseudomonas aeruginosa*. The following organisms are usually susceptible: *Escherichia coli*, *Klebsiella* species, *Enterobacter* species, *Morganella morganii*, *Proteus mirabilis*, indole-positive *Proteus* species, including *Proteus vulgaris*, *Haemophilus influenzae* (including ampicillin-resistant strains), *Streptococcus pneumoniae*, *Shigella flexneri* and *Shigella sonnei*. It should be noted, how-

ever, that there are little clinical data on the use of Septra I.V. Infusion in serious systemic infections due to *Haemophilus influenzae* and *Streptococcus pneumoniae*.
[See table above.]
Susceptibility Testing: The recommended quantitative disc susceptibility method may be used for estimating the susceptibility of bacteria to Septra.[3,4] With this procedure, a report from the laboratory of "Susceptible to trimethoprim and sulfamethoxazole" indicates that the infection is likely to respond to therapy with Septra. If the infection is confined to the urine, a report of "Intermediate susceptibility to trimethoprim and sulfamethoxazole" also indicates that the infection is likely to respond. A report of "Resistant to trimethoprim and sulfamethoxazole" indicates that the infection is unlikely to respond to therapy with Septra.

INDICATIONS AND USAGE

PNEUMOCYSTIS CARINII PNEUMONIA: Septra I.V. Infusion is indicated in the treatment of *Pneumocystis carinii* pneumonia in children and adults.
SHIGELLOSIS: Septra I.V. Infusion is indicated in the treatment of enteritis caused by susceptible strains of *Shigella flexneri* and *Shigella sonnei* in children and adults.
URINARY TRACT INFECTIONS: Septra I.V. Infusion is indicated in the treatment of severe or complicated urinary tract infections due to susceptible strains of *Escherichia coli*, *Klebsiella* species, *Enterobacter* species, *Morganella morganii*, and *Proteus* species when oral administration of Septra is not feasible and when the organism is not susceptible to single agent antibacterials effective in the urinary tract.
Although appropriate culture and susceptibility studies should be performed, therapy may be started while awaiting the results of these studies.

CONTRAINDICATIONS

Hypersensitivity to trimethoprim or sulfonamides. Patients with documented megaloblastic anemia due to folate deficiency. Pregnancy at term and during the nursing period, because sulfonamides pass the placenta and are excreted in the milk and may cause kernicterus. Infants less than two months of age.

WARNINGS

FATALITIES ASSOCIATED WITH THE ADMINISTRATION OF SULFONAMIDES, ALTHOUGH RARE, HAVE OCCURRED DUE TO SEVERE REACTIONS, INCLUDING STEVENS-JOHNSON SYNDROME, TOXIC EPIDERMAL NECROLYSIS, FULMINANT HEPATIC NECROSIS, AGRANULOCYTOSIS, APLASTIC ANEMIA, OTHER BLOOD DYSCRASIAS AND HYPERSENSITIVITY OF THE RESPIRATORY TRACT.
SEPTRA SHOULD BE DISCONTINUED AT THE FIRST APPEARANCE OF SKIN RASH OR ANY SIGN OF ADVERSE REACTION. Clinical signs, such as rash, sore throat, fever, arthralgia, cough, shortness of breath, pallor, purpura or jaundice may be early indications of serious reactions. In rare instances, a skin rash may be followed by more severe reactions, such as Stevens-Johnson syndrome, toxic epidermal necrolysis, hepatic necrosis or serious blood disorder. Complete blood counts should be done frequently in patients receiving sulfonamides.
SEPTRA SHOULD NOT BE USED IN THE TREATMENT OF STREPTOCOCCAL PHARYNGITIS. Clinical studies have documented that patients with group A β-hemolytic streptococcal tonsillopharyngitis have a greater incidence of bacteriologic failure when treated with Septra than do those patients treated with penicillin, as evidenced by failure to eradicate this organism from the tonsillopharyngeal area.
Contains sodium metabisulfite, a sulfite that may cause allergic-type reactions, anaphylactic symptoms and life-threatening or less severe asthmatic episodes in certain susceptible people. The overall prevalence of sulfite sensitivity in the general population is unknown and probably low. Sul-

Continued on next page

Burroughs Wellcome—Cont.

fite sensitivity is seen more frequently in asthmatic than in nonasthmatic people.

PRECAUTIONS

General: Septra should be given with caution to patients with impaired renal or hepatic function, to those with possible folate deficiency (e.g., the elderly, chronic alcoholics, patients receiving anticonvulsant therapy, patients with malabsorption syndrome, and patients in malnutrition states) and to those with severe allergy or bronchial asthma. In glucose-6-phosphate dehydrogenase-deficient individuals, hemolysis may occur. This reaction is frequently dose-related. Adequate fluid intake must be maintained in order to prevent crystalluria and stone formation. (See CLINICAL PHARMACOLOGY and DOSAGE AND ADMINISTRATION.)

Local irritation and inflammation due to extravascular infiltration of the infusion has been observed with Septra I.V. Infusion. If these occur the infusion should be discontinued and restarted at another site.

Use in the Elderly: There may be an increased risk of severe adverse reactions in elderly patients, particularly when complicating conditions exist, e.g., impaired kidney and/or liver function, or concomitant use of other drugs. Severe skin reactions, or generalized bone marrow suppression (see WARNINGS and ADVERSE REACTIONS sections) or a specific decrease in platelets (with or without purpura) are the most frequently reported severe adverse reactions in elderly patients. In those concurrently receiving certain diuretics, primarily thiazides, an increased incidence of thrombocytopenia with purpura has been reported. Appropriate dosage adjustments should be made for patients with impaired kidney function (see DOSAGE AND ADMINISTRATION section).

Use in the Treatment of *Pneumocystis carinii* Pneumonia in Patients with Acquired Immunodeficiency Syndrome (AIDS): The incidence of side effects, particularly rash, fever, leukopenia, and elevated aminotransferase (transaminase) values with Septra therapy in AIDS patients who are being treated for *Pneumocystis carinii* pneumonia has been reported to be greatly increased compared with the incidence normally associated with the use of Septra in non-AIDS patients.

Laboratory Tests: Appropriate culture and susceptibility studies should be performed before and throughout treatment. Complete blood counts should be done frequently in patients receiving Septra; if a significant reduction in the count of any formed blood element is noted, Septra should be discontinued. Urinalyses with careful microscopic examination and renal function tests should be performed during therapy, particularly for those patients with impaired renal function.

Drug Interactions: In elderly patients concurrently receiving certain diuretics, primarily thiazides, an increased incidence of thrombocytopenia with purpura has been reported. It has been reported that Septra may prolong the prothrombin time in patients who are receiving the anticoagulant warfarin. This interaction should be kept in mind when Septra is given to patients already on anticoagulant therapy, and the coagulation time should be reassessed.

Septra may inhibit the hepatic metabolism of phenytoin. Septra, given at a common clinical dosage, increased the phenytoin half-life by 39% and decreased the phenytoin metabolic clearance rate by 27%. When administering these drugs concurrently, one should be alert for possible excessive phenytoin effect.

Sulfonamides can also displace methotrexate from plasma protein binding sites, thus increasing free methotrexate concentrations.

Drug/Laboratory Test Interactions: Septra, specifically the trimethoprim component, can interfere with a serum methotrexate assay as determined by the competitive binding protein technique (CBPA) when a bacterial dihydrofolate reductase is used as the binding protein. No interference occurs, however, if methotrexate is measured by a radioimmunoassay (RIA).

The presence of trimethoprim and sulfamethoxazole may also interfere with the Jaffé alkaline picrate reaction assay for creatinine resulting in over-estimations of about 10% in the range of normal values.

Carcinogenesis, Mutagenesis, Impairment of Fertility:
Carcinogenesis: Long-term studies in animals to evaluate carcinogenic potential have not been conducted with Septra I.V. Infusion.

Mutagenesis: Bacterial mutagenic studies have not been performed with sulfamethoxazole and trimethoprim in combination. Trimethoprim was demonstrated to be non-mutagenic in the Ames assay. In studies at two laboratories no chromosomal damage was detected in cultured Chinese hamster ovary cells at concentrations approximately 500 times human plasma levels; at concentrations approximately 1000 times human plasma levels in these same cells a low level of chromosomal damage was induced at one of the laboratories.

No chromosomal abnormalities were observed in cultured human leukocytes at concentrations of trimethoprim up to 20 times human steady state plasma levels. No chromosomal effects were detected in peripheral lymphocytes of human subjects receiving 320 mg of trimethoprim in combination with up to 1600 mg of sulfamethoxazole per day for as long as 112 weeks.

Impairment of Fertility: Septra I.V. Infusion has not been studied in animals for evidence of impairment of fertility. However, studies in rats at oral dosages as high as 70 mg/kg trimethoprim plus 350 mg/kg sulfamethoxazole daily showed no adverse effects on fertility or general reproductive performance.

Pregnancy: *Teratogenic Effects:* Pregnancy Category C. In rats, oral doses of 533 mg/kg sulfamethoxazole or 200 mg/kg trimethoprim produced teratological effects manifested mainly as cleft palates. The highest dose which did not cause cleft palates in rats was 512 mg/kg sulfamethoxazole or 192 mg/kg trimethoprim when administered separately. In two studies in rats, no teratology was observed when 512 mg/kg of sulfamethoxazole was used in combination with 128 mg/kg of trimethoprim. In one study, however, cleft palates were observed in one litter out of 9 when 355 mg/kg of sulfamethoxazole was used in combination with 88 mg/kg of trimethoprim.

In some rabbit studies, an overall increase in fetal loss (dead and resorbed and malformed conceptuses) was associated with doses of trimethoprim 6 times the human therapeutic dose.

While there are no large, well-controlled studies on the use of trimethoprim and sulfamethoxazole in pregnant women, Brumfitt and Pursell[5], in a retrospective study, reported the outcome of 186 pregnancies during which the mother received either placebo or oral trimethoprim and sulfamethoxazole. The incidence of congenital abnormalities was 4.5% (3 of 66) in those who received placebo and 3.3% (4 of 120) in those receiving trimethoprim and sulfamethoxazole. There were no abnormalities in the 10 children whose mothers received the drug during the first trimester. In a separate survey, Brumfitt and Pursell also found no congenital abnormalities in 35 children whose mothers had received oral trimethoprim and sulfamethoxazole at the time of conception or shortly thereafter.

Because trimethoprim and sulfamethoxazole may interfere with folic acid metabolism, Septra I.V. Infusion should be used during pregnancy only if the potential benefit justifies the potential risk to the fetus.

Nonteratogenic Effects: See CONTRAINDICATIONS section.

Nursing Mothers: See CONTRAINDICATIONS section.

Pediatric Use: Septra I.V. Infusion is not recommended for infants younger than two months of age (see CONTRAINDICATIONS section).

ADVERSE REACTIONS

The most common adverse effects are gastrointestinal disturbances (nausea, vomiting, anorexia) and allergic skin reactions (such as rash and urticaria). **FATALITIES ASSOCIATED WITH THE ADMINISTRATION OF SULFONAMIDES, ALTHOUGH RARE, HAVE OCCURRED DUE TO SEVERE REACTIONS, INCLUDING STEVENS-JOHNSON SYNDROME, TOXIC EPIDERMAL NECROLYSIS, FULMINANT HEPATIC NECROSIS, AGRANULOCYTOSIS, APLASTIC ANEMIA, OTHER BLOOD DYSCRASIAS AND HYPERSENSITIVITY OF THE RESPIRATORY TRACT (SEE WARNINGS SECTION).** Local reaction, pain and slight irritation on I.V. administration are infrequent. Thrombophlebitis has rarely been observed.

Hematologic: Agranulocytosis, aplastic anemia, thrombocytopenia, leukopenia, neutropenia, hemolytic anemia, megaloblastic anemia, hypoprothrombinemia, methemoglobinemia, eosinophilia.

Allergic Reactions: Stevens-Johnson syndrome, toxic epidermal necrolysis, anaphylaxis, allergic myocarditis, erythema multiforme, exfoliative dermatitis, angioedema, drug fever, chills, Henoch-Schoenlein purpura, serum sickness-like syndrome, generalized allergic reactions, generalized skin eruptions, conjunctival and scleral injection, photosensitivity, pruritus, urticaria and rash. In addition, periarteritis nodosa and systemic lupus erythematosus have been reported.

Gastrointestinal: Hepatitis including cholestatic jaundice and hepatic necrosis, elevation of serum transaminase and bilirubin, pseudomembranous enterocolitis, pancreatitis, stomatitis, glossitis, nausea, emesis, abdominal pain, diarrhea, anorexia.

Genitourinary: Renal failure, interstitial nephritis, BUN and serum creatinine elevation, toxic nephrosis with oliguria and anuria, and crystalluria.

Neurologic: Aseptic meningitis, convulsions, peripheral neuritis, ataxia, vertigo, tinnitus, headache.

Psychiatric: Hallucinations, depression, apathy, nervousness.

Endocrine: The sulfonamides bear certain chemical similarities to some goitrogens, diuretics (acetazolamide and the thiazides) and oral hypoglycemic agents. Cross-sensitivity

may exist with these agents. Diuresis and hypoglycemia have occurred rarely in patients receiving sulfonamides.
Musculoskeletal: Arthralgia and myalgia.
Respiratory System: Pulmonary infiltrates, cough, shortness of breath.
Miscellaneous: Weakness, fatigue, insomnia.

OVERDOSAGE

Acute: Since there has been no extensive experience in humans with single doses of Septra I.V. Infusion in excess of 25 ml (400 mg trimethoprim and 2000 mg sulfamethoxazole), the maximum tolerated dose in humans is unknown. Signs and symptoms of overdosage reported with sulfonamides include anorexia, colic, nausea, vomiting, dizziness, headache, drowsiness and unconsciousness. Pyrexia, hematuria and crystalluria may be noted. Blood dyscrasias and jaundice are potential late manifestations of overdosage. Signs of acute overdosage with trimethoprim include nausea, vomiting, dizziness, headache, mental depression, confusion and bone marrow depression.

General principles of treatment include the administration of intravenous fluids if urine output is low and renal function is normal. Acidification of the urine will increase renal elimination of trimethoprim. The patient should be monitored with blood counts and appropriate blood chemistries, including electrolytes. If a significant blood dyscrasia or jaundice occurs, specific therapy should be instituted for these complications. Peritoneal dialysis is not effective and hemodialysis is only moderately effective in eliminating trimethoprim and sulfamethoxazole.

Chronic: Use of Septra I.V. Infusion at high doses and/or for extended periods of time may cause bone marrow depression manifested as thrombocytopenia, leukopenia, and/or megaloblastic anemia. If signs of bone marrow depression occur, the patient should be given leucovorin; 5 to 15 mg leucovorin daily has been recommended by some investigators.

Animal Toxicity: The LD_{50} of Septra I.V. Infusion in mice is 700 mg/kg or 7.3 ml/kg; in rats and rabbits the LD_{50} is > 500 mg /kg or > 5.2 ml/kg. The vehicle produced the same LD_{50} in each of these species as the active drug.

The signs and symptoms noted in mice, rats and rabbits with Septra I.V. Infusion or its vehicle at the high I.V. doses used in acute toxicity studies included ataxia, decreased motor activity, loss of righting reflex, tremors or convulsions, and /or respiratory depression.

DOSAGE AND ADMINISTRATION

CONTRAINDICATED IN INFANTS LESS THAN TWO MONTHS OF AGE. CAUTION—SEPTRA I.V. INFUSION MUST BE DILUTED IN 5% DEXTROSE IN WATER SOLUTION PRIOR TO ADMINISTRATION. DO NOT MIX SEPTRA I.V. INFUSION WITH OTHER DRUGS OR SOLUTIONS. RAPID INFUSION OR BOLUS INJECTION MUST BE AVOIDED.

DOSAGE

Children and Adults:
PNEUMOCYSTIS CARINII PNEUMONIA: Total daily dose is 15 to 20 mg/kg (based on the trimethoprim component) given in three to four equally divided doses every 6 to 8 hours for up to 14 days. One investigator noted that a total daily dose of 10 to 15 mg/kg was sufficient in 10 adult patients with normal renal function.[6]

SEVERE URINARY TRACT INFECTIONS AND SHIGELLOSIS: Total daily dose is 8 to 10 mg/kg (based on the trimethoprim component) given in two to four equally divided doses every 6, 8 or 12 hours for up to 14 days for severe urinary tract infections and 5 days for shigellosis. The maximum recommended daily dose is 60 ml per day.

For Patients with Impaired Renal Function: When renal function is impaired, a reduced dosage should be employed using the following table:

Creatinine Clearance (ml/min)	Recommended Dosage Regimen
Above 30	Use Standard Regimen
15–30	½ the Usual Regimen
Below 15	Use Not Recommended

Method of Preparation: Septra I.V. Infusion must be diluted. EACH 10 ML ADD-Vantage VIAL SHOULD BE ADDED TO 250 ML OF 5% DEXTROSE IN WATER AND USED WITHIN SIX (6) HOURS. EACH 5 ML ADD-Vantage VIAL SHOULD BE ADDED TO 100 ML OF 5% DEXTROSE IN WATER AND USED WITHIN SIX (6) HOURS. If upon visual inspection there is cloudiness or evidence of crystallization after mixing, the solution should be discarded and a fresh solution prepared.

DO NOT MIX SEPTRA I.V. INFUSION-5% DEXTROSE IN WATER WITH DRUGS OR SOLUTIONS IN THE SAME CONTAINER.

After diluting with 5% dextrose in water, the solution should not be refrigerated and should be administered within the specified time.

ADMINISTRATION

The solution should be given by intravenous infusion over a period of 60 to 90 minutes. Rapid infusion or bolus injections must be avoided. Septra I.V. Infusion should not be given intramuscularly.

INSTRUCTIONS FOR USE

To Open Diluent Container:

Peel overwrap from the corner and remove container. Some opacity of the plastic due to moisture absorption during the sterilization process may be observed. This is normal and does not affect the solution quality or safety. The opacity will diminish gradually.

To Assemble ADD-Vantage® Vial and Flexible Diluent Container:

(Use Aseptic Technique)

1. Remove the protective covers from the top of the vial and the vial port on the diluent container as follows:
   a. To remove the breakaway vial cap, swing the pull ring over the top of the vial and pull down far enough to start the opening (SEE FIGURE 1), then pull straight up to remove the cap. (SEE FIGURE 2.) **NOTE:** Once the breakaway cap has been removed, do not access vial with syringe.

Fig. 1

Fig. 2

   b. To remove the vial port cover, grasp the tab on the pull ring, pull up to break the three tie strings, then pull back to remove the cover. (SEE FIGURE 3.)
2. Screw the vial into the vial port until it will go no further. THE VIAL MUST BE SCREWED IN TIGHTLY TO ASSURE A SEAL. This occurs approximately ½ turn (180°) after the first audible click. (SEE FIGURE 4.) The clicking sound does not assure a seal; the vial must be turned as far as it will go. **NOTE:** Once vial is seated, do not attempt to remove. (SEE FIGURE 4.)
3. Recheck the vial to assure that it is tight by trying to turn it further in the direction of assembly.
4. Label appropriately.

Fig. 3

Fig. 4

To Prepare Admixture:

1. Squeeze the bottom of the diluent container gently to inflate the portion of the container surrounding the end of the drug vial.
2. With the other hand, push the drug vial down into the container telescoping the walls of the container. Grasp the inner cap of the vial through the walls of the container. (SEE FIGURE 5.)
3. Pull the inner cap from the drug vial. (SEE FIGURE 6.) Verify that the rubber stopper has been pulled out, allowing the drug and diluent to mix.
4. Mix container contents thoroughly and use within the specified time.

Fig. 5

Fig. 6

Preparation for Administration:

(Use Aseptic Technique)

1. Confirm the activation and admixture of vial contents.
2. Check for leaks by squeezing container firmly. If leaks are found, discard unit as sterility may be impaired.
3. Close flow control clamp of administration set.
4. Remove cover from outlet port at bottom of container.
5. Insert piercing pin of administration set into port with a twisting motion until the pin is firmly seated. **NOTE:** See full directions on administration set carton.
6. Lift the free end of the hanger loop on the bottom of the vial, breaking the two tie strings. Bend the loop outward to lock it in the upright position, then suspend container from hanger.
7. Squeeze and release drip chamber to establish proper fluid level in chamber.
8. Open flow control clamp and clear air from set. Close clamp.
9. Attach set to venipuncture device. If device is not indwelling, prime and make venipuncture.
10. Regulate rate of administration with flow control clamp.

WARNING

Do not use flexible container in series connections.

HOW SUPPLIED

5 ml ADD-Vantage® Vial, containing 80 mg trimethoprim (16 mg/ml) and 400 mg sulfamethoxazole (80 mg/ml) for infusion with 5% dextrose in water. Box of 10 (NDC-0081-0856-50).
10 ml ADD-Vantage® Vial containing 160 mg trimethoprim (16 mg/ml) and 800 mg sulfamethoxazole (80 mg/ml) for infusion with 5% dextrose in water. Box of 10 (NDC-0081-0856-47).
STORE AT 15°–25°C (59°–77°F).
DO NOT REFRIGERATE.
Also Available:
Septra I.V. Infusion 5 ml ampuls, containing 80 mg trimethoprim (16 mg/ml) and 400 mg sulfamethoxazole (80 mg/ml), box of 10; 5 ml vials, containing 80 mg trimethoprim (16 mg/ml) and 400 mg sulfamethoxazole (80 mg/ml), tray of 10; 10 ml multiple dose vials, containing 160 mg trimethoprim (16 mg/ml) and 800 mg sulfamethoxazole (80 mg/ml), tray of 10; 20 ml multiple dose vial, containing 320 mg trimethoprim (16 mg/ml) and 1600 mg sulfamethoxazole (80 mg/ml), box of 1.

REFERENCES

1. Grose WE, Bodey GP, Loo TL: Clinical Pharmacology of Intravenously Administered Trimethoprim-Sulfamethoxazole. *Antimicrob Agents Chemother 15*: 447–451, March 1979.
2. Siber GR, Gorham C, Durbin W, Lesko L, Levin MJ: Pharmacology of Intravenous Trimethoprim-Sulfamethoxazole in Children and Adults. Current Chemotherapy and Infectious Diseases, American Society for Microbiology, Washington, D.C., 1980, Vol. 1, pp. 691–692.
3. Bauer AW, Kirby WMM, Sherris JC, Turck M: Antibiotic Susceptibility Testing by Standardized Single Disk Method. *Am J Clin Path 45*: 493–496, April 1966.
4. Approved Standard ASM-2 Performance Standards for Antimicrobial Disc Susceptibility Test: National Committee for Clinical Laboratory Standards, 771 East Lancaster Avenue, Villanova, Pennsylvania 19085.
5. Brumfitt W and Pursell R: Trimethoprim/Sulfamethoxazole in the Treatment of Bacteriuria in Women. *J Infect Dis 128 (Suppl)*: S657–S663, Nov. 1973.
6. Winston DJ, Lau WK, Gale RP, Young LS: Trimethoprim-Sulfamethoxazole for the Treatment of *Pneumocystis carinii* pneumonia. *Ann Int Med 92*: 762–769, June 1980.
*Mfd. under U.S. Patent No. 3,956,327

SEPTRA® TABLETS   ℞
[sĕp'trah]
SEPTRA ® DS (Double Strength) TABLETS   ℞
SEPTRA® SUSPENSION   ℞
SEPTRA® GRAPE SUSPENSION   ℞
(Trimethoprim and Sulfamethoxazole)

DESCRIPTION

Septra (Trimethoprim and Sulfamethoxazole) is a synthetic antibacterial combination product. Each Septra Tablet contains 80 mg trimethoprim* and 400 mg sulfamethoxazole and the inactive ingredients docusate sodium, FD&C Red No. 40, magnesium stearate, povidone, and sodium starch glycolate.
Each Septra DS (double strength) Tablet contains 160 mg trimethoprim* and 800 mg sulfamethoxazole and the inactive ingredients docusate sodium, FD&C Red No. 40, magnesium stearate, povidone, and sodium starch glycolate.
Each teaspoonful (5 ml) of Septra Suspension contains 40 mg trimethoprim* and 200 mg sulfamethoxazole and the inactive ingredients alcohol 0.26%, methylparaben 0.1% and sodium benzoate 0.1% (added as preservatives), carboxymethylcellulose sodium, citric acid, FD&C Red No. 40 and Yellow No. 6, flavor, glycerin, microcrystalline cellulose, polysorbate 80, saccharin sodium, and sorbitol. Each teaspoonful (5 ml) of Septra Grape Suspension contains 40 mg trimethoprim* and 200 mg sulfamethoxazole and the inactive ingredients alcohol 0.26%, methylparaben 0.1% and sodium benzoate 0.1% (added as preservatives), carboxymethylcellulose sodium, citric acid, FD&C Red No. 40 and Blue No. 1, flavor, glycerin, microcrystalline cellulose, polysorbate 80, saccharin sodium, and sorbitol. Both tablet and suspension forms are for oral administration.
Trimethoprim is 2,4-diamino-5-(3,4,5-trimethoxybenzyl)-pyrimidine. It is a white to light yellow, odorless, bitter compound with a molecular weight of 290.3, and the molecular formula $C_{14}H_{18}N_4O_3$.
Sulfamethoxazole is N^1-(5-methyl-3-isoxazolyl)sulfanilamide. It is an almost white, odorless, tasteless compound with a molecular weight of 253.28, and the molecular formula $C_{10}H_{11}N_3O_3S$.

CLINICAL PHARMACOLOGY

Septra is rapidly absorbed following oral administration. Both sulfamethoxazole and trimethoprim exist in the blood as unbound, protein-bound and metabolized forms; sulfamethoxazole also exists as the conjugated form. The metabolism of sulfamethoxazole occurs predominately by N_4-acetylation, although the glucuronide conjugate has been identified. The principal metabolites of trimethoprim are the 1- and 3-oxides and the 3'- and 4'-hydroxy derivatives. The free forms of sulfamethoxazole and trimethoprim are considered to be the therapeutically active forms. Approximately 44% of trimethoprim and 70% of sulfamethoxazole are bound to plasma proteins. The presence of 10 mg percent sulfamethoxazole in plasma decreases the protein binding of trimethoprim by an insignificant degree; trimethoprim does not influence the protein binding of sulfamethoxazole.
Peak blood levels for the individual components occur 1 to 4 hours after oral administration. The mean serum half-lives of sulfamethoxazole and trimethoprim are 10 and 8 to 10 hours, respectively. However, patients with severely impaired renal function exhibit an increase in the half-lives of both components, requiring dosage regimen adjustment (see DOSAGE AND ADMINISTRATION section). Detectable amounts of trimethoprim and sulfamethoxazole are present in the blood 24 hours after drug administration. During administration of 160 mg trimethoprim and 800 mg sulfamethoxazole *b.i.d.*, the mean steady state plasma concentration of trimethoprim was 1.72 µg/ml. The steady state minimal plasma levels of free and total sulfamethoxazole were 57.4 µg/ml and 68.0 µg/ml, respectively. These steady state levels were achieved after three days of drug administration.[1]

Excretion of sulfamethoxazole and trimethoprim is primarily by the kidneys through both glomerular filtration and tubular secretion. Urine concentrations of both sulfamethox-

Continued on next page

Burroughs Wellcome—Cont.

azole and trimethoprim are considerably higher than are the concentrations in the blood. The average percentage of the dose recovered in urine from 0 to 72 hours after a single oral dose is 84.5% for total sulfonamide and 66.8% for free trimethoprim. Thirty percent of the total sulfonamide is excreted as free sulfamethoxazole, with the remaining as N_4-acetylated metabolite.[2] When administered together as Septra, neither sulfamethoxazole nor trimethoprim affects the urinary excretion pattern of the other.

Both trimethoprim and sulfamethoxazole distribute to sputum, vaginal fluid, and middle ear fluid; trimethoprim also distributes to bronchial secretion and both pass the placental barrier and are excreted in human milk.

Microbiology: Sulfamethoxazole inhibits bacterial synthesis of dihydrofolic acid by competing with *para*-aminobenzoic acid (PABA). Trimethoprim blocks the production of tetrahydrofolic acid from dihydrofolic acid by binding to and reversibly inhibiting the required enzyme, dihydrofolate reductase. Thus, Septra blocks two consecutive steps in the biosynthesis of nucleic acids and proteins essential to many bacteria.

In vitro studies have shown that bacterial resistance develops more slowly with Septra than with either trimethoprim or sulfamethoxazole alone.

In vitro serial dilution tests have shown that the spectrum of antibacterial activity of Septra includes the common urinary tract pathogens with the exception of *Pseudomonas aeruginosa*. The following organisms are usually susceptible: *Escherichia coli, Klebsiella* species, *Enterobacter* species, *Morganella morganii, Proteus mirabilis* and indole-positive *Proteus* species including *Proteus vulgaris*.

The usual spectrum of antimicrobial activity of Septra includes bacterial pathogens isolated from middle ear exudate and from bronchial secretions: *Haemophilus influenzae,* including ampicillin-resistant strains, and *Streptococcus pneumoniae. Shigella flexneri* and *Shigella sonnei* are also usually susceptible.

[See table below].

Susceptibility Testing: The recommended quantitative disc susceptibility method may be used for estimating the susceptibility of bacteria to Septra.[3,4] With this procedure, a report from the laboratory of "Susceptible to trimethoprim and sulfamethoxazole" indicates that the infection is likely to respond to therapy with Septra. If the infection is confined to the urine, a report of "Intermediate susceptibility to trimethoprim and sulfamethoxazole" also indicates that the infection is likely to respond. A report of "Resistant to trimethoprim and sulfamethoxazole" indicates that the infection is unlikely to respond to therapy with Septra.

INDICATIONS AND USAGE

URINARY TRACT INFECTIONS: For the treatment of urinary tract infections due to susceptible strains of the following organisms: *Escherichia coli, Klebsiella* species, *Enterobacter* species, *Morganella morganii, Proteus mirabilis,* and *Proteus vulgaris.* It is recommended that initial episodes of uncomplicated urinary tract infections be treated with a single effective antibacterial agent rather than the combination.

ACUTE OTITIS MEDIA: For the treatment of acute otitis media in children due to susceptible strains of *Streptococcus pneumoniae* or *Haemophilus influenzae* when in the judgment of the physician Septra offers some advantage over the use of other antimicrobial agents. To date, there are limited data on the safety of repeated use of Septra in children under two years of age. Septra is not indicated for prophylactic or prolonged administration in otitis media at any age.

ACUTE EXACERBATIONS OF CHRONIC BRONCHITIS IN ADULTS: For the treatment of acute exacerbations of chronic bronchitis due to susceptible strains of *Streptococcus pneumoniae* or *Haemophilus influenzae* when in the judgment of the physician, Septra offers some advantage over the use of a single antimicrobial agent.

SHIGELLOSIS: For the treatment of enteritis caused by susceptible strains of *Shigella flexneri* and *Shigella sonnei* when antibacterial therapy is indicated.

PNEUMOCYSTIS CARINII PNEUMONIA: For the treatment of documented *Pneumocystis carinii* pneumonia.

CONTRAINDICATIONS

Hypersensitivity to trimethoprim or sulfonamides. Patients with documented megaloblastic anemia due to folate deficiency. Pregnancy at term and during the nursing period, because sulfonamides pass the placenta and are excreted in the milk and may cause kernicterus. Infants less than two months of age.

WARNINGS

FATALITIES ASSOCIATED WITH THE ADMINISTRATION OF SULFONAMIDES, ALTHOUGH RARE, HAVE OCCURRED DUE TO SEVERE REACTIONS, INCLUDING STEVENS-JOHNSON SYNDROME, TOXIC EPIDERMAL NECROLYSIS, FULMINANT HEPATIC NECROSIS, AGRANULOCYTOSIS, APLASTIC ANEMIA, OTHER BLOOD DYSCRASIAS AND HYPERSENSITIVITY OF THE RESPIRATORY TRACT.

SEPTRA SHOULD BE DISCONTINUED AT THE FIRST APPEARANCE OF SKIN RASH OR ANY SIGN OF ADVERSE REACTION. Clinical signs, such as rash, sore throat, fever, arthralgia, cough, shortness of breath, pallor, purpura or jaundice may be early indications of serious reactions. In rare instances a skin rash may be followed by more severe reactions, such as Stevens-Johnson syndrome, toxic epidermal necrolysis, hepatic necrosis or serious blood disorder. Complete blood counts should be done frequently in patients receiving sulfonamides.

SEPTRA SHOULD NOT BE USED IN THE TREATMENT OF STREPTOCOCCAL PHARYNGITIS. Clinical studies have documented that patients with group A β-hemolytic streptococcal tonsillopharyngitis have a greater incidence of bacteriologic failure when treated with Septra than do those patients treated with penicillin, as evidenced by failure to eradicate this organism from the tonsillopharyngeal area.

PRECAUTIONS

General: Septra should be given with caution to patients with impaired renal or hepatic function, to those with possible folate deficiency (e.g., the elderly, chronic alcoholics, patients receiving anticonvulsant therapy, patients with malabsorption syndrome, and patients in malnutrition states) and to those with severe allergy or bronchial asthma. In glucose-6-phosphate dehydrogenase-deficient individuals, hemolysis may occur. This reaction is frequently dose-related. (See CLINICAL PHARMACOLOGY and DOSAGE AND ADMINISTRATION.)

Use in the Elderly: There may be an increased risk of severe adverse reactions in elderly patients, particularly when complicating conditions exist, e.g., impaired kidney and/or liver function, or concomitant use of other drugs. Severe skin reactions, or generalized bone marrow suppression (see WARNINGS and ADVERSE REACTIONS sections) or a specific decrease in platelets (with or without purpura) are the most frequently reported severe adverse reactions in elderly patients. In those concurrently receiving certain diuretics, primarily thiazides, an increased incidence of thrombocytopenia with purpura has been reported. Appropriate dosage adjustments should be made for patients with impaired kidney function (see DOSAGE AND AMDINISTRATION section).

Use in the Treatment of *Pneumocystis carinii* **Pneumonia in Patients with Acquired Immunodeficiency Syndrome (AIDS):** The incidence of side effects, particularly rash, fever, leukopenia, and elevated aminotransferase (transaminase) values with Septra therapy in AIDS patients who are being treated for *Pneumocystis carinii* pneumonia has been reported to be greatly increased compared with the incidence normally associated with the use of Septra in non-AIDS patients.

Information for Patients: Patients should be instructed to maintain an adequate fluid intake in order to prevent crystalluria and stone formation.

Laboratory Tests: Complete blood counts should be done frequently in patients receiving Septra; if a significant reduction in the count of any formed blood element is noted, Septra should be discontinued. Urinalysis with careful microscopic examination and renal function tests should be performed during therapy, particularly for those patients with impaired renal function.

Drug Interactions: In elderly patients concurrently receiving certain diuretics, primarily thiazides, an increased incidence of thrombocytopenia with purpura has been reported. It has been reported that Septra may prolong the prothrombin time in patients who are receiving the anticoagulant warfarin. This interaction should be kept in mind when Septra is given to patients already on anticoagulant therapy, and the coagulation time should be reassessed.

Septra may inhibit the hepatic metabolism of phenytoin. Septra, given at a common clinical dosage, increased the phenytoin half-life by 39% and decreased the phenytoin metabolic clearance rate by 27%. When administering these drugs concurrently, one should be alert for possible excessive phenytoin effect.

Sulfonamides can also displace methotrexate from plasma protein binding sites, thus increasing free methotrexate concentrations.

Drug/Laboratory Test Interactions: Septra, specifically the trimethoprim component, can interfere with a serum methotrexate assay as determined by the competitive binding protein technique (CBPA) when a bacterial dihydrofolate reductase is used as the binding protein. No interference occurs, however, if methotrexate is measured by a radioimmunoassay (RIA).

The presence of trimethoprim and sulfamethoxazole may also interfere with the Jaffé alkaline picrate reaction assay for creatinine resulting in over-estimations of about 10% in the range of normal values.

Carcinogenesis, Mutagenesis, Impairment of Fertility:
Carcinogenesis: Long-term studies in animals to evaluate carcinogenic potential have not been conducted with Septra. *Mutagenesis:* Bacterial mutagenic studies have not been performed with sulfamethoxazole and trimethoprim in combination. Trimethoprim was demonstrated to be non-mutagenic in the Ames assay. In studies at two laboratories no chromosomal damage was detected in cultured Chinese hamster ovary cells at concentrations approximately 500 times human plasma levels; at concentrations approximately 1000 times human plasma levels in this same cells a low level of chromosomal damage was induced at one of the laboratories. No chromosomal abnormalities were observed in cultured human leukocytes at concentrations of trimethoprim up to 20 times human steady state plasma levels. No chromosomal effects were detected in peripheral lymphocytes of human subjects receiving 320 mg of trimethoprim in combination with up to 1600 mg of sulfamethoxazole per day for as long as 112 weeks.

Impairment of Fertility: No adverse effects on fertility or general reproductive performance were observed in rats given oral dosages as high as 70 mg/kg/day trimethoprim plus 350 mg/kg/day sulfamethoxazole.

Pregnancy: *Teratogenic Effects:* Pregnancy Category C. In rats, oral doses of 533 mg/kg sulfamethoxazole or 200 mg/kg trimethoprim produced teratological effects manifested mainly as cleft palates. The highest dose which did not cause cleft palates in rats was 512 mg/kg sulfamethoxazole or 192 mg/kg trimethoprim when administered separately. In two studies in rats, no teratology was observed when 512 mg/kg of sulfamethoxazole was used in combination with 128 mg/kg of trimethoprim. In one study, however, cleft palates were observed in one litter out of 9 when 355 mg/kg of sulfamethoxazole was used in combination with 88 mg/kg of trimethoprim.

In some rabbit studies, an overall increase in fetal loss (dead and resorbed and malformed conceptuses) was associated with doses of trimethoprim 6 times the human therapeutic dose.

While there are no large, well-controlled studies on the use of trimethoprim and sulfamethoxazole in pregnant women, Brumfitt and Pursell[5], in a retrospective study, reported the outcome of 186 pregnancies during which the mother received either placebo or trimethoprim and sulfamethoxazole. The incidence of congenital abnormalities was 4.5% (3 of 66) in those who received placebo and 3.3% (4 of 120) in those receiving trimethoprim and sulfamethoxazole. There were no abnormalities in the 10 children whose mothers received the drug during the first trimester. In a separate survey, Brumfitt and Pursell also found no congenital abnormalities in 35 children whose mothers had received oral

REPRESENTATIVE MINIMUM INHIBITORY CONCENTRATION VALUES FOR SEPTRA SUSCEPTIBLE ORGANISMS
(MIC-μg/ml)

Bacteria	TMP Alone	SMX Alone	TMP/SMX (1:19) TMP	TMP/SMX (1:19) SMX
Escherichia coli	0.05–1.5	1.0–245	0.05–0.5	0.95–9.5
Proteus species (indole positive)	0.5–5.0	7.35–300	0.05–1.5	0.95–28.5
Morganella morganii	0.5–5.0	7.35–300	0.05–1.5	0.95–28.5
Proteus mirabilis	0.5–1.5	7.35–30	0.05–0.15	0.95–2.85
Klebsiella species	0.15–5.0	2.45–245	0.05–1.5	0.95–28.5
Enterobacter species	0.15–5.0	2.45–245	0.05–1.5	0.95–28.5
Haemophilus influenzae	0.15–1.5	2.85–95	0.015–0.15	0.285–2.85
Streptococcus pneumoniae	0.15–1.5	7.35–24.5	0.05–0.15	0.95–2.85
Shigella flexneri †	<0.01–0.04	<0.16–>320	<0.002–0.03	0.04–0.625
Shigella sonnei †	0.02–0.08	0.625–>320	0.004–0.06	0.08–1.25

TMP = Trimethoprim   SMX = Sulfamethoxazole

†Rudoy RC, Nelson JD, Haltalin KC. *Antimicrobial Agents and Chemotherapy* 5:439-43, 1974.

trimethoprim and sulfamethoxazole at the time of conception or shortly thereafter.

Because trimethoprim and sulfamethoxazole may interfere with folic acid metabolism, Septra should be used during pregnancy only if the potential benefit justifies the potential risk to the fetus.

Nonteratogenic Effects: See CONTRAINDICATIONS section.

Nursing Mothers: See CONTRAINDICATIONS section.

Pediatric Use: Septra is not recommended for infants younger than two months of age (see INDICATIONS AND USAGE and CONTRAINDICATIONS sections).

ADVERSE REACTIONS

The most common adverse effects are gastrointestinal disturbances (nausea, vomiting, anorexia) and allergic skin reactions (such as rash and urticaria). **FATALITIES ASSOCIATED WITH THE ADMINISTRATION OF SULFONAMIDES, ALTHOUGH RARE, HAVE OCCURRED DUE TO SEVERE REACTIONS, INCLUDING STEVENS-JOHNSON SYNDROME, TOXIC EPIDERMAL NECROLYSIS, FULMINANT HEPATIC NECROSIS, AGRANULOCYTOSIS, APLASTIC ANEMIA, OTHER BLOOD DYSCRASIAS AND HYPERSENSITIVITY OF THE RESPIRATORY TRACT (SEE WARNINGS SECTION).**

Hematologic: Agranulocytosis, aplastic anemia, thrombocytopenia, leukopenia, neutropenia, hemolytic anemia, megaloblastic anemia, hypoprothrombinemia, methemoglobinemia, eosinophilia.

Allergic Reactions: Stevens-Johnson syndrome, toxic epidermal necrolysis, anaphylaxis, allergic myocarditis, erythema multiforme, exfoliative dermatitis, angioedema, drug fever, chills, Henoch-Schoenlein purpura, serum sickness-like syndrome, generalized allergic reactions, generalized skin eruptions, photosensitivity, conjunctival and scleral injection, pruritus, urticaria and rash. In addition, periarteritis nodosa and systemic lupus erythematosus have been reported.

Gastrointestinal: Hepatitis including cholestatic jaundice and hepatic necrosis, elevation of serum transaminase and bilirubin, pseudomembranous enterocolitis, pancreatitis, stomatitis, glossitis, nausea, emesis, abdominal pain, diarrhea, anorexia.

Genitourinary: Renal failure, interstitial nephritis, BUN and serum creatinine elevation, toxic nephrosis with oliguria and anuria, and crystalluria.

Neurologic: Aseptic meningitis, convulsions, peripheral neuritis, ataxia, vertigo, tinnitus, headache.

Psychiatric: Hallucinations, depression, apathy, nervousness.

Endocrine: The sulfonamides bear certain chemical similarities to some goitrogens, diuretics (acetazolamide and the thiazides) and oral hypoglycemic agents. Cross-sensitivity may exist with these agents. Diuresis and hypoglycemia have occurred rarely in patients receiving sulfonamides.

Musculoskeletal: Arthralgia and myalgia.

Respiratory System: Pulmonary infiltrates, cough, shortness of breath.

Miscellaneous: Weakness, fatigue, insomnia.

OVERDOSAGE

Acute: The amount of a single dose of Septra that is either associated with symptoms of overdosage or is likely to be life-threatening has not been reported. Signs and symptoms of overdosage reported with sulfonamides include anorexia, colic, nausea, vomiting, dizziness, headache, drowsiness and unconsciousness. Pyrexia, hematuria and crystalluria may be noted. Blood dyscrasias and jaundice are potential late manifestations of overdosage. Signs of acute overdosage with trimethoprim include nausea, vomiting, dizziness, headache, mental depression, confusion and bone marrow depression.

General principles of treatment include the institution of gastric lavage or emesis; forcing oral fluids; and the administration of intravenous fluids if urine output is low and renal function is normal. Acidification of the urine will increase renal elimination of trimethoprim. The patient should be monitored with blood counts and appropriate blood chemistries, including electrolytes. If a significant blood dyscrasia or jaundice occurs, specific therapy should be instituted for these complications. Peritoneal dialysis is not effective and hemodialysis is only moderately effective in eliminating trimethoprim and sulfamethoxazole.

Chronic: Use of Septra at high doses and/or for extended periods of time may cause bone marrow depression manifested as thrombocytopenia, leukopenia and/or megaloblastic anemia. If signs of bone marrow depression occur, the patient should be given leucovorin; 5 to 15 mg leucovorin daily has been recommended by some investigators.

DOSAGE AND ADMINISTRATION

Not recommended for use in infants less than two months of age.

URINARY TRACT INFECTIONS AND SHIGELLOSIS IN ADULTS AND CHILDREN AND ACUTE OTITIS MEDIA IN CHILDREN:

Adults: The usual adult dosage in the treatment of urinary tract infections is one Septra DS (double strength) tablet, two

Septra tablets or four teaspoonfuls (20 ml) Septra Suspension every 12 hours for 10 to 14 days. An identical daily dosage is used for 5 days in the treatment of shigellosis.

Children: The recommended dose for children with urinary tract infections or acute otitis media is 8 mg/kg trimethoprim and 40 mg/kg sulfamethoxazole per 24 hours, given in two divided doses every 12 hours for 10 days. An identical daily dosage is used for 5 days in the treatment of shigellosis. The following table is a guideline for the attainment of this dosage:

Children: Two months of age or older

Weight		Dose—every 12 hours	
lb	kg	Teaspoonfuls	Tablets
22	10	1 (5 ml)	
44	20	2 (10 ml)	1
66	30	3 (15 ml)	1 ½
88	40	4 (20 ml)	2 (or 1 DS Tablet)

For patients with impaired renal function: When renal function is impaired, a reduced dosage should be employed using the following table:

Creatinine Clearance (ml/min)	Recommended Dosage Regimen
Above 30	Use Standard Regimen
15–30	½ the Usual Regimen
Below 15	Use Not Recommended

ACUTE EXACERBATIONS OF CHRONIC BRONCHITIS IN ADULTS: The usual adult dosage in the treatment of acute exacerbations of chronic bronchitis is one Septra DS (double strength) tablet, two Septra tablets or four teaspoonfuls (20 ml) Septra Suspension every 12 hours for 14 days.

PNEUMOCYSTIS CARINII PNEUMONIA:

The recommended dosage for patients with documented *Pneumocystis carinii* pneumonia is 20 mg/kg trimethoprim and 100 mg/kg sulfamethoxazole per 24 hours given in equally divided doses every 6 hours for 14 days. The following table is a guideline for the attainment of this dosage in children:

Weight		Dose—every 6 hours	
lb	kg	Teaspoonfuls	Tablets
18	8	1 (5 ml)	
35	16	2 (10 ml)	1
53	24	3 (15 ml)	1 ½
70	32	4 (20 ml)	2 (or 1 DS Tablet)

HOW SUPPLIED

TABLETS (pink, scored, round-shaped), containing 80 mg trimethoprim and 400 mg sulfamethoxazole—bottles of 100 (NDC 0081-0852-55) and 500 (NDC 0081-0852-70); unit dose pack of 100 (NDC 0081-0852-56). Imprint on tablets "SEPTRA" and "Y2B."

DS (DOUBLE STRENGTH) TABLETS (pink, scored, oval-shaped) containing 160 mg trimethoprim and 800 mg sulfamethoxazole—bottles of 100 (NDC 0081-0853-55) and 250 (NDC 0081-0853-65); unit dose pack of 100 (NDC 0081-0853-56); unit of use bottle of 20 with child-resistant cap (NDC 0081-0853-52). Imprint on tablets "SEPTRA DS" and "O2C."

ORAL SUSPENSIONS (pink, cherry flavored) containing 40 mg trimethoprim and 200 mg sulfamethoxazole in each teaspoonful (5 ml)—bottle of 1 pint (473 ml) (NDC 0081-0855-96); unit of use bottles of 20 ml—tray of 12 (NDC 0081-0855-93), 100 ml—box of 1 (NDC 0081-0855-09), 150 ml—tray of 6 (NDC 0081-0855-01), and 200 ml—tray of 6 (NDC 0081-0855-02) with child-resistant caps; and (purple, grape flavored) containing 40 mg trimethoprim and 200 mg sulfamethoxazole in each teaspoonful (5 ml)—bottle of 1 pint (473 ml) (NDC 0081-0854-96).

Tablets should be stored at 15°–30°C (59°–86°F) in a dry place and protected from light.

Suspension should be stored at 15°–25°C (59°–77°F) and protected from light.

Also available:

SEPTRA I.V. Infusion: 5 ml ampul, containing 80 mg trimethoprim (16 mg/ml) and 400 mg sulfamethoxazole (80 mg/ml), box of 10; 5 ml vial, containing 80 mg trimethoprim (16 mg/ml) and 400 mg sulfamethoxazole (80 mg/ml), tray of 10; 10 ml multiple dose vial, containing 160 mg trimethoprim (16 mg/ml) and 800 mg sulfamethoxazole (80 mg/ml), tray of 10; 20 ml multiple dose vial, containing 320 mg trimethoprim (16 mg/ml) and 1600 mg sulfamethoxazole (80 mg/ml), box of 1.

REFERENCES

1. Kremers P, Duvivier J and Heusghem C. Pharmacokinetic Studies of Co-Trimoxazole in Man after Single and Repeated Doses, *J. Clin Pharmacol 14:* 112–117, 1974.
2. Kaplan SA, *et al:* Pharmacokinetic Profile of Trimethoprim-Sulfamethoxazole in Man. *J Infect Dis 128:* S547–S554, November 1973.
3. Federal Register, *37:* 20527–20529, 1972.
4. Bauer AW, Kirby WMM, Sherris JC, Turck M: Antibiotic Susceptibility Testing by Standardized Single Disk Method. *Am J Clin Path 45:* 493–496, April 1966.
5. Brumfitt W and Pursell R: Trimethoprim/Sulfamethoxazole in the Treatment of Bacteriuria in Women. *J Infect Dis 128* (Suppl): S657–S663, November 1973.
* Mfd. under U.S. Patent No. 3,956,327
U.S. Patent No. 4,209,513 (Tablet)
Shown in Product Identification Section, page 408

Children's SUDAFED® Liquid
[*sū 'dah-fĕd "*]
Nasal Decongestant

(See PDR For Nonprescription Drugs)

SUDAFED® Cough Syrup
[*sū 'dah-fĕd "*]
Nasal Decongestant/Cough Suppressant/Expectorant

(See PDR For Nonprescription Drugs)

SUDAFED® SINUS Tablets and Caplets
[*sū 'dah-fĕd "*]
Analgesic/Nasal Decongestant

(See PDR For Nonprescription Drugs)
Shown in Product Identification Section, page 408

SUDAFED® Tablets 30 mg and 60 mg
[*sū 'dah-fĕd "*]
Nasal Decongestant

(See PDR For Nonprescription Drugs)
Shown in Product Identification Section, page 408

SUDAFED® PLUS Liquid and Tablets
[*sū 'dah-fĕd "*]
Nasal Decongestant/Antihistamine

(See PDR For Nonprescription Drugs)
Tablets shown in Product Identification Section, page 408

SUDAFED® 12 HOUR Capsules
[*sū 'dah-fĕd "*]
Nasal Decongestant

(See PDR For Nonprescription Drugs)
Shown in Product Identification Section, page 408

TABLOID® brand THIOGUANINE   ℞
[*tab 'loid*]
40 mg Scored Tablets

CAUTION: Tabloid brand thioguanine is a potent drug. It should not be used unless a diagnosis of acute nonlymphocytic leukemia has been adequately established and the responsible physician is knowledgeable in assessing response to chemotherapy.

DESCRIPTION

Tabloid brand thioguanine was synthesized and developed by Hitchings, Elion and associates at the Wellcome Research Laboratories. It is one of a large series of purine analogues which interfere with nucleic acid biosynthesis, and has been found active against selected human neoplastic diseases.[1] Thioguanine, known chemically as 2-amino-1,7-dihydro-6*H*-purine-6-thione, is an analogue of the nucleic acid constituent guanine, and is closely related structurally and functionally to Purinethol® (mercaptopurine).

Tabloid brand thioguanine is available in tablets for oral administration. Each scored tablet contains 40 mg thioguanine and the inactive ingredients gum acacia, lactose, magnesium stearate, potato starch, and stearic acid.

CLINICAL PHARMACOLOGY

Clinical studies have shown that the absorption of an oral dose of thioguanine in man is incomplete and variable, averaging approximately 30% of the administered dose (range: 14–46%).[2,3] Following oral administration of ^{35}S-6-

Continued on next page

Burroughs Wellcome—Cont.

thioguanine, total plasma radioactivity reached a maximum at eight hours and declined slowly thereafter. Parent drug represented only a very small fraction of the total plasma radioactivity at any time, being virtually undetectable throughout the period of measurements.

The oral administration of radiolabeled thioguanine revealed only trace quantities of parent drug in the urine. However, a methylated metabolite, 2-amino-6-methylthiopurine (MTG), appeared very early, rose to a maximum six to eight hours after drug administration, and was still being excreted after 12 to 22 hours. Radiolabeled sulfate appeared somewhat later than MTG but was the principal metabolite after eight hours. Thiouric acid and some unidentified products were found in the urine in small amounts.[3] Intravenous administration of ^{35}S-6-thioguanine disclosed a median plasma half-disappearance time of 80 minutes (range: 25–240 minutes) when the compound was given in single doses of 65 to 300 mg/m[2]. Although initial plasma levels of thioguanine did correlate with the dose level, there was no correlation between the plasma half-disappearance time and the dose.[2]

Thioguanine is incorporated into the DNA and the RNA of human bone marrow cells. Studies with intravenous ^{35}S-6-thioguanine have shown that the amount of thioguanine incorporated into nucleic acids is more than 100 times higher after five daily doses than after a single dose. With the 5-dose schedule, from one-half to virtually all of the guanine in the residual DNA was replaced by thioguanine.[2] Tissue distribution studies of ^{35}S-6-thioguanine in mice showed only traces of radioactivity in brain after oral administration. No measurements have been made of thioguanine concentrations in human cerebrospinal fluid, but observations on tissue distribution in animals, together with the lack of CNS penetration by the closely related compound, mercaptopurine, suggest that thioguanine does not reach therapeutic concentrations in the CSF.

Monitoring of plasma levels of thioguanine during therapy is of questionable value.[3] There is technical difficulty in determining plasma concentrations, which are seldom greater than 1 to 2 micrograms per ml after a therapeutic oral dose. More significantly, thioguanine enters rapidly into the anabolic and catabolic pathways for purines, and the active intracellular metabolites have appreciably longer half-lives than the parent drug. The biochemical effects of a single dose of thioguanine are evident long after the parent drug has disappeared from plasma. Because of this rapid metabolism of thioguanine to active intracellular derivatives, hemodialysis would not be expected to appreciably reduce toxicity of the drug.

Thioguanine competes with hypoxanthine and guanine for the enzyme hypoxanthine-guanine phosphoribosyltransferase (HGPRTase) and is itself converted to 6-thioguanylic acid (TGMP). This nucleotide reaches high intracellular concentrations at therapeutic doses. TGMP interferes at several points with the synthesis of guanine nucleotides. It inhibits de novo purine biosynthesis by pseudo-feedback inhibition of glutamine-5-phosphoribosylpyrophosphate amidotransferase—the first enzyme unique to the de novo pathway for purine ribonucleotide synthesis. TGMP also inhibits the conversion of inosinic acid (IMP) to xanthylic acid (XMP) by competition for the enzyme IMP dehydrogenase. At one time TGMP was felt to be a significant inhibitor of ATP:GMP phosphotransferase (guanylate kinase),[4] but recent results have shown this not to be so.[5]

Thioguanylic acid is further converted to the di- and tri-phosphates, thioguanosine diphosphate (TGDP) and thioguanosine triphosphate (TGTP) (as well as their 2'-deoxyribosyl analogues) by the same enzymes which metabolize guanine nucleotides.[6] Thioguanine nucleotides are incorporated into both the RNA and the DNA by phosphodiester linkages[2] and it has been argued that incorporation of such fraudulent bases contributes to the cytotoxicity of thioguanine.

Thus, thioguanine has multiple metabolic effects and at present it is not possible to designate one major site of action. Its tumor inhibitory properties may be due to one or more of its effects on (a) feedback inhibition of de novo purine synthesis; (b) inhibition of purine nucleotide interconversions; or (c) incorporation into the DNA and the RNA. The net consequence of its actions is a sequential blockade of the synthesis and utilization of the purine nucleotides.[4,6,7]

The catabolism of thioguanine and its metabolites is complex and shows significant differences between man and the mouse.[2,3] In both humans and mice, after oral administration of ^{35}S-6-thioguanine, urine contains virtually no detectable intact thioguanine. While deamination and subsequent oxidation to thiouric acid occurs only to a small extent in man, it is the main pathway in mice. The product of deamination by guanase, 6-thioxanthine is inactive, having negligible antitumor activity. This pathway of thioguanine inactivation is not dependent on the action of xanthine oxidase and an inhibitor of that enzyme (such as allopurinol), will not block the detoxification of thioguanine even though the inac-

tive 6-thioxanthine is normally further oxidized by xanthine oxidase to thiouric acid before it is eliminated. In man, methylation of thioguanine is much more extensive than in the mouse. The product of methylation, 2-amino-6-methylthiopurine, is also substantially less active and less toxic than thioguanine and its formation is likewise unaffected by the presence of allopurinol. Appreciable amounts of inorganic sulfate are also found in both murine and human urine, presumably arising from further metabolism of the methylated derivatives.

In some animal tumors, resistance to the effect of thioguanine correlates with the loss of HGPRTase activity and the resulting inability to convert thioguanine to thioguanylic acid. However, other resistance mechanisms, such as increased catabolism of TGMP by a nonspecific phosphatase, may be operative. Although not invariable, it is usual to find cross-resistance between thioguanine and its close analogue, Purinethol® (mercaptopurine).

INDICATIONS AND USAGE

a) Acute Nonlymphocytic Leukemias: Tabloid brand thioguanine is indicated for remission induction, remission consolidation, and maintenance therapy of acute nonlymphocytic leukemias.[8,9] The response to this agent depends upon the age of the patient (younger patients faring better than older), and whether thioguanine is used in previously treated or previously untreated patients. Reliance upon thioguanine alone is seldom justified for initial remission induction of acute nonlymphocytic leukemias because combination chemotherapy including thioguanine results in more frequent remission induction and longer duration of remission than thioguanine alone.

b) Other Neoplasms: Tabloid brand thioguanine is not effective in chronic lymphocytic leukemia, Hodgkin's lymphoma, multiple myeloma or solid tumors. Although thioguanine is one of several agents with activity in the treatment of the chronic phase of chronic myelogenous leukemia, more objective responses are observed with Myleran® (busulfan), and therefore busulfan is usually regarded as the preferred drug.

CONTRAINDICATIONS

Thioguanine should not be used in patients whose disease has demonstrated prior resistance to this drug. In animals and man, there is usually complete cross-resistance between Purinethol® (mercaptopurine) and Tabloid® brand thioguanine.

WARNINGS

SINCE DRUGS USED IN CANCER CHEMOTHERAPY ARE POTENTIALLY HAZARDOUS, IT IS RECOMMENDED THAT ONLY PHYSICIANS EXPERIENCED WITH THE RISKS OF THIOGUANINE AND KNOWLEDGEABLE IN THE NATURAL HISTORY OF ACUTE NONLYMPHOCYTIC LEUKEMIAS ADMINISTER THIS DRUG.

The most consistent, dose-related toxicity is bone marrow suppression. This may be manifest by anemia, leukopenia, thrombocytopenia, or any combination of these. Any one of these findings may also reflect progression of the underlying disease. Since thioguanine may have a delayed effect, it is important to withdraw the medication temporarily at the first sign of an abnormally large fall in any of the formed elements of the blood.

It is recommended that evaluation of the hemoglobin concentration or hematocrit; total white blood cell count and differential count; and quantitative platelet count be obtained frequently while the patient is on thioguanine therapy. In cases where the cause of fluctuations in the formed elements in the peripheral blood is obscure, bone marrow examination may be useful for the evaluation of marrow status. The decision to increase, decrease, continue or discontinue a given dosage of thioguanine must be based not only on the absolute hematologic values, but also upon the rapidity with which changes are occurring. In many instances, particularly during the induction phase of acute leukemia, complete blood counts will need to be done more frequently in order to evaluate the effect of the therapy. The dosage of thioguanine may need to be reduced when this agent is combined with other drugs whose primary toxicity is myelosuppression.

Myelosuppression is often unavoidable during the induction phase of adult acute nonlymphocytic leukemias if remission induction is to be successful. Whether or not this demands modification or cessation of dosage depends both upon the response of the underlying disease and a careful consideration of supportive facilities (granulocyte and platelet transfusions) which may be available. Life-threatening infections and bleeding have been observed as consequences of thioguanine-induced granulocytopenia and thrombocytopenia.

The effect of thioguanine on the immunocompetence of patients is unknown.

Pregnancy: "Pregnancy Category D": Drugs such as thioguanine are potential mutagens and teratogens. Thioguanine may cause fetal harm when administered to a pregnant woman. Thioguanine has been shown to be teratogenic in rats when given in doses five (5) times the human dose. When given to the rat on the 4th and 5th days of gestation, 13% of

surviving placentas did not contain fetuses, and 19% of offspring were malformed or stunted. The malformations noted included generalized edema, cranial defects and general skeletal hypoplasia, hydrocephalus, ventral hernia, situs inversus, and incomplete development of the limbs.[10] There are no adequate and well-controlled studies in pregnant women. If this drug is used during pregnancy, or if the patient becomes pregnant while taking the drug, the patient should be apprised of the potential hazard to the fetus. Women of childbearing potential should be advised to avoid becoming pregnant.

PRECAUTIONS

General: Although the primary toxicity of thioguanine is myelosuppression, other toxicities have occasionally been observed, particularly when thioguanine is used in combination with other cancer chemotherapeutic agents.

A few cases of jaundice have been reported in patients with leukemia receiving thioguanine. Among these were two adult male patients and four children with acute myelogenous leukemia and an adult male with acute lymphocytic leukemia who developed veno-occlusive hepatic disease while receiving chemotherapy for their leukemia.[11,12] Six patients had received cytarabine prior to treatment with thioguanine, and some were receiving other chemotherapy in addition to thioguanine when they became symptomatic. While veno-occlusive hepatic disease has not been reported in patients treated with thioguanine alone, it is recommended that thioguanine be withheld if there is evidence of toxic hepatitis or biliary stasis, and that appropriate clinical and laboratory investigations be initiated to establish the etiology of the hepatic dysfunction. Deterioration in liver function studies during thioguanine therapy should prompt discontinuation of treatment and a search for an explanation of the hepatotoxicity.

Information For Patients: Patients should be informed that the major toxicities of thioguanine are related to myelosuppression, hepatotoxicity and gastrointestinal toxicity. Patients should never be allowed to take the drug without medical supervision and should be advised to consult their physician if they experience fever, sore throat, jaundice, nausea, vomiting, signs of local infection, bleeding from any site, or symptoms suggestive of anemia. Women of childbearing potential should be advised to avoid becoming pregnant.

Laboratory Tests: It is advisable to monitor liver function tests (serum transaminases, alkaline phosphatase, bilirubin) at weekly intervals when first beginning therapy and at monthly intervals thereafter. It may be advisable to perform liver function tests more frequently in patients with known pre-existing liver disease or in patients who are receiving thioguanine and other hepatotoxic drugs. Patients should be instructed to discontinue thioguanine immediately if clinical jaundice is detected. (See WARNINGS section).

Drug Interactions: There is usually complete cross-resistance between Purinethol® (mercaptopurine) and Tabloid® brand thioguanine.

Carcinogenesis, Mutagenesis, Impairment of Fertility: In view of its action on cellular DNA, thioguanine is potentially mutagenic and carcinogenic, and consideration should be given to the theoretical risk of carcinogenesis when thioguanine is administered. (See WARNINGS section)

Pregnancy: Teratogenic Effects: Pregnancy Category D. See WARNINGS section.

Nursing Mothers: It is not known whether this drug is excreted in human milk. Because of the potential for tumorigenicity shown for thioguanine, a decision should be made whether to discontinue nursing or to discontinue the drug, taking into account the importance of the drug to the mother.

ADVERSE REACTIONS

The most frequent adverse reaction to thioguanine is myelosuppression. The induction of complete remission of acute myelogenous leukemia usually requires combination chemotherapy in dosages which produce marrow hypoplasia.[13] Since consolidation and maintenance of remission are also effected by multiple drug regimens whose component agents cause myelosuppression, pancytopenia is observed in nearly all patients. Dosages and schedules must be adjusted to prevent life-threatening cytopenias whenever these adverse reactions are observed.

Hyperuricemia frequently occurs in patients receiving thioguanine as a consequence of rapid cell lysis accompanying the antineoplastic effect. Adverse effects can be minimized by increased hydration, urine alkalinization, and the prophylactic administration of a xanthine oxidase inhibitor such as Zyloprim® (allopurinol). Unlike Purinethol® (mercaptopurine) and Imuran® (azathioprine), thioguanine may be continued in the usual dosage when allopurinol is used conjointly to inhibit uric acid formation.

Less frequent adverse reactions include nausea, vomiting, anorexia and stomatitis. Liver enzyme and other liver function studies are occasionally abnormal. If jaundice, hepatomegaly or anorexia with tenderness in the right hypochondrium occurs, thioguanine should be withheld until the exact etiology can be determined. There have been reports of veno-occlusive liver disease occuring in patients who received combination chemotherapy including thioguanine.[11,12] Intestinal necrosis and perforation have been reported also in patients who received multiple drug chemotherapy including thioguanine.

OVERDOSAGE

Signs and symptoms of overdosage may be immediate, such as nausea, vomiting, malaise, hypertension and diaphoresis; or delayed, such as myelosuppression and azotemia.[14] It is not known whether thioguanine is dialyzable. Hemodialysis is thought to be of marginal use due to the rapid intracellular incorporation of thioguanine into active metabolites with long persistence. The oral LD_{50} of thioguanine was determined to be 823 mg/kg $\pm$ 50.73 mg/kg and 740 mg/kg $\pm$ 45.24 mg/kg for male and female rats respectively.[15] Symptoms of overdosage may occur after a single dose of as little as 2.0 to 3.0 mg/kg thioguanine. As much as 35 mg/kg has been given in a single oral dose with reversible myelosuppression observed. There is no known pharmacologic antagonist of thioguanine. The drug should be discontinued immediately if unintended toxicity occurs during treatment. Severe hematologic toxicity may require supportive therapy with platelet transfusions for bleeding, and granulocyte transfusions and antibiotics if sepsis is documented. If a patient is seen immediately following an accidental overdosage of the drug, it may be useful to induce emesis.

DOSAGE AND ADMINISTRATION

Tabloid brand thioguanine is administered orally. The dosage which will be tolerated and effective varies according to the stage and type of neoplastic process being treated. Because the usual therapies for adult and childhood acute nonlymphocytic leukemias involve the use of thioguanine with other agents in combination, physicians responsible for administering these therapies should be experienced in the use of cancer chemotherapy and in the chosen protocol.

Ninety-six (59%) of one hundred sixty-three children with previously untreated acute nonlymphocytic leukemia obtained complete remission with a multiple drug protocol including thioguanine, prednisone, cytarabine, cyclophosphamide, and vincristine. Remission was maintained with daily thioguanine, four-day pulses of cytarabine and cyclophosphamide, and a single dose of vincristine every 28 days. The median duration of remission was 11.5 months.[8]

Fifty-three percent of previously untreated adults with acute nonlymphocytic leukemias attained remission following use of the combination of thioguanine and cytarabine according to a protocol developed at The Memorial Sloan-Kettering Cancer Center. A median duration of remission of 8.8 months was achieved with the multiple drug maintenance regimen which included thioguanine.[9]

On those occasions when single agent chemotherapy with thioguanine may be appropriate, the usual initial dosage for children and adults is approximately 2 mg/kg of body weight per day. If, after four weeks on this dosage, there is no clinical improvement and no leukocyte or platelet depression, the dosage may be cautiously increased to 3 mg/kg per day. The total daily dose may be given at one time.

The dosage of thioguanine used does not depend on whether or not the patient is receiving Zyloprim® (allopurinol); **this is in contradistinction to the dosage reduction which is mandatory when Purinethol® (mercaptopurine) or IMURAN® (azathioprine) is given simultaneously with allopurinol.**

Procedures for proper handling and disposal of anti-cancer drugs should be considered. Several guidelines on this subject have been published.[16-21]

There is no general agreement that all of the procedures recommended in the guidelines are necessary or appropriate.

HOW SUPPLIED

Greenish-yellow, scored tablets containing 40 mg thioguanine, imprinted with "WELLCOME" and "U3B" on each tablet; in bottle of 25 (NDC-0081-0880-25). Store at 15°-25°C (59°-77°F) in a dry place.

REFERENCES

1. Hitchings GH and Elion GB: The Chemistry and Biochemistry of Purine Analogs. *Ann NY Acad Sci* 60: 195–199, 1954.
2. LePage GA and Whitecar JP Jr.: Pharmacology of 6-thioguanine in Man. *Cancer Res 31:* 1627–1631, 1971.
3. Elion GB: Biochemistry and Pharmacology of Purine Analogues. *Fed Proc 26:* 898–904, 1967.
4. Miech RP, Parks RE, Jr., Anderson JH, Jr. and Sartorelli AC: An Hypothesis on the Mechanism of Action of 6-thioguanine. *Biochem Pharmacol* 16: 2222–2227, 1967.
5. Miller RL, Adamczyk DL, and Spector T: Reassessment of the Inter-Actions of Guanylate Kinase and 6-thioguanine 5'-phosphate. *Proc Am Assoc Cancer Res 18:* 6, 1977. Abstract.
6. Paterson ARP and Tidd DN: 6-Thiopurines. In: *Antineoplastic and Immunosuppressive Agents,* Part II. (Edited by AC Sartorelli and DG Johns.) Berlin, Springer-Verlag, 384–403, 1975.
7. Nelson JA, Carpenter JW, Rose LN, and Adamson DJ: Mechanisms of Action of 6-thioguanine, 6-mercaptopurine, and 8-azaguanine. *Cancer Res 35:* 2872–2878, 1975.
8. Chard RL, Finkelstein JZ, Sonley MJ, *et al.:* Increased Survival in Childhood Acute Nonlymphocytic Leukemia after Treatment with Prednisone, Cytosine Arabinoside, 6-thioguanine, Cyclophosphamide, and Oncovin (PATCO) Combination Chemotherapy. *Med Ped Oncol 4:* 263–273, 1978.
9. Mertelsmann R, Drapkin RL, Gee TS, *et al.:* Treatment of Acute Nonlymphocytic Leukemia in Adults. *Cancer 48:* 2136–2142, 1981.
10. Thiersch JB: Effect of 2-6 Diamino-purine (2-6 DP): 6 Chlorpurine (CIP) and Thioguanine (ThG) on Rat Litter *in utero. Proc Soc Exp Biol Med 94:* 40–43, 1957.
11. Griner PF, Elbadawi A, and Packman CH: Veno-Occlusive Disease of the Liver After Chemotherapy of Acute Leukemia. *Ann Intern Med 85:* 578–582, 1976.
12. Gill RA, Onstad GR, Cardamone JM, *et al.:* Hepatic Veno-Occlusive Disease Caused by 6-thioguanine. *Ann Intern Med 96:* 58–60, 1982.
13. Clarkson B, Dowling MD, Gee TS, *et al.:* Treatment of Acute Leukemia in Adults. *Cancer 36:* 775–795, 1975.
14. Presant CA, Denes AE, Klein L, *et al.:* Phase I and Preliminary Phase II Observations of High-dose Intermittent 6-thioguanine. *Cancer Treat Rep 64(10–11):* 1109–1113, 1980.
15. Unpublished data on file with Burroughs Wellcome Co.
16. Recommendations for the Safe Handling of Parenteral Antineoplastic Drugs. NIH Publications No. 83-2621. For sale by the Superintendent of Documents, U.S. Government Printing Office, Washington, D.C. 20402.
17. AMA Council Report. Guidelines for Handling Parenteral Antineoplastics. JAMA, March 15, 1985.
18. National Study Commission on Cytotoxic Exposure—Recommendations for Handling Cytotoxic Agents. Available from Louis P. Jeffrey, Sc.D., Director of Pharmacy Services, Rhode Island Hospital, 593 Eddy Street, Providence, Rhode Island 02902.
19. Clinical Oncological Society of Australia: Guidelines and recommendations for safe handling of antineoplastic agents. Med J Australia 1:426–428, 1983.
20. Jones R.B., et al. Safe handling of chemotherapeutic agents: A Report from the Mount Sinai Medical Center. Ca—A Cancer Journal for Clinicians Sept/Oct, 258–263, 1983.
21. American Society of Hospital Pharmacists technical assistance bulletin on handling cytotoxic drugs in hospitals. Am J Hosp Pharm 42:131–137, 1985.

Shown in Product Identification Section, page 408

TRACRIUM® INJECTION   ℞

[trā'krē"um]
(Atracurium Besylate)

This drug should be used only by adequately trained individuals familiar with its actions, characteristics, and hazards.

DESCRIPTION

Tracrium (atracurium besylate) is an intermediate-duration, nondepolarizing, skeletal muscle relaxant for intravenous administration. Atracurium besylate is designated as 2,2'-[pentamethylenebis(oxycarbonylethylene)]bis(1,2,3,4-tetrahydro-6,7-dimethoxy-2-methyl-1-veratrylisoquinolinium) dibenzenesulfonate. It has a molecular weight of 1243.49, and its molecular formula is $C_{65}H_{82}N_2O_{18}S_2$.

Atracurium besylate is a complex molecule containing four sites at which different stereochemical configurations can occur. The symmetry of the molecule, however, results in only ten, instead of sixteen, possible different isomers. The manufacture of atracurium besylate results in these isomers being produced in unequal amounts but with a consistent ratio. Those molecules in which the methyl group attached to the quaternary nitrogen projects on the opposite side to the adjacent substituted-benzyl moiety predominate by approximately 3:1.

Tracrium Injection is a sterile, non-pyrogenic aqueous solution. Each mL contains 10 mg atracurium besylate. The pH is adjusted to 3.25-3.65 with benzenesulfonic acid. The multiple dose vial contains 0.9% benzyl alcohol added as a preservative. Tracrium slowly loses potency with time at the rate of approximately 6% per *year* under refrigeration (5°C). Tracrium Injection should be refrigerated at 2° to 8°C (36° to 46°F) to preserve potency. Rate of loss in potency increases to approximately 5% per *month* at 25°C (77°F). Upon removal from refrigeration to room temperature storage conditions (25°C/77°F), use Tracrium Injection within 14 days even if rerefrigerated.

CLINICAL PHARMACOLOGY

Tracrium is a nondepolarizing skeletal muscle relaxant. Nondepolarizing agents antagonize the neurotransmitter action of acetylcholine by binding competitively with cholinergic receptor sites on the motor end-plate. This antagonism is inhibited, and neuromuscular block reversed, by acetylcholinesterase inhibitors such as neostigmine, edrophonium, and pyridostigmine.

Tracrium can be used most advantageously if muscle twitch response to peripheral nerve stimulation is monitored to assess degree of muscle relaxation.

The duration of neuromuscular blockade produced by Tracrium is approximately one-third to one-half the duration of blockade by d-tubocurarine, metocurine, and pancuronium at initially equipotent doses. As with other nondepolarizing neuromuscular blockers, the time to onset of paralysis decreases and the duration of maximum effect increases with increasing Tracrium doses.

The ED_{95} (dose required to produce 95% suppression of the muscle twitch response with balanced anesthesia) has averaged 0.23 mg/kg (0.11 to 0.26 mg/kg in various studies). An initial Tracrium dose of 0.4 to 0.5 mg/kg generally produces maximum neuromuscular blockade within 3 to 5 minutes of injection, with good or excellent intubation conditions within 2 to 2.5 minutes in most patients. Recovery from neuromuscular blockade (under balanced anesthesia) can be expected to begin approximately 20 to 35 minutes after injection. Under balanced anesthesia, recovery to 25% of control is achieved approximately 35 to 45 minutes after injection, and recovery is usually 95% complete approximately 60–70 minutes after injection. The neuromuscular blocking action of Tracrium is enhanced in the presence of potent inhalation anesthetics. Isoflurane and enflurane increase the potency of Tracrium and prolong neuromuscular blockade by approximately 35%; however, halothane's potentiating effect (approximately 20%) is marginal (see DOSAGE AND ADMINISTRATION section).

Repeated administration of maintenance doses of Tracrium has no cumulative effect on the duration of neuromuscular blockade if recovery is allowed to begin prior to repeat dosing. Moreover, the time needed to recover from repeat doses does not change with additional doses. Repeat doses can therefore be administered at relatively regular intervals with predictable results. After an initial dose of 0.4 to 0.5 mg/kg under balanced anesthesia, the first maintenance dose (suggested maintenance dose is 0.08 to 0.10 mg/kg) is generally required within 20 to 45 minutes, and subsequent maintenance doses are usually required at approximately 15 to 25 minute intervals.

Once recovery from Tracrium's neuromuscular blocking effects begins, it proceeds more rapidly than recovery from d-tubocurarine, metocurine, and pancuronium. Regardless of Tracrium dose, the time from start of recovery (from complete block) to complete (95%) recovery is approximately 30 minutes under balanced anesthesia, and approximately 40 minutes under halothane, enflurane or isoflurane. Repeated doses have no cumulative effect on recovery rate.

Reversal of neuromuscular blockade produced by Tracrium can be achieved with an anticholinesterase agent such as neostigmine, edrophonium, or pyridostigmine, in conjunction with an anticholinergic agent such as atropine or glycopyrrolate. Under balanced anesthesia, reversal can usually be attempted approximately 20 to 35 minutes after an initial Tracrium dose of 0.4 to 0.5 mg/kg, or approximately 10 to 30 minutes after a 0.08 to 0.10 mg/kg maintenance dose, when recovery of muscle twitch has started. Complete reversal is usually attained within 8–10 minutes of the administration of reversing agents. Rare instances of breathing difficulties, possibly related to incomplete reversal, have been reported following attempted pharmacologic antagonism of Tracrium-induced neuromuscular blockade. As with other agents in this class, the tendency for residual neuromuscular block is increased if reversal is attempted at deep levels of blockade or if inadequate doses of reversal agents are employed.

The pharmacokinetics of Tracrium in man are essentially linear within the 0.3 to 0.6 mg/kg dose range. The elimination half-life is approximately 20 minutes. THE DURATION OF NEUROMUSCULAR BLOCKADE PRODUCED BY TRACRIUM DOES NOT CORRELATE WITH PLASMA PSEUDOCHOLINESTERASE LEVELS AND IS NOT ALTERED BY THE ABSENCE OF RENAL FUNCTION. This is consistent with the results of *in vitro* studies which have shown that Tracrium is inactivated in plasma via two nonoxidative pathways: ester hydrolysis, catalyzed by nonspecific esterases; and Hofmann elimination, a nonenzymatic chemical process which occurs at physiological pH. Some placental transfer occurs in humans.

Radiolabel studies demonstrated that Tracrium undergoes extensive degradation in cats, and that neither kidney nor liver plays a major role in its elimination. Biliary and urinary excretion were the major routes of excretion of radioactivity (totaling > 90% of the labeled dose within 7 hours of dosing), of which Tracrium represented only a minor fraction. The metabolites in bile and urine were similar, including products of Hofmann elimination and ester hydrolysis.

Tracrium is a less potent histamine releaser than d-tubocurarine or metocurine. Histamine release is minimal with initial Tracrium doses up to 0.5 mg/kg, and hemodynamic

Continued on next page

Burroughs Wellcome—Cont.

changes are minimal within the recommended dose range. A moderate histamine release and significant falls in blood pressure have been seen following 0.6 mg/kg of Tracrium. The histamine and hemodynamic responses were poorly correlated. The effects were generally short-lived and manageable, but the possibility of substantial histamine release in sensitive individuals or in patients in whom substantial histamine release would be especially hazardous (e.g., patients with significant cardiovascular disease) must be considered.

It is not known whether the prior use of other nondepolarizing neuromuscular blocking agents has any effect on the activity of Tracrium. The prior use of succinylcholine decreases by approximately 2 to 3 minutes the time to maximum blockade induced by Tracrium, and may increase the depth of blockade. Tracrium should be administered only after a patient recovers from succinylcholine-induced neuromuscular blockade.

INDICATIONS AND USAGE
Tracrium is indicated, as an adjunct to general anesthesia, to facilitate endotracheal intubation and to provide skeletal muscle relaxation during surgery or mechanical ventilation.

CONTRAINDICATIONS
Tracrium is contraindicated in patients known to have a hypersensitivity to it.

WARNINGS
TRACRIUM SHOULD BE USED ONLY BY THOSE SKILLED IN AIRWAY MANAGEMENT AND RESPIRATORY SUPPORT. EQUIPMENT AND PERSONNEL MUST BE IMMEDIATELY AVAILABLE FOR ENDOTRACHEAL INTUBATION AND SUPPORT OF VENTILATION, INCLUDING ADMINISTRATION OF POSITIVE PRESSURE OXYGEN. ADEQUACY OF RESPIRATION MUST BE ASSURED THROUGH ASSISTED OR CONTROLLED VENTILATION. ANTICHOLINESTERASE REVERSAL AGENTS SHOULD BE IMMEDIATELY AVAILABLE.

DO NOT GIVE TRACRIUM BY INTRAMUSCULAR ADMINISTRATION.

Tracrium has no known effect on consciousness, pain threshold, or cerebration. It should be used only with adequate anesthesia.

Tracrium Injection, which has an acid pH, should not be mixed with alkaline solutions (e.g., barbiturate solutions) in the same syringe or administered simultaneously during intravenous infusion through the same needle. Depending on the resultant pH of such mixtures, Tracrium may be inactivated and a free acid may be precipitated.

PRECAUTIONS
General: Although Tracrium is a less potent histamine releaser than d-tubocurarine or metocurine, the possibility of substantial histamine release in sensitive individuals must be considered. Special caution should be exercised in administering Tracrium to patients in whom substantial histamine release would be especially hazardous (e.g., patients with clinically significant cardiovascular disease) and in patients with any history (e.g., severe anaphylactoid reactions or asthma) suggesting a greater risk of histamine release. In these patients, the recommended initial Tracrium dose is lower (0.3 to 0.4 mg/kg) than for other patients and should be administered slowly or in divided doses over one minute.

Since Tracrium has no clinically significant effects on heart rate in the recommended dosage range, it will not counteract the bradycardia produced by many anesthetic agents or vagal stimulation. As a result, bradycardia during anesthesia may be more common with Tracrium than with other muscle relaxants.

Tracrium may have profound effects in patients with myasthenia gravis, Eaton-Lambert syndrome, or other neuromuscular diseases in which potentiation of nondepolarizing agents has been noted. The use of a peripheral nerve stimulator is especially important for assessing neuromuscular blockade in these patients. Similar precautions should be taken in patients with severe electrolyte disorders or carcinomatosis.

Multiple factors in anesthesia practice are suspected of triggering malignant hyperthermia (MH), a potentially fatal hypermetabolic state of skeletal muscle. Halogenated anesthetic agents and succinylcholine are recognized as the principal pharmacologic triggering agents in MH-susceptible patients; however, since MH can develop in the absence of established triggering agents, the clinician should be prepared to recognize and treat MH in any patient scheduled for general anesthesia. Reports of MH have been rare in cases in which Tracrium has been used. In studies of MH-susceptible animals (swine) and in a clinical study of MH-susceptible patients, Tracrium did not trigger this syndrome.

Resistance to nondepolarizing neuromuscular blocking agents may develop in burn patients. Increased doses of nondepolarizing muscle relaxants may be required in burn patients and are dependent on the time elapsed since the burn injury and the size of the burn.

The safety of Tracrium has not been established in patients with bronchial asthma.

Drug Interactions: Drugs which may enhance the neuromuscular blocking action of Tracrium include: enflurane; isoflurane; halothane; certain antibiotics, especially the aminoglycosides and polymyxins; lithium; magnesium salts; procainamide; and quinidine.

If other muscle relaxants are used during the same procedure, the possibility of a synergistic or antagonist effect should be considered.

The prior administration of succinylcholine does not enhance the duration, but quickens the onset and may increase the depth of neuromuscular blockade induced by Tracrium. Tracrium should not be administered until a patient has recovered from succinylcholine-induced neuromuscular blockade.

Carcinogenesis, Mutagenesis, Impairment of Fertility: Carcinogenesis and fertility studies have not been performed. Atracurium was evaluated in a battery of three short-term mutagenicity tests. It was non-mutagenic in both the Ames Salmonella assay at concentrations up to 1000 μg/plate, and in a rat bone marrow cytogenicity assay at up to paralyzing doses. A positive response was observed in the mouse lymphoma assay under conditions (80 and 100 μg/mL, in the absence of metabolic activation) which killed over 80% of the treated cells; there was no mutagenicity at 60 μg/mL and lower, concentrations which killed up to half of the treated cells. A far weaker response was observed in the presence of metabolic activation at concentrations (1200 μg/mL and higher) which also killed over 80% of the treated cells.

Mutagenicity testing is intended to simulate chronic (years to lifetime) exposure in an effort to determine potential carcinogenicity. Thus, a single positive mutagenicity response for a drug used infrequently and/or briefly is of questionable clinical relevance.

Pregnancy: *Teratogenic Effects:* Pregnancy Category C. Tracrium has been shown to be potentially teratogenic in rabbits when given in doses up to approximately one-half the human dose. There are no adequate and well-controlled studies in pregnant women. Tracrium should be used during pregnancy only if the potential benefit justifies the potential risk to the fetus.

Tracrium was administered subcutaneously on days 6 through 18 of gestation to non-ventilated Dutch rabbits. Treatment groups were given either 0.15 mg/kg once daily or 0.10 mg/kg twice daily. Lethal respiratory distress occurred in two 0.15 mg/kg animals and in one 0.10 mg/kg animal, with transient respiratory distress or other evidence

of neuromuscular blockade occurring in 10 of 19 and in 4 of 20 of the 0.15 mg/kg and 0.10 mg/kg animals, respectively. There was an increased incidence of certain spontaneously occurring visceral and skeletal anomalies or variations in one or both treated groups when compared to non-treated controls. The percentage of male fetuses was lower (41% vs. 51%) and the post-implantation losses were increased (15% vs. 8%) in the group given 0.15 mg/kg once daily when compared to the controls; the mean numbers of implants (6.5 vs. 4.4) and normal live fetuses (5.4 vs. 3.8) were greater in this group when compared to the control group.

Labor and Delivery: It is not known whether muscle relaxants administered during vaginal delivery have immediate or delayed adverse effects on the fetus or increase the likelihood that resuscitation of the newborn will be necessary. The possibility that forceps delivery will be necessary may increase.

Tracrium (0.3 mg/kg) has been administered to 26 pregnant women during delivery by cesarean section. No harmful effects were attributable to Tracrium in any of the newborn infants, although small amounts of Tracrium were shown to cross the placental barrier. The possibility of respiratory depression in the newborn infant should always be considered following cesarean section during which a neuromuscular blocking agent has been administered. In patients receiving magnesium sulfate, the reversal of neuromuscular blockade may be unsatisfactory and Tracrium dose should be lowered as indicated.

Nursing Mothers: It is not known whether this drug is excreted in human milk. Because many drugs are excreted in human milk, caution should be exercised when Tracrium is administered to a nursing woman.

Pediatric Use: Safety and effectiveness in children below the age of 1 month have not been established.

ADVERSE REACTIONS
Observed in Controlled Clinical Studies: Tracrium was well tolerated and produced few adverse reactions during extensive clinical trials. Most adverse reactions were suggestive of histamine release. In studies including 875 patients, Tracrium was discontinued in only one patient (who required treatment for bronchial secretions), and six other patients required treatment for adverse reactions attributable to Tracrium (wheezing in one, hypotension in five). Of the five patients who required treatment for hypotension, three had a history of significant cardiovascular disease. The overall incidence rate for clinically important adverse reactions, therefore, was 7/875 or 0.8%. The table below includes all adverse reactions reported attributable to Tracrium during clinical trials with 875 patients.

[See table below left].

Most adverse reactions were of little clinical significance unless they were associated with significant hemodynamic changes. The table below summarizes the incidences of substantial vital sign changes noted during Tracrium clinical trials with 530 patients, without cardiovascular disease, in whom these parameters were assessed.

[See table above].

Observed in Clinical Practice: Based on initial clinical practice experience in approximately 3 million patients who received Tracrium in the U.S. and in the United Kingdom, spontaneously reported adverse reactions were uncommon (approximately 0.01–0.02%). The following adverse reactions are among the most frequently reported, but there are insufficient data to support an estimate of their incidence:
General: Allergic reactions (anaphylatic or anaphylactoid responses) which, in rare instances, were severe (e.g., cardiac arrest)
Musculoskeletal: Inadequate block, prolonged block
Cardiovascular: Hypotension, vasodilatation (flushing), tachycardia, bradycardia
Respiratory: Dyspnea, bronchospasm, laryngospasm
Integumentary: Rash, urticaria, reaction at injection site

OVERDOSAGE
There has been limited experience with Tracrium overdosage. The possibility of iatrogenic overdosage can be minimized by carefully monitoring muscle twitch response to peripheral nerve stimulation. Excessive doses of Tracrium can be expected to produce enhanced pharmacological ef-

---

PERCENT OF PATIENTS SHOWING ≥ 30% VITAL SIGN CHANGES FOLLOWING ADMINISTRATION OF TRACRIUM

Vital Sign Change	Initial Tracrium Dose (mg/kg)			
	0.00-0.30 (n = 365)	0.31-0.50* (n = 144)	≥ 0.60 (n = 21)	Total (n = 530)
Mean Arterial Pressure				
Increase	1.9%	2.8%	0%	2.1%
Decrease	1.1%	2.1%	14.3%	1.9%
Heart Rate				
Increase	1.6%	2.8%	4.8%	2.1%
Decrease	0.8%	0%	0%	0.6%

*Includes the recommended initial dosage range for most patients.

PERCENT OF PATIENTS REPORTING ADVERSE REACTIONS

Adverse Reaction	Initial Tracrium Dose (mg/kg)			
	0.00-0.30 (n = 485)	0.31-0.50* (n = 366)	≥ 0.60 (n = 24)	Total (n = 875)
Skin Flush	1.0%	8.7%	29.2%	5.0%
Erythema	0.6%	0.5%	0%	0.6%
Itching	0.4%	0%	0%	0.2%
Wheezing/Bronchial Secretions	0.2%	0.3%	0%	0.2%
Hives	0.2%	0%	0%	0.1%

*Includes the recommended initial dosage range for most patients.

fects. Overdosage may increase the risk of histamine release and cardiovascular effects, especially hypotension. If cardiovascular support is necessary, this should include proper positioning, fluid administration, and the use of vasopressor agents if necessary. The patient's airway should be assured, with manual or mechanical ventilation maintained as necessary. A longer duration of neuromuscular blockade may result from overdosage and a peripheral nerve stimulator should be used to monitor recovery. Recovery may be facilitated by administration of an anticholinesterase reversing agent such as neostigmine, edrophonium, or pyridostigmine, in conjunction with an anticholinergic agent such as atropine or glycopyrrolate. The appropriate package inserts should be consulted for prescribing information.

Three pediatric patients (3 weeks, 4 and 5 months of age) unintentionally received doses of 0.8 mg/kg to 1.0 mg/kg of Tracrium. The time to 25% recovery (50 to 55 minutes) following these doses, which were 5 to 6 times the ED_{95} dose, was moderately longer than the corresponding time observed following doses 2.0 to 2.5 times the Tracrium ED_{95} dose in infants (22 to 36 minutes). Cardiovascular changes were minimal. Nonetheless the possibility of cardiovascular changes must be considered in the case of overdose.

An adult patient (17 years of age) unintentionally received an initial dose of 1.3 mg/kg of Tracrium. The time from injection to 25% recovery (83 minutes) was approximately twice that observed following maximum recommended doses in adults (35–45 minutes). The patient experienced moderate hemodynamic changes (13% increase in mean arterial pressure and 27% increase in heart rate) which persisted for 40 minutes and did not require treatment.

The intravenous LD_{50}'s determined in non-ventilated male and female albino mice and male Wistar rats were 1.9, 2.01 and 1.31 mg/kg, respectively. Deaths occurred within 2 minutes and were caused by respiratory paralysis. The subcutaneous LD_{50} determined in non-ventilated male Wistar rats was 282.8 mg/kg. Tremors, ptosis, loss of reflexes and respiratory failure preceded death which occurred 45–120 minutes after injection.

DOSAGE AND ADMINISTRATION

To avoid distress to the patient, Tracrium should not be administered before unconsciousness has been induced. Tracrium should not be mixed in the same syringe, or administered simultaneously through the same needle, with alkaline solutions (e.g., barbiturate solutions).

Tracrium should be administered intravenously. DO NOT GIVE TRACRIUM BY INTRAMUSCULAR ADMINISTRATION. Intramuscular administration of Tracrium may result in tissue irritation and there are no clinical data to support this route of administration.

The use of a peripheral nerve stimulator to monitor muscle twitch suppression and recovery will permit the most advantageous use of Tracrium and minimize the possibility of overdosage.

Parenteral drug products should be inspected visually for particulate matter and discoloration prior to administration, whenever solution and container permit.

Bolus Doses for Intubation and Maintenance of Neuromuscular Blockade:

Adults: A Tracrium dose of 0.4 to 0.5 mg/kg (1.7 to 2.2 times the ED_{95}), given as an intravenous bolus injection, is the recommended initial dose for most patients. With this dose, good or excellent conditions for nonemergency intubation can be expected in 2 to 2.5 minutes in most patients, with maximum neuromuscular blockade achieved approximately 3 to 5 minutes after injection. Clinically required neuromuscular blockade generally lasts 20 to 35 minutes under balanced anesthesia. Under balanced anesthesia, recovery to 25% of control is achieved approximately 35 to 45 minutes after injection, and recovery is usually 95% complete approximately 60 minutes after injection.

Tracrium is potentiated by isoflurane or enflurane anesthesia. The same initial Tracrium dose of 0.4 to 0.5 mg/kg may be used for intubation prior to administration of these inhalation agents; however, if Tracrium is first administered under steady state of isoflurane or enflurane, the initial Tracrium dose should be reduced by approximately one-third, i.e., to 0.25 to 0.35 mg/kg, to adjust for the potentiating effects of these anesthetic agents. With halothane, which has only a marginal (approximately 20%) potentiating effect on Tracrium, smaller dosage reductions may be considered.

Tracrium doses of 0.08 to 0.10 mg/kg are recommended for maintenance of neuromuscular blockade during prolonged surgical procedures. The first maintenance dose will generally be required 20 to 45 minutes after the initial Tracrium injection, but the need for maintenance doses should be determined by clinical criteria. Because Tracrium lacks cumulative effects, maintenance doses may be administered at relatively regular intervals for each patient, ranging approximately from 15 to 25 minutes under balanced anesthesia, slightly longer under isoflurane or enflurane. Higher Tracrium doses (up to 0.2 mg/kg) permit maintenance dosing at longer intervals.

Children and Infants: No Tracrium dosage adjustments are required for pediatric patients two years of age or older. A

Tracrium dose of 0.3 to 0.4 mg/kg is recommended as the initial dose for infants (1 month to 2 years of age) under halothane anesthesia. Maintenance doses may be required with slightly greater frequency in infants and children than in adults.

Special Considerations: An initial Tracrium dose of 0.3 to 0.4 mg/kg, given slowly or in divided doses over one minute, is recommended for adults, children, or infants with significant cardiovascular disease and for adults, children, or infants with any history (e.g., severe anaphylactoid reactions or asthma) suggesting a greater risk of histamine release.

Dosage reductions must be considered also in patients with neuromuscular disease, severe electrolyte disorders, or carcinomatosis in which potentiation of neuromuscular blockade or difficulties with reversal have been demonstrated. There has been no clinical experience with Tracrium in these patients, and no specific dosage adjustments can be recommended. No Tracrium dosage adjustments are required for patients with renal disease.

An initial Tracrium dose of 0.3 to 0.4 mg/kg is recommended for adults following the use of succinylcholine for intubation under balanced anesthesia. Further reductions may be desirable with the use of potent inhalation anesthetics. The patient should be permitted to recover from the effects of succinylcholine prior to Tracrium administration. Insufficient data are available for recommendation of a specific initial Tracrium dose for administration following the use of succinylcholine in children and infants.

Use by Infusion: After administration of a recommended initial bolus dose of Tracrium (0.3 to 0.5 mg/kg), a diluted solution of Tracrium can be administered by continuous infusion to adults and children aged 2 or more years for maintenance of neuromuscular blockade during extended surgical procedures. Long-term intravenous infusion to support mechanical ventilation in the intensive care unit has not been studied sufficiently to support dosage recommendations.

Infusion of Tracrium should be individualized for each patient. The rate of administration should be adjusted according to the patient's response as determined by peripheral nerve stimulation. Accurate dosing is best achieved using a precision infusion device.

Infusion of Tracrium should be initiated only after early evidence of spontaneous recovery from the bolus dose. An initial infusion rate of 9 to 10 μg/kg/min may be required to rapidly counteract the spontaneous recovery of neuromuscular function. Thereafter, a rate of 5 to 9 μg/kg/min should be adequate to maintain continuous neuromuscular blockade in the range of 89 to 99% in most pediatric and adult patients under balanced anesthesia. Occasional patients may require infusion rates as low as 2 μg/kg/min or as high as 15 μg/kg/min.

The neuromuscular blocking effect of Tracrium administered by infusion is potentiated by enflurane or isoflurane and, to a lesser extent, by halothane. Reduction in the infusion rate of Tracrium should, therefore, be considered for patients receiving inhalation anesthesia. The rate of Tracrium infusion should be reduced by approximately one-third in the presence of steady-state enflurane or isoflurane anesthesia; smaller reductions should be considered in the presence of halothane.

In patients undergoing cardiopulmonary bypass with induced hypothermia, the rate of infusion of Tracrium required to maintain adequate surgical relaxation during hypothermia (25° to 28°C) has been shown to be approximately half the rate required during normothermia.

Spontaneous recovery from neuromuscular blockade following discontinuation of Tracrium infusion may be expected to proceed at a rate comparable to that following administration of a single bolus dose.

Tracrium infusion solutions may be prepared by admixing Tracrium Injection with an appropriate diluent such as 5% Dextrose Injection USP, 0.9% Sodium Chloride Injection USP, or 5% Dextrose and 0.9% Sodium Chloride Injection USP. Infusion solutions should be used within 24 hours of preparation. Unused solutions should be discarded. Solutions containing 0.2 mg/mL or 0.5 mg/mL Tracrium in the above diluents may be stored either under refrigeration or at room temperature for 24 hours without significant loss of potency. Care should be taken during admixture to prevent inadvertent contamination. Visually inspect prior to administration.

Spontaneous degradation of Tracrium has been demonstrated to occur more rapidly in lactated Ringer's solution than in 0.9% sodium chloride solution. Therefore, it is recommended that Lactated Ringer's Injection USP not be used as a diluent in preparing solutions of Tracrium for infusion.

The amount of infusion solution required per minute will depend upon the concentration of Tracrium in the infusion solution, the desired dose of Tracrium, and the patient's weight. The following tables provide guidelines for delivery, in mL/hr (equivalent to microdrops/min when 60 microdrops = 1 mL), of Tracrium solutions in concentrations of 0.2

mg/mL (20 mg in 100 mL) or 0.5 mg/mL (50 mg in 100 mL) with an infusion pump or a gravity flow device.

Tracrium (atracurium besylate) Infusion Rates for a Concentration of 0.2 mg/mL

Patient Weight (Kg)	Drug Delivery Rate (μg/kg/min)					
	5	6	7	8	9	10
	Infusion Delivery Rate (mL/hr)					
30	45	54	63	72	81	90
35	53	63	74	84	95	105
40	60	72	84	96	108	120
45	68	81	95	108	122	135
50	75	90	105	120	135	150
55	83	99	116	132	149	165
60	90	108	126	144	162	180
65	98	117	137	156	176	195
70	105	126	147	168	189	210
75	113	135	158	180	203	225
80	120	144	168	192	216	240
90	135	162	189	216	243	270
100	150	180	210	240	270	300

Tracrium (atracurium besylate) Infusion Rates for a Concentration of 0.5 mg/mL

Patient Weight (Kg)	Drug Delivery Rate (μg/kg/min)					
	5	6	7	8	9	10
	Infusion Delivery Rate (mL/hr)					
30	18	22	25	29	32	36
35	21	25	29	34	38	42
40	24	29	34	38	43	48
45	27	32	38	43	49	54
50	30	36	42	48	54	60
55	33	40	46	53	59	66
60	36	43	50	58	65	72
65	39	47	55	62	70	78
70	42	50	59	67	76	84
75	45	54	63	72	81	90
80	48	58	67	77	86	96
90	54	65	76	86	97	108
100	60	72	84	96	108	120

HOW SUPPLIED

Tracrium Injection, 10 mg atracurium besylate in each mL. 5 mL ampuls (50 mg atracurium besylate per ampul). Box of 10 (NDC 0081-0940-10).
10 mL Multiple Dose Vial (100 mg atracurium besylate per vial). Box of 10 (NDC 0081-0940-95).

STORAGE: Tracrium Injection should be refrigerated at 2° to 8°C (36° to 46°F) to preserve potency. DO NOT FREEZE. Upon removal from refrigeration to room temperature storage conditions (25°C/77°F), use Tracrium Injection within 14 days even if rerefrigerated.

U.S. Patent No. 4179507

VASOXYL® INJECTION   ℞
[väz"ox'ŭl]
(Methoxamine Hydrochloride)
20 mg in 1 ml

DESCRIPTION

Vasoxyl (methoxamine hydrochloride) Injection is a sterile solution for intravenous or intramuscular injection, made isotonic with sodium chloride. Each 1 ml ampul contains 20 mg methoxamine hydrochloride. Citric acid anhydrous 0.3% and sodium citrate 0.3% are added as buffers and potassium metabisulfite 0.1% is added as an antioxidant.

Methoxamine hydrochloride is a sympathomimetic amine. It has the empirical formula $C_{11}H_{17}NO_3 \cdot HCl$ and a molecular weight of 247.72. The drug is very soluble in water, soluble in ethanol, but practically insoluble in ether, benzene or chloroform. It is known chemically as α-(1-aminoethyl)-2,5-dimethoxybenzenemethanol hydrochloride.

CLINICAL PHARMACOLOGY

Vasoxyl is an alpha-receptor stimulant which produces a prompt and prolonged rise in blood pressure following parenteral administration. It is especially useful for maintaining blood pressure during operations under spinal anesthesia[1,2,3] and may also be used safely during general anesthesia. Vasoxyl does not increase the irritability of the cyclopropane-sensitized heart, making it useful during cyclopropane anesthesia.[4,5] Tachyphylaxis has not been a clinical problem.[1]

Continued on next page

Burroughs Wellcome—Cont.

The major pharmacological effect of Vasoxyl is a potent, prolonged pressor action following parenteral administration. Vasoxyl differs from most other sympathomimetic amines both in animals[4,6,7] and in man[1,8] by having a predominantly peripheral action and lacking inotropic and chronotropic effects. Vasoxyl has less arrhythmogenic potential than other sympathomimetic amines and rarely causes ventricular tachycardia, fibrillation, or increased sinoatrial rate.[4] On occasion, a decrease in rate occurs as blood pressure increases,[1,9,10] apparently caused by a carotid sinus reflex. This bradycardia can be abolished by atropine.[9] The pressor action appears to be due to peripheral vasoconstriction rather than a centrally mediated effect. Evidence for direct action of blood vessels is provided in part by the observation of intense constriction along the course of a vein into which Vasoxyl has been injected.[1] Vasoxyl also increases venous pressure.[8]

Following intravenous administration of Vasoxyl in dogs[11] and humans,[9,12] the peak pressor effect occurs within 0.5 to 2 minutes. In a group of human surgical patients,[13] the duration of the pressor effect following a single intravenous dose of 2 to 4 mg of Vasoxyl was 10 to 15 minutes. No clinical pharmacology studies are available concerning the onset and duration of action after administration of recommended intramuscular doses (10 to 15 mg). With administration of 10 to 40 mg Vasoxyl intramuscularly to patients, however, the peak effect occurs within 15 to 20 minutes, and the duration of action is approximately one and a half hours.[14]

Data from pharmacokinetic studies of Vasoxyl following either intravenous or intramuscular administration are not available.

INDICATIONS AND USAGE

Vasoxyl is intended for supporting, restoring or maintaining blood pressure during anesthesia (including cyclopropane anesthesia). It can be used to terminate some episodes of supraventricular tachycardia.

CONTRAINDICATIONS

Vasoxyl is contraindicated in patients with severe hypertension, or in patients who are hypersensitive to methoxamine.

WARNINGS

The use of Vasoxyl in patients receiving monoamine oxidase inhibitors, tricyclic antidepressants or oxytocic agents such as vasopressin or certain ergot alkaloids may result in potentiation of the pressor effect (See "Drug Interactions" under PRECAUTIONS).

Contains potassium metabisulfite, a sulfite that may cause allergic-type reactions including anaphylactic symptoms and life-threatening or less severe asthmatic episodes in certain susceptible people. The overall prevalence of sulfite sensitivity in the general population is unknown and probably low. Sulfite sensitivity is seen more frequently in asthmatic than in nonasthmatic people.

PRECAUTIONS

General: Vasoxyl, like other vasopressor agents, should be used with caution in patients with hyperthyroidism, bradycardia, partial heart block, myocardial disease, or severe arteriosclerosis. Caution should be exercised to avoid overdosage, preventing undesirable high blood pressure and/or bradycardia. Note: Bradycardia may be abolished with atropine (see OVERDOSAGE). Also, caution should be taken when Vasoxyl is used closely following the parenteral injection of ergot alkaloids to avoid an excessive rise in blood pressure.

Drug Interactions: The pressor effect of Vasoxyl may be markedly potentiated when Vasoxyl is used in conjunction with monoamine oxidase inhibitors, tricyclic antidepressants, vasopressin or ergot alkaloids such as ergotamine, ergonovine or methylergonovine. Therefore, when initiating pressor therapy in patients receiving these drugs the initial dose should be small and given with caution (see WARNINGS).

Drug/Laboratory Test Interactions: Vasoxyl may increase plasma cortisol and ACTH levels. Caution should be used when interpreting plasma cortisol and ACTH levels in a patient concurrently receiving Vasoxyl.[15,16]

Carcinogenesis, Mutagenesis, Impairment of Fertility: No long-term studies have been performed to evaluate the potential of Vasoxyl in these areas.

Pregnancy: _Teratogenic Effects:_ Pregnancy Category C: Vasoxyl has been shown to decrease uterine blood flow, decrease fetal heart rate and adversely affect the fetal acid-base status in pregnant ewes and monkeys at doses comparable to those used in humans. There are no adequate and well-controlled studies in pregnant women. There has been one report of a fetal death; the mother received Vasoxyl concomitantly with several other drugs. A direct causal relationship to Vasoxyl was not established. Vasoxyl should be used during pregnancy only if the potential benefit justifies the potential risk to the fetus.

Vasoxyl (2.5 mg I.V., 1 to 3 times over a 45 min. period) given to 7 pregnant ewes showed a significant deterioration in fetal acid-base status as evidenced by hypoxia, hypercarbia and metabolic acidosis.[17] An inverse relationship between pressor response to Vasoxyl and uteroplacental blood flow has been shown in 16 pregnant ewes studied at doses ranging from 0.025 mg/kg to 0.2 mg/kg.[18] Uterine blood flow was decreased at all doses, but no significant change in fetal blood gas or acid-base status was demonstrated. Vasoxyl administration to 4 fetuses (50 mcg/kg/min for 60 min) and to 4 ewes (25 mcg/kg/min for 30 min) was associated with a decrease in fetal heart rate and uterine blood flow.[19] Nine monkeys studied at an average Vasoxyl dose of 1.3 mg/kg administered over 57 min showed a decrease in uterine blood flow and a possible association with fetal asphyxia.[20]

Labor and Delivery: If vasopressor drugs are used to correct hypotension or added to the local anesthetic solution during labor and delivery, some oxytocic drugs (vasopressin, ergotamine, ergonovine, methylergonovine) may cause severe persistent hypertension (see WARNINGS and "Drug Interactions" under PRECAUTIONS).

"Note": In pregnant animals, Vasoxyl has been shown to decrease uterine blood flow, possibly resulting in fetal asphyxia. Uterine vasoconstriction and fetal bradycardia may also be produced. (See ADVERSE REACTIONS and "Pregnancy" under PRECAUTIONS.)

Nursing Mothers: It is not known whether this drug is excreted in human milk. Because many drugs are excreted in human milk, caution should be exercised when Vasoxyl is administered to a nursing woman.

Pediatric Use: Safety and effectiveness in children have not been established.

ADVERSE REACTIONS

The following adverse reactions have been observed, but there are insufficient data to support an estimate of their frequency:

Cardiovascular: Excessive blood pressure elevations particularly with high dosage, ventricular ectopic beats

Gastrointestinal: Nausea, vomiting (often projectile)

Central Nervous System: Headache (often severe), anxiety

Integumentary: Sweating, pilomotor response

Genitourinary: Uterine hypertonus, fetal bradycardia (see "Labor and Delivery" under PRECAUTIONS), urinary urgency

OVERDOSAGE

Overdosage of Vasoxyl may be manifested as an undesirable elevation in blood pressure and/or bradycardia. Should a clinically significant elevation of blood pressure occur that requires treatment, it may be immediately reversed with an alpha-adrenergic blocking agent (e.g. phentolamine). Bradycardia may be abolished by atropine.

DOSAGE AND ADMINISTRATION

Blood volume depletion should always be corrected before any vasopressor is administered. The usual intravenous dose of Vasoxyl for emergencies is 3 to 5 mg, injected slowly. Intravenous injection may be supplemented by intramuscular injections to provide a more prolonged effect. The usual intramuscular dose is 10 to 15 mg given shortly before or at the time of administering spinal anesthesia to prevent a fall in blood pressure. The tendency for the blood pressure to fall is greater with higher levels of spinal anesthesia, hence the dosage may be adjusted accordingly; 10 mg may be adequate at lower spinal levels while 15 to 20 mg may be required at high levels of spinal anesthesia. Repeated doses may be given if necessary, but time should be allowed for the previous dose to act (about 15 minutes, see CLINICAL PHARMACOLOGY). For cases of only moderate hypotension, 5 to 10 mg intramuscularly may be adequate.

For purposes of correcting a fall in blood pressure, an intramuscular injection of 10 to 15 mg of Vasoxyl may be given depending upon the degree of fall. In cases where the systolic pressure falls to 60 mmHg or less, or whenever an emergency exists, an intravenous injection of 3 to 5 mg Vasoxyl is indicated. This intravenous dose may be accompanied by 10 to 15 mg intramuscularly to provide more prolonged effect. For termination of episodes of supraventricular tachycardia not responsive to other modes of therapy, the usual dose of Vasoxyl is 10 mg intravenously, administered by slow push (i.e. 3 to 5 min).

Parenteral drug products should be inspected visually for particulate matter and discoloration prior to administration whenever solution and container permit.

HOW SUPPLIED

1 ml ampuls, containing 20 mg methoxamine hydrochloride. Box of 10 (NDC 0081-0957-10). Store at 15° to 30°C (59° to 86°F) and protect from light.

REFERENCES

1. King BD, Dripps RD: The use of methoxamine for maintenance of the circulation during spinal anesthesia. _Surg Gynecol Obstet_ 1950;90:659–665.
2. Kistler EM, Ruben JE: Methoxamine in 1 percent procaine as a prophylactic vasopressor in spinal anesthesia. _Arch Surg_ 1951;62:64–69.
3. Poe MF: Use of methoxamine hydrochloride as a pressor agent during spinal analgesia. _Anesthesiology_ 1952; 13:89–93.
4. Lahti RE, Brill IC, McCawley EL: The effect of methoxamine hydrochloride (Vasoxyl) on cardiac rhythm. _J Pharmacol Exp Ther_ 1955;115:268–274.
5. Stutzman JW, Pettinga FL, Fruggiero EJ: Cardiac effects of methoxamine (β-[2,5-dimethoxy-phenyl]-β-hydroxyisopropylamine HCl) and desoxyephedrine during cyclopropane anesthesia. _J Pharmacol Exp Ther_ 1949; 97:385–387.
6. West JW, Faulk AT, Guzman SV: Comparative study of effects of levarterenol and methoxamine in shock associated with acute myocardial ischemia in dogs. _Circ Res_ 1962;10:712–721.
7. Goldberg LI, Cotten M, Darby TD, Howell EV: Comparative heart contractile force effects of equipressor doses of several sympathomimetic amines. _J Pharmacol Exp Ther_ 1953;108:177–185.
8. Aviado DM, Wnuck AL: Mechanisms for cardiac slowing by methoxamine. _J Pharmacol Exp Ther_ 1957; 119:99–106.
9. Nathanson MH, Miller H: Clinical observations on a new epinephrin-like compound, methoxamine. _Am J Med Sci_ 1952;223:270–279.
10. Stanfield CA, Yu PN: Hemodynamic effects of methoxamine in mitral valve disease. _Circ Res_ 1960;8:859–864.
11. Imai S, Shigei T, Hashimoto K: Cardiac actions of methoxamine with special reference to its antagonist action to epinephrine. _Circ Res_ 1961;9:552–560.
12. _The Extra Pharmacopoeia, Martindale_ 28th Ed., Reynolds, JEF, ed., Pharmaceutical Press (London), pp.19.
13. Goldberg LI, Bloodwell RD, Braunwald E, _et al._ The direct effects of norepinephrine, epinephrine, and methoxamine on myocardial contractile force in man. _Circ_ 1960;22:1125–1132.
14. Data on File, Burroughs Wellcome Co.
15. Laurian L, Oberman Z, Hoerer E, _et al._: Low cortisol and growth hormone secretion in response to methoxamine administration in obese subjects. _Isr J Med Sci_ 1977;13:477–481.
16. Nakai Y, Imura H, Yoshimi T, Matsukura S: Adrenergic control mechanism for ACTH secretion in man. _Acta Endocrinol_ 1973;74:263–270.
17. Shnider SM, DeLorimier AA, Asling JH, Morishima HO: Vasopressors in obstetrics. II. Fetal hazards of methoxamine administration during obstetric spinal anesthesia. _Am J Obstet Gynecol_ 1970;106:680–686.
18. Ralston DH, Shnider SM, DeLorimier AA: Effects of equipotent ephedrine, metaraminol, mephentermine and methoxamine on uterine blood flow in the pregnant ewe. _Anesthesiology_ 1974;40:354–370.
19. Oakes GK, Ehrenkranz RA, Walker AM, _et al._: Effect of α-adrenergic agonist and antagonist infusion on the umbilical and uterine circulations of pregnant sheep. _Biol Neonate_ 1980;38:229–237.
20. Eng M, Berges PU, Ueland K, _et al._: The effects of methoxamine and ephedrine in normotensive pregnant primates. _Anesthesiology_ 1971;35:354–360.

VIROPTIC® OPHTHALMIC   ℞
[vī-rŏp'tĭk"]
SOLUTION, 1% Sterile
(Trifluridine)

DESCRIPTION

Viroptic is the brand name for trifluridine (also known as trifluorothymidine, F_3TdR, F_3T), an antiviral drug for topical treatment of epithelial keratitis caused by Herpes simplex virus. The chemical name of trifluridine is 2'-deoxy-5-(trifluoromethyl)uridine.

Viroptic sterile ophthalmic solution contains 1% trifluridine in an aqueous solution with acetic acid and sodium acetate (buffers), sodium chloride, and thimerosal 0.001% (added as a preservative).

CLINICAL PHARMACOLOGY

Trifluridine is a fluorinated pyrimidine nucleoside with _in vitro_ and _in vivo_ activity against Herpes simplex virus, types 1 and 2 and vacciniavirus. Some strains of Adenovirus are also inhibited _in vitro._

Trifluridine interferes with DNA synthesis in cultured mammalian cells. However, its antiviral mechanism of action is not completely known.

In vitro perfusion studies on excised rabbit corneas have shown that trifluridine penetrates the intact cornea as evidenced by recovery of parental drug and its major metabolite, 5-carboxy-2'-deoxyuridine, on the endothelial side of the cornea. Absence of the corneal epithelium enhances the penetration of trifluridine approximately two-fold.

Intraocular penetration of trifluridine occurs after topical instillation of Viroptic into human eyes. Decreased corneal integrity or stromal or uveal inflammation may enhance the penetration of trifluridine into the aqueous humor. Unlike the results of ocular penetration of trifluridine _in vitro_, 5-

carboxy-2'-deoxyuridine was not found in detectable concentrations within the aqueous humor of the human eye. Systemic absorption of trifluridine following therapeutic dosing with Viroptic appears to be negligible. No detectable concentrations of trifluridine or 5-carboxy-2'-deoxyuridine were found in the sera of adult healthy normal subjects who had Viroptic instilled into their eyes seven times daily for 14 consecutive days.

INDICATIONS AND USAGE

Viroptic (Trifluridine) Ophthalmic Solution, 1% is indicated for the treatment of primary keratoconjunctivitis and recurrent epithelial keratitis due to Herpes simplex virus, types 1 and 2. Viroptic is also effective in the treatment of epithelial keratitis that has not responded clinically to the topical administration of idoxuridine or when ocular toxicity or hypersensitivity to idoxuridine has occurred. In a smaller number of patients found to be resistant to topical vidarabine, Viroptic was also effective.

The clinical efficacy of Viroptic in the treatment of stromal keratitis and uveitis due to Herpes simplex virus or ophthalmic infections caused by vacciniavirus and Adenovirus has not been established by well-controlled clinical trials. Viroptic has not been shown to be effective in the prophylaxis of Herpes simplex virus keratoconjunctivitis and epithelial keratitis by well-controlled clinical trials. Viroptic is not effective against bacterial, fungal or chlamydial infections of the cornea or nonviral trophic lesions.

During controlled multicenter clinical trials, 92 of 97 (95%) patients (78 of 81 with dendritic and 14 of 16 with geographic ulcers) responded to Viroptic therapy as evidenced by complete corneal re-epithelialization within the 14 day therapy period. In these controlled studies, 56 of 75 (75%) patients (49 of 58 with dendritic and 7 of 17 with geographic ulcers) responded to idoxuridine therapy. The mean time to corneal re-epithelialization of dendritic ulcers (6 days) and geographic ulcers (7 days) was similar for both therapies. In other clinical studies, Viroptic was evaluated in the treatment of Herpes simplex virus keratitis in patients who were unresponsive or intolerant to the topical administration of idoxuridine or vidarabine. Viroptic was effective in 138 of 150 (92%) patients (109 of 114 with dendritic and 29 of 36 with geographic ulcers) as evidenced by corneal re-epithelialization. The mean time to corneal re-epithelialization was 6 days for patients with dendritic ulcers and 12 days for patients with geographic ulcers.

CONTRAINDICATIONS

Viroptic (Trifluridine) Ophthalmic Solution, 1%, is contraindicated for patients who develop hypersensitivity reactions or chemical intolerance to trifluridine.

WARNINGS

The recommended dosage and frequency of administration should not be exceeded (see DOSAGE AND ADMINISTRATION).

PRECAUTIONS

General: Viroptic (Trifluridine) Ophthalmic Solution, 1% should be prescribed only for patients who have a clinical diagnosis of herpetic keratitis.

Viroptic may cause mild local irritation of the conjunctiva and cornea when instilled but these effects are usually transient.

Although documented in vitro viral resistance to trifluridine has not been reported following multiple exposure to Viroptic, the possibility exists of viral resistance development.

Drug Interactions: The following drugs have been administered topically to the eye and concurrently with Viroptic in a limited number of patients without apparent evidence of adverse interaction: antibiotics—chloramphenicol, erythromycin, polymyxin B sulfate, bacitracin, gentamicin sulfate, tetracycline HCl, sodium sulfacetamide, neomycin sulfate; steroids—dexamethasone, dexamethasone sodium phosphate, prednisolone acetate, prednisolone sodium phosphate, hydrocortisone, fluorometholone; and other ophthalmic drugs—atropine sulfate, scopolamine hydrobromide, naphazoline hydrochloride, cyclopentolate hydrochloride, homatropine hydrobromide, pilocarpine, l-epinephrine hydrochloride, sodium chloride.

Carcinogenesis, Mutagenesis, Impairment of Fertility: *Mutagenic Potential.* Trifluridine has been shown to exert mutagenic, DNA-damaging and cell-transforming activities in various standard in vitro test systems, and clastogenic activity in Vicia faba cells.

Although the significance of these test results is not clear or fully understood, there exists the possibility that mutagenic agents may cause genetic damage in humans.

Oncogenic Potential. Lifetime carcinogenicity bioassays in rats and mice given daily subcutaneous doses of trifluridine have been performed. Rats tested at 1.5, 7.5 and 15 mg/kg/day had increased incidences of adenocarcinomas of the intestinal tract and mammary glands, hemangiosarcomas of the spleen and liver, carcinosarcomas of the prostate gland and granulosa-thecal cell tumors of the ovary. Mice were tested at 1, 5 and 10 mg/kg/day; those given 10 mg/kg/day trifluridine had significantly increased inci-

dences of adenocarcinomas of the intestinal tract and uterus. Those given 10 mg/kg/day also had a significantly increased incidence of testicular atrophy as compared to vehicle control mice.

Pregnancy: The drug should not be prescribed for pregnant women unless the potential benefits outweigh the potential risks.

Teratogenic Potential: Kury and Crosby[1] found that trifluridine was teratogenic when injected directly into the yolk sac of developing chick embryos. Itoi et al.[2] found that topical application of 1% trifluridine ophthalmic solution to the eyes of rabbits on days 6–18 of pregnancy produced no teratogenic effects. Trifluridine was not teratogenic when given subcutaneously to rats at doses up to 5.0 mg/kg/day although drug-induced fetal toxicity (delayed ossification of portions of the skeletal system) was observed at the 2.5 mg/kg/day dose level. Trifluridine was not teratogenic when given subcutaneously to rabbits at doses up to 5.0 mg/kg/day. Drug-induced fetal toxicity (delayed ossification of portions of the skeletal system) was observed at the 2.5 mg/kg/day dose level. A 1.0 mg/kg/day dose was considered to be a no-effect level in both rats and rabbits. Based upon these findings in animals, it is unlikely that Viroptic would cause embryonic or fetal damage if given in the recommended ophthalmic dosage to pregnant women. A safe dose, however, has not been established for the human embryo or fetus.

Nursing Mothers: It is unlikely that trifluridine is excreted in human milk after ophthalmic instillation of Viroptic because of the relatively small dosage (≤ 5.0 mg/day), its dilution in body fluids and its extremely short half-life (approximately 12 minutes). The drug should not be prescribed for nursing mothers unless the potential benefits outweigh the potential risks.

ADVERSE REACTIONS

The most frequent adverse reactions reported during controlled clinical trials were mild, transient burning or stinging upon instillation (4.6%) and palpebral edema (2.8%). Other adverse reactions in decreasing order of reported frequency were superficial punctate keratopathy, epithelial keratopathy, hypersensitivity reaction, stromal edema, irritation, keratitis sicca, hyperemia, and increased intraocular pressure.

OVERDOSAGE

Overdosage by ocular instillation is unlikely because any excess solution should be quickly expelled from the conjunctival sac.

Acute overdosage by accidental oral ingestion of Viroptic has not occurred. However, should such ingestion occur, the 75 mg dosage of trifluridine in a 7.5 mL bottle of Viroptic is not likely to produce adverse effects. Single intravenous doses of 15–30 mg/kg/day in children and adults with neoplastic disease produce reversible bone marrow depression as the only potentially serious toxic effect and only after 3–5 courses of therapy.[3] The acute oral LD_{50} in the mouse and rat was 4379 mg/kg or higher.

DOSAGE AND ADMINISTRATION

Instill one drop of Viroptic Ophthalmic Solution, 1% onto the cornea of the affected eye every two hours while awake for a maximum daily dosage of nine drops until the corneal ulcer has completely re-epithelialized. Following re-epithelialization, treatment for an additional seven days of one drop every four hours while awake for a minimum daily dosage of five drops is recommended.

If there are no signs of improvement after seven days of therapy or complete re-epithelialization has not occurred after 14 days of therapy, other forms of therapy should be considered. Continuous administration of Viroptic for periods exceeding 21 days should be avoided because of potential ocular toxicity.

HOW SUPPLIED

Viroptic Ophthalmic Solution, 1% is supplied as a sterile ophthalmic solution in a plastic Drop Dose® dispenser bottle of 7.5 mL. (NDC 0081-0968-02)

Store under refrigeration 2° to 8°C (36° to 46°F).

ANIMAL PHARMACOLOGY AND ANIMAL TOXICOLOGY

Corneal wound healing studies in rabbits showed that Viroptic did not significantly retard closure of epithelial wounds. However, mild toxic changes such as intracellular edema of the basal cell layer, mild thinning of the overlying epithelium and reduced strength of stromal wounds were observed.

Whereas instillation of Viroptic into rabbit eyes during a subchronic toxicity study produced some degree of corneal epithelial thinning, a 12-month chronic toxicity study in rabbits in which Viroptic was instilled into eyes in intermittent, multiple, full-therapy courses showed no drug-related changes in the cornea.

DoD NSN 6505-01-142-8314

REFERENCES

1. Kury G, Crosby RJ: The teratogenic effect of 5-trifluoromethyl-2'-deoxyuridine in chicken embryos. *Toxicol Appl Pharmacol* 1967;11:72–80.
2. Itoi M, Getter JW, Kaneko N, et al: Teratogenicities of ophthalmic drugs. I. Antiviral ophthalmic drugs. *Arch Ophthalmol* 1975;93:46–51.
3. Ansfield FJ, Ramirez G: Phase I and II studies of 2'-deoxy-5-(trifluoromethyl)-uridine (NSC-75520). *Cancer Chemother Rep* 1971; 55(pt 1):205–208.

WELLBUTRIN® Tablets   ℞
['wel 'byüt-trin]
(BUPROPION HYDROCHLORIDE)

DESCRIPTION

Wellbutrin (bupropion hydrochloride),* an antidepressant of the aminoketone class, is chemically unrelated to tricyclic, tetracyclic, or other known antidepressant agents. Its structure closely resembles that of diethylpropion; it is related to phenylethylamines. It is designated as 2-tert-butylamino-3'-chloropropiophenone hydrochloride. The molecular weight is 276.2. The empirical formula is $C_{13}H_{18}ClNO \cdot HCl$. Bupropion powder is white, crystalline, and highly soluble in water. It has a bitter taste and produces the sensation of local anesthesia on the oral mucosa. Wellbutrin is supplied for oral administration as 75 mg (yellow-gold) and 100 mg (red) film-coated tablets.

CLINICAL PHARMACOLOGY

Pharmacodynamics and Pharmacological Actions: The neurochemical mechanism of the antidepressant effect of bupropion is not known. Bupropion does not inhibit monoamine oxidase. Compared to classical tricyclic antidepressants, it is a weak blocker of the neuronal uptake of serotonin and norepinephrine; it also inhibits the neuronal reuptake of dopamine to some extent. Bupropion produces dose-related CNS stimulant effects in animals, as evidenced by increased locomotor activity, increased rates of responding in various schedule-controlled operant behavior tasks, and, at high doses, induction of mild stereotyped behavior. Bupropion causes convulsions in rodents and dogs at doses approximately tenfold the dose recommended as the human antidepressant dose.

Absorption, Distribution, Pharmacokinetics, Metabolism, and Elimination:

Oral bioavailability and single dose pharmacokinetics: In man, following oral administration of Wellbutrin, peak plasma bupropion concentrations are usually achieved within 2 hours, followed by a biphasic decline. The average half-life of the second (post-distributional) phase is approximately 14 hours, with a range of 8 to 24 hours. Six hours after a single dose, plasma bupropion concentrations are approximately 30% of peak concentrations. Plasma bupropion concentrations are dose-proportional following single doses of 100 to 250 mg; however, it is not known if the proportionality between dose and plasma level is maintained in chronic use.

The absolute bioavailability of Wellbutrin tablets in man has not been determined because an intravenous formulation for human use is not available. However, it appears likely that only a small proportion of any orally administered dose reaches the systemic circulation intact. For example, the absolute bioavailability of bupropion in animals (rats and dogs) ranges from 5–20%.

Metabolism: Following oral administration of 200 mg of ¹⁴C-bupropion, 87% and 10% of the radioactive dose were recovered in the urine and feces, respectively. However, the fraction of the oral dose of Wellbutrin excreted unchanged was only 0.5%, a finding documenting the extensive metabolism of bupropion.

Several of the known metabolites of bupropion are pharmacologically active, but their potency and toxicity relative to bupropion have not been fully characterized. However, because of their longer elimination half-lives, the plasma concentrations of at least two of the known metabolites can be expected, especially in chronic use, to be very much higher than the plasma concentration of bupropion. This is of potential clinical importance because factors or conditions altering metabolic capacity (e.g., liver disease, congestive heart failure, age, concomitant medications, etc.) or elimination may be expected to influence the degree and extent of accumulation of these active metabolites.

Furthermore, bupropion has been shown to induce its own metabolism in three animal species (mice, rats, and dogs) following subchronic administration. If induction also occurs in humans, the relative contribution of bupropion and its metabolites to the clinical effects of Wellbutrin may be changed in chronic use.

Continued on next page

Burroughs Wellcome—Cont.

Plasma and urinary metabolites so far identified include biotransformation products formed via reduction of the carbonyl group and/or hydroxylation of the *tert*- butyl group of bupropion. Four basic metabolites have been identified. They are the *erythro*- and *threo*- amino alcohols of bupropion, the *erythro*- amino diol of bupropion, and a morpholinol metabolite (formed from hydroxylation of the *tert*- butyl group of bupropion).

The morpholinol metabolite appears in the systemic circulation almost as rapidly as the parent drug following a single oral dose. Its peak level is three times the peak level of the parent drug; it has a half-life on the order of 24 hours; and its AUC 0–60 hrs is about 15 times that of bupropion.

The *threo*- amino alcohol metabolite has a plasma concentration-time profile similar to that of the morpholinol metabolite. The *erythro*-amino alcohol and the *erythro*- amino diol metabolites generally cannot be detected in the systemic circulation following a single oral dose of the parent drug. The morpholinol and the *threo*- amino alcohol metabolites have been found to be half as potent as bupropion in animal screening tests for antidepressant drugs.

During a chronic dosing study in 14 depressed patients with left ventricular dysfunction, it was found that there was substantial interpatient variability (two- to fivefold) in the trough steady-state concentrations of bupropion and the morpholinol and *threo*- amino alcohol metabolites. In addition, the steady-state plasma concentrations of these metabolites were 10–100 times the steady-state concentrations of the parent drug.

The effect of other disease states and altered organ function on the metabolism and/or elimination of bupropion has not been studied in detail. However, the elimination of the major metabolites of bupropion may be affected by reduced renal or hepatic function because they are moderately polar compounds and are likely to undergo conjugation in the liver prior to urinary excretion. The preliminary results of a comparative single-dose pharmacokinetic study in normal versus cirrhotic patients indicated that half-lives of the metabolites were prolonged by cirrhosis and that the metabolites accumulated to levels two to three times those in normals. The effect of age on plasma concentrations of bupropion and its metabolites has not been characterized.

In vitro tests show that bupropion is 80% or more bound to human albumin at plasma concentrations up to 800 micromolar (200 μg/mL).

INDICATIONS AND USAGE

Wellbutrin is indicated for the treatment of depression. A physician considering Wellbutrin for the management of a patient's first episode of depression should be aware that the drug may cause generalized seizures with an approximate incidence of 0.4% (4/1000). This incidence of seizures may exceed that of other marketed antidepressants by as much as fourfold. This relative risk is only an approximate estimate because no direct comparative studies have been conducted. The efficacy of Wellbutrin has been established in three placebo-controlled trials, including two of approximately three weeks duration in depressed inpatients, and one of approximately six weeks duration in depressed outpatients. The depressive disorder of the patients studied corresponds most closely to the Major Depression category of the APA Diagnostic and Statistical Manual III.

Major Depression implies a prominent and relatively persistent depressed or dysphoric mood that usually interferes with daily functioning (nearly every day for at least two weeks); it should include at least four of the following eight symptoms: change in appetite, change in sleep, psychomotor agitation or retardation, loss of interest in usual activities or decrease in sexual drive, increased fatigability, feelings of guilt or worthlessness, slowed thinking or impaired concentration, and suicidal ideation or attempts.

Effectiveness of Wellbutrin in long-term use, that is, for more than 6 weeks, has not been systematically evaluated in controlled trials. Therefore, the physician who elects to use Wellbutrin for extended periods should periodically reevaluate the long-term usefulness of the drug for the individual patient.

CONTRAINDICATIONS

Wellbutrin is contraindicated in patients with a seizure disorder. Wellbutrin is also contraindicated in patients with a current or prior diagnosis of bulimia or anorexia nervosa because of a higher incidence of seizures noted in such patients treated with Wellbutrin. The concurrent administration of Wellbutrin and a monoamine oxidase (MAO) inhibitor is contraindicated. At least 14 days should elapse between discontinuation of an MAO inhibitor and initiation of treatment with Wellbutrin. Wellbutrin is contraindicated in patients who have shown an allergic response to it.

WARNINGS

SEIZURES: Wellbutrin is associated with seizures in approximately 0.4% (4/1000) of patients treated at doses up to 450 mg/day. This incidence of seizures may exceed that of other marketed antidepressants by as much as fourfold. This relative risk is only an approximate estimate because no direct comparative studies have been conducted. The estimated seizure incidence for Wellbutrin increases almost tenfold between 450 and 600 mg/day, which is twice the usually required daily dose (300 mg) and one and one-third the maximum recommended daily dose (450 mg). Given the wide variability among individuals and their capacity to metabolize and eliminate drugs, this disproportionate increase in seizure incidence with dose incrementation calls for caution in dosing.

During the pre-approval evaluation period, 25 among approximately 2400 patients treated with Wellbutrin experienced seizures. At the time of seizure, 7 patients were receiving daily doses of 450 mg or below, for an incidence of 0.33% (3/1000) within the recommended dose range. Twelve (12) patients experienced seizures at 600 mg per day (2.3% incidence); 6 additional patients had seizures at daily doses between 600 and 900 mg (2.8% incidence). A separate, prospective study was conducted to determine the incidence of seizure during an 8 week treatment exposure in approximately 3200 additional patients who received daily doses of up to 450 mg. Patients were permitted to continue treatment beyond 8 weeks if clinically indicated. Eight (8) seizures occurred during the initial 8 week treatment period and 5 seizures were reported in patients continuing treatment beyond 8 weeks, resulting in a total seizure incidence of 0.4%.

The risk of seizure appears to be strongly associated with dose and the presence of predisposing factors. A significant predisposing factor (e.g., history of head trauma or prior seizure, CNS tumor, concomitant medications that lower seizure threshold, etc.) was present in approximately one-half of the patients experiencing a seizure. Sudden and large increments in dose may contribute to increased risk. While many seizures occurred early in the course of treatment, some seizures did occur after several weeks at fixed dose.

Recommendations for reducing the risk of seizure: Retrospective analysis of clinical experience gained during the development of Wellbutrin suggests that the risk of seizure may be minimized if (1) the total daily dose of Wellbutrin does *not* exceed 450 mg, (2) the daily dose is administered t.i.d., with each single dose *not* to exceed 150 mg to avoid high peak concentrations of bupropion and/or its metabolites, and (3) the rate of incrementation of dose is very gradual. Extreme caution should be used when Wellbutrin is (1) administered to patients with a history of seizure, cranial trauma, or other predisposition(s) toward seizure, or (2) prescribed with other agents (e.g., antipsychotics, other antidepressants, etc.) or treatment regimens (e.g., abrupt discontinuation of a benzodiazepine) that lower seizure threshold.

Potential for Hepatotoxicity: In rats receiving large doses of bupropion chronically, there was an increase in incidence of hepatic hyperplastic nodules and hepatocellular hypertrophy. In dogs receiving large doses of bupropion chronically, various histologic changes were seen in the liver, and laboratory tests suggesting mild hepatocellular injury were noted. Although scattered abnormalities in liver function tests were detected in patients participating in clinical trials, there is no clinical evidence that bupropion acts as a hepatotoxin in humans.

PRECAUTIONS

General:

Agitation and Insomnia: A substantial proportion of patients treated with Wellbutrin experience some degree of increased restlessness, agitation, anxiety, and insomnia, especially shortly after initiation of treatment. In clinical studies, these symptoms were sometimes of sufficient magnitude to require treatment with sedative/hypnotic drugs. In approximately 2% of patients, symptoms were sufficiently severe to require discontinuation of Wellbutrin treatment.

Psychosis, Confusion, and Other Neuropsychiatric Phenomena: Patients treated with Wellbutrin have been reported to show a variety of neuropsychiatric signs and symptoms including delusions, hallucinations, psychotic episodes, confusion, and paranoia. Because of the uncontrolled nature of many studies, it is impossible to provide a precise estimate of the extent of risk imposed by treatment with Wellbutrin. In several cases, neuropsychiatric phenomena abated upon dose reduction and/or withdrawal of treatment.

Activation of Psychosis and/or Mania: Antidepressants can precipitate manic episodes in Bipolar Manic Depressive patients during the depressed phase of their illness and may activate latent psychosis in other susceptible patients. Wellbutrin is expected to pose similar risks.

Altered Appetite and Weight: A weight loss of greater than 5 pounds occurred in 28% of Wellbutrin patients. This incidence is approximately double that seen in comparable patients treated with tricyclics or placebo. Furthermore, while 34.5% of patients receiving tricyclic antidepressants gained weight, only 9.4% of patients treated with Wellbutrin did. Consequently, if weight loss is a major presenting sign of a patient's depressive illness, the anorectic and/or weight reducing potential of Wellbutrin should be considered.

Suicide: The possibility of a suicide attempt is inherent in depression and may persist until significant remission occurs. Accordingly, prescriptions for Wellbutrin should be written for the smallest number of tablets consistent with good patient management.

Use in Patients with Systemic Illness: There is no clinical experience establishing the safety of Wellbutrin in patients with a recent history of myocardial infarction or unstable heart disease. Therefore, care should be exercised if it is used in these groups. Wellbutrin was well tolerated in patients who had previously developed orthostatic hypotension while receiving tricyclic antidepressants.

Because bupropion HCl and its metabolites are almost completely excreted through the kidney and metabolites are likely to undergo conjugation in the liver prior to urinary excretion, treatment of patients with renal or hepatic impairment should be initiated at reduced dosage as bupropion and its metabolites may accumulate in such patients beyond concentrations expected in patients without renal or hepatic impairment. The patient should be closely monitored for possible toxic effects of elevated blood and tissue levels of drug and metabolites.

Information for Patients: Physicians are advised to discuss the following issues with patients:

Patients should be instructed to take Wellbutrin in equally divided doses three or four times a day to minimize the risk of seizure.

Patients should be told that any CNS-active drug like Wellbutrin may impair their ability to perform tasks requiring judgment or motor and cognitive skills. Consequently, until they are reasonably certain that Wellbutrin does not adversely affect their performance they should refrain from driving an automobile or operating complex, hazardous machinery.

Patients should be told that the use and cessation of use of alcohol may alter the seizure threshold, and, therefore, that the consumption of alcohol should be minimized, and, if possible, avoided completely.

Patients should be advised to inform their physician if they are taking or plan to take any prescription or over-the-counter drugs. Concern is warranted because Wellbutrin and other drugs may affect each other's metabolism.

Patients should be advised to notify their physician if they become pregnant or intend to become pregnant during therapy.

Drug Interactions: No systematic data have been collected on the consequences of the concomitant administration of Wellbutrin and other drugs. However, animal data suggest that Wellbutrin may be an inducer of drug metabolizing enzymes. This may be of potential clinical importance because the blood levels of co-administered drugs may be altered.

Alternatively, because bupropion is extensively metabolized, the co-administration of other drugs may affect its clinical activity. In particular, care should be exercised when administering drugs known to affect hepatic drug metabolizing enzyme systems (e.g., carbamazepine, cimetidine, phenobarbital, phenytoin).

Studies in animals demonstrate that the acute toxicity of bupropion is enhanced by the MAO inhibitor phenelzine (see CONTRAINDICATIONS).

Limited clinical data suggest a higher incidence of adverse experiences in patients receiving concurrent administration of Wellbutrin and L-dopa. Administration of Wellbutrin to patients receiving L-dopa concurrently should be undertaken with caution, using small initial doses and small gradual dose increases.

Concurrent administration of Wellbutrin and agents which lower seizure threshold should be undertaken only with extreme caution (see WARNINGS). Low initial dosing and small gradual dose increases should be employed.

Carcinogenesis, Mutagenesis, Impairment of Fertility: Lifetime carcinogenicity studies were performed in rats and mice at doses up to 300 and 150 mg/kg/day, respectively. In the rat study there was an increase in nodular proliferative lesions of the liver at doses of 100 to 300 mg/kg/day; lower doses were not tested. The question of whether or not such lesions may be precursors of neoplasms of the liver is currently unresolved. Similar liver lesions were not seen in the mouse study, and no increase in malignant tumors of the liver and other organs was seen in either study.

Bupropion produced a borderline positive response (2–3 times control mutation rate) in some strains in the Ames bacterial mutagenicity test, and a high oral dose (300, but not 100 or 200 mg/kg) produced a low incidence of chromosomal aberrations in rats. The relevance of these results in estimating the risk of human exposure to therapeutic doses is unknown.

A fertility study was performed in rats; no evidence of impairment of fertility was encountered at oral doses up to 300 mg/kg/day.

Pregnancy: *Teratogenic Effects:* Pregnancy Category B: Reproduction studies have been performed in rabbits and rats at doses up to 15–45 times the human daily dose and have revealed no definitive evidence of impaired fertility or harm to the fetus due to bupropion. (In rabbits, a slightly increased incidence of fetal abnormalities was seen in two studies, but there was no increase in any specific abnormality). There are no adequate and well-controlled studies in pregnant women. Because animal reproduction studies are not always predictive of human response, this drug should be used during pregnancy only if clearly needed.

Labor and Delivery: The effect of Wellbutrin on labor and delivery in humans is unknown.

Nursing Mothers: Because of the potential for serious adverse reactions in nursing infants from Wellbutrin, a decision should be made whether to discontinue nursing or to discontinue the drug, taking into account the importance of the drug to the mother.

Pediatric Use: The safety and effectiveness of Wellbutrin in individuals under 18 years old have not been established.

Use in the Elderly: Wellbutrin has not been systematically evaluated in older patients.

ADVERSE REACTIONS

(See also WARNINGS and PRECAUTIONS) Adverse events commonly encountered in patients treated with Wellbutrin are agitation, dry mouth, insomnia, headache/migraine, nausea/vomiting, constipation, and tremor.

Adverse events were sufficiently troublesome to cause discontinuation of Wellbutrin treatment in approximately ten percent of the 2400 patients and volunteers who participated in the product's pre-approval clinical trials. The more common events causing discontinuation include neuropsychiatric disturbances (3.0%), primarily agitation and abnormalities in mental status; gastrointestinal disturbances (2.1%), primarily nausea and vomiting; neurological disturbances (1.7%), primarily seizures, headaches, and sleep disturbances; and dermatologic problems (1.4%), primarily rashes. It is important to note, however, that many of these events occurred at doses that exceed the recommended daily dose. Accurate estimates of the incidence of adverse events associated with the use of any drug are difficult to obtain. Estimates are influenced by drug dose, detection technique, setting, physician judgments, etc. Consequently, the table below is presented solely to indicate the relative frequency of adverse events reported in representative controlled clinical studies conducted to evaluate the safety and efficacy of Wellbutrin under relatively similar conditions of daily dosage (300–600 mg), setting, and duration (3–4 weeks). The figures cited cannot be used to predict precisely the incidence of untoward events in the course of usual medical practice where patient characteristics and other factors must differ from those which prevailed in the clinical trials. These incidence figures also cannot be compared with those obtained from other clinical studies involving related drug products as each group of drug trials is conducted under a different set of conditions.

Finally, it is important to emphasize that the tabulation does not reflect the relative severity and/or clinical importance of the events. A better perspective on the serious adverse events associated with the use of Wellbutrin is provided in the WARNINGS and PRECAUTIONS sections.
[See table above].

Other events observed during the entire pre-approval evaluation of Wellbutrin: During its pre-approval assessment, Wellbutrin was evaluated in almost 2400 subjects. The conditions and duration of exposure to Wellbutrin varied greatly and a substantial proportion of the experience was gained in open and uncontrolled clinical settings. During this experience, numerous adverse events were reported; however, without appropriate controls, it is impossible to determine with certainty which events were or were not caused by Wellbutrin. The following enumeration is organized by organ system and describes events in terms of their relative frequency of reporting in the data base. Events of major clinical importance are also described in the WARNINGS and PRECAUTIONS sections of the labeling.

The following definitions of frequency are used: Frequent adverse events are defined as those occurring in at least 1/100 patients. Infrequent adverse events are those occurring in 1/100 to 1/1000 patients, while rare events are those occurring in less than 1/1000 patients.

Cardiovascular: Frequent was edema; infrequent were chest pain, EKG abnormalities (premature beats and nonspecific ST-T changes), and shortness of breath/dyspnea; and rare were pallor and phlebitis.

Dermatologic: Frequent were nonspecific rashes; infrequent were alopecia and dry skin; rare were change in hair color and hirsutism.

Endocrine: Infrequent was gynecomastia; rare were glycosuria and hormone level change.

Gastrointestinal: Infrequent were dysphagia, thirst disturbance, and liver damage/jaundice; rare were rectal complaints, colitis, G.I. bleeding, and intestinal perforation.

Genitourinary: Frequent was nocturia; infrequent were vaginal irritation, testicular swelling, urinary tract infection, painful erection, and retarded ejaculation; rare were dysuria, enuresis, urinary incontinence, menopause, ovarian disorder, pelvic infection, cystitis, dyspareunia, and painful ejaculation.

TREATMENT EMERGENT ADVERSE EXPERIENCE INCIDENCE IN PLACEBO-CONTROLLED CLINICAL TRIALS*
(Percent of Patients Reporting)

Adverse Experience	Wellbutrin Patients (n = 323)	Placebo Patients (n = 185)	Adverse Experience	Wellbutrin Patients (n = 323)	Placebo Patients (n = 185)
CARDIOVASCULAR			Dry Mouth	27.6	18.4
Cardiac Arrhythmias	5.3	4.3	Excessive Sweating	22.3	14.6
Dizziness	22.3	16.2	Headache/Migraine	25.7	22.2
Hypertension	4.3	1.6	Impaired Sleep Quality	4.0	1.6
Hypotension	2.5	2.2	Increased Salivary Flow	3.4	3.8
Palpitations	3.7	2.2	Insomnia	18.6	15.7
Syncope	1.2	0.5	Muscle Spasms	1.9	3.2
Tachycardia	10.8	8.6	Pseudoparkinsonism	1.5	1.6
DERMATOLOGIC			Sedation	19.8	19.5
Pruritus	2.2	0.0	Sensory Disturbance	4.0	3.2
Rash	8.0	6.5	Tremor	21.1	7.6
GASTROINTESTINAL			**NEUROPSYCHIATRIC**		
Anorexia	18.3	18.4	Agitation	31.9	22.2
Appetite Increase	3.7	2.2	Anxiety	3.1	1.1
Constipation	26.0	17.3	Confusion	8.4	4.9
Diarrhea	6.8	8.6	Decreased Libido	3.1	1.6
Dyspepsia	3.1	2.2	Delusions	1.2	1.1
Nausea/Vomiting	22.9	18.9	Disturbed Concentration	3.1	3.8
Weight Gain	13.6	22.7	Euphoria	1.2	0.5
Weight Loss	23.2	23.2	Hostility	5.6	3.8
GENITOURINARY			**NONSPECIFIC**		
Impotence	3.4	3.1	Fatigue	5.0	8.6
Menstrual Complaints	4.7	1.1	Fever/Chills	1.2	0.5
Urinary Frequency	2.5	2.2	**RESPIRATORY**		
Urinary Retention	1.9	2.2	Upper Respiratory		
MUSCULOSKELETAL			Complaints	5.0	11.4
Arthritis	3.1	2.7	**SPECIAL SENSES**		
NEUROLOGICAL			Auditory Disturbance	5.3	3.2
Akathisia	1.5	1.1	Blurred Vision	14.6	10.3
Akinesia/Bradykinesia	8.0	8.6	Gustatory Disturbance	3.1	1.1
Cutaneous Temperature Disturbance	1.9	1.6			

* Events reported by at least 1% of Wellbutrin patients are included.

Hematologic/Oncologic: Rare was lymphadenopathy.

Neurological: (see WARNINGS) Frequent were ataxia/incoordination, seizure, myoclonus, dyskinesia, and dystonia; infrequent were mydriasis, vertigo, and dysarthria; and rare were EEG abnormality, abnormal neurological exam, impaired attention, and sciatica.

Neuropsychiatric: (see PRECAUTIONS) Frequent were mania/hypomania, increased libido, hallucinations, decrease in sexual function, and depression; infrequent were memory impairment, depersonalization, psychosis, dysphoria, mood instability, paranoia, formal thought disorder, and frigidity; rare was suicidal ideation.

Oral Complaints: Frequent was stomatitis; infrequent were toothache, bruxism, gum irritation, and oral edema; rare was glossitis.

Respiratory: Infrequent were bronchitis and shortness of breath/dyspnea; rare were epistaxis and rate or rhythm disorder.

Special Senses: Infrequent were visual disturbance; rare was diplopia.

Nonspecific: Frequent were flu-like symptoms; infrequent was nonspecific pain; rare were body odor, surgically related pain, infection, medication reaction and overdose.

Post-Approval Reports: The following additional events were rarely observed (less than 1/1000 patients) post-approval.

Cardiovascular: Flushing and myocardial infarction.
Dermatologic: Acne.
Gastrointestinal: Stomach ulcer.
Hematologic/Oncologic: Anemia and pancytopenia.
Neurological: Aphasia.
Musculoskeletal: Musculoskeletal chest pain.
Respiratory: Pneumonia and pulmonary embolism.

DRUG ABUSE AND DEPENDENCE

Humans: Controlled clinical studies conducted in normal volunteers, in subjects with a history of multiple drug abuse, and in depressed patients showed some increase in motor activity and agitation/excitement.

In a population of individuals experienced with drugs of abuse, a single dose of 400 mg Wellbutrin produced mild amphetamine-like activity as compared to placebo on the morphine-benzedrine subscale of the Addiction Research Center Index (ARCI) and a score intermediate between placebo and amphetamine on the Liking Scale of the ARCI. These scales measure general feelings of euphoria and drug desirability. Findings in clinical trials, however, are not known to predict the abuse potential of drugs reliably. Nonetheless, evidence from single dose studies does suggest that the recommended daily dosage of bupropion when administered in divided doses is not likely to be especially reinforcing to amphetamine or stimulant abusers. However, higher doses, which could not be tested because of the risk of seizure, might be modestly attractive to those who abuse stimulant drugs.

Animals: Studies in rodents have shown that bupropion exhibits some pharmacologic actions common to psychostimulants, including increases in locomotor activity and the production of a mild stereotyped behavior and increases in rates of responding in several schedule-controlled behavior paradigms. Drug discrimination studies in rats showed stimulus generalization between bupropion and amphetamine and other psychostimulants. Rhesus monkeys have been shown to self-administer bupropion intravenously.

OVERDOSAGE

Lethal doses in animals: In rats, the acute oral LD_{50} values were 607 mg/kg (males) and 482 mg/kg (females). Respective values for mice were 544 mg/kg and 636 mg/kg. Signs of acute toxicity included labored breathing, salivation, arched back, ptosis, ataxia, and convulsions.

Human overdose experience: There has been limited clinical experience with overdosage of Wellbutrin. Thirteen overdoses occurred during clinical trials. Twelve patients ingested 850 to 4200 mg and recovered without significant sequelae. Another patient who ingested 9000 mg of Wellbutrin and 300 mg of tranylcypromine experienced a grand mal seizure and recovered without further sequelae.

Management of overdose: Following suspected overdose, hospitalization is advised. If the patient is conscious, vomiting should be induced by syrup of ipecac. Activated charcoal also may be administered every 6 hours during the first 12 hours after ingestion. Baseline laboratory values should be obtained. Electrocardiogram and EEG monitoring also are recommended for the next 48 hours. Adequate fluid intake should be provided.

If the patient is stuporous, comatose, or convulsing, airway intubation is recommended prior to undertaking gastric lavage. Although there is little clinical experience with lavage following an overdose of Wellbutrin, it is likely to be of benefit within the first 12 hours after ingestion since absorption of the drug may not yet be complete.

While diuresis, dialysis, or hemoperfusion are sometimes used to treat drug overdosage, there is no experience with their use in the management of Wellbutrin overdose. Because diffusion of Wellbutrin from tissue to plasma may be slow, dialysis may be of minimal benefit several hours after overdose.

Based on studies in animals, it is recommended that seizures be treated with an intravenous benzodiazepine preparation and other supportive measures, as appropriate.

Further information about the treatment of overdoses may be available from a poison control center.

DOSAGE AND ADMINISTRATION

General Dosing Considerations: It is particularly important to administer Wellbutrin in a manner most likely to minimize the risk of seizure (see WARNINGS). Increases in

Continued on next page

Burroughs Wellcome—Cont.

dose should not exceed 100 mg/day in a 3 day period. Gradual escalation in dosage is also important if agitation, motor restlessness, and insomnia, often seen during the initial days of treatment, are to be minimized. If necessary, these effects may be managed by temporary reduction of dose or the short-term administration of an intermediate to long-acting sedative hypnotic. A sedative hypnotic usually is not required beyond the first week of treatment. Insomnia may also be minimized by avoiding bedtime doses. If distressing, untoward effects supervene, dose escalation should be stopped.

No single dose of Wellbutrin should exceed 150 mg. Wellbutrin should be administered t.i.d., preferably with at least 6 hours between successive doses.

Usual Dosage for Adults: The usual adult dose is 300 mg/day, given t.i.d. Dosing should begin at 200 mg/day, given as 100 mg b.i.d. Based on clinical response, this dose may be increased to 300 mg/day, given as 100 mg t.i.d., no sooner than 3 days after beginning therapy (see table below). [See table below].

Increasing the Dosage Above 300 mg/Day: As with other antidepressants, the full antidepressant effect of Wellbutrin may not be evident until 4 weeks of treatment or longer. An increase in dosage, up to a maximum of 450 mg/day, given in divided doses of not more than 150 mg each, may be considered for patients in whom no clinical improvement is noted after several weeks of treatment at 300 mg/day. Dosing above 300 mg/day may be accomplished using the 75 or 100 mg tablets. The 100 mg tablet must be administered q.i.d. with at least 4 hours between successive doses, in order not to exceed the limit of 150 mg in a single dose. Wellbutrin should be discontinued in patients who do not demonstrate an adequate response after an appropriate period of treatment at 450 mg/day.

Elderly Patients: In general, older patients are known to metabolize drugs more slowly and to be more sensitive to the anticholinergic, sedative, and cardiovascular side effects of antidepressant drugs. Clinical trials enrolled several hundred patients 60 years of age and older. The experience with these patients and younger ones was similar.

Maintenance: The lowest dose that maintains remission is recommended. Although it is not known how long the patient should remain on Wellbutrin, it is generally recognized that acute episodes of depression require several months or longer of antidepressant drug treatment.

HOW SUPPLIED

Wellbutrin (bupropion hydrochloride) Tablets are supplied as 75 mg (yellow-gold) round, biconvex tablets printed "WELLBUTRIN" and "75," bottles of 100 (NDC 0081-0177-55); and 100 mg (red) round, biconvex tablets printed "WELLBUTRIN" and "100," bottles of 100 (NDC 0081-0178-55).

Store at 15°–25°C (59°–77°F).

*U.S. Patent No. 3819706
U.S. Patent No. 3885046 (Use Patent)
Shown in Product Identification Section, page 408

WELLCOVORIN® TABLETS   ℞
[wĕl″kō-vor′ĭn]
(Leucovorin Calcium)

DESCRIPTION

Wellcovorin (leucovorin calcium) Tablets contain either 5 mg or 25 mg leucovorin as the calcium salt of N-[4-[[(2-amino-5-formyl-1, 4, 5, 6, 7, 8-hexahydro-4-oxo-6-pteridinyl)-methyl] amino]benzoyl]-L-glutamic acid and the inactive ingredients corn starch, FD&C Yellow No. 6 Lake (25 mg tablet only), lactose, povidone, and magnesium stearate. This is equivalent to 5.40 mg or 27.01 mg of anhydrous leucovorin calcium.

Leucovorin is a water soluble vitamin in the folate group; it is useful as an antidote to drugs which act as folic acid antagonists. These tablets are intended for oral administration only.

CLINICAL PHARMACOLOGY

Leucovorin is a mixture of the diastereoisomers of the 5-formyl derivative of tetrahydrofolic acid. The biologically active component of the mixture is the (-)-L-isomer, known as *Citrovorum factor*, or (-)-folinic acid. Leucovorin does *not* require reduction by the enzyme dihydrofolate reductase in order to participate in reactions utilizing folates as a source

of "one-carbon" moieties. Following oral administration, leucovorin is rapidly absorbed and enters the general body pool of reduced folates.[1] The increase in plasma and serum folate activity (determined microbiologically with *Lactobacillus casei*) seen after oral administration of leucovorin is predominantly due to 5-methyltetrahydrofolate.[1,2,3,4,5]

Twenty normal men were given a single, oral 15 mg dose (7.5 mg/m^2) of leucovorin calcium and serum folate concentrations were assayed with *L casei*.[6] Mean values observed ($\pm$ one standard error) were:[4]

a) Time to peak serum folate concentration: 1.72 ± 0.08 hrs.
b) Peak serum folate concentration achieved: 268 ± 18 ng/ml.
c) Serum folate half-disappearance time: 3.5 hours.

Oral tablets yielded areas under the serum folate concentration-time curves (AUC's) that were 12% greater than equal amounts of leucovorin given intramuscularly and equal to the same amounts given intravenously.

INDICATIONS AND USAGE

Wellcovorin (leucovorin calcium) is indicated for the prophylaxis and treatment of undesired hematopoietic effects of folic acid antagonists (see WARNINGS).

CONTRAINDICATIONS

Leucovorin is improper therapy for pernicious anemia and other megaloblastic anemias secondary to the lack of vitamin B$_{12}$. A hematologic remission may occur while neurologic manifestations remain progressive.

WARNINGS

In the treatment of accidental overdosage of folic acid antagonists, leucovorin should be administered as promptly as possible. As the time interval between antifolate administration (e.g. methotrexate [MTX]) and leucovorin rescue increases, leucovorin's effectiveness in counteracting hematologic toxicity diminishes.

Leucovorin may enhance the toxicity of fluorouracil. Deaths from severe enterocolitis, diarrhea, and dehydration have been reported in elderly patients receiving leucovorin and fluorouracil.[7] Concomitant granulocytopenia and fever were present in some but not all of the patients.

PRECAUTIONS

General: Following chemotherapy with folic acid antagonists, parenteral administration of leucovorin is preferable to oral dosing if there is a possibility that the patient may vomit and not absorb the leucovorin. In the presence of pernicious anemia a hematologic remission may occur while neurologic manifestations remain progressive. Leucovorin has no effect on other established toxicities of MTX, such as the nephrotoxicity resulting from drug precipitation in the kidney.

Drug Interactions: Folic acid in large amounts may counteract the antiepileptic effect of phenobarbital, phenytoin and primidone, and increase the frequency of seizures in susceptible children.

Leucovorin may enhance the toxicity of fluorouracil (see WARNINGS).

Pregnancy: *Teratogenic Effects:* Pregnancy Category C. Animal reproduction studies have not been conducted with leucovorin. It is also not known whether leucovorin can cause fetal harm when administered to a pregnant woman or can affect reproduction capacity. Leucovorin should be given to a pregnant woman only if clearly needed.

Nursing Mothers: It is not known whether this drug is excreted in human milk. Because many drugs are excreted in human milk, caution should be exercised when leucovorin is administered to a nursing mother.

Pediatric Use: See "Drug Interactions."

ADVERSE REACTIONS

Allergic sensitization has been reported following both oral and parenteral administration of folic acid.

OVERDOSAGE

Excessive amounts of leucovorin may nullify the chemotherapeutic effect of folic acid antagonists.

DOSAGE AND ADMINISTRATION

Leucovorin is a specific antidote for the hematopoietic toxicity of methotrexate and other strong inhibitors of the enzyme dihydrofolate reductase. Leucovorin rescue must begin within 24 hours of antifolate administration. A conventional leucovorin rescue dosage schedule is 10 mg/m^2 orally or parenterally followed by 10 mg/m^2 orally every six hours for seventy-two hours. If, however, at 24 hours following methotrexate administration the serum creatinine is increased by 50% or greater than the premethotrexate serum creatinine,

the leucovorin dose should be immediately increased to 100 mg/m^2 every three hours until the serum methotrexate level is below 5×10^{-8} M.[8,9]

The recommended dose of leucovorin to counteract hematologic toxicity from folic acid antagonists with less affinity for mammalian dihydrofolate reductase than methotrexate (i.e. trimethoprim, pyrimethamine) is substantially less and 5 to 15 mg of leucovorin per day has been recommended by some investigators.[10,11,12]

HOW SUPPLIED

5 mg (off-white) scored tablets containing 5 mg leucovorin as the calcium salt imprinted with "WELLCOVORIN" and "R3C"; bottles of 20 (NDC 0081-0631-20) and 100 (NDC 0081-0631-55); unit dose pack of 50 (NDC 0081-0631-35).

25 mg (peach) scored tablets containing 25 mg leucovorin as the calcium salt imprinted with "WELLCOVORIN" and "T3C"; bottle of 25 (NDC 0081-0632-25); and Unit Dose Rescue Pak of 10 (NDC 0081-0632-13).

Store at 15°–30°C (59°–86°F) in a dry place and protect from light and moisture.

REFERENCES

1. Nixon PF and Bertino JR: Effective Absorption and Utilization of Oral Formyltetrahydrofolate in Man. *N Engl J Med* 286 (4):175–179, Jan. 27, 1972.
2. Ratanasthien K, Blair JA, Leeming RJ, Cooke WT and Melikian V: Folates in Human Serum. *J Clin Pathol* 27:875–879, 1974.
3. Mehta BM, Gisolfi AL, Hutchison DJ, Nirenberg A, Kellick MG and Rosen G: Serum Distribution of Citrovorum Factor and 5-methyltetrahydrofolate Following Oral and I.M. Administration of Calcium Leucovorin in Normal Adults. *Cancer Treat Rep* 62 (3):345–350. Mar. 1978.
4. Data on file, Medical Division, Burroughs Wellcome Co., Research Triangle Park, N.C. 27709, USA.
5. Whitehead VM, Pratt R, Viallet A and Cooper BA: Intestinal Conversion of Folinic Acid to 5-methyltetrahydrofolate in Man. *Br J Haematol* 22 :63–72, 1972.
6. Herbert V: Aseptic Addition for *Lactobacillus casei* Assay of Folate Activity in Human Serum. *J Clin Path* 19 :12–16, 1966.
7. Grem JL, Shoemaker DD, Petrelli NJ, et al: Severe and Fatal Toxic Effects Observed in Treatment with High- and Low-Dose Leucovorin Plus 5-Fluorouracil for Colorectal Carcinoma. *Cancer Treat Rep* 71:1122, 1987.
8. Bleyer WA: The Clinical Pharmacology of Methotrexate. *Cancer*, 41 (1):36–51, 1978.
9. Frei E, Blum RH, Pitman SW, *et al:* High Dose Methotrexate with Leucovorin Rescue: Rationale and Spectrum of Antitumor Activity. *Am J Med*, 68: 370–376, 1980.
10. Golde DW, Bersch N, Quan SG: Trimethoprim and Sulphamethoxazole Inhibition of Haematopoiesis *in Vitro*. *Br J Haematol*, 40 (3):363–367, 1978.
11. Steinberg SE, Campbell CL, Rabinovitch PS, *et al:* The Effect of Trimethoprim/Sulfamethoxazole on Friend Erythroleukemia Cells. *Blood*, 55 (3):501–504, 1980.
12. Mahmoud AAF and Warren KS: Algorithms in the Diagnosis and Management of Exotic Disease. XX. Toxoplasmosis. *J Infect Dis*, 135 (3):493–496, 1977.
Shown in Product Identification Section, page 408

ZOVIRAX® Capsules   ℞
[zō″vī′răx]
(Acyclovir)

DESCRIPTION

Zovirax is the brand name for acyclovir, an antiviral drug. Zovirax Capsules are a formulation for oral administration. Each capsule of Zovirax contains 200 mg of acyclovir and the inactive ingredients corn starch, lactose, magnesium stearate, and sodium lauryl sulfate. The capsule shell consists of gelatin, FD&C Blue No. 2, and titanium dioxide. May contain one or more parabens. Printed with edible black ink.

The chemical name of acyclovir is 9-[(2-hydroxyethoxy)methyl]guanine.

Acyclovir is a white, crystalline powder with a molecular weight of 225 daltons, and a maximum solubility in water of 2.5 mg/ml at 37°C.

CLINICAL PHARMACOLOGY

Acyclovir is a synthetic acyclic purine nucleoside analogue with *in vitro* inhibitory activity against Herpes simplex types 1 and 2 (HSV-1 and HSV-2), varicella-zoster, Epstein-Barr and cytomegalovirus. In cell cultures, the inhibitory activity of acyclovir for Herpes simplex virus is highly selective. Cellular thymidine kinase does not effectively utilize acyclovir as a substrate. Herpes simplex virus-coded thymidine kinase, however, converts acyclovir into acyclovir monophosphate, a nucleotide analogue. The monophosphate is further converted into diphosphate by cellular guanylate kinase and into triphosphate by a number of cellular enzymes.[1] Acy-

Dosing Regimen

Treatment Day	Total Daily Dose	Tablet Strength	Number of Tablets		
			Morning	Midday	Evening
1	200 mg	100 mg	1	0	1
4	300 mg	100 mg	1	1	1

clovir triphosphate interferes with Herpes simplex virus DNA polymerase and inhibits viral DNA replication. Acyclovir triphosphate also inhibits cellular α-DNA polymerase, but to a lesser degree. *In vitro*, acyclovir triphosphate can be incorporated into growing chains of DNA by viral DNA polymerase and to a much smaller extent by cellular α-DNA polymerase.[2] When incorporation occurs, the DNA chain is terminated.[3] Acyclovir is preferentially taken up and selectively converted to the active triphosphate form by herpesvirus-infected cells. Thus, acyclovir is much less toxic *in vitro* for normal uninfected cells because: 1) less is taken up; 2) less is converted to the active form; 3) cellular α-DNA polymerase is less sensitive to the effects of the active form.

Microbiology: The quantitative relationship between the *in vitro* susceptibility of Herpes simplex virus to acyclovir and the clinical response to therapy has not been established in man. Sensitivity results, expressed as the concentration of drug required to inhibit by 50% the growth of virus in a tissue culture ("ID_{50} value") vary greatly depending upon the particular assay used,[4] the cell type employed,[5] and the laboratory performing the test. Using a dye-uptake method in Vero cells,[6] which gives ID_{50} values approximately 5- to 10-fold higher than plaque reduction assays, 1417 isolates (553 HSV-1 and 864 HSV-2) from approximately 500 patients were examined over a 5-year period.[7] It must be emphasized that neither the patients nor the isolates were randomly selected and, therefore, do not represent the general population. Isolates obtained from patients who continued to shed virus during or after acyclovir therapy were selected for assay; a smaller number were examined from all patients in a given clinical study.

These assays found that 90% of HSV-1 isolates were sensitive to ≤ 0.9 μg/ml acyclovir and 50% of all isolates were sensitive to ≤ 0.2 μg/ml acyclovir. For HSV-2 isolates, 90% were sensitive to ≤ 2.2 μg/ml and 50% of all isolates were sensitive to ≤ 0.7 μg/ml of acyclovir. Isolates with significantly diminished sensitivity were found in 44 patients.

All of the less sensitive viruses obtained from patients to date have been the result of alterations in the thymidine kinase enzyme[8-13] and were not the result of changes in the viral DNA polymerase.

Pharmacokinetics: The pharmacokinetics of acyclovir after oral administration have been evaluated in 5 clinical studies involving 38 adult patients. In 14 immunocompromised patients with Herpes simplex or varicella zoster infection given Zovirax Capsules in doses of 200 or 400 mg every 4 hours, 6 times daily for 5 days, the bioavailability was estimated to be 15-20%. In this study, steady-state plasma levels were reached by the second day of dosing. Mean steady-state peak and trough concentrations following the 200 mg dose were 0.56 μg/ml (0.38 to 0.74 μg/ml) and 0.29 μg/ml (0.18 to 0.42 μg/ml), respectively, and following the 400 mg dose were 1.2 μg/ml (0.75 to 1.7 μg/ml) and 0.62 μg/ml (0.14 to 0.90 μg/ml). When 6 normal volunteers received 200 mg acyclovir as a solution every 4 hours, 5 times daily, similar mean steady-state peak and trough concentrations (0.62 μg/ml and 0.30 μg/ml) were achieved.

A single oral dose bioavailability study in 23 normal volunteers showed that Zovirax Capsules 200 mg are bioequivalent to 200 mg acyclovir in aqueous solution. In another study in 6 volunteers, the influence of food on the absorption of acyclovir was not apparent.

Following oral administration of Zovirax Capsules 200 mg, the mean acyclovir plasma half-life in 14 patients with normal renal function was 3.3 hours. The mean renal excretion of unchanged drug accounts for 14.4% (8.6 to 19.8%) of the orally administered dose. The only urinary metabolite (identified by high performance liquid chromatography) is 9-[(carboxymethoxy)methyl]guanine.

The half-life and total body clearance of acyclovir are dependent on renal function. A dosage adjustment is recommended for patients with creatinine clearance ≤ 10 ml/min/1.73 m^2 (see DOSAGE AND ADMINISTRATION).

Orally administered acyclovir in pediatric and neonatal patients has not yet been fully studied.

INDICATIONS AND USAGE

Zovirax Capsules are indicated for the treatment of initial episodes and the management of recurrent episodes of genital herpes in certain patients.

The severity of disease is variable depending upon the immune status of the patient, the frequency and duration of episodes, and the degree of cutaneous or systemic involvement. These factors should determine patient management, which may include symptomatic support and counseling only, or the institution of specific therapy. The physical, emotional and psycho-social difficulties posed by herpes infections as well as the degree of debilitation, particularly in immunocompromised patients, are unique for each patient, and the physician should determine therapeutic alternatives based on his or her understanding of the individual patient's needs. Thus Zovirax Capsules are not appropriate in treating all genital herpes infections. The following guidelines may be useful in weighing the benefit/risk considerations in specific disease categories:

First Episodes (primary and nonprimary infections—commonly known as initial genital herpes):

Double-blind, placebo-controlled studies[14,15,16] have demonstrated that orally administered Zovirax significantly reduced the duration of acute infection (detection of virus in lesions by tissue culture) and lesion healing. The duration of pain and new lesion formation was decreased in some patient groups. The promptness of initiation of therapy and/or the patient's prior exposure to Herpes simplex virus may influence the degree of benefit from therapy. Patients with mild disease may derive less benefit than those with more severe episodes. In patients with extremely severe episodes, in which prostration, central nervous system involvement, urinary retention or inability to take oral medication require hospitalization and more aggressive management, therapy may be best initiated with intravenous Zovirax.

Recurrent Episodes:

Double-blind, placebo-controlled studies[13,17,18,19] in patients with frequent recurrences (6 or more episodes per year) have shown that Zovirax Capsules given for 4 to 6 months prevented or reduced the frequency and/or severity of recurrences in greater than 95% of patients. Clinical recurrences were prevented in 40 to 75% of patients. Some patients experienced increased severity of the first episode following cessation of therapy; the severity of subsequent episodes and the effect on the natural history of the disease are still under study.

The safety and efficacy of orally administered acyclovir in the suppression of frequent episodes of genital herpes have been established only for up to 6 months. Chronic suppressive therapy is most appropriate when, in the judgement of the physician, the benefits of such a regimen outweigh known or potential adverse effects. In general, Zovirax Capsules should not be used for the suppression of recurrent disease in mildly affected patients. Unanswered questions concerning the human relevance of *in vitro* mutagenicity studies and reproductive toxicity studies in animals given very high doses of acyclovir for short periods (see Carcinogenesis, Mutagenesis, Impairment of Fertility) should be borne in mind when designing long-term management for individual patients. Discussion of these issues with patients will provide them the opportunity to weigh the potential for toxicity against the severity of their disease. Thus, this regimen should be considered only for appropriate patients and only for six months until the results of ongoing studies allow a more precise evaluation of the benefit/risk assessment of prolonged therapy.

Limited studies[19,20] have shown that there are certain patients for whom intermittent short-term treatment of recurrent episodes is effective. This approach may be more appropriate than a suppressive regimen in patients with infrequent recurrences.

Immunocompromised patients with recurrent herpes infections can be treated with either intermittent or chronic suppressive therapy. Clinically significant resistance, although rare, is more likely to be seen with prolonged or repeated therapy in severely immunocompromised patients with active lesions.

Diagnosis:

The cutaneous vesicular lesions associated with Herpes simplex virus infections are often characteristic in appearance. However, other etiologic agents may cause similar lesions. Proof of herpesvirus infection rests on viral isolation and identification in tissue culture. Several other laboratory tests, however, can be used to establish presumptive evidence of herpesvirus infection. Smears prepared from lesion exudates or scrapings may be stained with Wright or Giemsa stains and examined for the presence of multinucleated giant cells (Tzanck preparation)[21]; this method is not specific for Herpes simplex virus infection. Smears may also be reacted in other test systems for herpes.

CONTRAINDICATIONS

Zovirax Capsules are contraindicated for patients who develop hypersensitivity or intolerance to the components of the formulation.

WARNINGS

Zovirax Capsules are intended for oral ingestion only.

PRECAUTIONS

General: Zovirax has caused decreased spermatogenesis at high doses in some animals and mutagenesis in some acute studies at high concentrations of drug (see PRECAUTIONS—Carcinogenesis, Mutagenesis, Impairment of Fertility). The recommended dosage and length of treatment should not be exceeded (see DOSAGE AND ADMINISTRATION).

Exposure of Herpes simplex isolates to acyclovir *in vitro* can lead to the emergence of less sensitive viruses. The possibility of the appearance of less sensitive viruses in man must be borne in mind when treating patients. The relationship between the *in vitro* sensitivity of Herpes simplex virus to acyclovir and clinical response to therapy has yet to be established (see CLINICAL PHARMACOLOGY—Microbiology).

Because of the possibility that less sensitive virus may be selected in patients who are receiving acyclovir, all patients should be advised to take particular care to avoid potential transmission of virus if active lesions are present while they are on therapy. In severely immunocompromised patients, the physician should be aware that prolonged or repeated courses of acyclovir may result in selection of resistant viruses which may not fully respond to continued acyclovir therapy.

Information for Patients: Educational material is being provided to pharmacists and other health care professionals to give to patients. It contains, in part, the following information:

Genital herpes is a sexually transmitted disease and patients should avoid intercourse when visible lesions are present because of the risk of infecting intimate partners. Zovirax Capsules are for oral ingestion only. Medication should not be shared with others. The prescribed dosage should not be exceeded. Zovirax Capsules do not eliminate latent viruses. Some patients experience increased severity of the first episode following cessation of therapy; the severity of subsequent episodes and the effect on the natural history of the disease are still under study.

There are still unanswered questions concerning reproductive/gonadal toxicity and mutagenesis; long-term studies are continuing. Decreased sperm production has been seen at high doses in some animals; preliminary analysis of a study using 400 mg or 1000 mg of Zovirax per day for six months in humans did not show similar findings. Chromosomal breaks were seen *in vitro* after brief exposure to high concentrations. Some other currently marketed medications also cause chromosomal breaks, and the significance of this finding is unknown.

Patients are instructed to consult with their physician if: they do not receive sufficient relief in the frequency and severity of their recurrences, they experience severe or troublesome adverse reactions, they become pregnant or intend to become pregnant, they wish to breastfeed while taking Zovirax Capsules, or they have any other questions.

Drug Interactions: Co-administration of probenecid with intravenous acyclovir has been shown to increase the mean half-life and the area under the concentration-time curve. Urinary excretion and renal clearance were correspondingly reduced.

Carcinogenesis, Mutagenesis, Impairment of Fertility: Acyclovir was tested in lifetime bioassays in rats and mice at single daily doses of 50, 150 and 450 mg/kg given by gavage. There was no statistically significant difference in the incidence of tumors between treated and control animals, nor did acyclovir shorten the latency of tumors. In 2 *in vitro* cell transformation assays, used to provide preliminary assessment of potential oncogenicity in advance of these more definitive life-time bioassays in rodents, conflicting results were obtained. Acyclovir was positive at the highest dose used in one system and the resulting morphologically transformed cells formed tumors when inoculated into immunosuppressed, syngeneic, weanling mice. Acyclovir was negative in another transformation system considered less sensitive.

In acute studies, there was an increase, not statistically significant, in the incidence of chromosomal damage at maximum tolerated parenteral doses of 100 mg/kg acyclovir in rats but not Chinese hamsters; higher doses of 500 and 1000 mg/kg were clastogenic in Chinese hamsters. In addition, no activity was found after 5 days dosing in a dominant lethal study in mice. In 6 of 11 microbial and mammalian cell assays, no evidence of mutagenicity was observed. At 3 loci in a Chinese hamster ovary cell line, the results were inconclusive. In 2 mammalian cell assays (human lymphocytes and L5178Y mouse lymphoma cells *in vitro*), positive responses for mutagenicity and chromosomal damage occurred, but only at concentrations at least 400 times the acyclovir plasma levels achieved in man.

Acyclovir has not been shown to impair fertility or reproduction in mice (450 mg/kg/day, p.o.) or in rats (25 mg/kg/day, s.c.). At 50 mg/kg/day s.c. in the rat, there was a statistically significant increase in post-implantation loss, but no concomitant decrease in litter size. In female rabbits treated subcutaneously with acyclovir subsequent to mating, there was a statistically significant decrease in implantation efficiency but no concomitant decrease in litter size at a dose of 50 mg/kg/day. No effect upon implantation efficiency was observed when the same dose was administered intravenously. In a rat peri- and postnatal study at 50 mg/kg/day s.c., there was a statistically significant decrease in the group mean numbers of corpora lutea, total implantation sites and live fetuses in the F_1 generation. Although not statistically significant, there was also a dose related decrease in group mean numbers of live fetuses and implantation sites at 12.5 mg/kg/day and 25 mg/kg/day, s.c. The intravenous administration of 100 mg/kg/day, a dose known to cause obstructive nephropathy in rabbits, caused a significant increase in fetal resorptions and a corresponding decrease in litter size. However, at a maximum tolerated intravenous dose of 50

Continued on next page

Burroughs Wellcome—Cont.

mg/kg/day in rabbits, there were no drug-related reproductive effects.

Intraperitoneal doses of 320 or 80 mg/kg/day acyclovir given to rats for 1 and 6 months, respectively, caused testicular atrophy. Testicular atrophy was persistent through the 4-week postdose recovery phase after 320 mg/kg/day; some evidence of recovery of sperm production was evident 30 days postdose. Intravenous doses of 100 and 200 mg/kg/day acyclovir given to dogs for 31 days caused aspermatogenesis. Testicles were normal in dogs given 50 mg/kg/day i.v. for one month.

Pregnancy: _Teratogenic Effects:_ Pregnancy Category C. Acyclovir was not teratogenic in the mouse (450 mg/kg/day, p.o.), rabbit (50 mg/kg/day, s.c. and i.v.) or in standard tests in the rat (50 mg/kg/day, s.c.). In a non-standard test in rats, fetal abnormalities, such as head and tail anomalies, were observed following subcutaneous administration of acyclovir at very high doses associated with toxicity to the maternal rat. The clinical relevance of these findings is uncertain.[22] There are no adequate and well-controlled studies in pregnant women. Acyclovir should not be used during pregnancy unless the potential benefit justifies the potential risk to the fetus. Although acyclovir was not teratogenic in standard animal studies, the drug's potential for causing chromosome breaks at high concentration should be taken into consideration in making this determination.

Nursing Mothers: It is not known whether this drug is excreted in human milk. Because many drugs are excreted in human milk, caution should be exercised when Zovirax is administered to a nursing woman. In nursing mothers, consideration should be given to not using acyclovir treatment or discontinuing breastfeeding.

Pediatric Use: Safety and effectiveness in children have not been established.

ADVERSE REACTIONS

Short-Term Administration: The most frequent adverse reactions reported during clinical trials of treatment with Zovirax Capsules were nausea and/or vomiting in 8 of 298 patient treatments (2.7%) and headache in 2 of 298 (0.6%). Nausea and/or vomiting occurred in 2 of 287 (0.7%) patients who received placebo.

Less frequent adverse reactions, each of which occurred in 1 of 298 patient treatments with Zovirax Capsules (0.3%), included diarrhea, dizziness, anorexia, fatigue, edema, skin rash, leg pain, inguinal adenopathy, medication taste and sore throat.

Long-Term Administration: The most frequent adverse reactions reported in clinical trials of continuous (up to 6 months) administration of Zovirax Capsules for the prevention of recurrences were headache in 33 of 251 Zovirax-treated patients (13.1%), diarrhea in 22 of 251 (8.8%), nausea and/or vomiting in 20 of 251 (8.0%), vertigo in 9 of 251 (3.6%), and arthralgia in 9 of 251 (3.6%). Of the control patients receiving either placebo or intermittent treatment of recurrences with Zovirax, headache was reported in 14 of 163 (8.6%), diarrhea in 7 of 163 (4.3%), and nausea and/or vomiting in 14 of 163 (8.6%).

Less frequent adverse reactions, each of which occurred in less than 3% of the 251 patients treated with Zovirax (see number of patients in parentheses), included skin rash (7), insomnia (4), fatigue (4), fever (4), palpitations (1), sore throat (2), superficial thrombophlebitis (1), muscle cramps (2), pars planitis (1), menstrual abnormality (4), acne (3), lymphadenopathy (2), irritability (1), accelerated hair loss (1), and depression (1).

OVERDOSAGE

No acute massive overdosage of Zovirax Capsules has been reported. Doses as high as 800 mg 6 times daily for 5 days have been administered to humans without acute untoward effects. This should not be construed as a recommended dosage for patients with more severe herpes. Peak plasma concentrations have reached 10.0 μg/ml.

Precipitation of acyclovir in renal tubules may occur when the solubility (2.5 mg/ml) in the intratubular fluid is exceeded. Renal lesions considered to be related to obstruction of renal tubules by precipitated drug crystals occurred in the following species: rats treated with i.v. and i.p. doses of 20 mg/kg/day for 21 and 31 days, respectively, and at s.c. doses of 100 mg/kg/day for 10 days; rabbits at s.c. and i.v. doses of 50 mg/kg/day for 13 days; and dogs at i.v. doses of 100 mg/kg/day for 31 days. A 6 hr hemodialysis results in a 60% decrease in plasma acyclovir concentration. Data concerning peritoneal dialysis are incomplete but indicate that this method may be significantly less efficient in removing acyclovir from the blood. In the event of acute renal failure and anuria, the patient may benefit from hemodialysis until renal function is restored (see DOSAGE AND ADMINISTRATION).

DOSAGE AND ADMINISTRATION

Treatment of initial genital herpes: One 200 mg capsule every 4 hours, while awake, for a total of 5 capsules daily for 10 days (total 50 capsules).

Chronic suppressive therapy for recurrent disease: One 200 mg capsule 3 times daily for up to 6 months. Some patients may require more drug, up to one 200 mg capsule 5 times daily for up to 6 months.

Intermittent Therapy: One 200 mg capsule every 4 hours, while awake, for a total of 5 capsules daily for 5 days (total 25 capsules). Therapy should be initiated at the earliest sign or symptom (prodrome) of recurrence.

Patients With Acute or Chronic Renal Impairment: Comprehensive pharmacokinetic studies have been completed following intravenous acyclovir infusions in patients with renal impairment. Based on these studies, a dosage adjustment is recommended for patients with creatinine clearance ≤ 10 ml/min/1.73 m². For these patients, a 200 mg dose every 12 hours is recommended.

HOW SUPPLIED

Zovirax Capsules (blue, opaque cap and body with a dark blue band) containing 200 mg acyclovir and printed with "Wellcome ZOVIRAX 200"—Bottles of 100 (NDC 0081-0991-55), and unit dose pack of 100 (NDC 0081-0991-56).

Store at 15° to 25°C (59° to 77°F) and protect from light and moisture.

REFERENCES

1. Miller, W.H. and Miller, R.L. J. Biol. Chem. 255(15):7204–7207, 1980.
2. Furman, P.A. _et al._ J. Virol. 32(1):72–77, 1979.
3. Derse, D. _et al._ J. Biol. Chem. 256(22): 11447–11451, 1981.
4. Barry, D.W. and Blum, M.R. In: Recent Advances in Clinical Pharmacology. Turner P. and Shand D.G. eds., 57–80, 1983.
5. DeClerq, E. Antimicrob. Agents Chemother. 21: 661–3, 1982.
6. McLaren, C., _et al._ Antiviral Res. 3: 223–34, 1983.
7. Barry, D.W. and Nusinoff-Lehrman, S. Pharmacological and Clinical Approaches to Herpes Viruses and Virus Chemotherapy. Oiso, Japan, September 10–13, 1984.
8. Dekker, C., _et al._ J. Antimicrob. Chemother. 12(B): 137–152, 1983.
9. Sibrack, C.D., _et al._ J. Infect. Dis. 146: 673–82, 1982.
10. Crumpacker, C.S., _et al._ N. Engl. J. Med. 306: 343–6, 1982.
11. Wade, J.C., _et al._ Ann. Int. Med. 96: 265–9, 1982.
12. Burns, W.H., _et al._ Lancet: 421–3, 1982.
13. Straus, S.E., _et al._ N. Engl. J. Med. 310: 1545–50, 1984.
14. Bryson, Y.J., _et al._ N. Engl. J. Med. 308(16): 916–921, 1983.
15. Mertz, G.J., _et al._ J.A.M.A. 252(9): 1147–1151, 1984.
16. Nilsen, A.E., _et al._ Lancet. 8298: 571–573, 1982.
17. Douglas, J.M. _et al._ N. Engl. J. Med. 310(24): 1551–1556, 1984.
18. Mindel, A., _et al._ Lancet: 8394: 57–59, 1984.
19. Data on File, Burroughs Wellcome Co.
20. Reichman, R.C., _et al._ J.A.M.A. 251(16) 2103–2107, 1984.
21. Naib, Z.M., _et al._ Cancer Res. 33:1452–1463, 1973.
22. Stahlmann R, Klug S, Lewandowski C, _et al,_ **Infection:** 15(4): 261-262, 1987.

U.S. Patent No. 4199574

Shown in Product Identification Section, page 408

ZOVIRAX® Ointment 5%   ℞
[zō″vī′răx]
(Acyclovir)

DESCRIPTION

Zovirax is the brand name for acyclovir, an antiviral drug active against herpes viruses. Zovirax Ointment 5% is a formulation for topical administration. Each gram of Zovirax Ointment 5% contains 50 mg of acyclovir in a polyethylene glycol (PEG) base.

The chemical name of acyclovir is 9-[(2-hydroxyethoxy)methyl]guanine.

Acyclovir is a white, crystalline powder with a molecular weight of 225 Daltons, and a maximum solubility in water of 1.3 mg/ml.

CLINICAL PHARMACOLOGY

Acyclovir is a synthetic acyclic purine nucleoside analogue with _in vitro_ inhibitory activity against Herpes simplex types 1 and 2 (HSV-1 and HSV-2), varicella-zoster, Epstein-Barr and cytomegalovirus. In cell cultures, the inhibitory activity of acyclovir for Herpes simplex virus is highly selective. Cellular thymidine kinase does not effectively utilize acyclovir as a substrate. Herpes simplex virus-coded thymidine kinase, however, converts acyclovir into acyclovir monophosphate, a nucleotide. The monophosphate is further converted into diphosphate by cellular guanylate kinase and into triphosphate by a number of cellular enzymes.[1] Acyclovir triphosphate interferes with Herpes simplex virus DNA polymerase and inhibits viral DNA replication. Acyclovir tri-

phosphate also inhibits cellular α-DNA polymerase but to a lesser degree. _In vitro_, acyclovir triphosphate can be incorporated into growing chains of DNA by viral DNA polymerase and to a much smaller extent by cellular α-DNA polymerase.[2] When incorporation occurs, the DNA chain is terminated.[3] Acyclovir is preferentially taken up and selectively converted to the active triphosphate form by herpesvirus-infected cells. Thus, acyclovir is much less toxic _in vitro_ for normal uninfected cells because: 1) less is taken up; 2) less is converted to the active form; 3) cellular α-DNA polymerase is less sensitive to the effects of the active form.

The relationship between _in vitro_ susceptibility of Herpes simplex virus to antiviral drugs and clinical response has not been established. The techniques and cell culture types used for determining _in vitro_ susceptibility may influence the results obtained. Using a quantitative assay to determine the acyclovir concentration producing 50% inhibition of viral cytopathic effect (ID$_{50}$), 28 HSV-1 clinical isolates had a mean ID$_{50}$ of 0.17 μg/ml and 32 HSV-2 clinical isolates had a mean ID$_{50}$ of 0.46 μg/ml.[*] Results from other studies using different assays have yielded mean ID$_{50}$ values for clinical HSV-1 isolates of 0.018, 0.03 and 0.043 μg/ml and for clinical HSV-2 isolates of 0.027, 0.36 and 0.03 μg/ml, respectively.[4,5,6]

Two clinical pharmacology studies were performed with Zovirax Ointment 5% in adult immunocompromised patients, at risk of developing mucocutaneous Herpes simplex virus infections or with localized varicella-zoster infections. These studies were designed to evaluate the dermal tolerance, systemic toxicity and percutaneous absorption of acyclovir.

In one of these studies, which included 16 inpatients, the complete ointment or its vehicle were randomly administered in a dose of 1 cm strips (25 mg acyclovir) four times a day for seven days to an intact skin surface area of 4.5 square inches. No local intolerance, systemic toxicity or contact dermatitis were observed. In addition, no drug was detected in blood and urine by radioimmunoassay (sensitivity, 0.01 μg/ml).

The other study included eleven patients with localized varicella-zoster. In this uncontrolled study, acyclovir was detected in the blood of 9 patients and in the urine of all patients tested. Acyclovir levels in plasma ranged from < 0.01 to 0.28 μg/ml in eight patients with normal renal function, and from < 0.01 to 0.78 μg/ml in one patient with impaired renal function. Acyclovir excreted in the urine ranged from < 0.02 to 9.4 percent of the daily dose. Therefore, systemic absorption of acyclovir after topical application is minimal.

INDICATIONS AND USAGE

Zovirax (Acyclovir) Ointment 5% is indicated in the management of initial herpes genitalis and in limited nonlife-threatening mucocutaneous Herpes simplex virus infections in immunocompromised patients. In clinical trials of initial herpes genitalis, Zovirax Ointment 5% has shown a decrease in healing time and in some cases a decrease in duration of viral shedding and duration of pain. In studies in immunocompromised patients with mainly herpes labialis, there was a decrease in duration of viral shedding and a slight decrease in duration of pain.

By contrast, in studies of recurrent herpes genitalis and of herpes labialis in nonimmunocompromised patients, there was no evidence of clinical benefit; there was some decrease in duration of viral shedding.

Diagnosis: Whereas mucocutaneous lesions associated with Herpes simplex infections are often characteristic, the finding of multinucleated giant cells in smears prepared from lesion exudate or scrapings may assist in the diagnosis.[7] Positive cultures for Herpes simplex virus offer a reliable means for confirmation of the diagnosis. In genital herpes, appropriate examinations should be performed to rule out other sexually transmitted diseases.

CONTRAINDICATIONS

Zovirax Ointment 5% is contraindicated for patients who develop hypersensitivity or chemical intolerance to the components of the formulation.

WARNINGS

Zovirax Ointment 5% is intended for cutaneous use only and should not be used in the eye.

PRECAUTIONS

General: The recommended dosage, frequency of applications, and length of treatment should not be exceeded (see DOSAGE AND ADMINISTRATION). There exist no data which demonstrate that the use of Zovirax Ointment 5% will either prevent transmission of infection to other persons or prevent recurrent infections when applied in the absence of signs and symptoms. Zovirax Ointment 5% should not be used for the prevention of recurrent HSV infections. Although clinically significant viral resistance associated with the use of Zovirax Ointment 5% has not been observed, this possibility exists.

Drug Interactions: Clinical experience has identified no interactions resulting from topical or systemic administration of other drugs concomitantly with Zovirax Ointment 5%.

Carcinogenesis, Mutagenesis, Impairment of Fertility: Acyclovir was tested in lifetime bioassays in rats and mice at single daily doses of 50, 150 and 450 mg/kg/day given by gavage. These studies showed no statistically significant difference in the incidence of benign and malignant tumors produced in drug-treated as compared to control animals, nor did acyclovir induce the occurrence of tumors earlier in drug-treated animals as compared to controls. In 2 *in vitro* cell transformation assays, used to provide preliminary assessment of potential oncogenicity in advance of these more definitive lifetime bioassays in rodents, conflicting results were obtained. Acyclovir was positive at the highest dose used in one system and the resulting morphologically transformed cells formed tumors when inoculated into immunosuppressed, syngeneic, weanling mice. Acyclovir was negative in another transformation system.

No chromosome damage was observed at maximum tolerated parenteral doses of 100 mg/kg acyclovir in rats or Chinese hamsters; higher doses of 500 and 1000 mg/kg were clastogenic in Chinese hamsters. In addition, no activity was found in a dominant lethal study in mice. In 9 of 11 microbial and mammalian cell assays, no evidence of mutagenicity was observed. In 2 mammalian cell assays (human lymphocytes and L5178Y mouse lymphoma cells *in vitro*), positive response for mutagenicity and chromosomal damage occurred, but only at concentrations at least 1000 times the plasma levels achieved in man following topical application.

Acyclovir does not impair fertility or reproduction in mice at oral doses up to 450 mg/kg/day or in rats at subcutaneous doses up to 25 mg/kg/day. In rabbits given a high dose of acyclovir (50 mg/kg/day, s.c.), there was a statistically significant decrease in implantation efficiency.

Pregnancy: *Teratogenic Effects.* Pregnancy Category C. Acyclovir was not teratogenic in the mouse (450 mg/kg/day, p.o.), rabbit (50 mg/kg/day, s.c. and i.v.) or in standard tests in the rat (50 mg/kg/day, s.c.). In a non-standard test in rats, fetal abnormalities, such as head and tail anomalies, were observed following subcutaneous administration of acyclovir at very high doses associated with toxicity to the maternal rat. The clinical relevance of these findings is uncertain.[8] There are no adequate and well-controlled studies in pregnant women. Acyclovir should not be used during pregnancy unless the potential benefit justifies the potential risk to the fetus.

Nursing Mothers: It is not known whether this drug is excreted in human milk. Because many drugs are excreted in human milk, caution should be exercised when Zovirax is administered to a nursing woman.

ADVERSE REACTIONS

Because ulcerated genital lesions are characteristically tender and sensitive to any contact or manipulation, patients may experience discomfort upon application of ointment. In the controlled clinical trials, mild pain (including transient burning and stinging) was reported by 103 (28.3%) of 364 patients treated with acyclovir and by 115 (31.1%) of 370 patients treated with placebo; treatment was discontinued in 2 of these patients. Other local reactions among acyclovir-treated patients included pruritis in 15 (4.1%), rash in 1 (0.3%) and vulvitis in 1 (0.3%). Among the placebo-treated patients, pruritus was reported by 17 (4.6%) and rash by 1 (0.3%).

In all studies, there was no significant difference between the drug and placebo group in the rate or type of reported adverse reactions nor were there any differences in abnormal clinical laboratory findings.

OVERDOSAGE

Overdosage by topical application of Zovirax Ointment 5% is unlikely because of limited transcutaneous absorption (see Clinical Pharmacology).

DOSAGE AND ADMINISTRATION

Apply sufficient quantity to adequately cover all lesions every 3 hours 6 times per day for 7 days. The dose size per application will vary depending upon the total lesion area but should approximate a one-half inch ribbon of ointment per 4 square inches of surface area. A finger cot or rubber glove should be used when applying Zovirax to prevent autoinoculation of other body sites and transmission of infection to other persons. **Therapy should be initiated as early as possible following onset of signs and symptoms.**

HOW SUPPLIED

Zovirax Ointment 5% is supplied in 15 g tubes (NDC 0081-0993-94) and 3 g tubes (NDC 0081-0993-41). Each gram contains 50 mg acyclovir in a polyethylene glycol base. Store at 15°–25°C (59°–77°F) in a dry place.

ANIMAL PHARMACOLOGY AND ANIMAL TOXICOLOGY

Topical treatment of guinea pigs with 10% acyclovir in polyethylene glycol ointment for three weeks did not result in cutaneous irritation or systemic toxicity. Also, a wide variety of animal tests by parenteral routes demonstrated that acyclovir has a low order of toxicity.

Acyclovir did not cause dermal sensitization in guinea pigs.

REFERENCES

1. Miller WH and Miller RL. *J Biol Chem* 255 (15):7204–7207, 1980.
2. Furman PA et al. *J Virol* 32 (1):72–77, 1979.
3. Derse D et al. *J Biol Chem* 256 (22): 11447–11451, 1981.
4. Collins P and Bauer DJ. *J Antimicrob Chemother* 5 :431–436, 1979.
5. Crumpacker CS et al. *Antimicrob Agents Chemother* 15 :642–645, 1979.
6. De Clercq E et al. *J Infect Dis* 141 :563–574, 1980.
7. Naib ZM et al. *Cancer Res* 33 :1452–1463, 1973.
8. Stahlmann R, Klug S, Lewandowski C, et al. *Infection:* 15(4): 261-262, 1987.
*Data on file at Burroughs Wellcome Co.

U.S. Patent No. 4199574

ZOVIRAX® Sterile Powder   ℞
[zō″vī′răx]
(Acyclovir Sodium)
FOR INTRAVENOUS INFUSION ONLY

DESCRIPTION

Zovirax is the brand name for acyclovir, an antiviral drug active against herpesviruses. Zovirax Sterile Powder is a formulation for intravenous administration. Each 10 mL vial of Zovirax Sterile Powder contains 549 mg of sterile lyophilized acyclovir sodium equivalent to 500 mg of acyclovir. Each 20 mL vial of Zovirax Sterile Powder contains 1098 mg of sterile lyophilized acyclovir sodium equivalent to 1000 mg of acyclovir.

The chemical name of acyclovir sodium is 9-[(2-hydroxyethoxy)methyl]guanine sodium.

Acyclovir sodium is a white, crystalline powder with a molecular weight of 247 daltons, and a solubility in water exceeding 100 mg/mL. Recommended reconstitution with 10 mL diluent per vial yields 50 mg/mL acyclovir (pH approximately 11). Further dilution in any appropriate intravenous solution must be performed before infusion (see Method of Preparation). At physiologic pH, acyclovir exists as the un-ionized form with a molecular weight of 225 daltons and a maximum solubility of 2.5 mg/mL at 37°C.

CLINICAL PHARMACOLOGY

Acyclovir is a synthetic acyclic purine nucleoside analogue with *in vitro* and *in vivo* inhibitory activity against Herpes simplex, varicella-zoster, Epstein-Barr and cytomegalovirus. In cell cultures, the inhibitory activity of acyclovir for Herpes simplex virus is highly selective. Cellular thymidine kinase does not effectively utilize acyclovir as a substrate. Herpes simplex virus-coded thymidine kinase, however, converts acyclovir into acyclovir monophosphate, a nucleotide analogue. The monophosphate is further converted into diphosphate by cellular guanylate kinase and into triphosphate by a number of cellular enzymes.[1] Acyclovir triphosphate interferes with Herpes simplex virus DNA polymerase and inhibits viral DNA replication. Acyclovir triphosphate also inhibits cellular α-DNA polymerase but to a lesser degree. *In vitro*, acyclovir triphosphate can be incorporated into growing chains of DNA by viral DNA polymerase and to a much smaller extent by cellular α-DNA polymerase.[2] When incorporation occurs, the DNA chain is terminated.[3] Acyclovir is preferentially taken up and selectively converted to the active triphosphate form by herpesvirus-infected cells. Thus, acyclovir is much less toxic *in vitro* for normal uninfected cells because: 1) less is taken up; 2) less is converted to the active form; 3) cellular α-DNA polymerase is less sensitive to the effects of the active form.

The relationship between *in vitro* susceptibility of Herpes simplex virus to antiviral drugs and clinical response has not been established. The techniques and cell types used for determining *in vitro* susceptibility may influence the results obtained. With a quantitative assay to determine the acyclovir concentration producing 50% inhibition of viral cytopathic effect (ID_{50}), 28 HSV-1 clinical isolates had a mean ID_{50} of 0.17 μg/mL and 32 HSV-2 clinical isolates had a mean ID_{50} of 0.46 μg/mL. Results from other studies using different assays have yielded mean ID_{50} values for clinical HSV-1 isolates of 0.018, 0.03 and 0.043 μg/mL and for clinical HSV-2 isolates of 0.027, 0.36 and 0.03 μg/mL, respectively.[4,5,6]

Pharmacokinetics: The pharmacokinetics of acyclovir has been evaluated in 95 patients (9 studies). Results were obtained in adult patients with normal renal function during Phase I/II studies after single doses ranging from 0.5 to 15 mg/kg and after multiple doses ranging from 2.5 to 15 mg/kg every 8 hours. Pharmacokinetics was also determined in pediatric patients with normal renal function ranging in age from 1 to 17 years at doses of 250 mg/M² or 500 mg/M² every 8 hours. In these studies, dose-independent pharmacokinetics is observed in the range of 0.5 to 15 mg/kg. Proportionality between dose and plasma levels is seen after single doses or at steady state after multiple dosing.[7] When Zovirax was administered to adults at 5 mg/kg (approximately 250

mg/M²) by 1-hr infusions every 8 hours, mean steady-state peak and trough concentrations of 9.8 μg/mL (5.5 to 13.8 μg/mL) and 0.7 μg/mL (0.2 to 1.0 μg/mL), respectively, were achieved. Similar concentrations are achieved in children over 1 year of age when doses of 250 mg/M² are given every 8 hours. Concentrations achieved in the cerebrospinal fluid are approximately 50% of plasma values. Plasma protein binding is relatively low (9% to 33%) and drug interactions involving binding site displacement are not anticipated.[7]

Renal excretion of unchanged drug by glomerular filtration and tubular secretion is the major route of acyclovir elimination accounting for 62 to 91% of the dose as determined by ^{14}C-labelled drug. The only major urinary metabolite detected is 9-carboxymethoxymethylguanine. This may account for up to 14.1% of the dose in patients with normal renal function. An insignificant amount of drug is recovered in feces and expired CO_2 and there is no evidence to suggest tissue retention.[7] However, postmortem examinations have shown that acyclovir is widely distributed in tissues and body fluids including brain, kidney, lung, liver, muscle, spleen, uterus, vaginal mucosa, vaginal secretions, cerebrospinal fluid and herpetic vesicular fluid.

In a Phase I study in 3 adult volunteers, 1 g of probenecid was administered orally prior to a single 1-hour 5 mg/kg intravenous infusion of acyclovir. The acyclovir half-life and area under the plasma concentration-time curve increased by 18 and 40%, respectively, compared to a control infusion of acyclovir without probenecid. The mean urinary excretion of acyclovir decreased from 79% to 69% of the dose indicating that probenecid can influence the renal excretion of acyclovir.[8]

The half-life and total body clearance of acyclovir is dependent on renal function as shown below.[7]

Creatinine Clearance (mL/min/1.73M²)	Half-Life (hr)	Total Body Clearance (mL/min/1.73M²)
> 80	2.5	327
50–80	3.0	248
15–50	3.5	190
0 (Anuric)	19.5	29

Zovirax was administered at a dose of 2.5 mg/kg to 6 adult patients with severe renal failure. The peak and trough plasma levels during the 47 hours preceding hemodialysis were 8.5 μg/mL and 0.7 μg/mL, respectively.

Consult DOSAGE AND ADMINISTRATION section for recommended adjustments in dosing based upon creatinine clearance.

The half-life and total body clearance of acyclovir in pediatric patients over 1 year of age is similar to those in adults with normal renal function (see DOSAGE AND ADMINISTRATION).

INDICATIONS AND USAGE

Zovirax Sterile Powder is indicated for the treatment of initial and recurrent mucosal and cutaneous Herpes simplex (HSV-1 and HSV-2) infections in immunocompromised adults and children. It is also indicated for severe initial clinical episodes of herpes genitalis in patients who are not immunocompromised.

These indications are based on the results of several double-blind, placebo-controlled studies which evaluated the drug's effect on virus excretion, complete healing of lesions, and relief of pain.

Herpes Simplex Infections in Immunocompromised Patients
A multicenter trial of Zovirax Sterile Powder at a dose of 250 mg/M² every 8 hours (750 mg/M²/day) for 7 days was conducted in 97 immunocompromised patients with oro-facial, esophageal, genital and other localized infections (50 treated with Zovirax and 47 with placebo). Zovirax significantly decreased virus excretion, reduced pain, and promoted scabbing and rapid healing of lesions.[9,10,11]

Initial Episodes of Herpes Genitalis
A controlled trial was conducted in 28 patients with severe initial episodes of herpes genitalis with a Zovirax dosage of 5 mg/kg every 8 hours for 5 days (12 patients treated with Zovirax and 16 with placebo). Significant treatment effects were seen in elimination of virus from lesions and in reduction of healing times.[12]

In a similar study, 15 patients with initial episodes of genital herpes were treated with Zovirax 5 mg/kg every 8 hours for 5 days and 15 with placebo. Zovirax decreased the duration of viral excretion, new lesion formation, duration of vesicles and promoted more rapid healing of all lesions.[13]

Diagnosis
The use of appropriate laboratory diagnostic procedures will help to establish the etiologic diagnosis. Positive cultures for Herpes simplex virus offer a reliable means for confirmation of the diagnosis. In initial episodes of genital herpes, appropriate examinations should be performed to rule out other sexually transmitted diseases. Whereas cutaneous lesions

Continued on next page

Burroughs Wellcome—Cont.

associated with Herpes simplex infections are often characteristic, the finding of multinucleated giant cells in smears prepared from lesion exudate or scrapings may assist in the diagnosis.[14]

CONTRAINDICATIONS

Zovirax Sterile Powder is contraindicated for patients who develop hypersensitivity to the drug.

WARNINGS

Zovirax Sterile Powder is intended for intravenous infusion only, and should not be administered topically, intramuscularly, orally, subcutaneously, or in the eye. Intravenous infusions must be given over a period of at least 1 (one) hour to prevent renal tubular damage (see PRECAUTIONS and DOSAGE AND ADMINISTRATION).

PRECAUTIONS

General: The recommended dosage, frequency and length of treatment should not be exceeded (see DOSAGE AND ADMINISTRATION).

Although the aqueous solubility of acyclovir sodium (for infusion) is > 100 mg/mL, precipitation of acyclovir crystals in renal tubules can occur if the maximum solubility of free acyclovir (2.5 mg/mL at 37℃ in water) is exceeded or if the drug is administered by bolus injection. This complication causes a rise in serum creatinine and blood urea nitrogen (BUN), and a decrease in renal creatinine clearance. Ensuing renal tubular damage can produce acute renal failure.

Abnormal renal function (decreased creatinine clearance) can occur as a result of acyclovir administration and depends on the state of the patient's hydration, other treatments, and the rate of drug administration. Bolus administration of the drug leads to a 10% incidence of renal dysfunction, while in controlled studies, infusion of 5 mg/kg (250 mg/M^2) over an hour was associated with a lower frequency—4.6%. Concomitant use of other nephrotoxic drugs, pre-existing renal disease, and dehydration make further renal impairment with acyclovir more likely. In most instances, alterations of renal function were transient and resolved spontaneously or with improvement of water and electrolyte balance, drug dosage adjustment or discontinuation of drug administration. However, in some instances, these changes may progress to acute renal failure.

Administration of Zovirax by intravenous infusion must be accompanied by adequate hydration. Since maximum urine concentration occurs within the first 2 hours following infusion, particular attention should be given to establishing sufficient urine flow during that period in order to prevent precipitation in renal tubules.

When dosage adjustments are required they should be based on estimated creatinine clearance (See DOSAGE AND ADMINISTRATION).

Approximately 1% of patients receiving intravenous acyclovir have manifested encephalopathic changes characterized by either lethargy, obtundation, tremors, confusion, hallucinations, agitation, seizures or coma. Zovirax should be used with caution in those patients who have underlying neurologic abnormalities and those with serious renal, hepatic, or electrolyte abnormalities or significant hypoxia. It should also be used with caution in patients who have manifested prior neurologic reactions to cytotoxic drugs or those receiving concomitant intrathecal methotrexate or interferon.

Exposure of HSV isolates to acyclovir *in vitro* can lead to the emergence of less sensitive viruses. These viruses usually are deficient in thymidine kinase (required for acyclovir activation) and are less pathogenic in animals. Similar isolates have been observed in 6 severely immunocompromised patients during the course of controlled and uncontrolled studies of intravenously administered Zovirax. These occurred in patients with congenital severe combined immunodeficiencies or following bone marrow transplantation. The presence of these viruses was not associated with a worsening of clinical illness and, in some instances, the virus disappeared spontaneously. The possibility of the appearance of less sensitive viruses must be borne in mind when treating such patients. The relationship between the *in vitro* sensitivity of herpesviruses to acyclovir and clinical response to therapy has yet to be established.

Drug Interactions: Co-administration of probenecid with acyclovir has been shown to increase the mean half-life and the area under the concentration-time curve. Urinary excretion and renal clearance were correspondingly reduced. Clinical experience has identified no other significant interactions resulting from administration of other drugs concomitantly with Zovirax Sterile Powder.

Carcinogenesis, Mutagenesis, Impairment of Fertility: Acyclovir was tested in lifetime bioassays in rats and mice at single daily doses of 50, 150 and 450 mg/kg given by gavage. There was no statistically significant difference in the incidence of tumors between treated and control animals, nor did acyclovir appear to shorten the latency of tumors. In 2 *in vitro* cell transformation assays, used to provide preliminary assessment of potential oncogenicity in advance of these more definitive lifetime bioassays in rodents, conflicting results were obtained. Acyclovir was positive at the highest dose used in one system and the resulting morphologically transformed cells formed tumors when inoculated into immunosuppressed, syngeneic, weanling mice. Acyclovir was negative in another transformation system.

No chromosome damage was observed at maximum tolerated parenteral doses of 100 mg/kg acyclovir in rats or Chinese hamsters; higher doses of 500 and 1000 mg/kg were clastogenic in Chinese hamsters. In addition, no activity was found in a dominant lethal study in mice. In 9 of 11 microbial and mammalian cell assays, no evidence of mutagenicity was observed. In 2 mammalian cell assays (human lymphocytes and L5178Y mouse lymphoma cells *in vitro*), positive responses for mutagenicity and chromosomal damage occurred, but only at concentrations at least 25 times the acyclovir plasma levels achieved in man.

Acyclovir does not impair fertility or reproduction in mice at oral doses up to 450 mg/kg/day. In female rabbits treated subcutaneously with acyclovir subsequent to mating, there was a statistically significant decrease in implantation efficiency but no concomitant decrease in litter size at a dose of 50 mg/kg/day.

Pregnancy: Teratogenic Effects. Pregnancy Category C. Acyclovir was not teratogenic in the mouse (450 mg/kg/day, p.o.), rabbit (50 mg/kg/day, s.c. and i.v.) or in standard tests in the rat (50 mg/kg/day, s.c.).

Although maximum tolerated doses were tested in the teratology studies, the plasma levels obtained did not exaggerate maximum plasma levels that might occur with clinical use of intravenous acyclovir.

In a non-standard test in rats, fetal abnormalities, such as head and tail anomalies, were observed following subcutaneous administration of acyclovir at very high doses associated with toxicity to the maternal rat. The clinical relevance of these findings is uncertain.[15]

There have been no adequate and well-controlled studies in pregnant women. Acyclovir should be used during pregnancy only if the potential benefit justifies the potential risk to the fetus.

Nursing Mothers: It is not known whether this drug is excreted in human milk. Because many drugs are excreted in human milk, caution should be exercised when Zovirax is administered to a nursing woman.

ADVERSE REACTIONS

The most frequent adverse reactions reported during controlled clinical trials of Zovirax in 64 patients were inflammation or phlebitis at the injection site following infiltration of the I.V. fluid in 9 (14.0%), transient elevations of serum creatinine in 3 (4.7%), and rash or hives in 3 (4.7%). Less frequent adverse reactions were diaphoresis, hematuria, hypotension, headache and nausea, each of which occurred in 1 patient (1.6%). Of the 63 patients receiving placebo, 3 (4.8%) experienced inflammation/phlebitis and 3 (4.8%) experienced rash or itching. Hematuria and nausea were experienced by placebo recipients at the same frequency.

Among 51 immunocompromised patients, one, a bone marrow transplant recipient with pneumonitis, developed seizures, cerebral edema, coma and expired with changes consistent with cerebral anoxia on postmortem biopsy; another immunocompromised patient exhibited coarse tremor and clonus.

Additional adverse reactions were reported in uncontrolled trials. The most frequent adverse reaction was elevated serum creatinine. This occurred in 9.8 percent of patients, usually rapid (less than 10 minutes) intravenous infusion. Less frequent adverse experiences were thrombocytosis and jitters, each in 0.4% of patients.

Approximately 1% of patients receiving intravenous acyclovir have manifested encephalopathic changes characterized by either lethargy, obtundation, tremors, confusion, hallucinations, agitation, seizures or coma (see PRECAUTIONS).

OVERDOSAGE

Overdosage has been reported following administration of bolus injections, or inappropriately high doses, and in patients whose fluid and electrolyte balance was not properly monitored. This has resulted in elevations in BUN, serum creatinine and subsequent renal failure.

Precipitation of acyclovir in renal tubules may occur when the solubility (2.5 mg/mL) in the intratubular fluid is exceeded (see PRECAUTIONS). A six hour hemodialysis results in a 60% decrease in plasma acyclovir concentration. Data concerning peritoneal dialysis are incomplete but indicate that this method may be significantly less efficient in removing acyclovir from the blood. In the event of acute renal failure and anuria, the patient may benefit from hemodialysis until renal function is restored (see DOSAGE AND ADMINISTRATION).

DOSAGE AND ADMINISTRATION

CAUTION— RAPID OR BOLUS INTRAVENOUS AND INTRAMUSCULAR OR SUBCUTANEOUS INJECTION MUST BE AVOIDED.

Dosage: *MUCOSAL AND CUTANEOUS HERPES SIMPLEX (HSV-1 and HSV-2) INFECTIONS IN IMMUNOCOMPROMISED PATIENTS* —5 mg/kg infused at a constant rate over 1 hour, every 8 hours (15 mg/kg/day) for 7 days in adult patients with normal renal function. In children under 12 years of age, more accurate dosing can be attained by infusing 250 mg/M^2 at a constant rate over 1 hour, every 8 hours (750 mg/M^2/day) for 7 days.

SEVERE INITIAL CLINICAL EPISODES OF HERPES GENITALIS —The same dose given above—administered for 5 days.

Therapy should be initiated as early as possible following onset of signs and symptoms.

PATIENTS WITH ACUTE OR CHRONIC RENAL IMPAIRMENT: Refer to DOSAGE AND ADMINISTRATION section for recommended doses, and adjust the dosing interval as indicated in the table below.

Creatinine Clearance (mL/min/1.73M^2)	Dose (mg/kg)	Dosing Interval (hours)
>50	5	8
25–50	5	12
10–25	5	24
0–10	2.5	24

Hemodialysis: For patients who require dialysis, the mean plasma half-life of acyclovir during hemodialysis is approximately 5 hours. This results in a 60% decrease in plasma concentrations following a 6 hour dialysis period. Therefore, the patient's dosing schedule should be adjusted so that a dose is administered after each dialysis.

Method of Preparation: Each 10 mL vial contains acyclovir sodium equivalent to 500 mg of acyclovir. Each 20 mL vial contains acyclovir sodium equivalent to 1000 mg of acyclovir. The contents of the vial should be dissolved in Sterile Water for Injection as follows:

Contents of Vial	Amount of Diluent
500 mg	10 mL
1000 mg	20 mL

The resulting solution in each case contains 50 mg acyclovir per mL (pH approximately 11). Shake the vial well to assure complete dissolution before measuring and transferring each individual dose. DO NOT USE BACTERIOSTATIC WATER FOR INJECTION CONTAINING BENZYL ALCOHOL OR PARABENS.

Administration: The calculated dose should then be removed and added to any appropriate intravenous solution at a volume selected for administration during each 1 hour infusion. Infusion concentrations of approximately 7 mg/mL or lower are recommended. In clinical studies, the average 70 kg adult received approximately 60 mL of fluid per dose. Higher concentrations (e.g., 10 mg/mL) may produce phlebitis or inflammation at the injection site upon inadvertent extravasation. Standard, commercially available electrolyte and glucose solutions are suitable for intravenous administration; biologic or colloidal fluids (e.g., blood products, protein solutions, etc.) are not recommended.

Once in solution in the vial at a concentration of 50 mg/mL, the drug should be used within 12 hours. Once diluted for administration, each dose should be used within 24 hours. Refrigeration of reconstituted solutions may result in formation of a precipitate which will redissolve at room temperature.

HOW SUPPLIED

10 mL sterile vials, each containing acyclovir sodium equivalent to 500 mg of acyclovir, tray of 10 (NDC 0081-0995-01). 20 mL sterile vials, each containing acyclovir sodium equivalent to 1000 mg of acyclovir, tray of 10 (NDC 0081-0952-01). Store at 15° to 25℃ (59° to 77°F).

Also available: ZOVIRAX Ointment, 5% in 3 g and 15 g tubes (each gram contains 50 mg acyclovir in a polyethylene glycol base) and ZOVIRAX Capsules in bottles of 100 and unit dose pack of 100 (each capsule contains 200 mg acyclovir).

References

1. W.H. Miller and R.L. Miller, J. Biol. Chem. 225 (15): 7204–7207, 1980.
2. P.A. Furman, *et al.*, J. Virol. 32 (1): 72–77, 1979.
3. D. Derse, *et al.*, J. Biol. Chem. 256 (22): 11447–11451, 1981.
4. P. Collins and D.J. Bauer. J. Antimicrob. Chemother. 5 :431–436, 1979.

5. C.S. Crumpacker, *et al.*, Antimicrob. Agents Chemother. *15*:642–645, 1979.

6. E. De Clercq. *et al.*, J. Infect. Dis. *141*:563–574, 1980.

7. M.R. Blum, *et al.*, Am. J. Med. 73 (1A): 186–192, Jul. 20, 1982.

8. O.L. Laskin, *et al.*, Antimicrob. Agents Chemother. *21* (5): 804–807, May 1982.

9. C.D. Mitchell, *et al.*, Lancet *1* (8235): 1389–1392, Jun. 27, 1981.

10. J.C. Wade, *et al.*, Ann. Intern. Med. *96* (3): 265–269, Mar. 1982.

11. J.D. Meyers, *et al.*, Am. J. Med. *73* (1A): 229–235, Jul. 20, 1982.

12. Data on file, Burroughs Wellcome Co.

13. A. Mindel, *et al.*, Lancet *1* (8274): 697–700, Mar. 27, 1982.

14. Z.M. Naib, *et al.*, Cancer Res. *33* :1452–1463, 1973.

15. R. Stahlmann, S. Klug, C. Lewandowski, et al., *Infection*: 15(4):261-262, 1987.

ZYLOPRIM ®

[zī'lō-prĭm]
(Allopurinol)
**100 mg Scored Tablets and
300 mg Scored Tablets**

DESCRIPTION

Zyloprim (Allopurinol) is known chemically as 1,5-dihydro-4*H*-pyrazolo-[3,4-*d*]pyrimidin-4-one. It is a xanthine oxidase inhibitor which is administered orally. Each scored white tablet contains 100 mg allopurinol and the inactive ingredients lactose, magnesium stearate, potato starch, and povidone. Each scored peach tablet contains 300 mg allopurinol and the inactive ingredients corn starch, FD&C Yellow No. 6 Lake, lactose, magnesium stearate, and povidone. Its solubility in water at 37°C is 80.0 mg/dl and is greater in an alkaline solution.

CLINICAL PHARMACOLOGY

Zyloprim (allopurinol) acts on purine catabolism, without disrupting the biosynthesis of purines. It reduces the production of uric acid by inhibiting the biochemical reactions immediately preceding its formation.

Zyloprim is a structural analogue of the natural purine base, hypoxanthine. It is an inhibitor of xanthine oxidase, the enzyme responsible for the conversion of hypoxanthine to xanthine and of xanthine to uric acid, the end product of purine metabolism in man. Zyloprim is metabolized to the corresponding xanthine analogue, oxipurinol (alloxanthine), which also is an inhibitor of xanthine oxidase.

It has been shown that reutilization of both hypoxanthine and xanthine for nucleotide and nucleic acid synthesis is markedly enhanced when their oxidations are inhibited by Zyloprim and oxipurinol. This reutilization does not disrupt normal nucleic acid anabolism, however, because feedback inhibition is an integral part of purine biosynthesis. As a result of xanthine oxidase inhibition, the serum concentration of hypoxanthine plus xanthine in patients receiving Zyloprim for treatment of hyperuricemia is usually in the range of 0.3 to 0.4 mg/dl compared to a normal level of approximately 0.15 mg/dl. A maximum of 0.9 mg/dl of these oxypurines has been reported when the serum urate was lowered to less than 2 mg/dl by high doses of Zyloprim. These values are far below the saturation levels at which point their precipitation would be expected to occur (above 7 mg/dl).

The renal clearance of hypoxanthine and xanthine is at least 10 times greater than that of uric acid. The increased xanthine and hypoxanthine in the urine have not been accompanied by problems of nephrolithiasis. Xanthine crystalluria has been reported in only three patients. Two of the patients had Lesch-Nyhan syndrome, which is characterized by excessive uric acid production combined with a deficiency of the enzyme, hypoxanthine-guanine phosphoribosyltransferase (HGPRTase). This enzyme is required for the conversion of hypoxanthine, xanthine, and guanine to their respective nucleotides. The third patient had lymphosarcoma and produced an extremely large amount of uric acid because of rapid cell lysis during chemotherapy.

Zyloprim is approximately 90% absorbed from the gastrointestinal tract. Peak plasma levels generally occur at 1.5 hours and 4.5 hours for Zyloprim and oxipurinol respectively, and after a single oral dose of 300 mg Zyloprim, maximum plasma levels of about 3 µg/ml of Zyloprim and 6.5 µg/ml of oxipurinol are produced.

Approximately 20% of the ingested Zyloprim is excreted in the feces. Because of its rapid oxidation to oxipurinol and a renal clearance rate approximately that of glomerular filtration rate, Zyloprim has a plasma half-life of about 1–2 hours. Oxipurinol, however, has a longer plasma half-life (approximately 15.0 hours) and therefore effective xanthine oxidase inhibition is maintained over a 24-hour period with single daily doses of Zyloprim. Whereas Zyloprim is cleared essentially by glomerular filtration, oxipurinol is reabsorbed in the kidney tubules in a manner similar to the reabsorption of uric acid.

The clearance of oxipurinol is increased by uricosuric drugs, and as a consequence, the addition of a uricosuric agent reduces to some degree the inhibition of xanthine oxidase by oxipurinol and increases to some degree the urinary excretion of uric acid. In practice, the net effect of such combined therapy may be useful in some patients in achieving minimum serum uric acid levels provided the total urinary uric acid load does not exceed the competence of the patient's renal function.

Hyperuricemia may be primary, as in gout, or secondary to diseases such as acute and chronic leukemia, polycythemia vera, multiple myeloma, and psoriasis. It may occur with the use of diuretic agents, during renal dialysis, in the presence of renal damage, during starvation or reducing diets and in the treatment of neoplastic disease where rapid resolution of tissue masses may occur. Asymptomatic hyperuricemia is not an indication for Zyloprim treatment (see INDICATIONS AND USAGE).

Gout is a metabolic disorder which is characterized by hyperuricemia and resultant deposition of monosodium urate in the tissues, particularly the joints and kidneys. The etiology of this hyperuricemia is the overproduction of uric acid in relation to the patient's ability to excrete it. If progressive deposition of urates is to be arrested or reversed, it is necessary to reduce the serum uric acid level below the saturation point to suppress urate precipitation.

Administration of Zyloprim generally results in a fall in both serum and urinary uric acid within two to three days. The degree of this decrease can be manipulated almost at will since it is dose-dependent. A week or more of treatment with Zyloprim may be required before its full effects are manifested; likewise, uric acid may return to pretreatment levels slowly (usually after a period of seven to ten days following cessation of therapy). This reflects primarily the accumulation and slow clearance of oxipurinol. In some patients a dramatic fall in urinary uric acid excretion may not occur, particularly in those with severe tophaceous gout. It has been postulated that this may be due to the mobilization of urate from tissue deposits as the serum uric acid level begins to fall.

Zyloprim's action differs from that of uricosuric agents, which lower the serum uric acid level by increasing urinary excretion of uric acid. Zyloprim reduces both the serum and urinary uric acid levels by inhibiting the formation of uric acid. The use of Zyloprim to block the formation of urates avoids the hazard of increased renal excretion of uric acid posed by uricosuric drugs.

Zyloprim can substantially reduce serum and urinary uric acid levels in previously refractory patients even in the presence of renal damage serious enough to render uricosuric drugs virtually ineffective. Salicylates may be given conjointly for their antirheumatic effect without compromising the action of Zyloprim. This is in contrast to the nullifying effect of salicylates on uricosuric drugs.

Zyloprim also inhibits the enzymatic oxidation of mercaptopurine, the sulfur-containing analogue of hypoxanthine, to 6-thiouric acid. This oxidation, which is catalyzed by xanthine oxidase, inactivates mercaptopurine. Hence, the inhibition of such oxidation by Zyloprim may result in as much as a 75% reduction in the therapeutic dose requirement of mercaptopurine when the two compounds are given together.

INDICATIONS AND USAGE

THIS IS NOT AN INNOCUOUS DRUG. IT IS NOT RECOMMENDED FOR THE TREATMENT OF ASYMPTOMATIC HYPERURICEMIA.

Zyloprim (allopurinol) reduces serum and urinary uric acid concentrations. Its use should be individualized for each patient and requires an understanding of its mode of action and pharmacokinetics (see CLINICAL PHARMACOLOGY, CONTRAINDICATIONS, WARNINGS and PRECAUTIONS).

Zyloprim is indicated in:

(1) the management of patients with signs and symptoms of primary or secondary gout (acute attacks, tophi, joint destruction, uric acid lithiasis and/or nephropathy).

(2) the management of patients with leukemia, lymphoma and malignancies who are receiving cancer therapy which causes elevations of serum and urinary uric acid levels. Zyloprim treatment should be discontinued when the potential for overproduction of uric acid is no longer present.

(3) the management of patients with recurrent calcium oxalate calculi whose daily uric acid excretion exceeds 800 mg/day in male patients and 750 mg/day in female patients. Therapy in such patients should be carefully assessed initially and reassessed periodically to determine in each case that treatment is beneficial and that the benefits outweigh the risks.

CONTRAINDICATIONS

Patients who have developed a severe reaction to Zyloprim (allopurinol) should not be restarted on the drug.

WARNINGS

ZYLOPRIM (ALLOPURINOL) SHOULD BE DISCONTINUED AT THE FIRST APPEARANCE OF SKIN RASH OR OTHER SIGNS WHICH MAY INDICATE AN ALLERGIC REACTION. In some instances a skin rash may be followed by more severe hypersensitivity reactions such as exfoliative, urticarial and purpuric lesions as well as Stevens-Johnson syndrome (erythema multiforme exudativum), and/or generalized vasculitis, irreversible hepatotoxicity and on rare occasions death.

In patients receiving Purinethol® (mercaptopurine) or Imuran® (azathioprine), the concomitant administration of 300–600 mg of Zyloprim per day will require a reduction in dose to approximately one-third to one-fourth of the usual dose of mercaptopurine or azathioprine. Subsequent adjustment of doses of mercaptopurine or azathioprine should be made on the basis of therapeutic response and the appearance of toxic effects (see CLINICAL PHARMACOLOGY).

A few cases of reversible clinical hepatotoxicity have been noted in patients taking Zyloprim, and in some patients asymptomatic rises in serum alkaline phosphatase or serum transaminase have been observed. If anorexia, weight loss or pruritus develop in patients on Zyloprim, evaluation of liver function should be part of their diagnostic workup. In patients with pre-existing liver disease, periodic liver function tests are recommended during the early stages of therapy. Due to the occasional occurrence of drowsiness, patients should be alerted to the need for due precaution when engaging in activities where alertness is mandatory.

The occurrence of hypersensitivity reactions to Zyloprim may be increased in patients with decreased renal function receiving thiazides and Zyloprim concurrently. For this reason, in this clinical setting, such combinations should be administered with caution and patients should be observed closely.

PRECAUTIONS

General: An increase in acute attacks of gout has been reported during the early stages of Zyloprim (allopurinol) administration, even when normal or subnormal serum uric acid levels have been attained. Accordingly, maintenance doses of colchicine generally should be given prophylactically when Zyloprim is begun. In addition, it is recommended that the patient start with a low dose of Zyloprim (100 mg daily) and increase at weekly intervals by 100 mg until a serum uric acid level of 6 mg/dl or less is attained but without exceeding the maximum recommended dose (800 mg per day). The use of colchicine or anti-inflammatory agents may be required to suppress gouty attacks in some cases. The attacks usually become shorter and less severe after several months of therapy. The mobilization of urates from tissue deposits which cause fluctuations in the serum uric acid levels may be a possible explanation for these episodes. Even with adequate Zyloprim therapy, it may require several months to deplete the uric acid pool sufficiently to achieve control of the acute attacks.

A fluid intake sufficient to yield a daily urinary output of at least two liters and the maintenance of a neutral or, preferably, slightly alkaline urine are desirable to (1) avoid the theoretical possibility of formation of xanthine calculi under the influence of Zyloprim therapy and (2) help prevent renal precipitation of urates in patients receiving concomitant uricosuric agents.

Some patients with pre-existing renal disease or poor urate clearance have shown a rise in BUN during Zyloprim administration. Although the mechanism responsible for this has not been established, patients with impaired renal function should be carefully observed during the early stages of Zyloprim administration and dosage decreased or the drug withdrawn if increased abnormalities in renal function appear and persist.

Renal failure in association with Zyloprim administration has been observed among patients with hyperuricemia secondary to neoplastic diseases. Concurrent conditions such as multiple myeloma and congestive myocardial disease were present among those patients whose renal dysfunction increased after Zyloprim was begun. Renal failure is also frequently associated with gouty nephropathy and rarely with Zyloprim-associated hypersensitivity reactions. Albuminuria has been observed among patients who developed clinical gout following chronic glomerulonephritis and chronic pyelonephritis.

Patients with decreased renal function require lower doses of Zyloprim than those with normal renal function. Lower than recommended doses should be used to initiate therapy in any patients with decreased renal function and they should be observed closely during the early states of Zyloprim administration. In patients with severely impaired renal function or decreased urate clearance, the half-life of oxipurinol in the plasma is greatly prolonged. Therefore, a dose of 100 mg per day or 300 mg twice a week, or perhaps less, may be sufficient to maintain adequate xanthine oxidase inhibition to reduce serum urate levels.

Continued on next page

Burroughs Wellcome—Cont.

Bone marrow depression has been reported in patients receiving Zyloprim, most of whom received concomitant drugs with the potential for causing this reaction. This has occurred as early as six weeks to as long as six years after the initiation of Zyloprim therapy. Rarely a patient may develop varying degrees of bone marrow depression, affecting one or more cell lines, while receiving Zyloprim alone.

Information for Patients: Patients should be informed of the following:
(1) They should be cautioned to discontinue Zyloprim (allopurinol) and to consult their physician immediately at the first sign of a skin rash, painful urination, blood in the urine, irritation of the eyes, or swelling of the lips or mouth. (2) They should be reminded to continue drug therapy prescribed for gouty attacks since optimal benefit of Zyloprim may be delayed for two to six weeks. (3) They should be encouraged to increase fluid intake during therapy to prevent renal stones. (4) If a single dose of Zyloprim is occasionally forgotten, there is no need to double the dose at the next scheduled time. (5) There may be certain risks associated with the concomitant use of Zyloprim and dicumarol, sulfinpyrazone, mercaptopurine, azathioprine, ampicillin, amoxicillin and thiazide diuretics, and they should follow the instructions of their physician. (6) Due to the occasional occurrence of drowsiness, patients should take precautions when engaging in activities where alertness is mandatory. (7) Patients may wish to take Zyloprim after meals to minimize gastric irritation.

Laboratory Tests: The correct dosage and schedule for maintaining the serum uric acid within the normal range is best determined by using the serum uric acid as an index. In patients with pre-existing liver disease, periodic liver function tests are recommended during the early stages of therapy (see WARNINGS).
Zyloprim (allopurinol) and its primary active metabolite oxipurinol are eliminated by the kidneys; therefore, changes in renal function have a profound effect on dosage. In patients with decreased renal function or who have concurrent illnesses which can affect renal function such as hypertension and diabetes mellitus, periodic laboratory parameters of renal function, particularly BUN and serum creatinine or creatinine clearance, should be performed and the patient's Zyloprim dosage reassessed.
The prothrombin time should be reassessed periodically in the patients receiving dicumarol who are given Zyloprim.

Drug Interactions: In patients receiving Purinethol® (mercaptopurine) or Imuran® (azathioprine), the concomitant administration of 300-600 mg of Zyloprim (allopurinol) per day will require a reduction in dose to approximately one-third to one-fourth of the usual dose of mercaptopurine or azathioprine. Subsequent adjustment of doses of mercaptopurine or azathioprine should be made on the basis of therapeutic response and the appearance of toxic effects (see CLINICAL PHARMACOLOGY).
It has been reported that Zyloprim prolongs the half-life of the anticoagulant, dicumarol. The clinical basis of this drug interaction has not been established but should be noted when Zyloprim is given to patients already on dicumarol therapy.
Since the excretion of oxipurinol is similar to that of urate, uricosuric agents, which increase the excretion of urate, are also likely to increase the excretion of oxipurinol and thus lower the degree of inhibition of xanthine oxidase. The concomitant administration of uricosuric agents and Zyloprim has been associated with a decrease in the excretion of oxypurines (hypoxanthine and xanthine) and an increase in urinary uric acid excretion compared with that observed with Zyloprim alone. Although clinical evidence to date has not demonstrated renal precipitation of oxypurines in patients either on Zyloprim alone or in combination with uricosuric agents, the possibility should be kept in mind.
The reports that the concomitant use of Zyloprim and thiazide diuretics may contribute to the enhancement of allopurinol toxicity in some patients have been reviewed in an attempt to establish a cause-and-effect relationship and a mechanism of causation. Review of these case reports indicates that the patients were mainly receiving thiazide diuretics for hypertension and that tests to rule out decreased renal function secondary to hypertensive nephropathy were not often performed. In those patients in whom renal insufficiency was documented, however, the recommendation to lower the dose of Zyloprim was not followed. Although a causal mechanism and a cause-and-effect relationship have not been established, current evidence suggests that renal function should be monitored in patients on thiazide diuretics and Zyloprim even in the absence of renal failure, and dosage levels should be even more conservatively adjusted in those patients on such combined therapy if diminished renal function is detected.
An increase in the frequency of skin rash has been reported among patients receiving ampicillin or amoxicillin concurrently with Zyloprim compared to patients who are not re-

ceiving both drugs. The cause of the reported association has not been established.
Enhanced bone marrow suppression by cyclophosphamide and other cytotoxic agents has been reported among patients with neoplastic disease, except leukemia, in the presence of Zyloprim. However, in a well-controlled study of patients with lymphoma on combination therapy, Zyloprim did not increase the marrow toxicity of patients treated with cyclophosphamide, doxorubicin, bleomycin, procarbazine and/or mechlorethamine.
Tolbutamide's conversion to inactive metabolites has been shown to be catalyzed by xanthine oxidase from rat liver. The clinical significance, if any, of these observations is unknown.
Chlorpropamide's plasma half-life may be prolonged by Zyloprim, since Zyloprim and chlorpropamide may compete for excretion in the renal tubule. The risk of hypoglycemia secondary to this mechanism may be increased if Zyloprim and chlorpropamide are given concomitantly in the presence of renal insufficiency.

Drug/Laboratory Test Interactions: Zyloprim (allopurinol) is not known to alter the accuracy of laboratory tests.

Pregnancy: *Teratogenic Effects:* Pregnancy Category C. Reproductive studies have been performed in rats and rabbits at doses up to twenty times the usual human dose (5 mg/kg/day), and it was concluded that there was no impaired fertility or harm to the fetus due to Zyloprim (allopurinol). There is a published report of a study in pregnant mice given 50 or 100 mg/kg allopurinol intraperitoneally on gestation days 10 or 13. There were increased numbers of dead fetuses in dams given 100 mg/kg allopurinol but not in those given 50 mg/kg. There were increased numbers of external malformations in fetuses at both doses of allopurinol on gestation day 10 and increased numbers of skeletal malformations in fetuses at both doses on gestation day 13. It cannot be determined whether this represented a fetal effect or an effect secondary to maternal toxicity. There are, however, no adequate or well-controlled studies in pregnant women. Because animal reproduction studies are not always predictive of human response, this drug should be used during pregnancy only if clearly needed.
Experience with Zyloprim during human pregnancy has been limited partly because women of reproductive age rarely require treatment with Zyloprim. There are two unpublished reports and one published paper of women giving birth to normal offspring after receiving Zyloprim during pregnancy.

Nursing Mothers: Zyloprim (allopurinol) and oxipurinol have been found in the milk of a mother who was receiving Zyloprim. Since the effect of Zyloprim on the nursing infant is unknown, caution should be exercised when Zyloprim is administered to a nursing woman.

Pediatric Use: Zyloprim (allopurinol) is rarely indicated for use in children with the exception of those with hyperuricemia secondary to malignancy or to certain rare inborn errors of purine metabolism (see INDICATIONS and DOSAGE AND ADMINISTRATION).

ADVERSE REACTIONS

Data upon which the following estimates of incidence of adverse reactions are made are derived from experiences reported in the literature, unpublished clinical trials and voluntary reports since marketing of Zyloprim (allopurinol) began. Past experience suggested that the most frequent event following the initiation of allopurinol treatment was an increase in acute attacks of gout (average 6% in early studies). An analysis of current usage suggests that the incidence of acute gouty attacks has diminished to less than 1%. The explanation for this decrease has not been determined but may be due in part to initiating therapy more gradually (see PRECAUTIONS and DOSAGE AND ADMINISTRATION).
The most frequent adverse reaction to Zyloprim is skin rash. Skin reactions can be severe and sometimes fatal. Therefore, treatment with Zyloprim should be discontinued immediately if a rash develops (see WARNINGS). Some patients with the most severe reaction also had fever, chills, arthralgias, cholestatic jaundice, eosinophilia and mild leukocytosis or leukopenia. Among 55 patients with gout treated with Zyloprim for 3 to 34 months (average greater than 1 year) and followed prospectively, Rundles observed that 3% of patients developed a type of drug reaction which was predominantly a pruritic maculopapular skin eruption, sometimes scaly or exfoliative. However, with current usage, skin reactions have been observed less frequently than 1%. The explanation for this decrease is not obvious. The incidence of skin rash may be increased in the presence of renal insufficiency. The frequency of skin rash among patients receiving ampicillin or amoxicillin concurrently with Zyloprim has been reported to be increased (see PRECAUTIONS).

Most Common Reactions*
Probably Causally Related
Gastrointestinal: diarrhea, nausea, alkaline phosphatase increase, SGOT/SGPT increase

Metabolic and Nutritional: acute attacks of gout
Skin and Appendages: rash, maculopapular rash
*Early clinical studies and incidence rates from early clinical experience with Zyloprim suggested that these adverse reactions were found to occur at a rate of greater than 1%. The most frequent event observed was acute attacks of gout following the initiation of therapy. Analyses of current usage suggest that the incidence of these adverse reactions is now less than 1%. The explanation for this decrease has not been determined, but it may be due to following recommended usage (see ADVERSE REACTIONS introduction, INDICATIONS, PRECAUTIONS and DOSAGE AND ADMINISTRATION).

Incidence Less Than 1%
Probably Causally Related
Body as a whole: ecchymosis, fever, headache
Cardiovascular: necrotizing angiitis, vasculitis
Gastrointestinal: hepatic necrosis, granulomatous hepatitis, hepatomegaly, hyperbilirubinemia, cholestatic jaundice, vomiting, intermittent abdominal pain, gastritis, dyspepsia
Hemic and Lymphatic: thrombocytopenia, eosinophilia, leukocytosis, leukopenia
Musculoskeletal: myopathy, arthralgias
Nervous: peripheral neuropathy, neuritis, paresthesia, somnolence
Repiratory: epistaxis
Skin and Appendages: erythema multiforme exudativum (Stevens-Johnson syndrome), toxic epidermal necrolysis (Lyell's syndrome), hypersensitivity vasculitis, purpura, vesicular bullous dermatitis, exfoliative dermatitis, eczematoid dermatitis, pruritus, urticaria, alopecia, onycholysis, lichen planus
Special Senses: taste loss/perversion
Urogenital: renal failure, uremia (see PRECAUTIONS)

Incidence Less Than 1%
Causal Relationship Unknown
Body as a whole: malaise
Cardiovascular: pericarditis, peripheral vascular disease, thrombophlebitis, bradycardia, vasodilation
Endocrine: infertility (male), hypercalcemia, gynecomastia (male)
Gastrointestinal: hemorrhagic pancreatitis, gastrointestinal bleeding, stomatitis, salivary gland swelling, hyperlipidemia, tongue edema, anorexia
Hemic and Lymphatic: aplastic anemia, agranulocytosis, eosinophilic fibrohistiocytic lesion of bone marrow, pancytopenia, prothrombin decrease, anemia, hemolytic anemia, reticulocytosis, lymphadenopathy, lymphocytosis
Musculoskeletal: myalgia
Nervous: optic neuritis, confusion, dizziness, vertigo, foot drop, decrease in libido, depression, amnesia, tinnitus, asthenia, insomnia
Respiratory: bronchospasm, asthma, pharyngitis, rhinitis
Skin and Appendages: furunculosis, facial edema, sweating, skin edema
Special Senses: cataracts, macular retinitis, iritis, conjunctivitis, amblyopia
Urogenital: nephritis, impotence, primary hematuria, albuminuria

OVERDOSAGE

Massive overdosing or acute poisoning by Zyloprim (allopurinol) has not been reported.
In mice the 50% lethal dose (LD$_{50}$) is 160 mg/kg given intraperitoneally (i.p.) with deaths delayed up to five days and 700 mg/kg orally (p.o.) (approximately 140 times the usual human dose) with deaths delayed up to three days. In rats the acute LD$_{50}$ is 750 mg/kg i.p. and 6000 mg/kg p.o. (approximately 1200 times the human dose).
In the management of overdosage there is no specific antidote for Zyloprim. There has been no clinical experience in the management of a patient who has taken massive amounts of Zyloprim.
Both Zyloprim and oxipurinol are dialyzable; however, the usefulness of hemodialysis or peritoneal dialysis in the management of a Zyloprim overdose is unknown.

DOSAGE AND ADMINISTRATION

The dosage of Zyloprim (allopurinol) to accomplish full control of gout and to lower serum uric acid to normal or near-normal levels varies with the severity of the disease. The average is 200 to 300 mg per day for patients with mild gout and 400 to 600 mg per day for those with moderately severe tophaceous gout. The appropriate dosage may be administered in divided doses or as a single equivalent dose with the 300 mg tablet. Dosage requirements in excess of 300 mg should be administered in divided doses. The minimal effective dosage is 100 to 200 mg daily and the maximal recommended dosage is 800 mg daily. To reduce the possibility of flare-up of acute gouty attacks, it is recommended that the patient start with a low dose of Zyloprim (100 mg daily) and increase at weekly intervals by 100 mg until a serum uric acid level of 6 mg/dl or less is attained but without exceeding the maximal recommended dosage.
Normal serum urate levels are usually achieved in one to three weeks. The upper limit of normal is about 7 mg/dl for men and postmenopausal women and 6 mg/dl for premeno-

pausal women. Too much reliance should not be placed on a single uric acid determination since, for technical reasons, estimation of uric acid may be difficult. By selecting the appropriate dosage and, in certain patients, using uricosuric agents concurrently, it is possible to reduce serum uric acid to normal or, if desired, to as low as 2 to 3 mg/dl and keep it there indefinitely.

While adjusting the dosage of Zyloprim in patients who are being treated with colchicine and/or anti-inflammatory agents, it is wise to continue the latter therapy until serum uric acid has been normalized and there has been freedom from acute gouty attacks for several months.

In transferring a patient from a uricosuric agent to Zyloprim, the dose of the uricosuric agent should be gradually reduced over a period of several weeks and the dose of Zyloprim gradually increased to the required dose needed to maintain a normal serum uric acid level.

It should also be noted that Zyloprim is generally better tolerated if taken following meals. A fluid intake sufficient to yield a daily urinary output of at least two liters and the maintenance of a neutral or, preferably, slightly alkaline urine are desirable.

Since Zyloprim and its metabolites are primarily eliminated only by the kidney, accumulation of the drug can occur in renal failure, and the dose of Zyloprim should consequently be reduced. With a creatinine clearance of 10 to 20 ml/min, a daily dosage of 200 mg of Zyloprim is suitable. When the creatinine clearance is less than 10 ml/min the daily dosage should not exceed 100 mg. With extreme renal impairment (creatinine clearance less than 3 ml/min) the interval between doses may also need to be lengthened.

The correct size and frequency of dosage for maintaining the serum uric acid just within the normal range is best determined by using the serum uric acid level as an index.

For the prevention of uric acid nephropathy during the vigorous therapy of neoplastic disease, treatment with 600 to 800 mg daily for two or three days is advisable together with a high fluid intake. Otherwise similar considerations to the above recommendations for treating patients with gout govern the regulation of dosage for maintenance purposes in secondary hyperuricemia.

The dose of Zyloprim recommended for management of recurrent calcium oxalate stones in hyperuricosuric patients is 200 to 300 mg/day in divided doses or as the single equivalent. This dose may be adjusted up or down depending upon the resultant control of the hyperuricosuria based upon subsequent 24 hour urinary urate determinations. Clinical experience suggests that patients with recurrent calcium oxalate stones may also benefit from dietary changes such as the reduction of animal protein, sodium, refined sugars, oxalate-rich foods, and excessive calcium intake as well as an increase in oral fluids and dietary fiber.

Children, 6 to 10 years of age, with secondary hyperuricemia associated with malignancies may be given 300 mg Zyloprim daily while those under 6 years are generally given 150 mg daily. The response is evaluated after approximately 48 hours of therapy and a dosage adjustment is made if necessary.

HOW SUPPLIED

100 mg (white) scored, flat cylindrical tablets imprinted with "ZYLOPRIM 100" on a raised hexagon.
Bottles of 90 (NDC 0081-0996-19). 100 (NDC 0081-0996-55) and 1000 (NDC 0081-0996-75) and Unit Dose Pack of 100 (NDC 0081-0996-56).

Store at 15° to 25°C (59° to 77°F) in a dry place.

300 mg (peach) scored, flat, cylindrical tablets imprinted with "ZYLOPRIM 300" on a raised hexagon.
Bottles of 30 (NDC 0081-0998-30), 90 (NDC 0081-0998-19), 100 (NDC 0081-0998-55) and 500 (NDC 0081-0998-70) and Unit Dose Pack of 100 (NDC 0081-0998-56).

Store at 15° to 25°C (59° to 77°F) in a dry place and protect from light.

U.S. Patent No. 3,624,205 (Use Patent)
Shown in Product Identification Section, page 408

EDUCATIONAL MATERIAL

The following is a selected list of materials loaned free or available without charge to medical personnel or pharmacists. To order or obtain information regarding availability of continuing health-care education credit, contact your area Burroughs Wellcome Co. Representative or write: Burroughs Wellcome Co., Educational Services, 3030 Cornwallis Road, Research Triangle Park, NC 27709.

CONTINUING HEALTH-CARE EDUCATION MATERIAL AVAILABLE FROM BURROUGHS WELLCOME CO.

Wellcome Programs in Pharmacy
Wellcome Programs in Hospital Pharmacy

Video/Monograph Programs
New Advances: Atracurium by Infusion—MD
Anesthesia and Neuromuscular Blockade in Extracorporeal Shock Wave Lithotripsy
Anesthetic Considerations for Posterior Spinal Fusion
Anesthetic Considerations for Renal Transplant Surgery
Selected Monographs
Alkeran: A Perspective on Current Clinical Issues
Thiopurines in Cancer Chemotherapy
Assessing the Risk of Herpes in the Immunocomprised Patient—RN
Current Concepts in Leucovorin Therapy
IV Trimethoprim/Sulfamethoxazole in Clinical Practice—MD
Leucovorin Rescue: The Pharmacology and Clinical Use of Leucovorin in Antifolate Chemotherapy
Collections of Symposia Presentations Covering the Following Medical Topics
Proceedings of a Symposium on Atracurium
Learning Units—CE for Pharmacists/Nurses
Digoxin Learning Unit
Head Lice Infestation
Patient Instructions/Information
"Important Information Concerning Genital Herpes and Its Treatment"
"Head Lice: Patient Instructions"

C & M Pharmacal, Inc.
1519 E. EIGHT MILE ROAD
HAZEL PARK, MI 48030-2696

LACTISOL–C&M   ℞
[lăk'-tĭ-sŏl]
for the removal of benign epithelial growths such as common warts

DESCRIPTION
Salicylic acid 16.7%, Lactic acid 16.7% in an exclusive, quick-drying collodion-like vehicle.
NOTE: This entry does not represent full information regarding the use of this product. Write or call for full data: direct inquiry to Medical Information Dept.

HOW SUPPLIED
½ fl oz bottle with brush applicator NDC 00398-106-12.

POD-BEN-25-C&M   ℞
[päd-bĕn-25]
for the removal of warts (including condylomas)

DESCRIPTION
25% Podophyllin (Podophyllum Resin, American) in Tincture of Benzoin, USP.
NOTE: This entry does not represent full information regarding the use of this product. Write or call for full data: direct inquiry to Medical Information Dept.

HOW SUPPLIED
1 fl. oz. bottle (with data sheet). NDC 00398-087-01.
NOTE: Pod-Ben-25 is to be used (applied) only by the doctor. It is not to be dispensed to the patient.

VERR–CANTH–C&M   ℞
[vĕr-kănth]
for the removal of benign epithelial growths such as verruca vulgaris or molluscum contagiosum

DESCRIPTION
Cantharidin 0.7% in an exclusive collodion-like vehicle.
NOTE: This entry does not represent full information regarding the use of this product. Write or call for full data: direct inquiry to Medical Information Dept.

HOW SUPPLIED
7.5 cc bottle (with data sheet) NDC 00398-085-75.
NOTE: Verr-Canth is to be used (applied) only by the doctor. It is not to be dispensed to the patient.

VERREX–C&M   ℞
[vĕr-rĕks]
for the removal of benign epithelial growths such as common warts

DESCRIPTION
Salicylic acid 30.0%, podophyllin 10.0%, in an exclusive collodion-like vehicle.
NOTE: This entry does not represent full information regarding the use of this product. Write or call for full data: direct inquiry to Medical Information Dept.

HOW SUPPLIED
7.5 cc bottle with thin-tipped applicator. NDC 00398-080-75.

VERRUSOL–C&M   ℞
[vĕr'yŭ-sol]
for the removal of benign epithelial growths such as common warts

DESCRIPTION
Salicylic acid 30.0%, podophyllin 5.0%, cantharidin 1.0%, in an exclusive collodion-like vehicle.
NOTE: This entry does not represent full information regarding the use of this product. Write or call for full data: direct inquiry to Medical Information Dept.

HOW SUPPLIED
7.5 cc bottle (with data sheet) NDC 00398-081-75.
NOTE: Verrusol is to be used (applied) only by the doctor. It is not to be dispensed to the patient.

Campbell Laboratories Inc.
300 EAST 51st STREET
P.O. BOX 812, F.D.R. STATION
NEW YORK, NY 10150-0812

HERPECIN-L® Cold Sore Lip Balm   OTC
[her"puh-sin-el"]

PRODUCT OVERVIEW

KEY FACTS
HERPECIN-L Lip Balm is a convenient, easy-to-use treatment for perioral herpes simplex (HSV-I) infections.

MAJOR USES
HERPECIN-L not only treats cold sores, sun and fever blisters, but with prophylactic use, its sunscreens also protect to help prevent them. Users report early use at the prodromal stages of an attack will often abort the lesions and prevent scabbing. Prescribe: Apply "early and often".

SAFETY INFORMATION
For topical use only. No contraindications. A rare sensitivity to pyridoxine or the sunscreen may occur.

PRESCRIBING INFORMATION

HERPECIN-L® Cold Sore Lip Balm   OTC
[her"puh-sin-el"]

COMPOSITION
A soothing, emollient, cosmetically pleasant lip balm incorporating pyridoxine HCl; allantoin; the sunscreen, octyl p-(dimethylamino)-benzoate (Padimate O); and titanium dioxide in a balanced, acidic lipid system. (All ingredients appear on the package. Has no "caines", antibiotics, phenol or camphor.) (NDC 38083-777-31)

ACTIONS AND USES
HERPECIN-L® relieves dryness and chapping by providing a lipid barrier to help restore normal moisture balance to labial tissues. The sunscreen is effective in 2900-3200 AU range while titanium dioxide helps to block, scatter and reflect the sun's rays.

ADMINISTRATION
(1) Recurrent "cold sores, sun and fever blisters": Simply put, users report the sooner and more often applied, the better the results. Frequent sufferers report that with prophylactic use (B.I.D./P.R.N.), their attacks are fewer and less severe. Most recurrent herpes labialis patients are aware of the prodromal symptoms: tingling, itching, burning. At this stage, or if the lesion has already developed, HERPECIN-L should be applied liberally as often as convenient —at least every hour (qq. hor.). The prodrome will often persist and remind the patient to continue to reapply HERPECIN-L. (2) Outdoor sun/winter protection: Apply during and after exposure (and after swimming) and again at bedtime (h.s.). (3) Dry, chapped lips: Apply as needed.

NOTE
HERPECIN-L is for peri-oral use only; not for "canker sores" (aphthous stomatitis). Primary attacks, usually in children and young adults, are normally intra-oral and accompanied by foul breath, pain and fever. Lasting up to six weeks, they are resistant to most treatments. Adjunctive therapy for pain, fever and secondary infection may be indicated. Excessive chapping may be from mouth breathing.

ADVERSE REACTIONS
A few, rare instances of topical sensitivity to pyridoxine HCl (Vitamin B6) and/or the sunscreen have been reported. Discontinue use if allergic reaction develops.

Continued on next page

Campbell—Cont.

CONTRAINDICATIONS
HERPECIN-L does not contain any steroids. (Corticosteroids are normally contraindicated in *herpes* infections.)

HOW SUPPLIED
2.8 gm. swivel tubes. O.T.C.

SAMPLES AVAILABLE
Yes. (Please request on your professional letterhead.)

Carnrick Laboratories, Inc.
65 HORSE HILL ROAD
CEDAR KNOLLS, NJ 07927

AMEN®   ℞
[ā'men']
(medroxyprogesterone acetate
tablet USP 10 mg)

CAUTION
Federal Law Prohibits Dispensing Without Prescription

WARNING

THE USE OF PROGESTATIONAL AGENTS DURING THE FIRST FOUR MONTHS OF PREGNANCY IS NOT RECOMMENDED.

Progestational agents have been used beginning with the first trimester of pregnancy in an attempt to prevent habitual abortion or treat threatened abortion. There is no adequate evidence that such use is effective and there is evidence of potential harm to the fetus when such drugs are given during the first four months of pregnancy. Furthermore, in the vast majority of women, the cause of abortion is a defective ovum, which progestational agents could not be expected to influence. In addition, the use of progestational agents, with their uterine-relaxant properties, in patients with fertilized defective ova may cause a delay in spontaneous abortion. Therefore, the use of such drugs during the first four months of pregnancy is not recommended.

Several reports suggest an association between intrauterine exposure to female sex hormones and congenital anomalies, including congenital heart defects and limb reduction defects (Refs. 1–5). One study (Ref. 4) estimated a 4.7-fold increased risk of limb reduction defects in infants exposed in utero to sex hormones (oral contraceptives, hormone withdrawal test for pregnancy, or attempted treatment for threatened abortion). Some of these exposures were very short and involved only a few days of treatment. The data suggest that the risk of limb reduction defects in exposed fetuses is somewhat less than 1 in 1,000.

If the patient is exposed to Amen® during the first four months of pregnancy or if she becomes pregnant while taking this drug, she should be apprised of the potential risks to the fetus.

DESCRIPTION
Amen® (medroxyprogesterone acetate USP) is a derivative of progesterone. It is a white to off-white, odorless crystalline powder, stable in air, melting between 200° and 210° C. It is freely soluble in chloroform, soluble in acetone and in dioxane, sparingly soluble in alcohol and in methanol, slightly soluble in ether, and insoluble in water.
The chemical name for medroxyprogesterone acetate is Pregn-4-ene-3,20-dione,17-(acetyloxy)-6-methyl-, (6α)-.
The structural formula is:

Amen tablets contain FD&C Yellow No. 6 as a color additive.

ACTIONS
Amen® (medroxyprogesterone acetate), administered orally in the recommended dose to women with adequate endogenous estrogen, transforms proliferative endometrium into secretory endometrium. Androgenic and anabolic effects have been noted, but the drug is apparently devoid of significant estrogenic activity.

INDICATIONS
Amen® (medroxyprogesterone acetate) is indicated in secondary amenorrhea and abnormal uterine bleeding due to hormonal imbalance in the absence of organic pathology, such as submucous fibroids or uterine cancer.

CONTRAINDICATIONS
1. Thrombophlebitis, thromboembolic disorders, cerebral apoplexy or patients with a past history of these conditions. 2. Liver dysfunction or disease. 3. Known or suspected malignancy of breast or genital organs. 4. Undiagnosed vaginal bleeding. 5. Missed abortion. 6. As a diagnostic test for pregnancy. 7. Known sensitivity to medroxyprogesterone acetate.

WARNINGS
1. The physician should be alert to the earliest manifestations of thrombotic disorders (thrombophlebitis, cerebrovascular disorders, pulmonary embolism, and retinal thrombosis). Should any of these occur or be suspected, the drug should be discontinued immediately.
2. Beagle dogs treated with medroxyprogesterone acetate developed mammary nodules, some of which were malignant. Although nodules occasionally appeared in control animals, they were intermittent in nature, whereas the nodules in the drug treated animals were larger, more numerous, persistent, and there were some breast malignancies with metastases, their significance with respect to humans has not been established.
3. Discontinue medication pending examination if there is sudden partial or complete loss of vision, or if there is sudden onset of proptosis, diplopia or migraine. If examination reveals papilledema, or retinal vascular lesions, medication should be withdrawn.
Detectable amounts of progestin have been identified in the milk of mothers receiving the drug. The effect of this on the nursing infant has not been determined. Masculinization of the female fetus has occurred when progestins have been used in pregnant women.
4. Retrospective studies of morbidity and mortality in Great Britain and studies of morbidity in the United States have shown a statistically significant association between thrombophlebitis, pulmonary embolism, and cerebral thrombosis and embolism and the use of oral contraceptives. There have been three principal studies in Great Britain[6–8] leading to this conclusion and one[9] in this country. The estimate of the relative risk of thromboembolism in the study by Vessey and Doll[8] was about sevenfold, while Sartwell and Associates[9] in the United States found a relative risk of 4.4, meaning that the users are several times as likely to undergo thromboembolic disease without evident cause as non-users. The American study also indicated that the risk did not persist after discontinuation of administration, and that it was not enhanced by long continued administration. The American study was not designed to evaluate a difference between products.

PRECAUTIONS
1. The pretreatment physical examination should include special reference to breast and pelvic organs, as well as Papanicolaou smear.
2. Because this drug may cause some degree of fluid retention, conditions which might be influenced by this factor, such as epilepsy, migraine, asthma, cardiac or renal dysfunction require careful observation.
3. In cases of breakthrough bleeding, as in all cases of irregular bleeding per vaginum, nonfunctional causes should be borne in mind. In cases of undiagnosed vaginal bleeding adequate diagnostic measures are indicated.
4. Patients who have a history of psychic depression should be carefully observed and the drug discontinued if the depression recurs to a serious degree.
5. Any possible influence of prolonged progestin therapy on pituitary, ovarian, adrenal, hepatic or uterine functions awaits further study.
6. A decrease in glucose tolerance has been observed in a small percentage of patients on estrogen-progestin combination drugs. The mechanism of this decrease is obscure. For this reason, diabetic patients should be carefully observed while receiving progestin therapy.
7. The age of the patient constitutes no absolute limiting factor although treatment with progestins may mask the onset of the climacteric.
8. The pathologist should be advised of progestin therapy when relevant specimens are submitted.
9. Because of the occasional occurence of thrombotic disorders, (thrombophlebitis, pulmonary embolism, retinal thrombosis, and cerebrovascular disorders) in patients taking estrogen-progestin combinations and since the mechanism is obscure, the physician should be alert to the earliest manifestation of these disorders.
10. Information for the patient. See text of Patient Information which is printed at the end of this insert.

ADVERSE REACTIONS
The following adverse reactions have been associated with the use of medroxyprogesterone acetate.
Breast: In a few instances, breast tenderness or galactorrhea have occurred.

Pregnancy: A few cases of clitoral hypertrophy have been reported in new born females, whose mothers received medroxyprogesterone acetate during pregnancy. Prolonged postpartum bleeding, postabortal bleeding and missed abortion have been reported. (See WARNING box for possible adverse effects on the fetus).
Psychic: An occasional patient has experienced nervousness, insomnia, somnolence, fatigue or dizziness.
Thromboembolic phenomena: Thromboembolic phenomena including thrombophlebitis and pulmonary embolism have been reported.
Skin and mucous membranes: Sensitivity reactions ranging from pruritus, urticaria, angioneurotic edema to generalized rash and anaphylaxis have occasionally been reported. Acne, alopecia, or hirsutism have been reported in a few cases.
Gastrointestinal: Rarely, nausea has been reported. Jaundice, including neonatal jaundice, has been noted in a few instances.
Miscellaneous: Rare cases of headache and hyperpyrexia have been reported. The following adverse reactions have been observed in women taking progestins including medroxyprogesterone acetate: breakthrough bleeding; spotting; change in menstrual flow; amenorrhea; edema; change in weight (increase or decrease); changes in cervical erosion and cervical secretions; cholestatic jaundice; rash (allergic) with and without pruritus; melasma or chloasma; mental depression.
A statistically significant association has been demonstrated between use of estrogen-progestin combination drugs and the following serious adverse reactions; thrombophlebitis, pulmonary embolism and cerebral thrombosis and embolism. For this reason patients on progestin therapy should be carefully observed.
Although available evidence is suggestive of an association, such a relationship has been neither confirmed nor refuted for the following serious adverse reactions: neuro-ocular lesions, e.g., retinal thrombosis and optic neuritis.
The following adverse reactions have been observed in patients receiving estrogen-progestin combination drugs; rise in blood pressure in susceptible individuals; premenstrual-like syndrome; changes in libido; changes in appetite; cystitis-like syndrome; headache; nervousness; dizziness; fatigue; backache; hirsutism; loss of scalp hair; erythema multiforme; erythema nodosum; hemorrhagic eruption; itching. In view of these observations, patients on progestin therapy should be carefully observed.
Female fetal masculinization has been observed in patients receiving progestins. The following laboratory results may be altered by the use of estrogen-progestin combination drugs: Increased sulfobromophthalein and other hepatic function tests; Coagulation tests: increase in prothrombin factors VII, VIII, IX and X; Metyrapone test; Pregnanediol determination.

DOSAGE AND ADMINISTRATION
Secondary Amenorrhea—Amen®(medroxyprogesterone acetate) may be given in dosages of 5 to 10 mg daily for from 5 to 10 days. A dose for inducing an optimum secretory transformation of an endometrium that has been adequately primed with either endogenous or exogenous estrogen is 10 mg of Amen® daily for 10 days. In cases of secondary amenorrhea, therapy may be started at any time. Progestin withdrawal bleeding usually occurs within three to seven days after discontinuing therapy with Amen®.
Abnormal Uterine Bleeding Due to Hormonal Imbalance in the Absence of Organic Pathology—Beginning on the calculated 16th or 21st day of the menstrual cycle, 5 to 10 mg of Amen® may be given daily for from 5 to 10 days. To produce an optimum secretory transformation of an endometrium that has been adequately primed with either endogenous or exogenous estrogen, 10 mg of Amen® daily for 10 days beginning on the 16th day of the cycle is suggested. Progestin withdrawal bleeding usually occurs within three to seven days after discontinuing therapy with Amen®. Patients with a past history of recurrent episodes of abnormal uterine bleeding may benefit from planned menstrual cycling with Amen®.

REFERENCES
1. Gal, I., B. Kirman, and J. Stern, "Hormonal Pregnancy Tests and Congenital Malformation," Nature, 216:83, 1967.
2. Levy, E. P., A. Cohen, and F. C. Fraser, "Hormone Treatment During Pregnancy and Congenital Heart Defects," Lancet, 1:611, 1973.
3. Nora, J. and A. Nora, "Birth Defects and Oral Contraceptives," Lancet, 1:941, 1973.
4. Janerich, D. T., J. M. Piper, and D. M. Glebatis, "Oral Contraceptives and Congenital Limb-Reduction Defects," New England Journal of Medicine, 291:697, 1974.
5. Heinonen, O. P., D. Slone, R. R. Monson, E. B. Hook, and S. Shapiro, "Cardiovascular Birth Defects and Antenatal Exposure to Female Sex Hormones," New England Journal of Medicine, 296:67, 1977.

6. Royal College of General Practitioners; Oral Contraception and Thromboembolic Disease. J. Coll. Gen. Prac., 13:267–279, 1967.

7. Inman, W. H. W. and Vessey, M. P.: Investigation of Deaths From Pulmonary Coronary and Cerebral Thrombosis and Embolism in Women in Child-Bearing Age, Brit. Med. J., 2:193–199, 1968.

8. Vessey, M. P. and Doll, R.: Investigation of Relation Between Use of Oral Contraceptives and Thromboembolic Disease. A Further Report, Brit. Med. J., 2:651–657, 1969.

9. Sartwell, P. E., Masi, A. T., Arthes, G. R., Greene, R. R., and Smith, H. E.: Thromboembolism and Oral Contraceptives: An Epidemiological Case-Control Study, Am. J. Epidem., 90: 365–380, (Nov.) 1969.

Patient Information for Amen®—Warning for Women

There is an increased risk of birth defects in children whose mothers take this drug during the first four months of pregnancy.

Amen® is similar to the progesterone hormones naturally produced by the body. Progesterone and progesterone-like drugs are used to treat menstrual disorders, to test if the body is producing certain hormones, and to treat some forms of cancer in women.

They have been used as a test for pregnancy but such use is no longer considered safe because of possible damage to a developing baby. Also, more rapid methods for testing for pregnancy are now available.

These drugs have also been used to prevent miscarriage in the first few months of pregnancy. No adequate evidence is available to show that they are effective for this purpose and there is evidence of an increased risk of birth defects, such as heart or limb defects, if these drugs are taken during the first four months of pregnancy. Furthermore, most cases of early miscarriage are due to causes which could not be helped by these drugs.

The exact risk of taking this drug early in pregnancy and having a baby with a birth defect is not known. However, one study found that babies born to women who had taken sex hormones (such as progesterone-like drugs) during the first three months of pregnancy were 4 to 5 times more likely to have abnormalities of the arms or legs than if their mothers had not taken such drugs. Some of these women had taken these drugs for only a few days. The chance that an infant whose mother had taken this drug will have this type of defect is about 1 in 1,000.

If you take Amen® and later find you were pregnant when you took it, be sure to discuss this with your doctor as soon as possible.

HOW SUPPLIED

Two-layered peach and white scored tablet with "C" on one side and "AMEN" on the other. Amen® tablets containing 10 mg. of medroxyprogesterone acetate USP are available in bottles of 50 (NDC 0086-0049-05), 100 (NDC 0086-0049-10) and 1000 (NDC 0086-0049-90).

The most recent revision of this labeling is October 1988. Manufactured for Carnrick Laboratories, Inc.

Shown in Product Identification Section, page 408

BONTRIL® PDM   Ⓒ

[bŏn 'tril]

(phendimetrazine tartrate tablets, USP 35 mg)

HOW SUPPLIED

Three layered green, white and yellow tablet with 8648 on the scored side and the letter "C" on the other. Bontril® PDM tablets containing 35 mg of phendimetrazine tartrate are available in bottles of 100 (NDC 0086-0048-10) and 1,000 (NDC 0086-0048-90).

CAUTION

Federal law prohibits dispensing without prescription.
See product insert for complete information.
Manufactured for Carnrick Laboratories, Inc.

Shown in Product Identification Section, page 408

BONTRIL® SLOW-RELEASE   Ⓒ

[bŏn 'tril]

(brand of phendimetrazine tartrate slow–release capsules 105 mg

DESCRIPTION

Phendimetrazine tartrate, as the dextro isomer, has the chemical name of (+)-3,4-Dimethyl-2-phenylmorpholine Tartrate.
The structural formula is as follows:
[See Chemical Formula at top of next column].
Phendimetrazine tartrate is a white, odorless powder with a bitter taste. It is soluble in water, methanol and ethanol. Bontril Slow-Release capsules contain FD&C Yellow No. 6 as a color additive.

M.W. 341

ACTIONS

Phendimetrazine tartrate is a sympathomimetic amine with pharmacological activity similar to the prototype drugs of this class used in obesity, the amphetamines. Actions include central nervous system stimulation and elevation of blood pressure. Tachyphylaxis and tolerance have been demonstrated with all drugs of this class in which these phenomena have been looked for.

Drugs of this class used in obesity are commonly known as "anorectics" or "anorexigenics". It has not been established, however, that the action of such drugs in treating obesity is primarily one of appetite suppression. Other central nervous system actions or metabolic effects may be involved.

Adult obese subjects instructed in dietary management and treated with anorectic drugs lose more weight on the average than those treated with placebo and diet, as determined in relatively short term clinical trials.

The magnitude of increased weight loss of drug-treated patients over placebo-treated patients is only a fraction of a pound a week. The rate of weight loss is greatest in the first weeks of therapy for both drug and placebo subjects and tends to decrease in succeeding weeks. The possible origin of the increased weight loss due to the various drug effects is not established. The amount of weight loss associated with the use of an anorectic drug varies from trial to trial, and the increased weight loss appears to be related in part to variables other than the drug prescribed, such as the physician investigator, the population treated, and the diet prescribed. Studies do not permit conclusions as to the relative importance of the drug and non-drug factors on weight loss.

The natural history of obesity is measured in years, whereas the studies cited are restricted to a few weeks duration; thus, the total impact of drug-induced weight loss over that of diet alone must be considered clinically limited.

The active drug 105 mg of phendimetrazine tartrate in each capsule of this special slow-release dosage form approximates the action of three 35 mg non-time release doses taken at 4 hours intervals.

The major route of elimination is via the kidneys where most of the drug and metabolites are excreted. Some of the drug is metabolized to phenmetrazine and also phendimetrazine-N-oxide.

The average half-life of elimination when studied under controlled conditions is about 1.9 hours for the non-time and 9.8 hours for the slow-release dosage form. The absorption half-life of the drug from conventional non-time 35 mg phendimetrazine tablets is approximately the same. These data indicate that the slow-release product has a similar onset of action to the conventional non-time-release product and, in addition, has a prolonged therapeutic effect.

INDICATIONS

Phendimetrazine tartrate is indicated in the management of exogenous obesity as a short term adjunct (a few weeks) in a regimen of weight reduction based on caloric restriction. The limited usefulness of agents of this class (see ACTIONS) should be measured against possible risk factors inherent in their use such as those described below.

CONTRAINDICATIONS

Advanced arteriosclerosis, symptomatic cardiovascular disease, moderate and severe hypertension, hyperthyroidism, known hypersensitivity, or idiosyncrasy to the sympathomimetic amines. Agitated states. Patients with a history of drug abuse. Use in patients taking other CNS stimulants including monoamine oxidase inhibitors.

WARNINGS

Tolerance to the anorectic effect usually develops within a few weeks. When this occurs, the recommended dose should not be exceeded in an attempt to increase the effect; rather, the drug should be discontinued.

Use of phendimetrazine within 14 days following the administration of monoamine oxidase inhibitors may result in a hypertensive crisis.

Abrupt cessation of administration following prolonged high dosage results in extreme fatigue and depression. Because of the effect on the central nervous system phendimetrazine tartrate may impair the ability of the patient to engage in potentially hazardous activities such as operating machinery or driving a motor vehicle; the patient should therefore be cautioned accordingly.

PRECAUTIONS

Caution is to be exercised in prescribing phendimetrazine for patients with even mild hypertension.

Insulin requirements in diabetes mellitus may be altered in association with the use of phendimetrazine and the concomitant dietary regimen.

Phendimetrazine may decrease the hypotensive effect of guanethidine.

The least amount feasible should be prescribed or dispensed at one time in order to minimize the possibility of overdosage.

Usage in Pregnancy: Safe use in pregnancy has not been established. Until more information is available, phendimetrazine tartrate should not be taken by women who are or may become pregnant unless, in the opinion of the physician, the potential benefits outweigh the possible hazards.

Usage in Children: Phendimetrazine tartrate is not recommended for use in children under 12 years of age.

ADVERSE REACTIONS

Cardiovascular: Palpitation, tachycardia, elevation of blood pressure.

Central Nervous System: Overstimulation, restlessness, dizziness, insomnia, tremor, headache; rarely psychotic episodes at recommended doses, agitation, flushing, sweating, blurring of vision.

Gastrointestinal: Dryness of the mouth, diarrhea, constipation, nausea, stomach pain.

Genitourinary: Changes in libido, urinary frequency, dysuria.

DRUG ABUSE AND DEPENDENCE

Controlled Substance: Phendimetrazine is a Schedule III controlled substance.

Dependence: Phendimetrazine Tartrate is related chemically and pharmacologically to the amphetamines. Amphetamines and related stimulant drugs have been extensively abused, and the possibility of abuse of phendimetrazine should be kept in mind when evaluating the desirability of including a drug as part of a weight reduction program. Abuse of amphetamines and related drugs may be associated with intense psychological dependence and severe social dysfunction. There are reports of patients who have increased the dosage to many times that recommended. Abrupt cessation following prolonged high dosage administration results in extreme fatigue and mental depression; changes are also noted on the sleep EEG. Manifestations of chronic intoxication with anorectic drugs include severe dermatoses, marked insomnia, irritability, hyperactivity and personality changes. The most severe manifestation of chronic intoxications is psychosis, often clinically indistinguishable from schizophrenia.

OVERDOSAGE

Manifestations of acute overdosage may include restlessness, tremor, hyperreflexia, rapid respiration, confusion, assaultiveness, hallucinations, panic states.

Fatigue and depression usually follow the central stimulation.

Cardiovascular effects include arrhythmias, hypertension, or hypotension and circulatory collapse. Gastrointestinal symptoms include nausea, vomiting, diarrhea, and abdominal cramps. Poisoning may result in convulsions, coma, and death.

Management of acute intoxication is largely symptomatic and includes lavage and sedation with a barbiturate. Experience with hemodialysis or peritoneal dialysis is inadequate to permit recommendation in this regard.

Acidification of the urine increases phendimetrazine tartrate excretion.

Intravenous phentolamine (Regitine) has been suggested for possible acute, severe hypertension, if this complicates overdosage.

DOSAGE AND ADMINISTRATION

One Slow-Release Capsule (105 mg) in the morning, taken 30-60 minutes before the morning meal.

Phendimetrazine Tartrate is not recommended for use in children under twelve years of age.

HOW SUPPLIED

Phendimetrazine Slow-Release Capsules, 105 mg is supplied in bottles of 100 opaque green and clear yellow capsules, imprinted with the letter "C" and 8647. NDC # 0086-0047-10. Store at controlled room temperature, 15°–30°C(59°–86°F). The most recent revision of this labeling is Nov. 1988.

CAUTION

Federal law prohibits dispensing without prescription.
Manufactured for Carnrick Laboratories, Inc.
Shown in Product Identification Section, page 408

CAPITAL® and CODEINE SUSPENSION   Ⓒ

(acetaminophen and codeine phosphate oral suspension)

HOW SUPPLIED

CAPITAL® AND CODEINE SUSPENSION contains 120 mg of acetaminophen and 12 mg of codeine phosphate/5 mL and is given orally. CAPITAL® AND CODEINE SUSPEN-

Continued on next page

Carnrick—Cont.

SION is a fruit punch-flavored pink suspension available in 16 fluid oz. (473 mL) bottles, NDC 0086-0046-16.
SHAKE WELL BEFORE USING
Store at controlled room temperature 15°–30°C (59°–86°F). Dispense in tight, light-resistant glass container and label "Shake Well Before Using."

CAUTION

Federal law prohibits dispensing without prescription.
See product insert for complete information.
Manufactured for Carnrick Laboratories, Inc.
    Shown in Product Identification Section, page 408

HYDROCET® CAPSULES   Ⓒ

CAUTION

Federal law prohibits dispensing without prescription.

DESCRIPTION

Each Hydrocet® capsule contains:
Hydrocodone Bitartrate, USP .... 5 mg
(WARNING: May be habit forming.)
Acetaminophen, USP ....500 mg
Hydrocodone bitartrate is an opioid analgesic and antitussive and occurs as fine, white crystals or as a crystalline powder. It is affected by light. The chemical name is: 4,5α-epoxy-3-methoxy-17-methylmorphinan-6-one tartrate (1:1) hydrate (2:5). Its structure is as follows:

$$C_{18}H_{21}NO_3 \cdot C_4H_6O_6 \cdot 2\frac{1}{2} H_2O$$
M.W. 494.50

Acetaminophen, 4'-hydroxyacetanilide, is a nonopiate, nonsalicylate analgesic and antipyretic which occurs as a white, odorless crystalline powder possessing a slightly bitter taste. Its structure is as follows:

$$C_8H_9NO_2$$
M.W. 151.16

CLINICAL PHARMACOLOGY

Hydrocodone is a semisynthetic narcotic analgesic and antitussive with multiple actions qualitatively similar to those of codeine. Most of these involve the central nervous system and smooth muscle. The precise mechanism of action of hydrocodone and other opiates is not known, although it is believed to relate to the existence of opiate receptors in the central nervous system. In addition to analgesia, narcotics may produce drowsiness, changes in mood and mental clouding.
Radioimmunoassay techniques have recently been developed for the analysis of hydrocodone in human plasma. After a 10 mg oral dose of hydrocodone bitartrate, a mean peak serum drug level of 23.6 ng/ml and an elimination half-life of 3.8 hours were found.
The analgesic action of acetaminophen involves peripheral and central influences, but the specific mechanism is as yet undetermined. Antipyretic activity is mediated through hypothalamic heat regulating centers. Acetaminophen inhibits prostaglandin synthetase. Therapeutic doses of acetaminophen have negligible effects on the cardiovascular or respiratory systems; however, toxic doses may cause circulatory failure and rapid, shallow breathing. Acetaminophen is rapidly and almost completely absorbed from the gastrointestinal tract, producing maximum serum concentrations within 30 minutes to one hour. The plasma half-life in adults and children ranges from 0.90 hours to 3.25 hours with an average of approximately 2 hours. The drug distributes uniformly in most body fluids and is approximately 25% protein bound. Acetaminophen is conjugated in the liver, with less than 3% of the dose excreted unchanged in 24 hours. The primary metabolic pathway is conjugation to sulfate and glucuronide by-products. A minor oxidative pathway forms cysteine and mercapturic acid. These compounds are subsequently excreted by the kidneys into the urine.

INDICATIONS AND USAGE

For the relief of moderate to moderately severe pain.

CONTRAINDICATIONS

Hypersensitivity to acetaminophen or hydrocodone.

WARNINGS

Respiratory Depression: At high doses or in sensitive patients, hydrocodone may produce dose-related respiratory depression by acting directly on the brain stem respiratory center. Hydrocodone also affects the center that controls respiratory rhythm, and may produce irregular and periodic breathing.
Head Injury and Increased Intracranial Pressure: The respiratory depressant effects of narcotics and their capacity to elevate cerebrospinal fluid pressure may be markedly exaggerated in the presence of head injury, other intracranial lesions or a preexisting increase in intracranial pressure. Furthermore, narcotics produce adverse reactions which may obscure the clinical course of patients with head injuries.
Acute Abdominal Conditions: The administration of narcotics may obscure the diagnosis or clinical course of patients with acute abdominal conditions.

PRECAUTIONS

Special Risk Patients: As with any narcotic analgesic agent, HYDROCET® (Hydrocodone Bitartrate, USP 5 mg and Acetaminophen, USP 500 mg) capsules should be used with caution in elderly or debilitated patients and those with severe impairment of hepatic or renal function, hypothyroidism, Addison's disease, prostatic hypertrophy or urethral stricture. The usual precautions should be observed and the possibility of respiratory depression should be kept in mind.
Information for Patients: HYDROCET® (Hydrocodone Bitartrate, USP 5 mg and Acetaminophen, USP 500 mg) capsules like all narcotics, may impair the mental and/or physical abilities required for the performance of potentially hazardous tasks such as driving a car or operating machinery; patients should be cautioned accordingly.
Cough Reflex: Hydrocodone suppresses the cough reflex; as with all narcotics, caution should be exercised when HYDROCET® capsules are used postoperatively and in patients with pulmonary disease.
Drug Interactions: Patients receiving other narcotic analgesics, antipsychotics, antianxiety agents, or other CNS depressants (including alcohol) concomitantly with HYDROCET® capsules may exhibit an additive CNS depression. When combined therapy is contemplated, the dose of one or both agents should be reduced.
The use of MAO inhibitors or tricyclic antidepressants with hydrocodone preparations may increase the effect of either the antidepressant or hydrocodone.
The concurrent use of anticholinergics with hydrocodone may produce paralytic ileus.
Usage In Pregnancy:
Teratogenic Effects: Pregnancy Category C. Hydrocodone has been shown to be teratogenic in hamsters when given in doses 700 times the human dose. There are no adequate and well-controlled studies in pregnant women. HYDROCET® capsules should be used during pregnancy only if the potential benefit justifies the potential risk to the fetus.
Nonteratogenic Effects: Babies born to mothers who have been taking opioids regularly prior to delivery will be physically dependent. The withdrawal signs include irritability and excessive crying, tremors, hyperactive reflexes, increased respiratory rate, increased stools, sneezing, yawning, vomiting, and fever. The intensity of the syndrome does not always correlate with the duration of maternal opioid use or dose. There is no consensus on the best method of managing withdrawal. Chlorpromazine 0.7 to 1 mg/kg q6h, and paregoric 2 to 4 drops/kg q4h, have been used to treat withdrawal symptoms in infants. The duration of therapy is 4 to 28 days, with the dosage decreased as tolerated.
Labor and Delivery: As with all narcotics, administration of HYDROCET® capsules to the mother shortly before delivery may result in some degree of respiratory depression in the newborn, especially if higher doses are used.
Nursing Mothers: It is not known whether this drug is excreted in human milk. Because many drugs are excreted in human milk and because of the potential for serious adverse reactions in nursing infants from HYDROCET® (Hydrocodone Bitartrate, USP 5 mg and Acetaminophen, USP 500 mg) capsules, a decision should be made whether to discontinue nursing or to discontinue the drug, taking into account the importance of the drug to the mother.
Pediatric Use: Safety and effectiveness in children have not been established.

ADVERSE REACTIONS

The most frequently observed adverse reactions include lightheadedness, dizziness, sedation, nausea and vomiting. These effects seem to be more prominent in ambulatory than in nonambulatory patients and some of these adverse reactions may be alleviated if the patient lies down.
Other adverse reactions include:
Central Nervous System: Drowsiness, mental clouding, lethargy, impairment of mental and physical performance, anxiety, fear, dysphoria, psychic dependence, and mood changes.

Gastrointestinal System: The antiemetic phenothiazines are useful in suppressing the nausea and vomiting which may occur (see above); however, some phenothiazine derivatives seem to be antianalgesic and to increase the amount of narcotic required to produce pain relief, while other phenothiazines reduce the amount of narcotic required to produce a given level of analgesia. Prolonged administration of HYDROCET® capsules may produce constipation.
Genitourinary System: Ureteral spasm, spasm of vesical sphincters and urinary retention have been reported.
Respiratory Depression: Hydrocodone bitartrate may produce dose-related respiratory depression by acting directly on the brain stem respiratory center. Hydrocodone also affects the center that control respiratory rhythm, and may produce irregular and periodic breathing. If significant respiratory depression occurs, it may be antagonized by the use of naloxone hydrochloride. Apply other supportive measures when indicated.

DRUG ABUSE AND DEPENDENCE

HYDROCET® capsules are subject to the Federal Controlled Substances Act (Schedule III).
Psychic dependence, physical dependence, and tolerance may develop upon repeated administration of narcotics; therefore, HYDROCET® capsules should be prescribed and administered with caution. However, psychic dependence is unlikely to develop when HYDROCET® capsules are used for a short time for the treatment of pain.
Physical dependence, the condition in which continued administration of the drug is required to prevent the appearance of a withdrawal syndrome, assumes clinically significant proportions only after several weeks of continued narcotic use, although some mild degree of physical dependence may develop after a few days of narcotic therapy. Tolerance, in which increasingly large doses are required in order to produce the same degree of analgesia, is manifested initially by a shortened duration of analgesic effect, and subsequently by decreases in the intensity of analgesia. The rate of development of tolerance varies among patients.

OVERDOSAGE

Acetaminophen:
Signs and Symptoms: In acute acetaminophen overdosage, dose-dependent, potentially fatal hepatic necrosis is the most serious adverse effect. Renal tubular necrosis, hypoglycemic coma, and thrombocytopenia may also occur.
In adults, hepatic toxicity has rarely been reported with acute overdoses of less than 10 grams and fatalities with less than 15 grams. Importantly, young children seem to be more resistant than adults to the hepatotoxic effect of an acetaminophen overdose. Despite this, the measures outlined below should be initiated in any adult or child suspected of having ingested an acetaminophen overdose.
Early symptoms following a potentially hepatotoxic overdose may include: nausea, vomiting, diaphoresis and general malaise. Clinical and laboratory evidence of hepatic toxicity may not be apparent until 48 to 72 hours post-ingestion.
Treatment: The stomach should be emptied promptly by lavage or by induction of emesis with syrup of ipecac. Patients' estimates of the quantity of a drug ingested are notoriously unreliable. Therefore, if an acetaminophen overdose is suspected, a serum acetaminophen assay should be obtained as early as possible, but no sooner than four hours following ingestion. Liver function studies should be obtained initially and repeated at 24-hour intervals.
The antidote, N-acetylcysteine, should be administered as early as possible, preferably within 16 hours of the overdose ingestion for optimal results, but in any case, within 24 hours. Following recovery, there are no residual, structural or functional hepatic abnormalities.
Hydrocodone:
Signs and Symptoms: Serious overdose with hydrocodone is characterized by respiratory depression (a decrease in respiratory rate and/or tidal volume. Cheyne-Stokes respiration, cyanosis), extreme somnolence progressing to stupor or coma, skeletal muscle flaccidity, cold and clammy skin, and sometimes bradycardia and hypotension. In severe overdosage, apnea, circulatory collapse, cardiac arrest and death may occur.
Treatment: Primary attention should be given to the reestablishment of adequate respiratory exchange through provision of a patent airway and the institution of assisted or controlled ventilation. The narcotic antagonist naloxone is a specific antidote against respiratory depression which may result from overdosage or unusual sensitivity to narcotics, including hydrocodone. Therefore, an appropriate dose of naloxone hydrochloride (see package insert) should be administered, preferably by the intravenous route, and simultaneously with efforts at respiratory resuscitation. Since the duration of action of hydrocodone may exceed that of the antagonist, the patient should be kept under continued surveillance and repeated doses of the antagonist should be administered as needed to maintain adequate respiration.
An antagonist should not be administered in the absence of clinically significant respiratory or cardiovascular depression. Oxygen, intravenous fluids, vasopressors and other supportive measures should be employed as indicated.

Gastric emptying may be useful in removing unabsorbed drug.

DOSAGE AND ADMINISTRATION

Dosage should be adjusted according to the severity of the pain and the response of the patient. However, it should be kept in mind that tolerance to hydrocodone can develop with continued use and that the incidence of untoward effects is dose related.

The usual adult dosage is one or two capsules every four to six hours as needed for pain. The total 24 hour dose should not exceed 8 capsules.

HOW SUPPLIED

Blue and white, opaque capsules imprinted with the letter "C" and 8657.

Each capsule contains Hydrocodone Bitartrate, USP 5 mg (WARNING: MAY BE HABIT FORMING.) and Acetaminophen, USP 500 mg. Keep in tight, light resistant containers. Supplied in bottles of 100 capsules NDC 0086-0057-10. Store at controlled room temperature, 15°–30°C (59°–86°F). The most recent revision of this labeling is July 1989. Manufactured for Carnrick Laboratories, Inc.

Shown in Product Identification Section, page 408

MIDRIN® ℞
[mid'rin]

CAUTION
Federal law prohibits dispensing without prescription.

DESCRIPTION
Each red capsule with pink band contains Isometheptene Mucate 65 mg., Dichloralphenazone 100 mg., and Acetaminophen 325 mg.

Isometheptene Mucate is a white crystalline powder having a characteristic aromatic odor and bitter taste. It is an unsaturated aliphatic amine with sympathomimetic properties. Dichloralphenazone is a white, microcrystalline powder, with slight odor and tastes saline at first, becoming acrid. It is a mild sedative.

Acetaminophen, a non-salicylate, occurs as a white, odorless, crystalline powder possessing a slightly bitter taste.

Midrin capsules contain FD&C Yellow No. 6 as a color additive.

ACTIONS
Isometheptene Mucate, a sympathomimetic amine, acts by constricting dilated cranial and cerebral arterioles, thus reducing the stimuli that lead to vascular headaches. Dichloralphenazone, a mild sedative, reduces the patient's emotional reaction to the pain of both vascular and tension headaches. Acetaminophen raises the threshold to painful stimuli, thus exerting an analgesic effect against all types of headaches.

INDICATIONS
For relief of tension and vascular headaches.*

> * Based on a review of this drug (isometheptene mucate) by the National Academy of Sciences-National Research Council and/or other information, FDA has classified the other indication as "possibly" effective in the treatment of migraine headache.
> Final classification of the less-than-effective indication requires further investigation.

CONTRAINDICATIONS
Midrin is contraindicated in glaucoma and/or severe cases of renal disease, hypertension, organic heart disease, hepatic disease and in those patients who are on monoamine-oxidase (MAO) inhibitor therapy.

PRECAUTIONS
Caution should be observed in hypertension, peripheral vascular disease and after recent cardiovascular attacks.

ADVERSE REACTIONS
Transient dizziness and skin rash may appear in hypersensitive patients. This can usually be eliminated by reducing the dose.

DOSAGE AND ADMINISTRATION
FOR RELIEF OF MIGRAINE HEADACHE: The usual adult dosage is two capsules at once, followed by one capsule every hour until relieved, up to 5 capsules within a twelve hour period.

FOR RELIEF OF TENSION HEADACHE: The usual adult dosage is one or two capsules every four hours up to 8 capsules a day.

HOW SUPPLIED
Red capsules imprinted with pink band, the letter "C" and 86120. Bottles of 50 capsules, NDC 0086-0120-05. Bottles of 100 capsules, NDC 0086-0120-10. Store at controlled room temperature 15–30°C (59–86°F) in a dry place.

The most recent revision of this labeling is Nov. 1988.
Manufactured for Carnrick Laboratories, Inc.
Shown in Product Identification Section, page 408

MOTOFEN® ℞
Tablets
(difenoxin hydrochloride with atropine sulfate)
antidiarrheal

DESCRIPTION
Difenoxin hydrochloride, 1-(3-cyano-3,3-diphenylpropyl)-4-phenyl-4-piperidinecarboxylic acid monohydrochloride, is an orally administered antidiarrheal agent which is chemically related to the narcotic meperidine. Atropine sulfate is present to discourage deliberate overdosage.

Each five-sided dye free MOTOFEN tablet contains:

Difenoxin ....1.0 mg
as the hydrochloride
Warning—May be habit forming.
Atropine sulfate ....0.025 mg
Inactive ingredients: calcium stearate, cellulose, lactose, corn starch.
The structural formula is:

Difenoxin Hydrochloride

CLINICAL PHARMACOLOGY
Animal studies have shown that difenoxin hydrochloride manifests its antidiarrheal effect by slowing intestinal motility. The mechanism of action is by a local effect on the gastrointestinal wall.

Difenoxin is the principal active metabolite of diphenoxylate and is clinically effective at one fifth the mg dosage of diphenoxylate.

Following oral administration of MOTOFEN, difenoxin is rapidly and extensively absorbed. Mean peak plasma levels of approximately 160 ng/mL occurred within 40 to 60 minutes in most patients following an oral dose of 2mg. Plasma levels decline to less than 10% of their peak values within 24 hours and to less than 1% of their peak values within 72 hours. This decline parallels the appearance of difenoxin and its metabolites in the urine. Difenoxin is metabolized to an inactive hydroxylated metabolite. Both the drug and its metabolites are excreted, mainly as conjugates, in urine and feces.

INDICATIONS AND USAGE
MOTOFEN (difenoxin hydrochloride with atropine sulfate) is indicated as adjunctive therapy in the management of acute nonspecific diarrhea and acute exacerbations of chronic functional diarrhea.

CONTRAINDICATIONS
MOTOFEN is contraindicated in patients with diarrhea associated with organisms that penetrate the intestinal mucosa (toxigenic *E. coli*, *Salmonella* species, *Shigella*) and pseudomembranous colitis associated with broad spectrum antibiotics. Antiperistaltic agents should not be used in these conditions because they may prolong and/or worsen diarrhea.

MOTOFEN is *contraindicated in children under 2 years of age* because of the decreased margin of safety of drugs in this class in younger age groups.

MOTOFEN is contraindicated in patients with a known hypersensitivity to difenoxin, atropine, or any of the inactive ingredients, and in patients who are jaundiced.

WARNINGS
MOTOFEN IS *NOT* AN INNOCUOUS DRUG AND DOSAGE RECOMMENDATIONS SHOULD BE STRICTLY ADHERED TO. MOTOFEN IS NOT RECOMMENDED FOR CHILDREN UNDER 2 YEARS OF AGE. OVERDOSAGE MAY RESULT IN SEVERE RESPIRATORY DEPRESSION AND COMA, POSSIBLY LEADING TO PERMANENT BRAIN DAMAGE OR DEATH (SEE *OVERDOSAGE*). THEREFORE, KEEP THIS MEDICATION OUT OF THE REACH OF CHILDREN.

FLUID AND ELECTROLYTE BALANCE—THE USE OF MOTOFEN DOES NOT PRECLUDE THE ADMINISTRATION OF APPROPRIATE FLUID AND ELECTROLYTE THERAPY. DEHYDRATION, PARTICULARY IN CHILDREN, MAY FURTHER INFLUENCE THE VARIABILITY OF RESPONSE TO MOTOFEN AND MAY PREDISPOSE TO DELAYED DIFENOXIN INTOXICATION. DRUG-INDUCED INHIBITION OF PERISTALSIS MAY RESULT IN FLUID RETENTION IN THE COLON, AND THIS MAY FURTHER AGGRAVATE DEHYDRATION AND ELECTROLYTE IMBALANCE.

IF SEVERE DEHYDRATION OR ELECTROLYTE IMBALANCE IS MANIFESTED, MOTOFEN SHOULD BE WITHHELD UNTIL APPROPRIATE CORRECTIVE THERAPY HAS BEEN INITIATED.

Ulcerative Colitis—In some patients with acute ulcerative colitis, agents which inhibit intestinal motility or delay intestinal transit time have been reported to induce toxic megacolon. Consequently, patients with acute ulcerative colitis should be carefully observed and MOTOFEN therapy should be discontinued promptly if abdominal distention occurs or if other untoward symptoms develop.

Liver and Kidney Disease—MOTOFEN (difenoxin hydrochloride with atropine sulfate) should be used with extreme caution in patients with advanced hepatorenal disease and in all patients with abnormal liver function tests since hepatic coma may be precipitated.

Atropine—A subtherapeutic dose of atropine has been added to difenoxin hydrochloride to discourage deliberate overdosage. Usage of MOTOFEN in recommended doses is not likely to cause prominent anticholinergic side effects, but MOTOFEN should be avoided in patients in whom anticholinergic drugs are contraindicated. The warnings and precautions for use of anticholinergic agents should be observed. In children, signs of atropinism may occur even with recommended doses of MOTOFEN, particularly in patients with Down's Syndrome.

PRECAUTIONS
Information for Patients
CAUTION PATIENTS TO ADHERE STRICTLY TO RECOMMENDED DOSAGE SCHEDULES. THE MEDICATION SHOULD BE KEPT OUT OF REACH OF CHILDREN SINCE ACCIDENTAL OVERDOSAGE MAY RESULT IN SEVERE, EVEN FATAL, RESPIRATORY DEPRESSION.

MOTOFEN may produce drowsiness or dizziness. The patient should be cautioned regarding activities requiring mental alertness, such as driving or operating dangerous machinery.

Drug Interactions
Since the chemical structure of difenoxin hydrochloride is similar to meperidine hydrochloride, the concurrent use of MOTOFEN with monoamine oxidase inhibitors may, in theory, precipitate a hypertensive crisis.

MOTOFEN may potentiate the action of barbiturates, tranquilizers, narcotics, and alcohol. When these medications are used concomitantly with MOTOFEN, the patient should be closely monitored.

Diphenoxylate hydrochloride, from which the principal active metabolite difenoxin is derived, was found to inhibit the hepatic microsomal enzyme system at a dose of 2 mg/kg/day in studies conducted with male rats. Therefore, diphenoxin has the potential to prolong the biological half-lives of drugs for which the rate of elimination is dependent on the microsomal drug metabolizing enzyme system.

Carcinogenesis, Mutagenesis, Impairment of Fertility
No evidence of carcinogenesis was found in a long-term study of difenoxin hydrochloride/atropine in the rat.

No experiments have been conducted to determine the mutagenic potential of MOTOFEN. MOTOFEN did not significantly impair fertility in rats.

Pregnancy/Teratogenic Effects
Pregnancy Category C. Reproduction studies in rats and rabbits with doses up to 75 times the human therapeutic dose, on a mg/kg basis, demonstrated no evidence of teratogenesis due to MOTOFEN (difenoxin hydrochloride with atropine sulfate).

Pregnant rats receiving oral doses of difenoxin hydrochloride/atropine 20 times the maximum human dose had an increase in delivery time as well as a significant increase in the percent of stillbirths.

Neonatal survival in rats was also reduced with most deaths occurring within four days of delivery.

There are no well controlled studies in pregnant women. MOTOFEN should be used during pregnancy only if the potential benefit justifies the potential risk to the fetus.

Nursing Mothers
Because of the potential for serious adverse reactions in nursing infants from MOTOFEN, a decision should be made whether to discontinue nursing or to discontinue the drug, taking into account the importance of the drug to the mother.

Pediatric Use
SAFETY AND EFFECTIVENESS IN CHILDREN BELOW THE AGE OF 12 HAVE NOT BEEN ESTABLISHED. MOTOFEN IS CONTRAINDICATED IN CHILDREN UNDER 2 YEARS OF AGE. See OVERDOSAGE section for information on hazards from accidental poisoning in children.

ADVERSE REACTIONS
In view of the small amount of atropine present (0.025 mg/tablet), effects such as dryness of the skin and mucous membranes, flushing, hyperthermia, tachycardia and urinary retention are very unlikely to occur, except perhaps in children.

Continued on next page

Carnrick—Cont.

Many of the adverse effects reported during clinical investigation of MOTOFEN are difficult to distinguish from symptoms associated with the diarrheal syndrome. However, the following events were reported at the stated frequencies:
Gastrointestinal: Nausea, 1 in 15 patients; vomiting, 1 in 30 patients; dry mouth, 1 in 30 patients; epigastric distress, 1 in 100 patients; and constipation, 1 in 300 patients.
Central Nervous System: Dizziness and light-headedness, 1 in 20 patients; drowsiness, 1 in 25 patients; and headache, 1 in 40 patients; tiredness, nervousness, insomnia and confusion ranged from 1 in 200 to 1 in 600 patients.
Other less frequent reactions: Burning eyes and blurred vision occurred in a few cases.
The following adverse reactions have been reported in patients receiving chemically-related drugs: numbness of extremities, euphoria, depression, sedation, anaphylaxis, angioneurotic edema, urticaria, swelling of the gums, pruritus, toxic megacolon, paralytic ileus, pancreatitis, and anorexia.
THIS MEDICATION SHOULD BE KEPT IN A CHILD-RESISTANT CONTAINER AND OUT OF THE REACH OF CHILDREN SINCE AN OVERDOSAGE MAY RESULT IN SEVERE RESPIRATORY DEPRESSION AND COMA, POSSIBLY LEADING TO PERMANENT BRAIN DAMAGE OR DEATH.

DRUG ABUSE AND DEPENDENCE
MOTOFEN (difenoxin hydrochloride with atropine sulfate) tablets are a Schedule IV controlled substance.
Addiction to (dependence on) difenoxin hydrochloride is theoretically possible at high dosage. Therefore, the recommended dosage should not be exceeded. Because of the structural and pharmacological similarities of difenoxin hydrochloride to drugs with a definite addiction potential, MOTOFEN should be administered with considerable caution to patients who are receiving addicting drugs, to individuals known to be addiction prone, or to those in whom histories suggest may increase the dosage on their own initiative.

OVERDOSAGE
Diagnosis and Treatment
In the event of overdosage (initial signs may include dryness of the skin and mucous membranes, flushing, hyperthermia and tachycardia followed by lethargy or coma, hypotonic reflexes, nystagmus, pinpoint pupils and respiratory depression) gastric lavage, establishment of a patent airway and possibly mechanically assisted respiration are advised.
The narcotic antagonist naloxone may be used in the treatment of respiratory depression caused by narcotic analgesics or pharmacologically related compounds such as MOTOFEN tablets. When naloxone is administered intravenously, the onset of action is generally apparent within two minutes. Naloxone may also be administered subcutaneously or intramuscularly providing a slightly less rapid onset of action but a more prolonged effect.
To counteract respiratory depression caused by MOTOFEN overdosage, the following dosage schedule for naloxone should be followed:
Adult Dosage: The usual initial adult dose of naloxone is 0.4 mg (one mL) administered intravenously. If respiratory function does not adequately improve after the initial dose, the same IV dose may be repeated at two-to-three minute intervals.
Children: The usual adult dose of naloxone for children is 0.01 mg/kg of body weight administered intravenously and repeated at two-to-three minute intervals if necessary.
Since the duration of action of difenoxin hydrochloride is longer than that of naloxone, improvement of respiration following administration may be followed by recurrent respiratory depression. Consequently, continuous observation is necessary until the effect of difenoxin hydrochloride on respiration (which effect may persist for many hours) has passed. Supplemental intramuscular doses of naloxone may be utilized to produce a longer lasting effect. TREAT ALL POSSIBLE MOTOFEN OVERDOSAGES AS SERIOUS AND MAINTAIN MEDICAL OBSERVATION FOR AT LEAST 48 HOURS, PREFERABLY UNDER CONTINUOUS HOSPITAL CARE.
Although signs of overdosage and respiratory depression may not be evident soon after ingestion of difenoxin hydrochloride, respiratory depression may occur from 12 to 30 hours later.

DOSAGE AND ADMINISTRATION
The recommended starting dose of MOTOFEN tablets in adults is 2 tablets (2 mg), then 1 tablet (1 mg) after each loose stool or 1 tablet (1 mg) every 3 to 4 hours as needed, but the total dosage during any 24-hour treatment period should not exceed 8 tablets (8 mg). In the treatment of diarrhea, if clinical improvement is not observed in 48 hours, continued administration of this type medication is not recommended. For acute diarrheas and acute exacerbations of functional diarrhea, treatment beyond 48 hours is usually not necessary.

Studies in children below the age of 12 have been inadequate to evaluate the safety and effectiveness of MOTOFEN in this age group. MOTOFEN is contraindicated in children under 2 years of age.

HOW SUPPLIED
MOTOFEN® is available as a white, dye-free, five-sided, scored tablet with "8674" on the scored side and "C" on the other. Each tablet contains 1.0 mg difenoxin (as the hydrochloride salt) and 0.025 mg atropine sulfate. Supplied in bottles of 100 tablets (NDC 0086-0074-10).
Store at controlled room temperature, 15°–30°C (59°–86°F).
CAUTION: FEDERAL LAW PROHIBITS DISPENSING WITHOUT PRESCRIPTION
Manufactured for: Carnrick Laboratories, Inc.
1/88
Shown in Product Identification Section, page 408

NOLAHIST®
[nō 'lă-hist]
(phenindamine tartrate)
ANTIHISTAMINE
Allergy/Cold Tablets

DESCRIPTION
Each dye-free NOLAHIST® tablet contains:
Phenindamine Tartrate .... 25 mg

INDICATIONS
Temporarily relieves runny nose, sneezing, itching of the nose or throat, and itchy, watery eyes due to hay fever or other upper respiratory allergies or allergic rhinitis. Temporarily relieves runny nose and sneezing associated with the common cold.

WARNINGS
May cause excitability especially in children. Do not take this product if you have asthma, glaucoma, emphysema, chronic pulmonary disease, shortness of breath, difficulty in breathing, or difficulty in urination due to enlargement of the prostate gland unless directed by a doctor. May cause drowsiness; alcohol may increase the drowsiness effect. Avoid alcoholic beverages while taking this product. Use caution when driving a motor vehicle or operating machinery. May cause nervousness and insomnia in some individuals. As with any drug, if you are pregnant or nursing a baby, seek the advice of a health professional before using this product. Keep this and all medication out of the reach of children. In case of accidental overdose, seek professional assistance or contact a Poison Control Center immediately.

DIRECTIONS
Adults: oral dosage is one tablet every 4 to 6 hours, not to exceed six tablets in 24 hours, or as directed by a doctor. Children 6 to under 12 years of age: oral dosage is one-half tablet every 4 to 6 hours, not to exceed 3 tablets in 24 hours, or as directed by a doctor. Children under 6 years of age: consult a doctor.
TAMPER-RESISTANT PACKAGE FEATURE
Bottle of 100—If printed outer wrap is broken or removed, do not purchase.

HOW SUPPLIED
White, capsule-shaped, scored tablet inscribed with 8652 on one side and C logo on the other side in bottles of 100. Each tablet contains phenindamine tartrate 25 mg. (NDC 0086-0052-10) Store at 15°–30°C (59°–86°F) and keep away from light.
Manufactured for Carnrick Laboratories, Inc.   6/87
Shown in Product Identification Section, page 408

NOLAMINE®
[nō 'lă-mēn '] *

DESCRIPTION
Each timed release tablet contains:
Phenindamine tartrate .... 24 mg
Chlorpheniramine maleate .... 4 mg
Phenylpropanolamine hydrochloride .... 50 mg
Formulated to provide 8 to
12 hours of continuous relief.

CAUTION
Federal law prohibits dispensing without prescription.

INDICATIONS
As a nasal decongestant associated with the common cold, sinusitis, hay fever and other allergies.

CONTRAINDICATIONS
Hypersensitivity to any of the components. Contraindicated in concurrent MAO inhibitor therapy.

SIDE EFFECTS
Nervousness, insomnia, tremors, dizziness and drowsiness may occur occasionally.

PRECAUTIONS
Antihistamines may cause drowsiness and should be used with caution in patients who operate motor vehicles or dangerous machinery. Use with caution in patients with hypertension, cardiovascular disease, diabetes or hyperthyroidism. This product should be used with caution in patients with prostatic hypertrophy or glaucoma.

DOSAGE
Usual adult dose: Orally, one tablet every 8 hours. In mild cases, one tablet every 10 to 12 hours.

HOW SUPPLIED
Pink, timed release tablets coded C 86204 in bottles of 100 (NDC 0086-0204-10) and 250 (NDC 0086-0204-25). Store at room temperature.
Manufactured for Carnrick Laboratories, Inc.
Shown in Product Identification Section, page 408

NOLEX™ LA   ℞
(phenylpropanolamine hydrochloride/guaifenesin)

DESCRIPTION
Each NOLEX LA white, blue-speckled, oval, scored, long-acting tablet for oral administration contains:
phenylpropanolamine hydrochloride .... 75 mg
guaifenesin .... 400 mg
in a special base to provide a prolonged therapeutic effect. This product contains ingredients of the following therapeutic classes: decongestant and expectorant.
Phenylpropanolamine hydrochloride is a decongestant having the chemical name, benzenemethanol, α-(l-aminoethyl)-, hydrochloride (R*, S*), ($\pm$), with the following structure:

Guaifenesin is an expectorant having the chemical name, 1,2-propanediol, 3-(2-methoxyphenoxy)-, with the following structure:

CLINICAL PHARMACOLOGY
Phenylpropanolamine hydrochloride is an α-adrenergic receptor agonist (sympathomimetic) which produces vasoconstriction by stimulating α-receptors within the mucosa of the respiratory tract. Clinically, phenylpropanolamine shrinks swollen mucous membranes, reduces tissue hyperemia, edema, and nasal congestion, and increases nasal airway patency. Guaifenesin promotes lower respiratory tract drainage by thinning bronchial secretions, lubricates irritated respiratory tract membranes through increased mucous flow, and facilitates removal of viscous, inspissated mucus. As a result, sinus and bronchial drainage is improved, and dry, nonproductive coughs become more productive and less frequent.

INDICATIONS AND USAGE
NOLEX LA is indicated for the symptomatic relief of sinusitis, bronchitis, pharyngitis, and coryza when these conditions are associated with nasal congestion and viscous mucus in the lower respiratory tract.

CONTRAINDICATIONS
NOLEX LA is contraindicated in individuals with known hypersensitivity to sympathomimetics, severe hypertension, or in patients receiving monoamine oxidase inhibitors.

WARNINGS
Sympathomimetic amines should be used with caution in patients with hypertension, diabetes mellitus, heart disease, peripheral vascular disease, increased intraocular pressure, hyperthyroidism, or prostatic hypertrophy.

PRECAUTIONS
Information for Patients: Do not crush or chew NOLEX LA tablets prior to swallowing.
Drug Interactions: NOLEX LA should not be used in patients taking monoamine oxidase inhibitors or other sympathomimetics.
Drug/Laboratory Test Interactions: Guaifenesin has been reported to interfere with clinical laboratory determinations of urinary 5-hydroxyindoleacetic acid (5-HIAA) and urinary vanilmandelic acid (VMA).
Pregnancy: Pregnancy Category C. Animal reproduction studies have not been conducted with NOLEX LA. It is also not known whether NOLEX LA can cause fetal harm when administered to a pregnant woman or can affect reproduc-

tion capacity. NOLEX LA should be given to a pregnant woman only if clearly needed.

Nursing Mothers: It is not known whether the drugs in NOLEX LA are excreted in human milk. Because many drugs are excreted in human milk and because of the potential for serious adverse reactions in nursing infants, a decision should be made whether to discontinue nursing or to discontinue the product, taking into account the importance of the drug to the mother.

Pediatric Use: Safety and effectiveness of NOLEX LA tablets in children below the age of 6 have not been established.

ADVERSE REACTIONS
Possible adverse reactions include nervousness, insomnia, restlessness, headache, nausea, or gastric irritation. These reactions seldom, if ever, require discontinuation of therapy. Urinary retention may occur in patients with prostatic hypertrophy.

OVERDOSAGE
The treatment of overdosage should provide symptomatic and supportive care. If the amount ingested is considered dangerous or excessive, induce vomiting with ipecac syrup unless the patient is convulsing, comatose, or has lost the gag reflex, in which case perform gastric lavage using a large-bore tube. If indicated, follow with activated charcoal and a saline cathartic. Since the effects of NOLEX LA may last up to 12 hours, treatment should be continued for at least that length of time.

DOSAGE AND ADMINISTRATION
Adults and children 12 years of age and older—one tablet twice daily (every 12 hours); children 6 to under 12 years —one-half (½) tablet twice daily (every 12 hours). NOLEX LA is not recommended for children under 6 years of age. Tablets may be broken in half for ease of administration without affecting release of medication but should not be crushed or chewed prior to swallowing.

HOW SUPPLIED
NOLEX LA is available as a white, blue-speckled, oval, scored, long-acting tablet for oral administration. It is inscribed with "8673" on the scored side and "C" on the other. Each long-acting tablet contains phenylpropanolamine hydrochloride 75 mg and guaifenesin 400 mg. Supplied in bottles of 100 tablets (NDC 0086-0073-10).
Store at controlled room temperature, 15°–30°C (59°–86°F.)

CAUTION
Federal law prohibits dispensing without prescription.
Manufactured for Carnrick Laboratories, Inc.
6/88
Shown in Product Identification Section, page 408

PHRENILIN®   ℞
[fren 'i-lin]
and
PHRENILIN® FORTE   ℞

CAUTION
Federal Law Prohibits Dispensing Without Prescription

DESCRIPTION
PHRENILIN®: Each PHRENILIN® tablet, an analgesic-sedative combination for oral administration contains Butalbital, USP 50 mg (WARNING—May be habit forming), Acetaminophen, USP 325 mg.
PHRENILIN® FORTE: Each PHRENILIN® FORTE capsule, an analgesic-sedative combination for oral administration, contains Butalbital, USP 50 mg (WARNING—May be habit forming); Acetaminophen, USP 650 mg.

HO—⬡—NHCOCH₃

$C_8H_9NO_2$
M.W. 151.16

Acetaminophen
Acetaminophen, 4'-hydroxy-acetanilide, is a non-opiate, non-salicylate analgesic and antipyretic which occurs as a white, odorless, crystalline powder possessing a slightly bitter taste.

CH₂=CHCH₂ / (CH₃)₂CHCH₂ structure

$C_{11}H_{16}N_2O_3$
M.W. 224.26

Butalbital
Butalbital, 5-Allyl-5-isobutyl-barbituric acid, a white odorless crystalline powder having a slightly bitter taste, is a short to intermediate-acting barbiturate.

CLINICAL PHARMACOLOGY
Pharmacologically, PHRENILIN® and PHRENILIN® FORTE (Butalbital and Acetaminophen) combine the analgesic properties of acetaminophen with the anxiolytic and muscle relaxant properties of butalbital.

INDICATIONS AND USAGE
PHRENILIN® and PHRENILIN® FORTE are indicated for the relief of the symptom complex of tension (or muscle contraction) headache.

CONTRAINDICATIONS
Hypersensitivity to acetaminophen or barbiturates. Patients with porphyria.

PRECAUTIONS
General
Barbiturates should be administered with caution, if at all, to patients who are mentally depressed, have suicidal tendencies, or a history of drug abuse.
Elderly or debilitated patients may react to barbiturates with marked excitement, depression, and confusion. In some persons, barbiturates repeatedly produce excitement rather than depression.

Information for Patients
Practitioners should give the following information and instructions to patients receiving barbiturates.
A. The use of barbiturates carries with it an associated risk of psychological and/or physical dependence. The patient should be warned against increasing the dose of the drug without consulting a physician.
B. Barbiturates may impair mental and/or physical abilities required for the performance of potentially hazardous tasks (e.g., driving, operating machinery, etc.)
C. Alcohol should not be consumed while taking barbiturates. Concurrent use of the barbiturates with other CNS depressants (e.g., alcohol, narcotics, tranquilizers, and antihistamines) may result in additional CNS depressant effects.

Drug Interactions:
Patients receiving narcotic analgesics, antipsychotics, antianxiety agents, or other CNS depressants (including alcohol) concomitantly with PHRENILIN® or PHRENILIN® FORTE (Butalbital and Acetaminophen) may exhibit additve CNS depressant effects.

DRUGS	EFFECT
Butalbital w/coumarin anticoagulants	Decreased effect of anticoagulant because of increased metabolism resulting from enzyme induction.
Butalbital w/tricyclic antidepressants	Decreased blood levels of the antidepressant

Usage in Pregnancy:
Adequate studies have not been performed in animals to determine whether this drug affects fertility in males or females, has teratogenic potential or has other adverse effects on the fetus. There are no well-controlled studies in pregnant women. Although there is no clearly defined risk, one cannot exclude the possibility of infrequent or subtle damage to the human fetus. PHRENILIN® or PHRENILIN® FORTE should be used in pregnant women only when clearly needed.

Nursing Mothers:
The effects of PHRENILIN® or PHRENILIN® FORTE on infants of nursing mothers are not known. Barbiturates are excreted in the breast milk of nursing mothers. The serum levels in infants are believed to be insignificant with therapeutic doses.

Pediatric Use:
Safety and effectiveness in children below the age of 12 have not been established.

ADVERSE REACTIONS
The most frequent adverse reactions are drowsiness and dizziness. Less frequent adverse reactions are lightheadedness and gastrointestinal disturbances including nausea, vomiting, and flatulence.
Mental confusion or depression can occur due to intolerance or overdosage of butalbital.

DRUG ABUSE AND DEPENDENCE
Prolonged use of barbiturates can produce drug dependence, characterized by psychic dependence and tolerance. The abuse liability of PHRENILIN® or PHRENILIN® FORTE (Butalbital and Acetaminophen) is similar to that of other barbiturate-containing drug combinations. Caution should be exercised when prescribing medication for patients with a known propensity for taking excessive quantities of drugs, which is not uncommon in patients with chronic tension headache.

OVERDOSAGE
The toxic effects of acute overdosage of PHRENILIN® or PHRENILIN® FORTE are attributable mainly to its barbiturate component, and, to a lesser extent, acetaminophen.

Barbiturate
Symptoms: Drowsiness, confusion, coma; respiratory depression; hypotension; shock.
Treatment:
1. Maintenance of an adequate airway, with assisted respiration and oxygen administration as necessary.
2. Monitoring of vital signs and fluid balance.
3. If the patient is conscious and has not lost the gag reflex, emesis may be induced with ipecac. Care should be taken to prevent pulmonary aspiration of vomitus. After completion of vomiting, 30 grams of activated charcoal in a glass of water may be administered.
4. If emesis is contraindicated, gastric lavage may be performed with a cuffed endotracheal tube in place with the patient in the face down position. Activated charcoal may be left in the emptied stomach and a saline cathartic administered.
5. Fluid therapy and other standard treatment for shock, if needed.
6. If renal function is normal, forced diuresis may aid in the elimination of the barbiturate. Alkalinization of the urine increases renal excretion of some barbiturates, especially phenobarbital.
7. Although not recommended as a routine procedure, hemodialysis may be used in severe barbiturate intoxication or if the patient is anuric or in shock.

Acetaminophen
Signs and Symptoms: In acute acetaminophen overdosage, dose-dependent, potentially fatal hepatic necrosis is the most serious adverse effect. Renal tubular necrosis, hypoglycemic coma, and thrombocytopenia may also occur.
In adults, hepatic toxicity has rarely been reported with acute overdoses of less than 10 grams and fatalities with less than 15 grams. Importantly, young children seem to be more resistant than adults to the hepatoxic effect of an acetaminophen overdose.
Early symptoms following a potentially hepatotoxic overdose may include: nausea, vomiting, diaphoresis and general malaise. Clinical and laboratory evidence of hepatic toxicity may not be apparent until 48 to 72 hours post-ingestion.
Treatment: The stomach should be emptied promptly by lavage or by induction of emesis with syrup of ipecac. Patients estimates of the quantity of a drug ingested are notoriously unreliable. Therefore, if an acetaminophen overdose is suspected, a serum acetaminophen assay should be obtained as early as possible, but no sooner than four hours following ingestion. Liver function studies should be obtained initially and repeated at 24-hour intervals.
The antidote, N-acetylcysteine, should be administered as early as possible, preferably within 16 hours of the overdose ingestion for optimal results, but in any case, within 24 hours. Following recovery, there are no residual, structural or functional hepatic abnormalities.

DOSAGE AND ADMINISTRATION
PHRENILIN®: Oral: One or two tablets every four hours as needed. Do not exceed six tablets per day.
PHRENILIN® FORTE : Oral: One capsule every four hours as needed. Do not exceed six capsules per day.

HOW SUPPLIED
PHRENILIN®: Pale violet scored tablets with the letter "C" on one side and 8650 on the other, in bottles of 100 (NDC 0086-0050-10). Each tablet contains butalbital, USP 50 mg (WARNING: May be habit forming) and acetaminophen, USP 325 mg.
PHRENILIN® FORTE: Amethyst, opaque capsules imprinted with the letter "C" and 8656, in bottles of 100 (NDC 0086-0056-10). Each capsule contains butalbital, USP 50 mg (WARNING: May be habit forming) and acetaminophen USP 650 mg.
Store PHRENILIN® and PHRENILIN® FORTE (Butalbital and Acetaminophen) at controlled room temperature, 15°–30°C (59°–86°F) and dispense in tight container.
The most recent revision of this labeling is October, 1987.
Manufactured for Carnrick Laboratories, Inc.
Shown in Product Identification Section, page 408

PROPAGEST®
(Phenylpropanolamine HCl)
NASAL DECONGESTANT TABLETS

DESCRIPTION
Each tablet contains:
Phenylpropanolamine HCl .... 25 mg.

INDICATIONS
For the temporary relief of nasal congestion associated with the common cold, sinusitis, hay fever or other upper respiratory allergies.

DOSAGE
Adult oral dosage is one tablet every 4 hours not to exceed 6 tablets in 24 hours. Children 6 to under 12 years oral dosage

Continued on next page

Carnrick—Cont.

is one-half tablet every 4 hours not to exceed 3 tablets in 24 hours. For children under 6 years, there is no recommended dosage except under the advice and supervision of a doctor.

WARNINGS

Do not exceed recommended dosage because at higher doses nervousness, dizziness, sleeplessness, rapid pulse or high blood pressure may occur.

Do not take this product for more than 7 days. If symptoms do not improve or are accompanied by fever, consult a doctor. Do not take this product if you have heart disease, high blood pressure, thyroid disease, glaucoma, diabetes, or difficulty in urination due to enlargement of the prostate gland unless directed by a doctor.

As with any drug, if you are pregnant or nursing a baby, seek the advice of a health professional before using this product.

Keep this and all medication out of the reach of children. In case of accidental overdose, seek professional assistance or contact a Poison Control Center immediately.

Drug Interaction Precaution: Do not take this product if you are presently taking a prescription drug for high blood pressure or depression, without first consulting your doctor. Do not take this product concurrently with other medication except on the advice of a doctor.

TAMPER-RESISTANT PACKAGE FEATURE:
Bottle of 100—If printed outer wrap is broken or removed, do not purchase.

HOW SUPPLIED

White, oval, scored tablets with "C" logo containing 25 mg. phenylpropanolamine HCl in bottles of 100. (NDC 0086-0051-10). Keep tightly closed, away from light and store at room temperature.   1/89
Manufactured for Carnrick Laboratories, Inc.
Shown in Product Identification Section, page 408

SALFLEX®   ℞
(salsalate)
Tablets

DESCRIPTION

SALFLEX (salsalate) is a nonsteroidal anti-inflammatory agent for oral administration. Chemically, salsalate (salicyl-salicylic acid or 2-hydroxy-benzoic acid, 2-carboxyphenyl ester) is a dimer of salicylic acid; its structural formula is shown below.

Chemical Structure:

Each round, white, dye-free, film-coated SALFLEX tablet contains 500 mg salsalate.
Each oval, white, dye-free, film-coated SALFLEX tablet contains 750 mg salsalate. (See HOW SUPPLIED)

CLINICAL PHARMACOLOGY

Salsalate is insoluble in acid gastric fluids (<0.1 mg/ml at pH 1.0), but readily soluble in the small intestine where it is partially hydrolyzed to two molecules of salicylic acid. A significant portion of the parent compound is absorbed unchanged and undergoes rapid esterase hydrolysis in the body; its half-life is about one hour. About 13% is excreted through the kidneys as a glucuronide conjugate of the parent compound, the remainder as salicylic acid and its metabolites. Thus, the amount of salicylic acid available from SAL-FLEX (salsalate) is about 15% less than from aspirin, when the two drugs are administered on a salicylic acid molar equivalent basis (3.6 g salsalate/5 g aspirin). Salicylic acid biotransformation is saturated at anti-inflammatory doses of salsalate. Such capacity-limited biotransformation results in an increase in the half-life of salicylic acid from 3.5 to 16 or more hours. Thus, dosing with SALFLEX twice a day will satisfactorily maintain blood levels within the desired therapeutic range (10 to 30 mg/100 ml) throughout the 12-hour intervals. Therapeutic blood levels continue for up to 16 hours after the last dose. The parent compound does not show capacity-limited biotransformation, nor does it accumulate in the plasma on multiple dosing. Food slows the absorption of all salicylates including salsalate.

The mode of anti-inflammatory action of salsalate and other nonsteroidal anti-inflammatory drugs is not fully defined. Although salicylic acid (the primary metabolite of salsalate) is a weak inhibitor of prostaglandin synthesis in vitro, salsalate appears to selectively inhibit prostaglandin synthesis in vivo,[1] providing anti-inflammatory activity equivalent to aspirin[2] and indomethacin.[3] Unlike aspirin, salsalate does not inhibit platelet aggregation.[4]

The usefulness of salicylic acid, the active in vivo product of salsalate, in the treatment of arthritic disorders has been established.[5,6] In contrast to aspirin, salsalate causes no greater fecal gastrointestinal blood loss than placebo.[7]

INDICATIONS AND USAGE

SALFLEX (salsalate) is indicated for relief of the signs and symptoms of rheumatoid arthritis, osteoarthritis and related rheumatic disorders.

CONTRAINDICATIONS

SALFLEX is contraindicated in patients hypersensitive to salsalate.

WARNINGS

Reye Syndrome may develop in individuals who have chicken pox, influenza, or flu symptoms. Some studies suggest possible association between the development of Reye Syndrome and the use of medicines containing salicylate or aspirin. SALFLEX contains a salicylate and therefore is not recommended for use in patients with chicken pox, influenza or flu symptoms. See PRECAUTIONS.

PRECAUTIONS

General Precautions: Patients on treatment with SAL-FLEX should be warned not to take other salicylates so as to avoid potentially toxic concentrations. Great care should be exercised when SALFLEX is prescribed in the presence of chronic renal insufficiency or peptic ulcer disease. Protein binding of salicylic acid can be influenced by nutritional status, competitive binding of other drugs, and fluctuations in serum proteins caused by disease (rheumatoid arthritis, etc.). Although cross reactivity, including bronchospasm, has been reported occasionally with non-acetylated salicylates, including salsalate, in aspirin-sensitive patients,[8,9] salsalate is less likely than aspirin to induce asthma in such patients.[10]

Laboratory Tests: Plasma salicylic acid concentrations should be periodically monitored during long-term treatment with SALFLEX to aid maintenance of therapeutically effective levels: 10 to 30 mg/100 ml. Toxic manifestations are not usually seen until plasma concentrations exceed 30 mg/100 ml (see OVERDOSAGE). Urinary pH should also be regularly monitored: sudden acidification, as from pH 6.5 to 5.5, can double the plasma level, resulting in toxicity.

Drug Interactions: Salicylates antagonize the uricosuric action of drugs used to treat gout. ASPIRIN AND OTHER SALICYLATE DRUGS WILL BE ADDITIVE TO SALFLEX (salsalate) AND MAY INCREASE PLASMA CONCENTRATIONS OF SALICYLIC ACID TO TOXIC LEVELS. Drugs and foods that raise urine pH will increase renal clearance and urinary excretion of salicylic acid, thus lowering plasma levels; acidifying drugs or foods will decrease urinary excretion and increase plasma levels. Salicylates given concomitantly with anticoagulant drugs may predispose to systemic bleeding. Salicylates may enhance the hypoglycemic effect of oral antidiabetic drugs of the sulfonylurea class. Salicylate competes with a number of drugs for protein binding sites, notably penicillin, thiopental, thyroxine, triiodothyronine, phenytoin, sulfinpyrazone, naproxen, warfarin, methotrexate, and possibly corticosteroids.

Drug/Laboratory Test Interactions: Salicylate competes with thyroid hormone for binding to plasma proteins, which may be reflected in a depressed plasma T_4 value in some patients: thyroid function and basal metabolism are unaffected.

Carcinogenesis: No long-term animal studies have been performed with salsalate to evaluate its carcinogenic potential.

Use in Pregnancy: Pregnancy Category C: Salsalate and salicylic acid have been shown to be teratogenic and embryocidal in rats when given in doses 4 to 5 times the usual human dose. These effects were not observed at doses twice as great as the usual human dose. There are no adequate and well-controlled studies in pregnant women. SALFLEX should be used during pregnancy only if the potential benefit justifies the potential risk to the fetus.

Labor and Delivery: There exist no adequate and well-controlled studies in pregnant women. Although adverse effects on mother or infant have not been reported with salsalate use during labor, caution is advised when anti-inflammatory dosage is involved. However, other salicylates have been associated with prolonged gestation and labor, maternal and neonatal bleeding sequelae, potentiation of narcotic and barbiturate effects (respiratory or cardiac arrest in the mother), delivery problems and stillbirth.

Nursing Mothers: It is not known whether salsalate per se is excreted in human milk; salicylic acid, the primary metabolite of salsalate, has been shown to appear in human milk in concentrations approximating the maternal blood level. Thus the infant of a mother on SALFLEX therapy might ingest in mother's milk 30 to 80% as much salicylate per kg body weight as the mother is taking. Accordingly, caution should be exercised when SALFLEX (salsalate) is administered to a nursing woman.

Pediatric Use: Safety and effectiveness of SALFLEX use in children have not been established. (See WARNINGS section.)

ADVERSE REACTIONS

In two well-controlled clinical trials, the following reversible adverse experiences characteristic of salicylates were most commonly reported with salsalate (n = 280 pts; listed in descending order of frequency): tinnitus, nausea, hearing impairment, rash, and vertigo. These common symptoms of salicylates, i.e., tinnitus or reversible hearing impairment, are often used as a guide to therapy.

Although cause-and-effect relationships have not been established, spontaneous reports over a ten-year period have included the following additional medically significant adverse experiences: abdominal pain, abnormal hepatic function, anaphylactic shock, angioedema, bronchospasm, decreased creatinine clearance, diarrhea, G.I. bleeding, hepatitis, hypotension, nephritis and urticaria.

DRUG ABUSE AND DEPENDENCE

Drug abuse and dependence have not been reported with salsalate.

OVERDOSAGE

Death has followed ingestion of 10 to 30 g of salicylates in adults, but much larger amounts have been ingested without fatal outcome.

Symptoms: The usual symptoms of salicylism—tinnitus, vertigo, headache, confusion, drowsiness, sweating, hyperventilation, vomiting and diarrhea—will occur. More severe intoxication will lead to disruption of electrolyte balance and blood pH, and hyperthermia and dehydration.

Treatment: Further absorption of salsalate from the G.I. tract should be prevented by emesis (syrup of ipecac) and, if necessary, by gastric lavage.

Fluid and electrolyte imbalance should be corrected by the administration of appropriate I.V. therapy. Adequate renal function should be maintained. Hemodialysis or peritoneal dialysis may be required in extreme cases.

DOSAGE AND ADMINISTRATION

Adults: The usual dosage is 3000 mg daily, given in divided doses as follows:
1) two doses of two 750 mg tablets;
2) two doses of three 500 mg tablets; or
3) three doses of two 500 mg tablets.
Some patients, e.g., the elderly, may require a lower dosage to achieve therapeutic blood concentrations and to avoid the more common side effects such as auditory.

Alleviation of symptoms is gradual, and full benefit may not be evident for 3 to 4 days, when plasma salicylate levels have achieved steady state. There is no evidence for development of tissue tolerance (tachyphylaxis), but salicylate therapy may induce increased activity of metabolizing liver enzymes, causing a greater rate of salicyluric acid production and excretion, with a resultant increase in dosage requirement for maintenance of therapeutic serum salicylate levels.

Children: Dosage recommendations and indications for SALFLEX use in children have not been established.

HOW SUPPLIED

SALFLEX 500 mg tablets:
Each round, white, dye-free, film-coated SALFLEX tablet is inscribed with 8671 on one side and "C" on the other. Each tablet contains 500 mg salsalate and is available in bottles of 100 tablets (NDC 0086-0071-10).

SALFLEX 750 mg tablets:
Each oval, white, dye-free, film-coated SALFLEX tablet is inscribed with 8672 on the scored side and "C" on the other. Each tablet contains 750 mg salsalate and is available in bottles of 100 tablets (NDC 0086-0072-10) and 500 tablets (NDC 0086-0072-50).

Store at controlled room temperature, 15°–30°C (59°–86°F).
CAUTION: Federal law prohibits dispensing without prescription.

REFERENCES

1. Morris HG, Sherman NA, McQuain C., et al: Effects of Salsalate (Non-Acetylated) Salicylate and Aspirin (ASA) on Serum and Urine Prostaglandins in Man. Clin. Pharm. Therap. **33**:(2) 197, 1983.
2. April PA, Curran NJ, Ekholm BP, et al: Multicenter Comparative Study of Salsalate (SSA) vs Aspirin (ASA) in Rheumatoid Arthritis (RA), Arthritis Rheumatism **50**(4 supplement):S93, 1987.
3. Deodhar SD, McLeod MM, Dick WC, et al: A Short-Term Comparative Trial of Salsalate and Indomethacin in Rheumatoid Arthritis. Curr. Med. Res. Opin. **5**:185–188, 1987.
4. Estes D, Kaplan K: Lack of Platelet Effect With the Aspirin Analog, Salsalate, Arthritis and Rheumatism, **23**:1303–1307, 1980.
5. Dick C, Dick PH, Nuki G, et al: Effect of Anti-inflammatory Drug Therapy on Clearance of ^{133}Xe from Knee Joints of Patients with Rheumatoid Arthritis. British Med. J. **3**:278–280, 1969.

6. Dick WC, Grayson MF, Woodburn A, et al: Indices of Inflammatory Activity. Ann. of the Rheum. Dis. **29**:643–648, 1970.

7. Cohen, A: Fecal Blood Loss and Plasma Salicylate Study of Salicylsalicylic Acid and Aspirin. J. Clin. Pharmacol. **19**:242–247, 1979.

8. Chudwin DS, Strub M, Golden HE, et al: Sensitivity to Non-Acetylated Salicylates in a Patient with Asthma, Nasal Polyps, and Rheumatoid Arthritis. Annals of Allergy **57**:133–134, 1986.

9. Spector SL, Wangaard CH, Farr RS: Aspirin and Concomitant Idiosyncrasies in Adult Asthmatic Patients. J. Allergy Clin. Immunol. **64**:500–506, 1979.

10. Stevenson DD, Schrank PJ, Hougham AJ, et al: Salsalate Cross Sensitivity in Aspirin-Sensitive Asthmatics. J. Allergy Clin. Immunol. **81**:181, 1988.

June 1989

Shown in Product Identification Section, page 408

SINULIN®
Analgesic ● Antihistamine ● Decongestant

DESCRIPTION
SINULIN contains acetaminophen, an analgesic and antipyretic that relieves pain, sinus headache and reduces fever; phenylpropanolamine HCl, a decongestant that promotes nasal drainage and relieves sinus pressure; and chlorpheniramine maleate, an antihistamine that helps control allergic symptoms.

ACTIVE INGREDIENTS
Each tablet contains: acetaminophen 650 mg. (650 mg. is a nonstandard strength of acetaminophen per tablet compared to the established standard of 325 mg. acetaminophen per tablet), chlorpheniramine maleate 4 mg., phenylpropanolamine HCl 25 mg.

INDICATIONS
For the temporary relief of nasal and sinus congestion, runny nose, sneezing, itching of the nose or throat, itchy watery eyes, headache and fever associated with the common cold, sinusitis, hay fever or other upper respiratory allergies.

WARNINGS
Sinulin tablets contain FD&C Yellow No. 6 as a color additive.

Do not exceed recommended dosage because severe liver damage may occur and at higher doses, nervousness, dizziness, sleeplessness, rapid pulse or high blood pressure may occur.

Adults should not take this product for more than 7 days. Children 6 to under 12 years of age should not take this product for more than 5 days. If fever persists for more than 3 days, or recurs, consult a doctor. If symptoms persist, do not improve, or new ones occur, consult a doctor.

Do not take this product if you have high blood pressure, heart disease, diabetes, thyroid disease, glaucoma, asthma, emphysema, chronic pulmonary disease, shortness of breath, difficulty in breathing, or difficulty in urination due to enlargement of the prostate gland, or if you are presently taking a prescription drug for high blood pressure or depression, unless directed by a doctor.

This product may cause drowsiness; alcohol may increase the drowsiness effect. Avoid alcoholic beverages while taking this product. Use caution when driving a motor vehicle or operating machinery. May cause excitability especially in children.

If a rare sensitivity reaction occurs, discontinue use and consult a doctor.

As with any drug, if you are pregnant or nursing a baby, seek the advice of a health professional before using this product. Keep this and all medication out of the reach of children. In case of accidental overdose, seek professional assistance or contact a Poison Control Center immediately.

DRUG INTERACTION PRECAUTION
Do not take this product if you are presently taking a prescription drug for high blood pressure or depression without first consulting your doctor. Do not take this product concurrently with other medication except on the advice of a doctor.

DIRECTIONS
Adults: oral dosage is one tablet every 4 to 6 hours, or as directed by a doctor. Do not exceed 6 tablets in 24 hours.

Children 6 to under 12 years of age: oral dosage is one-half tablet every 4 to 6 hours, or as directed by a doctor. Do not exceed 3 tablets in 24 hours.

Children under 6 years of age: do not use unless directed by a doctor.

TAMPER-RESISTANT PACKAGE FEATURE
Bottles of 20's & 100's—If printed outer wrap is broken or removed, do not purchase. Blisters—Each tablet in sealed unit; do not use if tablet seal is broken.

HOW SUPPLIED
Peach color, scored tablets inscribed with 8666 on one side and C logo on the other. Bottles of 20 (NDC 0086-0066-02), 7 boxes of 24 blisters (NDC 0086-0066-24), and Bottles of 100 (NDC 0086-0066-10). Store at controlled room temperature (59°–86°F).   12/88

Manufactured for Carnrick Laboratories, Inc.

Shown in Product Identification Section, page 408

SKELAXIN®   ℞
brand of metaxalone

CAUTION
Federal law prohibits dispensing without prescription.

DESCRIPTION
Each pale rose, scored tablet contains: metaxalone, 400 mg. Skelaxin (metaxalone) has the following chemical structure and name:

5-[(3,4-dimethylphenoxy)methyl]-2 oxazolidinone

ACTIONS
The mechanism of action of metaxalone in humans has not been established, but may be due to general central nervous system depression. It has no direct action on the contractile mechanism of striated muscle, the motor end plate or the nerve fiber.

INDICATIONS
Skelaxin (metaxalone) is indicated as an adjunct to rest, physical therapy, and other measures for the relief of discomforts associated with acute, painful musculoskeletal conditions. The mode of action of this drug has not been clearly identified, but may be related to its sedative properties. Metaxalone does not directly relax tense skeletal muscles in man.

CONTRAINDICATIONS
Metaxalone is contraindicated in individuals who have shown hypersensitivity to the drug. Metaxalone should not be administered to patients with a known tendency to drug-induced, hemolytic, or other anemias. It is contraindicated in patients with significantly impaired renal or hepatic function.

PRECAUTIONS
Elevation in cephalin flocculation tests without concurrent changes in other liver function parameters have been noted. Hence, it is recommended that metaxalone be administered with great care to patients with pre-existing liver damage and that serial liver function studies be performed as required.

False-positive Benedict's tests, due to an unknown reducing substance, have been noted. A glucose-specific test will differentiate findings.

Pregnancy: Reproduction studies have been performed in rats and have revealed no evidence of impaired fertility or harm to the fetus due to metaxalone. Reactions reports from marketing experience have not revealed evidence of fetal injury, but such experience cannot exclude the possibility of infrequent or subtle damage to the human fetus. Safe use of metaxalone has not been established with regard to possible adverse effects upon fetal development. Therefore, metaxalone tablets should not be used in women who are or may become pregnant and particularly during early pregnancy unless in the judgment of the physician the potential benefits outweigh the possbile hazards.

Nursing Mothers: It is not known whether this drug is secreted in human milk. As a general rule, nursing should not be undertaken while a patient is on a drug since many drugs are excreted in human milk.

Pediatric Use: Safety and effectiveness in children 12 years of age and below have not been established.

ADVERSE REACTIONS
The most frequent reactions to metaxalone include nausea, vomiting, gastrointestinal upset, drowsiness, dizziness, headache, and nervousness or "irritability." Other adverse reactions are: hypersensitivity reaction, characterized by a light rash with or without pruritus; leukopenia; hemolytic anemia; jaundice.

DOSAGE
The recommended dose for adults and children over 12 years of age is two tablets (800 mg) three to four times a day.

MANAGEMENT OF OVERDOSAGE
Gastric lavage and supportive therapy as indicated. (When determining the LD_{50} in rats and mice, progressive sedation, hypnosis and finally respiratory failure were noted as the dosage increased. In dogs, no LD_{50} could be determined as the higher doses produced an emetic action in 15 to 30 minutes). No documented case of major toxicity has been reported.

HOW SUPPLIED
Skelaxin (metaxalone) is available as a 400 mg. pale rose tablet, inscribed with 8662 on the scored side and "C" on the other. Available in bottles of 100 (NDC 0086-0062-10). Store at Controlled Room Temperature, between 15°C and 30°C (59°F and 86°F).

     12/85

Manufactured for Carnrick Laboratories, Inc.

Shown in Product Identification Section, page 408

Center Laboratories
Division of EM Pharmaceuticals, Inc.
35 CHANNEL DRIVE
PORT WASHINGTON, NY 11050

EPIPEN®/EPIPEN® JR. Auto-Injectors   ℞
Epinephrine Auto-Injectors

Brief summary: Before prescribing, please consult package insert.

DESCRIPTION
The EpiPen Auto-Injectors contain 2 mL Epinephrine Injection for emergency intramuscular use. Each EpiPen Auto-Injector delivers a single dose of 0.3 mg epinephrine from Epinephrine Injection, USP, 1:1000 (0.3 mL) in a sterile solution. Each EpiPen Jr. Auto-Injector delivers a single dose of 0.15 mg epinephrine from Epinephrine Injection, USP, 1:2000 (0.3 mL) in a sterile solution. Each 0.3 mL also contains 1.8 mg sodium chloride, 0.5 mg sodium metabisulfite, hydrochloric acid to adjust pH, and Water for Injection. The pH range is 2.5–5.0.

CLINICAL PHARMACOLOGY
Epinephrine is a sympathommetic drug, acting on both alpha and beta receptors. It is the drug of choice for the emergency treatment of severe allergic reactions (Type I) to insect stings or bites, foods, drugs, and other allergens. It can also be used in the treatment of idiopathic or exercise-induced anaphylaxis. Epinephrine when given subcutaneously or intramuscularly has a rapid onset and short duration of action.

INDICATIONS AND USAGE
Epinephrine is indicated in the emergency treatment of allergic reactions (anaphylaxis) to insect stings or bites, foods, drugs and other allergens as well as idiopathic or exercise-induced anaphylaxis. The EpiPen Auto-Injector is intended for immediate self-administration by a person with a history of an anaphylactic reaction. Such reactions may occur within minutes after exposure and consist of flushing, apprehension, syncope, tachycardia, thready or unobtainable pulse associated with a fall in blood pressure, convulsions, vomiting, diarrhea and abdominal cramps, involuntary voiding, wheezing, dyspnea due to laryngeal spasm, pruritis, rashes, urticaria or angioedema. The EpiPen is designed as emergency supportive therapy only and is not a replacement or substitute for immediate medical or hospital care.

CONTRAINDICATIONS
There are no absolute contraindications to the use of epinephrine in a life-threatening situation.

WARNINGS
Epinephrine is light sensitive and should be stored in the tube provided. Store at room temperature (15°–30°C/59°–88°F). Do not refrigerate. Before using, check to make sure solution in Auto-Injector is not discolored.

Replace the Auto-Injector if the solution is discolored or contains a precipitate. Avoid possible inadvertent intravascular administration. Select an appropriate injection site such as the thigh. DO NOT INJECT INTO BUTTOCK. Large doses or accidental intravenous injection of epinephrine may result in cerebral hemorrhage due to sharp rise in blood pressure. DO NOT INJECT INTRAVENOUSLY. Rapid acting vasodilators can counteract the marked pressor effects of epinephrine.

Epinephrine is the preferred treatment for serious allergic or other emergency situations even though this product contains sodium metabisulfite, a sulfite that may in other products cause allergic-type reactions including anaphylactic symptoms or life-threatening or less severe asthmatic episodes in certain susceptible persons. The alternatives to using epinephrine in a life-threatening situation may not be satisfactory. The presence of a sulfite in this product should not deter administration of the drug for treatment of serious allergic or other emergency situations.

Continued on next page

Center—Cont.

PRECAUTIONS

Epinephrine is ordinarily administered with extreme caution to patients who have heart disease. Use of epinephrine with drugs that may sensitize the heart to arrhythmias, e.g., digitalis, mercurial diuretics, or quinidine, ordinarily is not recommended. Anginal pain may be induced by epinephrine in patients with coronary insufficiency. The effects of epinephrine may be potentiated by tricyclic antidepressants and monoamine oxidase inhibitors. Hyperthyroid individuals, individuals with cardiovascular disease, hypertension, or diabetes, elderly individuals, pregnant women, and children under 30 kg (66 lbs.) body weight may be theoretically at greater risk of developing adverse reactions after epinephrine administration. Despite these concerns, epinephrine is essential for the treatment of anaphylaxis. Therefore, patients with these conditions, and/or any other person who might be in a position to administer EpiPen or EpiPen Jr. to a patient experiencing anaphylaxis should be carefully instructed in regard to the circumstances under which this lifesaving medication should be used.

CARCINOGENESIS, MUTAGENESIS, IMPAIRMENT OF FERTILIY

Studies of epinephrine in animals to evaluate the carcinogenic and mutagenic potential or the effect on fertility have not been conducted.

USAGE IN PREGNANCY

Pregnancy Category C: Epinephrine has been shown to be teratogenic in rats when given in doses about 25 times the human dose. There are no adequate and well-controlled studies in pregnant women. Epinephrine should be used during pregnancy only if the potential benefit justifies the potential risk to the fetus.

PEDIATRIC USE

Epinephrine may be given safely to children at a dosage appropriate to body weight (see Dosage and Administration).

ADVERSE REACTIONS

Side effects of epinephrine may include palpitations, tachycardia, sweating, nausea and vomiting, respiratory difficulty, pallor, dizziness, weakness, tremor, headache, apprehension, nervousness and anxiety.

Cardiac arrhythmias may follow administration of epinephrine.

OVERDOSAGE

Overdosage or inadvertent intravascular injection of epinephrine may cause cerebral hemorrhage resulting from a sharp rise in blood pressure. Fatalities may also result from pulmonary edema because of peripheral vascular constriction together with cardiac stimulation.

DOSAGE AND ADMINISTRATION

Usual epinephrine adult dose for allergic emergencies is 0.3 mg. For pediatric use, the appropriate dosage may be 0.15 or 0.30 mg depending upon the body weight of the patient. However, the prescribing physician has the option of prescribing more or less than these amounts, based on careful assessment of each individual patient and recognizing the life-threatening nature of the reactions for which this drug is being prescribed. With severe persistant anaphylaxis, repeat injections with an additional EpiPen may be necessary.

HOW SUPPLIED

EpiPen and EpiPen Jr. Auto-Injectors are available singly or in packages of twelve.

CAUTION

Federal (U.S.A.) law prohibits dispensing without a prescription.

Issued: April 1988

Central Pharmaceuticals, Inc.
120 EAST THIRD STREET
SEYMOUR, IN 47274

AZDŌNE® TABLETS   ⒸⒾⒾⒾ ℞
[ăz ′dōn]

DESCRIPTION

Each tablet contains:

Hydrocodone Bitartrate	5 mg
(WARNING—May be habit forming)	
Aspirin	500 mg

Hydrocodone bitartrate is an opioid analgesic and antitussive and occurs as fine, white crystals or as a crystalline powder. It is affected by light. The chemical name is: 4,5α-epoxy-3-methoxy-17-methylmorphinan-6-one tartrate (1:1) hydrate (2:5). Its structure is as follows:

$C_{18}H_{21}NO_3 \cdot C_4H_6O_6 \cdot 2\frac{1}{2}H_2O$ M.W. 494.50

Aspirin, salicylic acid acetate, is a non-opiate salicylate analgesic, anti-inflammatory, and antipyretic which occurs as a white, crystalline tabular or needle-like powder and is odorless or has a faint odor. Its structure is as follows:

$C_9H_8O_4$ M.W. 180.16

Inactive Ingredients: D&C Red #7 Lake, Pregelatinized Starch and Stearic Acid.

CLINICAL PHARMACOLOGY

Hydrocodone: Hydrocodone is a semisynthetic narcotic analgesic and antitussive with multiple actions qualitatively similar to those of codeine. Most of these involve the central nervous system and smooth muscle. The precise mechanism of action of hydrocodone and other opiates is not known, although it is believed to relate to the existence of opiate receptors in the central nervous system. In addition to analgesia, narcotics may produce drowsiness, changes in mood and mental clouding.

Radioimmunoassay techniques have recently been developed for the analysis of hydrocodone in human plasma. After a 10 mg oral dose of hydrocodone bitartrate, a mean peak serum drug level of 23.6 ng/mL and an elimination half-life of 3.8 hours were found.

Aspirin: The analgesic, anti-inflammatory and anti-pyretic effects of aspirin are believed to result from inhibition of the synthesis of certain prostaglandins. Aspirin interferes with clotting mechanisms primarily by diminishing platelet aggregation; at high doses prothrombin synthesis can be inhibited.

Aspirin in solution is rapidly absorbed from the stomach and from the upper small intestine. About 50 percent of an oral dose is absorbed in 30 minutes and peak plasma concentrations are reached in about 40 minutes. Higher than normal stomach pH or the presence of food slightly delays absorption.

Once absorbed, aspirin is mainly hydrolyzed to salicylic acid and distributed to all body tissues and fluids, including fetal tissue, breast milk and the central nervous system (CNS). Highest concentrations are found in plasma, liver, renal cortex, heart and lung.

From 50 to 80 percent of salicylic acid and its metabolites in plasma are loosely bound to protein. The plasma half-life of total salicylate is about 3.0 hours, with a 650 mg dose. Higher dose of aspirin cause increases in plasma salicylate half-life. Almost all of a therapeutic dose of aspirin is excreted through the kidneys, either as salicylic acid or its metabolites. Renal clearance of salicylate is greatly augmented by an alkaline urine, as is produced by concurrent administration of sodium bicarbonate or potassium citrate.

Toxic salicylate blood levels are usually above 30 mg/100 ml. The single lethal dose of aspirin in normal adults is approximately 25–30 g, but patients have recovered from much larger doses with appropriate treatment.

INDICATIONS AND USAGE

For the relief of moderate to moderately severe pain.

CONTRAINDICATIONS

Hydrocodone Bitartrate and Aspirin Tablets are contraindicated under the following conditions:

(1) hypersensitivity or intolerance to hydrocodone or aspirin.

(2) severe bleeding, disorders of coagulation or primary hemostatis, including hemophilia, hypoprothrombinemia, von Willebrand's disease, thrombocytopenias, thrombasthenia and other ill-defined hereditary platelet dysfunctions, severe vitamin K deficiency and severe liver damage.

(3) anticoagulant therapy

(4) peptic ulcer, or other serious gastrointestinal lesions.

WARNINGS

Hydrocodone: Respiratory Depression: At high doses or in sensitive patients, hydrocodone may produce dose-related respiratory depression by acting directly on the brain stem respiratory center. Hydrocodone also affects the center that controls respiratory rhythm, and may produce irregular and periodic breathing.

Head Injury and Increased Intracranial Pressure: The respiratory depressant effects of narcotics and their capacity to elevate cerebrospinal fluid pressure may be markedly exaggerated in the presence of head injury, other intracranial lesions or a pre-existing increase in intracranial pressure. Furthermore, narcotics produce adverse reactions which may obscure the clinical course of patients with head injuries.

Acute Abdominal Conditions: The administration of narcotics may obscure the diagnosis or clinical course of patients with acute abdominal conditions.

Aspirin: Allergic Reactions: Therapeutic doses of aspirin can cause anaphylactic shock and other severe allergic reactions. A history of allergy is often lacking.

Bleeding: Significant bleeding can result from aspirin therapy in patients with peptic ulcer or other gastrointestinal lesions, and in patients with bleeding disorders. Aspirin administered preoperatively may prolong the bleeding time.

PRECAUTIONS

Special Risk Patients: As with any narcotic analgesic agent, Hydrocodone Bitartrate and Aspirin Tablets should be used with caution in elderly or debilitated patients and those with severe impairment of hepatic or renal function, gallbladder disease or gallstones, respiratory impairment, cardiac arrhythmias, inflammatory disorders of the gastrointestinal tract, hypothyroidism, Addison's disease, prostatic hypertrophy or urethral stricture, coagulation disorders, head injuries or acute abdominal conditions. The usual precautions should be observed and the possibility of respiratory depression should not be overlooked.

Precautions should be taken when administering salicylates to persons with known allergies. Hypersensitivity to aspirin is particularly likely in patients with nasal polyps, and relatively common with asthma.

Information for Patients: Hydrocodone Bitartrate and Aspirin Tablets, like all narcotics, may impair the mental and/or physical abilities required for the performance of potentially hazardous tasks such as driving a car or operating machinery; patients should be cautioned accordingly.

Cough Reflex: Hydrocodone suppresses the cough reflex; as with all narcotics, caution should be exercised when Hydrocodone Bitartrate and Aspirin Tablets are used postoperatively and in patients with pulmonary disease.

Laboratory Tests: Hypersensitivity to aspirin cannot be detected by skin testing or radioimmunoassay procedures.

Drug Interactions:

Hydrocodone: Patients receiving other narcotic analgesics, antipsychotics, antianxiety agents, or other CNS depressants (including alcohol) concomitantly with Hydrocodone Bitartrate and Aspirin Tablets may exhibit an additive CNS depression. When combined therapy is contemplated, the dose of one or both agents should be reduced.

The use of MAO inhibitors or tricyclic antidepressants with hydrocodone preparations may increase the effect of either the antidepressant or hydrocodone.

The concurrent use of anticholinergics with hydrocodone, as with all narcotics, may produce paralytic ileus.

Aspirin: Aspirin may <u>enhance</u> the effects of:

(1) oral anticoagulants, causing bleeding by inhibiting prothrombin formation in the liver and displacing anticoagulants from plasma protein binding sites.

(2) oral antidiabetic agents and insulin, causing hypoglycemia by contributing an additive effect, and by displacing the oral antidiabetic agents from secondary binding sites.

(3) 6-mercaptopurine and methotrexate, causing bone marrow toxicity and blood dyscrasias by displacing these drugs from secondary binding sites.

(4) non-steroidal anti-inflammatory agents, increasing the risk of peptic ulceration and bleeding by contributing additive effects.

(5) corticosteroids, potentiating anti-inflammatory effects by displacing steroids from protein binding sites. Aspirin intoxication may occur with corticosteroid withdrawal because steroids promote renal clearance of salicylates.

Aspirin may <u>diminish</u> the effects of uricosuric agents, such as probenecid and sulfinpyrazone, in the treatment of gout by competing for protein binding sites.

Drug/Laboratory Test Interactions:

Aspirin: Aspirin may interfere with the following laboratory determinations.

In blood: serum amylase, fasting blood glucose, carbon dioxide, cholesterol, protein, protein bound iodine, uric acid, prothrombin time, bleeding time, and spectrophotometric deterction of barbituates.

In urine: glucose, 5-hydroxyindoleacetic acid, Gerhardt ketone, vanillylmandelic acid (VMA), protein, uric acid, and diacetic acid.

Pregnancy:

Teratogenic Effects: Pregnancy Category C.

Hydrocodone: Hydrocodone has been shown to be teratogenic in hamsters when given in doses 700 times the human dose. There are no adequate and well-controlled studies in pregnant women. Hydrocodone Bitartrate and Aspirin Tablets should be used during pregnancy only if the potential benefit justifies the potential risk to the fetus.

Aspirin: Reproductive studies in rats and mice have shown aspirin to be teratogenic and embryocidal at four to six times the human therapeutic dose. Studies in pregnant women, however, have not shown that aspirin increases the risk of abnormalities when administered during the first trimester of pregnancy. In controlled studes involving 41,337 pregnant women and their offspring, there was no evidence that aspirin taken during pregnancy caused stillbirth, neonatal death or reduced birthweight. In controlled studies of 50,282 pregnant women and their offspring, aspirin administration in moderate and heavy doses during the first four months of pregnancy showed no teratogenic effect.

Nonteratogenic Effects:

Hydrocodone: Babies born to mothers who have been taking opioids regularly prior to delivery will be physically dependent. The withdrawal signs include irritability and excessive crying, tremors, hyperactive reflexes, increased respiratory rate, increased stools, sneezing, yawning, vomiting, and fever. The intensity of the syndrome does not always correlate with the duration of maternal opioid use or dose. There is no consensus on the best method of managing withdrawal. Chlorpromazine 0.7 to 1 mg/kg q6h, and paregoric 2 to 4 drops/kg q4h, have been used to treat withdrawal symptoms in infants. The duration of therapy is 4 to 28 days, with the dosage decreased as tolerated.

Aspirin: Therapeutic doses of aspirin in pregnant women close to term may cause bleeding in the mother, fetus, or neonate. During the last six months of pregnancy, regular use of aspirin in high dosess may prolong pregnancy and delivery.

Labor and Delivery: As with all narcotics, administration of Hydrocodone Bitartrate and Aspirin Tablets to the mother shortly before delivery may result in some degree of respiratory depression in the newborn, especially if higher doses are used. Ingestion of aspirin prior to delivery may prolong delivery or lead to bleeding in the mother or neonate.

Nursing Mothers: Aspirin is excreted in human milk in a small amount; the significance of its effect on nursing infants is not known. It is not known whether hydrocodone is excreted in human milk. Because many drugs are excreted in human milk and because of the potential for serious adverse reactions in nursing infants, a decision should be made whether to discontinue nursing or to discontinue the drug, taking into account the importance of the drug to the mother.

Pediatric Use: Safety and effectiveness in children have not been established.

ADVERSE REACTIONS

The most frequently observed adverse reactions include lightheadedness, dizziness, sedation, nausea and vomiting. These effects seem to be more prominent in ambulatory than in nonambulatory patients and some of these adverse reactions may be alleviated if the patient lies down.

Other adverse reactions include:

Central Nervous System:

Hydrocodone: Drowsiness, mental clouding, lethargy, impairment of mental and physical performance, anxiety, fear, dysphoria, psychic dependence, mood changes.

Aspirin: Headache, drowsiness and mental confusion can occur in response to chronic use of large doses.

Gastrointestinal System:

Hydrocodone: The antiemetic phenothiazines are useful in suppressing the nausea and vomiting which may occur (see above); however, some phenothiazine derivatives seem to be antianalgesic and to increase the amount of narcotic required to produce pain relief, while other phenothiazines reduce the amount of narcotic required to produce a given level of analgesia. Prolonged administration of hydrocodone bitartrate and aspirin tablets may produce constipation.

Aspirin: Some patients are unable to take aspirin or other salicylates without developing nausea or vomiting. Occasional patients respond to aspirin (usually large doses) with dyspepsia or heartburn, which may be accompanied by occult bleeding. Excessive bruising or bleeding is sometimes seen in patients with mild disorders of primary hemostasis who regularly use low doses of aspirin.

Prolonged use of aspirin can cause painless erosion of gastric mucosa, occult bleeding and, infrequently, iron-deficiency anemia. High doses of aspirin can exacerbate symptoms of peptic ulcer and, occasionally, cause extensive bleeding. Excessive bleeding can follow injury or surgery in patients with or without known bleeding disorders who have taken therapeutic doses of aspirin within the preceding 10 days. Hepatotoxicity has been reported in association with prolonged use of large doses of aspirin in patients with lupus erythematosus, rheumatoid arthritis and rheumatic disease.

Hematologic:

Aspirin: Bone marrow depression, manifested by weakness, fatigue or abnormal bruising or bleeding, has occasionally been reported with aspirin.

In patients with glucose-6-phosphate dehydrogenase deficiency, aspirin can cause a mild degree of hemolytic anemia.

Respiratory:

Hydrocodone: Hydrocodone bitartrate may produce dose-related respiratory depression by acting directly on the brain stem respiratory center. Hydrocodone also affects the center that controls respiratory rhythm, and may produce irregular and periodic breathing. If significant respiratory depression occurs, it may be antagonized by the use of naloxone hydrochloride. Apply other supportive measures when indicated.

Aspirin: Hyperpnea and hyperventilation can occur in response to chronic use of large doses.

Cardiovascular:

Aspirin: Tachycardia can occur in response to chronic use of large doses of aspirin.

Genitourinary:

Hydrocodone: Ureteral spasm, spasm of vesical sphincters and urinary retention have been reported.

Metabolic:

Aspirin: In hyperuricemic persons, low doses of aspirin may reduce the effectiveness of uricosuric therapy or precipitate an attack of gout.

Allergic:

Aspirin: Therapeutic doses of aspirin can induce mild or severe allergic reactions manifested by skin rashes, urticaria, angioedema, rhinorrhea, asthma, abdominal pain, nausea, vomiting, or anaphylactic shock. A history of allergy is often lacking, and allergic reactions may occur even in patients who have previously taken aspirin without any ill effects. Allergic reactions to aspirin are most likely to occur in patients with a history of allergic disease, especially in patients with nasal polyps or asthma.

Other:

Aspirin: Sweating and thirst can occur in response to chronic use of large doses of aspirin.

DRUG ABUSE AND DEPENDENCE

Hydrocodone Bitartrate and Aspirin Tablets are subject to the Federal Controlled Substance Act (Schedule Ⓘ).

Psychic dependence, physical dependence, and tolerance may develop upon repeated administration of narcotics; therefore, Hydrocodone Bitartrate and Aspirin Tablets should be prescribed and administered with caution. However, psychic dependence is unlikely to develop when Hydrocodone Bitartrate and Aspirin Tablets are used for a short time for the treatment of pain.

Physical dependence, the condition in which continued administration of the drug is required to prevent the appearance of a withdrawal syndrome, assumes clinically significant proportions only after several weeks of continued narcotic use, although some mild degree of physical dependence may develop after a few days of narcotic therapy. Tolerance, in which increasingly large doses are required in order to produce the same degree of analgesia, is manifested initially by shortened duration of analgesic effect, and subsequently by decreases in the intensity of analgesia. The rate of development of tolerance varies among patients.

OVERDOSAGE

Hydrocodone:

Signs and Symptoms: Serious overdose with hydrocodone is characterized by respiratory depression (a decrease in respiratory rate and/or tidal volume, Cheyne-Stokes respiration, cyanosis), extreme somnolence progressing to stupor or coma, skeletal muscle flaccidity, cold and clammy skin, and sometimes bradycardia and hypotension. In severe overdosage, apnea, circulatory collapse, cardiac arrest and death may occur.

Treatment: Primary attention should be given to the reestablishment of adequate respiratory exchange through provision of a patent airway and the institution of assisted or controlled ventilation. If significant respiratory depression occurs, it may be antagonized by the use of naloxone hydrochloride preferably intravenously (see package insert for dosage and full information. Naloxone promptly reverses the effects of morphine-like opioid antagonists such as hydrocodone. In patients who are physically dependent, small doses of naloxone may be sufficient not only to antagonize respiratory depression, but also to precipitate withdrawal phenomena. The dose of naloxone should therefore be adjusted accordingly in such patients. Since the duration of action of hydrocodone may exceed that of the antagonist, the patient

should be kept under continued surveillance and repeated doses of the antagonist should be administered as needed to maintain adequate respiration.

A narcotic antagonist should not be administered in the absence of clinically significant respiratory or cardiovascular depression. Oxygen, intravenous fluids, vasopressors and other supportive measures should be employed as indicated. Gastric emptying may be useful in removing unabsorbed drug.

Aspirin:

Signs and Symptoms: The most severe manifestations from aspirin result from cardiovascular and respiratory insufficiency secondary to acid-base and electrolyte disturbances, complicated by hyperthermia and dehydration.

Respiratory alkalosis is characteristic of the early phase of intoxication with aspirin while hyperventilation is occurring, but is quickly followed by metabolic acidosis in most people with severe intoxication.

Concentrations of aspirin in plasma above 30 mg/100 ml are associated with toxicity (see Clinical Pharmacology Section for information on factors influencing aspirin blood levels.) The single lethal dose of aspirin in adults is probably about 25–30 g, but is not known with certainty.

Hemodialysis and peritoneal dialysis can be performed to reduce the body aspirin content.

Treatment: Treatment consists primarily of supporting vital functions, increasing salicylate elimination, and correcting the acid-base imbalance due primarily to salicylism.

Gastric emptying (Syrup of Ipecac) and/or lavage is recommended as soon as possible after ingestion, even if the patient has vomited spontaneously. Administration of activated charcoal as a slurry is beneficial after lavage and/or emesis, if less than three hours have passed since ingestion. Charcoal adsorption should <u>not</u> be employed prior to emesis or lavage.

Severity of aspirin intoxication is determined by measuring the blood salicylate level. Acid-base status should be closely followed with serial blood gas and serum pH measurements. Fluid and electrolyte balance should also be regularly monitored.

In severe cases, hyperthermia and hypovolemia are the major immediate threats to life. Children should be sponged with tepid water. Replacement fluid should be administered intravenously and augmented with sufficient bicarbonate to correct acidosis, with monitoring of plasma electrolytes and pH, to promote alkaline diuresis of salicylate if renal function is normal. Complete control may also require infusion of glucose to control hypoglycemia.

In patients with renal insufficiency or in cases of life-threatening intoxication, dialysis is usually required. Peritoneal dialysis or exchange transfusion is indicated in infants and young children and hemodialysis in older patients.

DOSAGE AND ADMINISTRATION

Dosage should be adjusted according to the severity of the pain and the response of the patient. However, tolerance to hydrocodone can develop with continued use and the incidence of untoward effects is dose related.

The usual adult dosage is one or two tablets every four to six hours as needed for pain.

Hydrocodone Bitartrate and Aspirin Tablets should be taken with food or a full glass of milk or water to lessen gastric irritation.

HOW SUPPLIED

Flat, truncated oval, bisected mottled pink tablet containing 5 mg Hydrocodone Bitartrate (WARNING: May be habit formimg) and 500 mg of Aspirin. Each tablet is debossed with the Central logo on one side and the number 21 and the score on the other side.

Bottles of 100 tablets—NDC 0131-2821-37

Bottles of 1000 tablets—NDC 0131-2821-43

Storage: Store at controlled room temperature 15°–30°C (59°–86°F). Protect from moisture.

Dispense in a tight, light-resistant container as defined in the USP/NF with a child-resistant closure.

CAUTION

Federal law prohibits dispensing without prescription.

A Schedule Ⓘ Controlled Substance (Narcotic).

CENTRAL PHARMACEUTICALS, INC.

Seymour, Indiana 47274

Shown in Product Identification Section, page 408

CODICLEAR® DH SYRUP   Ⓘ ℞

[kō′dĭ-klēr″]

DESCRIPTION

A clear, colorless, sweet-tasting syrup for oral administration, which is alcohol-free, sugar-free and dye-free.

Continued on next page

Central—Cont.

Each teaspoonful (5 mL) contains:
Hydrocodone bitartrate.. 5 mg
  (Warning—May be habit forming)
Guaifenesin .... 100 mg
This product contains ingredients of the following therapeutic classes: antitussive and expectorant.

CAUTION
Federal law prohibits dispensing without prescription.

CLINICAL PHARMACOLOGY
Hydrocodone bitartrate is a potent antitussive which causes suppression of the cough reflex by a direct action on the cough center. Hydrocodone is approximately three times as potent as codeine on a weight basis, and has a higher addiction potential. Guaifenesin is used as an expectorant. It is thought to increase mucous flow in the lung by stimulation of gastric mucosal reflexes.

INDICATIONS
For the temporary relief of dry, non-productive cough associated with upper and lower respiratory tract congestion.

CONTRAINDICATIONS
Hypersensitivity to hydrocodone or guaifenesin. Hydrocodone is contraindicated in the presence of increased intracranial pressure and whenever ventilatory function is depressed.

WARNINGS
Hydrocodone can produce drug dependence and therefore has the potential for being abused. Codiclear DH should be prescribed and administered with the degree of caution appropriate for this type of product.

PRECAUTIONS
General: The hydrocodone in this product may exhibit additive effects with other CNS depressants, including alcohol. Respiratory depression can be a real hazard so caution should be used, especially in patients with chronic obstructive pulmonary disease.
Information for Patients: The hydrocodone may cause drowsiness and ambulatory patients who operate machinery or motor vehicles should be cautioned accordingly.
Drug Interactions: Patients receiving other narcotic analgesics, general anesthetics, phenothiazines, other tranquilizers, sedative hypnotics or other CNS depressants (including alcohol) concomitantly with hydrocodone may exhibit an additive CNS depression. When such combined therapy is contemplated the dose of one or both agents should be reduced. (See WARNINGS.)
Laboratory Interactions: The metabolite of guaifenesin has been found to produce an apparent increase in urinary 5-hydroxyindoleacetic acid, and guaifenesin therefore may interfere with the interpretation of this test for the diagnosis of carcinoid syndrome. Guaifenesin administration should be discontinued 24 hours prior to the collection of urine specimens for the determination of 5-hydroxyindoleacetic acid.
Usage in Pregnancy: Pregnancy Category C. Hydrocodone has been shown to be teratogenic in hamsters when given in doses 700 times the human dose. There are no adequate and well-controlled studies in pregnant women. CODICLEAR DH Syrup should be used during pregnancy only if the potential benefit justifies the potential risk to the fetus.

ADVERSE REACTIONS
Adverse reactions include drowsiness, lassitude, nausea, giddiness, constipation, respiratory depression and addiction.

DRUG ABUSE AND DEPENDENCE
This product is a Schedule III Controlled Sustance. Because of the hydrocodone content, some abuse might be expected. Psychic dependence, physical dependence and tolerance may develop upon repeated administration. It should be prescribed and administered with the degree of caution appropriate for this type product.

OVERDOSAGE
Symptoms of overdosage include respiratory depression, extreme somnolence progressing to stupor or coma, skeletal muscle flaccidity, cold and clammy skin and other symptoms common with narcotic overdosage.
Primary treatment consists of insuring adequate respiration th:ough provision of a patent airway and the institution of assisted or controlled ventilation. Naloxone hydrochloride should be administered in small intravenous doses (consult specific product labeling before use). In addition, oxygen, intravenous fluids, vasopressors and other supportive measures should be employed as indicated. Gastric emptying may be useful in removing unabsorbed drug. Activated charcoal may also be of benefit.

DOSAGE AND ADMINISTRATION
Usual Adult Dose—One teaspoonful (5 mL) after meals and at bedtime, not less than 4 hours apart (not to exceed 6 teaspoonful in a 24 hour period.) Treatment should be initiated with one teaspoonful and subsequent doses, up to a maximum single dose of 3 teaspoonsful, adjusted if required. Usual Children's Dose—Over 12 years: Initial dose 1 teaspoonful; maximum single dose, 2 teaspoonful. 2–12 years: Initial dose ½ teaspoonful: maximum single dose, 1 teaspoonful. Under 2 years: Narcotic antitussives are not recommended for use in children under 2 years of age. Children under 2 years may be more susceptible to the respiratory depressant effects of narcotics, including respiratory arrest, coma, and death. However, dosages based on hydrocodone, 0.3 mg/kg/24 hours divided into four equal doses have been suggested.

HOW SUPPLIED
Bottles of 4 fl. oz.—NDC 0131-5134-64
Bottles of one pint—NDC 0131-5134-70

CODIMAL® DH   ⚆ ℞
[kō'di-mahl"]
CODIMAL® DM
CODIMAL® PH   ℂ
CODIMAL® EXPECTORANT

DESCRIPTION
Each teaspoonful (5 mL) of CODIMAL DH contains: Hydrocodone Bitartrate 1.66 mg. (Warning—May be habit forming); Phenylephrine Hydrochloride 5.0 mg.; Pyrilamine Maleate 8.33 mg.
Each teaspoonful (5 mL) of CODIMAL DM contains: Dextromethorphan hydrobromide 10 mg.; Phenylephrine hydrochloride 5 mg.; Pyrilamine maleate 8.33 mg.; Alcohol 4%. Sugar-free.
Each teaspoonful (5 mL) of CODIMAL PH contains: Codeine Phosphate 10 mg. (Warning —May be habit forming); Phenylephrine Hydrochloride 5 mg.; Pyrilamine Maleate 8.33 mg. Each teaspoonful (5 mL) of CODIMAL EXPECTORANT contains: Phenylpropanolamine Hydrochloride 25 mg.; Guaifenesin 100 mg.

INDICATIONS
Temporary relief of cough, nasal congestion, and other symptoms associated with colds, or seasonal or perennial allergic vasomotor rhinitis (hay fever).

CONTRAINDICATIONS
Patients with severe hypertension, severe coronary artery disease, in patients on MAO inhibitors therapy, and in nursing mothers. Products containing pyrilamine maleate are contraindicated in patients with angle-closure glaucoma and urinary retention. Products containing codeine phosphate or hydrocodone bitartrate are contraindicated in patients with peptic ulcer disease. These products are also contraindicated in patients with a hypersensitivity to any of the ingredients.

WARNINGS
Caution should be exercised in patients with high blood pressure, heart disease, diabetes, thyroid disease, glaucoma or chronic pulmonary disease and may cause excitability, especially in children. At dosages higher than the recommended dose, nervousness, dizziness or sleeplessness may occur.

Products containing pyrilamine maleate, codeine phosphate, or hydrocodone bitartrate may exhibit additive effects with other CNS depressants, including alcohol. Codeine phosphate and hydrocodone bitartrate can produce drug dependence and therefore products containing either of these ingredients have the potential for being abused. Psychic dependence, physical dependence, and tolerance may develop upon repeated administration.
Information for Patients
Codeine phosphate, hydrocodone bitartrate, and pyrilamine maleate may cause drowsiness. Ambulatory patients using products containing any of these ingredients who operate machinery or motor vehicles should be cautioned accordingly.
Drug Interactions
MAO inhibitors and beta-adrenergic blockers may increases the effects of sympathomimetics. Sympathomimetics may reduce the antihypertensive effects of methyldopa, mecamylamine, reserpine, and veratrum alkaloids. Concurrent use of codeine or hydrocodone and antihistamines with alcohol and other CNS depressants may have an additive effect.
Pregnancy
Teratogenic Effects: Pregnancy Category C. Hydrocodone has been shown to be teratogenic in hamsters when given in doses 700 times the human doses. A study in rats and rabbits reported no teratogenic effects of codeine administered during the period of organogenesis in doses ranging from 5 to 120 mg/kg. In the rat, doses at the 120 mg/kg level, in the toxic range for the adult animal, were associated with an increase in embryo resorption at the time of implantation. In another study, a single 100 mg/kg dose of codeine administered to pregnant mice reportedly resulted in delayed ossification in the offspring. There are no adequate and well-controlled studies in pregnant women for any of these products. Therefore, they should be used during pregnancy only if the potential benefit justifies the potential risk to the fetus.
Nonteratogenic Effects: Dependence has been reported in newborns whose mothers took opiates regularly during pregnancy. Withdrawal signs include irritability and excessive crying, increased stools, sneezing, yawning, vomiting, and fever. The intensity of the syndrome does not always correlate with the duration of maternal opioid use or dose.

ADVERSE REACTIONS
Adverse reactions include drowsiness, lassitude, nausea, giddiness, dryness of mouth, blurred vision, cardiac palpitations, flushing, increased irritability or excitement (especially in children)

DOSAGE AND ADMINISTRATION
[See table below left].
Narcotic antitussives are not recommended for use in children under 2 years of age. Children under 2 years may be more susceptible to the respiratory depressant effects of narcotics, including respiratory arrest, coma, and death. However, dosages based on hydrocodone, 0.3 mg/kg/24 hours divided into four equal doses have been suggested.

HOW SUPPLIED
Codimal DH (Red Syrup)
4oz—NDC# 0131-5129-64
Pint—NDC# 0131-5129-70
Gallon—NDC# 0131-5129-72
Codimal DM (Yellow Syrup)
4oz—NDC# 0131-5131-64
Pint—NDC# 0131-5131-70
Gallon—NDC# 0131-5131-72
Codimal PH (Red Syrup)
4oz—NDC # 0131-5038-64
Pint—NDC # 0131-5038-70
Gallon—NDC # 0131-5038-72
Codimal Expectorant (Light Amber Syrup)
4oz—NDC # 0131-5133-64
Pint—NDC # 0131-5133-70

CODIMAL®-L.A. CAPSULES   ℞
[kō'di-mahl"]

DESCRIPTION
Each Extended Release Capsule contains:
Chlorpheniramine maleate .... 8 mg
Pseudoephedrine
  hydrochloride .... 120 mg
in a specially prepared base to provide prolonged action.

HOW SUPPLIED
No. 1 clear body, red cap printed with white Central logo and 40, filled with red, white, and blue beads.
Bottle of 100 Capsules-NDC 0131-4213-37
Bottle of 1000 Capsules-NDC 0131-4213-43
Shown in Product Identification Section, page 408

Product	Adults and Children over 12 years of age	Children 6–12 years	Children 2–6 years	
Codimal® DH ⚆	1–2 tsp q 4 h	1 tsp q 4 h	½ tsp q 4 h	
Codimal® DM	2 tsp q 4 h	1 tsp q 4 h	½ tsp q 4 h	
Codimal® PH ℂ	2 tsp q 4 h	1 tsp q 4 h	Age	Dose q4h
			2 yrs	1.5 ml
			3 yrs	1.75 ml
			4 yrs	2 ml
			5 yrs	2.25 ml
			6 yrs	2.5 ml
			For low-weight children:	
			0.5 ml/kg/day	
Codimal® Expectorant	1 tsp q 4 h	½ tsp q 4 h	¼ tsp q 4 h	

CO–GESIC® TABLETS ℞
(Hydrocodone Bitartrate and Acetaminophen Tablets)

DESCRIPTION
Each CO-GESIC® Tablet contains:
Hydrocodone Bitartrate* .... 5 mg
*WARNING: May be habit forming.
Acetaminophen .... 500 mg

DOSAGE AND ADMINISTRATION
Dosage should be adjusted according to the severity of the pain and the response of the patient. However, it should be kept in mind that tolerance to hydrocodone can develop with continued use and that the incidence of untoward effects is dose related.

The usual adult dosage is one or two tablets every four to six hours as needed for pain. The total 24 hour dose should not exceed 8 tablets.

HOW SUPPLIED
CO-GESIC® [Hydrocodone Bitartrate 5 mg (Warning: May be habit forming) and Acetaminophen 500 mg] Tablets are oval-shaped, white, scored compressed tablets debossed with 500 and 5 separated by bisect on one side and Central logo on the other.
Bottle of 100 tablets: NDC 0131-2104-37
Bottle of 500 tablets: NDC 0131-2104-41
Shown in Product Identification Section, page 408

MONO–GESIC® TABLETS ℞
[mon"o-je'zik]
(salsalate)
(salicylsalicylic acid)

DESCRIPTION
Each round, pink film-coated tablet contains:
Salsalate (salicylsalicylic acid) .... 500 mg
Each oval, pink film-coated tablet contains:
Salsalate (salicylsalicylic acid) .... 750 mg
(see **HOW SUPPLIED**)

Mono-Gesic® (Salsalate) is a non-steroidal anti-inflammatory agent for oral administration. Chemically, salsalate (salicylsalicylic acid or 2-hydroxy-benzoic acid 2-carboxyphenyl ester) is a dimer of salicylic acid. It is represented by the following formula:

$C_{14}H_{10}O_5$ M.W. 258.2

The ingredient in this product is of the following classes: non-steroidal anti-inflammatory agent and analgesic.

Inactive Ingredients: Colloidal Silicon Dioxide, Corn Starch, D&C Red #30 Lake, Hydroxypropyl Cellulose, Hydroxypropyl Methylcellulose, Microcrystalline Cellulose, Polyethylene Glycol, Propylene Glycol, Stearic Acid and Titanium Dioxide.

CLINICAL PHARMACOLOGY
Due to the poor solubility of salsalate in gastric fluid, most will pass through the stomach unhydrolyzed and unabsorbed. In the small intestine, it is partially hydrolyzed to two molecules of salicylic acid and rapidly and almost completely absorbed both as the parent compound and as salicylic acid. Salsalate is almost completely excreted in the urine with 7–13 percent of a single dose appearing as glucuronide conjugates of salsalate, less than 1 percent appearing as unchanged salsalate, and the remaining appearing as salicylic acid and its metabolites. The elimination half-life of salsalate is approximately one hour. However, salsalate produces more sustained serum salicylate levels than does acetylsalicylic acid. The reasons for this probably relate to the slower rate of hydrolysis of salsalate than acetylsalicylic acid.

The mode of action of salsalate and other non-steroidal anti-inflammatory drugs is unresolved. It does, however, appear to be involved with the inhibition of prostaglandin synthesis. Unlike aspirin, salsalate has not been associated with reactions causing asthmatic attacks in susceptible people. Also, it is not known to affect the platelet adhesiveness involved in the clotting mechanism and it causes little gastrointestinal blood loss as compared to other non-steroidal anti-inflammatory agents.

INDICATIONS AND USAGE
Mono-Gesic® is indicated for the temporary relief of symptoms of rheumatoid arthritis, osteoarthritis and related rheumatic disorders.

CONTRAINDICATIONS
Hypersensitivity to salsalate.

WARNINGS
Drugs of this class, salicylates, have been reported to be associated with the development of Reye Syndrome in children and teenagers with chicken pox, influenza, and influenza-like infections.

PRECAUTIONS
General: To avoid potentially toxic concentrations, the plasma salicylic acid levels should be monitored to maintain the therapeutically effective levels of 10 to 30 mg/100 mL. Changes in urinary pH can have significant effects on the plasma level of salicylic acid. Acidification can result in an increase in the plasma level resulting in toxicity while an increase in urinary pH will increase renal clearance and urinary excretion of salicylic acid, thus lowering plasma levels.

Information for Patients: Patients on long-term treatment should be warned not to take other salicylates. They should also be warned that if symptoms of overdosage, such as tinnitus, vertigo, headache, confusion, drowsiness, sweating, hyperventilation, vomiting or diarrhea appear, the drug should be stopped and physician notified.

Drug Interactions: Salicylates antagonize the uricosuric action of drugs used to treat gout. Salicylates will be additive to Mono-Gesic® and could increase plasma concentrations to toxic levels. Drugs and foods that raise urine pH will increase renal clearance and urinary excretion of salicylic acid, thus lowering plasma levels; acidifying drugs or foods will decrease urinary excretion and increase plasma levels. Salicylates may competitively displace anticoagulant drugs from plasma protein binding sites and thereby predispose to systemic bleeding. Salicylates may enhance the hypoglycemic effect of oral antidiabetic drugs of the sulfonylurea class. Salicylate competes with a number of drugs for protein binding sites, notably penicillin, thiopental, thyroxine, triiodothyronine, phenytoin, sulfapyrazone, naproxen, warfarin, methotrexate, and possibly corticosteroids.

Drug/Laboratory Test Interactions: Salicylate competes with thyroid hormone for binding to plasma proteins, which may be reflected in a depressed plasma T_4 value in some patients; thyroid function and basal metabolism are unaffected.

Carcinogenesis: No long-term animal studies have been performed with Mono-Gesic® to evaluate its carcinogenic potential; however, several such studies using aspirin and other salicylates have failed to demonstrate any association of these agents with cancerous cell changes.

Use in Pregnancy: Pregnancy Category C: Salsalate and salicylic acid have been shown to be teratogenic and embryocidal in rats when given in doses four to five times the usual human dose. These effects were not observed at doses twice as great as the usual human dose. There are no adequate and well-controlled studies in pregnant women. Mono-Gesic® should be used during pregnancy only if the potential benefit justifies the potential risk to the fetus.

Labor and Delivery: There are no adequate and well-controlled studies in pregnant women. Although adverse effects on mother or infant have not been reported with Mono-Gesic® use during labor, caution is advised when anti-inflammatory dosage is involved. However, other salicylates have been associated with prolonged gestation and labor, maternal and neonatal bleeding sequelae, potentiation of narcotic and barbiturate effects (respiratory or cardiac arrest in the mother), delivery problems and stillbirth.

Nursing Mothers: It is not known whether salsalate per se is excreted in human milk; salicylic acid, the primary metabolite of Mono-Gesic®, has been shown to appear in human milk in concentrations approximating the maternal blood level. Thus the infant of a mother on Mono-Gesic® therapy might ingest in mother's milk 30 to 80 percent as much salicylate per kg body weight as the mother is taking. Accordingly, caution should be exercised when Mono-Gesic® is administered to a nursing woman.

Pediatric Use: Safety and effectiveness in children have not been established.

ADVERSE REACTIONS
Adverse reactions are usually the result of overdosage and may include tinnitus and temporary hearing loss, vertigo, headache, confusion, drowsiness, sweating, hyperventilation, vomiting and diarrhea.

DRUG ABUSE AND DEPENDENCE
Drug abuse and dependence have not been reported with Mono-Gesic®.

OVERDOSAGE
IN ALL CASES OF SUSPECTED OVERDOSE, IMMEDIATELY CALL YOUR REGIONAL POISON CENTER and/or SEEK PROFESSIONAL ASSISTANCE. No deaths after overdosage have been reported for Mono-Gesic®. Death has followed ingestion of 10 to 30 g of other salicylates in adults, but much larger amounts have been ingested without fatal outcome.

Signs and Symptoms: The usual symptoms of salicylism (tinnitus, vertigo, headache, confusion, drowsiness, sweating, hyperventilation, vomiting and diarrhea) will occur. More severe intoxication will lead to disruption of electrolyte balance and blood pH, hyperthermia and dehydration.

Treatment: Further absorption of Mono-Gesic® from the G.I. tract should be prevented by emesis (syrup of ipecac) and, if necessary, by gastric lavage.

Fluid and electrolyte imbalance should be corrected by the administration of appropriate I.V. therapy. Adequate renal function should be maintained. Hemodialysis or peritoneal dialysis may be required in extreme cases.

DOSAGE AND ADMINISTRATION
Dosage should be adjusted according to the severity of the disease and the response of the patient. Response will be gradual and full benefits may not be evident for three to four days when plasma salicylate levels have achieved steady state.

The usual dosage is 3,000 mg daily, given in divided doses, such as two 750 mg tablets twice daily or two 500 mg tablets three times daily.

HOW SUPPLIED
MONO-GESIC® 500 mg tablets:
A round, pink, film-coated tablet debossed with Central logo on one side and 500 mg on the other side.
Bottles of 100 tablets—NDC 0131-2154-37
Bottles of 500 tablets—NDC 0131-2154-41
MONO-GESIC® 750 mg tablets:
An oval, pink, film-coated tablet debossed with Central logo on one side and 750 bisect mg on the other side.
Bottles of 100 tablets—NDC 0131-2164-37
Bottles of 500 tablets—NDC 0131-2164-41
Shown in Product Identification Section, page 408

NIFEREX® DAILY TABLETS OTC
[ni'fer"ex]

DESCRIPTION
Each tablet contains:

Vitamin A (as acetate)	5000	IU
Vitamin E (as dl-alpha tocopheryl)	30	IU
Vitamin C (as ascorbic acid)	60	mg
Folic Acid	0.4	mg
B_1 (as thiamine mononitrate)	1.5	mg
B_2 (as riboflavin)	1.7	mg
Niacinamide	20	mg
Pantothenic Acid	10	mg
Biotin	0.3	mg
B_6 (as pyrodoxine)	2	mg
B_{12} (as cyanocobalamin)	6	mcg
Vitamin D	400	IU
Calcium	259	mg
(as calcium carbonate and dicalcium phosphate)		
Iodine (as potassium iodide)	150	mcg
Iron (as polysaccharide-iron complex)	18	mg
Phosphorus (as dicalcium phosphate)	5.4	mg
Manganese (as manganese sulfate)	5	mg
Magnesium (as magnesium oxide)	100	mg
Zinc (as zinc sulfate)	15	mg
Copper (as copper sulfate)	2	mg

HOW SUPPLIED
Capsule shaped, lavendar film-coated tablet imprinted with 20 on one side and Central logo on other side.
Bottle of 100—NDC #0131-2210-32

NIFEREX® TABLETS/ELIXIR
[ni'fer"ex]
NIFEREX®-150 CAPSULES
NIFEREX® with VITAMIN C TABLETS
(polysaccharide-iron complex)

DESCRIPTION
NIFEREX is a highly water-soluble complex of iron and a low molecular weight polysaccharide. Each NIFEREX-150 Capsule contains 150 mg. elemental iron. Each NIFEREX Film Coated Tablet and each NIFEREX with Vitamin C Chewable Tablet contains 50 mg. elemental iron. In addition, each NIFEREX with Vitamin C tablet contains Ascorbic acid, U.S.P., 100 mg. and Sodium ascorbate, 168.75 mg. Each 5 ml. (teaspoonful) NIFEREX Elixir contains 100 mg. elemental iron, alcohol 10% (sugar free).

ACTION AND USES
NIFEREX is an easily assimilated source of iron for treatment of uncomplicated iron deficiency anemia. Because NIFEREX is a polysaccharide bound iron complex, it is relatively nontoxic and there are relatively few, if any, of the gastrointestinal side effects associated with iron therapy, thus permitting full therapeutic dosage (150 to 300 mg. ele-

Continued on next page

Central—Cont.

mental iron daily) in a single dose if desirable. There is no staining of teeth and no metallic aftertaste.

INDICATIONS

For treatment of uncomplicated iron deficiency anemia.

CONTRAINDICATIONS

In patients with hemochromatosis and hemosiderosis, and in those with a known hypersensitivity to any of the ingredients.

DOSAGE AND ADMINISTRATION

ADULTS: One or two NIFEREX-150 Capsules daily, or one or two NIFEREX or NIFEREX with Vitamin C Tablets twice daily, *or* one to two teaspoonfuls NIFEREX Elixir daily or as directed by a physician, . CHILDREN 6 to 12 years of age: One or two NIFEREX *or* one NIFEREX with Vitamin C Tablet daily, or one teaspoonful NIFEREX Elixir daily or as directed by a physician, Children 2 to 6 years of age: ½ teaspoonful NIFEREX Elixir daily or as directed by a physician, Children under 2 years: ¼ teaspoonful daily or as directed by a physician.

HOW SUPPLIED

Niferex-150 Capsules (No. 1 opaque brown cap, opaque orange body printed with white Central logo and Central logo, filled with brown beads)
Bottles of 100—NDC 0131-4220-37
Bottles of 1000—NDC 0131-4220-43
Niferex Elixir (dark brown liquid)
Bottles of 8 ounces—NDC 0131-5066-68
Niferex Tablets (round, brown film-coated)
Bottles of 100—NDC 0131-2200-37
Niferex with Vitamin C Tablets (round, brown, compressed, chewable tablet imprinted with Central logo)
Bottles of 50—NDC 0131-2202-34
Shown in Product Identification Section, page 408

NIFEREX®-150 FORTE CAPSULES ℞
[ni'fer"ex for'ta]
NIFEREX® FORTE ELIXIR ℞

DESCRIPTION

Each capsule Niferex®-150 Forte contains:
Iron (Elemental) .... 150 mg
  (as polysaccharide-iron complex)
Folic Acid .... 1 mg
Vitamin B₁₂ .... 25 mcg

Each teaspoon (5 ml) Niferex® Forte Elixir contains:
Iron (Elemental) .... 100 mg
  (as polysaccharide-iron complex)
Folic Acid .... 1 mg
Vitamin B₁₂ .... 25 mcg
Alcohol 10%
Sugar-Free

PRECAUTION

Folic acid, especially in doses above 0.1 mg–0.4 mg daily, may obscure pernicious anemia, in that hematologic remission may occur while neurological manifestations remain progressive.

DOSAGE AND ADMINISTRATION

Adults—one capsule or one teaspoonful of elixir daily or as prescribed by a physician.

HOW SUPPLIED

Niferex-150 Forte Capsules (No. 1 opaque red cap, opaque brown body printed with white Central logo and 44, filled with brown beads)
Bottle of 100—NDC 0131-4330-37
Bottle of 1000—NDC 0131-4330-43
Niferex Forte Elixir (dark brown liquid)
Bottle of 4 fl. oz.—NDC 0131-5065-64
Capsules Shown in Product Identification Section, page 408

NIFEREX®—PN TABLETS ℞
[ni'fer"ex]

DESCRIPTION

Each film-coated tablet contains:
Iron (Elemental) .... 60 mg
  (as polysaccharide-iron complex)
Folic acid .... 1 mg
Ascorbic acid .... 50 mg
  (as sodium ascorbate)
Cyanocobalamin (Vitamin B₁₂) .... 3 mcg
Vitamin A .... 4000 IU
Vitamin D .... 400 IU
Thiamine mononitrate .... 3 mg
Riboflavin .... 3 mg
Pyridoxine hydrochloride .... 2 mg
Niacinamide .... 10 mg

Calcium (as calcium carbonate) .... 125 mg
Zinc (as zinc sulfate) .... 18 mg
This product contains ingredients of the following therapeutic classes: vitamins and minerals.

INACTIVE INGREDIENTS

Acetylated Monoglycerides, Alcohol, Castor Oil, Corn Syrup, Ethyl Cellulose, F.D.&C. Blue #1 Lake, Ferric Chloride, Hydrogenated Vegetable Oil, Hydroxypropyl Cellulose, Hydroxypropyl Methylcellulose, Magnesium Stearate, Microcrystalline Cellulose, Polyethylene Glycol, Povidone, Shellac, Sodium Hydroxide, Sorbitol and Titanium Dioxide.

CLINICAL PHARMACOLOGY

This product is formulated to meet the needs of the pregnant or lactating patient with special consideration given to adequate amounts of hematopoietic factors, iron, folic acid and cyanocobalamin. Calcium (phosphorus-free) is also included in the formula to help supply the increased requirements of this mineral. The 60 mg of elemental iron is available in the form of Niferex® (polysaccharide-iron complex). This form of iron is especially useful in the pregnant patient because, although it is absorbed as well as ferrous sulfate, it does not produce the gastrointestinal irritation commonly associated with iron salts. In addition, folic acid and cyanocobalamin in therapeutic amounts are included to prevent or treat the significant number of pregnant patients who develop megaloblastic anemia of pregnancy.

INDICATIONS AND USAGE

For the prevention and/or treatment of dietary vitamin and mineral deficiencies associated with pregnancy and lactation.

CONTRAINDICATIONS

Hypersensitivity to any of the ingredients.

WARNINGS

Folic acid alone is improper therapy in the treatment of pernicious anemia and other megaloblastic anemias where vitamin B₁₂ is deficient.

PRECAUTIONS

Folic acid, especially in doses above 0.1 mg–0.4 mg daily may obscure pernicious anemia, in that hematologic remission may occur while neurological manifestations remain progressive.

ADVERSE REACTIONS

Allergic sensitization has been reported following both oral and parenteral administration of folic acid.

DOSAGE AND ADMINISTRATION

One tablet daily or as prescribed by a physician.

HOW SUPPLIED

(Oval, blue film coated tablet imprinted with 131/05)
Bottles of 100 tablets–NDC 0131-2209-37
Bottles of 1000 tablets–NDC 0131-2209-43
Shown in Product Identification Section, page 408

NIFEREX®-PN FORTE TABLETS ℞

DESCRIPTION

Each tablet contains:
Iron (Elemental) .... 60 mg
  (as polysaccharide-iron complex)
Vitamin A acetate .... 5000 IU
Vitamin D .... 400 IU
Vitamin E .... 30 IU
  (as dl-alpha-tocopheryl acetate)
Vitamin C (ascorbic acid) .... 80 mg
Folic acid .... 1 mg
Thiamine (vitamin B₁) .... 3 mg
  (as thiamine mononitrate)
Riboflavin (vitamin B₂) .... 3.4 mg
Vitamin B₆ (as pyridoxine hydrochloride) .... 4 mg
Niacinamide .... 20 mg
Vitamin B₁₂ (Cyanocobalamin) .... 12 mcg
Calcium (as calcium carbonate) .... 250 mg
Iodine (as potassium iodide) .... 0.2 mg
Magnesium (as magnesium oxide) .... 10 mg
Copper (as cupric oxide) .... 2 mg
Zinc (as zinc sulfate) .... 25 mg

HOW SUPPLIED

Capsule shaped, white film coated tablet imprinted with Central logo on one side and 1 bisect O on the other.
Bottles of 100 Tablets—NDC 0131-2309-37
Shown in Product Identification Section, page 408

PREDNICEN®–M 21-Pak ℞
[pred "ni-sen']
(Prednisone Tablets, USP)

DESCRIPTION

Each red-film-coated tablet imprinted with 131/07 contains:
Prednisone .... 5 mg

HOW SUPPLIED

Unit Pack 21 x 5 mg.—NDC # 0131-2228-81
Also Available in
Bottle of 100—NDC # 0131-2228-37
Bottle of 1000—NDC # 0131-2228-43

THEOCLEAR® L.A.–260 CAPSULES ℞
[the'ō-klēr"]
THEOCLEAR® L.A.–130 CAPSULES ℞
THEOCLEAR®–80 Syrup ℞
(theophylline anhydrous)

DESCRIPTION

THEOCLEAR L.A.-260 and THEOCLEAR L.A.-130: Each capsule contains 260 mg or 130 mg of theophylline anhydrous in a sustained release bead formulation.
THEOCLEAR-80: Each 15 mL (1 tablespoonful) contains 80 mg. Anhydrous Theophylline as the active ingredient. Other ingredients are saccharin sodium; tartaric acid; benzoic acid; citric acid; sorbitol; glycerin; propylene glycol; artificial flavor and purified water. This formulation provides an alcohol-free, dye-free, and sugar-free vehicle containing no corn by-products.

HOW SUPPLIED

Theoclear L.A.-260 Capsule (No. 0 clear cap, clear body printed with black Central logo and 260 mg, filled with white beads)
Bottle of 100—NDC 0131-4248-37
Bottle of 1000—NDC 0131-4248-43
Theoclear L.A.-130 Capsule (No. 1 clear cap, clear body printed with black Central logo and 130 mg, filled with white beads)
Bottle of 100—NDC 0131-4247-37
Theoclear-80 Syrup (Clear, colorless liquid with an anise odor)
One Pint—NDC 0131-5098-70
One Gallon—NDC 0131-5098-72
Capsules shown in Product Identification Section, page 408

Cetus Corporation
1400 FIFTY-THIRD STREET
EMERYVILLE, CA 94608

DOXORUBICIN Hydrochloride ℞
For Injection, USP
DOXORUBICIN Hydrochloride Injection
FOR INTRAVENOUS USE ONLY

WARNINGS

1. Severe local tissue necrosis will occur if there is extravasation during administration (See "DOSAGE AND ADMINISTRATION" Section). Doxorubicin must not be given by the intramuscular or subcutaneous route.
2. Serious irreversible myocardial toxicity with delayed congestive failure often unresponsive to any cardiac supportive therapy may be encountered as total dosage approaches 550 mg/m². This toxicity may occur at lower cumulative doses in patients with prior mediastinal irradiation or on concurrent cyclophosphamide therapy.
3. Dosage should be reduced in patients with impaired hepatic function.
4. Severe myelosuppression may occur.
5. Doxorubicin should be administered only under the supervision of a physician who is experienced in the use of cancer chemotherapeutic agents.

DESCRIPTION

Doxorubicin is a cytotoxic anthracycline antibiotic isolated from cultures of *Streptomyces peucetius* var. *caesius*. Doxorubicin consists of a naphthacenequinone nucleus linked through a glycosidic bond at ring atom 7 to an amino sugar, daunosamine.

Doxorubicin binds to nucleic acids, presumably by specific intercalation of the planar anthracycline nucleus with the DNA double helix. The anthracycline ring is lipophilic but the saturated end of the ring system contains abundant hydroxyl groups adjacent to the amino sugar, producing a hydrophilic center. The molecule is amphoteric, containing acidic functions in the ring phenolic groups and a basic function in the sugar amino group. It binds to cell membranes as well as plasma proteins.

It is supplied in the hydrochloride form as a sterile lyophilized powder containing lactose and as a sterile aqueous solution with sodium chloride for intravenous use.

Doxorubicin Hydrochloride for Injection, USP:
Each 10 mg lyophilized vial contains 10 mg of Doxorubicin Hydrochloride, USP and 50 mg of Lactose, NF.

Each 20 mg lyophilized vial contains 20 mg of Doxorubicin Hydrochloride, USP and 100 mg of Lactose, NF.

Each 50 mg lyophilized vial contains 50 mg of Doxorubicin Hydrochloride, USP and 250 mg of Lactose, NF.

Doxorubicin Hydrochloride Injection:

Each 2 mg/mL, 5 mL (10 mg) vial contains 10 mg Doxorubicin Hydrochloride, USP; Sodium Chloride 0/9% (to adjust tonicity) and Water for Injection q.s.; pH adjusted to 3 using Hydrochloric Acid.

Each 2 mg/mL, 10 mL (20 mg) vial contains 20 mg Doxorubicin Hydrochloride, USP; Sodium Chloride 0.9% (to adjust tonicity) and Water for Injection q.s.; pH adjusted to 3 using Hydrochloric Acid.

Each 2 mg/mL, 25 mL (50 mg) vial contains 50 mg Doxorubicin Hydrochloride, USP; Sodium Chloride 0.9% (to adjust tonicity) and Water for Injection q.s.; pH adjusted to 3 using Hydrochloric Acid.

CLINICAL PHARMACOLOGY

Though not completely elucidated, the mechanism of action of doxorubicin is related to its ability to bind to DNA and inhibit nucleic acid synthesis. Cell culture studies have demonstrated rapid cell penetration and perinucleolar chromatin binding, rapid inhibition of mitotic activity and nucleic acid synthesis, mutagenesis and chromosomal aberrations. Animal studies have shown activity in a spectrum of experimental tumors, immunosuppression, carcinogenic properties in rodents, induction of a variety of toxic effects, including delayed and progressive cardiac toxicity, myelosuppression in all species and atrophy to testes in rats and dogs. Pharmacokinetic studies show the intravenous administration of normal or radiolabeled doxorubicin is followed by rapid plasma clearance and significant tissue binding. Urinary excretion, as determined by fluorimetric methods, accounts for approximately 4 to 5% of the administered dose in five days. Biliary excretion represents the major excretion route, 40 to 50% of the administered dose being recovered in the bile or the feces in seven days. Impairment of liver function results in slower excretion, and consequently, increased retention and accumulation in plasma and tissues. Doxorubicin does not cross the blood brain barrier.

INDICATIONS AND USAGE

Injectable doxorubicin hydrochloride has been used successfully to produce regression in disseminated neoplastic conditions such as acute lymphoblastic leukemia, acute myeloblastic leukemia, Wilms' tumor, neuroblastoma, soft tissue and bone sarcomas, breast carcinoma, ovarian carcinoma, transitional cell bladder carcinoma, thyroid carcinoma, lymphomas of both Hodgkin and non-Hodgkin types, bronchogenic carcinoma in which the small cell histologic type is the most responsive compared to other cell types and gastric carcinoma.

A number of other solid tumors have also shown some responsiveness but in numbers too limited to justify specific recommendation. Studies to date have shown malignant melanoma, kidney carcinoma, large bowel carcinoma, brain tumors and metastases to the central nervous system not to be significantly responsive to doxorubicin therapy.

CONTRAINDICATIONS

Doxorubicin therapy should not be started in patients who have marked myelosuppression induced by previous treatment with other antitumor agents or by radiotherapy. Conclusive data are not available on pre-existing heart disease as a cofactor of increased risk of doxorubicin induced cardiac toxicity. Preliminary data suggest that in such cases cardiac toxicity may occur at doses lower than the recommended cumulative limit. It is therefore not recommended to start doxorubicin in such cases. Doxorubicin treatment is contraindicated in patients who received previous treatment with complete cumulative doses of doxorubicin and/or daunorubicin.

WARNINGS

Special attention must be given to the cardiac toxicity exhibited by doxorubicin. Although uncommon, acute left ventricular failure has occurred, particularly in patients who have received total dosage of the drug exceeding the currently recommended limit of 550 mg/m^2. This limit appears to be lower (400 mg/m^2) in patients who received radiotherapy to the mediastinal area or concomitant therapy with other potentially cardiotoxic agents such as cyclophosphamide. The total dose of doxorubicin administered to the individual patient should also take into account previous or concomitant therapy with related compounds such as daunorubicin. Congestive heart failure and/or cardiomyopathy may be encountered several weeks after discontinuation of doxorubicin therapy.

Cardiac failure is often not favorably affected by presently known medical or physical therapy for cardiac support. Early clinical diagnosis of drug induced heart failure appears to be essential for successful treatment with digitalis, diuretics, low salt diet and bed rest. Severe cardiac toxicity may occur precipitously without antecedent EKG changes. A baseline EKG and EKGs performed prior to each dose or course after 300 mg/m^2 cumulative dose has been given is

suggested. Transient EKG changes consisting of T-wave flattening, S-T depression and arrhythmias lasting for up to two weeks after a dose or course of doxorubicin are presently not considered indications for suspension of doxorubicin therapy. Doxorubicin cardiomyopathy has been reported to be associated with a persistent reduction in the voltage of the QRS wave, a prolongation of the systolic time interval and a reduction of the ejection fraction as determined by echocardiography or radionuclide angiography. None of these tests have yet been confirmed to consistently identify those individual patients that are approaching their maximally tolerated cumulative dose of doxorubicin. If test results indicate change in cardiac function associated with doxorubicin, the benefit of continued therapy must be carefully evaluated against the risk of producing irreversible cardiac damage. Acute life-threatening arrhythmias have been reported to occur during or within a few hours after doxorubicin hydrochloride administration.

There is a high incidence of bone marrow depression, primarily of leukocytes, requiring careful hematologic monitoring. With the recommended dosage schedule, leukopenia is usually transient, reaching its nadir at 10 to 14 days after treatment with recovery usually occurring by the 21st day. White blood cell counts as low as 1000/mm^3 are to be expected during treatment with appropriate doses of doxorubicin. Red blood cell and platelet levels should also be monitored since they may also be depressed. Hematologic toxicity may require dose reduction or suspension or delay of doxorubicin therapy. Persistent severe myelosuppression may result in superinfection or hemorrhage.

Doxorubicin may potentiate the toxicity of other anticancer therapies. Exacerbation of cyclophosphamide induced hemorrhagic cystitis and enhancement of the hepatotoxicity of 6-mercaptopurine have been reported. Radiation induced toxicity to the myocardium, mucosae, skin and liver have been reported to be increased by the administration of doxorubicin.

Toxicity to recommended doses of doxorubicin hydrochloride is enhanced by hepatic impairment, therefore, prior to the individual dosing, evaluation of hepatic function is recommended using conventional clinical laboratory tests such as SGOT, SGPT, alkaline phosphatase and bilirubin. (See "DOSAGE AND ADMINISTRATION" Section).

Necrotizing colitis manifested by typhlitis (cecal inflammation), bloody stools and severe and sometimes fatal infections have been associated with a combination of doxorubicin hydrochloride given by IV push daily for 3 days and cytarabine given by continuous infusion daily for 7 or more days.

On intravenous administration of doxorubicin, extravasation may occur with or without an accompanying stinging or burning sensation and even if blood returns well on aspiration of the infusion needle (See "DOSAGE AND ADMINISTRATION" Section). If any signs or symptoms of extravasation have occurred the injection or infusion should be immediately terminated and restarted in another vein.

Doxorubicin and related compounds have also been shown to have mutagenic and carcinogenic properties when tested in experimental models.

Usage in Pregnancy: Safe use of doxorubicin in pregnancy has not been established. Doxorubicin is embryotoxic and teratogenic in rats and embryotoxic and abortifacient in rabbits. Therefore, the benefits to the pregnant patient should be carefully weighed against the potential toxicity to fetus and embryo. The possible adverse effects on fertility in males and females in humans or experimental animals have not been adequately evaluated.

PRECAUTIONS

Initial treatment with doxorubicin requires close observation of the patient and extensive laboratory monitoring. It is recommended, therefore, that patients be hospitalized at least during the first phase of the treatment.

Like other cytotoxic drugs, doxorubicin may induce hyperuricemia secondary to rapid lysis of neoplastic cells. The clinician should monitor the patient's blood uric acid level and be prepared to use such supportive and pharmacologic measures as might be necessary to control this problem.

Doxorubicin imparts a red coloration to the urine for 1 to 2 days after administration and patients should be advised to expect this during active therapy.

Doxorubicin is not an anti-microbial agent.

ADVERSE REACTIONS

Dose limiting toxicities of therapy are myelosuppression and cardiotoxicity (See "WARNINGS" Section). Other reactions reported are:

Cutaneous: Reversible complete alopecia occurs in most cases. Hyperpigmentation of nailbeds and dermal creases, primarily in children, and onycholysis have been reported in a few cases. Recall of skin reaction due to prior radiotherapy has occurred with doxorubicin administration.

Gastrointestinal: Acute nausea and vomiting occurs frequently and may be severe. This may be alleviated by antiemetic therapy. Mucositis (stomatitis and esophagitis) may occur 5 to 10 days after administration. The effect may be severe leading to ulceration and represents a site of origin for severe infections. The dosage regimen consisting of ad-

ministration of doxorubicin on three successive days results in the greater incidence and severity of mucositis. Ulceration and necrosis of the colon, especially the cecum, may occur leading to bleeding or severe infections which can be fatal. This reaction has been reported in patients with acute nonlymphocytic leukemia treated with a 3-day course of doxorubicin combined with cytarabine. Anorexia and diarrhea have been occasionally reported.

Vascular: Phlebosclerosis has been reported especially when small veins are used or a single vein is used for repeated administration. Facial flushing may occur if the injection is given too rapidly.

Local: Severe cellulitis, vesication and tissue necrosis will occur if doxorubicin is extravasated during administration. Erythematous streaking along the vein proximal to the site of the injection has been reported (See "DOSAGE AND ADMINISTRATION" Section).

Hypersensitivity: Fever, chills and urticaria have been reported occasionally. Anaphylaxis may occur. A case of apparent cross sensitivity to lincomycin has been reported.

Other: Conjunctivitis and lacrimation occur rarely.

OVERDOSAGE

Acute overdosage with doxorubicin enhances the toxic effects of mucositis, leukopenia and thrombopenia. Treatment of acute overdosage consists of treatment of the severely myelosuppressed patient with hospitalization, antibiotics, platelet and granulocyte transfusions and symptomatic treatment of mucositis.

Chronic overdosage with cumulative doses exceeding 550 mg/m^2 increases the risk of cardiomyopathy and resultant congestive heart failure. Treatment consists of vigorous management of congestive heart failure with digitalis preparations and diuretics. The use of peripheral vasodilators has been recommended.

DOSAGE AND ADMINISTRATION

Care in the administration of doxorubicin hydrochloride will reduce the chance of perivenous infiltration. It may also decrease the chance of local reactions such as urticaria and erythematous streaking. On intravenous administration of doxorubicin, extravasation may occur with or without any accompanying stinging or burning sensation and even if blood returns well on aspiration of the infusion needle. If any signs or symptoms of extravasation have occurred, the injection or infusion should be immediately terminated and restarted in another vein. If it is known or suspected that subcutaneous extravasation has occurred, local infiltration with an injectable corticosteroid and flooding the site with normal saline has been reported to lessen the local reaction. Because of the progressive nature of extravasation reactions, the area of injection should be frequently examined and plastic surgery consultation obtained. If ulceration begins, early wide excision of the involved area should be considered.[1]

The most commonly used dosage schedule is 60 to 75 mg/m^2 as a single intravenous injection administered at 21-day intervals. The lower dose should be given to patients with inadequate marrow reserves due to old age, or prior therapy, or neoplastic marrow infiltration. An alternative dosage schedule is weekly doses of 20 mg/m^2 which has been reported to produce a lower incidence of congestive heart failure. Thirty (30) mg/m^2 on each of three successive days repeated every 4 weeks has also been used. Doxorubicin dosage must be reduced if the bilirubin is elevated as follows: serum bilirubin 1.2 to 3 mg/dL—give $\frac{1}{2}$ normal dose, > 3 mg/dL—give $\frac{1}{4}$ normal dose.

Reconstitution Directions: Doxorubicin Hydrochloride For Injection, USP 10 mg, 20 mg and 50 mg vials should be reconstituted with 5 mL, 10 mL and 25 mL respectively of 0.9% Sodium Chloride Injection, USP to give a final concentration of 2 mg/mL of doxorubicin hydrochloride. An appropriate volume of air should be withdrawn from the vial during reconstitution to avoid excessive pressure build-up. Bacteriostatic diluents are not recommended.

After adding the diluent, the vial should be shaken and the contents allowed to dissolve. The reconstituted solution is stable for 24 hours at room temperature and 48 hours under refrigeration, 2 to 8°C (36 to 46°F). It should be protected from exposure to sunlight and any unused solution should be discarded.

Note: Parenteral drug products should be inspected visually for particulate matter and discoloration prior to administration, whenever solution and container permit.

It is recommended that doxorubicin be slowly administered into a tubing of a freely running intravenous infusion of Sodium Chloride Injection, USP or 5% of Dextrose Injection, USP. The tubing should be attached to a Butterfly® needle inserted preferable into a large vein. If possible, avoid veins over joints or in extremities with compromised venous or lymphatic drainage. The rate of administration is dependent on the size of the vein and the dosage. However the dose should be administered in not less than 3 to 5 minutes. Local erythematous streaking along the vein as well as facial

Continued on next page

Cetus—Cont.

flushing may be indicative of too rapid an administration. A burning or stinging sensation may be indicative of perivenous infiltration and the infusion should be immediately terminated and restarted in another vein. Perivenous infiltration may occur painlessly.

Doxorubicin should not be mixed with heparin or fluorouracil since it has been reported that these drugs are incompatible to the extent that a precipitate may form. Until specific compatibility data are available, it is not recommended that doxorubicin be mixed with other drugs.

Doxorubicin has been used concurrently with other approved chemotherapeutic agents. Evidence is available that in some types of neoplastic disease combination chemotherapy is superior to single agents. The benefits and risks of such therapy continue to be elucidated.

Handling and Disposal: Skin reactions associated with doxorubicin have been reported. Caution in the handling and preparation of the powder and solution must be exercised and the use of gloves is recommended. If doxorubicin powder or solution contacts the skin or mucosae, immediately wash thoroughly with soap and water.

Procedures for proper handling and disposal of anti-cancer drugs should be considered. Several guidelines on this subject have been published.[2-7] There is no general agreement that all of the procedures recommended in the guidelines are necessary or appropriate .

HOW SUPPLIED

Doxorubicin Hydrochloride For Injection, USP is supplied as a sterile red-orange lyophilized powder in single-dose flip-top vials in the following package strengths:

NDC 53905-231-10: 10 mg vial; supplied in boxes of 10.
NDC 53905-232-06: 20 mg vial; supplied in boxes of 6.
NDC 53905-233-01: 50 mg vial; individually cartoned.
Store unreconstituted vial at controlled room temperature, 15 to 30°C (59 to 86°F). After reconstitution the solution is stable for 24 hours at room temperature and 48 hours under refrigeration, 2 to 8°C (36 to 46°F).
Protect from light. Retain in carton until time of use. Discard unused portion.
Doxorubicin Hydrochloride Injection is supplied in single-dose, flip-top vials, as a red-orange solution containing Doxorubicin Hydrochloride, USP 2 mg/mL in the following package strengths:

NDC 53905-235-10: 10 mg in 5 mL; supplied in boxes of 10.
NDC 53905-236-06: 20 mg in 10 mL; supplied in boxes of 6.
NDC 53905-237-01: 50 mg in 25 mL; individually cartoned.
Store Doxorubicin Hydrochloride Injection in a refrigerator, 2 to 8°C (36 to 46°F).
Protect from light. Retain in carton until time of use. Discard unused portion.
CAUTION—Federal law prohibits dispensing without prescription.

REFERENCES

1. Rudolph R, *et al*: Skin Ulcers Due to Adriamycin. *Cancer* 38: 1087–1094, Sept. 1976.
2. Recommendations for the Safe Handling of Parenteral Antineoplastic Drugs. NIH Publication No. 83-2621. For sale by the Superintendent of Documents, U.S. Government Printing Office, Washington, D.C. 20402.
3. AMA Council Report. Guidelines for Handling Parenteral Antineoplastics. *JAMA*, March 15, 1985.
4. National Study Commission on Cytotoxic Exposure-Recommendations for Handling Cytotoxic Agents. Available from Louis P. Jeffrey, Sc.D., Director of Pharmacy Services, Rhode Island Hospital, 593 Eddy Street, Providence, Rhode Island 02902.
5. Clinical Oncological Society of Australia: Guidelines and Recommendations for Safe Handling of Antineoplastic Agents. *Med J Australia* 1: 426–428, 1983.
6. Jones RB, *et al.* Safe Handling of Chemotherapeutic Agents: A Report From the Mount Sinai Medical Center. *CA-A Cancer Journal for Clinicians* Sept/Oct, 258–263, 1983.
7. American Society of Hospital Pharmacists Technical Assistance Bulletin on Handling Cytotoxic Drugs in Hospitals. *Am J Hosp Pharm* 42: 131–137, 1985.

MANUFACTURED BY:
Ben Venue Laboratories, Inc.
Bedford, OH 44146
DISTRIBUTED BY:
Cetus Corporation
1400 Fifty-Third Street
Emeryville, CA 94608

Issued January, 1989   NO-P-02

LEUCOVORIN Calcium for Injection   ℞

HOW SUPPLIED

Leucovorin Calcium for Injection is supplied in packs of ten individually boxed vials.

50 mg vial: NDC 53905-051-10. Each vial contains 50 mg leucovorin as the calcium salt and 45 mg sodium chloride.
100 mg vial: NDC 53905-052-10. Each vial contains 100 mg leucovorin as the calcium salt and 90 mg sodium chloride.
Revised November 1987   DO-P-01

Sterile VINBLASTINE Sulfate, USP   ℞

HOW SUPPLIED

Sterile Vinblastine Sulfate, USP is supplied in packs of ten individually-boxed vials containing 10 mg lyophilized vinblastine sulfate. NDC 53905-091-10.
Store vials in a refrigerator, 2 to 8°C (36 to 46°F) to assure extended stability.
After reconstitution with 10 mL Bacteriostatic Sodium Chloride Injection, USP (preserved with benzyl alcohol), solution may be kept in a refrigerator, 2 to 8°C (36 to 46°F) for 30 days without significant loss of potency.
CAUTION—Federal law prohibits dispensing without a prescription.
Revised November, 1988   CO-P-02

Cetylite Industries, Inc.
P.O. BOX CN6
9051 RIVER ROAD
PENNSAUKEN, NJ 08110

CETACAINE®   ℞
[set 'a-cane"]
TOPICAL ANESTHETIC

A BRAND OF
Benzocaine	14.0%
Butyl Aminobenzoate	2.0%
Tetracaine Hydrochloride	2.0%
Benzalkonium Chloride	0.5%
Cetyl Dimethyl Ethyl Ammonium Bromide	0.005%

In a bland water soluble base.

ACTION

Cetacaine produces anesthesia rapidly in approximately 30 seconds.

INDICATIONS

Cetacaine is a topical anesthetic indicated for the production of anesthesia of accessible mucous membrane.
Cetacaine Spray is indicated for use to control pain or gagging. Cetacaine in all forms is indicated for use to control pain.

DOSAGE AND ADMINISTRATION

Cetacaine Spray should be applied for approximately one second or less for normal anesthesia. Only limited quantity of Cetacaine is required for anesthesia and a spray in excess of 2 seconds is contraindicated. Average expulsion rate of residue from spray, at normal temperatures, is 200 mg. per second.
Tissue need not be dried prior to application of Cetacaine. Cetacaine should be applied directly to the site where pain control is required.
Cetacaine Liquid or Cetacaine Ointment may be applied with a cotton pledget or directly to tissue. Cotton pledget should not be held in position for extended periods of time, since local reactions to benzoate topical anesthetics are related to the length of time of application.

ADVERSE REACTIONS

Although systemic reactions to Cetacaine have not been reported, local reactions to benzoate topical anesthetics may be associated with the condition of the mucous membrane treated and the length of time of application. Dehydration of the epithelium or an escharotic effect may result from prolonged contact. Allergic reactions are known to occur in some patients with preparations containing benzocaine.
Usage in Pregnancy: Safe use of Cetacaine has not been established with respect to possible adverse effects upon fetal development. Therefore Cetacaine should not be used during early pregnancy, unless in the judgment of a physician the potential benefits outweigh the unknown hazards.
Routine precaution for the use of any topical anesthetic should be observed when Cetacaine is used.

CONTRAINDICATIONS

Cetacaine is not for injection.
Do not use on the eyes.
To avoid excessive systemic absorption, Cetacaine should not be applied to large areas of denuded or inflamed tissue.
Cetacaine should not be administered to patients who are hypersensitive to any of its ingredients.
Individual dosage of tetracaine hydrochloride in excess of 20 mg. is contraindicated. Cetacaine should not be used under dentures or cotton rolls, as retention of the active ingredients under a denture or cotton roll could possibly cause an escharotic effect.

Jetco-Spray® Cannula: The Jetco cannula for Cetacaine Spray is specially designed for accessibility and application of Cetacaine, at the required site of pain control.
The Jetco cannula is supplied in various sizes and shapes. The Jetco cannula is inserted firmly onto the protruding plastic tubing on each bottle of Cetacaine Spray.
The Jetco cannula may be removed and re-inserted as many times as required for cleansing or sterilization.

PACKAGING AVAILABLE

Spray—Flavored, Aerosol 56 gm, including propellant with one J4 cannula ....NDC 10223-0201-1
Medical Kit E—Flavored, Aerosol 56 gm, including propellant with two J4, one J6, one J8
cannula...NDC 10223-0201-3
Liquid—Flavored, 56 gm bottle..............NDC 10223-0202-1
Ointment—Flavored, 37 gm jar............NDC 10223-0210-1
Gel—29 gm in polyethylene tube ....NDC 10223-0215-1

CAUTION

Federal law prohibits dispensing Cetacaine without prescription.
Keep out of reach of children.

(REV. 5/88)

CETYLCIDE® SOLUTION
[see 'til-side"]

ACTIVE INGREDIENTS

Cetyl Dimethyl Ethyl Ammonium Bromide	6.5%
Alkyl (50% C_{12}, 30% C_{14}, 17% C_{16}, 3% C_{18}) Dimethyl Benzyl Ammonium Chloride	6.5%
Isopropyl Alcohol	13.0%
Inert Ingredients	**74.0%**
Total Ingredients	100.0%

Formulation Contains Sodium Nitrite
An Instrument and Hard Surface Disinfectant, EPA Approved for Use in Hospitals and Dental/Medical Operatories.
In known hard water areas, use distilled water. Clean instruments thoroughly... rinse free of all soap before immersion, and allow them to remain in CETYLCIDE solution 15 minutes. Germicides containing a Quaternary Ammonium derivative should not be relied on to destroy spore forming organisms, Mycobacterium tuberculosis or the etiologic agent of viral hepatitis. Thus, instruments suspected of such contamination should be sterilized by heat. Needles, hypodermic syringes, corroded instruments or those with deep narrow crevices, as well as hinged or defective plated instruments should be sterilized by heat. To maintain disinfection, they may then be immersed in CETYLCIDE solution. Change solution periodically.

DIRECTIONS

PER GALLON: 1 oz. (30 ml) Cetylcide to one gallon (3.785 liters) tap water.
Dilution Directions For Use Against Pseudomonas Aeruginosa
PER GALLON: 2 oz. (60 ml) Cetylcide to one gallon (3.785 liters) tap water.
PER QUART: ½ oz. (15 ml) Cetylcide to one quart (946 ml) tap water.

STORAGE AND DISPOSAL

Do not reuse container.
Rinse thoroughly before discarding in trash.

INDICATIONS AND USES

CETYLCIDE... when diluted as directed, is a potent germicidal solution combining high bactericidal and bacteriostatic action against many kinds of pathogenic bacteria. CETYLCIDE is stable in both concentrated and diluted form. When diluted for use as directed, CETYLCIDE makes a RUST-INHIBITING ● ODORLESS ● COLORLESS, highly efficient germicidal solution for the chemical disinfection of ALL METAL, RUBBER AND PLASTIC SURGICAL AND DENTAL INSTRUMENTS AND APPLIANCES.

CAUTION

KEEP OUT OF REACH OF CHILDREN. HARMFUL IF SWALLOWED. CAUSES SEVERE EYE AND SKIN IRRITATION. DO NOT GET IN THE EYES OR ON SKIN. IN CASE OF EYE OR SKIN CONTACT, FLUSH WITH PLENTY OF WATER. FOR EYES, GET MEDICAL ATTENTION. AVOID CONTAMINATION OF FOOD.

HOW SUPPLIED

32 OUNCE, 16 OUNCE AND 12 OUNCE BOTTLES.
EPA Reg. No. 3150-1
EPA Est. No. 3150-NJ-1   MADE IN U.S.A.
(REV. 5/89)

CIBA Consumer Pharmaceuticals
Division of CIBA-GEIGY
Corporation
RARITAN PLAZA III
EDISON, NJ 08837

FIBERALL® Chewable Tablets   OTC
[fīb'ber-al]
Lemon Creme Flavor

DESCRIPTION
Fiberall brand is a bulk forming non-irritant laxative which contains less than 1.5 grams of sugar. The active ingredient is polycarbophil, a bulk forming manmade fiber. The smooth gelatinous bulk formed by Fiberall brand encourages peristaltic activity and a more normal elimination of the bowel contents.
The recommended dose of one tablet contains 1 gram of polycarbophil. Inactive ingredients: crospovidone, dextrose, flavors, magnesium stearate and yellow 10 aluminum lake. Each dose contains less than 1 mg of sodium, 225 mg of calcium, virtually no potassium, and provides less than 6 calories.

INDICATIONS
Fiberall brand is indicated for the management of chronic constipation, temporary constipation caused by illness or pregnancy, in irritable bowel syndrome, and for constipation related to duodenal ulcer or diverticulosis. Fiberall brand is also indicated for stool softening in patients with hemorrhoids.

ACTIONS
After the tablet is chewed it readily disperses and acts without irritants or stimulants. Polycarbophil absorbs water in the gastrointestinal tract to form a gelatinous bulk which encourages a more normal bowel movement.

DOSAGE AND ADMINISTRATION
Adults and children 12 years and older: chew and swallow 1 tablet, 1–4 times a day. Children 2 to under 12 years: chew and swallow ½ tablet, 1–2 times a day. Children under 2: consult a physician. Drink a full glass (8 fl. oz.) of liquid with each dose. Additional liquid is helpful.

CONTRAINDICATIONS
Fecal impaction or intestinal obstruction. Any disease state in which consumption of extra calcium is contraindicated.

DRUG INTERACTIONS
This product contains calcium which may interact with some forms of TETRACYCLINE if taken concomitantly. The tetracycline product should be taken 1 hour before or 2–3 hours after taking Fiberall Tablet.

HOW SUPPLIED
Boxes containing 18 tablets.

FIBERALL® Fiber Wafers   OTC
[fī'ber-al]
Fruit & Nut

DESCRIPTION
Fiberall Fiber Wafers are a bulk forming non-irritant laxative. The active ingredient is refined hydrophilic mucilloid, a recognized dietary fiber extracted from the seed husk of blond psyllium seed (Plantago ovata). The smooth gelatinous bulk formed by Fiberall Wafers encourages peristaltic activity and a more normal elimination of the bowel contents. The recommended dose of (1) Fiberall Fiber Wafer contains 3.4g of psyllium hydrophilic mucilloid in a good tasting wafer form, of which approximately 2.2g is soluble fiber. One wafer equals one slightly rounded teaspoonful of Fiberall Powder. Inactive ingredients: baking powder, brown sugar, butter flavor, cinnamon, corn syrup, crisp rice, dried ground apricots, flour, glycerin, granulated sugar, granulated walnuts, lecithin, margarine, molasses, oats, salt, shortening, water and wheat bran. Fiberall Fiber Wafers contain approximately 79 calories and 54mg of sodium per serving.

INDICATIONS
Fiberall Fiber Wafers are indicated for the management of chronic constipation, temporary constipation caused by illness or pregnancy, irritable bowel syndrome, and for constipation related to duodenal ulcer or diverticulosis. Fiberall Wafers are also indicated for stool softening in patients with hemorrhoids after anorectal surgery.

ACTIONS
The homogenous high fiber formula of Fiberall Fiber Wafers, eaten with 8 oz. of a beverage of the patient's choice, acts without irritants or stimulants in the gastrointestinal tract.

DOSAGE AND ADMINISTRATIONS
The recommended daily dosage for adults is one to two Fiberall Fiber Wafers with a full 8 oz. glass of water or other liquid taken one to three times daily according to individual response. The recommended daily dose for children 6 to 12 years old is one-half the adult dose. An additional glass of liquid is recommended and generally provides optimal response. Maximum benefits are usually obtained after two or three days of regular use of Fiberall Fiber Wafers.

CONTRAINDICATIONS
Fecal impaction or intestinal obstruction.

PRECAUTION
As with any grain product, inhaled or ingested psyllium powder may cause an allergic reaction in individuals sensitive to it.

HOW SUPPLIED
Boxes containing 14 wafers.

FIBERALL® Fiber Wafers   OTC
[fī'ber-al]
Oatmeal Raisin

DESCRIPTION
Fiberall Fiber Wafers are a bulk forming non-irritant laxative. The active ingredient is refined hydrophilic mucilloid, a recognized dietary fiber extracted from the seed husk of blond psyllium seed (Plantago ovata). The smooth gelatinous bulk formed by Fiberall Fiber Wafers encourages peristaltic activity and a more normal elimination of the bowel contents.
The recommended dose of (1) Fiberall Fiber Wafer contains 3.4g of psyllium hydrophilic mucilloid in a good tasting wafer form of which approximately 2.2g is soluble fiber. One wafer equals one slightly rounded teaspoonful of powder.
Inactive ingredients: baking powder, cinnamon, cinnamon flavor, cloves, corn syrup, flour, glycerin, granulated sugar, lecithin, molasses, oats, raisins, shortening, water and wheat bran. Oatmeal Raisin Fiberall Fiber Wafers contain approximately 78 calories and 28mg of sodium per serving.

INDICATIONS
Fiberall Fiber Wafers are indicated for the management of chronic constipation, temporary constipation caused by illness or pregnancy, irritable bowel syndrome, and for constipation related to duodenal ulcer or diverticulosis. Fiberall Wafers are also indicated for stool softening in patients with hemorrhoids after anorectal surgery.

ACTIONS
The homogenous high fiber formula of Fiberall Fiber Wafers, eaten with 8 oz. of a beverage of the patient's choice, acts without irritants or stimulants in the gastrointestinal tract.

DOSAGE AND ADMINISTRATION
The recommended daily dosage for adults is one to two Fiberall Fiber Wafer with a full 8 oz. glass of water or other liquid taken one to three times daily according to the individual response. The recommended daily dose for children 6 to 12 years old is one-half the adult dose. An additional glass of liquid is recommended and generally provides optimal response. Maximum benefits are usually obtained after two or three days of regular use of Fiberall Fiber Wafers.

CONTRAINDICATIONS
Fecal impaction or intestinal obstruction.

PRECAUTION
As with any grain product, inhaled or ingested psyllium powder may cause an allergic reaction in individuals sensitive to it.

HOW SUPPLIED
Boxes containing 14 wafers.

FIBERALL® Powder, Natural Flavor   OTC
[fī'ber-al]

DESCRIPTION
Fiberall is a bulk forming non-irritant laxative which contains no sugar. The active ingredient is refined hydrophilic mucilloid, a recognized dietary fiber, extracted from the seed husk of blond psyllium seed (Plantago ovata). The smooth gelatinous bulk formed by Fiberall encourages peristaltic activity and a more normal elimination of the bowel contents.
The recommended dose of one slightly rounded teaspoonful (5g) contains 3.4g of psyllium hydrophilic mucilloid of which approximately 2.2g is soluble fiber. Inactive ingredients: citric acid, flavor, polysorbate 60 and wheat bran. Each dose contains less than 10mg of sodium, less than 60mg of potassium, and provides less than 6 calories.

INDICATIONS
Fiberall is indicated for the management of chronic constipation, temporary constipation caused by illness or pregnancy, in irritable bowel syndrome, and for constipation related to duodenal ulcer or diverticulosis. Fiberall is also indicated for stool softening in patients with hemorrhoids after anorectal surgery.

ACTIONS
The homogenous, high fiber formula of Fiberall is readily dispersed in liquids and acts without irritants or stimulants in the gastrointestinal tract.

DOSAGE AND ADMINISTRATION
The recommended daily dosage for adults is one slightly rounded teaspoonful (5g) stirred into an 8 oz. glass of cool water or other liquid and taken orally one to three times daily according to the individual response. The recommended daily dose for children 6 to 12 years old is one-half the adult dose. An additional glass of liquid is recommended and generally provides optimal response. Maximum benefits are usually obtained after two or three days of regular use of Fiberall brand.

CONTRAINDICATIONS
Fecal impaction or intestinal obstruction.

PRECAUTION
As with any grain product, inhaled or ingested psyllium powder may cause an allergic reaction in individuals sensitive to it.

HOW SUPPLIED
Powder, in 10, and 15 oz. containers.

FIBERALL® Powder, Orange Flavor   OTC
[fī'ber-al]

DESCRIPTION
Fiberall is a bulk forming non-irritant laxative which contains no sugar. The active ingredient is refined hydrophilic mucilloid, a recognized dietary fiber, extracted from the seed husk of blond psyllium seed (Plantago ovata). The smooth gelatinous bulk formed by Fiberall encourages peristaltic activity and a more normal elimination of the lower bowel contents.
The recommended dose of one slightly rounded teaspoonful (5.9g) contains 3.4g of psyllium hydrophilic mucilloid of which approximately 2.2g is soluble fiber. Inactive ingredients: beta-carotene, citric acid, flavors, polysorbate 60, saccharin, wheat bran and yellow #6 lake. Each dose contains less than 10mg of sodium, less than 60mg of potassium, and provides less than 10 calories.

INDICATIONS
Fiberall is indicated for the management of chronic constipation, temporary constipation caused by illness or pregnancy, in irritable bowel syndrome, and for constipation related to duodenal ulcer or diverticulosis. Fiberall is also indicated for stool softening in patients with hemorrhoids after anorectal surgery.

ACTIONS
The homogenous, high fiber formula of Fiberall is readily dispersed in liquids and acts without irritants or stimulants in the gastrointestinal tract.

DOSAGE AND ADMINISTRATION
The recommended daily dosage for adults is one slightly rounded teaspoonful (5.9g) stirred into an 8 oz. glass of cool water or other liquid and taken orally one to three times daily according to the individual response. The recommended daily dose for children 6 to 12 years old is one-half the adult dose. An additional glass of liquid is recommended and generally provides optimal response. Maximum benefits are usually obtained after two or three days of regular use of Fiberall brand.

CONTRAINDICATIONS
Fecal impaction or intestinal obstruction.

PRECAUTION
As with any grain product, inhaled or ingested psyllium powder may cause an allergic reaction in individuals sensitive to it.

HOW SUPPLIED
Powder, in 10, and 15 oz. containers.

SLOW FE®
Slow Release Iron Tablets

DESCRIPTION
SLOW FE supplies ferrous sulfate, for the treatment of iron deficiency and iron deficiency anemia with a significant reduction in the incidence of common iron side effects. The wax

Continued on next page

CIBA Consumer—Cont.

matrix delivery system of SLOW FE is designed to maximize the release of ferrous sulfate in the duodenum and the jejunum where it is best tolerated and absorbed. SLOW FE is clinically shown to significantly reduce constipation, diarrhea and abdominal discomfort when compared to regular iron tablets and a leading capsule.

FORMULA
Each tablet contains 160 mg. dried ferrous sulfate USP, equivalent to 50 mg. elemental iron. Also contains cetostearyl alcohol, colloidal silicon dioxide, hydroxypropyl methylcellulose, shellac, lactose, magnesium stearate, polyethylene glycol.

DOSAGE
ADULTS—one or two tablets daily or as recommended by a physician. A maximum of four tablets daily may be taken. CHILDREN—one tablet daily. Tablets must be swallowed whole.

WARNING
The treatment of any anemic condition should be under the advice and supervision of a physician. As oral iron products interfere with absorption of oral tetracycline antibiotics, these products should not be taken within two hours of each other. As with any drug, if you are pregnant or nursing a baby, seek the advice of a health professional before using this product.
Keep this and all medicines out of reach of children. In case of accidental overdose, contact your physician or poison control center immediately.
Tamper Resistant Packaging.

HOW SUPPLIED
Packages of 30, 60 and 100.
Shown in Product Identification Section, page 408

The full prescribing information for this CIBA Consumer product is contained herein and is that in effect as of September 1, 1989.

CIBA Pharmaceutical Company
Division of CIBA-GEIGY Corporation
SUMMIT, NJ 07901

To provide a convenient and accurate means of identifying CIBA solid dosage form products, a code number has been imprinted on all tablets and capsules. To help you quickly identify a CIBA Tablet or Capsule by its code number, a numerical listing of codes (with corresponding product names) and an alphabetical listing of products (with corresponding codes and list numbers) have been compiled below.

CIBA Code #	ALPHABETICAL LISTING		List Number
	Anturane® sulfinpyrazone USP		
41	TABLETS (white, single-scored) each containing 100 mg sulfinpyrazone USP	100s	1910
168	CAPSULES (green) each containing 200 mg sulfinpyrazone USP	100s	1920
	Apresazide® hydralazine HCl and hydrochlorothiazide		
139	CAPSULES 25/25 (light blue and white opaque), each containing 25 mg hydralazine HCl and 25 mg hydrochlorothiazide	100s	3131
149	CAPSULES 50/50 (pink and white opaque), each containing 50 mg hydralazine HCl and 50 mg hydrochlorothiazide	100s	3132
159	CAPSULES 100/50 (pink flesh and white opaque), each containing 100 mg hydralazine HCl and 50 mg hydrochlorothiazide	100s	3133
	Apresoline® hydrochloride hydralazine hydrochloride USP		
37	TABLETS, 10 mg (pale yellow, dry-coated)	100s	2629
	Consumer Pack	100s	2603
39	TABLETS, 25 mg (deep blue, dry-coated)	100s	2611
		1000s	2615
	Accu-Pak®	100s	2647
	Consumer Pack	100s	2606

73	TABLETS, 50 mg (light blue, dry-coated)	100s	2619
		1000s	2623
	Accu-Pak®	100s	2648
	Consumer Pack	100s	2643
101	TABLETS, 100 mg (peach, dry-coated)	100s	2638
	Apresoline®-Esidrix® hydralazine hydrochloride and hydrochlorothiazide		
129	TABLETS (orange, dry-coated), each containing 25 mg hydralazine hydrochloride and 15 mg hydrochlorothiazide	100s	3120
	Cytadren® aminoglutethamide USP		
24	TABLETS-250 mg (white, round, scored into quarters)	100s	2120
	Esidrix® hydrochlorothiazide USP		
22	TABLETS, 25 mg (pink, scored)	100s	4310
		1000s	4313
	Accu-Pak®	100s	4312
	Consumer Pack	100s	4325
46	TABLETS, 50 mg (yellow, scored)	100s	4315
		1000s	4318
	Accu-Pak®	100s	4317
	Consumer Pack	30s	4328
		60s	4331
		100s	4330
192	TABLETS, 100 mg (blue, scored)	100s	4340
	Esimil®		
47	TABLETS (white, scored), each containing 10 mg guanethidine monosulfate USP and 25 mg hydrochlorothiazide USP	100s	4503
	Consumer Pack	100s	4512
	Estraderm® 0.05 mg estradiol transdermal system		
2310	Package of 6 Patient Calendar Packs (8 systems per Patient Calendar Pack)		0922
	Package of 1 Patient Calendar Pack (24 systems per Patient Calendar Pack)		0921
	Estraderm® 0.1 mg estradiol transdermal system		
2320	Package of 6 Patient Calendar Packs (8 systems per Patient Calendar Pack)		0932
	Package of 1 Patient Calendar Pack (24 systems per Patient Calendar Pack)		0931
	Ismelin® sulfate guanethidine monosulfate		
49	TABLETS, 10 mg (pale yellow, scored)	100s	5010
	Consumer Pack	100s	5003
103	TABLETS, 25 mg (white, scored)	100s	5020
	Consumer Pack	100s	5026
	Lithobid® lithium carbonate USP		
65	TABLETS, 300 mg (peach-colored)	100s	0210
		1000s	0220
	Accu-Pak®	100s	0230
	Ludiomil® maprotiline hydrochloride USP		
110	TABLETS, 25 mg (oval, dark orange, coated)	100s	1710
	Accu-Pak®	100s	1714
26	TABLETS, 50 mg (round, dark orange, coated)	100s	1720
	Accu-Pak®	100s	1721
135	TABLETS, 75 mg (oval, white, coated)	100s	1730
	Accu-Pak®	100s	1732
	Metandren® methyltestosterone USP		
30	TABLETS, 10 mg (white, scored)	100s	1414
32	TABLETS, 25 mg (pale yellow, scored)	100s	1418

51	LINGUETS®, 5 mg (white)	100s	1432
64	LINGUETS®, 10 mg (yellow)	100s	1438
	Metopirone® metyrapone USP		
130	TABLETS, 250 mg (white, scored)	18s	5403
	Rimactane® rifampin USP		
154	CAPSULES, 300 mg (opaque scarlet and caramel)	30s	8903
		60s	8904
		100s	8901
	Rimactane®/INH Dual Pack rifampin USP & isoniazid USP		
8912	Each Dual Pack contains two Rimactane 300-mg CAPSULES and one INH 300-mg TABLET		8912
	Ritalin® hydrochloride Ⓒ methylphenidate hydrochloride USP		
07	TABLETS, 5 mg (yellow)	100s	7410
		500s	7412
		1000s	7414
03	TABLETS, 10 mg (pale green, scored)	100s	7416
		500s	7418
		1000s	7420
	Accu-Pak®	100s	7415
34	TABLETS, 20 mg (pale yellow, scored)	100s	7422
		1000s	7426
	Ritalin-SR® Ⓒ methylphenidate hydrochloride sustained-release tablets		
16	TABLETS, 20 mg (round, white, scored)	100s	7442
	Ser-Ap-Es®		
71	TABLETS (light salmon pink, dry-coated), each containing 0.1 mg reserpine, 25 mg hydralazine hydrochloride and 15 mg hydrochlorothiazide	100s	6610
		1000s	6612
	Accu-Pak®	100s	6605
	Consumer Pack	100s	6617
	Serpasil® reserpine USP		
35	TABLETS, 0.1 mg (white)	100s	7610
36	TABLETS, 0.25 mg (white, scored)	100s	7616
		1000s	7620
	Consumer Pack	100s	7607
	Serpasil®-Apresoline® reserpine and hydralazine hydrochloride		
40	TABLETS #1 (yellow, dry-coated), each containing 0.1 mg reserpine and 25 mg hydralazine hydrochloride	100s	7721
104	TABLETS #2 (yellow, dry-coated), each containing 0.2 mg reserpine and 50 mg hydralazine hydrochloride	100s	7709
	Serpasil®-Esidrix® reserpine and hydrochlorothiazide		
13	TABLETS #1 (light orange), each containing 0.1 mg reserpine and 25 mg hydrochlorothiazide	100s	7010
97	TABLETS #2 (light orange), each containing 0.1 mg reserpine and 50 mg hydrochlorothiazide	100s	7020
	Transderm Scōp® scopolamine		
4345	Package of 3 cartons (4 discs per carton)		5921

CIBA Code #	NUMERICAL LISTING		
	Ritalin® hydrochloride Ⓒ methylphenidate hydrochloride USP		
03	TABLETS, 10 mg (pale green, scored)		
07	TABLETS, 5 mg (yellow)		
	Serpasil®-Esidrix® reserpine and hydrochlorothiazide		
13	TABLETS #1 (light orange), each containing 0.1 mg reserpine and 25 mg hydrochlorothiazide		

Ritalin-SR® ℂ℩℩
methylphenidate hydrochloride sustained-release tablets
16   TABLETS, 20 mg (round, white, scored)
Esidrix®
hydrochlorothiazide USP
22   TABLETS, 25 mg (pink, scored)
Cytadren®
aminoglutethamide
24   TABLETS, 250 mg (white, round, scored into quarters)
Ludiomil®
maprotiline hydrochloride USP
26   TABLETS, 50 mg (round, dark orange, coated)
Metandren®
methyltestosterone USP
30   TABLETS, 10 mg (white, scored)
Metandren®
methyltestosterone USP
32   TABLETS, 25 mg (pale yellow, scored)
Ritalin® hydrochloride ℂ℩℩
methylphenidate hydrochloride USP
34   TABLETS, 20 mg (pale yellow, scored)
Serpasil®
reserpine USP
35   TABLETS, 0.1 mg (white)
36   TABLETS, 0.25 mg (white, scored)
Apresoline® hydrochloride
hydralazine hydrochloride USP
37   TABLETS, 10 mg (pale yellow, dry-coated)
39   TABLETS, 25 mg (deep blue, dry-coated)
Serpasil®-Apresoline®
reserpine and hydralazine hydrochloride
40   TABLETS #1 (yellow, dry-coated), each containing 0.1 mg reserpine and 25 mg hydralazine hydrochloride
Anturane®
sulfinpyrazone USP
41   TABLETS (white, single-scored) each containing 100 mg sulfinpyrazone USP
Esidrix®
hydrochlorothiazide USP
46   TABLETS, 50 mg (yellow, scored)
Esimil®
47   TABLETS (white, scored), each containing 10 mg guanethidine monosulfate and 25 mg hydrochlorothiazide
Ismelin® sulfate
guanethidine monosulfate
49   TABLETS, 10 mg (pale yellow, scored)
Metandren®
methyltestosterone USP
51   LINGUETS®, 5 mg (white)
Metandren®
methyltestosterone USP
64   LINGUETS®, 10 mg (yellow)
Lithobid®
lithium carbonate
65   TABLETS, 300 mg (peach colored)
Ser-Ap-Es®
71   TABLETS (light salmon pink, dry-coated), containing 0.1 mg reserpine, 25 mg hydralazine hydrochloride and 15 mg hydrochlorothiazide
Apresoline® hydrochloride
hydralazine hydrochloride USP
73   TABLETS, 50 mg (light blue, dry-coated)
Serpasil®-Esidrix®
reserpine and hydrochlorothiazide
97   TABLETS #2 (light orange), each containing 0.1 mg reserpine and 50 mg hydrochlorothiazide
Apresoline® hydrochloride
hydralazine hydrochloride USP
101   TABLETS, 100 mg (peach, dry-coated)
Ismelin® sulfate
guanethidine monosulfate
103   TABLETS, 25 mg (white, scored)
Serpasil®-Apresoline®
reserpine and hydralazine hydrochloride
104   TABLETS #2 (yellow, dry-coated), each containing 0.2 mg reserpine and 50 mg hydralazine hydrochloride
Ludiomil®
maprotiline hydrochloride USP
110   TABLETS, 25 mg (oval, dark orange coated)
Apresoline®-Esidrix®
hydralazine hydrochloride and hydrochlorothiazide
129   TABLETS (orange, dry-coated), each containing 25 mg hydralazine hydrochloride and 15 mg hydrochlorothiazide
Metopirone®
metyrapone USP
130   TABLETS, 250 mg (white, scored)

Ludiomil®
maprotiline hydrochloride USP
135   TABLETS, 75 mg (oval, white, coated)
Apresazide®
hydralazine HCl and hydrochlorothiazide
139   CAPSULES 25/25 (light blue and white opaque), each containing 25 mg hydralazine hydrochloride and 25 mg hydrochlorothiazide
149   CAPSULES 50/50 (pink and white opaque), each containing 50 mg hydralazine hydrochloride and 50 mg hydrochlorothiazide
Rimactane®
rifampin USP
154   CAPSULES, 300 mg (opaque scarlet and caramel)
Rimactane®/INH® Dual Pack
rifampin USP & isoniazid USP
8912   Each Dual Pack contains two Rimactane 300-mg CAPSULES and one INH 300-mg TABLET
Apresazide®
hydralazine HCl and hydrochlorothiazide
159   CAPSULES 100/50 (pink flesh and white opaque), each containing 100 mg hydralazine hydrochloride and 50 mg hydrochlorothiazide
Anturane®
sulfinpyrazone USP
168   CAPSULES (green) each containing 200 mg sulfinpyrazone USP
Esidrix®
hydrochlorothiazide USP
192   TABLETS, 100 mg (blue, scored)
Estraderm® 0.05 mg
estradiol transdermal system
2310   Package of 6 Patient Calendar Packs (8 systems per Patient Calendar Pack)
Estraderm® 0.1 mg
estradiol transdermal system
2320   Package of 6 Patient Calendar Packs (8 systems per Patient Calendar Pack)
Transderm Scōp®
scopolamine
4345   Package of 3 cartons (4 discs per carton)

ANTURANE®   ℞

[ann 'too-rain]
sulfinpyrazone USP
Tablets, Capsules

DESCRIPTION

Anturane, sulfinpyrazone USP, is a uricosuric agent available as 100-mg tablets and 200-mg capsules for oral administration. Its chemical name is 1,2-diphenyl-4-[2-(phenylsulfinyl)ethyl]-3,5-pyrazolidinedione.
Sulfinpyrazone USP is a white to off-white powder practically insoluble in water and in solvent hexane, soluble in alcohol and in acetone, and sparingly soluble in dilute alkali. Its molecular weight is 404.48.
Inactive Ingredients. Anturane tablets: Colloidal silicon dioxide, gelatin, lactose, magnesium stearate, starch, stearic acid, and talc.
Anturane capsules: D&C Red No. 33, D&C Yellow No. 10, FD&C Blue No. 1, gelatin, lactose, magnesium stearate, methylparaben, propylparaben, silicon dioxide, sodium lauryl sulfate, starch, stearic acid, talc, and titanium dioxide.

CLINICAL PHARMACOLOGY

Its pharmacologic activity is the potentiation of the urinary excretion of uric acid. It is useful for reducing the blood urate levels in patients with chronic tophaceous gout and acute intermittent gout, and for promoting the resorption of tophi.

INDICATIONS

Anturane is indicated for the treatment of:
1. Chronic gouty arthritis
2. Intermittent gouty arthritis

CONTRAINDICATIONS

Patients with an active peptic ulcer or symptoms of gastrointestinal inflammation or ulceration should not receive the drug.
The drug is contraindicated in patients with a history or the presence of:
1. Hypersensitivity to phenylbutazone or other pyrazoles
2. Blood dyscrasias

WARNINGS

Studies on the teratogenicity of pyrazole compounds in animals have yielded inconclusive results. Up to the present time, however, there have been no reported cases of human congenital malformation proved to be due to the use of the drug.
It is suggested that Anturane be used with caution in pregnant women, weighing the potential risks against the possible benefits.

PRECAUTIONS

As with all pyrazole compounds, patients receiving Anturane should be kept under close medical supervision and

periodic blood counts are recommended. It may be administered with care to patients with a history of healed peptic ulcer.
Recent reports have indicated that Anturane potentiates the action of certain sulfonamides, such as sulfadiazine and sulfisoxazole. In addition, other pyrazole compounds (phenylbutazone) have been observed to potentiate the hypoglycemic sulfonylurea agents, as well as insulin. In view of these observations, it is suggested that Anturane be used with caution in conjunction with sulfa drugs, the sulfonylurea hypoglycemic agents and insulin.
Because Anturane is a potent uricosuric agent, it may precipitate urolithiasis and renal colic, especially in the initial stages of therapy. For this reason, an adequate fluid intake and alkalinization of the urine are recommended. In cases with significant renal impairment, periodic assessment of renal function is indicated. Occasional cases of renal failure have been reported; but a cause-and-effect relationship has not always been clearly established.
Salicylates antagonize the uricosuric action of Anturane and for this reason their concomitant use is contraindicated in gouty arthritis.
Anturane may accentuate the action of coumarin-type anticoagulants and further depress prothrombin activity when these medications are employed simultaneously.

NOTE

Anturane has minimal anti-inflammatory effect and is not intended for the relief of an acute attack of gout.
In the initial stages of therapy, because of the marked ability of Anturane to mobilize urates, acute attacks of gouty arthritis may be precipitated.

ADVERSE REACTIONS

The most frequently reported adverse reactions with Anturane have been upper gastrointestinal disturbances. In these patients it is advisable to administer the drug with food, milk, or antacids. Despite this precaution, Anturane may aggravate or reactivate peptic ulcer.
Rash has been reported. In most instances, this reaction did not necessitate discontinuance of therapy. In general, Anturane has not been observed to affect electrolyte balance.
Blood dyscrasias (anemia, leukopenia, agranulocytosis, thrombocytopenia and aplastic anemia) have rarely been reported. There has also been a published report associating Anturane, administered concomitantly with other drugs including colchicine, with leukemia following long-term treatment of patients with gout. However, the circumstances involved in the two cases reported are such that a cause-and-effect relationship to Anturane has not been clearly established.

OVERDOSAGE

Symptoms: Nausea, vomiting, diarrhea, epigastric pain, ataxia, labored respiration, convulsions, coma. Possible symptoms, seen after overdosage with other pyrazolone derivatives: anemia, jaundice, ulceration.
Treatment: No specific antidote. Induce emesis; gastric lavage; supportive treatment (intravenous glucose infusions, analeptics).

DOSAGE AND ADMINISTRATION

Initial: 200–400 mg daily in two divided doses, with meals or milk, gradually increasing when necessary to full maintenance dosage in one week.
Maintenance: 400 mg daily, given in two divided doses, as above. This dosage may be increased to 800 mg daily, if necessary, and may sometimes be reduced to as low as 200 mg daily after the blood urate level has been controlled. Treatment should be continued without interruption even in the presence of acute exacerbations, which can be concomitantly treated with phenylbutazone or colchicine. Patients previously controlled with other uricosuric therapy may be transferred to Anturane at full maintenance dosage.

HOW SUPPLIED

Tablets 100 mg—round, white, scored (imprinted CIBA 41)
   Bottles of 100 ....NDC 0083-0041-30
Capsules 200 mg—green (imprinted Anturane 200 CIBA 168)
   Bottles of 100 ....NDC 0083-0168-30
Dispense in tight container (USP).

C87-5 (Rev. 2/87)

Shown in Product Identification Section, page 408

Continued on next page

The full prescribing information for each CIBA product is contained herein and is that in effect as of September 1, 1989

CIBA—Cont.

APRESAZIDE®   ℞
[a-press'a-zyde]
hydralazine hydrochloride and
hydrochlorothiazide
Capsules

> **WARNING**
>
> This fixed-combination drug is not indicated for initial therapy of hypertension. Hypertension requires therapy titrated to the individual patient. If the fixed combination represents the dosage so determined, its use may be more convenient in patient management. The treatment of hypertension is not static but must be reevaluated as conditions in each patient warrant.

DESCRIPTION

Apresazide, hydralazine hydrochloride and hydrochlorothiazide, is an antihypertensive-diuretic combination available as capsules for oral administration. Apresazide capsules of 25/25 contain 25 mg of hydralazine hydrochloride USP and 25 mg of hydrochlorothiazide USP; capsules of 50/50 contain 50 mg of hydralazine hydrochloride USP and 50 mg of hydrochlorothiazide USP; and capsules of 100/50 contain 100 mg of hydralazine hydrochloride USP and 50 mg of hydrochlorothiazide USP.

Hydralazine hydrochloride is 1-hydrazinophthalazine monohydrochloride.

Hydralazine hydrochloride USP is a white to off-white, odorless crystalline powder. It is soluble in water, slightly soluble in alcohol, and very slightly soluble in ether. It melts at about 275°C, with decomposition, and has a molecular weight of 196.64.

Hydrochlorothiazide is 6-chloro-3,4-dihydro-2H-1,2,4-benzothiadiazine-7-sulfonamide 1,1-dioxide.

Hydrochlorothiazide USP is a white, or practically white, practically odorless crystalline powder. It is freely soluble in sodium hydroxide solution, in n-butylamine, and in dimethylformamide; sparingly soluble in methanol; slightly soluble in water; and insoluble in ether, in chloroform, and in dilute mineral acids. Its molecular weight is 297.73.

Inactive Ingredients: D&C Red No. 33 and D&C Yellow No. 10 (100/50 capsules only); FD&C Blue No. 1 and FD&C Red No. 3 (25/25 and 50/50 capsules only); gelatin; magnesium stearate; silicon dioxide; sodium bisulfite; sodium lauryl sulfate; starch; and titanium dioxide.

CLINICAL PHARMACOLOGY

Hydralazine

Although the precise mechanism of action of hydralazine is not fully understood, the major effects are on the cardiovascular system. Hydralazine apparently lowers blood pressure by exerting a peripheral vasodilating effect through a direct relaxation of vascular smooth muscle. Hydralazine, by altering cellular calcium metabolism, interferes with the calcium movements within the vascular smooth muscle that are responsible for initiating or maintaining the contractile state. The peripheral vasodilating effect of hydralazine results in decreased arterial blood pressure (diastolic more than systolic); decreased peripheral vascular resistance; and an increased heart rate, stroke volume, and cardiac output. The preferential dilatation of arterioles, as compared to veins, minimizes postural hypotension and promotes the increase in cardiac output. Hydralazine usually increases renin activity in plasma, presumably as a result of increased secretion of renin by the renal juxtaglomerular cells in response to reflex sympathetic discharge. This increase in renin activity leads to the production of angiotensin II, which then causes stimulation of aldosterone and consequent sodium reabsorption. Hydralazine also maintains or increases renal and cerebral blood flow.

Hydrochlorothiazide

Thiazides affect the renal tubular mechanism of electrolyte reabsorption. At maximal therapeutic dosage, all thiazides are approximately equal in their diuretic potency. Thiazides increase excretion of sodium and chloride in approximately equivalent amounts. Natriuresis causes a secondary loss of potassium.

The mechanism of the antihypertensive effect of thiazides is unknown. Thiazides do not affect normal blood pressure.

Pharmacokinetics

Hydralazine. Hydralazine is rapidly absorbed after oral administration, and peak plasma levels are reached at 1–2 hours. Plasma levels decline with a half-life of 3–7 hours. Binding to human plasma protein is 87%. Plasma levels of hydralazine vary widely among individuals. Hydralazine is subject to polymorphic acetylation; slow acetylators generally have higher plasma levels of hydralazine and require lower doses to maintain control of blood pressure. Hydralazine undergoes extensive hepatic metabolism; it is excreted mainly in the form of metabolites in the urine.

Administration of hydralazine with food results in higher levels of the drug in plasma.

Hydrochlorothiazide. Onset of action of thiazides occurs in 2 hours and the peak effect at about 4 hours. The action persists for approximately 6–12 hours. Hydrochlorothiazide is rapidly absorbed, as indicated by peak concentrations 1–2.5 hours after oral administration. Plasma levels of the drug are proportional to dose; the concentration in whole blood is 1.6–1.8 times higher than in plasma. Thiazides are eliminated rapidly by the kidney. After oral administration of 25- to 100-mg doses, 72–97% of the dose is excreted in the urine, indicating dose-independent absorption. Hydrochlorothiazide is eliminated from plasma in a biphasic fashion with a terminal half-life of 10–17 hours. Plasma protein binding is 67.9%. Plasma clearance is 15.9–30.0 L/hr; volume of distribution is 3.6–7.8 L/kg.

Gastrointestinal absorption of hydrochlorothiazide is enhanced when administered with food. Absorption is decreased in patients with congestive heart failure, and the pharmacokinetics are considerably different in these patients.

INDICATIONS AND USAGE

Hypertension (see boxed **WARNING**).

CONTRAINDICATIONS

Hydralazine

Hypersensitivity to hydralazine; coronary artery disease; mitral valvular rheumatic heart disease.

Hydrochlorothiazide

Anuria; hypersensitivity to this or other sulfonamide-derived drugs.

WARNINGS

Hydralazine

In a few patients hydralazine may produce a clinical picture simulating systemic lupus erythematosus including glomerulonephritis. In such patients hydralazine should be discontinued unless the benefit-to-risk determination requires continued antihypertensive therapy with this drug. Signs and symptoms usually regress when the drug is discontinued, but residua have been detected many years later. Long-term treatment with steroids may be necessary. (See **PRECAUTIONS, Laboratory Tests.**)

Hydrochlorothiazide

Thiazides should be used with caution in patients with severe renal disease. In patients with renal disease, thiazides may precipitate azotemia. Cumulative effects of the drug may develop in patients with impaired renal function.

Thiazides should be used with caution in patients with impaired hepatic function or progressive liver disease, since minor alterations of fluid and electrolyte imbalance may precipitate hepatic coma.

Thiazides may add to or potentiate the action of other antihypertensive drugs. Potentiation occurs with ganglionic or peripheral adrenergic blocking drugs.

Sensitivity reactions are more likely to occur in patients with a history of allergy or bronchial asthma.

The possibility of exacerbation or activation of systemic lupus erythematosus has been reported.

PRECAUTIONS

General

Hydralazine. Myocardial stimulation produced by hydralazine can cause anginal attacks and ECG changes indicative of myocardial ischemia. The drug has been implicated in the production of myocardial infarction. It must, therefore, be used with caution in patients with suspected coronary artery disease.

The "hyperdynamic" circulation caused by hydralazine may accentuate specific cardiovascular inadequacies. For example, hydralazine may increase pulmonary artery pressure in patients with mitral valvular disease. The drug may reduce the pressor responses to epinephrine. Postural hypotension may result from hydralazine but is less common than with ganglionic blocking agents. It should be used with caution in patients with cerebral vascular accidents.

In hypertensive patients with normal kidneys who are treated with hydralazine, there is evidence of increased renal blood flow and a maintenance of glomerular filtration rate. In some instances where control values were below normal, improved renal function has been noted after administration of hydralazine. However, as with any antihypertensive agent, hydralazine should be used with caution in patients with advanced renal damage.

Peripheral neuritis, evidenced by paresthesia, numbness, and tingling, has been observed. Published evidence suggests that hydralazine has an antipyridoxine effect and that pyridoxine should be added to the regimen if symptoms develop.

Hydrochlorothiazide. All patients receiving thiazide therapy should be observed for clinical signs of fluid or electrolyte imbalance, namely hyponatremia, hypochloremic alkalosis, and hypokalemia (see **Laboratory Tests** and **Drug/Drug Interactions**). Warning signs are dryness of mouth, thirst, weakness, lethargy, drowsiness, restlessness, muscle pains or cramps, muscular fatigue, hypotension, oliguria, tachy-

cardia, and gastrointestinal disturbance, such as nausea or vomiting.

Hypokalemia may develop, especially in cases of brisk diuresis or severe cirrhosis.

Interference with adequate oral intake of electrolytes will also contribute to hypokalemia. Hypokalemia may be avoided or treated by the use of potassium supplements or foods with a high potassium content.

Any chloride deficit is generally mild and usually does not require specific treatment, except under extraordinary circumstances (as in liver disease or renal disease). Dilutional hyponatremia may occur in edematous patients in hot weather; appropriate therapy is water restriction, rather than administration of salt, except in rare instances when the hyponatremia is life-threatening. In cases of actual salt depletion, appropriate replacement is the therapy of choice.

Hyperuricemia may occur or frank gout may be precipitated in certain patients receiving thiazide therapy.

Latent diabetes may become manifest during thiazide administration (see **Drug/Drug Interactions**).

The antihypertensive effects of the drug may be enhanced in the postsympathectomy patient.

If progressive renal impairment becomes evident, withholding or discontinuing diuretic therapy should be considered.

Calcium excretion is decreased by thiazides. Pathological changes in the parathyroid gland with hypercalcemia and hypophosphatemia have been observed in a few patients on prolonged thiazide therapy. The common complications of hyperparathyroidism, such as renal lithiasis, bone resorption, and peptic ulceration, have not been seen.

Information for Patients

Patients should be informed of possible side effects and advised to take the medication regularly and continuously as directed.

Laboratory Tests

Hydralazine. Complete blood counts and antinuclear antibody titer determinations are indicated before and periodically during prolonged therapy with hydralazine even though the patient is asymptomatic. These studies are also indicated if the patient develops arthralgia, fever, chest pain, continued malaise, or other unexplained signs or symptoms. A positive antinuclear antibody titer requires that the physician carefully weigh the implications of the test results against the benefits to be derived from antihypertensive therapy with a combination drug containing hydralazine. Blood dyscrasias, consisting of reduction in hemoglobin and red cell count, leukopenia, agranulocytosis, and purpura, have been reported. If such abnormalities develop, therapy should be discontinued.

Hydrochlorothiazide. Initial and periodic determinations of serum electrolytes to detect possible electrolyte imbalance should be performed at appropriate intervals.

Serum and urine electrolyte determinations are particularly important when the patient is vomiting excessively or receiving parenteral fluids.

Drug/Drug Interactions

Hydralazine. MAO inhibitors should be used with caution in patients receiving hydralazine.

When other potent parenteral antihypertensive drugs, such as diazoxide, are used in combination with hydralazine, patients should be continously observed for several hours for any excessive fall in blood pressure. Profound hypotensive episodes may occur when diazoxide injections and hydralazine are used concomitantly.

Hydrochlorothiazide. Hypokalemia can sensitize or exaggerate the response of the heart to the toxic effects of digitalis (e.g., increased ventricular irritability).

Hypokalemia may develop during concomitant use of steroids or ACTH.

Insulin requirements in diabetic patients may be increased, decreased, or unchanged.

Thiazides may decrease arterial responsiveness to norepinephrine, but not enough to preclude effectiveness of the pressor agent for therapeutic use.

Thiazides may increase the responsiveness to tubocurarine.

Lithium renal clearance is reduced by thiazides, increasing the risk of lithium toxicity.

Drug/Laboratory Test Interactions

Thiazides may decrease serum levels of protein-bound iodine without signs of thyroid disturbance. Apresazide should be discontinued before tests for parathyroid function are made (See **General, Hydrochlorothiazide,** Calcium excretion).

Carcinogenesis, Mutagenesis, Impairment of Fertility

Hydralazine. In a lifetime study in Swiss albino mice, there was a statistically significant increase in the incidence of lung tumors (adenomas and adenocarcinomas) of both male and female mice given hydralazine continuously in their drinking water at a dosage of about 250 mg/kg per day (about 80 times the maximum recommended human dose). In a 2-year carcinogenicity study of rats given hydralazine by gavage at dosages of 15, 30, and 60 mg/kg per day (approximately 5 to 20 times the recommended human daily dose), microscopic examination of the liver revealed a small, but statistically significant, increase in benign neoplastic nodules in male and female rats from the high-dose group and in female rats from the intermediate-dose group. Benign interstitial cell tumors of the testes were also significantly increased in male rats from the high-dose group. The tumors observed are common in aged rats, and a significantly increased incidence was not observed until 18 months of treatment. Hydralazine was shown to be mutagenic in three bacterial tester strains in the Ames test, both with and without metabolic activation, and elicited DNA repair both in the Pol A^+/A^- *E. coli* bacterial assay system and in cultured rat hepatocytes. (Evidence of DNA damage in the hepatocyte repair test is considered a strong indication of covalent binding, an established property of carcinogens and mutagens.) In tests with rabbit hepatocytes that exhibit an acetylator polymorphism like that of humans, hydralazine elicited DNA repair with only those hepatocytes having a slow rate of acetylation, suggesting that individuals who are rapid acetylators may have a diminished genotoxic liability. No increase in mutagenic potential was revealed in the mouse lymphoma assay, host-mediated assay, nucleus anomaly test, or dominant lethal test.

The extent to which these findings indicate a risk to man is uncertain. While long-term clinical observation has not suggested that human cancer is associated with hydralazine use, epidemiologic studies have so far been insufficient to arrive at any conclusions.

Hydrochlorothiazide. Long-term carcinogenicity studies in animals have not been conducted with hydrochlorothiazide.

Pregnancy Category C

Animal reproduction studies have not been conducted with Apresazide.

Animal studies indicate that hydralazine is teratogenic in mice at 20–30 times the maximum daily human dose of 200–300 mg and possibly in rabbits at 10–15 times the maximum daily human dose, but that it is nonteratogenic in rats. Teratogenic effects observed were cleft palate and malformations of facial and cranial bones. A reproduction study in rats receiving hydrochlorothiazide, 250 mg/kg daily, 62.5 times the maximum daily human dose, has revealed no evidence of impaired fertility or harm to the fetus.

There are not adequate and well-controlled studies of Apresazide in pregnant women. However, thiazides cross the placental barrier and appear in cord blood, and there is a risk of fetal or neonatal jaundice, thrombocytopenia, and possibly other adverse reactions that have occurred in adults. Apresazide should be used during pregnancy only if the potential benefit justifies the potential risk to the fetus.

Nursing Mothers

It is not known whether hydralazine is excreted in human milk. Thiazides are excreted in human milk. Because of the potential for serious adverse reactions in nursing infants, a decision should be made whether to discontinue nursing or to discontinue the drug, taking into account the importance of the drug to the mother.

Pediatric Use

Safety and effectiveness of the combination drug in children have not been established.

ADVERSE REACTIONS

Adverse reactions are usually reversible upon reduction of dosage or discontinuation of Apresazide. Whenever adverse reactions are moderate or severe, it may be necessary to discontinue the drug.

The following adverse reactions have been observed, but there has not been enough systematic collection of data to support an estimate of their frequency.

Hydralazine

Common

Headache, anorexia, nausea, vomiting, diarrhea, palpitations, tachycardia, angina pectoris.

Less Frequent

Digestive: Constipation, paralytic ileus.

Cardiovascular: Hypotension, paradoxical pressor response, edema.

Respiratory: Dyspnea.

Neurologic: Peripheral neuritis, evidenced by paresthesia, numbness, and tingling; dizziness; tremors; muscle cramps; psychotic reactions characterized by depression, disorientation, or anxiety.

Genitourinary: Difficulty in urination.

Hematologic: Blood dyscrasias, consisting of reduction in hemoglobin and red cell count, leukopenia, agranulocytosis, purpura; lymphadenopathy; splenomegaly.

Hypersensitive Reactions: Rash, urticaria, pruritus, fever, chills, arthralgia, eosinophilia, and, rarely, hepatitis.

Other: Nasal congestion, flushing, lacrimation, conjunctivitis.

Hydrochlorothiazide

Digestive: Anorexia, gastric irritation, nausea, vomiting, cramping, diarrhea, constipation, jaundice (intrahepatic cholestatic), pancreatitis, sialadenitis.

Cardiovascular: Orthostatic hypotension (may be potentiated by alcohol, barbiturates, or narcotics).

Neurologic: Dizziness, vertigo, paresthesia, headache, xanthopsia.

Hematologic: Leukopenia, agranulocytosis, thrombocytopenia, aplastic anemia.

Hypersensitive Reactions: Purpura, photosensitivity, rash, urticaria, necrotizing angiitis, Stevens-Johnson syndrome.

Other: Hyperglycemia, glycosuria, hyperuricemia, muscle spasm, weakness, restlessness, transient blurred vision.

OVERDOSAGE

Acute Toxicity

Oral LD_{50}'s in rats (mg/kg): hydralazine, 173 and 187; hydrochlorothiazide, 2750.

Signs and Symptoms

Hydralazine. Signs and symptoms of overdosage include hypotension, tachycardia, headache, and generalized skin flushing.

Complications can include myocardial ischemia and subsequent myocardial infarction, cardiac arrhythmia, and profound shock.

Hydrochlorothiazide. The most prominent feature of poisoning is acute loss of fluid and electrolytes.

Cardiovascular: Tachycardia, hypotension, shock.

Neuromuscular: Weakness, confusion, dizziness, cramps of the calf muscles, paresthesia, fatigue, impairment of consciousness.

Digestive: Nausea, vomiting, thirst.

Renal: Polyuria, oliguria, or anuria (due to hemoconcentration).

Laboratory Findings: Hypokalemia, hyponatremia, hypochloremia, alkalosis: increased BUN (especially in patients with renal insufficiency).

Combined Poisoning: Signs and symptoms may be aggravated or modified by concomitant intake of antihypertensive medication, barbiturates, curare, digitalis (hypokalemia), corticosteroids, narcotics, or alcohol.

Treatment

There is no specific antidote.

The gastric contents should be evacuated, taking adequate precautions against aspiration and for protection of the airway. An activated charcoal slurry may be instilled if conditions permit. Dialysis may not be effective for elimination of Apresazide because of its plasma protein binding (see **CLINICAL PHARMACOLOGY**).

These manipulations may have to be omitted or carried out after cardiovascular status has been stabilized, since they might precipitate cardiac arrhythmias or increase the depth of shock.

Support of the cardiovascular system is of primary importance in suspected hydralazine overdosage. Shock should be treated with plasma expanders. The patient's legs should be kept raised and lost fluid and electrolytes (potassium, sodium) should be replaced. If possible, vasopressors should not be given, but if a vasopressor is required, care should be taken not to precipitate or aggravate cardiac arrhythmia. Tachycardia responds to beta blockers. Digitalization may be necessary, and renal function should be monitored and supported as required.

DOSAGE AND ADMINISTRATION

Dosage should be determined by individual titration (see boxed **WARNING**).

The usual dosage is one Apresazide capsule twice daily, the strength depending upon individual requirement following titration. For maintenance, the dosage should be adjusted to the lowest effective level.

When necessary, other antihypertensive agents such as sympathetic inhibitors may be added gradually in reduced dosages, and the effects should be watched carefully.

HOW SUPPLIED

Capsules 25/25—light blue and white opaque (imprinted APRESAZIDE® 25/25 CIBA 139)

25 mg of hydralazine hydrochloride and 25 mg of hydrochlorothiazide

Bottles of 100 .... NDC 0083-0139-30

Capsules 50/50—pink and white opaque (imprinted APRESAZIDE® 50/50 CIBA 149)

50 mg of hydralazine hydrochloride and 50 mg of hydrochlorothiazide

Bottles of 100 .... NDC 0083-0149-30

Capsules 100/50—flesh pink and white opaque (imprinted APRESAZIDE® 100/50 CIBA 159)

100 mg of hydralazine hydrochloride and 50 mg of hydrochlorothiazide

Bottles of 100 .... NDC 0083-0159-30

Samples, when available, are identified by the word *SAMPLE* appearing on each capsule.

Do not store above 86°F.

Dispense in tight, light-resistant container (USP).

C88-31 (Rev. 9/88)

Shown in Product Identification Section, page 408

APRESOLINE® hydrochloride   ℞

[*a-press'oh-leen*]

hydralazine hydrochloride USP

Tablets

DESCRIPTION

Apresoline, hydralazine hydrochloride USP, is an antihypertensive, available as 10-, 25-, 50-, and 100-mg tablets for oral administration. Its chemical name is 1-hydrazinophthalazine monohydrochloride.

Hydralazine hydrochloride USP is a white to off-white, odorless crystalline powder. It is soluble in water, slightly soluble in alcohol, and very slightly soluble in ether. It melts at about 275°C, with decomposition, and has a molecular weight of 196.64.

Inactive Ingredients: Acacia, D&C Yellow No. 10 (10-mg tablets), FD&C Blue No. 1 (25-mg and 50-mg tablets), FD&C Yellow No. 5 and FD&C Yellow No. 6 (100-mg tablets), lactose, magnesium stearate, mannitol, polyethylene glycol, sodium starch glycolate, starch and stearic acid.

CLINICAL PHARMACOLOGY

Although the precise mechanism of action of hydralazine is not fully understood, the major effects are on the cardiovascular system. Hydralazine apparently lowers blood pressure by exerting a peripheral vasodilating effect through a direct relaxation of vascular smooth muscle. Hydralazine, by altering cellular calcium metabolism, interferes with the calcium movements within the vascular smooth muscle that are responsible for initiating or maintaining the contractile state. The peripheral vasodilating effect of hydralazine results in decreased arterial blood pressure (diastolic more than systolic); decreased peripheral vascular resistance; and an increased heart rate, stroke volume, and cardiac output. The preferential dilatation of arterioles, as compared to veins, minimizes postural hypotension and promotes the increase in cardiac output. Hydralazine usually increases renin activity in plasma, presumably as a result of increased secretion of renin by the renal juxtaglomerular cells in response to reflex sympathetic discharge. This increase in renin activity leads to the production of angiotensin II, which then causes stimulation of aldosterone and consequent sodium reabsorption. Hydralazine also maintains or increases renal and cerebral blood flow.

Hydralazine is rapidly absorbed after oral administration, and peak plasma levels are reached at 1–2 hours. Plasma levels of apparent hydralazine decline with a half-life of 3–7 hours. Binding to human plasma protein is 87%. Plasma levels of hydralazine vary widely among individuals. Hydralazine is subject to polymorphic acetylation; slow acetylators generally have higher plasma levels of hydralazine and require lower doses to maintain control of blood pressure. Hydralazine undergoes extensive hepatic metabolism; it is excreted mainly in the form of metabolites in the urine.

INDICATIONS AND USAGE

Essential hypertension, alone or as an adjunct.

CONTRAINDICATIONS

Hypersensitivity to hydralazine; coronary artery disease; mitral valvular rheumatic heart disease.

WARNINGS

In a few patients hydralazine may produce a clinical picture simulating systemic lupus erythematosus including glomerulonephritis. In such patients hydralazine should be discontinued unless the benefit-to-risk determination requires continued antihypertensive therapy with this drug. Symptoms and signs usually regress when the drug is discontinued but residua have been detected many years later. Long-term treatment with steroids may be necessary. (See **PRECAUTIONS, Laboratory Tests.**)

PRECAUTIONS

General: Myocardial stimulation produced by Apresoline can cause anginal attacks and ECG changes of myocardial ischemia. The drug has been implicated in the production of myocardial infarction. It must, therefore, be used with caution in patients with suspected coronary artery disease.

The "hyperdynamic" circulation caused by Apresoline may accentuate specific cardiovascular inadequacies. For example, Apresoline may increase pulmonary artery pressure in patients with mitral valvular disease. The drug may reduce the pressor responses to epinephrine. Postural hypotension may result from Apresoline but is less common than with ganglionic blocking agents. It should be used with caution in patients with cerebral vascular accidents.

In hypertensive patients with normal kidneys who are treated with Apresoline, there is evidence of increased renal blood flow and a maintenance of glomerular filtration rate.

Continued on next page

The full prescribing information for each CIBA product is contained herein and is that in effect as of September 1, 1989

CIBA—Cont.

In some instances where control values were below normal, improved renal function has been noted after administration of Apresoline. However, as with any antihypertensive agent, Apresoline should be used with caution in patients with advanced renal damage.

Peripheral neuritis, evidenced by paresthesia, numbness, and tingling, has been observed. Published evidence suggests an antipyridoxine effect, and that pyridoxine should be added to the regimen if symptoms develop.

The Apresoline tablets (100 mg) contain FD&C Yellow No. 5 (tartrazine), which may cause allergic-type reactions (including bronchial asthma) in certain susceptible individuals. Although the overall incidence of FD&C Yellow No. 5 (tartrazine) sensitivity in the general population is low, it is frequently seen in patients who are also hypersensitive to aspirin.

Information for Patients: Patients should be informed of possible side effects and advised to take the medication regularly and continuously as directed.

Laboratory Tests: Complete blood counts and antinuclear antibody titer determinations are indicated before and periodically during prolonged therapy with hydralazine even though the patient is asymptomatic. These studies are also indicated if the patient develops arthralgia, fever, chest pain, continued malaise, or other unexplained signs or symptoms. A positive antinuclear antibody titer requires that the physician carefully weigh the implications of the test results against the benefits to be derived from antihypertensive therapy with hydralazine.

Blood dyscrasias, consisting of reduction in hemoglobin and red cell count, leukopenia, agranulocytosis, and purpura, have been reported. If such abnormalities develop, therapy should be discontinued.

Drug/Drug Interactions: MAO inhibitors should be used with caution in patients receiving hydralazine.

When other potent parenteral antihypertensive drugs, such as diazoxide, are used in combination with hydralazine, patients should be continuously observed for several hours for any excessive fall in blood pressure. Profound hypotensive episodes may occur when diazoxide injection and Apresoline are used concomitantly.

Drug/Food Interactions: Administration of hydralazine with food results in higher plasma levels.

Carcinogensis, Mutagenesis, Impairment of Fertility: In a lifetime study in Swiss albino mice, there was a statistically significant increase in the incidence of lung tumors (adenomas and adenocarcinomas) of both male and female mice given hydralazine continuously in their drinking water at a dosage of about 250 mg/kg per day (about 80 times the maximum recommended human dose). In a 2-year carcinogenicity study of rats given hydralazine by gavage at dose levels of 15, 30, and 60 mg/kg/day (approximately 5 to 20 times the recommended human daily dosage), microscopic examination of the liver revealed a small, but statistically significant, increase in benign neoplastic nodules in male and female rats from the high-dose group and in female rats from the intermediate-dose group. Benign interstitial cell tumors of the testes were also significantly increased in male rats from the high-dose group. The tumors observed are common in aged rats and a significantly increased incidence was not observed until 18 months of treatment. Hydralazine was shown to be mutagenic in bacterial systems (Gene Mutation and DNA Repair) and in one of two rat and one rabbit hepatocyte *in vitro* DNA repair studies. Additional *in vivo* and *in vitro* studies using lymphoma cells, germinal cells, and fibroblasts from mice, bone marrow cells from chinese hamsters and fibroblasts from human cell lines did not demonstrate any mutagenic potential for hydralazine.

The extent to which these findings indicate a risk to man is uncertain. While long-term clinical observation has not suggested that human cancer is associated with hydralazine use, epidemiologic studies have so far been insufficient to arrive at any conclusions.

Pregnancy Category C: Animal studies indicate that hydralazine is teratogenic in mice at 20–30 times the maximum daily human dose of 200–300 mg and possibly in rabbits at 10–15 times the maximum daily human dose, but that it is nonteratogenic in rats. Teratogenic effects observed were cleft palate and malformations of facial and cranial bones. There are no adequate and well-controlled studies in pregnant women. Although clinical experience does not include any positive evidence of adverse effects on the human fetus, hydralazine should be used during pregnancy only if the expected benefit justifies the potential risk to the fetus.

Nursing Mothers: It is not known whether this drug is excreted in human milk. Because many drugs are excreted in human milk, caution should be exercised when Apresoline is administered to a nursing woman.

Pediatric Use: Safety and effectiveness in children have not been established in controlled clinical trials, although there is experience with the use of Apresoline in children. The usual recommended oral starting dosage is 0.75 mg/kg of body weight daily in four divided doses. Dosage may be increased gradually over the next 3–4 weeks to a maximum of 7.5 mg/kg or 200 mg daily.

ADVERSE REACTIONS

Adverse reactions with Apresoline are usually reversible when dosage is reduced. However, in some cases it may be necessary to discontinue the drug.

The following adverse reactions have been observed, but there has not been enough systematic collection of data to support an estimate of their frequency.

Common: Headache, anorexia, nausea, vomiting, diarrhea, palpitations, tachycardia, angina pectoris.

Less Frequent: *Digestive:* constipation, paralytic ileus. *Cardiovascular:* hypotension, paradoxical pressor response, edema.

Respiratory: dyspnea.

Neurologic: peripheral neuritis, evidenced by paresthesia, numbness, and tingling; dizziness; tremors; muscle cramps; psychotic reactions characterized by depression, disorientation, or anxiety.

Genitourinary: difficulty in urination.

Hematologic: blood dyscrasias, consisting of reduction in hemoglobin and red cell count, leukopenia, agranulocytosis, purpura; lymphadenopathy; splenomegaly.

Hypersensitive Reactions: rash, urticaria, pruritus, fever, chills, arthralgia, eosinophilia, and, rarely, hepatitis.

Other: nasal congestion, flushing, lacrimation, conjunctivitis.

OVERDOSAGE

Acute Toxicity: No deaths due to acute poisoning have been reported.

Highest known dose survived: adults, 10 g orally.

Oral LD$_{50}$ in rats: 173 and 187 mg/kg.

Signs and Symptoms: Signs and symptoms of overdosage include hypotension, tachycardia, headache, and generalized skin flushing.

Complications can include myocardial ischemia and subsequent myocardial infarction, cardiac arrhythmia, and profound shock.

Treatment: There is no specific antidote.

The gastric contents should be evacuated, taking adequate precautions against aspiration and for protection of the airway. An activated charcoal slurry may be instilled if conditions permit. These manipulations may have to be omitted or carried out after cardiovascular status has been stabilized, since they might precipitate cardiac arrhythmias or increase the depth of shock.

Support of the cardiovascular system is of primary importance. Shock should be treated with plasma expanders. If possible, vasopressors should not be given, but if a vasopressor is required, care should be taken not to precipitate or aggravate cardiac arrhythmia. Tachycardia responds to beta blockers. Digitalization may be necessary, and renal function should be monitored and supported as required.

No experience has been reported with extracorporeal or peritoneal dialysis.

DOSAGE AND ADMINISTRATION

Initiate therapy in gradually increasing dosages; adjust according to individual response. Start with 10 mg four times daily for the first 2–4 days, increase to 25 mg four times daily for the balance of the first week. For the second and subsequent weeks, increase dosage to 50 mg four times daily. For maintenance, adjust dosage to the lowest effective levels.

The incidence of toxic reactions, particularly the L.E. cell syndrome, is high in the group of patients receiving large doses of Apresoline.

In a few resistant patients, up to 300 mg of Apresoline daily may be required for a significant antihypertensive effect. In such cases, a lower dosage of Apresoline combined with a thiazide and/or reserpine or a beta blocker may be considered. However, when combining therapy, individual titration is essential to ensure the lowest possible therapeutic dose of each drug.

HOW SUPPLIED

Tablets 10 mg—round, pale yellow, dry-coated (imprinted CIBA 37)

   Bottles of 100—NDC 0083-0037-30

   Bottles of 1000—NDC 0083-0037-40

   Consumer Pack—One Unit

   12 bottles—100 tablets each—NDC 0083-0037-65

Tablets 25 mg—round, deep blue, dry-coated (imprinted CIBA 39)

   Bottles of 100—NDC 0083-0039-30

   Bottles of 1000—NDC 0083-0039-40

   Consumer Pack—One Unit

   12 bottles—100 tablets each—NDC 0083-0039-65

   Accu-Pak®—Unit Dose (blister pack)

   Box of 100 (strips of 10)—NDC 0083-0039-32

Tablets 50 mg—round, light blue, dry-coated (imprinted CIBA 73)

   Bottles of 100—NDC 0083-0073-30

   Bottles of 1000—NDC 0083-0073-40

   Consumer Pack—One Unit

   12 bottles—100 tablets each—NDC 0083-0073-65

   Accu-Pak®—Unit Dose (blister pack)

   Box of 100 (strips of 10)—NDC 0083-0073-32

Tablets 100 mg—round, peach, dry-coated (imprinted CIBA 101)

   Bottles of 100—NDC 0083-0101-30

Samples, when available, are identified by the word *SAMPLE* appearing on each tablet.

Do not store above 86°F (30°C).

Dispense in tight, light-resistant container (USP).

C88-28 (Rev. 9/88)

Shown in Product Identification Section, page 408

APRESOLINE® hydrochloride   ℞

[a-press 'oh-leen]

hydralazine hydrochloride USP

Parenteral

DESCRIPTION

Apresoline, hydralazine hydrochloride USP, is an antihypertensive available in 1-ml ampuls for intravenous and intramuscular administration. Each milliliter of the sterile, colorless solution contains hydralazine hydrochloride USP, 20 mg; methylparaben NF, 0.65 mg; propylparaben NF, 0.35 mg; propylene glycol USP, 103.6 mg. The pH of the solution is 3.4–4.0. Hydralazine hydrochloride USP is 1-hydrazinophthalazine monohydrochloride.

Hydralazine hydrochloride USP is a white to off-white, odorless crystalline powder. It is soluble in water, slightly soluble in alcohol, and very slightly soluble in ether. It melts at about 275°C, with decomposition, and has a molecular weight of 196.64.

CLINICAL PHARMACOLOGY

Although the precise mechanism of action of hydralazine is not fully understood, the major effects are on the cardiovascular system. Hydralazine apparently lowers blood pressure by exerting a peripheral vasodilating effect through a direct relaxation of vascular smooth muscle. Hydralazine, by altering cellular calcium metabolism, interferes with the calcium movements within the vascular smooth muscle that are responsible for initiating or maintaining the contractile state. The peripheral vasodilating effect of hydralazine results in decreased arterial blood pressure (diastolic more than systolic); decreased peripheral vascular resistance; and an increased heart rate, stroke volume, and cardiac output. The preferential dilatation of arterioles, as compared to veins, minimizes postural hypotension and promotes the increase in cardiac output. Hydralazine usually increases renin activity in plasma, presumably as a result of increased secretion of renin by the renal juxtaglomerular cells in response to reflex sympathetic discharge. This increase in renin activity leads to the production of angiotensin II, which then causes stimulation of aldosterone and consequent sodium reabsorption. Hydralazine also maintains or increases renal and cerebral blood flow.

The average maximal decrease in blood pressure usually occurs 10–80 minutes after administration of parenteral Apresoline. No other pharamacokinetic data on parenteral Apresoline are available.

INDICATIONS AND USAGE

Severe essential hypertension when the drug cannot be given orally or when there is an urgent need to lower blood pressure.

CONTRAINDICATIONS

Hypersensitivity to hydralazine; coronary artery disease; mitral valvular rheumatic heart disease.

WARNINGS

In a few patients hydralazine may produce a clinical picture simulating systemic lupus erythematosus including glomerulonephritis. In such patients hydralazine should be discontinued unless the benefit-to-risk determination requires continued antihypertensive therapy with this drug. Symptoms and signs usually regress when the drug is discontinued but residua have been detected many years later. Long-term treatment with steroids may be necessary. (See **PRECAUTIONS, Laboratory Tests.**)

PRECAUTIONS

General: Myocardial stimulation produced by Apresoline can cause anginal attacks and ECG changes of myocardial ischemia. The drug has been implicated in the production of myocardial infarction. It must, therefore, be used with caution in patients with suspected coronary artery disease.

The "hyperdynamic" circulation caused by Apresoline may accentuate specific cardiovascular inadequacies. For example, Apresoline may increase pulmonary artery pressure in patients with mitral valvular disease. The drug may reduce the pressor responses to epinephrine. Postural hypotension may result from Apresoline but is less common than with ganglionic blocking agents. It should be used with caution in patients with cerebral vascular accidents.

In hypertensive patients with normal kidneys who are treated with Apresoline, there is evidence of increased renal blood flow and a maintenance of glomerular filtration rate.

In some instances where control values were below normal, improved renal function has been noted after administration of Apresoline. However, as with any antihypertensive agent, Apresoline should be used with caution in patients with advanced renal damage.

Peripheral neuritis, evidenced by paresthesia, numbness, and tingling, has been observed. Published evidence suggests an antipyridoxine effect, and that pyridoxine should be added to the regimen if symptoms develop.

Laboratory Tests: Complete blood counts and antinuclear antibody titer determinations are indicated before and periodically during prolonged therapy with hydralazine even though the patient is asymptomatic. These studies are also indicated if the patient develops arthralgia, fever, chest pain, continued malaise, or other unexplained signs or symptoms. A positive antinuclear antibody titer requires that the physician carefully weigh the implications of the test results against the benefits to be derived from antihypertensive therapy with hydralazine.

Blood dyscrasias, consisting of reduction in hemoglobin and red cell count, leukopenia, agranulocytosis, and purpura, have been reported. If such abnormalities develop, therapy should be discontinued.

Drug/Drug Interactions: MAO inhibitors should be used with caution in patients receiving hydralazine.

When other potent parenteral antihypertensive drugs, such as diazoxide, are used in combination with hydralazine, patients should be continuously observed for several hours for any excessive fall in blood pressure. Profound hypotensive episodes may occur when diazoxide injection and Apresoline are used concomitantly.

Carcinogenesis, Mutagenesis, Impairment of Fertility: In a lifetime study in Swiss albino mice, there was a statistically significant increase in the incidence of lung tumors (adenomas and adenocarcinomas) of both male and female mice given hydralazine continuously in their drinking water at a dosage of about 250 mg/kg per day (about 80 times the maximum recommended human dose). In a 2-year carcinogenicity study of rats given hydralazine by gavage at dose levels of 15, 30, and 60 mg/kg/day (approximately 5 to 20 times the recommended human daily dosage), microscopic examination of the liver revealed a small, but statistically significant, increase in benign neoplastic nodules in male and female rats from the high-dose group and in female rats from the intermediate-dose group. Benign interstitial cell tumors of the testes were also significantly increased in male rats from the high-dose group. The tumors observed are common in aged rats and a significantly increased incidence was not observed until 18 months of treatment. Hydralazine was shown to be mutagenic in bacterial systems (Gene Mutation and DNA Repair) and in one of two rat and one rabbit hepatocyte in vitro DNA repair studies. Additional in vivo and in vitro studies using lymphoma cells, germinal cells, and fibroblasts from mice, bone marrow cells from chinese hamsters and fibroblasts from human cell lines did not demonstrate any mutagenic potential for hydralazine.

The extent to which these findings indicate a risk to man is uncertain. While long-term clinical observation has not suggested that human cancer is associated with hydralazine use, epidemiologic studies have so far been insufficient to arrive at any conclusions.

Pregnancy Category C: Animal studies indicate that hydralazine is teratogenic in mice at 20–30 times the maximum daily human dose of 200–300 mg and possibly in rabbits at 10–15 times the maximum daily human dose, but that it is nonteratogenic in rats. Teratogenic effects observed were cleft palate and malformations of facial and cranial bones. There are no adequate and well-controlled studies in pregnant women. Although clinical experience does not include any positive evidence of adverse effects on the human fetus, hydralazine should be used during pregnancy only if the expected benefit justifies the potential risk to the fetus.

Nursing Mothers: It is not known whether this drug is excreted in human milk. Because many drugs are excreted in human milk, caution should be exercised when Apresoline is administered to a nursing woman.

Pediatric Use: Safety and effectiveness in children have not been established in controlled clinical trials, although there is experience with the use of Apresoline in children. The usual recommended parenteral dosage, administered intramuscularly or intravenously, is 1.7–3.5 mg/kg of body weight daily, divided into four to six doses.

ADVERSE REACTIONS

Adverse reactions with Apresoline are usually reversible when dosage is reduced. However, in some cases it may be necessary to discontinue the drug.

The following adverse reactions have been observed, but there has not been enough systematic collection of data to support an estimate of their frequency.

Common: Headache, anorexia, nausea, vomiting, diarrhea, palpitations, tachycardia, angina pectoris.

Less Frequent: *Digestive:* constipation, paralytic ileus. *Cardiovascular:* hypotension, paradoxical pressor response, edema.

Respiratory: dyspnea.
Neurologic: peripheral neuritis, evidenced by paresthesia, numbness, and tingling; dizziness; tremors; muscle cramps; psychotic reactions characterized by depression, disorientation, or anxiety.
Genitourinary: difficulty in urination.
Hematologic: blood dyscrasias, consisting of reduction in hemoglobin and red cell count, leukopenia, agranulocytosis, purpura; lymphadenopathy; splenomegaly.
Hypersensitive Reactions: rash, urticaria, pruritus, fever, chills, arthralgia, eosinophilia, and, rarely, hepatitis.
Other: nasal congestion, flushing, lacrimation, conjunctivitis.

OVERDOSAGE

Acute Toxicity: No deaths due to acute poisoning have been reported.
Highest known dose survived: adults, 10 g orally.
Oral LD_{50} in rats: 173 and 187 mg/kg.
Signs and Symptoms: Signs and symptoms of overdosage include hypotension, tachycardia, headache, and generalized skin flushing.
Complications can include myocardial ischemia and subsequent myocardial infarction, cardiac arrhythmia, and profound shock.
Treatment: There is no specific antidote.
Support of the cardiovascular system is of primary importance. Shock should be treated with plasma expanders. If possible, vasopressors should not be given, but if a vasopressor is required, care should be taken not to precipitate or aggravate cardiac arrhythmia. Tachycardia responds to beta blockers. Digitalization may be necessary, and renal function should be monitored and supported as required.
No experience has been reported with extracorporeal or peritoneal dialysis.

DOSAGE AND ADMINISTRATION

When there is urgent need, therapy in the hospitalized patient may be initiated intramuscularly or as a rapid intravenous bolus injection directly into the vein. Parenteral Apresoline should be used only when the drug cannot be given orally. The usual dose is 20–40 mg, repeated as necessary. Certain patients (especially those with marked renal damage) may require a lower dose. Blood pressure should be checked frequently. It may begin to fall within a few minutes after injection, with the average maximal decrease occurring in 10–80 minutes. In cases where there has been increased intracranial pressure, lowering the blood pressure may increase cerebral ischemia. Most patients can be transferred to oral Apresoline within 24–48 hours.
The product should be used immediately after the ampul is opened. It should not be added to infusion solutions. Apresoline hydrochloride parenteral may discolor upon contact with metal; discolored solutions should be discarded. Parenteral drug products should be inspected visually for particulate matter and discoloration prior to administration, whenever solution and container permit.

HOW SUPPLIED

Ampuls 1 ml, containing 20 mg of hydralazine hydrochloride
Cartons of 5 ampuls—NDC 0083-2626-05
See **Dosage and Administration.**
Store between 59° and 86°F (15°-30°C).
Dist. by:
CIBA Pharmaceutical Company
Division of CIBA-GEIGY Corporation
Summit, New Jersey 07901
C86-15 (Rev. 4/86)

APRESOLINE®-ESIDRIX® ℞
[a-press 'oh-leen ess 'a-dricks]
hydralazine hydrochloride and hydrochlorothiazide Combination Tablets

---

WARNING
This fixed-combination drug is not indicated for initial therapy of hypertension. Hypertension requires therapy titrated to the individual patient. If the fixed combination represents the dosage so determined, its use may be more convenient in patient management. The treatment of hypertension is not static but must be reevaluated as conditions in each patient warrant.

DESCRIPTION

Apresoline-Esidrix is an antihypertensive-diuretic combination, available as tablets containing hydralazine hydrochloride USP, 25 mg, and hydrochlorothiazide USP, 15 mg, for oral administration.
Hydralazine hydrochloride is 1-hydrazinophthalazine monohydrochloride.
Hydralazine hydrochloride USP is a white to off-white, odorless crystalline powder. It is soluble in water, slightly soluble in alcohol, and very slightly soluble in ether. It melts at

about 275°C, with decomposition, and has a molecular weight of 196.64.
Hydrochlorothiazide is 6-chloro-3,4-dihydro-2H-1,2,4-benzothiadiazine-7-sulfonamide 1,1-dioxide.
Hydrochlorothiazide USP is a white, or practically white, practically odorless crystalline powder. It is slightly soluble in water; freely soluble in sodium hydroxide solution, in n-butylamine, and in dimethylformamide; sparingly soluble in methanol; and insoluble in ether, in chloroform, and in dilute mineral acids. Its molecular weight is 297.73.
Inactive Ingredients: Acacia, FD&C Yellow No. 6, lactose, polyethylene glycol, starch, stearic acid and sucrose.

CLINICAL PHARMACOLOGY

Hydralazine
Although the precise mechanism of action of hydralazine is not fully understood, the major effects are on the cardiovascular system. Hydralazine apparently lowers blood pressure by exerting a peripheral vasodilating effect through a direct relaxation of vascular smooth muscle. Hydralazine, by altering cellular calcium metabolism, interferes with the calcium movements within the vascular smooth muscle that are responsible for initiating or maintaining the contractile state. The peripheral vasodilating effect of hydralazine results in decreased arterial blood pressure (diastolic more than systolic); decreased peripheral vascular resistance; and an increased heart rate, stroke volume, and cardiac output. The preferential dilatation of arterioles, as compared to veins, minimizes postural hypotension and promotes the increase in cardiac output. Hydralazine usually increases renin activity in plasma, presumably as a result of increased secretion of renin by the renal juxtaglomerular cells in response to reflex sympathetic discharge. This increase in renin activity leads to the production of angiotensin II, which then causes stimulation of aldosterone and consequent sodium reabsorption. Hydralazine also maintains or increases renal and cerebral blood flow.

Hydrochlorothiazide
Thiazides affect the renal tubular mechanism of electrolyte reabsorption. At maximal therapeutic dosage, all thiazides are approximately equal in their diuretic potency. Thiazides increase excretion of sodium and chloride in approximately equivalent amounts. Natriuresis causes a secondary loss of potassium.
The mechanism of the antihypertensive effect of thiazides is unknown. Thiazides do not affect normal blood pressure.

Pharmacokinetics
The Apresoline-Esidrix tablet is bioequivalent to Apresoline (hydralazine) and Esidrix (hydrochlorothiazide) tablets administered simultaneously.
Hydralazine: Hydralazine is rapidly absorbed after oral administration, and peak plasma levels are reached at 1–2 hours. Plasma levels decline with a half-life of 3–7 hours. Binding to human plasma protein is 87%. Plasma levels of hydralazine vary widely among individuals. Hydralazine is subject to polymorphic acetylation; slow acetylators generally have higher plasma levels of hydralazine and require lower doses to maintain control of blood pressure. Hydralazine undergoes extensive hepatic metabolism; it is excreted mainly in the form of metabolites in the urine.
Administration of hydralazine with food results in higher levels of the drug in plasma.
Hydrochlorothiazide: Onset of action of thiazides occurs in 2 hours and the peak effect at about 4 hours. The action persists for approximately 6–12 hours. Hydrochlorothiazide is rapidly absorbed, as indicated by peak concentrations 1–2.5 hours after oral administration. Plasma levels of the drug are proportional to dose; the concentration in whole blood is 1.6–1.8 times higher than in plasma. Thiazides are eliminated rapidly by the kidney. After oral administration of 25- to 100-mg doses, 72–97% of the dose is excreted in the urine, indicating dose-independent absorption. Hydrochlorothiazide is eliminated from plasma in a biphasic fashion with a terminal half-life of 10–17 hours. Plasma protein binding is 67.9%. Plasma clearance is 15.9–30.0 L/hr; volume of distribution is 3.6–7.8 L/kg.
Gastrointestinal absorption of hydrochlorothiazide is enhanced when administered with food. Absorption is decreased in patients with congestive heart failure, and the pharmacokinetics are considerably different in these patients.

INDICATIONS AND USAGE
Hypertension (see boxed **WARNING**).

CONTRAINDICATIONS
Hydralazine
Hypersensitivity to hydralazine; coronary artery disease; mitral valvular rheumatic heart disease.

Continued on next page

CIBA—Cont.

Hydrochlorothiazide
Anuria; hypersensitivity to this or other sulfonamide-derived drugs.

WARNINGS

Hydralazine
In a few patients hydralazine may produce a clinical picture simulating systemic lupus erythematosus including glomerulonephritis. In such patients hydralazine should be discontinued unless the benefit-to-risk determination requires continued antihypertensive therapy with this drug. Signs and symptoms usually regress when the drug is discontinued, but residua have been detected many years later. Long-term treatment with steroids may be necessary. (See **PRECAUTIONS, Laboratory Tests.**)

Hydrochlorothiazide
Thiazides should be used with caution in patients with severe renal disease. In patients with renal disease, thiazides may precipitate azotemia. Cumulative effects of the drug may develop in patients with impaired renal function.
Thiazides should be used with caution in patients with impaired hepatic function or progressive liver disease, since minor alterations of fluid and electrolyte imbalance may precipitate hepatic coma.
Thiazides may add to or potentiate the action of other antihypertensive drugs. Potentiation occurs with ganglionic or peripheral adrenergic blocking drugs.
Sensitivity reactions are more likely to occur in patients with a history of allergy or bronchial asthma.
The possibility of exacerbation or activation of systemic lupus erythematosus has been reported.

PRECAUTIONS

General
Hydralazine: Myocardial stimulation produced by hydralazine can cause anginal attacks and ECG changes indicative of myocardial ischemia. The drug has been implicated in the production of myocardial infarction. It must, therefore, be used with caution in patients with suspected coronary artery disease.
The "hyperdynamic" circulation caused by hydralazine may accentuate specific cardiovascular inadequacies. For example, hydralazine may increase pulmonary artery pressure in patients with mitral valvular disease. The drug may reduce the pressor responses to epinephrine. Postural hypotension may result from hydralazine but is less common than with ganglionic blocking agents. It should be used with caution in patients with cerebral vascular accidents.
In hypertensive patients with normal kidneys who are treated with hydralazine, there is evidence of increased renal blood flow and a maintenance of glomerular filtration rate. In some instances where control values were below normal, improved renal function has been noted after administration of hydralazine. However, as with any antihypertensive agent, hydralazine should be used with caution in patients with advanced renal damage.
Peripheral neuritis, evidenced by paresthesia, numbness, and tingling, has been observed. Published evidence suggests that hydralazine has an antipyridoxine effect and that pyridoxine should be added to the regimen if symptoms develop.
Hydrochlorothiazide: All patients receiving thiazide therapy should be observed for clinical signs of fluid or electrolyte imbalance, namely hyponatremia, hypochloremic alkalosis, and hypokalemia (see **Laboratory Tests** and **Drug/Drug Interactions**). Warning signs are dryness of mouth, thirst, weakness, lethargy, drowsiness, restlessness, muscle pains or cramps, muscular fatigue, hypotension, oliguria, tachycardia, and gastrointestinal disturbance, such as nausea or vomiting.
Hypokalemia may develop, especially in cases of brisk diuresis or severe cirrhosis.
Interference with adequate oral intake of electrolytes will also contribute to hypokalemia. Hypokalemia may be avoided or treated by use of potassium supplements or foods with a high potassium content.
Any chloride deficit is generally mild and usually does not require specific treatment, except under extraordinary circumstances (as in liver disease or renal disease). Dilutional hyponatremia may occur in edematous patients in hot weather; appropriate therapy is water restriction, rather than administration of salt, except in rare instances when the hyponatremia is life-threatening. In cases of actual salt depletion, appropriate replacement is the therapy of choice.
Hyperuricemia may occur or frank gout may be precipitated in certain patients receiving thiazide therapy.
Latent diabetes may become manifest during thiazide administration (see **Drug/Drug Interactions**).
The antihypertensive effects of the drug may be enhanced in the postsympathectomy patient.
If progressive renal impairment becomes evident, withholding or discontinuing diuretic therapy should be considered.
Calcium excretion is decreased by thiazides. Pathological changes in the parathyroid gland with hypercalcemia and

hypophosphatemia have been observed in a few patients on prolonged thiazide therapy. The common complications of hyperparathyroidism, such as renal lithiasis, bone resorption, and peptic ulceration, have not been seen.
Information for Patients: Patients should be informed of possible side effects and advised to take the medication regularly and continuously as directed.

Laboratory Tests
Hydralazine: Complete blood counts and antinuclear antibody titer determinations are indicated before and periodically during prolonged therapy with hydralazine even though the patient is asymptomatic. These studies are also indicated if the patient develops arthralgia, fever, chest pain, continued malaise, or other unexplained signs or symptoms. A positive antinuclear antibody titer requires that the physician carefully weigh the implications of the test results against the benefits to be derived from antihypertensive therapy with a combination drug containing hydralazine.
Blood dyscrasias, consisting of reduction in hemoglobin and red cell count, leukopenia, agranulocytosis, and purpura, have been reported. If such abnormalities develop, therapy should be discontinued.
Hydrochlorothiazide: Initial and periodic determinations of serum electrolytes to detect possible electrolyte imbalance should be performed at appropriate intervals.
Serum and urine electrolyte determinations are particularly important when the patient is vomiting excessively or receiving parenteral fluids.

Drug/Drug Interactions
Hydralazine: MAO inhibitors should be used with caution in patients receiving hydralazine.
When other potent parenteral antihypertensive drugs, such as diazoxide, are used in combination with hydralazine, patients should be continuously observed for several hours for any excessive fall in blood pressure. Profound hypotensive episodes may occur when diazoxide injections and hydralazine are used concomitantly.
Hydrochlorothiazide: Hypokalemia can sensitize or exaggerate the response of the heart to the toxic effects of digitalis (e.g., increased ventricular irritability).
Hypokalemia may develop during concomitant use of steroids or ACTH.
Insulin requirements in diabetic patients may be increased, decreased, or unchanged.
Thiazides may decrease arterial responsiveness to norepinephrine, but not enough to preclude effectiveness of the pressor agent for therapeutic use.
Thiazides may increase the responsiveness to tubocurarine.
Lithium renal clearance is reduced by thiazides, increasing the risk of lithium toxicity.
There have been rare reports in the literature of hemolytic anemia occurring with the concomitant use of hydrochlorothiazide and methyldopa.
Concurrent administration of some non-steroidal anti-inflammatory agents may reduce the diuretic, natriuretic and antihypertensive effects of thiazide diuretics.

Drug/Laboratory Test Interactions
Thiazides may decrease serum levels of protein-bound iodine without signs of thyroid disturbance. Apresoline-Esidrix should be discontinued before tests for parathyroid function are made (See **General, Hydrochlorothiazide,** Calcium excretion).

Carcinogenesis, Mutagenesis, Impairment of Fertility
Hydralazine: In a lifetime study in Swiss albino mice, there was a statistically significant increase in the incidence of lung tumors (adenomas and adenocarcinomas) of both male and female mice given hydralazine continuously in their drinking water at a dosage of about 250 mg/kg per day (about 80 times the maximum recommended human dose). In a 2-year carcinogenicity study of rats given hydralazine by gavage at dose levels of 15, 30, and 60 mg/kg/day (approximately 5 to 20 times the recommended human daily dose), microscopic examination of the liver revealed a small, but statistically significant, increase in benign neoplastic nodules in male and female rats from the high-dose group and in female rats from the intermediate-dose group. Benign interstitial cell tumors of the testes were also significantly increased in male rats from the high-dose group. The tumors observed are common in aged rats and a significantly increased incidence was not observed until 18 months of treatment. Hydralazine was shown to be mutagenic in bacterial systems (Gene Mutation and DNA Repair) and in one of two rat and one rabbit hepatocyte *in vitro* DNA repair studies. Additional *in vivo* and *in vitro* studies using lymphoma cells, germinal cells, and fibroblasts from mice, bone marrow cells from chinese hamsters and fibroblasts from human cell lines did not demonstrate any mutagenic potential for hydralazine.
The extent to which these findings indicate a risk to man is uncertain. While long-term clinical observation has not suggested that human cancer is associated with hydralazine use, epidemiologic studies have so far been insufficient to arrive at any conclusions.
Hydrochlorothiazide: Long-term carcinogenicity studies in animals have not been conducted with Esidrix. Hydrochlorothiazide was not mutagenic in in vitro Ames mutagenicity

assay of Salmonella typhimurium strains TA 98, TA 100, TA 1535 and TA 1537 or in in vivo mutagenicity assays of mouse germinal cell chromosomes and chinese hamster bone marrow cell chromosomes. It was however, mutagenic in inducing nondisjunction (96% frequency) in diploid strains of Aspergillus nidulans.

Pregnancy Category C
Animal reproduction studies have not been conducted with Apresoline-Esidrix. Animal studies indicate that hydralazine is teratogenic in mice at 20–30 times the maximum daily human dose of 200–300 mg and possibly in rabbits at 10–15 times the maximum daily human dose, but that it is nonteratogenic in rats. Teratogenic effects observed were cleft palate and malformations of facial and cranial bones. A reproduction study in rats receiving hydrochlorothiazide, 250 mg/kg daily, 62.5 times the maximum daily human dose, has revealed no evidence of impaired fertility or harm to the fetus.
There are no adequate and well-controlled studies of Apresoline-Esidrix in pregnant women. However, thiazides cross the placental barrier and appear in cord blood, and there is a risk of fetal or neonatal jaundice, thrombocytopenia, and possibly other adverse reactions that have occurred in adults. Apresoline-Esidrix should be used during pregnancy only if the potential benefit justifies the potential risk to the fetus.
Nursing Mothers: It is not known whether hydralazine is excreted in human milk. Thiazides are excreted in human milk. Because of the potential for serious adverse reactions in nursing infants, a decision should be made whether to discontinue nursing or to discontinue the drug, taking into account the importance of the drug to the mother.
Pediatric Use: Safety and effectiveness of the combination drug in children have not been established.

ADVERSE REACTIONS

Adverse reactions are usually reversible upon reduction of dosage or discontinuation of Apresoline-Esidrix. Whenever adverse reactions are moderate or severe, it may be necessary to discontinue the drug.
The following adverse reactions have been observed, but there has not been enough systematic collection of data to support an estimate of their frequency.

Hydralazine
Common: Headache, anorexia, nausea, vomiting, diarrhea, palpitations, tachycardia, angina pectoris.
Less Frequent: *Digestive:* constipation, paralytic ileus.
Cardiovascular: hypotension, paradoxical pressor response, edema.
Respiratory: dyspnea.
Neurologic: peripheral neuritis, evidenced by paresthesia, numbness, and tingling; dizziness; tremors; muscle cramps; psychotic reactions characterized by depression, disorientation, or anxiety.
Genitourinary: difficulty in urination.
Hematologic: blood dyscrasias, consisting of reduction in hemoglobin and red cell count, leukopenia, agranulocytosis, purpura; lymphadenopathy; splenomegaly.
Hypersensitive Reactions: rash, urticaria, pruritus, fever, chills, arthralgia, eosinophilia, and, rarely, hepatitis.
Other: nasal congestion, flushing, lacrimation, conjunctivitis.
Hydrochlorothiazide: *Digestive:* anorexia, gastric irritation, nausea, vomiting, cramping, diarrhea, constipation, jaundice (intrahepatic cholestatic), pancreatitis, sialadenitis.
Cardiovascular: orthostatic hypotension (may be potentiated by alcohol, barbiturates, or narcotics).
Neurologic: dizziness, vertigo, paresthesia, headache, xanthopsia.
Hematologic: leukopenia, agranulocytosis, thrombocytopenia, aplastic anemia.
Hypersensitive Reactions: purpura, photosensitivity, rash, urticaria, necrotizing angiitis, Stevens-Johnson syndrome.
Other: hyperglycemia, glycosuria, hyperuricemia, muscle spasm, weakness, restlessness, transient blurred vision.

OVERDOSAGE

Acute Toxicity: No deaths due to acute poisoning with Apresoline-Esidrix have been reported.
Oral LD_{50}'s in rats (mg/kg): hydralazine, 173 and 187; hydrochlorothiazide, 2750.
Signs and Symptoms
Hydralazine: Signs and symptoms of overdosage include hypotension, tachycardia, headache, and generalized skin flushing.
Complications can include myocardial ischemia and subsequent myocardial infarction, cardiac arrhythmia, and profound shock.
Hydrochlorothiazide: The most prominent feature of poisoning is acute loss of fluid and electrolytes.
Cardiovascular: tachycardia, hypotension, shock.
Neuromuscular: weakness, confusion, dizziness, cramps of the calf muscles, paresthesia, fatigue, impairment of consciousness.

Digestive: nausea, vomiting, thirst.
Renal: polyuria, oliguria, or anuria (due to hemoconcentration).
Laboratory Findings: hypokalemia, hyponatremia, hypochloremia, alkalosis; increased BUN (especially in patients with renal insufficiency).
Combined Poisoning: Signs and symptoms may be aggravated or modified by concomitant intake of antihypertensive medication, barbiturates, curare, digitalis (hypokalemia), corticosteroids, narcotics, or alcohol.
Treatment: There is no specific antidote.
The gastric contents should be evacuated, taking adequate precautions against aspiration and for protection of the airway. An activated charcoal slurry may be instilled if conditions permit. Dialysis may not be effective for elimination of Apresoline-Esidrix because of its plasma protein binding (see **CLINICAL PHARMACOLOGY**).
These manipulations may have to be omitted or carried out after cardiovascular status has been stabilized, since they might precipitate cardiac arrhythmias or increase the depth of shock.
Support of the cardiovascular system is of primary importance in suspected hydralazine overdosage. Shock should be treated with plasma expanders. The patient's legs should be kept raised and lost fluid and electrolytes (potassium, sodium) should be replaced. If possible, vasopressors should not be given, but if a vasopressor is required, care should be taken not to precipitate or aggravate cardiac arrhythmia. Tachycardia responds to beta blockers. Digitalization may be necessary, and renal function should be monitored and supported as required.

DOSAGE AND ADMINISTRATION

Dosage should be determined by individual titration (see boxed **WARNING**).
The usual dosage is one tablet three times daily (maximal dosage is two tablets three times daily). For maintenance, dosage should be adjusted to the lowest effective level.
When necessary, other antihypertensive agents such as sympathetic inhibitors may be added gradually in reduced dosages and the effects should be watched carefully.

HOW SUPPLIED

Tablets —round, orange, dry-coated (imprinted CIBA 129) 25 mg of hydralazine hydrochloride and 15 mg of hydrochlorothiazide
Bottles of 100—NDC 0083-0129-30
Do not store above 86°F (30°C).
Dispense in tight, light-resistant container (USP).
C88-35 (Rev. 11/88)
Shown in Product Identification Section, page 408

CIBACALCIN®   ℞
calcitonin-human for injection
Syringes

DESCRIPTION

Cibacalcin, calcitonin-human for injection, is a synthetic polypeptide hormone consisting of 32 amino acids in the same linear sequence as found in naturally occurring human calcitonin.
All amino acids are in their optically active L configuration.
Cibacalcin is a white to off-white amorphous powder containing 3 moles of hydrochloric acid, bound to the basic peptide groups, and up to 8% (w/w) acetic acid and 10% (w/w) water. It is soluble in water, in physiological saline, in dilute acid, and in dilute base; sparingly soluble in methanol; and practically insoluble in chloroform. Its molecular formula is $C_{151}H_{226}N_{40}O_{45}S_3 \cdot 3HCl$ which corresponds to a molecular weight of 3527.2.
Cibacalcin is available in double-chambered, disposable, vial syringes for subcutaneous administration. The double-chambered syringes contain calcitonin-human for injection, 0.5 mg, and mannitol, 20 mg, in sterile, lyophilized form in one chamber, and a 1-ml solution of 30 mg of mannitol in Water for Injection in the other chamber.

CLINICAL PHARMACOLOGY

Calcitonins are polypeptide hormones secreted by the parafollicular or C-cells of the thyroid gland in mammals and by the ultimobranchial gland of birds and fish.
The precise physiologic functions of the calcitonins have not been completely defined; they appear to play a role in the regulation of calcium and bone metabolism. When Cibacalcin is given to normal subjects, serum calcium is lowered and urinary excretion of calcium, phosphorus, and sodium increases. Cibacalcin has also been shown to inhibit the pancreatic secretion of enzymes and gastric secretion during acute administration. The significance of these effects during chronic therapy, however, has not been investigated.
The metabolic clearance rate of exogenously administered immunoreactive Cibacalcin in normal subjects has been determined to be 8.4 ± 1.1 ml/kg per min. The half-life is 1.02 hours after single, subcutaneous doses of 0.5 mg. Evidence to date indicates that the kidney is the principal organ

responsible for its degradation, with only small fractions of the parent substance (0.1%) appearing in the urine.
In Paget's disease (osteitis deformans), Cibacalcin causes a decrease in serum alkaline phosphatase and in urinary hydroxyproline excretion. Among 44 patients in clinical studies who had one or more determinations of serum alkaline phosphatase and 29 patients who had one or more determinations of urinary hydroxyproline during the first year of therapy, the following mean percent reductions from baseline were observed:

	Mean % Reduction (n*)	
Time Interval†	Serum Alkaline Phosphatase	Urinary Hydroxyproline
1–3 months	23.4(30)	21.4(20)
4–6 months	41.0(22)	47.4(12)
7–12 months	44.7(25)	56.1(14)

† Duration of treatment at time of observation
* Number of patients evaluated at each time interval
The mean reduction in serum alkaline phosphatase at the final visit compared to baseline for these patients was 36.1% (mean duration of treatment = 18.5 months) and for urinary hydroxyproline was 37.5% (mean duration of treatment = 21.2 months).
In a limited number of studies, patients treated with Cibacalcin have been reported to show radiological evidence of bone remodeling towards normal, including healing of lytic lesions. Serial biopsies of Pagetic bone indicate a decrease in the number of osteoclasts per square millimeter of bone during treatment.
The risk of diminishing effectiveness as a result of antibody formation or hypersensitivity reactions is less with Cibacalcin than with nonhuman forms of the hormone.
Long-term treatment (up to ten or more years in a few patients) with Cibacalcin has not been limited by antibody-mediated resistance.
Cibacalcin has been shown to be effective in patients who have developed resistance to nonhuman calcitonins.

INDICATIONS AND USAGE

Cibacalcin is indicated for the treatment of symptomatic Paget's disease of bone.
The effectiveness of Cibacalcin was demonstrated primarily in patients with moderate-to-severe disease characterized by multiple bone involvement and elevations of serum alkaline phosphatase and urinary hydroxyproline excretion.
Although reduction of serum alkaline phosphatase and urinary hydroxyproline excretion usually occurs within 3 months after initiation of treatment, maximum reductions may not occur until after 6–24 months of continuous treatment.
Cibacalcin has been reported to cause subjective relief of bone pain and tenderness and a reduction in elevated skin temperature over the affected skeletal areas in some patients.

CONTRAINDICATIONS

None known.

WARNINGS

Since Cibacalcin is a protein, the possibility of a systemic allergic reaction should not be disregarded. Therefore, appropriate materials for the emergency treatment of such a reaction should be available.
The incidence of osteogenic sarcoma is known to be increased in Paget's disease. Pagetic lesions, with or without therapy, may appear by X-ray to progress markedly, possibly with some loss of definition of periosteal margins. Such lesions must be evaluated carefully to differentiate them from osteogenic sarcoma.

PRECAUTIONS

General
The administration of Cibacalcin could lead to hypocalcemic tetany, under special circumstances. Calcium for parenteral administration should be available during the first few administrations of Cibacalcin.
Information for Patients
Patients and other persons who may administer Cibacalcin should receive careful instruction in sterile-injection techniques.
Carcinogenesis, Mutagenesis, Impairment of Fertility
No long-term carcinogenicity studies have been conducted with Cibacalcin.
Pregnancy Category C
Animal reproduction studies have not been conducted with Cibacalcin. However, salmon calcitonin has been shown to cause a decrease in fetal birth weight in rabbits when given in doses 14–56 times the dose recommended for human use. Calcitonin does not cross the placental barrier. This finding may be due to metabolic effects of the drug on the pregnant animal. It is also not known whether Cibacalcin can cause fetal harm when administered to a pregnant woman or can affect reproduction capacity. Cibacalcin should be given to a pregnant woman only if clearly needed.

Nursing Mothers
It is not known whether this drug is excreted in human milk. Because Cibacalcin is a peptide and subject to digestion in the gastrointestinal tract, it is unlikely that active drug will be absorbed by the nursing infant. However, studies of drug activity after ingestion have not been done in nursing infants and caution should be exercised when Cibacalcin is administered to a nursing woman. Calcitonin has been shown to inhibit lactation in animals.
Pediatric Use
The use of Cibacalcin has been reported in the rare disorders of bone in children referred to as juvenile Paget's disease. However, the safety and effectiveness of Cibacalcin in children have not been established.

ADVERSE REACTIONS

The adverse reaction rates listed below are based on studies that included a large proportion of patients with histories of unresponsiveness to nonhuman calcitonins, a number of whom also had displayed intolerance to those calcitonins.
Gastrointestinal: Nausea, with or without vomiting, was noted in about 14% to 21% of patients treated with the recommended dose of Cibacalcin. Anorexia, diarrhea, epigastric discomfort, or abdominal pain were reported in a few patients. Nausea improved in the majority of patients with continued therapy.
Dermatologic/Hypersensitivity: Flushing of face, ears, or hands occurred within minutes of injection in 16% to 21% of patients treated with the recommended dose. Flushing improved in the majority of patients with continued therapy. Skin rashes were reported rarely.
Genitourinary: Increased frequency of urination was noted in about 5% to 10% of patients.
Metabolic: Mild tetanic symptoms were reported rarely during Cibacalcin therapy. One patient developed asymptomatic mild hypercalcemia during a study.
Miscellaneous: Rare side effects included chills, chest pressure, weakness, headache, tenderness of palms and soles, dizziness, nasal congestion, shortness of breath, metallic taste, and paresthesia.

OVERDOSAGE

Dosages greater than 1 mg per day have not been administered chronically. In animals, single doses as high as 1,000 mg/kg produced no mortality or functional or structural organ changes.

DOSAGE AND ADMINISTRATION

The recommended starting dosage of Cibacalcin is 0.5 mg daily, given subcutaneously.
Some patients may obtain sufficient clinical and biochemical improvement with a dosage of 0.5 mg two or three times weekly or 0.25 mg daily.
As an aid in evaluating the efficacy of Cibacalcin, determination of serum alkaline phosphatase and urinary hydroxyproline excretion should be performed prior to initiation of therapy, during the first three months and at intervals (approximately 3–6 months) during chronic treatment.
Adjustments in dose should be guided by clinical and radiological evidence, as well as changes in serum alkaline phosphatase and urinary hydroxyproline excretion.
Side effects such as nausea and flushing may be minimized by administration at bedtime. Dose adjustment (e.g. from 0.5 mg to 0.25 mg) may also be helpful in this regard.
More severe cases (e.g., when there is evidence of mechanically weak bones with osteolytic lesions) may require dosages of up to 1 mg daily (0.5 mg twice daily).
Treatment should be continued for 6 months; if symptoms have been relieved, therapy may be discontinued until symptoms or radiologic signs recur. Biochemical parameters will relapse on cessation of therapy and should not be relied on as the basis for a decision to restart therapy with Cibacalcin. The double-chambered syringe is intended primarily for subcutaneous administration by the patient. Reconstituted material should be used within 6 hours.
Note: **Parenteral drug products should be inspected visually for particulate matter and discoloration prior to administration, whenever solution and container permit.**
When the dosage is 0.25 mg (one-half of the solution), the remainder of the drug solution is to be discarded.

HOW SUPPLIED

Double-chambered syringes —each contains 0.5 mg of calcitonin-human for injection and 20 mg of mannitol, in sterile, lyophilized form, in one chamber and a 1-ml solution of 30 mg of mannitol in Water for Injection in the other chamber.
Unit Dose (blister pack)
Cartons of 5 syringes ....NDC 0083-6485-05
Do not store above 77°F (25°C). Protect from light.

Continued on next page

The full prescribing information for each CIBA product is contained herein and is that in effect as of September 1, 1989

CIBA—Cont.

Reconstituted material should be used within 6 hours.
No refrigeration required.

C87-50 (Rev. 2/88)

Information for the Patient
CIBACALCIN®
Calcitonin-human for injection
How to Prepare for Injection

1. Remove the foil covering from the double-chambered syringe.

2. Holding the barrel of the syringe, push it into the vial as far as it will go. Do not hold the plunger. If the red plastic collar positioned between the vial and the syringe is visible, then the syringe has **not** been pushed into the vial as far as it will go.

3. Hold the unit vertically as illustrated (vial up). Press firmly upward on the plunger as far as it will go, so the water in the syringe enters the vial containing the dry powder. Shake **gently** to mix. Whenever possible, inspect injectable products before use. If particles or discoloration are present, do not use.

4. Pull the plunger **slowly** to the black line on the barrel of the syringe for a 0.25 mg dose. Withdraw the entire solution into the syringe for a 0.5 mg dose.
When the dosage of 0.25 mg (one-half of the solution) is used, the remainder of the drug solution in the vial is to be discarded.

5. Carefully pull the vial away from the syringe. Pointing syringe upward, tap barrel with fingertips to force any air bubbles to the surface. Push **gently** on plunger to expel air. Stop pushing when you see droplets of liquid at tip of needle.

How to Inject

1. Clean the injection site by wiping firmly with a sterile alcohol swab. Make certain the skin is dry before injecting.

2. Hold the syringe in your hand, the way you would a pencil.
3. Using the thumb and index finger of your free hand, pinch up a two-inch fold of skin at the injection site.
4. Quickly plunge the needle all the way into the fold of skin, making sure the syringe is held at about a 60° angle. Let go of the skin fold with your free hand.

5. To check that the needle is not in a blood vessel, hold the syringe steady with your free hand and use the other hand to pull back slightly on the plunger.

6. If blood appears in the syringe, remove the needle, discard the double-chambered syringe, and begin again with a new unit.
7. If no blood appears, inject the medication by **slowly** pushing down on the plunger.

8. When you finish injecting the medication, take a fresh alcohol swab and press it against the skin with your free hand, as you quickly pull the needle out with your other hand. Remove the needle at the same 60° angle at which you inserted it.

9. Gently rub the injection site with an alcohol swab to promote absorption of Cibacalcin.
10. Replace needle in used vial and bend both units back and forth until needle is broken. Discard entire unit.

Injection Sites
The figures below show the usual sites for your daily injection of Cibacalcin.

Front   Rear

- Carefully follow your doctor's instructions for injection
- Always remember to use a **different** injection site each day
- To help you remember which sites you have already used, you may find it helpful to keep a daily record
- If you have any questions, be sure to speak to your doctor

Whenever possible, inspect injectable drug products for particles and discoloration before you use them.
Do not store above 77°F (25°C). Protect from light.
Once the solution has been made, it should be used within 6 hours.
No refrigeration required.

C87-51 (Rev. 2/88)

Dist. by:
CIBA Pharmaceutical Company
Division of CIBA-GEIGY Corporation
Summit, New Jersey 07901

CYTADREN® Tablets   ℞
[*sight 'a-dren*]
aminoglutethimide tablets USP

DESCRIPTION

Cytadren, aminoglutethimide tablets USP, is an inhibitor of adrenocortical steroid synthesis, available as 250-mg tablets for oral administration. Its chemical name is 3-(4-aminophenyl)-3-ethyl-2, 6-piperidinedione.
Aminoglutethimide USP is a fine, white or creamy white, crystalline powder. It is very slightly soluble in water, and readily soluble in most organic solvents. It forms water-soluble salts with strong acids. Its molecular weight is 232.28.
Inactive Ingredients. Cellulose compounds, colloidal silicon dioxide, starch, stearic acid, and talc.

CLINICAL PHARMACOLOGY

Cytadren inhibits the enzymatic conversion of cholesterol to Δ^5-pregnenolone, resulting in a decrease in the production of adrenal glucocorticoids, mineralocorticoids, estrogens, and androgens.
Cytadren blocks several other steps in steroid synthesis, including the C-11, C-18, and C-21 hydroxylations and the hydroxylations required for the aromatization of androgens to estrogens, mediated through the binding of Cytadren to cytochrome P-450 complexes.
A decrease in adrenal secretion of cortisol is followed by an increased secretion of pituitary adrenocorticotropic hormone (ACTH), which will overcome the blockade of adrenocortical steroid synthesis by Cytadren. The compensatory increase in ACTH secretion can be suppressed by the simultaneous administration of hydrocortisone. Since Cytadren increases the rate of metabolism of dexamethasone but not that of hydrocortisone, the latter is preferred as the adrenal glucocorticoid replacement.
Although Cytadren inhibits the synthesis of thyroxine by the thyroid gland, the compensatory increase in thyroid-stimulating hormone (TSH) is frequently of sufficient magnitude to overcome the inhibition of thyroid synthesis due to Cytadren. In spite of an increase in TSH, Cytadren has not been associated with increased prolactin secretion.
Note: Cytadren was marketed previously as an anticonvulsant but was withdrawn from marketing for that indication in 1966 because of the effects on the adrenal gland.

Pharmacokinetics

Cytadren is rapidly and completely absorbed after oral administration. In 6 healthy male volunteers, maximum plasma levels of Cytadren averaged 5.9 µg/ml at a median of 1.5 hours after ingestion of two 250-mg tablets. The bioavailability of tablets is equivalent to equal doses given as a solution. After ingestion of a single oral dose, 34–54% is excreted in the urine as unchanged drug during the first 48 hours, and an additional fraction as the N-acetyl derivative.

The half-life of Cytadren in normal volunteers given single oral doses averaged 12.5 ± 1.6 hours.

Upon withdrawal of therapy with Cytadren, the ability of the adrenal glands to synthesize steroid returns, usually within 72 hours.

INDICATIONS AND USAGE

Cytadren is indicated for the suppression of adrenal function in selected patients with Cushing's syndrome. Morning levels of plasma cortisol in patients with adrenal carcinoma and ectopic ACTH-producing tumors were reduced on the average to about one half of the pretreatment levels, and in patients with adrenal hyperplasia to about two thirds of the pretreatment levels, during 1–3 months of therapy with Cytadren. Data available from the few patients with adrenal adenoma suggest similar reductions in plasma cortisol levels. Measurements of plasma cortisol showed reductions to at least 50% of baseline or to normal levels in one third or more of the patients studied, depending on diagnostic groups and time of measurement.

Because Cytadren does not affect the underlying disease process, it is used primarily as an interim measure until more definitive therapy such as surgery can be undertaken or in cases where such therapy is not appropriate. Only small numbers of patients have been treated for longer than 3 months. A decreased effect or "escape phenomenon" seems to occur more frequently in patients with pituitary-dependent Cushing's syndrome, probably because of increasing ACTH levels in response to decreasing glucocorticoid levels. Cytadren should be used only in those patients who are responsive to treatment.

CONTRAINDICATIONS

Cytadren is contraindicated in those patients with serious forms, and/or severe manifestations, of hypersensitivity to glutethimide or aminoglutethimide.

WARNINGS

Cytadren may cause adrenocortical hypofunction, especially under conditions of stress, such as surgery, trauma, or acute illness. Patients should be carefully monitored and given hydrocortisone and mineralocorticoid supplements as indicated. Dexamethasone should not be used. (See PRECAUTIONS, Drug Interactions.)

Cytadren also may suppress aldosterone production by the adrenal cortex and may cause orthostatic or persistent hypotension. The blood pressure should be monitored in all patients at appropriate intervals. Patients should be advised of the possible occurrence of weakness and dizziness as symptoms of hypotension, and of measures to be taken should they occur.

The effects of Cytadren may be potentiated if it is taken in combination with alcohol.

Cytadren can cause fetal harm when administered to a pregnant woman. In the earlier experience with the drug in about 5000 patients, two cases of pseudohermaphroditism were reported in female infants whose mothers were treated with Cytadren and concomitant anticonvulsants. Normal pregnancies have also occurred in patients treated with Cytadren.

When administered to rats at doses ½ and 1¼ times the maximum daily human dose, Cytadren caused a decrease in fetal implantation, an increase in fetal deaths, and a variety of teratogenic effects. The compound also caused pseudohermaphroditism in rats treated with approximately 3 times the maximum daily human dose. If this drug must be used during pregnancy, or if the patient becomes pregnant while taking the drug, the patient should be apprised of the potential hazard to the fetus.

PRECAUTIONS

General

This drug should be administered only by physicians familiar with its use and hazards. Therapy should be initiated in a hospital. (See DOSAGE AND ADMINISTRATION.)

Information for Patients

Patients should be warned that drowsiness may occur and that they should not drive, operate potentially dangerous machinery, or engage in other activities that may become hazardous because of decreased alertness.

Patients should also be warned of the possibility of hypotension and its symptoms (see WARNINGS).

Laboratory Tests

Hypothyroidism may occur in association with Cytadren; hence, appropriate clinical observations should be made and laboratory studies of thyroid function performed as indicated. Supplementary thyroid hormone may be required.

Hematologic abnormalities in patients receiving Cytadren have been reported (see ADVERSE REACTIONS). Therefore, baseline hematologic studies should be performed, followed by periodic hematologic evaluation.

Since elevations in SGOT, alkaline phosphatase, and bilirubin have been reported, appropriate clinical observations and regular laboratory studies should be performed before and during therapy.

Serum electrolyte levels should be determined periodically.

Drug Interactions

Cytadren accelerates the metabolism of dexamethasone; therefore, if glucocorticoid replacement is needed, hydrocortisone should be prescribed.

Aminoglutethimide diminishes the effect of coumarin and warfarin.

Carcinogenesis, Mutagenesis, Impairment of Fertility

Long-term carcinogenicity studies in animals and mutagenicity studies have not been performed with Cytadren. Cytadren affects fertility in female rats (see WARNINGS). The relevance of these findings to humans is not known.

Pregnancy Category D

See WARNINGS.

Nursing Mothers

It is not known whether this drug is excreted in human milk. Because many drugs are excreted in human milk and because of the potential for serious adverse reactions in nursing infants from Cytadren, a decision should be made whether to discontinue nursing or to discontinue the drug, taking into account the importance of the drug to the mother.

Pediatric Use

Safety and effectiveness in children have not been established (see CLINICAL STUDIES IN CHILDREN).

ADVERSE REACTIONS

Untoward effects have been reported in about 2 out of 3 patients with Cushing's syndrome who were treated for 4 or more weeks with Cytadren as the only adrenocortical suppressant.

The most frequent and reversible side effects were drowsiness (approximately 1 in 3 patients), morbilliform skin rash (1 in 6 patients), nausea and anorexia (each approximately 1 in 8 patients), and dizziness (about 1 in 20 patients). The dizziness was possibly caused by lowered vascular resistance or orthostasis. These reactions often disappear spontaneously with continued therapy.

Other Effects Observed

Hematologic: Single instances of neutropenia, leukopenia (patient received concomitant *o,p′*-DDD), pancytopenia (patient received concomitant 5-fluorouracil), and agranulocytosis occurred in 4 of 27 patients with Cushing's syndrome caused by adrenal carcinoma who were treated for at least 4 weeks. In 1 patient with adrenal hyperplasia, hemoglobin levels and hematocrit decreased during the course of treatment with Cytadren. From the earlier experience with the drug used as an anticonvulsant in 1,214 patients, transient leukopenia was the only hematologic effect and was reported once; Coombs'-negative hemolytic anemia also occurred once. In approximately 300 patients with nonadrenal malignancy, 1 in 25 showed some degree of anemia, and 1 in 150 developed pancytopenia during treatment with Cytadren.

Endocrine: Adrenal insufficiency occurred in about 1 in 30 patients with Cushing's syndrome who were treated with Cytadren for 4 or more weeks. This insufficiency tended to involve glucocorticoids as well as mineralocorticoids. Hypothyroidism is occasionally associated with thyroid enlargement and may be detected or confirmed by measuring plasma levels of the thyroid hormone. Masculinization and hirsutism have occasionally occurred in females, as has precocious sexual development in males.

Central Nervous System: Headache was reported in about 1 in 20 patients.

Cardiovascular: Hypotension, occasionally orthostatic, occurred in 1 in 30 patients receiving Cytadren. Tachycardia occurred in 1 in 40 patients.

Gastrointestinal and Liver: Vomiting occurred in 1 in 30 patients. Isolated instances of abnormal findings on liver function tests were reported. Suspected hepatotoxicity occurred in less than 1 in 1000 patients.

Skin: In addition to rash (1 in 6 patients, and often reversible with continued therapy), pruritus was reported in 1 in 20 patients. These may be allergic or hypersensitive reactions. Urticaria has occurred rarely.

Miscellaneous: Fever was reported in several patients who were treated with Cytadren for less than 4 weeks; some of these patients also received other drugs. Myalgia occurred in 1 in 30 patients.

OVERDOSAGE

Acute Toxicity

No deaths due to overdosage with Cytadren have been reported.

The highest known doses that have been survived are 7 g (33-year-old woman) and 7.5–10.0 g (16-year-old girl).

Oral LD_{50}'s (mg/kg): rats, 1800; dogs, >100. Intravenous LD_{50}'s (mg/kg): rats, 156; dogs > 100.

Signs and Symptoms

An acute overdose with Cytadren may reduce the production of steroids in the adrenal cortex to a degree that is clinically relevant. The following manifestations may be expected:

Respiratory Function: Respiratory depression, hyperventilation.

Cardiovascular System: Hypotension, hypovolemic shock due to dehydration.

Central Nervous System/Muscles: Somnolence, lethargy, coma, ataxia, dizziness, fatigue. (Extreme weakness has been reported with divided doses of 3 g daily.)

Gastrointestinal System: Nausea, vomiting.

Renal Function: Loss of sodium and water.

Laboratory Findings: Hyponatremia, hypochloremia, hyperkalemia, hypoglycemia.

The signs and symptoms of acute overdosage with Cytadren may be aggravated or modified if alcohol, hypnotics, tranquilizers, or tricyclic antidepressants have been taken at the same time.

Treatment

Symptomatic treatment of overdosage is recommended.

Since aminoglutethimide and glutethimide are chemically related, measures that have been used in successfully removing glutethimide from the body might be useful in removing aminoglutethimide.

Gastric lavage and unspecified supportive treatment have been employed. Full consciousness following deep coma was regained 40 hours or less after ingestion of 3 or 4 g without lavage. No evidence of hematologic, renal, or hepatic effects was subsequently found.

Close monitoring should be provided, and appropriate measures taken to support vital functions, if necessary.

If deficiency of circulating glucocorticoid develops, an intravenous infusion of a soluble hydrocortisone preparation (100 mg of hydrocortisone sodium succinate in 500 ml of isotonic sodium chloride solution) and 50 ml of 40% glucose solution should be given within 3 hours. After the initial infusion is completed, an intravenous administration of hydrocortisone, 10 mg per hour, should be continued until the patient is able to take oral cortisone.

If hypovolemia or hypotension occurs, an intravenous administration of norepinephrine, 10 mg, in 500 ml of isotonic sodium chloride should be administered according to the patient's needs and response. After rehydration, 500 ml of plasma or blood should be given for maintenance of sufficient circulatory volume.

Dialysis may be considered in severe intoxication.

DOSAGE AND ADMINISTRATION

Adults

Treatment should be instituted in a hospital until a stable dosage regimen is achieved. Therapy should be initiated with 250 mg orally four times daily, preferably at 6-hour intervals. Adrenocortical response should be followed by careful monitoring of plasma cortisol levels until the desired level of suppression is achieved. If the level of cortisol suppression is inadequate, the dosage may be increased in increments of 250 mg daily at intervals of 1–2 weeks to a total daily dose of 2 g. Dose reduction or temporary discontinuation of therapy may be required in the event of adverse effects, including extreme drowsiness, severe skin rash, or excessively low cortisol levels. If a skin rash persists for longer than 5–8 days or becomes severe, the drug should be discontinued. It may be possible to reinstate therapy at a lower dosage following the disappearance of a mild or moderate rash. Mineralocorticoid replacement (e.g., fludrocortisone) may be necessary. If glucocorticoid replacement therapy is needed, 20–30 mg of hydrocortisone orally in the morning will replace endogenous secretion.

HOW SUPPLIED

Tablets 250 mg — white, round, scored into quarters (imprinted CIBA 24)

Bottles of 100 ....NDC 0083-0024-30

Protect from light.

Dispense in tight, light-resistant container (USP).

CLINICAL STUDIES IN CHILDREN

Clinical investigations included 9 patients aged 2½ to 16 years; 4 of these were aged 10 or less. Seven of the patients received other therapies (drugs or irradiation) either with Cytadren or within a short period before initiation of therapy with Cytadren. Diagnoses included 5 patients with adrenal carcinoma, 3 with adrenal hyperplasia, and 1 with ectopic ACTH-producing tumor. Duration of treatment ranged from 3 days to 6½ months. Dosages ranged from 0.375 g to 1.5 g daily. In general, smaller doses were used for younger patients; for example, a 2½-year-old received 0.5–0.75 g daily, a 3½-year-old received 0.5 g daily, and all others over 10 years of age received 0.75–1.5 g daily. Results are difficult

Continued on next page

The full prescribing information for each CIBA product is contained herein and is that in effect as of September 1, 1989

CIBA—Cont.

to evaluate because of the concomitant therapy, duration of therapy, or inadequate laboratory documentation. Most patients did show decreases in plasma or urinary steroids at some time during treatment, but these may have been due to other therapeutic modalities or their combinations.

C85-51 (Rev. 11/85)

Shown in Product Identification Section, page 408

DESFERAL®
[*des 'fer-all*]   ℞
deferoxamine mesylate USP
Vials

DESCRIPTION

Desferal, deferoxamine mesylate USP, is an iron-chelating agent, available in vials for intramuscular, subcutaneous, and intravenous administration. Each vial contains 500 mg of deferoxamine mesylate USP in sterile, lyophilized form. Deferoxamine mesylate is N-[5-[3-[(5-aminopentyl) hydroxycarbamoyl]propionamido]-pentyl]-3-[[5-(N-hydroxyacetamido)-pentyl]carbamoyl] propionohydroxamic acid monomethanesulfonate (salt).

Deferoxamine mesylate USP is a white to off-white powder. It is freely soluble in water and slightly soluble in methanol. Its molecular weight is 656.79.

CLINICAL PHARMACOLOGY

Desferal chelates iron by forming a stable complex that prevents the iron from entering into further chemical reactions. It readily chelates iron from ferritin and hemosiderin but not readily from transferrin; it does not combine with the iron from cytochromes and hemoglobin. Desferal does not cause any demonstrable increase in the excretion of electrolytes or trace metals. Theoretically, 100 parts by weight of Desferal is capable of binding approximately 8.5 parts by weight of ferric iron.

Desferal is metabolized principally by plasma enzymes, but the pathways have not yet been defined. The chelate is readily soluble in water and passes easily through the kidney, giving the urine a characteristic reddish color. Some is also excreted in the feces via the bile.

INDICATIONS AND USAGE

Desferal is indicated for the treatment of acute iron intoxication and of chronic iron overload due to transfusion-dependent anemias.

Acute Iron Intoxication

Desferal is an adjunct to, and not a substitute for, standard measures used in treating acute iron intoxication, which may include the following: induction of emesis with syrup of ipecac; gastric lavage; suction and maintenance of a clear airway; control of shock with intravenous fluids, blood, oxygen, and vasopressors; and correction of acidosis.

Chronic Iron Overload

Desferal can promote iron excretion in patients with secondary iron overload from multiple transfusions (as may occur in the treatment of some chronic anemias, including thalassemia). Long-term therapy with Desferal slows accumulation of hepatic iron and retards or eliminates progression of hepatic fibrosis.

Iron mobilization with Desferal is relatively poor in patients under the age of 3 years with relatively little iron overload. The drug should ordinarily not be given to such patients unless significant iron mobilization (e.g., 1 mg or more of iron per day) can be demonstrated.

Desferal is not indicated for the treatment of primary hemochromatosis, since phlebotomy is the method of choice for removing excess iron in this disorder.

CONTRAINDICATIONS

Desferal is contraindicated in patients with severe renal disease or anuria, since the drug and the iron chelate are excreted primarily by the kidney.

WARNINGS

Ocular and auditory disturbances have been reported when Desferal was administered over prolonged periods of time, at high doses, or in patients with low ferritin levels. The ocular disturbances observed have been blurring of vision; cataracts after prolonged administration in chronic iron overload; decreased visual acuity including visual loss; impaired peripheral, color, and night vision; and retinal pigmentary abnormalities. The auditory abnormalities reported have been tinnitus and hearing loss including high frequency sensorineural hearing loss. In most cases, both ocular and auditory disturbances were reversible upon immediate cessation of treatment. Slit-lamp examinations performed in patients treated with Desferal for acute iron intoxication have not revealed cataracts.

Visual acuity tests, slit-lamp examinations, funduscopy and audiometry are recommended periodically in patients treated for prolonged periods of time. Toxicity is more likely to be reversed if symptoms or test abnormalities are detected early.

PRECAUTIONS

General

Flushing of the skin, urticaria, hypotension, and shock have occurred in a few patients when Desferal was administered by rapid intravenous injection. THEREFORE, DESFERAL SHOULD BE GIVEN INTRAMUSCULARLY OR BY SLOW SUBCUTANEOUS OR INTRAVENOUS INFUSION.

Iron overload increases susceptibility of patients to Yersinia enterocolitica infections. In some rare cases, treatment with Desferal has enhanced this susceptibility, resulting in generalized infections by providing this bacteria with a siderophore otherwise missing. In such cases, Desferal treatment should be discontinued until the infection is resolved.

In patients undergoing hemodialysis while receiving Desferal, there have been rare reports of fungal infections (i.e., mucormycosis) that have sometimes been fatal; however, a causal relationship to the drug has not been established.

Information for Patients

Patients should be informed that occasionally their urine may show a reddish discoloration.

Carcinogenesis, Mutagenesis, Impairment of Fertility

Long-term carcinogenicity studies in animals have not been performed with Desferal.

Cytotoxicity may occur, since Desferal has been shown to inhibit DNA synthesis *in vitro.*

Pregnancy Category C

Delayed ossification in mice and skeletal anomalies in rabbits were observed after Desferal was administered in daily doses up to 4.5 times the maximum daily human dose. No adverse effects were observed in similar studies in rats. There are no adequate and well-controlled studies in pregnant women. Desferal should be used during pregnancy only if the potential benefit justifies the potential risk to the fetus.

Nursing Mothers

It is not known whether this drug is excreted in human milk. Because many drugs are excreted in human milk, caution should be exercised when Desferal is administered to a nursing woman.

Pediatric Use

Safety and effectiveness in children under the age of 3 years have not been established (see **INDICATIONS AND USAGE**).

ADVERSE REACTIONS

The following adverse reactions have been observed, but there are not enough data to support an estimate of their frequency.

Skin: Localized irritation and pain, swelling and induration, pruritus, erythema, wheal formation.

Hypersensitive Reactions: Generalized erythema (rash), urticaria, anaphylactic reaction.

Cardiovascular: Tachycardia, hypotension, shock.

Digestive: Abdominal discomfort, diarrhea.

Special Senses: Ocular and auditory disturbances (see **WARNINGS**).

Other: Dysuria, leg cramps, fever.

OVERDOSAGE

Acute Toxicity

Intravenous LD_{50}'s (mg/kg): mice, 287; rats, 329.

Signs and Symptoms

Since Desferal is available only for parenteral administration, acute poisoning is unlikely to occur. However, tachycardia, hypotension, and gastrointestinal symptoms have occasionally developed in patients who received overdoses of Desferal.

Treatment

There is no specific antidote.

Signs and symptoms of overdosage may be eliminated by reducing the dosage.

Desferal is readily dialyzable.

DOSAGE AND ADMINISTRATION

Acute Iron Intoxication

Intramuscular Administration

This route is preferred and should be used for ALL PATIENTS NOT IN SHOCK.

Dosage. A dose of 1.0 g should be administered initially. This may be followed by 500 mg (one vial) every 4 hours for two doses. Depending upon the clinical response, subsequent doses of 500 mg may be administered every 4–12 hours. The total amount administered should not exceed 6.0 g in 24 hours.

Preparation of Solution. Desferal is dissolved by adding 2 ml of Sterile Water for Injection to each vial, resulting in a solution of 250 mg/ml. The drug should be completely dissolved before the solution is withdrawn. Desferal is then administered intramuscularly. See *NOTE* below.

Intravenous Administration

THIS ROUTE SHOULD BE USED ONLY FOR PATIENTS IN A STATE OF CARDIOVASCULAR COLLAPSE AND THEN ONLY BY SLOW INFUSION. THE RATE OF INFUSION SHOULD NOT EXCEED 15 MG/KG PER HOUR.

Dosage: An initial dose of 1.0 g should be administered at a rate NOT TO EXCEED 15 mg/kg per hour. This may be followed by 500 mg every 4 hours for two doses. Depending upon the clinical response, subsequent doses of 500 mg may be administered every 4–12 hours. The total amount administered should not exceed 6.0 g in 24 hours.

As soon as the clinical condition of the patient permits, intravenous administration should be discontinued and the drug should be administered intramuscularly.

Preparation of Solution. Desferal is dissolved by adding 2 ml of Sterile Water for Injection to each vial, resulting in a solution of 250 mg/ml. The drug should be completely dissolved before the solution is withdrawn. The solution is then added to physiologic saline, glucose in water, or Ringer's lactate solution and administered at a rate NOT TO EXCEED 15 mg/kg per hour. See *NOTE* below.

Chronic Iron Overload

The more effective of the following routes of administration must be chosen on an individual basis for each patient.

Intramuscular Administration

A daily dose of 0.5–1.0 g should be administered intramuscularly. In addition, 2.0 g should be administered intravenously with each unit of blood transfused; however, Desferal should be administered separately from the blood. The rate of intravenous infusion must not exceed 15 mg/kg per hour.

Subcutaneous Administration

A daily dose of 1.0–2.0 g (20–40 mg/kg per day) should be administered over 8–24 hours, utilizing a small portable pump capable of providing continuous mini-infusion. The duration of infusion must be individualized. In some patients, as much iron will be excreted after a short infusion of 8–12 hours as with the same dose given over 24 hours. *Preparation of Solution for Subcutaneous or Intramuscular Administration.* Desferal is dissolved by adding 2.0 ml of Sterile Water for Injection to each vial, resulting in a solution of 250 mg/ml. The drug should be completely dissolved before the solution is withdrawn into the syringe to be used for administration. See *NOTE* below.

NOTE: Parenteral drug products should be inspected visually for particulate matter and discoloration prior to administration, whenever solution and container permit.

Desferal reconstituted with Sterile Water for Injection may be stored under sterile conditions and protected from light at room temperature for not longer than 1 week.

Reconstituting Desferal in solvents or under conditions other than indicated may result in precipitation. Turbid solutions should not be used.

HOW SUPPLIED

Vials —each containing 500 mg of sterile, lyophilized deferoxamine mesylate

     Cartons of 4 vials ....NDC 0083-3801-04

                                 C87-30 (Rev. 8/87)

Dist. by:
CIBA Pharmaceutical Company
Division of CIBA-GEIGY Corporation
Summit, New Jersey 07901

ESIDRIX®
[*ess 'a-dricks*]   ℞
hydrochlorothiazide USP

DESCRIPTION

Esidrix, hydrochlorothiazide USP, is a diuretic and antihypertensive available as 25-mg, 50-mg, and 100-mg tablets for oral administration. Its chemical name is 6-chloro-3,4-dihydro-2H-1,2,4-benzothiadiazine-7-sulfonamide 1,1-dioxide.

Hydrochlorothiazide USP is a white, or practically white, practically odorless, crystalline powder. It is slightly soluble in water, freely soluble in sodium hydroxide solution, in *n*-butylamine and in dimethylformamide, sparingly soluble in methanol, and insoluble in ether, in chloroform, and in dilute mineral acids. Its molecular weight is 297.73.

Inactive Ingredients: Colloidal silicon dioxide, D&C Yellow No. 10 (50-mg tablets), FD&C Blue No. 1 (100-mg tablets), FD&C Red No. 3 and FD&C Yellow No. 6 (25-mg tablets), lactose, starch, stearic acid, and sucrose.

CLINICAL PHARMACOLOGY

Thiazides affect the renal tubular mechanism of electrolyte reabsorption. At maximal therapeutic dosage all thiazides are approximately equal in their diuretic potency. Thiazides increase excretion of sodium and chloride in approximately equivalent amounts. Natriuresis causes a secondary loss of potassium.

The mechanism of the antihypertensive effect of thiazides is unknown. Thiazides do not affect normal blood pressure. Onset of action of thiazides occurs in 2 hours and the peak effect at about 4 hours. Its action persists for approximately 6 to 12 hours. Thiazides are eliminated rapidly by the kidney.

INDICATIONS AND USAGE

Hypertension

In the management of hypertension either as the sole therapeutic agent or to enhance the effect of other antihypertensive drugs in the more severe forms of hypertension.

Edema
As adjunctive therapy in edema associated with congestive heart failure, hepatic cirrhosis, and corticosteroid and estrogen therapy.

Esidrix has also been found useful in edema due to various forms of renal dysfunction, such as the nephrotic syndrome, acute glomerulonephritis, and chronic renal failure.

Usage in Pregnancy: The routine use of diuretics in an otherwise healthy woman is inappropriate and exposes mother and fetus to unnecessary hazard. Diuretics do not prevent development of toxemia of pregnancy, and there is no satisfactory evidence that they are useful in the treatment of developed toxemia.

Edema during pregnancy may arise from pathological causes or from the physiologic and mechanical consequences of pregnancy. Thiazides are indicated in pregnancy when edema is due to pathologic causes, just as they are in the absence of pregnancy (however, see **PRECAUTIONS, Pregnancy**). Dependent edema in pregnancy, resulting from restriction of venous return by the expanded uterus, is properly treated through elevation of the lower extremities and use of support hose; use of diuretics to lower intravascular volume in this case is illogical and unnecessary. There is hypervolemia during normal pregnancy which is not harmful to either the fetus or the mother (in the absence of cardiovascular disease) but which is associated with edema, including generalized edema, in the majority of pregnant women. If this edema produces discomfort, increased recumbency will often provide relief. In rare instances, this edema may cause extreme discomfort which is not relieved by rest. In these cases, a short course of diuretics may provide relief and may be appropriate.

CONTRAINDICATIONS
Anuria; hypersensitivity to this or other sulfonamide-derived drugs.

WARNINGS
Use with caution in severe renal disease. In patients with renal disease, thiazides may precipitate azotemia. Cumulative effects of the drug may develop in patients with impaired renal function.

Thiazides should be used with caution in patients with impaired hepatic function or progressive liver disease, since minor alterations of fluid and electrolyte imbalance may precipitate hepatic coma.

Thiazides may add to or potentiate the action of other antihypertensive drugs. Potentiation occurs with ganglionic or peripheral adrenergic blocking drugs.

Sensitivity reactions are more likely to occur in patients with a history of allergy or bronchial asthma.

The possibility of exacerbation or activation of systemic lupus erythematosus has been reported.

PRECAUTIONS
General
All patients receiving thiazide therapy should be observed for clinical signs of fluid or electrolyte imbalance: namely, hyponatremia, hypochloremic alkalosis, and hypokalemia (see **Laboratory Tests** and **Drug/Drug Interactions**). Warning signs are dryness of mouth, thirst, weakness, lethargy, drowsiness, restlessness, muscle pains or cramps, muscular fatigue, hypotension, oliguria, tachycardia, and gastrointestinal disturbance such as nausea or vomiting.

Hypokalemia may develop, especially with brisk diuresis or when severe cirrhosis is present.

Interference with adequate oral intake of electrolytes will also contribute to hypokalemia. Hypokalemia may be avoided or treated by use of potassium supplements or foods with a high potassium content.

Any chloride deficit is generally mild and usually does not require specific treatment except under extraordinary circumstances (as in liver disease or renal disease). Dilutional hyponatremia may occur in edematous patients in hot weather; appropriate therapy is water restriction rather than administration of salt, except in rare instances when the hyponatremia is life-threatening. In actual salt depletion, appropriate replacement is the therapy of choice.

Hyperuricemia may occur or frank gout may be precipitated in certain patients receiving thiazide therapy.

Latent diabetes may become manifest during thiazide administration (see **Drug/Drug Interactions**).

The antihypertensive effects of the drug may be enhanced in the postsympathectomy patient.

If progressive renal impairment becomes evident, withholding or discontinuing diuretic therapy should be considered. Calcium excretion is decreased by thiazides. Pathological changes in the parathyroid gland with hypercalcemia and hypophosphatemia have been observed in a few patients on prolonged thiazide therapy. The common complications of hyperparathyroidism such as renal lithiasis, bone resorption, and peptic ulceration have not been seen.

Information for Patients
Patients should be informed of possible side effects and advised to take the medication regularly and continuously as directed.

Laboratory Tests
Initial and periodic determinations of serum electrolytes to detect possible electrolyte imbalance should be performed at appropriate intervals.

Serum and urine electrolyte determinations are particularly important when the patient is vomiting excessively or receiving parenteral fluids.

Drug/Drug Interactions
Hypokalemia can sensitize or exaggerate the response of the heart to the toxic effects of digitalis (e.g., increased ventricular irritability).

Hypokalemia may develop during concomitant use of steroids or ACTH.

Insulin requirements in diabetic patients may be increased, decreased, or unchanged.

Thiazides may decrease arterial responsiveness to norepinephrine. This diminution is not sufficient to preclude effectiveness of the pressor agent for therapeutic use.

Thiazide drugs may increase the responsiveness to tubocurarine.

Lithium renal clearance is reduced by thiazides, increasing the risk of lithium toxicity.

There have been rare reports in the literature of hemolytic anemia occurring with the concomitant use of hydrochlorothiazide and methyldopa.

Concurrent administration of some nonsteroidal anti-inflammatory agents may reduce the diuretic, natriuretic and antihypertensive effects of thiazide diuretics.

Drug/Laboratory Test Interactions
Thiazides may decrease serum PBI levels without signs of thyroid disturbance.

Thiazides should be discontinued before carrying out tests for parathyroid function (see **PRECAUTIONS, General**, calcium excretion).

Carcinogenesis, Mutagenesis, Impairment of Fertility
Long-term carcinogenicity studies in animals have not been conducted with Esidrix. Hydrochlorothiazide was not mutagenic in in vitro Ames mutagenicity assay of *Salmonella typhimurium* strains TA 98, TA 100, TA 1535 and TA 1537 or in in vivo mutagenicity assays of mouse germinal cell chromosomes and Chinese hamster bone marrow cell chromosomes. It was however, mutagenic in inducing nondisjunction (96% frequency) in diploid strains of *Aspergillus nidulans.*

Pregnancy Category B
A reproduction study in rats receiving hydrochlorothiazide, 250 mg/kg/day, 62.5 times the maximum daily human dosage, has revealed no evidence of impaired fertility or harm to the fetus. There are, however, no adequate and well-controlled studies of Esidrix in pregnant women. Because animal reproduction studies are not always predictive of human response, Esidrix should be used during pregnancy only if clearly needed.

Nonteratogenic Effects. Thiazides cross the placental barrier and appear in cord blood, and there is a risk of fetal or neonatal jaundice, thrombocytopenia, and possibly other adverse reactions that have occurred in adults.

Nursing Mothers
Thiazides are excreted in breast milk. Because of the potential for serious adverse reactions in nursing infants, a decision should be made whether to discontinue nursing or to discontinue Esidrix, taking into account the importance of the drug to the mother.

Pediatric Use
Safety and effectiveness in children have not been established.

ADVERSE REACTIONS
Adverse reactions are usually reversible upon reduction of dosage or discontinuation of Esidrix. Whenever adverse reactions are moderate or severe, it may be necessary to discontinue the drug.

The following adverse reactions have been observed, but there has not been enough systematic collection of data to support an estimate of their frequency. Consequently the reactions are categorized by organ systems and are listed in decreasing order of severity and not frequency.

Digestive: Pancreatitis, jaundice (intrahepatic cholestatic), sialadenitis, vomiting, diarrhea, cramping, nausea, gastric irritation, constipation, anorexia.

Cardiovascular: Orthostatic hypotension (may be potentiated by alcohol, barbiturates, or narcotics).

Neurologic: Vertigo, dizziness, transient blurred vision, headache, paresthesia, xanthopsia, weakness, restlessness.

Musculoskeletal: Muscle spasm.

Hematologic: Aplastic anemia, agranulocytosis, leukopenia, thrombocytopenia.

Metabolic: Hyperglycemia, glycosuria, hyperuricemia.

Hypersensitive Reactions: Necrotizing angiitis, Stevens-Johnson syndrome, purpura, urticaria, rash, photosensitivity.

OVERDOSAGE
Acute Toxicity
No deaths due to acute poisoning with Esidrix have been reported.

Highest known doses ingested: children, 500 mg (14-year-old girl); young children, 125 mg (2½-year-old child).

Oral LD$_{50}$ in rats: > 2750 mg/kg.

Signs and Symptoms
The most prominent feature of poisoning with Esidrix is acute loss of fluid and electrolytes.

Cardiovascular: Tachycardia, hypotension, shock.

Neuromuscular: Weakness, confusion, dizziness, cramps of the calf muscles, paresthesia, fatigue, impairment of consciousness.

Gastrointestinal: Nausea, vomiting, thirst.

Renal: Polyuria, oliguria or anuria (due to hemoconcentration).

Laboratory findings: Hypokalemia, hyponatremia, hypochloremia, alkalosis, increased BUN (especially in patients with renal insufficiency).

Combined poisoning: Signs and symptoms may be aggravated or modified by concomitant intake of antihypertensive medication, barbiturates, curare, digitalis (hypokalemia), corticosteroids, narcotics, or alcohol.

Treatment
There is no specific antidote.

Elimination of the drug: Induction of vomiting, gastric lavage.

Measures to reduce absorption: Activated charcoal.

Hypotension, shock: The patient's legs should be kept raised, and lost fluid and electrolytes (potassium, sodium) should be replaced.

Surveillance: Fluid and electrolyte balance (especially serum potassium) and renal function should be monitored until conditions become normal.

DOSAGE AND ADMINISTRATION
Therapy should be individualized according to patient response. Dosage should be titrated to gain maximal therapeutic response as well as the minimal dose possible to maintain that therapeutic response.

ADULTS
Hypertension
To Initiate Therapy: Usual dosage is 50–100 mg daily. May be given as a single dose every morning.

Maintenance: After a week dosage may be adjusted downward to as little as 25 mg a day, or upward. Rarely patients may require up to 200 mg daily in divided doses.

Combined Therapy: When necessary, other antihypertensive agents may be added cautiously. Since this drug potentiates the antihypertensive effect of other agents, such additions should be gradual. Dosages of ganglionic blockers in particular should be halved initially.

Edema
To Initiate Diuresis: 25 to 200 mg daily for several days, or until dry weight is attained.

Maintenance: 25 to 100 mg daily or intermittently depending on the patient's response. A few refractory patients may require up to 200 mg daily.

INFANTS AND CHILDREN
The usual pediatric dosage is administered twice daily. The total daily dosage for infants up to 2 years of age: 12.5 to 37.5 mg; for children 2 to 12 years of age: 37.5 to 100 mg. Dosages should be based on body weight at the rate of 1 mg per pound, but infants below 6 months of age may require 1.5 mg per pound.

HOW SUPPLIED
Tablets 25 mg—round, pink, scored (imprinted CIBA 22)
　　Bottles of 100 .... NDC 0083-0022-30
　　Bottles of 1000 .... NDC 0083-0022-40
　Consumer Pack—One Unit
　　12 bottles—100 tablets each .... NDC 0083-0022-65
　Accu-Pak® Unit Dose (blister pack)
　　Box of 100 (strips of 10) .... NDC 0083-0022-32
Tablets 50 mg—round, yellow, scored (imprinted CIBA 46)
　　Bottles of 100 .... NDC 0083-0046-30
　　Bottles of 1000 .... NDC 0083-0046-40
　Consumer Pack—One Unit
　　12 bottles—30 tablets each .... NDC 0083-0046-82
　　12 bottles—60 tablets each .... NDC 0083-0046-73
　　12 bottles—100 tablets each .... NDC 0083-0046-65
　Accu-Pak® Unit Dose (blister pack)
　　Box of 100 (strips of 10) .... NDC 0083-0046-32
Tablets 100 mg—round, blue, scored (imprinted CIBA 192)
　　Bottles of 100 .... NDC 0083-0192-30
Dispense in tight, light-resistant container (USP).
C87-13 (Rev. 11/87)
　　　Shown in Product Identification Section, page 408

Continued on next page

The full prescribing information for each CIBA product is contained herein and is that in effect as of September 1, 1989

CIBA—Cont.

ESIMIL®   ℞
[ess'a-mill]
guanethidine monosulfate USP 10 mg
hydrochlorothiazide USP 25 mg
Combination Tablets

WARNING

This fixed-combination drug is not indicated for initial therapy of hypertension. Hypertension requires therapy titrated to the individual patient. If the fixed combination represents the dosage so determined, its use may be more convenient in patient management. The treatment of hypertension is not static, but must be reevaluated as conditions in each patient warrant.

DESCRIPTION

Esimil is an antihypertensive-diuretic combination, available as tablets for oral administration. Each tablet contains Ismelin (guanethidine monosulfate USP), 10 mg, and Esidrix (hydrochlorothiazide USP), 25 mg.

Guanethidine monosulfate is [2-(hexahydro-1(2H)-azocinyl) ethyl]guanidine sulfate 1:1.

Guanethidine monosulfate USP is a white to off-white crystalline powder with a molecular weight of 296.38. It is very soluble in water, sparingly soluble in alcohol and practically insoluble in chloroform.

Hydrochlorothiazide is 6-chloro-3,4-dihydro-2H-1,2,4-benzothiadiazine-7-sulfonamide 1,1-dioxide.

Hydrochlorothiazide USP is a white, or practically white, practically odorless crystalline powder. It is slightly soluble in water; freely soluble in sodium hydroxide solution, in n-butylamine, and in dimethylformamide; sparingly soluble in methanol; and insoluble in ether, in chloroform, and in dilute mineral acids. Its molecular weight is 297.73.

Inactive Ingredients: Colloidal silicon dioxide, lactose, starch, stearic acid, and sucrose.

CLINICAL PHARMACOLOGY

Guanethidine

Guanethidine acts at the sympathetic neuroeffector junction by inhibiting or interfering with the release and/or distribution of the chemical mediator (presumably the catecholamine norepinephrine), rather than acting at the effector cell by inhibiting the association of the transmitter with its receptors. In contrast to ganglionic blocking agents, guanethidine suppresses equally the responses mediated by alpha- and beta-adrenergic receptors but does not produce parasympathetic blockade. Since sympathetic blockade results in modest decreases in peripheral resistance and cardiac output, guanethidine lowers blood pressure in the supine position. It further reduces blood pressure by decreasing the degree of vasoconstriction that normally results from reflex sympathetic nervous activity upon assumption of the upright posture, thus reducing venous return and cardiac output more. The inhibition of sympathetic venoconstrictive mechanisms results in venous pooling of blood. Therefore, the effect of guanethidine is especially pronounced when the patient is standing. Both the systolic and diastolic pressures are reduced.

Other actions at the sympathetic nerve terminal include depletion of norepinephrine. Once it gains access to the neuron, guanethidine accumulates within the intraneuronal storage vesicles and causes depletion of norepinephrine stores within the nerve terminal. Prolonged oral administration of guanethidine produces a denervation sensitivity of the neuroeffector junction, probably resulting from the chronic reduction in norepinephrine released by the sympathetic nerve endings. Systemic responses to catecholamines released from the adrenal medulla are not prevented and may even be augmented as a result of this denervation sensitivity. A paradoxical hypertensive crisis may occur if guanethidine is given to patients with pheochromocytoma or if norepinephrine is given to a patient receiving the drug.

Due to its poor lipid solubility, guanethidine does not readily cross the blood-brain barrier. In contrast to most neural blocking agents, guanethidine does not appear to suppress plasma renin activity in many patients.

Pharmacokinetics

The pharmacokinetics of guanethidine are complex. The amount of drug in plasma and in urine is linearly related to dose, although large differences occur between individuals because of variation in absorption and metabolism. Adrenergic blockade occurs with a minimum concentration in plasma of 8 ng/ml; this concentration is achieved in different individuals with doses of 10-50 mg per day at steady state. Guanethidine is eliminated because of extensive tissue binding. After chronic oral administration, the initial phase of elimination with a half-life of 1.5 days is followed by a second phase of elimination with a half-life of 4-8 days. The renal clearance of guanethidine is 56 ml/min. Guanethidine

is converted by the liver to three metabolites, which are excreted in the urine. The metabolites are pharmacologically less active than guanethidine.

Hydrochlorothiazide

Thiazides affect the renal tubular mechanism of electrolyte reabsorption. At maximal therapeutic dosage, all thiazides are approximately equal in their diuretic potency. Thiazides increase excretion of sodium and chloride in approximately equivalent amounts. Natriuresis causes a secondary loss of potassium.

The mechanism of the antihypertensive effect of thiazides is unknown. Thiazides do not affect normal blood pressure.

Pharmacokinetics

The onset of action of thiazides occurs in 2 hours, and the peak effect at about 4 hours. The action persists for approximately 6–12 hours. Hydrochlorothiazide is rapidly absorbed, as indicated by peak plasma concentrations 1–2.5 hours after oral administration. Plasma levels of the drug are proportional to dose; the concentration in whole blood is 1.6–1.8 times higher than in plasma. Thiazides are eliminated rapidly by the kidney. After oral administration of 25- to 100-mg doses of hydrochlorothiazide, 72–97% of the dose is excreted in the urine, indicating dose-independent absorption. Hydrochlorothiazide is eliminated from plasma in a biphasic fashion with a terminal half-life of 10–17 hours. Plasma protein binding is 67.9%. Plasma clearance is 15.9–30.0 L/hr; volume of distribution is 3.6–7.8 L/kg.

Gastrointestinal absorption of hydrochlorothiazide is enhanced when administered with food. Absorption is decreased in patients with congestive heart failure, and the pharmacokinetics are considerably different in these patients.

INDICATIONS

Esimil is indicated for the treatment of hypertension (see boxed **WARNING**).

CONTRAINDICATIONS

Guanethidine

Known or suspected pheochromocytoma; hypersensitivity; frank congestive heart failure not due to hypertension; use of MAO inhibitors.

Hydrochlorothiazide

Anuria; hypersensitivity to this or other sulfonamide-derived drugs.

WARNINGS

Guanethidine and hydrochlorothiazide are potent drugs and their use can lead to disturbing and serious clinical problems. Physicians should be familiar with both drugs and their combination before prescribing, and patients should be warned not to deviate from instructions.

Guanethidine

Orthostatic hypotension can occur frequently and patients should be properly instructed about this potential hazard. Fainting spells may occur unless the patient is forewarned to sit or lie down with the onset of dizziness or weakness. Postural hypotension is most marked in the morning and is accentuated by hot weather, alcohol, or exercise. Dizziness or weakness may be particularly bothersome during the initial period of dosage adjustment and with postural changes, such as arising in the morning. The potential occurrence of these symptoms may require alteration of previous daily activity. The patient should be cautioned to avoid sudden or prolonged standing or exercise while taking the drug.

Inhibition of ejaculation has been reported in animals (see **PRECAUTIONS, Carcinogenesis, Mutagenesis, Impairment of Fertility**) as well as in men given guanethidine. This effect, which results from the sympathetic blockade caused by the drug's action, is reversible after guanethidine has been discontinued for several weeks. The drug does not cause parasympathetic blockade, and erectile potency is usually retained during administration of guanethidine. The possible occurrence of inhibition of ejaculation should be kept in mind when considering the use of guanethidine in men of reproductive age.

If possible, therapy should be withdrawn 2 weeks prior to surgery to reduce the possibility of vascular collapse and cardiac arrest during anesthesia. If emergency surgery is indicated, preanesthetic and anesthetic agents should be administered cautiously in reduced dosage. Oxygen, atropine, vasopressors, and adequate solutions for volume replacement should be ready for immediate use to counteract vascular collapse in the surgical patient. Vasopressors should be used only with extreme caution, since guanethidine augments responsiveness to exogenously administered norepinephrine and vasopressors; specifically, blood pressure may rise and cardiac arrhythmias may be produced.

Hydrochlorothiazide

Thiazides should be used with caution in patients with severe renal disease. In patients with renal disease, thiazides may precipitate azotemia. Cumulative effects of the drug may develop in patients with impaired renal function.

Thiazides should be used with caution in patients with impaired hepatic function or progressive liver disease, since minor alterations of fluid and electrolyte imbalance may precipitate hepatic coma.

Thiazides may add to or potentiate the action of other antihypertensive drugs. Potentiation occurs with ganglionic or peripheral adrenergic blocking drugs.

Sensitivity reactions are more likely to occur in patients with a history of allergy or bronchial asthma.

The possibility of exacerbation or activation of systemic lupus erythematosus has been reported.

PRECAUTIONS

General

Guanethidine. Dosage requirements may be reduced in the presence of fever.

Special care should be exercised when treating patients with a history of bronchial asthma; asthmatic patients are more apt to be hypersensitive to catecholamine depletion, and their condition may be aggravated.

The effects of guanethidine are cumulative over long periods; initial doses should be small and increased gradually in small increments.

Guanethidine should be used very cautiously in hypertensive patients with: renal disease and nitrogen retention or rising BUN levels, since decreased blood pressure may further compromise renal function; coronary insufficiency or recent myocardial infarction; and cerebrovascular disease, especially with encephalopathy.

Guanethidine should not be given to patients with severe cardiac failure except with extreme caution, since guanethidine may interfere with the compensatory role of the adrenergic system in producing circulatory adjustment in patients with congestive heart failure.

Patients with incipient cardiac decompensation should be watched for weight gain or edema.

Guanethidine should be used cautiously in patients with a history of peptic ulcer or other chronic disorders that may be aggravated by a relative increase in parasympathetic tone.

Hydrochlorothiazide. All patients receiving thiazide therapy should be observed for clinical signs of fluid or electrolyte imbalance, namely hyponatremia, hypochloremic alkalosis, and hypokalemia (see **Laboratory Tests** and **Drug/Drug Interactions**). Warning signs are dryness of mouth, thirst, weakness, lethargy, drowsiness, restlessness, muscle pains or cramps, muscular fatigue, hypotension, oliguria, tachycardia, and gastrointestinal disturbance, such as nausea or vomiting.

Hypokalemia may develop, especially in cases of brisk diuresis or severe cirrhosis.

Interference with adequate oral intake of electrolytes will also contribute to hypokalemia. Hypokalemia may be avoided or treated by use of potassium supplements or foods with a high potassium content.

Any chloride deficit is generally mild and usually does not require specific treatment, except under extraordinary circumstances (as in liver disease or renal disease). Dilutional hyponatremia may occur in edematous patients in hot weather; appropriate therapy is water restriction, rather than administration of salt, except in rare instances when the hyponatremia is life-threatening. In cases of actual salt depletion, appropriate replacement is the therapy of choice. Hyperuricemia may occur or frank gout may be precipitated in certain patients receiving thiazide therapy.

Latent diabetes may become manifest during thiazide administration (see **Drug/Drug Interactions**).

The antihypertensive effects of the drug may be enhanced in the postsympathectomy patient.

If progressive renal impairment becomes evident, withholding or discontinuing diuretic therapy should be considered.

Calcium excretion is decreased by thiazides. Pathological changes in the parathyroid gland with hypercalcemia and hypophosphatemia have been observed in a few patients on prolonged thiazide therapy. The common complications of hyperparathyroidism, such as renal lithiasis, bone resorption, and peptic ulceration, have not been seen.

Information for Patients

The patient should be advised to take this medication exactly as directed. If the patient misses a dose, he or she should be told to take only the next scheduled dose (without doubling it).

The patient should be advised to avoid sudden or prolonged standing or exercise and to arise slowly, especially in the morning, to reduce the orthostatic hypotensive effects of dizziness, lightheadedness, or fainting.

The patient should be cautioned about ingesting alcohol, since it aggravates the orthostatic hypotensive effects of guanethidine.

Male patients should be advised that guanethidine may interfere with ejaculation.

Laboratory Tests

Hydrochlorothiazide. Initial and periodic determinations of serum electrolytes to detect possible electrolyte imbalance should be performed at appropriate intervals.

Serum and urine electrolyte determinations are particularly important when the patient is vomiting excessively or receiving parenteral fluids.

Drug/Drug Interactions

Guanethidine. Concurrent use of guanethidine and rauwolfia derivatives may cause excessive postural hypotension, bradycardia, and mental depression.

Both digitalis and guanethidine slow the heart rate.

Amphetamine-like compounds, stimulants (e.g., ephedrine, methylphenidate), tricyclic antidepressants (e.g., amitriptyline, imipramine, desipramine) and other psychopharmacologic agents (e.g., phenothiazines and related compounds), as well as oral contraceptives, may reduce the hypotensive effect of guanethidine.

MAO inhibitors should be discontinued for at least 1 week before starting therapy with guanethidine.

Hydrochlorothiazide. Hypokalemia can sensitize or exaggerate the response of the heart to the toxic effects of digitalis (e.g., increased ventricular irritability).

Hypokalemia may develop during concomitant use of steroids or ACTH.

Insulin requirements in diabetic patients may be increased, decreased, or unchanged.

Thiazides may decrease arterial responsiveness to norepinephrine, but not enough to preclude effectiveness of the pressor agent for therapeutic use.

Thiazides may increase the responsiveness to tubocurarine.

Lithium renal clearance is reduced by thiazides, increasing the risk of lithium toxicity.

There have been rare reports in the literature of hemolytic anemia occurring with the concomitant use of hydrochlorothiazide and methyldopa.

Concurrent administration of some non-steroidal anti-inflammatory agents may reduce the diuretic, natriuretic and antihypertensive effects of thiazide diuretics.

Drug/Laboratory Test Interactions

Thiazides may decrease serum levels of protein-bound iodine without signs of thyroid disturbance. Esimil should be discontinued before tests for parathyroid function are made (see **General, Hydrochlorothiazide,** Calcium excretion).

Carcinogenesis, Mutagenesis, Impairment of Fertility

Long-term carcinogenicity studies in animals have not been conducted with Esimil.

Guanethidine: While inhibition of sperm passage and accumulation of sperm debris have been reported in rats and rabbits after several weeks of administration of guanethidine, 5 or 10 mg/kg per day, subcutaneously or intraperitoneally, recovery of ejaculatory function and fertility has been demonstrated in rats given guanethidine intramuscularly, 25 mg/kg per day, for 8 weeks. Inhibition of ejaculation has also been reported in men (see **WARNINGS** and **ADVERSE REACTIONS**). This effect, which is attributable to the sympathetic blockade caused by the drug, is reversible several weeks after discontinuance of the drug.

Hydrochlorothiazide: Hydrochlorothiazide was not mutagenic in in vitro Ames Mutagenicity assay of Salmonella typhimurium strains TA 98, TA 100, TA 1535 and TA 1537 or in in vivo mutagenicity assays of mouse germinal cell chromosomes and Chinese hamster bone marrow cell chromosomes. It was however, mutagenic in inducing nondisjunction (96% frequency) in diploid strains of Aspergillus nidulans.

Pregnancy Category B

A reproduction study performed in rats receiving doses at least 150 times the average daily human dose of Esimil has revealed no evidence of impaired fertility or harm to the fetus due to this drug.

There are no adequate and well-controlled studies of Esimil in pregnant women. Because animal reproduction studies are not always predictive of human response, this drug should be used during pregnancy only if clearly needed.

Nonteratogenic Effects. Thiazides cross the placental barrier and appear in cord blood, and there is a risk of fetal or neonatal jaundice, thrombocytopenia, and possibly other adverse reactions that have occurred in adults.

Nursing Mothers

Guanethidine is excreted in breast milk in very small quantity. Thiazides are also excreted in breast milk. Because of the potential for serious adverse reactions in nursing infants, a decision should be made whether to discontinue nursing or to discontinue Esimil, taking into account the importance of the drug to the mother.

Pediatric Use

Safety and effectiveness of the combination drug in children have not been established.

ADVERSE REACTIONS

Whenever adverse reactions are moderate or severe, it may be necessary to reduce the dosage of Esimil, discontinue the drug, or administer the individual active components, reducing the dosage of either guanethidine or hydrochlorothiazide.

The following adverse reactions have been observed, but there are not enough data to support an estimate of their frequency. Consequently the reactions are categorized by organ system and are listed in decreasing order of severity and not frequency.

Guanethidine

Digestive: Diarrhea, which may be severe at times and necessitate discontinuance of medication; vomiting; nausea; increased bowel movements; dry mouth; parotid tenderness.

Cardiovascular: Chest pains (angina); bradycardia; a tendency toward fluid retention and edema with occasional development of congestive heart failure.

Respiratory: Dyspnea; asthma in susceptible individuals; nasal congestion.

Neurologic: Syncope resulting from either postural or exertional hypotension; dizziness; blurred vision; muscle tremor; ptosis of the lids; mental depression; chest paresthesias; weakness; lassitude; fatigue.

Muscular: Myalgia.

Genitourinary: Rise in BUN; urinary incontinence; inhibition of ejaculation; nocturia.

Metabolic: Weight gain.

Skin and Appendages: Dermatitis; scalp hair loss.

Although a causal relationship has not been established, a few instances of blood dyscrasias (anemia, thrombocytopenia, and leukopenia) and of priapism or impotence have been reported.

Hydrochlorothiazide

Digestive: Pancreatitis, jaundice (intrahepatic cholestatic), sialadenitis, vomiting, diarrhea, cramping, nausea, gastric irritation, constipation, anorexia.

Cardiovascular: Orthostatic hypotension (may be potentiated by alcohol, barbiturates, or narcotics).

Neurologic: Vertigo, dizziness, transient blurred vision, headache, paresthesia, xanthopsia, weakness, restlessness.

Musculoskeletal: Muscle spasm.

Hematologic: Aplastic anemia, agranulocytosis, leukopenia, thrombocytopenia.

Metabolic: Hyperglycemia, glycosuria, hyperuricemia.

Hypersensitive Reactions: Necrotizing angiitis, Stevens-Johnson syndrome, purpura, urticaria, rash, photosensitivity.

OVERDOSAGE

Acute Toxicity

No deaths due to acute poisoning with Esimil have been reported.

Oral LD$_{50}$'s in rats (mg/kg): guanethidine, 1262; hydrochlorothiazide, 2750.

Signs and Symptoms

Guanethidine. Postural hypotension (with dizziness, blurred vision, and possibly syncope when standing), shock, and bradycardia are most likely to occur; diarrhea (possibly severe), nausea, and vomiting may also occur. Unconsciousness is unlikely if adequate blood pressure and cerebral perfusion can be maintained by placing the patient in the supine position and by administering other treatment as required.

Hydrochlorothiazide. The most prominent feature of poisoning is acute loss of fluid and electrolytes.

Cardiovascular: Tachycardia, hypotension, shock.

Neuromuscular: Weakness, confusion, dizziness, cramps of the calf muscles, paresthesia, fatigue, impairment of consciousness.

Digestive: Nausea, vomiting, thirst.

Renal: Polyuria, oliguria, or anuria (due to hemoconcentration).

Laboratory Findings: Hypokalemia, hyponatremia, hypochloremia, alkalosis; increased BUN (especially in patients with renal insufficiency).

Combined Poisoning: Signs and symptoms may be aggravated or modified by concomitant intake of antihypertensive medication, barbiturates, digitalis (hypokalemia), corticosteroids, narcotics, or alcohol.

Treatment

There is no specific antidote.

The stomach contents should be evacuated. An activated charcoal slurry should be instilled and laxative given, if conditions permit.

If hypotension or shock occurs, the patient's legs should be kept raised, and lost fluid and electrolytes (potassium, sodium) should be replaced. Renal function should be monitored until conditions become normal.

In sinus bradycardia, atropine should be administered.

In previously normotensive patients, treatment has consisted essentially of restoring blood pressure and heart rate to normal by keeping the patient in the supine position. Normal homeostatic control usually returns gradually over a 72-hour period in these patients.

In previously hypertensive patients, particularly those with impaired cardiac reserve or other cardiovascular-renal disease, intensive treatment may be required to support vital functions and to control cardiac irregularities that might be present. The supine position must be maintained; if vasopressors are required, they must be used with extreme caution, since guanethidine may increase responsiveness, causing a rise in blood pressure and development of cardiac arrhythmias.

Diarrhea, if severe or persistent, should be treated with anticholinergic agents to reduce intestinal hypermotility, and hydration and electrolyte balance should be maintained. Since guanethidine is excreted slowly, cardiovascular and renal function should be monitored for a few days.

DOSAGE AND ADMINISTRATION

Dosage should be determined by individual titration (see boxed **WARNING**).

The usual dosage of Esimil is two tablets daily. Depending upon the degree of hypertension, the patient should be started on the lowest possible dose (usually one tablet daily) and the dose gradually increased at weekly intervals until the desired response is obtained. Blood pressure should be recorded with the patient in the supine position and again after 10 minutes of standing. Dosage should be increased only if the standing blood pressure has not been reduced to desired levels. Dosage adjustment should be made at not less than weekly intervals; maximal dosage should not exceed four tablets daily. If additional effect is desirable, guanethidine tablets may be supplemented individually.

Before starting therapy with Esimil, at least 1 week should elapse after MAO inhibitors (see **CONTRAINDICATIONS**) or ganglionic blockers are discontinued.

When Esimil is to be substituted for other antihypertensive agents, the change should be made gradually. In general, dosage of the agent to be discontinued should be halved, and Esimil should be started at one tablet daily. This schedule should be followed for at least 1 week; then, dosage of the previous therapy may be halved again and the dosage of Esimil increased to two tablets daily. At the next weekly interval, the previously used drugs can generally be discontinued. The dosage of Esimil should be titrated at weekly intervals, as mentioned above.

Patients receiving more than 75 mg of guanethidine alone may do well on a smaller dose if also given hydrochlorothiazide. Because of the ratio of the combination, these patients are probably not candidates for Esimil.

HOW SUPPLIED

Tablets—round, white, scored (imprinted CIBA 47)
  10 mg guanethidine monosulfate
  25 mg hydrochlorothiazide
  Bottles of 100 ....NDC 0083-0047-30
  Consumer Pack—One Unit
   12 bottles—
   100 tablets each ....NDC 0083-0047-65
Dispense in tight container (USP)   C87-47 (Rev. 11/87)
Shown in Product Identification Section, page 408

ESTRADERM®   ℞
[ess-tra-derm]
estradiol transdermal system
Continuous delivery for twice-weekly
application

ESTROGENS HAVE BEEN REPORTED TO INCREASE THE RISK OF ENDOMETRIAL CARCINOMA.
Three independent case control studies have reported an increased risk of endometrial cancer in postmenopausal women exposed to exogenous estrogens for more than 1 year. This risk was independent of the other known risk factors for endometrial cancer. These studies are further supported by the finding that incidence rates of endometrial cancer have increased sharply since 1969 in eight different areas of the United States with population-based cancer-reporting systems, an increase which may be related to the rapidly expanding use of estrogens during the last decade.
The three case control studies reported that the risk of endometrial cancer in estrogen users was about 4.5–13.9 times greater that in nonusers. The risk appears to depend both on duration of treatment and on estrogen dose. In view of these findings, when estrogens are used for the treatment of menopausal symptoms, the lowest dose that will control symptoms should be utilized and medication should be discontinued as soon as possible. When prolonged treatment is medically indicated, the patient should be reassessed on at least a semiannual basis to determine the need for continued therapy. Although the evidence must be considered preliminary, one study suggests that cyclic administration of low doses of estrogen may carry less risk than continuous administration; it therefore appears prudent to utilize such a regimen.
Close clinical surveillance of all women taking estrogens is important. In all cases of undiagnosed persistent

Continued on next page

The full prescribing information for each CIBA product is contained herein and is that in effect as of September 1, 1989

CIBA—Cont.

or recurring abnormal vaginal bleeding, adequate diagnostic measures should be undertaken to rule out malignancy.

There is no evidence at present that "natural" estrogens are more or less hazardous than "synthetic" estrogens at equiestrogenic doses.

ESTROGENS SHOULD NOT BE USED DURING PREGNANCY.

The use of female sex hormones, both estrogens and progestogens, during early pregnancy may seriously damage the offspring. It has been shown that women who had been exposed *in utero* to diethylstilbestrol, a nonsteroidal estrogen, have an increased risk of developing in later life a form of vaginal or cervical cancer that is ordinarily extremely rare. This risk has been estimated as not greater than 4 per 1000 exposures. Furthermore, a high percentage of such exposed women (30–90%) have been found to have vaginal adenosis, epithelial changes of the vagina and cervix. Although these changes are histologically benign, it is not known whether they are precursors of malignancy. Although similar data on the use of other estrogens are not available, it cannot be presumed they would not induce similar changes.

Several reports suggest an association between intrauterine exposure to female sex hormones and congenital anomalies, including congenital heart defects and limb-reduction defects. One case control study estimated a 4.7-fold increased risk of limb-reduction defects in infants who had been exposed *in utero* to sex hormones (oral contraceptives, hormone withdrawal tests for pregnancy, or attempted treatment for threatened abortion). Some of these exposures were very short and involved only a few days of treatment. The data suggest that the risk of limb-reduction defects in exposed fetuses is somewhat less than 1 per 1000.

In the past, female sex hormones have been used during pregnancy in an attempt to treat threatened or habitual abortion. There is considerable evidence that estrogens are ineffective for these indications, and there is no evidence from well-controlled studies that progestogens are effective for these uses.

If Estraderm is used during pregnancy, or if the patient becomes pregnant while taking this drug, she should be apprised of the potential risks to the fetus and of the advisability of continuation of the pregnancy.

DESCRIPTION

Estraderm, estradiol transdermal system, is designed to release 17β-estradiol through a rate-limiting membrane continuously upon application to intact skin.

Two systems are available to provide nominal *in vivo* delivery of 0.05 or 0.1 mg of estradiol per day via skin of average permeability (interindividual variation in skin permeability is approximately 20%). Each corresponding system having a contact surface area of 10 or 20 cm² contains 4 or 8 mg of estradiol USP and 0.3 or 0.6 ml of alcohol USP, respectively. The composition of the systems per unit area is identical. Estradiol USP (17β-estradiol) is a white, crystalline powder, chemically described as estra-1,3,5(10)-triene-3, 17β-diol. The Estraderm system comprises four layers. Proceeding from the visible surface toward the surface attached to the skin, these layers are (1) a transparent polyester film, (2) a drug reservoir of estradiol USP and alcohol USP gelled with hydroxypropyl cellulose, (3) an ethylene-vinyl acetate copolymer membrane, and (4) an adhesive formulation of light mineral oil and polyisobutylene. A protective liner (5) of siliconized polyethylene terephthalate film is attached to the adhesive surface and must be removed before the system can be used.

(1) Backing
(2) Drug Reservoir
(3) Control Membrane
(4) Adhesive Layer
(5) Protective Liner

The active component of the system is estradiol. The remaining components of the system are pharmacologically inactive. Alcohol is also released from the system during use.

CLINICAL PHARMACOLOGY

The Estraderm system releases estradiol, the major estrogenic hormone secreted by the human ovary. Estraderm provides systemic estrogen replacement therapy. Among numerous effects, estradiol is largely responsible for the development and maintenance of the female reproductive system and of secondary sexual characteristics. It promotes growth and development of the vagina, uterus, fallopian tubes, and breasts. Indirectly, estradiol contributes to the shaping of the skeleton, to the maintenance of tone and elasticity of urogenital structures, to changes in the epiphyses of

the long bones that allow for the pubertal growth spurt and its termination, to the growth of axillary and pubic hair, and to the pigmentation of the nipples and genitals.

In the anovulatory cycle estrogen is the primary determinant in the onset of menstruation. Estradiol also affects the release of pituitary gonadotropins.

Loss of ovarian estradiol secretion after menopause can result in instability of thermoregulation, causing hot flushes associated with sleep disturbance and excessive sweating, and urogenital atrophy, causing dyspareunia and urinary incontinence. Estradiol replacement therapy alleviates many of these symptoms of estradiol deficiency in the menopausal woman. It has not been determined that the currently recommended doses of Estraderm are appropriate for the treatment or prevention of postmenopausal osteoporosis.

Orally administered estradiol is rapidly metabolized by the liver to estrone and its conjugates, giving rise to higher circulating levels of estrone than estradiol. In contrast, the skin metabolizes estradiol only to a small extent. Therefore, transdermal administration produces therapeutic serum levels of estradiol with lower circulating levels of estrone and estrone conjugates, and requires smaller total doses than does oral therapy. Because estradiol has a short half-life (~1 hour), transdermal administration of estradiol allows a rapid decline in blood levels after an Estraderm system is removed, e.g., in a cycling regimen.

In a study using transdermally administered estradiol, 0.1 mg daily, plasma levels increased by 66 pg/ml resulting in an average plasma level of 73 pg/ml. There were no significant increases in the concentration of renin substrate or other hepatic proteins (sex-hormone-binding globulin, thyroxine-binding globulin and corticosteroid-binding globulin).

Pharmacokinetics

Administration of Estraderm produces mean serum concentrations of estradiol comparable to those produced by a daily oral administration of estradiol at about 20 times the daily transdermal dose. In single-application studies in 14 postmenopausal women using Estraderm systems that provided 0.05 and 0.1 mg of exogenous estradiol per day, these systems produced increased blood levels within 4 hours and maintained respective mean serum estradiol concentrations of 32 and 67 pg/ml above baseline over the application period. At the same time, increases in estrone serum concentration averaged only 9 and 27 pg/ml above baseline, respectively. Serum concentrations of estradiol and estrone returned to preapplication levels within 24 hours after removal of the system. The estimated daily urinary output of estradiol conjugates increased 5 to 10 times the baseline values and returned to near baseline within 2 days after removal of the system.

By comparison, estradiol (2 mg per day) administered orally to postmenopausal women resulted in increases in mean serum concentration of 59 pg/ml of estradiol and 302 pg/ml of estrone above baseline on the third consecutive day of dosing. Urinary output of estradiol conjugates increased to about 100 times the baseline values and did not approach baseline until 7–8 days after the last dose.

In a 3-week multiple-application study of 14 postmenopausal women in which Estraderm 0.05 was applied twice weekly, the mean increments in steady-state serum concentration were 30 pg/ml for estradiol and 12 pg/ml for estrone. Urinary output of estradiol conjugates returned to baseline within 3 days after removal of the last (6th) system, indicating little or no estrogen accumulation in the body.

INDICATIONS AND USAGE

Estraderm is indicated for the treatment of the following: moderate-to-severe vasomotor symptoms associated with menopause; female hypogonadism; female castration; primary ovarian failure; and atrophic conditions caused by deficient endogenous estrogen production, such as atrophic vaginitis and kraurosis vulvae.

CONTRAINDICATIONS

Estrogens should not be used in women or men with any of the following conditions:

1. known or suspected cancer of the breast;
2. known or suspected estrogen-dependent neoplasia;
3. known or suspected pregnancy (see Boxed Warning);
4. undiagnosed abnormal genital bleeding;
5. active thrombophlebitis or thromboembolic disorders;
6. history of thrombophlebitis, thrombosis, or thromboembolic disorders associated with previous estrogen use.

WARNINGS

1. *Induction of Malignant Neoplasms.* Long-term continuous administration of natural and synthetic estrogens in certain animal species increases the frequency of carcinomas of the breast, cervix, vagina, and liver. There are now reports that estrogens increase the risk of carcinoma of the endometrium in humans. (See Boxed Warning.)

At the present time, there is no satisfactory evidence that estrogens given to postmenopausal women increase the risk of breast cancer, although a recent long-term followup of a single physician's practice has raised this possibility. Because of the animal data, there is a need for caution in prescribing estrogens for women with a strong family his-

tory of breast cancer or who have breast nodules, fibrocystic disease, or abnormal mammograms.

2. *Gallbladder Disease.* A recent study has reported a two- to threefold increase in the risk of surgically confirmed gallbladder disease in postmenopausal women receiving oral estrogens, similar to the twofold increase previously noted in users of oral contraceptives.

3. *Effects Similar to Those Caused by Estrogen-Progestogen Oral Contraceptives.* There are several serious adverse effects of oral contraceptives and other high-dose oral estrogen treatments, most of which have not, up to now, been documented as consequences of postmenopausal estrogen replacement therapy. This may reflect the comparatively low doses of estrogen used in postmenopausal women.

a. *Thromboembolic Disease.* It is now well established that users of oral contraceptives have an increased risk of various thromboembolic and thrombotic vascular diseases, such as thrombophlebitis, pulmonary embolism, stroke, and myocardial infarction. Cases of retinal thrombosis, mesenteric thrombosis, and optic neuritis have been reported in oral contraceptive users. There is evidence that the risk of several of these adverse reactions is related to the dose of the drug. An increased risk of post-surgery thromboembolic complications has also been reported in users of oral contraceptives. If feasible, estrogen should be discontinued at least 4 weeks before surgery of the type associated with an increased risk of thromboembolism, or during periods of prolonged immobilization.

While an increased rate of thromboembolic and thrombotic disease in postmenopausal users of estrogens has not been found, this does not rule out the possibility that such an increase may be present or that subgroups of women who have underlying risk factors or who are receiving relatively large doses of estrogens may have increased risk. Therefore, estrogens should not be used in persons with active thrombophlebitis or thromboembolic disorders, and they should not be used in persons with a history of such disorders in association with estrogen use. They should be used with caution in patients with cerebral vascular or coronary artery disease and only for those in whom estrogens are clearly needed.

Large doses of estrogen (5 mg conjugated estrogens per day), comparable to those used to treat cancer of the prostate and breast, have been shown in a large prospective clinical trial in men to increase the risk of nonfatal myocardial infarction, pulmonary embolism, and thrombophlebitis. When estrogen doses of this size are used, any of the thromboembolic and thrombotic adverse effects associated with oral contraceptive use should be considered a clear risk.

b. *Hepatic Adenoma.* Benign hepatic adenomas have been associated with the use of oral contraceptives. Although benign and rare, these tumors may rupture and cause death from intra-abdominal hemorrhage. Such lesions have not yet been reported in association with other estrogen or progestogen preparations, but they should be considered if abdominal pain and tenderness, abdominal mass, or hypovolemic shock occurs in patients receiving estrogen. Hepatocellular carcinoma has also been reported in women taking estrogen-containing oral contraceptives. The causal relationship of this malignancy to these drugs is not known.

c. *Elevated Blood Pressure.* Women using oral contraceptives sometimes experience increased blood pressure which, in most cases, returns to normal upon discontinuing the drug. There is now a report that this may occur with use of oral estrogens in the menopause and blood pressure should be monitored with estrogen use, especially if high doses are used. Ethinyl estradiol and conjugated estrogens have been shown to increase renin substrate. In contrast to these oral estrogens, transdermally administered estradiol does not affect renin substrate.

d. *Glucose Tolerance.* A worsening of glucose tolerance has been observed in a significant percentage of patients on estrogen-containing oral contraceptives. For this reason, diabetic patients should be carefully observed while receiving estrogen.

4. *Hypercalcemia.* Administration of high doses of estrogens may lead to severe hypercalcemia in patients with breast cancer and bone metastases. If hypercalcemia occurs, use of the drug should be stopped and appropriate measures should be taken to reduce the serum calcium level.

PRECAUTIONS
General

1. A complete medical and family history should be taken before initiation of any estrogen therapy. The pretreatment and periodic physical examinations should include special reference to blood pressure, breasts, abdomen, and pelvic organs, as well as a cervical Papanicolaou test. As a general rule, estrogen should not be prescribed for longer than 1 year without another physical examination being performed.

2. Because estrogens may cause some degree of fluid retention, careful observation is required when conditions

that might be influenced by this factor are present (e.g., asthma, epilepsy, migraine, and cardiac or renal dysfunction).

3. Certain patients may develop undesirable manifestations of excessive estrogenic stimulation, such as uterine bleeding, mastodynia, etc.

4. Prolonged administration of unopposed estrogen therapy has been reported to increase the risk of endometrial hyperplasia in some patients. Estrogens should be used with caution in patients who have or have had endometriosis.

5. Studies of the addition of a progestin for 7 or more days of a cycle of estrogen administration have reported a lowered incidence of endometrial hyperplasia. Morphological and biochemical studies of endometrium suggest that 12 to 13 days of progestin are needed to provide maximal maturation of the endometrium and to eliminate any hyperplastic changes. Whether this will provide protection from endometrial carcinoma has not been clearly established. There are possible additional risks that may be associated with the inclusion of progestin in estrogen replacement regimens. The potential risks include adverse effects on carbohydrate and lipid metabolism. The choice of progestin and dosage may be important in minimizing these adverse effects.

6. Oral contraceptives appear to be associated with an increased incidence of mental depression. Although it is not clear whether this is due to the estrogenic or progestogenic component of the contraceptive, patients with a history of depression should be carefully observed.

7. Preexisting uterine leiomyomata may increase in size during prolonged estrogen use. If this occurs, estrogen therapy should be discontinued while the cause is investigated.

8. In patients with a history of jaundice during pregnancy, there is an increased risk that jaundice will recur with the use of estrogen-containing oral contraceptives. If jaundice develops in any patient receiving estrogen, the medication should be discontinued while the cause is investigated.

9. Estrogens may be poorly metabolized in patients with impaired liver function and should be administered with caution in such patients.

10. Because the prolonged use of estrogens influences the metabolism of calcium and phosphorus, estrogens should be used with caution in patients with metabolic bone diseases associated with hypercalcemia and in patients with renal insufficiency.

Information for Patients
See Patient Package Insert printed below.
Drug/Laboratory Test Interactions
The results of certain endocrine and liver function tests may be affected by estrogen-containing oral contraceptives. The following changes have been observed with large doses of oral estrogen:

1. increased sulfobromophthalein retention;
2. increased prothrombin time; increased factors VII, VIII, IX, and X; decreased antithrombin 3; increased norepinephrine-induced platelet aggregability;
3. increased thyroxine-binding globulin (TBG), leading to increased circulating total thyroid hormone (T_4) as measured by column or radioimmunoassay; free T_3 resin uptake is decreased, reflecting the elevated TBG; free T_4 concentration is unaltered; TBG was not affected in clinical trials of Estraderm;
4. reduced response to the metyrapone test;
5. reduced serum folate concentration;
6. increased serum triglyceride and phospholipid concentration, and decreased pregnanediol excretion.

The pathologist should be informed that the patient is receiving estrogen therapy when relevant specimens are submitted.

Carcinogenesis, Mutagenesis, Impairment of Fertility
See WARNINGS and Boxed Warning.
Long-term continuous administration of natural and synthetic estrogens in certain animal species increases the frequency of carcinomas of the breast, cervix, vagina, and liver.

Pregnancy Category X
See CONTRAINDICATIONS and Boxed Warning.
Estrogens should not be used during pregnancy.

Nursing Mothers
As a general principle, the administration of any drug to nursing mothers should be done only when clearly necessary since many drugs are excreted in human milk.

ADVERSE REACTIONS
See WARNINGS and Boxed Warning regarding potential adverse effects on the fetus, induction of malignant neoplasms, increased incidence of gallbladder disease, and adverse effects similar to those of oral contraceptives, including thromboembolism.
The most commonly reported adverse reaction to Estraderm in clinical trials was redness and irritation at the application site. This occurred in about 17% of the women treated and caused approximately 2% to discontinue therapy. Reports of rash have been rare.

The following additional adverse reactions have been reported with estrogenic therapy, including oral contraceptives:
Genitourinary System: Breakthrough bleeding, spotting, change in menstrual flow; increase in size of uterine fibromyomata; change in cervical erosion and amount of cervical secretion.
Endocrine: Breast tenderness, breast enlargement.
Gastrointestinal: Nausea, vomiting; abdominal cramps, bloating; cholestatic jaundice have been observed with oral estrogen therapy.
Eyes: Steepening of corneal curvature; intolerance to contact lenses.
Central Nervous System: Headache, migraine, dizziness.
Miscellaneous: Change in weight, edema, change in libido.

OVERDOSAGE
Numerous reports of ingestion of large doses of estrogen-containing oral contraceptives by young children indicate that acute serious ill effects do not occur. Overdosage with estrogen may cause nausea, and withdrawal bleeding may occur in females.

DOSAGE AND ADMINISTRATION
The adhesive side of the Estraderm system should be placed on a clean, dry area of the skin on the trunk of the body, preferably the abdomen. *Estraderm should not be applied to the breasts.* The sites of application should be rotated, with an interval of at least 1 week allowed between applications to a particular site. The area selected should not be oily, damaged, or irritated. The waistline should be avoided, since tight clothing may rub the system off. The system should be applied immediately after opening the pouch and removing the protective liner. The system should be pressed firmly in place with the palm of the hand for about 10 seconds, making sure there is good contact, especially around the edges. In the unlikely event that a system should fall off, the same system may be reapplied. If necessary, a new system may be applied. In either case, the original treatment schedule should be continued.

Initiation of Therapy
Treatment is usually initiated with Estraderm 0.05 applied to the skin twice weekly. The dose should be adjusted as necessary to control symptoms.
In women who are not currently taking oral estrogens, treatment with Estraderm can be initiated at once. In women who are currently taking oral estrogen, treatment with Estraderm can be initiated 1 week after withdrawal of oral therapy or sooner if symptoms reappear before the week's end.
Clinical responses (relief of symptoms) at the lowest effective dose should generally be the guide for establishing administration of Estraderm for those indications in which symptoms are observable. Attempts to taper or discontinue medication should be made at 3- to 6-month intervals.

Therapeutic Regimen
Therapy with Estraderm is usually administered on a cyclic schedule (e.g., 3 weeks of therapy followed by 1 week without) especially in women who have not undergone a hysterectomy.

HOW SUPPLIED
Estraderm 0.05 (estradiol transdermal system)—each 10 cm^2 system contains 4 mg of estradiol USP for nominal* delivery of 0.05 mg of estradiol per day
Patient Calendar Pack of 8 systems ....
                NDC 0083-2310-08
Carton of 6 Patient Calendar Packs of 8 Systems ....
                NDC 0083-2310-62
Carton of 1 Patient Calendar Pack of 24 Systems ....
                NDC 0083-2310-24
Estraderm 0.1 (estradiol transdermal system—each 20 cm^2 system contains 8 mg of estradiol USP for nominal* delivery of 0.1 mg of estradiol per day
Patient Calendar Pack of 8 Systems ....NDC 0083-2320-08
Carton of 6 Patient Calendar Packs of 8 Systems ....
                NDC 0083-2320-62
Carton of 1 Patient Calendar Pack of 24 Systems ....
                NDC 0083-2320-24

*See DESCRIPTION.
Do not store above 86°F (30°C).
Do not store unpouched. Apply immediately upon removal from the protective pouch.
                C88-23 (Rev. 8/88)

Information for the Patient
ESTRADERM ®
Generic name:
estradiol transdermal system pronounced ess-tra-DYE-all

INTRODUCTION
Your doctor has prescribed Estraderm for the treatment of your menopausal symptoms. During menopause, production of estrogen hormones by your body decreases well below the amounts normally produced during your fertile years. In many women this decrease in estrogen production causes uncomfortable symptoms, most noticeably hot flushes and

sleep disturbance. Estrogens can be given to reduce or eliminate these symptoms.
The Estraderm system that your doctor has prescribed for you releases small amounts of estradiol through the skin in a continuous way. Estradiol is the same hormone that your ovaries produce abundantly before menopause. The dose of estradiol you require will depend upon your individual response. The dose is adjusted by the size of the Estraderm system used; the systems are available in two sizes.
This leaflet will provide you with general information about estrogens and with specific information about the Estraderm system. Please read it carefully. If you want to know more, you should ask your doctor for more information.

INFORMATION ABOUT ESTRADERM
How Estraderm Works
Estraderm contains estradiol. When applied to the skin as directed below, the Estraderm system releases estradiol, which flows through the skin into the bloodstream.
How and Where to Apply Estraderm
Each Estraderm system is individually sealed in a protective pouch. Tear open this pouch at the indentation (do not use scissors) and remove the system. Bubbles in the system are normal.

A stiff protective liner covers the adhesive side of the system—the side that will be placed against your skin. This liner must be removed before applying the system. Slide the protective liner sideways between your thumb and index finger. Then hold the system at one edge. Remove the protective liner and discard it. Try to avoid touching the adhesive.

Apply the adhesive side of the system to a clean, dry area of the skin on the trunk of your body, preferably the abdomen. *Do not apply Estraderm to your breasts.* The sites of application should be rotated, with an interval of at least 1 week allowed between applications to a particular site. The area selected should not be oily, damaged, or irritated. Avoid the waistline, since tight clothing may rub the system off. Apply the system immediately after opening the pouch and removing the protective liner. Press the system firmly in place with the palm of your hand for about 10 seconds, making sure there is good contact, especially around the edges.
The Estraderm system should be worn continuously until it is time to replace it with a new system. You may wish to experiment with different locations when applying a new system, to find ones that are most comfortable for you and where clothing will not rub on the system.
When to Apply Estraderm
The Estraderm system should be changed twice weekly. Your Estraderm package contains a dial on the back to help you remember a schedule. Turn the dial to the days on which you and your doctor decide you should apply a new system, and lock it there. Always change the system on the 2 days of the week shown on the dial.

When changing the system, remove the used Estraderm and discard it. Any adhesive that might remain on your skin can be easily rubbed off. Then place the new Estraderm on a different skin site. (The same skin site should not be used again for at least 1 week after removal of the system.)
Please note: Contact with water when you are bathing, swimming, or showering will not affect the system. In the unlikely event that a system should fall off, put this same system back on and continue to follow your original treatment schedule. If necessary, you may apply a new system but continue to follow your original schedule.
Benefits of Treatment With Estraderm
The simple application of Estraderm twice weekly offers relief of the symptoms of menopause. Small quantities of the naturally occurring hormone estradiol are absorbed through

Continued on next page

CIBA—Cont.

the skin from the Estraderm system, ensuring a continuous supply of circulating hormone in the body.

When estradiol is administered through your skin, the drug does not undergo the rapid chemical changes in the liver and stomach that would occur if you were taking it by mouth. There is no medical evidence that the use of any estrogen during menopause will keep you feeling young, keep your skin soft, or relieve nervousness.

PRECAUTIONS

The use of estrogens has benefits, but it has risks as well. Before using Estraderm, be sure to tell your doctor if you are pregnant. **ESTROGENS SHOULD NOT BE USED DURING PREGNANCY.** Also tell your doctor if you have ever had any of the following: cancer of the breast or uterus, unusual vaginal bleeding, endometriosis, or abnormal blood clotting. Your doctor may decide that Estraderm should not be used under these conditions.

Also tell your doctor if you have or have ever had high blood pressure, heart or kidney disease, asthma, skin allergy, epilepsy, migraine, diabetes, or depression. This information will help your doctor decide whether you should use Estraderm.

You should tell your doctor if any of the following occur while using Estraderm; any irregular bleeding; breast tenderness, enlargement, or lumps; pain or heaviness in the legs or chest; severe headache, dizziness, or changes in vision; or skin irritation, redness, or rash.

INFORMATION ABOUT ESTROGENS

Estrogens in the Menopause

Menopause occurs either naturally in the course of a woman's life or sooner if the ovaries are removed by surgery. During menopause—which usually occurs between the ages of 45 and 55—there is a decrease in estrogen production by the ovaries. In many women this decrease causes unpleasant symptoms such as a feeling of warmth in the face, neck, and chest, or sudden intense episodes of heat and sweating throughout the body (called "hot flashes" or "hot flushes"). Some women may also develop other changes: impaired bladder control and alterations in the vagina (such as dryness) that cause discomfort during and after intercourse.

Estrogens can be prescribed to treat menopausal symptoms. Some women have no symptoms or only mild ones and do not need estrogens; others may need estrogens for a few months; and others will need treatment for longer periods. Usually treatment is cyclical and includes days when no estrogen is given. Other drugs called progestins, are sometimes given to offset the effects of estrogens on the lining of the uterus. You may wish to discuss the risks and benefits of such treatment with your doctor.

Possible Risks and Discomforts From Treatment With Estrogens

The risk of endometrial cancer (cancer of the lining of the uterus) is greater in estrogen users than in nonusers. (If you have had your uterus removed by a total hysterectomy, this would not be a risk for you.) Recent studies have shown that this increased risk depends on estrogen dose, duration of treatment, and treatment regimen.

Despite numerous studies, there has been no definite link established between estrogen use and breast cancer. Nevertheless, women with a family history of breast cancer, or with breast nodules, fibrocystic breast disease (lumps), or abnormal mammograms should consult with their doctor before taking estrogens.

In certain animals treated with estrogen, cancer of the cervix, vagina, and liver occurred more frequently.

The following effects have also been reported in women taking estrogens: nausea (the most common side effect), retention of fluid, gallbladder disease, abnormal blood clotting, migraine, elevated serum calcium, growth of benign fibroid tumors in the uterus, jaundice, darkening of the skin, defects in the fetus, and liver tumors. Redness, irritation, or rash may occur at the site of Estraderm application.

Breast tenderness and excessive vaginal secretions may occur when the dose of estrogen administered is too high.

Based on a review of your medical needs, your doctor has prescribed Estraderm for you. Use it only as directed and do not give it to anyone else. Your doctor should reexamine you at least annually.

Do not store above 86°F (30°C).

Do not store unpouched. Apply immediately upon removal from the protective pouch.

C87-2 (Rev. 2/87)
C88-23/C87-2 (Rev. 8/88)

Shown in Product Identification Section, page 408

INH isoniazid USP   ℞
Tablets

> ### WARNING
> Severe and sometimes fatal hepatitis associated with isoniazid therapy may occur and may develop even after many months of treatment. The risk of developing hepatitis is age related. Approximate case rates by age are: 0 per 1,000 for persons under 20 years of age, 3 per 1,000 for persons in the 20–34 year age group, 12 per 1,000 for persons in the 35–49 year age group, 23 per 1,000 for persons in the 50–64 year age group, and 8 per 1,000 for persons over 65 years of age. The risk of hepatitis is increased with daily consumption of alcohol. Precise data to provide a fatality rate for isoniazid-related hepatitis is not available; however, in a U.S. Public Health Service Surveillance Study of 13,838 persons taking isoniazid, there were 8 deaths among 174 cases of hepatitis. Therefore, patients given isoniazid should be carefully monitored and interviewed at monthly intervals. Serum transaminase concentration becomes elevated in about 10–20 percent of patients, usually during the first few months of therapy but it can occur at any time. Usually enzyme levels return to normal despite continuance of drug but in some cases progressive liver dysfunction occurs. Patients should be instructed to report immediately any of the prodromal symptoms of hepatitis, such as fatigue, weakness, malaise, anorexia, nausea, or vomiting. If these symptoms appear or if signs suggestive of hepatic damage are detected, isoniazid should be discontinued promptly, since continued use of the drug in these cases has been reported to cause a more severe form of liver damage.
>
> Patients with tuberculosis should be given appropriate treatment with alternative drugs. If isoniazid must be reinstituted, it should be reinstituted only after symptoms and laboratory abnormalities have cleared. The drug should be restarted in very small and gradually increasing doses and should be withdrawn immediately if there is any indication of recurrent liver involvement. Preventive treatment should be deferred in persons with acute hepatic diseases.

DESCRIPTION

INH, isoniazid USP, is an antibiotic available as 300-mg tablets for oral administration. It is available in Dual Packs of Rimactane® rifampin USP/INH containing one 300-mg tablet of INH and two 300-mg capsules of Rimactane. Isoniazid is isonicotinic acid hydrazide.

Isoniazid USP is colorless or white crystals or white crystalline powder. It is odorless and slowly affected by exposure to air and light. It is freely soluble in water, sparingly soluble in alcohol, and slightly soluble in chloroform and in ether. Its molecular weight is 137.14.

Inactive Ingredients. Cellulose compounds, colloidal silicon dioxide, sodium starch glycolate, and stearic acid.

CLINICAL PHARMACOLOGY

Isoniazid acts against actively growing tubercle bacilli. Within 1 to 2 hours after oral administration isoniazid produces peak blood levels which decline to 50% or less within 6 hours. It diffuses readily into all body fluids (cerebrospinal, pleural, and ascitic fluids), tissues, organs, and excreta (saliva, sputum, and feces). The drug also passes through the placental barrier and into milk in concentrations comparable to those in the plasma. From 50 to 70% of a dose of isoniazid is excreted in the urine in 24 hours.

Isoniazid is metabolized primarily by acetylation and dehydrazination. The rate of acetylation is genetically determined. Approximately 50% of Blacks and Caucasians are "slow inactivators" and the rest are rapid inactivators; the majority of Eskimos and Orientals are "rapid inactivators." The rate of acetylation does not significantly alter the effectiveness of isoniazid. However, slow acetylation may lead to higher blood levels of the drug, and thus an increase in toxic reactions.

Pyridoxine (B_6) deficiency is sometimes observed in adults with high doses of isoniazid and is considered probably due to its competition with pyridoxal phosphate for the enzyme apotryptophanase.

INDICATIONS AND USAGE

For all forms of tuberculosis in which organisms are susceptible.

For preventive therapy for the following groups, in order of priority:

1. Household members and other close associates of persons with recently diagnosed tuberculous disease.
2. Positive tuberculin skin test reactors with findings on the chest roentgenogram consistent with nonprogressive tuberculous disease, in whom there are neither positive bacteriologic findings nor a history of adequate chemotherapy.

---

3. Newly infected persons.
4. Positive tuberculin skin test reactors in the following special clinical situations: prolonged therapy with adrenocorticosteroids; immunosuppressive therapy; some hematologic and reticuloendothelial diseases, such as leukemia or Hodgkin's disease; diabetes mellitus; silicosis; after gastrectomy.
5. Other positive tuberculin reactors under 35 years of age. The risk of hepatitis must be weighed against the risk of tuberculosis in positive tuberculin reactors over the age of 35. However, the use of isoniazid is recommended for those with the additional risk factors listed above (1–4) and on an individual basis in situations where there is likelihood of serious consequences to contacts who may become infected.

CONTRAINDICATIONS

Isoniazid is contraindicated in patients who develop severe hypersensitivity reactions, including drug-induced hepatitis. Previous isoniazid-associated hepatic injury: severe adverse reactions to isoniazid, such as drug fever, chills, and arthritis; acute liver disease of any etiology.

WARNINGS

See the boxed warning.

PRECAUTIONS

All drugs should be stopped and an evaluation made at the first sign of a hypersensitivity reaction. If isoniazid therapy must be reinstituted, the drug should be given only after symptoms have cleared. The drug should be restarted in very small and gradually increasing doses and should be withdrawn immediately if there is any indication of recurrent hypersensitivity reaction.

Use of isoniazid should be carefully monitored in the following:

1. Patients who are receiving phenytoin concurrently. Isoniazid may decrease the excretion of phenytoin or may enhance its effects. To avoid phenytoin intoxication, appropriate adjustment of the anticonvulsant should be made.
2. Daily users of alcohol. Daily ingestion of alcohol may be associated with a higher incidence of isoniazid hepatitis.
3. Patients with current chronic liver disease or severe renal dysfunction.

Ophthalmologic examinations (including ophthalmoscopy) should be done *before* INH is started and periodically thereafter, even without occurrence of visual syptoms.

Usage in Pregnancy and Lactation

It has been reported that in both rats and rabbits, isoniazid may exert an embryocidal effect when administered orally during pregnancy, although no isoniazid-related congenital anomalies have been found in reproduction studies in mammalian species (mice, rats, and rabbits). Isoniazid should be prescribed during pregnancy only when therapeutically necessary. The benefit of preventive therapy should be weighed against a possible risk to the fetus. Preventive treatment generally should be started after delivery because of the increased risk of tuberculosis for new mothers.

Since isoniazid is known to cross the placental barrier and to pass into maternal breast milk, neonates and breast-fed infants of isoniazid-treated mothers should be carefully observed for any evidence of adverse effects.

Carcinogenesis

Isoniazid has been reported to induce pulmonary tumors in a number of strains of mice.

ADVERSE REACTIONS

The most frequent reactions are those affecting the nervous system and the liver.

Nervous system reactions: Peripheral neuropathy is the most common toxic effect. It is dose-related, occurs most often in the malnourished and in those predisposed to neuritis (eg, alcoholics and diabetics), and is usually preceded by paresthesias of the feet and hands. The incidence is higher in "slow inactivators."

Other neurotoxic effects, which are uncommon with conventional doses, are convulsions, toxic encephalopathy, optic neuritis and atrophy, memory impairment, and toxic psychosis.

Gastrointestinal reactions: Nausea, vomiting, epigastric distress.

Hepatic reactions: Elevated serum transaminases (SGOT; SGPT), bilirubinemia, bilirubinuria, jaundice and occasionally severe and sometimes fatal hepatitis. The common prodromal symptoms are anorexia, nausea, vomiting, fatigue, malaise, and weakness. Mild and transient elevation of serum transaminase levels, occurs in 10 to 20 percent of persons taking isoniazid. The abnormality usually occurs in the first 4 to 6 months of treatment but can occur at any time during therapy. In most instances, enzyme levels return to normal with no necessity to discontinue medication. In occasional instances, progressive liver damage occurs, with accompanying symptoms. In these cases, the drug should be discontinued immediately. The frequency of progressive liver damage increases with age. It is rare in persons under 20, but occurs in up to 2.3 percent of those over 50 years of age.

Hematologic reactions: Agranulocytosis; hemolytic, sideroblastic, or aplastic anemia; thrombocytopenia; and eosinophilia.

Hypersensitivity reactions: Fever, skin eruptions (morbilliform, maculopapular, purpuric, or exfoliative), lymphadenopathy and vasculitis.

Metabolic and endocrine reactions: Pyridoxine deficiency, pellagra, hyperglycemia, metabolic acidosis, and gynecomastia.

Miscellaneous reactions: Rheumatic syndrome and systemic lupus erythematosus-like syndrome.

OVERDOSAGE

Signs and Symptoms

Isoniazid overdosage produces signs and symptoms within 30 minutes to 3 hours after ingestion. Nausea, vomiting, dizziness, slurring of speech, blurring of vision, and visual hallucinations (including bright colors and strange designs), are among the early manifestations. With marked overdosage, respiratory distress and CNS depression, progressing rapidly from stupor to profound coma, are to be expected, along with severe, intractable seizures. Severe metabolic acidosis, acetonuria, and hyperglycemia are typical laboratory findings.

Treatment

Untreated or inadequately treated cases of gross isoniazid overdosage can terminate fatally, but good response has been reported in most patients brought under adequate treatment within the first few hours after drug ingestion. Secure the airway and establish adequate respiratory exchange. Gastric lavage within the first 2 to 3 hours is advised, but should not be attempted until convulsions are under control. To control convulsions administer I.V. short-acting barbiturates and I.V. pyridoxine (usually 1 mg/1mg isoniazid ingested).

Obtain blood samples for immediate determination of gases, electrolytes, BUN, glucose, etc.; type and crossmatch blood in preparation for possible hemodialysis.

Rapid control of metabolic acidosis is fundamental to management. Give I.V. sodium bicarbonate at once and repeat as needed, adjusting subsequent dosage on the basis of laboratory findings (ie, serum sodium, pH, etc.).

Forced osmotic diuresis must be started early and should be continued for some hours after clinical improvement to hasten renal clearance of drug and help prevent relapse; monitor fluid intake and output.

Hemodialysis is advised for severe cases; if this is not available, peritoneal dialysis can be used along with forced diuresis.

Along with measures based on initial and repeated determination of blood gases and other laboratory tests as needed, utilize meticulous respiratory and other intensive care to protect against hypoxia, hypotension, aspiration pneumonitis, etc.

DOSAGE AND ADMINISTRATION [See also INDICATIONS]:

NOTE—For preventive therapy of tuberculous infection it is recommended that physicians be familiar with the joint recommendations of the American Thoracic Society, American Lung Association, and the Center for Disease Control, as published in the American Review of Respiratory Diseases Vol. 110, No. 3, September 1974, or CDC's Morbidity and Mortality Weekly Report, Vol. 24, No. 8, February 22, 1975.

For treatment of active tuberculosis

Isoniazid is used in conjunction with other effective antituberculous agents.

If the bacilli become resistant, therapy must be changed to agents to which the bacilli are susceptible.

Usual oral dosage

Adults: 5 mg/kg up to 300 mg daily in a single dose.

Infants and children: 10–20 mg/kg depending on severity of infection, (up to 300–500 mg daily) in a single dose.

For preventive therapy

Adults: 300 mg/day in a single dose.

Infants and children: 10 mg/kg (up to 300 mg daily) in a single dose.

Continuous administration of isoniazid for a sufficient period is an essential part of the regimen because relapse rates are higher if chemotherapy is stopped prematurely. In the treatment of tuberculosis, resistant organisms may multiply and the emergence of resistant organisms during the treatment may necessitate a change in the regimen.

Concomitant administration of pyridoxine (B$_6$) is recommended in the malnourished and in those predisposed to neuropathy (eg, alcoholics and diabetics).

HOW SUPPLIED

Tablets, 300 mg (white, scored); available as Rimactane® rifampin USP/INH Dual Pack containing 30 INH Tablets and 60 Rimactane 300-mg Capsules.

NDC 0083-8912-23

Protect from heat, light and moisture (Rimactane/INH Dual Pack).

C87-32 (Rev. 8/87)

ISMELIN® sulfate ℞

[*iz 'mel-lin*]

guanethidine monosulfate

Tablets

DESCRIPTION

Ismelin, guanethidine monosulfate, is an antihypertensive, available as tablets of 10 mg and 25 mg for oral administration. Each 10-mg and 25-mg tablet contains guanethidine monosulfate equivalent to 10 mg and 25 mg of guanethidine sulfate, USP. Its chemical name is [2-(hexahydro-1(2*H*)-azocinyl)ethyl]guanidine sulfate 1:1.

Guanethidine monosulfate is a white to off-white crystalline powder with a molecular weight of 296.38. It is very soluble in water, sparingly soluble in alcohol, and practically insoluble in chloroform.

Inactive ingredients: Calcium stearate, colloidal silicon dioxide, D&C Yellow No. 10 (10-mg tablets), lactose, starch, stearic acid, and sucrose.

CLINICAL PHARMACOLOGY

Ismelin acts at the sympathetic neuroeffector junction by inhibiting or interfering with the release and/or distribution of the chemical mediator (presumably the catecholamine norepinephrine), rather than acting at the effector cell by inhibiting the association of the transmitter with its receptors. In contrast to ganglionic blocking agents, Ismelin suppresses equally the responses mediated by alpha- and beta-adrenergic receptors but does not produce parasympathetic blockade. Since sympathetic blockade results in modest decreases in peripheral resistance and cardiac output, Ismelin lowers blood pressure in the supine position. It further reduces blood pressure by decreasing the degree of vasoconstriction that normally results from reflex sympathetic nervous activity upon assumption of the upright posture, thus reducing venous return and cardiac output more. The inhibition of sympathetic venoconstrictive mechanisms results in venous pooling of blood. Therefore, the effect of Ismelin is especially pronounced when the patient is standing. Both the systolic and diastolic pressures are reduced.

Other actions at the sympathetic nerve terminal include depletion of norepinephrine. Once it gains access to the neuron, Ismelin accumulates within the intraneuronal storage vesicles and causes depletion of norepinephrine stores within the nerve terminal. Prolonged oral administration of Ismelin produces a denervation sensitivity of the neuroeffector junction, probably resulting from the chronic reduction in norepinephrine released by the sympathetic nerve endings. Systemic responses to catecholamines released from the adrenal medulla are not prevented and may even be augmented as a result of this denervation sensitivity. A paradoxical hypertensive crisis may occur if Ismelin is given to patients with pheochromocytoma or if norepinephrine is given to a patient receiving the drug.

Due to its poor lipid solubility, Ismelin does not readily cross the blood-brain barrier. In contrast to most neural blocking agents, Ismelin does not appear to suppress plasma renin activity in many patients.

Pharmacokinetics

The pharmacokinetics of Ismelin are complex. The amount of drug in plasma and in urine is linearly related to dose, although large differences occur between individuals because of variation in absorption and metabolism. Adrenergic blockade occurs with a minimum concentration in plasma of 8 ng/ml; this concentration is achieved in different individuals with dosages of 10–50 mg/day at steady state. Ismelin is eliminated slowly because of extensive tissue binding. After chronic oral administration, the initial phase of elimination with a half-life of 1.5 days is followed by a second phase of elimination with a half-life of 4–8 days. The renal clearance of Ismelin is 56 ml/min. Ismelin is converted by the liver to three metabolites, which are excreted in the urine. The metabolites are pharmacologically less active than Ismelin.

INDICATIONS AND USAGE

Ismelin is indicated for the treatment of moderate and severe hypertension, either alone or as an adjunct, and for the treatment of renal hypertension, including that secondary to pyelonephritis, renal amyloidosis, and renal artery stenosis.

CONTRAINDICATIONS

Known or suspected pheochromocytoma; hypersensitivity; frank congestive heart failure not due to hypertension; use of monoamine oxidase (MAO) inhibitors.

WARNINGS

Ismelin is a potent drug and its use can lead to disturbing and serious clinical problems. Before prescribing, physicians should familiarize themselves with the details of its use and warn patients not to deviate from instructions.

Orthostatic hypotension can occur frequently, and patients should be properly instructed about this potential hazard. Fainting spells may occur unless the patient is forewarned to sit or lie down with the onset of dizziness or weakness. Postural hypotension is most marked in the morning and is accentuated by hot weather, alcohol, or exercise. Dizziness or weakness may be particularly bothersome during the initial period of dosage adjustment and with postural changes, such as arising in the morning. The potential occurrence of these symptoms may require alteration of previous daily activity. The patient should be cautioned to avoid sudden or prolonged standing or exercise while taking the drug.

Inhibition of ejaculation has been reported in animals (see PRECAUTIONS, Carcinogenesis, Mutagenesis, Impairment of Fertility) as well as in men given Ismelin. This effect, which results from the sympathetic blockade caused by the drug's action, is reversible after Ismelin has been discontinued for several weeks. The drug does not cause parasympathetic blockade, and erectile potency is usually retained during administration of Ismelin. The possible occurrence of inhibition of ejaculation should be kept in mind when considering the use of guanethidine in men of reproductive age. If possible, therapy should be withdrawn 2 weeks prior to surgery to reduce the possibility of vascular collapse and cardiac arrest during anesthesia. If emergency surgery is indicated, preanesthetic and anesthetic agents should be administered cautiously in reduced dosage. Oxygen, atropine, vasopressors, and adequate solutions for volume replacement should be ready for immediate use to counteract vascular collapse in the surgical patient. Vasopressors should be used only with extreme caution, since Ismelin augments responsiveness to exogenously administered norepinephrine and vasopressors; specifically, blood pressure may rise and cardiac arrhythmias may be produced.

PRECAUTIONS

General

Dosage requirements may be reduced in the presence of fever.

Special care should be exercised when treating patients with a history of bronchial asthma; asthmatic patients are more apt to be hypersensitive to catecholamine depletion, and their condition may be aggravated.

The effects of Ismelin are cumulative over long periods; initial doses should be small and increased gradually in small increments.

Ismelin should be used very cautiously in hypertensive patients with renal disease and nitrogen retention or rising BUN levels, since decreased blood pressure may further compromise renal function, coronary insufficiency or recent myocardial infarction, and cerebrovascular disease, especially with encephalopathy.

Ismelin should not be given to patients with severe cardiac failure except with extreme caution, since Ismelin may interfere with the compensatory role of the adrenergic system in producing circulatory adjustment in patients with congestive heart failure.

Patients with incipient cardiac decompensation should be watched for weight gain or edema, which may be averted by the concomitant administration of a thiazide.

Ismelin should be used cautiously in patients with a history of peptic ulcer or other chronic disorders that may be aggravated by a relative increase in parasympathetic tone.

Information for Patients

The patient should be advised to take Ismelin exactly as directed. If the patient misses a dose, he or she should be told to take only the next scheduled dose (without doubling it).

The patient should be advised to avoid sudden or prolonged standing or exercise and to arise slowly, especially in the morning, to reduce the orthostatic hypotensive effects of dizziness, lightheadedness, or fainting.

The patient should be cautioned about ingesting alcohol, since it aggravates the orthostatic hypotensive effects of Ismelin.

Male patients should be advised that guanethidine may interfere with ejaculation.

Drug Interactions

Concurrent use of Ismelin and rauwolfia derivatives may cause excessive postural hypotension, bradycardia, and mental depression.

Both digitalis and Ismelin slow the heart rate.

Thiazide diuretics enhance the antihypertensive action of Ismelin (see DOSAGE AND ADMINISTRATION).

Amphetamine-like compounds, stimulants (e.g., ephedrine, methylphenidate), tricylic antidepressants (e.g., amitriptyline, imipramine, desipramine) and other psychopharmacologic agents (e.g., phenothiazines and related compounds), as well as oral contraceptives, may reduce the hypotensive effect of Ismelin.

MAO inhibitors should be discontinued for at least 1 week before starting therapy with Ismelin.

Continued on next page

The full prescribing information for each CIBA product is contained herein and is that in effect as of September 1, 1989

CIBA—Cont.

Carcinogenesis, Mutagenesis, Impairment of Fertility
Long-term carcinogenicity studies in animals have not been conducted with Ismelin.

While inhibition of sperm passage and accumulation of sperm debris have been reported in rats and rabbits after several weeks of administration of Ismelin, 5 or 10 mg/kg per day, subcutaneously or intraperitoneally recovery of ejaculatory function and fertility has been demonstrated in rats given Ismelin intramuscularly, 25 mg/kg per day, for 8 weeks. Inhibition of ejaculation has also been reported in men (see **WARNINGS** and **ADVERSE REACTIONS**). This effect, which is attributable to the sympathetic blockade caused by the drug, is reversible several weeks after discontinuance of the drug.

Pregnancy Category C
Animal reproduction studies have not been conducted with Ismelin. It is also not known whether Ismelin can cause fetal harm when administered to a pregnant woman or can affect reproduction capacity. Ismelin should be given to a pregnant woman only if clearly needed.

Nursing Mothers
Ismelin is excreted in breast milk in very small quantity. Caution should be exercised when Ismelin is administered to a nursing woman.

Pediatric Use
Safety and effectiveness in children have not been established.

ADVERSE REACTIONS
The following adverse reactions have been observed, but there are not enough data to support an estimate of their frequency. Consequently the reactions are categorized by organ system and are listed in decreasing order of severity and not frequency.
Digestive: Diarrhea, which may be severe at times and necessitate discontinuation of medication; vomiting, nausea, increased bowel movements; dry mouth, parotid tenderness.
Cardiovascular: Chest pains (angina); bradycardia, a tendency toward fluid retention and edema with occasional development of congestive heart failure.
Respiratory: Dyspnea; asthma in susceptible individuals; nasal congestion.
Neurologic: Syncope resulting from either postural or exertional hypotension; dizziness; blurred vision; muscle tremor; ptosis of the lids; mental depression; chest paresthesias; weakness; lassitude; fatigue.
Muscular: Myalgia.
Genitourinary: Rise in BUN; urinary incontinence; inhibition of ejaculation; nocturia.
Metabolic: Weight gain.
Skin and Appendages: Dermatitis; scalp hair loss.
Although a causal relationship has not been established, a few instances of blood dyscrasias (anemia, thrombocytopenia, and leukopenia) and of priapism or impotence have been reported.

OVERDOSAGE
Acute Toxicity
No deaths due to acute poisoning have been reported. Oral LD_{50} in rats: 1262 mg/kg.
Signs and Symptoms
Postural hypotension (with dizziness, blurred vision, and possibly syncope when standing), shock, and bradycardia are most likely to occur, diarrhea (possibly severe), nausea and vomiting may also occur. Unconsciousness is unlikely if adequate blood pressure and cerebral perfusion can be maintained by placing the patient in the supine position and by administering other treatment as required.
Treatment
There is no specific antidote.
Treatment should consist of gastric lavage. An activated charcoal slurry should be instilled and laxatives given, if conditions permit.
In sinus bradycardia, atropine should be administered.
In previously normotensive patients, treatment has consisted essentially of restoring blood pressure and heart rate to normal by keeping the patient in the supine position. Normal homeostatic control usually returns gradually over a 72-hour period in these patients.
In previously hypertensive patients, particularly those with impaired cardiac reserve or other cardiovascular-renal disease, intensive treatment may be required to support vital functions and to control cardiac irregularities that might be present. The supine position must be maintained; if vasopressors are required, they must be used with extreme caution, since Ismelin may increase responsiveness, causing a rise in blood pressure and development of cardiac arrhythmias.
Diarrhea, if severe or persistent, should be treated with anticholinergic agents to reduce intestinal hypermotility; hydration and electrolyte balance should be maintained.
Since Ismelin is excreted slowly, cardiovascular and renal function should be monitored for a few days.

DOSAGE AND ADMINISTRATION
Better control may be obtained, especially in the initial phases of treatment, if the patient can have his blood pressure recorded regularly at home.
Ambulatory Patients
Initial doses should be small (10 mg) and increased gradually, depending upon the patient's response. Ismelin has a long duration of action; therefore, dosage increases should not be made more often than every 5–7 days, unless the patient is hospitalized.
Blood pressure should be measured in the supine position, after standing for 10 minutes, and immediately after exercise if feasible. Dosage may be increased only if there has been no decrease in the standing blood pressure from previous levels. The average daily dose is 25–50 mg; only one dose a day is usually required.

Dosage Chart for Ambulatory Patients

Visits (Intervals of 5–7 Days)	Daily Dose
Visit 1 (Patient may be started on 10-mg tablets)	10 mg
Visit 2	20 mg
Visit 3 (Patient may be changed to 25-mg tablets whenever convenient)	30 mg
	(three 10-mg tablets)
	or 37.5 mg
	(one and one-half 25-mg tablets)
Visit 4	50 mg
Visit 5 and subsequent	Dosage may be increased by 12.5 mg or 25 mg if necessary.

The dosage should be reduced in any of the following situations: (1) normal supine pressure (2) excessive orthostatic fall in pressure (3) severe diarrhea.
Hospitalized Patients
Initial oral dose is 25–50 mg, increased by 25 mg or 50 mg daily or every other day as indicated. This higher dosage is possible because hospitalized patients can be watched carefully. Unless absolutely impossible, the standing blood pressure should be measured regularly. Patients should not be discharged from the hospital until the effect of the drug on the standing blood pressure is known. Patients should be told about the possibility of orthostatic hypotension and warned not to get out of bed without help during the period of dosage adjustment.
Combination Therapy
Ismelin may be added gradually to thiazides and/or hydralazine. Thiazide diuretics enhance the effectiveness of Ismelin and may reduce the incidence of edema. When thiazide diuretics are added to the regimen in patients taking Ismelin, it is usually necessary to reduce the dosage of Ismelin. After control is established, the dosage of all drugs should be reduced to the lowest effective level.
Note: When Ismelin is replacing MAO inhibitors, at least 1 week should elapse before commencing treatment with Ismelin (see **CONTRAINDICATIONS**). If ganglionic blockers have not been discontinued before Ismelin is started, they should be gradually withdrawn to prevent a spiking blood pressure response during the transfer period.

HOW SUPPLIED
Tablets 10 mg—round, pale yellow, scored (imprinted CIBA 49)
Bottles of 100 ....NDC 0083-0049-30
Consumer Pack—One Unit
　12 bottles—100 tablets each ....NDC 0083-0049-65
Tablets 25 mg—round, white, scored (imprinted CIBA 103)
Bottles of 100 ....NDC 0083-0103-30
Consumer Pack—One Unit
　12 bottles—100 tablets each ....NDC 0083-0103-65
Dispense in tight container (USP).

C88-24 (Rev. 8/88)

Shown in Product Identification Section, page 408

LITHOBID®　　　　　　　　　　　　　　　　　　℞
[*lith 'oh-bidd*]
lithium carbonate USP
slow-release tablets

CIBALITH–S® Syrup　　　　　　　　　　　　　℞
[*see 'ba-lith-ess*]
lithium citrate syrup USP
For Control of Manic Episodes in Manic-Depressive Psychosis
Caution: Federal law prohibits dispensing without prescription

---

> **WARNING**
> Lithium toxicity is closely related to serum lithium levels, and can occur at doses close to therapeutic levels. Facilities for prompt and accurate serum lithium determinations should be available before initiating therapy.

DESCRIPTION
Lithobid and Cibalith-S are two different forms of an antimanic medication for oral administration. Lithobid is a film-coated, slow-release, 300-mg lithium carbonate tablet. This slowly dissolving, film-coated tablet is designed to give lower serum lithium peaks than obtained with conventional oral lithium dosage forms.

Lithium carbonate USP is a white, granular, odorless powder, which is sparingly soluble in water and very slightly soluble in alcohol. It dissolves, with effervescence, in dilute mineral acids. Its molecular formula is Li_2CO_3, and its molecular weight is 73.89.

Cibalith-S is lithium citrate syrup containing 8 mEq of lithium per 5 ml, equivalent to the amount in 300 mg of lithium carbonate.

Lithium citrate is prepared in solution from lithium hydroxide and citric acid in a ratio approximating dilithium citrate.

Inactive Ingredients. Lithobid tablets 300 mg: Calcium stearate, carnauba wax, cellulose compounds, FD&C Blue No. 1 Aluminum Lake, FD&C Red No. 3 Aluminum Lake, FD&C Yellow No. 6 Aluminum Lake, povidone, propylene glycol, sodium chloride, sodium lauryl sulfate, sodium starch glycolate, sorbitol, and titanium dioxide.

Cibalith-S syrup. Citric acid, raspberry flavor, alcohol 0.3% v/v, purified water, sodium benzoate, sodium saccharin, and sorbitol.

INDICATIONS
Lithium is indicated in the treatment of manic episodes of manic-depressive illness. Maintenance therapy prevents or diminishes the intensity of subsequent episodes in those manic-depressive patients with a history of mania.

Typical symptoms of mania include pressure of speech, motor hyperactivity, reduced need for sleep, flight of ideas, grandiosity, elation, poor judgment, aggressiveness, and possibly hostility. When given to a patient experiencing a manic episode, lithium may produce a normalization of symptomatology within 1 to 3 weeks.

WARNINGS
Lithium should generally not be given to patients with significant renal or cardiovascular disease, severe debilitation or dehydration, or sodium depletion, and to patients receiving diuretics, since the risk of lithium toxicity is very high in such patients. If the psychiatric indication is life-threatening, and if such a patient fails to respond to other measures, lithium treatment may be undertaken with extreme caution, including daily serum lithium determinations and adjustment to the usually low doses ordinarily tolerated by these individuals. In such instances, hospitalization is a necessity.

Lithium toxicity is closely related to serum lithium levels, and can occur at doses close to the therapeutic levels (see DOSAGE AND ADMINISTRATION).

Lithium therapy has been reported in some cases to be associated with morphologic changes in the kidneys. The relationship between such changes and renal function has not been established.

Outpatients and their families should be warned that the patient must discontinue lithium therapy and contact his physician if such clinical signs of lithium toxicity as diarrhea, vomiting, tremor, mild ataxia, drowsiness, or muscular weakness occur.

Lithium may impair mental and/or physical abilities. Caution patients about activities requiring alertness (e.g., operating vehicles or machinery).

Lithium may prolong or potentiate the effects of neuromuscular blocking agents, such as decamethonium, pancuronium, and succinylcholine. Therefore, neuromuscular blocking agents should be given with caution to patients receiving lithium.

Combined use of haloperidol and lithium: An encephalopathic syndrome (characterized by weakness; lethargy; fever; tremulousness and confusion; extrapyramidal symptoms; leukocytosis; elevated serum enzymes, BUN, and fasting blood sugar), followed by irreversible brain damage, has occurred in a few patients treated with lithium plus haloperidol. A causal relationship between these events and the concomitant administration of lithium and haloperidol has not been established. However, patients receiving such combined therapy should be monitored closely for early evidence of neurological toxicity, and treatment discontinued promptly if such signs appear. The possibility of similar adverse interactions with other antipsychotic medications exists. In addition, concurrent use of lithium with chlorpromazine and possibly other phenothiazines decreases serum chlorpromazine levels as much as 40%.

Usage in Pregnancy: Adverse effects on nidation in rats, embryo viability in mice, and metabolism *in vitro* of rat testis and human spermatozoa have been attributed to lithium, as have teratogenicity in submammalian species and cleft palates in mice.

There are lithium birth registries in the United States and elsewhere; however there are at the present time insufficient data to determine the effects of lithium on human fetuses. Therefore, at this point, lithium should not be used in pregnancy, especially the first trimester, unless in the opinion of the physician, the potential benefits outweigh the possible hazards.

Usage in Nursing Mothers: Lithium is excreted in human milk. Nursing should not be undertaken during lithium therapy except in rare and unusual circumstances where, in the view of the physician, the potential benefits to the mother outweigh possible hazards to the child.

Usage in Children: Since information regarding the safety and effectivenss of lithium in children under 12 years of age is not available, its use in such patients is not recommended at this time (see OVERDOSAGE).

PRECAUTIONS

The ability to tolerate lithium is greater during the acute manic phase and decreases when manic symptoms subside (see DOSAGE AND ADMINISTRATION).

The distribution space of lithium approximates that of total body water. Lithium is primarily excreted in urine with insignificant excretion in feces. Renal excretion of lithium is proportional to its plasma concentration. The half-elimination time of lithium is approximately 24 hours. Lithium decreases sodium reabsorption by the renal tubules which could lead to sodium depletion. Therefore, it is essential for the patient to maintain a normal diet, including salt, and an adequate fluid intake (2500–3000 ml) at least during the initial stabilization period. Decreased tolerance to lithium has been reported to ensue from protracted sweating or diarrhea and, if such occur, supplemental fluid and salt should be administered.

In addition to sweating and diarrhea, concomitant infection with elevated temperatures may also necessitate a temporary reduction or cessation of medication.

Previously existing underlying disorders do not necessarily constitute a contraindication to lithium treatment; where hypothyroidism exists, careful monitoring of thyroid function during lithium stabilization and maintenance allows for correction of changing thyroid parameters, if any, where hypothyroidism occurs during lithium stabilization and maintenance, supplemental thyroid treatment may be used.

Drug Interactions: Concomitant administration of carbamazepine and lithium may increase the risk of neurotoxic side effects.

Aminophylline, caffeine, dyphylline, oxtriphylline, sodium bicarbonate, or theophylline used concurrently may decrease the therapeutic effect of lithium because of its increased urinary excretion.

Concurrent use of diuretics, especially thiazides, with lithium may provoke lithium toxicity due to reduced renal clearance.

Concurrent extended use of iodide preparations, especially potassium iodide, with lithium may produce hypothyroidism.

Indomethacin and piroxicam have been reported to increase significantly steady state plasma lithium levels. In some cases, lithium toxicity has resulted from such interactions. There is also some evidence that other non-steroidal, anti-inflammatory agents may have a similar effect. When such combinations are used, increased monitoring of plasma lithium levels is recommended (see WARNINGS).

ADVERSE REACTIONS

Adverse reactions are seldom encountered at serum lithium levels below 1.5 mEq/l, except in the occasional patient sensitive to lithium. Mild-to-moderate toxic reactions may occur at levels from 1.5–2.5 mEq/l, and moderate-to-severe reactions may be seen at levels from 2.0–2.5 mEq/l, depending upon individual response to the drug.

Fine hand tremor, polyuria and mild thirst may occur during initial therapy for the acute manic phase, and may persist throughout treatment. Transient and mild nausea and general discomfort may also appear during the first few days of lithium administration.

These side effects are an inconvenience rather than a disabling condition, and usually subside with continued treatment or a temporary reduction or cessation of dosage. If persistent, a cessation of dosage is indicated.

Diarrhea, vomiting, drowsiness, muscular weakness and lack of coordination may be early signs of lithium intoxication, and can occur at lithium levels below 2.0 mEq/l. At higher levels, giddiness, ataxia, blurred vision, tinnitus and a large output of dilute urine may be seen. Serum lithium levels above 3.0 mEq/l may produce a complex clinical picture involving multiple organs and organ systems. Serum lithium levels should not be permitted to exceed 2.0 mEq/l during the acute treatment phase.

The following toxic reactions have been reported and appear to be related to serum lithium levels, including levels within the therapeutic range.

Neuromuscular: tremor, muscle hyperirritability (fasciculations, twitching, clonic movements of whole limbs), ataxia, choreoathetotic movements, hyperactive deep tendon reflexes.

Central Nervous System: blackout spells, epileptiform seizures, downbeat nystagmus, acute dystonia, slurred speech, dizziness, vertigo, incontinence of urine or feces, somnolence, psychomotor retardation, restlessness, confusion, stupor, coma. Cases of pseudotumor cerebri (increased intracranial pressure and papilledema) have been

reported with lithium use. If undetected, this condition may result in enlargement of the blind spot, constriction of visual fields, and eventual blindness due to optic atrophy. If this syndrome occurs, lithium should be discontinued if clinically possible.

Cardiovascular: cardiac arrhythmia, hypotension, peripheral circulatory collapse.

Gastrointestinal: anorexia, nausea, vomiting, diarrhea.

Genitourinary: albuminuria, oliguria, polyuria, glycosuria.

Dermatologic: drying and thinning of hair, anesthesia of skin, chronic folliculitis, xerosis cutis, alopecia, exacerbation of psoriasis.

Autonomic Nervous System: blurred vision, dry mouth.

Miscellaneous: fatigue, lethargy, tendency to sleep, dehydration, weight loss, transient scotomata.

Thyroid Abnormalities: euthyroid goiter and/or hypothyroidism (including myxedema) accompanied by lower T_3 and T_4. I_{131} iodine uptake may be elevated (see PRECAUTIONS). Paradoxically, rare cases of hyperthyroidism have been reported.

EEG Changes: diffuse slowing, widening of frequency spectrum, potentiation and disorganization of background rhythm.

EKG Changes: reversible flattening, isoelectricity or inversion of T-waves.

Miscellaneous reactions unrelated to dosage are: transient electroencephalographic and electrocardiographic changes, leukocytosis, headache, diffuse nontoxic goiter with or without hypothyroidism, transient hyperglycemia, generalized pruritus, with or without rash, cutaneous ulcers, albuminuria, worsening of organic brain syndromes, excessive weight gain, edematous swelling of ankles or wrists, metallic taste, and thirst or polyuria, sometimes resembling diabetes insipidus.

A single report has been received of the development of painful discoloration of fingers and toes and coldness of the extremities within one day of the starting of treatment of lithium. The mechanism through which these symptoms (resembling Raynaud's Syndrome) developed is not known. Recovery followed discontinuance.

DOSAGE AND ADMINISTRATION

Acute Mania: Optimal patient response can usually be established and maintained with the following dosages:

Lithobid	900 mg b.i.d. or 600 mg t.i.d. (1800 mg per day)
Cibalith-S	10 ml (2 teaspoons) (16 mEq of lithium) t.i.d.

Such doses will normally produce an effective serum lithium level ranging between 1.0 and 1.5 mEq/l. Dosage must be individualized according to serum levels and clinical response. Regular monitoring of the patient's clinical state and of serum lithium levels is necessary. Serum levels should be determined twice per week during the acute phase, and until the serum level and clinical condition of the patient have been stabilized.

Long-Term Control: The desirable serum lithium levels are 0.6 to 1.2 mEq/l. Dosage will vary from one individual to another, but usually the following dosages will maintain this level:

Lithobid	900 mg to 1200 mg per day given in two or three divided doses.
Cibalith-S	5 ml (1 teaspoon) (8mEq of lithium) t.i.d. or q.i.d.

Serum lithium levels in uncomplicated cases receiving maintenance therapy during remission should be monitored at least every two months. Patients abnormally sensitive to lithium may exhibit toxic signs at serum levels of 1.0 to 1.5 mEq/l. Elderly patients often respond to reduced dosage, and may exhibit signs of toxicity at serum levels ordinarily tolerated by other patients.

N.B.: Blood samples for serum lithium determinations should be drawn immediately prior to the next dose when lithium concentrations are relatively stable (i.e., 8–12 hours after previous dose). Total reliance must not be placed on serum levels alone. Accurate patient evaluation requires both clinical and laboratory analysis.

Lithobid slow-release tablets must be swallowed whole and never crushed or chewed.

OVERDOSAGE

The toxic levels for lithium are close to the therapeutic levels. It is therefore important that patients and their families be cautioned to watch for early toxic symptoms and to discontinue the drug and inform the physician should they occur. There has been a report of a transient syndrome of acute dystonia and hyperreflexia occurring in a 15 kg child who ingested 300 mg of lithium carbonate. Toxic symptoms are listed in detail under ADVERSE REACTIONS.

Treatment: No specific antidote for lithium poisoning is known. Early symptoms of lithium toxicity can usually be treated by reduction or cessation of dosage of the drug and resumption of the treatment at a lower dose after 24 to 48 hours. In severe cases of lithium poisoning, the first and fore-

most goal of treatment consists of elimination of this ion from the body.

Treatment is essentially the same as that used in barbiturate poisoning: 1) gastric lavage 2) correction of fluid and electrolyte imbalance and 3) regulation of kidney functioning. Urea, mannitol, and aminophylline all produce significant increases in lithium excretion. Hemodialysis is an effective and rapid means of removing the ion from the severely toxic patient. Infection prophylaxis, regular chest x-rays, and preservation of adequate respiration are essential.

HOW SUPPLIED

Lithobid, lithium carbonate
Tablets—slow-release 300 mg—peach-colored (imprinted CIBA 65)

Bottles of 100	NDC 0083-0065-30
Bottles of 1000	NDC 0083-0065-40

Accu-Pak® Unit Dose (blister pack)

Box of 100 (strips of 10)	NDC 0083-0065-32

Store between 59°–86°F (15°–30°C).
Protect from moisture.

Cibalith-S, lithium citrate
Syrup—sugar-free, raspberry flavored, 8 mEq of lithium per 5 ml, equivalent to the amount in 300 mg of lithium carbonate.

Bottles of 480 ml	NDC 0083-6565-76

Store between 59°–86°F (15°–30°C).
Dispense in tight container (USP).

C87-21 (Rev. 6/87)

Dist. by:
CIBA Pharmaceutical Co.
Division of CIBA-GEIGY Corporation
Summit, New Jersey 07901
Shown in Product Identification Section, page 409

LUDIOMIL®   ℞
[loó-dee-oh-mill]
(maprotiline hydrochloride)
Tablets

DESCRIPTION

Ludiomil, maprotiline hydrochloride USP, is a tetracyclic antidepressant, available as 25-mg, 50-mg and 75-mg tablets for oral administration. Its chemical name is N-methyl-9,10-ethanoanthracene-9(10H)-propylamine hydrochloride.

Maprotiline hydrochloride USP is a fine, white to off-white, practically odorless crystalline powder. It is freely soluble in methanol and in chloroform, slightly soluble in water, and practically insoluble in isooctane. Its molecular weight is 313.87.

Inactive Ingredients. Calcium phosphate, cellulose compounds, colloidal silicon dioxide, FD&C Yellow No. 6 Aluminum Lake (25-mg and 50-mg tablets), lactose, magnesium stearate, povidone, shellac, starch, stearic acid, talc, and titanium dioxide.

CLINICAL PHARMACOLOGY

The mechanism of action of Ludiomil is not precisely known. It does not act primarily by stimulation of the central nervous system and is not a monoamine oxidase inhibitor. The postulated mechanism of Ludiomil is that it acts primarily by potentiation of central adrenergic synapses by blocking reuptake of norepinephrine at nerve endings. This pharmacologic action is thought to be responsible for the drug's antidepressant and anxiolytic effects.

The mean time to peak is 12 hours. The half-life of elimination averages 51 hours.

Steady-state levels measured prior to the morning dose on a one-dosage regimen are summarized as follows:

Regimen	Average Minimum Concentration ng/ml	95% Confidence Limits ng/ml
50 mg x 3 daily	238	181–295

INDICATIONS AND USAGE

Ludiomil is indicated for the treatment of depressive illness in patients with depressive neurosis (dysthymic disorder) and manic-depressive illness, depressed type (major depressive disorder). Ludiomil is also effective for the relief of anxiety associated with depression.

CONTRAINDICATIONS

Ludiomil is contraindicated in patients hypersensitive to Ludiomil and in patients with known or suspected seizure disorders. It should not be given concomitantly with monoamine oxidase (MAO) inhibitors. A minimum of 14 days should be allowed to elapse after discontinuation of MAO inhibitors before treatment with Ludiomil is initiated. Ef-

Continued on next page

CIBA—Cont.

fects should be monitored with gradual increase in dosage until optimum response is achieved. The drug is not recommended for use during the acute phase of myocardial infarction.

WARNINGS

Seizures have been associated with the use of Ludiomil.
Most of the seizures have occurred in patients without a known history of seizures. However, in some of these cases, other confounding factors were present, including concomitant medications known to lower the seizure threshold, rapid escalation of the dosage of Ludiomil, and dosage that exceeded the recommended therapeutic range. The incidence of direct reports is less than $\frac{1}{10}$ of 1%. The risk of seizures may be increased when Ludiomil is taken concomitantly with phenothiazines, when the dosage of benzodiazepines is rapidly tapered in patients receiving Ludiomil or when the recommended dosage of Ludiomil is exceeded. While a cause-and-effect relationship has not been established, the risk of seizures in patients treated with Ludiomil may be reduced by (1) initiating therapy at a low dosage, (2) maintaining the initial dosage for 2 weeks before raising it gradually in small increments as necessitated by the long half-life of Ludiomil (average 51 hours), and (3) keeping the dosage at the minimally effective level during maintenance therapy. (See **DOSAGE AND ADMINISTRATION**.)

Extreme caution should be used when this drug is given to:
—patients with a history of myocardial infarction;
—patients with a history or presence of cardiovascular disease because of the possibility of conduction defects, arrhythmias, myocardial infarction, strokes and tachycardia.

PRECAUTIONS

General: The possibility of suicide in seriously depressed patients is inherent in their illness and may persist until significant remission occurs. Therefore, patients must be carefully supervised during all phases of treatment with Ludiomil, and prescriptions should be written for the smallest number of tablets consistent with good patient management.

Hypomanic or manic episodes have been known to occur in some patients taking tricyclic antidepressant drugs, particularly in patients with cyclic disorders. Such occurrences have also been noted, rarely, with Ludiomil.

Prior to elective surgery, Ludiomil should be discontinued for as long as clinically feasible, since little is known about the interaction between Ludiomil and general anesthetics. Ludiomil should be administered with caution in patients with increased intraocular pressure, history of urinary retention, or history of narrow-angle glaucoma because of the drug's anticholinergic properties.

Information for Patients: Patients should be warned of the association between seizures and the use of Ludiomil. Moreover, they should be informed that this association is enhanced in patients with a known history of seizures and in those patients who are taking certain other drugs. (See **WARNINGS**.)

Warn patients to exercise caution about potentially hazardous tasks, or operating automobiles or machinery since the drug may impair mental and/or physical abilities.

Ludiomil may enhance the response to alcohol, barbiturates, and other CNS depressants, requiring appropriate caution of administration.

Laboratory Tests: Ludiomil should be discontinued if there is evidence of pathological neutrophil depression. Leukocyte and differential counts should be performed in patients who develop fever and sore throat during therapy.

Drug Interactions: Close supervision and careful adjustment of dosage are required when administering Ludiomil concomitantly with anticholinergic or sympathomimetic drugs because of the possibility of additive atropine-like effects.

Concurrent administration of Ludiomil with electroshock therapy should be avoided because of the lack of experience in this area.

Caution should be exercised when administering Ludiomil to hyperthyroid patients or those on thyroid medication because of the possibility of enhanced potential for cardiovascular toxicity of Ludiomil.

Ludiomil should be used with caution in patients receiving guanethidine or similar agents since it may block the pharmacologic effects of these drugs.

The risk of seizures may be increased when Ludiomil is taken concomitantly with phenothiazines or when the dosage of benzodiazepines is rapidly tapered in patients receiving Ludiomil.

Because of the pharmacologic similarity of Ludiomil to the tricyclic antidepressants, the plasma concentration of Ludiomil may be increased when the drug is given concomitantly with cimetidine, as has occurred with tricyclic antidepressants. Adjustment of the dosage of Ludiomil may therefore

be necessary in such cases both when cimetidine therapy is initiated and when it is discontinued.
(See **Information for Patients**.)

Carcinogenesis, Mutagenesis, Impairment of Fertility: Carcinogenicity and chronic toxicity studies have been conducted in laboratory rats and dogs. No drug- or dose-related occurrence of carcinogenesis was evident in rats receiving daily oral doses up to 60 mg/kg of Ludiomil for eighteen months or in dogs receiving daily oral doses up to 30 mg/kg of Ludiomil for one year. In addition, no evidence of mutagenic activity was found in offspring of female mice mated with males treated with up to 60 times the maximum daily human dose.

Pregnancy Category B: Reproduction studies have been performed in female laboratory rabbits, mice, and rats at doses up to 1.3, 7, and 9 times the maximum daily human dose respectively and have revealed no evidence of impaired fertility or harm to the fetus due to Ludiomil. There are, however, no adequate and well-controlled studies in pregnant women. Because animal reproduction studies are not always predictive of human response, this drug should be used during pregnancy only if clearly needed.

Labor and Delivery: Although the effect of Ludiomil on labor and delivery is unknown, caution should be exercised as with any drug with CNS depressant action.

Nursing Mothers: Ludiomil is excreted in breast milk. At steady state, the concentrations in milk correspond closely to the concentrations in whole blood. Caution should be exercised when Ludiomil is administered to a nursing woman.

Pediatric Use: Safety and effectiveness in children below the age of 18 have not been established.

ADVERSE REACTIONS

The following adverse reactions have been noted with Ludiomil and are generally similar to those observed with tricyclic antidepressants.

Cardiovascular: Rare occurrences of hypotension, hypertension, tachycardia, palpitation, arrhythmia, heart block, and syncope have been reported with Ludiomil.

Psychiatric: Nervousness (6%), anxiety (3%), insomnia (2%), and agitation (2%); rarely, confusional states (especially in the elderly), hallucinations, disorientation, delusions, restlessness, nightmares, hypomania, mania, exacerbation of psychosis, decrease in memory, and feelings of unreality.

Neurological: Drowsiness (16%), dizziness (8%), tremor (3%), and, rarely, numbness, tingling, motor hyperactivity, akathisia, seizures, EEG alterations, tinnitus, extrapyramidal symptoms, ataxia, and dysarthria.

Anticholinergic: Dry mouth (22%), constipation (6%), and blurred vision (4%); rarely, accommodation disturbances, mydriasis, urinary retention, and delayed micturition.

Allergic: Rare instances of skin rash, petechiae, itching, photosensitization, edema, and drug fever.

Gastrointestinal: Nausea (2%) and, rarely, vomiting, epigastric distress, diarrhea, bitter taste, abdominal cramps and dysphagia.

Endocrine: Rare instances of increased or decreased libido, impotence, and elevation or depression of blood sugar levels.

Other: Weakness and fatigue (4%) and headache (4%); rarely, altered liver function, jaundice, weight loss or gain, excessive perspiration, flushing, urinary frequency, increased salivation, nasal congestion and alopecia.

Note: Although there have been only isolated reports of the following adverse reactions with Ludiomil, its pharmacologic similarity to tricyclic antidepressants requires that each reaction be considered when administering Ludiomil.
—Bone marrow depression, including agranulocytosis, eosinophilia, purpura, and thrombocytopenia, myocardial infarction, stroke, peripheral neuropathy, sublingual adenitis, black tongue, stomatitis, paralytic ileus, gynecomastia in the male, breast enlargement and galactorrhea in the female, and testicular swelling.

Post-Introduction Reports: Several voluntary reports of interstitial pneumonitis, which were in some cases associated with eosinophilia and increased liver enzymes, have been received since market introduction. However, there is no clear causal relationship.

OVERDOSAGE

Animal Oral LD$_{50}$: The oral LD$_{50}$ of Ludiomil is 600–750 mg/kg in mice, 760–900 mg/kg in rats, > 1000 mg/kg in rabbits, > 300 mg/kg in cats, and > 30 mg/kg in dogs.

Signs and Symptoms: Data dealing with overdosage in humans are limited with only a few cases on record. Symptoms are drowsiness, tachycardia, ataxia, vomiting, cyanosis, hypotension, shock, restlessness, agitation, hyperpyrexia, muscle rigidity, athetoid movements, mydriasis, cardiac arrhythmias, impaired cardiac condition. In severe cases, loss of consciousness and generalized convulsions may occur. Since congestive heart failure has been seen with overdosages of tricyclic antidepressants, it should be considered with Ludiomil overdosage.

Treatment: There is no specific antidote. Induced emesis and gastric lavage are recommended. It may be helpful to leave the tube in the stomach with irrigation and continual

aspiration of stomach contents possibly promoting more rapid elimination of the drug from the body. The room should be darkened, allowing only minimal external stimulation to reduce the tendency to convulsions.

Since it has been reported that physostigmine increases the risk of seizures, its use is not recommended in cases of overdosage with Ludiomil.

Hyperirritability and convulsions may be treated with carefully titrated parenteral barbiturates. Barbiturates should not be employed, however, if drugs that inhibit monoamine oxidase have also been taken by the patient in overdosage or in recent therapy. Similarly, barbiturates may induce respiratory depression, particularly in children. It is therefore advisable to have equipment available for artificial ventilation and resuscitation when barbiturates are employed. Paraldehyde may be used effectively in some children to counteract muscular hypertonus and convulsions with less likelihood of causing respiratory depression.

Shock (circulatory collapse) should be treated with supportive measures such as intravenous fluids, oxygen, and corticosteroids.

Hyperpyrexia should be controlled by whatever means available, including ice packs if necessary.

Signs of congestive heart failure may be satisfactorily treated by rapid digitalization.

Dialysis is of little value because of the low plasma concentration of this drug.

DOSAGE AND ADMINISTRATION

A single daily dose is an alternative to divided daily doses. Therapeutic effects are sometimes seen within 3 to 7 days, although as long as 2 to 3 weeks are usually necessary.

Initial Adult Dosage: An initial dosage of 75 mg daily is suggested for outpatients with mild-to-moderate depression. However, in some patients, particularly the elderly, an initial dosage of 25 mg daily may be used. Because of the long half-life of Ludiomil, the initial dosage should be maintained for two weeks. The dosage may then be increased gradually in 25-mg increments as required and tolerated. In most outpatients a maximum dose of 150 mg daily will result in therapeutic efficacy. It is recommended that this dose not be exceeded except in the most severely depressed patients. In such patients, dosage may be gradually increased to a maximum of 225 mg.

More severely depressed, hospitalized patients should be given an initial daily dose of 100 mg to 150 mg which may be gradually increased as required and tolerated. Most hospitalized patients with moderate-to-severe depression respond to a daily dosage of 150 mg although dosages as high as 225 mg may be required in some cases. Daily dosage of 225 mg should not be exceeded.

Elderly Patients: In general, lower dosages are recommended for patients over 60 years of age. Dosages of 50 mg to 75 mg daily are usually satisfactory as maintenance therapy for elderly patients who do not tolerate higher amounts.

Maintenance: Dosage during prolonged maintenance therapy should be kept at the lowest effective level. Dosage may be reduced to levels of 75 mg to 150 mg daily during such periods, with subsequent adjustment depending on therapeutic response.

HOW SUPPLIED

Tablets 25 mg —oval, dark orange, scored, coated (imprinted CIBA 110)
  Bottle of 100..NDC 0083-0110-30
  Accu-Pak® Unit Dose (blister pack)
    Box of 100 (strips of 10)....................NDC 0083-0110-32
Tablets 50 mg —round, dark orange, scored, coated (imprinted CIBA 26)
  Bottle of 100..NDC 0083-0026-30
  Accu-Pak® Unit Dose (blister pack)
    Box of 100 (strips of 10)....................NDC 0083-0026-32
Tablets 75 mg —oval, white, scored, coated (imprinted 135 CIBA)
  Bottle of 100..NDC 0083-0135-30
  Accu-Pak® Unit Dose (blister pack)
    Box of 100 (strips of 10)....................NDC 0083-0135-32
Dispense in tight container (USP).

C88-21 (Rev. 8/88)
Shown in Product Identification Section, page 409

METANDREN®   ℞
[meh-tan 'dren]
(methyltestosterone USP)
Linguets® (buccal tablets)
Tablets

DESCRIPTION

Metandren, methyltestosterone USP, is a synthetic androgenic steroid available as 5-mg and 10-mg Linguets for absorption through the buccal mucosa and as 10-mg and 25-mg tablets for oral administration. Its chemical name is 17β-hydroxy-17-methylandrost-4-en-3-one.

Methyltestosterone USP occurs as white or creamy white, odorless, and slightly hygroscopic crystals or crystalline pow-

der. It is practically insoluble in water; soluble in alcohol, in methanol, in ether, and in other organic solvents; and sparingly soluble in vegetable oils. Its molecular weight is 302.46.
Inactive Ingredients. Metandren Tablets: FD&C Yellow #5 (25-mg tablets), lactose, magnesium stearate, starch, sucrose, and talc.

Metandren Linguets: Acacia, FD&C Yellow #5 (10-mg linguets), lactose, magnesium stearate, mannitol, starch, sucrose, talc, and tragacanth.

CLINICAL PHARMACOLOGY

Endogenous androgens are responsible for the normal growth and development of the male sex organs and for maintenance of secondary sex characteristics. These effects include the growth and maturation of the prostate, seminal vesicles, penis, and scrotum; the development of male hair distribution, such as beard, pubic, chest, and axillary hair; laryngeal enlargement; vocal cord thickening; alterations in body musculature; and fat distribution. Drugs in this class also cause retention of nitrogen, sodium, potassium, and phosphorus, and decreased urinary excretion of calcium. Androgens have been reported to increase protein anabolism and decrease protein catabolism. Nitrogen balance is improved only when there is sufficient intake of calories and protein.

Androgens are responsible for the growth spurt of adolescence and for the eventual termination of linear growth, which is brought about by fusion of the epiphyseal growth centers. In children, exogenous androgens accelerate linear growth rates but may cause a disproportionate advancement in bone maturation. Use over long periods may result in fusion of the epiphyseal growth centers and termination of the growth process. Androgens have been reported to stimulate the production of red blood cells by enhancing the production of erythropoietic stimulating factor.

During exogenous administration of androgens, endogenous testosterone release is inhibited through feedback inhibition of pituitary luteinizing hormone (LH). At large doses of exogenous androgens, spermatogenesis may also be suppressed through feedback inhibition of pituitary follicle-stimulating hormone (FSH).

There is a lack of substantial evidence that androgens are effective in fractures, surgery, convalescence, and functional uterine bleeding.

Pharmacokinetics

Metandren is well absorbed, at a rate depending on the route of administration. Peak serum concentrations are attained about 1 hour after administration of a Linguet and about 2 hours after administration of a tablet.

The synthetic androgens, including methyltestosterone, are extensively metabolized by the liver, and they have a longer half-life than testosterone. They are more suitable than testosterone for oral administration.

After oral administration of a 10-mg tablet of Metandren in healthy human subjects, the serum concentration reaches a peak of about 30 ng/ml within 1–2 hours, then declines biphasically with half-lives of approximately 1 hour initially, changing to approximately 3.5 hours within 3–4 hours after dosage.

The bioavailability of Metandren Linguets approaches twice that of an equal dose of tablets, probably because the hepatic circulation is bypassed with sublingual administration.

About 10% of unchanged drug is recovered from the urine and feces. The major metabolic pathways of methyltestosterone are reduction of ring A, hydroxylation, and conjugation. The apparent elimination half-life averages 2.5–3 hours.

INDICATIONS AND USAGE

Males

Metandren is indicated for replacement therapy in conditions associated with a deficiency or absence of endogenous testosterone:

a. Primary hypogonadism—testicular failure due to cryptorchidism, bilateral torsion, orchitis, or vanishing testis syndrome; or orchidectomy.

b. Hypogonadotropic hypogonadism—idiopathic gonadotropin or LH-RH deficiency, or pituitary-hypothalamic injury from tumors, trauma, or radiation.

If the above conditions occur prior to puberty, androgen replacement therapy will be needed during the adolescent years for development of secondary sex characteristics. Prolonged androgen treatment will be required to maintain the sex characteristics in these males and in those who develop testosterone deficiency after puberty.

c. Metandren may be used to stimulate puberty in carefully selected males with clearly delayed puberty. These patients usually have a familial pattern of delayed puberty that is not secondary to a pathological disorder; puberty is expected to occur spontaneously at a relatively late date. Brief treatment with conservative doses may occasionally be justified in these patients if they do not respond to psychological support. The potential adverse effect on bone maturation should be discussed with the patient and his parents prior to androgen administration. An x-ray of the hand and wrist to determine bone age should be obtained every 6 months to assess the effect of treatment on the epiphyseal centers (see **WARNINGS** and **PRECAUTIONS, Pediatric Use**).

d. Metandren is indicated for the treatment of impotence and male climacteric symptoms, when these are secondary to androgen deficiency.

Females

Metandren may be used secondarily in women with advancing inoperable metastatic (skeletal) mammary cancer who are 1–5 years postmenopausal. Primary goals of therapy in these women include ablation of the ovaries. Other methods of counteracting estrogen activity are adrenalectomy, hypophysectomy, and antiestrogen therapy. Treatment with Metandren has also been used in premenopausal women with breast cancer who have benefited from oophorectomy and are considered to have a hormone-responsive tumor. Judgment concerning androgen therapy should be made by an oncologist with expertise in this field.

Metandren has been used for the management of postpartum breast pain and engorgement. There is no satisfactory evidence that this drug prevents or suppresses lactation.

CONTRAINDICATIONS

Metandren is contraindicated in men with carcinoma of the breast or with known or suspected carcinoma of the prostate, in women who are or may become pregnant, and in prepuberal males and females except those males with clearly delayed puberty as detailed in the **INDICATIONS AND USAGE** section, **Males**, c. When administered to pregnant women, androgens cause virilization of the external genitalia of the female fetus. This virilization includes clitoromegaly, abnormal vaginal development, and fusion of genital folds to form a scrotum-like structure. The degree of masculinization is related to the amount of drug given and the age of the fetus, and is most likely to occur in the female fetus when the drugs are given in the first trimester. If the patient becomes pregnant while taking these drugs, she should be apprised of the potential hazard to the fetus.

WARNINGS

In patients with breast cancer, androgen therapy may cause hypercalcemia by stimulating osteolysis. In this case, the drug should be discontinued.

Prolonged use of high doses of androgens has been associated with the development of peliosis hepatis and hepatic neoplasms including hepatocellular carcinoma (see **PRECAUTIONS, Carcinogenesis**). Peliosis hepatis can be a life-threatening or fatal complication.

Cholestatic hepatitis and jaundice occur with 17α-alkyl androgens at a relatively low dose. If cholestatic hepatitis with jaundice appears or if liver function tests become abnormal, the androgen should be discontinued and the etiology should be determined. Drug-induced jaundice is reversible when the medication is discontinued.

Geriatric patients treated with androgens may be at an increased risk for the development of prostatic hypertrophy, with resultant urinary obstruction, and prostatic carcinoma. Males, especially the elderly, may become overly stimulated. Oligospermia and reduced ejaculatory volume may occur after prolonged administration or excessive dosage.

Edema with or without congestive heart failure may be a serious complication in patients with preexisting cardiac, renal, or hepatic disease. In addition to discontinuation of the drug, diuretic therapy may be required.

Gynecomastia frequently develops and occasionally persists in patients being treated for hypogonadism.

Hypersensitivity may occur.

Androgen therapy should be used cautiously in healthy males with delayed puberty. The effect on bone maturation should be monitored by assessing bone age of the wrist and hand every 6 months. In children, androgen treatment may accelerate bone maturation without producing compensatory gain in linear growth. This adverse effect may result in compromised adult stature. The younger the child, the greater the risk of compromising final mature height.

Women should be observed for signs of virilization (deepening of the voice, hirsutism, acne, clitoromegaly, and menstrual irregularities). Discontinuation of drug therapy at the time mild virilism becomes evident is necessary to prevent irreversible virilization. Some effects, such as voice changes, may not be reversible even when the drug is stopped. Such virilization is usual following androgen use at high doses. The physician should discuss with the patient being treated for breast carcinoma whether she is willing to tolerate this potential effect of the therapy.

In general, when any of these effects appear, androgen therapy should be stopped; if resumption of therapy is considered necessary, a lower dose should be utilized.

PRECAUTIONS

General

The Metandren Linguets® of 10 mg and tablets of 25 mg contain FD&C Yellow No. 5 (tartrazine), which may cause allergic-type reactions (including bronchial asthma) in certain susceptible individuals. Although the overall incidence of FD&C Yellow No. 5 (tartrazine) sensitivity in the general population is low, it is frequently seen in patients who are also hypersensitive to aspirin.

Information for Patients

The physician should instruct patients to report any of the following side effects of androgens:

Adult or Adolescent Males: Too frequent or persistent erections of the penis.
Females: Hoarseness, acne, changes in menstrual periods, or more hair on the face.
All Patients: Any nausea, vomiting, changes in skin color, or ankle swelling.

Laboratory Tests

Women with disseminated breast carcinoma should have frequent determinations of urine and serum calcium levels during the course of androgen therapy (see **WARNINGS**).

Because of the hepatotoxicity associated with the use of 17α-alkyl androgens, liver function tests should be obtained periodically.

Periodic (every 6 months) x-ray examinations of bone age should be made during treatment of prepubertal males to determine the rate of bone maturation and the effects of androgen therapy on the epiphyseal centers.

Hemoglobin and hematocrit should be checked periodically for polycythemia in patients who are receiving high doses of androgens.

Drug/Drug Interactions

Anticoagulants. C-17-substituted derivatives of testosterone, such as methandrostenolone, have been reported to decrease the anticoagulant requirements of patients receiving oral anticoagulants. Patients receiving oral anticoagulant therapy require close monitoring, especially when androgen therapy is started or stopped.

Oxyphenbutazone. Concurrent administration of oxyphenbutazone and androgens may result in elevated serum levels of oxyphenbutazone.

Insulin. In diabetic patients, the metabolic effects of androgens may decrease blood glucose levels and insulin requirements.

Drug/Laboratory Test Interactions

Androgens may decrease levels of thyroxine-binding globulin, resulting in decreased total T_4 serum levels and increased resin uptake of T_3 and T_4. Free-thyroid hormone levels remain unchanged, however, and there is no clinical evidence of thyroid dysfunction.

Carcinogenesis

Animal Data. No long-term carcinogenicity or reproduction studies in animals have been performed with Metandren. There is no information on mutagenesis. However, testosterone has been tested by subcutaneous injection and implantation in mice and rats. The implant induced cervical-uterine tumors in mice, which metastasized in some cases. There is suggestive evidence that injection of testosterone into some strains of female mice increases their susceptibility to hepatoma. Testosterone is also known to increase the number of tumors and decrease the degree of differentiation of chemically induced carcinomas of the liver in rats.

Human Data. There are rare reports of hepatocellular carcinoma in patients receiving long-term therapy with androgens in high doses. Withdrawal of the drugs did not lead to regression of the tumors in all cases.

Geriatric patients treated with androgens may be at an increased risk for the development of prostatic hypertrophy and prostatic carcinoma.

Pregnancy Category X

See **CONTRAINDICATIONS**.

Nursing Mothers

It is not known whether androgens are excreted in human milk. Because many drugs are excreted in human milk and because of the potential for serious adverse reactions in nursing infants from androgens, a decision should be made whether to discontinue nursing or to discontinue the drug, taking into account the importance of the drug to the mother.

Pediatric Use

Androgen therapy should be prescribed very cautiously for use in males with clearly delayed puberty and only by specialists who are aware of the adverse effects on bone maturation. Skeletal maturation must be monitored every 6 months by an x-ray of the hand and wrist (see **INDICATIONS AND USAGE** and **WARNINGS**).

ADVERSE REACTIONS

Endocrine and Urogenital: In females, the most common side effects are amenorrhea and other menstrual irregularities, inhibition of gonadotropin secretion, and virilization, including deepening of the voice and clitoral enlargement. The latter usually is not reversible after androgens are discontinued. When administered to a pregnant woman, androgens cause virilization of the external genitalia of the female fetus (see **CONTRAINDICATIONS**).

Continued on next page

The full prescribing information for each CIBA product is contained herein and is that in effect as of September 1, 1989

CIBA—Cont.

In males, gynecomastia and excessive frequency and duration of penile erections may occur. Oligospermia may occur at high dosages (see **CLINICAL PHARMACOLOGY**).

Skin and Appendages: Hirsutism, male pattern of baldness, acne, and hypersensitivity including skin manifestations.

Fluid and Electrolyte Disturbances: Retention of sodium, chloride, water, potassium, and inorganic phosphates; and hypercalcemia, especially in immobile patients and those with metastatic breast carcinoma.

Gastrointestinal: Nausea, cholestatic jaundice, alterations in liver functions; and, rarely, hepatocellular neoplasms and peliosis hepatis (see **WARNINGS**).

Hematologic: Suppression of clotting factors II, V, VII, and X; bleeding in patients on concomitant anticoagulant therapy; and polycythemia.

Nervous System: Increased or decreased libido, headache, anxiety, depression, and generalized paresthesia.

Metabolic: Increased serum cholesterol.

Miscellaneous: Stomatitis with buccal preparations and, rarely, anaphylactoid reactions.

OVERDOSAGE

There have been no reports of acute overdosage with the androgens.

DOSAGE AND ADMINISTRATION

The suggested dosage for androgens varies, depending on the age, sex, and diagnosis of the individual patient. Dosage and duration of therapy are adjusted according to the patient's response and the appearance of adverse reactions. Suggested average daily dosages are given in the chart. Daily requirements are best administered in divided doses.

Note: Linguets have approximately twice the potency of the orally ingested hormone.

Males

Various dosage regimens have been used to induce pubertal changes in hypogonadal males. Some experts have advocated lower dosages initially, gradually increasing the dose as puberty progresses, with or without a decrease in maintenance levels. Other experts emphasize that higher dosages are needed to induce pubertal changes and that lower dosages can be used for maintenance after puberty. The chronological and skeletal ages must be taken into consideration, both in determining the initial dosage and in adjusting it.

Dosages used in delayed puberty generally are in the lower ranges of those given in the chart and are given for a limited duration, for example, 4–6 months.

Females

Women with metastatic breast carcinoma must be followed closely because androgen therapy occasionally appears to accelerate the disease.

Guideline dosages of androgens for use in the palliative treatment of women with metastatic breast carcinoma are also given in the chart.

INDICATION	AVERAGE DAILY DOSE	
Males	*Linguets*	*Tablets*
Hypogonadism	5–20 mg	10–40 mg
Male climacteric and male impotence	5–20 mg	10–40 mg
Cryptorchidism—postpubertal	15 mg	30 mg
Females		
Postpartum breast pain and engorgement (3–5 days)	40 mg	80 mg
Breast cancer	100 mg	200 mg

Administration of Linguets

Linguets should not be swallowed, since the hormone is meant to be absorbed through the mucous membranes. The Linguet should be placed in the upper or lower buccal pouch between the gum and cheek. The patient should avoid eating, drinking, chewing, or smoking while the Linguet is in place. Proper oral hygienic measures are particularly important after the use of Linguets.

HOW SUPPLIED

Linguets®️ 5 mg—capsule shaped, white (imprinted CIBA 51), for buccal administration

   Bottles of 100 ....NDC 0083-0051-30

Linguets®️ 10 mg—capsule shaped, yellow (imprinted CIBA 64), for buccal administration

   Bottles of 100 ....NDC 0083-0064-30

Tablets 10 mg—round, white, scored (imprinted CIBA 30)

   Bottles of 100 ....NDC 0083-0030-30

Tablets 25 mg—round, yellow, scored (imprinted CIBA 32)

   Bottles of 100 ....NDC 0083-0032-30

Dispense in tight, light-resistant container (USP).

                       C85-62 (Rev. 11/85)

Shown in Product Identification Section, page 409

METOPIRONE®️   ℞

[met-oh-pie 'rone]

metyrapone USP

Tablets

Diagnostic Test of Pituitary Adrenocorticotropic Function

DESCRIPTION

Metopirone, metyrapone USP, is an inhibitor of endogenous adrenal corticosteroid synthesis, available as 250-mg tablets for oral administration. Its chemical name is 2-methyl-1,2-di-3-pyridyl-1-propanone.

Metyrapone USP is a white to light amber, fine, crystalline powder, having a characteristic odor. It is sparingly soluble in water, and soluble in methanol and in chloroform. It forms water-soluble salts with acids. Its molecular weight is 226.28.

Inactive Ingredients: Calcium phosphate, colloidal silicon dioxide, gelatin, and magnesium stearate.

CLINICAL PHARMACOLOGY

The pharmacological effect of Metopirone is to reduce cortisol and corticosterone production by inhibiting the 11-β-hydroxylation reaction in the adrenal cortex. Removal of the strong inhibitory feedback mechanism exerted by cortisol results in an increase in adrenocorticotropic hormone (ACTH) production by the pituitary. With continued blockade of the enzymatic steps leading to production of cortisol and corticosterone, there is a marked increase in adrenocortical secretion of their immediate precursors, 11-deoxycortisol and desoxycorticosterone, which are weak suppressors of ACTH release, and a corresponding elevation of these steroids in the plasma and of their metabolites in the urine. These metabolites are readily determined by measuring urinary 17-hydroxycorticosteroids (17-OHCS) or 17-ketogenic steroids (17-KGS). Because of these actions, Metopirone is used as a diagnostic test, with urinary 17-OHCS measured as an index of pituitary ACTH responsiveness. Metopirone may also suppress biosynthesis of aldosterone, resulting in a mild natriuresis.

The response to Metopirone does not occur immediately. Following oral administration, peak steroid excretion occurs during the subsequent 24-hour period. Metopirone is absorbed rapidly and well when administered orally as prescribed. Plasma concentrations during the period of treatment are 0.5–1 μg/ml. The major biotransformation is reduction of the ketone to an alcohol and conjugation of metyrapone and reduced metyrapone to the corresponding glucuronides. The apparent half-life of elimination averages 1–2.5 hours. Within 2 days after initiation of treatment, about 40% of the administered dose is excreted in the urine, mostly in the form of glucuronides.

INDICATIONS AND USAGE

A diagnostic drug for testing hypothalamic-pituitary ACTH function.

CONTRAINDICATIONS

Adrenal cortical insufficiency, hypersensitivity to Metopirone.

WARNINGS

Metopirone may induce acute adrenal insufficiency in patients with reduced adrenal secretory capacity.

PRECAUTIONS

General

Ability of adrenals to respond to exogenous ACTH should be demonstrated before Metopirone is employed as a test. In the presence of hypo- or hyperthyroidism, response to the Metopirone test may be subnormal.

Laboratory Tests

See **INTERPRETATION.**

Drug Interactions

All corticosteroid therapy must be discontinued prior to and during testing with Metopirone.

The metabolism of Metopirone is accelerated by phenytoin; therefore, results of the test may be inaccurate in patients taking phenytoin within two weeks before. A subnormal response may occur in patients on estrogen therapy.

Carcinogenesis, Mutagenesis, Impairment of Fertility

Long-term carcinogenicity and reproduction studies in animals have not been conducted.

Pregnancy Category C

A subnormal response to Metopirone may occur in pregnant women. Animal reproduction studies have not been conducted with Metopirone. The Metopirone test was administered to 20 pregnant women in their second and third trimester of pregnancy and evidence was found that the fetal pituitary responded to the enzymatic block. It is not known if Metopirone can affect reproduction capacity. Metopirone should be given to a pregnant woman only if clearly needed.

Nursing Mothers

It is not known whether this drug is excreted in human milk. Because many drugs are excreted in human milk, a decision should be made whether a woman undergoing the Metopirone test should discontinue nursing for the duration of the test.

Pediatric Use

See **DOSAGE AND ADMINISTRATION.**

ADVERSE REACTIONS

Gastrointestinal System: Nausea, abdominal discomfort

Central Nervous System: Headache, dizziness, sedation

Dermatologic System: Allergic rash

Hematologic System: Rarely, decreased white blood cell count or bone marrow depression.

OVERDOSE

Acute Toxicity

One case has been recorded in which a 6-year-old girl died after two doses of Metopirone, 2 g.

Oral LD$_{50}$ in animals (mg/kg): rats, 521; maximum tolerated intravenous dose in one dog, 300.

Signs and Symptoms

The clinical picture of poisoning with Metopirone is characterized by gastrointestinal symptoms and by signs of acute adrenocortical insufficiency.

Cardiovascular System: Cardiac arrhythmias, hypotension, dehydration.

Nervous System and Muscles: Anxiety, confusion, weakness, impairment of consciousness.

Gastrointestinal System: Nausea, vomiting, epigastric pain, diarrhea.

Laboratory Findings: Hyponatremia, hypochloremia, hyperkalemia.

Combined Poisoning

In patients under treatment with insulin or oral antidiabetics, the signs and symptoms of acute poisoning with Metopirone may be aggravated or modified.

Treatment

There is no specific antidote. Besides general measures to eliminate the drug and reduce its absorption, a large dose of hydrocortisone should be administered at once, together with saline and glucose infusions.

Surveillance: For a few days blood pressure and fluid and electrolyte balance should be monitored.

DOSAGE AND ADMINISTRATION

Day 1: Control period—Collect 24-hour urine for measurement of 17-OHCS or 17-KGS.

Day 2: ACTH test to determine the ability of adrenals to respond—Standard ACTH test such as infusion of 50 units ACTH over 8 hours and measurement of 24-hour urinary steroids. If results indicate adequate response, the Metopirone test may proceed.

Day 3–4: Rest period.

Day 5: Administration of Metopirone:

Recommended with milk or snack.

Adults: 750 mg orally, every 4 hours for 6 doses. A single dose is approximately equivalent to 15 mg/kg.

Children: 15 mg/kg orally every 4 hours for 6 doses. A minimal single dose of 250 mg is recommended.

Day 6: After administration of Metopirone— Determination of 24-hour urinary steroids for effect.

INTERPRETATION

ACTH Test

The normal 24-hour urinary excretion of 17-OHCS ranges from 3 to 12 mg. Following continuous intravenous infusion of 50 units ACTH over a period of 8 hours, 17-OHCS excretion increases to 15 to 45 mg per 24 hours.

Metopirone

Normal response: In patients with a normally functioning pituitary, administration of Metopirone is followed by a two-to four-fold increase of 17-OHCS excretion or doubling of 17-KGS excretion.

Subnormal response: Subnormal response in patients without adrenal insufficiency is indicative of some degree of impairment of pituitary function, either panhypopituitarism or partial hypopituitarism (limited pituitary reserve).

1. *Panhypopituitarism* is readily diagnosed by the classical clinical and chemical evidences of hypogonadism, hypothyroidism, and hypoadrenocorticism. These patients usually have subnormal basal urinary steroid levels. Depending upon the duration of the disease and degree of adrenal atrophy, they may fail to respond to exogenous ACTH in the normal manner. Administration of Metopirone is not essential in the diagnosis, but if given, it will not induce an appreciable increase in urinary steroids.

2. *Partial hypopituitarism* or limited pituitary reserve is the more difficult diagnosis as these patients do not present the classical signs and symptoms of hypopituitarism. Measurements of target organ functions often are normal under basal conditions. The response to exogenous ACTH is usually normal, producing the expected rise of urinary steroids (17-OHCS or 17-KGS). The response, however, to Metopirone is *subnormal;* that is, no significant increase in 17-OHCS or 17-KGS excretion occurs.

This failure to respond to metyrapone may be interpreted as evidence of impaired pituitary-adrenal reserve. In view of the normal response to exogenous ACTH, the failure to respond to metyrapone is inferred to be related to a defect in the CNS-pituitary mechanisms which normally regulate ACTH secretions. Presumably the ACTH secreting mechanisms of these individuals are already working at their maximal rates to meet everyday conditions and possess limited "reserve" capacities to secrete additional ACTH either in response to stress or to decreased cortisol levels occurring as a result of metyrapone administration.

Subnormal response in patients with Cushing's syndrome is suggestive of either autonomous adrenal tumors that suppress the ACTH-releasing capacity of the pituitary or nonendocrine ACTH-secreting tumors.

Excessive response: An excessive excretion of 17-OHCS or 17-KGS after administration of Metopirone is suggestive of Cushing's syndrome associated with adrenal hyperplasia. These patients have an elevated excretion of urinary corticosteroids under basal conditions and will often, but not invariably, show a "supernormal" response to ACTH and also to Metopirone, excreting more than 35 mg per 24 hours of either 17-OHCS or 17-KGS.

HOW SUPPLIED

Tablets 250 mg—round, white, scored (imprinted CIBA 130)
Bottles of 18 ....NDC 0083-0130-11
Dispense in tight, light-resistant container (USP).
C86-6 (Rev. 3/86)
Shown in Product Identification Section, page 409

NUPERCAINAL®
[new-purr-cayne'ull]
Hemorrhoidal and Anesthetic Ointment
Pain-Relief Cream

CAUTION
Nupercainal products are not for prolonged or extensive use and should never be applied in or near the eyes.
Consult labels before using.
Keep this and all medications out of reach of children.
NUPERCAINAL SHOULD NOT BE SWALLOWED. SWALLOWING OR USE OF A LARGE QUANTITY IS HAZARDOUS, PARTICULARLY TO CHILDREN. CONSULT A PHYSICIAN OR POISON CONTROL CENTER IMMEDIATELY. IF THE SYMPTOM BEING TREATED DOES NOT SUBSIDE OR RASH, IRRITATION, SWELLING, PAIN, BLEEDING OR OTHER SYMPTOMS DEVELOP OR INCREASE, DISCONTINUE USE AND CONSULT A PHYSICIAN.

INDICATIONS

Nupercainal Ointment and Cream are fast-acting, long-lasting pain relievers that you can use for a number of painful skin conditions. **Nupercainal Hemorrhoidal and Anesthetic Ointment** is for hemorrhoids as well as for general use. **Nupercainal Pain-Relief Cream** is for general use only. The Cream is half as strong as the Ointment.

How to use Nupercainal Anesthetic Ointment (for general use). This soothing Ointment helps lubricate dry, inflamed skin and gives fast, temporary relief of pain, itching and burning. It is recommended for sunburn, nonpoisonous insect bites, minor burns, cuts, and scratches. DO NOT USE THIS PRODUCT IN OR NEAR YOUR EYES.

Apply to affected areas gently. If necessary, cover with a light dressing for protection. Do not use more than 1 ounce of Ointment in a 24-hour period for an adult, do not use more than one-quarter of an ounce in a 24-hour period for a child. If irritation develops, discontinue use and consult your doctor.

How to use Nupercainal Hemorrhoidal and Anesthetic Ointment for fast, temporary relief of pain and itching due to hemorrhoids (also known as piles).

Remove cap from tube and set it aside. Attach the white plastic applicator to the tube. Squeeze the tube until you see the Ointment begin to come through the little holes in the applicator. Using your finger, lubricate the applicator with the Ointment. Now insert the entire applicator gently into the rectum. Give the tube a good squeeze to get enough Ointment into the rectum for comfort and lubrication. Remove applicator from rectum and wipe it clean. Apply additional Ointment to anal tissues to help relieve pain, burning, and itching. For best results use Ointment morning and night and after each bowel movement. After each use detach applicator, and wash it off with soap and water. Put cap back on tube before storing. In case of rectal bleeding, discontinue use and consult your doctor.

Pain-Relief Cream for general use. This Cream is particularly effective for fast, temporary relief of pain and itching associated with sunburn, cuts, scrapes, scratches, minor burns, and nonpoisonous insect bites. DO NOT USE THIS PRODUCT IN OR NEAR YOUR EYES. Apply liberally to affected area and rub in gently. This Cream is water-washable, so be sure to reapply after bathing, swimming or sweating. If irritation develops, discontinue use and consult your doctor.

Nupercainal Hemorrhoidal and Anesthetic Ointment contains 1% dibucaine USP. Also contains acetone sodium bisulfite, lanolin, light mineral oil, purified water, and white petrolatum. Available in tubes of 1 and 2 ounces. Store at 59°–86°F.

Nupercainal Pain-Relief Cream contains 0.5% dibucaine USP. Also contains acetone sodium bisulfite, fragrance, glycerin, potassium hydroxide, purified water, stearic acid, and trolamine. Available in 1½ ounce tubes.

Dibucaine USP is officially classified as a "topical anesthetic" and is one of the strongest and longest lasting of all pain relievers. It is not a narcotic.

C86-62 (Rev. 12/86)

Distributed by:
CIBA CONSUMER PHARMACEUTICALS
EDISON, NEW JERSEY 08837

NUPERCAINAL®
[new-purr-cayne'ull]
Suppositories

CAUTION
Nupercainal Suppositories are not for prolonged or extensive use. Contact with the eyes should be avoided.
Consult labels before using.
Keep this and all medications out of reach of children.
NUPERCAINAL SUPPOSITORIES SHOULD NOT BE SWALLOWED. SWALLOWING CAN BE HAZARDOUS, PARTICULARLY TO CHILDREN. IN THE EVENT OF ACCIDENTAL SWALLOWING CONSULT A PHYSICIAN OR POISON CONTROL CENTER IMMEDIATELY.

INDICATIONS

Nupercainal Suppositories are for the temporary relief from itching, burning, and discomfort due to hemorrhoids or other anorectal disorders.

How to use Nupercainal Suppositories for hemorrhoids (also known as piles) or other anorectal disorders.

Tear off one suppository along the perforated line. Remove foil wrapper. Insert the suppository, rounded end first, well into the anus until you can feel it moving into your rectum. For best results, use one suppository after each bowel movement and as needed, but not to exceed 6 in a 24-hour period. Each suppository is sealed in its own foil packet to reduce danger of leakage when carried in pocket or purse. **To prevent melting, do not store above 86°F (30°C).**

Nupercainal Suppositories contain 2.4 gram cocoa butter and .25 gram zinc oxide. Also contains acetone sodium bisulfite and bismuth subgallate.

C86-42 (Rev. 9/86)

Distributed by:
CIBA CONSUMER PHARMACEUTICALS
EDISON, NEW JERSEY 08837

PRISCOLINE® hydrochloride   ℞
[priss'coe-leen]
tolazoline hydrochloride USP
Ampuls

DESCRIPTION

Priscoline, tolazoline hydrochloride USP, is a peripheral vasodilator available in ampuls for intravenous administration. Each milliliter of sterile, aqueous solution contains tolazoline hydrochloride USP, 25 mg; anhydrous chlorobutanol NF, 5 mg; tartaric acid ACS, 6.5 mg; and hydrous sodium citrate USP, 6.5 mg. Tolazoline hydrochloride is 4,5-dihydro-2-(phenylmethyl)-1H-imidazole monohydrochloride.

Tolazoline hydrochloride USP is a white to off-white crystalline powder. Its solutions are slightly acid to litmus. It is freely soluble in water and in alcohol. Its molecular weight is 196.68.

CLINICAL PHARMACOLOGY

Priscoline is a direct peripheral vasodilator with moderate competitive alpha-adrenergic blocking activity. It decreases peripheral resistance and increases venous capacitance. It has the following additional actions: (1) sympathomimetic, including cardiac stimulation; (2) parasympathomimetic, including gastrointestinal tract stimulation that is blocked by atropine; and (3) histamine-like, including stimulation of gastric secretion and peripheral vasodilatation. Priscoline given intravenously produces vasodilatation, primarily due to a direct effect on vascular smooth muscle, and cardiac stimulation; the blood pressure response depends on the relative contributions of the two effects. Priscoline usually reduces pulmonary arterial pressure and vascular resistance. In neonates the half-life of Priscoline ranges from 3 to 10 hours.

INDICATIONS AND USAGE

Priscoline is indicated for the treatment of persistent pulmonary hypertension of the newborn ("persistent fetal circulation") when systemic arterial oxygenation cannot be satisfactorily maintained by usual supportive care (supplemental oxygen and/or mechanical ventilation).

Priscoline should be used in a highly supervised setting, where vital signs, oxygenation, acid-base status, fluid, and electrolytes can be monitored and maintained.

CONTRAINDICATIONS

Priscoline is contraindicated in patients with hypersensitivity to tolazoline.

WARNINGS

Priscoline stimulates gastric secretion and may activate stress ulcers. Through this mechanism, it can produce significant hypochloremic alkalosis. Pretreatment of infants with antacids may prevent gastrointestinal bleeding.

Patients should be observed closely for signs of systemic hypotension, and supportive therapy should be instituted if needed.

In patients with mitral stenosis, parenterally administered Priscoline may produce a rise or fall in pulmonary artery pressure and total pulmonary resistance; therefore, it must be used with caution in patients with known or suspected mitral stenosis.

PRECAUTIONS

General: The effects of Priscoline on pulmonary vessels may be pH dependent. Acidosis may decrease the effect of Priscoline.

Carcinogenesis, Mutagenesis, Impairment of Fertility: Long-term carcinogenicity studies in animals have not been performed with Priscoline.

Pregnancy Category C: Animal reproduction studies have not been conducted with Priscoline. It is also not known whether Priscoline can cause fetal harm when administered to a pregnant woman or can affect reproduction capacity. Priscoline should be given to a pregnant woman only if clearly needed.

Nursing Mothers: It is not known whether this drug is excreted in human milk. Because many drugs are excreted in human milk, caution should be exercised when Priscoline is administered to a nursing woman.

ADVERSE REACTIONS

The following adverse reactions have been observed, but there are insufficient data to support an estimate of their frequency:

Cardiovascular: Hypotension, tachycardia, cardiac arrhythmias, hypertension, pulmonary hemorrhage.

Digestive and Hepatic: Gastrointestinal hemorrhage, nausea, vomiting, diarrhea, hepatitis.

Skin: Flushing, increased pilomotor activity with tingling or chilliness, rash.

Hematologic: Thrombocytopenia, leukopenia.

Renal: Edema, oliguria, hematuria.

OVERDOSAGE

Acute Toxicity
Oral LD$_{50}$'s (mg/kg): mice, 400; rats, 1200.

Signs and Symptoms
Signs and symptoms of overdosage may include increased pilomotor activity, peripheral vasodilatation, skin flushing, and, in rare instances, hypotension and shock.

Treatment
In treating hypotension, it is most important to place the patient's head low and administer intravenous fluids. Epinephrine should not be used, since large doses of Priscoline may cause "epinephrine reversal" (further reduction in blood pressure, followed by an exaggerated rebound).

DOSAGE AND ADMINISTRATION

An initial dose of 1 to 2 mg/kg, via scalp vein, followed by an infusion of 1 to 2 mg/kg per hour have usually resulted in significant increases in arterial oxygen. There is very little experience with infusions lasting beyond 36 to 48 hours. Response, if it occurs, can be expected within 30 minutes after the initial dose.

Note: Parenteral drug products should be inspected visually for particulate matter and discoloration prior to administration, whenever solution and container permit.

HOW SUPPLIED

Ampuls—4 ml—each milliliter contains 25 mg of tolazoline hydrochloride.
Carton of 4 ampuls .... NDC 0083-6732-04
Store between 15° and 30°C (59°–86°F). Protect from light.
C85-26 (Rev. 3/85)

Continued on next page

CIBA—Cont.

PRIVINE®
[pri-veen ']
0.05% Nasal Solution
0.05% Nasal Spray

CAUTION
Do not use Privine if you have glaucoma. Privine is an effective nasal decongestant **when you use it in the recommended dosage.** If you use too much, too long, or too often, Privine may be harmful to your nasal mucous membranes and cause burning, stinging, sneezing or an increased runny nose. Do not use Privine by mouth.

Keep this and all medications out of the reach of children. Do not use Privine with children under 12 years of age, except with the advice and supervision of a doctor.

OVERDOSAGE IN YOUNG CHILDREN MAY CAUSE MARKED SEDATION AND IF SEVERE, EMERGENCY TREATMENT MAY BE NECESSARY.

IF NASAL STUFFINESS PERSISTS AFTER 3 DAYS OF TREATMENT, DISCONTINUE USE AND CONSULT A DOCTOR.

Privine is a nasal decongestant that comes in two forms: Nasal Solution (in a bottle with a dropper) and Nasal Spray (in a plastic squeeze bottle). Both are for prompt and prolonged relief of nasal congestion due to common colds, sinusitis, hay fever, etc.

How to use Nasal Solution. Squeeze rubber bulb to fill dropper with proper amount of medication. For best results, tilt head as far back as possible and put two drops of solution into your right nostril. Then lean head forward, inhaling and turning your head to the left. Refill dropper by squeezing bulb. Now tilt head as far back as possible and put two drops of solution into your left nostril. Then lean head forward, inhaling, and turning your head to the right.

Use only 2 drops in each nostril. Do not repeat this dosage more than every 3 hours.

The Privine dropper bottle is designed to make administration of the proper dosage easy and to prevent accidental overdosage. Privine will not cause sleeplessness so you may use it before going to bed.

IMPORTANT
After use, be sure to rinse the dropper with very hot water. This helps prevent contamination of the bottle with bacteria from nasal secretions. Use of the dispenser by more than one person may spread infection.

NOTE
Privine Nasal Solution may be used on contact with glass, plastic, stainless steel and specially treated metals used in atomizers. Do not let the solution come in contact with reactive metals, especially aluminum. If solution becomes discolored, it should be discarded.

How to use Nasal Spray. For best results do **not** shake the plastic squeeze bottle.

Remove cap. With head held upright, spray twice into each nostril. Squeeze the bottle sharply and firmly while sniffing through the nose.

For best results use every 4 to 6 hours. Do not use more often than every 3 hours.

Avoid overdosage. Follow directions for use carefully.

Privine Nasal Solution contains 0.05% naphazoline hydrochloride, USP. It also contains benzalkonium chloride, disodium edetate dihydrate, hydrochloric acid, purified water, sodium chloride, and trolamine. It is available in bottles of .66 fl oz (20 ml) with dropper and bottles of 16 fl oz (473 ml). Privine Nasal Spray contains 0.05% naphazoline hydrochloride, USP. It also contains benzalkonium chloride, disodium edetate dihydrate, hydrochloric acid, purified water, sodium chloride, and trolamine. It is available in plastic squeeze bottles of ½ fl oz (15 ml).

Store the nasal solution and nasal spray between 59°–86°F.
C86-43 (Rev. 9/86)

Distributed by:
CIBA CONSUMER PHARMACEUTICALS
Edison, New Jersey 08837

REGITINE®   ℞
[rej 'a-teen]
phentolamine mesylate USP
Vials

DESCRIPTION
Regitine, phentolamine mesylate USP, is an antihypertensive, available in vials for intravenous and intramuscular administration. Each vial contains phentolamine mesylate USP, 5 mg, and mannitol USP, 25 mg, in sterile, lyophilized form.

Phentolamine mesylate is 4,5-dihydro-2-[N-(m -hydroxyphenyl)-N-(p -methylphenyl)aminomethyl]-1H -imidazole 1:1 methanesulfonate.

Phentolamine mesylate USP is a white or off-white, odorless crystalline powder with a molecular weight of 377.46. Its solutions are acid to litmus. It is freely soluble in water and in alcohol, and slightly soluble in chloroform. It melts at about 178°C.

CLINICAL PHARMACOLOGY
Regitine produces an alpha-adrenergic block of relatively short duration. It also has direct, but less marked, positive inotropic and chronotropic effects on cardiac muscle and vasodilator effects on vascular smooth muscle.

Regitine has a half-life in the blood of 19 minutes following intravenous administration. Approximately 13% of a single intravenous dose appears in the urine as unchanged drug.

INDICATIONS AND USAGE
Regitine is indicated for the prevention or control of hypertensive episodes that may occur in a patient with pheochromocytoma as a result of stress or manipulation during preoperative preparation and surgical excision.

Regitine is indicated for the prevention or treatment of dermal necrosis and sloughing following intravenous administration or extravasation of norepinephrine.

Regitine is also indicated for the diagnosis of pheochromocytoma by the Regitine blocking test.

CONTRAINDICATIONS
Myocardial infarction, history of myocardial infarction, coronary insufficiency, angina, or other evidence suggestive of coronary artery disease; hypersensitivity to phentolamine or related compounds.

WARNINGS
Myocardial infarction, cerebrovascular spasm, and cerebrovascular occlusion have been reported to occur following the administration of Regitine, usually in association with marked hypotensive episodes.

For screening tests in patients with hypertension, the generally available urinary assay of catecholamines or other biochemical assays have largely replaced the Regitine and other pharmacological tests for reasons of accuracy and safety. None of the chemical or pharmacological tests is infallible in the diagnosis of pheochromocytoma. The Regitine blocking test is not the procedure of choice and should be reserved for cases in which additional confirmatory evidence is necessary and the relative risks involved in conducting the test have been considered.

PRECAUTIONS
General
Tachycardia and cardiac arrhythmias may occur with the use of Regitine or other alpha-adrenergic blocking agents. When possible, administration of cardiac glycosides should be deferred until cardiac rhythm returns to normal.

Drug Interactions
See **DOSAGE AND ADMINISTRATION,** Diagnosis of pheochromocytoma, *Preparation.*

Carcinogenesis, Mutagenesis, Impairment of Fertility
Long-term carcinogenicity studies, mutagenicity studies, and fertility studies have not been conducted with Regitine.

Pregnancy Category C
Administration of Regitine to pregnant rats and mice at oral doses 24–30 times the usual daily human dose (based on a 60-kg human) resulted in slightly decreased growth and slight skeletal immaturity of the fetuses. Immaturity was manifested by increased incidence of incomplete or unossified calcanei and phalangeal nuclei of the hind limb and of incompletely ossified sternebrae. At oral doses 60 times the usual daily human dose (based on a 60-kg human), a slightly lower rate of implantation was found in the rat. Regitine did not affect embryonic or fetal development in the rabbit at oral doses 20 times the usual daily human dose (based on a 60-kg human). No teratogenic or embryotoxic effects were observed in the rat, mouse, or rabbit studies.

There are no adequate and well-controlled studies in pregnant women. Regitine should be used during pregnancy only if the potential benefit justifies the potential risk to the fetus.

Nursing Mothers
It is not known whether this drug is excreted in human milk. Because many drugs are excreted in human milk and because of the potential for serious adverse reactions in nursing infants from Regitine, a decision should be made whether to discontinue nursing or to discontinue the drug, taking into account the importance of the drug to the mother.

Pediatric Use
See **DOSAGE AND ADMINISTRATION.**

ADVERSE REACTIONS
Acute and prolonged hypotensive episodes, tachycardia, and cardiac arrhythmias have been reported. In addition, weakness, dizziness, flushing, orthostatic hypotension, nasal stuffiness, nausea, vomiting, and diarrhea may occur.

OVERDOSAGE
Acute Toxicity
No deaths due to acute poisoning with Regitine have been reported.

Oral LD$_{50}$'s (mg/kg): mice, 1000; rats, 1250.

Signs and Symptoms
Overdosage with Regitine is characterized chiefly by cardiovascular disturbances, such as arrhythmias, tachycardia, hypotension, and possibly shock. In addition, the following might occur: excitation, headache, sweating, pupillary contraction, visual disturbances; nausea, vomiting, diarrhea; hypoglycemia.

Treatment
There is no specific antidote.

A decrease in blood pressure to dangerous levels or other evidence of shocklike conditions should be treated vigorously and promptly. The patient's legs should be kept raised and a plasma expander should be administered. If necessary, intravenous infusion of norepinephrine, titrated to maintain blood pressure at the normotensive level, and all available supportive measures should be included. Epinephrine should not be used, since it may cause a paradoxical reduction in blood pressure.

DOSAGE AND ADMINISTRATION
The reconstituted solution should be used upon preparation and should not be stored.
Note: Parenteral drug products should be inspected visually for particulate matter and discoloration prior to administration, whenever solution and container permit.

1. Prevention or control of hypertensive episodes in the patient with pheochromocytoma.
For preoperative reduction of elevated blood pressure, 5 mg of Regitine (1 mg for children) is injected intravenously or intramuscularly 1 or 2 hours before surgery, and repeated if necessary.

During surgery, Regitine (5 mg for adults, 1 mg for children) is administered intravenously as indicated, to help prevent or control paroxysms of hypertension, tachycardia, respiratory depression, convulsions, or other effects of epinephrine intoxication. (Postoperatively, norepinephrine may be given to control the hypotension that commonly follows complete removal of a pheochromocytoma.)

2. Prevention or treatment of dermal necrosis and sloughing following intravenous administration or extravasation of norepinephrine.
For Prevention: 10 mg of Regitine is added to each liter of solution containing norepinephrine. The pressor effect of norepinephrine is not affected.
For Treatment: 5–10 mg of Regitine in 10 ml of saline is injected into the area of extravasation within 12 hours.

3. Diagnosis of pheochromocytoma—Regitine blocking test.
The test is most reliable in detecting pheochromocytoma in patients with sustained hypertension and least reliable in those with paroxysmal hypertension. False-positive tests may occur in patients with hypertension without pheochromocytoma.

a. Intravenous
Preparation
The **CONTRAINDICATIONS, WARNINGS,** and **PRECAUTIONS** sections should be reviewed. Sedatives, analgesics, and all other medications except those that might be deemed essential (such as digitalis and insulin) are withheld for at least 24 hours, and preferably 48–72 hours, prior to the test. Antihypertensive drugs are withheld until blood pressure returns to the untreated, hypertensive level. This test is not performed on a patient who is normotensive.
Procedure
The patient is kept at rest in the supine position throughout the test, preferably in a quiet, darkened room. Injection of Regitine is delayed until blood pressure is stabilized, as evidenced by blood pressure readings taken every 10 minutes for at least 30 minutes.

Five milligrams of Regitine is dissolved in 1 ml of Sterile Water for Injection. The dose for adults is 5 mg; for children, 1 mg.

The syringe needle is inserted into the vein, and injection is delayed until pressor response to venipuncture has subsided. Regitine is injected rapidly. Blood pressure is recorded immediately after injection, at 30-second intervals for the first 3 minutes, and at 60-second intervals for the next 7 minutes.
Interpretation
A positive response, suggestive of pheochromocytoma, is indicated when the blood pressure is reduced more than 35 mm Hg systolic and 25 mm Hg diastolic. A typical positive response is a reduction in pressure of 60 mm Hg systolic and 25 mm Hg diastolic. Usually, maximal effect is evident within 2 minutes after injection. A return to preinjection pressure commonly occurs within 15–30 minutes but may occur more rapidly.

If blood pressure decreases to a dangerous level, the patient should be treated as outlined under **OVERDOSAGE.**
A positive response should always be confirmed by other diagnostic procedures, preferably by measurement of urinary catecholamines or their metabolites.

A negative response is indicated when the blood pressure is elevated, unchanged, or reduced less than 35 mm Hg systolic and 25 mm Hg diastolic after injection of Regitine. A negative reponse to this test does not exclude the diagnosis of pheochromocytoma, especially in patients with paroxysmal hypertension in whom the incidence of false-negative responses is high.

b. Intramuscular

If the intramuscular test for pheochromocytoma is preferred, preparation is the same as for the intravenous test. Five milligrams of Regitine is then dissolved in 1 ml of Sterile Water for Injection. The dose for adults is 5 mg intramuscularly; for children, 3 mg. Blood pressure is recorded every 5 minutes for 30–45 minutes following injection. A positive response is indicated when the blood pressure is reduced 35 mm Hg systolic and 25 mm Hg diastolic, or more, within 20 minutes following injection.

HOW SUPPLIED

Vials—each containing 5 mg of phentolamine mesylate USP and 25 mg of mannitol USP, in lyophilized form
Cartons of 2 .... NDC 0083-6830-02
Cartons of 6 .... NDC 0083-6830-06
The reconstituted solution should be used upon preparation and should not be stored.
Store between 59° and 86°F.
Dist. by:
CIBA Pharmaceutical Company
Division of CIBA-GEIGY Corporation
Summit, NJ 07901

C85-2 (Rev. 8/85)

RIMACTANE®   ℞
[re-mack 'tayne]
rifampin USP

DESCRIPTION

Rimactane, rifampin USP , is a semisynthetic antibiotic derivative of rifamycin B, available as 300-mg capsules for oral administration. It is also available in Dual Packs containing two 300-mg capsules of Rimactane and one 300-mg tablet of INH®, isoniazid USP. Rimactane is 3-[[4-methyl-1-piperazinyl)imino] methyl] rifamycin.
Rifampin USP is a red-brown crystalline powder. It is very slightly soluble in water, freely soluble in chloroform, and soluble in ethyl acetate and in methanol. Its molecular weight is 822.95.
Inactive Ingredients: FD&C Blue No. 1, FD&C Red No. 40, FD&C Yellow No. 6, gelatin, lactose, magnesium stearate, methylparaben, propylparaben, silicon dioxide, sodium lauryl sulfate, starch, talc, and titanium dioxide.

ACTIONS

Rimactane inhibits DNA-dependent RNA polymerase activity in susceptible cells. Specifically, it interacts with bacterial RNA polymerase but does not inhibit the mammalian enzyme. This is the mechanism of action by which Rimactane exerts its therapeutic effect. Rimactane cross resistance has only been shown with other rifamycins.
Peak blood levels in normal adults vary widely from individual to individual. Peak levels occur between 2 and 4 hours following the oral administration of a 600-mg dose. The average peak value is 7 mcg/ml; however, the peak level may vary from 4 to 32 mcg/ml.
In normal subjects the $T\frac{1}{2}$ (biological half-life) of Rimactane in blood is approximately 3 hours. Elimination occurs mainly through the bile and, to a much lesser extent, the urine.

INDICATIONS

Pulmonary Tuberculosis

In the initial treatment and in the retreatment of pulmonary tuberculosis, Rimactane must be used in conjunction with at least one other antituberculous drug.
Frequently used regimens have been the following:
   isoniazid and Rimactane
   ethambutol and Rimactane
   isoniazid, ethambutol, and Rimactane
Neisseria Meningitidis Carriers

Rimactane is indicated for the treatment of asymptomatic carriers of *N. meningitidis* to eliminate meningococci from the nasopharynx.
Rimactane is not indicated for the treatment of meningococcal infection.
To avoid the indiscriminate use of Rimactane, diagnostic laboratory procedures, including serotyping and susceptibility testing, should be performed to establish the carrier state and the correct treatment. In order to preserve the usefulness of Rimactane in the treatment of asymptomatic meningococcal carriers, it is recommended that the drug be reserved for situations in which the risk of meningococcal meningitis is high.
Both in the treatment of tuberculosis and in the treatment of meningococcal carriers, small numbers of resistant cells, present within large populations of susceptible cells, can rapidly become the predominating type. Since rapid emergence of resistance can occur, culture and susceptibility tests should be performed in the event of persistent positive cultures.

CONTRAINDICATIONS

A history of previous hypersensitivity reaction to any of the rifamycins.

WARNINGS

Rifampin has been shown to produce liver dysfunction. There have been fatalities associated with jaundice in patients with liver disease or receiving rifampin concomitantly with other hepatotoxic agents. Since an increased risk may exist for individuals with liver disease, benefits must be weighed carefully against the risk of further liver damage. Periodic liver function monitoring is mandatory.
The possibility of rapid emergence of resistant meningococci restricts the use of Rimactane to short-term treatment of the asymptomatic carrier state. Rimactane is not to be used for the treatment of meningococcal disease.
Several studies of tumorigenicity potential have been done in rodents. In one strain of mice known to be particularly susceptible to the spontaneous development of hepatomas, rifampin given at a level 2–10 times the maximum dosage used clinically, resulted in a significant increase in the occurrence of hepatomas in female mice of this strain after one year of administration. There was no evidence of tumorigenicity in the males of this strain, in males or females of another mouse strain, or rats.

Usage in Pregnancy

Although rifampin has been reported to cross the placental barrier and appear in cord blood, the effect of Rimactane, alone or in combination with other antituberculous drugs, on the human fetus is not known. An increase in congenital malformations, primarily spina bifida and cleft palate, has been reported in the offspring of rodents given oral doses of 150-250 mg/kg/day of rifampin during pregnancy.
The possible teratogenic potential in women capable of bearing children should be carefully weighed against the benefits of therapy.

PRECAUTIONS

Rimactane is not recommended for intermittent therapy; the patient should be cautioned against intentional or accidental interruption of the daily dosage regimen since rare renal hypersensitivity reactions have been reported when therapy was resumed in such cases.
Rifampin has been observed to increase the requirements for anticoagulant drugs of the coumarin type. The cause of this phenomenon is unknown. In patients receiving anticoagulants and rifampin concurrently, it is recommended that the prothrombin time be performed daily or as frequently as necessary to establish and maintain the required dose of anticoagulant.
Urine, feces, saliva, sputum, sweat, and tears may be colored red-orange by rifampin and its metabolites. Soft contact lenses may be permanently stained. Individuals to be treated should be made aware of these possibilities.
It has been reported that the reliability of oral contraceptives may be affected in some patients being treated for tuberculosis with rifampin in combination with at least one other antituberculous drug. In such cases, alternative contraceptive measures may need to be considered.
Rifampin has been reported to diminish the effects of concurrently administered methadone, oral hypoglycemics, corticosteroids, dapsone, digitalis preparations and to reduce the bioavailability and efficacy of verapamil. Appropriate dosage adjustments may be necessary if indicated by the patient's clinical condition.
When rifampin is taken in combination with PAS, decreased rifampin serum levels may result. Therefore, the drugs should be given at least 4 hours apart.
Therapeutic levels of rifampin have been shown to inhibit standard assays for serum folate and vitamin B_{12}. Alternative methods must be considered when determining folate and vitamin B_{12} concentrations in the presence of rifampin.
Since rifampin has been reported to cross the placental barrier and appear in cord blood, neonates of rifampin-treated mothers should be carefully observed for any evidence of adverse effects. Rifampin is excreted in breast milk.

ADVERSE REACTIONS

Gastrointestinal disturbances such as heartburn, epigastric distress, anorexia, nausea, vomiting, gas, cramps, and diarrhea have been noted in some patients. Rarely, pseudomembranous enterocolitis has been reported. Headache, drowsiness, fatigue, ataxia, dizziness, inability to concentrate, mental confusion, visual disturbances, muscular weakness, fever, pains in extremities, generalized numbness, and menstrual disturbances have also been noted.
Hypersensitivity reactions have been reported. Encountered occasionally have been pruritus, urticaria, rash, pemphigoid reaction, eosinophilia, sore mouth, sore tongue, and exudative conjunctivitis. Rarely, hepatitis or a shock-like syndrome with hepatic involvement and abnormal liver function tests have been reported. Transient abnormalities in liver function tests (eg, elevations in serum bilirubin, BSP, alkaline phosphatase, serum transaminases) have also been observed. The BSP test should be performed prior to the morning dose of rifampin to avoid false-positive results.

Thrombocytopenia, transient leukopenia, hemolytic anemia, and decreased hemoglobin have been observed. Thrombocytopenia has occurred when rifampin and ethambutol were administered concomitantly according to an intermittent dose schedule twice weekly and in high doses.
Elevations in BUN and serum uric acid have occurred. Rarely, hemolysis, hemoglobinuria, hematuria, renal insufficiency or acute renal failure have been reported and are generally considered to be hypersensitivity reactions. These have usually occurred during intermittent therapy or when treatment was resumed following intentional or accidental interruption of a daily dosage regimen and were reversible when rifampin was discontinued and appropriate therapy instituted.
Although rifampin has been reported to have an immunosuppressive effect in some animal experiments, available human data indicate that this has no clinical significance.

DOSAGE AND ADMINISTRATION

It is recommended that Rimactane be administered once daily, either one hour before or two hours after a meal.
Data are not available for determination of dosage for children under 5.
Pulmonary Tuberculosis

Adults: 600 mg (two 300-mg Capsules) in a single daily administration.
Children: 10 to 20 mg/kg, not to exceed 600 mg/day.
In the treatment of pulmonary tuberculosis, Rimactane must be used in conjunction with at least one other antituberculous agent. In general, therapy should be continued until bacterial conversion and maximal improvement have occurred.
Meningococcal Carriers

It is recommended that Rimactane be administered once daily for four consecutive days in the following doses:
Adults: 600 mg (two 300-mg Capsules) in a single daily administration.
Children: 10 to 20 mg/kg, not to exceed 600 mg/day.
Susceptibility Testing

Pulmonary Tuberculosis: Rifampin susceptibility powders are available for both direct and indirect methods of determining the susceptibility of strains of mycobacteria. The MICs of susceptible clinical isolates when determined in 7H10 or other non-egg-containing media have ranged from 0.1 to 2 mcg/ml.
Meningococcal Carriers: Susceptibility discs containing 5 mcg rifampin are available for susceptibility testing of *N. meningitidis.*
Quantitative methods that require measurement of zone diameters give the most precise estimates of antibiotic susceptibility. One such procedure[1] has been recommended for use with discs for testing susceptibility to rifampin. Interpretations correlate zone diameters from the disc test with MIC (minimal inhibitory concentration) values for rifampin. A range of MIC's from 0.1 to 1 mcg/ml has been found *in vitro* for susceptible strains of *N. meningitidis.* With this procedure, a report from the laboratory of "resistant" indicates that the organism is not likely to be eradicated from the nasopharynx of asymptomatic carriers.

OVERDOSAGE

Signs and Symptoms

Nausea, vomiting, and increasing lethargy will probably occur within a short time after ingestion; actual unconsciousness may occur with severe hepatic involvement. Brownish-red or orange discoloration of the skin, urine, sweat, saliva, tears, and feces is proportional to amount ingested.
Liver enlargement, possibly with tenderness, can develop within a few hours after severe overdosage and jaundice may develop rapidly. Hepatic involvement may be more marked in patients with prior impairment of hepatic function. Other physical findings remain essentially normal.
Direct and total bilirubin levels may increase rapidly with severe overdosage; hepatic enzyme levels may be affected, especially with prior impairment of hepatic function. A direct effect upon hemopoietic system, electrolyte levels, or acid-base balance is unlikely.
Treatment

Since nausea and vomiting are likely to be present, gastric lavage is probably preferable to induction of emesis. Activated charcoal slurry instilled into the stomach following evacuation of gastric contents can help absorb any remaining drug in G.I. tract. Antiemetic medication may be required to control severe nausea/vomiting.
Active diuresis (with measured intake and output) will help promote excretion of the drug. Bile drainage may be indicated in presence of serious impairment of hepatic function

Continued on next page

The full prescribing information for each CIBA product is contained herein and is that in effect as of September 1, 1989

CIBA—Cont.

lasting more than 24–48 hours; under these circumstances, extracorporeal hemodialysis may be required.

In patients with previously adequate hepatic function, reversal of liver enlargement and impaired hepatic excretory function probably will be noted within 72 hours, with rapid return toward normal thereafter.

HOW SUPPLIED

Capsules 300 mg—opaque, scarlet, caramel (imprinted CIBA 154)

Bottles of 30 ....NDC 0083-0154-26
Bottles of 60 ....NDC 0083-0154-29
Bottles of 100 ....NDC 0083-0154-30

Keep tightly closed. Protect from heat and moisture.
Dispense in tight, light-resistant container (USP).

Also available—Rimactane®/INH® (isoniazid USP) Dual Pack. Each Dual Pack contains two Rimactane 300-mg capsules and one INH 300-mg tablet.

Cartons of 30 Dual Packs
(60 Rimactane capsules and
30 INH tablets).......................................NDC 0083-8912-23

Store between 59°–86°F (15°–30°C). Protect from light and moisture.

REFERENCE

1. Bauer AW, Kirby WMM, Sherris JC, et al: Antibiotic susceptibility testing by a standardized single disk method. *Am J Clin Path* 1966;45:493–496.

C89-7 (Rev. 3/89)
Shown in Product Identification Section, page 409

RITALIN® hydrochloride   Ⓒ
[*rit'ah-lin*]
methylphenidate hydrochloride
tablets USP

RITALIN-SR®   Ⓒ
methylphenidate hydrochloride USP
sustained-release tablets

DESCRIPTION

Ritalin, methylphenidate hydrochloride USP, is a mild central nervous system (CNS) stimulant, available as tablets of 5, 10, and 20 mg for oral administration; Ritalin-SR is available as sustained-release tablets of 20 mg for oral administration. Methylphenidate hydrochloride is methyl α-phenyl-2-piperidineacetate hydrochloride.

Methylphenidate hydrochloride USP is a white, odorless, fine crystalline powder. Its solutions are acid to litmus. It is freely soluble in water and in methanol, soluble in alcohol, and slightly soluble in chloroform and in acetone. Its molecular weight is 269.77.

Inactive Ingredients. Ritalin tablets: D&C Yellow No. 10 (5-mg and 20-mg tablets), FD&C Green No. 3 (10-mg tablets), lactose, magnesium stearate, polyethylene glycol, starch (5-mg and 10-mg tablets), sucrose, talc, and tragacanth (20-mg tablets).

Ritalin-SR tablets: Cellulose compounds, cetostearyl alcohol, lactose, magnesium stearate, mineral oil, povidone, titanium dioxide, and zein.

CLINICAL PHARMACOLOGY

Ritalin is a mild central nervous system stimulant.

The mode of action in man is not completely understood, but Ritalin presumably activates the brain stem arousal system and cortex to produce its stimulant effect.

There is neither specific evidence which clearly establishes the mechanism whereby Ritalin produces its mental and behavioral effects in children, nor conclusive evidence regarding how these effects relate to the condition of the central nervous system.

Ritalin in the SR tablets is more slowly but as extensively absorbed as in the regular tablets. Relative bioavailability of the SR tablet compared to the Ritalin tablet, measured by the urinary excretion of Ritalin major metabolite (α-phenyl-2-piperidine acetic acid) was 105% (49–168%) in children and 101% (85–152%) in adults. The time to peak rate in children was 4.7 hours (1.3–8.2 hours) for the SR tablets and 1.9 hours (0.3–4.4 hours) for the tablets. An average of 67% of SR tablet dose was excreted in children as compared to 86% in adults.

INDICATIONS

Attention Deficit Disorders, Narcolepsy

Attention Deficit Disorders (previously known as Minimal Brain Dysfunction in Children). Other terms being used to describe the behavioral syndrome below include: Hyperkinetic Child Syndrome, Minimal Brain Damage, Minimal Cerebral Dysfunction, Minor Cerebral Dysfunction.

Ritalin is indicated as an integral part of a total treatment program which typically includes other remedial measures (psychological, educational, social) for a stabilizing effect in children with a behavioral syndrome characterized by the following group of developmentally inappropriate symp-

---

toms: moderate-to-severe distractibility, short attention span, hyperactivity, emotional lability, and impulsivity. The diagnosis of this syndrome should not be made with finality when these symptoms are only of comparatively recent origin. Nonlocalizing (soft) neurological signs, learning disability, and abnormal EEG may or may not be present, and a diagnosis of central nervous system dysfunction may or may not be warranted.

Special Diagnostic Considerations

Specific etiology of this syndrome is unknown, and there is no single diagnostic test. Adequate diagnosis requires the use not only of medical but of special psychological, educational, and social resources.

Characteristics commonly reported include: chronic history of short attention span, distractibility, emotional lability, impulsivity, and moderate-to-severe hyperactivity; minor neurological signs and abnormal EEG. Learning may or may not be impaired. The diagnosis must be based upon a complete history and evaluation of the child and not solely on the presence of one or more of these characteristics.

Drug treatment is not indicated for all children with this syndrome. Stimulants are not intended for use in the child who exhibits symptoms secondary to environmental factors and/or primary psychiatric disorders, including psychosis. Appropriate educational placement is essential and psychosocial intervention is generally necessary. When remedial measures alone are insufficient, the decision to prescribe stimulant medication will depend upon the physician's assessment of the chronicity and severity of the child's symptoms.

CONTRAINDICATIONS

Marked anxiety, tension, and agitation are contraindications to Ritalin, since the drug may aggravate these symptoms. Ritalin is contraindicated also in patients known to be hypersensitive to the drug, in patients with glaucoma, and in patients with motor tics or with a family history or diagnosis of Tourette's syndrome.

WARNINGS

Ritalin should not be used in children under six years, since safety and efficacy in this age group have not been established.

Sufficient data on safety and efficacy of long-term use of Ritalin in children are not yet available. Although a causal relationship has not been established, suppression of growth (ie, weight gain, and/or height) has been reported with the long-term use of stimulants in children. Therefore, patients requiring long-term therapy should be carefully monitored.

Ritalin should not be used for severe depression of either exogenous or endogenous origin. Clinical experience suggests that in psychotic children, administration of Ritalin may exacerbate symptoms of behavior disturbance and thought disorder.

Ritalin should not be used for the prevention or treatment of normal fatigue states.

There is some clinical evidence that Ritalin may lower the convulsive threshold in patients with prior history of seizures, with prior EEG abnormalities in absence of seizures, and, very rarely, in absence of history of seizures and no prior EEG evidence of seizures. Safe concomitant use of anticonvulsants and Ritalin has not been established. In the presence of seizures, the drug should be discontinued.

Use cautiously in patients with hypertension. Blood pressure should be monitored at appropriate intervals in all patients taking Ritalin, especially those with hypertension.

Symptoms of visual disturbances have been encountered in rare cases. Difficulties with accommodation and blurring of vision have been reported.

Drug Interactions

Ritalin may decrease the hypotensive effect of guanethidine. Use cautiously with pressor agents and MAO inhibitors.

Human pharmacologic studies have shown that Ritalin may inhibit the metabolism of coumarin anticoagulants, anticonvulsants (phenobarbital, diphenylhydantoin, primidone), phenylbutazone, and tricyclic antidepressants (imipramine, desipramine). Downward dosage adjustments of these drugs may be required when given concomitantly with Ritalin.

Usage in Pregnancy

Adequate animal reproduction studies to establish safe use of Ritalin during pregnancy have not been conducted. Therefore, until more information is available, Ritalin should not be prescribed for women of childbearing age unless, in the opinion of the physician, the potential benefits outweigh the possible risks.

Drug Dependence

Ritalin should be given cautiously to emotionally unstable patients, such as those with a history of drug dependence or alcoholism, because such patients may increase dosage on their own initiative.

Chronically abusive use can lead to marked tolerance and psychic dependence with varying degrees of abnormal behavior. Frank psychotic episodes can occur, especially with parenteral abuse. Careful supervision is required during drug withdrawal, since severe depression

---

as well as the effects of chronic overactivity can be unmasked. Long-term follow-up may be required because of the patient's basic personality disturbances.

PRECAUTIONS

Patients with an element of agitation may react adversely; discontinue therapy if necessary.

Periodic CBC, differential, and platelet counts are advised during prolonged therapy.

Drug treatment is not indicated in all cases of this behavioral syndrome and should be considered only in light of the complete history and evaluation of the child. The decision to prescribe Ritalin should depend on the physician's assessment of the chronicity and severity of the child's symptoms and their appropriateness for his/her age. Prescription should not depend solely on the presence of one or more of the behavioral characteristics.

When these symptoms are associated with acute stress reactions, treatment with Ritalin is usually not indicated.

Long-term effects of Ritalin in children have not been well established.

ADVERSE REACTIONS

Nervousness and insomnia are the most common adverse reactions but are usually controlled by reducing dosage and omitting the drug in the afternoon or evening. Other reactions include hypersensitivity (including skin rash, urticaria, fever, arthralgia, exfoliative dermatitis, erythema multiforme with histopathological findings of necrotizing vasculitis, and thrombocytopenic purpura); anorexia; nausea; dizziness; palpitations; headache; dyskinesia; drowsiness; blood pressure and pulse changes, both up and down; tachycardia; angina; cardiac arrhythmia; abdominal pain; weight loss during prolonged therapy. There have been rare reports of Tourette's syndrome. Toxic psychosis has been reported. Although a definite causal relationship has not been established, the following have been reported in patients taking this drug: leukopenia and/or anemia; transient depressed mood, a few instances of scalp hair loss.

In children, loss of appetite, abdominal pain, weight loss during prolonged therapy, insomnia, and tachycardia may occur more frequently; however, any of the other adverse reactions listed above may also occur.

DOSAGE AND ADMINISTRATION

Dosage should be individualized according to the needs and responses of the patient.

Adults

Tablets: Administer in divided doses 2 or 3 times daily, preferably 30 to 45 minutes before meals. Average dosage is 20 to 30 mg daily. Some patients may require 40 to 60 mg daily. In others, 10 to 15 mg daily will be adequate. Patients who are unable to sleep if medication is taken late in the day should take the last dose before 6 p.m.

SR Tablets: Ritalin-SR tablets have a duration of action of approximately 8 hours. Therefore, Ritalin-SR tablets may be used in place of Ritalin tablets when the 8-hour dosage of Ritalin-SR corresponds to the titrated 8-hour dosage of Ritalin. Ritalin-SR tablets must be swallowed whole and never crushed or chewed.

Children (6 years and over)

Ritalin should be initiated in small doses, with gradual weekly increments. Daily dosage above 60 mg is not recommended.

If improvement is not observed after appropriate dosage adjustment over a one-month period, the drug should be discontinued.

Tablets: Start with 5 mg twice daily (before breakfast and lunch) with gradual increments of 5 to 10 mg weekly.

SR Tablets: Ritalin-SR tablets have a duration of action of approximately 8 hours. Therefore, Ritalin-SR tablets may be used in place of Ritalin tablets when the 8-hour dosage of Ritalin-SR corresponds to the titrated 8-hour dosage of Ritalin. Ritalin-SR tablets must be swallowed whole and never crushed or chewed.

If paradoxical aggravation of symptoms or other adverse effects occur, reduce dosage, or, if necessary, discontinue the drug.

Ritalin should be periodically discontinued to assess the child's condition. Improvement may be sustained when the drug is either temporarily or permanently discontinued.

Drug treatment should not and need not be indefinite and usually may be discontinued after puberty.

OVERDOSAGE

Signs and symptoms of acute overdosage, resulting principally from overstimulation of the central nervous system and from excessive sympathomimetic effects, may include the following: vomiting, agitation, tremors, hyperreflexia, muscle twitching, convulsions (may be followed by coma), euphoria, confusion, hallucinations, delirium, sweating, flushing, headache, hyperpyrexia, tachycardia, palpitations, cardiac arrhythmias, hypertension, mydriasis, and dryness of mucous membranes.

Treatment consists of appropriate supportive measures. The patient must be protected against self-injury and against

external stimuli that would aggravate overstimulation already present. If signs and symptoms are not too severe and the patient is conscious, gastric contents may be evacuated by induction of emesis or gastric lavage. In the presence of severe intoxication, use a carefully titrated dosage of a *short-acting* barbiturate *before* performing gastric lavage.
Intensive care must be provided to maintain adequate circulation and respiratory exchange; external cooling procedures may be required for hyperpyrexia.
Efficacy of peritoneal dialysis or extracorporeal hemodialysis for Ritalin overdosage has not been established.

HOW SUPPLIED

Tablets 5 mg—round, yellow (imprinted CIBA 7)

Bottles of 100	NDC 0083-0007-30
Bottles of 500	NDC 0083-0007-35
Bottles of 1000	NDC 0083-0007-40

Tablets 10 mg —round, pale green, scored (imprinted CIBA 3)

Bottles of 100	NDC 0083-0003-30
Bottles of 500	NDC 0083-0003-35
Bottles of 1000	NDC 0083-0003-40
Accu-Pak® Unit Dose (blister pack)	
Box of 100 (strips of 10)	NDC 0083-0003-32

Tablets 20 mg—round, pale yellow, scored (imprinted CIBA 34)

Bottles of 100	NDC 0083-0034-30
Bottles of 1000	NDC 0083-0034-40

Protect from light.
Dispense in tight, light-resistant container (USP).
SR Tablets 20 mg —round, white, coated (imprinted CIBA 16)

Bottles of 100	NDC 0083-0016-30

Note: SR Tablets are color-additive free.
Do not store above 86°F (30°C). Protect from moisture.
Dispense in tight, light-resistant container (USP).

C88-34 (Rev. 9/88)

Shown in Product Identification Section, page 409

SER-AP-ES®   ℞
[*su-rapp 'ess*]
reserpine 0.1 mg
hydralazine hydrochloride 25 mg
hydrochlorothiazide 15 mg
Combination Tablets

> **WARNING**
> This fixed-combination drug is not indicated for initial therapy of hypertension. Hypertension requires therapy titrated to the individual patient. If the fixed combination represents the dosage so determined, its use may be more convenient in patient management. The treatment of hypertension is not static but must be reevaluated as conditions in each patient warrant.

DESCRIPTION

Ser-Ap-Es is an antihypertensive-diuretic combination, available as tablets for oral administration. Each tablet contains Serpasil (reserpine USP), 0.1 mg; Apresoline (hydralazine hydrochloride USP), 25 mg; and Esidrix (hydrochlorothiazide USP), 15 mg.
Reserpine is methyl 18β-hydroxy-11, 17α-dimethoxy-3β, 20α-yohimban-16β-carboxylate 3,4,5-trimethoxybenzoate (ester).
Reserpine USP, a pure crystalline alkaloid of rauwolfia, is a white or pale buff to slightly yellowish, odorless crystalline powder. It darkens slowly on exposure to light, but more rapidly when in solution. It is insoluble in water, freely soluble in acetic acid and in chloroform, slightly soluble in benzene, and very slightly soluble in alcohol and in ether. Its molecular weight is 608.69.
Hydralazine hydrochloride is 1-hydrazinophthalazine monohydrochloride.
Hydralazine hydrochloride USP is a white to off-white, odorless crystalline powder. It is soluble in water, slightly soluble in alcohol, and very slightly soluble in ether. It melts at about 275°C, with decomposition, and has a molecular weight of 196.64.
Hydrochlorothiazide is 6-chloro-3,4-dihydro-$2H$-1,2,4-benzothiadiazine-7-sulfonamide 1,1-dioxide.
Hydrochlorothiazide USP is a white, or practically white, practically odorless crystalline powder. It is slightly soluble in water; freely soluble in sodium hydroxide solution, in *n*-butylamine, and in dimethylformamide; sparingly soluble in methanol; and insoluble in ether, in chloroform, and in dilute mineral acids. Its molecular weight is 297.73.
Inactive Ingredients: Acacia, FD&C Blue No. 1, FD&C Green No. 3, FD&C Red No. 40, FD&C Yellow No. 6, lactose, polyethylene glycol, starch, stearic acid and sucrose.

CLINICAL PHARMACOLOGY

Reserpine: Reserpine depletes stores of catecholamines and 5-hydroxytryptamine in many organs, including the brain

and adrenal medulla. Most of its pharmacological effects have been attributed to this action. Depletion is slower and less complete in the adrenal medulla than in other tissues. The depression of sympathetic nerve function results in a decreased heart rate and a lowering of arterial blood pressure. The sedative and tranquilizing properties of reserpine are thought to be related to depletion of catecholamines and 5-hydroxytryptamine from the brain.
Reserpine, like other rauwolfia compounds, is characterized by slow onset of action and sustained effects. Both cardiovascular and central nervous system effects may persist for a period of time following withdrawal of the drug.
Mean maximum plasma levels of 1.54 ng/ml were attained after a median of 3.5 hours in six normal subjects receiving a single oral dose of four 0.25-mg Serpasil tablets. Bioavailability was approximately 50% of that of a corresponding intravenous dose. Plasma levels of reserpine after intravenous administration declined with a mean half-life of 33 hours. Reserpine is extensively bound (96%) to plasma proteins. No definitive studies on the human metabolism of reserpine have been made.
Hydralazine: Although the precise mechanism of action of hydralazine is not fully understood, the major effects are on the cardiovascular system. Hydralazine apparently lowers blood pressure by exerting a peripheral vasodilating effect through a direct relaxation of vascular smooth muscle. Hydralazine, by altering cellular calcium metabolism, interferes with the calcium movements within the vascular smooth muscle that are responsible for initiating or maintaining the contractile state.
The peripheral vasodilating effect of hydralazine results in decreased arterial blood pressure (diastolic more than systolic); decreased peripheral vascular resistance; and an increased heart rate, stroke volume, and cardiac output. The preferential dilatation of arterioles, as compared to veins, minimizes postural hypotension and promotes the increase in cardiac output. Hydralazine usually increases renin activity in plasma, presumably as a result of increased secretion of renin by the renal juxtaglomerular cells in response to reflex sympathetic discharge. This increase in renin activity leads to the production of angiotensin II, which then causes stimulation of aldosterone and consequent sodium reabsorption. Hydralazine also maintains or increases renal and cerebral blood flow.
Hydralazine is rapidly absorbed after oral administration, and peak plasma levels are reached at 1–2 hours. Plasma levels decline with a half-life of 3–7 hours. Binding to human plasma protein is 87%. Plasma levels of hydralazine vary widely among individuals. Hydralazine is subject to polymorphic acetylation; slow acetylators generally have higher plasma levels of hydralazine and require lower doses to maintain control of blood pressure. Hydralazine undergoes extensive hepatic metabolism; it is excreted mainly in the form of metabolites in the urine.
Administration of hydralazine with food results in higher levels of the drug in plasma.
Hydrochlorothiazide: Thiazides affect the renal tubular mechanism of electrolyte reabsorption. At maximal therapeutic dosage, all thiazides are approximately equal in their diuretic potency. Thiazides increase excretion of sodium and chloride in approximately equivalent amounts. Natriuresis causes a secondary loss of potassium.
The mechanism of the antihypertensive effect of thiazides is unknown. Thiazides do not affect normal blood pressure.
The onset of action of thiazides occurs in 2 hours, and the peak effect at about 4 hours. The action persists for approximately 6–12 hours. Hydrochlorothiazide is rapidly absorbed, as indicated by peak plasma concentrations 1–2.5 hours after oral administration. Plasma levels of the drug are proportional to dose; the concentration in whole blood is 1.6–1.8 times higher than in plasma. Thiazides are eliminated rapidly by the kidney. After oral administration of 25- to 100-mg doses of hydrochlorothiazide, 72–97% of the dose is excreted in the urine, indicating dose-independent absorption. Hydrochlorothiazide is eliminated from plasma in a biphasic fashion with a terminal half-life of 10–17 hours. Plasma protein binding is 67.9%. Plasma clearance is 15.9–30.0 L/hr; volume of distribution is 3.6–7.8 L/kg.
Gastrointestinal absorption of hydrochlorothiazide is enhanced when administered with food. Absorption is decreased in patients with congestive heart failure, and the pharmacokinetics are considerably different in these patients.

INDICATIONS AND USAGE

Hypertension (see boxed **WARNING**).

CONTRAINDICATIONS

Reserpine: Hypersensitivity to reserpine; mental depression (especially with suicidal tendencies); active peptic ulcer, ulcerative colitis; patients receiving electroconvulsive therapy.
Hydralazine: Hypersensitivity to hydralazine; coronary artery disease; mitral valvular rheumatic heart disease.
Hydrochlorothiazide: Anuria; hypersensitivity to this or other sulfonamide-derived drugs.

WARNINGS

Reserpine: Extreme caution should be exercised in treating patients with a history of mental depression. The drug should be discontinued at the first sign of despondency, early morning insomnia, loss of appetite, impotence, or self-deprecation. Drug-induced depression may persist for several months after drug withdrawal and may be severe enough to result in suicide.
Hydralazine: In a few patients hydralazine may produce a clinical picture simulating systemic lupus erythematosus including glomerulonephritis. In such patients hydralazine should be discontinued unless the benefit-to-risk determination requires continued antihypertensive therapy with this drug. Signs and symptoms usually regress when the drug is discontinued, but residua have been detected many years later. Long-term treatment with steroids may be necessary. (See **PRECAUTIONS, Laboratory Tests.**)
Hydrochlorothiazide: Thiazides should be used with caution in patients with severe renal disease. In patients with renal disease, thiazides may precipitate azotemia. Cumulative effects of the drug may develop in patients with impaired renal function.
Thiazides should be used with caution in patients with impaired hepatic function or progressive liver disease, since minor alterations of fluid and electrolyte imbalance may precipitate hepatic coma.
Thiazides may add to or potentiate the action of other antihypertensive drugs. Potentiation occurs with ganglionic or peripheral adrenergic blocking drugs.
Sensitivity reactions are more likely to occur in patients with a history of allergy or bronchial asthma.
The possibility of exacerbation or activation of systemic lupus erythematosus has been reported.

PRECAUTIONS

General

Reserpine: Since reserpine increases gastrointestinal motility and secretion, it should be used cautiously in patients with a history of peptic ulcer, ulcerative colitis, or gallstones (biliary colic may be precipitated).
Caution should be exercised when treating hypertensive patients with renal insufficiency, since they adjust poorly to lowered blood pressure levels.
Preoperative withdrawal of reserpine does not assure that circulatory instability will not occur. It is important that the anesthesiologist be aware of the patient's drug intake and consider this in the overall management, since hypotension has occurred in patients receiving rauwolfia preparations. Anticholinergic and adrenergic drugs (e.g., metaraminol, norepinephrine) have been employed to treat adverse vagocirculatory effects.
Hydralazine: Myocardial stimulation produced by hydralazine can cause anginal attacks and ECG changes indicative of myocardial ischemia. The drug has been implicated in the production of myocardial infarction. It must, therefore, be used with caution in patients with suspected coronary artery disease.
The "hyperdynamic" circulation caused by hydralazine may accentuate specific cardiovascular inadequacies. For example, hydralazine may increase pulmonary artery pressure in patients with mitral valvular disease. The drug may reduce the pressor responses to epinephrine. Postural hypotension may result from hydralazine but is less common than with ganglionic blocking agents. It should be used with caution in patients with cerebral vascular accidents.
In hypertensive patients with normal kidneys who are treated with hydralazine, there is evidence of increased renal blood flow and a maintenance of glomerular filtration rate. In some instances where control values were below normal, improved renal function has been noted after administration of hydralazine. However, as with any antihypertensive agent, hydralazine should be used with caution in patients with advanced renal damage.
Peripheral neuritis, evidenced by paresthesia, numbness, and tingling, has been observed. Published evidence suggests that hydralazine has an antipyridoxine effect and that pyridoxine should be added to the regimen if symptoms develop.
Hydrochlorothiazide: All patients receiving thiazide therapy should be observed for clinical signs of fluid or electrolyte imbalance, namely hyponatremia, hypochloremic alkalosis, and hypokalemia (see **Laboratory Tests** and **Drug/Drug Interactions**). Warning signs are dryness of mouth, thirst, weakness, lethargy, drowsiness, restlessness, muscle pains or cramps, muscular fatigue, hypotension, oliguria, tachycardia, and gastrointestinal disturbance, such as nausea or vomiting.
Hypokalemia may develop, especially in cases of brisk diuresis or severe cirrhosis.

Continued on next page

The full prescribing information for each CIBA product is contained herein and is that in effect as of September 1, 1989

CIBA—Cont.

Interference with adequate oral intake of electrolytes will also contribute to hypokalemia. Hypokalemia may be avoided or treated by use of potassium supplements or foods with a high potassium content.

Any chloride deficit is generally mild and usually does not require specific treatment, except under extraordinary circumstances (as in liver disease or renal disease). Dilutional hyponatremia may occur in edematous patients in hot weather; appropriate therapy is water restriction, rather than administration of salt, except in rare instances when the hyponatremia is life-threatening. In cases of actual salt depletion, appropriate replacement is the therapy of choice. Hyperuricemia may occur or frank gout may be precipitated in certain patients receiving thiazide therapy.

Latent diabetes may become manifest during thiazide administration (see **Drug/Drug Interactions**).

The antihypertensive effects of the drug may be enhanced in the postsympathectomy patient.

If progressive renal impairment becomes evident, withholding or discontinuing diuretic therapy should be considered. Calcium excretion is decreased by thiazides. Pathological changes in the parathyroid gland with hypercalcemia and hypophosphatemia have been observed in a few patients on prolonged thiazide therapy. The common complications of hyperparathyroidism, such as renal lithiasis, bone resorption, and peptic ulceration, have not been seen.

Information for Patients: Patients should be informed of possible side effects and advised to take the medication regularly and continuously as directed.

Laboratory Tests

Hydralazine: Complete blood counts and antinuclear antibody titer determinations are indicated before and periodically during prolonged therapy with hydralazine even though the patient is asymptomatic. These studies are also indicated if the patient develops arthralgia, fever, chest pain, continued malaise, or other unexplained signs or symptoms. A positive antinuclear antibody titer requires that the physician carefully weigh the implications of the test results against the benefits to be derived from antihypertensive therapy with a combination drug containing hydralazine. Blood dyscrasias, consisting of reduction in hemoglobin and red cell count, leukopenia, agranulocytosis, and purpura, had been reported. If such abnormalities develop, therapy should be discontinued.

Hydrochlorothiazide: Initial and periodic determinations of serum electrolytes to detect possible electrolyte imbalance should be performed at appropriate intervals.

Serum and urine electrolyte determinations are particularly important when the patient is vomiting excessively or receiving parenteral fluids.

Drug/Drug Interactions

Reserpine: MAO inhibitors should be avoided or used with extreme caution.

Reserpine should be used cautiously with digitalis and quinidine, since cardiac arrhythmias have occurred with rauwolfia preparations.

Hydralazine: MAO inhibitors should be used with caution in patients receiving hydralazine.

When other potent parenteral antihypertensive drugs, such as diazoxide, are used in combination with hydralazine, patients should be continuously observed for several hours for any excessive fall in blood pressure. Profound hypotensive episodes may occur when diazoxide injections and hydralazine are used concomitantly.

Hydrochlorothiazide: Hypokalemia can sensitize or exaggerate the response of the heart to the toxic effects of digitalis (e.g., increased ventricular irritability).

Hypokalemia may develop during concomitant use of steroids or ACTH.

Insulin requirements in diabetic patients may be increased, decreased, or unchanged.

Thiazides may decrease arterial responsiveness to norepinephrine, but not enough to preclude effectiveness of the pressor agent for therapeutic use.

Thiazides may increase the responsiveness to tubocurarine.

Lithium renal clearance is reduced by thiazides, increasing the risk of lithium toxicity.

There have been rare reports in the literature of hemolytic anemia occurring with the concomitant use of hydrochlorothiazide and methyldopa.

Concurrent administration of some nonsteroidal anti-inflammatory agents may reduce the diuretic, natriuretic and antihypertensive effects of thiazide diuretics.

Drug/Laboratory Test Interactions: Thiazides may decrease serum levels of protein-bound iodine without signs of thyroid disturbance. Ser-Ap-Es should be discontinued before tests for parathyroid function are made (see **General, Hydrochlorothiazide,** Calcium excretion).

Carcinogenesis, Mutagenesis, Impairment of Fertility

Reserpine. *Animal Tumorigenicity:* Rodent studies have shown that reserpine is an animal tumorigen, causing an increased incidence of mammary fibroadenomas in female

mice, malignant tumors of the seminal vesicles in male mice, and malignant adrenal medullary tumors in male rats. These findings arose in 2-year studies in which the drug was administered in the feed at concentrations of 5 and 10 ppm—about 100 to 300 times the usual human dose. The breast neoplasms are thought to be related to reserpine's prolactin-elevating effect. Several other prolactin-elevating drugs have also been associated with an increased incidence of mammary neoplasia in rodents.

The extent to which these findings indicate a risk to humans is uncertain. Tissue culture experiments show that about one third of human breast tumors are prolactin-dependent *in vitro,* a factor of considerable importance if the use of the drug is contemplated in a patient with previously detected breast cancer. The possibility of an increased risk of breast cancer in reserpine users has been studied extensively; however, no firm conclusion has emerged. Although a few epidemiologic studies have suggested a slightly increased risk (less than twofold in all studies except one) in women who have used reserpine, other studies of generally similar design have not confirmed this. Epidemiologic studies conducted using other drugs (neuroleptic agents) that, like reserpine, increase prolactin levels and therefore would be considered rodent mammary carcinogens have not shown an association between chronic administration of the drug and human mammary tumorigenesis. While long-term clinical observation has not suggested such an association, the available evidence is considered too limited to be conclusive at this time. An association of reserpine intake with pheochromocytoma or tumors of the seminal vesicles has not been explored.

Hydralazine: In a lifetime study in Swiss albino mice, there was a statistically significant increase in the incidence of lung tumors (adenomas and adenocarcinomas) of both male and female mice given hydralazine continuously in their drinking water at a dosage of about 250 mg/kg per day (about 80 times the maximum recommended human dose). In a 2-year carcinogenicity study of rats given hydralazine by gavage at dose levels of 15, 30, and 60 mg/kg/day (approximately 5 to 20 times the recommended human daily dosage), microscopic examination of the liver revealed a small, but statistically significant, increase in benign neoplastic nodules in male and female rats from the high-dose group and in female rats from the intermediate-dose group. Benign interstitial cell tumors of the testes were also significantly increased in male rats from the high-dose group. The tumors observed are common in aged rats and a significantly increased incidence was not observed until 18 months of treatment. Hydralazine was shown to be mutagenic in bacterial systems (Gene Mutation and DNA Repair) and in one of two rats and one rabbit hepatocyte *in vitro* DNA repair studies. Additional *in vivo* and *in vitro* studies using lymphoma cells germinal cells, and fibroblasts from mice, bone marrow cells from chinese hamsters and fibroblasts from human cell lines did not demonstrate any mutagenic potential for hydralazine.

The extent to which these findings indicate a risk to man is uncertain. While long-term clinical observation has not suggested that human cancer is associated with hydralazine use, epidemiologic studies have so far been insufficient to arrive at any conclusions.

Hydrochlorothiazide: Long-term carcinogenicity studies in animals have not been conducted with Esidrix. Hydrochlorothiazide was not mutagenic in in vitro Ames mutagenicity assay of Salmonella typhimurium strains TA 98, TA 100, TA 1535 and TA 1537 or in in vivo mutagenicity assays of mouse germinal cell chromosomes and chinese hamster bone marrow cell chromosomes. It was however, mutagenic in inducing nondisjunction (96% frequency) in diploid strains of Aspergillus nidulans.

Pregnancy Category C: Animal reproduction studies have not been conducted with Ser-Ap-Es. Reserpine administered parenterally has been shown to be teratogenic in rats at doses up to 2 mg/kg and to have an embryocidal effect in guinea pigs given dosages of 0.5 mg daily. Animal studies indicate that hydralazine is teratogenic in mice at 20–30 times the maximum daily human dose of 200–300 mg and possibly in rabbits at 10–15 times the maximum daily human dose, but that it is nonteratogenic in rats. Teratogenic effects observed were cleft palate and malformations of facial and cranial bones. A reproduction study in rats receiving hydrochlorothiazide, 250 mg/kg daily, 62.5 times the maximum daily human dose, has revealed no evidence of impaired fertility or harm to the fetus.

There are no adequate and well-controlled studies of Ser-Ap-Es in pregnant women. Ser-Ap-Es should be used during pregnancy only if the potential benefit justifies the potential risk to the fetus.

Nonteratogenic Effects: Reserpine crosses the placental barrier, and increased respiratory tract secretions, nasal congestion, cyanosis, and anorexia may occur in neonates of mothers treated with reserpine. Thiazides also cross the placental barrier and appear in cord blood, and there is a risk of fetal or neonatal jaundice, thrombocytopenia, and possibly other adverse reactions that have occurred in adults.

Nursing Mothers: Reserpine is excreted in maternal breast milk, and increased respiratory tract secretions, nasal con-

gestion, cyanosis, and anorexia may occur in breast-fed infants. Thiazides are also excreted in breast milk. Because of the potential for serious adverse reactions in nursing infants and the potential for tumorigenicity shown for reserpine in animal studies, a decision should be made whether to discontinue nursing or to discontinue Ser-Ap-Es, taking into account the importance of the drug to the mother.

Pediatric Use: Safety and effectiveness of the combination drug in children have not been established.

ADVERSE REACTIONS

Adverse reactions are usually reversible upon reduction of dosage or discontinuation of Ser-Ap-Es. Whenever adverse reactions are moderate or severe, it may be necessary to discontinue the drug.

The following adverse reactions have been observed, but there has not been enough systematic collection of data to support an estimate of their frequency. Consequently the reactions are categorized by organ system and are listed in decreasing order of severity and not frequency.

Reserpine: The following have been observed with rauwolfia preparations:

Digestive: Vomiting, diarrhea, nausea, anorexia, dryness of mouth, hypersecretion.

Cardiovascular: Arrhythmias (particularly when used concurrently with digitalis or quinidine), syncope, angina-like symptoms, bradycardia, edema.

Respiratory: Dyspnea, epistaxis, nasal congestion.

Neurologic: Rare parkinsonian syndrome and other extrapyramidal tract symptoms; dizziness; headache; paradoxical anxiety; depression; nervousness; nightmares; dull sensorium; drowsiness.

Musculoskeletal: Muscular aches.

Genitourinary: Pseudolactation, impotence, dysuria, gynecomastia, decreased libido, breast engorgement.

Metabolic: Weight gain.

Special Senses: Deafness, optic atrophy, glaucoma, uveitis, conjunctival injection.

Hypersensitive Reactions: Purpura, rash, pruritus.

Hydralazine: *Digestive:* Hepatitis, paralytic ileus, vomiting, diarrhea, nausea, constipation, anorexia.

Cardiovascular: Angina pectoris, hypotension, paradoxical pressor response, tachycardia, palpitations, edema, flushing.

Respiratory: Dyspnea, nasal congestion.

Neurologic: Psychotic reactions characterized by depression, disorientation, or anxiety; peripheral neuritis, evidenced by paresthesia, numbness, and tingling; tremors; dizziness; headache.

Musculoskeletal: Muscle cramps, arthralgia.

Genitourinary: Difficulty in urination.

Hematologic: Blood dyscrasias, consisting of reduction in hemoglobin and red cell count, leukopenia, agranulocytosis; lymphadenopathy; splenomegaly; eosinophilia.

Special Senses: Conjunctivitis, lacrimation.

Hypersensitive Reactions: Purpura, fever, urticaria, rash, pruritus, chills.

Hydrochlorothiazide: *Digestive:* Pancreatitis, jaundice (intrahepatic cholestatic), sialadenitis, vomiting, diarrhea, cramping, nausea, gastric irritation, constipation, anorexia.

Cardiovascular: Orthostatic hypotension (may be potentiated by alcohol, barbiturates, or narcotics).

Neurologic: Vertigo, dizziness, transient blurred vision, headache, paresthesia, xanthopsia, weakness, restlessness.

Musculoskeletal: Muscle spasm.

Hematologic: Aplastic anemia, agranulocytosis, leukopenia, thrombocytopenia.

Metabolic: Hyperglycemia, glycosuria, hyperuricemia.

Hypersensitive Reactions: Necrotizing angiitis, Stevens-Johnson syndrome, purpura, urticaria, rash, photosensitivity.

OVERDOSAGE

Acute Toxicity: No deaths due to acute poisoning with Ser-Ap-Es have been reported.

Oral LD_{50}'s in animals (mg/kg): rats, 397; mice, 272.

Signs and Symptoms

Reserpine. The clinical picture of acute poisoning is characterized chiefly by signs and symptoms due to the reflex parasympathomimetic effect of reserpine.

Impairment of consciousness may occur and may range from drowsiness to coma, depending upon the severity of overdosage. Flushing of the skin, conjunctival injection, and pupillary constriction are to be expected. Hypotension, hypothermia, central respiratory depression, and bradycardia may develop in cases of severe overdosage. Increased salivary and gastric secretion and diarrhea may also occur.

Hydralazine. Signs and symptoms of overdosage include hypotension, tachycardia, headache, and generalized skin flushing.

Complications can include myocardial ischemia and subsequent myocardial infarction, cardiac arrhythmia, and profound shock.

Hydrochlorothiazide. The most prominent feature of poisoning is acute loss of fluid and electrolytes.

Cardiovascular: Tachycardia, hypotension, shock.

Neuromuscular: Weakness, confusion, dizziness, cramps of the calf muscles, paresthesia, fatigue, impairment of consciousness.

Digestive: Nausea, vomiting, thirst.

Renal: Polyuria, oliguria, or anuria (due to hemoconcentration).

Laboratory Findings: Hypokalemia, hyponatremia, hypochloremia, alkalosis; increased BUN (especially in patients with renal insufficiency).

Combined Poisoning: Signs and symptoms may be aggravated or modified by concomitant intake of antihypertensive medication, barbiturates, digitalis (hypokalemia), corticosteroids, narcotics, or alcohol.

Treatment: There is no specific antidote.

The gastric contents should be evacuated, taking adequate precautions against aspiration and for protection of the airway. An activated charcoal slurry may be instilled if conditions permit. Dialysis may not be effective for elimination of Ser-Ap-Es because of its plasma protein binding (see **CLINICAL PHARMACOLOGY**).

These manipulations may have to be omitted or carried out after cardiovascular status has been stabilized, since they might precipitate cardiac arrhythmias or increase the depth of shock.

If hypotension or shock occurs, the patient's legs should be kept raised and lost fluid and electrolytes (potassium, sodium) should be replaced.

Support of the cardiovascular system is of primary importance in suspected hydralazine overdosage. If possible, vasopressors should not be given, but if a vasopressor is required, care should be taken not to precipitate or aggravate cardiac arrhythmia. Tachycardia responds to beta blockers. Digitalization may be necessary.

If hypotension is severe enough to require treatment with a vasopressor, one having a direct action upon vascular smooth muscle (e.g., phenylephrine, levarterenol, metaraminol) should be used to treat the symptomatic effects of reserpine overdosage.

Fluid and electrolyte balance (especially serum potassium) and renal function should be monitored until conditions become normal. Since reserpine is long-acting, the patient should be observed carefully for at least 72 hours.

DOSAGE AND ADMINISTRATION

Dosage should be determined by individual titration (see boxed **WARNING**). The usual dosage is one to two tablets three times daily.

Since the antihypertensive effects of reserpine are not immediately apparent, maximal reduction in blood pressure from a given dosage may not occur for 2 weeks. For maintenance, dosage should be adjusted to the lowest requirement of the individual patient.

When necessary, more potent antihypertensives may be added gradually in dosages reduced by at least 50%; the effects should be carefully observed.

HOW SUPPLIED

Tablets —round, light-salmon pink, dry-coated (imprinted CIBA 71) 0.1 mg of reserpine, 25 mg of hydralazine hydrochloride, 15 mg of hydrochlorothiazide

   Bottles of 100—NDC 0083-0071-30

   Bottles of 1000—NDC 0083-0071-40

Consumer Pack—One Unit

   12 bottles—100 tablets each—NDC 0083-0071-65

Accu-Pak® Unit Dose (blister pack)

   Box of 100 (strips of 10)—NDC 0083-0071-32

Do not store above 86°F (30°C).

Dispense in tight, light-resistant container (USP).

C87-14 (Rev. 11/87)

Shown in Product Identification Section, page 409

SERPASIL®   ℞

[sir'pah-sill]

reserpine USP

Tablets

DESCRIPTION

Serpasil, reserpine USP, is an antihypertensive, available as 0.1-mg and 0.25-mg tablets for oral administration. Its chemical name is methyl 18β-hydroxy-11,17α-dimethoxy-3β,20α-yohimban-16β-carboxylate 3,4,5-trimethoxybenzoate (ester). Reserpine USP, a pure crystalline alkaloid of rauwolfia, is a white or pale buff to slightly yellowish, odorless crystalline powder. It darkens slowly on exposure to light, but more rapidly when in solution. It is insoluble in water, freely soluble in acetic acid and in chloroform, slightly soluble in benzene, and very slightly soluble in alcohol and in ether. Its molecular weight is 608.69.

Inactive Ingredients. Lactose, magnesium stearate, polyethylene glycol, starch, sucrose, talc, and tragacanth (0.1-mg tablets).

CLINICAL PHARMACOLOGY

Serpasil depletes stores of catecholamines and 5-hydroxytryptamine in many organs, including the brain and adrenal medulla. Most of its pharmacological effects have been attributed to this action. Depletion is slower and less complete in the adrenal medulla than in other tissues.

The depression of sympathetic nerve function results in a decreased heart rate and a lowering of arterial blood pressure. The sedative and tranquilizing properties of Serpasil are thought to be related to depletion of catecholamines and 5-hydroxytryptamine from the brain.

Serpasil, like other rauwolfia compounds, is characterized by slow onset of action and sustained effects. Both cardiovascular and central nervous system effects may persist for a period of time following withdrawal of the drug.

Mean maximum plasma levels of 1.54 ng/ml were attained after a median of 3.5 hours in six normal subjects receiving a single oral dose of four 0.25-mg Serpasil tablets. Bioavailability was approximately 50% of that of a corresponding intravenous dose. Plasma levels of reserpine after intravenous administration declined with a mean half-life of 33 hours. Reserpine is extensively bound (96%) to plasma proteins. No definitive studies on the human metabolism of reserpine have been made.

INDICATIONS AND USAGE

Mild essential hypertension; also useful as adjunctive therapy with other antihypertensive agents in the more severe forms of hypertension; relief of symptoms in agitated psychotic states (e.g., schizophrenia), primarily in those individuals unable to tolerate phenothiazine derivatives or in those who also require antihypertensive medication.

CONTRAINDICATIONS

Known hypersensitivity, mental depression (especially with suicidal tendencies), active peptic ulcer, ulcerative colitis, and patients receiving electroconvulsive therapy.

WARNINGS

Extreme caution should be exercised in treating patients with a history of mental depression. Discontinue the drug at first sign of despondency, early morning insomnia, loss of appetite, impotence, or self-deprecation. Drug-induced depression may persist for several months after drug withdrawal and may be severe enough to result in suicide.

PRECAUTIONS

General

Since Serpasil increases gastrointestinal motility and secretion, it should be used cautiously in patients with a history of peptic ulcer, ulcerative colitis, or gallstones (biliary colic may be precipitated).

Caution should be exercised when treating hypertensive patients with renal insufficiency, since they adjust poorly to lowered blood pressure levels.

Preoperative withdrawal of reserpine does not assure that circulatory instability will not occur. It is important that the anesthesiologist be aware of the patient's drug intake and consider this in the overall management, since hypotension has occurred in patients receiving rauwolfia preparations. Anticholinergic and/or adrenergic drugs (e.g., metaraminol, norepinephrine) have been employed to treat adverse vagocirculatory effects.

Information for Patients

Patients should be informed of possible side effects and advised to take the medication regularly and continuously as directed.

Drug Interactions

MAO inhibitors should be avoided or used with extreme caution.

Serpasil should be used cautiously with digitalis and quinidine, since cardiac arrhythmias have occurred with rauwolfia preparations.

Concomitant use of Serpasil with other antihypertensive agents necessitates careful titration of dosage with each agent.

Carcinogenesis, Mutagenesis, Impairment of Fertility

Animal Tumorigenicity. Rodent studies have shown that reserpine is an animal tumorigen, causing an increased incidence of mammary fibroadenomas in female mice, malignant tumors of the seminal vesicles in male mice, and malignant adrenal medullary tumors in male rats. These findings arose in 2-year studies in which the drug was administered in the feed at concentrations of 5 and 10 ppm—about 100 to 300 times the usual human dose. The breast neoplasms are thought to be related to reserpine's prolactin-elevating effect. Several other prolactin-elevating drugs have also been associated with an increased incidence of mammary neoplasia in rodents.

The extent to which these findings indicate a risk to humans is uncertain. Tissue culture experiments show that about one third of human breast tumors are prolactin-dependent *in vitro,* a factor of considerable importance if the use of the drug is contemplated in a patient with previously detected breast cancer. The possibility of an increased risk of breast cancer in reserpine users has been studied extensively; however, no firm conclusion has emerged. Although a few epidemiologic studies have suggested a slightly increased risk (less than twofold in all studies except one) in women who have used reserpine, other studies of generally similar design have not confirmed this. Epidemiologic studies conducted using other drugs (neuroleptic agents) that, like reserpine, increase prolactin levels and therefore would be considered rodent mammary carcinogens have not shown an association between chronic administration of the drug and human mammary tumorigenesis. While long-term clinical observation has not suggested such an association, the available evidence is considered too limited to be conclusive at this time. An association of reserpine intake with pheochromocytoma or tumors of the seminal vesicles has not been explored.

Pregnancy Category C

Reserpine administered parenterally has been shown to be teratogenic in rats at doses up to 2 mg/kg and to have an embryocidal effect in guinea pigs given dosages of 0.5 mg daily.

There are no adequate and well-controlled studies of Serpasil in pregnant women. Serpasil should be used during pregnancy only if the potential benefit justifies the potential risk to the fetus.

Nonteratogenic Effects. Reserpine crosses the placental barrier, and increased respiratory tract secretions, nasal congestion, cyanosis, and anorexia may occur in neonates of reserpine-treated mothers.

Nursing Mothers

Reserpine is excreted in maternal breast milk, and increased respiratory tract secretions, nasal congestion, cyanosis, and anorexia may occur in breast-fed infants. Because of the potential for adverse reactions in nursing infants and the potential for tumorigenicity shown for reserpine in animal studies, a decision should be made whether to discontinue nursing or to discontinue the drug, taking into account the importance of the drug to the mother.

Pediatric Use

Safety and effectiveness in children have not been established by means of controlled clinical trials, although there is experience with the use of Serpasil in children. (See **DOSAGE AND ADMINISTRATION.**) Because of adverse effects such as emotional depression and lability, sedation, and stuffy nose, Serpasil is not usually recommended as a step-2 drug in the treatment of hypertension in children.

ADVERSE REACTIONS

The following adverse reactions have been observed with rauwolfia preparations, but there has not been enough systematic collection of data to support an estimate of their frequency. Consequently the reactions are categorized by organ system and are listed in decreasing order of severity and not frequency.

Digestive: Vomiting, diarrhea, nausea, anorexia, dryness of mouth, hypersecretion.

Cardiovascular: Arrhythmias (particularly when used concurrently with digitalis or quinidine), syncope, angina-like symptoms, bradycardia, edema.

Respiratory: Dyspnea, epistaxis, nasal congestion.

Neurologic: Rare parkinsonian syndrome and other extrapyramidal tract symptoms; dizziness; headache; paradoxical anxiety; depression; nervousness; nightmares; dull sensorium; drowsiness.

Musculoskeletal: Muscular aches.

Genitourinary: Pseudolactation, impotence, dysuria, gynecomastia, decreased libido, breast engorgement.

Metabolic: Weight gain.

Special Senses: Deafness, optic atrophy, glaucoma, uveitis, conjunctival injection.

Hypersensitive Reactions: Purpura, rash, pruritus.

OVERDOSAGE

Acute Toxicity

No deaths due to acute poisoning with reserpine have been reported.

Highest known doses survived: children, 1000 mg (age and sex not specified); young children, 200 mg (20-month-old boy).

Oral LD$_{50}$'s in animals (mg/kg): rat, 2993; mouse, 47 and 500.

Signs and Symptoms

The clinical picture of acute poisoning is characterized chiefly by signs and symptoms due to the reflex parasympathomimetic effect of reserpine.

Impairment of consciousness may occur and may range from drowsiness to coma, depending upon the severity of overdosage. Flushing of the skin, conjunctival injection, and pupillary constriction are to be expected. Hypotension, hypothermia, central respiratory depression, and bradycardia may develop in cases of severe overdosage. Increased salivary and gastric secretion and diarrhea may also occur.

Continued on next page

CIBA—Cont.

Treatment

There is no specific antidote.

Stomach contents should be evacuated, taking adequate precautions against aspiration and for protection of the airway. Activated charcoal slurry should be instilled.

The effects of reserpine overdosage should be treated symptomatically. If hypotension is severe enough to require treatment with a vasopressor, one having a direct action upon vascular smooth muscle (e.g., phenylephrine, levarterenol, metaraminol) should be used. Since reserpine is long-acting, the patient should be observed carefully for at least 72 hours, and treatment administered as required.

DOSAGE AND ADMINISTRATION

Hypertension

In the average patient not receiving other antihypertensive agents, the usual initial dosage is 0.5 mg daily for 1 or 2 weeks. For maintenance, reduce to 0.1–0.25 mg daily. Higher dosages should be used cautiously, because occurrence of serious mental depression and other side effects may increase considerably.

Psychiatric Disorders

The usual initial dosage is 0.5 mg daily, but may range from 0.1 mg to 1.0 mg. Adjust dosage upward or downward according to the patient's response.

Children

Serpasil is not recommended for use in children (see **PRECAUTIONS, Pediatric Use**). If it is to be used in treating a child, the usual recommended starting dose is 20 μg/kg daily. The maximum recommended dose is 0.25 mg (total) daily.

HOW SUPPLIED

Tablets 0.1 mg—round, white (imprinted CIBA 35)

Bottles of 100 ....NDC 0083-0035-30

Tablets 0.25 mg—round, white, scored (imprinted CIBA 36)

Bottles of 100 ....NDC 0083-0036-30

Bottles of 1000 ....NDC 0083-0036-40

Consumer Pack—One Unit

12 bottles—100 tablets each ....NDC 0083-0036-65

Protect from light.

Dispense in tight, light-resistant container (USP).

C87-48 (Rev. 11/87)

Shown in Product Identification Section, page 409

SERPASIL®–APRESOLINE®　　℞

[sir′pah-sill a-press′oh-leen]

reserpine and hydralazine hydrochloride

Combination Tablets

WARNING

This fixed-combination drug is not indicated for initial therapy of hypertension. Hypertension requires therapy titrated to the individual patient. If the fixed combination represents the dosage so determined, its use may be more convenient in patient management. The treatment of hypertension is not static but must be reevaluated as conditions in each patient warrant.

DESCRIPTION

Serpasil-Apresoline is an antihypertensive combination, available as tablets for oral administration. Tablets #1 contain reserpine USP, 0.1 mg, and hydralazine hydrochloride USP, 25 mg; tablets #2 contain reserpine USP, 0.2 mg, and hydralazine hydrochloride USP, 50 mg.

Reserpine is methyl 18β-hydroxy-$11,17\alpha$-dimethoxy-3β, 20α-yohimban-16β-carboxylate,3,4,5-trimethoxybenzoate (ester).

Reserpine USP, a pure crystalline alkaloid of rauwolfia, is a white or pale buff to slightly yellowish, odorless crystalline powder. It darkens slowly on exposure to light, but more rapidly when in solution. It is insoluble in water, freely soluble in acetic acid and in chloroform, slightly soluble in benzene, and very slightly soluble in alcohol and in ether. Its molecular weight is 608.69.

Hydralazine hydrochloride is 1-hydrazinophthalazine monohydrochloride.

Hydralazine hydrochloride USP is a white to off-white, odorless crystalline powder. It is soluble in water, slightly soluble in alcohol, and very slightly soluble in ether. It melts at about 275°C, with decomposition, and has a molecular weight of 196.64.

Inactive Ingredients: FD&C Yellow No. 5, lactose, magnesium stearate, polyethylene glycol, starch, sucrose, talc and tragacanth.

CLINICAL PHARMACOLOGY

Reserpine

Reserpine depletes stores of catecholamines and 5-hydroxytryptamine in many organs, including the brain and adrenal medulla. Most of its pharmacological effects have been attributed to this action. Depletion is slower and less complete in the adrenal medulla than in other tissues.

The depression of sympathetic nerve function results in a decreased heart rate and a lowering of arterial blood pressure. The sedative and tranquilizing properties of reserpine are thought to be related to depletion of catecholamines and 5-hydroxytryptamine from the brain.

Reserpine, like other rauwolfia compounds, is characterized by slow onset of action and sustained effects. Both cardiovascular and central nervous system effects may persist for a period of time following withdrawal of the drug.

Mean maximum plasma levels of 1.54 ng/ml were attained after a median of 3.5 hours in six normal subjects receiving a single oral dose of four 0.25-mg Serpasil tablets. Bioavailability was approximately 50% of that of a corresponding intravenous dose. Plasma levels of reserpine after intravenous administration declined with a mean half-life of 33 hours. Reserpine is extensively bound (96%) to plasma proteins. No definitive studies on the human metabolism of reserpine have been made.

Hydralazine

Although the precise mechanism of action of hydralazine is not fully understood, the major effects are on the cardiovascular system. Hydralazine apparently lowers blood pressure by exerting a peripheral vasodilating effect through a direct relaxation of vascular smooth muscle. Hydralazine, by altering cellular calcium metabolism, interferes with the calcium movements within the vascular smooth muscle that are responsible for initiating or maintaining the contractile state. The peripheral vasodilating effect of hydralazine results in decreased arterial blood pressure (diastolic more than systolic); decreased peripheral vascular resistance; and an increased heart rate, stroke volume, and cardiac output. The preferential dilatation of arterioles, as compared to veins, minimizes postural hypotension and promotes the increase in cardiac output. Hydralazine usually increases renin activity in plasma, presumably as a result of increased secretion of renin by the renal juxtaglomerular cells in response to reflex sympathetic discharge. This increase in renin activity leads to the production of angiotensin II, which then causes stimulation of aldosterone and consequent sodium reabsorption. Hydralazine also maintains or increases renal and cerebral blood flow.

Hydralazine is rapidly absorbed after oral administration, and peak plasma levels are reached at 1–2 hours. Plasma levels decline with a half-life of 3–7 hours. Binding to human plasma protein is 87%. Plasma levels of hydralazine vary widely among individuals. Hydralazine is subject to polymorphic acetylation; slow acetylators generally have higher plasma levels of hydralazine and require lower doses to maintain control of blood pressure. Hydralazine undergoes extensive hepatic metabolism; it is excreted mainly in the form of metabolites in the urine.

Administration of hydralazine with food results in higher levels of the drug in plasma.

INDICATIONS AND USAGE

Hypertension (see boxed **WARNING**).

CONTRAINDICATIONS

Reserpine

Hypersensitivity to reserpine; mental depression or history of mental depression (especially with suicidal tendencies); active peptic ulcer, ulcerative colitis; patients receiving electroconvulsive therapy.

Hydralazine

Hypersensitivity to hydralazine; coronary artery disease; mitral valvular rheumatic heart disease.

WARNINGS

Reserpine

Reserpine may cause mental depression. Recognition of depression may be difficult because this condition may often be disguised by somatic complaints. The drug should be discontinued at first signs of depression such as despondency, early morning insomnia, loss of appetite, impotence, or self-deprecation. Drug-induced depression may persist for several months after drug withdrawal and may be severe enough to result in suicide.

Hydralazine

In a few patients hydralazine may produce a clinical picture simulating systemic lupus erythematosus including glomerulonephritis. In such patients hydralazine should be discontinued unless the benefit-to-risk determination requires continued antihypertensive therapy with this drug. Signs and symptoms usually regress when the drug is discontinued, but residua have been detected many years later. Long-term treatment with steroids may be necessary. (See **PRECAUTIONS, Laboratory Tests.**)

PRECAUTIONS

General

The Serpasil-Apresoline tablets (#1 and #2) contain FD&C Yellow No. 5 (tartrazine) which may cause allergic-type reactions (including bronchial asthma) in certain susceptible individuals. Although the overall incidence of FD&C Yellow No. 5 (tartrazine) sensitivity in the general population is low, it is frequently seen in patients who also have aspirin hypersensitivity.

Reserpine. Since reserpine increases gastrointestinal motility and secretion, it should be used cautiously in patients with a history of peptic ulcer, ulcerative colitis, or gallstones (biliary colic may be precipitated).

Caution should be exercised when treating hypertensive patients with renal insufficiency, since they adjust poorly to lowered blood pressure levels.

Preoperative withdrawal of reserpine does not assure that circulatory instability will not occur. It is important that the anesthesiologist be aware of the patient's drug intake and consider this in the overall management, since hypotension has occurred in patients receiving rauwolfia preparations. Anticholinergic and adrenergic drugs (e.g., metaraminol, norepinephrine) have been employed to treat adverse vagocirculatory effects.

Hydralazine. Myocardial stimulation produced by hydralazine can cause anginal attacks and ECG changes indicative of myocardial ischemia. The drug has been implicated in the production of myocardial infarction. It must, therefore, be used with caution in patients with suspected coronary artery disease.

The "hyperdynamic" circulation caused by hydralazine may accentuate specific cardiovascular inadequacies. For example, hydralazine may increase pulmonary artery pressure in patients with mitral valvular disease. The drug may reduce the pressor response to epinephrine. Postural hypotension may result from hydralazine but is less common than with ganglionic blocking agents. It should be used with caution in patients with cerebral vascular accidents.

In hypertensive patients with normal kidneys who are treated with hydralazine, there is evidence of increased renal blood flow and a maintenance of glomerular filtration rate. In some instances where control values were below normal, improved renal function has been noted after administration of hydralazine. However, as with any antihypertensive agent, hydralazine should be used with caution in patients with advanced renal damage.

Peripheral neuritis, evidenced by paresthesia, numbness, and tingling, has been observed. Published evidence suggests that hydralazine has an antipyridoxine effect and that pyridoxine should be added to the regimen if symptoms develop.

Information for Patients

Patients should be informed of possible side effects and advised to take the medication regularly and continuously as directed.

Laboratory Tests

Hydralazine. Complete blood counts and antinuclear antibody titer determinations are indicated before and periodically during prolonged therapy with hydralazine even though the patient is asymptomatic. These studies are also indicated if the patient develops arthralgia, fever, chest pain, continued malaise, or other unexplained signs or symptoms. A positive antinuclear antibody titer requires that the physician carefully weigh the implications of the test results against the benefits to be derived from antihypertensive therapy with a combination drug containing hydralazine. Blood dyscrasias, consisting of reduction in hemoglobin and red cell count, leukopenia, agranulocytosis, and purpura, have been reported. If such abnormalities develop, therapy should be discontinued.

Drug Interactions

MAO inhibitors should be avoided or used with extreme caution.

Reserpine should be used cautiously with digitalis and quinidine, since cardiac arrhythmias have occurred with rauwolfia preparations.

When other potent parenteral antihypertensive drugs, such as diazoxide, are used in combination with hydralazine, patients should be continuously observed for several hours for any excessive fall in blood pressure. Profound hypotensive episodes may occur when diazoxide injection and hydralazine are used concomitantly.

Carcinogenesis, Mutagenesis, Impairment of Fertility

Reserpine. Animal Tumorigenicity: Rodent studies have shown that reserpine is an animal tumorigen, causing an increased incidence of mammary fibroadenomas in female mice, malignant tumors of the seminal vesicles in male mice, and malignant adrenal medullary tumors in male rats. These findings arose in 2-year studies in which the drug was administered in the feed at concentrations of 5 and 10 ppm—about 100 to 300 times the usual human dose. The breast neoplasms are thought to be related to reserpine's prolactin-elevating effect. Several other prolactin-elevating drugs have also been associated with an increased incidence of mammary neoplasia in rodents.

The extent to which these findings indicate a risk to humans is uncertain. Tissue culture experiments show that about one third of human breast tumors are prolactin-dependent *in vitro*, a factor of considerable importance if the use of the drug is contemplated in a patient with previously detected breast cancer. The possibility of an increased risk of breast cancer in reserpine users has been studied extensively; however, no firm conclusion has emerged. Although a few epidemiologic studies have suggested a slightly increased risk (less than twofold in all studies except one) in women who have used reserpine, other studies of generally similar design have not confirmed this. Epidemiologic studies conducted using other drugs (neuroleptic agents) that, like reserpine, increase prolactin levels and therefore would be considered rodent mammary carcinogens, have not shown an association between chronic administration of the drug and human mammary tumorigenesis. While long-term clinical observation has not suggested such an association, the available evidence is considered too limited to be conclusive at this time. An association of reserpine intake with pheochromocytoma or tumors of the seminal vesicles has not been explored.

Hydralazine. In a lifetime study in Swiss albino mice, there was a statistically significant increase in the incidence of lung tumors (adenomas and adenocarcinomas) of both male and female mice given hydralazine continuously in their drinking water at a dosage of about 250 mg/kg per day (about 80 times the maximum recommended human dose). In a 2-year carcinogenicity study of rats given hydralazine by gavage at dose levels of 15, 30, and 60 mg/kg/day (approximately 5 to 20 times the recommended human daily dosage), microscopic examination of the liver revealed a small, but statistically significant, increase in benign neoplastic nodules in male and female rats from the high-dose group and in female rats from the intermediate-dose group. Benign interstitial cell tumors of the testes were also significantly increased in male rats from the high-dose group. The tumors observed are common in aged rats and a significantly increased incidence was not observed until 18 months of treatment. Hydralazine was shown to be mutagenic in bacterial systems (Gene Mutation and DNA Repair) and in one of two rats and one rabbit hepatocyte *In vitro* DNA repair studies. Additional *in vivo* and *in vitro* studies using lymphoma cells, germinal cells, and fibroblasts from mice, bone marrow cells from chinese hamsters and fibroblasts from human cell lines did not demonstrate any mutagenic potential for hydralazine.

The extent to which these findings indicate a risk to man is uncertain. While long-term clinical observation has not suggested that human cancer is associated with hydralazine use, epidemiologic studies have so far been insufficient to arrive at any conclusions.

Pregnancy Category C
Animal reproduction studies have not been conducted with Serpasil-Apresoline. Reserpine administered parenterally has been shown to be teratogenic in rats at doses up to 2 mg/kg and to have an embryocidal effect in guinea pigs given dosages of 0.5 mg daily. Animal studies indicate that hydralazine is teratogenic in mice at 20–30 times the maximum daily human dose of 200–300 mg and possibly in rabbits at 10–15 times the maximum daily human dose, but that it is nonteratogenic in rats. Teratogenic effects observed were cleft palate and malformations of facial and cranial bones. There are no adequate and well-controlled studies of Serpasil-Apresoline in pregnant women. Serpasil-Apresoline should be used during pregnancy only if the potential benefit justifies the potential risk to the fetus.
Nonteratogenic Effects. Reserpine crosses the placental barrier, and increased respiratory tract secretions, nasal congestion, cyanosis, and anorexia may occur in neonates of mothers treated with reserpine.

Nursing Mothers
Reserpine is excreted in maternal breast milk, and increased respiratory tract secretions, nasal congestion, cyanosis, and anorexia may occur in breast-fed infants. Because of the potential for serious adverse reactions in nursing infants and the potential for tumorigenicity shown for reserpine in animal studies, a decision should be made whether to discontinue nursing or to discontinue Serpasil-Apresoline, taking into account the importance of the drug to the mother.

Pediatric Use
Safety and effectiveness of the combination drug in children have not been established.

ADVERSE REACTIONS
Adverse reactions are usually reversible upon reduction of dosage or discontinuation of Serpasil-Apresoline. Whenever adverse reactions are moderate or severe, it may be necessary to discontinue the drug.
The following adverse reactions have been observed, but there has not been enough systematic collection of data to support an estimate of their frequency. Consequently the reactions are categorized by organ system and are listed in decreasing order of severity and not frequency.
Reserpine
The following have been observed with rauwolfia preparations:
Digestive: Vomiting, diarrhea, nausea, anorexia, dryness of mouth, hypersecretion.
Cardiovascular: Arrhythmias (particularly when used concurrently with digitalis or quinidine), syncope, angina-like symptoms, bradycardia, edema.
Respiratory: Dyspnea, epistaxis, nasal congestion.
Neurologic: Rare parkinsonian syndrome and other extrapyramidal tract symptoms; dizziness; headache; paradoxical

anxiety; depression; nervousness; nightmares; dull sensorium; drowsiness.
Musculoskeletal: Muscular aches.
Genitourinary: Pseudolactation, impotence, dysuria, gynecomastia, decreased libido, breast engorgement.
Metabolic: Weight gain.
Special Senses: Deafness, optic atrophy, glaucoma, uveitis, conjunctival injection.
Hypersensitive Reactions: Purpura, rash, pruritus.
Hydralazine
Digestive: Hepatitis, paralytic ileus, vomiting, diarrhea, nausea, constipation, anorexia.
Cardiovascular: Angina pectoris, hypotension, paradoxical pressor response, tachycardia, palpitations, edema, flushing.
Respiratory: Dyspnea, nasal congestion.
Neurologic: Psychotic reactions characterized by depression, disorientation, or anxiety; peripheral neuritis, evidenced by paresthesia, numbness, and tingling; tremors; dizziness; headache.
Musculoskeletal: Muscle cramps, arthralgia.
Genitourinary: Difficulty in urination.
Hematologic: Blood dyscrasias, consisting of reduction in hemoglobin and red cell count, leukopenia, agranulocytosis, lymphadenopathy; splenomegaly; eosinophilia.
Special Senses: Conjunctivitis, lacrimation.
Hypersensitive Reactions: Purpura, fever, urticaria, rash, pruritus, chills.

OVERDOSAGE
Acute Toxicity
No deaths due to acute poisoning with Serpasil-Apresoline have been reported.
Oral LD_{50}'s in animals (mg/kg): rats, 261; mice, 218.
Signs and Symptoms
Reserpine. The clinical picture of acute poisoning is characterized chiefly by signs and symptoms due to the reflex parasympathomimetic effect of reserpine.
Impairment of consciousness may occur and may range from drowsiness to coma, depending upon the severity of overdosage. Flushing of the skin, conjunctival injection, and pupillary constriction are to be expected. Hypotension, hypothermia, central respiratory depression, and bradycardia may develop in cases of severe overdosage. Increased salivary and gastric secretion and diarrhea may also occur.
Hydralazine. Signs and symptoms of overdosage include hypotension, tachycardia, headache, and generalized skin flushing.
Complications can include myocardial ischemia and subsequent myocardial infarction, cardiac arrhythmia, and profound shock.
Treatment
There is no specific antidote.
The gastric contents should be evacuated, taking adequate precautions against aspiration and for protection of the airway. An activated charcoal slurry may be instilled if conditions permit. Dialysis may not be effective for elimination of Serpasil-Apresoline because of its plasma protein binding (see **CLINICAL PHARMACOLOGY**).
These manipulations may have to be omitted or carried out after cardiovascular status has been stabilized, since they might precipitate cardiac arrhythmias or increase the depth of shock.
Support of the cardiovascular system is of primary importance in suspected hydralazine overdosage. Shock should be treated with plasma expanders. If possible, vasopressors should not be given, but if a vasopressor is required, care should be taken not to precipitate or aggravate cardiac arrhythmia. A vasopressor having direct action upon vascular smooth muscle (e.g., phenylephrine, levarterenol, metaraminol) should be used to treat the symptomatic effects of reserpine overdosage. Tachycardia responds to beta blockers. Digitalization may be necessary, and renal function should be monitored and supported as required. Since reserpine is long-acting, the patient should be observed carefully for at least 72 hours.

DOSAGE AND ADMINISTRATION
Dosage should be determined by individual titration (see boxed **WARNING**).
Step 1. Therapy should be started with reserpine alone, at an average dosage of 0.5 mg daily and continued for at least 1 week. If results prove satisfactory—as they will in many cases—no other medication is required. For maintenance, the dosage should be reduced to 0.25 mg, or less, daily.
Step 2. Should more than the therapeutic action of reserpine be indicated, therapy with one Serpasil-Apresoline tablet #2 (reserpine, 0.2 mg/hydralazine hydrochloride, 50 mg) four times daily should be initiated.
When reduction of dosage is indicated, one Serpasil-Apresoline tablet #1 (reserpine, 0.1 mg/hydralazine hydrochloride, 25 mg) four times daily should be used.
Side effects associated with hydralazine (headache, tachycardia, palpitations) are seldom encountered when the patient has been "primed" with reserpine before combination therapy is begun. Should side effects appear, however, reduction

of dosage to one tablet #1 two to four times daily for a few days will usually alleviate them.
In cases where further individualization of dosage is necessary, the adjustment may be made by increasing or decreasing the dosage of reserpine and/or hydralazine.
For maintenance, daily dosage of hydralazine should probably not exceed 200 mg, nor should the dosage of reserpine exceed 1 mg.
Patients on Hydralazine
Patients already on this drug may be given a combination tablet as required. With the addition of reserpine, it is usually possible to reduce the dose of hydralazine.

HOW SUPPLIED
Tablets #1—round, yellow, dry-coated (imprinted CIBA 40) 0.1 mg reserpine, 25 mg hydralazine hydrochloride
Bottles of 100 .... NDC 0083-0040-30
Do not store above 86°F (30°C)
Tablets #2—round, yellow, dry-coated (imprinted CIBA 104) 0.2 mg reserpine, 50 mg hydralazine hydrochloride
Bottles of 100 .... NDC 0083-0104-30
Do not store above 86°F (30°C)
Dispense in tight, light-resistant container (USP).
C86-53 (Rev. 9/86)
Shown in Product Identification Section, page 409

SERPASIL®–ESIDRIX®   ℞
[*sir'pah-sill ess'ah-dricks*]
reserpine and hydrochlorothiazide
Combination Tablets

WARNING
This fixed-combination drug is not indicated for initial therapy of hypertension. Hypertension requires therapy titrated to the individual patient. If the fixed combination represents the dosage so determined, its use may be more convenient in patient management. The treatment of hypertension is not static but must be reevaluated as conditions in each patient warrant.

DESCRIPTION
Serpasil-Esidrix is an antihypertensive-diuretic combination, available as tablets for oral administration. Tablets #1 contain reserpine USP, 0.1 mg, and hydrochlorothiazide USP, 25 mg; tablets #2 contain reserpine USP, 0.1 mg, and hydrochlorothiazide USP, 50 mg.
Reserpine is methyl 18β-hydroxy-11,17α-dimethoxy-3β, 20α-yohimban-16β-carboxylate 3,4,5-trimethoxybenzoate (ester).
Reserpine USP, a pure crystalline alkaloid of rauwolfia, is a white or pale buff to slightly yellowish, odorless crystalline powder. It darkens slowly on exposure to light, but more rapidly when in solution. It is insoluble in water, freely soluble in acetic acid and in chloroform, slightly soluble in benzene, and very slightly soluble in alcohol and in ether. Its molecular weight is 608.69.
Hydrochlorothiazide is 6-chloro-3,4-dihydro-2*H*-1,2,4-benzothiadiazine-7-sulfonamide 1,1-dioxide.
Hydrochlorothiazide USP is a white, or practically white, practically odorless crystalline powder. It is slightly soluble in water; freely soluble in sodium hydroxide solution, in *n*-butylamine, and in dimethylformamide; sparingly soluble in methanol; and insoluble in ether, in chloroform, and in dilute mineral acids. Its molecular weight is 297.73.
Inactive Ingredients: FD&C Yellow No. 5, FD&C Yellow No. 6, lactose, magnesium stearate, starch and sucrose.

CLINICAL PHARMACOLOGY
Reserpine: Reserpine depletes stores of catecholamines and 5-hydroxytryptamine in many organs, including the brain and adrenal medulla. Most of its pharmacological effects have been attributed to this action. Depletion is slower and less complete in the adrenal medulla than in other tissues. The depression of sympathetic nerve function results in a decreased heart rate and a lowering of arterial blood pressure. The sedative and tranquilizing properties of reserpine are thought to be related to depletion of catecholamines and 5-hydroxytryptamine from the brain.
Reserpine, like other rauwolfia compounds, is characterized by slow onset of action and sustained effects. Both cardiovascular and central nervous system effects may persist for a period of time following withdrawal of the drug.
Mean maximum plasma levels of 1.54 ng/ml were attained after a median of 3.5 hours in six normal subjects receiving a single oral dose of four 0.25-mg Serpasil tablets. Bioavailability was approximately 50% of that of a corresponding intra-

Continued on next page

CIBA—Cont.

venous dose. Plasma levels of reserpine after intravenous administration declined with a mean half-life of 33 hours. Reserpine is extensively bound (96%) to plasma proteins. No definitive studies on the human metabolism of reserpine have been made.

Hydrochlorothiazide: Thiazides affect the renal tubular mechanism of electrolyte reabsorption. At maximal therapeutic dosage, all thiazides are approximately equal in their diuretic potency. Thiazides increase excretion of sodium and chloride in approximately equivalent amounts. Natriuresis causes a secondary loss of potassium.

The mechanism of the antihypertensive effect of thiazides is unknown. Thiazides do not affect normal blood pressure.

The onset of action of thiazides occurs in 2 hours and the peak effect at about 4 hours. The action persists for approximately 6–12 hours. Hydrochlorothiazide is rapidly absorbed, as indicated by peak plasma concentrations 1–2.5 hours after oral administration. Plasma levels of the drug are proportional to dose; the concentration in whole blood is 1.6–1.8 times higher than in plasma. Thiazides are eliminated rapidly by the kidney. After oral administration of 25- to 100-mg doses, 72–97% of the dose is excreted in the urine, indicating dose-independent absorption. Hydrochlorothiazide is eliminated from plasma in a biphasic fashion, with a terminal half-life of 10–17 hours. Plasma protein binding is 67.9%. Plasma clearance is 15.9–30.0 L/hr; volume of distribution is 3.6–7.8 L/kg.

Gastrointestinal absorption of hydrochlorothiazide is enhanced when administered with food. Absorption is decreased in patients with congestive heart failure, and the pharmacokinetics are considerably different in these patients.

INDICATIONS AND USAGE

Hypertension (see boxed **WARNING**).

CONTRAINDICATIONS

Reserpine: Hypersensitivity to reserpine; mental depression (especially with suicidal tendencies); active peptic ulcer, ulcerative colitis; patients receiving electroconvulsive therapy.

Hydrochlorothiazide: Anuria; hypersensitivity to this or other sulfonamide-derived drugs.

WARNINGS

Reserpine: Extreme caution should be exercised in treating patients with a history of mental depression. The drug should be discontinued at the first sign of despondency, early morning insomnia, loss of appetite, impotence, or self-deprecation. Drug-induced depression may persist for several months after drug withdrawal and may be severe enough to result in suicide.

Hydrochlorothiazide: Thiazides should be used with caution in patients with severe renal disease. In patients with renal disease, thiazides may precipitate azotemia. Cumulative effects of the drug may develop in patients with impaired renal function.

Thiazides should be used with caution in patients with impaired hepatic function or progressive liver disease, since minor alterations of fluid and electrolyte imbalance may precipitate hepatic coma.

Thiazides may add to or potentiate the action of other antihypertensive drugs. Potentiation occurs with ganglionic or peripheral adrenergic blocking drugs.

Sensitivity reactions are more likely to occur in patients with a history of allergy or bronchial asthma.

The possibility of exacerbation or activation of systemic lupus erythematosus has been reported.

PRECAUTIONS

General

The Serpasil-Esidrix tablets (#1 and #2) contain FD&C Yellow No. 5 (tartrazine) which may cause allergic-type reactions (including bronchial asthma) in certain susceptible individuals. Although the overall incidence of FD&C Yellow No. 5 (tartrazine) sensitivity in the general population is low, it is frequently seen in patients who also have aspirin hypersensitivity.

Reserpine: Since reserpine increases gastrointestinal motility and secretion, it should be used cautiously in patients with a history of peptic ulcer, ulcerative colitis, or gallstones (biliary colic may be precipitated).

Caution should be exercised when treating hypertensive patients with renal insufficiency, since they adjust poorly to lowered blood pressure levels.

Preoperative withdrawal of reserpine does not assure that circulatory instability will not occur. It is important that the anesthesiologist be aware of the patient's drug intake and consider this in the overall management, since hypotension has occurred in patients receiving rauwolfia preparations. Anticholinergic and adrenergic drugs (e.g., metaraminol, norepinephrine) have been employed to treat adverse vagocirculatory effects.

Hydrochlorothiazide: All patients receiving thiazide therapy should be observed for clinical signs of fluid or electrolyte imbalance, namely hyponatremia, hypochloremic alkalosis, and hypokalemia (see **Laboratory Tests** and **Drug/Drug Interactions**). Warning signs are dryness of mouth, thirst, weakness, lethargy, drowsiness, restlessness, muscle pains or cramps, muscular fatigue, hypotension, oliguria, tachycardia, and gastrointestinal disturbance, such as nausea or vomiting.

Hypokalemia may develop, especially in cases of brisk diuresis or severe cirrhosis.

Interference with adequate oral intake of electrolytes will also contribute to hypokalemia. Hypokalemia may be avoided or treated by use of potassium supplements or foods with a high potassium content.

Any chloride deficit is generally mild and usually does not require specific treatment, except under extraordinary circumstances (as in liver disease or renal disease). Dilutional hyponatremia may occur in edematous patients in hot weather; appropriate therapy is water restriction, rather than administration of salt, except in rare instances when the hyponatremia is life-threatening. In cases of actual salt depletion, appropriate replacement is the therapy of choice. Hyperuricemia may occur or frank gout may be precipitated in certain patients receiving thiazide therapy.

Latent diabetes may become manifest during thiazide administration (see **Drug/Drug Interactions**).

The antihypertensive effects of the drug may be enhanced in the postsympathectomy patient.

If progressive renal impairment becomes evident, withholding or discontinuing diuretic therapy should be considered. Calcium excretion is decreased by thiazides. Pathological changes in the parathyroid gland with hypercalcemia and hypophosphatemia have been observed in a few patients on prolonged thiazide therapy. The common complications of hyperparathyroidism, such as renal lithiasis, bone resorption, and peptic ulceration, have not been seen.

Information for Patients: Patients should be informed of possible side effects and advised to take the medication regularly and continously as directed.

Laboratory Tests

Hydrochlorothiazide: Initial and periodic determinations of serum electrolytes to detect possible electrolyte imbalance should be performed at appropriate intervals.

Serum and urine electrolyte determinations are particularly important when the patient is vomiting excessively or receiving parenteral fluids.

Drug/Drug Interactions

Reserpine: MAO inhibitors should be avoided or used with extreme caution.

Reserpine should be used cautiously with digitalis and quinidine, since cardiac arrhythmias have occurred with rauwolfia preparations.

Hydrochlorothiazide: Hypokalemia can sensitize or exaggerate the response of the heart to the toxic effects of digitalis (e.g., increased ventricular irritability).

Hypokalemia may develop during concomitant use of steroids or ACTH.

Insulin requirements in diabetic patients may be increased, decreased, or unchanged.

Thiazides may decrease arterial responsiveness to norepinephrine, but not enough to preclude effectiveness of the pressor agent for therapeutic use.

Thiazides may increase the responsiveness to tubocurarine.

Lithium renal clearance is reduced by thiazides, increasing the risk of lithium toxicity.

There have been rare reports in the literature of hemolytic anemia occurring with the concomitant use of hydrochlorothiazide and methyldopa.

Concurrent administration of some nonsteroidal anti-inflammatory agents may reduce the diuretic, natriuretic and antihypertensive effects of thiazide diuretics.

Drug/Laboratory Test Interactions: Thiazides may decrease serum levels of protein-bound iodine without signs of thyroid disturbance. Serpasil-Esidrix should be discontinued before carrying out tests for parathyroid function (see **General, Hydrochlorothiazide**, Calcium excretion).

Carcinogenesis, Mutagenesis, Impairment of Fertility

Reserpine. Animal Tumorigenicity: Rodent studies have shown that reserpine is an animal tumorigen, causing an increased incidence of mammary fibroadenomas in female mice, malignant tumors of the seminal vesicles in male mice, and malignant adrenal medullary tumors in male rats. These findings arose in 2-year studies in which the drug was administered in the feed at concentrations of 5 and 10 ppm—about 100 to 300 times the usual human dose. The breast neoplasms are thought to be related to reserpine's prolactin-elevating effect. Several other prolactin-elevating drugs have also been associated with an increased incidence of mammary neoplasia in rodents.

The extent to which these findings indicate a risk to humans is uncertain. Tissue culture experiments show that about one third of human breast tumors are prolactin-dependent in vitro, a factor of considerable importance if the use of the drug is contemplated in a patient with previously detected breast cancer. The possibility of an increased risk of breast cancer in reserpine users has been studied extensively; however, no firm conclusion has emerged. Although a few epidemiologic studies have suggested a slightly increased risk (less than twofold in all studies except one) in women who have used reserpine, other studies of generally similar design have not confirmed this. Epidemiologic studies conducted using other drugs (neuroleptic agents) that, like reserpine, increase prolactin levels and therefore would be considered rodent mammary carcinogens, have not shown an association between chronic administration of the drug and human mammary tumorigenesis. While long-term clinical observation has not suggested such an association, the available evidence is considered too limited to be conclusive at this time. An association of reserpine intake with pheochromocytoma or tumors of the seminal vesicles has not been explored.

Hydrochlorothiazide: Long-term carcinogenicity studies in animals have not been conducted with Esidrix. Hydrochlorothiazide was not mutagenic in in vitro Ames mutagenicity assay of Salmonella typhimurium strains TA 98, TA 100, TA 1535 and TA 1537 or in in vivo mutagenicity assays of mouse germinal cell chromosomes and chinese hamster bone marrow cell chromosomes. It was however, mutagenic in inducing nondisjuction (96% frequency) in diploid strains of Aspergillus nidulans.

Pregnancy Category C: Animal reproduction studies have not been conducted with Serpasil-Esidrix. Reserpine administered parenterally has been shown to be teratogenic in rats at doses up to 2 mg/kg and to have an embryocidal effect in guinea pigs given dosages of 0.5 mg daily. A reproduction study in rats receiving hydrochlorothiazide, 250 mg/kg daily, 62.5 times the maximum daily human dose, has revealed no evidence of impaired fertility or harm to the fetus. There are no adequate and well-controlled studies of Serpasil-Esidrix in pregnant women. Serpasil-Esidrix should be used during pregnancy only if the potential benefit justifies the potential risk to the fetus.

Nonteratogenic Effects. Reserpine crosses the placental barrier, and increased respiratory tract secretions, nasal congestion, cyanosis, and anorexia may occur in neonates of mothers treated with reserpine. Thiazides also cross the placental barrier and appear in cord blood, and there is a risk of fetal or neonatal jaundice, thrombocytopenia, and possibly other adverse reactions that have occurred in adults.

Nursing Mothers: Reserpine is excreted in maternal breast milk, and increased respiratory tract secretions, nasal congestion, cyanosis, and anorexia may occur in breast-fed infants. Thiazides are also excreted in breast milk. Because of the potential for serious adverse reactions in nursing infants and the potential for tumorigenicity shown for reserpine in animal studies, a decision should be made whether to discontinue nursing or to discontinue Serpasil-Esidrix, taking into account the importance of the drug to the mother.

Pediatric Use: Safety and effectiveness of the combination drug in children have not been established.

ADVERSE REACTIONS

Adverse reactions are usually reversible upon reduction of dosage or discontinuation of Serpasil-Esidrix. Whenever adverse reactions are moderate or severe, it may be necessary to discontinue the drug.

The following adverse reactions have been observed, but there has not been enough systematic collection of data to support an estimate of their frequency. Consequently the reactions are categorized by organ systems and are listed in decreasing order of severity and not frequency.

Reserpine: The following have been observed with rauwolfia preparations:

Digestive: Vomiting, diarrhea, nausea, anorexia, dryness of mouth, hypersecretion.

Cardiovascular: Arrhythmias (particularly when used concurrently with digitalis or quinidine), syncope, angina-like symptoms, bradycardia, edema.

Respiratory: Dyspnea, epistaxis, nasal congestion.

Neurologic: Rare parkinsonian syndrome and other extrapyramidal tract symptoms; dizziness; headache; paradoxical anxiety; depression; nervousness; nightmares; dull sensorium; drowsiness.

Musculoskeletal: Muscular aches.

Genitourinary: Pseudolactation, impotence, dysuria, gynecomastia, decreased libido, breast engorgement.

Metabolic: Weight gain.

Special Senses: Deafness, optic atrophy, glaucoma, uveitis, conjunctival injection.

Hypersensitive Reactions: Purpura, rash, pruritus.

Hydrochlorothiazide: *Digestive:* Pancreatitis, jaundice (intrahepatic cholestatic), sialadenitis, vomiting, diarrhea, cramping, nausea, gastric irritation, constipation, anorexia.

Cardiovascular: Orthostatic hypotension (may be potentiated by alcohol, barbiturates, or narcotics).

Neurologic: Vertigo, dizziness, transient blurred vision, headache, paresthesia, xanthopsia, weakness, restlessness.

Musculoskeletal: Muscle spasm.

Hematologic: Aplastic anemia, agranulocytosis, leukopenia, thrombocytopenia.

Metabolic: Hyperglycemia, glycosuria, hyperuricemia.

Hypersensitive Reactions: Necrotizing angiitis, Stevens-Johnson syndrome, purpura, urticaria, rash, photosensitivity.

OVERDOSAGE

Acute Toxicity: No deaths due to acute poisoning with the combination drug have been reported.

Oral LD_{50}'s in animals (mg/kg): (reserpine) rats, 2993; mice, 47 and 500; (hydrochlorothiazide) rats, 2750.

Signs and Symptoms:

Reserpine. The clinical picture of acute poisoning is characterized chiefly by signs and symptoms due to the reflex parasympathomimetic effect of reserpine.

Impairment of consciousness may occur and may range from drowsiness to coma, depending upon the severity of overdosage. Flushing of the skin, conjunctival injection, and pupillary constriction are to be expected. Hypotension, hypothermia, central respiratory depression, and bradycardia may develop in cases of severe overdosage. Increased salivary and gastric secretion and diarrhea may also occur.

Hydrochlorothiazide. The most prominent feature of poisoning is acute loss of fluid and electrolytes.

Cardiovascular: Tachycardia, hypotension, shock.

Neuromuscular: Weakness, confusion, dizziness, cramps of the calf muscles, paresthesia, fatigue, impairment of consciousness.

Digestive: Nausea, vomiting, thirst.

Renal: Polyuria, oliguria, or anuria (due to hemoconcentration).

Laboratory Findings: Hypokalemia, hyponatremia, hypochloremia, alkalosis; increased BUN (especially in patients with renal insufficiency).

Combined Poisoning: Signs and symptoms may be aggravated or modified by concomitant intake of antihypertensive medication, barbiturates, curare, digitalis (hypokalemia), corticosteroids, narcotics, or alcohol.

Treatment: There is no specific antidote.

Stomach contents should be evacuated, taking adequate precautions against aspiration and for protection of the airway. An activated charcoal slurry should be instilled if conditions permit. Dialysis may not be effective for elimination of Serpasil-Esidrix because of its plasma protein binding (see **CLINICAL PHARMACOLOGY**).

The effects of reserpine overdosage should be treated symptomatically. If hypotension or shock occurs, the patient's legs should be kept raised and lost fluid and electrolytes (potassium, sodium) should be replaced. If hypotension is severe enough to require treatment with a vasopressor, one having a direct action upon vascular smooth muscle (e.g., phenylephrine, levarterenol, metaraminol) should be used.

Fluid and electrolyte balance (especially serum potassium) and renal function should be monitored until conditions become normal. Since reserpine is long-acting, the patient should be observed carefully for at least 72 hours.

DOSAGE AND ADMINISTRATION

Dosage should be determined by individual titration (see boxed **WARNING**).

The usual dosage is two Serpasil-Esidrix #2 Tablets daily in single or divided doses. For patients requiring less hydrochlorothiazide, Serpasil-Esidrix #1 Tablets should be substituted.

Since the antihypertensive effects of reserpine are not immediately apparent, maximal reduction in blood pressure from a given dosage may not occur for 2 weeks. For maintenance, dosage should be reduced to the lowest effective level; as little as one tablet daily may suffice.

When necessary, more potent antihypertensive agents may be added gradually in reduced dosages. The effects should be watched carefully.

HOW SUPPLIED

Tablets #1—round, light orange (imprinted CIBA 13) 0.1 mg of reserpine, 25 mg of hydrochlorothiazide Bottles of 100—NDC 0083-0013-30

Tablets #2—round, light orange (imprinted CIBA 97) 0.1 mg of reserpine, 50 mg of hydrochlorothiazide Bottles of 100—NDC 0083-0097-30

Protect from light.

Dispense in tight, light-resistant container (USP).

C87-15 (Rev. 11/87)

Shown in Product Identification Section, page 409

TRANSDERM SCŌP® ℞

[*trans-derm scōpe*]

scopolamine

(formerly Transderm-V)

Transdermal Therapeutic System

Programmed delivery *in vivo* of 0.5 mg of scopolamine over 3 days

This product is now marketed by CIBA Consumer Pharmaceuticals, Division of CIBA-GEIGY Corporation.

PRODUCT OVERVIEW

KEY FACTS

The active ingredient in the Transderm Scōp system is scopolamine, a belladonna alkaloid. The transdermal system contains 1.5 mg of scopolamine and is designed to deliver 0.5 mg of scopolamine at an approximately constant rate to the systemic circulation over the 3-day lifetime of the system.

MAJOR USES

Transderm Scōp system has proved to be clinically effective for the prevention of nausea and vomiting associated with motion sickness in adults when applied to the skin in the postauricular area.

SAFETY INFORMATION

Transderm Scōp system is contraindicated for patients with known hypersensitivity to scopolamine or any of the components of the adhesive matrix making up the therapeutic system, or in patients with glaucoma.

Before prescribing, please consult full prescribing information below.

PRESCRIBING INFORMATION

TRANSDERM SCŌP® ℞

[*trans-derm scōpe*]

scopolamine

(formerly Transderm-V)

Transdermal Therapeutic System

DESCRIPTION

The Transderm Scōp system is a circular flat disc designed for continuous release of scopolamine following application to an area of intact skin on the head, behind the ear. Clinical evaluation has demonstrated that the system provides effective antiemetic and antinauseant actions when tested against motion-sickness stimuli in adults. The Transderm Scōp system is a film 0.2 mm thick and 2.5 cm^2, with four layers. Proceeding from the visible surface towards the surface attached to the skin, these layers are: (1) a backing layer of tan-colored, aluminized, polyester film; (2) a drug reservoir of scopolamine, mineral oil, and polyisobutylene; (3) a microporous polypropylene membrane that controls the rate of delivery of scopolamine from the system to the skin surface; and (4) an adhesive formulation of mineral oil, polyisobutylene, and scopolamine. A protective peel strip of siliconized polyester, which covers the adhesive layer, is removed before the system is used. The inactive components, mineral oil (12.4 mg) and polyisobutylene (11.4 mg), are not released from the system.

Cross section of the system:

Backing Layer
Drug Reservoir
Rate-Controlling Membrane
Contact Adhesive
Protective Peel Strip

Release-Rate Concept: The Transderm Scōp system contains 1.5 mg of scopolamine. The system is programmed to deliver 0.5 mg of scopolamine at an approximately constant rate to the systemic circulation over the 3-day lifetime of the system. An initial priming dose of scopolamine, released from the adhesive layer of the system, saturates the skin binding sites and rapidly brings the plasma concentration of scopolamine to the required steady-state level. A continuous controlled release of scopolamine, which flows from the drug reservoir through the rate-controlling membrane, maintains the plasma level constant.

CLINICAL PHARMACOLOGY

The sole active agent of Transderm Scōp is scopolamine, a belladonna alkaloid with well-known pharmacological properties. The drug has a long history of oral and parenteral use for central anticholinergic activity, including prophylaxis of motion sickness. The mechanism of action of scopolamine in the central nervous system (CNS) is not definitely known but may include anticholinergic effects. The ability of scopolamine to prevent motion-induced nausea is believed to be associated with inhibition of vestibular input to the CNS, which results in inhibition of the vomiting reflex. In addition, scopolamine may have a direct action on the vomiting center within the reticular formation of the brain stem. Applied to the postauricular skin, Transderm Scōp provides for a gradual release of scopolamine from an adhesive matrix of mineral oil and polyisobutylene.

INDICATIONS AND USAGE

Transderm Scōp is indicated for prevention of nausea and vomiting associated with motion sickness in adults. The disc should be applied only to skin in the postauricular area.

Clinical Results: Transderm Scōp provides antiemetic protection within several hours following application of the disc behind the ear. In 195 adult subjects of different racial origins who participated in clinical efficacy studies at sea or in a controlled motion environment, there was a 75% reduction in the incidence of motion-induced nausea and vomiting. Transderm Scōp provided significantly greater protection than that obtained with oral dimenhydrinate.

CONTRAINDICATIONS

Transderm Scōp should not be used in patients with known hypersensitivity to scopolamine or any of the components of the adhesive matrix making up the therapeutic system, or in patients with glaucoma.

WARNINGS

Transderm Scōp should not be used in children and should be used with special caution in the elderly. See **PRECAUTIONS.**

Since drowsiness, disorientation, and confusion may occur with the use of scopolamine, patients should be warned of the possibility and cautioned against engaging in activities that require mental alertness, such as driving a motor vehicle or operating dangerous machinery.

Potentially alarming idiosyncratic reactions may occur with ordinary therapeutic doses of scopolamine.

PRECAUTIONS

General

Scopolamine should be used with caution in patients with pyloric obstruction, or urinary bladder neck obstruction. Caution should be exercised when administering an antiemetic or antimuscarinic drug to patients suspected of having intestinal obstruction.

Transderm Scōp should be used with special caution in the elderly or in individuals with impaired metabolic, liver, or kidney functions, because of the increased likelihood of CNS effects.

Information for Patients

Since scopolamine can cause temporary dilation of the pupils and blurred vision if it comes in contact with the eyes, patients should be strongly advised to wash their hands thoroughly with soap and water immediately after handling the disc.

Patients should be advised to remove the disc immediately and contact a physician in the unlikely event that they experience symptoms of acute narrow-angle glaucoma (pain in and reddening of the eyes accompanied by dilated pupils). Patients should be warned against driving a motor vehicle or operating dangerous machinery. A patient brochure is available.

Drug Interactions

Scopolamine should be used with care in patients taking drugs, including alcohol, capable of causing CNS effects. Special attention should be given to drugs having anticholinergic properties, e.g., belladonna alkaloids, antihistamines (including meclizine), and antidepressants.

Carcinogenesis, Mutagenesis, Impairment of Fertility

No long-term studies in animals have been performed to evaluate carcinogenic potential. Fertility studies were performed in female rats and revealed no evidence of impaired fertility or harm to the fetus due to scopolamine hydrobromide administered by daily subcutaneous injection. In the highest-dose group (plasma level approximately 500 times the level achieved in humans using a transdermal system), reduced maternal body weights were observed.

Pregnancy Category C

Teratogenic studies were performed in pregnant rats and rabbits with scopolamine hydrobromide administered by daily intravenous injection. No adverse effects were recorded in the rats. In the rabbits, the highest dose (plasma level approximately 100 times the level achieved in humans using a transdermal system) of drug administered had a marginal embryotoxic effect. Transderm Scōp should be used during pregnancy only if the anticipated benefit justifies the potential risk to the fetus.

Nursing Mothers

It is not known whether scopolamine is excreted in human milk. Because many drugs are excreted in human milk, caution should be exercised when Transderm Scōp is administered to a nursing woman.

Pediatric Use

Children are particularly susceptible to the side effects of belladonna alkaloids. Transderm Scōp should not be used in children because it is not known whether this system will release an amount of scopolamine that could produce serious adverse effects in children.

ADVERSE REACTIONS

The most frequent adverse reaction to Transderm Scōp is dryness of the mouth. This occurs in about two thirds of the people. A less frequent adverse reaction is drowsiness, which occurs in less than one sixth of the people. Transient impairment of eye accommodation, including blurred vision and dilation of the pupils, is also observed.

The following adverse reactions have also been reported on infrequent occasions during the use of Transderm Scōp: disorientation; memory disturbances; dizziness; restlessness; hallucinations; confusion; difficulty urinating; rashes and erythema; acute narrow-angle glaucoma; and dry, itchy, or red eyes.

Continued on next page

CIBA—Cont.

Drug Withdrawal: Symptoms including dizziness, nausea, vomiting, headache and disturbances of equilibrium have been reported in a few patients following discontinuation of the use of the Transderm Scōp system. These symptoms have occurred most often in patients who have used the systems for more than three days.

OVERDOSAGE
Overdosage with scopolamine may cause disorientation, memory disturbances, dizziness, restlessness, hallucinations, or confusion. Should these symptoms occur, the Transderm Scōp disc should be immediately removed. Appropriate parasympathomimetic therapy should be initiated if these symptoms are severe.

DOSAGE AND ADMINISTRATION
Initiation of Therapy: One Transderm Scōp disc (programmed to deliver 0.5 mg of scopolamine over 3 days) should be applied to the hairless area behind one ear at least 4 hours before the antiemetic effect is required. Only one disc should be worn at any time.

Handling: After the disc is applied on dry skin behind the ear, the hands should be washed thoroughly with soap and water and dried. Upon removal of the disc, it should be discarded, and the hands and application site washed thoroughly with soap and water and dried, to prevent any traces of scopolamine from coming into direct contact with the eyes. (A patient brochure is available.)

Continuation of Therapy: Should the disc become displaced, it should be discarded, and a fresh one placed on the hairless area behind the other ear. If therapy is required for longer than 3 days, the first disc should be discarded, and a fresh one placed on the hairless area behind the other ear.

HOW SUPPLIED
The Transderm Scōp system is a tan-colored disc, 2.5 cm², on a clear, oversized, hexagonal peel strip, which is removed prior to use.

Each Transderm Scōp system contains 1.5 mg of scopolamine and is programmed to deliver *in vivo* 0.5 mg of scopolamine over 3 days.

Transderm Scōp is available in packages of four discs. Each disc is foil wrapped. Patient instructions are included.

1 Package (4 discs) ....NDC 0083-4345-04
The system should be stored between 59° - 86°F (15° - 30°C).

C88-5 (Rev. 2/88)

Information for the Patient About—

TRANSDERM SCŌP®
Generic Name: scopolamine,
pronounced skoe-POL-a-meen
(formerly Transderm-V)
Transdermal Therapeutic System

The Transderm Scōp system helps to prevent the nausea and vomiting of motion sickness for up to 3 days. It is an adhesive disc that you place behind your ear several hours before you travel. Wear only one disc at any time.

Be sure to wash your hands thoroughly with soap and water immediately after handling the disc, so that any drug that might get on your hands will not come into contact with your eyes.

Avoid drinking alcohol while using Transderm Scōp. Also, be careful about driving or operating any machinery while using the system because the drug might make you drowsy.

DO NOT USE TRANSDERM SCŌP IF YOU ARE ALLERGIC TO SCOPOLAMINE OR HAVE GLAUCOMA.
TRANSDERM SCŌP SHOULD NOT BE USED IN CHILDREN AND SHOULD BE USED WITH SPECIAL CAUTION IN THE ELDERLY.

How the Transderm Scōp System Works
A group of nerve fibers deep inside the ear helps people keep their balance. For some people, the motion of ships, airplanes, trains, automobiles, and buses increases the activity of these nerve fibers. This increased activity causes the *dizziness, nausea, and vomiting* of motion sickness. People may have one, some, or all of these symptoms.

Transderm Scōp contains the drug scopolamine, which helps reduce the activity of the nerve fibers in the inner ear. When a Transderm Scōp disc is placed on the skin behind one of the ears, scopolamine passes through the skin and into the bloodstream. One disc may be kept in place for 3 days if needed.

Precautions
Before using Transderm Scōp be sure to tell your doctor if you—
- Are pregnant or nursing (or planning to become pregnant)
- Have (or have had) glaucoma (increased pressure in the eyeball)
- Have (or have had) any metabolic, liver, or kidney disease
- Have any obstructions of the stomach or intestine
- Have trouble urinating or any bladder obstruction
- Have any skin allergy or have had a skin reaction such as a rash or redness to any drug, especially scopolamine, or chemical or food substance.

Any of these conditions could make Transderm Scōp unsuitable for you. Also tell your doctor if you are taking any other medicines.

In the unlikely event that you experience pain in the eye and reddened whites of the eye, which may be accompanied by widening of the pupil and blurred vision, remove the disc immediately and consult your physician. As indicated below under Side Effects, widening of the pupils and blurred vision without pain or reddened whites of the eye is usually temporary and not serious.

Transderm Scōp should not be used in children. The safety of its use in children has not been determined. Children and the elderly may be particularly sensitive to the effects of scopolamine.

Side Effects
The most common side effect experienced by people using Transderm Scōp is dryness of the mouth. This occurs in about two thirds of the people. A less frequent side effect is drowsiness, which occurs in less than one sixth of the people. Temporary blurring of vision and dilation (widening) of the pupils may occur, especially if the drug is on your hands and comes in contact with the eyes. On infrequent occasions, disorientation, memory disturbances, dizziness, restlessness, hallucinations, confusion, difficulty urinating, skin rashes or redness, and dry, itchy, or red eyes and eye pain have been reported. If these effects do occur, remove the disc and call your doctor. Since drowsiness, disorientation, and confusion may occur with the use of scopolamine, be careful driving or operating any dangerous machinery, especially when you first start using the drug system.

Drug Withdrawal: Symptoms including dizziness, nausea, vomiting, headache and disturbances of equilibrium have been reported in a few people following discontinuation of the Transderm Scōp system. These symptoms have occurred most often in people who have used the systems for more than three days. We recommend that you consult your doctor if these symptoms occur.

How to Use Transderm Scōp
Transderm Scōp should be stored between 59° - 86°F (15° - 30°C) until you are ready to use it.
1. Plan to apply one Transderm Scōp disc at least 4 hours before you need it. **Wear only one disc at any time.**
2. Select a hairless area of skin behind one ear, taking care to avoid any cuts or irritations. Wipe the area with a clean, dry tissue.
3. Peel the package open and remove the disc (Figure 1).

(Figure 1)

4. Remove the clear plastic six-sided backing from the round system. Try not to touch the adhesive surface on the disc with your hands (Figure 2).

system
disposable backing

(Figure 2)

5. Firmly apply the adhesive surface (metallic side) to the dry area of skin behind the ear so that the tan-colored side is showing (Figure 3). Make good contact, especially around the edge. Once you have placed the disc behind your ear, do not move it for as long as you want to use it (up to 3 days).

tan-colored system

(Figure 3)

6. *Important:* **After the disc is in place, be sure to wash your hands thoroughly with soap and water to remove any scopolamine. If this drug were to contact your eyes, it could cause temporary blurring of vision and dilation (widening) of the pupils (the dark circles in the center of your eyes). This is not serious unless accompanied by eye pain and redness (see Precautions), and your pupils should return to normal.**
7. Remove the disc after 3 days and throw it away. (You may remove it sooner if you are no longer concerned about motion sickness). After removing the disc, be sure to wash your hands and the area behind your ear thoroughly with soap and water.
8. If you wish to control nausea for longer than 3 days, *remove* the first disc after 3 days, and place a new one *behind the other ear*, repeating instructions 2 to 7.
9. Keep the disc dry, if possible, to prevent it from falling off. Limited contact with water, however, as in bathing or swimming, will not affect the system. In the unlikely event that the disc falls off, throw it away and put a new one behind the other ear.

This leaflet presents a summary of information about Transderm Scōp. If you would like more information or if you have any questions, ask your doctor or pharmacist. A more technical leaflet is available, written for your doctor. If you would like to read the leaflet, ask your pharmacist to show you a copy. You may need the help of your doctor or pharmacist to understand some of the information.

Dist. by:
CIBA Consumer Pharmaceuticals
Division of CIBA-GEIGY Corp.
Summit, NJ 07901

C88-6 (Rev. 2/88)
Shown in Product Identification Section, page 409

VIOFORM®
[*vye-oh-form*]
(clioquinol USP)
Antifungal/Antibacterial Ointment and Cream

Listed in USP, a Medicare designated compendium.

DESCRIPTION
Vioform is 5-chloro-7-iodo-8-quinolinol—an effective antifungal and antibacterial agent—available as 3% *Ointment* and 3% *Cream.*

INDICATIONS AND DIRECTIONS FOR USE
A soothing antifungal and antibacterial preparation for the treatment of inflamed conditions of the skin, such as eczema, athlete's foot and other fungal infections.

Apply to the affected area 2 or 3 times a day or use as directed by physician.

CAUTION
Do not use in children under 2 years of age.
May prove irritating to sensitized skin in rare cases. If this should occur, discontinue treatment and consult physician.
May stain.
KEEP OUT OF REACH OF CHILDREN.

HOW SUPPLIED
Ointment, 3% clioquinol in a petrolatum base; tubes of 1 ounce.
Cream, 3% clioquinol in a water-washable base; tubes of 1 ounce.
Do not store above 86°F.

C86-8 (Rev. 2/86)

VIOFORM®-HYDROCORTISONE   ℞
[*vye-oh-form*]
(clioquinol USP and hydrocortisone USP)

DESCRIPTION
Vioform-Hydrocortisone, a topical compound for dermatologic use, combines the antifungal and antibacterial actions of clioquinol and the anti-inflammatory and antipruritic effects of hydrocortisone to provide broad control of acute and chronic dermatoses. It is available as *Cream, Ointment,* or *Lotion* containing 3% clioquinol and 1% hydrocortisone and as *Mild Cream* and *Mild Ointment* containing 3% clioquinol and 0.5% hydrocortisone.
Vioform is 5-chloro-7-iodo-8-quinolinol.
Hydrocortisone is 11β,17,21-trihydroxypregn-4-ene-3,20-dione.

ACTIONS
In vitro studies have demonstrated that Vioform effectively inhibits the growth of various mycotic organisms such as Microsporons, Trichophytons, and Candida albicans and gram positive cocci such as staphylococci and enterococci. The role of steroids in alleviating the inflammation and pruritus associated with many dermatoses has been well established.

INDICATIONS

Based on a review of this drug by the National Academy of Sciences-National Research Council and/or other information, FDA has classified the indications as follows:

"Possibly" effective: Contact or atopic dermatitis; impetiginized eczema; nummular eczema; infantile eczema; endogenous chronic infectious dermatitis; stasis dermatitis; pyoderma; nuchal eczema and chronic eczematoid otitis externa; acne urticata; localized or disseminated neurodermatitis; lichen simplex chronicus; anogenital pruritus (vulvae, scroti, ani); folliculitis; bacterial dermatoses; mycotic dermatoses such as tinea (capitis, cruris, corporis, pedis); moniliasis; intertrigo. Final classification of the less-than-effective indications requires further investigation.

CONTRAINDICATIONS

Hypersensitivity to Vioform-Hydrocortisone, or any of its ingredients or related compounds; lesions of the eye; tuberculosis of the skin; most viral skin lesions (including herpes simplex, vaccinia, and varicella).
Vioform should not be used in children under 2 years of age.

WARNINGS

This product is not for ophthalmic use.
In the presence of systemic infections, appropriate systemic antibiotics should be used.
Usage in Pregnancy: Although topical steroids have not been reported to have an adverse effect on pregnancy, the safety of their use in pregnant women has not been absolutely established. In laboratory animals, increases in incidence of fetal abnormalities have been associated with exposure of gestating females to topical corticosteroids, in some cases at rather low dosage levels. Therefore, drugs of this class should not be used extensively on pregnant patients in large amounts or for prolonged periods of time.

PRECAUTIONS

May prove irritating to sensitized skin in rare cases. If irritation occurs, discontinue therapy. Staining of skin and fabrics may occur. Additionally, there are rare reports of discoloration of hair and nails.
Signs and symptoms of systemic toxicity, electrolyte imbalance, or adrenal suppression have not been reported with Vioform-Hydrocortisone. Nevertheless, the possibility of suppression of the pituitary-adrenal axis during therapy should be kept in mind, especially when the drug is used under occlusive dressings, for a prolonged period, or for treating extensive cutaneous areas since significant absorption of corticosteroid may occur under these conditions, particularly in children and infants.
Vioform may be absorbed through the skin and interfere with thyroid function tests. If such tests are contemplated, wait at least one month between discontinuation of therapy and performance of these tests. The ferric chloride test for phenylketonuria (PKU) can yield a false-positive result if Vioform is present in the diaper or urine.
Prolonged use may result in overgrowth of nonsusceptible organisms requiring appropriate therapy.

ADVERSE REACTIONS

There have been a few reports of rash and hypersensitivity. The following local adverse reactions have been reported with topical corticosteroids, especially under occlusive dressings: burning; itching; irritation; dryness; folliculitis; hypertrichosis; acneiform eruptions; hypopigmentation; perioral dermatitis; allergic contact dermatitis; maceration of the skin; secondary infection; skin atrophy; striae; miliaria. Discontinue therapy if any untoward reaction occurs.

DOSAGE AND ADMINISTRATION

Apply a thin layer to the affected parts 3 or 4 times daily. The *Cream*, because of its slight drying effect, is primarily useful for moist, weeping lesions; the *Lotion* is particularly suitable for application behind the ears and in intertriginous areas of the body; the *Ointment* is best used for dry lesions accompanied by thickening and scaling of the skin.
The *Mild Cream* and *Mild Ointment* should be used when treating lesions involving extensive body areas or less severe dermatoses.

HOW SUPPLIED

Cream, 3% clioquinol and 1% hydrocortisone in a water-washable base containing stearyl alcohol, cetyl alcohol, stearic acid, petrolatum, sodium lauryl sulfate, and glycerin in water; tubes of 5 and 20 Gm.
Ointment, 3% clioquinol and 1% hydrocortisone in a petrolatum base; tubes of 20 Gm.
Lotion, 3% clioquinol and 1% hydrocortisone in a water-washable base containing stearic acid, cetyl alcohol, lanolin, propylene glycol, sorbitan trioleate, polysorbate 60, triethanolamine, methylparaben, propylparaben, and perfume Flora in water; plastic squeeze bottles of 15 ml.

Mild Cream, 3% clioquinol and 0.5% hydrocortisone in a water-washable base containing stearyl alcohol, cetyl alcohol, stearic acid, petrolatum, sodium lauryl sulfate, and glycerin in water; tubes of ½ and 1 ounce.
Mild Ointment, 3% clioquinol and 0.5% hydrocortisone in a petrolatum base; tubes of 1 ounce.
Do not store above 86°F.

C86-9 (Rev. 2/86)

Colgate-Hoyt Laboratories
Division of Colgate-Palmolive Co.
1 COLGATE WAY
CANTON, MA 02021 U.S.A.

LURIDE® Drops   ℞
brand of Sodium Fluoride

DESCRIPTION

Each ml. (18 drops) contains 2.25 mg fluoride ion (F^-) from 4.97 mg sodium fluoride (NaF), approximately 0.125 mg F per drop. For use as a dental caries preventive in children. Sugar-free. Saccharin-free.

CLINICAL PHARMACOLOGY

Sodium fluoride acts systemically (before tooth eruption) and topically (post-eruption) by increasing tooth resistance to acid dissolution, by promoting remineralization, and by inhibiting the cariogenic microbial process.

INDICATIONS AND USAGE

It has been established that ingestion of fluoridated drinking water (1 ppm F) during the period of tooth development results in a significant decrease in the incidence of dental caries.[1] LURIDE Drops was developed to provide systemic fluoride for use as a supplement in infants and children from birth to age 3 and older, living in areas where the drinking water fluoride level does not exceed 0.7 ppm.

CONTRAINDICATIONS

Do not use in areas where the drinking water exceeds 0.7 ppm F.

WARNINGS

See "Contraindications" above. As in the case of all medications, keep out of reach of children. Contains FD&C Yellow No. 6.

PRECAUTIONS

See "Overdosage" section below. Incompatibility of fluoride with dairy foods has been reported due to formation of calcium fluoride which is poorly absorbed.

ADVERSE REACTIONS

Allergic rash and other idiosyncrasies have been rarely reported.

OVERDOSAGE

Prolonged daily ingestion of excessive fluoride will result in varying degrees of dental fluorosis. (The total amount of sodium fluoride in a bottle of 30 ml LURIDE Drops (67.5 mg F) conforms with the recommendations of the American Dental Association for the maximum to be dispensed at one time for safety purposes.)

DOSAGE[2] AND ADMINISTRATION

Invert bottle vertically for proper drop delivery.

F-Content of Drinking Water	Daily Dosage		
	Birth to Age 2	Age 2–3	Age 3–12
<0.3 ppm	2 drops	4 drops	8 drops
0.3–0.7 ppm	One-half above dosage.		
>0.7 ppm	Fluoride supplements contraindicated.		

LURIDE Drops may be administered orally undiluted or mixed with fluids.

HOW SUPPLIED

Squeeze-bottles of 30 ml. (peach flavor—NDC#0126-0003-31)

CAUTION

Federal (U.S.A.) law prohibits dispensing without prescription.

REFERENCES

1. *Accepted Dental Therapeutics*, Ed. 40, American Dental Association, Chicago, 1984, p. 399–402.
2. Ibid., p. 401; American Academy of Pediatrics, Pediatrics 63:150–152, 1979.

LURIDE® Lozi–Tabs® Tablets   ℞
brand of Sodium Fluoride
  Full–strength 1.0 mg F
  Luride–SF (no artificial flavor or color)
    1.0 mg F
  Half–strength 0.5 mg F
  Quarter–strength 0.25 mg F

DESCRIPTION

LURIDE® brand of sodium fluoride Lozi-Tabs® brand of lozenge/chewable tablets for use as a dental caries preventive in children. Sugar-free. Saccharin-free. Erythrosine (FDC Red dye #3)-free.
Each LURIDE 1.0 mg F tablet (full-strength) contains 1.0 mg fluoride (F) from 2.2 mg sodium fluoride (NaF).
Each LURIDE -SF 1.0 mg F tablet (SF for Special Formula: no artificial color or flavor) contains 1.0 mg F from 2.2 mg NaF.
Each LURIDE 0.5 mg F tablet (half-strength) contains 0.5 mg F from 1.1 mg NaF.
Each Luride 0.25 mg F tablet (quarter-strength) contains 0.25 mg F from 0.55 mg NaF.

CLINICAL PHARMACOLOGY

Sodium fluoride acts systemically (before tooth eruption) and topically (post-eruption) by increasing tooth resistance to acid dissolution, by promoting remineralization, and by inhibiting the cariogenic microbial process.

INDICATIONS AND USAGE

It is well established that ingestion of fluoridated drinking water (1 ppm F) during the period of tooth development results in a significant decrease in the incidence of dental caries.[1] LURIDE tablets were developed to provide fluoride for children living in areas where the water fluoride level is 0.7 ppm or less.

CONTRAINDICATIONS

LURIDE and LURIDE-SF 1.0 mg F tablets are contraindicated when the F-content of drinking water is 0.3 ppm or more and should not be administered to children under age 3. LURIDE 0.5 mg F and .25 mg F tablets are contraindicated when the F-content of drinking water exceeds 0.7 ppm.

WARNINGS

Do not use LURIDE or LURIDE-SF 1.0 mg F tablets for children under age 3, nor in areas where the F-content of the drinking water is 0.3 ppm or more. Do not use LURIDE 0.5 mg F or LURIDE 0.25 mg F in areas where the F-content of the drinking water is more than 0.7 ppm. As in the case of all medications, keep out of reach of children. LURIDE 1.0 mg F Orange Flavor and LURIDE 0.25 mg F contain FD&C Yellow No. 6.

PRECAUTIONS

See "Overdosage" section below. Incompatibility of fluoride with dairy foods has been reported due to formation of calcium fluoride which is poorly absorbed.

ADVERSE REACTIONS

Allergic rash and other idiosyncrasies have been rarely reported.

OVERDOSAGE

Prolonged daily ingestion of excessive fluoride will result in varying degrees of dental fluorosis. (The total amount of sodium fluoride in a bottle of 120 LURIDE tablets (all strengths) conforms with the recommendations of the American Dental Association for the maximum to be dispensed at one time for safety purposes.)

DOSAGE[2] AND ADMINISTRATION

F-Content of Drinking Water	Daily Dosage (F ion)		
	Birth to Age 2	Age 2–3	Age 3–12
<0.3 ppm	0.25 mg	0.5 mg	1.0 mg.
0.3–0.7 ppm	One-half above dosages.		
>0.7 ppm	Fluoride supplements contra-indicated.		

One tablet daily, to be dissolved in the mouth or chewed before swallowing, preferably at bedtime after brushing teeth.

HOW SUPPLIED

[See table on next page].

CAUTION

Federal (U.S.A.) law prohibits dispensing without prescription.

REFERENCES

1. *Accepted Dental Therapeutics*, Ed. 40, American Dental Association, Chicago, 1984, p. 399–402.
2. Ibid., p. 401; American Academy of Pediatrics, Pediatrics 63:150–152, 1979
   Shown in Product Identification Section, page 409

Continued on next page

Colgate-Hoyt—Cont.

LURIDE

Strength (F ion)	Tablets per Bottle	Flavor	NDC Number 0126-
1.0mg F (full-strength)	120	cherry assorted[1] SF[2]	0006-21 0143-21 0007-21
	1000*	cherry assorted[1]	0006-10 0143-10
	5000*	cherry	0006-51
0.5mg F (half-strength)	120	grape	0014-21
	1200*	grape	0014-81
0.25mg F (quarter-strength)	120	vanilla	0186-21

(1) cherry, orange, lemon, lime
(2) Special Formula: no artificial flavor or coloring
* FOR DISPENSING ONLY

ORABASE® HCA   ℞
Oral Paste

DESCRIPTION
ORABASE® HCA is an adrenocorticoid topical dental paste for application to the oral mucosa. Each gram contains hydrocortisone acetate 5mg (0.5%) in a paste vehicle containing pectin, gelatin, sodium carboxymethylcellulose dispersed in a plasticized hydrocarbon gel composed of 5% polyethylene in mineral oil, flavored with imitation vanilla.
Hydrocortisone acetate is also known as cortisol acetate.
Structural formula: Pregn-4-ene-3,20-dione,21-(acetyloxy)-11,17 dihydroxy-, (11β)-.

CLINICAL PHARMACOLOGY
Hydrocortisone acetate is a natural corticosteroid and possesses properties of an anti-inflammatory, antipruritic, and vasoconstrictive nature. The paste acts as an adhesive vehicle for applying the active medication to oral tissues. The protective action of the adhesive vehicle may serve to reduce oral irritation.
The mechanism of anti-inflammatory activity of the topical corticosteroids is unclear. Various laboratory methods, including vasoconstrictor assays, are used to compare and predict potencies and/or clinical efficacies of the topical corticosteroids. There is some evidence to suggest that a recognizable correlation exists between vasoconstrictor potency and therapeutic efficacy in man.
Once absorbed, topical corticosteroids are handled through pharmacokinetic pathways similar to systemically administered corticosteroids. Corticosteroids are bound to plasma proteins in varying degrees. Corticosteroids are metabolized primarily in the liver and are then excreted by the kidneys. Some of the topical corticosteroids and their metabolites are also excreted into the bile.

INDICATIONS AND USAGE
Indicated for adjunctive treatment and for temporary relief of symptoms associated with oral inflammatory lesions and ulcerative lesions resulting from trauma.

CONTRAINDICATIONS
Topical corticosteroids are contraindicated in those patients with a history of hypersensitivity to any of the components of the preparation.

PRECAUTIONS
General: Systemic absorption of topical corticosteroids has produced reversible hypothalamic-pituitary-adrenal (HPA) axis suppression, manifestations of Cushing's syndrome, hyperglycemia, and glucosuria in some patients. Conditions which augment systemic absorption include the application of the more potent steroids, use over large surface areas, and prolonged use.
Therefore, patients receiving a large dose of a potent topical steroid applied to a large surface area should be evaluated periodically for evidence of HPA axis suppression by using the urinary free cortisol and ACTH stimulation tests. If HPA axis suppression is noted, an attempt should be made to withdraw the drug or to reduce the frequency of application. Recovery of HPA axis function is generally prompt and complete upon discontinuation of the drug. Infrequently, signs and symptoms of steroid withdrawal may occur, requiring supplemental systemic corticosteroids.
Children may absorb proportionally larger amounts of topical corticosteroids and thus be more susceptible to systemic toxicity (See PRECAUTIONS-Pediatric Use).
If irritation develops, topical corticosteroids should be discontinued and appropriate therapy instituted.

In the presence of infections, the use of an appropriate antifungal or antibacterial agent should be instituted. If a favorable response does not occur promptly, the corticosteroid should be discontinued until the infection has been adequately controlled.
Information for the Patient: Patients using topical corticosteroids should receive the following information and instructions:
1. This medication is to be used as directed by the dentist or physician. Avoid contact with the eyes.
2. Patients should be advised not to use this medication for any disorder other than for which it was prescribed.
3. The treated area should not be bandaged or otherwise covered or wrapped as to be occlusive unless directed by the dentist or physician.
4. Patients should report any signs of local adverse reactions especially under occlusive dressing.
Laboratory Tests: The following tests may be helpful in evaluating the HPA axis suppression:
Urinary free cortisol test
ACTH stimulation test
Carcinogenesis, Mutagenesis, and Impairment of Fertility: Long-term animal studies have not been performed to evaluate the carcinogenic potential or the affect on fertility of topical corticosteroids.
Studies to determine mutagenicity with hydrocortisone have revealed negative results.
Pregnancy Category C: Corticosteroids are generally teratogenic in laboratory animals when administered systemically at relatively low dosage levels. The more potent corticosteroids have been shown to be teratogenic after dermal application in laboratory animals. There are no adequate and well-controlled studies in pregnant women on teratogenic effects from topically applied corticosteroids. Therefore, topical corticosteroids should be used during pregnancy only if the potential benefit justifies the potential risk to the fetus. Drugs of this class should not be used extensively on pregnant patients, in large amounts, or for prolonged periods of time.
Nursing Mothers: It is not known whether topical administration of corticosteroids could result in sufficient systemic absorption to produce detectable quantities in breast milk. Systemically administered corticosteroids are secreted into breast milk in quantities not likely to have a deleterious effect on the infant. Nevertheless, caution should be exercised when topical corticosteroids are administered to a nursing woman.
Pediatric Use: Pediatric patients may demonstrate greater susceptibility to topical corticosteroid-induced HPA axis suppression and Cushing's syndrome than mature patients. Hypothalamic-pituitary-adrenal (HPA) axis suppression, Cushing's syndrome, and intracranial hypertension have been reported in children receiving topical corticosteroids. Manifestations of adrenal suppression in children include linear growth retardation, delayed weight gain, low plasma cortisol levels, and absence of response to ACTH stimulation. Manifestations of intracranial hypertension include bulging fontanelles, headaches, and bilateral papilledema. Adminstration of topical corticosteroids to children should be limited to the least amount compatible with an effective therapeutic regimen. Chronic corticosteroid therapy may interfere with the growth and development of children.

ADVERSE REACTIONS
The following local adverse reactions are reported infrequently with topical corticosteroids. These reactions are listed in an approximate decreasing order of occurrence:
Burning
Itching
Irritation
Dryness
Hypopigmentation
Perioral dermatitis

Allergic contact dermatitis
Secondary infection
Striae
Miliaria

OVERDOSAGE
Topically applied corticosteroids can be absorbed in sufficient amounts to produce systemic effects (See PRECAUTIONS).

DOSAGE AND ADMINISTRATION
Dab, *do not rub,* on the lesion until the paste adheres. (Rubbing this preparation on lesions may result in a granular, gritty sensation.) After application, a smooth, slippery film develops.
Usual adult dose: Topical, to the oral mucous membrane, 2 or 3 times a day following meals and at bedtime.
Usual pediatric dose: Dosage has not been established.

HOW SUPPLIED
Net weight 5 Gm. tubes (NDC#0126-0101-45) and 0.75 Gm. patient starter packets in boxes of 100 (NDC#0126-0101-01).

CAUTION
Federal (U.S.A.) law prohibits dispensing without a prescription.

Keep Out of Reach of Children

PHOS-FLUR® Oral Rinse/Supplement   ℞
brand of Acidulated Phosphate Fluoride

DESCRIPTION
Each teaspoonful (5 ml) contains 1.0 mg fluoride ion (F^-) from 2.2 mg sodium fluoride (NaF), in a 0.1 Molar phosphate solution at pH 4, for use as a dental caries preventive in children. Cherry, orange, lime–sugar and saccharin free. Cinnamon–contains saccharin but is sugar free.

CLINICAL PHARMACOLOGY
Sodium fluoride acts systemically (before tooth eruption) and topically (post-eruption) by increasing tooth resistance to acid dissolution, by promoting remineralization, and by inhibiting the cariogenic microbial process. Acidulation provides greater topical fluoride uptake by dental enamel than neutral solutions.[1] Phosphate protects enamel from demineralization by the acidulated formulation (common ion effect).[1]

INDICATIONS AND USAGE
It has been well established that ingestion of fluoridated drinking water (1 ppm F) during the period of tooth development results in a significant decrease in the incidence of dental caries.[2] PHOS-FLUR was developed to provide topical and systemic fluoride for use as a rinse/supplement (rinse-and-swallow) in children age 3 and older living in areas where the water fluoride level does not exceed 0.7 ppm. Where the drinking water contains more than 0.7 ppm F, PHOS-FLUR provides benefits as a topical fluoride dental rinse only (rinse-and-expectorate) for children age 6 and older.[3] Pioneering clinical studies on PHOS-FLUR were published by Frankl et al.[4] and Aasenden et al.[5] in 1972.

CONTRAINDICATIONS
DO NOT SWALLOW in areas where the F-content of drinking water exceeds 0.7 ppm, nor in children under age 3.

WARNINGS
Do not use as a rinse in children under age 6. Do not use as a supplement in children under age 3, nor in areas where the drinking water exceeds 0.7 ppm F. As in the case of all medications, keep out of reach of children. Orange Flavor contains FD&C Yellow No. 6.

PRECAUTIONS
See "Overdosage" section below. Incompatibility of systemic fluoride with dairy foods has been reported due to formation of calcium fluoride which is poorly absorbed.

ADVERSE REACTIONS
Allergic reactions and other idiosyncrasies have been rarely reported.

OVERDOSAGE
Prolonged daily ingestion of excessive fluoride will result in varying degrees of dental fluorosis. (The total amount of sodium fluoride in a bottle of 500ml PHOS-FLUR Rinse/Supplement conforms to the recommendations of the American Dental Association for the maximum to be dispensed at one time for safety purposes).

DOSAGE AND ADMINISTRATION
As A Daily Dental Rinse—Children age 6 and over, preferably at bedtime after thoroughly brushing the teeth, rinse one teaspoonful (5 ml) or two teaspoonfuls (10 ml) vigorously around and between teeth for one minute, then expectorate.
As A Daily Supplement—Children age 3 and over, in areas where the drinking water contains less than 0.3 ppm F, rinse one teaspoonful (5 ml) as above and swallow. When drinking water contains 0.3 to 0.7 ppm F, inclusive, reduce dosage to ½ teaspoonful.

HOW SUPPLIED

Bottles of	Flavors	NDC# 0126
250 ml	cherry	0129-99
500 ml	cherry	0129-46
	cinnamon	0126-46
	lime	0017-46
	orange	0128-46
1 gallon	cherry	0129-28

CAUTION

Federal (U.S.A.) law prohibits dispensing without prescription.

REFERENCES

[1]F. Brudevold et al. Arch. Oral Biol. 8:167–177, 1963. [2]Accepted Dental Therapeutics, American Dental Association, Chicago, 1984, p. 399–402. [3]Ibid., p. 399–402. [4]S.N. Frankl, S. Fleisch, and R. P. Diodati. J.A.D.A. 85:882–886, 1972. [5]R. Aasenden, P.F. DePaola, and F. Brudevold. Arch. Oral Biol. 17:1705–1714, 1972.

POINT–TWO® Dental Rinse
brand of Sodium Fluoride   ℞

DESCRIPTION

0.2% sodium fluoride (NaF) in a mint-flavored, neutral aqueous solution containing 6% alcohol. For weekly use as a caries preventive in children.

CLINICAL PHARMACOLOGY

Topical application of sodium fluoride increases tooth resistance to acid dissolution, promotes remineralization, and inhibits the cariogenic microbial process.

INDICATIONS AND USAGE

It has been established that weekly rinsing with a neutral 0.2% sodium fluoride solution protects against dental caries in children.[1] POINT-TWO Rinse was developed to provide a ready-to-use, flavored preparation for convenient administration and favorable compliance.

CONTRAINDICATIONS

None. (May be used whether drinking water is fluoridated or not, since **topical** fluoride cannot produce fluorosis).

WARNINGS

DO NOT SWALLOW. Do not use in children under age 6, since younger children frequently cannot perform the rinse process without significant swallowing. As in the case of all medications, keep out of reach of children.

PRECAUTIONS

Not for systemic use. (Each 5 ml contains 5 mg fluoride ion).

ADVERSE REACTIONS

In patients with mucositis, gingival tissues may be hypersensitive to flavor or alcohol present in formulation.

OVERDOSAGE

In the event a dose is accidentally swallowed, nausea and/or vomiting may result (treat with milk or antacids).

DOSAGE AND ADMINISTRATION[2]

Children age 6 to 12, one teaspoonful (5 ml); over age 12, 2 teaspoonfuls (10 ml). Once a week, preferably at bedtime after thoroughly brushing the teeth, rinse vigorously around and between the teeth for one minute, then expectorate. DO NOT SWALLOW. For maximum benefit, do not eat, drink, or rinse mouth for at least 30 minutes afterwards.

HOW SUPPLIED

Bottles of 8 fl. oz. with child-resistant closure. (Mint—NDC #0126-0178-99)
Gallon (with pump dispenser) (Mint—NDC #0126-0178-28)

CAUTION

Federal (U.S.A.) law prohibits dispensing without prescription.

REFERENCES

[1]Accepted Dental Therapeutics, Ed. 40, American Dental Association, Chicago, 1984, p. 404–405. [2]Ibid. p. 405.

PREVIDENT® Brush-On Gel
brand of Neutral Sodium Fluoride   ℞

DESCRIPTION

Self-topical neutral fluoride containing 1.1% sodium fluoride for use as a dental caries preventive in children and adults. This prescription product is not a dentifrice.

CLINICAL PHARMACOLOGY

Frequent topical applications to the teeth with preparations having a relatively high fluoride content increase tooth resistance to acid dissolution and enhance penetration of the fluoride ion into tooth enamel.

INDICATIONS AND USAGE

It is well established that 1.1% sodium fluoride is safe and extraordinarily effective as a caries preventive when applied frequently with mouthpiece applicators[1-4]. PreviDent Brush-On Gel in a squeeze-tube is a particularly convenient dosage form which permits the application of a thin ribbon of gel onto a toothbrush as well as a mouthpiece tray.

CONTRAINDICATIONS

None (May be used in areas where drinking water is fluoridated or not, because topical fluoride cannot produce fluorosis).

WARNINGS

As with all medications, keep out of reach of children. Use in children under age 6 requires special supervision to prevent repeated swallowing of gel which could cause dental fluorosis. Fruit Sherbet Flavor contains FD&C Yellow No. 6.

OVERDOSE

Accidental ingestion of a usual treatment dose (1-2 mgF) is not harmful.

DOSAGE AND ADMINISTRATION

Adults and children 6 years of age and older. Apply daily a thin ribbon of gel to the teeth with a toothbrush or mouth-trays, for at least one minute preferably at bedtime, after brushing with toothpaste. After use, expectorate gel and rinse mouth thoroughly.

HOW SUPPLIED

2 oz plastic tubes and 0.8 oz plastic tubes.
2 oz   Fresh mint flavor—NDC #0126-0088-02
      Cool lime flavor—NDC #0126-0089-02
      Very berry flavor—NDC #0126-0288-02
      Bing cherry flavor—NDC #0126-0290-02
      Fruit sherbet flavor—NDC #0126-0289-02
0.8 oz   Very berry flavor—NDC #0126-0288-82
      Fruit sherbet flavor—NDC #0126-0289-82
      Fresh mint flavor—NDC #0126-0088-82
      Bing cherry flavor—NDC #0126-0290-82

CAUTION

Federal (U.S.A.) law prohibits dispensing without prescription.

REFERENCES

1. Accepted Dental Therapeutics, Ed. 40, ADA, Chicago, p. 405-407, 1984.
2. Englander HR, Keyes PH and Gestwicki M: JADA 75:638-644, 1967.
3. Englander HR et al: JADA 78:783-787, 1969.
4. Englander HR et al: JADA 82:354-358, 1971.

THERA–FLUR® Topical Gel–Drops
brand of Acidulated Phosphate Fluoride   ℞
THERA–FLUR®–N Topical Gel–Drops
brand of Neutral Sodium Fluoride   ℞

DESCRIPTION

THERA-FLUR (acidulated) gel-drops contains 0.5% fluoride ion (F⁻) from 1.1% sodium fluoride (NaF) in a lime-flavored aqueous solution containing 0.1 Molar phosphate at pH 4.5. THERA-FLUR-N (neutral) also contains 0.5% (F⁻) from 1.1% NaF, but with no acid phosphate, nor artificial flavor or color, at neutral pH. For daily self-topical use as a dental caries preventive.

CLINICAL PHARMACOLOGY

Frequent topical applications to the teeth with preparations having a relatively high fluoride content increase tooth resistance to acid dissolution and enhance penetration of the fluoride ion into tooth enamel.

INDICATIONS AND USAGE

It is well established that 1.1% sodium fluoride is a safe and effective caries preventive when applied frequently with mouthpiece applicators.[1] Pioneering clinical studies with THERA-FLUR and THERA-FLUR-N Gel-Drops in schoolchildren were conducted by Englander et al.[2,3,4]
Both neutral and acidulated phosphate fluoride gels have been effective in controlling rampant dental decay which frequently follows xerostomia-producing radiotherapy of tumors in the head and neck region.[5,6]

CONTRAINDICATIONS

None (May be used in areas where drinking water is fluoridated or not, because **topical** fluoride cannot produce fluorosis).

WARNINGS

As with all medications, keep out of reach of children.

PRECAUTIONS

Laboratory tests indicate that use of acidulated fluoride may cause dulling of porcelain and ceramic restorations. Therefore, THERA-FLUR-N (neutral) is recommended for this type of patient.

ADVERSE REACTIONS

In patients with mucositis, gingival tissues may be hypersensitive to the acidity of THERA-FLUR, but will tolerate THERA-FLUR-N (neutral).

OVERDOSAGE

Accidental ingestion of a usual treatment dose (2–4 mg F) is not harmful.

DOSAGE AND ADMINISTRATION

Age 6 and older. For daily use with applicators supplied by the dentist.[2] Apply 4 to 8 drops as required to cover inner surface of each applicator. Spread gel-drops with tip of bottle. Place applicators over upper and lower teeth at the same time. Bite down lightly for 6 minutes. Remove applicators and rinse mouth. Clean applicators with cold water.

HOW SUPPLIED

24 ml plastic squeeze bottles.

		NDC# 0126-
THERA-FLUR (lime flavor)	24ml	0048-54
THERA-FLUR-N (no artificial flavor or color)	24ml	0196-54

CAUTION

Federal (U.S.A.) law prohibits dispensing without prescription.

REFERENCES

[1]Accepted Dental Therapeutics, Ed.40, American Dental Association, Chicago, 1984, p. 405–407. [2]H. R. Englander, P. H. Keyes, and M. Gestwicki. J.A.D.A. 75:638-644, 1967. [3]H. R. Englander et al. J.A.D.A. 78:783-787, 1969. [4]H. R. Englander et al. J.A.D.A. 82:354-358, 1971. [5]E. Johansen and T. O. Olsen in "Continuing Evaluation of the Use of Fluorides" (AAAS Selected Symposium 11), Westview Press, Boulder, CO, 1979, p.66. [6]S. Dreizen et al. J. Dent. Res. 56:99-104, 1977.

Connaught Laboratories, Inc.
SWIFTWATER, PA 18370

DIPHTHERIA AND TETANUS TOXOIDS AND PERTUSSIS VACCINE ADSORBED USP (FOR PEDIATRIC USE)   ℞

Caution: Federal (U.S.A.) law prohibits dispensing without prescription.

DESCRIPTION

Diphtheria and Tetanus Toxoids and Pertussis Vaccine Adsorbed USP, for intramuscular use, combines diphtheria and tetanus toxoids, adsorbed with pertussis vaccine in a sterile isotonic sodium chloride solution containing sodium phosphate to control pH; each 0.5 ml injection contains not more than 0.25 mg of aluminum added in the form of aluminum potassium sulfate. Thimerosal (mercury derivative) 1:10,000 is added as a preservative. The vaccine, in suspension, is a turbid liquid, whitish in color. Each single dose of 0.5 ml is formulated to contain 6.7 Lf units of diphtheria toxoid and 5 Lf units of tetanus toxoid. The total human immunizing dose (the first three 0.5 ml doses given) contains an estimate of 12 units of pertussis vaccine.[1] Each component of the vaccine — diphtheria, tetanus and pertussis — meets the required potency standards.

CLINICAL PHARMACOLOGY

Simultaneous immunization against diphtheria, tetanus, and pertussis during infancy and childhood has been a routine practice in the United States since the late 1940s. This practice has played a major role in markedly reducing the incidence rates of cases and deaths from each of these diseases.[2]

DIPHTHERIA

Cornyebacterium diphtheriae may cause both a localized and a generalized disease. The systemic intoxication is caused by diphtheria exotoxin, an extracellular protein metabolite of toxigenic strains of *C. diphtheriae*.
At one time, diphtheria was common in the United States. More than 200,000 cases, primarily among children, were reported in 1921. Approximately 5%–10% of cases were fatal; the highest case-fatality ratios were in the very young and the elderly. Reported cases of diphtheria of all types declined from 306 in 1975 to 59 in 1979; most were cutaneous diphtheria reported from a single state. After 1979, cutaneous diphtheria was no longer reportable. From 1980 to 1983, only 15 cases of respiratory diphtheria were reported; 11 occurred among persons 20 years of age or older.[2]
The current rarity of diphtheria in the United States is due primarily to the high level of appropriate immunization among children (96% of children entering school have received three or more doses of Diphtheria and Tetanus Tox-

Continued on next page

The simultaneous administration of DTP, oral polio virus vaccine (OPV), and/or measles-mumps-rubella vaccine (MMR) has resulted in seroconversion rates and rates of side effects similar to those observed when the vaccines are administered separately.[2,10] Therefore, if there is any doubt that a vaccine recipient will return for further vaccine doses, the ACIP recommends the simultaneous administration of all vaccines appropriate to the age and previous vaccination status of the recipient. This would especially include the simultaneous administration of DTP, OPV, and MMR to such persons at 15 months of age or older.[2]

PRECAUTIONS
GENERAL
Epinephrine Injection (1:1000) must be immediately available should an acute anaphylactic reaction occur due to any component of the vaccine.

Prior to an injection of any vaccine, all known precautions should be taken to prevent side reactions. This includes a review of the patient's history with respect to possible sensitivity and any previous adverse reactions to the vaccine or similar vaccines (see CONTRAINDICATIONS), and a current knowledge of the literature concerning the use of the vaccine under consideration.

The vial of vaccine should be vigorously shaken to ensure a proper suspension of the antigen and adjuvant.

Special care should be taken to ensure that the injection does not enter a blood vessel.

A separate sterile syringe and needle or a sterile disposable unit should be used for each individual patient to prevent transmission of hepatitis or other infectious agents from one person to another.

PEDIATRIC USE
THIS VACCINE IS RECOMMENDED FOR IMMUNIZING CHILDREN 6 WEEKS THROUGH 6 YEARS (UP TO THE SEVENTH BIRTHDAY) OF AGE ONLY. Do NOT administer to persons 7 years of age and older.
INFORMATION FOR PATIENT
Parents should be fully informed of the benefits and risks of immunization with DTP.

Prior to administration of any dose of DTP, the parent or guardian should be asked about the recent health status of the infant or child to be injected.

The physician should inform the parents or guardian about the significant adverse reactions that need to be monitored.

As part of the infant's or child's immunization record, informed consent should be obtained and recorded. The lot number and manufacturer of the vaccine administered should be recorded in the event of the occurrence of any symptoms and/or signs of an adverse reaction. Vaccine information sheets are available from the CDC or the State Health Department which may serve as guidelines.

WHEN AN INFANT OR CHILD IS RETURNED FOR THE NEXT DOSE IN THE SERIES, THE PARENT SHOULD BE QUESTIONED CONCERNING OCCURRENCE OF ANY SYMPTOMS AND/OR SIGNS OF AN ADVERSE REACTION AFTER PREVIOUS DOSE (see CONTRAINDICATIONS; ADVERSE REACTIONS).

ADVERSE REACTIONS
Not all adverse events following administration of DTP are causally related to DTP vaccine.

Adverse reactions which may be local and include pain, erythema, heat, edema and induration with or without tenderness, are common after the administration of vaccines containing diphtheria, tetanus, or pertussis antigens. Some data suggest that febrile reactions are more likely to occur in those who have experienced such responses after prior doses.[11] However, these observations were not noted by Barkin, R.M., et al.[12] Occasionally, a nodule may be palpable at the injection site of adsorbed products for several weeks. Sterile abscesses at the site of injection have been reported (6–10 per million doses).

Mild systemic reactions, such as fever, drowsiness, fretfulness, and anorexia, occur quite frequently. These reactions are significantly more common following DTP than following DT, are usually self-limited, and need no therapy other than, perhaps, symptomatic treatment (e.g., antipyretics).[2] Rash, allergic reactions, and respiratory difficulties, including apnea, have been observed.

Moderate to severe systemic events, such as fever of 40.5°C (105°F) or higher, persistent, inconsolable crying lasting 3 hours or more, unusual high-pitched crying, collapse, or convulsions, occur relatively infrequently. More severe neurologic complications, such as a prolonged convulsion or an encephalopathy, occasionally fatal, have been reported to be associated with DTP administration.[2]

Approximate rates for adverse events following receipt of DTP vaccine (regardless of dose number in the series) are indicated in Table 1.[2,13,14]

The frequency of local reactions and fever following DTP vaccination is significantly higher with increasing numbers of doses of DTP, while other mild to moderate systemic reactions (e.g., fretfulness, vomiting) are significantly less frequent.[13] If local redness of 2.5 cm or greater occurs, the likelihood of recurrence after another DTP dose increases significantly.[11]

In the National Childhood Encephalopathy Study (NCES), a large, case-control study in England,[14] children 2–35 months of age with serious, acute neurologic disorders, such as encephalopathy or complicated convulsion(s), were more likely to have received DTP in the 7 days preceding onset than their age-, sex-, and neighborhood-matched controls. Among children known to be neurologically normal before entering the study, the relative risk (estimated by odds ratio) of a neurologic illness occurring within the 7-day period following receipt of DTP dose, compared to children not receiving DTP vaccine in the 7-day period before onset of their illness, was 3.3 (p < 0.001). Within this 7-day period, the risk was significantly increased for immunized children only within 3 days of vaccination (relative risk 4.2, p < 0.001). The relative risk for illness occurring 4–7 days after vaccination was 2.1 (0.05 < p < 0.1). The attributable risk estimates for a serious acute neurologic disorder within 7 days after DTP vaccine (regardless of outcome) was one in 110,000 doses of DTP, and for a permanent neurologic deficit, one in 310,000 doses. No specific clinical syndrome was identified. Overall, DTP vaccine accounted for only a small proportion of cases of serious neurologic disorders reported in the population studied.[2] Although there are uncertainties in the reported studies, recent data suggest that infants and young children who have had previous convulsions (whether febrile or nonfebrile) are more likely to have seizures following DTP than those without such histories.[2,15]

Rarely, an anaphylactic reaction (i.e., hives, swelling of the mouth, difficulty breathing, hypotension, or shock) has been reported after receiving preparations containing diphtheria, tetanus, and/or pertussis antigens.[2]

Arthus-type hypersensitivity reactions, characterized by severe local reactions (generally starting 2–8 hours after an injection), may follow receipt of tetanus toxoid, particularly in adults who have received frequent (e.g., annual) boosters of tetanus toxoid. A few cases of peripheral neuropathy have been reported following tetanus toxoid administration, although a causal relationship has not been established.[2]

Sudden infant death syndrome (SIDS) has occurred in infants following administration of DTP. A large case-control study of SIDS in the United States showed that receipt of DTP was not causally related to SIDS.[16] It should be recognized that the first three primary immunizing doses of DTP are usually administered to infants 2–6 months old and that approximately 85% of SIDS cases occur at ages 1–6 months, with the peak incidence occurring at 6 weeks–4 months of age. By chance alone, some SIDS victims can be expected to have recently received vaccine.[2]

Onset of infantile spasms has occurred in infants who have recently received DTP or DT. Analysis of data from the NCES on children with infantile spasms showed that receipt of DTP or DT was not causally related to infantile spasms.[17] The incidence of onset of infantile spasms increases at 3–9 months of age, the time period in which the second and third doses of DTP are generally given. Therefore, some cases of infantile spasms can be expected to be related by chance to recent receipt of DTP.[2]

TABLE 1.[2] Adverse events occurring within 48 hours of DTP Immunizations

Event	Frequency*
Local	
Redness	$^1/_3$ doses
Swelling	$^2/_5$ doses
Pain	$^1/_2$ doses
Mild/moderate systemic	
Fever > 38°C (100.4°F)	$^1/_2$ doses
Drowsiness	$^1/_3$ doses
Fretfulness	$^1/_2$ doses
Vomiting	$^1/_{15}$ doses
Anorexia	$^1/_5$ doses
More serious systemic	
Persistent, inconsolable crying (duration ≥ 3 hours)	$^1/_{100}$ doses
High-pitched, unusual cry	$^1/_{900}$ doses
Fever ≥ 40.5°C (≥ 105°F)	$^1/_{330}$ doses
Collapse (hypotonic-hyporesponsive (episode)	$^1/_{1,750}$ doses
Convulsions (with or without fever)	$^1/_{1,750}$ doses
Acute encephalopathy†	$^1/_{110,000}$ doses
Permanent neurologic deficit†	$^1/_{310,000}$ doses

* Number of adverse events per total number of doses regardless of dose number in DTP series.

† Occurring within 7 days of DTP immunization.

Reporting of Adverse Events
Reporting by parents and patients of all adverse events occurring within 4 weeks of antigen administration should be encouraged. Adverse events that require a visit to a health-care provider should be reported by health-care providers to manufacturers and local or state health departments. The information will be forwarded to an appropriate federal agency (the Office of Biologics Research and Review, FDA, or CDC).[2]

The following illnesses have been reported as temporally associated with the vaccine; neurological complications[18] including cochlear lesion,[19] brachial plexus neuropathies,[19,20] paralysis of the radial nerve,[21] paralysis of the recurrent nerve,[19] accommodation paresis, and EEG disturbances with encephalopathy.[13] In the differential diagnosis of polyradiculoneuropathies following administration of a vaccine containing tetanus toxoid, tetanus toxoid should be considered as a possible etiology.[22]

DOSAGE AND ADMINISTRATION
Parenteral drug products should be inspected visually for extraneous particulate matter and/or discoloration prior to administration whenever solution and container permit. If these conditions exist, vaccine should not be administered.

Epinephrine Injection (1:1000) must be immediately available should an acute anaphylactic reaction occur due to any component of the vaccine.

SHAKE VIAL WELL *before withdrawing each dose. Vaccine contains a bacterial suspension. Vigorous agitation is required to resuspend the contents of the vial.*

Inject 0.5 ml intramuscularly. The vastus lateralis (mid-thigh laterally) is the preferred injection site for infants. The gluteus maximus should be avoided due to the potential for damage to the sciatic nerve. During the course of primary immunization, injections should not be made more than once at the same site.

Do NOT administer this product subcutaneously. Special care should be taken to ensure that the injection does not enter a blood vessel.

This vaccine is recommended for children 6 weeks through 6 years of age (up to seventh birthday) ideally beginning when the infant is 6 weeks to 2 months of age in accordance with the following schedules indicated in Table 2.[2]

[See table left].

Persons 7 years of age and older must NOT be immunized with Pertussis Vaccine.

HOW SUPPLIED
Vial, 7.5 ml — Product No. 49281-280-84

STORAGE
Store between 2°– 8°C (35°– 46°F). DO NOT FREEZE. Temperature extremes may adversely affect resuspendability of this vaccine.

REFERENCES
1. Code of Federal Regulations, 21CFR620.4(g), 1985
2. Recommendation of the Immunization Practices Advisory Committee. Diphtheria, Tetanus, and Pertussis: Guidelines for vaccine prophylaxis and other preventive measures. MMWR 34:405–426, 1985

TABLE 2.[2] Routine diphtheria, tetanus, and pertussis immunization schedule summary for children under 7 years old — United States, 1985*

Dose	Age/Interval†	Product
Primary 1	6 weeks old or older	DTP†£
Primary 2	4–8 weeks after first dose§	DTP£
Primary 3	4–8 weeks after second dose§	DTP£
Primary 4	6–12 months after third dose§	DTP£
Booster	4–6 years old, before entering kindergarten or elementary school (not necessary if fourth primary immunizing dose administered on or after fourth birthday)	DTP£
Additional boosters	Every 10 years after last dose	Td

* Important details are in the text.

† Customarily begun at 8 weeks of age, with second and third doses given at 8-week intervals.

§ Prolonging the interval does not require restarting series.

£ DT, if pertussis vaccine is contraindicated. If the child is 1 year of age or older at the time the primary dose is given, a third dose 6–12 months after the second completes primary immunization with DT.

Continued on next page

Connaught—Cont.

3. Manclark, C.R., et al: Pertussis. In R. Germanier (ed), Bacterial Vaccines Academic Press Inc., NY 69–106, 1984

4. Hinman, A.R., et al: Pertussis and pertussis vaccine. Reanalysis of benefits, risks, and costs. JAMA 251:3109–3113, 1984

5. Aoyama, T., et al: Efficacy of an acellular pertussis vaccine in Japan. J Pediatr 107:180–183, 1985

6. Sato, Y., et al: Development of a pertussis component vaccine in Japan. Lancet 122–126, 1984

7. Report of the Committee on Infectious Diseases. Immunization of premature infants. American Academy of Pediatrics, 1982

8. Bernbaum, J.C., et al: Response of preterm infants to diphtheria-tetanus-pertussis immunizations. J Pediatr 107:184–188, 1985

9. Wilson, G.S.: The Hazards of Immunization. Provocation poliomyelitis. 270–274, 1967

10. Deforest, A., et al: Simultaneous administration of MMR, OPV and DTP vaccines. Presented at the 24th Interscience Conference on Antimicrobial Agents and Chemotherapy, Washington, DC (abstract #86). October, 1984

11. Baraff, L., et al: DTP—associated reactions: An analysis by injection site, manufacturer, prior reactions and dose. Pediatr 73:31, 1984

12. Barkin, R.M., et al: Diphtheria-pertussis-tetanus vaccine: Reactogenicity of commercial products. Pediatr 63:256, 1979

13. Cody, C.L., et al: Nature and rates of adverse reactions associated with DTP and DT immunizations in infants and children. Pediatr 68: 650–660, 1981

14. Miller, D.L., et al: Pertussis immunization and serious acute neurological illness in children. Br Med J [Clin Res] 282: 1595–1599, 1981

15. CDC. Adverse events following immunization surveillance. Surveillance Report No. 1, 1979–1982 (August 1984)

16. Hoffman, H.J.: SIDS and DTP. 17th Immunization Conference Proceedings, Atlanta, GA: Centers for Disease Control: 79–88, 1982

17. Bellman, M.H., et al: Infantile spasms and pertussis immunization. Lancet, i: 1031–1034, 1983

18. Fenichel, G.M., Neurological complications of immunization. Ann Neurol 12:119–128, 1982

19. Wilson, G.S.: The Hazards of Immunization. Allergic manifestations: Post-vaccinal neuritis. 153–156, 1967

20. Tsairis, P., et al: Natural history of brachial plexus neuropathy. Arch Neurol 27: 109–117, 1972

21. Blumstein, G.I., et al: Peripheral neuropathy following Tetanus toxoid administration. JAMA 198:1030–1031, 1966

22. Schlenska, G.K.: Unusual neurological complications following tetanus toxoid administration. J Neurol 215:299–302, 1977.

Product Information
as of July, 1986
0906

ProHIBiT®   ℞
HAEMOPHILUS b CONJUGATE VACCINE
(Diphtheria Toxoid-Conjugate)

Caution: Federal (U.S.A.) law prohibits dispensing without prescription.

DESCRIPTION
ProHIBiT®, Haemophilus b Conjugate Vaccine (Diphtheria Toxoid-Conjugate), for intramuscular use, is a sterile solution, prepared from the purified capsular polysaccharide, a polymer of ribose, ribitol and phosphate (PRP) of the Eagen *Haemophilus influenzae* type b strain covalently bound to diphtheria toxoid (D) and dissolved in sodium phosphate buffered isotonic sodium chloride solution. The polysaccharide-protein conjugate molecule is referred to as PRP-D. Thimerosal (mercury derivative) 1:10,000 is added as a preservative. The vaccine is a clear, colorless solution. Each single dose of 0.5 ml is formulated to contain 25 mcg of purified capsular polysaccharide and 18 mcg of diphtheria toxoid protein.

CLINICAL PHARMACOLOGY
Haemophilus influenzae type b (Haemophilus b) is a leading cause of serious systemic bacterial disease in the United States. It is the most common cause of bacterial meningitis, accounting for an estimated 12,000 cases annually, primarily among children under 5 years of age. The mortality rate is 5%, and neurologic sequelae are observed in as many as 25%–35% of survivors.[1] Most cases of *Haemophilus influenzae* meningitis among children are caused by capsular strains of type b, although this capsular type represents only one of the six types known for this species. In addition to bacterial meningitis, Haemophilus b is responsible for other invasive diseases, including epiglottitis, sepsis, cellulitis, septic arthritis, osteomyelitis, pericarditis, and pneumonia.[1] In the United States, approximately one of every 1,000 children under 5 years of age develops systemic Haemophilus b disease each year, and a child's cumulative risk of developing systemic Haemophilus b disease at some time during the first 5 years of life is about one in 200. Attack rates peak between 6 months and 1 year of age and decline thereafter.[1] Approximately 30%–38% of Haemophilus b disease occurs among children 18 months of age or older, and 15%–25% occurs above 24 months of age.[2,3,4] Incidence rates of Haemophilus b disease are increased in certain high-risk groups, such as Native Americans (both American Indian and Eskimos), blacks, individuals of lower socioeconomic status, and patients with asplenia, sickle cell disease, Hodgkin's disease, and antibody deficiency syndromes.[1,4] Recent studies also have suggested that the risk of acquiring primary Haemophilus b disease for children under 5 years of age appears to be greater for those who attend day-care facilities than for those who do not.[5,6]

The potential for person-to-person transmission of the organism among susceptible individuals has been recognized. Studies of secondary spread of disease in household contacts of index patients have shown a substantially increased risk among exposed household contacts under 4 years of age.[7] In addition, numerous clusters of cases in day-care facilities have been reported, and recent studies suggest that secondary attack rates in day-care classroom contacts of a primary case also may be increased.[8,9] Adults can be colonized with *Haemophilus influenzae* type b from children infected with the organism.[10]

In 1974, a randomized controlled trial was conducted in Finland, which allowed the evaluation of clinical efficacy of a non-conjugated Haemophilus type b polysaccharide vaccine in children 3–71 months of age.[11] Approximately 98,000 children, half of whom received the Haemophilus b vaccine, were enrolled in the field trial and followed for a 4-year period for the occurrence of Haemophilus b disease. Among children 18–71 months of age, 90% protective efficacy (95% confidence limits, 55%–98%) in prevention of all forms of invasive Haemophilus b disease was demonstrated for the 4-year follow-up period.

Based on evidence from this 1974 Finnish efficacy trial, from passive protection in the infant rat model, and from experience with agammaglobulinemic children, an antibody concentration of ≥ 0.15 mcg/ml has been correlated with protection.[11,12,13,14] In three-week post-vaccination serum in the 1974 Finnish trial, antibody levels of ≥ 1 mcg/ml were correlated with long-term protection.[11]

The development of stable humoral immunity requires the recognition of foreign material by at least two separate sets of lymphocytes. These sets are the B-lymphocytes which are precursors of antibody forming cells, and the T-lymphocytes which can modulate the function of B-cells. Some antigens such as polysaccharides are capable of stimulating B-cells directly to produce antibody (T-independent). The responses to many other antigens are augmented by helper T-lymphocytes (T-dependent).[15] ProHIBiT utilizes a new technology, covalent bonding of the capsular polysaccharide of *Haemophilus influenzae* type b to diphtheria toxoid, to produce an antigen which is postulated to convert the T-independent antigen into a T-dependent antigen.[16,17] The protein carries both its own antigenic determinants and those of the covalently bound polysaccharide. As a result of the conjugation to protein, the polysaccharide is postulated to be presented as a T-dependent antigen resulting in both an enhanced antibody response and an immunologic memory. In studies for functional activity, anti-capsular antibodies induced by ProHIBiT had bactericidal activity, opsonic activity and were also active in passive protection assays.[18,19,20]

In studies conducted with ProHIBiT in several locations throughout the U.S., the antibody responses of 18–26 month old children were measured. (Table 1)[18] In other studies, the antibody responses to licensed Haemophilus b polysaccharide vaccines were measured in a comparable age group. (Table 1)[18] The data shown in Table 1 were obtained from sera tested in one laboratory using a single radioimmunoassay (RIA). Mean antibody levels induced by ProHIBiT in children 18–20 months of age are 30-fold higher than those induced by polysaccharide vaccines in the same age group.[18] The RIA procedure used by Connaught Laboratories, Inc. to estimate antibody responses to the Haemophilus b vaccines has been shown to correlate with the assay used by the Finland National Public Health Institute.[21] Antibody levels (≥ 1.0 mcg/ml) estimated by the Finnish assay were correlated with protection.[11]
[See table below].

Following immunization of 16–24 month old children with a single dose of ProHIBiT, eighty-nine percent (109/123) had antibody levels ≥ 0.15 mcg/ml 12 months post immunization, compared to 93% 1 month post vaccination.[18]

A group of 36 patients with sickle cell disease (SS, SC, S-thalassemia), aged 1.5 to 5.0 years (mean 3.3 years), was immunized with ProHIBiT. All produced titers of ≥ 0.15 mcg/ml and 94% produced titers of ≥ 1.0 mcg/ml.[18,22]

INDICATIONS AND USAGE
ProHIBiT is indicated for the routine immunization of children 18 months to 5 years of age against invasive diseases caused by *Haemophilus influenzae* type b. As with other vaccines, several days following administration of ProHIBiT are required for protective levels of antibody to be attained.
A booster dose of ProHIBiT is *not* required.
ProHIBiT will not protect against *Haemophilus influenzae* other than type b or other microorganisms that cause meningitis or septic disease.
No impairment of the immune response to the individual antigens was demonstrated when ProHIBiT and Diphtheria and Tetanus Toxoids and Pertussis Vaccine Adsorbed (DTP) were given at the same time at separate sites.[23]
Because the safety and efficacy of ProHIBiT have not been established in children less than 18 months of age. ProHIBiT is not indicated for use in this age group at this time. Studies to establish the safety and efficacy of ProHIBiT in children less than 18 months of age are ongoing.[24]
ProHIBiT IS NOT RECOMMENDED FOR USE IN CHILDREN YOUNGER THAN 18 MONTHS OF AGE.

CONTRAINDICATIONS
HYPERSENSITIVITY TO ANY COMPONENT OF THE VACCINE, INCLUDING THIMEROSAL AND DIPHTHERIA TOXOID, IS A CONTRAINDICATION TO USE OF THIS VACCINE.

WARNINGS
If ProHIBiT is used in persons with malignancies or those receiving immunosuppressive therapy or who are otherwise immunocompromised, the expected immune response may not be obtained.
As with any vaccine, ProHIBiT may not protect 100% of individuals receiving the vaccine.

PRECAUTIONS
GENERAL
As with the injection of any biological material, Epinephrine Injection (1:1000) should be available for immediate use should an anaphylactic or other allergic reaction occur.
Prior to an injection of any vaccine, all known precautions should be taken to prevent adverse reactions. This includes a review of the patient's history with respect to possible hypersensitivity to the vaccine or similar vaccines.
Any febrile illness or acute infection is reason to delay the use of ProHIBiT.
As reported with Haemophilus b to polysaccharide vaccine,[25] cases of Haemophilus b disease may occur in the week after vaccination, prior to the onset of the protective effects of the vaccine.
Special care should be taken to ensure that the injection does not enter a blood vessel.
A separate, sterile syringe and needle or a sterile disposable unit should be used for each individual patient to prevent

TABLE 1
Immunogenicity Studies of ProHIBiT and Polysaccharide Vaccines*[18]

Vaccine	Age Group	No. of Subjects	Anti-Polysaccharide GMT (mcg/ml) Pre	Anti-Polysaccharide GMT (mcg/ml) Post	% Subjects Responding with ≥ 1.0 mcg/ml**
ProHIBiT	18–21 Mo.	173	0.025	2.85	75%
	22–26 Mo.	37	0.021	2.96	73%
POLYSACCHARIDE	18–20 Mo.	51	0.021	0.100	24%
	24–27 Mo.	84	0.035	0.520	43%

* Only subjects whose sera had preimmunization levels ≤ 0.60 mcg/ml were included in this analysis.

** A subset of these data was obtained from a randomized comparison of the two vaccines, in which the percentage of children 18–20 months of age responding with ≥ 1.0 mcg/ml was 75% for ProHIBiT (n = 12) and 27% for the polysaccharide (n = 11).

transmission of hepatitis or other infectious agents from one person to another.

ALTHOUGH SOME IMMUNE RESPONSE TO THE DIPHTHERIA TOXOID COMPONENT MAY OCCUR, IMMUNIZATION WITH ProHIBiT DOES NOT SUBSTITUTE FOR ROUTINE DIPHTHERIA IMMUNIZATION.

CARCINOGENESIS, MUTAGENESIS, IMPAIRMENT OF FERTILITY

ProHIBiT has not been evaluated for its carcinogenic, mutagenic potential or impairment of fertility.

PREGNANCY

REPRODUCTIVE STUDIES — PREGNANCY CATEGORY C

Animal reproduction studies have not been conducted with ProHIBiT. It is also not known whether ProHIBiT can cause fetal harm when administered to a pregnant woman or can affect reproduction capacity. ProHIBiT is NOT recommended for use in a pregnant woman.

ADVERSE REACTIONS

When ProHIBiT alone was given to over 1,000 adults and children, no serious adverse reactions were observed.[17,18,26] Thrombocytopenia was seen in one adult but a causative relationship was not established.

When ProHIBiT was given with DTP and Inactivated Poliovirus Vaccine to 30,000 young infants, the rate and extent of serious adverse reactions were not different from those seen when DTP was administered alone. Allergic reactions such as urticaria were infrequently observed.[18,24]

Selected adverse reactions following vaccination with ProHIBiT (without DTP) in subjects 16–24 months of age are summarized in Table 2.

TABLE 2
Percentage of Subjects 16–24 Months Of Age
Developing Local Reactions or Fever to One
Dose of Haemophilus b Conjugate Vaccine
(Diphtheria Toxoid-Conjugate)[18]

	No. of Subjects*	Reaction % 6 Hours	24 Hours	48 Hours
Fever >38.3℃	281	1.1	2.1	1.8
Erythema	285	—	2.5	0.4
Induration	285	—	1.0	0.4
Tenderness	285	—	4.6	0.7

*Not all subjects had measurements at all time periods. Other adverse reactions temporally associated with administration of ProHIBiT including diarrhea, vomiting, and crying were reported at a frequency of ≤1.2%.[26]

Adverse reactions in clinical evaluations among 689 children, 7–14 months of age, 24 hours after receiving a single dose of ProHIBiT, were observed and compared to 139 children who received a saline placebo. There were no significant differences in the reaction rates for fever, erythema, induration, and tenderness between the two groups.[18]

DOSAGE AND ADMINISTRATION

Parenteral drug products should be inspected visually for extraneous particulate matter and/or discoloration prior to administration whenever solution and container permit. If these conditions exist, vaccine should not be administered.

ProHIBiT is indicated for children 18 months to 5 years of age. The immunizing dose is a single injection of 0.5 ml given intramuscularly in the outer aspect area of the vastus lateralis (mid-thigh) or deltoid.

Each 0.5 ml dose contains 25 mcg of purified capsular polysaccharide and 18 mcg of conjugated diphtheria toxoid protein.

Before injection, the skin over the site to be injected should be cleansed with a suitable germicide. After insertion of the needle, aspirate to ensure that the needle has not entered a blood vessel.

DO NOT INJECT INTRAVENOUSLY.

HOW SUPPLIED

Vial, 1 Dose (5 per package) — Product No. 49281-541-01
Vial, 5 Dose — Product No. 49281-541-05
Vial, 10 Dose — Product No. 49281-541-10

STORAGE

Store between 2°– 8℃ (35°– 46°F). DO NOT FREEZE.

REFERENCES

1. Recommendation of the Immunization Practices Advisory Committee. Polysaccharide vaccine for prevention of *Haemophilus influenzae* type b disease. MMWR 34:201–205, 1985
2. Cochi, S.L., et al: Immunization of U.S. children with *Hemophilus influenzae* type b polysaccharide vaccine: A cost-effectiveness model of strategy assessment. JAMA 253:521–529, 1985
3. Murphy, T.V., et al: Prospective surveillance of *Haemophilus influenzae* type b disease in Dallas County, Texas, and in Minnesota. Pediatr 79:173–179, 1987
4. Broome, C.V.: Epidemiology of *Haemophilus influenzae* type b infections in the United States. Pediatr Infect Dis J 6:779–782, 1987
5. Istre, G.R., et al: Risk factors for primary invasive *Haemophilus influenzae* disease: Increased risk from day care attendance and school-aged household members. J Pediatr 106: 190–195, 1985
6. Redmond, S.R., et al:*Hemophilus influenzae* type b disease. An epidemiologic study with special reference to day-care centers. JAMA 252: 2581–2584, 1984
7. CDC. Prevention of secondary cases of *Haemophilus influenzae* type b disease. MMWR 31:672–680, 1982
8. Murphy, T.V., et al: County-wide surveillance of invasive *Haemophilus* infections: Risk of associated cases in child care programs (CCPs). Twenty-third Interscience Conference on Antimicrobial Agents and Chemotherapy (Abstract #788) 229, 1983
9. Fleming, D., et al: *Haemophilus influenzae* b (Hib) disease—secondary spread in day care. Twenty-fourth International Conference on Antimicrobial Agents and Chemotherapy (Abstract #967) 261, 1984
10. Michaels, R.H., et al: Pharyngeal colonization with *Haemophilus influenzae* type b: A longitudinal study of families with a child with meningitis or epiglottitis due to *H. Influenzae* type b. J Infec Dis 136: 222–227, 1977
11. Peltola, H., et al: Prevention of Hemophilus influenzae type b bacteremic infections with the capsular polysaccharide vaccine. N Engl J Med 310: 1561–1566, 1984
12. Smith, D.H., et al: Responses of children immunized with the capsular polysaccharide of *Hemophilus influenzae*, type b. Pediatr 52:637–644, 1973
13. Robbins, J.B., et al: Quantitative measurement of "natural" and immunization-induced *Haemophilus influenzae* type b capsular polysaccharide antibodies. Pediatr Res 7:103–110, 1973
14. Robbins, J.B., et al: A review of the efficacy trials with *Haemophilus influenzae* type b polysaccharide vaccine. In: Sell, S.H., Wright, P.E. eds. *Haemophilus influenzae*. New York: Elsevier Science Publishing Co. 255–263, 1982
15. Benacerraf, B., et al: Textbook of Immunology. Cellular interactions. Williams and Wilkins, p. 22, 1979
16. Schneerson, R., et al: Preparation, characterization, and immunogenicity of *Haemophilus influenzae* type b polysaccharide-protein conjugates. J Exp Med 152: 361–376, 1980
17. Lepow, M.L., et al: Safety and immunogenicity of *Haemophilus influenzae* type b polysaccharide diphtheria toxoid conjugate vaccine in infants 9 to 15 months of age. J Pediatr 106: 185, 1985
18. Unpublished data available from Connaught Laboratories, Inc.
19. Granoff, D.M., et al: Immunogenicity of *Haemophilus influenzae* type b polysaccharide-diphtheria toxoid conjugate vaccine in adults. J Pediatr 105: 22–27, 1984
20. Cates, K.L.: Serum opsonic activity for *Haemophilus influenzae* type b in infants immunized with polysaccharide-protein conjugate vaccines. J Infec Dis 152: 1076–1077, 1985
21. Greenberg, D.P., et al: Variability in quantitation of *Haemophilus influenza* type b anticapsular antibody (anti-PRP) by radioimmunoassay (RIA). Twenty-sixth Interscience Conference on Antimicrobial Agents and Chemotherapy (Abstract #209) 133, 1986
22. Frank, A.L., et al: *H. influenzae* b immunization of children with sickle cell diseases. Pediatr Res Vol 21, #4, (Abstract #906), 1987
23. Hendley, J.O., et al: Immunogenicity of *Haemophilus influenzae* type b capsular polysaccharide vaccines in 18-month-old infants. Pediatr 80:351–354, 1987
24. Eskola, J., et al: Efficacy of *Haemophilus influenzae* type b polysaccharide — diphtheria toxoid conjugate vaccine in infancy. N Engl J Med 317:717–722, 1987
25. FDA Workshop on Haemophilus b polysaccharide vaccine—A Preliminary Report, MMWR 36:529–531, 1987
26. Berkowitz, C.D., et al: Safety and immunogenicity of *Haemophilus influenzae* type b polysaccharide and polysaccharide diphtheria toxoid conjugate vaccines in children 15 to 24 months of age. J Pediatr 110:509–514, 1987

Product information
as of December, 1987
0585

Products are
listed alphabetically
in the
PINK SECTION.

Consolidated Midland Corp.
195 EAST MAIN STREET
BREWSTER, NY 10509

ACTIBINE® ℞
Brand of Yohimbine hydrochloride

DESCRIPTION

Yohimbine is a 3α-15α-20β-17α-hydroxy Yohimbine-16α-carboxylic acid methyl ester. The alkaloid is found in Rubaceae and related trees. Also in Rauwolfia Serpentina (L) Benth. Each compressed tablet contains 5 mg of Yohimbine Hydrochloride.

ACTION

Yohimbine blocks presynaptic alpha-2 adrenergic receptors. Its action on peripheral blood vessels resembles that of reserpine though it is weaker and of short duration. Yohimbine's periperal autonomic nervous system effect is to increase parasympathetic (cholinergic) and decrease sympathetic (adrenergic) activity. It is to be noted that in male sexual performance, erection is linked to cholinergic activity and to alpha-2 adrenergic blockade which may theoretically result in increased penile inflow, decreased penile outflow or both. Yohimbine exerts a stimulation action on the mood and may increase anxiety. Such actions have not been adequately studied or related to dosage although they appear to require high doses of the drug. Yohimbine has a mild anti-diuretic action, probably via stimulation of hypothalmic centers and release of posterior pituitary hormone.

Reportedly, Yohimbine exerts no significant influence on cardiac stimulation and other effects mediated by β-adrenergic receptors, its effect on blood pressure, if any, would be to lower it; however, no adequate studies are at hand to quantitate this effect in terms of Yohimbine dosage.

INDICATIONS

No claims are made by the manufacturer for effectiveness in any indications. At present there is a growing interest among urologists to use Yohimbine HCl experimentally for the treatment and for the diagnostic classification of certain types of male erectile impotence. Yohimbine is a sympathicolytic agent.

CONTRAINDICATION

Renal diseases, and patient's sensitive to the drug. In view of the limited and inadequate information at hand, no precise tabulation can be offered of additional contra-indications.

WARNING

Generally, this drug is not proposed for use in females and certainly must not be used during pregnancy. Neither is this drug proposed for use in pediatric, geriatric or cardio-renal patients with gastric or duodenal ulcer history. Nor should it be used in conjunction with mood-modifying drugs such as antidepressants, or in psychiatric patients in general.

ADVERSE REACTIONS

Yohimbine readily penetrates the (CNS) and produces a complex pattern of responses in lower doses than required to produce peripheral α-adrenergic blockade. These include, antidiuresis, a general picture of central excitation including elevation of blood pressure and heart rate increased motor activity, irritability and tremor. Sweating, nausea and vomiting are common after parenteral administration of the drug. Also dizziness, headache, skin flushing reported when used orally.

DOSAGE AND ADMINISTRATION

Experimental dosage reported in treatment of erectile impotence: 1 tablet (5 mg) 4 times a day, to adult males taken orally. Occasional side effects reported with dosage are nausea, dizziness or nervousness. In the event of side effects dosage is to be reduced to ½ tablet 4 times a day, followed by gradual increases to 1 tablet 4 times a day. Reported therapy not more than 10 weeks.

HOW SUPPLIED

Oral tablets of Actibin 5 mg in bottles of 100's, U.D. (Unit Dose) 100's, and 1000's.

Products are cross-indexed by
generic and chemical names
in the
YELLOW SECTION

Cook-Waite Laboratories, Inc.

90 PARK AVENUE
NEW YORK, NEW YORK 10016

CARBOCAINE® ℞
hydrochloride 3% Injection
(mepivacaine hydrochloride
injection, USP)

CARBOCAINE® ℞
hydrochloride 2%
with NEO–COBEFRIN®
1:20,000 Injection
(mepivacaine hydrochloride
and levonordefrin injection, USP)

THESE SOLUTIONS ARE INTENDED FOR DENTAL USE ONLY.

DESCRIPTION

Carbocaine hydrochloride (mepivacaine hydrochloride), a tertiary amine used as a local anesthetic, is 1-methyl-2′, 6′-pipecoloxylidide monohydrochloride with the following structural formula:

It is a white, crystalline, odorless powder soluble in water, but very resistant to both acid and alkaline hydrolysis.
Neo-Cobefrin (levonordefrin), a sympathomimetic amine used as a vasoconstrictor in local anesthetic solutions, is (−)-α-(1-Aminoethyl)-3, 4-dihydroxybenzyl alcohol with the following structural formula:

It is a white or buff-colored crystalline solid, freely soluble in aqueous solutions of mineral acids, but practically insoluble in water.
DENTAL CARTRIDGES MAY NOT BE AUTOCLAVED.
CARBOCAINE hydrochloride 3% Injection and CARBOCAINE hydrochloride 2% with Neo-Cobefrin 1:20.000 Injection are sterile solutions for injection.

COMPOSITION

Each ml contains:	2%	3%
mepivacaine hydrochloride	20.0 mg	30.0 mg
levonordefrin	0.05 mg	—
sodium chloride	4.0 mg	3.0 mg
acetone sodium bisulfite not more than	2.0 mg	—
water for injection, qs ad	1.0 ml	1.0 ml

The pH of the 2% cartridge solution is adjusted between 3.3 and 5.5 with NaOH or HCl.
The pH of the 3% cartridge solution is adjusted between 4.5 and 6.8 with NaOH or HCl.

CLINICAL PHARMACOLOGY

CARBOCAINE stabilizes the neuronal membrane and prevents the initiation and transmission of nerve impulses, thereby effecting local anesthesia.
CARBOCAINE is rapidly metabolized, with only a small percentage of the anesthetic (5 to 10 per cent) being excreted unchanged in the urine. CARBOCAINE, because of its amide structure, is not detoxified by the circulating plasma esterases. The liver is the principal site of metabolism, with over 50 per cent of the administered dose being excreted into the bile as metabolites. Most of the metabolized mepivacaine is probably resorbed in the intestine and then excreted into the urine since only a small percentage is found in the feces. The principal route of excretion is via the kidney. Most of the anesthetic and its metabolites are eliminated within 30 hours. It has been shown that hydroxylation and N-demethylation, which are detoxification reactions, play important roles in the metabolism of the anesthetic. Three metabolites of mepivacaine have been identified from adult humans: two phenols, which are excreted almost exclusively as their glucuronide conjugates, and the N-demethylated compound (2′,6′-pipecoloxylidide).
The onset of action is rapid (30 to 120 seconds in the upper jaw; 1 to 4 minutes in the lower jaw) and CARBOCAINE hydrochloride 3% without vasoconstrictor will ordinarily provide operating anesthesia of 20 minutes in the upper jaw and 40 minutes in the lower jaw.
CARBOCAINE hydrochloride 2% with Neo-Cobefrin 1:20,000 provides anesthesia of longer duration for more prolonged procedures, 1 hour to 2.5 hours in the upper jaw and 2.5 hours to 5.5 hours in the lower jaw.
CARBOCAINE does not ordinarily produce irritation or tissue damage.
Neo-Cobefrin is a sympathomimetic amine used as a vasoconstrictor in local anesthetic solutions. It has pharmacologic activity similar to that of epinephrine but it is more stable than epinephrine. In equal concentrations, Neo-Cobefrin is less potent than epinephrine in raising blood pressure, and as a vasoconstrictor.

INDICATIONS AND USAGE

CARBOCAINE is indicated for production of local anesthesia for dental procedures by infiltration or nerve block in adults and children.

CONTRAINDICATIONS

Mepivacaine is contraindicated in patients with a known hypersensitivity to amide type local anesthetics.

WARNINGS

RESUSCITATIVE EQUIPMENT AND DRUGS SHOULD BE IMMEDIATELY AVAILABLE. (See Adverse Reactions). Reactions resulting in fatality have occurred on rare occasions with the use of local anesthetics, even in the absence of a history of hypersensitivity.
Fatalities may occur with use of local anesthetics in the head and neck region as the result of retrograde arterial flow to vital CNS areas even when maximum recommended doses are observed. The practitioner should be alert to early evidences of alteration in sensorium or vital signs.
The solution which contains a vasoconstrictor should be used with extreme caution for patients whose medical history and physical evaluation suggest the existence of hypertension, arteriosclerotic heart disease, cerebral vascular insufficiency, heart block, thyrotoxicosis and diabetes, etc.
Carbocaine hydrochloride 2% with Neo-Cobefrin 1:20,000 injection (mepivacaine hydrochloride and levonordefrin injection, USP) contains acetone sodium bisulfite, a sulfite that may cause allergic-type reactions including anaphylactic symptoms and life-threatening or less severe asthmatic episodes in certain susceptible people. The overall prevalence of sulfite sensitivity in the general population is unknown and probably low. Sulfite sensitivity is seen more frequently in asthmatic than in nonasthmatic people.
Carbocaine hydrochloride 3% injection (mepivacaine hydrochloride injection, USP) IS SULFITE FREE.

PRECAUTIONS

The safety and effectiveness of mepivacaine depend upon proper dosage, correct technique, adequate precautions, and readiness for emergencies.
The lowest dose that results in effective anesthesia should be used to avoid high plasma levels and possible adverse effects.
Injection of repeated doses of mepivacaine may cause significant increase in blood levels with each repeated dose due to slow accumulation of the drug or its metabolites, or due to slower metabolic degradation than normal.
Tolerance varies with the status of the patient. Debilitated, elderly patients, acutely ill patients, and children should be given reduced doses commensurate with their weight and physical status.
Mepivacaine should be used with caution in patients with a history of severe disturbances of cardiac rhythm or heart block.
INJECTIONS SHOULD ALWAYS BE MADE SLOWLY WITH ASPIRATION TO AVOID INTRAVASCULAR INJECTION AND THEREFORE SYSTEMIC REACTION TO BOTH LOCAL ANESTHETIC AND VASOCONSTRICTOR.
If sedatives are employed to reduce patient apprehension, use reduced doses, since local anesthetic agents, like sedatives, are central nervous system depressants which in combination may have an additive effect. Young children should be given minimal doses of each agent.
Changes in sensorium such as excitation, disorientation, drowsiness, may be early indications of a high blood level of the drug and may occur following inadvertent intravascular administration or rapid absorption of mepivacaine.
Local anesthetic procedures should be used with caution when there is inflammation and/or sepsis in the region of the proposed injection.
Information for Patients: The patient should be cautioned against loss of sensation and possibility of biting trauma should the patient attempt to eat or chew gum prior to return of sensation.
Drug Interactions: The solution which contains a vasoconstrictor should also be used with extreme caution in patients receiving drugs known to produce blood pressure alterations (i.e., MAO inhibitors, tricyclic anti-depressants, phenothiazines, etc.) as either sustained hypotension or hypertension may occur.
Solutions containing a vasoconstrictor should be used cautiously in the presence of diseases which may adversely affect the patient's cardiovascular system. Serious cardiac arrhythmias may occur if preparations containing a vasoconstrictor are employed in patients during or following the administration of potent inhalation anesthetics.

Mepivacaine SHOULD BE USED WITH CAUTION IN PATIENTS WITH KNOWN DRUG ALLERGIES AND SENSITIVITIES. A thorough history of the patient's prior experience with mepivacaine or other local anesthetics as well as concomitant or recent drug use should be taken (see Contraindications). Patients allergic to methylparaben or para-aminobenzoic acid derivatives (procaine, tetracaine, benzocaine, etc.) have not shown cross-sensitivity to agents of the amide type such as mepivacaine. Since mepivacaine is metabolized in the liver and excreted by the kidneys, it should be used cautiously in patients with liver and renal disease.
Carcinogenesis, Mutagenesis, Impairment of Fertility: Studies of CARBOCAINE hydrochloride in animals to evaluate the carcinogenic and mutagenic potential or the effect on fertility have not been conducted.
Pregnancy Category C: Animal reproduction studies have not been conducted with this solution. It is also not known whether this solution can cause fetal harm when administered to a pregnant woman or can effect reproduction capacity. This solution should be given to a pregnant woman only if clearly needed.
Nursing Mothers: It is not known whether this drug is excreted in human milk. Because many drugs are excreted in human milk, caution should be exercised when this solution is administered to a nursing woman.
Pediatric Use: Great care must be exercised in adhering to safe concentrations and dosages for pedodontic administration (see Dosage and Administration).

ADVERSE REACTIONS

Systemic adverse reactions involving the central nervous system and the cardiovascular system usually result from high plasma levels due to excessive dosage, rapid absorption, or inadvertent intravascular injection.
A small number of reactions may result from hypersensitivity, idiosyncrasy or diminished tolerance to normal dosage on the part of the patient.
Reactions involving the *central nervous system* are characterized by excitation and/or depression. Nervousness, dizziness, blurred vision, or tremors may occur followed by drowsiness, convulsions, unconsciousness, and possibly respiratory arrest. Since excitement may be transient or absent, the first manifestations may be drowsiness merging into unconsciousness and respiratory arrest.
Cardiovascular reactions are depressant. They may be the result of direct drug effect or more commonly in dental practice, the result of vasovagal reaction, particularly if the patient is in the sitting position. Failure to recognize premonitory signs such as sweating, feeling of faintness, changes in pulse or sensorium may result in progressive cerebral hypoxia and seizure or serious cardiovascular catastrophe. Management consists of placing the patient in the recumbent position and administration of oxygen. Vasoactive drugs such as ephedrine or methoxamine may be administered intravenously.
Allergic reactions are rare and may occur as a result of sensitivity to the local anesthetic and are characterized by cutaneous lesions of delayed onset or urticaria, edema and other manifestations of allergy. The detection of sensitivity by skin testing is of limited value. As with other local anesthetics, anaphylactoid reactions to CARBOCAINE have occurred rarely. The reaction may be abrupt and severe and is not usually dose related. Localized puffiness and swelling may occur.

OVERDOSAGE

Treatment of a patient with toxic manifestations consists of assuring and maintaining a patent airway and supporting ventilation (respiration) as required. This usually will be sufficient in the management of most reactions. Should a convulsion persist despite ventilatory therapy, small increments of anticonvulsive agents may be given intravenously, such as benzodiazepine (e.g., diazepam) or ultrashort-acting barbiturates (e.g., thiopental or thiamylal) or short-acting barbiturate (e.g., pentobarbital or secobarbital). Cardiovascular depression may require circulatory assistance with intravenous fluids and/or vasopressor (e.g., ephedrine) as dictated by the clinical situation. Allergic reactions should be managed by conventional means.
IV and SC LD_{50}'s in mice for CARBOCAINE hydrochloride 3% are 33 and 258 mg/kg respectively. The acute IV and SC LD_{50}'s in mice for CARBOCAINE hydrochloride 2% with Neo-Cobefrin 1:20,000 are 30 and 184 mg/kg respectively.

DOSAGE AND ADMINISTRATION

As with all local anesthetics, the dose varies and depends upon the area to be anesthetized, the vascularity of the tissues, individual tolerance and the technique of anesthesia. The lowest dose needed to provide effective anesthesia should be administered. For specific techniques and procedures refer to standard dental manuals and textbooks.
For infiltration and block injections in the upper or lower jaw, the average dose of 1 cartridge will usually suffice.
Each cartridge contains 1.8 ml (36 mg of 2% or 54 mg of 3%). Five cartridges (180 mg of the 2% solution or 270 mg of the 3% solution) are usually adequate to effect anesthesia of the entire oral cavity. Whenever a larger dose seems to be neces-

sary for an extensive procedure, the maximum dose should be calculated according to that patient's weight. A dose of up to 3 mg per pound of body weight may be administered. At any single dental sitting the total dose for all injected sites should not exceed 400 mg in adults.

The maximum pediatric dose should be *carefully calculated*

Maximum Dose for Children =

$$\frac{\text{Child's Weight (lbs.)}}{150} \times \frac{\text{Maximum Recommended Dose}}{\text{for Adults (400 mg)}}$$

The following table, approximating these calculations, may also be used as a guide. This table is based upon a recommended maximum for larger children of 5 cartridges (the maximum recommended adult dose) during any single dental sitting, regardless of the child's weight or (for 2% mepivacaine) calculated maximum amount of drug:
[See table above].

When using CARBOCAINE for infiltration or regional block anesthesia, injection should always be made slowly and with frequent aspiration.

Any unused portion of a cartridge should be discarded.

Parenteral drug products should be inspected visually for particulate matter and discoloration prior to administration, whenever solution and container permit.

DISINFECTION OF CARTRIDGES

As in the case of any cartridge, the diaphragm should be disinfected before needle puncture. The diaphragm should be thoroughly swabbed with either pure 91% isopropyl alcohol or 70% ethyl alcohol, USP just prior to use. Many commercially available alcohol solutions contain ingredients which are injurious to container components, and therefore, should not be used. Cartridges should not be immersed in any solution.

HOW SUPPLIED

Both formulas are available in 1.8 ml cartridges, containers of 50, to fit the Carpule® Aspirator.

The 2% solution should be stored at controlled room temperature, between 15° and 30°C (59° and 86°F).

2% solution	Code 0101	NDC 0961-0010-04
3% solution	Code 0201	NDC 0961-0020-04

Marketed by
COOK-WAITE LABORATORIES, INC.
Mfd. by Sterling Drug Inc.
New York, NY 10016
Carbocaine and Neo-Cobefrin are the registered trademarks of Sterling Drug Inc.

For full prescribing information on the medical use of CARBOCAINE, see Winthrop Pharmaceuticals product listing in this publication.

MARCAINE® hydrochloride 0.5%   ℞
with epinephrine 1:200,000 (as bitartrate)
brand of bupivacaine and epinephrine injection, USP
THIS SOLUTION IS INTENDED FOR DENTAL USE

DESCRIPTION

Bupivacaine hydrochloride is 1-butyl-2′, 6′-pipecoloxylidide hydrochloride, a white crystalline powder that is freely soluble in 95 per cent ethanol, soluble in water, and slightly soluble in chloroform or acetone. It has the following structural formula:

Epinephrine is (-)-3,4-Dihydroxy-α-[(methylamino)methyl] benzyl alcohol. It has the following structural formula:

MARCAINE is available in a sterile isotonic solution with epinephrine (as bitartrate) 1:200,000. Solutions of MARCAINE containing epinephrine may not be autoclaved. MARCAINE is related chemically and pharmacologically to the aminoacyl local anesthetics. It is a homologue of mepivacaine and is chemically related to lidocaine. All three of these anesthetics contain an amide linkage between the aromatic nucleus and the amino or piperidine group. They differ in this respect from the procaine-type local anesthetics, which have an ester linkage.

Maximum Allowable Dosage

	3% Mepivacaine (Plain)		2% Mepivacaine 1:20,000 Levonordefrin	
	3 mg/lb. (270 mg. max.)		3 mg/lb. (180 mg. max.)	
Weight (lb.)	Mg.	Number of Cartridges	Mg.	Number of Cartridges
20	60	1.1	60	1.6
30	90	1.7	90	2.5
40	120	2.2	120	3.3
50	150	2.8	150	4.2
60	180	3.3	180	5.0
80	240	4.4	180	5.0
100	270	5.0	180	5.0
120	270	5.0	180	5.0

Adapted from Malamed, Stanley F: Handbook of medical emergencies in the dental office, ed. 2, St. Louis, 1982. The C.V. Mosby Co.

CLINICAL PHARMACOLOGY

MARCAINE stabilizes the neuronal membrane and prevents the initiation and transmission of nerve impulses, thereby effecting local anesthesia.

The onset of action following dental injections is usually 2 to 10 minutes and anesthesia may last two or three times longer than lidocaine and mepivacaine for dental use, in many patients up to 7 hours. The duration of anesthetic effect is prolonged by the addition of epinephrine 1:200,000. It has also been noted that there is a period of analgesia that persists after the return of sensation, during which time the need for strong analgesic is reduced.

After injection of MARCAINE for caudal, epidural or peripheral nerve block in man, peak levels of MARCAINE In the blood are reached in 30 to 45 minutes, followed by a decline to insignificant levels during the next three to six hours. Because of its amide structure, MARCAINE is not detoxified by plasma esterases but is detoxified, via conjugation with glucuronic acid, in the liver. When administered in recommended doses and concentrations, MARCAINE does not ordinarily produce irritation or tissue damage, and does not cause methemoglobinemia.

Systemic absorption of local anesthetics produces effects on the cardiovascular and central nervous systems (CNS). At blood concentrations achieved with normal therapeutic doses, changes in cardiac conduction, excitability, refractoriness, contractility, and peripheral vascular resistance are minimal. However, toxic blood concentrations depress cardiac conduction and excitability, which may lead to atrioventricular block, ventricular arrhythmias, and cardiac arrest, sometimes resulting in fatalities. In addition, myocardial contractility is depressed and peripheral vasodilation occurs, leading to decreased cardiac output and arterial blood pressure. Recent clinical reports and animal research suggest that these cardiovascular changes are more likely to occur after unintended intravascular injection of bupivacaine. Therefore, incremental dosing is necessary.

Following systemic absorption, local anesthetics can produce central nervous system stimulation, depression, or both. Apparent central stimulation is manifested as restlessness, tremors and shivering progressing to convulsions, followed by depression and coma progressing ultimately to respiratory arrest. However, the local anesthetics have a primary depressant effect on the medulla and on higher centers. The depressed stage may occur without a prior excited state.

INDICATIONS AND USAGE

MARCAINE is indicated for the production of local anesthesia for dental procedures by infiltration injection or nerve block in adults.

MARCAINE is not recommended for children.

CONTRAINDICATION

MARCAINE is contraindicated in patients with a known hypersensitivity to it or to any local anesthetic agent of the amide type or to other components of MARCAINE solutions.

WARNINGS

LOCAL ANESTHETICS SHOULD BE EMPLOYED ONLY BY CLINICIANS WHO ARE WELL VERSED IN DIAGNOSIS AND MANAGEMENT OF DOSE-RELATED TOXICITY AND OTHER ACUTE EMERGENCIES WHICH MIGHT ARISE FROM THE BLOCK TO BE EMPLOYED, AND THEN ONLY AFTER INSURING THE *IMMEDIATE* AVAILABILITY OF OXYGEN, OTHER RESUSCITATIVE DRUGS, CARDIOPULMONARY RESUSCITATIVE EQUIPMENT, AND THE PERSONNEL RESOURCES NEEDED FOR PROPER MANAGEMENT OF TOXIC REACTIONS AND RELATED EMERGENCIES. (See also ADVERSE REACTIONS and PRECAUTIONS.) DELAY IN PROPER MANAGEMENT OF DOSE-RELATED TOXICITY, UNDERVENTILATION FROM ANY CAUSE, AND/OR ALTERED SENSITIVITY MAY LEAD TO THE DEVEL-

OPMENT OF ACIDOSIS, CARDIAC ARREST AND, POSSIBLY, DEATH.

Small doses of local anesthetics injected into the head and neck area, as small as nine to eighteen milligrams, may produce adverse reactions similar to systemic toxicity seen with unintentional intravascular injections of larger doses. Confusion, convulsions, respiratory depression, and/or respiratory arrest, cardiovascular stimulation or depression and cardiac arrest have been reported. Reactions resulting in fatalities have occurred on rare occasions. In a few cases, resuscitation has been difficult or impossible despite apparently adequate preparation and appropriate management. These reactions may be due to intra-arterial injection of the local anesthetic with retrograde flow to the cerebral circulation. Patients receiving these blocks should have their circulation and respiration monitored and be constantly observed. Resuscitative equipment and personnel for treating adverse reactions should be immediately available. Dosage recommendations should not be exceeded (See DOSAGE AND ADMINISTRATION).

It is essential that aspiration for blood or cerebrospinal fluid (where applicable) be done prior to injecting any local anesthetic, both the original dose and all subsequent doses, to avoid intravascular injection. However, a negative aspiration does *not* ensure against an intravascular injection.

Reactions resulting in fatality have occurred on rare occasions with the use of local anesthetics, even in the absence of a history of hypersensitivity.

This solution which contains a vasoconstrictor should be used with extreme caution for patients whose medical history and physical evaluation suggest the existence of hypertension, arteriosclerotic heart disease, cerebral vascular insufficiency, heart block, thyrotoxicosis and diabetes, etc., as well as patients receiving drugs likely to produce alterations in blood pressure.

MARCAINE with epinephrine 1:200,000 or other vasopressors should not be used concomitantly with ergot-type oxytocic drugs, because a severe persistent hypertension may occur. Likewise, solutions of MARCAINE containing a vasoconstrictor, such as epinephrine, should be used with extreme caution in patients receiving monoamine oxidase inhibitors (MAOI) or antidepressants of the triptyline or imipramine types, because severe prolonged hypertension may result.

Until further experience is gained in children younger than 12 years, administration of MARCAINE in this age group is not recommended.

Contains sodium metabisulfite, a sulfite that may cause allergic-type reactions including anaphylactic symptoms and life-threatening or less severe asthmatic episodes in certain susceptible people. The overall prevalence of sulfite sensitivity in the general population is unknown and probably low. Sulfite sensitivity is seen more frequently in asthmatic than in nonasthmatic people.

PRECAUTIONS

The safety and effectiveness of local anesthetics depend upon proper dosage, correct technique, adequate precautions, and readiness for emergencies.

The lowest dosage that gives effective anesthesia should be used in order to avoid high plasma levels and serious systemic side effects. Injection of repeated doses of MARCAINE may cause significant increase in blood levels with each additional dose, due to accumulation of the drug or its metabolites or due to slow metabolic degradation. Tolerance varies with the status of the patient. Debilitated, elderly patients and acutely ill patients should be given reduced doses commensurate with age and physical condition.

Because of the long duration of anesthesia, when MARCAINE 0.5% with epinephrine is used for dental injections, patients should be cautioned about the possibility of inadvertent trauma to tongue, lips, and buccal mucosa and advised

Continued on next page

Cook-Waite—Cont.

not to chew solid foods or test the anesthetized area by biting or probing.

Changes in sensorium such as excitation, disorientation, drowsiness, may be early indications of a high blood level of the drug and may occur following inadvertent intravascular administration or rapid absorption of MARCAINE.

Solutions containing a vasoconstrictor should be used cautiously in areas with limited blood supply, in the presence of diseases that may adversely affect the patient's cardiovascular system, or in patients with peripheral vascular disease. Caution is advised in administration of repeat doses of MARCAINE to patients with severe liver disease.

Local anesthetic procedures should be used with caution when there is inflammation and/or sepsis in the region of the proposed injection.

Drug Interactions: See WARNINGS concerning solutions containing a vasoconstrictor.

If sedatives are employed to reduce patient apprehension, use reduced doses, since local anesthetic agents, like sedatives, are central nervous system depressants which in combination may have an additive effect.

MARCAINE should be used cautiously in persons with known drug allergies or sensitivities, particularly to the amide-type local anesthetics.

Serious dose-related cardiac arrhythmias may occur if preparations containing a vasoconstrictor such as epinephrine are employed in patients during or following the administration of chloroform, halothane, cyclopropane, trichloroethylene, or other related agents. In deciding whether to use these products concurrently in the same patient, the combined action of both agents upon the myocardium, the concentration and volume of vasoconstrictor used, and the time since injection, when applicable, should be taken into account.

INFORMATION FOR PATIENTS: When appropriate, the dentist should discuss information including adverse reactions in the package insert for MARCAINE.

Clinically Significant Drug Interactions: The administration of local anesthetic solutions containing epinephrine or norepinephrine to patients receiving monoamine oxidase inhibitors or tricyclic antidepressants may produce severe, prolonged hypertension. Concurrent use of these agents should generally be avoided. In situations when concurrent therapy is necessary, careful patient monitoring is essential. Concurrent administration of vasopressor drugs and of ergot-type oxytocic drugs may cause severe, persistent hypertension or cerebrovascular accidents.

Phenothiazines and butyrophenones may reduce or reverse the pressor effect of epinephrine.

Carcinogenesis, Mutagenesis, Impairment of Fertility: Long-term studies in animals of most local anesthetics including bupivacaine to evaluate the carcinogenic potential have not been conducted. Mutagenic potential or the effect on fertility has not been determined. There is no evidence from human data that MARCAINE may be carcinogenic or mutagenic or that it impairs fertility.

Pregnancy Category C: Decreased pup survival in rats and an embryocidal effect in rabbits have been observed when bupivacaine hydrochloride was administered to these species in doses comparable to nine and five times respectively the maximum recommended daily human dose (400 mg). There are no adequate and well-controlled studies in pregnant women of the effect of bupivacaine on the developing fetus. Bupivacaine hydrochloride should be used during pregnancy only if the potential benefit justifies the potential risk to the fetus. This does not exclude the use of MARCAINE at term for obstetrical anesthesia or analgesia.

Nursing Mothers: It is not known whether local anesthetic drugs are excreted in human milk. Because many drugs are excreted in human milk, caution should be exercised when local anesthetics are administered to a nursing woman.

Pediatric Use: Until further experience is gained in children younger than 12 years, administration of MARCAINE in this age group is not recommended.

ADVERSE REACTIONS

Reactions to MARCAINE are characteristic of those associated with other amide-type local anesthetics. A major cause of adverse reactions to this group of drugs is excessive plasma levels, which may be due to overdosage, inadvertent intravascular injection, or slow metabolic degradation. Excessive plasma levels of the amide-type local anesthetics cause systemic reactions involving the central nervous system and the cardiovascular system. The *central nervous system effects* are characterized by excitation or depression. The first manifestation may be nervousness, dizziness, blurred vision, or tremors, followed by drowsiness, convulsions, unconsciousness, and possibly respiratory arrest. Since excitement may be transient or absent, the first manifestation may be drowsiness, sometimes merging into unconsciousness and respiratory arrest. Other central nervous system effects may be nausea, vomiting, chills, constriction of the pupils, or tinnitus. The *cardiovascular manifestations* of excessive

plasma levels may include depression of the myocardium, blood pressure changes (usually hypotension), and cardiac arrest. *Allergic reactions,* which may be due to hypersensitivity, idiosyncrasy, or diminished tolerance, are characterized by cutaneous lesions (e.g., urticaria), edema, and other manifestations of allergy. Detection of sensitivity by skin testing is of doubtful value.

Transient facial swelling and puffiness may occur near the injection site.

Treatment of Reactions: Toxic effects of local anesthetics require symptomatic treatment: there is no specific cure. The dentist should be prepared to maintain an airway and to support ventilation with oxygen and assisted or controlled respiration as required. Supportive treatment of the cardiovascular system includes intravenous fluids and, when appropriate, vasopressors (preferably those that stimulate the myocardium). Convulsions may be controlled with oxygen and intravenous administration, in small increments, of a barbiturate, as follows: preferably, an ultrashort-acting barbiturate such as thiopental or thiamylal; if this is not available, a short-acting barbiturate (e.g. secobarbital or pentobarbital) or diazepam. Intravenous barbiturates or anticonvulsant agents should only be administered by those familiar with their use.

DOSAGE AND ADMINISTRATION

As with all local anesthetics, the dosage varies and depends upon the area to be anesthetized, the vascularity of the tissues, the number of neuronal segments to be blocked, individual tolerance, and the technique of anesthesia. The lowest dosage needed to provide effective anesthesia should be administered. For specific techniques and procedures refer to standard textbooks.

The 0.5% concentration with epinephrine is recommended for infiltration and block injection in the maxillary and mandibular area when a longer duration of local anesthetic action is desired, such as for oral surgical procedures generally associated with significant postoperative pain. The average dose of 1.8 ml (9 mg) per injection site will usually suffice; an occasional second dose of 1.8 ml (9 mg) may be used if necessary to produce adequate anesthesia after making allowance for 2 to 10 minutes onset time (see Clinical Pharmacology). The lowest effective dose should be employed and time should be allowed between injections; it is recommended that the total dose for all injection sites, *spread out* over a single dental sitting, should not ordinarily exceed 90 mg for a healthy adult patient (ten 1.8 ml injections of 0.5% MARCAINE with epinephrine). Injections should be made slowly and with frequent aspirations. Until further experience is gained, MARCAINE in dentistry is not recommended for children younger than 12 years.

Parenteral drug products should be inspected visually for particulate matter and discoloration prior to administration, whenever solution and container permit.

HOW SUPPLIED

Store at 25 C. May be stored for brief periods during shipment at temperatures not to exceed 30 C.

0.5% MARCAINE hydrochloride with epinephrine 1:200,000 (as bitartrate)—Sterile isotonic solutions containing sodium chloride. Each 1 ml contains 5 mg bupivacaine hydrochloride and 0.0091 mg epinephrine bitartrate, with 0.5 mg sodium metabisulfite, 0.001 ml monothioglycerol, and 2 mg ascorbic acid as antioxidants, 0.0017 ml 60% sodium lactate buffer, and 0.1 mg edetate calcium disodium as stabilizer. The pH of these solutions is adjusted with sodium hydroxide or hydrochloric acid. Solutions of MARCAINE that contain epinephrine should not be autoclaved and should be protected from light. Do not use if solution is discolored or contains a precipitate.

This solution is available in 1.8 ml cartridges, containers of 50, to fit the Carpule® Aspirator.

Code 6301　　　　　　　　　　NDC 0961-1230-50

Marketed by
Cook-Waite Laboratories, Inc.
Mfg. by Sterling Drug Inc.
New York, NY 10016
MARCAINE is the registered trademark of Sterling Drug Inc.

For full prescribing information on the medical use of Marcaine, see Winthrop Pharmaceuticals product listing in this publication.

Products are cross-indexed by
generic and chemical names in the
YELLOW SECTION

Curatek Pharmaceuticals
1965 PRATT BOULEVARD
ELK GROVE VILLAGE, IL 60007

METROGEL®　　　　　　　　　　　℞
(metronidazole)
0.75% Topical Gel
FOR TOPICAL USE ONLY
(NOT FOR OPHTHALMIC USE)

DESCRIPTION

METROGEL contains metronidazole, USP, at a concentration of 7.5 mg per gram (0.75%) in a gelled, purified water solution, containing methyl and propyl parabens, propylene glycol, carbomer 940, and edetate disodium. Metronidazole is classified therapeutically as an antiprotozoal and antibacterial agent. Chemically, metronidazole is named 2-methyl-5-nitro-1H-Imidazole-1-ethanol and has the following structure:

CLINICAL PHARMACOLOGY

Bioavailability studies on the topical administration of 1 gram of METROGEL to the face (7.5 mg of metronidazole) of 10 rosacea patients showed a maximum serum concentration of 66 nanograms per milliliter in one patient. This concentration is approximately 100 times less than concentrations afforded by a single 250 mg oral tablet. The serum metronidazole concentrations were below the detectable limits of the assay at the majority of time points in all patients. Three of the patients had no detectable serum concentrations of metronidazole at any time point. The mean dose of gel applied during clinical studies was 600 mg which represents 4.5 mg of metronidazole per application. Therefore, under normal usage levels, the formulation affords minimal serum concentrations of metronidazole.

The mechanisms by which METROGEL acts in reducing inflammatory lesions of rosacea are unknown, but may include an anti-bacterial and/or an anti-inflammatory effect.

INDICATIONS AND USAGE

METROGEL is indicated for topical application in the treatment of inflammatory papules, pustules, and erythema of rosacea.

CONTRAINDICATIONS

METROGEL is contraindicated in individuals with a history of hypersensitivity to metronidazole, parabens, or other ingredients of the formulations.

PRECAUTIONS

Because of the minimal absorption of metronidazole and consequently its insignificant plasma concentration after topical administration, the adverse experiences reported with the oral form of the drug have not been reported with METROGEL.

General

METROGEL has been reported to cause tearing of the eyes. Therefore, contact with the eyes should be avoided. If a reaction suggesting local irritation occurs, patients should be directed to use the medication less frequently, discontinue use temporarily, or discontinue use until further instructions. Metronidazole is a nitroimidazole and should be used with care in patients with evidence of, or history of, blood dyscrasia.

Information for the Patient

This medication is to be used as directed by the physician. It is for external use only. Avoid contact with the eyes.

Drug Interactions

Drug interactions are less likely with topical administration but should be kept in mind when METROGEL is prescribed for patients who are receiving anticoagulant treatment. Oral metronidazole has been reported to potentiate the anticoagulant effect of coumarin and warfarin resulting in a prolongation of prothrombin time.

Carcinogenesis: Tumorigenicity in Rodents

Metronidazole has shown evidence of carcinogenic activity in a number of studies involving chronic, oral administration in mice and rats but not in studies involving hamsters. These studies have not been conducted with 0.75% metronidazole gel, which would result in significantly lower systemic blood levels than oral formulations.

Mutagenicity Studies

Although metronidazole has shown mutagenic activity in a number of *in vitro* bacterial assay systems, studies in mammals (*in vivo*) have failed to demonstrate a potential for genetic damage.

Pregnancy: Pregnancy Category B

There has been no experience to date with the use of METROGEL in pregnant patients. Metronidazole crosses the placental barrier and enters the fetal circulation rapidly. No fetotoxicity was observed after oral metronidazole in rats or mice. However, because animal reproduction studies are not always predictive of human response and since oral metronidazole has been shown to be a carcinogen in some rodents, this drug should be used during pregnancy only if clearly needed.

Nursing Mothers

After oral administration, metronidazole is secreted in breast milk in concentrations similar to those found in the plasma. Even though METROGEL blood levels are significantly lower than those achieved after oral metronidazole, a decision should be made whether to discontinue nursing or to discontinue the drug, taking into account the importance of the drug to the mother.

Pediatric Use

Safety and effectiveness in children have not been established.

ADVERSE REACTIONS

Adverse conditions reported include watery (tearing) eyes if the gel is applied too closely to this area, transient redness, and mild dryness, burning, and skin irritation. None of the side effects exceeded an incidence of 2% of patients.

OVERDOSAGE

There is no human experience with overdosage of METROGEL. The acute oral toxicity of the METROGEL formulation was determined to be greater than 5 g/kg (the highest dose given) in albino rats.

DOSAGE AND ADMINISTRATION

Apply and rub in a thin film of METROGEL twice daily, morning and evening, to entire affected areas after washing. Significant therapeutic results should be noticed within three weeks. Clinical studies have demonstrated continuing improvement through nine weeks of therapy.

Areas to be treated should be cleansed before application of METROGEL. Patients may use cosmetics after application of METROGEL.

HOW SUPPLIED

METROGEL (0.75% metronidazole) is supplied in a 1 oz. (28.4 g) aluminum tube—NDC 55326-100-21.

Caution: Federal law prohibits dispensing without a prescription.

STORE AT CONTROLLED ROOM TEMPERATURES: 59° to 86° F; 15° to 30° C.

Issued 10/88

©1988

Daniels Pharmaceuticals, Inc.
2517 25TH AVENUE NORTH
ST. PETERSBURG, FL 33713-3999

LEVOXINE®   ℞
LEVOTHYROXINE SODIUM FOR INJECTION
LYOPHILIZED
For parenteral administration after reconstitution.

DESCRIPTION

Levothyroxine Sodium for Injection contains synthetic crystalline levothyroxine sodium (L-thyroxine). L-thyroxine is the principal hormone secreted by the normal thyroid gland. Chemically, L-thyroxine is designated as L-tyrosine, O-(4-hydroxy-3,5-diiodophenyl)-3,5-diiodo-, monosodium salt, hydrate.

The structural formula is:

The empirical formula is: $C_{15}H_{10}I_4NNaO_4 \cdot xH_2O$

Levothyroxine Sodium for Injection is a sterile lyophilized powder. Each vial contains levothyroxine sodium 200 mcg or 500 mcg, mannitol, 10 mg, tribasic sodium phosphate anhydrous, 0.7 mg. sodium hydroxide may have been used to adjust pH.

For intravenous or intramuscular administration after reconstitution with 2 mL (200 mcg strength) or 5 mL (500 mcg strength) of 0.9% Sodium Chloride Injection, USP, or Bacteriostatic Sodium Chloride Injection, USP, with benzyl alcohol, only. The resulting solution contains 100 mcg/mL.

CLINICAL PHARMACOLOGY

Levothyroxine sodium, taken orally, provides hormone that is absorbed readily from the gastrointestinal tract. Levothyroxine Sodium for Injection is effective by any parenteral route. Following absorption, the synthetic L-thyroxine pro-

vided by levothyroxine sodium cannot be distinguished from L-thyroxine that is secreted endogenously. Each is bound to the same serum proteins forming a reservoir of circulating L-thyroxine.

Levothyroxine sodium will provide L-thyroxine (T_4) as a substrate for physiologic deiodination to L-triiodothyronine (T_3). Therefore, patients taking properly adjusted doses of levothyroxine sodium will demonstrate normal blood levels of L-triiodothyronine even when the thyroid gland has been removed surgically or destroyed by radioiodine. Administration of levothyroxine sodium alone will result in complete physiologic thyroid replacement.

INDICATIONS AND USAGE

Levothyroxine sodium serves as specific replacement therapy for reduced or absent thyroid function of any etiology. Levothyroxine Sodium for Injection can be used intravenously whenever a rapid onset of effect is critical, and either intravenously or intramuscularly in hypothyroid patients whenever the oral route is precluded for long periods of time.

CONTRAINDICATIONS

There are no absolute contraindications to levothyroxine sodium therapy. Relative contraindications include acute myocardial infarction, uncorrected adrenal insufficiency and thyrotoxicosis (see WARNINGS).

> **WARNINGS**
>
> **Drugs with thyroid hormone activity, alone or together with other therapeutic agents, have been used for the treatment of obesity. In euthyroid patients, doses within the range of daily hormonal requirements are ineffective for weight reduction. Larger doses may produce serious or even life threatening manifestations of toxicity, particularly when given in association with sympathomimetic amines such as those used for anorectic effects.**

Patients with cardiovascular diseases warrant particularly close attention during the restoration of normal thyroid function by any thyroid drug. In such cases, low initial dosage increased by small increments is indicated. Occasionally, the cardiovascular capacity of the patient is so compromised that the metabolic demands of the normal thyroid state cannot be met. Clinical judgment will then dictate a less-than-complete restoration of thyroid status.

Endocrine disorders such as diabetes mellitus, adrenal insufficiency (Addison's disease), hypopituitarism and diabetes insipidus are characterized by signs and symptoms which may be diminished in severity or obscured by hypothyroidism. Levothyroxine sodium therapy for such patients may aggravate the intensity of previously obscured symptoms and require appropriate adjustment of therapeutic measures directed at these concomitant disorders.

Thyroid replacement may potentiate the effects of anticoagulants. Patients on anticoagulant therapy should have frequent prothrombin determinations when instituting thyroid replacement to gauge the need to reduce anticoagulant dosage.

PRECAUTIONS

Overdosage with any thyroid drug may produce the signs and symptoms of thyrotoxicosis, but resistance to such factitious thyrotoxicosis is the general rule.

Close observation of the patient following administration of Levothyroxine Sodium for Injection is advised, and appropriate adjustment of repeated dosage is recommended.

ADVERSE REACTIONS

Adverse reactions are due to overdosage and are those of induced hyperthyroidism.

DOSAGE AND ADMINISTRATION

Levothyroxine Sodium for Injection by intravenous or intramuscular routes can be substituted for the oral dosage form when ingestion of levothyroxine sodium tablets is precluded for long periods of time. The initial parenteral dosage should be approximately one half of the oral dosage of levothyroxine sodium tablets. Close observation of the patient, with individual adjustment of the dosage as needed, is recommended. For most adults, a final dosage of 100 mcg (0.1 mg) to 200 mcg (0.2 mg) of levothyroxine sodium tablets daily will provide adequate thyroid replacement, and only occasionally will patients require larger doses. Failure to respond adequately to a daily oral intake of 400 mcg (0.4 mg) or more is rare and should prompt reconsideration of the diagnosis of hypothyroidism, special investigation of the patient in terms of malabsorption of L-thyroxine from the gastrointestinal tract or evaluation of patient compliance to therapy.

The concomitant appearance of other diseases, especially cardiovascular diseases, usually dictates a replacement regimen with initial doses smaller than 100 mcg/day (0.1 mg). In otherwise healthy adults with relatively recent onset of hypothyroidism, full replacement doses of 150 mcg (0.15 mg) or 200 mcg (0.2 mg) have been instituted immediately with-

out untoward effect and with good therapeutic response. General experience, however, favors a more cautious approach on view of the possible presence of subclinical disorders of the cardiovascular system or other endocrinopathies. The age and general physical condition of the patient and the severity and duration of hypothyroid symptoms determine the starting dose and the rate of incremental dosage increase leading to a final maintenance dosage. In the elderly patient with long standing disease, evidence of myxedematous infiltration and symptomatic, functional or electrocardiographic evidence of cardiovascular dysfunction, the starting dose may be as little as 25 mcg (0.025 mg) per day. Further, incremental increases of 25 mcg (0.025 mg) per day may be instituted at three to four week intervals depending on patient response. Conversely, otherwise healthy adults may be started at higher daily doses and raised to a full replacement dose in two to three weeks. Clearly it is the physician's judgment of the severity of the disease and close observation of patient response which determine the rate and extent of dosage increase.

Appropriate laboratory tests are beneficial in monitoring thyroid replacement therapy. Although measurements of normal blood levels of thyroxine in patients on oral replacement regimens frequently coincide with clinical impressions of normal thyroid status, higher than normal levels occur occasionally and should not be considered evidence of overdosage per se. In all cases, clinical impressions of the well-being of the patient take precedence over laboratory determinations of appropriate individual dosage.

In infants and children, there is a great urgency to achieve full thyroid replacement because of the critical importance of thyroid hormone in sustaining growth and maturation. Despite the smaller body size, the dosage needed to sustain a full rate of growth, development and general thriving is higher in the child than in the adult.

The recommended daily replacement dosage of levothyroxine sodium in childhood is 0–1 years: 9 mcg/kg; 1–5 years: 6 mcg/kg; 6–10 years: 4 mcg/kg; 11–20 years: 3 mcg/kg. Dose is administered once daily only. Optimal maintenance levels should be adjusted individually to obtain normal serum T_3, T_4, free T_4 index and Thyroid Stimulating Hormone (TSH) values after several weeks of therapy for hypothyroidism. The patients clinical status is most important and some patients may be clinically euthyroid with individual laboratory values that are not within normal range (i.e. elevated total T_4 with normal T_3). An exception may be seen in congenital hypothyroidism where elevated serum TSH values may persist for the first 2–3 years of life despite normalization of free T_4 measurements. In such cases, it generally is recommended that maintenance of normal serum free T_4 values alone should be considered therapeutically sufficient.

In myxedema coma or stupor, without concomitant severe heart disease, 200 to 500 mcg of Levothyroxine Sodium for Injection may be administered intravenously as a solution containing 100 mcg/mL DO NOT ADD TO OTHER INTRAVENOUS FLUIDS. Although the patient may show evidence of increased responsivity within six to eight hours, full therapeutic effect may not be evident until the following day. An additional 100 to 300 mcg or more may be given on the second day if evidence of significant and progressive improvement has not occurred. Levothyroxine Sodium for Injection produces a predictable increase in the reservoir level of hormone with a seven day half-life. This usually precludes the need for multiple injections but continued daily administration of lesser amounts parenterally should be maintained until the patient is fully capable of accepting a daily oral dose. A daily maintenance dose of 50 to 100 mcg parenterally should suffice to maintain the euthyroid state, once established.

In the presence of concomitant heart disease, the sudden administration of such large doses of L-thyroxine intravenously is clearly not without its cardiovascular risks. Under such circumstances, intravenous therapy should not be undertaken without weighing the alternative risks of the myxedema coma and the cardiovascular disease. Clinical judgment in this situation may dictate smaller intravenous doses of Levothyroxine Sodium for Injection.

Parenteral drug products should be inspected visually for particulate matter and discoloration prior to administration, whenever the solution and container permit.

HOW SUPPLIED

Sterile 10 mL vials containing Levothyroxine Sodium for Injection 200 mcg or 500 mcg, lyophilized in the final containers with 10 mg Mannitol, USP and 0.7 mg tribasic sodium phosphate anhydrous. pH may have been adjusted with sodium hydroxide.

DIRECTIONS FOR RECONSTITUTION

Reconstitute the lyophilized levothyroxine sodium by aseptically adding 2 mL (200 mcg strength) or 5 mL (500 mcg strength) of 0.9% Sodium Chloride Injection, USP, or Bacteriostatic Sodium Chloride Injection, USP with benzyl alcohol, only. Shake vial to insure complete mixing. Use immedi-

Continued on next page

Daniels—Cont.

ately after reconstitution. Do not add to other intravenous fluids. Discard any unused portion.
Store at 15°–30° C (59°–86° F).

CAUTION
Federal law prohibits dispensing without prescription.
Literature Revised: July 1989
Product No.: 0732-10, 0835-10

Mfd. by Steris Laboratories, Inc.
Phoenix, Arizona 85043 USA

LEVOXINE®   ℞
(LEVOTHYROXINE SODIUM TABLETS, USP)
FOR ORAL ADMINISTRATION

DESCRIPTION
Each LEVOXINE (Levothyroxine Sodium, USP) tablet contains synthetic crystalline levothyroxine sodium (L-thyroxine). L-thyroxine is the principal hormone secreted by the normal thyroid gland. Chemically, L-thyroxine is designated as L-tyrosine, 0-(4-hydroxy-3, 5-diidophenyl) - 3,5-diiodo-, monosodium salt, hydrate. The molecular formula is $C_{15}H_{10}I_4N$ Na O_4 and the structural formula is:

CLINICAL PHARMACOLOGY
The principal effect of thyroid hormones is to increase the metabolic rate of body tissues.
The thyroid hormones are also concerned with growth and development of tissues in the young.
The major thyroid hormones are L-thyroxine (T_4) and L-triiodothyronine (T_3). The amounts of T_4 and T_3 released from the normally functioning thyroid gland are regulated by the amount of thyrotropin (TSH) secreted from the anterior pituitary gland. T_4 is the major component of normal thyroid gland excretions and is therefore the primary determinant of normal thyroid functions. T_4 acts as a substrate for physiologic deiodination to T_3 in the peripheral tissues. The physiologic effects of thyroid hormones are mediated at the cellular level primarily by T_3.
LEVOXINE (L-thyroxine) tablets taken orally provide T_4 which upon absorption can not be distinguished from T_4 that is secreted endogenously.

INDICATIONS AND USAGE
LEVOXINE (L-thyroxine) tablets are indicated as replacement or supplemental therapy for diminished or absent thyroid function (e.g., cretinism, myxedema, nontoxic goiter or hypothyroidism generally, including the hypothyroid state in children, in pregnancy and in the elderly) resulting from functional deficiency, primary atrophy, from partial or complete absence of the gland or from the effects of surgery, radiation or antithyroid agents. Therapy must be maintained continuously to control the symptoms of hypothyroidism.

CONTRAINDICATIONS
L-thyroxine therapy is contraindicated in thyrotoxicosis, acute myocardial infarction and uncorrected adrenal insufficiency.

WARNINGS

Drugs with thyroid hormone activity, alone or together with other therapeutic agents, have been used for the treatment of obesity. In euthyroid patients, doses within the range of daily hormonal requirements are ineffective for weight reduction. Larger doses may produce serious or even life-threatening manifestations of toxicity, particularly when given in association with sympathomimetic amines such as those used for their anorectic effects.

PRECAUTIONS
General—Caution must be exercised in the administration of this drug to patients with cardiovascular disease. Development of chest pains or other aggravation of the cardiovascular disease requires a reduction of dosage.
Information for the Patient—Patients on thyroid preparations and parents of children on thyroid therapy should be informed that:
1. Replacement therapy is to be taken essentially for life, with the exception of cases of transient hypothyroidism, usually associated with thyroiditis, and in those patients receiving a therapeutic trial of the drug.
2. They should immediately report during the course of therapy any signs or symptoms of thyroid hormone toxicity, e.g., chest pain, increased pulse rate, palpitations, exces-

sive sweating, heat intolerance, nervousness, or any other unusual event.
3. In case of concomitant diabetes mellitus, the daily dosage of antidiabetic medication may need readjustment as thyroid hormone replacement is achieved. If thyroid medication is stopped, a downward readjustment of the dosage of insulin or oral hypoglycemic agent may be necessary to avoid hypoglycemia. At all times, close monitoring of urinary glucose levels is mandatory in such patients.
4. In case of concomitant oral anticoagulant therapy, the prothrombin time should be measured frequently to determine if the dosage of oral anticoagulants is to be readjusted.
5. Partial loss of hair may be experienced by children in the first few months of thyroid therapy, but this is usually a transient phenomenon and later recovery is usually the rule.
Laboratory Tests—The patient's response to thyroid replacement may be followed by laboratory tests such as serum thyroxine (T_4), serum triiodothyronine (T_3), free thyroxine index and thyroid stimulating hormone (TSH) blood levels.
Drug Interactions—In patients with diabetes mellitus, addition of thyroid hormone therapy may cause an increase in the required dosage of insulin or oral hypoglycemic agents. Therefore, patients with diabetes mellitus should be observed closely for possible changes in antidiabetic dosage requirements.
Patients stabilized on oral anticoagulants who are found to require thyroid replacement therapy should be watched very closely when therapy is started. If a patient is truly hypothyroid, it is likely that a reduction in anticoagulant dosage will be required. No special precautions appear to be necessary when oral anticoagulant therapy is begun in a patient already stabilized on maintance thyroid replacement therapy. Cholestyramine binds both T_4 and T_3 in the intestine, thus impairing absorption of these thyroid hormones. In vitro studies indicate that the binding is not easily removed. Therefore, four to five hours should elapse between administration of cholestyramine and thyroid hormones.
Estrogens tend to increase serum thyroxine-binding globulin (TBg). In patients with a non-functioning thyroid gland who are receiving thyroid replacement therapy, free thyroxine may be decreased when estrogens are started thus increasing thyroid requirements. However, if the patient's thyroid gland has sufficient function the decreased free thyroxine will result in a compensatory increase in thyroxine output by the thyroid. Therefore, patients without a functioning thyroid gland who are on thyroid replacement therapy may need to increase their thyroid dose if estrogens or estrogen containing oral contraceptives are given.
Drug/Laboratory Test Interactions—The following drugs or moieties are known to interfere with laboratory tests performed on patients taking thyroid hormone: androgens, corticosteroids, estrogens, oral contraceptives containing estrogens, iodine-containing preparations, and the numerous preparations containing salicylates.
1. Changes in TBg concentration should be taken into consideration in the interpretation of T_4 and T_3 values. In such cases, the unbound (free) hormone should be measured. Pregnancy, estrogens, and estrogen-containing oral contraceptives increase TBg concentrations. TBg may also be increased during infectious hepatitis. Decreases in TBg concentrations are observed in nephrosis, acromegaly, and after androgen or corticosteroid therapy. Familial hyper- or hypo-thyroxine-binding-globulinemias have been described. The incidence of TBg deficiency approximates 1 in 9000. The binding of thyroxine by thyroid-binding prealbumin (TBPA) is inhibited by salicylates.
2. Medical or dietary iodine interferes with all in vivo tests of radio-iodine uptake, producing low uptakes which may not be reflective of a true decrease in hormone synthesis.
3. The persistence of clinical and laboratory evidence of hypothyroidism in spite of adequate dosage replacement indicates either poor patient compliance, poor absorption, excessive fecal loss, or inactivity of the preparation. Intracellular resistance to thyroid hormone is quite rare.
Carcinogenesis, Mutagenesis, And Impairment Of Fertility—A reportedly apparent association between prolonged thyroid therapy and breast cancer has not been confirmed and patients on thyroid for established indications should not discontinue therapy. No confirmatory long-term studies in animals have been performed to evaluate carcinogenic potential, mutagenicity, or impairment of fertility in either males or females.
Pregnancy—Category A—Thyroid hormones do not readily cross the placental barrier. The clinical experience to date does not indicate any adverse effect on fetuses when thyroid hormones are administered to pregnant women. On the basis of current knowledge, thyroid replacement therapy to hypothyroid women should not be discontinued during pregnancy.
Nursing Mothers—Minimal amounts of thyroid hormones are excreted in human milk. Thyroid is not associated with serious adverse reactions and does not have a known tumorigenic potential. However, caution should be exercised when thyroid is administered to a nursing woman.

Pediatric Use—Pregnant mothers provide little or no thyroid hormone to the fetus. The incidence of congenital hypothyroidism is relatively high (1:4,000) and the hypothyroid fetus would not derive any benefit from the small amounts of hormone crossing the placental barrier. Routine determinations of serum (T_4) and/or TSH is strongly advised in neonates in view of the deleterious effects of thyroid deficiency on growth and development.
Treatment should be initiated immediately upon diagnosis, and maintained for life, unless transient hypothyroidism is suspected; in which case, therapy may be interrupted for 2 to 8 weeks after the age of 3 years to reassess the condition. Cessation of therapy is justified in patients who have maintained a normal TSH during those 2 to 8 weeks.

ADVERSE REACTIONS
Adverse reactions are due to overdosage and are those of induced hyperthyroidism.
OVERDOSAGE—Excessive dosage of thyroid medication may result in symptoms of hyperthyroidism. Since, however, the effects do not appear at once, the symptoms may not appear for one to three weeks after the dosage regimen is begun. The most common signs and symptoms of overdosage are weight loss, palpitation, nervousness, diarrhea or abdominal cramps, sweating, tachycardia, cardiac arrhythmias, angina pectoris, tremors, headache, insomnia, intolerance to heat and fever. If symptoms of overdosage appear, discontinue medication for several days and reinstitute treatment at a lower dosage level.
Laboratory tests such as serum T_4, serum T_3 and the free thyroxine index will be elevated during the period of overdosage.
Complications as a result of the induced hypermetabolic state may include cardiac failure and death due to arrhythmia or failure.
TREATMENT OF OVERDOSAGE—Dosage should be reduced or therapy temporarily discontinued if signs and symptoms of overdosage appear. Treatment may be reinstituted at a lower dosage. In normal individuals, normal hypothalamic pituitary-thyroid axis function is restored in 6 to 8 weeks after thyroid suppression.
Treatment of acute massive thyroid hormone overdosage is aimed at reducing gastrointestinal absorption of the drugs and counteracting central and peripheral effects, mainly those of increased sympathetic activity. Vomiting may be induced initially if further gastrointestinal absorption can reasonably be prevented and barring contraindications such as coma, convulsions, or loss of the gagging reflex. Treatment is symptomatic and supportive. Oxygen may be administered and ventilation maintained. Cardiac glycosides may be indicated if congestive heart failure develops. Measures to control fever, hypoglycemia, or fluid loss should be instituted if needed. Antiadrenergic agents, particularly propranolol, have been used advantageously in the treatment of increased sympathetic activity. Propranolol may be administered intravenously at a dosage of 1 to 3 mg over a 10 minute period or orally, 80 to 160 mg/day, especially when no contraindications exist for its use.

DOSAGE AND ADMINISTRATION
The goal of therapy should be the restoration of euthyroidism as judged by clinical response and confirmed by appropriate laboratory tests such as serum thyroxine (T_4), serum triiodothyronine (T_3), free thyroxine index and thyroid stimulating hormone (TSH) blood levels. The age and general condition of the patient and the severity and duration of hypothyroid symptoms determine the starting dosage and the rate of incremental dosage increase leading to a final maintenance dosage.
In otherwise healthy adults, the recommended initial dosage is 25 to 100 mcg (0.025 to 0.1 mg) daily, while the predicted full maintenance dose of 100 to 200 mcg (0.1 to 0.2 mg) daily may be achieved in two to three weeks.
In the elderly patient with long standing disease, evidence of myxedema, or evidence of cardiovascular dysfunction, the initial dose may be as little as 12.5 mcg (0.0125 mg) per day. Incremental increases of 25 mcg (0.025 mg) per day at 3 to 4 week intervals may be instituted depending on patient response. It is the physician's judgment of the severity of the disease and close observation of patient response which determine the rate and extent of dosage increase.
In infants and children there is a great urgency to achieve full thyroid replacement because of the critical importance of thyroid hormone in sustaining growth and maturation. Despite the smaller body size, the dosage needed to sustain a full rate of growth, development and general thriving is higher in the child than in the adult. The recommended daily replacement dosage of L-thyroxine in childhood is: 0–6 months: 5–6 mcg/kg; 6–12 months: 5–6 mcg/kg; 1–5 years: 3–5 mcg/kg; 6–12 years: 4–5 mcg/kg of body weight daily.

DOSAGE FORMS AVAILABLE
LEVOXINE (L-thyroxine) tablets are supplied as oval, color coded, potency marked tablets in 11 strengths: 12½ mcg (0.0125 mg)—maroon, 25 mcg (0.025 mg)—orange, 50 mcg (0.05 mg)—white, 75 mcg (0.075 mg)—purple, 100 mcg (0.1 mg)—yellow, 112 mcg (0.112 mg)—rose, 125 mcg (0.125

mg)—brown, 150 mcg (0.15 mg)—blue, 175 mcg (0.175 mg)—turquoise, 200 mcg (0.2 mg)—pink and 300 mcg (0.3 mg)—green, in bottles of 100 and 1000, and unit dose in cartons of 100 (10 strips of 10 tablets) 200 mcg and 500 mcg injectable (see injectable package insert).
Revised March 1989

TUSSIGON® Tablets   ©
(hydrocodone bitartrate and homatropine methylbromide)

DESCRIPTION
Tussigon contains hydrocodone (dihydrocodeinone) bitartrate, a semisynthetic centrally-acting narcotic antitussive. Homatropine methylbromide is included in a subtherapeutic amount to discourage deliberate overdosage.
Each TUSSIGON tablet contains:
Hydrocodone Bitartarte USP... 5 mg
    WARNING: May be habit forming
Homatropine Methylbromide USP.............................. 1.5 mg
The hydrocodone component is 4,5α-epoxy-3-methoxy-17-methylmorphinan-6-one tartrate (1:1) hydrate (2.5), a fine white crystal or crystalline powder which is derived from the opium alkaloid, thebaine, has a molecular weight of (494.50) and may be represented by the following structural formula:

$$C_{18}H_{21}NO_3C_4H_6O_6 \cdot 2\tfrac{1}{2}H_2O$$
Hydrocodone Bitartrate

Homatropine methylbromide is 8-azonia-bicyclo(3,2,1)octane, 3-[(hydroxyphenyl-acetyl)oxy]-8, 8 dimethyl-, bromide-endo- a white crystal or fine white crystalline powder, with a molecular weight of (370.29).

$$C_{17}H_{24}BrNO_3$$
Homatropine Methylbromide

CLINICAL PHARMACOLOGY
Hydrocodone is a semisynthetic narcotic antitussive and analgesic with multiple actions qualitatively similar to those of codeine. The precise mechanism of action of hydrocodone and other opiates is not known; however, hydrocodone is believed to act directly on the cough center. In excessive doses, hydrocodone like other opium derivatives, will depress respiration. The effects of hydrocodone in therapeutic doses on the cardiovascular system are insignificant. Hydrocodone can produce miosis, euphoria, physical and psychological dependence.
Following a 10 mg oral dose of hydrocodone administered to five adult male subjects, the mean peak concentration was 23.6 ± 5.2 ng/ml. Maximum serum levels were achieved at 1.3 ± 0.3 hours and the half-life was determined to be 3.8 ± 0.3 hours. Hydrocodone exhibits a complex pattern of metabolism including 0-demethylation, N-demethylation and 6-keto reduction to the corresponding 6-α and 6-β-hydroxymetabolites.

INDICATION AND USAGE
TUSSIGON is indicated for the symptomatic relief of cough.

CONTRAINDICATIONS
TUSSIGON should not be administered to patients who are hypersensitive to hydrocodone or homatropine methylbromide.

WARNINGS
May be habit forming. Hydrocodone can produce drug dependence of the morphine type and, therefore, has the potential for being abused. Psychic dependence, physical dependence and tolerance may develop upon repeated administration of TUSSIGON and it should be prescribed and administered with the same degree of caution appropriate to the use of other narcotic drugs (See DRUG ABUSE AND DEPENDENCE).
Respiratory Depression: TUSSIGON produces dose-related respiratory depression by directly acting on brain stem respiratory centers. If respiratory depression occurs, it may be antagonized by the use of naloxone hydrochloride and other supportive measures when indicated.
Head Injury And Increased Intracranial Pressure: The respiratory depression properties of narcotics and their capac-

ity to elevate cerebrospinal fluid pressure may be markedly exaggerated in the presence of head injury, other intracranial lesions, or a pre-existing increase in intracranial pressure. Furthermore, narcotics produce adverse reactions which may obscure the clinical course of patients with head injuries.
Acute Abdominal Conditions: The administration of TUSSIGON or other narcotics may obscure the diagnosis or clinical course of patients with acute abdominal conditions.
Pediatric Use: In young children, as well as adults, the respiratory center is sensitive to the depressant action of narcotic cough suppressants in a dose-dependent manner. Benefit to risk ratio should be carefully considered especially in children with respiratory embarrassment (e.g., croup).

PRECAUTIONS
General: Before prescribing medication to suppress or modify cough, it is important to ascertain that the underlying cause of cough is identified, that modification of cough does not increase the risk of clinical or physiological complications, and that appropriate therapy for the primary disease is provided.
Special Risk Patients: TUSSIGON should be given with caution to certain patients such as the elderly or debilitated, and those with severe impairment of hepatic or renal functions, hypothyroidism, Addison's disease, prostatic hypertrophy or urethral stricture, asthma, and narrow-angle glaucoma.
Information For Patients: Hydrocodone may impair the mental and/or physical abilities required for the performance of potentially hazardous tasks such as driving a car or operating machinery. The patient using TUSSIGON should be cautioned accordingly.
Drug Interactions: Patients receiving narcotics, antihistamines, antipsychotics, antianxiety agents or other CNS depressants (including alcohol) concomitantly with TUSSIGON may exhibit an additive CNS depression. When combined therapy is contemplated, the dose of one or both agents should be reduced.
The use of MAO inhibitors or tricyclic antidepressants with hydrocodone preparations may increase the effect of either the antidepressants or hydrocodone.
Carcinogenesis, Mutagenesis, Impairment of Fertility: Studies of TUSSIGON in animals to evaluate the carcinogenic and mutagenic potential and the effect on fertility have not been conducted.
Pregnancy:
Teratogenic Effects: Pregnancy Category C; Animal reproduction studies have not been conducted with TUSSIGON. It is also not known whether TUSSIGON can cause fetal harm when administered to a pregnant woman or can affect reproduction capacity. TUSSIGON should be given to a pregnant woman only if clearly needed.
Nonteratogenic Effects: Babies born to mothers who have been taking opioids regularly prior to delivery will be physically dependent. The withdrawal signs include: irritability and excessive crying, tremors, hyperactive reflexes, increased respiratory rate, increased stools, sneezing, yawning, vomiting and fever. The intensity of the syndrome does not always correlate with the duration of maternal opioid use or dose.
Labor and Delivery: As with all narcotics, administration of TUSSIGON to the mother shortly before delivery may result in some degree of respiratory depression in the newborn, especially if higher doses are used.
Nursing Mothers: It is not known whether this drug is excreted in human milk. Because many drugs are excreted in human milk and because of the potential for serious adverse reactions in nursing infants from TUSSIGON, a decision should be made whether to discontinue nursing or to discontinue the drug, taking into account the importance of the drug to the mother.
Pediatric Use: Safety and effectiveness of TUSSIGON in children under six have not been established.

ADVERSE REACTIONS
Central Nervous System: Sedation, drowsiness, mental clouding, lethargy, impairment of mental and physical performance, anxiety, fear, dysphoria, dizziness, psychic dependence, mood changes.
Gastrointestinal System: Nausea and vomiting may occur; they are more frequent in ambulatory than in recumbent patients. Prolonged administration of TUSSIGON may produce constipation.
Genitourinary System: Ureteral spasm, spasm of vesicle sphincters and urinary retention have been reported with opiates.
Respiratory Depression: TUSSIGON may produce dose-related respiratory depression by acting directly on brain stem respiratory centers (see OVERDOSAGE).
Dermatological: Skin rash, pruritus.

DRUG ABUSE AND DEPENDENCE
TUSSIGON is a Schedule III narcotic. Psychic dependence, physical dependence and tolerance may develop upon repeated administration of narcotics; therefore, TUSSIGON should be prescribed and administered with caution. How-

ever, psychic dependence is unlikely to develop when TUSSIGON is used for a short time for the treatment of cough. Physical dependence, the condition in which continued administration of the drug is required to prevent the appearance of a withdrawal syndrome, assume clinically significant proportions only after several weeks of continued oral narcotic use, although some mild degree of physical dependence may develop after a few days of narcotic therapy.

OVERDOSAGE
Signs and Symptoms: Serious overdosage with hydrocodone is characterized by respiratory depression (a decrease in respiratory rate and/or tidal volume, Cheyne-Stokes respiration, cyanosis), extreme somnolence progressing to stupor or coma, skeletal muscle flaccidity, cold and clammy skin and sometimes bradycardia and hypotension. In severe overdosage apnea, circulatory collapse, cardiac arrest and death may occur. The ingestion of very large amounts of TUSSIGON may, in addition, result in acute homatropine intoxication.
Treatment: Primary attention should be given to the reestablishment of adequate respiratory exchange through provision of a patent airway and the institution of assisted or controlled ventilation. The narcotic antagonist naloxone hydrochloride is a specific antidote for respiratory depression which may result from overdosage or unusual sensitivity to narcotics including hydrocodone. Therefore, an appropriate dose of naloxone hydrochloride should be administered, preferably by the intravenous route, simultaneously with efforts at respiratory resuscitation. For further information, see full prescribing information for naloxone hydrochloride. An antagonist should not be administered in the absence of clinically significant respiratory depression. Oxygen, intravenous fluids, vasopressors and other supportive measures should be employed as indicated. Gastric emptying may be useful in removing unabsorbed drug.

DOSAGE AND ADMINISTRATION
Adult: One (1) tablet every 4 to 6 hours as needed; do not exceed six (6) tablets in 24 hours.
Children 6 to 12 years of age: One-half (½) tablet every 4 to 6 hours as needed, do not exceed three (3) tablets in 24 hours.

HOW SUPPLIED
Each blue, scored tablet contains 5 mg hydrocodone bitartrate and 1.5 mg homatropine methylbromide and is available in:
Bottles of 100 NDC 0689-0082-01
Bottles of 500 NDC 0689-0082-05
Store at controlled room temperature 15°–30°C (59°–86°F). Oral prescription where permitted by state law.
Revised 4/89

Dayton Laboratories, Inc.
**3307 N.W. 74TH AVENUE
MIAMI, FL 33122**

FLATULEX
Simethicone plus Activated Charcoal

DESCRIPTION
Flatulex is a uniquely constructed tablet for the control and elimination of flatulence. It contains two active ingredients: Simethicone and Activated Charcoal. The tablets are constructed so that the 2 actives are independent of each other; Simethicone in a coated form for release in the stomach and Activated Charcoal in an enteric coated form for release in the intestine. This unique delivery system ensures that the Simethicone is released in the stomach while the Charcoal safely traverses the stomach to the intestine without being neutralized by acid.

ACTIONS
Simethicone (polydimethylsiloxane) is a surface active agent which acts as a dispersant of gas bubbles by reducing the surface tension of the bubbles, thus destroying mucosal pockets of gas which cause distress. It does not absorb gas per se, or reduce the quantity of gas present. This is done by movement of the gas into the intestine. Simethicone is not active in the intestine.
Activated Charcoal is a gas absorbent of high capacity. Its highly porous surface absorbs and adsorbs gases, poorly soluble substances, and toxins. It is widely used as a detoxicant. Activated Charcoal reduces the volume of intestinal gas, providing relief of symptoms and reducing or eliminating flatulence. It also absorbs microbial metabolites and toxins which may generate gas, thus reducing gas production, especially of hydrogen and methane. Charcoal is not effective in the stomach, due to absorption of HCl, which has a neutralizing effect. Flatulex is sodium-free, and safe, since ingredients are not absorbed into the bloodstream.

Continued on next page

Dayton—Cont.

INDICATIONS
For relief of stomach gas, intestinal gas, and flatulence.

CONTRAINDICATIONS
No known contraindications other than hypersensitivity to Simethicone or Activated Charcoal.

PRECAUTIONS
Drug interaction: Activated Charcoal may absorb medication(s) while in the digestive tract. May cause temporary blackening of the stool. Do not exceed recommended dosage.

ADVERSE REACTIONS
No adverse reactions to this product have been reported.

DOSAGE
One tablet three times daily, preferably after meals. One tablet may be taken at bedtime to provide overnight relief.

HOW SUPPLIED
Each DUAL-COATED tablet contains
OUTER LAYER (for gastric release)
Simethicone ....80 mg.
INNER LAYER (for intestinal release)
Activated Charcoal ....250 mg.
Supplied in bottles of 100
NDC #52041-028-15

Delmont Laboratories, Inc.
P.O. BOX AA
SWARTHMORE, PA 19081

STAPHAGE LYSATE (SPL)®　　　　　　　　℞
[staf'faj lĭ'sāt]
BACTERIAL ANTIGEN MADE FROM
STAPHYLOCOCCUS

DESCRIPTION
STAPHAGE LYSATE (SPL)® is a whole culture vaccine, in solution, of two strains of lysed *Staphylococcus aureus*, Serologic Types I & III, specially selected for their broad antigenic spectrum.

HOW SUPPLIED
1-ml ampules, boxes of 10 (NDC 48532-0299-2), for subcutaneous, aerosol, topical, and oral use; 10-ml multiple-dose vials (NDC 48532-0299-1) for aerosol, topical, and oral use.
For complete prescribing information and literature, please write, or call (215) 543-3365 or 543-2747.

Dermaide Research Corp.
P.O. BOX 562
PALOS HEIGHTS, IL 60463

DERMAIDE® ALOE CREAM
[der'maid al"o cream]

ACTIVE INGREDIENT
Aloe Vera Jel

INACTIVE INGREDIENTS
Mineral oil; stearic acid; petrolatum; cetyl alcohol; glycerin; triethenolamine; propylparaben; methyl paraben; imidazolidinyl urea.

ACTIONS
Dermaide Aloe Cream is a soothing moisturizer for dry itchy skin, minor burns and sunburn, minor cuts, scrapes and mild skin irritations.

WARNINGS
If relief is not evident, consult your physician. Certain people may be allergic. If any skin reaction occurs, discontinue its use and wash off with soap and water.

PRECAUTION
Certain individuals may be allergic. If area become red and itchy, discontinue its use and wash off with soap and water.

DIRECTIONS
Wash and rinse the affected area thoroughly with luke warm water, apply Dermaide Aloe Cream generously over the affected area and continue to apply as often as necessary to keep the affected area covered.

HOW SUPPLIED
4 oz. jar.

REFERENCES
Robson, MC, Heggers J, Hagstrom WJ: Myth, Magic, Witchcraft or Fact? Aloe Vera Revisted*, 1982; JBCR 3(2): 157–163.
McCauley R, Hing D, Robson M, Heggers J: Frostbite Injuries: A Rational Approach Based on The Pathophysiology, J Trau 1983; 23(2): 143–147
Prostanoid derivatives and their influence on thermal injury, Sixth International Congress on Burns, International Society for Burn Injuries, San Francisco, CA August 31, 1982.
Raine TJ, London MD, Goluch L, Heggers JP, Robson MC: Antiprostaglandins and antithromboxanes in the treatment of frostbite. Surg. Forum 31:557–59, 1980.
Heggers JP, Pinless GR, Robson MC: Dermaide Aloe Gel: Comparison of antimicrobial effects. J. Amer. Med. Technol. 41:293–94, 1979.
The Good Old Remedies for Frostbite. Emer Med 16(20) 80–82, 1984.
Shown in Product Identification Section, page 409

Dermik Laboratories, Inc.
920A HARVEST DRIVE
BLUE BELL, PA 19422

ANTHRA-DERM® Ointment　　　　　　　℞
[anthra-derm]
(anthralin) 1%, ½%, ¼%, ¹⁄₁₀%
FOR TOPICAL USE ONLY

DESCRIPTION
Each gram of Anthra-Derm® (anthralin) Ointment ¹⁄₁₀%, ¼%, ½% and 1.0% contains 1 mg, 2.5 mg, 5 mg and 10 mg, respectively, of anthralin in a base consisting of mineral oil and white petrolatum. Anthralin is an anti-psoriatic agent with cytostatic, irritant and weak antimicrobial properties.

CLINICAL PHARMACOLOGY
Although the exact mechanism of anthralin's activity is unknown, there is experimental evidence that anthralin binds DNA, inhibiting synthesis of nucleic protein, and thus reduces mitotic activity.
Absorption in man has not been determined. However, based on a study in piglets it would appear to be quite low.

INDICATIONS AND USAGE
For the topical treatment of psoriasis.

CONTRAINDICATIONS
Anthra-Derm® (anthralin) Ointment is contraindicated in patients with acute psoriasis or where inflammation is present, and in those patients with a history of hypersensitivity to any of the ingredients.

WARNINGS
Although no renal, hepatic or hematologic abnormalities have been reported as a result of topical application of Anthra-Derm® (anthralin) Ointment, caution is advised in patients with renal disease. Patients with renal disease and those having extensive and prolonged applications should have periodic urine tests for albuminuria. Discontinue use if sensitivity reactions occur.

PRECAUTIONS
General: When redness is observed on adjacent normal skin, reduce frequency of application. For external use only. Do not apply to face, genitalia or intertriginous areas. Wash hands thoroughly and carefully after using. Keep out of the reach of children. Anthralin is a tumor-promoting agent in 2-stage carcinogenesis on mouse skin. However, there have not been any reports of such effects in humans at the usual dosages.
Pregnancy: Pregnancy Category C. Animal reproduction studies have not been conducted with anthralin. It is also not known whether anthralin can cause fetal harm when administered to a pregnant woman or can affect reproduction capacity. Anthra-Derm® Ointment should be given to a pregnant woman only if clearly needed.
Nursing mothers: It is not known whether this drug is excreted in human milk. Because many drugs are excreted in human milk and because of the potential for tumorigenicity shown for anthralin in animal studies, a decision should be made whether to discontinue nursing or to discontinue the drug, taking into account the importance of the drug to the mother.
Pediatric use: Safety and effectiveness in children have not been established.

ADVERSE REACTIONS
Irritation of normal skin is the most frequently reported adverse reaction. Anthra-Derm® may stain skin, hair, or fabrics.

DOSAGE AND ADMINISTRATION
The usual dosage regimen begins with the lowest concentration (¹⁄₁₀%) and is gradually increased until the desired effect is obtained. Apply in a thin layer to affected areas once or twice daily, or as directed by a physician.

HOW SUPPLIED
Anthra-Derm® (anthralin) Ointment ¹⁄₁₀% (NDC 0066-0010-15), ¼% (NDC 0066-0025-15), ½% (NDC 0066-0050-15) and 1.0% (NDC-0066-0100-15) is available in 1.5 oz (42.5 g) tubes.

5 BENZAGEL®　　　　　　　　　　　　℞
[ben-za-jel]
(5% benzoyl peroxide) and
10 BENZAGEL®　　　　　　　　　　　℞
(10% benzoyl peroxide)
MICROGEL™ FORMULA
Acne Gels

DESCRIPTION
Each gram of 5 Benzagel® and 10 Benzagel® contains 50 mg and 100 mg respectively, of benzoyl peroxide in a gel vehicle of purified water, carbomer 940, sodium hydroxide, docusate sodium, fragrance and alcohol 14%.
Benzoyl peroxide is an antibacterial and keratolytic agent.

CLINICAL PHARMACOLOGY
Benzoyl peroxide is an antibacterial agent which has been shown to be effective against *Propionibacterium acnes*. This action is believed to be responsible for its usefulness in acne. One study in the rhesus monkey demonstrated a percutaneous absorption of about 1.8 μg per cm^2 of benzoyl peroxide or 45% of the applied dose in a 24-hour period. The absorbed benzoyl peroxide was completely converted in the skin to benzoic acid.

INDICATION AND USAGE
5 & 10 Benzagel® may be used alone topically for mild to moderate acne and as an adjunct in acne treatment regimens which might include retinoic acid products, systemic antibiotics, and/or sulfur and salicylic acid-containing preparations. The active ingredient, benzoyl peroxide, exerts a desquamative and antibacterial action. It provides mild peeling and keratolytic activity.

CONTRAINDICATIONS
Benzagel® should not be used by patients having known sensitivity to benzoyl peroxide or any of its components.

WARNINGS
If itching, redness, burning, swelling or undue dryness occurs, discontinue use.

PRECAUTIONS
For external use only. Not for ophthalmic use. Keep away from eyes and mucosae. Very fair individuals should begin with a single application at bedtime allowing overnight medication. May bleach colored fabrics. Keep this and all medications out of the reach of children.
Carcinogenesis, Mutagenesis and Impairment of Fertility—Long-term studies in animals have not been performed to evaluate carcinogenic potential.
Pregnancy Category C—Animal reproduction studies have not been conducted with benzoyl peroxide. It is also not known whether benzoyl peroxide can cause fetal harm when administered to a pregnant woman or can affect reproduction capacity. Benzoyl peroxide should be given to a pregnant woman only if clearly needed.
Nursing Mothers—It is not known whether this drug is excreted in human milk. Because many drugs are excreted in human milk, caution should be exercised when benzoyl peroxide is administered to a nursing woman.
Pediatric Use: Safety and effectiveness in children under the age of 12 have not been established.

ADVERSE REACTIONS
Irritation and contact dermatitis are the most frequent side reactions to benzoyl peroxide.

DOSAGE AND ADMINISTRATION
Wash and dry affected areas prior to application. Apply sparingly one or more times daily.

HOW SUPPLIED
5 & 10 Benzagel® are available in 1.5 oz (42.5 g) and 3 oz (85 g) plastic tubes; 5 Benzagel® contains 50 mg benzoyl peroxide per gram and 10 Benzagel® contains 100 mg benzoyl peroxide per gram.
5-Benzagel 1.5 oz NDC 0066-0430-15
5-Benzagel 3.0 oz NDC 0066-0430-30
10-Benzagel 1.5 oz NDC 0066-0431-15
10 Benzagel 3.0 oz NDC 0066-0431-30

CAUTION
Federal law prohibits dispensing without prescription.

BENZAMYCIN® Topical Gel ℞
[ben'za-mi"sin]
(erythromycin—benzoyl peroxide)

PRODUCT OVERVIEW
KEY FACTS
Benzamycin® is a topical gel containing 3% erythromycin and 5% benzoyl peroxide. Erythromycin is an antibiotic and benzoyl peroxide is an antibacterial and keratolytic agent.

MAJOR USES
Benzamycin® is indicated for the topical control of acne vulgaris.

SAFETY INFORMATION
Benzamycin® is contraindicated in patients with a history of hypersensitivity to erythromycin, benzoyl peroxide, or any of the other listed ingredients. Avoid contact with eyes and mucous membranes. Concomitant topical acne therapy should be used with caution. Adverse reactions may include dryness, erythema, and pruritus.

PRESCRIBING INFORMATION
BENZAMYCIN® Topical Gel ℞
[ben'za-mi"sin]
(erythromycin—benzoyl peroxide)
Reconstitute Before Dispensing

DESCRIPTION
Each gram of Benzamycin® (erythromycin—benzoyl peroxide) topical gel contains, as dispensed, 30 mg (3%) of erythromycin and 50 mg (5%) of benzoyl peroxide in a gel vehicle of purified water, carbomer 940, alcohol 22%, sodium hydroxide, docusate sodium and fragrance.
Erythromycin ($C_{37}H_{67}NO_{13}$) is produced by a strain of *Streptomyces erythraeus* and belongs to the macrolide group of antibiotics.
Benzoyl peroxide ($C_{14}H_{10}O_4$), is an antibacterial and keratolytic agent.

CLINICAL PHARMACOLOGY
Erythromycin is a bacteriostatic macrolide antibiotic, but may be bactericidal in high concentrations. Although the mechanism by which erythromycin acts in reducing inflammatory lesions of acne vulgaris is unknown, it is presumably due to its antibiotic action. Antagonism has been demonstrated between clindamycin and erythromycin.
Benzoyl peroxide is an antibacterial agent which has been shown to be effective against *Propionibacterium acnes,* an anaerobe found in sebaceous follicles and comedones. The antibacterial action of benzoyl peroxide is believed to be due to the release of active oxygen. Benzoyl peroxide has a keratolytic and desquamative effect which may also contribute to its efficacy.
Benzoyl peroxide has been shown to be absorbed by the skin where it is converted to benzoic acid.

INDICATIONS AND USAGE
Benzamycin® Topical Gel is indicated for the topical control of acne vulgaris.

CONTRAINDICATIONS
Benzamycin® Topical Gel is contraindicated in those patients with a history of hypersensitivity to erythromycin, benzoyl peroxide or any of the other listed ingredients.

PRECAUTIONS
General—For external use only. Not for ophthalmic use. Avoid contact with eyes and mucous membranes. Concomitant topical acne therapy should be used with caution because a possible cumulative irritancy effect may occur, especially with peeling, desquamating or abrasive agents. If severe irritation develops, discontinue use and institute appropriate therapy.
The use of antibiotic agents may be associated with the overgrowth of antibiotic-resistant organisms. If this occurs, administration of this drug should be discontinued and appropriate measures taken.
Information for Patients—Patients using Benzamycin® Topical Gel should receive the following information and instructions:
1. Benzamycin® Topical Gel is for external use only. Avoid contact with the eyes and mucous membranes.
2. Patients should not use any other topical acne preparation unless otherwise directed by physician.
3. Benzamycin® Topical Gel may bleach hair or colored fabric.
4. If excessive irritation or dryness should occur, patient should discontinue medication and consult physician.
5. Discard product after 3 months and obtain fresh material.
Carcinogenesis, Mutagenesis and Impairment of Fertility: Long-term studies in animals have not been performed to evaluate carcinogenic potential or the effect on fertility.
Pregnancy Category C: Animal reproduction studies have not been conducted with Benzamycin® Topical Gel. It is also not known whether Benzamycin® Topical Gel can

cause fetal harm when administered to a pregnant woman or can affect reproduction capacity. Benzamycin® Topical Gel should be given to a pregnant woman only if clearly needed.
Nursing Mothers: It is not known whether this drug is excreted in human milk. Because many drugs are excreted in human milk, caution should be exercised when Benzamycin® Topical Gel is administered to a nursing woman.
Pediatric Use: Safety and effectiveness in children under the age of 12 have not been established.

ADVERSE REACTIONS
Adverse reactions which may occur include dryness, erythema and pruritus. Of a total of 153 patients treated with Benzamycin® Topical Gel during clinical trials, 4 patients experienced adverse reactions, of whom three experienced dryness and one an urticarial reaction which responded well to symptomatic treatment.

DOSAGE AND ADMINISTRATION
Benzamycin® Topical Gel should be applied twice daily, morning and evening, or as directed by physician, to affected areas after the skin is thoroughly washed, rinsed with warm water and gently patted dry.
How Supplied and Dispensing Information: Benzamycin® Topical Gel is supplied in a package containing 20 g of benzoyl peroxide gel and a plastic vial containing 0.8 g of active erythromycin powder. Prior to dispensing, tap vial gently until powder flows freely, add 3 mL of ethyl alcohol (to the mark) to vial and shake well to dissolve erythromycin. Add this solution to gel and stir until homogeneous in appearance (1–1½ minutes). Benzamycin® Topical Gel should then be stored under refrigeration. Place a 3-month expiration date on the label.
Benzamycin® Topical Gel (NDC 0066-0510-23), as dispensed, is 23.3 g net weight.
Note: *Prior* to reconstitution, store at room temperature. *After* reconstitution, store in a cold place, preferably in a refrigerator. Do not freeze. Keep tightly closed. Keep out of the reach of children.
U.S. Patent Nos. 4,387,107 and 4,497,794. Other Patents Pending.

CAUTION
Federal law prohibits dispensing without prescription.

FLORONE® ℞
[flŏr-ōhn]
(brand of diflorasone diacetate cream and diflorasone diacetate ointment 0.05%)
Not For Ophthalmic Use

PRODUCT OVERVIEW
KEY FACTS
Florone® is a topical corticosteroid containing 0.05% diflorasone diacetate in an emulsified, hydrophilic cream and in an ointment with an emollient, occlusive base. Florone® Ointment contains no propylene glycol.

MAJOR USES
Florone® is indicated for the relief of the inflammatory and pruritic manifestations of corticosteroid-responsive dermatoses.

SAFETY INFORMATION
Florone® is contraindicated in patients with a history of hypersensitivity to any of its components. Systemic absorption of topical corticosteroids has produced reversible HPA axis suppression. Therefore, patients receiving a large dose applied to a large area or under an occusive dressing should be evaluated periodically. The most common adverse reactions are burning, itching, irritation, and dryness.

PRESCRIBING INFORMATION
FLORONE® ℞
[flŏr-ōhn]
(brand of diflorasone diacetate cream and diflorasone diacetate ointment 0.05%)
Not For Ophthalmic Use

DESCRIPTION
Each gram of FLORONE Cream and FLORONE Ointment contains 0.5 mg diflorasone diacetate in a cream or ointment base.
Chemically, diflorasone diacetate is: 6α, 9α-difluoro-11β, 17,21-trihydroxy-16β-methylpregna-1,4-diene-3,20-dione 17,21 diacetate.
FLORONE Cream contains diflorasone diacetate in an emulsified and hydrophilic cream base consisting of propylene glycol, stearic acid, polysorbate 60, sorbitan monostearate and monooleate, sorbic acid, citric acid and water. The corticosteroid is formulated as a solution in the vehicle using 15 percent propylene glycol to optimize drug delivery.
FLORONE Ointment contains diflorasone diacetate in an emollient, occlusive base consisting of polyoxypropylene 15-stearyl ether, stearic acid, lanolin alcohol and white petrolatum.

CLINICAL PHARMACOLOGY
Topical corticosteroids share anti-inflammatory, antipruritic and vasoconstrictive actions.
The mechanism of anti-inflammatory activity of the topical corticosteroids is unclear. Various laboratory methods, including vasoconstrictor assays, are used to compare and predict potencies and/or clinical efficacies of the topical corticosteroids. There is some evidence to suggest that a recognizable correlation exists between vasoconstrictor potency and therapeutic efficacy in man.
Pharmacokinetics: The extent of percutaneous absorption of topical corticosteroids is determined by many factors including the vehicle, the integrity of the epidermal barrier and the use of occlusive dressings.
Topical corticosteroids can be absorbed from normal intact skin. Inflammation and/or other disease processes in the skin increase percutaneous absorption. Occlusive dressings substantially increase the percutaneous absorption of topical corticosteroids. Thus, occlusive dressings may be a valuable therapeutic adjunct for treatment of resistant dermatoses. (See DOSAGE AND ADMINISTRATION).
Once absorbed through the skin, topical corticosteroids are handled through pharmacokinetic pathways similar to systemically administered corticosteroids. Corticosteroids are bound to plasma proteins in varying degrees. They are metabolized primarily in the liver and are then excreted by the kidneys. Some of the topical corticosteroids and their metabolites are also excreted into the bile.

INDICATIONS AND USAGE
Topical corticosteroids are indicated for relief of the inflammatory and pruritic manifestations of corticosteroid-responsive dermatoses.

CONTRAINDICATIONS
Topical steroids are contraindicated in those patients with a history of hypersensitivity to any of the components of the preparation.

PRECAUTIONS
General:
Systemic absorption of topical corticosteroids has produced reversible hypothalamic-pituitary-adrenal (HPA) axis suppression, manifestations of Cushing's syndrome, hyperglycemia, and glucosuria in some patients.
Conditions which augment systemic absorption include the application of the more potent steroids, use over large surface areas, prolonged use, and the addition of occlusive dressings.
Therefore, patients receiving a large dose of a potent topical steroid applied to a large surface area or under an occlusive dressing should be evaluated periodically for evidence of HPA axis suppression by using the urinary free cortisol and ACTH stimulation tests. If HPA axis suppression is noted, an attempt should be made to withdraw the drug, to reduce the frequency of application, or to substitute a less potent steroid.
Recovery of HPA axis function is generally prompt and complete upon discontinuation of the drug. Infrequently, signs and symptoms of steroid withdrawal may occur, requiring supplemental systemic corticosteroids.
Children may absorb proportionally larger amounts of topical corticosteroids and thus be more susceptible to systemic toxicity. (See PRECAUTIONS—Pediatric Use)
If irritation develops, topical corticosteroids should be discontinued and appropriate therapy instituted.
In the presence of dermatological infections, the use of an appropriate antifungal or antibacterial agent should be instituted. If a favorable response does not occur promptly, the corticosteroid should be discontinued until the infection has been adequately controlled.
Information for the Patient: Patients using topical corticosteroids should receive the following information and instructions:
1. This medication is to be used as directed by the physician. It is for external use only. Avoid contact with the eyes.
2. Patients should be advised not to use this medication for any disorder other than for which it was prescribed.
3. The treated skin area should not be bandaged or otherwise covered or wrapped as to be occlusive unless directed by the physician.
4. Patients should report any signs of local adverse reactions especially under occlusive dressing.
5. Parents of pediatric patients should be advised not to use tight-fitting diapers or plastic pants on a child being treated in the diaper area, as these garments may constitute occlusive dressings.
Laboratory Tests: The following tests may be helpful in evaluating the HPA axis suppression:
Urinary free cortisol test
ACTH stimulation test
Carcinogenesis, Mutagenesis, and Impairment of Fertility: Long-term animal studies have not been performed to evalu-

Continued on next page

Dermik—Cont.

ate the carcinogenic potential or the effect on fertility of topical corticosteroids.

Studies to determine mutagenicity with prednisolone and hydrocortisone have revealed negative results.

Pregnancy Category C: Corticosteroids are generally teratogenic in laboratory animals when administered systemically at relatively low dosage levels. The more potent corticosteroids have been shown to be teratogenic after dermal application in laboratory animals. There are no adequate and well-controlled studies in pregnant women on teratogenic effects from topically applied corticosteroids. Therefore, topical corticosteroids should be used during pregnancy only if the potential benefit justifies the potential risk to the fetus. Drugs of this class should not be used extensively on pregnant patients, in large amounts, or for prolonged periods of time.

Nursing Mothers: It is not known whether topical administration of corticosteroids could result in sufficient systemic absorption to produce detectable quantities in breast milk. Systemically administered corticosteroids are secreted into breast milk in quantities **not** likely to have a deleterious effect on the infant. Nevertheless, caution should be exercised when topical corticosteroids are administered to a nursing woman.

Pediatric Use *Pediatric patients may demonstrate greater susceptibility to topical corticosteroid-induced HPA axis suppression and Cushing's syndrome than mature patients because of a larger skin surface area to body weight ratio.*

Hypothalamic-pituitary-adrenal (HPA) axis suppression, Cushing's syndrome, and intracranial hypertension have been reported in children receiving topical corticosteroids. Manifestations of adrenal suppression in children include linear growth retardation, delayed weight gain, low plasma cortisol levels, and absence of response to ACTH stimulation. Manifestations of intracranial hypertension include bulging fontanelles, headaches, and bilateral papilledema.

Administration of topical corticosteroids to children should be limited to the least amount compatible with an effective therapeutic regimen. Chronic corticosteroid therapy may interfere with the growth and development of children.

ADVERSE REACTIONS

The following local adverse reactions have been reported with topical corticosteroids, but may occur more frequently with the use of occlusive dressings. These reactions are listed in an approximate decreasing order of occurrence:

1. Burning
2. Itching
3. Irritation
4. Dryness
5. Folliculitis
6. Hypertrichosis
7. Acneiform eruptions
8. Hypopigmentation
9. Perioral dermatitis
10. Allergic contact dermatitis
11. Maceration of the skin
12. Secondary infection
13. Skin atrophy
14. Striae
15. Miliaria

OVERDOSAGE

Topically applied corticosteroids can be absorbed in sufficient amounts to produce systemic effects (See PRECAUTIONS).

DOSAGE AND ADMINISTRATION

Topical corticosteroids are generally applied to the affected area as a thin film from one to four times daily depending on the severity of the condition.

Occlusive dressings may be used for the management of psoriasis or recalcitrant conditions.

If an infection develops, the use of occlusive dressings should be discontinued and appropriate antimicrobial therapy instituted.

HOW SUPPLIED

FLORONE Cream is available as follows:

  15 gram tube   NDC 0066-0074-17
  30 gram tube   NDC 0066-0074-31
  60 gram tube   NDC 0066-0074-60

FLORONE Ointment is available as follows:

  15 gram tube   NDC 0066-0075-17
  30 gram tube   NDC 0066-0075-31
  60 gram tube   NDC 0066-0075-60

CAUTION Federal law prohibits dispensing without prescription.

FLORONE E®   ℞

[*flōr-ōhn E*]
brand of diflorasone diacetate
emollient cream
0.05%
Not For Ophthalmic Use

DESCRIPTION

Each gram of **florone E** Emollient Cream contains 0.5 mg diflorasone diacetate in a cream base.

Chemically, diflorasone diacetate is: 6α, 9α-difluoro-11β, 17, 21-trihydroxy-16β-methyl-pregna-1,4-diene-3,20-dione 17,21 diacetate.

Each gram of **florone E** Emollient Cream contains 0.5 mg diflorasone diacetate in a hydrophilic vanishing cream base of propylene glycol, stearyl alcohol, cetyl alcohol, sorbitan monostearate, polysorbate 60, mineral oil and purified water.

CLINICAL PHARMACOLOGY

Topical corticosteroids share anti-inflammatory, antipruritic and vasoconstrictive actions.

The mechanism of anti-inflammatory activity of the topical corticosteroids is unclear. Various laboratory methods, including vasoconstrictor assays, are used to compare and predict potencies and/or clinical efficacies of the topical corticosteroids. There is some evidence to suggest that a recognizable correlation exists between vasoconstrictor potency and therapeutic efficacy in man.

PHARMACOKINETICS

The extent of percutaneous absorption of topical corticosteroids is determined by many factors including the vehicle, the integrity of the epidermal barrier, and the use of occlusive dressings.

Topical corticosteroids can be absorbed from normal intact skin. Inflammation and/or other disease processes in the skin increase percutaneous absorption. Occlusive dressings substantially increase the percutaneous absorption of topical corticosteroids. Thus, occlusive dressings may be a valuable therapeutic adjunct for treatment of resistant dermatoses. (See DOSAGE AND ADMINISTRATION.)

Once absorbed through the skin, topical corticosteroids are handled through pharmacokinetic pathways similar to systemically administered corticosteroids. Corticosteroids are bound to plasma proteins in varying degrees. They are metabolized primarily in the liver and are then excreted by the kidneys. Some of the topical corticosteroids and their metabolites are also excreted into the bile.

INDICATIONS AND USAGE

Topical corticosteroids are indicated for relief of the inflammatory and pruritic manifestations of corticosteroid-responsive dermatoses.

CONTRAINDICATIONS

Topical steroids are contraindicated in those patients with a history of hypersensitivity to any of the components of the preparation.

PRECAUTIONS

General: Systemic absorption of topical corticosteroids has produced reversible hypothalamic-pituitary-adrenal (HPA) axis suppression, manifestations of Cushing's syndrome, hyperglycemia, and glucosuria in some patients.

Conditions which augment systemic absorption include the application of the more potent steroids, use over large surface areas, prolonged use, and the addition of occlusive dressings.

Therefore, patients receiving a large dose of a potent steroid applied to a large surface area or under an occlusive dressing should be evaluated periodically for evidence of HPA axis suppression by using the urinary free cortisol and ACTH stimulation tests. If HPA axis suppression is noted, an attempt should be made to withdraw the drug, to reduce the frequency of application, or to substitute a less potent steroid.

Recovery of HPA axis function is generally prompt and complete upon discontinuation of the drug. Infrequently, signs and symptoms of steroid withdrawal may occur, requiring supplemental systemic corticosteroids.

Children may absorb proportionally larger amounts of topical corticosteroids and thus be more susceptible to systemic toxicity. (See PRECAUTIONS—Pediatric Use.)

If irritation develops, topical corticosteroids should be discontinued and appropriate therapy instituted.

In the presence of dermatological infections, the use of an appropriate antifungal or antibacterial agent should be instituted. If a favorable response does not occur promptly, the corticosteroid should be discontinued until the infection has been adequately controlled.

Information for the Patient: Patients using topical corticosteroids should receive the following information and instructions:

1. This medication is to be used as directed by the physician. It is for external use only. Avoid contact with the eyes.

2. Patients should be advised not to use this medication for any disorder other than for which it was prescribed.
3. The treated skin area should not be bandaged or otherwise covered or wrapped as to be occlusive unless directed by the physician.
4. Patients should report any signs of local adverse reactions especially under occlusive dressing.
5. Parents of pediatric patients should be advised not to use tight-fitting diapers or plastic pants on a child being treated in the diaper area, as these garments may constitute occlusive dressings.

Laboratory Tests: The following tests may be helpful in evaluating the HPA axis suppression:

  Urinary free cortisol test
  ACTH stimulation test

Carcinogenesis, Mutagenesis, and Impairment of Fertility: Long-term animal studies have not been performed to evaluate the carcinogenic potential or the effect on fertility of topical corticosteroids.

Studies to determine mutagenicity with prednisolone and hydrocortisone have revealed negative results.

Pregnancy Category C: Corticosteroids are generally teratogenic in laboratory animals when administered systemically at relatively low dosage levels. The more potent corticosteroids have been shown to be teratogenic after dermal application in laboratory animals. There are no adequate and well-controlled studies in pregnant women on teratogenic effects from topically applied corticosteroids. Therefore, topical corticosteroids should be used during pregnancy only if the potential benefit justifies the potential risk to the fetus.

Nursing Mothers: It is not known whether topical administration of corticosteroids could result in sufficient systemic absorption to produce detectable quantities in breast milk. Systemically administered corticosteroids are secreted into breast milk in quantities **not** likely to have a deleterious effect on the infant. Nevertheless, caution should be exercised when topical corticosteroids are administered to a nursing woman.

Pediatric Use: *Pediatric patients may demonstrate greater susceptibility to topical corticosteroid-induced HPA axis suppression and Cushing's syndrome than mature patients because of a larger skin surface area to body weight ratio.*

Hypothalmic-pituitary-adrenal (HPA) axis suppression, Cushing's syndrome, and intracranial hypertension have been reported in children receiving topical corticosteroids. Manifestations of adrenal suppression in children include linear growth retardation, delayed weight gain, low plasma cortisol levels, and absence of response to ACTH stimulation. Manifestations of intracranial hypertension include bulging fontanelles, headaches, and bilateral papilledema.

Administration of topical corticosteroids to children should be limited to the least amount compatible with an effective therapeutic regimen. Chronic corticosteroid therapy may interfere with the growth and development of children.

ADVERSE REACTIONS

The following local adverse reactions have been reported with topical corticosteroids, but may occur more frequently with the use of occlusive dressings. These reactions are listed in an approximate decreasing order of occurrence:

1. Burning
2. Itching
3. Irritation
4. Dryness
5. Folliculitis
6. Hypertrichosis
7. Acneiform eruptions
8. Hypopigmentation
9. Perioral dermatitis
10. Allergic contact dermatitis
11. Maceration of the skin
12. Secondary infection
13. Skin atrophy
14. Striae
15. Miliaria

OVERDOSAGE

Topically applied corticosteroids can be absorbed in sufficient amounts to produce systemic effects (See PRECAUTIONS.)

DOSAGE AND ADMINISTRATION

florone E Emollient Cream should be applied to the affected areas as a thin film from one to three times daily depending on the severity or resistant nature of the condition.

Occlusive dressings may be used for the management of psoriasis or recalcitrant conditions.

If an infection develops, the use of occlusive dressings should be discontinued and appropriate antimicrobial therapy instituted.

HOW SUPPLIED

florone E Emollient Cream is available in the following size tubes:

15 gram	NDC 0066-0072-17
30 gram	NDC 0066-0072-31
60 gram	NDC 0066-0072-60

Store at controlled room temperature 15°–30° C (59°–86° F).
Caution: Federal law prohibits dispensing without prescription.

HYTONE® Cream ½%

(See PDR For Nonprescription Drugs)

HYTONE® Cream, Lotion and Ointment   ℞
[hi-tōne]
(hydrocortisone)

PRODUCT OVERVIEW
KEY FACTS
Hytone® contains 1% and 2½% Hydrocortisone and is available in a cream, a lotion, and an ointment.

MAJOR USES
Hytone® is indicated for the relief of the inflammatory and pruritic manifestations of corticosteroid-responsive dermatoses.

SAFETY INFORMATION
Hytone® is contraindicated in patients with a history of hypersensitivity to any of its components. Systemic absorption of topical corticosteroids has produced reversible HPA axis suppression. Therefore, patients receiving a large dose applied to a large area or under an occlusive dressing should be evaluated periodically. The most common adverse reactions are burning, itching, irritation, and dryness.

PRESCRIBING INFORMATION
HYTONE® Cream, Lotion and Ointment   ℞
[hi-tōne]
(hydrocortisone)

DESCRIPTION
Cream —Each gram of 1% and 2½% Cream contains 10 mg or 25 mg, respectively, of hydrocortisone in a water-washable base of purified water, propylene glycol, glyceryl monostearate SE, cholesterol and related sterols, isopropyl myristate, polysorbate 60, cetyl alcohol, sorbitan monostearate, polyoxyl 40 stearate and sorbic acid.
Lotion —Each ml of 1% and 2½% Lotion contains 10 mg or 25 mg, respectively, of hydrocortisone in a vehicle consisting of carbomer 940, propylene glycol, polysorbate 40, propylene glycol stearate, cholesterol and related sterols, isopropyl myristate, sorbitan palmitate, cetyl alcohol, triethanolamine, sorbic acid, simethicone and purified water.
Ointment —Each gram of 1% and 2½% contains 10 mg or 25 mg, respectively, of hydrocortisone in a topical emollient base of mineral oil, white petrolatum and sorbitan sesquioleate.
Chemically, hydrocortisone is 11, 17, 21-trihydroxypregn-4-ene 3, 20-dione.
The topical corticosteroids including hydrocortisone, constitute a class of primarily synthetic steroids used as anti-inflammatory and antipruritic agents.

CLINICAL PHARMACOLOGY
Topical corticosteroids share anti-inflammatory, antipruritic and vasoconstrictive actions. The mechanism of anti-inflammatory activity of the topical corticosteroids is unclear. Various laboratory methods, including vasoconstrictor assays, are used to compare and predict potencies and/or clinical efficacies of the topical corticosteroids. There is some evidence to suggest that a recognizable correlation exists between vasoconstrictor potency and therapeutic efficacy in man.
Pharmacokinetics
The extent of percutaneous absorption of topical corticosteroids is determined by many factors including the vehicle, the integrity of the epidermal barrier, and the use of occlusive dressings.
Topical corticosteroids can be absorbed from normal intact skin. Inflammation and/or other disease processes in the skin increase percutaneous absorption. Occlusive dressings substantially increase the percutaneous absorption of topical corticosteroids. Thus, occlusive dressings may be a valuable therapeutic adjunct for treatment of resistant dermatoses.
(See *DOSAGE AND ADMINISTRATION.*)
Once absorbed through the skin, topical corticosteroids are handled through pharmacokinetic pathways similar to systemically administered corticosteroids. Corticosteroids are bound to plasma proteins in varying degrees. Corticosteroids are metabolized primarily in the liver and are then excreted by the kidneys. Some of the topical corticosteroids and their metabolites are also excreted into the bile.

INDICATIONS AND USAGE
Topical corticosteroids are indicated for the relief of the inflammatory and pruritic manifestations of corticosteroid-responsive dermatoses.

CONTRAINDICATIONS
Topical corticosteroids are contraindicated in those patients with a history of hypersensitivity to any of the components of the preparation.

PRECAUTIONS
General — Systemic absorption of topical corticosteroids has produced reversible hypothalamic-pituitary-adrenal (HPA) axis suppression, manifestations of Cushing's syndrome, hyperglycemia, and glucosuria in some patients.
Conditions which augment systemic absorption include the application of the more potent steroids, use over large surface areas, prolonged use, and the addition of occlusive dressings.
Therefore, patients receiving a large dose of a potent topical steroid applied to a large surface area or under an occlusive dressing should be evaluated periodically for evidence of HPA axis suppression by using the urinary free cortisol and ACTH stimulation tests. If HPA axis suppression is noted, an attempt should be made to withdraw the drug, to reduce the frequency of application, or to substitute a less potent steroid.
Recovery of HPA axis function is generally prompt and complete upon discontinuation of the drug. Infrequently, signs and symptoms of steroid withdrawal may occur, requiring supplemental systemic corticosteroids.
Children may absorb proportionally larger amounts of topical corticosteroids and thus be more susceptible to systemic toxicity (See PRECAUTIONS—Pediatric Use).
If irritation develops, topical corticosteroids should be discontinued and appropriate therapy instituted.
In the presence of dermatological infections, the use of an appropriate antifungal or antibacterial agent should be instituted. If a favorable response does not occur promptly, the corticosteroid should be discontinued until the infection has been adequately controlled.
Information for the Patient — Patients using topical corticosteroids should receive the following information and instructions:
1. This medication is to be used as directed by the physician. It is for external use only. Avoid contact with the eyes.
2. Patients should be advised not to use this medication for any disorder other than for which it was prescribed.
3. The treated skin area should not be bandaged or otherwise covered or wrapped as to be occlusive unless directed by the physician.
4. Patients should report any signs of local adverse reactions, especially under occlusive dressing.
5. Parents of pediatric patients should be advised not to use tight-fitting diapers or plastic pants on a child being treated in the diaper area, as these garments may constitute occlusive dressings.
Laboratory Tests — The following tests may be helpful in evaluating the HPA axis suppression:
  Urinary free cortisol test
  ACTH stimulation test
Carcinogenesis, Mutagenesis, and Impairment of Fertility — Long-term animal studies have not been performed to evaluate the carcinogenic potential or the effect on fertility of topical corticosteroids.
Studies to determine mutagenicity with prednisolone and hydrocortisone have revealed negative results.
Pregnancy Category C — Corticosteroids are generally teratogenic in laboratory animals when administered systemically at relatively low dosage levels. The more potent corticosteroids have been shown to be teratogenic after dermal application in laboratory animals. There are no adequate and well-controlled studies in pregnant women on teratogenic effects from topically applied corticosteroids. Therefore, topical corticosteroids should be used during pregnancy only if the potential benefit justifies the potential risk to the fetus. Drugs of this class should not be used extensively on pregnant patients, in large amounts, or for prolonged periods of time.
Nursing Mothers — It is not known whether topical administration of corticosteroids could result in sufficient systemic absorption to produce detectable quantities in breast milk. Systemically administered corticosteroids are secreted into breast milk in quantities *not* likely to have a deleterious effect on the infant. Nevertheless, caution should be exercised when topical corticosteroids are administered to a nursing woman.
Pediatric Use —Pediatric patients may demonstrate greater susceptibility to topical corticosteroid-induced HPA axis suppression and Cushing's syndrome than mature patients because of a larger skin surface area to body weight ratio.
Hypothalamic-pituitary-adrenal (HPA) axis suppression, Cushing's syndrome, and intracranial hypertension have been reported in children receiving topical corticosteroids. Manifestations of adrenal suppression in children include linear growth retardation, delayed weight gain, low plasma

cortisol levels, and absence of response to ACTH stimulation. Manifestations of intracranial hypertension include bulging fontanelles, headaches, and bilateral papilledema.
Administration of topical corticosteroids to children should be limited to the least amount compatible with an effective therapeutic regimen. Chronic corticosteroid therapy may interfere with the growth and development of children.

ADVERSE REACTIONS
The following local adverse reactions are reported infrequently with topical corticosteroids, but may occur more frequently with the use of occlusive dressings. These reactions are listed in an approximate decreasing order of occurrence:

Burning	Perioral dermatitis
Itching	Allergic contact dermatitis
Irritation	Maceration of the skin
Dryness	Secondary infection
Folliculitis	Skin atrophy
Hypertrichosis	Striae
Acneiform	Miliaria
eruptions	
Hypopigmentation	

OVERDOSAGE
Topically applied corticosteroids can be absorbed in sufficient amounts to produce systemic effects (See PRECAUTIONS).

DOSAGE AND ADMINISTRATION
Topical corticosteroids are generally applied to the affected area as a thin film from two to four times daily depending on the severity of the condition. Occlusive dressings may be used for the management of psoriasis or recalcitrant conditions.
If an infection develops, the use of occlusive dressings should be discontinued and appropriate antimicrobial therapy instituted.

HOW SUPPLIED
Cream —2½% - tube 1 oz NDC 0066-0095-01; 1% - tube 1 oz NDC 0066-0083-01 and jar 4 oz NDC 0066-0083-04; ½% - tube 1 oz (OTC) NDC 0066-0182-01.
Lotion —2½% - bottle 2 fl oz NDC 0066-0098-02; 1% - bottle 4 fl oz NDC 0066-0090-04.
Ointment —2 ½% - tube 1 oz NDC 0066-0085-01; 1% - tube 1 oz NDC 0066-0087-01.

CAUTION
Federal law prohibits dispensing without prescription.

LOROXIDE® Acne Lotion

(See PDR For Nonprescription Drugs)

PSORCON™   ℞
[sŏr-kon]
brand of diflorasone diacetate ointment
0.05%
Not For Ophthalmic Use

PRODUCT OVERVIEW
KEY FACTS
Psorcon® is a potent (Class I) topical corticosteroid containing 0.05% diflorasone diacetate in an optimized base.

MAJOR USES
Psorcon® is indicated for the relief of the inflammatory and pruritic manifestations of corticosteroid-responsive dermatoses.

SAFETY INFORMATION
Psorcon® is contraindicated in patients with a history of hypersensitivity to any of its components. Systemic absorption of topical corticosteroids has produced reversible HPA axis suppression. Therefore, patients receiving a large dose applied to a large area or under an occlusive dressing should be evaluated periodically. The most common adverse reactions are burning, itching, irritation, and dryness.

PRESCRIBING INFORMATION
PSORCON™   ℞
[sŏr-kon]
brand of diflorasone diacetate ointment
0.05%
Not For Ophthalmic Use

DESCRIPTION
Each gram of **psorcon** Ointment contains 0.5 mg diflorasone diacetate in an ointment base.
Chemically, diflorasone diacetate is 6α, 9α-difluoro-11β, 17, 21 -trihydroxy-16β-methylpregna-1, 4-diene-3, 20-dione 17,21 diacetate.

Continued on next page

Dermik—Cont.

Each gram of **psorcon** Ointment contains 0.5 mg diflorasone diacetate in an ointment base of propylene glycol, glyceryl monostearate and white petrolatum.

CLINICAL PHARMACOLOGY
Topical corticosteroids share anti-inflammatory, antipruritic and vasoconstrictive actions.

The mechanism of anti-inflammatory activity of the topical corticosteroids is unclear. Various laboratory methods, including vasoconstrictor assays, are used to compare and predict potencies and/or clinical efficacies of the topical corticosteroids. There is some evidence to suggest that a recognizable correlation exists between vasoconstrictor potency and therapeutic efficacy in man.

Pharmacokinetics
The extent of percutaneous absorption of topical corticosteroids is determined by many factors including the vehicle, the integrity of the epidermal barrier, and the use of occlusive dressings.

Topical corticosteroids can be absorbed from normal intact skin. Inflammation and/or other disease processes in the skin increase percutaneous absorption. Occlusive dressings substantially increase the percutaneous absorption of topical corticosteroids. Thus, occlusive dressings may be a valuable therapeutic adjunct for treatment of resistant dermatoses. (See DOSAGE AND ADMINISTRATION.)

Once absorbed through the skin, topical corticosteroids are handled through pharmacokinetic pathways similar to systemically administered corticosteroids. Corticosteroids are bound to plasma proteins in varying degrees. They are metabolized primarily in the liver and are then excreted by the kidneys. Some of the topical corticosteroids and their metabolites are also excreted into the bile.

INDICATIONS AND USAGE
Topical corticosteroids are indicated for relief of the inflammatory and pruritic manifestations of corticosteroid-responsive dermatoses.

CONTRAINDICATIONS
Topical steroids are contraindicated in those patients with a history of hypersensitivity to any of the components of the preparation.

PRECAUTIONS
General
Systemic absorption of topical corticosteroids has produced reversible hypothalamic-pituitary-adrenal (HPA) axis suppression, manifestations of Cushing's syndrome, hyperglycemia, and glucosuria in some patients.

Conditions which augment systemic absorption include the application of the more potent steroids, use over large surface areas, prolonged use, and the addition of occlusive dressings.

Therefore, patients receiving a large dose of a potent topical steroid applied to a large surface area or under an occlusive dressing should be evaluated periodically for evidence of HPA axis suppression by using the urinary free cortisol and ACTH stimulation tests. If HPA axis suppression is noted, an attempt should be made to withdraw the drug, to reduce the frequency of application, or to substitute a less potent steroid.

Recovery of HPA axis function is generally prompt and complete upon discontinuation of the drug. Infrequently, signs and symptoms of steroid withdrawal may occur, requiring supplemental systemic corticosteroids.

Children may absorb proportionally larger amounts of topical corticosteroids and thus be more susceptible to systemic toxicity. (See PRECAUTIONS—Pediatric Use.)

If irritation develops, topical corticosteroids should be discontinued and appropriate therapy instituted.

In the presence of dermatological infections, the use of an appropriate antifungal or antibacterial agent should be instituted. If a favorable response does not occur promptly, the corticosteroid should be discontinued until the infection has been adequately controlled.

Information for the Patient
Patients using topical corticosteroids should receive the following information and instructions:
1. This medication is to be used as directed by the physician. It is for external use only. Avoid contact with the eyes.
2. Patients should be advised not to use this medication for any disorder other than for which it was prescribed.
3. The treated skin area should not be bandaged or otherwise covered or wrapped as to be occlusive unless directed by the physician.
4. Patients should report any signs of local adverse reactions especially under occlusive dressing.
5. Parents of pediatric patients should be advised not to use tight-fitting diapers or plastic pants on a child being treated in the diaper area, as these garments may constitute occlusive dressings.

Laboratory Tests
The following tests may be helpful in evaluating the HPA axis suppression:
   Urinary free cortisol test
   ACTH stimulation test

Carcinogenesis, Mutagenesis, and Impairment of Fertility
Long-term animal studies have not been performed to evaluate the carcinogenic potential or the effect on fertility of topical corticosteroids.

Studies to determine mutagenicity with prednisolone and hydrocortisone have revealed negative results.

Pregnancy Category C
Corticosteroids are generally teratogenic in laboratory animals when administered systemically at relatively low dosage levels. The more potent corticosteroids have been shown to be teratogenic after dermal application in laboratory animals. There are no adequate and well-controlled studies in pregnant women on teratogenic effects from topically applied corticosteroids. Therefore, topical corticosteroids should be used during pregnancy only if the potential benefit justifies the potential risk to the fetus.

Nursing Mothers
It is not known whether topical administration of corticosteroids could result in sufficient systemic absorption to produce detectable quantities in breast milk. Systemically administered corticosteroids are secreted into breast milk in quantities **not** likely to have a deleterious effect on the infant. Nevertheless, caution should be exercised when topical corticosteroids are administered to a nursing woman.

Pediatric Use
Pediatric patients may demonstrate greater susceptibility to topical corticosteroid-induced HPA axis suppression and Cushing's syndrome than mature patients because of a large skin surface area to body weight ratio.

Hypothalamic-pituitary-adrenal (HPA) axis suppression, Cushing's syndrome, and intracranial hypertension have been reported in children receiving topical corticosteroids. Manifestations of adrenal suppression in children include linear growth retardation, delayed weight gain, low plasma cortisol levels, and absence of response to ACTH stimulation. Manifestations of intracranial hypertension include bulging fontanelles, headaches, and bilateral papilledema.

Administration of topical corticosteroids to children should be limited to the least amount compatible with an effective therapeutic regimen. Chronic corticosteroid therapy may interfere with the growth and development of children.

ADVERSE REACTIONS
The following local adverse reactions have been reported with topical corticosteroids, but may occur more frequently with the use of occlusive dressings. These reactions are listed in approximate decreasing order of occurrence.
1. Burning
2. Itching
3. Irritation
4. Dryness
5. Folliculitis
6. Hypertrichosis
7. Acneiform eruptions
8. Hypopigmentation
9. Perioral dermatitis
10. Allergic contact dermatitis
11. Maceration of the skin
12. Secondary infection
13. Skin atrophy
14. Striae
15. Miliaria

OVERDOSAGE
Topically applied corticosteroids can be absorbed in sufficient amounts to produce systemic effects. (See PRECAUTIONS.)

DOSAGE AND ADMINISTRATION
psorcon Ointment should be applied to the affected area as a thin film from one to three times daily depending on the severity or resistant nature of the condition.

Occlusive dressings may be used for the management of psoriasis or recalcitrant conditions.

If an infection develops, the use of occlusive dressings should be discontinued and appropriate antimicrobial therapy initiated.

HOW SUPPLIED
psorcon Ointment 0.05% is available in the following size tubes:

15 gram	NDC 0066-0071-17
30 gram	NDC 0066-0071-31
60 gram	NDC 0066-0071-60

Store at controlled room temperature 15°–30°C (59°–80°F).

CAUTION
Federal law prohibits dispensing without prescription.

SHEPARD'S® Cream Lotion

(See PDR For Nonprescription Drugs)

SHEPARD'S® Moisturizing Soap

(See PDR For Nonprescription Drugs)

SHEPARD'S® Skin Cream

(See PDR For Nonprescription Drugs)

SULFACET-R® Acne Lotion   ℞
[*sul-fa-set*]
(sodium sulfacetamide 10% and sulfur 5%)

PRODUCT OVERVIEW
KEY FACTS
Sulfacet-R® contains sodium sulfacetamide 10% and sulfur 5% in a flesh-tinted lotion. Sodium sulfacetamide is an antibacterial, while sulfur acts as a keratolytic agent.

MAJOR USES
Sulfacet-R® is indicated in the topical control of acne vulgaris, acne rosacea, and seborrheic dermatitis.

SAFETY INFORMATION
Sulfacet-R® is contraindicated in patients with a known hypersensitivity to sulfonamides, sulfur, or any other of its ingredients. It should not be used in patients with kidney disease. Although rare, sensitivity to sodium sulfacetamide may occur. It contains sodium bisulfite which may cause allergic-type reactions. Sulfacet-R® may cause local irritation. If irritation develops, discontinue use of the product.

PRESCRIBING INFORMATION
SULFACET-R® Acne Lotion   ℞
[*sul-fa-set*]
(sodium sulfacetamide 10% and sulfur 5%)

DESCRIPTION
Each mL of Sulfacet-R® Acne Lotion (sodium sulfacetamide 10% and sulfur 5%) as dispensed, contains 100 mg of sodium sulfacetamide and 50 mg of sulfur in a tinted lotion of purified water, alkylaryl sulfonic acid salts, hydroxyethylcellulose, propylene glycol, xanthan gum, lauric myristic diethanolamide, polyoxyethylene laurate, butylparaben, methylparaben, silicone emulsion, talc, zinc oxide, titanium dioxide, attapulgite, iron oxides, pH buffers and 2-bromo-2-nitropropane-1, 3-diol.

Sodium sulfacetamide is a sulfonamide with antibacterial activity while sulfur acts as a keratolytic agent. Chemically sodium sulfacetamide is N'-[(4-aminophenyl)sulfonyl]-acetamide, monosodium salt, monohydrate.

CLINICAL PHARMACOLOGY
The most widely accepted mechanism of action of sulfonamides is the Woods-Fildes theory which is based on the fact that sulfonamides act as competitive antagonists to para-aminobenzoic acid (PABA), an essential component for bacterial growth. While absorption through intact skin has not been determined, sodium sulfacetamide is readily absorbed from the gastrointestinal tract when taken orally and excreted in the urine, largely unchanged. The biological half-life has variously been reported as 7 to 12.8 hours.

The exact mode of action of sulfur in the treatment of acne is unknown, but it has been reported that it inhibits the growth of *p. acnes* and the formation of free fatty acids.

INDICATIONS
Sulfacet-R® is indicated in the topical control of acne vulgaris, acne rosacea and seborrheic dermatitis.

CONTRAINDICATIONS
Sulfacet-R® Acne Lotion is contraindicated for use by patients having known hypersensitivity to sulfonamides, sulfur, or any other component of this preparation. Sulfacet-R® Acne Lotion is not to be used by patients with kidney disease.

WARNINGS
Although rare, sensitivity to sodium sulfacetamide may occur. Therefore, caution and careful supervision should be observed when prescribing this drug for patients who may be prone to hypersensitivity to topical sulfonamides. Systemic toxic reactions such as agranulocytosis, acute hemolytic anemia, purpura hemorrhagica, drug fever, jaundice and contact dermatitis indicate hypersensitivity to sulfonamides. Particular caution should be employed if areas of denuded or abraded skin are involved. Contains sodium bisulfite, a sulfite that may cause allergic-type reactions including anaphylactic symptoms and life-threatening or less severe asthmatic episodes in certain susceptible people. The overall prevalence of sulfite sensitivity in the general population is unknown and probably low. Sulfite sensitivity is seen more frequently in asthmatic than in nonasthmatic people.

Dermik—Cont.

ZETAR® EMULSION (Coal Tar)   ℞
[zē-tar]

DESCRIPTION
Zetar® Emulsion, coal tar, is a liquid for topical application, following dilution in aqueous media. Each ml contains 300 mg whole coal tar in polysorbates. It is a topical anti-eczematic. The complete chemical composition of coal tar has not been ascertained; components are grouped into six categories: aromatic hydrocarbons, acidic phenolic compounds, cyclic nitrogen compounds, organic sulfur compounds, nonacidic phenolics and nonbasic nitrogen compounds.

CLINICAL PHARMACOLOGY
There is no confirmed scientific evidence as to the clinical pharmacologic effects of coal tar. Its actions in humans have been reported in the literature as antiseptic, antipruritic, antiparasitic, antifungal, antibacterial, keratoplastic and antiacanthotic. Vasoconstrictive activity of coal tar has also been reported.

INDICATIONS AND USAGE
Zetar® Emulsion is indicated for the relief of symptoms associated with generalized, persistent dermatoses such as psoriasis, eczema, atopic dermatitis and seborrheic dermatitis.

CONTRAINDICATIONS
Not to be used on open or infected lesions.

WARNINGS
Application of coal tar may elicit a pustular eruption or a cyst (epidermal) like reaction.
Patients who have previously exhibited sensitivity to tars must be under careful and continuous supervision by the physician.

PRECAUTIONS
For external (topical) use only. Keep away from the eyes. When used in the bath, add lukewarm water (not hot water). For 72 hours following treatment with coal tar, patients should avoid exposure to either direct sunlight or sunlamps (ultra-violet A and/or B) unless directed by physician, as this drug may photoactivate the skin. Prior to exposure to sunlight, completely remove all tar from skin. Sensitization or dermatitis may occur after prolonged use. If irritation develops or increases, discontinue use and consult physician. Keep out of the reach of children.
While no known drug interactions have been reported pertaining to the clinical use of this drug in patients, the concomitant use of drugs with phototoxic and/or photoactivating potential is not recommended (i.e. tetracyclines, psoralens, topical retinoic acid).
Carcinogenesis—Coal tar applied to the skin of mice resulted in an increase in epidermal carcinomas. Painting rabbit ears with coal tar appears to increase self-limiting keratoacanthomas. To date, existing reports do not suggest an increased incidence of skin cancer in psoriatics treated with coal tar.
Pregnancy Category C—Animal reproduction studies have not been conducted with Zetar® Emulsion (coal tar). It is also not known whether Zetar® Emulsion can cause fetal harm when administered to a pregnant woman or can affect reproduction capacity. Zetar® Emulsion should be given to a pregnant woman only if clearly needed.
Nursing Mothers—It is not known whether this drug is excreted in human milk. Because of the tumorigenicity shown for coal tar in animal studies, a decision should be made whether to discontinue nursing or to discontinue the drug, taking into account the importance of the drug to the mother.

ADVERSE REACTIONS
Application of coal tar may result in superficial folliculitis. Patients hypersensitive to coal tar may exhibit a pustular or keratocystic response.

DOSAGE AND ADMINISTRATION
Add 3 to 5 teaspoonfuls of Zetar® Emulsion to a bath of lukewarm water. This is mixed throughout the bath. The patient immerses in the bath for 15 to 20 minutes. The interval recommended between dosing is from once-a-day to once every third day, and usual duration of treatment is 30 to 45 days.
If the physician decides to administer supplemental ultraviolet irradiation (Goeckerman treatment) to the patient (ultraviolet B; A or A/B), this may be accomplished between 2 and 72 hours. A determination of minimal erythemal dosage (MED) should be made for each patient; initial irradiation should be suberythemal, not to exceed MED.
Compounding: Zetar® Emulsion (coal tar) may be utilized in compounding prescriptions in aqueous based vehicles requiring coal tar. Each ml of Zetar® Emulsion contains 300 mg whole coal tar.

HOW SUPPLIED
Zetar® Emulsion (coal tar) is available in 6 fl oz (177 ml) plastic bottles. The strength of the preparation is 300 mg coal tar/mL.
SHAKE WELL before each use. No special handling or storage conditions are required.

CAUTION
Federal law prohibits dispensing without prescription

ZETAR® SHAMPOO
[zē-tar]

(See PDR For Nonprescription Drugs)

The Dial Corporation
15101 N. SCOTTSDALE ROAD
SCOTTSDALE, AZ 85254-2199

LUROSCRUB®   OTC
[lur'o-scrub]
Antimicrobial Skin Cleanser

DESCRIPTION
LUROSCRUB is an antimicrobial skin cleanser possessing bactericidal activity. LUROSCRUB contains 4% w/w chlorhexidine gluconate, a chemically unique hexamethylenebis biguanide with inactive ingredients: fragrance, isopropyl alcohol 4%, purified water, and other ingredients, in a mild, sudsing base adjusted to pH 4.5–6.8 for optimal activity and stability.

ACTION
LUROSCRUB is bactericidal on contact. It has antiseptic activity and a persistent antimicrobial effect with rapid bactericidal activity against a wide range of microorganisms, including gram positive and gram negative bacteria such as *Pseudomonas aeruginosa*, also yeasts and molds. The effectiveness of LUROSCRUB is not significantly reduced by the presence of organic matter, such as blood.[1] LUROSCRUB prevents skin infection thereby reducing the risk of cross-infection.

INDICATIONS
LUROSCRUB is indicated for use as a surgical scrub, a health-care personnel handwash, a skin wound cleanser and a general skin cleanser.

SAFETY
The extensive use of chlorhexidene gluconate for over 20 years outside the United States has produced no evidence of absorption of the compound through intact skin. The potential for producing skin reactions is extremely low. LUROSCRUB can be used many times a day without causing irritation, dryness or discomfort. Experimental studies indicate that when used for cleaning superficial wounds, LUROSCRUB will neither cause additional tissue injury nor delay healing.

WARNINGS
FOR EXTERNAL USE ONLY. KEEP OUT OF EYES, EARS AND MOUTH. CHLORHEXIDINE GLUCONATE SHOULD NOT BE USED AS A PREOPERATIVE SKIN PREPARATION OF THE PERIOBITAL OR EYELID AREAS. Misuse of products containing chlorhexidine gluconate has been reported to cause serious and permanent eye injury when it has been permitted to enter the eye during surgical procedures. If LUROSCRUB should contact these areas, rinse out promptly and thoroughly with water. Chlorhexidine has been reported to cause deafness when instilled in the middle ear through perforated eardrums. Avoid contact with meninges. LUROSCRUB should not be used by any persons who have a sensitivity to it or its components. Irritation, sensitization and generalized allergic reactions have been reported with chlorhexidine-containing products, especially in the genital areas. If adverse reactions occur, discontinue use immediately and if severe, contact a physician. Keep this and all drugs out of the reach of children. In case of accidental ingestion, seek professional assistance or contact a Poison Control Center immediately.
Accidental ingestion: Chlorhexidine gluconate taken orally is poorly absorbed. Treat with gastric lavage using milk, egg white, gelatin or mild soap. Employ supportive measures as appropriate.
Avoid excessive heat (above 104°F).

DIRECTIONS FOR USE
SURGICAL HAND SCRUB:
Wet hands and forearms with water. Scrub for 3 minutes with about 5 ml. of LUROSCRUB and a wet brush, paying particular attention to the nails, cuticles, and interdigital spaces. A separate nail cleaner may be used. Rinse thoroughly. Wash for an additional 3 minutes with 5 ml. of LUROSCRUB and rinse under running water. Dry thoroughly.
HEALTH CARE PERSONNEL HAND WASH:
Wet hands with water. Dispense about 5 ml. of LUROSCRUB into cupped hands and wash in a vigorous manner for 15 seconds. Rinse and dry thoroughly.
SKIN WOUND AND GENERAL SKIN CLEANSING:
Wounds which involve more than the superficial layers of the skin should not be routinely treated with LUROSCRUB. LUROSCRUB should not be used for repeated general skin cleansing of large body areas except in those patients whose underlying condition makes it necessary to reduce the bacterial population of the skin. To use, thoroughly rinse the area to be cleansed with water. Apply the minimum amount of LUROSCRUB necessary to cover the skin or wound area and wash gently. Rinse again thoroughly.

HOW SUPPLIED
For general handwashing locations: 4 oz squeeze bottles with dispenser caps and 12 oz pump bottles. For surgical scrub areas: 1 gallon and 32 oz plastic disposable bottles. These bottles are designed for use with standard wall dispensers, and can accommodate either hand pump or foot pump mechanisms. NDC 54012-284.

REFERENCES
1. Lowbury, E. J. L. and Lilly, H. A.: The Effect of Blood on Disinfection of Surgeon's Hands. Brit. J. Surg. 61:19–21 (Jan.) 1974.

Dista Products Company
Division of Eli Lilly and Company
LILLY CORPORATE CENTER
INDIANAPOLIS, IN 46285

LEGEND

Hyporets®—*Disposable Syringes, Dista*
Identi-Code®—*Formula Identification Code, Dista*
Identi-Dose®—*Unit Dose Medication, Dista*
Pulvules®—*Filled Gelatin Capsules, Dista*
℞Pak—*Prescription Package, Dista*

IDENTI-CODE® Index
(formula identification code, Dista)
Provides Positive Product Identification

A letter-number symbol, a 4-digit number, the name of the product, the strength of the product, or a combination of these appears on each Dista capsule and tablet and on each label of pediatric liquids and powders for oral suspension. The letter/number or 4-digit number identifies the product.

**Identi-
Code® Product Name**

CO3-C22 (Coated Tablets)

CO3 Ilotycin®
    Composition (Each Enteric-Coated Tablet): Erythromycin, USP, 250 mg
C19 Mi-Cebrin®
    Composition (Each Coated Tablet): Thiamine (vitamin B_1), 10 mg; riboflavin (vitamin B_2), 5 mg; pyridoxine (vitamin B_6), 1.7 mg; pantothenic acid, 10 mg; niacinamide, 30 mg; vitamin B_{12} (activity equivalent), 3 mcg; ascorbic acid (vitamin C), 100 mg; dl-alpha tocopheryl acetate (vitamin E), 5.5 IU (5.5 mg); vitamin A, 10,000 IU (3 mg); vitamin D, 400 IU (10 mcg); contains also (approximately): iron (as ferrous sulfate), 15 mg; copper (as the sulfate), 1 mg; iodine (as potassium iodide), 0.15 mg; manganese (as the glycerophosphate), 1 mg; magnesium (as the hydroxide), 5 mg; zinc (as the chloride), 1.5 mg
C20 Mi-Cebrin T®
    Composition (Each Coated Tablet): Thiamine mononitrate (vitamin B_1), 15 mg; riboflavin (vitamin B_2), 10 mg; pyridoxine hydrochloride (vitamin B_6), 2 mg; pantothenic acid (as calcium pantothenate), 10 mg; niacinamide, 100 mg; vitamin B_{12} (activity equivalent), 7.5 mcg; ascorbic acid (vitamin C), 150 mg; dl-alpha tocopheryl acetate (vitamin E), 5.5 IU (5.5 mg); vitamin A, 10,000 IU (3 mg); vitamin D, 400 IU (10 mcg); contains also (approximately): iron (as ferrous sulfate), 15 mg; copper (as the sulfate), 1 mg; iodine (as potassium iodide), 0.15 mg; manganese (as the glycerophos-

phate), 1 mg; magnesium (as the hydroxide), 5 mg; zinc (as the chloride), 1.5 mg

C22 Becotin®-T

Composition (Each Coated Tablet): Thiamine mononitrate (vitamin B₁), 15 mg; riboflavin (vitamin B₂), 10 mg; pyridoxine hydrochloride (vitamin B₆), 5 mg; niacinamide, 100 mg; pantothenic acid (as calcium pantothenate), 20 mg; vitamin B₁₂ (activity equivalent), 4 mcg; ascorbic acid (vitamin C) (as sodium ascorbate), 300 mg

---

F62-H77 (Pulvules®)

F62 Becotin®

Composition (Each Pulvule®): Thiamine hydrochloride (vitamin B₁), 10 mg; riboflavin (vitamin B₂), 10 mg; pyridoxine (vitamin B₆), 4.1 mg; niacinamide, 50 mg; pantothenic acid, 25 mg; vitamin B₁₂ (activity equivalent), 1 mcg

F77 Becotin® with Vitamin C

Composition (Each Pulvule®): Thiamine hydrochloride (vitamin B₁), 10 mg; riboflavin (vitamin B₂), 10 mg; pyridoxine (vitamin B₆), 4.1 mg; niacinamide, 50 mg; pantothenic acid, 25 mg; vitamin B₁₂ (activity equivalent), 1 mcg; ascorbic acid (vitamin C), 150 mg

3055 Cinobac®

Composition (Each Pulvule®): Cinoxacin, USP, 250 mg

3056 Cinobac®

Composition (Each Pulvule®): Cinoxacin, USP, 500 mg

3105 Prozac®

Composition (Each Pulvule®): fluoxetine hydrochloride, 20 mg (equiv. to fluoxetine)

3123 Co-Pyronil 2®

Composition (Each Pulvule®): chlorpheniramine maleate, 4 mg; pseudoephedrine hydrochloride, 60 mg

---

H07 Ilosone®

Composition (Each Pulvule®): Erythromycin Estolate, USP, 125 mg (equiv. to erythromycin)

H09 Ilosone®

Composition (Each Pulvule®): Erythromycin Estolate, USP, 250 mg (equiv. to erythromycin)

H69 Keflex®

Composition (Each Pulvule®): Cephalexin, USP, 250 mg

H71 Keflex®

Composition (Each Pulvule®): Cephalexin, USP, 500 mg

℞H74 Valmid®

Composition (Each Pulvule®): Ethinamate, USP, 500 mg

H76 Nalfon® 200

Composition (Each Pulvule®): Fenoprofen Calcium, USP, 200 mg (equiv. to fenoprofen)

H77 Nalfon®

Composition (Each Pulvule®): Fenoprofen Calcium, USP, 300 mg (equiv. to fenoprofen)

U05-U60 (Compressed Tablets)

U05 Ilosone® Chewable

Composition (Each Compressed Tablet): Erythromycin Estolate, USP, 125 mg (equiv. to erythromycin)

U25 Ilosone® Chewable

Composition (Each Compressed Tablet): Erythromycin Estolate, USP, 250 mg (equiv. to erythromycin)

U26 Ilosone®

Composition (Each Compressed Tablet): Erythromycin Estolate, USP, 500 mg (equiv. to erythromycin)

U59 Nalfon®

Composition (Each Compressed Tablet): Fenoprofen Calcium, USP, 600 mg (equiv. to fenoprofen)

U60 Keflex®

Composition (Each Compressed Tablet): Cephalexin, 1 mg

4142 Keftab®

Composition (Each Compressed Tablet): Cephalexin Hydrochloride, 250 mg (equiv. to cephalexin)

4143 Keftab®

Composition (Each Compressed Tablet): Cephalexin Hydrochloride, 500 mg (equiv. to cephalexin)

4202 Keflet®

Composition (Each Tablet): Cephalexin, 250 mg

4203 Keflet®

Composition (Each Tablet): Cephalexin, 500 mg

W14-W68 (Miscellaneous)

W14 Cordran® Tape

Composition: Flurandrenolide, USP, 4 mcg/sq cm

W15 Ilosone® Liquid, Oral Suspension

Composition: Each 5 ml contain erythromycin estolate equivalent to 125 mg erythromycin (USP).

W17 Ilosone® Liquid, Oral Suspension

Composition: Each 5 ml contain erythromycin estolate equivalent to 250 mg erythromycin (USP).

W18 Ilosone® Ready-Mixed Drops

Composition: Each ml contains erythromycin estolate equivalent to 100 mg erythromycin (USP).

W21 Keflex®, for Oral Suspension

Composition (When Mixed as Directed): Each 5 ml contain 125 mg cephalexin (USP).

W22 Keflex®, for Pediatric Drops

Composition (When Mixed as Directed): Each ml contains 100 mg cephalexin (USP).

W68 Keflex®, for Oral Suspension

Composition (When Mixed as Directed): Each 5 ml contain 250 mg cephalexin (USP).

UNIT-DOSE PACKAGING

Identi-Dose® (unit dose medication, Dista) Closed-circuit control of medication from pharmacy to nurse to patient and return. Simplifies counting and dispensing whether in single-unit or prescription-size quantities. Fits into any dispensing system for ready identification and legibility, better inventory control, protection from contamination, easier handling and recording under Medicare, prevention of drug loss through pilferage or spilling, better control of Federal Controlled Substances, and less chance of medication errors. The following products are available through normal channels of supply:

Identi-Dose®
Pulvules®
No.
375 Ilosone®, 250 mg
402 Keflex®, 250 mg
403 Keflex®, 500 mg
Tablets
No.
1790 Mi-Cebrin®
1807 Mi-Cebrin T®
1896 Keflex®, 1 g
Miscellaneous
No.
M-201 Keflex®, for Oral Suspension, 125 mg/5 ml
M-202 Keflex®, for Oral Suspension, 250 mg/5 ml

CINOBAC®   ℞
[sĭn ′ō-băk]
(cinoxacin)
Capsules, USP

DESCRIPTION

Cinobac® (Cinoxacin, USP, Dista) is a synthetic antibacterial agent for oral administration. It is 1-ethyl-1,4-dihydro-4-oxo-[1,3] dioxolo[4,5-g]cinnoline-3-carboxylic acid and occurs as white or very light-yellow, needle-shaped crystals. Cinobac is available as 250- and 500-mg Pulvules®. These Pulvules also contain D&C Yellow No. 10, FD&C Blue No. 1, FD&C Red No. 3, FD&C Yellow No. 6, gelatin, starch, titanium dioxide, and other inactive ingredients. Examples of antibacterial drugs in the quinolone class include nalidixic acid and norfloxacin.

CLINICAL PHARMACOLOGY

Cinoxacin is rapidly absorbed after oral administration. In fluorometric assay, a 500-mg dose produced a peak serum concentration of 15 mg/L, which declined to approximately 1 to 2 mg/L 6 hours after administration, as determined by fluorometric assay. A 500-mg dose produced an average urine concentration of approximately 300 mg/L during the first 4 hours and approximately 100 mg/L during the second 4-hour period. These urine concentrations are many times greater than the minimal inhibitory concentration (MIC) of cinoxacin for most gram-negative organisms commonly found in urinary tract infections.

Ninety-seven percent of a 500-mg oral dose of radiolabeled cinoxacin was recovered in the urine within 24 hours, 60% of which was present as unaltered cinoxacin and the remainder as inactive metabolic products.

The presence of food did not affect the total absorption of cinoxacin. Peak serum concentrations were reduced, but the 24-hour urinary recovery of antibacterial activity was unaltered. The mean serum half-life is 1.5 hours.

Microbiology—Cinoxacin has in vitro activity against a wide variety of aerobic gram-negative bacilli, particularly strains of *Enterobacteriaceae*. In vitro tests demonstrate that cinoxacin is bactericidal. The mode of action has been shown to be inhibition of bacterial DNA replication. It is active within the range of urinary pH.

Cinoxacin is active against most strains of the following organisms: *Escherichia coli*, *Klebsiella* sp (including *Klebsiella pneumoniae*), *Enterobacter* sp, *Proteus mirabilis*, and *Proteus vulgaris*.

Cinoxacin is not active against *Pseudomonas*, enterococci, or staphylococci. Cross-resistance with nalidixic acid has been demonstrated. Bacterial resistance to cinoxacin has been reported in less than 4% of patients treated with recommended doses; however, bacterial resistance to cinoxacin has not been shown to be transferable via R-factor.

Susceptibility Tests—Quantitative methods give the most precise estimates of susceptibility to antibacterial drugs. For purposes of judging susceptibility of bacterial isolates to cinoxacin, minimal inhibitory concentration and disk test breakpoints were established on the basis of (1) human drug bioavailability studies and (2) test results obtained with normally susceptible strains compared with results from resistant strains. The breakpoints have been verified by comparison with results of the clinical trials with cinoxacin.

One quantitative method, a standardized disk test, has been recommended.* Reports from the laboratory giving results of the standardized test using the 100-μg cinoxacin disk should be interpreted according to the following criteria:

Organisms producing zones of ≥ 19 mm are classified as susceptible, whereas those producing zones of 15 to 18 mm are classified as having intermediate susceptibility. Organisms in either of these categories are likely to respond to therapy if the infection is confined to the urinary tract. Organisms producing zones of ≤ 14 mm are reported as resistant, a test result that indicates that other therapy should be selected.

Certain strains of *Enterobacteriaceae* exhibit heterogeneity of resistance to cinoxacin. These strains produce isolated colonies within the inhibition zone. When such strains are encountered, the clear inhibition zone should be measured *within* the isolated colonies.

Dilution methods for determining susceptibility are also used, and results are reported as the minimal drug concentration that inhibits microbial growth (MIC).

If the MIC is ≤ 16 mg/L, the microorganism is considered "susceptible"; if > 16 mg/L and < 64 mg/L, it is "intermediate"; and it is "resistant" if the MIC is ≥ 64 mg/L.

---

* Approved Standard ASM-2 Performance Standards for Antimicrobial Disk Susceptibility Tests; National Committee for Clinical Laboratory Standards, 771 East Lancaster Avenue, Villanova, Pennsylvania 19085.

INDICATIONS AND USAGE

Cinobac® (Cinoxacin, USP, Dista) is indicated for the treatment of initial and recurrent urinary tract infections in adults caused by the following susceptible microorganisms: *E coli*, *P mirabilis*, *P vulgaris*, *Klebsiella* sp (including *K pneumoniae*), and *Enterobacter* sp.

Cinobac is effective in preventing urinary tract infections for up to 5 months in women with a history of recurrent urinary tract infections.

In vitro susceptibility testing should be performed prior to administration of the drug and, when clinically indicated, during treatment.

CONTRAINDICATION

Cinobac® (Cinoxacin, USP, Dista) is contraindicated in patients with a history of hypersensitivity to cinoxacin or other quinolones.

WARNINGS

The use of cinoxacin in prepubertal children and pregnant women is not recommended. The oral administration of a single 250-mg/kg dose of cinoxacin caused lameness in immature dogs. Histologic examination of the weight-bearing joints of these dogs revealed permanent lesions of the cartilage. Related drugs (eg, nalidixic acid and norfloxacin) also produce erosions of the cartilage in weight-bearing joints and other signs of arthropathy in immature animals of various species.

PRECAUTIONS

General—Since Cinobac® (Cinoxacin, USP, Dista) is eliminated primarily by the kidney, the usual dosage should be lower in patients with reduced renal function (*see* Dosage

Continued on next page

Dista—Cont.

and Administration). Administration of Cinobac is not recommended for anuric patients.

Cinobac should be used with caution in patients with a history of hepatic disease.

Pregnancy—Pregnancy Category C—Reproduction studies have been performed in rats and rabbits at doses up to 10 times the daily human dose and have revealed no evidence of impaired fertility or harm to the fetus due to cinoxacin. There are, however, no adequate and well-controlled studies in pregnant women. **Since cinoxacin, like other drugs in its class, causes arthropathy in immature animals, its use during pregnancy is not recommended** (see **Warnings**).

Nursing Mothers—It is not known whether cinoxacin is excreted in human milk. Because other drugs in this class are excreted in human milk and because of the potential for serious adverse reactions from cinoxacin in nursing infants, a decision that takes into account the importance of the drug to the mother should be made either to discontinue nursing or to discontinue the drug.

Pediatric Use—Cinoxacin is not recommended for use in prepubertal children (see Warnings).

ADVERSE REACTIONS

In clinical studies involving 1,118 patients, the following adverse effects were considered to be related to cinoxacin therapy:

Gastrointestinal—Nausea was reported most commonly and occurred in less than 3 in 100 patients. Other side effects, occurring less frequently (1 in 100), were anorexia, vomiting, abdominal cramps/pain, perverse taste, and diarrhea.

Central Nervous System—The most frequent side effects were headache and dizziness, reported by 1 in 100 patients. Other adverse reactions possibly related to Cinobac® (Cinoxacin, USP, Dista) include insomnia, drowsiness, tingling sensation, perineal burning, photophobia, and tinnitus. These were reported by less than 1 in 100 patients.

Hypersensitivity—Rash, urticaria, pruritus, edema, angioedema, and eosinophilia were reported by less than 3 in 100 patients. Rare cases of anaphylactoid reactions have been reported. Toxic epidermal necrolysis has been reported very rarely.

Hematologic—Rare reports of thrombocytopenia.

Laboratory values that were reported to be abnormal were, in order of frequency, BUN (1 in 100) and SGOT, SGPT, serum creatinine, alkaline phosphatase, and reduction in hematocrit/hemoglobin (each less than 1 in 100).

Although not observed in the 1,118 patients treated with cinoxacin, the following side effects have been reported for other drugs in the same pharmacologically active and chemically related class: restlessness, nervousness, change in color perception, difficulty in focusing, decrease in visual acuity, double vision, weakness, constipation, erythema and bullae, feelings of disorientation or agitation or acute anxiety, palpitation, soreness of the gums, joint stiffness, swelling of the extremities, and toxic psychosis or convulsions (rare).

All adverse reactions observed with drugs in this class were reversible.

OVERDOSAGE

Signs and Symptoms—Symptoms following an overdose of cinoxacin may include anorexia, nausea, vomiting, epigastric distress, and diarrhea. The severity of the epigastric distress and the diarrhea are dose related. Headache, dizziness, insomnia, photophobia, tinnitus, and a tingling sensation have been reported in some patients. If other symptoms are present, they are probably secondary to an underlying disease state, an allergic reaction, or the ingestion of a second medication with toxicity.

Treatment—To obtain up-to-date information about the treatment of overdose, a good resource is your certifed Regional Poison Control Center. Telephone numbers of certified poison control centers are listed in the *Physicians' Desk Reference (PDR)*. In managing overdosage, consider the possibility of multiple drug overdoses, interaction among drugs, and unusual drug kinetics in your patient.

Patients who have ingested an overdose of cinoxacin should be kept well hydrated to prevent crystalluria.

Protect the patient's airway and support ventilation and perfusion. Meticulously monitor and maintain, within acceptable limits, the patient's vital signs, blood gases, serum electrolytes, etc. Absorption of drugs from the gastrointestinal tract may be decreased by giving activated charcoal, which, in many cases, is more effective than emesis or lavage; consider charcoal instead of or in addition to gastric emptying. Repeated doses of charcoal over time may hasten elimination of some drugs that have been absorbed. Safeguard the patient's airway when employing gastric emptying or charcoal.

Forced diuresis, peritoneal dialysis, hemodialysis, or charcoal hemoperfusion have not been established as beneficial for an overdose of cinoxacin.

DOSAGE AND ADMINISTRATION

The usual adult dosage for the treatment of urinary tract infections is 1 g daily, administered orally in 2 or 4 divided doses (500 mg b.i.d. or 250 mg q.i.d. respectively) for 7 to 14 days. Although susceptible organisms may be eradicated within a few days after therapy has begun, the full treatment course is recommended.

Impaired Renal Function—When renal function is impaired, a reduced dosage must be employed. After an initial dose of 500 mg, a maintenance dosage schedule should be used (see table).

MAINTENANCE DOSAGE GUIDE
FOR PATIENTS WITH RENAL
IMPAIRMENT

Creatinine Clearance (mL/min/1.73 m²)	Renal Function	Dosage
>80	Normal	500 mg b.i.d.
	Mild	250 mg
80–50	Impairment	t.i.d.
	Moderate	250 mg
50–20	Impairment	b.i.d.
	Marked	250 mg
<20	Impairment	q.d.

Administration of Cinobac® (Cinoxacin, USP, Dista) to anuric patients is not recommended.

When only serum creatinine is available, the following formula (based on sex, weight, and age of the patient) may be used to convert this value into creatinine clearance.

The serum creatinine should represent a steady state of renal function.

Males: $\dfrac{\text{Weight (kg) x (140} - \text{age)}}{72 \text{ x serum creatinine}}$

Females: 0.9 x male value

Preventive Therapy—A single dose of 250 mg at bedtime for up to 5 months has been shown to be effective in women with a history of recurrent urinary tract infections.

HOW SUPPLIED

Pulvules:

   250 mg, orange and green (No. 3055)—(40s) NDC 0777-3055-40.

   500 mg, orange and green (No. 3056)—(50s) NDC 0777-3056-50.

ANIMAL PHARMACOLOGY

Crystalluria, sometimes associated with secondary urinary tract pathology, occurs in laboratory animals treated orally with cinoxacin. In the rhesus monkey, crystalluria (without urinary tract pathology) has been noted at doses as low as 50 mg/kg/day (lowest dose tested). Cinoxacin-related crystalluria has not been observed in humans receiving twice the recommended daily dosage.

Cinoxacin and related drugs have been shown to cause arthropathy in immature animals of most species tested (see Warnings).

Some drugs of this class have been shown to have oculotoxic potential. Cinoxacin administered to cats at high dosages (200 mg/kg/day) resulted in retinal degeneration and other ocular changes. The dog appeared to be somewhat resistant to these effects, but high dosages (500 mg/kg/day) resulted in mild retinal atrophy. No cinoxacin-related ocular changes were noted in rabbit, rat, monkey, or human studies. (In one of the studies involving the monkey, cinoxacin was administered for 1 year at 10 times the recommended clinical dose.)

[020289]

Shown in Product Identification Section, page 409

CORDRAN® and   ℞
CORDRAN® SP
[kŏr 'drăn]
(flurandrenolide) USP

CORDRAN®-N
[kŏr 'drăn ĕn]
**(neomycin sulfate with flurandrenolide)
USP**

DESCRIPTION

Cordran® (Flurandrenolide, USP, Dista) is a potent corticosteroid intended for topical use. It occurs as white to off-white, fluffy, crystalline powder and is odorless. Flurandrenolide is practically insoluble in water and in ether. One g dissolves in 72 mL of alcohol and in 10 mL of chloroform. The molecular weight of Cordran is 436.52.

The chemical name of flurandrenolide is Pregn-4-ene-3, 20-dione, 6-fluoro 11,21 dihydroxy-16, 17-[(1-methylethylidene)bis (oxy)]-, (6α, 11β, 16α)-; its empirical formula is $C_{24}H_{33}FO_6$.

Each g of Cream Cordran® SP (Flurandrenolide Cream, USP, Dista) contains 0.5 mg (0.05%) or 0.25 mg (0.025%) flurandrenolide in an emulsified base composed of cetyl alcohol, citric acid, mineral oil, polyoxyl 40 stearate, propylene glycol, sodium citrate, stearic acid, and purified water.

Each g of Ointment Cordran® (Flurandrenolide Ointment, USP, Dista) contains 0.5 mg (0.05%) or 0.25 mg (0.025%) flurandrenolide in a base composed of white wax, cetyl alcohol, sorbitan sesquioleate, and white petrolatum.

Each mL of Lotion Cordran® (Flurandrenolide Lotion, USP, Dista) contains 0.5 mg (1.145 μmol) (0.05%) flurandrenolide in an oil-in-water emulsion base composed of glycerin, cetyl alcohol, stearic acid, glyceryl monostearate, mineral oil, polyoxyl 40 stearate, menthol, benzyl alcohol, and purified water.

Each g of Cordran-N cream contains 0.5 mg (0.05%) flurandrenolide and 5 mg neomycin sulfate (equivalent to 3.5 mg neomycin base) in a base composed of stearic acid, cetyl alcohol, mineral oil, polyoxyl 40 stearate, ethylparaben, glycerin, and purified water.

Each g of Cordran-N ointment contains 0.5 mg (0.05%) flurandrenolide and 5 mg neomycin sulfate (equivalent to 3.5 mg neomycin base) in a base composed of white wax, cetyl alcohol, sorbitan sesquioleate, and white petrolatum.

CLINICAL PHARMACOLOGY

Cordran® (Flurandrenolide, USP, Dista) is primarily effective because of its anti-inflammatory, antipruritic, and vasoconstrictive actions.

The mechanism of the anti-inflammatory effect of topical corticosteroids is not completely understood. Various laboratory methods, including vasoconstrictor assays, are used to compare and predict potencies and/or clinical efficacies of the topical corticosteroids. There is some evidence to suggest that a recognizable correlation exists between vasoconstrictor potency and therapeutic efficacy in man. Corticosteroids with anti-inflammatory activity may stabilize cellular and lysosomal membranes. There is also the suggestion that the effect on the membranes of lysosomes prevents the release of proteolytic enzymes and, thus, plays a part in reducing inflammation.

Evaporation of water from the lotion vehicle produces a cooling effect which is often desirable in the treatment of acutely inflamed or weeping lesions.

Pharmacokinetics—The extent of percutaneous absorption of topical corticosteroids is determined by many factors, including the vehicle, the integrity of the epidermal barrier, and the use of occlusive dressings.

Topical corticosteroids can be absorbed from normal intact skin. Inflammation and/or other disease processes in the skin increase percutaneous absorption. Occlusive dressings substantially increase the percutaneous absorption of topical corticosteroids. Thus, occlusive dressings may be a valuable therapeutic adjunct for treatment of resistant dermatoses (see Dosage and Administration).

Once absorbed through the skin, topical corticosteroids are handled through pharmacokinetic pathways similar to those of systemically administered corticosteroids. Corticosteroids are bound to plasma proteins in varying degrees. Corticosteroids are metabolized primarily in the liver and then excreted in the kidneys. Some of the topical corticosteroids and their metabolites are also excreted into the bile.

The addition of neomycin in Cordran-N broadens the usefulness of Cordran so that dermatoses complicated by actual skin infections may be treated more effectively and with safety.

INDICATIONS AND USAGE

Cordran® (Flurandrenolide, USP, Dista) is indicated for the relief of the inflammatory and pruritic manifestations of corticosteroid-responsive dermatoses.

Cordran-N is indicated for the treatment of corticosteroid-responsive dermatoses with secondary infection. It has not been demonstrated that this steroid-antibiotic combination provides greater benefit than the steroid component alone after seven days of treatment (see Warning).

CONTRAINDICATIONS

Topical corticosteroids are contraindicated in patients with a history of hypersensitivity to any of the components of these preparations.

WARNING

Because of the concern of nephrotoxicity and ototoxicity associated with neomycin, this combination product should not be used over a wide area or for extended periods of time.

PRECAUTIONS

General—Systemic absorption of topical corticosteroids has produced reversible hypothalamic-pituitary-adrenal (HPA) axis suppression, manifestations of Cushing's syndrome, hyperglycemia, and glucosuria in some patients.

Conditions that augment systemic absorption include application of the more potent steroids, use over large surface areas, prolonged use, and the addition of occlusive dressings. Therefore, patients receiving a large dose of a potent topical steroid applied to a large surface area or under an occlusive dressing should be evaluated periodically for evidence of HPA axis suppression by using urinary-free cortisol and ACTH stimulation tests. If HPA axis suppression is noted, an attempt should be made to withdraw the drug, to reduce the frequency of application, or to substitute a less potent steroid.

Recovery of HPA axis function is generally prompt and complete upon discontinuation of the drug. Infrequently, signs and symptoms of steroid withdrawal may occur, so that supplemental systemic corticosteroids are required.

Children may absorb proportionately larger amounts of topical corticosteroids and thus be more susceptible to systemic toxicity (*see* Usage in Children under Precautions).

If irritation develops, topical corticosteroids should be discontinued and appropriate therapy instituted.

In the presence of dermatologic infections, the use of an appropriate antifungal or antibacterial agent should be instituted. If a favorable response does not occur promptly, Cordran® (Flurandrenolide, USP, Dista) should be discontinued until the infection has been adequately controlled.

Prolonged use of neomycin preparations may result in the overgrowth of nonsusceptible organisms. If this occurs, appropriate measures should be taken.

There are articles in the current medical literature that indicate an increase in the prevalence of persons who are sensitive to neomycin.

These products are not for ophthalmic use.

Information for the Patient —Patients using topical corticosteroids should receive the following information and instructions.

1. This medication is to be used as directed by the physician. It is for external use only. Avoid contact with the eyes.
2. Patients should be advised not to use this medication for any disorder other than that for which it was prescribed.
3. The treated skin area should not be bandaged or otherwise covered or wrapped in order to be occlusive unless the patient is directed to do so by the physician.
4. Patients should report any signs of local adverse reactions, especially under occlusive dressing.
5. Parents of pediatric patients should be advised not to use tight-fitting diapers or plastic pants on a child being treated in the diaper area, because these garments may constitute occlusive dressings.

Laboratory Tests —The following tests may be helpful in evaluating the HPA axis suppression:

    Urinary-free cortisol test
    ACTH stimulation test

Carcinogenesis, Mutagenesis, and Impairment of Fertility —Long-term animal studies have not been performed to evaluate the carcinogenic potential or the effect on fertility of topical corticosteroids.

Studies to determine mutagenicity with prednisolone and hydrocortisone have revealed negative results.

Usage in Pregnancy —*Pregnancy Category C* —Corticosteroids are generally teratogenic in laboratory animals when administered systemically at relatively low dosage levels. The more potent corticosteroids have been shown to be teratogenic after dermal application in laboratory animals. There are no adequate and well-controlled studies in pregnant women on teratogenic effects from topically applied corticosteroids. Therefore, topical corticosteroids should be used during pregnancy only if the potential benefit justifies the potential risk to the fetus. Drugs of this class should not be used extensively for pregnant patients or in large amounts or for prolonged periods of time.

Nursing Mothers —It is not known whether topical administration of corticosteroids could result in sufficient systemic absorption to produce detectable quantities in breast milk. Systemically administered corticosteroids are secreted into breast milk in quantities *not* likely to have a deleterious effect on the infant. Nevertheless, caution should be exercised when topical corticosteroids are administered to a nursing woman.

Usage in Children —Pediatric patients may demonstrate greater susceptibility to topical corticosteroid-induced HPA axis suppression and Cushing's syndrome than do mature patients because of a larger skin surface area to body weight ratio.

Hypothalamic-pituitary-adrenal (HPA) axis suppression, Cushing's syndrome, and intracranial hypertension have been reported in children receiving topical corticosteroids. Manifestations of adrenal suppression in children include linear growth retardation, delayed weight gain, low plasma cortisol levels, and absence of response to ACTH stimulation. Manifestations of intracranial hypertension include bulging fontanelles, headaches, and bilateral papilledema.

Administration of topical corticosteroids to children should be limited to the least amount compatible with an effective therapeutic regimen. Chronic corticosteroid therapy may interfere with the growth and development of children.

ADVERSE REACTIONS

The following local adverse reactions are reported infrequently with topical corticosteroids but may occur more frequently with the use of occlusive dressings. These reactions are listed in an approximate decreasing order of occurrence:

Burning
Itching
Irritation
Dryness
Folliculitis
Hypertrichosis
Acneiform eruptions
Hypopigmentation
Perioral dermatitis
Allergic contact dermatitis

The following may occur more frequently with occlusive dressings:

Maceration of the skin
Secondary infection
Skin atrophy
Striae
Miliaria

Topical neomycin has been reported to cause allergic contact dermatitis, ototoxicity, and nephrotoxicity.

OVERDOSAGE

Topically applied corticosteroids can be absorbed in sufficient amounts to produce systemic effects (*see* Precautions).

DOSAGE AND ADMINISTRATION

Topical corticosteroids are generally applied to the affected area as a thin film 1 to 4 times daily, depending on the severity of the condition.

For moist lesions, a small quantity of the cream or lotion should be rubbed gently into the affected areas 2 or 3 times a day. For dry, scaly lesions, the ointment is applied as a thin film to affected areas 2 or 3 times daily.

Occlusive dressings may be used for the management of psoriasis or recalcitrant conditions.

If an infection develops, the use of occlusive dressings should be discontinued and appropriate antimicrobial therapy instituted.

Use with Occlusive Dressings

The technique of occlusive dressings (for management of psoriasis and other persistent dermatoses) is as follows:

1. Remove as much as possible of the superficial scaling before applying Cream Cordran® SP (Flurandrenolide, USP, Dista) or Ointment or Lotion Cordran. Soaking in a bath will help soften the scales and permit easier removal by brushing, picking, or rubbing.
2. Rub Cream Cordran SP or Ointment or Lotion Cordran thoroughly into the affected areas.
3. Cover with an occlusive plastic film, such as polyethylene, Saran Wrap™, or Handi-Wrap®. (When Cream Cordran SP or Lotion Cordran is used, added moisture may be provided by placing a slightly dampened cloth or gauze over the lesion before the plastic film is applied.)
4. Seal the edges to adjacent normal skin with tape or hold in place by a gauze wrapping.
5. For convenience, the patient may remove the dressing during the day. The dressing should then be reapplied each night.
6. For daytime therapy, the condition may be treated by rubbing Cream Cordran SP or Ointment or Lotion Cordran sparingly into the affected areas.
7. In more resistant cases, leaving the dressing in place for 3 to 4 days at a time may result in a better response.
8. Thin polyethylene gloves are suitable for treatment of the hands and fingers; plastic garment bags may be utilized for treating lesions on the trunk or buttocks. A tight shower cap is useful in treating lesions on the scalp.

Occlusive Dressings Have the Following Advantages —1. Percutaneous penetration of the corticosteroid is enhanced.

2. Medication is concentrated on the areas of skin where it is most needed.

3. This method of administration frequently is more effective in very resistant dermatoses than is the conventional application of Cordran® (Flurandrenolide, USP, Dista).

Precautions to Be Observed in Therapy with Occlusive Dressings —Treatment should be continued for at least a few days after clearing of the lesions. If it is stopped too soon, a relapse may occur. Reinstitution of treatment frequently will cause remission.

Because of the increased hazard of secondary infection from resistant strains of staphylococci among hospitalized patients, it is suggested that the use of occlusive plastic films for corticosteroid therapy in such cases be restricted.

Generally, occlusive dressings should not be used on weeping, or exudative, lesions.

When large areas of the body are covered, thermal homeostasis may be impaired. If elevation of body temperature occurs, use of the occlusive dressing should be discontinued.

Rarely, a patient may develop miliaria, folliculitis, or a sensitivity to either the particular dressing material or a combination of Cordran® (Flurandrenolide, USP, Dista) and the occlusive dressing. If miliaria or folliculitis occurs, use of the occlusive dressing should be discontinued. Treatment by inunction with a corticosteroid such as Cordran may be continued. If the sensitivity is caused by the particular material of the dressing, substitution of a different material may be tried.

Warnings —Some plastic films are readily flammable. Patients should be cautioned against the use of any such material.

When plastic films are used on infants and children, the persons caring for the patients must be reminded of the danger of suffocation if the plastic material accidentally covers the face.

HOW SUPPLIED

℞ Cordran® *(Flurandrenolide, USP), 0.05%, Lotion No. M-128,* in 15-ml (NDC 0777-2352-47) and 60-ml (NDC 0777-2352-97) plastic squeeze bottles. *Avoid freezing.*

℞ Cordran® *(Flurandrenolide, USP), 0.025%, Ointment No. 79,* in 30-g (NDC 0777-1824-67) and 60-g (NDC 0777-1824-97) tubes and in 225-g (NDC 0777-1824-88) jars.

℞ Cordran® *(Flurandrenolide, USP), 0.05%, Ointment No. 85,* in 15-g (NDC 0777-1826-47), 30-g (NDC 0777-1826-67), and 60-g (NDC 0777-1826-97) tubes and in 225-g (NDC 0777-1826-88) jars.

℞ Cordran® SP *(Flurandrenolide, USP), 0.025%, Cream No. 9,* in 30-g (NDC 0777-6034-67) and 60-g (NDC 0777-6034-97) tubes and in 225-g (NDC 0777-6034-88) jars.

℞ Cordran® SP *(Flurandrenolide, USP), 0.05%, Cream No. 11,* in 15-g (NDC 0777-6035-47), 30-g (NDC 0777-6035-67), and 60-g (NDC 0777-6035-97) tubes and in 225-g (NDC 0777-6035-88) jars.

℞ Cordran ®-N *(Neomycin Sulfate and Flurandrenolide, USP), Cream No. 12,* in 15 (NDC 0777-1884-47), 30 (NDC 0777-1884-67), and 60-g (NDC 0777-1884-97) tubes.

℞ Cordran ®-N *(Neomycin Sulfate and Flurandrenolide, USP), Ointment No. 86,* in 15 (NDC 0777-1827-47), 30 (NDC 0777-1827-67), and 60-g (NDC 0777-1827-97) tubes.

[081688]

CORDRAN® TAPE   ℞

[kŏr'drăn tāp]
(flurandrenolide tape)
USP

DESCRIPTION

Cordran Tape is a transparent, inconspicuous, plastic surgical tape, impervious to moisture. It contains Cordran® (Flurandrenolide, USP, Dista), a potent corticosteroid for topical use. *See also* under Cordran and Cordran SP.

Each square centimeter contains 4 μg (0.00916 μmol) flurandrenolide uniformly distributed in the adhesive layer. The tape is made of a thin, matte-finish polyethylene film that is slightly elastic and highly flexible.

The adhesive is a synthetic copolymer of acrylate ester and acrylic acid that is free from substances of plant origin. The pressure-sensitive adhesive surface is covered with a protective paper liner to permit handling and trimming before application.

CLINICAL PHARMACOLOGY

Cordran® (Flurandrenolide, USP, Dista) is primarily effective because of its anti-inflammatory, antipruritic, and vasoconstrictive actions.

See also under Cordran and Cordran SP.

The tape serves as both a vehicle and an occlusive dressing. Retention of insensible perspiration by the tape results in hydration of the stratum corneum and improved diffusion of the medication. The skin is protected from scratching, rubbing, desiccation, and chemical irritation. The tape acts as a mechanical splint to fissured skin. Since it prevents removal of the medication by washing or the rubbing action of clothing, the tape formulation provides a sustained action.

Pharmacokinetics —See under Cordran and Cordran SP.

INDICATIONS AND USAGE

For relief of the inflammatory and pruritic manifestations of corticosteroid-responsive dermatoses, particularly dry, scaling localized lesions.

CONTRAINDICATIONS

Topical corticosteroids are contraindicated in patients with a history of hypersensitivity to any of the components of this preparation.

Use of Cordran® Tape (Flurandrenolide Tape, USP, Dista) is not recommended for lesions exuding serum or in intertriginous areas.

PRECAUTIONS, ADVERSE REACTIONS, and OVERDOSAGE

See under Cordran and Cordran SP.

DOSAGE AND ADMINISTRATION

Occlusive dressings may be used for the management of psoriasis or recalcitrant conditions.

If an infection develops, the use of occlusive dressings should be discontinued and appropriate antimicrobial therapy instituted.

Replacement of the tape every 12 hours produces the lowest incidence of adverse reactions, but it may be left in place for 24 hours if it is well tolerated and adheres satisfactorily. When necessary, the tape may be used at night only and removed during the day.

If ends of the tape loosen prematurely, they may be trimmed off and replaced with fresh tape.

Continued on next page

Dista—Cont.

The directions given below are included on a separate package insert for the patient to follow unless otherwise instructed by the physician.

Application of Cordran Tape

IMPORTANT: Skin should be clean and <u>dry</u> before tape is applied. Tape should always be cut, never torn.

DIRECTIONS FOR USE:
1. Prepare skin as directed by your physician or as follows: Gently clean the area to be covered to remove scales, crusts, dried exudates, and any previously used ointments or creams. A germicidal soap or cleanser should be used to prevent the development of odor under the tape. Shave or clip the hair in the treatment area to allow good contact with the skin and comfortable removal. If shower or tub bath is to be taken, it should be completed before the tape is applied. The skin should be dry before application of the tape.
2. Remove tape from package and cut a piece slightly larger than area to be covered. Round off corners.
3. Pull white paper from transparent tape. Be careful that tape does not stick to itself.
4. Apply tape, keeping skin smooth; press tape into place.
REPLACEMENT OF TAPE:
Unless instructed otherwise by your physician, replace tape after 12 hours. Cleanse skin and allow it to dry for 1 hour before applying new tape.
IF IRRITATION OR INFECTION DEVELOPS, REMOVE TAPE AND CONSULT PHYSICIAN.

HOW SUPPLIED

(℞) Cordran® Tape (Flurandrenolide Tape, USP), M-170, 4 μg flurandrenolide/sq cm, in Small Rolls 24 inches long and 3 inches wide (60 cm x 7.5 cm) (NDC 0777-2314-24) and in Large Rolls 80 inches long and 3 inches wide (200 cm x 7.5 cm) (NDC 0777-2314-28), in single packages.
Directions for the patient are included in each package.
[081688]
Cordran Tape is manufactured by Minnesota Mining and Mfg. Co., St. Paul, Minnesota 55101, for Dista Products Company.

ILOSONE®　　　　　　　　　　　　　　　　　℞
[ĭ′lō-sŏn]
(erythromycin estolate)
USP

WARNING

Hepatic dysfunction with or without jaundice has occurred, chiefly in adults, in association with erythromycin estolate administration. It may be accompanied by malaise, nausea, vomiting, abdominal colic, and fever. In some instances, severe abdominal pain may simulate an abdominal surgical emergency.
If the above findings occur, discontinue Ilosone® (Erythromycin Estolate, USP, Dista) promptly.
Ilosone is contraindicated for patients with a known history of sensitivity to this drug and for those with preexisting liver disease.

DESCRIPTION

Erythromycin is produced by a strain of *Streptomyces erythraeus* and belongs to the macrolide group of antibiotics. It is basic and readily forms salts with acids. The base, the stearate salt, and the esters are poorly soluble in water and are suitable for oral administration.
Ilosone® (Erythromycin Estolate, USP, Dista) is the lauryl sulfate salt of the propionyl ester of erythromycin.
The Pulvules® contain 250 mg erythromycin estolate. They also contain FD&C Red No. 3, FD&C Yellow No. 6, gelatin, iron oxides, magnesium stearate, mineral oil, silica gel, talc, titanium dioxide, and other inactive ingredients.
The chewable tablets contain 125 mg or 250 mg erythromycin estolate. They also contain cellulose, citric acid, FD&C Red No. 40, flavors, magnesium stearate, mannitol, saccharin, sodium chloride, sodium citrate, stearic acid, and sucrose.
The tablets contain 500 mg erythromycin estolate. They also contain cornstarch, D&C Red No. 30, D&C Yellow No. 10, FD&C Red No. 3, magnesium stearate, povidone, titanium dioxide, and other inactive ingredients.
The suspensions contain 125 mg or 250 mg of erythromycin estolate per 5 mL. The drops contain 5 mg/drop of erythromycin estolate. The suspensions and drops also contain carboxymethylcellulose, cellulose, citric acid, edetate calcium disodium, flavors, methylparaben, propylparaben,

silicone, sodium chloride, sodium citrate, sodium lauryl sulfate, sucrose, and water. The 125-mg suspension also contains butylparaben and FD&C Yellow No. 6. The 250-mg suspension also contains butylparaben and FD&C Red No. 40, and the drops also contain FD&C Yellow No. 6.

ACTIONS

Erythromycin inhibits protein synthesis without affecting nucleic acid synthesis. Some strains of *Haemophilus influenzae* and staphylococci have demonstrated resistance to erythromycin. Some strains of *H. influenzae* that are resistant in vitro to erythromycin alone are susceptible to erythromycin and sulfonamides used concomitantly. Culture and susceptibility testing should be done. If the Bauer-Kirby method of disk susceptibility testing is used, a 15-μg erythromycin disk should give a zone diameter of at least 18 mm when tested against an erythromycin-susceptible organism.
Orally administered erythromycin estolate is readily and reliably absorbed. Because of acid stability, serum levels are comparable whether the estolate is taken in the fasting state or after food. After a single 250-mg dose, blood concentrations average 0.29, 1.2, and 1.2 mg/L respectively at 2, 4, and 6 hours. Following a 500-mg dose, blood concentrations average 3, 1.9, and 0.7 mg/L respectively at 2, 6, and 12 hours. After oral administration, serum antibiotic levels consist of erythromycin base and propionyl erythromycin ester. The propionyl ester continuously hydrolyzes to the base form of erythromycin to maintain an equilibrium ratio of approximately 20% base and 80% ester in the serum.
After absorption, erythromycin diffuses readily into most body fluids. In the absence of meningeal inflammation, low concentrations are normally achieved in the spinal fluid, but passage of the drug across the blood-brain barrier increases in meningitis. In the presence of normal hepatic function, erythromycin is concentrated in the liver and excreted in the bile; the effect of hepatic dysfunction on excretion of erythromycin by the liver into the bile is not known. After oral administration, less than 5% of the administered dose can be recovered as the active form in the urine.
Erythromycin crosses the placental barrier, but fetal plasma levels are low.

INDICATIONS

Streptococcus pyogenes (Group A β-hemolytic)—Upper and lower respiratory tract, skin, and soft-tissue infections of mild to moderate severity.
Injectable penicillin G benzathine is considered by the American Heart Association to be the drug of choice in the treatment and prevention of streptococcal pharyngitis and in long-term prophylaxis of rheumatic fever.
When oral medication is preferred for treating these conditions, penicillin G or V or erythromycin is the alternate drug of choice.
The importance of the patient's strict adherence to the prescribed dosage regimen must be stressed when oral medication is given. A therapeutic dose should be administered for at least 10 days.
Alpha-Hemolytic Streptococci (viridans group)—Although no controlled clinical efficacy trials have been conducted, oral erythromycin has been suggested by the American Heart Association and American Dental Association for prophylactic use against bacterial endocarditis in patients hypersensitive to penicillin who have congenital heart disease or rheumatic or other acquired valvular heart disease when they undergo dental procedures and surgical procedures of the upper respiratory tract.[1] Erythromycin is not suitable for such prophylaxis prior to genitourinary or gastrointestinal tract surgery.
Note: When selecting antibiotics for the prevention of bacterial endocarditis, the physician or dentist should read the full joint statement of the American Heart Association and the American Dental Association.[1]
Staphylococcus aureus—Acute infections of skin and soft tissue which are mild to moderately severe. Resistance may develop during treatment.
Streptococcus (Diplococcus) pneumoniae—Infections of the upper respiratory tract (eg, otitis media, pharyngitis) and lower respiratory tract (eg, pneumonia) of mild to moderate severity.
Mycoplasma pneumoniae (Eaton Agent, PPLO)—In the treatment of respiratory tract infections due to this organism.
H. influenzae—May be used concomitantly with adequate doses of sulfonamides in treating upper respiratory tract infections of mild to moderate severity. Not all strains of this organism are susceptible at the erythromycin concentrations ordinarily achieved (see appropriate sulfonamide labeling for prescribing information).
Treponema pallidum—Erythromycin is an alternate choice of treatment for primary syphilis in penicillin-allergic patients. In primary syphilis, spinal-fluid examinations should be done before treatment and as part of follow-up after therapy.
Corynebacterium diphtheriae—As an adjunct to antitoxin, to prevent establishment of carriers, and to eradicate the organism in carriers.

C. minutissimum—In the treatment of erythrasma.
Entamoeba histolytica—In the treatment of intestinal amebiasis only. Extraenteric amebiasis requires treatment with other agents.
Listeria monocytogenes—Infections due to this organism.
Bordetella pertussis—Erythromycin is effective in eliminating the organism from the nasopharynx of infected individuals, rendering them noninfectious. Some clinical studies suggest that erythromycin may be helpful in the prophylaxis of pertussis in exposed susceptible individuals.
Legionnaires' Disease—Although no controlled clinical efficacy studies have been conducted, in vitro and limited preliminary clinical data suggest that erythromycin may be effective in treating Legionnaires' disease.
Chlamydia trachomatis—Erythromycins are indicated for treatment of the following infections caused by *C. trachomatis:* conjunctivitis of the newborn, pneumonia of infancy, urogenital infections during pregnancy (see Warnings). When tetracyclines are contraindicated or not tolerated, erythromycin is indicated for the treatment of adults with uncomplicated urethral, endocervical, or rectal infections due to *C. trachomatis*.[2]

CONTRAINDICATION

Erythromycin is contraindicated in patients with known hypersensitivity to this antibiotic.

WARNINGS

(See boxed Warning.) The administration of erythromycin estolate has been associated with the infrequent occurrence of cholestatic hepatitis. Laboratory findings have been characterized by abnormal hepatic function test values, peripheral eosinophilia, and leukocytosis. Symptoms may include malaise, nausea, vomiting, abdominal cramps, and fever. Jaundice may or may not be present. In some instances, severe abdominal pain may simulate the pain of biliary colic, pancreatitis, perforated ulcer, or an acute abdominal surgical problem. In other instances, clinical symptoms and results of liver function tests have resembled findings in extrahepatic obstructive jaundice.
Initial symptoms have developed in some cases after a few days of treatment but generally have followed 1 or 2 weeks of continuous therapy. Symptoms reappear promptly, usually within 48 hours after the drug is readministered to sensitive patients. The syndrome seems to result from a form of sensitization, occurs chiefly in adults, and has been reversible when medication is discontinued.
Pseudomembranous colitis has been reported with virtually all broad-spectrum antibiotics (including macrolides, semisynthetic penicillins, and cephalosporins); therefore, it is important to consider its diagnosis in patients who develop diarrhea in association with the use of antibiotics. Such colitis may range in severity from mild to life-threatening.
Treatment with broad-spectrum antibiotics alters the normal flora of the colon and may permit overgrowth of clostridia. Studies indicate that a toxin produced by *Clostridium difficile* is one primary cause of antibiotic-associated colitis. Mild cases of pseudomembraneous colitis usually respond to drug discontinuance alone. In moderate to severe cases, management should include sigmoidoscopy, appropriate bacteriologic studies, and fluid, electrolyte, and protein supplementation. When the colitis does not improve after the drug has been discontinued, or when it is severe, oral vancomycin is the drug of choice for antibiotic-associated pseudomembranous colitis produced by *C. difficile*. Other causes of colitis should be ruled out.
Usage in Pregnancy—Safety of this drug for use during pregnancy has not been established. Therefore, the physician should consider carefully the benefits and risks of use of this drug during pregnancy.

PRECAUTIONS

Since erythromycin is excreted principally by the liver, caution should be exercised in administering the antibiotic to patients with impaired hepatic function.
Surgical procedures should be performed when indicated.
Drug Interactions—The use of erythromycin in patients who are receiving high doses of theophylline may be associated with an increase in serum theophylline levels and potential theophylline toxicity. In case of theophylline toxicity and/or elevated serum theophylline levels, the dose of theophylline should be reduced while the patient is receiving concomitant erythromycin therapy.
There have been reports of excessive prolongation of prothrombin times in patients receiving erythromycin concurrently with chronic warfarin therapy. Such patients, particularly the elderly, who generally exhibit slower warfarin clearance, may be at risk for developing bleeding due to this interaction. In patients receiving erythromycin during chronic treatment with warfarin, prothrombin times should be monitored closely and warfarin dosage adjusted accordingly.
The use of erythromycin in patients concurrently taking drugs metabolized by the cytochrome P-450 system may be associated with elevations in serum levels of these other drugs. There have been reports of interactions of erythromycin with carbamazepine, cyclosporine, hexobarbital, pheny-

toin, and alfentanil. Serum concentrations of drugs metabolized by the cytochrome P-450 system should be monitored closely in patients concurrently receiving erythromycin.

ADVERSE REACTIONS

The most frequent side effects of erythromycin preparations are gastrointestinal (eg, abdominal cramping and discomfort) and are dose related. Nausea, vomiting, and diarrhea occur infrequently with usual oral doses.

During prolonged or repeated therapy, there is a possibility of overgrowth of nonsusceptible bacteria or fungi. If such infections arise, the drug should be discontinued and appropriate therapy instituted.

Mild allergic reactions, such as urticaria and other skin rashes, have occurred. Serious allergic reactions, including anaphylaxis, have been reported.

There have been isolated reports of reversible hearing loss occurring chiefly in patients with renal insufficiency and in patients receiving high doses of erythromycin.

Rarely, erythromycin has been associated with the production of ventricular arrhythmias, including ventricular tachycardia and torsade des pointes, in individuals with prolonged QT intervals.

OVERDOSAGE

Signs and Symptoms—Symptoms of oral overdose of erythromycin estolate may include nausea, vomiting, epigastric distress, and diarrhea. The severity of the epigastric distress and the diarrhea are dose related. Hearing loss, with or without tinnitus and vertigo, may occur, especially in patients with renal insufficiency.

Treatment—To obtain up-to-date information about the treatment of overdose, a good resource is your certified Regional Poison Control Center. Telephone numbers of certified poison control centers are listed in the *Physicians's Desk Reference (PDR)*. In managing overdosage, consider the possibility of multiple drug overdoses, interaction among drugs, and unusual drug kinetics in your patient.

Unless 5 times the normal dose of erythromycin estolate has been ingested, gastrointestinal decontamination should not be necessary. An accidental ingestion of erythromycin should not be predicted to have minimal toxicity unless there is a good approximation of how much was ingested and unless only a single medication was involved.

Protect the patient's airway and support ventilation and perfusion. Meticulously monitor and maintain, within acceptable limits, the patient's vital signs, blood gases, serum electrolytes, etc. Absorption of drugs from the gastrointestinal tract may be decreased by giving activated charcoal, which, in many cases, is more effective than emesis or lavage; consider charcoal instead of or in addition to gastric emptying. Repeated doses of charcoal over time may hasten elimination of some drugs that have been absorbed. Safeguard the patient's airway when employing gastric emptying or charcoal.

Forced diuresis, peritoneal dialysis, hemodialysis, or charcoal hemoperfusion have not been established as beneficial for an overdose of erythromycin estolate.

DOSAGE AND ADMINISTRATION

Adults—The usual dosage is 250 mg every 6 hours. This may be increased up to 4 g or more/day according to the severity of the infection.

Children—Age, weight, and severity of the infection are important factors in determining the proper dosage. The usual regimen is 30 to 50 mg/kg/day in divided doses. For more severe infections, this dosage may be doubled.

If administration is desired on a twice-a-day schedule in either adults or children, ½ of the total daily dose may be given every 12 hours.

Twice-a-day dosing is not recommended when doses larger than 1 g daily are administered.

Streptococcal Infections—For the treatment of streptococcal pharyngitis and tonsillitis, the usual dosage range is 20 to 50 mg/kg/day in divided doses.

Body Weight	Total Daily Dose
10 kg or less (less than 25 lb)	250 mg
11–18 kg (25–40 lb)	375 mg
18–25 kg (40–55 lb)	500 mg
25–36 kg (55–80 lb)	750 mg
36 kg or more (more than 80 lb)	1,000 mg (adult dose)

In the treatment of group A β-hemolytic streptococcal infections, a therapeutic dosage of erythromycin should be administered for at least 10 days. In continuous prophylaxis of streptococcal infections in persons with a history of rheumatic heart disease, the dosage is 250 mg twice a day.

For prophylaxis against bacterial endocarditis[1] in penicillin-allergic patients with congenital heart disease or rheumatic or other acquired valvular heart disease when undergoing dental procedures or surgical procedures of the upper respiratory tract, the dosage schedule for adults is 1 g (20 mg/kg

for children) orally 1 hour before the procedure and then 500 mg (10 mg/kg for children) orally 6 hours later.

Primary Syphilis—A regimen of 20 g of erythromycin estolate in divided doses over a period of 10 days has been shown to be effective in the treatment of primary syphilis.

Dysenteric Amebiasis—Dosage for adults is 250 mg 4 times daily for 10 to 14 days; for children, 30 to 50 mg/kg/day in divided doses for 10 to 14 days.

Pertussis—Although optimum dosage and duration have not been established, the dosage of erythromycin utilized in reported clinical studies was 40 to 50 mg/kg/day, given in divided doses for 5 to 14 days.

Legionnaires' Disease—Although optimum doses have not been established, doses utilized in reported clinical data were those recommended above (1 to 4 g erythromycin estolate daily in divided doses).

Conjunctivitis of the Newborn Caused by C. trachomatis —Oral erythromycin suspension, 50 mg/kg/day in 4 divided doses for at least 2 weeks.[2]

Pneumonia of Infancy Caused by C. trachomatis —Although the optimum duration of therapy has not been established, the recommended therapy is oral erythromycin suspension, 50 mg/kg/day in 4 divided doses for at least 3 weeks.[2]

Urogenital Infections During Pregnancy Due to C. trachomatis—Although the optimum dose and duration of therapy have not been established, the suggested treatment is erythromycin, 500 mg orally 4 times a day for at least 7 days. For women who cannot tolerate this regimen, a decreased dose of 250 mg orally 4 times a day should be used for at least 14 days.[2]

For adults with uncomplicated urethral, endocervical, or rectal infections caused by *C. trachomatis* in whom tetracyclines are contraindicated or not tolerated: 500 mg orally 4 times a day for at least 7 days.[2]

REFERENCES

1. American Heart Association: Prevention of bacterial endocarditis. *Circulation*, 1984; 70:1123A.
2. Sexually Transmitted Diseases Treatment Guidelines 1982. Centers for Disease Control, Morbidity and Mortality Weekly Report, US Department of Health and Human Services, Atlanta, 1982; 31 (suppl): 355.

HOW SUPPLIED

(℞) Pulvules, ivory and red

250 mg* (No. 375)—(24s) NDC 0777-0809-24; (100s) NDC 0777-0809-02; (ID†100) NDC 0777-0809-33

(℞) Tablets, specially coated, light-pink (capsule-shaped, scored)

500 mg* (No. 1863)—(50s) NDC 0777-2126-50

(℞) Tablets, chewable, light-pink

125 mg* (No. 1834)—(50s) NDC 0777-2105-50
250 mg* (No. 1865)—(50s) NDC 0777-2125-50

Store at controlled room temperature, 59° to 86°F (15° to 30°C).

(℞) Liquid, Oral Suspension

125 mg*/5 mL, orange-flavored vehicle (M-148)‡—(100 mL) NDC 0777-2315-48; (16 fl oz) NDC 0777-2315-05
250 mg*/5 mL, cherry-flavored vehicle (M-153)‡—(100 mL) NDC 0777-2317-48; (16 fl oz) NDC 0777-2317-05

(℞) Ready-Mixed Drops, Oral Suspension

100 mg*/mL, 5 mg*/drop (M-159)‡—(10 mL) NDC 0777-2318-37

---

* Equivalent to erythromycin.
† Identi-Dose= (unit dose medication, Dista).
‡ Shake well before using. Refrigerate to maintain optimum taste.

[020789]

*Identi-Code® symbol.
Shown in Product Identification Section, page 409

ILOTYCIN®   ℞

[ī-lō-tī'-sĭn]
(erythromycin)
Ophthalmic Ointment, USP
and Tablets, USP
(Enteric-Coated)

DESCRIPTION

Erythromycin is produced by a strain of *Streptomyces erythraeus* and belongs to the macrolide group of antibiotics. It is basic and readily forms salts with acids. The base, the stearate salt, and the esters are poorly soluble in water and are suitable for oral administration.

Each gram of the ophthalmic ointment contains erythromycin, USP, 5 mg, in a sterile ophthalmic base of mineral oil and white petrolatum. The ⅛-oz tamper-resistant tubes also contain methylparaben and propylparaben. The special sterile ophthalmic ointment base flows freely over the conjunctiva.

Tablets Ilotycin® (Erythromycin, USP. Dista) are specially coated to protect the contents from the inactivating effect of

gastric acid and to permit efficient absorption of the antibiotic in the small intestine.

Each enteric-coated tablet contains 250 mg erythromycin. Each tablet also contains carboxymethyl cellulose, cellulose, dibasic calcium phosphate, hydroxypropyl cellulose, iron oxide, magnesium stearate, stearic acid, silicon dioxide, titanium dioxide, and other inactive ingredients.

ACTIONS

See under Ilosone®.

Tablets Ilotycin® (Erythromycin, USP, Dista) are well absorbed and may be given without regard to meals.

INDICATIONS AND USAGE

Ophthalmic Ointment

For the treatment of superficial ocular infections involving the conjunctiva and/or cornea caused by organisms susceptible to Ilotycin® (Erythromycin, USP, Dista).

For prophylaxis of ophthalmia neonatorum due to *Neisseria gonorrhoeae* or *Chlamydia trachomatis*. The Centers for Disease Control (USPHS) and the Committee on Drugs, the Committee on Fetus and Newborn, and the Committee on Infectious Diseases of the American Academy of Pediatrics recommend 1% silver nitrate solution in single-dose ampoules or single-use tubes of an ophthalmic ointment containing 0.5% erythromycin or 1% tetracycline as "effective and acceptable regimens for prophylaxis of gonococcal ophthalmia neonatorum."[1] (For infants born to mothers with clinically apparent gonorrhea, intravenous or intramuscular injections of aqueous crystalline penicillin G should be given: a single dose of 50,000 units for term infants or 20,000 units for infants of low birth weight. Topical prophylaxis alone is inadequate for these infants.[1]) Ophthalmic Ointment Ilotycin also has been effective for prevention of neonatal conjunctivitis due to *C. trachomatis*,[2] a condition that may develop one to several weeks after delivery in infants of mothers whose birth canals harbor the organism.

Tablets

Streptococcus pyogenes (Group A β-hemolytic)—Upper and lower respiratory tract, skin, and soft-tissue infections of mild to moderate severity.

Injectable penicillin G benzathine is considered by the American Heart Association to be the drug of choice in the treatment and prevention of streptococcal pharyngitis and in long-term prophylaxis of rheumatic fever.

When oral medication is preferred for treating the above-mentioned conditions, penicillin G or V or erythromycin is the alternate drug of choice.

The importance of the patient's strict adherence to the prescribed dosage regimen must be stressed when oral medication is given. A therapeutic dose should be administered for at least 10 days.

Alpha-Hemolytic Streptococci (viridans group)—Although no controlled clinical efficacy trials have been conducted, oral erythromycin has been suggested by the American Heart Association and the American Dental Association for use in a regimen for prophylaxis against bacterial endocarditis in patients hypersensitive to penicillin who have congenital heart disease or rheumatic or other acquired valvular heart disease when they undergo dental procedures and surgical procedures of the upper respiratory tract.[3] Erythromycin is not suitable for such prophylaxis prior to genitourinary or gastrointestinal tract surgery.

Note: When selecting antibiotics for the prevention of bacterial endocarditis, the physician or dentist should read the full joint statement of the American Heart Association and the American Dental Association.[3]

Staphylococcus aureus—Acute infections of skin and soft tissue which are mild to moderately severe. Resistance may develop during treatment.

S. (Diplococcus) pneumoniae—Infections of the upper respiratory tract (eg, otitis media, pharyngitis) and lower respiratory tract (eg, pneumonia) of mild to moderate severity.

Mycoplasma pneumoniae (Eaton Agent, PPLO)—In the treatment of respiratory tract infections due to this organism.

H. influenzae—May be used concomitantly with adequate doses of sulfonamides in treating upper respiratory tract infections of mild to moderate severity. Not all strains of this organism are susceptible at the erythromycin concentrations ordinarily achieved (see appropriate sulfonamide labeling for prescribing information).

Treponema pallidum—Erythromycin is an alternate choice of treatment for primary syphilis in penicillin-allergic patients. In primary syphilis, spinal-fluid examinations should be done before treatment and as part of follow-up after therapy.

Corynebacterium diphtheriae—As an adjunct to antitoxin, to prevent establishment of carriers, and to eradicate the organism in carriers.

C. minutissimum—In the treatment of erythrasma.

Entamoeba histolytica—In the treatment of intestinal amebiasis only. Extraenteric amebiasis requires treatment with other agents.

Continued on next page

Dista—Cont.

Listeria monocytogenes —Infections due to this organism.

Neisseria gonorrhoeae —In female patients with a history of sensitivity to penicillin, a parenteral erythromycin (such as the gluceptate) may be administered in conjunction with an oral erythromycin as alternate therapy in acute pelvic inflammatory disease caused by *N. gonorrhoeae*. In the treatment of gonorrhea, patients suspected of having concomitant syphilis should have microscopic examinations (by immunofluorescence or darkfield) before receiving erythromycin and monthly serologic tests for a minimum of 4 months.

Bordetella pertussis —Erythromycin is effective in eliminating the organism from the nasopharynx of infected individuals and in rendering them noninfectious. Some clinical studies suggest that erythromycin may be helpful in the prophylaxis of pertussis in exposed susceptible individuals.

Legionnaires' Disease —Although no controlled clinical efficacy studies have been conducted, in vitro and limited preliminary clinical data suggest that erythromycin may be effective in treating Legionnaires' disease.

Chlamydia trachomatis —Erythromycins are indicated for treatment of the following infections caused by *C. trachomatis*: conjunctivitis of the newborn, pneumonia of infancy, urogenital infections during pregnancy (*see* Warnings). When tetracyclines are contraindicated or not tolerated, erythromycin is indicated for the treatment of adults with uncomplicated urethral, endocervical, or rectal infections due to *C. trachomatis*.[4]

CONTRAINDICATION

Erythromycin is contraindicated in patients with known hypersensitivity to this antibiotic.

WARNINGS

Tablets

Usage in Pregnancy —Safety of this drug for use during pregnancy has not been established. Therefore, the physician should consider carefully the benefits and risks of the use of this drug during pregnancy.

Pseudomembranous colitis has been reported with virtually all broad-spectrum antibiotics (including macrolides, semisynthetic penicillins, and cephalosporins); therefore, it is important to consider its diagnosis in patients who develop diarrhea in association with the use of antibiotics. Such colitis may range in severity from mild to life-threatening.

Treatment with broad-spectrum antibiotics alters the normal flora of the colon and may permit overgrowth of clostridia. Studies indicate that a toxin produced by *Clostridium difficile* is one primary cause of antibiotic-associated colitis. Mild cases of pseudomembranous colitis usually respond to drug discontinuance alone. In moderate to severe cases, management should include sigmoidoscopy, appropriate bacteriologic studies, and fluid, electrolyte, and protein supplementation. When the colitis does not improve after the drug has been discontinued, or when it is severe, oral vancomycin is the drug of choice for antibiotic-associated pseudomembranous colitis produced by *C. difficile*. Other causes of colitis should be ruled out.

PRECAUTIONS

Ophthalmic Ointment

General—The use of antimicrobial agents may be associated with the overgrowth of antibiotic-resistant organisms; in such a case, antibiotic administration should be stopped and appropriate measures taken.

Usage in Pregnancy—Pregnancy Category B—Reproduction studies have been performed in rats, mice, and rabbits using erythromycin and its various salts and esters, at doses which were several multiples of the usual human dose. No evidence of impaired fertility or harm to the fetus that appeared related to erythromycin was reported in these studies. There are, however, no adequate and well-controlled studies in pregnant women. Because animal reproductive studies are not always predictive of human response, the erythromycins should be used during pregnancy only if clearly needed.

Prediatric Use—See Indications and Usage and Dosage and Administration.

Tablets

Surgical procedures should be performed when indicated. Since erythromycin is excreted principally by the liver, caution should be exercised in administering the antibiotic to patients with impaired hepatic function. There have been reports of hepatic dysfunction, with or without jaundice, occurring in patients taking oral erythromycin products.

Drug Interactions —The use of erythromycin in patients who are receiving high doses of theophylline may be associated with an increase in serum theophylline levels and potential theophylline toxicity. In case of theophylline toxicity and/or elevated serum theophylline levels, the dose of theophylline should be reduced while the patient is receiving concomitant erythromycin therapy.

There have been reports of excessive prolongation of prothrombin times in patients receiving erythromycin concurrently with chronic warfarin therapy. Such patients, particularly the elderly, who generally exhibit slower warfarin clearance, may be at risk for developing bleeding due to this interaction. In patients receiving erythromycin during chronic treatment with warfarin, prothrombin times should be monitored closely and warfarin dosage adjusted accordingly.

The use of erythromycin in patients concurrently taking drugs metabolized by the cytochrome P450 system may be associated with elevations in serum levels of these other drugs. There have been reports of interactions of erythromycin with carbamapezine,[5] cyclosporine,[6] hexobarbital,[7] and phenytoin.[8] Serum concentrations of drugs metabolized by the cytochrome P450 system should be monitored closely in patients concurrently receiving erythromycin.

ADVERSE REACTIONS

Ophthalmic Ointment

As with any other medicament intended for topical use, there is always the possibility that sensitivity reactions will occur in certain individuals. If such reactions develop, the medication should be discontinued. Eye irritation has been infrequently reported.

Tablets

The most frequent side effects of erythromycin preparations are gastrointestinal (eg, abdominal cramping and discomfort) and are dose related. Nausea, vomiting, and diarrhea occur infrequently with usual oral doses.

During prolonged or repeated therapy, there is a possibility of overgrowth of nonsusceptible bacteria or fungi. If such infections arise, the drug should be discontinued and appropriate therapy instituted.

Mild allergic reactions, such as urticaria and other skin rashes, have occurred. Serious allergic reactions, including anaphylaxis, have been reported.

There have been isolated reports of reversible hearing loss occurring chiefly in patients with renal insufficiency and in patients receiving high doses of erythromycin.

Rarely, erythromycin has been associated with the production of ventricular arrhythmias, including ventricular tachycardia and torsade des pointes, in individuals with prolonged QT intervals.

OVERDOSAGE

Signs and Symptoms—Symptoms of oral overdose of erythromycin estolate may include nausea, vomiting, epigastric distress, and diarrhea. The severity of the epigastric distress and the diarrhea are dose related. Hearing loss, with or without tinnitus and vertigo, may occur, especially in patients with renal insufficiency.

Treatment—To obtain up-to-date information about the treatment of overdose, a good resource is your certified Regional Poison Control Center. Telephone numbers of certified poison control centers are listed in the *Physicians's Desk Reference (PDR)*. In managing overdosage, consider the possibility of multiple drug overdoses, interaction among drugs, and unusual drug kinetics in your patient.

Unless 5 times the normal dose of erythromycin estolate has been ingested, gastrointestinal decontamination should not be necessary. However, minimal toxicity should not be assumed in the case of accidental ingestion of erythromycin unless there is a good approximation of how much was ingested and only a single medication was involved.

Protect the patient's airway and support ventilation and perfusion. Meticulously monitor and maintain, within acceptable limits, the patient's vital signs, blood gases, serum electrolytes, etc. Absorption of drugs from the gastrointestinal tract may be decreased by giving activated charcoal, which, in many cases, is more effective than emesis or lavage; consider charcoal instead of or in addition to gastric emptying. Repeated doses of charcoal over time may hasten elimination of some drugs that have been absorbed. Safeguard the patient's airway when employing gastric emptying or charcoal.

Forced diuresis, peritoneal dialysis, hemodialysis, or charcoal hemoperfusion have not been established as beneficial for an overdose of erythromycin.

DOSAGE AND ADMINISTRATION

In the treatment of external ocular infections, Ophthalmic Ointment Ilotycin® (Erythromycin, USP, Dista) should be applied directly to the infected structure one or more times daily, depending on the severity of the infection.

For prophylaxis of neonatal gonococcal or chlamydial conjunctivitis, a ribbon of ointment approximately 0.5 to 1 cm in length should be instilled into each conjunctival sac. The ointment should not be flushed from the eye following instillation. A new tube should be used for each infant. Infants born by cesarean section as well as those delivered by the vaginal route should receive prophylaxis.

Tablets Ilotycin® (Erythromycin, USP, Dista) are well absorbed whether given immediately after meals or between meals on an empty stomach.

Adults —The usual dosage is 250 mg every 6 hours. This may be increased up to 4 g or more/day according to the severity of the infection.

Children —Age, weight, and severity of the infection are important factors in determining the proper dosage. The usual regimen is 30 to 50 mg/kg/day in divided doses. For more severe infections, this dosage may be doubled.

If administration is desired on a twice-a-day schedule in either adults or children, one-half of the total daily dose may be given every 12 hours.

Streptococcal Infections —In the treatment of group A β-hemolytic streptococcal infections, a therapeutic dosage of erythromycin should be administered for at least 10 days. In continuous prophylaxis of streptococcal infections in persons with a history of rheumatic heart disease, the dosage is 250 mg twice a day.

For prophylaxis against bacterial endocarditis[3] in patients with congenital heart disease or rheumatic or other acquired valvular heart disease when undergoing dental procedures or surgical procedures of the upper respiratory tract, the dosage schedule for adults is 1 g (20 mg/kg for children) orally one and one-half to 2 hours before the procedure and then 500 mg (10 mg/kg for children) orally every 6 hours for 8 doses.

Primary Syphilis —30 to 40 g given in divided doses over a period of 10 to 15 days.

Acute Pelvic Inflammatory Disease Caused by N. gonorrhoeae—Ilotycin® Gluceptate (Sterile Erythromycin Gluceptate, USP, Dista), 500 mg intravenously every 6 hours for at least 3 days, followed by Ilotycin, 250 mg every 6 hours for 7 days.

Dysenteric Amebiasis —250 mg 4 times daily for 10 to 14 days for adults; 30 to 50 mg/kg/day in divided doses for 10 to 14 days for children.

Pertussis —Although optimum dosage and duration of treatment have not been established, the dosage of erythromycin utilized in reported clinical studies was 40 to 50 mg/kg/day, given in divided doses for 5 to 14 days.

Legionnaires' Disease —Although optimum doses have not been established, doses utilized in reported clinical data were those recommended above (1 to 4 g erythromycin base daily in divided doses).

Conjunctivitis of the Newborn Caused by C. trachomatis —Oral erythromycin suspension, 50 mg/kg/day in 4 divided doses for at least 2 weeks.[4]

Pneumonia of Infancy Caused by C. trachomatis —Although the optimum duration of therapy has not been established, the recommended therapy is oral erythromycin suspension, 50 mg/kg/day in 4 divided doses for at least 3 weeks.[4]

Urogenital Infections during Pregnancy Due to C. trachomatis —Although the optimum dose and duration of therapy have not been established, the suggested treatment is erythromycin, 500 mg orally 4 times a day for at least 7 days. For women who cannot tolerate this regimen, a decreased dose of 250 mg orally 4 times a day should be used for at least 14 days.[4]

For adults with uncomplicated urethral, endocervical, or rectal infections caused by *C. trachomatis* in whom tetracyclines are contraindicated or not tolerated: 500 mg orally 4 times a day for at least 7 days.[4]

REFERENCES

1. American Academy of Pediatrics: Prophylaxis and treatment of neonatal gonococcal infections, *Pediatrics* 1980; 65:1047.
2. Hammerschlag MR, et al.: Erythromycin ointment for ocular prophylaxis of neonatal chlamydial infection. *JAMA* 1980; 244:2291.
3. American Heart Association: Prevention of bacterial endocarditis. *Circulation* 1984; 70:1123A.
4. Sexually Transmitted Diseases Treatment Guidelines 1982. Centers for Disease Control, Morbidity and Mortality Weekly Report, US Department of Health and Human Services, Atlanta, 1982; 31 (suppl) 355.
5. Wroblewski BA, et al.: Carbamapezine-erythromycin interaction, *JAMA* 1986; 255:1165–1167.
6. Ptachcinski RJ, et al: Effect of erythromycin on cyclosporine levels *N Engl J Med* 1985; 313:1416–1417.
7. Ludden TM: Pharmacokinetic interactions of the macrolide antibiotics, *Clin Pharmacokinet* 1985; 10:63–79.
8. Bachmann K, et al: Single dose phenytoin clearance during erythromycin treatment. *Res Commun Chem Pathol Pharmacol* 1984; 46:207–217.

HOW SUPPLIED

(℞) Ophthalmic Ointment, 5 mg/g (No. 52) (⅛-oz tamper-resistant tubes), NDC 0777-1863-17; (ID24*—1-g plastic containers) NDC 0777-1863-52

Store at controlled room temperature, 59° to 86°F (15° to 30°C).

(℞) Tablets (enteric-coated), orange (CO3*)
250 mg (No. 23)—(100s) NDC 0777-0303-02; (500s) NDC 0777-0303-03

Keep tightly closed. Store at 59° to 86°F. Dispense in a tight, light-resistant container.

---

* Identi-Dose® (unit dose medication, Dista)

[070788]

ILOTYCIN® GLUCEPTATE ℞
[ĭ-lō-tī'sĭn gloo-sĕp'tāt]
(erythromycin gluceptate)
Sterile, USP
Intravenous

DESCRIPTION

Erythromycin is produced by a strain of *Streptomyces erythraeus* and belongs to the macrolide group of antibiotics. It is basic and readily forms a salt when combined with an acid.

ACTIONS

See under Ilosone®.

Intravenous injection of 200 mg of erythromycin produces peak serum levels of 3 to 4 mg/L at 1 hour and 0.5 mg/L at 6 hours.

From 12 to 15% of intravenously administered erythromycin is excreted in active form in the urine.

INDICATIONS

Streptococcus pyogenes (Group A β-hemolytic)—Upper and lower respiratory tract, skin, and soft-tissue infections of mild to moderate severity.

Injectable penicillin G benzathine is considered by the American Heart Association to be the drug of choice in the treatment and prevention of streptococcal pharyngitis and in long-term prophylaxis of rheumatic fever.

Staphylococcus aureus—Acute infections of skin and soft tissue that are mild to moderately severe. Resistance may develop during treatment.

Streptococcus (Diplococcus) pneumoniae—Infections of the upper respiratory tract (eg, otitis media and pharyngitis) and lower respiratory tract (eg, pneumonia) of mild to moderate severity.

Mycoplasma pneumoniae (Eaton Agent, PPLO)—In the treatment of respiratory tract infections due to this organism.

Haemophilus influenzae—May be used concomitantly with adequate doses of sulfonamides in treating upper respiratory tract infections of mild to moderate severity. Not all strains of this organism are susceptible at the erythromycin concentrations ordinarily achieved (see appropriate sulfonamide labeling for prescribing information).

Corynebacterium diphtheriae—As an adjunct to antitoxin.

Listeria monocytogenes—Infections due to this organism.

Neisseria gonorrhoeae—In female patients with a history of sensitivity to penicillin, a parenteral erythromycin (such as the gluceptate) may be administered in conjunction with an oral erythromycin as alternate therapy in acute pelvic inflammatory disease caused by *N. gonorrhoeae*. In the treatment of gonorrhea, patients suspected of having concomitant syphilis should have microscopic examinations (by immunofluorescence or darkfield) before receiving erythromycin and monthly serologic tests for a minimum of 4 months.

Legionnaires' Disease—Although no controlled clinical efficacy studies have been conducted, in vitro and limited preliminary clinical data suggest that erythromycin may be effective in treating Legionnaires' disease.

CONTRAINDICATION

Intravenous erythromycin is contraindicated in patients with known hypersensitivity to this antibiotic.

WARNINGS

See under Ilotycin®.

PRECAUTIONS

Surgical procedures should be performed when indicated.

Side effects following the use of intravenous erythromycin are rare. Occasional venous irritation has been encountered, but if the injection is given slowly, in dilute solution, preferably by continuous intravenous infusion over 20 to 60 minutes, pain and vessel trauma are minimized.

Since erythromycin is excreted principally by the liver, caution should be exercised in administering the antibiotic to patients with impaired hepatic function.

Drug Interactions—See under Ilotycin®.

ADVERSE REACTIONS

Allergic reactions, ranging from urticaria and mild skin eruptions to anaphylaxis, have occurred with intravenously administered erythromycin.

During prolonged or repeated therapy, there is a possibility of overgrowth of nonsusceptible bacteria or fungi. If such infections arise, the drug should be discontinued and appropriate therapy instituted.

Variations in liver function have been observed following daily doses at high levels or after prolonged therapy. Hepatic function tests should be performed when such therapy is given.

Reversible hearing loss associated with the intravenous infusion of 4 g or more/day of erythromycin has been reported rarely.

Rarely, erythromycin has been associated with the production of ventricular arrhythmias, including ventricular tachycardia and torsade des pointes, in individuals with prolonged QT intervals.

OVERDOSAGE

Signs and Symptoms—Experience with overdosage of Ilotycin® Gluceptate (Erythromycin Gluceptate, USP, Dista) is limited. Alterations in liver function tests and reversible hearing loss are possible, especially in patients with renal insufficiency.

Treatment—To obtain up-to-date information about the treatment of overdose, a good resource is your certified Regional Poison Control Center. Telephone numbers of certified poison control centers are listed in the *Physicians' Desk Reference (PDR)*. In managing overdosage, consider the possibility of multiple drug overdoses, interaction among drugs, and unusual drug kinetics in your patient.

Protect the patient's airway and support ventilation and perfusion. Meticulously monitor and maintain, within acceptable limits, the patient's vital signs, blood gases, serum electrolytes, etc.

Forced diuresis, peritoneal dialysis, hemodialysis, or charcoal hemoperfusion have not been established as beneficial for an overdose of erythromycin gluceptate.

DOSAGE AND ADMINISTRATION

Prepare the initial solution of Ilotycin® Gluceptate (Erythromycin Gluceptate, USP, Dista) by (1) adding at least 10 mL of Sterile Water for Injection to the 500-mg vial or at least 20 mL of Sterile Water for Injection to the 1-g vial of Ilotycin Gluceptate and (2) shaking the vial until all of the drug is dissolved.

It is important that the product be diluted only *with Sterile Water for Injection without preservatives.*

After reconstitution, the sterile solutions should be stored in a refrigerator and used within 7 days.

When all of the drug is dissolved, the solution may then be added to 0.9% Sodium Chloride Injection or to 5% Dextrose in Water to give 1 g/liter for slow, continuous infusion. IV fluid admixtures with a pH below 5.5 tend to lose potency rapidly. Therefore, such solutions should be administered completely within 4 hours after dilution.

If the period of administration is prolonged, the pH of the infusion fluid should be buffered to neutrality with a sterile agent such as Neut® (Sodium Bicarbonate 4% Additive Solution, Abbott) or Buff™ (Phosphate-Carbonate Buffer, Travenol). For administration of the antibiotic in 500 or 1,000 mL of 5% Dextrose in Water, add 1 ampoule full-strength Buff or 5 mL of Neut; for administration of the antibiotic in the same volumes of 0.9% Sodium Chloride Injection, add 1 ampoule half-strength Buff or 5 mL of Neut. These solutions should be completely administered within 24 hours after dilution.

If the medication is to be given in 100 to 250 mL of fluid by a volume control set such as Metriset® (McGaw), Volu-Trole® "B" (Cutter), Soluset® (Abbott), or Buretrol® (Baxter-Travenol), the IV fluid should be buffered in its primary container before being added to the volumetric administration set.

If the medication is to be given by intermittent injection, one-fourth of the total daily dose can be given in 20 to 60 minutes by slow intravenous injection of 250 to 500 mg in 100 to 250 mL of 0.9% Sodium Chloride Injection or 5% Dextrose in Water. Injection should be sufficiently slow to avoid pain along the vein.

The recommended IV dosage for severe infections in adults and children is 15 to 20 mg/kg of body weight/day. Higher doses (up to 4 g/day) may be given in very severe infections. Continuous infusion is preferable, but administration in divided doses at intervals of no more than every 6 hours is also effective.

For treatment of acute pelvic inflammatory disease caused by *N. gonorrhoeae*, administer 500 mg Ilotycin Gluceptate intravenously every 6 hours for at least 3 days, followed by 250 mg Ilotycin® (Erythromycin Tablets, USP, Dista) every 6 hours for 7 days.

Patients receiving intravenous erythromycin should be changed to the oral dosage form as soon as possible.

For Treatment of Legionnaires' Disease—Although optimum doses have not been established, doses utilized in reported clinical data were those recommended above (1 to 4 g daily in divided doses).

HOW SUPPLIED

(℞) Vials Ilotycin® Gluceptate (Sterile Erythromycin Gluceptate, USP), IV, rubber-stoppered (Dry Powder): No. 538, 500 mg (equivalent to erythromycin), 30-mL size (NDC 0777-1409-01); and No. 646, 1 g (equivalent to erythromycin), 30-mL size (NDC 0777-1441-01), in singles (10 per carton).

[020789]

KEFLET® ℞
[kĕf'lĕt]
(cephalexin tablets)
USP

DESCRIPTION

Tablets Keflet® (Cephalexin, USP, Dista) contain the active ingredient cephalexin, which is a semisynthetic cephalosporin antibiotic intended for oral administration. It is 7-(D-α-amino-α-phenylacetamido)-3-methyl-3-cephem-4-carboxylic acid, monohydrate.

The nucleus of cephalexin is related to that of other cephalosporin antibiotics. The compound is a zwitterion; ie, the molecule contains both a basic and an acidic group. The isoelectric point of cephalexin in water is approximately 4.5 to 5. The crystalline form of cephalexin which is available is a monohydrate. It is a white crystalline solid having a bitter taste. Solubility in water is low at room temperature; 1 or 2 mg/mL may be dissolved readily, but higher concentrations are obtained with increasing difficulty.

The cephalosporins differ from penicillins in the structure of the bicyclic ring system. Cephalexin has a D-phenylglycyl group as substituent at the 7-amino position and an unsubstituted methyl group at the 3-position.

Each tablet contains cephalexin monohydrate equivalent to 250 mg, 500 mg, or 1 g of cephalexin. The tablets also contain cornstarch, D & C Yellow No. 10, F D & C Blue No. 1, magnesium stearate, povidone, titanium dioxide, and other ingredients. The 250-mg tablet also contains F D & C Red No. 40, and the 500-mg tablet also contains F D & C Yellow No. 6. The 1-g tablet also contains F D & C Blue No. 2 and F D & C Yellow No. 6.

CLINICAL PHARMACOLOGY

Human Pharmacology—Keflet® (Cephalexin Tablets, USP, Dista) is acid stable and may be given without regard to meals. It is rapidly absorbed after oral administration. Following doses of 250 mg, 500 mg, and 1 g, average peak serum levels of approximately 9, 18, and 32 mg/L respectively were obtained at 1 hour. Measurable levels were present 6 hours after administration. Cephalexin is excreted in the urine by glomerular filtration and tubular secretion. Studies showed that over 90% of the drug was excreted unchanged in the urine within 8 hours. During this period, peak urine concentrations following the 250-mg, 500-mg, and 1-g doses were approximately 1,000, 2,200, and 5,000 mg/L respectively.

Microbiology—In vitro tests demonstrate that the cephalosporins are bactericidal because of their inhibition of cell-wall synthesis. Cephalexin is active against the following organisms in vitro:

> β-hemolytic streptococci
> Staphylococci, including coagulase-positive, coagulase-negative, and penicillinase-producing strains
> *Streptococcus (Diplococcus) pneumoniae*
> *Escherichia coli*
> *Proteus mirabilis*
> *Klebsiella* sp
> *Haemophilus influenzae*
> *Moraxella (Branhamella) catarrhalis*

Note—Most strains of enterococci (*Enterococcus faecalis* [formerly *Streptococcus faecalis*]) and a few strains of staphylococci are resistant to cephalexin. It is not active against most strains of *Enterobacter* sp, *Morganella morganii* (formerly *Proteus morganii*), and *Proteus vulgaris*. It has no activity against *Pseudomonas* or *Acinetobacter* (formerly *Mima* and *Herellea*) sp. When tested by in vitro methods, staphylococci exhibit cross-resistance between cephalexin and methicillin-type antibiotics.

Disk Susceptibility Tests—Quantitative methods that require measurement of zone diameters give the most precise estimates of antibiotic susceptibility. One such procedure* has been recommended for use with disks for testing susceptibility to cephalothin. Interpretations correlate zone diameters of the disk test with MIC values for cephalexin. With this procedure, a report from the laboratory of "resistant" indicates that the infecting organism is not likely to respond to therapy. A report of "intermediate susceptibility" suggests that the organism would be susceptible if the infection is confined to the urine, in which high antibiotic levels can be obtained, or if high dosage is used in other types of infection.

* Bauer AW, Kirby WMM, Sherris JC, et al: Antibiotic susceptibility testing by a standardized single disk method. *Am J Clin Pathol* 1966;45:493; Standardized disk susceptibility test. *Federal Register* 1974;39:19182–19184.

INDICATIONS AND USAGE

Keflet® (Cephalexin Tablets, USP, Dista) is indicated for the treatment of the following infections when caused by susceptible strains of the designated microorganisms:

> Respiratory tract infections caused by *S pneumoniae* and group A β-hemolytic streptococci (Penicillin is the usual drug of choice in the treatment and prevention of streptococcal infections, including the prophylaxis of rheumatic fever. Keflet is generally effective in the eradication of streptococci from the nasopharynx; however, substantial data establishing the efficacy of Keflet in the subsequent prevention of rheumatic fever are not available at present.)
>
> Otitis media due to *S pneumoniae*, *H influenzae*, staphylococci, streptococci, and *M catarrhalis*

Continued on next page

Dista—Cont.

Skin and skin-structure infections caused by staphylococci and/or streptococci

Bone infections caused by staphylococci and/or *P mirabilis*

Genitourinary tract infections, including acute prostatitis, caused by *E coli*, *P mirabilis*, and *Klebsiella* sp

Note—Culture and susceptibility tests should be initiated prior to and during therapy. Renal function studies should be performed when indicated.

CONTRAINDICATION

Keflex® (Cephalexin Tablets, USP, Dista) is contraindicated in patients with known allergy to the cephalosporin group of antibiotics.

WARNINGS

BEFORE CEPHALEXIN THERAPY IS INSTITUTED, CAREFUL INQUIRY SHOULD BE MADE CONCERNING PREVIOUS HYPERSENSITIVITY REACTIONS TO CEPHALOSPORINS AND PENICILLIN. CEPHALOSPORIN C DERIVATIVES SHOULD BE GIVEN CAUTIOUSLY TO PENICILLIN-SENSITIVE PATIENTS.

SERIOUS ACUTE HYPERSENSITIVITY REACTIONS MAY REQUIRE EPINEPHRINE AND OTHER EMERGENCY MEASURES.

There is some clinical and laboratory evidence of partial cross-allergenicity of the penicillins and the cephalosporins. Patients have been reported to have had severe reactions (including anaphylaxis) to both drugs.

Any patient who has demonstrated some form of allergy, particularly to drugs, should receive antibiotics cautiously. No exception should be made with regard to Keflet® (Cephalexin Tablets, USP, Dista).

Pseudomembranous colitis has been reported with virtually all broad-spectrum antibiotics (including macrolides, semisynthetic penicillins, and cephalosporins); therefore, it is important to consider its diagnosis in patients who develop diarrhea in association with the use of antibiotics. Such colitis may range in severity from mild to life-threatening.

Treatment with broad-spectrum antibiotics alters the normal flora of the colon and may permit overgrowth of clostridia. Studies indicate that a toxin produced by *Clostridium difficile* is one primary cause of antibiotic-associated colitis. Mild cases of pseudomembranous colitis usually respond to drug discontinuance alone. In moderate to severe cases, management should include sigmoidoscopy, appropriate bacteriologic studies, and fluid, electrolyte, and protein supplementation. When the colitis does not improve after the drug has been discontinued, or when it is severe, oral vancomycin is the drug of choice for antibiotic-associated pseudomembranous colitis produced by *C difficile*. Other causes of colitis should be ruled out.

Usage in Pregnancy—Safety of this product for use during pregnancy has not been established.

PRECAUTIONS

General—Patients should be followed carefully so that any side effects or unusual manifestations of drug idiosyncrasy may be detected. If an allergic reaction to Keflet® (Cephalexin Tablets, USP, Dista) occurs, the drug should be discontinued and the patient treated with the usual agents (eg, epinephrine or other pressor amines, antihistamines, or corticosteroids).

Prolonged use of Keflet may result in the overgrowth of nonsusceptible organisms. Careful observation of the patient is essential. If superinfection occurs during therapy, appropriate measures should be taken.

Positive direct Coombs' tests have been reported during treatment with the cephalosporin antibiotics. In hematologic studies or in transfusion cross-matching procedures when antiglobulin tests are performed on the minor side or in Coombs' testing of newborns whose mothers have received cephalosporin antibiotics before parturition, it should be recognized that a positive Coombs' test may be due to the drug.

Keflet should be administered with caution in the presence of markedly impaired renal function. Under such conditions, careful clinical observation and laboratory studies should be made because safe dosage may be lower than that usually recommended.

Indicated surgical procedures should be performed in conjunction with antibiotic therapy.

As a result of administration of Keflet, a false-positive reaction for glucose in the urine may occur. This has been observed with Benedict's and Fehling's solutions and also with Clinitest® tablets but not with Tes-Tape® (Glucose Enzymatic Test Strip, USP, Lilly).

Broad-spectrum antibiotics should be prescribed with caution in individuals with a history of gastrointestinal disease, particularly colitis.

Usage in Pregnancy—Pregnancy Category B—The daily oral administration of cephalexin to rats in doses of 250 or 500 mg/kg prior to and during pregnancy, or to rats and mice during the period of organogenesis only, had no adverse effect on fertility, fetal viability, fetal weight, or litter size.

Note that the safety of cephalexin during pregnancy in humans has not been established.

Cephalexin showed no enhanced toxicity in weanling and newborn rats as compared with adult animals. Nevertheless, because the studies in humans cannot rule out the possibility of harm, Keflet should be used during pregnancy only if clearly needed.

Nursing Mothers—The excretion of cephalexin in the milk increased up to 4 hours after a 500-mg dose; the drug reached a maximum level of 4 mg/L, then decreased gradually, and had disappeared 8 hours after administration. Caution should be exercised when Keflet is administered to a nursing woman.

ADVERSE REACTIONS

Gastrointestinal—Symptoms of pseudomembranous colitis may appear either during or after antibiotic treatment. Nausea and vomiting have been reported rarely. The most frequent side effect has been diarrhea. It was very rarely severe enough to warrant cessation of therapy. Dyspepsia and abdominal pain have also occurred. As with some penicillins and some other cephalosporins, transient hepatitis and cholestatic jaundice have been reported rarely.

Hypersensitivity—Allergic reactions in the form of rash, urticaria, angioedema, and, rarely, erythema multiforme, Stevens-Johnson syndrome, or toxic epidermal necrolysis have been observed. These reactions usually subsided upon discontinuation of the drug. Anaphylaxis has also been reported.

Other reactions have included genital and anal pruritus, genital moniliasis, vaginitis and vaginal discharge, dizziness, fatigue, headache, agitation, confusion, hallucinations, arthralgia, arthritis, and joint disorder. Reversible interstitial nephritis has been reported rarely. Eosinophilia, neutropenia, thrombocytopenia, and slight elevations in SGOT and SGPT have been reported.

OVERDOSAGE

Signs and Symptoms—Symptoms of oral overdose may include nausea, vomiting, epigastric distress, diarrhea, and hematuria. If other symptoms are present, they are probably secondary to an underlying disease state, an allergic reaction, or toxicity due to ingestion of a second medication.

Treatment—To obtain up-to-date information about the treatment of overdose, a good resource is your certified Regional Poison Control Center. Telephone numbers of certified poison control centers are listed in the *Physicians' Desk Reference (PDR)*. In managing overdosage, consider the possibility of multiple drug overdoses, interaction among drugs, and unusual drug kinetics in your patient.

Unless 5 to 10 times the normal dose of cephalexin has been ingested, gastrointestinal decontamination should not be necessary.

Protect the patient's airway and support ventilation and perfusion. Meticulously monitor and maintain, within acceptable limits, the patient's vital signs, blood gases, serum electrolytes, etc. Absorption of drugs from the gastrointestinal tract may be decreased by giving activated charcoal, which, in many cases, is more effective than emesis or lavage; consider charcoal instead of or in addition to gastric emptying. Repeated doses of charcoal over time may hasten elimination of some drugs that have been absorbed. Safeguard the patient's airway when employing gastric emptying or charcoal.

Forced diuresis, peritoneal dialysis, hemodialysis, or charcoal hemoperfusion have not been established as beneficial for an overdose of cephalexin; however, it would be extremely unlikely that one of these procedures would be indicated.

The oral LD$_{50}$ of cephalexin in rats is 5,000 mg/kg.

DOSAGE AND ADMINISTRATION

Keflet® (Cephalexin Tablets, USP, Dista) is administered orally.

Adults—The adult dosage ranges from 1 to 4 g daily in divided doses. The usual adult dose is 250 mg every 6 hours. For the following infections, a dosage of 500 mg may be administered every 12 hours: streptococcal pharyngitis, skin and skin-structure infections, and uncomplicated cystitis in patients over 15 years of age. Cystitis therapy should be continued for 7 to 14 days. For more severe infections or those caused by less susceptible organisms, larger doses may be needed. If daily doses of Keflet greater than 4 g are required, parenteral cephalosporins, in appropriate doses, should be considered.

Children—The usual recommended daily dosage for children is 25 to 50 mg/kg in divided doses. For streptococcal pharyngitis in patients over 1 year of age and for skin and skin-structure infections, the total daily dose may be divided and administered every 12 hours.

In severe infections, the dosage may be doubled.

In the therapy of otitis media, clinical studies have shown that a dosage of 75 to 100 mg/kg/day in 4 divided doses is required.

In the treatment of β-hemolytic streptococcal infections, a therapeutic dosage of Keflet should be administered for at least 10 days.

HOW SUPPLIED

(℞) Tablets (capsule-shaped):

250 mg,* light blue-green (No. 4202)—(100s) NDC 0777-4202-02
500 mg,* dark green (No. 4203)—(100s) NDC 0777-4203-02
1 g,* dark green (No. 1896)—(24s) NDC 0777-2160-24; (ID†100) NDC 0777-2160-33

* Equivalent to cephalexin.
† Identi-Dose® (unit dose medication, Dista).

Store at controlled room temperature, 59° to 86°F (15° to 30°C).

[080888]

KEFTAB®   ℞
[kĕf'tăb]
(cephalexin hydrochloride)

DESCRIPTION

Keftab® (Cephalexin Hydrochloride, Dista) is a semisynthetic cephalosporin antibiotic intended for oral administration. Chemically, it is designated 7-(D-α-amino-α-phenylacetamido)-3-methyl-3-cephem-4-carboxylic acid, hydrochloride monohydrate.

The nucleus of cephalexin hydrochloride is related to that of other cephalosporin antibiotics. The compound is the hydrochloride salt of cephalexin. The isoelectric point of cephalexin in water is appropriately 4.5 to 5.

Cephalexin hydrochloride is in crystalline form and is a monohydrate. It is a white, crystalline solid having a bitter taste. Solubility in water is high at room temperature; greater than 10 mg/mL may be dissolved readily.

The cephalosporins differ from penicillins in the structure of the bicyclic ring system. Cephalexin has a D-phenylglycyl group as substituent at the 7-amino position and an unsubstituted methyl group at the 3-position.

Each tablet contains cephalexin hydrochloride equivalent to 250 mg or 500 mg cephalexin. The tablets also contain D & C Yellow No. 10, F D & C Blue No. 1, magnesium stearate, silicon dioxide, stearic acid, sucrose, and titanium dioxide. The 250-mg tablet also contains F D & C Blue No. 2, and the 500-mg tablet also contains F D & C Red No. 40.

CLINICAL PHARMACOLOGY

Human Pharmacology—Keftab® (Cephalexin Hydrochloride, Dista) is acid stable and may be given without regard to meals. It is rapidly absorbed after oral administration. Following doses of 250 mg and 500 mg, average peak serum levels of approximately 9 and 18 mg/L respectively were obtained at 1 hour and declined to 1.6 and 3.4 mg/L respectively at 3 hours. Measurable levels were present 6 hours after administration. Cephalexin is excreted in the urine by glomerular filtration and tubular secretion. Studies showed that approximately 70% of the drug was excreted unchanged in the urine within 12 hours. During the first 6 hours, average urine concentrations following the 250-mg and 500-mg doses were approximately 200 mg/L (range, 54 to 663) and 500 mg/L (range, 137 to 1,306) respectively. The average serum half-life is 1.1 hours.

Microbiology—In vitro tests demonstrate that the cephalosporins are bactericidal because of their inhibition of cell-wall synthesis. Keftab is active against the following organisms in vitro:

β-hemolytic streptococci
Staphylococcus aureus, including penicillinase-producing strains
Streptococcus pneumoniae (formerly *Diplococcus pneumoniae*)
Escherichia coli
Proteus mirabilis
Klebsiella sp
Haemophilus influenzae
Moraxella (Branhamella) catarrhalis

Note—Most strains of enterococci (formerly *Streptococcus faecalis*) and a few strains of staphylococci are resistant to Keftab. When tested by in vitro methods, staphylococci exhibit cross-resistance between Keftab and methicillin-type antibiotics. Keftab is not active against most strains of *Enterobacter* sp, *Morganella morganii* (formerly *Proteus morganii*), *Serratia* sp, and *Proteus vulgaris*. It has no activity against *Pseudomonas* or *Acinetobacter* sp.

Disk Susceptibility Tests—Quantitative methods that require measurement of zone diameters give the most precise estimates of antibiotic susceptibility. One such procedure[1] has been recommended for use with cephalosporin-class (cephalothin) disks for testing susceptibility to cephalexin. The currently accepted zone diameter interpretations for the cephalothin disks[1] are appropriate for determining susceptibility to cephalexin. Interpretations correlate zone diameters of the disk test with MIC values for cephalexin. With this procedure, a report from the laboratory of "resistant" indicates a zone diameter of 14 mm or less and that the infecting organism is not likely to respond to therapy. A report of "susceptibility" indicates a zone diameter of 18 mm or greater. A report of "intermediate susceptibility" indicates zone diameters between 15 and 17 mm and suggests that the organism would be susceptible if the infection is confined to the urine, in which high antibiotic levels can be obtained, or if high dosage is used in other types of infection.

Standardized procedures require use of control organisms.[1] The 30-μg cephalothin disk should give zone diameters between 18 and 23 mm and 25 and 37 mm for the reference strains *E coli* ATCC 25922 and *S aureus* ATCC 25923 respectively.

1. 21 CFR 460.1, *Federal Register* 1987; 838–842.

INDICATIONS AND USAGE

Keftab® (Cephalexin Hydrochloride, Dista) is indicated for the treatment of the following infections when caused by susceptible strains of the designated microorganisms:

Respiratory tract infections caused by *S pneumoniae* and group A β-hemolytic streptococci (Penicillin is the usual drug of choice in the treatment and prevention of streptococcal infections, including the prophylaxis of rheumatic fever. Keftab is generally effective in the eradication of streptococci from the nasopharynx; however, data establishing the efficacy of Keftab in the subsequent prevention of rheumatic fever are not available at present.)

Skin and skin structure infections caused by *S aureus* and/or β-hemolytic streptococci.

Bone infections caused by *S aureus* and/or *P mirabilis.*

Genitourinary tract infections, including acute prostatitis, caused by *E coli, P mirabilis,* and *Klebsiella* sp.

Note—Culture and susceptibility tests should be initiated prior to and during therapy. Renal function studies should be performed when indicated.

CONTRAINDICATION

Keftab® (Cephalexin Hydrochloride, Dista) is contraindicated in patients with known allergy to the cephalosporin group of antibiotics.

WARNINGS

BEFORE CEPHALEXIN THERAPY IS INSTITUTED, CAREFUL INQUIRY SHOULD BE MADE CONCERNING PREVIOUS HYPERSENSITIVITY REACTIONS TO CEPHALOSPORINS AND PENICILLIN. CEPHALOSPORIN C DERIVATIVES SHOULD BE GIVEN CAUTIOUSLY TO PENICILLIN-SENSITIVE PATIENTS.

SERIOUS ACUTE HYPERSENSITIVITY REACTIONS MAY REQUIRE EPINEPHRINE AND OTHER EMERGENCY MEASURES.

There is some clinical and laboratory evidence of partial cross-allergenicity of the penicillins and the cephalosporins. Patients have been reported to have had severe reactions (including anaphylaxis) to both drugs.

Any patient who has demonstrated some form of allergy, particularly to drugs, should receive antibiotics cautiously. No exception should be made with regard to Keftab® (Cephalexin Hydrochloride, Dista).

Pseudomembraneous colitis has been reported with virtually all broad-spectrum antibiotics (including macrolides, semisynthetic penicillins, and cephalosporins); therefore, it is important to consider its diagnosis in patients who develop diarrhea in association with the use of antibiotics. Such colitis may range in severity from mild to life-threatening.

Treatment with broad-spectrum antibiotics alters the normal flora of the colon and may permit overgrowth of clostridia. Studies indicate that a toxin produced by *Clostridium difficile* is one primary cause of antibiotic-associated colitis. Mild cases of pseudomembranous colitis usually respond to drug discontinuance alone. In moderate to severe cases, management should include sigmoidoscopy, appropriate bacteriologic studies, and fluid, electrolyte, and protein supplementation. When the colitis does not improve after the drug has been discontinued or when it is severe, oral vancomycin is the drug of choice for antibiotic-associated pseudomembranous colitis produced by *C. difficile.* Other causes of colitis should be ruled out.

Usage in Pregnancy—Safety of this product for use during pregnancy has not been established.

PRECAUTIONS

General—Patients should be followed carefully so that any side effects or unusual manifestations of drug idiosyncrasy may be detected. If an allergic reaction to Keftab® (Cephalexin Hydrochloride, Dista) occurs, the drug should be discontinued and the patient treated with the usual agents (eg, epinephrine or other pressor amines, antihistamines, or corticosteroids).

Prolonged use of Keftab may result in the overgrowth of nonsusceptible organisms. Careful observation of the patient is essential. If superinfection occurs during therapy, appropriate measures should be taken.

Positive direct Coombs' tests have been reported during treatment with the cephalosporin antibiotics. In hematologic studies or in transfusion cross-matching procedures when antiglobulin tests are performed on the minor side or in Coombs' testing of newborns whose mothers have received cephalosporin antibiotics before parturition, it should be recognized that a positive Coombs' test may be due to the drug.

Keftab should be administered with caution in the presence of markedly impaired renal function. Under such conditions, careful clinical observation and laboratory studies should be made because safe dosage may be lower than that usually recommended.

As a result of administration of Keftab, a false-positive reaction for glucose in the urine may occur. This has been observed with Benedict's and Fehling's solutions and also with Clinitest® tablets but not with Tes-Tape® (Glucose Enzymatic Test Strip, USP, Lilly).

Broad-spectrum antibiotics should be prescribed with caution in individuals with a history of gastrointestinal disease, particularly colitis.

Pregnancy—*Pregnancy Category B*—Reproduction studies have been performed on rats in doses of 250 or 500 mg/kg/day and have revealed no evidence of impaired fertility or harm to the fetus due to cephalexin. There are, however, no adequate and well-controlled studies in pregnant women. Because animal reproduction studies are not always predictive of human response, this drug should be used during pregnancy only if clearly needed.

Nursing Mothers—The excretion of cephalexin in the milk increased up to 4 hours after a 500-mg dose; the drug reached a maximum level of 4 mg/L, then decreased gradually, and had disappeared 8 hours after administration. A decision should be considered to discontinue nursing temporarily during therapy with Keftab.

Pediatric Use—Safety and effectiveness in children have not been established.

ADVERSE REACTIONS

Gastrointestinal—Symptoms of pseudomembranous colitis may appear either during or after antibiotic treatment. Nausea and vomiting have been reported rarely. The most frequent side effect has been diarrhea. It was very rarely severe enough to warrant cessation of therapy. Dyspepsia and abdominal pain have also occurred. As with some penicillins and some other cephalosporins, transient hepatitis and cholestatic jaundice have been reported rarely.

Hypersensitivity—Allergic reactions in the form of rash, urticaria, angioedema, and, rarely, erythema multiforme, Stevens-Johnson syndrome, or toxic epidermal necrolysis have been observed. These reactions usually subsided upon discontinuation of the drug. Anaphylaxis has also been reported.

Other reactions have included genital and anal pruritus, genital moniliasis, vaginitis and vaginal discharge, dizziness, fatigue, headache, agitation, confusion, hallucinations, arthralgia, arthritis, and joint disorder. Reversible interstitial nephritis has been reported rarely. Eosinophilia, neutropenia, thrombocytopenia, and slight elevations in aspartate aminotransferase (AST, SGOT) and alanine aminotransferase (ALT, SGPT) have been reported.

In addition to the adverse reactions listed above that have been observed in patients treated with Keftab® (Cephalexin Hydrochloride, Dista), the following adverse reactions and altered laboratory tests have been reported for cephalosporin-class antibiotics:

> *Adverse Reactions*—Allergic reactions, including fever, colitis, renal dysfunction, toxic nephropathy, and hepatic dysfunction, including cholestasis.

> Several cephalosporins have been implicated in triggering seizures, particularly in patients with renal impairment when the dosage was not reduced (*see* Indications and Usage and Precautions, General). If seizures associated with drug therapy should occur, the drug should be discontinued. Anticonvulsant therapy can be given if clinically indicated.

> *Altered Laboratory Tests*—Increased prothrombin time, increased BUN, increased creatinine, increased alkaline phosphatase, and leukopenia.

OVERDOSAGE

Signs and Symptoms—Symptoms of oral overdose may include nausea, vomiting, epigastric distress, diarrhea, and hematuria. If other symptoms are present, they are probably secondary to an underlying disease state, an allergic reaction, or toxicity due to ingestion of a second medication.

Treatment—To obtain up-to-date information about the treatment of overdose, a good resource is your certified Regional Poison Control Center. Telephone numbers of certified poison control centers are listed in the *Physicians' Desk Reference (PDR).* In managing overdosage, consider the possibility of multiple drug overdoses, interaction among drugs, and unusual drug kinetics in your patient.

Unless 5 to 10 times the normal dose of cephalexin has been ingested, gastrointestinal decontamination should not be necessary.

Protect the patient's airway and support ventilation and perfusion. Meticulously monitor and maintain, within acceptable limits, the patient's vital signs, blood gases, serum electrolytes, etc. Absorption of drugs from the gastrointestinal tract may be decreased by giving activated charcoal, which, in many cases, is more effective than emesis or lavage; consider charcoal instead of or in addition to gastric emptying. Repeated doses of charcoal over time may hasten elimination of some drugs that have been absorbed. Safeguard the patient's airway when employing gastric emptying or charcoal.

Forced diuresis, peritoneal dialysis, hemodialysis, or charcoal hemoperfusion have not been established as beneficial for an overdose of cephalexin; however, it would be extremely unlikely that one of these procedures would be indicated.

The oral LD_{50} of cephalexin in rats is 5,000 mg/kg.

DOSAGE AND ADMINISTRATION

Keftab® (Cephalexin Hydrochloride, Dista) is administered orally.

The adult dosage ranges from 1 to 4 g daily in divided doses. For the following infections, a dosage of 500 mg may be administered every 12 hours: streptococcal pharyngitis, skin and skin structure infections, and uncomplicated cystitis. Cystitis therapy should be continued for 7 to 14 days. For other infections, the usual dose is 250 mg every 6 hours. For more severe infections or those caused by less susceptible organisms, larger doses may be needed. If daily doses of Keftab greater than 4 g are required, parenteral cephalosporins, in appropriate doses, should be considered.

HOW SUPPLIED

Tablets (elliptical-shaped):
   250 mg* (light-green) (No. 4142)—(100s) NDC 0777-4142-02
   500 mg* (dark-green) (No. 4143)—(100s) NDC 0777-4143-02

Store at controlled room temperature, 59° to 86°F (15° to 30°C).

* Equivalent to cephalexin.

[080888]

Shown in Product Identification Section, page 409

NALFON®   ℞

[nǎl'fŏn]

NALFON® 200
(fenoprofen calcium)
USP

DESCRIPTION

Nalfon® (Fenoprofen Calcium, USP, Dista) is a nonsteroidal, anti-inflammatory, antiarthritic drug. Pulvules® Nalfon contain fenoprofen calcium as the dihydrate in an amount equivalent to 200 mg or 300 mg of fenoprofen. They also contain cellulose, gelatin, iron oxides, silicone, titanium dioxide, and other inactive ingredients. The 300-mg Pulvules also contain D & C Yellow No. 10 and F D & C Yellow No. 6. Tablets Nalfon contain fenoprofen calcium as the dihydrate in an amount equivalent to 600 mg of fenoprofen. They also contain amberlite, calcium phosphate, cornstarch, D & C Yellow No. 10, F D & C Yellow No. 6, magnesium stearate, and stearic acid.

Chemically, Nalfon is an arylacetic acid derivative.

Nalfon is a white crystalline powder. At 25°C, it dissolves to a 15 mg/mL solution in alcohol (95%). It is slightly soluble in water and insoluble in benzene.

The pK_a of Nalfon is 4.5 at 25°C.

CLINICAL PHARMACOLOGY

Nalfon® (Fenoprofen Calcium, USP, Dista) is a nonsteroidal, anti-inflammatory, antiarthritic drug that also possesses analgesic and antipyretic activities. Its exact mode of action is unknown, but it is thought that prostaglandin synthetase inhibition is involved. Nalfon has been shown to inhibit prostaglandin synthetase isolated from bovine seminal vesicles. Reproduction studies in rats have shown Nalfon to be associated with prolonged labor and difficult parturition when given during late pregnancy. Evidence suggests that this may be due to decreased uterine contractility resulting from the inhibition of prostaglandin synthesis. Its action is not mediated through the adrenal gland.

Fenoprofen shows anti-inflammatory effects in rodents by inhibiting the development of redness and edema in acute inflammatory conditions and by reducing soft-tissue swelling and bone damage associated with chronic inflammation. It exhibits analgesic activity in rodents by inhibiting the writhing response caused by the introduction of an irritant into the peritoneal cavities of mice and by elevating pain thresholds that are related to pressure in edematous hindpaws of rats. In rats made febrile by the subcutaneous administration of brewer's yeast, fenoprofen produces antipyretic action. These effects are characteristic of nonsteroidal, anti-inflammatory, antipyretic, analgesic drugs.

The results in humans confirmed the anti-inflammatory and analgesic actions found in animals. The emergence and degree of erythemic response were measured in adult male volunteers exposed to ultraviolet irradiation. The effects of Nalfon, aspirin, and indomethacin were each compared with

Continued on next page

Dista—Cont.

those of a placebo. All 3 drugs demonstrated antierythemic activity.

In patients with rheumatoid arthritis, the anti-inflammatory action of Nalfon has been evidenced by relief of pain, increase in grip strength, and reductions in joint swelling, duration of morning stiffness, and disease activity (as assessed by both the investigator and the patient). The anti-inflammatory action of Nalfon has also been evidenced by increased mobility (ie, a decrease in the number of joints having limited motion).

The use of Nalfon® (Fenoprofen Calcium, USP, Dista) in combination with gold salts or corticosteroids has been studied in patients with rheumatoid arthritis. The studies, however, were inadequate in demonstrating whether further improvement is obtained by adding Nalfon to maintenance therapy with gold salts or steroids. Whether or not Nalfon used in conjunction with partially effective doses of a corticosteroid has a "steroid-sparing" effect is unknown.

In patients with osteoarthritis, the anti-inflammatory and analgesic effects of Nalfon have been demonstrated by reduction in tenderness as a response to pressure and reductions in night pain, stiffness, swelling, and overall disease activity (as assessed by both the patient and the investigator). These effects have also been demonstrated by relief of pain with motion and at rest and increased range of motion in involved joints.

In patients with rheumatoid arthritis and osteoarthritis, clinical studies have shown Nalfon to be comparable to aspirin in controlling the aforementioned measures of disease activity, but mild gastrointestinal reactions (nausea, dyspepsia) and tinnitus occurred less frequently in patients treated with Nalfon than in aspirin-treated patients. It is not known whether Nalfon causes less peptic ulceration than does aspirin.

In patients with pain, the analgesic action of Nalfon has produced a reduction in pain intensity, an increase in pain relief, improvement in total analgesia scores, and a sustained analgesic effect.

Under fasting conditions, Nalfon is rapidly absorbed, and peak plasma levels of 50 mg/L are achieved within 2 hours after oral administration of 600-mg doses. Good dose proportionality was observed between 200-mg and 600-mg doses in fasting male volunteers. The plasma half-life is approximately 3 hours. About 90% of a single oral dose is eliminated within 24 hours as fenoprofen glucuronide and 4'-hydroxy-fenoprofen glucuronide, the major urinary metabolites of fenoprofen. Fenoprofen is highly bound (99%) to albumin. The concomitant administration of antacid (containing both aluminum and magnesium hydroxide) does not interfere with absorption of Nalfon.

There is less suppression of collagen-induced platelet aggregation with single doses of Nalfon than there is with aspirin.

INDICATIONS AND USAGE

Nalfon® (Fenoprofen Calcium, USP, Dista) is indicated for relief of the signs and symptoms of rheumatoid arthritis and osteoarthritis. It is recommended for the treatment of acute flare-ups and exacerbations and for the long-term management of these diseases.

Nalfon is also indicated for the relief of mild to moderate pain.

CONTRAINDICATIONS

Nalfon® (Fenoprofen Calcium, USP, Dista) is contraindicated in patients who have shown hypersensitivity to it.

The drug should not be administered to patients with a history of significantly impaired renal function.

Nalfon should not be given to patients in whom aspirin and other nonsteroidal anti-inflammatory drugs induce the symptoms of asthma, rhinitis, or urticaria, because cross-sensitivity to these drugs occurs in a high proportion of such patients.

WARNINGS

Risk of GI Ulceration, Bleeding, and Perforation with NSAID Therapy—Serious gastrointestinal toxicity, such as bleeding, ulceration, and perforation, can occur at any time, with or without warning symptoms, in patients treated chronically with NSAID therapy. Although minor upper gastrointestinal problems, such as dyspepsia, are common, usually developing early in therapy, physicians should remain alert for ulceration and bleeding in patients treated chronically with NSAIDs, even in the absence of previous GI tract symptoms. In patients observed in clinical trials of several months' to 2 years' duration, symptomatic upper GI ulcers, gross bleeding, or perforation appeared to occur in approximately 1% of patients treated for 3 to 6 months, and in about 2% to 4% of patients treated for 1 year. Physicians should inform patients about the signs and/or symptoms of serious GI toxicity and what steps to take if they occur.

Studies to date have not identified any subset of patients not at risk of developing peptic ulceration and bleeding. Except for a prior history of serious GI events and other risk facts known to be associated with peptic ulcer disease, such as

alcoholism, smoking, etc, no risk factors (eg, age, sex) have been associated with increased risk. Elderly or debilitated patients seem to tolerate ulceration or bleeding less well than other individuals, and most spontaneous reports of fatal GI events are in this population. Studies to date are inconclusive concerning the relative risk of various NSAIDs in causing such reactions. High doses of any NSAID probably carry a greater risk of these reactions, although controlled clinical trials showing this do not exist in most cases. In considering the use of relatively large doses (within the recommended dosage range), sufficient benefit should be anticipated to offset the potential increased risk of GI toxicity.

Since Nalfon® (Fenoprofen Calcium, USP, Dista) has been marketed, there have been reports of genitourinary tract problems in patients taking it. The most frequently reported problems have been episodes of dysuria, cystitis, hematuria, interstitial nephritis, and nephrotic syndrome. This syndrome may be preceded by the appearance of fever, rash, arthralgia, oliguria, and azotemia and may progress to anuria. There may also be substantial proteinuria, and, on renal biopsy, electron microscopy has shown foot process fusion and T-lymphocyte infiltration in the renal interstitium. Early recognition of the syndrome and withdrawal of the drug have been followed by rapid recovery. Administration of steroids and the use of dialysis have also been included in the treatment. Because a syndrome with some of these characteristics has also been reported with other nonsteroidal anti-inflammatory drugs, it is recommended that patients who have had these reactions with other such drugs not be treated with Nalfon. In patients with possibly compromised renal function, periodic renal function examinations should be done.

PRECAUTIONS

General—Renal Effects—There have been reports of acute interstitial nephritis and nephrotic syndrome (see Contraindications and Warnings).

A second form of renal toxicity has been seen in patients with prerenal conditions leading to a reduction in renal blood flow or blood volume, in which renal prostaglandins play a supportive role in the maintenance of renal perfusion. In these patients, administration of an NSAID may cause a dose-dependent reduction in prostaglandin formation and may precipitate overt renal decompensation at any time. Patients at greatest risk for this reaction are those with impaired renal function, heart failure, liver dysfunction, those taking diuretics, and the elderly. Discontinuation of NSAID therapy is typically followed by recovery to the pretreatment state.

Since Nalfon® (Fenoprofen Calcium, USP, Dista) is eliminated primarily by the kidneys, patients with possibly compromised renal function (such as the elderly) should be closely monitored; for such patients, it may be anticipated that a lower daily dosage will avoid excessive drug accumulation.

Miscellaneous—Peripheral edema has been observed in some patients taking Nalfon® (Fenoprofen Calcium, USP, Dista); therefore, Nalfon should be used with caution in patients with compromised cardiac function or hypertension. The possibility of renal involvement should be considered. Studies to date have not shown changes in the eyes attributable to the administration of Nalfon. However, adverse ocular effects have been observed with other anti-inflammatory drugs. Eye examinations, therefore, should be performed if visual disturbances occur in patients taking Nalfon.

Caution should be exercised by patients whose activities require alertness if they experience central-nervous-system side effects while taking Nalfon.

Since the safety of Nalfon has not been established in patients with impaired hearing, these patients should have periodic tests of auditory function during prolonged therapy with Nalfon.

Information for Patients—Nalfon, like other drugs of its class, is not free of side effects. The side effects of these drugs can cause discomfort and, rarely, there are more serious side effects, such as gastrointestinal bleeding, which may result in hospitalization and even fatal outcomes.

NSAIDs (Nonsteroidal Anti-Inflammatory Drugs) are often essential agents in the management of arthritis and have a major role in the treatment of pain, but they also may be commonly employed for conditions which are less serious. Physicians may wish to discuss with their patients the potential risks (see Warnings, Precautions, and Adverse Reactions sections) and likely benefits of NSAID treatment, particularly when the drugs are used for less serious conditions where treatment without NSAIDs may represent an acceptable alternative to both the patient and physician.

Laboratory Tests—In chronic studies in rats, high doses of Nalfon caused elevation of serum transaminase and hepatocellular hypertrophy. In clinical trials, some patients developed elevation of serum transaminase, LDH, and alkaline phosphatase that persisted for some months and usually, but not always, declined despite continuation of the drug. The significance of this is unknown. It is recommended, therefore, that Nalfon be discontinued if any significant liver abnormality occurs.

As with other nonsteroidal anti-inflammatory drugs, borderline elevations in 1 or more liver tests may occur in up to 15% of patients. These abnormalities may progress, may remain essentially unchanged, or may be transient with continued therapy. The SGPT (ALT) test is probably the most sensitive indicator of liver dysfunction. Meaningful (ie, 3 times the upper limit of normal) elevations of SGPT or SGOT (AST) occurred in controlled clinical trials in less than 1% of patients. A patient with symptoms and/or signs suggesting liver dysfunction, or in whom an abnormal liver test has occurred, should be evaluated for evidence of the more severe hepatic reactions while using Nalfon. Severe hepatic reactions, including jaundice and cases of fatal hepatitis, have been reported with Nalfon, as with other nonsteroidal anti-inflammatory drugs. Although such reactions are rare, if liver tests continue to be abnormal or worsen, if clinical signs and symptoms consistent with liver disease develop, or if systemic manifestations occur (eg, eosinophilia and rash), Nalfon should be discontinued.

Patients with initial low hemoglobin values who are receiving long-term therapy with Nalfon should have a hemoglobin determination made at reasonable intervals.

Nalfon decreases platelet aggregation and may prolong bleeding time. Patients who may be adversely affected by prolongation of the bleeding time should be carefully observed when Nalfon is administered.

Because serious GI tract ulceration and bleeding can occur without warning symptoms, physicians should follow chronically treated patients for the signs and symptoms of ulceration and bleeding and should inform them of the importance of this follow-up (see Risk of GI Ulceration, Bleeding, and Perforation with NSAID Therapy *under* Warnings).

Laboratory Test Interactions—Amerlex-M kit assay values of total and free triiodothyronine in patients receiving Nalfon have been reported as falsely elevated on the basis of a chemical cross-reaction that directly interferes with the assay. Thyroid-stimulating hormone, total thyroxine, and thyrotropin-releasing hormone response are not affected.

Drug Interactions—The coadministration of aspirin decreases the biologic half-life of fenoprofen because of an increase in metabolic clearance that results in a greater amount of hydroxylated fenoprofen in the urine. Although the mechanism of interaction between fenoprofen and aspirin is not totally known, enzyme induction and displacement of fenoprofen from plasma albumin binding sites are possibilities. Because Nalfon® (Fenoprofen Calcium, USP, Dista) has not been shown to produce any additional effect beyond that obtained with aspirin alone and because aspirin increases the rate of excretion of Nalfon, the concomitant use of Nalfon and salicylates is not recommended.

Chronic administration of phenobarbital, a known enzyme inducer, may be associated with a decrease in the plasma half-life of fenoprofen. When phenobarbital is added to or withdrawn from treatment, dosage adjustment of Nalfon may be required.

In vitro studies have shown that fenoprofen, because of its affinity for albumin, may displace from their binding sites other drugs that are also albumin bound, and this may lead to drug interaction. Theoretically, fenoprofen could likewise be displaced. Patients receiving hydantoin, sulfonamides, or sulfonylureas should be observed for increased activity of these drugs and, therefore, signs of toxicity from these drugs. In patients receiving coumarin-type anticoagulants, the addition of Nalfon to therapy could prolong the prothrombin time. Patients receiving both drugs should be under careful observation. Patients treated with Nalfon may be resistant to the effects of loop diuretics.

In patients receiving Nalfon and a steroid concomitantly, any reduction in steroid dosage should be gradual in order to avoid the possible complications of sudden steroid withdrawal.

Usage in Pregnancy—Safe use of Nalfon during pregnancy and lactation has not been established; therefore, administration to pregnant patients and nursing mothers is not recommended. Reproduction studies have been performed in rats and rabbits. When fenoprofen was given to rats during pregnancy and continued until the time of labor, parturition was prolonged. Similar results have been found with other nonsteroidal anti-inflammatory drugs that inhibit prostaglandin synthetase.

Usage in Children—Fenoprofen calcium is not recommended for use in children because documented clinical experience has been insufficient to establish safety and a suitable dosage regimen in the pediatric age group.

ADVERSE REACTIONS

During clinical studies for rheumatoid arthritis or osteoarthritis, complaints were compiled from a checklist of potential adverse reactions, and the following data emerged. These encompass observations in 6,768 patients, including 188 observed for at least 52 weeks. During short-term studies for analgesia, the incidence of adverse reactions was markedly lower than that seen in longer-term studies.

INCIDENCE GREATER THAN 1%
Probable Causal Relationship
Digestive System —During clinical trials with Nalfon®
(Fenoprofen Calcium, USP, Dista), the most common adverse
reactions were gastrointestinal in nature and occurred in
about 14% of patients. In descending order of frequency,
these reactions included dyspepsia,* constipation,* nausea,*
vomiting,* abdominal pain, anorexia, occult blood in the
stool, diarrhea, flatulence, and dry mouth.
The drug was discontinued because of adverse gastrointestinal reactions in less than 2% of patients.
Nervous System —The most frequent adverse neurologic
reactions were headache and somnolence, which occurred in
about 15% of patients. Dizziness,* tremor, confusion, and
insomnia were noted less frequently.
Nalfon was discontinued in less than 0.5% of patients because of these side effects.
Skin and Appendages —Pruritus,* rash, increased sweating,
and urticaria.
Nalfon was discontinued in about 1% of patients because of
an adverse effect related to the skin.
Special Senses —Tinnitus, blurred vision, and decreased
hearing.
Nalfon was discontinued in less than 0.5% of patients because of adverse effects related to the special senses.
Cardiovascular —Palpitations* and tachycardia.
Nalfon was discontinued in about 0.5% of patients because of
adverse cardiovascular reactions.
Miscellaneous —Nervousness,* asthenia,* dyspnea, fatigue,
and malaise.

---

* Reactions in 3% to 9% of patients treated with Nalfon.
(Those reactions occurring in less than 3% of the patients are
unmarked.)
INCIDENCE LESS THAN 1%
Probable Causal Relationship
The following adverse reactions, occurring in less than 1% of
patients, were reported in controlled clinical trials and voluntary reports made since Nalfon® (Fenoprofen Calcium,
USP, Dista) was initially marketed. The probability of a causal relationship exists between Nalfon and these adverse
reactions:
Digestive System —Gastritis, peptic ulcer with/without perforation, and gastrointestinal hemòrrhage. Increases in alkaline phosphatase, LDH, and SGOT, jaundice, and cholestatic hepatitis were observed (*see* Precautions).
Genitourinary Tract —Dysuria, cystitis, hematuria, oliguria,
azotemia, anuria, interstitial nephritis, nephrosis, and papillary necrosis (*see* Warnings).
Hypersensitivity —Angioedema (angioneurotic edema).
Hematologic —Purpura, bruising, hemorrhage, thrombocytopenia, hemolytic anemia, aplastic anemia, agranulocytosis, and pancytopenia.
Miscellaneous —Peripheral edema and anaphylaxis.
INCIDENCE LESS THAN 1%
Causal Relationship Unknown
Other reactions have been reported but occurred in circumstances in which a causal relationship could not be established. However, with these rarely reported reactions, the
possibility of such a relationship cannot be excluded. Therefore, these observations are listed to alert the physician.
Skin and Appendages —Exfoliative dermatitis, toxic epidermal necrolysis, Stevens-Johnson syndrome, and alopecia.
Digestive System —Aphthous ulcerations of the buccal mucosa, metallic taste, and pancreatitis.
Cardiovascular —Atrial fibrillation, pulmonary edema, electrocardiographic changes, and supraventricular tachycardia.
Nervous System —Depression, disorientation, seizures, and
trigeminal neuralgia.
Special Senses —Burning tongue, diplopia, and optic neuritis.
Miscellaneous —Personality change, lymphadenopathy,
mastodynia, and fever.

OVERDOSAGE

Signs and Symptoms —Symptoms of oral overdose appear
within several hours and generally involve the gastrointestinal and central nervous system. They include dyspepsia,
nausea, vomiting, abdominal pain, dizziness, headache,
ataxia, tinnitus, tremor, drowsiness, and confusion. Hyperpyrexia, tachycardia, hypotension, and acute renal failure
may occur rarely following overdose. Respiratory depression
and metabolic acidosis have also been reported following
overdose with certain NSAIDs.
Treatment —To obtain up-to-date information about the
treatment of overdose, a good resource is your certified Regional Poison Control Center. Telephone numbers of certified poison control centers are listed in the *Physicians' Desk
Reference (PDR)*. In managing overdosage, consider the possibility of multiple drug overdoses, interaction among drugs,
and unusual drug kinetics in your patient.
Protect the patient's airway and support ventilation and
perfusion. Meticulously monitor and maintain, within acceptable limits, the patient's vital signs, blood gases, serum
electrolytes, etc. Absorption of drugs from the gastrointesti-

nal tract may be decreased by giving activated charcoal,
which, in many cases, is more effective than emesis or lavage; consider charcoal instead of or in addition to gastric
emptying. Repeated doses of charcoal over time may hasten
elimination of some drugs that have been absorbed. Safeguard the patient's airway when employing gastric emptying or charcoal.
Alkalinization of the urine, forced diuresis, peritoneal dialysis, hemodialysis, and charcoal hemoperfusion do not enhance systemic drug elimination.

DOSAGE AND ADMINISTRATION

Analgesia —For the treatment of mild to moderate pain, the
recommended dosage is 200 mg every 4 to 6 hours, as needed.
Rheumatoid Arthritis and Osteoarthritis —The suggested
dosage is 300 to 600 mg 3 or 4 times a day. The dose should be
tailored to the needs of the patient and may be increased or
decreased depending on the severity of the symptoms. Dosage adjustments may be made after initiation of drug therapy or during exacerbations of the disease. Total daily dosage should not exceed 3,200 mg.
If gastrointestinal complaints occur, Nalfon® (Fenoprofen
Calcium, USP, Dista) may be administered with meals or
with milk. Although the total amount absorbed is not affected, peak blood levels are delayed and diminished.
Patients with rheumatoid arthritis generally seem to require larger doses of Nalfon than do those with osteoarthritis. The smallest dose that yields acceptable control should
be employed.
Although improvement may be seen in a few days in many
patients, an additional 2 to 3 weeks may be required to gauge
the full benefits of therapy.

HOW SUPPLIED

(R) Pulvules:
   200 mg* (white and ocher) (No. 415)—(Identi-Code† H76)
   (RxPak‡ of 100) NDC 0777-0876-02
   300 mg* (yellow and ocher) (No. 416)—(Identi-Code H77)
   (RxPak of 100) NDC 0777-0877-02; (500s) NDC 0777-0877-
   03
Tablets (DISTA imprinted on one side, NALFON on other
side):
   600 mg* (yellow, paracapsule-shaped, scored) (No.
   1900)—(Identi-Code U59) (RxPak of 100) NDC 0777-2159-
   02; (500s) NDC 0777-2159-03

---

* Equivalent to fenoprofen.
† Identi-Code® (formula identification code, Dista).
‡ All RxPaks (prescription packages, Dista) have safey clo-
sures.
Store at controlled room temperature, 59° to 86°F (15° to
30°C).

[100588]

Shown in Product Identification Section, page 409

PROZAC®   ℞
[prō′zăk]
(fluoxetine hydrochloride)
PULVULES®

DESCRIPTION

Prozac® (Fluoxetine Hydrochloride, Dista) is an antidepressant for oral administration; it is chemically unrelated to
tricyclic, tetracyclic, or other available antidepressant
agents. It is designated (±)-N-methyl-3-phenyl-3-[(α,α,α-
trifluoro-p-tolyl)-oxy]-propylamine hydrochloride and has
the empirical formula of $C_{17}H_{18}F_3NO \cdot HCl$. Its molecular
weight is 345.79. The structural formula is:

$$F_3C{-}\bigcirc{-}O{-}CH{-}(CH_2)_2{-}NH{-}CH_3 \cdot HCl$$

Fluoxetine hydrochloride is a white to off-white crystalline
solid with a solubility of 50 mg/mL in water.
Each Pulvule® contains fluoxetine hydrochloride equivalent to 20 mg (64.7 μmoles) of fluoxetine. It also contains F D
& C Blue No. 1, gelatin, iron oxide, silicone, starch, titanium
dioxide, and other inactive ingredients.

CLINICAL PHARMACOLOGY

Pharmacodynamics —The antidepressant action of fluoxetine is presumed to be linked to its inhibition of CNS neuronal uptake of serotonin. Studies at clinically relevant doses
in man have demonstrated that fluoxetine blocks the uptake
of serotonin, but not of norepinephrine, into human platelets. Studies in animals also suggest that fluoxetine is a
much more potent uptake inhibitor of serotonin than of norepinephrine.
Antagonism of muscarinic, histaminergic, and α₁-adrenergic
receptors has been hypothesized to be associated with various anticholinergic, sedative, and cardiovascular effects of

classical tricyclic antidepressant drugs. Fluoxetine binds to
these and other membrane receptors from brain tissue much
less potently in vitro than do the tricyclic drugs.
Absorption, Distribution, Metabolism, and Excretion:
Systemic Bioavailability—In man, following a single oral 40-
mg dose, peak plasma concentrations of fluoxetine from 15 to
55 ng/mL are observed after 6 to 8 hours.
Food does not appear to affect the systemic bioavailability of
fluoxetine, although it may delay its absorption inconse-
quentially. Thus, fluoxetine may be administered with or
without food.
Protein Binding—Over the concentration range from 200 to
1,000 ng/mL, approximately 94.5% of fluoxetine is bound in
vitro to human serum proteins, including albumin and α₁-
glycoprotein. The interaction between fluoxetine and other
highly protein-bound drugs has not been fully evaluated but
may be important (*see* Precautions).
Metabolism—Fluoxetine is extensively metabolized in the
liver to norfluoxetine and a number of other, unidentified
metabolites. The only identified active metabolite, norfluoxetine, is formed by demethylation of fluoxetine. In animal models, norfluoxetine's potency and selectivity as a serotonin uptake blocker are essentially equivalent to fluoxetine's. The primary route of elimination appears to be hepatic metabolism to inactive metabolites excreted by the
kidney.
Clinical Issues Related to Metabolism/Elimination —The
complexity of the metabolism of fluoxetine has several
consequences that may potentially affect fluoxetine's clinical use.
Accumulation and Slow Elimination—The relatively slow
elimination of fluoxetine (elimination half-life of 2 to 3 days)
and its active metabolite, norfluoxetine (elimination half-life
of 7 to 9 days), assures significant accumulation of these active species in chronic use. After 30 days of dosing at 40
mg/day, plasma concentrations of fluoxetine in the range of
91 to 302 ng/mL and norfluoxetine in the range of 72 to 258
ng/mL have been observed. Plasma concentrations of fluoxetine were higher than those predicted by single-dose studies,
presumably because fluoxetine's metabolism is not proportional to dose. Norfluoxetine, however, appears to have linear pharmacokinetics. Its mean terminal half-life after a
single dose was 8.6 days and after multiple dosing was 9.3
days.
Thus, even if patients are given a fixed dose, steady-state
plasma concentrations are only achieved after continuous
dosing for weeks. Nevertheless, plasma concentrations do
not appear to increase without limit. Specifically, patients
receiving fluoxetine at doses of 40 to 80 mg/day over periods
as long as 3 years exhibited, on average, plasma concentrations similar to those seen among patients treated for 4 or 5
weeks.
The long elimination half-lives of fluoxetine and norfluoxetine assure that, even when dosing is stopped, active drug
substance will persist in the body for weeks. This is of potential consequence when drug discontinuation is required or
when drugs are prescribed that might interact with fluoxetine and norfluoxetine following the discontinuation of Pro-
zac® (Fluoxetine Hydrochloride, Dista).
Liver Disease—As might be predicted from its primary site
of metabolism, liver impairment can affect the elimination
of fluoxetine. The elimination half-life of fluoxetine was prolonged in a study of cirrhotic patients, with a mean of 7.6
days compared to the range of 2 to 3 days seen in subjects
without liver disease; norfluoxetine elimination was also
delayed, with a mean duration of 12 days for cirrhotic patients compared to the range of 7 to 9 days in normal subjects. This suggests that the use of fluoxetine in patients with
liver disease must be approached with caution. If fluoxetine
is administered to patients with liver disease, a lower or less
frequent dose should be used (*see* Precautions and Dosage
and Administration).
Renal Disease—In single-dose studies, the pharmacokinetics
of fluoxetine and norfluoxetine were similar among subjects
with all levels of impaired renal function, including anephric
patients on chronic hemodialysis. However, with chronic
administration, additional accumulation of fluoxetine or its
metabolites (possibly including some not yet identified) may
occur in patients with severely impaired renal function, and
use of a lower or less frequent dose is advised (*see* Precautions).
Age—The effects of age upon the metabolism of fluoxetine
have not been fully explored. The disposition of single doses
of fluoxetine in healthy elderly subjects (greater than 65
years of age) did not differ significantly from that in younger
normal subjects. However, given the long half-life and non-
linear disposition of the drug, a single-dose study is not adequate to rule out the possibility of altered pharmacokinetics
in the elderly, particularly if they have systemic illness or
are receiving multiple drugs for concomitant diseases.

INDICATIONS AND USAGE

Prozac® (Fluoxetine Hydrochloride, Dista) is indicated for
the treatment of depression. The efficacy of Prozac was es-

Continued on next page

Dista—Cont.

tablished in 5- and 6-week trials with depressed outpatients whose diagnoses corresponded most closely to the DSM-III category of major depressive disorder.

A major depressive episode implies a prominent and relatively persistent depressed or dysphoric mood that usually interferes with daily functioning (nearly every day for at least 2 weeks); it should include at least 4 of the following 8 symptoms: change in appetite, change in sleep, psychomotor agitation or retardation, loss of interest in usual activities or decrease in sexual drive, increased fatigue, feelings of guilt or worthlessness, slowed thinking or impaired concentration, and a suicide attempt or suicidal ideation.

The antidepressant action of Prozac in hospitalized depressed patients has not been adequately studied.

The effectiveness of Prozac in long-term use, that is, for more than 5 to 6 weeks, has not been systematically evaluated in controlled trials. Therefore, the physician who elects to use Prozac for extended periods should periodically reevaluate the long-term usefulness of the drug for the individual patient.

CONTRAINDICATIONS

Prozac® (Fluoxetine Hydrochloride, Dista) is contraindicated in patients known to be hypersensitive to it.

WARNINGS

Monoamine Oxidase Inhibitors —Data on the effects of the combined use of fluoxetine and MAO inhibitors are limited. Their combined use should be avoided. Based on experience with the combined administration of MAOIs and tricyclics, at least 14 days should elapse between discontinuation of an MAO inhibitor and initiation of treatment with fluoxetine. Because of the long half-lives of fluoxetine and its active metabolite, at least 5 weeks (approximately 5 half-lives of norfluoxetine) should elapse between discontinuation of fluoxetine and initiation of therapy with a MAOI. Administration of an MAOI within 5 weeks of discontinuation of fluoxetine may increase the risk of serious events. While a causal relationship to fluoxetine has not been established, death has been reported to occur following the initiation of MAOI therapy shortly after discontinuation of fluoxetine.

Rash and Accompanying Events —During premarketing testing of more than 5,600 US patients given fluoxetine, approximately 4% developed a rash and/or urticaria. Among these cases, almost a third were withdrawn from treatment because of the rash and/or systemic signs or symptoms associated with the rash. Clinical findings reported in association with rash include fever, leukocytosis, arthralgias, edema, carpal tunnel syndrome, respiratory distress, lymphadenopathy, proteinuria, and mild transaminase elevation. Most patients improved promptly with discontinuation of fluoxetine and/or adjunctive treatment with antihistamines or steroids, and all patients experiencing these events were reported to recover completely.

Two patients are known to have developed a serious cutaneous systemic illness. In neither patient was there an unequivocal diagnosis, but 1 was considered to have a leukocytoclastic vasculitis, and the other, a severe desquamating syndrome that was considered variously to be a vasculitis or erythema multiforme. Several other patients have had systemic syndromes suggestive of serum sickness.

Since the introduction of Prozac, systemic events, possibly related to vasculitis, have developed in patients with rash. Although these events are rare, they may be serious, involving the lung, kidney, or liver. Death has been reported to occur in association with these systemic events.

Whether these systemic events and rash have a common underlying cause or are due to different etiologies or pathogenic processes is not known. Upon the appearance of rash, Prozac should be discontinued.

PRECAUTIONS

General —Anxiety and Insomnia—Anxiety, nervousness, and insomnia were reported by 10% to 15% of patients treated with Prozac® (Fluoxetine Hydrochloride, Dista). These symptoms led to drug discontinuation in 5% of patients treated with Prozac.

Altered Appetite and Weight—Significant weight loss, especially in underweight depressed patients, may be an undesirable result of treatment with Prozac.

In controlled clinical trials, approximately 9% of patients treated with Prozac experienced anorexia. This incidence is approximately sixfold that seen in placebo controls. A weight loss of greater than 5% of body weight occurred in 13% of patients treated with Prozac compared to 4% of placebo- and 3% of tricyclic-antidepressant-treated patients. However, only rarely have patients been discontinued from treatment with Prozac because of weight loss.

Activation of Mania/Hypomania—During premarketing testing, hypomania or mania occurred in approximately 1% of fluoxetine-treated patients. Activation of mania/hypomania has also been reported in a small proportion of patients with Major Affective Disorder treated with other marketed antidepressants.

Seizures—Twelve patients among more than 6,000 evaluated worldwide in the course of premarketing development of fluoxetine experienced convulsions (or events described as possibly having been seizures), a rate of 0.2% that appears to be similar to that associated with other marketed antidepressants. Prozac should be introduced with care in patients with a history of seizures.

Suicide—The possibility of a suicide attempt is inherent in depression and may persist until significant remission occurs. Close supervision of high-risk patients should accompany initial drug therapy. Prescriptions for Prozac should be written for the smallest quantity of capsules consistent with good patient management, in order to reduce the risk of overdose.

The Long Elimination Half-Lives of Fluoxetine and Its Metabolites—Because of the long elimination half-lives of the parent drug (2 to 3 days) and its major active metabolite (7 to 9 days), changes in dose will not be fully reflected in plasma for several weeks, affecting both strategies for titration to final dose and withdrawal from treatment (see Clinical Pharmacology and Dosage and Administration).

Use in Patients with Concomitant Illness—Clinical experience with Prozac® (Fluoxetine Hydrochloride, Dista) in patients with concomitant systemic illness is limited. Caution is advisable in using Prozac in patients with diseases or conditions that could affect metabolism or hemodynamic responses.

Fluoxetine has **not** been evaluated or used to any appreciable extent in patients with a recent history of myocardial infarction or unstable heart disease. Patients with these diagnoses were systematically excluded from clinical studies during the product's premarket testing. However, the electrocardiograms of 312 patients who received Prozac in double-blind trials were retrospectively evaluated; no conduction abnormalities that resulted in heart block were observed. The mean heart rate was reduced by approximately 3 beats/min.

In subjects with cirrhosis of the liver, the clearances of fluoxetine and its active metabolite, norfluoxetine, were decreased, thus increasing the elimination half-lives of these substances. A lower or less frequent dose should be used in patients with cirrhosis.

Since fluoxetine is extensively metabolized, excretion of unchanged drug in urine is a minor route of elimination. However, until adequate numbers of patients with severe renal impairment have been evaluated during chronic treatment with fluoxetine, it should be used with caution in such patients.

In patients with diabetes, Prozac may alter glycemic control. Hypoglycemia has occurred during therapy with Prozac, and hyperglycemia has developed following discontinuation of the drug. As is true with many other types of medication when taken concurrently by patients with diabetes, insulin and/or oral hypoglycemic dosage may need to be adjusted when therapy with Prozac is instituted or discontinued.

Interference with Cognitive and Motor Performance—Any psychoactive drug may impair judgment, thinking, or motor skills, and patients should be cautioned about operating hazardous machinery, including automobiles, until they are reasonably certain that the drug treatment does not affect them adversely.

Information for Patients —Physicians are advised to discuss the following issues with patients for whom they prescribe Prozac:

Because Prozac may impair judgment, thinking, or motor skills, patients should be advised to avoid driving a car or operating hazardous machinery until they are reasonably certain that their performance is not affected.

Patients should be advised to inform their physician if they are taking or plan to take any prescription or over-the-counter drugs or alcohol.

Patients should be advised to notify their physician if they become pregnant or intend to become pregnant during therapy.

Patients should be advised to notify their physician if they are breast-feeding an infant.

Patients should be advised to notify their physician if they develop a rash or hives.

Laboratory Tests —There are no specific laboratory tests recommended.

Drug Interactions —As with all drugs, the potential for interaction by a variety of mechanisms (ie, pharmacodynamic, pharmacokinetic drug inhibition or enhancement, etc) is a possibility (see Accumulation and Slow Elimination under Clinical Pharmacology).

Tryptophan—Five patients receiving Prozac® (Fluoxetine Hydrochloride, Dista) in combination with tryptophan experienced adverse reactions, including agitation, restlessness, and gastrointestinal distress.

Monoamine Oxidase Inhibitors—See Warnings.

Other Antidepressants—There have been greater than 2-fold increases of previously stable plasma levels of other antidepressants when Prozac has been administered in combination with these agents (see Accumulation and Slow Elimination under Clinical Pharmacology).

Diazepam Clearance—The half-life of concurrently administered diazepam may be prolonged in some patients (see Accu-

mulation and Slow Elimination *under* Clinical Pharmacology).

Potential Effects of Coadministration of Drugs Highly Bound to Plasma Proteins—Because fluoxetine is tightly bound to plasma protein, the administration of fluoxetine to a patient taking another drug which is tightly bound to protein (eg, Coumadin, digitoxin) may cause a shift in plasma concentrations potentially resulting in an adverse effect. Conversely, adverse effects may result from displacement of protein-bound fluoxetine by other tightly bound drugs (see Accumulation and Slow Elimination *under* Clinical Pharmacology).

CNS-Active Drugs—The risk of using Prozac in combination with other CNS-active drugs has not been systematically evaluated. Consequently, caution is advised if the concomitant administration of Prozac and such drugs is required (see Accumulation and Slow Elimination *under* Clinical Pharmacology).

Electroconvulsive Therapy—There are no clinical studies establishing the benefit of the combined use of ECT and fluoxetine. A single report of a prolonged seizure in a patient on fluoxetine has been reported.

Carcinogenesis, Mutagenesis, Impairment of Fertility —There is no evidence of carcinogenicity, mutagenicity, or impairment of fertility with Prozac.

The dietary administration of fluoxetine to rats and mice for 2 years at levels equivalent to approximately 7.5 and 9.0 times the maximum human dose (80 mg) respectively produced no evidence of carcinogenicity.

Fluoxetine and norfluoxetine have been shown to have no genotoxic effects based on the following assays: bacterial mutation assay, DNA repair assay in cultured rat hepatocytes, mouse lymphoma assay, and in vivo sister chromatid exchange assay in Chinese hamster bone marrow cells.

Two fertility studies conducted in rats at doses of approximately 5 and 9 times the maximum human dose (80 mg) indicated that fluoxetine had no adverse effects on fertility. A slight decrease in neonatal survival was noted, but this was probably associated with depressed maternal food consumption and suppressed weight gain.

Pregnancy —Teratogenic Effects —Pregnancy Category B: Reproduction studies have been performed in rats and rabbits at doses 9 and 11 times the maximum daily human dose (80 mg) respectively and have revealed no evidence of harm to the fetus due to Prozac® (Fluoxetine Hydrochloride, Dista). There are, however, no adequate and well-controlled studies in pregnant women. Because animal reproduction studies are not always predictive of human response, this drug should be used during pregnancy only if clearly needed.

Labor and Delivery —The effect of Prozac on labor and delivery in humans is unknown.

Nursing Mothers —It is not known whether and, if so, in what amount this drug or its metabolites are excreted in human milk. Because many drugs are excreted in human milk, caution should be exercised when Prozac is administered to a nursing woman.

Usage in Children —Safety and effectiveness in children have not been established.

Use in the Elderly —Prozac has not been systematically evaluated in older patients; however, several hundred elderly patients have participated in clinical studies with Prozac, and no unusual adverse age-related phenomena have been identified. However, these data are insufficient to rule out possible age-related differences during chronic use, particularly in elderly patients who have concomitant systemic illnesses or who are receiving concomitant drugs.

Hyponatremia —Several cases of hyponatremia (some with serum sodium lower than 110 mmol/L) have been reported. The hyponatremia appeared to be reversible when Prozac was discontinued. Although these cases were complex with varying possible etiologies, some were possibly due to the syndrome of inappropriate antidiuretic hormone secretion (SIADH). The majority of these occurrences have been in older patients and in patients taking diuretics or who are otherwise volume depleted.

ADVERSE REACTIONS

Commonly Observed —The most commonly observed adverse events associated with the use of Prozac® (Fluoxetine Hydrochloride, Dista) and not seen at an equivalent incidence among placebo-treated patients were: nervous system complaints, including anxiety, nervousness, and insomnia; drowsiness and fatigue or asthenia; tremor; sweating; gastrointestinal complaints, including anorexia, nausea, and diarrhea; and dizziness or lightheadedness.

Associated with Discontinuation of Treatment —Fifteen percent of approximately 4,000 patients who received Prozac in US premarketing clinical trials discontinued treatment due to an adverse event. The more common events causing discontinuation included: psychiatric (5.3%), primarily nervousness, anxiety, and insomnia; digestive (3.0%), primarily nausea; nervous system (1.6%), primarily dizziness; body as a whole (1.5%), primarily asthenia and headache; and skin (1.4%), primarily rash and pruritus.

Incidence in Controlled Clinical Trials —The table that follows enumerates adverse events that occurred at a frequency of 1% or more among patients treated with Prozac who participated in controlled trials comparing Prozac with placebo. The prescriber should be aware that these figures cannot be used to predict the incidence of side effects in the course of usual medical practice where patient characteristics and other factors differ from those that prevailed in the clinical trials. Similarly, the cited frequencies cannot be compared with figures obtained from other clinical investigations involving different treatments, uses, and investigators. The cited figures, however, do provide the prescribing physician with some basis for estimating the relative contribution of drug and nondrug factors to the side-effect incidence rate in the population studied.

[See table right].

Other Events Observed During the Premarketing Evaluation of Prozac® (Fluoxetine Hydrochloride, Dista)—During clinical testing in the US, multiple doses of Prozac were administered to approximately 5,600 subjects. Untoward events associated with this exposure were recorded by clinical investigators using descriptive terminology of their own choosing. Consequently, it is not possible to provide a meaningful estimate of the proportion of individuals experiencing adverse events without first grouping similar types of untoward events into a limited (ie, reduced) number of standardized event categories.

In the tabulations which follow, a standard COSTART Dictionary terminology has been used to classify reported adverse events. The frequencies presented, therefore, represent the proportion of the 5,600 individuals exposed to Prozac who experienced an event of the type cited on at least 1 occasion while receiving Prozac. All reported events are included except those already listed in tables, those COSTART terms so general as to be uninformative, and those events where a drug cause was remote. It is important to emphasize that, although the events reported did occur during treatment with Prozac, they were not necessarily caused by it. Events are further classified within body system categories and enumerated in order of decreasing frequency using the following definitions: frequent adverse events are defined as those occurring on 1 or more occasions in at least 1/100 patients; infrequent adverse events are those occurring in 1/100 to 1/1,000 patients; rare events are those occurring in less than 1/1,000 patients.

Body as a Whole—*Frequent:* chills; *Infrequent:* chills and fever, cyst, face edema, hangover effect, jaw pain, malaise, neck pain, neck rigidity, and pelvic pain; *Rare:* abdomen enlarged, cellulitis, hydrocephalus, hypothermia, LE syndrome, moniliasis, and serum sickness.

Cardiovascular System—*Infrequent:* angina pectoris, arrhythmia, hemorrhage, hypertension, hypotension, migraine, postural hypotension, syncope, and tachycardia; *Rare:* AV block (first-degree), bradycardia, bundle-branch block, cerebral ischemia, myocardial infarct, thrombophlebitis, vascular headache, and ventricular arrhythmia.

Digestive System—*Frequent:* increased appetite; *Infrequent:* aphthous stomatitis, dysphagia, eructation, esophagitis, gastritis, gingivitis, glossitis, liver function tests abnormal, melena, stomatitis, thirst; *Rare:* bloody diarrhea, cholecystitis, cholelithiasis, colitis, duodenal ulcer, enteritis, fecal incontinence, hematemesis, hepatitis, hepatomegaly, hyperchlorhydria, increased salivation, jaundice, liver tenderness, mouth ulceration, salivary gland enlargement, stomach ulcer, tongue discoloration, and tongue edema.

Endocrine System—*Infrequent:* hypothyroidism; *Rare:* goiter and hyperthyroidism.

Hemic and Lymphatic System—*Infrequent:* anemia and lymphadenopathy; *Rare:* bleeding time increased, blood dyscrasia, leukopenia, lymphocytosis, petechia, purpura, sedimentation rate increased, and thrombocythemia.

Metabolic and Nutritional—*Frequent:* weight loss; *Infrequent:* generalized edema, hypoglycemia, peripheral edema, and weight gain; *Rare:* dehydration, gout, hypercholesteremia, hyperglycemia, hyperlipemia, hypoglycemic reaction, hypokalemia, hyponatremia, and iron deficiency anemia.

Musculoskeletal System—*Infrequent:* arthritis, bone pain, bursitis, tenosynovitis, and twitching; *Rare:* bone necrosis, chondrodystrophy, muscle hemorrhage, myositis, osteoporosis, pathologic fracture, and rheumatoid arthritis.

Nervous System—*Frequent:* abnormal dreams and agitation; *Infrequent:* abnormal gait, acute brain syndrome, akathisia, amnesia, apathy, ataxia, buccoglossal syndrome, CNS stimulation, convulsion, delusions, depersonalization, emotional lability, euphoria, hallucinations, hostility, hyperkinesia, hypesthesia, incoordination, libido increased, manic reaction, neuralgia, neuropathy, paranoid reaction, psychosis, and vertigo; *Rare:* abnormal electroencephalogram, antisocial reaction, chronic brain syndrome, circumoral paresthesia, CNS depression, coma, dysarthria, dystonia, extrapyramidal syndrome, hypertonia, hysteria, myoclonus, nystagmus, paralysis, reflexes decreased, stupor, and torticollis.

Respiratory System—*Frequent:* bronchitis, rhinitis, and yawn; *Infrequent:* asthma, epistaxis, hiccup, hyperventilation, and pneumonia; *Rare:* apnea, hemoptysis, hypoxia, larynx edema, lung edema, lung fibrosis/alveolitis, and pleural effusion.

TREATMENT-EMERGENT ADVERSE EXPERIENCE INCIDENCE IN PLACEBO-CONTROLLED CLINICAL TRIALS

Body System/ Adverse Event*	Percentage of Patients Reporting Event Prozac† (N=1,730)	Placebo (N=799)	Body System/ Adverse Event*	Percentage of Patients Reporting Event Prozac† (N=1,730)	Placebo (N=799)
Nervous			**Body as a Whole**		
Headache	20.3	15.5	Asthenia	4.4	1.9
Nervousness	14.9	8.5	Infection, viral	3.4	3.1
Insomnia	13.8	7.1	Pain, limb	1.6	1.1
Drowsiness	11.6	6.3	Fever	1.4	—
Anxiety	9.4	5.5	Pain, chest	1.3	1.1
Tremor	7.9	2.4	Allergy	1.2	1.1
Dizziness	5.7	3.3	Influenza	1.2	1.5
Fatigue	4.2	1.1	**Respiratory**		
Sedated	1.9	1.3	Upper respiratory infection	7.6	6.0
Sensation disturbance	1.7	2.0	Flu-like syndrome	2.8	1.9
Libido, decreased	1.6	—	Pharyngitis	2.7	1.3
Light-headedness	1.6	—	Nasal congestion	2.6	2.3
Concentration, decreased	1.5	—	Headache, sinus	2.3	1.8
Digestive			Sinusitis	2.1	2.0
Nausea	21.1	10.1	Cough	1.6	1.6
Diarrhea	12.3	7.0	Dyspnea	1.4	—
Mouth dryness	9.5	6.0	**Cardiovascular**		
Anorexia	8.7	1.5	Hot flushes	1.8	1.0
Dyspepsia	6.4	4.3	Palpitations	1.3	1.4
Constipation	4.5	3.3	**Musculoskeletal**		
Pain, abdominal	3.4	2.9	Pain, back	2.0	2.4
Vomiting	2.4	1.3	Pain, joint	1.2	1.1
Taste change	1.8	—	Pain, muscle	1.2	1.0
Flatulence	1.6	1.1	**Urogenital**		
Gastroenteritis	1.0	1.4	Menstruation, painful	1.9	1.4
Skin and Appendages			Sexual dysfunction	1.9	—
Sweating, excessive	8.4	3.8	Frequent micturition	1.6	—
Rash	2.7	1.8	Urinary tract infection	1.2	—
Pruritus	2.4	1.4	**Special Senses**		
			Vision disturbance	2.8	1.8

* Events reported by at least 1% of patients treated with Prozac are included.
† Prozac® (Fluoxetine Hydrochloride Dista).
—Incidence less than 1%.

Skin and Appendages—*Infrequent:* acne, alopecia, contact dermatitis, dry skin, herpes simplex, maculopapular rash, and urticaria; *Rare:* eczema, erythema multiforme, fungal dermatitis, herpes zoster, hirsutism, psoriasis, purpuric rash, pustular rash, seborrhea, skin discoloration, skin hypertrophy, subcutaneous nodule, and vesiculobullous rash.

Special Senses—*Infrequent:* amblyopia, conjunctivitis, ear pain, eye pain, mydriasis, photophobia, and tinnitus; *Rare:* blepharitis, cataract, corneal lesion, deafness, diplopia, eye hemorrhage, glaucoma, iritis, ptosis, strabismus, and taste loss.

Urogenital System—*Infrequent:* abnormal ejaculation, amenorrhea, breast pain, cystitis, dysuria, fibrocystic breast, impotence, leukorrhea, menopause, menorrhagia, ovarian disorder, urinary incontinence, urinary retention, urinary urgency, urination impaired, and vaginitis; *Rare:* abortion, albuminuria, breast enlargement, dyspareunia, epididymitis, female lactation, hematuria, hypomenorrhea, kidney calculus, metrorrhagia, orchitis, polyuria, pyelonephritis, pyuria, salpingitis, urethral pain, urethritis, urinary tract disorder, urolithiasis, uterine hemorrhage, uterine spasm, and vaginal hemorrhage.

Postintroduction Reports—Voluntary reports of adverse events temporally associated with Prozac that have been received since market introduction and which may have no causal relationship with the drug include the following: vaginal bleeding after drug withdrawal, hyperprolactinemia, thrombocytopenia, and confusion.

DRUG ABUSE AND DEPENDENCE

Controlled Substance Class—Prozac® (Fluoxetine Hydrochloride, Dista) is not a controlled substance.

Physical and Psychologic Dependence—Prozac has not been systematically studied, in animals or humans, for its potential for abuse, tolerance, or physical dependence. While the premarketing clinical experience with Prozac did not reveal any tendency for a withdrawal syndrome or any drug-seeking behavior, these observations were not systematic, and it is not possible to predict on the basis of this limited experience the extent to which a CNS-active drug will be misused, diverted, and/or abused once marketed. Consequently, physicians should carefully evaluate patients for history of drug abuse and follow such patients closely, observing them for signs of misuse or abuse of Prozac (eg, development of tolerance, incrementation of dose, drug-seeking behavior).

OVERDOSAGE

Human Experience—As of December 1987, there were 2 deaths among approximately 38 reports of acute overdose with fluoxetine, either alone or in combination with other drugs and/or alcohol. One death involved a combined overdose with approximately 1,800 mg of fluoxetine and an undetermined amount of maprotiline. Plasma concentrations of fluoxetine and maprotiline were 4.57 mg/L and 4.18 mg/L, respectively. A second death involved 3 drugs yielding plasma concentrations as follows: fluoxetine, 1.93 mg/L; norfluoxetine, 1.10 mg/L; codeine, 1.80 mg/L; temazepam, 3.80 mg/L.

One other patient who reportedly took 3,000 mg of fluoxetine experienced 2 grand mal seizures that remitted spontaneously without specific anticonvulsant treatment (see Management). The actual amount of drug absorbed may have been less due to vomiting.

Nausea and vomiting were prominent in overdoses involving higher fluoxetine doses. Other prominent symptoms of overdose included agitation, restlessness, hypomania, and other signs of CNS excitation. Except for the 2 deaths noted above, all other overdose cases recovered without residua.

Animal Experience—Studies in animals do not provide precise or necessarily valid information about the treatment of human overdose. However, animal experiments can provide useful insights into possible treatment strategies.

The oral LD_{50} in rats and mice was found to be 452 and 248 mg/kg, respectively. Acute high oral doses produced hyperirritability and convulsions in several animal species.

Among 6 dogs purposely overdosed with oral fluoxetine, 5 experienced grand mal seizures. Seizures stopped immediately upon the bolus intravenous administration of a standard veterinary dose of diazepam. In this short-term study, the lowest plasma concentration at which a seizure occurred was only twice the maximum plasma concentration seen in humans taking 80 mg/day chronically.

In a separate single-dose study, the ECG in dogs given high doses did not reveal prolongation of the PR, QRS, or QT in-

Continued on next page

Dista—Cont.

tervals. Tachycardia and an increase in blood pressure were observed. Consequently, the value of the ECG in predicting cardiac toxicity is unknown. Nonetheless, the ECG should ordinarily be monitored in cases of human overdose (*see* Management).

Management of Overdose—Establish and maintain an airway; ensure adequate oxygenation and ventilation. Activated charcoal, which may be used with sorbitol, may be as effective as emesis or lavage or more so and should be considered in treating overdose.

Cardiac and vital signs monitoring is recommended, along with general symptomatic and supportive measures. Based on experience in animals, which may not be relevant to humans, fluoxetine-induced seizures which fail to remit spontaneously may respond to diazepam.

There are no specific antidotes for Prozac® (Fluoxetine Hydrochloride, Dista).

Due to the large volume of distribution of Prozac, forced diuresis, dialysis, hemoperfusion, and exchange transfusion are unlikely to be of benefit.

In managing overdosage, consider the possibility of multiple drug involvement. The physician should consider contacting a poison control center on the treatment of any overdose.

DOSAGE AND ADMINISTRATION

Initial Treatment—In controlled trials used to support the efficacy of fluoxetine, patients were administered morning doses ranging from 20 mg to 80 mg/day. Recent studies suggest that 20 mg/day may be sufficient to obtain a satisfactory antidepressant response. Consequently, a dose of 20 mg/day, administered in the morning, is recommended as the initial dose.

A dose increase may be considered after several weeks if no clinical improvement is observed. Doses above 20 mg/day should be administered on a b.i.d. schedule (ie, morning and noon) and should not exceed a maximum dose of 80 mg/day. As with other antidepressants, the full antidepressant effect may be delayed until 4 weeks of treatment or longer.

As with many other medications, a lower or less frequent dosage should be used in patients with renal and/or hepatic impairment. A lower or less frequent dosage should also be considered for patients, such as the elderly, with concurrent disease or on multiple medications.

Maintenance/Continuation/Extended Treatment—There is no body of evidence available to answer the question of how long the patient treated with fluoxetine should remain on it. It is generally agreed among expert psychopharmacologists (circa 1987) that acute episodes of depression require several months or longer of sustained pharmacologic therapy. Whether the dose of antidepressant needed to induce remission is identical to the dose needed to maintain and/or sustain euthymia is unknown.

HOW SUPPLIED

(℞) Pulvules: 20 mg,* green and off-white (No. 3105)—(100s) NDC 0777-3105-02

Store at controlled room temperature, 59° to 86°F (15° to 30°C).

---

*Equivalent to fluoxetine.

Animal Toxicology: Phospholipids are increased in some tissues of mice, rats, and dogs given fluoxetine chronically. This effect is reversible after cessation of fluoxetine treatment. Phospholipid accumulation in animals has been observed with many cationic amphiphilic drugs, including fenfluramine, imipramine, and ranitidine. The significance of this effect in humans is unknown.

[062089]

Shown in Product Identification Section, page 409

VALMID®   Ⓒⱽ

[văl 'mĭd]
(ethinamate)
Capsules, USP

DESCRIPTION

Valmid® (Ethinamate, USP, Dista) is 1-ethinyl-cyclohexyl-carbamate. It is a nonirritating, colorless, faintly bitter, stable crystalline powder with a melting point of 96°-98° C. Valmid is relatively insoluble in water but quite soluble in many alcohols and oils.

Each Pulvule® contains 500 mg ethinamate. These Pulvules also contain F D & C Blue No. 1, F D & C Red No. 3, gelatin, silicone, sodium bicarbonate, sodium carboxymethyl starch, sodium lauryl sulfate, titanium dioxide, and other inactive ingredients.

Valmid is a hypnotic agent for oral administration. Its site and mechanism of action are unknown.

CLINICAL PHARMACOLOGY

Valmid® (Ethinamate, USP, Dista) is rapidly absorbed after oral administration. Following a single oral dose of 1 g, peak plasma levels are reached in approximately 36 minutes and

---

decline to negligible values over the next 8 hours. Approximately 36% of the administered dose appears in the urine within 24 hours. The effect of multiple doses and prolonged administration on pharmacodynamics and pharmacokinetics is not known.

INDICATIONS AND USAGE

Valmid® (Ethinamate, USP, Dista) is a short-acting hypnotic. It has not been sufficiently well studied with currently available sleep laboratory techniques to delimit its value in specific types of insomnia. Valmid is best used for limited periods. Should insomnia persist, drug-free intervals of 1 week or more should elapse before re-treatment is considered. Attempts should be made to find alternative nondrug therapy for chronic insomnia. The prolonged administration of Valmid is not recommended, since it has not been shown to be effective for a period of more than 7 days.

CONTRAINDICATION

Valmid® (Ethinamate, USP, Dista) is contraindicated in patients with known hypersensitivity to the drug.

WARNINGS

Patients receiving Valmid® (Ethinamate, USP, Dista) should be cautioned about possible additive effects when it is taken in combination with alcohol or other CNS depressants. Patients should be cautioned against becoming involved in hazardous occupations requiring complete mental alertness, such as operating machines or driving a motor vehicle, shortly after ingestion of the drug.

PRECAUTIONS

Drug Interactions—If Valmid® (Ethinamate, USP, Dista) is to be administered in combination with other drugs known to have a hypnotic or CNS-depressant effect, consideration should be given to the potential additive effects.

Carcinogenesis—Long-term studies in animals have *not* been performed to evaluate carcinogenic potential.

Usage in Pregnancy—Pregnancy Category C—Animal reproduction studies have not been conducted with Valmid. It is also not known whether the drug can cause fetal harm when administered to a pregnant woman or can affect reproduction capacity. Valmid should be given to a pregnant woman only if clearly needed.

Nursing Mothers—It is not known whether this drug is excreted in human milk. Because many drugs are excreted in human milk, caution should be exercised when Valmid is administered to a nursing woman.

Usage in Children—Safety and effectiveness in children below the age of 15 years have not been established.

ADVERSE REACTIONS

Rare cases of thrombocytopenic purpura and drug idiosyncrasy with fever have been reported. Paradoxical excitement in children, mild gastrointestinal symptoms, and skin rashes have occurred after the use of Valmid® (Ethinamate, USP, Dista).

DRUG ABUSE AND DEPENDENCE

Controlled Substance—Valmid® (Ethinamate, USP, Dista) is a Schedule IV drug.

Dependence—Drug dependence characterized by both a psychologic and a physical dependence has occurred when Valmid has been taken at higher than recommended doses for prolonged intervals. It is, therefore, desirable to exercise caution in administering Valmid to individuals who are addiction-prone and to those whose history suggests that they may increase dosage on their own initiative. It is advisable to limit repeated prescriptions without adequate medical supervision.

In the event that an individual has established dependence on Valmid, withdrawal must be accomplished with extreme care. Abrupt withdrawal may cause a typical abstinence syndrome accompanied by convulsions. Withdrawal may be accomplished by hospitalizing the patient and reducing the addictive daily dose at a rate of 500 to 1,000 mg every 2 or 3 days. Psychiatric follow-up is indicated.

OVERDOSAGE

Signs and Symptoms—The onset of symptoms following toxic oral exposure to ethinamate may occur as early as 15 minutes following ingestion. Ethinamate has a half-life of 2.5 hours. The manifestations of ethinamate overdose may include CNS depression, respiratory depression, hypothermia, and hypotension. Other findings may include absent or depressed reflexes and erythematous or hemorrhagic blisters (primarily at pressure points). Following massive exposure to ethinamate, pulmonary edema, circulatory collapse with loss of peripheral vascular tone, and cardiac arrest may occur. Ethinamate may interfere with hepatic function resulting in transient jaundice.

Treatment—To obtain up-to-date information about the treatment of overdose, a good resource is your certified Regional Poison Control Center. Telephone numbers of certified poison control centers are listed in the *Physicians' Desk Reference (PDR)*. In managing overdosage, consider the possibility of multiple drug overdoses, interaction among drugs, and unusual drug kinetics in your patient.

The initial intervention in an ethinamate overdose is to establish an airway and ensure oxygenation and ventilation. Resuscitative measures should be initiated promptly. If the patient is hypotensive, consider giving intravenous fluids, raising the legs, or administering pharmacologic agents. Protect the patient's airway and support ventilation and perfusion. Meticulously monitor and maintain, within acceptable limits, the patient's vital signs, blood gases, serum electrolytes, etc. Absorption of drugs from the gastrointestinal tract may be decreased by giving activated charcoal, which, in many cases, is more effective than emesis or lavage; consider charcoal instead of or in addition to gastric emptying. Repeated doses of charcoal over time may hasten elimination of some drugs that have been absorbed. Safeguard the patient's airway when employing gastric emptying or charcoal.

Forced diuresis has not been established as beneficial for an overdosage of ethinamate. Peritoneal dialysis, hemodialysis, or charcoal hemoperfusion are effective in treating this overdose. These procedures should be reserved for patients with life-threatening toxicity who have not responded to supportive care or more conservative treatments.

DOSAGE AND ADMINISTRATION

For insomnia, 1 or 2 Pulvules (500 mg or 1 g) of Valmid® (Ethinamate, USP, Dista) should be taken 20 minutes before retiring.

Special Patient Population—Since the risk of oversedation, dizziness, confusion, and/or ataxia substantially increases with the administration of large doses of sedatives and hypnotics in the elderly and debilitated, it is recommended that a dose of a single 500-mg Pulvule be given to such individuals. Should this dose prove to be ineffective, clinical judgment must weigh the risk of increasing the dosage against the potential hazards mentioned above.

HOW SUPPLIED

(Ⓒⱽ) *Pulvules No. 399, Valmid ® (Ethinamate Capsules, USP), H74,* 500 mg* (No. 0, Light-Blue Opaque Body, Blue Opaque Cap), in bottles of 100 (NDC 0777-0874-02).   [042888]

Shown in Product Identification Section, page 409

---

*Identi-Code® symbol.

Doctors' Recommended Pharmaceutical Products
**9400 BRIGHTON WAY
SUITE 414
BEVERLY HILLS, CA 90210**

DOCTORS' RECOMMENDED BEST   OTC
MultiVitamins and Minerals

EACH TABLET CONTAINS:	Quantity	U.S. RDA Adults & Children 4 years & older
Vitamin A	5000 I.U.	(100%)
(as Acetate and Beta Carotene)		
Vitamin E	30 I.U.	(100%)
(as dl-Alpha Tocopheryl Acetate)		
Vitamin C	90 mg	(100%)
(as Ascorbic Acid)		
Folic Acid	400 mcg	(100%)
Vitamin B1	2.25 mg	(100%)
(as Thiamine Mononitrate)		
Vitamin B2	2.6 mg	(153%)
(as Riboflavin)		
Niacinamide	20 mg	(100%)
Vitamin B6	3 mg	(150%)
(as Pyridoxine Hydrochloride)		
Vitamin B12	9 mcg	(150%)
(as Cyanocobalamin)		
Vitamin D	400 I.U.	(100%)
Biotin	45 mcg	(15%)
Pantothenic Acid	10 mg	(100%)
(as Calcium Pantothenate)		
Calcium	162 mg	(16%)
(as Dibasic Calcium Phosphate)		
Phosphorus	125 mg	(13%)
(as Dibasic Calcium Phosphate)		
Iodine	150 mcg	(100%)
(as Potassium Iodide)		
Iron	27 mg	(150%)
(as Ferrous Fumarate)		
Magnesium	100 mg	(25%)
(as Magnesium Oxide)		
Copper	2 mg	(100%)
(as Cupric Oxide)		
Zinc	15 mg	(100%)
(as Zinc Oxide)		
Manganese	5 mg	*
(as Manganese Sulfate)		
Potassium	30 mg	*
(as Potassium Chloride)		

Chloride	27.2 mg	*
(as Potassium Chloride)		
Chromium	25 mcg	*
(as Chromium Chloride)		
Molybdenum	25 mcg	*
(as Sodium Molybdate)		
Selium	25 mcg	*
(as Sodium Selenate)		
Vitamin K1	25 mcg	*
(as Phytonadione)		

* No U.S. RDA established.

INDICATIONS

BEST is recommended for adults who need additional vitamin supplements and iron; women with heavy menstrual periods; adults who diet or exercise a lot; adults with fever or stressful psychological conditions.

RECOMMENDED DAILY INTAKE

Adults, 1 tablet as indicated by clinical need.
Keep this and all other medications out of the reach of children.

HOW SUPPLIED

Bottles of 100.
Store at room temperature.

DOCTORS' RECOMMENDED ℞
HIGH POTENCY THERAPEUTIC
MultiVitamins and Minerals

EACH TABLET CONTAINS:	Quantity
Vitamin A	5000 I.U.
(as Acetate and Beta Carotene)	
Vitamin E	30 I.U.
(as dl-Alpha Tocopheryl Acetate)	
Vitamin C	500 mg
(as Ascorbic Acid)	
Folic Acid	0.8 mg
Vitamin B1	20 mg
(as Thiamine Mononitrate)	
Vitamin B2	20 mg
(as Riboflavin)	
Niacin	100 mg
(as Niacinamide)	
Vitamin B6	25 mg
(as Pyridoxine Hydrochloride)	
Vitamin B12	50 mcg
(as Cyanocobalamin)	
Biotin	0.15 mg
Pantothenic Acid	25 mg
(as Calcium Pantothenate)	
Iron	27 mg
(as Ferrous Fumarate)	
Chromium	0.1 mg
(as Chromium Nitrate)	
Magnesium	50 mg
(as Magnesium Oxide)	
Manganese	5 mg
(as Manganese Dioxide)	
Copper	3 mg
(as Cupric Oxide)	
Zinc	22.5 mg
(as Zinc Oxide)	

INDICATIONS

High Potency Therapeutic is recommended for the following: Pregnant or lactating women; women on birth control; renal failure or dialysis patients; alcoholics or patients with malnutrition; patients with fever or infection; patients with diabetes or gastrointestinal problems.

RECOMMENDED DAILY INTAKE

Adults, 1 tablet as indicated by clinical need.
Keep this and all other medications out of the reach of children.

HOW SUPPLIED

Child-resistant bottles of 100.
Store at 59° to 86°F.

CAUTION

Federal law prohibits dispensing without a prescription.
Shown in Product Identification Section, page 409

Products are cross-indexed by
generic and chemical names
in the
YELLOW SECTION

Dorsey Pharmaceuticals

FOR DORSEY PRESCRIPTION PRODUCTS, PLEASE SEE SANDOZ PHARMACEUTICALS CORPORATION LISTING.

Du Pont Pharmaceuticals
E.I. duPont de Nemours & Co. (Inc.)
WILMINGTON, DE 19898

BRETYLOL® ℞
[*bre'tĭ-lol"*]
(bretylium tosylate)
INJECTION

For Intravenous or Intramuscular Use

DESCRIPTION

BRETYLOL (bretylium tosylate) Injection is an antifibrillatory and antiarrhythmic agent, intended for intravenous or intramuscular use.
The chemical structure is:

$$C_{18}H_{24}BrNO_3S$$

Mol. Wt. 414.39

BRETYLOL is a white, crystalline powder with an extremely bitter taste. It is freely soluble in water and alcohol. Each mL of sterile, non-pyrogenic solution contains 50 mg bretylium tosylate in Water for Injection, USP. The pH is adjusted when necessary, with dilute hydrochloric acid or sodium hydroxide. BRETYLOL contains no preservative.

CLINICAL PHARMACOLOGY

BRETYLOL (bretylium tosylate) is a bromobenzyl quaternary ammonium compound which selectively accumulates in sympathetic ganglia and their postganglionic adrenergic neurons where it inhibits norepinephrine release by depressing adrenergic nerve terminal excitability.
BRETYLOL also suppresses ventricular fibrillation and ventricular arrhythmias. The mechanisms of the antifibrillatory and antiarrhythmic actions of BRETYLOL are not established. In efforts to define these mechanisms, the following electrophysiologic actions of BRETYLOL have been demonstrated in animal experiments:

1. Increase in ventricular fibrillation threshold.
2. Increase in action potential duration and effective refractory period without changes in heart rate.
3. Little effect on the rate of rise or amplitude of the cardiac action potential (Phase 0) or in resting membrane potential (Phase 4) in normal myocardium. However, when cell injury slows the rate of rise, decreases amplitude, and lowers resting membrane potential, BRETYLOL transiently restores these parameters toward normal.
4. In canine hearts with infarcted areas BRETYLOL decreases the disparity in action potential duration between normal and infarcted regions.
5. Increase in impulse formation and spontaneous firing rate of pacemaker tissue as well as increased ventricular conduction velocity.

The restoration of injured myocardial cell electrophysiology toward normal, as well as the increase of the action potential duration and effective refractory period without changing their ratio to each other, may be important factors in suppressing re-entry of aberrant impulses and decreasing induced dispersion of local excitable states.
BRETYLOL induces a chemical sympathectomy-like state which resembles a surgical sympathectomy. Catecholamine stores are not depleted by BRETYLOL, but catecholamine effects on the myocardium and on peripheral vascular resistance are often seen shortly after administration because BRETYLOL causes an early release of norepinephrine from the adrenergic postganglionic nerve terminals. Subsequently, BRETYLOL blocks the release of norepinephrine in response to neuron stimulation. Peripheral adrenergic blockade regularly causes orthostatic hypotension but has less effect on supine blood pressure. The relationship of adrenergic blockade to the antifibrillatory and antiarrhythmic actions of BRETYLOL is not clear. In a study in patients with frequent ventricular premature beats, peak plasma concentration of BRETYLOL and peak hypotensive effects were seen within one hour of intramuscular administration, presumably reflecting adrenergic postganglionic blockade. However, suppression of premature ventricular beats was not maximal until 6–9 hours after dosing, when mean plasma concentration had declined to less than one-half of peak

level. This suggests a slower mechanism, other than neuronal blockade, was involved in suppression of the arrhythmia. On the other hand, antifibrillatory effects can be seen within minutes of an intravenous injection, suggesting that the effect on the myocardium may occur quite rapidly.
BRETYLOL has a positive inotropic effect on the myocardium, but it is not yet certain whether this effect is direct or is mediated by catecholamine release.
BRETYLOL is eliminated intact by the kidneys. No metabolites have been identified following administration of BRETYLOL in man and laboratory animals. In man, approximately 70 to 80% of a ^{14}C-labelled intramuscular dose is excreted in the urine during the first 24 hours, with an additional 10% excreted over the next three days.
The terminal half-life in four normal volunteers averaged 7.8 ± 0.6 hrs (range 6.9–8.1). In one patient with a creatinine clearance of 21.0 ml/min x 1.73 m^2, the half-life was 16 hours. In one patient with a creatinine clearance of 1.0 ml/min x 1.73 m^2 the half-life was 31.5 hours. During hemodialysis, this patient's arterial and venous BRETYLOL concentrations declined rapidly, resulting in a half-life of 13 hours. During dialysis there was a two-fold increase in total BRETYLOL clearance.

Effect on Heart Rate: There is sometimes an initial small increase in heart rate when BRETYLOL is administered, but this is an inconsistent and transient occurrence.
Hemodynamic Effects: Following intravenous administration of 5 mg/kg of BRETYLOL to patients with acute myocardial infarction, there was a mild increase in arterial pressure, followed by a modest decrease, remaining within normal limits throughout. Pulmonary artery pressures, pulmonary capillary wedge pressure, right atrial pressure, cardiac index, stroke volume index, and stroke work index were not significantly changed. These hemodynamic effects were not correlated with antiarrhythmic activity.
Onset of Action: Suppression of ventricular fibrillation is rapid, usually occurring within minutes following intravenous administration. Suppression of ventricular tachycardia and other ventricular arrhythmias develops more slowly, usually 20 minutes to 2 hours after parenteral administration.

INDICATIONS

BRETYLOL is indicated in the prophylaxis and therapy of ventricular fibrillation.
BRETYLOL is also indicated in the treatment of life-threatening ventricular arrhythmias, such as ventricular tachycardia, that have failed to respond to adequate doses of a first-line antiarrhythmic agent, such as lidocaine.
Use of BRETYLOL should be limited to intensive care units, coronary care units or other facilities where equipment and personnel for constant monitoring of cardiac arrhythmias and blood pressure are available.
Following injection of BRETYLOL there may be a delay of 20 minutes to 2 hours in the onset of antiarrhythmic action, although it appears to act within minutes in ventricular fibrillation. The delay in effect appears to be longer after intramuscular than after intravenous injection.

CONTRAINDICATIONS

There are no contraindications to use in treatment of ventricular fibrillation or life-threatening refractory ventricular arrhythmias.

WARNINGS

1. **Hypotension**
   Administration of BRETYLOL regularly results in postural hypotension, subjectively recognized by dizziness, light-headedness, vertigo or faintness. Some degree of hypotension is present in about 50% of patients while they are supine. Hypotension may occur at doses lower than those needed to suppress arrhythmias.

   > Patients should be kept in the supine position until tolerance to the hypotensive effect of BRETYLOL develops. Tolerance occurs unpredictably but may be present after several days.

   Hypotension with supine systolic pressure greater than 75 mm Hg need not be treated unless there are associated symptoms. If supine systolic pressure falls below 75 mm Hg, an infusion of dopamine or norepinephrine may be used to raise blood pressure. When catecholamines are administered, a dilute solution should be employed and blood pressure monitored closely because the pressor effects of the catecholamines are enhanced by BRETYLOL. Volume expansion with blood or plasma and correction of dehydration should be carried out where appropriate.

2. **Transient Hypertension and Increased Frequency of Arrhythmias**
   Due to the initial release of norepinephrine from adrenergic postganglionic nerve terminals by BRETYLOL, transient hypertension or increased frequency of pre-

Continued on next page

Du Pont Pharm.—Cont.

mature ventricular contractions and other arrhythmias may occur in some patients.

3. **Caution During Use with Digitalis Glycosides**
The initial release of norepinephrine caused by BRETY-LOL may aggravate digitalis toxicity. When a life-threatening cardiac arrhythmia occurs in a digitalized patient, BRETYLOL should be used only if the etiology of the arrhythmia does not appear to be digitalis toxicity and other antiarrhythmic drugs are not effective. Simultaneous initiation of therapy with digitalis glycosides and BRETYLOL (bretylium tosylate) should be avoided.

4. **Patients with Fixed Cardiac Output**
In patients with fixed cardiac output (i.e., severe aortic stenosis or severe pulmonary hypertension) BRETY-LOL should be avoided since severe hypotension may result from a fall in peripheral resistance without a compensatory increase in cardiac output. If survival is threatened by the arrhythmia, BRETYLOL may be used but vasoconstrictive catecholamines should be given promptly if severe hypotension occurs.

PRECAUTIONS
General
1. **Dilution for Intravenous Use**
BRETYLOL should be diluted (one part BRETYLOL with four parts of Dextrose Injection, USP or Sodium Chloride Injection, USP) prior to intravenous use. Rapid intravenous administration may cause severe nausea and vomiting. Therefore, the diluted solution should be infused over a period greater than 8 minutes. In treating existing ventricular fibrillation BRETYLOL should be given as rapidly as possible and may be given without dilution.

2. **Use Various Sites for Intramuscular Injection**
When injected intramuscularly, not more than 5 mL should be given in a site, and injection sites should be varied since repeated intramuscular injection into the same site may cause atrophy and necrosis of muscle tissue, fibrosis, vascular degeneration and inflammatory changes.

3. **Reduce Dosage in Impaired Renal Function**
Since BRETYLOL is excreted principally via the kidney, the dosage interval should be increased in patients with impaired renal function. See 'Clinical Pharmacology' section for information on the effect of reduced renal function on half-life.

Drug Interactions
1. Digitalis toxicity may be aggravated by the initial release of norepinephrine caused by BRETYLOL.
2. The pressor effects of catecholamines such as dopamine or norepinephrine are enhanced by BRETYLOL. When catecholamines are administered, dilute solutions should be used and blood pressure should be monitored closely. (See Warnings.)
3. Although there is little published information on concomitant administration of lidocaine and BRETYLOL, these drugs are often administered concurrently without any evidence of interactions resulting in adverse effects or diminished efficacy.

Carcinogenesis, Mutagenesis, Impairment of Fertility
No data are available on potential for carcinogenicity, mutagenicity or impairment of fertility in animals or humans.

Pregnancy Category C
Animal reproduction studies have not been conducted with bretylium tosylate. It is also not known whether bretylium tosylate can cause harm when administered to a pregnant woman or can affect reproduction capacity. Bretylium tosy-late should be given to pregnant women only if clearly needed.

Pediatric Use
The safety and efficacy of this drug in children has not been established. BRETYLOL has been administered to a limited number of pediatric patients, but such use has been inadequate to define fully proper dosage and limitations for use.

ADVERSE REACTIONS
Hypotension and postural hypotension have been the most frequently reported adverse reactions (see Warnings section). Nausea and vomiting occurred in about three percent of patients, primarily when BRETYLOL was administered rapidly by the intravenous route (see Precautions section). Vertigo, dizziness, light-headedness and syncope, which sometimes accompanied postural hypotension, were reported in about 7 patients in 1000.

Bradycardia, increased frequency of premature ventricular contractions, transitory hypertension, initial increase in arrhythmias (see Warnings section), precipitation of anginal attacks, and sensation of substernal pressure have also been reported in a small number of patients, i.e., approximately 1–2 patients in 1000.

Renal dysfunction, diarrhea, abdominal pain, hiccups, erythematous macular rash, flushing, hyperthermia, confusion, paranoid psychosis, emotional lability, lethargy, generalized tenderness, anxiety, shortness of breath, diaphoresis, nasal stuffiness and mild conjunctivitis, have been reported in about 1 patient in 1000. The relationship of BRETYLOL administration to these reactions has not been clearly established.

OVERDOSAGE
In the presence of life threatening arrhythmias, underdosing with BRETYLOL probably presents a greater risk to the patient than potential overdosage. However, one case of accidental overdose has been reported in which a rapidly injected intravenous bolus of 30 mg/kg was given instead of an intended 10 mg/kg dose during an episode of ventricular tachycardia. Marked hypertension resulted, followed by protracted refractory hypotension. The patient expired 18 hours later in asystole, complicated by renal failure and aspiration pneumonitis. Bretylium serum levels were 8,000 ng/mL.

The exaggerated hemodynamic response was attributed to the rapid injection of a very large dose while some effective circulation was still present. Neither the total dose nor the serum levels observed in this patient are in themselves associated with toxicity. Total doses of 30 mg/kg are not unusual and do not cause toxicity when given incrementally during cardio-pulmonary resuscitation procedures. Similarly, patients maintained on chronic BRETYLOL therapy have had documented serum levels of 12,000 ng/mL. These levels were achieved after sequential dosage increases over time with no apparent ill effects.

If BRETYLOL is overdosed and symptoms of toxicity develop, administration of nitroprusside or another short acting intravenous antihypertensive agent should be considered for the treatment of the hypertensive response. Long acting drugs that might potentiate the subsequent hypotensive effects of BRETYLOL should not be used. Hypotension should be treated with appropriate fluid therapy and pressor agents such as dopamine or norepinephrine. Dialysis is probably not useful in the treatment of BRETYLOL overdose.

DOSAGE AND ADMINISTRATION
BRETYLOL is to be used clinically only for treatment of life-threatening ventricular arrhythmias under constant electrocardiographic monitoring. The clinical use of BRETYLOL is for short-term use only. Patients should either be kept supine during the course of BRETYLOL therapy or be closely observed for postural hypotension. The optimal dose schedule for parenteral administration of BRETYLOL has not been determined. There is comparatively little experience with dosages greater than 40 mg/kg/day, although such doses have been used without apparent adverse effects. The following schedule is suggested.

A. **For immediately Life-threatening Ventricular Arrhythmias such as Ventricular Fibrillation or Hemodynamically Unstable Ventricular Tachycardia:**
Administer undiluted BRETYLOL at a dosage of 5 mg/kg of body weight by rapid intravenous injection. Other usual cardiopulmonary resuscitative procedures, including electrical cardioversion, should be employed prior to and following the injection in accordance with good medical practice. If ventricular fibrillation persists, the dosage may be increased to 10 mg/kg and repeated as necessary.

For continuous suppression, dilute BRETYLOL with Dextrose Injection, USP or Sodium Chloride Injection, USP using the table below and administer the diluted solution as a constant infusion of 1 to 2 mg BRETYLOL per minute. When administering BRETYLOL (or any potent medication) by continuous intravenous infusion, it is advisable to use a precision volume control device. An alternative maintenance schedule is to infuse the diluted solution at a dosage of 5 to 10 mg BRETYLOL per kg body weight, over a period greater than 8 minutes, every 6 hours. More rapid infusion may cause nausea and vomiting.

B. **Other Ventricular Arrhythmias:**
1. Intravenous Use: **BRETYLOL must be diluted as described above before intravenous use.**
Administer the diluted solution at a dosage of 5 to 10 mg BRETYLOL per kg of body weight by intravenous infusion over a period greater than 8 minutes. More rapid infusion may cause nausea and vomiting. Subsequent doses may be given at 1 to 2 hour intervals if the arrhythmia persists.
For maintenance therapy, the same dosage may be administered every 6 hours, or a constant infusion of 1 to 2 mg BRETYLOL per minute may be given.
[See table below left].
2. For intramuscular Injection: **Do not dilute BRETYLOL prior to intramuscular injection.** Inject 5 to 10 mg BRETYLOL per kg of body weight. Subsequent doses may be given at 1 to 2 hour intervals if the arrhythmia persists. Thereafter maintain the same dosage every 6 to 8 hours.
Intramuscular injection should not be made directly into or near a major nerve, and the site of injection should be varied on repeated injection.

As soon as possible, and when indicated, patients should be changed to an oral antiarrhythmic agent for maintenance therapy.

HOW SUPPLIED
NDC 0094-0012-10: 10 mL ampul containing 500 mg bretylium tosylate individually boxed in cartons of 20.

NDC 0094-0012-37: 10 mL prefilled syringe containing 500 mg bretylium tosylate packaged in cartons of 5.

NDC 0094-0012-71: 10 mL single use vial containing 500 mg bretylium tosylate individually boxed in cartons of 20.

NDC 0094-0012-79: 20 mL single use vial containing 1 g bretylium tosylate packaged in cartons of 20.

Caution: Federal (USA) law prohibits dispensing without prescription.

Du Pont Pharmaceuticals
E.I. du Pont de Neumours & Co.
Wilmington, Delaware 19898
January, 1989   A43106

Suggested BRETYLOL Admixture Dilutions and Administration Rates for Continuous Infusion Maintenance Therapy Arranged in Descending Order of Concentration

Amount of BRETYLOL	Volume of IV Fluid*	Final Volume	Final Conc. (mg/mL)	Dose mg/min	Microdrops per min	mL/hr
FOR FLUID RESTRICTED PATIENTS:						
500 mg (10 mL)	50 mL	60 mL	8.3	1.0	7	7
				1.5	11	11
				2.0	14	14
2 g (40 mL)	500 mL	540 mL	3.7	1.0	16	16
1 g (20 mL)	250 mL	270 mL	3.7	1.5	24	24
				2.0	32	32
1 g (20 mL)	500 mL	520 mL	1.9	1.0	32	32
500 mg (10 mL)	250 mL	260 mL	1.9	1.5	47	47
				2.0	63	63

*IV fluid may be either Dextrose Injection, USP or Sodium Chloride Injection, USP.

BREVIBLOC® INJECTION   ℞
[brě'vĭ-blok]
(esmolol hydrochloride)
10 mL Ampul—2.5 g

NOT FOR DIRECT INTRAVENOUS INJECTION. AMPUL MUST BE DILUTED PRIOR TO ITS INFUSION (SEE DOSAGE AND ADMINISTRATION SECTION).

10 mL Single Dose Vial - 100 mg

DESCRIPTION
BREVIBLOC® (esmolol HCl) is a beta$_1$ selective (cardioselective) adrenergic receptor blocking agent with a very short duration of action (elimination half-life is approximately 9 minutes). Esmolol HCl is:
(±)-Methyl p-[2-hydroxy-3-(isopropylamino) propoxy] hydrocinnamate hydrochloride and has the following structure:
[See Chemical Formula at top of next page].
Esmolol HCl has the emperical formula $C_{16}H_{26}NO_4Cl$ and a molecular weight of 331.8. It has one asymmetric center and exists as an enantiomeric pair.

Esmolol HCl is a white to off-white crystalline powder. It is a relatively hydrophilic compound which is very soluble in water and freely soluble in alcohol. Its partition coefficient (octanol/water) at pH 7.0 is 0.42 compared to 17.0 for propranolol.

BREVIBLOC® (esmolol HCl) INJECTION is a clear, colorless to light yellow, sterile, nonpyrogenic solution. 2.5 g, 10 mL Ampul - Each mL contains 250 mg esmolol HCl in 25% Propylene Glycol, USP, 25% Alcohol, USP and Water for Injection, USP; buffered with 17.0 mg Sodium Acetate, USP, and 0.00715 mL Glacial Acetic Acid, USP. Sodium hydroxide and/or hydrochloric acid added, as necessary, to adjust pH to 3.5-5.5.

100 mg, 10 mL Single Dose Vial - Each mL contains 10 mg esmolol HCl and Water for Injection, USP; buffered with 2.8 mg Sodium Acetate, USP, and 0.546 mg Glacial Acetic Acid, USP. Sodium hydroxide and/or hydrochloric acid added, as necessary, to adjust pH to 4.5-5.5.

CLINICAL PHARMACOLOGY

BREVIBLOC® (esmolol HCl) is a beta$_1$ selective (cardioselective) adrenergic receptor blocking agent with rapid onset, a very short duration of action, and no significant intrinsic sympathomimetic or membrane stabilizing activity at therapeutic dosages. Its elimination half-life after intravenous infusion is approximately 9 minutes. BREVIBLOC® inhibits the beta$_1$ receptors located chiefly in cardiac muscle, but this preferential effect is not absolute and at higher doses it begins to inhibit beta$_2$ receptors located chiefly in the bronchial and vascular musculature.

Pharmacokinetics and Metabolism

BREVIBLOC® (esmolol HCl) is rapidly metabolized by hydrolysis of the ester linkage, chiefly by the esterases in the cytosol of red blood cells and not by plasma cholinesterases or red cell membrane acetylcholinesterase. Total body clearance in man was found to be about 20 L/kg/hr, which is greater than cardiac output; thus the metabolism of BREVIBLOC® is not limited by the rate of blood flow to metabolizing tissues such as the liver or affected by hepatic or renal blood flow. BREVIBLOC® has a rapid distribution half-life of about 2 minutes and an elimination half-life of about 9 minutes.

Using an appropriate loading dose, steady-state blood levels of BREVIBLOC® for dosages from 50–300 mcg/kg/min are obtained within five minutes. (Steady-state is reached in about 30 minutes without the loading dose.) Steady-state blood levels of BREVIBLOC® increase linearly over this dosage range and elimination kinetics are dose-independent over this range. Steady-state blood levels are maintained during infusion but decrease rapidly after termination of the infusion. Because of its short half-life, blood levels of BREVIBLOC® can be rapidly altered by increasing or decreasing the infusion rate and rapidly eliminated by discontinuing the infusion.

Consistent with the high rate of blood-based metabolism of BREVIBLOC®, less than 2% of the drug is excreted unchanged in the urine. Within 24 hours of the end of infusion, approximately 73–88% of the dosage has been accounted for in the urine as the acid metabolite of BREVIBLOC®.

Metabolism of BREVIBLOC® results in the formation of the corresponding free acid and methanol. The acid metabolite has been shown in animals to have about 1/1500th the activity of esmolol and in normal volunteers its blood levels do not correspond to the level of beta blockade. The acid metabolite has an elimination half-life of about 3.7 hours and is excreted in the urine with a clearance approximately equivalent to the glomerular filtration rate. Excretion of the acid metabolite is significantly decreased in patients with renal disease, with the elimination half-life increased to about ten-fold that of normals, and plasma levels considerably elevated.

Methanol blood levels, monitored in subjects receiving BREVIBLOC® for up to 6 hours at 300 mcg/kg/min and 24 hours at 150 mcg/kg/min, approximated endogenous levels and were less than 2% of levels usually associated with methanol toxicity.

BREVIBLOC® has been shown to be 55% bound to human plasma protein, while the acid metabolite is only 10% bound.

Pharmacodynamics

Clinical pharmacology studies in normal volunteers have confirmed the beta blocking activity of BREVIBLOC® (esmolol HCl), showing reduction in heart rate at rest and during exercise, and attenuation of isoproterenol-induced increases in heart rate. Blood levels of BREVIBLOC® have been shown to correlate with extent of beta blockade. After termination of infusion, substantial recovery from beta blockade is observed in 10–20 minutes.

In human electrophysiology studies, BREVIBLOC® produced effects typical of a beta blocker: a decrease in the heart rate, increase in sinus cycle length, prolongation of the sinus node recovery time, prolongation of the AH interval during

normal sinus rhythm and during atrial pacing, and an increase in antegrade Wenckebach cycle length.

In patients undergoing radionuclide angiography, BREVIBLOC®, at dosages of 200 mcg/kg/min, produced reductions in heart rate, systolic blood pressure, rate pressure product, left and right ventricular ejection fraction and cardiac index at rest, which were similar in magnitude to those produced by intravenous propranolol (4 mg). During exercise, BREVIBLOC® produced reductions in heart rate, rate pressure product and cardiac index which were also similar to those produced by propranolol, but produced a significantly larger fall in systolic blood pressure. In patients undergoing cardiac catheterization, the maximum therapeutic dose of 300 mcg/kg/min of BREVIBLOC® produced similar effects, and, in addition, there were small, clinically insignificant, increases in the left ventricular end diastolic pressure and pulmonary capillary wedge pressure. At thirty minutes after the discontinuation of BREVIBLOC® infusion, all of the hemodynamic parameters had returned to pretreatment levels.

The relative cardioselectivity of BREVIBLOC® was demonstrated in 10 mildly asthmatic patients. Infusions of BREVIBLOC® (100, 200 and 300 mcg/kg/min) produced no significant increases in specific airway resistance compared to placebo. At 300 mcg/kg/min, BREVIBLOC® produced slightly enhanced bronchomotor sensitivity to dry air stimulus. These effects were not clinically significant, and BREVIBLOC® was well tolerated by all patients. Six of the patients also received intravenous propranolol, and at a dosage of 1 mg, two experienced significant, symptomatic bronchospasm requiring bronchodilator treatment. One other propranolol-treated patient also experienced dry air-induced bronchospasm. No adverse pulmonary effects were observed in patients with COPD who received therapeutic dosages of BREVIBLOC® for treatment of supraventricular tachycardia (51 patients) or in perioperative settings (32 patients).

Supraventricular Tachycardia

In two multicenter, randomized, double-blind, controlled comparisons of BREVIBLOC® (esmolol HCl) with placebo and propranolol, maintenance doses of 50 to 300 mcg/kg/min of BREVIBLOC® were found to be more effective than placebo and about as effective as propranolol, 3–6 mg given by bolus injections, in the treatment of supraventricular tachycardia, principally atrial fibrillation and atrial flutter. The majority of these patients developed their arrhythmias postoperatively. About 60–70% of the patients treated with BREVIBLOC® had a desired therapeutic effect (either a 20% reduction in heart rate, a decrease in heart rate to less than 100 bpm, or rarely conversion to NSR) and about 95% of those who responded did so at a dosage of 200 mcg/kg/min or less. The average effective dosage of BREVIBLOC® was approximately 100–115 mcg/kg/min in the two studies. Other multicenter baseline-controlled studies gave essentially similar results. In the comparison with propranolol, about 50% of patients in both the BREVIBLOC® and propanolol groups were on concomitant digoxin. Response rates were slightly higher with both beta blockers in the digoxin-treated patients.

In all studies significant decreases of blood pressure occurred in 20–50% of patients, identified either as adverse reaction reports by investigators, or by observation of systolic pressure less than 90 mmHg or diastolic pressure less than 50 mmHg. The hypotension was symptomatic (mainly diaphosesis or dizziness) in about 12% of patients, and therapy was discontinued in about 11% of patients, about half of whom were symptomatic. In comparison to propanolol, hypotension was about three times as frequent with BREVIBLOC®, 53% vs. 17%. The hypotension was rapidly reversible with decreased infusion rate or after discontinuation of therapy with BREVIBLOC®. For both BREVIBLOC® and propranolol, hypotension was reported less frequently in patients receiving concomitant digoxin.

INDICATIONS AND USAGE

Supraventricular Tachycardia

BREVIBLOC® (esmolol HCl) is indicated for the rapid control of ventricular rate in patients with atrial fibrillation or atrial flutter in perioperative, postoperative, or other emergent circumstances where short term control of ventricular rate with a short-acting agent is desirable. BREVIBLOC® is also indicated in noncompensatory sinus tachycardia where, in the physician's judgment, the rapid heart rate requires intervention. BREVIBLOC® is not intended for use in chronic settings where transfer to another agent is anticipated.

CONTRAINDICATIONS

BREVIBLOC® (esmolol HCl) is contraindicated in patients with sinus bradycardia, heart block greater than first degree, cardiogenic shock or overt heart failure (see Warnings).

WARNINGS

Hypotension: In clinical trials 20–50% of patients treated with BREVIBLOC® (esmolol HCl) have experienced hypotension, generally defined as systolic pressure less than 90 mmHg and/or diastolic pressure less than 50 mmHg. About 12% of the patients have been symptomatic (mainly diapho-

resis or dizziness). Hypotension can occur at any dose but is dose-related so that doses beyond 200 mcg/kg/min are not recommended. Patients should be closely monitored, especially if pretreatment blood pressure is low. Decrease of dose or termination of infusion reverses hypotension, usually within 30 minutes.

Cardiac Failure: Sympathetic stimulation is necessary in supporting circulatory function in congestive heart failure, and beta blockade carries the potential hazard of further depressing myocardial contractility and precipitating more severe failure. Continued depression of the myocardium with beta blocking agents over a period of time can, in some cases, lead to cardiac failure. At the first sign or symptom of impending cardiac failure, the dosage should be reduced or BREVIBLOC® should be withdrawn. Although this dosage adjustment or withdrawal may be sufficient because of the short elimination half-life of BREVIBLOC®, specific treatment may also be considered. (see Overdosage.)

Bronchospastic Diseases: PATIENTS WITH BRONCHOSPASTIC DISEASES SHOULD, IN GENERAL, NOT RECEIVE BETA BLOCKERS. Because of its relative beta$_1$ selectivity and titrability, BREVIBLOC® may be used with caution in patients with bronchospastic diseases. However, since beta$_1$ selectivity is not absolute, BREVIBLOC® should be carefully titrated to obtain the lowest possible effective dose. In the event of bronchospasm, the infusion should be terminated immediately; a beta$_2$ stimulating agent may be administered if conditions warrant but should be used with particular caution as patients already have rapid ventricular rates.

Diabetes Mellitus and Hypoglycemia: BREVIBLOC® should be used with caution in diabetic patients requiring a beta blocking agent. Beta blockers may mask tachycardia occurring with hypoglycemia, but other manifestations such as dizziness and sweating may not be significantly affected.

PRECAUTIONS

General

Infusion concentrations of 20 mg/mL were associated with more serious venous irritation, including thrombophlebitis, than concentrations of 10 mg/mL. Extravasation of 20 mg/mL may lead to a serious local reaction and possible skin necrosis. Concentrations greater than 10 mg/mL or infusion into small veins or through a butterfly catheter should be avoided.

Because the acid metabolite of BREVIBLOC® is primarily excreted unchanged by the kidney, BREVIBLOC® (esmolol HCl) should be administered with caution to patients with impaired renal function. The elimination half-life of the acid metabolite was prolonged ten-fold and the plasma level was considerably elevated in patients with end-stage renal disease.

Drug Interactions

Catecholamine-depleting drugs, e.g., reserpine, may have an additive effect when given with beta blocking agents. Patients treated concurrently with BREVIBLOC® and a catecholamine depletor should therefore be closely observed for evidence of hypotension or marked bradycardia, which may result in vertigo, syncope, or postural hypotension.

A study of interaction between BREVIBLOC® and warfarin showed that concomitant administration of BREVIBLOC® and warfarin does not alter warfarin plasma levels. BREVIBLOC® concentrations were equivocally higher when given with warfarin, but this is not likely to be clinically important.

When digoxin and BREVIBLOC® (esmolol HCl) were concomitantly administered intravenously to normal volunteers, there was a 10–20% increase in digoxin blood levels at some time points. Digoxin did not affect BREVIBLOC® pharmacokinetics. When intravenous morphine and BREVIBLOC® were concomitantly administered in normal subjects, no effect on morphine blood levels was seen, but BREVIBLOC® steady-state blood levels were increased by 46% in the presence of morphine. No other pharmacokinetic parameters were changed.

The effect of BREVIBLOC® on the duration of succinylcholine-induced neuromuscular blockade was studied in patients undergoing surgery. The onset of neuromuscular blockade by succinylcholine was unaffected by BREVIBLOC®, but the duration of neuromuscular blockade was prolonged from 5 minutes to 8 minutes.

Although the interactions observed in these studies do not appear to be of major clinical importance, BREVIBLOC® should be titrated with caution in patients being treated concurrently with digoxin, morphine, succinylcholine or warfarin.

Carcinogenesis, Mutagenesis, Impairment of Fertility

Because of its short term usage no carcinogenicity, mutagenicity or reproductive performance studies have been conducted with BREVIBLOC®.

Pregnancy Category C

Teratogenicity studies in rats at intravenous dosages of BREVIBLOC® up to 3000 mcg/kg/min (ten times the maximum human maintenance dosage) for 30 minutes daily produced no evidence of maternal toxicity, embryotoxicity or

Continued on next page

Du Pont Pharm.—Cont.

teratogenicity, while a dosage of 10,000 mcg/kg/min produced maternal toxicity and lethality. In rabbits, intravenous dosages up to 1000 mcg/kg/min for 30 minutes daily produced no evidence of maternal toxicity, embryotoxicity or teratogenicity, while 2500 mcg/kg/min produced minimal maternal toxicity and increased fetal resorptions.

There are no adequate and well controlled studies in pregnant women. BREVIBLOC® should be used during pregnancy only if the potential benefit justifies the potential risk to the fetus.

Nursing Mothers
It is not known whether BREVIBLOC® is excreted in human milk, however, caution should be exercised when BREVIBLOC® is administered to a nursing woman.

Pediatric Use
The safety and effectiveness of BREVIBLOC® in children have not been established.

ADVERSE REACTIONS

Supraventricular Tachycardia
The following adverse reaction rates are based on use of BREVIBLOC® (esmolol HCl) in almost 400 clinical trial patients with supraventricular tachycardia. In addition, over 600 patients have been exposed in clinical studies of other conditions. The most important adverse effect has been hypotension (see Warnings). Most adverse effects have been mild and transient.

Cardiovascular—Symptomatic hypotension (diaphoresis, dizziness) occurred in 12% of patients, and therapy was discontinued in 11%, about half of whom were symptomatic. Asymptomatic hypotension occurred in about 25% of patients. Hypotension resolved during BREVIBLOC® infusion in 63% of these patients and within 30 minutes after discontinuation of infusion in 80% of the remaining patients. Diaphoresis accompanied hypotension in 10% of patients. Peripheral ischemia occurred in approximately 1% of patients. Pallor, flushing, bradycardia (heart rate less than 50 beats per minute), chest pain, syncope, pulmonary edema and heart block have each been reported in less than 1% of patients. In two patients without supraventricular tachycardia but with serious coronary artery disease (post inferior myocardial infarction or unstable angina), severe bradycardia/sinus pause/asystole has developed, reversible in both cases with discontinuation of treatment.

Central Nervous System—Dizziness has occurred in 3% of patients; somnolence in 3%, confusion, headache, and agitation in about 2%, and fatigue in about 1% of patients. Paresthesia, asthenia, depression, abnormal thinking, anxiety, anorexia, lightheadedness and grand mal seizures were reported in less than 1% of patients.

Respiratory—Bronchospasm, wheezing, dyspnea, nasal congestion, rhonchi, and rales have each been reported in less than 1% of patients.

Gastrointestinal—Nausea was reported in 7% of patients. Vomiting has occurred in about 1% of patients. Dyspepsia, constipation, dry mouth, and abdominal discomfort have each occurred in less than 1% of patients. Taste perversion has also been reported.

Skin (Infusion Site)—Infusion site reactions including inflammation and induration were reported in about 8% of patients. Edema, erythema, skin discoloration, burning at the infusion site, thrombophlebitis, and local skin necrosis from extravasation have each occurred in less than 1% of patients.

Miscellaneous—Each of the following has been reported in less than 1% of patients: Urinary retention, speech disorder, abnormal vision, midscapular pain, rigors, and fever.

OVERDOSAGE

Acute Toxicity
A few cases of massive accidental overdosage of BREVIBLOC® (esmolol HCl) have occurred due to errors in dilution. These intravenous bolus doses of BREVIBLOC® of 5000–6250 mcg/kg over 1–2 minutes have produced hypotension, bradycardia, drowsiness and loss of consciousness. The effects have resolved within 10 minutes, in some cases with administration of a pressor agent.

Because of its approximately 9-minute elimination half-life, the first step in the management of toxicity should be to discontinue BREVIBLOC® infusion. Then, based on the observed clinical effects, the following general measures should also be considered:

Bradycardia: Intravenous administration of atropine or another anticholinergic drug.

Bronchospasm: Intravenous administration of a beta$_2$ stimulating agent and/or a theophylline derivative.

Cardiac Failure: Intravenous administration of a diuretic and/or digitalis glycoside. In shock resulting from inadequate cardiac contractility, intravenous administration of dopamine, dobutamine, isoproterenol, or amrinone may be considered.

Symptomatic Hypotension:
Intravenous administration of fluids and/or pressor agents.

DOSAGE AND ADMINISTRATION

2.5 g AMPUL
THE 2.5 g AMPUL IS NOT FOR DIRECT INTRAVENOUS INJECTION. THIS DOSAGE FORM IS A CONCENTRATED, POTENT DRUG WHICH MUST BE DILUTED PRIOR TO ITS INFUSION. BREVIBLOC® SHOULD NOT BE ADMIXED WITH SODIUM BICARBONATE. BREVIBLOC® SHOULD NOT BE MIXED WITH OTHER DRUGS PRIOR TO DILUTION IN A SUITABLE INTRAVENOUS FLUID. (See Compatibility Section below.)

Dilution: Aseptically prepare a 10 mg/mL infusion, by adding two 2.5 g ampuls to a 500 mL container, or one 2.5 g ampul to a 250 mL container, of a compatible intravenous solution listed below. (Remove overage prior to dilution as appropriate). This yields a final concentration of 10 mg/mL. The diluted solution is stable for at least 24 hours at room temperature. Note: Concentrations of BREVIBLOC® greater than 10 mg/mL are likely to produce irritation on continued infusion (see Precautions). BREVIBLOC® has, however, been well tolerated when administered via a central vein.

100 mg VIAL
This dosage form is prediluted to provide a ready-to-use 10 mg/mL concentration recommended for BREVIBLOC® intravenous administration. It may be used to administer the appropriate BREVIBLOC® loading dosage infusions by hand-held syringe while the maintenance infusion is being prepared.

Supraventricular Tachycardia
In the treatment of supraventricular tachycardia, responses to BREVIBLOC® usually (over 95%) occur within the range of 50 to 200 mcg/kg/min. The average effective dosage is approximately 100 mcg/kg/min although dosages as low as 25 mcg/kg/min have been adequate in some patients. Dosages as high as 300 mcg/kg/min have been used, but these provide little added effect and an increased rate of adverse effects, and are not recommended. Dosage of BREVIBLOC® in supraventricular tachycardia must be individualized by titration in which each step consists of a loading dosage followed by a maintenance dosage.

To initiate treatment of a patient with supraventricular tachycardia, administer a loading dosage infusion of 500 mcg/kg/min of BREVIBLOC® for one minute followed by a 4 min maintenance infusion of 50 mcg/kg/min. If an adequate therapeutic effect is not observed within five minutes, repeat the same loading dosage and follow with a maintenance infusion increased to 100 mcg/kg/min.

Continue titration procedure as above, repeating loading infusion (500 mcg/kg/min for 1 minute), increasing maintenance infusion by increments of 50 mcg/kg/min (for 4 minutes). As the desired heart rate or a safety end-point (e.g., lowered blood pressure) is approached, omit the loading infusion and reduce incremental dose in maintenance infusion from 50 mcg/kg/min to 25 mcg/kg/min or lower. Also, if desired, increase interval between titration steps from 5 to 10 minutes.

This specific dosage regimen has not been studied intraoperatively and, because of the time, required for titration, may not be optimal for intraoperative use.

Maintenance dosages above 200 mcg/kg/min have not been shown to have significantly increased benefits, and the safety of dosages above 300 mcg/kg/min has not been studied.

In the event of an adverse reaction, the dosage of BREVIBLOC® may be reduced or discontinued. If a local infusion site reaction develops, an alternative infusion site should be used and caution should be taken to prevent extravasation. The use of butterfly needles should be avoided.

Abrupt cessation of BREVIBLOC® in patients has not been reported to produce the withdrawal effects which may occur with abrupt withdrawal of beta blockers following chronic use in coronary artery disease (CAD) patients. However, caution should still be used in abruptly discontinuing infusions of BREVIBLOC® in CAD patients.

After achieving an adequate control of the heart rate and a stable clinical status in patients with supraventricular tachycardia, transition to alternative antiarrhythmic agents such as propranolol, digoxin, or verapamil, may be accomplished. A recommended guideline for such a transition is given below but the physician should carefully consider the labeling instructions for the alternative agent selected:

Alternative Agent	Dosage
Propranolol hydrochloride	10–20 mg q 4–6 h
Digoxin	0.125–0.5 mg q 6 h
	(p.o. or i.v.)
Verapamil	80 mg q 6 h

The dosage of BREVIBLOC® should be reduced as follows:
1. Thirty minutes following the first dose of the alternative agent, reduce the infusion rate of BREVIBLOC® by one-half (50%).
2. Following the second dose of the alternative agent, monitor the patient's response and if satisfactory control is maintained for the first hour, discontinue BREVIBLOC®.

The use of infusions of BREVIBLOC® up to 24 hours has been well documented; in addition, limited data from 24–48 hrs (N=48) indicate that BREVIBLOC® is well tolerated up to 48 hours.

Compatibility with Commonly Use Intravenous Fluids
BREVIBLOC® (esmolol HCl) INJECTION was tested for compatibility with ten commonly used intravenous fluids at a final concentration of 10 mg esmolol HCl per mL. BREVIBLOC® INJECTION was found to be compatible with the following solutions and was stable for at least 24 hours at controlled room temperature or under refrigeration:

- Dextrose (5) Injection, USP
- Dextrose (5%) in Lactated Ringer's Injection
- Dextrose (5%) in Ringer's Injection
- Dextrose (5%) and Sodium Chloride (0.45%) Injection, USP
- Dextrose (5%) and Sodium Chloride (0.9%) Injection, USP
- Lactated Ringer's Injection, USP
- Potassium Chloride (40 mEq/liter) in Dextrose (5%) Injection, USP
- Sodium Chloride (0.45%) Injection, USP
- Sodium Chloride (0.9%) Injection, USP

BREVIBLOC® INJECTION was NOT compatible with Sodium Bicarbonate (5%) Injection, USP.

Note: Parenteral drug products should be inspected visually for particulate matter and discoloration prior to administration, whenever solution and container permit.

HOW SUPPLIED
NDC 0094-0015-71, 100 mg - 10 mL vial, Box of 20
NDC 0094-0025-18, 2.5 g - 10 mL ampul, Box of 10
STORE AT CONTROLLED ROOM TEMPERATURE (59°–86°F, 15°–30°C). Freezing does not adversely affect the product, but exposure to elevated temperatures should be avoided.

Du Pont Pharmaceuticals
E. I. du Pont de Nemours & Co.
Wilmington, Delaware 19898
Date: April, 1989　　　　　　　　　　　　　　　　　A43107

CALCIPARINE®　　　　　　　　　　　　　　　　℞
[cal-ci'pŭ-rin]
(heparin calcium)
INJECTION

For Subcutaneous and IV Use

DESCRIPTION
Heparin is a heterogenous group of straight-chain anionic mucopolysaccharides, called glycosaminoglycans having anticoagulant properties. Although others may be present, the main sugars occurring in heparin are: (1) α-L-iduronic acid 2-sulfate, (2) 2-deoxy-2-sulfamino-α-D-glucose 6-sulfate, (3) β-D-glucuronic acid, (4) 2-acetamido-2-deoxy-α-D-glucose, and (5) α-L-iduronic acid. These sugars are present in decreasing amounts, usually in the order (2)> (1)> (4)> (3)> (5), and are joined by glycosidic linkages, forming polymers of varying sizes. Heparin is strongly acidic because of its content of covalently linked sulfate and carboxylic acid groups. In heparin calcium, the acidic protons of the sulfate units are replaced by calcium ions.

Structure of Heparin Calcium (representative subunits):

Calciparine (heparin calcium injection) is a sterile solution of heparin calcium derived from porcine intestinal mucosa, standardized for anticoagulant activity. It is to be administered by intravenous or deep subcutaneous routes. The potency is determined by a biological assay using a USP reference standard based on units of heparin activity per milligram. Each mL of Calciparine contains 25,000 USP heparin units in Water for Injection. Calcium hydroxide and/or hydrochloric acid may have been added during manufacture to adjust pH to approximately 7.

CLINICAL PHARMACOLOGY
Heparin inhibits reactions that lead to the clotting of blood and the formation of fibrin clots both in vitro and in vivo. Heparin acts at multiple sites in the normal coagulation system. Small amounts of heparin in combination with antithrombin III (heparin cofactor) can inhibit thrombosis by inactivating activated Factor X and inhibiting the conversion of prothrombin to thrombin. Once active thrombosis has developed, larger amounts of heparin can inhibit further coagulation by inactivating thrombin and preventing the

conversion of firbrinogen to fibrin. Heparin also prevents the formation of a stable fibrin clot by inhibiting the activation of the fibrin stabilizing factor.

Bleeding time is usually unaffected by heparin. Clotting time is prolonged by full therapeutic doses of heparin; in most cases, it is not measurably affected by low doses of heparin. Peak plasma levels of heparin are achieved 2–4 hours following subcutaneous administration, although there are considerable individual variations. Loglinear plots of heparin plasma concentrations with time for a wide range of dose levels are linear which suggests the absence of zero order processes. Liver and the reticulo-endothelial system are the site of biotransformation. The biphasic elimination curve, a rapidly declining alpha phase ($t_{1/2} = 10$ minutes) and after the age of 40 a slower beta phase, indicates uptake in organs. The absence of a relationship between anticoagulant half-life and concentration half-life may reflect factors such as protein binding of heparin.

Heparin does not have fibrinolytic activity; therefore, it will not lyse existing clots.

INDICATIONS AND USAGE

Calciparine is indicated for:
Anticoagulant therapy in prophylaxis and treatment of venous thrombosis and its extension;
In a low-dose regimen for prevention of postoperative deep venous thrombosis and pulmonary embolism in patients undergoing major abdomino-thoracic surgery or who for other reasons are at risk of developing thromboembolic disease (see DOSAGE AND ADMINISTRATION);
Prophylaxis and treatment of pulmonary embolism;
Atrial fibrillation with embolization;
Diagnosis and treatment of acute and chronic consumption coagulopathies (disseminated intravascular coagulation);
Prevention of clotting in arterial and heart surgery;
Prophylaxis and treatment of peripheral arterial embolism;
As an anticoagulant in blood transfusions, extracorporeal circulation, and dialysis procedures and in blood samples for laboratory purposes.

CONTRAINDICATIONS

Heparin calcium should not be used in patients:
With severe thrombocytopenia;
In whom suitable blood coagulation tests—e.g., the whole-blood clotting time, partial thromboplastin time, etc.—cannot be performed at appropriate intervals (this contraindication refers to full-dose heparin; there is usually no need to monitor coagulation parameters in patients receiving low-dose heparin);
With an uncontrollable active bleeding state (see WARNINGS), except when this is due to disseminated intravascular coagulation.

WARNINGS

Heparin is not intended for intramuscular use.
Hypersensitivity: Patients with documented hypersensitivity to heparin should be given the drug only in clearly life-threatening situations.
Hemorrhage: Hemorrhage can occur at virtually any site in patients receiving heparin. An unexplained fall in hematocrit, fall in blood pressure, or any other unexplained symptom should lead to serious consideration of a hemorrhagic event.

Heparin calcium should be used with extreme caution in disease states in which there is increased danger of hemorrhage. Some of the conditions in which increased danger of hemorrhage exists are:
Cardiovascular—Subacute bacterial endocarditis. Severe hypertension.
Surgical—During and immediately following (a) spinal tap or spinal anesthesia or (b) major surgery, especially involving the brain, spinal cord, or eye.
Hematologic—Conditions associated with increased bleeding tendencies, such as hemophilia, thrombocytopenia, and some vascular purpuras.
Gastrointestinal—Ulcerative lesions and continuous tube drainage of the stomach or small intestine.
Other—Menstruation, liver disease with impaired hemostasis.
Coagulation Testing: When Calciparine is administered in therapeutic amounts, its dosage should be regulated by frequent blood coagulation tests. If the coagulation test is unduly prolonged or if hemorrhage occurs, Calciparine should be discontinued promptly (see OVERDOSAGE).
Thrombocytopenia: Thrombocytopenia has been reported to occur in patients receiving heparin with a reported incidence of 0 to 30%. Mild thrombocytopenia (count greater than 100,000/mm³) may remain stable or reverse even if heparin is continued. However, thrombocytopenia of any degree should be monitored closely. If the count falls below 100,000/mm³ or if recurrent thrombosis develops (see White Clot Syndrome, PRECAUTIONS), Calciparine should be discontinued. If continued heparin therapy is essential, administration of heparin from a different organ source can be reinstituted with caution.

PRECAUTIONS

1. *General:*
a. White Clot Syndrome:
Rare patients on heparin may develop new thrombus formation in association with thrombocytopenia resulting from irreversible aggregation of platelets induced by heparin, the so-called "white clot syndrome." The process may lead to severe thromboembolic complications like skin necrosis, gangrene of the extremities, myocardial infarction, pulmonary embolism, and stroke. Therefore, heparin administration should be promptly discontinued if a patient develops new thrombosis in association with thrombocytopenia.
b. Heparin Resistance:
Increased resistance to heparin is frequently encountered in fever, thrombosis, thrombophlebitis, infections with thrombosing tendencies, myocardial infarction, cancer and in postsurgical patients.
c. Increased Risk in Older Women:
A higher incidence of bleeding has been reported in women over 60 years of age.
2. *Laboratory Tests:*
Periodic platelet counts, hematocrits, and tests for occult blood in stool are recommended during the entire course of heparin therapy, regardless of the route of administration (see DOSAGE AND ADMINISTRATION).
3. *Drug Interactions:*
Oral anticoagulants: Calciparine may prolong the one-stage prothrombin time. Therefore, when Calciparine is given with dicumarol or warfarin sodium, a period of at least 5 hours after the last intravenous dose or 24 hours after the last subcutaneous dose should elapse before blood is drawn if a valid prothrombin time is to be obtained.
Platelet Inhibitors: Coadministration of drugs which interfere with platelet aggregation (the main hemostatic defense of heparinized patients) result in an additive or synergistic pharmacologic activity and can result in an increased risk of bleeding. They should be used with caution in patients receiving heparin calcium; these include:
Penicillins: High doses of parenteral penicillins should be avoided during coadministration of heparin.
Cephalosporins, especially those that possess methylthiotetrazole side chain (moxolactam, cefamandole, cefotetan and cefoperazone).
Salicylates, non-steroidal anti-inflammatory drugs, dextran and both ionic and non-ionic contrast media agents.
Other interactions: Patients receiving intravenous nitroglycerin require higher doses of heparin for effective anticoagulation. On stopping nitroglycerin therapy, the partial thromboplastin time (PTT) can rise markedly, unless the heparin dosage is decreased. Close monitoring of the PTT is required to maintain adequate anticoagulant effect whenever these drugs are used in combination and to avoid excessive bleeding when therapy with nitroglycerin is terminated or the dosage decreased.
Antibiotics: Interactions between heparin and streptomycin, neomycin, polymxin B and M, gentamicin, erythromycin and tetracyclines can result in the loss of antimicrobial activity of the antibiotic, loss of anticoagulant effect of heparin or both.
Phenothiazines, ascorbic acid, nicotine, antihistamines and digitaloids antagonize the antithrombotic activity of heparin.
4. *Drug/Laboratory Tests Interactions:*
Hyperaminotransferasemia:
Significant elevations of aminotransferase (SGOT [S-AST] and SGPT [S-ALT]) levels have occurred in a high percentage of patients (and healthy subjects) who have received heparin. Since aminotransferase determinations are important in the differential diagnosis of myocardial infarction, liver disease, and pulmonary emboli, rises that might be caused by drugs (like heparin) should be interpreted with caution.
5. *Carcinogenesis, Mutagenesis, Impairment of Fertility:*
No long-term studies in animals have been performed to evaluate carcinogenic potential of heparin. Also, no reproduction studies in animals have been performed concerning mutagenesis or impairment of fertility.
6. *Pregnancy:*
Teratogenic Effects: Pregnancy Category C. Animal reproduction studies have not been conducted with heparin calcium. It is also not known whether heparin calcium can cause fetal harm when administered to a pregnant woman or can affect reproduction capacity. Calciparine should be given to a pregnant woman only if clearly needed.
Nonteratogenic Effects: Heparin does not cross the placental barrier.
7. *Nursing Mothers:*
Heparin is not excreted in human milk.
8. *Pediatric Use:*
See DOSAGE AND ADMINISTRATION.

ADVERSE REACTIONS

1. Hemorrhage.
Hemorrhage from any tissue or organ is the chief complication that may result from heparin therapy (see WARNINGS). The signs and symptoms will vary according to the location and extent of bleeding and may present as paralysis, headache, chest, abdomen, joint or other pain, shortness of breath, difficult breathing or swallowing, unexplained swelling or unexplained shock. An overly prolonged clotting time or minor bleeding during therapy can usually be controlled by withdrawing the drug (see OVERDOSAGE). *It should be appreciated that gastrointestinal or urinary tract bleeding during anticoagulant therapy may indicate the presence of an underlying occult lesion.* Bleeding can occur at any site but certain specific hemorrhagic complications may be difficult to detect:
a. Adrenal hemorrhage, with resultant acute adrenal insufficiency, has occurred during anticoagulant therapy. Therefore, such treatment should be discontinued in patients who develop signs and symptoms of acute adrenal hemorrhage and insufficiency. Intiation of corrective therapy should not depend on laboratory confirmation of the diagnosis, since any delay in an acute situation may result in the patient's death.
b. Ovarian (corpus luteum) hemorrhage developed in a number of women of reproductive age receiving short- or long-term anticoagulant therapy. This complication if unrecognized may be fatal.
c. Retroperitoneal hemorrhage.
2. Local Irritation.
Local irritation, erythema, mild pain, hematoma or ulceration may follow deep subcutaneous (intrafat) injection of heparin calcium. These complications are much more common after intramuscular use, and such use is not recommended.
3. Hypersensitivity.
Generalized hypersensitivity reactions have been reported, with chills, fever, and urticaria as the most usual manifestations, and asthma, rhinitis, lacrimation, headache, nausea and vomiting, and anaphylactoid reactions, including shock, occurring more rarely. Itching and burning, especially on the plantar site of the feet, may occur.
Thrombocytopenia has been reported to occur in patients receiving heparin with a reported incidence of 0–30%. While often mild and of no obvious clinical significance, such thrombocytopenia can be accompanied by severe thromboembolic complications such as skin necrosis, gangrene of the extremities, myocardial infarction, pulmonary embolism, and stroke. (See WARNINGS, PRECAUTIONS).
Certain episodes of painful, ischemic, and cyanosed limbs have in the past been attributed to allergic vasopastic reactions. Whether these are in fact identical to the thrombocytopenia associated complications remains to be determined.
4. Miscellaneous
Osteoporosis following long-term administration of high-doses of heparin, cutaneous necrosis after systemic administration, suppression of aldosterone synthesis, delayed transient alopecia, priapism, and rebound hyperlipemia on discontinuation of heparin calcium have also been reported.
Significant elevations of aminotransferase (SGOT [S-AST] and SGPT [S-ALT]) levels have occurred in a high percentage of patients (and healthy subjects) who have received heparin.

OVERDOSAGE

Symptoms: Bleeding is the chief sign of heparin overdosage. Nosebleeds, blood in urine or tarry stools may be noted as the first sign of bleeding. Easy bruising or petechial formations may precede frank bleeding.
Treatment: Neutralization of heparin effect:
When clinical circumstances (bleeding) require reversal of heparinization, protamine sulfate (1% solution) by slow infusion will neutralize heparin calcium. *No more than 50 mg should be administered, very slowly, in any 10 minute period.* Each mg of protamine sulfate neutralizes approximately 100 USP heparin units. The amount of protamine required decreases over time as heparin is metabolized. Although the metabolism of heparin is complex, it may, for the purpose of choosing a protamine dose, be assumed to have a half-life of about ½ hour after intravenous injection.
Administration of protamine sulfate can cause severe hypotensive and anaphylactoid reactions. Because fatal reactions often resembling anaphylaxis have been reported, the drug should be given only when resuscitation techniques and treatment of anaphylactoid shock are readily available. For additional information the labeling of Protamine Sulfate Injection, USP products should be consulted.

DOSAGE AND ADMINISTRATION

Parenteral drug products should be inspected visually for particulate matter and discoloration prior to administration, whenever solution and container permit. Slight discoloration does not alter potency.
When heparin is added to an infusion solution for continuous intravenous administration, the container should be inverted at least six times to insure adequate mixing and prevent pooling of the heparin in the solution.

Continued on next page

Du Pont Pharm.—Cont.

Calciparine (heparin calcium) is not effective by oral administration and should be given by intermittent intravenous injection, intravenous infusion, or deep subcutaneous (intrafat, i.e., above the iliac crest or abdominal fat layer) injection. *The intramuscular route of administration should be avoided because of the frequent occurrence of hematoma at the injection site.*

The dosage of Calciparine should be adjusted according to the patient's coagulation test results. When heparin is given by continuous intravenous infusion, the coagulation time should be determined approximately every 4 hours in the early stages of treatment. When the drug is administered intermittently by intravenous injection, coagulation tests should be performed before each injection during the early stages of treatment and at appropriate intervals thereafter. Dosage is considered adequate when the activated partial thromboplastin time (APTT) is 1.5 to 2 times normal or when the whole blood clotting time is elevated approximately 2.5 to 3 times the control value. After deep subcutaneous (intrafat) injections, tests for adequacy of dosage are best performed on samples drawn 4–6 hours after the injections. Periodic platelet counts, hematocrits, and tests for occult blood in stool are recommended during the entire course of heparin therapy, regardless of the route of administration.

Converting to Oral Anticoagulant: When an oral anticoagulant of the coumarin or similar type is to be begun in patients already receiving Calciparine, baseline and subsequent tests of prothrombin activity must be determined at a time when heparin activity is too low to affect the prothrombin time. This is about 5 hours after the last I.V. bolus and 24 hours after the last subcutaneous dose. If continuous I.V. heparin infusion is used, prothrombin time can usually be measured at any time.

In converting from Calciparine to an oral anticoagulant, the dose of the oral anticoagulant should be the usual initial amount and thereafter prothrombin time should be determined at the usual intervals. To ensure continuous anticoagulation, it is advisable to continue full Calciparine therapy for several days after the prothrombin time has reached the therapeutic range. Calciparine therapy may then be discontinued without tapering.

Therapeutic Anticoagulant Effect
with Full-Dose Calciparine

Although dosage must be adjusted for the individual patient according to the results of suitable laboratory tests, the following dosage schedules may be used as guidelines:

[See table below]

Pediatric Use Follow recommendations of appropriate pediatric reference texts. In general, the following dosage schedule may be used as a guideline:

   Initial Dose: 50 units/kg (I.V. drip)
   Maintenance Dose: 100 units/kg (I.V. drip) every four hours, or 20,000 units/M²/24 hours continuously

Surgery of the Heart and Blood Vessels Patients undergoing total body perfusion for open-heart surgery should receive an initial dose of not less than 150 units of heparin calcium per kilogram of body weight. Frequently, a dose of 300 units per kilogram is used for procedures estimated to last less than 60 minutes or 400 units per kilogram for those estimated to last longer than 60 minutes.

Low-Dose Prophylaxis of Postoperative Thromboembolism: A number of well-controlled clinical trials have demonstrated that low-dose heparin prophylaxis, given just prior to and after surgery, will reduce the incidence of postoperative deep vein thrombosis in the legs (as measured by the I–125 fibrinogen technique and venography) and of clinical pulmonary embolism. The most widely used dosage has been 5,000 units 2 hours before surgery and 5,000 units every 8 to 12

hours thereafter for 7 days or until the patient is fully ambulatory, whichever is longer. The heparin is given by deep subcutaneous (intrafat, i.e., above the iliac crest or abdominal fat layer) injection with a fine (25 to 26 gauge) needle to minimize tissue trauma. A concentrated solution of Calciparine (heparin calcium) is recommended. Such prophylaxis should be reserved for patients over the age of 40 who are undergoing major surgery. Patients with bleeding disorders and those having brain or spinal cord surgery, spinal anesthesia, eye surgery, or potentially sanguineous operations should be excluded, as should patients receiving oral anticoagulants or platelet-active drugs (see WARNINGS). The value of such prophylaxis in hip surgery has not been established. The possibility of increased bleeding during surgery or postoperatively should be borne in mind. If such bleeding occurs, discontinuance of Calciparine and neutralization with protamine sulfate are advisable. If clinical evidence of thromboembolism develops despite low-dose prophylaxis, full therapeutic doses of anticoagulants should be given unless contraindicated. Prior to initiating heparinization, the physician should rule out bleeding disorders by appropriate history and laboratory tests, and appropriate coagulation tests should be repeated just prior to surgery. Coagulation tests values should be normal or only slightly elevated at these times.

Extracorporeal Dialysis Follow equipment manufacturers' operating directions carefully.

Blood Transfusion: Addition of 400 to 600 USP units per 100 mL of whole blood is usually employed to prevent coagulation. Usually, 7,500 USP units of heparin calcium are added to 100 mL of 0.9% Sodium Chloride Injection, USP (or 75,000 USP units per 1,000 mL of 0.9% Sodium Chloride Injection, USP) and mixed; from this sterile solution, 6 to 8 mL are added per 100 mL of whole blood.

Laboratory Samples: Addition of 70 to 150 units of heparin calcium per 10 to 20 mL sample of whole blood is usually employed to prevent coagulation of the sample. Leukocyte counts should be performed on heparinized blood within 2 hours after addition of the Calciparine. Heparinized blood should not be used for isoagglutinin, complement, or erythrocyte fragility tests or platelet counts.

Clearing Intermittent Infusion (Heparin Lock) Sets: To prevent clot formation in a heparin lock set following its proper insertion, dilute heparin solution (Heparin Lock Flush Solution, USP) is injected via the injection hub in a quantity sufficient to fill the entire set to the needle tip. This solution should be replaced each time the heparin lock is used. Aspirate before administering any solution via the lock in order to confirm patency and location of needle or catherter tip. If the drug to be administered is incompatible with heparin, the entire heparin lock set should be flushed with sterile water or normal saline before and after the medication is administered; following the second flush, the dilute heparin solution may be reinstilled into the set. The set manufacturer's instructions should be consulted for specifics concerning the heparin lock set in use at a given time.

NOTE: Since repeated injections of small doses of heparin can alter tests for activated partial thromboplastin time (APTT), a baseline value for APTT should be obtained prior to insertion of a heparin lock set.

HOW SUPPLIED

Calciparine (heparin calcium injection) is available as follows:

Calciparine 5,000 USP heparin units, 0.2 mL pre-filled disposable syringe, carton of 10, NDC 0094-0030-02.

Calciparine 12,500 USP heparin units, 0.5 mL ampule with sterile syringe and attached needle, carton of 10, NDC 0094-0030-05.

Calciparine 20,000 USP heparin units, 0.8 mL ampule with sterile syringe and attached needle, carton of 10, NDC 0094-0030-08.

Distributed by
Du Pont Pharmaceuticals
E. I. du Pont de Neumours & Co.
Wilmington, Delaware 19898
Under license from Choay Laboratories Inc.
New York, NY
April, 1989   A43159

COUMADIN®   ℞
[ku 'ma-din]
(Crystalline Warfarin Sodium, U.S.P.)
TABLETS

DESCRIPTION

COUMADIN® (crystalline warfarin sodium), a vitamin K dependent factor anticoagulant, is chemically crystalline sodium warfarin isopropanol clathrate. The crystallization of warfarin sodium virtually eliminates trace impurities present in amorphous warfarin sodium, thus achieving a crystalline product of the highest purity. Warfarin is the coined generic name for 3-(α-Acetonylbenzyl)-4-hydroxycoumarin. Its empirical formula is $C_{19}H_{15}NaO_4$ and its structural formula may be represented by the following:

Warfarin sodium crystalline occurs as a white, odorless, crystalline powder, is discolored by light and is very soluble in water; freely soluble in alcohol; very slightly soluble in chloroform and in ether.

COUMADIN Tablets for oral use also contain:

All strengths:	Lactose, starch and other ingredients
2 mg:	FD&C Blue 2 and FD&C Red 40
2½ mg:	FD&C Blue 1 and D&C Yellow 10
5 mg:	FD&C Red 3 and FD&C Yellow 6
7½ mg:	D&C Yellow 10 and FD&C Yellow 6
10 mg:	Dye Free

CLINICAL PHARMACOLOGY

COUMADIN and other coumarin anticoagulants act by inhibiting the synthesis of vitamin K dependent coagulation factors. The resultant **in vivo** effect is a sequential depression of Factors VII, IX, X and II. The degree of depression is dependent upon the dosage administered. Anticoagulants have no direct effect on an established thrombus, nor do they reverse ischemic tissue damage. However, once a thrombosis has occurred, anticoagulant treatment aims to prevent further extension of the formed clot and prevents secondary thromboembolic complications which may result in serious and possible fatal sequelae.

After oral administration, absorption is essentially complete, and maximal plasma concentrations are reached in 1 to 9 hours. Approximately 97% is bound to albumin within the plasma. COUMADIN usually produces its anticoagulant effect in 36 to 72 hours, and its duration of action may persist for 4 to 5 days, thus producing a smooth, long lasting response curve. COUMADIN is metabolized by hepatic, microsomal enzymes to inactive metabolites that are excreted into the bile, reabsorbed and excreted into the urine.

INDICATIONS AND USAGE

COUMADIN is indicated for the prophylaxis and/or treatment of venous thrombosis and its extension, pulmonary embolism, atrial fibrillation with embolization, and as an adjunct in the prophylaxis of systemic embolism after myocardial infarction.

CONTRAINDICATIONS

Anticoagulation is contraindicated in any localized or general physical condition or personal circumstance in which the hazard of hemorrhage might be greater than the potential clinical benefits of anticoagulation, such as:

Pregnancy—COUMADIN is contraindicated in women who are or may become pregnant because the drug passes through the placental barrier and may cause fatal hemorrhage to the fetus in utero. Furthermore, there have been reports of birth malformations in children born to mothers who have been treated with warfarin during pregnancy. Women of childbearing potential who are candidates for anticoagulant therapy should be carefully evaluated and the indications critically reviewed with the patient. If the patient becomes pregnant while taking this drug, she should be apprised of the potential risks to the fetus, and the possibility of termination of the pregnancy should be discussed in light of those risks.

Hemorrhagic tendencies or blood dyscrasias.

Recent or contemplated surgery of: (1) central nervous system; (2) eye; (3) traumatic surgery resulting in large open surfaces.

Bleeding tendencies associated with active ulceration or overt bleeding of: (1) gastrointestinal, genitourinary or

METHOD OF ADMINISTRATION	FREQUENCY	RECOMMENDED DOSE*
Deep Subcuatneous (Intrafat) Injection A different site should be used for each injection to prevent the development of massive hematoma.	Initial Dose	5,000 units by I.V. injection, followed by 10,000–20,000 units of a concentrated solution, subcutaneously
	Every 8 hours or Every 12 hours	8,000–10,000 units of a concentrated solution 15,000–20,000 units of a concentrated solution
Intermittent Intravenous Injection	Initial dose	10,000 units, either undiluted or in 50–100 mL of 0.9% Sodium Chloride Injection, USP
	Every 4 to 6 Hours	5,000–10,000 units, either undiluted or in 50–100 mL of 0.9% Sodium Chloride Injection, USP
Continuous Intravenous Infusion	Initial Dose	5,000 units by I.V. Injection
	Continuous	20,000–40,000 units/24 hours in 1,000 mL of 0.9% Sodium Chloride Injection, USP (or in any compatible solution) for infusion

*Based on 150-lb. (68-kg) patient.

respiratory tracts; (2) cerebrovascular hemorrhage; (3) aneurysms–cerebral, dissecting aorta; (4) pericarditis and pericardial effusions; (5) bacterial endocarditis.

Threatened abortion, eclampsia and preeclampsia.

Inadequate laboratory facilities or unsupervised senility, alcoholism, psychosis; or lack of patient cooperation.

Spinal puncture and other diagnostic or therapeutic procedures with potential for uncontrollable bleeding.

Miscellaneous: major regional, lumbar block anesthesia and malignant hypertension.

WARNINGS

The most serious risks associated with anticoagulant therapy with sodium warfarin are hemorrhage in any tissue or organ and, less frequently, necrosis and/or gangrene of skin and other tissues. The risk of hemorrhage is related to the level of intensity and the duration of anticoagulant therapy. Hemorrhage and necrosis have in some cases been reported to result in death or permanent disability. Necrosis appears to be associated with local thrombosis and usually appears within a few days of the start of anticoagulant therapy. In severe cases of necrosis, treatment through debridement or amputation of the affected tissue, limb, breast or penis has been reported. Careful diagnosis is required to determine whether necrosis caused by an underlying disease. Warfarin therapy should be discontinued when warfarin is suspected to be the cause of developing necrosis and heparin therapy may be considered for anticoagulation. Although various treatments have been attempted, no treatment for necrosis has been considered uniformly effective. See below for information on predisposing conditions. These and other risks associated with anticoagulant therapy must be weighed against the risk of thrombosis or embolization in untreated cases.

COUMADIN is a potent drug with a half-life of $2\frac{1}{2}$ days; therefore its effects may become more pronounced as daily maintenance doses overlap. It cannot be emphasized too strongly that treatment of each patient is a highly individualized matter. Dosage should be controlled by periodic determinations of prothrombin time or other suitable coagulation tests. Determinations of whole blood clotting and bleeding times are not effective measures for control of therapy. Heparin prolongs the one-stage prothrombin time. When heparin and COUMADIN are administered concomitantly, refer to CONVERSION FROM HEPARIN THERAPY for recommendations.

Caution should be observed when COUMADIN is administered in any situation or in the presence of any predisposing condition where added risk of hemorrhage or necrosis is present.

Anticoagulation therapy with COUMADIN may enhance the release of atheroma plaque emboli, which may cause the Purple Toe Syndrome. These atheroma emboli may produce systemic complications. Discontinuing COUMADIN therapy is recommended. The condition has been reported to be reversible.

Administration of anticoagulants in the following conditions will be based upon clinical judgment in which the risks of anticoagulant therapy are weighed against the risk of thrombosis or embolization in untreated cases. The following may be associated with these increased risks:

Lactation—COUMADIN appears in the milk of nursing mothers in an inactive form. Infants nursed by COUMADIN treated mothers had no change in prothrombin times. Effects in premature infants have not been evaluated.

Severe to moderate hepatic or renal insufficiency.

Infectious diseases or disturbances of intestinal flora— sprue, antibiotic therapy.

Trauma which may result in internal bleeding.

Surgery or trauma resulting in large exposed raw surfaces.

Indwelling catheters.

Severe to moderate hypertension.

Known or suspected deficiency in protein C—This hereditary or acquired condition, which should be suspected if there is a history of recurrent episodes of thromboembolic disorders in the patient or in the family, has been associated with an increased risk of developing necrosis following warfarin administration. Tissue necrosis may occur in the absence of protein C deficiency. It has been reported that concurrent anticoagulation therapy with heparin for 5 to 7 days during initiation of therapy with COUMADIN may minimize the incidence of this reaction. Warfarin therapy should be discontinued when warfarin is suspected to be the cause of developing necrosis and heparin therapy may be considered for anticoagulation.

Miscellaneous: polycythemia vera, vasculitis, severe diabetes, severe allergic and anaphylactic disorders.

Patients with congestive heart failure may become more sensitive to COUMADIN, thereby requiring more frequent laboratory monitoring, and reduced doses of COUMADIN. Concurrent use of anticoagulants with streptokinase or urokinase is not recommended and may be hazardous. (Please note recommendations accompanying these preparations.)

PRECAUTIONS

Periodic determination of prothrombin time or other suitable coagulation test is essential.

Numerous factors, alone or in combination, including travel, changes in diet, environment, physical state and medication may influence response of the patient to anticoagulants. It is generally good practice to monitor the patient's response with additional prothrombin time determinations in the period immediately after discharge from the hospital, and whenever other medications are initiated, discontinued or taken haphazardly. The following factors are listed for your reference; however, other factors may also affect the anticoagulant response.

The following factors, alone or in combination, may be responsible for INCREASED PT response.

ENDOGENOUS FACTORS:

cancer	hepatic disorders–
collagen disease	infectious hepatitis
congestive heart failure	jaundice
diarrhea	hyperthyroidism
elevated temperature	poor nutritional state
	steatorrhea
	vitamin K deficiency

EXOGENOUS FACTORS:

alcohol†	ibuprofen
allopurinol	indomethacin
aminosalicylic acid	influenza virus vaccine
amiodarone HCl	mefenamic acid
anabolic steroids	methyldopa
anesthetics, inhalation	methylphenidate
antibiotics	metronidazole
bromelains	miconazole
chloral hydrate†	monoamine oxidase inhibitors
chlorpropamide	nalidixic acid
chymotrypsin	naproxen
cimetidine	narcotics, prolonged
clofibrate	pentoxifylline
COUMADIN overdosage	phenylbutazone
dextran	phenytoin
dextrothyroxine	pyrazolones
diazoxide	quinidine
diflunisal	quinine
diuretics†	ranitidine†
disulfiram	salicylates
ethacrynic acid	sulfinpyrazone
fenoprofen	sulfonamides, long acting
glucagon	sulindac
hepatotoxic drugs	tamoxifen
	thyroid drugs
	tolbutamide
	trimethoprim/sulfamethoxazole

also: other medications affecting blood elements which may modify hemostasis
    dietary deficiencies
    prolonged hot weather
    unreliable prothrombin time determinations
†Increased and decreased prothrombin time responses have been reported.

The following factors, alone or in combination, may be responsible for DECREASED PT response:

ENDOGENOUS FACTORS:

edema
hereditary coumarin resistance
hyperlipemia
hypothyroidism

EXOGENOUS FACTORS:

adrenocortical steroids	ethchlorvynol
alcohol†	glutethimide
aminoglutethimide	griseofluvin
antacids	haloperidol
antihistamines	meprobamate
barbiturates	oral contraceptives
carbamazepine	paraldehyde
chloral hydrate†	primidone
chlordiazepoxide	ranitidine†
cholestyramine	rifampin
COUMADIN underdosage	trazadone
diuretics†	vitamin C

also: diet high in vitamin K
unreliable PT determinations
†Increased and decreased prothrombin time responses have been reported.

Because a patient may be exposed to a combination of the above factors, the net effect of COUMADIN on PT response may be unpredictable. More frequent PT monitoring is therefore advisable. Medications of unknown interaction with coumarins are best regarded with caution. When these medications are started or stopped, more frequent PT monitoring is advisable. Coumarins may also affect the action of other drugs. Hypoglycemic agents (chlorpropamide and tolbutamide) and anticonvulsants (phenytoin and phenobarbital) may accumulate in the body as a result of interference with either their metabolism or excretion.

Special Risk Patients: Caution should be observed when warfarin sodium is administered to certain patients such as the elderly or debilitated or when administered in any situation or physical condition where added risk of hemorrhage is present.

Information for Patients: The objective of anticoagulant therapy is to control the coagulation mechanism so that thrombosis is prevented, while avoiding spontaneous bleeding. Effective therapeutic levels with minimal complications are in part dependent upon cooperative and well-instructed patients who communicate effectively with their physician. Various COUMADIN patient educational guides are available to physicians on request. Patients should be advised: Strict adherence to prescribed dosage schedule is necessary. Do not take or discontinue any other medication, except on advice of physician. Avoid alcohol, salicylates (e.g. aspirin), large amounts of green leafy vegetables and/or drastic changes in dietary habits, which may affect COUMADIN therapy. COUMADIN may cause a red-orange discoloration of alkaline urine. The patient should notify the physician if any illness, such as diarrhea, infection or fever develops or if any unusual symptoms, such as pain, swelling or discomfort appear or if prolonged bleeding from cuts, increased menstrual flow or vaginal bleeding, nosebleeds or bleeding of gums from brushing, unusual bleeding or bruising, red or dark brown urine, red or tar black stools or diarrhea occurs.

Carcinogenesis, Mutagenesis, Impairment of Fertility: Carcinogenicity and mutagenicity studies have not been performed with COUMADIN. The reproductive effects of COUMADIN have not been evaluated.

Use in Pregnancy: Pregnancy Category X–"See CONTRAINDICATIONS."

Pediatric Use: Safety and effectiveness in children below the age of 18 have not been established.

ADVERSE REACTIONS

Potential adverse reactions to COUMADIN (crystalline warfain sodium) may include:

- Hemorrhage from any tissue or organ. This is a consequence of the anticoagulant effect. The signs and symptoms will vary according to the location and degree or extent of the bleeding. Hemorrhagic complications may present as paralysis; headache, chest, abdomen, joint or other pain; shortness of breath, difficult breathing or swallowing; unexplained swelling; or unexplained shock. Therefore, the possibility of hemorrhage should be considered in evaluating the condition of any anticoagulated patient with complaints which do not indicate an obvious diagnosis. Bleeding during anticoagulant therapy does not always correlate with prothrombin activity. (See OVERDOSAGE–Treatment.)

  Bleeding which occurs when the prothrombin time is within the therapeutic range warrants diagnostic investigation since it may unmask a previously unsuspected lesion, e.g. tumor, ulcer, etc.

- Necrosis of skin and other tissues. (See WARNINGS.)

- Other adverse reactions are infrequent and consist of alopecia, urticaria, dermatitis, fever, nausea, diarrhea, abdominal cramping, a syndrome called "purple toes", cholestatic hepatic injury, and hypersensitivity reactions.

- Priapism has been associated with anticoagulant administration, however, a causal relationship has not been established.

OVERDOSAGE

Signs and Symptoms: Suspected or overt abnormal bleeding (i.e., appearance of blood in stools or urine, hematuria, excessive menstrual bleeding, melena, petechiae, excessive bruising or persistent oozing from superficial injuries) are early manifestations of anticoagulation beyond a safe and satisfactory level.

Treatment: Excessive anticoagulation, with or without bleeding, may be controlled by discontinuing COUMADIN therapy and if necessary, by administration of oral or parenteral vitamin K_1. (Please see recommendations accompanying vitamin K_1 preparations prior to use.)

Such use of vitamin K_1 reduces response to subsequent COUMADIN therapy. Patients may return to a pretreatment thrombotic status following the rapid reversal of a prolonged PT. Resumption of COUMADIN administration reverses the effect of vitamin K, and a therapeutic PT can again be obtained by careful dosage adjustment. If rapid anticoagulation is indicated, heparin may be preferable for initial therapy.

If minor bleeding progresses to major bleeding, give 5 to 25 mg (rarely up to 50 mg) parenteral vitamin K_1. In emergency situations of severe hemorrhage, clotting factors can be returned to normal by administering 200 to 500 ml of fresh whole blood or fresh frozen plasma, or by giving commercial Factor IX complex. Purified Factor IX preparations should not be used because they cannot increase the levels of prothrombin, Factor VII and Factor X which are also depressed along with the levels of Factor IX as a result of COUMADIN treatment. Packed red blood cells may also be given if signifi-

Continued on next page

Du Pont Pharm.—Cont.

cant blood loss has occurred. Infusions of blood or plasma should be monitored carefully to avoid precipitating pulmonary edema in elderly patients or patients with heart disease.

DOSAGE AND LABORATORY CONTROL

ADMINISTRATION The administration and dosage of COUMADIN must be individualized for each patient according to the particular patient's sensitivity to the drug. The dosage should be adjusted based upon the results of the one stage prothrombin time (PT). Different thromboplastin reagents vary substantially in their responsiveness to sodium warfarin–induced effects on prothrombin time. To define the appropriate therapeutic regimen it is important to be familiar with the sensitivity of the thromboplastin reagent used in the laboratory and its relationship to the International Reference Preparation (IRP)*, a sensitive thromboplastin reagent prepared from human brain.

Early clinical studies of oral anticoagulants, which formed the basis for recommended therapeutic ranges of 1.5 to 2.5 times control PT, used sensitive human brain thromboplastin. When using the less sensitive rabbit brain thromboplastins commonly employed in PT assays today, adjustments must be made to the targeted PT range that reflect this decrease in sensitivity. Available clinical evidence indicates that prolongation of the prothrombin time 1.2 to 1.5 times control, when measuring with the less sensitive thromboplastin reagents, is sufficient for prophylaxis and treatment of venous thromboembolism and minimizes the risk of hemorrhage associated with more prolonged PT values. In cases where the risk of thromboembolism is great, such as in patients with recurrent systemic embolism, a PT of 1.5 to 2.0 times control should be maintained. A ratio of greater than 2.0 appears to provide no additional therapeutic benefit in most patients and is associated with a higher risk of bleeding.

The proceedings and recommendations of the 1986 National Conference on Antithrombotic Therapy[1-3] review and evaluate issues related to oral anticoagulant therapy and the sensitivity of thromboplastin reagents and provide additional guidelines for defining the appropriate therapeutic regimen. *A system of standardizing the prothrombin time in oral anticoagulant control was introduced by the World Health Organization in 1983. It is based upon the determination of an International Normalized Ratio (INR) which provides a common basis for communication of PT results and interpretations of therapeutic ranges. The INR is derived from calibrations of commercial thromboplastin reagents against a sensitive human brain thromboplastin, the International Reference Preparation (IRP). For the three commercial rabbit brain thromboplastins, currently used in North America, a PT ratio of 1.3 to 2.0 is equivalent to an INR of 2.0 to 4.0. For other thromboplastins, the INR can be calculated as:*

$$INR = (observed\ PT\ ratio)^{ISI}$$

where the ISI (International Sensitivity Index) is the calibration factor and is available from the manufacturers of the thromboplastin reagent.[4]

Initial Dosage COUMADIN therapy is commonly started above anticipated maintenance dosage levels. A commonly used regimen for COUMADIN is 10 mg/day for 2 to 4 days; with daily dosage adjustments based on the results of PT determinations. Use of a large loading dose (i.e., 30 mg) may increase the incidence of hemorrhagic and other complications, does not offer more rapid protection against thrombi formation, and is not recommended. Lower doses are recommended for elderly and/or debilitated patients and patients with increased sensitivity (see PRECAUTIONS section of this package insert).

Maintenance—Most patients are satisfactorily maintained at a dose of 2 to 10 mg daily. Flexibility of dosage is provided by breaking scored tablets in half. The individual dose and interval should be gauged by the patient's prothrombin response.

Duration of Therapy—The duration of therapy in each patient should be individualized. In general, anticoagulant therapy should be continued until the danger of thrombosis and embolism has passed.

LABORATORY CONTROL The prothrombin time (PT) reflects the depression of vitamin K dependent Factors VII, IX, X and II. There are several modifications of the one-stage PT and the physician should become familiar with the specific method used in his laboratory. The degree of anticoagulation indicated by any range of prothrombin times may be altered by the type of thromboplastin used; the appropriate therapeutic range must be based on the experience of each laboratory. The PT should be determined daily after the administration of the initial dose until PT results stabilize in the therapeutic range. Intervals between subsequent PT determinations should be based upon the physicians judgment of the patient's reliability and response to COUMADIN in order to maintain the individual within the therapeutic range. Acceptable intervals for PT determinations are normally within the range of one to four weeks. To ensure adequate

control, it is recommended that additional prothrombin time tests are done when other warfarin products are interchanged with COUMADIN.

TREATMENT DURING DENTISTRY AND SURGERY The management of patients who undergo dental and surgical procedures requires close liaison between attending physicians, surgeons and dentists. In patients who must be anticoagulated prior to, during, or immediately following dental or surgical procedures, adjusting the dosage of COUMADIN to maintain the PT at the low end of the therapeutic range, may safely allow for continued anticoagulation. The operative site should be sufficiently limited and accessible to permit the effective use of local procedures for hemostasis. Under these conditions, dental and surgical procedures may be performed without undue risk of hemorrhage.

CONVERSION FROM HEPARIN THERAPY Since the onset of the COUMADIN effect is delayed, heparin is preferred initially for rapid anticoagulation. Conversion to COUMADIN may begin concomitantly with heparin therapy or may be delayed 3 to 6 days. As heparin may affect the PT, patients receiving both heparin and COUMADIN should have blood for PT determination, drawn at least:

• 5 hours after the last IV bolus dose of heparin, or
• 4 hours after cessation of a continuous IV infusion of heparin, or
• 24 hours after the last subcutaneous heparin injection.

When COUMADIN has produced the desired therapeutic range or prothrombin activity, heparin may be discontinued. I.M. injections should be confined to the upper extremities which permits easy access for manual compression, inspections for bleeding and use of pressure bandages.

HOW SUPPLIED

Tablets: COUMADIN (crystalline warfarin sodium, USP). For oral use, single scored, imprinted numerically in bottles with potencies and colors as follows:

	100's	1000's
2 mg lavender	NDC 0056-0170-70	NDC 0056-0170-90
2½ mg green	NDC 0056-0176-70	NDC 0056-0176-90
5 mg peach	NDC 0056-0172-70	NDC 0056-0172-90
7½ mg yellow	NDC 0056-0173-70	
10 mg white	NDC 0056-0174-70	

Also available in Hospital Unit-Dose blister package of 100:

2 mg	NDC 0056-0170-75
2½ mg	NDC 0056-0176-75
5 mg	NDC 0056-0172-75
7½ mg	NDC 0056-0173-75
10 mg	NDC 0056-0174-75

COUMADIN oral tablet is available in 2, 2½, 5, 7½ and 10 mg of crystalline warfarin sodium with one face inscribed with the word COUMADIN, single scored and imprinted numerically with the 2, 2½, 5, 7½ and 10 superimposed, and on the other face inscribed with the Du Pont logo. Protect from light. Store in carton until contents have been used.

REFERENCES

1. Sackett, D.L.: Rules of Evidence and Clinical Recommendations on the Use of Antithrombotic Agents. Chest, ACCP-NHLBI National Conference on Antithrombotic Therapy, Vol. 89, No. 2, pp. 2s–3s, 1986.
2. Hirsh, J., Deykin, D., Poller, L.: "Therapeutical Range" for Oral Anticoagulant Therapy. Chest, ACCP-NHLBI National Conference on Antithrombolic Therapy,. Vol. 89, No. 2, pp. 11s–15s, 1986.
3. Hirsh, J.: Is the Dose of Warfarin Prescribed by American Physicians Unnessarily High? Arch Int Med, Vol. 147, pp. 769–771, 1987.
4. Poller, L.: Laboratory Control of Anticoagulant Therapy. Seminars in Thrombosis and Hemostasis, Vol. 12, No. 1, pp. 13–19, 1986.

COUMADIN® is a Registered U.S. Trademark of E.I. du Pont de Nemours & Co.

6136-12 April, 1989

Shown in Product Identification Section, page 409

HESPAN®   ℞

[hes′pan]
**(6% hetastarch in
0.9% sodium chloride injection)**

DESCRIPTION

HESPAN (6% hetastarch in 0.9% sodium chloride injection) is a sterile, nonpyrogenic solution. The composition of each 100 mL is as follows:

Hetastarch	6.0 g
Sodium Chloride, USP	0.9 g
Water for Injection, USP	qs

pH adjusted with Sodium Hydroxide
Concentration of Electrolytes (mEq/Liter): Sodium 154, Chloride 154
pH: Approx. 5.5
Hetastarch is an artifical colloid derived from a waxy starch composed almost entirely of amylopectin. Hydroxyethyl

ether groups are introduced into the glucose units of the starch and the resultant material is hydrolyzed to yield a product with a molecular weight suitable for use as a plasma volume expander and erythrocyte sedimenting agent. Hetastarch is characterized by its molar substitution, and also by its molecular weight. The molar substitution is 0.7 which means hetastarch has 7 hydroxyethyl groups for every 10 glucose units. The weight average molecular weight is approximately 480,000 with a range of 400,000 to 550,000 and with 80% of the polymers falling between the range of 30,000 and 2,400,000. Hydroxyethyl groups are attached by ether linkage primarily at C-2 of the glucose unit and to a lesser extent at C-3 and C-6. The polymerized glucose units are joined primarily by 1–4 linkages with occasional 1–6 branching linkages. The degree of branching is approximately 1:20 which means that there is one 1–6 branch for every 20 glucose monomer units.

The chemical name for hetastarch is hydroxyethyl starch. The structural formula is as follows:

Amylopectin derivative in which R_2, R_3, and R_6 are H or CH_2CH_2OH, or R_6 is a branching point in the starch polymer connected through a 1–6 linkage to additional α-D-glucopyranosyl units.

HESPAN is a clear, pale yellow to amber solution. Exposure to prolonged adverse storage conditions may result in a change to a turbid deep brown or the formation of a crystalline precipitate. Do not use the solution if these conditions are evident.

CLINICAL PHARMACOLOGY

The plasma volume expansion produced by HESPAN approximate those of 5% human albumin. Intravenous infusion of HESPAN results in expansion of plasma volume that decreases over the succeeding 24 to 36 hours. The degree of plasma volume expansion and improvement in hemodynamic state depend upon the patient's intravascular status. Hetastarch molecules below 50,000 molecular weight are rapidly eliminated by renal excretion. A single dose of approximately 500 mL of HESPAN (approximately 30 g) results in elimination in the urine of approximately 33% of the dose within 24 hours. This is a variable process but generally results in an intravascular hetastarch concentration of less than 10% of the total dose injected by two weeks. The hydroxyethyl group is not cleaved by the body, but remains intact and attached to glucose units when excreted. Significant quantities of glucose are not produced as hydroxyethylation prevents complete metabolism of the smaller polymers.

The addition of HESPAN to whole blood increases the erythrocyte sedimentation rate. Therefore, HESPAN is used to improve the efficiency of granulocyte collection by centrifugal means.

INDICATIONS AND USAGE

HESPAN is indicated in the treatment of hypovolemia when plasma volume expansion is desired. It is not a substitute for blood or plasma.

The adjunctive use of HESPAN in leukapheresis has also been shown to be safe and efficacious in improving the harvesting and increasing the yield of granulocytes by centrifugal means.

CONTRAINDICATIONS

HESPAN is contraindicated in patients with known hypersensitivity to hydroxyethyl starch, or with bleeding disorders, or with congestive heart failure where volume overload is a potential problem. HESPAN should not be used in renal disease with oliguria or anuria not related to hypovolemia.

WARNINGS

Usage in Plasma Volume Expansion
Large volumes may alter the coagulation mechanism. Thus, administration of HESPAN may result in transient prolongation of prothrombin, partial thromboplastin and clotting times. With administration of large doses, the physician should also be alert to the possibility of transient prolongation of bleeding time.

Hematocrit may be decreased and plasma proteins diluted excessively by administration of large volumes of HESPAN. Administration of packed red cells, platelets, and fresh frozen plasma should be considered if excessive dilution occurs. Use over extended periods: HESPAN has not been adequately evaluated to establish its safety in situations other than leukapheresis that require frequent use of colloidal solutions over extended periods. Certain conditions may affect the safe use of HESPAN on a chronic basis. For example, in patients with subarachnoid hemorrhage where HESPAN is used repeatedly over a period of days for the prevention of cerebral vasospasm, significant clinical bleeding may occur.

Usage in Leukapheresis

Slight declines in platelet counts and hemoglobin levels have been observed in donors undergoing repeated leukapheresis procedures using HESPAN due to the volume expanding effects of HESPAN and to the collection of platelets and erythrocytes. Hemoglobin levels usually return to normal within 24 hours. Hemodilution by HESPAN and saline may also result in 24 hour declines of total protein, albumin, calcium and fibrinogen values. None of these decreases are to a degree recognized to be clinically significant risks to healthy donors.

PRECAUTIONS

General

Regular and frequent clinical evaluation and complete blood counts (CBC) are necessary for proper monitoring of HESPAN use during leukapheresis. If the frequency of leukapheresis is to exceed the guidelines for whole blood donation, you may wish to consider the following additional studies: total leukocyte and platelet counts, leukocyte differential count, hemoglobin and hematocrit, prothrombin time (PT), and partial thromboplastin time (PTT) tests.

The possibility of circulatory overload should be kept in mind. Caution should be used when the risk of pulmonary edema and/or congestive heart failure is increased. Special care should be exercised in patients who have impaired renal clearance since this is the principal way in which hetastarch is eliminated.

Indirect bilirubin levels of 8.3 mg/mL (normal 0.0–7.0 mg/mL) have been reported in 2 out of 20 normal subjects who received multiple HESPAN infusions. Total bilirubin was within normal limits at all times; indirect bilirubin returned to normal by 96 hours following the final infusion. The significance, if any, of these elevations is not known; however, caution should be observed before administering HESPAN to patients with a history of liver disease.

HESPAN has been reported to produce hypersensitivity reactions such as wheezing and urticaria. However, hetastarch has not been observed to stimulate antibody formation. If hypersensitivity effects occur, they are readily controlled by discontinuation of the drug and, if necessary, administration of an antihistaminic agent.

Elevated serum amylase levels may be observed temporarily following administration of HESPAN, although no association with pancreatitis has been demonstrated.

Carcinogenesis, mutagenesis, impairment of fertility.

Long-term studies of animals have not been performed to evaluate the carcinogenic potential of hetastarch.

Teratogenic Effects

Pregnancy Category C. Animal reproduction studies have not been conducted with HESPAN. It is also not known whether HESPAN can cause fetal harm when administered to a pregnant woman or can affect reproduction capacity. HESPAN should be given to a pregnant woman only if clearly needed.

Nursing Mothers

It is not known whether hetastarch is excreted in human milk. Because many drugs are excreted in human milk, caution should be exercised when HESPAN is administered to a nursing woman.

Pediatric Use

The safety and effectiveness of HESPAN in children have not been established.

ADVERSE REACTIONS

The following have been reported: vomiting, fever, chills, pruritus, submaxillary and parotid glandular enlargement, mild influenza-like symptoms, headaches, muscle pains, peripheral edema of the lower extremities, anaphylactoid reactions (periorbital edema, urticaria, wheezing) bleeding due to hemodilution (see Warnings), and circulatory overload and pulmonary edema (see Precautions).

DOSAGE AND ADMINISTRATION

Dosage for Acute Use in Plasma Volume Expansion

HESPAN is administered by intravenous infusion only. Total dosage and rate of infusion depend upon the amount of blood or plasma lost and the resultant hemoconcentration. In adults, the amount usually administered is 500 to 1000 mL. Doses of more than 1500 mL per day for the typical 70 kg patient (approximately 20 mL per kg of body weight) are usually not required, although higher doses have been reported in postoperative and trauma patients where severe blood loss has occurred.

Dosage in Leukapheresis

250 to 700 mL of HESPAN to which citrate anticoagulant has been added is typically administered by aseptic addition to the input line of the centrifugation apparatus at a ratio of 1:8 to 1:13 to venous whole blood. The HESPAN and citrate should be thoroughly mixed to assure effective anticoagulation of blood as it flows through the leukapheresis machine. Parenteral drug products should be inspected for particulate matter and discoloration prior to administration whenever solution and container permit.

The safety and compatibility of other additives have not been established.

HOW SUPPLIED

Exposure of pharmaceutical products to heat should be minimized. Avoid excessive heat. Protect from freezing. It is recommended that the product be stored at room temperature (25°C); however, brief exposure up to 40°C does not adversely affect the product.

HESPAN is supplied sterile and nonpyrogenic in 500 mL intravenous plastic infusion containers (NDC 0094-0037-44) and 500 mL intravenous glass bottles (NDC 0094-0037-05).

CAUTION

Federal (USA) law prohibits dispensing without prescription.

Directions for Use (Plastic Container)

Caution: Before administering to the patient, review these directions:

Visual Checking

1. Do not remove the plastic infusion container from its overwrap until immediately before use.
2. While the overwrap is intact, identify the solution (HESPAN), lot number, and expiration date.
3. Check that the solution is clear.
4. Inspect the intact unit for signs of obvious damage. If present, the unit should not be used.

Removal of Overwrap

To open overwrap, tear at any notch located at either end of unit. After removing overwrap, check for minute leaks by squeezing container firmly. If leaks are found, discard unit as sterility may be impaired.

Preparation for Administration (Use aseptic technique)

1. Close flow control clamp of administration set.
2. Twist off plug from port designated "Infusion Set Port."
3. Insert spike of infusion set into port with a twisting motion until the set is firmly seated.
4. Suspend container from hanger.
5. Follow manufacturer's recommended procedures for the administration set.
6. Discontinue administration and notify physician immediately if patient exhibits signs of adverse reactions.

Directions for Use (Glass Bottles)

Caution: Before administering to the patient, review these instructions:

1. Inspect each container before use. Read the label. Identify the solution (HESPAN), lot number and expiration date, and that label name agrees with the abbreviated name stamped on closure. Check the security of bail and band.
2. Invert container and carefully inspect the solution in good light for cloudiness, haze, or particulate matter; check the bottle for cracks or other damage. In checking for cracks, do not be confused by normal surface mold marks and seams on bottom and sides of bottle. These are not flaws. Look instead for bright reflections that have depth and penetrate into the wall of the bottle. Reject any such bottle.
3. Check for vacuum, first by confirming the presence of depressions in the latex disk and then by audible hiss when the disk is removed. Reject any container that does not meet these criteria.
4. Discontinue administration and notify physician immediately if patient exhibits signs of adverse reactions.

Distributed by
Du Pont Pharmaceuticals
E. I. du Pont de Nemours & Co.
Wilmington, Delaware 19898
Revised: April, 1989
A43095

HYCODAN®

[hī-kō-dan]

(hydrocodone bitartrate and homatropine methylbromide)
Tablets and Syrup

DESCRIPTION

HYCODAN contains hydrocodone (dihydrocodeinone) bitartrate, a semisynthetic centrally-acting narcotic antitussive. Homatropine methylbromide is included in a subtherapeutic amount to discourage deliberate overdosage.

Each HYCODAN tablet or teaspoonful (5 ml) contains:

Hydrocodone bitartrate, USP .... 5 mg
WARNING: May be habit forming.
Homatropine methylbromide, USP .... 1.5 mg

HYCODAN tablets also contain: calcium phosphate dibasic, colloidal silicon dioxide, lactose, magnesium stearate, starch and stearic acid.

HYCODAN syrup: caramel coloring, FD&C Red 40, liquid sugar, methylparaben, propylparaben, sorbitol solution and wild cherry imitation flavor.

The hydrocodone component is 4,5α-epoxy-3-methoxy-17-methylmorphinan-6-one tartrate (1:1) hydrate (2:5), a fine white crystal or crystalline powder, which is derived from the opium alkaloid, thebaine, has a molecular weight of

---

(494.50), and may be represented by the following structural formula:

$$C_{18}H_{21}NO_3 \cdot C_4H_6O_6 \cdot 2\,1/2H_2O$$
HYDROCODONE BITARTRATE

$$C_{17}H_{24}BrNO_3$$
HOMATROPINE METHYLBROMIDE

Homatropine methylbromide is 8-Azoniabicyclo [3.2.1]octane,3-[(hydroxyphenylacetyl)oxy]-8,8-dimethyl-, bromide, endo-; a white crystal or fine white crystalline powder, with a molecular weight of (370.29).

CLINICAL PHARMACOLOGY

Hydrocodone is a semisynthetic narcotic antitussive and analgesic with multiple actions qualitatively similar to those of codeine. The precise mechanism of action of hydrocodone and other opiates is not known; however, hydrocodone is believed to act directly on the cough center. In excessive doses, hydrocodone, like other opium derivatives, will depress respiration. The effects of hydrocodone in therapeutic doses on the cardiovascular system are insignificant. Hydrocodone can produce miosis, euphoria, physical and physiological dependence.

Following a 10 mg oral dose of hydrocodone administered to five adult male subjects, the mean peak concentration was 23.6 ± 5.2 ng/ml. Maximum serum levels were achieved at 1.3 ± 0.3 hours and the half-life was determined to be 3.8 ± 0.3 hours. Hydrocodone exhibits a complex pattern of metabolism including O-demethylation, N-demethylation and 6-keto reduction to the corresponding 6-α- and 6-β- hydroxy metabolites.

INDICATIONS AND USAGE

HYCODAN is indicated for the symptomatic relief of cough.

CONTRAINDICATIONS

HYCODAN should not be administered to patients who are hypersensitive to hydrocodone or homatropine methylbromide.

WARNINGS

May be habit forming. Hydrocodone can produce drug dependence of the morphine type and, therefore, has the potential for being abused. Psychic dependence, physical dependence and tolerance may develop upon repeated administration of HYCODAN and it should be prescribed and administered with the same degree of caution appropriate to the use of other narcotic drugs (See DRUG ABUSE AND DEPENDENCE).

Respiratory Depression: HYCODAN produces dose-related respiratory depression by directly acting on brain stem respiratory centers. If respiratory depression occurs, it may be antagonized by the use of naloxone hydrochloride and other supportive measures when indicated.

Head Injury And Increased Intracranial Pressure: The respiratory depression properties of narcotics and their capacity to elevate cerebrospinal fluid pressure may be markedly exaggerated in the presence of head injury, other intracranial lesions or a pre-existing increase in intracranial pressure. Furthermore, narcotics produce adverse reactions which may obscure the clinical course of patients with head injuries.

Acute Abdominal Conditions: The administration of HYCODAN or other narcotics may obscure the diagnosis or clinical course of patients with acute abdominal conditions.

Pediatric Use: In young children, as well as adults, the respiratory center is sensitive to the depressant action of narcotic cough suppressants in a dose-dependent manner. Benefit to risk ratio should be carefully considered especially in children with respiratory embarrassment (e.g., croup).

Continued on next page

Du Pont Pharm.—Cont.

PRECAUTIONS

General: Before prescribing medication to suppress or modify cough, it is important to ascertain that the underlying cause of cough is identified, that modification of cough does not increase the risk of clinical or physiological complications, and that appropriate therapy for the primary disease is provided.

Special Risk Patients: HYCODAN should be given with caution to certain patients such as the elderly or debilitated, and those with severe impairment of hepatic or renal functions, hypothyroidism, Addison's disease, prostatic hypertrophy or urethral stricture, asthma, and narrow-angle glaucoma.

Information For Patients: Hydrocodone may impair the mental and/or physical abilities required for the performance of potentially hazardous tasks such as driving a car or operating machinery. The patient using HYCODAN should be cautioned accordingly.

Drug Interactions: Patients receiving narcotics, antihistamines, antipsychotics, antianxiety agents or other CNS depressants (including alcohol) concomitantly with HYCODAN may exhibit an additive CNS depression. When combined therapy is contemplated, the dose of one or both agents should be reduced. The use of MAO inhibitors or tricyclic antidepressants with hydrocodone preparations may increase the effect of either the antidepressant or hydrocodone.

Carcinogenesis, Mutagenesis, Impairment Of Fertility: Studies of HYCODAN in animals to evaluate the carcinogenic and mutagenic potential and the effect on fertility have not been conducted.

Pregnancy:

Teratogenic Effects: Pregnancy Category C: Animal reproduction studies have not been conducted with HYCODAN. It is also not known whether HYCODAN can cause fetal harm when administered to a pregnant woman or can affect reproduction capacity. HYCODAN should be given to a pregnant woman only if clearly needed.

Nonteratogenic Effects: Babies born to mothers who have been taking opioids regularly prior to delivery will be physically dependent. The withdrawal signs include irritability and excessive crying, tremors, hyperactive reflexes, increased respiratory rate, increased stools, sneezing, yawning, vomiting and fever. The intensity of the syndrome does not always correlate with the duration of maternal opioid use or dose.

Labor and Delivery: As with all narcotics, administration of HYCODAN to the mother shortly before delivery may result in some degree of respiratory depression in the newborn, especially if higher doses are used.

Nursing Mothers: It is not known whether this drug is excreted in human milk. Because many drugs are excreted in human milk and because of the potential for serious adverse reactions in nursing infants from HYCODAN, a decision should be made whether to discontinue nursing or to discontinue the drug, taking into account the importance of the drug to the mother.

Pediatric Use: Safety and effectiveness of HYCODAN in children under six have not been established.

ADVERSE REACTIONS

Central Nervous System: Sedation, drowsiness, mental clouding, lethargy, impairment of mental and physical performance, anxiety, fear, dysphoria, dizziness, psychic dependence, mood changes.

Gastrointestinal System: Nausea and vomiting may occur; they are more frequent in ambulatory than in recumbent patients. Prolonged administration of HYCODAN may produce constipation.

Genitourinary System: Ureteral spasm, spasm of vesicle sphincters and urinary retention have been reported with opiates.

Respiratory Depression: HYCODAN may produce dose-related respiratory depression by acting directly on brain stem respiratory centers (see OVERDOSAGE).

Dermatological: Skin rash, pruritus.

DRUG ABUSE AND DEPENDENCE

HYCODAN is a Schedule III narcotic. Psychic dependence, physical dependence and tolerance may develop upon repeated administration of narcotics; therefore, HYCODAN should be prescribed and administered with caution. However, psychic dependence is unlikely to develop when HYCODAN is used for a short time for the treatment of cough. Physical dependence, the condition in which continued administration of the drug is required to prevent the appearance of a withdrawal syndrome, assumes clinically significant proportions only after several weeks of continued oral narcotic use, although some mild degree of physical dependence may develop after a few days of narcotic therapy.

OVERDOSAGE

Signs and Symptoms: Serious overdosage with hydrocodone is characterized by respiratory depression (a decrease in respiratory rate and/or tidal volume, Cheyne-Stokes respiration, cyanosis), extreme somnolence progressing to stupor or coma, skeletal muscle flaccidity, cold and clammy skin, and sometimes bradycardia and hypotension. In severe overdosage apnea, circulatory collapse, cardiac arrest and death may occur. The ingestion of very large amounts of HYCODAN may, in addition, result in acute homatropine intoxication.

Treatment: Primary attention should be given to the reestablishment of adequate respiratory exchange through provision of a patent airway and the institution of assisted or controlled ventilation. The narcotic antagonist naloxone hydrochloride is a specific antidote for respiratory depression which may result from overdosage or unusual sensitivity to narcotics including hydrocodone. Therefore, an appropriate dose of naloxone hydrochloride should be administered, preferably by the intravenous route, simultaneously with efforts at respiratory resuscitation. For further information, see full prescribing information for naloxone hydrochloride. An antagonist should not be administered in the absence of clinically significant respiratory depression. Oxygen, intravenous fluids, vasopressors and other supportive measures should be employed as indicated. Gastric emptying may be useful in removing unabsorbed drug.

DOSAGE AND ADMINISTRATION

Adults: One (1) tablet or one (1) teaspoonful (5 ml) of the syrup every 4 to 6 hours as needed; do not exceed six (6) tablets or six (6) teaspoonfuls in 24 hours.

Children 6 to 12 years of age: One-half ($\frac{1}{2}$) tablet or one-half ($\frac{1}{2}$) teaspoonful (2.5 ml) of the syrup every 4 to 6 hours as needed; do not exceed three (3) tablets or three (3) teaspoonfuls in 24 hours.

HOW SUPPLIED

As white tablets with one face scored and inscribed HYCODAN, and the other inscribed with Du Pont name is available in:

Bottles of 100	NDC 0056-0042-70
Bottles of 500	NDC 0056-0042-85

As a clear red colored, wild cherry flavored syrup in:

Bottles of one pint	NDC 0056-0234-16
Bottles of one gallon	NDC 0056-0234-82

Store at controlled room temperature (59°–86° F, 15°–30° C). Oral prescription where permitted by state law.
HYCODAN® is a Registered Trademark of E. I. du Pont de Nemours & Co. (Inc.)
NARCAN® is a Registered Trademark of Du Pont Pharmaceuticals, Inc.
6014–16

Shown in Product Identification Section, page 409

HYCOMINE®   ⒸⒾⒾⒾ
[hĭ-ko-mēn]
Pediatric Syrup

HYCOMINE®   ⒸⒾⒾⒾ
Syrup

DESCRIPTION

Hycomine® contains hydrocodone (dihydrocodeinone) bitartrate, a semi-synthetic centrally-acting narcotic antitussive and phenylpropanolamine hydrochloride, a sympathomimetic amine decongestant for oral administration.

	Hycomine® Pediatric Syrup	Hycomine® Syrup
Each teaspoonful (5 ml) contains:		
Hydrocodone bitartrate, U.S.P.	2.5 mg	5 mg
WARNING: May be habit forming		
Phenylpropanolamine hydrochloride, U.S.P.	12.5 mg	25 mg

Also, HYCOMINE®, both strengths, contain: artificial cherry flavor, glycerin, methylparaben, propylparaben, saccharin sodium, and sorbitol solution. HYCOMINE® Pediatric Syrup contains: D&C Yellow 10 and FD&C Green 3. HYCOMINE® Syrup: FD&C Red 40 and FD&C Yellow 6.

CLINICAL PHARMACOLOGY

Clinical trials have proven hydrocodone bitartrate to be an effective antitussive agent which is pharmacologically 2 to 8 times as potent as codeine. At equi-effective doses, its sedative action is greater than codeine. The precise mechanism of action of hydrocodone and other opiates is not known, however, hydrocodone is believed to act by directly depressing the cough center. In excessive doses, hydrocodone, like other opium derivatives, will depress respiration. The effects of hydrocodone in therapeutic doses on the cardiovascular system is insignificant. The constipation effects of hydrocodone are much weaker than that of morphine and no stronger than that of codeine. Hydrocodone can produce miosis, euphoria, physical and psychological dependence. At therapeutic antitussive doses, it does exert analgesic effects. Following a 10 mg oral dose of hydrocodone administered to five adult male subjects, the mean peak concentration was 23.6 ± 5.2 ng/ml. Maximum serum levels were achieved at 1.3 ± 0.3 hours and the half-life was determined to be 3.8 ± 0.3 hours. Hydrocodone exhibits a complex pattern of metabolism including O-demethylation, N-demethylation and 6-keto reduction to the corresponding 6-α- and 6-β-hydroxy-metabolites.

Phenylpropanolamine effects its vasoconstrictor activity by releasing noradrenaline from sympathetic nerve endings, and from direct stimulation of α-adrenoreceptors of blood vessels.

INDICATIONS AND USAGE

Hycomine® is indicated for the symptomatic relief of cough and nasal congestion.

CONTRAINDICATIONS

Hycomine® is contraindicated in patients hypersensitive to hydrocodone or phenylpropanolamine, and in patients on concurrent MAO inhibitor therapy. Patients known to be hypersensitive to other opioids or sympathomimetic amines may exhibit cross sensitivity to Hycomine®. Phenylpropanolamine is contraindicated in patients with heart disease, hypertension, diabetes or hyperthyroidism. Hydrocodone is contraindicated in the presence of an intracranial lesion associated with increased intracranial pressure; and whenever ventilatory function is depressed.

WARNINGS

May be habit forming. Hydrocodone can produce drug dependence of the morphine type and, therefore, has the potential for being abused. Psychic dependence, physical dependence and tolerance may develop upon repeated administration of Hycomine® and it should be prescribed and administered with the same degree of caution appropriate to the use of other narcotic drugs (See DRUG ABUSE AND DEPENDENCE).

Respiratory Depression: Hycomine® produces dose-related respiratory depression by directly acting on brain stem respiratory centers. If respiratory depression occurs, it may be antagonized by the use of Narcan® (naloxone hydrochloride) and other supportive measures when indicated.

Head Injury and Increased Intracranial Pressure: The respiratory depression properties of narcotics and their capacity to elevate cerebrospinal fluid pressure may be markedly exaggerated in the presence of head injury, other intracranial lesions or a preexisting increase in intracranial pressure. Furthermore, narcotics produce adverse reactions which may obscure the clinical course of patients with head injuries.

Acute Abdominal Conditions: The administration of Hycomine® or other narcotics may obscure the diagnosis or clinical course of patients with acute abdominal conditions.

Phenylpropanolamine: Hypertensive crises can occur with concurrent use of phenylpropanolamine and monoamine oxidase (MAO) inhibitors, indomethacin or with beta-blockers and methyldopa.

If a hypertensive crisis occurs, these drugs should be discontinued immediately and therapy to lower blood pressure should be instituted immediately. Fever should be managed by means of external cooling.

PRECAUTIONS

Before prescribing medication to suppress or modify cough, it is important to ascertain that the underlying cause of cough is identified, that modification of cough does not increase the risk of clinical or physiologic complications, and that appropriate therapy for the primary disease is provided.

Usage in Ambulatory Patients: Hydrocodone, like all narcotics, may impair the mental and/or physical abilities required for the performance of potentially hazardous tasks such as driving a car or operating machinery; phenylpropanolamine may produce a rapid pulse, dizziness or palpitations; patients should be cautioned accordingly.

Drug Interactions: Patients receiving other narcotic analgesics, general anesthetics, phenothiazines, other tranquilizers, sedative-hypnotics or other CNS depressants (including alcohol) concomitantly with hydrocodone may exhibit an additive CNS depression. When such combined therapy is contemplated, the dose of one or both agents should be reduced. The use of phenylpropanolamine with other sympathomimetic amines and MAO inhibitors may produce an additive elevation of blood pressure (See WARNINGS).

Carcinogenesis, Mutagenesis, Impairment of Fertility: Carcinogenicity, mutagenicity and reproduction studies have not been conducted with Hycomine®.

Usage in Pregnancy: Pregnancy Category C: Animal reproduction studies have not been conducted with Hycomine®. It is also not known whether Hycomine® can cause fetal harm when administered to a pregnant woman or can affect reproductive capacity. Hycomine® should be given to a pregnant woman only if clearly needed.

Nonteratogenic Effects: Babies born to mothers who have been taking opioids regularly prior to delivery will be physically dependent. The withdrawal signs include irritability and excessive crying, tremors, hyperactive reflexes, increased respiratory rate, increased stools, sneezing, yawning, vomiting and fever. The intensity of the syndrome does not always correlate with the duration of maternal opioid use or dose. There is no consensus on the best method of managing withdrawal. Chlorpromazine 0.7–1.0 mg/kg q 6 h, phenobarbital 2 mg/kg q 6 h, and paregoric 2–4 drops/kg q 4 h, have been used to treat withdrawal symptoms in infants. The duration of therapy is 4 to 28 days, with the dosages decreased as tolerated.

Nursing Mothers: It is not known whether this drug is excreted in human milk. Because many drugs are excreted in human milk and because of the potential for serious adverse reactions in nursing infants from Hycomine®, a decision should be made whether to discontinue nursing or discontinue the drug, taking into account the importance of the drug to the mother.

Usage in Patients Below the Age of 6 Years: Safety and effectiveness in this group have not been established.

ADVERSE REACTIONS

Respiratory System: Hydrocodone produces dose-related respiratory depression by acting directly on brain stem respiratory centers.

Cardiovascular System: Hypertension, postural hypotension, tachycardia and palpitations.

Genitourinary System: Ureteral spasm, spasm of vesical sphincters and urinary retention have been reported with opiates.

Central Nervous System: Sedation, drowsiness, mental clouding, lethargy, impairment of mental and physical performance, anxiety, fear, dysphoria, dizziness, psychic dependence, mood changes and blurred vision.

Gastrointestinal System: Nausea and vomiting occur more frequently in ambulatory than in recumbent patients.

DRUG ABUSE AND DEPENDENCE

Special care should be exercised in prescribing hydrocodone for emotionally unstable patients and for those with a history of drug misuse. Such patients should be closely supervised when long-term therapy is contemplated.

Hycomine® is a Schedule III narcotic. Psychic dependence, physical dependence, and tolerance may develop upon repeated administration of narcotics; therefore, Hycomine® should always be prescribed and administered with caution. Physical dependence is the condition in which continued administration of the drug is required to prevent the appearance of a withdrawal syndrome.

Patients physically dependent on opioids will develop an abstinence syndrome upon abrupt discontinuation of the opioid or following the administration of a narcotic antagonist. The character and severity of the withdrawal symptoms are related to the degree of physical dependence. Manifestations of opioid withdrawal are similar to but milder than that of morphine and include lacrimation, rhinorrhea, yawning, sweating, restlessness, dilated pupils, anorexia, gooseflesh, irritability and tremor. In more severe forms, nausea, vomiting, intestinal spasm and diarrhea, increased heart rate and blood pressure, chills, and pains in bones and muscles of the back and extremities may occur. Peak effects will usually be apparent at 48 to 72 hours.

Treatment of withdrawal is usually managed by providing sufficient quantities of an opioid to suppress severe withdrawal symptoms and then gradually reducing the dose of opioid over a period of several days.

OVERDOSAGE

Signs and Symptoms: Serious overdosage with Hycomine® is characterized by respiratory depression (a decrease in respiratory rate and/or tidal volume, Cheyne-Stokes respiration, cyanosis), extreme somnolence progressing to stupor or coma, skeletal muscle flaccidity, cold and clammy skin, and sometimes bradycardia and hypotension. In severe overdosage apnea, circulatory collapse, cardiac arrest, and death may occur.

The signs and symptoms of overdosage of the individual components of Hycomine® may be modified in varying degrees by the presence of other active ingredients. Overdosage with phenylpropanolamine alone may result in tremor, restlessness, increased motor activity, agitation and hallucinations.

Treatment: Primary attention should be given to the reestablishment of adequate respiratory exchange through provision of a patent airway and the institution of assisted or controlled ventilation. The narcotic antagonist naloxone hydrochloride (NARCAN®) is a specific antidote against respiratory depression which may result from overdosage or unusual sensitivity to narcotics including hydrocodone. Therefore, an appropriate dose of naloxone hydrochloride should be administered (Usual initial dose: 0.4 mg–2 mg; usual initial child dose: 0.01 mg/kg body weight. For further information see NARCAN® full prescribing information.) preferably by the intravenous route, simultaneously with efforts at respiratory resuscitation. Since the duration of action of hydrocodone may exceed that of the antagonist, the patient should be kept under continued surveillance and repeated doses of the antagonist should be administered as

needed to maintain adequate respiration. Oxygen, intravenous fluids, vasopressors and other supportive measures should be employed as indicated.

Gastric emptying may be useful in removing unabsorbed drug. Activated charcoal may be of benefit.

DOSAGE AND ADMINISTRATION

Usual Dosage:

	Hycomine® Pediatric Syrup	Hycomine® Syrup
Adults	—	1 tsp. (5 ml)
Children		
6 to 12 years	1 tsp. (5 ml)	—

After meals and at bedtime, not less than 4 hours apart (not to exceed 6 teaspoonfuls in a 24 hour period).

HOW SUPPLIED

Hycomine® Syrup is available as an orange-colored, fruit-flavored syrup in bottles as follows:
    One Pint: NDC 0056-0246-16
    One Gallon: NDC 0056-0246-82

Hycomine® Pediatric Syrup is available as a green-colored, fruit-flavored syrup in bottles as follows:
    One Pint: NDC 0056-0247-16

Store at controlled room temperature (59°–86°F, 15°–30°C). Oral prescription where permitted by state law.

Hycomine® is a Registered U.S. Trademark of E. I. du Pont de Nemours & Co. (Inc.)

Narcan® is a Registered U.S. Trademark of Du Pont Pharmaceuticals, Inc.

6153-2   July, 1985

HYCOMINE® COMPOUND   Ⓒ
[hĭ-ko-mĕn kom'pound]

DESCRIPTION

HYCOMINE Compound tablets contain hydrocodone (dihydrocodeinone) bitartrate, a semi-synthetic centrally-acting narcotic antitussive; chlorpheniramine maleate, an antihistamine; phenylephrine hydrochloride, a sympathomimetic amine decongestant; acetaminophen, an analgesic/antipyretic; and caffeine, a centrally-acting stimulant; for oral administration.

Each HYCOMINE Compound tablet contains:
Hydrocodone bitartrate U.S.P. .... 5 mg
    WARNING: May be habit forming
Chlorpheniramine maleate U.S.P. .... 2 mg
Phenylephrine hydrochloride U.S.P. .... 10 mg
Acetaminophen U.S.P. .... 250 mg
Caffeine, Anhydrous, U.S.P. .... 30 mg
HYCOMINE Compound tablets also contain: cherry flavor, colloidal silicon dioxide, FD&C Red 40, magnesium stearate, microcrystalline cellulose, povidone and starch.

CLINICAL PHARMACOLOGY

Clinical trials have proven hydrocodone bitartrate to be an effective antitussive agent which is pharmacologically 2 to 8 times as potent as codeine. At equi-effective doses, its sedative action is greater than codeine. The precise mechanism of action of hydrocodone and other opiates is not known, however, hydrocodone is believed to act by directly depressing the cough center. In excessive doses hydrocodone, like other opium derivatives, will depress respiration. The effects of hydrocodone in therapeutic doses on the cardiovascular system is insignificant. The constipation effects of hydrocodone are much weaker than that of morphine and no stronger than that of codeine. Hydrocodone can produce miosis, euphoria, physical and psychological dependence. At therapeutic antitussive doses, it does exert analgesic effects. Following a 10 mg oral dose of hydrocodone administered to five adult male human subjects, the mean peak concentration was 23.6 ± 5.2 ng/ml. Maximum serum levels were achieved at 1.3 ± 0.3 hours and the half-life was determined to be 3.8 ± 0.3 hours. Hydrocodone exhibits a complex pattern of metabolism including O-demethylation, N-demethylation and 6-keto reduction to the corresponding 6-α- and 6-β-hydroxymetabolites.

Chlorpheniramine maleate is a competitive H_1-receptor histamine blocking drug, thereby counteracting the effects of histamine release associated with allergic manifestations of upper respiratory tract inflammatory disorders. H_1-blocking drugs inhibit the actions of histamine on smooth muscle, capillary permeability, and can both stimulate and depress the central nervous system. Phenylephrine hydrochloride effects its vasoconstrictor activity by releasing noradrenaline from sympathetic nerve endings, and from direct stimulation of α-adrenoreceptors in blood vessels. Acetaminophen is an antipyretic and peripherally acting analgesic. Caffeine is a central nervous system stimulant.

INDICATIONS AND USAGE

HYCOMINE Compound is indicated for the symptomatic relief of cough, nasal congestion, and discomfort associated with upper respiratory tract infections.

CONTRAINDICATIONS

HYCOMINE Compound is contraindicated in patients hypersensitive to any component of the drug, and concurrent MAO inhibitor therapy. Patients known to be hypersensitive to other opioids, antihistamines, or sympathomimetic amines may exhibit cross sensitivity with HYCOMINE Compound. Phenylephrine is contraindicated in patients with heart disease, hypertension, diabetes or hyperthyroidism. Hydrocodone is contraindicated in the presence of an intracranial lesion associated with increased intracranial pressure; and whenever ventilatory function is depressed.

WARNINGS

May be habit forming. Hydrocodone can produce drug dependence of the morphine type and therefore has the potential for being abused. Psychic dependence, physical dependence and tolerance may develop upon repeated administration of HYCOMINE Compound and it should be prescribed and administered with the same degree of caution appropriate to the use of other narcotic drugs. (See DRUG ABUSE AND DEPENDENCE).

Respiratory Depression: HYCOMINE Compound produces dose-related respiratory depression by directly acting on brain stem respiratory centers. If respiratory depression occurs, it may be antagonized by the use of NARCAN® (naloxone hydrochloride) and other supportive measures when indicated.

Head Injury and Increased Intracranial Pressure: The respiratory depressant properties of narcotics and their capacity to elevate cerebrospinal fluid pressure may be markedly exaggerated in the presence of head injury, other intracranial lesions or a pre-existing increase in intracranial pressure. Furthermore, narcotics produce adverse reactions which may obscure the clinical course of patients with head injuries.

Acute abdominal conditions: The administration of HYCOMINE Compound or other narcotics may obscure the diagnosis or clinical course of patients with acute abdominal conditions.

Phenylephrine: Hypertensive crises can occur with concurrent use of phenylephrine and monoamine oxidase (MAO) inhibitors, indomethacin or with beta-blockers and methyldopa.

If a hypertensive crisis occurs these drugs should be discontinued immediately and therapy to lower blood pressure should be instituted immediately. Fever should be managed by means of external cooling.

Chlorpheniramine: Antihistamines may produce drowsiness or excitation, particularly in children and elderly patients.

PRECAUTIONS

Before prescribing medication to suppress or modify cough, it is important to ascertain that the underlying cause of cough is identified, that modification of cough does not increase the risk of clinical or physiologic complications, and that appropriate therapy for the primary disease is provided.

Usage in Ambulatory Patients: Hydrocodone, like all narcotics, and antihistamines such as chlorpheniramine maleate, may impair the mental and/or physical abilities required for the performance of potentially hazardous tasks such as driving a car or operating machinery; phenylephrine may produce a rapid pulse, dizziness or palpitations; patients should be cautioned accordingly.

Drug Interactions: Patients receiving other narcotic analgesics, general anesthetics, phenothiazines, other tranquilizers, sedative-hypnotics or other CNS depressants (including alcohol) concomitantly with hydrocodone may exhibit an additive CNS depression. When such combined therapy is contemplated, the dose of one or both agents should be reduced. The use of phenylephrine with other sympathomimetic amines and MAO inhibitors may produce an additive elevation of blood pressure. MAO inhibitors may prolong the anticholinergic effects of antihistamines. (See WARNINGS).

Carcinogenesis, mutagenesis, impairment of fertility: Carcinogenicity, mutagenicity, and reproduction studies have not been conducted with HYCOMINE Compound.

Usage in Pregnancy: Pregnancy Category C. Animal reproduction studies have not been conducted with HYCOMINE Compound. It is also not known whether HYCOMINE Compound can cause fetal harm when administered to a pregnant woman or can affect reproductive capacity. HYCOMINE Compound should be given to a pregnant woman only if clearly needed.

Nonteratogenic effects: Babies born to mothers who have been taking opioids regularly prior to delivery will be physically dependent. The withdrawal signs include irritability and excessive crying, tremors, hyperactive reflexes, increased respiratory rate, increased stools, sneezing, yawning, vomiting and fever. The intensity of the syndrome does not always correlate with the duration of maternal opioid use or dose. Chlorpromazine 0.7–1.0 mg/kg q 6 h, phenobarbital 2 mg/kg q 6 h, and paregoric 2–4 drops/kg q 4 h, have been used to treat withdrawal symptoms in infants. The du-

Continued on next page

Du Pont Pharm.—Cont.

ration of therapy is 4 to 28 days, with the dosages decreased as tolerated.

Nursing mothers: It is not known whether this drug is excreted in human milk. Because many drugs are excreted in human milk and because of the potential for serious adverse reactions in nursing infants from HYCOMINE Compound, a decision should be made whether to discontinue nursing or discontinue the drug, taking into account the importance of the drug to the mother.

Pediatric use: Safety and effectiveness in children below the age of 2 years have not been established.

ADVERSE REACTIONS

Respiratory System: Hydrocodone produces dose-related respiratory depression by acting directly on brain stem respiratory centers.

Cardiovascular System: Hypertension, postural hypotension, tachycardia and palpitations.

Genitourinary System: Ureteral spasm, spasm of vesical sphincters and urinary retention have been reported with opiates.

Central Nervous System: Sedation, drowsiness, mental clouding, lethargy, impairment of mental and physical performance, anxiety, fear, dysphoria, dizziness, psychic dependence, mood changes, and blurred vision.

Gastrointestinal System: Nausea and vomiting occur more frequently in ambulatory than in recumbent patients.

DRUG ABUSE AND DEPENDENCE

Special care should be exercised in prescribing hydrocodone for emotionally unstable patients and for those with a history of drug misuse. Such patients should be closely supervised when long-term therapy is contemplated. HYCOMINE Compound is a Schedule III narcotic. Psychic dependence, physical dependence, and tolerance may develop upon repeated administration of narcotics; therefore, HYCOMINE Compound should always be prescribed and administered with caution. Physical dependence is the condition in which continued administration of the drug is required to prevent the appearance of a withdrawal syndrome. Patients physically dependent on opioids will develop an abstinence syndrome upon abrupt discontinuation of the opioid or following the administration of a narcotic antagonist. The character and severity of the withdrawal symptoms are related to the degree of physical dependence. Manifestations of opioid withdrawal are similar to but milder than that of morphine and include lacrimation, rhinorrhea, yawning, sweating, restlessness, dilated pupils, anorexia, gooseflesh, irritability and tremor. In more severe forms, nausea, vomiting, intestinal spasms and diarrhea, increased heart rate and blood pressure, chills, and pains in bones and muscles of the back and extremities may occur. Peak effects will usually be apparent at 48 to 72 hours.

Treatment of withdrawal is usually managed by providing sufficient quantities of an opioid to suppress **severe** withdrawal symptoms and then gradually reducing the dose of opioid over a period of several days.

OVERDOSAGE

The signs and symptoms of overdosage of the individual components of HYCOMINE Compound may be modified in varying degrees by the presence of other active ingredients. Overdosage with phenylephrine alone may result in tremor, restlessness, increased motor activity, agitation and hallucinations.

Acetaminophen

Signs and Symptoms: In acute acetaminophen overdosage, dose-dependent, potentially fatal hepatic necrosis is the most serious adverse effect. Renal tubular necrosis, hypoglycemic coma and thrombocytopenia may also occur.

Acetaminophen in massive overdosage may cause hepatic toxicity in some patients. In cases of suspected overdose, you may wish to call your regional poison center for assistance in diagnosis and for directions in the use of N-acetylcysteine as an antidote.

In adults, hepatic toxicity has rarely been reported with acute overdoses of less than 10 grams and fatalities with less than 15 grams. Importantly, young children seem to be more resistant than adults to the hepatotoxic effect of an acetaminophen overdose. Despite this, the measures outlined below should be initiated in any adult or child suspected of having ingested an acetaminophen overdose.

Early symptoms following a potentially hepatotoxic overdose may include nausea, vomiting, diaphoresis and general malaise. Clinical and laboratory evidence of hepatic toxicity may not be apparent until 48 to 72 hours post-ingestion.

Treatment: The stomach should be emptied promptly by lavage or by induction of emesis with syrup of ipecac. Patient's estimates of the quantity of a drug ingested are notoriously unreliable. Therefore, if an acetaminophen overdose is suspected, a serum acetaminophen assay should be obtained as early as possible, but no sooner than four hours following ingestion. Liver function studies should be obtained initially and repeated at 24-hour intervals.

The antidote, N-acetylcysteine should be administered as early as possible, preferably within 16 hours of the overdose ingestions for optimal results, but in any case, within 24 hours. Following recovery, there are no residual structural or functional hepatic abnormalities.

Hydrocodone

Signs and Symptoms: Serious overdosage with hydrocodone is characterized by respiratory depression (a decrease in respiratory rate and/or tidal volume, Cheyne-Stokes respiration, cyanosis), extreme somnolence progressing to stupor or coma, skeletal muscle flaccidity, cold and clammy skin, and sometimes bradycardia and hypotension. In severe overdosage apnea, circulatory collapse, cardiac arrest and death may occur.

Treatment: Primary attention should be given to the reestablishment of adequate respiratory exchange through provision of a patent airway and the institution of assisted or controlled ventilation. The narcotic antagonist naloxone hydrochloride is a specific antidote for respiratory depression which may result from overdosage or unusual sensitivity to narcotics including hydrocodone. Therefore, an appropriate dose of naloxone hydrochloride should be administered, preferably by the intravenous route, simultaneously with efforts at respiratory resuscitation. For further information, see full prescribing information for naloxone hydrochloride. An antagonist should not be administered in the absence of clinically significant respiratory depression. Oxygen, intravenous fluids, vasopressors and other supportive measures should be employed as indicated. Gastric emptying may be useful in removing unabsorbed drug. Activated charcoal may be of benefit.

DOSAGE AND ADMINISTRATION

Usual dosage, not less than 4 hours apart:
Adults: 1 tablet 4 times a day.
Children: 6 to 12 years: 1/2 tablet 4 times a day.

HOW SUPPLIED

HYCOMINE® Compound is available as a coral pink, scored tablet in bottles as follows:

Bottles of 100	NDC 0056-0048-70
Bottles of 500	NDC 0056-0048-85

Store at controlled room temperature (59°–86° F, 15°–30° C)
Oral prescription where permitted by State Law.
HYCOMINE® is a Registered U.S. Trademark of E. I. du Pont de Nemours & Co. (Inc.)
NARCAN® is a Registered U.S. Trademark of Du Pont Pharmaceuticals, Inc.
6015-11

HYCOTUSS®   Ⓒ
[hī-kō-tus]
Expectorant

DESCRIPTION

HYCOTUSS Expectorant Syrup contains hydrocodone (dihydrocodeinone) bitartrate, a semi-synthetic centrally-acting narcotic antitussive and guaifenesin, an expectorant for oral administration.

Each teaspoonful (5 ml) contains:
Hydrocodone bitartrate U.S.P. .... 5 mg
     WARNING: May be habit forming
Guaifenesin U.S.P. .... 100 mg
Alcohol U.S.P. .... 10% v/v
HYCOTUSS Expectorant Syrup also contains: artificial butterscotch flavor, FD&C Red 40, FD&C Yellow 6, glycerin, liquid sugar, methylparaben, propylparaben, saccharin sodium, and sorbitol solution.

CLINICAL PHARMACOLOGY

Clinical trials have proven hydrocodone bitartrate to be an effective antitussive agent which is pharmacologically 2 to 8 times as potent as codeine. At equi-effective doses, its sedative action is greater than codeine. The precise mechanism of action of hydrocodone and other opiates is not known, however, hydrocodone is believed to act by directly depressing the cough center. In excessive doses hydrocodone, like other opium derivatives, can depress respiration. The effects of hydrocodone in therapeutic doses on the cardiovascular system is insignificant. The constipation effects of hydrocodone are much weaker than that of morphine and no stronger than that of codeine. Hydrocodone can produce miosis, euphoria, physical and psychological dependence. At therapeutic antitussive doses, it does exert analgesic effects. Following a 10 mg oral dose of hydrocodone administered to five male human subjects, the mean peak concentration was 23.6 ± 5.2 ng/ml. Maximum serum levels were achieved at 1.3 ± 0.3 hours and half-life was determined to be 3.8 ± 0.3 hours. Hydrocodone exhibits a complex pattern of metabolism including O-demethylation, N-demethylation and 6-keto reduction to the corresponding 6-α- and 6-β-hydroxymetabolites.

The exact mechanism of action is not established but guaifenesin is believed to act by stimulating receptors in the gastric mucosa that initiates a reflex secretion of respiratory tract fluid, thereby increasing the volume and decreasing the viscosity of bronchial secretions. Studies with guaifenesin indicate that it is rapidly absorbed from the gastrointestinal tract and has a half-life of one hour.

INDICATIONS AND USAGE

HYCOTUSS Expectorant is indicated for the symptomatic relief of irritating non-productive cough associated with upper and lower respiratory tract congestion.

CONTRAINDICATIONS

HYCOTUSS Expectorant is contraindicated in patients hypersensitive to hydrocodone or guaifenesin. Patients known to be hypersensitive to other opioids may exhibit cross sensitivity to HYCOTUSS Expectorant. Hydrocodone is contraindicated in the presence of an intracranial lesion associated with increased intracranial pressure; and whenever ventilatory function is depressed.

WARNINGS

May be habit forming. Hydrocodone can produce drug dependence of the morphine type and therefore has the potential for being abused. Psychic dependence, physical dependence and tolerance may develop upon repeated administration of HYCOTUSS Expectorant and it should be prescribed and administered with the same degree of caution appropriate to the use of other narcotic drugs (See DRUG ABUSE AND DEPENDENCE).

Respiratory Depression: HYCOTUSS Expectorant produces dose-related respiratory depression by directly acting on the brain stem respiratory centers. If respiratory depression occurs, it may be antagonized by the use of NARCAN® (naloxone hydrochloride) and other supportive measures when indicated.

Head Injury and Increased Intracranial Pressure: The respiratory depressant properties of narcotics and their capacity to elevate cerebrospinal fluid pressure may be markedly exaggerated in the presence of head injury, other intracranial lesions or a pre-existing increase in intracranial pressure. Furthermore, narcotics produce adverse reactions which may obscure the clinical course of patients with head injuries.

Acute Abdominal Conditions: The administration of HYCOTUSS Expectorant or other opioids may obscure the diagnosis or clinical course of patients with acute abdominal conditions.

PRECAUTIONS

Before prescribing medication to suppress or modify cough, it is important to ascertain that the underlying cause of cough is identified, that modification of cough does not increase the risk of clinical or physiologic complications, and that appropriate therapy for the primary disease is provided.

Usage in Ambulatory Patients: Hydrocodone, like all narcotics, may impair the mental and/ or physical abilities required for the performance of potentially hazardous tasks such as driving a car or operating machinery, and patients should be warned accordingly.

Drug Interactions: Patients receiving other narcotic analgesics, general anesthetics, phenothiazines, other tranquilizers, sedative hypnotics or other CNS depressants (including alcohol) concomitantly with hydrocodone may exhibit an additive CNS depression. When such combined therapy is contemplated, the dose of one or both agents should be reduced. (See WARNINGS).

Laboratory Interactions: The metabolite of guaifenesin has been found to produce an apparent increase in urinary 5-hydroxyindoleacetic acid, and guaifenesin therefore may interfere with the interpretation of this test for the diagnosis of carcinoid syndrome. Guaifenesin administration should be discontinued 24 hours prior to the collection of urine specimens for the determination of 5-hydroxyindoleacetic acid.

Carcinogenesis, mutagenesis, impairment of fertility: Carcinogenicity, mutagenicity and reproduction studies have not been conducted with HYCOTUSS Expectorant.

Usage in Pregnancy: Pregnancy Category C. Animal reproduction studies have not been conducted with HYCOTUSS Expectorant. It is also not known whether HYCOTUSS Expectorant can cause fetal harm when administered to a pregnant woman or can affect reproductive capacity. HYCOTUSS Expectorant should be given to a pregnant woman only if clearly needed.

Nonteratogenic effects: Babies born to mothers who have been taking opioids regularly prior to delivery will be physically dependent. The withdrawal signs include irritability and excessive crying, tremors, hyperactive reflexes, increased respiratory rate, increased stools, sneezing, yawning, vomiting and fever. The intensity of the syndrome does not always correlate with the duration of maternal opioid use or dose. There is no consensus on the best method of managing withdrawal. Chlorpromazine 0.7–1.0 mg/kg q 6 h, phenobarbital 2 mg/kg q 6 h, and paregoric 2–4 drops/kg q 4 h, have been used to treat withdrawal symptoms in infants. The duration of therapy is 4 to 28 days, with the dosages decreased as tolerated.

Nursing mothers: It is not known whether this drug is excreted in human milk. Because many drugs are excreted in human milk and because of the potential for serious adverse reactions in nursing infants from HYCOTUSS Expectorant, a decision should be made whether to discontinue nursing or discontinue the drug, taking into account the importance of the drug to the mother.

ADVERSE REACTIONS

Respiratory System: Hydrocodone produces dose-related respiratory depression by acting directly on brain stem respiratory centers.

Cardiovascular System: Hypertension, postural hypotension and palpitations.

Genitourinary System: Ureteral spasm, spasm of vesical sphinchters and urinary retention have been reported with opiates.

Central Nervous System: Sedation, drowsiness, mental clouding, lethargy, impairment of mental and physical performance, anxiety, fear, dysphoria, dizziness, psychic dependence, mood changes and blurred vision.

Gastrointestinal System: Nausea and vomiting occur more frequently in ambulatory than in recumbent patients.

DRUG ABUSE AND DEPENDENCE

Special care should be exercised in prescribing hydrocodone for emotionally unstable patients and for those with a history of drug misuse. Such patients should be closely supervised when long-term therapy is contemplated.

HYCOTUSS Expectorant is a Schedule III narcotic. Psychic dependence, physical dependence and tolerance may develop upon repeated administration of narcotics; therefore, HYCOTUSS Expectorant should always be prescribed and administered with caution. Physical dependence is the condition in which continued administration of the drug is required to prevent the appearance of a withdrawal syndrome.

Patients physically dependent on opioids will develop an abstinence syndrome upon abrupt discontinuation of the opioid or following the administration of a narcotic antagonist. The character and severity of the withdrawal symptoms are related to the degree of physical dependence. Manifestations of opioid withdrawal are similar to but milder than that of morphine and include lacrimation, rhinorrhea, yawning, sweating, restlessness, dilated pupils, anorexia, gooseflesh, irritability and tremor. In more severe forms, nausea, vomiting, intestinal spasm and diarrhea, increased heart rate and blood pressure, chills, and pains in bones and muscles of the back and extremities may occur. Peak effects will usually be apparent at 48 to 72 hours.

Treatment of withdrawal is usually managed by providing sufficient quantities of an opioid to suppress **severe** withdrawal symptoms and then gradually reducing the dose of opioid over a period of several days.

OVERDOSAGE

Signs and Symptoms: Serious overdosage with HYCOTUSS Expectorant is characterized by respiratory depression (a decrease in respiratory rate and/or tidal volume, Cheyne-Stokes respiration, cyanosis), extreme somnolence progressing to stupor or coma, skeletal muscle flaccidity, cold and clammy skin, and sometimes bradycardia and hypotension. In severe overdosage apnea, circulatory collapse, cardiac arrest, and death may occur.

Treatment: Primary attention should be given to the reestablishment of adequate respiratory exchange through provision of a patent airway and the institution of assisted or controlled ventilation. The narcotic antagonist naloxone hydrochloride is a specific antidote for respiratory depression which may result from overdosage or unusual sensitivity to narcotics including hydrocodone. Therefore, an appropriate dose of naloxone hydrochloride should be administered, preferably by the intravenous route, simultaneously with efforts at respiratory resuscitation. For further information, see full prescribing information for naloxone hydrochloride. An antagonist should not be administered in the absence of clinically significant respiratory depression. Oxygen, intravenous fluids, vasopressors and other supportive measures should be employed as indicated. Gastric emptying may be useful in removing unabsorbed drug. Activated charcoal may be of benefit.

DOSAGE AND ADMINISTRATION

Usual Adult Dose: One teaspoonful (5 ml) after meals and at bedtime, not less than 4 hours apart (not to exceed 6 teaspoonsful in a 24 hour period). Treatment should be initiated with one teaspoonful and subsequent doses, up to a maximum single dose of 3 teaspoonsful, adjusted if required.

Usual Children's Dose:

Over 12 years: Initial dose 1 teaspoonful; maximum single dose, 2 teaspoonsful.

6 to 12 years: Initial dose ½ teaspoonful; maximum single dose, 1 teaspoonful.

HOW SUPPLIED

HYCOTUSS Expectorant is available as an orange-colored, butterscotch flavored syrup in bottles as follows:

One pint: NDC 0056-0235-16

Store at controlled room temperature (59°–86° F, 15°–30° C). Oral prescription as permitted by State Law.

HYCOTUSS® is a Registered U.S. Trademark of E.I. du Pont de Nemours & Co. (Inc.)

NARCAN® is a Registered U.S. Trademark of Du Pont Pharmaceuticals, Inc.

6131-5

INTROPIN® ℞

[in-trō'pin]

(dopamine HCl injection, USP)

DESCRIPTION

INTROPIN (dopamine HCl injection, USP) is a clear, practically colorless, aqueous, additive solution for intravenous infusion after dilution. Each mL contains either 40 mg, 80 mg or 160 mg dopamine hydrochloride, USP (equivalent to 32.3 mg, 64.6 mg and 129.2 mg dopamine base, respectively) in Water for Injection, USP containing 1% sodium metabisulfite, NF as an antioxidant. Hydrochloric acid or sodium hydroxide added to adjust pH when necessary. The solution is sterile and non-pyrogenic. The pH is 2.5-4.5. Dopamine HCl, a naturally-occurring catecholamine, is an inotropic vasopressor agent. Its chemical name is 3,4 dihydroxyphenethylamine hydrochloride and its chemical structure is:

$$HO-\text{(ring)}-CH_2CH_2NH_2 \cdot HCl$$

$C_8H_{11}NO_2 \cdot HCl$ Mol. Wt. 189.65

Dopamine HCl is sensitive to alkalis, iron salts and oxidizing agents. **INTROPIN must be diluted in an appropriate, sterile parenteral solution** (see Dosage and Administration section) **before intravenous administration.**

ACTIONS

INTROPIN exerts an inotropic effect on the myocardium resulting in an increased cardiac output. INTROPIN produces less increase in myocardial oxygen consumption than isoproterenol and its use is usually not associated with a tachyarrhythmia. Clinical studies indicate that INTROPIN usually increases systolic and pulse pressure with either no effect or a slight increase in diastolic pressure. Total peripheral resistance at low and intermediate therapeutic doses is usually unchanged. Blood flow to peripheral vascular beds may decrease while mesenteric flow increases. INTROPIN has also been reported to dilate the renal vasculature presumptively by activation of a "dopaminergic" receptor. This action is accompanied by increases in glomerular filtration rate, renal blood flow, and sodium excretion. An increase in urinary output produced by dopamine is usually not associated with a decrease in osmolality of the urine.

INDICATIONS

INTROPIN is indicated for the correction of hemodynamic imbalances present in the shock syndrome due to myocardial infarctions, trauma, endotoxic septicemia, open heart surgery, renal failure, and chronic cardiac decompensation as in congestive failure.

Where appropriate, restoration of blood volume with a suitable plasma expander or whole blood should be instituted or completed prior to administration of INTROPIN.

Patients most likely to respond adequately to INTROPIN are those in whom physiological parameters, such as urine flow, myocardial function, and blood pressure, have not undergone profound deterioration. Multiclinic trials indicate that the shorter the time interval between onset of signs and symptoms and initiation of therapy with volume correction and INTROPIN, the better the prognosis.

Poor Perfusion of Vital Organs—Urine flow appears to be one of the better diagnostic signs by which adequacy of vital organ perfusion can be monitored. Nevertheless, the physician should also observe the patient for signs of reversal of confusion or comatose condition. Loss of pallor, increase in toe temperature, and/or adequacy of nail bed capillary filling may also be used as indices of adequate dosage. Clinical studies have shown that when INTROPIN is administered before urine flow has diminished to levels approximately 0.3 mL/minute, prognosis is more favorable. Nevertheless, in a number of oliguric or anuric patients, administration of INTROPIN has resulted in an increase in urine flow which in some cases reached normal levels. INTROPIN may also increase urine flow in patients whose output is within normal limits and thus may be of value in reducing the degree of preexisting fluid accumulation. It should be noted that at doses above those optimal for the individual patient, urine flow may decrease, necessitating reduction of dosage. Concurrent administration of INTROPIN and diuretic agents may produce an additive or potentiating effect.

Low Cardiac Output—Increased cardiac output is related to the direct inotropic effect of INTROPIN on the myocardium. Increased cardiac output at low or moderate doses appears to be related to a favorable prognosis. Increase in cardiac output has been associated with either static or decreased systemic vascular resistance (SVR). Static or decreased SVR associated with low or moderate increments in cardiac output is believed to be a reflection of differential effects on spe-

---

cific vascular beds with increased resistance in peripheral beds (e.g. femoral) and concomitant decreases in mesenteric and renal vascular beds. Redistribution of blood flow parallels these changes so that an increase in cardiac output is accompanied by an increase in mesenteric and renal blood flow. In many instances the renal fraction of the total cardiac output has been found to increase. The increase in cardiac output produced by INTROPIN is not associated with substantial decreases in systemic vascular resistance as may occur with isoproterenol.

Hypotension—Hypotension due to inadequate cardiac output can be managed by administration of low to moderate doses of INTROPIN, which have little effect on SVR. At high therapeutic doses, the alpha adrenergic activity of INTROPIN becomes more prominent and thus may correct hypotension due to diminished SVR. As in the case of other circulatory decompensation states, prognosis is better in patients whose blood pressure and urine flow have not undergone profound deterioration. Therefore, it is suggested that the physician administer INTROPIN as soon as a definite trend toward decreased systolic and diastolic pressure becomes evident.

CONTRAINDICATIONS

INTROPIN should not be used in patients with pheochromocytoma.

WARNINGS

INTROPIN should not be administered in the presence of uncorrected tachyarrhythmias or ventricular fibrillation.

Do **NOT** add INTROPIN to any alkaline diluent solution, since the drug is inactivated in alkaline solution.

Patients who have been treated with monoamine oxidase (MAO) inhibitors prior to the administration of INTROPIN will require substantially reduced dosage. Dopamine is metabolized by MAO, and inhibition of this enzyme prolongs and potentiates the effect of INTROPIN. The starting dose in such patients should be reduced to at least one-tenth ($\frac{1}{10}$) of the usual dose.

Contains sodium metabisulfite, a sulfite that may cause allergic-type reactions including anaphylactic symptoms and life-threatening or less severe asthmatic episodes in certain susceptible people. The overall prevalence of sulfite sensitivity in the general population is unknown, and probably low. Sulfite sensitivity is seen more frequently in asthmatic than in nonasthmatic people.

PRECAUTIONS: General

Avoid Hypovolemia—Prior to treatment with INTROPIN, hypovolemia should be fully corrected, if possible, with either whole blood or plasma as indicated.

Decreased Pulse Pressure—If a disproportionate rise in the diastolic pressure (i.e., a marked decrease in the pulse pressure) is observed in patients receiving INTROPIN, the infusion rate should be decreased and the patient observed carefully for further evidence of predominant vasoconstrictor activity, unless such an effect is desired.

Extravasation—INTROPIN should be infused into a large vein whenever possible to prevent the possibility of extravasation into tissue adjacent to the infusion site. Extravasation may cause necrosis and sloughing of surrounding tissue. Large veins of the antecubital fossa are preferred to veins in the dorsum of the hand or ankle. Less suitable infusion sites should be used only if the patient's condition requires immediate attention. The physician should switch to more suitable sites as rapidly as possible. The infusion site should be continuously monitored for free flow.

Occlusive Vascular Disease—Patients with a history of occlusive vascular disease (for example, atherosclerosis, arterial embolism, Raynaud's disease, cold injury, diabetic endarteritis, and Buerger's disease) should be closely monitored for any changes in color or temperature of the skin in the extremities. If a change in skin color or temperature occurs and is thought to be the result of compromised circulation to the extremities, the benefits of continued INTROPIN infusion should be weighed against the risk of possible necrosis. This condition may be reversed by either decreasing or discontinuing the rate of infusion.

IMPORTANT—Antidote for Peripheral Ischemia: To prevent sloughing and necrosis in ischemic areas, the area should be infiltrated as soon as possible with 10 to 15 mL. of saline solution containing from 5 to 10 mg of Regitine® (brand of phentolamine), an adrenergic blocking agent. A syringe with a fine hypodermic needle should be used, and the solution liberally infiltrated throughout the ischemic area. Sympathetic blockade with phentolamine causes immediate and conspicuous local hyperemic changes if the area is infiltrated within 12 hours. Therefore, <u>phentolamine should be given as soon as possible</u> after the extravasation is noted.

Avoid Cyclopropane or Halogenated Hydrocarbon Anesthetics—Cyclopropane or halogenated hydrocarbon anes-

Continued on next page

Du Pont Pharm.—Cont.

thetics increase cardiac autonomic irritability and therefore may sensitize the myocardium to the action of certain intravenously administered catecholamines. This interaction appears to be related both to pressor activity and to beta adrenergic stimulating properties of these catecholamines. Therefore, as with certain other catecholamines, and because of the theoretical arrhythmogenic potential, INTROPIN should be used with EXTREME CAUTION in patients inhaling cyclopropane or halogenated hydrocarbon anesthetics.

Careful Monitoring Required—Close monitoring of the following indices—urine flow, cardiac output and blood pressure—during INTROPIN (dopamine HCl injection, USP) infusion is necessary as in the case of any adrenergic agent.

Pregnancy—Pregnancy Category C. Animal studies have revealed no evidence of teratogenic effects from INTROPIN. In one study, administration of INTROPIN to pregnant rats resulted in a decreased survival rate of the newborn and a potential for cataract formation in the survivors. There are no adequate and well-controlled studies in pregnant women. INTROPIN should be used during pregnancy only if the potential benefit justifies the potential risk to the fetus.

Pediatric Use—Safety and effectiveness in children have not been established.

ADVERSE REACTIONS

The most frequent adverse reactions observed in clinical evaluation of INTROPIN included ectopic beats, nausea, vomiting, tachycardia, anginal pain, palpitation, dyspnea, headache, hypotension, and vasoconstriction. Other adverse reactions which have been reported infrequently were aberrant conduction, bradycardia, piloerection, widened QRS complex, azotemia, and elevated blood pressure.

DOSAGE AND ADMINISTRATION

WARNING: This is a potent drug: It must be diluted before administration to patient.

Suggested Dilution—Transfer contents of one or more ampuls, vials or additive syringes by aseptic technique to either a 250 mL or 500 mL bottle of one of the following sterile intravenous solutions:

1) Sodium Chloride Injection, USP
2) Dextrose (5%) Injection, USP
3) Dextrose (5%) and Sodium Chloride (0.9%) Injection, USP
4) 5% Dextrose in 0.45% Sodium Chloride Solution
5) Dextrose (5%) in Lactated Ringer's Solution
6) Sodium Lactate (1/6 Molar) Injection, USP
7) Lactated Ringer's Injection, USP

INTROPIN has been found to be stable for a minimum of 24 hours after dilution in the sterile intravenous solutions listed above. However, as with all intravenous admixtures, dilution should be made just prior to administration.

Do **NOT** add INTROPIN Injection to Sodium Bicarbonate or other alkaline intravenous solutions, since the drug is inactivated in alkaline solution.

Rate of Administration—INTROPIN, after dilution, is administered intravenously through a suitable intravenous catheter or needle. An i.v. drip chamber or other suitable metering device is essential for controlling the rate of flow in drops/minute. Each patient must be individually titrated to the desired hemodynamic and/or renal response with INTROPIN. In titrating to the desired increase in systolic blood pressure, the optimum dosage rate for renal response may be exceeded, thus necessitating a reduction in rate after the hemodynamic condition is stablized.

Administration at rates greater than 50 mcg/kg/minute have safely been used in advanced circulatory decompensation states. If unnecessary fluid expansion is of concern, adjustment of drug concentration may be preferred over increasing the flow rate of a less concentrated dilution.

Suggested Regimen:

1. When appropriate, increase blood volume with whole blood or plasma until central venous pressure is 10 to 15 cm H_2O or pulmonary wedge pressure is 14–18 mm Hg.

2. Begin administration of diluted solution at doses of 2–5 mcg/kg/minute INTROPIN in patients who are likely to respond to modest increments of heart force and renal perfusion.

In more seriously ill patients, begin administration of diluted solution at doses of 5 mcg/kg/minute INTROPIN and increase gradually using 5 to 10 mcg/kg/minute increments up to 20 to 50 mcg/kg/minute as needed. If doses of INTROPIN in excess of 50 mcg/kg/minute are required, it is suggested that urine output be checked frequently. Should urine flow begin to decrease in the absence of hypotension, reduction of INTROPIN dosage should be considered. Multiclinic trials have shown that more than 50% of the patients were satisfactorily maintained on doses of INTROPIN less than 20 mcg/kg/minute. In patients who do not respond to these doses with adequate arterial pressures or urine flow, additional increments of INTROPIN may be employed in an effort to produce an appropriate arterial pressure and central perfusion.

3. Treatment of all patients requires constant evaluation of therapy in terms of the blood volume, augmentation of myocardial contractility, and distribution of peripheral perfusion. Dosage of INTROPIN should be adjusted according to the patient's response, with particular attention to diminution of established urine flow rate, increasing tachycardia or development of new dysrhythmias as indices for decreasing or temporarily suspending the dosage.

4. As with all potent intravenously administered drugs, care should be taken to control the rate of administration so as to avoid inadvertent administration of a bolus of drug.

OVERDOSAGE

In case of accidental overdosage, as evidenced by excessive blood pressure elevation, reduce rate of administration or temporarily discontinue INTROPIN until patient's condition stabilizes. Since the duration of action of INTROPIN is quite short, no additional remedial measures are usually necessary. If these measures fail to stabilize the patient's condition, use of the short-acting alpha adrenergic blocking agent, phentolamine, should be considered.

HOW SUPPLIED

—200 mg (5 mL containing 40 mg dopamine HCl, USP per mL)
NDC 0094-0040-05—Ampul
NDC 0094-0040-06—Single-dose vial (color coded white)
NDC 0094-0040-07—RAP-ADD® Additive Syringe (color coded white)
—400 mg (5 mL containing 80 mg dopamine HCl, USP per mL)
NDC 0094-0046-06—Single-dose vial (color coded green)
NDC 0094-0046-07—RAP-ADD® Additive Syringe (color coded green)
—800 mg (5 mL containing 160 mg dopamine HCl, USP per mL)
NDC 0094-0047-06—Single-dose vial (color coded yellow)
NDC 0094-0047-07—RAP-ADD® Additive Syringe (color coded yellow)

WARNING

NOT FOR DIRECT INTRAVENOUS INJECTION. MUST BE DILUTED BEFORE USE.

INSTRUCTIONS FOR USE: RAP-ADD® Additive Syringe

1. Firmly grasp cap with one hand and needle shroud with the other. Twist-pull to remove cap.

2. Twist pull needle guard free

3. Place needle on center of target area and push fully into place.

4. Using firm pressure, hold syringe and press pushrod in to activate syringe and discharge contents. Since an internal membrane is used to preserve sterility, resistance will be felt during initial activation until membrane is ruptured.

5. Remove syringe after use and dispose of in proper manner.

Du Pont Pharmaceuticals
E. I. du Pont de Nemours & Co.
Wilmington, Delaware 19898
March, 1989   A43109

MOBAN®

[mŏ'ban]
(molindone hydrochloride)

DESCRIPTION

MOBAN (molindone hydrochloride) is a dihydroindolone compound which is not structurally related to the phenothiazines, the butyrophenones or the thioxanthenes.

MOBAN is 3-ethyl-6, 7-dihydro-2-methyl-5-(morpholinomethyl) indol-4 (5H)-one hydrochloride. It is a white to off-white crystalline powder, freely soluble in water and alcohol and has a molecular weight of 312.67.

MOBAN Tablets also contain:
All strengths: calcium sulfate, lactose, magnesium stearate, microcrystalline cellulose and povidone.
- 5 mg: alginic acid, colloidal silicon dioxide and FD&C Yellow 6.
- 10 mg: alginic acid, colloidal silicon dioxide, FD&C Blue 2 and FD&C Red 40.
- 25 mg: alginic acid, colloidal silicon dioxide, D&C Yellow 10, FD&C Blue 2, and FD&C Yellow 6.
- 50 mg: FD&C Blue 2 and starch.
- 100 mg: FD&C Blue 2, FD&C Yellow 6 and sodium starch glycolate.

MOBAN Concentrate contains: alcohol, artificial cherry flavor, artificial cover flavor, edetate disodium, glycerin, liquid sugar, methylparaben, propylparaben, sodium metabisulfite, sorbitol solution, and hydrochloric acid reagent grade for pH adjustment.

MOLINDONE HYDROCHLORIDE

ACTIONS

MOBAN (molindone hydrochloride) has a pharmacological profile in laboratory animals which predominantly resembles that of major tranquilizers causing reduction of spontaneous locomotion and aggressiveness, suppression of a conditioned response and antagonism of the bizarre stereotyped behavior and hyperactivity induced by amphetamines. In addition, MOBAN antagonizes the depression caused by the tranquilizing agent tetrabenazine.

In human clinical studies tranquilization is achieved in the absence of muscle relaxing or incoordinating effects. Based on EEG studies, MOBAN exerts its effect on the ascending reticular activating system.

Human metabolic studies show MOBAN (molindone hydrochloride) to be rapidly absorbed and metabolized when given orally. Unmetabolized drug reached a peak blood level at 1.5 hours. Pharmacological effect from a single oral dose persists for 24-36 hours. There are 36 recognized metabolites with less than 2-3% unmetabolized MOBAN being excreted in urine and feces.

INDICATIONS

MOBAN is indicated for the management of the manifestations of psychotic disorders. The antipsychotic efficacy of MOBAN was established in clinical studies which enrolled newly hospitalized and chronically hospitalized, acutely ill, schizophrenic patients as subjects.

CONTRAINDICATIONS

MOBAN (molindone hydrochloride) is contraindicated in severe central nervous system depression (alcohol, barbiturates, narcotics, etc.) or comatose states, and in patients with known hypersensitivity to the drug.

WARNINGS

Tardive Dyskinesia: Tardive dyskinesia, a syndrome consisting of potentially irreversible, involuntary, dyskinetic movements may develop in patients treated with neuroleptic (antipsychotic) drugs. Although the prevalence of the syndrome appears to be highest among the elderly, especially elderly women, it is impossible to rely upon prevalence estimates to predict, at the inception of neuroleptic treatment, which patients are likely to develop the syndrome. Whether neuroleptic drug products differ in their potential to cause tardive dyskinesia is unknown.

Both the risk of developing the syndrome and the likelihood that it will become irreversible are believed to increase as the duration of treatment and the total cumulative dose of neuroleptic drugs administered to the patient increase. However, the syndrome can develop, although much less commonly, after relatively brief treatment periods at low doses. There is no known treatment for established cases of tardive dyskinesia, although the syndrome may remit, partially or completely, if neuroleptic treatment is withdrawn. Neuroleptic treatment, itself, however, may suppress (or partially suppress) the signs and symptoms of the syndrome and thereby may possibly mask the underlying disease process. The effect that symptomatic suppression has upon the long-term course of the syndrome is unknown.

Given these considerations, neuroleptics should be prescribed in a manner that is most likely to minimize the occurrence of tardive dyskinesia. Chronic neuroleptic treatment should generally be reserved for patients who suffer from a chronic illness that, 1) is known to respond to neuroleptic drugs, and 2) for whom alternative, equally effective, but potentially less harmful treatments are *not* available or appropriate. In patients who do require chronic treatment, the smallest dose and the shortest duration of treatment producing a satisfactory clinical response should be sought. The need for continued treatment should be reassessed periodically.

If signs and symptoms of tardive dyskinesia appear in a patient on neuroleptics, drug discontinuation should be considered. However, some patients may require treatment despite the presence of the syndrome.

(For further information about the description of tardive dyskinesia and its clinical detection, please refer to the section on Adverse Reactions.)

Neuroleptic Malignant Syndrome (NMS)
A potentially fatal symptom complex sometimes referred to as Neuroleptic Malignant Syndrome (NMS) has been reported in association with antipsychotic drugs. Clinical manifestations of NMS are hyperpyrexia, muscle rigidity, altered mental status and evidence of autonomic instability (irregular pulse or blood pressure, tachycardia, diaphoresis, and cardiac dysrhythmias).

The diagnostic evaluation of patients with this syndrome is complicated. In arriving at a diagnosis, it is important to identify cases where the clinical presentation includes both serious medical illness (e.g., pneumonia, systemic infection, etc.) and untreated or inadequately treated extrapyramidal signs and symptoms (EPS). Other important considerations in the differential diagnosis include central anticholinergic toxicity, heat stroke, drug fever and primary central nervous system (CNS) pathology.

The management of NMS should include, 1) immediate discontinuation of antipsychotic drugs and other drugs not essential to concurrent therapy, 2) intensive symptomatic treatment and medical monitoring, and 3) treatment of any concomitant serious medical problems for which specific treatments are available. There is no general agreement about specific pharmacological treatment regimens for uncomplicated NMS.

If a patient requires antipsychotic drug treatment after recovery from NMS, the potential reintroduction of drug therapy should be carefully considered. The patient should be carefully monitored, since recurrences of NMS have been reported.

Usage in Pregnancy: Studies in pregnant patients have not been carried out. Reproduction studies have been performed in the following animals:

Pregnant Rats oral dose—	
no adverse effect	20 mg/kg/day—10 days
no adverse effect	40 mg/kg/day—10 days
Pregnant Mice oral dose—	
slight increase resorptions	20 mg/kg/day—10 days
slight increase resorptions	40 mg/kg/day—10 days
Pregnant Rabbits oral dose—	
no adverse effect	5 mg/kg/day—12 days
no adverse effect	10 mg/kg/day—12 days
no adverse effect	20 mg/kg/day—12 days

Animal reproductive studies have not demonstrated a teratogenic potential. The anticipated benefits must be weighed against the unknown risks to the fetus if used in pregnant patients.

Nursing Mothers: Data are not available on the content of MOBAN (molindone hydrochloride) in the milk of nursing mothers:

Usage in Children: Use of MOBAN (molindone hydrochloride) in children below the age of twelve years is not recommended because safe and effective conditions for its usage have not been established.

MOBAN has not been shown effective in the management of behavioral complications in patients with mental retardation.

Sulfites Sensitivity: MOBAN Concentrate contains sodium metabisulfite, a sulfite that may cause allergic-type reactions including anaphylactic symptoms and life-threatening or less severe asthmatic episodes in certain susceptible people. The overall prevalence of sulfite sensitivity in the general population is unknown and probably low. Sulfite sensi-

tivity is seen more frequently in asthmatic than in nonasthmatic people.

PRECAUTIONS
Some patients receiving MOBAN (molindone hydrochloride) may note drowsiness initially and they should be advised against activities requiring mental alertness until their response to the drug has been established.

Increased activity has been noted in patients receiving MOBAN. Caution should be exercised where increased activity may be harmful.

MOBAN does not lower the seizure threshold in experimental animals to the degree noted with more sedating antipsychotic drugs. However, in humans convulsive seizures have been reported in a few instances.

The physician should be aware that this tablet preparation contains calcium sulfate as an excipient and that calcium ions may interfere with the absorption of preparations containing phenytoin sodium and tetracyclines.

MOBAN has an antiemetic effect in animals. A similar effect may occur in humans and may obscure signs of intestinal obstruction or brain tumor.

Neuroleptic drugs elevate prolactin levels; the elevation persists during chronic administration. Tissue culture experiments indicate that approximately one-third of human breast cancers are prolactin dependent in vitro, a factor of potential importance if the prescription of these drugs is contemplated in a patient with a previously detected breast cancer. Although disturbances such as galactorrhea, amenorrhea, gynecomastia, and impotence have been reported, the clinical significance of elevated serum prolactin levels is unknown for most patients. An increase in mammary neoplasms has been found in rodents after chronic administration of neuroleptic drugs. Neither clinical studies nor epidemiologic studies conducted to date, however, have shown an association between chronic administration of these drugs and mammary tumorigenesis; the available evidence is considered too limited to be conclusive at this time.

ADVERSE REACTIONS
CNS Effects
The most frequently occurring effect is initial drowsiness that generally subsides with continued usage of the drug or lowering of the dose.

Noted less frequently were depression, hyperactivity and euphoria.

Neurological
Extrapyramidal Reactions
Extrapyramidal reactions noted below may occur in susceptible individuals and are usually reversible with appropriate management.

Akathisia
Motor restlessness may occur early.

Parkinson Syndrome
Akinesia, characterized by rigidity, immobility and reduction of voluntary movements and tremor, have been observed. Occurrence is less frequent than akathisia.

Dystonic Syndrome
Prolonged abnormal contractions of muscle groups occur infrequently. These symptoms may be managed by the addition of a synthetic antiparkinson agent (other than L-dopa), small doses of sedative drugs, and/or reduction in dosage.

Tardive Dyskinesia
Neuroleptic drugs are known to cause a syndrome of dyskinetic movements commonly referred to as tardive dyskinesia. The movements may appear during treatment or upon withdrawal of treatment and may be either reversible or irreversible (i.e., persistent) upon cessation of further neuroleptic administration.

The syndrome is known to have a variable latency for development and the duration of the latency cannot be determined reliably. It is thus wise to assume that any neuroleptic agent has the capacity to induce the syndrome and act accordingly until sufficient data has been collected to settle the issue definitively for a specific drug product. In the case of neuroleptics known to produce the irreversible syndrome, the following has been observed:

Tardive dyskinesia has appeared in some patients on long-term therapy and has also appeared after drug therapy has been discontinued. The risk appears to be greater in elderly patients on high-dose therapy, especially females. The symptoms are persistent and in some patients appear to be irreversible. The syndrome is characterized by rhythmical involuntary movements of the tongue, face, mouth or jaw (e.g., protrusion of tongue, puffing of cheeks, puckering of mouth, chewing movements). There may be involuntary movements of extremities.

There is no known effective treatment of tardive dyskinesia; antiparkinsonism agents usually do not alleviate the symptoms of this syndrome. It is suggested that all antipsychotic agents be discontinued if these symptoms appear. Should it be necessary to reinstitute treatment, or increase the dosage of the agent, or switch to a different antipsychotic agent, the syndrome may be masked. It has been reported that fine vermicular movements of the tongue may be an early sign of

the syndrome and if the medication is stopped at that time the syndrome may not develop (See WARNINGS).

Autonomic Nervous System
Occasionally blurring of vision, tachycardia, nausea, dry mouth and salivation have been reported. Urinary retention and constipation may occur particularly if anticholinergic drugs are used to treat extrapyramidal symptoms. One patient being treated with MOBAN experienced priapism which required surgical intervention, apparently resulting in residual impairment of erectile function.

Laboratory Tests
There have been rare reports of leucopenia and leucocytosis. If such reactions occur, treatment with MOBAN may continue if clinical symptoms are absent. Alterations of blood glucose, B.U.N., and red blood cells have not been considered clinically significant.

Metabolic and Endocrine Effects
Alteration of thyroid function has not been significant. Amenorrhea has been reported infrequently. Resumption of menses in previously amenorrheic women has been reported. Initially heavy menses may occur. Galactorrhea and gynecomastia have been reported infrequently. Increase in libido has been noted in some patients. Impotence has not been reported. Although both weight gain and weight loss have been in the direction of normal or ideal weight, excessive weight gain has not occurred with MOBAN.

Hepatic Effects
There have been rare reports of clinically significant alterations in liver function in association with MOBAN use.

Cardiovascular
Rare, transient, non-specific T wave changes have been reported on E.K.G. Association with a clinical syndrome has not been established. Rarely has significant hypotension been reported.

Ophthalmological
Lens opacities and pigmentary retinopathy have not been reported where patients have received MOBAN (molindone hydrochloride). In some patients, phenothiazine induced lenticular opacities have resolved following discontinuation of the phenothiazine while continuing therapy with MOBAN.

Skin
Early, non-specific skin rash, probably of allergic origin, has occasionally been reported. Skin pigmentation has not been seen with MOBAN usage alone.

MOBAN (molindone hydrochloride) has certain pharmacological similarities to other antipsychotic agents. Because adverse reactions are often extensions of the pharmacological activity of a drug, all of the known pharmacological effects associated with other antipsychotic drugs should be kept in mind when MOBAN is used. Upon abrupt withdrawal after prolonged high dosage an abstinence syndrome has not been noted.

DOSAGE AND ADMINISTRATION
Initial and maintenance doses of MOBAN (molindone hydrochloride) should be individualized.

Initial Dosage Schedule
The usual starting dosage is 50-75 mg/day.
— Increase to 100 mg/day in 3 or 4 days.
— Based on severity of symptomatology, dosage may be titrated up or down depending on individual patient response.
— An increase to 225 mg/day may be required in patients with severe symptomatology.
Elderly and debilitated patients should be started on lower dosage.

Maintenance Dosage Schedule
1. Mild-5 mg-15 mg three or four times a day.
2. Moderate-10 mg-25 mg three or four times a day.
3. Severe-225 mg/day may be required.

DRUG INTERACTIONS
Potentiation of drugs administered concurrently with MOBAN (molindone hydrochloride) has not been reported. Additionally, animal studies have not shown increased toxicity when MOBAN is given concurrently with representative members of three classes of drugs (i.e., barbiturates, chloral hydrate and antiparkinson drugs).

MANAGEMENT OF OVERDOSAGE
Symptomatic, supportive therapy should be the rule.
Gastric lavage is indicated for the reduction of absorption of MOBAN (molindone hydrochloride) which is freely soluble in water.

Since the adsorption of MOBAN (molindone hydrochloride) by activated charcoal has not been determined, the use of this antidote must be considered of theoretical value.

Emesis in a comatose patient is contraindicated. Additionally, while the emetic effect of apomorphine is blocked by MOBAN in animals, this blocking effect has not been determined in humans.

A significant increase in the rate of removal of unmetabolized MOBAN from the body by forced diuresis, peritoneal or renal dialysis would not be expected. (Only 2% of a single

Continued on next page

Du Pont Pharm.—Cont.

ingested dose of MOBAN is excreted unmetabolized in the urine). However, poor response of the patient may justify use of these procedures.

While the use of laxatives or enemas might be based on general principles, the amount of unmetabolized MOBAN in feces is less than 1%. Extrapyramidal symptoms have responded to the use of diphenhydramine (Benadryl*), Amantadine HCl (Symmetrel®) and the synthetic anticholinergic antiparkinson agents, (i.e., Artane*, Cogentin*, Akineton*).

HOW SUPPLIED

As tablets in bottles of 100 with potencies and colors as follows:

5 mg orange	NDC 0056-0072-70
10 mg lavender	NDC 0056-0073-70
25 mg light green	NDC 0056-0074-70
50 mg blue	NDC 0056-0076-70
100 mg tan	NDC 0056-0077-70

As a concentrate containing 20 mg molindone hydrochloride per ml in 4 oz. (120 ml) bottles, NDC 0056-0460-04.
Store at controlled room temperature (59°–86°F, 15°–30°C).
* Benadryl-Trademark, Parke-Davis and Co.
* Artane-Trademark, Lederle Laboratories
* Cogentin-Trademark, Merck Sharp & Dohme
* Akineton-Trademark, Knoll Pharmaceutical Co.
* Symmetrel-Trademark of E. I. du Pont de Nemours & Co. (Inc.)
MOBAN® is a registered U.S. Trademark of E.I. du Pont de Nemours & Co. (Inc.)

6145-11 Feb. 1989

Shown in Product Identification Section, page 409

NARCAN® INJECTION   ℞
[nar'kan]
(naloxone hydrochloride)
Narcotic Antagonist

DESCRIPTION

NARCAN (naloxone hydrochloride), a narcotic antagonist, is a synthetic congener of oxymorphone. In structure it differs from oxymorphone in that the methyl group on the nitrogen atom is replaced by an allyl group.
Naloxone hydrochloride occurs as a white to slightly off-white powder, and is soluble in water, in dilute acids, and in strong alkali; slightly soluble in alcohol; practically insoluble in ether and in chloroform.
NARCAN injection is available as a sterile solution for intravenous, intramuscular and subcutaneous administration in three concentrations, 0.02 mg, 0.4 mg and 1.0 mg of naloxone hydrochloride per ml. One ml of the 0.02 mg and 0.4 mg strengths contains 8.6 mg of sodium chloride. One ml of the 1.0 mg strength contains 8.35 mg of sodium chloride. One ml of all strengths also contains 2.0 mg of methylparaben and propylparaben as preservatives in a ratio of 9 to 1. pH is adjusted to 3.5 ± 0.5 with hydrochloric acid.
NARCAN injection is also available in a paraben-free formulation in two concentrations: 0.02 mg and 0.4 mg of naloxone hydrochloride per ml. One ml of each strength contains 9.0 mg of sodium chloride. pH is adjusted to 3.5 ± 0.5 with hydrochloric acid.

CLINICAL PHARMACOLOGY

NARCAN (naloxone hydrochloride) prevents or reverses the effects of opioids including respiratory depression, sedation and hypotension. Also, it can reverse the psychotomimetic and dysphoric effects of agonist-antagonists such as pentazocine.
NARCAN (naloxone hydrochloride) is an essentially pure narcotic antagonist, i.e., it does not possess the "agonistic" or morphine-like properties characteristic of other narcotic antagonists; NARCAN does not produce respiratory depression, psychotomimetic effects or pupillary constriction. In the absence of narcotics or agonistic effects of other narcotic antagonists it exhibits essentially no pharmacologic activity. NARCAN has not been shown to produce tolerance nor to cause physical or psychological dependence.
In the presence of physical dependence on narcotics NARCAN will produce withdrawal symptoms.
Mechanisms of Action: While the mechanism of action of NARCAN is not fully understood, the preponderance of evidence suggests that NARCAN antagonizes the opioid effects by competing for the same receptor sites.
When NARCAN is administered intravenously the onset of action is generally apparent within two minutes; the onset of action is only slightly less rapid when it is administered subcutaneously or intramuscularly. The duration of action is dependent upon the dose and route of administration of NARCAN. Intramuscular administration produces a more prolonged effect than intravenous administration. The requirement for repeat doses of NARCAN, however, will also be dependent upon the amount, type and route of administration of the narcotic being antagonized.

Following parenteral administration NARCAN is rapidly distributed in the body. It is metabolized in the liver, primarily by glucuronide conjugation and excreted in urine. In one study the serum half-life in adults ranged from 30 to 81 minutes (mean 64 ± 12 minutes). In a neonatal study the mean plasma half-life was observed to be 3.1 ± 0.5 hours.

INDICATIONS AND USAGE

NARCAN is indicated for the complete or partial reversal of narcotic depression, including respiratory depression, induced by opioids including natural and synthetic narcotics, propoxyphene, methadone and certain narcotic-antagonist analgesics: nalbuphine, pentazocine and butorphanol. NARCAN is also indicated for the diagnosis of suspected acute opioid overdosage.

CONTRAINDICATIONS

NARCAN is contraindicated in patients known to be hypersensitive to it.

WARNINGS

NARCAN should be administered cautiously to persons including newborns of mothers who are known or suspected to be physically dependent on opioids. In such cases an abrupt and complete reversal of narcotic effects may precipitate an acute abstinence syndrome.
The patient who has satisfactorily responded to NARCAN should be kept under continued surveillance and repeated doses of NARCAN should be administered, as necessary, since the duration of action of some narcotics may exceed that of NARCAN.
NARCAN is not effective against respiratory depression due to non-opioid drugs. Reversal of buprenorphine-induced respiratory depression may be incomplete. If an incomplete response occurs, respirations should be mechanically assisted.

PRECAUTIONS

In addition to NARCAN, other resuscitative measures such as maintenance of a free airway, artificial ventilation, cardiac massage, and vasopressor agents should be available and employed when necessary to counteract acute narcotic poisoning.
Several instances of hypotension, hypertension, ventricular tachycardia and fibrillation, and pulmonary edema have been reported. These have occurred in postoperative patients most of whom had pre-existing cardiovascular disorders or received other drugs which may have similar adverse cardiovascular effects. Although a direct cause and effect relationship has not been established, NARCAN should be used with caution in patients with pre-existing cardiac disease or patients who have received potentially cardiotoxic drugs.
Carcinogenesis, Mutagenesis, Impairment of Fertility: Carcinogenicity and mutagenicity studies have not been performed with NARCAN. Reproductive studies in mice and rats demonstrated no impairment of fertility.
Use in Pregnancy: Pregnancy Catagory B: Reproduction studies performed in mice and rats at doses up to 1,000 times the human dose, revealed no evidence of impaired fertility or harm to the fetus due to NARCAN. There are, however, no adequate and well controlled studies in pregnant women. Because animal reproduction studies are not always predictive of human response, NARCAN should be used during pregnancy only if clearly needed.
Nursing Mothers: It is not known whether NARCAN is excreted in human milk. Because many drugs are excreted in human milk, caution should be exercised when NARCAN is administered to a nursing woman.

ADVERSE REACTIONS

Abrupt reversal of narcotic depression may result in nausea, vomiting, sweating, tachycardia, increased blood pressure, tremulousness, seizures and cardiac arrest. In postoperative patients, larger than necessary dosage of NARCAN may result in significant reversal of analgesia, and in excitement. Hypotension, hypertension, ventricular tachycardia and fibrillation, and pulmonary edema have been associated with the use of NARCAN postoperatively (see PRECAUTIONS & USAGE IN ADULTS-POSTOPERATIVE NARCOTIC DEPRESSION).

OVERDOSAGE

There is no clinical experience with NARCAN overdosage in humans.
In the mouse and rat the intravenous LD_{50} is 150 ± 5 mg/kg and 109 ± 4 mg/kg respectively. In acute subcutaneous toxicity studies in newborn rats the LD_{50} (95% CL) is 260 (228-296) mg/kg. Subcutaneous injection of 100 mg/kg/day in rats for 3 weeks produced only transient salivation and partial ptosis following injection: no toxic effects were seen at 10 mg/kg/day for 3 weeks.

DOSAGE AND ADMINISTRATION

NARCAN (naloxone hydrochloride) may be administered intravenously, intramuscularly, or subcutaneously. The most rapid onset of action is achieved by intravenous administration and it is recommended in emergency situations. Since the duration of action of some narcotics may exceed that of NARCAN the patient should be kept under continued

surveillance and repeated doses of NARCAN should be administered, as necessary.
Intravenous Infusion: NARCAN may be diluted for intravenous infusion in normal saline or 5% dextrose solutions. The addition of 2 mg of NARCAN in 500 ml of either solution provides a concentration of 0.004 mg/ml. Mixtures should be used within 24 hours. After 24 hours, the remaining unused solution must be discarded. The rate of administration should be titrated in accordance with the patient's response. Parenteral drug products should be inspected visually for particulate matter and discoloration prior to administration whenever solution and container permit. NARCAN should not be mixed with preparations containing bisulfite, metabisulfite, long-chain or high molecular weight anions, or any solution having an alkaline pH. No drug or chemical agent should be added to NARCAN unless its effect on the chemical and physical stability of the solution has first been established.

USAGE IN ADULTS

Narcotic Overdose—Known or Suspected: An initial dose of 0.4 mg to 2 mg of NARCAN may be administered intravenously. If the desired degree of counteraction and improvement in respiratory functions is not obtained, it may be repeated at 2 to 3 minute intervals. If no response is observed after 10 mg of NARCAN have been administered, the diagnosis of narcotic induced or partial narcotic induced toxicity should be questioned. Intramuscular or subcutaneous administration may be necessary if the intravenous route is not available.
Postoperative Narcotic Depression: For the partial reversal of narcotic depression following the use of narcotics during surgery, smaller doses of NARCAN are usually sufficient. The dose of NARCAN should be titrated according to the patient's response. For the initial reversal of respiratory depression, NARCAN should be injected in increments of 0.1 to 0.2 mg intravenously at two to three minute intervals to the desired degree of reversal i.e. adequate ventilation and alertness without significant pain or discomfort. Larger than necessary dosage of NARCAN may result in significant reversal of analgesia and increase in blood pressure. Similarly, too rapid reversal may induce nausea, vomiting, sweating or circulatory stress.
Repeat doses of NARCAN may be required within one to two hour intervals depending upon the amount, type (i.e., short or long acting) and time interval since last administration of narcotic. Supplemental intramuscular doses have been shown to produce a longer lasting effect.

USAGE IN CHILDREN

Narcotic Overdose—Known or Suspected: The usual initial dose in children is 0.01 mg/kg body weight given I.V. If this dose does not result in the desired degree of clinical improvement, a subsequent dose of 0.1 mg/kg body weight may be administered. If an I.V. route of administration is not available, NARCAN may be administered I.M. or S.C. in divided doses. If necessary, NARCAN can be diluted with sterile water for injection.
Postoperative Narcotic Depression: Follow the recommendations and cautions under **Adult Postoperative Depression.** For the initial reversal of respiratory depression NARCAN should be injected in increments of 0.005 mg to 0.01 mg intravenously at two to three minute intervals to the desired degree of reversal.

USAGE IN NEONATES

Narcotic-Induced Depression: The usual initial dose is 0.01 mg/kg body weight administered I.V., I.M., or S.C. This dose may be repeated in accordance with adult administration guidelines for postoperative narcotic depression.

HOW SUPPLIED

NARCAN (naloxone hydrochloride) for intravenous, intramuscular and subcutaneous administration is available as:

0.4 mg/ml	1 ml ampul-box of 10	NDC 0590-0365-10
	1 ml disposable prefilled syringe-box of 10	NDC 0590-0365-15
	10 ml vial-box of 1	NDC 0590-0365-05
0.4 mg/ml		
(paraben-free)	1 ml ampul-box of 10	NDC 0590-0358-10
1.0 mg/ml	2 ml ampul-box of 10	NDC 0590-0368-10
1.0 mg/ml	10 ml vial-box of 1	NDC 0590-0368-05
1.0 mg/ml	1 ml disposable prefilled syringe-box of 10	NDC 0590-0368-15
1.0 mg/ml	2 ml disposable prefilled syringe-box of 10	NDC 0590-0368-13
1.0 mg/ml		
(paraben-free)	2 ml ampul-box of 10	NDC 0590-0377-10
0.02 mg/ml	2 ml ampul-box of 10	NDC 0590-0367-10
0.02 mg/ml		
(paraben-free)	2 ml ampul-box of 10	NDC 0590-0359-10

Store at controlled room temperature (59°–86°F, 15°–30°C).
NARCAN® is a Registered U.S. Trademark of Du Pont Pharmaceuticals, Inc.   6108-10 Feb. 1989

Shown in Product Identification Section, page 409

NUBAIN®   ℞
[nū'bān]
(nalbuphine hydrochloride)

DESCRIPTION

NUBAIN® (nalbuphine hydrochloride) is a synthetic narcotic agonist-antagonist analgesic of the phenanthrene series. It is chemically related to both the widely used narcotic antagonist, naloxone, and the potent narcotic analgesic, oxymorphone.

NALBUPHINE HYDROCHLORIDE

Nalbuphine hydrochloride is (-)-17-(cyclobutylmethyl)-4, 5α-epoxymorphinan-3,6α, 14-triol, hydrochloride.

NUBAIN® is available in two concentrations, 10 mg and 20 mg of nalbuphine hydrochloride per ml. Both strengths contain 0.94% sodium citrate hydrous, 1.26% citric acid anhydrous, 0.1% sodium metabisulfite, and 0.2% of a 9:1 mixture of methylparaben and propylparaben as preservatives; pH is adjusted, if necessary, with hydrochloric acid. The 10 mg/ml strength contains 0.1% sodium chloride.

NUBAIN is also available in a sulfite and paraben-free formulation in two concentrations, 10 mg and 20 mg of nalbuphine hydrochloride per ml. One ml of each strength contains 0.94% sodium citrate hydrous, 1.26% citric acid anhydrous; pH is adjusted, if necessary, with hydrochloric acid. The 10 mg/ml strength contains 0.2% sodium chloride.

ACTIONS

NUBAIN is a potent analgesic. Its analgesic potency is essentially equivalent to that of morphine on a milligram basis. Its onset of action occurs within 2 to 3 minutes after intravenous administration, and in less than 15 minutes following subcutaneous or intramuscular injection. The plasma half-life of nalbuphine is 5 hours and in clinical studies the duration of analgesic activity has been reported to range from 3 to 6 hours.

The narcotic antagonist activity of NUBAIN is one-fourth as potent as nalorphine and 10 times that of pentazocine.

INDICATIONS

NUBAIN (nalbuphine hydrochloride) is indicated for the relief of moderate to severe pain. NUBAIN can also be used as a supplement to balanced anesthesia, for preoperative and postoperative analgesia, and for obstetrical analgesia during labor and delivery.

CONTRAINDICATIONS

NUBAIN should not be administered to patients who are hypersensitive to it.

WARNINGS

NUBAIN should be administered as a supplement to general anesthesia only by persons specifically trained in the use of intravenous anesthetics and management of the respiratory effects of potent opioids.

Naloxone, resuscitative and intubation equipment and oxygen should be readily available.

Drug Dependence NUBAIN has been shown to have a low abuse potential. When compared with drugs which are not mixed agonist-antagonists, it has been reported that nalbuphine's potential for abuse would be less than that of codeine and propoxyphene. Psychological and physical dependence and tolerance may follow the abuse or misuse of nalbuphine. Therefore, caution should be observed in prescribing it for emotionally unstable patients, or for individuals with a history of narcotic abuse. Such patients should be closely supervised when long-term therapy is contemplated.

Care should be taken to avoid increases in dosage or frequency of administration which in susceptible individuals might result in physical dependence.

Abrupt discontinuation of NUBAIN following prolonged use has been followed by symptoms of narcotic withdrawal, i.e., abdominal cramps, nausea and vomiting, rhinorrhea, lacrimation, restlessness, anxiety, elevated temperature and piloerection.

Use in Ambulatory Patients NUBAIN may impair the mental or physical abilities required for the performance of potentially dangerous tasks such as driving a car or operating machinery. Therefore, NUBAIN should be administered with caution to ambulatory patients who should be warned to avoid such hazards.

Use in Emergency Procedures Maintain patient under observation until recovered from NUBAIN effects that would affect driving or other potentially dangerous tasks.

Use in Children Clinical experience to support administration to patients under 18 years is not available at present.

Use in Pregnancy (other than labor) Safe use of NUBAIN in pregnancy has not been established. Although animal reproductive studies have not revealed teratogenic or embryotoxic effects, nalbuphine should only be administered to pregnant women when, in the judgment of the physician, the potential benefits outweigh the possible hazards.

Use During Labor and Delivery NUBAIN can produce respiratory depression in the neonate. It should be used with caution in women delivering premature infants.

Head Injury and Increased Intracranial Pressure The possible respiratory depressant effects and the potential of potent analgesics to elevate cerebrospinal fluid pressure (resulting from vasodilation following CO_2 retention) may be markedly exaggerated in the presence of head injury, intracranial lesions or a pre-existing increase in intracranial pressure. Furthermore, potent analgesics can produce effects which may obscure the clinical course of patients with head injuries. Therefore, NUBAIN should be used in these circumstances only when essential, and then should be administered with extreme caution.

Interaction With Other Central Nervous System Depressants Although NUBAIN possesses narcotic antagonist activity, there is evidence that in nondependent patients it will not antagonize a narcotic analgesic administered just before, concurrently, or just after an injection of NUBAIN. Therefore, patients receiving a narcotic analgesic, general anesthetics, phenothiazines, or other tranquilizers, sedatives, hypnotics, or other CNS depressants (including alcohol) concomitantly with NUBAIN may exhibit an additive effect. When such combined therapy is contemplated, the dose of one or both agents should be reduced.

Sulfites Sensitivity: NUBAIN contains sodium metabisulfite, a sulfite that may cause allergic-type reactions including anaphylactic symptoms and life-threatening or less severe asthmatic episodes in certain susceptible people. The overall prevalence of sulfite sensitivity in the general population is unknown and probably low. Sulfite sensitivity is seen more frequently in asthmatic than in nonasthmatic people.

PRECAUTIONS

Impaired Respiration At the usual adult dose of 10 mg/70 kg, NUBAIN causes some respiratory depression approximately equal to that produced by equal doses of morphine. However, in contrast to morphine, respiratory depression is not appreciably increased with higher doses of NUBAIN. Respiratory depression induced by NUBAIN can be reversed by NARCAN® (naloxone hydrochloride) when indicated. NUBAIN should be administered with caution at low doses to patients with impaired respiration (e.g., from other medication, uremia, bronchial asthma, severe infection, cyanosis or respiratory obstructions).

Impaired Renal or Hepatic Function Because NUBAIN is metabolized in the liver and excreted by the kidneys, patients with renal or liver dysfunction may over-react to customary doses. Therefore, in these individuals, NUBAIN should be used with caution and administered in reduced amounts.

Myocardial Infarction As with all potent analgesics, NUBAIN should be used with caution in patients with myocardial infarction who have nausea or vomiting.

Biliary Tract Surgery As with all narcotic analgesics, NUBAIN should be used with caution in patients about to undergo surgery of the biliary tract since it may cause spasm of the sphincter of Oddi.

Cardiovascular System During evaluation of NUBAIN in anesthesia, a higher incidence of bradycardia has been reported in patients who did not receive atropine pre-operatively or in the pre-operative period.

ADVERSE REACTIONS

The most frequent adverse reaction in 1066 patients treated with NUBAIN is sedation 381(36%).

Less frequent reactions are: sweaty/clammy 99(9%), nausea/vomiting 68(6%), dizziness/ vertigo 58(5%), dry mouth 44(4%), and headache 27(3%).

Other adverse reactions which may occur (reported incidence of 1% or less) are:

CNS Effects Nervousness, depression, restlessness, crying, euphoria, floating, hostility, unusual dreams, confusion, faintness, hallucinations, dysphoria, feeling of heaviness, numbness, tingling, unreality. The incidence of psychotomimetic effects, such as unreality, depersonalization, delusions, dysphoria and hallucinations has been shown to be less than that which occurs with pentazocine.

Cardiovascular Hypertension, hypotension, bradycardia, tachycardia, pulmonary edema.

Gastrointestinal Cramps, dyspepsia, bitter taste.

Respiration Depression, dyspnea, asthma.

Dermatological Itching, burning, urticaria.

Miscellaneous Speech difficulty, urinary urgency, blurred vision, flushing and warmth.

DOSAGE AND ADMINISTRATION

The usual recommended adult dose is 10 mg for a 70 kg individual, administered subcutaneously, intramuscularly or intravenously; this dose may be repeated every 3 to 6 hours as necessary. Dosage should be adjusted according to the severity of the pain, physical status of the patient, and other medications which the patient may be receiving. (See Interaction with Other Central Nervous System Depressants under WARNINGS). In non-tolerant individuals, the recommended single maximum dose is 20 mg, with a maximum total daily dose of 160 mg.

The use of NUBAIN as a supplement to balanced anesthesia requires larger doses than those recommended for analgesia. Induction doses of NUBAIN range from 0.3 mg/kg to 3.0 mg/kg intravenously to be administered over a 10 to 15 minute period with maintenance doses of 0.25 to 0.50 mg/kg in single intravenous administrations as required. The use of NUBAIN may be followed by respiratory depression which can be reversed with the narcotic antagonist NARCAN® (naloxone hydrochloride).

Patients Dependent on Narcotics Patients who have been taking narcotics chronically may experience withdrawal symptoms upon the administration of NUBAIN. If unduly troublesome, narcotic withdrawal symptoms can be controlled by the slow intravenous administration of small increments of morphine, until relief occurs. If the previous analgesic was morphine, meperidine, codeine, or other narcotic with similar duration of activity, one-fourth of the anticipated dose of NUBAIN can be administered initially and the patient observed for signs of withdrawal, i.e., abdominal cramps, nausea and vomiting, lacrimation, rhinorrhea, anxiety, restlessness, elevation of temperature or piloerection. If untoward symptoms do not occur, progressively larger doses may be tried at appropriate intervals until the desired level of analgesia is obtained with NUBAIN.

Management of Overdosage The immediate intravenous administration of NARCAN® (naloxone hydrochloride) is a specific antidote. Oxygen, intravenous fluids, vasopressors and other supportive measures should be used as indicated. The administration of single doses of 72 mg of NUBAIN subcutaneously to eight normal subjects has been reported to have resulted primarily in symptoms of sleepiness and mild dysphoria.

HOW SUPPLIED

NUBAIN® (nalbuphine hydrochloride) injection for intramuscular, subcutaneous, or intravenous use is available in:
NDC 0590-0385-10
   10 mg/ml, 1 ml ampuls (box of 10)
NDC 0590-0386-01
   10 mg/ml, 10 ml vials (box of 1)
NDC 0590-0395-10
   (sulfite/paraben-free) 10 mg/ml, 1 ml ampuls (box of 10)
NDC 0590-0396-10
   20 mg/ml, 1 ml ampuls (box of 10)
NDC 0590-0396-15
   20 mg/ml, 1 ml disposable pre-filled syringes (box of 10)
NDC 0590-0399-01
   20 mg/ml, 10 ml vials (box of 1)
NDC 0590-0398-10
   (sulfite/paraben-free) 20 mg/ml, 1 ml ampuls (box of 10)
Also available in Military Depot:
10 mg/ml, 1 ml box of 10
   NSN 6505-01-115-9852
10 mg/ml, 10 ml box of 1
   NSN 6505-01-117-9690
Store At Controlled Room Temperature (59°–86°F, 15°–30°C).
NUBAIN® is a Registered U.S. Trademark of E.I. du Pont de Nemours & Co. (Inc.)
NARCAN® is a Registered U.S. Trademark of DuPont Pharmaceuticals, Inc.
6109-10   Rev. March 1989

Shown in Product Identification Section, page 409

NUMORPHAN®   Ⓒ
[nū-mor'fan]
(oxymorphone hydrochloride)
injection

DESCRIPTION

NUMORPHAN® (oxymorphone hydrochloride), a semisynthetic narcotic substitute for morphine, is a potent analgesic.

Oxymorphone hydrochloride is 4,5α-Epoxy-3, 14-dihydroxy-17-methylmorphinan-6-one hydrochloride.

Oxymorphone hydrochloride occurs as a white or slightly off-white, odorless powder, sparingly soluble in alcohol and ether, but freely soluble in water.

NUMORPHAN injection is available in two concentrations, 1 mg and 1.5 mg of oxymorphone hydrochloride per ml. Both strengths contain sodium chloride 0.8% with methylparaben 0.18%, propylparaben 0.02% and sodium dithionite 0.1%, as preservatives. pH is adjusted with sodium hydroxide.

ACTIONS

NUMORPHAN (oxymorphone hydrochloride) is a potent narcotic analgesic. Administered parenterally, 1 mg of

Continued on next page

Du Pont Pharm.—Cont.

NUMORPHAN is approximately equivalent in analgesic activity to 10 mg of morphine sulfate.

The onset of action is rapid; initial effects are usually perceived within 5 to 10 minutes. Its duration of action is approximately 3 to 6 hours.

NUMORPHAN produces mild sedation and causes little depression of the cough reflex. These properties make it particularly useful in postoperative patients.

INDICATIONS

NUMORPHAN (oxymorphone hydrochloride) is indicated for the relief of moderate to severe pain. This drug is also indicated parenterally for preoperative medication, for support of anesthesia, for obstetrical analgesia, and for relief of anxiety in patients with dyspnea associated with acute left ventricular failure and pulmonary edema.

CONTRAINDICATIONS

Safe use of NUMORPHAN (oxymorphone hydrochloride) in children under 12 years of age has not been established. This drug should not be used in patients known to be hypersensitive to morphine analogs.

WARNINGS

May be habit forming. As with other narcotic drugs, tolerance and addiction may develop. The addicting potential of the drug appears to be about the same as for morphine. Like other narcotic-containing medications, NUMORPHAN is subject to the Federal Controlled Substances Act.

Interaction with other central nervous system depressants: Patients receiving other narcotic analgesics, general anesthetics, phenothiazines, other tranquilizers, sedatives, hypnotics or other CNS depressants (including alcohol) concomitantly with NUMORPHAN may exhibit an additive CNS depression. When such combined therapy is contemplated, the dose of one or both agents should be reduced.

Safe use in pregnancy has not been established (relative to possible adverse effects on fetal development). As with other analgesics, the use of NUMORPHAN (oxymorphone hydrochloride) in pregnancy, in nursing mothers, or in women of child-bearing potential requires that the possible benefits of the drug be weighed against the possible hazards to the mother and the child.

Sulfites Sensitivity: NUMORPHAN contains sodium dithionite, a sulfite that may cause allergic-type reactions including anaphylactic symptoms and life-threatening or less severe asthmatic episodes in certain susceptible people. The overall prevalence of sulfite sensitivity in the general population is unknown and probably low. Sulfite sensitivity is seen more frequently in asthmatic than in nonasthmatic people.

PRECAUTIONS

The same care and caution should be taken when administering NUMORPHAN (oxymorphone hydrochloride) as when other potent narcotic analgesics are used. It should be borne in mind that some respiratory depression may occur as with all potent narcotics especially when other analgesic and/or anesthetic drugs with depressant action have been given shortly before administration of NUMORPHAN.

The respiratory depressant effects of narcotics and their capacity to elevate cerebrospinal fluid pressure may be markedly exaggerated in the presence of head injury, other intracranial lesions or a pre-existing increase in intracranial pressure. Furthermore narcotics produce adverse reactions which may obscure the clinical course of patients with head injuries.

As with other analgesics, caution must also be exercised in elderly and debilitated patients and in patients who are known to be sensitive to central nervous system depressants, such as those with cardiovascular, pulmonary, or hepatic disease, in hypothyroidism (myxedema), acute alcoholism, delirium tremens, convulsive disorders, bronchial asthma and kyphoscoliosis. Debilitated and elderly patients and those with severe liver diseases should receive smaller doses of NUMORPHAN (oxymorphone hydrochloride).

ADVERSE REACTIONS

As with all potent narcotic analgesics, possible side effects include drowsiness, nausea, vomiting, miosis, itching, dysphoria, light-headedness, and headache. Respiratory depression may occur with oxymorphone as with other narcotics.

DOSAGE AND ADMINISTRATION

Usual Adult Dosage of NUMORPHAN (oxymorphone hydrochloride) Injection: Subcutaneous or intramuscular administration: initially 1 mg to 1.5 mg, repeated every 4 to 6 hours as needed. Intravenous: 0.5 mg initially. In nondebilitated patients the dose can be cautiously increased until satisfactory pain relief is obtained. For analgesia during labor 0.5 mg to 1 mg intramuscularly is recommended.

MANAGEMENT OF OVERDOSAGE

Signs Pond Symptoms: Serious overdosage with NUMORPHAN is characterized by respiratory depression (a decrease in respiratory rate and/or tidal volume, Cheyne-Stokes res-

piration, cyanosis), extreme somnolence progressing to stupor or coma, skeletal muscle flaccidity, cold and clammy skin, and sometimes bradycardia and hypotension. In severe overdosage, apnea, circulatory collapse, cardiac arrest and death may occur.

Treatment: Primary attention should be given to the reestablishment of adequate respiratory exchange through provision of a patent airway and the institution of assisted or controlled ventilation. The narcotic antagonist naloxone hydrochloride (NARCAN®) is a specific antidote against respiratory depression which may result from overdosage or unusual sensitivity to narcotics including oxymorphone. Therefore, an appropriate dose of naloxone hydrochloride should be administered (usual initial adult dose: 0.4–2 mg) preferably by the intravenous route and simultaneously with efforts at respiratory resuscitation. Since the duration of action of oxymorphone may exceed that of the antagonist, the patient should be kept under continued surveillance and repeated doses of the antagonist should be administered as needed to maintain adequate respiration.

Oxygen, intravenous fluids, vasopressors and other supportive measures should be employed as indicated.

HOW SUPPLIED

For Injection: DEA Order Form Required
1 mg/ml 1 ml ampuls (box of 10)
  NDC 0590-0370-10
1.5 mg/ml 1 ml ampuls (box of 10)
  NDC 0590-0373-10
10 ml multiple dose vial (box of 1)
  NDC 0590-0374-01
Store at controlled room temperature (59°–86°F, 15°–30°C). Protect from excessive light.

Numorphan® is a Registered U.S. Trademark of E.I. du Pont de Nemours & Co. (Inc.)

NARCAN® is a Registered U.S. Trademark of DuPont Pharmaceuticals, Inc.

6110-4 Jan 1989

NUMORPHAN®   C⅟ ℞
(oxymorphone hydrochloride)
RECTAL SUPPOSITORIES
Narcotic
Analgesic

DESCRIPTION

NUMORPHAN (oxymorphone hydrochloride), a semi-synthetic narcotic substitute for morphine, is a potent analgesic. Oxymorphone hydrochloride occurs as a white or slightly off-white, odorless powder, sparingly soluble in alcohol and ether, but freely soluble in water.

The NUMORPHAN rectal suppository is available in a concentration of 5 mg of oxymorphone hydrochloride in a base consisting of polyethylene glycol 1000 and polyethylene glycol 3350.

ACTIONS

NUMORPHAN (oxymorphone hydrochloride) is a potent narcotic analgesic. Administered parenterally, 1 mg of NUMORPHAN is approximately equivalent in analgesic activity to 10 mg of morphine sulfate.

The onset of action of parenterally administered NUMORPHAN is rapid; initial effects are usually perceived within 5 to 10 minutes. Its duration of action is approximately 3 to 6 hours.

NUMORPHAN produces mild sedation and causes little depression of the cough reflex. These properties make it particularly useful in postoperative patients.

INDICATIONS

For the relief of moderate to severe pain.

CONTRAINDICATIONS

Safe use of NUMORPHAN (oxymorphone hydrochloride) in children under 12 years of age has not been established. This drug should not be used in patients known to be hypersensitive to morphine analogs.

WARNINGS

May be habit forming. As with other narcotic drugs, tolerance and addiction may develop. The addicting potential of the drug appears to be about the same as for morphine. Like other narcotic-containing medications, NUMORPHAN is subject to the Federal Controlled Substances Act.

Interaction with other central nervous system depressants: Patients receiving other narcotic analgesics, general anesthetics, phenothiazines, other tranquilizers, sedatives, hypnotics or other CNS depressants (including alcohol) concomitantly with NUMORPHAN may exhibit an additive CNS depression. When such combined therapy is contemplated, the dose of one or both agents should be reduced.

Safe use in pregnancy has not been established (relative to possible adverse effects on fetal development). As with other potent analgesics the use of NUMORPHAN (oxymorphone hydrochloride) in pregnancy, in nursing mothers, or in women of child-bearing potential requires that the possible

benefits of the drug be weighed against the possible hazards to the mother and child.

PRECAUTIONS

The same care and caution should be taken when administering NUMORPHAN (oxymorphone hydrochloride) as when other potent narcotic analgesics are used. It should be borne in mind that some respiratory depression may occur as with all potent narcotics especially when other analgesic and/or anesthetic drugs with depressant action have been given shortly before administration of NUMORPHAN.

The respiratory depressant effects of narcotics and their capacity to elevate cerebrospinal fluid pressure may be markedly exaggerated in the presence of head injury, other intracranial lesions or a pre-existing increase in intracranial pressure. Furthermore, narcotics produce adverse reactions which may obscure the clinical course of patients with head injuries.

As with other analgesics, caution must also be exercised in elderly and debilitated patients and in patients who are known to be sensitive to central nervous system depressants, such as those with cardiovascular, pulmonary, or hepatic disease, in hypothyroidism (myxedema), acute alcoholism, delirium tremens, convulsive disorders, bronchial asthma and kyphoscoliosis. Debilitated and elderly patients and those with severe liver diseases should receive smaller doses of NUMORPHAN.

ADVERSE REACTIONS

As with all potent narcotic analgesics, possible side effects include drowsiness, nausea, vomiting, miosis, itching, dysphoria, light-headedness, and headache. Respiratory depression may occur with oxymorphone as with other narcotics.

DOSAGE AND ADMINISTRATION

Usual Adult Dosage of NUMORPHAN (oxymorphone hydrochloride) Rectal Suppositories: One suppository, 5 mg, every 4 to 6 hours. In nondebilitated patients the dose can be cautiously increased until satisfactory pain relief is obtained.

MANAGEMENT OF OVERDOSAGE

Signs and Symptoms: Serious overdosage with NUMORPHAN is characterized by respiratory depression, (a decrease in respiratory rate and/or tidal volume, Cheyne-Stokes respiration, cyanosis), extreme somnolence progressing to stupor or coma, skeletal muscle flaccidity, cold and clammy skin, and sometimes bradycardia and hypotension. In severe overdosage, apnea, circulatory collapse, cardiac arrest and death may occur.

Treatment: Primary attention should be given to the reestablishment of adequate respiratory exchange through provision of a patent airway and the institution of assisted or controlled ventilation. The narcotic antagonist naloxone hydrochloride (NARCAN®) is a specific antidote against respiratory depression which may result from overdosage or unusual sensitivity to narcotics including oxymorphone. Therefore, an appropriate dose of naloxone hydrochloride should be administered (usual initial adult dose: 0.4 mg-2 mg) preferably by the intravenous route and simultaneously with efforts at respiratory resuscitation. Since the duration of action of oxymorphone may exceed that of the antagonist, the patient should be kept under continued surveillance and repeated doses of the antagonist should be administered as needed to maintain adequate respiration.

Oxygen, intravenous fluids, vasopressors and other supportive measures should be employed as indicated.

HOW SUPPLIED

Rectal Suppositories: DEA Order Form Required
5 mg, wrapped in gold foil, box of 6
Store under refrigeration (36°–46°F, 2°–8°C).

NUMORPHAN® is a Registered U.S. Trademark of E.I. du Pont de Nemours & Co. (Inc.)

NARCAN® is a Registered U.S. Trademark of Du Pont Pharmaceuticals, Inc.

6111-2/Rev. July, 1985

Shown in Product Identification Section, page 409

PENTASPAN®   ℞
(10% pentastarch in 0.9% sodium chloride injection)

DESCRIPTION

PENTASPAN (10% pentastarch in 0.9% sodium chloride injection) is a sterile, nonpyrogenic solution. The composition of each 100 mL is as follows:

Pentastarch .... 10.0 g
Sodium Chloride USP .... 0.9 g
Water for Injection USP .... qs
pH adjusted with Sodium Hydroxide
Concentration of Electrolytes (mEq/Liter): Sodium 154, Chloride 154
pH: Approx. 5.0; Calculated osmolarity: Approx. 326 mOsM

Pentastarch is an artificial colloid derived from a waxy starch composed almost entirely of amylopectin. Hydroxyethyl ether groups are introduced into the glucose units of the starch and the resultant material is hydrolyzed to yield a product with a molecular weight suitable for use as an erythrocyte sedimenting agent. Pentastarch is characterized by its molar substitution, and also by its molecular weight. The degree of substitution is 0.45 which means pentastarch has 45 hydroxyethyl groups for every 100 glucose units. The weight average molecular weight of pentastarch is approximately 264,000 with a range of 150,000 to 350,000 and with 80% of the polymers falling between 10,000 and 2,000,000. Hydroxyethyl groups are attached by an ether linkage primarily at C-2 of the glucose unit and to a lesser extent at C-3 and C-6. The polymer resembles glycogen, and the polymerized glucose units are joined primarily by 1–4 linkages with occasional 1–6 branching linkages. The degree of branching is approximately 1:20 which means that there is one 1–6 branch for every 20 glucose monomer units.

The chemical name for pentastarch is hydroxyethyl starch. The structural formula is as follows:

Amylopectin derivative in which R_2, R_3, and R_6 are H or CH_2CH_2OH, or R_6 is a branching point in the starch polymer connected through a 1–6 linkage to additional α-D-glucopyranosyl units.

PENTASPAN is a clear, pale yellow to amber solution. Exposure to prolonged adverse storage conditions may result in a change to a turbid deep brown or the formation of a crystalline precipitate. Do not use the solution if these conditions are evident.

CLINICAL PHARMACOLOGY

The addition of PENTASPAN to whole blood increases the erythrocyte sedimentation rate. Therefore, 10% pentastarch in 0.9% sodium chloride injection is used to improve the efficiency of leukocyte collection by centrifugal means.

Pentastarch molecules below 50,000 molecular weight are rapidly eliminated by renal excretion. A single dose of approximately 500 mL of PENTASPAN (approximately 50 g) results in elimination in the urine of approximately 70% of the dose within 24 hours, and approximately 80% of the dose within one week. An additional 5–6% of the pentastarch dose is recovered in the leukapheresis collection bag. The remaining 12–15% (approximately 6.8 g) of an administered dose is presumed to undergo slower elimination. This is a variable process but generally results in an intravascular pentastarch concentration below the level of detection by one week. The hydroxyethyl group is not cleaved by the body, but remains intact and attached to glucose units when excreted.

The colloidal properties of the related product HESPAN® (6% hetastarch in 0.9% sodium chloride injection) approximate those of 5% human albumin. Intravenous infusion of HESPAN results in expansion of plasma volume that decreases over the succeeding 24 to 36 hours. Similar, although reduced duration, volume expansion may be expected to occur following use of PENTASPAN (10% pentastarch in 0.9% sodium chloride injection) in leukapheresis procedures.

INDICATIONS AND USAGE

10% pentastarch in 0.9% sodium chloride injection is indicated as an adjunct in leukapheresis, to improve the harvesting and increase the yield of leukocytes by centrifugal means.

CONTRAINDICATIONS

PENTASPAN is contraindicated in donors with known hypersensitivity to hydroxyethyl starch, or with bleeding disorders, or with congestive heart failure where volume overload is a potential problem. PENTASPAN should not be used in renal disease with oliguria or anuria.

WARNINGS

Slight declines in platelet counts and hemoglobin levels have been observed in donors undergoing repeated leukapheresis procedures using HESPAN due to the volume expanding effects of HESPAN and to the collection of platelets and erythrocytes. Hemoglobin levels usually return to normal within 24 hours. Similar effects may be expected with PENTASPAN. Hemodilution by PENTASPAN and saline may also result in 24 hour declines of total protein, albumin, calcium and fibrinogen values. None of these decreases are to a degree recognized to be clinically significant risks to healthy donors.

Large volumes of PENTASPAN may slightly alter the coagulation mechanisms; *i.e.*, transient prolongation of prothrombin, partial thromboplastin and clotting times. The physician should also be alert to the possibility of transient prolongation of bleeding time.

PRECAUTIONS
General
Regular and frequent clinical evaluation and complete blood counts (CBC) are necessary for proper monitoring of PENTASPAN use during leukapheresis. If the frequency of leukapheresis is to exceed the guidelines for whole blood donation, you may wish to consider the following additional studies: total leukocyte and platelet counts, leukocyte differential count, hemoglobin and hematocrit, prothrombin time (PT), and partial thromboplastin time (PTT) tests.

The possibility of circulatory overload should be kept in mind. Caution should be used when the risk of pulmonary edema and/or congestive heart failure is increased. Special care should be exercised in patients who have impaired renal clearance since this is the principal way in which pentastarch is eliminated.

The serum chemistries of sixteen normal volunteers who were given 500 to 2000 mL infusions of PENTASPAN were essentially unchanged pre- and post-infusion, except for dilutional effects. However, indirect bilirubin levels of 8.3 mg/L (normal 0–7 mg/L) have been reported in 2 out of 20 normal subjects who received multiple HESPAN infusions. Total bilirubin was within normal limits at all times; indirect bilirubin returned to normal by 96 hours following the final infusion. The significance, if any, of these elevations is not known; however, caution should be observed before administering PENTASPAN to patients with a history of liver disease.

PENTASPAN has been reported to produce hypersensitivity reactions such as wheezing and urticaria. However, pentastarch has not been observed to stimulate antibody formation. If hypersensitivity effects occur, they are readily controlled by discontinuation of the drug and, if necessary, administration of an antihistaminic agent.

Elevated serum amylase levels may be observed temporarily following administration of PENTASPAN, although no association with pancreatitis has been demonstrated.

Carcinogenesis, mutagenesis, impairment of fertility—
Long-term studies in animals have not been performed to evaluate the carcinogenic potential of pentastarch.

Teratogenic Effects—
Pregnancy Category C. PENTASPAN has been shown to be embryocidal in New Zealand rabbits and in Swiss Mice when given in doses 5 times the human dose. There are no adequate and well-controlled clinical studies using pentastarch in pregnant women. PENTASPAN should be used during pregnancy only if the potential benefits justify the potential risk to the fetus.

PENTASPAN (10% pentastarch in 0.9% sodium chloride injection) was administered to mated New Zealand rabbits and Swiss Mice with intravenous doses of 10, 20, and 40 mL/kg/day during the period of gestation. The results demonstrated that at 10 and 20 mL/kg/day pentastarch produced no higher incidence of teratogenicity or embryotoxicity in either species than normal saline did in control animals. At 40 mL/kg/day, however, pentastarch increased the number of resorptions and minor visceral anomalies (diffuse edema of the trunk and extremities and diffuse whitish color of the heart, lungs, liver, and kidneys) in rabbits and reduced nidation in the mouse.

Nursing mothers—
It is not known whether pentastarch is excreted in human milk. Because many drugs are excreted in human milk, caution should be exercised when PENTASPAN is administered to a nursing woman.

Pediatric use—
The safety and effectiveness of PENTASPAN in children have not been established.

ADVERSE REACTIONS

The following have been reported in association with the use of PENTASPAN in leukapheresis: headache, diarrhea, nausea, weakness, temporary weight gain, insomnia, fatigue, fever, edema, paresthesia, acne, malaise, shakiness, dizziness, chest pain, chills, nasal congestion, anxiety, and increased heart rate. It is uncertain whether they are attributable to the drug, the procedure, additional adjunctive medication, or some combination of these factors.

DOSAGE AND ADMINISTRATION

250 to 700 mL of PENTASPAN to which citrate anticoagulant has been added is typically administered by aseptic addition to the input line of the centrifugation apparatus at a ratio of 1:8 to 1:13 to venous whole blood. The bottle containing PENTASPAN and citrate should be thoroughly mixed to assure effective anticoagulation of blood as it flows through the leukapheresis machine.

Parenteral drug products should be inspected visually for particulate matter and discoloration prior to administration whenever solution and container permit.

The safety and compatibility of other additives have not been established.

HOW SUPPLIED
NDC 0094-0077-95: PENTASPAN® (10% pentastarch in 0.9% sodium chloride injection) is supplied sterile and non-pyrogenic in 500 mL intravenous infusion bottles. Protect from freezing. It is recommended that the product be stored at room temperature (25°C); however, brief exposure up to 40°C does not adversely affect the product.

CAUTION
Federal (U.S.A.) law prohibits dispensing without prescription.

Directions for Use
Caution: Before administering to patient, perform the following checks:

1. Each container should be inspected before use. Read the label. Insure solution is the one ordered, is within the expiration date, and that label name agrees with the abbreviated name stamped on closure. Check the security of bail and band.

2. Invert container and carefully inspect the solution in good light for cloudiness, haze, or particulate matter; check the bottle for cracks or other damage. In checking for cracks, do not be confused by normal surface mold marks and seams on bottom and sides of bottle. These are not flaws. Look instead for bright reflections that have depth and penetrate into the wall of the bottle. Reject any such bottle.

3. Check for vacuum, first by confirming the presence of depressions in the latex disk and then by audible hiss when the disk is removed. Reject any container that does not meet these criteria.

4. After admixtures and during administration, reinspect solution as frequently as possible. If any evidence of solution contamination or instability is found or if the patient exhibits any signs of fever or chills or other reaction not readily explainable, discontinue administration immediately and notify physician.

Distributed by
Du Pont Pharmaceuticals
E.I. du Pont de Nemours and Company
Wilmington, Delaware 19898
Manufactured by
Kendall McGaw
Laboratories, Inc.
Irvine CA USA 92714-5895
Sept. 1987

PERCOCET®   ℞
[perk 'o-set]
(oxycodone and acetaminophen tablets, USP)

DESCRIPTION
Each tablet of PERCOCET contains:

Oxycodone hydrochloride .... 5 mg†
   WARNING: May be habit forming
Acetaminophen, USP .... 325 mg
† 5 mg oxycodone HCl is equivalent to 4.4815 mg of oxycodone.

PERCOCET Tablets also contain: microcrystalline cellulose, povidone, pregelatinized starch, stearic acid and other ingredients.

Acetaminophen occurs as a white, odorless crystalline powder, possessing a slightly bitter taste.

The oxycodone component is 14-hydroxydihydrocodeinone, a white, odorless crystalline powder having a saline, bitter taste. It is derived from the opium alkaloid thebaine, and may be represented by the following structural formula:

CLINICAL PHARMACOLOGY

The principal ingredient, oxycodone, is a semisynthetic narcotic analgesic with multiple actions qualitatively similar to those of morphine; the most prominent of these involve the central nervous system and organs composed of smooth muscle. The principal actions of therapeutic value of the oxycodone in PERCOCET are analgesia and sedation.

Oxycodone is similar to codeine and methadone in that it retains at least one-half of its analgesic activity when administered orally.

Acetaminophen is a non-opiate, non-salicylate analgesic and antipyretic.

INDICATIONS AND USAGE

PERCOCET is indicated for the relief of moderate to moderately severe pain.

CONTRAINDICATIONS

PERCOCET should not be administered to patients who are hypersensitive to oxycodone or acetaminophen.

Continued on next page

Du Pont Pharm.—Cont.

WARNINGS

Drug Dependence: Oxycodone can produce drug dependence of the morphine type and, therefore, has the potential for being abused. Psychic dependence, physical dependence and tolerance may develop upon repeated administration of PERCOCET, and it should be prescribed and administered with the same degree of caution appropriate to the use of other oral narcotic-containing medications. Like other narcotic-containing medications, PERCOCET is subject to the Federal Controlled Substances Act (Schedule II).

PRECAUTIONS

General

Head Injury and Increased Intracranial Pressure: The respiratory depressant effects of narcotics and their capacity to elevate cerebrospinal fluid pressure may be markedly exaggerated in the presence of head injury, other intracranial lesions or a pre-existing increase in intracranial pressure. Furthermore, narcotics produce adverse reactions which may obscure the clinical course of patients with head injuries.

Acute Abdominal Conditions: The administration of PERCOCET or other narcotics may obscure the diagnosis or clinical course in patients with acute abdominal conditions.

Special Risk Patients: PERCOCET should be given with caution to certain patients such as the elderly or debilitated, and those with severe impairment of hepatic or renal function, hypothyroidism, Addison's disease, and prostatic hypertrophy or urethral stricture.

Information for Patients Oxycodone may impair the mental and/or physical abilities required for the performance of potentially hazardous tasks such as driving a car or operating machinery. The patient using PERCOCET should be cautioned accordingly.

Drug Interaction Patients receiving other narcotic analgesics, general anesthetics, phenothiazines, other tranquilizers, sedative-hypnotics or other CNS depressants (including alcohol) concomitantly with PERCOCET may exhibit an additive CNS depression. When such combined therapy is contemplated, the dose of one or both agents should be reduced.

The use of MAO inhibitors or tricyclic antidepressants with oxycodone preparations may increase the effect of either the antidepressant or oxycodone.

The concurrent use of anticholinergics with narcotics may produce paralytic ileus.

Usage In Pregnancy Pregnancy Category C: Animal reproductive studies have not been conducted with PERCOCET. It is also not known whether PERCOCET can cause fetal harm when administered to a pregnant woman or can affect reproductive capacity. PERCOCET should not be given to a pregnant woman unless in the judgment of the physician, the potential benefits outweigh the possible hazards.

Nonteratogenic Effects: Use of narcotics during pregnancy may produce physical dependence in the neonate.

Labor and Delivery: As with all narcotics, administration of PERCOCET to the mother shortly before delivery may result in some degree of respiratory depression in the newborn and the mother, especially if higher doses are used.

Nursing Mothers It is not known whether PERCOCET is excreted in human milk. Because many drugs are excreted in human milk, caution should be exercised when PERCOCET is administered to a nursing woman.

Pediatric Use Safety and effectiveness in children have not been established.

ADVERSE REACTIONS

The most frequently observed adverse reactions include light headedness, dizziness, sedation, nausea and vomiting. These effects seem to be more prominent in ambulatory than in nonambulatory patients, and some of these adverse reactions may be alleviated if the patient lies down.

Other adverse reactions include euphoria, dysphoria, constipation, skin rash and pruritus. At higher doses, oxycodone has most of the disadvantages of morphine including respiratory depression.

DRUG ABUSE AND DEPENDENCE

PERCOCET Tablets are a Schedule II controlled substance. Oxycodone can produce drug dependence and has the potential for being abused. (See WARNINGS.)

OVERDOSAGE

Acetaminophen

Signs and Symptoms: In acute acetaminophen overdosage, dose-dependent, potentially fatal hepatic necrosis is the most serious adverse effect. Renal tubular necrosis, hypoglycemic coma and thrombocytopenia may also occur.

In adults, hepatic toxicity has rarely been reported with acute overdoses of less than 10 grams and fatalities with less than 15 grams. Importantly, young children seem to be more resistant than adults to the hepatotoxic effect of an acetaminophen overdose. Despite this, the measures outlined below

should be initiated in any adult or child suspected of having ingested an acetaminophen overdose.

Early symptoms following a potentially hepatotoxic overdose may include: nausea, vomiting, diaphoresis and general malaise. Clinical and laboratory evidence of hepatic toxicity may not be apparent until 48 to 72 hours post-ingestion.

Treatment: The stomach should be emptied promptly by lavage or by induction of emesis with syrup of ipecac. Patient's estimates of the quantity of a drug ingested are notoriously unreliable. Therefore, if an acetaminophen overdose is suspected, a serum acetaminophen assay should be obtained as early as possible, but no sooner than four hours following ingestion. Liver function studies should be obtained initially and repeated at 24-hour intervals.

The antidote, N-acetylcysteine, should be administered as early as possible, and within 16 hours of the overdose ingestions for optimal results, but in any case, within 24 hours. Following recovery, there are no residual, structural, or functional hepatic abnormalities.

Oxycodone

Signs and Symptoms: Serious overdose with oxycodone is characterized by respiratory depression (a decrease in respiratory rate and or tidal volume, Cheyne-Stokes respiration, cyanosis), extreme somnolence progressing to stupor or coma, skeletal muscle flaccidity, cold and clammy skin, and sometimes bradycardia and hypotension. In severe overdosage, apnea, circulatory collapse, cardiac arrest and death may occur.

Treatment: Primary attention should be given to the reestablishment of adequate respiratory exchange through provision of a patent airway and the institution of assisted or controlled ventilation. The narcotic antagonist naloxone hydrochloride (Narcan®) is a specific antidote against respiratory depression which may result from overdosage or unusual sensitivity to narcotics, including oxycodone. Therefore, an appropriate dose of naloxone hydrochloride (usual initial adult dose 0.4 mg to 2 mg) should be administered preferably by the intravenous route, and simultaneously with efforts at respiratory resuscitation (see package insert). Since the duration of action of oxycodone may exceed that of the antagonist, the patient should be kept under continued surveillance and repeated doses of the antagonist should be administered as needed to maintain adequate respiration. An antagonist should not be administered in the absence of clinically significant respiratory or cardiovascular depression. Oxygen, intravenous fluids, vasopressors and other supportive measures should be employed as indicated.

Gastric emptying may be useful in removing unabsorbed drug.

DOSAGE AND ADMINISTRATION

Dosage should be adjusted according to the severity of the pain and the response of the patient. It may occasionally be necessary to exceed the usual dosage recommended below in cases of more severe pain or in those patients who have become tolerant to the analgesic effect of narcotics. PERCOCET is given orally. The usual adult dose is one tablet every 6 hours as needed for pain.

HOW SUPPLIED

PERCOCET, supplied as a white tablet, with one face scored and inscribed PERCOCET, and the other inscribed with Du Pont name is available in:

Bottles of 100	NDC 0060-0127-70
Bottles of 500	NDC 0060-0127-85
Hospital Blister Pack of 25	NDC 0060-0127-65
(in units of 250 and 1000 tablets)	

Store at controlled room temperature (59°–86°F, 15°–30°C).
DEA Order Form Required
Du Pont Pharmaceuticals Caribe, Inc.
Subsidiary of E.I. du Pont de Nemours & Co. (Inc.)
P.O. Box 12
Manati, Purto Rico 00701
PERCOCET® is a Registered Trademark of DuPont Pharmaceuticals Caribe, Inc.
NARCAN® is a Registered U.S. Trademark of DuPont Pharmaceuticals, Inc.

6090-8 Rev. March 1989
Shown in Product Identification Section, page 409

---

†PERCODAN®   Ⓒ
[perk 'o-dan]
(oxycodone and aspirin)
†PERCODAN®-DEMI
Tablets
(oxycodone and aspirin)

DESCRIPTION

Each tablet of PERCODAN® contains:
Oxycodone hydrochloride .... 4.50 mg
  WARNING: May be habit forming
Oxycodone terephthalate .... 0.38 mg
  WARNING: May be habit forming

Aspirin, U.S.P. .... 325 mg
PERCODAN Tablets also contain: D&C Yellow 10, FD&C Yellow 6, microcrystalline cellulose and starch.
Each tablet of PERCODAN®-Demi contains:
Oxycodone hydrochloride .... 2.25 mg
  WARNING: May be habit forming
Oxycodone terephthalate .... 0.19 mg
  WARNING: May be habit forming
Aspirin, U.S.P. .... 325 mg
PERCODAN-Demi Tablets also contain: FD&C Blue 2, FD&C Red 3, microcrystalline cellulose and starch.
The oxycodone component is 14-hydroxydihydrocodeinone, a white odorless crystalline powder which is derived from the opium alkaloid, thebaine.

ACTIONS

The principal ingredient, oxycodone, is a semisynthetic narcotic analgesic with multiple actions qualitatively similar to those of morphine; the most prominent of these involve the central nervous system and organs composed of smooth muscle. The principal actions of therapeutic value of the oxycodone in PERCODAN® and PERCODAN®-Demi are analgesia and sedation.

Oxycodone is similar to codeine and methadone in that it retains at least one half of its analgesic activity when administered orally.

PERCODAN® and PERCODAN®-Demi also contain the non-narcotic antipyretic-analgesic, aspirin.

INDICATIONS

For the relief of moderate to moderately severe pain.

CONTRAINDICATIONS

Hypersensitivity to oxycodone or aspirin.

WARNINGS

Drug Dependence: Oxycodone can produce drug dependence of the morphine type and, therefore, has the potential for being abused. Psychic dependence, physical dependence and tolerance may develop upon repeated administration of PERCODAN® and PERCODAN®-Demi, and it should be prescribed and administered with the same degree of caution appropriate to the use of other oral narcotic-containing medications. Like other narcotic-containing medications, PERCODAN® and PERCODAN®-Demi are subject to the Federal Controlled Substances Act.

Usage in ambulatory patients: Oxycodone may impair the mental and/or physical abilities required for the performance of potentially hazardous tasks such as driving a car or operating machinery. The patient using PERCODAN® and PERCODAN®-Demi should be cautioned accordingly.

Interaction with other central nervous system depressants: Patients receiving other narcotic analgesics, general anesthetics, phenothiazines, other tranquilizers, sedative-hypnotics or other CNS depressants (including alcohol) concomitantly with PERCODAN® and PERCODAN®-Demi may exhibit an additive CNS depression. When such combined therapy is contemplated, the dose of one or both agents should be reduced.

Usage in pregnancy: Safe use in pregnancy has not been established relative to possible adverse effects on fetal development. Therefore, PERCODAN® and PERCODAN®-Demi should not be used in pregnant women unless, in the judgment of the physician, the potential benefits outweigh the possible hazards.

Usage in children: PERCODAN® should not be administered to children. PERCODAN®-Demi, containing half the amount of oxycodone, can be considered. (See Dosage and Administration for PERCODAN®-Demi).

Reye Syndrome is a rare but serious disease which can follow flu or chicken pox in children and teenagers. While the cause of Reye Syndrome is unknown, some reports claim aspirin (or salicylates) may increase the risk of developing this disease.

Salicylates should be used with caution in the presence of peptic ulcer or coagulation abnormalities.

PRECAUTIONS

Head injury and increased intracranial pressure: The respiratory depressant effects of narcotics and their capacity to elevate cerebrospinal fluid pressure may be markedly exaggerated in the presence of head injury, other intracranial lesions or a pre-existing increase in intracranial pressure. Furthermore, narcotics produce adverse reactions which may obscure the clinical course of patients with head injuries.

Acute abdominal conditions: The administration of PERCODAN® and PERCODAN®-Demi or other narcotics may obscure the diagnosis or clinical course in patients with acute abdominal conditions.

Special risk patients: PERCODAN® and PERCODAN®-Demi should be given with caution to certain patients such as the elderly or debilitated, and those with severe impairment of hepatic or renal function, hypothyroidism, Addison's disease, and prostatic hypertrophy or urethral stricture.

ADVERSE REACTIONS

The most frequently observed adverse reactions include light headedness, dizziness, sedation, nausea and vomiting. These effects seem to be more prominent in ambulatory than in nonambulatory patients, and some of these adverse reactions may be alleviated if the patient lies down.

Other adverse reactions include euphoria, dysphoria, constipation and pruritus.

DRUG ABUSE AND DEPENDENCE

PERCODAN® and PERCODAN®-Demi tablets are a Schedule II controlled substance. Oxycodone can produce drug dependence and has the potential for being abused. (See WARNINGS)

DOSAGE AND ADMINISTRATION

Dosage should be adjusted according to the severity of the pain and the response of the patient. It may occasionally be necessary to exceed the usual dosage recommended below in cases of more severe pain or in those patients who have become tolerant to the analgesic effect of narcotics. PERCODAN® and PERCODAN®-Demi are given orally.

PERCODAN®: The usual adult dose is one tablet every 6 hours as needed for pain.

PERCODAN®-Demi: Adults—One or two tablets every six hours. Children 12 years and older—One-half tablet every six hours. Children 6 to 12 years—One-quarter tablet every six hours. PERCODAN®-Demi is not indicated for children under 6 years of age.

DRUG INTERACTIONS

The CNS depressant effects of PERCODAN® and PERCODAN®-Demi may be additive with that of other CNS depressants. See WARNINGS.

Aspirin may enhance the effect of anticoagulants and inhibit the uricosuric effects of uricosuric agents.

MANAGEMENT OF OVERDOSAGE

Signs and Symptoms: Serious overdose with PERCODAN® or PERCODAN®-Demi is characterized by respiratory depression (a decrease in respiratory rate and/or tidal volume, Cheyne-Stokes respiration, cyanosis), extreme somnolence progressing to stupor or coma, skeletal muscle flaccidity, cold and clammy skin, and sometimes bradycardia and hypotension. In severe overdosage, apnea, circulatory collapse, cardiac arrest and death may occur. The ingestion of very large amounts of PERCODAN® or PERCODAN®-Demi may, in addition, result in acute salicylate intoxication.

Treatment: Primary attention should be given to the reestablishment of adequate respiratory exchange through provision of a patent airway and the institution of assisted or controlled ventilation. The narcotic antagonist naloxone hydrochloride (NARCAN®) is a specific antidote against respiratory depression which may result from overdosage or unusual sensitivity to narcotics, including oxycodone. Therefore, an appropriate dose of naloxone hydrochloride should be administered (usual initial adult dose: 0.4 mg–2 mg) preferably by the intravenous route, simultaneously with efforts at respiratory resuscitation. Since the duration of action of oxycodone may exceed that of the antagonist, the patient should be kept under continued surveillance and repeated doses of the antagonist should be administered as needed to maintain adequate respiration.

Oxygen, intravenous fluids, vasopressors and other supportive measures should be employed as indicated.

Gastric emptying may be useful in removing unabsorbed drug.

HOW SUPPLIED

Percodan®—As yellow, scored tablets, available in:

Bottles of 100	NDC 0060-0135-70
Bottles of 500	NDC 0060-0135-85
Bottles of 1000	NDC 0060-0135-90
Hospital blister pack of 25	NDC 0060-0135-65
(available in units of 250 and 1000)	

Also available in Military Depot:

Btl's of 100 NSN 6505-01-030-9493

Blister Pack (250) NSN 6505-01-030-9492

Percodan®-Demi—As pink, scored tablets available in:

Bottles of 100	NDC 0060-0136-70

Store At Controlled Room Temperature (59°–86°F, 15°–30°C).

DEA Order Form Required

Shown in Product Identification Section, page 409

PERCODAN is a registered U.S. trademark of DuPont Pharmaceuticals Caribe, Inc.

†Products of DuPont Pharmaceuticals Caribe, Inc.

NARCAN is a Registered U.S. Trademark of DuPont Pharmaceuticals, Inc.

6117-6/6118-6

SYMMETREL®   ℞
[sim 'e-trel"]
(amantadine hydrochloride)

DESCRIPTION

SYMMETREL is designated generically as amantadine hydrochloride and chemically as 1-adamantanamine hydrochloride.

Amantadine hydrochloride is a stable white or nearly white crystalline powder, freely soluble in water and soluble in alcohol and in chloroform.

Amantadine hydrochloride has pharmacological actions as both an anti-Parkinson and an antiviral drug.

SYMMETREL is available in capsules and syrup.

SYMMETREL capsules contain: FD&C Red 40, gelatin, glycerin, hydrogenated vegetable oil, lecithin, methylparaben, propylparaben, soybean oil, titanium dioxide, vegetable shortening, white printing ink, and yellow wax.

SYMMETREL syrup contains: artificial raspberry flavor, citric acid, methylparaben, propylparaben, and sorbitol solution.

CLINICAL PHARMACOLOGY

SYMMETREL is readily absorbed, is not metabolized, and is excreted unchanged in the urine by glomerular filtration and tubular secretion.

After oral administration of a single dose of 100 mg, maximum blood levels are reached, based on the mean time of the peak urinary excretion rate, in approximately 4 hours; the peak excretion rate is approximately 5 mg/hr; the mean half-life of the excretion rate approximates 15 hours.

Compared with otherwise healthy adult individuals, the clearance of SYMMETREL is significantly reduced in adult patients with renal insufficiency. The elimination of half-life increases two to three fold when creatinine clearance is less than 40 ml/min./1.73m^2 and averages eight days in patients on chronic maintenance hemodialysis.

The renal clearance of SYMMETREL is reduced and plasma levels are increased in otherwise healthy elderly patients age 65 years and older. The drug plasma levels in elderly patients receiving 100 mg daily have been reported to approximate those determined in younger adults taking 200 mg daily. Whether these changes are due to the normal decline in renal function or other age related factors is not known.

The mechanism of action of SYMMETREL in the treatment of Parkinson's disease and drug-induced extrapyramidal reactions is not known. It has been shown to cause an increase in dopamine release in the animal brain. The drug does not possess anticholinergic activity in animal tests at doses similar to those used clinically. The antiviral activity of SYMMETREL against influenza A virus is not completely understood. The mode of action of SYMMETREL appears to be the prevention of the release of infectious viral nucleic acid into the host cell. SYMMETREL does not appear to interfere with the immunogenicity of inactivated influenza A virus vaccine.

INDICATIONS AND USAGE

Parkinson's Disease/Syndrome: SYMMETREL is indicated in the treatment of idiopathic Parkinson's disease (Paralysis Agitans), postencephalitic parkinsonism, and symptomatic parkinsonism which may follow injury to the nervous system by carbon monoxide intoxication, it is indicated in those elderly patients believed to develop parkinsonism in association with cerebral arteriosclerosis. In the treatment of Parkinson's disease, SYMMETREL is less effective than levodopa, (-)-3-(3,4-dihydroxyphenyl)-L-alanine, and its efficacy in comparison with the anticholinergic antiparkinson drugs has not yet been established.

Drug-Induced Extrapyramidal Reactions: SYMMETREL is indicated in the treatment of drug-induced extrapyramidal reactions. Although anticholinergic-type side effects have been noted with SYMMETREL when used in patients with drug-induced extrapyramidal reactions, there is a lower incidence of these side effects than that observed with the anticholinergic antiparkinson drugs.

Influenza A Virus Respiratory Tract Illness:

Prophylaxis: SYMMETREL (amantadine hydrochloride) is indicated in the prevention or chemoprophylaxis of influenza A virus illness. SYMMETREL should be considered especially for high risk individuals, close household or hospital ward contacts of index cases, immunocompromised patients, health care and community services personnel. In the prophylaxis of influenza early vaccination as periodically recommended by the Centers for Disease Control's Immunization Practices Advisory Committee is the method of choice. When early vaccination is not feasible, or when the vaccine is contraindicated or not available, SYMMETREL can be used for chemoprophylaxis against influenza A virus illness.

Because SYMMETREL does not appear to suppress antibody response, it can be used chemoprophylactically in conjunction with inactivated influenza A virus vaccine until protective antibody responses develop.

Treatment: SYMMETREL is also indicated in the treatment of uncomplicated respiratory tract illness caused by influenza A virus strains. There are as yet no well-controlled clinical studies demonstrating treatment with SYMMETREL will avoid the development of influenza A virus pneumonitis or other complications in high risk patients.

There is no clinical evidence indicating that SYMMETREL is effective in the prophylaxis or treatment of viral respiratory tract illnesses other than those caused by influenza A virus strains.

CONTRAINDICATIONS:

SYMMETREL is contraindicated in patients with known hypersensitivity to the drug.

WARNINGS:

Patients with a history of epilepsy or other "seizures" should be observed closely for possible increased seizure activity. Patients with a history of congestive heart failure or peripheral edema should be followed closely as there are patients who developed congestive heart failure while receiving SYMMETREL.

Patients with Parkinson's disease improving on SYMMETREL should resume normal activities gradually and cautiously, consistent with other medical considerations, such as the presence of osteoporosis or phlebothrombosis.

Patients receiving SYMMETREL who note central nervous system effects or blurring of vision should be cautioned against driving or working in situations where alertness and adequate motor coordination are important.

PRECAUTIONS:

SYMMETREL (amantadine hydrochloride) should not be discontinued abruptly since a few patients with Parkinson's disease experienced a parkinsonian crisis, i.e., a sudden marked clinical deterioration when this medication was suddenly stopped. The dose of anticholinergic drugs or of SYMMETREL should be reduced if atropine-like effects appear when these drugs are used concurrently.

Because SYMMETREL is not metabolized and is mainly excreted in the urine, it accumulates in the plasma and in the body when renal function declines. Thus, the dose of SYMMETREL should be reduced in patients with renal impairment and in individuals who are 65 years of age or older. The dose of SYMMETREL may need careful adjustment in patients with congestive heart failure, peripheral edema, or orthostatic hypotension.

Occasional instances of reversible elevation of liver enzyme levels have been reported. Care should be exercised when administering SYMMETREL to patients with liver disease, a history of recurrent eczematoid rash, or to patients with psychosis or severe psychoneurosis not controlled by chemotherapeutic agents. Careful observation is required when SYMMETREL is administered concurrently with central nervous system stimulants.

No long-term studies in animals have been performed to evaluate the carcinogenic potential of SYMMETREL. The mutagenic potential of the drug has not yet been determined in experimental systems.

Pregnancy Category C: SYMMETREL (amantadine hydrochloride) has been shown to be embryotoxic and teratogenic in rats at 50 mg/kg/day, about 12 times the recommended human dose, but not at 37 mg/kg/day. Embryotoxic and teratogenic drug effects were not seen in rabbits which received up to 25 times the recommended human dose. There are no adequate and well-controlled studies in pregnant women. SYMMETREL should be used during pregnancy only if the potential benefit justifies the potential risk to the embryo or the fetus.

Nursing Mothers: SYMMETREL is excreted in human milk. Caution should be exercised when SYMMETREL is administered to a nursing woman.

Pediatric Use: The safety and efficacy of SYMMETREL in newborn infants, and infants below the age of 1 year have not been established.

ADVERSE REACTIONS:

The adverse reactions reported most frequently (5–10%) are: nausea, dizziness (lightheadedness), and insomnia.

Less frequently (1–5%) reported adverse reactions are: depression, anxiety and irritability, hallucinations, confusion, anorexia, dry mouth, and constipation, ataxia, livedo reticularis, peripheral edema, orthostatic hypotension and headache.

Infrequently (0.1–1%) occurring adverse reactions are: congestive heart failure, psychosis, urinary retention, dyspnea, fatigue, skin rash, vomiting, weakness, slurred speech and visual disturbance.

Rare (less than 0.1%) occurring adverse reactions are: instances of convulsion, leukopenia, neutropenia, eczematoid dermatitis and oculogyric episodes.

Continued on next page

Du Pont Pharm.—Cont.

OVERDOSAGE:

There is no specific antidote. Death has been reported from a major overdose. However, slowly administered intravenous physostigmine in 1 and 2 mg doses in an adult[1] at 1 to 2 hour intervals and 0.5 mg doses in a child[2] at 5 to 10 minute intervals up to a maximum of 2 mg/hour have been reported to be effective in the control of central nervous system toxicity caused by amantadine hydrochloride. For acute overdosing, general supportive measures should be employed along with immediate gastric lavage or induction of emesis. Fluids should be forced, and if necessary, given intravenously. Hemodialysis does not remove significant amounts of SYMMETREL; in patients with renal failure, a four hour hemodialysis removed 7 to 15 mg after a single 300 mg oral dose.[3] The pH of the urine has been reported to influence the excretion rate of SYMMETREL. Since the excretion rate of SYMMETREL increases rapidly when the urine is acidic, the administration of urine acidifying drugs may increase the elimination of the drug from the body. The blood pressure, pulse, respiration and temperature should be monitored. The patient should be observed for hyperactivity and convulsions; if required, sedation, and anticonvulsant therapy should be administered. The patient should be observed for the possible development of arrhythmias and hypotension; if required, appropriate antiarrhythmic and antihypotensive therapy should be given. The blood electrolytes, urine pH and urinary output should be monitored. If there is no record of recent voiding, catheterization should be done. The possibility of multiple drug ingestion by the patient should be considered.

[1] D.F. Casey, N. Engl. J. Med. 298:516, 1978.
[2] C.D. Berkowitz, J. Pediatr. 95:144, 1979.
[3] V.W. Horadam, et al., Ann. Intern. Med. 94:454, 1981.

DOSAGE AND ADMINISTRATION

Dosage for Parkinsonism:

Adult: The usual dose of SYMMETREL (amantadine hydrochloride) is 100 mg twice a day when used alone. SYMMETREL has an onset of action usually within 48 hours.

The initial dose of SYMMETREL is 100 mg daily for patients with serious associated medical illnesses or who are receiving high doses of other antiparkinson drugs. After one to several weeks at 100 mg once daily, the dose may be increased to 100 mg twice daily, if necessary.

Occasionally, patients whose responses are not optimal with SYMMETREL at 200 mg daily may benefit from an increase up to 400 mg daily in divided doses. However, such patients should be supervised closely by their physicians.

Patients initially deriving benefit from SYMMETREL not uncommonly experience a fall-off of effectiveness after a few months. Benefit may be regained by increasing the dose to 300 mg daily. Alternatively, temporary discontinuation of SYMMETREL for several weeks, followed by reinitiation of the drug, may result in regaining benefit in some patients. A decision to use other antiparkinson drugs may be necessary.

Dosage for Concomitant Therapy

Some patients who do not respond to anticholinergic antiparkinson drugs may respond to SYMMETREL. When SYMMETREL or anticholinergic antiparkinson drugs are each used with marginal benefit, concomitant use may produce additional benefit.

When SYMMETREL and levodopa are initiated concurrently, the patient can exhibit rapid therapeutic benefits. SYMMETREL should be held constant at 100 mg daily or twice daily while the daily dose of levodopa is gradually increased to optimal benefit.

When SYMMETREL is added to optimal well-tolerated doses of levodopa, additional benefit may result, including smoothing out the fluctuations in improvement which sometimes occur in patients on levodopa alone. Patients who require a reduction in their usual dose of levodopa because of development of side effects may possibly regain lost benefit with the addition of SYMMETREL.

Dosage for Drug-Induced Extrapyramidal Reactions:

Adult: The usual dose of SYMMETREL (amantadine hydrochloride) is 100 mg twice a day. Occasionally, patients whose responses are not optimal with SYMMETREL at 200 mg daily may benefit from an increase up to 300 mg daily in divided doses.

Dosage for Prophylaxis of Influenza A Virus Illness and Treatment of Uncomplicated Influenza A Virus Illness:

Normal Renal Function:

Adult: The adult daily dosage of SYMMETREL (amantadine hydrochloride) is 200 mg: two 100 mg capsules (or four teaspoonfuls of syrup) as a single daily dose, or the daily dosage may be split into one capsule of 100 mg (or two teaspoonfuls of syrup) twice a day. If central nervous system effects develop on once-a-day dosage, a split dosage schedule may reduce such complaints. In persons 65 years of age or older, the daily dosage of SYMMETREL is 100 mg.

Children: 1 yr.–9 yrs. of age: The total daily dose should be calculated on the basis of 2 to 4 mg/lb/day (4.4 to 8.8 mg/kg/day), but not to exceed 150 mg per day.

9 yrs.–12 yrs. of age: The total daily dose is 200 mg given as one capsule of 100 mg (or two teaspoonfuls of syrup) twice a day.

IMPAIRED RENAL FUNCTION: Depending upon creatinine clearance, the following dosage adjustments are recommended:

Creatinine Clearance (ml/min./1.73m²)	Symmetrel Dosage
30–50	200 mg 1st day and 100 mg each day thereafter
15–29	200 mg 1st day followed by 100 mg on alternate days
<15	200 mg every 7 days

The recommended dosage for patients on hemodialysis is 200 mg every 7 days.

Prophylactic dosing should be started in anticipation of an influenza A outbreak and before or after contact with individuals with influenza A virus respiratory tract illness. SYMMETREL should be continued daily for at least 10 days following a known exposure. If SYMMETREL is used chemoprophylactically in conjunction with inactivated influenza A virus vaccine until protective antibody responses develop, then it should be administered for 2 to 3 weeks after the vaccine has been given. When inactivated influenza A virus vaccine is unavailable or contraindicated, SYMMETREL should be administered for up to 90 days in case of possible repeated and unknown exposures. Treatment of influenza A virus illness should be started as soon as possible, preferably within 24 to 48 hours, after onset of signs and symptoms, and should be continued for 24 to 48 hours after the disappearance of signs and symptoms.

HOW SUPPLIED

SYMMETREL (amantadine hydrochloride) is available as capsules (each red, soft gelatin capsule contains 100 mg amantadine hydrochloride) in:
Bottles of 100 NDC 0056-0105-70
Bottles of 500 NDC 0056-0105-85
Hospital Unit-Dose Blister Package of 100 NDC 0056-0105-75
As a syrup (each 5 ml (1 teaspoonful) contains 50 mg amantadine hydrochloride) in:
16 oz. (480 ml) bottles NDC 0056-0205-16.
Store at controlled room temperature (59°–86°F, 15°–30°C).
CAPSULES MANUFACTURED BY
R.P. Scherer—North America
St. Petersburg, Florida 33702
FOR
DuPont Pharmaceuticals
E.I. duPont de Nemours & Co. (Inc.)
Wilmington, Delaware 19898
SYMMETREL® is a Registered U.S. Trademark of E.I. du Pont de Nemours & Co., (Inc.)

6043-21/Rev. June 1988

Shown in Product Identification Section, page 410

TREXAN™   ℞
[treks'an]
(naltrexone hydrochloride)

DESCRIPTION

TREXAN (naltrexone hydrochloride), an opioid antagonist, is a synthetic congener of oxymorphone, and is technically, therefore, a thebaine derivative. However, it has no opioid agonist properties. Naltrexone differs in structure from oxymorphone in that the methyl group on the nitrogen atom is replaced by a cyclopropylmethyl group. TREXAN (naltrexone hydrochloride) is also related to the potent opioid antagonist, naloxone, or n-allylnoroxymorphone (NARCAN®).

TREXAN (naltrexone hydrochloride) is a white, crystalline compound. The hydrochloride salt is soluble in water to the extent of about 100 mg/cc. TREXAN is available in scored tablets containing 50 mg of naltrexone hydrochloride.

TREXAN Tablets also contain: alginic acid, FD&C Yellow 6, microcrystalline cellulose, stearic acid, and sugar.

CLINICAL PHARMACOLOGY

Pharmacodynamic actions: TREXAN (naltrexone hydrochloride) is a pure opioid antagonist. It markedly attenuates or completely blocks, reversibly, the subjective effects of intravenously administered opioids. [In this context, the term opioid is used to describe 1) classic morphine-like agonists and 2) analgesics possessing agonist and antagonist activity (e.g., butorphanol, nalbuphine and pentazocine).]

When co-administered with morphine, on a chronic basis, TREXAN blocks the physical dependence to morphine and presumably other opioids.

TREXAN has few, if any, intrinsic actions besides its opioid blocking properties. However, it does produce some pupillary constriction, by an unknown mechanism.

The administration of TREXAN is not associated with the development of tolerance or dependence.

In subjects physically dependent on opioids, TREXAN will precipitate withdrawal symptomatology.

Clinical studies indicate that 50 mg of TREXAN will block the pharmacologic effects of 25 mg of intravenously administered heroin for periods as long as 24 hours. Other data suggest that doubling the dose of TREXAN provides blockade for 48 hours, and tripling the dose of TREXAN provides blockade for about 72 hours.

While the mechanism of action is not fully understood, the preponderance of evidence suggests that TREXAN blocks the effects of opioids by competitive binding (i.e., analogous to competitive inhibition of enzymes) at opioid receptors. This makes the blockade produced potentially surmountable.

Bioavailability/Pharmacokinetics: Following oral administration, TREXAN (naltrexone hydrochloride) is subject to extensive "first pass" hepatic metabolism (its major route of elimination) with approximately 95% of the absorbed drug being converted to several metabolites. The major metabolite, 6-β-naltrexol, like TREXAN, is believed to be a pure antagonist and may contribute to the pharmacological blockade of opioid receptors. A minor metabolite is 2-hydroxy-3-methoxy-6-β-naltrexol. TREXAN and its metabolites are also conjugated to form additional metabolic products. TREXAN and its metabolites are excreted primarily by the kidney, with fecal excretion being a minor elimination pathway. The urinary excretion of unchanged TREXAN accounts for less than 1% of an oral dose; urinary excretion of unchanged and conjugated 6-β-naltrexol accounts for approximately 38% of an oral dose. The pharmacokinetic profile of TREXAN suggests that TREXAN and its metabolites undergo enterohepatic recycling.

Following the administration of 50 mg TREXAN tablets to 24 healthy adult male volunteers, the C_{max} for TREXAN and its major metabolite, 6-β-naltrexol were 8.6 ng/ml and 99.3 ng/ml, respectively. The maximum concentration (C_{max}), area under the curve (AUC), and amount excreted in the urine for both TREXAN and 6-β-naltrexol increased proportionally as the amount of TREXAN administered increased from 50 mg to 200 mg. The time to maximum concentration (T_{max}) is one hour for both TREXAN and 6-β-naltrexol. The mean elimination half-life (T-½) values for TREXAN and 6-β-naltrexol are 3.9 hours and 12.9 hours, respectively. The mean elimination half-life (T-½) and time to maximum concentration (T_{max}) for TREXAN and 6-β-naltrexol are independent of dose. TREXAN does not accumulate during chronic dosing. As predicted by its longer half-life, plasma levels of 6-β-naltrexol increase by 40% during chronic TREXAN dosing.

The total body clearance of TREXAN is 1.5 L/min, which approximates liver blood flow, and suggests TREXAN is a highly extracted compound. A renal clearance of 127 ml/min for TREXAN suggests it is solely cleared by glomerular filtration. A renal clearance of 283 ml/min for 6-β-naltrexol suggests an additional renal tubular secretory mechanism. The volume of distribution for TREXAN following intravenous administration is estimated to be 1350 liters. In vitro tests with human plasma show TREXAN to be 21% bound to plasma protein over the therapeutic dose range.

In a relative bioavailability study in 24 healthy adult male volunteers, TREXAN tablets were found to be bioequivalent to TREXAN syrup; no differences were observed for C_{max}, AUC, and urinary excretion. As expected, the time to maximum concentration (T_{max}) occurred slightly earlier for the syrup (0.6 hours) than for the tablet (1.0 hr).

INDICATIONS AND USAGE

TREXAN (naltrexone hydrochloride) is indicated to provide blockade of the pharmacologic effects of exogenously administered opioids as an adjunct to the maintenance of the opioid free-state in detoxified formerly opioid-dependent individuals.

There are no data that demonstrate an unequivocally beneficial effect of TREXAN on rates of recidivism among detoxified, formerly opioid-dependent individuals.

CONTRAINDICATIONS

TREXAN is contraindicated in:
1) Patients receiving opioid analgesics.
2) Opioid dependent patients.
3) Patients in acute opioid withdrawal (see WARNINGS).
4) Any individual who has failed to pass the NARCAN challenge. (See DOSAGE AND ADMINISTRATION section)
5) Any individual who has a positive urine screen for opioids.
6) Any individual with a history of sensitivity to TREXAN (naltrexone hydrochloride). It is not known if there is any cross-sensitivity with naloxone or other phenanthrene containing opioids.
7) Any individual with acute hepatitis or liver failure.

WARNINGS

Hepatotoxicity:

> **TREXAN has the capacity to cause dose related hepatocellular injury.**

Prior to making a decision to initiate treatment with TREXAN, the physician should establish whether the patient has subclinical liver injury or disease. (See PRECAUTIONS; Laboratory Tests). TREXAN is contraindicated in acute hepatitis or liver failure, but its use even in patients with evidence of less severe liver disease or a history of recent liver disease must be carefully considered in light of its hepatotoxic potential.

The evidence that identified TREXAN as a hepatotoxin was not obtained in studies involving its use at the doses recommended for opiate blockade, where the changes in serum levels of liver enzymes seen were similar to those present at baseline in the study population. However, the margin of separation between the apparently safe and the hepatotoxic doses appears to be only five-fold or less.

Evidence of TREXAN's hepatotoxic potential is derived primarily from a placebo controlled study in which TREXAN was administered to obese subjects at a dose approximately five-fold that recommended for the blockade of opiate receptors (300 mg per day). In the study, 5 of 26 TREXAN recipients developed elevations of serum transaminases (i.e., peak SGPT values ranging from a low of 121 to a high of 532; or 3 to 19 times their baseline values) after three to eight weeks of treatment. Although the patients involved were generally clinically asymptomatic and the transaminase levels of all patients on whom follow-up was obtained returned to (or toward) baseline values in a matter of weeks, the lack of any transaminase elevations of similar magnitude in any of the 24 placebo patients in the same study is persuasive evidence that TREXAN is a direct (i.e., not an idiosyncratic) hepatotoxin. This conclusion is also supported by evidence from other placebo controlled studies in which exposure to TREXAN at doses from one to two-fold the amount recommended for opiate blockade consistently produced more numerous and more significant elevations of serum transaminases than did placebo, and reports of transaminase elevations in 3 of 9 patients with Alzheimer's Disease who received TREXAN (up to 300 mg/day) for 5 to 8 weeks in a open clinical trial.

Unintended Precipitation of Abstinence: To prevent occurrence of an acute abstinence syndrome, or exacerbation of a pre-existing sub-clinical abstinence syndrome, patients should remain opioid-free for a minimum of 7–10 days before starting TREXAN. Since the absence of an opioid drug in the urine is often not sufficient proof that a patient is opioid-free, a NARCAN challenge should be employed to exclude the possibility of precipitating a withdrawal reaction following administration of TREXAN. The NARCAN challenge test is described in the DOSAGE AND ADMINISTRATION section. While TREXAN is a potent antagonist with a prolonged pharmacologic effect (24 to 72 hours), the blockade produced by TREXAN is surmountable. This is useful in patients who may require analgesia, but poses a potential risk to individuals who attempt, on their own, to overcome the blockade by administering large amounts of exogenous opioids. Indeed, any attempt by a patient to overcome the antagonism by taking opioids is very dangerous and may lead to a fatal overdose. Injury may arise because the plasma concentration of exogenous opioids attained immediately following their acute administration may be sufficient to overcome the competitive receptor blockade. As a consequence, the patient may be in immediate danger of suffering life endangering opioid intoxication (e.g., respiratory arrest, circulatory collapse). Also, lesser amounts of exogenous opioids may prove dangerous if they are taken in a manner (i.e. relatively long after the last dose of naltrexone) and in an amount so that they persist in the body longer than effective concentrations of naltrexone and its metabolites. Patients should be told of the serious consequences of surmounting the opiate blockade. See Information for Patients section.

PRECAUTIONS

General:

Actions Suggested When Reversal of TREXAN Blockade is Required: In an emergency situation requiring analgesia which can only be achieved with opioids, the amount of opioid required may be greater than usual, and the resulting respiratory depression may be deeper and more prolonged. No methods to reverse overdose have been established by controlled clinical trials; therefore in such circumstances, a rapidly acting analgesic which minimizes respiratory depression is preferred. The amount of analgesic administered should be titrated to the needs of the patient.

Additionally, non-receptor mediated actions may occur (e.g., facial swelling, itching, generalized erythema presumably due to histamine release).

Irrespective of the drug chosen to reverse TREXAN (naltrexone hydrochloride) blockade, the patient should be monitored closely by appropriately trained personnel in a hospital setting.

Actions Suggested When Withdrawal is Accidentally Precipitated With TREXAN: Severe opioid withdrawal syndromes precipitated by the accidental ingestion of TREXAN have been reported in opioid-dependent individuals. Symptoms of withdrawal have usually appeared within five minutes of ingestion of TREXAN and have lasted for up to 48 hours. Mental status changes including confusion, somnolence and visual hallucinations have occurred. Significant fluid losses from vomiting and diarrhea have required intravenous fluid administration. In all cases patients were closely monitored and therapy tailored to meet individual requirements.

Interference With the Action of Narcotic Containing Drug Product: Patients taking TREXAN may not benefit from opioid containing medicines, such as cough and cold preparations, antidiarrheal preparations, and opioid analgesics. Where a non-opioid containing alternative is available, it should be used.

Information for Patients: It is suggested that the prescribing physician relate the following information to patients being treated with TREXAN:

You have been prescribed TREXAN (naltrexone hydrochloride) as part of the comprehensive treatment for your drug dependence. You should carry identification to alert medical personnel to the fact that you are taking TREXAN. A TREXAN medication card may be obtained from your physician and can be used for this purpose. Carrying the identification card should help to ensure that you can obtain adequate treatment in an emergency. If you require medical treatment be sure to tell the treating physician that you are receiving TREXAN therapy.

You should take TREXAN as directed by your physician. If you attempt to self-administer heroin or any other opiate drug, in small doses, you will not perceive any effect. Most important, however, if you attempt to self-administer large doses of heroin or any other narcotic, you may die or sustain serious injury, including coma.

Laboratory tests: Tests designed to detect hepatic injury should be obtained prior to initiation of TREXAN therapy and periodically thereafter. (See "WARNINGS" section on Hepatotoxicity).

Periodic testing of all patients after initiation of treatment is critical if the occurrence of TREXAN induced liver damage is to be detected at the earliest possible time. Evaluations, using appropriate batteries of tests to detect liver injury are recommended on a monthly basis during the first six months of use; thereafter, clinical judgment about the frequency of monitoring must be relied upon.

Laboratory tests which may be used for the separation and detection of morphine, methadone or quinine in the urine and with which TREXAN does not interfere include thin-layer, gas-liquid, and high pressure liquid chromatographic methods.

Carcinogenesis, Mutagenesis and Impairment of Fertility:

Carcinogenesis: In a two-year carcinogenicity study in rats, there were small increases in the numbers of mesotheliomas in males, and tumors of vascular origin in both sexes. The number of tumors were within the range seen in historical control groups, except for the vascular tumors in females, where the 4% incidence exceeded the historical maximum of 2%.

Mutagenesis: A total of twenty-two distinct tests were performed using bacterial, mammalian, and tissue culture systems. All tests were negative except for weakly positive findings in the Drosophila recessive lethal assay and non-specific DNA repair tests with *E. coli*. The significance of these findings is undetermined.

Impairment of Fertility: TREXAN (100 mg/kg, approximately 140 times the human therapeutic dose) caused a significant increase in pseudopregnancy in the rat. A decrease in the pregnancy rate of mated female rats also occurred. The relevance of these observations to human fertility is not known.

Pregnancy: Category C. TREXAN has been shown to have an embryocidal effect in the rat and rabbit when given in doses approximately 140 times the human therapeutic dose. This effect was demonstrated in rats dosed with TREXAN (100 mg/kg) prior to and throughout gestation, and rabbits treated with 60 mg/kg of TREXAN during the period of organogenesis.

There are no adequate and well-controlled studies in pregnant women. TREXAN should be used in pregnancy only when the potential benefit justifies the potential risk to the fetus.

LABOR AND DELIVERY

Whether or not TREXAN affects the duration of labor and delivery is unknown.

NURSING MOTHERS

Whether or not TREXAN is excreted in human milk is unknown. Because many drugs are excreted in human milk, caution should be exercised when TREXAN is administered to a nursing mother.

PEDIATRIC USE

The safe use of TREXAN in subjects younger than 18 years old has not been established.

ADVERSE REACTIONS

While extensive clinical studies evaluating the use of TREXAN in detoxified, formerly opioid dependent individuals failed to identify any single, serious untoward risk of TREXAN use, placebo controlled studies employing up to five-fold higher doses of TREXAN (up to 300 mg per day) than that recommended for use in opiate receptor blockade have shown that TREXAN causes hepatocellular injury in a substantial proportion of patients exposed at this higher dose. (See WARNINGS and PRECAUTIONS: Laboratory Tests).

Aside from this finding, however, available evidence does not incriminate TREXAN, used at any dose, as a cause of any other serious untoward event for the patient who is "opioid free." It is critical to recognize that TREXAN can precipitate or exacerbate abstinence signs and symptoms in any individual who is not completely free of exogenous opioids.

TREXAN used at the doses recommended to produce opiate receptor blockade does not appear to be the cause of any of the numerous adverse events and abnormal laboratory findings, including liver function abnormalities, that were observed in the course of the clinical trials that enrolled individuals with a history of both alcohol and substance abuse. In the one placebo controlled trial intended to assess the effects of opiate receptor blockade on drug abuse recidivism, observed untoward events and laboratory abnormalities occurred with nearly equal frequency among placebo and TREXAN recipients. In all open studies, the untoward events observed (e.g., lymphocytosis, transaminase elevations, GI disturbances) were findings that would be anticipated in any similar population not treated with naltrexone. Supporting this judgment, many of the abnormalities detected during the course of the clinical trials were present at baseline, and in some instances, baseline abnormalities, including transaminase elevations, improved or returned to normal during the course of treatment with naltrexone.

In summary, among opioid free individuals, TREXAN administration at the recommended dose has not been associated with a predictable profile of serious adverse or untoward events. However, as mentioned above, among individuals using opioids, TREXAN may cause serious reactions (see CONTRAINDICATIONS, WARNINGS, DOSAGE AND ADMINISTRATION).

Events other than hepatocellular injury reported during clinical testing:

The following adverse reactions have been reported both at baseline and during the TREXAN medication period at an incidence rate of more than 10%:

Difficulty sleeping, anxiety, nervousness, abdominal pain/-cramps, nausea and/or vomiting, low energy, joint and muscle pain, and headache.

The incidence was less than 10% for:

Loss of appetite, diarrhea, constipation, increased thirst, increased energy, feeling down, irritability, dizziness, skin rash, delayed ejaculation, decreased potency, and chills.

The following events occurred in less than 1% of subjects:

Respiratory: nasal congestion, itching, rhinorrhea, sneezing, sore throat, excess mucus or phlegm, sinus trouble, heavy breathing, hoarseness, cough, shortness of breath.

Cardiovascular: nose bleeds, phlebitis, edema, increased blood pressure, non-specific ECG changes, palpitations, tachycardia.

Gastrointestinal: excessive gas, hemorrhoids, diarrhea, ulcer.

Musculoskeletal: painful shoulders, legs or knees; tremors, twitching.

Genitourinary: increased frequency of or discomfort during urination; increased or decreased sexual interest.

Dermatologic: oily skin, pruritus, acne, athlete's foot, cold sores, alopecia.

Psychiatric: depression, paranoia; fatigue, restlessness, confusion, disorientation, hallucinations, nightmares, bad dreams.

Special senses: eyes-blurred, burning, light sensitive, swollen, aching, strained; ears "clogged", aching, tinnitus.

General: increased appetite, weight loss, weight gain, yawning, somnolence, fever, dry mouth, head "pounding", inguinal pain, swollen glands, "side" pains, cold feet, "hot spells."

Lethargy and somnolence have been reported following dosing of TREXAN (naltrexone hydrochloride) and thioridazine.

Laboratory tests: With the exception of liver test abnormalities in investigator studies (See WARNINGS, PRECAUTIONS, etc.), results of laboratory tests, like adverse reaction reports, have not shown consistent patterns of abnormalities that can be attributed to treatment with TREXAN.

In the trials evaluating TREXAN for the blockade of opiate receptors, abnormal liver function tests and lymphocytosis were the two most common categories of abnormalities reported. As noted earlier, these abnormalities are common among populations of parenteral opioid users and alcoholics. As is the case with the untoward events described above, a large proportion of patients had abnormal laboratory tests at

Continued on next page

Du Pont Pharm.—Cont.

baseline, further supporting the conclusion that the abnormalities observed are not attributable to TREXAN.

Idiopathic thrombocytopenic purpura was reported in one patient who may have been sensitized to TREXAN in a previous course of treatment with TREXAN. The condition cleared without sequelae after discontinuation of TREXAN and corticosteroid treatment.

DRUG ABUSE AND DEPENDENCE

TREXAN is a pure opioid antagonist. It does not lead to physical or psychological dependence. Tolerance to the opioid antagonist effect is not known to occur.

OVERDOSAGE

There is no clinical experience with TREXAN overdosage in humans. In one study, subjects who received 800 mg daily TREXAN for up to one week showed no evidence of toxicity. In the mouse, rat and guinea pig, the oral LD_{50}s were 1,100 ± 96 mg/kg; 1,450 ± 265 mg/kg; and 1,490 ± 102 mg/kg, respectively.

In acute toxicity studies in the mouse, rat, and dog, cause of death was due to clonic-tonic convulsions and/or respiratory failure.

TREATMENT OF OVERDOSAGE

Consideration should be given to contacting a poison control center for the most up-to-date information.

In view of the lack of actual experience in the treatment of TREXAN overdose, patients should be treated symptomatically in a closely supervised environment.

DOSAGE AND ADMINISTRATION

Induction of TREXAN Therapy: DO NOT ATTEMPT TREATMENT UNTIL NARCAN CHALLENGE IS NEGATIVE (see below). Initiate treatment with TREXAN using the following guidelines:

1. Treatment should not be attempted until the patient has remained opioid-free for 7–10 days. Self-reporting of abstinence from opioids should be verified by analysis of the patient's urine for absence of opioids. The patient should not be manifesting withdrawal signs or reporting withdrawal symptoms.
2. A NARCAN challenge test (see below) should be administered to the patient. If signs of opioid withdrawal are still observed following NARCAN challenge, treatment with TREXAN should not be attempted. The NARCAN challenge can be repeated in 24 hours.
3. Treatment should be initiated carefully, slowly increasing the dose of TREXAN administered. This can be accomplished by administration of 25 mg of TREXAN initially. The patient should be observed for 1 hour. If no withdrawal signs occur, the patient may be given the rest of the daily dose.

NARCAN Challenge Test: The NARCAN challenge test should *not* be performed in a patient showing clinical signs or symptoms of opioid withdrawal, or in a patient whose urine contains opioids.

The NARCAN challenge test may be administered by either the intravenous or subcutaneous routes.

Intravenous challenge: Following appropriate screening of the patient, 0.8 mg of NARCAN should be drawn into a sterile syringe. If the intravenous route of administration is selected, 0.2 mg of NARCAN should be injected, and while the needle is in the patient's vein, the patient should be observed for 30 seconds for evidence of withdrawal signs or symptoms. If there is no evidence of withdrawal, the remaining 0.6 mg of NARCAN should be injected, and the patient observed for an additional period of 20 minutes for signs and symptoms of withdrawal.

Subcutaneous challenge: If the subcutaneous route is selected, 0.8 mg should be administered subcutaneously, and the patient observed for signs and symptoms of withdrawal for 45 minutes.

Conditions and technique for observation of patient: During the appropriate period of observation, the patient's vital signs should be monitored and the patient should be monitored for signs of withdrawal. It is also important to question the patient carefully. The signs and symptoms of opioid withdrawal include, but are not limited to, the following:

WITHDRAWAL SIGNS: stuffiness or running nose, tearing, yawning, sweating, tremor, vomiting or piloerection.

WITHDRAWAL SYMPTOMS: feeling of temperature change, joint or bone and muscle pain, abdominal cramps, skin crawling, etc.

Interpretation of the Challenge: Warning: the elicitation of the enumerated signs or symptoms indicates a potential risk for the subject, and TREXAN should not be administered. If no signs or symptoms of withdrawal are observed, elicited, or reported, TREXAN MAY BE ADMINISTERED. If there is any doubt in the observer's mind that the patient is not in an opioid-free state, or is in continuing withdrawal, NARCAN should be readministered as follows:

Confirmatory rechallenge (if necessary): 1.6 mg of NARCAN should be injected intravenously and the patient again ob-

served for signs and symptoms of withdrawal. If none are present, TREXAN may be administered. If signs and symptoms of withdrawal are present, administration of TREXAN should be delayed until repeated NARCAN challenge indicates the patient is no longer at risk.

Maintenance Treatment: Once the patient has been started on TREXAN, 50 mg every 24 hours will produce adequate clinical blockade of the actions of parenterally administered opioids (i.e., this dose will block the effects of a 25 mg intravenous heroin challenge). A flexible approach to a dosing regimen may be employed. Thus, patients may receive 50 mg of TREXAN every weekday with a 100 mg dose on Saturday or patients may receive 100 mg every other day, or 150 mg every third day. While the degree of opioid blockade may be somewhat reduced by using higher doses at longer dosing intervals, improved patient compliance may result from dosing every 48–72 hours.

Several of the clinical studies reported in the literature have employed the following dosing regimen: 100 mg on Monday, 100 mg on Wednesday, and 150 mg on Friday. This dosing schedule appeared to be acceptable to many TREXAN patients successfully maintaining their opioid free state.

HOW SUPPLIED

TREXAN tablets are available in 50 mg round tablets, scored imprinted with DuPont on one side and TREXAN on the other. Bottles of 50 tablets (NDC 0056-0080-50).

Additional medical information may be obtained from Du Pont Pharmaceuticals by calling 1-800-441-9861. In Delaware, call 302-992-3273. For medical emergencies, call 1-212-340-4494 or your Regional Poison Control Center.

NARCAN® is a Registered U.S. Trademark of Du Pont Pharmaceuticals, Inc.

TREXAN™ is a U.S. Trademark of E.I. du Pont de Nemours & Co. (Inc.).

6162-3/Rev. Dec., 1988
Shown in Product Identification Section, page 410

TRIDIL®   ℞
[tri 'dil]
(nitroglycerin)

FOR INTRAVENOUS USE ONLY. NOT FOR DIRECT INTRAVENOUS INJECTION. TRIDIL® MUST BE DILUTED IN DEXTROSE (5%) INJECTION, USP OR SODIUM CHLORIDE (0.9%) INJECTION, USP PRIOR TO ITS INFUSION (SEE DOSAGE AND ADMINISTRATION SECTION). THE ADMINISTRATION SET USED FOR INFUSION WILL AFFECT THE AMOUNT OF TRIDIL DELIVERED TO THE PATIENT. (SEE WARNINGS, AND DOSAGE AND ADMINISTRATION SECTIONS).

CAUTION SEVERAL PREPARATIONS OF NITROGLYCERIN FOR INJECTION ARE AVAILABLE. THEY DIFFER IN CONCENTRATION AND/OR VOLUME PER VIAL. WHEN SWITCHING FROM ONE PRODUCT TO ANOTHER ATTENTION MUST BE PAID TO THE DILUTION AND DOSAGE AND ADMINISTRATION INSTRUCTIONS.

DESCRIPTION

TRIDIL (nitroglycerin) is a clear, practically colorless additive solution for intravenous infusion after dilution. Each mL of TRIDIL 5 mg contains 0.5 mg Nitroglycerin with 4.5 mg Lactose, USP; 10% Alcohol, USP; and 13.8 mg Monobasic Sodium Phosphate, USP as a buffer in Water for Injection, USP. Each mL of TRIDIL 25 mg, TRIDIL 50 mg, or Tridil 100 mg contains 5 mg Nitroglycerin in 30% Alcohol, USP; 30% Propylene Glycol, USP; and Water for Injection, USP.

The solution is sterile, nonpyrogenic, and nonexplosive. TRIDIL, an organic nitrate, is a vasodilator. The chemical name for nitroglycerin is 1,2,3 propanetriol, trinitrate and its chemical structure is:

$$CH_2 - ONO_2$$
$$CH - ONO_2$$
$$CH_2 - ONO_2$$

$C_3H_5N_3O_9$ MOL. WT. 227.09

CLINICAL PHARMACOLOGY

Relaxation of vascular smooth muscle is the principal pharmacologic action of TRIDIL (nitroglycerin). Although venous effects predominate, nitroglycerin produces, in a dose-related manner, dilation of both arterial and venous beds. Dilation of the post-capillary vessels, including large veins, promotes peripheral pooling of blood and decreases venous return to the heart, reducing left ventricular end-diastolic pressure (pre-load). Arteriolar relaxation reduces systemic vascular resistance and arterial pressure (afterload). Myocardial oxygen consumption or demand (as measured by the pressure-rate product, tension-time index and stroke work index) is decreased by both the arterial and venous effects of nitroglycerin, and a more favorable supply-demand ratio can be achieved.

Therapeutic doses of intravenous nitroglycerin reduce systolic, diastolic and mean arterial blood pressure. Effective coronary perfusion pressure is usually maintained, but can be compromised if blood pressure falls excessively or increased heart rate decreases diastolic filling time.

Elevated central venous and pulmonary capillary wedge pressures, pulmonary vascular resistance and systemic vascular resistance are also reduced by nitroglycerin therapy. Heart rate is usually slightly increased, presumably a reflex response to the fall in blood pressure. Cardiac index may be increased, decreased, or unchanged. Patients with elevated left ventricular filling pressure and systemic vascular resistance values in conjunction with a depressed cardiac index are likely to experience an improvement in cardiac index. On the other hand, when filling pressures and cardiac index are normal, cardiac index may be slightly reduced by intravenous nitroglycerin.

Nitroglycerin is widely distributed in the body with an apparent volume of distribution of approximately 200 liters in adult male subjects, and is rapidly metabolized to dinitrates and mononitrates, with a short half-life estimated at 1–4 minutes. This results in a low plasma concentration after intravenous infusion. At plasma concentrations of between 50 and 500 ng/mL, the binding of nitroglycerin to plasma proteins is approximately 60%, while that of 1,2 dinitroglycerin and 1,3 dinitroglycerin is 60% and 30% respectively. The activity and half-life of the dinitroglycerin metabolites are not well characterized. The mononitrate is not active.

INDICATIONS AND USAGE

TRIDIL is indicated for:
1. **Control of blood pressure in perioperative hypertension,** i.e., hypertension associated with surgical procedures, especially cardiovascular procedures, such as the hypertension seen during intratracheal intubation, anesthesia, skin incision, sternotomy, cardiac bypass, and in the immediate postsurgical period.
2. **Congestive Heart Failure Associated with Acute Myocardial Infarction.**
3. **Treatment of Angina Pectoris** in patients who have not responded to recommended doses of organic nitrates and/or a beta blocker.
4. **Production of controlled hypotension during surgical procedures.**

CONTRAINDICATIONS

TRIDIL should not be administered to individuals with:
1. A known hypersensitivity to nitroglycerin or a known idiosyncratic reaction to organic nitrates.
2. Hypotension or uncorrected hypovolemia, as the use of TRIDIL in such states could produce severe hypotension or shock.
3. Increased intracranial pressure (e.g., head trauma or cerebral hemorrhage).
4. Constrictive pericarditis and pericardial tamponade.

WARNINGS

1. Nitroglycerin readily migrates into many plastics. To avoid absorption of nitroglycerin into plastic parenteral solution containers, the dilution and storage of TRIDIL for intravenous infusion should be made only in *glass* parenteral solution bottles.
2. Some filters absorb nitroglycerin; they should be avoided.
3. Forty to 80% of the total amount of nitroglycerin in the final diluted solution for infusion is absorbed by the polyvinyl chloride (PVC) tubing of the intravenous administration sets currently in general use. The higher rates of absorption occur when flow rates are low, nitroglycerin concentrations are high, and the administration set is long. Although the rate of loss is highest during the early phase of infusion (when flow rates are lowest) the loss is neither constant nor self-limiting; consequently no simple calculation or correction can be performed to convert the theoretical infusion rate (based on the concentration of the infusion solution) to the actual delivery rate.

Because of this problem, Tridilset® i.v. administration set and TRIDILSET V.I.P.® volumetric infusion pump connector set were devloped to minimize the loss of TRIDIL. TRIDILSET or TRIDILSET V.I.P. are recommended for infusions of TRIDIL (see DOSAGE AND ADMINISTRATION). DOSING INSTRUCTIONS MUST BE FOLLOWED WITH CARE. IT SHOULD BE NOTED THAT WHEN TRIDILSET/TRIDILSET V.I.P. IS USED, THE CALCULATED DOSE WILL BE DELIVERED TO THE PATIENT BECAUSE THE LOSS OF TRIDIL DUE TO ABSORPTION IN STANDARD PVC TUBING WILL BE KEPT TO A MINIMUM. NOTE THAT THE DOSAGES COMMONLY USED IN PUBLISHED STUDIES UTILIZED GENERAL-USE PVC ADMINISTRATION SETS AND RECOMMENDED DOSES BASED ON THIS EXPERIENCE ARE TOO HIGH WHEN TRIDILSET/TRIDILSET V.I.P. IS USED.

PRECAUTIONS

TRIDIL (nitroglycerin) should be used with caution in patients with severe liver or renal disease. Safety of intracoronary injection of this preparation has not been shown.

TRIDIL DILUTION AND ADMINISTRATION TABLE

TRIDILSET ADMIXTURE FLOW RATE MICRO DROPS/MIN=ML/HR	**DILUTE** 5 MG TRIDIL IN 100 ML OR 25 MG TRIDIL IN 500 ML	5 MG TRIDIL IN 50 ML OR 25 MG TRIDIL IN 250 ML OR 50 MG TRIDIL IN 500 ML	10 MG TRIDIL IN 50 ML OR 50 MG TRIDIL IN 250 ML OR 100 MG TRIDIL IN 500 ML	100 MG TRIDIL IN 250 ML OR 200 MG TRIDIL IN 500 ML
	TO YIELD			
	50 MCG/ML	100 MCG/ML	200 MCG/ML	400 MCG/ML
	TRIDIL ADMINISTRATION RATE MCG I.V. NITROGLYCERIN/MIN			
3	—	5	10	20
6	5	10	20	40
12	10	20	40	80
24	20	40	80	160
48	40	80	160	320
72	60	120	240	480
96	80	160	320	640

Excessive hypotension, especially for prolonged periods of time, must be avoided because of possible deleterious effects on the brain, heart, liver, and kidney from poor perfusion and the attendant risk of ischemia, thrombosis, and altered function of these organs. Paradoxical bradycardia and increased angina pectoris may accompany nitroglycerin-induced hypotension. Patients with normal or low pulmonary capillary wedge pressure are especially sensitive to the hypotensive effects of TRIDIL. If pulmonary capillary wedge pressure is being monitored, it will be noted that a fall in wedge pressure precedes the onset of arterial hypotension, and the pulmonary capillary wedge pressure is thus a useful guide to safe titration of the drug.

Drug Interactions
Patients receiving intravenous nitroglycerin require higher doses of heparin for effective anticoagulation. On stopping nitroglycerin therapy, the partial thromboplastin time (PTT) can rise markedly, unless the heparin dosage is decreased. Close monitoring of the PTT is required to maintain adequate anticoagulant effect whenever these drugs are used in combination and to avoid excessive bleeding when therapy with nitroglycerin is terminated or the dosage decreased.

Carcinogenesis, mutagenesis, impairment of fertility
No long-term studies in animals were performed to evaluate carcinogenic potential of TRIDIL.

Pregnancy
Category C. Animal reproduction studies have not been conducted with TRIDIL. It is also not known whether TRIDIL can cause fetal harm when administered to a pregnant woman or can affect reproduction capacity. TRIDIL should be given to a pregnant woman only if clearly needed.

Nursing Mothers
It is not known whether nitroglycerin is excreted in human milk. Because many drugs are excreted in human milk, caution should be exercised when TRIDIL is administered to a nursing woman.

Pediatric Use
The safety and effectiveness of TRIDIL in children have not been established.

ADVERSE REACTIONS
The most frequent adverse reaction in patients treated with TRIDIL is headache, which occurs in approximately 2% of patients. Other adverse reactions occuring in less than 1% of patients are the following: tachycardia, nausea, vomiting, apprehension, restlessness, muscle twitching, retrosternal discomfort, palpitations, dizziness and abdominal pain.
The following additional adverse reactions have been reported with the oral and/or topical use of nitroglycerin: cutaneous flushing, weakness and occasionally drug rash or exfoliative dermatitis.

OVERDOSAGE
Accidental overdosage of TRIDIL may result in severe hypotension and reflex tachycardia which can be treated by elevating the legs and decreasing or temporarily terminating the infusion until the patient's condition stabilizes. Since the duration of the hemodynamic effects following TRIDIL administration is quite short, additional corrective measures are usually not required. However, if further therapy is indicated, administration of an intravenous alpha adrenergic agonist (e.g. methoxamine or phenylephrine) should be considered.

DOSAGE AND ADMINISTRATION
NOT FOR DIRECT INTRAVENOUS INJECTION
TRIDIL IS A CONCENTRATED, POTENT DRUG WHICH MUST BE DILUTED IN DEXTROSE (5%) INJECTION, USP OR SODIUM CHLORIDE (0.9%) INJECTION, USP PRIOR TO ITS INFUSION. TRIDIL SHOULD NOT BE ADMIXED WITH OTHER DRUGS.

1. Initial Dilution:
Aseptically transfer the contents of one TRIDIL ampul or vial (containing 25 or 50 mg of nitroglycerin) into a 500 mL *glass* bottle of either Dextrose (5%) Injection, USP or Sodium Chloride Injection (0.9%), USP. This yields a final concentration of 50 or 100 mcg/mL. Diluting 5 mg TRIDIL into 100 mL will also yield a final concentration of 50 mcg/mL.

2. Maintenance Dilution:
It is important to consider the fluid requirements of the patient as well as the expected duration of infusion in selecting the appropriate dilution of TRIDIL® (nitroglycerin).
After the initial dosage titration, the concentration of the admixture solution may be increased, if necessary, to limit fluids given to the patient. The TRIDIL concentration should not exceed 400 mcg/mL. See chart.
[See table above].
Note: If the concentration is adjusted, it is imperative to flush TRIDILSET®/TRIDILSET V.I.P.® before a new concentration is utilized. The dead-space of the set is approximately 15 mL, and depending on the flow rate it could take from 10 minutes to 3 hours for the new concentration to reach the patient if the set were not flushed.
Invert the glass parenteral bottle several times following admixture to assure uniform dilution of TRIDIL. When stored in *glass* containers, the diluted solution is physically and chemically stable for up to 48 hours at room temperature, and up to seven days under refrigeration.
Dosage is affected by the type of container and administration set used. See WARNINGS.
Although the usual starting adult dose range reported in clinical studies was 25 mcg/min or more, these studies used PVC ADMINISTRATION SETS. THE USE OF NON-ABSORBING TUBING WILL RESULT IN THE NEED FOR REDUCED DOSES.
If a peristaltic action infusion pump is used, a TRIDILSET i.v. administration set should be selected. As the TRIDILSET drip chamber delivers approximately 60 microdrops/mL, the TRIDIL DILUTION AND ADMINISTRATION TABLE may be used to calculate TRIDIL dilution and admixture flow rate in microdrops/minute to achieve the desired TRIDIL administration rate. If a volumetric infusion pump is used, a TRIDILSET V.I.P. volumetric infusion pump connector set should be selected. The TRIDIL DILUTION AND ADMINISTRATION TABLE may still be used; however, admixture flow rate will be determined directly by the infusion pump and is independent of the drop size of the TRIDILSET V.I.P. drip chamber, which is approximately 15 drops/mL. Thus, the reference to "MICRODROPS/MIN" is not applicable and the corresponding flow rate in ML/HR should be used to determine pump settings. NOTE: the TRIDILSET V.I.P. is not intended for use as an i.v. administration set independent of a volumetric infusion pump.
The dosage for TRIDILSET/TRIDILSET V.I.P. should initially be 5 mcg/min delivered through an infusion pump capable of exact and constant delivery of the drug. Subsequent titration must be adjusted to the clinical situation, with dose increments becoming more cautious as partial response is seen. Initial titration should be in 5 mcg/min increments with increases every 3–5 minutes until some response is noted. If no response is seen at 20 mcg/min, increments of 10 and later 20 mcg/min can be used. Once a partial blood pressure response is observed, the dose increase should be reduced and the interval between increases should be lengthened. Some patients with normal or low left ventricular filling pressures or pulmonary capillary wedge pressure (e.g. angina patients without other complications) may be hypersensitive to the effects of TRIDIL and may respond fully to doses as small as 5 mcg/min. These patients require especially careful titration and monitoring.

There is no fixed optimum dose of TRIDIL. Due to variations in the responsiveness of individual patients to the drug, each patient must be titrated to the desired level of hemodynamic function. Therefore, continuous monitoring of physiologic parameters (e.g. blood pressure and heart rate in all patients, other measurement such as pulmonary capillary wedge pressure, as appropriate MUST BE PERFORMED to achieve the correct dose. Adequate systemic blood pressure and coronary perfusion pressure must be maintained.

HOW SUPPLIED
NDC 0094-0073-10, 5 mg-10 mL ampul.
NDC 0094-0085-05, 25 mg-5 mL ampul.
NDC 0094-0085-86, 25 mg-5 mL single use vial.
NDC 0094-0090-10, 50 mg-10 mL ampul.
NDC 0094-0090-66, 50 mg-10 mL single use vial.
NDC 0094-0095-79, 100 mg-20 mL single use vial.
Protect from freezing.
Du Pont Pharmaceuticals
E. I. du Pont de Nemours & Co.
Wilmington, Delaware 19898
Date: April, 1989   A43111

VALPIN® 50   ℞
[*val 'pin*]
anisotropine methylbromide 50 mg

DESCRIPTION
VALPIN® 50 is anisotropine methylbromide, a quaternary ammonium salt which differs chemically from atropine and most other anticholinergics in the substitution of an aliphatic for an aromatic side chain in the acid moiety of the ester.
Chemically, VALPIN® 50 is 2-propyl pentanoyl tropinium methylbromide. Its stability both to acid and alkaline hydrolysis minimizes inactivation.
VALPIN 50 Tablets also contain: colloidal silicon dioxide, FD&C Blue 2, FD&C Yellow 6, magnesium stearate, microcrystalline cellulose, starch, stearic acid and sugar.

ACTIONS
VALPIN® 50 inhibits gastric acid secretion and reduces gastrointestinal motility.

INDICATIONS
For use as adjunctive therapy in the treatment of peptic ulcer.
AS WITH ALL ANTICHOLINERGICS, IT SHOULD BE NOTED THAT AT THE PRESENT TIME THERE IS LACK OF CONCURRENCE AS TO THEIR VALUE IN THE TREATMENT OF GASTRIC ULCER. IT HAS NOT BEEN SHOWN CONCLUSIVELY WHETHER ANTICHOLINERGIC DRUGS AID IN THE HEALING OF A PEPTIC ULCER, DECREASE THE RATE OF RECURRENCES OR PREVENT COMPLICATION.

CONTRAINDICATIONS
Glaucoma; obstructive uropathy (for example, bladder neck obstruction due to prostatic hypertrophy); obstructive disease of the gastrointestinal tract (as in achalasia, pyloroduodenal stenosis, etc.); paralytic ileus, intestinal atony of the elderly or debilitated patient; unstable cardiovascular status in acute hemorrhage; severe ulcerative colitis; toxic megacolon complicating ulcerative colitis; myasthenia gravis.

WARNINGS
Use in Pregnancy Since the safety of these preparations in pregnancy, lactation or in women of child-bearing age has not been established, use of the drugs in such patients re-

Continued on next page

Du Pont Pharm.—Cont.

quires that the potential benefits of the drug be weighed against possible hazards to the mother and child.

In the presence of a high environmental temperature, heat prostration can occur with drug use (fever and heat stroke due to decreased sweating).

Diarrhea may be an early symptom of incomplete intestinal obstruction, especially in patients with ileostomy or colostomy. In this instance treatment with this drug would be inappropriate and possibly harmful.

VALPIN® 50 may produce drowsiness or blurred vision. In this event, the patient should be warned not to engage in activities requiring mental alertness such as operating a motor vehicle or other machinery or perform hazardous work while taking this drug.

PRECAUTIONS

Use with caution in patients with:
—Autonomic neuropathy.
—Hepatic or renal disease.
— Ulcerative colitis—large doses may suppress intestinal motility to the point of producing a paralytic ileus and the use of this drug may precipitate or aggravate the serious complication of toxic megacolon.
—Hyperthyroidism, coronary heart disease, congestive heart failure, cardiac arrhythmias, hypertension and non-obstructing prostatic hypertrophy.
— Hiatal hernia associated with reflux esophagitis since anticholinergic drugs may aggravate this condition.

It should be noted that the use of anticholinergic drugs in the treatment of gastric ulcer may produce a delay in gastric emptying time and may complicate such therapy (antral stasis).

Do not rely on the use of the drug in the presence of complication of biliary tract disease.

Investigate any tachycardia before giving anticholinergic (atropine-like) drugs since they may increase the heart rate. With overdosage, a curare-like action may occur.

ADVERSE REACTIONS

Anticholinergic drugs produce certain effects which may be physiologic or toxic depending upon the individual patient's response. The physician must delineate these.

Adverse reactions may include xerostomia; urinary hesitancy and retention; blurred vision and tachycardia; palpitations; mydriasis; cycloplegia; increased ocular tension; loss of taste; headaches; nervousness; drowsiness; weakness; dizziness; insomnia; nausea; vomiting; impotence; suppression of lactation; constipation; bloated feeling; severe allergic reaction or drug idiosyncrasies including anaphylaxis; urticaria and other dermal manifestations; some degree of mental confusion and/or excitement especially in elderly persons. Decreased sweating is another adverse reaction that may occur.

DOSAGE AND ADMINISTRATION

To be effective dosage must be titrated to individual patient needs. Usual adult dosage—VALPIN® 50 mg tablet; one tablet 3 times daily.

MANAGEMENT OF OVERDOSAGE

While overdosage intoxication with anisotropine methylbromide has not been reported, theoretically it could occur since anisotropine methylbromide is an anticholinergic drug. When anticholinergic drugs are taken in sufficient overdose to produce severe symptoms, prompt treatment should be instituted. If the drug has been taken orally, gastric lavage and other measures to limit intestinal absorption should be initiated without delay. Physostigmine administered parenterally may be necessary for treatment of the serious manifestations of intoxication. Additionally, symptomatic therapy, including oxygen, sedatives, and control of hyperthermia may be necessary.

HOW SUPPLIED

VALPIN® 50: 50 mg anisotropine methylbromide in each scored, beige tablet.
Bottles of 100 tablets NDC 0056-0161-70
Store at controlled room temperature (59°–86°F, 15°–30°C).

Animal Pharmacology and Toxicology: VALPIN® 50 (anisotropine methylbromide) is a relatively non-toxic drug. In dogs, mice, rats and guinea pigs both acute toxic and chronic toxic dose-levels are at many times in excess of the clinically useful range.

Both in vitro and oral in vivo data in mice and rats indicate that VALPIN® 50 (anisotropine methylbromide) is at least 2 or 3 times as potent as homatropine methylbromide in antispasmodic action while it is less than two-thirds as active in mydriatic effect. It has less than one-fiftieth of the mydriatic activity of atropine sulfate. In inhibition of salivary flow, VALPIN® 50 (anisotropine methylbromide) is one-fifth as active as homatropine methylbromide and only one-hundredth as active as atropine sulfate. This pharmacologic profile is consistent with relative specificity of action on the gastrointestinal smooth muscle and the lesser tendency to produce side effects.

VALPIN® is a registered U.S. trademark of E.I. duPont de Nemours & Co. (Inc.)
6083-9

ZYDONE®   ⒸⒾⒾⒾ
[zī"dōn']
(Hydrocodone Bitartrate and Acetaminophen)
Capsules

DESCRIPTION

Each ZYDONE capsule contains:
Hydrocodone Bitartrate .... 5 mg
WARNING: May be habit forming
Acetaminophen... 500 mg
Hydrocodone Bitartrate is an opioid analgesic and antitussive and occurs as fine, white crystals or as a crystalline powder. It is affected by light. The chemical name is: 4,5α-epoxy-3-methoxy-17-methylmorphinan-6-one tartrate (1:1) hydrate (2:5). Its structure is as follows:

$$C_{18}H_{21}NO_3 \cdot C_4H_6O_6 \cdot 2\tfrac{1}{2}H_2O \qquad M.W.\ 494.50$$

Acetaminophen, 4'-hydroxyacetanilide, is a non-opiate, non-salicylate analgesic and antipyretic which occurs as a white, odorless crystalline powder possessing a slightly bitter taste. Its structure is as follows:

$$C_8H_9NO_2 \qquad M.W.\ 151.16$$

CLINICAL PHARMACOLOGY

Hydrocodone is a semisynthetic narcotic analgesic and antitussive with multiple actions qualitatively similar to those of codeine. Most of these involve the central nervous system and smooth muscle. The precise mechanism of action of hydrocodone and other opiates is not known, although it is believed to relate to the existence of opiate receptors in the central nervous system. In addition to analgesia, narcotics may produce drowsiness, changes in mood and mental clouding.

Radioimmunoassay techniques have recently been developed for the analysis of hydrocodone in human plasma. After a 10 mg oral dose of hydrocodone bitartrate, a mean peak serum drug level of 23.6 ng/ml and an elimination half-life of 3.8 hours were found.

The analgesic action of acetaminophen involves peripheral and central influences, but the specific mechanism is as yet undetermined. Antipyretic activity is mediated through hypothalamic heat regulating centers. Acetaminophen inhibits prostaglandin synthetase. Therapeutic doses of acetaminophen have negligible effects on the cardiovascular or respiratory systems; however, toxic doses may cause circulatory failure and rapid, shallow breathing. Acetaminophen is rapidly and almost completely absorbed from the gastrointestinal tract, producing maximum serum concentrations within 30 minutes to one hour. The plasma half-life in adults and children ranges from 0.90 hours to 3.25 hours with an average of approximately 2 hours. The drug distributes uniformly in most body fluids and is approximately 25% protein bound. Acetaminophen is conjugated in the liver, with less than 3% of the dose excreted unchanged in 24 hours. The primary metabolic pathway is conjugation to sulfate and glucuronide by-products. A minor oxidative pathway forms cysteine and mercapturic acid. These compounds are subsequently excreted by the kidneys into the urine.

INDICATIONS AND USAGE

For the relief of moderate to moderately severe pain.

CONTRAINDICATIONS

Hypersensitivity to acetaminophen or hydrocodone.

WARNINGS

Respiratory Depression: At high doses or in sensitive patients, hydrocodone may produce dose-related respiratory depression by acting directly on brain stem respiratory centers. Hydrocodone also affects centers that control respiratory rhythm, and may produce irregular and periodic breathing.

Head Injury and Increased Intracranial Pressure: The respiratory depressant effects of narcotics and their capacity to elevate cerebrospinal fluid pressure may be markedly exaggerated in the presence of head injury, other intracranial lesions or a preexisting increase in intracranial pressure. Furthermore, narcotics produce adverse reactions which

may obscure the clinical course of patients with head injuries.

Acute Abdominal Conditions: The administration of narcotics may obscure the diagnosis or clinical course of patients with acute abdominal conditions.

PRECAUTIONS

Special Risk Patients: As with any narcotic analgesic agent, Hydrocodone Bitartrate and Acetaminophen Capsules should be used with caution in elderly or debilitated patients and those with severe impairment of hepatic or renal function, hypothyroidism, Addison's disease, prostatic hypertrophy or urethral stricture. The usual precautions should be observed and the possibility of respiratory depression should be kept in mind.

Information for Patients: ZYDONE Capsules, like all narcotics, may impair the mental and/or physical abilities required for the performance of potentially hazardous tasks such as driving a car or operating machinery; patients should be cautioned accordingly.

Cough Reflex: Hydrocodone suppresses the cough reflex; as with all narcotics, caution should be exercised when ZYDONE Capsules are used postoperatively and in patients with pulmonary disease.

Drug Interactions: Patients receiving other narcotic analgesics, antipsychotics, antianxiety agents, or other CNS depressants (including alcohol) concomitantly with ZYDONE Capsules may exhibit an additive CNS depression. When combined therapy is contemplated, the dose of one or both agents should be reduced.

The use of MAO inhibitors or tricyclic antidepressants with hydrocodone preparations may increase the effect of either the antidepressant or hydrocodone.

The concurrent use of anticholinergics with hydrocodone may produce paralytic ileus.

Usage in Pregnancy: Teratogenic Effects: Pregnancy Category C. Hydrocodone has been shown to be teratogenic in hamsters when given in doses 700 times the human dose. There are no adequate and well-controlled studies in pregnant women. Hydrocodone Bitartrate and Acetaminophen Capsules should be used during pregnancy only if the potential benefit justifies the potential risk to the fetus.

Nonteratogenic Effects: Babies born to mothers who have been taking opioids regularly prior to delivery will be physically dependent. The withdrawal signs include irritability and excessive crying, tremors, hyperactive reflexes, increased respiratory rate, increased stools, sneezing, yawning, vomiting, and fever. The intensity of the syndrome does not always correlate with the duration of maternal opioid use or dose. There is no consensus on the best method of managing withdrawal. Chlorpromazine 0.7 to 1.0 mg/kg q6h, and paregoric 2 to 4 drops/kg q4h, have been used to treat withdrawal symptoms in infants. The duration of therapy is 4 to 28 days, with the dosage decreased as tolerated.

Labor and Delivery: As with all narcotics, administration of ZYDONE Capsules to the mother shortly before delivery may result in some degree of respiratory depression in the newborn, especially if higher doses are used.

Nursing Mothers: It is not known whether this drug is excreted in human milk. Because many drugs are excreted in human milk and because of the potential for serious adverse reactions in nursing infants from ZYDONE Capsules, a decision should be made whether to discontinue nursing or to discontinue the drug, taking into account the importance of the drug to the mother.

Pediatric Use: Safety and effectiveness in children have not been established.

ADVERSE REACTIONS

The most frequently observed adverse reactions include lightheadedness, dizziness, sedation, nausea and vomiting. These effects seem to be more prominent in ambulatory than in nonambulatory patients and some of these adverse reactions may be alleviated if the patient lies down.
Other adverse reactions include:

Central Nervous System: Drowsiness, mental clouding, lethargy, impairment of mental and physical performance, anxiety, fear, dysphoria, psychic dependence, mood changes.

Gastrointestinal System: The antiemetic phenothiazines are useful in suppressing the nausea and vomiting which may occur (see above); however, some phenothiazine derivatives seem to be antianalgesic and to increase the amount of narcotic required to produce pain relief, while other phenothiazines reduce the amount of narcotic required to produce a given level of analgesia. Prolonged administration of ZYDONE (Hydrocodone Bitartrate and Acetaminophen) Capsules may produce constipation.

Genitourinary System: Ureteral spasm, spasm of vesical sphincters and urinary retention have been reported.

Respiratory Depression: Hydrocodone Bitartrate may produce dose-related respiratory depression by acting directly on the brain stem respiratory center. Hydrocodone also affects the center that controls respiratory rhythm, and may produce irregular and periodic breathing. If significant respiratory depression occurs, it may be antagonized by the use of naloxone hydrochloride. Apply other supportive measures when indicated.

DRUG ABUSE AND DEPENDENCE

ZYDONE Capsules are subject to the Federal Controlled Substance Act (Schedule III). Psychic dependence, physical dependence, and tolerance may develop upon repeated administration of narcotics; therefore, ZYDONE Capsules should be prescribed and administered with caution. However, psychic dependence is unlikely to develop when ZYDONE Capsules are used for a short time for the treatment of pain.

Physical dependence, the condition in which continued administration of the drug is required to prevent the appearance of a withdrawal syndrome, assumes clinically significant proportions only after several weeks of continued narcotic use, although some mild degree of physical dependence may develop after a few days of narcotic therapy. Tolerance, in which increasingly large doses are required in order to produce the same degree of analgesia, is manifested initially by a shortened duration of analgesic effect, and subsequently by decreases in the intensity of analgesia. The rate of development of tolerance varies among patients.

OVERDOSAGE

Hydrocodone: Signs and Symptoms: Serious overdose with hydrocodone is characterized by respiratory depression (a decrease in respiratory rate and/or tidal volume, Cheyne-Stokes respiration, cyanosis), extreme somnolence progressing to stupor or coma, skeletal muscle flaccidity, cold and clammy skin, and sometimes bradycardia and hypotension. In severe overdosage, apnea, circulatory collapse, cardiac arrest and death may occur.

Treatment: Primary attention should be given to the reestablishment of adequate respiratory exchange through provision of a patent airway and the institution of assisted or controlled ventilation. The narcotic antagonist naloxone is a specific antidote against respiratory depression which may result from overdosage or unusual sensitivity to narcotics. Including hydrocodone. Therefore, an appropriate dose of naloxone hydrochloride (see package insert) should be administered, preferably by the intravenous route,, and simultaneously with efforts at respiratory resuscitation. Since the duration of action of hydrocodone may exceed that of the antagonist, the patient should be kept under continued surveillance and repeated doses of the antagonist should be administered as needed to maintain adequate respiration.

An antagonist should not be administered in the absence of clinically significant respiratory or cardiovascular depression. Oxygen, intravenous fluids, vasopressors and other supportive-measures should be employed as indicated.

Gastric emptying may be useful in removing unabsorbed drug.

Acetaminophen: Signs and symptoms: In acute acetaminophen overdosage, dose-dependent, potentially fatal hepatic necrosis is the most serious adverse effect. Renal tubular necrosis, hypoglycemic coma and thrombocytopenia may also occur.

In adults, hepatic toxicity has rarely been reported with acute overdoses of less than 10 grams and fatalities with less than 15 grams. Importantly, young children seem to be more resistant than adults to the hepatotoxic effect of an acetaminophen overdose. Despite this, the measures outlined below should be initiated in any adult or child suspected of having ingested an acetaminophen overdose.

Early symptoms following a potentially hepatotoxic overdose may include: nausea, vomiting, diaphoresis and general malaise. Clinical and laboratory evidence of hepatic toxicity may not be apparent under 48 to 72 hours post-ingestion.

Treatment: The stomach should be emptied promptly by lavage or by induction of emesis with syrup of ipecac. Patients' estimates of the quantity of a drug ingested are notoriously unreliable. Therefore, if an acetaminophen overdose is suspected, a serum acetaminophen assay should be obtained as early as possible, but no sooner than four hours following ingestion. Liver function studies should be obtained initially and repeated at 24-hour intervals.

The antidote, N-acetylcysteine, should be administered as early as possible, preferably within 16 hours of the overdose ingestion for optimal results, but in any case within 24 hours. Following recovery, there are no residual, structural or functional hepatic abnormalities.

DOSAGE AND ADMINISTRATION

Dosage should be adjusted according to the severity of the pain and the response of the patient. However, it should be kept in mind that tolerance to hydrocodone can develop with continued use and that the incidence of untoward effects is dose related.

The usual adult dose is one or two capsules every four to six hours as needed for pain. The total 24 hour dose should not exceed eight capsules.

HOW SUPPLIED

ZYDONE (Hydrocodone Bitratrate 5 mg and Acetaminophen 500 mg) is a white, hard gelatin capsule with red band. Each capsule is imprinted in red, DU PONT ZYDONE.

Bottles of 100: NDC 0056-0091-70

Storage: Store at controlled room temperature 15°–30°C (59°–86°F).

CAUTION: Federal law prohibits dispensing without prescription.

Manufactured by
D.M. Graham Laboratories, Inc., Hobart, New York 13788
for
DuPont Pharmaceuticals
E.I. duPont de Nemours & Co. (Inc.)
Wilmington, Delaware 19898

ZYDONE™ is a U.S. Trademark of E.I. duPont de Nemours & Co. (Inc.)

6173-4/Rev. April, 1988
Shown in Product Identification Section, page 410

EDUCATIONAL MATERIAL

BREVIBLOC®

Films/Slides/Videos

"Dosing and Administration of BREVIBLOC® in the Critical Care Setting." This 15-minute video describes the dosing and administration of esmolol in the ICU/CCU setting. It features medical professionals from Cedars-Sinai Medical Center, Los Angeles, California. Available in ½" VHS video.

COUMADIN ®

Books/Booklets/Brochures

"COUMADIN Patient Aid." This patient aid kit is designed to increase patient compliance and understanding of COUMADIN therapy. The kit includes an easy-to-understand patient guide, a dosing calendar, and a wallet card. No charge to physicians, pharmacists, patients, and others involved with the management of patients on COUMADIN. Call 1-800-341-4004 for copies.

Films/Slides/Video

"Using COUMADIN® Safely and Effectively." This 11½ minute, ½-inch VHS video is designed to be shown by the physician to his patients on COUMADIN® in order to increase patient compliance and understanding of COUMADIN® therapy. Single copies can be ordered at no charge by calling 1-800-341-4004.

An audiocassette is also available as a patient give-away of the "Using COUMADIN® Safely and Effectively" video.

Pictures/Charts

"COUMADIN Drug Interaction Chart." A 8½" × 11" chart highlighting the drugs which can increase or decrease the effects of COUMADIN is available at no charge to physicians, pharmacists, and other healthcare professionals.

"COUMADIN Patient Anticoagulant Record Charts." These packs of 8½" × 11" charts provide a convenient way to record patient prothrombin times and COUMADIN doses. Available at no charge to physicians, pharmacists, and other healthcare professionals involved with the management of patients on COUMADIN therapy.

PERCODAN®/PERCOCET®/ZYDONE®

Books/Booklets/Brochures

"How to talk to your Doctor about acute pain." An educational aid to help patients be more specific in describing acute pain. No charge publication. Call 1 (800) 527-2601.

"Coping with Pain at Home." An educational aid to help cancer patients with acute or chronic pain caused by malignancy. No charge publication. Call 1 (800) 527-2601.

"The Proper Management of Acute Pain in the Primary Care Setting." Four physician pain specialists, a pharmacologist and a pain center coordinator discuss evaluation and treatment options for patients who present with acute pain in the office setting. No charge publication. Write to Du Pont Pharmaceuticals and ask for H-07602 or call 1 (800) 527-2601.

"The Proper Management of Acute Pain in the Postoperative Setting." Two orthopedic surgeons, a general surgeon, an anesthesiologist and a nursing director discuss evaluation and treatment options for patients with postoperative pain. No charge publication. Write Du Pont Pharmaceuticals and ask for H-07614 or call 1 (800) 527-2601.

SYMMETREL®

"Cause of Death: Influenza" examines the deadly impact of influenza, the sixth leading cause of death in the U.S. Opening with a historical documentary on influenza in the 20th century the program features a panel discussion of leading infectious disease experts, moderated by Jim Hartz. Case histories of influenza in the family and the community are included along with myths and truths about influenza prevention and treatment. Strategies for clinical practice offer practical guidance to the medical professional. A one-hour videotape is available in VHS, ¾-inch or BETA formats at no charge to healthcare professional by calling the West

Glen Films Video Loan Library, (212) 921-2800. Ask for "Du Pont's Cause of Death: Influenza" videotape.

Dura Pharmaceuticals, Inc.
P.O. BOX 2209
RAMONA, CA 92065-0938

DURA-GEST®   ℞

DESCRIPTION

Each Dura-Gest gray and white capsule for oral administration contains:
Phenylephrine hydrochloride .... 5 mg.
Phenylpropanolamine hydrochloride .... 45 mg.
Guaifenesin .... 200 mg.

HOW SUPPLIED

DURA-GEST gray and white capsules are imprinted with DURA-GEST and 51479005.
NDC 51479-005-01 Bottle of 100
NDC 51479-005-05 Bottle of 500
Dispense in tight containers as defined in USP/NF.
Store between 15°–30°C (59°–86°F).
Dispense in child resistant containers.

DURA-TAP/PD® CAPSULES   ℞

DESCRIPTION

Each Dura-Tap/PD opaque blue and clear capsule containing white beads for oral administration contains:
Chlorpheniramine Maleate .... 4 mg.
Pseudoephedrine Hydrochloride .... 60 mg.
in a special base to provide prolonged action.

HOW SUPPLIED

Dura-Tap/PD is available as a opaque blue and clear capsule containing white beads imprinted with 51479007.
NDC 51479-007-01 Bottle of 100
Dispense in tight containers as defined in USP/NF.
Store between 15°–30°C (59°–86°F).
Dispense in child-resistant containers.

DURA-VENT® TABLETS   ℞

DESCRIPTION

Each Dura-Vent white, scored tablet for oral administration contains:
Phenylpropanolamine Hydrochloride .... 75 mg.
Guaifenesin .... 600 mg.
in a special base to provide prolonged action.

HOW SUPPLIED

Dura-Vent is available as a white, scored tablet imprinted with 7.5.
NDC 51479-006-01 Bottle of 100
NDC 51479-006-06 Bottle of 600
Dispense in tight containers as defined in USP/NF.
Store between 15°–30°C (59°–86°F).
Dispense in child-resistant containers.

DURA-VENT/A® CAPSULES   ℞

DESCRIPTION

Each Dura-Vent/A clear capsule containing white beads for oral administration contains:
Phenylpropanolamine Hydrochloride .... 75 mg.
Chlorpheniramine Maleate .... 10 mg.
in a special base to provide prolonged action.

HOW SUPPLIED

Dura-Vent/A is available as a clear capsule containing white beads imprinted with Dura-Vent/A and 51479002.
NDC 51479-002-01 Bottle of 100
Dispense in tight containers as defined in USP/NF.
Store between 15°–30°C (59°–86°F).
Dispense in child-resistant containers.

DURA-VENT/DA® TABLETS   ℞

DESCRIPTION

Each Dura-Vent/DA light brown, scored tablet for oral administration contains:
Chlorpheniramine Maleate .... 8 mg.
Phenylephrine Hydrochloride .... 20 mg.
Methscopolamine Nitrate .... 2.5 mg.
in a special base to provide prolonged action.

Continued on next page

Dura—Cont.

HOW SUPPLIED

Dura-Vent/DA is available as a light brown, scored tablet imprinted with S-103.
NDC 51479-008-01 Bottle of 100
Dispense in tight containers as defined in USP/NF.
Store between 15°–30°C (59°–86°F).
Dispense in child-resistant containers.

FENESIN™ TABLETS   ℞

DESCRIPTION

Each light blue, scored, sustained-release tablet for oral administration contains:
Guaifenesin .... 600 mg.
in a special base to provide prolonged action.

HOW SUPPLIED

Fenesin is available as a light blue, scored tablet imprinted wiht DURA/009.
NDC 51479-009-01 Bottle of 100
NDC 51479-009-06 Bottle of 600
Dispense in tight containers as defined in USP/NF.
Store between 15°–30°C (59°–86°F).
Dispense in child-resistant containers.

Duramed Pharmaceuticals, Inc.
5040 LESTER ROAD
CINCINNATI, OH 45213

PRODUCT LIST

NDC No. 51285	STRENGTH	PKG. SIZES	CODE IMPRINT ON PRODUCT
	Aminophylline Tablets		℞
223	100 mg	100, 1000	223
224	200 mg	100, 1000	224
	Chlorpropamide Tablets		℞
252	100 mg	100, 1000	252
251	250 mg	100, 1000	251
	Clonidine HCl Tablets		℞
211	0.1 mg	100, 1000	01
212	0.2 mg	100, 1000	02
213	0.3 mg	100, 1000	03
	Conjugated Estrogens Tablets		℞
235	0.3 mg	100	30
236	0.625 mg	100, 1000	31
237	1.25 mg	100, 1000	32
238	2.5 mg	100	34
	Cyproheptadine HCl Tablets		℞
246	4 mg	100, 1000	246
	Diazepam Tablets		©/℞
621	2 mg	100, 500, 1000	15
622	5 mg	100, 500, 1000	622
623	10 mg	100, 500, 1000	623
	Dipyridamole Tablets		℞
255	25 mg	100, 1000	25
257	50 mg	100, 1000	50
258	75 mg	100, 1000	75
	Duratex Capsules		℞
293	5/45/200 mg	100	293
	Haloperidol Tablets		℞
225	0.5 mg	100, 1000	225
226	1 mg	100, 1000	226
227	2 mg	100, 1000	227
228	5 mg	100, 500	228
229	10 mg	100, 500	229
230	20 mg	100, 500	230
	Hydroxyzine Pamoate Capsules		℞
265	25 mg	100, 500	265
266	50 mg	100, 500	266
267	100 mg	100, 500	267
	Indomethacin Capsules		℞
275	25 mg	100, 1000	275
	Iodur w/Codeine Liquid		©/℞
705	30/10 mg	pt.	—
	Iodur DM Liquid		℞
706	30/10 mg	pt.	—
	Iodur Elixir Liquid		℞
707	60 mg	pt.	—
	Isoniazid Tablets		℞
274	100 mg	100, 1000	274
277	300 mg	30, 100, 1000	277
	Methyldopa Tablets		℞
371	250 mg	100, 1000	371
372	500 mg	100, 500	372

	Methylprednisolone Tablets			℞
301	4 mg	100, 21 pk	301	
	Phentermine HCl Capsules			©/℞
651	30 mg	100, 1000	651	
	Phenylpropanolamine HCl and Guaifenesin Long-Acting Tablets			℞
294	75/400 mg	100, 500	294	
295	75/400 mg	100, 500	295	
	Prednisone Tablets			℞
311	5 mg	100, 1000	311	
312	10 mg	100, 1000	312	
313	20 mg	100, 1000	313	
	Prochlorperazine Maleate Tablets			℞
314	5 mg	100, 1000	314	
315	10 mg	100, 1000	315	
316	25 mg	100	316	
	Propranolol HCl Tablets			℞
321	10 mg	100, 1000	10	
322	20 mg	100, 1000	20	
323	40 mg	100, 1000	40	
320	60 mg	100	60	
324	80 mg	100, 500	80	
319	90 mg	100	90	
	Propranolol HCl and Hydrochlorothiazide Tablets			℞
332	40/25 mg	100	332	
333	80/25 mg	100	333	
	Temazepam Capsules			©/℞
660	15 mg	100, 500	660	
661	30 mg	100, 500	661	
	Tolazamide Tablets			℞
325	100 mg	100, 500	325	
326	250 mg	100, 200, 1000	326	
327	500 mg	100, 500	327	
	Trifluoperazine HCl Tablets			℞
351	1 mg	100, 1000	11	
352	2 mg	100, 1000	12	
353	5 mg	100, 1000	13	
354	10 mg	100, 1000	14	

Note: All code imprints have the ႟ logo on the product.

Elder Pharmaceuticals Inc.
See ICN PHARMACEUTICALS, INC.

Elkins-Sinn, Inc.
A subsidiary of A. H. Robins Company
2 ESTERBROOK LANE
CHERRY HILL, NJ 08003-4099

Elkins-Sinn's DOSETTE® line offers a broad spectrum of injectable products in a variety of unit-of-use containers— DOSETTE® vials, DOSETTE® ampuls, DOSETTE® syringes, and DOSETTE® cartridge-needle units. Easily adaptable to any hospital pharmacy set-up, the DOSETTE® system combines easily identifiable, clearly printed product labeling with space-conserving packaging. Each DOSETTE® container is characterized by product name and strength in large, bold-faced type, important usage and storage data, lot identification number, and expiration date. Elkins-Sinn also produces a vast number of multiple dose vials. Listed below are the major ESI products. For a complete catalog and price list, direct inquiries to Marketing Services. For specific product information, direct inquiries to the Professional Services Department.

AMINOCAPROIC ACID INJECTION, USP
250 mg/mL   20 mL Multiple Dose Vial
AMINOPHYLLINE INJECTION, USP (Preservative-Free)
250 mg/10 mL   10 mL Single Use Vial
250 mg/10 mL   10 mL Dosette Ampul
500 mg/20 mL   20 mL Single Use Vial
500 mg/20 mL   20 mL Dosette Ampul
AMPICILLIN SODIUM, USP (Sterile Powder)
250 mg   Single Use Vial
500 mg   Single Use Vial
500 mg   100 mL Piggyback Vial
1 gram   Single Use Vial
1 gram   100 mL Piggyback Vial
2 gram   Single Use Vial
2 gram   100 mL Piggyback Vial
10 gram   Pharmacy Bulk Package
ATROPINE SULFATE INJECTION, USP
400 mcg/mL   1 mL Dosette Vial
(0.4 mg, 1/150 gr)
400 mcg/mL   1 mL Dosette Ampul
(0.4 mg, 1/150 gr)
400 mcg/mL   20 mL Multiple Dose Vial
(0.4 mg, 1/150 gr)
1 mg/mL (1/60 gr)   1 mL Dosette Vial
BRETYLIUM TOSYLATE INJECTION (Preservative-Free)
500 mg/10mL   10 mL Dosette Ampul
500 mg/10mL   10 mL Single Use Vial

CALCIUM GLUCONATE INJECTION, USP
10% (1 g/10 mL)   10 mL Dosette Ampul
CHLORPROMAZINE HYDROCHLORIDE INJECTION, USP
25 mg/mL   1 mL Dosette Ampul
50 mg/2 mL   2 mL Dosette Ampul
CLINDAMYCIN PHOSPHATE INJECTION, USP
300 mg/2 mL   2 mL Single Dose Vial
600 mg/4 mL   4 mL Single Dose Vial
900 mg/6 mL   6 mL Single Dose Vial
9 gram/60 mL (150 mg/mL)   Pharmacy Bulk Package
CODEINE PHOSPHATE INJECTION, USP
30 mg/mL   1 mL Dosette Vial
60 mg/mL   1 mL Dosette Vial
CYANOCOBALAMIN INJECTION, USP
1 mg/mL (1000 mcg)   1 mL Dosette Vial
1 mg/mL (1000 mcg)   10 mL Multiple Dose Vial
1 mg/mL (1000 mcg)   30 mL Multiple Dose Vial
CYCLOPHOSPHAMIDE FOR INJECTION, USP
100 mg   Single Use Vial
200 mg   Single Use Vial
500 mg   Single Use Vial
1 gram   Single Use Vial
DEXAMETHASONE SODIUM PHOSPHATE INJECTION, USP
4 mg/mL   1 mL Dosette Vial
4 mg/mL   1 mL Dosette Syringe
4 mg/mL   5 mL Multiple Dose Vial
4 mg/mL   30 mL Multiple Dose Vial
10 mg/mL   1 mL Dosette Vial
10 mg/mL   1 mL Dosette Syringe
10 mg/mL   10 mL Multiple Dose Vial
DEXTROSE INJECTION, USP
10%   17 mL fill in 20 mL Vial
DIAZEPAM INJECTION, USP
5 mg/mL   2 mL Dosette Ampul
10 mg/2 mL   2 mL Dosette Ampul
10 mg/2 mL   10 mL Multiple Dose Vial
5 mg/mL   1 mL Dosette Syringe
10 mg/2 mL   2 mL Dosette Syringe
DIAZEPAM INJECTION, USP
DOSETTE CARTRIDGE NEEDLE UNITS
5 mg/mL   1 mL Dosette Cartridge
10 mg/2 mL   2 mL Dosette Cartridge
DIGOXIN INJECTION, USP
500 mcg/2 mL (0.5 mg)   2 mL Dosette Ampul
DIPHENHYDRAMINE HYDROCHLORIDE INJECTION, USP (High Potency)
50 mg/mL   1 mL Dosette Vial
DOPAMINE HYDROCHLORIDE INJECTION, USP
200 mg/5 mL   5 mL Dosette Ampul
200 mg/5 mL   5 mL Single Use Vial
400 mg/5 mL   5 mL Dosette Ampul
400 mg/5 mL   5 mL Single Use Vial
DOXYCYCLINE HYCLATE FOR INJECTION, USP
100 mg   Single Use Vial
DURAMORPH® (Morphine Sulfate Injection, USP) (Preservative-Free for Epidural & Intrathecal Administration)
5 mg/10 mL (0.5 mg/mL)   10 mL Dosette Ampul
10 mg/10 mL (1 mg/mL)   10 mL Dosette Ampul
EPINEPHRINE INJECTION, USP
1 mg/mL (1:1000)   1 mL Dosette Ampul
ERYTHROMYCIN LACTOBIONATE FOR INJECTION, USP
500 mg   Multiple Dose Vial
1 gram   Multiple Dose Vial
500 mg   100 mL Piggyback Vial
FENTANYL CITRATE INJECTION, USP (Preservative-Free)
100 mcg/2 mL   2 mL Dosette Ampul
(0.05 mg/mL)
250 mcg/5 mL   5 mL Dosette Ampul
(0.05 mg/mL)
500 mcg/10 mL   10 mL Dosette Ampul
(0.05 mg/mL)
1000 mcg/20 mL   20 mL Dosette Ampul
(0.05 mg/mL)
FUROSEMIDE INJECTION, USP (Preservative-Free)
20 mg/2 mL   2 mL Dosette Ampul
20 mg/2 mL   2 mL Single Use Vial
40 mg/4 mL   4 mL Dosette Ampul
40 mg/4 mL   4 mL Single Use Vial
100 mg/10 mL   10 mL Dosette Ampul
100 mg/10 mL   10 mL Single Use Vial
GENTAMICIN SULFATE INJECTION, USP
20 mg/2 mL   2 mL Dosette Vial
(10 mg/mL—Pediatric)
80 mg/2 mL   2 mL Dosette Vial
(40 mg/mL)
800 mg/20 mL   20 mL Multiple Dose Vial
(40 mg/mL)
GENTAMICIN SULFATE INJECTION, USP
DOSETTE CARTRIDGE NEEDLE UNITS
60 mg/1.5 mL   1.5 mL Dosette Cartridge
80 mg/2 mL   2 mL Dosette Cartridge
HEPARIN SODIUM INJECTION, USP (Porcine Derived)
1,000 Units/mL   1 mL Dosette Vial

1,000 Units/mL	10 mL Multiple Dose Vial
1,000 Units/mL	30 mL Multiple Dose Vial
5,000 Units/mL	1 mL Dosette Vial
5,000 Units/mL	10 mL Multiple Dose Vial
10,000 Units/mL	1 mL Dosette Vial
10,000 Units/mL	4 mL Multiple Dose Vial

HEPARIN SODIUM INJECTION, USP (Porcine Derived)
DOSETTE CARTRIDGE NEEDLE UNITS

1,000 Units/1 mL	1 mL Dosette Cartridge
5,000 Units/0.5 mL	0.5 mL Dosette Cartridge
5,000 Units/1 mL	1 mL Dosette Cartridge
10,000 Units/1 mL	1 mL Dosette Cartridge

HEP-LOCK® (Heparin Lock Flush Solution, USP)

10 Units/mL	1 mL Dosette Vial
10 Units/mL	2 mL Dosette Vial
10 Units/mL	10 mL Multiple Dose Vial
10 Units/mL	30 mL Multiple Dose Vial
100 Units/mL	1 mL Dosette Vial
100 Units/mL	2 mL Dosette Vial
100 Units/mL	10 mL Multiple Dose Vial
100 Units/mL	30 mL Multiple Dose Vial

HEP-LOCK® (Heparin Lock Flush Solution, USP)
DOSETTE CARTRIDGE NEEDLE UNITS

10 Units/1 mL	1 mL Dosette Cartridge
25 Units/2.5 mL	2.5 mL Dosette Cartridge
100 Units/1 mL	1 mL Dosette Cartridge
250 Units/2.5 mL	2.5 mL Dosette Cartridge

HEP-LOCK® U/P (Preservative-Free Heparin Lock Flush Solution, USP)

10 Units/mL	1 mL Dosette Vial
100 Units/mL	1 mL Dosette Vial

HYDROMORPHONE HYDROCHLORIDE INJECTION, USP

2 mg/mL	1 mL Dosette Vial
2 mg/mL	20 mL Multiple Dose Vial

HYDROXYZINE HYDROCHLORIDE INJECTION, USP

25 mg/mL	1 mL Dosette Vial
50 mg/mL	1 mL Dosette Vial
100 mg/2 mL	2 mL Dosette Vial
50 mg/mL	10 mL Multiple Dose Vial

ISOPROTERENOL HYDROCHLORIDE INJECTION, USP
(Refrigeration not required)

0.2 mg/mL (1:5000)	5 mL Dosette Ampul

LEUCOVORIN CALCIUM FOR INJECTION (Lyophilized)

50 mg	Single Use Vial

LIDOCAINE HYDROCHLORIDE INJECTION, USP
(Preserved)

1% (10 mg/mL)	30 mL Multiple Dose Vial
1% (10 mg/mL)	50 mL Multiple Dose Vial
2% (20 mg/mL)	30 mL Multiple Dose Vial
2% (20 mg/mL)	50 mL Multiple Dose Vial

LIDOCAINE HYDROCHLORIDE INJECTION, USP
(Preservative-Free, Single Use)

1% (10 mg/mL)	5 mL Single Use Vial
2% (20 mg/mL)	5 mL Single Use Vial

LIDOCAINE HYDROCHLORIDE AND EPINEPHRINE INJECTION, USP   (1:100,000)
(Refrigeration not required)

1% (10 mg/mL)	30 mL Multiple Dose Vial
2% (20 mg/mL)	30 mL Multiple Dose Vial

MEPERIDINE HYDROCHLORIDE INJECTION, USP

25 mg/mL	1 mL Dosette Vial
25 mg/mL	1 mL Dosette Ampul
50 mg/mL	1 mL Dosette Vial
50 mg/mL	1 mL Dosette Ampul
75 mg/mL	1 mL Dosette Vial
75 mg/mL	1 mL Dosette Ampul
100 mg/mL	1 mL Dosette Vial
100 mg/mL	1 mL Dosette Ampul

METHYLDOPATE HYDROCHLORIDE INJECTION, USP

250 mg/5 mL	5 mL Single Use Vial
500 mg/10 mL	10 mL Single Use Vial

METRONIDAZOLE REDI-INFUSION™
(Preservative-Free, Single Use)

500 mg/100 mL	100 mL Single Use Vial
(5 mg/mL with secondary IV infusion set)	
500 mg/100 mL	100 mL Single Use Vial
(5 mg/mL without secondary IV infusion set)	
500 mg/100 mL (5 mg/mL)	100 mL Plastic Bag

MORPHINE SULFATE INJECTION, USP

5 mg/mL (¹/₁₂ gr)	1 mL Dosette Vial
8 mg/mL (¹/₈ gr)	1 mL Dosette Vial
8 mg/mL (¹/₈ gr)	1 mL Dosette Ampul
10 mg/mL (¹/₆ gr)	1 mL Dosette Vial
10 mg/mL (¹/₆ gr)	1 mL Dosette Ampul
10 mg/mL (¹/₆ gr)	10 mL Multiple Dose Vial
15 mg/mL (¹/₄ gr)	1 mL Dosette Vial
15 mg/mL (¹/₄ gr)	1 mL Dosette Ampul
15 mg/mL (¹/₄ gr)	20 mL Multiple Dose Vial

NALOXONE HYDROCHLORIDE INJECTION, USP

400 mcg/mL	1 mL Dosette Vial
(0.4 mg/mL)	
400 mcg/mL	1 mL Dosette Ampul
(0.4 mg/mL)	
400 mcg/mL	10 mL Multiple Dose Vial
(0.4 mg/mL)	

NEOSTIGMINE METHYLSULFATE INJECTION, USP

1:1000 (1 mg/mL)	10 mL Multiple Dose Vial
1:2000 (0.5 mg/mL)	10 mL Multiple Dose Vial

PANCURONIUM BROMIDE INJECTION

2 mg/mL	2 mL Dosette Vial
2 mg/mL	2 mL Dosette Ampul
2 mg/mL	5 mL Dosette Ampul
2 mg/mL	5 mL Single Use Vial
1 mg/mL	10 mL Multiple Dose Vial

PHENOBARBITAL SODIUM INJECTION, USP

65 mg/mL (1 gr)	1 mL Dosette Vial
130 mg/mL (2 gr)	1 mL Dosette Vial

PHENYLEPHRINE HYDROCHLORIDE INJECTION, USP

10 mg/mL	1 mL Dosette Vial

PHENYTOIN SODIUM INJECTION, USP

100 mg/2 mL (50 mg/mL)	2 mL Dosette Vial
100 mg/2 mL (50 mg/mL)	2 mL Dosette Ampul
250 mg/5 mL (50 mg/mL)	5 mL Single Use Vial
250 mg/5 mL (50 mg/mL)	5 mL Dosette Ampul

PROCAINAMIDE HYDROCHLORIDE INJECTION, USP

500 mg/mL (1 gram/2 mL)	2 mL Multiple Dose Vial
100 mg/mL (1 gram/10 mL)	10 mL Multiple Dose Vial

PROCHLORPERAZINE EDISYLATE INJECTION, USP

10 mg/2 mL	2 mL Dosette Ampul

PROMETHAZINE HYDROCHLORIDE INJECTION, USP

25 mg/mL	1 mL Dosette Ampul
50 mg/mL	1 mL Dosette Ampul

PROTAMINE SULFATE INJECTION, USP
(Preservative-Free)
(Refrigeration not required)

50 mg/5 mL	5 mL Dosette Ampul
250 mg/25 mL	25 mL Single Use Vial

SODIUM CHLORIDE INJECTION, USP (Preservative-Free, Single Use)

0.9%	2 mL Dosette Vial
0.9%	5 mL Dosette Ampul
0.9%	10 mL Dosette Ampul

SODIUM CHLORIDE INJECTION, BACTERIOSTATIC, USP
(Preserved with 0.9% Benzyl Alcohol)

0.9%	30 mL Multiple Dose Vial
0.9%	2 mL Dosette Cartridge

SODIUM NITROPRUSSIDE, STERILE, USP

50 mg	Single Use Vial

SOTRADECOL® (Sodium Tetradecyl Sulfate Injection)

1%	2 mL Dosette Ampul
3%	2 mL Dosette Ampul

STERILE EMPTY VIAL

20 mL	20 mL Vial

SULFAMETHOXAZOLE & TRIMETHOPRIM CONCENTRATE FOR INJECTION, USP

80 mg/mL Sulfamethoxazole with 16 mg/mL Trimethoprim	5 mL Dosette Vial
80 mg/mL Sulfamethoxazole with 16 mg/mL Trimethoprim	5 mL Single Use Vial
80 mg/mL Sulfamethoxazole with 16 mg/mL Trimethoprim	10 mL Single Use Vial
80 mg/mL Sulfamethoxazole with 16 mg/mL Trimethoprim	30 mL Multiple Use Vial

THIAMINE HYDROCHLORIDE INJECTION, USP

100 mg/mL	1 mL Dosette Vial

VANCOMYCIN HYDROCHLORIDE, STERILE, USP

500 mg Vial	
1 gram Vial	

WATER FOR INJECTION, STERILE, USP (Preservative-Free)

	10 mL Dosette Ampul

WATER FOR INJECTION, BACTERIOSTATIC, USP
(Preserved with 0.9% Benzyl Alcohol)

	30 mL Multiple Dose Vial

DURAMORPH® ℃

[dūr "a 'mŏrf]
(morphine sulfate injection, USP)
Preservative-Free

PRODUCT OVERVIEW

KEY FACTS

Preservative-free DURAMORPH® is a sterile, pyrogen-free, isobaric solution free of antioxidants, preservatives or other potentially neurotoxic additives, and is intended for intravenous, epidural or intrathecal administration as a narcotic analgesic.

MAJOR USES

DURAMORPH® is used for the management of pain not responsive to non-narcotic analgesics. Administered epidurally or intrathecally, it provides pain relief for extended periods without attendant loss of motor, sensory or sympathetic function.

SAFETY INFORMATION

The most serious side effect is respiratory depression. When administered epidurally or intrathecally, patient monitoring should be continued for at least 24 hours after each dose since delayed respiratory depression may occur.

DURAMORPH® ℃

[dūr "a 'mŏrf]
(morphine sulfate injection, USP)
Preservative-free

DESCRIPTION

Morphine is the most important alkaloid of opium and is a phenanthrene derivative. It is available as the sulfate, having the following structural formula:

7,8 Didehydro-4,5-epoxy-17-methyl-(5α,6α)-
morphinan-3,6-diol
sulfate (2:1)
(salt), pentahydrate

$(C_{17}H_{19}NO_3)_2 \cdot H_2SO_4 \cdot 5H_2O$ Molecular weight is 758.83 Preservative-free DURAMORPH® (Morphine Sulfate Injection, USP) is a sterile, pyrogen-free, isobaric solution free of antioxidants, preservatives or other potentially neurotoxic additives, and is intended for intravenous, epidural or intrathecal administration as a narcotic analgesic. Each milliliter contains morphine sulfate 0.5 mg or 1 mg (Warning: May Be Habit Forming) and sodium chloride 9 mg in Water for Injection, pH range is 2.5–6.5. Ampuls are sealed under nitrogen. Each Dosette® ampul is intended for SINGLE USE ONLY. Discard any unused portion. DO NOT HEAT-STERILIZE.

CLINICAL PHARMACOLOGY

Morphine exerts its primary effects on the central nervous system and organs containing smooth muscle. Pharmacologic effects include analgesia, drowsiness, alteration in mood (euphoria), reduction in body temperature (at low doses), dose-related depression of respiration, interference with adrenocortical response to stress (at high doses), reduction in peripheral resistance with little or no effect on cardiac index and miosis.

Morphine, as other opioids, acts as an agonist interacting with stereospecific and saturable binding sites/receptors in the brain, spinal cord and other tissues. These sites have been classified as μ receptors and are widely distributed throughout the central nervous system being present in highest concentration in the limbic system (frontal and temporal cortex, amygdala and hippocampus), thalamus, striatum, hypothalamus, midbrain and laminae I, II, IV and V of the dorsal horn in the spinal cord. It has been postulated that exogenously administered morphine exerts its analgesic effect, in part, by altering the central release of neurotransmitter from afferent nerves sensitive to noxious stimuli. Peripheral threshold or responsiveness to noxious stimuli is unaffected leaving monosynaptic reflexes such as the patellar or the Achilles tendon reflex intact.

Autonomic reflexes are not affected by epidural or intrathecal morphine, however, morphine exerts spasmogenic effects on the gastrointestinal tract that result in decreased peristaltic activity.

Central nervous system effects of intravenously administered morphine sulfate are influenced by ability to cross the blood-brain barrier.

The delay in the onset of analgesia following epidural or intrathecal injection may be attributed to its relatively poor lipid solubility (i.e., an oil/water partition coefficient of 1.42), and its slow access to the receptor sites. The hydrophilic character of morphine may also explain its retention in the CNS and its slow release into the systemic circulation, resulting in a prolonged effect.

Nausea and vomiting may be prominent and are thought to be the result of central stimulation of the chemoreceptor trigger zone. Histamine release is common; allergic manifestations of urticaria and, rarely, anaphylaxis may occur. Bronchoconstriction may occur either as an idiosyncratic reaction or from large dosages.

Approximately one-third of intravenous morphine is bound to plasma proteins. Free morphine is rapidly redistributed in parenchymatous tissues. The major metabolic pathway is through conjugation with glucuronic acid in the liver. Elimination half-life is approximately 1.5 to 2 hours in healthy volunteers. For intravenously administered morphine, 90% is excreted in the urine within 24 hours and traces are detectable in urine up to 48 hours. About 7–10% of administered morphine eventually appears in the feces as conjugated morphine.

Peak serum levels following epidural or intrathecal administration of DURAMORPH® are reached within 30 minutes in most subjects and decline to very low levels during the

Continued on next page

Elkins-Sinn—Cont.

next 2 to 4 hours. The onset of action occurs in 15 to 60 minutes following epidural administration or intrathecal administration; analgesia may last up to 24 hours. Due to this extended duration of action, sustained pain relief can be provided with lower daily doses (by these two routes) than are usually required with intravenous or intramuscular morphine administration.

INDICATIONS AND USAGE

Preservative-free DURAMORPH® is a systemic narcotic analgesic for administration by the intravenous, epidural or intrathecal routes. It is used for the management of pain not responsive to non-narcotic analgesics. Morphine sulfate, administered epidurally or intrathecally, provides pain relief for extended periods without attendant loss of motor, sensory or sympathetic function.

CONTRAINDICATIONS

DURAMORPH® is contraindicated in those medical conditions which would preclude the administration of opioids by the intravenous route—allergy to morphine or other opiates, acute bronchial asthma, upper airway obstruction.
Administration of morphine by the epidural or intrathecal route is contraindicated in the presence of infection at the injection site, anticoagulant therapy, bleeding diathesis, parenterally administered corticosteroids within a two week period or other concomitant drug therapy or medical condition which would contraindicate the technique of epidural or intrathecal analgesia.

WARNINGS

DURAMORPH® administration should be limited to use by those familiar with the management of respiratory depression, and in the case of epidural or intrathecal administration, familiar with the techniques and patient management problems associated with epidural or intrathecal drug administration. Because epidural administration has been associated with lessened potential for immediate or late adverse effects than intrathecal administration, the epidural route should be used whenever possible. Rapid intravenous administration may result in chest wall rigidity. FACILITIES WHERE DURAMORPH® IS ADMINISTERED MUST BE EQUIPPED WITH RESUSCITATIVE EQUIPMENT, OXYGEN, NALOXONE INJECTION, AND OTHER RESUSCITATIVE DRUGS. WHEN THE EPIDURAL OR INTRATHECAL ROUTE OF ADMINISTRATION IS EMPLOYED, PATIENTS MUST BE OBSERVED IN A FULLY EQUIPPED AND STAFFED ENVIRONMENT FOR AT LEAST 24 HOURS.
SEVERE RESPIRATORY DEPRESSION UP TO 24 HOURS FOLLOWING EPIDURAL OR INTRATHECAL ADMINISTRATION HAS BEEN REPORTED.
Morphine sulfate may be habit forming. (See DRUG ABUSE AND DEPENDENCE.)

PRECAUTIONS

General
Preservative-free DURAMORPH® (Morphine Sulfate Injection, USP) should be administered with extreme caution in aged or debilitated patients, in the presence of increased intracranial/intraocular pressure and in patients with head injury. Pupillary changes (miosis) may obscure the course of intracranial pathology. Care is urged in patients who have a decreased respiratory reserve (e.g., emphysema, severe obesity, kyphoscoliosis).
Seizures may result from high doses. Patients with known seizure disorders should be carefully observed for evidence of morphine-induced seizure activity.
It is recommended that administration of DURAMORPH® by the epidural or intrathecal routes be limited to the lumbar area. Intrathecal use has been associated with a higher incidence of respiratory depression than epidural use.
Smooth muscle hypertonicity may result in biliary colic, difficulty in urination and possible urinary retention requiring catheterization. Consideration should be given to risks inherent in urethral catheterization, e.g., sepsis, when epidural or intrathecal administration is considered, especially in the perioperative period.
Elimination half-life may be prolonged in patients with reduced metabolic rates and with hepatic or renal dysfunction. Hence, care should be exercised in administering morphine in these conditions, particularly with repeated dosing.
Patients with reduced circulating blood volume, impaired myocardial function or on sympatholytic drugs should be observed carefully for orthostatic hypotension, particularly in transport.
Patients with chronic obstructive pulmonary disease and patients with acute asthmatic attack may develop acute respiratory failure with administration of morphine. Use in these patients should be reserved for those whose conditions require endotracheal intubation and respiratory support or control of ventilation.

DRUG INTERACTIONS
Depressant effects of morphine are potentiated by either concomitant administration or in the presence of other CNS

depressants such as alcohol, sedatives, antihistaminics or psychotropic drugs (e.g., MAO inhibitors, phenothiazines, butyrophenones and tricyclic antidepressants). Premedication or intra-anesthetic use of neuroleptics with morphine may increase the risk of respiratory depression.

CARCINOGENESIS, MUTAGENESIS, IMPAIRMENT OF FERTILITY
Studies of morphine sulfate in animals to evaluate the carcinogenic and mutagenic potential or the effect on fertility have not been conducted.

PREGNANCY
Teratogenic Effects—Pregnancy Category C. Animal reproduction studies have not been conducted with morphine. It is also not known whether morphine sulfate can cause fetal harm when administered to a pregnant woman or can affect reproduction capacity. Morphine sulfate should be given to a pregnant woman only if clearly needed.
Nonteratogenic Effects. Infants born from mothers who have been taking morphine chronically may exhibit withdrawal symptoms.

LABOR AND DELIVERY
Intravenous morphine readily passes into the fetal circulation and may result in respiratory depression in the neonate. Naloxone and resuscitative equipment should be available for reversal of narcotic-induced respiratory depression in the neonate. In addition, intravenous morphine may reduce the strength, duration and frequency of uterine contraction resulting in prolonged labor.
Epidurally and intrathecally administered morphine readily passes into the fetal circulation and may result in respiratory depression of the neonate. Controlled clinical studies have shown that epidural administration has little or no effect on the relief of labor pain.
However, studies have suggested that in most cases 0.2 to 1 mg of morphine intrathecally provides adequate pain relief with little effect on the duration of first stage labor. The second stage labor, though, may be prolonged if the parturient is not encouraged to bear down. A continuous intravenous infusion of naloxone, 0.6 mg/hr, for 24 hours after intrathecal injection may be employed to reduce the incidence of potential side effects.

NURSING MOTHERS
Morphine is excreted in maternal milk. Effect on the nursing infant is not known.

PEDIATRIC USE
Safety and effectiveness in children have not been established.

ADVERSE REACTIONS
The most serious side effect is respiratory depression. Because of delay in maximum CNS effect with intravenously administered drug (30 min), rapid administration may result in overdosing. Bolus administration by the epidural or intrathecal route may result in early respiratory depression due to direct venous redistribution of morphine to the respiratory centers in the brain. Late (up to 24 hours) onset of acute respiratory depression has been reported with administration by the epidural or intrathecal route and is believed to be the result of rostral spread. Reports of respiratory depression following intrathecal administration have been more frequent, but the dosage used in most of these cases has been considerably higher than that recommended. This depression may be severe and could require intervention. (See WARNINGS and OVERDOSAGE.) Even without clinical evidence of ventilatory inadequacy, a diminished CO_2 ventilation response may be noted for up to 22 hours following epidural or intrathecal administration.
While low doses of intravenously administered morphine have little effect on cardiovascular stability, high doses are excitatory, resulting from sympathetic hyperactivity and increase in circulating catecholamines. Excitation of the central nervous system resulting in convulsions may accompany high doses of morphine given intravenously. Dysphoric reactions may occur and toxic psychoses have been reported. Epidural or intrathecal administration is accompanied by a high incidence of pruritus which is dose related but not confined to site of administration. Nausea and vomiting are frequently seen in patients following morphine administration. Urinary retention which may persist for 10–20 hours following single epidural or intrathecal administration has been reported in approximately 90% of males. Incidence is somewhat lower in females. Patients may require catheterization. (See PRECAUTIONS.) Pruritus, nausea/vomiting and urinary retention frequently can be alleviated by the intravenous administration of low doses of naloxone (0.2 mg). Tolerance and dependence to chronically administered morphine, by whatever route, is known to occur. (See DRUG ABUSE AND DEPENDENCE.)
Miscellaneous side effects include constipation, headache, anxiety, depression of cough reflex, interference with thermal regulation and oliguria. Evidence of histamine release such as urticaria, wheals and/or local tissue irritation may occur. In general, side effects are amenable to reversal by narcotic antagonists. NALOXONE INJECTION AND RESUSCITATIVE EQUIPMENT SHOULD BE IMMEDIATELY AVAILABLE FOR ADMINISTRATION IN CASE

OF LIFE-THREATENING OR INTOLERABLE SIDE EFFECTS.

DRUG ABUSE AND DEPENDENCE

CONTROLLED SUBSTANCE
Morphine sulfate is a Schedule II substance under the Drug Enforcement Administration classification.
ABUSE
Morphine has recognized abuse and dependence potential.
DEPENDENCE
Cerebral and spinal receptors may develop tolerance/dependence independently, as a function of local dosage. Care must be taken to avert withdrawal in those patients who have been maintained on parenteral/oral narcotics when epidural or intrathecal administration is considered. Withdrawal may occur following chronic epidural or intrathecal administration, as well as the development of tolerance to morphine by these routes. (See Nonteratogenic Effects under PREGNANCY.)

OVERDOSAGE
Overdosage is characterized by respiratory depression with or without concomitant CNS depression. Since respiratory arrest may result either through direct depression of the respiratory center or as the result of hypoxia, primary attention should be given to the establishment of adequate respiratory exchange through provision of a patent airway and institution of assisted or controlled ventilation. The narcotic antagonist naloxone is a specific antidote. Naloxone (usually 0.4 mg) should be administered intravenously, simultaneously with respiratory resuscitation. *As the duration of effect of naloxone is considerably shorter than that of epidural or intrathecal morphine, repeated administration may be necessary.* Patients should be closely observed for evidence of renarcotization. *Note: Respiratory depression may be delayed in onset up to 24 hours* following epidural or intrathecal administration. In painful conditions, reversal of narcotic effect may result in acute onset of pain and release of catecholamines. Careful administration of naloxone may permit reversal of side effects without affecting analgesia. Parenteral administration of narcotics in patients receiving epidural or intrathecal morphine may result in overdosage.

DOSAGE AND ADMINISTRATION
Preservative-free DURAMORPH® (Morphine Sulfate Injection, USP) is intended for intravenous, epidural or intrathecal administration.
INTRAVENOUS ADMINISTRATION
Dosage: The initial dose of morphine should be 2 mg to 10 mg/70 kg of body weight. Patients under the age of 18; no information available.
EPIDURAL ADMINISTRATION
DURAMORPH® SHOULD BE ADMINISTERED EPIDURALLY ONLY BY PHYSICIANS EXPERIENCED IN THE TECHNIQUES OF EPIDURAL ADMINISTRATION AND WHO ARE THOROUGHLY FAMILIAR WITH THE LABELING. IT SHOULD BE ADMINISTERED ONLY IN SETTINGS WHERE ADEQUATE PATIENT MONITORING IS POSSIBLE. RESUSCITATIVE EQUIPMENT AND A SPECIFIC ANTAGONIST (NALOXONE INJECTION) SHOULD BE IMMEDIATELY AVAILABLE FOR THE MANAGEMENT OF RESPIRATORY DEPRESSION AS WELL AS COMPLICATIONS WHICH MIGHT RESULT FROM INADVERTENT INTRATHECAL OR INTRAVASCULAR INJECTION. [NOTE: INTRATHECAL DOSAGE IS USUALLY 1/10 THAT OF EPIDURAL DOSAGE.] PATIENT MONITORING SHOULD BE CONTINUED FOR AT LEAST 24 HOURS AFTER EACH DOSE, SINCE DELAYED RESPIRATORY DEPRESSION MAY OCCUR.
Proper placement of a needle or catheter in the epidural space should be verified before DURAMORPH® is injected. Acceptable techniques for verifying proper placement include: a) aspiration to check for absence of blood or cerebrospinal fluid, or b) administration of 5 mL (3 mL in obstetric patients) of 1.5% UNPRESERVED Lidocaine and Epinephrine (1:200,000) Injection and then observe the patient for lack of tachycardia (this indicates that vascular injection has *not* been made) and lack of sudden onset of segmental anesthesia (this indicates that intrathecal injection has *not* been made).
Epidural Adult Dosage: Initial injection of 5 mg in the lumbar region may provide satisfactory pain relief for up to 24 hours. If adequate pain relief is not achieved within one hour, careful administration of incremental doses of 1 to 2 mg at intervals sufficient to assess effectiveness may be given. No more than 10 mg/24 hr should be administered. Thoracic administration has been shown to dramatically increase the incidence of early and late respiratory depression even at doses of 1 to 2 mg.
For continuous infusion an initial dose of 2 to 4 mg/24 hours is recommended. Further doses of 1 to 2 mg may be given if pain relief is not achieved initially.
Aged or debilitated patients—Administer with extreme caution. (See PRECAUTIONS.) Doses of less than 5 mg may provide satisfactory pain relief for up to 24 hours.
Epidural Pediatric Use: No information on use in pediatric patients is available.

INTRATHECAL ADMINISTRATION

> **NOTE: INTRATHECAL DOSAGE IS USUALLY 1/10 THAT OF EPIDURAL DOSAGE.**

DURAMORPH® SHOULD BE ADMINISTERED INTRATHECALLY ONLY BY PHYSICIANS EXPERIENCED IN THE TECHNIQUES OF INTRATHECAL ADMINISTRATION AND WHO ARE THOROUGHLY FAMILIAR WITH THE LABELING. IT SHOULD BE ADMINISTERED ONLY IN SETTINGS WHERE ADEQUATE PATIENT MONITORING IS POSSIBLE. RESUSCITATIVE EQUIPMENT AND A SPECIFIC ANTAGONIST (NALOXONE INJECTION) SHOULD BE IMMEDIATELY AVAILABLE FOR THE MANAGEMENT OF RESPIRATORY DEPRESSION AS WELL AS COMPLICATIONS WHICH MIGHT RESULT FROM INADVERTENT INTRAVASCULAR INJECTION. **PATIENT MONITORING SHOULD BE CONTINUED FOR AT LEAST 24 HOURS AFTER EACH DOSE, SINCE DELAYED RESPIRATORY DEPRESSION MAY OCCUR.** RESPIRATORY DEPRESSION (BOTH EARLY AND LATE ONSET) HAS OCCURRED MORE FREQUENTLY FOLLOWING INTRATHECAL ADMINISTRATION.

Intrathecal Adult Dosage: A single injection of 0.2 to 1 mg may provide satisfactory pain relief for up to 24 hours. (CAUTION: THIS IS ONLY 0.4 TO 2 ML OF THE 5 MG/10 ML AMPUL OR 0.2 TO 1 ML OF THE 10 MG/10 ML AMPUL OF DURAMORPH®). DO NOT INJECT INTRATHECALLY MORE THAN 2 ML OF THE 5 MG/10 ML AMPUL OR 1 ML OF THE 10 MG/10 ML AMPUL USE IN THE LUMBAR AREA ONLY IS RECOMMENDED. Repeated intrathecal injections of DURAMORPH® are not recommended. A constant intravenous infusion of naloxone, 0.6 mg/hr, for 24 hours after intrathecal injection may be used to reduce the incidence of potential side effects.

Aged or debilitated patients—Administer with extreme caution. (See PRECAUTIONS.) A lower dosage is usually satisfactory.

Repeat Dosage: If pain recurs, alternative routes of administration should be considered, since experience with repeated doses of morphine by the intrathecal route is limited.

Intrathecal Pediatric Use: No information on use in pediatric patients is available.

Parenteral drug products should be inspected for particulate matter and discoloration prior to administration, whenever solution and container permit. Do not use if color is darker than pale yellow, if it is discolored in any other way or if it contains a precipitate.

HOW SUPPLIED

Preservative-free DURAMORPH® (Morphine Sulfate Injection, USP) is available in amber DOSETTE® ampuls for intravenous, epidural or intrathecal administration:

5 mg/10 mL (0.5 mg/mL) packaged in 10s (NDC 0641-1112-33)

10 mg/10 mL (1 mg/1 mL) packaged in 10s (NDC 0641-1114-33)

STORAGE

Protect from light Store in carton at controlled room temperature, 15° to 30°C (59° to 86°F) until ready to use. DURAMORPH® contains no preservative. DISCARD ANY UNUSED PORTION. DO NOT HEAT-STERILIZE.

* * * *

Additional inserts may be obtained by contacting the Professional Services Department.

Revised October 1988

Manufactured by

ELKINS-SINN, INC., Cherry Hill, NJ 08003-4099

A subsidiary of A. H. Robins Company

SOTRADECOL®   ℞

[sō'trah "de'kol"]

(Sodium Tetradecyl Sulfate)

For Intravenous Use Only

DESCRIPTION

Sodium tetradecyl sulfate is an anionic surfactant which occurs as a white, waxy solid. The structural formula is as follows:

$$CH_3(CH_2)_3CH(CH_2)_2CHOSONa$$

with $CH_2CH(CH_3)_2$ and C_2H_5 substituents and two O double bonds

$C_{14}H_{29}NaSO_4$

7-Ethyl-2-methyl-4-hendecanol sulfate sodium salt

M.W. 316.44

Sotradecol® (Sodium Tetradecyl Sulfate Injection) is a sterile nonpyrogenic solution for intravenous use as a sclerosing agent. Each mL contains sodium tetradecyl sulfate 10 mg or 30 mg, benzyl alcohol 0.02 mL and dibasic sodium phosphate, anhydrous 0.72 mg in Water for Injection. pH 7.9; monobasic sodium phosphate and/or sodium hydroxide added, if needed, for pH adjustment.

CLINICAL PHARMACOLOGY

Sotradecol® (Sodium Tetradecyl Sulfate Injection) is a mild sclerosing agent. Intravenous injection causes intima inflammation and thrombus formation. This usually occludes the injected vein. Subsequent formation of fibrous tissue results in partial or complete vein obliteration.

INDICATIONS AND USAGE

Indicated in the treatment of small uncomplicated varicose veins of the lower extremities that show simple dilation with competent valves. The benefit-to-risk ratio should be considered in selected patients who are great surgical risks due to conditions such as old age.

CONTRAINDICATIONS

Contraindicated in previous hypersensitivity reactions to the drug; in acute superficial thrombophlebitis; significant valvular or deep vein incompetence; huge superficial veins with wide open communications to deeper veins; phlebitis migrans; acute cellulitis; allergic conditions; acute infections; varicosities caused by abdominal and pelvic tumors unless the tumor has been removed; bedridden patients; such uncontrolled systemic diseases as diabetes, toxic hyperthyroidism, tuberculosis, asthma, neoplasm, sepsis, blood dyscrasias and acute respiratory or skin diseases.

WARNINGS

Since severe adverse local effects, including tissue necrosis, may occur following extravasation, Sotradecol® (Sodium Tetradecyl Sulfate Injection), should be administered only by a physician familiar with proper injection technique. Extreme care in needle placement and using the minimal effective volume at each injection site are, therefore, important. Allergic reactions have been reported. Therefore, as a precaution against anaphylactoid shock, it is recommended that 0.5 mL of Sotradecol® be injected into a varicosity, followed by observation of the patient for several hours before administration of a second or larger dose. The possibility of an anphylactoid reaction should be kept in mind, and the physician should be prepared to treat it appropriately. In extreme emergencies, 0.25 mL of 1:1000 Epinephrine Injection (0.25 mg) intravenously should be used and side reactions controlled with antihistamines.

PRECAUTIONS

General

Venous sclerotherapy should not be undertaken if tests, such as the Trendelenberg and Perthes, and angiography show significant valvular or deep venous incompetence. The physician should bear in mind the fact that injection necrosis is likely to result from extravascular injection of sclerosing agents.

Extreme caution must be exercised in the presence of underlying arterial disease such as marked peripheral arteriosclerosis or thromboangiitis obliterans (Buerger's Disease).

The drug should only be administered by physicians who are familiar with an acceptable injection technique. Because of the danger of thrombosis extension into the deep venous system, thorough preinjection evaluation for valvular competency should be carried out and slow injections with a small amount (not over 2 mL) of the preparation should be injected into the varicosity. In particular, deep venous patency must be determined by angiography and/or the Perthes test before sclerotherapy is undertaken.

Embolism may occur as much as four weeks after injection of sodium tetradecyl sulfate.

The incidence of recurrence is low if the patient wears elastic stockings.

DRUG INTERACTIONS

No well-controlled studies have been performed on patients taking antiovulatory agents. The physician must use judgment and evaluate any patient taking antiovulatory drugs prior to initiating treatment with Sotradecol® (Sodium Tetradecyl Sulfate Injection). (See ADVERSE REACTIONS.) Heparin should not be included in the same syringe as Sotradecol® since the two are incompatible.

CARCINOGENESIS, MUTAGENESIS, IMPAIRMENT OF FERTILITY

When tested in the L5178YTK$^{+/-}$ mouse lymphoma assay, sodium tetradecyl sulfate did not induce a dose-related increase in the frequency of thymidine kinase-deficient mutants and, therefore, was judged to be nonmutagenic in this system. However, no long-term animal carcinogenicity studies with sodium tetradecyl sulfate have been performed.

PREGNANCY

Teratogenic Effects—Pregnancy Category C. Adequate reproduction studies have not been performed in animals to determine whether this drug affects fertility in males or females, has teratogenic potential, or has other adverse effects on the fetus. There are no well-controlled studies in pregnant women, but investigational and marketing experience does not include any positive evidence of adverse effects on the fetus. Although there is no clearly defined risk, such experience cannot exclude the possibility of infrequent or subtle damage to the human fetus.

NURSING MOTHERS

It is not known whether this drug is excreted in human milk. Because many drugs are excreted in human milk, caution should be exercised when Sodium Tetradecyl Sulfate Injection is administered to a nursing woman.

ADVERSE REACTIONS

Local reactions consisting of pain, urticaria or ulceration may occur at the site of injection. A permanent discoloration, usually small and hardly noticeable but which may be objectionable from a cosmetic viewpoint, may remain along the path of the sclerosed vein segment. Sloughing and necrosis of tissue may occur following extravasation of the drug. Systemic reactions, except for allergic ones, have been slight. These include headache, nausea and vomiting. Allergic reactions such as hives, asthma, hayfever and anaphylactoid shock have been reported. (See WARNINGS.)

One death has been reported in a patient who received Sotradecol® (Sodium Tetradecyl Sulfate Injection) and who had been receiving an antiovulatory agent.

Another death (fatal pulmonary embolism) has been reported in a 36-year-old female treated with sodium tetradecyl *acetate* and who was **not** taking oral contraceptives.

DOSAGE AND ADMINISTRATION

For intravenous use only. Do not use if precipitated or discolored. The strength of solution required depends on the size and degree of varicosity. In general, the 1% solution will be found most useful with the 3% solution preferred for larger varicosities. The dosage should be kept small, using 0.5 to 2 mL (preferably 1 mL maximum) for each injection, and the maximum single treatment should not exceed 10 mL.

Parenteral drug products should be inspected visually for particulate matter and discoloration prior to administration, whenever solution and container permit.

HOW SUPPLIED

Sotradecol® (Sodium Tetradecyl Sulfate Injection)

1%—2 mL DOSETTE® ampuls packaged in 5s (NDC 0641-1514-34)

3%—2 mL DOSETTE® ampuls packaged in 5s (NDC 0641-1516-34)

STORAGE

Store at controlled room temperature 15°–30°C (59°–86°F).

ANIMAL TOXICOLOGY

The intravenous LD$_{50}$ of sodium tetradecyl sulfate in mice was reported to be 90 ± 5 mg/kg.

In the rat, the acute intravenous LD$_{50}$ of sodium tetradecyl sulfate was estimated to be between 72 mg/kg and 108 mg/kg.

Purified sodium tetradecyl sulfate was found to have an LD$_{50}$ of 2 g/kg when administered orally by stomach tube as a 25% aqueous solution to rats. In rats given 0.15 g/kg in drinking water for 30 days, no appreciable toxicity was seen although some growth inhibition was discernible.

* * * *

Additional package inserts may be obtained by contacting the Professional Services Department.

Revised October 1988

Manufactured by

ELKINS-SINN, INC., Cherry Hill, NJ 08003-4099

A subsidiary of A.H. Robins Company

Everett Laboratories, Inc.
76 FRANKLIN STREET
EAST ORANGE, NEW JERSEY 07017

FLORVITE Chewable Tablets 0.5 mg & 1 mg   ℞
Children's Vitamins + Fluoride

SUPPLIED

Multiflavored chewable tablets in bottles of 100 and 1000.

FLORVITE Drops 0.25 mg & 0.5 mg   ℞
Children's Vitamins + Fluoride

SUPPLIED

Bottles of 50 ml.

FLORVITE + IRON Drops 0.25 mg   ℞
FLORVITE + IRON Chewable Tablets   ℞
0.5 mg & 1 mg
Children's Vitamins + Iron + Fluoride

SUPPLIED

Bottles of 50 mL and tablets 100.

Continued on next page

Everett—Cont.

LIBIDINAL™ ZE CAPS   OTC
Soft Gel Capsules

EACH CAPSULE CONTAINS:
Zinc Gluconate 75 mg., Vitamin E 200 I.U.

SUPPLIED
Bottles of 60 sugar and salt free capsules.

REPAN Tablets—REPAN Capsules   ℞

EACH TABLET AND EACH CAPSULE CONTAINS:
Butalbital 50 mg.
(Warning: May be habit forming.), Caffeine (Anhydrus) 40 mg., Acetaminophen 325 mg.

SUPPLIED
Bottles of 100 tablets imprinted EVERETT and 162.
Bottles of 100 two-tone blue capsules imprinted EVERETT.

STROVITE PLUS Tablets   ℞
Therapeutic Multivitamin Mineral Supplement
Sugar Free

SUPPLIED
Bottles of 100 imprinted EVERETT and 0201.

TUSSAFED DROPS & SYRUP
Antitussive-Decongestant-Antihistamine

Each dropperful (A) & each teaspoonful (B) contains:

	A	B
Dextromethorphan	4 mg	15 mg
Pseudoephedrine	25 mg	60 mg
Carbinoxamine	2 mg	4 mg

VITAFOL Syrup   ℞
Vitamins, Minerals, Iron, Folic Acid Supplement
Sugar and Alcohol Free

SUPPLIED
Bottles of 16 oz.

VITAFOL Tablets   ℞
Vitamins, Minerals, Iron, Folic Acid Supplement
Sugar Free

SUPPLIED
Bottles of 100 and 1000 tablets imprinted EVERETT and 0072.

Ferndale Laboratories, Inc.
780 W. EIGHT MILE ROAD
FERNDALE, MI 48220

ANALPRAM–HC® CREAM   ℞
Rectal Cream

DESCRIPTION
Contains Hydrocortisone acetate 1% and Pramoxine HCl 1% in a washable, nongreasy base containing stearic acid, cetyl alcohol, aquaphor, isopropyl palmitate, polyoxyl 40 stearate, propylene glycol, potassium sorbate 0.1%, sorbic acid 0.1%, trieth anolamine lauryl sulfate and water.

ACTIONS
Hydrocortisone acetate is a corticosteroid. Topically, it is primarily effective because of its anti-inflammatory, anti-pruritic and vaso-constrictive actions. Pramoxine hydrochloride is a topical anesthetic which provides temporary relief from itching and pain.

INDICATIONS AND USAGE
Topical corticosteroids are indicated for the relief of the inflammatory and pruritic manifestations of corticosteroid-responsive dermatoses of the anal region.

CONTRAINDICATIONS
Topical steroids are contraindicated in viral diseases of the skin, such as varicella and vaccinia. Topical steroids are contraindicated in those patients with a history of hypersensitivity to any of the components of the preparation. Topical steroids should not be used when circulation is markedly impaired.

PRECAUTIONS
If irritation develops, the product should be discontinued and appropriate therapy instituted. In the presence of an infection, the use of appropriate antifungal or antibacterial agents should be instituted. If a favorable response does not occur promptly, the corticosteroid should be discontinued until the infection has been adequately controlled. If extensive areas are treated or if the occlusive technique is used, the possibility exists of increased systemic absorption of the corticosteroid and suitable precautions should be taken. The product is not for opthalmic use.

WARNINGS
USAGE IN PREGNANCY: Although topical steroids have not been reported to have an adverse effect on the fetus, the safety of their use in pregnant females has not absolutely been established. Therefore, they should not be used extensively on pregnant patients, or in large amounts, or for prolonged periods of time.

CAUTION
Federal law prohibits dispensing without prescription.

ADVERSE REACTIONS
The following local adverse reactions have been reported with topical corticosteroids, especially under occlusive dressings.
Burning, Itching, Irritation, Dryness, Folliculitis, Hypertrichosis, Acneiform eruptions, Hypopigmentation, Perioral dermatitis, Allergic Contact Dermatitis, Maceration of the skin, Secondary infection, Skin atrophy, Striae, and Miliaria.

DOSAGE AND ADMINISTRATION
Apply to affected area 3 or 4 times daily.

HOW SUPPLIED
ANALPRAM-HC® Cream is supplied in a 1 oz. tube with six (6) rectal applicators.

KRONOFED–A® Kronocaps   ℞
Dye–Free
Decongestant plus Antihistamine

Each sustained release, white and clear capsule contains:
Pseudoephedrine HCl ....120 mg
Chlorpheniramine Maleate .... 8 mg

KRONOFED–A–JR® Kronocaps   ℞
Dye–Free
Decongestant plus Antihistamine

Each sustained release, white and clear capsule contains:
Pseudoephedrine HCl ....60 mg
Chlorpheniramine Maleate .... 4 mg

INDICATIONS
For temporary relief of upper respiratory and nasal congestion associated with the common cold, hay fever and allergies, sinusitis and vasomotor and allergic rhinitis.

CONTRAINDICATIONS
Severe hypertension or severe cardiac disease. Sensitivity to antihistamines or sympathomimetic agents.

PRECAUTIONS
Use with caution in patients with hyperthyroidism. Patients susceptible to the soporific effects of chlorpheniramine should be warned against driving or operating of machinery which requires complete mental alertness.

PREGNANCY
Pregnancy Category C: Animal reproduction studies have not been conducted with KRONOFED-A® medications. It is also not known whether KRONOFED-A® medications can cause fetal harm when administered to a pregnant woman or can affect reproduction capacity. KRONOFED-A® medications should be given to a pregnant woman only if clearly needed.
Nursing Mothers: Due to the possible passage of pseudoephedrine and chlorpheniramine into breast milk, and, because of the higher than usual risk for infants from sympathomimetic amines and antihistamines, the benefit to the mother vs. the potential risk should be considered and a decision should be made whether to discontinue nursing or to discontinue the drug.

CAUTION
Federal law prohibits dispensing without prescription.

DOSAGE
Kronofed-A® Capsules: Adults and children over 12 years of age—1 capsule every 12 hours. Kronofed-A-JR® Capsules: Children 6–12 years of age—1 capsule every 12 hours. Adults 1 or 2 capsules every 12 hours.

HOW SUPPLIED
Bottles of 100 and 500 Capsules.

PRAMOSONE® CREAM, LOTION AND OINTMENT   ℞

DESCRIPTION
Pramosone® Cream: Contains Hydrocortisone acetate 0.5%, 1% or 2.5% and Pramoxine HCl 1% in a hydrophilic base containing stearic acid, cetyl alcohol, aquaphor, isopropyl palmitate, polyoxyl 40 stearate, propylene glycol, potassium sorbate 0.1%, sorbic acid 0.1%, triethanolamine lauryl sulfate and water.
Pramosone® Lotion: Contains Hydrocortisone acetate 0.5%, 1% or 2.5% and Pramoxine HCl 1% in a base containing forlan-L, cetyl alcohol, stearic acid, di-isopropyl adipate, polyoxyl 40 stearate, silicon, triethanolamine, glycerine, polyvinylpyrolidone, potassium sorbate 0.1%, sorbic acid 0.1% and water.
Pramosone® Ointment: Contains Hydrocortisone acetate 1% or 2.5% and Pramoxine HC1 1% in an emollient ointment base containing Sorbitan sesquioleate, Water, Aquaphor and White petrolatum.

ACTIONS
Hydrocortisone acetate is a corticosteroid. Topically, it is primarily effective because of its anti-inflammatory, anti-pruritic and vaso-constrictive actions. Pramoxine hydrochloride is a topical anesthetic which provides temporary relief from itching and pain.

INDICATIONS AND USAGE
Topical corticosteroids are indicated for the relief of the inflammatory and pruritic manifestations of corticosteroid-responsive dermatoses.

CONTRAINDICATIONS
Topical steroids are contraindicated in viral diseases of the skin, such as varicella and vaccinia. Topical steroids are contraindicated in those patients with a history of hypersensitivity to any of the components of the preparation. Topical steroids should not be used when circulation is markedly impaired.

PRECAUTIONS
If irritation develops, the product should be discontinued and appropriate therapy instituted. In the presence of an infection, the use of appropriate antifungal or antibacterial agents should be instituted. If a favorable response does not occur promptly, the corticosteroid should be discontinued until the infection has been adequately controlled. If extensive areas are treated or if the occlusive technique is used, the possibility exists of increased systemic absorption of the corticosteroid and suitable precautions should be taken. The product is not for opthalmic use.

WARNINGS
USAGE IN PREGNANCY: Although topical steroids have not been reported to have an adverse effect on the fetus, the safety of their use in pregnant females has not absolutely been established. Therefore, they should not be used extensively on pregnant patients, or in large amounts, or for prolonged periods of time.

CAUTION
Federal law prohibits dispensing without prescription.

ADVERSE REACTIONS
The following local adverse reactions have been reported with topical corticosteroids, especially under occlusive dressings.
Burning, Itching, Irritation, Dryness, Folliculitis, Hypertrichosis, Acneiform eruptions, Hypopigmentation, Perioral dermatitis, Allergic Contact Dermatitis, Maceration of the skin, Secondary infection, Skin atrophy, Striae, and Miliaria.

DOSAGE AND ADMINISTRATION
Apply to affected area 3 or 4 times daily.

HOW SUPPLIED
CREAM: ½%, 1% or 2½% in 1 oz. tubes, 4 oz. jars and lb. jars. LOTION: ½% or 1% in 2 fl. oz., 4 fl. oz. and 8 fl. oz. dispenser bottles. 2½% in 2 fl. oz. dispenser bottles. OINTMENT: 1% or 2½% in 1 oz. tubes, 4 oz. jars and lb. jars.

PRAX® CREAM AND LOTION*
(Pramoxine HCl 1% in an emollient hydrophilic base)

AVAILABLE
CREAM: 1 oz. tubes, 4 oz. jars and lb. jars. LOTION: 15 mL., 120 mL., and 240 mL. dispenser bottles.
*Additional information available upon request.

Products are cross-indexed by
generic and chemical names in the
YELLOW SECTION

Ferring Laboratories, Inc.
75 MONTEBELLO ROAD
SUFFERN, NY 10901

SECRETIN–FERRING ℞

HOW SUPPLIED
Secretin-Ferring is supplied as a lyophilized sterile powder in 10 ml vials containing 75 CU. The unreconstituted product should be stored at −20° C (freezer). However, the biological activity of Secretin-Ferring will not be significantly decreased by storage at 25° C or below for up to 3 weeks. Expiration date is marked on the label.
NDC 55566-1075-1

The Fielding Company
2384 CENTERLINE INDUSTRIAL DRIVE
ST. LOUIS, MO 63146

GERIMED® Tablets

DESCRIPTION
A multivitamin-multimineral supplement useful as adjunctive therapy in osteoporosis. Provides a balanced ratio of calcium and phosphorus (2.8 to 1) with adequate Vitamin D for proper absorption.
Each tablet contains:

			U.S. RDA
Dibasic Calcium Phosphate	600	mg.	*
Calcium Carbonate	500	mg.	*
Vitamin A	5000	I. U.	100%
Vitamin D	400	I. U.	100%
Vitamin E	30	I. U.	100%
Vitamin C	120	mg.	200%
Thiamine B₂	3	mg.	200%
Riboflavin B₂	3	mg.	176%
Niacinamide	25	mg.	100%
Pyridoxine B₆	2	mg.	100%
Vitamin B₁₂	6	mcg.	100%
Magnesium	50	mg.	11%
Zinc	15	mg.	100%

*Total Calcium	370	mg.	37%
*Total Phosphorus	130	mg.	13%
Calcium/Phosphorus ratio 2.8 - 1			

DOSAGE
One tablet daily, or as prescribed by the physician.
HOW SUPPLIED
Bottle of 60 tablets.
NDC 0421-0080-60

IROSPAN® Tablets/Capsules

Each tablet or capsule contains:
Ferrous Sulfate (exsic.)	200 mg.
Ascorbic Acid (Vit. C)	150 mg.

DESCRIPTION
Irospan is a unique presentation of sustained release ferrous sulfate and ascorbic acid. Irospan is of particular value during pregnancy and lactation providing excellent tolerance and absorption.
DOSAGE
One tablet or capsule daily or as prescribed by the physician.
HOW SUPPLIED
Irospan Tablets—bottles of 100.
Irospan Capsules—bottles of 60.

LURLINE® PMS Tablets

Each tablet contains:
Acetaminophen	500 mg.
Pamabrom	25 mg.
Pyridoxine	50 mg.

DESCRIPTION
Lurline PMS is a safe and effective approach for relief of the multi-symptom complex of premenstrual syndrome. The medication combines an analgesic, a mild diuretic and pyridoxine, representing a safe first line treatment.
Lurline PMS contains no hormones, no sedatives and is aspirin free.
DOSAGE
Start Lurline PMS at the first sign of pain or discomfort, usually 7 to 10 days before menses. Usual dosage is one tablet 3 or 4 times daily. Do not exceed the maximum dose of 8 tablets a day.

HOW SUPPLIED
Lurline PMS—bottles of 24. NDC 0421-8787-24
Lurline PMS—bottles of 100. NDC 0421-8787-50
Physician samples and literature available.

METRIC® 21 ℞
(metronidazole)

DESCRIPTION
An antiprotozoal and antibacterial agent for use in the treatment of trichomoniasis in both the female and male patient.
HOW SUPPLIED
Metric 21 (250 mg) in bottles of 100.
NDC 0421-8282-01

NESTABS® FA Tablets ℞
Prenatal Tablets

DESCRIPTION
East tablet contains:

			U.S. RDA
Vitamin A	5000	Units	100%
Vitamin D	400	Units	100%
Vitamin E	30	Units	100%
Vitamin C	120	mg.	200%
Folic Acid	1	mg.	125%
Thiamine	3	mg.	176%
Riboflavin	3	mg.	125%
Niacinamide	20	mg.	100%
Pyridoxine	3	mg.	120%
Vitamin B12	8	mcg.	100%
Calcium Carbonate	500	mg.	15%
Iodine	150	mcg.	100%
Ferrous Fumarate	110	mg.	200%
Zinc	15	mg.	100%

A comprehensive vitamin-mineral supplement expressly formulated for use during pregnancy and lactation.
DOSAGE
One tablet daily, or as prescribed by the physician.
PRECAUTION
Folic acid may obscure pernicious anemia in that hematologic remission can occur while neurological manifestations remain progressive.
HOW SUPPLIED
Bottles of 100 tablets.
NDC 0421-1594-01

Fisons Consumer Health
Fisons Corporation
P.O. Box 1212
ROCHESTER, NY 14603

ALLEREST®
[al 'e-rest]
Tablets, Children's Chewable Tablets, Headache Strength Tablets, Sinus Pain Formula Tablets, No Drowsiness Tablets, Eye Drops, 12 Hour Caplets and 12 Hour Nasal Spray

(See PDR For Nonprescription Drugs)

AMERICAINE®
[a-mer 'i-kān]
Hemorrhoidal Ointment, Topical Anesthetic Spray and Ointment

(See PDR For Nonprescription Drugs)

CaldeCORT®
[kal 'de-cort]
Hydrocortisone Multi-Purpose Anti-Itch Cream and Spray

(See PDR For Nonprescription Drugs)

CaldeCORT Light®
[kal 'de-cort līt]
Hydrocortisone in a Light Moisturizing Creme with Aloe

(See PDR For Nonprescription Drugs)

CALDESENE®
[kal 'de-sēn]
Medicated Powder and Ointment

(See PDR For Nonprescription Drugs)

CRUEX®
[kru 'ex]
Antifungal Powder, Spray Powder and Cream

(See PDR For Nonprescription Drugs)

DESENEX®
[dess 'i-nex]
Antifungal Powder, Spray Powder, Cream, Ointment, Liquid and Penetrating Foam

(See PDR For Nonprescription Drugs)

SINAREST®
[sĭn 'a-rest]
Tablets, Extra Strength Tablets, No Drowsiness Tablets and 12 Hour Nasal Spray

(See PDR For Nonprescription Drugs)

Fisons Corporation
P.O. BOX 1710
ROCHESTER, NY 14603

In addition to the products described in this section, Fisons also distributes the following products. On these and all Fisons products, information may be obtained by addressing Fisons Corporation, P.O. Box 1710, Rochester, NY 14603.

Adapin® Capsules ℞
(doxepin HCl)
10 mg, 25 mg, 50 mg, 75 mg, 100 mg Bottles of 100 and 1000
150 mg Bottle of 50

Americaine® Anesthetic Lubricant ℞
(benzocaine)
1 oz tube and 144 × 2.5 gm Packet

Biphetamine® Capsules Ⓒ
(amphetamine/dextroamphetamine)
12½ mg and 20 mg Bottles of 100

Ergomar® Sublingual Tablets ℞
(ergotamine tartrate tablets, USP)
2 mg Vials of 20

Hylorel® Tablets ℞
(guanadrel sulfate)
10 mg and 25 mg Bottles of 100

Ionamin® Capsules Ⓒ
(phentermine resin)
15 mg and 30 mg Bottles of 100 and 400

K-Norm® Capsules ℞
(potassium chloride)
10 mEq (750 mg) Bottles of 100 and 500

Kolyum® ℞
(potassium gluconate/potassium chloride)
Pints, Gallons, and Powder Packets

Somophyllin® CRT Capsules ℞
(theophylline controlled release capsules)
100 mg, 200 mg, 250 mg, 300 mg, Bottles of 100

Somophyllin®-DF Oral Liquid ℞
(aminophylline oral solution, USP)
105 mg/5 ml 8 fl oz Bottle

Somophyllin® Oral Liquid ℞
(aminophylline oral solution, USP)
105 Mg/5 ml Bottles of 8 oz and 32 oz

Somophyllin® Rectal Solution ℞
(aminophylline enema, USP)
300 mg/5 ml
3 fl oz Bottle with syringe and 18 rectal tips
5 fl oz Bottle with syringe and 30 rectal tips

Somophyllin®-T Capsules ℞
(theophylline capsules)
100 mg, 200 mg, 250 mg Bottles of 100

Zaroxolyn® Tablets ℞
(metolazone)
2.5 mg, 5 mg, 10 mg, Bottles of 100, 500, 1000, and Unit Dose 100

Continued on next page

Information on Fisons' products appearing in these pages is current as of May, 1989. For further information, please consult the package insert currently accompanying the product, or Fisons Corporation, P.O. Box 1710, Rochester, NY 14603, (716) 475-9000.

Fisons—Cont.

AMERICAINE® OTIC   ℞
(benzocaine)
Topical Anesthetic Ear Drops

DESCRIPTION

AMERICAINE Otic, topical anesthetic ear drops, contains benzocaine 20% (w/w) in a water soluble base of glycerin 1% (w/w) and polyethylene glycol 300 with benzethonium chloride 0.1% as a preservative.

Benzocaine, a local anesthetic, is chemically ethyl p-aminobenzoate, $C_9H_{11}NO_2$, with a molecular weight of 165.19 and has the following structural formula:

CLINICAL PHARMACOLOGY

Benzocaine reversibly stabilizes the neuronal membrane which decreases its permeability to sodium ions. Depolarization of the neuronal membrane is inhibited thereby blocking the initiation and conduction of nerve impulses.

INDICATIONS AND USAGE

AMERICAINE Otic is indicated for relief of pain and pruritis in acute congestive and serous otitis media, acute swimmer's ear, and other forms of otitis externa.

CONTRAINDICATIONS

In the presence of a perforated tympanic membrane or ear discharge.

Known allergy or hypersensitivity to benzocaine.

WARNINGS

Indiscriminate use of anesthetic ear drops may mask symptoms of fulminating infection of the middle ear.

PRECAUTIONS

General: Medication should be discontinued if sensitivity or irritation occurs.

Carcinogenesis, Mutagenesis, Impairment of Fertility: Long-term studies in animals or humans to evaluate the carcinogenic and mutagenic potential or the effect on fertility have not been conducted.

Pregnancy Category C: Animal reproduction studies have not been conducted with AMERICAINE Otic. It is also not known whether AMERICAINE Otic can cause fetal harm when administered to a pregnant woman or can affect reproduction capacity. AMERICAINE Otic should be given to a pregnant woman only if clearly needed.

Nursing Mothers: It is not known whether this drug is excreted in human milk. Because many drugs are excreted in human milk, caution should be exercised when AMERICAINE Otic is administered to a nursing woman.

Pediatric Use: Do not use in infants under 1 year of age.

ADVERSE REACTIONS

Contact dermatitis and/or hypersensitivity to benzocaine can cause burning, stinging, pruritis, tenderness, erythema, rash, urticaria and edema. Rarely, benzocaine may induce methemoglobinemia causing respiratory distress and cyanosis. Intravenous methylene blue is the specific therapy for this condition.

DOSAGE AND ADMINISTRATION

Instill 4–5 drops of AMERICAINE Otic in the external auditory canal, then insert a cotton pledget into the meatus. Application may be repeated every one to two hours if necessary.

Keep bottle tightly closed. Store at 59°–86°F (15°–30°C).

HOW SUPPLIED

AMERICAINE (benzocaine) Otic, topical anesthetic ear drops, is available in ½ fl. oz. dropper-top bottles (NDC 0585-0377-51).

Caution: Federal law prohibits dispensing without prescription.

Marketed by
Fisons Pharmaceuticals
Prescription Products
Rochester, NY 14623
2/89
©FISONS CORPORATION 1989

IMFERON®   ℞
[ĭm ′fer-ŏn]
(iron dextran injection, USP)

WARNING

> THE PARENTERAL USE OF COMPLEXES OF IRON AND CARBOHYDRATES HAS RESULTED IN ANAPHYLACTIC-TYPE REACTIONS. DEATHS ASSOCIATED WITH SUCH ADMINISTRATION HAVE BEEN REPORTED. THEREFORE, IMFERON SHOULD BE USED ONLY IN THOSE PATIENTS IN WHOM THE INDICATIONS HAVE BEEN CLEARLY ESTABLISHED AND LABORATORY INVESTIGATIONS CONFIRM AN IRON DEFICIENT STATE NOT AMENABLE TO ORAL IRON THERAPY.

DESCRIPTION

IMFERON (iron dextran injection, USP) is a dark brown, slightly viscous sterile liquid complex of ferric oxyhydroxide and low molecular weight dextran derivative in approximately 0.9% w/v sodium chloride for intravenous or intramuscular use. It contains the equivalent of 50 mg elemental iron (as an iron dextran complex) per mL. The pH of the solution is between 5.2 and 6.5. The multiple dose vial also contains 0.5% w/v phenol (for intramuscular use only).

Electron microscopy has shown the molecule to have an inner electron-dense FeOOH core with a diameter approximating 3 nm and an outer plastic (moldable) dextran shell with a diameter of approximately 13 nm. Almost all the iron (98–99%) is present as a stable ferric-dextran complex. The remaining iron represents a very weak ferrous complex.

Therapeutic Class: Hematinic

CLINICAL PHARMACOLOGY

General: After intramuscular injection, iron dextran is absorbed from the injection site into the capillaries and the lymphatic system. Circulating iron dextran is removed from the plasma by cells of the reticuloendothelial system, which split the complex into its components of iron and dextran. The iron is immediately bound to the available protein moieties to form hemosiderin or ferritin, the physiological forms of iron, or to a lesser extent to transferrin. This iron which is subject to physiological control replenishes hemoglobin and depleted iron stores.

Dextran, a polyglucose, is either metabolized or excreted. Negligible amounts of iron are lost via the urinary or alimentary pathways after administration of iron dextran. When iron dextran is administered during hemodialysis only negligible amounts may cross the dialysis membranes.

The major portion of intramuscular injections of iron dextran is absorbed within 72 hours; most of the remaining iron is absorbed over the ensuing 3 to 4 weeks. Staining from inadvertent deposition of iron dextran in subcutaneous and/or cutaneous tissues usually resolves or fades within several weeks or months; in some rare instances, however, such stains have been reported to persist for several years.

Various studies involving intravenously administered [59Fe] iron dextran to iron deficient subjects, some of whom had coexisting diseases, have yielded half-life values ranging from 5 hours to more than 20 hours. The 5-hour value was determined for [59Fe] iron dextran from a study that used laboratory methods to separate the circulating [59Fe] iron dextran from the transferrin-bound [59Fe]. The 20-hour value reflects a half-life determined by measuring total [59Fe], both circulating and bound. It should be understood that these half-life values do not represent clearance of iron from the body. Iron is not easily eliminated from the body and accumulation of iron can be toxic.

INDICATIONS

Intravenous or intramuscular injections of iron dextran are indicated for treatment of patients with documented iron deficiency in whom oral administration is unsatisfactory or impossible.

CONTRAINDICATIONS

Hypersensitivity to the product. All anemias not associated with iron deficiency.

WARNINGS

See Boxed WARNING.

A risk of carcinogenesis may attend the intramuscular injection of iron-carbohydrate complexes. Such complexes have been found under experimental conditions to produce sarcoma when large doses or small doses injected repeatedly at the same site were given to rats, mice, and rabbits, and possibly in hamsters.

The long latent period between the injection of a potential carcinogen and the appearance of a tumor makes it impossible to measure accurately the risk in man. There have, however, been several reports in the literature describing tumors at the injection site in humans who had previously received intramuscular injections of iron-carbohydrate complexes.

Large intravenous doses, such as used with total dose infusions (TDI), have been associated with an increased incidence of adverse effects. The adverse effects frequently are delayed (1–2 days) reactions typified by one or more of the following symptoms: arthralgia, backache, chills, dizziness, moderate to high fever, headache, malaise, myalgia, nausea, and vomiting. The onset is usually 24–48 hours after administration and symptoms generally subside within 3–4 days (such symptoms have been well recognized since iron dextran was first used). These symptoms have also been reported following intramuscular injection and usually subside within 3–7 days. The etiology of these reactions is not known. The potential for a delayed reaction must be considered when estimating the risk/benefit of treatment.

The maximum intravenous daily dose should not exceed 2 mL undiluted iron dextran.

This preparation should be used with extreme care in patients with serious impairment of liver function.

It should not be used during the acute phase of infectious kidney disease.

Patients with rheumatoid arthritis may have an acute exacerbation of joint pain and swelling following the intravenous administration of IMFERON.

PRECAUTIONS

General: Unwarranted therapy with parenteral iron will cause excess storage of iron with the consequent possibility of exogenous hemosiderosis. Such iron overload is particularly apt to occur in patients with hemoglobinopathies and other refractory anemias that might be erroneously diagnosed as iron deficiency anemias.

IMFERON should be used with caution in individuals with histories of significant allergies and/or asthma.

Epinephrine should be immediately available in the event of acute hypersensitivity reactions. (Usual adult dose: 0.5 mL of a 1:1000 solution, by subcutaneous or intramuscular injection.) Note: Patients using beta-blocking agents may not respond adequately to epinephrine. Isoproterenol or similar beta-agonist agents may be required in these patients.

Reports in the literature from countries outside the United States (in particular, New Zealand) have suggested that the use of intramuscular iron dextran in neonates has been associated with an increased incidence of gram-negative sepsis, primarily due to *E. coli*. This effect from the use of IMFERON in the United States has not been reported.

Information for Patients: Patients should be advised of the potential adverse reactions associated with the use of IMFERON.

Drug/Laboratory Test Interactions: Large doses of iron dextran (5 mL or more) have been reported to give a brown color to serum from a blood sample drawn 4 hours after administration.

The drug may cause falsely elevated values of serum bilirubin and falsely decreased values of serum calcium.

Serum iron determinations by colorimetric assays may not be meaningful for 3 weeks following the administration of iron dextran, particularly after large intravenous doses.

Serum ferritin peaks approximately 7 to 9 days after an intravenous dose of IMFERON and slowly returns to normal after about 3 weeks.

Examination of the bone marrow for iron stores may not be meaningful for prolonged periods following iron dextran therapy because residual iron dextran may remain in the reticuloendothelial cells.

Prolongation of the partial thromboplastin time has been reported to occur after intravenous administration of iron dextran when the blood sample for the test is mixed with anticoagulant citrate dextrose solution, USP. This interference apparently does not occur when anticoagulant sodium citrate solution, USP is used. Blood-typing and cross-matching are not affected by iron dextran.

Bone scans involving 99mTc-diphosphonate have been reported to show a dense, crescentic area of activity in the buttocks, following the contour of the iliac crest, 1 to 6 days after intramuscular injections of IMFERON.

Bone scans with 99mTc-labeled bone seeking agents, in the presence of high serum ferritin levels or following iron dextran infusions, have been reported to show reduction of bony uptake, marked renal activity, and excessive blood pool and soft tissue accumulation.

Caution should be used in interpreting results of serum iron measurements when blood samples are obtained within 1 or 2 weeks of administration of large doses of IMFERON.

Carcinogenesis, Mutagenesis, Impairment of Fertility: See WARNINGS.

Pregnancy: Pregnancy Category C. IMFERON has been shown to be teratogenic and embryocidal in mice, rats, rabbits, dogs, and monkeys when given in doses of about 3* times the maximum human dose. No consistent adverse fetal effects were observed in mice, rats, rabbits, dogs and monkeys at doses of 50 mg iron/kg or less. Fetal and maternal toxicity has been reported in monkeys at a total intravenous dose of 90 mg iron/kg over a 14 day period. Similar effects were observed in mice and rats on administration of a single dose of 125 mg iron/kg. Fetal abnormalities in rats and dogs were observed at doses of 250 mg iron/kg and higher. The animals used in these tests were not iron deficient. There are no adequate and well-controlled studies in pregnant women. IMFERON should be used during pregnancy only if the potential benefit justifies the potential risk to the fetus.

Placental Transfer: Various animal studies and studies in pregnant humans have demonstrated inconclusive results with respect to the placental transfer of iron dextran as iron dextran. It appears that some iron does reach the fetus, but the form in which it crosses the placenta is not clear.

Nursing Mothers: Caution should be exercised when IMFERON is administered to a nursing woman. Only traces of unmetabolized iron dextran are excreted in human milk.

Pediatric Usage: Not recommended for use in infants under 4 months of age (see DOSAGE AND ADMINISTRATION).

---

*The human dose presented here is the total iron required for treating an iron deficient state in a representative patient. The calculation represents a 50 kg patient with a hemoglobin value of 8 g/dL requiring 30 mL of IMFERON or 1500 mg iron—equivalent to 30 mg/kg.

ADVERSE REACTIONS

Severe/fatal: Anaphylactic reactions have been reported with the use of IMFERON; on rare occasions these reactions have been fatal. Such reactions, which occur most often within the first several minutes of administration, have been generally characterized by sudden onset of respiratory difficulty and/or cardiovascular collapse. The incidence of these acute hypersensitivity reactions has been estimated between 0.2% to 0.3%. (See boxed WARNING and PRECAUTIONS, *General*, pertaining to immediate availability of epinephrine.)

Mild/moderate: Delayed reactions (see WARNINGS). The incidence of delayed reactions reported in a longitudinal study of patients given multiple intravenous injections of IMFERON, usually 5 mL or greater, was approximately 8% (4% of the total number of injections given).

Other systemic/local: Isolated or multiple signs/symptoms with varying severity have been reported.

Cardiovascular: Chest pain, shock, hypotension, tachycardia, flushing.

(Flushing and hypotension may occur from too rapid injections by the I.V. route.)

Dermatologic: Urticaria, pruritus, purpura, rash.

Gastrointestinal: Abdominal pain, nausea, vomiting, diarrhea.

Hematologic/lymphatic: Leucocytosis, lymphadenopathy (generally inguinal and associated with I.M. injections).

Musculoskeletal/soft tissue: Arthralgia, arthritis (may represent reactivation in patients with quiescent rheumatoid arthritis—see PRECAUTIONS, *General*), myalgia, including backache; abscess formation (sterile); necrosis; atrophy/fibrosis (I.M. injection site); cellulitis, swelling; brown skin and/or underlying tissue discoloration (staining) (See CLINICAL PHARMACOLOGY), soreness or pain at or near intramuscular injection sites, which in some isolated instances was reported to persist for over a year; variable degree of inflammation; local phlebitis at or near I.V. injection site.

Neurologic: Convulsions (may accompany anaphylaxis), syncope, headache, weakness, paresthesia, febrile episodes, chills.

Respiratory: Bronchospasm, dyspnea.

Urologic: Hematuria.

Miscellaneous: Febrile episodes, sweating, chills.

OVERDOSAGE

Overdosage with IMFERON is unlikely to be associated with any acute manifestations. Excessive doses of IMFERON beyond the requirements for restoration of hemoglobin and replenishment of iron stores, may lead to hemosiderosis. Periodic monitoring of serum ferritin levels may be helpful in recognizing a deleterious progressive accumulation of iron resulting from impaired uptake of iron from the reticuloendothelial system in concurrent medical conditions such as chronic renal failure, Hodgkins disease, and rheumatoid arthritis. The LD_{50} of IMFERON is not less than 500 mg/kg in the mouse.

Dialysis: A study of [59Fe] iron dextran utilizing isotonic saline in a 4-hour in vitro dialysis run, indicated that less than 0.5% of the injected radiolabeled iron dextran traversed the dialysis membrane.

DOSAGE AND ADMINISTRATION

Oral iron should be discontinued prior to administration of IMFERON.

DOSAGE

I. *Iron Deficiency Anemia*

Periodic hematologic determination (hemoglobin and hematocrit) is a simple and accurate technique for monitoring hematological response, and should be used as a guide in therapy. It should be recognized that iron storage may lag behind the appearance of normal blood morphology. Serum iron, total iron binding capacity (TIBC) and percent saturation of transferrin are other important tests for detecting and monitoring the iron deficient state.

After administration of iron dextran complex, evidence of a therapeutic response can be seen in a few days as an increase in the reticulocyte count. If there has not been a 1 gram per 100 mL rise in hemoglobin within 2 weeks of starting iron dextran therapy, the diagnosis of iron deficiency anemia should be reviewed.

Although serum ferritin is usually a good guide to body iron stores, the correlation of body iron stores and serum ferritin may not be valid in patients on chronic renal dialysis who are also receiving iron dextran complex.

Although there are significant variations in body build and weight distribution among males and females, the accompanying table and formulae represent a convenient means for estimating the total iron required. This total iron requirement reflects the amount of iron needed to restore hemoglobin concentration to normal or near normal levels plus an additional allowance to provide adequate replenishment of iron stores in most individuals with moderately or severely reduced levels of hemoglobin. It should be remembered that iron deficiency anemia will not appear until essentially all iron stores have been depleted. Therapy, thus, should aim at not only replenishment of hemoglobin iron but iron stores as well.

Factors contributing to the formula are shown below.

$$\frac{\text{mg blood iron}}{\text{lb body weight}} = \frac{\text{mL blood}}{\text{lb body weight}} \times \frac{\text{g hemoglobin}}{\text{mL blood}} \times \frac{\text{mg iron}}{\text{g hemoglobin}}$$

a) Blood volume .... 7.0% body weight
b) Normal hemoglobin (males and females)
     over 15 kg (33 lbs.) .... 14.8 g/100 mL
     15 kg (33 lbs.) or less .... 12.0 g/100 mL
c) Iron content of hemoglobin 0.34%
d) Weight

Based on the above factors, individuals with normal hemoglobin levels will have approximately 35 mg of blood iron per kilogram of body weight (16 mg/lb).

Note: The table and accompanying formulae are applicable for dosage determinations only in patients with iron deficiency anemia; they are not to be used for dosage determinations in patients requiring iron replacement for blood loss.

TOTAL DOSE OF IMFERON IN ML
Observed Hemoglobin g/dL

Body Weight		3	4	5	6	7	8	9	10
kg	lb								
5	11	3	3	3	2	2	2	2	1
10	22	6	6	5	5	4	4	3	3
15	33	9	9	8	7	7	6	5	4
20	44	15	14	13	12	11	10	10	9
25	55	19	18	17	15	14	13	12	11
30	66	23	21	20	19	17	16	14	13
35	77	27	25	23	22	20	18	17	15
40	88	30	29	27	25	23	21	19	17
45	99	34	32	30	28	26	24	21	19
50	110	38	36	33	31	29	26	24	21
55	121	42	39	37	34	31	29	26	24
60	132	46	43	40	37	34	31	29	26
65	143	50	46	43	40	37	34	31	28
70	154	53	50	47	43	40	37	33	30
75	165	56	53	49	45	42	38	35	31
80	176	59	55	51	48	44	40	36	32
85	187	62	58	54	50	46	42	37	33
90	198	65	60	56	52	47	43	39	35
95	209	67	63	58	54	49	45	40	36
100	220	70	66	61	56	51	46	42	37
105	231	73	68	63	58	53	48	43	38
110	242	76	71	65	60	55	50	44	39
115	253	79	73	68	62	57	51	46	40
120	264	81	76	70	64	59	53	47	41

Dosage was calculated using the formula: Dose = 0.0476 × W × (Normal H − Observed H) + 1 mL per 5 kg to a maximum of 14 mL for iron stores.

Adults and Children over 15 kg (33 pounds):
See Dosage Table.

The total dose required may be calculated. If the patient's body weight in kilograms is W and the hemoglobin level is H g/dL:

Dose of IMFERON in mL required = 0.0476 × W × (14.8 − H) + iron stores.

Add 1 mL IMFERON for each 5 kg body weight to provide for the replenishment of iron stores to a maximum of 14 mL. For weight in pounds use the factor 0.0216.

Children 5–15 kg (11–33 pounds):
See Dosage Table.

Alternatively the total dose may be calculated.

IMFERON should not normally be given in the first four months of life. If the child's body weight in kilograms is W and hemoglobin level is H g/dL:

Dose of IMFERON required in mL = 0.0476 × W × (12 − H) + iron stores.

Add 1 mL IMFERON for each 5 kg body weight to provide for the replenishment of iron stores to a maximum of 14 mL. For weight in pounds use the factor 0.0216.

II. *Iron Replacement for Blood Loss*

Some individuals sustain blood losses on an intermittent or repetitive basis. Such blood losses may occur periodically in patients with hemorrhagic diatheses (familial telangiectasia; hemophilia; gastrointestinal bleeding) and on a repetitive basis from the procedures such as renal hemodialysis. Iron therapy in these patients should be directed toward replacement of the equivalent amount of iron represented in the lost blood. The table and formula presented under iron deficiency anemia are *not* applicable for simple iron replacement values.

Quantitative estimates of the individual's periodic blood loss and hematocrit during the bleeding episode provide a convenient method for the calculation of the required iron dose. The formula shown below is based on the approximation that 1 mL of normocytic, normochromic red cells contain 1 mg of elemental iron:

Replacement iron (in mg) = Blood loss (in mL) × hematocrit
Example: Blood loss of 500 mL with 20% hematocrit
     Replacement iron = 500 × 0.20 = 100 mg
     IMFERON dose = $\frac{100\ mg}{50}$ = 2 mL

Administration

The total amount of IMFERON required for the treatment of *iron deficiency anemia* or *iron replacement for blood loss* is determined from the table or appropriate formula. (See **Dosage**.)

I. *Intravenous Injection*

Prior to receiving their first intravenous IMFERON therapeutic dose, all patients should be given an intravenous *test dose* of 0.5 mL. Although anaphylactic reactions known to occur following IMFERON administration are usually evident within a few minutes, or sooner, it is recommended that a period of an hour or longer elapse before the remainder of the initial therapeutic dose is given.

Individual doses of 2 mL or less may be given on a daily basis until the calculated total amount required has been reached. IMFERON is given undiluted and *slowly* (1 mL or less per minute).

II. *Intramuscular Injection*

Prior to receiving their first intramuscular IMFERON therapeutic dose, all patients should be given an intramuscular *test dose* of 0.5 mL, administered in the same recommended test site and by the same technique as described below. Although anaphylactic reactions known to occur following IMFERON administration are usually evident within a few minutes or sooner, it is recommended that at least an hour or longer elapse before the remainder of the initial therapeutic dose is given.

If no adverse reactions are observed, IMFERON can be given according to the following schedule until the calculated total amount required has been reached. Each day's dose should ordinarily not exceed 0.5 mL (25 mg of iron) for infants under 5 kg (11 lbs.); 1.0 mL (50 mg of iron) for children under 10 kg (22 lbs.); and 2.0 mL (100 mg of iron) for other patients. Daily doses larger than these have been associated with an increased number of reports of delayed reactions and should be utilized only in those situations where the potential benefits clearly outweigh the increased risk. A daily dose of 5 mL should not be exceeded.

IMFERON should be injected only into the muscle mass of the upper outer quadrant of the buttock—never into the arm or other exposed areas—and should be injected deeply, with a 2-inch or 3-inch 19 or 20 gauge needle. If the patient is standing, he/she should be bearing his/her weight on the leg opposite the injection site, or if in bed, he/she should be in the lateral position with injection site uppermost. To avoid injection or leakage into the subcutaneous tissue, a Z-track technique (displacement of the skin laterally prior to injection) is recommended.

NOTE: Do not mix IMFERON with other medications or add to parenteral nutrition solutions for intravenous infusion.

HOW SUPPLIED

For intramuscular or intravenous use:
     2 mL ampules, boxes of 10:
     NDC 0585-2226-10
For intramuscular use ONLY:
     10 mL multiple dose vial containing
     0.5% phenol as a preservative, boxes of 2:
     NDC 0585-3226-20

Store at room temperature, preferably below 86°F. Do not freeze. Keep out of the reach of children.

CAUTION: Federal law prohibits dispensing without prescription.

® Registered trademark of Fisons plc   Revised 12/86
Made in England

Continued on next page

Information on Fisons' products appearing in these pages is current as of May, 1989. For further information, please consult the package insert currently accompanying the product, or Fisons Corporation, P.O. Box 1710, Rochester, NY 14603, (716) 475-9000.

Fisons—Cont.

INTAL® Capsules ℞
(cromolyn sodium for inhalation, USP)
For Inhalation Only
For Use With The SPINHALER®
TURBO-INHALER

DESCRIPTION
Chemically, cromolyn sodium is the disodium salt of 1,3-bis (2-carboxychromon-5-yloxy)-2-hydroxypropane.
Please see package insert for complete instructions.

INTAL® Inhaler ℞
[ĭn′tăl]
(cromolyn sodium inhalation aerosol)

DESCRIPTION
The active ingredient of INTAL Inhaler is cromolyn sodium. Cromolyn sodium is the disodium salt of 1,3 bis (2-carboxy-chromon-5-yloxy)-2-hydroxypropane. Cromolyn sodium has a molecular weight of 512.34. Cromolyn sodium is soluble in water.
The molecular structure of cromolyn sodium is:

INTAL Inhaler is a metered dose aerosol unit for oral inhalation containing micronized cromolyn sodium, sorbitan trioleate with dichlorotetrafluoroethane and dichlorodifluoromethane as propellants. Each metered spray delivers to the patient approximately 800 mcg of cromolyn sodium. Each 8.1 g canister delivers at least 112 metered sprays (56 doses); each 14.2 g canister delivers at least 200 metered sprays (100 doses).
Pharmacological Category: Mast cell stabilizer/antiallergic.
Therapeutic Category: Prophylactic antiasthmatic; reduces bronchial hyperreactivity.

CLINICAL PHARMACOLOGY
In vitro and *in vivo* animal studies have shown that cromolyn sodium inhibits sensitized mast cell degranulation which occurs after exposure to specific antigens. Cromolyn sodium acts by inhibiting the release of mediators from mast cells. Studies show that cromolyn sodium indirectly blocks calcium ions from entering the mast cell, thereby preventing mediator release.
Cromolyn sodium inhibits both the immediate and non-immediate bronchoconstrictive reactions to inhaled antigen. Cromolyn sodium also attenuates bronchospasm caused by exercise, toluene diisocyanate, aspirin, cold air, sulfur dioxide and environmental pollutants, at least in some patients. Cromolyn sodium has no intrinsic bronchodilator, antihistaminic or anti-inflammatory activity.
After administration of cromolyn sodium capsules by inhalation, approximately 8% of the total dose administered is absorbed and rapidly excreted unchanged, approximately equally divided between urine and bile. The remainder of the dose is either exhaled or deposited in the oropharynx, swallowed, and excreted via the alimentary tract.

INDICATIONS AND USAGE
INTAL Inhaler is a prophylactic agent indicated in the management of patients with bronchial asthma.
In patients whose symptoms are sufficiently frequent to require a continuous program of medication, INTAL Inhaler is given by inhalation on a regular daily basis (see Dosage and Administration). The effect of INTAL Inhaler is usually evident after several weeks of treatment, although some patients show an almost immediate response.
If improvement occurs, it will ordinarily occur within the first 4 weeks of administration as manifested by a decrease in the severity of clinical symptoms of asthma, or in the need for concomitant therapy, or both.
In patients who develop acute bronchoconstriction in response to exposure to exercise, toluene diisocyanate, environmental pollutants, known antigens, etc., INTAL Inhaler should be used shortly before exposure to the precipitating factor, i.e., within 10–15 minutes but not more than 60 minutes (see Dosage and Administration). INTAL Inhaler may be effective in relieving bronchospasm in some, but not all, patients with exercise induced bronchospasm.

CONTRAINDICATIONS
INTAL Inhaler is contraindicated in those patients who have shown hypersensitivity to cromolyn sodium or other components.

WARNINGS
INTAL Inhaler has no role in the treatment of an acute attack of asthma, especially status asthmaticus. Severe anaphylactic reactions can occur after cromolyn sodium administration. The recommended dosage should be decreased in patients with decreased renal or hepatic function. INTAL Inhaler should be discontinued if the patient develops eosinophilic pneumonia (or pulmonary infiltrates with eosinophilia). Because of the propellants in this preparation, it should be used with caution in patients with coronary artery disease or a history of cardiac arrhythmias.

PRECAUTIONS
General: In view of the biliary and renal routes of excretion for cromolyn sodium, consideration should be given to decreasing the dosage or discontinuing the administration of the drug in patients with impaired renal or hepatic function. Occasionally, patients may experience cough and/or bronchospasm following cromolyn sodium inhalation. At times, patients who develop bronchospasm may not be able to continue administration despite prior bronchodilator administration. Rarely, very severe bronchospasm has been encountered.
Carcinogenesis, Mutagenesis, Impairment of Fertility: Long term studies in mice (12 months intraperitoneal treatment followed by 6 months observation), hamsters (12 months intraperitoneal treatment followed by 12 months observation), and rats (18 months subcutaneous treatment) showed no neoplastic effect of cromolyn sodium.
No evidence of chromosomal damage or cytotoxicity was obtained in various mutagenesis studies.
No evidence of impaired fertility was shown in laboratory animal reproduction studies.
Pregnancy: Pregnancy Category B. Reproduction studies with cromolyn sodium administered parenterally to pregnant mice, rats, and rabbits in doses up to 338 times the human clinical doses produced no evidence of fetal malformations. Adverse fetal effects (increased resorptions and decreased fetal weight) were noted only at the very high parenteral doses that produced maternal toxicity. There are, however, no adequate and well-controlled studies in pregnant women. Because animal reproduction studies are not always predictive of human response, this drug should be used during pregnancy only if clearly needed.
Drug Interaction During Pregnancy: Cromolyn sodium and isoproterenol were studied following subcutaneous injections in pregnant mice. Cromolyn sodium alone in doses of 60 to 540 mg/kg (38 to 338 times the human dose) did not cause significant increases in resorptions or major malformations. Isoproterenol alone at a dose of 2.7 mg/kg (90 times the human dose) increased both resorptions and malformations. The addition of cromolyn sodium (338 times the human dose) to isoproterenol (90 times the human dose) appears to have increased the incidence of both resorptions and malformations.
Nursing Mothers: It is not known whether this drug is excreted in human milk, therefore, caution should be exercised when INTAL Inhaler is administered to a nursing woman and the attending physician must make a benefit/risk assessment in regard to its use in this situation.
Pediatric Use: Safety and effectiveness in children below the age of 5 years have not been established. For young children unable to utilize the Inhaler, INTAL Nebulizer Solution (cromolyn sodium inhalation, USP) is recommended. Because of the possibility that adverse effects of this drug could become apparent only after many years, a benefit/risk consideration of the long-term use of INTAL Inhaler is particularly important in pediatric patients.

ADVERSE REACTIONS
In controlled clinical studies of INTAL Inhaler, the most frequently reported adverse reactions attributed to cromolyn sodium treatment were: Throat irritation or dryness, Bad taste, Cough, Wheeze, Nausea.
The most frequently reported adverse reactions attributed to other forms of cromolyn sodium (on the basis of reoccurrence following readmicistration) involve the respiratory tract and are: bronchospasm [sometimes severe, associated with a precipitous fall in pulmonary function (FEV$_1$)], cough, laryngeal edema (rare), nasal congestion (sometimes severe), pharyngeal irritation and wheezing.
Adverse reactions which occur infrequently and are associated with administration of the drug are: anaphylaxis, angioedema, dizziness, dysuria and urinary frequency, joint swelling and pain, lacrimation, nausea and headache, rash, swollen parotid gland, urticaria, pulmonary infiltrates with eosinophilia, substernal burning, and myopathy.
The following adverse reactions have been reported as rare events and it is unclear whether they are attributable to the drug: anemia, exfoliative dermatitis, hemoptysis, hoarseness, myalgia, nephrosis, periarteritic vasculitis, pericarditis, peripheral neuritis, photodermatitis, sneezing, drowsiness, nasal itching, nasal bleeding, nasal burning, serum sickness, stomach ache, polymyositis, vertigo, and liver disease.

OVERDOSAGE
No action other than medical observation should be necessary.

DOSAGE AND ADMINISTRATION
For management of bronchial asthma in adults and children (5 years of age and over) who are able to use the Inhaler, the usual starting dosage is two metered sprays inhaled four times daily at regular intervals. This dose should not be exceeded. Not all patients will respond to the recommended dose and there is evidence to suggest, at least in younger patients, that a lower dose may provide efficacy.
Patients with chronic asthma should be advised that the effect of INTAL Inhaler therapy is dependent upon its administration at regular intervals, as directed. INTAL Inhaler should be introduced into the patient's therapeutic regimen when the acute episode has been controlled, the airway has been cleared and the patient is able to inhale adequately.
For the prevention of acute bronchospasm which follows exercise, exposure to cold dry air or environmental agents, the usual dose is inhalation of two metered dose sprays shortly, i.e., 10–15 minutes but not more than 60 minutes, before exposure to the precipitating factor.
INTAL INHALER THERAPY IN RELATION TO OTHER TREATMENTS FOR ASTHMA: Non-steroidal agents: INTAL Inhaler should be **added** to the patient's existing treatment regimen (e.g., bronchodilators). When a clinical response to INTAL Inhaler is evident, usually within two to four weeks, and if the asthma is under good control, an attempt may be made to decrease concomitant medication usage gradually.
If concomitant medications are eliminated or required on no more than a prn basis, the frequency of administration of INTAL Inhaler may be titrated downward to the lowest level consistent with the desired effect. The usual decrease is from four to three to two inhalations of two sprays per day. It is important that the dosage be reduced gradually to avoid exacerbation of asthma. It is emphasized that in patients whose dosage has been titrated to fewer than four inhalations per day, an increase in the dosage of INTAL Inhaler and the introduction of, or increase in, symptomatic medications may be needed if the patient's clinical condition deteriorates.
Corticosteroids: In patients chronically receiving corticosteroids for the management of bronchial asthma, the dosage should be maintained following the introduction of INTAL Inhaler. If the patient improves, an attempt to decrease corticosteroids should be made. Even if the corticosteroid-dependent patient fails to show symptomatic improvement following INTAL Inhaler administration, the potential to reduce corticosteroids may nonetheless be present. Thus, gradual tapering of corticosteroid dosage may be attempted. It is important that the dose be reduced slowly, maintaining close supervision of the patient to avoid an exacerbation of asthma.
It should be borne in mind that prolonged corticosteroid therapy frequently causes an impairment in the activity of the hypothalamo-pituitary-adrenal axis and a reduction in the size of the adrenal cortex. A potentially critical degree of impairment or insufficiency may persist asymptomatically for some time even after gradual discontinuation of adrenocortical steroids. Therefore, if a patient is subjected to significant stress, such as a severe asthmatic attack, surgery, trauma or severe illness while being treated or within one year (occasionally up to two years) after corticosteroid treatment has been terminated, consideration should be given to reinstituting corticosteroid therapy. When respiratory function is impaired, as may occur in severe exacerbation of asthma, a temporary increase in the amount of corticosteroids may be required to regain control of the patient's asthma.
It is particularly important that great care be exercised if for any reason cromolyn sodium is withdrawn in cases where its use has permitted a reduction in the maintenance dose of corticosteroids. In such cases, continued close supervision of the patient is essential since there may be sudden reappearance of severe manifestations of asthma which will require immediate therapy and possible reintroduction of corticosteroids.

HOW SUPPLIED
INTAL Inhaler, 8.1 g or 14.2 g canister, box of one. Supplied with inhalation adapter and patient instructions.
NDC 0585-0675-01   14.2 g canister
NDC 0585-0675-02   8.1 g canister
Store between 2°–30°C (36°–86°F). Contents under pressure. Do not puncture or incinerate. Keep out of the reach of children.

CAUTION
Federal law prohibits dispensing without prescription.
Manufactured for:
Fisons Pharmaceuticals
Rochester, NY 14623

By:
Riker Laboratories
One Morley Street
Loughborough, England LE11 1EP
Made in England   Revised 7/86
®Registered Trademark of Fisons plc

MYKROX™   ℞
[mǐ'krahks]
(metolazone)
TABLETS
Product formerly called MICROX®

DO NOT INTERCHANGE
MYKROX™ TABLETS ARE A RAPIDLY AVAILABLE FORMULATION OF METOLAZONE FOR ORAL ADMINISTRATION. MYKROX TABLETS AND OTHER FORMULATIONS OF METOLAZONE THAT SHARE ITS MORE RAPID AND COMPLETE BIOAVAILABILITY ARE NOT THERAPEUTICALLY EQUIVALENT TO ZAROXOLYN® TABLETS AND OTHER FORMULATIONS OF METOLAZONE THAT SHARE ITS SLOW AND INCOMPLETE BIOAVAILABILITY. FORMULATIONS BIOEQUIVALENT TO MYKROX AND FORMULATIONS BIOEQUIVALENT TO ZAROXOLYN SHOULD NOT BE INTERCHANGED FOR ONE ANOTHER.

DESCRIPTION
Metolazone has the molecular formula $C_{16}H_{16}ClN_3O_3S$, the chemical name 7-chloro-1,2,3,4-tetrahydro-2-methyl-3-(2-methylphenyl)-4-oxo-6-quinazoline-sulfonamide, and a molecular weight of 365.83. The structural formula is:

Metolazone is only sparingly soluble in water, but more soluble in plasma, blood, alkali and organic solvents.
Other ingredients in MYKROX Tablets: dibasic calcium phosphate, magnesium stearate, microcrystalline cellulose, pregelatinized starch, sodium starch glycolate.

CLINICAL PHARMACOLOGY
MYKROX is a quinazoline diuretic, with properties generally similar to the thiazide diuretics. The actions of MYKROX (metolazone) result from interference with the renal tubular mechanism of electrolyte reabsorption. MYKROX acts primarily to inhibit sodium reabsorption at the cortical diluting site and to a lesser extent in the proximal convoluted tubule. Sodium and chloride ions are excreted in approximately equivalent amounts. The increased delivery of sodium to the distal-tubular exchange site results in increased potassium excretion. MYKROX does not inhibit carbonic anhydrase. A proximal action has been shown in humans by increased excretion of phosphate and magnesium ions, and by a markedly increased fractional excretion of sodium in patients with severely compromised glomerular filtration. This action has been demonstrated in animals by micropuncture studies.
The antihypertensive mechanism of action of metolazone is not fully understood but is presumed to be related to its saluretic and diuretic properties.
In two double-blind, controlled clinical trials of MYKROX Tablets, the maximum effect on mean blood pressure was achieved within 2 weeks of treatment and showed some evidence of an increased response at 1 mg compared to ½ mg. There was no indication of an increased response with 2 mg. After six weeks of treatment, the mean fall in serum potassium was 0.42 mEq/L at ½ mg, 0.66 mEq/L at 1 mg and 0.7 mEq/L at 2 mg. Serum uric acid increased by 1.1 to 1.4 mg/dl at increasing doses. There were small falls in serum sodium and chloride and a 1.3–2.1 mg/dl increase in BUN at increasing doses.
The rate and extent of absorption of metolazone from MYKROX Tablets were equivalent to those from an oral solution of metolazone. Peak blood levels are obtained within 2 to 4 hours of oral administration with an elimination half-life of approximately 14 hours. MYKROX Tablets have been shown to produce blood levels that are dose proportional between ½–2 mg. Steady state blood levels are usually reached in 4–5 days.
In contrast, other formulations of metolazone produce peak blood concentrations approximately 8 hours following oral administration; absorption continues for an additional 12 hours.

INDICATIONS AND USAGE
MYKROX Tablets are indicated for the treatment of hypertension, alone or in combination with other antihypertensive drugs of a different class.

MYKROX TABLETS HAVE NOT BEEN EVALUATED FOR THE TREATMENT OF CONGESTIVE HEART FAILURE OR FLUID RETENTION DUE TO RENAL OR HEPATIC DISEASE AND THE CORRECT DOSAGE FOR THESE CONDITIONS AND OTHER EDEMA STATES HAS NOT BEEN ESTABLISHED.
SINCE A SAFE AND EFFECTIVE DIURETIC DOSE HAS NOT BEEN ESTABLISHED, MYKROX TABLETS SHOULD NOT BE USED WHEN DIURESIS IS DESIRED.
Usage in Pregnancy
The routine use of diuretics in an otherwise healthy woman is inappropriate and exposes mother and fetus to unnecessary hazard. Diuretics do not prevent development of toxemia of pregnancy, and there is no evidence that they are useful in the treatment of developed toxemia (see PRECAUTIONS).
Edema during pregnancy may arise from pathologic causes or from the physiologic and mechanical consequences of pregnancy. MYKROX is not indicated for the treatment of edema in pregnancy. Dependent edema in pregnancy resulting from restriction of venous return by the expanded uterus is properly treated through elevation of the lower extremities and use of support hose; use of diuretics to lower intravascular volume in this case is illogical and unnecessary. There is hypervolemia during normal pregnancy which is harmful to neither the fetus nor the mother (in the absence of cardiovascular disease), but which is associated with edema, including generalized edema, in the majority of pregnant women. If this edema produces discomfort, increased recumbency will often provide relief. In rare instances, this edema may cause extreme discomfort which is not relieved by rest. In these cases, a short course of diuretics may be appropriate.

CONTRAINDICATIONS
Anuria, hepatic coma or pre-coma, known allergy or hypersensitivity to metolazone.

WARNINGS
Rapid Onset Hyponatremia
Rarely, the rapid onset of severe hyponatremia and/or hypokalemia has been reported following initial doses of thiazide and nonthiazide diuretics. When symptoms consistent with electrolyte imbalance appear rapidly, drug should be discontinued and supportive measures should be initiated immediately. Parenteral electrolytes may be required. Appropriateness of therapy with this class of drugs should be carefully reevaluated.
Hypokalemia
Hypokalemia may occur, with consequent weakness, cramps, and cardiac dysrhythmias. Serum potassium should be determined at regular intervals, and dose reduction, potassium supplementation or addition of a potassium sparing diuretic instituted whenever indicated. Hypokalemia is a particular hazard in patients who are digitalized or who have or have had a ventricular arrhythmia; dangerous or fatal arrhythmias may be precipitated. Hypokalemia is dose related.
Lithium
In general, diuretics should not be given concomitantly with lithium because they reduce its renal clearance and add a high risk of lithium toxicity. Read prescribing information for lithium preparations before use of such concomitant therapy.
Concomitant Therapy
Furosemide: Unusually large or prolonged losses of fluids and electrolytes may result when metolazone is administered concomitantly to patients receiving furosemide (see DRUG INTERACTIONS).
Other Antihypertensive Drugs: When MYKROX Tablets are used with other antihypertensive drugs, particular care must be taken to avoid excessive reduction of blood pressure, especially during initial therapy.
Cross-Allergy
Cross-allergy, while not reported to date, theoretically may occur when MYKROX Tablets are given to patients known to be allergic to sulfonamide-derived drugs, thiazides, or quinethazone.

PRECAUTIONS
DO NOT INTERCHANGE
MYKROX TABLETS ARE A RAPIDLY AVAILABLE FORMULATION OF METOLAZONE FOR ORAL ADMINISTRATION. MYKROX TABLETS AND OTHER FORMULATIONS OF METOLAZONE THAT SHARE ITS MORE RAPID AND COMPLETE BIOAVAILABILITY ARE NOT THERAPEUTICALLY EQUIVALENT TO ZAROXOLYN TABLETS AND OTHER FORMULATIONS OF METOLAZONE THAT SHARE ITS SLOW AND INCOMPLETE BIOAVAILABILITY. FORMULATIONS BIOEQUIVALENT TO MYKROX AND FORMULATIONS BIOEQUIVALENT TO ZAROXOLYN SHOULD NOT BE INTERCHANGED FOR ONE ANOTHER.
A. GENERAL:
Fluid and Electrolytes
All patients receiving therapy with MYKROX Tablets should have serum electrolyte measurements done at appropriate intervals and be observed for clinical signs of fluid

and/or electrolyte imbalance: namely, hyponatremia, hypochloremic alkalosis, and hypokalemia. In patients with severe edema accompanying cardiac failure or renal disease, a low-salt syndrome may be produced, especially with hot weather and a low-salt diet. Serum and urine electrolyte determinations are particularly important when the patient has protracted vomiting, severe diarrhea, or is receiving parenteral fluids. Warning signs of imbalance are: dryness of mouth, thirst, weakness, lethargy, drowsiness, restlessness, muscle pains or cramps, muscle fatigue, hypotension, oliguria, tachycardia, and gastrointestinal disturbances such as nausea and vomiting. Hyponatremia may occur at any time during long term therapy and, on rare occasions, may be life threatening.
The risk of hypokalemia is increased when larger doses are used, when diuresis is rapid, when severe liver disease is present, when corticosteroids are given concomitantly, when oral intake is inadequate or when excess potassium is being lost extrarenally, such as with vomiting or diarrhea.
Glucose Tolerance
Metolazone may raise blood glucose concentrations possibly causing hyperglycemia and glycosuria in patients with diabetes or latent diabetes.
Hyperuricemia
MYKROX regularly causes an increase in serum uric acid and can occasionally precipitate gouty attacks even in patients without a prior history of them.
Azotemia
Azotemia, presumably pre-renal azotemia, may be precipitated during the administration of MYKROX Tablets. If azotemia and oliguria worsen during treatment of patients with severe renal disease, MYKROX Tablets should be discontinued.
Renal Impairment
Use caution when administering MYKROX Tablets to patients with severely impaired renal function. As most of the drug is excreted by the renal route, accumulation may occur.
Orthostatic Hypotension
Orthostatic hypotension may occur; this may be potentiated by alcohol, barbiturates, narcotics, or concurrent therapy with other antihypertensive drugs. In controlled clinical trials, 1.4% of patients treated with MYKROX Tablets (½ mg) had orthostatic hypotension; this effect was not reported in the placebo group.
Hypercalcemia
Use of other diuretics has been associated on rare occasions with pathological changes in the parathyroid glands. This possibility should be considered with clinical use of MYKROX Tablets. Hypercalcemia has been noted in a few patients treated with metolazone.
Systemic Lupus Erythematosus
Thiazide diuretics have exacerbated or activated systemic lupus erythematosus and this possibility should be considered with MYKROX (metolazone) Tablets.
B. INFORMATION FOR PATIENTS:
Patients should be informed of possible adverse effects, advised to take the medication as directed and promptly report any possible adverse reactions to the treating physician.
C. DRUG INTERACTIONS:
Diuretics
Furosemide and probably other loop diuretics given concomitantly with metolazone can cause unusually large or prolonged losses of fluid and electrolytes (see WARNINGS).
Other Antihypertensives
When MYKROX Tablets are used with other antihypertensive drugs, care must be taken, especially during initial therapy. Dosage adjustments of other antihypertensives may be necessary.
Alcohol, Barbiturates, and Narcotics
The hypotensive effects of these drugs may be potentiated by the volume contraction that may be associated with metolazone therapy.
Digitalis Glycosides
Diuretic-induced hypokalemia can increase the sensitivity of the myocardium to digitalis. Serious arrhythmias can result.
Corticosteroids or ACTH
May increase the risk of hypokalemia and increase salt and water retention.
Lithium
Serum lithium levels may increase (see WARNINGS).
Curariform Drugs
Diuretic-induced hypokalemia may enhance neuromuscular blocking effects of curariform drugs (such as tubocurarine)—the most serious effect would be respiratory depression which could proceed to apnea. Accordingly, it may be advis-

Continued on next page

Information on Fisons' products appearing in these pages is current as of May, 1989. For further information, please consult the package insert currently accompanying the product, or Fisons Corporation, P.O. Box 1710, Rochester, NY 14603, (716) 475-9000.

Fisons—Cont.

able to discontinue MYKROX Tablets three days before elective surgery.

Salicylates and Other Non-Steroidal Anti-Inflammatory Drugs
May decrease the antihypertensive effects of MYKROX Tablets.

Sympathomimetics
Metolazone may decrease arterial responsiveness to norepinephrine, but this diminution is not sufficient to preclude effectiveness of the pressor agent for therapeutic use.

Insulin and Oral Antidiabetic Agents
See Glucose Tolerance under GENERAL PRECAUTIONS

Methenamine
Efficacy may be decreased due to urinary alkalizing effect of metolazone.

D. DRUG/LABORATORY TEST INTERACTIONS: None reported.

E. CARCINOGENESIS, MUTAGENESIS, IMPAIRMENT OF FERTILITY: Mice and rats given metolazone for $1\frac{1}{2}$ to 2 years at daily doses of 2, 10 and 50 mg/kg (approximately 100, 500, and 2,500 times the recommended maximum daily dose of MYKROX 1 mg given to a 50 kg person) showed no evidence that metolazone caused an increased number of tumors. The small number of animals examined histologically and poor survival in the mice limit the conclusions that can be reached from these studies.

Reproductive performance has been evaluated in mice and rats. There is no evidence that metolazone possesses the potential for altering reproductive capacity in mice. In a rat study, in which males were treated orally with metolazone at doses of 2, 10 and 50 mg/kg for 127 days prior to mating with untreated females, an increased number of resorption sites was observed in dams mated with males from the 50 mg/kg group. In addition, the fetal weight of offspring was decreased and the pregnancy rate was reduced in dams mated with males from the 10 and 50 mg/kg groups.

F. PREGNANCY
Teratogenic Effects—Pregnancy Category B.
Reproduction studies performed in mice, rabbits and rats treated during the appropriate periods of gestation at doses up to 50 mg/kg/day (2,500 times the recommended maximum daily dose of MYKROX) have revealed no evidence of harm to the fetus due to metolazone. There are, however, no adequate and well-controlled studies in pregnant women. Because animal reproduction studies are not always predictive of human response, MYKROX Tablets should be used during pregnancy only if clearly needed. Metolazone crosses the placental barrier and appears in cord blood.

Non-Teratogenic Effects
The use of MYKROX Tablets in pregnant women requires that the anticipated benefit be weighed against possible hazards to the fetus. These hazards include fetal or neonatal jaundice, thrombocytopenia, and possibly other adverse reactions which have occurred in the adult. It is not known what effect the use of the drug during pregnancy has on the later growth, development and functional maturation of the child. No such effects have been reported with metolazone.

G. LABOR AND DELIVERY: Based on clinical studies in which women received metolazone in late pregnancy until the time of delivery, there is no evidence that the drug has any adverse effects on the normal course of labor or delivery.

H. NURSING MOTHERS: Metolazone appears in breast milk. Because of the potential for serious adverse reactions in nursing infants from metolazone, a decision should be made whether to discontinue nursing or to discontinue the drug, taking into account the importance of the drug to the mother.

I. PEDIATRIC USE: Safety and effectiveness of MYKROX Tablets in children have not been established, and such use is not recommended.

ADVERSE REACTIONS

Adverse experience information is available from more than 14 years of accumulated marketing experience with other formulations of metolazone for which reliable quantitative information is lacking and from controlled clinical trials with MYKROX from which incidences can be calculated.
In controlled clinical trials with MYKROX, adverse experiences resulted in discontinuation of therapy in 6.7–6.8% of patients given $\frac{1}{2}$ to 1 mg of MYKROX.
Adverse experiences occurring in controlled clinical trials with MYKROX with an incidence of > 2%, whether or not considered drug-related, are summarized in the following table.

Incidence of Adverse Experiences
Volunteered or Elicited
(by Patient in Percent)*

	MYKROX n=226†
Dizziness (lightheadedness)	10.2
Headaches	9.3
Muscle Cramps	5.8
Fatigue (malaise, lethargy, lassitude)	4.4
Joint Pain, swelling	3.1
Chest Pain (precordial discomfort)	2.7

* Percent of patients reporting an adverse experience one or more times.

† All doses combined ($\frac{1}{2}$, 1 and 2 mg).

Some of the adverse effects reported in association with MYKROX also occur frequently in untreated hypertensive patients, such as headache and dizziness, which occurred in 14.8 and 7.4% of patients in a smaller parallel placebo group. The following adverse effects were reported in less than 2% of the MYKROX treated patients.

Cardiovascular: Cold extremities, edema, orthostatic hypotension, palpitations.

Central and Peripheral Nervous System: Anxiety, depression, dry mouth, impotence, nervousness, neuropathy, weakness, "weird" feeling.

Dermatological: Pruritus, rash, skin dryness.

Eyes, Ears, Nose, Throat: Cough, epistaxis, eye itching, sinus congestion, sore throat, tinnitus.

Gastrointestinal: Abdominal discomfort (pain, bloating), bitter taste, constipation, diarrhea, nausea, vomiting.

Genitourinary: Nocturia.

Musculoskeletal: Back pain.

Other Adverse Experiences:
Adverse experiences reported with other marketed metolazone formulations and most thiazide diuretics, for which quantitative data are not available, are listed in decreasing order of severity within body systems. Several are single or rare occurrences.

Cardiovascular—excessive volume depletion, hemoconcentration, venous thrombosis.

Central and Peripheral Nervous System—syncope, paresthesia, drowsiness, restlessness (sometimes resulting in insomnia).

Dermatological/Hypersensitivity—necrotizing angiitis (cutaneous vasculitis), purpura, dermatitis, photosensitivity, urticaria.

Gastrointestinal—hepatitis, intrahepatic cholestatic jaundice, pancreatitis, anorexia.

Hematologic—aplastic (hypoplastic) anemia, agranulocytosis, leukopenia.

Metabolic—hypokalemia, hyponatremia, hyperuricemia, hypochloremia, hypochloremic alkalosis, hyperglycemia, glycosuria, increase in serum urea nitrogen (BUN) or creatinine, hypophosphatemia.

Musculoskeletal—acute gouty attacks.

Other—transient blurred vision, chills.

In addition, rare adverse experiences reported in association with similar antihypertensive-diuretics but not reported to date for metolazone include: sialadenitis, xanthopsia, respiratory distress (including pneumonitis), thrombocytopenia and anaphylactic reactions. These experiences could occur with clinical use of metolazone.

OVERDOSAGE

Intentional overdosage has been reported rarely with metolazone and similar diuretic drugs.

Signs and Symptoms
Orthostatic hypotension, dizziness, drowsiness, syncope, electrolyte abnormalities, hemoconcentration and hemodynamic changes due to plasma volume depletion may occur. In some instances depressed respiration may be observed. At high doses, lethargy of varying degree may appear and may progress to coma within a few hours. The mechanism of CNS depression with thiazide overdosage is unknown. Also, GI irritation and hypermotility may occur. Temporary elevation of BUN has been reported, especially in patients with impairment of renal function. Serum electrolyte changes and cardiovascular and renal function should be closely monitored.

Treatment
There is no specific antidote available but immediate evacuation of the stomach contents is advised. Dialysis is not likely to be effective. Care should be taken when evacuating the gastric contents to prevent aspiration, especially in the stuporous or comatose patient. Supportive measures should be initiated as required to maintain hydration, electrolyte balance, respiration and cardiovascular and renal function.

DOSAGE AND ADMINISTRATION

Therapy should be individualized according to patient response.
For initial treatment of mild to moderate hypertension, the recommended dose is one MYKROX Tablet ($\frac{1}{2}$ mg) once daily, usually in the morning. If patients are inadequately controlled with one $\frac{1}{2}$ mg tablet, the dose can be increased to two MYKROX Tablets (1 mg) once a day. An inrease in hypokalemia may occur. Doses larger than one mg do not give increased effectiveness.
The same dose titration is necessary if MYKROX Tablets are to be substituted for other dosage forms of metolazone in the treatment of hypertension.
If blood pressure is not adequately controlled with two MYKROX Tablets alone, the dose should not be increased; rather,

another antihypertensive agent with a different mechanism of action should be added to therapy with MYKROX Tablets.

HOW SUPPLIED

MYKROX (metolazone) Tablets, $\frac{1}{2}$ mg: White, flat-faced, round tablets embossed, MYKROX on one side and, $\frac{1}{2}$, on reverse side.
Bottles of 100 NDC 0585-0847-71
Bottles of 500 NDC 0585-0847-85
Bottles of 1000 NDC 0585-0847-90
Store at room temperature. Dispense in a tight, light-resistant container.
Caution: Federal law prohibits dispensing without prescription.
9/88

NASALCROM® NASAL SOLUTION   ℞
[nāz ′ŭl-krōm ″]
(cromolyn sodium nasal solution, USP)

DESCRIPTION

Each milliliter of NASALCROM® Nasal Solution (cromolyn sodium nasal solution, USP) contains 40 mg cromolyn sodium in purified water with 0.01% benzalkonium chloride to preserve and 0.01% EDTA (edetate disodium) to stabilize the solution. NASALCROM possesses a natural pH of 4.5–6.5 and negligible titratable acidity. Chemically, cromolyn sodium is the disodium salt of 1,3-bis(2-carboxychromon-5-yloxy)-2-hydroxypropane.
The molecular structure is:

Pharmacologic Category: Mast cell stabilizer/ antiallergic.
Therapeutic Category: Antiallergic.
After priming the delivery system for NASALCROM, each actuation of the unit delivers a metered spray containing 5.2 mg of cromolyn sodium. The contents of one bottle delivers at least 100 sprays (13 mL bottle) or 200 sprays (26 mL bottle).

CLINICAL PHARMACOLOGY

In vitro and *in vivo* animal studies have shown that cromolyn sodium inhibits the degranulation of sensitized mast cells which occurs after exposure to specific antigens. Cromolyn sodium inhibits the release of histamine and SRS-A (the slow-reacting substance of anaphylaxis). Rhinitis induced by the inhalation of specific antigens can be inhibited to varying degrees by pretreatment with NASALCROM.
Another activity demonstrated *in vitro* is the capacity of cromolyn sodium to inhibit the degranulation of non-sensitized rat mast cells by phospholipase A and the subsequent release of chemical mediators. An additional *in vitro* study showed that cromolyn sodium did not inhibit the enzymatic activity of released phospholipase A on its specific substrate. Cromolyn sodium has no intrinsic bronchodilator, antihistaminic or anti-inflammatory activity.
Cromolyn sodium is poorly absorbed from the gastrointestinal tract. After instillation of NASALCROM, less than 7% of the total dose administered is absorbed and is rapidly excreted unchanged in the bile and urine. The remainder of the dose is expelled from the nose, or swallowed and excreted via the alimentary tract.

INDICATIONS

NASALCROM is indicated for the prevention and treatment of the symptoms of allergic rhinitis.

CONTRAINDICATIONS

NASALCROM is contraindicated in those patients who have shown hypersensitivity to any of the ingredients.

PRECAUTIONS

General: Some patients may experience transient nasal stinging and/or sneezing immediately following instillation of NASALCROM. Except in rare occurrences, these experiences have not caused discontinuation of therapy.
In view of the biliary and renal routes of excretion for cromolyn sodium, consideration should be given to decreasing the dosage or discontinuing the administration of the drug in patients with impaired renal or hepatic function.
Carcinogenesis, Mutagenesis, and Impairment of Fertility: Long term studies in mice (12 months intraperitoneal treatment followed by 6 months observation), hamsters (12 months intraperitoneal treatment followed by 12 months observation), and rats (18 months subcutaneous treatment) showed no neoplastic effect of cromolyn sodium.
No evidence of chromosomal damage or cytotoxicity was obtained in various mutagenesis studies.
No evidence of impaired fertility was shown in laboratory animal reproduction studies.
Pregnancy: Pregnancy Category B. Reproduction studies with cromolyn sodium administered parenterally to pregnant mice, rats, and rabbits in doses up to 338 times the human clinical doses produced no evidence of fetal malforma-

tions. Adverse fetal effects (increased resorptions and decreased fetal weight) were noted only at the very high parenteral doses that produced maternal toxicity. There are, however, no adequate and well-controlled studies in pregnant women. Because animal reproduction studies are not always predictive of human response, this drug should be used during pregnancy only if clearly needed.

Drug Interaction During Pregnancy: Cromolyn sodium and isoproterenol were studied following subcutaneous injections in pregnant mice. Cromolyn sodium alone in doses of 60 to 540 mg/kg (38 to 338 times the human dose) did not cause significant increases in resorptions or major malformations. Isoproterenol alone at a dose of 2.7 mg/kg (90 times the human dose) increased both resorptions and malformations. The addition of cromolyn sodium (338 times the human dose) to isoproterenol (90 times the human dose) appears to have increased the incidence of both resorptions and malformations.

Nursing Mothers: It is not known whether this drug is excreted in human milk. Because many drugs are excreted in human milk, caution should be exercised when NASALCROM is administered to a nursing woman.

Pediatric Use: Safety and effectiveness in children below the age of 6 years have not been established.

ADVERSE REACTIONS

The most frequent adverse reactions occurring in the 430 patients included in the clinical trials with NASALCROM were sneezing (1 in 10 patients), nasal stinging (1 in 20), nasal burning (1 in 25), and nasal irritation (1 in 40). Headaches and bad taste were reported in about 1 in 50 patients. Epistaxis, postnasal drip, and rash were reported in less than one percent of the patients. One patient in the clinical trials developed anaphylaxis.

Adverse reactions which have occurred in the use of other cromolyn sodium formulations for inhalation include angioedema, joint pain and swelling, urticaria, cough, and wheezing. Other reactions reported rarely are serum sickness, periarteritic vasculitis, polymyositis, pericarditis, photodermatitis, exfoliative dermatitis, peripheral neuritis, and nephrosis.

DOSAGE AND ADMINISTRATION

The dose for adults and children 6 years and older is one spray in each nostril 3–4 times daily at regular intervals. If needed, this dose may be increased to one spray to each nostril 6 times daily. The patient should be instructed to clear the nasal passages before administering the spray and should inhale through the nose during administration.

In the management of seasonal (pollenotic) rhinitis, and for prevention of rhinitis caused by exposure to other types of specific inhalant allergens, treatment with NASALCROM will be more effective if started prior to expected contact with the offending allergen. Treatment should be continued throughout the period of exposure, i.e., until the pollen season is over or until exposure to the offending allergen is terminated.

In the management of perennial allergic rhinitis, the effects of treatment with NASALCROM may become apparent only after two to four weeks of treatment. The concomitant use of antihistamine and/or nasal decongestant may be necessary during the initial phase of treatment, but the need for this type of medication should diminish and may be eliminated when the full benefit of NASALCROM is achieved.

HOW SUPPLIED

NASALCROM is available in bottles of 13 mL and 26 mL. Each fully assembled unit consists of a pump unit and actuator with cover in position on the bottle of nasal solution. The amount of cromolyn sodium in each bottle is: 13 mL -520 mg (40 mg/mL); 26 mL -1040 mg (40 mg/mL). NASALCROM should be stored at controlled room temperature between 15° and 30°C (59° and 86°F).

NDC 0585-0671-03 13 mL bottle (fully assembled unit)
NDC 0585-0671-04 26 mL bottle (fully assembled unit)

CAUTION

Federal law prohibits dispensing without prescription.
®Registered Trademark of Fisons plc

Rev.9/88

OPTICROM® 4%   ℞
[op 'ti-krŏm]
Ophthalmic Solution
(cromolyn sodium ophthalmic solution, USP)

DESCRIPTION

Each milliliter of OPTICROM 4% Ophthalmic Solution (cromolyn sodium ophthalmic solution, USP) contains 40 mg cromolyn sodium in purified water with 0.01% benzalkonium chloride to preserve and 0.1% EDTA (edetate disodium, USP) to stabilize the solution. OPTICROM is a clear, colorless, sterile solution with a pH of 4.0–7.0. It is intended for topical administration to the eye.

Chemically, cromolyn sodium is the disodium salt of 1,3-bis(2-carboxychromon-5-yloxy)-2-hydroxypropane. Its chemical structure is:

Pharmacologic Category: Mast cell stabilizer
Therapeutic Category: Antiallergic

CLINICAL PHARMACOLOGY

In vitro and *in vivo* animal studies have shown that cromolyn sodium inhibits the degranulation of sensitized mast cells which occurs after exposure to specific antigens. Cromolyn sodium acts by inhibiting the release of histamine and SRS-A (slow-reacting substance of anaphylaxis) from the mast cell. Another activity demonstrated *in vitro* is the capacity of cromolyn sodium to inhibit the degranulation of non-sensitized rat mast cells by phospholipase A and the subsequent release of chemical mediators. Another study showed that cromolyn sodium did not inhibit the enzymatic activity of released phospholipase A on its specific substrate.

Cromolyn sodium has no intrinsic vasoconstrictor, antihistaminic or anti-inflammatory activity.

Cromolyn sodium is poorly absorbed. When multiple doses of cromolyn sodium ophthalmic solution are instilled into normal rabbit eyes, less than 0.07% of the administered dose of cromolyn sodium is absorbed into the systemic circulation (presumably by way of the eye, nasal passages, buccal cavity and gastrointestinal tract). Trace amounts (less than 0.01%) of the cromolyn sodium dose penetrate into the aqueous humor and clearance from this chamber is virtually complete within 24 hours after treatment is stopped.

In normal volunteers, analysis of drug excretion indicates that approximately 0.03% of cromolyn sodium is absorbed following administration to the eye.

A study on corneal epithelial wound healing in albino rabbits failed to demonstrate any significant difference in the rate of corneal re-epithelialization between cromolyn sodium ophthalmic solution, sterile saline solution, no treatment and an ophthalmic corticosteroid.

INDICATIONS AND USAGE

OPTICROM is indicated in the treatment of certain allergic ocular disorders referred to by the terms vernal keratoconjunctivitis, vernal conjunctivitis, giant papillary conjunctivitis, vernal keratitis, and allergic keratoconjunctivitis. The etiologic factors are unknown, but common airborne allergens and contact lenses have been implicated.[1]

Symptomatic response to therapy (decreased itching, tearing, redness and discharge) is usually evident within a few days, but longer treatment for up to six weeks is sometimes required. Once symptomatic improvement has been established, therapy should be continued for as long as needed to sustain improvement.

If required, corticosteroids may be used concomitantly with OPTICROM.

Users of soft (hydrophilic) contact lenses should refrain from wearing lenses while under treatment with OPTICROM (see **Contraindications**). Wear can be resumed within a few hours after discontinuation of the drug.

CONTRAINDICATIONS

OPTICROM is contraindicated in those patients who have shown hypersensitivity to cromolyn sodium or to any of the other ingredients.

As with all ophthalmic preparations containing benzalkonium chloride, patients are advised not to wear soft contact lenses during treatment with OPTICROM.

PRECAUTIONS

General: Patients may experience a transient stinging or burning sensation following application of OPTICROM. The recommended frequency of administration should not be exceeded. The dose for adults and children is 1–2 drops in each eye 4–6 times a day at regular intervals.

Carcinogenesis, Mutagenesis, and Impairment of Fertility: Long term studies in mice (12 months intraperitoneal treatment followed by six months observation), hamsters (12 months intraperitoneal treatment followed by 12 months observation), and rats (18 months subcutaneous treatment) showed no neoplastic effect of cromolyn sodium.

No evidence of chromosomal damage or cytotoxicity was obtained in various mutagenesis studies.

No evidence of impaired fertility was shown in laboratory animal reproduction studies.

Pregnancy: Pregnancy Category B. Reproduction studies with cromolyn sodium administered parenterally to pregnant mice, rats and rabbits in doses up to 338 times the human clinical doses produced no evidence of fetal malformations. Adverse fetal effects (increased resorption and decreased fetal weight) were noted only at the very high parenteral doses that produced maternal toxicity. There are, however, no adequate and well controlled studies in pregnant women. Because animal reproduction studies are not always predictive of human response, this drug should be used during pregnancy only if clearly needed.

Nursing Mothers: It is not known whether this drug is excreted in human milk. Because many drugs are excreted in human milk, caution should be exercised when OPTICROM is administered to a nursing woman.

Pediatric Use: Safety and effectiveness in children below the age of 4 years have not been established.

ADVERSE REACTIONS

The most frequently reported adverse reaction attributed to the use of OPTICROM, on the basis of reoccurrence following readministration, is transient ocular stinging or burning upon instillation.

The following adverse reactions have been reported as infrequent events. It is unclear whether they are attributable to the drug: conjunctival injection, watery eyes, itchy eyes, dryness around the eye, puffy eyes, eye irritation, styes.

DOSAGE AND ADMINISTRATION

The dose for adults and children is 1–2 drops in each eye 4–6 times a day at regular intervals. One drop contains approximately 1.6 mg cromolyn sodium.

Patients should be advised that the effect of OPTICROM therapy is dependent upon its administration at regular intervals, as directed.

HOW SUPPLIED

OPTICROM is supplied as 10 ml of solution in an opaque polyethylene eye drop bottle.
NDC 0585-0680-01   10 ml bottle
Keep tightly closed and out of the reach of children. Store below 30°C (86°F) and protect from direct sunlight.

CAUTION

Federal law prohibits dispensing without prescription.

REFERENCE

[1] Allansmith MR, Abelson MB. Ocular Allergies. In: The Cornea, ed. by G Smolin, RA Thoft. Little, Brown and Co., Boston/Toronto, 1983; 231–43.
® Registered trademark of Fisons plc
Made in England   Revised 11/85

PEDIAPRED®   ℞
[pĕd 'ē-uh-pred]
(prednisolone sodium phosphate, USP)
ORAL LIQUID

DESCRIPTION

PEDIAPRED Oral Liquid is a dye free, colorless to light straw colored, raspberry flavored solution. Each 5 mL (teaspoonful) of PEDIAPRED contains 6.7 mg prednisolone sodium phosphate (5 mg prednisolone base) in a palatable, aqueous vehicle.

Prednisolone sodium phosphate occurs as white or slightly yellow, friable granules or powder. It is freely soluble in water; soluble in methanol; slightly soluble in alcohol and in chloroform; and very slightly soluble in acetone and in dioxane. The chemical name of prednisolone sodium phosphate is pregna-1,4-diene-3,20-dione,11,17-dihydroxy-21-(phosphonooxy)-, disodium salt, (11β)-. Its chemical structure is:

Pharmacological Category: Glucocorticoid

CLINICAL PHARMACOLOGY

Prednisolone is a synthetic adrenocortical steroid drug with predominantly glucocorticoid properties. Some of these properties reproduce the physiological actions of endogenous glucocorticosteroids, but others do not necessarily reflect any of the adrenal hormones' normal functions; they are seen only after administration of large therapeutic doses of the drug. The pharmacological effects of prednisolone which are due to its glucocorticoid properties include: promotion of gluconeogenesis; increased deposition of glycogen in the liver; inhibition of the utilization of glucose; anti-insulin activity; increased catabolism of protein; increased lipolysis; stimulation of fat synthesis and storage; increased glomerular filtration rate and resulting increase in urinary excretion

Continued on next page

Fisons—Cont.

of urate (creatinine excretion remains unchanged); and increased calcium excretion.

Depressed production of eosinophils and lymphocytes occurs, but erythropoiesis and production of polymorphonuclear leukocytes are stimulated. Anti-inflammatory processes (edema, fibrin deposition, capillary dilatation, migration of leukocytes and phagocytosis) and the later stages of wound healing (capillary proliferation, deposition of collagen, cicatrization) are inhibited. Prednisolone can stimulate secretion of various components of gastric juice. Stimulation of the production of corticotropin may lead to suppression of endogenous corticosteroids. Prednisolone has slight mineralocorticoid activity, whereby entry of sodium into cells and loss of intracellular potassium is stimulated. This is particularly evident in the kidney, where rapid ion exchange leads to sodium retention and hypertension.

Prednisolone is rapidly and well absorbed from the gastrointestinal tract following oral administration. PEDIAPRED Oral Liquid produces a 20% higher peak plasma level of prednisolone which occurs approximately 15 minutes earlier than the peak seen with tablet formulations. Prednisolone is 70–90% protein-bound in the plasma and it is eliminated from the plasma with a half-life of 2 to 4 hours. It is metabolized mainly in the liver and excreted in the urine as sulfate and glucuronide conjugates.

INDICATIONS AND USAGE

PEDIAPRED Oral Liquid is indicated in the following conditions:

1. **Endocrine Disorders**
   Primary or secondary adrenocortical insufficiency (hydrocortisone or cortisone is the first choice; synthetic analogs may be used in conjunction with mineralocorticoids where applicable; in infancy mineralocorticoid supplementation is of particular importance); congenital adrenal hyperplasia; hypercalcemia associated with cancer; nonsuppurative thyroiditis

2. **Rheumatic Disorders**
   As adjunctive therapy for short term administration (to tide the patient over an acute episode or exacerbation) in: psoriatic arthritis; rheumatoid arthritis, including juvenile rheumatoid arthritis (selected cases may require low dose maintenance therapy); ankylosing spondylitis; acute and subacute bursitis; acute nonspecific tenosynovitis; acute gouty arthritis; post-traumatic osteoarthritis; synovitis of osteoarthritis; epicondylitis

3. **Collagen Diseases**
   During an exacerbation or as maintenance therapy in selected cases of: systemic lupus erythematosus; systemic dermatomyositis (polymyositis); acute rheumatic carditis

4. **Dermatologic Diseases**
   Pemphigus; bullous dermatitis herpetiformis; severe erythema multiforme (Stevens-Johnson syndrome); exfoliative dermatitis; mycosis fungoides; severe psoriasis; severe seborrheic dermatitis

5. **Allergic States**
   Control of severe or incapacitating allergic conditions intractable to adequate trials of conventional treatment in: seasonal or perennial allergic rhinitis; bronchial asthma; contact dermatitis; atopic dermatitis; serum sickness; drug hypersensitivity reactions

6. **Ophthalmic Diseases**
   Severe acute and chronic allergic and inflammatory processes involving the eye and its adnexa such as: allergic conjunctivitis; keratitis; allergic corneal marginal ulcers; herpes zoster ophthalmicus; iritis and iridocyclitis; chorioretinitis; anterior segment inflammation; diffuse posterior uveitis and choroiditis; optic neuritis; sympathetic ophthalmia

7. **Respiratory Diseases**
   Symptomatic sarcoidosis; Loeffler's syndrome not manageable by other means; berylliosis; fulminating or disseminated pulmonary tuberculosis when used concurrently with appropriate antituberculous chemotherapy; aspiration pneumonitis

8. **Hematologic Disorders**
   Idiopathic thrombocytopenic purpura in adults; secondary thrombocytopenia in adults; acquired (autoimmune) hemolytic anemia; erythroblastopenia (RBC anemia); congenital (erythroid) hypoplastic anemia

9. **Neoplastic Diseases**
   For palliative management of: leukemias and lymphomas in adults; acute leukemia of childhood

10. **Edematous States**
    To induce a diuresis or remission of proteinuria in the nephrotic syndrome, without uremia, of the idiopathic type or that due to lupus erythematosus

11. **Gastrointestinal Diseases**
    To tide the patient over a critical period of the disease in: ulcerative colitis; regional enteritis

12. **Nervous System**
    Acute exacerbations of multiple sclerosis

13. **Miscellaneous**
    Tuberculous meningitis with subarachnoid block or impending block when used concurrently with appropriate antituberculous chemotherapy; trichinosis with neurologic or myocardial involvement

CONTRAINDICATIONS
Systemic fungal infections.

WARNINGS
In patients on corticosteroid therapy subjected to unusual stress, increased dosage of rapidly acting corticosteroids before, during and after the stressful situation is indicated. Corticosteroids may mask some signs of infection, and new infections may appear during their use. There may be decreased resistance and inability to localize infection when corticosteroids are used.

Prolonged use of corticosteroids may produce posterior subcapsular cataracts, glaucoma with possible damage to the optic nerves, and may enhance the establishment of secondary ocular infections due to fungi or viruses.

Average and large doses of hydrocortisone or cortisone can cause elevation of blood pressure, salt and water retention, and increased excretion of potassium. These effects are less likely to occur with the synthetic derivatives except when used in large doses. Dietary salt restriction and potassium supplementation may be necessary. All corticosteroids increase calcium excretion. **While on corticosteroid therapy patients should not be vaccinated against smallpox. Other immunization procedures should not be undertaken in patients who are on corticosteroids, especially on high doses, because of possible hazards of neurological complications and a lack of antibody response.**

The use of prednisolone in active tuberculosis should be restricted to those cases of fulminating or disseminated tuberculosis in which the corticosteroid is used for the management of the disease in conjunction with an appropriate antituberculous regimen.

If corticosteroids are indicated in patients with latent tuberculosis or tuberculin reactivity, close observation is necessary as reactivation of the disease may occur. During prolonged corticosteroid therapy these patients should receive chemoprophylaxis.

PRECAUTIONS

General: Drug-induced secondary adrenocortical insufficiency may be minimized by gradual reduction of dosage. This type of relative insufficiency may persist for months after discontinuation of therapy; therefore, in any situation of stress occurring during that period, hormone therapy should be reinstituted. Since mineralocorticoid secretion may be impaired, salt and/or a mineralocorticoid should be administered concurrently.

There is an enhanced effect of corticosteroids in patients with hypothyroidism and in those with cirrhosis.

Corticosteroids should be used cautiously in patients with ocular herpes simplex because of possible corneal perforation.

The lowest possible dose of corticosteroid should be used to control the condition under treatment, and when reduction in dosage is possible, the reduction should be gradual.

Psychic derangements may appear when corticosteroids are used, ranging from euphoria, insomnia, mood swings, personality changes, and severe depression, to frank psychotic manifestations. Also, existing emotional instability or psychotic tendencies may be aggravated by corticosteroids.

Aspirin should be used cautiously in conjunction with corticosteroids in hypoprothrombinemia.

Steroids should be used with caution in nonspecific ulcerative colitis, if there is a probability of impending perforation, abscess or other pyogenic infection; diverticulitis; fresh intestinal anastomoses; active or latent peptic ulcer; renal insufficiency; hypertension; osteoporosis; and myasthenia gravis.

Growth and development of infants and children on prolonged corticosteroid therapy should be carefully observed.

Although controlled clinical trials have shown corticosteroids to be effective in speeding the resolution of acute exacerbations of multiple sclerosis, they do not show that they affect the ultimate outcome or natural history of the disease. The studies do show that relatively high doses of corticosteroids are necessary to demonstrate a significant effect. (See DOSAGE AND ADMINISTRATION.)

Since complications of treatment with glucocorticoids are dependent on the size of the dose and the duration of treatment, a risk/benefit decision must be made in each individual case as to dose and duration of treatment and as to whether daily or intermittent therapy should be used.

Information for Patients: Patients should be warned not to discontinue the use of PEDIAPRED abruptly or without medical supervision, to advise any medical attendants that they are taking PEDIAPRED and to seek medical advice at once should they develop fever or other signs of infection.

Drug Interactions: Drugs such as barbiturates which induce hepatic microsomal drug metabolizing enzyme activity may enhance metabolism of prednisolone and require that the dosage of PEDIAPRED be increased.

Pregnancy: Pregnancy Category C—Prednisolone has been shown to be teratogenic in many species when given in doses equivalent to the human dose. There are no adequate and well controlled studies in pregnant women. PEDIAPRED should be used during pregnancy only if the potential benefit justifies the potential risk to the fetus. Animal studies in which prednisolone has been given to pregnant mice, rats and rabbits have yielded an increased incidence of cleft palate in the offspring.

Nursing Mothers: Prednisolone is excreted in breast milk, but only to a small (less than 1% of the administered dose) and probably clinically insignificant extent. Caution should be exercised when PEDIAPRED is administered to a nursing woman.

ADVERSE REACTIONS

Fluid and Electrolyte Disturbances
Sodium retention; fluid retention; congestive heart failure in susceptible patients; potassium loss; hypokalemic alkalosis; hypertension

Musculoskeletal
Muscle weakness; steroid myopathy; loss of muscle mass; osteoporosis; vertebral compression fractures; aseptic necrosis of femoral and humeral heads; pathologic fracture of long bones

Gastrointestinal
Peptic ulcer with possible perforation and hemorrhage; pancreatitis; abdominal distention; ulcerative esophagitis

Dermatologic
Impaired wound healing; thin fragile skin; petechiae and ecchymoses; facial erythema; increased sweating; may suppress reactions to skin tests

Metabolic
Negative nitrogen balance due to protein catabolism

Neurological
Convulsions; increased intracranial pressure with papilledema (pseudotumor cerebri) usually after treatment; vertigo; headache

Endocrine
Menstrual irregularities; development of cushingoid state; secondary adrenocortical and pituitary unresponsiveness, particularly in times of stress, as in trauma, surgery or illness; suppression of growth in children; decreased carbohydrate tolerance; manifestations of latent diabetes mellitus; increased requirements for insulin or oral hypoglycemic agents in diabetes

Ophthalmic
Posterior subcapsular cataracts; increased intraocular pressure; glaucoma; exophthalmos

OVERDOSAGE

The effects of accidental ingestion of large quantities of prednisolone over a very short period of time have not been reported, but prolonged use of the drug can produce mental symptoms, moon face, abnormal fat deposits, fluid retention, excessive appetite, weight gain, hypertrichosis, acne, striae, ecchymosis, increased sweating, pigmentation, dry scaly skin, thinning scalp hair, increased blood pressure, tachycardia, thrombophlebitis, decreased resistance to infection, negative nitrogen balance with delayed bone and wound healing, headache, weakness, menstrual disorders, accentuated menopausal symptoms, neuropathy, fractures, osteoporosis, peptic ulcer, decreased glucose tolerance, hypokalemia, and adrenal insufficiency. Hepatomegaly and abdominal distention have been observed in children.

Treatment of acute overdosage is by immediate gastric lavage or emesis. For chronic overdosage in the face of severe disease requiring continuous steroid therapy the dosage of prednisolone may be reduced only temporarily, or alternate day treatment may be introduced.

DOSAGE AND ADMINISTRATION

The initial dosage of PEDIAPRED may vary from 5 mL to 60 mL (5 to 60 mg prednisolone base) per day depending on the specific disease entity being treated. In situations of less severity lower doses will generally suffice while in selected patients higher initial doses may be required. The initial dosage should be maintained or adjusted until a satisfactory response is noted. If after a reasonable period of time there is a lack of satisfactory clinical response, PEDIAPRED should be discontinued and the patient transferred to other appropriate therapy. **IT SHOULD BE EMPHASIZED THAT DOSAGE REQUIREMENTS ARE VARIABLE AND MUST BE INDIVIDUALIZED ON THE BASIS OF THE DISEASE UNDER TREATMENT AND THE RESPONSE OF THE PATIENT.** After a favorable response is noted, the proper maintenance dosage should be determined by decreasing the initial drug dosage in small decrements at appropriate time intervals until the lowest dosage which will maintain an adequate clinical response is reached. It should be kept in mind that constant monitoring is needed in regard to drug dosage. Included in the situations which may make dosage adjustments necessary are changes in clinical status secondary to remissions or exacerbations in the disease process, the patient's individual drug responsiveness, and the effect of patient exposure to stressful situations not directly related to the disease entity under treatment; in this latter situation it may be necessary to increase the dosage of PEDIAPRED for a period of time consistent with the patient's condition. If after long term therapy the drug is to be stopped, it is recommended that it be withdrawn gradually rather than abruptly.

In the treatment of acute exacerbations of multiple sclerosis daily doses of 200 mg of prednisolone for a week followed by 80 mg every other day or 4 to 8 mg dexamethasone every other day for one month have been shown to be effective. For the purpose of comparison, the following is the equivalent milligram dosage of the various glucocorticoids: cortisone, 25; hydrocortisone, 20; prednisolone, 5; prednisone, 5; methylprednisolone, 4; triamcinolone, 4; paramethasone, 2; betamethasone, 0.75; dexamethasone, 0.75. These dose relationships apply only to oral or intravenous administration of these compounds. When these substances or their derivatives are injected intramuscularly or into joint spaces, their relative properties may be greatly altered.

HOW SUPPLIED

PEDIAPRED Oral Liquid is a colorless to light straw colored solution containing 6.7 mg prednisolone sodium phosphate (5 mg prednisolone base) per 5 mL (teaspoonful).

NDC 0585-2250-01   4 fl oz bottle

Store at room temperature. Do not refrigerate. Keep tightly closed and out of the reach of children.

CAUTION

Federal law prohibits dispensing without prescription.
® Registered trademark of Fisons Corporation.

Revised 5/89

PENNTUSS®   ℭ
(controlled release codeine polistirex with chlorpheniramine polistirex)
[pĕn 'tuhs]

DESCRIPTION

Provides 12-hour relief of cough. Each teaspoonful (5 mL) contains codeine polistirex (Warning: May be habit forming) equivalent to 10 mg of codeine base, plus chlorpheniramine polistirex equivalent to 4 mg of chlorpheniramine maleate.
Other Ingredients: Ethylcellulose, Flavor, High Fructose Corn Syrup, Methylparaben, Polyethylene Glycol 3350, Polysorbate 80, Pregelatinized Starch, Propylene Glycol, Propylparaben, Red 33, Sucrose, Vegetable Oil, Water, Xanthan Gum.

INDICATIONS

Temporarily controls cough due to minor throat and bronchial irritation as may occur with the common cold or inhaled irritants. Temporarily alleviates runny nose and relieves sneezing, itching of the nose or throat, and itchy, watery eyes due to hay fever or other upper respiratory allergies (allergic rhinitis). Temporarily relieves runny nose and reduces sneezing associated with the common cold.

WARNINGS

Prescribe with caution to children who have a chronic pulmonary disease, shortness of breath, or who are taking other drugs. Use with caution in patients with persistent or chronic cough such as occurs with smoking, asthma, or emphysema, or if cough is accompanied by excessive phlegm (mucus). Caution is also advised when prescribing this drug to patients with asthma, glaucoma, emphysema, chronic pulmonary disease, shortness of breath, difficulty in breathing, or difficulty in urination due to enlargement of the prostate gland. May cause excitability especially in children. May cause or aggravate constipation. May cause marked drowsiness; alcohol may increase the drowsiness effect. Patients should be advised to avoid alcoholic beverages and to use caution when driving a motor vehicle or operating machinery while taking this product.

DIRECTIONS

INVERT BOTTLE, SHAKE VIGOROUSLY BEFORE USING. Adults and children 12 years of age and over: 2 to 3 teaspoonfuls every 12 hours; not to exceed 6 teaspoonfuls in 24 hours, or as directed by a physician. Children 6 to under 12: 1 teaspoonful every 12 hours; not to exceed 2 teaspoonfuls in 24 hours, or as directed by a physician. Children under 6: Use only under the advice and supervision of a physician.

HOW SUPPLIED

4 fl. oz. bottles (NDC #0585-0818-38)
Pint bottles (NDC# 0585-0818-67)
Store at 59°–86°F.

TUSSIONEX®   ℭ
[tus 'e-uh-nex]
Pennkinetic®
Extended-Release Suspension

DESCRIPTION

Each teaspoonful (5 mL) of TUSSIONEX Pennkinetic Extended-Release Suspension contains hydrocodone polistirex equivalent to 10 mg of hydrocodone bitartrate (Warning: May be habit-forming) and chlorpheniramine polistirex equivalent to 8 mg of chlorpheniramine maleate. TUSSIONEX Pennkinetic Extended-Release Suspension provides up to 12-hour relief per dose. Hydrocodone is a centrally-acting narcotic antitussive. Chlorpheniramine is an antihistamine. TUSSIONEX Pennkinetic Extended-Release Suspension is for oral use only.
Hydrocodone Polistirex: sulfonated styrene-divinylbenzene copolymer complex with 4,5α-epoxy-3-methoxy-17-methylmorphinan-6-one.
Chlorpheniramine Polistirex: sulfonated styrene-divinylbenzene copolymer complex with 2-[p -chloro-α-[2-(dimethylamino)ethyl]-benzyl]pyridine.
Other ingredients in TUSSIONEX Pennkinetic Extended-Release Suspension: Ascorbic Acid; D&C Yellow No. 10; Ethylcellulose; FD&C Yellow No. 6; Flavor; High Fructose Corn Syrup; Methylparaben; Polyethylene Glycol 3350; Polysorbate 80; Pregelatinized Starch; Propylene Glycol; Propylparaben; Sucrose; Vegetable Oil; Water; Xanthan Gum.

CLINICAL PHARMACOLOGY

Hydrocodone is a semisynthetic narcotic antitussive and analgesic with multiple actions qualitatively similar to those of codeine. The precise mechanism of action of hydrocodone and other opiates is not known; however, hydrocodone is believed to act directly on the cough center. In excessive doses, hydrocodone, like other opium derivatives, will depress respiration. The effects of hydrocodone in therapeutic doses on the cardiovascular system are insignificant. Hydrocodone can produce miosis, euphoria, physical and psychological dependence.
Chlorpheniramine is an antihistamine drug (H₁ receptor antagonist) that also possesses anticholinergic and sedative activity. It prevents released histamine from dilating capillaries and causing edema of the respiratory mucosa.
Hydrocodone release from TUSSIONEX Pennkinetic Extended-Release Suspension is controlled by the Pennkinetic System, an extended-release drug delivery system which combines an ion-exchange polymer matrix with a diffusion rate-limiting permeable coating. Chlorpheniramine release is prolonged by use of an ion-exchange polymer system.
Following multiple dosing with TUSSIONEX Pennkinetic Extended-Release Suspension, hydrocodone mean (S.D.) peak plasma concentrations of 22.8 (5.9) ng/mL occurred at 3.4 hours. Chlorpheniramine mean (S.D.) peak plasma concentrations of 58.4 (14.7) ng/mL occurred at 6.3 hours following multiple dosing. Peak plasma levels obtained with an immediate-release syrup occurred at approximately 1.5 hours for hydrocodone and 2.8 hours for chlorpheniramine. The plasma half-lives of hydrocodone and chlorpheniramine have been reported to be approximately 4 and 16 hours, respectively.

INDICATIONS AND USAGE

TUSSIONEX Pennkinetic Extended-Release Suspension is indicated for relief of cough and upper repiratory symptoms associated with allergy or a cold.

CONTRAINDICATIONS

Known allergy or sensitivity to hydrocodone or chlorpheniramine.

WARNINGS

Respiratory Depression: As with all narcotics, TUSSIONEX Pennkinetic Extended-Release Suspension produces dose-related respiratory depression by directly acting on brain stem respiratory centers. Caution should be exercised when TUSSIONEX Pennkinetic Extended-Release Suspension is used postoperatively and in patients with pulmonary disease. If respiratory depression occurs, it may be antagonized by the use of naloxone hydrochloride and other supportive measures when indicated (see OVERDOSAGE).
Head Injury and Increased Intracranial Pressure: The respiratory depressant effects of narcotics and their capacity to elevate cerebrospinal fluid pressure may be markedly exaggerated in the presence of head injury, other intracranial lesions or a pre-existing increase in intracranial pressure. Furthermore, narcotics produce adverse reactions which may obscure the clinical course of patients with head injuries.
Acute Abdominal Conditions: The administration of narcotics may obscure the diagnosis or clinical course of patients with acute abdominal conditions.
Pediatric Use: In young children, as well as adults, the respiratory center is sensitive to the depressant action of narcotic cough suppressants in a dose-dependent manner. Benefit to risk ratio should be carefully considered especially in

children with respiratory embarrassment (e.g., croup). See PRECAUTIONS.

PRECAUTIONS

General: Caution is advised when prescribing this drug to patients with narrow-angle glaucoma, asthma or prostatic hypertrophy.
Special Risk Patients: As with any narcotic agent, TUSSIONEX Pennkinetic Extended-Release Suspension should be used with caution in elderly or debilitated patients and those with severe impairment of hepatic or renal function, hypothyroidism, Addison's disease, prostatic hypertrophy or urethral stricture. The usual precautions should be observed and the possibility of respiratory depression should be kept in mind.
Information for Patients: As with all narcotics, TUSSIONEX Pennkinetic Extended-Release Suspension may produce marked drowsiness and impair the mental and/or physical abilities required for the performance of potentially hazardous tasks such as driving a car or operating machinery; patients should be cautioned accordingly.
Drug Interactions: Patients receiving narcotics, antihistaminics, antipsychotics, antianxiety agents or other CNS depressants (including alcohol) concomitantly with TUSSIONEX Pennkinetic Extended-Release Suspension may exhibit an additive CNS depression. When combined therapy is contemplated, the dose of one or both agents should be reduced.
The use of MAO inhibitors or tricyclic antidepressants with hydrocodone preparations may increase the effect of either the antidepressant or hydrocodone.
Carcinogenesis, Mutagenesis, Impairment of Fertility: Carcinogenicity, mutagenicity and reproductive studies have not been conducted with TUSSIONEX Pennkinetic Extended-Release Suspension.
Pregnancy
Teratogenic Effects—Pregnancy Category C: Animal reproduction studies have not been conducted with TUSSIONEX Pennkinetic Extended-Release Suspension. It is also not known whether TUSSIONEX Pennkinetic Extended-Release Suspension can cause fetal harm when administered to a pregnant woman or can affect reproduction capacity. TUSSIONEX Pennkinetic Extended-Release Suspension should be given to a pregnant woman only if clearly needed.
Nonteratogenic Effects: Babies born to mothers who have been taking opioids regularly prior to delivery will be physically dependent. The withdrawal signs include irritability and excessive crying, tremors, hyperactive reflexes, increased respiratory rate, increased stools, sneezing, yawning, vomiting and fever. The intensity of the syndrome does not always correlate with the duration of maternal opioid use or dose.
Labor and Delivery: As with all narcotics, administration of TUSSIONEX Pennkinetic Extended-Release Suspension to the mother shortly before delivery may result in some degree of respiratory depression in the newborn, especially if higher doses are used.
Nursing Mothers: It is not known whether this drug is excreted in human milk. Because many drugs are excreted in human milk and because of the potential for serious adverse reaction in nursing infants from TUSSIONEX Pennkinetic Extended-Release Suspension, a decision should be made whether to discontinue nursing or to discontinue the drug, taking into account the importance of the drug to the mother.
Pediatric Use: Safety and effectiveness of TUSSIONEX Pennkinetic Extended-Release Suspension in children under six have not been established.

ADVERSE REACTIONS

Central Nervous System: Sedation, drowsiness, mental clouding, lethargy, impairment of mental and physical performance, anxiety, fear, dysphoria, dizziness, psychic dependence, mood changes.
Gastrointestinal System: Nausea and vomiting may occur; they are more frequent in ambulatory than in recumbent patients. Prolonged administration of TUSSIONEX Pennkinetic Extended-Release Suspension may produce constipation.
Genitourinary System: Ureteral spasm, spasm of vesicle sphincters and urinary retention have been reported with opiates.
Respiratory Depression: TUSSIONEX Pennkinetic Extended-Release Suspension may produce dose-related respiratory depression by acting directly on brain stem respiratory centers (see OVERDOSAGE).

Continued on next page

Fisons—Cont.

DRUG ABUSE AND DEPENDENCE
TUSSIONEX Pennkinetic Extended-Release Suspension is a Schedule III narcotic. Psychic dependence, physical dependence and tolerance may develop upon repeated administration of narcotics; therefore, TUSSIONEX Pennkinetic Extended-Release Suspension should be prescribed and administered with caution. However, psychic dependence is unlikely to develop when TUSSIONEX Pennkinetic Extended-Release Suspension is used for a short time for the treatment of cough. Physical dependence, the condition in which continued administration of the drug is required to prevent the appearance of a withdrawal syndrome, assumes clinically significant proportions only after several weeks of continued oral narcotic use, although some mild degree of physical dependence may develop after a few days of narcotic therapy.

OVERDOSAGE
Signs and Symptoms: Serious overdosage with hydrocodone is characterized by respiratory depression (a decrease in respiratory rate and/or tidal volume, Cheyne-Stokes respiration, cyanosis), extreme somnolence progressing to stupor or coma, skeletal muscle flaccidity, cold and clammy skin, and sometimes bradycardia and hypotension. In severe overdosage apnea, circulatory collapse, cardiac arrest and death may occur. The manifestations of chlorpheniramine overdosage may vary from central nervous system depression to stimulation.

Treatment: Primary attention should be given to the reestablishment of adequate respiratory exchange through provision of a patent airway and the institution of assisted or controlled ventilation. The narcotic antagonist naloxone hydrochloride is a specific antidote for respiratory depression which may result from overdosage or unusual sensitivity to narcotics including hydrocodone. Therefore, an appropriate dose of naloxone hydrochloride should be administered, preferably by the intravenous route, simultaneously with efforts at respiratory resuscitation. Since the duration of action of hydrocodone in this formulation may exceed that of the antagonist, the patient should be kept under continued surveillance and repeated doses of the antagonist should be administered as needed to maintain adequate respiration. For further information, see full prescribing information for naloxone hydrochloride. An antagonist should not be administered in the absence of clinically significant respiratory depression. Oxygen, intravenous fluids, vasopressors and other supportive measures should be employed as indicated. Gastric emptying may be useful in removing unabsorbed drug.

DOSAGE AND ADMINISTRATION
Shake well before using.
Adults: 1 teaspoonful (5 mL) every 12 hours; do not exceed 2 teaspoonfuls in 24 hours.
Children 6–12: ½ teaspoonful every 12 hours; **do not exceed 1 teaspoonful in 24 hours.**

HOW SUPPLIED
TUSSIONEX Pennkinetic Extended-Release Suspension is a gold-colored suspension available in bottles of one pint (473 mL) (NDC 0585-0548-67) and 900 mL (NDC 0585-0548-91). Shake well. Dispense in a well-closed container. Store at 59°–86°F (15°–30°C).
Caution: Federal law prohibits dispensing without prescription.

Rev. 10/88

EDUCATIONAL MATERIAL

Booklets:
"Asthma Answer Book"—written in lay terminology outlining asthma, medications, triggers, etc. Available in Spanish. (Free)
"New Asthma Patient Kit"—contains an Asthma Answer Book, a patient diary and a therapy evaluation card. (Free)
"How to Use Metered Dose Inhalers"—written in lay terminology outlining the proper use of metered dose inhalers. (Free)
"Your Allergic Nose"—written in lay terminology outlining allergic rhinitis, causes and prevention. (Free)
"Your Allergic Eyes"—written in lay terminology outlining allergic eye disorders, causes and their prevention. (Free)
Monographs—for Intal®, Mykrox™, Nasalcrom® and Opticrom®. (Free)

Pictures—Charts:
Instructional Wall Charts—for Intal® capsules via Spinhaler®, Intal® Nebulizer Solution and Intal® Inhaler. (Free)

Samples:
Intal® Inhaler, Intal® Nebulizer Solution, Intal® Capsules, Mykrox™, Nasalcrom® Sample Pack, Opticrom® Sample Pack. Available in limited quantities.

C. B. Fleet Co., Inc.
**4615 MURRAY PL.
LYNCHBURG, VA. 24502-2235**

FLEET® BABYLAX®   OTC

ACTIVE INGREDIENT
Glycerin (USP)

INDICATIONS
For temporary relief of constipation in young children. Children under 2 years old, consult physician.

ACTIONS
This product generally produces a bowel movement within 30 minutes. The exact mode of action of glycerin administered rectally as a laxative is not known. It has been suggested that glycerin causes dehydration of exposed tissues to produce an irritant effect which results in a laxative response.

WARNINGS
For rectal use only. Glycerin administered rectally may produce rectal discomfort or a burning sensation in some individuals. If use results in unusual pain or side effects, consult a physician.

GENERAL LAXATIVE WARNINGS
Do not use a laxative product when nausea, vomiting or abdominal pain are present unless directed by a physician. If you have noticed a sudden change in bowel habits that persists over two weeks, consult a physician before using a laxative. Laxative products should not be used longer than one week except under a physician's advice. Frequent or prolonged use of laxatives may result in dependence. Rectal bleeding or failure to have a bowel movement after use of a laxative may indicate a serious condition; discontinue use and consult a physician. Keep this and all drugs out of the reach of children. In case of accidental ingestion, seek professional assistance or contact a Poison Control Center immediately.

DOSAGE AND ADMINISTRATION
REMOVE PROTECTIVE SHIELD FROM TIP BEFORE ADMINISTERING.
Children under 2 years old: consult physician. Children 2–6 years of age: 1 rectal applicator containing 4 ml. of glycerin as needed or as directed by physician. Hold unit upright. Gently insert stem with tip pointing toward navel. Squeeze unit until nearly all liquid is expelled. Remove tip from rectum. Note: A small amount of liquid will remain in unit. Store and use at room temperature.

HOW SUPPLIED
Six 4 ml. rectal applicators per package.

IS THIS PRODUCT OTC
Yes.

FLEET® BISACODYL ENEMA   OTC
(bisacodyl U.S.P.)

COMPOSITION
Each 30 ml (delivered dose) contains 10 mg. of bisacodyl, U.S.P. suspended in an aqueous medium. The FLEET® Bisacodyl Enema unit, with a 2-inch prelubricated Comfortip®, contains 1¼ fl. oz. of enema suspension in a ready-to-use plastic squeeze bottle. Designed for quick, convenient administration by nurse or patient according to instructions. Disposable after single use.

ACTION AND USES
FLEET® Bisacodyl Enema is a contact laxative acting directly on the colonic mucosa to produce peristalsis. FLEET® Bisacodyl Enema actually produces peristalsis and evacuation of the large intestine by stimulating sensory nerve endings in the colonic mucosa to produce parasympathetic reflexes. FLEET® Bisacodyl Enema is very effective usually producing an evacuation within 15 minutes to 1 hour. FLEET® Bisacodyl Enema may be used whenever a laxative or enema is indicated. It is useful as a laxative for occasional relief of constipation, in bowel cleansing in preparation before X-ray and endoscopic examination.

WARNINGS
Do not use a laxative product when nausea, vomiting, or abdominal pain is present unless directed by a physician. If you have noticed a sudden change in bowel habits that persists over a period of 2 weeks, consult a physician before using a laxative. Rectal bleeding or failure to have a bowel movement after use of a laxative may indicate a serious condition.

Discontinue use and consult a physician. Laxative products should not be used longer than 1 week unless directed by a physician. Frequent or prolonged use of a laxative may result in dependence. Keep this and all drugs out of the reach of children. In case of accidental ingestion, seek professional assistance or contact a Poison Control Center immediately.

DOSAGE AND ADMINISTRATION
SHAKE BEFORE USING.
REMOVE PROTECTIVE SHIELD FROM TIP BEFORE ADMINISTERING.
Adults—one unit or as directed by a physician. **Precaution:** Do not administer to children under 2 years of age. **Administration:** Preferred position—Lying on left side with left knee slightly bent and the right leg drawn up, or knee-chest position. Rubber diaphragm at base of tube prevents accidental leakage and assures controlled flow of the enema solution. May be used at room temperature.

PROFESSIONAL ADMINISTRATION
See FLEET® Ready-to-Use Enema.

HOW SUPPLIED
FLEET® Bisacodyl Enema is supplied in 1¼ fl. oz. ready-to-use squeeze bottle.

IS THIS PRODUCT OTC
Yes.

LITERATURE AVAILABLE
Professional literature mailed on request.

FLEET® ENEMA   OTC

COMPOSITION
Each 118 ml (delivered dose) contains 19 g. sodium biphosphate and 7 g. sodium phosphate. The FLEET® Enema unit, with a 2-inch, pre-lubricated Comfortip®, contains 4½ fl. oz. of enema solution in a hand-size plastic squeeze bottle. Designed for quick, convenient administration by nurse or patient according to instructions. Disposable after single use.

ACTION AND USES
FLEET Enema is useful as a laxative in the relief of constipation, and as a bowel evacuant for a variety of diagnostic, surgical, and therapeutic indications. Used as directed, FLEET Enema provides thorough yet safe cleansing action and induces complete emptying of the left colon usually within 2 to 15 minutes without pain or spasm. FLEET Enema may be used for the occasional relief of constipation; as a routine enema; for cleansing of the colon in preparation for rectal examination; preoperative cleansing and general postoperative care; to help relieve fecal or barium impaction.

GENERAL LAXATIVE WARNINGS
Do not use laxative products when nausea, vomiting, or abdominal pain is present. If you notice a sudden change in bowel habits that persists over a period of 2 weeks, consult a physician. Rectal bleeding or failure to have a bowel movement after use of a laxative may indicate a serious condition. Discontinue use and consult a physician. Laxative products should not be used longer than 1 week unless directed by a physician. Frequent or prolonged use of a laxative may result in dependence. As with any drug, if you are pregnant or nursing a baby, seek the advice of a health professional before using this product. Keep this and all drugs out of the reach of children. In case of accidental ingestion or overdose, seek professional assistance or contact a Poison Control Center immediately.

PROFESSIONAL USE WARNINGS
Do not use in patients with congenital megacolon, imperforate anus or congestive heart failure as hypernatremic dehydration may occur. Use with caution in patients with impaired renal function, heart disease, or pre-existing electrolyte disturbances (such as dehydration or those secondary to the use of diuretics) or in patients on calcium channel blockers, diuretics or other medications which may affect electrolyte levels — or where colostomy exists, as hypocalcemia, hyperphosphatemia, hypernatremia and acidosis may occur. Calcium and phosphorous levels should be carefully monitored. Since FLEET® Ready-To-Use Enema contains sodium phosphate and sodium biphosphate, there is a risk of acute elevation of sodium concentration in the serum and consequent dehydration, particularly in children with megacolon or any other condition where there is retention of enema solution. Additional fluids by mouth are recommended where appropriate (Fonkalsrud, E. and Keen, J.: "Hypernatremic Dehydration Hypertonic Enemas in Congenital Megacolon," *JAMA* 199:584–586, 1967. Zumoff, B. and Hellman, L.: "Rectal Absorption of Sodium from Hypertonic Sodium Phosphate Solutions," data on file, C. B. Fleet Company, Inc. Gilman, A., Goodman, L., Gilman, A., eds., *The Pharmacological Basis of Therapeutics*, Sixth Edition, 1980, p. 1005.) In addition, elevated levels of serum phosphates and decreased levels of serum calcium have been reported in patients with renal disease (and with prolonged use). (McConnell, T. H., "Fatal Hypocalcemia from Phosphate Absorption from Lax-

ative Preparation," *JAMA*, 216:147–148, 1971.) If any of these complications occur following administration of Fleet® Ready-To-Use Enema or if the enema solution is retained, immediate corrective action should be taken to restore electrolyte balance with appropriate fluid replacements and continued monitoring of calcium and phosphorus levels.

PRECAUTIONS

DO NOT ADMINISTER 4½ oz. ADULT SIZE TO CHILDREN UNDER 12 YEARS OF AGE. DO NOT ADMINISTER 2¼ OZ CHILDREN'S SIZE TO CHILDREN UNDER 2 YEARS OF AGE. IF AFTER THE ENEMA SOLUTION IS ADMINISTERED THERE IS NO RETURN OF LIQUID, CONTACT A PHYSICIAN IMMEDIATELY AS DEHYDRATION COULD OCCUR.

ADMINISTRATION AND DOSAGE

REMOVE PROTECTIVE SHIELD FROM TIP BEFORE ADMINISTERING.
Preferred position: Lying on left side with left knee slightly bent and the right leg drawn up, or knee-chest position. Dosage: Adults, 4 fl. oz. Rubber diaphragm at base of tube prevents accidental leakage and assures controlled flow of the enema solution. May be used at room temperature. Each 118 ml. (delivered dose) contains 4.4 g. sodium.

PROFESSIONAL DOSAGE AND ADMINISTRATION

Fleet® Ready-To-Use 4½ oz. Adult Size Enema should not be used in children under 12 years of age. In those cases where complications are reported, infants and young children are often involved. Fleet® Ready-To-Use Enema for Children should be used with caution in children of any age. Careful consideration of the use of enemas in general in children is recommended. The adult size enema should not be used in children under 12 years of age. For children 2 to 12 years of age, use Fleet® Ready-To-Use Enema for Children, which contains a dosage of one-half the adult size enema. For children less than 2 years of age, Fleet® Glycerin Suppositories for Children should be used.
Proper and safe use of Fleet® Ready-To-Use Enema also requires that the product be administered according to the Directions for Use. Health care professionals should remember, when administering the product, to *gently* insert the enema into the rectum with steady pressure with the tip pointing toward the navel. Care during insertion is necessary due to lack of sensory innervation of the rectum. Once inserted, squeeze the bottle until nearly all the liquid is expelled. If resistance is encountered on insertion of the nozzle or in administering the solution, the procedure should be discontinued. Forcing the enema can result in perforation and/or abrasion of the rectum.

HOW SUPPLIED

FLEET® Enema is supplied in a 4½ fl. oz. ready-to-use squeeze bottle. Children's size, 2¼ fl. oz.

IS THIS PRODUCT OTC

Yes.

LITERATURE AVAILABLE

Professional literature mailed on request.

FLEET® MINERAL OIL ENEMA   OTC

COMPOSITION

The FLEET Mineral Oil Enema unit, with a 2-inch, prelubricated Comfortip®, contains 4½ fl.oz. (133 ml.) mineral oil USP in a hand-size plastic squeeze bottle.

ACTION AND INDICATIONS

Serves to soften and lubricate hard stools, easing their passage without irritating the mucosa. Results approximate a normal bowel movement in that only the rectum, sigmoid, and part or all of the descending colon are evacuated. Indicated for relief of fecal impaction; valuable in relief of constipation when straining must be avoided (in hypertension, coronary occlusion, proctologic procedures, postoperative care); for removal of barium sulfate residues from the colon after barium administration for GI series or outlining the left atrium; to obtain the laxative benefits of mineral oil while avoiding possible untoward effects of oral administration such as (1) interference with intestinal absorption of fat-soluble vitamins A, D, E and K and other nutrients (2) danger of systemic absorption (3) possible risk of lipid pneumonia due to aspiration.

WARNINGS

Do not use laxative products when nausea, vomiting, abdominal pain is present unless directed by a physician. If you have noticed a sudden change in bowel habits that persists over a period of 2 weeks, consult a physician. Rectal bleeding or failure to have a bowel movement after use of a laxative may indicate a serious condition. Discontinue use and consult a physician. Laxative products should not be used longer than 1 week unless directed by a physician. Frequent and prolonged use of enemas may result in dependence. Keep this and all drugs out of the reach of children. In case of acci-

dental ingestion, seek professional assistance or contact a Poison Control Center immediately.

PRECAUTIONS

DO NOT ADMINISTER TO CHILDREN UNDER 2 YEARS OF AGE.

ADMINISTRATION AND DOSAGE

REMOVE PROTECTIVE SHIELD FROM TIP BEFORE ADMINISTERING.
For rectal administration only. Ready-to-use unit permits easy, rapid administration by physician, nurse, or patient; disposable after single use.

PROFESSIONAL DOSAGE AND ADMINISTRATION

Fleet® Ready-To-Use Mineral Oil Enema should not be used in children under 2 years of age. Fleet® Ready-To-Use Mineral Oil Enema should be used with caution in children of any age. Careful consideration of the use of enemas in general in children is recommended.
Proper and safe use of Fleet® Ready-To-Use Mineral Oil Enema also requires that the product be administered according to the Directions for Use. Health care professionals should remember, when administering the product, to gently insert the enema into the rectum with steady pressure with the tip pointing toward the naval. Care during insertion is necessary due to lack of sensory innervation of the rectum. Once inserted, squeeze the bottle until nearly all the liquid is expelled. If resistance is encountered on insertion of the nozzle or in administering the solution, the procedure should be discontinued. Forcing the enema can result in perforation and/or abrasion of the rectum.

HOW SUPPLIED

FLEET Mineral Oil Enema is supplied in 4½ fl.oz. ready-to-use squeeze bottle.

IS THIS PRODUCT OTC

Yes.

FLEET® PHOSPHO®-SODA   OTC
Buffered Laxative

COMPOSITION

Each 100 ml. of regular or flavored PHOSPHO-SODA contains 48 g. sodium biphosphate and 18 g. sodium phosphate in a stable, buffered aqueous solution.

INDICATIONS

For relief of occasional constipation or for preparing the colon for x-ray or other endoscopic examination.

ACTION AND USES

Versatile in action as a gentle laxative or purgative, according to dosage. This product produces a bowel movement in ½ to 6 hours.

CONTRAINDICATIONS

DO NOT USE THIS PRODUCT IF YOU HAVE KIDNEY DISEASE OR ARE ON A LOW SALT DIET UNLESS DIRECTED BY A PHYSICIAN.

PROFESSIONAL USE WARNINGS

Do not use in patients with congenital megacolon or congestive heart failure, as hypernatremic dehydration may occur. Use with caution in patients with impaired renal function as hypocalcemia, hyperphosphatemia, hypernatremia and acidosis may occur. Since FLEET® Phospho®-Soda contains sodium phosphate and sodium biphosphate, there is a risk of acute elevation of sodium concentration in the serum and consequent dehydration, particularly in children with megacolon. Additional fluids by mouth are recommended where appropriate. (Fonkalsrud, E. and Keen, J.: "Hypernatremic Dehydration Hypertonic Enemas in Congenital Megacolon," *JAMA* 199:584–586, 1967. Zumoff, B. and Hellman, L.: "Rectal Absorption of Sodium from Hypertonic Sodium Phosphate Solutions," data on file, C. B. Fleet Company, Inc. Gilman, A., Goodman, L., Gilman, A., eds., *The Pharmacological Basis of Therapeutics*, Sixth Edition, 1980, p. 1005.) In addition, elevated levels of serum phosphates and decreased levels of serum calcium have been reported in patients with renal disease (and with prolonged use). (McConnell, T. H., "Fatal Hypocalcemia from Phosphate Absorption from Laxative Preparation," *JAMA*, 216:147–148, 1971.) If any of these complications occurs following administration of Fleet® Phospho®-Soda, immediate corrective action should be taken to restore electrolyte balance with appropriate fluid replacements. Calcium and phosphorous levels should be carefully monitored.

GENERAL LAXATIVE WARNINGS

Do not use a laxative product when nausea, vomiting, or abdominal pain is present unless directed by a physician. If you have noticed a sudden change in bowel habits that persists over a period of 2 weeks, consult a physician before using a laxative. Rectal bleeding or failure to have a bowel movement may indicate a serious condition. Discontinue use and consult a physician. Laxative products should not be used longer than 1 week unless directed by a physician. Frequent

or prolonged use of a laxative may result in dependence on laxatives. Each recommended dose (4 teaspoonfuls) contains 96.4 milliequivalents of sodium. DO NOT USE THIS PRODUCT IF YOU ARE ON A LOW SALT DIET OR IF YOU HAVE KIDNEY DISEASE UNLESS DIRECTED BY A DOCTOR. SERIOUS SIDE EFFECTS FROM OVERDOSAGE MAY OCCUR. Keep this and all drugs out of the reach of children. In case of accidental overdose or ingestion, seek professional assistance or contact a Poison Control Center immediately. As with any drug, if you are pregnant or nursing a baby, seek the advice of a health professional before using this product.

ADMINISTRATION AND DOSAGE

Best taken on an empty stomach. **Dilute recommended dosage with one-half glass (4 oz.) cool water. Drink, then follow with one glass (8 oz.) cool water.** Most effective when taken upon rising, at least 30 minutes before a meal, or at bedtime for overnight action.
DOSAGE: DO NOT EXCEED RECOMMENDED DOSAGE, AS SERIOUS SIDE EFFECTS MAY OCCUR.
Adults: Purgative: 3 tablespoons (45 ml). Laxative: 4 teaspoonfuls (20 ml). Children 10 and over: Laxative: 2 teaspoonfuls (10 ml). Children 6 to 9: Laxative: 1 teaspoonful (5 ml). DO NOT GIVE TO CHILDREN UNDER 6 YEARS OF AGE.
Each teaspoonful (5 ml) contains: Active Ingredients: Sodium Biphosphate 2.4 g and Sodium Phosphate 0.9 g.

HOW SUPPLIED

Regular or Flavored, in bottles of 1½, 3, and 8 fl. oz.

IS THIS PRODUCT OTC

Yes.

FLEET® PREP KITS   OTC
Bowel Evacuant

DESCRIPTION

FLEET® Prep Kit No. 1 contains:
1. FLEET® Phospho®-Soda—1½ fl. oz. Ingredients: Each teaspoonful (5 ml) contains : Active Ingredients: Sodium Biphosphate 2.4 Gm. and Sodium Phosphate 0.9 Gm.
2. FLEET® Bisacodyl—4 laxative tablets. Ingredients: Each enteric-coated tablet contains Bisacodyl, USP, 5 mg.
3. FLEET® Bisacodyl—1 laxative suppository. Ingredients: Bisacodyl, USP, 10 mg.
4. 1 Patient Instruction Sheet.
FLEET® Prep Kit No. 2 contains:
1. FLEET® Phospho®-Soda—1½ fl. oz.
2. FLEET® Bisacodyl—4 tablets.
3. FLEET® Bagenema—1. Ingredients: Liquid castile soap ⅔ fl. oz.
4. 1 Patient Instruction Sheet.
FLEET® Prep Kit No. 3 contains:
1. FLEET® Phospho®-Soda—1½ fl. oz.
2. FLEET® Bisacodyl—4 tablets.
3. FLEET® Bisacodyl Enema—1 laxative enema. Ingredients: 1–30 ml. dose containing 10 mg. of Bisacodyl.
4. 1 Patient Instruction Sheet.
FLEET® Prep Kit No. 4 contains:
1. FLEET® Flavored Castor Oil Emulsion-1½ fl. oz. Ingredients: Each tablespoonful (15 ml.) contains: Active Ingredients: Castor Oil U.S.P. 10 ml.
2. FLEET® Bisacodyl—4 tablets.
3. FLEET® Bisacodyl—1 suppository.
4. 1 Patient Instruction Sheet.
FLEET® Prep Kit No. 5 contains:
1. FLEET® Flavored Castor Oil Emulsion-1½ fl. oz.
2. FLEET® Bisacodyl—4 tablets.
3. FLEET® Bagenema—1.
4. 1 Patient Instruction Sheet.
FLEET® Prep Kit No. 6 contains:
1. FLEET® Flavored Castor Oil Emulsion-1½ fl. oz.
2. FLEET® Bisacodyl—4 tablets.
3. FLEET® Bisacodyl Enema—30 ml.
4. 1 Patient Instruction Sheet.

ACTIONS

Bowel Cleansing System

INDICATIONS

For use as part of a bowel cleansing regiment in preparation of the colon for radiology (prior to barium enemas or I.V.P.'s), surgery, and many proctologic and colonoscopic procedures.

WARNINGS

Each recommended dose ((1½ fl. oz.) (45 ml)) of Phospho®-Soda contains 216.9 milli-equivalents (meq) of sodium. Persons on a low salt diet or with kidney disease should consult a health professional before use.

Continued on next page

Fleet—Cont.

Castor oil affects the small intestine, and regular use may cause excessive loss of water and body salts which can have debilitating effects.

GENERAL LAXATIVE WARNINGS

Do not use a laxative product when nausea, vomiting, or abdominal pain is present unless directed by a physician. If you have noticed a sudden change in bowel habits that persists over a period of 2 weeks, consult a doctor before using a laxative. Rectal bleeding or failure to have a bowel movement may indicate a serious condition. Discontinue use and consult a physician. Laxative products should not be used longer than 1 week unless directed by a physician. Frequent or prolonged use of a laxative may result in dependence on laxatives. Keep this and all drugs out of the reach of children. In case of accidental overdose or ingestion, seek professional assistance or contact a Poison Control Center immediately.

PROFESSIONAL USE WARNINGS

Do not use in patients with congenital megacolon or congestive heart failure as hypernatremic dehydration may occur. Use with caution in patients with impaired renal function or where colostomy exists as hypocalcemia, hyperphosphatemia, hypernatremia and acidosis may occur. Since FLEET® Phospho®-Soda contains sodium phosphate and sodium biphosphate, there is a risk of acute elevation of sodium concentration in the serum and consequent dehydration, particularly in children with megacolon. Additional fluids by mouth are recommended where appropriate. (Fonkalsrud, E. and Keen, J.: "Hypernatremic Dehydration Hypertonic Enemas in Congenital Megacolon," JAMA 199:584–586, 1967. Zumoff, B. and Hellman, L.: "Rectal Absorption of Sodium from Hypertonic Sodium Phosphate Solutions," data on file, C. B. Fleet Company, Inc. Gilman, A., Goodman, L., Gilman, A., eds., The Pharmacological Basis of Therapeutics, Sixth Edition, 1980, p. 1005.) In addition, elevated levels of serum phosphates and decreased levels of serum calcium have been reported in patients with renal disease (and with prolonged use). (McConnell, T. H., "Fatal Hypocalcemia from Phosphate Absorption from Laxative Preparation," JAMA, 216:147–148, 1971.) If any of these complications occur following administration of FLEET® Phospho®-Soda, immediate corrective action should be taken to restore electrolyte balance with appropriate fluid replacements. Calcium and phosphorous levels should be carefully monitored. **See individual listings (Fleet® Phospho-Soda, Fleet® Bisacodyl Enema and Fleet® Flavored Castor Oil Emulsion) for additional warnings.**
THESE KITS SHOULD NOT BE USED BY PATIENTS UNDER 6 YEARS OF AGE.

DOSAGE AND ADMINISTRATION
SEE PATIENT INSTRUCTION SHEET FOR 12, 24, AND 48 HOUR PREPARATION SCHEDULE IN EACH KIT.

HOW SUPPLIED
See "Description" for contents of each kit.
Shipping Unit: 48 FLEET® Prep Kits per carton.
For full prescribing information on specific products, see individual listings (FLEET® Phospho®-Soda, FLEET® Bisacodyl Enema and FLEET® Flavored Castor Oil Emulsion).

IS THIS PRODUCT OTC
Yes.

LITERATURE AVAILABLE
Yes.

FLEET® FLAVORED CASTOR OIL EMULSION   OTC
(Stimulant Laxative)

INGREDIENTS
Each tablespoonful (15 ml.) contains:
ACTIVE INGREDIENTS
Castor Oil U.S.P. 10 ml.

INDICATIONS
For the occasional relief of constipation and preparation of the colon for x-ray and endoscopic examination. (See FLEET® Prep Kit listings.)

ACTIONS
Works directly on the small intestine to promote bowel movement. This product usually produces a bowel movement in 6 to 12 hours.

WARNINGS
Do not use laxative products when nausea, vomiting or abdominal pain is present unless directed by a physician. If you have noticed a sudden change in bowel habits that persists over a period of 2 weeks, consult a physician before using a laxative. Laxative products should not be used longer than 1 week unless directed by a physician. Frequent or prolonged

use of a laxative may result in a dependence on laxatives. Rectal bleeding or failure to have a bowel movement may indicate a serious condition. Discontinue use and consult a physician. Castor oil affects the small intestine and regular use may cause excessive loss of water and body salts, which can have a debilitating effect. Keep this and all drugs out of the reach of children. In case of accidental overdose, seek professional assistance or contact a Poison Control Center immediately. As with any drug, if you are pregnant or nursing a baby, seek the advice of a health professional before using this product.

DOSAGE AND ADMINISTRATION
Fleet® Flavored Castor Oil Emulsion Stimulant Laxative is best taken on an empty stomach. **Shake well before use.** Follow recommended dosage with one full glass of cool water. (Fleet® Flavored Castor Oil Emulsion may be chilled to enhance taste.) Avoid freezing.
Adults: Purgative: 6 tablespoonfuls (90 ml). Laxative: 3 tablespoonfuls (45 ml.) Children 2 to 12 years: 1 tablespoonful (15 ml.) Children up to 2 years: up to 1 teaspoonful (5 ml.) or as directed by a physician.

HOW SUPPLIED
Bottles of 1½ and 3 fl. oz.

IS THIS PRODUCT OTC
Yes.

FLEET® RELIEF   OTC
Anesthetic Hemorrhoidal Ointment

ACTIVE INGREDIENT
Pramoxine Hydrochloride 1%

INDICATIONS
For the temporary relief of itching, burning and pain associated with hemorrhoids or other anorectal disorders.

ACTIONS
Pramoxine hydrochloride is a topical anesthetic proven to be safe and effective in clinical tests. Delivered in a water soluble base that is greaseless, stainless, and odorless, it begins to work immediately to relieve hemorrhoidal discomforts.

WARNING
In case of bleeding, consult a physician promptly. Certain persons can develop allergic reactions to ingredients in this product. If the symptom being treated does not subside or redness, irritation, swelling, pain, itching or other symptoms develop or increase, within 7 days, discontinue use and consult a physician. Do not exceed recommended daily dosage except under the supervision of a physician. If introduction of this product into the rectum causes additional pain, stop use and consult physician promptly. As with any drug, if you are pregnant or nursing a baby, seek the advice of a health professional before using this product. The safety of this product has not been established for use by pregnant women or nursing mothers. Keep this and all drugs out of the reach of children. In case of accidental ingestion, seek professional assistance or contact a Poison Control Center immediately.

DOSAGE AND ADMINISTRATION
When practical, wash the anorectal area with mild soap and warm water and rinse off all soap before application of this product. Disposable Pre-filled Applicator—REMOVE PROTECTIVE SHIELD FROM TIP BEFORE ADMINISTERING. Gently insert prelubricated stem into the rectum. Squeeze gently until applicator is empty. Remove and discard unit. Use one unit as needed each morning and night and after bowel movements. Do not exceed 5 applications in 24 hours. Tube—Apply Fleet Relief Ointment generously to the affected area up to 5 times daily. If accompanying applicator is used, attach to tube and lubricate with small amount of ointment. Insert gently into rectum and squeeze tube. Cleanse applicator after each use.

HOW SUPPLIED
Six 4 ml. rectal applicators per package or single one ounce tube with applicator.

IS THIS PRODUCT OTC
Yes.

SUMMER'S EVE®   OTC
MEDICATED DOUCHE

ACTIVE INGREDIENT
Povidone-iodine provided as a .30 percent solution when packet and sanitized fluid are mixed.

INDICATIONS
For temporary relief of minor vaginal irritation and itching. Clinically effective in a program of treatment for vaginal moniliasis, vaginales vaginitis and non-specific vaginitis due to Candida albicans, Trichomonas vaginalis, and Gardnerella vaginalis.

ACTIONS
Povidone-iodine is an effective broad spectrum anti-microbial agent used in treatment of both gram negative and gram positive bacteria, fungi, yeast, and protozoa.

WARNINGS
DOUCHING DOES NOT PREVENT PREGNANCY. Do not use during pregnancy or if nursing a baby except with the approval of a physician. If douching results in pain, soreness, itching, excessive dryness, or irritation, stop douching. If symptoms persist consult a physician. If minor irritation has not improved after 1 week of use, consult a physician. Women with iodine sensitivity should not use this product. The use of iodine as a douche may cause a transient rise of serum protein-bound iodine. Keep this and all drugs out of the reach of children. In case of accidental ingestion, seek professional assistance or contact a Poison Control Center immediately.

DOSAGE AND ADMINISTRATION
Dosage is contained in a single-unit concentrate packet to be added to 4.5 fluid ounces of sanitized solution supplied in a disposable unit. Remove the sanitary overwrap. Unscrew nozzle cap. Carefully open medicated packet and pour contents into bottle. Screw nozzle cap back on to bottle. Swirl gently to assure complete mixing. Pull up the flexible nozzle until it clicks and locks, and Summer's Eve® Medicated Douche is ready to use. After use, the unit is discarded. Use once daily for seven days even if symptoms disappear.

HOW SUPPLIED
4.5 fluid ounce single pack with one 0.14 fluid ounce medicated packet or twin pack containing two 4.5 fluid ounce units and two 0.14 fluid ounce packets.

IS THIS PRODUCT OTC
Yes.

Fleming & Company
1600 FENPARK DR.
FENTON, MO 63026

AEROLATE SR & JR & III Capsules   R
(theophylline, anhydrous T.D.)

AEROLATE LIQUID
(theophylline, anhydrous)

COMPOSITION
Contains theophylline 4 grs. (260 mg) as SR, 2 grs (130 mg) as JR, 1 gr. as III (65 mg), in red/clear capsules. Liquid has 150 mg theophylline/15cc in a non-sugar, non-alcoholic, non-saccharin tangerine flavored base.

ACTION AND USES
Timed action pellets by-pass stomach to prevent gastric upset. Bronchodilation is achieved through bowel absorption only. Liquid is for the acute attack primarily.

ADMINISTRATION AND DOSAGE
One capsule every 12 hours. Every 8 hours in severe attacks. Liquid—adults—40 ml (2.5 tablespoonfuls) for acute attack. Children—0.25 ml/lb. Maintainance therapy—adults—for the first 6 doses, 25 ml (1.5 tablespoonfuls) before breakfast, at 3 p.m., at bedtime. Then 15 ml doses at above times. Children—0.15ml/lb. at these times, then 0.1ml/lb per dose.

SIDE EFFECTS
Nausea, vomiting, epigastric or substernal pain, palpitation, headache, dizziness may occur.

HOW SUPPLIED
Capsules in bottles of 100.
Liquid in pints and gallons.

CHLOR-3   OTC

DESCRIPTION
Medical condiment containing sodium chloride 50%; potassium chloride 30%; magnesium chloride 20%.

INDICATIONS AND USAGE
To reduce sodium intake for patients on diuretics; for potential hypertensives and cardiacs.
To encourage physicians to recommend a condiment to replace "table salt" for family use and gourmet cooking.

HOW SUPPLIED
Shaker 8 oz. plastic bottles.

CONGESS SR & JR Capsules   ℞
Expectorant/Decongestant T.D.

COMPOSITION
Contains guaifenesin 250 mgs/pseudoephedrine 120 mgs as SR; guaifenesin 125 mgs/pseudoephedrine 60 mgs as JR in blue/pink capsules.

ACTION AND USES
To loosen mucus plugs in upper respiratory tract and congestion in acute pulmonary disorders, and in coughing. Nasal decongestion and alleviation of bronchospasm is also achieved up to 12 hrs. that accompany most coughs, especially during the nocturnal period.

INDICATIONS
Nasal congestion, sinusitis, acute aerotitis media, bronchial asthma, serous otitis media, and symptoms of the common cold.

DOSAGE
Adults and children over 12 yrs. one SR capsule every 12 hrs. Under 12 yrs. one JR capsule as prescribed by physician.

PRECAUTION AND SIDE EFFECTS
Use with care in severe hypertension, heart disease, hyperthyroidism, diabetes. Low grade sensitivity to drugs may be experienced.

CONTRAINDICATIONS
Prostatic hypertrophy, patients receiving MAO inhibitors.

HOW SUPPLIED
Plastic bottles of 100 and 1000 capsules.

EXTENDRYL   ℞
T.D. Capsules SR & JR, Syrup and Tablets

Each timed action SR capsule contains phenylephrine HCl 20 mg; methscopolamine nitrate 2.5 mg; chlorpheniramine maleate 8 mg. The JR potency is exactly half-strength. Green/red color for both. Each 5 cc of root beer flavored syrup and tablet contains: phenylephrine HCl 10 mg; methscopolamine nitrate 1.25 mg; chlorpheniramine maleate 2 mg.

ACTION AND USES
Antihistaminic-decongestant for relief of respiratory congestion; allergic rhinitis; allergic skin reactions of urticaria and angioedema.

ADMINISTRATION AND DOSAGE
Capsules—one every 12 hrs of the SR for adults; one JR every 12 hrs for children 6–12 yrs. Syrup-two teaspoonfuls every 4 hrs for adults; children 1 teaspoonful every 4 hrs. Tablets—adults two and children one every 4 hrs. Do not exceed 4 doses in 24 hrs.
Children under 6 yrs. as recommended by a physician.

PRECAUTIONS
Withdraw therapy if drowsiness occurs. Patients are cautioned against driving or operating mechanical devices.

CONTRAINDICATIONS
Glaucoma, cardiac disease, hyperthyroidism and hypertension.

HOW SUPPLIED
Capsules and tablets in bottles of 100 and 1000. Syrup in pints and gallons.

IMPREGON Concentrate   OTC

ACTIVE INGREDIENT
Tetrachlorosalicylanilide 2%

INDICATIONS
Diaper Rash Relief, 'Staph' control, Mold inhibitor.

ACTIONS
This is a bacteriostatic/fungistatic agent for home usage and hospital usage.

WARNINGS
Impregon should not be exposed to direct sunlight for long periods after applications.

PRECAUTION
Addition of bleach prior to diaper treatment negates application effects.

DOSAGE AND ADMINISTRATION
One capful (5ml) per gallon of water to impregnate diapers in the diaper pail. Dilutions for many home areas accompany the full package.

NOTE
For disposable-type diapers, add one teaspoonful to 8 oz of water to a 'Windex-type' sprayer. Spray middle half area of diapers until damp, and allow to dry before using, to prevent rashes.

HOW SUPPLIED
Four ounce amber plastic bottles.

MAGONATE Liquid
(magnesium gluconate)

FORMULA
Each dye-free 5ml has 54mg magnesium as the gluconate in a very low sugary mixed melon flavored base, as the equivalent to two Magonate tablets.

INDICATIONS
Alcoholism; digitalis toxicity; cardiac arrhythmias; extrinsic asthma; dysmenorrhea; eclampsia; hypertension; insomnia; muscle twitching; tremors; anxiety; pancreatitis, and toxicity of chemotherapy.

DOSAGE
Adults and children over 12 yrs.—mid-morning, mid-afternoon and mid-evening—one tsp.
Children under 12—one-half tsp (50 drops) t.i.d.
Children 1–6—one-quarter tsp. (25 drops) t.i.d.

HOW SUPPLIED
Plastic pints and gallons.

MARBLEN
(calcium and magnesium carbonates)
ANTACID SUSPENSIONS AND TABLET

(See PDR For Nonprescription Drugs)

NEPHROCAPS   ℞
Dialysis Vitamin Supplement

DESCRIPTION
Each black oval gelatin 'liquid' capsule provides:
Thiamin 1.5 mg; Riboflavin 1.7 mg; Niacin 20 mg; Pantothenic acid 5 mg; Biotin 150 mcg; Cyanocobalamin 6 mcg; Pyridoxin 10 mg; Ascorbic acid 100 mg and Folic acid 1.0 mg.

INDICATIONS
The wasting syndrome in chronic renal failure; uremia; impaired metabolic functions of the kidney.

DOSAGE
One capsule daily. On dialysis days, one Nephrocap must be taken after treatment.

SUPPLIED
Plastic bottles of 100 only.

NEPHROX SUSPENSION
(aluminum hydroxide)
Antacid Suspension

(See PDR For Nonprescription Drugs)

NICOTINEX Elixir
nicotinic acid

(See PDR For Nonprescription Drugs)

OCEAN-A/S Nasal Spray

COMPOSITION
Each 20cc bottle contains 0.0192mg atropine sulfate.

ACTION AND USES
For 'post nasal drip'; snoring due to mucus formation; smokers cough due to irritants.

ADMINISTRATION AND DOSAGE
Two sprays in each nostril t.i.d. & h.s. for 'p.n.d.' and cough; two sprays at 7 p.m. and h.s. for snoring.

HOW SUPPLIED
20cc bottles only.

OCEAN MIST
(buffered isotonic saline)

(See PDR For Nonprescription Drugs)

PIMA Syrup   ℞
(potassium iodide)

COMPOSITION
Contains KI 5 grs./tsp., in a black raspberry flavored base.

ACTION AND USES
An expectorant in the symptomatic treatment of chronic pulmonary diseases where tenacious mucus complicates the problem, including bronchial asthma, bronchitis and pulmonary emphysema.

ADMINISTRATION AND DOSAGE
Children—one half to one tsp. and adults one or two tsp. every 4-6 hours.

SIDE EFFECTS
May include gastrointestinal upset, metallic taste, minor skin eruptions, nausea, vomiting and epigastric pain. Therapy should be withdrawn.

PRECAUTIONS
In patients sensitive to iodides, in hyperthyroidism, and in rare cases iodine-induced goiter may occur.

HOW SUPPLIED
Plastic pints and gallons.

PURGE
(flavored castor oil)

(See PDR For Nonprescription Drugs)

RUM–K   ℞
(potassium chloride 15% conc.)

DESCRIPTION
Each 10 ml. contains 1.5 Gm. potassium chloride (20 mEq) in a butter/rum synthetic flavored base that is alcohol and sugar free.

INDICATIONS
Hypokalemic-hypochloremic alkalosis; digitalis toxicity; hypokalemia prevention secondary to corticosteroid or diuretic administration.

CONTRAINDICATIONS
Impaired renal function, untreated Addison's Disease, acute dehydration, heat cramps, hyperkalemia.

PRECAUTIONS
Do not use in patients with low urinary output or renal decompensation. Potassium replacements vary and should be individualized. Patients should be checked frequently, ECG and plasma K^+ levels should be made. High serum concentrations of K^+ cause death thru cardiac depression, arrhythmias or arrest. Use with caution in cardiac disease.

ADVERSE REACTIONS
Vomiting, nausea, abdominal discomfort, diarrhea may occur. Symptoms and signs of potassium overdose include paresthesias of extremities, flaccid paralysis, listlessness, fall in blood pressure, weakness and heaviness of the legs, cardiac arrhythmias and heart block. Hyperkalemia may cause ECG changes as disappearance of the P wave, widening and slurring of QRS complex, changes of the S-T segment, tall peaked T waves.

DOSAGE AND ADMINISTRATION
Adults—two teaspoonsful (10ml) in 4–6 oz water 2 to 4 times daily after meals to supply 40–80 mEq of elemental potassium and chloride. Larger doses may be required and administered under close supervision due to possible potassium intoxication or saline laxative effect.

HOW SUPPLIED
2 oz; 4 oz; pints and gallons.

S-P-T   ℞
(Pork thyroid "liquid" capsules USP)

COMPOSITION
S-P-T is prepared by special process from cleaned, fresh pork thyroid glands, deprived of connective tissue, defatted and suspended in soy bean oil and encapsulated in gelatin for greater oral absorption. The active hormones (T4 and T3) are available in their natural state in a ratio of approximately 2.5:1, as in humans, to insure therapeutic availability. Capsules are standardized by USP method for iodine content and also biologically to insure 100% metabolic potency.

ACTION
To increase metabolic rate of body tissues. S-P-T is replacement therapy for diminished or absent thyroid function. Effect develops slowly and is fully reached in 10—14 days per grain increase in most instances.

INDICATIONS
As replacement therapy in hypothyroidism, cretinism, myxedema, and after surgery following complete thyroidectomy.

CONTRAINDICATIONS
In thyrotoxicosis, angina pectoris, myocardial infarction and hypertension unless complicated by hypothyroidism, and uncorrected adrenal insufficiency.

Continued on next page

Fleming—Cont.

PRECAUTION AND SIDE EFFECTS

Overdosage may cause tachycardia, angina pectoris, diarrhea, nervousness, sweating, headache and increased pulse action. In most cases, reduction of dosage overcomes side effects.

DOSAGE AND ADMINISTRATION

Patients should be titrated starting at lower levels and increasing by 1 gr every 2 weeks until mild thyromimetic effects are noted. Then lower the dose to the level at which the patient felt best, as patients vary widely as to thyroid need.

> **WARNINGS**
>
> Drugs with thyroid hormone activity, alone or together with other therapeutic agents, have been used for the treatment of obesity. In euthyroid patients, doses within the range of daily hormonal requirements are ineffective for weight reduction. Larger doses may produce serious or even life-threatening manifestations of toxicity, particularly when given in association with sympathomimetic amines such as those used for their anorectic effects.

HOW SUPPLIED

As 1 gr (green); 2 gr (brown); 3 gr (red); 5 gr (black) gelatin sealed capsules in bottles of 100 and 1000.

Fluoritab Corporation
P.O. BOX 507
TEMPERANCE, MICHIGAN 48182-0507

FLUORITAB® ℞
[*floor 'a tab*]
sodium fluoride (active ingredient)

DESCRIPTION AND USES

FLUORITAB dietary fluoride products contain sodium fluoride and no other active ingredients. FLUORITAB TABLETS and FLUORITAB LIQUID provide optimum fluoride in areas where the drinking water fluoride level does not exceed 0.7 ppm. FLUORITAB dietary fluoride products are for use as a tooth development agent and prevention against dental caries in children. Fluoride combines with calcium to form the apatite molecule of teeth and bone to form fluorapatite crystals.

ADMINISTRATION AND DOSAGE

Fluoride must be taken on a continual basis throughout the period of tooth formation. FLUORITAB TABLETS may be swallowed quickly, permitted to dissolve in the mouth or chewed, which may provide maximum surface benefit to tooth enamel. FLUORITAB LIQUID can be dropped directly into the mouth or added to any liquid.
Water supplies with 0.3 ppm fluoride and less require fluoride supplements that provide the child with $\frac{1}{2}$ mg of F per day from birth to 3 years of age and 1 mg of F per day from 3 years of age up. Water supplies with 0.3 to 0.7 ppm fluoride require $\frac{1}{4}$ mg of F and $\frac{1}{2}$ of F dosage per day for children under 3 and over 3 respectively.

CONTRAINDICATIONS

Dietary fluoride supplements should not be used where water with 0.7 ppm of fluoride is available.

OVERDOSAGE

Excess fluoride is to be avoided, as it may cause dental fluorosis (mottling of the teeth).

HOW SUPPLIED

FLUORITAB TABLETS contain 1 mg of fluoride per tablet. They are scored for easy dividing. FLUORITAB TABLET flavors are dye-free original pineapple and cherry. FLUORITAB TABLETS are available in bottles of 100, 1000*, and 5000*. FLUORITAB LIQUID is available in 19 ml, 475 drop, squeeze type dropper bottles. Each FLUORITAB LIQUID drop contains 0.25 mg of fluoride. FLUORITAB LIQUID contains no artificial flavor or coloring.
*FOR DISPENSING ONLY

PRODUCT IDENTIFICATION

FLUORITAB products have the "FLUORITAB" name on all packages.

REMARKS

FLUORITAB dietary sodium fluoride products were given American Dental Association acceptance in July 1958. FLUORITAB CORPORATION markets only fluoride supplements.

LITERATURE AVAILABLE

Educational folders, direct ordering information, and prescription instructions will be sent free, on request.

Forest Pharmaceuticals, Inc.
(Subsidiary of Forest Laboratories, Inc.)
2510 METRO BLVD.
ST. LOUIS, MO 63043

AEROBID® ℞
(flunisolide)
Inhaler system
For oral inhalation only

PRODUCT OVERVIEW

KEY FACTS

The active component of the Aerobid Inhaler System is flunisolide which is an anti-inflammatory steroid. Each metered inhalation delivers about 250 mcg of flunisolide. Clinical studies indicate that recommended doses confer topical therapeutic activity on bronchial mucosa with minimal evidence of systemic action. Patients have been able to tolerate significant decreases in their systemic steroid dosages while using flunisolide.

MAJOR USES

Aerobid Inhaler System is to be used in patients who need chornic corticosteroid therapy in order to control their bronchial asthma symptoms.

SAFETY INFORMATION

Contraindicated in patients who are allergic to any of the ingredients used in the formilation of Aerobid. This product is not to be used in the primary treatment of status asthmaticus or other serious, acute episodes of asthma. Because Aerobid is not regarded as a bronchodilator, it should not be employed for rapid relief of bronchospasm.

PRESCRIBING INFORMATION

AEROBID® ℞
(flunisolide)
Inhaler system
For oral inhalation only

DESCRIPTION

Flunisolide, the active component of **AeroBid** Inhaler System, is an anti-inflammatory steroid having the chemical name 6α-fluoro-11β, 16α, 17, 21-tetrahydroxypregna-1, 4-diene-3, 20-dione cyclic-16, 17-acetal with acetone. It has the following structure:

Flunisolide is a white to creamy white crystalline powder with a molecular weight of 434.49. It is soluble in acetone, sparingly soluble in chloroform, slightly soluble in methanol, and practically insoluble in water. It has a melting point of about 245°C.
AeroBid Inhaler is delivered in a metered-dose aerosol system containing a microcrystalline suspension of flunisolide as the hemihydrate in propellants (trichloromonofluoromethane, dichlorodifluoromethane and dichlorotetrafluoroethane) with sorbitan trioleate as a dispersing agent. Each activation delivers approximately 250 mcg of flunisolide to the patient. One **AeroBid** Inhaler System is designed to deliver at least 100 metered inhalations.

CLINICAL PHARMACOLOGY

Flunisolide has demonstrated marked anti-inflammatory and anti-allergic activity in classical test systems. It is a corticosteroid that is several hundred times more potent in animal anti-inflammatory assays than the cortisol standard. The molar dose of each activation of flunisolide in this preparation is approximately 2½ to 7 times that of comparable inhaled corticosteroid products marketed for the same indication. The dose of flunisolide delivered per activation in this preparation is 10 times that per activation of Nasalide® (flunisolide) nasal solution. Clinical studies have shown therapeutic activity on bronchial mucosa with minimal evidence of systemic activity at recommended doses.
After oral inhalation of 1 mg flunisolide, total systemic availability was 40%. The flunisolide that is swallowed is rapidly and extensively converted to the 6β-OH metabolite and to water-soluble conjugates during the first pass through the liver. This offers a metabolic explanation for the low sys-

temic activity of oral flunisolide itself since the metabolite has low corticosteroid potency (on the order of the cortisol standard). The inhaled flunisolide absorbed through the bronchial tree is converted to the same metabolites. Repeated inhalation of 2.0 mg of flunisolide per day (the maximum recommended dose) for 14 days did not show accumulation of the drug in plasma. The plasma half-life of flunisolide is approximately 1.8 hours.
The following observations relevant to systemic absorption were made in clinical studies. In one uncontrolled study a statistically significant decrease in responsiveness to metyrapone was noted in 15 adult steroid-independent patients treated with 2.0 mg of flunisolide per day (the maximum recommended dose) for 3 months. A small but statistically significant drop in eosinophils from 11.5% to 7.4% of total circulating leucocytes was noted in another study in children who were not taking oral corticosteroids simultaneously. A 5% incidence of menstrual disturbances was reported during open studies, in which there were no control groups for comparison.
Aerosol administration of flunisolide 2.0 mg twice daily for one week to 6 healthy male subjects revealed neither suppression of adrenal function as measured by early morning cortisol levels nor impairment of HPA axis function as determined by insulin hypoglycemia tests.
Controlled clinical studies have included over 500 patients with asthma, among them 150 children age 6 and over. More than 120 patients have been treated in open trials for two years or more. No significant adrenal suppression attributed to flunisolide was seen in these studies.
Significant decreases of systemic steroid dosages have been possible in flunisolide-treated patients. Asthma patients have had further symptomatic improvement with flunisolide treatment even while reducing concomitant medication.

INDICATIONS AND USAGE

AeroBid Inhaler is indicated only for patients who require chronic treatment with corticosteroids for control of the symptoms of bronchial asthma. Such patients would include those already receiving systemic corticosteroids, and selected patients who are inadequately controlled on a non-steroid regimen and in whom steroid therapy has been withheld because of concern over potential adverse effects.
As with any topically applied medication, flunisolide is absorbed through the mucous membrane and is systemically available. For these reasons, **AeroBid** Inhaler should be used with caution for initial therapy and the recommended dosage should not be exceeded. When the drug is used chronically at 2 mg/day, patients should be monitored periodically for effects on the hypothalamic-pituitary-adrenal axis.
AeroBid Inhaler is NOT indicated:
1. For relief of asthma that can be controlled by bronchodilators and other non-steroid medications.
2. In patients who require systemic corticosteroid treatment infrequently.
3. In the treatment of non-asthmatic bronchitis.
Insufficient information is available to warrant use in children under the age of 6.

CONTRAINDICATIONS

AeroBid Inhaler is contraindicated in the primary treatment of status asthmaticus or other acute episodes of asthma where intensive measures are required. Hypersensitivity to any of the ingredients of this preparation contraindicates its use.

> **WARNINGS**
>
> Particular care is needed in patients who are transferred from systemically active corticosteroids to **AeroBid** Inhaler because deaths due to adrenal insufficiency have occurred in asthmatic patients during and after transfer from systemic corticosteroids to aerosol corticosteroids. After withdrawal from systemic corticosteroids, a number of months are required for recovery of hypothalamic-pituitary-adrenal (HPA) function. During this period of HPA suppression, patients may exhibit signs and symptoms of adrenal insufficiency when exposed to trauma, surgery or infections, particularly gastroenteritis. Although **AeroBid** Inhaler may provide control of asthmatic symptoms during these episodes, it does NOT provide the systemic steroid that is necessary for coping with these emergencies.
> During periods of stress or a severe asthmatic attack, patients who have been withdrawn from systemic corticosteroids should be instructed to resume systemic steroids (in large doses) immediately and to contact their physician for further instruction. These patients should also be instructed to carry a warning card indicating that they may need supplementary systemic steroids during periods of stress or a severe asthma attack. To assess the risk of adrenal insufficiency in emergency situations, routine tests of adrenal cortical function, including measurement of early morning resting cortisol levels, should be performed periodically in all patients. An early morning resting cortisol level may be

accepted as normal if it falls at or near the normal mean level.

Localized infections with *Candida albicans* or *Aspergillus niger* have occurred in the mouth and pharynx and occasionally in the larynx. Positive cultures for oral *Candida* may be present in up to 34% of patients. Although the frequency of clinically apparent infection is considerably lower, these infections may require treatment with appropriate antifungal therapy or discontinuance of treatment with **AeroBid** inhaler.

AeroBid Inhaler is not to be regarded as a bronchodilator and is not indicated for rapid relief of bronchospasm. Patients should be instructed to contact their physician immediately when episodes of asthma that are not responsive to bronchodilators occur during the course of treatment. During such episodes, patients may require therapy with systemic corticosteroids.

There is no evidence that control of asthma can be achieved by administration of the drug in amounts greater than the recommended doses, which appear to be the therapeutic equivalent of approximately 10 mg/day of oral prednisone. Theoretically, the use of inhaled corticosteroids with alternate day prednisone systemic treatment should be accompanied by more HPA suppression than a therapeutically equivalent regimen of either alone.

Transfer of patients from systemic steroid therapy to **AeroBid** Inhaler may unmask allergic conditions previously suppressed by the systemic steroid therapy, e.g., rhinitis, conjunctivitis, and eczema.

PRECAUTIONS

General: Because of the relatively high molar dose of flunisolide per activation in this preparation, and because of the evidence suggesting higher levels of systemic absorption with flunisolide than with other comparable inhaled corticosteroids (see CLINICAL PHARMACOLOGY section), patients treated with **AeroBid** should be observed carefully for any evidence of systemic corticosteroid effect, including suppression of bone growth in children. Particular care should be taken in observing patients post-operatively or during periods of stress for evidence of a decrease in adrenal function. During withdrawal from oral steroids, some patients may experience symptoms of systemically active steroid withdrawal, e.g., joint and/or muscular pain, lassitude and depression, despite maintenance or even improvement of respiratory function (See DOSAGE AND ADMINISTRATION for details).

In responsive patients, flunisolide may permit control of asthmatic symptoms without suppression of HPA function. Since flunisolide is absorbed into the circulation and can be systemically active, the beneficial effects of **AeroBid** Inhaler in minimizing or preventing HPA dysfunction may be expected only when recommended dosages are not exceeded. The long-term effects of the drug in human subjects are still unknown. In particular, the local effects of the agent on developmental or immunologic processes in the mouth, pharynx, trachea, and lung are unknown. There is also no information about the possible long-term systemic effects of the agent.

The potential effects of the drug on acute, recurrent, or chronic pulmonary infections, including active or quiescent tuberculosis, are not known. Similarly, the potential effects of long-term administration of the drug on lung or other tissues are unknown.

Pulmonary infiltrates with eosinophilia may occur in patients on **AeroBid** Inhaler therapy. Although it is possible that in some patients this state may become manifest because of systemic steroid withdrawal when inhalational steroids are administered, a causative role for the drug and/or its vehicle cannot be ruled out.

Information for Patients

There is no evidence that better control of asthma can be achieved by the administration of **AeroBid** Inhaler in amounts greater than the recommended doses; higher doses may induce adrenal suppression.

Since the relief from **AeroBid** Inhaler depends on its regular use and on proper inhalation technique, patients must be instructed to take inhalations at regular intervals. They should also be instructed in the correct method of use (See Patient instruction Leaflet).

Patients receiving bronchodilators by inhalation should be advised to use the bronchodilator before **AeroBid** Inhaler in order to enhance penetration of flunisolide into the bronchial tree. After use of an aerosol bronchodilator, several minutes should elapse before using the **AeroBid** Inhaler. Patients whose systemic corticosteroids have been reduced or withdrawn should be instructed to carry a warning card indicating that they may need supplemental systemic steroids during periods of stress or a severe asthmatic attack that is not responsive to bronchodilators.

An illustrated leaflet of patient instructions for proper use accompanies each **AeroBid** Inhaler System.

CONTENTS UNDER PRESSURE

Do not puncture. Do not use or store near heat or open flame. Exposure to temperatures above 120°F (49°C) may cause con-

tainer to explode. Never throw container into fire or incinerator. Keep out of reach of children.

Carcinogenesis: Long-term studies were conducted in mice and rats using oral administration to evaluate the carcinogenic potential of the drug. There was an increase in the incidence of pulmonary adenomas in mice, but not in rats. Female rats receiving the highest oral dose had an increased incidence of mammary adenocarcinoma compared to control rats. An increased incidence of this tumor type has been reported for other corticosteroids.

Impairment of Fertility: Female rats receiving high doses of flunisolide (200 mcg/kg/day) showed some evidence of impaired fertility. Reproductive performance in the low (8 mcg/kg/day) and mid-dose (40 mcg/kg/day) groups was comparable to controls.

Pregnancy: Pregnancy Category C. As with other corticosteroids, flunisolide has been shown to be teratogenic in rabbits and rats at doses of 40 and 200 mcg/kg/day respsectively. It was also fetotoxic in these animal reproductive studies. There are no adequate and well-controlled studies in pregnant women. Flunisolide should be used during pregnancy only if the potential benefit justifies the potential risk to the fetus.

Nursing Mothers: It is not known whether this drug is excreted in human milk. Because other corticosteroids are excreted in human milk, caution should be exercised when flunisolide is administered to nursing women.

ADVERSE REACTIONS

Adverse events reported in controlled clinical trials and long-term open studies in 514 patients treated with **AeroBid** are described below. Of those patients, 463 were treated for 3 months or longer, 407 for 6 months or longer, 287 for 1 year or longer, and 122 for 2 years or longer.

Musculoskeletal reactions were reported in 35% of steroid-dependent patients in whom the dose of oral steroid was being tapered. This is a well-known effect of steroid withdrawal.

Incidence 10% or greater:
Gastrointestinal: diarrhea (10%), nausea and/or vomiting (25%), upset stomach (10%)
General: flu (10%)
Mouth and Throat: sore throat (20%)
Nervous system: headache (25%)
Respiratory: cold symptoms (15%), nasal congestion (15%), upper respiratory infection (25%)
Special Senses: unpleasant taste (10%)

Incidence 3–9%
Cardiovascular: palpitations
Gastrointestinal: abdominal pain, heartburn
General: chest pain, decreased appetite, edema, fever
Mouth and Throat: *Candida* infection
Nervous System: dizziness, irritability, nervousness, shakiness
Reproductive: menstrual disturbances
Respiratory: chest congestion, cough*, hoarseness, rhinitis, runny nose, sinus congestion, sinus drainage, sinus infection, sinusitis, sneezing, sputum, wheezing*
Skin: eczema, itching (pruritus), rash
Special Senses: ear infection, loss of smell or taste

Incidence 1–3%
General: chills, increased appetite and weight gain, malaise, peripheral edema, sweating, weakness
Cardiovascular: hypertension, tachycardia
Gastrointestinal: constipation, dyspepsia, gas
Hemic/Lymph: capillary fragility, enlarged lymph nodes
Mouth and Throat: dry throat, glossitis, mouth irritation, pharyngitis, phlegm, throat irritation
Nervous System: anxiety, depression, faintness, fatigue, hyperactivity, hypoactivity, insomnia, moodiness, numbness, vertigo
Respiratory: bronchitis, chest tightness*, dyspnea, epistaxis, head stuffiness, laryngitis, nasal irritation, pleurisy, pneumonia, sinus discomfort
Skin: acne, hives, or urticaria
Special Senses: blurred vision, earache, eye discomfort, eye infection

Incidence less than 1%, judged by investigators as possibly or probably drug related: abdominal fullness, shortness of breath.

---

*The incidences as shown of cough, wheezing, and chest tightness were judged by investigators to be possibly or probably drug-related. In placebo-controlled trials, the *overall* incidences of these adverse events (regardless of investigators' judgment of drug relationship) were similar for drug and placebo-treated groups. They may be related to the vehicle or delivery system.

DOSAGE AND ADMINISTRATION

The **AeroBid** Inhaler System is for oral inhalation only.
Adults: The recommended starting dose is 2 inhalations twice daily morning and evening for a total daily dose of 1 mg. The maximum daily dose should not exceed 4 inhalations twice a day for a total daily dose of 2 mg. When the drug is used chronically at 2 mg/day, patients should be moni-

tored periodically for effects on the hypothalamic-pituitary-adrenal axis.

Children: For children 6–15 years of age, two inhalations may be administered twice daily for a total daily dose of 1 mg. Higher doses have not been studied. Insufficient information is available to warrant use in children under age 6. With chronic use, children should be monitored for growth as well as for effects on the HPA axis.

Rinsing the mouth after inhalation is advised. Patients receiving bronchodilators by inhalation should be advised to use the bronchodilator before **AeroBid** Inhaler in order to enhance penetration of flunisolide into the bronchial tree. After use of an aerosol bronchodilator, several minutes should elapse before use of the **AeroBid** inhaler to reduce the potential toxicity from the inhaled fluorocarbon propellants in the two aerosols.

Different considerations must be given to the following groups of patients in order to obtain the full therapeutic benefit of **AeroBid** Inhaler.

Patients not receiving systemic steroids: The use of **AeroBid** Inhaler is straightforward in patients who are inadequately controlled with non-steroid medications but in whom systemic steroid therapy has been withheld because of concern over potential adverse reactions. In patients who respond to the drug, an improvement in pulmonary function is usually apparent within one to four weeks after the start of treatment.

Patients receiving systemic steroids: In those patients dependent on systemic steroids, transfer to **AeroBid** and subsequent management may be more difficult because recovery from impaired adrenal function is usually slow. Such suppression has been known to last for up to 12 months. Clinical studies, however, have demonstrated that **AeroBid** may be effective in the management of these asthmatic patients and may permit replacement or significant reduction in the dosage of systemic corticosteroids.

Inhaled corticosteroids generally are not recommended for chronic use with alternate day prednisone regimens (see WARNINGS).

The patient's asthma should be reasonably stable before treatment with **AeroBid** Inhaler is started. Initially, the aerosol should be used concurrently with the patient's usual maintenance dose of systemic steroid. After approximately one week, gradual withdrawal of the systemic steroid is started by reducing the daily or alternate daily dose. The next reduction is made after an interval of one or two weeks, depending on the response of the patient. Generally, these decrements should not exceed 2.5 mg of prednisone or its equivalent. A slow rate of withdrawal cannot be overemphasized. During withdrawal, some patients may experience symptoms of systemically active steroid withdrawal, e.g., joint and/or muscular pain, lassitude and depression, despite maintenance or even improvement of respiratory function. Such patients should be encouraged to continue with the Inhaler but should be watched carefully for objective signs of adrenal insufficiency, such as hypotension and weight loss. If evidence of adrenal insufficiency occurs, the systemic steroid dose should be boosted temporarily and thereafter further withdrawal should continue more slowly. *During periods of stress or a severe asthma attack, transfer patients will require supplementary treatment with systemic steroids.* Exacerbations of asthma that occur during the course of treatment with **AeroBid** Inhaler should be treated with a short course of systemic steroid that is gradually tapered as these symptoms subside. There is no evidence that control of asthma can be achieved by administration of the drug in amounts greater than the recommended doses.

HOW SUPPLIED

AeroBid (flunisolide) Inhaler System is available in canisters of 100 metered inhalations. NDC 0456-0672-99
Caution: FEDERAL LAW PROHIBITS DISPENSING WITHOUT PRESCRIPTION.
Revised 2/87

Shown in Product Identification Section, page 410

AEROCHAMBER®
Aerosol Holding Chamber for Use With Metered-Dose Inhalers

Before using your *AeroChamber* Aerosol Holding Chamber, please read this leaflet carefully and follow these instructions.

The *AeroChamber* is a device that attaches to a metered-dose aerosol inhaler (MDI) prescribed by your doctor.

The purpose of the *AeroChamber* is to hold the aerosol drug particles released from the metered-dose inhaler for a few seconds, thus allowing you to inhale the medication after spraying the MDI.

Continued on next page

Forest Pharmaceuticals—Cont.

INSTRUCTIONS

1 Remove caps from inhaler and mouthpiece of *AeroChamber*.

2 Insert inhaler mouthpiece into wider, rubber-sealed end of *AeroChamber*.

3 Shake vigorously 3 or 4 times.

4 Place *AeroChamber* mouthpiece in mouth and close lips.

5 Spray one puff from inhaler into the *AeroChamber*.

6 Then breathe in slowly and fully (take about five seconds for this step).
7 Hold breath for 5–10 seconds.
8 Repeat Steps 3 to 7 as instructed by your doctor.

Alternative Inhalation Method

For small children, or if any difficulty is encountered, an alternative method for taking medication with the *AeroChamber* is as follows:

1 Put the *AeroChamber* into child's mouth and have child breathe slowly in and out continuously from the *AeroChamber* for 20–30 seconds.

2 While child is still breathing from the *AeroChamber*, and after 3 or 4 breaths, spray the drug from the metered-dose inhaler into the *AeroChamber*.
3 Have child continue breathing from the *AeroChamber* for 3 or 4 breaths after the drug has been discharged into the *AeroChamber*.
4 If child is breathing through the nose only, it may be necessary to pinch the nose gently while child breathes from the *AeroChamber*.

PROBLEMS

If you breathe out first while using the *AeroChamber*, the medication is not lost and will be breathed in with your next breath, but do not wait more than 3 seconds between breaths. If you are unable to press down on the metered-dose inhaler with your fingers (Step 5) due to weakness or a handicap: After the metered-dose inhaler has been inserted into the *AeroChamber*, press the top of the metered-dose inhaler against any flat surface such as the underside of a table and then immediately put the *AeroChamber* into your mouth and inhale slowly and deeply as above (Step 6).

CLEANING Warning—Do Not Disassemble

The *AeroChamber* is made of medical grade plastic and has only one moving part—the flap valve. With repeated use, powder will accumulate in the *AeroChamber* and around the valve. This may eventually interfere with effective use. We suggest washing the metered-dose inhaler mouthpiece and *AeroChamber* approximately once a week. Warm tap water passing through the back is best, followed by drying with a soft lint-free cloth or leaving the *AeroChamber* overnight to air dry.
With time the flap valve may harden and start to curl. If this happens, the *AeroChamber* will not work properly, and we suggest you replace the *AeroChamber*.

TECHNICAL INFORMATION

This apparently simple device is a product of considerable medical research and engineering. It was developed in a leading medical center.
The holding chamber selectively removes large aerosol medication particles that normally deposit in the mouth and throat while allowing the smaller treatment particles to pass through the valve into the lung. This provides effective treatment and helps to reduce unwanted side effects.
The one-way valve allows you to inhale at your own rate. You will not have to time your inhalation in coordination with the spraying of the puff.
This new aerosol holding chamber can help you inhale your aerosol medication more reliably. Should you have any problem using the *AeroChamber*, please contact your doctor or pharmacist.

BIBLIOGRAPHY

Berenberg MJ, Baigelman W, Cupples LA, Pearce L. Comparison of metered-dose inhaler attached to an aerochamber with updraft nebulizer for the administration of metaproterenol in hospitalized patients. *J Asthma* 22: 87–92, 1985.
Corr D, Dolovich M, McCormack D, Ruffin R, Obminski G, Newhouse M. Design and characteristics of a portable breath-actuated particle size selective medical aerosol inhaler. *J Aerosol Sci* 13: 1–7, 1982.
Corr D, Dolovich M, McCormach D, Ruffin R, Obminski G, Newhouse M. The AEROCHAMBER: A new demand-inhalation device for delivery of aerosolized drugs. *Am Rev Respir Dis* 121 (Part 2): 123, 1980.
Rachelefsky GS, Rohr AS, Wo J, Gracey V, et al. Use of a tube spacer to improve the efficacy of a metered-dose inhaler in asthmatic children. *AJDC* vol. 140, Nov. 1986.
Salzman GA, Pyszczynski DR: Oral pharyngeal candidiasis in patients treated with beclomethasone dipropionate delivered by metered-dose inhaler alone and with aerochamber. *Chest* (ACCP Special Issue) 88: 53S, 1985.

Manufactured by Monaghan Medical Corporation Plattsburgh NY
Distributed by FOREST PHARMACEUTICALS, INC.
Subsidiary of Forest Laboratories, Inc.
St. Louis, MO 63043

Shown in Product Identification Section, page 410

AEROCHAMBER® with *Mask*

INSTRUCTIONS FOR USE OF AEROCHAMBER WITH *MASK*

This product and your metered dose inhaler (MDI) should be used only as directed by a physician.

1. Remove cap from Metered Dose Inhaler (also called MDI or inhaler).

2. Insert the inhaler mouthpiece into the soft rubber ring at the open end of the AeroChamber.

3. Shake vigorously three or four times.

4. Apply mask to face so that both nose and mouth are covered. Diaphragm should move with each breath, indicating a good seal. This is ESSENTIAL because leaks will prevent medication from being adequately delivered.

5. Spray one puff into AeroChamber.

6. Keep the mask in place for at least 6 breaths (diaphragm should move with each breath).
7. Repeat steps 3 to 6 as instructed by your doctor.
8. Remove MDI from AeroChamber with *Mask* for storage.

CLEANING

The AeroChamber with *Mask* is made of medical grade plastic and has only one moving part—the flap valve. With repeated use, powder will accumulate in the AeroChamber and around the valve. This may eventually interfere with effective use. We suggest washing the metered dose inhaler mouthpiece and AeroChamber approximately once a week. Warm tap water passing through the back is best, followed by drying with a soft lint-free cloth or leaving the AeroChamber overnight to air dry.
With time the flap valve may harden and start to curl. If this happens, the AeroChamber will not work properly, and should be replaced.

TECHNICAL INFORMATION

This apparently simple device is a product of considerable medical research and engineering. It was developed in a leading medical center.
The valve holding chamber selectively removes large aerosol particles that normally deposit in the mouth and throat while allowing the smaller treatment particles to pass into the lungs. This provides effective treatment and helps to reduce unwanted side effects.

This new device helps to deliver aerosol medication to the lungs more reliably. Should you have any problem using the AeroChamber, please contact your doctor.

Manufactured by Monaghan Medical Corporation, Plattsburgh, NY
Distributed by:
FOREST PHARMACEUTICALS, INC.
Subsidiary of Forest Laboratories, Inc.
St. Louis, MO 63043-9979
© Forest Laboratories, Inc.   AWM-002-88   Patent Pending

Pharmacist: Detach here and give instructions to patient.
IMPORTANT INFORMATION

Package insert dosing instructions should be consulted for all metered dose inhalers (MDIs) when used with AeroChamber with *Mask*. Dosage and administration recommendations vary for different MDIs, and the limitations and conditions of use for each product should be considered before utilizing this device, particularly with younger and older patients.

BIBLIOGRAPHY

Conner WT, Dolovich MB, Frame R, Newhouse MT: Salbutamol administration to children under three by means of a mask and aerochamber. *J Clin Invest Med* 8:A179, 1985.

Rachelefsky GS, Rohr AS, Wo J et al: Use of a tube spacer to improve the efficacy of a metered-dose inhaler in asthmatic children. *AJDC* 140, 1986.

Salzman GA, Pyszczynski DR: Oral pharyngeal candidiasis in patients treated with beclomethasone dipropionate delivered by metered-dose inhaler alone and with AeroChamber. *J Allergy Clin Immunol* 81:424–428, 1988.

Sly RM, Barbera JM, Middleton HB, Eby DM: Delivery of albuterol aerosol by aerochamber to young children. *Ann Allergy* 60:403–406, 1988.

Manufactured by Monaghan Medical Corporation Plattsburgh, NY
Distributed by:

FOREST PHARMACEUTICALS, INC.
Subsidiary of Forest Laboratories, Inc.
St. Louis, MO 63043-9979
© Forest Laboratories, Inc.   AWM-002-88   Patent Pending

Shown in Product Identification Section, page 410

AMBENYL® Cough Syrup   © ℞
[ăm 'bĕn-il]

DESCRIPTION
Each 5 ml of AMBENYL Cough Syrup contains:
Codeine phosphate
  (Warning—May be habit-forming) .... 10 mg
Bromodiphenhydramine hydrochloride .... 12.5 mg
Alcohol, 5%
AMBENYL Cough Syrup also contains citric acid, D&C Red #33, ethyl alcohol, flavor, glucose liquid, glycerin, menthol, sodium citrate, sucrose, vanillin, water, and has a pH between 5.0 and 6.0.
Chemically, codeine phosphate is morphinan-6-ol,7,8-didehydro-4,5-epoxy -3- methoxy-17-methyl-,(5α,6α)-, phosphate (1:1)(salt),hemihydrate and bromodiphenhydramine hydrochloride is ethanamine,2-[(4-bromophenyl) phenylmethoxy]-N,N-dimethyl-, hydrochloride. The structural formulas are:

codeine phosphate

bromodiphenhydramine
hydrochloride

AMBENYL Cough Syrup is for oral administration.

CLINICAL PHARMACOLOGY
CODEINE: Codeine exerts its antitussive activity by depressing the medullary (brain) cough center, thereby raising its threshold for incoming cough impulses.
Codeine resembles morphine both structurally and pharmacologically, but its actions at the doses of codeine used therapeutically are milder, with less sedation, respiratory depression, and gastrointestinal, urinary, and pupillary effects. Codeine produces an increase in biliary tract pressure, but less than morphine or meperidine.
Codeine has good antitussive activity, although less than that of morphine at equal doses. It is used in preference to morphine, because side effects are infrequent at the usual antitussive dose of codeine.
Codeine may cause nausea and vomiting by stimulating the chemoreceptor trigger zone (CTZ); however, it may also depress the vomiting center, so that subsequent doses are unlikely to produce vomiting. Nausea is minimal after usual oral doses of codeine.
Codeine causes histamine release, which may also produce dilation of cutaneous blood vessels, with resultant flushing of the face and neck, pruritus, and sweating.
Codeine is readily absorbed from the gastrointestinal tract following oral administration. Codeine is metabolized primarily in the liver by enzymes of the endoplasmic reticulum, where it undergoes O-demethylation, N-demethylation, and partial conjugation with glucuronic acid. The drug is excreted primarily in the urine largely as inactive metabolites and small amounts of free and conjugated morphine. Negligible amounts of codeine and its metabolites are found in the feces.
The cough-depressing action, in animal studies, was observed to occur 15 minutes after oral administration of co-

deine, peak action at 45 to 60 minutes after ingestion. The duration of action, which is dose-dependent, usually did not exceed three hours.
BROMODIPHENHYDRAMINE: Antihistamines competitively antagonize various physiological effects of histamine including increased capillary permeability and dilatation, the formation of edema, the "flare" and "itch" response, and gastrointestinal and respiratory smooth-muscle constriction. Within the vascular tree, antihistamines inhibit both the vasoconstrictor and vasodilator effects of histamine. Depending on the dose, antihistamines can produce CNS stimulation or depression. Most antihistamines exhibit central and / or peripheral anticholinergic activity.
Antihistamines are well absorbed following oral administration. Many antihistamines achieve peak blood levels within two to five hours following oral administration.
Tissue distribution of the antihistamines in humans has not been established. Diphenhydramine hydrochloride and probably other antihistamines cross the placenta.
Antihistamines appear to be metabolized in the liver chiefly via mono- and didemethylation and glucuronide conjugation. Antihistamine metabolites and small amounts of unchanged drug are excreted in the urine. Small amounts of the drugs may also be excreted in breast milk.

INDICATIONS AND USAGE
AMBENYL is indicated for temporary relief of upper respiratory symptoms and coughs associated with allergies or the common cold.

CONTRAINDICATIONS
Use in Newborn or Premature Infants: This drug should *not* be used in newborn or premature infants.
AMBENYL Cough Syrup is contraindicated in patients with known hypersensitivity to codeine phosphate, bromodiphenhydramine hydrochloride, and any other drugs of similar chemical structures.

WARNINGS
Antihistamines should be used with considerable caution in patients with:
Narrow angle glaucoma
Stenosing peptic ulcer
Pyloroduodenal obstruction
Symptomatic prostatic hypertrophy
Bladder neck obstruction
Overdoses of antihistamines may cause hallucinations, convulsions or death, especially in infants and children (See **OVERDOSAGE**). Therapeutic doses of antihistamines can produce excitation or drowsiness.
AMBENYL Cough Syrup may have additive effects with alcohol and other CNS depressants (see **PRECAUTIONS:** Drug Interactions).
Patients should be warned about engaging in activities requiring mental alertness such as driving a car or operating appliances, machinery, etc.
Antihistamines are more likely to cause dizziness, sedation, and hypotension in elderly patients.
Dosage of codeine **should not be increased** if cough fails to respond; an unresponsive cough should be reevaluated in five days or sooner for possible underlying pathology, such as foreign body or lower respiratory tract disease.
Respiratory depression leading to arrest, coma, and death has occurred with the use of codeine antitussives in young children, particularly in the under-one-year infants whose ability to deactivate the drug is not fully developed.
Administration of codeine may be accompanied by histamine release resulting in flushing of the face and neck, pruritus, and sweating. It should be used with caution in atopic children.
Narcotics, including codeine, may produce adverse reactions which may obscure the clinical course of patients with head injuries.
Asthma and Other Respiratory Conditions: Cough suppressants, including codeine, should not be used in asthmatic patients (see **CONTRAINDICATIONS**). Nor should they be used in acute febrile illness associated with productive cough or in chronic respiratory disease where interference with ability to clear the tracheobronchial tree of secretions would have a deleterious effect on the patient's respiratory function.
Hypotensive Effect: Codeine may produce orthostatic hypotension in ambulatory patients.

PRECAUTIONS
General: Bromodiphenhydramine has an atropine-like action and, therefore, should be used with caution in patients with:
History of bronchial asthma
Increased intraocular pressure
Hyperthyroidism
Cardiovascular disease
Hypertension
At near toxic doses antihistamines can cause hallucinations. They have been abused by some patients to produce intoxication.
The drug abuse and dependence potential of antihistamines remains to be determined.

Codeine should be administered with caution and the initial dose reduced in patients with acute abdominal pathology, convulsive disorders, significant renal or hepatic impairment, fever, hypothyroidism, ulcerative colitis, prostatic hypertrophy, and in the very young or elderly or debilitated individual.
Information for Patients: AMBENYL Cough Syrup may cause marked drowsiness or may impair the mental and/or physical abilities required for the performance of potentially hazardous tasks, such as driving a vehicle or operating machinery. Ambulatory patients should be told to avoid engaging in such activities until it is known that they do not become drowsy or dizzy from the use of this product.
Codeine, unlike other narcotic analgesics, may produce orthostatic hypotension in some ambulatory patients.
Patients should report any involuntary muscle movements or unusual sensitivity to light.
Patients should be questioned regarding a history of glaucoma, peptic ulcer, urinary retention, or pregnancy before starting therapy with AMBENYL Cough Syrup.
Patients should be told the sedative effects may be additive if alcohol, sleeping pills, sedatives, or tranquilizers are taken with AMBENYL Cough Syrup.
AMBENYL Cough Syrup may cause drowsiness, dizziness, dry mouth, blurred vision, weakness, nausea, headache, or nervousness in some patients.
Patients should be told to store this medicine in a tightly closed container in a dry, cool place away from heat or direct sunlight and out of the reach of children.
Drug Interactions: AMBENYL Cough Syrup may potentiate the effects of other narcotics, general anesthetics, tranquilizers, sedatives and hypnotics, tricyclic antidepressants, MAO inhibitors, alcohol, and other CNS depressants.
Also, the prominent anticholinergic effects of the tricyclic antidepressants and monoamine oxidase (MAO) inhibitors are additive with those produced by other drugs having a similar action, including antihistamines, and may prolong and intensify the anticholinergic effects of antihistamines. This could result in a toxic confusional and delirious state in the elderly. Bromodiphenhydramine should be used with caution in patients receiving tricyclic antidepressants or MAO inhibitors such as isocarboxazid, pargyline hydrochloride, phenelzine sulfate, tranylcypromine sulfate and other drugs which do not achieve their therapeutic effect by MAO inhibition, but which, nevertheless are powerful MAO inhibitors, eg, Furoxone, procarbazine hydrochloride.
Carcinogenesis, Mutagenesis, Impairment of Fertility: No long-term studies in animals were performed to evaluate the carcinogenic potential of AMBENYL Cough Syrup.
Pregnancy: Pregnancy Category C. Animal reproduction studies have not been conducted with AMBENYL Cough Syrup. It is also not known whether AMBENYL Cough Syrup can cause fetal harm when administered to a pregnant woman or can affect reproduction capacity. AMBENYL Cough Syrup should be given to a pregnant woman only if clearly needed.
Nursing Mothers: Because of the potential for serious adverse reactions in nursing infants, from maternal ingestion of AMBENYL Cough Syrup, a decision should be made whether to discontinue nursing or to discontinue the drug, taking into account the importance of the drug to the mother.
Pediatric Use: Safety and effectiveness in children below the age of six have not been established.

ADVERSE REACTIONS
The most frequent adverse reactions are highlighted:

General	Urticaria, drug rash, anaphylactic shock, photosensitivity, excessive perspiration, chills, dryness of mouth, nose, and throat.
Cardiovascular System	Hypotension, headache, palpitations, tachycardia, extrasystoles.
Hematologic System	Hemolytic anemia, thrombocytopenia, agranulocytosis.
Nervous System	**Sedation, sleepiness, dizziness, disturbed coordination,** fatigue, confusion, restlessness, excitation, nervousness, tremor, irritability, insomnia, euphoria, paresthesia, blurred vision, diplopia, vertigo, tinnitus, acute labyrinthitis, hysteria, neuritis, convulsions.
Gastrointestinal System	**Epigastric distress, constipation,** anorexia, nausea, vomiting, diarrhea.
Genitourinary System	Urinary frequency, difficult urination, urinary retention.

Continued on next page

Forest Pharmaceuticals—Cont.

Respiratory System	**Thickening of bronchial secretions,** tightness of chest and wheezing, nasal stuffiness.

DRUG ABUSE AND DEPENDENCE

AMBENYL with codeine is a schedule V controlled substance. Codeine can produce drug dependence of the morphine type and, therefore, has the potential for being abused. Psychic dependence, physical dependence, and tolerance may develop upon repeated administration of this drug, and it should be prescribed and administered with the same degree of caution appropriate to the user of other oral narcotic-containing medications. Like other narcotic-containing medications, the drug is subject to the Federal Controlled Substances Act.

OVERDOSAGE

Serious overdosage with codeine is characterized by respiratory depression (a decrease in respiratory rate and/or tidal volume, Cheyne-Stokes respiration, cyanosis), extreme somnolence progressing to stupor or coma, skeletal muscle flaccidity, cold and clammy skin, and sometimes bradycardia and hypotension. The triad of coma, pinpoint pupils, and respiratory depression is strongly suggestive of opiate poisoning. In severe overdosage, particularly by the intravenous route, apnea, circulatory collapse, cardiac arrest, and death may occur. Bromodiphenhydramine is additive to the depressant effects of codeine.

It is difficult to determine what constitutes a standard toxic or lethal dose. However, the lethal oral dose of codeine in an adult is reported to be in the range of 0.5 to 1.0 gram. Infants and children are believed to be relatively more sensitive to opiates on a body weight basis. It is estimated that 5 mg/kg could be fatal in children. Elderly patients are also comparatively intolerant to opiates.

Antihistamine overdosage reactions may vary from CNS depression to stimulation. In children, stimulation predominates initially in a syndrome which may include excitement, hallucinations, ataxia, incoordination, muscle twitching, athetosis, hyperthermia, cyanosis, convulsions, tremors, and hyperreflexia followed by postictal depression and cardiorespiratory arrest. Convulsions in children may be preceded by mild depression. Dry mouth, fixed dilated pupils, flushing of the face, and fever are common. In adults, CNS depression, ranging from drowsiness to coma, is more common. The convulsant dose of antihistamines lies near the lethal dose. Convulsions indicate a poor prognosis.

In both children and adults, coma and cardiovascular collapse may occur. Deaths are reported especially in infants and children.

There is no specific therapy for acute overdosage with antihistamines. The latent period from ingestion to appearance of toxic effects is characteristically short (one-half to two hours). General symptomatic and supportive measures should be instituted promptly and maintained for as long as necessary.

Since overdoses of other classes of drugs (ie, tricyclic antidepressants) may also present anticholinergic symptomatology, appropriate toxicological analysis should be performed as soon as possible to identify the causative agent.

In the conscious patient, vomiting should be induced even though it may have occurred spontaneously. If vomiting cannot be induced, gastric lavage is indicated. Adequate precautions must be taken to protect against aspiration, especially in infants and children. Charcoal slurry or other suitable agents should be instilled into the stomach after vomiting or lavage. Saline cathartics or milk of magnesia may be of additional benefit.

In the unconscious patient, the airway should be secured with a cuffed endotracheal tube before attempting to evacuate the gastric contents. Intensive supportive and nursing care is indicated, as for any comatose patient.

If breathing is significantly impaired, maintenance of an adequate airway and mechanical support of respiration is the most effective means of providing adequate oxygenation. Hypotension is an early sign of impending cardiovascular collapse and should be treated vigorously. Although general supportive measures are important, specific treatment with intravenous infusion of vasopressor titrated to maintain adequate blood pressure may be necessary.

Do not use CNS stimulants.

Convulsions should be controlled by careful administration of diazepam or a short-acting barbiturate, repeated as necessary. Physostigmine may also be considered for use in controlling centrally mediated convulsions.

Ice packs and cooling sponge baths, not alcohol, can aid in reducing the fever commonly seen in children.

The LD_{50} (single oral dose) of bromodiphenhydramine is 366 mg/kg in the mouse and 602 mg/kg in the rat.

DOSAGE AND ADMINISTRATION

DOSAGE SHOULD BE INDIVIDUALIZED ACCORDING TO THE NEEDS AND THE RESPONSE OF THE PATIENT.

Adults—one or two teaspoonfuls every four to six hours, not to exceed 12 teaspoonfuls in 24 hours. Children (total intake of codeine phosphate should not exceed 1 mg/kg/24 hours) —Six to under 12 years of age—one-half to one teaspoonful every six hours.

Not recommended for use in children under 6 years of age.

HOW SUPPLIED

AMBENYL Cough Syrup is red and is supplied in 4 fl. oz. (NDC 0456-0681-04), 1 pint (NDC 0456-0681-16), and 1 gallon (NDC 0456-0681-28) bottles. Store at controlled room temperature 15°–30°C (59°–86°F).

Revised 2/88

AMBENYL®-D   OTC
[ăm ′bĕ-nĭl]
Decongestant Cough Formula

Antitussive-Expectorant-Nasal Decongestant

Two teaspoonfuls (10 ml) contain the following active ingredients:

Guaifenesin (glyceryl guaiacolate) .... 200 mg
Pseudoephedrine hydrochloride .... 60 mg
Dextromethorphan hydrobromide .... 30 mg
Also contains 9.5% alcohol, citric acid, FD&C Blue #1, FD&C Red #40, flavors, glycerin, menthol, methylparaben, saccharin sodium, sodium chloride, sorbitol solution, sucrose, and water.

HOW SUPPLIED

AMBENYL-D Decongestant Cough Formula is supplied in a 4-fl-oz bottle (NDC 0456-0682-04).

Issued 5/85

ANTILIRIUM   ℞
(physostigmine salicylate)

DESCRIPTION

ANTILIRIUM (Physostigmine Salicylate) is a derivative of the Calabar bean, and its active moiety, physostigmine, is also known as eserine.

It is soluble in water and a 0.5% aqueous solution has a pH of 5.8.

ANTILIRIUM Injection is available in 2 ml ampuls, each ml containing 1 mg of Physostigmine Salicylate in a vehicle composed of sodium bisulfite 0.1%, benzyl alcohol 2.0% as a preservative in water for injection.

CLINICAL PHARMACOLOGY

ANTILIRIUM is a reversible anticholinesterase which effectively increases the concentration of acetylcholine at the sites of cholinergic transmission. The action of acetylcholine is normally very transient because of its hydrolysis by the enzyme, acetylcholinesterase. ANTILIRIUM inhibits the destructive action of acetylcholinesterase and thereby prolongs and exaggerates the effect of the acetylcholine.

ANTILIRIUM contains a tertiary amine and easily penetrates the blood brain barrier, while an anticholinesterase, such as neostigmine, which has a quaternary ammonium ion is not capable of crossing the barrier. ANTILIRIUM can reverse both central and peripheral anticholinergia. The anticholinergic syndrome has both central and peripheral signs and symptoms. Central toxic effects include anxiety, delirium, disorientation, hallucinations, hyper-activity and seizures. Severe poisoning may produce coma, medullary paralysis and death. Peripheral toxicity is characterized by tachycardia, hyperpyrexia, mydriasis, vasodilatation, urinary retention, diminution of gastrointestinal motility, decrease of secretion in salivary and sweat glands, and loss of secretions in the pharynx, bronchi, and nasal passages.

Dramatic reversal of the effects of anticholinergic symptoms can be expected in minutes after the intravenous administration of ANTILIRIUM, if the diagnosis is correct and the patient has not suffered anoxia or other insult. The duration of action of ANTILIRIUM is relatively short, approx. 45 to 60 minutes.

Numerous drugs and some plants produce the anticholinergic syndrome either directly or as a side effect; this undesirable or potentially dangerous phenomenon may be brought about by either therapeutic doses or overdoses of the drugs. Such drugs include among others, atropine, other derivatives of the belladonna alkaloids, tricyclic antidepressants, phenothiazines, and antihistamines.

INDICATIONS AND USAGES

To reverse the effect upon the central nervous system, caused by clinical or toxic dosages of drugs capable of producing the anticholinergic syndrome.

CONTRAINDICATIONS

ANTILIRIUM should not be used in the presence of asthma, gangrene, diabetes, cardiovascular disease, mechanical obstruction of the intestine or urogenital tract or any vagotonic state, and in patients receiving choline esters or depolarizing neuromuscular blocking agents (decamethonium succinylcholine).

For post-anesthesia, the concomitant use of atropine with the physostigmine salicylate is not recommended, since the atropine antagonizes the action of physostigmine.

WARNINGS

Contains sodium metabisulfite), a sulfite that may cause allergic-type reactions including anaphylactic symptoms and life-threatening or less severe asthmatic episodes in certain susceptible people. The overall prevalence of sulfite sensitivity in the general population is unknown and probably low. Sulfite sensitivity is seen more frequently in asthmatic than in non-asthmatic people.

If excessive symptoms of salivation, emesis, urination and defecation occur, the use of ANTILIRIUM should be terminated. If excessive sweating or nausea occur, the dosage should be reduced.

Intravenous administration should be a slow, controlled rate, no more than 1 mg per minute (see dosage). Rapid administration can cause bradycardia, hypersalivation leading to respiratory difficulties and possible convulsions.

An overdosage of ANTILIRIUM can cause a cholinergic crisis.

PRECAUTIONS

Because of the possibility of hypersensitivity in an occasional patient, atropine sulfate injection should always be at hand since it is an antagonist and antidote for physostigmine.

USAGE IN PREGNANCY

Safe use in pregnancy and lactation has not been established; therefore, use in pregnant women, nursing mothers or women who may become pregnant requires that possible benefits be weighed against possible hazards to mother and child.

ADVERSE REACTIONS

Nausea, vomiting and salivation; can be offset by reducing dosage. Bradycardia and convulsions, if intravenous administration is too rapid. See DOSAGE AND ADMINISTRATION.

OVERDOSAGE

Can cause a cholinergic crisis. Appropriate antidote is atropine sulfate.

DOSAGE AND ADMINISTRATION

Post Anesthesia Care: 0.5 to 1.0 mg intramuscularly or intravenously. INTRAVENOUS ADMINISTRATION SHOULD BE AT A SLOW CONTROLLED RATE OF NO MORE THAN 1 MG PER MINUTE. Dosage may be repeated at intervals of 10 to 30 minutes if desired patient response is not obtained.

Overdosages of Drugs That Cause Anticholinergia: 2.0 mg intramuscularly or intravenously AT SLOW CONTROLLED RATE (SEE ABOVE). Dosage may be repeated if life threatening signs, such as arrhythmia, convulsions or coma occurs.

Pediatric Dosage: Recommended dosage is .02 mg/kg, intramuscularly or by slow intravenous injection, no more than 0.5 mg per minute. If the toxic effects persist, and there is no sign of cholinergic effects, the dosage may be repeated at 5 to 10 minute intervals until a therapeutic effect is obtained or a maximum dose of 2 mg is attained.

IN ALL CASES OF POISONING, THE USUAL SUPPORTIVE MEASURES SHOULD BE UNDERTAKEN.

HOW SUPPLIED

Ampuls, 2 ml packed 12 per box, 1 mg per ml NDC-0456-1037-12.

CAUTION

Federal law prohibits dispensing without prescription.

BANCAP HC® CAPSULES   ©℞

DESCRIPTION

Each hard gelatin capsule contains:
Hydrocodone Bitartrate ....5 mg
   (WARNING: May be habit forming)
Acetaminophen ....500 mg
This product also contains FD&C Yellow No. 6
Hydrocodone bitartrate is an opioid analgesic and antitussive and occurs as fine, white crystals or as a crystalline powder. It is affected by light. The chemical name is: 4,5α-epoxy-3-methoxy-17-methylmorphinan-6-one tartrate (1:1) hydrate (2:5). its structure is as follows:

$C_{18}H_{21}NO_3 \cdot C_4H_6O_6 \cdot 2\frac{1}{2}H_2O$ M.W. 494.50

Acetaminophen, 4'-hydroxyacetanilide, is a non-opiate, non-salicylate analgesic and antipyretic which occurs as a white, odorless crystalline power possessing a slightly bitter taste. Its structure is as follows:

HO—⟨benzene ring⟩—NHCOCH$_3$

$C_8H_9NO_2$ 151.16

CLINICAL PHARMACOLOGY

Hydrocodone is a semisynthetic narcotic analgesic and antitussive with multiple actions qualitatively similar to those of codeine. Most of these involve the central nervous system and smooth muscle. The precise mechanism of action of hydrocodone and other opiates is not known, although it is believed to relate to the existence of opiate receptors in the central nervous system. In additon to analgesia, narcotics may produce drowsiness, changes in mood and mental clouding.

Radioimmunoassay techniques have recently been developed for the analysis of hydrocodone in human plasma. After a 10 mg oral dose of hydrocodone bitartrate, a mean peak serum drug level of 23.6 ng/ml and an elimination half-life of 3.8 hours were found.

The analgesic action of acetaminophen involves peripheral and central influences, but the specific mechanism is as yet undetermined. Antipyretic activity is mediated through hypothalamic heat regulating centers. Acetaminophen inhibits prostaglandin synthetase. Therapeutic doses of acetaminophen have negligible effects on the cardiovascular or respiratory systems; however, toxic doses may cause circulatory failure and rapid, shallow breathing. Acetaminophen is rapidly and almost completely absorbed from the gastrointestinal tract, producing maximum serum concentrations within 30 minutes to one hour. The plasma half-life in adults and children ranges from 0.90 hours to 3.25 hours with an average of approximately 2 hours. The drug distributes uniformly in most body fluids and is approximately 25% protein bound. Acetaminophen is conjugated in the liver, with less than 3% of the dose excreted unchanged in 24 hours. The primary metabolic pathway is conjugation to sulfate and glucuronide by-products. A minor oxidative pathway forms cysteine and mercapturic acid. These compounds are subsequently excreted by the kidneys into the urine.

INDICATIONS AND USAGE

For the relief of moderate to moderately severe pain.

CONTRAINDICATIONS

Hypersensitivity to acetaminophen or hydrocodone.

WARNINGS

Respiratory Depression: At high doses or in sensitive patients, hydrocodone may produce dose-related respiratory depression by acting directly on brain stem respiratory centers. Hydrocodone also affects centers that control respiratory rhythm, and may produce irregular and periodic breathing.

Head Injury and Increased Intracranial Pressure: The respiratory depressant effects of narcotics and their capacity to elevate cerebrospinal fluid pressure may be markedly exaggerated in the presence of head injury, other intracranial lesions or a preexisting increase in intracranial pressure. Furthermore, narcotics produce adverse reactions which may obscure the clinical course of patients with head injuries.

Acute Abdominal Conditions: The administration of narcotics may obscure the diagnosis or clinical course of patients with acute abdominal conditions.

PRECAUTIONS

Special Risk Patients: As with any narcotic analgesic agent, BANCAP HC Capsules should be used with caution in elderly or debilitated patients and those with severe impairment of hepatic or renal function, hypothyroidism, Addison's disease, prostatic hypertrophy or urethral stricture. The usual precautions should be observed and the possibility of respiratory depression should be kept in mind.

Information for Patients: BANCAP HC Capsules like all narcotics, may impair the mental and/or physical abilities required for the performance of potentially hazardous tasks such as driving a car or operating machinery; patients should be cautioned accordingly.

Cough Reflex: Hydrocodone suppresses the cough reflex; as with all narcotics, caution should be exercised when BANCAP HC Capsules are used postoperatively and in patients with pulmonary disease.

Drug Interactions: Patients receiving other narcotic analgesics, antipsychotics, antianxiety agents, or other CNS depressants (including alcohol) concomitantly with BANCAP HC Capsules may exhibit an additive CNS depression. When combined therapy is contemplated, the dose of one or both agents should be reduced.

The use of MAO inhibitors or tricyclic antidepressants with hydrocodone preparations may increase the effect of either the antidepressant or hydrocodone.

The concurrent use of anticholinergics with hydrocodone may produce paralytic ileus.

Usage in Pregnancy: Teratogenic Effects: Pregnancy Category C. Hydrocodone has been shown to be teratogenic in hamsters when given in doses 700 times the human dose. There are no adequate and well-controlled studies in pregnant women. BANCAP HC Capsules should be used during pregnancy only if the potential benefit justifies the potential risk to the fetus.

Nonteratogenic Effects: Babies born to mothers who have been taking opioids regularly prior to delivery will be physically dependent. The withdrawal signs include irritability and excessive crying, tremors, hyperactive reflexes, increased respiratory rate, increased stools, sneezing, yawning, vomiting, and fever. The intensity of the syndrome does not always correlate with the duration of maternal opioid use or dose. There is no consensus on the best method of managing withdrawal. Chlorpromazine 0.7 to 1.0 mg/kg q6h, and paregoric 2 to 4 drops/kg q4h, have been used to treat withdrawal symptoms in infants. The duration of therapy is 4 to 28 days, with the dosage decreased as tolerated.

Labor and Delivery: As with all narcotics, administration of BANCAP HC Capsules to the mother shortly before delivery may result in some degree of respiratory depression in the newborn, especially if higher doses are used.

Nursing Mothers: It is not known whether this drug is excreted in human milk. Because many drugs are excreted in human milk and because of the potential for serious adverse reactions in nursing infants from BANCAP HC Capsules, a decision should be made whether to discontinue nursing or to discontinue the drug, taking into account the importance of the drug to the mother.

Pediatric Use: Safety and effectiveness in children have not been established.

ADVERSE REACTIONS

Central Nervous System: Sedation, drowsiness, mental clouding, lethargy, impairment of mental and physical performance, anxiety, fear, dysphoria, dizziness, psychic dependence, mood changes.

Gastrointestinal System: Nausea and vomiting may occur; they are more frequent in ambulatory than in recumbent patients. The antiemetic phenothiazines are useful in suppressing these effects; however, some phenothiazine derivatives seem to be antianalgesic and to increase the amount of narcotic required to produce pain relief, while other phenothiazines reduce the amount of narcotic required to produce a given level of analgesia. Prolonged administration of BANCAP HC Capsules may produce constipation.

Genitourinary System: Ureteral spasm, spasm of vesical sphincters and urinary retention have been reported.

Respiratory Depression: BANCAP HC Capsules may produce dose-related respiratory depression by acting directly on brain stem respiratory centers. Hydrocodone also affects centers that control respiratory rhythm, and may produce irregular and periodic breathing. If significant respiratory depression occurs, it may be antagonized by the use of naloxone hydrochloride. Apply other supportive measures when indicated.

Drug Abuse and Dependence: BANCAP HC Capsules are subject to the Federal Controlled Substances Act (Schedule III). Psychic dependence, physical dependence, and tolerance may develop upon repeated administration of narcotics; therefore, BANCAP HC Capsules should be prescribed and administered with caution. However, psychic dependence is unlikely to develop when BANCAP HC Capsules are used for a short time for the treatment of pain.

Physical dependence, the condition in which continued administration of the drug is required to prevent the appearance of a withdrawal syndrome, assumes clinically significant proportions only after several weeks of continued narcotic use, although some mild degree of physical dependence may develop after a few days of narcotic therapy. Tolerance, in which increasingly large doses are required in order to produce the same degree of analgesia, is manifested initially by a shortened duration of analgesic effect, and subsequently by decreases in the intensity of analgesia. The rate of development of tolerance varies among patients.

OVERDOSAGE

Acetaminophen:

Signs and Symptoms: In acute acetaminophen overdosage, dose-dependent, potentially fatal hepatic necrosis is the most serious adverse effect. Renal tubular necrosis, hypoglycemic coma, and thrombocytopenia may also occur.

In adults, hepatic toxicity has rarely been reported with acute overdoses of less than 10 grams and fatalities with less than 15 grams. Importantly, young children seem to be more resistant than adults to the hepatotoxic effect of an acetaminophen overdose. Despite this, the measures outlined below should be initiated in any adult or child suspected of having ingested an acetaminophen overdose.

Early symptoms following a potentially hepatotoxic overdose may include: nausea, vomiting, diaphoresis and general malaise. Clinical and laboratory evidence of hepatic toxicity may not be apparent until 48 to 72 hours post-ingestion.

Treatment: The stomach should be emptied promptly by lavage or by induction of emesis with syrup of ipecac. Patients' estimates of the quantity of a drug ingested are notoriously unreliable. Therefore, if an acetaminophen overdose is suspected, a serum acetaminophen assay should be obtained as early as possible, but no sooner than four hours following ingestion. Liver function studies should be obtained initially and repeated at 24-hour intervals.

The antidote, N-acetylcysteine, should be administered as early as possible, and within 16 hours of the overdose ingestion for optimal results, but in any case, within 24 hours. Following recovery, there are no residual, structural or functional hepatic abnormalities.

Hydrocodone: Signs and Symptoms: Serious overdose with hydrocodone is characterized by respiratory depression (a decrease in respiratory rate and/or tidal volume, Cheyne-Stokes respiration, cyanosis), extreme somnolence progressing to stupor or coma, skeletal muscle flaccidity, cold and clammy skin, and sometimes bradycardia and hypotension. In severe overdosage, apnea, circulatory collapse, cardiac arrest and death may occur.

Treatment: Primary attention should be given to the reestablishment of adequate respiratory exchange through provision of a patent airway and the institution of assisted or controlled ventilation. The narcotic antagonist, naloxone is a specific antidote against respiratory depression which may result from overdosage or unusual sensitivity to narcotics, including hydrocodone. Therefore, an appropriate dose of naloxone hydrochloride should be administered, preferably by the intravenous route, and simultaneously with efforts at respiratory resuscitation. Since the duration of action of hydrocodone may exceed that of the antagonist, the patient should be kept under continued surveillance and repeated doses of the antagonist should be administered as needed to maintain adequate respiration.

An antagonist should not be administered in the absence of clinically significant respiratory or cardiovascular depression. Oxygen, intravenous fluids, vasopressors and other supportive measures should be employed as indicated. Gastric emptying may be useful in removing unabsorbed drug.

DOSAGE AND ADMINISTRATION

Dosage should be adjusted according to the severity of the pain and the response of the patient. However, it should be kept in mind that tolerance to hydrocodone can develop with continued use and that the incidence of untoward effects is dose related.

Oral: The usual adult dosage is one or two capsules every four to six hours as needed for pain. The total 24 hour dose should not exceed 8 capsules.

HOW SUPPLIED

Bancap HC (Hydrocodone Bitartrate 5 mg and Acetaminophen 500 mg) Capsules are black and red capsules imprinted FOREST 610. They are supplied as:
Bottles of 100—NDC 0456-0610-01
Bottles of 500—NDC 0456-0610-02
Unit Dose package of 25—NDC 0456-0610-45
Store at controlled room temperature 15°–30°C (59°–86°F).
CAUTION: Federal law prohibits dispensing without prescription.
Revised MARCH 88

Shown in Product Identification Section, page 410

DALALONE D.P.® INJECTION   ℞
(Dexamethasone acetate suspension)
Equivalent to Dexamethasone 16 mg/ml

PRODUCT OVERVIEW

KEY FACTS

Dalalone D.P. injection is a synthetic, long-acting, depot adrenocorticosteroid agent that provides a prompt onset of action. Each ml of suspension contains 16 mg of dexamethasone. It may be administered via intramuscular, intra-articular, or soft tissue injection, but must not be given intravenously or intralesionally.

MAJOR USES

Dexamethasone, a fluorinated derivative of prednisolone, is used primarily for its potent anti-inflammatory effects in disorders of many organ systems and other diseases responsive to glucocorticosteroids. At equipotent anti-inflammatory doses, dexamethasone almost lacks the sodium-retaining property of hydrocortisone.

SAFETY INFORMATION

Contraindicated in patients with systemic fungal infections. Corticosteroids can mask signs of existing or new infection. Repeated injections at the same site are to be avoided, as are subcutaneous injections, and injections into the deltoid muscle.

Continued on next page

Forest Pharmaceuticals—Cont.

<u>PRESCRIBING</u> <u>INFORMATION</u>

DALALONE D.P.® INJECTION   ℞
(Dexamethasone acetate suspension)
Equivalent to Dexamethasone 16 mg/ml

NOT FOR INTRAVENOUS OR INTRALESIONAL USE
FOR INTRAMUSCULAR, INTRA-ARTICULAR AND
SOFT TISSUE USE

DESCRIPTION
Dexamethasone acetate, a synthetic adrenocortical steroid, is a white to practically white, odorless powder. It is a practically insoluble ester of dexamethasone.

It has a molecular weight of 434.5 and its empirical formula is $C_{24}H_{31}FO_6$.

Dexamethasone Acetate suspension is a sterile white suspension that settles on standing, but is easily resuspended by mild shaking.

Each ml. contains: Dexamethasone Acetate equivalent to Dexamethasone 16 mg., Sodium Chloride 6.67 mg., Creatinine 5 mg., Edetate Disodium 0.5 mg., Carboxymethylcellulose Sodium 5 mg., Polysorbate 80 - 0.75 mg., Benzyl Alcohol 9 mg., Sodium Bisulfite 1 mg. as preservatives in Water for Injection q.s., Sodium Hydroxide to adjust pH.

CLINICAL PHARMACOLOGY
Dexamethasone Acetate suspension is a long-acting, repository adrenocorticosteroid preparation with a prompt onset of action. It is suitable for intramuscular or local injection, but not when an immediate effect of short duration is desired.

Naturally occurring glucocorticoids (hydrocortisone and cortisone), which also have salt-retaining properties, are used as replacement therapy in adrenocortical deficiency states. Their synthetic analogs, including dexamethasone, are primarily used for their potent anti-inflammatory effects in disorders of many organ systems.

Glucocorticoids cause profound and varied metabolic effects. In addition, they modify the body's immune responses to diverse stimuli.

At equipotent anti-inflammatory doses, dexamethasone almost completely lacks the sodium-retaining property of hydrocortisone.

INDICATIONS AND USAGE
A. Intramuscular administration. When oral therapy is not feasible and the strength, dosage form, and route of administration of the drug reasonably lend the preparation to the treatment of the condition, those products labeled for intramuscular use are indicated as follows:

1. Endocrine disorders
Primary or secondary adrenocortical insufficiency (hydrocortisone or cortisone is the drug of choice; synthetic analogs may be used in conjunction with mineralocorticoids where applicable; in infancy, mineralocorticoid supplementation is of particular importance).

Acute adrenocortical insufficiency (hydrocortisone or cortisone is the drug of choice; mineralocorticoid supplementation may be necessary, particularly when synthetic analogs are used).

Preoperatively and in the event of serious trauma or illness, in patients with known adrenal insufficiency or when adrenocortical reserve is doubtful.

Shock unresponsive to conventional therapy if adrenocortical insufficiency exists or is suspected.

Congenital adrenal hyperplasia.
Nonsuppurative thyroiditis.
Hypercalcemia associated with cancer.

2. Rheumatic disorders
As adjunctive therapy for short-term administration (to tide the patient over an acute episode or exacerbation) in:
Post-traumatic osteoarthritis
Synovitis of osteoarthritis
Rheumatoid arthritis, including juvenile rheumatoid arthritis (selected cases may require low-dose maintenance therapy).
Acute and subacute bursitis
Epicondylitis
Acute nonspecific tenosynovitis
Acute gouty arthritis
Psoriatic arthritis
Ankylosing spondylitis

3. Collagen diseases
During an exacerbation or as maintenance therapy in selected cases of:
Systemic lupus erythematosus
Acute rheumatic carditis

4. Dermatologic diseases
Pemphigus
Severe erythema multiforme (Stevens-Johnson syndrome)
Exfoliative dermatitis
Bullous dermatitis herpetiformis

Severe seborrheic dermatitis
Severe psoriasis
Mycosis fungoides.

5. Allergic states
Control of severe or incapacitating allergic conditions intractable to adequate trials of conventional treatment in:
Bronchial asthma
Contact dermatitis
Atopic dermatitis
Serum sickness
Seasonal or perennial allergic rhinitis
Drug hypersensitivity reactions
Urticarial transfusion reactions
Acute noninfectious laryngeal edema (epinephrine is the drug of first choice).

6. Ophthalmic diseases
Severe acute and chronic allergic and inflammatory processes involving the eye, such as:
Herpes zoster ophthalmicus
Iritis, Iridocyclitis
Chorioretinitis
Diffuse posterior uveitis and choroiditis
Optic neuritis
Sympathetic ophthalmia
Anterior segment inflammation
Allergic conjunctivitis
Allergic corneal marginal ulcers

7. Gastrointestinal diseases
To tide the patient over a critical period of disease in:
Ulcerative colitis—(Systemic therapy)
Regional enteritis—(Systemic therapy)

8. Respiratory diseases
Symptomatic sarcoidosis
Berylliosis
Fulminating or disseminated pulmonary tuberculosis when used concurrently with appropriate antituberculous chemotherapy.
Loeffler's syndrome not manageable by other means.
Aspiration pneumonitis.

9. Hematologic disorders
Acquired (autoimmune) hemolytic anemia
Idiopathic thrombocytopenic purpura in adults (I.V. only; I.M. administration is contraindicated)
Secondary thrombocytopenia in adults
Erythroblastopenia (RBC anemia)
Congenital (erythroid) hypoplastic anemia.

10. Neoplastic diseases
For palliative management of leukemias and lymphomas in adults
Acute leukemia of childhood.

11. Edematous state
To induce diuresis or remission of proteinuria in the nephrotic syndrome without uremia, of the idiopathic type, or that due to lupus erythematosus.

12. Miscellaneous
Tuberculous meningitis with subarachnoid block or impending block when used concurrently with appropriate antituberculous chemotherapy.
Trichinosis with neurologic or myocardial involvement
Diagnostic testing of adrenocortical hyperfunction.

B. By intra-articular or soft tissue injection as adjunctive therapy for short-term administration (to tide the patient over an acute episode of exacerbation) in:
Synovitis of osteoarthritis
Rheumatoid arthritis
Acute and subacute bursitis
Acute gouty arthritis
Epicondylitis
Acute nonspecific tenosynovitis
Post-traumatic osteoarthritis

CONTRAINDICATION
Systemic fungal infections.

WARNINGS
Contains sodium metabisulfite, a sulfite that may cause allergic-type reactions including anaphylactic symptoms and life-threatening or less severe asthmatic episodes in certain susceptible people.

The overall prevalence of sulfite sensitivity in the general population is unknown and probably low. Sulfite sensitivity is seen more frequently in asthmatic than in non-asthmatic people.

DO NOT INJECT INTRAVENOUSLY. In patients on corticosteroid therapy subjected to any unusual stress, increased dosage of rapidly acting corticosteroids before, during, and after the stressful situation is indicated.

Corticosteroids may mask some signs of infection, and new infections may appear during their use. There may be decreased resistance and inability to localize infection when corticosteroids are used.

Prolonged use of corticosteroids may produce posterior subcapsular cataracts, glaucoma with possible damage to the optic nerves, and may enhance the establishment of secondary ocular infections due to fungi or viruses.

Usage in pregnancy. Since adequate human reproduction studies have not been done with corticosteroids, the use of these drugs in pregnancy, nursing mothers, or women of childbearing potential requires that the possible benefits of the drug be weighed against the potential hazards to the mother and embryo or fetus. Infants born of mothers who have received substantial doses of corticosteroids during pregnancy should be carefully observed for signs of hypoadrenalism.

Average and large doses of cortisone or hydrocortisone can cause elevation of blood pressure, salt and water retention, and increased excretion of potassium. These effects are less likely to occur with the synthetic derivatives except when used in large doses. Dietary salt restriction and potassium supplementation may be necessary. All corticosteroids increase calcium excretion.

While on corticosteroid therapy patients should not be vaccinated against smallpox. Other immunization procedures should not be undertaken in patients who are on corticosteroids, especially in high doses, because of possible hazards of neurologic complications and lack of antibody response.

If corticosteroids are indicated in patients with latent tuberculosis or tuberculin reactivity, close observation is necessary as reactivation of the disease may occur. During prolonged corticosteroid therapy, these patients should receive chemoprophylaxis.

Because rare instances of anaphylactoid reactions have occurred in patients receiving parenteral corticosteroid therapy, appropriate precautionary measures should be taken prior to administration, especially when the patient has a history of allergy to any drug.

Corticosteroids may suppress reaction to skin tests.

Repository adrenocorticosteroid preparations may cause atrophy at the site of injection. To minimize the likelihood and/or severity of atrophy, do not inject subcutaneously, avoid injection into the deltoid muscle, and avoid repeated intramuscular injections into the same site if possible. Dosage in children under 12 has not been established.

PRECAUTIONS
Dexamethasone Acetate suspension is not recommended as initial therapy in acute, life-threatening situations.

This product, like many other steroid formulations, is sensitive to heat. Therefore, it should not be autoclaved when it is desirable to sterilize the exterior of the vial.

Drug-induced secondary adrenocortical insufficiency may be minimized by gradual reduction of dosage. This type of relative insufficiency may persist for months after discontinuation of therapy; therefore, in any situation of stress occurring during that period, hormone therapy should be reinstituted. If the patient is receiving steroids already, the dosage may have to be increased. Since mineralocorticoid secretion may be impaired, salt and/or a mineralocorticoid should be administered concurrently.

There is an enhanced effect of corticosteroids in patients with hypothyroidism and in those with cirrhosis.

Corticosteroids should be used cautiously in patients with ocular herpes simplex for fear of corneal ulceration and perforation.

Psychic derangements may appear when corticosteroids are used, ranging from euphoria, insomnia, mood swings, personality changes, and severe depression to frank psychotic manifestations. Also, existing emotional instability or psychotic tendencies may be aggravated by corticosteroids.

Aspirin should be used cautiously in conjunction with corticosteroids in hypoprothrombinemia.

Steroids should be used with caution in nonspecific ulcerative colitis, if there is a probability of impending perforation, abscess or other pyogenic infection, also in diverticulitis, fresh intestinal anastomoses, active or latent peptic ulcer, renal insufficiency, hypertension, osteoporosis, and myasthenia gravis. Fat embolism has been reported as a possible complication of hypercortisonism.

An ulcer regimen including an antacid should be considered as a prophylactic measure during prolonged therapy.

Growth and development of infants and children on prolonged corticosteroid therapy should be carefully followed.

Steroids may increase or decrease motility and number of spermatozoa in some patients.

Since phenytoin, phenobarbital, ephedrine and rifampin may alter cortisol metabolism, glucocorticoid dosage adjustments may be required when any of these substances is started or stopped.

The prothrombin time should be checked frequently in patients who are receiving corticosteroids and coumarin anticoagulants at the same time because of reports that corticosteroids have altered the response to these anticoagulants. There are some reports of potentiation; others of inhibition.

Intra-articular injection of a corticosteroid may produce systemic as well as local effects.

Appropriate examination of any joint fluid present is necessary to exclude a septic process.

A marked increase in pain accompanied by local swelling, further restriction of joint motion, fever, and malaise are suggestive of septic arthritis. If this complication occurs and the diagnosis of sepsis is confirmed, appropriate antimicrobial therapy should be instituted.

Local injection of a steroid into an infected site is to be avoided.

Corticosteroids should not be injected into unstable joints. Patients should be impressed strongly with the importance of not over-using joints in which symptomatic benefit has been obtained as long as the inflammatory process remains active.

ADVERSE REACTIONS

Fluid and electrolyte disturbances:
Sodium retention
Fluid retention
Congestive heart failure in susceptible patients
Potassium loss
Hypokalemic alkalosis
Hypertension
Hypotensive or shock-like reaction
Musculoskeletal:
Muscle weakness
Steroid myopathy
Loss of muscle mass
Osteoporosis
Vertebral compression fractures
Aseptic necrosis of femoral and humeral heads
Pathologic fracture of long bones
Gastrointestinal:
Peptic ulcer with possible subsequent perforation and hemorrhage
Pancreatitis
Abdominal distention
Ulcerative esophagitis
Dermatologic:
Impaired wound healing
Thin fragile skin
Petechiae and ecchymoses
Erythema
Increased sweating
Other cutaneous reactions
Neurologic:
Convulsions
Increased intracranial pressure with papilledema (pseudotumor cerebri) usually after treatment
Vertigo
Headache
Endocrine:
Menstrual irregularities
Development of cushingoid state
Suppression of growth in children
Secondary adrenocortical and pituitary unresponsiveness, particularly in times of stress, as in trauma, surgery or illness
Decreased carbohydrate tolerance
Manifestations of latent diabetes mellitus
Increased requirements for insulin or oral hypoglycemic agents in diabetics
Ophthalmic:
Posterior subcapsular cataracts
Increased intraocular pressure
Glaucoma
Exophthalmos
Metabolic:
Negative nitrogen balance due to protein catabolism
Other:
Hypersensitivity
Thromboembolism
Weight gain
Increased appetite
Nausea
Malaise
The following **additional** adverse reactions are related to parenteral corticosteroid therapy:
Rare instances of blindness associated with intralesional therapy around the face and head
Hyperpigmentation or hypopigmentation
Subcutaneous and cutaneous atrophy
Sterile abscess
Postinjection flare (following intra-articular use)
Charcot-like arthropathy
Scarring
Induration
Inflammation
Paresthesia
Ecchymosis
Delayed pain or soreness
Muscle twitching, ataxia, hiccups, and nystagmus have been reported in low incidence after injection of Dexamethasone Acetate suspension

DRUG ABUSE AND DEPENDENCE
(See WARNINGS section).

OVERDOSAGE
(See ADVERSE REACTION section).

DOSAGE AND ADMINISTRATION
Dosage Requirements Are Variable and Must Be Individualized on the Basis of the Disease Under Treatment and the Response of the Patient.
Dosage in children under 12 has not been established.
Intramuscular Injection
Dosage ranges from 0.5 to 1 ml., equivalent to 8 to 16 mg. of dexamethasone. If further treatment is needed, dosage may be repeated at intervals of 1 to 3 weeks.
Intra-articular and Soft Tissue Injection
The dose varies, depending on the location and the severity of inflammation. The usual dose is 0.25 to 1 ml., equivalent to 4 to 16 mg. of dexamethasone. If further treatment is needed, dosage may be repeated at intervals of 1 to 3 weeks.
PROTECT FROM LIGHT, STORE AT CONTROLLED ROOM TEMPERATURE 59°–86° F. (15°–30° C). DO NOT PERMIT TO FREEZE. SENSITIVE TO HEAT—DO NOT AUTOCLAVE.
CAUTION: Federal law prohibits dispensing without prescription.
Literature Revised: **May 1982**

HOW SUPPLIED
Multiple dose vials of 5 ml, each ml containing dexamethasone acetate equivalent to dexamethasone 16 mg., NDC 0456-1097-05.
Also single dose vials of 1 ml., NDC 0456-1097-41.

DURAPHYL™   ℞
(anhydrous theophylline)
Theophylline Controlled Release Tablets

HOW SUPPLIED
Duraphyl (Theophylline Anhydrous) is available as 100 mg, 200 mg, and 300 mg controlled release tablets having the following identification characteristics:
Duraphyl 300 mg: capsule shaped, white, scored tablets, imp. FOREST/300. Available in bottles of 100 (NDC 0456-0634-01).
Duraphyl 200 mg: capsule shaped, white, bisected tablets, imp. FOREST/200. Available in bottles of 100 (NDC 0456-0633-01).
Duraphyl 100 mg: round concave, white, bisected tablets, imp. FOREST/100. Available in bottles of 100 (NDC 0456-0632-01).

STORAGE
Store at controlled room temperature 15°–30°C (59°–86°F). Dispense in tight containers.

CAUTION
Federal law prohibits dispensing without prescription.

ELIXOPHYLLIN®   ℞
[ĕ″lĭx·ŏff′fĭl·ĭn]
(theophylline anhydrous)
Capsules

ELIXOPHYLLIN® SR   ℞
(theophylline anhydrous)
Capsules

ELIXOPHYLLIN®   ℞
(theophylline anhydrous)
Elixir

DESCRIPTION
Elixophyllin® Capsules are available as Soft Gelatin Capsules intended for oral administration, containing 100 and 200 mg of Theophylline Anhydrous.
Each Elixophyllin® Capsule also contains the following inactive ingredients: gelatin, glycerin, methylparaben and sorbitol.
Elixophyllin® (theophylline anhydrous) SR Capsules
Elixophyllin® SR Capsules are designed to provide a prolonged therapeutic effect.
125 mg capsule—Each white, opaque, dye-free capsule contains 125 mg anhydrous theophylline.
250 mg capsule—Each clear, dye-free capsule contains 250 mg anhydrous theophylline.
Elixophyllin® (theophylline anhydrous) Elixir
ELIXOPHYLLIN Elixir is available as a liquid intended for oral administration, containing 80 mg of theophylline anhydrous and 20% alcohol in each 15 ml (tablespoonful).
ELIXOPHYLLIN Elixir also contains the following inactive ingredients: citric acid, FD&C Red #40, flavoring agent, glycerin, saccharin sodium and purified water. Elixophyllin Elixir has a pH of 3.0–4.0.
Theophylline is a bronchodilator structurally classified as a xanthine derivative. It occurs as a white, odorless, crystalline powder having a bitter taste. Theophylline anhydrous has the chemical name, 1H- Purine-2, 6-dione, 3,7-dihydro-1,3-dimethyl-, and is represented by the following structural formula:

ANHYDROUS THEOPHYLLINE

CLINICAL PHARMACOLOGY
Theophylline directly relaxes the smooth muscle of the bronchial airways and pulmonary blood vessels, thus acting mainly as a bronchodilator and smooth muscle relaxant. The drug also produces other actions typical of the xanthine derivatives: Coronary vasodilation, cardiac stimulant, diuretic, cerebral stimulant and skeletal muscle stimulant. It has also been demonstrated that aminophylline has a potent effect on diaphragmatic contractility in normal persons and may then be capable of reducing fatigability and thereby improve contractility in patients with chronic obstructive airways disease. The exact mode of action remains unsettled. Although theophylline does cause inhibition of phosphodiesterase with a resultant increase in intracellular cyclic AMP, other agents similarly inhibit the enzyme producing a rise of cyclic AMP but are unassociated with any demonstrable bronchodilation. Other mechanisms proposed include an effect on translocation of intracellular calcium; prostaglandin antagonism; stimulation of catecholamines endogenously; inhibition of cyclic guanosine monophosphate metabolism and adenosine receptor antagonism. None of these mechanisms has been proved, however.
In vitro, theophylline has been shown to act synergistically with beta agonists and there are now available data which do demonstrate an additive effect *in vivo* with combined use. Apparently, no development of tolerance occurs with chronic use of theophylline.
Pharmacokinetics:
The half-life of theophylline is influenced by a number of known variables. It may be prolonged in chronic alcoholics, particularly those with liver disease (cirrhosis or alcoholic liver disease), in patients with congestive heart failure, and in those patients taking certain other drugs (see **PRECAUTIONS, Drug Interactions**). Newborns and neonates have extremely slow clearance rates compared to older infants and children, i.e., those over 1 year. Older children have rapid clearance rates while most non-smoking adults have clearance rates between these two extremes. In premature neonates the decreased clearance is related to oxidative pathways that have yet to be established.

THEOPHYLLINE ELIMINATION CHARACTERISTICS

	Range	Half-life (in hours) Mean
Children	1 - 9	3.7
Adults	3 - 15	7.7

In cigarette smokers (1-2 packs/day) the mean half-life is 4-5 hours, much shorter than in non-smokers. The increase in clearance associated with smoking is presumably due to stimulation of the hepatic metabolic pathway by components of cigarette smoke. The duration of this effect after cessation of smoking is unknown but may require 6 months to 2 years before the rate approaches that of the non-smoker.

INDICATIONS AND USAGE
For relief and/or prevention of symptoms of asthma and reversible bronchospasm associated with chronic bronchitis and emphysema.

CONTRAINDICATIONS
This product is contraindicated in individuals who have shown hypersensitivity to its components. It is also contraindicated in patients with active peptic ulcer disease, and in individuals with underlying seizure disorders. (Unless receiving appropriate anti-convulsant medication).

WARNINGS
Serum levels above 20 mcg/mL are rarely found after appropriate administration of the recommended doses. However, in individuals in whom theophylline plasma clearance is reduced *for any reason,* even conventional doses may result in increased serum levels and potential toxicity. Reduced theophylline clearance has been documented in the following readily indentifiable groups: 1) patients with impaired liver function; 2) patients over 55 years of age, particularly males and those with chronic lung disease; 3) those with cardiac failure from any cause; 4) patients with sustained high fever; 5) neonates and infants under 1 year of age; and 6) those patients taking certain drugs (see **PRECAUTIONS, Drug Interactions**). Frequently, such patients have markedly prolonged theophylline serum levels following discontinuation of the drug.
Reduction of dosage and laboratory monitoring is especially appropriate in the above individuals.

Continued on next page

Forest Pharmaceuticals—Cont.

Serious side effects such as ventricular arrhythmias, convulsions or even death may appear as the first sign of toxicity without any previous warning. Less serious signs of theophylline toxicity (i.e., nausea and restlessness) may occur frequently when initiating therapy, but are usually transient; when such signs are persistent during maintenance therapy, they are often associated with serum concentrations above 20 mcg/mL.

Stated differently; *serious toxicity is not reliably preceded by less severe side effects.* A serum concentration measurement is the only reliable method of predicting potentially life-threatening toxicity.

Many patients who require theophylline exhibit tachycardia due to their underlying disease process so that the cause/effect relationship to elevated serum theophylline concentrations may not be appreciated.

Theophylline products may cause dysrhythmia and/or worsen pre-existing arrhythmias and any significant change in rate and/or rhythm warrants monitoring and further investigation.

Studies in laboratory animals (minipigs, rodents, and dogs) recorded the occurrence of cardiac arrhythmias and sudden death (with histologic evidence of myocardial necrosis) when beta-agonists and methylxanthines were administered concurrently. The significance of these findings when applied to humans is currently unknown.

PRECAUTIONS

General:
On the average, theophylline half-life is shorter in cigarette and marijuana smokers than in non-smokers, but smokers can have half-lives as long as non-smokers. Elixophyllin® Elixir should not be administered concurrently with other xanthine medications. Use with caution in patients with hypoxemia, hypertension or those with history of peptic ulcer. Theophylline preparations should be used cautiously in patients with history of peptic ulcer, since they may occasionally act as a local irritant to the G.I. tract; gastrointestinal symptoms, however, are more commonly centrally mediated and associated with serum drug concentrations over 20 mcg/mL.

Information for Patients:
The importance of taking only the prescribed dose and time interval between doses should be reinforced.

Laboratory Tests:
Serum levels should be monitored periodically to determine the theophylline level associated with observed clinical response and as the method of predicting toxicity. For such measurements, the serum sample should be obtained at the time of peak concentration, 1 to 2 hours after administration for immediate release products. It is important that the patient will not have missed or taken additional doses during the previous 48 hours and that dosing intervals will have been reasonably equally spaced. DOSAGE ADJUSTMENT BASED ON SERUM THEOPHYLLINE MEASUREMENTS WHEN THESE INSTRUCTIONS HAVE NOT BEEN FOLLOWED MAY RESULT IN RECOMMENDATIONS THAT PRESENT RISK OF TOXICITY TO THE PATIENT.

Drug Interactions:
Drug-Drug: Toxic synergism with ephedrine has been documented and may occur with some other sympathomimetic bronchodilators. In addition, the following drug interactions have been demonstrated:
Theophylline with:

Allopurinol (high-dose)	Increased serum theophylline levels
Cimetidine	Increased serum theophylline levels
Erythromycin, Troleandomycin	Increased serum theophylline levels
Lithium carbonate	Increased renal excretion of lithium
Oral Contraceptives	Increased serum theophylline levels
Phenytoin	Decreased theophylline and phenytoin serum levels
Rifampin	Decreased serum theophylline levels

Drug-Laboratory Test Interactions: Currently available analytical methods, including high pressure liquid chromatography and immunoassay techniques for measuring serum theophylline levels are specific. Metabolites and other drugs generally do not affect the results. Other new analytic methods are also now in use. The physician should be aware of the laboratory method used and whether other drugs will interfere with the assay for theophylline.

Carcinogenesis, Mutagenesis and Impairment of Fertility:
Long-term carcinogenicity studies have not been performed with theophylline.

Chromosome-breaking activity was detected in human cell cultures at concentrations of theophylline up to 50 times the therapeutic serum concentration in humans. Theophylline was not mutagenic in the dominant lethal assay in male mice given theophylline intraperitoneally in doses up to 30 times the maximum daily human oral dose.

Studies to determine the effect on fertility have not been performed with theophylline.

Pregnancy: Category C—Animal reproduction studies have not been conducted with theophylline. It is not known whether theophylline can cause fetal harm when administered to a pregnant woman or can affect reproduction capacity. Xanthines should be given to a pregnant woman only if clearly needed.

Nursing Mothers: Theophylline is distributed into breast milk and may cause irritability or other signs of toxicity in nursing infants. Because of the potential of serious adverse reactions in nursing infants from theophylline, a decision should be made whether to discontinue nursing or to discontinue the drug, taking into account the importance of the drug to the mother.

Pediatric Use: Sufficient numbers of infants under the age of 1 year have not been studied in clinical trials to support use in this age group; however, there is evidence recorded that the use of dosage recommendations for older infants and young children (16 mg/kg/24 hours) may result in the development of toxic serum levels. Such findings very probably reflect differences in the metabolic handling of the drug related to absent or undeveloped enzyme systems. Consequently, the use of the drug in this age group should carefully consider the associated benefits and risks. If used, the maintenance dose must be conservative and in accord with the following guidelines:
Initial Maintenance Dosage:
Premature Infants:
Up to 24 days postnatal age—1.0 mg/kg q 12h
Beyond 24 days postnatal age—1.5 mg/kg q 12h
Infants 6 to 52 weeks:
$[(0.2 \times \text{age in weeks}) + 5.0] \times$ kg body wt = 24 hour dose in mg.
Up to 26 weeks, divide into q8h dosing intervals.
From 26-52 weeks, divide into q6h dosing intervals.
Final Dosage should be guided by serum concentration after a steady state (no further accumulation of drug) has been achieved.

ADVERSE REACTIONS

The following adverse reactions have been observed, but there has not been enough systematic collection of data to support an estimate of their frequency. The most consistent adverse reactions are usually due to overdosage.
1. *Gastrointestinal:* nausea, vomiting, epigastric pain, hematemesis, diarrhea.
2. *Central nervous system:* headaches, irritability, restlessness, insomnia, reflex hyperexcitability, muscle twitching, clonic and tonic generalized convulsions.
3. *Cardiovascular:* palpitations, tachycardia, extrasystoles, flushing, hypotension, circulatory failure, ventricular arrhythmias.
4. *Respiratory:* tachypnea.
5. *Renal:* potentiation of diuresis.
6. *Others:* alopecia, hyperglycemia, inappropriate ADH syndrome, rash.

OVERDOSAGE

Management:
It is suggested that the management principles (consistent with the clinical status of the patient when first seen) outlined below be instituted and that simultaneously contact with a Regional Poison Control Center be established. In this way both updated information and individualization regarding required therapy may be provided.
1. When potential oral overdose is established and seizure has not occured:
a) If patient is alert and seen within the early hours after ingestion, induction of emesis may be of value. Gastric lavage has been demonstrated to be of no value in influencing outcome in patients who present more than 1 hour after ingestion.
b) Administer a cathartic. Sorbitol solution is reported to be of value.
c) Administer repeated dose of activated charcoal and monitor theophylline serum levels.
d) Prophylactic administration of phenobarbital has been shown to increase the seizure threshold in laboratory animals, and administration of this drug can be considered.
2. If patient presents with a seizure:
a) Establish an airway.
b) Administer oxygen.
c) Treat the seizure with intravenous diazepam, 0.1 to 0.3 mg/kg up to 10 mg. If seizures cannot be controlled, the use of general anesthesia should be considered.
d) Monitor vital signs, maintain blood pressure and provide adequate hydration.
3. If post-seizure coma is present:
a) Maintain airway and oxygenation.
b) If a result of oral medication, follow above recommendations to prevent absorption of the drug, but intubation and lavage will have to be performed instead of inducing emesis, and the cathartic and charcoal will need to be introduced via a large bore gastric lavage tube.
c) Continue to provide full supportive care and adequate hydration until the drug is metabolized. In general, drug metabolism is sufficiently rapid so as not to warrant dialysis. If repeated, oral activated charcoal is ineffective (as noted by stable or raising serum levels) charcoal hemoperfusion may be indicated.

DOSAGE AND ADMINISTRATION

Effective use of theophylline (i.e., the concentration of drug in the serum associated with optimal benefit and minimal risk of toxicity) is considered to occur when the theophylline concentration is maintained from 10 to 20 mcg/mL. The early studies from which these levels were derived were carried out in patients immediately or shortly after recovery from acute exacerbations of their disease (some hospitalized with status asthmaticus).

Although the 20 mcg/mL level remains appropriate as a critical value (above which toxicity is more likely to occur) for safety purposes, additional data are now available which indicate that the serum theophylline concentrations required to produce maximum physiologic benefit may, in fact, fluctuate with the degree of bronchospasm present and are variable. Therefore, the physician should individualize the range appropriate to the patient's requirements based on both symptomatic response and improvement in pulmonary function. It should be stressed that serum theophylline concentrations maintained at the upper level of the 10 to 20 mcg/mL range may be associated with potential toxicity when facts known to reduce theophylline clearance are operative. (See WARNINGS).

If it is not possible to obtain serum level determinations, restrictions of the daily dose (in otherwise healthy adults) to not greater than 13 mg/kg/day, to a maximum of 900 mg, in divided doses will result in relatively few patients exceeding serum levels of 20 mcg/mL and the resultant greater risk of toxicity.

Caution should be exercised for younger children who cannot complain of minor side effects. Older adults, those with cor pulmonale, congestive heart failure, and/or liver disease may have unusually low dosage requirements and thus may experience toxicity at the maximal dosage recommended below.

Theophylline does not distribute into fatty tissue. Dosage should be calculated on the basis of lean (ideal) body weight where mg/kg doses are presented.

Frequency of Dosing: When immediate release products with rapid absorption are used, dosing to maintain serum levels generally requires administration every 6 hours. This is particularly true in children, but dosing intervals up to 8 hours may be satisfactory in adults since they eliminate the drug at a slower rate. Some children, and adults requiring higher than average doses (those having rapid rates of clearance, e.g., half-lives of under 6 hours) may benefit and be more effectively controlled during chronic therapy when given products with sustained-release characteristics since these provide longer dosing intervals and/or less fluctuation in serum concentration between dosing.

Dosage guidelines are approximations only and the wide range of theophylline clearance between individuals (particularly those with concomitant disease) makes indiscriminate usage hazardous.

Dosage Guidelines:
I. Acute symptoms of bronchospasm requiring rapid attainment of theophylline serum levels for bronchodilation.
NOTE: Status asthmaticus should be considered a medical emergency and is defined as that degree of bronchospasm which is not rapidly responsive to usual doses of conventional bronchodilators. Optimal therapy for such patients frequently requires both *additional medication,* parenterally administered, and *close monitoring,* preferably in an intensive care setting.
A. Patients not currently receiving theophylline products.

	Theophylline Dosage	
	Oral Loading	Maintenance
Children age: 1 to 9 years	5mg/kg	4mg/kg q 6 hours
Children age: 9 to 16 years and smokers	5mg/kg	3mg/kg q 6 hours
Otherwise healthy non-smoking adults	5mg/kg	3mg/kg q 8 hours
Older patients and patients with cor pulmonale	5mg/kg	2mg/kg q 8 hours
Patients with congestive heart failure	5mg/kg	1-2mg/kg q 12 hours

B. Patients currently receiving theophylline products: Determine, where possible, the time, amount, dosage form, and route of administration of the last dose the patient received.
The loading dose for theophylline is based on the principle that each 0.5 mg/kg of theophylline administered as a loading dose will result in a 1.0 mcg/mL increase in

serum theophylline concentration. Ideally, the loading should be deferred if a serum theophylline concentration can be obtained rapidly.

If this is not possible, the clinician must exercise judgement in selecting a dose based on the potential for benefit and risk. When there is sufficient respiratory distress to warrant a small risk, then 2.5 mg/kg of theophylline administered in a rapidly absorbed form is likely to increase serum concentration by approximately 5 mcg/mL. If the patient is not experiencing theophylline toxicity, this is unlikely to result in dangerous adverse effects.

Subsequent to the decision regarding use of a loading dose for this group of patients, the maintenance dosage recommendations are the same as those described above.

II. Chronic Therapy

A. Initiating Therapy with an Immediate-Release Product:

It is recommended that the appropriate dosage be established using an immediate-release preparation. A dosage form which allows small incremental doses is desirable for initiating therapy. A liquid preparation should be considered for children to permit easier and more accurate dosage adjustment. Slow clinical titration is generally preferred to help assure acceptance and safety of the medication and to allow the patient to develop tolerance to transient caffeine-like side effects.

Initial Dose:	*16 mg/kg/24 hours or 400 mg/24 hours (whichever is less) of theophylline in divided doses at 6 or 8 hour intervals.*
Increasing Dose:	The above dosage may be increased in approximately 25 percent increments at 3 day intervals so long as the drug is tolerated; until clinical response is satisfactory or the maximum dose as indicated in section III (below) is reached. The serum concentration may be checked at these intervals, but at a minimum, should be determined at the end of this adjustment period. It is important that no patient be maintained on any dosage that is not tolerated. When instructing patients to increase dosage according to the schedule above, they should be told not to take a subsequent dose if apparent side effects occur and to resume therapy at a lower dose once adverse effects have disappeared.

III. Maximum Dose of Theophylline where the Serum Concentration is not measured:

WARNING: DO NOT ATTEMPT TO MAINTAIN ANY DOSE THAT IS NOT TOLERATED.

Not to exceed the following: (or 900 mg, whichever is less)

Age 1–9 years	24 mg/kg/day
Age 9–12 years	20 mg/kg/day
Age 12–16 years	18 mg/kg/day
Age 16 years and older	13 mg/kg/day

IV. Measurement of Serum Theophylline Concentrations During Chronic Therapy:

If the above maximum doses are to be maintained or exceeded, serum theophylline measurement is essential. (see PRECAUTIONS, Laboratory Tests, for guidance).

V. Final Adjustment of Dosage:

Dosage adjustment after serum theophylline measurement

If serum theophylline is:		*Directions:*
Within desired range		Maintain dosage if tolerated.
Too high	20 to 25 mcg/mL	Decrease doses by about 10% and recheck serum level after 3 days.
	25 to 30 mcg/mL	Skip the next dose and decrease subsequent doses by about 25%. Recheck serum level after 3 days.
	Over 30 mcg/mL	Skip next 2 doses and decrease subsequent doses by 50%. Recheck serum level after 3 days.
Too low		Increase dosage by 25% at 3 day intervals until either the desired serum concentration and/or clinical response is achieved. The total daily dose may need to be administered at more frequent intervals if symptoms occur repeatedly at the end of a dosing interval.

The serum concentration may be rechecked at appropriate intervals, but at least at the end of any adjustment period. When the patient's condition is otherwise clinically stable and none of the recognized factors which alter elimination are present, measurement of serum levels need be repeated only every 6 to 12 months.

HOW SUPPLIED

Elixophyllin® (brand of theophylline anhydrous) 100 mg Capsules are one piece, opaque capsules imprinted with FOREST 642. They are supplied as:

Bottles of 100 ....NDC 0456-0642-01

ELIXOPHYLLIN® (brand of theophylline anhydrous) 200 mg Capsules are one piece, opaque, capsules imprinted with FOREST 643. They are supplied as:

Bottles of 100 ....NDC 0456-0643-01
Bottles of 500 ....NDC 0456-0643-02
Unit Dose boxes
of 100 ....NDC 0456-0643-63

Elixophyllin® SR Capsules

125 mg Capsules
Bottles of 100 ....NDC 0456-0646-01
Bottles of 1000 ....NDC 0456-0646-00
Unit Dose Boxes
of 100 ....NDC 0456-0646-63

250 mg Capsules
Bottles of 100 ....NDC 0456-0647-01
Bottles of 1000 ....NDC 0456-0647-00
Unit Dose Boxes
of 100 ....NDC 0456-0647-63

ELIXOPHYLLIN® Elixir is a clear red solution with a mixed fruit flavor. Each tablespoonful (15 mL) contains 80 mg anhydrous theophylline.

ELIXOPHYLLIN® Elixir is available in bottles of
473 mL ....NDC 0456-0644-16
946 mL ....NDC 0456-0644-32
3785 mL ....NDC 0456-0644-28

ELIXOPHYLLIN®-GG   ℞

[ē ″lĭx-off′fĭl-ĭn gēē-gēē]
(theophylline-guaifenesin)
ORAL LIQUID

DESCRIPTION

Each 15 mL (tablespoonful) of ELIXOPHYLLIN®-GG (brand of theophylline-guaifenesin) Oral Liquid contains 100 mg anhydrous theophylline and 100 mg guaifenesin (glyceryl guaiacolate) in a cherry-berry flavored non-alcoholic liquid. ELIXOPHYLLIN®-GG Oral Liquid contains no sugar or dye.

Theophylline, a xanthine bronchodilator, is a white, odorless, crystalline powder having a bitter taste. Guaifenesin, a guaiacol compound is a white to slightly yellow crystalline powder with a bitter, aromatic taste.

ANHYDROUS THEOPHYLLINE

GUAIFENESIN

ELIXOPHYLLIN®-GG Oral Liquid also contains the following inactive ingredients: citric acid, flavoring agent, glycerin, methylparaben, propylene glycol, propylparaben, sorbitol and water.

CLINICAL PHARMACOLOGY

Theophylline:

Theophylline directly relaxes the smooth muscle of the bronchial airways and pulmonary blood vessels, thus acting mainly as a bronchodilator and smooth muscle relaxant. The drug also produces other actions typical of the xanthine derivatives: coronary vasodilation, cardiac stimulation, diuresis, cerebral stimulation, and skeletal muscle stimulation. The actions of theophylline may be medicated through inhibition of phosphodiesterase and a resultant increase in intracellular cyclic AMP. *In vivo* studies indicate that xanthines improve the contractile properties of the diaphragm in normal human subjects.

In vitro, theophylline has been shown to act synergistically with beta agonists that increase intracellular cyclic AMP through the stimulation of adenyl cyclase, but synergism has not been demonstrated in patient studies. More data are needed to determine if theophylline and beta agonists have a clinically important additive effect *in vivo*.

Apparently, tolerance does not develop with chronic use of theophylline.

Pharmacokinetics:

The half-life of theophylline is influenced by a number of known variables. It is prolonged in patients suffering from

chronic alcoholism, impaired hepatic or renal function, congestive heart failure, and in patients receiving macrolide antibiotics or cimetidine. Older adults (over age 55) and patients with chronic obstructive pulmonary disease, with or without cor pulmonale, may also have much slower clearance rates. For such patients, the theophylline half-life may exceed 24 hours.

Newborns and neonates have extremely slow clearance rates compared to older infants (over 6 months) and children, and may also have a theophylline half-life of over 24 hours. High fever for prolonged periods may also reduce the rate of theophylline elimination in adults as well as children.

THEOPHYLLINE ELIMINATION CHARACTERISTICS

	Theophylline Clearance Rates (mean ± S.D.)	Half-life Average (mean ± S.D.)
Children (over 6 months of age)	1.45 ± 0.58 ml/kg/min	3.7 ± 1.1 hr
Adult non-smokers uncomplicated asthma	0.65 ± 0.19 ml/kg/min	8.7 ± 2.2 hr

The half-life of theophylline in smokers (1 to 2 packs/day) averages 4 to 5 hours, much shorter than the half-life in non-smokers which averages 7 to 9 hours. The increase in theophylline clearance caused by smoking is probably the result of induction of drug-metabolizing enzymes that do not readily normalize after cessation of smoking. It appears that 3 months to 2 years may be necessary for normalization of the effect of smoking on theophylline pharmacokinetics.

Guaifenesin:

Guaifenesin exerts its expectorant action by reducing the viscosity of bronchial secretions, thereby increasing the efficiency of the cough reflex and of ciliary action in removing accumulated secretions from the trachea and bronchi. Unlike many other expectorants, guaifenesin rarely causes gastric irritation.

INDICATIONS

For relief and/or prevention of symptoms of asthma and reversible bronchospasm associated with chronic bronchitis and of emphysema.

CONTRAINDICATIONS

This product is contraindicated in individuals who have shown hypersensitivity to its components.

WARNINGS

Status asthmaticus should be considered a medical emergency and is that degree of bronchospasm which is not rapidly responsive to usual doses of conventional bronchodilators. Optimal therapy for such patients frequently requires both *additional medication*, parenterally administered, and *close monitoring*, preferably in an intensive care setting. Although increasing the dose of theophylline may bring about relief, such treatment may be associated with toxicity. The likelihood of such toxicity developing increases significantly when the serum theophylline concentration exceeds 20 µg/ml. Therefore, determination of serum theophylline levels is recommended to assure maximum benefit without excessive risk.

Serum levels about 20 µg/ml are rarely found after appropriate administration of the recommended doses. However, in individuals in whom theophylline plasma clearance is reduced *for any reason*, even conventional doses may result in increased serum levels and potential toxicity. Reduced theophylline clearance has been documented in the following readily identifiable groups: 1) patients with impaired renal or liver function; 2) patients over 55 years of age, particularly males and those with chronic lung disease; 3) those with cardiac failure from any cause; 4) neonates; and 5) those patients taking certain drugs (macrolide antibiotics or cimetidine). Decreased clearance of theophylline may be associated with either influenza immunization or active infection with influenza.

Reduction of dosage and laboratory monitoring is especially appropriate in the above individuals.

Less serious signs of theophylline toxicity, ie nausea and restlessness, may appear in up to 50% of patients. Unfortunately, serious side effects such as ventricular arrhythmias, convulsions or even death may appear as the first sign of toxicity without any previous warning. Stated differently; *serious toxicity is not reliably preceded by less severe side effects.*

Many patients who require theophylline may exhibit tachycardia due to their underlying disease process so that the cause/effect relationship to elevated serum theophylline concentrations may not be appreciated.

Theophylline products may cause arrhythmia and/or worsen pre-existing arrhythmias. Any significant change in cardiac rate and/or rhythm warrants monitoring and further investigation.

Continued on next page

Forest Pharmaceuticals—Cont.

PRECAUTIONS

General:
Theophylline half-life is shorter in smokers than in non-smokers.Therefore, smokers may require larger or more frequent doses. Theophylline should not be administered concurrently with other xanthine medications. Use with caution in patients with severe cardiac disease, severe hypoxemia, hypertension, hyperthyroidism, acute myocardial injury, cor pulmonale, congestive heart failure, liver disease, in the elderly (especially males), and in neonates. In particular, great caution should be used in giving theophylline to patients with congestive heart failure. Frequently such patients have markedly prolonged theophylline serum levels with theophylline persisting in serum for long periods following discontinuation of the drug.

Use theophylline cautiously in patients with history of peptic ulcer. Theophylline may occasionally act as a local irritant to the G.I. tract although gastrointestinal symptoms are more commonly centrally mediated and are associated with serum drug concentrations over 20 μg/ml.

Information for Patients:
The physician should reinforce the importance of taking only the prescribed dose and the time interval between doses. If necessary, taking the drug with food may help avoid local irritation of the G.I. tract.

Drug Interactions:
Toxic synergism with ephedrine has been documented and may occur with some other sympathomimetic bronchodilators. In addition, the following drug interactions have been demonstrated:

DRUG	EFFECT
Aminophylline with lithium carbonate	Increased excretion of lithium carbonate
Aminophylline with propranolol	Antagonism of propranolol effect
Theophylline with cimetidine	Increased theophylline blood levels
Theophylline with troleandomycin, erythromycin	Increased theophylline blood levels

Drug-Laboratory Test Interactions:
Guaifenesin has been shown to produce a color interference with certain clinical laboratory determinations of 5-hydroxy-indoleacetic acid (5-HIAA) and vanillylmandelic acid (VMA). When plasma levels of theophylline are measured by spectrophotometric methods, coffee, tea, cola beverages, chocolate, and acetaminophen contribute to falsely high values.

Carcinogenesis, Mutagenesis, and Impairment of Fertility:
Long-term animal studies have not been performed to evaluate the carcinogenic potential, mutagenic potential, or the effect on fertility of xanthine compounds.

Pregnancy:
Category C-Animal reproduction studies have not been conducted with theophylline. It is not known whether theophylline can cause fetal harm when administered to a pregnant woman or can affect reproduction capacity. Xanthines should be administered to a pregnant woman only if clearly indicated.

Nursing Mothers:
It has been reported that theophylline distributes readily into breast milk and may cause adverse effects in the infant. Caution must be used if prescribing xanthines to a nursing mother taking into account the risk-benefit of this therapy.

Pediatric Use:
Due to the marked variation in theophylline metabolism in infants under 6 months of age, this drug is not recommended for this age group.

ADVERSE REACTIONS
The most consistent adverse reactions are usually due to overdose and are:

1. *Gastrointestinal:* nausea, vomiting, epigastric pain, hematemesis, diarrhea.
2. *Central nervous system:* headaches, irritability, restlessness, insomnia, reflex hyperexcitability, muscle twitching, clonic and tonic generalized convulsions.
3. *Cardiovascular:* palpitations, tachycardia, extrasystoles, flushing hypotension, circulatory failure, ventricular arrhythmias.
4. *Respiratory:* tachypnea.
5. *Renal:* albuminuria, increased excretion of renal tubular and red blood cells, potentiation of diuresis.
6. *Others:* hyperglycemia and inappropriate ADH secretion, rash.

OVERDOSAGE

Management:
If potential oral overdose is established and seizure has not occurred:
A. Induce vomiting.
B. Administer a cathartic (this is particularly important if sustained-release preparations have been taken).
C. Administer activated charcoal.
If patient is having a seizure:
A. Establish an airway.
B. Administer oxygen.
C. Treat the seizure with intravenous diazepam, 0.1 to 0.3 mg/kg up to 10 mg.
D. Monitor vital signs, maintain blood pressure and provide adequate hydration.
Postseizure Coma:
A. Maintain airway and oxygenation.
B. If a result of oral medication, follow above recommendations to prevent absorption of the drug, but intubation and lavage will have to be performed instead of inducing emesis, and the cathartic and charcoal will need to be introduced via a large bore gastric lavage tube.
C. Continue to provide full supportive care and adequate hydration while waiting for the drug to be metabolized. In general, the drug is rapidly metabolized so as not to warrant consideration of dialysis. However, if serum levels exceed 50μg/ml, charcoal hemoperfusion may be indicated.

DOSAGE AND ADMINISTRATION
For most patients, *effective use* of theophylline, ie, associated with optimal likelihood of benefit combined with minimal risk of toxicity, is considered to occur when serum levels are maintained between 10 and 20 μg/ml. Levels above 20 μg/ml may produce toxicity, and in a small number of patients, toxicity may even be seen with serum levels between 15 and 20 μg/ml, particulary during initiation of therapy. There is considerable variation from patient to patient in the dosage required to achieve and maintain therapeutic and safe levels, primarily due to variable rates of elimination. Therefore, it is not only essential to individualize the dosage but to titrate and monitor serum levels when possible. When serum concentration cannot be obtained, restriction of dosage to the amounts and intervals recommended in the guidelines listed below becomes essential. Dosage should be calculated on the basis of lean (ideal) body weight where mg/kg doses are presented. Theophylline does not distribute into fatty tissue. Giving theophylline with food may prevent some

local gastric irritation. Although absorption is slower, it is still complete.

Frequency of Dosing: Dosing to maintain serum levels generally requires administration every 6 hours. This is particularly true in children, but dosing intervals up to 8 hours may be satisfactory in adults, since they eliminate the drug at a slower rate. Average maintenance dosage following theophyllinization*

Child 6 mos. to 9 yrs. (55 lbs):	1 tablespoonful (15 ml) q6h
Child 9-16 (75 lbs):	1 tablespoonful (15 ml) q6h
(110 lbs):	1½ tablespoonfuls (22.5 ml) q6h
(145 lbs):	2 tablespoonfuls (30 ml) q6h
Adult (150 lbs):	2 tablespoonfuls (30 ml) q8h

*Dosage must be individualized—see chart below left .
Dosage guidelines are approximations only and the wide range of theophylline clearance between individuals (particularly those with concomitant disease) makes indiscriminate usage hazardous.

As a practical consideration, it is not always possible to obtain serum level determinations. Under such conditions, the daily dose (in otherwise healthy adults) should not be greater than 16 mg/kg/day of anhydrous theophylline in divided doses. This will result in relatively few patients exceeding a serum level of 20μg/ml and the resultant risk of toxicity.

Dosage Guidelines:
I. Acute Symptoms of Asthma Requiring Rapid Theophyllinization:
  A. Patients not currently receiving theophylline products. Dosage recommendations are for theophylline anhydrous.
[See table below left].
  B. Patients currently receiving theophylline products: Determine, where possible, the time, amount, dosage form, and route of administration of the patient's last dose.
The loading dose for theophylline is based on the principle that each 0.5 mg/kg of theophylline administered as a loading dose will result in a 1.0 μg/ml increase in serum theophylline concentration. Ideally the loading dose should be deferred if a serum theophylline concentration can be obtained rapidly.
If this is not possible, the clinician must exercise judgment in selecting a dose based on the potential for benefit and risk. When there is sufficient respiratory distress to warrant a small risk, then 2.5 mg/kg of theophylline administered in a rapidly absorbed form is likely to increase serum concentration by approximatley 5 μg/ml. If the patient is not experiencing theophylline toxicity, this is unlikely to result in dangerous adverse effects. Subsequent to modifying the loading dose for this group of patients, the maintenance dosage recommendations are the same as those described above.
II. Chronic Therapy
Theophylline administration is a treatment of first choice for the management of chronic asthma (to prevent symptoms and maintain patient airways). Slow titration is generally preferred to assure acceptance and safety of the medication.

Initial Dose:	16 mg/kg 24 hr or 400 mg/24 hr (whichever is less) of anhydrous theophylline in divided doses at 6 or 8 hour intervals.
Increasing Dose:	The above dosage may be increased in approximately 25% increments at 2 to 3 day intervals so long as the drug is tolerated, until the maximum dose indicated in section III (below) is reached.

III. Maximum Dose of Theophylline Where the Serum Concentration is not Measured:
WARNING: DO NOT ATTEMPT TO MAINTAIN ANY DOSE THAT IS NOT TOLERATED.

	Not to exceed the following:
Age <9 years	24 mg/kg/day
Age 9-12 years	20 mg/kg/day
Age 12-16 years	18 mg/kg/day
Age >16 years	13 mg/kg/day OR 900 mg (WHICHEVER IS LESS)

NOTE: Use ideal body weight for obese patients.

IV. Measurement of Serum Theophylline Concentrations During Chronic Therapy:
If the above maximum doses are to be maintained or exceeded, serum theophylline measurement is recommended. The serum sample should be obtained at the time of peak absorption, 1 to 2 hours after administration for immediate-release products, and 4 hours after dosing for most sustained-release formulations. It is im-

	Oral Loading:	Followed by:	Maintenance:
1. Children 6 months to 9 yrs.	6 mg/kg	4 mg/kg q4h × 3 doses	4 mg/kg q6h
2. Children 9–16 yrs. and young adult smokers	6 mg/kg	3 mg/kg q4h × 3 doses	3 mg/kg q6h
3. Otherwise healthy non-smoking adults	6 mg/kg	3 mg/kg q6h × 2 doses	3 mg/kg q8h
4. Older patients and patients with cor pulmonale	6 mg/kg	2 mg/kg q6h × 2 doses	2 mg/kg q8h
5. Patients with congestive heart failure	6 mg/kg	2 mg/kg q8h × 2 doses	1–2 mg/kg q12h

portant that the patient will have missed no doses during the previous 48 hours and that dosing intervals will have been reasonably typical with no added doses during that period. DOSAGE ADJUSTMENT BASED ON SERUM THEOPHYLLINE MEASUREMENTS WHEN THESE INSTRUCTIONS HAVE NOT BEEN FOLLOWED MAY RESULT IN RECOMMENDATIONS THAT PRESENT RISK OF TOXICITY TO THE PATIENT.

V. Final Adjustment of Dosage: (See Table I)

Table I—Dosage adjustment after serum theophylline measurement

If serum theophylline		Directions:
Within normal limits	10 to 20 µg/ml	Maintain dosage if tolerated. Recheck serum theophylline concentration at 6 to 12 month intervals.*
Too high	20 to 25 µg/ml	Decrease doses by about 10%. Recheck serum theophylline concentration at 6 to 12 month intervals.*
	25 to 30 µg/ml	Skip next dose and decrease subsequent doses by about 25%. Recheck serum theophylline.
	Over 30 µg/ml	Skip next 2 doses and decrease subsequent doses by about 50%. Recheck serum theophylline.
Too low	7.5 to 10 µg/ml	Increase dose by about 25%.** Recheck serum theophylline concentration at 6 to 12 month intervals.*
	5 to 7.5 µg/ml	Increase dose by about 25% to the nearest dose increment and recheck serum theophylline for guidance in further dosage adjustment. Another increase will probably be needed, but this provides a safety check.

*Finer adjustments in dosage may be needed for some patients.
**The total daily dose may need to be administered at more frequent intervals if symptoms occur repeatedly at the end of a dosing interval.
1. From the J Resp Dis, 1981; 2(7):16

Caution should be exercised in younger children who cannot complain of minor side effects. Older adults, those with cor pulmonale, congestive heart failure, and/or liver disease may have unusually low dosage requirements and thus may experience toxicity at the maximal dosage recommended above. It is important that no patient be maintained on any dosage that is not tolerated. In instructing patients to increase dosage according to the schedule above, they should be instructed not to take a subsequent dose if apparent side effects occur and to resume therapy at a lower dose once adverse effects have disappeared.

HOW SUPPLIED

ELIXOPHYLLIN®-GG Oral Liquid is a clear, colorless, cherry-berry flavored non-alcoholic liquid. Each tablespoonful (15 ml) contains 100 mg anhydrous theophylline and 100 mg guaifenesin.
ELIXOPHYLLIN®-GG Oral Liquid is available in bottles of:
237 mL ....NDC 0456-0648-08
473 mL ....NDC 0456-0648-16

RECOMMENDED STORAGE

Product should be stored at controlled room temperature 15–30°C (59–86°F).
Revised 7-87

ELIXOPHYLLIN-KI®   ℞
(brand of theophylline anhydrous and potassium iodide) Elixir

(PLEASE REFER TO ELIXOPHYLLIN® [THEOPHYLLINE ANHYDROUS] ELIXIR FOR COMPLETE INFORMATION ON THEOPHYLLINE.)

DESCRIPTION
Each 15 mL (tablespoonful) of ELIXOPHYLLIN-KI® (brand of theophylline anhydrous and potassium iodide) Elixir con-

tains 80 mg anhydrous theophylline and 130 mg potassium iodide.
Theophylline, a xanthine bronchodilator, is a white, odorless, crystalline powder having a bitter taste. Potassium iodide is either colorless or white cubical crystals, or a white powder. Theophylline is represented by the following structural formula:

ANHYDROUS THEOPHYLLINE

ELIXOPHYLLIN-KI® Elixir also contains the following inactive ingredients; alcohol 10%, anise oil, citric acid, coloring agent, flavoring agents, glycerin, saccharin sodium, sodium bisulfite, sucrose and water.

CLINICAL PHARMACOLOGY
Potassium iodide acts as an expectorant by liquefying tenacious bronchial secretions.

INDICATIONS
For excessive tenacious mucus in chronic asthma, severe chronic and allergic bronchitis and chronic pulmonary emphysema.

WARNINGS
Status asthmaticus should be considered a medical emergency and is that degree of bronchospasm which is not rapidly responsive to usual doses of conventional bronchodilators. Optimal therapy for such patients frequently requires both *additional medication*, parenterally administered, and *close monitoring*, preferably in an intensive care setting. Although increasing the dose of theophylline may bring about relief, such treatment may be associated with toxicity. The likelihood of such toxicity developing increases significantly when the serum theophylline concentration exceeds 20µg/mL. Therefore, determination of serum theophylline levels is recommended to assure maximum benefit without excessive risk.
Serum levels above 20µg/mL are rarely found after appropriate administration of the recommended doses. However, in individuals in whom theophylline plasma clearance is reduced *for any reason*, even conventional doses may result in increased serum levels and potential toxicity. Reduced theophylline clearance has been documented in the following readily identifiable groups: 1) patients with impaired renal or liver function; 2) patients over 55 years of age, particularly males and those with chronic lung disease; 3) those with cardiac failure from any cause; and 4) those patients taking certain drugs (macrolide antibiotics or cimetidine). Decreased clearance of theophylline may be associated with either influenza immunization or active infection with influenza.
Reduction of dosage and laboratory monitoring is especially appropriate in the above individuals.
Less serious signs of theophylline toxicity, ie nausea and restlessness, may appear in up to 50% of patients. Unfortunately, serious side effects such as ventricular arrhythmias, convulsions or even death may appear as the first sign of toxicity without any previous warning. Stated differently; *serious toxicity is not reliably preceded by less severe side effects.*
Many patients who require theophylline may exhibit tachycardia due to their underlying disease process so that the cause/effect relationship to elevated serum theophylline concentrations may not be appreciated.
Theophylline products may cause arrhythmia and/or worsen pre-existing arrhythmias. Any significant change in cardiac rate and/or rhythm warrants monitoring and further investigation.
Potassium iodide can cause fetal harm when administered to a pregnant woman. Because of the possible development of fetal goiter, if this drug is used during pregnancy or if the patient becomes pregnant while taking it, the patient should be apprised of the potential hazard to the fetus.
Contains sodium bisulfite, a sulfite that may cause allergic-type reactions including anaphylactic symptoms and life-threatening or less severe asthmatic episodes in certain susceptible people. The overall prevalence of sulfite sensitivity in the general population is unknown and probably low. Sulfite sensitivity is seen more frequently in asthmatic than in non-asthmatic people.

PRECAUTIONS
Occasionally, persons are markedly sensitive to iodides and care should be used in administering ELIXOPHYLLIN-KI® Elixir for the first time. Caution is recommended in patients sensitive to iodides and in patients receiving potassium sparing diuretics or potassium supplements.
Drug Interactions

Potassium iodide with lithium carbonate	Increased hypothyroid and goitrogenic effect

Potassium Iodide—Thyroid function tests may be altered by iodides. As with any potassium containing medication, the potential for developing hyperkalemia is increased.
Since iodides are also secreted in human milk, caution must be used when prescribing ELIXOPHYLLIN-KI® Elixir to a nursing mother, taking into account the risk-benefit of this therapy.
Usage in Children:
Since safety and effectiveness in children have not been established it is recommended that ELIXOPHYLLIN-KI® Elixir not be used in children under 12 years of age.

ADVERSE REACTIONS
Potassium Iodide—Thyroid adenoma, goiter and myxedema are possible side effects of potassium iodide.
Hypersensitivity to iodides may be manifested by angioneurotic edema, cutaneous and mucosal hemorrhages, and symptoms resembling serum sickness, such as fever, arthralgia, lymph node enlargement and eosinophilia.
Iodism or chronic iodine poisoning may occur during prolonged treatment. The symptoms of iodism include: a metallic taste, soreness of the mouth, increased salivation, coryza, sneezing and swelling of the eyelids. There may be a severe headache, productive cough, pulmonary edema and swelling and tenderness of the salivary glands. Acneform skin lesions are seen in the seborrheic areas. Severe and sometimes fatal skin eruptions may develop. Gastric disturbance and diarrhea are common. If iodism appears, the drug should be withdrawn and the patient given appropriate supportive therapy.

HOW SUPPLIED
ELIXOPHYLLIN-KI® Elixir is a clear yellowish amber solution with an anise aroma. Each tablespoonful (15 ml) contains 80 mg anhydrous theophylline and 130 mg potassium iodide.
ELIXOPHYLLIN-KI® Elixir is available in bottles of:
237 ml ....NDC 0456-0645-08

RECOMMENDED STORAGE
Product should be stored at controlled room temperature 15–30°C (59 –86°F).
Dispense in tight container.

ESGIC®   ℞
[es 'jik]
(butalbital, acetaminophen and caffeine)
CAPSULES, TABLETS

PRODUCT OVERVIEW

KEY FACTS
Esgic is a combination product that provides analgesia, muscle relaxation, and anti-anxiety activity. Each tablet or capsule contains 50 mg of butalbital, 325 mg of acetaminophen, and 40 mg of caffeine.

MAJOR USES
Esgic is used to relieve the symptoms that accompany tension or muscle contraction headache.

SAFETY INFORMATION
Contraindicated in patients who are allergic to barbiturates, acetaminophen, or caffeine, and in those who have porphyria. Esgic should be prescribed cautiously for patients who have a tendency to use excessive quantities of drugs, a potential characteristic of chronic tension headache sufferers. Barbiturates can also alter the metabolism of other drugs. Concomitant administration of Esgic and other CNS depressants can augment CNS depression.

PRESCRIBING INFORMATION
ESGIC®   ℞
[es 'jik]
(butalbital, acetaminophen and caffeine)
CAPSULES, TABLETS

DESCRIPTION
Each Esgic® tablet or capsule for oral administration contains:
Butalbital*   50 mg.
(isobutylallylbarbituric acid)
*Warning: May be habit forming
Acetaminophen   325 mg.
Caffeine anhydrous   40 mg.
Butalbital, 5-allyl-5-isobutylbarbituric acid, a white, odorless crystalline powder having a slightly bitter taste, is a short to intermediate-acting barbiturate. Its structure is as follows:

$C_{11}H_{16}N_2O_3$ M.W. 224.26

Continued on next page

Forest Pharmaceuticals—Cont.

Acetaminophen, 4'-hydroxyacetanilide, is a non-opiate, non-salicylate analagesic and antipyretic which occurs as a white, odorless crystalline powder possessing a slightly bitter taste. Its structure is as follows:

$C_8H_9NO_2$ M.W. 151.16

Caffeine, 1, 3, 7-trimethylxanthine, is a central nervous system stimulant, which occurs as a white powder or white glistening needles. It also has a bitter taste. Its structure is a follows:

$C_8H_{10}N_4O_2$ M.W. 194.19

CLINICAL PHARMACOLOGY

Pharmacologically, Esgic® combines the analgesic properties of acetaminophen-caffeine with the anxiolytic and muscle relaxant properties of butalbital.

INDICATIONS AND USAGE

Esgic® is indicated for the relief of the symptom complex of tension (or muscle contraction) headache.

CONTRAINDICATIONS

Hypersensitivity to acetaminophen, caffeine, or barbiturates. Patients with porphyria.

PRECAUTIONS

General:
Barbiturates should be administered with caution, if at all, to patients who are mentally depressed, have suicidal tendencies, or a history of drug abuse.
Elderly or debilitated patients may react to barbiturates with marked excitement, depression, and confusion. In some persons, barbiturates repeatedly produce excitement rather than depression.

Information for Patients
Practitioners should give the following information and instructions to patients receiving barbiturates.
A. The use of barbiturates carries with it an associated risk of psychological and/or physical dependence. The patient should be warned against increasing the dose of the drug without consulting a physician.
B. Barbiturates may impair mental and/or physical abilities required for the performance of potentially hazardous tasks (e.g., driving, operating machinery, etc.).
C. Alcohol should not be consumed while taking barbiturates. Concurrent use of the barbiturates with other CNS depressants (e.g., alcohol, narcotics, tranquilizers, and antihistamines) may result in additional CNS depressant effects.

Drug Interactions:
Patients receiving narcotic analgesics, antipsychotics, antianxiety agents, or other CNS depressants (including alcohol) concomitantly with Esgic® (Butalbital 50 mg [WARNING: May be habit forming], Acetaminophen 325 mg, and Caffeine anhydrous 40 mg) may exhibit additive CNS depressant effects.

Drugs	Effect
Butalbital with coumarin anticoagulants	Decreased effect of anticoagulants because of increased metabolism resulting from enzyme induction.
Butalbital with tricyclic antidepressants	Decreased blood levels of the antidepressant.

Usage in Pregnancy:
Adequate studies have not been performed in animals to determine whether this drug affects fertility in males or females, has teratogenic potential or has other adverse effects on the fetus. There are no well-controlled studies in pregnant women. Although there is no clearly defined risk, one cannot exclude the possibility of infrequent or subtle damage to the human fetus. Esgic® should be used in pregnant women only when clearly needed.

Nursing Mothers:
The effects of Esgic® on infants of nursing mothers are not known.
Barbiturates are excreted in the breast milk of nursing mothers. The serum levels of infants are believed to be insignificant with therapeutic doses.

Pediatric Use:
Safety and effectiveness in children below the age of 12 have not been established.

ADVERSE REACTIONS

The most frequent adverse reactions are drowsiness and dizziness. Less frequent adverse reactions are lightheadedness and gastrointestinal disturbances including nausea, vomiting and flatulence. Mental confusion or depression can occur due to intolerance or overdosage of butalbital.

DRUG ABUSE AND DEPENDENCE

Prolonged use of barbiturates can produce drug dependence, characterized by psychic dependence and tolerance. The abuse liability of Esgic® is similar to that of other barbiturate-containing drug combinations. Caution should be exercised when prescribing medication for patients with a known propensity for taking excessive quantities of drugs, which is not uncommon in patients with chronic tension headache.

OVERDOSAGE

The toxic effects of acute overdosage of Esgic® are attributable mainly to its barbiturate component, and, to a lesser extent, acetaminophen. Because toxic effects of caffeine occur in very high dosages only, the possibility of significant caffeine toxicity from Esgic® overdosage is unlikely.

Barbiturate:
Signs and Symptoms: Drowsiness, confusion, coma; respiratory depression; hypotension; shock.
Treatment:
1. Maintenance of an adequate airway, with assisted respiration and oxygen administration as necessary.
2. Monitoring of vital signs and fluid balance.
3. If the patient is conscious and has not lost the gag reflex, emesis may be induced with ipecac. Care should be taken to prevent pulmonary aspiration of vomitus. After completion of vomiting, 30 grams activated charcoal in a glass of water may be administered.
4. If emesis is contraindicated, gastric lavage may be performed with a cuffed endotracheal tube in place with the patient in the face down position. Activated charcoal may be left in the emptied stomach and a saline cathartic administered.
5. Fluid therapy and other standard treatment for shock, if needed.
6. If renal function is normal, forced diuresis may aid in the elimination of the barbiturate. Alkalinization of the urine increases renal excretion of some barbiturates, especially phenobarbital.
7. Although not recommended as a routine procedure, hemodialysis may be used in severe barbiturate intoxications or if the patient is anuric or in shock.

Acetaminophen:
Signs and Symptoms: In acute acetaminophen overdosage, dose-dependent, potentially fatal hepatic necrosis is the most serious adverse effect. Renal tubular necrosis, hypoglycemic coma, and thrombocytopenia may also occur.
In adults, hepatic toxicity has rarely been reported with acute overdoses of less than 10 grams and fatalities with less than 15 grams. Importantly, young children seem to be more resistant than adults to the hepatotoxic effect of an acetaminophen overdose.
Early symptoms following a potentially hepatotoxic overdose may include: nausea, vomiting, diaphoresis and general malaise. Clinical and laboratory evidence of hepatic toxicity may not be apparent until 48 to 72 hours post-ingestion.
Treatment: The stomach should be emptied promptly by lavage or by induction of emesis with syrup of ipecac. Patients' estimates of the quantity of a drug ingested are notoriously unreliable. Therefore, if an acetaminophen overdose is suspected, a serum acetaminophen assay should be obtained as early as possible, but no sooner than four hours following ingestion. Liver function studies should be obtained initially and repeated at 24-hour intervals.
The antidote, N-acetylcysteine, should be administered as early as possible, preferably within 16 hours of the overdose ingestion for optimal results, but in any case, within 24 hours. Following recovery, there are no residual, structural or functional hepatic abnormalities.

DOSAGE AND ADMINISTRATION

Oral: One or two capsules/tablets every four hours as needed. Do not exceed 6 capsules/tablets per day.

HOW SUPPLIED

Esgic® (Butalbital 50 mg [WARNING—May be habit forming], Acetaminophen 325 mg and Caffeine anhydrous 40 mg) Tablets are white, round compressed, scored tablets imprinted with FOREST on one side and 630 on the opposite side. They are supplied as :
Bottles of 100—NDC 0456-0630-01
Bottles of 500—NDC 0456-0630-02
Esgic® (Butalbital 50 mg [WARNING—May be habit forming], Acetaminophen 325 mg and Caffeine anhydrous 40 mg) Capsules are white, opaque capsules imprinted with FOREST on one side and 631 on the opposite side. They are supplied as:
Bottles of 100—NDC 0456-0631-01
Store at controlled room temperature 15°–30°C (59°–86°F). Protect from moisture. Dispense in a tight container as defined in the USP/NF.
CAUTION: Federal law prohibits dispensing without prescription.
Revised 588
Shown in Product Identification Section, page 410

ESGIC® WITH CODEINE   CⅢ ℞
[es 'jik]

PRODUCT OVERVIEW

KEY FACTS

Esgic with Codeine is a combination product that provides analgesia, muscle relaxation, and anti-anxiety activity. Each capsule contains 50 mg of butalbital, 325 mg of acetaminophen, 40 mg of caffeine, and 30 mg of codeine phosphate.

MAJOR USES

Esgic with Codeine is used to relieve moderate to moderately severe pain in conditions where additional muscle relaxant or anti-anxiety properties would be beneficial. The product may also be used to control the symptoms of severe tension or muscle contraction headache.

SAFETY INFORMATION

Contraindicated in patients who are allergic to barbiturates, acetaminophen, caffeine, or codeine, and in those with porphyria. Patients with head injuries, increased intracranial pressure, or acute abdominal conditions are not good candidates for treatment with the product. Barbiturates can alter the metabolism of other drugs. Concurrent administration of Esgic with Codeine and sedative-hypnotics, alcohol, or other CNS depressants can potentiate respiratory and CNS depression.

PRESCRIBING INFORMATION

ESGIC® WITH CODEINE   CⅢ ℞
[es 'jik]
Caution: Federal law prohibits dispensing without prescription.

DESCRIPTION

Each ESGIC® with Codeine capsule for oral administration contains:
Butalbital* .... 50 mg
*Warning: May be habit forming
Acetaminophen ....325 mg
Caffeine anhydrous .... 40 mg
Codeine Phosphate* .... 30 mg
*Warning: May be habit forming
Butalbital, 5-allyl-5-isobutylbarbituric acid, a white, odorless, crystalline powder having a slightly bitter taste, is a short to intermediate-acting barbiturate. Its structure is as follows:

$C_{11}H_{16}N_2O_3$ M.W. 224.26

Acetaminophen, 4'-hydroxyacetanilide, is a non-opiate, non-salicylate analgesic and antipyretic which occurs as a white, odorless crystalline powder possessing a slightly bitter taste. Its structure is as follows:

$C_8H_9NO_2$ M.W. 151.16

Caffeine, 1,3,7-trimethylxanthine, is a central nervous system stimulant, which occurs as a white powder or white glistening needles. It also has a bitter taste. Its structure is as follows:

$C_8H_{16}N_4O_2$ M.W. 194.19

Codeine Phosphate, methylmorphine phosphate, is a white, odorless crystalline powder, freely soluble in water. It effloresces slowly in dry air and is affected by light. Codeine Phosphate is an opiate analgesic and antitussive. Its structure is as follows:

$N-CH_3$

$\cdot H_3PO_4 \cdot \frac{1}{2} H_2O$

CH_3O O OH

$C_{18}H_{24}NO_7P$ M.W. 397.37

CLINICAL PHARMACOLOGY

Pharmacologically, ESGIC® with Codeine combines the analgesic properties of acetaminophen, caffeine, and codeine with the anxiolytic and muscle relaxant properties of butalbital.

PHARMACOKINETICS

Butalbital

Butalbital is well absorbed from the gastrointestinal tract and is expected to distribute to most of the tissues in the body. Barbiturates in general may appear in milk and readily cross the placental barrier. They are bound to plasma and tissue proteins to a varying degree and binding increases directly as a function of lipid solubility.

The onset and duration of action, which is related to the rate at which the barbiturates are redistributed throughout the body, varies among persons and in the same person from time to time. Butalbital has a duration of action from 3 to 6 hours.

Barbiturates are metabolized primarily by the hepatic microsomal enzyme system and the metabolic products as well as the unchanged drug are primarily excreted in the urine, and less commonly, in the feces. The inactve metabolites of the barbiturates are excreted as conjugates of glucuronic acid.

Acetaminophen

Acetaminophen is rapidly and almost completely absorbed from the gastrointestinal tract, producing maximum serum concentrations within 30 minutes to one hour. The plasma half-life varies from one to four hours. Acetaminophen is relatively uniformly distributed throughout most body fluids and is approximately 25% protein bound. Approximately 90 to 95% of a dose is metabolized in the liver, primarily by conjugation with glucuronic acid, sulfuric acid, and cysteine. An intermediate metabolite is hepatotoxic. Excretion is renal; primarily as conjugates. About 3% of a dose may be excreted unchanged.

Codeine

Codeine is readily absorbed from the gastrointestinal tract, and is rapidly distributed from blood to body tissues. During distribution it is taken up preferentially by parenchymatous organs such as liver, spleen and kidney. It passes the blood-brain barrier and is found in fetal tissue and breast milk. The drug is not bound to plasma proteins nor does it accumulate in body tissues.

The elimination of codeine is primarily through the kidney. The plasma half-life is about 2.5–3 hours. The urinary excretion products represent about 90% of the dose within 24 hours and consist of free and glucuronide-conjugated codeine [about 70%], free and conjugated norcodeine [about 10%], free and conjugated morphine [about 10%], normorphine [under 4%] and hydrocodone [<1%]. The remainder of the dose appears in the feces.

Caffeine

Like most xanthines, caffeine is rapidly absorbed and distributed in all body tissues and fluids, including the CNS, fetal tissues and breast milk.

Caffeine is cleared rapidly through metabolism and excretion in the urine. The plasma half-life is about 3 hours. Hepatic biotransformation prior to excretion results in about equal amounts of 1-methylxanthine and 1-methyluric acid.

INDICATIONS AND USAGE

For the relief of moderate to moderately severe pain.

For the relief of moderate to moderately severe pain where additional muscle relaxant, and/or anxiolytic actions are desired such as in sprains/strains, fractures, displaced disc, back pain, etc.

For the relief of moderate to moderately severe pain where additional muscle relaxant, and/or anxiolytic actions are desired in surgical aftercare.

For the relief of the symptom complex of tension [or muscle contraction] headache where the severity would require the additional analgesic benefit of codeine.

CONTRAINDICATIONS

Hypersensitivity to acetaminophen, caffeine, barbiturates, or codeine. Patients with porphyria.

PRECAUTIONS

1. General

Head injury and increased intracranial pressure. The respiratory depressant effects of narcotics and their capacity to elevate cerebrospinal fluid pressure may be markedly exaggerated in the presence of head injury, other intracranial lesions or a pre-existing increase in intracranial pressure. Furthermore, narcotics produce adverse reactions which may obscure the clinical course of patients with head injuries.

Acute abdominal conditions. The administration of products containing codeine or other narcotics may obscure the diagnosis or clinical course in patients with acute abdominal conditions.

Special risk patients: ESGIC® with Codeine should be given with caution to certain patients such as the elderly or debilitated, and those with severe impairment of hepatic or renal function, hypothyroidism, Addison's disease, and prostatic hypertrophy or urethral stricture.

Barbiturates should be administered with caution, if at all, to patients who are mentally depressed, have suicidal tendencies or a history of drug abuse.

Elderly or debilitated patients may react to barbiturates with marked excitement, depression, and confusion. In some persons, barbiturates repeatedly produce excitement rather than depression.

2. Information for the Patient

Practitioners should give the following information and instructions to patients receiving barbiturates and codeine.

a. The use of codeine and butalbital carries with it an associated risk of psychological and/or physical dependence. The patient should be warned against increasing the dose of the drug without consulting a physician. Patients should take ESGIC® with Codeine only for as long as prescribed, in the amounts prescribed, and no more frequently than prescribed.

b. Barbiturates and codeine may impair mental and/or physical abilities required for the performance of potentially hazardous tasks [e.g., driving, operating machinery, etc.]

c. Central Nervous System depressant effects of butalbital and codeine may be additive with those of other CNS depressants. Concurrent use with sedative-hypnotics or alcohol should be avoided. When such combined therapy is necessary, the dose of one or more agents may need to be reduced to avoid respiratory depression.

d. Keep medication out of reach of children; overdose is especially dangerous in young children.

3. Drug Interactions

Patients receiving other narcotic analgesics, antipsychotics, antianxiety agents, or other CNS depressants [including alcohol] concomitantly with ESGIC® with Codeine [Butalbital 50 mg (Warning: May be habit forming), Acetaminophen 325 mg, Caffeine 40 mg, Codeine Phosphate 30 mg (Warning: May be habit forming)] may exhibit additive CNS depressant effects.

Barbiturates do not impair normal hepatic function, but have been shown to induce liver microsomal enzymes, thus increasing and/or altering the metabolism of barbiturates and other drugs.

DRUGS	EFFECT
Butalbital with coumarin anticoagulants	Decreased effect of anticoagulant because of increased metabolism resulting from enzyme induction.
Codeine with anticholiergics	May produce paralytic ileus

4. Usage in Pregnancy

Category C. Adequate studies have not been performed in animals to determine whether this drug affects fertility in males or females, has teratogenic potential or has other adverse effects on the fetus. There are no well-controlled studies in pregnant women. Although there is no clearly defined risk, one cannot exclude the possibility of infrequent or subtle damage to the human fetus. ESGIC® with Codeine capsules should be used in pregnant women only when clearly needed.

5. Nursing Mothers

The effects of ESGIC® with Codeine capsules on infants of nursing mothers are not known. Codeine, caffeine, and barbiturates are excreted in the breast milk of nursing mothers. Caution should be exercised when ESGIC® with Codeine is administered to a nursing woman.

6. Pediatric Use

Safety and effectiveness in children below the age of 12 have not been established.

ADVERSE REACTIONS

Nausea, vomiting, constipation, dizziness, weakness, drowsiness, and lethargy are the most common side effects. Overdosage is primarily manifested by drowsiness.

DRUG ABUSE AND DEPENDENCE

ESGIC® with Codeine is controlled by the Drug Enforcement Administration and is classified under Schedule III.

Codeine

Codeine can produce drug dependence of the morphine type, and therefore has the potential for being abused. Psychic dependence, physical dependence and tolerance may develop upon repeated administration and it should be prescribed and administered with the same degree of caution appropriate to the use of other oral narcotic medications.

Butalbital

Barbiturates may be habit forming: Tolerance, psychological dependence, and physical dependence may occur especially following prolonged use of high doses of barbiturates. The average daily dose for the barbiturate addict is usually about 1,500 mg. As tolerance to barbiturates develops, the amount needed to maintain the same level of intoxication increases; tolerance to a fatal dosage, however, does not increase more than two-fold. As this occurs, the margin between an intoxication dosage and fatal dosage becomes smaller. The lethal dose of a barbiturate is far less if alcohol or any other CNS depressant is also ingested. Major withdrawal symptoms [convulsions and delirium] may occur within 16 hours and last up to 5 days after abrupt cessation of these drugs. Intensity of withdrawal symptoms gradually declines over a period of approximately 15 days.

Treatment of barbiturate dependence consists of cautious and gradual withdrawal of the drug. Barbiturate-dependent patients can be withdrawn by using a number of different withdrawal regimens. One method involves initiating treatment at the patient's regular dosage level and gradually decreasing the daily dosage as tolerated by the patient.

OVERDOSAGE

The toxic effects of acute overdosage of ESGIC® with Codeine are attributable mainly to its barbiturate and codeine components, and, to a lesser extent, acetaminophen. Because toxic effects of caffeine occur in very high dosages only, the possibility of significant caffeine toxicity from ESGIC® with Codeine overdosage is unlikely.

Barbiturates

Symptoms:

Drowsiness, confusion, coma; respiratory depression; hypotension; shock.

Treatment:

1. Maintenance of an adequate airway, with assisted respiration and oxygen administration as necessary.
2. Monitoring of vital signs and fluid balance.
3. If the patient is conscious and has not lost the gag reflex, emesis may be induced with ipecac. Care should be taken to prevent pulmonary aspiration of vomitus. After completion of vomiting, 30 grams of activated charcoal in a glass of water may be administered.
4. If emesis is contraindicated, gastric lavage may be performed with a cuffed endotracheal tube in place with the patient in the face down position. Activated charcoal may be left in the emptied stomach and a saline cathartic administered.
5. Fluid therapy and other standard treatment for shock, if needed.
6. If renal function is normal, forced diuresis may aid in the elimination of the barbiturate. Alkalinization of the urine increases renal excretion of some barbiturates.
7. Although not recommended as a routine procedure, hemodialysis may be used in severe barbiturate intoxications or if the patient is anuric or in shock.

Acetaminophen

Signs and Symptoms:

Acetaminophen in massive overdosage may cause hepatic toxicity in some patients. In cases of suspected overdose, you may wish to call your regional poison center for assistance in diagnosis and for directions in the use of N-acetylcysteine as an antidote.

In adults, hepatic toxicity has rarely been reported with acute overdoses of less than 10 grams and fatalities with less than 15 grams. Importantly, young children seem to be more resistant than adults to the hepatotoxic effect of an acetaminophen overdose.

Early symptoms following a potentially hepatotoxic overdose may include: nausea, vomiting, diaphoresis and general malaise. Clinical and laboratory evidence of hepatic toxicity may not be apparent until 48 to 72 hours post-ingestion.

Treatment:

The stomach should be emptied promptly by lavage or by induction of emesis with syrup of ipecac. Patients' estimates of the quantity of a drug ingested are notoriously unreliable. Therefore, if an acetaminophen overdose is suspected, a serum acetaminophen assay should be obtained as early as possible, but no sooner than four hours following ingestion.

Continued on next page

Forest Pharmaceuticals—Cont.

Liver function studies should be obtained initially and repeated at 24-hour intervals.

The antidote, N-acetylcysteine, should be administered as early as possible, preferably within 16 hours of the overdose ingestion for optimal results, but in any case, within 24 hours. Following recovery, there are no residual, structural or functional hepatic abnormalities.

Codeine

Signs and Symptoms:

Serious overdose with codeine is characterized by respiratory depression [a decrease in respiratory rate and/or total volume, Cheyne-Stokes respiration, cyanosis], extreme somnolence progressing to stupor or coma, skeletal muscle flaccidity, cold and clammy skin, and sometimes bradycardia and hypotension. In severe overdosage, apnea, circulatory collapse, cardiac arrest ans death may occur.

Treatment:

Primary attention should be given to the reestablishment of adequate respiratory exchange through provision of a patent airway and the institution of assisted or controlled ventilation. The narcotic antagonist naloxone is a specific antidote against respiratory depression which may result from overdosage or unusual sensitivity to narcotics, including codeine. Therefore, an appropriate dose of naloxone should be administered, preferably by the intravenous route, and simultaneously with efforts at respiratory resuscitation. Since the duration of action of codeine may exceed that of the antagonist, the patient should be kept under continued surveillance and repeated doses of the antagonist should be administered as needed to maintain adequate respiration.

Gastric emptying may be useful in removing unabsorbed drug.

DOSAGE AND ADMINISTRATION

One or two capsules every 4 to 6 hours, repeated if necessary up to six capsules per day, as directed by physician.

HOW SUPPLIED

ESGIC® with Codeine [Butalbital 50mg (Warning: May be habit forming), Acetaminophen 325mg, Caffeine anhydrous 40 mg and Codeine Phosphate 30 mg (Warning: May be habit forming)] Capsules are black and blue capsules imprinted with FOREST on one half and 677 on the other half.

They are supplied as:

Bottles of 100—NDC 0456-0677-01

CAUTION:　Federal law prohibits dispensing without prescription.

Shown in Product Information Section, page 410

FEOSTAT Tablets　　　　　　　　　　　　　　OTC
FEOSTAT Suspension
FEOSTAT Drops
(Ferrous Fumarate)

FEOSTAT Tablets
Each chocolate-flavored chewable tablet contains:
　Ferrous fumarate ....100 mg.
　　(Elemental iron ....33 mg.)

FEOSTAT Suspension
Each 5 cc. (teaspoonful) contains:
　Ferrous fumarate ....100 mg.
　　(Elemental iron ....33 mg.)

FEOSTAT Drops
Each 12 drops (0.6 cc.) contains:
　Ferrous fumarate ....45 mg.
　　(Elemental iron ....15 mg.)

HOW SUPPLIED

Suspension: 8 ounce bottle; NDC-0456-0373-08.
Drops: 2 ounce bottle; NDC-0456-0374-21.
Tablets:
Bottle of 100, NDC-0456-0372-01.
Bottle of 1000, NDC-0456-0372-00.

IODO-NIACIN® TABLETS　　　　　　　　　　℞

DESCRIPTION

Each controlled action tablet contains:
Potassium Iodide ....135 mg
Niacinamide Hydroiodide ....25 mg

HOW SUPPLIED

Bottles of 100, NDC 0456-0295-01.
Bottles of 500, NDC 0456-0295-02.

KAY CIEL®　　　　　　　　　　　　　　　　℞
[kā'sēēl"]
(potassium chloride)
Oral Solution 10%

KAY CIEL®　　　　　　　　　　　　　　　　℞
(potassium chloride)
Powder

DESCRIPTION

ORAL SOLUTION—

Each 15 ml (tablespoonful) contains 1.5 g (20 mEq) potassium chloride in a palatable base.

KAY CIEL® Oral Solution also contains the following inactive ingredients; alcohol 4%, coloring agent, flavoring agent, methylparaben, propylparaben, saccharin sodium and water. Contains no sugar.

POWDER—

Each packet contains 1.5 g (20 mEq) potassium chloride. KAY CIEL® Powder also contains the following inactive ingredients; coloring agents, flavoring agent and saccharin sodium. Contains no sugar.

INDICATIONS

Treatment and prevention of potassium deficiency occurring especially during thiazide diuretic or corticosteroid therapy, digitalis intoxication, low dietary intake of potassium, or as a result of excessive vomiting and diarrhea and for correction of associated hypochloremic alkalosis.

CONTRAINDICATIONS

Impaired renal function, untreated Addison's Disease, dehydration, heat cramps and hyperkalemia.

WARNINGS

Do not use excessively.

PRECAUTIONS

Administer with caution and adjust to requirements of individual patient. Patient should be checked frequently, periodic ECG recorded and/or plasma potassium levels determined. Use with caution in patients with cardiac disease. In hypokalemic states, attention should be directed toward correction of frequently associated hypochloremic alkalosis.
PATIENTS SHOULD BE CAUTIONED TO ADHERE TO DILUTION INSTRUCTIONS TO ASSURE AGAINST GASTRO-INTESTINAL INJURY.
Contains FD&C Yellow No. 6 (Sunset Yellow) as a color additive.

ADVERSE REACTIONS

Potassium intoxication indicated by listlessness, mental confusion, paresthesia of the extremities, weakness of the legs, flaccid paralysis, fall in blood pressure, cardiac depression, arrhythmias, arrest and heartblock. Vomiting, nausea, abdominal discomfort and diarrhea may occur.

DOSAGE AND ADMINISTRATION

Oral Solution —One tablespoonful (15 ml supplying 20 mEq) **diluted** in 4 ounces cold water or fruit juice twice daily (preferably after a meal), or as directed by physician.
Powder—Contents of 1 packet dissolved in 4 ounces cold water or fruit juice twice daily (preferably after a meal), or as directed by physician.

OVERDOSAGE

In case of excessive use resulting in hyperkalemia or potassium intoxication, discontinue use of potassium chloride and/or take other steps to lower serum levels if indicated.

HOW SUPPLIED

Oral Solution in bottles of:
　118 ml..NDC 0456-0661-04
　473 ml..NDC 0456-0661-16
　3785 ml..NDC 0456-0661-28
Powder in boxes of:
　30 packets ....NDC 0456-0662-70
　100 packets ....NDC 0456-0662-71
Revised 4-86

PEDAMETH® CAPSULE　　　　　　　　　　℞
PEDAMETH® LIQUID　　　　　　　　　　　℞
(racemethionine)

COMPOSITION

CAPSULES—200 mg. racemethionine.
LIQUID—75 mg. racemethionine per 5 cc. (teaspoon) in a fruit flavored base.

HOW SUPPLIED

PEDAMETH® (racemethionine) is available in 200 mg. Capsules in bottles of 50 (NDC 0456-0355-50) and 500 (NDC 0456-0355-02) and as 75 mg. per 5 ml. Liquid in bottles of 16 fluid ounces (NDC 0456-1039-16).

PYOCIDIN-OTIC®　　　　　　　　　　　　　℞
[pī"ō-cī'dĭn ō'tĭk"]
(polymyxin B-hydrocortisone)
Sterile Otic Solution

DESCRIPTION

Each ml contains 10,000 USP units of polymyxin B sulfate and 5 mg hydrocortisone in a vehicle containing propylene glycol and water. Sodium hydroxide or hydrochloric acid may have been added to adjust pH.

ACTIONS

Polymyxin B sulfate is effective against the gram-negative *Pseudomonas aeruginosa*, one of the most resistant microorganisms commonly causing otitis externa. The addition of hydrocortisone to the antibiotic affords an anti-inflammatory effect and relief against allergic manifestations and reduces the possibility of sensitivity and tissue reaction.

INDICATIONS

For the treatment of superficial bacterial infections of the external auditory canal caused by organisms susceptible to the action of the antibiotic.

CONTRAINDICATIONS

This product is contraindicated in those individuals who have shown hypersensitivity to any of its components, and in herpes simplex, vaccinia and varicella. Perforated tympanic membrane is considered a contraindication to the use of any medication in the external ear canal.

WARNINGS

Discontinue promptly if sensitization or irritation occurs. As with other antibiotic preparations, prolonged treatment may result in overgrowth of nonsusceptible organisms and fungi.
If the infection is not improved after one week, cultures and susceptibility tests should be repeated to verify the identity of the organism and to determine whether therapy should be changed.
Patients who prefer to warm the medication before using should be cautioned against heating the solution above body temperature, in order to avoid loss of potency.

PRECAUTIONS

If sensitization or irritation occurs, medication should be discontinued promptly.

DOSAGE AND ADMINISTRATION

The external auditory canal should be thoroughly cleaned and dried with a sterile cotton applicator.
For adults, 4 drops of the solution should be instilled into the affected ear 3 or 4 times daily. For infants and children, 3 drops are suggested because of the smaller capacity of the ear canal.
The patient should lie with the affected ear upward and then the drops should be instilled. This position should be maintained for 5 minutes to facilitate penetration of the drops into the ear canal. Repeat, if necessary, for the opposite ear. If preferred, a cotton wick may be inserted into the canal and then the cotton may be saturated with the solution. This wick should be kept moist by adding further solution every four hours. The wick should be replaced at least once every 24 hours.

HOW SUPPLIED

10 ml bottle with sterile dropper
NDC 0456-0663-10

RECOMMENDED STORAGE

Product should be stored at controlled room temperature 15°-30°C (59°-86°F).
Revised 2/88

SUS-PHRINE®　　　　　　　　　　　　　　　℞
[sŭs'frĭn"]
(brand of epinephrine)
1:200
Aqueous Suspension for
Subcutaneous Injection

DESCRIPTION

Each ml of Sus-Phrine® (brand of epinephrine) Suspension contains 5 mg epinephrine in a sterile aqueous vehicle containing ascorbic acid 10 mg and thioglycolic acid 6.6 mg (as sodium salts), phenol 5 mg and glycerin (USP) 325 mg. Sodium hydroxide is added to adjust the pH. Approximately 80% of the total epinephrine is in suspension.
SUS-PHRINE® (brand of epinephrine) is sulfite free.

CLINICAL PHARMACOLOGY

Sus-Phrine® Suspension (epinephrine) acts at both the alpha and beta receptor sites. Beta stimulation provides bronchodilator action by relaxing bronchial muscle. Alpha stimulation increases vital capacity by relieving congestion of the bronchial mucosa and by constricting pulmonary vessels. Recent studies in laboratory animals (minipigs, rodents, and dogs) recorded the occurrence of cardiac arrhythmias and sudden death (with histologic evidence of myocardial necrosis) when beta agonists and methylxanthines were administered concurrently. The significance of these findings when applied to humans is currently unknown.

Sus-Phrine® Suspension (epinephrine) provides both rapid and sustained epinephrine activity. The rapid action is due to the epinephrine in solution, while the sustained activity is due to the crystalline epinephrine free base in suspension.

INDICATIONS

For the symptomatic treatment of bronchial asthma, and reversible bronchospasm associated with chronic bronchitis and emphysema.

CONTRAINDICATIONS

Hypersensitivity to any of the components.
Narrow angle glaucoma, shock, cerebral arteriosclerosis and organic heart disease. Epinephrine is also contraindicated during general anesthesia with halogenated hydrocarbons or cyclopropane, and in local anesthesia of certain areas, e.g., fingers, toes, because of the danger of vasoconstriction producing sloughing of tissue, and in labor because the drug may delay the second stage.

WARNINGS (epinephrine)

SUS-PHRINE (epinephrine) SUSPENSION SHOULD NOT BE EMPLOYED TO CORRECT DRUG-INDUCED HYPOTENSION.

Administer with caution to elderly people; those with cardiovascular disease, diabetes, hypertension or hyperthyroidism; in psychoneurotic individuals and in pregnancy. Administer with extreme caution to patients with long-standing bronchial asthma and emphysema who have developed degenerative heart disease.

Cardiac arrhythmias may follow administration of epinephrine.

Anginal pain may be induced when coronary insufficiency is present.

PRECAUTIONS

DO NOT USE IF PRODUCT IS DISCOLORED. Discoloration indicates the oxidation of epinephrine and possible loss of potency.

Use of Sus-Phrine® (eprinephrine) Suspension with digitalis, mercurial diuretics or other drugs that sensitize the heart to arrhythmias is not recommended.

Sus-Phrine® Suspension (epinephrine) should not be administered concomitantly with other sympathomimetic agents, since their combined effects on the cardiovascular system may be deleterious to the patient.

The effects of epinephrine may be potentiated by tricyclic antidepressants; sodium L-thyroxine, and certain antihistamines (eg, diphenhydramine, tripelennamine or chlorpheniramine).

ADVERSE REACTIONS

In some individuals, restlessness, anxiety, headache, tremor, weakness, dizziness, pallor, respiratory difficulties, palpitation, nausea and vomiting may occur. These reactions may be exaggerated in hyperthyroidism. Occlusion of the central retinal artery and shock have also been reported.

Also, urticaria, wheal and hemorrhage at the site of injection may occur. Repeated injections at the same site may result in necrosis from vascular constriction.

Tolerance to epinephrine may occur with prolonged use.

OVERDOSAGE

Overdosage or inadvertent intravenous injection may cause cerebrovascular hemorrhage resulting from the sharp rise in blood pressure. Fatalities may also result from pulmonary edema because of peripheral constriction and cardiac stimulation produced. Rapidly acting vasodilators such as nitrites, or alpha blocking agents may counteract the marked pressor effects. Cardiac arrhythmias may be countered by administering rapidly acting antiarrhythmic or beta blocking agents.

DOSAGE AND ADMINISTRATION

NOTE: INJECT SUBCUTANEOUSLY.

It is suggested that Sus-Phrine® (epinephrine) Suspension be administered with a tuberculin syringe and a 26 gauge, ½ inch needle.

A small initial test dose may be administered subcutaneously as a possible aid in determining patient sensitivity to epinephrine.

Site of injection should be varied to avoid necrosis at the site of injection.

Each time before withdrawing Sus-Phrine® (epinephrine) Suspension into syringe, **shake vial or ampul thoroughly** to disperse particles and obtain a uniform suspension. Inject promptly subcutaneously to avoid settling of suspension in the syringe.

Adults:

Adult dosage range is 0.1 to 0.3 mL depending on patient response.

Subsequent doses should be administered only when necessary and not more frequently than every six hours.

Infants 1 month to 2 years and Children 2 to 12 years:

Pediatric dose is 0.005 mL/kg (2.2 lb) body weight injected subcutaneously.

FOR CHILDREN 30 kg OR LESS MAXIMUM SINGLE DOSE IS 0.15 mL

Subsequent doses should be administered only when necessary and not more frequently than every six hours.

CLINICAL STUDIES

Controlled studies comparing the effectiveness of Sus-Phrine® (epinephrine) Suspension 1:200 and an aqueous solution of epinephrine 1:1000 were conducted in both pediatric and adult asthmatics. The studies demonstrated rapid bronchodilator activity following administration of either Sus-Phrine® (epinephrine) Suspension or epinephrine 1:1000; however during the 6 hour study period, a greater improvement in FEV_1 and $FEF_{25-75\%}$ was observed 4 to 6 hours subsequent to Sus-Phrine® (epinephrine) Suspension administration. Improvement in Wright Peak Expiratory Flow Rate was greater for Sus-Phrine® (epinephrine) Suspension than epinephrine 1:1000 3 to 8 hours following administration (10 hour study duration).

HOW SUPPLIED

In boxes of:
12 × 0.3 mL ampuls..................................NDC 0456-0664-12
25 × 0.3 mL ampuls..................................NDC 0456-0664-34
5.0 mL multiple dose vial.........................NDC 0456-0664-05
Store under refrigeration. Do not freeze. Do not expose to temperature above 30° C (86°F).

TESSALON®   ℞
(benzonatate USP)

PRODUCT OVERVIEW

KEY FACTS

Tessalon is a nonnarcotic, oral antitussive agent. It contains 100 mg of benzonatate per Perle. Chemically related to tetracaine and other topical anesthetics, Tessalon diminishes the cough reflex by anesthetizing the stretch receptors in the respiratory passages, lungs, and pleura.

MAJOR USES

Tessalon is used for the symptomatic relief of cough.

SAFETY INFORMATION

Contraindicated in patients who are allergic to benzonatate or related compounds. Tessalon should not be chewed or allowed to dissolve in the mouth.

PRESCRIBING INFORMATION

TESSALON®   ℞
(benzonatate USP)

DESCRIPTION

TESSALON®, a nonnarcotic oral antitussive agent, is 2, 5, 8, 11, 14, 17, 20, 23, 26-nonaoxaoctacosan-28-yl p-(butylamino) benzoate; with a molecular weight of 603.7.

$$CH_3(CH_2)_2CH_2NH\text{---}\langle\bigcirc\rangle\text{---}COOCH_2CH_2(OCH_2CH_2)_8OCH_3$$
$$C_{30}H_{53}NO_{11}$$

Each TESSALON Perle contains:
Benzonatate, USP .... 100 mg
TESSALON Perles also contain: D&C Yellow 10, gelatin, glycerin, methylparaben and propylparaben.

CLINICAL PHARMACOLOGY

TESSALON acts peripherally by anesthetizing the stretch receptors located in the respiratory passages, lungs, and pleura by dampening their activity and thereby reducing the cough reflex at its source. It begins to act within 15 to 20 minutes and its effect lasts for 3 to 8 hours. TESSALON has no inhibitory effect on the respiratory center in recommended dosage.

INDICATIONS AND USAGE

TESSALON is indicated for the symptomatic relief of cough.

CONTRAINDICATIONS

Hypersensitivity to benzonatate or related compounds.

PRECAUTIONS

Information for patients: Release of TESSALON from the perle in the mouth can produce a temporary local anesthesia of the oral mucosa and choking could occur. Therefore, the perles should be swallowed without chewing.

Usage in Pregnancy: Pregnancy Category C. Animal reproduction studies have not been conducted with TESSALON. It is also not known whether TESSALON can cause fetal harm when administered to a pregnant woman or can affect reproduction capacity. TESSALON should be given to a pregnant woman only if clearly needed.

Nursing mothers: It is not known whether this drug is excreted in human milk. Because many drugs are excreted in

human milk caution should be exercised when TESSALON is administered to a nursing woman.

Carcinogenesis, mutagenesis, impairment of fertility: Carcinogenicity, mutagenicity, and reproduction studies have not been conducted with TESSALON.

ADVERSE REACTIONS

Sedation, headache, mild dizziness, pruritus and skin eruptions, nasal congestion, constipation, nausea, gastrointestinal upset, sensation of burning in the eyes, a vague "chilly" sensation, numbness in the chest, and hypersensitivity have been reported.

OVERDOSAGE

No clinically significant cases have been reported, to our knowledge. The drug is chemically related to tetracaine and other topical anesthetics and shares various aspects of their pharmacology and toxicology. Drugs of this type are generally well absorbed after ingestion.

Signs and Symptoms

If perles are chewed or dissolved in the mouth, oropharyngeal anesthesia will develop rapidly. CNS stimulation may cause restlessness and tremors which may proceed to clonic convulsions followed by profound CNS depression.

Treatment

Evacuate gastric contents and administer copious amounts of activated charcoal slurry. Even in the conscious patient, cough and gag reflexes may be so depressed as to necessitate special attention to protection against aspiration of gastric contents and orally administered materials.

Convulsions should be treated with a short-acting barbiturate given intravenously and carefully titrated for the smallest effective dosage.

Intensive support of respiration and cardiovascular-renal function is an essential feature of the treatment of severe intoxication from overdosage.

Do not use CNS stimulants.

DOSAGE AND ADMINISTRATION

Adults and Children over 10: Usual dose is one 100 mg perle t.i.d. as required. If necessary, up to 6 perles daily may be given.

HOW SUPPLIED

Perles, 100 mg (yellow); bottles of 100 NDC 0456-0688-01.
Store at controlled room temperature (59°–86°F, 15°–30°C).

Manufactured by
R.P. Scherer-North America
St. Petersburg, Florida 33702
for
Forest Pharmaceuticals, Inc.
Subsidiary of Forest Laboratories, Inc.
St. Louis, MO 63043-9979
Shown in Product Indentification Section, page 410

Fujisawa SmithKline Corp.
401 CITY AVENUE
SUITE 300
BALA CYNWYD, PA 19004

CEFIZOX®   ℞
brand of sterile ceftizoxime sodium
and ceftizoxime sodium injection

DESCRIPTION

Cefizox (sterile ceftizoxime sodium, FSK) is a sterile, semisynthetic, broad-spectrum, beta-lactamase resistant cephalosporin antibiotic for parenteral (I.V., I.M.) administration. It is the sodium salt of [6R-[6α, 7 β(Z)]]-7-[[(2,3-dihydro-2-imino-4-thiazolyl) (methoxyimino) acetyl] amino]-8-oxo-5-thia-1-azabicyclo [4.2.0] oct-2-ene-2-carboxylic acid. Its sodium content is approximately 60 mg. (2.6 mEq.) per gram of ceftizoxime activity. Structurally it is:

Sterile ceftizoxime sodium is a white to pale yellow crystalline powder.

'Cefizox' is supplied in vials equivalent to 1 gram, 2 grams or 10 grams of ceftizoxime, and in "Piggyback" Vials for intravenous admixture equivalent to 1 gram or 2 grams of ceftizcxime.

'Cefizox', equivalent to 1 gram or 2 grams of ceftizoxime, is also supplied as a frozen, sterile, nonpyrogenic solution of ceftizoxime sodium in an iso-osmotic diluent in plastic containers. After thawing, the solution is intended for intravenous use.

Continued on next page

Fujisawa SmithKline—Cont.

The plastic container is fabricated from specially formulated polyvinyl chloride. Solutions in contact with the plastic container can leach out certain of its chemical components in very small amounts within the expiration period, e.g., di 2-ethylhexyl phthalate (DEHP), up to 5 parts per million. However, the safety of the plastic has been confirmed in tests in animals according to the USP biological tests for plastic containers as well as by tissue culture toxicity studies.

CLINICAL PHARMACOLOGY

The table below demonstrates the serum levels and duration of Cefizox (sterile ceftizoxime sodium, FSK) following intramuscular administration of 500 mg. and 1.0 gram doses respectively to normal volunteers.
[See table below].
Following intravenous administration of 1.0, 2.0 and 3.0 gram doses of 'Cefizox' to normal volunteers, the following serum levels were obtained:
[See table above right].
A serum half-life of approximately 1.7 hours was observed after intravenous or intramuscular administration.
'Cefizox' is 30% protein bound.
'Cefizox' is not metabolized, and is excreted virtually unchanged by the kidneys in 24 hours. This provides a high urinary concentration. Concentrations greater than 6,000 mcg./mL. have been achieved in the urine by 2 hours after a 1 gram dose of 'Cefizox' intravenously. Probenecid slows tubular secretion and produces even higher serum levels, increasing the duration of measurable serum concentrations.
'Cefizox' achieves therapeutic levels in various body fluids, e.g., cerebrospinal fluid (in patients with inflamed meninges), bile, surgical wound fluid, pleural fluid, aqueous humor, ascitic fluid, peritoneal fluid, prostatic fluid and saliva, and the following body tissues: heart, gallbladder, bone, biliary, peritoneal, prostatic and uterine.
In clinical experience to date, no disulfiram-like reactions have been reported with Cefizox (sterile ceftizoxime sodium, FSK).

Microbiology

The bactericidal action of 'Cefizox' results from inhibition of cell-wall synthesis. 'Cefizox' is highly resistant to a broad spectrum of beta-lactamases (penicillinase and cephalosporinase), including Richmond types I, II, III, TEM, and IV, produced by both aerobic and anaerobic gram-positive and gram-negative organisms. 'Cefizox' is active against a wide range of gram-positive and gram-negative organisms, and is usually active against the following organisms in vitro and in clinical situations (see Indications and Usage):

Gram-Positive Aerobes:
Staphylococcus sp. including penicillinase and nonpenicillinase producing S. aureus and S. epidermidis. Note: Methicillin-resistant staphylococci are resistant to cephalosporins, including ceftizoxime.
Streptococcus sp. including S. pneumoniae (formerly D. pneumoniae) and S. pyogenes.
Note: 'Cefizox' is usually inactive in vitro against most strains of enterococci, e.g., S. faecalis.

Gram-Negative Aerobes:

Kiebsiella sp. including K. pneumoniae	Serratia sp. including S. marcescens
Escherichia coli	Enterobacter sp.
Proteus mirabilis	Pseudomonas sp. including Ps. aeruginosa
Proteus vulgaris	
Morganella morganii (formerly Proteus morganii) and	Haemophilus sp. including ampicillin-resistant strains of H. influenzae
Providencia rettgeri (formerly Proteus rettgeri)	Neisseria gonorrhoeae

Anaerobes:

Bacteroides sp. including B. fragilis	Anaerobic cocci including Peptococcus sp. Peptostreptococcus sp.

'Cefizox' is usually active against strains of Acinetobacter sp.
Cefizox (sterile ceftizoxime sodium, FSK) is usually active against the following organisms in vitro, but the clinical significance of these data has not been established:

Gram-Positive Aerobes:
Corynebacterium diphtheriae

Gram-Negative Aerobes:

Shigella sp.	Moraxella sp.
Providencia stuartii	Pasteurella multocida
Salmonella sp.	Neisseria meningitidis
Aeromonas hydrophila	Citrobacter sp.
Yersinia enterocolitica	

Anaerobes:

Actinomyces sp.	Fusobacterium sp.
Veillonella sp.	Bifidobacterium sp.
Eubacterium sp.	Propionibacterium sp.
Clostridium sp.	

(Note: Most strains of C. difficile are resistant.)

Susceptibility Testing

Quantitative methods that require measurement of zone diameters give the most precise estimate of antibiotic susceptibility. One such procedure* has been recommended for use with disks to test susceptibility to ceftizoxime.
Reports from the laboratory giving results of the standard single-disk susceptibility test with a 30 mcg. ceftizoxime disk should be interpreted according to the following criteria (with the exception of Ps. aeruginosa):

Susceptible organisms produce zones of 20 mm. or greater, indicating that the test organism is likely to respond to therapy.

Organisms that produce zones of 15 to 19 mm. are expected to be susceptible if high dosage is used or if the infection is confined to tissues and fluids (e.g., urine) in which high antibiotic levels are attained.

Resistant organisms produce zones of 14 mm. or less, indicating that other therapy should be selected.

Organisms should be tested with the 'Cefizox' disk, since 'Cefizox' has been shown by in vitro tests to be active against certain strains found resistant when other beta-lactam disks are used.

Susceptibility Testing for Pseudomonas in Urinary Tract Infections

Most strains of Ps. aeruginosa are moderately susceptible to Cefizox (sterile ceftizoxime sodium, FSK). 'Cefizox' achieves high levels in the urine (greater than 6,000 mcg./mL. at 2 hours with 1 gram I.V.) and therefore the following zone sizes should be used when testing 'Cefizox' for treatment of urinary tract infections caused by Ps. aeruginosa:

Susceptible organisms produce zones of 20 mm. or greater, indicating that the test organism is likely to respond to therapy.

Organisms that produce zones of 11 to 19 mm. are expected to be susceptible when the infection is confined to the urinary tract in which high antibiotic levels are attained.

Resistant organisms produce zones of 10 mm. or less, indicating that other therapy should be selected.

A bacterial isolate may be considered susceptible if the MIC value for 'Cefizox' is equal to or less than 16 mcg./mL. Organisms are considered moderately susceptible if the MIC is greater than 16 mcg./mL. but less than 64 mcg./mL. Organisms are considered resistant if the MIC is 64 mcg./mL. or greater. For most organisms the MBC value for 'Cefizox' is the same as the MIC value.

The standardized quality control procedure requires use of control organisms. The 30 mcg. ceftizoxime disk should give the zone diameters listed below for the quality control strains.

Organism	ATCC	Zone Size Range
E. coli	25922	30–36 mm.
S. aureus	25923	27–35 mm.
Ps. aeruginosa	27853	12–17 mm.

INDICATIONS AND USAGE

Cefizox (sterile ceftizoxime sodium, FSK) is indicated in the treatment of infections due to susceptible strains of the microorganisms listed below:

LOWER RESPIRATORY TRACT INFECTIONS caused by Streptococcus sp. including S. pneumoniae (formerly D. pneumoniae), but excluding enterococci; Klebsiella sp.; Proteus mirabilis; Escherichia coli; Haemophilus influenzae including ampicillin-resistant strains; Staphylococcus aureus (penicillinase and nonpenicillinase producing); Serratia sp.; Enterobacter sp.; and Bacteroides sp.

URINARY TRACT INFECTIONS caused by Staphylococcus aureus (penicillinase and nonpenicillinase producing); Escherichia coli; Pseudomonas sp. including Ps. aeruginosa; Proteus mirabilis; P. vulgaris; Providencia rettgeri (formerly Proteus rettgeri) and Morganella morganii (formerly Proteus morganii); Klebsiella sp.; Serratia sp. including S. marcescens; Enterobacter sp.

GONORRHEA. Uncomplicated cervical and urethral gonorrhea caused by Neisseria gonorrhoeae.

INTRA-ABDOMINAL INFECTIONS caused by Escherichia coli; Staphylococcus epidermidis; Streptococcus sp. (excluding enterococci); Enterobacter sp.; Klebsiella sp.; Bacteroides sp. including B. fragilis; and anaerobic cocci, including Peptococcus sp. and Peptostreptococcus sp.

SEPTICEMIA caused by Streptococcus sp. including S. pneumoniae (formerly D. pneumoniae), but excluding enterococci; Staphylococcus aureus (penicillinase and nonpenicillinase producing); Escherichia coli; Bacteroides sp. including B. fragilis; Klebsiella sp.; and Serratia sp.

SKIN AND SKIN STRUCTURE INFECTIONS caused by Staphylococcus aureus (penicillinase and nonpenicillinase producing); Staphylococcus epidermidis; Escherichia coli; Klebsiella sp.; Streptococcus sp. including Streptococcus pyogenes (group A beta-hemolytic), but excluding enterococci; Proteus mirabilis; Serratia sp.; Enterobacter sp.; Bacteroides sp. including B. fragilis; and anaerobic cocci, including Peptococcus sp. and Peptostreptococcus sp.

BONE AND JOINT INFECTIONS caused by Staphylococcus aureus (penicillinase and nonpenicillinase producing); Streptococcus sp. (excluding enterococci); Proteus mirabilis; Bacteroides sp.; and anaerobic cocci, including Peptococcus sp. and Peptostreptococcus sp.

MENINGITIS caused by Haemophilus influenzae. 'Cefizox' has also been used successfully in the treatment of a limited number of pediatric and adult cases of meningitis caused by Streptococcus pneumoniae.

'Cefizox' has been effective in the treatment of seriously ill, compromised patients, including those who were debilitated, immunosuppressed or neutropenic.

Infections caused by aerobic gram-negative and by mixtures of organisms resistant to other cephalosporins, aminoglycosides, or penicillins have responded to treatment with 'Cefizox'.

Because of the serious nature of some urinary tract infections due to Ps. aeruginosa and because many strains of Pseudomonas species are only moderately susceptible to 'Cefizox', higher dosage is recommended. Other therapy should be instituted if the response is not prompt.

Susceptibility studies on specimens obtained prior to therapy should be used to determine the response of causative organisms to 'Cefizox'. Therapy with 'Cefizox' may be initiated pending results of the studies; however, treatment should be adjusted according to study findings. In serious infections 'Cefizox' has been used concomitantly with aminoglycosides (see Precautions). Before using 'Cefizox' concomitantly with other antibiotics, the prescribing information for those agents should be reviewed for contraindications, warnings, precautions and adverse reactions. Renal function should be carefully monitored.

CONTRAINDICATIONS

Cefizox (sterile ceftizoxime sodium, FSK) is contraindicated in patients who have known allergy to the drug.

WARNINGS

BEFORE THERAPY WITH CEFIZOX (STERILE CEFTIZOXIME SODIUM, FSK) IS INSTITUTED, CAREFUL INQUIRY SHOULD BE MADE TO DETERMINE WHETHER THE PATIENT HAS HAD PREVIOUS HYPERSENSITIVITY REACTIONS TO CEPHALOSPORINS, PENICILLINS, OR OTHER DRUGS. THIS PRODUCT SHOULD BE GIVEN CAUTIOUSLY TO PENICILLIN-SENSITIVE PATIENTS. ANTIBIOTICS SHOULD BE ADMINISTERED WITH CAUTION TO ANY PATIENT WHO HAS DEMONSTRATED SOME FORM OF ALLERGY, PARTICULARLY TO DRUGS. SERIOUS ACUTE HYPERSENSITIVITY REACTIONS MAY REQUIRE EPINEPHRINE AND OTHER EMERGENCY MEASURES.
Pseudomembranous colitis has been reported with the use of cephalosporins (and other broad-spectrum antibiotics);

Serum Concentrations After Intravenous Administration
Serum Concentration (mcg./mL.)

Dose	5 mins.	10 mins.	30 mins.	1 hr.	2 hrs.	4 hrs.	8 hrs.
1.0 gram	ND	ND	60.5	38.9	21.5	8.4	1.4
2.0 grams	131.8	110.9	77.5	53.6	33.1	12.1	2.0
3.0 grams	221.1	174.0	112.7	83.9	47.4	26.2	4.8

ND = Not Done

Serum Concentrations After Intramuscular Administration
Serum Concentration (mcg./mL.)

Dose	½ hr.	1 hr.	2 hrs.	4 hrs.	6 hrs.	8 hrs.
500 mg.	13.3	13.7	9.2	4.8	1.9	.0.7
1.0 gram	36.0	39.0	31.0	15.0	6.0	3.0

therefore, it is important to consider its diagnosis in patients who developed diarrhea in association with antibiotic use.

Treatment with broad-spectrum antibiotics alters normal flora of the colon and may permit overgrowth of *Clostridia*. Studies indicate a toxin produced by *Clostridium difficile* is one primary cause of antibiotic-associated colitis. Cholestyramine and colestipol resins have been shown to bind the toxin *in vitro*.

Mild cases of colitis may respond to drug discontinuance alone.

Moderate to severe cases should be managed with fluid, electrolyte and protein supplementation as indicated.

When the colitis is not relieved by drug discontinuance or when it is severe, oral vancomycin is the treatment of choice for antibiotic-associated pseudomembranous colitis produced by *C. difficile*. Other causes of colitis should also be considered.

PRECAUTIONS

General: As with all broad-spectrum antibiotics, Cefizox (sterile ceftizoxime sodium, FSK) should be prescribed with caution in individuals with a history of gastrointestinal disease, particularly colitis.

Although 'Cefizox' has not been shown to produce an alteration in renal function, renal status should be evaluated, especially in seriously ill patients receiving maximum dose therapy. As with any antibiotic, prolonged use may result in overgrowth of nonsusceptible organisms. Careful observation is essential; appropriate measures should be taken if superinfection occurs.

Drug Interactions: Although the occurrence has not been reported with 'Cefizox', nephrotoxicity has been reported following concomitant administration of other cephalosporins and aminoglycosides.

Pregnancy: (Category B.) Reproduction studies have been performed in rats and rabbits and have revealed no evidence of impaired fertility or harm to the fetus due to 'Cefizox'. There are, however, no adequate and well-controlled studies in pregnant women. Because animal reproduction studies are not always predictive of human response, this drug should be used during pregnancy only if clearly needed.

Labor and Delivery: Safety of 'Cefizox' use during labor and delivery has not been established.

Nursing Mothers: 'Cefizox' is excreted in human milk in low concentrations. Caution should be exercised when 'Cefizox' is administered to a nursing woman.

Infants and Children: Safety and efficacy in infants from birth to six months of age have not been established. In children six months of age and older, treatment with 'Cefizox' has been associated with transient elevated levels of eosinophils, SGOT, SGPT and CPK (creatine phosphokinase). The CPK elevation may be related to I.M. administration.

ADVERSE REACTIONS

Ceftizoxime is generally well tolerated. The *most* frequent adverse reactions (*greater than* 1% but less than 5%) are:

Hypersensitivity—Rash, pruritus, fever.

Hepatic—Transient elevation in SGOT, SGPT and alkaline phosphatase.

Hematologic—Transient eosinophilia, thrombocytosis. Some individuals have developed a positive Coombs test.

Local—Injection site—Burning, cellulitis, phlebitis with I.V. administration, pain, induration, tenderness, paresthesia.

The *less* frequent adverse reactions (*less than* 1%) are:

Hypersensitivity—Numbness has been reported rarely.

Hepatic—Elevation of bilirubin has been reported rarely.

Renal—Transient elevations of BUN and creatinine have been occasionally observed with ceftizoxime.

Hematologic—Anemia, leukopenia, neutropenia and thrombocytopenia have been reported rarely.

Genitourinary—Vaginitis has rarely occurred.

Gastrointestinal—Diarrhea; nausea and vomiting have been reported occasionally.

Symptoms of pseudomembranous colitis can appear during or after antibiotic treatment. (See Warnings section.)

DOSAGE AND ADMINISTRATION

The usual adult dosage is 1 or 2 grams of Cefizox (sterile ceftizoxime sodium, FSK) every 8 to 12 hours. Proper dosage and route of administration should be determined by the condition of the patient, severity of the infection and susceptibility of the causative organisms.

[See table above.]

Because of the serious nature of urinary tract infections due to *Ps. aeruginosa* and because many strains of *Pseudomonas* species are only moderately susceptible to 'Cefizox', higher dosage is recommended. Other therapy should be instituted if the response is not prompt.

A single, 1 gram I.M. dose is the usual dose for treatment of uncomplicated gonorrhea.

The intravenous route may be preferable for patients with bacterial septicemia, localized parenchymal abscesses (such as intra-abdominal abscess), peritonitis, or other severe or life-threatening infections.

In those with normal renal function, the intravenous dosage for such infections is 2 to 12 grams of Cefizox (sterile ceftizoxime sodium, FSK) daily. In conditions such as bacterial septi-

---

General Guidelines for Dosage of 'Cefizox'

Type of Infection	Daily Dose (Grams)	Frequency and Route
Uncomplicated Urinary Tract	1	500 mg. q12h I.M. or I.V.
Other Sites	2–3	1 gram q8–12h I.M. or I.V.
Severe or Refractory	3–6	1 gram q8h I.M. or I.V. 2 grams q8–12h I.M.* or I.V.
Life-Threatening†	9–12	3–4 grams q8h I.V.

*When administering 2 gram I.M. doses, the dose should be divided and given in different large muscle masses.
†In life-threatening infections dosages up to 2 grams every 4 hours have been given.

---

cemia, 6 to 12 grams/day may be given initially by the intravenous route for several days, and the dosage may then be gradually reduced according to clinical response and laboratory findings.

Pediatric Dosage Schedule

	Unit Dose	Frequency
Children 6 months and older	50 mg./kg.	q6-8h

Dosage may be increased to a total daily dose of 200 mg./kg. (not to exceed the maximum adult dose for serious infection).

Impaired Renal Function

Modification of 'Cefizox' dosage is necessary in patients with impaired renal function. Following an initial loading dose of 500 mg.–1.0 gram I.M. or I.V., the maintenance dosing schedule shown below should be followed. Further dosing should be determined by therapeutic monitoring, severity of the infection and susceptibility of the causative organisms.

When only the serum creatinine level is available, creatinine clearance may be calculated from the following formula. The serum creatinine level should represent current renal function at the steady state.

Males

$$Clcr = \frac{Weight\ (kg.) \times (140 - age)}{72 \times serum\ creatinine\ (mg./100\ mL.)}$$

Females 0.85 of the above values

In patients undergoing hemodialysis no additional supplemental dosing is required following hemodialysis; however, dosing should be timed so that the patient receives the dose (according to the table below) at the end of the dialysis.

Dosage in Adults with Reduced Renal Function

Creatinine Clearance mL./min.	Renal Function	Less Severe Infections	Life-Threatening Infections
79–50	Mild impairment	500 mg. q8h	0.75 gram– 1.5 grams q8h
49–5	Moderate to severe impairment	250 mg.– 500 mg. q12h	0.5 gram– 1.0 gram q12h
4–0	Dialysis patients	500 mg. q48h or 250 mg. q24h	0.5 gram– 1.0 gram q48h or 0.5 gram q24h

Preparation of Parenteral Solution
RECONSTITUTION

I.M. Administration: Reconstitute with Sterile Water for Injection. SHAKE WELL.

Vial Size	Diluent to Be Added	Approx. Avail. Vol.	Approx. Avg. Concentration
1 gram	3.0 mL.	3.7 mL.	270 mg./mL.
2 grams*	6.0 mL.	7.4 mL.	270 mg./mL.

* When administering 2 gram I.M. doses, the dose should be divided and given in different large muscle masses.

I.V. Administration: Reconstitute with Sterile Water for Injection. SHAKE WELL.

Vial Size	Diluent to Be Added	Approx. Avail. Vol.	Approx. Avg. Concentration
1 gram	10 mL.	10.7 mL.	95 mg./mL.
2 grams	20 mL.	21.4 mL.	95 mg./mL.

These solutions of Cefizox (sterile ceftizoxime sodium, FSK) are stable 24 hours at room temperature or 96 hours if refrigerated (5°C.).

Parenteral drug products should be inspected visually for particulate matter prior to administration. If particulate matter is evident in reconstituted fluids, then the drug solu-

---

tion should be discarded. Reconstituted solutions may range from yellow to amber without changes in potency.

Pharmacy Bulk Vials: For I.M. or I.V. direct injection, add Sterile Water for Injection according to table below. SHAKE WELL. For I.V. intermittent or continuous infusion, add Sterile Water for Injection according to table below. SHAKE WELL. Add to parenteral fluids listed below under I.V. Administration.

Vial Size	Diluent to Be Added	Approx. Avail. Vol.	Approx. Avg. Concentration
10 grams	30 mL.	37 mL.	1 gram/3.5 mL.
	45 mL.	51 mL.	1 gram/5 mL.

These reconstituted solutions of 'Cefizox' are stable 24 hours at room temperature or 96 hours if refrigerated (5°C.).

"Piggyback" Vials: Reconstitute with 50 to 100 mL. of Sodium Chloride Injection or any other I.V. solution listed below. SHAKE WELL.

Administer with primary I.V. fluids, as a single dose. These solutions of 'Cefizox' are stable 24 hours at room temperature or 96 hours if refrigerated (5°C.).

A solution of 1 gram 'Cefizox' in 13 mL. Sterile Water for Injection is isotonic.

I.M. Injection: Inject well within the body of a relatively large muscle. Aspiration is necessary to avoid inadvertent injection into a blood vessel. When administering 2 gram I.M. doses, the dose should be divided and given in different large muscle masses.

I.V. Administration: Direct (bolus) injection, slowly over 3 to 5 minutes, directly or through tubing for patients receiving parenteral fluids (see list below). Intermittent or continuous infusion, dilute reconstituted 'Cefizox' in 50 to 100 mL. of one of the following solutions:

Sodium Chloride Injection
5% or 10% Dextrose Injection
5% Dextrose and 0.9%, 0.45%, or 0.2% Sodium Chloride Injection
Ringer's Injection
Lactated Ringer's Injection
Invert Sugar 10% in Sterile Water for Injection
5% Sodium Bicarbonate in Sterile Water for Injection
5% Dextrose in Lactated Ringer's Injection (only when reconstituted with 4% Sodium Bicarbonate Injection)

In these fluids 'Cefizox' is stable 24 hours at room temperature or 96 hours if refrigerated (5°C.).

DIRECTIONS FOR USE OF CEFIZOX (CEFTIZOXIME SODIUM, FSK) PLASTIC CONTAINERS

'Cefizox' supplied as a frozen, sterile, nonpyrogenic solution in plastic containers is to be administered either as a continuous or intermittent infusion.

Thaw container at room temperature. After thawing, check for minute leaks by squeezing bag firmly. If leaks are found, discard solution as sterility may be impaired. Additives should not be introduced into this solution. Do not use if the solution is cloudy or precipitated or if the seal is not intact. After thawing, the solution is stable for 24 hours at room temperature or 10 days if stored under refrigeration (5°C.). DO NOT REFREEZE.

Use sterile equipment. It is recommended that the intravenous administration apparatus be replaced at least once every 48 hours.

CAUTION: Do not use plastic containers in series connections. Such use could result in air embolism due to residual air being drawn from the primary container before administration of the fluid from the secondary container is complete.

Preparation for administration:

1. Suspend container from eyelet support.
2. Remove plastic protector from outlet port at bottom of container.
3. Attach administration set. Refer to complete directions accompanying set.

HOW SUPPLIED

Cefizox (sterile ceftizoxime sodium, FSK)—supplied in vials equivalent to 1 gram or 2 grams of ceftizoxime; in Pharmacy Bulk Vials equivalent to 10 grams of ceftizoxime; and in

Continued on next page

Fujisawa SmithKline—Cont.

"Piggyback" Vials for I.V. admixture equivalent to 1 gram or 2 grams of ceftizoxime.
Note: Unreconstituted Cefizox (sterile ceftizoxime sodium, FSK) should be protected from excessive light, and stored at controlled room temperature (59°–86°F.) in the original package until used.
Cefizox (ceftizoxime sodium injection, FSK) as a frozen, sterile, nonpyrogenic solution in plastic containers—supplied in 50 mL. single-dose containers equivalent to 1 gram or 2 grams of ceftizoxime in 5% Dextrose (D5W). Do not store above −20°C.
'Cefizox' supplied as a frozen, sterile, nonpyrogenic solution in plastic containers is manufactured for Fujisawa Smith-Kline Corporation by Baxter Healthcare Corporation, Deerfield, IL 60015.

---

*Am. J. Clin. Pathol. 45:493, 1966; Federal Register 39:19182–19184, 1974.
DATE OF ISSUANCE SEPT. 1987
©Smith Kline &French Laboratories, 1987
Div. of SmithKline Beecham Corporation
Manufactured for **Fujisawa SmithKline Corp.**
by Fujisawa Pharmaceutical Co., Ltd., Osaka, Japan.
Filled and distributed by Smith Kline &French Laboratories,
Division of SmithKline Beecham Corporation.
Philadelphia, PA 19101
    Shown in Product Identification Section, page 430

VAGISTAT®   ℞
vaginal ointment
(tioconazole 6.5%)

DESCRIPTION
Tioconazole, 1-[2-[(2-chloro-3-thienyl)methoxy]-2(2,4-dichlorophenyl)ethyl]-1H-imidazole, is a topical antifungal agent. Its chemical formula is $C_{16}H_{13}Cl_3N_2OS$ with a molecular weight of 387.7. The structural formula is given below:

VAGISTAT (tioconazole 6.5%) is formulated in a base of white soft paraffin and aluminum magnesium silicate with butylated hydroxyanisole (BHA) added as a preservative. Each applicator-full of VAGISTAT provides approximately 4.6 grams of ointment containing 300 mg of tioconazole.

CLINICAL PHARMACOLOGY
Tioconazole is a broad-spectrum antifungal agent that inhibits the growth of human pathogenic yeasts. Tioconazole exhibits fungicidal activity *in vitro* against *Candida albicans*, other species of the genus *Candida*, and against *Torulopsis glabrata*.
Pharmacokinetics: Systemic absorption of tioconazole after a single intravaginal application of VAGISTAT in nonpregnant patients is negligible.

INDICATIONS AND USAGE
VAGISTAT is indicated for the local treatment of vulvo-vaginal candidiasis (moniliasis). As VAGISTAT has been shown to be effective only for candidal vulvo-vaginitis, the diagnosis should be confirmed by KOH smears and/or cultures. Other pathogens commonly associated with vulvo-vaginitis should be ruled out by appropriate methods.
Studies have shown that women taking oral contraceptives have a cure rate similar to those not taking such agents when treated with VAGISTAT.
Safety and effectiveness in pregnant and diabetic patients have not been established (see Precautions).

CONTRAINDICATIONS
VAGISTAT is contraindicated in individuals who have been shown to be sensitive to imidazole antifungal agents or to other components of the ointment.

PRECAUTIONS
General: VAGISTAT is intended for intravaginal administration only. Applicators should be opened just prior to administration to prevent contamination. Administration of VAGISTAT just prior to bedtime may be preferred. If clinical symptoms persist, appropriate microbiological tests should be repeated to rule out other pathogens and to confirm the diagnosis.
Carcinogenesis: No long term studies in animals have been performed to evaluate the carcinogenic potential of tioconazole.

Mutagenesis: Tioconazole did not demonstrate mutagenic activity at the levels examined in tests at either the chromosomal or subchromosomal level.
Impairment of Fertility: No impairment of fertility was seen in male rats administered tioconazole hydrochloride in oral doses up to 150 mg/kg/day.
However, there was evidence of preimplantation loss in female rats at oral dose levels above 35 mg/kg/day.
Pregnancy—Pregnancy Category C: Tioconazole hydrochloride had no adverse effects on fetal viability or growth when administered orally to pregnant rats at doses of 55, 110, and 165 mg/kg/day during the period of organogenesis. A drug-related increase in the incidence of dilated ureters, hydroureters, and hydronephrosis observed in the fetuses of this study was transient and no longer evident in pups raised to 21 days of age. These effects did not occur following intravaginal administration of approximately 10 mg/kg/day in a 2% cream. There was no evidence of major structural anomalies. No embryotoxic or teratogenic effects were observed in rabbits receiving oral dose levels as high as 165 mg/kg/day or daily intravaginal application of approximately 2–3 mg/kg in a 2% tioconazole cream during organogenesis. Tioconazole hydrochloride, like other azole antimycotic agents, causes dystocia in rats when treatment is extended through parturition. Associated effects in rats include prolongation of pregnancy, *in utero* deaths, and impaired pup survival. The "no-effect" level for this phenomenon is 20 mg/kg/day orally and approximately 9 mg/kg/day intravaginally. No effect on parturition occurred in rabbits at 50 mg/kg/day orally.
There are no adequate and well-controlled studies in pregnant women. VAGISTAT (tioconazole 6.5%) should be used during pregnancy only if the potential benefit justifies the potential risk to the fetus.
Nursing Mothers: It is not known whether this drug is excreted in human milk. Because many drugs are excreted in human milk, nursing should be temporarily discontinued while VAGISTAT is administered.
Pediatric Use: Safety and effectiveness in children have not been established.

ADVERSE REACTIONS
The incidence of adverse reactions to VAGISTAT is based on clinical trials involving 1000 patients. Burning and itching were the most frequent side effects occurring in approximately 6% and 5% of the patients, respectively. In most instances these did not interfere with the course of therapy. There were occasional reports (less than 1%) of other side effects including irritation, discharge, vulvar edema and swelling, vaginal pain, dysuria, nocturia, dyspareunia, dryness of vaginal secretions, desquamation, and burning sensation.

DOSAGE AND ADMINISTRATION
VAGISTAT has been found to be effective as a single dose treatment for vulvo-vaginal candidiasis. Using the pre-filled applicator, insert one applicator-full intravaginally. Administration of VAGISTAT just prior to bedtime may be preferred.

HOW SUPPLIED
VAGISTAT is supplied in a ready to use pre-filled single dose vaginal applicator. Each applicator-full will deliver approximately 4.6 grams of VAGISTAT containing 65 mg of tioconazole per gram of ointment. Store at controlled room temperature (59°–86° F).
       Fujisawa SmithKline
Manufactured for Fujisawa SmithKline Corp.,
Philadelphia, PA 19004 by Pfizer Canada, Inc.,
Arnprior, Ontario, Canada.
NDC 57317-001-01   Issued June 1989

Gebauer Chemical Company
9410 ST. CATHERINE AVE.
CLEVELAND, OH 44104

ETHYL CHLORIDE, U.S.P.   ℞
(Chloroethane)

INDICATIONS AND USAGE
Ethyl Chloride is a vapocoolant intended for topical application to control pain associated with minor surgical procedures (such as lancing boils, or incision and drainage of small abscesses), athletic injuries, injections, and for treatment of myofascial pain, restricted motion, and muscle spasm.

PRECAUTIONS
Inhalation of Ethyl Chloride should be avoided as it may produce narcotic and general anesthetic effects, and may produce deep anesthesia or fatal coma with respiratory or cardiac arrest. Ethyl Chloride is flammable and should never be used in the presence of an open flame, or electrical cautery equipment. When used to produce local freezing of tissues, adjacent skin areas should be protected by application

of petrolatum. The thawing process may be painful, and freezing may lower local resistance to infection and delay healing.

ADVERSE REACTIONS
Cutaneous sensitization may occur, but appears to be extremely rare. Freezing can occasionally alter pigmentation.

CONTRAINDICATIONS
Ethyl Chloride is contraindicated in individuals with a history of hypersensitivity to it.

WARNINGS
For external use only.
Skin absorption of Ethyl Chloride can occur; no cases of chronic poisoning have been reported. Ethyl Chloride is known as a liver and kidney toxin; long term exposure may cause liver or kidney damage.
Contents under pressure. Store in a cool place. Do not store above 120°F.

DOSAGE AND ADMINISTRATION
To apply Ethyl Chloride from metal tube, invert nozzle 12 inches (30 cm.) above the treatment area. Open adjustable dispensing valve until the spray flows freely.
To apply Ethyl Chloride from amber bottle with dispenseal valve, invert over the treatment area approximately 12 inches (30 cm.) away from site of application. Open dispenseal spring valve completely allowing Ethyl Chloride to flow in a stream from the bottle.
1. TOPICAL ANESTHESIA IN MINOR SURGERY
The operative site should be cleansed with a suitable antiseptic. Apply petrolatum to protect the adjacent area. Spray Ethyl Chloride for a few seconds to the point of frost formation, when the tissue becomes white. Avoid prolonged spraying of skin beyond this state. The anesthetic action of Ethyl Chloride rarely lasts more than a few seconds to a minute. Therefore, the incision should be made promptly when the tissue becomes white. Reapply as needed.
2. SPORTS INJURIES
The pain of bruises, contusions, abrasions, swelling, and minor sprains may be controlled with Ethyl Chloride.
Spray affected area for a few seconds until the tissue begins to frost and turn white. Avoid spraying of skin beyond this state. Use as you would ice. The amount of cooling depends on the dosage. The smallest dose needed to produce the desired effect should be used. Dosage varies with the nozzle size and duration of application.
Determine the extent of injury (fracture, sprain, etc.). The anesthetic effect of Ethyl Chloride rarely lasts more than a few seconds to a minute. This time interval is usually sufficient to help reduce or relieve the initial trauma of the injury.
3. FOR PRE-INJECTION ANESTHESIA
Prepare syringe and have it ready. Cleanse skin with antiseptic, if alcohol, wait for it to dry. Spray skin with Ethyl Chloride from a distance of about 12 inches (30 cm.) continuously for 3 to 5 seconds; do not frost skin. Quickly set down bottle and pick up syringe. Watch liquid film of spray on skin and just as it dries, introduce needle quickly with skin taut.
4. SPRAY and STRETCH TECHNIQUE for MYOFASCIAL PAIN
Ethyl Chloride may be used as a counterirritant in the management of myofascial pain, restricted motion, and muscle spasm. Clinical conditions that may respond to Ethyl Chloride include low back pain (due to muscle spasm), acute stiff neck, torticollis, acute bursitis of the shoulder, muscle spasm associated with osteoarthritis, tight hamstring, sprained ankle, masseter muscle spasm, certain types of headache, and referred pain due to irritated trigger point. Relief of pain facilitates early mobilization in restoration of muscle function. The Spray and Stretch technique is a therapeutic system which involves three stages. EVALUATION, SPRAYING, and STRETCHING.
The therapeutic value of Spray and Stretch becomes most effective when the practitioner has mastered all stages and applies them in the proper sequence.
I. EVALUATION
During the evaluation phase the cause of pain is determined as local spasm or an irritated trigger point. The method of applying the spray to a muscle spasm differs slightly from application to a trigger point. A trigger point is a deep hypersensitive localized spot in a muscle which causes a referred pain pattern. With trigger points the source of pain is seldom the site of the pain. A trigger point may be detected by a snapping palpation over the muscle causing the muscle in which the irritated trigger point is situated to "jump".
II. SPRAYING
A. Patients should assume a comfortable position.
B. Take precautions to cover the patient's eyes, nose, mouth, if spraying near face.
C. Hold bottle in an upside down position 12 to 18 inches (30 to 45 cm.) away from the treatment surface allowing the jet stream of vapocoolant to meet the skin at an acute angle to lessen the shock of impact.
D. The spray is directed in parallel sweeps 1.5 to 2 cm. apart. The rate of spraying is approximately 10 cm/sec. and is

continued until the entire muscle has been covered. The number of sweeps is determined by the size of the muscle. In the case of the trigger point, the spray should be applied over the trigger point through and over the reference zone. In the case of muscle spasm, the spray should be applied from origin to insertion.

III. STRETCHING

During application of the spray, the muscle is passively stretched. Force is gradually increased with successive sweeps, and the slack is smoothly taken up as the muscle relaxes, establishing a new stretch length.

Reaching the full normal length of the muscle is necessary to completely inactivate trigger points and relieve pain.

After rewarming, the procedure may be repeated as necessary. Moist heat should be applied for 10 to 15 minutes following treatment. For lasting benefit, any factors that perpetuate the trigger mechanism must be eliminated.

HOW SUPPLIED

100 gram metal tube.................................(NDC 0386-0001-05)
4 ounce amber glass bottle:
Fine Spray...(NDC 0386-0001-04)
Medium Spray.......................................(NDC 0386-0001-03)
Coarse Spray..(NDC 0386-0001-02)
"Spra Pak"..(NDC 0386-0001-01)

CAUTION

Federal law prohibits dispensing without a prescription.

FLUORI–METHANE®   ℞
(Dichlorodifluoromethane 15%
Trichloromonofluoromethane 85%)

INDICATIONS AND USAGE

Fluori-Methane Spray is a vapocoolant intended for topical application in the management of myofascial pain, restricted motion, and muscle spasm, and for the control of pain associated with injections.

Clinical conditions that may respond to Spray and Stretch include low back pain (due to muscle spasm), acute stiff neck, torticollis, muscle spasm associated with osteoarthritis, ankle sprain, tight hamstring, masseter muscle spasm, certain types of headache, and referred pain due to trigger points. Relief of pain facilitates early mobilization in restoration of muscle function.

PRECAUTIONS

Care should be taken to minimize inhalation of vapors, especially with application around head or neck. Avoid contact with eyes. Fluori-Methane should not be applied to the point of frost formation.

ADVERSE REACTIONS

Cutaneous sensitization may occur, but appears to be extremely rare. Freezing can occasionally alter pigmentation.

CONTRAINDICATIONS

Fluori-Methane is contraindicated in individuals with a history of hypersensitivity to dichlorodifluoromethane, and/or trichloromonofluoromethane.

WARNINGS

For external use only.

Dichlorodifluoromethane and trichloromonofluoromethane are not classified as carcinogens. Based on animal studies and human experience, these fluorocarbons pose no hazard to man relative to systemic toxicity, carcinogenicity, mutagenicity, or teratogenicity when occupational exposures are below 1000 p.p.m. over an 8 hour time weighted average. Contents under pressure. Store in a cool place. Do not store above 120°F.

DOSAGE AND ADMINISTRATION

To apply Fluori-Methane, invert the bottle over the treatment area approximately 12 inches (30 cm.) away from site of application. Open dispenseal spring valve completely, allowing the liquid to flow in a stream from the bottle.

1. SPRAY and STRETCH TECHNIQUE for MYOFASCIAL PAIN

Spray and stretch technique is a therapeutic system which involves three stages: EVALUATION, SPRAYING, and STRETCHING.

The therapeutic value of Spray and Stretch becomes most effective when the practitioner has mastered all stages and applies them in proper sequence.

I. EVALUATION

During the evaluation phase the cause of pain is determined as local spasm or an irritated trigger point. The method of applying the spray to a muscle spasm differs slightly from application to a trigger point. A trigger point is a deep hypersensitive localized spot in a muscle which causes a referred pain pattern. With trigger points the source of pain is seldom the site of the pain. A trigger point may be detected by snapping palpation over the muscle causing the muscle in which the irritated trigger point is situated to "jump".

II. SPRAYING

A. Patients should assume a comfortable poisition.

B. Take precautions to cover the patient's eyes, nose, mouth, if spraying near face.

C. Hold bottle in an upside down position 12 to 18 inches (30 to 45 cm.) away from the treatment surface allowing the jet stream of vapocoolant to meet the skin at an acute angle to lessen the shock of impact.

D. The spray is directed in parallel sweeps 1.5 to 2 cm. apart. The rate of spraying is approximately 10 cm/sec. and is continued until the entire muscle has been covered. The number of sweeps is determined by the size of the muscle. In the case of trigger point, the spray should be applied over the trigger point through and over the reference zone. In the case of muscle spasm, the spray should be applied from origin to insertion.

III. STRETCHING

During application of the spray, the muscle is passively stretched. Force is gradually increased with successive sweeps, and the slack is smoothly taken up as the muscle relaxes, establishing a new stretch length.

Reaching the full normal length of the muscle is necessary to completely inactivate trigger points and relieve pain.

After rewarming, the procedure may be repeated as necessary. Moist heat should be applied for 10 to 15 minutes following treatment.

For lasting benefit, any factors that perpetuate the trigger mechanism must be eliminated.

2. PRE-INJECTION ANESTHESIA

Prepare syringe and have it ready. Cleanse skin with antiseptic, if alcohol, wait for it to dry. Spray skin with Fluori-Methane, from a distance of about 12 inches (30 cm.) continuously for 3 to 5 seconds; do not frost the skin. Quickly set down bottle and pick up syringe. Watch liquid film of spray on skin and just as it dries, introduce needle quickly with skin taut.

HOW SUPPLIED

4 ounce amber glass bottle.
Calibrated Fine Spray............................(NDC 0386-0003-04)
Calibrated Medium Spray.......................(NDC 0386-0003-05)

CAUTION

Federal law prohibits dispensing without a prescription.

FLURO–ETHYL®   ℞
(Ethyl Chloride, U.S.P., 25%
Dichlorotetrafluoroethane, N.F., 75%)

INDICATIONS and USAGE

Fluro-Ethyl is a topical refrigerant anesthetic intended to control the pain associated with minor surgical procedures, dermabrasion, injections, contusions and minor strains.

PRECAUTIONS

Inhalation of Fluro-Ethyl should be avoided as it may produce narcotic and general anesthetic effects, and may produce deep anesthesia, or fatal coma with respiratory or cardiac arrest. When used to produce local freezing of tissues, adjacent skin areas should be protected by application of petrolatum. The thawing process may be painful, and freezing may lower local resistance to infection and delay healing.

ADVERSE REACTIONS

Cutaneous sensitization may occur, but appears to be extremely rare. Freezing can occasionally alter pigmentation. Frostbite may occur.

CONTRAINDICATIONS

Fluro-Ethyl is contraindicated in individuals with a history of hypersensitivity to Ethyl Chloride or Dichlorotetrafluoroethane. Fluro-Ethyl should not be used on patients having vascular impairment of the extremities.

WARNINGS

For external use only.

The components of Fluro-Ethyl are not listed as carcinogens by IARC, NTP or OSHA. Based on animal studies and human experiences this mixture poses no hazard to man relative to systemic toxicity, carcinogenicity, mutagenicity, or teratogenicity when occupational exposures are below its recommended exposure limits.

Skin absorption of Ethyl Chloride can occur; no cases of chronic poisoning have been reported. Ethyl Chloride is known as a liver and kidney toxin; long term exposure may cause liver or kidney damage.

Fluro-Ethyl can cause frostbite.

Contents under pressure. Store in a cool place, do not store above 120°F.

DOSAGE and ADMINISTRATION

To apply Fluro-Ethyl, invert the container over the treatment area approximately 2 to 4 inches (5-10cm) from the site of application. Press gently on side of the spray valve allowing the liquid to emerge as a fine mist spray.

1. TOPICAL ANESTHESIA IN MINOR SURGERY

The operative site should be cleansed with a suitable antiseptic. Apply petrolatum to protect the adjacent area. Spray Fluro-Ethyl for a few seconds to the point of frost formation, when the tissue becomes white. Avoid prolonged spraying of skin beyond this state. The anesthetic action of Fluro-Ethyl rarely lasts more than a few seconds to a minute. Therefore, the incision should be made promptly when the tissue becomes white. Reapply as needed.

2. DERMABRASION

The operative site should be cleansed with a suitable antiseptic. Apply petrolatum to protect adjacent areas. Take precautions to cover the patient's eyes, nose, mouth, if spraying near the face. To firm the skin and numb the dermabrasion site, spray treatment area for 20 to 30 seconds prior to starting the dermabrasion procedure. Reapply as necessary during the procedure to maintain desired skin firmness.

3. FOR PRE-INJECTION ANESTHESIA

Prepare syringe and have it ready. Cleanse skin with antiseptic, if alcohol, wait for it to dry. Spray skin with Fluro-Ethyl from a distance of about 4 inches (10 cm.) continuously for 2 to 3 seconds; do not frost skin. Quickly set down can and pick up syringe. Watch liquid film of spray on skin and just as it dries, introduce needle quickly with skin taut.

4. CONTUSIONS and MINOR STRAINS

The pain of bruises, contusions, and minor sprains may be controlled with Fluro-Ethyl.

Spray affected area from a distance of 6 to 12 inches (15 to 30 cm.) for a few seconds until the tissue begins to frost and turn white. Avoid spraying of skin beyond this state. Use as you would ice. The amount of cooling depends on the dosage. The smallest dose needed to produce the desired effect should be used.

Determine the extent of injury (fracture, sprain, etc.). The anesthetic effect of Fluro-Ethyl rarely lasts more than a few seconds to a minute. This time interval is usually sufficient to help reduce or relieve the initial trauma of the injury.

HOW SUPPLIED

Net weight 9 ounce aerosol spray can (NDC 0386-0002-09)

CAUTION

Federal law prohibits dispensing without a prescription.

EDUCATIONAL MATERIAL

For supporting educational materials contact Gebauer Chemical Company.

GEIGY Pharmaceuticals
Division of CIBA-GEIGY Corporation
ARDSLEY, NY 10502

GY-CODE® INDEX

Geigy Pharmaceuticals has established a Drug Identity Code System entitled GY-CODE. This system affords a convenient and accurate means of uniquely identifying each Geigy solid dosage form on which the GY-CODE number and the name "Geigy" appear. The GY-CODE number also appears as part of the National Drug Code number.

GY-CODE NUMBER	PROD. DESCRIPTION		NATIONAL DRUG CODE
14 Butazolidin® Tablets			
	phenylbutazone USP	100 mg	
	Red, film-coated tablets		
	100's		0028-0014-01
	1000's		0028-0014-10
	100's Unit Dose Pkg.		0028-0014-61
20 Tofranil-PM® Capsules			
	imipramine pamoate	75 mg	
	Coral-colored capsules		
	30's		0028-0020-26
	100's		0028-0020-01
	1000's		0028-0020-10
	100's Unit Dose Pkg.		0028-0020-61
22 Tofranil-PM® Capsules			
	imipramine pamoate	150 mg	
	Coral-colored capsules		
	30's		0028-0022-26
	100's		0028-0022-01
	100's Unit Dose Pkg.		0028-0022-61
23 Lioresal® Tablets			
	baclofen	10 mg	
	White, oval, scored tablets		
	100's		0028-0023-01
	100's Unit Dose Pkg.		0028-0023-61

Continued on next page

The full prescribing information for each GEIGY product is contained herein and is that in effect as of September 1, 1989

Geigy—Cont.

32 Tofranil® Tablets
imipramine hydrochloride USP

                                   10 mg
Triangular, coral-colored,
   coated tablets
   100's   0028-0032-01
   1000's   0028-0032-10

33 Lioresal® Tablets
baclofen   20 mg
White, capsule shaped, scored tablets
   100's   0028-0033-01
   100's Unit Dose Pkg.   0028-0033-61

40 Tofranil-PM® Capsules
imipramine pamoate   100 mg
Dark yellow/coral-colored capsules
   30's   0028-0040-26
   100's   0028-0040-01

42 Constant-T® Tablets
theophylline (anhydrous)   200 mg
Light pink, oval, scored tablets
   100's   0028-0042-01
   100's Unit Dose Pkg.   0028-0042-61
   Gy-Pak® 60's
     One Unit (12 × 60)   0028-0042-73
     Six Units (72 × 60)   0028-0042-73

44 Butazolidin® Capsules
phenylbutazone USP   100 mg
Orange/white capsules
   100's   0028-0044-01
   1000's   0028-0044-10
   100's Unit Dose Pkg.   0028-0044-61
   Gy-Pak® 100's
     One Unit (12 × 100)   0028-0044-65
     Six Units (72 × 100)   0028-0044-65

45 Tofranil-PM® Capsules
imipramine pamoate   125 mg
Light yellow/coral-colored capsules
   30's   0028-0045-26
   100's   0028-0045-01

48 PBZ-SR® Tablets
tripelennamine hydrochloride

                                   100 mg
Lavender-colored tablets
   100's   0028-0048-01

51 Lopressor® Tablets
metoprolol tartrate   50 mg
Light red, capsule-shaped, scored tablets
   100's   0028-0051-01
   1000's   0028-0051-10
   100's Unit Dose Pkg.   0028-0051-61
   Gy-Pak® 60's
     One Unit (12 × 60)   0028-0051-73
     Six Units (72 × 60)   0028-0051-73
   Gy-Pak® 100's
     One Unit (12 × 100)   0028-0051-65
     Six Units (72 × 100)   0028-0051-65

52 Tegretol® Chewable Tablets
carbamazepine USP   100 mg
Round, red-speckled, pink, single-scored tablets
   100's   0028-0052-01
   100's Unit Dose Pkg.   0028-0052-61

57 Constant-T® Tablets
theophylline (anhydrous)   300 mg
Light blue, oval, scored tablets
   100's   0028-0057-01
   100's Unit Dose Pkg.   0028-0057-61
   Gy-Pak® 60's
     One Unit (12 × 60)   0028-0057-73
     Six Units (72 × 60)   0028-0057-73

25 Voltaren® Tablets
diclofenac sodium   25 mg
Yellow, biconvex with beveled edges, enteric-coated
   60's   0028-0058-60
   100's   0028-0058-01
   100's Unit Dose Pkg.   0028-0058-61

27 Tegretol® Tablets
carbamazepine USP   200 mg
White, single-scored tablets
   100's   0028-0027-01
   1000's   0028-0027-10
   100's Unit Dose Pkg.   0028-0027-61
   Gy-Pak® 100's
     One Unit (12 × 100)   0028-0027-65
     Six Units (72 × 100)   0028-0027-65

71 Lopressor® Tablets
metoprolol tartrate   100 mg
Light blue, capsule-shaped, scored tablets
   100's   0028-0071-01
   1000's   0028-0071-10
   100's Unit Dose Pkg.   0028-0071-61

Gy-Pak® 60's
     One Unit (12 × 60)   0028-0071-73
     Six Units (72 × 60)   0028-0071-73
Gy-Pak® 100's
     One Unit (12 × 100)   0028-0071-65
     Six Units (72 × 100)   0028-0071-65

72 Brethine® Tablets
terbutaline sulfate USP   2.5 mg
Oval, white, scored tablets
   100's   0028-0072-01
   1000's   0028-0072-10
   100's Unit Dose Pkg.   0028-0072-61
   Gy-Pak® 100's
     One Unit (12 × 100)   0028-0072-65
     Six Units (72 × 100)   0028-0072-65

105 Brethine® Tablets
terbutaline sulfate USP   5 mg
Round, scored, white tablets
   100's   0028-0105-01
   1000's   0028-0105-10
   100's Unit Dose Pkg.   0028-0105-61
   Gy-Pak® 100's
     One unit (12 × 100)   0028-0105-65
     Six units (72 × 100)   0028-0105-65

108 Lamprene® Capsules
clofazimine   50 mg
Brown, spherical capsules
   100's   0028-0108-01

109 Lamprene® Capsules
clofazimine   100 mg
Brown, oblong capsules
   100's   0028-0109-01

111 PBZ® Tablets
tripelennamine hydrochloride USP   25 mg
Round, white, scored tablets
   100's   0028-0111-01

117 PBZ® Tablets
tripelennamine hydrochloride USP

                                   50 mg
Round, white, scored tablets
   100's   0028-0117-01
   1000's   0028-0117-10

136 Tofranil® Tablets
imipramine hydrochloride USP

                                   50 mg
Coral-colored (white Geigy imprint) coated tablets
   100's   0028-0136-01
   1000's   0028-0136-10
   100's Unit Dose Pkg.   0028-0136-61
   Gy-Pak® 100's
     One unit (12 × 100)   0028-0136-65
     Six units (72 × 100)   0028-0136-65

140 Tofranil® Tablets
imipramine hydrochloride USP

                                   25 mg
Coral-colored (black Geigy imprint) coated tablets
   100's   0028-0140-01
   1000's   0028-0140-10
   100's Unit Dose Pkg.   0028-0140-61
   Gy-Pak® 100's
     One unit (12 × 100)   0028-0140-65
     Six units (72 × 100)   0028-0140-65

50 Voltaren® Tablets
diclofenac sodium   50 mg
Light brown, biconvex with beveled edges, enteric-coated
   60's   0028-0162-60
   100's   0028-0162-01
   1000's   0028-0162-10
   100's Unit Dose Pkg.   0028-0162-61

75 Voltaren® Tablets
diclofenac sodium   75 mg
White, biconvex with beveled edges, enteric-coated
   60's   0028-0164-60
   100's   0028-0164-01
   1000's   0028-0164-10
   100's Unit Dose Pkg.   0028-0164-61

6114 Otrivin® Nasal Drops (0.1%)
xylometazoline hydrochloride USP
   20 ml   0028-6114-58

6116 Otrivin® Pediatric (0.05%)
xylometazoline hydrochloride USP
   20 ml   0028-6116-58

6118 Otrivin® Spray (0.1%)
xylometazoline hydrochloride USP
   15 ml   0028-6118-57

6925 PBZ® Elixir
Per 5-ml teaspoon:
tripelennamine citrate
     USP   37.5 mg
     (equivalent to 25 mg
       tripelennamine hydrochloride)
   473 ml   0028-6925-16

6946 PBZ® Antihistamine Cream
tripelennamine hydrochloride
Cream 2% (water-washable base)
   1 oz   0028-6946-76

BRETHAIRE®   ℞
[breth-air´]
terbutaline sulfate USP inhaler
Bronchodilator Aerosol
For Oral Inhalation Only

DESCRIPTION
The active ingredient of Brethaire is terbutaline sulfate USP, α-[(tert-butylamino)methyl]-3,5-dihydroxybenzyl alcohol sulfate (2:1) (salt), a relatively selective beta$_2$-adrenergic bronchodilator.

Terbutaline sulfate USP is a white to gray-white crystalline powder. It is odorless or has a faint odor of acetic acid. It is soluble in water and in 0.1N hydrochloric acid, slightly soluble in methanol, and insoluble in chloroform. Its molecular weight is 548.65.

Brethaire is a metered-dose dispenser containing micronized terbutaline sulfate in a suspension of the following composition:

	7.5-ml (10.5-g) Canister
terbutaline sulfate USP	0.075 g
sorbitan trioleate	0.105 g
trichloromonofluoromethane NF	2.58 g
dichlorotetrafluoroethane NF	2.58 g
dichlorodifluoromethane NF	5.16 g

Each actuation delivers 0.20 mg of terbutaline sulfate from the mouthpiece (0.25 mg valve delivery). Each canister provides about 300 inhalations.

CLINICAL PHARMACOLOGY
Brethaire is a beta-adrenergic-receptor agonist that has been shown by in vitro and in vivo studies in animals to exert a preferential effect on beta$_2$-adrenergic receptors such as those located in bronchial smooth muscle. However, controlled clinical studies in patients who were administered the drug have not revealed a preferential beta$_2$-adrenergic effect.

It has been postulated that beta-adrenergic agonists produce many of their pharmacologic effects by activation of adenyl cyclase, the enzyme that catalyzes the conversion of adenosine triphosphate to cyclic adenosine monophosphate.

Terbutaline sulfate by inhaler has been shown in controlled clinical studies to relieve bronchospasm associated with chronic obstructive pulmonary disease such as asthma, chronic bronchitis, and emphysema. This action was manifested by a clinically significant improvement in pulmonary function as demonstrated by an increase in FEV$_1$ of 15% or more in some patients. Terbutaline sulfate by inhaler also produced clinically significant increases in peak expiratory flow rate and instantaneous flow rates at 75, 50, and 25% of vital capacity. There were also clinically significant reductions in functional residual capacity, residual volume, and airway resistance in some patients. Clinically significant improvement in pulmonary function occurred within 5 to 30 minutes in most patients after administration of the drug. The response was well established by 5 minutes and the maximal effect usually occurred between 1 and 2 hours in most patients. Significant bronchodilator activity has been observed to persist for 3 to 4 hours after dosing in many patients in 3-month repetitive-dose studies. With continued administration of Brethaire, the duration of effectiveness decreases in most patients.

INDICATIONS AND USAGE
Brethaire is indicated for the relief of bronchospasm in patients with reversible obstructive airway disease.

In controlled clinical trials the onset of improvement in pulmonary function was within 5 to 30 minutes. These studies also showed that maximum improvement in pulmonary function occurred at 120 minutes following two inhalations of Brethaire and that clinically significant improvement (i.e., 15% increase in FEV$_1$/predicted FEV$_1$) generally continued for 3 to 4 hours in most patients. In some studies there was a significant decrease in improvement of pulmonary function noted with continued administration of terbutaline sulfate aerosol. Continued effectiveness of Brethaire was demonstrated over a 14-week period in some patients in these clinical trials. Some patients with asthma, in single-dose studies only, have shown a therapeutic response that was still apparent at 6 hours.

CONTRAINDICATIONS
Brethaire is contraindicated in patients with a history of hypersensitivity to any of its components.

WARNINGS
As with other adrenergic aerosols, the potential for paradoxical bronchospasm should be kept in mind. If it occurs, the preparation should be discontinued immediately and alternative therapy instituted.

Fatalities have been reported in association with excessive use of inhaled sympathomimetic drugs. The exact cause of death is unknown.

The contents of Brethaire are under pressure. Do not puncture the container. Do not use or store it near heat or open flame. Exposure to temperatures above 120°F may cause bursting. Never throw the container into a fire or incinerator. Keep it out of children's reach.

PRECAUTIONS

General: Terbutaline sulfate is a sympathomimetic amine and, as such, should be used with caution in patients with cardiovascular disorders, including coronary insufficiency and hypertension, in patients with hyperthyroidism or diabetes mellitus, and in patients who are unusually responsive to sympathomimetic amines.

Large doses of intravenous terbutaline sulfate have been reported to aggravate preexisting diabetes and ketoacidosis. Aerosol terbutaline sulfate is not indicated for tocolysis.

Although there have been no reports concerning the use of aerosol terbutaline sulfate during labor and delivery, it has been reported that high doses of terbutaline sulfate administered intravenously inhibit uterine contractions. Although this effect is extremely unlikely as a consequence of aerosol use, it should be kept in mind.

Information for Patients: The action of Brethaire may last up to 6 hours, and therefore, it should not be used more frequently than recommended. Patients should not increase the number or frequency of doses without consulting the physician. If symptoms get worse, patients should consult their physician promptly. While taking Brethaire, patients should not take other inhaled medicines that have not been prescribed by the physician.

See illustrated **Instructions for Patients.**

Drug Interactions: Other sympathomimetic aerosol bronchodilators or epinephrine should not be used concomitantly with terbutaline sulfate. Terbutaline sulfate should be administered with caution to patients being treated with monoamine oxidase inhibitors or tricyclic antidepressants, since the action of terbutaline sulfate on the vascular system may be potentiated.

Beta-receptor-blocking agents and terbutaline sulfate inhibit the effect of each other.

Carcinogenesis, Mutagenesis, Impairment of Fertility: A 2-year oral carcinogenesis bioassay of terbutaline sulfate (50, 500, 1000, and 2000 mg/kg, corresponding to 1042, 10,417, 20,833, and 41,667 times the recommended daily adult dose) in Sprague-Dawley rats revealed drug-related changes in the female genital system. Female rats showed drug-related increases in leiomyomas of the mesovarium: 3 (5%) at 50 mg/kg, 17 (28%) at 500 mg/kg, 21 (35%) at 1000 mg/kg, and 23 (38%) at 2000 mg/kg, which were significant at the three highest levels. None occurred in female controls. The incidence of ovarian cysts was significantly elevated at all dose levels except at 2000 mg/kg, and hyperplasia of the mesovarium was increased significantly at 500 and 2000 mg/kg.

A 21-month oral (feeding) study of terbutaline sulfate (5, 50, and 200 mg/kg, corresponding to 104, 1042, and 4167 times the recommended daily adult dose) in the mouse revealed no evidence of carcinogenicity.

Studies of terbutaline sulfate have not been conducted to determine mutagenic potential.

A Segment 1 oral reproduction study of terbutaline sulfate (up to 50 mg/kg corresponding to 1042 times the maximum clinical dose) in the rat revealed no adverse effects on fertility.

Pregnancy Category B: Reproduction studies have been performed in rats and rabbits at doses up to 1042 times the human dose and have revealed no evidence of impaired fertility or harm to the fetus due to terbutaline sulfate. There are, however, no adequate and well-controlled studies in pregnant women. Because animal reproduction studies are not always predictive of human response, this drug should be used during pregnancy only if clearly needed. For use in labor and delivery, see **Precautions, General.**

Nursing Mothers: It is not known whether this drug is excreted in human milk. Because many drugs are excreted in human milk, caution should be exercised when terbutaline sulfate is administered to a nursing woman.

Pediatric Use: Safety and effectiveness in children below the age of 12 years have not been established.

ADVERSE REACTIONS

The adverse reactions of terbutaline sulfate are similar to those of other sympathomimetic agents. A 14-week double-blind study compared terbutaline sulfate and isoproterenol aerosols in 259 asthmatic patients. The results of this study showed that the incidence of cardiovascular effects was as follows: palpitations, none with terbutaline and fewer than 1 per 100 with isoproterenol; tachycardia, about 3 per 100 with terbutaline and about 2 per 100 with isoproterenol; and increased blood pressure, fewer than 1 per 100 with terbutaline and about 2 per 100 with isoproterenol. In the same study, both drugs caused headache and nausea or digestive disorder in fewer than 10 patients per 100, tremor or nervousness in fewer than 5 patients per 100, and drowsiness in fewer than 5 patients per 100. About 4% of patients receiving terbutaline and about 1% of patients receiving isoproterenol had dysrhythmias. In addition, terbutaline sulfate, like other sympathomimetic agents, can cause adverse reactions such as angina, dyspnea and wheezing, vomiting, vertigo, central stimulation, insomnia, unusual taste, and drying or irritation of the oropharynx. Significantly more patients experienced dyspnea or wheezing, or both, after terbutaline than after isoproterenol administration. ECG changes such as sinus pause, atrial premature beats, AV block, ventricular premature beats, ST-T-wave depression, T-wave inversion, sinus bradycardia, and atrial escape beat with aberrant conduction were described after terbutaline administration. ECG changes were similar in frequency after isoproterenol administration.

OVERDOSAGE

Overdosage experience is limited. Excessive adrenergic-receptor stimulation may augment the signs and symptoms listed under **ADVERSE REACTIONS** and may be accompanied by other adrenergic effects. In the case of terbutaline overdosage, the patient should be treated symptomatically for the sympathomimetic overdosage with careful consideration given to the appropriateness of any chosen therapy and to the possible effect on the patient's underlying disease state.

DOSAGE AND ADMINISTRATION

The usual dosage for adults and children 12 years and older is two inhalations separated by a 60-second interval, repeated every 4 to 6 hours. Dosing should not be repeated more often than every 4 to 6 hours. The use of Brethaire can be continued as medically indicated to control recurring bouts of bronchospasm. During this time most patients gain optimal benefit from regular use of the inhaler. Safe usage for periods extending over several years has been documented.

If a previously effective dosage regimen fails to provide the usual relief, medical advice should be sought immediately, as this is often a sign of seriously worsening asthma, which would require reassessment of therapy.

HOW SUPPLIED

Brethaire contains 75 mg of terbutaline sulfate as a micronized powder in an inert propellant. This is sufficient medication for about 300 actuations. Each actuation delivers approximately 0.20 mg of terbutaline sulfate from the mouthpiece (0.25 mg valve delivery).

Brethaire canister with mouthpiece, 7.5 ml (10.5 g)
....NDC 0028-5557-88

Brethaire canister refill, 7.5 ml (10.5 g)
....NDC 0028-5557-87

Do not store above 86°F.
Dispense with enclosed instructions for use.
Federal law prohibits dispensing without a prescription.
U.S. Patent No. 3,937,838

C85-67 (Rev. 11/85)

Dist. by:
GEIGY Pharmaceuticals
Division of CIBA-GEIGY Corporation
Ardsley, New York 10502
Shown in Product Identification Section, page 410

BRETHANCER® ℞
[breth-anc'er]
spacer-inhaler

The Brethancer spacer-inhaler is recommended for patients with difficulty coordinating conventional aerosol inhalers, so those patients may derive greater therapeutic benefit from their medication.

Although aerosol medications offer patients the benefits of rapidity of action, many patients have difficulty coordinating inhalation with aerosol activation. With Brethancer, the patient no longer requires this coordination but can inhale the aerosolized drug from the spacer tube after the canister is activated.

Unlike other devices designed to aid in the proper use of aerosol medications, Brethancer is compact and easy to carry in its closed form. The Brethancer has three interlocking and telescoping plastic components which, when extended, assist in improving the use of aerosol medications. Opening the device is accomplished in one motion, which simplifies use by the patient. As an additional feature, the breathing hole is closed when the Brethancer is telescoped, which prevents foreign matter from entering the unit.

The Brethancer unit will accommodate any of several currently available prescription aerosol bronchodilator medications.

The patient's inhalation technique should be checked regularly. See the patient package insert for operating instructions.

PATIENT PACKAGE INSERT—DIRECTIONS FOR USE PLEASE READ THESE INSTRUCTIONS BEFORE USING THE BRETHANCER.®

1. Remove the metal aerosol canister from the plastic mouthpiece, if so packaged.
2. Place the metal canister in the Brethancer so the narrow metal tip of the canister is inserted securely in the center hole of the Brethancer.
3. Shake well.
4. When opening Brethancer, do not push in the yellow plastic mouthpiece flap that appears behind the mouth hole of the gold outer section. Doing so can damage the unit and block the flow of medication when it is used.
   Open the Brethancer by pulling firmly on the open end, so that all three sections are fully extended. Turn the light yellow section upwards until it locks in the upright position.

Open the spacer

DO NOT USE Brethancer if the mouthpiece flap is not fully opened *or* if you cannot see all the way through the inside of the fully extended and locked unit to the lightest colored inner section.

5. Place the open, dark yellow end of the Brethancer to your mouth and breathe out.

Breathe out

6. Press down on the canister one time.

Release one dose

7. Then breathe in through the Brethancer, and try to hold your breath for a count of 10 before breathing out again. It is not necessary to press down on the canister and to breathe in at the same time.

Breathe in and hold your breath

8. If another dose is needed, repeat steps 5 to 7.
   To close the Brethancer completely, first press lightly on the sides of the middle yellow section and slide inside the dark yellow section. Then press lightly on the arrow on the bottom of the light yellow section and collapse all three sections together.

To close

Continued on next page

The full prescribing information for each GEIGY product is contained herein and is that in effect as of September 1, 1989

Geigy—Cont.

To close

PLEASE NOTE: Incorrectly closing Brethancer can damage it.

At least once a week, remove the canister and wash the extended Brethancer unit in hot water to keep the unit clean. Be sure to use the Brethancer correctly so the inhaled drug reaches the lungs and produces its full effect. The Brethancer allows both time and distance for the aerosol to form a fine mist of small drug particles, which are carried into the lungs by the inhaled air. The Brethancer makes inhalation of the drug almost fail-safe.

Mfd by: Perlos, Finland
Dist. by: GEIGY Pharmaceuticals
Division of CIBA-GEIGY Corporation
Ardsley, New York 10502

C88-30 (Rev. 10/88)

BRETHINE®   ℞

[breth-een ']
terbutaline sulfate USP
Tablets of 5 mg
Tablets of 2.5 mg

DESCRIPTION

Brethine, terbutaline sulfate USP, is a bronchodilator available as tablets of 2.5 mg (2.05 mg of the free base) and 5 mg (4.1 mg of the free base) for oral administration. Terbutaline sulfate is α [(tert-Butylamino) methyl]-3,5 dihydroxybenzyl alcohol sulfate (2:1) (salt).
Terbutaline sulfate USP is a white to gray-white crystalline powder. It is odorless or has a faint odor of acetic acid. It is soluble in water and in 0.1N hydrochloric acid, slightly soluble in methanol, and insoluble in chloroform. Its molecular weight is 548.65.
Inactive Ingredients. Cellulose compounds, lactose, magnesium stearate, povidone, and starch.

ACTIONS

Brethine is a β-adrenergic receptor agonist which has been shown by *in vitro* and *in vivo* pharmacological studies in animals to exert a preferential effect on β_2-adrenergic receptors such as those located in bronchial smooth muscle. Controlled clinical studies in patients who were administered the drug orally have revealed proportionally greater changes in pulmonary function parameters than in heart rate or blood pressure. While this *suggests* a relative preference for the β_2 receptor in man, the usual cardiovascular effects commonly associated with sympathomimetic agents were also observed with Brethine.
Brethine has been shown in controlled clinical studies to relieve bronchospasm in chronic obstructive pulmonary disease.
This action is manifested by a clinically significant increase in pulmonary function as demonstrated by an increase of 15% or more in FEV_1 and in $FEF_{25-75\%}$. Following administration of Brethine tablets, a measurable change in flow rate is usually observed in 30 minutes, and a clinically significant improvement in pulmonary function occurs at 60–120 minutes. The maximum effect usually occurs within 120-180 minutes. Brethine also produces a clinically significant decrease in airway and pulmonary resistance which persists for at least four hours or longer. Significant bronchodilator action, as measured by various pulmonary function determinations (airway resistance, $FEF_{25-75\%}$, or PEFR), has been demonstrated in some studies for periods up to eight hours. Clinical studies were conducted in which the effectiveness of Brethine was evaluated in comparison with ephedrine over periods up to three months. Both drugs continued to produce significant improvement in pulmonary function throughout this period of treatment.

INDICATIONS

Brethine is indicated as a bronchodilator for bronchial asthma and for reversible bronchospasm which may occur in association with bronchitis and emphysema.

CONTRAINDICATIONS

Brethine is contraindicated when there is known hypersensitivity to sympathomimetic amines.

WARNINGS

Usage in Pregnancy: Animal reproductive studies have been negative with respect to adverse effects on fetal development. The safe use of Brethine has not, however, been established in human pregnancy. As with any medication, the use of the drug in pregnancy, lactation, or women of childbearing potential requires that the expected therapeutic benefit of the drug be weighed against its possible hazards to the mother or child.
Usage in Pediatrics: Brethine tablets are not presently recommended for children below the age of 12 years due to insufficient clinical data in this pediatric group.

PRECAUTIONS

Brethine should be used with caution in patients with diabetes, hypertension, hyperthyroidism, and a history of seizures. Large doses of intravenous terbutaline sulfate have been reported to aggravate preexisting diabetes and ketoacidosis.
As with other sympathomimetic bronchodilator agents, Brethine should be administered cautiously to cardiac patients, especially those with associated arrhythmias.
The concomitant use of Brethine with other sympathomimetic agents is not recommended, since their combined effect on the cardiovascular system may be deleterious to the patient. However, this does not preclude the use of an aerosol bronchodilator of the adrenergic stimulant type for the relief of an acute bronchospasm in patients receiving chronic oral Brethine therapy.
Terbutaline sulfate is not indicated for tocolysis. Serious adverse reactions may occur following administration of parenteral terbutaline sulfate to women in labor. In the mother, these include increased heart rate, transient hyperglycemia, transient hypokalemia, and possibly pulmonary edema. Increased fetal heart rate and neonatal hypoglycemia may occur as a result of maternal parenteral administration.

ADVERSE REACTIONS

Commonly observed side effects include nervousness and tremor. Other reported reactions include headache, increased heart rate, palpitations, drowsiness, nausea, vomiting, sweating, and muscle cramps. These reactions are generally transient in nature and usually do not require treatment. The frequency of these side effects appears to diminish with continued therapy. In general, all the side effects observed are characteristic of those commonly seen with sympathomimetic amines.

DOSAGE AND ADMINISTRATION

The usual oral dose of Brethine for adults is 5 mg administered at approximately six-hour intervals, three times daily, during the hours the patient is usually awake. If side effects are particularly disturbing, the dose may be reduced to 2.5 mg three times daily, and still provide a clinically significant improvement in pulmonary function. A dose of 2.5 mg, three times daily, also is recommended for children in the 12- to 15-year group. Brethine is not recommended at present for use in children below the age of 12 years. In adults, a total dose of 15 mg should not be exceeded in a 24-hour period. In children, a total dose of 7.5 mg should not be exceeded in a 24-hour period.

OVERDOSAGE

Overdosage experience is limited. Excessive beta-adrenergic receptor stimulation may augment the signs or symptoms listed under **ADVERSE REACTIONS** and they may be accompanied by other adrenergic effects. Treat the alert patient who has taken excessive oral medication by emptying the stomach by means of induced emesis, followed by gastric lavage. In the unconscious patient, secure the airway with a cuffed endotracheal tube before beginning lavage (do not induce emesis). Instillation of activated charcoal slurry may help reduce absorption of terbutaline sulfate. Maintain adequate respiratory exchange. Provide cardiac and respiratory support as needed. Continue observation until symptom-free.

HOW SUPPLIED

Tablets 2.5 mg—oval, white, scored (imprinted Geigy 72)
Bottles of 100 ....NDC 0028-0072-01
Bottles of 1000 ....NDC 0028-0072-10
Gy-Pak®—One Unit
12 bottles—100 tablets each ....NDC 0028-0072-65
Unit Dose (blister pack)
Box of 100 (strips of 10) ....NDC 0028-0072-61
Tablets 5 mg—round, white, scored (imprinted Geigy 105)
Bottles of 100 ....NDC 0028-0105-01
Bottles of 1000 ....NDC 0028-0105-10
Gy-Pak®—one Unit
12 bottles—100 tablets each ....NDC 0028-0105-65
Unit Dose (blister pack)
Box of 100 (strips of 10) ....NDC 0028-0105-61
Store at controlled room temperature 59°-86°F (15°-30°C).
Dispense in tight, light-resistant container (USP).

C85-56 (Rev. 11/85)
Shown in Product Identification Section, page 410

BRETHINE®   ℞

[breth-een ']
terbutaline sulfate Injection USP
Ampuls
A sterile aqueous solution for subcutaneous injection.

DESCRIPTION

Brethine, terbutaline sulfate injection USP, is a β-adrenergic agonist bronchodilator available as a sterile, nonpyrogenic, aqueous solution in ampuls, for subcutaneous administration. Each milliliter of solution contains 1 mg of terbutaline sulfate USP (0.82 mg of the free base); sodium chloride ACS, for isotonicity; and hydrochloric acid ACS, for adjustment to a target pH of 4. Terbutaline sulfate is $(\pm)$-α-[(tert-butylamino)methyl]-3,5-dihydroxybenzyl alcohol sulfate (2:1) (salt). The empirical formula is $(C_{12}H_{19}NO_3)_2 \cdot H_2SO_4$
Terbutaline sulfate USP is a white to gray-white crystalline powder. It is odorless or has a faint odor of acetic acid. It is soluble in water and in 0.1N hydrochloric acid, slightly soluble in methanol, and insoluble in chloroform. Its molecular weight is 548.65.

CLINICAL PHARMACOLOGY

Brethine is a β-adrenergic receptor agonist. In vitro and in vivo studies in animals have shown that Brethine exerts a preferential effect on β_2-adrenergic receptors. While it is recognized that β_2-adrenergic receptors are the predominant receptors in bronchial smooth muscle, recent data indicate that there is a population of β_2-receptors in the human heart, existing in a concentration between 10–50%. The precise function of these, however, is not yet established (see WARNINGS). Controlled clinical studies in patients given Brethine subcutaneously have not revealed a preferential β_2-adrenergic effect.
The pharmacologic effects of β-adrenergic agonists, including Brethine, are at least in part attributable to stimulation through β-adrenergic receptors of intracellular adenylcyclase, the enzyme which catalyzes the conversion of adenosine triphosphate (ATP) to cyclic 3', 5'-adenosine monophosphate (cAMP). Increased cAMP levels are associated with relaxation of bronchial smooth muscle and inhibition of release of mediators of immediate hypersensitivity from cells, especially from mast cells.
Controlled clinical studies have shown that Brethine relieves bronchospasm in acute and chronic obstructive pulmonary disease by significantly increasing pulmonary flow rates (e.g., an increase of 15% or more in FEV_1). After subcutaneous administration of 0.25 mg of Brethine, a measurable change in flow rate usually occurs within 5 minutes, and a clinically significant increase in FEV_1 occurs within 15 minutes. The maximum effect usually occurs within 30–60 minutes, and clinically significant bronchodilator activity may continue for 1.5 to 4 hours. The duration of clinically significant improvement is comparable to that observed with equimilligram doses of epinephrine.
Recent studies in laboratory animals (minipigs, rodents, and dogs) recorded the occurrence of cardiac arrhythmias and sudden death (with histological evidence of necrosis) when β-agonists and methylxanthines were administered concurrently. The significance of these findings when applied to humans is currently unknown.

Pharmacokinetics

After subcutaneous administration of 0.25 mg of terbutaline sulfate to two male subjects, peak terbutaline serum concentrations of 5.2 and 5.3 ng/ml were observed at about 20 minutes after dosing. Further studies are needed to confirm these results.
Elimination half-life of the drug in 10 of 14 patients was approximately 2.9 hr after subcutaneous administration, but longer elimination half-lives (between 6–14 hr) were found in the other 4 patients. About 90% of the drug was excreted in the urine at 96 hr after subcutaneous administration, with about 60% of this being unchanged drug. It appears that the sulfate conjugate is a major metabolite of terbutaline and urinary excretion is the primary route of elimination.

INDICATIONS AND USAGE

Brethine is indicated for the prevention and reversal of bronchospasm in patients with bronchial asthma and reversible bronchospasm associated with bronchitis and emphysema.

CONTRAINDICATIONS

Brethine is contraindicated in patients known to be hypersensitive to sympathomimetic amines or any component of this drug product.

WARNINGS

There have been rare reports of seizures in patients receiving terbutaline; seizures did not recur in these patients after the drug was discontinued.
Controlled clinical studies and other clinical experience have shown that Brethine, like other β-adrenergic agonists, can produce a significant cardiovascular effect in some patients, as measured by pulse rate, blood pressure, symptoms, and/or ECG changes.

PRECAUTIONS

General

Since Brethine is a sympathomimetic amine, it should be used with caution in patients with cardiovascular disorders, including ischemic heart disease, hypertension, and cardiac arrhythmias; in patients with hyperthyroidism or diabetes mellitus; and in patients who are unusually responsive to sympathomimetic amines or who have convulsive disorders. Significant changes in systolic and diastolic blood pressure can be expected to occur in some patients after use of any β-adrenergic bronchodilator.

Immediate hypersensitivity reactions and exacerbations of bronchospasm have been reported after terbutaline administration.

Terbutaline sulfate should not be used for tocolysis.

Drug Interactions

The concomitant use of Brethine with other sympathomimetic agents is not recommended, since the combined effect on the cardiovascular system may be deleterious to the patient.

β-adrenergic agonists should be administered with caution to patients being treated with monoamine oxidase inhibitors or tricyclic antidepressants, since the action of β-adrenergic agonists on the vascular system may be potentiated.

Carcinogenesis, Mutagenesis, Impairment of Fertility

In a 2-year oral study in the rat, terbutaline sulfate caused a significant dose-related increase in the incidence of benign leiomyomas of the mesovarium at doses corresponding to 5,000, 50,000, 100,000, and 200,000 times the maximum recommended human subcutaneous dose (0.01 mg/kg). The relevance of these findings to humans is not known. An 18-month oral study in mice revealed no evidence of tumorigenicity at doses up to 200 mg/kg (20,000 times the maximum recommended human subcutaneous dose). Mutagenicity studies have not been performed. A reproduction study in rats at oral doses up to 5000 times the maximum subcutaneous dose (0.01 mg/kg) revealed no evidence of impaired fertility.

Pregnancy Category B

Reproduction studies performed in mice, rats, or rabbits at doses up to 1500 times the subcutaneous maximum daily human dose of 0.01 mg/kg have revealed no evidence of impaired fertility or harm to the fetus due to Brethine. Increased levels of maternal and fetal blood glucose have been observed after intravenous administration of terbutaline to near-term pregnant baboons at doses up to 4 times the maximum recommended human subcutaneous dose.

There are, however, no adequate and well-controlled studies in pregnant women. Because animal reproduction studies are not always predictive of human response, this drug should be used during pregnancy only if clearly needed. Administration of the drug under these conditions requires careful benefit-to-risk determination.

Labor and Delivery

Terbutaline sulfate should not be used for tocolysis. Serious adverse reactions may occur after administration of terbutaline sulfate to women in labor. In the mother, these include increased heart rate, transient hyperglycemia, hypokalemia, cardiac arrhythmias, pulmonary edema, and myocardial ischemia. Increased fetal heart rate and neonatal hypoglycemia may occur as a result of maternal administration.

Nursing Mothers

It is not known whether this drug is excreted in human milk. Therefore, Brethine should be used during nursing only if the potential benefit justifies the possible risk to the newborn.

Pediatric Use

Brethine is not recommended for patients under the age of 12 years because of insufficient clinical data to establish safety and effectiveness.

ADVERSE REACTIONS

Adverse reactions observed with Brethine are similar to those commonly seen with other sympathomimetic agents. All these reactions are transient in nature and usually do not require treatment.

The following table compares adverse reactions seen in patients treated with terbutaline sulfate injection (0.25 mg and 0.5 mg) with those seen in patients treated with epinephrine injection (0.25 mg and 0.5 mg), during eight double-blind crossover studies involving a total of 214 patients. [See table above right].

OVERDOSAGE

Acute Toxicity

Intravenous LD_{50}'s (mg/kg): rats, 61.5; mice, 48.4. Oral LD_{50} in rats is > 5000 mg/kg.

Signs and Symptoms

Excessive β-adrenergic receptor stimulation may augment the signs and symptoms listed under ADVERSE REACTIONS.

Treatment

There is no specific antidote. Treatment consists of discontinuation of Brethine along with the institution of appropriate symptomatic therapy.

Percent Incidence of Adverse Reactions

Reaction	Terbutaline 0.25 mg N=77	Terbutaline 0.5 mg N=205	Epinephrine 0.25 mg N=153	Epinephrine 0.5 mg N=61
Central Nervous System				
Tremors	7.8%	38.0%	16.3%	18.0%
Nervousness	16.9%	30.7%	8.5%	31.1%
Dizziness	1.3%	10.2%	7.8%	3.3%
Headache	7.8%	8.8%	3.3%	9.8%
Drowsiness	11.7%	9.8%	14.4%	8.2%
Cardiovascular				
Palpitations	7.8%	22.9%	7.8%	29.5%
Tachycardia	1.3%	1.5%	2.6%	0.0%
Respiratory				
Dyspnea	0.0%	2.0%	2.0%	0.0%
Chest Discomfort	1.3%	1.5%	2.6%	0.0%
Gastrointestinal				
Nausea/Vomiting	1.3%	3.9%	1.3%	11.5%
Systemic				
Weakness	1.3%	0.5%	2.6%	1.6%
Flushed Feeling	0.0%	2.4%	1.3%	0.0%
Sweating	0.0%	2.4%	0.0%	0.0%
Pain at Injection Site	2.6%	0.5%	2.6%	1.6%

Note: Some patients received more than one dosage strength of terbutaline sulfate and epinephrine. In addition, there were reports of anxiety, muscle cramps, and dry mouth (<0.5%).

DOSAGE AND ADMINISTRATION

Ampuls should be used only for subcutaneous administration and not intravenous infusion. Sterility and accurate dosing cannot be assured if the ampuls are not used in accordance with DOSAGE AND ADMINISTRATION.

The usual subcutaneous dose of Brethine is 0.25 mg injected into the lateral deltoid area. If significant clinical improvement does not occur within 15–30 minutes, a second dose of 0.25 mg may be administered. If the patient then fails to respond within another 15–30 minutes, other therapeutic measures should be considered. The total dose within 4 hours should not exceed 0.5 mg.

Note: Parenteral drug products should be inspected visually for particulate matter and discoloration prior to administration, whenever solution and container permit.

HOW SUPPLIED

Ampuls 1 mg/ml—The drug is supplied at a volume of 1 ml contained in a 2 ml clear glass ampul. Each ampul contains 1 mg of Brethine per 1 ml of solution; 0.25 ml of solution will provide the usual clinical dose of 0.25 mg. Ampuls are expiration-dated.

Box of 10 ampuls ....NDC 0028-7507-23
Box of 100 ampuls ....NDC 0028-7507-01

Keep at controlled room temperature 59°–86°F (15°–30°C). Protect from light by storing ampuls in original carton until dispensed. Do not use if solution is discolored.

C89-4 (Rev. 2/89)

Shown in Product Identification Section, page 410

BUTAZOLIDIN®

[bew-ta-zahl 'eh-dinn]
phenylbutazone USP
Tablets
Capsules

Because of the increased risk of agranulocytosis and aplastic anemia (see **ADVERSE REACTIONS**), Butazolidin is not recommended as initial therapy for any of its indications. It should be used only after other nonsteroidal anti-inflammatory drugs have been tried and found unsatisfactory. Butazolidin cannot be considered a simple analgesic and should never be administered casually. If it is used, the following cautions should be observed:

1. Therapy should not be initiated until a careful detailed history is taken and complete physical and laboratory examinations, including an examination of red cells, white cells and platelets, have been made. These examinations should be repeated if any signs or symptoms suggesting blood dyscrasia appear.
2. Patients should be told to discontinue use of the drug and report to the physician immediately any sign of:
a. Fever, sore throat, or lesions in the mouth (symptoms of blood dyscrasia);
b. Dyspepsia, epigastric pain; symptoms of anemia; unusual bleeding or bruising; black or tarry stools, or other evidence of intestinal ulceration;
c. Skin rashes;
d. Significant weight gain or edema.
3. The risk of aplastic anemia is greater in women, in the elderly of both sexes, and with chronic therapy, but

even short-term exposure of healthy young persons can result in fatal aplastic anemia.

4. A trial period of 1 week of therapy is considered adequate to determine the therapeutic effect of the drug. In the absence of a favorable response, therapy should be discontinued.
a. In patients 60 years and over, the drug should be restricted to short-term treatment periods only—if possible, 1 week maximum.
5. If long-term treatment is necessary, the lowest possible effective dose should be used, and patients should be adequately warned (see **Information for Patients**) and closely monitored.

DESCRIPTION

Butazolidin, phenylbutazone USP, is a nonsteroidal, anti-inflammatory agent, available as 100-mg tablets and capsules for oral administration. Phenylbutazone is 4-butyl-1,2-diphenyl-3,5-pyrazolidinedione.

Phenylbutazone USP is a white to off-white, odorless crystalline powder. It is very slightly soluble in water; freely soluble in acetone and in ether; soluble in alcohol. Its molecular weight is 308.38.

Butazolidin is closely related chemically and pharmacologically, including toxic effects, to the pyrazole compounds aminopyrine and antipyrine.

Inactive Ingredients (Butazolidin Tablets 100 mg): cellulose compounds, D&C Red No. 7 Lake, D&C Yellow No. 10 Aluminum Lake, magnesium stearate, starch and titanium dioxide.

(Butazolidin Capsules 100 mg): D&C Yellow No. 10, FD&C Red No. 3, gelatin, magnesium stearate, silicon dioxide, sodium bisulfite, sodium lauryl sulfate, starch and titanium dioxide.

CLINICAL PHARMACOLOGY

Butazolidin is a nonsalicylate, nonsteroidal, anti-inflammatory drug. It has anti-inflammatory, antipyretic, analgesic and mild uricosuric properties that produce symptomatic relief but do not alter the disease process.

The exact mechanism of the anti-inflammatory effects of Butazolidin has not been elucidated, but clinical pharmacology studies have shown that Butazolidin inhibits certain factors believed to be involved in the inflammatory process. These processes are (1) prostaglandin synthesis; (2) leukocyte migration; (3) release and activity of lysosomal enzymes.

Pharmacokinetics: Butazolidin is rapidly absorbed after oral administration and distributed partially into an extravascular compartment, with about one third remaining in plasma. About 98% of the drug in plasma is bound to albumin.

After administration of single 100-, 300-, and 600-mg doses, the mean elimination half-life is approximately 77 (54–99) hours (n = 6). There is a linear relationship between dose and area-under-the-curve.

After the administration of three 100-mg tablets, a peak plasma concentration of 43.3 mg/L is attained within 2.5 ± 1.4 hours. Elimination half-lives corresponding to the appar-

Continued on next page

The full prescribing information for each GEIGY product is contained herein and is that in effect as of September 1, 1989

Geigy—Cont.

ent elimination rate constant in each subject do not differ greatly for the first and last doses administered.

The pharmacokinetics of single doses of Butazolidin can be described by a two-compartment open model. Steady-state plasma concentrations of phenylbutazone are about four times higher than the peak concentration after the first single dose.

Steady-state plasma concentrations of the major, active metabolite, oxyphenbutazone, are about 50% of those of phenylbutazone. Less than 2% of the dose appears in the urine as oxyphenbutazone.

At steady state, 61% of ^{14}C-labelled Butazolidin can be recovered from the urine and 27% from the feces. However, only about 1% of total urinary radioactivity is eliminated in the urine as unchanged drug. The sum of nonconjugated urinary metabolites (oxyphenbutazone, γ-hydroxyphenylbutazone, p,γ-dihydroxyphenylbutazone) and phenylbutazone itself amounts to only about 10%. About 40% of the drug (total urinary radioactivity) is excreted in the urine as the C-4 glucuronide of phenylbutazone and an additional 12% is the C-4 glucuronide of γ-hydroxyphenylbutazone.

INDICATIONS AND USAGE

Butazolidin is indicated for the relief of symptoms associated with the following conditions, but only after other therapeutic measures, including other nonsteroidal, anti-inflammatory drugs, have been tried and found unsatisfactory: active ankylosing spondylitis, acute gouty arthritis, active rheumatoid arthritis, and acute attacks of degenerative joint disease of the hips and knees.

CONTRAINDICATIONS

Butazolidin is contraindicated in patients with a hypersensitivity to phenylbutazone or oxyphenbutazone, and in patients who have a bronchospastic reaction to aspirin or other nonsteroidal anti-inflammatory drugs.

WARNINGS

Hematologic: Butazolidin can cause aplastic anemia and agranulocytosis (see **ADVERSE REACTIONS**).

If patients develop any signs or symptoms suggesting a blood cell dyscrasia, then an examination of red cells, white cells, and platelets should be performed. If there is any significant change in the total leukocyte count, relative decrease in granulocytes, appearance of immature forms, or fall in hematocrit or platelet count, treatment with this drug should be discontinued immediately and a complete hematologic investigation should be made. Hematologic toxicity may occur shortly after initiation of therapy or after prolonged treatment; it may develop abruptly or gradually and may become apparent days or weeks after cessation of therapy. It is manifested by the appearance of anemia, leukopenia, thrombocytopenia, or clinically significant hemorrhagic diathesis.

Gastrointestinal Effects: Risk of G.I. Ulcerations, Bleeding, and Perforation with NSAID Therapy:

Serious gastrointestinal toxicity such as bleeding, ulceration, and perforation can occur at any time, with or without warning symptoms, in patients treated chronically with NSAID therapy. Although minor upper gastrointestinal problems, such as dyspepsia, are common, usually developing early in therapy, physicians should remain alert for ulceration and bleeding in patients treated chronically with NSAIDs even in the absence of previous G.I. tract symptoms. In patients observed in clinical trials of several months to 2 years duration, symptomatic upper G.I. ulcers, gross bleeding, or perforation appear to occur in approximately 1% of patients treated for 3–6 months, and in about 2–4% of patients treated for 1 year. Physicians should inform patients about the signs and/or symptoms of serious G.I. toxicity and what steps to take if they occur.

Studies to date have not identified any subset of patients not at risk of developing peptic ulceration and bleeding. Except for a prior history of serious G.I. events and other risk factors known to be associated with peptic ulcer disease, such as alcoholism, smoking, etc., no risk factors (e.g., age, sex) have been associated with increased risk. Elderly or debilitated patients seem to tolerate ulceration or bleeding less well than other individuals and most spontaneous reports of fatal G.I. events are in this population. Studies to date are inconclusive concerning the relative risk of various NSAIDs in causing such reactions. High doses of any NSAID probably carry a greater risk of these reactions, although controlled clinical trials showing this do not exist in most cases. In considering the use of relatively large doses (within the recommended dosage range), sufficient benefit should be anticipated to offset the potential increased risk of G.I. toxicity.

Hepatic: As with other nonsteroidal anti-inflammatory drugs, borderline elevations of values measured by one or more liver tests may occur in up to 15% of patients. These abnormalities may progress, may remain essentially unchanged, or may be transient with continued therapy. The SGPT (ALT) test is probably the most sensitive indicator of liver dysfunction. Meaningful elevations (three times the

upper limit of normal) of SGPT or SGOT (AST) have occurred in controlled clinical trials in less than 1% of patients. A patient with symptoms and/or signs suggesting liver dysfunction, or in whom abnormal liver test results have occurred, should be evaluated for evidence of the development of more severe hepatic reactions while on therapy with Butazolidin. Severe hepatic reactions, including jaundice and cases of fatal hepatitis, have been reported with Butazolidin as with other nonsteroidal anti-inflammatory drugs. Although such reactions are rare, if abnormal liver tests persist or worsen, if clinical signs and symptoms consistent with liver disease develop, or if systemic manifestations (eosinophilia, rash, etc.) occur, therapy with Butazolidin should be discontinued.

Respiratory: Like other drugs that inhibit prostaglandin synthetase activity, such as aspirin and sulfinpyrazone, Butazolidin may precipitate acute episodes of asthmatic attacks in patients with asthma (see **CONTRAINDICATIONS**).

PRECAUTIONS

General: Because serious adverse reactions or aggravation of existing medical problems can occur and have been reported, Butazolidin should be used with caution in patients with incipient cardiac failure; blood dyscrasias; pancreatitis; parotitis; stomatitis; polymyalgia rheumatica; temporal arteritis; severe renal, cardiac and hepatic disease; and in patients with a history of peptic ulcer disease or with symptoms of gastrointestinal inflammation or active ulceration, inflammatory bowel disease or Crohn's disease.

Renal Effects: As with other nonsteroidal anti-inflammatory drugs, long-term administration of phenylbutazone to animals has resulted in renal papillary necrosis and other abnormal renal pathology. In humans, there have been reports of acute interstitial nephritis with hematuria, proteinuria, and occasionally nephrotic syndrome.

A second form of renal toxicity has been seen in patients with prerenal conditions leading to a reduction in renal blood flow or blood volume, where the renal prostaglandins have a supportive role in the maintenance of renal perfusion. In these patients, administration of an NSAID may cause a dose-dependent reduction in prostaglandin formation and may precipitate overt renal decompensation. Patients at greatest risk of this reaction are those with impaired renal function, heart failure, liver dysfunction, those taking diuretics, and the elderly. Discontinuation of NSAID therapy is typically followed by recovery to the pretreatment state. Patients with significantly impaired renal function should be closely monitored; a lower daily dose should be anticipated to avoid excessive drug accumulation.

Patients reporting visual disturbances while receiving the drug should discontinue treatment and have an ophthalmologic examination, because ophthalmic adverse reactions have been reported (see **ADVERSE REACTIONS**, *Special Senses*).

Butazolidin increases sodium retention. As with other nonsteroidal anti-inflammatory drugs, Butazolidin should be used with caution in patients with whom fluid retention would aggravate an underlying condition such as severe cardiac or renal disease.

From age 40 on, the possibility of adverse reactions increases, and therefore Butazolidin should be used with commensurately greater care in these patients.

Information for Patients: Butazolidin, like other drugs of its class, is not free of side effects. The side effects of these drugs can cause discomfort and, rarely, more serious side effects, such as blood disorders and gastrointestinal bleeding, which may result in hospitalization and even fatal outcomes. Patients should be told to discontinue use of the drug and report to the physician immediately any sign of fever, sore throat, or lesions in the mouth (symptoms of blood dyscrasia); dyspepsia and epigastric pain; symptoms of anemia; unusual bleeding or bruising; black or tarry stools or other evidence of intestinal ulceration; skin rashes; or significant weight gain or edema. Patients should also be warned not to exceed the recommended dosage, since this may lead to toxic effects.

Physicians should discuss with their patients the potential risks (see WARNINGS, PRECAUTIONS, and ADVERSE REACTIONS) and likely benefits of Butazolidin treatment.

Laboratory Tests: Therapy should not be initiated until a careful detailed history is taken and complete physical and laboratory examinations, including an examination of red cells, white cells, and platelets, have been made. These examinations should also be made if any signs or symptoms appear suggesting depression of the formed blood elements.

Because serious G.I. tract ulceration and bleeding can occur without warning symptoms, physicians should follow patients for the signs and symptoms of ulceration and bleeding and should inform them of the importance of this follow-up (see WARNINGS, *Risk of G.I. Ulcerations, Bleeding, and Perforation with NSAID Therapy*).

Drug/Drug Interactions (see **CONTRAINDICATIONS**.)

Butazolidin competitively displaces other drugs, e.g., other anti-inflammatory agents, oral anticoagulants, oral antidiabetics, sulfonamides, sodium valproate, and phenytoin, from serum-binding sites. The activity, duration of effect, and

toxicity of the displaced drugs may thus be increased. Butazolidin accentuates the prothrombin depression produced by coumarin-type anticoagulants. When administered alone, Butazolidin does not affect prothrombin activity.

Butazolidin may induce the hepatic microsomal metabolism of dicoumarol, amidopyrine, digitoxin, hexobarbital, and cortisone. Conversely, it may inhibit the metabolism of phenytoin.

Concomitant administration of phenylbutazone and phenytoin may result in increased serum levels of phenytoin which could lead to increased phenytoin toxicity.

Inducers of hepatic microsomal enzymes, e.g., barbiturates, promethazine, chlorpheniramine, rifampin, and corticosteroids (prednisone), may decrease the half-life of Butazolidin. The effects of methotrexate, insulin, antidiabetic and sulfonamide drugs may be potentiated by Butazolidin. Butazolidin increases the serum concentration of lithium by increasing tubular reabsorption, and it reduces the renal clearance of sulfonylureas.

Methylphenidate is reported to prolong the half-life of Butazolidin and to increase the serum level of oxyphenbutazone. Cholestyramine reduces the enteral absorption of Butazolidin.

Drug/Laboratory Test Interactions: Butazolidin reduces iodine uptake by the thyroid and may interfere with laboratory tests of thyroid function. (Thyroid hyperplasia, goiters, and hypothyroidism have also been reported; see **ADVERSE REACTIONS**.)

Carcinogenesis, Mutagenesis, Impairment of Fertility

Long-term carcinogenicity studies in animals have not been performed with Butazolidin.

An increased incidence of chromosome anomalies has been reported in cultured leukocyte cells from patients receiving therapeutic doses of phenylbutazone. In other similar studies in humans and horses, results were inconclusive or negative. In Chinese-hamster fibroblast cells *in vitro*, chromosome aberrations were induced at a concentration of phenylbutazone exceeding 20 times the human plasma level of 43 mg/L. In mice, Chinese hamsters, and rats given up to 33 times the maximum daily human dose of phenylbutazone, no evidence of mutagenic activity or adverse effects on fertility was found. Phenylbutazone was not mutagenic in bacteria or fungi.

Pregnancy Category C: Reproduction studies in rats and rabbits given Butazolidin in oral doses up to 16 times the maximum daily human dose have revealed no evidence of teratogenicity due to Butazolidin. However, slightly reduced litter sizes were observed after oral or subcutaneous administration of phenylbutazone to pregnant rats or rabbits; an increase in stillbirths and a reduced survival of offspring were observed after oral administration of 3.5 times the maximum daily human dose of phenylbutazone to rats during late pregnancy and lactation.

There are no adequate and well-controlled studies in pregnant women. However, Butazolidin may appear in cord blood. Butazolidin should be used during pregnancy only if the potential benefit justifies the potential risk to the fetus.

Nursing Mothers: Butazolidin is excreted in breast milk in small quantity. Because of the potential for serious adverse reactions in nursing infants from Butazolidin, a decision should be made whether to discontinue nursing or to discontinue use of the drug, taking into account the importance of the drug to the mother.

Pediatric Use: Safety and effectiveness in children 14 years of age or younger have not been established.

ADVERSE REACTIONS

Aplastic anemia and agranulocytosis are the most serious adverse reactions that have been reported with use of Butazolidin. An incidence of 2.2 deaths from aplastic anemia and agranulocytosis per 100,000 exposures to Butazolidin was reported by Inman, in a review of all deaths in England and Wales from October 1974 through September 1975 in which aplastic anemia or agranulocytosis was considered a primary or contributing cause of death. The study found an increased risk with long-term use and use in elderly patients, especially women, with a rate of 6.5 deaths per 100,000 elderly women (over age 65). These data, while generated under conditions of use which differ from those presently recommended in the United States, indicate the need for careful consideration in any contemplated long-term use or use in the elderly.

The following adverse reactions have been reported with phenylbutazone and oxyphenbutazone:

Incidence Greater Than 1%

Gastrointestinal (see **WARNINGS**): Abdominal discomfort and distress (3–9%); nausea; dyspepsia, including indigestion and heartburn.

Dermatologic: Rash.

Cardiovascular/Fluid and Electrolyte: Edema, water retention (3–9%).

Incidence Less Than 1%—(Causal Relationship Probable)

Hematologic (see **WARNINGS**): Aplastic anemia; agranulocytosis; bone marrow depression; thrombocytopenia; pancytopenia; leukopenia; anemia; hemolytic anemia.

Gastrointestinal (see **WARNINGS**): Vomiting; abdominal distention with flatulence; constipation; diarrhea; esophagitis; gastritis; salivary gland enlargement; stomatitis, sometimes with ulceration; ulceration and perforation of the intestinal tract, including acute and reactivated peptic ulcer; exacerbation of inflammatory bowel disease or Crohn's disease; anemia due to occult gastrointestinal bleeding; hepatitis.

Hypersensitive Reactions: Urticaria; anaphylactic shock; arthralgia; fever; vasculitis; Lyell's syndrome; serum sickness; Stevens-Johnson syndrome; activation of systemic lupus erythematosus; aggravation of temporal arteritis.

Dermatologic: Pruritus; erythema nodosum; erythema multiforme; nonthrombocytopenic purpura.

Cardiovascular/Fluid and Electrolyte: Sodium and chloride retention; fluid retention and plasma dilution; congestive heart failure; metabolic acidosis; respiratory alkalosis; hypertension; pericarditis; interstitial myocarditis.

Renal: Hematuria; proteinuria; ureteral obstruction with uric acid crystals; anuria; glomerulonephritis; acute tubular necrosis; cortical necrosis; renal stones; nephrotic syndrome; impaired renal function and renal failure; interstitial nephritis.

Central Nervous System: Headache; drowsiness; agitation; confusional states and lethargy; tremors; numbness; weakness.

Endocrine-Metabolic: Hyperglycemia.

Special Senses, Otic: Hearing loss; tinnitus.

Incidence Less Than 1%—(Causal Relationship Unknown)

Hematologic: Leukemia. (There have been reports associating phenylbutazone with leukemia. However, the circumstances involved in these reports are such that a causal relationship to the drug has not been clearly established.)

Special Senses, Ocular (see **PRECAUTIONS, General**): Blurred vision; optic neuritis; toxic amblyopia; scotomata; retinal detachment; retinal hemorrhage; oculomotor palsy.

Endocrine-Metabolic: Thyroid hyperplasia; goiters associated with hyperthyroidism and hypothyroidism (see **PRECAUTIONS, Drug/Laboratory Test Interactions**); pancreatitis.

OVERDOSAGE

Acute Toxicity: The lowest known lethal doses are 14 g (45-year-old man) and 2 g (3-year-old child). The highest known doses that have been survived are 40 g (20-year-old man) and 5 g (3-year-old boy). Oral LD₅₀'s (mg/kg): mice, 650; rats, 364; guinea pigs, 1220.

Signs and Symptoms: The first signs and symptoms, referable chiefly to the stomach and the nervous system, appear 1 to 2 hours after ingestion of the overdose in children and somewhat later in adults.

The signs and symptoms of phenylbutazone poisoning can be summarized as follows:

Mild poisoning
  Nausea, abdominal pain, drowsiness
Severe poisoning
  Early onset
    Upper abdominal pain, nausea, vomiting, hematemesis, diarrhea, restlessness, dizziness, agitation, hallucinations, psychosis, coma, convulsions (more prevalent in children), hyperpyrexia, electrolyte disturbances, hyperventilation, alkalosis or acidosis, respiratory arrest, hypotension, hypertension, cyanosis.
  Late onset (2–7 days)
    Acute renal failure, edema, hematuria, oliguria, abnormal laboratory test results, jaundice, electrocardiographic abnormalities, cardiac arrest, blood dyscrasias (anemia, thrombocytopenia, leukopenia, leukocytosis, hypoprothrombinemia).

Abnormalities evident on laboratory tests after overdosage may include respiratory or metabolic acidosis, impaired hepatic or renal function, and abnormalities of formed blood elements.

Treatment: There is no specific antidote.

In the alert patient, the stomach should be emptied promptly by induced emesis followed by lavage. In the obtunded patient, the airway should be secured with a cuffed endotracheal tube before lavage; emesis should not be induced. Adequate respiratory exchange should be maintained; respiratory stimulants should not be used. Shock should be treated with appropriate supportive measures. Seizures should be controlled with intravenous diazepam or short-acting barbiturates. Hemoperfusion has been used as an adjunct to supportive therapy in cases with poor prognosis.

DOSAGE AND ADMINISTRATION

Butazolidin should be used at the smallest effective dosage that provides rapid relief of severe symptoms. If a favorable symptomatic response to treatment is not obtained after 1 week, use of the drug should be discontinued. When a favorable therapeutic response has been obtained, the dosage should be reduced and the therapy discontinued as soon as possible.

In elderly patients (60 years and over), every effort should be made to discontinue therapy on, or as soon as possible after,

the seventh day, because of the increased risk of severe or fatal toxic reactions in this age group.

The drug should be taken with milk or with meals so that the possibility of gastric upset will be minimized.

In selecting the appropriate dosage, the physician should consider the patient's age, weight, general health, and any other factors that may influence the patient's response to the drug.

Rheumatoid Arthritis, Ankylosing Spondylitis, and Acute Attacks of Degenerative Joint Disease:

Initial Dosage: The initial daily dosage in adult patients is 300–600 mg in three to four divided doses. Maximum therapeutic response is usually obtained with a total daily dose of 400 mg. A trial period of 1 week of therapy is considered adequate to determine the therapeutic effect of the drug; in the absence of a favorable response, therapy should be discontinued.

Maintenance Dosage: When improvement is obtained, the dosage should be promptly decreased to the minimum effective level necessary to maintain relief and not exceeding 400 mg daily, because of the possibility of cumulative toxicity. A satisfactory clinical response may be obtained with daily doses as low as 100–200 mg.

Acute Gouty Arthritis: Satisfactory results may be obtained after an initial dose of 400 mg followed by doses of 100 mg every 4 hours. The articular inflammation usually subsides within 4 days. Treatment should not be continued longer than 1 week.

HOW SUPPLIED

Tablets 100 mg —round, red, film-coated (imprinted Geigy 14)
Bottles of 100 ....NDC 0028-0014-01
Bottles of 1000 ....NDC 0028-0014-10
Unit Dose (blister pack)
Box of 100 (strips of 10) ....NDC 0028-0014-61
Capsules 100 mg —orange and white (imprinted Geigy 44 on one portion and Butazolidin® 100 mg on the other portion)
Bottles of 100 ....NDC 0028-0044-01
Unit Dose (blister pack)
Box of 100 (strips of 10) ....NDC 0028-0044-61
Dispense in tight, light-resistant container (USP).
C89-14 (Rev. 4/89)

Shown in Product Identification Section, page 410

CONSTANT–T®
[*kahn-stant 'tee ' *]
theophylline (anhydrous) USP
Sustained-Action Tablets
Tablets
200 mg
300 mg

DESCRIPTION

Constant-T, theophylline (anhydrous) USP, is a xanthine bronchodilator available as sustained-action tablets of 200 mg and 300 mg for oral administration. Its chemical name is 3,7-Dihydro-1,3-dimethyl-1*H*-purine-2,6-dione.

Theophylline (anhydrous) USP is a white, odorless crystalline powder having a bitter taste. It is stable in air. It is freely soluble in solutions of alkali hydroxides and in ammonia; sparingly soluble in alcohol, in chloroform, and in ether; and slightly soluble in water but more soluble in hot water. Its molecular weight is 180.17.

Inactive Ingredients. Cellulose compound, FD&C Blue No. 1 (300-mg tablets), FD&C Red No. 3 (200-mg tablets), lactose, magnesium stearate, povidone, and stearic acid.

ACTIONS

The pharmacologic actions of Constant-T are as a bronchodilator, pulmonary vasodilator and smooth muscle relaxant, since the drug directly relaxes the smooth muscle of the bronchial airways and pulmonary blood vessels. Theophylline also possesses other actions typical of the xanthine derivatives: coronary vasodilator, diuretic, cardiac stimulant, cerebral stimulant and skeletal muscle stimulant. The actions of theophylline may be mediated through inhibition of phosphodiesterase and a resultant increase in intracellular cyclic AMP which could mediate smooth muscle relaxation. No development of tolerance appears to occur with chronic use of theophylline.

The half-life is shortened with cigarette smoking and prolonged in alcoholism, reduced hepatic or renal function, congestive heart failure, and in patients receiving certain antibiotics (see **Drug Interactions**). High fever for prolonged periods may decrease theophylline elimination. Children over six months of age have rapid clearances with average half-lives of approximately 3–5 hours. Newborn infants have extremely slow clearances and half-lives exceeding 24 hours. Older adults with chronic obstructive pulmonary disease, any patients with cor pulmonale or other causes of heart failure, and patients with liver pathology may have much lower clearances with half-lives that exceed 24 hours. The half-life of theophylline in smokers (1–2 packs per day) aver-

ages 4–5 hours; the half-life in nonsmokers averages 7–9 hours.

In single-dose studies, adjusting the data to dosing equivalent to 8 mg/kg body weight, Constant-T produced mean peak theophylline blood levels of 9.1 ± 0.7 μg/ml at 5.0 ± 1.2 hours with the 200-mg dosage form, and 9.8 ± 0.9 μg/ml at 4.6 ± 0.9 hours with the 300-mg dosage form. In a multidose, steady-state, 5-day study, Constant-T achieved constant intrasubject theophylline levels with an average peak-trough difference of only 3.4 μg/ml. This is indicative of smooth and stable maintenance therapeutic theophylline levels throughout a 12-hour dosing interval.

INDICATIONS

Symptomatic relief and/or prevention of asthma and reversible bronchospasm associated with chronic bronchitis and emphysema.

CONTRAINDICATIONS

Constant-T is contraindicated in individuals who have shown hypersensitivity to any of its components or to xanthine derivatives.

WARNINGS

Excessive theophylline doses may be associated with toxicity; serum theophylline levels should be monitored to assure maximum benefit with minimum risk. Incidence of toxicity increases at serum levels greater than 20 μg/ml. High blood levels of theophylline resulting from conventional doses are correlated with clinical manifestations of toxicity in: patients with lowered body plasma clearances; patients with liver dysfunction or chronic obstructive lung disease, and patients who are older than 55 years of age, particularly males. There are often no early signs of less serious theophylline toxicity such as nausea and restlessness, which may appear in up to 50% of patients prior to onset of convulsions. Ventricular arrhythmias or seizures may be the first signs of toxicity. Many patients who have higher theophylline serum levels exhibit a tachycardia. Theophylline products may worsen preexisting arrhythmias.

Usage in Pregnancy: Safe use in pregnancy has not been established relative to possible adverse effects on fetal development, but neither have adverse effects on fetal development been established. This is, unfortunately, true for most antiasthmatic medications. Therefore, use of theophylline in pregnant women should be balanced against the risk of uncontrolled asthma.

PRECAUTIONS

CONSTANT-T TABLETS SHOULD NOT BE CHEWED OR CRUSHED. Theophyllines should not be administered concurrently with other xanthine medications. It should be used with caution in patients with severe cardiac disease, severe hypoxemia, hypertension, hyperthyroidism, acute myocardial injury, cor pulmonale, congestive heart failure, liver disease and in the elderly, particularly males, and in neonates. Great caution should be used in giving theophylline to patients in congestive heart failure since these patients show markedly prolonged theophylline blood level curves. Use theophylline cautiously in patients with history of peptic ulcer. Theophylline may occasionally act as a local irritant to GI tract although gastrointestinal symptoms are more commonly central and associated with high serum concentrations above 20 μg/ml.

ADVERSE REACTIONS

The most consistent adverse reactions are usually due to overdose and are:

Gastrointestinal: Nausea, vomiting, epigastric pain, hematemesis, diarrhea.

Central Nervous System: Headaches, irritability, restlessness, insomnia, reflex hyperexcitability, muscle twitching, clonic and tonic generalized convulsions.

Cardiovascular: Palpitation, tachycardia, extrasystoles, flushing, hypotension, circulatory failure, life-threatening ventricular arrhythmias.

Respiratory: Tachypnea.

Renal: Albuminuria, increased excretion of renal tubular cells and red blood cells; potentiation of diuresis.

Others: Hyperglycemia and inappropriate ADH syndrome.

Drug/Drug Interactions:

Drug	Effect
Theophylline with Furosemide	Increased Diuresis
Theophylline with Hexamethonium	Decreased Chronotropic Effect
Theophylline with Reserpine	Tachycardia
Theophylline with Cyclamycin (TAO), Erythromycin, or Lincomycin	Increased Theophylline Blood Levels

Continued on next page

Geigy—Cont.

Drug/Food Interactions:
Constant-T has not been adequately studied to determine whether its bioavailability is altered when it is given with food.

Available data suggest that drug administration at the time of food ingestion may influence the absorption characteristics of some or all theophylline controlled-release products resulting in serum values different from those found after administration in the fasting state.

A drug-food effect, if any, would likely have its greatest clinical significance when high theophylline serum levels are being maintained and/or when large single doses (greater than 13 mg/kg or 900 mg) of a controlled-release theophylline product are given. The influence of the type and amount of food on performance of controlled-release theophylline products is under study at this time.

OVERDOSAGE
Management:
A. If potential oral overdose is established and seizure has not occurred:
   1) Induce vomiting.
   2) Administer a cathartic (this is particularly important if sustained-release preparations have been taken).
   3) Administer activated charcoal.
B. If patient is having a seizure:
   1) Establish an airway.
   2) Administer O₂.
   3) Treat the seizure with intravenous diazepam, 0.1 to 0.3 mg/kg up to 10 mg.
   4) Monitor vital signs, maintain blood pressure and provide adequate hydration.
C. Postseizure coma:
   1) Maintain airway and oxygenation.
   2) If a result of oral medication, follow above recommendations to prevent absorption of the drug, but intubation and lavage will have to be performed instead of inducing emesis, and the cathartic and charcoal will need to be introduced via a large-bore gastric lavage tube.
   3) Continue to provide full supportive care and adequate hydration while waiting for drug to be metabolized. In general, the drug is metabolized sufficiently rapidly so as to not warrant consideration of dialysis.

DOSAGE AND ADMINISTRATION
Therapeutic serum levels associated with optimal likelihood for benefit and minimal risk of toxicity are considered to be between 10 and 20 µg/ml. There is a great variation from patient to patient in dosage needed in order to achieve a therapeutic blood level due to variable rates of elimination. Because of this wide variation from patient to patient, and the relatively narrow therapeutic range, dosage must be individualized. Constant-T has not been adequately studied for its bioavailability when administered with food (see PRECAUTIONS, Drug/Food Interactions).

THE AVERAGE INITIAL CHILDREN'S (15 to 20 kg) DOSE IS ONE-HALF OF A CONSTANT-T 200-mg TABLET q12h.
THE AVERAGE INITIAL CHILDREN'S (20 to 25 kg) DOSE IS ONE-HALF (150 mg) OF A CONSTANT-T 300-mg TABLET q12h.
THE AVERAGE INITIAL ADULT AND CHILDREN'S (OVER 25 kg) DOSE IS ONE CONSTANT-T 200-mg TABLET q12h.

If the desired response is not achieved with the above AVERAGE INITIAL DOSAGE recommendations, and there are no adverse reactions, the dose may be increased, after 3 days, to the following MAXIMUM DOSE WITHOUT MEASUREMENT OF SERUM CONCENTRATION.

MAXIMUM DOSE WITHOUT MEASUREMENT OF SERUM CONCENTRATION

	Dose Per Interval
Children (15–20 kg)	150 mg q12h
Children (20–25 kg)	200 mg q12h
Children (25–35 kg)	250 mg q12h
Adults and Children (over 35 kg)	300 mg q12h

If increased dose is not tolerated because of headaches or stomach upset (nausea, vomiting, diarrhea, etc.), decrease dose to AVERAGE INITIAL DOSE. If tolerated, the dose may be increased, after 3 days, to the following MINIMUM DOSE REQUIRING MEASUREMENT OF SERUM CONCENTRATION.

MINIMUM DOSE REQUIRING MEASUREMENT OF SERUM CONCENTRATION

	Dose Per Interval
Children (15–20 kg)	200 mg q12h
Children (20–30 kg)	250 mg q12h
Children (30–35 kg)	300 mg q12h
Children (35–40 kg)	350 mg q12h
Adults and Children (over 40 kg)	400 mg q12h

CHECK SERUM CONCENTRATION BETWEEN 3 AND 8 HOURS AFTER A DOSE WHEN NONE HAVE BEEN MISSED OR ADDED FOR AT LEAST 3 DAYS.
If serum theophylline concentration is between 10 and 20 µg/ml, maintain dose, if tolerated. RECHECK SERUM THEOPHYLLINE CONCENTRATION AT 6- TO 12-MONTH INTERVALS.*
* Finer adjustments in dosage may be needed for some patients.
Take the following action if the serum theophylline concentration is too high.
20 to 25 µg/ml—Decrease dose by 50 mg q12h.
25 to 30 µg/ml—Skip next dose and decrease subsequent doses by 25% to the nearest 50 mg q12h.
Over 30 µg/ml—Skip next 2 doses and decrease subsequent doses by 50% to nearest 50 mg q12h. RECHECK SERUM THEOPHYLLINE CONCENTRATION.
Take the following action if the serum theophylline concentration is too low.
7.5 to 10 µg/ml—Increase dose by 25% to the nearest 50 mg.†
5 to 7.5 µg/ml—Increase dose by 25% to the nearest 50 mg and RECHECK SERUM THEOPHYLLINE FOR GUIDANCE IN FURTHER DOSAGE ADJUSTMENT.
† Dividing the daily dosage into 3 doses administered at 8-hour intervals may be indicated if symptoms occur repeatedly at the end of a dosing interval.
DOSAGE ADJUSTMENT, BASED ON SERUM THEOPHYLLINE CONCENTRATION MEASUREMENTS WHEN THESE INSTRUCTIONS HAVE NOT BEEN FOLLOWED. MAY RESULT IN RECOMMENDATIONS THAT PRESENT RISK OF TOXICITY TO THE PATIENT.

HOW SUPPLIED
Sustained-Action Tablets 200 mg—light pink, oval, scored (imprinted Geigy 42)
   Bottles of 100 ....NDC 0028-0042-01
Unit Dose (blister pack)
   Box of 100 (strips of 10) ....NDC 0028-0042-61
Sustained-Action Tablets 300 mg—light blue, oval, scored (imprinted Geigy 57)
   Bottles of 100 ....NDC 0028-0057-01
Unit Dose (blister pack)
   Box of 100 (strips of 10) ....NDC 0028-0057-61
Do not store above 86°F (30°C). Protect from moisture.
Dispense in tight, light-resistant container (USP).

C85-57 (Rev. 11/85)

Dist. by:
GEIGY Pharmaceuticals
Div. of CIBA-GEIGY Corp.
Ardsley, New York 10502
Shown in Product Identification Section, page 410

LAMPRENE®   ℞
clofazimine
Capsules

DESCRIPTION
Lamprene, clofazimine, is an antileprosy agent available as capsules for oral administration. Each capsule contains 50 mg or 100 mg of micronized clofazimine suspended in an oil-wax base. Clofazimine is a substituted iminophenazine bright-red dye. Its chemical name is 3-(p -chloroanilino)-10-(p -chlorophenyl)-2, 10-dihydro-2-isopropyliminophenazine. Clofazimine is a reddish-brown powder. It is readily soluble in benzene; soluble in chloroform; poorly soluble in acetone and in ethyl acetate; sparingly soluble in methanol and in ethanol; and virtually insoluble in water. Its molecular weight is 473.4.
Inactive Ingredients. Beeswax, butylated hydroxytoluene, citric acid, ethyl vanillin, gelatin, glycerin, iron oxide, lecithin, p-methoxy acetophenone, parabens, plant oils, propylene glycol.

CLINICAL PHARMACOLOGY
Lamprene exerts a slow bactericidal effect on *Mycobacterium leprae* (Hansen's bacillus). Lamprene inhibits mycobacterial growth and binds preferentially to mycobacterial DNA. Lamprene also exerts anti-inflammatory properties in controlling erythema nodosum leprosum reactions. However, its precise mechanisms of action are unknown.
Pharmacokinetics
Lamprene has a variable absorption rate in leprosy patients, ranging from 45–62% after oral administration. The average serum concentrations in leprosy patients treated with 100 mg and 300 mg daily were 0.7 µg/ml and 1.0 µg/ml, respectively. After ingestion of a single dose of 300 mg, elimination of unchanged Lamprene and its metabolites in a 24-hour urine collection was negligible. Lamprene is retained in the human body for a long time. The half-life of Lamprene following repeated oral doses is estimated to be at least 70 days. Part of the ingested drug recovered from the feces may represent excretion via the bile. A small amount is also eliminated in the sputum, sebum, and sweat.
Lamprene is highly lipophilic and tends to be deposited predominantly in fatty tissue and in cells of the reticuloendothelial system. It is taken up by macrophages throughout the body. In autopsies performed on leprosy patients, clofazimine crystals were found predominantly in the mesenteric lymph nodes, adrenals, subcutaneous fat, liver, bile, gall bladder, spleen, small intestine, muscles, bones, and skin.
Microbiology
Measurement of the minimum inhibitory concentration (MIC) of Lamprene against leprosy bacilli *in vitro* is not yet feasible. In the mouse footpad system, the multiplication of *M. leprae* is inhibited by introducing 0.0001–0.001% Lamprene in the diet. Although bacterial killing may begin shortly after starting the drug, it cannot be measured in biopsy tissues taken from patients for mouse footpad studies until approximately 50 days after the start of therapy. Lamprene does not show cross-resistance with dapsone or rifampin.
The following *in vitro* data are available, but their clinical significance is unknown. Lamprene has been shown *in vitro* to inhibit *M. avium* and *M. bovis* at concentrations of approximately 0.1–1.0 µg/ml. The MIC for *M. avium-intracellulare* isolated from patients with acquired immuno-deficiency syndrome (AIDS) ranged from 1.0 to 5.0 µg/ml. With a few exceptions, microorganisms other than mycobacteria are not inhibited by Lamprene.

INDICATIONS AND USAGE
Lamprene is indicated in the treatment of lepromatous leprosy, including dapsone-resistant lepromatous leprosy and lepromatous leprosy complicated by erythema nodosum leprosum. Lamprene has not been demonstrated to be effective in the treatment of other leprosy-associated inflammatory reactions.
Combination drug therapy has been recommended for initial treatment of multibacillary leprosy to prevent the development of drug resistance.

CONTRAINDICATIONS
There are no known contraindications.

WARNINGS
Severe abdominal symptoms (see below) have necessitated exploratory laparotomies in some patients receiving Lamprene. Rare reports have included splenic infarction, bowel obstruction, and gastrointestinal bleeding. There have also been reports of death following severe abdominal symptoms. Autopsies have revealed crystalline deposits of clofazimine in various tissues including the intestinal mucosa, liver, spleen, and mesenteric lymph nodes.
Lamprene should be used with caution in patients who have gastrointestinal problems such as abdominal pain and diarrhea. Dosages of Lamprene of more than 100 mg daily should be given for as short a period as possible and only under close medical supervision. If a patient complains of colicky or burning pain in the abdomen, nausea, vomiting, or diarrhea, the dose should be reduced, and if necessary, the interval between doses should be increased, or the drug should be discontinued.

PRECAUTIONS
General
Physicians should be aware that skin discoloration due to Lamprene may result in depression. Two suicides have been reported in patients receiving Lamprene. For skin dryness and ichthyosis, oil can be applied to the skin.
Information for Patients
Patients should be warned that Lamprene may cause a discoloration of the skin from red to brownish black, as well as discoloration of the conjunctivae, lacrimal fluid, sweat, sputum, urine, and feces. Patients should be advised that skin discoloration, although reversible, may take several months or years to disappear after the conclusion of therapy with Lamprene.
Patients should be told to take Lamprene with meals.
Drug Interactions
Preliminary data which suggest that dapsone may inhibit the anti-inflammatory activity of Lamprene have not been confirmed. If leprosy-associated inflammatory reactions develop in patients being treated with dapsone and clofazimine, it is still advisable to continue treatment with both drugs.
Carcinogenesis, Mutagenesis, Impairment of Fertility
Long-term carcinogenicity studies in animals have not been conducted with Lamprene. Results of mutagenicity studies (Ames test) were negative. There was some evidence of impaired fertility in one study in rats treated at a dose 25 times the usual human dose; the number of offspring was reduced and there was a lower proportion of implantations.
Pregnancy Category C
Lamprene was not teratogenic in laboratory animals at dose levels equivalent to 8 times (rabbit) and 25 times (rat) the usual human daily dose. However, there was evidence of

fetotoxicity in the mouse at 12-25 times the human dose, i.e., retardation of fetal skull ossification, increased incidence of abortions and stillbirths, and impaired neonatal survival. The skin and fatty tissue of offspring became discolored approximately 3 days after birth, which was attributed to the presence of Lamprene in the maternal milk.

It has been found that Lamprene crosses the human placenta. The skin of infants born to women who had received the drug during pregnancy was found to be deeply pigmented at birth. No evidence of teratogenicity was found in these infants. There are no adequate and well-controlled studies in pregnant women. Lamprene should be used during pregnancy only if the potential benefit justifies the risk to the fetus.

Nursing Mothers
Lamprene is excreted in the milk of nursing mothers. Lamprene should not be administered to a nursing woman unless clearly indicated.

Pediatric Use
Safety and effectiveness in children have not been established. Several cases of children treated with Lamprene have been reported in the literature.

ADVERSE REACTIONS
In general, Lamprene is well tolerated when administered in dosages no greater than 100 mg daily. The most consistent adverse reactions are usually dose related and are usually reversible when Lamprene is discontinued.

Adverse Reactions Occuring in More Than 1% of Patients
Skin: Pigmentation from pink to brownish-black in 75–100% of the patients within a few weeks of treatment; ichthyosis and dryness (8–28%); rash and pruritus (1–5%).
Gastrointestinal: Abdominal and epigastric pain, diarrhea, nausea, vomiting, gastrointestinal intolerance (40–50%).
Ocular: Conjunctival and corneal pigmentation due to clofazimine crystal deposits; dryness; burning; itching; irritation.
Other: Discoloration of urine, feces, sputum, sweat; elevated blood sugar; elevated ESR.

Adverse Reactions Occurring in Less Than 1% of Patients
Skin: Phototoxicity, erythroderma, acneiform eruptions, monilial cheilosis.
Gastrointestinal: Bowel obstruction (see WARNINGS), gastrointestinal bleeding (see WARNINGS), anorexia, constipation, weight loss, hepatitis, jaundice, eosinophilic enteritis, enlarged liver.
Ocular: Diminished vision.
Nervous: Dizziness, drowsiness, fatigue, headache, giddiness, neuralgia, taste disorder.
Psychiatric: Depression secondary to skin discoloration; two suicides have been reported.
Laboratory: Elevated levels of albumin, serum bilirubin, and AST (SGOT); eosinophilia; hypokalemia.
Other: Splenic infarction (see WARNINGS), thromboembolism, anemia, cystitis, bone pain, edema, fever, lymphadenopathy, vascular pain.

OVERDOSAGE
No specific data are available on the treatment of overdosage with Lamprene. However, in case of overdose, the stomach should be emptied by inducing vomiting or by gastric lavage, and supportive symptomatic treatment should be employed.

DOSAGE AND ADMINISTRATION
Lamprene should be taken with meals.
Lamprene should be used preferably in combination with one or more other antileprosy agents to prevent the emergence of drug resistance.
For the treatment of proven dapsone-resistant leprosy, Lamprene should be given at a dosage of 100 mg daily in combination with one or more other antileprosy drugs for 3 years, followed by monotherapy with 100 mg of Lamprene daily. Clinical improvement usually can be detected between the first and third months of treatment and is usually clearly evident by the sixth month.
For dapsone-sensitive multibacillary leprosy, a combination therapy with two other antileprosy drugs is recommended. The triple-drug regimen should be given for at least 2 years and continued, if possible, until negative skin smears are obtained. At this time, monotherapy with an appropriate antileprosy drug can be instituted.
The treatment of erythema nodosum leprosum reactions depends on the severity of symptoms. In general, the basic antileprosy treatment should be continued, and if nerve injury or skin ulceration is threatened, corticosteriods should be given. Where prolonged corticosteroid therapy becomes necessary, Lamprene administered at dosages of 100 mg to 200 mg daily for up to 3 months may be useful in eliminating or reducing corticosteroid requirements. Dosages above 200 mg daily are not recommended, and the dosage should be tapered to 100 mg daily as quickly as possible after the reactive episode is controlled. The patient must remain under medical surveillance.
For advice about combination drug regimens, contact the USPHS Gillis W. Long Hansen's Disease Center, Carville, LA (504-642-7771).

HOW SUPPLIED
Capsules 50 mg—brown, spherical
Bottles of 100 ....NDC 0028-0108-01
Capsules 100 mg—brown, oblong (imprinted GEIGY GM)
Bottles of 100 ....NDC 0028-0109-01
Do not store above 86°F. Protect from moisture.
Dispense in tight container (USP).

C87-25 (Rev. 9/87)

Dist. by:
GEIGY Pharmaceuticals
Division of CIBA-GEIGY Corporation
Ardsley, New York 10502
Shown in Product Identification Section, page 410

LIORESAL®   Tablets ℞
[lye-oar'eh-sal]
baclofen USP   10 mg
Muscle Relaxant, Antispastic   20 mg ℞

DESCRIPTION
Lioresal, baclofen USP, is a muscle relaxant and antispastic, available as 10-mg and 20-mg tablets for oral administration. Its chemical name is 4-amino-3-(4-chlorophenyl) butanoic acid.
Baclofen USP is a white to off-white, odorless or practically odorless crystalline powder, with a molecular weight of 213.66. It is slightly soluble in water, very slightly soluble in methanol, and insoluble in chloroform.
Inactive Ingredients. Cellulose compounds, magnesium stearate, povidone, and starch.

ACTIONS
The precise mechanism of action of Lioresal is not fully known. Lioresal is capable of inhibiting both monosynaptic and polysynaptic reflexes at the spinal level, possibly by hyperpolarization of afferent terminals, although actions at supraspinal sites may also occur and contribute to its clinical effect. Although Lioresal is an analog of the putative inhibitory neurotransmitter gamma-aminobutyric acid (GABA), there is no conclusive evidence that actions on GABA systems are involved in the production of its clinical effects. In studies with animals, Lioresal has been shown to have general CNS depressant properties as indicated by the production of sedation with tolerance, somnolence, ataxia, and respiratory and cardiovascular depression. Lioresal is rapidly and extensively absorbed and eliminated. Absorption may be dose-dependent, being reduced with increasing doses. Lioresal is excreted primarily by the kidney in unchanged form and there is relatively large intersubject variation in absorption and/or elimination.

INDICATIONS
Lioresal is useful for the alleviation of signs and symptoms of spasticity resulting from multiple sclerosis, particularly for the relief of flexor spasms and concomitant pain, clonus, and muscular rigidity.
Patients should have reversible spasticity so that Lioresal treatment will aid in restoring residual function.
Lioresal may also be of some value in patients with spinal cord injuries and other spinal cord diseases.
Lioresal is not indicated in the treatment of skeletal muscle spasm resulting from rheumatic disorders.
The efficacy of Lioresal in stroke, cerebral palsy, and Parkinson's disease has not been established and, therefore, it is not recommended for these conditions.

CONTRAINDICATIONS
Hypersensitivity to baclofen.

WARNINGS
a. *Abrupt Drug Withdrawal:* Hallucinations and seizures have occurred on abrupt withdrawal of Lioresal. Therefore, except for serious adverse reactions, the dose should be reduced slowly when the drug is discontinued.
b. *Impaired Renal Function:* Because Lioresal is primarily excreted unchanged through the kidneys, it should be given with caution, and it may be necessary to reduce the dosage.
c. *Stroke:* Lioresal has not significantly benefited patients with stroke. These patients have also shown poor tolerability to the drug.
d. *Pregnancy:* Lioresal has been shown to increase the incidence of omphaloceles (ventral hernias) in fetuses of rats given approximately 13 times the maximum dose recommended for human use, at a dose which caused significant reductions in food intake and weight gain in dams. This abnormality was not seen in mice or rabbits. There was also an increased incidence of incomplete sternebral ossification in fetuses of rats given approximately 13 times the maximum recommended human dose, and an increased incidence of unossified phalangeal nuclei of forelimbs and hindlimbs in fetuses of rabbits given approximately 7 times the maximum recommended human dose. In mice, no teratogenic effects were observed, although reductions in mean fetal weight with consequent delays in skeletal ossification were present when dams were given 17 or 34

times the human daily dose. There are no studies in pregnant women. Lioresal should be used during pregnancy only if the benefit clearly justifies the potential risk to the fetus.

PRECAUTIONS
Safe use of Lioresal in children under age 12 has not been established, and it is, therefore, not recommended for use in children.
Because of the possibility of sedation, patients should be cautioned regarding the operation of automobiles or other dangerous machinery, and activities made hazardous by decreased alertness. Patients should also be cautioned that the central nervous system effects of Lioresal may be additive to those of alcohol and other CNS depressants.
Lioresal should be used with caution where spasticity is utilized to sustain upright posture and balance in locomotion or whenever spasticity is utilized to obtain increased function.
In patients with epilepsy, the clinical state and electroencephalogram should be monitored at regular intervals, since deterioration in seizure control and EEG have been reported occasionally in patients taking Lioresal.
It is not known whether this drug is excreted in human milk. As a general rule, nursing should not be undertaken while a patient is on a drug since many drugs are excreted in human milk.
A dose-related increase in incidence of ovarian cysts and a less marked increase in enlarged and /or hemorrhagic adrenal glands was observed in female rats treated chronically with Lioresal.
Ovarian cysts have been found by palpation in about 4% of the multiple sclerosis patients that were treated with Lioresal for up to one year. In most cases these cysts disappeared spontaneously while patients continued to receive the drug. Ovarian cysts are estimated to occur spontaneously in approximately 1% to 5% of the normal female population.

ADVERSE REACTIONS
The most common is transient drowsiness (10–63%). In one controlled study of 175 patients, transient drowsiness was observed in 63% of those receiving Lioresal compared to 36% of those in the placebo group. Other common adverse reactions are dizziness (5–15%), weakness (5–15%) and fatigue (2–4%). Others reported:
Neuropsychiatric: Confusion (1–11%), headache (4–8%), insomnia (2–7%); and, rarely, euphoria, excitement, depression, hallucinations, paresthesia, muscle pain, tinnitus, slurred speech, coordination disorder, tremor, rigidity, dystonia, ataxia, blurred vision, nystagmus, strabismus, miosis, mydriasis, diplopia, dysarthria, epileptic seizure.
Cardiovascular: Hypotension (0–9%). Rare instances of dyspnea, palpitation, chest pain, syncope.
Gastrointestinal: Nausea (4–12%), constipation (2–6%); and, rarely, dry mouth, anorexia, taste disorder, abdominal pain, vomiting, diarrhea, and positive test for occult blood in stool.
Genitourinary: Urinary frequency (2–6%); and, rarely, enuresis, urinary retention, dysuria, impotence, inability to ejaculate, nocturia, hematuria.
Other: Instances of rash, pruritus, ankle edema, excessive perspiration, weight gain, nasal congestion.
Some of the CNS and genitourinary symptoms may be related to the underlying disease rather than to drug therapy.
The following laboratory tests have been found to be abnormal in a few patients receiving Lioresal: increased SGOT, elevated alkaline phosphatase, and elevation of blood sugar.

OVERDOSAGE
Signs and Symptoms: Vomiting, muscular hypotonia, drowsiness, accommodation disorders, coma, respiratory depression, and seizures.
Treatment: In the alert patient, empty the stomach promptly by induced emesis followed by lavage. In the obtunded patient, secure the airway with a cuffed endotracheal tube before beginning lavage (do not induce emesis). Maintain adequate respiratory exchange, do not use respiratory stimulants.

DOSAGE AND ADMINISTRATION
The determination of optimal dosage requires individual titration. Start therapy at a low dosage and increase gradually until optimum effect is achieved (usually between 40–80 mg daily).
The following dosage titration schedule is suggested:
5 mg t.i.d. for 3 days
10 mg t.i.d. for 3 days
15 mg t.i.d. for 3 days
20 mg t.i.d. for 3 days

Continued on next page

The full prescribing information for each GEIGY product is contained herein and is that in effect as of September 1, 1989

Geigy—Cont.

Thereafter additional increases may be necessary but the total daily dose should not exceed a maximum of 80 mg daily (20 mg q.i.d.).

The lowest dose compatible with an optimal response is recommended. If benefits are not evident after a reasonable trial period, patients should be slowly withdrawn from the drug (see **WARNINGS** *Abrupt Drug Withdrawal*).

HOW SUPPLIED

Tablets 10 mg —oval, white, scored (imprinted GEIGY 23)

Bottles of 100 ....NDC 0028-0023-01

Unit Dose (blister pack)

Box of 100 (strips of 10) ....NDC 0028-0023-61

Tablets 20 mg —capsule shaped, white, scored (imprinted GEIGY 33)

Bottles of 100 ....NDC 0028-0033-01

Unit Dose (blister pack)

Box of 100 (strips of 10)   NDC 0028-0033-61

Samples, when available, are identified by the word *Sample* appearing on each tablet.

Do not store above 86°F (30°C).

Dispense in tight container (USP).

C88-29 (Rev. 9/88)

Shown in Product Identification Section, page 410

LOPRESSOR®   ℞

metoprolol tartrate USP
Tablets
Ampuls
Prefilled syringes

DESCRIPTION

Lopressor, metoprolol tartrate, is a selective beta₁-adrenoreceptor blocking agent, available as 50- and 100-mg tablets for oral administration and in 5-ml ampuls or 5-ml prefilled syringes for intravenous administration. Each ampul or prefilled syringe contains a sterile solution of metoprolol tartrate USP, 5 mg, and sodium chloride USP, 45 mg. Metoprolol tartrate is 1-(isopropylamino)-3-[*p*-(2-methoxyethyl) phenoxy]-2-propanol (2:1) *dextro* -tartrate salt.

Metoprolol tartrate is a white, practically odorless, crystalline powder with a molecular weight of 684.82. It is very soluble in water; freely soluble in methylene chloride, in chloroform, and in alcohol; slightly soluble in acetone; and insoluble in ether.

Inactive Ingredients: Cellulose compounds, colloidal silicon dioxide, D&C Red No. 30 aluminum lake (50-mg tablets), FD&C Blue No. 2 aluminum lake (100-mg tablets), lactose, magnesium stearate, polyethylene glycol, propylene glycol, povidone, sodium starch glycolate, talc, and titanium dioxide.

CLINICAL PHARMACOLOGY

Lopressor is a beta-adrenergic receptor blocking agent. *In vitro* and *in vivo* animal studies have shown that it has a preferential effect on beta₁ adrenoreceptors, chiefly located in cardiac muscle. This preferential effect is not absolute, however, and at higher doses, Lopressor also inhibits beta₂ adrenoreceptors, chiefly located in the bronchial and vascular musculature.

Clinical pharmacology studies have confirmed the beta-blocking activity of metoprolol in man, as shown by (1) reduction in heart rate and cardiac output at rest and upon exercise, (2) reduction of systolic blood pressure upon exercise, (3) inhibition of isoproterenol-induced tachycardia, and (4) reduction of reflex orthostatic tachycardia.

Relative beta₁ selectivity has been confirmed by the following: (1) In normal subjects, Lopressor is unable to reverse the beta₂-mediated vasodilating effects of epinephrine. This contrasts with the effect of nonselective (beta₁ plus beta₂) beta blockers, which completely reverse the vasodilating effects of epinephrine. (2) In asthmatic patients, Lopressor reduces FEV₁ and FVC significantly less than a nonselective beta blocker, propranolol, at equivalent beta₁-receptor blocking doses.

Lopressor has no intrinsic sympathomimetic activity, and membrane-stabilizing activity is detectable only at doses much greater than required for beta blockade. Lopressor crosses the blood-brain barrier and has been reported in the CSF in a concentration 78% of the simultaneous plasma concentration. Animal and human experiments indicate that Lopressor slows the sinus rate and decreases AV nodal conduction.

In controlled clinical studies, Lopressor has been shown to be an effective antihypertensive agent when used alone or as concomitant therapy with thiazide-type diuretics, at dosages of 100–450 mg daily. In controlled, comparative, clinical studies, Lopressor has been shown to be as effective an antihypertensive agent as propranolol, methyldopa, and thia-

zide-type diuretics, and to be equally effective in supine and standing positions.

The mechanism of the antihypertensive effects of beta-blocking agents has not been elucidated. However, several possible mechanisms have been proposed: (1) competitive antagonism of catecholamines at peripheral (especially cardiac) adrenergic neuron sites, leading to decreased cardiac output; (2) a central effect leading to reduced sympathetic outflow to the periphery; and (3) suppression of renin activity.

By blocking catecholamine-induced increases in heart rate, in velocity and extent of myocardial contraction, and in blood pressure, Lopressor reduces the oxygen requirements of the heart at any given level of effort, thus making it useful in the long-term management of angina pectoris. However, in patients with heart failure, beta-adrenergic blockade may increase oxygen requirements by increasing left ventricular fiber length and end-diastolic pressure.

Although beta-adrenergic receptor blockade is useful in the treatment of angina and hypertension, there are situations in which sympathetic stimulation is vital. In patients with severely damaged hearts, adequate ventricular function may depend on sympathetic drive. In the presence of AV block, beta blockade may prevent the necessary facilitating effect of sympathetic activity on conduction. Beta₂-adrenergic blockade results in passive bronchial constriction by interfering with endogenous adrenergic bronchodilator activity in patients subject to bronchospasm and may also interfere with exogenous bronchodilators in such patients.

In controlled clinical trials, Lopressor, administered two or four times daily, has been shown to be an effective antianginal agent, reducing the number of angina attacks and increasing exercise tolerance. The dosage used in these studies ranged from 100 to 400 mg daily. A controlled, comparative, clinical trial showed that Lopressor was indistinguishable from propranolol in the treatment of angina pectoris.

In a large (1,395 patients randomized), double-blind, placebo-controlled clinical study, Lopressor was shown to reduce 3-month mortality by 36% in patients with suspected or definite myocardial infarction.

Patients were randomized and treated as soon as possible after their arrival in the hospital, once their clinical condition had stabilized and their hemodynamic status had been carefully evaluated. Subjects were ineligible if they had hypotension, bradycardia, peripheral signs of shock, and/or more than minimal basal rales as signs of congestive heart failure. Initial treatment consisted of intravenous followed by oral administration of Lopressor or placebo, given in a coronary care or comparable unit. Oral maintenance therapy with Lopressor or placebo was then continued for 3 months. After this double-blind period, all patients were given Lopressor and followed up to 1 year.

The median delay from the onset of symptoms to the initiation of therapy was 8 hours in both the Lopressor and placebo treatment groups. Among patients treated with Lopressor, there were comparable reductions in 3-month mortality for those treated early (≤ 8 hours) and those in whom treatment was started later. Significant reductions in the incidence of ventricular fibrillation and in chest pain following initial intravenous therapy were also observed with Lopressor and were independent of the interval between onset of symptoms and initiation of therapy.

The precise mechanism of action of Lopressor in patients with suspected or definite myocardial infarction is not known.

In this study, patients treated with metoprolol received the drug both very early (intravenously) and during a subsequent 3-month period, while placebo patients received no beta-blocker treatment for this period. The study thus was able to show a benefit from the overall metoprolol regimen but cannot separate the benefit of very early intravenous treatment from the benefit of later beta-blocker therapy. Nonetheless, because the overall regimen showed a clear beneficial effect on survival without evidence of an early adverse effect on survival, one acceptable dosage regimen is the precise regimen used in the trial. Because the specific benefit of very early treatment remains to be defined however, it is also reasonable to administer the drug orally to patients at a later time as is recommended for certain other beta blockers.

Pharmacokinetics

In man, absorption of Lopressor is rapid and complete. Plasma levels following oral administration, however, approximate 50% of levels following intravenous administration, indicating about 50% first-pass metabolism.

Plasma levels achieved are highly variable after oral administration. Only a small fraction of the drug (about 12%) is bound to human serum albumin. Elimination is mainly by biotransformation in the liver, and the plasma half-life ranges from approximately 3 to 7 hours. Less than 5% of an oral dose of Lopressor is recovered unchanged in the urine; the rest is excreted by the kidneys as metabolites that appear to have no clinical significance. The systemic availability and half-life of Lopressor in patients with renal failure do not differ to a clinically significant degree from those in normal subjects. Consequently, no reduction in dosage is usually needed in patients with chronic renal failure.

Significant beta-blocking effect (as measured by reduction of exercise heart rate) occurs within 1 hour after oral administration, and its duration is dose-related. For example, a 50% reduction of the maximum registered effect after single oral doses of 20, 50, and 100 mg occurred at 3.3, 5.0, and 6.4 hours, respectively, in normal subjects. After repeated oral dosages of 100 mg twice daily, a significant reduction in exercise systolic blood pressure was evident at 12 hours.

Following intravenous administration of Lopressor, the urinary recovery of unchanged drug is approximately 10%. When the drug was infused over a 10-minute period, in normal volunteers, maximum beta blockade was achieved at approximately 20 minutes. Doses of 5 mg and 15 mg yielded a maximal reduction in exercise-induced heart rate of approximately 10% and 15%, respectively. The effect on exercise heart rate decreased linearly with time at the same rate for both doses, and disappeared at approximately 5 hours and 8 hours for the 5-mg and 15-mg doses, respectively.

Equivalent maximal beta-blocking effect is achieved with oral and intravenous doses in the ratio of approximately 2.5:1.

There is a linear relationship between the log of plasma levels and reduction of exercise heart rate. However, antihypertensive activity does not appear to be related to plasma levels. Because of variable plasma levels attained with a given dose and lack of a consistent relationship of antihypertensive activity to dose, selection of proper dosage requires individual titration.

In several studies of patients with acute myocardial infarction, intravenous followed by oral administration of Lopressor caused a reduction in heart rate, systolic blood pressure, and cardiac output. Stroke volume, diastolic blood pressure, and pulmonary artery end diastolic pressure remained unchanged.

In patients with angina pectoris, plasma concentration measured at 1 hour is linearly related to the oral dose within the range of 50 to 400 mg. Exercise heart rate and systolic blood pressure are reduced in relation to the logarithm of the oral dose of metoprolol. The increase in exercise capacity and the reduction in left ventricular ischemia are also significantly related to the logarithm of the oral dose.

INDICATIONS AND USAGE

Hypertension

Lopressor tablets are indicated for the treatment of hypertension. They may be used alone or in combination with other antihypertensive agents.

Angina Pectoris

Lopressor is indicated in the long-term treatment of angina pectoris.

Myocardial Infarction

Lopressor ampuls, prefilled syringes, and tablets are indicated in the treatment of hemodynamically stable patients with definite or suspected acute myocardial infarction to reduce cardiovascular mortality. Treatment with intravenous Lopressor can be initiated as soon as the patient's clinical condition allows (see **DOSAGE AND ADMINISTRATION, CONTRAINDICATIONS,** and **WARNINGS**). Alternatively, treatment can begin within 3 to 10 days of the acute event (see **DOSAGE AND ADMINISTRATION**).

CONTRAINDICATIONS

Hypertension and Angina

Lopressor is contraindicated in sinus bradycardia, heart block greater than first degree, cardiogenic shock, and overt cardiac failure (see **WARNINGS**).

Myocardial Infarction

Lopressor is contraindicated in patients with a heart rate < 45 beats/min; second- and third-degree heart block; significant first-degree heart block (P-R interval ≥ 0.24 sec); systolic blood pressure < 100 mmHg; or moderate-to-severe cardiac failure (see **WARNINGS**).

WARNINGS

Hypertension and Angina

Cardiac Failure: Sympathetic stimulation is a vital component supporting circulatory function in congestive heart failure, and beta blockade carries the potential hazard of further depressing myocardial contractility and precipitating more severe failure. In hypertensive and angina patients who have congestive heart failure controlled by digitalis and diuretics, Lopressor should be administered cautiously. Both digitalis and Lopressor slow AV conduction.

In Patients Without a History of Cardiac Failure: Continued depression of the myocardium with beta-blocking agents over a period of time can, in some cases, lead to cardiac failure. At the first sign or symptom of impending cardiac failure, patients should be fully digitalized and/or given a diuretic. The response should be observed closely. If cardiac failure continues, despite adequate digitalization and diuretic therapy, Lopressor should be withdrawn.

Ischemic Heart Disease: Following abrupt cessation of therapy with certain beta-blocking agents, exacerbations of angina pectoris and, in some cases, myocardial infarction have occurred. When discontinuing chronically administered Lopressor, particularly in patients with ischemic heart disease, the dosage should be gradually reduced over a period of 1–2 weeks and the patient should be carefully monitored. If angina markedly worsens or acute coronary insufficiency develops, Lopressor administration should be reinstated promptly, at least temporarily, and other measures appropriate for the management of unstable angina should be taken. Patients should be warned against interruption or discontinuation of therapy without the physician's advice. Because coronary artery disease is common and may be unrecognized, it may be prudent not to discontinue Lopressor therapy abruptly even in patients treated only for hypertension.

Bronchospastic Diseases: PATIENTS WITH BRONCHOSPASTIC DISEASES SHOULD, IN GENERAL, NOT RECEIVE BETA-BLOCKERS. Because of its relative beta$_1$ selectivity, however, Lopressor may be used with caution in patients with bronchospastic disease who do not respond to, or cannot tolerate, other antihypertensive treatment. Since beta$_1$ selectivity is not absolute, a beta$_2$-stimulating agent should be administered concomitantly, and the lowest possible dose of Lopressor should be used. In these circumstances it would be prudent initially to administer Lopressor in smaller doses three times daily, instead of larger doses two times daily, to avoid the higher plasma levels associated with the longer dosing interval. (See DOSAGE AND ADMINISTRATION.)

Major Surgery: The necessity or desirability of withdrawing beta-blocking therapy prior to major surgery is controversial; the impaired ability of the heart to respond to reflex adrenergic stimuli may augment the risks of general anesthesia and surgical procedures.

Lopressor, like other beta blockers, is a competitive inhibitor of beta-receptor agonists, and its effects can be reversed by administration of such agents, e.g., dobutamine or isoproterenol. However, such patients may be subject to protracted severe hypotension. Difficulty in restarting and maintaining the heart beat has also been reported with beta blockers.

Diabetes and Hypoglycemia: Lopressor should be used with caution in diabetic patients if a beta-blocking agent is required. Beta blockers may mask tachycardia occurring with hypoglycemia, but other manifestations such as dizziness and sweating may not be significantly affected.

Thyrotoxicosis: Beta-adrenergic blockade may mask certain clinical signs (e.g., tachycardia) of hyperthyroidism. Patients suspected of developing thyrotoxicosis should be managed carefully to avoid abrupt withdrawal of beta blockade, which might precipitate a thyroid storm.

Myocardial Infarction
Cardiac Failure: Sympathetic stimulation is a vital component supporting circulatory function, and beta blockade carries the potential hazard of depressing myocardial contractility and precipitating or exacerbating minimal cardiac failure.

During treatment with Lopressor, the hemodynamic status of the patient should be carefully monitored. If heart failure occurs or persists despite appropriate treatment, Lopressor should be discontinued.

Bradycardia: Lopressor produces a decrease in sinus heart rate in most patients; this decrease is greatest among patients with high initial heart rates and least among patients with low initial heart rates. Acute myocardial infarction (particularly inferior infarction) may in itself produce significant lowering of the sinus rate. If the sinus rate decreases to < 40 beats/min, particularly if associated with evidence of lowered cardiac output, atropine (0.25–0.5 mg) should be administered intravenously. If treatment with atropine is not successful, Lopressor should be discontinued, and cautious administration of isoproterenol or installation of a cardiac pacemaker should be considered.

AV Block: Lopressor slows AV conduction and may produce significant first- (P-R interval ≥ 0.26 sec), second-, or third-degree heart block. Acute myocardial infarction also produces heart block.

If heart block occurs, Lopressor should be discontinued and atropine (0.25–0.5 mg) should be administered intravenously. If treatment with atropine is not successful, cautious administration of isoproterenol or installation of a cardiac pacemaker should be considered.

Hypotension: If hypotension (systolic blood pressure ≤ 90 mmHg) occurs, Lopressor should be discontinued, and the hemodynamic status of the patient and the extent of myocardial damage carefully assessed. Invasive monitoring of central venous, pulmonary capillary wedge, and arterial pressures may be required. Appropriate therapy with fluids, positive inotropic agents, balloon counterpulsation, or other treatment modalities should be instituted. If hypotension is associated with sinus bradycardia or AV block, treatment should be directed at reversing these (see above).

Bronchospastic Diseases: PATIENTS WITH BRONCHOSPASTIC DISEASES SHOULD, IN GENERAL, NOT RECEIVE BETA BLOCKERS. Because of its relative beta$_1$ selectivity, Lopressor may be used with extreme caution in patients

with bronchospastic disease. Because it is unknown to what extent beta$_2$-stimulating agents may exacerbate myocardial ischemia and the extent of infarction, these agents should *not* be used prophylactically. If bronchospasm not related to congestive heart failure occurs, Lopressor should be discontinued. A theophylline derivative or a beta$_2$ agonist may be administered cautiously, depending on the clinical condition of the patient. Both theophylline derivatives and beta$_2$ agonists may produce serious cardiac arrhythmias.

PRECAUTIONS
General
Lopressor should be used with caution in patients with impaired hepatic function.

Information for Patients
Patients should be advised to take Lopressor regularly and continuously, as directed, with or immediately following meals. If a dose should be missed, the patient should take only the next scheduled dose (without doubling it). Patients should not discontinue Lopressor without consulting the physician.

Patients should be advised (1) to avoid operating automobiles and machinery or engaging in other tasks requiring alertness until the patient's response to therapy with Lopressor has been determined; (2) to contact the physician if any difficulty in breathing occurs; (3) to inform the physician or dentist before any type of surgery that he or she is taking Lopressor.

Laboratory Tests
Clinical laboratory findings may include elevated levels of serum transaminase, alkaline phosphatase, and lactate dehydrogenase.

Drug Interactions
Catecholamine-depleting drugs (e.g., reserpine) may have an additive effect when given with beta-blocking agents. Patients treated with Lopressor plus a catecholamine depletor should therefore be closely observed for evidence of hypotension or marked bradycardia, which may produce vertigo, syncope, or postural hypotension.

Carcinogenesis, Mutagenesis, Impairment of Fertility
Long-term studies in animals have been conducted to evaluate carcinogenic potential. In 2-year studies in rats at three oral dosage levels of up to 800 mg/kg per day, there was no increase in the development of spontaneously occurring benign or malignant neoplasms of any type. The only histologic changes that appeared to be drug related were an increased incidence of generally mild focal accumulation of foamy macrophages in pulmonary alveoli and a slight increase in biliary hyperplasia. Neither finding represents symptoms of a known disease entity in man. In a 21-month study in Swiss albino mice at three oral dosage levels of up to 750 mg/kg per day, benign lung tumors (small adenomas) occurred more frequently in female mice receiving the highest dose than in untreated control animals. There was no increase in malignant or total (benign plus malignant) lung tumors, nor in the overall incidence of tumors or malignant tumors. This 21-month study was repeated in CD-1 mice, and no statistically or biologically significant differences were observed between treated and control mice of either sex for any type of tumor. All mutagenicity tests performed (a dominant lethal study in mice, chromosome studies in somatic cells, a Salmonella/mammalian-microsome mutagenicity test, and a nucleus anomaly test in somatic interphase nuclei) were negative. No evidence of impaired fertility due to Lopressor was observed in a study performed in rats at doses up to 55.5 times the maximum daily human dose of 450 mg.

Pregnancy Category C
Lopressor has been shown to increase postimplantation loss and decrease neonatal survival in rats at doses up to 55.5 times the maximum daily human dose of 450 mg. Distribution studies in mice confirm exposure of the fetus when Lopressor is administered to the pregnant animal. These studies have revealed no evidence of impaired fertility or teratogenicity. There are no adequate and well-controlled studies in pregnant women. Because animal reproduction studies are not always predictive of human response, this drug should be used during pregnancy only if clearly needed.

Nursing Mothers
Lopressor is excreted in breast milk in very small quantity. An infant consuming 1 liter of breast milk daily would receive a dose of less than 1 mg of the drug. Caution should be exercised when Lopressor is administered to a nursing woman.

Pediatric Use
Safety and effectiveness in children have not been established.

ADVERSE REACTIONS
Hypertension and Angina
Most adverse effects have been mild and transient.
Central Nervous System: Tiredness and dizziness have occurred in about 10 of 100 patients. Depression has been reported in about 5 of 100 patients. Mental confusion and short-term memory loss have been reported. Headache, nightmares, and insomnia have also been reported.

Cardiovascular: Shortness of breath and bradycardia have occurred in approximately 3 of 100 patients. Cold extremities; arterial insufficiency, usually of the Raynaud type; palpitations; congestive heart failure; peripheral edema; and hypotension have been reported in about 1 of 100 patients. (See CONTRAINDICATIONS, WARNINGS, and PRECAUTIONS.)

Respiratory: Wheezing (bronchospasm) and dyspnea have been reported in about 1 of 100 patients (see WARNINGS).
Gastrointestinal: Diarrhea has occurred in about 5 of 100 patients. Nausea, dry mouth, gastric pain, constipation, flatulence, and heartburn have been reported in about 1 of 100 patients.
Hypersensitive Reactions: Pruritus or rash have occurred in about 5 of 100 patients. Worsening of psoriasis has also been reported
Miscellaneous: Peyronie's disease has been reported in fewer than 1 of 100,000 patients. Musculoskeletal pain, blurred vision, and tinnitus have also been reported.
There have been rare reports of reversible alopecia, agranulocytosis, and dry eyes. Discontinuation of the drug should be considered if any such reaction is not otherwise explicable. The oculomucocutaneous syndrome associated with the beta blocker practolol has not been reported with Lopressor.

Myocardial Infarction
Central Nervous System: Tiredness has been reported in about 1 of 100 patients. Vertigo, sleep disturbances, hallucinations, headache, dizziness, visual disturbances, confusion, and reduced libido have also been reported, but a drug relationship is not clear.
Cardiovascular: In the randomized comparison of Lopressor and placebo described in the CLINICAL PHARMACOLOGY section, the following adverse reactions were reported:

	Lopressor	Placebo
Hypotension	27.4%	23.2%
(systolic BP < 90 mmHg)		
Bradycardia	15.9%	6.7%
(heart rate < 40 beats/min)		
Second- or	4.7%	4.7%
third-degree heart block		
First-degree	5.3%	1.9%
heart block (P-R ≥ 0.26 sec)		
Heart failure	27.5%	29.6%

Respiratory: Dyspnea of pulmonary origin has been reported in fewer than 1 of 100 patients.
Gastrointestinal: Nausea and abdominal pain have been reported in fewer than 1 of 100 patients.
Dermatologic: Rash and worsened psoriasis have been reported, but a drug relationship is not clear.
Miscellaneous: Unstable diabetes and claudication have been reported, but a drug relationship is not clear.

Potential Adverse Reactions
A variety of adverse reactions not listed above have been reported with other beta-adrenergic blocking agents and should be considered potential adverse reactions to Lopressor.
Central Nervous System: Reversible mental depression progressing to catatonia; an acute reversible syndrome characterized by disorientation for time and place, short-term memory loss, emotional lability, slightly clouded sensorium, and decreased performance on neuropsychometrics.
Cardiovascular: Intensification of AV block (See CONTRAINDICATIONS).
Hematologic: Agranulocytosis, nonthrombocytopenic purpura, thrombocytopenic purpura.
Hypersensitive Reactions: Fever combined with aching and sore throat, laryngospasm, and respiratory distress.

OVERDOSAGE
Acute Toxicity
Several cases of overdosage have been reported, some leading to death.
Oral LD$_{50}$'s (mg/kg): mice, 1158–2460; rats, 3090–4670.
Signs and Symptoms
Potential signs and symptoms associated with overdosage with Lopressor are bradycardia, hypotension, bronchospasm, and cardiac failure.
Treatment
There is no specific antidote.
In general, patients with acute or recent myocardial infarction may be more hemodynamically unstable than other patients and should be treated accordingly (see WARNINGS, Myocardial Infarction).
On the basis of the pharmacologic actions of Lopressor, the following general measures should be employed:
Elimination of the Drug: Gastric lavage should be performed.

Continued on next page

The full prescribing information for each GEIGY product is contained herein and is that in effect as of September 1, 1989

Geigy—Cont.

Bradycardia: Atropine should be administered. If there is no response to vagal blockade, isoproterenol should be administered cautiously.

Hypotension: A vasopressor should be administered, e.g., levarterenol or dopamine.

Bronchospasm: A beta$_2$-stimulating agent and/or a theophylline derivative should be administered.

Cardiac Failure: A digitalis glycoside and diuretic should be administered. In shock resulting from inadequate cardiac contractility, administration of dobutamine, isoproterenol, or glucagon may be considered.

DOSAGE AND ADMINISTRATION

Hypertension

The dosage of Lopressor should be individualized. Lopressor should be taken with or immediately following meals.

The usual initial dosage is 100 mg daily in single or divided doses, whether used alone or added to a diuretic. The dosage may be increased at weekly (or longer) intervals until optimum blood pressure reduction is achieved. In general, the maximum effect of any given dosage level will be apparent after 1 week of therapy. The effective dosage range is 100 to 450 mg per day. Dosages above 450 mg per day have not been studied. While once-daily dosing is effective and can maintain a reduction in blood pressure throughout the day, lower doses (especially 100 mg) may not maintain a full effect at the end of the 24-hour period, and larger or more frequent daily doses may be required. This can be evaluated by measuring blood pressure near the end of the dosing interval to determine whether satisfactory control is being maintained throughout the day. Beta$_1$ selectivity diminishes as the dose of Lopressor is increased.

Angina Pectoris

The dosage of Lopressor should be individualized. Lopressor should be taken with or immediately following meals.

The usual initial dosage is 100 mg daily, given in two divided doses. The dosage may be gradually increased at weekly intervals until optimum clincial response has been obtained or there is pronounced slowing of the heart rate. The effective dosage range is 100 to 400 mg per day. Dosages above 400 mg per day have not been studied. If treatment is to be discontinued, the dosage should be reduced gradually over a period of 1–2 weeks. (See **WARNINGS.**)

Myocardial Infarction

Early Treatment: During the early phase of definite or suspected acute myocardial infarction, treatment with Lopressor can be initiated as soon as possible after the patient's arrival in the hospital. Such treatment should be initiated in a coronary care or similar unit immediately after the patient's hemodynamic condition has stabilized.

Treatment in this early phase should begin with the intravenous administration of three bolus injections of 5 mg of Lopressor each; the injections should be given at approximately 2-minute intervals. During the intravenous administration of Lopressor, blood pressure, heart rate, and electrocardiogram should be carefully monitored.

In patients who tolerate the full intravenous dose (15 mg), Lopressor tablets, 50 mg every 6 hours, should be initiated 15 minutes after the last intravenous dose and continued for 48 hours. Thereafter, patients should receive a maintenance dosage of 100 mg twice daily (see **Late Treatment** below). Patients who appear not to tolerate the full intravenous dose should be started on Lopressor tablets either 25 mg or 50 mg every 6 hours (depending on the degree of intolerance) 15 minutes after the last intravenous dose or as soon as their clinical condition allows. In patients with severe intolerance, treatment with Lopressor should be discontinued (see **WARNINGS**).

Late Treatment: Patients with contraindications to treatment during the early phase of suspected or definite myocardial infarction, patients who appear not to tolerate the full early treatment, and patients in whom the physician wishes to delay therapy for any other reason should be started on Lopressor tablets, 100 mg twice daily, as soon as their clinical condition allows. Therapy should be continued for at least 3 months. Although the efficacy of Lopressor beyond 3 months has not been conclusively established, data from studies with other beta blockers suggest that treatment should be continued for 1–3 years.

Note: Parenteral drug products should be inspected visually for particulate matter and discoloration prior to administration, whenever solution and container permit.

HOW SUPPLIED

Tablets 50 mg —capsule-shaped, biconvex, pink, scored (imprinted GEIGY on one side and 51 twice on the scored side)

Bottles of 100 .... NDC 0028-0051-01
Bottles of 1000 .... NDC 0028-0051-10

Gy-Pak®—One Unit
  12 bottles—60 tablets each .... NDC 0028-0051-73
  12 bottles—100 tablets each .... NDC 0028-0051-65

Unit Dose (blister pack)
  Box of 100 (strips of 10) .... NDC 0028-0051-61

Tablets 100 mg —capsule-shaped, biconvex, light blue, scored (imprinted GEIGY on one side and 71 twice on the scored side)

Bottles of 100 .... NDC 0028-0071-01
Bottles of 1000 .... NDC 0028-0071-10

Gy-Pak®—One Unit
  12 bottles—60 tablets each .... NDC 0028-0071-73
  12 bottles—100 tablets each .... NDC 0028-0071-65

Unit Dose (blister pack)
  Box of 100 (strips of 10) .... NDC 0028-0071-61

Samples, when available, are identified by the word *SAMPLE* appearing on each tablet.

Store at controlled room temperature and protect from moisture.

Dispense in tight, light-resistant container (USP).

Ampuls 5 ml —each containing 5 mg of metoprolol tartrate

  Tray of 4 packs of 3 ampuls .... NDC 0028-4201-33
Protect from light.

Prefilled Syringes 5 ml—each containing 5 mg of metoprolol tartrate

  Box of 12 syringes .... NDC 0028-4202-12
Protect from light.

C88-41 (Rev. 12/88)
Shown in Product Identification Section, page 410

LOPRESSOR HCT®   ℞
metoprolol tartrate USP and hydrochlorothiazide USP
50/25 Tablets
100/25 Tablets
100/50 Tablets
Beta Blocker/Diuretic Antihypertensive

DESCRIPTION

Lopressor HCT has the antihypertensive effect of Lopressor®, metoprolol tartrate, a selective beta$_1$-adrenoreceptor blocking agent, and the antihypertensive and diuretic actions of hydrochlorothiazide. It is available as tablets for oral administration. The 50/25 tablets contain 50 mg of metoprolol tartrate USP and 25 mg of hydrochlorothiazide USP; the 100/25 tablets contain 100 mg of metoprolol tartrate USP and 25 mg of hydrochlorothiazide USP; and the 100/50 tablets contain 100 mg of metoprolol tartrate USP and 50 mg of hydrochlorothiazide USP.

Metoprolol tartrate is 1-isopropylamino-3-[p-(2-methoxyethyl)phenoxy]-2-propanol 2:1 *dextro*-tartrate salt.

Metoprolol tartrate is a white, practically odorless, crystalline powder with a molecular weight of 684.82. It is readily soluble in chloroform, in methylene chloride, and in water; soluble in ethanol; and sparingly soluble in acetone.

Hydrochlorothiazide is 6-chloro-3,4-dihydro-2H-1,2,4-benzothiadiazine-7-sulfonamide, 1,1-dioxide.

Hydrochlorothiazide USP is a white, or practically white, practically odorless, crystalline powder. It is freely soluble in sodium hydroxide solution, in n-butylamine, and in dimethylformamide; sparingly soluble in methanol; slightly soluble in water; and insoluble in ether, in chloroform, and in dilute mineral acids. Its molecular weight is 297.73.

Inactive Ingredients: Cellulose compounds, colloidal silicon dioxide, D&C Yellow No. 10 (100/50-mg tablets), FD&C Blue No. 1 (50/25-mg tablets), FD&C Red No. 3 and FD&C Yellow No. 6 (100/25-mg tablets), lactose, magnesium stearate, povidone, sodium starch glycolate, starch, stearic acid, and sucrose.

CLINICAL PHARMACOLOGY

Lopressor

Lopressor is a beta-adrenergic receptor blocking agent. *In vitro* and *in vivo* animal studies have shown that it has a preferential effect on beta$_1$ adrenoreceptors, chiefly located in cardiac muscle. This preferential effect is not absolute, however, and at higher doses, Lopressor also inhibits beta$_2$ adrenoreceptors, chiefly located in the bronchial and vascular musculature.

Clinical pharmacology studies have confirmed the beta-blocking activity of metoprolol in man, as shown by (1) reduction in heart rate and cardiac output at rest and upon exercise, (2) reduction of systolic blood pressure upon exercise, (3) inhibition of isoproterenol-induced tachycardia, and (4) reduction of reflex orthostatic tachycardia.

Relative beta$_1$ selectivity has been confirmed by the following: (1) In normal subjects, Lopressor is unable to reverse the beta$_2$-mediated vasodilating effects of epinephrine. This contrasts with the effect of nonselective (beta$_1$ plus beta$_2$) beta blockers, which completely reverse the vasodilating effects of epinephrine. (2) In asthmatic patients, Lopressor reduces FEV$_1$ and FVC significantly less than a nonselective beta blocker, propranolol at equivalent beta$_1$-receptor blocking doses.

Lopressor has no intrinsic sympathomimetic activity and only weak membrane-stabilizing activity. Lopressor crosses the blood-brain barrier and has been reported in the CSF in a concentration 78% of the simultaneous plasma concentra-

tion. Animal and human experiments indicate that Lopressor slows the sinus rate and decreases AV nodal conduction. In controlled clinical studies, Lopressor has been shown to be an effective antihypertensive agent when used alone or as concomitant therapy with thiazide-type diuretics, at dosages of 100–450 mg daily. In controlled, comparative, clinical studies, Lopressor has been shown to be as effective as an antihypertensive agent as propranolol, methyldopa, and thiazide-type diuretics, and to be equally effective in supine and standing positions.

The mechanism of the antihypertensive effects of beta-blocking agents has not been elucidated. However, several possible mechanisms have been proposed: (1) competitive antagonism of catecholamines at peripheral (especially cardiac) adrenergic neuron sites, leading to decreased cardiac output; (2) a central effect leading to reduced sympathetic outflow to the periphery; and (3) suppression of renin activity.

In man, absorption of Lopressor is rapid and complete. Plasma levels following oral administration, however, approximate 50% of levels following intravenous administration, indicating about 50% first-pass metabolism. Plasma levels achieved are highly variable after oral administration. Only a small fraction of the drug (about 12%) is bound to human serum albumin. Elimination is mainly by biotransformation in the liver, and the plasma half-life ranges from approximately 3 to 7 hours. Less than 5% of an oral dose of Lopressor is recovered unchanged in the urine; the rest is excreted by the kidneys as metabolites that appear to have no clinical significance. The systemic availability and half-life of Lopressor in patients with renal failure do not differ to a clinically significant degree from those in normal subjects. Consequently, no reduction in dosage is usually needed in patients with chronic renal failure.

Significant beta-blocking effect (as measured by reduction of exercise heart rate) occurs within 1 hour after oral administration, and its duration is dose-related. For example, a 50% reduction of the maximum registered effect after single oral doses of 20, 50, and 100 mg occurred at 3.3, 5.0, and 6.4 hours, respectively, in normal subjects. After repeated oral dosages of 100 mg twice daily, a significant reduction in exercise systolic blood pressure was evident at 12 hours.

There is a linear relationship between the log of plasma levels and reduction of exercise heart rate. However, antihypertensive activity does not appear to be related to plasma levels. Because of variable plasma levels attained with a given dose and lack of a consistent relationship of antihypertensive activity to dose, selection of proper dosage requires individual titration.

Hydrochlorothiazide

Thiazides affect the renal tubular mechanism of electrolyte reabsorption. At maximal therapeutic dosage, all thiazides are approximately equal in their diuretic potency. Thiazides increase excretion of sodium and chloride in approximately equivalent amounts. Natriuresis causes a secondary loss of potassium.

The mechanism of the antihypertensive effect of thiazides is unknown. Thiazides do not affect normal blood pressure. The onset of action of thiazides occurs in 2 hours and the peak effect at about 4 hours. The action persists for approximately 6–12 hours. Hydrochlorothiazide is rapidly absorbed, as indicated by peak plasma concentrations 1–2.5 hours after oral administration. Plasma levels of the drug are proportional to dose; the concentration in whole blood is 1.6–1.8 times higher than in plasma. Thiazides are eliminated rapidly by the kidney. After oral administration of 25- to 100-mg doses, 72–97% of the dose is excreted in the urine, indicating dose-independent absorption. Hydrochlorothiazide is eliminated from plasma in a biphasic fashion with a terminal half-life of 10–17 hours. Plasma protein binding is 67.9%. Plasma clearance is 15.9–30.0 L/hr; volume of distribution is 3.6–7.8 L/kg.

Gastrointestinal absorption of hydrochlorothiazide is enhanced when administered with food. Absorption is decreased in patients with congestive heart failure, and the pharmacokinetics are considerably different in these patients.

INDICATIONS AND USAGE

Lopressor HCT is indicated for the management of hypertension.

This fixed-combination drug is not indicated for initial therapy of hypertension. If the fixed combination represents the dose titrated to the individual patient's needs, therapy with the fixed combination may be more convenient than with the separate components.

CONTRAINDICATIONS

Lopressor

Lopressor is contraindicated in sinus bradycardia, heart block greater than first degree, cardiogenic shock, and overt cardiac failure (see **WARNINGS**).

Hydrochlorothiazide

Hydrochlorothiazide is contraindicated in patients with anuria or hypersensitivity to this or other sulfonamide-derived drugs (see **WARNINGS**).

WARNINGS

Lopressor

Cardiac Failure. Sympathetic stimulation is a vital component supporting circulatory function in congestive heart failure, and beta blockade carries the potential hazard of further depressing myocardial contractility and precipitating more severe failure. In hypertensive patients who have congestive heart failure controlled by digitalis and diuretics, Lopressor should be administered cautiously. Both digitalis and Lopressor slow AV conduction.

In Patients Without a History of Cardiac Failure. Continued depression of the myocardium with beta-blocking agents over a period of time can, in some cases, lead to cardiac failure. At the first sign or symptom of impending cardiac failure, patients should be fully digitalized and/or given a diuretic. The response should be observed closely. If cardiac failure continues, despite adequate digitalization and diuretic therapy, Lopressor should be withdrawn.

Ischemic Heart Disease. Following abrupt cessation of therapy with certain beta-blocking agents, exacerbations of angina pectoris and, in some cases, myocardial infarction have been reported. Even in the absence of overt angina pectoris, when discontinuing therapy, Lopressor should not be withdrawn abruptly, and patients should be cautioned against interruption of therapy without the physician's advice (see PRECAUTIONS, Information for Patients).

Bronchospastic Diseases. **PATIENTS WITH BRONCHOSPASTIC DISEASES SHOULD, IN GENERAL, NOT RECEIVE BETA BLOCKERS. Because of its relative beta₁ selectivity, however, Lopressor may be used with caution in patients with bronchospastic disease who do not respond to, or cannot tolerate, other antihypertensive treatment. Since beta₁ selectivity is not absolute, a beta₂-stimulating agent should be administered concomitantly, and the lowest possible dose of Lopressor should be used. In these circumstances it would be prudent initially to administer Lopressor in smaller doses three times daily, instead of larger doses two times daily, to avoid the higher plasma levels associated with the longer dosing interval. (See DOSAGE AND ADMINISTRATION.)**

Major Surgery. The necessity or desirability of withdrawing beta-blocking therapy prior to major surgery is controversial; the impaired ability of the heart to respond to reflex adrenergic stimuli may augment the risks of general anesthesia and surgical procedures.

Lopressor, like other beta blockers, is a competitive inhibitor of beta-receptor agonists, and its effects can be reversed by administration of such agents, e.g., dobutamine or isoproterenol. However, such patients may be subject to protracted severe hypotension. Difficulty in restarting and maintaining the heart beat has also been reported with beta blockers.

Diabetes and Hypoglycemia. Lopressor should be used with caution in diabetic patients if a beta-blocking agent is required. Beta blockers may mask tachycardia occurring with hypoglycemia, but other manifestations such as dizziness and sweating may not be significantly affected. Selective beta blockers do not potentiate insulin-induced hypoglycemia and, unlike nonselective beta blockers, do not delay recovery of blood glucose to normal levels.

Thyrotoxicosis. Beta-adrenergic blockade may mask certain clinical signs (e.g., tachycardia) or hyperthyroidism. Patients suspected of developing thyrotoxicosis should be managed carefully to avoid abrupt withdrawal of beta blockade, which might precipitate a thyroid storm.

Hydrochlorothiazide

Thiazides should be used with caution in patients with severe renal disease. In patients with renal disease, thiazides may precipitate azotemia. Cumulative effects of the drug may develop in patients with impaired renal function.

Thiazides should be used with caution in patients with impaired hepatic function or progressive liver disease, since minor alterations of fluid and electrolyte imbalance may precipitate hepatic coma.

Thiazides may add to or potentiate the action of other antihypertensive drugs. Potentiation occurs with ganglionic or peripheral adrenergic blocking drugs.

Sensitivity reactions are more likely to occur in patients with a history of allergy or bronchial asthma.

The possibility of exacerbation or activation of systemic lupus erythematosus has been reported.

PRECAUTIONS

General

Lopressor. Lopressor should be used with caution in patients with impaired hepatic function.

Hydrochlorothiazide. All patients receiving thiazide therapy should be observed for clinical signs of fluid or electrolyte imbalance, namely hyponatremia, hypochloremic alkalosis, and hypokalemia (see Laboratory Tests and Drug/Drug Interactions). Warning signs are dryness of mouth, thirst, weakness, lethargy, drowsiness, restlessness, muscle pains or cramps, muscular fatigue, hypotension, oliguria, tachycardia, and gastrointestinal disturbance, such as nausea or vomiting.

Hypokalemia may develop, especially in cases of brisk diuresis or severe cirrhosis.

Interference with adequate oral intake of electrolytes will also contribute to hypokalemia. Hypokalemia may be avoided or treated by the use of potassium supplements or foods with a high potassium content.

Any chloride deficit is generally mild and usually does not require specific treatment, except under extraordinary circumstances (as in liver disease or renal disease). Dilutional hyponatremia may occur in edematous patients in hot weather; appropriate therapy is water restriction, rather than administration of salt, except in rare instances when the hyponatremia is life-threatening. In cases of actual salt depletion, appropriate replacement is the therapy of choice.

Hyperuricemia may occur or frank gout may be precipitated in certain patients receiving thiazide therapy.

Latent diabetes may become manifest during thiazide administration (see Drug/Drug Interactions).

The antihypertensive effects of the drug may be enhanced in the postsympathectomy patient.

If progressive renal impairment becomes evident, withholding or discontinuing diuretic therapy should be considered.

Calcium excretion is decreased by thiazides. Pathological changes in the parathyroid gland with hypercalcemia and hypophosphatemia have been observed in a few patients on prolonged thiazide therapy. The common complications of hyperparathyroidism, such as renal lithiasis, bone resorption, and peptic ulceration, have not been seen.

Information for Patients

Patients should be advised to take Lopressor HCT regularly and continuously, as directed, with or immediately following meals. If a dose should be missed, the patient should take only the next scheduled dose (without doubling it). Patients should not discontinue Lopressor HCT without consulting the physician.

Patients should be advised (1) to avoid operating automobiles and machinery or engaging in other tasks requiring alertness until the patient's response to therapy with Lopressor has been determined; (2) to contact the physician if any difficulty in breathing occurs; (3) to inform the physician or dentist before any type of surgery that he or she is taking Lopressor HCT.

Laboratory Tests

Lopressor. Clinical laboratory findings may include elevated levels of serum transaminase, alkaline phosphatase, and lactate dehydrogenase.

Hydrochlorothiazide. Initial and periodic determinations of serum electrolytes to detect possible electrolyte imbalance should be performed at appropriate intervals.

Serum and urine electrolyte determinations are particularly important when the patient is vomiting excessively or receiving parenteral fluids.

Drug/Drug Interactions

Lopressor. Catecholamine-depleting drugs (e.g., reserpine) may have an additive effect when given with beta-blocking agents. Patients treated with Lopressor plus a catecholamine depletor should therefore be closely observed for evidence of hypotension or marked bradycardia, which may produce vertigo, syncope, or postural hypotension.

Hydrochlorothiazide. Hypokalemia can sensitize or exaggerate the response of the heart to the toxic effects of digitalis (e.g., increased ventricular irritability).

Hypokalemia may develop during concomitant use of steroids or ACTH.

Insulin requirements in diabetic patients may be increased, decreased, or unchanged.

Thiazides may decrease arterial responsiveness to norepinephrine, but not enough to preclude effectiveness of the pressor agent for therapeutic use.

Thiazides may increase the responsiveness to tubocurarine.

Lithium renal clearance is reduced by thiazides, increasing the risk of lithium toxicity.

There have been rare reports in the literature of hemolytic anemia occurring with the concomitant use of hydrochlorothiazide and methyldopa.

Concurrent administration of some nonsteroidal antiinflammatory agents may reduce the diuretic, natriuretic and antihypertensive effects of thiazide diuretics.

Drug/Laboratory Test Interactions

Hydrochlorothiazide. Thiazides may decrease serum levels of protein-bound iodine without signs of thyroid disturbance. Thiazides should be discontinued before tests for parathyroid function are made. (See General, *Hydrochlorothiazide*, Calcium excretion.)

Carcinogenesis, Mutagenesis, Impairment of Fertility

Lopressor. Long-term studies in animals have been conducted to evaluate carcinogenic potential. In 2-year studies in rats at three oral dosage levels of up to 800 mg/kg per day, there was no increase in the development of spontaneously occurring benign or malignant neoplasms of any type. The only histologic changes that appeared to be drug related were an increased incidence of generally mild focal accumulation of foamy macrophages in pulmonary alveoli and a slight increase in biliary hyperplasia. Neither finding represents symptoms of a known disease entity in man. In a 21-month study in Swiss albino mice at three oral dosage levels of up to 750 mg/kg per day, benign lung tumors (small adenomas) occurred more frequently in female mice receiving the

highest dose than in untreated control animals. There was no increase in malignant or total (benign plus malignant) lung tumors, nor in the overall incidence of tumors or malignant tumors. This 21-month study was repeated in CD-1 mice, and no statistically or biologically significant differences were observed between treated and control mice of either sex for any type of tumor.

All mutagenicity tests performed (a dominant lethal study in mice, chromosome studies in somatic cells, a *Salmonella/mammalian-microsome* mutagenicity test, and a nucleus anomaly test in somatic interphase nuclei) were negative. No evidence of impaired fertility due to Lopressor was observed in a study performed in rats at doses up to 55.5 times the maximum daily human dose of 450 mg.

Hydrochlorothiazide. Long-term carcinogenicity studies in animals have not been conducted. Hydrochlorothiazide was not mutagenic in in vitro Ames mutagenicity assay of *Salmonella typhimurium* strains TA 98, TA 100, TA 1535 and TA 1537 or in in vivo mutagenicity assays of mouse germinal cell chromosomes and Chinese hamster bone marrow cell chromosomes. It was however, mutagenic in inducing nondisjunction (96% frequency) in diploid strains of *Aspergillus nidulans*.

Pregnancy Category C

Lopressor has been shown to increase postimplantation loss and decrease neonatal survival in rats at doses up to 55.5 times the maximum daily human dose of 450 mg. Distribution studies in mice confirm exposure of the fetus when Lopressor is administered to the pregnant animal. These studies have revealed no evidence of impaired fertility or teratogenicity.

A reproduction study with hydrochlorothiazide has been performed in rats at doses 62.5 times the maximum daily human dose and has revealed no evidence of impaired fertility or teratogenicity due to hydrochlorothiazide.

There are, however, no adequate and well-controlled studies in pregnant women with Lopressor HCT. Because animal reproduction studies are not always predictive of human response, this drug should be used during pregnancy only if clearly needed.

Nonteratogenic Effects. Thiazides cross the placental barrier and appear in cord blood, and there is a risk of fetal or neonatal jaundice, thrombocytopenia, and possibly other adverse reactions that have occurred in adults.

Nursing Mothers

Lopressor is excreted in breast milk in very small quantity. An infant consuming 1 liter of breast milk daily would receive a dose of metoprolol of less than 1 mg. Thiazides are also excreted in breast milk. If the use of Lopressor HCT is deemed essential, the patient should stop nursing.

Pediatric Use

Safety and effectiveness in children have not been established.

ADVERSE REACTIONS

Lopressor HCT

The following adverse reactions were reported in controlled clinical studies of the combination of Lopressor and hydrochlorothiazide.

Body as a Whole: Fatigue or lethargy and flu syndrome have each been reported in about 10 in 100 patients.

Nervous System: Dizziness or vertigo, drowsiness or somnolence, and headache have each occurred in about 10 in 100 patients. Nightmare has occurred in 1 in 100 patients.

Cardiovascular: Bradycardia has occurred in about 6 in 100 patients. Decreased exercise tolerance and dyspnea have each occurred in about 1 of 100 patients.

Digestive: Diarrhea, digestive disorder, dry mouth, nausea or vomiting, and constipation have each occurred in about 1 in 100 patients.

Metabolic and Nutritional: Hypokalemia has occurred in fewer than 10 in 100 patients. Edema, gout, and anorexia have each occurred in 1 in 100 patients.

Special Senses: Blurred vision, tinnitus, and earache have each been reported in 1 in 100 patients.

Skin: Sweating and purpura have each occurred in 1 in 100 patients.

Urogenital: Impotence has occurred in 1 in 100 patients.

Musculoskeletal: Muscle pain has occurred in 1 in 100 patients.

Lopressor

Most adverse effects have been mild and transient.

Central Nervous System: Tiredness and dizziness have occurred in about 10 of 100 patients. Depression has been reported in about 5 of 100 patients. Mental confusion and short-term memory loss have been reported. Headache, nightmares, and insomnia have also been reported, but a drug relationship is not clear.

Continued on next page

The full prescribing information for each GEIGY product is contained herein and is that in effect as of September 1, 1989

Geigy—Cont.

Cardiovascular: Shortness of breath and bradycardia have occurred in approximately 3 of 100 patients. Cold extremities; arterial insufficiency, usually of the Raynaud type; palpitations; and congestive heart failure have been reported. (See **CONTRAINDICATIONS, WARNINGS,** and **PRECAUTIONS**).
Respiratory: Wheezing (bronchospasm) has been reported in fewer than 1 of 100 patients (see **WARNINGS**).
Gastrointestinal: Diarrhea has occurred in about 5 of 100 patients. Nausea, gastric pain, constipation, flatulence, and heartburn have been reported in 1 of 100, or fewer, patients.
Hypersensitive Reactions: Pruritus has occurred in fewer than 1 of 100 patients. Rash has been reported.
Miscellaneous: Peyronie's disease has been reported in fewer than 1 of 100,000 patients. Alopecia has been reported. The oculomucocutaneous syndrome associated with the beta blocker practolol has not been reported with Lopressor.

Potential Adverse Reactions

A variety of adverse reactions not listed above have been reported with other beta-adrenergic blocking agents and should be considered potential adverse reactions to Lopressor.
Central Nervous System: Reversible mental depression progressing to catatonia; visual disturbances; hallucinations; an acute reversible syndrome characterized by disorientation for time and place, short-term memory loss, emotional lability, slightly clouded sensorium, and decreased performance on neuropsychometrics.
Cardiovascular: Intensification of AV block (see **CONTRAINDICATIONS**).
Hematologic: Agranulocytosis, nonthrombocytopenic purpura, thrombocytopenic purpura.
Hypersensitive Reactions: Fever combined with aching and sore throat, laryngospasm, and respiratory distress.

Hydrochlorothiazide

Gastrointestinal: Anorexia, gastric irritation, nausea, vomiting, cramping, diarrhea, constipation, jaundice (intrahepatic cholestatic), pancreatitis, sialadenitis.
Cardiovascular: Orthostatic hypotension (may be potentiated by alcohol, barbiturates, or narcotics).
Neurologic: Dizziness, vertigo, paresthesia, headache, xanthopsia.
Hematologic: Leukopenia, agranulocytosis, thrombocytopenia, aplastic anemia.
Hypersensitive Reactions: Purpura, photosensitivity, rash, urticaria, necrotizing angiitis, Stevens-Johnson syndrome, other hypersensitive reactions.
Other: Hyperglycemia, glycosuria, hyperuricemia, muscle spasm, weakness, restlessness, transient blurred vision.

OVERDOSAGE

Acute Toxicity

Several cases of overdosage with Lopressor have been reported, some leading to death. No deaths have been reported with hydrochlorothiazide.
Oral LD_{50}'s (mg/kg): mice, 1158 (Lopressor); rats, 3090 (Lopressor), 2750 (hydrochlorothiazide).

Signs and Symptoms

Lopressor. Potential signs and symptoms associated with overdosage with Lopressor are bradycardia, hypotension, bronchospasm, and cardiac failure.
Hydrochlorothiazide. The most prominent feature of poisoning is acute loss of fluid and electrolytes.
Cardiovascular: Tachycardia, hypotension, shock.
Neuromuscular: Weakness, confusion, dizziness, cramps of the calf muscles, paresthesia, fatigue, impairment of consciousness.
Digestive: Nausea, vomiting, thirst.
Renal: Polyuria, oliguria, or anuria (due to hemoconcentration).
Laboratory Findings: Hypokalemia, hyponatremia, hypochloremia, alkalosis; increased BUN (especially in patients with renal insufficiency).
Combined Poisoning: Signs and symptoms may be aggravated or modified by concomitant intake of antihypertensive medication, barbiturates, curare, digitalis (hypokalemia), corticosteroids, narcotics, or alcohol.

Treatment

There is no specific antidote.
On the basis of the pharmacologic actions of Lopressor and hydrochlorothiazide, the following general measures should be employed:
Elimination of the Drug: Inducement of vomiting, gastric lavage, and activated charcoal.
Bradycardia: Atropine should be administered. If there is no response to vagal blockade, isoproterenol should be administered cautiously.
Hypotension: The patient's legs should be elevated, and lost fluid and electrolytes (potassium, sodium) should be replaced. A vasopressor should be administered, e.g., levarterenol or dopamine.
Bronchospasm: A $beta_2$-stimulating agent and/or a theophylline derivative should be administered.

Cardiac Failure: A digitalis glycoside and diuretic should be administered. In shock resulting from inadequate cardiac contractility, administration of dobutamine, isoproterenol, or glucagon may be considered.
Surveillance: Fluid and electrolyte balance (especially serum potassium) and renal function should be monitored until conditions become normal.

DOSAGE AND ADMINISTRATION

Dosage should be determined by individual titration (see **INDICATIONS AND USAGE**).
Hydrochlorothiazide is usually given at a dosage of 25 to 100 mg per day. The usual initial dosage of Lopressor is 100 mg daily in single or divided doses. Dosage may be increased gradually until optimum blood pressure control is achieved. The effective dosage range is 100 to 450 mg per day. While once-daily dosing is effective and can maintain a reduction in blood pressure throughout the day, lower doses (especially 100 mg) may not maintain a full effect at the end of the 24-hour period, and larger or more frequent daily doses may be required. This can be evaluated by measuring blood pressure near the end of the dosing interval to determine whether satisfactory control is being maintained throughout the day. $Beta_1$ selectivity diminishes as dosage of Lopressor is increased.
The following dosage schedule may be used to administer from 100 to 200 mg of Lopressor per day and from 25 to 50 mg of hydrochlorothiazide per day:

Lopressor HCT	Dosage
Tablets of 50/25	2 tablets per day in single or divided doses
Tablets of 100/25	1 to 2 tablets per day in single or divided doses
Tablets of 100/50	1 tablet per day in single or divided doses

Dosing regimens that exceed 50 mg of hydrochlorothiazide per day are not recommended. When necessary, another antihypertensive agent may be added gradually, beginning with 50% of the usual recommended starting dose to avoid an excessive fall in blood pressure.

HOW SUPPLIED

Tablets 50/25—capsule-shaped, white and blue, scored (imprinted Geigy on one side and 35 twice on the scored side) 50 mg of metoprolol tartrate and 25 mg of hydrochlorothiazide
Bottles of 100 .... NDC 0028-0035-01
Tablets 100/25—capsule-shaped, white and pink, scored (imprinted Geigy on one side and 53 twice on the scored side) 100 mg of metoprolol tartrate and 25 mg of hydrochlorothiazide
Bottles of 100 .... NDC 0028-0053-01
Tablets 100/50—capsule-shaped, white and yellow, scored (imprinted Geigy on one side and 73 twice on the scored side) 100 mg of metoprolol tartrate and 50 mg of hydrochlorothiazide
Bottles of 100 .... NDC 0028-0073-01
Samples, when available, are identified by the word *Sample* appearing on each tablet.
Store between 59°–86°F (15°–30°C). Protect from moisture.
Dispense in tight, light-resistant container (USP).
C88-42 (Rev. 12/88)
Shown in Product Identification Section, page 410

OTRIVIN®
xylometazoline hydrochloride USP
Nasal Spray and Nasal Drops 0.1%
Pediatric Nasal Drops 0.05%

One application provides rapid and long-lasting relief of nasal congestion for up to 10 hours.
Quickly clears stuffy noses due to common cold, sinusitis, hay fever.
Nasal congestion can make life miserable—you can't breathe, smell, taste, or sleep comfortably. That is why Otrivin is so helpful. It clears away that stuffy feeling, usually within 5 to 10 minutes, and your head feels clear for hours.
Otrivin has been prescribed by doctors for many years. Here is how you use it:
Nasal Spray 0.1%—Spray 2 or 3 times into each nostril every 8-10 hours. With head upright, squeeze sharply and firmly while inhaling (sniffing) through the nose.

Nasal Drops 0.1%—for adults and children 12 years and older. Put 2 or 3 drops into each nostril every 8 to 10 hours.

Tilt head as far back as possible. Immediately bend head forward toward knees, hold a few seconds, then return to upright position.
Do not give Nasal Spray 0.1% or Nasal Drops 0.1% to children under 12 years except under the advice and supervision of a physician.

Pediatric Nasal Drops 0.05%—for children 2 to 12 years of age. Put 2 or 3 drops into each nostril every 8 to 10 hours. Tilt head as far back as possible. Immediately bend head forward toward knees, hold a few seconds, then return to upright position.
Do not give this product to children under 2 years except under the advice and supervision of a physician.

Otrivin Nasal Spray/Nasal Drops contain 0.1% xylometazoline hydrochloride, USP. Also contains benzalkonium chloride, potassium chloride, potassium phosphate monobasic, purified water, sodium chloride and sodium phosphate dibasic.
They are available in an unbreakable plastic spray package of $\frac{1}{2}$ fl oz (15ml) and in a plastic dropper bottle of .66 fl oz (20ml).
Otrivin Pediatric Nasal Drops contain 0.05% xylometazoline hydrochloride, USP. Also contains benzalkonium chloride, potassium chloride, potassium phosphate monobasic, purified water, sodium chloride and sodium phosphate dibasic. It is available in a plastic dropper bottle of .66 fl oz (20ml).

WARNINGS

Do not exceed recommended dosage, because symptoms such as burning, stinging, sneezing, or increase of nasal discharge may occur. Do not use this product for more than 3 days. If symptoms persist, consult a physician. The use of this dispenser by more than one person may cause infection.
Keep this and all medicines out of the reach of children. In case of accidental ingestion, seek professional assistance or contact a Poison Control Center immediately.
C86-44 (Rev. 9/86)
Distributed by CIBA CONSUMER PHARMACEUTICALS EDISON, NEW JERSEY 08837

PBZ–SR®   ℞
tripelennamine hydrochloride USP
Extended-Release Tablets

DESCRIPTION

PBZ-SR, tripelennamine hydrochloride USP, is an antihistamine for oral administration available as 100-mg extended-release tablets that provide a gradual and prolonged release of drug from the wax matrix.

Tripelennamine hydrochloride is 2-[Benzyl[2-(dimethylamino)ethyl]amino] pyridine monohydrochloride.
Tripelennamine hydrochloride USP is a white, crystalline powder. Its solutions are practically neutral to litmus. It is freely soluble in water, in alcohol, and in chloroform; slightly soluble in acetone; and insoluble in benzene, in ether, and in ethyl acetate. Its molecular weight is 291.82.

Inactive Ingredients: Cellulose compounds, cetostearyl alcohol, D&C Red No. 30 lake, FD&C Blue No. 2 lake, magnesium stearate, mineral oil, titanium dioxide, and zein.

ACTIONS
Antihistamines are competitive antagonists of histamine, which also produce central nervous system effects (both stimulant and depressant) and peripheral anticholinergic, atropine-like effects (e.g., drying).

INDICATIONS
Perennial and seasonal allergic rhinitis; vasomotor rhinitis; allergic conjunctivitis due to inhalant allergens and foods; mild, uncomplicated allergic skin manifestations of urticaria and angioedema; amelioration of allergic reactions to blood or plasma; dermographism; anaphylactic reactions as adjunctive therapy to epinephrine and other standard measures after the acute manifestations have been controlled.

CONTRAINDICATIONS
PBZ-SR should not be used in premature infants, neonates, or nursing mothers; patients receiving MAO inhibitors; patients with narrow-angle glaucoma, stenosing peptic ulcer, symptomatic prostatic hypertrophy, bladder neck obstruction, pyloroduodenal obstruction, lower respiratory tract symptoms (including asthma), or hypersensitivity to tripelennamine or related compounds.

WARNINGS
Antihistamines often produce drowsiness and may reduce mental alertness in children and adults. Patients should be warned about engaging in activities requiring mental alertness (e.g., driving a car, operating machinery or hazardous appliances). In elderly patients, approximately 60 years or older, antihistamines are more likely to cause dizziness, sedation and hypotension. Patients should be warned that the central nervous system effects of PBZ-SR may be additive with those of alcohol and other CNS depressants (e.g., hypnotics, sedatives, tranquilizers, antianxiety agents).
Antihistamines may produce excitation, particularly in children.

Usage in Pregnancy: Although no tripelennamine-related teratogenic potential or other adverse effects on the fetus have been observed in limited animal reproduction studies, the safe use of this drug in pregnancy or during lactation has not been established. Therefore, the drug should not be used during pregnancy or lactation unless, in the judgment of the physician, the expected benefits outweigh the potential hazards.

Usage in Children: In infants and children particularly, antihistamines in overdosage may produce hallucinations, convulsions and/or death.

PRECAUTIONS
PBZ-SR, like other antihistamines, has atropine-like, anticholinergic activity and should be used with caution in patients with increased intraocular pressure, hyperthyroidism, cardiovascular disease, hypertension, or history of bronchial asthma.

ADVERSE REACTIONS
The most frequent adverse reactions to antihistamines are sedation or drowsiness; sleepiness; dryness of the mouth, nose, and throat; thickening of bronchial secretions; dizziness; disturbed coordination; epigastric distress.
Other adverse reactions which may occur are: fatigue; chills; confusion; restlessness; excitation; hysteria; nervousness; irritability; insomnia; euphoria; anorexia; nausea; vomiting; diarrhea; constipation; hypotension; tightness in the chest; wheezing; blurred vision; diplopia; vertigo; tinnitus; convulsions; headache; palpitations; tachycardia; extrasystoles; nasal stuffiness; urinary frequency; difficult urination; urinary retention; leukopenia; hemolytic anemia; thrombocytopenia; agranulocytosis; aplastic anemia; allergic or hypersensitivity reactions, including drug rash, urticaria, anaphylactic shock, and photosensitivity. Although the following may have been reported to occur in association with some antihistamines, they have not been known to result from the use of PBZ-SR: excessive perspiration, tremor, paresthesias, acute labyrinthitis, neuritis and early menses.

DOSAGE AND ADMINISTRATION
Dosage should be individualized according to the needs and response of the patient.
Adults: One 100-mg PBZ-SR tablet in the morning and one in the evening is generally adequate. In difficult cases, one 100-mg PBZ-SR tablet every 8 hours may be required.
Children: PBZ-SR tablets are not intended for use in children.
Note: PBZ-SR extended-release tablets must be swallowed whole and never crushed or chewed.

OVERDOSAGE
Signs and Symptoms: The greatest danger from acute overdosage with antihistamines is their central nervous system effects which produce depression and/or stimulation.
In children, stimulation predominates initially in a syndrome which may include excitement, hallucinations, ataxia, incoordination, athetosis, and convulsions followed by postictal depression. Dry mouth, fixed dilated pupils, flushing of the face, and fever are common and resemble the syndrome of atropine poisoning. In adults, CNS depression (i.e., drowsiness, coma) is more common. CNS stimulation is rare; fever and flushing are uncommon.
In both children and adults, there can be a terminal deepening of coma and cardiovascular collapse; death can occur, especially in infants and children.
Treatment: There is no specific therapy for acute overdosage with antihistamines. General symptomatic and supportive measures should be instituted promptly and maintained for as long as necessary.
In the conscious patient, vomiting should be induced even though it may have occurred spontaneously. If vomiting cannot be induced, gastric lavage is indicated. Adequate precautions must be taken to protect against aspiration, especially in infants and children. Charcoal slurry or other suitable agent should be instilled into the stomach after vomiting or lavage. Saline cathartics or milk of magnesia may be of additional benefit.
In the unconscious patient, the airway should be secured with a cuffed endotracheal tube before attempting to evacuate the gastric contents. Intensive supportive and nursing care is indicated, as for any comatose patient.
If breathing is significantly impaired, maintenance of an adequate airway and mechanical support of respiration is the safest and most effective means of providing for adequate oxygenation of tissues to prevent hypoxia (especially brain hypoxia during convulsions).
Hypotension is an early sign of impeding cardiovascular collapse and should be treated vigorously. Although general supportive measures are important, specific treatment with intravenous infusion of a vasopressor (e.g., levarterenol bitartrate) titrated to maintain adequate blood pressure may be necessary.
Do *not* use CNS stimulants.
Convulsions should be controlled by careful titration of a short-acting barbiturate, repeated as necessary.
Ice packs and cooling sponge baths can aid in reducing the fever commonly seen in children.

HOW SUPPLIED
Tablets (extended-release) 100 mg—round, lavender (imprinted Geigy 48)
Bottles of 100 ....NDC 0028-0048-01
Store at controlled room temperature (15°–30°C) (59°–86°F). Protect from moisture.
Dispense in tight container (USP).

C87-36 (Rev. 10/87)
Shown in Product Identification Section, page 410

PBZ®   ℞
tripelennamine hydrochloride
Tablets USP
tripelennamine citrate Elixir USP

Listed in USP, a Medicare designated compendium.

DESCRIPTION
PBZ, an antihistamine for oral administration, is available as tripelennamine hydrochloride USP, and tripelennamine citrate USP. PBZ *tablets* contain 25 mg and 50 mg of the hydrochloride salt. PBZ *elixir* contains 37.5 mg of the citrate salt per 5 ml. Tripelennamine hydrochloride is 2-]Benzyl[2-(dimethylamino)ethyl]amino]pyridine monohydrochloride.
Tripelennamine hydrochloride USP is a white, crystalline powder. Its solutions are practically neutral to litmus. It is freely soluble in water, in alcohol, and in chloroform; slightly soluble in acetone; and insoluble in benzene, in ether, and in ethyl acetate. Its molecular weight is 291.82.
Tripelennamine citrate is 2-[Benzyl[2-(dimethylamino) ethyl]amino]pyridine citrate (1:1).
Tripelennamine citrate USP is a white, crystalline powder. Its solutions are acid to litmus. It is freely soluble in water and in alcohol, very slightly soluble in ether, and practically insoluble in benzene and in chloroform. It melts at about 107°C and has a molecular weight of 447.49.
Inactive ingredients (PBZ Tablets 25 mg): Lactose, magnesium stearate, polyethylene glycol, starch, sucrose and talc.
(PBZ Tablets 50 mg): Acacia, lactose, magnesium stearate, polyethylene glycol, talc and tragacanth.
(PBZ citrate Elixir): Alcohol (12% [v/v]), D&C Green No. 5, flavoring, glycerin, purified water and sucrose.

ACTIONS
Antihistamines are competitive antagonists of histamine, which also produce central nervous system effects (both stimulant and depressant) and peripheral anticholinergic, atropine-like effects (e.g., drying).

INDICATIONS
Perennial and seasonal allergic rhinitis; vasomotor rhinitis; allergic conjunctivitis due to inhalant allergens and foods; mild, uncomplicated allergic skin manifestations of urticaria and angioedema; amelioration of allergic reactions to blood or plasma; dermographism; anaphylactic reactions as adjunctive therapy to epinephrine and other standard measures after the acute manifestations have been controlled.

CONTRAINDICATIONS
PBZ should not be used in premature infants, neonates, or nursing mothers; patients receiving MAO inhibitors; patients with narrow-angle glaucoma, stenosing peptic ulcer, symptomatic prostatic hypertrophy, bladder neck obstruction, pyloroduodenal obstruction, lower respiratory tract symptoms (including asthma), or hypersensitivity to tripelennamine or related compounds.

WARNINGS
Antihistamines often produce drowsiness and may reduce mental alertness in children and adults. Patients should be warned about engaging in activities requiring mental alertness (e.g., driving a car, operating machinery or hazardous appliances). In elderly patients, approximately 60 years or older, antihistamines are more likely to cause dizziness, sedation and hypotension.
Patients should be warned that the central nervous system effects of PBZ may be additive with those of alcohol and other CNS depressants (e.g., hypnotics, sedatives, tranquilizers, antianxiety agents).
Antihistamines may produce excitation, particularly in children.

Usage in Pregnancy
Although no tripelennamine-related teratogenic potential or other adverse effects on the fetus have been observed in limited animal reproduction studies, the safe use of this drug in pregnancy or during lactation has not been established. Therefore, the drug should not be used during pregnancy or lactation unless, in the judgment of the physician, the expected benefits outweigh the potential hazards.

Usage in Children
In infants and children particularly, antihistamines in overdosage may produce hallucinations, convulsions and/or death.

PRECAUTIONS
PBZ, like other antihistamines, has atropine-like, anticholinergic activity and should be used with caution in patients with increased intraocular pressure, hyperthyroidism, cardiovascular disease, hypertension, or history of bronchial asthma.

ADVERSE REACTIONS
The most frequent adverse reactions to antihistamines are sedation or drowsiness; sleepiness; dryness of the mouth, nose, and throat; thickening of bronchial secretions; dizziness; disturbed coordination; epigastric distress.
Other adverse reactions which may occur are: fatigue; chills; confusion; restlessness; excitation; hysteria; nervousness; irritability; insomnia; euphoria; anorexia; nausea; vomiting; diarrhea; constipation; hypotension; tightness in the chest; wheezing; blurred vision; diplopia; vertigo; tinnitus; convulsions; headache; palpitations; tachycardia; extrasystoles; nasal stuffiness; urinary frequency; difficult urination; urinary retention; leukopenia; hemolytic anemia; thrombocytopenia; agranulocytosis; aplastic anemia; allergic or hypersensitivity reactions, including drug rash, urticaria, anaphylactic shock, and photosensitivity. Although the following may have been reported to occur in association with some antihistamines, they have not been known to result from the use of PBZ: excessive perspiration, tremor, paresthesias, acute labyrinthitis, neuritis and early menses.

DOSAGE AND ADMINISTRATION
Dosage should be individualized.
Usual Adult Dose: 25 to 50 mg every four to six hours. As little as 25 mg may control symptoms, but as much as 600 mg daily may be given in divided doses, if necessary.
Children and Infants: 5 mg/kg/24 hours or 150 mg/m^2/24 hours divided into four to six doses. Do not exceed maximum total dose of 300 mg/24 hours.
Note: Recommended dosages are based on the hydrochloride salt; each ml of Elixir (tripelennamine citrate) is equivalent to 5 mg tripelennamine hydrochloride.

OVERDOSAGE
Signs and Symptoms
The greatest danger from acute overdosage with antihistamines is their central nervous system effects which produce depression and/or stimulation.

Continued on next page

The full prescribing information for each GEIGY product is contained herein and is that in effect as of September 1, 1989

Geigy—Cont.

In children, stimulation predominates initially in a syndrome which may include excitement, hallucinations, ataxia, incoordination, athetosis, and convulsions followed by postictal depression. Dry mouth, fixed dilated pupils, flushing of the face, and fever are common and resemble the syndrome of atropine poisoning.

In adults, CNS depression (i.e., drowsiness, coma) is more common. CNS stimulation is rare; fever and flushing are uncommon.

In both children and adults, there can be a terminal deepening of coma and cardiovascular collapse, death can occur, especially in infants and children.

Treatment

There is no specific therapy for acute overdosage with antihistamines. General symptomatic and supportive measures should be instituted promptly and maintained for as long as necessary.

In the conscious patient, vomiting should be induced even though it may have occurred spontaneously. If vomiting cannot be induced, gastric lavage is indicated. Adequate precautions must be taken to protect against aspiration, especially in infants and children. Charcoal slurry or other suitable agent should be instilled into the stomach after vomiting or lavage. Saline cathartics or milk of magnesia may be of additional benefit.

In the unconscious patient, the airway should be secured with a cuffed endotracheal tube before attempting to evacuate the gastric contents. Intensive supportive and nursing care is indicated, as for any comatose patient.

If breathing is significantly impaired, maintenance of an adequate airway and mechanical support of respiration is the safest and most effective means of providing for adequate oxygenation of tissues to prevent hypoxia (especially brain hypoxia during convulsions).

Hypotension is an early sign of impending cardiovascular collapse and should be treated vigorously. Although general supportive measures are important, specific treatment with intravenous infusion of a vasopressor (e.g., levarterenol bitartrate) titrated to maintain adequate blood pressure may be necessary.

Do *not* use CNS stimulants.

Convulsions should be controlled by careful titration of a short-acting barbiturate, repeated as necessary.

Ice packs and cooling sponge baths can aid in reducing the fever commonly seen in children.

HOW SUPPLIED

Tablets 25 mg—round, white to off-white, biconvex (scored on one side and imprinted Geigy 111 on the other side)
    Bottles of 100 ....NDC 0028-0111-01
Tablets 50 mg—round, white to off-white, biconvex (scored on one side and imprinted Geigy 117 on the other side)
    Bottles of 100 ....NDC 0028-0117-01
    Bottles of 1000 ....NDC 0028-0117-10
Elixir—green, cinnamon-flavored—37.5 mg tripelennamine citrate USP (equivalent to 25 mg tripelennamine hydrochloride) per 5 ml
Bottles of 473 ml..NDC 0028-6925-16
Dispense in tight, light-resistant container.

C85-53 (Rev. 8/85)
Shown in Product Identification Section, page 410

TEGRETOL® ℞
[*teg'rit-tall*]
carbamazepine USP
Chewable Tablets of 100 mg—red-speckled, pink
Tablets of 200 mg—pink

WARNING
APLASTIC ANEMIA AND AGRANULOCYTOSIS HAVE BEEN REPORTED IN ASSOCIATION WITH THE USE OF TEGRETOL. DATA FROM A POPULATION-BASED CASE CONTROL STUDY DEMONSTRATE THAT THE RISK OF DEVELOPING THESE REACTIONS IS 5-8 TIMES GREATER THAN IN THE GENERAL POPULATION. HOWEVER, THE OVERALL RISK OF THESE REACTIONS IN THE UNTREATED GENERAL POPULATION IS LOW, APPROXIMATELY SIX PATIENTS PER ONE MILLION POPULATION PER YEAR FOR AGRANULOCYTOSIS AND TWO PATIENTS PER ONE MILLION POPULATION PER YEAR FOR APLASTIC ANEMIA.
ALTHOUGH REPORTS OF TRANSIENT OR PERSISTENT DECREASED PLATELET OR WHITE BLOOD CELL COUNTS ARE NOT UNCOMMON IN ASSOCIATION WITH THE USE OF TEGRETOL, DATA ARE NOT AVAILABLE TO ESTIMATE ACCURATELY THEIR INCIDENCE OR OUTCOME. HOWEVER, THE VAST MAJORITY OF THE CASES OF LEUKOPENIA HAVE NOT PROGRESSED TO THE MORE SERIOUS CONDITIONS OF APLASTIC ANEMIA OR AGRANULOCYTOSIS.
BECAUSE OF THE VERY LOW INCIDENCE OF AGRANULOCYTOSIS AND APLASTIC ANEMIA, THE VAST MAJORITY OF MINOR HEMATOLOGIC CHANGES OBSERVED IN MONITORING OF PATIENTS ON TEGRETOL ARE UNLIKELY TO SIGNAL THE OCCURRENCE OF EITHER ABNORMALITY. NONETHELESS, COMPLETE PRETREATMENT HEMATOLOGICAL TESTING SHOULD BE OBTAINED AS A BASELINE. IF A PATIENT IN THE COURSE OF TREATMENT EXHIBITS LOW OR DECREASED WHITE BLOOD CELL OR PLATELET COUNTS, THE PATIENT SHOULD BE MONITORED CLOSELY. DISCONTINUATION OF THE DRUG SHOULD BE CONISIDERED IF ANY EVIDENCE OF SIGNIFICANT BONE MARROW DEPRESSION DEVELOPS.

Before prescribing Tegretol, the physician should be thoroughly familiar with the details of this prescribing information, particularly regarding use with other drugs, especially those which accentuate toxicity potential.

DESCRIPTION
Tegretol, carbamazepine USP, is an anticonvulsant and specific analgesic for trigeminal neuralgia, available as chewable tablets of 100 mg and tablets of 200 mg for oral administration. Its chemical name is 5H-dibenz[b,f]azepine-5-carboxamide.
Carbamazepine USP is a white to off-white powder, practically insoluble in water and soluble in alcohol and in acetone. Its molecular weight is 236.27.
Inactive Ingredients. Colloidal silicon dioxide, FD&C Red No. 3 (chewable tablets only), FD&C Red No. 40 (200-mg tablets only) flavoring (chewable tablets only), gelatin, glycerin, magnesium stearate, sodium starch glycolate (chewable tablets only), starch, stearic acid, and sucrose (chewable tablets only).

CLINICAL PHARMACOLOGY
In controlled clinical trials, Tegretol has been shown to be effective in the treatment of psychomotor and grand mal seizures, as well as trigeminal neuralgia.
It has demonstrated anticonvulsant properties in rats and mice with electrically and chemically induced seizures. It appears to act by reducing polysynaptic responses and blocking the posttetanic potentiation. Tegretol greatly reduces or abolishes pain induced by stimulation of the infraorbital nerve in cats and rats. It depresses thalamic potential and bulbar and polysynaptic reflexes, including the linguomandibular reflex in cats. Tegretol is chemically unrelated to other anticonvulsants or other drugs used to control the pain of trigeminal neuralgia. The mechanism of action remains unknown.
Tegretol tablets are adequately absorbed after oral administration at a slower rate than a solution, thus avoiding undesirably high peak concentrations. Tegretol in blood is 76% bound to plasma proteins. Plasma levels of Tegretol are variable and may range from 0.5–25 µg/ml, with no apparent relationship to the daily intake of the drug. Usual adult therapeutic levels are between 4 and 12 µg/ml. Following oral administration, serum levels peak at 4 to 5 hours. The CSF/serum ratio is 0.22, similar to the 22% unbound Tegretol in serum. Because Tegretol may induce its own metabolism, the half-life is also variable. Initial half-life values range from 25–65 hours, with 12–17 hours on repeated doses. Tegretol is metabolized in the liver. After oral administration of ^{14}C-carbamazepine, 72% of the administered radioactivity was found in the urine and 28% in the feces. This urinary radioactivity was composed largely of hydroxylated and conjugated metabolites, with only 3% of unchanged Tegretol. Transplacental passage of Tegretol is rapid (30 to 60 minutes), and the drug is accumulated in fetal tissues, with higher levels found in liver and kidney than in brain and lungs.

INDICATIONS AND USAGE
Epilepsy: Tegretol is indicated for use as an anticonvulsant drug. Evidence supporting efficacy of Tegretol as an anticonvulsant was derived from active drug-controlled studies that enrolled patients with the following seizure types:
1. Partial seizures with complex symptomatology (psychomotor, temporal lobe). Patients with these seizures appear to show greater improvement than those with other types.
2. Generalized tonic-clonic seizures (grand mal).
3. Mixed seizure patterns which include the above, or other partial or generalized seizures.
Absence seizures (petit mal) do not appear to be controlled by Tegretol (see PRECAUTIONS General).
Trigeminal Neuralgia: Tegretol is indicated in the treatment of the pain associated with true trigeminal neuralgia. Beneficial results have also been reported in glossopharyngeal neuralgia.
This drug is not a simple analgesic and should not be used for the relief of trivial aches or pains.

CONTRAINDICATIONS
Tegretol should not be used in patients with a history of previous bone marrow depression, hypersensitivity to the drug, or known sensitivity to any of the tricyclic compounds, such as amitriptyline, desipramine, imipramine, protriptyline, nortriptyline, etc. Likewise, on theoretical grounds its use with monoamine oxidase inhibitors is not recommended. Before administration of Tegretol, MAO inhibitors should be discontinued for a minimum of fourteen days, or longer if the clinical situation permits.

WARNINGS
Patients with a history of adverse hematologic reaction to any drug may be particularly at risk.
Severe dermatologic reactions including toxic epidermal necrolysis (Lyell's syndrome) and Stevens-Johnson syndrome, have been reported with Tegretol. These reactions have been extremely rare. However, a few fatalities have been reported.
Tegretol has shown mild anticholinergic activity; therefore, patients with increased intraocular pressure should be closely observed during therapy.
Because of the relationship of the drug to other tricyclic compounds, the possibility of activation of a latent psychosis and, in elderly patients, of confusion or agitation should be borne in mind.

PRECAUTIONS
General: Before initiating therapy, a detailed history and physical examination should be made.
Tegretol should be used with caution in patients with a mixed seizure disorder that includes atypical absence seizures, since in these patients Tegretol has been associated with increased frequency of generalized convulsions (see INDICATIONS AND USAGE).
Therapy should be prescribed only after critical benefit-to-risk appraisal in patients with a history of cardiac, hepatic or renal damage, adverse hematologic reaction to other drugs, or interrupted courses of therapy with Tegretol.
Information for Patients: Patients should be made aware of the early toxic signs and symtpoms of a potential hematologic problem, such as fever, sore throat, ulcers in the mouth, easy bruising, petechial or purpuric hemorrhage, and should be advised to report to the physician immediately if any such signs or symptoms appear.
Since dizziness and drowsiness may occur, patients should be cautioned about the hazards of operating machinery or automobiles or engaging in other potentially dangerous tasks.
Laboratory Tests: Complete pretreatment blood counts, including platelets and possibly reticulocytes and serum iron, should be obtained as a baseline. If a patient in the course of treatment exhibits low or decreased white blood cell or platelet counts, the patient should be monitored closely. Discontinuation of the drug should be considered if any evidence of significant bone marrow depression develops.
Baseline and periodic evaluations of liver function, particularly in patients with a history of liver disease, must be performed during treatment with this drug since liver damage may occur. The drug should be discontinued immediately in cases of aggravated liver dysfunction or active liver disease.
Baseline and periodic eye examinations, including slit-lamp, funduscopy and tonometry, are recommended since many phenothiazines and related drugs have been shown to cause eye changes.
Baseline and periodic complete urinalysis and BUN determinations are recommended for patients treated with this agent because of observed renal dysfunction.
Monitoring of blood levels (see CLINICAL PHARMACOLOGY) has increased the efficacy and safety of anticonvulsants. This monitoring may be particularly useful in cases of dramatic increase in seizure frequency and for verification of compliance. In addition, measurement of drug serum levels may aid in determining the cause of toxicity when more than one medication is being used.
Thyroid function tests have been reported to show decreased values with Tegretol administered alone.
Hyponatremia has been reported in association with Tegretol use, either alone or in combination with other drugs.
Drug Interactions: The simultaneous administration of phenobarbital, phenytoin, or primidone, or a combination of two, produces a marked lowering of serum levels of Tegretol. The half-lives of phenytoin, warfarin, doxycycline, and theophylline were significantly shortened when administered concurrently with Tegretol. Haloperidol serum levels may be reduced when the drug is administered with Tegretol. The doses of these drugs may therefore have to be increased when Tegretol is added to the therapeutic regimen.
Concomitant administration of Tegretol with erythromycin, cimetidine, propoxyphene, isoniazid or calcium channel blockers has been reported to result in elevated plasma levels of carbamazepine resulting in toxicity in some cases. Also, concomitant administration of carbamazepine and lithium may increase the risk of neurotoxic side effects.
Alterations of thyroid function have been reported in combination therapy with other anticonvulsant medications.

Breakthrough bleeding has been reported among patients receiving concomitant oral contraceptives and their reliability may be adversely affected.

Carcinogenesis, Mutagenesis, Impairment of Fertility: Carbamazepine, when administered to Sprague-Dawley rats for two years in the diet at doses of 25, 75, and 250 mg/kg/day, resulted in a dose-related increase in the incidence of hepatocellular tumors in females and of benign interstitial cell adenomas in the testes of males.

Carbamazepine must, therefore, be considered to be carcinogenic in Sprague-Dawley rats. Bacterial and mammalian mutagenicity studies using carbamazepine produced negative results. The significance of these findings relative to the use of carbamazepine in humans is, at present, unknown.

Pregnancy Category C: Tegretol has been shown to have adverse effects in reproduction studies in rats when given orally in dosages 10–25 times the maximum human daily dosage of 1200 mg. In rat teratology studies, 2 of 135 offspring showed kinked ribs at 250 mg/kg and 4 of 119 offspring at 650 mg/kg showed other anomalies (cleft palate, 1; talipes, 1; anophthalmos, 2). In reproduction studies in rats, nursing offspring demonstrated a lack of weight gain and an unkempt appearance at a maternal dosage level of 200 mg/kg.

There are no adequate and well-controlled studies in pregnant women. Tegretol should be used during pregnancy only if the potential benefit justifies the potential risk to the fetus.

Retrospective case reviews suggest that, compared with monotherapy, there may be a higher prevalence of teratogenic effects associated with the use of anticonvulsants in combination therapy. Therefore, monotherapy is recommended for pregnant women.

It is important to note that anticonvulsant drugs should not be discontinued in patients in whom the drug is administered to prevent major seizures because of the strong possibility of precipitating status epilepticus with attendant hypoxia and threat to life. In individual cases where the severity and frequency of the seizure disorder are such that removal of medication does not pose a serious threat to the patient, discontinuation of the drug may be considered prior to and during pregnancy, although it cannot be said with any confidence that even minor seizures do not pose some hazard to the developing embryo or fetus.

Labor and Delivery: The effect of Tegretol on human labor and delivery is unknown.

Nursing Mothers: During lactation, concentration of Tegretol in milk is approximately 60% of the maternal plasma concentration.

Because of the potential for serious adverse reactions in nursing infants from carbamazepine, a decision should be made whether to discontinue nursing or to discontinue the drug, taking into account the importance of the drug to the mother.

Pediatric Use: Safety and effectiveness in children below the age of 6 years have not been established.

ADVERSE REACTIONS

If adverse reactions are of such severity that the drug must be discontinued, the physician must be aware that abrupt discontinuation of any anticonvulsant drug in a responsive epileptic patient may lead to seizures or even status epilepticus with its life-threatening hazards.

The most severe adverse reactions have been observed in the hemopoietic system (see boxed WARNING), the skin and the cardiovascular system.

The most frequently observed adverse reactions, particularly during the initial phases of therapy, are dizziness, drowsiness, unsteadiness, nausea, and vomiting. To minimize the possibility of such reactions, therapy should be initiated at the low dosage recommended.

The following additional adverse reactions have been reported:

Hemopoietic System: Aplastic anemia, agranulocytosis, pancytopenia, bone marrow depression, thrombocytopenia, leukopenia, leukocytosis, eosinophilia.

Skin: Pruritic and erythematous rashes, urticaria, toxic epidermal necrolysis (Lyell's syndrome) (see WARNINGS), Stevens-Johnson syndrome (see WARNINGS), photosensitivity reactions, alterations in skin pigmentation, exfoliative dermatitis, erythema multiforme and nodosum, purpura, aggravation of disseminated lupus erythematosus, alopecia, and diaphoresis. In certain cases, discontinuation of therapy may be necessary.

Cardiovascular System: Congestive heart failure, edema, aggravation of hypertension, hypotension, syncope and collapse, aggravation of coronary artery disease, arrhythmias and AV block, primary thrombophlebitis, recurrence of thrombophlebitis, and adenopathy or lymphadenopathy. Some of these cardiovascular complications have resulted in fatalities. Myocardial infarction has been associated with other tricyclic compounds.

Liver: Abnormalities in liver function tests, cholestatic and hepatocellular jaundice, hepatitis.

Respiratory System: Pulmonary hypersensitivity characterized by fever, dyspnea, pneumonitis or pneumonia.

Genitourinary System: Urinary frequency, acute urinary retention, oliguria with elevated blood pressure, azotemia, renal failure, and impotence. Albuminuria, glycosuria, elevated BUN and microscopic deposits in the urine have also been reported.

Testicular atrophy occurred in rats receiving Tegretol orally from 4 to 52 weeks at dosage levels of 50 to 400 mg/kg/day. Additionally, rats receiving Tegretol in the diet for two years at dosage levels of 25, 75, and 250 mg/kg/day had a dose-related incidence of testicular atrophy and aspermatogenesis. In dogs, it produced a brownish discoloration, presumably a metabolite, in the urinary bladder at dosage levels of 50 mg/kg and higher. Relevance of these findings to humans is unknown.

Nervous System: Dizziness, drowsiness, disturbances of coordination, confusion, headache, fatigue, blurred vision, visual hallucinations, transient diplopia, oculomotor disturbances, nystagmus, speech disturbances, abnormal involuntary movements, peripheral neuritis and paresthesias, depression with agitation, talkativeness, tinnitus, and hyperacusis.

There have been reports of associated paralysis and other symptoms of cerebral arterial insufficiency, but the exact relationship of these reactions to the drug has not been established.

Digestive System: Nausea, vomiting, gastric distress and abdominal pain, diarrhea, constipation, anorexia, and dryness of the mouth and pharynx, including glossitis and stomatitis.

Eyes: Scattered, punctate, cortical lens opacities, as well as conjunctivitis have been reported. Although a direct causal relationship has not been established, many phenothiazines and related drugs have been shown to cause eye changes.

Musculoskeletal System: Aching joints and muscles and leg cramps.

Metabolism: Fever and chills. Inappropriate antidiuretic hormone (ADH) secretion syndrome has been reported. Cases of frank water intoxication, with decreased serum sodium (hyponatremia) and confusion, have been reported in association with Tegretol use (see PRECAUTIONS, Laboratory Tests).

Other: Isolated cases of a lupus erythematosus-like syndrome have been reported. There have been occasional reports of elevated levels of cholesterol, HDL cholesterol and triglycerides in patients taking anticonvulsants.

DRUG ABUSE AND DEPENDENCE

No evidence of abuse potential has been associated with Tegretol, nor is there evidence of psychological or physical dependence in humans.

OVERDOSAGE

Acute Toxicity: Lowest known lethal dose: adults, > 60 g (39-year-old man).

Highest known doses survived: adults, 30 g (31-year-old woman); children, 10 g (6-year-old boy); small children, 5 g (3-year-old girl).

Oral LD_{50} in animals (mg/kg): mice, 1100–3750; rats, 3850–4025; rabbits, 1500–2680; guinea pigs, 920.

Signs and Symptoms:
The first signs and symptoms appear after 1–3 hours. Neuromuscular disturbances are the most prominent. Cardiovascular disorders are generally milder, and severe cardiac complications occur only when very high doses (> 60 g) have been ingested.

Respiration: Irregular breathing, respiratory depression.

Cardiovascular System: Tachycardia, hypotension or hypertension, shock, conduction disorders.

Nervous System and Muscles: Impairment of consciousness ranging in severity to deep coma. Convulsions, especially in small children. Motor restlessness, muscular twitching, tremor, athetoid movements, opisthotonos, ataxia, drowsiness, dizziness, mydriasis, nystagmus, adiadochokinesia, ballism, psychomotor disturbances, dysmetria. Initial hyperreflexia, followed by hyporeflexia.

Gastrointestinal Tract: Nausea, vomiting.

Kidneys and Bladder: Anuria or oliguria, urinary retention.

Laboratory Findings: Isolated instances of overdosage have included leukocytosis, reduced leukocyte count, glycosuria and acetonuria. EEG may show dysrhythmias.

Combined Poisoning: When alcohol, tricyclic antidepressants, barbiturates or hydantoins are taken at the same time, the signs and symptoms of acute poisoning with Tegretol may be aggravated or modified.

Treatment:
The prognosis in cases of severe poisoning is critically dependent upon prompt elimination of the drug, which may be achieved by inducing vomiting, irrigating the stomach, and by taking appropriate steps to diminish absorption. If these measures cannot be implemented without risk on the spot, the patient should be transferred at once to a hospital, while ensuring that vital functions are safeguarded. There is no specific antidote.

Elimination of the Drug: Induction of vomiting. Gastric lavage. Even when more than 4 hours have elapsed following ingestion of the drug, the stomach should be repeatedly irrigated, especially if the patient has also consumed alcohol.

Measures to Reduce Absorption: Activated charcoal, laxatives.

Measures to Accelerate Elimination: Forced diuresis. Dialysis is indicated only in severe poisoning associated with renal failure. Replacement transfusion is indicated in severe poisoning in small children.

Respiratory Depression: Keep the airways free; resort, if necessary, to endotracheal intubation, artificial respiration, and administration of oxygen.

Hypotension, Shock: Keep the patient's legs raised and administer a plasma expander. If blood pressure fails to rise despite measures taken to increase plasma volume, use of vasoactive substances should be considered.

Convulsions: Diazepam or barbiturates.

Warning: Diazepam or barbiturates may aggravate respiratory depression (especially in children), hypotension, and coma. However, barbiturates should not be used if drugs that inhibit monoamine oxidase have also been taken by the patient either in overdosage or in recent therapy (within one week).

Surveillance: Respiration, cardiac function (ECG monitoring), blood pressure, body temperature, pupillary reflexes, and kidney and bladder function should be monitored for several days.

Treatment of Blood Count Abnormalities: If evidence of significant bone marrow depression develops, the following recommendations are suggested: (1) stop the drug, (2) perform daily CBC, platelet and reticulocyte counts, (3) do a bone marrow aspiration and trephine biopsy immediately and repeat with sufficient frequency to monitor recovery. Special periodic studies might be helpful as follows: (1) white cell and platelet antibodies, (2) ^{59}Fe—ferrokinetic studies, (3) peripheral blood cell typing, (4) cytogenetic studies on marrow and peripheral blood, (5) bone marrow culture studies for colony-forming units, (6) hemoglobin electrophoresis for A_2 and F hemoglobin, and (7) serum folic acid and B_{12} levels. A fully developed aplastic anemia will require appropriate, intensive monitoring and therapy, for which specialized consultation should be sought.

DOSAGE AND ADMINISTRATION

Monitoring of blood levels has increased the efficacy and safety of anticonvulsants (see PRECAUTIONS Laboratory Tests). Dosage should be adjusted to the needs of the individual patient. A low initial daily dosage with a gradual increase is advised. As soon as adequate control is achieved, the dosage may be reduced very gradually to the minimum effective level. Tablets should be taken with meals.

Epilepsy (see INDICATIONS AND USAGE).

Adults and children over 12 years of age—Initial: 200 mg b.i.d. Increase at weekly intervals by adding up to 200 mg per day using a t.i.d. or q.i.d. regimen until the best response is obtained. Dosage should generally not exceed 1000 mg daily in children 12 to 15 years of age, and 1200 mg daily in patients above 15 years of age. Doses up to 1600 mg daily have been used in adults in rare instances. *Maintenance:* Adjust dosage to the minimum effective level, usually 800–1200 mg daily.

Children 6–12 years of age—Initial: 100 mg b.i.d. Increase at weekly intervals by adding 100 mg per day using a t.i.d. or q.i.d. regimen until the best response is obtained. Dosage should generally not exceed 1000 mg. *Maintenance:* Adjust dosage to the minimum effective level, usually 400–800 mg daily.

Combination Therapy: Tegretol may be used alone or with other anticonvulsants. When added to existing anticonvulsant therapy, the drug should be added gradually while the other anticonvulsants are maintained or gradually decreased, except phenytoin, which may have to be increased. (see PRECAUTIONS, Drug Interactions and Pregnancy Category C).

Trigeminal Neuralgia (see INDICATIONS AND USAGE).

Initial: 100 mg b.i.d. on the first day for a total daily dose of 200 mg. This daily dose may be increased by up to 200 mg a day using increments of 100 mg every 12 hours only as needed to achieve freedom from pain. Do not exceed 1200 mg daily.

Maintenance: Control of pain can be maintained in most patients with 400 mg to 800 mg daily. However, some patients may be maintained on as little as 200 mg daily, while others may require as much as 1200 mg daily. At least once every 3 months throughout the treatment period, attempts should be made to reduce the dose to the minimum effective level or even to discontinue the drug.

Continued on next page

The full prescribing information for each GEIGY product is contained herein and is that in effect as of September 1, 1989

Geigy—Cont.

HOW SUPPLIED

Chewable Tablets 100 mg —round, red-speckled, pink, single-scored (imprinted Tegretol on one side and 52 twice on the scored side)

Bottles of 100 .... NDC 0028-0052-01
Unit Dose (blister pack)
  Box of 100
  (strips of 10) .... NDC 0028-0052-61

Tablets 200 mg —capsule-shaped, pink, single-scored (imprinted Tegretol on one side and 27 twice on the scored side)

Bottles of 100 .... NDC 0028-0027-01
Bottles of 1000 .... NDC 0028-0027-10
Gy-Pak® —One Unit
  12 bottles—100 tablets each .... NDC 0028-0027-65
Unit Dose (blister pack)
  Box of 100
  (strips of 10) .... NDC 0028-0027-61

Samples, when available, are identified by the word *SAMPLE* appearing on each tablet.
Protect from moisture.
Dispense in tight container (USP).
Also available as: Tegretol suspension 100 mg/5 ml, in 450 ml bottles.

C88-27 (Rev. 12/88)
Shown in Product Identification Section, page 410

TEGRETOL® Suspension   ℞
[teg'rit-tall]
carbamazepine USP
Suspension of 100 mg/5 ml

WARNING

APLASTIC ANEMIA AND AGRANULOCYTOSIS HAVE BEEN REPORTED IN ASSOCIATION WITH THE USE OF TEGRETOL. DATA FROM A POPULATION-BASED CASE CONTROL STUDY DEMONSTRATE THAT THE RISK OF DEVELOPING THESE REACTIONS IS 5–8 TIMES GREATER THAN IN THE GENERAL POPULATION. HOWEVER, THE OVERALL RISK OF THESE REACTIONS IN THE UNTREATED GENERAL POPULATION IS LOW, APPROXIMATELY SIX PATIENTS PER ONE MILLION POPULATION PER YEAR FOR AGRANULOCYTOSIS AND TWO PATIENTS PER ONE MILLION POPULATION PER YEAR FOR APLASTIC ANEMIA.
ALTHOUGH REPORTS OF TRANSIENT OR PERSISTENT DECREASED PLATELET OR WHITE BLOOD CELL COUNTS ARE NOT UNCOMMON IN ASSOCIATION WITH THE USE OF TEGRETOL, DATA ARE NOT AVAILABLE TO ESTIMATE ACCURATELY THEIR INCIDENCE OR OUTCOME. HOWEVER, THE VAST MAJORITY OF THE CASES OF LEUKOPENIA HAVE NOT PROGRESSED TO THE MORE SERIOUS CONDITIONS OF APLASTIC ANEMIA OR AGRANULOCYTOSIS.
BECAUSE OF THE VERY LOW INCIDENCE OF AGRANULOCYTOSIS AND APLASTIC ANEMIA, THE VAST MAJORITY OF MINOR HEMATOLOGIC CHANGES OBSERVED IN MONITORING OF PATIENTS ON TEGRETOL ARE UNLIKELY TO SIGNAL THE OCCURRENCE OF EITHER ABNORMALITY. NONETHELESS, COMPLETE PRETREATMENT HEMATOLOGICAL TESTING SHOULD BE OBTAINED AS A BASELINE. IF A PATIENT IN THE COURSE OF TREATMENT EXHIBITS LOW OR DECREASED WHITE BLOOD CELL OR PLATELET COUNTS, THE PATIENT SHOULD BE MONITORED CLOSELY. DISCONTINUATION OF THE DRUG SHOULD BE CONSIDERED IF ANY EVIDENCE OF SIGNIFICANT BONE MARROW DEPRESSION DEVELOPS.

Before prescribing Tegretol, the physician should be thoroughly familiar with the details of this prescribing information, particularly regarding use with other drugs, especially those which accentuate toxicity potential.

DESCRIPTION

Tegretol, carbamazepine USP, is an anticonvulsant and specific analgesic for trigeminal neuralgia, available as a suspension of 100 mg/5 ml (teaspoon). It is also available as chewable tablets of 100 mg, and as tablets of 200 mg for oral administration. Its chemical name is 5H-dibenz[b,f]azepine-5-carboxamide.
Carbamazepine USP is a white to off-white powder, practically insoluble in water and soluble in alcohol and in acetone. Its molecular weight is 236.27.
Inactive Ingredients (Suspension). Citric acid, FD&C Yellow No. 6, flavoring, polymer, potassium sorbate, propylene glycol, purified water, sorbitol, sucrose, and xanthan gum.

CLINICAL PHARMACOLOGY

In controlled clinical trials, Tegretol has been shown to be effective in the treatment of psychomotor and grand mal seizures, as well as trigeminal neuralgia.
It has demonstrated anticonvulsant properties in rats and mice with electrically and chemically induced seizures. It appears to act by reducing polysynaptic responses and blocking the posttetanic potentiation. Tegretol greatly reduces or abolishes pain induced by stimulation of the infraorbital nerve in cats and rats. It depresses thalamic potential and bulbar and polysynaptic reflexes, including the linguomandibular reflex in cats. Tegretol is chemically unrelated to other anticonvulsants or other drugs used to control the pain of trigeminal neuralgia. The mechanism of action remains unknown.
In clinical studies both suspension and conventional tablet delivered equivalent amounts of drug to the systemic circulation. However, the suspension was absorbed somewhat faster than the tablet. Following a b.i.d. dosage regimen, the suspension has higher peak levels and lower trough levels than those obtained from the tablet formulation for the same dosage regimen. On the other hand, following a t.i.d. dosage regimen, Tegretol suspension affords steady-state plasma levels comparable to Tegretol tablets given b.i.d. when administered at the same total mg daily dose. Tegretol in blood is 76% bound to plasma proteins. Plasma levels of Tegretol are variable and may range from 0.5–25 μg/ml, with no apparent relationship to the daily intake of the drug. Usual adult therapeutic levels are between 4 and 12 μg/ml. Following chronic oral administration of suspension, plasma levels peak at approximately 1.5 hours compared to 4 to 5 hours after administration of oral tablets. The CSF/serum ratio is 0.22, similar to the 22% unbound Tegretol in serum.
Because Tegretol may induce its own metabolism, the half-life is also variable. Initial half-life values range from 25–65 hours, with 12–17 hours on repeated doses. Tegretol is metabolized in the liver. After oral administration of ^{14}C-carbamazepine, 72% of the administered radioactivity was found in the urine and 28% in the feces. This urinary radioactivity was composed largely of hydroxylated and conjugated metabolites, with only 3% of unchanged Tegretol. Transplacental passage of Tegretol is rapid (30 to 60 minutes), and the drug is accumulated in fetal tissues, with higher levels found in liver and kidney than in brain and lungs.

INDICATIONS AND USAGE

Epilepsy: Tegretol is indicated for use as an anticonvulsant drug. Evidence supporting efficacy of Tegretol as an anticonvulsant was derived from active drug-controlled studies that enrolled patients with the following seizure types:
1. Partial seizures with complex symptomatology (psychomotor, temporal lobe). Patients with these seizures appear to show greater improvement than those with other types.
2. Generalized tonic-clonic seizures (grand mal).
3. Mixed seizure patterns which include the above, or other partial or generalized seizures.
Absence seizures (petit mal) do not appear to be controlled by Tegretol (see PRECAUTIONS General).
Trigeminal Neuralgia: Tegretol is indicated in the treatment of the pain associated with true trigeminal neuralgia. Beneficial results have also been reported in glossopharyngeal neuralgia.
This drug is not a simple analgesic and should not be used for the relief of trivial aches or pains.

CONTRAINDICATIONS

Tegretol should not be used in patients with a history of previous bone marrow depression, hypersensitivity to the drug, or known sensitivity to any of the tricyclic compounds, such as amitriptyline, desipramine, imipramine, protriptyline, nortriptyline, etc. Likewise, on theoretical grounds its use with monoamine oxidase inhibitors is not recommended. Before administration of Tegretol, MAO inhibitors should be discontinued for a minimum of fourteen days, or longer if the clinical situation permits.

WARNINGS

Patients with a history of adverse hematologic reaction to any drug may be particularly at risk.
Severe dermatologic reactions including toxic epidermal necrolysis (Lyell's syndrome) and Stevens-Johnson syndrome, have been reported with Tegretol. These reactions have been extremely rare. However, a few fatalities have been reported.
Tegretol has shown mild anticholinergic activity; therefore, patients with increased intraocular pressure should be closely observed during therapy.
Because of the relationship of the drug to other tricyclic compounds, the possibility of activation of a latent psychosis and, in elderly patients, of confusion or agitation should be borne in mind.

PRECAUTIONS

General: Before initiating therapy, a detailed history and physical examination should be made.

Tegretol should be used with caution in patients with a mixed seizure disorder that includes atypical absence seizures, since in these patients Tegretol has been associated with increased frequency of generalized convulsions (see INDICATIONS AND USAGE).
Therapy should be prescribed only after critical benefit-to-risk appraisal in patients with a history of cardiac, hepatic or renal damage, adverse hematologic reaction to other drugs, or interrupted courses of therapy with Tegretol.
Since a given dose of Tegretol suspension will produce higher peak levels than the same dose given as the tablet, it is recommended that patients given the suspension be started on lower doses and increased slowly to avoid unwanted side effects (see DOSAGE AND ADMINISTRATION).
Information for Patients: Patients should be made aware of the early toxic signs and symptoms of a potential hematologic problem, such as fever, sore throat, ulcers in the mouth, easy bruising, petechial or purpuric hemorrhage, and should be advised to report to the physician immediately if any such signs or symptoms appear.
Since dizziness and drowsiness may occur, patients should be cautioned about the hazards of operating machinery or automobiles or engaging in other potentially dangerous tasks.
Laboratory Tests: Complete pretreatment blood counts, including platelets and possibly reticulocytes and serum iron, should be obtained as a baseline. If a patient in the course of treatment exhibits low or decreased white blood cell or platelet counts, the patient should be monitored closely. Discontinuation of the drug should be considered if any evidence of significant bone marrow depression develops.
Baseline and periodic evaluations of liver function, particularly in patients with a history of liver disease, must be performed during treatment with this drug since liver damage may occur. The drug should be discontinued immediately in cases of aggravated liver dysfunction or active liver disease.
Baseline and periodic eye examinations, including slit-lamp, funduscopy and tonometry, are recommended since many phenothiazines and related drugs have been shown to cause eye changes.
Baseline and periodic complete urinalysis and BUN determinations are recommended for patients treated with this agent because of observed renal dysfunction.
Monitoring of blood levels (see CLINICAL PHARMACOLOGY) has increased the efficacy and safety of anticonvulsants. This monitoring may be particularly useful in cases of dramatic increase in seizure frequency and for verification of compliance. In addition, measurement of drug serum levels may aid in determining the cause of toxicity when more than one medication is being used.
Thyroid function tests have been reported to show decreased values with Tegretol administered alone.
Hyponatremia has been reported in association with Tegretol use, either alone or in combination with other drugs.
Drug Interactions: The simultaneous administration of phenobarbital, phenytoin, or primidone, or a combination of two, produces a marked lowering of serum levels of Tegretol. The half-lives of phenytoin, warfarin, doxycycline, and theophylline were significantly shortened when administered concurrently with Tegretol. Haloperidol serum levels may be reduced when the drug is administered with Tegretol. The doses of these drugs may therefore have to be increased when Tegretol is added to the therapeutic regimen.
Concomitant administration of Tegretol with erythromycin, cimetidine, propoxyphene, isoniazid or calcium channel blockers has been reported to result in elevated plasma levels of carbamazepine resulting in toxicity in some cases. Also, concomitant administration of carbamazepine and lithium may increase the risk of neurotoxic side effects.
Alterations of thyroid function have been reported in combination therapy with other anticonvulsant medications.
Breakthrough bleeding has been reported among patients receiving concomitant oral contraceptives and their reliability may be adversely affected.
Carcinogenesis, Mutagenesis, Impairment of Fertility: Carbamazepine, when administered to Sprague-Dawley rats for two years in the diet at doses of 25, 75, and 250 mg/kg/day, resulted in a dose-related increase in the incidence of hepatocellular tumors in females and of benign interstitial cell adenomas in the testes of males.
Carbamazepine must, therefore, be considered to be carcinogenic in Sprague-Dawley rats. Bacterial and mammalian mutagenicity studies using carbamazepine produced negative results. The significance of these findings relative to the use of carbamazepine in humans is, at present, unknown.
Pregnancy Category C: Tegretol has been shown to have adverse effects in reproduction studies in rats when given orally in dosages 10–25 times the maximum human daily dosage of 1200 mg. In rat teratology studies, 2 of 135 offspring showed kinked ribs at 250 mg/kg and 4 of 119 offspring at 650 mg/kg showed other anomalies (cleft palate, 1; talipes, 1; anophthalmos, 2). In reproduction studies in rats, nursing offspring demonstrated a lack of weight gain and an unkempt appearance at a maternal dosage level of 200 mg/kg.

There are no adequate and well-controlled studies in pregnant women. Tegretol should be used during pregnancy only if the potential benefit justifies the potential risk to the fetus.

Retrospective case reviews suggest that, compared with monotherapy, there may be a higher prevalence of teratogenic effects associated with the use of anticonvulsants in combination therapy. Therefore, monotherapy is recommended for pregnant women.

It is important to note that anticonvulsant drugs should not be discontinued in patients in whom the drug is administered to prevent major seizures because of the strong possibility of precipitating status epilepticus with attendant hypoxia and threat to life. In individual cases where the severity and frequency of the seizure disorder are such that removal of medication does not pose a serious threat to the patient, discontinuation of the drug may be considered prior to and during pregnancy, although it cannot be said with any confidence that even minor seizures do not pose some hazard to the developing embryo or fetus.

Labor and Delivery: The effect of Tegretol on human labor and delivery is unknown.

Nursing Mothers: During lactation, concentration of Tegretol in milk is approximately 60% of the maternal plasma concentration.

Because of the potential for serious adverse reactions in nursing infants from carbamazepine, a decision should be made whether to discontinue nursing or to discontinue the drug, taking into account the importance of the drug to the mother.

Pediatric Use: Safety and effectiveness in children below the age of 6 years have not been established.

ADVERSE REACTIONS

If adverse reactions are of such severity that the drug must be discontinued, the physician must be aware that abrupt discontinuation of any anticonvulsant drug in a responsive epileptic patient may lead to seizures or even status epilepticus with its life-threatening hazards.

The most severe adverse reactions have been observed in the hemopoietic system (see boxed WARNING), the skin and the cardiovascular system.

The most frequently observed adverse reactions, particularly during the initial phases of therapy, are dizziness, drowsiness, unsteadiness, nausea, and vomiting. To minimize the possibility of such reactions, therapy should be initiated at the low dosage recommended.

The following additional adverse reactions have been reported:

Hemopoietic System: Aplastic anemia, agranulocytosis, pancytopenia, bone marrow depression, thrombocytopenia, leukopenia, leukocytosis, eosinophilia.

Skin: Pruritic and erythematous rashes, urticaria, toxic epidermal necrolysis (Lyell's syndrome) (see WARNINGS), Stevens-Johnson syndrome (see WARNINGS), photosensitivity reactions, alterations in skin pigmentation, exfoliative dermatitis, erythema multiforme and nodosum, purpura, aggravation of disseminated lupus erythematosus, alopecia, and diaphoresis. In certain cases, discontinuation of therapy may be necessary.

Cardiovascular System: Congestive heart failure, edema, aggravation of hypertension, hypotension, syncope and collapse, aggravation of coronary artery disease, arrhythmias and AV block, primary thrombophlebitis, recurrence of thrombophlebitis, and adenopathy or lymphadenopathy.

Some of these cardiovascular complications have resulted in fatalities. Myocardial infarction has been associated with other tricyclic compounds.

Liver: Abnormalities in liver function tests, cholestatic and hepatocellular jaundice, hepatitis.

Respiratory System: Pulmonary hypersensitivity characterized by fever, dyspnea, pneumonitis or pneumonia.

Genitourinary System: Urinary frequency, acute urinary retention, oliguria with elevated blood pressure, azotemia, renal failure, and impotence. Albuminuria, glycosuria, elevated BUN and microscopic deposits in the urine have also been reported.

Testicular atrophy occurred in rats receiving Tegretol orally from 4 to 52 weeks at dosage levels of 50 to 400 mg/kg/day. Additionally, rats receiving Tegretol in the diet for two years at dosage levels of 25, 75, and 250 mg/kg/day had a dose-related incidence of testicular atrophy and aspermatogenesis. In dogs, it produced a brownish discoloration, presumably a metabolite, in the urinary bladder at dosage levels of 50 mg/kg and higher. Relevance of these findings to humans is unknown.

Nervous System: Dizziness, drowsiness, disturbances of coordination, confusion, headache, fatigue, blurred vision, visual hallucinations, transient diplopia, oculomotor disturbances, nystagmus, speech disturbances, abnormal involuntary movements, peripheral neuritis and paresthesias, depression with agitation, talkativeness, tinnitus, and hyperacusis.

There have been reports of associated paralysis and other symptoms of cerebral arterial insufficiency, but the exact relationship of these reactions to the drug has not been established.

Digestive System: Nausea, vomiting, gastric distress and abdominal pain, diarrhea, constipation, anorexia, and dryness of the mouth and pharynx, including glossitis and stomatitis.

Eyes: Scattered punctate cortical lens opacities, as well as conjunctivitis, have been reported. Although a direct causal relationship has not been established, many phenothiazines and related drugs have been shown to cause eye changes.

Musculoskeletal System: Aching joints and muscles, and leg cramps.

Metabolism: Fever and chills. Inappropriate antidiuretic hormone (ADH) secretion syndrome has been reported. Cases of frank water intoxication, with decreased serum sodium (hyponatremia) and confusion, have been reported in association with Tegretol use (see PRECAUTIONS, Laboratory Tests).

Other: Isolated cases of a lupus etythematosus-like syndrome have been reported. There have been occasional reports of elevated levels of cholesterol, HDL cholesterol and triglycerides in patients taking anticonvulsants.

DRUG ABUSE AND DEPENDENCE

No evidence of abuse potential has been associated with Tegretol, nor is there evidence of psychological or physical dependence in humans.

OVERDOSAGE

Acute Toxicity

Lowest known lethal dose: adults, > 60 g (39-year-old man). Highest known doses survived; adults, 30 g (31-year-old woman); children, 10 g (6-year-old boy); small children, 5 g (3-year-old girl).

Oral LD_{50} in animals (mg/kg): mice, 1100–3750; rats 3850–4025; rabbits, 1500–2680; guinea pigs, 920.

Signs and Symptoms

The first signs and symptoms appear after 1–3 hours. Neuromuscular disturbances are the most prominent. Cardiovascular disorders are generally milder, and severe cardiac complications occur only when very high doses (> 60 g) have been ingested.

Respiration: Irregular breathing, respiratory depression.

Cardiovascular System: Tachycardia, hypotension or hypertension, shock, conduction disorders.

Nervous System and Muscles: Impairment of consciousness ranging in severity to deep coma. Convulsions, especially in small children. Motor restlessness, muscular twitching, tremor, athetoid movements, opisthotonos, ataxia, drowsiness, dizziness, mydriasis, nystagmus, adiadochokinesia, ballism, psychomotor disturbances, dysmetria. Initial hyperreflexia, followed by hyporeflexia.

Gastrointesinal Tract: Nausea, vomiting.

Kidneys and Bladder: Anuria or oliguria, urinary retention.

Laboratory Findings: Isolated instances of overdosage have included leukocytosis, reduced leukocyte count, glycosuria and acetonuria. EEG may show dysrhythmias.

Combined Poisoning: When alcohol, tricyclic antidepressants, barbiturates or hydantoins are taken at the same time, the signs and symptoms of acute poisoning with Tegretol may be aggravated or modified.

Treatment

The prognosis in cases of severe poisoning is critically dependent upon prompt elimination of the drug, which may be achieved by inducing vomiting, irrigating the stomach, and by taking appropriate steps to diminish absorption. If these measures cannot be implemented without risk on the spot, the patient should be transferred at once to a hospital, while ensuring that vital functions are safeguarded. There is no specific antidote.

Elimination of the Drug: Induction of vomiting. Gastric lavage. Even when more than 4 hours have elapsed following ingestion of the drug, the stomach should be repeatedly irrigated, especially if the patient has also consumed alcohol.

Measures to Reduce Absorption: Activated charcoal, laxatives.

Measures to Accelerate Elimination: Forced diuresis. Dialysis is indicated only in severe poisoning associated with renal failure. Replacement transfusion is indicated in severe poisoning in small children.

Respiratory Depression: Keep the airways free; resort, if necessary, to endotracheal intubation, artificial respiration, and administration of oxygen.

Hypotension, Shock: Keep the patient's legs raised and administer a plasma expander. If blood pressure fails to rise despite measures taken to increase plasma volume, use of vasoactive substances should be considered.

Convulsions: Diazepam or barbiturates.

Warning: Diazepam or barbiturates may aggravate respiratory depression (especially in children), hypotension, and coma. However, barbiturates should not be used if drugs that inhibit monoamine oxidase have also been taken by the patient either in overdosage or in recent therapy (within one week).

Surveillance: Respiration, cardiac function (ECG monitoring), blood pressure, body temperature, pupillary reflexes, and kidney and bladder function should be monitored for several days.

Treatment of Blood Count Abnormalities: If evidence of significant bone marrow depression develops, the following recommendations are suggested: (1) stop the drug, (2) perform daily CBC, platelet and reticulocyte counts, (3) do a bone marrow aspiration and trephine biopsy immediately and repeat with sufficient frequency to monitor recovery. Special periodic studies might be helpful as follows: (1) white cell and platelet antibodies, (2) ^{59}Fe—ferrokinetic studies, (3) peripheral blood cell typing, (4) cytogenetic studies on marrow and peripheral blood, (5) bone marrow culture studies for colony-forming units, (6) hemoglobin electrophoresis for A_2 and F hemoglobin, and (7) serum folic acid and B_{12} levels. A fully developed aplastic anemia will require appropriate, intensive monitoring and therapy, for which specialized consultation should be sought.

DOSAGE AND ADMINISTRATION

[See table above].

Monitoring of blood levels has increased the efficacy and safety of anticonvulsants (see PRECAUTIONS Laboratory Tests). Dosage should be adjusted to the needs of the individual patient. A low initial daily dosage with a gradual increase is advised. As soon as adequate control is achieved, the dosage may be reduced very gradually to the minimum effective level. Medication should be taken with meals.

Since a given dose of Tegretol suspension will produce higher peak levels than the same dose given as the tablet, it is recommended to start with low doses (children 6–12 years: ½ teaspoon q.i.d.) and to increase slowly to avoid unwanted side effects.

Conversion of patients from oral Tegretol tablets to Tegretol suspension: Patients should be converted by administering the same number of mg per day in smaller, more frequent doses (i.e., b.i.d. tablets to t.i.d. suspension).

Epilepsy (see INDICATIONS AND USAGE).

Children 6–12 years of age—Initial: ½ teaspoon q.i.d. (200 mg per day). Increase at weekly intervals by adding up to one teaspoon (100 mg) per day using a t.i.d. or q.i.d. regimen until the optimal response is obtained. Dosage generally should not exceed 1000 mg daily. *Maintenance:* Adjust dosage to the minimum effective level, usually 400–800 mg daily.

Adults and children over 12 years of age—Initial: one teaspoon q.i.d. (400 mg per day). Increase at weekly intervals by adding up to two teaspoons (200 mg) per day using a t.i.d. or q.i.d. regimen until the optimal response is obtained. Dosage generally should not exceed 1000 mg daily in children 12 to 15 years of age, and 1200 mg daily in patients above 15 years of age. Doses up to 1600 mg daily have been used in adults in rare instances. *Maintenance:* Adjust dosage to the minimum effective level, usually 800–1200 mg daily.

Tegretol Suspension Dosage Information
100 mg = 1 teaspoon

	Epilepsy		Trigeminal Neuralgia
Dose	6–12 Years of Age	Over 12 Years of Age	
Initial	½ teaspoon q.i.d. (200 mg/d)	1 teaspoon q.i.d. (400 mg/d)	½ teaspoon q.i.d. (200 mg/d)
Subsequent	Add up to 1 teaspoon (100 mg) per day at weekly intervals, t.i.d. or q.i.d.	Add up to 2 teaspoons (200 mg) per day at weekly intervals, t.i.d. or q.i.d.	Add up to 2 teaspoons (200 mg) per day q.i.d.
Maximum	1000 mg/24 hrs	1000 mg/24 hr: 12–15 yrs 1200 mg/24 hr: over 15 yrs 1600 mg/24 hr: adults, in rare instances	1200 mg/24 hrs

Continued on next page

The full prescribing information for each GEIGY product is contained herein and is that in effect as of September 1, 1989

Geigy—Cont.

Combination Therapy: Tegretol may be used alone or with other anticonvulsants. When added to existing anticonvulsant therapy, the drug should be added gradually while the other anticonvulsants are maintained or gradually decreased, except phenytoin, which may have to be increased (see PRECAUTIONS, Drug Interactions and Pregnancy Category C).

Trigeminal Neuralgia (see INDICATIONS AND USAGE).
Initial: ½ teaspoon q.i.d. on the first day for a total daily dose of 200 mg. This daily dose may be increased by up to 200 mg (two teaspoons) a day in increments of 50 mg (½ teaspoon) q.i.d. only as needed to achieve freedom from pain. Do not exceed 1200 mg daily.
Maintenance: Control of pain can be maintained in most patients with 400 mg to 800 mg daily. However, some patients may be maintained on as little as 200 mg daily, while others may require as much as 1200 mg daily. At least once every 3 months throughout the treatment period, attempts should be made to reduce the dose to the minimum effective level or even to discontinue the drug.

HOW SUPPLIED

Suspension 100 mg/5 ml (teaspoon) —yellow-orange, citrus-vanilla flavored
Bottles of 450 ml ....NDC 0028-7019-16
Shake well before using.
Do not store above 86°F.
Dispense in tight, light-resistant container (USP).
Also available as: chewable tablets of 100 mg, and as tablets of 200 mg for oral administration.
                                C88-26 (Rev. 12/88)
Shown in Product Identification Section, page 410

TOFRANIL®   ℞

[*toe-fray'nill*]
imipramine hydrochloride USP
Ampuls, 2 cc
For intramuscular administration

Each 2 cc ampul contains: imipramine hydrochloride USP, 25 mg; ascorbic acid, 2 mg; sodium bisulfite, 1 mg; sodium sulfite, anhydrous, 1 mg

DESCRIPTION

Tofranil, imipramine hydrochloride USP, the original tricyclic antidepressant, is a member of the dibenzazepine group of compounds. It is designated 5-[3-(dimethylamino)propyl] - 10, 11-dihydro-5H-dibenz[b,f] azepine monohydrochloride. Imipramine hydrochloride USP is a white to off-white, odorless, or practically odorless crystalline powder. It is freely soluble in water and in alcohol, soluble in acetone, and insoluble in ether and in benzene. Its molecular weight is 316.87.

CLINICAL PHARMACOLOGY

The mechanism of action of Tofranil is not definitely known. However, it does not act primarily by stimulation of the central nervous system. The clinical effect is hypothesized as being due to potentiation of adrenergic synapses by blocking uptake of norepinephrine at nerve endings. The mode of action of the drug in controlling childhood enuresis is thought to be apart from its antidepressant effect.

INDICATIONS

Depression: For the relief of symptoms of depression. Endogenous depression is more likely to be alleviated than other depressive states. One to three weeks of treatment may be needed for optimal therapeutic effects are evident.

CONTRAINDICATIONS

The concomitant use of monoamine oxidase inhibiting compounds is contraindicated. Hyperpyretic crises or severe convulsive seizures may occur in patients receiving such combinations. The potentiation of adverse effects can be serious, or even fatal. When it is desired to substitute Tofranil in patients receiving a monoamine oxidase inhibitor, as long an interval should elapse as the clinical situation will allow, with a minimum of 14 days. Initial dosage should be low and increases should be gradual and cautiously prescribed.
The drug is contraindicated during the acute recovery period after a myocardial infarction. Patients with a known hypersensitivity to this compound should not be given the drug. The possibility of cross-sensitivity to other dibenzazepine compounds should be kept in mind.

WARNINGS

Children: A dose of 2.5 mg/kg/day of imipramine hydrochloride should not be exceeded in childhood. ECG changes of unknown significance have been reported in pediatric patients with doses twice this amount.
Extreme caution should be used when this drug is given to: patients with cardiovascular disease because of the possibility of conduction defects, arrhythmias, congestive heart failure, myocardial infarction, strokes and tachycardia. These patients require cardiac surveillance at all dosage levels of the drug;

patients with increased intraocular pressure, history of urinary retention, or history of narrow-angle glaucoma because of the drug's anticholinergic properties;
hyperthyroid patients or those on thyroid medication because of the possibility of cardiovascular toxicity;
patients with a history of seizure disorder because this drug has been shown to lower the seizure threshold;
patients receiving guanethidine, clonidine, or similar agents, since imipramine hydrochloride may block the pharmacologic effects of these drugs;
patients receiving methylphenidate hydrochloride.
Since methylphenidate hydrochloride may inhibit the metabolism of imipramine hydrochloride, downward dosage adjustment of imipramine hydrochloride may be required when given concomitantly with methylphenidate hydrochloride.
Tofranil may enhance the CNS depressant effects of alcohol. Therefore, it should be borne in mind that the dangers inherent in a suicide attempt or accidental overdosage with the drug may be increased for the patient who uses excessive amounts of alcohol. (See **PRECAUTIONS.**)
Since imipramine hydrochloride may impair the mental and/or physical abilities required for the performance of potentially hazardous tasks, such as operating an automobile or machinery, the patient should be cautioned accordingly.
Contains sodium sulfite and sodium bisulfite, that may cause allergic-type reactions including anaphylactic symptoms and life-threatening or less severe asthmatic episodes in certain susceptible people. The overall prevalence of sulfite sensitivity in the general population is unknown and probably low. Sulfite sensitivity is seen more frequently in asthmatic than in nonasthmatic people.

PRECAUTIONS

An ECG recording should be taken prior to the initiation of larger-than-usual doses of imipramine hydrochloride and at appropriate intervals thereafter until steady state is achieved. (Patients with any evidence of cardiovascular disease require cardiac surveillance at all dosage levels of the drug. See **WARNINGS.**) Elderly patients and patients with cardiac disease or a prior history of cardiac disease are at special risk of developing the cardiac abnormalities associated with the use of imipramine hydrochloride.
It should be kept in mind that the possibility of suicide in seriously depressed patients is inherent in the illness and may persist until significant remission occurs. Such patients should be carefully supervised during the early phase of treatment with imipramine hydrochloride, and may require hospitalization. Prescriptions should be written for the smallest amount feasible.
Hypomanic or manic episodes may occur, particularly in patients with cyclic disorders.
Such reactions may necessitate discontinuation of the drug. If needed, imipramine hydrochloride may be resumed in lower dosage when these episodes are relieved.
Administration of a tranquilizer may be useful in controlling such episodes.
An activation of the psychosis may occasionally be observed in schizophrenic patients and may require reduction of dosage and the addition of a phenothiazine.
Concurrent administration of imipramine hydrochloride with electroshock therapy may increase the hazards; such treatment should be limited to those patients for whom it is essential, since there is limited clinical experience.
Usage During Pregnancy and Lactation:
Animal reproduction studies have yielded inconclusive results. (See also **ANIMAL PHARMACOLOGY & TOXICOLOGY.**)
There have been no well-controlled studies conducted with pregnant women to determine the effect of imipramine hydrochloride on the fetus. However, there have been clinical reports of congenital malformations associated with the use of the drug. Although a causal relationship between these effects and the drug could not be established, the possibility of fetal risk from the maternal ingestion of imipramine hydrochloride cannot be excluded. Therefore, imipramine hydrochloride should be used in women who are or might become pregnant only if the clinical condition clearly justifies potential risk to the fetus.
Limited data suggest that imipramine hydrochloride is likely to be excreted in human breast milk. As a general rule, a woman taking a drug should not nurse since the possibility exists that the drug may be excreted in breast milk and be harmful to the child.
Usage in Children: The effectiveness of the drug in children for conditions other than nocturnal enuresis given orally has not been established.
Patients should be warned that imipramine hydrochloride may enhance the CNS depressant effects of alcohol. (See **WARNINGS.**)
Imipramine hydrochloride should be used with caution in patients with significantly impaired renal or hepatic function.

Patients who develop a fever and a sore throat during therapy with imipramine hydrochloride should have leukocyte and differential blood counts performed. Imipramine hydrochloride should be discontinued if there is evidence of pathological neutrophil depression.
Prior to elective surgery, imipramine hydrochloride should be discontinued for as long as the clinical situation will allow.
In occasional susceptible patients or in those receiving anticholinergic drugs (including antiparkinsonism agents) in addition, the atropine-like effects may become more pronounced (e.g., paralytic ileus).
Close supervision and careful adjustment of dosage is required when imipramine hydrochloride is administered concomitantly with anticholinergic drugs.
Avoid the use of preparations, such as decongestants and local anesthetics, which contain any sympathomimetic amine (e.g., epinephrine, norepinephrine), since it has been reported that tricyclic antidepressants can potentiate the effects of catecholamines.
Caution should be exercised when imipramine hydrochloride is used with agents that lower blood pressure.
Imipramine hydrochloride may potentiate the effects of CNS depressant drugs.
The plasma concentration of imipramine may increase when the drug is given concomitantly with cimetidine, and adjustment of the dosage of imipramine may therefore be necessary both when cimetidine therapy is initiated and when it is discontinued.
Patients taking imipramine hydrochloride should avoid excessive exposure to sunlight since there have been reports of photosensitization.
Both elevation and lowering of blood sugar levels have been reported with imipramine hydrochloride use.

ADVERSE REACTIONS

Note: Although the listing which follows includes a few adverse reactions which have not been reported with this specific drug, the pharmacological similarities among the tricyclic antidepressant drugs require that each of the reactions be considered when imipramine is administered.
Cardiovascular: Orthostatic hypotension, hypertension, tachycardia, palpitation, myocardial infarction, arrhythmias, heart block, ECG changes, precipitation of congestive heart failure, stroke.
Psychiatric: Confusional states (especially in the elderly) with hallucinations, disorientation, delusions; anxiety, restlessness, agitation; insomnia and nightmares; hypomania; exacerbation of psychosis.
Neurological: Numbness, tingling, paresthesias of extremities; incoordination, ataxia, tremors; peripheral neuropathy; extrapyramidal symptoms; seizures, alterations in EEG patterns; tinnitus.
Anticholinergic: Dry mouth, and, rarely, associated sublingual adenitis; blurred vision, disturbances of accommodation, mydriasis; constipation, paralytic ileus; urinary retention, delayed micturition, dilation of the urinary tract.
Allergic: Skin rash, petechiae, urticaria, itching, photosensitization; edema (general or of face and tongue); drug fever; cross-sensitivity with desipramine.
Hematologic: Bone marrow depression including agranulocytosis; eosinophilia; purpura; thrombocytopenia.
Gastrointestinal: Nausea and vomiting, anorexia, epigastric distress, diarrhea; peculiar taste, stomatitis, abdominal cramps, black tongue.
Endocrine: Gynecomastia in the male; breast enlargement and galactorrhea in the female; increased or decreased libido, impotence; testicular swelling; elevation or depression of blood sugar levels; inappropriate antidiuretic hormone (ADH) secretion syndrome.
Other: Jaundice (simulating obstructive); altered liver function; weight gain or loss; perspiration; flushing; urinary frequency; drowsiness, dizziness, weakness and fatigue; headache; parotid swelling; alopecia; proneness to falling.
Withdrawal Symptoms: Though not indicative of addiction, abrupt cessation of treatment after prolonged therapy may produce nausea, headache and malaise.

DOSAGE AND ADMINISTRATION

Initially, up to 100 mg/day intramuscularly in divided doses. Parenteral administration should be used only for starting therapy in patients unable or unwilling to use oral medication. The oral form should supplant the injectable as soon as possible.
Lower dosages are recommended for elderly patients and adolescents. Lower dosages are also recommended for outpatients as compared to hospitalized patients who will be under close supervision. Dosage should be initiated at a low level and increased gradually, noting carefully the clinical response and any evidence of intolerance. Following remission, oral maintenance medication may be required for a longer period of time, at the lowest dose that will maintain remission.

OVERDOSAGE

Children have been reported to be more sensitive than adults to an acute overdosage of imipramine hydrochloride. An acute overdose of any amount in infants or young children, especially, must be considered serious and potentially fatal.

Signs and Symptoms: These may vary in severity depending upon factors such as the amount of drug absorbed, the age of the patient, and the interval between drug ingestion and the start of treatment. Blood and urine levels of imipramine may not reflect the severity of poisoning; they have chiefly a qualitative rather than quantitative value, and are unreliable indicators in the clinical management of the patient.

CNS abnormalities may include drowsiness, stupor, coma, ataxia, restlessness, agitation, hyperactive reflexes, muscle rigidity, athetoid and choreiform movements, and convulsions.

Cardiac abnormalities may include arrhythmia, tachycardia, ECG evidence of impaired conduction, and signs of congestive failure.

Respiratory depression, cyanosis, hypotension, shock, vomiting, hyperpyrexia, mydriasis, and diaphoresis may also be present.

Treatment: Because CNS involvement, respiratory depression and cardiac arrhythmia can occur suddenly, hospitalization and close observation are necessary, even when the amount ingested is thought to be small or the initial degree of intoxication appears slight or moderate. All patients with ECG abnormalities should have continuous cardiac monitoring for at least 72 hours and be closely observed until well after cardiac status has returned to normal; relapses may occur after apparent recovery.

The *slow* intravenous administration of physostigmine salicylate has been reported to reverse most of the cardiovascular and CNS effects of overdosage with tricyclic antidepressants. In adults, 1 to 3 mg has been reported to be effective. In children, start with 0.5 mg and repeat at 5-minute intervals to determine the minimum effective dose; do not exceed 2 mg. Because of the short duration of action of physostigmine, repeat the effective dose at 30- to 60-minute intervals, as necessary. Avoid rapid injection to reduce the possibility of physostigmine-induced convulsions.

In the alert patient, empty the stomach promptly by induced emesis followed by lavage. In the obtunded patient, secure the airway with a cuffed endotracheal tube before beginning lavage (do not induce emesis). Continue lavage for 24 hours or longer, depending on the apparent severity of intoxication. Use normal or half-normal saline to avoid water intoxication, especially in children. Instillation of activated charcoal slurry may help reduce absorption of imipramine.

Minimize external stimulation to reduce the tendency to convulsions. If anticonvulsants are necessary, diazepam, short-acting barbiturates, paraldehyde or methocarbamol may be useful. Do not use barbiturates if MAO inhibitors have been taken recently.

Maintain adequate respiratory exchange. Do not use respiratory stimulants.

Shock should be treated with supportive measures, such as intravenous fluids, oxygen and corticosteroids. Digitalis may increase conduction abnormalities and further irritate an already sensitized myocardium. If congestive heart failure necessitates rapid digitalization, particular care must be exercised.

Hyperpyrexia should be controlled by whatever external means are available, including ice packs and cooling sponge baths, if necessary.

Hemodialysis, peritoneal dialysis, exchange transfusions and forced diuresis have been generally reported as ineffective because of the rapid fixation of imipramine in tissues. Blood and urine levels of imipramine may not correlate with the degree of intoxication, and are unreliable indicators in the clinical management of the patient.

HOW SUPPLIED

Ampuls 2 ml—*For intramuscular administration only*
  25 mg imipramine hydrochloride, 2 mg ascorbic acid, 1 mg sodium bisulfite, 1 mg sodium sulfite
  Boxes of 10 ....NDC 0028-0065-23
Note: Upon storage, minute crystals may form in some ampuls. This has no influence on the therapeutic efficacy of the preparation, and the crystals redissolve when the affected ampuls are immersed in hot tap water for 1 minute.

ANIMAL PHARMACOLOGY & TOXICOLOGY

A. *Acute:* Oral LD$_{50}$ ranges are as follows:
Rat   355 to 682 mg/kg
Dog   100 to 215 mg/kg
Depending on the dosage in both species, toxic signs proceeded progressively from depression, irregular respiration and ataxia to convulsions and death.

B. *Reproduction/Teratogenic:* The overall evaluation may be summed up in the following manner:

Oral: Independent studies in three species (rat, mouse and rabbit) revealed that when Tofranil is administered orally in doses up to approximately $2\frac{1}{2}$ times the maximum human dose in the first 2 species and up to 25 times the maximum human dose in the third species, the drug is essentially free from teratogenic potential. In the three species studied, only one instance of fetal abnormality occurred (in the rabbit) and

in that study there was likewise an abnormality in the control group. However, evidence does exist from the rat studies that some systemic and embryotoxic potential is demonstrable. This is manifested by reduced litter size, a slight increase in the stillborn rate and a reduction in the mean birth weight.

Parenteral: In contradistinction to the oral data, Tofranil does exhibit a slight but definite teratogenic potential when administered by the subcutaneous route. Drug effects on both the mother and fetus in the rabbit are manifested in higher resorption rates and decrease in mean fetal birth weights, while teratogenic findings occurred at a level of 5 times the maximum human dose. In the mouse, teratogenicity occurred at $1\frac{1}{2}$ and $6\frac{1}{2}$ times the maximum human dose, but no teratogenic effects were seen at levels 3 times the maximum human dose. Thus, in the mouse, the findings are equivocal.

C87-4 (Rev. 2/87)

Dist. by:
GEIGY Pharmaceuticals
Division of CIBA-GEIGY Corporation
Ardsley, New York 10502

TOFRANIL®   ℞

[*toe-fray'nill*]
imipramine hydrochloride USP
Tablets of 10 mg
Tablets of 25 mg
Tablets of 50 mg
For oral administration

DESCRIPTION

Tofranil, imipramine hydrochloride USP, the original tricyclic antidepressant, is a member of the dibenzazepine group of compounds. It is designated 5-[3-(Dimethylamino)propyl] - 10, 11-dihydro-5H-dibenz[b,f] azepine Monohydrochloride. Imipramine hydrochloride USP is a white to off-white, odorless, or practically odorless crystalline powder. It is freely soluble in water and in alcohol, soluble in acetone, and insoluble in ether and in benzene. Its molecular weight is 316.87.
Inactive Ingredients. Calcium phosphate, cellulose compounds, docusate sodium, iron oxides, magnesium stearate, polyethylene glycol, povidone, sodium starch glycolate, sucrose, talc and titanium dioxide.

CLINICAL PHARMACOLOGY

The mechanism of action of Tofranil is not definitely known. However, it does not act primarily by stimulation of the central nervous system. The clinical effect is hypothesized as being due to potentiation of adrenergic synapses by blocking uptake of norepinephrine at nerve endings. The mode of action of the drug in controlling childhood enuresis is thought to be apart from its antidepressant effect.

INDICATIONS

Depression: For the relief of symptoms of depression. Endogenous depression is more likely to be alleviated than other depressive states. One to three weeks of treatment may be needed before optimal therapeutic effects are evident.
Childhood Enuresis: May be useful as temporary adjunctive therapy in reducing enuresis in children aged 6 years and older, after possible organic causes have been excluded by appropriate tests. In patients having daytime symptoms of frequency and urgency, examination should include voiding cystourethrography and cystoscopy, as necessary. The effectiveness of treatment may decrease with continued drug administration.

CONTRAINDICATIONS

The concomitant use of monoamine oxidase inhibiting compounds is contraindicated. Hyperpyretic crises or severe convulsive seizures may occur in patients receiving such combinations. The potentiation of adverse effects can be serious, or even fatal. When it is desired to substitute Tofranil in patients receiving a monoamine oxidase inhibitor, as long an interval should elapse as the clinical situation will allow, with a minimum of 14 days. Initial dosage should be low and increases should be gradual and cautiously prescribed.
The drug is contraindicated during the acute recovery period after a myocardial infarction. Patients with a known hypersensitivity to this compound should not be given the drug. The possibility of cross-sensitivity to other dibenzazepine compounds should be kept in mind.

WARNINGS

Children: A dose of 2.5 mg/kg/day of Tofranil should not be exceeded in childhood. ECG changes of unknown significance have been reported in pediatric patients with doses twice this amount.
Extreme caution should be used when this drug is given to: patients with cardiovascular disease because of the possibility of conduction defects, arrhythmias, congestive heart failure, myocardial infarction, strokes and tachycardia. These patients require cardiac surveillance at all dosage levels of the drug;

patients with increased intraocular pressure, history of urinary retention, or history of narrow-angle glaucoma because of the drug's anticholinergic properties;

hyperthyroid patients or those on thyroid medication because of the possibility of cardiovascular toxicity;

patients with a history of seizure disorder because this drug has been shown to lower the seizure threshold;

patients receiving guanethidine, clonidine, or similar agents, since Tofranil may block the pharmacologic effects of these drugs;

patients receiving methylphenidate hydrochloride. Since methylphenidate hydrochloride may inhibit the metabolism of Tofranil, downward dosage adjustment of imipramine hydrochloride may be required when given concomitantly with methylphenidate hydrochloride.

Tofranil may enhance the CNS depressant effects of alcohol. Therefore, it should be borne in mind that the dangers inherent in a suicide attempt or accidental overdosage with the drug may be increased for the patient who uses excessive amounts of alcohol. (See **PRECAUTIONS**.)

Since Tofranil may impair the mental and/or physical abilities required for the performance of potentially hazardous tasks, such as operating an automobile or machinery, the patient should be cautioned accordingly.

PRECAUTIONS

An ECG recording should be taken prior to the initiation of larger-than-usual doses of Tofranil and at appropriate intervals thereafter until steady state is achieved. (Patients with any evidence of cardiovascular disease require cardiac surveillance at all dosage levels of the drug. See **WARNINGS**.)

Elderly patients and patients with cardiac disease or a prior history of cardiac disease are at special risk of developing the cardiac abnormalities associated with the use of Tofranil.

It should be kept in mind that the possibility of suicide in seriously depressed patients is inherent in the illness and may persist until significant remission occurs. Such patients should be carefully supervised during the early phase of treatment with Tofranil, and may require hospitalization. Prescriptions should be written for the smallest amount feasible.

Hypomanic or manic episodes may occur, particularly in patients with cyclic disorders. Such reactions may necessitate discontinuation of the drug. If needed, Tofranil may be resumed in lower dosage when these episodes are relieved. Administration of a tranquilizer may be useful in controlling such episodes.

An activation of the psychosis may occasionally be observed in schizophrenic patients and may require reduction of dosage and the addition of a phenothiazine.

Concurrent administration of Tofranil with electroshock therapy may increase the hazards; such treatment should be limited to those patients for whom it is essential, since there is limited clinical experience.

Usage During Pregnancy and Lactation:
Animal reproduction studies have yielded inconclusive results. (See also **ANIMAL PHARMACOLOGY & TOXICOLOGY**.)

There have been no well-controlled studies conducted with pregnant women to determine the effect of Tofranil on the fetus. However, there have been clinical reports of congenital malformations associated with the use of the drug. Although a causal relationship between these effects and the drug could not be established, the possibility of fetal risk from the maternal ingestion of Tofranil cannot be excluded. Therefore, Tofranil should be used in women who are or might become pregnant only if the clinical condition clearly justifies potential risk to the fetus.

Limited data suggest that Tofranil is likely to be excreted in human breast milk. As a general rule, a woman taking a drug should not nurse since the possibility exists that the drug may be excreted in breast milk and be harmful to the child.

Usage in Children: The effectiveness of the drug in children for conditions other than nocturnal enuresis has not been established.

The safety and effectiveness of the drug as temporary adjunctive therapy for nocturnal enuresis in children less than 6 years of age has not been established.

The safety of the drug for long-term, chronic use as adjunctive therapy for nocturnal enuresis in children 6 years of age or older has not been established; consideration should be given to instituting a drug-free period following an adequate therapeutic trial with a favorable response.

A dose of 2.5 mg/kg/day should not be exceeded in childhood. ECG changes of unknown significance have been reported in pediatric patients with doses twice this amount.

Patients should be warned that Tofranil may enhance the CNS depressant effects of alcohol. (See **WARNINGS**.)

Continued on next page

The full prescribing information for each GEIGY product is contained herein and is that in effect as of September 1, 1989

Geigy—Cont.

Tofranil should be used with caution in patients with significantly impaired renal or hepatic function.

Patients who develop a fever and a sore throat during therapy with Tofranil should have leukocyte and differential blood counts performed. Tofranil should be discontinued if there is evidence of pathological neutrophil depression.

Prior to elective surgery, Tofranil should be discontinued for as long as the clinical situation will allow.

In occasional susceptible patients or in those receiving anticholinergic drugs (including antiparkinsonism agents) in addition, the atropine-like effects may become more pronounced (e.g., paralytic ileus).

Close supervision and careful adjustment of dosage is required when Tofranil is administered concomitantly with anticholinergic drugs.

Avoid the use of preparations, such as decongestants and local anesthetics, which contain any sympathomimetic amine (e.g., epinephrine, norepinephrine), since it has been reported that tricyclic antidepressants can potentiate the effects of catecholamines.

Caution should be exercised when Tofranil is used with agents that lower blood pressure.

Tofranil may potentiate the effects of CNS depressant drugs. The plasma concentration of Tofranil may increase when the drug is given concomitantly with cimetidine, and adjustment of the dosage of Tofranil may therefore be necessary both when cimetidine therapy is initiated and when it is discontinued.

Patients taking Tofranil should avoid excessive exposure to sunlight since there have been reports of photosensitization. Both elevation and lowering of blood sugar levels have been reported with Tofranil use.

ADVERSE REACTIONS

Note: Although the listing which follows includes a few adverse reactions which have not been reported with this specific drug, the pharmacological similarities among the tricyclic antidepressant drugs require that each of the reactions be considered when Tofranil is administered.

Cardiovascular: Orthostatic hypotension, hypertension, tachycardia, palpitation, myocardial infarction, arrhythmias, heart block, ECG changes, precipitation of congestive heart failure, stroke.

Psychiatric: Confusional states (especially in the elderly) with hallucinations, disorientation, delusions; anxiety, restlessness, agitation; insomnia and nightmares; hypomania; exacerbation of psychosis.

Neurological: Numbness, tingling, paresthesias of extremities; incoordination, ataxia, tremors; peripheral neuropathy; extrapyramidal symptoms; seizures, alterations in EEG patterns; tinnitus.

Anticholinergic: Dry mouth, and, rarely, associated sublingual adenitis; blurred vision, disturbances of accommodation, mydriasis; constipation, paralytic ileus; urinary retention, delayed micturition, dilation of the urinary tract.

Allergic: Skin rash, petechiae, urticaria, itching, photosensitization; edema (general or of face and tongue); drug fever; cross-sensitivity with desipramine.

Hematologic: Bone marrow depression including agranulocytosis; eosinophilia; purpura; thrombocytopenia.

Gastrointestinal: Nausea and vomiting, anorexia, epigastric distress, diarrhea; peculiar taste, stomatitis, abdominal cramps, black tongue.

Endocrine: Gynecomastia in the male; breast enlargement and galactorrhea in the female; increased or decreased libido, impotence; testicular swelling; elevation or depression of blood sugar levels; inappropriate antidiuretic hormone (ADH) secretion syndrome.

Other: Jaundice (simulating obstructive); altered liver function; weight gain or loss; perspiration; flushing; urinary frequency; drowsiness; dizziness, weakness and fatigue; headache; parotid swelling; alopecia; proneness to falling.

Withdrawal Symptoms: Though not indicative of addiction, abrupt cessation of treatment after prolonged therapy may produce nausea, headache and malaise.

Note: In enuretic children treated with imipramine hydrochloride the most common adverse reactions have been nervousness, sleep disorders, tiredness, and mild gastrointestinal disturbances. These usually disappear during continued drug administration or when dosage is decreased. Other reactions which have been reported include constipation, convulsions, anxiety, emotional instability, syncope, and collapse. All of the adverse reactions reported with adult use should be considered.

DOSAGE AND ADMINISTRATION

Depression: Lower dosages are recommended for elderly patients and adolescents. Lower dosages are also recommended for outpatients as compared to hospitalized patients who will be under close supervision. Dosage should be initiated at a low level and increased gradually, noting carefully the clinical response and any evidence of intolerance. Following remission, maintenance medication may be required

for a longer period of time, at the lowest dose that will maintain remission.

Usual Adult Dose:

Hospitalized patients — Initially, 100 mg/day in divided doses gradually increased to 200 mg/day as required. If no response after two weeks, increase to 250–300 mg/day.

Outpatients—Initially, 75 mg/day increased to 150 mg/day. Dosages over 200 mg/day are not recommended. Maintenance, 50–150 mg/day.

Adolescent and geriatric patients—Initially, 30–40 mg/day; it is generally not necessary to exceed 100 mg/day.

Childhood Enuresis: Initially, an oral dose of 25 mg/day should be tried in children aged 6 and older. Medication should be given one hour before bedtime. If a satisfactory response does not occur within one week, increase the dose to 50 mg nightly in children under 12 years; children over 12 may receive up to 75 mg nightly. A daily dose greater than 75 mg does not enhance efficacy and tends to increase side effects. Evidence suggests that in early night bedwetters, the drug is more effective given earlier and in divided amounts, i.e., 25 mg in midafternoon, repeated at bedtime. Consideration should be given to instituting a drug-free period following an adequate therapeutic trial with a favorable response. Dosage should be tapered off gradually rather than abruptly discontinued; this may reduce the tendency to relapse. Children who relapse when the drug is discontinued do not always respond to a subsequent course of treatment.

A dose of 2.5 mg/kg/day should not be exceeded. ECG changes of unknown significance have been reported in pediatric patients with doses twice this amount.

The safety and effectiveness of Tofranil as temporary adjunctive therapy for nocturnal enuresis in children less than 6 years of age has not been established.

OVERDOSAGE

Children have been reported to be more sensitive than adults to an acute overdosage of imipramine hydrochloride. An acute overdose of any amount in infants or young children, especially, must be considered serious and potentially fatal.

Signs and Symptoms: These may vary in severity depending upon factors such as the amount of drug absorbed, the age of the patient, and the interval between drug ingestion and the start of treatment. Blood and urine levels of Tofranil may not reflect the severity of poisoning; they have chiefly a qualitative rather than quantitative value, and are unreliable indicators in the clinical management of the patient.

CNS abnormalities may include drowsiness, stupor, coma, ataxia, restlessness, agitation, hyperactive reflexes, muscle rigidity, athetoid and choreiform movements, and convulsions.

Cardiac abnormalities may include arrhythmia, tachycardia, ECG evidence of impaired conduction, and signs of congestive failure.

Respiratory depression, cyanosis, hypotension, shock, vomiting, hyperpyrexia, mydriasis, and diaphoresis may also be present.

Treatment: Because CNS involvement, respiratory depression and cardiac arrhythmia can occur suddenly, hospitalization and close observation are necessary, even when the amount ingested is thought to be small or the initial degree of intoxication appears slight or moderate. All patients with ECG abnormalities should have continuous cardiac monitoring for at least 72 hours and be closely observed until well after cardiac status has returned to normal; relapses may occur after apparent recovery.

The *slow* intravenous administration of physostigmine salicylate has been reported to reverse most of the cardiovascular and CNS effects of overdosage with tricyclic antidepressants. In adults, 1 to 3 mg has been reported to be effective. In children, start with 0.5 mg and repeat at 5-minute intervals to determine the minimum effective dose; do not exceed 2 mg. Because of the short duration of action of physostigmine, repeat the effective dose at 30- to 60-minute intervals, as necessary. Avoid rapid injection to reduce the possibility of physostigmine-induced convulsions.

In the alert patient, empty the stomach promptly by induced emesis followed by lavage. In the obtunded patient, secure the airway with a cuffed endotracheal tube before beginning lavage (do not induce emesis). Continue lavage for 24 hours or longer, depending on the apparent severity of intoxication. Use normal or half-normal saline to avoid water intoxication, especially in children. Instillation of activated charcoal slurry may help reduce absorption of imipramine.

Minimize external stimulation to reduce the tendency to convulsions. If anticonvulsants are necessary, diazepam, short-acting barbiturates, paraldehyde or methocarbamol may be useful.

Do not use barbiturates if MAO inhibitors have been taken recently.

Maintain adequate respiratory exchange. Do not use respiratory stimulants.

Shock should be treated with supportive measures, such as intravenous fluids, oxygen and corticosteroids. Digitalis may increase conduction abnormalities and further irritate an already sensitized myocardium. If congestive heart failure

necessitates rapid digitalization, particular care must be exercised.

Hyperpyrexia should be controlled by whatever external means are available, including ice packs and cooling sponge baths, if necessary.

Hemodialysis, peritoneal dialysis, exchange transfusions and forced diuresis have been generally reported as ineffective because of the rapid fixation of Tofranil in tissues. Blood and urine levels of Tofranil may not correlate with the degree of intoxication, and are unreliable indicators in the clinical management of the patient.

HOW SUPPLIED

Tablets 10 mg — triangular, coral, sugar-coated (imprinted black Geigy 32)

    Bottles of 100 ....NDC 0028-0032-01

    Bottles of 1000 ....NDC 0028-0032-10

Tablets 25 mg — round, biconvex, coral, sugar-coated (imprinted black Geigy 140)

    Bottles of 100 ....NDC 0028-0140-01

    Bottles of 1000 ....NDC 0028-0140-10

    Gy-Pak®—One Unit

      12 bottles - 100 tablets each

                        ....NDC 0028-0140-65

    Unit Dose (blister pack)

      Box of 100 (strips of 10)

                        ....NDC 0028-0140-61

Tablets 50 mg — round, biconvex, coral, sugar-coated (imprinted black Geigy 136)

    Bottles of 100 ....NDC 0028-0136-01

    Bottles of 1000 ....NDC 0028-0136-10

    Gy-Pak®—One Unit

      12 bottles - 100 tablets each

                        ....NDC 0028-0136-65

    Unit Dose (blister pack)

      Box of 100 (strips of 10)

                        ....NDC 0028-0136-61

Store at controlled room temperature 15°–30°C (59°–86°F).

Dispense in tight container (USP).

ANIMAL PHARMACOLOGY & TOXICOLOGY

A. *Acute:* Oral LD_{50} ranges are as follows:

Rat	355 to 682 mg/kg
Dog	100 to 215 mg/kg

Depending on the dosage in both species, toxic signs proceeded progressively from depression, irregular respiration and ataxia to convulsions and death.

B. *Reproduction/Teratogenic:* The overall evaluation may be summed up in the following manner:

Oral: Independent studies in three species (rat, mouse and rabbit) revealed that when Tofranil is administered orally in doses up to approximately 2½ times the maximum human dose in the first 2 species and up to 25 times the maximum human dose in the third species, the drug is essentially free from teratogenic potential. In the three species studied, only one instance of fetal abnormality occurred (in the rabbit) and in that study there was likewise an abnormality in the control group. However, evidence does exist from the rat studies that some systemic and embryotoxic potential is demonstrable. This is manifested by reduced litter size, a slight increase in the stillborn rate and a reduction in the mean birth weight.

C85-59 (Rev. 11/85)

Shown in Product Identification Section, page 410

For full prescribing information on Enuresis, please refer to Tofranil® imipramine hydrochloride USP, on page 992.

TOFRANIL–PM® ℞
[toe-fray'nill]
imipramine pamoate
Capsules of 75 mg
Capsules of 100 mg
Capsules of 125 mg
Capsules of 150 mg
For oral administration

Each 75-mg capsule contains imipramine pamoate equivalent to 75 mg of imipramine hydrochloride.
Each 100-mg capsule contains imipramine pamoate equivalent to 100 mg of imipramine hydrochloride.
Each 125-mg capsule contains imipramine pamoate equivalent to 125 mg of imipramine hydrochloride.
Each 150-mg capsule contains imipramine pamoate equivalent to 150 mg of imipramine hydrochloride.

DESCRIPTION
Tofranil-PM, imipramine pamoate, is a tricyclic antidepressant, available as capsules for oral administration. The 75-, 100-, 125-, and 150-mg capsules contain imipramine pamoate equivalent to 75, 100, 125, and 150 mg of imipramine hydrochloride.
Imipramine pamoate is 5-(3-[dimethylamino]propyl]-10,11-dihydro-5H-dibenz [b,f] azepine 4,4'-methylenebis-(3-hydroxy-2-naphthoate) (2:1).
Imipramine pamoate is a fine, yellow, tasteless and odorless powder. It is soluble in ethanol, in acetone, in ether, in chloroform, and in carbon tetrachloride, and is insoluble in water. Its molecular weight is 949.21.
Inactive Ingredients: D&C Red No. 28, edetate calcium disodium, FD&C Blue No. 1, FD&C Yellow No. 6, gelatin, magnesium stearate, parabens, sodium lauryl sulfate, sodium propionate, starch, talc, and titanium dioxide.

CLINICAL PHARMACOLOGY
The mechanism of action of imipramine is not definitely known. However, it does not act primarily by stimulation of the central nervous system. The clinical effect is hypothesized as being due to potentiation of adrenergic synapses by blocking uptake of norepinephrine at nerve endings.

INDICATIONS
For the relief of symptoms of depression. Endogenous depression is more likely to be alleviated than other depressive states. One to three weeks of treatment may be needed before optimal therapeutic effects are evident.

CONTRAINDICATIONS
The concomitant use of monoamine oxidase inhibiting compounds is contraindicated. Hyperpyretic crises or severe convulsive seizures may occur in patients receiving such combinations. The potentiation of adverse effects can be serious, or even fatal. When it is desired to substitute Tofranil-PM in patients receiving a monoamine oxidase inhibitor, as long an interval should elapse as the clinical situation will allow, with a minimum of 14 days. Initial dosage should be low and increases should be gradual and cautiously prescribed.
The drug is contraindicated during the acute recovery period after a myocardial infarction. Patients with a known hypersensitivity to this compound should not be given the drug. The possibility of cross-sensitivity to other dibenzazepine compounds should be kept in mind.

WARNINGS
Extreme caution should be used when this drug is given to:
patients with cardiovascular disease because of the possibility of conduction defects, arrhythmias, congestive heart failure, myocardial infarction, strokes and tachycardia. These patients require cardiac surveillance at all dosage levels of the drug;
patients with increased intraocular pressure, history of urinary retention, or history of narrow-angle glaucoma because of the drug's anticholinergic properties;
hyperthyroid patients or those on thyroid medication because of the possibility of cardiovascular toxicity;
patients with a history of seizure disorder because this drug has been shown to lower the seizure threshold;
patients receiving guanethidine, clonidine, or similar agents, since imipramine pamoate may block the pharmacologic effects of these drugs;
patients receiving methylphenidate hydrochloride. Since methylphenidate hydrochloride may inhibit the metabolism of imipramine pamoate, downward dosage adjustment of imipramine pamoate may be required when given concomitantly with methylphenidate hydrochloride.
Since imipramine pamoate may impair the mental and/or physical abilities required for the performance of potentially hazardous tasks, such as operating an automobile or machinery, the patient should be cautioned accordingly.

Tofranil-PM may enhance the CNS depressant effects of alcohol. Therefore, it should be borne in mind that the dangers inherent in a suicide attempt or accidental overdosage with the drug may be increased for the patient who uses excessive amounts of alcohol. (See **PRECAUTIONS.**)
Usage in Children: Tofranil-PM should not be used in children of any age because of the increased potential for acute overdosage due to the high unit potency (75 mg, 100 mg, 125 mg and 150 mg). Each capsule contains imipramine pamoate equivalent to 75 mg, 100 mg, 125 mg or 150 mg imipramine hydrochloride.

PRECAUTIONS
An ECG recording should be taken prior to the initiation of larger-than-usual doses of imipramine pamoate and at appropriate intervals thereafter until steady state is achieved. (Patients with any evidence of cardiovascular disease require cardiac surveillance at all dosage levels of the drug. See **WARNINGS.**) Elderly patients and patients with cardiac disease or a prior history of cardiac disease are at special risk of developing the cardiac abnormalities associated with the use of imipramine pamoate. It should be kept in mind that the possibility of suicide in seriously depressed patients is inherent in the illness and may persist until significant remission occurs. Such patients should be carefully supervised during the early phase of treatment with imipramine pamoate and may require hospitalization. Prescriptions should be written for the smallest amount feasible.
Hypomanic or manic episodes may occur, particularly in patients with cyclic disorders. Such reactions may necessitate discontinuation of the drug. If needed, imipramine pamoate may be resumed in lower dosage when these episodes are relieved. Administration of a tranquilizer may be useful in controlling such episodes.
An activation of the psychosis may occasionally be observed in schizophrenic patients and may require reduction of dosage and the addition of a phenothiazine.
Concurrent administration of imipramine pamoate with electroshock therapy may increase the hazards; such treatment should be limited to those patients for whom it is essential, since there is limited clinical experience.

Usage During Pregnancy and Lactation:
Animal reproduction studies have yielded inconclusive results. (See also **ANIMAL PHARMACOLOGY & TOXICOLOGY.**)
There have been no well-controlled studies conducted with pregnant women to determine the effect of imipramine on the fetus. However, there have been clinical reports of congenital malformations associated with the use of the drug. Although a causal relationship between these effects and the drug could not be established, the possibility of fetal risk from the maternal ingestion of imipramine cannot be excluded. Therefore, imipramine should be used in women who are or might become pregnant only if the clinical condition clearly justifies potential risk to the fetus.
Limited data suggest that imipramine is likely to be excreted in human breast milk. As a general rule, a woman taking a drug should not nurse since the possibility exists that the drug may be excreted in breast milk and be harmful to the child.
Patients should be warned that imipramine pamoate may enhance the CNS depressant effects of alcohol. (See **WARNINGS.**)
Imipramine pamoate should be used with caution in patients with significantly impaired renal or hepatic function.
Patients who develop a fever and a sore throat during therapy with imipramine pamoate should have leukocyte and differential blood counts performed. Imipramine pamoate should be discontinued if there is evidence of pathological neutrophil depression.
Prior to elective surgery, imipramine pamoate should be discontinued for as long as the clinical situation will allow.
In occasional susceptible patients or in those receiving anticholinergic drugs (including antiparkinsonism agents) in addition, the atropine-like effects may become more pronounced (e.g., paralytic ileus). Close supervision and careful adjustment of dosage is required when imipramine pamoate is administered concomitantly with anticholinergic drugs.
Avoid the use of preparations, such as decongestants and local anesthetics, which contain any sympathomimetic amine (e.g., epinephrine, norepinephrine), since it has been reported that tricyclic antidepressants can potentiate the effects of catecholamines.
Caution should be exercised when imipramine pamoate is used with agents that lower blood pressure.
Imipramine pamoate may potentiate the effects of CNS depressant drugs.
The plasma concentration of imipramine may increase when the drug is given concomitantly with cimetidine, and adjustment of the dosage of imipramine may therefore be necessary both when cimetidine therapy is initiated and when it is discontinued.
Patients taking imipramine pamoate should avoid excessive exposure to sunlight since there have been reports of photosensitization.

Both elevation and lowering of blood sugar levels have been reported with imipramine pamoate use.

ADVERSE REACTIONS
Note: Although the listing which follows includes a few adverse reactions which have not been reported with this specific drug, the pharmacological similarities among the tricyclic antidepressant drugs require that each of the reactions be considered when imipramine is administered.
Cardiovascular: Orthostatic hypotension, hypertension, tachycardia, palpitation, myocardial infarction, arrhythmias, heart block, ECG changes, precipitation of congestive heart failure, stroke.
Psychiatric: Confusional states (especially in the elderly) with hallucinations, disorientation, delusions; anxiety, restlessness, agitation; insomnia and nightmares; hypomania; exacerbation of psychosis.
Neurological: Numbness, tingling, paresthesias of extremities; incoordination, ataxia, tremors; peripheral neuropathy; extrapyramidal symptoms; seizures, alterations in EEG patterns; tinnitus.
Anticholinergic: Dry mouth, and, rarely, associated sublingual adenitis; blurred vision, disturbances of accommodation, mydriasis; constipation, paralytic ileus; urinary retention, delayed micturition, dilation of the urinary tract.
Allergic: Skin rash, petechiae, urticaria, itching, photosensitization; edema (general or of face and tongue); drug fever; cross-sensitivity with desipramine.
Hematologic: Bone marrow depression including agranulocytosis; eosinophilia; purpura; thrombocytopenia.
Gastrointestinal: Nausea and vomiting, anorexia, epigastric distress, diarrhea; peculiar taste, stomatitis, abdominal cramps, black tongue.
Endocrine: Gynecomastia in the male; breast enlargement and galactorrhea in the female; increased or decreased libido, impotence; testicular swelling; elevation or depression of blood sugar levels; inappropriate antidiuretic hormone (ADH) secretion syndrome.
Other: Jaundice (simulating obstructive); altered liver function; weight gain or loss; perspiration; flushing; urinary frequency; drowsiness, dizziness, weakness and fatigue; headache; parotid swelling; alopecia; proneness to falling.
Withdrawal Symptoms: Though not indicative of addiction, abrupt cessation of treatment after prolonged therapy may produce nausea, headache and malaise.

DOSAGE AND ADMINISTRATION
The following recommended dosages for Tofranil-PM should be modified as necessary by the clinical response and any evidence of intolerance.
Initial Adult Dosage:
Outpatients—Therapy should be initiated at 75 mg/day. Dosage may be increased to 150 mg/day which is the dose level at which optimum response is usually obtained. If necessary, dosage may be increased to 200 mg/day.
Dosage higher than 75 mg/day may also be administered on a once-a-day basis after the optimum dosage and tolerance have been determined. The daily dosage may be given at bedtime. In some patients it may be necessary to employ a divided-dose schedule.
As with all tricyclics, the antidepressant effect of imipramine may not be evident for one to three weeks in some patients.
Hospitalized Patients—Therapy should be initiated at 100–150 mg/day and may be increased to 200 mg/day. If there is no response after two weeks, dosage should be increased to 250–300 mg/day.
Dosage higher than 150 mg/day may also be administered on a once-a-day basis after the optimum dosage and tolerance have been determined. The daily dosage may be given at bedtime. In some patients it may be necessary to employ a divided-dose schedule.
As with all tricyclics, the antidepressant effect of imipramine may not be evident for one to three weeks in some patients.
Adult Maintenance Dosage: Following remission, maintenance medication may be required for a longer period of time at the lowest dose that will maintain remission after which the dosage should gradually be decreased.
The usual maintenance dosage is 75–150 mg/day. The total daily dosage can be administered on a once-a-day basis, preferably at bedtime. In some patients it may be necessary to employ a divided-dose schedule.

Continued on next page

The full prescribing information for each GEIGY product is contained herein and is that in effect as of September 1, 1989

Geigy—Cont.

In cases of relapse due to premature withdrawal of the drug, the effective dosage of imipramine should be reinstituted.

Adolescent and Geriatric Patients: Therapy in these age groups should be initiated with Tofranil®, brand of imipramine hydrochloride, tablets at a total daily dosage of 25–50 mg, since Tofranil-PM capsules are not available in these strengths. Dosage may be increased according to response and tolerance, but it is generally unnecessary to exceed 100 mg/day in these patients. Tofranil-PM capsules may be used when total daily dosage is established at 75 mg or higher. The total daily dosage can be administered on a once-a-day basis, preferably at bedtime. In some patients it may be necessary to employ a divided-dose schedule.

As with all tricyclics, the antidepressant effect of imipramine may not be evident for one to three weeks in some patients.

Adolescent and geriatric patients can usually be maintained at lower dosage. Following remission, maintenance medication may be required for a longer period of time at the lowest dose that will maintain remission after which the dosage should gradually be decreased.

The total daily maintenance dosage can be administered on a once-a-day basis, preferably at bedtime. In some patients it may be necessary to employ a divided-dose schedule.

In cases of relapse due to premature withdrawal of the drug, the effective dosage of imipramine should be reinstituted.

OVERDOSAGE

Children have been reported to be more sensitive than adults to an acute overdosage of imipramine pamoate. An acute overdose of any amount in infants or young children, especially, must be considered serious and potentially fatal.

Signs and Symptoms: These may vary in severity depending upon factors such as the amount of drug absorbed, the age of the patient, and the interval between drug ingestion and the start of treatment. Blood and urine levels of imipramine may not reflect the severity of poisoning; they have chiefly a qualitative rather than a quantitative value, and are unreliable indicators in the clinical management of the patient.

CNS abnormalities may include drowsiness, stupor, coma, ataxia, restlessness, agitation, hyperactive reflexes, muscle rigidity, athetoid and choreiform movements, and convulsions.

Cardiac abnormalities may include arrhythmia, tachycardia, ECG evidence of impaired conduction, and signs of congestive failure.

Respiratory depression, cyanosis, hypotension, shock, vomiting, hyperpyrexia, mydriasis, and diaphoresis may also be present.

Treatment: Because CNS involvement, respiratory depression and cardiac arrhythmia can occur suddenly, hospitalization and close observation are necessary, even when the amount ingested is thought to be small or the initial degree of intoxication appears slight or moderate. All patients with ECG abnormalities should have continuous cardiac monitoring for at least 72 hours and be closely observed until well after cardiac status has returned to normal; relapses may occur after apparent recovery.

The *slow* intravenous administration of physostigmine salicylate has been reported to reverse most of the cardiovascular and CNS effects of overdosage with tricyclic antidepressants. In adults, 1 to 3 mg has been reported to be effective. In children, start with 0.5 mg and repeat at 5-minute intervals to determine the minimum effective dose; do not exceed 2 mg. Because of the short duration of action of physostigmine, repeat the effective dose at 30- to 60-minute intervals, as necessary. Avoid rapid injection to reduce the possibility of physostigmine-induced convulsions.

In the alert patient, empty the stomach promptly by induced emesis followed by lavage. In the obtunded patient, secure the airway with a cuffed endotracheal tube before beginning lavage (do not induce emesis). Continue lavage for 24 hours or longer, depending on the apparent severity of intoxication. Use normal or half-normal saline to avoid water intoxication, especially in children. Instillation of activated charcoal slurry may help reduce absorption of imipramine.

Minimize external stimulation to reduce the tendency to convulsions. If anticonvulsants are necessary, diazepam, short-acting barbiturates, paraldehyde or methocarbamol may be useful. Do not use barbiturates if MAO inhibitors have been taken recently.

Maintain adequate respiratory exchange. Do not use respiratory stimulants.

Shock should be treated with supportive measures, such as intravenous fluids, oxygen and corticosteroids. Digitalis may increase conduction abnormalities and further irritate an already sensitized myocardium. If congestive heart failure necessitates rapid digitalization, particular care must be exercised.

Hyperpyrexia should be controlled by whatever external means are available, including ice packs and cooling sponge baths, if necessary.

Hemodialysis, peritoneal dialysis, exchange transfusions and forced diuresis have been generally reported as ineffective because of the rapid fixation of imipramine in tissues. Blood and urine levels of imipramine may not correlate with the degree of intoxication, and are unreliable indicators in the clinical management of the patient.

HOW SUPPLIED

Capsules 75 mg — coral (imprinted Geigy 20) equivalent to 75 mg imipramine hydrochloride

    Bottles of 30 ....NDC 0028-0020-26
    Bottles of 100 ....NDC 0028-0020-01
    Bottles of 1000 ....NDC 0028-0020-10
    Unit Dose (blister pack)
      Box of 100 (strips of 10)

    ....NDC 0028-0020-61

Capsules 100 mg — dark yellow/coral (imprinted Geigy 40) equivalent to 100 mg imipramine hydrochloride

    Bottles of 30 ....NDC 0028-0040-26
    Bottles of 100 ....NDC 0028-0040-01

Capsules 125 mg — light yellow/coral (imprinted Geigy 45) equivalent to 125 mg imipramine hydrochloride

    Bottles of 30 ....NDC 0028-0045-26
    Bottles of 100 ....NDC 0028-0045-01

Capsules 150 mg — coral (imprinted Geigy 22) equivalent to 150 mg imipramine hydrochloride

    Bottles of 30 ....NDC 0028-0022-26
    Bottles of 100 ....NDC 0028-0022-01
    Unit Dose (blister pack)
      Box of 100 (strips of 10)

    ....NDC 0028-0022-61

Do not store above 86°F (30°C).

Dispense in tight container (USP).

ANIMAL PHARMACOLOGY & TOXICOLOGY

A. *Acute:* Oral LD$_{50}$:

Mouse		2185 mg/kg
Rat	(F)	1142 mg/kg
	(M)	1807 mg/kg
Rabbit		1016 mg/kg
Dog		693 mg/kg (Emesis ED$_{50}$)

B. *Subacute:*

Two three-month studies in dogs gave evidence of an adverse drug effect on the testes, but only at the highest dose level employed, i.e., 90 mg/kg (10 times the maximum human dose). Depending on the histological section of the testes examined, the findings consisted of a range of degenerative changes up to and including complete atrophy of the seminiferous tubules, with spermatogenesis usually arrested. Human studies show no definitive effect on sperm count, sperm motility, sperm morphology or volume of ejaculate.

Rat

One three-month study was done in rats at dosage levels comparable to those of the dog studies. No adverse drug effect on the testes was noted in this study, as confirmed by histological examination.

C. *Reproduction/Teratogenic:*

Oral: Imipramine pamoate was fed to male and female albino rats for 28 weeks through two breeding cycles at dose levels of 15 mg/kg/day and 40 mg/kg/day (equivalent to 2½ and 7 times the maximum human dose). No abnormalities which could be related to drug administration were noted in gross inspection. Autopsies performed on pups from the second breeding likewise revealed no pathological changes in organs or tissues; however, a decrease in mean litter size from both matings was noted in the drug-treated groups and significant growth suppression occurred in the nursing pups of both sexes in the high group as well as in the females of the low-level group. Finally, the lactation index (pups weaned divided by number left to nurse) was significantly lower in the second litter of the high-level group.

                                            C88-10 (Rev. 3/88)

Shown in Product Identification Section, page 410

VOLTAREN®   ℞
diclofenac sodium
Enteric-Coated Tablets

DESCRIPTION

Voltaren, diclofenac sodium, is a nonsteroidal, anti-inflammatory phenylacetic acid derivative, designated chemically as sodium [o-[(2,6-dichlorophenyl)amino]phenyl] acetate. Diclofenac sodium is a faintly yellow-white to light beige, virtually odorless, slightly hygroscopic crystalline powder. It is freely soluble in methanol, sparingly soluble in water, very slightly soluble in acetonitrile, and insoluble in chloroform and in 0.1N hydrochloric acid. Its molecular weight is 318.14. In water, diclofenac sodium has a single dissociation constant (pKa) of 4.0.

Voltaren is available as enteric-coated tablets of 25 mg, 50 mg, and 75 mg for oral administration.

Inactive Ingredients. Cellulose acetate phthalate, colloidal silicon dioxide (25-mg and 50-mg enteric-coated tablets only), diethyl phthalate, hydroxypropyl methylcellulose, iron oxide (25-mg and 50-mg enteric-coated tablets only), lactose, magnesium stearate, microcrystalline cellulose, povidone, shellac, sodium starch glycolate (75-mg enteric-coated tablets only), starch (25-mg and 50-mg enteric-coated tablets only), talc (75-mg enteric-coated tablets only), titanium dioxide.

CLINICAL PHARMACOLOGY

Pharmacology

In pharmacologic studies, Voltaren has shown anti-inflammatory, analgesic, and antipyretic activity. As with other nonsteroidal anti-inflammatory agents, its mode of action is not known; however, its ability to inhibit prostaglandin synthesis may be involved in the anti-inflammatory effect.

Pharmacokinetics

Voltaren is completely absorbed from the gastrointestinal tract after fasting oral administration, with peak plasma levels occurring in 2–3 hours. However, due to first-pass metabolism only about 50% of the absorbed dose is systemically available. The mean terminal half-life in plasma is approximately 2 hours, but early elimination is much more rapid. Area under the plasma concentration curve (AUC) is dose-proportional within the range of 25 mg to 150 mg. Peak plasma levels are less than dose-proportional and are approximately 1.0, 1.5, and 2 mcg/ml for 25-mg, 50-mg, and 75-mg doses, respectively. Clearance and volume of distribution were about 350 ml/min and 550 ml/kg, respectively. After repeated oral administration of 50 mg b.i.d., Voltaren did not accumulate in plasma. The degree of accumulation of diclofenac metabolites is unknown. Some of the metabolites may have activity. More than 99% of diclofenac is reversibly bound to human plasma albumin.

Voltaren is eliminated through metabolism and subsequent urinary and biliary excretion of the glucuronide and the sulfate conjugates of the metabolites. Approximately 65% of the dose is excreted in the urine, and approximately 35% in the bile.

Conjugates of the principal metabolite, 4'-hydroxy-diclofenac, account for 20–30% of the dose excreted in the urine and for 10–20% of the dose excreted in the bile. Conjugates of three other metabolites (5-hydroxy-,3'-hydroxy-, and 4',5-dihydroxy-diclofenac) together account for 10–20% of the dose excreted in the urine and for small amounts excreted in the bile. Conjugates of unchanged diclofenac account for 5–10% of the dose excreted in the urine and for less than 5% excreted in the bile. Little or no unchanged unconjugated drug is excreted. It is not known whether there is genetic polymorphism in the enzymes responsible for metabolism of diclofenac.

The extent of absorption of Voltaren is not significantly affected when the drug is taken with food; however, there is usually a delay in the onset of absorption of 1 to 4.5 hours, with delays as long as 10 hours in some patients. There is also a reduction in peak plasma levels.

A 4-week study comparing plasma level profiles of diclofenac (50 mg b.i.d.) in younger (26–46) versus older (66–81) adults did not show differences between age groups (10 patients per age group).

Single-dose studies of the effects of renal function impairment (50 mg intravenously) or hepatic impairment (100 mg oral solution) have been performed in small numbers of patients. To date no differences in the pharmacokinetics of diclofenac have been detected in patients with renal or hepatic impairment.

In patients with renal impairment (N=5, creatinine clearance 3 to 42 ml/min), AUC values and elimination rates were comparable to those in healthy subjects.

In patients with biopsy-confirmed cirrhosis or chronic active hepatitis (variably elevated transaminases and mildly elevated bilirubins, N=10), diclofenac concentrations and urinary elimination values were comparable to those in healthy subjects.

Voltaren diffuses into and out of the synovial fluid. Diffusion into the joint occurs during the first 4 hours following a dose, while plasma levels are higher than those in synovial fluid, after which the process reverses and synovial fluid levels are slightly higher than plasma levels. It is not known whether diffusion into the joint plays a role in the effectiveness of Voltaren.

In healthy subjects, the daily administration of 150 mg of Voltaren for 3 weeks resulted in a mean fecal blood loss less than that observed with 3.0 g of aspirin daily. In repeated-dose studies, mean fecal blood loss with 150 mg of Voltaren was also less than that observed with 750 mg of naproxen or 150 mg of indomethacin. Repeated-dose endoscopic studies in normal volunteers showed that daily doses of 75 mg or 100 mg of Voltaren for 1 week caused fewer gastric lesions, and those that did occur had lower scores than those which occurred following 500 mg daily doses of naproxen. The clinical significance of these findings is unknown since there is no evidence available to indicate that diclofenac is less likely than other drugs of its class to cause serious gastrointestinal lesions when used in chronic therapy.

In patients with rheumatoid arthritis, Voltaren has been administered safely in combination with gold or corticosteroids.

INDICATIONS AND USAGE

Voltaren is indicated for acute and chronic treatment of the signs and symptoms of rheumatoid arthritis, osteoarthritis, and ankylosing spondylitis.

CONTRAINDICATIONS

Voltaren is contraindicated in patients with hypersensitivity to it. Voltaren should not be given to patients in whom Voltaren, aspirin, or other nonsteroidal anti-inflammatory drugs induce asthma, urticaria, or other allergic-type reactions because severe, rarely fatal, anaphylactic-like reactions to Voltaren have been reported in such patients.

WARNINGS

Gastrointestinal Effects

Peptic ulceration and gastrointestinal bleeding have been reported in patients receiving Voltaren. Physicians and patients should therefore remain alert for ulceration and bleeding in patients treated chronically with diclofenac sodium, even in the absence of previous G.I. tract symptoms. It is recommended that patients be maintained on the lowest dose of diclofenac sodium possible consistent with achieving a satisfactory therapeutic response.

Risk of G.I. Ulcerations, Bleeding, and Perforation with NSAID Therapy: Serious gastrointestinal toxicity such as bleeding, ulceration, and perforation can occur at any time, with or without warning symptoms, in patients treated chronically with NSAID therapy. Although minor upper gastrointestinal problems, such as dyspepsia, are common, usually developing early in therapy, physicians should remain alert for ulceration and bleeding in patients treated chronically with NSAIDs even in the absence of previous G.I. tract symptoms. In patients observed in clinical trials of several months to 2 years duration, symptomatic upper G.I. ulcers, gross bleeding, or perforation appear to occur in approximately 1% of patients treated for 3–6 months, and in about 2–4% of patients treated for 1 year. Physicians should inform patients about the signs and/or symptoms of serious G.I. toxicity and what steps to take if they occur.

Studies to date have not identified any subset of patients not at risk of developing peptic ulceration and bleeding. Except for a prior history of serious G.I. events and other risk factors known to be associated with peptic ulcer disease, such as alcoholism, smoking, etc., no risk factors (e.g., age, sex) have been associated with increased risk. Elderly or debilitated patients seem to tolerate ulceration or bleeding less well than other individuals and most spontaneous reports of fatal G.I. events are in this population. Studies to date are inconclusive concerning the relative risk of various NSAIDs in causing such reactions. High doses of any NSAID probably carry a greater risk of these reactions, although controlled clinical trials showing this do not exist in most cases. In considering the use of relatively large doses (within the recommended dosage range), sufficient benefit should be anticipated to offset the potential increased risk of G.I. toxicity.

Hepatic Effects

As with other nonsteroidal anti-inflammatory drugs, elevations of one or more liver tests may occur during Voltaren therapy. These laboratory abnormalities may progress, may remain unchanged, or may be transient with continued therapy. Borderline elevations, (i.e., 1.2–3 times the upper limit of normal [ULN]), or greater elevations of transaminases occurred in about 15% of Voltaren-treated patients. The SGPT (ALT) test is probably the most sensitive indicator of liver injury. In clinical trials, meaningful elevations (i.e., more than 3 times the ULN) of SGOT (SGPT was not measured in all studies) occurred in about 2% of approximately 5700 patients at some time during Voltaren treatment. In a large, open, controlled trial, meaningful elevations of SGOT and/or SGPT occurred in about 4% of 3700 patients treated for 2–6 months, including marked elevations (i.e., more than 8 times the ULN) in about 1% of the 3700 patients. In that open-label study, a lower incidence of borderline (1.2–3 times the ULN), moderate (3–8 times the ULN), and marked (> 8 times the ULN) elevations of SGOT or SGPT was observed in patients randomized to other NSAIDs. Transaminase elevations were seen more frequently in patients with osteoarthritis than in those with rheumatoid arthritis (see ADVERSE REACTIONS).

Transaminase elevations were reversible on cessation of therapy, and among 51 patients in all studies with marked elevations, signs and symptoms of liver disease occurred in only 3 cases, and only 1 patient developed jaundice. Most patients with borderline elevations did not have therapy interrupted; transaminase elevations in most of these cases disappeared or did not progress. There were no identifying features to distinguish those patients who developed marked elevations from those who did not.

In addition to the enzyme elevations seen in clinical trials, rare cases of severe hepatic reactions, including jaundice and fatal fulminant hepatitis, have been reported in foreign marketing experience.

Because severe hepatotoxicity may develop without a prodrome of distinguishing symptoms, physicians should measure transaminases periodically in patients receiving long-term therapy with Voltaren. The optimum times for making

the first and subsequent transaminase measurements are not known. In the largest U.S. trial (open-label), which involved 3700 patients monitored first at 8 weeks and 1200 patients monitored again at 24 weeks, almost all meaningful elevations in transaminases were detected before patients became symptomatic. In 42 of the 51 patients in all trials who developed marked transaminase elevations, abnormal tests occurred during the first 2 months of therapy with Voltaren. Based on this experience the first transaminase measurement should be made no later than 8 weeks after the start of Voltaren treatment. As with other NSAIDs, if abnormal liver tests persist or worsen, if clinical signs and/or symptoms consistent with liver disease develop, or if systemic manifestations occur (e.g., eosinophilia, rash, etc.), Voltaren should be discontinued.

To minimize the possibility that hepatic injury will become severe between transaminase measurements, physicians should inform patients of the warning signs and symptoms of hepatotoxicity (e.g., nausea, fatigue, lethargy, pruritus, jaundice, right upper quadrant tenderness and "flu-like" symptoms), and the appropriate action to take should these signs and symptoms appear.

PRECAUTIONS

General

Allergic Reactions: As with other nonsteroidal anti-inflammatory drugs, allergic reactions including anaphylaxis, have been reported with Voltaren. Specific allergic manifestations consisting of swelling of eyelids, lips, pharynx and larynx, urticaria, asthma, and bronchospasm, sometimes with a concomitant fall in blood pressure (severe at times) have been observed in clinical trials and/or the foreign marketing experience with Voltaren. Anaphylaxis has been reported rarely from foreign sources; in U.S. clinical trials with Voltaren in over 6000 patients, 1 case of anaphylaxis was reported. In controlled clinical trials, allergic reactions have been observed at an incidence of 0.5%. These reactions can occur without prior exposure to the drug.

Fluid Retention and Edema: Fluid retention and edema have been observed in some patients taking Voltaren. Therefore, as with other nonsteroidal anti-inflammatory drugs, Voltaren should be used with caution in patients with a history of cardiac decompensation, hypertension, or other conditions predisposing to fluid retention.

Renal Effects: As a class, nonsteroidal anti-inflammatory drugs have been associated with renal papillary necrosis and other abnormal renal pathology in long-term administration to animals. Papillary necrosis was observed only in 1 animal study with diclofenac, a 4-week study in baboons in which the drug was administered intramuscularly. In oral studies some evidence of renal toxicity was noted but papillary necrosis was not reported.

A second form of renal toxicity generally associated with nonsteroidal anti-inflammatory drugs is seen in patients with conditions leading to a reduction in renal blood flow or blood volume, where renal prostaglandins have a supportive role in the maintenance of renal perfusion. In these patients, administration of a nonsteroidal anti-inflammatory drug results in a dose-dependent decrease in prostaglandin synthesis and, secondarily, in a reduction of renal blood flow, which may precipitate overt renal failure. Patients at greatest risk of this reaction are those with impaired renal function, heart failure, liver dysfunction, those taking diuretics, and the elderly. Discontinuation of nonsteroidal anti-inflammatory drug therapy is typically followed by recovery to the pretreatment state.

Cases of significant renal failure in patients receiving Voltaren have been reported from postmarketing experience, but were not observed in over 4,000 patients in clinical trials during which serum creatinines and BUNs were followed serially. There were only 7 patients (0.18%) whose serum creatinines and concurrent serum BUNs were greater than 2.0 mg/dl and 40 mg/dl, respectively, while on diclofenac (mean rise in the 7 patients; creatinine 1.5 mg/dl and BUN 20 mg/dl). It is not yet clear whether this low incidence of renal impairment in clinical trials, plus the observation of less renal toxicity than is usual in rodents, will translate into a significant reduction of the risk of renal failure in susceptible patients in widespread use.

Since Voltaren metabolites are eliminated primarily by the kidneys, patients with significantly impaired renal function should be more closely monitored than subjects with normal renal function.

Porphyria: The use of diclofenac in patients with hepatic porphyria should be avoided. To date, 1 patient has been described in whom diclofenac probably triggered a clinical attack of porphyria. The postulated mechanism for causing such attacks by diclofenac, as well as some other NSAIDs, is through stimulation of the porphyrin precursor delta-aminolevulinic acid (ALA, demonstrated in rats).

Information for Patients

Voltaren, like other drugs of its class, is not free of side effects. The side effects of these drugs can cause discomfort and, rarely, there are more serious side effects, such as gastrointestinal bleeding, which may result in hospitalization and even fatal outcomes.

NSAIDs are often essential agents in the management of arthritis, but they also may be commonly employed for conditions which are less serious.

Physicians may wish to discuss with their patients the potential risks (see WARNINGS, PRECAUTIONS, and ADVERSE REACTIONS) and likely benefits of NSAID treatment, particularly when the drugs are used for less serious conditions where treatment without NSAIDs may represent an acceptable alternative to both the patient and physician.

Laboratory Tests

Because serious G.I. tract ulceration and bleeding can occur without warning symptoms, physicians should follow chronically treated patients for the signs and symptoms of ulceration and bleeding and should inform them of the importance of this follow-up (see WARNINGS, *Risk of G.I. Ulcerations, Bleeding, and Perforation with NSAID Therapy*).

Drug Interactions

Aspirin: Concomitant administration of Voltaren and aspirin is not recommended because Voltaren is displaced from its binding sites during the concomitant administration of aspirin, resulting in lower plasma concentrations, peak plasma levels, and AUC values.

Anticoagulants: While studies have not shown Voltaren to interact with anticoagulants of the warfarin type, caution should be exercised, nonetheless, since interactions have been seen with other NSAIDs. Because prostaglandins play an important role in hemostasis, and NSAIDs affect platelet function as well, concurrent therapy with all NSAIDs, including Voltaren, and warfarin requires close monitoring of patients to be certain that no change in their anticoagulant dosage is required.

Digoxin, Methotrexate, Cyclosporine: Voltaren, like other NSAIDs, through effects on renal prostaglandins, may cause increased toxicity of certain drugs. Digoxin and methotrexate serum levels may be elevated as well as cyclosporine's nephrotoxicity. Patients receiving these drugs who are started on, or are given increased doses of, Voltaren or any other NSAID, and particularly those patients with altered renal function, should be observed for the development of the specific toxicities of these drugs. In the case of digoxin, serum levels should be monitored.

Lithium: Voltaren decreases lithium renal clearance and increases lithium plasma levels. In patients taking Voltaren and lithium concomitantly, lithium toxicity may develop.

Oral Hypoglycemics: Voltaren does not alter glucose metabolism in normal subjects nor are the effects of oral hypoglycemic agents altered by the concomitant administration of Voltaren. There are rare reports, however, from postmarketing experiences of changes in effects in insulin or oral hypoglycemic agents in the presence of diclofenac which necessitated changes in the doses of such agents. Both hypo- and hyperglycemic effects have been reported. A direct causal relationship has not been established, but physicians should consider the possibility that diclofenac may alter a diabetic patient's response to insulin or oral hypoglycemic agents.

Diuretics: Voltaren and other NSAIDs can inhibit the activity of diuretics. Concomitant treatment with potassium-sparing diuretics may be associated with increased serum potassium levels.

Other Drugs: In small groups of patients (7–10/interaction study), the concomitant administration of azathioprine, gold, chloroquine, D-penicillamine, prednisolone, doxycycline, or digitoxin did not significantly affect the peak levels and AUC values of Voltaren.

Protein Binding

In vitro, Voltaren interferes minimally or not at all with the protein binding of salicylic acid (20% decrease in binding), tolbutamide, prednisolone (10% decrease in binding), or warfarin. Benzylpenicillin, ampicillin, oxacillin, chlortetracycline, doxycycline, cephalothin, erythromycin, and sulfamethoxazole have no influence in vitro on the protein binding of Voltaren in human serum.

Drug/Laboratory Test Interactions

Effect on Blood Coagulation: Voltaren increases platelet aggregation time but does not affect bleeding time, plasma thrombin clotting time, plasma fibrinogen, or factors V and VII to XII. Statistically significant changes in prothrombin and partial thromboplastin times have been reported in normal volunteers. The mean changes were observed to be less than 1 second in both instances, however, and are unlikely to be clinically important. Voltaren is a prostaglandin synthetase inhibitor, however, and all drugs that inhibit prostaglandin synthesis interfere with platelet function to some degree; therefore, patients who may be adversely affected by such an action should be carefully observed.

Continued on next page

Geigy—Cont.

Carcinogenesis, Mutagenesis, Impairment of Fertility

Long-term carcinogenicity studies in rats given Voltaren up to 2 mg/kg/day (approximately the human dose) have revealed no significant increases in tumor incidence.

There was a slight increase in benign mammary fibroadenomas in mid-dose females (high-dose females had excessive mortality), but the increase was not significant for this common rat tumor. Voltaren did not show mutagenic potential in various mutagenicity studies including the Ames test. Voltaren administered to male and female rats at 4 mg/kg/day did not affect fertility. A 2-year mouse carcinogenicity study is underway.

Teratogenic Effects

Pregnancy Category B: Reproduction studies have been performed in mice given Voltaren (up to 20 mg/kg/day) and in rats and rabbits given Voltaren (up to 10 mg/kg/day), and have revealed no evidence of teratogenicity despite the induction of maternal toxicity and fetal toxicity. In rats, maternally toxic doses were associated with dystocia, prolonged gestation, reduced fetal weights and growth, and reduced fetal survival. Voltaren has been shown to cross the placental barrier in mice and rats.

There are no adequate and well-controlled studies in pregnant women. Voltaren should be used during pregnancy only if the benefits to the mother justify the potential risk to the fetus. Because of the known effects of prostaglandin-inhibiting drugs on the fetal cardiovascular system (closure of ductus arteriosus), use of Voltaren during late pregnancy should be avoided.

Labor and Delivery

The effects of Voltaren on labor and delivery in pregnant women are unknown. However, as with other nonsteroidal anti-inflammatory drugs, it is possible that Voltaren may inhibit uterine contraction.

Nursing Mothers

Voltaren has been found in the milk of nursing mothers. As with other drugs that are excreted in milk, Voltaren is not recommended for use in nursing women.

Pediatric Use

Dosage recommendations and indications for use in children have not been established.

ADVERSE REACTIONS

Adverse reaction information is derived from blinded-controlled and open-label clinical trials and worldwide marketing experience. In the description below, rates of the more common events represent clinical study results; rarer events are derived principally from marketing experience and publications, and accurate rate estimates are generally impossible.

The incidence of common adverse reactions (greater than 1%) is based upon controlled clinical trials in 1543 patients treated up to 13 weeks. By far the most common adverse effects were gastrointestinal symptoms, most of them minor, occurring in about 20%, and leading to discontinuation in about 3%, of patients. Peptic ulcer or G.I. bleeding occurred in clinical trials in less than 1% of approximately 1800 patients during their first 3 months of diclofenac treatment and in less than 2% of approximately 800 patients followed for 1 year. The only control group with sufficient patients for comparison received aspirin and only for the first 30 days of treatment. Comparative rates were 0.2% for peptic ulcer or G.I. bleeding in approximately 2000 diclofenac-treated patients and 0.6% in approximately 600 aspirin-treated patients.

In double-blind trials there were fewer minor gastrointestinal complaints in 1227 patients treated with Voltaren than in 721 patients treated with aspirin, 22% vs 33% (compared to 13% on placebo).

Gastrointestinal symptoms were followed in frequency by central nervous system side effects such as headache (7%) and dizziness (3%).

Meaningful (exceeding 3 times the upper limit of normal) elevations of SGPT (ALT) or SGOT (AST) occurred at an overall rate of about 2% during the first 2 months of Voltaren treatment. Unlike aspirin, where elevations occur more frequently in patients with rheumatoid arthritis, these elevations were more frequently observed in patients with osteoarthritis (2.6%) than in patients with rheumatoid arthritis (0.7%). Marked elevations (exceeding 8 times the upper limit of normal) were seen in about 1% of patients treated for 2–6 months (see WARNINGS).

The following adverse reactions were reported in patients treated with Voltaren:

Incidence Greater Than 1% (All derived from clinical trials.)

Digestive: Abdominal pain or cramps,* constipation,* diarrhea,* indigestion,* nausea,* abdominal distention, liver test abnormalities, flatulence, PUB, i.e., peptic ulcer, with or without bleeding and/or perforation, or bleeding without ulcer (see above and also WARNINGS).

Central Nervous System: Headache,* dizziness.

Metabolic/Nutritional: Fluid retention.*

Skin and Appendages: Rash, pruritus.

Special Senses: Tinnitus.

*Incidence, 3% to 9% (incidence of unmarked reactions is 1–3%)

Incidence Less Than 1%—Causal Relationship Probable (Adverse reactions reported only in the literature, not seen in clinical trials, are considered rare and are italicized.)

Digestive: Bloody diarrhea, melena, hepatitis, jaundice, vomiting, aphthous stomatitis, appetite change, dry mouth and mucous membranes, *colitis.*

Hematologic/Lymphatic: Leukopenia, thrombocytopenia, hemoglobin decrease, epistaxis, purpura, *agranulocytosis, aplastic anemia.*

Respiratory: Asthma.

Cardiovascular: Congestive heart failure, hypertension.

Skin and Appendages: Urticaria, eczema, dermatitis, alopecia, photosensitivity, *bullous eruption, Stevens-Johnson syndrome, erythema multiforme major, allergic purpura.*

Urogenital: Azotemia, proteinuria, *acute renal failure, oliguria, interstitial nephritis, nephrotic syndrome, papillary necrosis.*

Hypersensitivity: Swelling of lips and tongue, laryngeal edema, anaphylactoid reactions, angioedema, *anaphylaxis.*

Central Nervous System: Drowsiness, depression, insomnia, anxiety, irritability.

Special Senses: Blurred vision, scotoma, diplopia, taste disorder, reversible hearing loss.

Body as a Whole: Malaise.

Incidence Less Than 1%—Causal Relationship Unknown (Adverse reactions reported only in the literature, not seen in clinical trials, are considered rare and are italicized.)

Skin and Appendages: Exfoliative dermatitis.

Cardiovascular: Myocardial infarction, palpitations, chest pain, premature ventricular contractions, tachycardia.

Hypersensitivity: Edema of the pharynx.

Digestive: Esophageal lesions.

Urogenital: Vaginal bleeding, hematuria, nocturia, impotence, urinary frequency.

Respiratory: Dyspnea, hyperventilation.

Endocrine: Hypoglycemia, *flushing.*

Central Nervous System: Paresthesia, convulsions, memory disturbances, nightmares, tremor, tic, *disorientation, psychotic reaction, abnormal coordination.*

Special Senses: Amblyopia, night blindness, vitreous floaters.

Body as a Whole: Excess perspiration, *bruising, weight loss.*

OVERDOSAGE

Worldwide reports on overdosage with diclofenac cover 27 cases. In 10 of these 27 cases, diclofenac was the only drug taken; all of these patients recovered. The highest dose of diclofenac was 2.5 g in a 20-year-old male who suffered acute renal failure as a consequence, and who was treated with three dialysis sessions and recovered in 2 days. The next highest dose was 2.35 g in a 17-year-old girl who experienced vomiting and drowsiness. A dose of 2.0 g of diclofenac was taken by a woman of unspecified age who remained asymptomatic.

Animal LD$_{50}$'s show a wide range of susceptibilities to acute overdosage with primates being more resistant to acute toxicity than rodents (LD$_{50}$ in mg/kg—rats, 55; dogs, 500; monkeys, 3200).

In case of acute overdosage it is recommended that the stomach be emptied by vomiting or lavage. Forced diuresis may theoretically be beneficial because the drug is excreted in the urine. The effect of dialysis or hemoperfusion in the elimination of Voltaren (99% protein bound, see CLINICAL PHARMACOLOGY) remains unproven. In addition to supportive measures, the use of oral activated charcoal may help to reduce the absorption and reabsorption of Voltaren.

DOSAGE AND ADMINISTRATION

Voltaren may be administered as 25-mg, 50-mg, and 75-mg enteric-coated tablets. Patients should be generally maintained on the lowest dosage of Voltaren consistent with achieving a satisfactory therapeutic response.

In osteoarthritis, the recommended dosage is 100–150 mg/day in divided doses, 50 mg b.i.d. or t.i.d., or 75 mg b.i.d. Dosages above 150 mg/day have not been studied in patients with osteoarthritis.

In rheumatoid arthritis, the recommended dosage is 150–200 mg/day in divided doses, 50 mg t.i.d. or q.i.d., or 75 mg b.i.d. Dosages above 200 mg/day have not been studied in patients with rheumatoid arthritis.

In ankylosing spondylitis, the recommended dosage is 100–125 mg/day, administered as 25 mg q.i.d. with an extra 25 mg dose at bedtime if necessary. Dosages above 125 mg/day have not been studied in patients with ankylosing spondylitis.

HOW SUPPLIED

Enteric-Coated Tablets 25 mg—yellow, round, biconvex with beveled edges (imprinted VOLTAREN 25)

Bottles of 60..NDC 0028-0058-60
Bottles of 100..NDC 0028-0058-01
Unit Dose (blister pack)
   Box of 100 (strips of 10)....................NDC 0028-0058-61
Enteric-Coated Tablets 50 mg—light brown, round, biconvex with beveled edges (imprinted VOLTAREN 50)
Bottles of 60..NDC 0028-0162-60
Bottles of 100..NDC 0028-0162-01
Bottles of 1000......................................NDC 0028-0162-10
Unit Dose (blister pack)
   Box of 100 (strips of 10)....................NDC 0028-0162-61
Enteric-Coated Tablets 75 mg—white, round, biconvex with beveled edges (imprinted VOLTAREN 75)
Bottles of 60..NDC 0028-0164-60
Bottles of 100..NDC 0028-0164-01
Bottles of 1000......................................NDC 0028-0164-10
Unit Dose (blister pack)
   Box of 100 (strips of 10)....................NDC 0028-0164-61

Samples, when available, are identified by the word *SAMPLE* appearing on each enteric-coated tablet.
Do not store above 86°F. Protect from moisture.
Dispense in tight container (USP).

C88-36 (Rev. 10/88)

Shown in Product Identification Section, page 410

GenDerm Corporation
425 HUEHL ROAD
NORTHBROOK, IL 60062

OCCLUSAL®   ℞

[ō-kloo'sal]

(Salicylic Acid, U.S.P., 17%)

DESCRIPTION

Occlusal is a topical preparation containing 17% Salicylic Acid, U.S.P., in a polyacrylic vehicle containing acrylates copolymer, butyl acetate, dibutyl phthalate, isopropyl alcohol and polyvinyl butyral. The pharmacologic activity of Occlusal is generally attributed to the keratolytic action of Salicylic Acid. The structural formula of Salicylic Acid is:

CLINICAL PHARMACOLOGY

Although the exact mode of action of Salicylic Acid in the treatment of warts is not known, its activity appears to be associated with its keratolytic action which results in mechanical removal of epidermal cells infected with wart viruses.

INDICATIONS AND USAGE

Occlusal is indicated in the treatment and removal of common warts and plantar warts.

CONTRAINDICATIONS

Occlusal should not be used by diabetics or patients with impaired blood circulation. Occlusal should not be used on moles, birthmarks, unusual warts with hair growing from them, or warts on the face.

PRECAUTIONS

Occlusal is for external use only. Do not permit Occlusal to contact eyes or mucous membranes. If contact with eyes or mucous membranes occurs, immediately flush with water for 15 minutes. Occlusal should not be allowed to contact normal skin surrounding wart. Treatment should be discontinued if excessive irritation occurs. Occlusal is flammable and should be kept away from fire or flame. Keep bottle tightly capped when not in use.

ADVERSE REACTIONS

A localized irritant reaction may occur if Occlusal is applied to the normal skin surrounding the wart. Any irritation may normally be controlled by temporarily discontinuing use of Occlusal, and by applying the medication only to the wart site when treatment is resumed.

DOSAGE AND ADMINISTRATION

Prior to application of Occlusal, soak wart in warm water for five minutes. Remove any loosened tissue by gently rubbing with a brush, wash cloth, or emery board. Dry thoroughly. Using the brush applicator supplied, apply twice to affected area, allowing the first application to dry before applying the second. Treatment should be once a day and should continue as directed by physician. Be careful not to apply to surrounding skin.

Clinically visible improvement will normally occur during the first two to four weeks of therapy. Maximum resolution may be expected after six to twelve weeks of drug use.

HOW SUPPLIED

½ fl. oz. bottle with brush applicator, (NDC 52761-121-15).
U.S. Patent No. 4588590

OCCLUSAL®–HP   ℞
[ŏ-kloo'sal]
(Salicylic Acid, U.S.P.)
26% Solution in a
Polyacrylic Vehicle
HIGH POTENCY WART REMOVER
FOR TOPICAL USE

DESCRIPTION

Occlusal-HP is a topical preparation containing 26% Salicylic Acid, U.S.P., in a polyacrylic vehicle containing acrylates copolymer, butyl acetate, dibutyl phthalate, isopropyl alcohol and polyvinyl butyral. The pharmacologic activity of Occlusal-HP is generally attributed to the keratolytic action of Salicylic Acid. The structural formula of Salicylic Acid is:

CLINICAL PHARMACOLOGY

Although the exact mode of action of Salicylic Acid in the treatment of warts is not known, its activity appears to be associated with its keratolytic action which results in mechanical removal of epidermal cells infected with wart viruses.

INDICATIONS AND USAGE

Occlusal-HP is indicated in the treatment and removal of common warts and plantar warts.

CONTRAINDICATIONS

Occlusal-HP should not be used by diabetics or patients with impaired blood circulation. Occlusal-HP should not be used on moles, birthmarks, unusual warts with hair growing from them, or warts on the face.

PRECAUTIONS

Occlusal-HP is for external use only. Do not permit Occlusal-HP to contact eyes or mucous membranes. If contact with eyes or mucous membranes occurs, immediately flush with water for 15 minutes. Occlusal-HP should not be allowed to contact normal skin surrounding wart. Treatment should be discontinued if excessive irritation occurs. Occlusal-HP is flammable and should be kept away from fire or flame. Keep bottle tightly capped when not in use.

ADVERSE REACTIONS

A localized irritant reaction may occur if Occlusal-HP is applied to the normal skin surrounding the wart. Any irritation may normally be controlled by temporarily discontinuing use of Occlusal-HP, and by applying the medication only to the wart site when treatment is resumed.

DOSAGE AND ADMINISTRATION

Prior to application of Occlusal-HP, soak wart in warm water for five minutes. Remove any loosened tissue by gently rubbing with a brush, wash cloth, or emery board. Dry thoroughly. Using the brush applicator supplied, apply twice to the entire wart surface, allowing the first application to dry before applying the second. Treatment should be once or twice a day and should continue as directed by physician. Be careful not to apply to surrounding skin.
Clinically visible improvement will normally occur during the first or second week of therapy. Maximum resolution may be expected after four to six weeks of drug use.

HOW SUPPLIED

10 ml amber bottle with brush applicator (NDC 52761-135-10).
U.S. Patent No. 4588590

OVIDE™ Lotion   ℞
[ŏ-vĭd]
(Malathion) 0.5% (w/v)

DESCRIPTION

OVIDE (malathion) Lotion is a liquid for topical application to the hair and scalp as a lousicide and ovicide. Each mL contains 0.005 mg of malathion in a vehicle of isopropyl alcohol (78%), terpineol, dipentene and pine needle oil. Malathion insecticide, has a molecular weight of 330.36 represented by $C_{10}H_{19}O_6PS_2$ and depicted as:

CLINICAL PHARMACOLOGY

Malathion is lousicidal and ovicidal *in vitro*. Louse eggs succumb to 3 seconds of exposure to 0.062% malathion in acetone and lice to about 0.003% respectively. Resistance to malathion could not be induced.
Human safety studies included a 21-day cumulative irritancy and others undertaken to determine the potential for contact sensitization, phototoxicity, and photo-contact sensitization. Application of OVIDE Lotion showed no evidence of sensitization and a very low level of irritation.

INDICATIONS AND USAGE

OVIDE Lotion is indicated for the treatment of head lice and their ova.

CONTRAINDICATIONS

OVIDE Lotion should not be used by individuals with known sensitivity to OVIDE Lotion or to any of its components.

WARNINGS

This product is flammable and open flames or hair dryers should be avoided to allow the hair to dry naturally and uncovered.

PRECAUTIONS

If accidentally placed in the eye, flush immediately with water.
Carcinogenesis, Mutagenesis and Fertility—Malathion is neither carcinogenic in male or female F344 rats after 2 years feeding with up to 4000 ppm (0.4%) nor is it tumorigenic in Osborn-Mendel rats or B6C3F1 mice after a similar feeding for 80 weeks with 8,000 ppm (0.8%) and 16,000 ppm (1.6%) respectively. Tests for mutagenicity have not been conducted.
Pregnancy Category B—There was no evidence of teratogenicity in studies utilizing single i.p. injections of malathion at 600 and 900 mg/kg in pregnant rats or oral dosing with up to 300 mg/kg on days 6 through 15 of gestation. A reproduction study in rats failed to show any gross fetal abnormalities attributable to feeding malathion up to 2,500 ppm in the diet during a three-generation evaluation period. These studies employed at least 50 to 70 times the adult human topical dose.
Because animal reproduction studies are not always predictive of human response, this drug should be used during pregnancy only if clearly needed.
Nursing Mothers—Malathion in an acetone vehicle has been reported to be absorbed through human skin only to the extent of 8% of the applied dose. However, percutaneous absorption from the OVIDE Lotion formulation has not been studied and it is not known whether malathion is excreted in human milk. Caution should be exercised when OVIDE Lotion is administered to the nursing mother.

ADVERSE REACTIONS

Irritation of the scalp has been reported.

OVERDOSAGE

Consideration should be given as part of the treatment program to the high concentration of isopropyl alcohol in the vehicle.
Malathion, although a weaker cholinesterase inhibitor and therefore safer than other organophosphates, may be expected to exhibit the same symptoms of cholinesterase depletion after accidental ingestion orally. Vomiting should be induced promptly or the stomach lavaged with 5% sodium bicarbonate solution.
Severe respiratory distress is the major and most serious symptom of organophosphate poisoning requiring artificial respiration and large doses of i.m. or i.v. atropine. The usual starting dose of atropine is 1 to 4 mg with supplementation hourly as needed to counteract the symptoms of cholinesterase depletion. Repeat analyses of serum and RBC cholinesterase assist in establishing the diagnosis and formulating a long-range prognosis.

DOSAGE AND ADMINISTRATION

1. Sprinkle OVIDE Lotion on DRY hair and rub gently until the scalp is thoroughly moistened. Pay special attention to the back of the head and neck.
2. Allow to dry naturally—use no heat and leave uncovered.
3. After 8–12 hours, the hair should be washed with a non-medicated shampoo.
4. Rinse and use a fine-toothed comb to remove dead lice and eggs.
5. If required, repeat with second application of OVIDE Lotion in 7 to 9 days.
Further treatment is generally not necessary. Other family members should be evaluated to determine if infested and if so, receive treatment.

HOW SUPPLIED

OVIDE (malathion) Lotion in bottles of 2 fl oz (59 mL)
NDC 52761-637-02.
Store at controlled room temperature 15°–30°C (59°–86°F).
Caution: Federal law prohibits dispensing without prescription.
Rev. May, 1989

PENTRAX®
[pen'trax]
Tar Shampoo with Fractar®

DESCRIPTION

Pentrax Tar Shampoo contains 8.75% Fractar (equal to 4.3% crude coal tar), a standardized tar extract, a blend of highly concentrated detergents, and conditioning agents. Spectrophotometric standardization, based on hydrocarbon analysis, assures uniform therapeutic activity from batch to batch. Pentrax Tar Shampoo does not contain parabens or other preservatives. Pentrax Tar Shampoo contains the highest concentration of coal tar currently available. Fractar consists of the desirable crude coal tar fractions without undesirable residues. It has excellent lathering qualities and leaves hair clean and manageable.

ACTION AND INDICATIONS

Coal tar helps correct abnormalities of keratinization by decreasing epidermal proliferation and dermal infiltration. Pentrax Tar Shampoo is indicated for relief of itching, irritation, redness, flaking and/or scaling associated with dandruff, seborrheic dermatitis, cradle cap or psoriasis.

WARNINGS

FOR EXTERNAL USE ONLY. Avoid contact with the eyes—if this happens, rinse thoroughly with water. Do not use for prolonged periods without consulting a physician. If condition worsens or does not improve after regular use of this product as directed, consult a physician.

ACTIVE INGREDIENTS

Fractar, a patented extract of coal tar, equivalent to coal tar 4.3%.

INACTIVE INGREDIENTS

Cocamide DEA, Dioctyl sodium sulfosuccinate, Isopropyl myristate, Lauramide oxide, Laureth-23, PEG-8, Sodium lauryl sulfate and Squalane.

DIRECTIONS

Massage into wet hair and scalp to produce a lather. Rinse. Reapply liberally allowing lather to remain on hair up to 10 minutes. Rinse thoroughly. For best results, use at least twice a week or as directed by a physician.

HOW SUPPLIED

4 fl. oz. plastic bottle (NDC 52761-665-04) and
8 fl. oz. plastic bottle (NDC 52761-665-08)

PRAMEGEL®
[pram'eh-gel]
Antipruritic

DESCRIPTION

PrameGel is an antipruritic containing pramoxine hydrochloride 1% and menthol 0.5% in a water soluble emollient base with a naturally derived humectant. PrameGel is propylene glycol, paraben and fragrance free.

INDICATIONS

PrameGel provides prompt temporary relief of itching associated with eczemas (including poison ivy and poison oak), insect bites, heat rash, sunburn, and other pruritic skin conditions, as well as for external anal itching.

WARNINGS

FOR EXTERNAL USE ONLY. Avoid contact with the eyes. If itching worsens or if symptoms persist for more than 7 days, advise your physician. Keep this and all medications out of the reach of children.

ACTIVE INGREDIENTS

Pramoxine hydrochloride 1% and menthol 0.5%.

INACTIVE INGREDIENTS

Benzyl alcohol, Carbomer 940, Methyl gluceth-20, SD Alcohol 40, Sodium hydroxide and Water.

DIRECTIONS

Adults and children 2 years of age and older: Apply PrameGel liberally to affected area 3 to 4 times daily. Children under 2 years of age: As directed by your physician.

HOW SUPPLIED

4 fl. oz. plastic bottle (NDC 52761-395-04).

SALAC®
[sal'ak]
Acne Medication-Cleanser

DESCRIPTION

SalAc is an acne medication-cleanser containing 2% salicylic acid in a surfactant blend especially formulated to remove excess sebum.

Continued on next page

GenDerm—Cont.

INDICATIONS
For the management of acne. Helps prevent new comedones papules, and pustules.

PRECAUTIONS
For External Use Only. Keep Cleanser Out of Eyes. Keep Out of Reach of Children. If undue skin irritation develops or increases, adjust usage schedule or consult your physician.

ACTIVE INGREDIENTS
Salicylic acid 2%

INACTIVE INGREDIENTS
Benzyl Alcohol, Lauramide DEA, PEG-7 Glyceryl Cocoate, Polystyrene Dispersion, Purified Water, Sodium C_{14-16} Olefin Sulfonate and Sodium Chloride.

DIRECTIONS
Wash affected area 2–3 times daily. Lather with warm water, massage into skin, rinse, and dry.

HOW SUPPLIED
6 fl. oz. plastic bottle (NDC 52761-077-06).

ZOSTRIX®
[zos'trix]
(Capsaicin 0.025%)
Topical Analgesic Cream

PRODUCT OVERVIEW
KEY FACTS
Zostrix cream contains capsaicin which works via localized depletion of substance P, an endogenous neuropeptide involved in the transmission of pain impulses.

MAJOR USES
Zostrix cream is applied to the skin only after the zoster lesions have healed. Zostrix has proven to be clinically effective in controlling the pain in patients with a history of post-herpetic neuralgia.

SAFETY INFORMATION
Patients may experience a warm, stinging, or burning sensation at the site of application, especially during the initial 24 to 72 hours of use. This effect is related to the pharmacologic action.

PRESCRIBING INFORMATION
ZOSTRIX®
[zos'trix]
(Capsaicin 0.025%)
Topical Analgesic Cream

DESCRIPTION
Zostrix cream contains capsaicin .025% in an emollient base. Capsaicin is a natural chemical derived from plants of the Solanaceae family with the chemical name trans-8-methyl-N-vanillyl-6-nonenamide. Capsaicin is a white crystalline powder with a molecular weight of 305.4. It is practically insoluble in water but very soluble in alcohol, ether, and chloroform.

ACTION AND INDICATIONS
Although the precise mechanism of action of capsaicin is not fully understood, current evidence suggests that capsaicin renders skin insensitive to pain by depleting and preventing reaccumulation of substance P in peripheral sensory neurons. Substance P is thought to be the principal chemomediator of pain impulses from the periphery to the central nervous system.
Zostrix cream is indicated for the temporary relief of pain (neuralgia) following Herpes Zoster infections after open skin lesions have healed.

WARNINGS
FOR EXTERNAL USE ONLY. Avoid getting in eyes or on broken or irritated skin. Do not bandage tightly. If condition worsens, or does not improve after 28 days, discontinue use of this product and consult your physician.

DIRECTIONS
Adults and children 2 years of age or older: Apply Zostrix to affected area 3 or 4 times daily. Zostrix may cause transient burning on application. This burning usually disappears in 24–72 hours and is observed more frequently when application schedules of less than 3 or 4 times daily are utilized. After Zostrix is applied with the fingers, the hands should be washed immediately afterwards.

HOW SUPPLIED
1½ oz. tubes (NDC 52761-552-45)
U.S. Patents No. 4486450, 5536404

Genentech, Inc.
460 POINT SAN BRUNO BLVD.
SOUTH SAN FRANCISCO, CA 94080

ACTIVASE® ℞
Alteplase, recombinant

DESCRIPTION
ACTIVASE®, Alteplase, is a tissue plasminogen activator produced by recombinant DNA technology. It is a sterile, purified glycoprotein of 527 amino acids. It is synthesized using the complementary DNA (cDNA) for natural human tissue-type plasminogen activator obtained from a human melanoma cell line. The manufacturing process involves the secretion of the enzyme, alteplase, into the culture medium by an established mammalian cell line (Chinese Hamster Ovary cells) into which the cDNA for alteplase has been genetically inserted.
ACTIVASE® is a sterile, white to off-white, lyophilized powder for intravenous administration after reconstitution with Sterile Water for Injection, USP. The quantitative composition of the lyophilized product is:

50 mg (29 million IU) Vial	20 mg (11.6 million IU) Vial
Alteplase 50 mg (29 million IU)	Alteplase 20 mg (11.6 million IU)
L-Arginine 1.7 g	L-Arginine 0.7 g
Phosphoric Acid 0.5 g	Phosphoric Acid 0.2 g
Polysorbate 80, less than 4 mg	Polysorbate 80, less than 1.6 mg

Phosphoric acid and/or sodium hydroxide may be used prior to lyophilization for pH adjustment.
Biological potency is determined by an *in vitro* clot lysis assay and is expressed in International Units as tested against the WHO standard. The specific activity of ACTIVASE® is 580,000 IU/mg.

CLINICAL PHARMACOLOGY
ACTIVASE® is an enzyme (serine protease) which has the property of fibrin-enhanced conversion of plasminogen to plasmin. It produces limited conversion of plasminogen in the absence of fibrin. When introduced into the systemic circulation at pharmacologic concentration, ACTIVASE® binds to fibrin in a thrombus and converts the entrapped plasminogen to plasmin. This initiates local fibrinolysis with limited systemic proteolysis. Following administration of 100 mg ACTIVASE®, there is a decrease (16–36%) in circulating fibrinogen.[1,2] In a controlled trial, 8 of 73 patients (11%) receiving ACTIVASE® (1.25 mg/kg body weight over 3 hours) experienced a decrease in fibrinogen to below 100 mg/dL.[2]
ACTIVASE® is cleared rapidly from circulating plasma at a rate of 550–680 mL/min. ACTIVASE® is cleared primarily by the liver. More than 50% of ACTIVASE® present in plasma is cleared within 5 minutes after the infusion has been terminated, and approximately 80% is cleared within 10 minutes.
Coronary occlusion due to a thrombus is present in the infarct-related coronary artery in approximately 80% of patients experiencing a transmural myocardial infarction evaluated within four hours of onset of symptoms.[3,4]
In patients studied in a controlled trial with coronary angiography at 90 and 120 minutes following infusion of ACTIVASE®, Alteplase, recombinant, infarct artery patency was observed in 71% and 85% of patients (n=85), respectively.[2] In a second study, where patients received coronary angiography prior to and following infusion of ACTIVASE® within six hours of the onset of symptoms, reperfusion of the obstructed vessel occurred within 90 minutes after the commencement of therapy in 71% of 83 patients.[1]
In a double blind, randomized trial (138 patients) comparing ACTIVASE® to placebo, patients infused with ACTIVASE® within 4 hours of onset of symptoms experienced improved left ventricular function at day 10 compared to the placebo group, when ejection fraction was measured by gated blood pool scan (53.2% versus 46.4%, p=0.018). Relative to baseline (day 1) values, the net changes in ejection fraction were +3.6% and −4.7% for the treated and placebo group, respectively (p=0.0001). Also documented was a reduced incidence of clinical congestive heart failure in the treated group (14%) compared to the placebo group (33%) (p=0.009).[5]
In a second double blind randomized trial (145 patients) comparing ACTIVASE® to placebo, patients infused with ACTIVASE® within 2.5 hours of onset of symptoms experienced improved left ventricular function at a mean of 21 days compared to the placebo group, when ejection fraction was measured by gated blood pool scan (52% versus 48%, p=0.08) and by contrast ventriculogram (61% versus 54%, p=0.006). Although the contribution of ACTIVASE® alone is unclear, the incidence of nonischemic cardiac complica-

tions when taken as a group (i.e., congestive heart failure, pericarditis, atrial fibrillation, conduction disturbance) was reduced when compared to those patients treated with placebo (p <0.01).[6]
In a double blind randomized trial (5013 patients) comparing ACTIVASE® to placebo (ASSET study), patients infused with ACTIVASE® within five hours of the onset of symptoms of acute myocardial infarction experienced improved 30-day survival compared to those treated with placebo. At one month the overall mortality rates were 7.2% for the ACTIVASE® treated group and 9.8% for the placebo treated group (p=0.001).[7,8] This benefit was maintained at 6 months for ACTIVASE® treated patients (10.4%) compared to those treated with placebo (13.1%) (p=0.008).[8]
In a second double blind randomized trial (721 patients) comparing ACTIVASE® to placebo, patients infused with ACTIVASE® within five hours of the onset of symptoms experienced improved ventricular function 10–22 days after treatment compared to the placebo group, when global ejection fraction was measured by contrast ventriculography (50.7% versus 48.5%, p=0.01). Patients treated with ACTIVASE® had a 19% reduction in infarct size, as measured by cumulative release of HBDH (α-hydroxybutyrate dehydrogenase) activity compared to placebo treated patients (p=0.001). Patients treated with ACTIVASE® had significantly fewer episodes of cardiogenic shock (p=0.02), ventricular fibrillation (p<0.04) and pericarditis (p=0.01) compared to patients treated with placebo. Mortality at 21 days in ACTIVASE® treated patients was reduced to 3.7% compared to 6.3% in placebo treated patients (1p=0.05).[9] Although these data do not demonstrate unequivocally a significant reduction in mortality for this study, they do indicate a trend that is supported by the results of the ASSET study.

INDICATIONS AND USAGE
Acute Myocardial Infarction
ACTIVASE® is indicated for use in the management of acute myocardial infarction (AMI) in adults for the lysis of thrombi obstructing coronary arteries, the reduction of infarct size, the improvement of ventricular function following AMI, the reduction of the incidence of congestive heart failure and the reduction of mortality associated with AMI. Treatment should be initiated as soon as possible after the onset of AMI symptoms (see CLINICAL PHARMACOLOGY).

CONTRAINDICATIONS
Because thrombolytic therapy increases the risk of bleeding, ACTIVASE® is contraindicated in the following situations: ● Active internal bleeding ● History of cerebrovascular accident ● Recent (within two months) intracranial, or intraspinal, surgery or trauma (see WARNINGS) ● Intracranial neoplasm, arteriovenous malformation, or aneurysm ● Known bleeding diathesis ● Severe uncontrolled hypertension.

WARNINGS
Bleeding: The most common complication encountered during ACTIVASE® therapy is bleeding. The type of bleeding associated with thrombolytic therapy can be divided into two broad categories: ● Internal bleeding, involving the gastrointestinal tract, genitourinary tract, retroperitoneal or intracranial sites ● Superficial or surface bleeding, observed mainly at invaded or disturbed sites (e.g., venous cutdowns, arterial punctures, sites of recent surgical intervention).
The concomitant use of heparin anticoagulation may contribute to the bleeding. Some of the hemorrhagic episodes occurred one or more days after the effects of ACTIVASE® had dissipated, but while heparin therapy was continuing.
As fibrin is lysed during ACTIVASE®, Alteplase, recombinant, therapy, bleeding from recent puncture sites may occur. Therefore, thrombolytic therapy requires careful attention to all potential bleeding sites (including catheter insertion sites, arterial and venous puncture sites, cutdown sites and needle puncture sites).
Intramuscular injections and nonessential handling of the patient should be avoided during treatment with ACTIVASE®. Venipunctures should be performed carefully and only as required.
Should an arterial puncture be necessary during an infusion of ACTIVASE®, it is preferable to use an upper extremity vessel that is accessible to manual compression. Pressure should be applied for at least 30 minutes, a pressure dressing applied and the puncture site checked frequently for evidence of bleeding.
Should serious bleeding (not controllable by local pressure) occur, the infusion of ACTIVASE® and any concomitant heparin should be terminated immediately.
Each patient being considered for therapy with ACTIVASE® should be carefully evaluated and anticipated benefits weighed against potential risks associated with therapy.
In the following conditions, the risks of ACTIVASE® therapy may be increased and should be weighed against the anticipated benefits: ● Recent (within 10 days) major surgery, e.g., coronary artery bypass graft, obstetrical delivery,

organ biopsy, previous puncture of noncompressible vessels • Cerebrovascular disease • Recent gastrointestinal or genitourinary bleeding (within 10 days) • Recent trauma (within 10 days) • Hypertension: systolic BP ≥ 180 mm Hg and/or diastolic BP ≥ 110 mm Hg • High likelihood of left heart thrombus, e.g., mitral stenosis with atrial fibrillation • Acute pericarditis • Subacute bacterial endocarditis • Hemostatic defects including those secondary to severe hepatic or renal disease • Significant liver dysfunction • Pregnancy • Diabetic hemorrhagic retinopathy, or other hemorrhagic ophthalmic conditions • Septic thrombophlebitis or occluded AV cannula at seriously infected site • Advanced age, i.e., over 75 years old • Patients currently receiving oral anticoagulants, e.g., warfarin sodium • Any other condition in which bleeding constitutes a significant hazard or would be particularly difficult to manage because of its location.

Arrhythmias: Coronary thrombolysis may result in arrhythmias associated with reperfusion. These arrhythmias (such as sinus bradycardia, accelerated idioventricular rhythm, ventricular premature depolarizations, ventricular tachycardia) are not different from those often seen in the ordinary course of acute myocardial infarction and may be managed with standard antiarrhythmic measures. It is recommended that antiarrhythmic therapy for bradycardia and/or ventricular irritability be available when infusions of ACTIVASE®, Alteplase, are administered.

PRECAUTIONS

General: Standard management of myocardial infarction should be implemented concomitantly with ACTIVASE® treatment. Noncompressible arterial puncture must be avoided (i.e., internal jugular and subclavian punctures should be avoided to minimize bleeding from noncompressible sites). Arterial and venous punctures should be minimized. In the event of serious bleeding, ACTIVASE® and heparin should be discontinued immediately. Heparin effects can be reversed by protamine.

Readministration: There is no experience with readministration of ACTIVASE®. If an anaphylactoid reaction occurs, the infusion should be discontinued immediately and appropriate therapy initiated.

Although sustained antibody formation in patients receiving one dose of ACTIVASE® has not been documented, readministration should be undertaken with caution. Detectable levels of antibody (a single point measurement) were reported in one patient but subsequent antibody test results were negative.

Laboratory Tests: During ACTIVASE® therapy, if coagulation tests and/or measures of fibrinolytic activity are performed, the results may be unreliable unless specific precautions are taken to prevent *in vitro* artifacts. ACTIVASE® is an enzyme that when present in blood in pharmacologic concentrations remains active under *in vitro* conditions. This can lead to degradation of fibrinogen in blood samples removed for analysis. Collection of blood samples in the presence of aprotinin (150–200 units/mL) can to some extent mitigate this phenomenon.

Drug Interactions: The interaction of ACTIVASE® with other cardioactive drugs has not been studied. In addition to bleeding associated with heparin and vitamin K antagonists, drugs that alter platelet function (such as acetylsalicylic acid, dipyridamole) may increase the risk of bleeding if administered prior to, during or after ACTIVASE® therapy.

Use of Anticoagulants: Heparin has been administered concomitantly with and following infusions of ACTIVASE® to reduce the risk of rethrombosis. Because either heparin or ACTIVASE® alone may cause bleeding complications, careful monitoring for bleeding is advised, especially at arterial puncture sites.

Pregnancy (Category C): Animal reproduction studies have not been conducted with ACTIVASE®. It is also not known whether ACTIVASE® can cause fetal harm when administered to a pregnant woman or can affect reproduction capacity. ACTIVASE® should be given to a pregnant woman only if clearly needed.

Pediatric Use: Safety and effectiveness of ACTIVASE® in children has not been established.

Carcinogenesis, Mutagenesis, Impairment of Fertility: Long-term studies in animals have not been performed to evaluate the carcinogenic potential or the effect on fertility. Short-term studies, which evaluated tumorigenicity of ACTIVASE® and effect on tumor metastases in rodents, were negative.

Studies to determine mutagenicity (Ames test) and chromosomal aberration assays in human lymphocytes were negative at all concentrations tested. Cytotoxicity, as reflected by a decrease in mitotic index, was evidenced only after prolonged exposure and only at the highest concentrations tested.

Nursing Mothers: It is not known whether ACTIVASE® is excreted in human milk. Because many drugs are excreted in human milk, caution should be exercised when ACTIVASE®, Alteplase, is administered to a nursing woman.

ADVERSE REACTIONS

Bleeding: The most frequent adverse reaction associated with ACTIVASE®, Alteplase, recombinant, is bleeding. The type of bleeding associated with thrombolytic therapy can be divided into two broad categories: • Internal bleeding, involving the gastrointestinal tract, genitourinary tract, retroperitoneal or intracranial sites • Superficial or surface bleeding, observed mainly at invaded or disturbed sites (e.g., venous cutdowns, arterial punctures, sites of recent surgical intervention).

The following incidence of significant bleeding (estimated as > 250 cc blood loss) has been reported in studies in over 800 patients treated at all doses:

	Total Dose ≤ 100 mg	Total Dose > 100 mg
gastrointestinal	5%	5%
genitourinary	4%	4%
ecchymosis	1%	<1%
retroperitoneal	<1%	<1%
epistaxis	<1%	<1%
gingival	<1%	<1%

The incidence of intracranial bleeding (ICB) in patients treated with ACTIVASE® is as follows:

Dose	Number of Patients	%
100 mg	3272	0.4
150 mg	1779	1.3
1–1.4 mg/kg	237	0.4

These data indicate that a dose of 150 mg of ACTIVASE® should not be used because it has been associated with an increase in intracranial bleeding.

Recent data indicate that the incidence of stroke in 6 randomized double blind placebo controlled trials[2,5-10] is not significantly different in the ACTIVASE® treated patients compared to those treated with placebo (37/3161, 1.2% versus 27/3092, 0.9%, respectively) (p=0.26).

Should serious bleeding in a critical location (intracranial, gastrointestinal, retroperitoneal, pericardial) occur, ACTIVASE® therapy should be discontinued immediately, along with any concomitant therapy with heparin.

Fibrin which is part of the hemostatic plug formed at needle puncture sites will be lysed during ACTIVASE® therapy. Therefore, ACTIVASE® therapy requires careful attention to potential bleeding sites, e.g., catheter insertion sites, arterial puncture sites.

Allergic Reactions: No serious or life-threatening allergic reactions have been reported. Other mild hypersensitivity reactions such as urticaria have been observed occasionally.

Other Adverse Reactions: Other adverse reactions have been reported, principally nausea and/or vomiting, hypotension, and fever. These reactions are frequent sequelae of myocardial infarction and may or may not be attributable to ACTIVASE® therapy.

DOSAGE AND ADMINISTRATION

Administer ACTIVASE® as soon as possible after the onset of symptoms.

ACTIVASE® is for intravenous administration only.

The recommended dose is 100 mg administered as 60 mg (34.8 million IU) in the first hour (of which 6 to 10 mg is administered as a bolus over the first 1–2 minutes), 20 mg (11.6 million IU) over the second hour, and 20 mg (11.6 million IU) over the third hour. For smaller patients (less than 65 kg), a dose of 1.25 mg/kg administered over 3 hours, as described above, may be used.[11]

A DOSE OF 150 MG OF ACTIVASE®, ALTEPLASE, SHOULD NOT BE USED BECAUSE IT HAS BEEN ASSOCIATED WITH AN INCREASE IN INTRACRANIAL BLEEDING.

Although the use of anticoagulants and antiplatelet drugs during and following administration of ACTIVASE® has not been shown to be of unequivocal benefit, heparin has been administered concomitantly for 24 hours or longer in more than 90% of patients. Aspirin and/or dipyridamole have been given either during and/or following heparin treatment.

Reconstitution and Dilution: DO NOT USE IF VACUUM IS NOT PRESENT.

ACTIVASE® should be reconstituted by aseptically adding the appropriate volume of the accompanying Sterile Water for Injection, USP, to the vial. It is important that ACTIVASE® be reconstituted only with Sterile Water for Injection, USP, without preservatives. Do not use Bacteriostatic Water for Injection, USP. The reconstituted preparation results in a colorless to pale yellow transparent solution containing ACTIVASE® 1.0 mg/mL at approximately pH 7.3. The osmolality of this solution is approximately 215 mOsm/kg.

Reconstitution should be carried out using a large bore needle (e.g., 18 gauge), directing the stream of Sterile Water for Injection, USP into the lyophilized cake. Slight foaming upon reconstitution is not unusual; standing undisturbed for

several minutes is usually sufficient to allow dissipation of any large bubbles.

Because ACTIVASE® contains no antibacterial preservatives, it should be reconstituted immediately before use. The solution may be used for intravenous administration within 8 hours following reconstitution when stored between 2–30°C. Before further dilution or administration the product should be visually inspected for particulate matter and discoloration prior to administration whenever solution and container permit.

ACTIVASE® may be administered as reconstituted at 1.0 mg/mL. As an alternative, the reconstituted solution may be diluted further immediately before administration in an equal volume of 0.9% Sodium Chloride Injection, USP or 5% Dextrose Injection, USP to yield a concentration of 0.5 mg/mL. Either polyvinyl chloride bags or glass bottles are acceptable. ACTIVASE® is stable for up to 8 hours in these solutions at room temperature. Exposure to light has no effect on the stability of these solutions. Excessive agitation during dilution should be avoided; mixing should be accomplished with gentle swirling and/or slow inversion. Do not use other infusion solutions, e.g., Sterile Water for Injection, USP or preservative-containing solutions for further dilution.

No other medication should be added to infusion solutions containing ACTIVASE®, Alteplase. Any unused infusion solution should be discarded.

HOW SUPPLIED

ACTIVASE®is supplied as a sterile, lyophilized powder in 20 mg and 50 mg vials containing vacuum.

Each 20 mg ACTIVASE® vial (11.6 million IU) is packaged with diluent for reconstitution. (20 mL Sterile Water for Injection, USP): NDC 50242-044-12.

Each 50 mg ACTIVASE® vial (29.0 million IU) is packaged with diluent for reconstitution. (50 mL Sterile Water for Injection, USP): NDC 50242-044-13.

Storage: Store lyophilized ACTIVASE® at controlled room temperature not to exceed 30°C (86°F), or under refrigeration (2–8°C/36–46°F). Protect the lyophilized material during extended storage from excessive exposure to light. Do not use beyond the expiration date stamped on the vial.

REFERENCES

1. Mueller, H., Rao, A.K., Forman, S.A., et al., Thrombolysis in Myocardial Infarction (TIMI): Comparative Studies of Coronary Reperfusion and Systemic Fibrinogenolysis with Two Forms of Recombinant Tissue-Type Plasminogen Activator. J. Am. Coll. Card. 10: 479–490, 1987.
2. Topol, E.J., Morriss, D.C., Smalling, R.W., et al., A Multicenter, Randomized, Placebo-Controlled Trial of a New Form of Intravenous Recombinant Tissue-Type Plasminogen Activator (Activase®) in Acute Myocardial Infarction. J. Am. Coll. Card. 9: 1205–1213, 1987.
3. De Wood, M.A., Spores, J., Notske, R., et al., Prevalence of Total Coronary Occlusion during the Early Hours of Transmural Myocardial Infarction. New Eng. J. Med. 303: 897–902, 1980.
4. Chesebro, J.H., Knatterud, G., Roberts, R., et al., Thrombolysis in Myocardial Infarction (TIMI) Trial, Phase I: A Comparison between Intravenous Tissue Plasminogen Activator and Intravenous Streptokinase. Circulation 76, No. 1, 142–154, July, 1987.
5. Guerci, A.D., Gerstenblith, G., Brinker, J.A., et al., A Randomized Trial of Intravenous Tissue Plasminogen Activator for Acute Myocardial Infarction with Subsequent Randomization of Elective Coronary Angioplasty. New Eng. J. Med. 317: 1613–1618, 1987.
6. O'Rourke, M., Baron, D., Keogh, A., et al., Limitation of Myocardial Infarction by Early Infusion of Recombinant Tissue-Plasminogen Activator. Circulation 77: 1311–1315, 1988.
7. Wilcox, R.G., von der Lippe, G., Olsson, C.G., et al., Trial of Tissue Plasminogen Activator for Mortality Reduction in Acute Myocardial Infarction: ASSET. Lancet 2: 525–530, 1988.
8. Hampton, J.R., The University of Nottingham, Personal Communication.
9. Van de Werf, F., Arnold, A.E.R., et al., Effect of Intravenous Tissue-Plasminogen Activator on Infarct Size, Left Ventricular Function and Survival in Patients with Acute Myocardial Infarction. Br. Med. J. 297: 1374–1379, 1988.
10. National Heart Foundation of Australia Coronary Thrombolysis Group: Coronary Thrombolysis and Myocardial Infarction Salvage by Tissue Plasminogen Activator Given up to 4 Hours After Onset of Myocardial Infarction. Lancet 1: 203–207, 1988.
11. Califf, R.M., Stump, D., Thornton, D., et al., Hemorrhagic Complications After Tissue Plasminogen Activator (t-PA) Therapy for Acute Myocardial Infarction. Circulation 76: IV-1, 1987.

Continued on next page

Genentech—Cont.

ACTIVASE®, Alteplase, recombinant
Manufactured by
GENENTECH®, INC.
460 Point San Bruno Boulevard
South San Francisco, CA 94080
April, 1989
G48005-R2
For further information, call 1-800-821-8590.
Shown in Product Identification Section, page 410

PROTROPIN®
(somatrem for injection)   ℞

DESCRIPTION
Protropin is the Genentech trademark for somatrem, a polypeptide hormone which is of recombinant DNA origin. Protropin has 192 amino acid residues and a molecular weight of about 22,000 daltons. The product contains the identical sequence of 191 amino acids constituting pituitary-derived human growth hormone plus an additional amino acid, methionine, on the N-terminus of the molecule. Protropin growth hormone is synthesized in a special laboratory strain of **E. coli** bacteria which has been modified by the addition of the gene for human growth hormone production. Protropin growth hormone, a sterile, white, lyophilized powder, is intended for intramuscular or subcutaneous administration after reconstitution with Bacteriostatic Water for Injection, USP (Benzyl Alcohol Preserved).
The quantitative composition of the lyophilized drug per vial is:

Somatrem 5.0 mg (approximately 13 IU)
Mannitol 40.0 mg
Sodium Phosphates 1.7 mg
(Monobasic Sodium Phosphate 0.1 mg and
Dibasic Sodium Phosphate 1.6 mg)

Phosphoric acid may be used for pH adjustment.
Protropin growth hormone is a highly purified preparation. Biological potency is determined by measuring the increase in body weight induced in hypophysectomized rats.
Bacteriostatic Water for Injection, USP (Benzyl Alcohol Preserved) is a sterile water for injection packaged in a multiple dose vial. It contains an antimicrobial preservative. Each mL contains 0.9 percent benzyl alcohol. The pH is 4.5–7.0.

CLINICAL PHARMACOLOGY
Linear Growth
The primary and most intensively studied action of Protropin (somatrem for injection) is the stimulation of linear growth. This effect is demonstrated in patients lacking adequate endogenous growth hormone production.
In vitro, preclinical, and clinical testing has demonstrated that Protropin growth hormone is therapeutically equivalent to somatropin (human growth hormone, pituitary origin). Short term clinical studies in normal adults show equivalent pharmacokinetics. Treatment of growth hormone deficient children with Protropin growth hormone results in an increase in growth rate and somatomedin-C levels similar to that seen with somatropin therapy.
Other actions that have been demonstrated for Protropin (somatrem for injection) and/or somatropin include:
A. Tissue Growth
1. **Skeletal Growth.** Protropin (somatrem for injection) stimulates skeletal growth in patients with growth hormone deficiency. The measurable increase in body length after administration of somatropin results from its effect on the epiphyseal growth plates of long bones. Studies *in vitro* have shown that the incorporation of sulfate into proteoglycans is not due to a direct effect of somatropin, but rather is accomplished by a mediator called somatomedin-C. Somatomedin-C is low in the serum of growth hormone deficient children but increases during treatment with Protropin (somatrem for injection).
2. **Cell Growth.** It has been shown that the total number of skeletal muscle cells is markedly decreased in short-stature children lacking endogenous growth hormone compared with normal children. Treatment with somatropin results in an increase in both the number and the size of muscle cells.
3. **Organ Growth.** Somatropin influences the size of internal organs and it also increases red cell mass.
B. Protein Metabolism
Linear growth is facilitated in part by increased cellular protein synthesis. This is reflected by nitrogen retention as demonstrated by a decline in urinary nitrogen excretion and blood urea nitrogen following the initiation of somatropin therapy. Treatment with Protropin (somatrem for injection) results in a similar decline in blood urea nitrogen.

C. Carbohydrate Metabolism
Both somatropin and Protropin (somatrem for injection) have been found to influence carbohydrate metabolism. It is recognized that children with hypopituitarism sometimes experience fasting hypoglycemia. In normal healthy subjects, large doses of Protropin growth hormone may impair glucose tolerance. Administration of either somatropin or Protropin to normal adults resulted in an increase in serum insulin levels. Although the precise mechanism by which somatropin and Protropin induce insulin resistance is presently not known, it is attributed to a decrease in insulin sensitivity. An increase in serum glucose levels is observed during treatment with somatropin.
D. Lipid Metabolism
In growth hormone deficient subjects long term administration of somatropin often results in a general reduction in body fat stores. Acute administration of somatropin to humans results in lipid mobilization. Nonesterified fatty acids increase in plasma within two hours of somatropin administration.
E. Mineral Metabolism
The retention of total body potassium and phosphorus which is induced by somatropin administration is thought to be due to cell growth. Sodium retention also occurs.
Serum levels of inorganic phosphate increase in patients with growth hormone deficiency after somatropin or Protropin (somatrem for injection) therapy due to metabolic activity associated with bone growth as well as increased tubular reabsorption of phosphate by the kidney. Serum calcium is not significantly altered in patients treated with either somatropin or Protropin.
Although calcium excretion in the urine is increased, there is a simultaneous increase in calcium absorption from the intestine.
F. Connective Tissue Metabolism
Somatropin stimulates the synthesis of chondroitin sulfate and collagen as well as the urinary excretion of hydroxyproline.

INDICATIONS AND USAGE
Protropin (somatrem for injection) is indicated only for the long term treatment of children who have growth failure due to a lack of adequate endogenous growth hormone secretion. Other etiologies of short stature should be excluded.

CONTRAINDICATIONS
Protropin (somatrem for injection) should not be used in subjects with closed epiphyses.
Protropin growth hormone should not be used in patients with active neoplasia. Intracranial lesions must be inactive and antitumor therapy complete prior to instituting therapy. Protropin growth hormone should be discontinued if there is evidence of recurrent tumor growth.
Protropin growth hormone, when reconstituted with Bacteriostatic Water for Injection, USP (Benzyl Alcohol Preserved) should not be used in patients with a known sensitivity to benzyl alcohol.

WARNINGS
Benzyl alcohol as a preservative in Bacteriostatic Water for Injection has been associated with toxicity in newborns. When administering Protropin to newborns, reconstitute with Water for Injection, USP. USE ONLY ONE DOSE PER VIAL AND DISCARD THE UNUSED PORTION.

PRECAUTIONS
Protropin (somatrem for injection) should be used only by physicians experienced in the diagnosis and management of patients with pituitary growth hormone deficiency.
Patients with growth hormone deficiency secondary to an intracranial lesion should be examined frequently for progression or recurrence of the underlying disease process.
Because Protropin may induce a state of insulin resistance, patients should be observed for evidence of glucose intolerance.
Concomitant glucocorticoid therapy may inhibit the growth promoting effect of Protropin growth hormone. Patients with coexisting ACTH deficiency should have their glucocorticoid replacement dose carefully adjusted to avoid an inhibitory effect on growth.
Hypothyroidism may develop during Protropin treatment. Untreated hypothyroidism prevents optimal response to Protropin growth hormone. Therefore, patients should have periodic thyroid function tests and should be treated with thyroid hormone when indicated.
Leukemia has been reported in a small number of growth hormone deficient patients, treated with growth hormone. On the basis of current evidence, experts cannot conclude that growth hormone therapy is responsible for these occurrences. If there is any risk to an individual patient, it is minimal.
Slipped capital femoral epiphysis may occur more frequently in patients with endocrine disorders. Physicians and parents should be alert to the development of a limp or complaints of hip or knee pain in Protropin-treated patients.

As for any protein, a systemic allergic reaction may occur. See WARNINGS for use of Bacteriostatic Water for Injection, USP (Benzyl Alcohol Preserved) in newborns.

ADVERSE REACTIONS
A. Protropin (somatrem for injection)
Approximately 30 percent of all Protropin treated patients developed persistent antibodies to growth hormone.
In patients who had been previously treated with pituitary-derived growth hormone, one of twenty-two subjects developed persistent antibodies to growth hormone in response to Protropin (somatrem for injection) therapy. In children not previously treated with any exogenous growth hormone approximately 40 percent developed persistent antibodies to growth hormone.
In general, the growth hormone antibodies are not neutralizing and do not interfere with the growth response to Protropin growth hormone. One of eighty-four subjects treated with Protropin growth hormone for 6 to 36 months developed antibodies associated with high binding capacities and failed to respond to treatment with Protropin growth hormone.
In addition to an evaluation of compliance with treatment program and thyroid status, testing for antibodies to human growth hormone should be carried out in any patient who fails to respond to therapy.
Additional short term immunologic and renal function studies were carried out in a group of patients after approximately two years of treatment to detect other potential adverse effects of antibodies to growth hormone. The antibody was determined to be of the IgG class; no antibodies to growth hormone of the IgE class were detected. Testing included immune complex determination, measurement of total hemolytic complement and specific complement components, and immunochemical analyses. No adverse effects of growth hormone antibody formation were observed.
These findings are supported by a toxicity study conducted in a primate model in which a similar antibody response to growth hormone was observed. Protropin (somatrem for injection), administered to monkeys by intramuscular injection at doses of 125 and 625 μg/kg t.i.w. was compared to pituitary-human growth hormone at the same doses and with placebo over a period of 90 days. Most monkeys treated with high-dose Protropin growth hormone developed persistent antibodies at week four. There were no biologically significant drug related changes in standard laboratory variables. Histopathologic examination of the kidney and other selected organs (pituitary, lungs, liver and pancreas) showed no treatment related toxicity. There was no evidence of immune complexes or immune complex toxicity when the kidney was also examined for the presence of immune complexes and possible toxic effects of immune complexes by immunohistochemistry and electron microscopy.
B. Bacteriostatic Water for Injection, USP (Benzyl Alcohol Preserved)
Toxicity in newborns has been associated with benzyl alcohol as a preservative (see WARNINGS).

OVERDOSAGE
The recommended dosage of up to 0.1 mg (0.26 IU) per kg body weight three times per week should not be exceeded due to the potential risk of side effects.

DOSAGE AND ADMINISTRATION
The Protropin (somatrem for injection) dosage must be individualized for each patient. A dosage and schedule of up to 0.1 mg/kg (0.26 IU/kg) body weight administered three times per week (t.i.w.) by intramuscular or subcutaneous injection is recommended.
After the dose has been determined, reconstitute each 5 mg vial with 1–5 mL of Bacteriostatic Water for Injection, USP (Benzyl Alcohol Preserved) only. For use in newborns see WARNINGS. The pH of Protropin (somatrem for injection) after reconstitution is approximately 7.8.
To prepare the Protropin solution, inject the Bacteriostatic Water for Injection, USP (Benzyl Alcohol Preserved) into the vial of Protropin growth hormone, aiming the stream of liquid against the glass wall. Then swirl the product vial with a **GENTLE** rotary motion until the contents are completely dissolved. **DO NOT SHAKE.** Because Protropin growth hormone is a protein, shaking can result in a cloudy solution. Immediately after reconstitution, the Protropin solution should be clear. Occasionally, after refrigeration, you may notice that small colorless particles of protein are present in the Protropin solution. This is not unusual for proteins like Protropin growth hormone. If the solution is cloudy immediately after reconstitution or refrigeration the contents **MUST NOT** be injected. Before and after injections the septum of the vial should be wiped with an antiseptic solution to prevent contamination of the contents after repeated needle insertions. It is recommended that Protropin growth hormone be administered using sterile, disposable syringes and needles. The syringes should be of small enough volume that

the prescribed dose can be drawn from the vial with reasonable accuracy.

STORAGE

Protropin (somatrem for injection), before and after reconstitution with Bacteriostatic Water for Injection, USP (Benzyl Alcohol Preserved), must be stored at 2° to 8°C/36° to 46°F (refrigerator).

Reconstituted vials should be used within 14 days after reconstitution.

Avoid freezing the reconstituted vial of Protropin growth hormone and the Bacteriostatic Water for Injection, USP (Benzyl Alcohol Preserved).

Expiration dates are stated on the labels.

HOW SUPPLIED

Protropin (somatrem for injection) is supplied as 5 mg (approximately 13 IU) of lyophilized, sterile somatrem per vial. There are two vials of Protropin (somatrem for injection) and one 10 mL multiple dose vial of Bacteriostatic Water for Injection, USP (Benzyl Alcohol Preserved) per carton. NDC 50242-015-02.

Protropin (somatrem for injection) Manufactured by:
Genentech, Inc.
460 Point San Bruno Boulevard
South San Francisco, CA 94080
Bacteriostatic Water for Injection, USP (Benzyl Alcohol Preserved) Manufactured for:
Genentech, Inc.
G40053-R6
Revised May 1989
PROTROPIN®
(somatrem for injection)
From Genentech®, Inc.

Shown in Product Identification Section, page 410

Geneva Generics, Inc.
2599 W. MIDWAY BLVD.
BROOMFIELD, CO 80020

NDC # 0781-	PRODUCT	
1552	Acetaminophen/Codeine Tablets 300mg./15mg.	©III/℞
1752	Acetaminophen/Codeine Tablets 300mg./30mg.	©III/℞
1654	Acetaminophen/Codeine Tablets 300mg./60mg.	©III/℞
1080	Allopurinol Tablets 100mg.	℞
1082	Allopurinol Tablets 300mg.	℞
1214	Aminophylline Tablets 100mg.	℞
1318	Aminophylline Tablets 200mg.	℞
1486	Amitriptyline HCl Tablets 10mg.	℞
1487	Amitriptyline HCl Tablets 25mg.	℞
1488	Amitriptyline HCl Tablets 50mg.	℞
1489	Amitriptyline HCl Tablets 75mg.	℞
1490	Amitriptyline HCl Tablets 100mg.	℞
1491	Amitriptyline HCl Tablets 150mg.	℞
1435	Butalbital Compound Tablets	©III/℞
1050	Carisoprodol Tablets	℞
2938	Cefadroxil Capsules 500mg.	℞
6407	Cefadroxil Oral Suspension 125mg.	℞
6507	Cefadroxil Oral Suspension 250mg.	℞
6607	Cefadroxil Oral Suspension 500mg.	℞
2531	Cephalexin Capsules 250mg.	℞
2532	Cephalexin Capsules 500mg.	℞
7028	Cephalexin Suspension 125mg.	℞
7029	Cephalexin Suspension 250mg.	℞
2080	Chlordiazepoxide HCl Capsules 5mg.	©IV/℞
2082	Chlordiazepoxide HCl Capsules 10mg.	©IV/℞
2084	Chlordiazepoxide HCl Capsules 25mg.	©IV/℞
2602	Chlorpheniramine Maleate S.R. Capsules 8mg.	℞
1140	Chlorpheniramine Maleate Tablets 4mg.	℞
4007	Chlorpromazine HCl Concentrate 30mg./mL	℞
4009	Chlorpromazine HCl Concentrate 100mg./mL	℞
4017	Chlorpromazine HCl Syrup 10mg./5mL	℞
1715	Chlorpromazine HCl Tablets 10mg.	℞
1716	Chlorpromazine HCl Tablets 25mg.	℞
1717	Chlorpromazine HCl Tablets 50mg.	℞
1718	Chlorpromazine HCl Tablets 100mg.	℞
1719	Chlorpromazine HCl Tablets 200mg.	℞
1613	Chlorpropamide Tablets 100mg.	℞
1623	Chlorpropamide Tablets 250mg.	℞
2580	Clinoxide Capsules	℞
1471	Clonidine HCl Tablets 0.1mg.	℞
1472	Clonidine HCl Tablets 0.2mg.	℞
1473	Clonidine HCl Tablets 0.3mg.	℞
1132	Conjugated Estrogens Tablets 0.3mg.	℞

1135	Conjugated Estrogens Tablets 0.625mg.	℞
1835	Conjugated Estrogens Tablets 1.25mg.	℞
1625	Conjugated Estrogens Tablets 2.5mg.	℞
1576	Decongestant S.R. Tablets	℞
1482	Diazepam Tablets 2mg.	©IV/℞
1483	Diazepam Tablets 5mg.	©IV/℞
1484	Diazepam Tablets 10mg.	©IV/℞
2066	Dicyclomine Capsules 10mg.	℞
1935	Dicyclomine Tablets 20mg.	℞
2458	Diphenhydramine HCl Capsules 25 mg.	℞
2498	Diphenhydramine HCl Capsules 50mg.	℞
1890	Dipyridamole Tablets 25mg.	℞
1678	Dipyridamole Tablets 50mg.	℞
1478	Dipyridamole Tablets 75mg.	℞
1600	Disobrom Tablets	℞
2800	Doxepin HCl Capsules 10mg.	℞
2801	Doxepin HCl Capsules 25mg.	℞
2802	Doxepin HCl Capsules 50mg.	℞
2803	Doxepin HCl Capsules 75mg.	℞
2804	Doxepin HCl Capsules 100mg.	℞
1990	Ergoloid Mesylates Tablets 0.5mg., Sublingual	℞
1155	Ergoloid Mesylates Tablets 1.0mg., Oral	℞
1255	Ergoloid Mesylates Tablets 1.0mg., Sublingual	℞
6302	Furosemide Oral Solution 10mg.	℞
1818	Furosemide Tablets 20mg.	℞
1966	Furosemide Tablets 40mg.	℞
1446	Furosemide Tablets 80mg.	℞
1732	Hydralazine HCl Tablets 10mg.	℞
1733	Hydralazine HCl Tablets 25mg.	℞
1734	Hydralazine HCl Tablets 50mg.	℞
1480	Hydrochlorothiazide Tablets 25mg.	℞
1481	Hydrochlorothiazide Tablets 50mg.	℞
1735	Hydrochlorothiazide Tablets 100mg.	℞
1606	Hydrocodone Bitartrate/Acetaminophen Tablets 5mg./500mg.	©III/℞
6570	Hydroxyzine HCl Syrup	℞
1332	Hydroxyzine HCl Tablets 10mg.	℞
1334	Hydroxyzine HCl Tablets 25mg.	℞
1336	Hydroxyzine HCl Tablets 50mg.	℞
1343	H.H.R. (Hydralazine HCl/Hydrochlorothiazide/Reserpine) Tablets	℞
1352	Ibuprofen Tablets 400mg.	℞
1362	Ibuprofen Tablets 600mg.	℞
1363	Ibuprofen Tablets 800mg.	℞
1762	Imipramine HCl Tablets 10mg.	℞
1764	Imipramine HCl Tablets 25mg.	℞
1766	Imipramine HCl Tablets 50mg.	℞
2325	Indomethacin Capsules 25mg.	℞
2350	Indomethacin Capsules 50mg.	℞
2153	Indomethacin S.R. Capsules 75mg.	℞
1515	Isosorbide Dinitrate Tablets 2.5mg., Sublingual	℞
1565	Isosorbide Dinitrate Tablets 5mg., Sublingual	℞
1635	Isosorbide Dinitrate Tablets 5mg., Oral	℞
1556	Isosorbide Dinitrate Tablets 10mg., Oral	℞
1695	Isosorbide Dinitrate Tablets 20mg., Oral	℞
2520	Isosorbide Dinitrate S.R. Capsules 40mg.	℞
1417	Isosorbide Dinitrate S.R. Tablets 40mg.	℞
1840	Isoxsuprine HCl Tablets 10mg.	℞
1842	Isoxsuprine HCl Tablets 20mg.	℞
2100	Lithium Carbonate Capsules 300mg.	℞
1262	Lonox (Diphenoxylate HCl/Atropine Sulfate) Tablets	©V/℞
1403	Lorazepam Tablets 0.5mg.	©IV/℞
1404	Lorazepam Tablets 1mg.	©IV/℞
1405	Lorazepam Tablets 2mg.	©IV/℞
1905	L-Thyroxine Sodium Tablets 0.1mg.	℞
1908	L-Thyroxine Sodium Tablets 0.15mg.	℞
1910	L-Thyroxine Sodium Tablets 0.2mg.	℞
1913	L-Thyroxine Sodium Tablets 0.3mg.	℞
1680	Medroxyprogesterone Acetate Tablets 10mg.	℞
1388	Meprobamate Tablets 200mg.	©IV/℞
1410	Meprobamate Tablets 400mg.	©IV/℞
1760	Methocarbamol Tablets 500mg.	℞
1750	Methocarbamol Tablets 750mg.	℞
1317	Methyldopa Tablets 125mg.	℞
1320	Methyldopa Tablets 250mg.	℞
1322	Methyldopa Tablets 500mg.	℞
1809	Methyldopa/Hydrochlorothiazide Tablets 250mg./15mg.	℞
1819	Methyldopa/Hydrochlorothiazide Tablets 250mg./25mg.	℞
1843	Methyldopa/Hydrochlorothiazide Tablets 500mg./30mg.	℞
1853	Methyldopa/Hydrochlorothiazide Tablets 500mg./50mg.	℞
6301	Metoclopramide HCl Syrup 5mg.	℞

1301	Metoclopramide HCl Tablets 10mg.	℞
2718	Nitroglycerin S.R. Capsules 2.5mg.	℞
2786	Nitroglycerin S.R. Capsules 6.5mg.	℞
2798	Nitroglycerin S.R. Capsules 9mg.	℞
2809	Oxazepam Capsules 10mg.	©IV/℞
2810	Oxazepam Capsules 15mg.	©IV/℞
2811	Oxazepam Capsules 30mg.	©IV/℞
2000	Papaverine HCl S.R. Capsules 150mg.	℞
1091	Phenobarbital Tablets 15mg.	℞
1110	Phenobarbital Tablets 30mg.	℞
2415	Phentermine HCl Capsules 30mg.	℞
2211	Prazosin HCl Capsules 1mg.	℞
2212	Prazosin HCl Capsules 2mg.	℞
2213	Prazosin HCl Capsules 5mg.	℞
1495	Prednisone Tablets 5mg.	℞
1500	Prednisone Tablets 10mg.	℞
1485	Prednisone Tablets 20mg.	℞
1450	Prednisone Tablets 50mg.	℞
1040	Primidone Tablets 50mg.	℞
1021	Probenecid Tablets 0.5gm.	℞
1830	Promethazine HCl Tablets 25mg.	℞
1832	Promethazine HCl Tablets 50mg.	℞
1378	Propoxphene HCl/Acetaminophen Tablets 65mg./650mg.	©IV/℞
2140	Propoxyphene HCl Capsules 65mg.	©IV/℞
2367	Propoxyphene HCl/Aspirin & Caffeine Capsules 65mg./389mg./32.4mg.	©IV/℞
1720	Propoxyphene Napsylate/Acetaminophen Tablets 100mg./650mg.	©IV/℞
1344	Propranolol HCl Tablets 10mg.	℞
1354	Propranolol HCl Tablets 20mg.	℞
1364	Propranolol HCl Tablets 40mg.	℞
1374	Propranolol HCl Tablets 60mg.	℞
1384	Propranolol HCl Tablets 80mg.	℞
1339	Propylthiouracil Tablets 50mg.	℞
1804	Quinidine Gluconate S.R. Tablets 324mg.	℞
1900	Quinidine Sulfate Tablets 200mg.	℞
1902	Quinidine Sulfate Tablets 300mg.	℞
1105	Relaxadon Tablets	℞
2427	Resaid S.R. Capsules	℞
1096	Reserpine Tablets 0.25mg.	℞
1086	Reserpine Tablets 0.1mg.	℞
1108	Salsalate Tablets 500mg.	℞
1109	Salsalate Tablets 750mg.	℞
1816	Sodium Fluoride Tablets 2.2mg.	℞
1599	Spironolactone Tablets 25mg.	℞
1149	Spironolactone/Hydrochlorothiazide Tablets 25mg./25mg.	℞
6063	Sulfamethoxazole/Trimethoprim Suspension 200mg./40mg.	℞
1063	Sulfamethoxazole/Trimethoprim DS Tablets 800mg./160mg.	℞
1062	Sulfamethoxazole/Trimethoprim S.S. Tablets 400mg./80mg.	℞
1045	Sulfasalazine Tablets 500mg.	℞
1153	Tamine S.R. Tablets	℞
2201	Temazepam Capsules 15mg.	©IV/℞
2202	Temazepam Capsules 30mg.	©IV/℞
2529	Tetracycline HCl Capsules 250 mg.	℞
2466	Tetracycline HCl Capsules 500mg.	℞
6181	Tetracycline HCl Syrup	℞
1003	Theophylline S.R. Tablets 100mg.	℞
1004	Theophylline S.R. Tablets 200mg.	℞
1005	Theophylline S.R. Tablets 300mg.	℞
1604	Thioridazine HCl Tablets 10mg.	℞
1614	Thioridazine HCl Tablets 15mg.	℞
1624	Thioridazine HCl Tablets 25mg.	℞
1634	Thioridazine HCl Tablets 50mg.	℞
1644	Thioridazine HCl Tablets 100mg.	℞
1664	Thioridazine HCl Tablets 150mg.	℞
1674	Thioridazine HCl Tablets 200mg.	℞
1704	Tolbutamide Tablets 500mg.	℞
1807	Trazodone HCl Tablets 50mg.	℞
1808	Trazodone HCl Tablets 100mg.	℞
2715	Triamterene/Hydrochlorothiazide Capsules 50mg./25mg.	℞
1008	Triamterene/Hydrochlorothiazide Tablets 75mg./50mg.	℞
4045	Trifluoperazine HCl Concentrate 10mg.	℞
1030	Trifluoperazine HCl Tablets 1mg.	℞
1032	Trifluoperazine HCl Tablets 2mg.	℞
1034	Trifluoperazine HCl Tablets 5mg.	℞
1036	Trifluoperazine HCl Tablets 10mg.	℞
1965	Trihexyphenidyl HCl Tablets 2mg.	℞
1960	Trihexyphenidyl HCl Tablets 5mg.	℞
1503	ULR-LA (Phenylpropanolamine HCl/Guaifenesin) Tablets 75mg./400mg.	℞
1016	Verapamil HCl Tablets 80mg.	℞
1017	Verapamil HCl Tablets 120mg.	℞

Geriatric Pharm. Corp.
16820 RIDGE VIEW DRIVE
BROOKFIELD, WI 53005

B-C-BID™ CAPSULES
B Complex with Vitamin C
SUSTAINED RELEASE
BY MICRODIALYSIS DIFFUSION

COMPOSITION
Each capsule contains: Vitamin B-1 15 mg., Vitamin B-2 10 mg., Vitamin B-6 5 mg., Niacinamide 50 mg., Calcium Pantothenate 10 mg., Vitamin C 300 mg., and Vitamin B-12 (Cyanocobalamin) 5 mcg.
Medication is released at a smooth, continuous, predictable rate dependent only upon the presence of fluid in the G.I. tract, and not dependent on pH and other variables. *No regurgitation; no after-taste.*
On b.i.d. dosage, this smooth, continuous release of B-C-BID's essential vitamins frees your patient from the "peak and valley" effect of ordinary capsules or tablets.

DOSAGE
For continuous 24 hour therapy, one capsule after breakfast and one after supper.

SUPPLIED
Bottles of 30, 100, and 500 (NDC #249-1153-01,-02 and -03).

BILEZYME™   ℞
[bī′le zīm]
Bile Acids and Digestive Enzymes

COMPOSITION
Each BILEZYME tablet contains 30 mg. of Gerilase (Standardized Amylolytic Enzyme derived from Aspergillus oryzae), 6 mg. of Geriprotase (Standardized Proteolytic Enzyme derived from Carica papaya), 200 mg. Dehydrocholic Acid (a choleretic) and 50 mg. Desoxycholic Acid (a cholagogue). Not enteric coated.

SUPPLIED
Bottles of 42, 100 and 500 (NDC #249-1110-01, -02, and 03).

CAL-BID™
Calcium Supplement with Vitamin C and D Added

COMPOSITION

Each tablet contains:	Quantity:	% USRDA:
Vitamin C (ascorbic acid)	100 mg.	167
Vitamin D	125 IU	31.25
Calcium Carbonate*	625 mg.	25

(*equivalent to 250 mg. elemental Calcium)

SUPPLIED
As bottles of 100 (NDC #249-1168-02).

CAL-PLUS™ TABLETS
High Potency Calcium Supplement

COMPOSITION
Each tablet contains Calcium Carbonate, 1500 mg. (equivalent to 600 mg. elemental Calcium or 60% USRDA).

SUPPLIED
As bottles of 100 and 500 (NDC #249-1170-02 and -03).

CEVI-BID™ Capsules (500 mg. Vitamin C)
SUSTAINED RELEASE
BY MICRO-DIALYSIS DIFFUSION

COMPOSITION
Each CEVI-BID capsule contains 500 mg. Vitamin C.

ACTION AND USES
For treatment of Vitamin C deficiency. CEVI-BID maintains optimal blood levels of Vitamin C around the clock on b.i.d. dosage, and avoids "peak and valley" effects of ordinary Vitamin C tablets. Medication is released at a smooth, continuous, predictable rate dependent only upon the presence of fluid in the G.I. tract and independent of pH or other variables.

DOSAGE
For continuous 24 hour therapy, one capsule after breakfast and one after supper.

SUPPLIED
Bottles of 30, 100 and 500. (NDC #249-1161-01, -02 and -03).

CEVI-FER™ CAPSULES   ℞
Hematinic with 300 mg Vitamin C
SUSTAINED RELEASE BY
MICRO-DIALYSIS DIFFUSION

COMPOSITION
CEVI-FER capsules contain *Ferrous Fumarate 60 mg. (Equivalent to 20 mg. elemental iron), *Ascorbic Acid 300 mg., Folic Acid 1 mg.
*Prepared in a special base for prolonged therapeutic effect. Ferrous fumarate and ascorbic acid are released at a smooth, continuous, predictable rate dependent only upon the presence of fluid in the G.I. tract; not dependent on the variable digestive processes.

INDICATIONS
Cevi-Fer Capsules is a high potency formulation of Iron, Ascorbic Acid, and Folic Acid and is intended for use as:
1) intensive therapy for the acute and/or severe iron deficiency anemia where a high intake of elemental iron is required.
2) a maintenance hematinic for those patients needing a daily iron supplement to maintain normal hemoglobin levels.
3) prevention of concomitant folic acid deficiency in adults.
4) especially indicated in geriatric patients who are on special diets or suffer from nutritional anemias.
5) folic acid is effective in the treatment of megaloblastic anemias due to a deficiency of folic acid (as may be seen in tropical or nontropical sprue) and in anemias of nutritional origin, pregnancy, infancy, or childhood.

ACTIONS AND USES
The Ferrous form of iron is better absorbed and utilized than the ferric form. Absorption of iron can occur along the entire length of the alimentary tract, but is greatest in the duodenum and becomes progressively less distal.
The stomach being acid, keeps the iron salts in Ferrous state. Reducing agents such as Ascorbic Acid increase iron absorption.
In Cevi-Fer's special sustained release pattern, Ferrous Fumarate and the Ascorbic Acid will be released over a 12 hour period.
The advantage of having Ferrous Fumarate present in a Sustained Release pellet formulation is that it provides high levels of elemental iron with a low incidence of gastric distress.
300 mg. of Sustained Release Ascorbic Acid serves to maintain the iron in a more absorbable Ferrous state.
Studies have found that large doses of Ascorbic Acid tend to enhance iron absorption.

CONTRAINDICATIONS
Folic acid, (pteroylglutamic acid), is contraindicated in patients with untreated and uncomplicated pernicious anemia, and in those with anaphylactic sensitivity to folic acid. Iron therapy is contraindicated in patients with hemachromatosis, iron storage disease or the potential for iron storage disease due to chronic hemolytic anemia (e.g., inherited anomalies of hemoglobin structure or synthesis and/or red cell enzyme deficiencies, etc.), pyridoxine responsive anemia, or cirrhosis of the liver.

WARNINGS
Pernicious anemia should be ruled out before starting treatment. While folic acid corrects the blood picture of pernicious anemia, it does not ameliorate the attendant neurologic involvement.
Resistance to treatment may be due to depressed hematopoiesis, alcoholism, the presence of antimetabolic drugs and to deficiencies of vitamins.
Iron deficiency anemia may be due to occult blood loss, the cause of which should be determined and treated appropriately. Prolonged therapeutic use of iron salts may produce iron storage disease.

PRECAUTIONS
Folic acid in doses above 0.1 mg. daily may obscure pernicious anemia, in that hematologic remission may occur while neurological manifestations remain progressive.
Folic acid (pteroylglutamic acid) microbiological blood assays are invalidated by the administration of most antibiotics, methotrexate, and pyrimethamine. Folic acid is not effective in reversing the toxic effects of methotrexate. Folinic acid (5-formyl-5,6,7,8-tetrahydrofolic acid) must be used in this situation. Black tarry stools may be due to either occult G.I. bleeding or iron therapy, or both.

ADVERSE REACTIONS
Allergic sensitivity reactions and gastrointestinal disturbances may occur.

DOSAGE AND ADMINISTRATION
One capsule after breakfast and supper for two weeks in severe anemias, then one capsule a day. Not to be administered to children under 12 years of age.

OVERDOSAGE
The average human lethal dose of iron is about 200 to 250 mg. iron/kg. body weight. In the case of a 4 kg. infant, this is about 800 mg. iron or about (2) grams anhydrous ferrous sulfate or ferrous fumarate.

WARNING
Keep out of the reach of children. In case of accidental overdose, seek professional assistance or contact a poison control center immediately. Protect from heat and moisture.

HOW SUPPLIED
Available in bottles of 30 and 100 capsules (NDC #'s 249-1166-01 and -02).

CAUTION
Federal law prohibits dispensing without a prescription.

GERITONIC™ LIQUID
Elixir with Vitamin B Complex and Iron

COMPOSITION

Each teaspoonful (5 cc.) contains:		
Iron (from Ferric Ammonium Citrate)	35	mg.
Thiamine Hydrochloride (Vitamin B-1)	1	mg.
Riboflavin (Vitamin B-2)	1	mg.
Niacinamide	10	mg.
Vitamin B-12 (Cyanacobalamin)	3	mcg.
Pyridoxine Hydrochloride (Vitamin B-6)	0.1	mg.
Magnesium (from Magnesium Sulfate)	1	mg.
Manganese (from Manganese Sulfate)	0.5	mg.
Calcium (from Calcium Glycerophosphate)	10	mg.
Phosphorus (from Calcium Glycerophosphate)	8	mg.
Potassium (from Potassium Sulfate)	1	mg.
Alcohol (by volume)	20	%

In a base of Yeast Concentrate and Liver Fraction 1

SUPPLIED
8 ounce bottles (NDC# 249-1118-01).

GUSTASE®
Gastrointestinal Enzyme Tablets

COMPOSITION
Each GUSTASE tablet contains GERILASE (standardized amylolytic enzyme) 30 mg., GERIPROTASE (standardized proteolytic enzyme) 6 mg., GERICELLULASE (standardized cellulolytic enzyme) 2 mg. Not enteric coated.

SUPPLIED
Bottles of 42 and 100 (NDC #249-1120-01 and 02).

GUSTASE PLUS™   ℞
Gastrointestinal Enzyme Tablets with Phenobarbital

COMPOSITION
Each GUSTASE PLUS tablet contains Phenobarbital, 8 mg.; Homatrophine Methylbromide, 2.5 mg.; Gerilase (standardized amylolytic enzyme) 30 mg.; Geriprotase (standardized proteolytic enzyme) 6 mg.; Gericellulase (standardized cellulytic enzyme) 2 mg. Not enteric coated.

SUPPLIED
Bottles of 42 and 100 (NDC #249-1121-01 and -02).

ISO-BID® CAPSULES 40 mg.   ℞
SUSTAINED RELEASE BY
MICRO-DIALYSIS DIFFUSION

COMPOSITION
Each ISO-BID SUSTAINED-MEDICATION CAPSULE contains 40 mg. Isosorbide Dinitrate. Medication is released at a smooth, continuous, predictable rate dependent only upon the presence of fluid in the G.I. tract; not dependent on the variable digestive processes.

SUPPLIED
Bottles of 30, 100, and 500 (NDC #249-1164-01, -02 and -03).

NIA–BID VIA MICRO-DIALYSIS DIFFUSION ℞
(Niacin, USP (Nicotinic Acid) 400 mg.)
Sustained release base to provide prolonged activity

DESCRIPTION
[Nicotinamide Adenine Dinucleotide Phosphate (NADP), sometimes called Triphosphopyridine Nucleotide (TPN)]. Niacin in addition to its functions as a vitamin, exerts several distinctive pharmacologic effects which vary according to the dosage level employed. Niacin in large doses causes a reduction in serum lipids. The exact mechanism of this action is unknown.

INDICATIONS AND USAGE
As adjunctive therapy in addition to diet and other measures in the treatment of hypercholesterolemia and hyperbetalipoproteinemia. Because NIA-BID has prolonged release, it minimizes flushing, pruritus and gastrointestinal irritation and permits adequate dosage with maximum patient cooperation.

NOTICE
It has not been established whether Niacin induced lowering of serum cholesterol or triglyceride levels has a beneficial effect, no effect, or a detrimental effect on the morbidity or mortality due to atherosclerosis including coronary heart disease. Investigations now in progress may yield an answer to this question.

CONTRAINDICATIONS
Niacin is contraindicated in patients with hepatic dysfunction or in patients with active acute peptic ulcer.

WARNINGS
Use of niacin in pregnancy, during lactation, or in women of child-bearing age requires that the potential benefits of niacin should be weighed against its possible hazards to the mother and child. Although fetal abnormalities have not been reported with niacin, its use as an antilipidemic agent requires high dosages, and animal reproduction or teratology studies have not been done. There are insufficient studies done for usage in children.

PRECAUTIONS
Patients with gall bladder disease, or those with a past history of jaundice, liver disease or peptic ulcer should be observed closely while taking the niacin. Frequent monitoring of liver function tests and blood glucose should be performed during therapy to ascertain that the niacin has no adverse effects on these organ systems. Diabetic or potential diabetic patients should be observed closely in the event of decreased tolerance. Adjustment of diet and/or hypoglycemic therapy may be necessary. Antihypertensive drugs of the adrenergic-blocking type may have an additive vasodilating effect and produce postural hypotension. Elevated uric acid levels have occurred; therefore, use with caution in patients predisposed to gout.

ADVERSE REACTIONS
Severe flushing, decreased glucose tolerance, activation of peptic ulcer, abnormal liver function tests, jaundice, gastrointestinal disorders, dry skin, kerotosis nigricans-pruritus, hyperuricemia, toxic amblyopia, hypotension, transient headache.

DOSAGE AND ADMINISTRATION
The dose and frequency for the administration of NIA-BID should be adjusted to the response of the patient. Slow build-up of dosage in gradual increments is recommended to observe efficacy and/or adverse effects. One or two capsules three times a day is the usual dosage. The maximum dosage is 8 g per day.

HOW SUPPLIED
NIA-BID 400 mg sustained action capsules are available in bottles of 100, NDC #249-1130-02. No dietary supplement can replace the need for sound nutritional practice—supervised by a physician or qualified health professional.

EDUCATIONAL MATERIAL

Brochures and samples available on all Geriatric Phamaceutical Products.

Products are
listed alphabetically
in the
PINK SECTION.

Glaxo Dermatology
Division of Glaxo Inc.
FIVE MOORE DRIVE
RESEARCH TRIANGLE PARK, NC 27709

ACLOVATE® ℞
[a΄klō-vāt΄΄]
(alclometasone dipropionate)
Cream, 0.05%
Ointment, 0.05%
For Dermatologic Use Only—
Not for Ophthalmic Use.
TEMOVATE® ℞
[tem΄ō-vāt΄΄]
(clobetasol propionate)
Cream, 0.05%
Ointment, 0.05%
(potency expressed as clobetasol propionate)
For Dermatologic Use Only—
Not for Ophthalmic Use.

DESCRIPTION
Aclovate® Cream and Ointment contain alclometasone dipropionate for dermatologic use. Alclometasone dipropionate is a synthetic corticosteroid with anti-inflammatory activity.
Chemically, alclometasone dipropionate is 7α-chloro-11β,17,21-trihydroxy-16α-methylpregna-1, 4-diene-3,20-dione 17,21-dipropionate.
Alclometasone dipropionate has the empirical formula $C_{28}H_{37}ClO_7$ and a molecular weight of 521. It is a white powder, insoluble in water, slightly soluble in propylene glycol, and moderately soluble in hexylene glycol.
Aclovate Cream contains alclometasone dipropionate 0.5 mg/g in a hydrophilic, emollient cream base of propylene glycol, white petrolatum, cetearyl alcohol, glyceryl stearate, PEG 100 stearate, ceteth-20, monobasic sodium phosphate, chlorocresol, phosphoric acid, and purified water.
Aclovate Ointment contains alclometasone dipropionate 0.5 mg/g in an ointment base of hexylene glycol, white wax, propylene glycol stearate, and white petrolatum.
Temovate® Cream and Ointment contain the active compound clobetasol propionate, a synthetic corticosteroid, for topical dermatologic use. Clobetasol, an analog of prednisolone, has a high degree of glucocorticoid activity and a slight degree of mineralocorticoid activity.
Chemically, clobetasol propionate is 21-chloro-9-fluoro-11β, 17-dihydroxy-16β-methylpregna-1, 4-diene-3, 20-dione, 17-propionate.
Clobetasol propionate has the empirical formula $C_{25}H_{32}ClFO_5$ and a molecular weight of 467. It is a white to cream-colored crystalline powder insoluble in water.
Temovate Cream contains clobetasol propionate 0.5 mg/g in a cream base of propylene glycol, glyceryl monostearate, cetostearyl alcohol, glyceryl stearate, PEG 100 stearate, white wax, chlorocresol, sodium citrate, citric acid monohydrate, and purified water.
Temovate Ointment contains clobetasol propionate 0.5 mg/g in a base of propylene glycol, sorbitan sesquioleate, and white petrolatum.

CLINICAL PHARMACOLOGY
The corticosteroids are a class of compounds comprising steroid hormones secreted by the adrenal cortex and their synthetic analogs. In pharmacologic doses, corticosteroids are used primarily for their anti-inflammatory and/or immunosuppressive effects. Topical corticosteroids such as alclometasone dipropionate and clobetasol propionate are effective in the treatment of corticosteroid-responsive dermatoses primarily because of their anti-inflammatory, antipruritic, and vasoconstrictive actions. However, while the physiologic, pharmacologic, and clinical effects of the corticosteroids are well known, the exact mechanisms of their actions in each disease are uncertain.
Corticosteroids alclometasone dipropionate and clobetasol propionate have been shown to have topical (dermatologic) and systemic pharmacologic and metabolic effects characteristic of this class of drugs.
Pharmacokinetics: The extent of percutaneous absorption of topical corticosteroids, including alclometasone dipropionate and clobetasol propionate, is determined by many factors, including the vehicle, the integrity of the epidermal barrier, and the use of occlusive dressings (see DOSAGE AND ADMINISTRATION).
Topical corticosteroids can be absorbed from normal intact skin. A study utilizing a radio-labelled alclometasone dipropionate *ointment* formulation was performed to measure systemic absorption and excretion. Results indicated that approximately 3% of the steroid was absorbed during eight hours of contact with intact skin of normal volunteers.
Inflammation and/or other disease processes in the skin may increase percutaneous absorption. Occlusive dressings substantially increase the percutaneous absorption of topical corticosteroids. Thus, occlusive dressings may be a valu-

able therapeutic adjunct for treatment of resistant dermatoses with alclometasone dipropionate (see DOSAGE AND ADMINISTRATION).
The effects of Aclovate® (alclometasone dipropionate) Cream and Ointment on the hypothalamic-pituitary-adrenal (HPA) axis were studied under exaggerated conditions. In one study, Aclovate Ointment was applied to 30% of the body twice daily for seven days, and occlusive dressings were used in selected patients either 12 hours or 24 hours daily. In another study, Aclovate Cream was applied to 80% of the body surface of normal subjects twice daily for 21 days with daily 12-hour periods of whole body occlusion. Average plasma and urinary free cortisol levels and urinary levels of 17-hydroxysteroids were slightly decreased (about 10%), suggesting slight suppression of the HPA axis under the exaggerated conditions of these studies.
Once absorbed through the skin, topical corticosteroids enter pharmacokinetic pathways similarly to systemically administered corticosteroids. Corticosteroids are bound to plasma proteins in varying degrees. Corticosteroids are metabolized primarily in the liver and are then excreted by the kidneys. Some of the topical corticosteroids, including alclometasone dipropionate and clobetasol propionate and their metabolites, are also excreted into the bile.

INDICATIONS AND USAGE
Aclovate® (alclometasone dipropionate) Cream and Ointment are indicated for relief of the inflammatory and pruritic manifestations of corticosteroid-response dermatoses.
Temovate® (clobetasol propionate) Cream and Ointment are indicated for short-term treatment of inflammatory and pruritic manifestations of moderate to severe corticosteroid-responsive dermatoses. Treatment beyond two consecutive weeks is not recommended, and the total dosage should not exceed 50 g per week because of the potential for the drug to suppress the HPA axis. These products are not recommended for use in children under 12 years of age.

CONTRAINDICATIONS
Aclovate® (alclometasone dipropionate) Cream and Ointment and Temovate® (clobetasol propionate) Cream and Ointment are contraindicated in patients who are hypersensitive to alclometasone dipropionate, clobetasol propionate, to other corticosteroids, or any ingredient in these preparations.

PRECAUTIONS
Temovate® (clobetasol propionate) is a highly potent topical corticosteroid that has been shown to suppress the HPA axis at doses as low as 2 g per day.
General: Systemic absorption of topical corticosteroids has resulted in reversible HPA axis suppression, manifestations of Cushing's syndrome, hyperglycemia, and glucosuria in some patients.
Conditions that augment systemic absorption include the application of the more potent steroids, use over large surface areas, prolonged use, and the addition of occlusive dressings.
Therefore, patients receiving a large dose of a potent topical steroid, such as Temovate, applied to a large surface area should be evaluated periodically for evidence of HPA axis suppression by using the urinary free cortisol and ACTH stimulation tests. If HPA axis suppression is noted, an attempt should be made to withdraw the drug, to reduce the frequency of application, or to substitute a less potent steroid.
Recovery of HPA axis function is generally prompt and complete upon discontinuation of the drug. Infrequently, signs and symptoms of steroid withdrawal may occur, requiring supplemental systemic corticosteroids.
Children may absorb proportionally larger amounts of topical corticosteroids and thus be more susceptible to systemic toxicity (see PRECAUTIONS: Pediatric Use).
If irritation develops, topical corticosteroids should be discontinued and appropriate therapy instituted.
In the presence of dermatologic infections, the use of an appropriate antifungal or antibacterial agent should be instituted. If a favorable response does not occur promptly, the corticosteroid should be discontinued until the infection has been adequately controlled.
Certain areas of the body, such as the face, groin, and axillae, are more prone to atrophic changes than other areas of the body following treatment with corticosteroids. Frequent observation of the patient is important if these areas are to be treated.
As with other potent topical corticosteroids, Temovate Cream and Ointment should not be used in the treatment of rosacea and perioral dermatitis. Topical corticosteroids in general should not be used in the treatment of acne.
Information for Patients: Patients using Aclovate® (alclometasone dipropionate) should receive the following information and instructions:
1. This medication is to be used as directed by the physician. It is for external use only. Avoid contact with the eyes.

Continued on next page

Glaxo Derm.—Cont.

2. This medication should not be used for any disorder other than that for which it was prescribed.
3. The treated skin area should not be bandaged or otherwise covered or wrapped as to be occlusive unless directed by the physician.
4. Patients should report any signs of local adverse reactions, especially under occlusive dressings, to the physician.
5. Parents of pediatric patients should be advised not to use tight-fitting diapers or plastic pants on a child being treated in the diaper area, as these garments may constitute occlusive dressings.

Patients using Temovate should receive the following information and instructions:

1. This medication is to be used as directed by the physician and should not be used longer than the prescribed time period. It is for external use only. Avoid contact with the eyes.
2. This medication should not be used for any disorder other than that for which it was prescribed.
3. The treated skin area should not be bandaged or otherwise covered or wrapped so as to be occlusive.
4. Patients should report any signs of local adverse reactions to the physician.

Laboratory Tests: The following tests may be helpful in evaluating HPA axis suppression, although Aclovate was shown not to produce HPA axis suppression: Urinary free cortisol test and ACTH stimulation test.

Carcinogenesis, Mutagenesis, Impairment of Fertility: Long-term animal studies have not been peformed to evaluate the carcinogenic potential or the effect on fertility of topical corticosteroids.

Studies to determine mutagenicity with prednisolone have revealed negative results.

Pregnancy: *Teratogenic Effects: Pregnancy Category C:* Corticosteroids are generally teratogenic in laboratory animals when administered systemically at relatively low dosage levels. The more potent corticosteroids have been shown to be teratogenic in animals after dermal application. Clobetasol propionate has not been tested for teratogenicity by this route; however, it appears to be fairly well absorbed percutaneously, and when administered subcutaneously, it proved to be a relatively potent teratogen in both the rabbit and the mouse.

There are no adequate and well-controlled studies of the teratogenic effects of topically applied corticosteroids in pregnant women. Therefore, topical corticosteroids should be used during pregnancy only if the potential benefit justifies the potential risk to the fetus. Drugs of this class should not be used extensively on pregnant patients, in large amounts, or for prolonged periods of time.

Nursing Mothers: It is not known whether topical administration of corticosteroids could result in sufficient systemic absorption to produce detectable quantities in breast milk. Systemically administered corticosteroids are secreted into breast milk in quantities not likely to have a deleterious effect on the infant. Nevertheless, caution should be exercised when topical corticosteroids are prescribed for a nursing woman.

Pediatric Use: Use of Temovate Cream and Ointment in children under 12 years of age is not recommended.

Pediatric patients may demonstrate greater susceptibility to topical corticosteroid-induced HPA axis suppression and Cushing's syndrome than mature patients because of a larger skin surface area to body weight ratio.

HPA axis suppression, Cushing's syndrome, and intracranial hypertension have been reported in children receiving topical corticosteroids. Manifestations of adrenal suppression in children include linear growth retardation, delayed weight gain, low plasma cortisol levels, and absence of response to ACTH stimulation. Manifestations of intracranial hypertension include bulging fontanelles, headaches, and bilateral papilledema.

Administration of topical corticosteroids to children should be limited to the least amount compatible with an effective therapeutic regimen. Chronic corticosteroid therapy may interfere with the growth and development of children.

ADVERSE REACTIONS

The following local adverse reactions have been reported with Aclovate® (alclometasone dipropionate) Cream: itching occurred in about 2 per 100 patients; burning, erythema, dryness, irritation, and papular rashes occurred in about 1 per 100 patients.

The following local adverse reactions have been reported with Aclovate Ointment: itching or burning, 1 per 200 patients; erythema, 2 per 1,000 patients.

Temovate® (clobetasol propionate) Cream and Ointment are generally well tolerated when used for two-week treatment periods.

The most frequent adverse reactions reported for Temovate Cream have been local and have included burning sensation in 4 of 421 patients and stinging sensation in 3 of 421 patients. Less frequent adverse reactions were itching, skin atrophy, and cracking and fissuring of the skin, which occurred in 1 of 421 patients.

The most frequent adverse events reported for Temovate Ointment have been local and have included burning sensation, irritation, and itching. These occurred in 2 of 366 patients. Less frequent adverse reactions were stinging, cracking, erythema, folliculitis, numbness of fingers, skin atrophy, and telangiectasia, which occurred in 1 of 366 patients.

The following local adverse reactions are reported infrequently when topical corticosteroids are used as recommended. These reactions are listed in an approximately decreasing order of occurrence: burning, itching, irritation, dryness, folliculitis, hypertrichosis, acneiform eruptions, hypopigmentation, perioral dermatitis, allergic contact dermatitis, maceration of the skin, secondary infection, skin atrophy, striae, and miliaria. Systemic absorption of topical corticosteroids has produced reversible HPA axis suppression, manifestations of Cushing's syndrome, hyperglycemia, and glucosuria in some patients. In rare instances, treatment (or withdrawal of treatment) of psoriasis with corticosteroids is thought to have provoked the pustular form of the disease.

OVERDOSAGE

Topically applied Aclovate® (alclometasone dipropionate) and Temovate® (clobetasol propionate) can be absorbed in sufficient amounts to produce systemic effects (see PRECAUTIONS).

DOSAGE AND ADMINISTRATION

Apply a thin film of Aclovate® (alclometasone dipropionate) Cream or Ointment to the affected skin areas two or three times daily; massage gently until the medication disappears. Occlusive dressings may be used for the management of refractory lesions of psoriasis and other deep-seated dermatoses, such as localized neurodermatitis (lichen simplex chronicus).

Evaporation from the skin is reduced by use of the hydration technique with occlusive dressing as follows:

1. Cover the lesion with a thick layer of Aclovate Cream or Ointment and a light gauze dressing, then cover the area with a pliable plastic film.
2. Seal the edges to the normal skin by adhesive tape or other means.
3. Leave the dressing in place one to four days and repeat the procedure three or four times as needed.

With this method of treatment, marked improvement is often seen in a few days.

If an infection develops, the use of occlusive dressings should be discontinued and appropriate antimicrobial therapy instituted.

A thin layer of Temovate® (clobetasol propionate) Cream or Ointment should be applied with gentle rubbing to the affected skin areas twice daily, once in the morning and once at night.

Temovate Cream and Ointment are potent; therefore, treatment must be limited to 14 consecutive days, and amounts greater than 50 g per week should not be used.

Temovate Cream and Ointment are not to be used with occlusive dressings.

HOW SUPPLIED

Aclovate® (alclometasone dipropionate) Cream, 0.05% is supplied in 15-g (NDC 0173-0401-00) and 45-g (NDC 0173-0401-01) tubes.

Aclovate Ointment, 0.05% is supplied in 15-g (NDC 0173-0402-00) and 45-g (NDC 0173-0402-01) tubes.

Store between 2° and 30°C (36° and 86°F).

Temovate® (clobetasol propionate) Cream, 0.05% is supplied in 15-g (NDC 0173-0375-73), 30-g (NDC 0173-0375-72), and 45-g (NDC 0173-0375-01) tubes.

Temovate Ointment, 0.05% is supplied in 15-g (NDC 0173-0376-73), 30-g (NDC 0173-0376-72), and 45-g (NDC 0173-0371-01) tubes.

Store between 15° and 30°C (59° and 86°F). Temovate Cream should not be refrigerated.

Shown in Product Identification Section, page 410

OXISTAT® Cream, 1%*   ℞
(oxiconazole nitrate)
*Potency expressed as oxiconazole.
For Topical Use Only

DESCRIPTION

Oxistat® (oxiconazole nitrate) Cream contains the active compound oxiconazole nitrate, a broad-spectrum antifungal, for topical dermatologic use.

Chemically, oxiconazole nitrate is 2',4'-dichloro-2-imidazol-1-ylacetophenone (Z)-(O-(2,4-dichlorobenzyl)oxime), mononitrate, with the empirical formula $C_{18}H_{13}ON_3Cl_4 \cdot HNO_3$, a molecular weight of 492.16, and the following structural formula:

[See Chemical Formula at top of next column].

Oxiconazole nitrate is a nearly white crystalline powder, soluble in methanol; sparingly soluble in ethanol, chloroform, and acetone; and very slightly soluble in water.

Oxistat Cream contains 10 mg/g oxiconazole as oxiconazole nitrate in a white to off-white, opaque cream base of purified water, white petrolatum, stearyl alcohol, propylene glycol, polysorbate 60, cetyl alcohol, and benzoic acid 0.2% as a preservative.

CLINICAL PHARMACOLOGY

Five hours after application of 2.5 mg/cm^2 of oxiconazole nitrate cream onto human skin, the concentration of oxiconazole nitrate was demonstrated to be 16.2 μmol in the epidermis, 3.64 μmol in the upper corneum, and 1.29 μmol in the deeper corneum. Systemic absorption of oxiconazole nitrate appears to be low. Less than 0.3% of the applied dose was recovered in the urine of volunteer subjects up to five days after application. Feces were not analyzed for the drug and it is not known whether the absorption is higher than that estimated by recovery of drug in urine.

Microbiology: The fungicidal activity of oxiconazole results primarily from the inhibition of ergosterol synthesis, which is needed for cytoplasmic membrane integrity. It has *in vitro* activity against a wide range of organisms.

In vitro, oxiconazole is active against many strains of clinical isolates of the following dermatophytic organisms: *Trichophyton rubrum* and *Trichophyton mentagrophytes*. Oxiconazole has been shown to be active against the following microorganisms *in vitro*; however, clinical efficacy has not been established: *Trichophyton tonsurans, Trichophyton violaceum, Microsporum canis, Microsporum audouini, Microsporum gypseum, Epidermophyton floccosum, Candida albicans,* and *Malassezia furfur*.

INDICATIONS AND USAGE

Oxistat® Cream is indicated for the topical treatment of the following dermal infections: tinea pedis, tinea cruris, and tinea corporis due to *T rubrum* and *T mentagrophytes*.

CONTRAINDICATIONS

Oxistat® Cream is contraindicated in individuals who have shown hypersensitivity to any of its components.

WARNINGS

Oxistat® Cream is not for ophthalmic use.

PRECAUTIONS

General: If a reaction suggesting sensitivity or chemical irritation should occur with the use of Oxistat® Cream, treatment should be discontinued and appropriate therapy instituted. Oxistat Cream is for external use only. Avoid introduction of Oxistat Cream into the eyes.

Carcinogenesis, Mutagenesis, Impairment of Fertility: Although no long-term studies in animals have been performed to evaluate carcinogenic potential, no evidence of mutagenic effect was found in two mutation assays (Ames test and Chinese hamster V79 *in vitro* cell mutation assay) or in two cytogenetic assays (human peripheral blood lymphocyte *in vitro* chromosome aberration assay and *in vivo* micronucleus assay in mice.)

Reproductive studies revealed no impairment of fertility in rats at oral doses of 3 mg/kg/day in females and 15 mg/kg/day in males. However, at doses above this level, the following effects were observed: a reduction in the fertility parameters of males and females; a reduction in the number of sperm in vaginal smears; extended estrous cycle; and a decrease in mating frequency.

Pregnancy: *Teratogenic Effects: Pregnancy Category B:* Reproduction studies have been performed in rabbits, rats, and mice at oral doses up to 100, 150, and 200 mg/kg/day, respectively, and revealed no evidence of harm to the fetus due to oxiconazole nitrate. There are, however, no adequate and well-controlled studies in pregnant women. Because animal reproduction studies are not always predictive of human response, this drug should be used during pregnancy only if clearly needed.

Nursing Mothers: Since oxiconazole is excreted in human milk, caution should be exercised when the drug is administered to a nursing woman. Although human data relating concentrations of oxiconazole in milk were not obtained, after subcutaneous administration of 5 mg/kg to female rats, the milk:plasma ratio at 1.5 to 12 hours was in the range of 3.0 to 8.0.

ADVERSE REACTIONS

During clinical trials, 41 (4.3%) of 955 patients treated with oxiconazole nitrate 1% cream reported adverse reactions, including itching (1.6%), burning (1.4%), irritation (0.4%), erythema (0.2%), maceration (0.1%), and fissuring (0.1%).

OVERDOSAGE
Animal studies have shown oxiconazole nitrate to be a central nervous system depressant and tissue irritant when administered orally or by injection.

DOSAGE AND ADMINISTRATION
Oxistat® Cream should be applied to cover affected areas once daily (in the evening) in patients with tinea pedis, tinea corporis, and tinea cruris. Tinea corporis and tinea cruris should be treated for two weeks and tinea pedis for one month to reduce the possibility of recurrence. If a patient shows no clinical improvement after the treatment period, the diagnosis should be reviewed.

HOW SUPPLIED
Oxistat® Cream, 1% is supplied in 15-g (NDC 0173-0423-00) and 30-g (NDC 0173-0423-01) tubes.
Store between 15° and 30° C (50° and 86° F).
Shown in Product Identification Section, page 410

Glaxo Pharmaceuticals
Division of Glaxo Inc.
FIVE MOORE DRIVE
RESEARCH TRIANGLE PARK, NC 27709

ETHAMOLIN® ℞
(ethanolamine oleate)
Injection, 5%
For Local Intravenous Use Only

DESCRIPTION
Ethamolin® (ethanolamine oleate) Injection is a mild sclerosing agent. Chemically it is $C_{17}H_{33}COOH \cdot NH_2CH_2CH_2OH$. It has the following structure:

The empirical formula is $C_{20}H_{41}NO_3$, representing a molecular weight of 343.55.
Ethamolin Injection consists of ethanolamine, a basic substance, which when combined with oleic acid forms a clear, straw to pale yellow colored, deliquescent oleate. The pH ranges from 8.0 to 9.0.
Ethamolin Injection is a sterile, apyrogenic, aqueous solution containing in each ml approximately 50 mg ethanolamine oleate with benzyl alcohol 2% by volume as preservative.

CLINICAL PHARMACOLOGY
When injected intravenously, Ethamolin® (ethanolamine oleate) Injection acts primarily by irritation of the intimal endothelium of the vein and produces a sterile dose-related inflammatory response. This results in fibrosis and occlusion of the vein. Ethamolin Injection also rapidly diffuses through the venous wall and produces a dose-related extravascular inflammatory reaction.
The oleic acid component of the Ethamolin injection is responsible for the inflammatory response, and may also activate coagulation *in vivo* by release of tissue factor and activation of Hageman factor. The ethanolamine component, however, may inhibit fibrin clot formation by chelating calcium, so that a procoagulant action of Ethamolin has not been demonstrated.
After injection, Ethamolin disappears from the injection site within five minutes via the portal vein. When volumes larger than 20 ml are injected, some Ethamolin also flows into the azygos vein through the periesophageal vein. In human autopsy studies it was found that within four days after injection there is neutrophil infiltration of the esophageal wall and hemorrhage within six days. Granulation tissue is first seen at ten days, red thrombi obliterating the varices by twenty days, and sclerosis of the varices by two and a half months. The time course of these findings suggests that sclerosis of esophageal varices will be a delayed rather than an immediate effect of the drug.
The minimum lethal dose of Ethamolin Injection administered intravenously to rabbits is 130 mg/kg.
In dogs, Ethamolin injected into the right atrium at a dose of 1 ml/kg over one minute has been shown to increase extravascular lung water. The maximum recommended human dose is 20 ml, or 0.4 ml/kg for a 50-kg person. The concentration of Ethamolin reaching the lung in human treatment will be less than in the dog studies, but pleural effusions, pulmonary edema, pulmonary infiltration, and pneumonitis have been reported in clinical trials, and minimizing the total per session dose, especially in patients with concomitant cardiopulmonary disease, is recommended (see PRECAUTIONS).

INDICATIONS AND USAGE
Ethamolin® Injection is indicated for the treatment of patients with esophageal varices that have recently bled, to prevent rebleeding.
Ethamolin is not indicated for the treatment of patients with esophageal varices that have not bled. There is no evidence that treatment of this population decreases the likelihood of bleeding.
Sclerotherapy with Ethamolin has no beneficial effect upon portal hypertension, the cause of esophageal varices, so that recanalization and collateralization may occur, necessitating reinjection.

CONTRAINDICATIONS
Ethamolin® Injection should not be administered to subjects with a known hypersensitivity to ethanolamine, oleic acid, or ethanolamine oleate.

WARNINGS
Ethamolin® Injection should be used in pregnant women only when clearly needed (see PRECAUTIONS).
The practice of injecting varicosities of the leg with Ethamolin Injection is not supported by adequately controlled clinical trials. Therefore, such use is not recommended.

PRECAUTIONS
Fatal anaphylactic shock was reported following Injection of a larger than normal volume of Ethamolin® Injection into a male who had a known allergic disposition. Although there are only three known reports of anaphylaxis, the possibility of an anaphylactic reaction should be kept in mind, and the physician should be prepared to treat it appropriately. In extreme emergencies, 0.25 ml of a 1:10,000 intravenous solution of epinephrine (0.25 mg) should be used and allergic reactions should be controlled with antihistamines.
Acute renal failure with spontaneous recovery followed injection of 15 to 20 ml of Ethamolin Injection into two women. The physician should bear in mind that severe injection necrosis may result from direct injection of sclerosing agents, especially if excessive volumes are used. At least one fatal case of extensive esophageal necrosis and death has been reported. The drug should be administered by physicians who are familiar with an acceptable injection technique.
Patients in Child Class C are more likely to develop esophageal ulceration than those in Classes A and B. Complications of ulceration, necrosis, and delayed esophageal perforation appear to occur more frequently when Ethamolin® (ethanolamine oleate) Injection is injected submucosally. This route is not recommended.
In patients with concomitant cardiorespiratory disease, careful monitoring and minimization of the total dose per session is recommended.
Fatal aspiration pneumonia has occurred in elderly patients undergoing esophageal variceal sclerotherapy with Ethamolin Injection. This adverse event appears to be procedure-related rather than drug-related, but as aspiration of blood and/or stomach contents is not uncommon in patients with bleeding esophageal varices, special precautions should be taken to prevent its occurrence, especially in the elderly and critically ill subjects.
Pregnancy: *Teratogenic Effects: Pregnancy Category C:* Animal reproduction studies have not been conducted with Ethamolin Injection. It is also not known whether Ethamolin Injection can cause fetal harm when administered to a pregnant woman or can affect reproduction capacity. Ethamolin Injection should be given to a pregnant woman only if clearly needed.
Nursing Mothers: It is not known whether this drug is excreted in human milk. Because many drugs are excreted in human milk, caution should be exercised when Ethamolin Injection is administered to a nursing woman.
Pediatric Use: Safety and effectiveness in children have not been established.

ADVERSE REACTIONS
The reported frequency of complications/adverse events per injection session was 13%. The most common complications were pleural effusion/infiltration (2.1%), esophageal ulcer (2.1%), pyrexia (1.8%), retrosternal pain (1.6%), esophageal stricture (1.3%), and pneumonia (1.2%).
Other adverse local esophageal reactions have also been reported at rates of 0.1% to 0.4%, including esophagitis, tearing of the esophagus, sloughing of the mucosa overlying the injected varix, ulceration, stricture, necrosis, periesophageal abscess and perforation (see PRECAUTIONS). These complications appear to be dependent upon the dose and the patient's clinical state.
Bacteremia has been observed in patients following injection of esophageal varices with Ethamolin. Pyrexia and retrosternal pain are not infrequently observed during the post-injection period. Fatal aspiration pneumonia has occurred in patients with esophageal varices who underwent Ethamolin® Injection sclerotherapy (see PRECAUTIONS). Anaphylactic shock and acute renal failure with spontaneous recovery have occurred (see PRECAUTIONS).

Spinal cord paralysis due to occlusion of the anterior spinal artery has been reported in one child eight hours after Ethamolin sclerotherapy.

OVERDOSAGE
Overdosage of Ethamolin® Injection can result in severe intramural necrosis of the esophagus. Complications resulting from such overdosage have resulted in death.

DOSAGE AND ADMINISTRATION
Local Ethamolin® (ethanolamine oleate) Injection sclerotherapy of esophageal varices should be performed by physicians who are familiar with an acceptable technique. The usual intravenous dose is 1.5 to 5 ml per varix. The maximum total dose per treatment session should not exceed 20 ml. Patients with significant liver dysfunction (Child Class C) or concomitant cardiopulmonary disease should usually receive less than the recommended maximum dose. Submucosal injections are not recommended as they are reportedly more likely to result in ulceration at the site of injection.
To obliterate the varix, injections may be made at the time of the acute bleeding episode and then after one week, six weeks, three months, and six months as indicated.
Note: Parenteral drug products should be inspected visually for particulate matter and discoloration before administration whenever solution and container permit.

HOW SUPPLIED
Ethamolin Injection, 5% is available in 2-ml ampules in boxes of 10 (NDC 0173-0397-38).
Store at Controlled Room Temperature, 15°–30°C (59°–86°F). Protect from light.
Shown in Product Identification Section, page 410

FORTAZ® ℞
[*for' taz*]
(ceftazidime for injection, Glaxo)
FORTAZ® ℞
(ceftazidime sodium injection)

For Intravenous or Intramuscular Use

DESCRIPTION
Ceftazidime is a semisynthetic, broad-spectrum, beta-lactam antibiotic for parenteral administration. It is the pentahydrate of Pyridinium, 1-[[7-[[(2-amino-4-thiazolyl)[(1-carboxy-1-methylethoxy) imino]acetyl] amino]-2-carboxy -8- oxo-5-thia -1- azabicyclo[4.2.0]oct-2-en-3-yl]methyl]-, hydroxide, inner salt, [6R-[6α,7β(Z)]]. It has the following structure:

Fortaz® (ceftazidime for injection) is a sterile, dry, powdered mixture of ceftazidime pentahydrate and sodium carbonate. The sodium carbonate at a concentration of 118 mg/g of ceftazidime activity has been admixed to facilitate dissolution. The total sodium content of the mixture is approximately 54 mg (2.3 mEq)/g of ceftazidime activity. Fortaz in sterile crystalline form is supplied in vials equivalent to 500 mg, 1 g, 2 g, or 6 g anhydrous ceftazidime. Solutions of Fortaz range in color from light yellow to amber, depending upon the diluent and volume used. The pH of freshly constituted solutions usually ranges from 5 to 8.
Fortaz® (ceftazidime sodium injection) is available as a frozen, iso-osmotic, sterile, nonpyrogenic solution with 1 or 2 g of ceftazidime as ceftazidime sodium premixed with approximately 2.2 or 1.6 g, respectively, of dextrose hydrous, USP. Dextrose has been added to adjust the osmolality. Sodium hydroxide is used to adjust pH and neutralize ceftazidime pentahydrate free acid to the sodium salt. The pH may have been adjusted with hydrochloric acid. Solutions of premixed Fortaz range in color from light yellow to amber. The solution is intended for intravenous use after thawing to room temperature. The osmolality of the solution is approximately 300 mOsml/kg, and the pH of thawed solutions ranges from 5 to 7.5.
The plastic container is fabricated from a specially designed multilayer plastic, PL 2040. Solutions are in contact with the polyethylene layer of this container and can leach out certain chemical components of the plastic in very small amounts within the expiration period. The suitability of the plastic has been confirmed in tests in animals according to USP biological tests for plastic containers as well as by tissue culture toxicity studies.

CLINICAL PHARMACOLOGY
After intravenous administration of 500-mg and 1-g doses of ceftazidime over five minutes to normal adult male volunteers, mean peak serum concentrations of 45 and 90 mcg/ml,

Continued on next page

Glaxo Pharm.—Cont.

respectively, were achieved. After intravenous infusion of 500-mg, 1-g, and 2-g doses of ceftazidime over 20 to 30 minutes to normal adult male volunteers, mean peak serum concentrations of 42, 69, and 170 mcg/ml, respectively, were achieved. The average serum concentrations following intravenous infusion of 500-mg, 1-g, and 2-g doses to these volunteers over an eight-hour interval are given in Table 1.

Table 1

Ceftazidime IV Dosage	Serum Concentrations (mcg/ml)				
	0.5 h	1 h	2 h	4 h	8 h
500 mg	42	25	12	6	2
1 g	60	39	23	11	3
2 g	129	75	42	13	5

The absorption and elimination of ceftazidime were directly proportional to the size of the dose. The half-life following intravenous administration was approximately 1.9 hours. Less than 10% of ceftazidime was protein bound. The degree of protein binding was independent of concentration. There was no evidence of accumulation of ceftazidime in the serum in individuals with normal renal function following multiple intravenous doses of 1 and 2 g every eight hours for ten days. Following intramuscular administration of 500-mg and 1-g doses of ceftazidime to normal adult volunteers, the mean peak serum concentrations were 17 and 39 mcg/ml, respectively, at approximately one hour. Serum concentrations remained above 4 mcg/ml for six and eight hours after the intramuscular administration of 500-mg and 1-g doses, respectively. The half-life of ceftazidime in these volunteers was approximately two hours.

The presence of hepatic dysfunction had no effect on the pharmacokinetics of ceftazidime in individuals administered 2 g intravenously every eight hours for five days. Therefore, a dosage adjustment from the normal recommended dosage is not required for patients with hepatic dysfunction, provided renal function is not impaired.

Approximately 80% to 90% of an intramuscular or intravenous dose of ceftazidime is excreted unchanged by the kidneys over a 24-hour period. After the intravenous administration of single 500-mg or 1-g doses, approximately 50% of the dose appeared in the urine in the first two hours. An additional 20% was excreted between two and four hours after dosing, and approximately another 12% of the dose appeared in the urine between four and eight hours later. The elimination of ceftazidime by the kidneys resulted in high, therapeutic concentrations in the urine.

The mean renal clearance of ceftazidime was approximately 100 ml/min. The calculated plasma clearance of approximately 115 ml/min indicated nearly complete elimination of ceftazidime by the renal route. Administration of probenecid before dosing had no effect on the elimination kinetics of ceftazidime. This suggested that ceftazidime is eliminated by glomerular filtration and is not actively secreted by renal tubular mechanisms.

Since ceftazidime is eliminated almost solely by the kidneys, its serum half-life is significantly prolonged in patients with impaired renal function. Consequently, dosage adjustments in such patients as described in the DOSAGE AND ADMINISTRATION section are suggested.

Therapeutic concentrations of ceftazidime are achieved in the following body tissues and fluids.
[See table below].

Microbiology: Ceftazidime is bactericidal in action, exerting its effect by inhibition of enzymes responsible for cell-wall synthesis. A wide range of gram-negative organisms is susceptible to ceftazidime in vitro, including strains resistant to gentamicin and other aminoglycosides. In addition, ceftazidime has been shown to be active against gram-positive organisms. It is highly stable to most clinically important beta-lactamases, plasmid or chromosomal, which are produced by both gram-negative and gram-positive organisms, and consequently is active against many strains resistant to ampicillin and other cephalosporins.

Ceftazidime has been shown to be active against the following organisms both in vitro and in clinical infections (see INDICATIONS AND USAGE).

Aerobes, Gram-negative: Pseudomonas spp (including Pseudomonas aeruginosa); Klebsiella spp (including Klebsiella pneumoniae); Proteus mirabilis; Proteus vulgaris; Escherichia coli; Enterobacter spp, including Enterobacter cloacae and Enterobacter aerogenes; Citrobacter spp, including Citrobacter freundii and Citrobacter diversus; Serratia spp; Haemophilus influenzae, including ampicillin-resistant strains; and Neisseria meningitidis.

Aerobes, Gram-positive: Staphylococcus aureus, including penicillinase- and non-penicillinase-producing strains; Streptococcus pyogenes (group A beta-hemolytic streptococci); Streptococcus agalactiae (group B streptococci); and Streptococcus pneumoniae.

Anaerobes: Bacteroides spp (NOTE: many strains of Bacteroides fragilis are resistant).

Ceftazidime has also been shown to demonstrate in vitro activity against the following organisms, although its clinical significance is not known: Staphylococcus epidermidis; Morganella morganii (formerly Proteus morganii); Providencia spp (including Providencia rettgeri, formerly Proteus rettgeri); Acinetobacter spp; Salmonella spp; Clostridium spp (not including Clostridium difficile); Peptococcus spp; Peptostreptococcus spp; Neisseria gonorrhoeae; Haemophilus parainfluenzae; Yersinia enterocolitica; and Shigella spp.

Ceftazidime and the aminoglycosides have been shown to be synergistic in vitro against P aeruginosa and the Enterobacteriaceae. Ceftazidime and carbenicillin have also been shown to be synergistic in vitro against P aeruginosa.

Ceftazidime is not active in vitro against methicillin-resistant staphylococci; Streptococcus faecalis and many other enterococci; Listeria monocytogenes; Campylobacter spp; or C difficile.

Susceptibility Tests: *Diffusion Techniques:* Quantitative methods that require measurement of zone diameters give an estimate of antibiotic susceptibility. One such procedure[1-3] has been recommended for use with disks to test susceptibility to ceftazidime.

Reports from the laboratory giving results of the standard single-disk susceptibility test with a 30-mcg ceftazidime disk should be interpreted according to the following criteria:

Susceptible organisms produce zones of 18 mm or greater, indicating that the test organism is likely to respond to therapy.

Organisms that produce zones of 15 to 17 mm are expected to be susceptible if high dosage is used or if the infection is confined to tissues and fluids (eg, urine) in which high antibiotic levels are attained.

Resistant organisms produce zones of 14 mm or less, indicating that other therapy should be selected.

Organisms should be tested with the ceftazidime disk since ceftazidime has been shown by in vitro tests to be active against certain strains found resistant when other beta-lactam disks are used.

Standardized procedures require the use of laboratory control organisms. The 30-mcg ceftazidime disk should give zone diameters between 25 and 32 mm for E coli ATCC 25922. For P aeruginosa ATCC 27853, the zone diameters should be between 22 and 29 mm. For S aureus ATCC 25923, the zone diameters should be between 16 and 20 mm.

Dilution Techniques: In other susceptibility testing procedures, eg, ICS agar dilution or the equivalent, a bacterial isolate may be considered susceptible if the minimum inhibitory concentration (MIC) value for ceftazidime is not more than 16 mcg/ml. Organisms are considered resistant to ceftazidime if the MIC is equal to or greater than 64 mcg/ml. Organisms having an MIC value of less than 64 mcg/ml but greater than 16 mcg/ml are expected to be susceptible if high dosage is used or if the infection is confined to tissues and fluids (eg, urine) in which high antibiotic levels are attained. As with standard diffusion methods, dilution procedures require the use of laboratory control organisms. Standard ceftazidime powder should give MIC values in the range of 4 to 16 mcg/ml for S aureus ATCC 25923. For E coli ATCC 25922, the MIC range should be between 0.125 and 0.5 mcg/ml. For P aeruginosa ATCC 27853, the MIC range should be between 0.5 and 2 mcg/ml.

INDICATIONS AND USAGE

Fortaz® (ceftazidime for injection/ceftazidime sodium injection) is indicated for the treatment of patients with infections caused by susceptible strains of the designated organisms in the following diseases:

1. **Lower Respiratory Tract Infections,** including pneumonia, caused by P aeruginosa and other Pseudomonas spp; H influenzae, including ampicillin-resistant strains; Klebsiella spp; Enterobacter spp; P mirabilis; E coli; Serratia spp; Citrobacter spp; S pneumoniae; and S aureus (methicillin-susceptible strains).

2. **Skin and Skin Structure Infections** caused by P aeruginosa; Klebsiella spp; E coli; Proteus spp, including P mirabilis and indole-positive Proteus; Enterobacter spp; Serratia spp; S aureus (methicillin-susceptible strains); and S pyogenes (group A beta-hemolytic streptococci).

3. **Urinary Tract Infections,** both complicated and uncomplicated, caused by P aeruginosa; Enterobacter spp; Proteus spp, including P mirabilis and indole-positive Proteus; Klebsiella spp; and E coli.

4. **Bacterial Septicemia,** caused by P aeruginosa; Klebsiella spp; H influenzae; E coli; Serratia spp; S pneumoniae; and S aureus (methicillin-susceptible strains).

5. **Bone and Joint Infections** caused by P aeruginosa; Klebsiella spp; Enterobacter spp; and S aureus (methicillin-susceptible strains).

6. **Gynecologic Infections,** including endometritis, pelvic cellulitis, and other infections of the female genital tract caused by E coli.

7. **Intra-abdominal Infections,** including peritonitis caused by E coli, Klebsiella spp, and S aureus (methicillin-susceptible strains) and polymicrobial infections caused by aerobic and anaerobic organisms and Bacteroides spp (many strains of B fragilis are resistant).

8. **Central Nervous System Infections,** including meningitis, caused by H influenzae and Neisseria meningitidis. Fortaz has also been used successfully in a limited number of cases of meningitis due to P aeruginosa and S pneumoniae.

Specimens for bacterial cultures should be obtained before therapy in order to isolate and identify causative organisms and to determine their susceptibility to ceftazidime. Therapy may be instituted before results of susceptibility studies are known; however, once these results become available, the antibiotic treatment should be adjusted accordingly.

Fortaz may be used alone in cases of confirmed or suspected sepsis. Fortaz has been used successfully in clinical trials as empiric therapy in cases where various concomitant therapies with other antibiotics have been used.

Fortaz may also be used concomitantly with other antibiotics, such as aminoglycosides, vancomycin, and clindamycin; in severe and life-threatening infections; and in the immunocompromised patient. When such concomitant treatment is appropriate, prescribing information in the labeling for the other antibiotics should be followed. The dose depends on the severity of the infection and the patient's condition.

CONTRAINDICATIONS

Fortaz® (ceftazidime for injection/ceftazidime sodium injection) is contraindicated in patients who have shown hypersensitivity to ceftazidime or the cephalosporin group of antibiotics.

WARNINGS

BEFORE THERAPY WITH FORTAZ® (ceftazidime for injection/ceftazidime sodium injection) IS INSTITUTED, CAREFUL INQUIRY SHOULD BE MADE TO DETERMINE WHETHER THE PATIENT HAS HAD PREVIOUS HYPERSENSITIVITY REACTIONS TO CEFTAZIDIME, CEPHALOSPORINS, PENICILLINS, OR OTHER DRUGS.

Table 2: Ceftazidime Concentrations in Body Tissues and Fluids

Tissue or Fluid	Dose/ Route	No. of Patients	Time of Sample Post-dose	Average Tissue or Fluid Level (mcg/ml or mcg/g)
Urine	500 mg IM	6	0–2 h	2,100.0
	2 g IV	6	0–2 h	12,000.0
Bile	2 g IV	3	90 min	36.4
Synovial fluid	2 g IV	13	2 h	25.6
Peritoneal fluid	2 g IV	8	2 h	48.6
Sputum	1 g IV	8	1 h	9.0
Cerebrospinal fluid	2 g q8h IV	5	120 min	9.8
(inflamed meninges)	2 g q8h IV	6	180 min	9.4
Aqueous humor	2 g IV	13	1–3 h	11.0
Blister fluid	1 g IV	7	2–3 h	19.7
Lymphatic fluid	1 g IV	7	2–3 h	23.4
Bone	2 g IV	8	0.67 h	31.1
Heart muscle	2 g IV	35	30–280 min	12.7
Skin	2 g IV	22	30–180 min	6.6
Skeletal muscle	2 g IV	35	30–280 min	9.4
Myometrium	2 g IV	31	1–2 h	18.7

ANTIBIOTICS SHOULD BE ADMINISTERED WITH CAUTION TO ANY PATIENT WHO HAS DEMONSTRATED SOME FORM OF ALLERGY, PARTICULARLY TO DRUGS. THIS PRODUCT SHOULD BE GIVEN WITH CAUTION TO PATIENTS WITH TYPE 1 HYPERSENSITIVITY REACTIONS TO PENICILLIN. IF AN ALLERGIC REACTION TO FORTAZ OCCURS, DISCONTINUE TREATMENT WITH THE DRUG. SERIOUS ACUTE HYPERSENSITIVITY REACTIONS MAY REQUIRE EPINEPHRINE AND OTHER EMERGENCY MEASURES.

Pseudomembranous colitis has been reported with the use of ceftazidime, other cephalosporins, and broad-spectrum antibiotics; therefore, it is important to consider this diagnosis in patients who develop diarrhea in association with antibiotic use.

Treatment with broad-spectrum antibiotics alters normal flora of the colon and may permit overgrowth of clostridia. Studies indicate a toxin produced by *C difficile* is one primary cause of antibiotic-associated colitis.

Mild cases of colitis may respond to drug discontinuation alone. Moderate to severe cases should be managed with fluid, electrolyte, and protein supplementation as indicated. When the colitis is not relieved by drug discontinuation or when it is severe, oral vancomycin is the treatment of choice for antibiotic-associated pseudomembranous colitis produced by *C difficile*. Other causes of colitis should also be considered.

PRECAUTIONS

Fortaz® (ceftazidime for injection/ceftazidime sodium injection) has not been shown to be nephrotoxic; however, because high and prolonged serum antibiotic concentrations can occur from usual doses in patients with transient or persistent reduction of urinary output because of renal insufficiency, the total daily dosage should be reduced when ceftazidime is administered to such patients to avoid the clinical consequences, eg, seizures, of elevated levels of antibiotics (see DOSAGE AND ADMINISTRATION). Continued dosage should be determined by degree of renal impairment, severity of infection, and susceptibility of the causative organisms.

As with other antibiotics, prolonged use of Fortaz may result in overgrowth of nonsusceptible organisms. Repeated evaluation of the patient's condition is essential. If superinfection occurs during therapy, appropriate measures should be taken.

Fortaz should be prescribed with caution in individuals with a history of gastrointestinal disease, particularly colitis.

Drug Interactions: Nephrotoxicity has been reported following concomitant administration of cephalosporins with aminoglycoside antibiotics or potent diuretics such as furosemide. Renal function should be carefully monitored, especially if higher dosages of the aminoglycosides are to be administered or if therapy is prolonged, because of the potential nephrotoxicity and ototoxicity of aminoglycosidic antibiotics. Nephrotoxicity and ototoxicity were not noted when Fortaz was given alone in clinical trials.

Carcinogenesis, Mutagenesis, Impairment of Fertility: Long-term studies in animals have not been performed to evaluate carcinogenic potential. However, a mouse Micronucleus test and an Ames test were both negative for mutagenic effects.

Pregnancy: *Teratogenic Effects: Pregnancy Category B:* Reproduction studies have been performed in mice and rats at doses up to 40 times the human dose and have revealed no evidence of impaired fertility or harm to the fetus due to Fortaz. There are, however, no adequate and well-controlled studies in pregnant women. Because animal reproduction studies are not always predictive of human response, this drug should be used during pregnancy only if clearly needed.

Nursing Mothers: Ceftazidime is excreted in human milk in low concentrations. Caution should be exercised when Fortaz is administered to a nursing woman.

ADVERSE REACTIONS

Fortaz® (ceftazidime for injection/ceftazidime sodium injection) is generally well tolerated. The incidence of adverse reactions associated with the administration of Fortaz was low in clinical trials. The most common were local reactions following intravenous injection and allergic and gastrointestinal reactions. Other adverse reactions were encountered infrequently. No disulfiram-like reactions were reported.

The following adverse effects from clinical trials were considered to be either related to ceftazidime therapy or were of uncertain etiology:

Local Effects, reported in less than 2% of patients, were phlebitis and inflammation at the site of injection (1 in 69 patients).

Hypersensitivity Reactions, reported in 2% of patients, were pruritus, rash, and fever. Immediate reactions, generally manifested by rash and/or pruritus, occurred in 1 in 285 patients. Angioedema and anaphylaxis (bronchospasm and/or hypotension) have been reported very rarely.

Gastrointestinal Symptoms, reported in less than 2% of patients, were diarrhea (1 in 78), nausea (1 in 156), vomiting (1

in 500), and abdominal pain (1 in 416). Onset of pseudomembranous colitis symptoms may occur during or after antibiotic treatment (see WARNINGS).

Central Nervous System Reactions (less than 1%) include headache, dizziness, and paresthesia. Seizures have been reported with several cephalosporins, including ceftazidime (see PRECAUTIONS).

Less Frequent Adverse Events (less than 1%) were candidiasis (including oral thrush) and vaginitis.

Laboratory Test Changes noted during Fortaz clinical trials were transient and included: eosinophilia (1 in 13), positive Coombs' test without hemolysis (1 in 23), thrombocytosis (1 in 45), and slight elevations in one or more of the hepatic enzymes, aspartate aminotransferase (AST, SGOT) (1 in 16), alanine aminotransferase (ALT, SGPT) (1 in 15), LDH (1 in 18), GGT (1 in 19), and alkaline phosphatase (1 in 23). As with some other cephalosporins, transient elevations of blood urea, blood urea nitrogen, and/or serum creatinine were observed occasionally. Transient leukopenia, neutropenia, agranulocytosis, thrombocytopenia, and lymphocytosis were seen very rarely.

In addition to the adverse reactions listed above that have been observed in patients treated with ceftazidime, the following adverse reactions and altered laboratory tests have been reported for cephalosporin class antibiotics:

> *Adverse Reactions:* Urticaria, Stevens-Johnson syndrome, erhthema multiforme, toxic epidermal necrolysis, colitis, renal dysfunction, toxic nephropathy, hepatic dysfunction including cholestasis, aplastic anemia, hemolytic anemia, hemorrhage.

> *Altered Laboratory Tests:* Prolonged prothrombin time, false positive test for urinary glucose, elevated bilirubin, pancytopenia.

DOSAGE AND ADMINISTRATION

Dosage: The usual adult dosage is 1 g administered intravenously or intramuscularly every eight to 12 hours. The dosage and route should be determined by the susceptibility of the causative organisms, the severity of infection, and the condition and renal function of the patient.

The guidelines for dosage of Fortaz® (ceftazidime for injection/ceftazidime sodium injection) are listed in Table 3. The following dosage schedule is recommended.

[See table above].

Impaired Hepatic Function: No adjustment in dosage is required for patients with hepatic dysfunction.

Impaired Renal Function: Ceftazidime is excreted by the kidneys, almost exclusively by glomerular filtration. Therefore, in patients with impaired renal function (glomerular filtration rate [GFR] <50 ml/min), it is recommended that the dosage of ceftazidime be reduced to compensate for its slower excretion. In patients with suspected renal insufficiency, an initial loading dose of 1 g of ceftazidime may be given. An estimate of GFR should be made to determine the appropriate maintenance dose. The recommended dosage is presented in Table 4.

Table 3: Recommended Dosage Schedule

	Dose	Frequency
Adults		
Usual recommended dosage	**1 g IV or IM**	**q8-12h**
Uncomplicated urinary tract infections	250 mg IV or IM	q12h
Bone and joint infections	2 g IV	q12h
Complicated urinary tract infections	500 mg IV or IM	q8-12h
Uncomplicated pneumonia; mild skin and skin structure infections	500 mg–1 g IV or IM	q8h
Serious gynecologic and intra-abdominal infections	2 g IV	q8h
Meningitis	2 g IV	q8h
Very severe life-threatening infections, especially in immunocompromised patients	2 g IV	q8h
Pseudomonal lung infections in patients with cystic fibrosis with normal renal function*	30–50 mg/kg IV to a maximum of 6 g/day	q8h
Neonates (0–4 weeks)	30 mg/kg IV	q12h
Infants and children (1 month–12 years)	30–50 mg/kg IV to a maximum of 6 g/day†	q8h

* Although clinical improvement has been shown, bacteriological cures cannot be expected in patients with chronic respiratory disease and cystic fibrosis.
† The higher dose should be reserved for immunocompromised children or children with cystic fibrosis or meningitis.

Table 4: Recommended Maintenance Doses of Fortaz in Renal Insufficiency

NOTE: IF THE DOSE RECOMMENDED IN TABLE 3 ABOVE IS LOWER THAN THAT RECOMMENDED FOR PATIENTS WITH RENAL INSUFFICIENCY AS OUTLINED IN TABLE 4, THE LOWER DOSE SHOULD BE USED.

Creatinine Clearance (ml/min)	Recommended Unit Dose of Ceftazidime	Frequency of Dosing
50–31	1 g	q12h
30–16	1 g	q24h
15–6	500 mg	q24h
<5	500 mg	q48h

When only serum creatinine is available, the following formula (Cockcroft's equation)[4] may be used to estimate creatinine clearance. The serum creatinine should represent a steady state of renal function:

Males:
$$\text{Creatinine clearance (ml/min)} = \frac{\text{Weight (kg)} \times (140 - \text{age})}{72 \times \text{serum creatinine (mg/dl)}}$$

Females: $0.85 \times$ male value

In patients with severe infections who would normally receive 6 g of ceftazidime daily were it not for renal insufficiency, the unit dose given in the table above may be increased by 50% or the dosing frequency increased appropriately. Further dosing should be determined by therapeutic monitoring, severity of the infection, and susceptibility of the causative organism.

In children as for adults, the creatinine clearance should be adjusted for body surface area or lean body mass and the dosing frequency reduced in cases of renal insufficiency.

In patients undergoing hemodialysis, a loading dose of 1 g is recommended, followed by 1 g after each hemodialysis period.

Fortaz can also be used in patients undergoing intraperitoneal dialysis and continuous ambulatory peritoneal dialysis. In such patients, a loading dose of 1 g of ceftazidime may be given, followed by 500 mg every 24 hours. In addition to intravenous use, Fortaz can be incorporated in the dialysis fluid at a concentration of 250 mg for 2 L of dialysis fluid.

Note: Generally Fortaz should be continued for two days after the signs and symptoms of infection have disappeared, but in complicated infections longer therapy may be required.

Administration: Fortaz may be given intravenously or by deep intramuscular injection into a large muscle mass such as the upper outer quadrant of the gluteus maximus or lateral part of the thigh.

Intramuscular Administration: For intramuscular administration, Fortaz should be constituted with one of the following diluents: Sterile Water for Injection, Bacteriostatic Water for Injection, or 0.5% or 1% Lidocaine Hydrochloride Injection. Refer to Table 5.

Intravenous Administration: The IV route is preferable for patients with bacterial septicemia, bacterial meningitis, peritonitis, or other severe or life-threatening infections, or

Continued on next page

Glaxo Pharm.—Cont.

for patients who may be poor risks because of lowered resistance resulting from such debilitating conditions as malnutrition, trauma, surgery, diabetes, heart failure, or malignancy, particularly if shock is present or pending.

For direct intermittent intravenous administration, constitute Fortaz as directed in Table 5 with Sterile Water for Injection. Slowly inject directly into the vein over a period of three to five minutes or give through the tubing of an administration set while the patient is also receiving one of the compatible intravenous fluids (see COMPATIBILITY AND STABILITY).

For intravenous infusion, constitute the 1- or 2-g Infusion Pack with 100 ml of Sterile Water for Injection or one of the compatible intravenous fluids listed under the COMPATIBILITY AND STABILITY section. Alternatively, constitute the 500-mg, 1-g, or 2-g vial and add an appropriate quantity of the resulting solution to an IV container with one of the compatible intravenous fluids.

Intermittent intravenous infusion with a Y-type administration set can be accomplished with compatible solutions. However, during infusion of a solution containing ceftazidime, it is desirable to discontinue the other solution.

[See table below.]

All vials of Fortaz as supplied are under reduced pressure. When Fortaz is dissolved, carbon dioxide is released and a positive pressure develops. For ease of use please follow the recommended techniques of constitution described on the detachable Instructions for Constitution section of the package insert.

Solutions of Fortaz, like those of most beta-lactam antibiotics, should not be added to solutions of aminoglycoside antibiotics because of potential interaction.

However, if concurrent therapy with Fortaz and an aminoglycoside is indicated, each of these antibiotics can be administered separately to the same patient.

Directions for Use of Fortaz Frozen in Galaxy™ Plastic Containers: Fortaz supplied as a frozen, sterile, iso-osmotic, nonpyrogenic solution in plastic containers is to be administered after thawing either as a continuous or intermittent intravenous infusion. Do not force thaw by immersion in water baths or by microwave irradiation. The thawed solution is stable for 24 hours at room temperature or for seven days if stored under refrigeration. **Do not Refreeze.**

Thaw container at room temperature (25°C) or under refrigeration (5°C). Components of the solution may precipitate in the frozen state and will dissolve upon reaching room temperature with little or no agitation. Potency is not affected. Mix after solution has reached room temperature. Check for minute leaks by squeezing bag firmly. Discard bag if leaks are found as sterility may be impaired. Do not add supplementary medication. Do not use unless solution is clear and seal is intact.

Use sterile equipment.

Caution: Do not use plastic containers in series connections. Such use could result in air embolism due to residual air being drawn from the primary container before administration of the fluid from the secondary container is complete.

Preparation for Administration:
1. Suspend container from eyelet support.
2. Remove protector from outlet port at bottom of container.
3. Attach administration set. Refer to complete directions accompanying set.

COMPATIBILITY AND STABILITY

Intramuscular: Fortaz® (ceftazidime for injection), when constituted as directed with Sterile Water for Injection, Bacteriostatic Water for Injection, or 0.5% or 1% Lidocaine Hydrochloride Injection, maintains satisfactory potency for 24 hours at room temperature or for seven days under refrigeration. Solutions in Sterile Water for Injection that are frozen immediately after constitution in the original container are

stable for three months when stored at −20°C. Once thawed, solutions should not be refrozen. Thawed solutions may be stored for up to eight hours at room temperature or for four days in a refrigerator.

Intravenous: Fortaz, when constituted as directed with Sterile Water for Injection, maintains satisfactory potency for 24 hours at room temperature or for seven days under refrigeration. Solutions in Sterile Water for Injection in the infusion vial or in 0.9% Sodium Chloride Injection in Viaflex® small volume containers that are frozen immediately after constitution are stable for six months when stored at −20°C. Do not force thaw by immersion in water baths or by microwave irradiation. Once thawed, solutions should not be refrozen. Thawed solutions may be stored for up to 24 hours at room temperature or for seven days in a refrigerator. More concentrated solutions in Sterile Water for Injection in the original container that are frozen immediately after constitution are stable for three months when stored at -20°C. Once thawed, solutions should not be refrozen. Thawed solutions may be stored for up to eight hours at room temperature or for four days in a refrigerator.

Fortaz is compatible with the more commonly used intravenous infusion fluids. Solutions at concentrations between 1 and 40 mg/ml in 0.9% Sodium Chloride Injection; 0.16 M Sodium Lactate Injection; 5% Dextrose Injection; 5% Dextrose and 0.225% Sodium Chloride Injection; 5% Dextrose and 0.45% Sodium Chloride Injection; 5% Dextrose and 0.9% Sodium Chloride Injection; 10% Dextrose Injection; Ringer's Injection, USP; Lactated Ringer's Injection, USP; 10% Invert Sugar in Water for Injection; and Normosol®-M in 5% Dextrose Injection may be stored for up to 24 hours at room temperature or for seven days if refrigerated.

Fortaz is less stable in Sodium Bicarbonate Injection than in other intravenous fluids. It is not recommended as a diluent.

Solutions of Fortaz in 5% Dextrose and 0.9% Sodium Chloride Injection are stable for at least six hours at room temperature in plastic tubing, drip chambers, and volume control devices of common intravenous infusion sets.

Ceftazidime at a concentration of 4 mg/ml has been found compatible for 24 hours at room temperature or for seven days under refrigeration in 0.9% Sodium Chloride Injection or 5% Dextrose Injection when admixed with: cefuroxime sodium (Zinacef®) 3 mg/ml; Heparin 10 or 50 U/ml; or Potassium Chloride 10 or 40 mEq/L.

Vancomycin solution exhibits a physical incompatibility when mixed with a number of drugs including ceftazidime. The likelihood of precipitation with ceftazidime is dependent on the concentrations of vancomycin and ceftazidime present. It is therefore recommended, when both drugs are to be administered by intermittent intravenous infusion, that they be given separately, flushing the intravenous lines (with one of the compatible intravenous fluids) between the administration of these two agents.

Note: Parenteral drug products should be inspected visually for particulate matter before administration whenever solution and container permit.

As with other cephalosporins, Fortaz powder, as well as solutions, tends to darken depending on storage conditions; within the stated recommendations, however, product potency is not adversely affected.

HOW SUPPLIED

Fortaz® (ceftazidime for injection) in the dry state should be stored between 15° and 30° C (59° and 86°F) and protected from light. Fortaz is a dry, white to off-white powder supplied in vials and infusion packs as follows:

NDC 0173-0377-31 500-mg* Vial (Tray of 25)
NDC 0173-0378-35 1-g* Vial (Tray of 25)
NDC 0173-0379-34 2-g* Vial (Tray of 10)
NDC 0173-0380-32 1-g* Infusion Pack (Tray of 10)

NDC 0173-0381-32 2-g* Infusion Pack (Tray of 10)
NDC 0173-0382-37 6-g* Pharmacy Bulk Package (Tray of 6)
Fortaz® (ceftazidime sodium injection) frozen as a premixed solution of ceftazidime sodium should not be stored above −20° C. Fortaz is supplied frozen in 50-ml, single-dose, plastic containers as follows:
NDC 0173-0412-00 1-g* Plastic Container
NDC 0713-0413-00 2-g* Plastic Container
*Equivalent to anhydrous ceftazidime.

REFERENCES: 1. Bauer AW, Kirby WMM, Sherris JC, et al: Antibiotic susceptibility testing by a standardized single disc method. *Am J Clin Pathol* 1966;45:493. 2. National Committee for Clinical Laboratory Standards, Approved Standard: Performance Standards for Antimicrobial Disc Susceptibility Tests (M2-A3), December, 1984. 3. Standardized disc susceptibility test. *Federal Register* 1974;39(May 30):19182-19184. 4. Cockcroft DW, Gault MH: Prediction of creatinine clearance from serum creatinine. *Nephron* 1976;16:31-41.

Fortaz is a registered trademark of Glaxo.
Galaxy is a trademark of Baxter International Inc.
Viaflex is a registered trademark of Baxter International Inc.

Shown in Product Identification Section, pages 410 & 411

ZANTAC® Injection   ℞
[*zan'tak*]
(ranitidine hydrochloride)
ZANTAC® Injection Premixed   ℞
(ranitidine hydrochloride)

DESCRIPTION

The active ingredient in Zantac® Injection and Zantac® Injection Premixed, ranitidine hydrochloride, is a histamine H_2-receptor antagonist. Chemically, it is N[2-[[[5-[(dimethylamino)-methyl]-2-furanyl]methyl]thio]ethyl]-N'-methyl-2-nitro-1,1-ethenediamine, hydrochloride.

The empirical formula is $C_{13}H_{22}N_4O_3S.HCl$, representing a molecular weight of 350.87.

Ranitidine hydrochloride is a white to pale yellow, granular substance that is soluble in water.

Zantac Injection is a clear, colorless to yellow, nonpyrogenic liquid that tends to darken slightly without adversely affecting potency. The pH of the injection solution is 6.7 to 7.3.

Sterile Injection for IM or IV Administration: Each 1 ml of aqueous solution contains ranitidine 25 mg (as the hydrochloride); phenol 5 mg as preservative; and 0.96 mg monobasic potassium phosphate and 2.4 mg dibasic sodium phosphate as buffers.

A pharmacy bulk package is a container of a sterile preparation for parenteral use that contains many single doses. The contents are intended for use in a pharmacy admixture program and are restricted to the preparation of admixtures for intravenous infusion.

Sterile Premixed Solution for IV Administration in Single-dose Flexible Plastic Containers: Each 100 ml contains ranitidine hydrochloride equivalent to 50 mg ranitidine, sodium chloride 450 mg, and citric acid 30 mg and dibasic sodium phosphate 180 mg as buffers in water for injection. It contains no preservatives. The osmolarity of this solution is 180 mOsm/L (approx.), and the pH is 6.7 to 7.3.

The flexible plastic container is fabricated from a specially formulated, nonplasticized, thermoplastic co-polyester (CR3). Water can permeate from inside the container into the overwrap but not in amounts sufficient to affect the solution significantly. Solutions inside the plastic container also can leach out certain of the chemical components in very small amounts before the expiration period is attained. However, the safety of the plastic has been confirmed by tests in animals according to USP biological standards for plastic containers.

CLINICAL PHARMACOLOGY

Zantac® (ranitidine hydrochloride) is a competitive, reversible inhibitor of the action of histamine at the histamine H_2-receptors, including receptors on the gastric cells. Zantac does not lower serum Ca^{++} in hypercalcemic states. Zantac is not an anticholinergic agent.

Antisecretory Activity:

1. Effects on Acid Secretion: Zantac Injection inhibits basal gastric acid secretion as well as gastric acid secretion stimulated by betazole and pentagastrin, as shown in the following table:

[See table on top next page].

In a group of ten known hypersecretors, ranitidine plasma levels of 71, 180, and 376 ng/ml inhibited basal acid secretion by 76%, 90%, and 99.5%, respectively.

It appears that basal- and betazole-stimulated secretions are most sensitive to inhibition by Zantac, while pentagastrin-stimulated secretion is more difficult to suppress.

2. Effects on Other Gastrointestinal Secretions:

Pepsin: Zantac does not affect pepsin secretion. Total pepsin output is reduced in proportion to the decrease in volume of gastric juice.

Intrinsic Factor: Zantac has no significant effect on pentagastrin-stimulated intrinsic factor secretion.

Table 5: Preparation of Fortaz Solutions

Size	Amount of Diluent to be Added (ml)	Approximate Available Volume (ml)	Approximate Ceftazidime Concentration (mg/ml)
Intramuscular			
500-mg vial	1.5	1.8	280
1-g vial	3.0	3.6	280
Intravenous			
500-mg vial	5.0	5.3	100
1-g vial	10.0	10.6	100
2-g vial	10.0	11.5	170
Infusion Pack			
1-g vial	100*	100	10
2-g vial	100*	100	20
Pharmacy Bulk Package			
6-g vial	26	30	200

*Note: Addition should be in two stages (see Instructions for Constitution in the package insert).

Serum Gastrin: Zantac has little or no effect on fasting or postprandial serum gastrin.

Other Pharmacologic Actions:

a. Gastric bacterial flora—increase in nitrate-reducing organisms, significance not known.

b. Prolactin levels—no effect in recommended oral or IV dosage, but small, transient, dose-related increases in serum prolactin have been reported after IV bolus injections of 100 mg or more.

c. Other pituitary hormones—no effect on serum gonadotropins, TSH, or GH. Possible impairment of vasopressin release.

d. No change in cortisol, aldosterone, androgen, or estrogen levels.

e. No antiandrogenic action.

f. No effect on count, motility, or morphology of sperm.

Pharmacokinetics: Serum concentrations necessary to inhibit 50% of stimulated gastric acid secretion are estimated to be 36 to 94 ng/ml. Following single intravenous or intramuscular 50-mg doses, serum concentrations of Zantac are in this range for six to eight hours.

Following intravenous injection, approximately 70% of the dose is recovered in the urine as unchanged drug. Renal clearance averages 530 ml/min, with a total clearance of 760 ml/min. The volume of distribution is 1.4 L/kg, and the elimination half-life is 2 to 2.5 hours.

Four patients with clinically significant renal function impairment (creatinine clearance 25 to 35 ml/min) administered 50 mg of ranitidine IV had an average plasma half-life of 4.8 hours, a ranitidine clearance of 29 ml/min, and a volume of distribution of 1.76 L/kg. In general, these parameters appear to be altered in proportion to creatinine clearance (see DOSAGE AND ADMINISTRATION).

Zantac is absorbed very rapidly after intramuscular injection. Mean peak levels of 576 ng/ml occur within 15 minutes or less following a 50-mg intramuscular dose. Absorption from intramuscular sites is virtually complete, with a bioavailability of 90% to 100% compared with intravenous administration. Following oral administration, the relative bioavailability of Zantac Tablets is 50%.

In man, the N-oxide is the principal metabolite in the urine; however, this amounts to less than 4% of the dose. Other metabolites are the S-oxide (1%) and the desmethyl ranitidine (1%). The remainder of the administered dose is found in the stool.

Studies in patients with hepatic dysfunction (compensated cirrhosis) indicate that there are minor, but clinically insignificant, alterations in ranitidine half-life, distribution, clearance, and bioavailability.

Serum protein binding averages 15%.

Clinical Trials: *Duodenal Ulcer:* In a multicenter, double-blind, controlled US study of endoscopically diagnosed duodenal ulcers, earlier healing was seen in the patients treated with oral Zantac as shown in the following table:

[See table below].

In these studies, patients treated with oral Zantac reported a reduction in both daytime and nocturnal pain, and they also consumed less antacid than the placebo-treated patients. [See table on bottom next page.]

Pathological Hypersecretory Conditions (such as Zollinger-Ellison syndrome): Zantac inhibits gastric acid secretion and reduces occurrence of diarrhea, anorexia, and pain in patients with pathological hypersecretion associated with Zollinger-Ellison syndrome, systemic mastocytosis, and other pathological hypersecretory conditions (eg, postoperative, "short-gut" syndrome, idiopathic). Use of oral Zantac was followed by healing of ulcers in 8 of 19 (42%) patients who were intractable to previous therapy.

INDICATIONS AND USAGE

Zantac® (ranitidine hydrochloride) Injection and Zantac® (ranitidine hydrochloride) Injection Premixed are indicated in some hospitalized patients with pathological hypersecretory conditions or intractable duodenal ulcers, or as an alternative to the oral dosage form for short-term use in patients who are unable to take oral medication.

CONTRAINDICATIONS

Zantac® (ranitidine hydrochloride) Injection and Zantac® (ranitidine hydrochloride) Injection Premixed are contraindicated for patients known to have hypersensitivity to the drug.

Effect of IV Zantac on Gastric Acid Secretion

	Time after Dose, h	% Inhibition of Gastric Acid Output by IV Dose, mg		
		20 mg	60 mg	100 mg
Betazole	Up to 2	93	99	99
Pentagastrin	Up to 3	47	66	77

PRECAUTIONS

General: 1. Symptomatic response to Zantac® (ranitidine hydrochloride) therapy does not preclude the presence of gastric malignancy.

2. Since Zantac is excreted primarily by the kidney, dosage should be adjusted in patients with impaired renal function (see DOSAGE AND ADMINISTRATION). Caution should be observed in patients with hepatic dysfunction since Zantac is metabolized in the liver.

3. In controlled studies in normal volunteers, elevations in SGPT have been observed when H_2-antagonists have been administered intravenously at greater than recommended doses for five days or longer. Therefore, it seems prudent in patients receiving IV ranitidine at doses greater than or equal to 100 mg qid for periods of five days or longer to monitor SGPT daily (from day 5) for the remainder of IV therapy.

4. Bradycardia in association with rapid administration of Zantac Injection has been reported rarely, usually in patients with factors predisposing to cardiac rhythm disturbances. Recommended rates of administration should not be exceeded (see DOSAGE AND ADMINISTRATION).

Laboratory Tests: False-positive tests for urine protein with Multistix® may occur during Zantac therapy, and therefore testing with sulfosalicylic acid is recommended.

Drug Interactions: Although Zantac has been reported to bind weakly to cytochrome P-450 *in vitro*, recommended doses of the drug do not inhibit the action of the cytochrome P-450-linked oxygenase enzymes in the liver. However, there have been isolated reports of drug interactions that suggest that Zantac may affect the bioavailability of certain drugs by some mechanism as yet unidentified (eg, a pH-dependent effect on absorption or a change in volume of distribution).

Carcinogenesis, Mutagenesis, Impairment of Fertility: There was no indication of tumorigenic or carcinogenic effects in lifespan studies in mice and rats at oral doses up to 2,000 mg/kg/day.

Ranitidine was not mutagenic in standard bacterial tests *(Salmonella, Escherichia coli)* for mutagenicity at concentrations up to the maximum recommended for these assays.

In a dominant lethal assay, a single oral dose of 1,000 mg/kg to male rats was without effect on the outcome of two matings per week for the next nine weeks.

Pregnancy: *Teratogenic Effects: Pregnancy Category B:* Reproduction studies have been performed in rats and rabbits at oral doses up to 160 times the human oral dose and have revealed no evidence of impaired fertility or harm to the fetus due to Zantac. There are, however, no adequate and well-controlled studies in pregnant women. Because animal reproduction studies are not always predictive of human response, this drug should be used during pregnancy only if clearly needed.

Nursing Mothers: Zantac is secreted in human milk. Caution should be exercised when Zantac is administered to a nursing woman.

Pediatric Use: Safety and effectiveness in children have not been established.

Use in Elderly Patients: Ulcer healing rates in elderly patients (65 to 82 years of age) treated with oral Zantac were no different from those in younger age groups. The incidence rates for adverse events and laboratory abnormalities were also not different from those seen in other age groups.

ADVERSE REACTIONS

Transient pain at the site of intramuscular injection has been reported. Transient local burning or itching has been reported with intravenous administration of Zantac® (ranitidine hydrochloride).

The following have been reported as events in clinical trials or in the routine management of patients treated with oral or parenteral Zantac. The relationship to Zantac therapy has been unclear in many cases. Headache, sometimes severe, seems to be related to Zantac administration.

Central Nervous System: Rarely, malaise, dizziness, somnolence, insomnia, and vertigo. Rare cases of reversible mental confusion, agitation, depression, and hallucinations have been reported, predominantly in severely ill elderly patients.

Rare cases of reversible blurred vision suggestive of a change in accomodation have been reported.

Cardiovascular: As with other H_2-blockers, rare reports of arrhythmias such as tachycardia, bradycardia, asystole, atrioventricular block, and premature ventricular beats.

Gastrointestinal: Constipation, diarrhea, nausea/vomiting, abdominal discomfort/pain, and rare reports of pancreatitis.

Hepatic: In normal volunteers, SGPT values were increased to at least twice the pretreatment levels in 6 of 12 subjects receiving 100 mg qid IV for seven days, and in 4 of 24 subjects receiving 50 mg qid IV for five days. With oral administration there have been occasional reports of hepatitis, hepatocellular or hepatocanalicular or mixed, with or without jaundice. These were usually reversible.

Musculoskeletal: Rare reports of arthralgias.

Hematologic: Blood count changes (leukopenia, granulocytopenia, and thrombocytopenia) have occurred in a few patients. These were usually reversible. Rare cases of agranulocytosis, pancytopenia, sometimes with marrow hypoplasia, and aplastic anemia have been reported.

Endocrine: Controlled studies in animals and man have shown no stimulation of any pituitary hormone by Zantac and no antiandrogenic activity, and cimetidine-induced gynecomastia and impotence in hypersecretory patients have resolved when Zantac has been substituted. However, occasional cases of gynecomastia, impotence, and loss of libido have been reported in male patients receiving Zantac, but the incidence did not differ from that in the general population.

Integumentary: Rash, including rare cases suggestive of mild erythema multiforme, and, rarely, alopecia.

Other: Rare cases of hypersensitivity reactions (eg, bronchospasm, fever, rash, eosinophilia), anaphylaxis, angioneurotic edema, and small increases in serum creatinine.

OVERDOSAGE

There is no experience to date with deliberate overdosage. Clinical monitoring and supportive therapy should be employed.

Studies in dogs receiving doses of Zantac® (ranitidine hydrochloride) in excess of 225 mg/kg/day have shown muscular tremors, vomiting, and rapid respiration. Single oral doses of 1,000 mg/kg in mice and rats were not lethal. Intravenous LD_{50} values in mice and rats were 77 and 83 mg/kg, respectively.

DOSAGE AND ADMINISTRATION

Parenteral Administration: In some hospitalized patients with pathological hypersecretory conditions or intractable duodenal ulcers, or in patients who are unable to take oral medication, Zantac® (ranitidine hydrochloride) may be administered parenterally according to the following recommendations:

Intramuscular Injection: 50 mg (2 ml) every six to eight hours. (No dilution necessary.)

Intravenous Injection: 50 mg (2 ml) every six to eight hours. Dilute Zantac Injection, 50 mg, in 0.9% Sodium Chloride Injection or other compatible IV solution (see Stability) to a total volume of 20 ml and inject over a period of not less than five minutes.

Intermittent Intravenous Infusion: 50 mg (2 ml) every six to eight hours. Dilute Zantac Injection, 50 mg, in 100 ml of 5% Dextrose Injection or other compatible IV solution (see Stability) or use one 100-ml flexible plastic container of Zantac Injection Premixed solution, 50 mg, in 0.45% sodium chloride and infuse over 15 to 20 minutes. (No dilution necessary.) In some patients it may be necessary to increase dosage. When this is necessary, the increases should be made by more frequent administration of a 50-mg dose, but generally should not exceed 400 mg per day.

Zantac Injection Premixed in Flexible Plastic Containers: Instructions for Use: To Open: Tear outer wrap at notch and remove solution container. Check for minute leaks by squeezing container firmly. If leaks are found, discard unit as sterility may be impaired.

Preparation for Administration: Use aseptic technique.

1. Close flow control clamp of administration set.
2. Remove cover from outlet port at bottom of container.
3. Insert piercing pin of administration set into port with a twisting motion until the pin is firmly seated. NOTE: See full directions on administration set carton.
4. Suspend container from hanger.
5. Squeeze and release drip chamber to establish proper fluid level in chamber during infusion of Zantac® (ranitidine hydrochloride) Injection Premixed.

	Oral Zantac*		Oral Placebo*	
	Number Entered	Healed/ Evaluable	Number Entered	Healed/ Evaluable
Outpatients				
Week 2	195	69/182 (38%)†	188	31/164 (19%)
Week 4		137/187 (73%)†		76/168 (45%)

*All patients were permitted prn antacids for relief of pain.   †p < 0.0001

Continued on next page

% = Life-Table estimate
* = p < 0.05 (Zantac vs comparator)
RAN = Ranitidine (Zantac)
PLC = Placebo

As with other H_2-antagonists, the factors responsible for the significant reduction in the prevalence of duodenal ulcers include prevention of recurrence of ulcers, more rapid healing of ulcers that may occur during maintenance therapy, or both.

Gastric Ulcer: In a multicenter, double-blind, controlled US study of endoscopically diagnosed gastric ulcers, earlier healing was seen in the patients treated with Zantac as shown in the following table:

	Zantac*		Placebo*	
	Number Entered	Healed/ Evaluable	Number Entered	Healed/ Evaluable
Outpatients				
Week 2	92	16/83 (19%)	94	10/83 (12%)
Week 6		50/73 (68%)†		35/69 (51%)

*All patients were permitted prn antacids for relief of pain.
† p = 0.009

In this multicenter trial, significantly more patients treated with Zantac became pain-free during therapy.

Pathological Hypersecretory Conditions (such as Zollinger-Ellison syndrome): Zantac inhibits gastric acid secretion and reduces occurrence of diarrhea, anorexia, and pain in patients with pathological hypersecretion associated with Zollinger-Ellison syndrome, systemic mastocytosis, and other pathological hypersecretory conditions (eg, postoperative, "short-gut" syndrome, idiopathic). Use of Zantac was followed by healing of ulcers in 8 of 19 (42%) patients who were intractable to previous therapy.

Gastroesophageal Reflux Disease (GERD): In two multicenter, double-blind, placebo-controlled, six-week trials performed in the United States and Europe, Zantac was more effective than placebo for the relief of heartburn and other symptoms associated with GERD. Ranitidine-treated patients consumed significantly less antacid than did placebo-treated patients.

The US trial indicated that Zantac significantly reduced the frequency of heartburn attacks and severity of heartburn pain within one to two weeks after starting therapy. The improvement was maintained throughout the six-week trial period. Moreover, patient response rates demonstrated that the effect on heartburn extends through both the day and night time periods.

In patients with endoscopically verified reflux esophagitis before treatment, those treated with Zantac had a somewhat higher incidence of healing at six weeks than did placebo-treated patients.

INDICATIONS AND USAGE

Zantac® (ranitidine hydrochloride) is indicated in:
1. Short-term treatment of active duodenal ulcer. Most patients heal within four weeks. Studies available to date have not assessed the safety of ranitidine in uncomplicated duodenal ulcer for periods of more than eight weeks.
2. Maintenance therapy for duodenal ulcer patients at reduced dosage after healing of acute ulcers. No placebo-controlled comparative studies have been carried out for periods of longer than one year.
3. The treatment of pathological hypersecretory conditions (eg, Zollinger-Ellison syndrome and systemic mastocytosis).
4. Short-term treatment of active, benign gastric ulcer. Most patients heal within six weeks and the usefulness of further treatment has not been demonstrated. Studies available to date have not assessed the safety of ranitidine in uncomplicated, benign gastric ulcer for periods of more than six weeks.
5. Treatment of gastroesophageal reflux disease. Symptomatic relief commonly occurs within one or two weeks after starting therapy. Therapy for longer than six weeks has not been studied.
In active duodenal ulcer; active, benign gastric ulcer; hypersecretory states; and GERD, concomitant antacids should be given as needed for relief of pain.

Table I

	Zantac*		Placebo*	
	Number Entered	Healed/ Evaluable	Number Entered	Healed/ Evaluable
Outpatients				
Week 2	195	69/182 (38%)†	188	31/164 (19%)
Week 4		137/187 (73%)†		76/168 (45%)

*All patients were permitted prn antacids for relief of pain.   †p < 0.0001

CONTRAINDICATIONS
Zantac® (ranitidine hydrochloride) is contraindicated for patients known to have hypersensitivity to the drug.

PRECAUTIONS
General: 1. Symptomatic response to Zantac® (ranitidine hydrochloride) therapy does not preclude the presence of gastric malignancy.
2. Since Zantac is excreted primarily by the kidney, dosage should be adjusted in patients with impaired renal function (see DOSAGE AND ADMINISTRATION). Caution should be observed in patients with hepatic dysfunction since Zantac is metabolized in the liver.
Laboratory Tests: False-positive tests for urine protein with Multistix® may occur during Zantac therapy, and therefore testing with sulfosalicylic acid is recommended.
Drug Interactions: Although Zantac has been reported to bind weakly to cytochrome P-450 *in vitro*, recommended doses of the drug do not inhibit the action of the cytochrome P-450-linked oxygenase enzymes in the liver. However, there have been isolated reports of drug interactions that suggest that Zantac may affect the bioavailability of certain drugs by some mechanism as yet unidentified (eg, a pH-dependent effect on absorption or a change in volume of distribution).
Carcinogenesis, Mutagenesis, Impairment of Fertility: There was no indication of tumorigenic or carcinogenic effects in lifespan studies in mice and rats at doses up to 2,000 mg/kg/day.
Ranitidine was not mutagenic in standard bacterial tests (*Salmonella, Escherichia coli*) for mutagenicity at concentrations up to the maximum recommended for these assays.
In a dominant lethal assay, a single oral dose of 1,000 mg/kg to male rats was without effect on the outcome of two matings per week for the next nine weeks.
Pregnancy: *Teratogenic Effects: Pregnancy Category B:* Reproduction studies have been performed in rats and rabbits at doses up to 160 times the human dose and have revealed no evidence of impaired fertility or harm to the fetus due to Zantac. There are, however, no adequate and well-controlled studies in pregnant women. Because animal reproduction studies are not always predictive of human response, this drug should be used during pregnancy only if clearly needed.
Nursing Mothers: Zantac is secreted in human milk. Caution should be exercised when Zantac is administered to a nursing mother.
Pediatric Use: Safety and effectiveness in children have not been established.
Use in Elderly Patients: Ulcer healing rates in elderly patients (65 to 82 years of age) were no different from those in younger age groups. The incidence rates for adverse events and laboratory abnormalities were also not different from those seen in other age groups.

ADVERSE REACTIONS
The following have been reported as events in clinical trials or in the routine management of patients treated with Zantac® (ranitidine hydrochloride). The relationship to Zantac therapy has been unclear in many cases. Headache, sometimes severe, seems to be related to Zantac administration.
Central Nervous System: Rarely, malaise, dizziness, somnolence, insomnia, and vertigo. Rare cases of reversible mental confusion, agitation, depression, and hallucinations have been reported, predominantly in severely ill elderly patients. Rare cases of reversible blurred vision suggestive of a change in accommodation have been reported.
Cardiovascular: As with other H_2-blockers, rare reports of arrhythmias such as tachycardia, bradycardia, atrioventricular block, and premature ventricular beats.
Gastrointestinal: Constipation, diarrhea, nausea/vomiting, abdominal discomfort/pain, and rare reports of pancreatitis.
Hepatic: In normal volunteers, SGPT values were increased to at least twice the pretreatment levels in 6 of 12

subjects receiving 100 mg qid IV for seven days, and in 4 of 24 subjects receiving 50 mg qid IV for five days. With oral administration there have been occasional reports of hepatitis, hepatocellular or hepatocanalicular or mixed, with or without jaundice. These were usually reversible.
Musculoskeletal: Rare reports of arthralgias.
Hematologic: Blood count changes (leukopenia, granulocytopenia, and thrombocytopenia) have occurred in a few patients. These were usually reversible. Rare cases of agranulocytosis, pancytopenia, sometimes with marrow hypoplasia, and aplastic anemia have been reported.
Endocrine: Controlled studies in animals and man have shown no stimulation of any pituitary hormone by Zantac and no antiandrogenic activity, and cimetidine-induced gynecomastia and impotence in hypersecretory patients have resolved when Zantac has been substituted. However, occasional cases of gynecomastia, impotence, and loss of libido have been reported in male patients receiving Zantac, but the incidence did not differ from that in the general population.
Integumentary: Rash, including rare cases suggestive of mild erythema multiforme, and, rarely, alopecia.
Other: Rare cases of hypersensitivity reactions (eg, bronchospasm, fever, rash, eosinophilia), anaphylaxis, angioneurotic edema, and small increases in serum creatinine.

OVERDOSAGE
There is no experience to date with deliberate overdosage. The usual measures to remove unabsorbed material from the gastrointestinal tract, clinical monitoring, and supportive therapy should be employed.
Studies in dogs receiving doses of Zantac® (ranitidine hydrochloride) in excess of 225 mg/kg/day have shown muscular tremors, vomiting, and rapid respiration. Single oral doses of 1,000 mg/kg in mice and rats were not lethal. Intravenous LD_{50} values in mice and rats were 77 and 83 mg/kg, respectively.

DOSAGE AND ADMINISTRATION
Active Duodenal Ulcer: The current recommended adult oral dosage of Zantac® (ranitidine hydrochloride) for duodenal ulcer is 150 mg or 10 ml (2 teaspoonfuls equivalent to 150 mg of ranitidine) twice daily. An alternate dosage of 300 mg or 20 ml (4 teaspoonfuls equivalent to 300 mg of ranitidine) once daily at bedtime can be used for patients in whom dosing convenience is important. The advantages of one treatment regimen compared to the other in a particular patient population have yet to be demonstrated (see Clinical Trials: *Active Duodenal Ulcer*). Smaller doses have been shown to be equally effective in inhibiting gastric acid secretion in US studies, and several foreign trials have shown that 100 mg bid is as effective as the 150-mg dose.
Antacid should be given as needed for relief of pain (see CLINICAL PHARMACOLOGY: Pharmacokinetics).
Maintenance Therapy: The current recommended adult oral dosage is 150 or 10 ml (2 teaspoonfuls equivalent to 150 mg of ranitidine) at bedtime.
Pathological Hypersecretory Conditions (such as Zollinger-Ellison syndrome): The current recommended adult oral dosage is 150 mg or 10 ml (2 teaspoonfuls equivalent to 150 mg of ranitidine) twice a day. In some patients it may be necessary to administer Zantac 150-mg doses more frequently. Doses should be adjusted to individual patient needs, and should continue as long as clinically indicated. Doses up to 6 g/day have been employed in patients with severe disease.
Benign Gastric Ulcer: The current recommended adult oral dosage is 150 mg or 10 ml (2 teaspoonfuls equivalent to 150 mg of ranitidine) twice a day.
GERD: The current recommended adult oral dosage is 150 mg or 10 ml (2 teaspoonfuls equivalent to 150 mg of ranitidine) twice a day.
Dosage Adjustment for Patients with Impaired Renal Function: On the basis of experience with a group of subjects with severely impaired renal function treated with Zantac, the recommended dosage in patients with a creatinine clearance less than 50 ml/min is 150 mg or 10 ml (2 teaspoonfuls equivalent to 150 mg of ranitidine) every 24 hours. Should the patient's condition require, the frequency of dosing may be increased to every 12 hours or even further with caution. Hemodialysis reduces the level of circulating ranitidine. Ideally, the dosage schedule should be adjusted so that

Table II

	Mean Daily Doses of Antacid	
	Ulcer Healed	Ulcer Not Healed
Zantac	0.06	0.71
Placebo	0.71	1.43

Continued on next page

Glaxo Pharm.—Cont.

the timing of a scheduled dose coincides with the end of hemodialysis.

HOW SUPPLIED

Zantac® 150 Tablets (ranitidine hydrochloride equivalent to 150 mg of ranitidine) are white tablets embossed with "Zantac 150" on one side and "Glaxo" on the other. They are available in bottles of 60 tablets (NDC 0173-0344-42) and unit dose packs of 100 tablets (NDC 0173-0344-47).
Zantac® 300 Tablets (ranitidine hydrochloride equivalent to 300 mg of ranitidine) are yellow, capsule-shaped tablets embossed with "Zantac 300" on one side and "Glaxo" on the other. They are available in bottles of 30 tablets (NDC 0173-0393-40) and unit dose packs of 100 tablets (NDC 0173-0393-47).

Store between 15° and 30°C (59° and 86°F) in a dry place. Protect from light. Replace cap securely after each opening.
Zantac® Syrup, a clear, peppermint-flavored liquid, contains 16.8 mg of ranitidine hydrochloride equivalent to 15 mg of ranitidine per 1 ml in bottles of 16 fluid ounces (one pint) (NDC 0173-0383-54).

Store between 4° and 25°C (39° and 77°F). Dispense in tight, light-resistant containers as defined in the USP/NF.
Shown in Product Identification Section, page 411

ZINACEF®   ℞
[zin 'ah-sef]
(sterile cefuroxime sodium, Glaxo)
ZINACEF®   ℞
(cefuroxime sodium injection)

DESCRIPTION

Cefuroxime is a semisynthetic, broad-spectrum cephalosporin antibiotic for parenteral administration. It is the sodium salt of (6R, 7R)-3-carbəmoyloxymethyl-7-[Z-2-methoxyimino-2-(fur-2-yl) acetamido]ceph-3-em-4-carboxylate.
Zinacef® (sterile cefuroxime sodium/cefuroxime sodium injection) contains approximately 54.2 mg (2.4 mEq) of sodium per gram of cefuroxime activity.
Zinacef® (sterile cefuroxime sodium) in sterile crystalline form is supplied in vials equivalent to 750 mg, 1.5 g. or 7.5 g of cefuroxime as cefuroxime sodium. Solutions of Zinacef range in color from light yellow to amber, depending on the concentration and diluent used. The pH of freshly constituted solutions usually ranges from 6 to 8.5.
Zinacef® (cefuroxime sodium injection) is available as a frozen, iso-osmotic, sterile, nonpyrogenic solution with 750 mg or 1.5 g cefuroxime as cefuroxime sodium. Approximately 1.4 g dextrose hydrous, USP has been added to the 750-mg dose to adjust the osmolality. Sodium citrate hydrous, USP has been added as a buffer (300 mg and 600 mg to the 750-mg and 1.5-g doses, respectively). Zinacef contains approximately 111 mg (4.8 mEq) and 222 mg (9.7 mEq) of sodium in the 750-mg and 1.5-g doses, respectively. The pH has been adjusted with hydrochloric acid and may have been adjusted with sodium hydroxide. Solutions of premixed Zinacef range in color from light yellow to amber. The solution is intended for intravenous use after thawing to room temperature. The osmolality of the solution is approximately 300 mOsmol/kg, and the pH of thawed solutions ranges from 5.0 to 7.5.
The plastic container is fabricated from a specially designed multilayer plastic, PL 2040. Solutions are in contact with the polyethylene layer of this container and can leach out certain chemical components of the plastic in very small amounts within the expiration period. The suitabilty of the plastic has been confirmed in tests in animals according to USP biological tests for plastic containers as well as by tissue culture toxicity studies.

CLINICAL PHARMACOLOGY

After intramuscular injection of a 750-mg dose of cefuroxime to normal volunteers, the mean peak serum concentration was 27 mcg/ml. The peak occurred at approximately 45 minutes (range, 15 to 60 minutes). Following intravenous doses of 750 mg and 1.5 g, serum concentrations were approximately 50 and 100 mcg/ml, respectively, at 15 minutes. Therapeutic serum concentrations of approximately 2 mcg/ml or more were maintained for 5.3 hours and eight hours or more, respectively. There was no evidence of accumulation of cefuroxime in the serum following intravenous administration of 1.5-g doses every eight hours to normal volunteers. The serum half-life after either intramuscular or intravenous injections is approximately 80 minutes.
Approximately 89% of a dose of cefuroxime is excreted by the kidneys over an eight-hour period, resulting in high urinary concentrations.
Following the intramuscular administration of a 750-mg single dose, urinary concentrations averaged 1,300 mcg/ml during the first eight hours. Intravenous doses of 750 mg and 1.5 g produced urinary levels averaging 1,150 and 2,500 mcg/ml, respectively, during the first eight-hour period.

The concomitant oral administration of probenecid with cefuroxime slows tubular secretion, decreases renal clearance by approximately 40%, increases the peak serum level by approximately 30%, and increases the serum half-life by approximately 30%. Cefuroxime is detectable in therapeutic concentrations in pleural fluid, joint fluid, bile, sputum, bone, cerebrospinal fluid (in patients with meningitis), and aqueous humor.
Cefuroxime is approximately 50% bound to serum protein.
Microbiology: Cefuroxime has *in vitro* activity against a wide range of gram-positive and gram-negative organisms, and it is highly stable in the presence of beta-lactamases of certain gram-negative bacteria. The bactericidal action of cefuroxime results from inhibition of cell-wall synthesis. Cefuroxime is usually active against the following organisms *in vitro.*
Aerobes, Gram-negative: *Haemophilus influenzae* (including ampicillin-resistant strains); *Haemophilus parainfluenzae; Moraxella (Branhamella) catarrhalis* (including ampicillin- and cephalothin-resistant strains); *Neisseria gonorrhoeae* (including penicillinase- and non-penicillinase-producing strains); *Neisseria meningitidis; Escherichia coli; Klebsiella* spp (including *Klebsiella pneumoniae*); *Enterobacter* spp; *Citrobacter* spp; *Salmonella* spp; *Shigella* spp; *Proteus mirabilis; Proteus inconstans* (formerly *Providencia inconstans*); *Providencia rettgeri* (formerly *Proteus rettgeri*); and *Morganella morganii* (formerly *Proteus morganii*).
Some strains of *M morganii, Enterobacter cloacae,* and *Citrobacter* spp have been shown by *in vitro* tests to be resistant to cefuroxime and other cephalosporins.
Aerobes, Gram-positive: Staphylococcus aureus (including penicillinase- and non-penicillinase-producing strains); *Staphylococcus epidermidis; Streptococcus pyogenes* (and other streptococci); and *Streptococcus pneumoniae* (formerly *Diplococcus pneumoniae*).
Certain strains of enterococci, eg, *Streptococcus faecalis,* are resistant.
Anaerobes: Gram-positive and gram-negative cocci (including *Peptococcus* and *Peptostreptococcus* spp); gram-positive bacilli (including *Clostridium* spp); and gram-negative bacilli (including *Bacteroides* and *Fusobacterium* spp). Most strains of *Bacteroides fragilis* are resistant.
Pseudomonas and *Campylobacter* spp, *Acinetobacter calcoaceticus* (formerly *Mima* and *Herellea* spp), and most strains of *Serratia* and *Proteus vulgaris* are resistant to most cephalosporins. Methicillin-resistant staphylococci, *Clostridium difficile,* and *Listeria monocytogenes* are resistant to cefuroxime.
Susceptibility Tests: *Diffusion Techniques:* Quantitative methods that require measurement of zone diameters give an estimate of antibiotic susceptibility. One such procedure[1-3] has been recommended for use with disks to test susceptibility to cefuroxime. Interpretation involves correlation of the diameters obtained in the disk test with minimum inhibitory concentration (MIC) values for cefuroxime.
Reports from the laboratory giving results of the standard single-disk susceptibility test with a 30-mcg cefuroxime disk should be interpreted according to the following criteria:
   Susceptible organisms produce zones of 18 mm or greater, indicating that the test organism is likely to respond to therapy.
   Organisms that produce zones of 15 to 17 mm are expected to be susceptible if high dosage is used or if the infection is confined to tissues and fluids (eg, urine) in which high antibiotic levels are attained.
   Resistant organisms produce zones of 14 mm or less, indicating that other therapy should be selected.
For gram-positive isolates, the test can be performed with either the cephalosporin-class disk (30 mcg of cephalothin) or the cefuroxime disk (30 mcg of cefuroxime), and a zone of 18 mm or greater indicates a cefuroxime-susceptible organism.
Gram-negative organisms should be tested with the cefuroxime disk (using the above criteria), since cefuroxime has been shown by *in vitro* tests to have activity against certain strains of Enterobacteriaceae found resistant when tested with the cephalosporin-class disk. Gram-negative organisms having zones of less than 18 mm around the cephalothin disk are not necessarily of intermediate susceptibility or resistant to cefuroxime.
The cefuroxime disk should not be used for testing susceptibility to other cephalosporins.
Standardized procedures require the use of laboratory control organisms. The 30-mcg cefuroxime disk should give zone diameters between 27 and 35 mm for *S aureus* ATCC 25923. For *E coli* ATCC 25922, the zone diameters should be between 20 and 26 mm.
Dilution Techniques: A bacterial isolate may be considered susceptible if the MIC value for cefuroxime is not more than 16 mcg/ml. Organisms are considered resistant if the MIC is greater than 32 mcg/ml.
As with standard diffusion methods, dilution procedures require the use of laboratory control organisms. Standard cefuroxime powder should give MIC values in the range of 0.5 and 2 mcg/ml for *S aureus* ATCC 25923. For *E coli* ATCC 25922, the MIC range should be between 2 and 8 mcg/ml.

INDICATIONS AND USAGE

Zinacef® (sterile cefuroxime sodium/cefuroxime sodium injection) is indicated for the treatment of patients with infections caused by susceptible strains of the designated organisms in the following diseases:
1. **Lower Respiratory Tract Infections,** including pneumonia, caused by *S pneumoniae* (formerly *D pneumoniae*), *H influenzae* (including ampicillin-resistant strains), *Klebsiella* spp, *S aureus* (penicillinase- and non-penicillinase-producing), *S pyogenes,* and *E coli.*
2. **Urinary Tract Infections** caused by *E coli* and *Klebsiella* spp.
3. **Skin and Skin Structure Infections** caused by *S aureus* (penicillinase- and non-penicillinase-producing), *S pyogenes, E coli, Klebsiella* spp, and *Enterobacter* spp.
4. **Septicemia** caused by *S aureus* (penicillinase- and non-penicillinase-producing), *S pneumoniae, E coli, H influenzae* (including ampicillin-resistant strains), and *Klebsiella* spp.
5. **Meningitis** caused by *S pneumoniae, H influenzae* (including ampicillin-resistant strains), *N meningitidis,* and *S aureus* (penicillinase- and non-penicillinase-producing).
6. **Gonorrhea:** Uncomplicated and disseminated gonococcal infections due to *N gonorrhoeae* (penicillinase- and non-penicillinase-producing strains) in both males and females.
7. **Bone and Joint Infections** caused by *S aureus* (including penicillinase- and non-penicillinase-producing strains).
Clinical microbiological studies in skin and skin structure infections frequently reveal the growth of susceptible strains of both aerobic and anaerobic organisms. Zinacef has been used successfully in these mixed infections in which several organisms have been isolated. Appropriate cultures and susceptibility studies should be performed to determine the susceptibility of the causative organisms to Zinacef.
Therapy may be started while awaiting the results of these studies; however, once these results become available, the antibiotic treatment should be adjusted accordingly. In certain cases of confirmed or suspected gram-positive or gram-negative sepsis or in patients with other serious infections in which the causative organism has not been identified, Zinacef may be used concomitantly with an aminoglycoside (see PRECAUTIONS). The recommended doses of both antibiotics may be given depending on the severity of the infection and the patient's condition.
Prevention: The preoperative prophylactic administration of Zinacef may prevent the growth of susceptible disease-causing bacteria and thereby may reduce the incidence of certain postoperative infections in patients undergoing surgical procedures (eg, vaginal hysterectomy) that are classified as clean-contaminated or potentially contaminated procedures. Effective prophylactic use of antibiotics in surgery depends on the time of administration. Zinacef should usually be given one-half to one hour before the operation to allow sufficient time to achieve effective antibiotic concentrations in the wound tissues during the procedure. The dose should be repeated intraoperatively if the surgical procedure is lengthy.
Prophylactic administration is usually not required after the surgical procedure ends and should be stopped within 24 hours. In the majority of surgical procedures, continuing prophylactic administration of any antibiotic does not reduce the incidence of subsequent infections but will increase the possibility of adverse reactions and the development of bacterial resistance.
The perioperative use of Zinacef has also been effective during open heart surgery for surgical patients in whom infections at the operative site would present a serious risk. For these patients it is recommended that Zinacef therapy be continued for at least 48 hours after the surgical procedure ends. If an infection is present, specimens for culture should be obtained for the identification of the causative organism and appropriate antimicrobial therapy should be instituted.

CONTRAINDICATIONS

Zinacef® (sterile cefuroxime sodium/cefuroxime sodium injection) is contraindicated in patients with known allergy to the cephalosporin group of antibiotics.

WARNINGS

BEFORE THERAPY WITH ZINACEF® (sterile cefuroxime sodium/cefuroxime sodium injection) IS INSTITUTED, CAREFUL INQUIRY SHOULD BE MADE TO DETERMINE WHETHER THE PATIENT HAS HAD PREVIOUS HYPERSENSITIVITY REACTIONS TO CEPHALOSPORINS, PENICILLINS, OR OTHER DRUGS. THIS PRODUCT SHOULD BE GIVEN CAUTIOUSLY TO PENICILLIN-SENSITIVE PATIENTS. ANTIBIOTICS SHOULD BE ADMINISTERED WITH CAUTION TO ANY PATIENT WHO HAS DEMONSTRATED SOME FORM OF ALLERGY, PARTICULARLY TO DRUGS. IF AN ALLERGIC REACTION TO ZINACEF OCCURS, DISCONTINUE THE DRUG. SERIOUS ACUTE HYPERSENSITIVITY REACTIONS MAY REQUIRE EPINEPHRINE AND OTHER EMERGENCY MEASURES.

Pseudomembranous colitis has been reported with the use of cephalosporins (and other broad-spectrum antibiotics); therefore, it is important to consider its diagnosis in patients who develop diarrhea in association with antibiotic use.

Treatment with broad-spectrum antibiotics alters normal flora of the colon and may permit overgrowth of clostridia. Studies indicate a toxin produced by *C difficile* is one primary cause of antibiotic-associated colitis. Cholestyramine and colestipol resins have been shown to bind the toxin *in vitro*.

Mild cases of colitis may respond to drug discontinuation alone. Moderate to severe cases should be managed with fluid, electrolyte, and protein supplementation as indicated. When the colitis is not relieved by drug discontinuation or when it is severe, oral vancomycin is the treatment of choice for antibiotic-associated pseudomembranous colitis produced by *C difficile*. Other causes of colitis should also be considered.

PRECAUTIONS

Although Zinacef® (sterile cefuroxime sodium/cefuroxime sodium injection) rarely produces alterations in kidney function, evaluation of renal status during therapy is recommended, especially in seriously ill patients receiving the maximum doses. Cephalosporins should be given with caution to patients receiving concurrent treatment with potent diuretics as these regimens are suspected of adversely affecting renal function.

The total daily dose of Zinacef should be reduced in patients with transient or persistent renal insufficiency (see DOSAGE AND ADMINISTRATION), because high and prolonged serum antibiotic concentrations can occur in such individuals from usual doses.

As with other antibiotics, prolonged use of Zinacef may result in overgrowth of nonsusceptible organisms. Careful observation of the patient is essential. If superinfection occurs during therapy, appropriate measures should be taken.

Broad-spectrum antibiotics should be prescribed with caution in individuals with a history of gastrointestinal disease, particularly colitis.

Nephrotoxicity has been reported following concomitant administration of aminoglycoside antibiotics and cephalosporins.

Drug/Laboratory Test Interactions: A false-positive reaction for glucose in the urine may occur with copper reduction tests (Benedict's or Fehling's solution or with Clinitest® tablets), but not with enzyme-based tests for glycosuria (eg, Tes-Tape®). As a false-negative result may occur in the ferricyanide test, it is recommended that either the glucose oxidase or hexokinase method be used to determine blood plasma glucose levels in patients receiving Zinacef.

Cefuroxime does not interfere with the assay of serum and urine creatinine by the alkaline picrate method.

Carcinogenesis, Mutagenesis, Impairment of Fertility: Although no long-term studies in animals have been performed to evaluate carcinogenic potential, no mutagenic potential of cefuroxime was found in standard laboratory tests.

Reproductive studies revealed no impairment of fertility in animals.

Pregnancy: *Teratogenic Effects: Pregnancy Category B:* Reproduction studies have been performed in mice and rabbits at doses up to 60 times the human dose and have revealed no evidence of impaired fertility or harm to the fetus due to cefuroxime. There are, however, no adequate and well-controlled studies in pregnant women. Because animal reproduction studies are not always predictive of human response, this drug should be used during pregnancy only if clearly needed.

Nursing Mothers: Since cefuroxime is excreted in human milk, caution should be exercised when Zinacef is administered to a nursing woman.

Pediatric Use: Safety and effectiveness in children below 3 months of age have not been established. Accumulation of other members of the cephalosporin class in newborn infants (with resulting prolongation of drug half-life) has been reported.

ADVERSE REACTIONS

Zinacef® (sterile cefuroxime sodium/cefuroxime sodium injection) is generally well tolerated. The most common adverse effects have been local reactions following intravenous administration. Other adverse reactions have been encountered only rarely.

Local Reactions: Thrombophlebitis has occurred with intravenous administration in 1 in 60 patients.

Gastrointestinal: Gastrointestinal symptoms occurred in 1 in 150 patients and included diarrhea (1 in 220 patients) and nausea (1 in 440 patients). Onset of pseudomembranous colitis symptoms may occur during or after antibiotic treatment (see WARNINGS).

Hypersensitivity Reactions: Hypersensitivity reactions have been reported in less than 1% of the patients treated with Zinacef and include rash (1 in 125). Pruritus, urticaria, and positive Coombs' test each occurred in less than 1 in 250 patients, and, as with other cephalosporins, rare cases of ana-

Table 2: Preparation of Solution and Suspension

Strength	Amount of Diluent to be Added (ml)		Volume to be Withdrawn	Approximate Cefuroxime Concentration (mg/ml)
750-mg Vial	3.0	(IM)	Total*	220
750-mg Vial	8.0	(IV)	Total	90
1.5-g Vial	16.0	(IV)	Total	90
750-mg Infusion Pack	100	(IV)	—	7.5
1.5-g Infusion Pack	100	(IV)	—	15
7.5-g Pharmacy Bulk Package	77	(IV)	Amount Needed†	95

*Note: Zinacef is a suspension at IM concentrations.
†8 ml of solution contains 750 mg of cefuroxime; 16 ml of solution contains 1.5 g of cefuroxime.

phylaxis, erythema multiforme, and Stevens-Johnson syndrome have occurred.

Blood: A decrease in hemoglobin and hematocrit has been observed in 1 in 10 patients and transient eosinophilia in 1 in 14 patients. Less common reactions seen were transient neutropenia (less than 1 in 100 patients) and leukopenia (1 in 750 patients). A similar pattern and incidence was seen with other cephalosporins used in controlled studies.

Hepatic: Transient rise in SGOT and SGPT (1 in 25 patients), alkaline phosphatase (1 in 50 patients), LDH (1 in 75 patients), and bilirubin (1 in 500 patients) levels has been noted.

Kidney: Elevations in serum creatinine and/or blood urea nitrogen and a decreased creatinine clearance have been observed, but their relationship to cefuroxime is unknown.

In addition to the adverse reactions listed above that have been observed in patients treated with cefuroxime, the following adverse reactions and altered laboratory tests have been reported for cephalosporin class antibiotics:

Adverse Reactions: Toxic epidermal necrolysis, fever, vomiting, abdominal pain, colitis, vaginitis including vaginal candidiasis, toxic nephropathy, hepatic dysfunction including cholestasis, aplastic anemia, hemolytic anemia, hemorrhage.

Several cephalosporins have been implicated in triggering seizures, particularly in patients with renal impairment when the dosage was not reduced (see DOSAGE AND ADMINISTRATION). If seizures associated with drug therapy should occur, the drug should be discontinued. Anticonvulsant therapy can be given if clinically indicated.

Altered Laboratory Tests: Prolonged prothrombin time, pancytopenia, agranulocytosis, thrombocytopenia.

DOSAGE AND ADMINISTRATION

Dosage: *Adults:* The usual adult dosage range for Zinacef® (sterile cefuroxime sodium/cefuroxime sodium injection) is 750 mg to 1.5 g every eight hours, usually for five to ten days. In uncomplicated urinary tract infections, skin and skin structure infections, disseminated gonococcal infections, and uncomplicated pneumonia, a 750-mg dose every eight hours is recommended. In severe or complicated infections, a 1.5-g dose every eight hours is recommended.

In bone and joint infections, a 1.5-g dose every eight hours is recommended. In clinical trials, surgical intervention was performed when indicated as an adjunct to Zinacef therapy. A course of oral antibiotics was administered when appropriate following the completion of parenteral administration of Zinacef.

In life-threatening infections or infections due to less susceptible organisms, 1.5 g every six hours may be required. In bacterial meningitis, the dose should not exceed 3 g every eight hours. The recommended dose for uncomplicated gonococcal infection is 1.5 g given intramuscularly as a single dose at two different sites together with 1 g of oral probenecid. For preventive use for clean-contaminated or potentially contaminated surgical procedures, a 1.5-g dose administered intravenously just before surgery (approximately one-half to one hour before the initial incision) is recommended. Thereafter, give 750 mg intravenously or intramuscularly every eight hours when the procedure is prolonged.

For preventive use during open heart surgery, a 1.5-g dose administered intravenously at the induction of anesthesia and every 12 hours thereafter for a total of 6 g is recommended.

Impaired Renal Function: A reduced dosage must be employed when renal function is impaired. Dosage should be determined by the degree of renal impairment and the susceptibility of the causative organism (see Table 1).

Table 1: Dosage of Zinacef in Adults with Reduced Renal Function

Creatinine Clearance (ml/min)	Dose	Frequency
>20	750 mg–1.5 g	q8h
10–20	750 mg	q12h
<10	750 mg	q24h*

* Since Zinacef is dialyzable, patients on hemodialysis should be given a further dose at the end of the dialysis.

When only serum creatinine is available, the following formula[4] (based on sex, weight, and age of the patient) may be used to convert this value into creatinine clearance. The serum creatinine should represent a steady state of renal function.

Males: Creatinine Clearance (ml/min) =
$$\frac{\text{Weight (kg)} \times (140 - \text{age})}{72 \times \text{serum creatinine (mg/dl)}}$$

Females: 0.85 × male value

Note: As with antibiotic therapy in general, administration of Zinacef should be continued for a minimum of 48 to 72 hours after the patient becomes asymptomatic or after evidence of bacterial eradication has been obtained; a minimum of ten days of treatment is recommended in infections caused by *S pyogenes* in order to guard against the risk of rheumatic fever or glomerulonephritis; frequent bacteriologic and clinical appraisal is necessary during therapy of chronic urinary tract infection and may be required for several months after therapy has been completed; persistent infections may require treatment for several weeks; and doses smaller than those indicated above should not be used. In staphylococcal and other infections involving a collection of pus, surgical drainage should be carried out where indicated.

Infants and Children Above 3 Months of Age: Administration of 50 to 100 mg/kg/day in equally divided doses every six to eight hours has been successful for most infections susceptible to cefuroxime. The higher dose of 100 mg/kg/day (not to exceed the maximum adult dose) should be used for the more severe or serious infections.

In bone and joint infections, 150 mg/kg/day (not to exceed the maximum adult dose) is recommended in equally divided doses every eight hours. In clinical trials a course of oral antibiotics was administered to children following the completion of parenteral administration of Zinacef.

In cases of bacterial meningitis, larger doses of Zinacef are recommended, 200 to 240 mg/kg/day intravenously in divided doses every six to eight hours.

In children with renal insufficiency, the frequency of dosage should be modified consistent with the recommendations for adults.

Preparation of Solution and Suspension: The directions for preparing Zinacef for both intravenous and intramuscular use are summarized in Table 2.

For Intramuscular Use: Each 750-mg vial of Zinacef should be constituted with 3 ml of Sterile Water for Injection. Shake gently to disperse and withdraw completely the resulting suspension for injection.

For Intravenous Use: Each 750-mg vial should be constituted with 8 ml of Sterile Water for Injection. Withdraw completely the resulting solution for injection.

Each 1.5-g vial should be constituted with 16 ml of Sterile Water for Injection, and the solution should be completely withdrawn for injection.

The 7.5-g Pharmacy Bulk vial should be constituted with 77 ml of Sterile Water for Injection; each 8 ml of the resulting solution contains 750 mg of cefuroxime.

Each 750-mg and 1.5-g infusion pack should be constituted with 100 ml of Sterile Water for Injection, 5% Dextrose Injection, 0.9% Sodium Chloride Injection, or any of the solutions listed under the Intravenous portion of the COMPATIBILITY AND STABILITY section.

[See table above].

Administration: After constitution, Zinacef may be given intravenously or by deep intramuscular injection into a large muscle mass (such as the gluteus or lateral part of the thigh). Prior to injecting intramuscularly, aspiration is necessary to avoid inadvertent injection into a blood vessel.

Intravenous Administration: The intravenous route may be preferable for patients with bacterial septicemia or other severe or life-threatening infections or for patients who may be poor risks because of lowered resistance, particularly if shock is present or impending.

For direct intermittent intravenous administration, slowly inject the solution into a vein over a period of three to five

Continued on next page

Glaxo Pharm.—Cont.

minutes or give it through the tubing system by which the patient is also receiving other intravenous solutions.

For intermittent intravenous infusion with a Y-type administration set, dosing can be accomplished through the tubing system by which the patient may be receiving other intravenous solutions. However, during infusion of the solution containing Zinacef, it is advisable to temporarily discontinue administration of any other solutions at the same site.

For continuous intravenous infusion, a solution of Zinacef may be added to an intravenous infusion pack containing one of the following fluids: 0.9% Sodium Chloride Injection; 5% Dextrose Injection; 10% Dextrose Injection; 5% Dextrose and 0.9% Sodium Chloride Injection; 5% Dextrose and 0.45% Sodium Chloride Injection; or 0.16 M Sodium Lactate Injection.

Solutions of Zinacef, like those of most beta-lactam antibiotics, should not be added to solutions of aminoglycoside antibiotics because of potential interaction.

However, if concurrent therapy with Zinacef and an aminoglycoside is indicated, each of these antibiotics can be administered separately to the same patient.

Directions for Use of Zinacef® Frozen in Galaxy™ Plastic Containers: Zinacef supplied as a frozen, sterile, iso-osmotic, nonpyrogenic solution in plastic containers is to be administered after thawing either as a continuous or intermittent intravenous infusion. The thawed solution of the premixed product is stable for 28 days if stored under refrigeration (5° C) or for 24 hours at room temperature (25° C). **Do not refreeze.**

Thaw container at room temperature (25°C) or under refrigeration. (5°C) Do not force thaw by immersion in water baths or by microwave irradiation. Components of the solution may precipitate in the frozen state and will dissolve upon reaching room temperature with little or no agitation. Potency is not affected. Mix after solution has reached room temperature. Check for minute leaks by squeezing bag firmly. Dicard bag if leaks are found as sterility may be impaired. Do not add supplementary medication. Do not use unless solution is clear and seal is intact.

Use sterile equipment.

Caution: Do not use plastic containers in series connections. Such use could result in air embolism due to residual air being drawn from the primary container before administration of the fluid from the secondary container is complete.

Preparation for Administration:

1. Suspend container from eyelet support.
2. Remove protector from outlet part of bottom of container.
3. Attach administration set. Refer to complete directions accompanying set.

COMPATIBILITY AND STABILITY

Intramuscular: When constituted as directed with Sterile Water for Injection, suspensions of Zinacef® (sterile cefuroxime sodium) for intramuscular injection maintain satisfactory potency for 24 hours at room temperature and for 48 hours under refrigeration (5°C).

After the periods mentioned above any unused suspensions should be discarded.

Intravenous: When the 750-mg, 1.5-g, and 7.5-g Pharmacy Bulk vials are constituted as directed with Sterile Water for Injection, the Zinacef solutions for intravenous administration maintain satisfactory potency for 24 hours at room temperature and for 48 hours (750-mg and 1.5-g vials) or seven days (7.5-g Pharmacy Bulk vial) under refrigeration (5°C). More dilute solutions, such as 750 mg or 1.5 g plus 100 ml of Sterile Water for Injection, 5% Dextrose Injection, or 0.9% Sodium Chloride Injection, also maintain satisfactory potency for 24 hours at room temperature and for seven days under refrigeration.

These solutions may be further diluted to concentrations of between 1 and 30 mg/ml in the following solutions and will lose not more than 10% activity for 24 hours at room temperature or for at least seven days under refrigeration: 0.9% Sodium Chloride Injection; 0.16 M Sodium Lactate Injection; Ringer's Injection, USP; Lactated Ringer's Injection, USP; 5% Dextrose and 0.9% Sodium Chloride Injection; 5% Dextrose Injection; 5% Dextrose and 0.45% Sodium Chloride Injection; 5% Dextrose and 0.225% Sodium Chloride Injection; 10% Dextrose Injection; and 10% Invert Sugar in Water for Injection.

Unused solutions should be discarded after the time periods mentioned above.

Zinacef has also been found compatible for 24 hours at room temperature when admixed in intravenous infusion with Heparin (10 and 50 U/ml) in 0.9% Sodium Chloride Injection and Potassium Chloride (10 and 40 mEq/L) in 0.9% Sodium Chloride Injection. Sodium Bicarbonate Injection, USP is not recommended for the dilution of Zinacef.

Frozen Stability: Constitute the 750-mg, 1.5-g, or 7.5-g vial as directed for IV administration in Table 2. Immediately withdraw the total contents of the 750-mg or 1.5-g vial or 8 or 16 ml from the 7.5-g bulk vial and add to a Baxter Viaflex® Mini-bag™ containing 50 or 100 ml of 0.9% Sodium Chlo-

ride Injection or 5% Dextrose Injection and freeze. Frozen solutions are stable for six months when stored at -20°C. Frozen solutions should be thawed at room temperature and not refrozen. Do not force thaw by immersion in water baths or by microwave irradiation. Thawed solutions may be stored for up to 24 hours at room temperature or seven days in a refrigerator.

Note: Parenteral drug products should be inspected visually for particulate matter and discoloration before administration whenever solution and container permit.

As with other cephalosporins, however, Zinacef powder, as well as solutions and suspensions, tends to darken, depending on storage conditions, without adversely affecting product potency.

Directions for Dispensing: *Pharmacy Bulk Package—Not for Direct Infusion:* The pharmacy bulk package is for use in a pharmacy admixture service only under a laminar flow hood. Entry into the vial must be made with a sterile transfer set or other sterile dispensing device, and the contents dispensed in aliquots using aseptic technique. The use of syringe and needle is not recommended as it may cause leakage (see DOSAGE AND ADMINISTRATION). AFTER INITIAL WITHDRAWAL USE ENTIRE CONTENTS OF VIAL PROMPTLY. ANY UNUSED PORTION MUST BE DISCARDED WITHIN 24 HOURS.

HOW SUPPLIED

Zinacef® (sterile cefuroxime sodium) in the dry state should be stored between 15° and 30°C (59° and 86°F) and protected from light. Zinacef is a dry, white to off-white powder supplied in vials and infusion packs as follows:

NDC 0173-0352-31 750-mg* Vial (Tray of 25)
NDC 0173-0354-35 1.5-g* Vial (Tray of 25)
NDC 0173-0353-32 750-mg* Infusion Pack (Tray of 10)
NDC 0173-0356-32 1.5-g* Infusion Pack (Tray of 10)
NDC 0173-0400-00 7.5-g* Pharmacy Bulk Package (Tray of 6)
Zinacef frozen as a premixed solution of cefuroxime sodium should not be stored above −20° C. Zinacef is supplied frozen in 50-ml, single-dose, plastic containers as follows:
NDC 0173-0424-00 750-mg* Plastic Container (Carton of 24)
NDC 0173-0425-00 1.5-g* Plastic Container (Carton of 24)
*Equivalent to cefuroxime.

REFERENCES

1. Bauer AW, Kirby WMM, Sherris JC, et al: Antibiotic susceptibility testing by a standardized single disc method. *Am J Clin Pathol* 1966;45:493.
2. National Committee for Clinical Laboratory Standards, Approved Standard: Performance Standards for Antimicrobial Disc Susceptibility Tests (M2-A3), December, 1984.
3. Standardized disc susceptibility test. *Federal Register* 1974;39(May 30):19182–19184.
4. Cockcroft DW, Gault MH: Prediction of creatinine clearance from serum creatinine. *Nephron* 1976;16:31–41.
Zinacef is a registered trademark of Glaxo.
Galaxy is a trademark of Baxter International Inc.
Viaflex is a registered trademark of Baxter International Inc.

Shown in Product Identification Section, page 411

Glenbrook Laboratories
Division of Sterling Drug Inc.
90 PARK AVENUE
NEW YORK, NY 10016

BAYER® CHILDREN'S COLD TABLETS

ACTIVE INGREDIENTS

Each tablet contains phenylpropanolamine HCl 3.125 mg, aspirin 1¼ gr. (81 mg). The tablets are orange flavored and chewable.

INACTIVE INGREDIENTS

Colloidal Silicon Dioxide, Compressible Sugar, Ethylcellulose, FD&C Red #3, Red #40 and FD&C Yellow #6, Flavor, Mannitol, Microcrystalline Cellulose, Povidone, Saccharin Sodium, Starch, Stearic Acid.

ACTION AND USES

Bayer Children's Cold Tablets combine two effective ingredients: a gentle decongestant to relieve nasal congestion and ease breathing, and genuine Bayer Aspirin to reduce fever and relieve minor aches and pains of colds.

ADMINISTRATION AND DOSAGE

The following dosage is provided in the packaging:

Age (yrs)	Weight (lbs)	Dosage
3 up to 6	32–45	2 tabs
6 up to 12	46–83	4 tabs
12 & over	84 & over	8 tabs

Indicated dosage may be repeated every four hours up to but not more than five times a day. Larger dosage may be prescribed by your physician. For easy administration, tablets

may be chewed, dissolved or swallowed whole. Follow with liquid.

CONTRAINDICATIONS

Side effects at higher doses may include nervousness, dizziness, sleeplessness. To be used with caution in presence of high blood pressure, heart disease, diabetes, asthma, or thyroid disease.

CAUTION

Do not exceed recommended dosage. For larger or more frequent doses, or for children under 3, consult a physician. If symptoms persist or are accompanied by high fever or vomiting, consult your physician before continuing use.

WARNINGS

Children and teenagers should not use this medicine for chicken pox or flu symptoms before a doctor is consulted about Reye Syndrome, a rare but serious illness reported to be associated with aspirin. Keep this and all drugs out of the reach of children. In case of accidental overdose, seek professional assistance or contact a poison control center immediately. As with any drug, if you are pregnant or nursing a baby, seek the advice of a health professional before using this product.

HOW SUPPLIED

NDC 12843-181-01, bottles of 30 tablets with child-resistant safety closure. Samples available on request
Shown in Product Identification Section, page 411

BAYER® CHILDREN'S COUGH SYRUP

ACTIVE INGREDIENTS

Each 5 ml (1 tsp.) contains phenylpropanolamine HCl 9 mg and dextromethorphan hydrobromide 7.5 mg.

INACTIVE INGREDIENTS

Alcohol 5%, Caramel, Flavor, Glycerin, Liquid Glucose, Parabens, Purified Water, Saccharin Sodium, Sorbitol Solution. May also contain Sodium Chloride. Cherry flavored.

ACTION AND USES

Bayer Children's Cough Syrup combines two effective ingredients in a syrup with a very appealing cherry flavor: a gentle nasal decongestant and a cough suppressant. It is nonnarcotic, and contains no chloroform or red dyes.

ADMINISTRATION AND DOSAGE

The following dosage is provided on the packaging:
Dosage: For children under 2 consult physician.

Age (yrs)	Weight (lbs)	Dosage
2 up to 6	27–45	1 tsp.
6 up to 12	46–83	2 tsp.
12 & over	84 & over	4 tsp.

Dose may be repeated every 4 hrs., not more than 4 times/day.

CONTRAINDICATIONS AND PRECAUTIONS

To be used with caution in presence of high blood pressure, heart disease, diabetes, asthma, or thyroid disease.
Caution: Consult your physician if cough persists for more than 7 days or if cough is accompanied by high fever since either may be signs of a serious condition.

WARNINGS

Do not give this product to children under 2 years of age or exceed recommended dosage, unless directed by a physician. Keep this and all drugs out of the reach of children. In case of accidental overdose, seek professional assistance or contact a poison control center immediately. As with any drug, if you are pregnant or nursing a baby, seek the advice of a health professional before using this product.

HOW SUPPLIED

NDC 12843-401-02, 3.0 oz. bottles. Samples available on request.
Shown in Product Identification Section, page 411

CHILDREN'S BAYER® CHEWABLE ASPIRIN
Aspirin (Acetylsalicylic Acid)

ACTIVE INGREDIENTS

Bayer Children's Chewable Aspirin-Aspirin 1¼ grains (81 mg) per orange flavored chewable tablet.

INACTIVE INGREDIENTS

Dextrose excipient, FD&C Yellow #6, flavor, saccharin sodium, starch.

ACTIONS AND USES

Analgesic, antipyretic, anti-inflammatory, antiplatelet. For effective, gentle relief of painful discomforts, sore throat; fever of colds; headache; teething pain, toothache, and other minor aches and pains.

WARNINGS

Children and teenagers should not use this medicine for chicken pox or flu symptoms before a doctor is consulted about Reye Syndrome, a rare but serious illness reported to be associated with aspirin. Keep this and all drugs out of the reach of children. In case of accidental overdose, seek professional assistance or contact a poison control center immediately. As with any drug, if you are pregnant or nursing a baby, seek the advice of a health professional before using this product.

ADMINISTRATION AND DOSAGE

The following dosages are those provided in the packaging, as appropriate for self-medication.

Children's Dose: To be administered only under adult supervision. For children under 3 consult physician.

Age (Years)	Weight (Lbs.)	Dosage
Under 3 consult a physician		
3 up to 4	32 to 35	2 tablets
4 up to 6	36 to 45	3 tablets
6 up to 9	46 to 65	4 tablets
9 up to 11	66 to 76	5 tablets
11 up to 12	77 to 83	6 tablets
12 and over	84 and over	8 tablets

Indicated dosage may be repeated every four hours up to but not more than five times a day. Larger dosage may be prescribed by a physician.

Ways to Administer: CHEW then follow with a half glass of water, milk or fruit juice.
SWALLOW WHOLE with a half a glass of water, milk or fruit juice.
DISSOLVE ON TONGUE follow with a half a glass of water, milk or fruit juice.
DISSOLVE TABLET in a little water, milk or fruit juice and drink the solution.
CRUSHED in a teaspoonful of water—followed with part of a glass of water.
HOW SUPPLIED: Bayer Children's Chewable Aspirin 1¼ grains (81 mg)—
NDC 12843-131-05, bottle of 36 tablets with child resistant safety closure.
Samples available on request.
Shown in Product Identification Section, page 411

GENUINE BAYER® ASPIRIN
Aspirin (Acetylsalicylic Acid)
Tablets and Caplets

ACTIVE INGREDIENTS:
Each Bayer-Aspirin contains Aspirin 5 grains (325 mg) in a thin, inert, hydroxypropyl methylcellulose coating for easier swallowing. This is not an enteric coating and does not alter the onset of action of Genuine Bayer Aspirin.

INACTIVE INGREDIENTS
Starch and Triacetin.

ACTIONS AND USES
Analgesic, antipyretic, anti-inflammatory, antiplatelet. For relief of headache; painful discomfort and fever of colds and flu; sore throats; muscular aches and pains; temporary relief of minor pains of arthritis, rheumatism, bursitis, lumbago, sciatica; toothache, teething pains, and pain following dental procedures; neuralgia and neuritic pain; functional menstrual pain; sleeplessness when caused by minor painful discomfort; painful discomfort and fever accompanying immunizations.

CAUTION
If pain persists for more than 10 days, or redness is present, or in conditions affecting children under 12 years of age, consult a physician immediately.

WARNINGS
Children and teenagers should not use this medicine for chicken pox or flu symptoms before a doctor is consulted about Reye Syndrome, a rare but serious illness reported to be associated with aspirin. Keep this and all drugs out of the reach of children. In case of accidental overdose, seek professional assistance or contact a poison control center immediately. As with any drug, if you are pregnant or nursing a baby, seek the advice of a health professional before using this product.

ADMINISTRATION AND DOSAGE
The following dosages are those provided in the packaging, as appropriate for self-medication. Larger or more frequent dosage may be necessary as appropriate to the condition or needs of the patient.
The hydroxypropyl methylcellulose coating makes Genuine Bayer Aspirin particularly appropriate for those who must take frequent doses of aspirin and for those who have difficulty in swallowing uncoated tablets and caplets.
Usual Adult Dose: One or two tablets/caplets with water. May be repeated every four hours as necessary up to 12 tablets/caplets a day.

FOR ANTIPLATELET USE:
RECURRENT TIA
There is evidence that aspirin is safe and effective for reducing the risk of recurrent transient ischemic attacks or stroke in men who have had transient ischemia of the brain due to fibrin platelet emboli:
There is no evidence that aspirin is effective in reducing TIA's in women, or that it is of benefit in the treatment of completed strokes in men or women. Patients presenting with signs and symptoms of TIA's should have a complete medical and neurologic evaluation. Consideration should be given to other disorders which resemble TIA's.
It is important to evaluate and treat, if appropriate, other diseases associated with TIA's and stroke, such as hypertension and diabetes.
DOSAGE: The recommended dosage for this new indication is 1,300 mg/day (650 mg twice/day or 325 mg four times a day).

PRECAUTIONS
A complete medical and neurologic evaluation should be performed on the male patient with recurrent TIA prior to instituting antiplatelet therapy with aspirin. The differential diagnosis should include consideration of disorders that resemble TIA's. An assessment of the presence and need for treatment of other diseases associated with TIA's or stroke, such as diabetes and hypertension, should be made.

IN MI PROPHYLAXIS
Aspirin is indicated to reduce the risk of death and/or non-fatal myocardial infarction in patients with a previous infarction or unstable angina pectoris.

CLINICAL TRIALS
The indication is supported by the results of six, large, randomized multicenter, placebo-controlled studies (1–6) by the word-studies involving 10,816, predominantly male, post-myocardial infarction (MI) patients and one randomized placebo-controlled study (7) by the word study of 1,266 men with unstable angina. Therapy with aspirin was begun at intervals after the onset of acute MI varying from less than 3 days to more than 5 years and continued for periods of from less than one year to four years. In the unstable angina study, treatment was started within 1 month after the onset of unstable angina and continued for 12 weeks and complicating conditions, such as congestive heart failure, were not included in the study.
Aspirin therapy in MI patients was associated with about a 20 percent reduction in the risk of subsequent death and/or non-fatal reinfarction, a median absolute decrease of 3 percent from the 12 to 22 percent event rates in the placebo groups. In aspirin-treated unstable angina patients the reduction in risk was about 50 percent, a reduction in event rate of 5 percent from the 10 percent rate in the placebo group over the 12 weeks of the study.
Daily dosage of aspirin in the post-myocardial infarction studies was 300 mg in one study and 900—1500 mg in five studies. A dose of 325 mg was used in the study of unstable angina.

ADVERSE REACTIONS
Gastrointestinal Reactions: Doses of 1000 mg per day of aspirin caused gastrointestinal symptoms and bleeding that in some cases were clinically significant. In the largest post-infarction study (the Aspirin Myocardial Infarction Study (AMIS) trial with 4,500 people), the percentage incidences of gastrointestinal symptoms for the aspirin (1000 mg of a standard, solid-tablet formulation) and placebo-treated subjects, respectively, were: stomach pain (14.5%; 4.4%); heartburn (11.9%; 4.8%); nausea and/or vomiting (7.6%; 2.1%) hospitalization for GI disorder (4.9%; 3.5%). In the AMIS and other trials, aspirin treated patients had increased rates of gross gastrointestinal bleeding. Symptoms and signs of gastrointestinal irritation were not significantly increased in subjects treated for unstable angina with buffered aspirin in solution.

CARDIOVASCULAR AND BIOCHEMICAL
In the AMIS trial, the dosage of 1000 mg per day of aspirin was associated with small increases in systolic blood pressure (BP) (average 1.5 to 2.1 mm) and diastolic BP (0.5 to 0.6 mm), depending upon whether maximal or last available readings were used. Blood urea nitrogen and uric acid levels were also increased, but by less than 1.0 mg%. Subjects with marked hypertension or renal insufficiency had been excluded from the trial so that the clinical importance of these observations for such subjects or for any subjects treated over more prolonged periods is not known. It is recommended that patients placed on long-term aspirin treatment, even at doses of 300 mg per day, be seen at regular intervals to assess changes in these measurements.

SODIUM IN BUFFERED ASPIRIN FOR SOLUTION FORMULATIONS
One tablet daily of buffered aspirin in solution adds 553 mg of sodium to that in the diet and may not be tolerated by patients with active sodium-retaining states such as congestive heart or renal failure. This amount of sodium adds about 30

percent to the 70 to 90 meq intake suggested as appropriate for dietary treatment of essential hypertension in the 1984 Report of the Joint National Committee on Detection, Evaluation, and Treatment of High Blood Pressure.[8]

DOSAGE AND ADMINISTRATION
Although most of the studies used dosages exceeding 300 mg, two trials used only 300 mg, daily and pharmacologic data indicate that this dose inhibits platelet function fully. Therefore, 300 mg or a conventional 325 mg aspirin dose daily, is a reasonable routine dose that would minimize gastrointestinal adverse reactions. This use of aspirin applies to both solid, oral dosage forms (buffered and plain aspirin) and buffered aspirin in solution.

REFERENCES
(1) Elwood, P.C., et al., A Randomized Controlled Trial of Acetylsalicylic Acid in the Secondary Prevention of Mortality from Myocardial Infarction, *British Medical Journal*, 1:436–440, 1974.
(2) The Coronary Drug Project Research Group, "Aspirin in Coronary Heart Disease," *Journal of Chronic Disease*, 29:625–642, 1976.
(3) Breddin, K., et al., "Secondary Prevention of Myocardial Infarction: A Comparison of Acetylsalicylic Acid, Phenprocoumon or Placebo," *Homeostasis*, 470:263–258, 1979.
(4) Aspirin Myocardial Infarction Study Research Group, "A Randomized, Controlled Trial of Aspirin in Persons Recovered from Myocardial Infarction," *Journal American Medical Association* 245:661–669, 1980.
(5) Elwood, P.C., and Sweetnam P.M., "Aspirin and Secondary Mortality after Myocardial Infarction," *Lancet*, pp. 1313–1315, December 22–29, 1979.
(6) The Persantine-Aspirin Reinfarction Study Research Group, "Persantine and Aspirin in Coronary Heart Disease," *Circulation*, 62: 449–460, 1980.
(7) Lewis, H.D., et al., "Protective Effects of Aspirin Against Acute Myocardial Infarction and Death in Men with Unstable Angina. Results of a Veterans Administration Cooperative Study," *New England Journal of Medicine* 309:396–403, 1983.
(8) "1984 Report of the Joint National Committee on Detection, Evaluation and Treatment of High Blood Pressure," U.S. Department of Health and Human Services and United States Public Health Service, National Institutes of Health.

HOW SUPPLIED
Genuine Bayer Aspirin 5 grains (325 mg)—
NDC 12843-101-10, packs of 12 tablets
NDC 12843-101-11, bottles of 24 tablets
NDC 12843-101-17, bottles of 50 tablets
NDC 12843-101-12, bottles of 100 tablets
NDC 12843-101-20, bottles of 200 tablets
NDC 12843-101-13, bottles of 300 tablets
NDC 12843-102-38, bottles of 50 caplets
NDC 12843-102-39, bottles of 100 caplets
NDC 12843-102-20, bottles of 200 caplets
Child resistant safety closures on 12's, 24's, 50's, 200's, 300's tablets and 50's and 200's caplets. Bottles of 100's tablets and caplets available without safety closure for households without small children.
Samples available on request.
Shown in Product Identification Section, page 411

MAXIMUM BAYER® ASPIRIN
Aspirin (Acetylsalicylic Acid)
Tablets and Caplets

ACTIVE INGREDIENTS
Maximum Bayer Aspirin — Aspirin 500 mg (7.7 grains) contains a thin, inert, hydroxypropyl methylcellulose coating for easier swallowing. This is not an enteric coating and does not alter the onset of action of Bayer Aspirin.

INACTIVE INGREDIENTS
Starch and Triacetin.

ACTIONS AND USES
Analgesic, antipyretic, anti-inflammatory. For relief of headache; painful discomfort and fever of colds and flu; sore throats; muscular aches and pains; temporary relief of minor pains of arthritis, rheumatism, bursitis, lumbago, sciatica; toothache, teething pains, and pain following dental procedures; neuralgia and neuritic pain; functional menstrual pain; sleeplessness when caused by minor painful discomforts; painful discomfort and fever accompanying immunizations.

CAUTION
If pain persists for more than 10 days or redness is present, or in conditions affecting children under 12 years of age, consult a physician immediately.

WARNINGS
Children and teenagers should not use this medicine for chicken pox or flu symptons before a doctor is consulted

Continued on next page

Glenbrook—Cont.

about Reye Syndrome, a rare but serious illness reported to be associated with aspirin. Keep this and all drugs out of the reach of children. In case of accidental overdose, seek professional assistance or contact a poison control center immediately. As with any drugs, if you are pregnant or nursing a baby, seek the advice of a health professional before using this product.

ADMINISTRATION AND DOSAGE

The following dosages are those provided on the packaging, as appropriate for self-medication. Larger or more frequent dosage may be necessary as appropriate to the condition or needs of the patient.

The hydroxypropyl methylcellulose coating makes Maximum Bayer Aspirin particularly appropriate for those who must take frequent doses of aspirin and for those who have difficulty in swallowing uncoated tablets/caplets.

Maximum Bayer Aspirin — 500 mg (7.7 grains) tablets/caplets.

Usual Adult Dose: One or two tablets/caplets with water. May be repeated every four hours as necessary up to 8 tablets/caplets a day.

HOW SUPPLIED

Maximum Bayer Aspirin 500 mg (7.7 grains)
NDC 12843-161-53 bottles of 30 tablets
NDC 12843-161-56 bottles of 60 tablets
NDC 12843-161-58 bottles of 100 tablets
NDC 12843-202-30 bottles of 30 caplets
NDC 12843-202-56 bottles of 60 caplets
Child-resistant safety closures on 30's bottles of tablets and caplets, 60's bottles of caplets, and 100's bottles of tablets. Bottle of 60's tablets available without safety closure for households without small children.
Samples available on request.

Shown in Product Identification Section, page 411

8 HOUR BAYER®
TIMED-RELEASE ASPIRIN
Aspirin (acetylsalicylicacid)

ACTIVE INGREDIENTS

Each oblong white scored caplet contains 10 grains (650 mg) of aspirin in microencapsolated form.

INACTIVE INGREDIENTS

Guar Gum, Microcrystalline Cellulose, Starch and other ingredients.

INDICATIONS

8 Hour Bayer Timed-Release Aspirin is indicated for the temporary relief of low grade pain amenable to relief with salicylates, such as in rheumatoid arthritis, osteoarthritis, spondylitis, bursitis and other forms of rheumatism, as well as in many common musculoskeletal disorders. It possesses the same advantages for other types of prolonged aches and pains, such as minor injuries, dental pain and dysmenorrhea. Its long-lasting effectiveness should also make it valuable as an analgesic in simple headache, colds, grippe, flu and other similar conditions in which aspirin is indicated for symptomatic relief, either by itself or as an adjunct to specific therapy.

CAUTION

If pain persists for more than 10 days, or redness is present, or in conditions affecting children under 12 years, consult a physician immediately.

WARNINGS

Children and teenagers should not use this medicine for chicken pox or flu symptoms before a doctor is consulted about Reye Syndrome, a rare but serious illness reported to be associated with aspirin. Keep this and all drugs out of the reach of children. In case of accidental overdose, seek professional assistance or contact a poison control center immediately. As with any drug, if you are pregnant or nursing a baby, seek the advice of a health professional before using this product.

ADMINISTRATION AND DOSAGE

Two 8 Hour Bayer Timed-Release Aspirin caplets q. 8 h. provide effective long-lasting pain relief. This two-caplet (20 grain or 1300 mg) dose of timed-release aspirin promptly produces salicylate blood levels greater than those achieved by a 10-grain (650 mg) dose of regular aspirin, and in the second 4 hour period produces a salicylate blood level curve which approximates that of two successive 10-grain (650 mg) doses of regular aspirin at 4 hour intervals. The 10-grain (650 mg) scored 8 Hour Bayer Timed-Release Aspirin caplets permit administration of aspirin in multiples of 5 grains (325 mg) allowing individualization of dosage to meet the specific needs of the patient. For the convenience of patients on a regular aspirin dosage schedule, two 10-grain (650 mg) 8 Hour Bayer Timed-Release Aspirin caplets may be administered with water every 8 hours. Whenever necessary, two caplets (20 grains or 1300 mg) should be given before retiring to provide effective analgesic and anti-inflammatory action—for relief of pain throughout the night and lessening of stiffness upon arising. Do not exceed 6 caplets in 24 hours. 8 Hour Bayer Timed-Release Aspirin has been made in a special caplet to permit easy swallowing. However, for patients who do have difficulty, 8 Hour Bayer Timed-Release Aspirin caplets may be gently crumbled in the mouth and swallowed with water without loss of timed-release effect. There is no bitter "aspirin" taste. For children under 12, consult physician.

SIDE EFFECTS

Side effects encountered with regular aspirin may be encountered with 8 Hour Bayer Timed-Release Aspirin. Tinnitus and dizziness are the ones most frequently encountered.

CONTRAINDICATIONS AND PRECAUTIONS

8 Hour Bayer Timed-Release Aspirin is contraindicated in patients with marked aspirin hypersensitivity, and should be given with extreme caution to any patient with a history of adverse reaction to salicylates. It may cautiously be tried in patients intolerant to aspirin because of gastric irritation, but the usual precautions for any form of aspirin should be observed in patients with gastric ulcers, bleeding tendencies, asthma, or hypoprothrombinemia.

SUPPLIED

Caplets in Bottle of 30's   NDC 12843-191-72
Caplets in Bottle of 72's   NDC 12843-191-74
Caplets in Bottle of 125's   NDC 12843-191-76
All sizes packaged in child-resistant safety closure except 72's which is a size recommended for households without young children.
Samples available upon request.

Shown in Product Identification Section, page 411

HALEY'S M-O®

ACTIVE INGREDIENTS

A suspension of magnesium hydroxide in purified water plus mineral oil. Haley's M-O contains 304 mg per teaspoon (5 ml) of Magnesium Hydroxide and 1.25 ml of Mineral Oil.

INACTIVE INGREDIENTS

Purified water. For flavored Haley's M-O only, D&C Red #28, flavor, purified water, saccharin sodium.

INDICATIONS

For the relief of occasional constipation or irregularity accompanied by hemorrhoids.

ACTION AT LAXATIVE DOSAGE

Haley's M-O is a mild saline laxative which acts by drawing water into the gut, increasing intraluminal pressure, and increasing intestinal motility. This product generally produces bowel movement in $\frac{1}{2}$ to 6 hours.

ADMINISTRATION AND DOSAGE

As a laxative, especially for hemorrhoid sufferers, adults 1–2 tbsp. at bedtime and upon arising. For constipation relief, adults 2 tbsp. at bedtime and upon arising; children 6–12, minimum single dose; 1 tsp., maximum daily dose; 1 tbsp. For adults and children, as bowel function improves reduce dose gradually.

CAUTION

Do not take this product if you are presently taking a stool softener laxative unless directed by a doctor. Do not take with meals.

WARNINGS

Do not use laxative products when abdominal pain, nausea or vomiting are present unless directed by a doctor. If you have noticed a sudden change in bowel habits that persists over a period of 2 weeks, consult a doctor before using a laxative. Laxative products should not be used for a period longer than 1 week unless directed by a doctor. Rectal bleeding, or failure to have a bowel movement after use of a laxative may indicate a serious condition; discontinue use and consult your doctor. Do not administer to children under 6 years of age, to pregnant women, to bedridden patients, or to persons with difficulty swallowing. As with any drug, if you are nursing a baby, seek the advice of a health professional before using this product. Keep this and all drugs out of the reach of children. In case of accidental overdose, seek professional assistance or contact a poison control center immediately.

HOW SUPPLIED

Haley's M-O is available in regular and flavored liquids:
Regular
4 fl. oz. NDC 12843-350-45; 12 fl. oz. NDC 12843-350-46; 26 fl. oz. NDC 12843-350-47.
Flavored
4 fl. oz. NDC 12843-360-67; 12 fl. oz. NDC 12843-360-68; 26 fl. oz. NDC 12843-360-69.

Shown in Product Identification Section, page 411

REGULAR STRENGTH MIDOL®
MULTI-SYMPTOM FORMULA

ACTIVE INGREDIENTS

Each caplet contains: Acetaminophen 325 mg and Pyrilamine Maleate 12.5 mg.

INACTIVE INGREDIENTS

Croscarmellose Sodium Type A, Hydroxypropyl Methylcellulose, Magnesium Stearate, Microcrystalline Cellulose, Pregelatinized Starch and Triacetin.

ACTION AND USES

For relief of multiple symptoms suffered during menstrual cycle: cramps, bloating, headache, tension, irritability, and backache caused by menstrual discomfort.
Unlike general pain relievers, which contain only analgesics, Midol Regular Strength Multi-Symptom Formula has a unique combination of ingredients (an analgesic, tension and water retention reliever) specially formulated to give:
1. Relief from cramps, headaches, backaches and muscle aches.
2. Relief of irritability, anxiety and tension.
3. Relief from the discomforts of fluid retention and bloating.

CAUTION

May cause drowsiness. Use caution when driving or operating machinery. Alcohol, sedatives or tranquilizers may increase drowsiness.

WARNINGS

Keep this and all drugs out of the reach of children. In case of accidental overdose, seek professional assistance or contact a poison control center immediately. As with any drug, if you are pregnant or nursing a baby, seek the advice of a health professional before using this product.

DOSAGE

Take 2 caplets with water. Repeat every four hours as needed up to a maximum of 12 caplets per day. Under age 12; Consult your physician.

HOW SUPPLIED

White, capsule-shaped caplets.
NDC 12843-156-16, professional dispenser, 250 2-caplet Packets for sample use.
NDC 12843-156-17, bottle of 12 caplets
NDC 12843-156-18, bottle of 30 caplets
NDC 12843-156-19, bottles of 60 caplets
Child resistant safety closures on bottles of 12 and 60 Caplets.
Samples Supplied: Available on request.
Shown in Product Identification Section, page 411

MAXIMUM STRENGTH
MIDOL® PMS
Premenstrual Syndrome Formula

ACTIVE INGREDIENTS

Each caplet contains: Acetaminophen 500 mg, Pamabrom 25 mg, Pyrilamine Maleate 15 mg.

INACTIVE INGREDIENTS

Croscarmellose Sodium, Hydrogenated Vegetable Oil, Hydroxypropyl Methylcellulose, Magnesium Stearate, Microcrystalline Cellulose, Pregelatinized Starch, Talc and Triacetin.

ACTION AND USES

Relieves the symptoms of Premenstrual Syndrome (PMS). Contains maximum strength medication for all these premenstrual symptoms: tension, irritability, anxiety, bloating, water-weight gain, cramps, backache, and headache. Unlike general pain relievers, which contain only analgesics, Midol PMS contains a combination of ingredients (an analgesic, diuretic, and a tension reliever) for the physical and emotional symptoms associated with PMS.

DOSAGE

Take 2 caplets with water. Repeat every 4 hours as needed, up to a maximum of 8 caplets per day. Under age 12: Take under the advice of your physician.

CAUTION

May cause drowsiness. Use caution when driving or operating machinery. Alcohol, sedatives or tranquilizers may increase drowsiness.

WARNINGS: Keep this and all drugs out of the reach of children. In case of accidental overdose, seek professional assistance or contact a poison control center immediately. As with any drug, if you are pregnant or nursing a baby, seek the advice of a health professional before using this product.

HOW SUPPLIED

White capsule shaped caplets.
NDC 12843-163-46, bottles of 16 caplets
NDC 12843-163-47, bottles of 32 caplets
Child-resistant safety closure on bottles of 32 caplets.
Samples Supplied: Available upon request.
Shown in Product Identification Section, page 411

MAXIMUM STRENGTH MIDOL®
MULTI-SYMPTOM FORMULA

ACTIVE INGREDIENTS
Each caplet contains Acetaminophen 500 mg and Pyrilamine Maleate 15 mg.

INACTIVE INGREDIENTS
Croscarmellose Sodium Type A, Hydroxypropyl Methylcellulose, Magnesium Stearate, Microcrystalline Cellulose, Pregelatinized Starch and Triacetin.

ACTION AND USES
Maximum strength medication for the relief of multiple symptoms suffered during menstrual cycle: cramps, bloating, headache, tension, irritability and backache caused by menstrual discomfort.
Unlike general pain relievers, which contain only analgesics, Midol Maximum Strength Multi-Symptom Formula has a unique combination of ingredients (an analgesic, tension reliever and water retention reliever) specially formulated to give
1. Maximum strength relief from cramps, plus relief of headaches, backaches and muscle aches.
2. Maximum relief of irritability, anxiety and tension.
3. Maximum relief from the discomforts of fluid retention, bloating and water-weight gain.

CAUTION
May cause drowsiness. Use caution when driving or operating machinery. Alcohol, sedatives or tranquilizers may increase drowsiness.

WARNINGS
Keep this and all drugs out of the reach of children. In case of accidental overdose, seek professional assistance or contact a poison control center immediately. As with any drug, if you are pregnant or nursing a baby, seek the advice of a health professional before using this product.

DOSAGE
Take 2 caplets with water. Repeat every 4 hours, as needed, up to a maximum of 8 caplets per day.
Under age 12: Consult your physician.

HOW SUPPLIED
White capsule-shaped caplets.
NDC 12843-157-16, professional dispenser, 250 2-caplet Packets for sample use.
NDC 12843-157-17, bottles of 8 caplets
NDC 12843-157-18, bottles of 16 caplets
NDC 12843-157-19, bottles of 32 caplets
Child-resistant safety closures on bottles of 8 and 32 caplets.
Samples Supplied: Available upon request.
Shown in Product Identification Section, page 411

MIDOL® 200 ADVANCED CRAMP FORMULA
Ibuprofen Tablets, USP
Menstrual Pain/Cramp Reliever

WARNING
ASPIRIN SENSITIVE PATIENTS. Do not take this product if you have had a severe allergic reaction to aspirin, e.g.—asthma, swelling, shock or hives, because even though this product contains no aspirin or salicylates, cross-reactions may occur in patients allergic to aspirin.

INDICATIONS
For the temporary relief of painful menstrual cramps (Dysmenorrhea); also headaches, backaches and muscular aches and pains associated with Premenstrual Syndrome.

DIRECTIONS
Adults: Take 1 tablet every 4 to 6 hours at the onset of menstrual symptoms and while pain persists. If pain does not respond to 1 tablet, 2 tablets may be used but do not exceed 6 tablets in 24 hours, unless directed by a doctor. The smallest effective dose should be used. Take with food or milk if occasional and mild heartburn, upset stomach, or stomach pain occurs with use. Consult a doctor if these symptoms are more than mild or if they persist. Children: Do not give this product to children under 12 except under the advice and supervision of a doctor.

WARNINGS
Do not take for pain for more than 10 days unless directed by a doctor. If pain persists or gets worse, or if new symptoms occur, consult a doctor. These could be signs of serious illness. If you are under a doctor's care for any serious condition, consult a doctor before taking this product. As with aspirin and acetaminophen, if you have any condition which requires you to take prescription drugs or if you have had any problems or serious side effects from taking any non-prescription pain reliever, do not take this product without first discussing it with your doctor. If you experience any symptoms which are unusual or seem unrelated to the condition for which you took ibuprofen, consult a doctor before taking any more of it. Although ibuprofen is indicated for the same conditions as aspirin and acetaminophen, it should not be taken with them except under a doctor's direction. Do not combine this product with any other ibuprofen-containing product. As with any drug, if you are pregnant or nursing a baby, seek the advice of a health professional before using this product. **IT IS ESPECIALLY IMPORTANT NOT TO USE IBUPROFEN DURING THE LAST 3 MONTHS OF PREGNANCY UNLESS SPECIFICALLY DIRECTED TO DO SO BY A DOCTOR BECAUSE IT MAY CAUSE PROBLEMS IN THE UNBORN CHILD OR COMPLICATIONS DURING DELIVERY.** Keep this and all drugs out of the reach of children. In case of accidental overdose, seek professional assistance or contact a poison control center immediately. Ibuprofen is used for the relief of painful menstrual cramps and the pain associated with Premenstrual Syndrome. Ibuprofen has been proven more effective in relieving menstrual pain and cramps than aspirin and is gentler on the stomach. Ibuprofen had been widely prescribed for years and is now available in nonprescription strength.

ACTIVE INGREDIENTS
Each tablet contains ibuprofen USP 200 mg.

INACTIVE INGREDIENTS
Calcium Phosphate, Cellulose, Magnesium Stearate, Silicon Dioxide, Sodium Lauryl Sulfate, Sodium Starch Glycolate, Stearic Acid, Titanium Dioxide.
Store at room temperature; avoid excessive heat 40°C (104°F).

HOW SUPPLIED
White tablets NDC 12843-154-50, bottles of 16 tablets.
NDC 12843-154-51, bottles of 32 tablets.
Child-resistant safety closure on bottles of 32 tablets.

SAMPLES SUPPLIED
Available upon request.
Shown in Product Identification Section on page 411

CHILDREN'S PANADOL®
Acetaminophen Chewable Tablets, Liquid, Drops

DESCRIPTION
Each Children's PANADOL Chewable Tablet contains 80 mg acetaminophen in a fruit flavored sugar-free tablet. Children's PANADOL Acetaminophen Liquid is fruit flavored, red in color, and is alcohol-free, sugar-free and aspirin-free. Each ½ teaspoonful contains 80 mg of acetaminophen. Infant's PANADOL Drops are fruit flavored, red in color, and are alcohol-free, sugar-free and aspirin-free. Each 0.8 ml (one calibrated dropper full) contains 80 mg acetaminophen.

ACTIONS AND INDICATIONS
Acetaminophen, the active ingredient in PANADOL, is the analgesic/antipyretic most widely recommended by pediatricians for fast, effective relief of children's fevers. It also relieves the aches and pains of colds and flu, earaches, headaches, teething, immunizations, tonsillectomy, and childhood illnesses.
Children's PANADOL Tablets, Liquid, and Drops are aspirin-free and contain no alcohol or sugar. The pleasant tasting formulations are not likely to upset or irritate children's stomachs.

USUAL DOSAGE
Dosing is based on single doses in the range of 10–15 mg/kg body weight. Doses may be repeated every four hours up to 4 or 5 times daily, but not to exceed 5 doses in 24 hours. To be administered to children under 2 years only on the advice of a physician.
Infant's Panadol Drops: 0–3 mos., 6–11 lbs., ½ dropperful (0.4ml); 4–11 mos., 12–17 lbs., 1 dropperful (0.8ml); 12–23 mos., 18–23 lbs., 1½ droppersful (1.2ml); 2–3 yrs., 24–35 lbs., 2 droppersful (1.6ml); 4–5 yrs., 36–47 lbs., 3 droppersfuls (2.4ml); 6–8 yrs., 48–59 lbs., 4 dropperfuls (3.2ml). May be repeated every 4 hours, up to 5 times in a 24 hour period. May be administered alone or mixed with formula, milk, juice, cereal, etc.
Children's Panadol Liquid: (a special 3 teaspoon cup for accurate measurement is provided). 0–3 mos., 6–11 lbs., ¼ teaspoonful; 4–11 mos., 12–17 lbs., ½ teaspoonful; 12–23 mos., 18–23 lbs., ¾ teaspoonful; 2–3 yrs., 24–35 lbs., 1 teaspoonful; 4–5 yrs., 36–47 lbs., 1½ teaspoonfuls; 6–8 yrs., 48–59 lbs., 2 teaspoonfuls; 9–10 yrs., 60–71 lbs., 2½ teaspoonfuls; 11–12 yrs., 72–95 lbs., 3 teaspoonfuls. May be repeated every 4 hours up to 5 times in a 24 hour period. May be administered alone or mixed with formula, milk, juice, cereal, etc.
Children's Panadol Chewable Tablets: 2–3 yrs., 24–35 lbs., 2 tablets; 4–5 yrs., 36–47 lbs., 3 tablets; 6–8 yrs., 48–59 lbs., 4 tablets; 9–10 yrs., 60–71 lbs., 5 tablets; 11–12 yrs., 72–95 lbs., 6 tablets. May be repeated every 4 hours, up to 5 times in a 24 hour period.

WARNINGS
Since Children's PANADOL Acetaminophen Chewable Tablets, Liquid, and Drops are available without a prescription as an analgesic/antipyretic, the following appears on the package labels: "WARNINGS: Do not take this product for more than 5 days. If symptoms persist or new ones occur, consult a physician. If fever persists for more than 3 days, or recurs, consult a physician. Keep this and all drugs out of the reach of children. In case of accidental overdose, seek professional assistance or contact a poison control center immediately. High fever, severe or persistent sore throat, cough, headache, nausea or vomiting may be serious; consult a physician."
Tamper Resistant: Children's PANADOL Acetaminophen Chewable Tablets packaging provides tamper resistant features on both the outer carton and bottle. The following copy appears on the end flaps of this carton—"Purchase only if carton end flaps are sealed." The following copy appears on the bottle—"Use only if printed seal under cap is intact." Children's PANADOL Liquid and Drops provide tamper resistant features on the carton. The following copy appears on the carton—"Purchase only if Red Tear Tape and Plastic Overwrap are intact" and bottle "Use only if Carton Overwrap and Red Tear Tape Are Intact."

COMPOSITION
Tablets: Active Ingredients: Acetaminophen. Inactive Ingredients: D&C Red #28, FD&C Red #40, Flavor, Mannitol, Saccharin Sodium, Starch, Stearic Acid and other ingredients.
Liquid: Active Ingredients: Acetaminophen. Inactive Ingredients: Benzoic Acid, FD&C Red #40, Flavor, Glycerin, Polyethylene Glycol, Potassium Sorbate, Propylene Glycol, Purified Water, Saccharin Sodium, Sorbitol Solution. May also contain Sodium Chloride or Sodium Hydroxide.
Drops: Active Ingredients: Acetaminophen. Inactive Ingredients: Citric Acid, FD&C Red #40, Flavors, Glycerin, Parabens, Polyethylene Glycol, Propylene Glycol, Purified Water, Saccharin Sodium, Sodium Chloride, Sodium Citrate.

HOW SUPPLIED
Chewable Tablets (colored pink and scored)—bottles of 30. Liquid (colored red)—bottles of 2 fl. oz. and 4 fl. oz. Drops (colored red)—bottles of ½ oz. (15 ml).
All packages listed above have child resistant safety caps and tamper resistant features.
Samples available on request.
Shown in Product Identification Section, page 411

JUNIOR STRENGTH PANADOL®

DESCRIPTION
Each Junior Strength PANADOL® caplet contains 160 mg of acetaminophen.

ACTIONS AND INDICATIONS
Acetaminophen, the active ingredient in Junior Strength PANADOL®, is the analgesic/antipyretic most widely recommended by pediatricians for fast, effective relief of children's fevers. It also relieves the aches and pains of colds and flu, earaches, headaches, teething, immunizations, tonsillectomy, menstrual discomfort, and childhood illness. Junior Strength PANADOL® caplets are aspirin-free, sugar-free.

USUAL DOSAGE
2–3 yrs., 24–35 lbs., 1 caplet; 4–5 yrs., 36–47 lbs., 1½ caplets; 6–8 yrs., 48–59 lbs., 2 caplets; 9–10 yrs., 60–71 lbs., 2½ caplets; 11–12 yrs., 72–95 lbs., 3 caplets; over 12 yrs., 96 lbs., and over, 4 caplets. Dosage may be repeated every 4 hours, up to 5 times in a 24 hour period.

INACTIVE INGREDIENTS
Hydroxypropyl Methylcellulose, Potassium Sorbate, Povidone, Pregelatinized Starch, Starch, Stearic Acid, Talc, Triacetin.

WARNINGS
If symptoms persist or new ones occur, consult a physician. If fever persists for more than 3 days, or recurs, consult a physician. Do not take this product for more than 5 days. Keep this and all drugs out of the reach of children. In case of accidental overdose, seek professional assistance or contact a poison control center immediately. As with any drug, if you are pregnant, or nursing a baby, seek the advice of a health professional before using this product.

HOW SUPPLIED
Swallowable caplets (white)—blister-pack of 30. Package has child resistant and tamper resistant features.
NDC 12843-216-14.
Samples available on request.
Shown in Product Identification Section, page 411

MAXIMUM STRENGTH PANADOL®
Tablets and Caplets

DESCRIPTION
Active Ingredients: Each Maximum Strength PANADOL micro-thin coated tablet and caplet contains acetaminophen

Continued on next page

Glenbrook—Cont.

500 mg. Inactive Ingredients: Hydroxypropyl Methylcellulose, Potassium Sorbate, Povidone, Pregelatinized Starch, Starch, Stearic Acid, Talc, Triacetin.

ACTIONS
PANADOL acetaminophen has been clinically proven as a fast, effective analgesic (pain reliever) and antipyretic (fever reducer). PANADOL acetaminophen is a non-aspirin product designed to provide relief without stomach upset. Its patented micro-thin coating makes each 500 mg tablet or caplet easy to swallow.

INDICATIONS
For the temporary relief from pain of headaches, colds or flu, sinusitis, backaches, muscle aches, and menstrual discomfort. Also to reduce fever and for temporary relief of minor arthritis pain and headache.

PRECAUTIONS
If a rare sensitivity reaction occurs, the drug should be stopped. PANADOL acetaminophen has rarely been found to produce any side effects. It is usually well tolerated by aspirin sensitive patients.
Severe recurrent pain or high continued fever may indicate a serious condition. Under these circumstances consult a physician.

WARNING
As with other products available without prescription, the following appears on the label of PANADOL acetaminophen: Do not give to children under 12 or use for more than 10 days unless directed by a physician. Keep this and all drugs out of the reach of children. In case of accidental overdose, seek professional assistance or contact a poison control center immediately. As with any drug, if you are pregnant or nursing a baby, seek the advice of a health professional before using this product.

USUAL DOSAGE
Adults: Two tablets or caplets every 4 hours as needed. Do not exceed 8 tablets or caplets in 24 hours unless directed by a physician.

OVERDOSAGE
In massive overdosage acetaminophen may cause hepatic toxicity in some patients. Clinical and laboratory evidence of overdosage may be delayed up to 7 days. Under circumstances of suspected overdose, contact your regional poison control center immediately.

HOW SUPPLIED
Tablets and caplets (white, micro-thin coated, imprinted "PANADOL" and "500"). Tablets packaged in tamper-evident bottles of 30 and 60. Caplets packaged in tamper-evident bottles of 24, 50.
Samples available on request.
Shown in Product Identification Section, page 411

PHILLIPS'® LAXCAPS®

ACTIVE INGREDIENTS
A combination of phenolphthalein (90 mg) and Docusate Sodium (83 mg) per gelatin capsule.

INACTIVE INGREDIENTS
FD&C Blue #1, Red #3, Red #40 and Yellow #6, Gelatin, Glycerin, PEG 400 and 3350, Propylene Glycol and Sorbitol.

INDICATIONS
For relief of occasional constipation (irregularity).

ACTION
Phenolphthalein is a stimulant laxative which increases the peristaltic activity of the intestine. Docusate Sodium is a stool softener which allows easier passage of the stool. This product generally produces bowel movement in 6 to 12 hours.

ADMINISTRATION AND DOSAGE
Adults and children 12 and over take one (1) or two (2) capsules daily with a full glass (8 ounce) of liquid, or as directed by a physician. For children under 12, consult your physician.

WARNINGS
Do not take any laxative if abdominal pain, nausea, vomiting, change in bowel habits persisting for over 2 weeks, rectal bleeding or kidney disease are present. Laxative products should not be used for a period longer than one week, unless directed by a physician. If there is a failure to have a bowel movement after use, discontinue and consult your doctor. If a skin rash appears do not take this or any other preparation which contains phenolphthalein. Keep this and all drugs out of the reach of children. In case of accidental overdose, seek professional assistance or contact a Poison Control Center immediately. As with any drug, if you are pregnant or nurs-

ing a baby, seek the advice of a health professional before using this product.

HOW SUPPLIED
Blister packs for safety:
8's NDC 12843-384-18
24's NDC 12843-384-19
Shown in Product Identification Section, page 411

PHILLIPS'® MILK OF MAGNESIA

ACTIVE INGREDIENTS
A suspension of magnesium hydroxide in purified water meeting all USP specifications. Phillips' Milk of Magnesia contains 405 mg per teaspoon (5 ml) of Magnesium Hydroxide.

INACTIVE INGREDIENTS
Purified water, and for Mint Flavored Phillips Milk of Magnesia only—Flavor, Mineral Oil and Saccharin Sodium.

INDICATIONS
For relief of occasional constipation (irregularity) relief of acid indigestion, sour stomach and heartburn.

ACTION AT LAXATIVE DOSAGE
Phillips' Milk of Magnesia is a mild saline laxative which acts by drawing water into the gut, increasing intraluminal pressure, and increasing intestinal motility. This product generally produces bowel movement in ½ to 6 hours.
AT ANTACID DOSAGE: Phillips' Milk of Magnesia is an effective acid neutralizer.

ADMINISTRATION AND DOSAGE
As a laxative, adults and children 12 years and older, 2–4 tbsp.; children 6–11, 1–2 tbsps.; children 2–5, 1–3 tsps. followed by a full glass (8 oz.) of liquid. Children under 2, consult a physician.
As an antacid, 1–3 tsps. with a little water, up to four times a day, or as directed by your physician.

CAUTIONS
Antacids may interact with certain prescription drugs. If you are taking a prescription drug do not take this product without checking with your physician.

LAXATIVE WARNINGS
Do not take any laxative if abdominal pain, nausea, vomiting, change in bowel habits persisting for over 2 weeks, rectal bleeding, or kidney disease are present. Laxative products should not be used for a period longer than 1 week, unless directed by a doctor. If there is a failure to have a bowel movement after use, discontinue and consult your doctor.

ANTACID WARNINGS
Do not take more than the maximum recommended daily dosage in a 24 hour period (See Directions), or use the maximum dosage of this product for more than two weeks, or use this product if you have kidney disease, except under the advice and supervision of a physician. May have laxative effect.

GENERAL WARNINGS
As with any drug, if you are pregnant or nursing a baby, seek the advice of a health professional before using this product. Keep this and all drugs out of reach of children. In case of accidental overdose, seek professional assistance or contact a poison control center immediately.

HOW SUPPLIED
Phillips' Milk of Magnesia is available in regular and mint flavor in bottles of:
Regular
4 fl. oz. NDC 12843-353-01, 12 fl. oz. NDC 12843-353-02, 26 fl. oz. NDC 12843-353-03.
Mint
4 fl. oz. NDC 12843-363-04, 12 fl. oz. NDC 12843-363-05, 26 fl. oz. NDC 12843-363-06.
Also available in tablet form.
Shown in Product Identification Section, page 411

PHILLIPS'® MILK OF MAGNESIA TABLETS

ACTIVE INGREDIENTS
Each Tablet contains 311 mg of Magnesium Hydroxide.

INACTIVE INGREDIENTS
Flavor, Starch, Sucrose. Product description not USP.

INDICATIONS
For relief of acid indigestion, sour stomach, heartburn and occasional constipation (irregularity).

ACTIONS
At Laxative Dosage: Phillips' Milk of Magnesia Tablets offer the same mild saline laxative ingredient as liquid Phillips' Milk of Magnesia in a convenient, chewable tablet form. It acts by drawing water into the gut, increasing intraluminal

pressure, and increasing intestinal motility. This product generally produces bowel movement in ½ to 6 hours.
At Antacid Dosage: Phillips' Milk of Magnesia Tablets are effective acid neutralizers.

ADMINISTRATION AND DOSAGE
As an Antacid, adults chew thoroughly 2 to 4 tablets up to 4 times a day. Children 7 to 14 years, 1 tablet up to 4 times a day or as directed by a physician.
As a laxative, adults and children 12 years of age and older chew thoroughly 6 to 8 tablets. Children 6 to 11, 3 to 4 tablets; children 2 to 5, 1 to 2 tablets, preferably before bedtime and follow with a full glass (8 oz.) of liquid. Children under 2, consult a physician.

LAXATIVE WARNINGS
Do not take any laxative if abdominal pain, nausea, vomiting, change in bowel habits (that persists for over 2 weeks), rectal bleeding, or kidney disease are present. Laxative products should not be used for a period longer than 1 week, unless directed by a doctor. If there is a failure to have a bowel movement after use, discontinue and consult your doctor.

ANTACID WARNINGS
Do not take more than the maximum recommended daily dosage in a 24 hour period (See Directions), or use the maximum dosage of this product for more than two weeks, or use this product if you have kidney disease, except under the advice and supervision of a physician. May have laxative effect.

GENERAL WARNINGS
As with any drug, if you are pregnant or nursing a baby, seek the advice of a health professional before using this product. Keep this and all drugs out of reach of children. In case of accidental overdose, seek professional assistance or contact a poison control center immediately.

HOW SUPPLIED
Phillips' Milk of Magnesia Tablets are available in a mint flavor in bottles of:
Blister packed 24's. NDC 12843-373-19, Bottle of 100. NDC-12843-373-12, Bottle of 200. NDC 12843-373-09.
Also available in liquid form.
Shown in Product Identification Section, page 411

STRI-DEX® REGULAR STRENGTH PADS and
STRI-DEX® MAXIMUM STRENGTH PADS
STRI-DEX® REGULAR STRENGTH BIG PADS
STRI-DEX® MAXIMUM STRENGTH BIG PADS

ACTIVE INGREDIENTS:
Stri-Dex® Regular Strength: Salicylic Acid 0.5%, Alcohol 28% by volume.

INACTIVE INGREDIENTS
Citric Acid, Fragrance, Purified Water, Simethicone Emulsion, Sodium Carbonate, Sodium Dodecylbenzenesulfonate, Sodium Xylenesulfonate.
Stri-Dex® Maximum Strength: Salicylic Acid 2.0%, SD Alcohol 40 44% by volume.

INACTIVE INGREDIENTS
Ammonium Xylenesulfonate, Citric Acid, Fragrance, Purified Water, Simethicone Emulsion, Sodium Carbonate, Sodium Dodecylbenzenesulfonate.

INDICATIONS
For the treatment of acne. Reduces the number of acne pimples and blackheads, and allows the skin to heal. Helps prevent new acne pimples from forming.

DIRECTIONS
Cleanse the skin thoroughly before using medicated pad. Use the pad to wipe the entire affected area one to three times daily. Because excessive drying of the skin may occur, start with one application daily, then gradually increase to two or three times daily if needed or as directed by a doctor.

WARNING
FOR EXTERNAL USE ONLY. Using other topical acne medications at the same time or immediately following use of this product may increase dryness or irritation of the skin. If this occurs, only one medication should be used unless directed by a doctor.
Persons with very sensitive skin or known allergy to salicylic acid should not use this medication. If irritation or excessive dryness and/or peeling occurs, reduce frequency of use or dosage. If excessive itching, dryness, redness, or swelling occurs, discontinue use. If these symptoms persist, consult a physician promptly.
Keep away from eyes, lips, and other mucous membranes. Keep this and all drugs out of reach of children. In the case of accidental ingestion, seek professional assistance or contact a Poison Control Center immediately.

DOSAGE AND ADMINISTRATION

See Labeling instructions for use.

HOW SUPPLIED

Stri-Dex Regular Strength is available in
NDC 12843-087-13—Porta-Pak Refillable Plastic container consisting of 12 pads, 2″ in diameter.
NDC 12843-087-07—Plastic jar consisting of 42 pads, 2″ in diameter.
NDC 12843-087-08—Plastic jar consisting of 75 pads, 2″ in diameter.
NDC 12843-087-04—Stri-Dex Big Pads in a plastic jar consisting of 42 pads, 2⅞″ in diameter.
Stri-Dex Maximum Strength is available in:
NDC 12843-097-12—Porta-Pak Refillable Plastic container consisting of 12 pads, 2″ in diameter.
NDC 12843-097-09—Plastic jar consisting of 42 pads, 2″ in diameter.
NDC 12843-097-11—Plastic jar consisting of 75 pads, 2″ in diameter.
NDC 12843-097-03—Stri-Dex Big Pads in a plastic jar consisting of 42 pads, 2⅞″ in diameter.

VANQUISH® Analgesic Caplets

ACTIVE INGREDIENTS

Each caplet contains aspirin 227 mg, acetaminophen 194 mg, caffeine 33 mg, dried aluminum hydroxide gel 25 mg, magnesium hydroxide 50 mg.

INACTIVE INGREDIENTS

Acacia, Colloidal Silicon Dioxide, Hydrogenated Vegetable Oil, Microcrystalline Cellulose, Powdered Cellulose, Sodium Lauryl Sulfate, Starch, Talc.

ACTION AND USES

A buffered analgesic, antipyretic for relief of headache; muscular aches and pains; neuralgia and neuritic pain; toothache; pain following dental procedures; for painful discomforts and fever of colds and flu; sinusitis; functional menstrual pain, headache and pain due to cramps; temporary relief from minor pains of arthritis, rheumatism, bursitis, lumbago, sciatica.

CAUTION

If pain persists for more than 10 days, or redness is present or in conditions affecting children under 12 years of age, consult a physician immediately.

WARNINGS

Children and teenagers should not use this medicine for chicken pox or flu symptoms before a doctor is consulted about Reye Syndrome, a rare but serious illness reported to be associated with aspirin. Keep this and all drugs out of the reach of children. In case of accidental overdose, seek professional assistance or contact a poison control center immediately. As with any drug, if you are pregnant or nursing a baby, seek the advice of a health professional before using this product.

USUAL ADULT DOSAGE

Two caplets with water. May be repeated every four hours if necessary up to 12 tablets per day. Larger or more frequent doses may be prescribed by physician if necessary.

CONTRAINDICATIONS

Hypersensitivity to salicylates and acetaminophen.
(To be used with caution during anticoagulant therapy or in asthmatic patients).

HOW SUPPLIED

White, capsule-shaped caplets in bottles of:
  30 Caplets NDC 12843-171-44
  60 Caplets NDC 12843-171-46
  100 Caplets NDC 12843-171-48
Samples available on request.
Shown in Product Identification Section, page 411

IDENTIFICATION PROBLEM?
Consult PDR's
Product Identification Section
where you'll find over 1700
products pictured actual size
and in full color.

Glenwood, Inc.
83 N. SUMMIT STREET
TENAFLY, NJ 07670

BICHLORACETIC ACID® KAHLENBERG ℞
Dichloroacetic Acid—Topical

HOW SUPPLIED

Bichloracetic Acid® Kahlenberg
Complete Treatment Kit, NDC 0516-1004-11
Restocking Unit, NDC 0516-1006-77, 75 ml. bottle
Replenishment Unit, NDC 0516-1007-11, 10 ml. bottle

CALPHOSAN® ℞
(calcium glycerophosphate/calcium lactate)
calcium/phosphorus solution in metabolic disorders involving low calcium

COMPOSITION

CALPHOSAN is a specially processed solution containing calcium glycerophosphate and calcium lactate. CALPHOSAN is isotonic, with a pH of about 7 or somewhat above. (Other calcium solutions are usually quite acid, with pH values of 4.5 to 5.5). Each 10 ml. CALPHOSAN contains calcium glycerophosphate 50 mg. and calcium lactate 50 mg. in a physiological solution of sodium chloride, with 0.25% phenol as a preservative.

ADVANTAGES

Intramuscular injections of CALPHOSAN raise blood serum calcium levels, do not raise the calcium levels above normal. Of conspicuous importance, intramuscular injections of CALPHOSAN are without pain, inflammatory reactions or sloughing.

INDICATIONS

Wherever calcium is indicated or in conditions associated with hypocalcemia.

ADMINISTRATION

10 ml. 1 to 4 times weekly or as determined by the physician.

USE IN PREGNANCY

Safety for use in pregnancy or during Lactation has not been established.

CONTRAINDICATIONS

Hypercalcemia; and in view of the fact that hypercalcemia is associated with sarcoidosis and bone metastasis of neoplastic processes, it should not be used in those conditions. As there is a similarity in the actions of calcium and digitalis on the contractility and excitability of the heart muscle, CALPHOSAN is contraindicated in fully digitalized patients. **Do not use intramuscularly in infants and young children.**

AVAILABILITY

10 ml. vials in boxes of 12's—NDC 0516-0060-80 and 60 ml. multiple dose vials—NDC 0516-0060-60.

MYOTONACHOL™ ℞
Bethanechol Chloride—Oral USP

HOW SUPPLIED

Myotonachol.
    10 mg. tablets, flat, NDC 0516-0021-01 in bottles of 100s.
    25 mg. tablets, flat, NDC 0516-0022-01 in bottles of 100s.

POTABA® ℞
Systemic ANTIFIBROSIS THERAPY

PRODUCT OVERVIEW

KEY FACTS

Potaba® (Aminobenzoate Potassium) is considered a member of the vitamin B complex. It has been suggested that the antifibrotic action of Potaba® is due to its mediation of increased oxygen uptake at the tissue level.

MAJOR USES

Potaba® offers a means of treatment of serious and often chronic entities, such as scleroderma and Peyronie's Disease.

SAFETY INFORMATION

Contraindicated in patients taking sulfonamides. Anorexia, nausea, fever and rash have occurred infrequently and subside with omission of the drug. Often, desensitization can be accomplished and treatment resumed.

PRODUCT ILLUSTRATION

POTABA 54	POTABA 51
500 mg TABLET	500 mg CAPSULE

2.0 grams

PRESCRIBING INFORMATION

POTABA® ℞
Systemic ANTIFIBROSIS THERAPY

FORMULA

POTABA is chemically Aminobenzoate Potassium, U.S.P.

> ### INDICATIONS
> Based on a review of this drug by the National Academy of Sciences-National Research Council and/or other information, FDA has classified the indications as follows:
> "Possibly" effective: Potassium aminobenzoate is possibly effective in the treatment of scleroderma, dermatomyositis, morphea, linear scleroderma, pemphigus, and Peyronie's disease.
> Final classification of the less-than-effective indications requires further investigation.

ADVANTAGES

POTABA offers a means of treatment of serious and often chronic entities involving fibrosis and nonsuppurative inflammation.

PHARMACOLOGY

P-Aminobenzoate is considered a member of the vitamin B complex. Small amounts are found in cereal, eggs, milk and meats. Detectable amounts are normally present in human blood, spinal fluid, urine, and sweat. PABA is a component of several biologically important systems, and it participates in a number of fundamental biological processes. It has been suggested that the antifibrosis action of POTABA is due to its mediation of increased oxygen uptake at the tissue level. Fibrosis is believed to occur from either too much serotonin or too little monoamine oxidase activity over a period of time. Monoamine oxidase requires an adequate supply of oxygen to function properly. By increasing oxygen supply at the tissue level POTABA may enhance MAO activity and prevent or bring about regression of fibrosis.

CLINICAL USES

PEYRONIE'S DISEASE: 21 patients with Peyronie's disease were placed on POTABA therapy for periods ranging from 3 months to 2 years. Pain disappeared from 16 of 16 cases in which it had been present. There was objective improvement in penile deformity in 10 of 17 patients, and decrease in plaque size in 16 of 21. The authors suggest that this medication offers no hazard of further local injury as may result from other therapy. There were no significant untoward effects encountered on long term POTABA therapy.

SCLERODERMA: Of 135 patients with diffuse systemic sclerosis treated with POTABA every patient but one has shown softening of the involved skin if treatment has been continued for 3 months or longer. The responses have been reported in a number of publications. The treatment program consists of systemic antifibrosis therapy with POTABA, physical therapy, including deep breathing exercises and dynamic traction splints where indicated, and bethanechol chloride (MYOTONACHOL, Glenwood) for relief of dysphagia as well as small doses of reserpine for amelioration of Raynaud's phenomena.

DERMATOMYOSITIS: Five patients with scleroderma and 2 with dermatomyositis were treated with POTABA. There was striking clinical improvement in each patient. Doses of 15-20 grams per day were well tolerated, and patients were easily able to take these doses.

MORPHEA and LINEAR SCLERODERMA: All 14 patients with localized forms of scleroderma placed on long-term POTABA treatment showed softening of the sclerotic component of their disorder. Treatment is particularly indicated in patients where persistent compressive sclerosis may contribute even greater disfigurement or functional embarrassment from secondary pressure atrophy.

DOSAGE AND ADMINISTRATION

The average adult daily dose of POTABA is 12 grams, usually given in four to six divided doses. Tablets and capsules 0.5 gram are given at the rate of 4 tablets or capsules 6 times daily, or 6 given four times daily, usually with meals, and at

Continued on next page

Glenwood—Cont.

bed-time with a snack. Tablets must be dissolved in an adequate amount of liquid to prevent gastrointestinal upset. POTABA Envules contain 2 grams pure drug each, and 6 Envules are given for a total of 12 grams POTABA daily. POTABA Powder is used to prepare solutions, which are kept refrigerated, but for no longer than one week. 100 grams POTABA powder make 1 quart of 10% solution when dissolved in potable tap water. Children are given 1 gram POTABA daily in divided doses for each 10 lbs. of body weight.

SIDE EFFECTS

Anorexia, nausea, fever and rash have occurred infrequently and subside with omission of the drug. Often, desensitization can be accomplished and treatment resumed.

USE IN PREGNANCY

Safety for use in pregnancy or during lactation has not been established.

PRECAUTIONS

Should anorexia or nausea occur, therapy is interrupted until the patient is eating normally again. This permits prompt subsidence of symptoms and also avoids the possible development of hypoglycemia. Give cautiously to patients with renal disease. If a hypersensitivity reaction should occur, POTABA should be stopped.

CONTRAINDICATIONS

POTABA should not be administered to patients taking sulfonamides.

HOW SUPPLIED

POTABA Capsules—0.5 gm.
NDC 0516-0051-25 Bottle of 250
NDC 0516-0051-10 Bottle of 1000
POTABA Tablets—0.5 gm.
NDC 0516-0054-01 Bottle of 100
NDC 0516-0054-10 Bottle of 1000
POTABA Envules—2 gm.
NDC 0516-0052-50 Box of 50
POTABA Powder, pure
NDC 0516-0053-01 Bottle of 100 gms.
NDC 0516-0053-16 Bottle of 1 lb.
    Shown in Product Identification Section, page 411

PRIMER® Unna Boot

COMPOSITION

Zinc Oxide, Acacia, Glycerin, Castor Oil and White Petrolatum. No preservatives.

ACTIONS AND USES

Treatment of venous insufficiency conditions such as stasis ulcers.

ADMINISTRATION AND DOSAGE

The combination of PRIMER and TENSOPLAST elastic adhesive bandage produces a flexible cast boot. Apply the PRIMER over the entire lower leg, starting immediately behind the toes and continue up to the knee. Apply the elastic bandage over the PRIMER using firm evenly distributed pressure. Continue bandaging until the PRIMER is completely covered. The treatment is ambulatory and the patient should be encouraged to walk as much as possible. Change bandage at least once a week for the first two or three weeks, then every two or three weeks until healing is complete.

PRECAUTIONS

If skin sensitivity or irritation develops discontinue use and consult a physician.

HOW SUPPLIED

3″ × 10 yards—Unna Boot-List No. 300-1
NDC 0516-1410-30
4″ × 10 yards—Unna Boot-List No. 400-1
NDC 0516-1410-40

YODOXIN®
210 mg. & 650 mg. Tablets
(IODOQUINOL TABLETS U.S.P.)

PRODUCT OVERVIEW

KEY FACTS

Yodoxin (Iodoquinol) is amebicidal against the cyst and trophozoite forms of Entaemoeba histolytica. Yodoxin® contains 64% organically bound iodine.

MAJOR USES

Yodoxin® is used in the treatment of intestinal amebiasis.

SAFETY INFORMATION

Contraindicated in patients with hepatic damage and in patients with known hypersensitivity to iodine and 8-

hydroxyquinolines. Long term use of this drug should be avoided as optic neuritis, optic atrophy and peripheral neuropathy have been reported following prolonged high dosage with halogenated 8-hydroxyquinolines.

PRODUCT ILLUSTRATION

210 mg   650 mg

PRESCRIBING INFORMATION

YODOXIN®   ℞
210 mg. & 650 mg. Tablets
(IODOQUINOL TABLETS U.S.P.)

DESCRIPTION

Iodoquinol is of a light yellowish to tan color, nearly odorless and stable in air. The compound is practically insoluble in water, and sparingly soluble in most other solvents. It contains 64 per cent organically bound iodine.

ACTION

Iodoquinol is amebicidal against Entamoeba histolytica and is considered effective against the trophozoite and cyst forms.

INDICATIONS

Iodoquinol is used in the treatment of intestinal amebiasis.

CONTRAINDICATIONS

Known hypersensitivity to iodine and 8-hydroxyquinolines. Contraindicated in patients with hepatic damage.

WARNINGS

Optic neuritis, optic atrophy, and peripheral neuropathy have been reported following prolonged high dosage therapy with halogenated 8-hydroxyquinolines. Long term use of this drug should be avoided.

USE IN PREGNANCY

Safety for use in pregnancy or during lactation has not been established.

PRECAUTIONS

Iodoquinol should be used with caution in patients with thyroid disease.
Protein-bound serum iodine levels may be increased during treatment with iodoquinol and therefore interfere with certain thyroid function tests. These effects may persist for as long as six months after discontinuation of therapy. Discontinue the drug if hypersensitivity reactions occur.

ADVERSE REACTIONS

Skin: various forms of skin eruptions (acneiform papular and pustular; bullae; vegetating of tuberous iododerma), urticaria and pruritus. Gastrointestinal: nausea, vomiting, abdominal cramps, diarrhea, and pruritus ani.
Fever, chills, headache, vertigo and enlargement of thyroid have been reported. Optic neuritis, optic atrophy and peripheral neuropathy have been reported in association with prolonged high-dosage 8-hydroxyquinoline therapy.

DOSAGE AND ADMINISTRATION

Usual adult dose: (210 mg. each) 3 tablets three times daily, after meals for 20 days. Children 6 to 12 years: (210 mg. each) 2 tablets, t.i.d. Children under 6: (210 mg. each) one tablet per 15 pounds of body weight. Usual adult dose: (650 mg. each) one tablet three times a day for twenty days, to be taken after meals. Children (650 mg. each): For twenty days, 40 mg. per Kg. of body weight daily divided into 3 doses, not to exceed 1.95 grams in 24 hours, for 20 days.

HOW SUPPLIED

YODOXIN Tablets—210 mg.
NDC-0516-0092-01 Bottle of 100
NDC-0516-0092-10 Bottle of 1000
YODOXIN Tablets—650 mg.
NDC-0516-0093-01 Bottle of 100
NDC-0516-0093-10 Bottle of 1000

STORAGE

Store at Controlled Room Temperature 15–30°C. (59–86°F.)

CAUTION

Federal law prohibits dispensing without prescription.

Products are cross-indexed by
generic and chemical names in the
YELLOW SECTION

Graham-Field, Inc.
400 RABRO DRIVE EAST
HAUPPAUGE, NY 11788

GRAFCO® SILVER NITRATE APPLICATORS

COMPOSITION

Wooden applicator stick tipped with Silver Nitrate and Potassium Nitrate.

INDICATIONS

Used for cauterization of wounds and for removing granulation tissue and warts. Caustic if applied to mucous membranes.

DIRECTIONS

Employed in solid form or in solution. For use, the tip is moistened with water and applied to the area to be treated until the desired effect is obtained.

CAUTION

Do not apply in or near eyes. Continuous use of Silver Nitrate may cause permanent discoloration at the site of application.

HOW SUPPLIED

Dispenser tube pack (3 sizes available)
Length 6″, 100 applicators/tube
Length 12″, 100 applicators/tube
Length 18″ Individually packaged. For use with sigmoidoscope.

MEDICOPASTE® BANDAGE
3″ and 4″ Medicopaste® Bandage
Medicopaste® Bandage w/Calamine
3″ and 4″ Unna's Boot Dressing

COMPOSITION

Zinc Oxide, Glycerine, Gelatine (and Calamine).

INDICATIONS

Compression treatment of venous insufficiencies of the lower extremities requiring protection and support. To be used in the treatment of venous stasis ulcers, edema, eczema and postfracture foot conditions.

DIRECTIONS

Detailed instructions for application are supplied on each box.

CAUTION

If skin sensitivity or irritation develops, discontinue use and consult a physician.

HOW SUPPLIED

3″ and 4″ gauze bandage by 10 yards. Each carton contains one medicated bandage sealed in polyethylene bag. Available in standard and Calamine formulation.

Gray Pharmaceutical Co.
100 CONNECTICUT AVENUE
NORWALK, CT 06856

X-PREP® LIQUID
[ĕx ′prep]
(standardized extract of senna fruit)

ACTION AND USES

An easy-to-administer, palatable, highly effective bowel evacuant for the preparation of the intestinal tract prior to G.I. and urological radiography as well as colonoscopy, sigmoidoscopy and other diagnostic bowel procedures. In addition, X-PREP Liquid may be used for preparation of the bowel prior to elective colon surgery. Permits excellent visualization without residual oil droplets. X-PREP Liquid is fully prepared in a single dose container—all the patient has to do is drink the contents of one small bottle (2½ fl. oz.). Good patient cooperation is ensured because of highly pleasant taste. Predictable effectiveness helps reduce or eliminate the need for enemas prior to radiography.

CONTRAINDICATIONS

Acute surgical abdomen.

WARNINGS

Do not use this product unless directed by a physician. Do not use when abdominal pain, nausea or vomiting is present.

CAUTION

In diabetic patients, the physician should be aware of the sugar content of X-PREP Liquid (50 grams per 2½ fl. oz. dose).

ADVERSE REACTIONS

As with all potent purgatives, some patients may experience abdominal discomfort and nausea; vomiting is rare.

ADMINISTRATION AND DOSAGE

For adults: Entire contents of X-PREP Liquid bottle should be taken between 2:00 and 4:00 p.m. on the day prior to diagnostic procedure or elective colon surgery. Patients should be advised to expect a thorough, strong bowel action to begin approximately six hours later. After X-PREP Liquid is taken, diet should be confined to clear fluids.

X-PREP Liquid has proved to be effective following the above regimen. However, at physician's discretion, X-PREP Liquid may be given in divided doses, particularly to elderly or debilitated patients. The following split dosage regimens are equally effective: (1) One-half (½) of the contents of the bottle is taken at bedtime two days prior to diagnostic procedure. On day prior to examination, remaining contents of bottle is taken, also at bedtime. OR (2) On the day prior to examination, one-half (½) contents of bottle is taken at noon and the remaining one-half (½) at 4:00 p.m.

Some physicians prefer the hydration method, with 24-hour liquid diet and consumption of several extra glasses of water during this period, prior to the administration of X-PREP Liquid. Morning enema is optional. X-PREP Liquid may be successfully combined with adjunctive laxative suppositories or citrate of magnesia

HOW SUPPLIED

2½ fl. oz. bottles (alcohol 7% by volume), each providing a single, complete adult dose.

Also Available—Two X-PREP® Bowel Evacuant Kits.

Kit #1 contains: Two SENOKOT-S® Tablets (standardized senna concentrate and docusate sodium), one bottle of X-PREP Liquid 2½ fl. oz., and one RECTOLAX® Suppository (bisacodyl 10 mg), plus easy-to-follow patient instructions for hydration, clear liquid diet, and the correct time-sequence for administering the above laxatives.

Kit #2 contains: One dose CITRALAX® Granules 1.06 oz. (effervescent citrate/sulfate of magnesia), one bottle of X-PREP Liquid 2½ fl. oz., and one RECTOLAX Suppository (bisacodyl 10 mg), plus easy-to-follow patient instructions.

Guardian Chemical
a division of United-Guardian, Inc.
P.O. Box 2500
SMITHTOWN, N.Y. 11787

CLORPACTIN® WCS-90
[klor-pak'tin]
(brand of sodium oxychlorosene)

COMPOSITION
Stabilized organic derivative of hypochlorous acid. A white, water soluble powder with a characteristic smell of hypochlorous acid. Active chlorine derived from calcium hypochlorite: 3–4%.

ACTION AND USES
For use as a topical antiseptic for treating localized infections, particularly when resistant organisms are present. Complete spectrum (bacteria, fungi, viruses, mold, yeast and spores); effective in cases of antibiotic resistance; nontoxic and non-allergenic in use concentrations.

ADMINISTRATION AND DOSAGE
Applied by irrigation, instillations, spray, soaks or wet compresses, preferably thoroughly cleansing with gravity flow irrigation or syringe to provide copious quantities of fresh solution to remove the organic wastes and debris from the site of the involvement. Also for preoperative skin preparation and postoperative protection. Generally applied as the 0.4% solution in water, or isotonic saline, but as the 0.1% to 0.2% in Urology and Ophthalmology.

CONTRAINDICATIONS
The use of this product is contraindicated where the site of the infection is not exposed to the direct contact with the solution. Not for systemic use.

HOW SUPPLIED
In boxes containing 5 x 2 gram bottles.

LUBRASEPTIC® JELLY
[loo-bra"sep'tik]

COMPOSITION
Active ingredients: Aryl phenols, as phenyl phenol 0.1%, Alkyl phenols, as amyl phenol 0.02%, in water miscible form as an acid complex. Phenyl mercuric nitrate 0.007%.

USES
For urethral instillation, prior to insertion of cystoscopes or sounds; for urethral dilations in the case of strictures. For proctologic use, in cases of hemorrhoids, or for post-hemorrhoidectomies, to provide increased comfort between and during the passage of stools. For endotracheal intubation. For use whenever a sterile water soluble lubricant is required: on cystoscopes and proctoscopes, in urological, rectal, and vaginal examinations or for use as a sterile dressing on burns, abrasions, and decubitus ulcers (bedsores).

PRECAUTIONS AND SIDE EFFECTS
No serious side effects or contraindications are known. Urethral instillation, in some individuals, may cause a temporary burning or stinging sensation but this usually disappears in several minutes. Excessive pressure should be avoided when instilling where strictures may exist.

HOW SUPPLIED
In boxes containing 24 sterile packets each with a 10 gram "bellows" shaped tube of jelly and a urethral Disposatip.

pHos-pHaid® R
[fos'fād]
(brand of urinary acidifier)

COMPOSITION
Each 0.5 Gm. tablet contains ammonium biphosphate, 190 mg., sodium biphosphate, 200 mg., and sodium acid pyrophosphate, 110 mg. pH: approximately 4.5. Sodium content: less than one grain per tablet.

ACTION AND USES
pHos-pHaid is a highly effective urinary acidifier which, in conjunction with an acid ash diet, can decrease the urinary pH to a 5–5.5 level. Useful in increasing the solubility of calcium in the urine to assist in preventing formation of calculi in the urinary tract.

ADMINISTRATION AND DOSAGE
In conjunction with an acidifying diet, the recommended dosage is two 0.5 Gm. tablets, followed by a glass of water, t.i.d. Occasionally, higher dosage is required and may be employed when necessary.

SIDE EFFECTS
Occasional hyperacidity, particularly where gastritis or ulceration exists, and/or occasional nausea have been observed in some patients on a high dosage level. This may be decreased or eliminated by the use of the Enteric-Coated tablets. Excessive doses may also act as a saline cathartic and cause diarrhea. In such cases dosage should be decreased until the symptoms disappear. In cases of severe or extensive renal damage, pHos-pHaid should be administered with caution.

HOW SUPPLIED
In color-coded tablets, either regular or Enteric- Coated.

Size	Type	Packaged	Color
0.5 Gm.	Reg.	90 & 500	Blue
0.5 Gm.	Ent.-Coat	90 & 500	Orange

LITERATURE AVAILABLE
Literature on pHospHaid and Acid Ash Diet Sheets are available to physicians on request.

RENACIDIN® R
[ren "a-sē'din]

COMPOSITION
Active Ingredients (in a 300 gram bottle): Citric acid, anhydrous, 156–171 grams; D-gluconic acid (primarily as the lactone), 21–30 grams. Inert Ingredients: Purified magnesium hydroxycarbonate, 75–87 grams; Magnesium Acid Citrate ($MgHC_6H_5O_7$), 9–15 grams; Calcium (as the carbonate), 2–6 grams; Water, combined and free, 17–21 grams.

ACTION AND USES
For use in preparing solutions for irrigating indwelling urethral catheters and the urinary bladder in order to dissolve or prevent formation of calcifications.

ADMINISTRATION AND DOSAGE
As a 10% solution (sterile) in distilled water. Irrigation is carried out with 1-2 ounces, b.i.d. or t.i.d. by means of a small, sterile, rubber syringe.

SIDE EFFECTS
Only occasionally will a patient complain of some temporary pain or burning sensation from this procedure, in which case use of the solution should be discontinued.

CONTRAINDICATIONS
It is contraindicated for therapy or preventive therapy above the ureteral-vesical junction; therefore it is contraindicated for ureteral catheters, nephrostomy or pyelostomy tubes or renal lavage for dissolving calculi. Contraindicated for biliary calculi.

HOW SUPPLIED
In bottles containing 300 grams; also in boxes containing six 25 gram bottles.

GynoPharma Inc.
50 DIVISION STREET
SOMERVILLE, NJ 08876

NORCEPT–E® 1/35•21 R
NORCEPT–E® 1/35•28 R
[nōr-cĕpt']
(Norethindrone and Ethinyl Estradiol Tablets USP)

PRODUCT OVERVIEW

KEY FACTS
NORCEPT-E®1/35·21 and NORCEPT-E®1/35·28 Tablets are a combination oral contraceptive. Each white tablet contains 1 mg of the progestational compound, norethindrone, together with 35 mcg of the estrogenic compound, ethinyl estradiol. Oral contraceptives are highly effective. The pregnancy rate in women using conventional combination oral contraceptives is generally reported as less than 1 pregnancy per 100 woman years.

Combination oral contraceptives act primarily through the mechanism of gonadotrophin suppression due to the estrogenic and progestational activity of the ingredients.

MAJOR USES
NORCEPT-E®1/35·21 and NORCEPT-E 1/35·28 is indicated for the prevention of pregnancy in women who elect to use oral contraceptive as a method of contraception. To achieve maximum contraceptive effectiveness, NORCEPT-E®Tablets must be taken exactly as directed (the first white tablet is taken on the first Sunday after menstruation begins and at intervals not exceeding 24 hours).

SAFETY INFORMATION

> Cigarette smoking increases the risk of serious cardiovascular side effects from oral contraceptive use. This risk increases with age and with heavy smoking (15 or more cigarettes per day) and is quite marked in women over 35 years of age. Women who use oral contraceptives should be strongly advised not to smoke.

The use of oral contraceptives is associated with increased risk of several serious conditions including thromboembolism, stroke, myocardial infarction, hepatic adenoma, gallbladder disease, hypertension. Practitioners prescribing oral contraceptives should be familiar with the information relating to these risks.

PRESCRIBING INFORMATION

NORCEPT–E® 1/35•21 R
NORCEPT–E® 1/35•28 R
[nōr-cĕpt']
(Norethindrone and Ethinyl Estradiol Tablets USP)

DESCRIPTION
NORCEPT-E® 1/35·21 Tablets (Norethindrone and Ethinyl Estradiol Tablets USP) are a conbination oral contraceptive. Each NORCEPT-E® 1/35·21 Tablet contains 1 mg of the progestational compound, norethindrone (17-hydroxy-19-nor-17α-pregn-4-en-20-yn-3-one) together with 35 mcg of the estrogenic compound, ethinyl estradiol (19-nor-17α-pregna-1,3,5 (10)-trien-20-yne-3, 17-diol). Inactive ingredients: colloidal silicon dioxide, gelatin, lactose, magnesium stearate, starch (corn and potato), and talc.

NORCEPT-E® 1/35·28 Tablets (Norethindrone and Ethinyl Estradiol Tablets USP) are a conbination oral contraceptive. Each white NORCEPT-E® 1/35·28 Tablet contains 1 mg of the progestational compound, norethindrone (17-hydroxy-19-nor-17α-pregn-4-en-20-yn-3-one) together with 35 mcg of the estrogenic compound, ethinyl estradiol (19-nor-17α-pregna-1,3,5 (10)-trien-20-yne-3, 17-diol). Inactive ingredients: colloidal silicon dioxide, gelatin, lactose, magnesium stearate, starch (corn and potato), and talc. Each green tablet contains the following inert ingredients: colloidal silicon dioxide, FD&C Blue No. 1, FD&C Yellow No. 10, gelatin, lactose, magnesium stearate, starch (corn and potato) and talc.

Norethindrone

Continued on next page

GynoPharma—Cont.

Ethinyl Estradiol

CLINICAL PHARMACOLOGY

Combination oral contraceptives act by suppression of gonadotropins. Although the primary mechanism of this action is inhibition of ovulation, other alterations include changes in the cervical mucus (which increase the difficulty of sperm entry into the uterus) and the endometrium (which reduce the likelihood of implantation).

INDICATIONS AND USAGE

NORCEPT-E® 1/35·21 and NORCEPT-E® 1/35·28 are indicated for the prevention of pregnancy in women who elect to use oral contraceptives as a method of contraception. Oral contraceptives are highly effective. Table I lists the typical accidental pregnancy rates for users of combination oral contraceptives and other methods of contraception. The efficacy of these contraceptive methods, except sterilization, depends upon the reliability with which they are used. Correct and consistent use of methods can result in lower failure rates.

TABLE I: LOWEST EXPECTED AND TYPICAL FAILURE RATES DURING THE FIRST YEAR OF CONTINUOUS USE OF A METHOD

% of Women Experiencing an Accidental Pregnancy in the First Year of Continuous Use

Method	Lowest Expected*	Typical**
(No contraception)	(89)	(89)
Oral contraceptives		3
combined	0.1	N/A***
progestin only	0.5	N/A***
Diaphragm with spermicidal cream or jelly	3	18
Spermicides alone (foam, creams, jellies and vaginal suppositories)	3	21
Vaginal sponge		
nulliparous	5	18
multiparous	>8	>28
IUD (medicated)	1	6#
Condom without spermicides	2	12
Periodic abstinence (all methods)	2–10	20
Female sterilization	0.2	0.4
Male sterilization	0.1	0.15

Adapted from J. Trussell and K. Kost: Table II, ref. #1.
* The authors' best guess of the percentage of women expected to experience an accidental pregnancy among couples who initiate a method (not necessarily for the first time) and who use it consistently and correctly during the first year if they do not stop for any other reason other than pregnancy.
** This term represents "typical" couples who initiate use of a method (not necessarily for the first time), who experience an accidental pregnancy during the first year if they do not stop for any other reason other than pregnancy.
*** N/A—Data not available
# Combined typical rate for both medicated and non-medicated IUD. The rate for medicated IUD alone is not available.

CONTRAINDICATIONS

Oral contraceptives should not be used in women who currently have the following conditions:
• Thrombophlebitis or thromboembolic disorders
• A past history of deep vein thrombophlebitis or thromboembolic disorders
• Cerebral vascular or coronary artery disease
• Known or suspected carcinoma of the breast
• Carcinoma of the endometrium or other known or suspected estrogen-dependent neoplasia
• Undiagnosed abnormal genital bleeding
• Cholestatic jaundice of pregnancy or jaundice with prior pill use

• Hepatic adenomas or carcinomas
• Known or suspected pregnancy

WARNINGS

> Cigarette smoking increases the risk of serious cardiovascular side effects from oral contraceptive use. This risk increases with age and with heavy smoking (15 or more cigarettes per day) and is quite marked in women over 35 years of age. Women who use oral contraceptives should be strongly advised not to smoke.

The use of oral contraceptives is associated with increased risk of several serious conditions including myocardial infarction, thromboembolism, stroke, hepatic neoplasia, and gallbladder disease, although the risk of serious morbidity or mortality is very small in healthy women without underlying risk factors. The risk of morbidity and mortality increases significantly in the presence of other underlying risk factors such as hypertension, hyperlipidemias, obesity and diabetes.

Practitioners prescribing oral contraceptives should be familiar with the following information relating to these risks. The information contained in this package insert is principally based on studies carried out in patients who used oral contraceptives with higher formulations of estrogens and progestogens than those in common use today. The effect of long term use of the oral contraceptives with lower formulations of both estrogens and progestogens remains to be determined.

Throughout this labeling, epidemiological studies reported are of two types: retrospective or case control studies and prospective or cohort studies. Case control studies provide a measure of the relative risk of a disease, namely, a *ratio* of the incidence of a disease among oral contraceptive users to that among nonusers. The relative risk does not provide information on the actual clinical occurrence of a disease. Cohort studies provide a measure of attributable risk, which is the *difference* in the incidence of disease between oral contraceptive users and nonusers. The attributable risk does provide information about the actual occurrence of a disease in the population (adapted from refs. 2 and 3 with the author's permission). For further information, the reader is referred to a text on epidemiological methods.

1. THROMBOEMBOLIC DISORDERS AND OTHER VASCULAR PROBLEMS

a. Myocardial Infarction

An increased risk of myocardial infarction has been associated with oral contraceptive use. This risk is primarily in smokers or women with other underlying risk factors for coronary artery disease such as hypertension, hypercholesterolemia, morbid obesity, and diabetes. The relative risk of heart attack for current oral contraceptive users has been estimated to be two to six[4–10]. The risk is very low under the age of 30.

Smoking in combination with oral contraceptive use has been shown to contribute substantially to the incidence of myocardial infarctions in women in their mid-thirties or older, with smoking accounting for the majority of excess cases[11]. Mortality rates associated with circulatory disease have been shown to increase substantially in smokers, especially in those 35 years of age and older among women who use oral contraceptives.

CIRCULATORY DISEASE MORTALITY
RATES PER 100,000
WOMAN YEARS BY AGE, SMOKING STATUS
AND ORAL CONTRACEPTIVE USE

TABLE II. (Adapted from P.M. Layde and V. Beral, ref. #12.)
Oral contraceptives may compound the effects of well-known risk factors, such as hypertension, diabetes, hyperlipidemias, age and obesity[13]. In particular, some progestogens are known to decrease HDL cholesterol and cause glucose intol-

erance, while estrogens may create a state of hyperinsulinism[14–18]. Oral contraceptives have been shown to increase blood pressure among users (see section 9 in WARNINGS). Similar effects on risk factors have been associated with an increased risk of heart disease. Oral contraceptives must be used with caution in women with cardiovascular disease risk factors.

b. Thromboembolism

An increased risk of thromboembolic and thrombotic disease associated with the use of oral contraceptives is well established. Case control studies have found the relative risk of users compared to non-users to be 3 for the first episode of superficial venous thrombosis, 4 to 11 for deep vein thrombosis or pulmonary embolism, and 1.5 to 6 for women with predisposing conditions for venous thromboembolic disease[2,3,19–24]. Cohort studies have shown the relative risk to be somewhat lower, about 3 for new cases and about 4.5 for new cases requiring hospitalization[25]. The risk of thromboembolic disease associated with oral contraceptives is not related to length of use and disappears after pill use is stopped[26].

A two- to four-fold increase in relative risk of post-operative thromboembolic complications has been reported with the use of oral contraceptives[9]. The relative risk of venous thrombosis in women who have predisposing conditions is twice that of women without such medical conditions[26]. If feasible, oral contraceptives should be discontinued at least four weeks prior to and for two weeks after elective surgery of a type associated with an increase in risk of thromboembolism and during and following prolonged immobilization. Since the immediate postpartum period is also associated with an increased risk of thromboembolism, oral contraceptives should be started no earlier than four weeks after delivery in women who elect not to breast feed.

c. Cerebrovascular diseases

Oral contraceptives have been shown to increase both the relative and attributable risks of cerebrovascular events (thrombotic and hemorrhagic strokes), although, in general, the risk is greatest among older (> 35 years), hypertensive women who also smoke. Hypertension was found to be a risk factor for both users and non-users, for both types of strokes, and smoking interacted to increase the risk for hemorrhagic stroke[27–29].

In a large study, the relative risk of thrombotic strokes has been shown to range from 3 for normotensive users to 14 for users with severe hypertension[30]. The relative risk of hemorrhagic stroke is reported to be 1.2 for non-smokers who used oral contraceptives, 2.6 for smokers who did not use oral contraceptives, 7.6 for smokers who used oral contraceptives, 1.8 for normotensive users and 25.7 for users with severe hypertension[30]. The attributable risk is also greater in older women[3].

d. Dose-related risk of vascular disease from oral contraceptives

A positive association has been observed between the amount of estrogen and progestogen in oral contraceptives and the risk of vascular disease[31–33]. A decline in serum high density lipoproteins (HDL) has been reported with many progestational agents[14–16]. A decline in serum high density lipoproteins has been associated with an increased incidence of ischemic heart disease. Because estrogens increase HDL cholesterol, the net effect of an oral contraceptive depends on a balance achieved between doses of estrogen and progestogen and the activity of the progestogen used in the contraceptive. The activity and amount of both hormones should be considered in the choice of an oral contraceptive.

Minimizing exposure to estrogen and progestogen is in keeping with good principles of therapeutics. For any particular estrogen/progestogen combination, the dosage regimen prescribed should be one which contains the least amount of estrogen and progestogen that is compatible with a low failure rate and the needs of the individual patient. New acceptors of oral contraceptives agents should be started on preparations containing 0.035 mg or less of estrogen.

e. Persistence of risk

There are two studies which have shown persistence of risk of vascular disease for ever-users of oral contraceptives. In a study in the United States, the risk of developing myocardial infarction after discontinuing oral contraceptives persists for at least 9 years for women 40–49 years who had used oral contraceptives for five or more years, but this increased risk was not demonstrated in other age groups[8]. In another study in Great Britain, the risk of developing cerebrovascular disease persisted for at least 6 years after discontinuation of oral contraceptives, although excess risk was very small[34]. However, both studies were performed with oral contraceptive formulations containing 50 micrograms or higher of estrogens.

2. ESTIMATES OF MORTALITY FROM CONTRACEPTIVE USE

One study gathered data from a variety of sources which have estimated the mortality risk associated with different methods of contraception at different ages (Table III). These estimates include the combined risk of death associated with contraceptive methods plus the risk attributable to pregnancy in the event of method failure. Each method of contraception has its specific benefits and risks. The study concluded that with the exception of oral contraceptive users 35 and older who smoke and 40 and older who do not smoke, mortality associated with all methods of birth control is low and below that associated with childbirth. However, smokers 35 and older and non-smokers 40 and older who use oral contraceptives have a significant increase in mortality higher than those using other methods of birth control. These facts must be weighed in conjunction with failure rates for other methods and the risk associated with subsequent pregnancy. (See Table I.)

[See table right].

3. CARCINOMA OF THE REPRODUCTIVE ORGANS

Numerous epidemiological studies have been performed on the incidence of breast, endometrial, ovarian, and cervical cancer in women using oral contraceptives. While there are conflicting reports the overall evidence in the literature suggests that use of oral contraceptives is not associated with an increase in the risk of developing breast cancer[36,38]. The Cancer and Steroid Hormone (CASH) study[36,79] also showed no latent effect on the risk of breast cancer for at least a decade following long term use. Some studies have shown a slightly increased relative risk of developing breast cancer[37,39-43].

Some studies suggest that oral contraceptive use has been associated with an increase in the risk of cervical intraepithelial neoplasia in some populations of women[45-48]. However, there continues to be controversy about the extent to which such findings may be due to differences in sexual behavior and other factors.

In spite of many studies of the relationship between oral contraceptive use and breast and cervical cancers, a cause and effect relationship has not been established.

4. HEPATIC NEOPLASIA

Benign hepatic adenomas are associated with oral contraceptive use, although the incidence of benign tumors is rare in the United States. Indirect calculations have estimated the attributable risk to be in the range of 3.3 cases/100,000 for users, a risk that increases after four or more years of use especially with oral contraceptives of higher dose.[49]. Rupture of benign, hepatic adenomas may cause death through intra-abdominal hemorrhage[50-51].

Studies from Britain have shown an increased risk of developing hepatocellular carcinoma[52-54] in long term (> 8 years) oral contraceptive users. However, these cancers are rare in the U.S. and the attributable risk (the excess incidence) of liver cancers in oral contraceptive users approaches less than one per million users.

5. OCULAR LESIONS

There have been clincial case reports of retinal thrombosis associated with the use of oral contraceptives. Oral contraceptives should be discontinued if there is unexplained partial or complete loss of vision; onset of proptosis or diplopia; papilledema; or retinal vascular lesions. Appropriate diagnostic and therapeutic measures should be undertaken immediately.

6. ORAL CONTRACEPTIVE USE BEFORE OR DURING EARLY PREGNANCY: RISK OF BIRTH DEFECTS

Extensive epidemiological studies have revealed no increased risk of birth defects in women who have used oral contraceptives prior to pregnancy[56,57]. The majority of recent studies also do not indicate a teratogenic effect, particularly in so far as cardiac anomalies and limb reduction defects are concerned[55,56,58,59], when taken inadvertently during early pregnancy.

The administration of oral contraceptives to induce withdrawal bleeding should not be used as a test for pregnancy. Oral contraceptives should not be used during pregnancy to treat threatened or habitual abortion.

It is recommended that for any patient who has missed two consecutive periods, pregnancy should be ruled out before continuing oral contraceptive use. If the patient has not adhered to the prescribed schedule, the possibility of pregnancy should be considered at the time of the first missed period. Oral contraceptive use should be discontinued until pregnancy is ruled out.

7. GALLBLADDER DISEASE

Earlier studies have reported an increased lifetime relative risk of gallbladder surgery in users of oral contraceptives and estrogens[60-61]. More recent studies, however, have shown that the relative risk of developing gallbladder disease among oral contraceptive users may be minimal[62-64]. The recent findings of minimal risk may be related to the use of oral contraceptive formulations containing lower hormonal doses of estrogens and progestogens.

8. CARBOHYDRATE AND LIPID METABOLIC EFFECTS

Oral contraceptives have been shown to cause a decrease in glucose intolerance in a significant percentage of users[17]. This effect has been shown to be directly related to estrogen dose[65]. Progestogens increase insulin secretion and create insulin resistance, this effect varying with different progestational agents[17,66]. However, in the non-diabetic woman, oral contraceptives appear to have no effect on fasting blood glucose[67]. Because of these demonstrated effects, prediabetic and diabetic women in particular should be carefully monitored while taking oral contraceptives.

TABLE III—ANNUAL NUMBER OF BIRTH-RELATED OR METHOD-RELATED DEATHS ASSOCIATED WITH CONTROL OF FERTILITY PER 100,000 NONSTERILE WOMEN, BY FERTILITY CONTROL METHOD ACCORDING TO AGE

Method of control and outcome	15–19	20–24	25–29	30–34	35–39	40–44
No fertility control methods*	7.0	7.4	9.1	14.8	25.7	28.2
Oral contraceptives non-smoker**	0.3	0.5	0.9	1.9	13.8	31.6
Oral contraceptives smoker**	2.2	3.4	6.6	13.5	51.1	117.2
IUD**	0.8	0.8	1.0	1.0	1.4	1.4
Condom*	1.1	1.6	0.7	0.2	0.3	0.4
Diaphragm/spermicide*	1.9	1.2	1.2	1.3	2.2	2.8
Periodic abstinence*	2.5	1.6	1.6	1.7	2.9	3.6

* Deaths are birth related
** Deaths are method related

Adapted from H.W. Ory, ref. #35.

A small proportion of women will have persistent hypertriglyceridemia while on the pill. As discussed earlier (see WARNINGS 1a. and 1d.), changes in serum triglycerides and lipoprotein levels have been reported in oral contraceptive users.

9. ELEVATED BLOOD PRESSURE

An increase in blood pressure has been reported in women taking oral contraceptives[68] and this increase is more likely in older oral contraceptive users[69] and with extended duration of continued use[61]. Data from the Royal College of General Practitioners[12] and subsequent randomized trials have shown that the incidence of hypertension increases with increasing progestational activity.

Women with a history of hypertension or hypertension-related diseases, or renal disease[70] should be encouraged to use another method of contraception. If women elect to use oral contraceptives, they should be monitored closely and if significant elevation of blood pressure occurs, oral contraceptives should be discontinued. For most women, elevated blood pressure will return to normal after stopping oral contraceptives, and there is no difference in the occurrence of hypertension between former and never users[68-71].

10. HEADACHE

The onset or exacerbation of migraine or development of headache with a new pattern which is recurrent, persistent or severe requires discontinuation of oral contraceptives and evaluation of the cause.

11. BLEEDING IRREGULARITIES

Breakthrough bleeding and spotting are sometimes encountered in patients on oral contraceptives, especially during the first three months of use. Nonhormonal causes should be considered and adequate diagnostic measures taken to rule out malignancy or pregnancy in the event of breakthrough bleeding, as in the case of any abnormal vaginal bleeding. If pathology has been excluded, time or a change to another formulation may solve the problem. In the event of amenorrhea, pregnancy should be ruled out.

An alteration in menstrual patterns is likely to occur in women using progestogen-only contraceptives The amount and duration of flow, cycle length, breakthrough bleeding, spotting and amenorrhea will probably be quite variable. Bleeding irregularities occur more frequently with the use of progestogen-only oral contraceptives than with the combinations and the dropout rate due to such conditions is higher. Some women may encounter post-pill amenorrhea or oligomenorrhea, especially when such a condition was preexistent.

12. ECTOPIC PREGNANCY

Ectopic as well as intrauterine pregnancy may occur in contraceptive failures. However, in progestogen-only oral contraceptive failures, the ratio of ectopic to intrauterine pregnancies is higher than in women who are not receiving oral contraceptives, since the drugs are more effective in preventing intrauterine than ectopic pregnancies.

PRECAUTIONS

General

1. PHYSICAL EXAMINATION AND FOLLOW UP

A complete medical history and physical examination should be taken prior to the initiation or reinstitution of oral contraceptives and at least annually during use of oral contraceptives. These physical examinations should include special reference to blood pressure, breasts, abdomen and pelvic organs, including cervical cytology, and relevant laboratory tests. In case of undiagnosed, persistent, or recurrent abnormal vaginal bleeding, appropriate diagnostic measures should be conducted to rule out malignancy. Women with a strong family history of breast cancer or who have breast nodules should be monitored with particular care.

2. LIPID DISORDERS

Women who are being treated for hyperlipidemias should be followed closely if they elect to use oral contraceptives. Some progestogens may elevate LDL levels and may render the control of hyperlipidemias more difficult.

3. LIVER FUNCTION

If jaundice develops in any woman receiving such drugs, the medication should be discontinued. Steroid hormones may be poorly metabolized in patients with impaired liver furction.

4. FLUID RETENTION

Oral contraceptives may cause some degree of fluid retention. They should be prescribed with caution, and only with careful monitoring, in patients with conditions which might be aggravated by fluid retention.

5. EMOTIONAL DISORDERS

Women with a history of depression should be carefully observed and the drug discontinued if depression recurs to a serious degree.

6. CONTACT LENSES

Contact lens wearers who develop visual changes or changes in lens tolerance should be assessed by an ophthalmologist.

7. DRUG INTERACTIONS

Reduced efficacy and increased incidence of breakthrough bleeding and menstrual irregularities have been associated with concomitant use of rifampin. A similar assocation, though less marked, has been suggested with barbiturates, phenylbutazone, phenytoin sodium, and possibly with griseofulvin, ampicillin and tetracyclines[72].

8. INTERACTIONS WITH LABORATORY TESTS

Certain endocrine and liver function tests and blood components may be affected by oral contraceptives:

a. Increased prothrombin and factors VII, VIII, IX, and X; decreased antithrombin 3; increased norepinephrine-induced platelet aggregability.

b. Increased thyroid binding globulin (TBG) leading to increased circulating total thyroid hormone, as measured by protein-bound iodine (PBI), T4 by column or by radio-immunoassay. Free T3 resin uptake is decreased, reflecting the elevated TBG, free T4 concentration is unaltered.

c. Other binding proteins may be elevated in serum.

d. Sex-binding globulins are increased and result in elevated levels of total circulating sex steroids and corticoids; however, free or biologically active levels remain unchanged.

e. Triglycerides may be increased.

f. Glucose tolerance may be decreased.

g. Serum folate levels may be depressed by oral contraceptive therapy. This may be of clinical significance if a woman becomes pregnant shortly after discontinuing oral contraceptives.

9. CARCINOGENESIS

See WARNINGS section.

10. PREGNANCY

Pregnancy Category X. See CONTRAINDICATIONS and WARNINGS sections.

11. NURSING MOTHERS

Small amounts of oral contraceptive steroids have been identified in the milk of nursing mothers and a few adverse effects on the child have been reported, including jaundice and breast enlargement. In addition, oral contraceptives given in the postpartum period may interfere with lactation by decreasing the quantity and quality of breast milk. If possible, the nursing mother should be advised not to use oral contraceptives but to use other forms of contraception until she has completely weaned her child.

12. INFORMATION FOR THE PATIENT

(See Patient Labeling printed below)

ADVERSE REACTIONS

An increased risk of the following serious adverse reactions has been associated with the use of oral contraceptives (see WARNINGS section):

- Thrombophlebitis and venous thrombosis with or without embolism
- Arterial thromboembolism
- Pulmonary embolism
- Myocardial infarction
- Cerebral hemorrhage

Continued on next page

GynoPharma—Cont.

- Cerebral thrombosis
- Hypertension
- Gallbladder disease
- Hepatic adenomas or benign liver tumors

The following adverse reactions have been reported in patients receiving oral contraceptives and are believed to be drug-related:

- Nausea
- Vomiting
- Gastrointestinal symptoms (such as abdominal cramps and bloating)
- Breakthrough bleeding
- Spotting
- Change in menstrual flow
- Amenorrhea
- Temporary infertility after discontinuation of treatment
- Edema
- Melasma which may persist
- Breast changes: tenderness, enlargement, and secretion
- Change in weight (increase or decrease)
- Change in cervical erosion and secretion
- Diminution in lactation when given immediately postpartum
- Cholestatic jaundice
- Migraine
- Rash (allergic)
- Mental depression
- Reduced tolerance to carbohydrates
- Vaginal candidiasis
- Change in corneal curvature (steepening)
- Intolerance to contact lenses

The following adverse reactions have been reported in users of oral contraceptives, and the association has been neither confirmed nor refuted:

- Pre-menstrual syndrome
- Cataracts
- Changes in appetite
- Cystitis-like syndrome
- Headache
- Nervousness
- Dizziness
- Hirsutism
- Loss of scalp hair
- Erythema multiforme
- Erythema nodosum
- Hemorrhagic eruption
- Vaginitis
- Porphyria
- Impaired renal function
- Hemolytic uremic syndrome
- Acne
- Changes in libido
- Colitis

OVERDOSAGE

Serious ill effects have not been reported following acute ingestion of large doses of oral contraceptives by young children. Overdosage may cause nausea, and withdrawal bleeding may occur in females.

NON-CONTRACEPTIVE HEALTH BENEFITS

The following non-contraceptive health benefits related to the use of combination oral contraceptives are supported by epidemiological studies which largely utilized oral contraceptive formulations containing estrogen doses exceeding 35 mcg of estrogen[73-78].

Effects on menses:
- increased menstrual cycle regularity
- decreased blood loss and decreased incidence of iron deficiency anemia
- decreased incidence of dysmenorrhea

Effects related to inhibition of ovulation:
- decreased incidence of functional ovarian cysts
- decreased incidence of ectopic pregnancies

Other effects:
- decreased incidence of fibroadenomas and fibrocystic disease of the breast
- decreased incidence of acute pelvic inflammatory disease
- decreased incidence of endometrial cancer
- decreased incidence of ovarian cancer

DOSAGE AND ADMINISTRATION

To achieve maximum contraceptive effectiveness, NORCEPT-E® Tablets must be taken exactly as directed and at intervals not exceeding 24 hours.

21-Day Regimen (Sunday Start)

When taking NORCEPT-E® 1/35·21, the first white tablet should be taken on the first Sunday after menstruation begins. If period begins on Sunday, the first white tablet is taken on that day and continued without interruption for 21 days. No tablets are taken for 7 days, then a new course is started (on Sunday) with one white tablet a day for 21 days. Contraceptive reliance should not be placed on these prod-

ucts until after the first 7 consecutive days of administration.

The use of NORCEPT-E® 1/35·21 for contraception may be initiated postpartum. When the tablets are administered during the postpartum period, the increased risk of throemboembolic disease associated with the postpartum period must be considered. (See CONTRAINDICATIONS and WARNINGS concerning thromboembolic disease.) The possibility of ovulation and conception prior to initiation of medication should be considered. If the patient misses more than one tablet, the patient should begin taking tablets again as soon as remembered and another method of conception used for the balance of that tablet cycle.

21-Day Regimen (Day 5 Start)

The dosage of NORCEPT-E® 1/35·21 for the initial cycle of therapy is one tablet administered daily from the 5th day through 25th day of the menstrual cycle, counting the first day of menstrual flow as "Day 1". The use of these products for contraception may be initiated postpartum. When the tablets are administered during the postpartum period, the increased risk of thromboembolic disease associated with the postpartum period must be considered. (See CONTRAINDICATIONS and WARNINGS concerning thromboebolic disease.) If NORCEPT-E® 1/35·21 is first taken later than the fifth day of the first menstrual cycle of medication or postpartum, contraceptive reliance should not be placed on these products until after the first 7 consecutive days of administration. For subsequent cycles, no tablets are taken for 7 days, then a new course is started of one tablet a day for 21 days. The dosage regimen then continues with 7 days of no medication, followed by 21 days of medication, instituting a three-weeks-on, one-week-off dosage regimen. The possibility of ovulation and conception prior to initiation of medication should be considered. If the patient misses more than one tablet, the patient should begin taking tablets again as soon as remembered and another method of contraception used for the balance of that tablet cycle.

28-Day Regimen (Sunday Start)

When taking NORCEPT-E® 1/35·28, the first white tablet should be taken on the first Sunday after menstruation begins. If period begins on Sunday, the first white tablet is taken on that day. If switching directly from another oral contraceptive, the first white tablet should be taken on the first Sunday after the last ACTIVE tablet of the previous product. Tablets are taken without interruption as follows: One white tablet daily for 21 days, then one green tablet daily for 7 days. After 28 tablets have been taken, a white tablet is then taken the next day (Sunday), etc. If first starting oral contraceptives more than 5 days from the onset of menses, contraceptive reliance should not be placed on these products until after the first 7 consecutive days of administration.

The use of NORCEPT-E® 1/35·28 for contraception may be initiated postpartum. When tablets are administered during the postpartum period, the increased risk of thromboembolic disease associated with the postpartum period must be considered. (See CONTRAINDICATIONS and WARNINGS concerning thromboembolic disease.) The possibility of ovulation and conception prior to initiation of medication should be considered. If the patient misses more than one tablet, the patient should begin taking tablets again as soon as remembered and another method of contraception used for the balance of that tablet cycle.

All Oral Contraceptives

Breakthrough bleeding, spotting, and amenorrhea are frequent reasons for patients discontinuing oral contraceptives. In breakthrough bleeding, as in all cases of irregular bleeding from the vagina, nonfunctional causes should be borne in mind. In undiagnosed persistent or recurrent abnormal bleeding from the vagina, adequate diagnostic measures are indicated to rule out pregnancy or malignancy. If pathology has been excluded, time or a change to another formulation may solve the problem. Changing to an oral contraceptive with a higher estrogen content, while potentially useful in minimizing menstrual irregularities, should be done only if necessary since this may increase the risk of thromboembolic disease.

Use of oral contraceptives in the event of a missed menstrual period:

1. If the patient has not adhered to the prescribed dosage regimen, the possibility of pregnancy should be considered after the first missed period and oral contraceptive use should be discontinued until pregnancy has been ruled out.
2. If the patient has adhered to the prescribed schedule and misses two consecutive periods, pregnancy should be ruled out before continuing oral contraceptive use.

HOW SUPPLIED

NORCEPT-E® 1/35·21 Tablets are supplied in a blister card containing 21 plain white unscored tablets. Each white tablet contains 1 mg of the progestational compound, norethindrone together with 35 mcg of the estrogenic compound, ethinyl estradiol. Each carton contains 6 blister cards. NDC 54765-035-21.

NORCEPT-E® 1/35·28 Tablets are supplied in a blister card containing 28 tablets, 21 plain white unscored norethindrone with ethinyl estradiol tablets and 7 plain green unscored tablets containing inert ingredients. Each white tablet contains 1 mg norethindrone and 35 mcg of ethinyl estradiol. Each carton contains 6 blister cards. NDC 54765-035-28.

REFERENCES

1. Reproduced with permission of the Population Council from J. Trussell and K. Kost: Contraceptive failure in the United States: A critical review of the literature. Studies in Family Planning, 18 (5), September–October 1987. 2. Stadel BV. Oral contraceptives and cardiovascular disease. (Pt. 1). N Engl J Med 1981; 305 :612–618. 3. Stadel BV. Oral contraceptives and cardiovascular disease. (Pt. 2.). N Engl J Med 1981; 305 :672–677. 4. Adam, SA, Thorogood M. Oral contraception and myocardial infarction revisited: the effects of new preparations and prescribing patterns. Br J Obstet Gynecol 1981; 88 :838–845. 5. Mann JI, Inman WH. Oral contraceptives and death from myocardial infarction. Br Med J 1975; 2(5965): 245–248. 6. Mann, JI, Vessey MP, Thorogood M, Doll R. Myocardial infarction in young women with special reference to oral contraceptive practice. Br Med J 1975 2(5956): 241–245. 7. Royal College of General Practitioners' Oral Contraception Study: Further analyses of mortality in oral contraceptive users. Lancet 1981; 1 :541–546. 8. Slone, D, Shapiro S, Kaufman DW, Rosenberg L, Miettinen OS, Stolley PD. Risk of myocardial infarction in relation to current and discontinued use of oral contraceptives. N Engl J Med 1981; 305 :420–424. 9. Vessey, MP. Female hormones and vascular disease: an epidemiological overview, Br J Fam Plann 1980; 6 :1–12. 10. Russell-Briefel RG, Ezzati TM, Fulwood R, Perlman JA, Murphy RS. Cardiovascular risk status and oral contraceptive use, United States, 1976–80. Prevent Med 1986; 15 :352–362. 11. Goldbaum GM, Kendrick JS, Hogelin GC, Gentry EM. The relative impact of smoking and oral contraceptive use on women in the United States. JAMA 1987; 258 :1339–1342. 12. Layde PM, Beral V. Further analyses of mortality in oral contraceptive users: Royal College General Practitioners' Oral Contraception Study. (Table 5) Lancet 1981; 1 :541–546. 13. Knopp, RH. Arteriosclerosis risk: the roles of oral contraceptives and postmenopausal estrogens. J Reprod Med 1986 31(9)(Supplement) :913–921. 14. Krauss RM, Roy S, Mishell DR, Casagrande J, Pike MC. Effects of two low-dose oral contraceptives on serum lipids and lipoproteins: Differential changes in high-density lipoproteins subclasses. Am J Obstet 1983 145 :446–452. 15. Wahl P, Walden C, Knopp R, Hoover J, Wallace R, Heiss G, Rifkind B. Effect of estrogen/progestin potency on lipid/lipoprotein cholesterol, N Engl J Med 1983; 308 :862–867. 16. Wynn V, Niththyananthan R. The effect of progestin in combined oral contraceptives on serum lipids with special reference to high-density lipoproteins. Am J Obstet Gynecol 1982; 142 :766–771. 17. Wynn V, Godsland I. Effects of oral contraceptives on carbohydrate metabolism. J Reprod Med 1986; 31(9)(Supplement) :892–897. 18. LaRosa JC. Atherosclerotic risk factors in cardiovascular disease. J Reprod Med 1986; 31(9)(Supplement) :906–912. 19. Inman WH, Vessey MP. Investigation of death from pulmonary, coronary, and cerebral thrombosis and embolism in women of child-bearing age. Br Med J 1968; 2(5599) :193–199. 20. Maquire MG, Tonascia J, Sartwell PE, Stolley PD, Tockman MS. Increased risk of thrombosis due to oral contraceptives: a further report. Am J Epidemiol 1979; 110(2) :188–195. 21. Pettiti DB, Wingerd J, Pellegrin F, Ramacharan S. Risk of vascular disease in women: smoking, oral contraceptives, noncontraceptive estrogens, and other factors, JAMA 1979; 242 :1150–1154. 22. Vessey MP, Doll R. Investigation of relation between use of oral contraceptives and thromboembolic disease. Br Med J 1968; 2(5599) :199–205. 23. Vessey MP, Doll R. Investigation of relation between use of oral contraceptives and thromboembolic disease: A further report. Br Med J 1969; 2(5658) :651–657. 24. Porter JB, Hunter JR, Danielson DA, Jick H, Stergachis A. Oral contraceptives and non-fatal vascular disease—recent experience. Obstet Gynecol 1982; 59(3) :299–302. 25. Vessey, M, Doll R, Peto R, Johnson B, Wiggins P. A long term follow-up study of women using different methods of contraception: an interim report. J Biosocial Sci 1976; 8 :375–427. 26. Royal College of General Practitioners: Oral contraceptives, venous thrombosis, and varicose veins. J Royal Coll Gen Prac 1978; 28 :393–399. 27. Collaborative Group for the Study of Stroke in Young Women: Oral contraception and increased risk of cerebral ischemia or thrombosis. N Engl J Med 1973; 288 :871–878. 28. Petitti DB, Wingerd J. Use of oral contraceptives, cigarette smoking, and risk of subarachnoid hemorrhage. Lancet 1978; 2 :234–236. 29. Inman WH. Oral contraceptives and fatal subarachnoid hemorrhage. Br Med J 1979; 2(6203) :1468–70. 30. Collaborative Group for the Study of Stroke in Young Women: Oral Contraceptives and stroke in young women: associated risk factors JAMA 1975 231 :718–722. 31. Inman WH, Vessey MP, Westerholm B, Engelund A. Thromboembolic disease and the steroidal content of oral contraceptives. A report to the Committee on Safety of Drugs. Br Med J 1970 2 :203–209. 32. Meade TW, Greenberg G, Thompson SG. Progestogens and cardiovascu-

lar reactions associated with oral contraceptives and a comparison of the safety of 50- and 35-mcg oestrogen preparations. Br Med J 1980; *280(6224)*:1157–1161. **33.** Kay, CR. Progestogens and arterial disease—evidence from the Royal College of General Practitioners' Study. Am J Obstet Gynecol 1982; *142* :762–765. **34.** Royal College of General Practitioners: Incidence of arterial disease among oral contraceptive users. J Royal Coll Gen Pract 1983; *33* :75–82. **35.** Ory, HW. Mortality associated with fertility and fertility control: 1983. Family Planning Perspectives 1983; *15* :50–56. **36.** The Cancer and Steroid Hormone Study of the Centers for Disease Control and the National Institute of Child Health and Human Development: Oral-contraceptive use and the risk of breast cancer. N Engl J Med 1986; *315* :405–411. **37.** Pike MC, Henderson BE, Krailo MD, Duke A, Roy S. Breast cancer in young women and use of oral contraceptives: possible modifying effect of formulation and age at use. Lancet 1983; *2* :926–929. **38.** Paul C, Skegg DG, Spears GFS , Kaldorf JM. Oral contraceptives and breast cancer: A national study. Br Med J 1986; *293* :723–725. **39.** Miller DR, Rosenberg L, Kaufman DW, Schottenfeld W, Stolley PD, Shapiro S. Breast cancer risk in relation to early oral contraceptive use. Obstet Gynecol 1986; *68* :863–868. **40.** Olson H, Olson KL, Moller TR, Ranstam J, Holm P. Oral contraceptive use and breast cancer in young women in Sweden (letter). Lancet 1985; *2* : 748–749. **41.** McPherson K, Vessey M, Neil A, Doll R, Jones L, Roberts M. Early contraceptive use and breast cancer: Results of another case-control study. Br J Cancer 1987; *56* :653–660. **42.** Huggins GR, Zucker PF. Oral contraceptives and neoplasia: 1987 update. Fertil Steril 1987; *47* :733–761. **43.** McPherson K, Drife JO. The pill and breast cancer: Why the uncertainty? Br Med J 1986; *293* :709–710. **44.** Shapiro S. Oral contraceptives—time to take stock. N Engl J Med 1987; *315* 450–451. **45.** Ory, H, Naib Z, Conger SB, Hatcher RA, Tyler CW. Contraceptive choice and prevalence of cervical dysplasia and carcinoma in situ. Am J Obstet Gynecol 1976; *124* :573–577. **46.** Vessey MP, Lawless M, McPherson, K Yeates D. Neoplasia of the cervix uteri and contraception: A possible adverse effect of the pill. Lancet 1983; *2* :930. **47.** Brinton LA, Huggins GR, Lehman HF, Malli K, Savitz DA, Trapido E, Rosenthal J, Hoover R. Long term use of oral contraceptives and risk of invasive cervical cancer. Int J Cancer 1986; *38* :339–344. **48.** WHO Collaborative Study of Neoplasia and Steroid Contraceptives: Invasive cervical cancer and combined oral contraceptives. Br Med J 1985; *290* :961–965. **49.** Rooks JB, Ory HW, Ishak KG, Strauss LT, Greenspan JR, Hill AP, Tyler CW. Epidemiology of hepatocellular adenoma: the role of oral contraceptive use. JAMA 1979; *242* :644–648. **50.** Bein NN, Goldsmith HS. Recurrent massive hemorrhage from benign hepatic tumors secondary to oral contraceptives. Br J Surg 1977; *64* :433–435. **51.** Klatskin G. Hepatic tumors: possible relationship to use of oral contraceptives. Gastroenterology 1977; *73* :386–394. **52.** Henderson BE, Preston-Martin S, Edmondson HA, Peters RL, Pike MC. Hepatocellular carcinoma and oral contraceptives. Br J Cancer 1983; *48* :437–440. **53.** Neuberger J, Forman D, Doll R, Williams R. Oral contraceptives and hepatocellular carcinoma, Br Med J 1986; *292* :1355–1357. **54.** Forman D, Vincent TJ, Doll R. Cancer of the liver and oral contraceptives. Br Med J 1986; *292* :1357–1361. **55.** Harlap S, Eldor J. Births following oral contraceptive failures. Obstet Gynecol 1980; *55* :447–452. **56.** Savolainen E, Saksela E, Saxen L. Teratogenic hazards of oral contraceptives analyzed in a national malformation register. Am J Obstet Gynecol 1981; *140* :521–524. **57.** Janerich DT, Piper JM, Glebatis DM. Oral contraceptives and birth defects. Am J Epidemiol 1980; *112* :73–79. **58.** Ferencz C, Matanoski GM, Wilson PD, Rubin JD, Neill CA, Gutberlet R. Maternal hormone therapy and congenital heart disease. Teratology 1980; *21* :225–239. **59.** Rothman KJ, Fyler DC, Goldbatt A, Kreidberg MB. Exogenous hormones and other drug exposures of children with congenital heart disease. Am J Epidemiol 1979; *109* :433–439. **60.** Boston Collaborative Drug Surveillance Program: Oral contraceptives and venous thromboembolic disease, surgically confirmed gallbladder disease, and breast tumors. Lancet 1973; *1*: 1399–1404. **61.** Royal College of General Practitioners: Oral Contraceptives and Health. New York, Pittman, 1974. **62.** Layde PM, Vessey MP, Yeates D. Risk of gallbladder disease: a cohort study of young women attending family planning clinics. J Epidemiol Community Health 1982; *36* : 274–278. **63.** Rome Group for the Epidemiology and Prevention of Cholelithiasis (GREPCO): Prevalence of gallstone disease in an Italian adult female population, Am J Epidemiol 1984; *119* :796–805. **64.** Strom BL, Tamragouri RT, Morse ML, Lazar ML, West SL, Stolley PD, Jones JK. Oral contraceptives and other risk factors for gallbladder disease. Clin Pharmacol Ther 1986; *39* :335–341. **65.** Wynn V, Adams PW, Godsland IF, Melrose J, Niththyananthan R, Oakley NW, Seedj A. Comparison of effects of different combined oral-contraceptive formulations on carbohydrate and lipid metabolism. Lancet 1979; *1* :1045–1049. **66.** Wynn V. Effect of progesterone and progestins on carbohydrate metabolism. In: Progesterone and Progestin. Bardin CW, Milgrom E, Mauvis-Jarvis P, eds. New York, Raven Press 1983, pp. 395–410. **67.** Perlman JA, Roussell-Briefel RG, Ezzati

TM, Lieberknecht G. Oral glucose tolerance and the potency of oral contraceptive progestogens. J Chronic Dis 1985; *38* :857–864. **68.** Royal College of General Practitioners' Oral contraception Study: Effect on hypertension and benign breast disease of progestogen component in combined oral contraceptives. Lancet 1977; *1* :624. **69.** Fisch IR, Frank J. Oral contraceptives and blood pressure. JAMA 1977 *237* :2499–2503. **70.** Laragh AJ: Oral contraceptive induced hypertension—Nine years later. Am J Obstet Gynecol 1976; *126* :141–147. **71.** Ramcharan S, Peritz E, Pellegrin FA, Williams WT. Incidence of hypertension in the Walnut Creek Contraceptive Drug Study cohort. In: Pharmacology of steroid contraceptive drugs. Garattini S, Berendes HW Eds. New York. Raven Press, 1977; pp. 277–288. (Monographs of the Mario Negri Institute for Pharmacological Research, Milan.) **72.** Stockley I. Interactions with oral contraceptives. J Pharm 1976; *216* :140–143. **73.** The Cancer and Steroid Hormone Study of the Centers for Disease Control and the National Institute of Child Health and Human Development: Oral contraceptive use and the risk of ovarian cancer. JAMA 1983; *249* :1596–1599. **74.** The Cancer and Steroid Hormone Study of the Centers for Disease Control and the National Institute of Child Health and Human Development: Combination oral contraceptive use and the risk of endometrial cancer. JAMA 1987; *257* :796–800. **75.** Ory HW. Functional ovarian cysts and oral contraceptives: negative association confirmed surgically. JAMA 1974; *228* :68–69. **76.** Ory HW, Cole P, Macmahon B, Hoover R. Oral contraceptives and reduced risk of benign breast disease. N Engl J Med 1976; *294* :41–422. **77.** Ory HW. The noncontraceptive health benefits from oral contraceptive use. Fam Plann Perspect 1982; *14* :182–184. **78.** Ory, HW, Forrest JD, Lincoln R. Making choices: Evaluating the health risks and benefits of birth control methods. New York, The Alan Guttmacher Institute, 1983, p.1. **79.** Schlesselman, J, Stadel BV, Murray P, Lai S. Breast cancer in relation to early use of oral contraceptives 1988; *259* :1828–1833.

BRIEF SUMMARY PATIENT PACKAGE INSERT

Oral contraceptives, also known as "birth control pills" or "the pill," are taken to prevent pregnancy and when taken correctly, have a failure rate of less than 1% per year when used without missing any pills. The typical failure rate of large numbers of pill users is less than 3% per year when women who miss pills are included. For most women oral contraceptives are also free of serious or unpleasant side effects. However, forgetting to take pills considerably increases the chances of pregnancy.

For the majority of women, oral contraceptives can be taken safely. But there are some women who are at high risk of developing certain serious diseases that can be fatal or may cause temporary or permanent disability. The risks associated with taking oral contraceptives increase significantly if you:
- Smoke
- are over the age of 40
- have high blood pressure, diabetes, high cholesterol
- have or have had clotting disorders, heart attack, stroke, angina pectoris, cancer of the breast or sex organs, jaundice or malignant or benign liver tumors.

You should not take the pill if you suspect you are pregnant or have unexplained vaginal bleeding.

> Cigarette smoking increases the risk of serious cardiovascular side effects from oral contraceptive use. This risk increases with age and with heavy smoking (15 or more cigarettes per day) and is quite marked in women over 35 years of age. Women who use oral contraceptives are strongly advised not to smoke.

Most side effects of the pill are not serious. The most common such effects are nausea, vomiting, bleeding between menstrual periods, weight gain, breast tenderness, and difficulty wearing contact lenses. These side effects, especially nausea and vomiting, may subside within the first three months of use.

The serious side effects of the pill occur very infrequently, especially if you are in good health and are young. However, you should know that the following medical conditions have been associated with or made worse by the pill:

1. Blood clots in the legs (thrombophlebitis), lungs (pulmonary embolism), stoppage or rupture of a blood vessel in the brain (stroke), blockage of blood vessels in the heart (heart attack or angina pectoris), or other organs of the body. As mentioned above, smoking increases the risk of heart attacks and strokes and subsequent serious medical consequences.

2. Liver tumors, which may rupture and cause severe bleeding. A possible but not definite association has been found with the pill and liver cancer. However, liver cancers are extremely rare. The chance of developing liver cancer from using the pill is thus even rarer.

3. High blood pressure, although blood pressure usually returns to normal when the pill is stopped.

The symptoms associated with these serious side effects are discussed in the detailed leaflet given to you with your supply of pills. Notify your doctor or health care provider if you notice any unusual physical disturbances while taking the pill. In addition, drugs such as rifampin, as well as some anticonvulsants and some antibiotics may decrease oral contraceptive effectiveness.

Studies to date of women taking the pill have not shown an increase in the incidence of cancer of the breast or cervix. There is, however, insufficient evidence to rule out the possibility that pills may cause such cancers.

Taking the combination pill provides some important noncontraceptive benefits. These include less painful menstruation, less menstrual blood loss and anemia, fewer pelvic infections, and fewer cancers of the ovary and the lining of the uterus.

Be sure to discuss any medical condition you may have with your health care provider. Your health care provider will take a medical and family history before prescribing oral contraceptives and will examine you. You should be reexamined at least once a year while taking oral contraceptives. Your pharmacist should have given you the detailed patient information labeling which gives you further information which you should read and discuss with your health care provider.

DETAILED PATIENT LABELING

PLEASE NOTE: This labeling is revised from time to time as important new medical information becomes available. Therefore, please review this labeling carefully.

The following oral contraceptive products contain a combination of an estrogen and progestogen, the two kinds of female hormones:

NORCEPT-E® 1/35·21 (Norethindrone and Ethinyl Estradiol Tablets USP) Each white tablet contains 1 mg norethindrone and 35 mcg ethinyl estradiol.

NORCEPT-E® 1/35·28 (Norethindrone and Ethinyl Estradiol Tablets USP) Each white tablet contains 1 mg norethindrone and 35 mcg ethinyl estradiol. Each green tablet contains inert ingredients.

INTRODUCTION

Any woman who considers using oral contraceptives (the birth control pill or the pill) should understand the benefits and risks of using this form of birth control. This patient labeling will give you much of the information you will need to make this decision and will also help you determine if you are at risk of developing any of the serious side effects of the pill. It will tell you how to use the pill properly so that it will be as effective as possible. However, this labeling is not a replacement for a careful discussion between you and your health care provider. You should discuss the information provided in this labeling with him or her, both when you first start taking the pill and during your revisits. You should also follow your health care provider's advice with regard to regular check-ups while you are on the pill.

EFFECTIVENESS OF ORAL CONTRACEPTIVES

Oral contraceptives or "birth control pills" or "the pill" are used to prevent pregnancy and are more effective than other non-surgical methods of birth control. When they are taken correctly, the chance of becoming pregnant is less than 1% (1 pregnancy per 100 women per year of use) when used perfectly, without missing any pills. Typical failure rates are actually 3% per year. The chance of becoming pregnant increases with each missed pill during a menstrual cycle.

In comparison, typical failure rates for other methods of birth control during the first year of use are as follows:

IUD: 6%
Diaphragm with spermicides: 18%
Spermicides alone: 21%
Vaginal sponge: 18 to 30%
Condom alone: 12%
Periodic abstinence: 20%
No methods: 89%

WHO SHOULD NOT TAKE ORAL CONTRACEPTIVES

> Cigarette smoking increases the risk of serious cardiovascular side effects from oral contraceptive use. This risk increases with age and with heavy smoking (15 or more cigarettes per day) and is quite marked in women over 35 years of age. Women who use oral contraceptives are strongly advised not to smoke.

Some women should not use the pill. For example, you should not take the pill if you are pregnant or think you may be pregnant. You should also not use the pill if you have any of the following conditions:
- A history of heart attack or stroke
- Blood clots in the legs (thrombophlebitis), lungs (pulmonary embolism), or eyes

Continued on next page

GynoPharma—Cont.

- A history of blood clots in the deep veins of your legs
- Chest pain (angina pectoris)
- Known or suspected breast cancer or cancer of the lining of the uterus, cervix or vagina
- Unexplained vaginal bleeding (until a diagnosis is reached by your doctor)
- Yellowing of the whites of the eyes or of the skin (jaundice) during pregnancy or during previous use of the pill
- Liver tumor (benign or cancerous)
- Known or suspected pregnancy

Tell your health care provider if you have ever had any of these conditions. Your health care provider can recommend a safer method of birth control.

OTHER CONSIDERATIONS BEFORE TAKING ORAL CONTRACEPTIVES

Tell your health care provider if you have or have had:
- Breast nodules, fibrocystic disease of the breast, or an abnormal breast x-ray or mammogram
- Diabetes
- Elevated cholesterol or triglycerides
- High blood pressure
- Migraine or other headaches or epilepsy
- Mental depression
- Gallbladder, heart, or kidney disease
- History of scanty or irregular menstrual periods

Women with any of these conditions should be checked often by their health care provider if they choose to use oral contraceptives.

Also, be sure to inform your doctor or health care provider if you smoke or are on any medications.

RISKS OF TAKING ORAL CONTRACEPTIVES

1. Risk of developing blood clots
Blood clots and blockage of blood vessels are the most serious side effects of taking oral contraceptives. In particular, a clot in the legs can cause thrombophlebitis and a clot that travels to the lungs can cause a sudden blocking of the vessel carrying blood to the lungs. Rarely, clots occur in the blood vessels of the eye and may cause blindness, double vision, or impaired vision.

If you take oral contraceptives and need elective surgery, need to stay in bed for a prolonged illness or have recently delivered a baby, you may be at risk of developing blood clots. You should consult your doctor about stopping oral contraceptives three to four weeks before surgery and not taking oral contraceptives for two weeks after surgery or during bed rest. You should also not take oral contraceptives soon after delivery of a baby. It is advisable to wait for at least four weeks after delivery if you are not breast feeding. If you are breast feeding, you should wait until you have weaned your child before using the pill. (See also the section on Breast Feeding in General Precautions.)

The risk of circulatory disease in oral contraceptive users may be higher in users of high dose pills and may be greater with longer duration of oral contraceptive use. In addition, some of these increased risks may continue for a number of years after stopping oral contraceptives. The risk of abnormal blood clotting increases with age in both users and nonusers of oral contraceptives, but the increased risk from the oral contraceptive appears to be present at all ages. For women aged 20 to 44 it is estimated that about 1 in 2,000 using oral contraceptives will be hospitalized each year because of abnormal clotting. Among nonusers in the same age group, about 1 in 20,000 would be hospitalized each year. For oral contraceptive users in general, it has been estimated that in women between the ages of 15 and 34 the risk of death due to a circulatory disorder is about 1 in 12,000 per year, whereas for nonusers the rate is about 1 in 50,000 per year. In the age group 35 to 44, the risk is estimated to be about 1 in 2,500 per year for oral contraceptive users and about 1 in 10,000 per year for nonusers.

2. Heart attacks and strokes
Oral contraceptives may increase the tendency to develop strokes (stoppage or rupture of blood vessels in the brain) and angina pectoris and heart attacks (blockage of blood vessels in the heart). Any of these conditions can cause death or disability.

Smoking greatly increases the possibility of suffering heart attacks and strokes. Furthermore, smoking and the use of oral contraceptives greatly increase the chances of developing and dying of heart disease.

3. Gallbladder disease
Oral contraceptive users probably have a greater risk than nonusers of having gallbladder disease, although this risk may be related to pills containing high doses of estrogens.

4. Liver tumors
In rare cases, oral contraceptives can cause benign but dangerous liver tumors. These benign liver tumors can rupture and cause fatal internal bleeding. In addition, a possible but not definite, association has been found with the pill and liver cancers in two studies, in which a few women who developed these very rare cancers were found to have used oral contraceptives for long periods. However, liver cancers are rare.

5. Cancer of the reproductive organs
There is, at present, no confirmed evidence that oral contraceptives increase the risk of cancer of the reproductive organs in human studies. While there is some conflict among studies regarding breast cancer and oral contraceptive use, the majority of studies have found no overall increase in the risk of developing breast cancer. However, women who use oral contraceptives and have a strong family history of breast cancer, or who have breast nodules or abnormal mammograms should be closely followed by their doctors.

Some studies have found an increase in the incidence of cancer of the cervix in women who use oral contraceptives. However, this finding may be related to factors other than the use of oral contraceptives.

ESTIMATED RISK OF DEATH FROM A BIRTH CONTROL METHOD OR PREGNANCY

All methods of birth control and pregnancy are associated with a risk of developing certain diseases which may lead to disability or death. An estimate of the number of deaths associated with different methods of birth control and pregnancy has been calculated and is shown in the following table. [See table below].

In the above table, the risk of death from any birth control method is less than the risk of childbirth, except for oral contraceptive users over the age of 35 who smoke and pill users over the age of 40 even if they do not smoke. It can be seen in the table that for women aged 15 to 39, the risk of death was highest with pregnancy (7–26 deaths per 100,000 women, depending on age). Among pill users who do not smoke, the risk of death was always lower than that associated with pregnancy for any age group, although over the age of 40, the risk increases to 32 deaths per 100,000 women, compared to 28 associated with pregnancy at that age. However, for pill users who smoke and are over the age of 35, the estimated number of deaths exceeds those for other methods of birth control. If a woman is over the age of 40 and smokes, her estimated risk of death is four times higher (117/100,000 women) than the estimated risk associated with pregnancy (28/100,000 women) in that age group.

Moreover, if you do not smoke and are under the age of 35, the possible risk of death from oral contraceptive use is extremely low when you consider the failure rate associated with other methods of contraception such as the condom or diaphragm and the resulting pregnancy-associated risk.

WARNING SIGNALS

If any of these adverse effects occur while you are taking oral contraceptives, call your doctor immediately:
- Sharp chest pain, coughing of blood, or sudden shortness of breath (indicating a possible clot in the lung)
- Pain in the calf (indicating a possible clot in the leg)
- Crushing chest pain or heaviness in the chest (indicating a possible heart attack)
- Sudden severe headache or vomiting, dizziness or fainting, disturbances of vision or speech, weakness, or numbness in an arm or leg (indicating a possible stroke)

- Sudden partial or complete loss of vision (indicating a possible clot in the eye)
- Breast lumps (indicating possible breast cancer or fibrocystic disease of the breast; ask your doctor or health care provider to show you how to examine your breasts)
- Severe pain or tenderness in the stomach area (indicating a possibly ruptured liver tumor)
- Difficulty in sleeping, weakness, lack of energy, fatigue, or change in mood (possibly indicating severe depression)
- Jaundice or a yellowing of the skin or eyeballs, accompanied frequently by fever, fatigue, loss of appetite, dark colored urine, or light colored bowel movements (indicating possible liver problems)

SIDE EFFECTS OF ORAL CONTRACEPTIVES

1. Vaginal bleeding
Irregular vaginal bleeding or spotting may occur while you are taking the pills. Irregular bleeding may vary from slight staining between menstrual periods to breakthrough bleeding which is a flow much like a regular period. Irregular bleeding occurs most often during the first few months of oral contraceptive use, but may also occur after you have been taking the pill for some time. Such bleeding may be temporary and usually does not indicate any serious problems. It is important to continue taking your pills on schedule. If the bleeding occurs in more than one cycle or lasts for more than a few days, talk to your doctor or health care provider.

2. Contact lenses
If you wear contact lenses and notice a change in vision or an inability to wear your lenses, contact your doctor or health care provider.

3. Fluid retention
Oral contraceptives may cause edema (fluid retention) with swelling of the fingers or ankles and may raise your blood pressure. If you experience fluid retention, contact your doctor or health care provider.

4. Melasma
A spotty darkening of the skin is possible, particularly of the face, which may persist.

5. Other side effects
Other side effects may include nausea and vomiting, change in appetite, headache, nervousness, depression, dizziness, loss of scalp hair, rash, and vaginal infections.

If any of these side effects bother you, call your doctor or health care provider.

GENERAL PRECAUTIONS

1. Missed periods and use of oral contraceptives before or during early pregnancy
There may be times when you may not menstruate regularly after you have completed taking a cycle of pills. If you have taken your pills regularly and miss one menstrual period, continue taking your pills for the next cycle but be sure to inform your health care provider before doing so. If you have not taken the pills daily as instructed and missed a menstrual period you may be pregnant. If you missed two consecutive menstrual periods you may be pregnant. Check with your health care provider immediately to determine whether you are pregnant. Do not continue to take oral contraceptives until you are sure you are not pregnant, but continue to use another method of contraception.

There is no conclusive evidence that oral contraceptive use is associated with an increase in birth defects, when taken inadvertently during early pregnancy. Previously, a few studies had reported that oral contraceptives might be associated with birth defects, but these findings have not been seen in more recent studies. Nevertheless, oral contraceptives or any other drugs should not be used during pregnancy unless clearly necessary and prescribed by your doctor. You should check with your doctor about risks to your unborn child of any medication taken during pregnancy.

2. While breast feeding
If you are breast feeding, consult your doctor before starting oral contraceptives. Some of the drug will be passed on to the child in the milk. A few adverse effects on the child have been reported, including yellowing of the skin (jaundice) and breast enlargement. In addition, oral contraceptives may decrease the amount and quality of your milk. If possible, do not use oral contraceptives while breast feeding. You should use another method of contraception since breast feeding provides only partial protection from becoming pregnant and this partial protection decreases significantly as you breast feed for longer periods of time. You should consider starting oral contraceptives only after you have weaned your child completely.

3. Laboratory tests
If you are scheduled for any laboratory tests, tell your doctor you are taking birth control pills. Certain blood tests may be affected by birth control pills.

4. Drug interactions
Certain drugs may interact with birth control pills to make them less effective in preventing pregnancy or cause an increase in breakthrough bleeding. Such drugs include rifampin, drugs used for epilepsy such as barbiturates (for example, phenobarbital) and phenytoin (Dilantin is one brand of

ANNUAL NUMBER OF BIRTH-RELATED OR METHOD-RELATED DEATHS ASSOCIATED WITH CONTROL OF FERTILITY PER 100,000 NONSTERILE WOMEN, BY FERTILITY CONTROL METHOD ACCORDING TO AGE

Method of control and outcome	15–19	20–24	25–29	30–34	35–39	40–44
No fertility control methods*	7.0	7.4	9.1	14.8	25.7	28.2
Oral contraceptives non-smoker**	0.3	0.5	0.9	1.9	13.8	31.6
Oral contraceptives smoker**	2.2	3.4	6.6	13.5	51.1	117.2
IUD**	0.8	0.8	1.0	1.0	1.4	1.4
Condom*	1.1	1.6	0.7	0.2	0.3	0.4
Diaphragm/spermicide*	1.9	1.2	1.2	1.3	2.2	2.8
Periodic abstinence*	2.5	1.6	1.6	1.7	2.9	3.6

* Deaths are birth-related
** Deaths are method-related

this drug), phenylbutazone (Butazolidin is one brand) and possibly certain antibiotics. You may need to use an additional method of contraception when you take drugs which can make oral contraceptives less effective.

HOW TO TAKE ORAL CONTRACEPTIVES

1. General Instructions

You must take your pill every day according to the instructions. Oral contraceptives are most effective if taken no more than 24 hours apart. Take your pill at the same time every day so that you are less likely to forget to take it. You will then maintain an effective dose of the oral contraceptive in your body.

NORCEPT-E® 1/35·21—21-Day Regimen. Unless your physician has instructed you differently, start with 1 tablet daily on the first Sunday after menstrual flow begins. If period begins on Sunday, take tablet on that day and continue without interruption for 21 days. Wait 7 days, then, whether menstrual bleeding has stopped or not, begin with the first tablet of your next new package of tablets. When you first begin to use the pill, you should use an additional method of protection until you have taken your first seven pills. Alternatively, counting the first day of menstrual flow as "Day 1", take one tablet daily the 5th day through the 25th day of the menstrual cycle. If the first tablet is taken later than the 5th day of the menstrual cycle, or postpartum, contraceptive reliance should not be placed on NORCEPT-E® until after the first 7 consecutive days of administration. Take a tablet the same time each day, preferably at bedtime, for 21 days, then wait for 7 days during which time a menstrual period usually occurs. Following this 7-day waiting period, start taking a tablet each day for the next 21 days, thus using the three-weeks-on, one-week-off dosage regimen.

NORCEPT-E® 1/35·28—28-Day Regimen. Unless your physician has instructed you differently, the first white tablet should be taken on the first Sunday after the menstrual period begins. If period begins on Sunday, begin taking a white tablet that day. If switching directly from another oral contraceptive, take the first white tablet on the first Sunday after your last ACTIVE tablet of the previous product. Take one white tablet at the same time each day for 21 consecutive days, then take one green tablet daily for 7 days, during which time your menstrual period usually occurs. When newly starting oral contraceptives, if the Sunday you begin NORCEPT-E® 1/35 is more than 5 days from the start of your menstrual period, it is important that you use another method of birth control until you have taken a white tablet daily for 7 consecutive days. After 28 tablets have been taken (last green tablet will always be taken on a Staurday), take the first white tablet from your next package the following day (Sunday) whether or not you are still menstruating. With the 28-day regimen, pills are taken every day of the year.

If your doctor has scheduled you for surgery, or you need prolonged bed rest, he or she may suggest that you stop taking the pill four weeks before surgery to avoid an increased risk of blood clots. It is also advisable not to start oral contraceptives sooner than four weeks after delivery of a baby.

2. If your forget to take your pill

Combination Oral Contraceptives

If you miss only one combination pill in a cycle, the chance of becoming pregnant is small. Take the missed pill as soon as you realize that you have forgotten it and continue to take your tablets for the rest of that cycle as directed. Since the risk of pregnancy increases with each additional pill you skip, it is very important that you take one pill a day. If you should miss more than one tablet, do not take those tablets missed, but begin taking tablets again as soon as remembered and use another method of contraception for the balance of that tablet cycle.

3. Pregnancy due to pill failure

The incidence of pill failure resulting in pregnancy is approximately one percent (ie, one pregnancy per 100 women per year) if taken every day as directed, but more typical failure rates are about 3%. If failure does occur, the risk to the fetus is minimal.

4. Pregnancy after stopping the pill

There may be some delay in becoming pregnant after you stop using oral contraceptives, especially if you had irregular menstrual cycles before you used oral contraceptives. It may be advisable to postpone conception until you begin menstruating regularly once you have stopped taking the pill and desire pregnancy.

There does not appear to be any increase in birth defects in newborn babies when pregnancy occurs soon after stopping the pill.

5. Overdosage

Serious ill effects have not been reported following ingestion of large doses of oral contraceptives by young children. Overdosage may cause nausea and withdrawal bleeding in females. In case of overdosage, contact your health care provider or pharmacist.

6. Other information

Your health care provider will take a medical and family history before prescribing oral contraceptives and will examine you. You should be reexamined at least once a year. Be sure to inform your health care provider if there is a family history of any of the conditions listed previously in this leaflet. Be sure to keep all appointments with your health care provider, because this is a time to determine if there are early signs of side effects of oral contraceptive use.

Do not use the drug for any condition other than the one for which it was prescribed. This drug has been prescribed specifically for you; do not give it to others who may want birth control pills.

HEALTH BENEFITS FROM ORAL CONTRACEPTIVES

In addition to preventing pregnancy, use of combination oral contraceptives may provide certain benefits. They are:

- menstrual cycles may become more regular
- blood flow during menstruation may be lighter and less iron may be lost. Therefore, anemia due to iron deficiency is less likely to occur.
- pain or other symptoms during menstruation may be encountered less frequently
- ectopic (tubal) pregnancy may occur less frequently
- noncancerous cysts or lumps in the breast may occur less frequently
- acute pelvic inflammatory disease may occur less frequently
- oral contraceptive use may provide some protection against developing two forms of cancer: cancer of the ovaries and cancer of the lining of the uterus

If you want more information about birth control pills, ask your doctor or pharmacist. They have a more technical leaflet called the Professional Labeling, which you may wish to read. The professional labeling is also published in a book entitled *Physicians' Desk Reference*, available in many book stores and public libaries.

Manufactured by Gedeon Richter
Budapest, Hungary
for
GynoPharma Inc.
Somerville, New Jersey 08876
Issued June 1989

PARAGARD® T380A   ℞
Intrauterine Copper Contraceptive

CAUTION: Federal law prohibits dispensing without prescription

NOTICE

You have received a Patient Information for an Informed Decision brochure that Federal Regulations (21 CFR 310.502) require you to furnish to each patient who is considering the use of the ParaGard®.

The Patient Information for an Informed Decision brochure contains information on the safety and efficacy of the ParaGard®. It also contains the Patient Consent. You must not insert the ParaGard® until:

- You have read this physician prescription labeling and are familiar with all the information it contains.
- You and the patient have read and she has initialed each section of the Patient Information for an Informed Decision brochure.
- You have counseled the patient and answered her questions about contraception, the ParaGard®, and the information in the brochure.
- You and the patient have reviewed and signed the Patient Consent.

The completely initialed and signed Patient Consent, should be retained with the patient's records and a second copy of the initialed and signed brochure given to the patient for her records.

DESCRIPTION: (labels) T 380A — Horizontal arms — Vertical arm — Threads — Flange — Insertion tube — Solid rod

DESCRIPTION

The polyethylene body of the ParaGard® is wound with approximately 176 mg of copper wire and carries a copper collar of approximately 66.5 mg of copper on each of its transverse arms. The exposed surface areas of copper are 380 ± 23 mm². The dimensions of the ParaGard® are 36 mm in the vertical direction and 32 mm in the horizontal direction. The tip of the vertical arm of the ParaGard® is enlarged to form a bulb having a diameter of 3 mm. The ParaGard® is equipped with a monofilament polyethylene thread which is tied through the bulb, resulting in two threads at the tip to aid in removal of the IUD. The ParaGard® contains barium sulfate to render it radiopaque.

The ParaGard® is packaged together with an insertion tube and plunger in a Tyvek®-polyethylene pouch and then sterilized. The insertion tube is equipped with a movable flange to aid in gauging the depth to which the insertion tube is inserted through the cervical canal and into the uterine cavity.

CLINICAL PHARMACOLOGY

Available data indicate that the contraceptive effectiveness of the ParaGard® is enhanced by copper being released continuously from the copper coil and sleeves into the uterine cavity. The exact mechanism by which metallic copper enhances the contraceptive effect of an IUD has not been conclusively demonstrated. Various hypotheses have been advanced, including interference with sperm transport, fertilization, and implantation. Clinical studies with copper-bearing IUDs also suggest that fertilization is prevented either due to an altered number or lack of viability of spermatozoa.

INDICATIONS AND USAGE

The ParaGard® is indicated for intrauterine contraception. The ParaGard® is recommended for women who *have had at least one child* and are in a stable, mutually monogamous relationship. The ParaGard® should not be kept in place longer than 48 months.

CONTRAINDICATIONS

The ParaGard® should not be inserted when one or more of the following conditions exist:

1. Pregnancy or suspicion of pregnancy.
2. Abnormalities of the uterus resulting in distortion of the uterine cavity.
3. Acute pelvic inflammatory disease or a history of pelvic inflammatory disease.
4. Postpartum endometritis or infected abortion in the past 3 months.
5. Known or suspected uterine or cervical malignancy, including unresolved, abnormal "Pap" smear.
6. Genital bleeding of unknown etiology.
7. Untreated acute cervicitis until infection is controlled.
8. Copper-containing IUDs should not be inserted in the presence of diagnosed Wilson's disease.
9. Known allergy to copper.
10. History of ectopic pregnancy.
11. Patient or her partner has multiple sexual partners.
12. Conditions associated with increased susceptibility to infections with microorganisms. Such conditions include, but are not limited to, leukemia, diabetes, acquired immune deficiency syndrome (AIDS) and those requiring chronic corticosteroid therapy.
13. Genital actinomycosis.
14. A previously inserted IUD that has not been removed.

WARNINGS

1. PREGNANCY

Long-term effects on the offspring when pregnancy occurs with the ParaGard® in place are unknown.

a. Septic Abortion

Reports indicate an increased incidence of septic abortion with septicemia, septic shock, and death in patients becoming pregnant with an IUD in place. Most of these reports have been associated with, but not limited to, the mid-trimester of pregnancy. In some cases, the initial symptoms have been insidious and not easily recognized. If pregnancy should occur with a an IUD *in situ*, the IUD should be removed if the string is visible and removal is easily accomplished. Of course, manipulation may result in spontaneous abortion. If removal proves to be difficult, or if threads are not visible, interruption of the pregnancy should be considered and offered as an option.

b. Continuation of Pregnancy

If the patient elects to maintain the pregnancy and the IUD remains *in situ*, she should be warned that there is an increased risk of spontaneous abortion and sepsis. In addition, she is at increased risk of premature labor and delivery. As a consequence of premature birth, the fetus is at increased risk of damage. She should be followed more closely than the usual obstetrical patient. The patient must be advised to report immediately all abnormal symptoms, such as flu-like syndrome, fever, abdominal cramping or pain, bleeding or vaginal discharge, because generalized symptoms of septicemia may be insidious.

2. ECTOPIC PREGNANCY

a. Although current data indicate that there is no increased risk of ectopic pregnancy in patients using the ParaGard® and some data suggest there may be a lower risk than the general population using no method of contraception, a pregnancy which occurs with the ParaGard® in

Continued on next page

GynoPharma—Cont.

place is more likely to be ectopic than a pregnancy occurring without the ParaGard®[1,2]. Therefore, patients who become pregnant while using the ParaGard® should be carefully evaluated for the possibility of an ectopic pregnancy.

b. Special attention should be directed to patients with delayed menses, slight metrorrhagia and/or unilateral pelvic pain, and to those patients who wish to terminate a pregnancy because of IUD failure, to determine whether ectopic pregnancy has occurred.

3. PELVIC INFECTION (PELVIC INFLAMMATORY DISEASE, PID)

The ParaGard® is contraindicated in the presence of PID or in women with a history of PID. Use of all IUDs, including the ParaGard®, has been associated with an increased incidence of PID. Therefore a decision to use the ParaGard® must include consideration of the risks of PID. The highest rate of PID occurs shortly after insertion and up to four months thereafter. Administration of prophylactic antibiotics has been reported as useful (see INSERTION PRECAUTIONS). PID can necessitate hysterectomy and can also lead to tubo-ovarian abscesses, tubal occlusion and infertility and tubal damage that can predispose to ectopic pregnancy. PID can result in peritonitis and, infrequently, in death. The effect of PID on fertility is especially important for women who may wish to have children at a later date.

a. **Women at special risk of PID**

The risk of PID appears to be greater for women who have multiple sexual partners and also for those women whose sexual partners have multiple sexual partners. Women who have had PID are at high risk for a recurrence or reinfection.

b. **PID warning to ParaGard® users**

All women who choose the ParaGard® must be informed prior to insertion that IUD use has been associated with an increased incidence of PID and that PID can necessitate hysterectomy, can cause tubal damage leading to ectopic pregnancy or infertility or, in infrequent cases, can cause death. Patients must be taught to recognize and report to their physician promptly any symptoms of pelvic inflammatory disease. These symptoms include development of menstrual disorders (prolonged or heavy bleeding), unusual vaginal discharge, abdominal or pelvic pain or tenderness, dyspareunia, chills, and fever.

c. **Asymptomatic PID**

PID may be asymptomatic but still result in tubal damage and its sequelae.[3,4]

d. **Treatment of PID**

Following diagnosis of PID, or suspected PID, bacteriologic specimens should be obtained and antibiotic therapy should be initiated promptly. Removal of the ParaGard® after initiation of antibiotic therapy is usually appropriate. Time should be allowed for therapeutic blood levels to be reached prior to removal. Guidelines for PID treatment are available from the Center for Disease Control (CDC), Atlanta, Georgia. A copy of the printed guidelines has been provided to you by GynoPharma Inc. The guidelines were established after deliberation by a group of experts and staff of the CDC, but they should not be construed as rules suitable for use in all patients. Adequate PID treatment requires the application of current standards of therapy prevailing at the time of occurrence of the infection with reference to the prescription labeling of the antibiotic selected.

Genital actinomycosis has been associated primarily with long-term IUD use. If it occurs, promptly institute appropriate antibiotic therapy and remove the ParaGard®.

4. EMBEDMENT

Partial penetration or embedment of the ParaGard® in the endometrium or myometrium can result in difficult removal. In some cases this can result in breakage of the IUD, necessitating surgical removal.

5. PERFORATION

Partial or total perforation of the uterine wall or cervix may occur with the use of the ParaGard®. Insertions into patients after abortion or delivery should occur when the uterus is fully involuted. There is an increased risk of perforation in women who are lactating. The possibility of perforation must be kept in mind during insertion and at the time of any subsequent examination. If perforation occurs, the ParaGard® should be removed as soon as feasible. A surgical procedure may be required. Abdominal adhesions, intestinal penetration, intestinal obstruction, and local inflammatory reaction with abscess formation and erosion of adjacent viscera may result if the ParaGard® is left in the peritoneal cavity. There are reports that there has been migration after insertion, apparently in the absence of perforation at insertion.

6. MEDICAL DIATHERMY

The use of medical diathermy (short-wave and microwave) in a patient with a metal-containing IUD may cause heat injury to the surrounding tissue. Therefore, medical diathermy to the abdominal and sacral areas should not be used on patients with a ParaGard® in place.

7. EFFECTS OF COPPER

Additional amounts of copper available to the body from the ParaGard® may precipitate symptoms in women with Wilson's disease. The incidence of Wilson's disease is approximately 1 in 200,000. The long-term effects of intrauterine copper to a child conceived in the presence of an IUD are unknown.

8. RISKS OF MORTALITY

The available data from a variety of sources have been analyzed to estimate the risk of death associated with various methods of contraception. The estimates of risk of death include the combined risk of the contraceptive method plus the risk of pregnancy or abortion in the event of method failure. The findings of the analysis are shown in Table I.[5] [See table below].

PRECAUTIONS

1. Patient Counseling

Prior to insertion, the physician, nurse, or other trained health professional must provide the patient with the Patient Information for an Informed Decision brochure. The patient should be given the opportunity to read the leaflet and discuss fully any questions she may have concerning the ParaGard® as well as other methods of contraception.

2. Patient Evaluation and Clinical Considerations

a. A complete medical and social history should be obtained to determine conditions that might influence the selection of an IUD. A physical examination should include a pelvic examination, "Pap" smear, and appropriate tests for any other forms of genital disease, such as gonococcal and chlamydial laboratory evaluations if indicated. The physician should determine that the patient is not pregnant.

b. The uterus should be carefully sounded prior to the insertion to determine the degree of patency of the endocervical canal and the internal os, and the direction and depth of the uterine cavity. In occasional cases, severe cervical stenosis may be encountered. Do not use excessive force to overcome this resistance.

c. The uterus should sound to a depth of 6 to 8 centimeters (cm). Insertion of an IUD into a uterine cavity measuring less than 6.5 cm by sounding may increase the incidence of expulsion, bleeding, and pain.

d. Physicians are cautioned that is is imperative for them to become thoroughly familiar with the instructions for use before attempting placement of the ParaGard®. To reduce the possibility of insertion in the presence of an existing undetermined pregnancy, the optimal time for insertion is the latter part of the menstrual period, or one or two days thereafter. The ParaGard® should not be inserted postpartum or postabortion until involution of the uterus is complete. The incidence of perforation and expulsion is greater if involution is not complete. Data also suggest that there may be an increased risk of perforation and expulsion if the woman is lactating.[6,7]

The ParaGard® should be placed at the fundus of the uterine cavity. Proper placement helps avoid partial or complete expulsion that could result in pregnancy. Contraceptive effectiveness is enhanced by proper placement.

e. Patients experiencing menorrhagia and/or metrorrhagia following IUD insertion may be at risk for the development of hypochromic microcytic anemia. Careful consideration of this risk must be given before insertion in patients with anemia or a history of menorrhagia or hypermenorrhea. Patients receiving anticoagulants or having a coagulopathy may have a greater risk of menorrhagia or hypermenorrhea.

f. Syncope, bradycardia, or other neurovascular episodes may occur during insertion or removal of IUDs, especially in patients with a previous disposition to these conditions or cervical stenosis.

g. Use of an IUD in patients with cervicitis should be postponed until treatment has eradicated the infection.

h. Patients with valvular or congenital heart disease are more prone to develop subacute bacterial endocarditis than patients who do not have valvular or congenital heart disease. Use of an IUD in these patients may represent a potential source of septic emboli. Patients with known congenital heart disease who may be at increased risk should be treated with appropriate antibiotics at the time of insertion.

i. Patients requiring chronic corticosteroid therapy should be carefully monitored for infection as a result of the insertion.

j. Since the ParaGard® may be partially or completely expelled, patients should be reexamined and evaluated shortly after the first postinsertion menses, but no later than 3 months afterwards. Thereafter, annual examination with appropriate evaluation, including a "Pap" smear, should be carried out. The ParaGard® should be kept in place no longer than 4 years.

k. The patient should be told that some bleeding or cramps may occur during the first few weeks after insertion. If these symptoms continue or are severe she should report them to her physician. She should be instructed on how to check to make certain that the threads still protrude from the cervix and cautioned that there is no contraceptive protection if the ParaGard® has been expelled. She should check frequently, at least after each menstrual period. She should be cautioned not to dislodge the ParaGard® by pulling on the thread. If a partial expulsion occurs, removal is indicated.

l. Rarely, a copper-induced urticarial allergic skin reaction may develop in women using a copper-containing IUD. If the symptoms of such an allergic response occur, the patient should be instructed to tell the consulting physician that a copper-containing device is being used.

3. Insertion Precautions

Because the presence of organisms capable of establishing PID cannot be determined by appearance, and because IUD insertion may be associated with introduction of vaginal bacteria into the uterus, clinicians may wish to consider the prophylactic administration of antibiotics. Regimens include doxycycline 200 mg orally one hour before insertion, or erythromycin 500 mg orally one hour before insertion and 500 mg orally six hours after insertion. The use of antibiotics in nursing mothers is not recommended. Before prescribing the above-mentioned antibiotics, refer to their prescription drug labeling and make certain that the patient is a suitable candidate for the drug.

4. Requirements for Continuation and Removal

a. The ParaGard® must be replaced before the end of the fourth year of use. There is no evidence of decreasing contraceptive efficacy with time before four years, but the contraceptive effectiveness at longer times has not been established; therefore, the patient should be informed of the known duration of contraceptive efficacy and be advised to return in 4 years for removal and possible insertion of a new ParaGard®.

b. The ParaGard® should be removed for the following medical reasons: menorrhagia- and/or metrorrhagia-producing anemia; pelvic infection; genital actinomycosis; intractable pelvic pain; dyspareunia; pregnancy; endometrial or cervical malignancy; uterine or cervical perforation; increase in length of the threads extending from the cervix, or any other indication of partial expulsion.

c. If the retrieval threads cannot be visualized, they may have retracted into the uterus or have been broken, or the ParaGard® may have been broken, or the ParaGard® may have been expelled. Localization may be made by feeling with a probe, X-ray, or sonography. When the physician elects to recover a ParaGard® with the threads not visible, the removal instructions should be reviewed.

5. Continuing Care of Patients Using ParaGard®

a. Any inquiries regarding pain, odorous discharge, bleeding, fever, genital lesions or sores, or a missed period should be promptly responded to and prompt examination is recommended.

b. If examination during visits subsequent to insertion reveals that the length of the threads has visibly or palpably changed from their length at time of insertion, the Para-

TABLE I—Annual Number of Birth-related or Method-related Deaths Associated with Control of Fertility per 100,000 Non-sterile Women, by Fertility Control Method According to Age

Method of control and outcome	15–19	20–24	25–29	30–34	35–39	40–44
No fertility control methods*	7.0	7.4	9.1	14.8	25.7	28.2
Oral contraceptives non-smokers**	0.3	0.5	0.9	1.9	13.8	31.6
Oral contraceptives smokers**	2.2	3.4	6.6	13.5	51.1	117.2
IUD**	0.8	0.8	1.0	1.0	1.4	1.4
Condom*	1.1	1.6	0.7	0.2	0.3	0.4
Diaphragm/spermicide*	1.9	1.2	1.2	1.3	2.2	2.8
Periodic abstinence*	2.5	1.6	1.6	1.7	2.9	3.6

* Deaths are birth related
** Deaths are method related

ParaGard®
Intrauterine Copper Contraceptive
NET CUMULATIVE RATES PER 100 ACCEPTORS
BY YEAR AND PARITY

	12 Mo.			24 Mo.			36 Mo.	48 Mo.
	Nulli-parous	Parous	All	Nulli-parous	Parous	All	All	All
Pregnancy	0.7	0.6	0.7	0.8	0.7	0.8	1.1	1.3
Expulsion	5.6	5.3	5.5	7.8	6.8	7.5	8.5	9.2
Medical	16.5	15.4	16.1	26.8	25.8	26.4	32.4	36.3
Continuation	73.5	72.0	73.0	55.5	50.2	53.6	40.3	31.8
No. Completed Year	1313	718	2032*	726	338	1064	293	153

*1 Woman with Parity Unrecorded
Cut Off Date: 1972 Admissions: December 31, 1976
1973–1975 Admissions: December 31, 1975

Gard® should be considered displaced and should be removed. A new ParaGard® may be inserted at that time or during the next menses or when it is certain that conception has not occurred. When the threads cannot be visualized by the physician, further investigation is necessary.

c. Since the ParaGard® may be partially or completely expelled, patients should be reexamined and evaluated shortly after the first postinsertion menses, but no later than 3 months afterwards. Thereafter, at least annual examination with appropriate evaluation, including a "Pap" smear, and if indicated, gonococcal and chlamydial laboratory evaluations, should be carried out. The ParaGard® should be kept in place no longer than 4 years.

d. In the event a pregnancy is confirmed during ParaGard® use, the following steps should be taken:

• Determine whether pregnancy is ectopic and take appropriate measures if it is.

• Inform patient of the risks of leaving an IUD *in situ* or removing it during pregnancy and of the lack of data on the long-term effects of the ParaGard® on the offspring of women who had it *in utero* during conception or gestation (see WARNINGS).

• If possible the ParaGard® should be removed after the patient has been warned of the risks of removal. If removal is difficult, the patient should be counseled about and offered pregnancy termination.

• If the ParaGard® is left in place, the patient's course should be followed closely.

ADVERSE REACTIONS

These adverse reactions are not listed in any order of frequency or severity.

Reported adverse reactions with intrauterine contraceptives include: endometritis; spontaneous abortion; septic abortion; septicemia; perforation of the uterus and cervix; embedment; fragmentation of the IUD; pelvic infection; tubo-ovarian abscess; tubal damage; vaginitis; leukorrhea; cervical erosion; pregnancy; ectopic pregnancy; fetal damage; difficult removal; complete or partial expulsion of the IUD, particularly in those patients with uteri measuring less than 6.5 cm by sounding; menstrual spotting; prolongation of menstrual flow; anemia; amenorrhea or delayed menses; pain and cramping; dysmenorrhea; backaches; dyspareunia; neurovascular episodes, including bradycardia and syncope secondary to insertion. Uterine perforation and IUD displacement into the abdomen have been followed by peritonitis, abdominal adhesions, intestinal penetration, intestinal obstruction, and cystic masses in the pelvis. (Certain of these adverse reactions can lead to loss of fertility, partial or total removal of reproductive organs, hormonal imbalance, or death). Urticarial allergic skin reaction may occur.

CLINICAL STUDIES

Different event rates have been reported with the use of different intrauterine contraceptives. Inasmuch as these rates are usually derived from separate studies conducted by different investigators in several populations, they cannot be compared with precision. Considerably different rates are likely to be obtained because event rates per unit of time tend to decrease as studies are extended, since more susceptible subjects discontinue due to expulsions, adverse reactions, or pregnancy, leaving the study population richer in less susceptible subjects. In clinical trials conducted in the United States by The Population Council[8,9,10], use-effectiveness of the ParaGard® as caculated by the life table method was determined as follows: (Rates are expressed as events per 100 women through 12, 24, 36, and 48 months of use). Data suggest a higher pregnancy rate in women under 20.[8,9] [See table above].

The lowest expected and typical failure rates during the first year of continuous use of all contraceptive methods are listed in Table II.[11]

TABLE II—Percentage of Women Experiencing an Accidental Pregnancy in the First Year of Continuous Use

Method	Lowest Expected*	Typical**
(No Contraception)	(89)	(89)
Oral Contraceptives		3.0
combined	0.1	N/A***
progestin only	0.5	N/A***
Diaphragm with spermicidal cream or jelly	3.0	18.0
Spermicides alone (foam, creams, jellies, and vaginal suppositories)	3.0	21.0
Vaginal Sponge		
nulliparous	5.0	18.0
multiparous	>8.0	>28.0
IUD (medicated)	1.0	6.0†
Condom		
without spermicides	3.0	12.0
Periodic abstinence		
(all methods)	2.0–8.0	20.0
Female sterilization	0.3	0.4
Male sterilization	0.1	0.15

* The authors' best guess of the percentage of women expected to experience an accidental pregnancy among couples who initiate a method (not necessarily for the first time) and who use it consistently and correctly during the first year if they do not stop for any other reason.

** This term represents "typical" couples who initiate use of a method (not necessarily for the first time), who experience an accidental pregnancy during the first year if they do not stop use for any other reason.

*** N/A—Data not available.

† Combined typical rate for both medicated and non-medicated IUD. The rate for the medicated IUD alone is not available.

HOW SUPPLIED

Available in cartons of one (NDC 54765-380-01) or five (NDC 54765-380-05) sterile units. Each ParaGard® is packaged in a Tyvek®-polyethylene pouch, together with an insertion tube and plunger rod.

INSTRUCTIONS FOR USE
PARAGARD®
Intrauterine Copper Contraceptive

THERE IS DEBATE AS TO HOW MANY IUD INSERTIONS CONSTITUTE ADEQUATE TRAINING FOR A CLINICIAN. IT IS PROBABLY WISE TO HAVE DONE 15–25 INSERTIONS UNDER SUPERVISION PRIOR TO INSERTING AN IUD UNSUPERVISED. A PRACTITIONER WITH ONLY 4–6 INSERTIONS WOULD PROBABLY NOT HAVE HAD ADEQUATE EXPERIENCE WITH DIFFICULT INSERTIONS.

The ParaGard® (Intrauterine Copper Contraceptive) represents a different design in intrauterine contraceptives. Physicians are, therefore, cautioned that they should become thoroughly familiar with instructions for insertion before attempting placement of the ParaGard®. The insertion technique is different in several respects from that employed with other intrauterine contraceptives and the physician should pay particular attention to the drawings and commentary accompanying these instructions.

A single ParaGard® is placed at the fundus of the uterine cavity.

The optimal time of insertion is during the latter part of the menstrual period, or one or two days thereafter. The cervical canal is relatively patent at this time and there is less chance that the patient may then be pregnant.

Present information indicates that the efficacy is retained for 4 years. Therefore, the ParaGard® must be removed and a new one inserted on or before 4 years from the date of insertion.

PRELIMINARY PREPARATION AND INSERTION

1. Before insertion, the patient must read and initial each section of the Patient Information Brochure for an Informed Decision; the medical and social history and counseling of the patient must be completed; and the Patient Consent must be signed by the patient and by the physician.

2. Refer to CONTRAINDICATIONS, WARNINGS, and PRECAUTIONS.

3. Pelvic examination is to be performed prior to insertion of the ParaGard®, including a cervical "Pap" smear, and gonococcal and chlamydial evaluations, if indicated, and any other necessary specific tests.

4. If appropriate, commence antibiotic prophylaxis one hour before insertion.

5. Use of aseptic technique during insertion is essential.

6. The endocervix should be cleansed with an antiseptic solution and a tenaculum applied to the cervix with downward traction for correction of the angulation as well as stabilization of the cervix.

7. With a speculum in place, gently insert a sterile sound to determine the depth and direction of the uterine canal. Be sure to determine the position of the uterus before insertion.

CAUTION

Any intrauterine procedure can result in severe pain, bradycardia, and syncope.

It is generally believed that perforations, if they occur, are encountered at the time of insertion, although the perforation may not be detected until some time later. The position of the uterus should be determined during the preinsertion examination. Great care must be exercised during the preinsertion sounding and subsequent insertion. No attempt should be made to force the insertion.

HOW TO INSERT ParaGard®
STEP 1

To minimize chance of introducing contamination, do not remove the ParaGard® from the inserter tube prior to placement in the uterus. Do not bend the arms of the ParaGard® earlier than 5 minutes before it is to be introduced into the uterus.

In the absence of sterile gloves, this can be accomplished without destroying sterility by folding the arms in the partially opened package. Place the partially opened package on a flat surface and the solid rod partially from the package so it will not interfere with assembly. Place thumb and index finger on top of package on ends of the horizontal arms. Push insertion tube against arms of ParaGard® as indicated by arrow in Fig. 1 to start arms folding.

Fig. 1

Complete the bending by bringing thumb and index finger together while using the other hand to maneuver the insertion tube to pick up the arms of the ParaGard® (Fig. 2). Insert no further than necessary to insure retention of the arms. Introduce the solid rod into the insertion tube from the bottom alongside the threads until it touches the bottom of the ParaGard®.

Fig. 2

STEP 2

Adjust the movable flange so that it indicates the depth to which the ParaGard® should be inserted and the direction in which the arms of the ParaGard® will open. At this point, make certain that the horizontal arms of the ParaGard® and the long axis of the flange lie in the same horizontal plane. Introduce the loaded inserter through the cervical canal and upwards until the ParaGard® lies in contact with the fundus. The movable flange should be at the cervix (Fig. 3).

DO NOT FORCE THE INSERTION.

Continued on next page

GynoPharma—Cont.

Fig. 3

STEP 3

To release the ParaGard®, withdraw the insertion tube not more than ½ inch while the solid rod is not permitted to move. This releases the arms of the ParaGard® (Fig. 4).

Retract

Stationary

Fig. 4

STEP 4

Withdraw the solid rod while holding the insertion tube stationary (Fig. 5).

Stationary

Retract

Fig. 5

STEP 5

Withdraw the insertion tube from the cervix. Be sure sufficient length of the threads are visible (1 in., or 2.5 cm) to facilitate checking for the presence of the ParaGard® (Fig. 6). Notation of length of the threads should be made in patient record.

Fig. 6

HOW TO REMOVE ParaGard®

To remove the ParaGard®, pull gently on the exposed threads. The arms of the ParaGard® will fold upward as it is withdrawn from the uterus. Even if removal proves difficult, the ParaGard® should not remain in the uterus after 4 years.

REFERENCES

1. World Health Organization's Special Programme of Research, Development and Research Training in Human Reproduction: A multinational case-control study of ectopic pregnancy. *Clin Reprod Fertil* 1985; 3:131–143.
2. Ory HW, Women's Health Study: Ectopic pregnancy and intrauterine contraceptive devices: New perspectives. *Obstet Gynecol* 1981; 57:137–144.
3. Cramer DW et al: Tubal infertility and the intrauterine device. *N Engl J Med* 1985; 312:941–947.
4. Daling JR et al: Primary tubal infertility in relation to the use of an intrauterine device. *N Engl J Med* 1985; 312:937–941.
5. Ory HW: Mortality associated with fertility and fertility control. *Fam Plann Perspect* 1983; 15:57–63.
6. Heartwell SF, Schlesselman S: Risk of uterine perforation among users of intrauterine devices. *Obstet Gynecol* 1983; 61:31–36.
7. Chi I-C, Kelly E: Is lactation a risk factor of IUD and sterilisation-related uterine perforations? A hypothesis. *Int J Gynaecol Obstet* 1984; 22:315–317.
8. Sivin, I, Stern J: Long-acting, more effective Copper T IUDs: A summary of US experience, 1970–1975, *Stud Fam Plann* 1979; 10:263–281.
9. Sivin I, Schmidt F: Effectiveness of IUDs: A review. *Contraception* 1987; 36:55–84.
10. Sivin I, Tatum HJ: Four years of experience with the TCu 380A intrauterine contraceptive device. *Fertil Steril* 1981; 36:159–163.
11. Trussell J, Kost K: Contraceptive failure in the United States: A critical review of the literature. *Stud Fam Plann* 1987; 18:237–283.

Patient Information for an Informed Decision

PARAGARD® T380A

Intrauterine Copper Contraceptive

Introduction

The ParaGard® is the third generation of a family of copper-bearing IUDs which have been used extensively around the world. It is the first to contain copper on both the arms and the stem of the T. Tested in more than 3,500 women in the United States, the ParaGard® is the product of over a decade of research involving an international group of scientists and family-planning specialists. However, as with all methods of contraception, its use is associated with some risk. The purpose of this brochure is to explain those risks to you.

Important Notice

To understand the risks and benefits of the ParaGard® (Intrauterine Copper Contraceptive) you will need to read and understand this entire brochure and discuss it with your doctor. It contains information vital to your health. A more technical leaflet is available which is written for the medical professional. If you would like to read that leaflet, ask your doctor for a copy. You may need his/her help to understand some of the information.

If you have difficulty understanding any of the technical terms in this brochure, check the glossary on page 11 and ask your doctor for clarification.

Intrauterine devices (IUDs) have been the subject of many personal injury lawsuits. Several IUD manufacturers have discontinued U.S. sales of their IUDs. Nevertheless, many doctors consider IUDs to be the best contraceptive choice for certain women. The ParaGard® is most appropriately used in women who have had at least one child and are in a stable, mutually monogamous relationship, and those who require a reversible form of contraception, whether or not they feel they have completed their family.

In addition to reading this brochure, you should also learn about other reversible birth control methods. One of these methods may be more suitable or safer for you than the ParaGard®. In order to make the appropriate decision, you must discuss your questions about the IUDs and other kinds of birth control with your doctor. Also, have the doctor explain to your satisfaction anything you do not understand in this brochure.

Under certain conditions you should not have the ParaGard® inserted; the risks to your health or your ability to bear children may be too great. Such conditions are described under *Special Risk Factors* and *What You Should Discuss With Your Doctor*. Even if none of these conditions applies to you, you may still experience serious problems while using the ParaGard® which will require immediate medical treatment. These medical problems could cause damage to your reproductive organs and the ability to bear children, or in some cases, could cause death. You may have to undergo major surgery, and you may become temporarily or permanently sterile (see *Special Risk Factors*). Prompt medical treatment, though absolutely necessary, may not be effective.

To become familiar with the danger signs of ParaGard® use, read *Side Effects, Adverse Reactions, and Warnings*. Always discuss these and other sections of the brochure with your doctor.

I have read this notice, and I understand it. In order to insure that I have read and understood this material, I must initial all sections of the brochure where indicated, and will discuss its contents with my doctor. I will not use the ParaGard® without fully understanding this information.

Signature

Date

DESCRIPTION

The ParaGard® (Intrauterine Copper Contraceptive) is a type of IUD that contains copper, and is inserted into the uterus (womb) to prevent pregnancy. Like all other contraceptives it is not 100% effective. (See *Effectiveness* for pregnancy rates.)

The ParaGard® is flexible and T-shaped with copper on both of the arms and stem of the T. The T itself is made of a flexible plastic material. The ParaGard® must be replaced

every 4 years, to maintain its contraceptive effectiveness. Two white threads extend from the base of the ParaGard®. They will extend into your vagina to indicate the presence of the ParaGard®, and aid in its removal. The ParaGard® (Intrauterine Copper Contraceptive) is 36 mm in the vertical direction and 32 mm in the horizontal direction.

The Copper in the ParaGard®

Available data indicate that the contraceptive effectiveness of ParaGard® is enhanced by copper released continuously from the IUD into the uterine cavity. The ParaGard® differs from earlier copper IUDs in that it contains copper on the stem and horizontal arms of the T. The placement of the copper on the arms of the ParaGard® increases effectiveness.

How the ParaGard® Acts as a Contraceptive

How the ParaGard® prevents pregnancy is not completely understood at the present time. Several theories have been suggested, including interference with sperm transport, fertilization, and implantation. Clinical studies with copper-bearing IUDs suggest that fertilization is affected either due to an altered number or lack of viability of spermatozoa. IUDs do not prevent ovulation (production and release of an egg by the ovary).

The ParaGard® does not always prevent ectopic pregnancy (pregnancy outside the uterus, sometimes called tubal pregnancy). Ectopic pregnancy can require surgery, and can make you unable to bear children; in some cases it can cause death. (See *Special Risk Factors for Ectopic Pregnancy*.)

I have read this section and understand it and have discussed it with my doctor.

Initials

Effectiveness

In clinical trials the incidence of unplanned pregnancies in women who have used the ParaGard® continuously for one year was less than 1 per 100 woman-years. This means that if 100 women use the ParaGard® for a period of one year, one of these women would become pregnant. Data suggest that the pregnancy rate is higher in women under 20. The typical failure rates for all methods of birth control during the first year are listed below in Table 1. The failure rate tabulated below for IUDs includes *all* IUDs combined.

Table 1

Typical Failure Rates for All Methods

Oral Contraceptives	less than 1%
IUD	up to 6%
Diaphragm with Spermicides	18%
Vaginal Sponge	18% to 30%
Condom alone	12%
Periodic abstinence	20%
No method	89%

Continuation Rates

In clinical trials 5 to 6 women out of 100 expelled the system during the first year. The number of women in the clinical trials who used the ParaGard® continuously for one year was 73 to 78 per 100 users. About 15% of the women who discontinue use during the first year do so for medical reasons, such as bleeding or pain, and about 6% discontinue because the IUD is expelled.

I have read this section and understand it and have discussed it with my doctor.

Initials

Lack of Contraceptive Effect After ParaGard® Removal

After discontinuation of ParaGard® use, its contraceptive effect on the uterus is reversed. Usually, but not always, a woman is able to become pregnant. In a study of 293 women, 78.4% of women seeking pregnancy became pregnant within a year following discontinuation.

I have read this section and understand it and have discussed it with my doctor.

Initials

Special Risk Factors

The conditions discussed below can significantly increase your chances of developing serious complications while using an IUD. Some of these conditions can necessitate surgery, can make you unable to have children, or can cause death. Read the information carefully and discuss it with your doctor.

Special Risk Factors for Pelvic Infection (Pelvic Inflammatory Disease)

Evidence indicates that ParaGard® users are more likely than other women to suffer a serious infection called pelvic inflammatory disease (PID), particularly in women with multiple sexual partners. PID is the medical term for infection in the upper pelvic area. This area includes the uterus (womb), fallopian tubes, ovaries, and surrounding tissues. (Vaginitis, a local infection of the vagina, is not PID, but may lead to it.) Studies indicate that the highest rate of PID occurs shortly after insertion and up to 4 months thereafter. PID can cause permanent blockage of the tubes; sterility; ectopic pregnancy; or, in infrequent cases, death. If you have now or have ever had PID, you must not use the ParaGard®. PID is an infection caused by gonorrhea, chlamydia, or other microscopic organisms. PID is frequently a sexually transmitted disease (STD or VD), and your chances of getting PID increase greatly if you have more than one sexual partner. Your risk of getting PID also increases if you have a sexual partner, who has sexual intercourse with others. If you are exposed to such situations, you have an increased risk of getting PID and must not use the ParaGard®. You should consider the use of a barrier method which may provide partial protection against sexually transmitted diseases. Treatment of PID may require surgical removal of your uterus (hysterectomy), tubes, and ovaries. Such surgery may have to be done on an emergency basis, and may result in death. Removing the ovaries may result in a lifelong need for hormonal treatments. Symptoms of PID include pelvic or lower abdominal pain, chills, fever, abnormal vaginal discharge, abnormal menstrual bleeding, or painful sexual intercourse. PID can occur even without these symptoms.

If you are using the ParaGard® and develop any of these symptoms, see your doctor as soon as possible. If you have PID, you should receive appropriate antibiotics promptly, and the IUD should be removed at the appropriate time. Failure to seek and receive prompt and adequate treatment will greatly increase the chances that you will become sterile, require surgery, or have life-threatening or fatal PID. Even prompt and adequate treatment cannot guarantee that these events will not occur.

Special Risk Factors for Ectopic Pregnancy
Ectopic pregnancy is an infrequent, but dangerous type of pregnancy that develops outside the uterus. Although current data indicate that the rate of ectopic pregnancy in patients using the ParaGard® is no higher, and some data suggest a lower rate than the general population, a pregnancy which occurs with the ParaGard® in place is more likely to be ectopic than a pregnancy occurring without the ParaGard®. If you have ever had an ectopic pregnancy, you have an increased risk of having another one. You also have an increased risk of an ectopic pregnancy if you have ever had certain types of infections. These infections include pelvic inflammatory disease (PID) or any venereal disease (VD) or sexually transmitted disease (STD) caused by, for example, gonorrhea or chlamydia. If you have ever had an ectopic pregnancy or these kinds of infections, you must not use the ParaGard®. Other contraceptive methods may be more suitable for you. Discuss this matter with your doctor.

Other Conditions That Increase Risk of Infection
Some conditions make you susceptible to infection during ParaGard® use or following ParaGard® insertion. These conditions include leukemia and acquired immune deficiency syndrome (AIDS). In addition, certain defects or diseases of the heart valves, such as rheumatic heart disease, and diabetes and long-term steroid therapy, make you more likely than other ParaGard® users to develop an infection which may involve the heart. If you have any of these conditions you should probably not use the ParaGard®.
I have read this section and understand it and have discussed it with my doctor.
_____ Initials

Side Effects
The following may occur while the ParaGard® is being inserted and while it is in place.
1. Pain, usually uterine cramps or low backache, occur at the time of insertion and may persist. (Pain and cramping may also occur at removal.) If pain is severe, becomes worse, or persists, contact your doctor.
2. Fainting may occur at the time of insertion or removal of the ParaGard®.
3. Some bleeding occurs following insertion in most women.
4. Partial or total perforation of the ParaGard® through the wall of the uterus may occur at the time of, or after, insertion. If you think the ParaGard® is displaced, check with your doctor (see *Warnings —tail or thread disappearance*). Perforation could result in abdominal adhesions, (scars) intestinal obstruction or penetration, inflammation, serious infection, and loss of contraceptive protection. Perforation and its complications may require surgery and, in infrequent cases, may result in serious illness or death.
5. Bleeding between menstrual periods may occur during the first 2 or 3 months after insertion. The first few menstrual periods after insertion may be heavier and longer than usual. If these conditions continue for longer than 2 or 3 months, consult your doctor.
6. Occasionally you may miss a menstrual period while using the ParaGard®. It is important to determine if you are pregnant; report this without delay to your doctor.

	Yes	No	Not Sure
Heart disease	☐	☐	☐
Heart murmur	☐	☐	☐
Hepatitis or severe liver disease	☐	☐	☐
Wilson's disease	☐	☐	☐
Diabetes	☐	☐	☐
Leukemia	☐	☐	☐
Fainting attacks	☐	☐	☐
Steroid therapy	☐	☐	☐
Anemia or blood clotting problems	☐	☐	☐
Current suspected or possible pregnancy	☐	☐	☐
Ectopic pregnancy (pregnancy outside of the uterus)	☐	☐	☐
Recent pregnancy	☐	☐	☐
Recent abortion or miscarriage	☐	☐	☐
Abnormalities of the uterus	☐	☐	☐
Bleeding between periods	☐	☐	☐
Cancer of the uterus (womb) or cervix	☐	☐	☐
Suspicious or abnormal Pap smear	☐	☐	☐
Prior IUD use	☐	☐	☐
IUD in place now	☐	☐	☐
Heavy menstrual flow	☐	☐	☐
Severe menstrual cramps	☐	☐	☐
Multiple sexual partners	☐	☐	☐
A sexual partner who has multiple sexual partners	☐	☐	☐
Pelvic infection (including pus in fallopian tubes)	☐	☐	☐
Infection of the uterus (womb) or cervix	☐	☐	☐
Genital sores or lesions	☐	☐	☐
Sexually transmitted disease (venereal disease), such as herpes, gonorrhea, chlamydia, or acquired immune deficiency syndrome (AIDS)	☐	☐	☐
Unexplained genital bleeding	☐	☐	☐
Uterine or pelvic surgery	☐	☐	☐
Vaginal discharge or infection	☐	☐	☐

7. The ParaGard® may come out of your uterus through the cervical opening. This is called expulsion, and is most likely to occur during the first 2 or 3 menstrual cycles following insertion. Expulsion leaves you unprotected against pregnancy. Refer to the section called *Directions for Use* for information on how to check to see if your ParaGard® has been expelled. If you think the ParaGard® has come out or has been displaced, use another birth control method, such as contraceptive vaginal foam, cream, or jelly, or condoms (rubbers), until you can be checked by your doctor. (These alternative methods are usually not as effective in preventing uterine pregnancy as the ParaGard®.) Call your doctor for an examination.
I have read this section and understand it and have discussed it with my doctor.
_____ Initials

What You Should Discuss With Your Doctor
Before you have the ParaGard® inserted, indicate below if you have ever had—or suspect you have ever had—any of the conditions listed below. Conditions listed are not necessarily contraindications.
[See table above].
Make certain you discuss any items you're not sure about.
I have read this section and understand it and have discussed it with my doctor.
_____ Initials

Adverse Reactions
The following adverse reactions have been reported and may be caused by the ParaGard®:
- Abdominal infection or adhesions (scar tissue)
- Anemia
- Backache
- Blood poisoning
- Bowel obstruction
- Cervical infection or erosion
- Cysts on ovaries and tubes
- Death
- Delayed menstruation
- Difficult removal
- Ectopic pregnancy
- Embedment (IUD surrounded by uterine tissue)
- Expulsion (IUD comes completely or partially out of the uterus)
- Fainting and pain at the time of insertion or removal
- Fragmentation (breakage) of the ParaGard®
- Infertility
- Spotting between periods
- Miscarriage
- Pain and cramps
- Painful intercourse
- Pelvic infection (PID), which may result in surgical removal of your reproductive organs, including hysterectomy
- Perforation of the uterus (womb) or cervix (IUD passes through uterine tissue)

- Pregnancy
- Prolonged or heavy menstrual flow
- Infected miscarriage followed, in some cases, by blood poisoning, which can lead to death
- Vaginal discharge
I have read this section and understand it and have discussed it with my doctor.
_____ Initials

Warnings
If you have the ParaGard® inserted, call your doctor immediately for any of the following reasons:
1. A missed period. This may mean you are pregnant and the ParaGard® should be removed.
2. Unexplained or abnormal vaginal bleeding or discharge. This could indicate a serious complication, such as an infection or ectopic pregnancy.
3. A delayed period followed by scanty or irregular bleeding. This could indicate an ectopic pregnancy.
4. Pelvic or lower abdominal pain or cramps or unexplained fever. Such symptoms could mean an ectopic pregnancy or infection has developed requiring immediate treatment.
5. Exposure to venereal disease (VD), also called sexually transmitted disease (STD). The use of the ParaGard® does not prevent venereal disease. If exposure to venereal disease is suspected, report for examination and treatment promptly. Failure to do so could result in serious pelvic infection.
6. Genital sores or lesions, or fever with vaginal discharge. These may indicate an infection.
7. Severe or prolonged menstrual bleeding. If the flow is heavier and lasts much longer than your usual menstrual flow, you may need to have the ParaGard® removed to prevent anemia.
8. Tail or thread disappearance or pain during sex. If you cannot feel the threads coming through the cervix, or have pain during sex, the ParaGard® may have been expelled or displaced, or may have perforated the uterus. If any of these has occurred, you are no longer protected from pregnancy. Use another birth control method, such as contraceptive vaginal foam, cream, or jelly, or condoms (rubbers) until you can be checked. (These alternative methods are not as effective against uterine pregnancy as the ParaGard®.) If perforation has occurred removal of the ParaGard® is necessary, usually by surgery.
9. Risk of death. Available data from a variety of sources have been analyzed to estimate the risk of death associated with various methods of contraception. The estimates of risk of death include the combined risk of the contraceptive method plus the risk of pregnancy or abortion in the event of method failure. The findings of the analysis are shown in Table 2.
[See table on next page].
I have read this section and understand it and have discussed it with my doctor.
_____ Initials

Continued on next page

GynoPharma—Cont.

How the ParaGard® is Inserted and Removed

Before insertion, your doctor will perform a pelvic examination. Its purpose is to determine the size, shape, and position of the uterus. An instrument called a speculum will hold your vagina open so that the cervix (the entrance to the uterus) can be seen. (You will probably feel pressure from the speculum throughout the insertion procedure.)

The cervix is then cleaned with an antiseptic solution and an instrument called a tenaculum is attached to it. This instrument assists in holding the uterus steady during insertion. You may feel pain or a pinching sensation as the tenaculum is attached. Then the doctor will guide a narrow instrument called a sound through the opening of the cervix into the uterus. The sound measures the depth and position of the uterus. You can expect to feel cramping similar to menstrual cramps as the sound is inserted and withdrawn.

Then your doctor will guide the ParaGard® (with the cross-arms of the T folded down) through the vagina and the cervix into the uterus.

As the ParaGard® is inserted, the arms of the T will unfold. During insertion you will have some pain or cramping. You may feel nauseated, weak, or faint. After the inserter is removed, the threads attached to the end of the ParaGard® will be clipped. The threads will extend into the vagina from the cervical opening. The tenaculum and speculum will then be removed. You may feel pain or pinching when the tenaculum is removed. You should remain lying down for a while and rise slowly to prevent fainting. During intercourse, neither you nor your partner should be aware of these threads. You should also not be aware of any other part of the ParaGard®. If you are, promptly follow the instructions under the heading, *Checking Your ParaGard®*, in the section *Directions for Use*.

When it is time to remove the ParaGard®, your doctor must remove it. Its removal may cause pain or cramping. The arms of the ParaGard® should fold upward as it is withdrawn from the uterus.

I have read this section and understand it and have discussed it with my doctor.

—————————
Initials

Directions for Use

Please read the following information and instructions carefully. Keep a copy of this brochure so that you may refer to it. If you have any questions, consult your doctor.

Checking Your ParaGard®

The ParaGard® can come out of the uterus (womb) without your knowing it. When this occurs, it is most often during or right after a menstrual period. Therefore at least after each menstrual period, check to make sure the threads can be felt at the cervix. You may check more often, and especially if you have some concern, or think you have an expulsion.

Follow these steps to make sure that the ParaGard® has not been expelled without your knowing it:
1. Wash your hands.
2. Squat down or seat yourself on the toilet.
3. Insert the index or middle finger high into your vagina and locate your cervix. The cervix is the mouth of the uterus (womb). It feels firm, like the tip of your nose.

4. Feel for the threads of the ParaGard®. The threads should extend from the cervix and be high in your vagina. The threads may be difficult to feel.
5. If you can feel the threads, the ParaGard® is probably, but not always, in place. You should not pull on the threads. Doing so may displace the ParaGard®.
6. If you cannot feel threads, or if you can feel the ParaGard® itself, it has probably been displaced from the uterus. Also, if you or your partner can feel the ParaGard® during intercourse, it is displaced. If so, you are not being protected against pregnancy. Until you can be examined, use another birth control method, such as a contraceptive vaginal foam, cream, or jelly, or condoms (rubbers). (These alternative methods are not as effective against uterine pregnancy as the ParaGard®.) Call your doctor for an examination.

Follow-up Visits to the Doctor
1. You should return to see your doctor as soon as possible after your first menstrual period following insertion of your IUD, but no later than 3 months after insertion. This will allow the doctor to check on the location of the ParaGard®.

2. The ParaGard® requires replacement every 4 years. Check with your doctor concerning an appointment to have the ParaGard® replaced or removed.
3. The ParaGard® should not interfere with the proper use of tampons and douches. You may want to discuss this with your doctor.

I have read this section and understand it and have discussed it with my doctor.

—————————
Initials

Special Warning About Uterine Pregnancy With the ParaGard® in Place

Some women become pregnant while using the ParaGard®. If you miss your menstrual period, or if you suspect you are pregnant, see your doctor right away. When a pregnancy continues with the ParaGard® in place, serious complications may occur, including severe blood infection, spontaneous miscarriage, infected miscarriage, and death. These may occur at any time during the pregnancy.

When the ParaGard® remains in the uterus during conception or pregnancy, the long-term effects on the child (or fetus) are not known. Under such conditions some birth defects have occurred. Their relationship to the ParaGard® has not been established but has been suggested.

If your doctor confirms that you are pregnant, the ParaGard® should be removed. Removal of the ParaGard® may cause a miscarriage. However, successful ParaGard® removal in pregnancy decreases the likelihood of subsequent complications.

In some cases removal of the ParaGard® may prove to be difficult. If so, you and your doctor should discuss at that time the question of continuing the pregnancy in view of the serious complications [described above] that may occur. In reaching a decision about termination of pregnancy, you should be aware that the risks associated with abortion increase with the length of time you have been pregnant.

If you continue your pregnancy with the ParaGard® in place, your physician will have to follow your course more closely than usual throughout your pregnancy. Be sure to report immediately to the doctor if you have any of the following symptoms or signs:
- Bleeding from the vagina
- Pelvic or lower abdominal pain or cramping
- Flu-like symptoms such as chills or fever
- Unusual vaginal discharge
- Ruptured membranes (your water breaks)
- Any other signs/symptoms which gives you concern

Any of these symptoms could indicate that you are having a miscarriage or that you are beginning, or about to begin, premature labor. Premature labor may lead to delivery of a premature infant. Premature infants have a higher chance of dying, mental retardation, cerebral palsy, or other serious medical problems. Additionally, infection can cause infertility or death. Therefore, report any symptoms without delay to your doctor, so that you can obtain immediate treatment.

I have read this section and understand it and have discussed it with my doctor.

—————————
Initials

Patient Consent

I have read this brochure in its entirety and discussed its contents with my doctor. My doctor has answered all my questions and has advised me of the risks and benefits associated with the use of the ParaGard®, with other forms of contraception, and with no form of contraception at all. I understand that while using the ParaGard® I may experience serious medical problems. These problems could lead to surgery, sterility, or death.

I have considered all factors and voluntarily choose to have the ParaGard® inserted by

Dr.———————————on date—————————

Patient Signature ——————————————————————

The patient has signed this brochure in my presence after I counseled her and answered all her questions.

—————————————————————
Doctor   Date

This ParaGard is scheduled for removal on————————

Glossary

Cervix —Lower portion of the uterus visible in the vagina
Conception —Same as implantation
Contraceptive —Means of preventing conception
Ectopic Pregnancy —Pregnancy outside of the uterus
Expel —To force out
Fallopian Tubes —Tubes which carry the egg from the ovary to the uterus
Fertilization —The process of the sperm penetrating the egg of the female
Genital —Organs concerned with reproduction
Implantation —Embedding of the fertilized egg into the wall of the uterus

Table 2
Annual Number of Birth-Related or Method-Related Deaths Associated With Control of Fertility per 100,000 Nonsterile Women, by Fertility Control Method, According to Age

Method of control and outcome	15–19	20–24	25–29	30–34	35–39	40–44
No fertility control methods*	7.0	7.4	9.1	14.8	25.7	28.2
Oral contraceptives, nonsmokers**	0.3	0.5	0.9	1.9	13.8	31.6
Oral contraceptives, smokers**	2.2	3.4	6.6	13.5	51.1	117.2
IUD**	0.8	0.8	1.0	1.0	1.4	1.4
Condom*	1.1	1.6	0.7	0.2	0.3	0.4
Diaphragm/spermicide*	1.9	1.2	1.2	1.3	2.2	2.8
Periodic abstinence*	2.5	1.6	1.6	1.7	2.9	3.6

* Deaths are birth related
** Deaths are method related

Intrauterine—Within the uterus

Microscopic—Can be seen only by using a microscope

Monogamous—Practicing sexual relations with only one partner

Ovary—Almond-shaped organ. One ovary is located on each side of the uterus. Produces and releases human eggs.

Ovulation—Release of an egg by the ovary

STD—Sexually transmitted disease—also called venereal disease

Spermatozoa—Male reproductive cells

Uterus (womb)—Pear-shaped organ, located deep in the pelvis, that contains and nourishes a fetus during pregnancy

VD—Venereal disease—also called sexually transmitted disease

Viability—Ability to live

Shown in Product Identification Section, page 411

Hauck Pharmaceuticals
Division of W. E. Hauck, Inc.
P.O. BOX 1065
ALPHARETTA, GA 30239-1065

CHLORAFED H.S. TIMECELLES*   ℞
(CHLORAFED HALF-STRENGTH)

COMPOSITION

Chlorpheniramine Maleate 4 mg.; Pseudoephedrine HCl 60 mg.
* In special time release beads.

SUPPLIED

Bottles of 100 and 500's.

CHLORAFED LIQUID   OTC
(Corn, Dye, Alcohol, Sugar Free)

COMPOSITION

Each 5 ml. of liquid contains: Chlorpheniramine Maleate 2 mg.; Pseudoephedrine HCl 30 mg.

SUPPLIED

4 oz. and pints.

CHLORAFED TIMECELLES*   ℞

COMPOSITION

Chlorpheniramine Maleate 8 mg.; Pseudoephedrine HCl 120 mg.;
*In special time release beads.

SUPPLIED

Bottles of 100 and 500.

DOLACET CAPSULES   ℃ ℞

COMPOSITION

Each imprinted capsule contains Hydrocodone Bitartrate 5 mg. (WARNING: May be habit forming) and Acetaminophen 500 mg.

SUPPLIED

Imprinted capsules in bottles of 100 and 500.

ENTUSS PEDIATRIC EXPECTORANT   ℃ ℞

COMPOSITION

Each 5 mL teaspoonful of Entuss Pediatric Expectorant contains Hydrocodone Bitartrate (**Warning:** May be habit forming) 2.5 mg, Pseudoephedrine Hydrochloride 30 mg, and Guaifenesin 100 mg.

SUPPLIED

Pints and 4 fl. oz. bottles.

ENTUSS TABLETS and LIQUID   ℃ ℞
(Sugar, Alcohol, Corn, Tartrazine Free)

COMPOSITION

Each tablet contains: Hydrocodone Bitartrate (WARNING: May be habit forming) 5 mg., Guaifenesin 300 mg. Each 5 ml. of liquid contains: Hydrocodone Bitartrate (WARNING: May be habit forming) 5 mg., Potassium Guaiacolsulfonate 300 mg.

SUPPLIED

Tablets—bottles of 100. Liquid—4 oz. and pints

ENTUSS–D LIQUID and TABLETS   ℃ ℞
(Sugar, Dye, Corn, Alcohol Free)

COMPOSITION

Each tablet contains Hydrocodone Bitartrate (WARNING: May be habit forming) 5 mg., Guaifenesin 300 mg. and Pseudoephedrine Hydrochloride 30 mg. Each 5 mL teaspoonful contains Hydrocodone Bitartrate (WARNING: May be habit forming) 5 mg and Pseudoephedrine Hydrochloride 30 mg.

SUPPLIED

Imprinted Tablets—Bottles of 100. Liquid—16 oz. bottles.

GASTROSED™ DROPS   ℞
(Sugar, Corn, Alcohol, Tartrazine Free)

COMPOSITION

GASTROSED Drops (oral Solution) contain Hyoscyamine Sulfate 0.125 mg/cc, in a green non-alcoholic aqueous solution.

SUPPLIED

In a 15 cc Dropper Bottle.

GASTROSED TABLETS   ℞
(Hyoscyamine Sulfate 0.125 mg.)

COMPOSITION

GASTROSED Tablets contain Hyoscyamine Sulfate 0.125 mg. They are green hexagonal-shaped scored tablets with HAUCK logo and 43797-007 imprint.

SUPPLIED

Bottles of 100.

HISTOR–D® TIMECELLES*   ℞

COMPOSITION

Chlorpheniramine Maleate 8 mg.; Phenylephrine Hydrochloride 20 mg.; Methscopolamine Nitrate 2.5 mg.
*In special time release beads.

SUPPLIED

Bottles of 100 and 500.

NIACELS™ CAPSULES   OTC
Niacin, USP (Nicotinic Acid) 400 mg.

COMPOSITION

NIACELS, formulated as sustained action capsules, contains 400 mg. of niacin in a specially prepared form to permit prolonged release.

SUPPLIED

Bottles of 100.

SINUFED TIMECELLES   ℞

COMPOSITION

Each imprinted capsule contains Pseudoephedrine hydrochloride 60 mg. in a special base to provide for prolonged action and Guaifenesin 300 mg. designed for immediate release for rapid action.

SUPPLIED

Imprinted capsules in bottles of 100.

SINUMIST–SR CAPSULETS®   ℞
(Guaifenesin)

COMPOSITION

Each green speckled capsule-shaped sustained release Capsulet® provides 600 mg guaifenesin.

SUPPLIED

Bottles of 100 imprinted Capsulets®.

WEHLESS–105 TIMECELLES   ℃ ℞

COMPOSITION

Each capsule contains: Phendimetrazine Tartrate 105 mg. in a sustained release base which lasts for 10 hours. Black and clear capsule imprinted WEHLESS T.C. 105 mg.

SUPPLIED

Bottles of 100.

Health Maintenance Programs, Inc.
7 WESTCHESTER PLAZA
ELMSFORD, NY 10523

ASCORBIC–B™
High Potency, Pure Crystalline Antioxidants and Vitamins

Each Capsule Contains:

Antioxidants/Vitamins	Quantity	%RDA
Ascorbic Acid/C	800 mg	1333%
Calcium Pantothenate/B-5	120 mg	1200%
Thiamine HCl/B-1	40 mg	2667%
Pyridoxine HCl/B-6	20 mg	1000%
Niacinamide/B-3	15 mg	75%
Niacin/B-3	5 mg	25%
Riboflavin/B-2	4 mg	235%
Cyanocobalamin/B-12	150 mcg	2500%

120 Capsules

CALCIUM–D™
Bone-Promoting Formulation with Calcium and Added Vitamin D to Enhance Absorption

Each Capsule Contains:

Antioxidants/Vitamins	Quantity	%RDA
Calcium as the Carbonate	250 mg	25%
Cholecalciferol/D3	125 IU	31%

90 Capsules

CALCIUM ENDURANCE PACKS™
Moderate-Dose Antioxidants and Vitamins plus High Dose Calcium, *without Glutathione*

- For moderately paced adults
- Regular work-outs
- Otherwise, similar to Performance Packs™
- Economic supplements because there is no glutathione

Each Packet Contains:

Antioxidants/Vitamins	Quantity	%RDA
1 Ascorbic-B/Yellow Cap		
Ascorbic Acid/C	800 mg	1333%
Calcium Pantothenate/B-5	120 mg	1200%
Thiamine HCl/B-1	40 mg	2667%
Pyridoxine HCl/B-6	20 mg	1000%
Niacinamide/B-3	15 mg	75%
Niacin/B-3	5 mg	25%
Riboflavin/B-2	4 mg	235%
Cyanocobalamin/B-12	150 mcg	2500%
2 Calcium-D/White Caps		
Calcium as the Carbonate	500 mg	50%
Cholecalciferol/D3	250 IU	63%
1 Carotene-E/Red Cap		
Beta Carotene	15 mg	—
DL-Alpha Tocopheryl Acetate/E	100 IU	333%

DIRECTIONS

Same as Performance Packs
30 Packets/120 Capsules

Continued on next page

Health Maintenance—Cont.

CALCIUM HEALTH PACKETS™
Moderate-Dose Antioxidants and Vitamins plus High Dose Calcium, with Glutathione

- For moderately paced adults
- Regular work-outs
- Otherwise, similar to Performance Packs™

Each Packet Contains:

Antioxidants/Vitamins	Quantity	%RDA
1 Ascorbic-B/Yellow Cap		
Ascorbic Acid/C	800 mg	1333%
Calcium Pantothenate/B-5	120 mg	1200%
Thiamine HCl/B-1	40 mg	2666%
Pyridoxine HCl/B-6	20 mg	1000%
Niacinamide/B-3	15 mg	75%
Niacin/B-3	5 mg	25%
Riboflavin/B-2	4 mg	235%
Cyanocobalamin/B-12	150 mcg	2500%
1 Combination/White Cap		
Calcium as the Carbonate	400 mg	40%
Ascorbic Acid/C	150 mg	250%
Glutathione	50 mg	—
Cholecalciferol/D3	125 IU	31%
1 Carotene-E/Red Cap		
Beta Carotene	15 mg	—
DL-Alpha Tocopheryl Acetate/E	100 IU	333%

DIRECTIONS
Same as Performance Packs™
45 Packets/135 Capsules

CAROTENE–E™
Antioxidant Formulation with Pure Beta Carotene in Pure Vitamin E. Nothing else is present. Body Prevents Overproducing Vit. A

Each Capsule Contains:

Antioxidants/Vitamins	Quantity	% RDA
Beta Carotene	15 mg	
DL-Alpha Tocopheryl Acetate/E	100 IU	333%

90 Capsules

ENDURANCE PACKS™
High-Dose Antioxidants and Vitamins plus Calcium, *without* Glutathione

- For active adults
- Regular work-outs
- Otherwise, similar to Performance Packs™
- Economic supplements because there is no glutathione

Each Packet Contains:

Antioxidants/Vitamins	Quantity	% RDA
2 Ascorbic-B/Yellow Caps		
Ascorbic Acid/C	1600 mg	2667%
Calcium Pantothenate/B-5	240 mg	2400%
Thiamine HCl/B-1	80 mg	5333%
Pyridoxine HCl/B-6	40 mg	2000%
Niacinamide/B-3	30 mg	150%
Niacin/B-3	10 mg	50%
Riboflavin/B-2	8 mg	471%
Cyanocobalamin/B-12	300 mcg	5000%
1 Calcium-D/White Cap		
Calcium as the Carbonate	250 mg	25%
Cholecalciferol/D3	125 IU	31%
1 Carotene-E/Red Cap		
Beta Carotene	15 mg	—
DL-Alpha Tocopheryl Acetate/E	100 IU	333%

DIRECTIONS
Same as Performance Packs
30 Packets/120 Capsules

FOR TWO™
Scientifically calculated, for pregnant/lactating women, to help provide the extra amounts of nutrients around the clock for mother and child

2 Capsules Contain:

Antioxidants/Vitamins	Quantity	RDA%
Retinyl Acetate/A	5000 IU	63%
Cholecalciferol/D3	400 IU	100%
Ascorbic Acid/C	120 mg	200%
Niacinamide/B-3	40 mg	200%
DL-Alpha Tocopheryl Acetate/E	30 IU	100%
Calcium Pantothenate/B-5	20 mg	200 %
Pyridoxine HCl/B-6	6 mg	240%
Riboflavin/B-2	4 mg	200%
Thiamine HCl/B-1	3400 mcg	200%
Folic Acid	800 mcg	100%
Cyanocobalamin/B-12	8 mcg	100%
MINERALS:		
Calcium as the Carbonate	600 mg	60%
Magnesium as the Sulfate	200 mg	50%
Iron as Ferrous Fumarate	36 mg	200%
Iodine as Potassium Iodide	150 mcg	100%

DIRECTIONS
One with breakfast and one at bedtime.
120 Capsules

GLUTATHIONE–C™
Pure Glutathione Antioxidant with Pure Crystalline Ascorbic Acid

Each Capsule Contains:

Antioxidants/Vitamins	Quantity	%RDA
Ascorbic Acid/C	200 mg	333%
Glutathione	50 mg	—

120 Capsules

GLUTATHIONE–FORTÉ™
New, high potency formula. Pure Glutathione Antioxidant, with Pure Crystalline Ascorbic Acid

Each Capsule Contains:

Antioxidants/Vitamins	Quantity	%RDA
Ascorbic Acid/C	750 mg	1250%
Glutathione	250 mg	—

40 Capsules

PERFORMANCE PACKS™
High-Dose Antioxidants and Vitamins plus Calcium, with Glutathione

- Supplements During: Weight Loss Programs and Other Stresses
- For very Active Adults
- Strenuous Exercise
- Late Night Work
- Extensive Travel

Each Packet Contains:

Antioxidants/Vitamins	Quantity	%RDA
2 Ascorbic-B/Yellow Caps		
Ascorbic Acid/C	1600 mg	2667%
Calcium Pantothenate/B-5	240 mg	2400%
Thiamine HCl/B-1	80 mg	5333%
Pyridoxine HCl/B-6	40 mg	2000%
Niacinamide	30 mg	150%
Niacin	10 mg	50%
Riboflavin/B-2	8 mg	471%
Cyanocobalamin/B-12	300 mcg	5000%
1 Combination/White Cap		
Ascorbic Acid/C	400 mg	667%
Calcium as the Carbonate	250 mg	25%
Glutathione	100 mg	—
Cholecalciferol/D3	125 IU	31%
1 Carotene-E/Red Cap		
Beta Carotene	15 mg	—
DL-Alpha Tocopheryl Acetate/E	100 IU	333%

DIRECTIONS
One packet after meals or snacks, 1 to 3 times a day
45 Packets/180 Capsules

PURE–E™
Antioxidant Formulation of Pure Vitamin E, as capsules or as liquid

Each 0.3 cc = 300 IU:

Antioxidants/Vitamins	Quantity	%RDA
DL-Alpha Tocopheryl, Acetate/E	300 IU	1000%
DL-Alpha Tocopheryl Acetate/E	600 IU	2000%

Two Ounces Liquid

Each Capsule Contains:

Antioxidants/Vitamins	Quantity	%RDA
DL-Alpha Tocopheryl Acetate/E	400 IU	1333%

90 Capsules

SENIORS™
Scientifically formulated, delicious supplements of powerful antioxidants, vitamins and minerals for senior citizens. Available as easy-chewable tablets or as packets that contain a great tasting powder that can be sprinkled on foods, or mixed in any liquid.

2 Tablets or 2 Packs Contain:

Antioxidants/Vitamins	Quantity	RDA%
Retinyl Acetate/A	5000 IU	100%
Ascorbic Acid/C	480 mg	800%
Cholecalciferol/D3	400 IU	100%
DL-Alpha Tocopheryl Acetate/E	120 IU	400%
Calcium Pantothenate/B-5	80 mg	800%
Thiamine No 3/B-1	40 mg	2667%
Pyridoxine HCl/B-6	40 mg	2000%
Niacinamide/B-3	40 mg	200%
Glutathione	20 mg	—
Riboflavin/B-2	4 mg	235%
Folic Acid	400 mcg	100%
Cyanocobalamin/B-12	100 mcg	1667%
Minerals:		
Calcium as the Carbonate	320 mg	32%
Magnesium as the Oxide	120 mg	30%

DIRECTIONS
One tablet or one packet of powder, at breakfast and one mid-afternoon.
60 Chewable tablets
60 Packets of powder

SUPERKIDS™
Scientifically developed, great tasting supplements. With extra water-soluble antioxidants and vitamins to help extend energy production.

Antioxidants/Vitamins	Children 2–4 yrs, 1 Tablet Contains: Quantity	RDA%	Over 4 yrs 2 Tablets: RDA%
Retinyl Acetate/A	2500 IU	100%	100%
Cholecalciferol/D3	200 IU	50%	100%
Ascorbic Acid/C	120 mg	300%	400%
Niacinamide/B-3	20 mg	222%	200%
DL-Alpha Tocopheryl Acetate	15 IU	150%	100%
Calcium Pantothenate/B-5	10 mg	200%	200%
Pyridoxine HCl/B-6	4 mg	571%	400%
Thiamine NO₃/B-1	3 mg	428%	400%
Riboflavin/B-2	2 mg	250%	235%
Folic Acid	50 mcg	25%	25%
Cyanocobalamin/B-12	6 mcg	200%	200%
Minerals:			
Iron as Ferrous Fumarate			
Copper as Cupric Oxide			
Zinc as the Oxide		Provides less than	
Manganese as the Sulfate		25% of RDA	

DIRECTIONS
Over 4 years old, one in the morning and one in the afternoon. 2-4 years old ½ tablet twice a day.
60 Chewable tablets

Herbert Laboratories
**A Division of Allergan, Inc.
2525 DUPONT DRIVE
IRVINE, CA 92715**

AEROSEB–DEX®   ℞
(dexamethasone) 0.01%
Topical Aerosol Spray

Contains:
dexamethasone 0.01%
SD Alcohol 40-2 ....59%
with: isopropyl myristate and propellant (butane).
Each 1 second of spray dispenses approximately 0.02 mg of dexamethasone.

HOW SUPPLIED
In a 58 g aerosol with applicator tube.* NDC 0023-0852-90
*U.S. Patent 3,730,182

AEROSEB–HC® ℞
(hydrocortisone) 0.5%
Topical Aerosol Spray

Contains:
hydrocortisone 0.5%
SD Alcohol 40-2 ....58%
with: isopropyl myristate and propellant (butane).
Each 1 second of spray dispenses approximately 1 mg of hydrocortisone.

HOW SUPPLIED
In a 58 g aerosol with applicator tube.* NDC 0023-0804-90
*U.S. Patent 3,730,182

AQUATAR®
Therapeutic Tar Gel

(See PDR For Nonprescription Drugs)

BLUBORO® Powder
Astringent Soaking Solution

(See PDR For Nonprescription Drugs)

DANEX®
Protein Enriched Dandruff Shampoo

(See PDR For Nonprescription Drugs)

ERYGEL® ℞
[är'ē-jel]
(erythromycin) 2%
Topical Gel

PRODUCT OVERVIEW

KEY FACTS
Proven topical erythromycin efficacy and safety. Easy to apply gel. Contains no propylene glycol, no acetone, no Laureth-4, no fragrance. Twenty-four month expiration dating.

MAJOR USES
Acne vulgaris.

SAFETY INFORMATION
Contraindicated in persons hypersensitive to erythromycin or its listed ingredients. Safe use in lactation or pregnancy has not been established.

PRESCRIBING INFORMATION

ERYGEL® ℞
[är'ē-jel]
(erythromycin) 2%
Topical Gel

DESCRIPTION
Erygel Topical Gel contains erythromycin. Erythromycin is a macrolide antibiotic obtained from cultures of *Streptomyces erythraeus*.
Contains: erythromycin, USP .... 2% (20 mg/g)
with: alcohol 92% and hydroxypropyl cellulose.

CLINICAL PHARMACOLOGY
The exact mechanism by which erythromycin reduces lesions of acne vulgaris is not fully known; however, the effect appears to be due in part to the antibacterial activity of the drug.

MICROBIOLOGY
Erythromycin appears to inhibit protein synthesis in susceptible organisms by reversibly binding to ribosomal subunits, thereby inhibiting translocation of aminoacyl transfer-RNA and inhibiting polypeptide synthesis. Antagonism has been demonstrated between erythromycin, lincomycin, chloramphenicol, and clindamycin.

INDICATIONS AND USAGE
Erygel is indicated for the topical treatment of acne vulgaris.

CONTRAINDICATIONS
Erygel is contraindicated in those individuals who have shown hypersensitivity to any of its components.

PRECAUTIONS
General: For topical use only; not for ophthalmic use. Concomitant topical acne therapy should be used with caution since a possible cumulative irritancy effect may occur, especially with the use of peeling, desquamating or abrasive agents.
Avoid contact with eyes and all mucous membranes. The use of antibiotic agents may be associated with the overgrowth of antibiotic-resistant organisms. If this occurs, discontinue use and take appropriate measures.
Carcinogenesis, mutagenesis, impairment of fertility: Animal studies to evaluate carcinogenic and mutagenic potential, or effects on fertility have not been performed with erythromycin.
Pregnancy Category B: There was no evidence of teratogenicity or any other adverse effect on reproduction in female rats fed erythromycin base (up to 0.25% of diet) prior to and during mating, during gestation and through weaning of two successive litters. There are, however, no adequate and well-controlled studies in pregnant women. Because animal reproduction studies are not always predictive of human response, this drug should be used in pregnancy only if clearly needed. Erythromycin has been reported to cross the placental barrier in humans, but fetal plasma levels are generally low.
Nursing Mothers: It is not known whether topically applied erythromycin is excreted in human milk. A decision should be made whether to discontinue nursing or to discontinue the drug, taking into account the importance of the drug to the mother.
Pediatric Use: Safety and effectiveness in children have not been established.

ADVERSE REACTIONS
The most common adverse reaction reported with Erygel was burning. The following have been reported occasionally: peeling, dryness, itching, erythema, and oiliness. Irritation of the eyes and tenderness of the skin have also been reported with the topical use of erythromycin. A generalized urticarial reaction, possibly related to the use of erythromycin, which required systemic steroid therapy has been reported.

DOSAGE AND ADMINISTRATION
Apply sparingly as a thin layer to affected area(s) twice a day, in the morning and the evening after the skin is thoroughly washed with soap and water and patted dry. The hands should be washed after application. If there has been no improvement after 6 to 8 weeks, or if the condition becomes worse, treatment should be discontinued, and the physician should be reconsulted. Spread the medication lightly rather than rubbing it in.

HOW SUPPLIED
Erygel® (erythromycin) 2% Topical Gel is supplied in plastic tubes in the following size: 30 g—NDC 0023-4312-30. Also available in a 60 g size with a 5 g travel size tube included: 65 g—NDC 0023-4312-65.
Note: FLAMMABLE. Keep away from heat and flame. Keep tube tightly closed. Store at room temperature.
Caution: Federal law prohibits dispensing without prescription.

ERYMAX® ℞
(erythromycin) 2% Topical Solution, USP

Contains: erythromycin .... 2% (20 mg/mL)
with: SD Alcohol 40-2 (66%), propylene glycol, and citric acid.

HOW SUPPLIED
Erymax® Topical Solution, USP is supplied in a 2 fl oz plastic bottle with optional Dab-O-Matic applicator and a 4 fl oz plastic bottle:
2 fl oz (59 mL)—NDC 0023-0540-02
4 fl oz (118 mL)—NDC 0023-0540-04

EXSEL® ℞
(selenium sulfide) 2.5%
Shampoo/Lotion

Contains:
selenium sulfide 2.5%
with: edetate disodium; bentonite; sodium dodecylbenzene sulfonate; sodium C14-16 olefin sulfonate; glyceryl ricinoleate; dimethicone copolyol; titanium dioxide; citric acid monohydrate; sodium phosphate monobasic, monohydrate; fragrance; and purified water.

HOW SUPPLIED
In 4 oz plastic bottles. Protect from heat. For external use only. Keep out of the reach of children. NDC 0023-0817-99

FLUONID® ℞
(fluocinolone acetonide)
Topical Solution 0.01%

Contains: fluocinolone acetonide 0.01%
with: propylene glycol and citric acid.

HOW SUPPLIED
Fluonid (fluocinolone acetonide)
Topical Solution 0.01%—20 mL and 60 mL plastic squeeze bottles. 20 mL NDC 0023-0878-20; 60 mL NDC 0023-0878-60.

FLUOROPLEX® ℞
(fluorouracil)
1% Topical Cream
and 1% Topical Solution

PRODUCT OVERVIEW

KEY FACTS
Effective treatment for multiple AK sites.
Provides effective treatment for both clinical and subclinical lesions.
As effective as 5% 5FU on the face.
Fluoroplex cream does not contain irritating parabens or propylene glycol.

MAJOR USES
Multiple actinic keratoses.

SAFETY INFORMATION
Contraindicated in persons hypersensitive to fluorouracil or its listed ingredients.
Contraindicated in pregnancy.
Prolonged exposure to sunlight or other forms of ultraviolet irradiation may increase intensity of reaction.
Adequate long-term studies in animals to evaluate carcinogenic potential have not been conducted with fluorouracil.

PRESCRIBING INFORMATION

FLUOROPLEX® ℞
(fluorouracil)
1% Topical Cream
and
1% Topical Solution

DESCRIPTION
Fluoroplex (fluorouracil) 1% Topical Cream and 1% Topical Solution are antineoplastic/antimetabolite products for dermatological use. Fluorouracil has the empirical formula $C_4H_3FN_2O_2$ and a molecular weight of 130.08. It is sparingly soluble in water and slightly soluble in alcohol. The pH is approximately 8.5 for Fluoroplex Topical Cream and 9.2 for Fluoroplex Topical Solution.
Chemical Name:
2,4(1*H*, 3*H*)-Pyrimidinedione,5-fluoro-.
Fluoroplex 1% Topical Cream contains:
fluorouracil 1.0%
with: benzyl alcohol, emulsifying wax, mineral oil, isopropyl myristate, sodium hydroxide and purified water.
Fluoroplex 1% Topical Solution contains:
fluorouracil 1.0%
with: propylene glycol, sodium hydroxide and/or hydrochloric acid to adjust the pH, and purified water.
Structural Formula:

fluorouracil

CLINICAL PHARMACOLOGY
There is evidence that fluorouracil (or its metabolites) blocks the methylation reaction of deoxyuridylic acid to thymidylic acid. In this fashion, fluorouracil interferes with the synthesis of deoxyribonucleic acid (DNA) and to a lesser extent inhibits the formation of ribonucleic acid (RNA).

INDICATIONS AND USAGE
Fluoroplex is indicated for the topical treatment of multiple actinic (solar) keratoses.

CONTRAINDICATIONS
Fluorouracil may cause fetal harm when administered to a pregnant woman. Fluorouracil has been shown to be teratogenic in mice and rats when injected intraperitoneally in doses of 20 mg/kg and above on day 9, 10, 11, 12, or 13 of gestation. Fluorouracil is contraindicated in women who are or may become pregnant. If this drug is used during pregnancy, or if the patient becomes pregnant while taking this drug, the patient should be apprised of the potential hazard to the fetus.
These products should not be used by patients who are allergic to any of their components.

WARNINGS
There exists the potential for a delayed hypersensitivity reaction to 5-fluorouracil. Patch testing to prove hypersensitivity may be inconclusive.[1]
If an occlusive dressing is used, there may be an increase in the incidence of inflammatory reactions in the adjacent normal skin.
The patient should avoid prolonged exposure to sunlight or other forms of ultraviolet irradiation during treatment with Fluoroplex, as the intensity of the reaction may be increased.

Continued on next page

Herbert—Cont.

PRECAUTIONS

General: There is a possibility of increased absorption through ulcerated or inflamed skin.

Information for patients: The medication should be applied with care near the eyes, nose and mouth. Excessive reaction in these areas may occur due to irritation from accumulation of drug. If Fluoroplex is applied with the fingers, the hands should be washed immediately afterward.

The reaction to Fluoroplex in treated areas may be unsightly during therapy, and, in some cases, for several weeks following cessation of therapy.

Laboratory Tests: To rule out the presence of a frank neoplasm, a biopsy should be made of those areas failing to respond to treatment or recurring after treatment.

Carcinogenesis, Mutagenesis, Impairment of Fertility: No studies have been conducted in animals or in humans to evaluate the potential of these effects.

Pregnancy: Teratogenic effects: Pregnancy Category X: See **CONTRAINDICATIONS** section.

Nursing mothers: It is not known whether this drug is excreted in human milk. Because many drugs are excreted in human milk, and because there is some systemic absorption of fluorouracil after topical administration (see **CLINICAL PHARMACOLOGY**), mothers should not nurse their infants while receiving this drug.

Pediatric use: Safety and effectiveness in children have not been established.

ADVERSE REACTIONS

Pain, pruritus, burning, irritation, inflammation, allergic contact dermatitis and telangiectasia have been reported. Occasionally, hyperpigmentation and scarring have also been reported.

OVERDOSAGE

Ordinarily, overdosage will not cause acute problems. If Fluoroplex® accidentally comes in contact with the eye(s), flush the eye(s) with water or normal saline. If Fluoroplex is accidentally ingested, induce emesis and gastric lavage. Administer symptomatic and supportive care as needed.

DOSAGE AND ADMINISTRATION

The patient should be instructed to apply sufficient medication to cover the entire face or other affected areas.

Apply medication twice daily with non-metallic applicator or fingertips and wash hands afterwards. A treatment period of 2–6 weeks is usually required.

Increasing the frequency of application and a longer period of administration with Fluoroplex may be required on areas other than the head and neck.

When Fluoroplex is applied to keratotic skin, a response occurs with the following sequence: erythema, usually followed by scaling, tenderness, erosion, ulceration, necrosis and re-epithelization. When the inflammatory reaction reaches the erosion, ulceration and necrosis stages, the use of the drug should be terminated. Responses may sometimes occur in areas which appear clinically normal. These may be sites of subclinical actinic (solar) keratosis which the medication is affecting.

HOW SUPPLIED

Fluoroplex (fluorouracil) 1% Topical Cream is available in 30 g tubes (NDC 0023-0812-30). On prescription only.

Fluoroplex (fluorouracil) 1% Topical Solution is available in 30 mL plastic dropper bottles (NDC 0023-0810-30). On prescription only.

Avoid freezing. Store at controlled room temperature (59°–86°F) in tight containers.

REFERENCE

1. Epstein E. Testing for 5-fluorouracil allergy: patch and intradermal tests. Contact Dermatitis 1984; 10:311.

Revised February 1987

Herbert Laboratories, Dermatology Division of **Allergan, Inc.,** Irvine, California 92713, U.S.A.
© Herbert Laboratories, Inc.
Printed in U.S.A.   7813   30-3/J

Gris–PEG®   ℞
(griseofulvin ultramicrosize)
Tablets, USP
125 mg; 250 mg

DESCRIPTION

Gris-PEG Tablets contain ultramicrosize crystals of griseofulvin, an antibiotic derived from a species of *Penicillium*. Each Gris-PEG Tablet contains:

griseofulvin ultramicrosize .... 125 mg
with: colloidal silicon dioxide, lactose, magnesium stearate; methylcellulose; methylparaben; polyethylene glycol 400 and 8000, polyvinylpolypyrrolidone; povidone; and titanium dioxide, or

griseofulvin ultramicrosize .... 250 mg
with: colloidal silicon dioxide; magnesium stearate; methylcellulose; methylparaben; polyethylene glycol 400 and 8000; povidone; sodium lauryl sulfate; and titanium dioxide.

ACTION

Microbiology—Griseofulvin is fungistatic with *in vitro* activity against various species of *Microsporum, Epidermophyton* and *trichophyton*. It has no effect on bacteria or other genera of fungi.

Human Pharmaocology—Following oral administration, griseofulvin is deposited in the keratin precursor cells and has a greater affinity for diseased tissue. The drug is tightly bound to the new keratin which becomes highly resistant to fungal invasions.

The efficiency of gastrointestinal absorption of ultramicrocrystalline griseofulvin is approximately one and one-half times that of the conventional microsize griseofulvin. This factor permits the oral intake of two-thirds as much ultramicrocrystalline griseofulvin as the microsize form. However, there is currently no evidence that this lower dose confers any significant clinical differences with regard to safety and/or efficacy.

INDICATIONS

Gris-PEG (griseofulvin ultramicrosize) is indicated for the treatment of the following ringworm infections; tinea corporis (ringworm of the body), tinea pedis (athlete's foot), tinea cruris (ringworm of the groin and thigh), tinea barbae (barber's itch), tinea capitis (ringworm of the scalp), and tinea unguium (onychomyocosis, ringworm of the nails), when caused by one or more of the following genera of fungi: *Trichophyton rubrum, Trichophytox tonsurans, Trichophyton mentagrophyies, Trichophyton interdigitalis, Trichophyton verrucosum, Trichophyton megnini, Trichophyton gallinae, Trichophyton crateriform, Trichophyton sulphureum, Trichophyton schoenlelni, Microsporum audouini, Microsporum canis, Microsporum gypseum* and *Epidermophyton floccosum.* Note: Prior to therapy, the type of fungi responsible for the infection should be identified. The use of the drug is not justified in minor or trivial infections which will repsond to topical agents alone. Griseofulvin is *not* effective in the following: bacterial infections, candidiasis (moniliasis), histoplasmosis, actinomycosis, sporotrichosis, chromoblastomycosis, coccidioidomycosis, North American blastomycosis, cryptococcosis (torulosis), tinea versicolor and nocardiosis.

CONTRAINDICATIONS

Two cases of conjoined twins have been reported since 1977 in patients taking griseofulvin during the first trimester of pregnancy. Griseofulvin should not be prescribed to pregnant patients. If the patient becomes pregnant while taking this drug, the patient should be apprised of the potential hazard to the fetus.

This drug is contraindicated in patients with porphyria or hepatocellular failure and in individuals with a history of hypersensitivity to griseofulvin.

WARNINGS

Prophylactic Usage—Safety and efficacy of griseofulvin for prophylaxis of fungal infections have not been established. *Animal Toxicology*—Chronic feeding of griseofulvin, at levels ranging from 0.5%–2.5% of the diet resulted in the development of liver tumors in several strains of mice, particularly in males. Smaller particle sizes result in an enhanced effect. Lower oral dosage levels have not been tested. Subcutaneous administration of relatively small doses of griseofulvin once a week during the first three weeks of life has also been reported to induce hepatomata in mice. Thyroid tumors, mostly adenomas but some carcinomas, have been reported in male rats receiving griseofulvin at levels of 2.0%, 1.0% and 0.2% of the diet, and in female rats receiving the two higher dose levels. Although studies in other animal species have not yielded evidence of tumorigenicity, these studies were not of adequate design to form a basis for conclusion in this regard. In subacute toxicity studies, orally administered griseofulvin produced hepatocellular necrosis in mice, but this has not been seen in other species. Disturbances in porphyrin metabolism have been reported in griseofulvin-treated laboratory animals. Griseofulvin has been reported to have a colchicine-like effect on mitosis and cocarcinogenicity with methylcholanthrene in cutaneous tumor induction in laboratory animals. *Usage in Pregnancy* —See CONTRAINDICATIONS section. *Animal Reproduction Studies* —It has been reported in the literature that griseofulvin was found to be embryotoxic and teratogenic on oral administration to pregnant rats. Pups with abnormalities have been reported in the litters of a few bitches treated with griseofulvin. Suppression of spermatogenesis has been reported to occur in rats, but investigation in man failed to confirm this.

PRECAUTIONS

Patients on prolonged therapy with any potent medication should be under close observation. Periodic monitoring of organ system function, including renal, hepatic and hematopoietic, should be done. Since griseofulvin is derived from species of *Penicillium*, the possibility of cross-sensitivity with

penicillin exists; however, known penicillin-sensitive patients have been treated without difficulty. Since a photosensitivity reaction is occasionally associated with griseofulvin therapy, patients should be warned to avoid exposure to intense natural or artificial sunlight. Lupus erythematosus or lupus-like syndromes have been reported in patients receiving griseofulvin. Griseofulvin decreases the activity of warfarin-type anticoagulants so that patients receiving these drugs concomitantly may require dosage adjustment of the anticoagulant during and after griseofulvin therapy. Barbiturates usually depress griseofulvin activity and concomitant administration may require a dosage adjustment of the antifungal agent. There have been reports in the literature of possible interactions between griseofulvin and oral contraceptives. The effect of alcohol may be potentiated by griseofulvin, producing such effects as tachycardia and flush.

ADVERSE REACTIONS

When adverse reactions occur, they are most commonly of the hypersensitivity type such as skin rashes, urticaria, and rarely, angioneurotic edema, and may necessitate withdrawal of therapy and appropriate countermeasures. Paresthesias of the hands and feet have been reported rarely after extended therapy. Other side effects reported occasionally are oral thrush, nausea, vomiting, epigastric distress, diarrhea, headache, fatigue, dizziness, insomnia, mental confusion, and impairment of performance of routine activities. Proteinuria and leukopenia have been reported rarely. Administration of the drug should be discontinued if granulocytopenia occurs. When rare, serious reactions occur with griseofulvin, they are usually associated with high dosages, long periods of therapy, or both.

DOSAGE AND ADMINISTRATION

Accurate diagnosis of the infecting organism is essential. Identification should be made either by direct microscopic examination of a mounting of infected tissue in a solution of potassium hydroxide or by culture on an appropriate medium. Medication must be continued until the infecting organism is completely eradicated as indicated by appropriate clinical or laboratory examination. Representative treatment periods are tinea capitis, 4 to 6 weeks; tinea corporis, 2 to 4 weeks; tinea pedis, 4 to 8 weeks; tinea unguium—depending on rate of growth—fingernails, at least 4 months; toenails, at least 6 months.

General measures in regard to hygiene should be observed to control sources of infection or reinfection. Concomitant use of appropriate topical agents is usually required, particularly in treatment of tinea pedis. In some forms of athlete's foot, yeasts and bacteria may be involved as well as fungi. Griseofulvin will not eradicate the bacterial or monllial infection.

Adults: Daily administration of 375 mg (as a single dose or in divided doses) will give a satisfactory response in most patients with tinea corporis, tinea cruris, and tinea capitis. For those fungal infections more difficult to eradicate, such as tinea pedis and tinea unguium, a divided dose of 750 mg is recommended.

Children: Approximately 3.3 mg per pound of body weight per day of ultramicrosize griseofulvin is an effective dose for most children. On this basis, the following dosage schedule is suggested; Children weighing 35–60 pounds—125 mg to 187.5 mg daily. Children weighing over 60 pounds—187.5 mg to 375 mg daily. Children 2 years of age and younger—dosage has not been established.

Clinical experience with griseofulvin in children with tinea capitis indicates that a single daily dose is effective. Clinical relapse will occur if the medication is not continued until the infecting organism is eradicated.

HOW SUPPLIED

Gris-PEG (griseofulvin ultramicrosize) Tablets, 125 mg, white, scored, elliptical-shaped, embossed "Gris-PEG" on one side and "125" on the other. Gris-PEG (griseofulvin ultramicrosize) Tablets, 250 mg, white, scored, capsule-shaped, embossed "Gris-PEG" on one side and "250" on the other. The 125 mg strength is available in bottles of 100 and 500 (NDC 0023-0763-04, and NDC 0023-0763-99 respectively). The 250 mg strength is available in bottles of 100, 250 and 500 (NDC 0023- 0773-04, NDC 0023-0773-25, and NDC 0023-0773-50 respectively). Both strengths are film-coated.

CAUTION

Federal law prohibits dispensing without prescription.

STORAGE

Store Gris-PEG tablets at controlled room temperature 15°–30°C (59°–86°F) in tight, light-resistant containers.

MAXIFLOR®   ℞
(diflorasone diacetate)
Cream, USP, 0.05%
Ointment, USP, 0.05%

DESCRIPTION

MAXIFLOR Cream contains 0.5 mg diflorasone diacetate, USP, in an emulsified and hydrophilic cream base consisting of propylene glycol, stearic acid, polysorbate 60, sorbitan monostearate and monooleate, sorbic acid, citric acid and water. The corticosteroid is formulated as a solution in the vehicle using 15 percent propylene glycol to optimize drug delivery.

MAXIFLOR Ointment contains 0.5 mg diflorasone diacetate, USP, in an emollient, occlusive base consisting of polyoxypropylene 15-stearyl ether, stearic acid, lanolin alcohol and white petrolatum.

HOW SUPPLIED

MAXIFLOR® (diflorasone diacetate) Cream, USP, 0.05% is available in collapsible tubes in the following sizes:
   15 gram NDC 0023-0766-15
   30 gram NDC 0023-0766-30
   60 gram NDC 0023-0766-60

MAXIFLOR® (diflorasone diacetate) Ointment, USP, 0.05% is available in collapsible tubes in the following sizes:
   15 gram NDC 0023-0770-15
   30 gram NDC 0023-0770-30
   60 gram NDC 0023-0770-60

NAFTIN®   ℞
(naftifine hydrochloride) 1%
Cream

Naftin Cream contains the synthetic, broad-spectrum, antifungal agent naftifine hydrochloride.
Naftin Cream is for topical use only.
Contains: Naftifine hydrochloride 1%
with benzyl alcohol, cetyl alcohol, cetyl esters wax, isopropyl myristate, polysorbate 60, purified water, sodium hydroxide, sorbitan monostearate, and stearyl alcohol. Hydrochloric acid may be added to adjust pH.

CLINICAL PHARMACOLOGY
Naftifine hydrochloride is a synthetic allylamine derivative. Naftifine hydrochloride has been shown to exhibit fungicidal activity *in vitro* against a broad spectrum of organisms including *Trichophyton rubrum, Trichophyton mentagrophytes, Trichophyton tonsurans, Epidermophyton floccosum, Microsporum canis, Microsporum audouini,* and *Microsporum gypseum;* and fungistatic activity against *Candida* species, including *Candida albicans.* Naftin Cream has only been shown to be clinically effective against the disease entities listed in the INDICATIONS AND USAGE section.
Although the exact mechanism of action against fungi is not known, naftifine hydrochloride appears to interfere with sterol biosynthesis by inhibiting the enzyme squalene 2,3-epoxidase. This inhibition of enzyme activity results in decreased amounts of sterols, especially ergosterol, and a corresponding accumulation of squalene in the cells.
Pharmacokinetics: *In vitro* and *in vivo* bioavailability studies have demonstrated that naftifine penetrates the stratum corneum in sufficient concentration to inhibit the growth of dermatophytes.
Following a single topical application of 1% naftifine cream to the skin of healthy subjects, systemic absorption of naftifine was approximately 6% of the applied does. Naftifine and/or its metabolites are excreted via the urine and feces with a half-life of approximately two to three days.

INDICATIONS AND USAGE
Naftin Cream is indicated for the topical application in the treatment of tinea pedis, tinea cruris and tinea corporis caused by the organisms *Tricophyton rubrum, Tricophyton mentagrophytes,* and *Epidermophyton floccosum.*

CONTRAINDICATIONS
Naftin Cream is contraindicated in individuals who have shown hypersensitivity to any of its components.

WARNING
Naftin Cream is for topical use only and not for ophthalmic use.

PRECAUTIONS
General: If irritation or sensitivity develops with the use of Naftin Cream, treatment should be discontinued and appropriate therapy instituted. For external use only. Diagnosis of the disease should be confirmed either by direct microscopic examination of a mounting of infected tissue in a solution of potassium hydroxide or by culture on an appropriate medium.
Information for patients: The patient should be told to:
1. Avoid the use of occlusive dressings or wrappings unless otherwise directed by the physician.
2. Keep Naftin Cream away from the eyes, nose, mouth and other mucous membranes.
Carcinogenesis, mutagenesis, impairment of fertility: Long-term animal studies to evaluate the carcinogenic potential have not been performed. *In vitro* and animal studies have not demonstrated any mutagenic effect or effect on fertility.
Pregnancy Category B: Reproduction studies have been performed in rats and rabbits (via oral administration) at doses 150 times or more the topical human doses and have revealed no significant evidence of impaired fertility or harm to the fetus due to naftifine. There are, however, no

adequate and well-controlled studies in pregnant women. Because animal reproduction studies are not always predictive of human response, this drug should be used during pregnancy only if clearly needed.
Nursing mothers: It is not known whether naftifine hydrochloride is excreted in human milk. Consideration should be given to discontinuing nursing temporarily while using Naftin® (naftifine hydrocyhloride) 1% Cream and for several days after the last application of Naftin Cream.
Pediatric use: Safety and effectiveness in children have not been established.

ADVERSE REACTIONS
During clinical trials with Naftin Cream, the incidence of adverse reactions was as follows: burning/stinging (6%), dryness (3%), erythema (2%), itching (2%), local irritation (2%).

DOSAGE AND ADMINISTRATION
A sufficient quantity of Naftin Cream should be gently massaged into the affected and surrounding skin areas twice a day, in the morning and evening. The hands should be washed after application.
Clinical improvement usually occurs within the first week of treatment. Treatment should be continued for one to two weeks after manifestations have subsided to assure healing and reduce the possibility of recurrence. If no clinical improvement is seen after four weeks of treatment with Naftin Cream, the patient should be re-evaluated.

HOW SUPPLIED
Naftin Cream is supplied in collapsible tubes in the following sizes.
15 g-NDC-0023-4126-15
30 g-NDC-0023-4126-30
Note: Store below 30°C (86°F).
Caution: Federal law prohibits dispensing without prescription.

February 1988

PENECORT®   ℞
(hydrocortisone)
Cream, USP, 1% and 2.5%
Topical Solution 1%

PENECORT Cream contains:
hydrocortisone, USP 1%, 2.5%
with: benzyl alcohol; petrolatum; stearyl alcohol; propylene glycol; isopropyl myristate; polyoxyl 40 stearate; carbomer 934; sodium lauryl sulfate; edetate disodium; sodium hydroxide to adjust the pH; and purified water.
PENECORT Ointment contains:
hydrocortisone, USP 2.5%
in a white petrolatum base.
PENECORT Topical Solution contains:
hydrocortisone, USP 1%
with: alcohol (57%); propylene glycol; benzyl alcohol; and purified water.

HOW SUPPLIED
PENECORT® (hydrocortisone):
Cream, USP, 1%—30 g and 60 g collapsible tubes: 30 g NDC 0023-0510-30; 60 g NDC 0023-0510-60
Cream, USP, 2.5%—30 g collapsible tubes: NDC 0023-0550-30
Topical Solution 1%—30 mL and 60 mL plastic bottles: 30 mL NDC 0023-0889-30; 60 mL NDC 0023-0889-60

PHOTOPLEX® Broad Spectrum Sunscreen Lotion

(See PDR For Nonprescription Drugs)

TAC™–3   ℞
(sterile triamcinolone acetonide suspension) 3mg/mL
NOT FOR INTRAVENOUS USE
FOR INTRALESIONAL AND INTRADERMAL USE

Contains: Each mL of aqueous suspension contains: Triamcinolone acetonide 3 mg; sodium chloride 2 mg; carboxymethylcellulose sodium 7.5 mg; polysorbate 80—0.4mg; with benzyl alcohol 0.9% as preservative; in water for injection q.s. Sodium hydroxide and/or hydrochloric acid may have been used to adjust pH.

HOW SUPPLIED
Multiple dose vials of 5 mL containing triamcinolone acetonide 3 mg/mL.
NDC 0023-0218-05.
Manufactured for HERBERT LABORATORIES
A Division of Allergan, Inc.
Irvine, California 92713, U.S.A.
by
Steris Laboratories Inc.
Phoenix, AZ 85043

TEMARIL®   ℞
(trimeprazine tartrate)
Tablets, Syrup and
Spansule® capsules
(sustained release capsules)

DESCRIPTION
'Temaril', available as trimeprazine tartrate, a phenothiazine derivative is 10-[3-(dimethylamino)-2-methylpropyl]-phenothiazine tartrate.
Trimeprazine tartrate is a white to off-white odorless, crystalline powder readily soluble in water.
Tablets—Each round, gray, coated tablet is imprinted HL and T41 and contains trimeprazine tartrate equivalent to 2.5 mg of trimeprazine. Inactive ingredients consist of acacia, calcium sulfate, FD&C Yellow No. 6, gelatin, iron oxide, mineral oil, starch, stearic acid, sucrose, talc, titanium dioxide and trace amounts of other inactive ingredients.
Syrup—Each 5 ml (one teaspoonful) of clear, red, raspberry/strawberry flavored liquid contains trimeprazine tartrate equivalent to 2.5 mg of trimeprazine, and alcohol, 5.7%. Inactive ingredients consist of citric acid, FD&C Green No. 3, FD&C Red No. 40, flavors, glycerin, saccharin sodium, sodium benzoate, sucrose and water.
Spansule® sustained release capsules—Each 'Spansule' sustained release capsule is so prepared that an initial dose is released promptly and the remaining medication is released gradually over a prolonged period. Each capsule, with opaque gray cap and natural body, is imprinted HL and T50 and contains trimeprazine tartrate equivalent to 5 mg of trimeprazine. Inactive ingredients consist of benzyl alcohol, cetylpyridinium chloride, FD&C Green No. 3, FD&C Red No. 40, FD&C Yellow No. 6, gelatin, glyceryl distearate, glyceryl monostearate, iron oxide, sodium lauryl sulfate, starch, sucrose, titanium dioxide, wax and trace amounts of other inactive ingredients.

ACTIONS
Temaril (trimeprazine tartrate), a phenothiazine, possesses antipruritic and antihistaminic properties with anticholinergic (drying) and sedative side effects.

INDICATIONS
Treatment of pruritic symptoms in urticaria. Relief of pruritic symptoms in a variety of allergic and non-allergic conditions including atopic dermatitis, neurodermatitis, contact dermatitis, pityriasis rosea, poison ivy dermatitis, eczematous dermatitis, pruritus ani and vulvae, and drug rash.

CONTRAINDICATIONS
Temaril (trimeprazine tartrate) is contraindicated: in comatose patients; in patients who have received large amounts of central nervous system depressants (alcohol, barbiturates, narcotics, etc.); in patients with bone marrow depression; in patients who have demonstrated an idiosyncrasy or hypersensitivity to 'Temaril' or other phenothiazines; in newborn or premature children; and in nursing mothers. It should not be used in children who are acutely ill and/or dehydrated, as there is an increased susceptibility to dystonias in such patients.

WARNINGS
Temaril® (trimeprazine tartrate) may impair the mental and/or physical ability required for the performance of potentially hazardous tasks, such as driving a vehicle or operating machinery. Similarly, it may impair mental alertness in children. The concomitant use of alcohol or other central nervous system depressants may have an additive effect. Patients should be warned accordingly.
'Temaril' should be used with extreme caution in patients with:
   Asthmatic attack
   Narrow-angle glaucoma
   Prostatic hypertrophy
   Stenosing peptic ulcer
   Pyloroduodenal obstruction
   Bladder neck obstruction
   Patients receiving monoamine oxidase inhibitors
Usage in Pregnancy: The safe use of 'Temaril' has not been established with respect to the possible adverse effects upon fetal development. Therefore, it should not be used in women of childbearing potential. Jaundice and prolonged extrapyramidal symptoms have been reported in infants whose mothers received phenothiazines during pregnancy.
Usage in Children: 'Temaril' should be used with caution in children who have a history of sleep apnea or a family history of sudden infant death syndrome (SIDS). It should also be used with caution in young children, in whom it may cause excitation.
Overdosage may produce hallucinations, convulsions and sudden death.
Usage in Elderly Patients (60 years or older): Elderly patients are more prone to develop the following side effects from phenothiazines:

Continued on next page

Herbert—Cont.

Hypotension
Syncope
Toxic confusional states
Extrapyramidal symptoms, especially parkinsonism
Excessive sedation

PRECAUTIONS

Temaril (trimeprazine tartrate) may significantly affect the actions of other drugs. It may increase, prolong or intensify the sedative action of central nervous system depressants such as anesthetics, barbiturates or alcohol. When 'Temaril' is administered concomitantly the dose of a narcotic or barbiturate should be reduced to ¼ or ½ the usual amount. In the patient with pain, receiving treatment with narcotics, excessive amounts of 'Temaril' may lead to restlessness and motor hyperactivity. 'Temaril' can block and even reverse the usual pressor effect of epinephrine.

'Temaril' should be used cautiously in persons with acute or chronic respiratory impairment, particularly children, as it may suppress the cough reflex.

This drug should be used cautiously in persons with cardiovascular disease, impairment of liver function, or those with a history of ulcer disease.

Since 'Temaril' has a slight antiemetic action, it may obscure signs of intestinal obstruction, brain tumor, or overdosage of toxic drugs.

Phenothiazines have been shown to elevate prolactin levels; the elevation persists during chronic administration. Tissue culture experiments indicate that approximately one-third of human breast cancers are prolactin-dependent in vitro, a factor of potential importance if the prescribing of these drugs is contemplated in a patient with a previously detected breast cancer. Although disturbances such as galactorrhea, amenorrhea, gynecomastia, and impotence have been reported, the clinical significance of elevated serum prolactin levels is unknown for most patients. An increase in mammary neoplasms has been found in rodents after chronic administration of neuroleptic drugs. Neither clinical nor epidemiologic studies conducted to date, however, have shown an association between chronic administration of these drugs and mammary tumorigenesis; the available evidence is considered too limited to be conclusive at this time.

Drugs which lower the seizure threshold, including phenothiazine derivatives, should not be used with Amipaque®.* As with other phenothiazine derivatives, 'Temaril' should be discontinued at least 48 hours before myelography, should not be resumed for at least 24 hours postprocedure, and should not be used for the control of nausea and vomiting occurring either prior to myelography or postprocedure.

ADVERSE REACTIONS

Temaril (trimeprazine tartrate) may produce adverse reactions attributable to both phenothiazines and antihistamines.

Note: Not all of the following adverse reactions have been reported with Temaril (trimeprazine tartrate); however, pharmacological similarities among the phenothiazine derivatives require that each be considered when 'Temaril' is administered. There have been occasional reports of sudden death in patients receiving phenothiazine derivatives chronically.

C.N.S. Effects: Drowsiness is the most common C.N.S. effect of this drug. Extrapyramidal reactions (opisthotonos, dystonia, akathisia, dyskinesia, parkinsonism) occur, particularly with high doses. (See Overdosage section for management of extrapyramidal symptoms). Hyperreflexia has been reported in the newborn when a phenothiazine was used during pregnancy. Other reported reactions include dizziness, headache, lassitude, tinnitus, incoordination, fatigue, blurred vision, euphoria, diplopia, nervousness, insomnia, tremors and grand mal seizures, excitation, catatonic-like states, neuritis and hysteria, oculogyric crises, disturbing dreams/nightmares, pseudoschizophrenia, and intensification and prolongation of the action of C.N.S. depressants (opiates, analgesics, antihistamines, barbiturates, alcohol), atropine, heat, organophosphorus insecticides.

Cardiovascular Effects: Postural hypotension is the most common cardiovascular effect of phenothiazines. Reflex tachycardia may be seen. Bradycardia, faintness, dizziness and cardiac arrest have been reported. ECG changes, including blunting of T waves and prolongation of the Q-T interval, may be seen.

Gastrointestinal: Anorexia, nausea, vomiting, epigastric distress, diarrhea, constipation, and dry mouth may occur. Increased appetite and weight gain have also been reported.

Genitourinary: Urinary frequency and dysuria, urinary retention, early menses, induced lactation, gynecomastia, decreased libido, inhibition of ejaculation and false positive pregnancy tests have been reported.

Respiratory: Thickening of bronchial secretions, tightness of the chest, wheezing and nasal stuffiness may occur.

Allergic Reactions: These include urticaria, dermatitis, asthma, laryngeal edema, angioneurotic edema, photosensi-

tivity, lupus erythematosus-like syndrome and anaphylactoid reactions.

Other Reported Reactions: Leukopenia, agranulocytosis, pancytopenia, hemolytic anemia, elevation of plasma cholesterol levels and thrombocytopenic purpura have been reported. Jaundice of the obstructive type has also been reported; it is usually reversible but chronic jaundice has been reported. Erythema, peripheral edema, and stomatitis have been reported. High or prolonged glucose tolerance curves, glycosuria, elevated spinal fluid proteins and reversed epinephrine effects may also occur.

Rare occurrences of neuroleptic malignant syndrome (NMS) have been reported in patients receiving phenothiazines. This syndrome is comprised of the symptom complex of hyperthermia, altered consciousness, muscular rigidity and autonomic dysfunction and is potentially fatal.

Long-Term Therapy Considerations: After prolonged phenothiazine administration at high dosage, pigmentation of the skin has occurred, chiefly in the exposed areas. Ocular changes consist of the appearance of lenticular and corneal opacities, epithelial keratopathies and pigmentary retinopathy. Vision may be impaired.

DOSAGE AND ADMINISTRATION

Tablets and Syrup:
Adults: Usual dosage is 2.5 mg q.i.d.
Children over three years: Usual dosage is 2.5 mg h.s., or t.i.d. if needed.
Children 6 months to 3 years: Usual dosage is 1.25 mg (½ teaspoonful of syrup) h.s., or t.i.d. if needed.
'Spansule' capsules:
Adults: Usual daily dosage is 1 capsule q12h.
Children over 6 years of age: 1 capsule daily.
This product form is not recommended for children under 6 years of age. Use tablets or syrup for their dosage flexibility. Because some side effects appear to be dose-related, it is important to use the lowest effective dosage.

DRUG INTERACTIONS

MAO inhibitors and thiazide diuretics prolong and intensify the anticholinergic effects of Temaril (trimeprazine tartrate). Combined use of MAO inhibitors and phenothiazines may result in hypertension and extrapyramidal reactions.
Narcotics: The C.N.S. depressant and analgesic effects of narcotics are potentiated by phenothiazines.
The following drugs may result in potentiation of phenothiazine effects:

Oral contraceptives
Progesterone
Reserpine
Nylidrin hydrochloride

MANAGEMENT OF OVERDOSAGE

Signs and symptoms of Temaril® (trimeprazine tartrate) overdosage range from mild depression of the central nervous system and cardiovascular system to profound hypotension, respiratory depression and unconsciousness. Stimulation may be evident, especially in children and geriatric patients. Atropine-like signs and symptoms—dry mouth, fixed, dilated pupils, flushing, etc.—as well as gastrointestinal symptoms may occur. The treatment of overdosage is essentially symptomatic and supportive. Early gastric lavage may be beneficial. **Do not administer emetics or attempt to induce vomiting because a dystonic reaction of the head or neck might result in aspiration of vomitus.** Extrapyramidal symptoms may be treated with anti-parkinsonism drugs, barbiturates, or Benadryl®.†

Avoid analeptics, which may cause convulsions. Severe hypotension usually responds to the administration of levarterenol or phenylephrine. EPINEPHRINE SHOULD NOT BE USED, since its use in a patient with partial adrenergic blockade may further lower the blood pressure. Additional measures include oxygen and intravenous fluids. Limited experience with dialysis indicates that it is not helpful.
Special note on 'Spansule' capsules—Since much of the 'Spansule' capsule medication is coated for gradual release, therapy directed at reversing the effects of the ingested drug and at supporting the patient should be continued for as long as overdosage symptoms remain. Saline cathartics are useful for hastening evacuation of pellets that have not already released medication.

HOW SUPPLIED

Tablets—2.5 mg in bottles of 100 and 1000; Single Unit Packages of 100 (intended for institutional use only).
Syrup—2.5 mg/5 mL (teaspoonful) and alcohol 5.7%, in 4 fl oz bottles.
'Spansule' capsules—5 mg in bottles of 50; Single Unit Packages of 100 (intended for institutional use only).

---

* metrizamide, Winthrop Pharmaceuticals.
† diphenhydramine hydrochloride, Parke-Davis.
Manufactured for
Herbert Laboratories

A Division of Allergan, Inc.
　　　　　　　　　by
SmithKline & French Laboratories
　　　　　Division of
SmithKline Beckman Corporation
Philadelphia, PA 19101

VANSEB® Cream and Lotion
Dandruff Shampoo

(See PDR For Nonprescription Drugs)

VANSEB-T® Cream and Lotion
Tar Dandruff Shampoo

(See PDR For Nonprescription Drugs)

Dow B. Hickam, Inc.
P.O. BOX 2006
SUGAR LAND, TX 77487-2006

GRANULEX　　　　　　　　　　　　　　℞

COMPOSITION
Each 0.82 cc. of medication delivered to the wound site contains Trypsin crystallized 0.1 mg., Balsam Peru 72.5 mg., Castor Oil 650.0 mg., and an emulsifier.

ACTION
Trypsin is intended for debridement of eschar and other necrotic tissue. It appears that in many instances removal of wound debris strengthens humoral defense mechanisms sufficiently to retard proliferation of local pathogens. Balsam Peru is an effective capillary bed stimulant used to increase circulation in the wound site area. Also, Balsam Peru has a mildly bactericidal action. Castor Oil is used to improve epithelialization by reducing premature epithelial desiccation and cornification. Also, it can act as a protective covering and aids in the reduction of pain.

INDICATIONS
For the treatment of decubitus ulcers, varicose ulcers, debridement of eschar, dehiscent wounds and sunburn.

USES
Granulex is in aerosol form which can be important to healing. It must be remembered, healing starts with a thin sheath of epithelium no more than a cell or two thick. Any rough movement or trauma can quickly destroy the healing tissue. Aerosols have the advantage of eliminating all extraneous physical contact with the wound. Granulex is easy to apply and quickly reduces odor frequently accompanying a decubitus ulcer. The wound may be left open or a wet bandage may be applied. As a suggestion; keep in mind wounds heal poorly in the presence of hemoglobin or zinc deficiency.

WARNING
Do not spray on fresh arterial clots. Avoid spraying in eyes. Flammable, do not expose to fire or open flame. Contents under pressure. Do not puncture or incinerate. Do not store at temperature above 120°F. Keep out of reach of children. Use only as directed. Intentional misuse by deliberately concentrating and inhaling the contents can be harmful or fatal.

DOSAGE
Apply a minimum of twice daily or as often as necessary. Shake well, press the aerosol valve and coat the wound rapidly but not excessively.

HOW SUPPLIED
2 oz. Aerosol NDC 0514-0001-01
4 oz. Aerosol NDC 0514-0001-02

UNIFIBER®　　　　　　　　　　　　　　　OTC
[yoo 'nĭ-fī 'bĕr]
Dietary Fiber Supplement

DESCRIPTION
UNIFIBER Dietary Fiber contains 75% powdered cellulose, a natural non-gelling fiber. Each 4 gram serving (1 Tablespoon) of UNIFIBER contains 3 grams dietary fiber; less than four calories; less than 1 gram carbohydrate; no protein, fat, cholesterol, or vitamins; trace quantities of minerals such as iron and calcium; and is sodium free and potassium free. In recent years the importance of dietary fiber in a healthy diet and its role in healthy bowel habits has been recognized. Americans have been advised to increase their daily fiber intake from about 11 grams per day to between 20 and 30 grams per day. The preferred approach to accomplish this is by increasing the intake of fiber-rich foods, but this is not always possible due to such reasons as poor dentition or palatability. In these cases, UNIFIBER can be mixed with soft foods, fruit juices, milk or other liquids to increase fiber intake without significantly altering a food's natural flavor or texture, or its nutritional content.

INGREDIENTS

UNIFIBER contains: Powdered Cellulose, Corn Syrup Solids and Xanthan Gum

USAGE

A balanced diet that includes adequate amounts of dietary fiber and liquids, plus daily physical activity, is important in maintaining healthy bowel function without laxatives. UNIFIBER provides a concentrated source of fiber for those unable to ingest adequate amounts of fiber-rich foods.

DIRECTIONS

Each tablespoon of UNIFIBER contains 3 grams of dietary fiber. For adults, stir one to two tablespoons once or twice per day into a glass of fruit juice, milk or water, or mix with soft foods such as applesauce, mashed potatoes or pudding. As with any healthful diet, adequate liquids should be included in the daily diet.

HOW SUPPLIED

UNIFIBER Dietary Fiber is supplied in 16 oz (113 servings), 9 oz (63 servings), and 5 oz (35 servings) canisters. UNIFIBER UNI-PACK available in boxes of 30, single serving (4 g) packets.

High Chemical Co.
Div. Day & Frick, Inc.
1760 N. HOWARD ST.
PHILADELPHIA, PA 19122

SARAPIN   ℞
[sar'a-pin]

COMPOSITION

An aqueous distillate of Sarracenia purpurea, pitcher plant, prepared for parenteral administration.

ACTION AND USES

Local injection therapy for the relief of pain of neuro-muscular or neuralgic origin.

ADMINISTRATION AND DOSAGE

Paravertebral nerve injection—2 to 10 cc. Local neuromuscular infiltration—5 to 10 cc.

SIDE EFFECTS
None.

PRECAUTIONS
Non-toxic.

CONTRAINDICATIONS
Local inflammation.

HOW SUPPLIED

One dozen 10 cc. ampuls NDC 10541-492-10 and 50 cc. multidose vials NDC 10541-492-50.

LITERATURE AVAILABLE

Booklet "SARAPIN, Injection Technique in Pain Control."

Hoechst-Roussel
Pharmaceuticals Inc.
SOMERVILLE, NJ 08876-1258

A/T/S®   ℞
(erythromycin)
2% Acne Topical Solution

DESCRIPTION

A/T/S® (erythromycin) is an antibiotic produced from a strain of Streptomyces erythraeus. It is basic and readily forms salts with acids. Each mL of A/T/S (erythromycin) topical solution contains 20 mg of erythromycin base in a vehicle consisting of alcohol USP (66%), propylene glycol USP, and citric acid USP to adjust pH.

ACTIONS

Although the mechanism by which A/T/S® (erythromycin) acts in reducing inflammatory lesions of acne vulgaris is unknown, it is presumably due to its antibiotic action.

INDICATIONS

A/T/S® (erythromycin) is indicated for the topical control of acne vulgaris.

CONTRAINDICATIONS

A/T/S® (erythromycin) is contraindicated in persons who have shown hypersensitivity to any of its ingredients.

WARNING

The safe use of A/T/S® (erythromycin) during pregnancy or lactation has not been established.

PRECAUTIONS

General: The use of antibiotic agents may be associated with the overgrowth of antibiotic-resistant organisms. If this occurs, administration of the drug should be discontinued and appropriate measures taken.

Information for Patients: A/T/S® is for external use only and should be kept away from the eyes, nose, mouth, and other mucous membranes. Concomitant topical acne therapy should be used with caution because a cumulative irritant effect may occur, especially with the use of peeling, desquamating, or abrasive agents.

Carcinogenesis, Mutagenesis, Impairment of Fertility: Long-term animal studies to evaluate carcinogenic potential, mutagenicity, or the effect on fertility of erythromycin have not been performed.

Pregnancy: Pregnancy Category C. Animal reproduction studies have not been conducted with erythromycin. It is also not known whether erythromycin can cause fetal harm when administered to a pregnant woman or can affect reproduction capacity. Erythromycin should be given to a pregnant woman only if clearly needed.

Nursing Mothers: Erythromycin is excreted in breast milk. Caution should be exercised when erythromycin is administered to a nursing woman.

ADVERSE REACTIONS

Adverse conditions reported with the use of erythromycin topical solutions include dryness, tenderness, pruritis, desquamation, erythema, oiliness, and burning sensation. Irritation of the eyes has also been reported. A case of generalized urticarial reaction, possibly related to the drug, which required the use of systemic steroid therapy has been reported.

Of a total of 90 patients exposed to A/T/S® during clinical effectiveness studies, 17 experienced some type of adverse effect. These included dry skin, scaly skin, pruritus, irritation of the eye, and burning sensation.

DOSAGE AND ADMINISTRATION

A/T/S® (erythromycin) Topical Solution should be applied to the affected area twice a day after the skin is thoroughly washed with warm water and soap and patted dry. Moisten the applicator or a pad with A/T/S®, then rub over the affected area. Acne lesions on the face, neck, shoulder, chest, and back may be treated in this manner.

HOW SUPPLIED

A/T/S® 2% Acne Topical Solution—60 mL
Store at controlled room temperature 59°–86°F (15°–30°C).
716000-4/86
Shown in Product Identification Section, page 411

CLAFORAN®   ℞
[kläf'or-an]
(cefotaxime sodium)*
Sterile and
Injection

DESCRIPTION

Sterile Claforan® (cefotaxime sodium) is a semisynthetic, broad spectrum cephalosporin antibiotic for parenteral administration. It is the sodium salt of 7-[2-(2-amino-4-thiazolyl) glyoxylamido]-3-(hydroxymethyl)-8-oxo-5-thia-1-azabicyclo [4.2.0] oct-2-ene-2-carboxylate 7²-(Z)-(O-methyloxime), acetate (ester). Claforan contains approximately 50.5 mg (2.2 mEq) of sodium per gram of cefotaxime activity. Solutions of Claforan range from very pale yellow to light amber depending on the concentration and the diluent used. The pH of the injectable solutions usually ranges from 5.0 to 7.5.

Claforan is supplied as a dry powder in conventional and ADD-Vantage® System compatible vials, infusion bottles, pharmacy bulk package bottles, and as a frozen, premixed injection in a buffered diluent solution in plastic containers. Claforan, equivalent to 1 gram and 2 grams cefotaxime, is supplied as frozen, premixed injections in plastic containers in 5% dextrose (containing dextrose hydrous, USP). The injections are buffered with sodium citrate hydrous, USP. The pH is adjusted with hydrochloric acid and may be adjusted with sodium hydroxide. The plastic container is fabricated from a specially formulated polyvinyl chloride. Solutions in contact with the plastic container can leach out certain of its chemical components in very small amounts within the expiration period, e.g., di-2-ethylhexyl phthalate (DEHP), up to 5 parts per million. However, the safety of the plastic has been confirmed in tests in animals according to

USP biological tests for plastic containers as well as by tissue culture toxicity studies.

CLINICAL PHARMACOLOGY

Following IM administration of a single 500 mg or 1 g dose of Claforan to normal volunteers, mean peak serum concentrations of 11.7 and 20.5 μg/mL respectively were attained within 30 minutes and declined with an elimination half-life of approximately 1 hour. There was a dose-dependent increase in serum levels after the IV administration of 500 mg, 1 g and 2 g of Claforan (38.9, 101.7, and 214.4 μg/mL respectively) without alteration in the elimination half-life. There is no evidence of accumulation following repetitive IV infusion of 1 g doses every 6 hours for 14 days as there are no alterations of serum or renal clearance. About 60% of the administered dose was recovered from urine during the first 6 hours following the start of the infusion.

Approximately 20–36% of an intravenously administered dose of ¹⁴C-cefotaxime is excreted by the kidney as unchanged cefotaxime and 15–25% as the desacetyl derivative, the major metabolite. The desacetyl metabolite has been shown to contribute to the bactericidal activity. Two other urinary metabolites (M_2 and M_3) account for about 20–25%. They lack bactericidal activity.

A single 50 mg/kg dose of Claforan was administered as an intravenous infusion over a 10- to 15-minute period to 29 newborn infants grouped according to birth weight and age. The mean half-life of cefotaxime in infants with lower birth weights ($\leq$ 1500 grams), regardless of age, was longer (4.6 hours) than the mean half-life (3.4 hours) in infants whose birth weight was greater than 1500 grams. Mean serum clearance was also smaller in the lower birth weight infants. Although the differences in mean half-life values are statistically significant for weight, they are not clinically important. Therefore, dosage should be based solely on age. (See **Dosage and Administration** section.)

Additionally, no disulfiram-like reactions were reported in a study conducted in 22 healthy volunteers administered Claforan and ethanol.

Microbiology

The bactericidal activity of cefotaxime sodium results from inhibition of cell wall synthesis. Cefotaxime sodium has *in vitro* activity against a wide range of gram-positive and gram-negative organisms. Claforan has a high degree of stability in the presence of beta-lactamases, both penicillinases and cephalosporinases, of gram-negative and gram-positive bacteria. Cefotaxime sodium has been shown to be a potent inhibitor of β-lactamases produced by certain gram-negative bacteria. Cefotaxime sodium is usually active against the following microorganisms both *in vitro* and in clinical infections (see **Indications and Usage**).

Aerobes, Gram-positive: *Staphylococcus aureus*, including penicillinase and non-penicillinase producing strains, *Staphylococcus epidermidis*, *Enterococcus* species, *Streptococcus pyogenes* (Group A beta-hemolytic streptococci), *Streptococcus agalactiae* (Group B streptococci), *Streptococcus pneumoniae* (formerly *Diplococcus pneumoniae*).

Aerobes, Gram-negative: *Citrobacter* species, *Enterobacter* species, *Escherichia coli*, *Haemophilus influenzae* (including ampicillin-resistant *H. influenzae*), *Haemophilus parainfluenzae*, *Klebsiella* species (including *K. pneumoniae*), *Neisseria gonorrhoeae* (including penicillinase and non-penicillinase producing strains), *Neisseria meningitidis*, *Proteus mirabilis*, *Proteus vulgaris*, *Proteus inconstans*, Group B, *Morganella morganii*, *Providencia rettgeri*, *Serratia* species, and *Acinetobacter* species.

NOTE: Many strains of the above organisms that are multiply resistant to other antibiotics, e.g., penicillins, cephalosporins, and aminoglycosides, are susceptible to cefotaxime sodium.

Cefotaxime sodium is active against some strains of *Pseudomonas aeruginosa*.

Anaerobes: *Bacteroides* species, including some strains of *B. fragilis*, *Clostridium* species (NOTE: Most strains of *C. difficile* are resistant), *Peptococcus* species, *Peptostreptococcus* species, and *Fusobacterium* species (including *F. nucleatum*).

Cefotaxime sodium is highly stable *in vitro* to four of the five major classes of β-lactamases described by Richmond et al., including type IIIa (TEM) which is produced by many gram-negative bacteria. The drug is also stable to β-lactamase (penicillinase) produced by staphylococci. In addition, cefotaxime sodium shows high affinity for penicillin-binding proteins in the cell wall, including PBP, Ib and III.

Cefotaxime sodium also demonstrates *in vitro* activity against the following microorganisms although clinical significance is unknown: *Salmonella* species (including *S. typhi*), *Providencia* species, and *Shigella* species.

Cefotaxime sodium and aminoglycosides have been shown to be synergistic *in vitro* against some strains of *Pseudomonas aeruginosa*.

Susceptibility Tests

Quantitative methods that require measurement of zone diameters give the most precise estimate of antibiotic suscep-

Continued on next page

Hoechst-Roussel—Cont.

tibility. One such procedure[1] has been recommended for use with discs to test susceptibility to cefotaxime sodium. Interpretation involves correlation of the diameters obtained in the disc test with minimum inhibitory concentration (MIC) values for cefotaxime sodium.

Reports from the laboratory giving results of the standardized single-disc susceptibility test using a 30-µg cefotaxime sodium disc should be interpreted according to the following criteria:

Susceptible organisms produce zones of 20 mm or greater, indicating that the tested organism is likely to respond to therapy.

Organisms that produce zones of 15 to 19 mm are expected to be susceptible if high dosage is used or if the infection is confined to tissues and fluids (e.g., urine) in which high antibiotic levels are attained.

Resistant organisms produce zones of 14 mm or less, indicating that other therapy should be selected.

Organisms should be tested with the cefotaxime sodium disc, since cefotaxime sodium has been shown by *in vitro* tests to be active against certain strains found resistant when other beta lactam discs are used. The cefotaxime sodium disc should not be used for testing susceptibility to other cephalosporins. Organisms having zones of less than 18 mm around the cephalothin disc are not necessarily of intermediate susceptibility or resistant to cefotaxime sodium.

A bacterial isolate may be considered susceptible if the MIC value for cefotaxime sodium is not more than 16 µg/mL. Organisms are considered resistant to cefotaxime sodium if the MIC is equal to or greater than 64 µg/mL. Organisms having an MIC value of less than 64 µg/mL but greater than 16µg/mL are expected to be susceptible if high dosage is used or if the infection is confined to tissues and fluids (e.g., urine) in which high antibiotic levels are attained.

INDICATIONS AND USAGE

Treatment

Claforan is indicated for the treatment of patients with serious infections caused by susceptible strains of the designated microorganisms in the diseases listed below.

(1) **Lower respiratory tract infections,** including pneumonia, caused by *Streptococcus pneumoniae* (formerly *Diplococcus pneumoniae*), *Streptococcus pyogenes* * (Group A streptococci) and other streptococci (excluding enterococci, e.g., *Streptococcus faecalis*), *Staphylococcus aureus* (penicillinase and non-penicillinase producing), *Escherichia coli, Klebsiella* species, *Haemophilus influenzae* (including ampicillin resistant strains), *Haemophilus parainfluenzae, Proteus mirabilis, Serratia marcescens**, *Enterobacter* species, indole positive *Proteus* and *Pseudomonas* species (including *P. aeruginosa*).

(2) **Genitourinary infections.** Urinary tract infections caused by *Enterococcus* species, *Staphylococcus epidermidis, Staphylococcus aureus** (penicillinase and non-penicillinase producing), *Citrobacter* species, *Enterobacter* species, *Escherichia coli, Klebsiella* species, *Proteus mirabilis, Proteus vulgaris**, *Proteus inconstans* Group B, *Morganella morganii**, *Providencia rettgeri**, and *Serratia marcescens,* and *Pseudomonas* species (including *P. aeruginosa*). Also, uncomplicated gonorrhea of single or multiple sites caused by *Neisseria gonorrhoeae,* including penicillinase producing strains.

(3) **Gynecologic infections,** including pelvic inflammatory disease, endometritis and pelvic cellulitis caused by *Staphylococcus epidermidis, Streptococcus* species, *Enterococcus* species, *Enterobacter* species*, *Klebsiella* species*, *Escherichia coli, Proteus mirabilis, Bacteroides* species (including *Bacteroides fragilis**), *Clostridium* species, and anaerobic cocci (including *Peptostreptococcus* species and *Peptococcus* species) and *Fusobacterium* species (including *F. nucleatum**).

(4) **Bacteremia/Septicemia** caused by *Escherichia coli, Klebsiella* species, *Serratia marcescens, Staphylococcus aureus,* and *Streptococcus* species (including *S. pneumoniae*).

(5) **Skin and skin structure infections** caused by *Staphylococcus aureus* (penicillinase and non-penicillinase producing), *Staphylococcus epidermidis, Streptococcus pyogenes* (Group A streptococci) and other streptococci, *Enterococcus* species, *Acinetobacter* species*, *Escherichia coli, Citrobacter* species (including *C. freundii**). *Enterobacter* species, *Klebsiella* species, *Proteus mirabilis, Proteus vulgaris**, *Morganella morganii, Providencia rettgeri**, *Pseudomonas* species, *Serratia marcescens, Bacteroides* species, and anaerobic cocci (including *Peptostreptococcus** species and *Peptococcus* species).

(6) **Intra-abdominal infections** including peritonitis caused by *Streptococcus* species*, *Escherichia coli, Klebsiella* species, *Bacteroides* species, and anaerobic cocci (including *Peptostreptococcus** species and *Peptococcus** species), *Proteus mirabilis**, and *Clostridium* species* .

(7) **Bone and/or joint infections** caused by *Staphylococcus aureus* (penicillinase and non-penicillinase producing

strains), *Streptococcus* species (including *S. pyogenes* *), *Pseudomonas* species (including *P. aeruginosa* *), and *Proteus mirabilis**.

(8) **Central nervous system infections,** e.g., meningitis and ventriculitis, caused by *Neisseria meningitidis, Haemophilus influenzae, Streptococcus pneumoniae, Klebsiella pneumoniae**, and *Escherichia coli**.

(*) Efficacy for this organism, in this organ system, has been studied in fewer than 10 infections.

Although many strains of enterococci (e.g., *S. faecalis*) and *Pseudomonas* species are resistant to cefotaxime sodium *in vitro,* Claforan has been used successfully in treating patients with infections caused by susceptible organisms.

Specimens for bacteriologic culture should be obtained prior to therapy in order to isolate and identify causative organisms and to determine their susceptibilities to Claforan. Therapy may be instituted before results of susceptibility studies are known; however, once these results become available, the antibiotic treatment should be adjusted accordingly.

In certain cases of confirmed or suspected gram-positive or gram-negative sepsis or in patients with other serious infections in which the causative organism has not been identified, Claforan may be used concomitantly with an aminoglycoside. The dosage recommended in the labeling of both antibiotics may be given and depends on the severity of the infection and the patient's condition. Renal function should be carefully monitored, especially if higher dosages of the aminoglycosides are to be administered or if therapy is prolonged, because of the potential nephrotoxicity and ototoxicity of aminoglycoside antibiotics. Some β-lactam antibiotics also have a certain degree of nephrotoxicity. Although, to date, this has not been noted when Claforan was given alone, it is possible that nephrotoxicity may be potentiated if Claforan is used concomitantly with an aminoglycoside.

Prevention

The administration of Claforan preoperatively reduces the incidence of certain infections in patients undergoing surgical procedures (e.g. abdominal or vaginal hysterectomy, gastrointestinal and genitourinary tract surgery) that may be classified as contaminated or potentially contaminated.

In patients undergoing cesarean section, intraoperative (after clamping the umbilical cord) and postoperative use of Claforan may also reduce the incidence of certain postoperative infections. See **Dosage and Administration** section.

Effective use for elective surgery depends on the time of administration. To achieve effective tissue levels, Claforan should be given ½ to 1½ hours before surgery. See **Dosage and Administration** section.

For patients undergoing gastrointestinal surgery, preoperative bowel preparation by mechanical cleansing as well as with a non-absorbable antibiotic (e.g., neomycin) is recommended.

If there are signs of infection, specimens for culture should be obtained for identification of the causative organism so that appropriate therapy may be instituted.

CONTRAINDICATIONS

Claforan is contraindicated in patients who have shown hypersensitivity to cefotaxime sodium or the cephalosporin group of antibiotics.

WARNINGS

BEFORE THERAPY WITH CLAFORAN IS INSTITUTED, CAREFUL INQUIRY SHOULD BE MADE TO DETERMINE WHETHER THE PATIENT HAS HAD PREVIOUS HYPERSENSITIVITY REACTIONS TO CEFOTAXIME SODIUM, CEPHALOSPORINS, PENICILLINS, OR OTHER DRUGS. THIS PRODUCT SHOULD BE GIVEN WITH CAUTION TO PATIENTS WITH TYPE 1 HYPERSENSITIVITY REACTIONS TO PENICILLIN. ANTIBIOTICS SHOULD BE ADMINISTERED WITH CAUTION TO ANY PATIENT WHO HAS DEMONSTRATED SOME FORM OF ALLERGY, PARTICULARLY TO DRUGS. IF AN ALLERGIC REACTION TO CLAFORAN OCCURS, DISCONTINUE TREATMENT WITH THE DRUG. SERIOUS HYPERSENSITIVITY REACTIONS MAY REQUIRE EPINEPHRINE AND OTHER EMERGENCY MEASURES.

Pseudomembranous colitis has been reported with the use of cephalosporins (and other broad spectrum antibiotics); therefore, it is important to consider its diagnosis in patients who develop diarrhea in association with antibiotic use.

Treatment with broad spectrum antibiotics alters normal flora of the colon and may permit overgrowth of Clostridia. Studies indicate a toxin produced by *Clostridium difficile* is one primary cause of antibiotic-associated colitis. Cholestyramine and colestipol resins have been shown to bind the toxin *in vitro.*

Mild cases of colitis may respond to drug discontinuance alone.

Moderate to severe cases should be managed with fluid, electrolyte, and protein supplementation as indicated.

When the colitis is not relieved by drug discontinuance or when it is severe, oral vancomycin is the treatment of choice for antibiotic-associated pseudomembranous colitis pro-

duced by *C. difficile.* Other causes of colitis should also be considered.

PRECAUTIONS

Claforan® (cefotaxime sodium) should be prescribed with caution in individuals with a history of gastrointestinal disease, particularly colitis.

Claforan has not been shown to be nephrotoxic; however, because high and prolonged serum antibiotic concentrations can occur from usual doses in patients with transient or persistent reduction of urinary output because of renal insufficiency, the total daily dosage should be reduced when Claforan is administered to such patients. Continued dosage should be determined by degree of renal impairment, severity of infection, and susceptibility of the causative organism. Although there is no clinical evidence supporting the necessity of changing the dosage of cefotaxime sodium in patients with even profound renal dysfunction, it is suggested that, until further data are obtained, the dose of cefotaxime sodium be halved in patients with estimated creatinine clearances of less than 20 mL/min/1.73 m[2].

When only serum creatinine is available, the following formula[2] (based on sex, weight, and age of the patient) may be used to convert this value into creatinine clearance. The serum creatinine should represent a steady state of renal function.

$$\frac{\text{Weight (kg)} \times (140 - \text{age})}{72 \times \text{serum creatinine}}$$

Males $72 \times$ serum creatinine

Females $0.85 \times$ above value

As with other antibiotics, prolonged use of Claforan may result in overgrowth of nonsusceptible organisms. Repeated evaluation of the patient's condition is essential. If superinfection occurs during therapy, appropriate measures should be taken.

Drug Interactions: Increased nephrotoxicity has been reported following concomitant administration of cephalosporins and aminoglycoside antibiotics.

Carcinogenesis, Mutagenesis: Long-term studies in animals have not been performed to evaluate carcinogenic potential. Mutagenic tests included a micronucleus and an Ames test. Both tests were negative for mutagenic effects.

Pregnancy (Category B): Reproduction studies have been performed in mice and rats at doses up to 30 times the usual human dose and have revealed no evidence of impaired fertility or harm to the fetus because of cefotaxime sodium. However, there are no well-controlled studies in pregnant women. Because animal reproductive studies are not always predictive of human response, this drug should be used during pregnancy only if clearly needed.

Nonteratogenic Effects: Use of the drug in women of childbearing potential requires that the anticipated benefit be weighed against the possible risks.

In perinatal and postnatal studies with rats, the pups in the group given 1200 mg/kg of Claforan were significantly lighter in weight at birth and remained smaller than pups in the control group during the 21 days of nursing.

Nursing Mothers: Claforan is excreted in human milk in low concentrations. Caution should be exercised when Claforan is administered to a nursing woman.

ADVERSE REACTIONS

Claforan is generally well tolerated. The most common adverse reactions have been local reactions following IM or IV injection. Other adverse reactions have been encountered infrequently.

The most frequent adverse reactions (greater than 1%) are:

Local (4.3%) - Injection site inflammation with IV administration. Pain, induration, and tenderness after IM injection.

Hypersensitivity (2.4%) - Rash, pruritus, fever, and eosinophilia.

Gastrointestinal (1.4%) - Colitis, diarrhea, nausea, and vomiting.

Symptoms of pseudomembranous colitis can appear during or after antibiotic treatment.

Nausea and vomiting have been reported rarely.

Less frequent adverse reactions (less than 1%) are:

Hemic and Lymphatic System - Granulocytopenia, transient leukopenia, eosinophilia, neutropenia and thrombocytopenia have been reported. Some individuals have developed positive direct Coombs Tests during treatment with the cephalosporin antibiotics.

Genitourinary System - Moniliasis, vaginitis.

Central Nervous System - Headache.

Liver - Transient elevations in SGOT, SGPT, serum LDH, and serum alkaline phosphatase levels have been reported.

Kidney - As with some other cephalosporins, transient elevations of BUN have been occasionally observed with Claforan.

DOSAGE AND ADMINISTRATION

Adults

Dosage and route of administration should be determined by susceptibility of the causative organisms, severity of the infection, and the condition of the patient (see table for dosage guideline). Claforan may be administered IM or IV after

reconstitution. Premixed Claforan Injection is intended for IV administration after thawing. The maximum daily dosage should not exceed 12 grams.
[See table right].
To prevent postoperative infection in contaminated or potentially contaminated surgery, the recommended dose is a single 1 gram IM or IV administered 30 to 90 minutes prior to start of surgery.

Cesarean Section Patients
The first dose of 1 gram is administered intravenously as soon as the umbilical cord is clamped. The second and third doses should be given as 1 gram intravenously or intramuscularly at 6 and 12 hours after the first dose.

Neonates, Infants and Children
The following dosage schedule is recommended:
Neonates (birth to 1 month):

0–1 week of age	50 mg/kg IV q 12 h
1–4 weeks of age	50 mg/kg IV q 8 h

It is not necessary to differentiate between premature and normal-gestational age infants.
Infants and Children (1 month to 12 years): For body weights less than 50 kg, the recommended daily dose is 50 to 180 mg/kg IM or IV of body weight divided into four to six equal doses. The higher dosages should be used for more severe or serious infections, including meningitis. For body weights 50 kg or more, the usual adult dosage should be used; the maximum daily dosage should not exceed 12 grams.
Impaired Renal Function - see **Precautions** section.
NOTE: As with antibiotic therapy in general, administration of Claforan should be continued for a minimum of 48 to 72 hours after the patient defervesces or after evidence of bacterial eradication has been obtained; a minimum of 10 days of treatment is recommended for infections caused by Group A beta-hemolytic streptococci in order to guard against the risk of rheumatic fever or glomerulonephritis; frequent bacteriologic and clinical appraisal is necessary during therapy of chronic urinary tract infection and may be required for several months after therapy has been completed; persistent infections may require treatment of several weeks and doses smaller than those indicated above should not be used.

PREPARATION OF CLAFORAN STERILE
Claforan for IM or IV administration should be reconstituted as follows:

Strength	Diluent (mL)	Withdrawable Volume (mL)	Approximate Concentration (mg/mL)
1g vial (IM)*	3	3.4	300
2g vial (IM)*	5	6.0	330
1g vial (IV)*	10	10.4	95
2g vial (IV)*	10	11.0	180
1g infusion	50–100	50–100	20–10
2g infusion	50–100	50–100	40–20
10g bottle	47	52.0	200
10g bottle	97	102.0	100

*in conventional vials

Shake to dissolve; inspect for particulate matter and discoloration prior to use. Solutions of Claforan range from light yellow to amber, depending on concentration, diluent used, and length and condition of storage.
For intramuscular use: Reconstitute VIALS with Sterile Water for Injection or Bacteriostatic Water for Injection as described above.
For intravenous use: Reconstitute VIALS with at least 10 mL of Sterile Water for Injection. Reconstitute INFUSION BOTTLES with 50 or 100 mL of 0.9% Sodium Chloride Injection or 5% Dextrose Injection. For other diluents, see **COMPATIBILITY and STABILITY** section.
Pharmacy Bulk Package: Reconstitute with 47 mL of diluent for an approximate concentration of 200 mg/mL or 97 mL of diluent for an approximate concentration of 100 mg/mL. Stock solutions may be further diluted for IV infusion with diluents as listed in **COMPATIBILITY and STABILITY** section.
NOTE: Solutions of Claforan must not be admixed with aminoglycoside solutions. If Claforan and aminoglycosides are to be administered to the same patient, they must be administered separately and not as mixed injection.
A SOLUTION OF 1 G CLAFORAN IN 14 ML OF STERILE WATER FOR INJECTION IS ISOTONIC.
IM Administration: As with all IM preparations, Claforan should be injected well within the body of a relatively large muscle such as the upper outer quadrant of the buttock (i.e., gluteus maximus); aspiration is necessary to avoid inadvertent injection into a blood vessel. Individual IM doses of 2 grams may be given if the dose is divided and is administered in different intramuscular sites.
IV Administration: The IV route is preferable for patients with bacteremia, bacterial septicemia, peritonitis, meningitis, or other severe or life-threatening infections, or for patients who may be poor risks because of lowered resistance resulting from such debilitating conditions as malnutrition, trauma, surgery, diabetes, heart failure, or malignancy, particularly if shock is present or impending.
For intermittent IV administration, a solution containing 1 gram or 2 grams in 10 mL of Sterile Water for Injection can

GUIDELINES FOR DOSAGE OF CLAFORAN

Type of Infection	Daily Dose (grams)	Frequency and Route
Gonorrhea	1	1 gram IM (single dose)
Uncomplicated infections	2	1 gram every 12 hours IM or IV
Moderate to severe infections	3–6	1–2 grams every 8 hours IM or IV
Infections commonly needing antibiotics in higher dosage (e.g., septicemia)	6–8	2 grams every 6–8 hours IV
Life-threatening infections	up to 12	2 grams every 4 hours IV

be injected over a period of three to five minutes. With an infusion system, it may also be given over a longer period of time through the tubing system by which the patient may be receiving other IV solutions. However, during infusion of the solution containing Claforan, it is advisable to discontinue temporarily the administration of other solutions at the same site.
For the administration of higher doses by continuous IV infusion, a solution of Claforan may be added to IV bottles containing the solutions discussed below.

Preparation of Premixed Claforan Injection in Plastic Container
Premixed Claforan Injection may be used directly after thawing at room temperature. Solutions range from very pale yellow to light amber. After thawing, check for minute leaks by squeezing bag firmly and inspect for particulate matter, discoloration and solution clarity. Discard if leaks are found or seal is not intact. Additives should not be introduced into this solution.
Use sterile equipment.
WARNING: Do not use plastic containers in series connections. Such use could result in air embolism due to residual air being drawn from the primary container before administration of the fluid from the secondary container is complete.
Preparation for administration:
1. Suspend container from eyelet support.
2. Remove plastic protector from outlet port at bottom of container.
3. Attach administration set. Refer to complete directions accompanying set.
After thawing, premixed Claforan Injection, 1 gram and 2 grams in 50 mL plastic containers may be used for continuous or intermittent intravenous infusion.

PREPARATION OF CLAFORAN STERILE IN ADD-VANTAGE® SYSTEM
Claforan Sterile 1 g or 2 g may be reconstituted in 50 mL or 100 mL of 5% Dextrose or 0.9% Sodium Chloride in the ADD-Vantage® diluent container. Refer to enclosed, separate INSTRUCTIONS FOR ADD-VANTAGE® SYSTEM.

COMPATIBILITY AND STABILITY
Solutions of Claforan Sterile reconstituted as described above (**Preparation of Claforan Sterile**) maintain satisfactory potency for 24 hours at room temperature (at or below 22℃), 10 days under refrigeration (at or below 5℃), and for at least 13 weeks frozen. Solutions may be stored in disposable glass or plastic syringes for 24 hours at room temperature (at or below 22℃), 5 days under refrigeration (at or below 5℃), and 13 weeks frozen.
Reconstituted solutions may be further diluted up to 1000 mL with the following solutions and maintain satisfactory potency for 24 hours at room temperature (at or below 22℃), and at least 5 days under refrigeration (at or below 5℃); 0.9% Sodium Chloride Injection; 5 or 10% Dextrose Injection; 5% Dextrose and 0.9% Sodium Chloride Injection; 5% Dextrose and 0.45% Sodium Chloride Injection; 5% Dextrose and 0.2% Sodium Chloride Injection; Lactated Ringer's Solution; Sodium Lactate Injection (M/6); 10% Invert Sugar Injection, 8.5% TRAVASOL® (Amino Acid) Injection without Electrolytes.
Solutions of Claforan Sterile reconstituted in 0.9% Sodium Chloride Injection or 5% Dextrose Injection in Viaflex® plastic containers maintain satisfactory potency for 24 hours at room temperature (at or below 22℃), 5 days under refrigeration (at or below 5℃) and 13 weeks frozen. Solutions of Claforan Sterile reconstituted in 0.9% Sodium Chloride Injection or 5% Dextrose Injection in the ADD-Vantage® flexible containers maintain satisfactory potency for 24 hours at room temperature (at or below 22℃). DO NOT FREEZE.
NOTE: Claforan solutions exhibit maximum stability in the pH 5–7 range. Solutions of Claforan should not be prepared with diluents having a pH above 7.5, such as Sodium Bicarbonate Injection.
Claforan supplied as premixed, frozen injection is stable for the expiration dating period as indicated on the label. Thawed solutions of premixed Claforan Injection in plastic containers are stable for 24 hours at room temperature (at or below 22℃) or for 10 days under refrigeration (at or below 5℃).
Frozen samples should not be heated but should be thawed at room temperature before use. After the periods mentioned

above, any unused solutions or frozen material should be discarded. DO NOT REFREEZE.

HOW SUPPLIED
Sterile Claforan is a dry off-white to pale yellow crystalline powder supplied in vials and bottles containing cefotaxime sodium as follows:
1 g cefotaxime (free acid equivalent) in vials in packages of 10 (NDC 0039-0018-10), packages of 25 (NDC 0039-0018-25), packages of 50 (NDC 0039-0018-50); infusion bottles in packages of 10 (NDC 0039-0018-11)
2 g cefotaxime (free acid equivalent) in vials in packages of 10 (NDC 0039-0019-10), in packages of 25 (NDC 0039-0019-25), in packages of 50 (NDC 0039-0019-50); infusion bottles in packages of 10 (NDC 0039-0019-11)
10 g cefotaxime (free acid equivalent) in bottles (NDC 0039-0020-01).
1 g cefotaxime (free acid equivalent) in ADD-Vantage® System vials in packages of 25 (NDC 0039-0023-25) and 50 (NDC 0039-0023-50).
2 g cefotaxime (free acid equivalent) in ADD-Vantage® System vials in packages of 25 (NDC 0039-0024-25) and 50 (NDC 0039-0024-50). ADD-Vantage® System diluents (5% Dextrose or 0.9% Sodium Chloride) are available from Abbott Laboratories.
NOTE: Claforan in the dry state should be stored below 30℃. The dry material as well as solutions tend to darken depending on storage conditions and should be protected from elevated temperatures and excessive light.
Premixed Claforan injection is supplied as a frozen, sterile, nonpyrogenic solution in 50 mL single dose plastic containers as follows:
1 g cefotaxime (free acid equivalent) in 5% dextrose solution in packages of 24 (NDC 0039-0043-50) 2B3518
2 g cefotaxime (free acid equivalent) in 5% dextrose solution in packages of 24 (NDC 0039-0044-50) 2B3519
NOTE: Premixed Claforan Injection in the frozen state should not be stored above −20℃.
Claforan injection supplied as a frozen, sterile, nonpyrogenic solution in plastic containers is manufactured for Hoechst-Roussel Pharmaceticals Inc., by Travenol Laboratories, Inc., Deerfield, IL 60015.

References:
1) Bauer, A.W.; Kirby, W.M.M.; Sherris, J.C.; and Turck, M.: Antibiotic Susceptibility Testing by a Standardized Single Disk Method, Am. J. Clin. Pathol., 45:493, 1966; Standardized Disc Susceptibility Test, Federal Register, 39:19182-4, 1974. National Committee for Clinical Laboratory Standards, Approved Standard: ASM-2, Performance Standards for Antimicrobial Disc Susceptibility Tests, July, 1975.
2) Cockcroft, D.W. and Gault, M.H.: Prediction of Creatinine Clearance from Serum Creatinine. Nephron 16:31-41, 1976.

CLAFORAN® REG TM ROUSSEL-UCLAF
VIAFLEX® REG TM BAXTER TRAVENOL LABS, INC.
ADD-Vantage REG TM ABBOTT LABORATORIES
Patent Pending
71789T-10/87
*U.S. Patent 4,152,432

DIAβETA®   ℞
(glyburide)*
Tablets 1.25, 2.5 and 5.0 mg

DESCRIPTION
Diaβeta® (glyburide) is an oral blood-glucose-lowering drug of the sulfonylurea class. It is a white, crystalline compound, formulated as tablets of 1.25 mg, 2.5 mg, and 5 mg strengths for oral administration. Diaβeta® tablets contain the active ingredient glyburide and the following inactive ingredients: dibasic calcium phosphate USP, magnesium stearate NF, microcrystalline cellulose NF, sodium alginate NF, talc USP. Diaβeta® 2.5 mg tablets also contain FD&C Red #40. Diaβeta® 5 mg tablets also contain D&C Yellow #10 and FD&C Blue #1.
Chemically, Diaβeta® (glyburide) is identified as 1-[p-[2-(5-chloro-O-anisamido)ethyl] phenyl] -sulfonyl] -3-cyclohexylurea. The structural formula is:
[See Chemical Formula at top of next page].

Continued on next page

Hoechst-Roussel—Cont.

The molecular weight is 493.99. The aqueous solubility of Diaβeta® (glyburide) increases with pH as a result of salt formation.

CLINICAL PHARMACOLOGY

Diaβeta® (glyburide) appears to lower the blood glucose acutely by stimulating the release of insulin from the pancreas, an effect dependent upon functioning beta cells in the pancreatic islets. The mechanism by which Diaβeta® (glyburide) lowers blood glucose during long-term administration has not been clearly established.

With chronic administration in Type II diabetic patients, the blood glucose lowering effect persists despite a gradual decline in the insulin secretory response to the drug. Extrapancreatic effects may play a part in the mechanism of action of oral sulfonylurea hypoglycemic drugs.

In addition to its blood glucose lowering actions, Diaβeta® (glyburide) produces a mild diuresis by enhancement of renal free water clearance. Clinical experience to date indicates an extremely low incidence of disulfiram-like reactions in patients while taking Diaβeta® (glyburide).

Pharmacokinetics

Single-dose studies with Diaβeta® (glyburide) in normal subjects demonstrate significant absorption within one hour, peak drug levels at about four hours, and low but detectable levels at twenty-four hours. Mean serum levels of glyburide, as reflected by areas under the serum concentration-time curve, increase in proportion to corresponding increases in dose. Multiple-dose studies with Diaβeta® (glyburide) in diabetic patients demonstrate drug level concentration-time curves similar to single-dose studies, indicating no build-up of drug in tissue depots. The decrease of glyburide in the serum of normal healthy individuals is biphasic, the terminal half-life being about 10 hours. In single-dose studies in fasting normal subjects, the degree and duration of blood glucose lowering is proportional to the dose administered and to the area under the drug level concentration-time curve. The blood glucose lowering effect persists for 24 hours following single morning doses in non-fasting diabetic patients. Under conditions of repeated administration in diabetic patients, however, there is no reliable correlation between blood drug levels and fasting blood glucose levels. A one-year study of diabetic patients treated with Diaβeta® (glyburide) showed no reliable correlation between administered dose and serum drug level.

The major metabolite of Diaβeta® (glyburide) is the 4-trans-hydroxy derivative. A second metabolite, the 3-cis-hydroxy derivative, also occurs. These metabolites contribute no significant hypoglycemic action since they are only weakly active ($\frac{1}{400}$th and $\frac{1}{40}$th, respectively, as glyburide) in rabbits.

Diaβeta® (glyburide) is excreted as metabolites in the bile and urine, approximately 50% by each route. This dual excretory pathway is qualitatively different from that of other sulfonylureas, which are excreted primarily in the urine.

Sulfonylurea drugs are extensively bound to serum proteins. Displacement from protein binding sites by other drugs may lead to enhanced hypoglycemic action. In vitro, the protein binding exhibited by Diaβeta® (glyburide) is predominantly non-ionic, whereas that of other sulfonylureas (chlorpropamide, tolbutamide, tolazamide) is predominantly ionic. Acidic drugs such as phenylbutazone, warfarin, and salicylates displace the ionic-binding sulfonylureas from serum proteins to a far greater extent than the non-ionic binding Diaβeta® (glyburide). It has not been shown that this difference in protein binding will result in fewer drug-drug interactions with Diaβeta® (glyburide) in clinical use.

INDICATIONS AND USAGE

Diaβeta® (glyburide) is indicated as an adjunct to diet to lower the blood glucose in patients with non-insulin-dependent diabetes mellitus (Type II) whose hyperglycemia cannot be controlled by diet alone.

In initiating treatment for non-insulin-dependent diabetes, diet should be emphasized as the primary form of treatment. Caloric restriction and weight loss are essential in the obese diabetic patient. Proper dietary management alone may be effective in controlling the blood glucose and symptoms of hyperglycemia. The importance of regular physical activity should also be stressed, and cardiovascular risk factors should be identified and corrective measures taken where possible.

If this treatment program fails to reduce symptoms and/or blood glucose, the use of an oral sulfonylurea or insulin should be considered. Use of Diaβeta® (glyburide) must be viewed by both the physician and patient as a treatment in addition to diet, and not as a substitute for diet or as a convenient mechanism for avoiding dietary restraint. Furthermore, loss of blood glucose control on diet alone may be transient, thus requiring only short-term administration of Diaβeta® (glyburide).

During maintenance programs, Diaβeta® (glyburide) should be discontinued if satisfactory lowering of blood glucose is no longer achieved. Judgments should be based on regular clinical and laboratory evaluations.

In considering the use of Diaβeta® (glyburide) in asymptomatic patients, it should be recognized that controlling the blood glucose in non-insulin dependent diabetes has not been definitely established to be effective in preventing the long-term cardiovascular or neural complications of diabetes.

CONTRAINDICATIONS

Diaβeta® (glyburide) is contraindicated in patients with:
1. Known hypersensitivity to the drug.
2. Diabetic ketoacidosis, with or without coma. This condition should be treated with insulin.

WARNINGS:

SPECIAL WARNING ON INCREASED RISK OF CARDIOVASCULAR MORTALITY

The administration of oral hypoglycemic drugs has been reported to be associated with increased cardiovascular mortality as compared to treatment with diet alone or diet plus insulin. This warning is based on the study conducted by the University Group Diabetes Program (UGDP), a long-term prospective clinical trial designed to evaluate the effectiveness of glucose-lowering drugs in preventing or delaying vascular complications in patients with non-insulin-dependent diabetes. The study involved 823 patients who were randomly assigned to one of four treatment groups (Diabetes, 19 (supp. 2): 747-830, 1970).

UGDP reported that patients treated for 5 to 8 years with diet plus a fixed dose of tolbutamide (1.5 grams per day) had a rate of cardiovascular mortality approximately 2$\frac{1}{2}$ times that of patients treated with diet alone. A significant increase in total mortality was not observed, but the use of tolbutamide was discontinued based on the increase in cardiovascular mortality, thus limiting the opportunity for the study to show an increase in overall mortality. Despite controversy regarding the interpretation of these results, the findings of the UGDP study provide an adequate basis for this warning. The patient should be informed of the potential risks and advantages of Diaβeta® (glyburide) and of alternative modes of therapy.

Although only one drug in the sulfonylurea class (tolbutamide) was included in this study, it is prudent from a safety standpoint to consider that this warning may also apply to other oral hypoglycemic drugs in this class, in view of their close similarities in mode of action and chemical structure.

PRECAUTIONS

General

Hypoglycemia: All sulfonylurea drugs are capable of producing severe hypoglycemia. Proper patient selection, dosage, and instructions are important to avoid hypoglycemic episodes. Renal or hepatic insufficiency may cause elevated blood levels of Diaβeta® (glyburide) and the latter may also diminish gluconeogenic capacity, both of which increase the risk of serious hypoglycemic reactions. Elderly, debilitated or malnourished patients, and those with adrenal or pituitary insufficiency are particularly susceptible to the hypoglycemic action of glucose-lowering drugs. Hypoglycemia may be difficult to recognize in the elderly, and in people who are taking beta-adrenergic blocking drugs. Hypoglycemia is more likely to occur when caloric intake is deficient, after severe or prolonged exercise, when alcohol is ingested, or when more than one glucose-lowering drug is used.

Loss of control of blood glucose: When a patient stabilized on any diabetic regimen is exposed to stress such as fever, trauma, infection, or surgery, a loss of control may occur. At such times, it may be necessary to discontinue Diaβeta® (glyburide) and administer insulin.

The effectiveness of any oral hypoglycemic drug, including Diaβeta® (glyburide), in lowering blood glucose to a desired level decreases in many patients over a period of time, which may be due to progression of the severity of the diabetes or to diminished responsiveness to the drug. This phenomenon is known as secondary failure, to distinguish it from primary failure in which the drug is ineffective in an individual patient when first given.

Information for Patients

Patients should be informed of the potential risks and advantages of Diaβeta® (glyburide) and of alternative modes of therapy. They should also be informed about the importance of adherence to dietary instructions, of a regular exercise program, and of regular testing of urine and/or blood glucose.

The risks of hypoglycemia, its symptoms and treatment, and conditions that predispose to its development should be explained to patients and responsible family members. Primary and secondary failure should also be explained.

Laboratory Tests

Blood and urine glucose should be monitored periodically. Measurement of glycosylated hemoglobin may be useful.

Drug Interactions

The hypoglycemic action of sulfonylureas may be potentiated by certain drugs including nonsteroidal anti-inflammatory agents and other drugs that are highly protein bound, salicylates, sulfonamides, chloramphenicol, probenecid, coumarins, monoamine oxidase inhibitors, and beta adrenergic blocking agents. When such drugs are administered to a patient receiving Diaβeta® (glyburide), the patient should be observed closely for hypoglycemia. When such drugs are withdrawn from a patient receiving Diaβeta® (glyburide), the patient should be observed closely for loss of control. Certain drugs tend to produce hyperglycemia and may lead to loss of control. These drugs include the thiazides and other diuretics, corticosteroids, phenothiazines, thyroid products, estrogens, oral contraceptives, phenytoin, nicotinic acid, sympathomimetics, calcium channel blocking drugs, and isoniazid. When such drugs are administered to a patient receiving Diaβeta® (glyburide), the patient should be closely observed for loss of control. When such drugs are withdrawn from a patient receiving Diaβeta® (glyburide), the patient should be observed closely for hypoglycemia.

A potential interaction between oral miconazole and oral hypoglycemic agents leading to severe hypoglycemia has been reported. Whether this interaction also occurs with the intravenous, topical or vaginal preparations of miconazole is not known.

Carcinogenesis, Mutagenesis, and Impairment of Fertility

Diaβeta® (glyburide) is non-mutagenic when studied in the Salmonella microsome test (Ames test) and in the DNA damage/alkaline elution assay. Studies in rats at doses up to 300 mg/kg/day for 18 months showed no carcinogenic effects.

Pregnancy

Teratogenic Effects: Pregnancy Category B

Reproduction studies have been performed in rats and rabbits at doses up to 500 times the human dose and have revealed no evidence of impaired fertility or harm to the fetus due to Diaβeta®(glyburide). There are, however, no adequate and well controlled studies in pregnant women. Because animal reproduction studies are not always predictive of human response, this drug should be used during pregnancy only if clearly needed.

Because recent information suggests that abnormal blood glucose levels during pregnancy are associated with a higher incidence of congenital abnormalities, many experts recommend that insulin be used during pregnancy to maintain blood glucose levels as close to normal as possible.

Nonteratogenic Effects

Prolonged severe hypoglycemia (4 to 10 days) has been reported in neonates born to mothers who were receiving a sulfonylurea drug at the time of delivery. This had been reported more frequently with the use of agents with prolonged half-lives. If Diaβeta® (glyburide) is used during pregnancy, it should be discontinued at least two weeks before the expected delivery date.

Nursing Mothers

Although it is not known whether Diaβeta® (glyburide) is excreted in human milk, some sulfonylureas are known to be excreted in human milk. Because the potential for hypoglycemia in nursing infants may exist, a decision should be made whether to discontinue nursing or to discontinue administering the drug, taking into account the importance of the drug to the mother. If Diaβeta® (glyburide) is discontinued and if diet alone is inadequate for controlling blood glucose, insulin therapy should be considered.

Pediatric Use: Safety and effectiveness in children have not been established.

ADVERSE REACTIONS

Hypoglycemia: See **Precautions** and **Overdosage** Sections.

Gastrointestinal Reactions: Cholestatic jaundice and hepatitis may occur rarely; Diaβeta® (glyburide) should be discontinued if this occurs. Liver function abnormalities, including isolated transaminase elevations, have been reported. Gastrointestinal disturbances, e.g., nausea, epigastric fullness, and heartburn, are the most common reactions and occur in 1.8% of treated patients. They tend to be dose-related and may disappear when dosage is reduced.

Dermatologic Reactions: Allergic skin reactions, e.g., pruritus, erythema, urticaria, and morbilliform or maculopapular eruptions, occur in 1.5% of treated patients. These may be transient and may disappear despite continued use of Diaβeta® (glyburide); if skin reactions persist, the drug should be discontinued.

Porphyria cutanea tarda and photosensitivity reactions have been reported with sulfonylureas.

Hematologic Reactions: Leukopenia, agranulocytosis, thrombocytopenia, hemolytic anemia, aplastic anemia, and pancytopenia have been reported with sulfonylureas.

Metabolic Reactions: Hepatic porphyria reactions have been reported with sulfonylureas; however, these have not been reported with Diaβeta® (glyburide). Disulfiram-like reactions have been reported very rarely with Diaβeta® (glyburide).

Cases of hyponatremia have been reported with glyburide and all other sulfonylureas, most often in patients who are on other medications or have medical conditions known to cause hyponatremia or increase release of antidiuretic hormone. The syndrome of inappropriate antidiuretic hormone (SIADH) secretion has been reported with certain other sulfonylureas, and it has been suggested that these sulfonylureas may augment the peripheral (antidiuretic) action of ADH and/or increase release of ADH.

OVERDOSAGE

Overdosage of sulfonylureas, including Diaβeta® (glyburide), can produce hypoglycemia. Mild hypoglycemic symptoms without loss of consciousness or neurologic findings should be treated aggressively with oral glucose and adjustments in drug dosage and/or meal patterns. Close monitoring should continue until the physician is assured that the patient is out of danger. Severe hypoglycemic reactions with coma, seizure, or other neurological impairment occur infrequently, but constitute medical emergencies requiring immediate hospitalization. If hypoglycemic coma is diagnosed or suspected, the patient should be given a rapid intravenous injection of concentrated (50%) glucose solution. This should be followed by a continuous infusion of a more dilute (10%) glucose solution at a rate that will maintain the blood glucose at a level above 100 mg/dL. Patients should be closely monitored for a minimum of 24 to 48 hours, since hypoglycemia may recur after apparent clinical recovery.

DOSAGE AND ADMINISTRATION

There is no fixed dosage regimen for the management of diabetes mellitus with Diaβeta® (glyburide) or any other hypoglycemic agent. In addition to the usual monitoring of urinary glucose, the patient's blood glucose must also be monitored periodically to determine the minimum effective dose for the patient; to detect primary failure, i.e., inadequate lowering of blood glucose at the maximum recommended dose of medication; and to detect secondary failure, i.e., loss of adequate blood glucose lowering response after an initial period of effectiveness. Glycosylated hemoglobin levels may also be of value in monitoring the patient's response to therapy.

Short-term administration of Diaβeta® (glyburide) may be sufficient during periods of transient loss of control in patients usually controlled well on diet.

1. Usual Starting Dose

The usual starting dose of Diaβeta® (glyburide) as initial therapy is 2.5–5 mg daily, administered with breakfast or the first main meal. Those patients who may be more sensitive to hypoglycemic drugs should be started at 1.25 mg daily. (See **Precautions** Section for patients at increased risk.) Failure to follow an appropriate dosage regimen may precipitate hypoglycemia. Patients who do not adhere to their prescribed dietary and drug regimen are more prone to exhibit unsatisfactory response to therapy. Transfer of patients from other oral antidiabetic regimens to Diaβeta® (glyburide) should be done conservatively and the initial daily dose should be 2.5 to 5 mg. When transferring patients from oral hypoglycemic agents other than chlorpropamide to Diaβeta® (glyburide), no transition period and no initial or priming dose is necessary. When transferring patients from chlorpropamide, particular care should be exercised during the first two weeks because the prolonged retention of chlorpropamide in the body and subsequent overlapping drug effects may provoke hypoglycemia.

Some Type II diabetic patients being treated with insulin may respond satisfactorily to Diaβeta® (glyburide). If the insulin dose is less than 20 units daily, substitution of Diaβeta® (glyburide) 2.5 to 5 mg as a single daily dose may be tried. If the insulin dose is between 20 and 40 units daily, the patient may be placed directly on Diaβeta® (glyburide) 5 mg daily as a single dose. If the insulin dose is more than 40 units daily, a transition period is required for conversion to Diaβeta® (glyburide). In these patients, insulin dosage is decreased by 50% and Diaβeta® (glyburide) 5 mg daily is started. Please refer to Usual Maintenance Dose for further explanation.

2. Usual Maintenance Dose

The usual maintenance dose is in the range of 1.25 to 20 mg daily, which may be given as a single dose or in divided doses (See Dosage Interval Section). Dosage increases should be made in increments of no more than 2.5 mg at weekly intervals based upon the patient's blood glucose response.

No exact dosage relationship exists between Diaβeta® (glyburide) and the other oral hypoglycemic agents. Although patients may be transferred from the maximum dose of other sulfonylureas, the maximum starting dose of 5 mg of Diaβeta® (glyburide) should be observed. A maintenance dose of 5 mg Diaβeta® (glyburide) provides approximately the same degree of blood glucose control as 250 to 375 mg chlorpropamide, 250 to 375 mg tolazamide,

500 to 750 mg acetohexamide, or 1000 to 1500 mg tolbutamide.

When transferring patients receiving more than 40 units of insulin daily, they may be started on a daily dose of Diaβeta® (glyburide) 5 mg concomitantly with a 50% reduction in insulin dose. Progressive withdrawal of insulin and increase of Diaβeta® (glyburide) in increments of 1.25 to 2.5 mg every 2 to 10 days is then carried out. During this conversion period when both insulin and Diaβeta® (glyburide) are being used, hypoglycemia may rarely occur. During insulin withdrawal, patients should test their urine for glucose and acetone at least three times daily and report results to their physician. The appearance of persistent acetonuria with glycosuria indicates that the patient is a Type I diabetic who requires insulin therapy.

3. Maximum Dose

Daily doses of more than 20 mg are not recommended.

4. Dosage Interval

Once-a-day therapy is usually satisfactory, based upon usual meal patterns and a 10 hour half-life of Diaβeta® (glyburide). Some patients, particularly those receiving more than 10 mg daily, may have a more satisfactory response with twice-a-day dosage.

In elderly patients, debilitated or malnourished patients, and patients with impaired renal or hepatic function, the initial and maintenance dosing should be conservative to avoid hypoglycemic reactions. (See **Precautions** Section.)

HOW SUPPLIED

Diaβeta® (glyburide) tablets are supplied as white, oblong, monogrammed, scored tablets of 1.25 mg in bottles of 50 (NDC 0039-0050-05); pink, oblong, monogrammed, scored tablets of 2.5 mg in bottles of 30 (NDC 0039-0051-03); bottles of 60 (NDC 0039-0051-06); bottles of 100 (NDC 0039-0051-10); and in Unit Dose Cartons of 100 (NDC 0039-0051-11); and light green, oblong monogrammed, scored tablets of 5 mg in bottles of 30 (NDC 0039-0052-03); bottles of 60 (NDC 0039-0052-06); bottles of 100 (NDC 0039-0052-10); bottles of 500 (NDC 0039-0052-50), bottles of 1000 (NDC 0039-0052-70); and in Unit Dose Cartons of 100 (NDC 0039-0052-11).

Store at controlled room temperature (59°–86°F).
Dispense in well-closed containers with safety closures.
Caution: Federal law prohibits dispensing without a prescription.
*U.S. Patents 3,454,635 and 3,507,954   751010-6/88
Shown in Product Identification Section, page 411

DOXIDAN®
[dox 'i-dan "]

(See PDR For Nonprescription Drugs)
Shown in Product Identification Section, page 411

FESTAL® II
[fes 'tal]

(See PDR For Nonprescription Drugs)
Shown in Product Identification Section, page 411

LASIX®   ℞
[la ' siks]
(furosemide)
Oral Solution
Tablets/Injection
Diuretic

WARNING

Lasix (furosemide) is a potent diuretic which, if given in excessive amounts, can lead to a profound diuresis with water and electrolyte depletion. Therefore, careful medical supervision is required, and dose and dose schedule have to be adjusted to the individual patient's needs. (See under "DOSAGE AND ADMINISTRATION.")

DESCRIPTION

Lasix (furosemide) is a diuretic which is an anthranilic acid derivative. Chemically, it is 4-chloro-N-furfuryl-5-sulfamoylanthranilic acid.

Lasix® (furosemide) tablets for oral administration contain furosemide as the active ingredient and the following inactive ingredients: lactose USP, magnesium stearate NF, starch NF and talc USP.

Lasix® (furosemide) injection 10 mg/mL is a sterile, non-pyrogenic solution in ampules and disposable syringes for intravenous and intramuscular injection.

Lasix® (furosemide) Oral Solution contains furosemide as the active ingredient and the following inactive ingredients: alcohol USP 11.5%, D&C Yellow #10, FD&C Yellow #6 as color additives, flavors, glycerin USP, parabens NF, purified water USP, sorbitol NF; sodium hydroxide NF added to adjust pH. Lasix® (furosemide) Oral Solution 10 mg/mL is an orange flavored liquid for oral administration. Furosemide is a white to off-white odorless crystalline powder. It is practi-

cally insoluble in water, sparingly soluble in alcohol, freely soluble in dilute alkali solutions and insoluble in dilute acids.

The structural formula is as follows:

CLINICAL PHARMACOLOGY

Investigations into the mode of action of Lasix (furosemide) have utilized micropuncture studies in rats, stop flow experiments in dogs, and various clearance studies in both humans and experimental animals. It has been demonstrated that Lasix (furosemide) inhibits primarily the absorption of sodium and chloride not only in the proximal and distal tubules but also in the loop of Henle. The high degree of efficacy is largely due to this unique site of action. The action on the distal tubule is independent of any inhibitory effect on carbonic anhydrase and aldosterone.

Recent evidence suggests that furosemide glucuronide is the only or at least the major bio-transformation product of furosemide in man. Furosemide is extensively bound to plasma proteins, mainly to albumin. Plasma concentrations ranging from 1 to 400 ug/mL are 91 to 99% bound in healthy individuals. The unbound fraction averages 2.3 to 4.1% at therapeutic concentrations.

The onset of diuresis following oral administration is within 1 hour. The peak effect occurs within the first or second hour. The duration of diuretic effect is 6 to 8 hours.

The onset of diuresis following intravenous administration is within 5 minutes and somewhat later after intramuscular administration. The peak effect occurs within the first half hour. The duration of diuretic effect is approximately 2 hours.

In fasted normal men, the mean bioavailability of furosemide from Lasix® (furosemide) Tablets and Lasix® (furosemide) Oral Solution is 64% and 60%, respectively, of that from an intravenous injection of the drug. Although furosemide is more rapidly absorbed from the oral solution (50 minutes) than from the tablet (87 minutes), peak plasma levels and area under the plasma concentration-time curves do not differ significantly. Peak plasma concentrations increase with increasing dose but times-to-peak do not differ among doses. The terminal half-life of furosemide is approximately 2 hours.

Significantly more furosemide is excreted in urine following the IV injection than after the tablet or oral solution. There are no significant differences between the two oral formulations in the amount of unchanged drug excreted in urine.

INDICATIONS AND USAGE

Edema—Lasix (furosemide) is indicated in adults, infants, and children for the treatment of edema associated with congestive heart failure, cirrhosis of the liver, and renal disease, including the nephrotic syndrome. Lasix (furosemide) is particularly useful when an agent with greater diuretic potential is desired.

Parenteral therapy should be reserved for patients unable to take oral medication or for patients in emergency clinical situations.

Lasix (furosemide) Injection is also indicated as adjunctive therapy in acute pulmonary edema. The intravenous administration of Lasix (furosemide) is indicated when a rapid onset of diuresis is desired, eg, in acute pulmonary edema. If gastrointestinal absorption is impaired or oral medication is not practical for any reason, Lasix (furosemide) is indicated by the intravenous or intramuscular route. Parenteral use should be replaced with oral Lasix (furosemide) as soon as practical.

Hypertension—Oral Lasix (furosemide) may be used in adults for the treatment of hypertension alone or in combination with other antihypertensive agents. Hypertensive patients who cannot be adequately controlled with thiazides will probably also not be adequately controlled with Lasix (furosemide) alone.

CONTRAINDICATIONS

Lasix® is contraindicated in patients with anuria and in patients with a history of hypersensitivity to furosemide.

WARNINGS

In patients with hepatic cirrhosis and ascites, Lasix® (furosemide) therapy is best initiated in the hospital. In hepatic coma and in states of electrolyte depletion therapy should not be instituted until the basic condition is improved. Sudden alterations of fluid and electrolyte balance in patients with cirrhosis may precipitate hepatic coma; therefore, strict observation is necessary during the period of diuresis. Supplemental potassium chloride and, if required, an aldosterone antagonist are helpful in preventing hypokalemia and metabolic alkalosis.

Continued on next page

Hoechst-Roussel—Cont.

If increasing azotemia and oliguria occur during treatment of severe progressive renal disease, Lasix® (furosemide) should be discontinued.

Cases of tinnitus and reversible or irreversible hearing impairment have been reported. Usually, reports indicate that Lasix® (furosemide) ototoxicity is associated with rapid injection, severe renal impairment, doses exceeding several times the usual recommended dose, or concomitant therapy with aminoglycoside antibiotics, ethacrynic acid, or other ototoxic drugs. If the physician elects to use high dose parenteral therapy, controlled intravenous infusion is advisable (for adults, an infusion rate not exceeding 4 mg Lasix® (furosemide) per minute has been used).

PRECAUTIONS

General

Excessive diuresis may cause dehydration and blood volume reduction with circulatory collapse and possible vascular thrombosis and embolism, particularly in elderly patients. As with any effective diuretic, electrolyte depletion may occur during Lasix® (furosemide) therapy, especially in patients receiving higher doses and restricted salt intake. Hypokalemia may develop with Lasix® (furosemide), especially with brisk diuresis, inadequate oral electrolyte intake, when cirrhosis is present, or during concomitant use of corticosteroids or ACTH. Digitalis therapy may exaggerate metabolic effects of hypokalemia, especially myocardial effects. All patients receiving Lasix® (furosemide) therapy should be observed for these signs or symptoms of fluid or electrolyte imbalance (hyponatremia, hypochloremic alkalosis or hypokalemia): dryness of mouth, thirst, weakness, lethargy, drowsiness, restlessness, muscle pains or cramps, muscular fatigue, hypotension, oliguria, tachycardia, arrhythmia, or gastrointestinal disturbances such as nausea and vomiting.

Increases in blood glucose and alterations in glucose tolerance tests (with abnormalities of the fasting and 2-hour postprandial sugar) have been observed, and rarely, precipitation of diabetes mellitus has been reported.

Asymptomatic hyperuricemia can occur and gout may rarely be precipitated.

The sorbitol present in the vehicle may cause diarrhea (especially in children) when higher doses of Lasix® (furosemide) Oral Solution are given.

Patients allergic to sulfonamides may also be allergic to Lasix® (furosemide).

The possibility exists of exacerbation or activation of systemic lupus erythematosus.

As with many other drugs, patients should be observed regularly for the possible occurrence of blood dyscrasias, liver damage, or other idiosyncratic reactions.

Information for Patients

Patients receiving Lasix® (furosemide) should be advised that they may experience symptoms from excessive fluid and/or electrolyte losses. The postural hypotension that sometimes occurs can usually be managed by getting up slowly. Potassium supplements and/or dietary measures may be needed to control or avoid hypokalemia.

Patients with diabetes mellitus should be told that furosemide may increase blood glucose levels and thereby affect urine glucose tests. The skin of some patients may be more sensitive to the effects of sunlight while taking furosemide.

Hypertensive patients should avoid medications that may increase blood pressure, including over-the-counter products for appetite suppression and cold symptoms.

Laboratory Tests

Serum electrolytes, CO_2 and BUN should be determined frequently during the first few months of Lasix® (furosemide) therapy and periodically thereafter.

Serum and urine electrolyte determinations are particularly important when the patient is vomiting profusely or receiving parenteral fluids. Abnormalities should be corrected or the drug temporarily withdrawn. Other medications may also influence serum electrolytes.

Reversible elevations of BUN may occur and are associated with dehydration, which should be avoided, particularly in patients with renal insufficiency.

Urine and blood glucose should be checked periodically in diabetics receiving Lasix® (furosemide), even in those suspected of latent diabetes.

Lasix® (furosemide) may lower serum calcium levels and tetany has been reported rarely. Accordingly, serum calcium levels should be determined periodically.

Drug Interactions

Lasix® (furosemide) may increase the ototoxic potential of aminoglycoside antibiotics, especially in the presence of impaired renal function. Except in life-threatening situations, avoid this combination.

Lasix® (furosemide) should not be used concomitantly with ethacrynic acid because of the possibility of ototoxicity.

Patients receiving high doses of salicylates concomitantly with Lasix® (furosemide), as in rheumatic disease, may experience salicylate toxicity at lower doses because of competitive renal excretory sites.

Lasix® (furosemide) has a tendency to antagonize the skeletal muscle relaxing effect of tubocurarine and may potentiate the action of succinylcholine.

Lithium generally should not be given with diuretics because they reduce lithium's renal clearance and add a high risk of lithium toxicity.

Lasix® (furosemide) may add to or potentiate the therapeutic effect of other antihypertensive drugs. Potentiation occurs with ganglionic or peripheral adrenergic blocking drugs.

Lasix® (furosemide) may decrease arterial responsiveness to norepinephrine. However, norepinephrine may still be used effectively.

Literature reports indicate that coadministration of indomethacin may reduce the natriuretic and antihypertensive effects of Lasix® (furosemide) in some patients by inhibiting prostaglandin synthesis. Indomethacin may also affect plasma renin levels, aldosterone excretion, and renin profile evaluation. Patients receiving both indomethacin and Lasix® (furosemide) should be observed closely to determine if the desired diuretic and/or antihypertensive effect of Lasix® (furosemide) is achieved.

Carcinogenesis, Mutagenesis, Impairment of Fertility

No carcinogenic or mutagenic studies have been conducted with Lasix® (furosemide).

Lasix® (furosemide) produced no impairment of fertility in male or female rats, at 100 mg/kg/day (the maximum effective diuretic dose in the rat and 8 times the maximal human dose of 600 mg/day).

Pregnancy

Pregnancy Category C. Furosemide has been shown to cause unexplained maternal deaths and abortions in rabbits at 2, 4 and 8 times the human dose. There are no adequate and well-controlled studies in pregnant women. Lasix® (furosemide) should be used during pregnancy only if the potential benefit justifies the potential risk to the fetus.

The effects of furosemide on embryonic and fetal development and on pregnant dams were studied in mice, rats and rabbits.

Furosemide caused unexplained maternal deaths and abortions in the rabbit at the lowest dose of 25 mg/kg (2 times the maximal recommended human dose of 600 mg/day). In another study, a dose of 50 mg/kg (4 times the maximal recommended human dose of 600 mg/day) also caused maternal deaths and abortions when administered to rabbits between Days 12 and 17 of gestation. In a third study, none of the pregnant rabbits survived a dose of 100 mg/kg. Data from the above studies indicate fetal lethality that can precede maternal deaths.

The results of the mouse study and one of the three rabbit studies also showed an increased incidence of hydronephrosis (distention of the renal pelvis and, in some cases, of the ureters) in fetuses derived from treated dams as compared to the incidence in fetuses from the control group.

Nursing Mothers

Because it appears in breast milk, caution should be exercised when Lasix® (furosemide) is administered to a nursing mother.

Pediatric Use

Renal calcifications (from barely visible on x-ray to staghorn) have occurred in some severely premature infants treated with intravenous Lasix® (furosemide) for edema due to patent ductus arteriosus and hyaline membrane disease. The concurrent use of chlorothiazide has been reported to decrease hypercalciuria and dissolve some calculi.

ADVERSE REACTIONS

Adverse reactions are categorized below by organ system and listed by decreasing severity.

Gastrointestinal System Reactions

1. pancreatitis
2. jaundice (intrahepatic cholestatic jaundice)
3. anorexia
4. oral and gastric irritation
5. cramping
6. diarrhea
7. constipation
8. nausea
9. vomiting

Central Nervous System Reactions

1. tinnitus and hearing loss
2. paresthesias
3. vertigo
4. dizziness
5. headache
6. blurred vision
7. xanthopsia

Hematologic Reactions

1. aplastic anemia (rare)
2. thrombocytopenia
3. agranulocytosis (rare)
4. leukopenia
5. anemia

Dermatologic-Hypersensitivity Reactions

1. necrotizing angiitis (vasculitis, cutaneous vasculitis)
2. exfoliative dermatitis
3. erythema multiforme
4. purpura
5. photosensitivity
6. urticaria
7. rash
8. pruritus

Cardiovascular Reaction

Orthostatic hypotension may occur and be aggravated by alcohol, barbiturates or narcotics.

Other Reactions

1. hyperglycemia
2. glycosuria
3. hyperuricemia
4. muscle spasm
5. weakness
6. restlessness
7. urinary bladder spasm
8. thrombophlebitis
9. transient injection site pain following intramuscular injection

Whenever adverse reactions are moderate or severe, Lasix® (furosemide) dosage should be reduced or therapy withdrawn.

OVERDOSAGE

The principal signs and symptoms of overdose with Lasix® (furosemide) are dehydration, blood volume reduction, hypotension, electrolyte imbalance, hypokalemia and hypochloremic alkalosis, and are extensions of its diuretic action. The acute toxicity of Lasix® (furosemide) has been determined in mice, rats and dogs. In all three, the oral LD_{50} exceeded 1000 mg/kg body weight, while the intravenous LD_{50} ranged from 300 to 680 mg/kg. The acute intragastric toxicity in neonatal rats is 7 to 10 times that of adult rats.

The concentration of Lasix® (furosemide) in biological fluids associated with toxicity or death is not known.

Treatment of overdose is supportive and consists of replacement of excessive fluid and electrolyte losses.

Serum electrolytes, carbon dioxide level and blood pressure should be determined frequently. Adequate drainage must be assured in patients with urinary bladder outlet obstruction (such as prostatic hypertrophy). Hemodialysis does not accelerate furosemide elimination.

DOSAGE AND ADMINISTRATION

Oral Administration

Edema

Therapy should be individualized according to patient response to gain maximal therapeutic response and to determine the minimal dose needed to maintain that response.

Adults—The usual initial dose of Lasix® (furosemide) is 20 to 80 mg given as a single dose. Ordinarily a prompt diuresis ensues. If needed, the same dose can be administered 6 to 8 hours later or the dose may be increased. The dose may be raised by 20 or 40 mg and given not sooner than 6 to 8 hours after the previous dose until the desired diuretic effect has been obtained. This individually determined single dose should then be given once or twice daily (eg, at 8 am and 2 pm). The dose of Lasix® (furosemide) may be carefully titrated up to 600 mg/day in patients with clinically severe edematous states.

Edema may be most efficiently and safely mobilized by giving Lasix® (furosemide) on 2 to 4 consecutive days each week.

When doses exceeding 80 mg/day are given for prolonged periods, careful clinical observation and laboratory monitoring are particularly advisable. (See **PRECAUTIONS: Laboratory Tests.**)

Infants and Children—The usual initial dose of oral Lasix® (furosemide) in infants and children is 2 mg/kg body weight, given as a single dose. If the diuretic response is not satisfactory after the initial dose, dosage may be increased by 1 or 2 mg/kg no sooner than 6 to 8 hours after the previous dose. Doses greater than 6 mg/kg body weight are not recommended.

For maintenance therapy in infants and children, the dose should be adjusted to the minimum effective level.

Hypertension

Therapy should be individualized according to the patient's response to gain maximal therapeutic response and to determine the minimal dose needed to maintain that therapeutic response.

Adults—The usual initial daily dose of Lasix® (furosemide) for hypertension is 80 mg, usually divided into 40 mg twice a day. Dosage should then be adjusted according to response. If response is not satisfactory, add other antihypertensive agents.

Changes in blood pressure must be carefully monitored when Lasix® (furosemide) is used with other antihypertensive drugs, especially during initial therapy. To prevent excessive drop in blood pressure, the dosage of other agents should be reduced by at least 50 percent when Lasix® (furosemide) is added to the regimen. As the blood pressure falls under the potentiating effect of Lasix® (furosemide), a further reduction in dosage or even discontinuation of other antihypertensive drugs may be necessary.

Parenteral Administration

Adults—Parenteral therapy with Lasix® (furosemide) injection should be used only in patients unable to take oral medication or in emergency situations and should be replaced with oral therapy as soon as practical.

Edema

The usual initial dose of Lasix® (furosemide) is 20 to 40 mg given as a single dose, injected intramuscularly or intravenously. The intravenous dose should be given slowly (1 to 2 minutes). Ordinarily a prompt diuresis ensues. If needed, another dose may be administered in the same manner 2 hours later or the dose may be increased. The dose may be raised by 20 mg and given not sooner than 2 hours after the previous dose until the desired diuretic effect has been obtained. This individually determined single dose should then be given once or twice daily.

Therapy should be individualized according to patient response to gain maximal therapeutic response and to determine the minimal dose needed to maintain that response. Close medical supervision is necessary. If the physician elects to use high dose parenteral therapy, add the Lasix® (furosemide) to either Sodium Chloride Injection USP, Lactated Ringer's Injection USP, or Dextrose (5%) Injection USP after pH has been adjusted to above 5.5, and administer as a controlled intravenous infusion at a rate not greater than 4 mg/min. Lasix® (furosemide) Injection is a buffered alkaline solution.

Acute Pulmonary Edema

The usual initial dose of Lasix® (furosemide) is 40 mg injected slowly intravenously (over 1 to 2 minutes). If a satisfactory response does not occur within 1 hour, the dose may be increased to 80 mg injected slowly intravenously (over 1 to 2 minutes).

If necessary, additional therapy (eg, digitalis, oxygen) may be administered concomitantly.

Infants and Children—Parenteral therapy should be used only in patients unable to take oral medication or in emergency situations and should be replaced with oral therapy as soon as practical.

The usual initial dose of Lasix® (furosemide) Injection (intravenously or intramuscularly) in infants and children is 1 mg/kg body weight and should be given slowly under close medical supervision. If the diuretic response to the initial dose is not satisfactory, dosage may be increased by 1 mg/kg not sooner than 2 hours after the previous dose, until the desired diuretic effect has been obtained. Doses greater than 6 mg/kg body weight are not recommended.

Lasix® (furosemide) Injection should be inspected visually for particulate matter and discoloration before administration. Do not use if solution is discolored.

HOW SUPPLIED

Lasix® (furosemide) Tablets 20 mg are supplied as white, oval, monogrammed tablets in Bottles of 100 (NDC 0039-0067-10), 500 (NDC 0039-0067-50), 1000 (NDC 0039-0067-70), and in Unit Dose Packs of 100 (NDC 0039-0067-11). The 20 mg tablets are imprinted with "Lasix® " on one side and "HOECHST" on the other.

Lasix® (furosemide) Tablets 40 mg are supplied as white, round, monogrammed, scored tablets in Bottles of 100 (NDC 0039-0060-10), 500 (NDC 0039-0060-50), 1000 (NDC 0039-0060-70), Unit Dose Packs of 100 (NDC 0039-0060-11), and in 25 Unit of Use Bottle packages of 30 (NDC 0039-0060-03), 60 (NDC 0039-0060-06), and 12 Unit of Use Bottle packages of 100 (NDC 0039-0060-13). The 40 mg tablets are imprinted with "Lasix®" on one side and the Hoechst logo on the other.

Lasix® (furosemide) Tablets 80 mg are supplied as white, round, monogrammed, facetted edge tablets in Bottles of 50 (NDC 0039-0066-05), 500 (NDC 0039-0066-50), and in Unit Dose Packs of 100 (NDC 0039-0066-11). The 80 mg tablets are imprinted with "Lasix® 80" on one side and the Hoechst logo on the other.

Note: Dispense in well-closed, light-resistant containers. Exposure to light might cause a slight discoloration. Discolored tablets should not be dispensed.

Lasix® (furosemide) Oral Solution 10 mg/mL is supplied as orange-flavored liquid in Bottles of 60 mL (accompanied by graduated dropper) (NDC 0039-0063-06) and Bottles of 120 mL (accompanied by graduated dispensing spoon) (NDC 0039-0063-40).

Note: Store at controlled room temperature (59°–86°F). Dispense in light-resistant containers. Discard opened bottle after 60 days.

Lasix® Injection, brand of furosemide, (10 mg/mL), is supplied as a sterile solution in 2 mL, 4 mL, and 10 mL amber ampules, single use vials, and in syringes.

Ampules:

2 mL 5's (NDC 0039-0061-15); 50's (NDC 0039-0061-05)
4 mL 5's (NDC 0039-0061-45); 25's (NDC 0039-0061-65)
10 mL 5's (NDC 0039-0061-08); 25's (NDC 0039-0061-25)

Syringes:

2 mL 5's (NDC 0039-0062-08)
4 mL 5's (NDC 0039-0064-08)
10 mL 5's (NDC 0039-0069-08)

Single Use Vials:

2 mL 25's (NDC 0039-0055-25)
4 mL 25's (NDC 0039-0056-25)
10 mL 25's (NDC 0039-0057-25)

Syringes supplied with 22 gauge x 1 ¼" needle.

To insure patient safety, this needle should be handled with care and should be destroyed and discarded if damaged in any manner. If cannula is bent, no attempt should be made to straighten.

To prevent needle-stick injuries, needles should not be recapped, purposely bent, or broken by hand.

Store at controlled room temperature (59°–86°F).
Do not use if solution is discolored.
Protect syringes from light. Do not remove syringes from individual package until time of use.
760010-7/86
763000-9/88
705060-7/86
Shown in Product Identification Section, pages 411 & 412

LOPROX®   ℞
[lo' prahks]
(ciclopirox olamine) Cream 1%
Lotion 1%

DESCRIPTION

Loprox® (ciclopirox olamine) Cream 1% and Lotion 1% are for topical use. Each gram of Loprox® (ciclopirox olamine) Cream 1% contains 10 mg ciclopirox olamine in a water miscible vanishing cream base consisting of purified water USP, octyldodecanol NF, mineral oil USP, stearyl alcohol NF, cetyl alcohol NF, cocamide DEA, polysorbate 60 NF, myristyl alcohol NF, sorbitan monostearate NF, lactic acid USP, and benzyl alcohol NF (1%) as preservative.

Each gram of Loprox® (ciclopirox olamine) Lotion 1% contains 10 mg of ciclopirox olamine in a water miscible lotion base consisting of purified water USP, cocamide DEA, octyldodecanol NF, mineral oil USP, stearyl alcohol NF, cetyl alcohol NF, polysorbate 60 NF, myristyl alcohol NF, sorbitan monostearate NF, lactic acid USP, and benzyl alcohol NF (1%) as preservative. Loprox® (ciclopirox olamine) Cream and Lotion contain a synthetic, broad-spectrum, antifungal agent ciclopirox olamine. The chemical name is 6-cyclohexyl-1-hydroxy-4-methyl-2(1 *H*)-pyridone, 2-aminoethanol salt.

The chemical structure is:

$$\text{OH} \quad \text{N} \quad \text{O} \qquad \cdot\ H_2NCH_2CH_2OH \qquad CH_3$$

Loprox® (ciclopirox olamine) Cream 1% and Lotion 1% have a pH of 7.

CLINICAL PHARMACOLOGY

Ciclopirox olamine is a broad-spectrum, antifungal agent that inhibits the growth of pathogenic dermatophytes, yeasts, and *Malassezia furfur*. Ciclopirox olamine exhibits fungicidal activity *in vitro* against isolates of *Trichophyton rubrum*, *Trichophyton mentagrophytes*, *Epidermophyton floccosum*, *Microsporum canis*, and *Candida albicans*.

Pharmacokinetic studies in men with radiolabeled 1% ciclopirox olamine solution in polyethylene glycol 400 showed an average of 1.3% absorption of the dose when it was applied topically to 750 cm^2 on the back followed by occlusion for 6 hours. The biological half-life was 1.7 hours and excretion occurred via the kidney. Two days after application only 0.01% of the dose applied could be found in the urine. Fecal excretion was negligible.

Penetration studies in human cadaverous skin from the back, with Loprox® (ciclopirox olamine) Cream 1% with tagged ciclopirox olamine showed the presence of 0.8 to 1.6% of the dose in stratum corneum 1.5 to 6 hours after application. The levels in the dermis were still 10 to 15 times above the minimum inhibitory concentrations.

Autoradiographic studies with human cadaverous skin showed that ciclopirox olamine penetrates into the hair and through the epidermis and hair follicles into the sebaceous glands and dermis, while a portion of the drug remains in the stratum corneum.

Draize Human Sensitization Assay, 21-Day Cumulative Irritancy study, Phototoxicity study, and Photo-Draize study conducted in a total of 142 healthy male subjects showed no contact sensitization of the delayed hypersensitivity type, no irritation, no phototoxicity, and no photo-contact sensitization due to Loprox® (ciclopirox olamine) Cream 1%.

In vitro penetration studies in frozen or fresh excised human cadaver and pig skin indicated that the penetration of Loprox® (ciclopirox olamine) Lotion 1% is equivalent to that of Loprox® (ciclopirox olamine) Cream 1%. Therapeutic equivalence of cream and lotion formulations also was indicated by studies of experimentally induced guinea pig and human trichophytosis.

INDICATIONS AND USAGE

Loprox® (ciclopirox olamine) Cream 1% and Lotion 1% are indicated for the topical treatment of the following dermal infections: tinea pedis, tinea cruris and tinea corporis due to *Trichophyton rubrum*, *Trichophyton mentagrophytes*, *Epidermophyton floccosum*, and *Microsporum canis;* cutaneous candidiasis (moniliasis) due to *Candida albicans;* and tinea (pityriasis) versicolor due to *Malassezia furfur*.

CONTRAINDICATIONS

Loprox® (ciclopirox olamine) Cream 1% and Lotion 1% are contraindicated in individuals who have shown hypersensitivity to any of its components.

WARNINGS

General: Loprox® (ciclopirox olamine) Cream 1% and Lotion 1% are not for ophthalmic use.

PRECAUTIONS

If a reaction suggesting sensitivity or chemical irritation should occur with the use of Loprox® (ciclopirox olamine) Cream 1% or Lotion 1%, treatment should be discontinued and appropriate therapy instituted.

Information for patients—The patient should be told to:

1. Use the medication for the full treatment time even though symptoms may have improved and notify the physician if there is no improvement after four weeks.
2. Inform the physician if the area of application shows signs of increased irritation (redness, itching, burning, blistering, swelling, oozing) indicative of possible sensitization.
3. Avoid the use of occlusive wrappings or dressings.

Carcinogenesis, mutagenesis, impairment of fertility:

A carcinogenicity study in female mice dosed cutaneously twice per week for 50 weeks followed by a 6-month drug-free observation period prior to necropsy revealed no evidence of tumors at the application site. Several mutagenic tests indicated no potential for mutagenesis.

Pregnancy Category B:

Reproduction studies have been performed in the mouse, rat, rabbit, and monkey, (via various routes of administration) at doses 10 times or more the topical human dose and have revealed no significant evidence of impaired fertility or harm to the fetus due to ciclopirox olamine. There are, however, no adequate or well-controlled studies in pregnant women. Because animal reproduction studies are not always predictive of human response this drug should be used during pregnancy only if clearly needed.

Nursing mothers:

It is not known whether this drug is excreted in human milk. Because many drugs are excreted in human milk, caution should be exercised when Loprox® (ciclopirox olamine) Cream 1% or Lotion 1% is administered to a nursing woman.

Pediatric use:

Safety and effectiveness in children below the age of 10 years have not been established.

ADVERSE REACTIONS

In all controlled clinical studies with 514 patients using Loprox® (ciclopirox olamine) Cream 1% and in 296 patients using the vehicle cream, the incidence of adverse reactions was low. This included pruritus at the site of application in one patient and worsening of the clinical signs and symptoms in another patient using ciclopirox olamine cream 1% and burning in one patient and worsening of the clinical signs and symptoms in another patient using the vehicle cream.

In the controlled clinical trial with 89 patients using Loprox® (ciclopirox olamine) Lotion 1% and 89 patients using the vehicle, the incidence of adverse reactions was low. Those considered possibly related to treatment or occurring in more than one patient were pruritus, which occurred in two patients using ciclopirox olamine lotion 1% and one patient using the lotion vehicle, and burning, which occurred in one patient using ciclopirox olamine lotion 1%.

DOSAGE AND ADMINISTRATION

Gently massage Loprox® (ciclopirox olamine) Cream 1% or Lotion 1% into the affected and surrounding skin areas twice daily, in the morning and evening. Clinical improvement with relief of pruritus and other symptoms usually occurs within the first week of treatment. If a patient shows no clinical improvement after four weeks of treatment with Loprox® (ciclopirox olamine) Cream 1% or Lotion 1%, the diagnosis should be redetermined. Patients with tinea versicolor usually exhibit clinical and mycological clearing after two weeks of treatment.

HOW SUPPLIED

Loprox® (ciclopirox olamine) Cream 1% is supplied in 15 gram, (NDC 0039-0009-15); 30 gram, (NDC 0039-0009-30); and 90 gram tubes, (NDC 0039-0009-90).

Loprox® (ciclopirox olamine) Lotion 1% is supplied in 30 mL bottles (NDC 0039-0008-30).

Shake lotion vigorously before each use.

Store at controlled room temperature (59°– 86°F).

Loprox® REG TM HOECHST AG   709000-2/89
U.S. Patent 3,883,545   708000-11/88

Shown in Product Identification Section, page 412

Continued on next page

Hoechst-Roussel—Cont.

STREPTASE®　　　　　　　　　　Ŗ
[strep'tās]
(streptokinase)

DESCRIPTION

Streptase®, Streptokinase, is a sterile, purified preparation of a bacterial protein elaborated by group C β-hemolytic streptococci. It is supplied as a lyophilized white powder containing 25 mg cross-linked gelatin polypeptides, 25 mg sodium L-glutamate, sodium hydroxide to adjust pH, and 100 mg Albumin (Human) per vial or infusion bottle as stabilizers. The preparation contains no preservatives and is intended for intravenous and intracoronary administration.

CLINICAL PHARMACOLOGY

Streptase®, Streptokinase, acts with plasminogen to produce an "activator complex" that converts plasminogen to the proteolytic enzyme plasmin. The $t_{1/2}$ of the activator complex is about 23 minutes; the complex is inactivated, in part, by antistreptococcal antibodies. The mechanism by which streptokinase is eliminated is unknown; no metabolites of streptokinase have been identified. Plasmin degrades fibrin clots as well as fibrinogen and other plasma proteins. Plasmin is inactivated by circulating inhibitors, such as α-2-plasmin inhibitor or α-2-macroglobulin. These inhibitors are rapidly consumed at high doses of streptokinase.
Intravenous infusion of Streptokinase is followed by increased fibrinolytic activity, which decreases plasma fibrinogen levels for 24 to 36 hours. The decrease in plasma fibrinogen is associated with decreases in plasma and blood viscosity and red blood cell aggregation. The hyperfibrinolytic effect disappears within a few hours after discontinuation, but a prolonged thrombin time may persist for up to 24 hours due to the decrease in plasma levels of fibrinogen and an increase in the amount of circulating fibrin(ogen) degradation products (FDP). Depending upon the dosage and duration of infusion of Streptokinase, the thrombin time will decrease to less than two times the normal control value within 4 hours, and return to normal by 24 hours.
Intravenous administration has been shown to reduce blood pressure and total peripheral resistance with a corresponding reduction in cardiac afterload. These expected responses were not studied with the intracoronary administration of Streptase®, Streptokinase. The quantitative benefit has not been evaluated.
Variable amounts of circulating antistreptokinase antibody are present in individuals as a result of recent streptococcal infections. The recommended dosage schedule usually obviates the need for antibody titration.
Two large randomized, placebo-controlled studies conducted with a 60 minute intravenous infusion of 1,500,000 IU of Streptase®, Streptokinase, for the treatment of acute myocardial infarction within 6 hours of the onset of symptoms have reported reductions in acute mortality from 20–25%.[1,2]
In the GISSI study, the reduction in mortality was time dependent; there was a 47% reduction in mortality among patients treated within one hour of the onset of chest pain, a 23% reduction among patients treated within three hours, and a 17% reduction among patients treated between three and six hours. There was also a reduction in mortality in patients treated between six and twelve hours from the onset of symptoms, but the reduction was not statistically significant.
One of eight smaller studies using a similar dosing schedule showed statistically significant reduction in mortality. When all of these studies were pooled, the overall decrease in mortality was approximately 23%. Results from pooling several studies using different dosages with long term infusion corroborate these observations.
In addition, studies measuring left ventricular ejection fraction (LVEF) at discharge showed the mean LVEFs were approximately 3–6 percentage points higher in the Streptase®, Streptokinase group when compared to the control group. This difference was statistically significant in some of the studies.[3,4] Furthermore, some studies reported greater improvement in LVEF among patients treated within three hours than in patients treated later.
The rate of reocclusion of the infarct-related vessel has been reported to be approximately 20%. The rate of reocclusion depends on dosage, additional anticoagulant therapy and residual stenosis. When the reinfarctions were evaluated in studies involving 8,800 Streptokinase treated patients, the overall rate was 3.8% (range 2–15%). In over 8,500 control patients, the rate of reinfarction was 2.4%.
Streptase®, Streptokinase, administered by the intracoronary route has resulted in thrombolysis usually within one hour, and ensuing reperfusion results in limitation of infarct size, improvement of cardiac function, and reduction of mortality.[5,6] LVEF was increased in patients treated with Streptokinase when compared to patients treated with conventional therapy. When the initial LVEF was low, the Streptokinase-treated patients showed greater improvement than

did the controls. Spontaneous reperfusion is known to occur and has been observed with angiography at various time points after infarction. Data from one study show that 73% of the Streptokinase-treated patients and 47% of the placebo-allocated patients reperfused during hospitalization.
Studies with thrombolytic therapy for pulmonary embolism show no significant difference in lung perfusion scan between the thrombolysis group and the heparin group at one-year follow-up. However, measurements of pulmonary capillary blood volumes and diffusing capacities at two weeks and one year after therapy indicate that a more complete resolution of thrombotic obstruction and normalization of pulmonary physiology was achieved with thrombolytic therapy, thus preventing the long term sequelae of pulmonary hypertension and pulmonary failure.[7]
The long term benefit of Streptase®, Streptokinase, therapy for deep vein thrombosis (DVT) has been evaluated venographically.[8] The combined results of five randomized studies show no residual thrombotic material in 60–75% of patients treated with Streptokinase versus only 10% of those treated with heparin. Thrombolytic therapy also preserves venous valve function in a majority of cases, thus avoiding the pathologic venous changes that produce the clinical postphlebitic syndrome which occurs in 90% of the DVT patients treated with heparin.
There is a time-related decrease in effectiveness when Streptase®, Streptokinase, is used in the management of peripheral arterial thromboembolism. When administered three to ten days after onset of obstruction, rates of clearance of 50–75% were reported.

INDICATIONS AND USAGE

Acute Evolving Transmural Myocardial Infarction

Streptase®, Streptokinase, is indicated for use in the management of acute myocardial infarction in adults, for the lysis of intracoronary thrombi, for the improvement of ventricular function, and reduction of mortality when administered by either the intravenous or intracoronary route. Earlier administration of Streptokinase is correlated with greater clinical benefit. (See CLINICAL PHARMACOLOGY section.)

Pulmonary Embolism

Streptase®, Streptokinase, is indicated for the lysis of objectively diagnosed (angiography or lung scan) pulmonary emboli, involving obstruction of blood flow to a lobe or multiple segments, with or without unstable hemodynamics.

Deep Vein Thrombosis

Streptase®, Streptokinase, is indicated for the lysis of objectively diagnosed (preferably ascending venography), acute, extensive thrombi of the deep veins such as those involving the popliteal and more proximal vessels.

Arterial Thrombosis or Embolism

Streptase®, Streptokinase, is indicated for the lysis of acute arterial thrombi and emboli. Streptokinase is not indicated for arterial emboli originating from the left side of the heart due to the risk of new embolic phenomena such as cerebral embolism.

Occlusion of Arteriovenous Cannulae

Streptase®, Streptokinase, is indicated as an alternative to surgical revision for clearing totally or partially occluded arteriovenous cannulae when acceptable flow cannot be achieved.

CONTRAINDICATIONS

Because thrombolytic therapy increases the risk of bleeding, Streptase®, Streptokinase, is contraindicated in the following situations:

- active internal bleeding
- recent (within 2 months) cerebrovascular accident, intracranial or intraspinal surgery (see WARNINGS)
- intracranial neoplasm
- severe uncontrolled hypertension

Streptokinase should not be administered to patients having experienced severe allergic reaction to the product.

WARNINGS

Bleeding

Streptase®, Streptokinase, will cause lysis of hemostatic fibrin deposits such as those occurring at sites of needle punctures, and bleeding may occur from such sites. In order to minimize the risk of bleeding during treatment with Streptokinase, venipunctures and physical handling of the patient should be performed carefully and as infrequently as possible, and intramuscular injections must be avoided.
Should arterial puncture be necessary during intravenous therapy, upper extremity vessels are preferable. Pressure should be applied for at least 30 minutes, a pressure dressing applied, and the puncture site checked frequently for evidence of bleeding.
In the following conditions the risks of therapy may be increased and should be weighed against the anticipated benefits.

- Recent (within 10 days) major surgery, obstetrical delivery, organ biopsy, previous puncture of noncompressible vessels

- Recent (within 10 days) serious gastrointestinal bleeding
- Recent (within 10 days) trauma including cardiopulmonary resuscitation
- Hypertension: systolic BP $\geq$ 180 mm Hg and/or diastolic BP $\geq$ 110 mm Hg
- High likelihood of left heart thrombus, e.g., mitral stenosis with atrial fibrillation
- Subacute bacterial endocarditis
- Hemostatic defects including those secondary to severe hepatic or renal disease
- Pregnancy
- Age $\geq$ 75 years
- Cerebrovascular disease
- Diabetic hemorrhagic retinopathy
- Septic thrombophlebitis or occluded AV cannula at seriously infected site
- Any other condition in which bleeding constitutes a significant hazard or would be particularly difficult to manage because of its location.

Should serious spontaneous bleeding (not controllable by local pressure) occur, the infusion of Streptase®, Streptokinase, should be terminated immediately and treatment instituted as described under ADVERSE REACTIONS.

Arrhythmias

Rapid lysis of coronary thrombi has been shown to cause reperfusion atrial or ventricular dysrhythmias requiring immediate treatment. Careful monitoring for arrhythmia is recommended during and immediately following administration of Streptase®, Streptokinase, for acute myocardial infarction.

Hypotension

Hypotension, sometimes severe, not secondary to bleeding or anaphylaxis has been observed during intravenous Streptase®, Streptokinase, infusion in 1% to 10% of patients. Patients should be monitored closely and, should symptomatic or alarming hypotension occur, appropriate treatment should be administered. This treatment may include a decrease in the intravenous Streptokinase infusion rate. Smaller hypotensive effects are common and have not required treatment.

Other

Non-cardiogenic pulmonary edema has been reported rarely in patients treated with Streptase®, Streptokinase. The risk of this appears greatest in patients who have large myocardial infarctions and are undergoing thrombolytic therapy by the intracoronary route.
Rarely, polyneuropathy has been temporally related to the use of Streptase®, Streptokinase.
Should pulmonary embolism or recurrent pulmonary embolism occur during Streptase®, Streptokinase, therapy, the originally planned course of treatment should be completed in an attempt to lyse the embolus. While pulmonary embolism may occasionally occur during Streptokinase treatment, the incidence is no greater than when patients are treated with heparin alone.

PRECAUTIONS

General

Because of the increased likelihood of resistance, due to antistreptokinase antibody, Streptase®, Streptokinase, may not be effective if administered between five days and six months of prior Streptokinase administration or streptococcal infections, such as streptococcal pharyngitis, acute rheumatic fever, or acute glomerulonephritis secondary to a streptococcal infection.

Laboratory Tests

Intravenous or Intracoronary Infusion for Myocardial Infarction. Intravenous administration of Streptase®, Streptokinase, will cause marked decreases in plasminogen and fibrinogen and increases in thrombin time (TT), activated partial thromboplastin time (APTT), and prothrombin time (PT). These changes may also occur in some patients with intracoronary administration of Streptokinase.
Intravenous Infusion for Other Indications. Before commencing thrombolytic therapy, it is desirable to obtain an activated partial thromboplastin time (APTT), a prothrombin time (PT), a thrombin time (TT), fibrinogen levels, and a hematocrit and platelet count. If heparin has been given, it should be discontinued and the TT or APTT should be less than twice the normal control value before thrombolytic therapy is started.
During the infusion, decreases in plasminogen and fibrinogen levels and an increase in the level of FDP (the latter two causing a prolongation in the clotting times of coagulation tests) will generally confirm the existence of a lytic state. Therefore, lytic therapy can be confirmed by performing the TT, APTT, PT, or fibrinogen levels approximately 4 hours after initiation of therapy.
If heparin is to be (re)instituted following the Streptase®, Streptokinase, infusion, the TT or APTT should be less than twice the normal control value (see manufacturer's prescribing information for proper use of heparin).

Drug Interactions

The interaction of Streptase®, Streptokinase, with other drugs has not been well studied.

Use of Anticoagulants and Antiplatelet Agents. Streptase®, Streptokinase, alone or in combination with antiplatelet agents and anticoagulants, may cause bleeding complications. Therefore, careful monitoring is advised.

Anticoagulation After Treatment for Myocardial Infarction. The administration of anticoagulant and/or antiplatelet drugs following administration of Streptase®, Streptokinase, appears to increase the risk of bleeding (see **ADVERSE REACTIONS**). These agents have been used in an attempt to prevent reocclusion of the target vessel. Use of anticoagulants following administration of Streptokinase has not yet been shown to be of unequivocal clinical benefit. Therefore, the use of anticoagulant regimens should be individualized.

Anticoagulation After IV Treatment for Other Indications. Continuous intravenous infusion of heparin, without a loading dose, has been recommended following termination of Streptase®, Streptokinase, infusion for treatment of pulmonary embolism or deep vein thrombosis to prevent rethrombosis. The effect of Streptokinase on thrombin time (TT) and activated partial thromboplastin time (APTT) will usually diminish within 3 to 4 hours after Streptokinase therapy, and heparin therapy without a loading dose can be initiated when the TT or the APTT is less than twice the normal control value.

Pregnancy
Pregnancy Category C. Animal reproduction studies have not been conducted with Streptase®, Streptokinase. It is also not known whether Streptokinase can cause fetal harm when administered to a pregnant woman or can affect reproduction capacity. Streptokinase should be given to a pregnant woman only if clearly needed.

Pediatric Use
Safety and effectiveness in children have not been established.

ADVERSE REACTIONS
The following adverse reactions have been associated with intravenous therapy and may also occur with intracoronary artery infusion:

Bleeding
The incidence of bleeding (major or minor) varied widely from study to study depending on dosage, patient population and concomitant therapy.

Minor bleeding can be anticipated mainly in invaded or disturbed sites. If such bleeding occurs, local measures should be taken to control the bleeding.

Severe internal bleeding involving gastrointestinal, genitourinary, retroperitoneal, or intracerebral sites has occurred and has resulted in fatalities. In three studies in which anticoagulation was optional following intravenous administration of Streptase®, Streptokinase, for acute myocardial infarction, the incidence of major bleeding ranged from 0.3%–6.2%. In 21 studies in which anticoagulation was compulsory, the incidence of major bleeding ranged from 0–16%. The overall incidence of major bleeding with high-dose intravenous infusion is 1.2%.

Major bleed rates are difficult to determine for other dosages and patient populations because of the different dosing and intervals of infusions. The rates reported appear to be within the ranges reported for intravenous administration in acute myocardial infarction.

Should uncontrollable bleeding occur, Streptokinase infusion should be terminated immediately. Slowing the rate of administration of Streptokinase will not help correct bleeding and may make it worse. If necessary, bleeding can be reversed and blood loss effectively managed with appropriate replacement therapy. Although the use of aminocaproic acid (ACA, AMICAR®) in humans as an antidote for Streptokinase has not been documented, in may be considered in an emergency situation.

Allergic Reactions
Anaphylactic and anaphylactoid reactions have been observed rarely in patients treated intravenously with Streptase®, Streptokinase. These ranged in severity from minor breathing difficulty to bronchospasm, periorbital swelling or angioneurotic edema. Other milder allergic effects such as urticaria, itching, flushing, nausea, headache and musculoskeletal pain have also been observed, as have delayed hypersensitivity reactions such as vasculitis and interstitial nephritis. Anaphylactic shock was reported in one study with an incidence rate of 0.1%.

Mild or moderate allergic reactions may be managed with concomitant antihistamine and/or corticosteroid therapy. Severe allergic reactions require immediate discontinuation of Streptase®, Streptokinase, with adrenergic, antihistamine, and/or corticosteroid agents administered intravenously as required.

Fever
Although Streptase®, Streptokinase, is nonpyrogenic in standard animal tests, recent reports in the literature have noted an incidence of fever ranging from 0 to 21% in patients treated intravenously with Streptokinase. Symptomatic treatment is usually sufficient to alleviate discomfort.

DOSAGE AND ADMINISTRATION

Acute Evolving Transmural Myocardial Infarction
Administer Streptokinase as soon as possible after onset of symptoms. The greatest benefit in mortality reduction was observed when Streptase®, Streptokinase, was administered within one hour; statistically significant benefits were observed up to six hours and some benefit was observed up to 12 hours without statistical significance. (See **CLINICAL PHARMACOLOGY**)

Route	Total Dose	Dosage/Duration
Intravenous infusion	1,500,000 IU	1,500,000 IU within 60 min.
Intracoronary infusion	140,000 IU	20,000 IU by bolus followed by 2,000 IU/min. for 60 min.

Pulmonary Embolism, Deep Vein Thrombosis, Arterial Thrombosis or Embolism
Streptase®, Streptokinase, treatment should be instituted as soon as possible after onset of the thrombotic event, preferably within 7 days. Any delay in instituting lytic therapy to evaluate the effect of heparin therapy decreases the potential for optimal efficacy. Since human exposure to streptococci is common, antibodies to Streptokinase are prevalent. Thus, a loading dose of Streptokinase sufficient to neutralize these antibodies is required. A dose of 250,000 IU of Streptokinase infused into a peripheral vein over 30 minutes has been found appropriate in over 90% of patients. Furthermore, if the thrombin time or any other parameter of lysis after 4 hours of therapy is not significantly different from the normal control level, discontinue Streptokinase because excessive resistance is present.

Indication	Loading Dose	IV Infusion Dosage/Duration
Pulmonary Embolism	250,000 IU/30 min	100,000 IU/hr for 24 hr (72 hrs if concurrent DVT is suspected)
Deep Vein Thrombosis	250,000 IU/30 min	100,000 IU/hr for 72 hr
Arterial Thrombosis or Embolism	250,000 IU/30 min	100,000 IU/hr for 24–72 hr

Arteriovenous Cannulae Occlusion
Before using Streptase®, Streptokinase, an attempt should be made to clear the cannula by careful syringe technique, using heparinized saline solution. If adequate flow is not reestablished, Streptokinase may be employed. Allow the effect of any pretreatment anticoagulants to diminish. Instill 250,000 IU Streptokinase in 2 ml of solution into each occluded limb of the cannula slowly. Clamp off cannula limb(s) for 2 hours. Observe the patient closely for possible adverse effects. After treatment, aspirate contents of infused cannula limb(s), flush with saline, reconnect cannula.

Reconstitution and Dilution
The protein nature and lyophilized form of Streptase®, Streptokinase, require careful reconstitution and dilution. Slight flocculation (described as thin translucent fibers) of reconstituted Streptokinase occurred occasionally during clinical trials but did not interfere with the safe use of the solution. The following reconstitution and dilution procedures are recommended:

Vials and Infusion Bottles
1. Slowly add 5 ml Sodium Chloride Injection, USP or Dextrose (5%) Injection, USP to the Streptase®, Streptokinase, vial, directing the diluent at the side of the vacuum-packed vial rather than into the drug powder.
2. Roll and tilt the vial gently to reconstitute. *Avoid shaking.* (Shaking may cause foaming.)
3. Withdraw the entire reconstituted contents of the vial; slowly and carefully dilute further to a total volume as

TABLE I
SUGGESTED DILUTIONS AND INFUSION RATES

DOSAGE	VIAL SIZE (IU)	TOTAL SOLUTION VOLUME	INFUSION RATE
I. *Acute Myocardial Infarction*			
A. *Intravenous Infusion*	1,500,000	45 ml	Infuse 45 ml within 60 minutes
B. *Intracoronary Infusion*	250,000	125 ml	
1. 20,000 IU bolus			1. Loading Dose of 10 ml
2. 2,000 IU/minute for 60 minutes			2. Then 60 ml/hour
II. *Pulmonary Embolism, Deep Vein Thrombosis, Arterial Thrombosis or Embolism Intravenous Infusion*			
A. 1. 250,000 IU loading dose over 30 minutes	1,500,000	90 ml	1. Infuse 30 ml/hour for 30 minutes
2. 100,000 IU/hour maintenance dose			2. Infuse 6 ml per hour
B. SAME	1,500,000 infusion bottle	45 ml	1. 15 ml/hour for 30 minutes 2. Infuse 3 ml per hour

recommended in Table I. Avoid shaking and agitation on dilution. (If necessary, total volume may be increased to a maximum of 500 ml in glass or 50 ml in plastic containers, and the infusion pump rate in Table I should be adjusted accordingly.) To facilitate setting the infusion pump rate, a total volume of 45 ml, or a multiple thereof, is recommended.

4. When diluting the 1,500,000 IU infusion bottle (50 ml), slowly add 5 ml Sodium Chloride Injection, USP, or Dextrose (5%) Injection, USP, directing it at the side of the bottle rather than into the drug powder. Roll and tilt the bottle gently to reconstitute. Avoid shaking as it may cause foaming. Add an additional 40 ml of diluent to the bottle, avoiding shaking and agitation. (Total Volume = 45 ml). Administer by infusion pump at the rate indicated in Table I.
5. Parenteral drug products should be inspected visually for particulate matter and discoloration prior to administration. (The Albumin (Human) may impart a slightly yellow color to the solution.)
6. The reconstituted solution can be filtered through a $0.8\mu m$ or larger pore size filter.
7. Because Streptase®, Streptokinase, contains no preservatives, it should be reconstituted immediately before use. The solution may be used for direct intravenous administration within eight hours following reconstitution if stored at 2–8°C (36–46°F).
8. Do not add other medication to the container of Streptase®, Streptokinase.

[See table above].

For Use in Arteriovenous Cannulae
Slowly reconstitute the contents of 250,000 IU Streptase®, Streptokinase, vacuum-packed vial with 2 ml Sodium Chloride Injection, USP or Dextrose (5%) Injection, USP.

HOW SUPPLIED
Streptase®, Streptokinase, is supplied as a lyophilized white powder in 50 ml infusion bottles (1,500,000 IU) or in 6.5 ml vials with a color-coded label corresponding to the amount of purified Streptokinase in each vial as follows:
green—250,000 IU
blue—750,000 IU
red—1,500,000 IU vials and infusion bottles.
Store unopened vials at controlled room temperature (15–30°C or 59–86°F). Unused reconstituted drug should be discarded.

REFERENCES
1. GISSI: Effectiveness of intravenous thrombolytic treatment in acute myocardial infarction. Lancet I: 397–402, 1986
2. ISIS Steering Committee: Intravenous streptokinase given within 0–4 hours of onset of myocardial infarction reduced mortality in ISIS-2. Lancet I: 502, 1987
3. White, H., Norris, R., Brown, M., et al: Effect of intravenous streptokinase on left ventricular function and early survival after acute myocardial infarction. N Engl J Med 317, 850–5, 1987
4. The I.S.A.M. Study Group: A prospective trial of intravenous streptokinase in acute myocardial infarction (I.S. A.M.). N Engl J Med 314: 1465–1471, 1986
5. Anderson, J., Marshall, H., Bray, B., et al: A randomized trial of intracoronary streptokinase in the treatment of acute myocardial infarction. N Engl J Med 308: 1312–18, 1983
6. Kennedy, J., Ritchie, J., Davis, K., Fritz, J.: Western Washington randomized trial of intracoronary streptokinase in acute myocardial infarction. N Engl J Med 309: 1477–82, 1983

Continued on next page

Hoechst-Roussel—Cont.

7. Sharma, G., Burleson, V., Sasahara, A.: Effect of thrombolytic therapy on pulmonary-capillary blood volume in patients with pulmonary embolism. N Engl J Med 303: 842–5, 1980

8. Arneson, H., Heilo, A., Jakobsen, E., et al: A prospective study of streptokinase and heparin in the treatment of venous thrombosis. Acta Med Scand 203: 457–463, 1978.

Manufactured by: Behringwerke AG
US License No. 97
785000   Revised 5/88
Distributed by: Hoechst-Roussel Pharmaceuticals Inc.
Somerville, NJ 08876

SURFAK®
[ser′ fak]
(docusate calcium USP)

(See PDR For Nonprescription Drugs)
Shown in Product Identification Section, page 412

TOPICORT®   R
[top′ i-kort ″]
(desoximetasone)
EMOLLIENT CREAM 0.25%

TOPICORT® LP
(desoximetasone)
EMOLLIENT CREAM 0.05%

TOPICORT® GEL
(desoximetasone) 0.05%
TOPICORT® OINTMENT
(desoximetasone) 0.25%

DESCRIPTION
Topicort® (desoximetasone) Emollient Cream 0.25%, Topicort® LP (desoximetasone) Emollient Cream 0.05%, Topicort® Gel (desoximetasone) 0.05%, and Topicort® Ointment (desoximetasone) 0.25% contain the active synthetic corticosteroid desoximetasone. The topical corticosteroids constitute a class of primarily synthetic steroids used as anti-inflammatory and anti-pruritic agents. Each gram of Topicort® (desoximetasone) Emollient Cream 0.25% contains 2.5 mg of desoximetasone in an emollient cream consisting of white petrolatum USP, purified water USP, isopropyl myristate NF, lanolin alcohols NF, mineral oil USP, cetostearyl alcohol NF, aluminum stearate and magnesium stearate.
Each gram of Topicort® LP (desoximetasone) Emollient Cream 0.05% contains 0.5 mg of desoximetasone in an emollient cream consisting of white petrolatum USP, purified water USP, isopropyl myristate NF, lanolin alcohols NF, mineral oil USP, cetostearyl alcohol NF, aluminum stearate, edetate disodium USP, lactic acid USP and magnesium stearate.
Each gram of Topicort® Gel (desoximetasone) 0.05% contains 0.5 mg desoximetasone in a gel consisting of purified water USP, SD alcohol 40 (20% w/w), isopropyl myristate NF, carbomer 940, trolamine NF, edetate disodium USP, and docusate sodium USP.
Each gram of Topicort® Ointment (desoximetasone) 0.25% contains 2.5 mg of desoximetasone in a base consisting of white petrolatum USP, propylene glycol USP, sorbitan sesquioleate, beeswax, fatty alcohol citrate, fatty acid pentaerythritol ester, aluminum stearate, citric acid, and butylated hydroxyanisole.
The chemical name of desoximetasone is Pregna-1, 4-diene-3, 20-dione, 9-fluoro-11, 21-dihydroxy-16-methyl-, (11β,16α)-. Desoximetasone has the empirical formula $C_{22}H_{29}FO_4$ and a molecular weight of 376.47. The CAS Registry Number is 382-67-2.
The chemical structure is:

CLINICAL PHARMACOLOGY
Topical corticosteroids share anti-inflammatory, anti-pruritic and vasoconstrictive actions.
The mechanism of anti-inflammatory activity of the topical corticosteroids is unclear. Various laboratory methods, including vasoconstrictor assays, are used to compare and predict potencies and/or clinical efficacies of the topical corticosteroids. There is some evidence to suggest that a recognizable correlation exists between vasoconstrictor potency and therapeutic efficacy in man.

Pharmacokinetics
The extent of percutaneous absorption of topical corticosteroids is determined by many factors including the vehicle, the integrity of the epidermal barrier, and the use of occlusive dressings.
Topical corticosteroids can be absorbed from normal intact skin. Inflammation and/or other disease processes in the skin increase percutaneous absorption. Occlusive dressings substantially increase the percutaneous absorption of topical corticosteroids. Thus, occlusive dressings may be a valuable therapeutic adjunct for treatment of resistant dermatoses.
Once absorbed through the skin, topical corticosteroids are handled through pharmacokinetic pathways similar to systemically administered corticosteroids. Corticosteroids are bound to plasma proteins in varying degrees. Corticosteroids are metabolized primarily in the liver and are then excreted by the kidneys. Some of the topical corticosteroids and their metabolites are also excreted into the bile.
Pharmacokinetic studies in men with Topicort® (desoximetasone) Emollient Cream 0.25% with tagged desoximetasone showed a total of $5.2\% \pm 2.9\%$ excretion in urine ($4.1\% \pm 2.3\%$) and feces ($1.1\% \pm 0.6\%$) and no detectable level (limit of sensitivity: 0.005 μg/mL) in the blood when it was applied topically on the back followed by occlusion for 24 hours. Seven days after application, no further radioactivity was detected in urine or feces. The half-life of the material was 15 ± 2 hours (for urine) and 17 ± 2 hours (for feces) between the third and fifth trial day.
Pharmacokinetic studies in men with Topicort® Ointment (desoximetasone) 0.25% with tagged desoximetasone showed no detectable level (limit of sensitivity: 0.003 μg/mL) in 1 subject and 0.004 and 0.006 μg/mL in the remaining 2 subjects in the blood when it was applied topically on the back followed by occlusion for 24 hours. The extent of absorption for the ointment was 7% based on radioactivity recovered from urine and feces. Seven days after application, no further radioactivity was detected in urine or feces.
Studies with other similarly structured steroids have shown that predominant metabolite reaction occurs through conjugation to form the glucuronide and sulfate ester.

INDICATIONS AND USAGE
Topicort® (desoximetasone) Emollient Cream 0.25%, Topicort® LP (desoximetasone) Emollient Cream 0.05%, Topicort® Gel (desoximetasone) 0.05% and Topicort® Ointment (desoximetasone) 0.25% are indicated for the relief of the inflammatory and pruritic manifestations of corticosteroid-responsive dermatoses.

CONTRAINDICATIONS
Topical corticosteroids are contraindicated in those patients with a history of hypersensitivity to any of the components of the preparation.

PRECAUTIONS
General
Systemic absorption of topical corticosteroids has produced reversible hypothalamic-pituitary-adrenal (HPA) axis suppression, manifestations of Cushing's syndrome, hyperglycemia, and glucosuria in some patients.
Conditions which augment systemic absorption include the application of the more potent steroids, use over large surface areas, prolonged use, and the addition of occlusive dressings.
Therefore, patients receiving a large dose of a potent topical steroid applied to a large surface area or under an occlusive dressing should be evaluated periodically for evidence of HPA axis suppression by using the urinary free cortisol and ACTH stimulation tests. If HPA axis suppression is noted, an attempt should be made to withdraw the drug, to reduce the frequency of application, or to substitute a less potent steroid.
Recovery of HPA axis function is generally prompt and complete upon discontinuation of the drug. Infrequently, signs and symptoms of steroid withdrawal may occur, requiring supplemental systemic corticosteroids.
Children may absorb proportionally larger amounts of topical corticosteroids and thus be more susceptible to systemic toxicity (See **Precautions—Pediatric Use**)
If irritation develops, topical corticosteroids should be discontinued and appropriate therapy instituted.
In the presence of dermatological infections, the use of an appropriate antifungal or antibacterial agent should be instituted. If a favorable response does not occur promptly, the corticosteroid should be discontinued until the infection has been adequately controlled.
Information for the Patient
Patients using topical corticosteroids should receive the following information and instructions:
1. This medication is to be used as directed by the physician. It is for external use only. Avoid contact with the eyes.
2. Patients should be advised not to use this medication for any disorder other than for which it was prescribed.
3. The treated skin area should not be bandaged or otherwise covered or wrapped as to be occlusive unless directed by the physician.
4. Patients should report any signs of local adverse reactions especially under occlusive dressing.
5. Parents of pediatric patients should be advised not to use tight-fitting diapers or plastic pants on a child being treated in the diaper area, as these garments may constitute occlusive dressings.
Laboratory Tests
The following tests may be helpful in evaluating the HPA axis suppression:
    Urinary free cortisol test
    ACTH stimulation test
Carcinogenesis, Mutagenesis, and Impairment of Fertility
Long-term animal studies have not been performed to evaluate the carcinogenic potential or the effect on fertility of topical corticosteroids.
Studies to determine mutagenicity with prednisolone and hydrocortisone have revealed negative results.
Pregnancy Category C
Corticosteroids are generally teratogenic in laboratory animals when administered systemically at relatively low dosage levels. The more potent corticosteroids have been shown to be teratogenic after dermal application in laboratory animals.
Desoximetasone has been shown to be teratogenic and embryotoxic in mice, rats, and rabbits when given by subcutaneous or dermal routes of administration in doses 3 to 30 times the human dose of Topicort® (desoximetasone) Emollient Cream 0.25% and Topicort® Ointment (desoximetasone) 0.25%, or 15 to 150 times the human dose of Topicort® LP (desoximetasone) Emollient Cream 0.05% and Topicort® Gel (desoximetasone) 0.05%.
There are no adequate and well-controlled studies in pregnant women on teratogenic effects from topically applied corticosteroids. Therefore, Topicort® (desoximetasone) Emollient Cream 0.25%, Topicort® LP (desoximetasone) Emollient Cream 0.05%, Topicort® Gel (desoximetasone) 0.05% and Topicort® Ointment (desoximetasone) 0.25% should be used during pregnancy only if the potential benefit justifies the potential risk to the fetus. Drugs of this class should not be used extensively on pregnant patients, in large amounts, or for prolonged periods of time.
Nursing Mothers
It is not known whether topical administration of corticosteroids could result in sufficient systemic absorption to produce detectable quantities in breast milk. Systemically administered corticosteroids are secreted into breast milk in quantities not likely to have a deleterious effect on the infant. Nevertheless, caution should be exercised when topical corticosteroids are administered to a nursing woman.
Pediatric Use
Pediatric patients may demonstrate greater susceptibility to topical corticosteroid-induced HPA axis suppression and Cushing's syndrome than mature patients because of a larger skin surface area to body weight ratio.
Hypothalamic-pituitary-adrenal (HPA) axis suppression, Cushing's syndrome, and intracranial hypertension have been reported in children receiving topical corticosteroids. Manifestations of adrenal suppression in children include linear growth retardation, delayed weight gain, low plasma cortisol levels, and absence of response to ACTH stimulation. Manifestations of intracranial hypertension include bulging fontanelles, headaches, and bilateral papilledema.
Administration of topical corticosteroids to children should be limited to the least amount compatible with an effective therapeutic regimen. Chronic corticosteroid therapy may interfere with the growth and development of children. The safety and effectiveness of Topicort® Ointment (desoximetasone) 0.25% in children below the age of 10 have not been established.

ADVERSE REACTIONS
The following local adverse reactions are reported infrequently with topical corticosteroids, but may occur more frequently with the use of occlusive dressings. These reactions are listed in an approximate decreasing order of occurrence:

Burning	Perioral dermatitis
Itching	Allergic contact dermatitis
Irritation	Maceration of the skin
Dryness	Secondary infection
Folliculitis	Skin Atrophy
Hypertrichosis	Striae
Acneiform eruptions	Miliaria
Hypopigmentation	

In controlled clinical studies the incidence of adverse reactions was low (0.8%) for Topicort® (desoximetasone) Emollient Cream 0.25% and included burning, folliculitis and folliculo-pustular lesions. The incidence of adverse reactions was also 0.8% for Topicort® LP (desoximetasone) Emollient Cream 0.05% and included pruritus, erythema, vesiculation and burning sensation. In controlled clinical studies the incidence of adverse reactions was low (0.3%) for Topicort®

Ointment (desoximetasone) 0.25% and consisted of development of comedones at the site of application.

OVERDOSAGE

Topically applied corticosteroids can be absorbed in sufficient amounts to produce systemic effects (See **Precautions**).

DOSAGE AND ADMINISTRATION

Apply a thin film of Topicort® (desoximetasone) Emollient Cream 0.25%, Topicort® LP (desoximetasone) Emollient Cream 0.05%, Topicort® Gel (desoximetasone) 0.05% or Topicort® Ointment (desoximetasone) 0.25% to the affected skin areas twice daily. Rub in gently.

HOW SUPPLIED

Topicort® (desoximetasone) Emollient Cream 0.25% is supplied in 15 gram, 60 gram, and 4 ounce tubes.
Topicort® LP (desoximetasone) Emollient Cream 0.05% is supplied in 15 gram and 60 gram tubes.
Topicort® Gel (desoximetasone) 0.05% is supplied in 15 gram and 60 gram tubes.
Topicort® Ointment (desoximetasone) 0.25% is supplied in 15 gram and 60 gram tubes.
Store at controlled room temperature (59°-86°F).
Topicort® REG TM Roussel Uclaf
711000-11/87
725000-1/86
714000-2/88

Shown in Product Identification Section, page 412

TRENTAL® ℞
(pentoxifylline)*
Tablets, 400 mg

DESCRIPTION

Trental® (pentoxifylline) tablets for oral administration contain 400 mg of the active drug and the following inactive ingredients: benzyl alcohol NF, FD&C Red #3, hydroxypropyl methylcellulose USP, magnesium stearate NF, polyethylene glycol NF, povidone USP, talc USP, titanium dioxide USP, and other ingredients in a controlled-release formulation. Trental® (pentoxifylline) is a trisubstituted xanthine derivative designated chemically as 1-(5-oxohexyl)-3, 7-dimethylxanthine that, unlike theophylline, is a hemorheologic agent, i.e. an agent that affects blood viscosity. Pentoxifylline is soluble in water and ethanol, and sparingly soluble in toluene.
The chemical structure is:

CLINICAL PHARMACOLOGY
Mode of Action

Pentoxifylline and its metabolites improve the flow properties of blood by decreasing its viscosity. In patients with chronic peripheral arterial disease, this increases blood flow to the affected microcirculation and enhances tissue oxygenation. The precise mode of action of pentoxifylline and the sequence of events leading to clinical improvement are still to be defined. Pentoxifylline administration has been shown to produce dose related hemorheologic effects, lowering blood viscosity, and improving erythrocyte flexibility. Tissue oxygen levels have been shown to be significantly increased by therapeutic doses of pentoxifylline in patients with peripheral arterial disease.

Pharmacokinetics and Metabolism

After oral administration in aqueous solution pentoxifylline is almost completely absorbed. It undergoes a first-pass effect and the various metabolites appear in plasma very soon after dosing. Peak plasma levels of the parent compound and its metabolites are reached within 1 hour. The major metabolites are Metabolite I (1-[5-hydroxyhexyl]-3,7-dimethylxanthine) and Metabolite V (1-[3-carboxypropyl]-3,-7-dimethylxanthine), and plasma levels of these metabolites are 5 and 8 times greater, respectively, than pentoxifylline.
Following oral administration of aqueous solutions containing 100 to 400 mg of pentoxifylline, the pharmacokinetics of the parent compound and Metabolite I are dose-related and not proportional (non-linear), with half-life and area under the blood-level time curve (AUC) increasing with dose. The elimination kinetics of Metabolite V are not dose-dependent. The apparent plasma half-life of pentoxifylline varies from 0.4 to 0.8 hours and the apparent plasma half-lives of its metabolites vary from 1 to 1.6 hours. There is no evidence of accumulation or enzyme induction (Cytochrome P$_{450}$) following multiple oral doses.
Excretion is almost totally urinary; the main biotransformation product is Metabolite V. Essentially no parent drug is found in the urine. Despite large variations in plasma levels of parent compound and its metabolites, the urinary recovery of Metabolite V is consistent and shows dose proportionality. Less than 4% of the administered dose is recovered in feces. Food intake shortly before dosing delays absorption of an immediate release dosage form but does not affect total absorption. The pharmacokinetics and metabolism of Trental® (pentoxifylline) have not been studied in patients with renal and/or hepatic dysfunction, but AUC was increased and elimination rate decreased in an older population (60–68 years) compared to younger individuals (22–30 years).
After administration of the 400 mg controlled-release Trental® (pentoxifylline) tablet, plasma levels of the parent compound and its metabolites reach their maximum within 2 to 4 hours and remain constant over an extended period of time. The controlled release of pentoxifylline from the tablet eliminates peaks and troughs in plasma levels for improved gastrointestinal tolerance.

INDICATIONS AND USAGE

Trental® (pentoxifylline) is indicated for the treatment of patients with intermittent claudication on the basis of chronic occlusive arterial disease of the limbs. Trental® (pentoxifylline) can improve function and symptoms but is not intended to replace more definitive therapy, such as surgical bypass, or removal of arterial obstructions when treating peripheral vascular disease.

CONTRAINDICATIONS

Trental® (pentoxifylline) should not be used in patients who have previously exhibited intolerance to this product or methylxanthines such as caffeine, theophylline, and theobromine.

PRECAUTIONS

General: Patients with chronic occlusive arterial disease of the limbs frequently show other manifestations of arteriosclerotic disease. Trental® (pentoxifylline) has been used safely for treatment of peripheral arterial disease in patients with concurrent coronary artery and cerebrovascular diseases, but there have been occasional reports of angina, hypotension, and arrhythmia. Controlled trials do not show that Trental® (pentoxifylline) causes such adverse effects more often than placebo, but, as it is a methylxanthine derivative, it is possible some individuals will experience such responses.

Drug Interactions: Although a causal relationship has not been established, there have been reports of bleeding and/or prolonged prothrombin time in patients treated with Trental® (pentoxifylline) with and without anticoagulants or platelet aggregation inhibitors. Patients on warfarin should have more frequent monitoring of prothrombin times, while patients with other risk factors complicated by hemorrhage (e.g., recent surgery, peptic ulceration) should have periodic examinations for bleeding including hematocrit and/or hemoglobin. Trental® (pentoxifylline) has been used concurrently with antihypertensive drugs, beta blockers, digitalis, diuretics, antidiabetic agents, and antiarrhythmics, without observed problems. Small decreases in blood pressure have been observed in some patients treated with Trental® (pentoxifylline); periodic systemic blood pressure monitoring is recommended for patients receiving concomitant antihypertensive therapy. If indicated, dosage of the antihypertensive agents should be reduced.

Carcinogenesis, Mutagenesis and Impairment of Fertility: Long-term studies of the carcinogenic potential of pentoxifylline were conducted in mice and rats by dietary administration of the drug at doses up to approximately 24 times (570 mg/kg) the maximum recommended human daily dose (MRHD) of 24 mg/kg for 18 months in mice and 18 months in rats with an additional 6 months without drug exposure in the latter. No carcinogenic potential for pentoxifylline was noted in the mouse study. In the rat study, there was a statistically significant increase in benign mammary fibroadenomas in females in the high dose group (24 × MRHD). The relevance of this finding to human use is uncertain since this was only a marginal statistically significant increase for a tumor that is common in aged rats. Pentoxifylline was devoid of mutagenic activity in various strains of *Salmonella* (Ames test) when tested in the presence and absence of metabolic activation.

Pregnancy: Category C. Teratogenic studies have been performed in rats and rabbits at oral doses up to about 25 and 10 times the maximum recommended human daily dose (MRHD) of 24 mg/kg, respectively. No evidence of fetal malformation was observed. Increased resorption was seen in rats at 25 times MRHD. There are, however, no adequate and well controlled studies in pregnant women. Because animal reproduction studies are not always predictive of human response. Trental® (pentoxifylline) should be used during pregnancy only if clearly needed.

Nursing Mothers: Pentoxifylline and its metabolites are excreted in human milk. Because of the potential for tumorigenicity shown for pentoxifylline in rats, a decision should be made whether to discontinue nursing or discontinue the drug, taking into account the importance of the drug to the mother.

Pediatric Use: Safety and effectiveness in children below the age of 18 years have not been established.

ADVERSE REACTIONS

Clinical trials were conducted using either controlled-release Trental® (pentoxifylline) tablets for up to 60 weeks or immediate-release Trental® (pentoxifylline) capsules for up to 24 weeks. Dosage ranges in the tablet studies were 400 mg bid to tid and in the capsule studies, 200–400 mg tid.
The table summarizes the incidence (in percent) of adverse reactions considered drug related, as well as the numbers of patients who received controlled-release Trental® (pentoxifylline) tablets, immediate-release Trental® (pentoxifylline) capsules, or the corresponding placebos. The incidence of adverse reactions was higher in the capsule studies (where dose related increases were seen in digestive and nervous system side effects) than in the tablet studies. Studies with the capsule include domestic experience, whereas studies with the controlled-release tablets were conducted outside the U.S. The table indicates that in the tablet studies few patients discontinued because of adverse effects.
[See table above].
Trental® (pentoxifylline) has been marketed in Europe and elsewhere since 1972. In addition to the above symptoms, the following have been reported spontaneously since marketing or occurred in other clinical trials with an incidence of less than 1%; the causal relationship was uncertain:
Cardiovascular—dyspnea, edema, hypotension.
Digestive—anorexia, cholecystitis, constipation, dry mouth/thirst.
Nervous—anxiety, confusion.
Respiratory—epistaxis, flu-like symptoms, laryngitis, nasal congestion.

INCIDENCE (%) OF SIDE EFFECTS

	Controlled-Release Tablets Commercially Available		Immediate-Release Capsules Used only for Controlled Clinical Trials	
	Trental®	Placebo	Trental®	Placebo
(Numbers of Patients at Risk)	(321)	(128)	(177)	(138)
Discontinued for Side Effect	3.1	0	9.6	7.2
CARDIOVASCULAR SYSTEM				
Angina/Chest pain	0.3	—	1.1	2.2
Arrhythmia/Palpitation	—	—	1.7	0.7
Flushing	—	—	2.3	0.7
DIGESTIVE SYSTEM				
Abdominal Discomfort	—	—	4.0	1.4
Belching/Flatus/Bloating	0.6	—	9.0	3.6
Diarrhea	—	—	3.4	2.9
Dyspepsia	2.8	4.7	9.6	2.9
Nausea	2.2	0.8	28.8	8.7
Vomiting	1.2	—	4.5	0.7
NERVOUS SYSTEM				
Agitation/Nervousness	—	—	1.7	0.7
Dizziness	1.9	3.1	11.9	4.3
Drowsiness	—	—	1.1	5.8
Headache	1.2	1.6	6.2	5.8
Insomnia	—	—	2.3	2.2
Tremor	0.3	0.8	—	—
Blurred Vision	—	—	2.3	1.4

Continued on next page

Hoechst-Roussel—Cont.

Skin and Appendages—brittle fingernails, pruritus, rash, urticaria, angioedema.
Special Senses—blurred vision, conjunctivitis, earache, scotoma.
Miscellaneous—bad taste, excessive salivation, leukopenia, malaise, sore throat/swollen neck glands, weight change.
A few rare events have been reported spontaneously worldwide since marketing in 1972. Although they occurred under circumstances in which a causal relationship with pentoxifylline could not be established, they are listed to serve as information for physicians: Cardiovascular—angina, arrhythmia, tachycardia; Digestive—hepatitis, jaundice, increased liver enzymes; and Hemic and Lymphatic—decreased serum fibrinogen, pancytopenia, aplastic anemia, purpura, thrombocytopenia.

OVERDOSAGE

Overdosage with Trental® (pentoxifylline) has been reported in children and adults. Symptoms appear to be dose related. A report from a poison control center on 44 patients taking overdoses of enteric-coated pentoxifylline tablets noted that symptoms usually occurred 4–5 hours after ingestion and lasted about 12 hours. The highest amount ingested was 80 mg/kg; flushing, hypotension, convulsions, somnolence, loss of consciousness, fever, and agitation occurred. All patients recovered.
In addition to symptomatic treatment and gastric lavage, special attention must be given to supporting respiration, maintaining systemic blood pressure, and controlling convulsions. Activated charcoal has been used to adsorb pentoxifylline in patients who have overdosed.

DOSAGE AND ADMINISTRATION

The usual dosage of Trental® (pentoxifylline) in controlled-release tablet form is one tablet (400 mg) three times a day with meals.
While the effect of Trental® (pentoxifylline) may be seen within 2 to 4 weeks, it is recommended that treatment be continued for at least 8 weeks. Efficacy has been demonstrated in double-blind clinical studies of 6 months duration. Digestive and central nervous system side effects are dose related. If patients develop these side effects it is recommended that the dosage be lowered to one tablet twice a day (800 mg/day). If side effects persist at this lower dosage, the administration of Trental® (pentoxifylline) should be discontinued.

HOW SUPPLIED

Trental® (pentoxifylline) is available for oral administration as 400 mg pink film-coated oblong tablets imprinted Trental®; supplied in Unit of Use bottles of 100 (NDC 0039-0078-10) and Unit Dose Packs of 100 (NDC 0039-0078-11).
Store at controlled room temperature (59°–86°F).
Dispense in well closed, light resistant containers.
Protect blisters from light.
*U.S. Patents 3,737,433 and 4,189,469   778010-2/88
Trental® REG TM Hoechst AG
Shown in Product Identification Section, page 412

Hollister-Stier

See MILES INC,
Pharmaceutical Division

Hyland Division

Baxter Healthcare Corporation

444 W. GLENOAKS BLVD.
GLENDALE, CA 91202-2936

AUTOPLEX® T   ℞
Anti-Inhibitor Coagulant Complex, Heat Treated

Supplied in single dose 30 ml vials (Hyland Factor VIII correctional activity is stated on label of each vial) with sterile diluent and needles for reconstitution and withdrawal. Heat treated at 60°C for 6 days (144 hours).

BUMINATE® 5%   ℞
Albumin (Human),
USP, 5% Solution

Supplied as a 5% solution in 250 ml and 500 ml bottles. For use with intravenous administration set.

BUMINATE® 25%   ℞
Albumin (Human),
USP, 25% Solution

Supplied as a 25% solution in 20 ml, 50 ml, and 100 ml vials. For use with intravenous administration set.

GAMMAGARD®   ℞
Immune Globulin
Intravenous (Human)

DESCRIPTION

Immune Globulin Intravenous (Human), GAMMAGARD®* is a sterile, dried, highly purified preparation of immunoglobulin G (IgG) which is derived from the cold ethanol fractionation process and is further purified using ultra-filtration and ion exchange adsorption. When reconstituted with the appropriate volume of diluent, this preparation contains approximately 50 mg of protein per mL, of which at least 90% is gamma globulin. The reconstituted product contains approximately 0.15 M sodium chloride and has a pH of 6.8 ± 0.4. Stabilizing agents are present in the following maximum amounts: 20 mg/mL glucose, 2 mg/mL polyethylene glycol (PEG), 0.3 M glycine, and 3 mg/mL Albumin (Human).
The manufacturing process for Immune Globulin Intravenous (Human), Gammagard, isolates IgG without additional chemical or enzymatic modification and the Fc portion is maintained intact. Immune Globulin Intravenous (Human), Gammagard contains all the IgG antibody activities which are present in the donor population. On the average, the distribution of IgG subclasses present in this product is the same as is present in normal plasma.[1] Immune Globulin Intravenous (Human), Gammagard contains only trace amounts of IgM and IgA.
Immune Globulin Intravenous (Human), Gammagard contains no preservative.
This product has been prepared from large pools of human plasma from which donors found to have elevated alanine aminotransferase (ALT) levels were excluded. Each unit of plasma used in the manufacture of this product has been found to be nonreactive for HBsAg by an FDA approved test.

CLINICAL PHARMACOLOGY

Immune Globulin Intravenous (Human), Gammagard contains a broad spectrum of IgG antibodies against bacterial and viral agents that are capable of opsonization and neutralization of microbes and toxins.
Peak levels of IgG are reached immediately after infusion of Immune Globulin Intravenous (Human), Gammagard. It has been shown that IgG is distributed relatively rapidly between plasma and extravascular fluid until approximately half of the total body pool is partitioned in the extravascular space. A rapid initial drop in serum levels is, therefore, to be expected.[2]
As a class, IgG survives longer *in vivo* than other serum proteins.[2,3] Studies show that the half-life of Immune Globulin Intravenous (Human), Gammagard is approximately 24 days. These findings are consistent with reports of a 21 to 25 day half-life for IgG.[2,3,4] The half-life of IgG can vary considerably from person to person, however. In particular, high concentrations of IgG and hypermetabolism associated with fever and infection have been seen to coincide with a shortened half-life of IgG.[2,3,4,5]

INDICATIONS AND USAGE
Immunodeficiencies
Primary
Immune Globulin Intravenous (Human), Gammagard is indicated for the treatment of primary immunodeficient states such as: congenital agammaglobulinemias, common variable immunodeficiency, Wiskott-Aldrich syndrome, and severe combined immunodeficiencies.[4,5] Immune Globulin Intravenous (Human), Gammagard is especially useful when high levels or rapid elevation of circulating IgG are desired or when intramuscular injections are contraindicated (e.g., small muscle mass).
B-cell Chronic Lymphocytic Leukemia
Immune Globulin Intravenous (Human) (IGIV), Gammagard is indicated for prevention of bacterial infections in patients with hypogammaglobulinemia and/or recurrent bacterial infections associated with B-cell Chronic Lymphocytic Leukemia (CLL). In a study of 81 patients, 41 of whom were treated with Immune Globulin Intravenous (Human), Gammagard, bacterial infections were significantly reduced in the treatment group.[6,7] In this study, the placebo group had approximately twice as many bacterial infections as the IGIV group. The median time to first bacterial infection for the IGIV group was greater than 365 days. By contrast, the time to first bacterial infection in the placebo group was 192 days. The number of viral and fungal infections, which were for the most part minor, was not statistically different between the two groups.
Idiopathic Thrombocytopenic Purpura (ITP)
When a rapid rise in platelet count is needed to control bleeding or to allow a patient with ITP to undergo surgery, the

administration of Immune Globulin Intravenous (Human), Gammagard should be considered. The efficacy of Immune Globulin Intravenous (Human), Gammagard has been demonstrated in a clinical study involving sixteen patients (twelve adults and four children) diagnosed with acute or chronic Idiopathic Thrombocytopenic Purpura (ITP). Each of the sixteen patients (100%) demonstrated an acute, clinically significant rise in platelet count (platelet count greater than 40,000/mm³) following the administration of Immune Globulin Intravenous (Human), Gammagard.
Ten of the sixteen patients (62%) exhibited a clinically significant rise in platelet count after only one 1 g/kg infusion; four patients (25%) exhibited this result after only two 1 g/kg infusions; and two patients exhibited this result after more than two 1 g/kg infusions. The rise in platelet count is generally rapid, occurring within 5 days. The rise, however, is transient and should not be considered curative. Platelet rises most often lasted 2 to 3 weeks, with a range of 12 days to 6 months. *It should be noted that childhood ITP may resolve spontaneously without treatment.*

CONTRAINDICATIONS
None known.

WARNINGS
Immune Globulin Intravenous (Human), Gammagard should only be administered intravenously. Other routes of administration have not been evaluated.
Immune Globulin Intravenous (Human), Gammagard contains very low quantities of IgA (not more than 10 μg/mL); nonetheless, it should be given with caution to patients with antibodies to IgA or selective IgA deficiencies.[5,8]

PRECAUTIONS
Drug Interactions
Admixtures of Immune Globulin Intravenous (Human), Gammagard with other drugs have not been evaluated. It is recommended that Immune Globulin Intravenous (Human), Gammagard be administered separately from other drugs or medication which the patient may be receiving.
Pregnancy Category C
Animal reproduction studies have not been conducted with Immune Globulin Intravenous (Human), Gammagard. It is also not known whether Immune Globulin Intravenous (Human), Gammagard can cause fetal harm when administered to a pregnant woman or can affect reproduction capacity. Immune Globulin Intravenous (Human), Gammagard should be given to a pregnant woman only if clearly needed.

ADVERSE REACTIONS
In general, adverse reactions to Immune Globulin Intravenous (Human) (IGIV), Gammagard in patients with congenital or acquired immunodeficiencies are similar in kind and frequency. The incidence of untoward reactions in these patients is low, although various minor reactions, such as headache, fatigue, chills, backache, leg cramps, lightheadedness, fever, urticaria, flushing, slight elevation of blood pressure, nausea and vomiting may occasionally occur. The incidence of these reactions directly attributable to the infusion of Immune Globulin Intravenous (Human), Gammagard during the clinical trials of primary immunodeficiencies was about 6%. In the study of patients with B-cell Chronic Lymphocytic Leukemia (CLL), the incidence was about 3%. Slowing or stopping the infusion usually allows the symptoms to disappear promptly.
During the clinical study of this product for treatment of Idiopathic Thrombocytopenic Purpura (ITP), the only side effect reported was headache which occurred in 12 of 16 patients. Oral antihistamines and analgesics alleviated the headache and were used as pretreatment for those patients requiring additional IGIV therapy. The remaining four patients did not report any side effects and did not require pretreatment.
Immediate anaphylactic and hypersensitivity reactions are a remote possibility. Epinephrine should be available for treatment of any acute anaphylactoid reaction. (See *Warnings*.)

DOSAGE AND ADMINISTRATION
Immunodeficiencies
For patients with primary immunodeficiencies, monthly doses of at least 100 mg/kg are recommended. Initially, patients may receive 200–400 mg/kg. As there are significant differences in the half-life of IgG among patients with primary immunodeficiencies, the frequency and amount of immunoglobulin therapy may vary from patient to patient. The proper amount can be determined by monitoring clinical response. The minimum serum concentration of IgG necessary for protection has not been established.
For patients with hypogammaglobulinemia and/or recurrent bacterial infections due to B-cell Chronic Lymphocytic Leukemia (CLL), a dose of 400 mg/kg every three to four weeks is recommended.
Idiopathic Thrombocytopenic Purpura (ITP)
For patients with acute or chronic Idiopathic Thrombocytopenic Purpura (ITP), a dose of 1 g/kg is recommended. The need for additional doses can be determined by clinical re-

sponse and platelet count. Up to three doses may be given on alternate days if required.

Rate of Administration

It is recommended that initially a rate of 0.5 mL/kg/Hr be used. If infusion at this rate causes the patient no distress, the administration rate may be gradually increased but should not exceed 4 mL/kg/Hr.

A rate of administration which is too rapid may cause flushing and changes in pulse rate and blood pressure. Slowing or stopping the infusion usually allows the symptoms to disappear promptly.

Administration

Immune Globulin Intravenous (Human), Gammagard should be administered as soon after reconstitution as possible. Administration should not begin more than 2 hours after reconstitution.

The reconstituted material should be at room temperature during administration.

Parenteral drug products should be inspected visually for particulate matter and discoloration prior to administration, whenever solution and container permit.

HOW SUPPLIED

Immune Globulin Intravenous (Human), Gammagard is supplied in either 0.5 g, 2.5 g, 5.0 g, or 10.0 g single use bottles. Each bottle of Immune Globulin Intravenous (Human), Gammagard is furnished with a suitable volume of Sterile Water for Injection, USP, and a transfer device. An administration set, which contains an integral airway and a 15 micron filter, is included with the 2.5 g, 5.0 g, and 10.0 g sizes.

STORAGE

Immune Globulin Intravenous (Human), Gammagard is to be stored at a temperature not to exceed 25°C (77°F). Freezing should be avoided to prevent the diluent bottle from breaking.

REFERENCES

1. Unpublished data in the files of Baxter Healthcare Corporation
2. Waldmann TA, Storber W: Metabolism of immunoglobulins. *Prog Allergy 13:* 1–110, 1969
3. Morell A, Riesen W: Structure, function and catabolism of immunoglobulins in *Immunohemotherapy.* Nydegger UE (ed), London, Academic Press, 1981, pp 17–26
4. Stiehm ER: Standard and special human immune serum globulins as therapeutic agents. *Pediatrics 63:* 301–319, 1979
5. Buckley RH: Immunoglobulin replacement therapy: Indications and contraindications for use and variable IgG levels achieved in *Immunoglobulins: Characteristics and Use of Intravenous Preparations.* Alving BM, Finlayson JS (eds), Washington, DC, U.S. Department of Health and Human Services, 1979, pp 3–8
6. Bunch C, Chapel HM, Rai K, et al: Intravenous Immune Globulin reduces bacterial infections in Chronic Lymphocytic Leukemia: A controlled randomized clinical trial, *Blood 70 Suppl 1:* 753, 1987
7. Cooperative Group for The Study Of Immunoglobulin in Chronic Lymphocytic Leukemia: Intravenous immunoglobulin for the prevention of infection in Chronic Lymphocytic Leukemia: A randomized, controlled clinical trial. *N Eng J Med 319:* 902–907, 1988
8. Burks AW, Sampson HA, Buckley RH: Anaphylactic reactions after gammaglobulin administration in patients with hypogammaglobulinemia: Detection of IgE antibodies to IgA. *N Eng J Med 314:* 560–564, 1986

BIBLIOGRAPHY

Bussel JB, Kimberly RP, Inman RD, *et al:* Intravenous gammaglobulin treatment of chronic idiopathic thrombocytopenic purpura. *Blood 62:* 480–486, 1983

HEMOFIL® M   ℞
Antihemophilic Factor (Human)
Method M, Monoclonal Purified

Supplied in single dose bottles. Each bottle is labeled with the potency in international Units, and is packaged together with 10 mL of Sterile Water for Injection, USP, double-ended needle, and a filter needle.

PROPLEX® T   ℞
Factor IX Complex, Heat Treated

Indicated for Factor VII and Factor IX deficiency and Factor VIII inhibitor therapy. Supplied in single dose 30 ml vials

(Factor IX and Factor VII content are stated on the label of each vial) with sterile diluent and needles for reconstitution and withdrawal. Heat treated at 60°C for 144 hours (6 days).

PROTENATE® 5%   ℞
Plasma Protein Fraction (Human),
USP, 5% Solution

Supplied as a 5% solution in 250 ml and 500 ml bottles. For use with intravenous administration set.

Hynson, Westcott & Dunning Products
**Becton Dickinson Microbiology Systems
Division of Becton Dickinson and Company
P.O. BOX 243
COCKEYSVILLE, MD 21030**

BAL IN OIL AMPULES   ℞
(Dimercaprol Injection, USP)

DESCRIPTION

Dimercaprol (2,3-dimercapto-1-propanol) is a colorless or almost colorless liquid, having a disagreeable, mercaptanlike odor. Each 1 ml sterile BAL in Oil contains 100 mg Dimercaprol in 200 mg benzyl benzoate and 700 mg peanut oil. The slight sediment which may be noticed in some ampules develops during sterilization. It is not an indication that the solution is deteriorating.

ACTION

Dimercaprol promotes the excretion of arsenic, gold and mercury in cases of poisoning. It is also used in combination with Edetate Calcium Disodium Injection, USP to promote the excretion of lead.

INDICATIONS

BAL in Oil (Dimercaprol Injection, USP) is indicated in the treatment of arsenic, gold and mercury poisoning. It is indicated in acute lead poisoning when used concomitantly with Edetate Calcium Disodium Injection, USP.

Dimercaprol Injection, USP is effective for use in acute poisoning by mercury salts if therapy is begun within one or two hours following ingestion. It is not very effective for chronic mercury poisoning.

Dimercaprol Injection, USP is of questionable value in poisoning caused by other heavy metals such as antimony and bismuth. It should not be used in iron, cadmium, or selenium poisoning because the resulting dimercaprol-metal complexes are more toxic than the metal alone, especially to the kidneys.

CONTRAINDICATIONS

BAL in Oil is contraindicated in most instances of hepatic insufficiency with the exception of postarsenical jaundice. The drug should be discontinued or used only with extreme caution if acute renal insufficiency develops during therapy.

WARNINGS

There may be local pain at the site of the injection. A reaction apparently peculiar to children is fever which may persist during therapy. It occurs in approximately 30% of children. A transient reduction of the percentage of polymorphonuclear leukocytes may also be observed.

PRECAUTIONS

Because the dimercaprol-metal complex breaks down easily in an acid medium, production of an alkaline urine affords protection to the kidney during therapy. Medicinal iron should not be administered to patients under therapy with BAL. Data is not available regarding the use of dimercaprol during pregnancy and it should not be used unless judged by the physician to be necessary in the treatment of life threatening acute poisoning.

ADVERSE REACTIONS

One of the most consistent responses to Dimercaprol Injection, USP is a rise in blood pressure accompanied by tachycardia. This rise is roughly proportional to the dose administered. Doses larger than those recommended may cause other transitory signs and symptoms in approximate order of frequency as follows: (1) nausea and, in some instances, vomiting; (2) headache; (3) a burning sensation in the lips, mouth and throat; (4) a feeling of constriction, even pain, in the throat, chest, or hands; (5) conjunctivitis, lacrimation, blepharal spasm, rhinorrhea, and salivation; (6) tingling of the hands; (7) a burning sensation in the penis; (8) sweating of the forehead, hands and other areas; (9) abdominal pain; and (10) occasional appearance of painful sterile abscesses. Many of the above symptoms are accompanied by a feeling of anxiety, weakness, and unrest and often are relieved by administration of an antihistamine.

DOSAGE AND ADMINISTRATION

By deep intramuscular injection only. For mild arsenic or gold poisoning, 2.5 mg/kg of body weight four times daily for two days, two times on the third day, and once daily thereafter for ten days; for severe arsenic or gold poisoning, 3 mg/kg every four hours for two days, four times on the third day, then twice daily thereafter for ten days. For mercury poisoning, 5 mg/kg initially, followed by 2.5 mg/kg one or two times daily for ten days. For acute lead encephalopathy 4 mg/kg body weight is given alone in the first dose and thereafter at four hour intervals in combination with Edetate Calcium Disodium Injection, USP administered at a separate site. For less severe poisoning the dose can be reduced to 3 mg/kg after the first dose. Treatment is maintained for two to seven days depending on clinical response. Successful treatment depends on beginning injections at the earliest possible moment and on the use of adequate amounts at frequent intervals. Other supportive measures should always be used in conjunction with BAL in Oil therapy.

HOW SUPPLIED

3 ml (100 mg/ml, ampules, box of 10, NDC 0011-8341-09).

LACTINEX® TABLETS AND GRANULES

(See PDR For Nonprescription Drugs)

ICI Pharma
**A Business Unit of ICI Americas Inc.
WILMINGTON, DE 19897 USA**

NOLVADEX® 10 mg Tablets   ℞
[nol'va-dex"]
(tamoxifen citrate)

DESCRIPTION

NOLVADEX (tamoxifen citrate) tablets for oral administration contain 15.2 mg of tamoxifen citrate, which is equivalent to 10 mg of tamoxifen. It is a nonsteroidal antiestrogen. Chemically, NOLVADEX is the trans-isomer of a triphenylethylene derivative. The chemical name is (Z) 2-[4-(1,2-diphenyl-1-butenyl) phenoxy]-N, N-dimethylethanamine 2-hydroxy-1,2,3-propanetricarboxylate (1:1).

Tamoxifen citrate has a molecular weight of 563.62, the pKa' is 8.85, the equilibrium solubility in water at 37°C is 0.5 mg/mL and in 0.02 N HCl at 37°C, it is 0.2 mg/mL.

NOLVADEX is intended only for oral administration; the tablets should be protected from heat and light.

Inactive ingredients: carboxymethylcellulose calcium, magnesium stearate, mannitol, starch.

CLINICAL PHARMACOLOGY

NOLVADEX is a nonsteroidal agent which has demonstrated potent antiestrogenic properties in animal test systems. The antiestrogenic effects may be related to its ability to compete with estrogen for binding sites in target tissues such as breast. Tamoxifen inhibits the induction of rat mammary carcinoma induced by dimethylbenzanthracene (DMBA), and causes the regression of already established DMBA-induced tumors. In this rat model, tamoxifen appears to exert its antitumor effects by binding to estrogen receptors.

In cytosols derived from human breast adenocarcinomas, tamoxifen competes with estradiol for estrogen receptor protein.

Preliminary pharmacokinetics in women using radiolabeled tamoxifen has shown that most of the radioactivity is slowly excreted in the feces, with only small amounts appearing in urine. The drug is excreted mainly as conjugates, with unchanged drug and hydroxylated metabolites accounting for 30% of the total.

Blood levels of total radioactivity following single oral doses of approximately 0.3 mg/kg reached peak values of 0.06–0.14 μg/mL at 4–7 hours after dosing, with only 20%–30% of the drug present as tamoxifen. There was an initial half-life of 7–14 hours with secondary peaks four or more days later. The prolongation of blood levels and fecal excretion is believed to be due to enterohepatic circulation.

Two studies (Hubay and NSABP B-09) demonstrated an improved disease-free survival following radical or modified radical mastectomy in postmenopausal women or women 50 years of age or older with surgically curable breast cancer with positive axillary nodes when NOLVADEX was added to adjuvant cytotoxic chemotherapy. In the Hubay study, NOLVADEX was added to 'low-dose' CMF (cyclophosphamide, methotrexate and fluorouracil). In the NSABP B-09 study, NOLVADEX was added to melphalan [L-phenylalanine mustard (P)] and fluorouracil (F).

Tumor hormone receptors may help predict which patients will benefit from the adjuvant therapy, but not all breast

Continued on next page

ICI Pharma—Cont.

cancer adjuvant NOLVADEX studies have shown a clear relationship between hormone receptor status and treatment effect. In the Hubay study, patients with a positive (more than 3 fmol) estrogen receptor were more likely to benefit. In the NASBP B-09 study in women age 50–59 years, only women with both estrogen and progesterone receptor levels 10 fmol or greater clearly benefited, while there was a nonstatistically significant trend toward adverse effect in women with both estrogen and progesterone receptor levels less than 10 fmol. In women age 60–70 years, there was a trend toward a beneficial effect of NOLVADEX without any clear relationship to estrogen or progesterone receptor status.

Three prospective studies (ECOG-1178, Toronto, NATO) using NOLVADEX adjuvantly as a single agent demonstrated an improved disease-free survival following total mastectomy and axillary dissection for postmenopausal women with positive axillary nodes compared to placebo/no treatment controls. The NATO study also demonstrated an overall survival benefit. These overall survival results have yet to be replicated.

Three prospective, randomized studies (Ingle, Pritchard, Buchanan) compared NOLVADEX to ovarian ablation (oophorectomy or ovarian irradiation) in premenopausal woman with advanced breast cancer. Although the objective response rate, time to treatment failure, and survival were similar with both treatments, the limited patient accrual prevented a demonstration of equivalence. In an overview analysis of survival data from the three studies, the hazard ratio for death (NOLVADEX/ovarian ablation) was 1.00 with two-sided 95% confidence intervals of 0.73 to 1.37. Elevated serum and plasma estrogens have been observed in premenopausal women receiving NOLVADEX. However, the data from the randomized studies do not suggest an adverse effect. A limited number of premenopausal patients with disease progression during NOLVADEX therapy responded to subsequent ovarian ablation.

INDICATIONS AND USAGE

NOLVADEX is effective in the treatment of metastatic breast cancer in women. In premenopausal women with metastatic breast cancer, NOLVADEX is an alternative to oophorectomy or ovarian ablation. Available evidence indicates that patients whose tumors are estrogen receptor positive are more likely to benefit from NOLVADEX therapy.

NOLVADEX is effective in delaying recurrence following total mastectomy and axillary dissection in postmenopausal women with breast cancer (T_{1-3}, N_1, M_0). The estrogen and progesterone receptor values may help to predict whether NOLVADEX therapy is likely to be beneficial. In some NOLVADEX adjuvant studies, most of the benefit to date has been in the subgroup with 4 or more positive axillary nodes.

CONTRAINDICATIONS

NOLVADEX is contraindicated in patients with known hypersensitivity to the drug.

WARNINGS

Pregnancy Category D: NOLVADEX may cause fetal harm when administered to a pregnant woman. Individuals should not become pregnant while taking NOLVADEX and should use barrier or nonhormonal contraceptive measures. Effects on reproductive functions are expected from the antiestrogenic properties of the drug. In reproductive studies in rats at dose levels equal to or below the human dose, nonteratogenic developmental skeletal changes were seen and were found to be reversible. In addition, in fertility studies in rats and in teratology studies in rabbits using doses at or below those used in humans, a lower incidence of embryo implantation and a higher incidence of fetal death or retarded in utero growth were observed, with slower learning behavior in some rat pups. The impairment of learning behavior did not achieve statistical significance in one study, and, in another study where significance was reported, this was obtained by comparing dosed animals with controls of another study. Several pregnant marmosets were dosed during organogene-

sis or in the last half of pregnancy. No deformations were seen, and although the dose was high enough to terminate pregnancy in some animals, those that did maintain pregnancy showed no evidence of teratogenic malformations. There are no adequate and well-controlled studies in pregnant women. There have been reports of spontaneous abortions, birth defects, fetal deaths, and vaginal bleeding. If this drug is used during pregnancy or the patient becomes pregnant while taking this drug, the patient should be apprised of the potential hazard to the fetus.

Ocular changes have been reported in a few patients who, as part of a clinical trial, were treated for periods greater than one year with NOLVADEX at doses at least four times the highest recommended daily dose of 40 mg. The ocular changes consist of retinopathy and, in some patients, there are also corneal changes and a decrease in visual acuity.

In addition, a few cases of ocular changes including visual disturbances, cataracts, corneal changes, and/or retinopathy have been reported in patients treated with NOLVADEX at recommended doses. It is uncertain if all of these effects are due to NOLVADEX. NOLVADEX has been observed to cause cataracts in rats after 6 months in studies at doses of 20 mg/kg/day (gavage) and higher.

As with other additive hormonal therapy (estrogens and androgens), hypercalcemia has been reported in some breast cancer patients with bone metastases within a few weeks of starting treatment with NOLVADEX. If hypercalcemia does occur, appropriate measures should be taken, and if severe, NOLVADEX should be discontinued.

PRECAUTIONS

General: NOLVADEX should be used cautiously in patients with existing leukopenia or thrombocytopenia. Observations of leukopenia and thrombocytopenia occasionally have been made, but it is uncertain if these effects are due to NOLVADEX therapy. Transient decreases in platelet counts, usually to 50,000–100,000/mm³, infrequently lower, have been occasionally reported in patients taking NOLVADEX for breast cancer. No hemorrhagic tendency has been recorded, and the platelet counts returned to normal levels even though treatment with NOLVADEX continued.

Laboratory Tests: Periodic complete blood counts, including platelet counts, may be appropriate.

Drug Interactions: When NOLVADEX is used in combination with coumarin-type anticoagulants, a significant increase in anticoagulant effect may occur. Where such coadministration exists, careful monitoring of the patient's prothrombin time is recommended.

Drug/Laboratory Testing Interactions: During postmarketing surveillance, T_4 elevations were reported for a few postmenopausal patients which may be explained by increases in thyroid binding globulin. These elevations were not accompanied by clinical hyperthyroidism.

Variations in the karyopyknotic index on vaginal smears and various degrees of estrogen effect on pap smears have been infrequently seen in postmenopausal patients given NOLVADEX.

In the postmarketing experience with NOLVADEX, infrequent cases of hyperlipidemias have been reported. Periodic monitoring of plasma triglycerides and cholesterol may be indicated in patients with preexisting hyperlipidemias.

Carcinogenesis: A conventional carcinogenesis study in rats, presently in progress, has revealed hepatocellular carcinomas at doses of 35 mg/kg/day (206.5 mg/m²) within 31–37 weeks and cataracts at doses of 20 and 35 mg/kg/day within six months. In addition, preliminary data from two independent reports of 6-month studies in rats reveal liver tumors which in one study are classified as malignant.

Endocrine changes in immature and mature mice were investigated in a 13-month study. Granulosa cell ovarian tumors and interstitial cell testicular tumors were found in mice receiving NOLVADEX, but not in the controls.

Mutagenesis: No genotoxic potential has been found in a battery of in vivo and in vitro tests with pro- and eukaryotic test systems with drug metabolizing systems present.

Impairment of Fertility
Fertility of female rats was decreased following administration of 0.04 mg/kg for two weeks prior to mating through day

7 of pregnancy. There was a decreased number of implantations, and all fetuses were found dead.

Following administration to rats of 0.16 mg/kg from days 7–17 of pregnancy, there were increased numbers of fetal deaths. Administration of 0.125 mg/kg to rabbits during days 6–18 of pregnancy resulted in abortion or premature delivery. Fetal deaths occurred at higher doses. There were no teratogenic changes in either rat or rabbit segment II studies. Several pregnant marmosets were dosed with 10 mg/kg/day either during organogenesis or in the last half of pregnancy. No deformations were seen, and although the dose was high enough to terminate pregnancy in some animals, those that did maintain pregnancy showed no evidence of teratogenic malformations. Rats given 0.16 mg/kg from day 17 of pregnancy to one day before weaning demonstrated increased numbers of dead pups at parturition. It was reported that some rat pups showed slower learning behavior, but this did not achieve statistical significance in one study, and in another study where significance was reported, this was obtained by comparing dosed animals with controls of another study.

The recommended daily human dose of 20–40 mg corresponds to 0.4–0.8 mg/kg for an average 50 kg woman.

Pregnancy Category D: See WARNINGS.

Nursing Mothers: It is not known whether this drug is excreted in human milk. Because many drugs are excreted in human milk and because of the potential for serious adverse reactions in nursing infants from NOLVADEX, a decision should be made whether to discontinue nursing or to discontinue the drug, taking into account the importance of the drug to the mother.

ADVERSE REACTIONS

Adverse reactions to NOLVADEX are relatively mild and rarely severe enough to require discontinuation of treatment. If adverse reactions are severe, it is sometimes possible to control them by a simple reduction of dosage without loss of control of the disease.

In patients treated with NOLVADEX for metastatic breast cancer, the most frequent adverse reactions are hot flashes, nausea, and vomiting. These may occur in up to one-fourth of patients.

Less frequently reported adverse reactions are vaginal bleeding, vaginal discharge, menstrual irregularities, and skin rash. Usually these have not been of sufficient severity to require dosage reduction or discontinuation of treatment.

Increased bone and tumor pain, and also local disease flare have occurred which are sometimes associated with a good tumor response. Patients with increased bone pain may require additional analgesics. Patients with soft tissue disease may have sudden increases in the size of preexisting lesions, sometimes associated with marked erythema within and surrounding the lesions, and/or the development of new lesions. When they occur, the bone pain or disease flare are seen shortly after starting NOLVADEX and generally subside rapidly.

Other adverse reactions which are seen infrequently are hypercalcemia, peripheral edema, distaste for food, pruritus vulvae, depression, dizziness, light-headedness, and headache.

There have been infrequent reports of thromboembolic events occurring during NOLVADEX therapy. Since for cancer patients in general, an increased incidence of thromboembolic events is known to occur, a causal relationship to NOLVADEX remains conjectural. An increased incidence has been reported when cytotoxins are combined with NOLVADEX.

Isolated cases of endometrial hyperplasia, endometrial polyps and endometrial carcinoma have been reported with NOLVADEX treatment. A definitive relationship to NOLVADEX therapy has not been established. Women taking NOLVADEX should be instructed to report abnormal vaginal bleeding which should be promptly investigated. Ovarian cysts have been observed in a small number of premenopausal patients with advanced breast cancer who have been treated with NOLVADEX.

Continued clinical studies have resulted in further information which better indicates the incidence of adverse reactions with NOLVADEX as compared to placebo.

In the Eastern Cooperative Oncology Group (ECOG) adjuvant breast cancer trial, NOLVADEX or placebo was administered for two years to patients following mastectomy. When compared to placebo, NOLVADEX showed a significantly higher incidence of hot flashes (19% versus 8% for placebo). The incidence of all other adverse reactions was similar in the two treatment groups with the exception of thrombocytopenia where the incidence for NOLVADEX was 10% versus 3% for placebo, an observation of borderline statistical significance.

[See table left].

In other adjuvant studies, Toronto and NOLVADEX Adjuvant Trial Organization (NATO), patients received either NOLVADEX or no therapy. In the Toronto study, hot flashes and nausea and/or vomiting were observed in 29% and 19% of patients respectively for NOLVADEX versus 1% and 0% in the untreated group. In the NATO trial, hot flashes, nau-

ECOG Adjuvant Trial
Number of Patients (%)

ADVERSE EFFECT	NOLVADEX (n=91)		Placebo (n=90)	
Pain	31	(34%)	34	(38%)
Abnormal renal function tests	22	(24%)	19	(21%)
Hot Flashes	17	(19%)	7	(8%)
Leukopenia	14	(15%)	16	(18%)
Nausea and/or Vomiting	13	(14%)	15	(17%)
Edema	10	(11%)	11	(12%)
Thrombocytopenia	9	(10%)	3	(3%)
Fatigue/Tiredness	9	(10%)	8	(9%)
Dyspnea	7	(8%)	6	(7%)
Anorexia	5	(6%)	4	(4%)
Cough	5	(6%)	7	(8%)

sea, and/or vomiting and vaginal bleeding were reported in 2.8%, 2.1%, and 2.0% of patients respectively for NOLVADEX versus 0.2% for each in the untreated group. The following table summarizes the incidence of adverse reactions reported at a frequency of 2% or greater from clinical trials (Ingle, Pritchard, Buchanan) which compared NOLVADEX therapy to ovarian ablation in premenopausal patients with metastatic breast cancer.
[See table right].

OVERDOSAGE

Acute overdosage in humans has not been reported. Signs observed at the highest doses following studies to determine LD_{50} in animals were respiratory difficulties and convulsions. No specific treatment for overdosage is known; treatment must be symptomatic.

DOSAGE AND ADMINISTRATION

One or two 10 mg tablets twice a day (morning and evening). In the three single-agent adjuvant NOLVADEX studies noted above (See Clinical Pharmacology), NOLVADEX was administered for two years. The optimal duration of adjuvant therapy is not known.

HOW SUPPLIED

Tablets containing tamoxifen as the citrate in an amount equivalent to 10 mg of tamoxifen (round, biconvex, uncoated, white tablet identified with NOLVADEX 600 debossed on one side and a cameo debossed on the other side) are supplied in bottles of 60 tablets and 250 tablets. Protect from heat and light. NDC 0310-0600.
Shown in Product Identification Section, page 412
Rev. T 05/89

SORBITRATE® ℞
[sorb´i-trate]
(Isosorbide Dinitrate)

DESCRIPTION
SORBITRATE (isosorbide dinitrate), an organic nitrate, is a vasodilator with effects on both arteries and veins.
Isosorbide dinitrate is a white, crystalline, odorless compound which is stable in air and in solution, has a melting point of 70°C and has an optical rotation of +134° (c = 1.0, alcohol, 20°C). Isosorbide dinitrate is freely soluble in organic solvents such as acetone, alcohol, and ether; but is only sparingly soluble in water.
The chemical name for isosorbide dinitrate is 1,4,3,6-dianhydrosorbitol-2,5-dinitrate.
Molecular Weight: 236.14
SORBITRATE is available as:

SORBITRATE SUBLINGUAL
2.5 mg Sublingual Tablet. Each tablet contains 2.5 mg of isosorbide dinitrate.
Inactive ingredients: lactose, magnesium stearate, starch.
5 mg Sublingual Tablet. Each tablet contains 5 mg of isosorbide dinitrate.
Inactive ingredients: lactose, magnesium stearate, Red 7, starch.
10 mg Sublingual Tablet. Each tablet contains 10 mg of isosorbide dinitrate.
Inactive ingredients: lactose, magnesium stearate, starch, Yellow 10.
SORBITRATE CHEWABLE
5 mg Chewable Tablet. Each tablet contains 5 mg of isosorbide dinitrate.
Inactive ingredients: Blue 1, confectioner's sugar, flavor, hydrogenated vegetable oil, magnesium stearate, mannitol, povidone, starch, Yellow 10.
10 mg Chewable Tablet. Each tablet contains 10 mg of isosorbide dinitrate.
Inactive ingredients: confectioner's sugar, flavor, hydrogenated vegetable oil, magnesium stearate, mannitol, povidone, starch, Yellow 10.
SORBITRATE ORAL
5 mg Oral Tablet. Each tablet contains 5 mg of isosorbide dinitrate.
Inactive ingredients: Blue 1, lactose, magnesium stearate, starch, Yellow 10.
10 mg Oral Tablet. Each tablet contains 10 mg of isosorbide dinitrate.
Inactive ingredients: lactose, magnesium stearate, starch, Yellow 10.
20 mg Oral Tablet. Each tablet contains 20 mg of isosorbide dinitrate.
Inactive ingredients: Blue 1, lactose, magnesium stearate, starch.
30 mg Oral Tablet. Each tablet contains 30 mg of isosorbide dinitrate.
Inactive ingredients: lactose, magnesium stearate, starch.
40 mg Oral Tablet. Each tablet contains 40 mg of isosorbide dinitrate.
Inactive ingredients: Blue 1, lactose, magnesium stearate, starch.

Adverse Reactions*	NOLVADEX All Effects Number of Patients (%) n=104		OVARIAN ABLATION All Effects Number of Patients (%) n=100	
Flush	34	(32.7)	46	(46)
Amenorrhea	17	(16.3)	69	(69)
Altered Menses	13	(12.5)	5	(5)
Oligomenorrhea	9	(8.7)	1	(1)
Bone Pain	6	(5.7)	6	(6)
Menstrual Disorder	6	(5.7)	4	(4)
Nausea	5	(4.8)	4	(4)
Cough/Coughing	4	(3.8)	1	(1)
Edema	4	(3.8)	1	(1)
Fatigue	4	(3.8)	1	(1)
Musculoskeletal Pain	3	(2.8)	0	(0)
Pain	3	(2.8)	4	(4)
Ovarian Cyst(s)	3	(2.8)	2	(2)
Depression	2	(1.9)	2	(2)
Abdominal Cramps	1	(1)	2	(2)
Anorexia	1	(1)	2	(2)

*Some patients had more than one adverse reaction.

SORBITRATE SA
Sustained Action Tablet. Each tablet contains 10 mg of isosorbide dinitrate in the outer coat and 30 mg in the inner core (sustained action base).
Inactive ingredients: carbomer 934P, ethylcellulose, lactose, magnesium stearate, polyethylene glycol, Yellow 10.

CLINICAL PHARMACOLOGY
The principal pharmacological action of isosorbide dinitrate is relaxation of vascular smooth muscle, producing a vasodilatory effect on both peripheral arteries and veins, with predominant effects on the latter. Dilation of the post-capillary vessels, including large veins, promotes peripheral pooling of blood and decreases venous return to the heart, thereby reducing left-ventricular end-diastolic pressure (preload). Arteriolar relaxation reduces systemic vascular resistance and arterial pressure (after-load).
The mechanism by which isosorbide dinitrate relieves angina pectoris is not fully understood. Myocardial oxygen consumption or demand (as measured by the pressure-rate product, tension-time index, and stroke-work index) is decreased by both the arterial and venous effects of isosorbide dinitrate and, presumably, a more favorable supply-demand ratio is achieved. While the large epicardial coronary arteries are also dilated by isosorbide dinitrate, the extent to which this contributes to relief of exertional angina is unclear.
Therapeutic doses of isosorbide dinitrate may reduce systolic, diastolic, and mean arterial blood pressures, especially in the upright posture. Effective coronary perfusion is usually maintained. The decrease in systemic blood pressure may result in reflex tachycardia, an effect which results in an unfavorable influence on myocardial oxygen demand. Hemodynamic studies indicate that isosorbide dinitrate may reduce the abnormally elevated left ventricular end-diastolic and pulmonary capillary wedge pressures that occur during an acute episode of angina pectoris.
Isosorbide dinitrate is metabolized by enzymatic denitration to the intermediate products isosorbide-2-mononitrate and isosorbide-5-mononitrate. Both metabolites have biological activity, especially the 5-mononitrate which is also the principal metabolite. The liver is a principal site of metabolism and isosorbide dinitrate is subject to a large first-pass effect. The systemic clearance of the drug following intravenous infusion is about 3.4 liters/min. Since the clearance exceeds hepatic blood flow, considerable extrahepatic metabolism must also occur.
The average bioavailability of isosorbide dinitrate is 59 and 22 percent following sublingual and oral administration, respectively. The terminal half-life is about 20 minutes, 60 minutes, and 4 hours following i.v., sublingual, and oral administration, respectively. The dependence of half-life on the route of administration is not understood. Over limited ranges of i.v. dosing, the pharmacokinetics of isosorbide dinitrate appear linear. However, both the 2- and 5-mononitrate metabolites have been shown to decrease the rate of disappearance of the dinitrate from the blood and the half-lives of isosorbide-5-mononitrate and isosorbide-2-mononitrate range from 4.0–5.6 and 1.5–3.1 hours, respectively.
The pharmacokinetics and/or bioavailability of isosorbide dinitrate during multiple dosing have not been well studied. Because the metabolites influence the clearance of isosorbide dinitrate, prediction of blood levels of parent compound to metabolites from single-dose studies is uncertain.

INDICATIONS AND USAGE
SORBITRATE (isosorbide dinitrate) is indicated for the treatment and prevention of angina pectoris. Controlled clinical trials have demonstrated that the sublingual, chewable, immediate release, and controlled release oral dosage forms of isosorbide dinitrate are effective in improving exercise tolerance in patients with angina pectoris. When single sublingual or chewable doses (5 mg) of isosorbide dinitrate were administered prophylactically to patients with angina pectoris in various clinical studies, duration of exercise until chest pain or fatigue was significantly improved for at least 45 minutes (and as long as 2 hours in some studies) following dosing. Similar studies after single oral (15 to 120 mg) and oral controlled-release (40 to 80 mg) doses of isosorbide dinitrate have shown significant improvement in exercise tolerance for up to 8 hours following dosing. The exercise electro-cardiographic evidence suggests that improved exercise tolerance with isosorbide dinitrate is not at the expense of greater myocardial ischemia. All dosage forms of isosorbide dinitrate may therefore be used prophylactically to decrease frequency and severity of anginal attacks and can be expected to decrease the need for sublingual nitroglycerin.
The sublingual and chewable forms of the drug are indicated for acute prophylaxis of angina pectoris when taken a few minutes before situations likely to provoke anginal attacks. Because of a slower onset of effect, the oral forms of isosorbide dinitrate are not indicated for acute prophylaxis.
In controlled clinical trials, chewable and sublingual isosorbide dinitrate were effective in relieving an acute attack of angina pectoris. Relief occurred with a mean time of 2.9 and 3.4 minutes (chewable and sublingual respectively) compared to relief of angina with a mean time of 1.9 minutes following sublingual nitroglycerin. Because of the more rapid relief of chest pain with sublingual nitroglycerin, the use of sublingual or chewable isosorbide dinitrate for aborting an acute anginal attack should be limited to patients intolerant or unresponsive to sublingual nitroglycerin.

CONTRAINDICATIONS
SORBITRATE is contraindicated in patients who have shown purported hypersensitivity or idiosyncrasy to it or other nitrates or nitrites.

WARNINGS
The benefits of SORBITRATE during the early days of an acute myocardial infarction have not been established. If one elects to use organic nitrates in early infarction, hemodynamic monitoring and frequent clinical assessment should be used because of the potential deleterious effects of hypotension.

PRECAUTIONS
General: Severe hypotensive response, particularly with upright posture, may occur with even small doses of SORBITRATE. The drug should therefore be used with caution in subjects who may have blood volume depletion from diuretic therapy or in subjects who have low systolic blood pressure (eg, below 90 mmHg). Paradoxical bradycardia and increased angina pectoris may accompany nitrate-induced hypotension.
Nitrate therapy may aggravate the angina caused by hypertrophic cardiomyopathy. Tolerance to this drug and cross-tolerance to other nitrates and nitrites may occur.
Marked symptomatic, orthostatic hypotension has been reported when calcium channel blockers and organic nitrates were used in combination. Dose adjustment of either class of agents may be necessary.
Tolerance to the vascular and antianginal effects of isosorbide dinitrate or nitroglycerin has been demonstrated in clinical trials, experience through occupational exposure, and in isolated tissue experiments in the laboratory. The importance of tolerance to the appropriate use of isosorbide dinitrate in the management of patients with angina pectoris has not been determined. However, one clinical trial using treadmill exercise tolerance (as an endpoint) found an 8-hour duration of action of oral isosorbide dinitrate following the first dose (after a 2-week placebo washout) and only a

Continued on next page

ICI Pharma—Cont.

2-hour duration of effect of the same dose after 1 week of repetitive dosing at conventional dosing intervals. On the other hand, several trials have been able to differentiate isosorbide dinitrate from placebo after 4 weeks of therapy, and in open trials, an effect seems detectable for as long as several months.

Tolerance clearly occurs in industrial workers continuously exposed to nitroglycerin. Moreover, physical dependence also occurs since chest pain, acute myocardial infarction, and even sudden death have occurred during temporary withdrawal of nitroglycerin from the workers. In clinical trials in angina patients, there are reports of anginal attacks being more easily provoked and of rebound in the hemodynamic effects soon after nitrate withdrawal. The relative importance of these observations to the routine, clinical use of isosorbide dinitrate is not known. However, it seems prudent to gradually withdraw patients from isosorbide dinitrate when the therapy is being terminated, rather than stopping the drug abruptly.

Information for Patients: Headache may occur during initial therapy with SORBITRATE. Headache is usually relieved by the use of standard headache remedies, or by lowering the dose, and tends to disappear after the first week or two of use.

Drug Interactions: Alcohol may enhance any marked sensitivity to the hypotensive effect of nitrates.

Isosorbide dinitrate acts directly on vascular smooth muscle; therefore, any other agent that depends on vascular smooth muscle as the final common path can be expected to have decreased or increased effect depending on the agent.

Carcinogenesis, Mutagenesis, Impairment of Fertility: No long-term studies in animals have been performed to evaluate the carcinogenic potential of this drug. A modified two-litter reproduction study in rats fed isosorbide dinitrate at 25 or 100 mg/kg/day did not reveal any effects on fertility or gestation or any remarkable gross pathology in any parent or offspring fed isosorbide dinitrate as compared with rats fed a basal-controlled diet.

Pregnancy Category C: Isosorbide dinitrate has been shown to cause a dose-related increase in embryotoxicity (increase in mummified pups) in rabbits at oral doses 35 and 150 times the maximum recommended human daily dose. There are no adequate and well-controlled studies in pregnant women. SORBITRATE should be used during pregnancy only if the potential benefit justifies the potential risk to the fetus.

Nursing Mothers: It is not known whether this drug is excreted in human milk. Because many drugs are excreted in human milk, caution should be exercised when SORBITRATE is administered to a nursing woman.

Pediatric Use: The safety and effectiveness of SORBITRATE in children has not been established.

ADVERSE REACTIONS

Adverse reactions, particularly headache and hypotension, are dose related. In clinical trials at various doses, the following have been observed.

Headache is the most common (reported incidence varies widely, apparently being dose related, with an average occurrence of about 25%) adverse reaction and may be severe and persistent. Cutaneous vasodilation with flushing may occur. Transient episodes of dizziness and weakness, as well as other signs of cerebral ischemia associated with postural hypotension, may occasionally develop (the incidence of reported symptomatic hypotension ranges from 2% to 36%). An occasional individual will exhibit marked sensitivity to the hypotensive effects of nitrates and severe responses (nausea, vomiting, weakness, restlessness, pallor, perspiration, and collapse) may occur even with the usual therapeutic dose. Drug rash and/or exfoliative dermatitis may occasionally occur. Nausea and vomiting appear to be uncommon.

OVERDOSAGE

Signs and Symptoms: These may include the following: a prompt fall in blood pressure, persistent and throbbing headache, vertigo, palpitation, visual disturbances, flushed and perspiring skin (later becoming cold and cyanotic), nausea and vomiting (possibly with colic and even bloody diarrhea), syncope (especially in the upright position), methemoglobinemia with cyanosis and anoxia, initial hyperpnea, dyspnea and slow breathing, slow pulse (dicrotic and intermittent), heart block, increased intracranial pressure with cerebral symptoms of confusion and moderate fever, paralysis and coma followed by clonic convulsions and possibly death due to circulatory collapse.

It is not known what dose of the drug is associated with symptoms of overdosing or what dose of the drug would be life-threatening. The acute oral LD_{50} of isosorbide dinitrate in rats was found to be approximately 1100 mg/kg of body weight. These animal experiments indicate that approximately 500 times the usual therapeutic dose would be required to produce such toxic symptoms in humans. It is not known whether the drug is dialyzable.

Treatment of Overdose: Prompt removal of the ingested material by gastric lavage is reasonable, but not documented to be useful. Keep the patient recumbent in a shock position and comfortably warm. Passive movements of the extremities may aid venous return. Administer oxygen and artificial respiration if necessary. If methemoglobinemia is present, administer methylene blue (1% solution), 1 to 2 mg/kg intravenously.

Methemoglobin: Case reports of clinically significant methemoglobinemia are rare at conventional doses of organic nitrates. The formation of methemoglobin is dose related and in the case of genetic abnormalities of hemoglobin that favor methemoglobin formation, even conventional doses of organic nitrate could produce harmful concentrations of methemoglobin.

WARNING

Epinephrine is ineffective in reversing the severe hypotensive events associated with overdose. It and related compounds are contraindicated in this situation.

DOSAGE AND ADMINISTRATION

For the treatment of angina pectoris, the usual starting dose for sublingual isosorbide dinitrate is 2.5 to 5 mg; and for chewable tablets, 5 mg.

Isosorbide dinitrate should be titrated upward until angina is relieved or side effects limit the dose. In ambulatory patients, the magnitude of the incremental dose increase should be guided by measurements of standing blood pressure.

The initial dosage of sublingual or chewable isosorbide dinitrate for acute prophylactic therapy in angina pectoris patients is generally 5 or 10 mg every 2 to 3 hours. Adequate, controlled clinical studies demonstrating the effectiveness of chronic maintenance therapy with these dosage forms have not been reported.

For the treatment of chronic stable angina pectoris, the usual starting dose for immediate-release oral (swallowed) tablets is 5 to 20 mg; and for controlled-release forms, 40 mg. For maintenance therapy, oral doses of 10 to 40 mg given every 6 hours; or oral controlled-release doses of 40 to 80 mg given every 8 to 12 hours is generally recommended. The extent to which development of tolerance should modify the dosage program has not been defined. **The oral controlled release forms of isosorbide dinitrate should not be chewed.**

HOW SUPPLIED

SORBITRATE Sublingual

2.5 mg Sublingual Tablets. (NDC-0310-0853) White, round tablets (identified front "S", reverse "853") are supplied in bottles of 100 and Unit Dose 100.

5 mg Sublingual Tablets. (NDC-0310-0760) Pink, round tablets (identified front "S", reverse "760") are supplied in bottles of 100 and Unit Dose 100.

10 mg Sublingual Tablets. (NDC-0310-0761) Yellow, round tablets (identified front "S", reverse "761") are supplied in bottles of 100 and Unit Dose 100.

SORBITRATE Chewable

5 mg Chewable Tablets. (NDC-0310-0810) Green, round, scored tablets (identified front "S", reverse "810") are supplied in bottles of 100, 500, and Unit Dose 100.

10 mg Chewable Tablets. (NDC-0310-0815) Yellow, round, scored tablets (identified front "S", reverse "815") are supplied in bottles of 100 and Unit Dose 100.

SORBITRATE Oral

5 mg Oral Tablets. (NDC-0310-0770) Green, oval-shaped, scored tablets (identified front "S", reverse "770") are supplied in bottles of 100, 500, and Unit Dose 100.

10 mg Oral Tablets. (NDC-0310-0780) Yellow, oval-shaped, scored tablets (identified front "S", reverse "780") are supplied in bottles of 100, 500, and Unit Dose 100.

20 mg Oral Tablets. (NDC-0310-0820) Blue, oval-shaped, scored tablets (identified front "S", reverse "820") are supplied in bottles of 100 and Unit Dose 100.

30 mg Oral Tablets. (NDC-0310-0773) White, oval-shaped, scored tablets (identified front "S", reverse "773") are supplied in bottles of 100 and Unit Dose 100.

40 mg Oral Tablets. (NDC-0310-0774) Light blue, oval-shaped, scored tablets (identified front "S", reverse "774") are supplied in bottles of 100 and Unit Dose 100.

SORBITRATE SA

40 mg Sustained Action Tablets. (NDC-0310-0880) Yellow, round, compression-coated tablets (identified front "S", reverse "880") are supplied in bottles of 100 and Unit Dose 100.

All forms of SORBITRATE should be stored in a dry place at room temperature. Avoid excessive heat (over 104°F/40°C).

Rev A   11/86

Shown in Product Identification Section, page 412

TENORETIC®   ℞
[ten "o-ret 'ic]
(atenolol and chlorthalidone)

DESCRIPTION

TENORETIC (atenolol and chlorthalidone) is for the treatment of hypertension. It combines the antihypertensive activity of two agents: a beta₁-selective (cardioselective) hydrophilic blocking agent (atenolol, TENORMIN®) and a monosulfonamyl diuretic (chlorthalidone).

Atenolol is Benzeneacetamide, 4-[2'-hydroxy-3'-[1-methylethyl) amino]propoxy]-.

Atenolol (free base) is a relatively polar hydrophilic compound with a water solubility of 26.5 mg/mL at 37°C. It is freely soluble in 1 N HCl (300 mg/mL at 25°C) and less soluble in chloroform (3 mg/mL at 25°C).

Chlorthalidone is 2-Chloro-5-(1-hydroxy-3-oxo-1-isoindolinyl) benzene sulfonamide.

Chlorthalidone has a water solubility of 12 mg/100 mL at 20°C.

Each TENORETIC 50 tablet contains:
    Atenolol (TENORMIN) ....50 mg
    Chlorthalidone ....25 mg

Each TENORETIC 100 tablet contains:
    Atenolol (TENORMIN) ....100 mg
    Chlorthalidone ....25 mg

Inactive ingredients: magnesium stearate, microcrystalline cellulose, povidone, sodium starch glycolate.

CLINICAL PHARMACOLOGY

Atenolol and chlorthalidone have been used singly and concomitantly for the treatment of hypertension. The antihypertensive effects of these agents are additive and studies have shown that there is no interference with bioavailability when these agents are given together in the single combination tablet. Therefore, this combination provides a convenient formulation for the concomitant administration of these two entities. In patients with more severe hypertension, TENORETIC may be administered with other antihypertensives such as vasodilators.

Atenolol: Atenolol is a beta₁-selective (cardioselective) beta-adrenergic receptor blocking agent without membrane stabilizing or intrinsic sympathomimetic (partial agonist) activities. This preferential effect is not absolute, however, and at higher doses, atenolol inhibits beta₂-adrenoreceptors, chiefly located in the bronchial and vascular musculature.

Pharmacodynamics: In standard animal or human pharmacological tests, beta-adrenoreceptor blocking activity of atenolol has been demonstrated by: 1) reduction in resting and exercise heart rate and cardiac output, 2) reduction of systolic and diastolic blood pressure at rest and on exercise, 3) inhibition of isoproterenol induced tachycardia, and 4) reduction in reflex orthostatic tachycardia.

A significant beta-blocking effect of atenolol, as measured by reduction of exercise tachycardia, is apparent within 1 hour following oral administration of a single dose. This effect is maximal at about 2 to 4 hours and persists for at least 24 hours. The effect at 24 hours is dose-related and also bears a linear relationship to the logarithm of plasma atenolol concentration. However, as has been shown for all beta-blocking agents, the antihypertensive effect does not appear to be related to plasma level.

In normal subjects, the beta₁-selectivity of atenolol has been shown by its reduced ability to reverse the beta₂-mediated vasodilating effect of isoproterenol as compared to equivalent beta-blocking doses of propranolol. In asthmatic patients, a dose of atenolol producing a greater effect on resting heart rate than propranolol resulted in much less increase in airway resistance. In a placebo-controlled comparison of approximately equipotent oral doses of several beta blockers, atenolol produced a significantly smaller decrease of FEV_1 than nonselective beta blockers such as propranolol and unlike those agents did not inhibit bronchodilation in response to isoproterenol.

Consistent with its negative chronotropic effect due to beta blockade of the SA node, atenolol increases sinus cycle length and sinus node recovery time. Conduction in the AV node is also prolonged. Atenolol is devoid of membrane stabilizing activity, and increasing the dose well beyond that producing beta blockade does not further depress myocardial contractility. Several studies have demonstrated a moderate (approximately 10%) increase in stroke volume at rest and exercise.

In controlled clinical trials, atenolol given as a single daily dose, was an effective antihypertensive agent providing 24-hour reduction of blood pressure. Atenolol has been studied in combination with thiazide-type diuretics and the blood pressure effects of the combination are approximately additive. Atenolol is also compatible with methyldopa, hydralazine, and prazosin, the combination resulting in a larger fall in blood pressure than with the single agents. The dose range of atenolol is narrow, and increasing the dose beyond 100 mg once daily is not associated with increased antihypertensive effect. The mechanisms of the antihypertensive effects of beta-blocking agents have not been established. Several mechanisms have been proposed and include: 1) competitive antagonism of catecholamines at peripheral (especially cardiac) adrenergic neuron sites, leading to decreased cardiac output, 2) a central effect leading to reduced sympathetic outflow to the periphery, and 3) suppression of renin activity. The results from long-term studies have not shown any diminution of the antihypertensive efficacy of atenolol with prolonged use.

Pharmacokinetics and Metabolism: In man, absorption of an oral dose is rapid and consistent but incomplete. Approximately 50% of an oral dose is absorbed from the gastrointestinal tract, the remainder being excreted unchanged in the feces. Peak blood levels are reached between 2 and 4 hours after ingestion. Unlike propranolol or metoprolol, but like nadolol, hydrophilic atenolol undergoes little or no metabolism by the liver and the absorbed portion is eliminated primarily by renal excretion. Atenolol also differs from propranolol in that only a small amount (6-16%) is bound to proteins in the plasma. This kinetic profile results in relatively consistent plasma drug levels with about a fourfold interpatient variation. There is no information as to the pharmacokinetic effect of atenolol on chlorthalidone.

The elimination half-life of atenolol is approximately 6 to 7 hours, and there is no alteration of the kinetic profile of the drug by chronic administration. Following doses of 50 mg or 100 mg, both beta-blocking and antihypertensive effects persist for at least 24 hours. When renal function is impaired, elimination of atenolol is closely related to the glomerular filtration rate; but, significant accumulation does not occur until the creatinine clearance falls below 35 mL/min/1.73 m². (See circular for atenolol [TENORMIN]).

Chlorthalidone: Chlorthalidone is a monosulfonamyl diuretic which differs chemically from thiazide diuretics in that a double ring system is incorporated in its structure. It is an oral diuretic with prolonged action and low toxicity. The diuretic effect of the drug occurs within 2 hours of an oral dose. It produces diuresis with greatly increased excretion of sodium and chloride. At maximal therapeutic dosage, chlorthalidone is approximately equal in its diuretic effect to comparable maximal therapeutic doses of benzothiadiazine diuretics. The site of action appears to be the cortical diluting segment of the ascending limb of Henle's loop of the nephron.

INDICATIONS AND USAGE

TENORETIC is indicated for the treatment of hypertension. This fixed-dose combination drug is not indicated for initial therapy of hypertension. If the fixed-dose combination represents the dose appropriate to the individual patient's needs, it may be more convenient than the separate components.

CONTRAINDICATIONS

TENORETIC is contraindicated in patients with: sinus bradycardia, heart block greater than first degree, cardiogenic shock, overt cardiac failure (see WARNINGS), anuria, hypersensitivity to this product or to sulfonamide-derived drugs.

WARNINGS

Cardiac Failure: Sympathetic stimulation is necessary in supporting circulatory function in congestive heart failure, and beta blockade carries the potential hazard of further depressing myocardial contractility and precipitating more severe failure. In hypertensive patients who have congestive heart failure controlled by digitalis and diuretics, TENORETIC should be administered cautiously. Both digitalis and atenolol slow AV conduction.

IN PATIENTS WITHOUT A HISTORY OF CARDIAC FAILURE, continued depression of the myocardium with beta-blocking agents over a period of time can, in some cases, lead to cardiac failure. At the first sign or symptom of impending cardiac failure, patients receiving TENORETIC should be digitalized and/or be given additional diuretic therapy. Observe the patient closely. If cardiac failure continues despite adequate digitalization and diuretic therapy, TENORETIC therapy should be withdrawn.

Renal and Hepatic Disease and Electrolyte Disturbances: Since atenolol is excreted via the kidneys, TENORETIC should be used with caution in patients with impaired renal function.

In patients with renal disease, thiazides may precipitate azotemia. Since cumulative effects may develop in the presence of impaired renal function, if progressive renal impairment becomes evident, TENORETIC should be discontinued. In patients with impaired hepatic function or progressive liver disease, minor alterations in fluid and electrolyte balance may precipitate hepatic coma. TENORETIC should be used with caution in these patients.

Ischemic Heart Disease: Although not yet reported with atenolol following abrupt cessation of therapy with certain beta-blocking agents in patients with coronary artery disease, exacerbations of angina pectoris and, in some cases, myocardial infarction have been reported. Therefore, such patients should be cautioned against interruption of therapy without the physician's advice. Even in the absence of overt angina pectoris, when discontinuation of TENORETIC is planned, the patient should be carefully observed and should

be advised to limit physical activity to a minimum. TENORETIC should be reinstated if withdrawal symptoms occur.

Bronchospastic Diseases: PATIENTS WITH BRONCHOSPASTIC DISEASE SHOULD, IN GENERAL, NOT RECEIVE BETA BLOCKERS. Because of its relative beta₁-selectivity, however, TENORETIC may be used with caution in patients with bronchospastic disease who do not respond to, or cannot tolerate, other antihypertensive treatment. Since beta₁-selectivity is not absolute, the lowest possible dose of TENORETIC should be used and a beta₂-stimulating agent (bronchodilator) should be made available. If dosage must be increased, dividing the dose should be considered in order to achieve lower peak blood levels.

Anesthesia and Major Surgery: As with all beta-receptor blocking drugs, it may be decided to withdraw TENORETIC before surgery. In this case, 48 hours should be allowed to elapse between the last dose and anesthesia. If treatment is continued, care should be taken when using anesthetic agents because of the risk of further depression of the myocardium.

Beta blockers are competitive inhibitors of beta-receptor agonists and their effects on the heart can be reversed by administration of such agents; eg, dobutamine or isoproterenol with caution (see section on OVERDOSAGE). Manifestations of excessive vagal tone (eg, profound bradycardia, hypotension) may be corrected with atropine (1-2 mg IV).

Metabolic and Endocrine Effects: TENORETIC may be used with caution in diabetic patients. Beta blockers may mask tachycardia occurring with hypoglycemia, but other manifestations such as dizziness and sweating may not be significantly affected. Atenolol does not potentiate insulin-induced hypoglycemia and, unlike nonselective beta blockers, does not delay recovery of blood glucose to normal levels. Insulin requirements in diabetic patients may be increased, decreased, or unchanged; latent diabetes mellitus may become manifest during chlorthalidone administration.

Beta-adrenergic blockade may mask certain clinical signs (eg, tachycardia) of hyperthyroidism. Abrupt withdrawal of beta blockade might precipitate a thyroid storm; therefore, patients suspected of developing thyrotoxicosis and from whom TENORETIC therapy is to be withdrawn should be monitored closely.

Because calcium excretion is decreased by thiazides, TENORETIC should be discontinued before carrying out tests for parathyroid function. Pathologic changes in the parathyroid glands, with hypercalcemia and hypophosphatemia, have been observed in a few patients on prolonged thiazide therapy; however, the common complications of hyperparathyroidism such as renal lithiasis, bone resorption, and peptic ulceration have not been seen.

Hyperuricemia may occur or acute gout may be precipitated in certain patients receiving thiazide therapy.

PRECAUTIONS

General:—Electrolyte and Fluid Balance Status: Periodic determination of serum electrolytes to detect possible electrolyte imbalance should be performed at appropriate intervals.

Patients should be observed for clinical signs of fluid or electrolyte imbalance, ie, hyponatremia, hypochloremic alkalosis, and hypokalemia. Serum and urine electrolyte determinations are particularly important when the patient is vomiting excessively or receiving parenteral fluids. Warning signs or symptoms of fluid and electrolyte imbalance include dryness of the mouth, thirst, weakness, lethargy, drowsiness, restlessness, muscle pains or cramps, muscular fatigue, hypotension, oliguria, tachycardia, and gastrointestinal disturbances such as nausea and vomiting.

Hypokalemia may develop, especially with brisk diuresis, when severe cirrhosis is present, or during concomitant use of corticosteroids or ACTH.

Interference with adequate oral electrolyte intake will also contribute to hypokalemia. Hypokalemia can sensitize or exaggerate the response of the heart to the toxic effects of digitalis (eg, increased ventricular irritability). Hypokalemia may be avoided or treated by use of potassium supplements or foods with a high potassium content.

Any chloride deficit during thiazide therapy is generally mild and usually does not require specific treatment except under extraordinary circumstances (as in liver disease or renal disease). Dilutional hyponatremia may occur in edematous patients in hot weather; appropriate therapy is water restriction rather than administration of salt except in rare instances when the hyponatremia is life-threatening. In actual salt depletion, appropriate replacement is the therapy of choice.

Drug Interactions: TENORETIC may potentiate the action of other antihypertensive agents used concomitantly. Patients treated with TENORETIC plus a catecholamine depletor (eg. reserpine) should be closely observed for evidence of hypotension and/or marked bradycardia which may produce vertigo, syncope, or postural hypotension.

Thiazides may decrease arterial responsiveness to norepinephrine. This diminution is not sufficient to preclude the

therapeutic effectiveness of norepinephrine. Thiazides may increase the responsiveness to tubocurarine.

Lithium generally should not be given with diuretics because they reduce its renal clearance and add a high risk of lithium toxicity. Read circulars for lithium preparations before use of such preparations with TENORETIC.

Should it be decided to discontinue therapy in patients receiving TENORETIC and clonidine concurrently, the TENORETIC should be discontinued several days before the gradual withdrawal of clonidine.

Other Precautions: In patients receiving thiazides, sensitivity reactions may occur with or without a history of allergy or bronchial asthma. The possible exacerbation or activation of systemic lupus erythematosus has been reported. The antihypertensive effects of thiazides may be enhanced in the postsympathectomy patient.

Carcinogenesis, Mutagenesis, Impairment of Fertility: Two long-term (maximum dosing duration of 18 or 24 months) rat studies and one long-term (maximum dosing duration of 18 months) mouse study with atenolol, each employing dose levels as high as 300 mg/kg/day or 150 times the maximum recommended human dose, did not indicate a carcinogenic potential in rodents.

Atenolol was negative in the mouse dominant lethal test, the Chinese hamster in vivo cytogenetic test and the Salmonella typhimurium back mutation test (Ames test), with or without metabolic activation.

Fertility of male or female rats (evaluated at dose levels as high as 200 mg/kg/day or 100 times the maximum recommended human dose) was unaffected by atenolol administration.

Animal Toxicology: Six month oral studies were conducted in rats and dogs using TENORETIC dosages up to 12.5 mg/kg/day (approximately 5 times the proposed maximum therapeutic dose). There were no functional or morphological abnormalities resulting from dosing either compound alone or together other than minor changes in heart rate, blood pressure, and urine chemistry, which were attributed to the known pharmacologic properties of atenolol and/or chlorthalidone.

Chronic studies of atenolol performed in animals have revealed the occurrence of vacuolation of epithelial cells of Brunner's glands in the duodenum of both male and female dogs at all tested dose levels (starting at 15 mg/kg/day or 7.5 times the maximum recommended human dose) and increased incidence of atrial degeneration of hearts of male rats at 300 mg but not 150 mg atenolol/kg/day (150 and 75 times the maximum recommended human dose, respectively).

Use in Pregnancy: Pregnancy Category C. TENORETIC was studied for teratogenic potential in the rat and rabbit. Doses of 10, 100, and 300 mg/kg/day were administered orally to pregnant rats, with no teratologic effects observed. Two studies were conducted in rabbits. In the first study, pregnant rabbits were dosed with 10, 100, or 200 mg/kg/day. No teratologic changes were noted; embryonic resorptions were observed at all dose levels (ranging from approximately 5 times to 100 times the maximum recommended human dose). In a second rabbit study, dosages were 5, 10, and 25 mg/kg/day. No teratogenic or embryotoxic effects were demonstrated. It is concluded that the no-effect level for embryonic resorptions is 25 mg/kg/day (approximately 12.5 times the maximum recommended human dose) or greater. TENORETIC should be used during pregnancy only if the potential benefit justifies the potential risk to the fetus.

Atenolol—Atenolol has been shown to produce a dose-related increase in embryo/fetal resorptions in rats at doses equal to or greater than 50 mg/kg or 25 or more times the maximum recommended human dose. Although similar effects were not seen in rabbits, the compound was not evaluated in rabbits at doses above 25 mg/kg or 12.5 times the maximum recommended human dose. There are no adequate and well-controlled studies in pregnant women.

Chlorthalidone—Thiazides cross the placental barrier and appear in cord blood. The use of chlorthalidone and related drugs in pregnant women requires that the anticipated benefits of the drug be weighed against possible hazards to the fetus. These hazards include fetal or neonatal jaundice, thrombocytopenia, and possibly other adverse reactions which have occurred in the adult.

Nursing Mothers: It is not established to what extent this drug is excreted in human milk. Since most drugs are excreted in human milk, nursing should not be undertaken by mothers receiving TENORETIC.

Pediatric Use: Safety and effectiveness in children have not been established.

ADVERSE REACTIONS

TENORETIC is usually well tolerated in properly selected patients. Most adverse effects have been mild and transient. The adverse effects observed for TENORETIC are essentially the same as those seen with the individual components.

Atenolol: The frequency estimates that follow were derived from controlled studies in which adverse reactions were ei-

Continued on next page

ICI Pharma—Cont.

ther volunteered by the patient (U.S. studies) or elicited, eg, by checklist (foreign studies). The reported frequency of elicited adverse effects was higher for both atenolol and placebo-treated patients than when these reactions were volunteered. Where frequency of adverse effects for atenolol and placebo is similar, causal relationship to atenolol is uncertain.

The data present these estimates in terms of percentages: first from the U.S. studies (volunteered side effects) and then from both U.S. and foreign studies (volunteered and elicited side effects).

U.S. Studies (% Atenolol -% Placebo):
CARDIOVASCULAR: bradycardia (3%-0%), cold extremities (0%-0.5%), postural hypotension (2%-1%), leg pain (0%-0.5%).
CENTRAL NERVOUS SYSTEM / NEUROMUSCULAR: dizziness (4%-1%), vertigo (2%-0.5%), light-headedness (1%-0%), tiredness (0.6%-0.5%), fatigue (3%-1%), lethargy (1%-0%), drowsiness (0.6%-0%), depression (0.6%-0.5%), dreaming (0%-0%).
GASTROINTESTINAL: diarrhea (2%-0%), nausea (4%-1%).
RESPIRATORY (See WARNINGS): wheeziness (0%-0%), dyspnea (0.6%-1%).

Totals U.S. and Foreign Studies:
CARDIOVASCULAR: bradycardia (3%-0%), cold extremities (12%-5%), postural hypotension (4%-5%), leg pain (3%-1%).
CENTRAL NERVOUS SYSTEM / NEUROMUSCULAR: dizziness (13%-6%), vertigo (2%-0.2%), light-headedness (3%-0.7%), tiredness (26%-13%), fatigue (6%-5%), lethargy (3%-0.7%), drowsiness (2%-0.5%), depression (12%-9%), dreaming (3%-1%).
GASTROINTESTINAL: diarrhea (3%-2%), nausea (3%-1%).
RESPIRATORY (see WARNINGS): wheeziness (3%-3%), dyspnea (6%-4%).
MISCELLANEOUS: There have been reports of skin rashes and/or dry eyes associated with the use of beta-adrenergic blocking drugs. The reported incidence is small and, in most cases the symptoms have cleared when treatment was withdrawn. Discontinuance of the drug should be considered if any such reaction is not otherwise explicable. Patients should be closely monitored following cessation of therapy.
Chlorthalidone: Cardiovascular: orthostatic hypotension; Gastrointestinal: anorexia, gastric irritation, vomiting, cramping, constipation, jaundice (intrahepatic cholestatic jaundice), pancreatitis; CNS: vertigo, paresthesias, xanthopsia; Hematologic: leukopenia, agranulocytosis, thrombocytopenia, aplastic anemia; Hypersensitivity: purpura, photosensitivity, rash, urticaria, necrotizing angiitis (vasculitis), (cutaneous vasculitis), Lyell's syndrome (toxic epidermal necrolysis); Miscellaneous: hyperglycemia, glycosuria, hyperuricemia, muscle spasm, weakness, restlessness. Clinical trials of TENORETIC conducted in the United States (89 patients treated with TENORETIC) revealed no new or unexpected adverse effects.
Potential Adverse Effects: In addition, a variety of adverse effects not observed in clinical trials with atenolol but reported with other beta-adrenergic blocking agents, should be considered potential adverse effects of atenolol. Nervous System: reversible mental depression progressing to catatonia, hallucinations, an acute reversible syndrome characterized by disorientation for time and place, short-term memory loss, emotional lability, slightly clouded sensorium, and decreased performance on neuropsychometrics; Cardiovascular: intensification of AV block (see CONTRAINDICATIONS); Gastrointestinal: mesenteric arterial thrombosis, ischemic colitis; Hematologic: agranulocytosis, nonthrombocytopenic purpura, thrombocytopenic purpura; Allergic: erythematous rash, fever combined with aching and sore throat, laryngospasm and respiratory distress; Miscellaneous: reversible alopecia, Peyronie's disease.
There have been reports of a syndrome comprising psoriasiform skin rash, conjunctivitis sicca, otitis, and sclerosing serositis attributed to the beta-adrenergic receptor blocking agent, practolol. This syndrome has not been reported with TENORETIC or TENORMIN (atenolol).
Clinical Laboratory Test Findings: Clinically important changes in standard laboratory parameters were rarely associated with the administration of TENORETIC. The changes in laboratory parameters were not progressive and usually were not associated with clinical manifestations. The most common changes were increases in uric acid and decreases in serum potassium.

OVERDOSAGE

No specific information is available with regard to overdosage to TENORETIC in humans. Treatment is symptomatic and supportive. Therapy with TENORETIC should be discontinued and the patient observed closely. Suggested measures include induction of emesis and/or gastric lavage, and correction of dehydration, electrolyte imbalance, and hypotension by established procedures.

Atenolol: To date, there is no known case of acute overdosage with atenolol. The most common effects expected with overdosage of a beta-adrenergic blocking agent are bradycardia, congestive heart failure, hypotension, bronchospasm, and hypoglycemia. Atenolol can be removed from the general circulation by hemodialysis. In addition to gastric lavage, the following therapeutic measures are suggested if warranted:
BRADYCARDIA: atropine or another anticholinergic drug.
HEART BLOCK (second or third degree): isoproterenol or transvenous cardiac pacemaker.
CONGESTIVE HEART FAILURE: conventional therapy.
HYPOTENSION (depending on associated factors): epinephrine rather than isoproterenol or norepinephrine may be useful in addition to atropine and digitalis.
BRONCHOSPASM: aminophylline, isoproterenol, or atropine.
HYPOGLYCEMIA: intravenous glucose.
ELECTROLYTE IMBALANCE: supportive treatment; where necessary, intravenous dextrose-saline with potassium, administered with caution.
Chlorthalidone: Symptoms of chlorthalidone overdose include nausea, weakness, dizziness, and disturbances of electrolyte balance.

DOSAGE AND ADMINISTRATION

DOSAGE MUST BE INDIVIDUALIZED (SEE INDICATIONS). Chlorthalidone is usually given at a dose of 25 mg daily; the usual initial dose of atenolol is 50 mg daily. Therefore, the initial dose should be one TENORETIC 50 tablet given once a day. If an optimal response is not achieved, the dosage should be increased to one TENORETIC 100 tablet given once a day.
When necessary, another antihypertensive agent may be added gradually beginning with 50% of the usual recommended starting dose to avoid an excessive fall in blood pressure.
Since atenolol is excreted via the kidneys, dosage should be adjusted in cases of severe impairment of renal function. No significant accumulation of atenolol occurs until creatinine clearance falls below 35 mL/min/1.73 m^2 (normal range is 100–150 mL/min/1.73 m^2), therefore, the following maximum dosages are recommended for patients with renal impairment.

Creatinine Clearance (mL/min/1.73 m^2)	Atenolol Elimination Half-life (hrs)	Maximum Dosage
15–35	16–27	50 mg daily
<15	>27	50 mg every other day

HOW SUPPLIED

TENORETIC 50 Tablets (atenolol 50 mg and chlorthalidone 25 mg) NDC 0310-0115 (white, round, biconvex, uncoated tablets with ICI on one side and 115 on the other side, bisected) are supplied in bottles of 100 tablets. TENORETIC 100 Tablets (atenolol 100 mg and chlorthalidone 25 mg) NDC 0310-0117 (white, round, biconvex, uncoated tablets with ICI on one side and 117 on the other side) are supplied in bottles of 100 tablets.
Protect from heat, light, and moisture. Dispense in well-closed, light-resistant container.

Shown in Product Identification Section, page 412
Rev A   12/86

TENORMIN®
[ten-or 'min]
(atenolol)   ℞

DESCRIPTION

TENORMIN (atenolol), a synthetic, beta$_1$-selective (cardioselective) adrenoreceptor blocking agent, may be chemically described as benzeneacetamide, 4-[2'-hydroxy-3'-[(1-methylethyl) amino] propoxy]-.
Atenolol (free base) has a molecular weight of 266. It is a relatively polar hydrophilic compound with a water solubility of 26.5 mg/mL at 37°C and a log partition coefficient (octanol/-water) of 0.23. It is freely soluble in 1N HCl (300 mg/mL at 25°C) and less soluble in chloroform (3 mg/mL at 25°C).
TENORMIN is available as 50 mg and 100 mg tablets for oral administration.
Inactive ingredients: magnesium stearate, microcrystalline cellulose, povidone, sodium starch glycolate.

CLINICAL PHARMACOLOGY

TENORMIN is a beta$_1$-selective (cardioselective) beta-adrenergic receptor blocking agent without membrane stabilizing or intrinsic sympathomimetic (partial agonist) activities. This preferential effect is not absolute, however, and at higher doses, TENORMIN inhibits beta$_2$-adrenoreceptors, chiefly located in the bronchial and vascular musculature.
Pharmacokinetics and Metabolism: In man, absorption of an oral dose is rapid and consistent but incomplete. Approximately 50% of an oral dose is absorbed from the gastrointestinal tract, the remainder being excreted unchanged in the feces. Peak blood levels are reached between 2 and 4 hours

after ingestion. Unlike propranolol or metoprolol, but like nadolol, TENORMIN undergoes little or no metabolism by the liver, and the absorbed portion is eliminated primarily by renal excretion. TENORMIN also differs from propranolol in that only a small amount (6%–16%) is bound to proteins in the plasma. This kinetic profile results in relatively consistent plasma drug levels with about a fourfold interpatient variation.
The elimination half-life of TENORMIN is approximately 6 to 7 hours and there is no alteration of the kinetic profile of the drug by chronic administration. Following doses of 50 mg or 100 mg, both beta-blocking and antihypertensive effects persist for at least 24 hours. When renal function is impaired, elimination of TENORMIN is closely related to the glomerular filtration rate; but, significant accumulation does not occur until the creatinine clearance falls below 35 mL/min/1.73 m^2.(See DOSAGE AND ADMINISTRATION.)
By blocking the positive chronotropic and inotropic effects of catecholamines and by decreasing blood pressure, atenolol generally reduces the oxygen requirements of the heart at any given level of effort, making it useful for many patients in the long-term management of angina pectoris. On the other hand, atenolol can increase oxygen requirements by increasing left ventricular fiber length and end diastolic pressure, particularly in patients with heart failure.
Pharmacodynamics.: In standard animal or human pharmacological tests, beta-adrenoreceptor blocking activity of TENORMIN has been demonstrated by: (1) reduction in resting and exercise heart rate and cardiac output, (2) reduction of systolic and diastolic blood pressure at rest and on exercise, (3) inhibition of isoproterenol-induced tachycardia, and (4) reduction in reflex orthostatic tachycardia.
A significant beta-blocking effect of TENORMIN, as measured by reduction of exercise tachycardia, is apparent within 1 hour following oral administration of a single dose. This effect is maximal at about 2 to 4 hours, and persists for at least 24 hours. The effect at 24 hours is dose-related and also bears a linear relationship to the logarithm of plasma TENORMIN concentration. However, as has been shown for all beta-blocking agents, the antihypertensive effect does not appear to be related to plasma level.
In normal subjects, the beta$_1$-selectivity of TENORMIN has been shown by its reduced ability to reverse the beta$_2$-mediated vasodilating effect of isoproterenol as compared to equivalent beta-blocking doses of propranolol. In asthmatic patients, a dose of TENORMIN producing a greater effect on resting heart rate than propranolol resulted in much less increase in airway resistance. In a placebo-controlled comparison of approximately equipotent oral doses of several beta blockers, TENORMIN produced a significantly smaller decrease of FEV$_1$ than nonselective beta blockers such as propranolol and, unlike those agents, did not inhibit bronchodilation in response to isoproterenol.
Consistent with its negative chronotropic effect due to beta blockade of the SA node, TENORMIN increases sinus cycle length and sinus node recovery time. Conduction in the AV node is also prolonged. TENORMIN is devoid of membrane-stabilizing activity, and increasing the dose well beyond that producing beta blockade does not further depress myocardial contractility. Several studies have demonstrated a moderate (approximately 10%) increase in stroke volume at rest and exercise.
In controlled clinical trials TENORMIN, given as a single daily dose, was an effective antihypertensive agent providing 24-hour reduction of blood pressure. TENORMIN has been studied in combination with thiazide-type diuretics and the blood pressure effects of the combination are approximately additive. TENORMIN is also compatible with methyldopa, hydralazine, and prazosin, the combination resulting in a larger fall in blood pressure than with the single agents. The dose range of TENORMIN is narrow and increasing the dose beyond 100 mg once daily is not associated with increased antihypertensive effect. The mechanisms of the antihypertensive effects of beta-blocking agents have not been established. Several possible mechanisms have been proposed and include: (1) competitive antagonism of catecholamines at peripheral (especially cardiac) adrenergic neuron sites, leading to decreased cardiac output, (2) a central effect leading to reduced sympathetic outflow to the periphery, and (3) suppression of renin activity. The results from long-term studies have not shown any diminution of the antihypertensive efficacy of TENORMIN with prolonged use.

INDICATIONS AND USAGE

Hypertension: TENORMIN is indicated in the management of hypertension. It may be used alone or concomitantly with other antihypertensive agents, particularly with a thiazide-type diuretic.
Angina Pectoris Due to Coronary Atherosclerosis: TENORMIN is indicated for the long-term management of patients with angina pectoris.

CONTRAINDICATIONS

TENORMIN is contraindicated in sinus bradycardia, heart block greater than first degree, cardiogenic shock, and overt cardiac failure (see WARNINGS).

WARNINGS

Cardiac Failure: Sympathetic stimulation is necessary in supporting circulatory function in congestive heart failure, and beta blockade carries the potential hazard of further depressing myocardial contractility and precipitating more severe failure. In hypertensive patients who have congestive heart failure controlled by digitalis and diuretics, TENORMIN (atenolol) should be administered cautiously. Both digitalis and atenolol slow AV conduction.

In Patients Without a History of Cardiac Failure: Continued depression of the myocardium with beta-blocking agents over a period of time can, in some cases, lead to cardiac failure. At the first sign or symptom of impending cardiac failure, patients should be fully digitalized and/or be given a diuretic and the response observed closely. If cardiac failure continues, despite adequate digitalization and diuresis, TENORMIN should be withdrawn. (See Dosage and Administration.)

Cessation of Therapy With TENORMIN: Patients with coronary artery disease, who are being treated with TENORMIN, should be advised against abrupt discontinuation of therapy. Severe exacerbation of angina and the occurrence of myocardial infarction and ventricular arrhythmias have been reported in angina patients following the abrupt discontinuation of therapy with other beta blockers. The last two complications may occur with or without preceding exacerbation of the angina pectoris. To date, there has been no report of myocardial infarction or severe angina upon withdrawal of TENORMIN, probably due to its long plasma half-life. Because of the problems encountered with other beta blockers, when discontinuation of TENORMIN is planned, the patients should be carefully observed and advised to limit physical activity to a minimum. If the angina worsens or acute coronary insufficiency develops, it is recommended that TENORMIN be promptly reinstituted, at least temporarily. (See Dosage and Administration.)

Bronchospastic Diseases: PATIENTS WITH BRONCHOSPASTIC DISEASE SHOULD, IN GENERAL, NOT RECEIVE BETA BLOCKERS. Because of its relative beta$_1$ selectivity, however, TENORMIN may be used with caution in patients with bronchospastic disease who do not respond to, or cannot tolerate, other antihypertensive treatment. Since beta$_1$selectivity is not absolute, the lowest possible dose of TENORMIN should be used with therapy initiated at 50 mg and a beta$_2$-stimulating agent (bronchodilator) should be made available. If dosage must be increased, dividing the dose should be considered in order to achieve lower peak blood levels.

Anesthesia and Major Surgery: As with all beta-receptor blocking drugs it may be decided to withdraw TENORMIN before surgery. In this case, 48 hours should be allowed to elapse between the last dose and anesthesia. If treatment is continued, care should be taken when using anesthetic agents which depress the myocardium such as ether, cyclopropane, and trichloroethylene.

TENORMIN, like other beta blockers, is a competitive inhibitor of beta-receptor agonists and its effects on the heart can be reversed by administration of such agents (eg, dobutamine or isoproterenol) with caution. (See section on OVERDOSAGE). Manifestations of excessive vagal tone (eg, profound bradycardia, hypotension) may be corrected with atropine (1–2 mg IV).

Diabetes and Hypoglycemia: TENORMIN should be used with caution in diabetic patients if a beta-blocking agent is required. Beta blockers may mask tachycardia occurring with hypoglycemia, but other manifestations such as dizziness and sweating may not be significantly affected. TENORMIN does not potentiate insulin-induced hypoglycemia and, unlike nonselective beta blockers, does not delay recovery of blood glucose to normal levels.

Thyrotoxicosis: Beta-adrenergic blockade may mask certain clinical signs (eg, tachycardia) of hyperthyroidism. Abrupt withdrawal of beta blockade might precipitate a thyroid storm; therefore, patients suspected of developing thyrotoxicosis from whom TENORMIN is to be withdrawn should be monitored closely. (See DOSAGE AND ADMINISTRATION).

PRECAUTIONS

Impaired Renal Function: The drug should be used with caution in patients with impaired renal function (see DOSAGE AND ADMINISTRATION).

Drug Interactions: Catecholamine-depleting drugs (eg, reserpine) may have an additive effect when given with beta-blocking agents. Patients treated with TENORMIN plus a catecholamine depletor should therefore be closely observed for evidence of hypotension and/or marked bradycardia

which may produce vertigo, syncope, or postural hypotension.

Should it be decided to discontinue therapy in patients receiving beta blockers and clonidine concurrently, the beta blocker should be discontinued several days before the gradual withdrawal of clonidine.

Carcinogenesis, Mutagenesis, Impairment of Fertility: Two long-term (maximum dosing duration of 18 or 24 months) rat studies and one long-term (maximum dosing duration of 18 months) mouse study, each employing dose levels as high as 300 mg/kg/day or 150 times the maximum recommended human dose, did not indicate a carcinogenic potential in rodents. Results of various mutagenicity studies support this finding.

Fertility of male or female rats (evaluated at dose levels as high as 200 mg/kg/day or 100 times the maximum recommended human dose) was unaffected by atenolol administration.

Animal Toxicology: Chronic studies performed in animals have revealed the occurrence of vacuolation of epithelial cells of Brunner's glands in the duodenum of both male and female dogs at all tested dose levels of atenolol (starting at 15 mg/kg/day or 7.5 times the maximum recommended human dose) and increased incidence of atrial degeneration of hearts of male rats at 300 mg but not 150 mg atenolol/kg/day (150 and 75 times the maximum recommended human dose, respectively).

USAGE IN PREGNANCY

Pregnancy Category C. Atenolol has been shown to produce a dose-related increase in embryo/fetal resorptions in rats at doses equal to or greater than 50 mg/kg/day or 25 or more times the maximum recommended human dose. Although similar effects were not seen in rabbits, the compound was not evaluated in rabbits at doses above 25 mg/kg/day or 12.5 times the maximum recommended human dose. There are no adequate and well-controlled studies in pregnant women. TENORMIN should be used during pregnancy only if the potential benefit justifies the potential risk to the fetus.

Nursing Mothers: Atenolol is excreted in human breast milk at a ratio of 1.5 to 6.8 when compared to the concentration in plasma. Caution should be exercised when TENORMIN is administered to a nursing woman.

Pediatric Use: Safety and effectiveness in children have not been established.

ADVERSE REACTIONS

Most adverse effects have been mild and transient. Frequency estimates were derived from controlled studies in which adverse reactions were either volunteered by the patient (U.S. studies) or elicited, eg, by checklist (foreign studies). The reported frequency of elicited adverse effects was higher for both TENORMIN and placebo-treated patients than when these reactions were volunteered. Where frequency of adverse effects for TENORMIN and placebo is similar, causal relationship to TENORMIN is uncertain.

The following adverse-reaction data present frequency estimates in terms of percentages: first from the U.S. studies (volunteered side effects) and then from both U.S. and foreign studies (volunteered and elicited side effects):

U.S. STUDIES (% ATENOLOL—% PLACEBO):
CARDIOVASCULAR: bradycardia (3%–0%), cold extremities (0%–0.5%), postural hypotension (2%–1%), leg pain (0%–0.5%)

CENTRAL NERVOUS SYSTEM/NEUROMUSCULAR: dizziness (4%–1%), vertigo (2%–0.5%), light-headedness (1%–0%), tiredness (0.6%–0.5%), fatigue (3%–1%), lethargy (1%–0%), drowsiness (0.6%–0%), depression (0.6%–0.5%), dreaming (0%–0%)

GASTROINTESTINAL: diarrhea (2%–0%), nausea (4%–1%)

RESPIRATORY (See WARNINGS): wheeziness (0%–0%), dyspnea (0.6%–1%)

TOTALS U.S. AND FOREIGN STUDIES:
CARDIOVASCULAR: bradycardia (3%–0%), cold extremities (12%–5%), postural hypotension (4%–5%), leg pain (3%–1%)

CENTRAL NERVOUS SYSTEM/NEUROMUSCULAR: dizziness (13%–6%), vertigo (2%–0.2%), light-headedness (3%–0.7%), tiredness (26%–13%), fatigue (6%–5%), lethargy (3%–0.7%), drowsiness (2%–0.5%), depression (12%–9%), dreaming (3%–1%)

GASTROINTESTINAL: diarrhea (3%–2%), nausea (3%–1%)

RESPIRATORY (see WARNINGS): wheeziness (3%–3%), dyspnea (6%–4%)

MISCELLANEOUS: There have been reports of skin rashes and/or dry eyes associated with the use of beta-adrenergic blocking drugs. The reported incidence is small, and in most cases, the symptoms have cleared when treatment was withdrawn. Discontinuance of the drug should be considered if any such reaction is not otherwise explicable. Patients should be closely monitored following cessation of therapy.

POTENTIAL ADVERSE EFFECTS

In addition, a variety of adverse effects have been reported with other beta-adrenergic blocking agents and may be considered potential adverse effects of TENORMIN.

HEMATOLOGIC: Agranulocytosis, nonthrombocytopenic purpura, thrombocytopenic purpura.

ALLERGIC: Fever, combined with aching and sore throat, laryngospasm, and respiratory distress.

CENTRAL NERVOUS SYSTEM: Reversible mental depression progressing to catatonia, visual disturbances, hallucinations, an acute reversible syndrome characterized by disorientation of time and place, short-term memory loss, emotional lability with slightly clouded sensorium, and decreased performance on neuropsychometrics.

GASTROINTESTINAL: Mesenteric arterial thrombosis, ischemic colitis.

OTHER: Reversible alopecia, Peyronie's disease, erythematous rash, Raynaud's phenomenon.

MISCELLANEOUS: The oculomucocutaneous syndrome associated with the beta blocker practolol has not been reported with TENORMIN during investigational use and foreign marketing experience. Furthermore, a number of patients who had previously demonstrated established practolol reactions were transferred to TENORMIN therapy with subsequent resolution or quiescence of the reaction.

OVERDOSAGE

To date, there is no known case of acute overdosage, and no specific information on emergency treatment of overdosage is available. The most common effects expected with overdosage of a beta-adrenergic blocking agent are bradycardia, congestive heart failure, hypotension, bronchospasm, and hypoglycemia.

In the case of overdosage, treatment with TENORMIN should be stopped and the patient carefully observed. TENORMIN can be removed from the general circulation by hemodialysis. In addition to gastric lavage, the following therapeutic measures are suggested if warranted:

BRADYCARDIA: Atropine or another anticholinergic drug.

HEART BLOCK (SECOND OR THIRD DEGREE): Isoproterenol or transvenous cardiac pacemaker.

CONGESTIVE HEART FAILURE: Conventional therapy.

HYPOTENSION (DEPENDING ON ASSOCIATED FACTORS): Epinephrine rather than isoproterenol or norepinephrine may be useful in addition to atropine and digitalis.

BRONCHOSPASM: Aminophylline, isoproterenol, or atropine.

HYPOGLYCEMIA: Intravenous glucose.

DOSAGE AND ADMINISTRATION

Hypertension: The initial dose of TENORMIN is 50 mg given as one tablet a day either alone or added to diuretic therapy. The full effect of this dose will usually be seen within one to two weeks. If an optimal response is not achieved, the dosage should be increased to TENORMIN 100 mg given as one tablet a day. Increasing the dosage beyond 100 mg a day is unlikely to produce any further benefit.

TENORMIN may be used alone or concomitantly with other antihypertensive agents including thiazide-type diuretics, hydralazine, prazosin, and alpha-methyldopa.

Angina Pectoris: The initial dose of TENORMIN (atenolol) is 50 mg given as one tablet a day. If an optimal response is not achieved within one week, the dosage should be increased to TENORMIN 100 mg given as one tablet a day. Some patients may require a dosage of 200 mg once a day for optimal effect.

Twenty-four hour control with once daily dosing is achieved by giving doses larger than necessary to achieve an immediate maximum effect. The maximum early effect on exercise tolerance occurs with doses of 50 to 100 mg, but at these doses the effect at 24 hours is attenuated, averaging about 50% to 75% of that observed with once a day oral doses of 200 mg.

Patients with Renal Impairment: Since TENORMIN is excreted via the kidneys, dosage should be adjusted in cases of severe impairment of renal function. No significant accumulation of TENORMIN occurs until creatinine clearance falls below 35 mL/min/1.73 m^2 (normal range is 100–150 mL/min/1.73 m^2); therefore, the following maximum dosages are recommended for patients with renal impairment:

Creatinine Clearance (mL/min/1.73m^2)	Atenolol Elimination Half-life (hrs.)	Maximum Dosage
15–35	16–27	50 mg daily
< 15	> 27	50 mg every other day

Patients on hemodialysis should be given 50 mg after each dialysis; this should be done under hospital supervision as marked falls in blood pressure can occur.

Cessation of Therapy: If withdrawal of TENORMIN therapy is planned, it should be achieved gradually over a period of about two weeks. Patients should be carefully observed and advised to limit physical activity to a minimum.

Continued on next page

ICI Pharma—Cont.

HOW SUPPLIED

Tablets of 50 mg atenolol, NDC 0310-0105 (round, flat, un-coated, white tablets identified with ICI debossed on one side and 105 debossed on the other side, bisected) are supplied in bottles of 100 tablets and unit dose packages of 100 tablets. Tablets of 100 mg atenolol, NDC 0310-0101 (round, flat, un-coated white tablets identified with ICI debossed on one side and 101 debossed on the other side) are supplied in bottles of 100 tablets and unit dose packages of 100 tablets.

Protect from heat, light, and moisture.

Rev A   11/86

Shown in Product Identification Section, page 412

ICN Pharmaceuticals, Inc.
ICN PLAZA
3300 HYLAND AVENUE
COSTA MESA, CA 92626

ANDROID–5®   ℞
Methyltestosterone Tablets (Buccal) USP, 5 mg

ANDROID–10®   ℞
Methyltestosterone Tablets (Oral) USP, 10 mg

ANDROID–25®   ℞
Methyltestosterone Tablets (Oral) USP, 25 mg

DESCRIPTION

Android 5, Android 10 and Android 25 contain methyltestosterone, USP, a synthetic androgen. Androgens are steriods that develop and maintain primary and secondary male sex characteristics. Android 10 and Android 25 are to be taken orally. Android 5 Buccal Tablets are NOT to be swallowed but are to be placed in the lower or upper buccal pouches. Androgens are derivatives of cyclopentanoperhydrophenanthrene. Endogenous androgens are C-19 steriods with a side chain at C-17, and with two angular methyl groups. Testosterone is the primary endogenous androgen. In their active form, all drugs in the class have a 17-beta-hydroxy group. 17-alpha alkylation (methyltestosterone) increases the pharmacological activity per unit weight compared to testosterone when given orally.

Methyltestosterone is the 17α-methyl derivative of testosterone, the true testicular hormone. Chemically, methyltestosterone is 17β-Hydroxy-17-methylandrost-4-en-3-one, with the empirical formula $C_{20}H_{30}O_2$, a molecular weight of 302.5.

Methyltestosterone is a white to creamy-white, odorless, slightly hygroscopic powder. It is practically insoluble in water, soluble in alcohol and other organic solvents.

Android 10 and Android 25 (Oral Tablets) contain 10 mg and 25 mg, respectively, of methyltestosterone, USP. Android 5 (Buccal Tablets) contain 5 mg methyltestosterone, USP.

Structural Formula and Chemical Name:

METHYLTESTOSTERONE

$C_{20}H_{30}O_2$ m.w. 302.46 (CAS-58-18-4)
17β-Hydroxy-17-methylandrost-4-en-3-one

CLINICAL PHARMACOLOGY

Endogenous androgens are responsible for the normal growth and development of the male sex organs and for maintenance of secondary sex characteristics. These effects include the growth and maturation of prostate, seminal vesicles, penis and scrotum; the development of male hair distribution, such as beard, pubic, chest and axillary hair; laryngeal enlargement, vocal chord thickening, alterations in body musculature and fat distribution. Drugs in this class also cause retention of nitrogen, sodium, potassium, phosphorus, and decreased urinary excretion of calcium. Androgens have been reported to increase protein anabolism and decrease protein catabolism. Nitrogen balance is improved only when there is sufficient intake of calories and protein. Androgens are responsible for the growth spurt of adolescence and eventual termination of linear growth which is brought about by fusion of the epiphyseal growth centers. In children, exogenous androgens accelerate linear growth rates, but may cause a disproportionate advancement in bone maturation. Use over long periods may result in fusion of the epiphyseal growth centers and termination of growth process. Androgens have been reported to stimulate the production of red blood cells by enhancing the production of erythropoietic stimulating factor.

During exogenous administration of androgens, endogenous testosterone release is inhibited through feedback inhibition of pituitary luteinizing hormone (LH). At large doses of exogenous androgens, spermatogenesis may also be suppressed through feedback inhibition of pituitary follicle stimulating hormone (FSH).

There is a lack of substantial evidence that androgens are effective in fractures, surgery, convalescence, and functional uterine bleeding.

Pharmacokinetics

Testosterone given orally is metabolized by the gut and 44 percent is cleared by the liver in the first pass. Oral doses as high as 400 mg per day are needed to achieve clinically effective blood levels for full replacement therapy. The synthetic androgen (methyltestosterone) is less extensively metabolized by the liver and has a longer half-life. It is more suitable than testosterone for oral administration.

Testosterone in plasma is 98 percent bound to a specific testosterone-estradiol binding globulin, and about 2 percent is free. Generally, the amount of this sex-hormone binding globulin in the plasma will determine the distribution of testosterone between free and bound forms, and the free testosterone concentration will determine its half-life.

About 90 percent of a dose of testosterone is excreted in the urine as glucuronic and sulfuric acid conjugates of testosterone and its metabolites; about 6 percent of a dose is excreted in the feces, mostly in the unconjugated form. Inactivation of testosterone occurs primarily in the liver. Testosterone is metabolized to various 17-keto steroids through two different pathways. There are considerable variations of the half-life of testosterone as reported in the literature, ranging from 10 to 100 minutes.

In many tissues the activity of testosterone appears to depend on reduction to dihydrotestosterone, which binds to cytosol receptor proteins. The steroid-receptor complex is transported to the nucleus where it initiates transcription events and cellular changes related to androgen action.

INDICATIONS AND USAGE

1. Males

Androgens are indicated for replacement therapy in conditions associated with a deficiency or absence of endogenous testosterone:

a. Primary hypogonadism (congenital or acquired)-testicular failure due to cryptorchidism, bilateral torsion, orchitis, vanishing testis syndrome or orchidectomy.

b. Hypogonadotropic hypogonadism (congenital or acquired)—idiopathic gonadotropin or LHRH deficiency, or pituitary-hypothalamic injury from tumors, trauma or radiation.

If the above conditions occur prior to puberty, androgen replacement therapy will be needed during the adolescent years for development of secondary sexual characteristics. Prolonged androgen treatment will be required to maintain sexual characteristics in these and other males who develop testosterone deficiency after puberty.

c. Androgens may be used to stimulate puberty in carefully selected males with clearly delayed puberty. These patients usually have a familial pattern of delayed puberty that is not secondary to a pathological disorder; puberty is expected to occur spontaneously at a relatively late date. Brief treatment with conservative doses may occasionally be justified in these patients if they do not respond to psychological support. The potential adverse effect on bone maturation should be discussed with the patient and parents prior to androgen administration. An X-ray of the hand and wrist to determine bone age should be obtained every 6 months to assess the effect of treatment on the epiphyseal centers (see WARNINGS).

2. Females

Androgens may be used secondarily in women with advancing inoperable metastatic (skeletal) mammary cancer who are 1 to 5 years postmenopausal. Primary goals of therapy in these women include ablation of the ovaries. Other methods of counteracting estrogen activity are adrenalectomy, hypophysectomy, and/or antiestrogen therapy. This treatment has also been used in premenopausal women with breast cancer who benefited from oophorectomy and are considered to have a hormone-responsive tumor. Judgment concerning androgen therapy should be made by an oncologist with expertise in this field.

Androgens, such as methyltestosterone, have been used for the management of postpartum breast pain and engorgement.

CONTRAINDICATIONS

Androgens are contraindicated in men with carcinomas of the breast or with known or suspected carcinomas of the prostate, and in women who are or may become pregnant. When administered to pregnant women, androgens cause virilization of the external genitalia of the female fetus. This virilization includes clitoromegaly, abnormal vaginal development, and fusion of genital folds to form a scrotal-like structure. The degree of masculinization is related to the amount of drug given and the age of the fetus, and is most likely to occur in the female fetus when the drugs are given

in the first trimester. If the patient becomes pregnant while taking these drugs, she should be apprised of the potential hazard to the fetus.

WARNINGS

In patients with breast cancer, androgen therapy may cause hypercalcemia by stimulating osteolysis. In this case, the drug should be discontinued.

Prolonged use of high doses of androgens have been associated with the development of peliosis hepatis and hepatic neoplasms including hepatocellular carcinoma (see PRECAUTIONS—Carcinogenesis). Peliosis hepatis can be a life-threatening or fatal complication.

Cholestatic hepatitis and jaundice occur with 17-alpha-alkylandrogens at a relatively low dose. If cholestatic hepatitis with jaundice appears or if liver function tests become abnormal, the androgen should be discontinued and the etiology should be determined. Drug-induced jaundice is reversible when the medication is discontinued.

Geriatric patients treated with androgens may be at an increased risk for the development of prostatic hypertropy and prostatic carcinoma.

Edema with or without congestive heart failure may be a serious complication in patients with preexisting cardiac, renal or hepatic disease. In addition to discontinuation of the drug, diuretic therapy may be required.

Gynecomastia frequently develops and occasionally persists in patients being treated for hypogonadism.

Androgen therapy should be used cautiously in healthy males with delayed puberty. The effect on bone maturation should be monitored by assessing bone age of the wrist and hand every 6 months. In children, androgen treatment may accelerate bone maturation without producing compensatory gain in linear growth. This adverse effect may result in compromised adult stature. The younger the child the greater the risk of compromising final mature height.

PRECAUTIONS

General

Women should be observed for signs of virilization (deepening of the voice, hirsutism, acne, clitoromegaly and menstrual irregularities). Discontinuation of drug therapy at the time of evidence of mild virilism is necessary to prevent irreversible virilization. Such virilization is usual following androgen use at high doses. A decision may be made by the patient and the physician that some virilization will be tolerated during treatment for breast carcinoma.

Information for the Patient:

The physician should instruct patients to report any of the following side effects of androgens:

    Adult or Adolescent Males: Too frequent or persistent erections of the penis.

    Women: Hoarseness, acne, changes in menstrual periods or more hair on the face.

    All Patients: Any nausea, vomiting, changes in skin color or ankle swelling.

Any male adolescent patient receiving androgens for delayed puberty should have bone development checked every six months.

Laboratory Tests:

1. Women with disseminated breast carcinoma should have frequent determination of urine and serum calcium levels during the course of androgen therapy. (See WARNINGS).

2. Because of the hepatotoxicity associated with the use of 17-alpha-alkylated androgens, liver function tests should be obtained periodically.

3. Periodic (every 6 months) x-ray examinations of bone age should be made during treatment of prepubertal males to determine the rate of bone maturation and the effects of androgen therapy on the epiphyseal centers.

4. Hemoglobin and hematocrit should be checked periodically for polycythemia in patients who are receiving high doses of androgens.

Drug Interactions:

1. Anticoagulants. C-17 substituted derivatives of testosterone, such as methandrostenolone, have been reported to decrease the anticoagulant requirements of patients receiving oral anticoagulants. Patients receiving oral anticoagulant therapy require close monitoring, especially when androgens are started or stopped.

2. Oxyphenbutazone. Concurrent administration of oxyphenbutazone and androgens may result in elevated serum levels of oxyphenbutazone.

3. Insulin. In diabetic patients the metabolic effects of androgens may decrease blood glucose and insulin requirements.

Drug/Laboratory Test Interferences:

Androgens may decrease levels of thyroxine-binding globulin, resulting in decreased total T_4 serum levels and increased resin uptake of T_3 and T_4. Free thyroid hormone levels remain unchanged, however, and there is no clinical evidence of thyroid dysfunction.

Carcinogenesis:

Animal Data. Testosterone has been tested by subcutaneous injection and implantation in mice and rats. The implant induced cervical-uterine tumors in mice, which metastasized in some cases. There is suggestive evidence that injection of testosterone into some strains of female mice increases their susceptibility to hepatoma. Testosterone is also known to increase the number of tumors and decrease the degree of differention of chemically induced carcinomas of the liver in rats.

Human Data. There are rare reports of hepatocellular carcinoma in patients receiving long-term therapy with androgens in high doses. Withdrawal of the drugs did not lead to regression of the tumors in all cases.

Geriatric patients treated with androgens may be at an increased risk for the development of prostatic hypertrophy and prostatic carcinoma.

Pregnancy: Teratogenic Effects: Pregnancy Category X (See Contraindications).

Nursing Mothers:

It is not known whether androgens are excreted in human milk. Because many drugs are excreted in human milk and because of the potential for serious adverse reactions in nursing infants from androgens, a decision should be made whether to discontinue nursing or to discontinue the drug, taking into account the importance of the drug to the mother.

Pediatric Use:

Androgen therapy should be used very cautiously in children and only by specialists who are aware of the adverse effects on bone maturation. Skeletal maturation must be monitored every six months by an x-ray of hand and wrist. (See INDICATIONS AND USAGE and WARNINGS.)

ADVERSE REACTIONS

Endocrine and Urogenital:

Female: The most common side effects of androgen therapy are amenorrhea and other menstrual irregularities, inhibition of gonadotropin secretion and virilization, including deepening of the voice and clitoral enlargement. The latter usually is not reversible after androgens are discontinued. When administered to a pregnant woman androgens cause virilization of external genitalia of the female fetus.

Male: Gynecomastia, and excessive frequency and duration of penile erections. Oligospermia may occur at high dosages (see CLINICAL PHARMACOLOGY).

Skin and appendages: Hirsutism, male pattern of baldness, and acne.

Fluid and Electrolyte Disturbances: Retention of sodium, chloride, water, potassium, calcium, and inorganic phosphates.

Gastrointestinal: Nausea, cholestatic jaundice, alterations in liver function tests, rarely hepatocellular neoplasms and peliosis hepatis.

Hematologic: Suppression of clotting factors, II, V, VII, and X, bleeding in patients on concomitant anticoagulant therapy, and polycythemia.

Nervous System: Increased or decreased libido, headache, anxiety, depression, and generalized paresthesia.

Metabolic: Increased serum cholesterol.

Miscellaneous: Stomatitis with buccal preparations; rarely anaphylactoid reactions.

OVERDOSAGE

There have been no reports of acute overdosage with the androgens.

DOSAGE AND ADMINISTRATION

The suggested dosage for androgens varies depending on the age, sex, and diagnosis of the individual patient. Dosage is adjusted according to the patient's response and the appearance of adverse reactions. See Table 1 for guidelines for replacement therapy in androgen-deficient males. Various dosage regimens have been used to induce pubertal changes in hypogonadal males: some experts have advocated lower dosages initially, gradually increasing the dose as puberty progresses, with or without a decrease to maintenance levels. Other experts emphasize that higher dosages are needed to induce pubertal changes and lower dosages can be used for maintenance after puberty. The chronological and skeletal ages must be taken into consideration, both in determining the initial dose and in adjusting the dose.

Dosages used in delayed puberty generally are in the lower ranges of those given in Table 1, and for a limited duration, for example 4 to 6 months.

Women with metastatic breast carcinoma must be followed closely because androgen therapy occasionally appears to accelerate the disease. Thus, many experts prefer to use the shorter acting androgen preparations rather than those with prolonged activity for treating breast carcinoma, particularly during the early stages of androgen therapy.

Guideline dosages of androgens for use in the palliative treatment of women with metastatic breast carcinoma are given in Table 2.

Suggested dosages of androgens for use in the prevention of postpartum breast pain and engorement are: methyltestosterone, buccal tablets 40 mg daily, or oral tablets 80 mg daily for 3 to 5 days after delivery.

Administration of Buccal Tablets: Android 5 Buccal Tablets should NOT be swallowed, since the hormone is meant to be absorbed through the oral mucous membranes. The effective buccal dose of methyltestosterone is approximately one-

TABLE 1
Guidelines for Androgen Replacement Therapy in the Male

Drug	Route	Dose	Frequency
Methyltestosterone	Oral	10-50 mg	Daily
	Buccal	5-25 mg	Daily

TABLE 2
Guidelines for Androgen Therapy in Breast Carcinoma in Females

Drug	Route	Dose	Frequency
Methyltestosterone	Oral	50-200 mg	Daily
	Buccal	25-100 mg	Daily

half that required when the drug is given orally. Place the buccal tablet in the upper or lower buccal pouch between the gum and cheek; let the tablet dissolve completely. Avoid eating, drinking, chewing, or smoking while the buccal tablet is in place. Proper oral hygienic measures (e.g., rinsing mouth with water) are particularly important after the use of buccal tablets.

[See table above].

HOW SUPPLIED

Android 5 mg Buccal Tablets are oblong white unscored tablets, imprinted BP 956, and are supplied in bottles of 60 tablets.

Android 10 mg Oral Tablets are square green unscored tablets, imprinted BP 958. and are supplied in bottles of 60 tablets..

Android 25 mg Oral Tablets are square yellow unscored tablets, imprinted BP 996, and are supplied in bottles of 60 tablets.

LITERATURE AVAILABLE

Samples.
Revised 1/87

BENOQUIN®   ℞

[ben'ō-kwin]

(Monobenzone USP 20% Cream)

Federal (U.S.A.) law prohibits dispensing without prescription.

DESCRIPTION

Each gram of Benoquin Cream contains 200 mg of monobenzone, USP, in a water-washable base consisting of purified water, cetyl alcohol, propylene glycol, sodium lauryl sulfate and beeswax.

CLINICAL PHARMACOLOGY

The mechanism of action of Benoquin is not fully understood. Denton et al. suggested that Benoquin may be converted to hydroquinone, which they found to inhibit the enzymatic oxidation of tyrosine to DOPA. Iijima and Watanabe suggested a direct action on tyrosinase. Another suggestion by Denton and his group was that Benoquin acts as an anti-oxidant to prevent SH-group oxidation so that more SH groups are available to inhibit tyrosinase. The primary role of inflammation in the depigmentation process was studied by Becker and Spencer who suggested that increased cell permeability allows Benoquin to enter the melanocyte to form an antigenic substance which attached to the melanin granule enters the dermis where antibodies are produced, remote positive patch-testing may result.

INDICATIONS AND USAGE

Benoquin Cream is indicated for final depigmentation in extensive vitiligo.

Benoquin Cream is not recommended for freckling, hyperpigmentation due to photosensitization following use of certain perfumes (berlock dermatitis), melasma (chloasma) of pregnancy, and hyperpigmentation following inflammation of the skin. Benoquin Cream is of no value in the treatment of cafe-au-lait spots, pigmented nevi, malignant melanoma, or pigment resulting from pigments other than melanin, including bile, silver, and artificial pigments.

CONTRAINDICATIONS

Prior history of sensitivity or allergic reaction to this product or any of its ingredients. The safety of topical monobenzone use during pregnancy or in children (12 years and under) has not been established.

WARNINGS

A. Benoquin Cream is a potent depigmenting agent, not a mild cosmetic bleach. Do not use except for final depigmentation in extensive vitiligo.

B. Keep this and all medication out of the reach of children. In case of accidental ingestion, call a physician or a poison control center immediately.

PRECAUTIONS

See Warnings.

A. Pregnancy Category C. Animal reproduction studies have not been conducted with topical monobenzone. It is also not known whether monobenzone can cause fetal harm when used topically on a pregnant woman or affect reproductive capacity. It is not known to what degree, if

any, topical monobenzone is absorbed systemically. Topical monobenzone should be used in pregnant women only when clearly indicated.

B. Nursing mothers. It is not known whether topical monobenzone is absorbed or excreted in human milk. Caution is advised when topical monobenzone is used by a nursing mother.

C. Pediatric usage. Safety and effectiveness in children below the age of 12 years have not been established.

ADVERSE REACTIONS

Occasional irritation, a burning sensation, or dermatitis may occur in which case medication should be discontinued and the physician notified immediately.

DOSAGE AND ADMINISTRATION

Benoquin should be applied to the pigmented area and rubbed in well two or three times daily or as directed by physician. There is no recommended dosage for children under 12 years of age except under the advice and supervision of a physician.

NOTE

Depigmentation is usually observed after one to four months of therapy. If satisfactory results have not been obtained within four months, treatment should be discontinued.

HOW SUPPLIED

BENOQUIN Cream, 20% in 1¼ oz. tubes (NDC 0187-0380-34).

BENOQUIN Cream should be stored at room temperature (15-30°C) (59-86°F)

ELDOPAQUE Forte® 4% Cream   ℞

[él-do-pāk " for'tā]

(Hydroquinone USP, 4%)

Skin Bleaching Cream With SunBlock

CAUTION: FEDERAL LAW (U.S.A.) PROHIBITS DISPENSING WITHOUT A PRESCRIPTION.

FOR EXTERNAL USE ONLY

DESCRIPTION

Each gram of Eldopaque Forte 4% Cream contains 40 mg of hydroquinone in a tinted sunblocking base of water, stearic acid, talc, PEG-40 stearate, PEG-25 propylene glycol stearate, propylene glycol, glyceryl stearate, iron oxides, mineral oil, squalane, disodium EDTA, sodium metabisulfite, and potassium sorbate.

CLINICAL PHARMACOLOGY

Topical application of hydroquinone produces a reversible depigmentation of the skin by inhibition of the enzymatic oxidation of tyrosine to 3, 4-dihydroxyphenylalanine (dopa) and suppression of other melanocyte metabolic processes. Exposure to sunlight or ultraviolet light will cause repigmentation which may be prevented by the sunblocking agents contained in Eldopaque Forte.

INDICATIONS AND USAGE

Eldopaque Forte 4% Cream is indicated for the gradual bleaching of hyperpigmented skin conditions such as chloasma, melasma, freckles, senile lentigines, and other unwanted areas of melanin hyperpigmentation.

CONTRAINDICATIONS

Prior history of sensitivity or allergic reaction to this product or any of its ingredients. The safety of topical hydroquinone use during pregnancy or in children (12 years and under) has not been established.

WARNINGS

A. CAUTION: Hydroquinone is a skin bleaching agent which may produce unwanted cosmetic effects if not used as directed. The physician should be familiar with the contents of this insert before prescribing or dispensing this medication.

B. Test for skin sensitivity before using Eldopaque Forte 4% Cream by applying a small amount to an unbroken patch of skin and check in 24 hours. Minor redness is not a contraindication, but where there is itching or vesicle formation or excessive inflammatory response, further treatment is not advised. Close patient supervision is recommended.

Continued on next page

ICN Pharmaceuticals—Cont.

Contact with the eyes should be avoided. If no bleaching or lightening effect is noted after 2 months of treatment use, Eldopaque Forte 4% Cream should be discontinued. Eldopaque Forte 4% Cream is formulated for use as a skin bleaching agent and should not be used for the prevention of sunburn.

C. Sunscreen use is an essential aspect of hydroquinone therapy because even minimal sunlight exposure sustains melanocytic activity. The sunscreens in Eldopaque Forte 4% Cream provide the necessary sun protection during skin bleaching therapy. After clearing and during maintenance therapy, sun exposure should be avoided on bleached skin by application of a sunscreen or sunblock agent, or protective clothing to prevent repigmentation.

D. Keep this and all medications out of the reach of children. In case of accidental ingestion, call a physician or a poison control center immediately.

E. WARNING: Contains sodium metabisulfite, a sulfite that may cause serious allergic type reactions (e.g. hives, itching, wheezing, anaphylaxis, severe asthma attacks) in certain susceptible persons.

PRECAUTIONS
SEE WARNINGS.

A. Pregnancy Category C. Animal reproduction studies have not been conducted with topical hydroquinone. It is also not known whether hydroquinone can cause fetal harm when used topically on a pregnant woman or affect reproductive capacity. It is not known to what degree, if any, topical hydroquinone is absorbed systemically. Topical hydroquinone should be used in women only when clearly indicated.

B. Nursing mothers. It is not known whether topical hydroquinone is absorbed or excreted in human milk. Caution is advised when topical hydroquinone is used by a nursing mother.

C. Pediatric usage. Safety and effectiveness in children below the age of 12 years have not been established.

ADVERSE REACTIONS
No systemic adverse reactions have been reported. Occasional hypersensitivity (localized contact dermatitis) may occur in which case the medication should be discontinued and the physician notified immediately.

OVERDOSAGE
There have been no systemic reactions from the use of topical hydroquinone or the sunblockers in Eldopaque Forte 4% Cream. However, treatment should be limited to relatively small areas of the body at one time since some patients experience a transient skin reddening and a mild burning sensation which does not preclude treatment.

DRUG DOSAGE AND ADMINISTRATION
A thin application of Eldopaque Forte 4% Cream should be applied to the affected area twice daily or as directed by a physician. Do not rub in. There is no recommendation for children under 12 years of age except under the advice and supervision of a physician.

HOW SUPPLIED
Eldopaque Forte 4% Cream is available as follows:

Size	NDC Number
0.5 ounce tube (15 grams)	0187-0395-35
1.0 ounce tube (30 grams)	0187-0395-31

Available without prescription for maintenance therapy: Eldopaque® (2% Hydroquinone) in ½ ounce (NDC 0187-0518-35) and 1 ounce (NDC 0187-0518-31) tubes.
Eldopaque Forte 4% Cream should be stored at room temperature (15-30°C) (59-86°F).

ELDOQUIN Forte® 4% Cream
[el'-dō-kwin" for'tā]
(Hydroquinone USP, 4%)
Skin Bleaching Cream

CAUTION: FEDERAL LAW (U.S.A.) PROHIBITS DISPENSING WITHOUT A PRESCRIPTION.
FOR EXTERNAL USE ONLY

DESCRIPTION
Each gram of Eldoquin Forte contains 40 mg of hydroquinone in a vanishing cream base of purified water, stearic acid, propylene glycol, poloxyl 40 stearate, propylene glycol monostearate, glyceryl monostearate, mineral oil, squalane, propylparaben and sodium metabisulfite.

CLINICAL PHARMACOLOGY
Topical application of hydroquinone produces a reversible depigmentation of the skin by inhibition of the enzymatic oxidation of tyrosine to 3, 4-dihydroxyphenylalanine (dopa) and suppression of the other melanocyte metabolic processes. Exposure to sunlight or ultraviolet light will cause repigmentation of the bleached areas.

INDICATIONS AND USAGE
Eldoquin Forte 4% Cream is indicated for the gradual bleaching of hyperpigmented skin conditions such as chloasma, melasma, freckles, senile lentigines, and other unwanted areas of melanin hyperpigmentation. It is intended for night-time use only since it contains no sunblocking agents. For daytime usage, Solaquin Forte™ 4% Cream or Eldopaque Forte® 4% Cream should be prescribed.

CONTRAINDICATIONS
Prior history of sensitivity or allergic reaction to this product or any of its ingredients. The safety of topical hydroquinone use during pregnancy or in children (12 years and under) has not been established.

WARNINGS
A. CAUTION: Hydroquinone is a skin bleaching agent which may produce unwanted cosmetic effects if not used as directed. The physician should be familiar with the contents of this insert before prescribing or dispensing this medication.

B. Test for skin sensitivity before using Eldoquin Forte 4% Cream by applying a small amount to an unbroken patch of skin and check in 24 hours. Minor redness is not a contraindication, but where there is itching or vesicle formation or excessive inflammatory response, further treatment is not advised. Close patient supervision is recommended.
Contact with the eyes should be avoided. If no bleaching or lightening effect is noted after 2 months of treatment, the medication should be discontinued.

C. There are no sunblocking or sunscreening agents in Eldoquin Forte 4% Cream and since minimal sunlight exposure may reverse the bleaching effect of this preparation, it should be used only at night or on areas of the body covered by protective clothing. During the daytime, sunblocking or broad spectrum sunscreen preparations or protective clothing should be used to prevent the bleached areas from repigmentation. For daytime bleaching of unwanted pigmented areas, the use of Solaquin Forte™ 4% Cream or Eldopaque Forte® 4% Cream should be considered.

D. Keep this and all medication out of the reach of children. In case of accidental ingestion, call a physician or a poison control center immediately.

E. WARNING: Contains sodium metabisulfite, a sulfite that may cause serious allergic type reactions (e.g. hives, itching, wheezing, anaphylaxis, serious asthma attacks) in certain susceptible persons.

PRECAUTIONS
SEE WARNINGS.

A. Pregnancy Category C. Animal reproduction studies have not been conducted with topical hydroquinone. It is also not known whether hydroquinone can cause fetal harm when used topically on a pregnant woman or affect reproductive capacity. It is not known to what degree, if any, topical hydroquinone is absorbed systemically. Topical hydroquinone should be used in women only when clearly indicated.

B. Nursing mothers. It is not known whether topical hydroquinone is absorbed or excreted in human milk. Caution is advised when topical hydroquinone is used by a nursing mother.

C. Pediatric usage. Safety and effectiveness in children below the age of 12 years have not been established.

ADVERSE REACTIONS
No systemic adverse reactions have been reported. Occasional hypersensitivity (localized contact dermatitis) may occur in which case the medication should be discontinued and the physician notified immediately.

OVERDOSAGE
There have been no systemic reactions from the use of topical hydroquinone in Eldoquin Forte 4% Cream. However, treatment should be limited to relatively small areas of the body at one time since some patients experience a transient skin reddening and a mild burning sensation which does not preclude treatment.

DRUG DOSAGE AND ADMINISTRATION
Eldoquin Forte 4% Cream should be applied to the affected area and rubbed in well twice daily or as directed by a physician. There is no recommended dosage for children under 12 years of age except under the advice and supervision of a physician.

HOW SUPPLIED
ELDOQUIN FORTE 4% Cream is available as follows:

Size	NDC Number
0.5 ounce tube (15 grams)	0187-0394-35
1.0 ounce tube (30 grams)	0187-0394-31

Available without prescription for maintenance therapy: Eldoquin® (2% Hydroquinone) in ½ ounce (NDC 0187-0382-35) and 1 ounce tubes (NDC 0187-0382-31); Eldoquin Lotion (2% Hydroquinone) in ½ ounce bottles (NDC 0187-0423-35).
Eldoquin Forte 4% Cream should be stored at room temperature (15-30°C) (59-86°F).

FOTOTAR® CREAM
[fōtō'tar]
2% Coal Tar USP
(Equivalent to 10% Coal Tar Solution, USP)
Therapeutic Coal Tar Cream
FOR EXTERNAL USE ONLY

DESCRIPTION
Fototar® Cream contains Eldotar® (equivalent to 2% Coal Tar USP), in an emollient moisturizing cream base containing purified water, white petrolatum, mineral oil, microcrystalline cellulose, PEG 8, stearyl alcohol, glyceryl stearate PEG 100 stearate blend, coceth 6, imidazolidinyl urea, methylparaben, and propylparaben.

CLINICAL PHARMACOLOGY
The mechanism of action of coal tar products is largely unknown. Coal tars have antiseptic qualities, because they contain many substituted phenols. Coal tars also act as mild irritants and have a keratoplastic and antipruritic action. Coal tars have a photosensitizing effect and have been used for years with sunlight or ultraviolet (UV) radiation (Goeckerman Therapy) for the treatment of psoriasis. Coal tars have been successfully used in the treatment of seborrhea, eczema, psoriasis, lichen simplex chronicus, and other chronic skin diseases with lichenification. Pharmaceutical compounding of the crude coal tars has not lessened their therapeutic effectiveness and has increased patient acceptability.

INDICATIONS
Fototar is indicated in chronic skin disorders that are responsive to coal tars such as psoriasis, infantile and atopic eczema, seborrhea, lichen simplex chronicus, and other chronic skin disorders exhibiting lichenification. Fototar is useful in the Goeckerman program (tars plus UV radiation) in the treatment of psoriasis or other conditions responding to this combined therapy.

CONTRAINDICATIONS
A. Fototar is contraindicated in patients with a history of sensitivity to this product or with a history of sensitivity to coal tar products.
B. Fototar should not be used on patients who have a disease characterized by photosensitivity such as lupus erythematosus or allergy to sunlight.

WARNINGS
A. Fototar should not be applied to inflamed or broken skin except on the advice of a physician.
B. Since Fototar is photosensitizing, care must be exercised in exposing the areas of application to excessive UV or sunlight for 24 hours. In the Goeckerman treatment of psoriasis or other skin conditions, care must be taken against overexposure of the areas of application during therapeutic UV radiation or subsequent to such treatment because serious burns may result. Sunscreening or sunblocking agents or protective clothing for at least 24 hours after treatment is recommended to protect the treated areas against additional UV exposure from sunlight.
C. Fototar contains a coal tar derivative. Coal tar preparations should not be used in patients with an exacerbation of psoriasis since this may precipitate total body exfoliation.
D. In psoriatic patients receiving Goeckerman therapy, care should be taken that Fototar application and/or subsequent sunlight exposure be avoided over normal skin since this may cause the appearance of new psoriatic lesions in areas of skin trauma (Koebner Phenomenon).
E. Contact with the eyes should be avoided.
F. Staining of clothing may occur which is normally removed by standard laundry methods. Use on the scalp may cause temporary staining of light colored hair.

PRECAUTIONS
A. Patients should be advised of the photosensitizing effect of Fototar.
B. Laboratory tests—none required.
C. Carcinogenesis. Skin cancer following the use of Fototar has not been seen. The use of crude coal tar combined with UV radiation in the production of skin cancer has been studied with conflicting results. Stern, et al, 1980, estimated an increased risk for such cancer in patients with high exposure to tar and ultraviolet radiation compared with those lacking high exposure. They recommended continued surveillance for tumors among psoriatic patients who receive long-term tar and/or UV radiation therapy. However, Pittelkow, et al, 1981, did a 25 year follow-up study on patients receiving combined crude coal tar and UV radiation for psoriasis at the Mayo Clinic and found the incidence of skin cancer not appreciably increased above the expected incidence for the general population, and concluded that this combined regimen (Goeck-

erman) could be used with minimal risk for skin cancer in the treatment of psoriasis.

D. Pregnancy Category C. Animal reproduction studies have not been conducted with Fototar. It is not known whether Fototar can cause fetal harm when administered to a pregnant woman or can affect reproductive capacity. Fototar should be given to a pregnant woman only if clearly indicated.

E. Nursing Mothers. The absorption of Fototar in nursing mothers has not been studied and caution should be exercised when Fototar is administered to a nursing woman.

F. Pediatric Use. Safety and effectiveness of Fototar in children have not been established.

ADVERSE REACTIONS

A. SEE WARNINGS

B. Chemical folliculitis has been observed in areas of skin which have received long term coal tar applications. This phenomenon has not been observed with the use of Fototar, but its possibility should be borne in mind. This reaction normally clears if coal tar is discontinued or frequency of application reduced.

OVERDOSAGE

A. SEE WARNINGS about use on normal skin.

B. If Fototar is accidentally ingested, call a physician or a poison control center for instructions.

DOSAGE AND ADMINISTRATION

Fototar should be rubbed in the desired area well prior to UV radiation. After several minutes, the excess cream remaining on the skin can be patted with paper tissues to remove the excess.

HOW SUPPLIED

Fototar is supplied in 3.0 ounce (85 gm) tubes (NDC 0187-0526-03) and in 1-lb. (453.6 gm) jars (NDC 0187-0526-05). Fototar Cream should be stored at room temperature (15–30°C) (59–86°F).

KATO®   ℞
[kay 'tō]
(potassium chloride for oral solution)
20 mEq (1.5 g. KCl)

DESCRIPTION

KATO® (potassium chloride for oral solution) is a pleasantly flavored spray-dried tomato powder containing 20 mEq potassium (equivalent to 1.5 g KCl) per 5.7-grams of powder (one dose). KATO® is a potassium replacement product. Each daily dose (2 packets) contains approximately 0.5 mEq sodium.

CLINICAL PHARMACOLOGY

As the principal intracellular cation of most body tissues, potassium is instrumental in physiological processes such as maintenance of intracellular tonicity, contractility of cardiac, skeletal, and smooth muscles, maintenance of renal function and transmission of nervous impulses.

Potassium depletion may occur when potassium intake is insufficient to compensate for potassium loss from the G.I. tract or via renal excretion. Such loss may slowly develop during prolonged oral diuretic therapy, in hyperaldosteronism, diabetic ketoacidosis, severe diarrhea, or where potassium intake is inadequate in patients receiving prolonged parenteral nutrition.

The potassium deficit is usually accompanied by chloride depletion and is manifested by hypokalemia and a hypochloremic metabolic alkalosis. Clinical symptoms and signs include weakness, fatigue, disturbances of cardiac rhythmicity (primarily ectopic beats), EKG changes (prominent U waves) and, in severe cases, flaccid paralysis and /or impaired urinary concentration.

Potassium chloride is therefore regarded as the appropriate potassium salt for use in correcting potassium depletion states associated with metabolic alkalosis.

INDICATIONS AND USAGE

KATO® is indicated for the treatment or prevention of potassium deficit, particularly when accompanied by hypochloremic alkalosis in conjunction with thiazide diuretic therapy, in digitalis intoxication, or as a result of long-term corticosteroid therapy, low dietary intake of potassium, or excessive vomiting or diarrhea.

CONTRAINDICATION

Potassium is contraindicated in patients with: severe renal impairment involving oliguria, anuria or azotemia, untreated Addison's disease, familial periodic paralysis, acute dehydration, heat cramps, and hyperkalemia from any cause.

WARNINGS

Potassium intoxication may result from overdosage or from the usual therapeutic dose in patients for whom the drug is contraindicated. Hyperkalemia, when detected, must be treated immediately because lethal levels can be reached in a few hours. (See Overdosage for treatment of hyperkalemia).

PRECAUTIONS

General: Patients receiving potassium supplementation should be monitored with periodic checks of plasma potassium levels.

A high plasma concentration of potassium ion may cause death through cardiac depression, arrhythmias or arrest. Therefore, the drug should be used with caution in patients with cardiac disease.

The drug should not be used in patients with low urinary output or renal decompensation because of the heightened likelihood of overdosage.

In rare circumstances (e.g. patients with renal tubular acidosis) potassium depletion may be associated with a hyperchloremic metabolic acidosis. In such patients, potassium depletion is appropriately corrected using potassium salts other than the chloride.

As with other concentrated potassium supplements. KATO® must be reconstituted with the proper amount of water (2 oz. for 1 packet) to avoid the possibility of gastrointestinal irritation.

DRUG INTERACTIONS

Concomitant administration of potassium chloride and a potassium-sparing diuretic (e.g. aldosterone antagonists or triamterene) can lead to severe hyperkalemia.

ADVERSE REACTIONS

Adverse reactions are related to the gastrointestinal system. Vomiting, diarrhea, nausea and abdominal discomfort may occur.

OVERDOSAGE

The symptoms and signs of potassium intoxication include paresthesias of the extremities, flaccid paralysis, listlessness, mental confusion, weakness and heaviness of the legs, fall in blood pressure, cardiac arrhythmias and heart block. Hyperkalemia may be associated with the following electrocardiographic abnormalities: disappearance of the P wave, widening and slurring of QRS complex, changes of the S-T segment and tall peaked T waves.

The drug is dialyzable.

Treatment of hyperkalemia includes: 1. Elimination of potassium-containing foods and medicaments. 2. Dextrose solution 10% or 25% containing 10 units of crystalline insulin per 20 g dextrose, given i.v. with a dose of 300 cc to 500 cc in an hour. 3. Adsorption and exchange of potassium using sodium or ammonium cycle cation exchange resin, orally or as retention enema. 4. Hemodialysis or peritonial dialysis. Warning: Digitalis toxicity can be precipitated by lowering the plasma potassium concentration too rapidly in digitalized patients.

DOSAGE AND ADMINISTRATION

The usual adult dose is 1 packet of KATO® (20 mEq potassium) mixed with 2 ounces of cold water twice daily. If possible it should stand for 15 minutes to allow the tomato powder to absorb moisture. The preparation should be taken with meals, if convenient. If not, drink ½ glass of water immediately after taking the medication. Larger doses may be required, but should be administered under close supervision because of the possibility of potassium intoxication.

The appropriate dosage of potassium for pediatric use may be calculated from the adult dosage according to relative total body weight.

HOW SUPPLIED

KATO® is available in cartons of 30 (NDC 0187-0112-03) and 120 (NDC 0187-0112-12) 5.7-gram unit dose packets (20 mEq potassium each). Store away from heat.

CAUTION: Federal (U.S.A.) law prohibits dispensing without prescription.

Rev. 6/85

LIPO–NICIN®/100 mg. Tablets
LIPO–NICIN®/250 mg. Tablets
LIPO–NICIN®/300 mg. Timed Release Capsules
Nicotinic Acid Supplement

COMPOSITION

LIPO-NICIN®/100 mg.
Each blue tablet contains:

Nicotinic Acid	100 mg.
Niacinamide	75 mg.
Ascorbic Acid (Vit. C)	150 mg.
Thiamine Hydrochloride (B-1)	25 mg.
Riboflavin (B-2)	2 mg.
Pyridoxine Hydrochloride (B-6)	10 mg.

LIPO-NICIN /250 mg.
Each yellow tablet contains:

Nicotinic Acid	250 mg.
Niacinamide	75 mg.
Ascorbic Acid (Vit. C)	150 mg.
Thiamine Hydrochloride (B-1)	25 mg.
Riboflavin (B-2)	2 mg.
Pyridoxine Hydrochloride (B-6)	10 mg.

LIPO-NICIN/300 mg. Timed Release
Each Clear Capsule Contains:

Nicotinic Acid	300 mg.
Ascorbic Acid (Vit. C)	150 mg.
Thiamine Hydrochloride (B-1)	25 mg.
Riboflavin (B-2)	2 mg.
Pyridoxine Hydrochloride (B-6)	10 mg.

USES

Lipo-Nicin is used in all those conditions in which Niacin (Nicotinic Acid) supplementation is indicated.

SIDE EFFECTS

Temporary flushing with heat and itching, in some cases followed by sweating, nausea and abdominal cramps. This reaction is usually transient. Nausea caused by high acidity can be relieved by nonabsorbable antacid.

CAUTIONS

Lipo-Nicin should not be used by persons with a known sensitivity to Niacin (Nicotinic Acid) and by persons with arterial bleeding, glaucoma, severe diabetes, impaired liver function, peptic ulcer, or by pregnant women.

SUGGESTED USE

LIPO-NICIN /100 mg.—1 tablet daily.
LIPO-NICIN /250 mg.—1 tablet daily.
LIPO-NICIN/300 mg.—1 capsule daily.

AVAILABLE

Bottles of 100.

LITERATURE AVAILABLE

Samples.

MESTINON® INJECTABLE   ℞
[mes 'tin-on]
(pyridostigmine bromide)

DESCRIPTION

Mestinon (pyridostigmine bromide) Injectable is an active cholinesterase inhibitor. Chemically, pyridostigmine bromide is 3-hydroxy-1-methylpyridinium bromide dimethylcarbamate. Its structural formula is:

Each ml contains 5 mg pyridostigmine bromide compounded with 0.2% parabens (methyl and propyl) as preservatives, 0.02% sodium citrate and pH adjusted to approximately 5.0 with citric acid and, if necessary, sodium hydroxide.

ACTIONS

Mestinon facilitates the transmission of impulses across the myoneural junction by inhibiting the destruction of acetylcholine by cholinesterase. Pyridostigmine is an analog of neostigmine (Prostigmin®) but differs from it clinically by having fewer side effects. Currently available data indicate that pyridostigmine may have a significantly lower degree and incidence of bradycardia, salivation and gastrointestinal stimulation. Animal studies using the injectable form of pyridostigmine and human studies using the oral preparation have indicated that pyridostigmine has a longer duration of action than does neostigmine measured under similar circumstances.

INDICATIONS

Mestinon Injectable is useful in the treatment of myasthenia gravis and as a reversal agent or antagonist to nondepolarizing muscle relaxants such as curariform drugs and gallamine triethiodide.

CONTRAINDICATIONS

Known hypersensitivity to anticholinesterase agents; intestinal and urinary obstructions of mechanical type.

WARNINGS

Mestinon Injectable should be used with particular caution in patients with bronchial asthma or cardiac dysrhythmias. Transient bradycardia may occur and be relieved by atropine sulfate. Atropine should also be used with caution in patients with cardiac dysrhythmias. When large doses of Mestinon are administered, as during reversal of muscle relaxants, the prior or simultaneous injection of atropine sulfate is advisable. Because of the possibility of hypersensitivity in an occasional patient, atropine and antishock medication should always be readily available.

As is true of all cholinergic drugs, overdosage of Mestinon may result in cholinergic crisis, a state characterized by increasing muscle weakness which, through involvement of the muscles of respiration, may lead to death. Myasthenic crisis due to an increase in the severity of the disease is also accompanied by extreme muscle weakness and thus may be

Continued on next page

ICN Pharmaceuticals—Cont.

difficult to distinguish from cholinergic crisis on a symptomatic basis. Such differentiation is extremely important, since increases in doses of Mestinon or other drugs in this class in the presence of cholinergic crisis or of a refractory or "insensitive" state could have grave consequences. Osserman and Genkins[1] indicate that the two types of crisis may be differentiated by the use of Tensilon® (edrophonium chloride) as well as by clinical judgment. The treatment of the two conditions obviously differs radically. Whereas the presence of *myasthenic crisis* requires more intensive anticholinesterase therapy, *cholinergic crisis*, according to Osserman and Genkins,[1] calls for the prompt withdrawal of all drugs of this type. The immediate use of atropine in cholinergic crisis is also recommended. A syringe containing 1 mg of atropine sulfate should be immediately available to be given in aliquots intravenously to counteract severe cholinergic reactions.

Atropine may also be used to abolish or obtund gastrointestinal side effects or other muscarinic reactions; but such use, by masking signs of overdosage, can lead to inadvertent induction of cholinergic crisis.

For detailed information on the management of patients with myasthenia gravis, the physician is referred to one of the excellent reviews such as those by Osserman and Genkins,[2] Grob[3] or Schwab.[4,5]

When used as an antagonist to nondepolarizing muscle relaxants, adequate recovery of voluntary respiration and neuromuscular transmission must be obtained prior to discontinuation of respiratory assistance and there should be continuous patient observation. Satisfactory recovery may be defined by a combination of clinical judgment, respiratory measurements and observation of the effects of peripheral nerve stimulation. If there is any doubt concerning the adequacy of recovery from the effects of the nondepolarizing muscle relaxant, artificial ventilation should be continued until all doubt has been removed.

Usage in Pregnancy: The safety of Mestinon during pregnancy or lactation in humans has not been established. Therefore, use of Mestinon in women who may become pregnant requires weighing the drug's potential benefits against its possible hazards to mother and child.

ADVERSE REACTIONS

The side effects of Mestinon are most commonly related to overdosage and generally are of two varieties, muscarinic and nicotinic. Among those in the former group are nausea, vomiting, diarrhea, abdominal cramps, increased peristalsis, increased salivation, increased bronchial secretions, miosis and diaphoresis. Nicotinic side effects are comprised chiefly of muscle cramps, fasciculation and weakness. Muscarinic side effects can usually be counteracted by atropine, but for reasons shown in the preceding section the expedient is not without danger. As with any compound containing the bromide radical, a skin rash may be seen in an occasional patient. Such reactions usually subside promptly upon discontinuance of the medication. Thrombophlebitis has been reported subsequent to intravenous administration.

DOSAGE AND ADMINISTRATION

For Myasthenia Gravis—To supplement oral dosage, pre- and postoperatively, during labor and postpartum, during myasthenic crisis, or whenever oral therapy is impractical, approximately 1/30th of the oral dose of Mestinon may be given parenterally, either by intramuscular or *very slow* intravenous injection. *The patient must be closely observed for cholinergic reactions, particularly if the intravenous route is used.*

For details regarding the management of myasthenic patients who are to undergo major surgical procedures, see the article by Foldes.[6]

Neonates of myasthenic mothers may have transient difficulty in swallowing, sucking and breathing. Injectable Mestinon may be indicated—by symptomatology and use of the Tensilon® (edrophonium chloride) test—until Mestinon Syrup can be taken. To date the world literature consists of less than 100 neonate patients.[7] Of these only 5 were treated with injectable pyridostigmine, with the vast majority of the remaining neonates receiving neostigmine. Dosage requirements of Mestinon Injectable are minute, ranging from 0.05 mg to 0.15 mg/kg of body weight given intramuscularly. It is important to differentiate between cholinergic and myasthenic crises in neonates. (See **WARNINGS**.)

Mestinon given parenterally one hour before completion of second stage labor enables patients to have adequate strength during labor and provides protection to infants in the immediate postnatal state. For further information on the use of Mestinon Injectable in neonates of myasthenic mothers, see the article by Namba.[7]

NOTE: For information on a diagnostic test for myasthenia gravis, and on the evaluation and stabilization of therapy, please see product information on Tensilon® (edrophonium chloride).

For Reversal of Nondepolarizing Muscle Relaxants: When Mestinon Injectable is given intravenously to reverse the action of muscle relaxant drugs, it is recommended that atropine sulfate (0.6 to 1.2 mg) also be given intravenously immediately prior to the Mestinon. Side effects, notably excessive secretions and bradycardia, are thereby minimized. Usually 10 or 20 mg of Mestinon will be sufficient for antagonism of the effects of the nondepolarizing muscle relaxants. Although full recovery may occur within 15 minutes in most patients, others may require a half hour or more. Satisfactory reversal can be evident by adequate voluntary respiration, respiratory measurements and use of a peripheral nerve stimulator device. It is recommended that the patient be well ventilated and a patent airway maintained until complete recovery of normal respiration is assured. Once satisfactory reversal has been attained, recurarization has not been reported. For additional information on the use of Mestinon for antagonism of nondepolarizing muscle relaxants see the article by Katz[8] and McNall.[9]

Failure of Mestinon Injectable to provide prompt (within 30 minutes) reversal may occur, *e.g.*, in the presence of extreme debilitation, carcinomatosis, or with concomitant use of certain broad spectrum antibiotics or anesthetic agents, notably ether. Under these circumstances ventilation must be supported by artificial means until the patient has resumed control of his respiration.

HOW SUPPLIED

Mestinon is available in 2-ml ampuls (boxes of 10) (NDC 0187-3010-10).

REFERENCES

1. K. E. Osserman and G. Genkins, *J.A.M.A.* 183: 97, 1963.
2. K. E. Osserman and G. Genkins, *New York State J. Med.*, 61: 2076, 1961.
3. D. Grob, *Arch. Intern. Med.*, 108: 615, 1961.
4. R. S. Schwab, *New Eng. J. Med.*, 268: 596, 1963.
5. R. S. Schwab, *New Eng. J. Med.*, 268: 717, 1963.
6. F. F. Foldes and P. McNall, *Anesthesiology*, 23: 837, 1962.
7. T. Namba *et al.*, *Pediatrics*, 45: 488, 1970.
8. R. L. Katz, *Anesthesiology*, 28: 528, 1967.
9. P. McNall *et al.*, *Anesthesia and Analgesia*, 48: 1026, 1969.
Manufactured for ICN Pharmaceuticals, Inc.
Costa Mesa, CA 92626
by Hoffmann-La Roche Inc.
Nutley, N.J. 07110
Rev. 3/89

MESTINON®   ℞
[*mes'tin-on*]
(pyridostigmine bromide)
TABLETS, SYRUP and
TIMESPAN® TABLETS

DESCRIPTION

Mestinon (pyridostigmine bromide) is an orally active cholinesterase inhibitor. Chemically, pyridostigmine bromide is 3-hydroxy-1-methylpyridinium bromide dimethylcarbamate. Mestinon is available in the following forms: Syrup containing 60 mg pyridostigmine bromide per teaspoonful in a vehicle containing 5% alcohol, glycerin, lactic acid, sodium benzoate, sorbitol, sucrose, FD&C Red No. 40, FD&C Blue No. 1, flavors and water. *Tablets* containing 60 mg pyridostigmine bromide; each tablet also contains lactose, silicon dioxide and stearic acid. *Timespan Tablets* containing 180 mg pyridostigmine bromide; each tablet also contains carnauba wax, corn-derived proteins, magnesium stearate, silica gel and tribasic calcium phosphate.

ACTIONS

Mestinon inhibits the destruction of acetylcholine by cholinesterase and thereby permits freer transmission of nerve impulses across the neuromuscular junction. Pyridostigmine is an analog of neostigmine (Prostigmin®), but differs from it in certain clinically significant respects; for example, pyridostigmine is characterized by a longer duration of action and fewer gastrointestinal side effects.

INDICATION

Mestinon is useful in the treatment of myasthenia gravis.

CONTRAINDICATIONS

Mestinon is contraindicated in mechanical intestinal or urinary obstruction, and particular caution should be used in its administration to patients with bronchial asthma. Care should be observed in the use of atropine for counteracting side effects, as discussed below.

WARNINGS

Although failure of patients to show clinical improvement may reflect underdosage, it can also be indicative of overdosage. As is true of all cholinergic drugs, overdosage of Mestinon may result in cholinergic crisis, a state characterized by increasing muscle weakness which, through involvement of the muscles of respiration, may lead to death. Myasthenic crisis due to an increase in the severity of the disease is also accompanied by extreme muscle weakness, and thus may be

difficult to distinguish from cholinergic crisis on a symptomatic basis. Such differentiation is extremely important, since increases in doses of Mestinon or other drugs of this class in the presence of cholinergic crisis or of a refractory or "insensitive" state could have grave consequences. Osserman and Genkins[1] indicate that the differential diagnosis of the two types of crisis may require the use of Tensilon® (edrophonium chloride) as well as clinical judgment. The treatment of the two conditions obviously differs radically. Whereas the presence of myasthenic crisis suggests the need for more intensive anticholinesterase therapy, the diagnosis of cholinergic crisis, according to Osserman and Genkins,[1] calls for the prompt *withdrawal* of all drugs of this type. The immediate use of atropine in cholinergic crisis is also recommended. Atropine may also be used to abolish or obtund gastrointestinal side effects or other muscarinic reactions; but such use, by masking signs of overdosage, can lead to inadvertent induction of cholinergic crisis.

For detailed information on the management of patients with myasthenia gravis, the physician is referred to one of the excellent reviews such as those by Osserman and Genkins,[2] Grob[3] or Schwab.[4,5]

Usage in Pregnancy: The safety of Mestinon during pregnancy or lactation in humans has not been established. Therefore, use of Mestinon in women who may become pregnant requires weighing the drug's potential benefits against its possible hazards to mother and child.

ADVERSE REACTIONS

The side effects of Mestinon are most commonly related to overdosage and generally are of two varieties, muscarinic and nicotinic. Among those in the former group are nausea, vomiting, diarrhea, abdominal cramps, increased peristalsis, increased salivation, increased bronchial secretions, miosis and diaphoresis. Nicotinic side effects are comprised chiefly of muscle cramps, fasciculation and weakness. Muscarinic side effects can usually be counteracted by atropine, but for reasons shown in the preceding section the expedient is not without danger. As with any compound containing the bromide radical, a skin rash may be seen in an occasional patient. Such reactions usually subside promptly upon discontinuance of the medication.

DOSAGE AND ADMINISTRATION

Mestinon is available in three dosage forms:

Syrup—raspberry-flavored, containing 60 mg pyridostigmine bromide per teaspoonful (5 ml). This form permits accurate dosage adjustment for children and "brittle" myasthenic patients who require fractions-of 60-mg doses. It is more easily swallowed, especially in the morning, by patients with bulbar involvement.

Conventional tablets—each containing 60 mg pyridostigmine bromide.

Timespan tablets—each containing 180 mg pyridostigmine bromide. This form provides uniformly slow release, hence prolonged duration of drug action; it facilitates control of myasthenic symptoms with fewer individual doses daily. The immediate effect of a 180-mg Timespan tablet is about equal to that of a 60-mg conventional tablet; however, its duration of effectiveness, although varying in individual patients, averages 2½ times that of a 60-mg dose.

Dosage: The size and frequency of the dosage must be adjusted to the needs of the individual patient.

Syrup and conventional tablets—The average dose is ten 60-mg tablets or ten 5-ml teaspoonfuls daily, spaced to provide maximum relief when maximum strength is needed. In severe cases as many as 25 tablets or teaspoonfuls a day may be required, while in mild cases one to six tablets or teaspoonfuls a day may suffice.

Timespan tablets—One to three 180-mg tablets, once or twice daily, will usually be sufficient to control symptoms; however, the needs of certain individuals may vary markedly from this average. The interval between doses should be at least six hours. For optimum control, it may be necessary to use the more rapidly acting regular tablets or syrup in conjunction with Timespan therapy.

Note: For information on a diagnostic test for myasthenia gravis, and for the evaluation and stabilization of therapy, please see product literature on Tensilon® (edrophonium chloride).

HOW SUPPLIED

Syrup, 60 mg pyridostigmine bromide per teaspoonful (5 ml) and 5% alcohol—bottles of 16 fluid ounces (1 pint) (NDC 0187-3010-20).

Tablets, scored, 60 mg pyridostigmine bromide each—bottles of 100 (NDC 0187-3010-30)and 500 (NDC 0187-3010-40).

Timespan tablets, scored, 180 mg pyridostigmine bromide each—bottles of 100 (NDC 0187-3010-50).

Note: Because of the hygroscopic nature of the Timespan tablets, mottling may occur. This does not affect their efficacy.

REFERENCES

1. K. E. Osserman and G. Genkins, *J.A.M.A.*, 183: 97, 1963.
2. K. E. Osserman and G. Genkins, *New York State J. Med.*, 61:2076, 1961.

3. D. Grob, *Arch. Intern. Med.*, 108 :615, 1961.
4. R. S. Schwab, *New England J. Med.*, 268 :596, 1963.
5. R. S. Schwab, *New England J. Med.*, 268 :717, 1963.
Manufactured for ICN Pharmaceuticals, Inc.
Costa Mesa, CA 92626
by Hoffmann-La Roche Inc.
Nutley, N.J. 07110
Rev. 3/89

OXSORALEN® LOTION 1%   ℞
[ox 'sore "a-len]
(methoxsalen USP, 1%)

CAUTION: FEDERAL (U.S.A.) LAW PROHIBITS DISPENS-
ING WITHOUT A PRESCRIPTION.
CAUTION: METHOXSALEN LOTION IS A POTENT TOPI-
CAL DRUG. READ ENTIRE BROCHURE BEFORE PRE-
SCRIBING OR USING THIS MEDICATION.
WARNING: METHOXSALEN LOTION IS A POTENT
DRUG CAPABLE OF PRODUCING SEVERE BURNS IF IM-
PROPERLY USED. IT SHOULD BE APPLIED ONLY BY A
PHYSICIAN UNDER CONTROLLED CONDITIONS FOR
LIGHT EXPOSURE AND SUBSEQUENT LIGHT SHIELDING.
THIS PREPARATION SHOULD NEVER BE DISPENSED TO
A PATIENT.

DESCRIPTION
Each ml of Oxsoralen Lotion contains 10 mg methoxsalen in
an inert vehicle containing alcohol (71% v/v), propylene
glycol, acetone, and purified water.
Methoxsalen is a naturally occurring substance found in the
seeds of the Ammi majus (Umbelliferae) plant; it belongs to a
group of compounds known as psoralens or furocoumarins.
The chemical name of methoxsalen is 9-methoxy-7H-furo(3,
2g) (1)-benzopyran-7-one. It has the following structure:

CLINICAL PHARMACOLOGY
The exact mechanism of action of methoxsalen with the epidermal melanocytes and keratinocytes is not known. Psoralens given orally are preferentially taken up by epidermal
cells (Artuc et al, 1979). The best known biochemical reaction
of methoxsalen is with DNA. Methoxsalen, upon photoactivation, conjugates and forms covalent bonds with DNA
which leads to the formation of both monofunctional (addition to a single strand of DNA) and bifunctional adducts
(crosslinking of psoralen to both strands of DNA) (Dall'Acqua et al, 1971). Reactions with proteins have also been described (Yoshikawa et al, 1979).
Methoxsalen acts as a photosensitizer. Topical application of
this drug and subsequent exposure to UVA, whether artificial or sunlight, can cause cell injury. If sufficient cell injury
occurs in the skin an inflammatory reaction will result. The
most obvious manifestation of this reaction is delayed erythema which may not begin for several hours and may not
peak for 2 to 3 days or longer. It is crucial to realize that the
length of time the skin remains sensitized or when the maximum erythema will occur is quite variable from person to
person. The erythematous reaction is followed over several
days or weeks by repair which is manifested by increased
melanization of the epidermis and thickening of the stratum
corneum. The exact mechanics are unknown but it has been
suggested melanocytes in the hair follicles are stimulated to
move up the follicle and to repopulate the epidermis. (Or-
tonne, et al, 1979)

INDICATIONS AND USAGE
As a topical repigmenting agent in vitiligo in conjunction
with controlled doses of ultraviolet A (320–400 nm) or sunlight.

CONTRAINDICATIONS
A. Patients exhibiting idiosyncratic reactions to psoralen
compounds or a history of sensitivity reactions to them.
B. Patients exhibiting melanoma or with a history of melanoma.
C. Patients exhibiting invasive skin carcinoma generally.
D. Patients with photosensitivity diseases such as porphyria, acute lupus erythematosus, xeroderma pigmentosum, etc.
E. Children under 12 since clinical studies to determine the
efficacy and safety of treatment in this age group have
not been done.

WARNINGS
A. Skin Burns
Serious skin burns from either UVA or sunlight (even
through window glass) can result if recommended exposure
schedule is exceeded and/or protective covering or sunscreens are not used. The blistering of the skin sometimes
encountered after UVA exposure generally heals without
complication or scarring. (Farrington Daniels, Jr, M.D., per-

sonal communication). Suitable covering of the area of application or a topical sunblock should follow the therapeutic
UVA exposure.
B. Carcinogenicity
1. Animal Studies. Topical methoxsalen has been reported
to be a potent photocarcinogen in certain strains of mice.
(Pathak et al 1959).
2. Human Studies. None of our clinical investigators reported skin cancers as a complication of topical treatment
for vitiligo. However, it is recommended that caution be exercised when the patient is fair-skinned or has a history of
prior coal tar UVA treatment, or has had ionizing radiation
or taken arsenical compounds. Such patients who subsequently have oral psoralen—UVA treatment (PUVA) are at
increased risk for developing skin cancer.
C. Concomitant Therapy
Special care should be exercised in treating patients who are
receiving concomitant therapy (either topically or systemically) with known photosensitizing agents such as anthralin,
coal tar or coal tar derivatives, griseofulvin, phenothiazines,
nalidixic acid, halogenated salicylanilides (bacteriostatic
soaps), sulfonamides, tetracyclines, thiazides, and certain
organic staining dyes such as methylene blue, toluidine blue,
rose bengal, and methyl orange.

PRECAUTIONS
A. This product should be applied only in small well defined
lesions and preferably on lesions which can be protected
by clothing or a sunscreen from subsequent exposure to
radiant UVA. If this product is used to treat vitiligo of
face or hands, be very emphatic when instructing patient to keep the treated areas protected from light by
use of protective clothing or sunscreening agents. The
area of application may be highly photosensitive for several days and may result in severe burn injury if exposed
to additional UVA or sunlight.
B. CARCINOGENESIS: See Warning Section
C. Pregnancy Category C. Animal reproduction studies
have not been conducted with topical methoxsalen. It is
also not known whether methoxsalen can cause fetal
harm when used topically on a pregnant woman or affect
reproductive capacity. It is not known to what degree, if
any, topical methoxsalen is absorbed systemically. Topical methoxsalen should be used in pregnant women only
when clearly indicated.
D. Nursing Mothers. It is not known whether topical methoxsalen is absorbed or excreted in human milk. Caution is advised when topical methoxsalen is used in a
nursing mother.
E. Pediatric Usage. Safety and effectiveness in children
below the age of 12 years have not been established.

ADVERSE REACTIONS
Systemic adverse reactions have not been reported. The most
common adverse reaction is severe burns of the treated area
from overexposure to UVA, including sunlight. TREAT-
MENT MUST BE INDIVIDUALIZED. Minor blistering of
the skin is not a contraindication to further treatment and
generally heals without incident. Treatment would be the
standard for burn therapy. Since 1953, many studies have
demonstrated the safety and effectiveness of topical methoxsalen and UVA for the treatment of vitiligo when used as
directed. (Lerner, A.B., et al, 1953) (Fitzpatrick, T.B., et al,
1966) (Fulton, James F. et al, 1969)

OVERDOSAGE
This does not apply to topical usage. In the unlikely event
that the lotion is ingested, standard procedures for poisoning
should be followed, including gastric lavage. Protection from
UVA or daylight for hours or days would also be necessary
and the patient kept in a darkened room.

ADMINISTRATION
The OXSORALEN® Lotion is applied to a well-defined area
of vitiligo by the physician and the area is then exposed to a
suitable source of UVA. Initial exposure time should be conservative and not exceed that which is predicted to be one-
half the minimal erythema dose. Treatment intervals should
be regulated by the erythema response; generally once a
week is recommended or less often depending on the results.
The hands and fingers of the person applying the medication
should be protected by gloves or finger cots to avoid photosensitization and possible burns.
Pigmentation may begin after a few weeks but significant
repigmentation may require up to 6 to 9 months of treatment. Periodic re-treatment may be necessary to retain all of
the new pigment. Idiopathic vitiligo is reversible but not
equally reversible in every patient. Treatment must be individualized. Repigmentation will vary in completeness, time
of onset, and duration. Repigmentation occurs more rapidly
in fleshy areas such as face, abdomen, and buttocks and less
rapidly over less fleshy areas such as the dorsum of the
hands or feet.

HOW SUPPLIED
Oxsoralen Lotion containing 1% methoxsalen (8-methoxp-
soralen) packaged in 1 ounce (30 ml) amber glass bottles
(NDC 0187-0402-31).

Oxsoralen Lotion 1% should be stored at room temperature
(15–30℃) (59–86℉).

OXSORALEN–ULTRA® CAPSULES   ℞
[ox '-sore "a-len]
(Methoxsalen, 10 mg)

CAUTION: FEDERAL LAW PROHIBITS DISPENSING
WITHOUT PRESCRIPTION.
CAUTION: METHOXSALEN IS A POTENT DRUG,
READ ENTIRE BROCHURE PRIOR TO PRESCRIBING OR
DISPENSING THIS MEDICATION.

> Methoxsalen with UV radiation should be used only by
> physicians who have special competence in the diagno-
> sis and treatment of psoriasis and who have special
> training and experience in photochemotherapy. The use
> of Psoralen and ultraviolet radiation therapy should be
> under constant supervision of such a physician. For the
> treatment of patients with psoriasis, photochemoth-
> erapy should be restricted to patients with severe, recal-
> citrant, disabling psoriasis which is not adequately re-
> sponsive to other forms of therapy, and only when the
> diagnosis has been supported by biopsy. Because of the
> possibilities of ocular damage, aging of the skin, and
> skin cancer (including melanoma), the patient should be
> fully informed by the physician of the risks inherent in
> this therapy.

> CAUTION: Oxsoralen-Ultra® should not be used
> interchangeably with regular Oxsoralen®. This new
> dosage form of methoxsalen exhibits significantly
> greater bioavailability and earlier photosensitization
> onset time than previous methoxsalen dosage forms.
> Patients should be treated in accordance with the do-
> simetry specifically recommended for this product. The
> minimum phototoxic dose (MPD) and phototoxic peak
> time after drug administration prior to onset of photo-
> chemotherapy with this dosage form should be deter-
> mined.

DESCRIPTION
Oxsoralen-Ultra (methoxsalen, 8-methoxpsoralen) Capsules, 10mg Methoxsalen is a naturally occurring photoac-
tive substance found in the seeds of the Ammi majus (Umbelliferae) plant. It belongs to a group of compounds known as
psoralens, or furocoumarins. The chemical name of methoxsalen is 9-methoxy-7H-furo [3,2-g] [1]benzopyran-7-one; it
has the following structure:

CLINICAL PHARMACOLOGY
The combination treatment regimen of psoralen (P) and ultraviolet radiation of 320–400 nm wavelength commonly
referred to as UVA is known by the acronym, PUVA. Skin
reactivity to UVA (320–400nm) radiation is markedly enhanced by the ingestion of methoxsalen. In a well controlled
bioavailability study, Oxsoralen-Ultra Capsules reached
peak drug levels in the blood of test subjects between 0.5 and
4 hours (Mean = 1.8 hours) as compared to between 1.5 and 6
hours (Mean = 3.0 hours) for regular Oxsoralen when administered with 8 ounces of milk. Peak drug levels were 2 to
3 fold greater when the overall extent of drug absorption was
approximately two fold greater for Oxsoralen-Ultra Capsules as compared to regular Oxsoralen Capsules. Detectable
methoxsalen levels were observed up to 12 hours post dose.
The drug half-life is approximately 2 hours. Photosensitivity
studies demonstrate a shorter time of peak photosensitivity
of 1.5 to 2.1 hours vs. 3.9 to 4.25 hours for regular Oxsoralen
capsules. In addition, the mean minimal erythema dose
(MED), J/cm^2, for the Oxsoralen-Ultra Capsules is substantially less than that required for regular Oxsoralen Capsules
(Levins et al., 1984 and private communication[1]).
Methoxsalen is reversibly bound to serum albumin and is
also preferentially taken up by epidermal cells (Artuc et al.,
1979[2]). At a dose which is six times larger than that used in
humans, it induces mixed function oxidases in the liver of
mice (Mandula et al., 1978[3]). In both mice and man, methoxsalen is rapidly metabolized. Approximately 95% of the drug
is excreted as a series of metabolites in the urine within 24
hours (Pathak et al., 1977[4]). The exact mechanism of action
of methoxsalen with the epidermal melanocytes and
keratinocytes is not known. The best known biochemical
reaction of methoxsalen is with DNA. Methoxsalen, upon
photoactivation, conjugates and forms covalent bonds with

Continued on next page

ICN Pharmaceuticals—Cont.

DNA which leads to the formation of both monofunctional (addition to a single strand of DNA) and bifunctional (cross-linking of psoralen to both strands of DNA) adducts (Dall' Acqua et al., 1971[5]; Cole, 1970[6]; Musajo et al., 1974[7]; Dall' Acqua et al., 1979[8]). Reactions with proteins have also been described (Yoshikawa, et al., 1979[9]).

Methoxsalen acts as a photosensitizer. Administration of the drug and subsequent exposure to UVA can lead to cell injury. Orally administered methoxsalen reaches the skin via the blood and UVA penetrates well into the skin. If sufficient cell injury occurs in the skin, an inflammatory reaction occurs. The most obvious manifestation of this reaction is delayed erythema, which may not begin for several hours and peaks at 48–72 hours. The inflammation is followed, over several days to weeks, by repair which is manifested by increased melanization of the epidermis and thickening of the stratum corneum. The mechanisms of therapy are not known. In the treatment of psoriasis, the mechanism is most often assumed to be DNA photodamage and resulting decrease in cell proliferation but other vascular, leukocyte, or cell regulatory mechanisms may also be playing some role. Psoriasis is a hyper-proliferative disorder and other agents known to be therapeutic for psoriasis are known to inhibit DNA systhesis.

INDICATIONS AND USAGE

Photochemotherapy (methoxsalen with long wave UVA radiation) is indicated for the symptomatic control of severe, recalcitrant, disabling psoriasis not adequately responsive to other forms of therapy and when the diagnosis has been supported by biopsy. Methoxsalen is intended to be administered only in conjunction with a schedule of controlled doses of long wave ultraviolet radiation.

CONTRAINDICATIONS

A. Patients exhibiting idiosyncratic reactions to psoralen compounds.
B. Patients possessing a specific history of light sensitive disease states should not initiate methoxsalen therapy except under special circumstances. Diseases associated with photosensitivity include lupus erythematosus, porphyria cutanea tarda, erythropoietic protoporphyria, variegate porphyria, xeroderma pigmentosum, and albinism.
C. Patients with melanoma or with a history of melanoma.
D. Patients with invasive squamous cell carcinomas.
E. Patients with aphakia, because of the significantly increased risk of retinal damage due to the absence of lenses.

WARNINGS—GENERAL

A. SKIN BURNING: Serious burns from either UVA or sunlight (even through window glass) can result if the recommended dosage of the drug and/or exposure schedules are exeeded.
B. CARCINOGENICITY:
1. ANIMAL STUDIES: Topical or intraperitoneal methoxsalen has been reported to be a potent photocarcinogen in albino mice and hairless mice (Hakim et al., 1960[10]). However, methoxsalen given by the oral route to Swiss albino mice suggests this agent exerts a protective effect against ultraviolet carcinogenesis; mice given 8-methoxypsoralen in their diet showed 38% ear tumors 180 days after the start of ultraviolet therapy compared to 62% for controls (O'Neal et al., 1957[11]).
2. HUMAN STUDIES: A 5.7 year prospective study of 1380 psoriasis patients treated with oral methoxsalen and ultraviolet A photochemotherapy (PUVA) demonstrated that the risk of cutaneous squamous-cell carcinoma developing at least 22 months following the first PUVA exposure was approximately 12.8 times higher in the high dose patients than in the low dose patients (Stern et al., 1979[12], Stern et al., 1980[13], and Stern et al., 1984[14]). The substantial dose-dependent increase was observed in patients with neither a prior history of skin cancer nor significant exposure to cutaneous carcinogens. Reduction in PUVA dosage significantly reduces the risk. No substantial dose related increase was noted for basal cell carcinoma according to Stern et al., 1984[14]. Increases appear greatest in patients who have pre-PUVA exposure to 1) prolonged tar and UVB treatment, 2) ionizing radiation, or 3) arsenic.
Roenigk et al., 1980[15], studied 690 patients for up to 4 years and found no increase in the risk of non-melanoma skin cancer, although patients in this cohort had significantly less exposure to PUVA than in the Stern et al. study. After 5 years, two of 1380 patients in the Stern et al. PUVA study have developed malignant melanoma. In addition, more than $\frac{1}{5}$ of the patients in this cohort have developed macular pigmented lesions on the buttocks. While there is no evidence that an increased risk of melanoma exists in PUVA treated patients, these observations indicate the need for continued evaluation of melanoma risk of PUVA treated patients.

In a study in Indian patients treated for 4 years for vitiligo, 12 percent developed keratoses, but not cancer, in the depigmented, vitiliginous areas (Mosher, 1980[16]). Clinically, the keratoses were keratotic papules, actinic keratosis-like macules, nonscaling dome-shaped papules, and lichenoid porokeratotic-like papules.

C. CATARACTOGENICITY:
1. ANIMAL STUDIES: Exposure to large doses of UVA causes cataracts in animals, and this effect is enhanced by the administration of methoxsalen (Cloud et al, 1960[17]; Cloud et al, 1961[18]; Freeman et al, 1969[19]).
2. HUMAN STUDIES: It has been found that the concentration of methoxsalen in the lens is proportional to the serum level. If the lens is exposed to UVA during the time methoxsalen is present in the lens, photochemical action may lead to irreversible binding of methoxsalen to proteins and the DNA components of the lens (Lerman et al, 1980[20]). However, if the lens is shielded from UVA, the methoxsalen will diffuse out of the lens in a 24 hour period (Lerman et al., 1980[20]). Patients should be told emphatically to wear UVA-absorbing, wrap-around sunglasses for the twenty-four (24) hour period following ingestion of methoxsalen, whether exposed to direct or indirect sunlight in the open or through a window glass. Among patients using proper eye protection, there is no evidence for a significantly increased risk of cataracts in association with PUVA therapy. (Stern et al., 1979[12]). Thirty-five of 1380 patients have developed cataracts in the five years since their first PUVA treatment. This incidence is comparable to that expected in a population of this size and age distribution. No relationship between PUVA dose and cataract risk in this group has been noted.

D. ACTINIC DEGENERATION: Exposure to sunlight and/or ultraviolet radiation may result in "premature aging" of the skin.

E. BASAL CELL CARCINOMAS: Patients exhibiting multiple basal cell carcinomas or having a history of basal cell carcinomas should be diligently observed and treated.

F. RADIATION THERAPY: Patients having a history of previous x-ray therapy or grenz ray therapy should be diligently observed for signs of carcinoma.

G. ARSENIC THERAPY: Patients having a history of previous arsenic therapy should be diligently observed for signs of carcinoma.

H. HEPATIC DISEASES: Patients with hepatic insufficiency should be treated with caution since hepatic biotransformation is necessary for drug urinary excretion.

I. CARDIAC DISEASES: Patients with cardiac diseases or others who may be unable to tolerate prolonged standing or exposure to heat stress should not be treated in a vertical UVA chamber.

J. TOTAL DOSAGE: The total cumulative dose of UVA that can be given over long periods of time with safety has not as yet been established.

K. CONCOMITANT THERAPY: Special care should be exercised in treating patients who are receiving concomitant therapy (either topically or systemically) with known photosensitizing agents such as anthralin, coal tar or coal tar derivatives, griseofulvin, phenothiazines, nalidixic acid, halogenated salicylanilides (bacteriostatic soaps), sulfonamides, tetracyclines, thiazides and certain organic staining dyes such as methylene blue, toluidine blue, rose bengal, and methyl orange.

PRECAUTIONS

A. GENERAL—APPLICABLE TO PSORIASIS TREATMENT
1. BEFORE METHOXSALEN INGESTION
Patients must not sunbathe during the 24 hours prior to methoxsalen ingestion and UV exposure. The presence of a sunburn may prevent an accurate evaluation of the patient's response to photochemotherapy.
2. AFTER METHOXSALEN INGESTION
a. UVA-absorbing wrap-around sunglasses should be worn during daylight for 24 hours after methoxsalen ingestion. The protective eyewear must be designed to prevent entry of stray radiation to the eyes, including that which may enter from the sides of the eyewear. The protective eyewear is used to prevent the irreversible binding of methoxsalen to the proteins and DNA components of the lens. Cataracts form when enough of the binding occurs. Visual discrimination should be permitted by the eyewear for patient well-being and comfort.
b. Patients must avoid sun exposure, even through window glass or cloud cover, for at least 8 hours after methoxsalen ingestion. If sun exposure cannot be avoided, the patient should wear protective devices such as a hat and gloves, and/or apply sunscreens which contain ingredients that filter out UVA radiation (e.g. sunscreens containing benzophenone and/or PABA esters which exhibit a sun protective factor equal to or greater than 15). These chemical sunscreens should be applied to all areas that might be exposed to the sun (including lips). Sunscreens should

not be applied to areas affected by psoriasis until after the patient has been treated in the UVA chamber.
3. DURING PUVA THERAPY
a. Total UVA-absorbing/blocking goggles mechanically designed to give maximal ocular protection must be worn. Failure to do so may increase the risk of cataract formation. A reliable radiometer can be used to verify elimination of UVA transmission through the goggles.
b. Abdominal skin, breasts, genitalia, and other sensitive areas should be protected for approximately $\frac{1}{3}$ of the initial exposure time until tanning occurs.
c. Unless affected by disease, male genitalia should be shielded.
4. AFTER COMBINED METHOXSALEN/UVA THERAPY
a. UVA-absorbing wrap-around sunglasses should be worn during daylight for 24 hours after combined methoxsalen/UVA therapy.
b. Patients should not sunbathe for 48 hours after therapy. Erythema and/or burning due to photochemotherapy and sunburn due to sun exposure are additive.

B. INFORMATION FOR PATIENTS: See accompanying Patient Package Insert.

C. LABORATORY TESTS:
1. Patients should have an ophthalmologic examination prior to start of therapy, and thence yearly.
2. Patients should have routine laboratory tests prior to the start of therapy and at regular periods thereafter if patients are on extended treatments.

D. DRUG INTERACTIONS: See Warnings Section.

E. CARCINOGENESIS: See Warnings Section.

F. PREGNANCY:
Pregnancy Category C. Animal reproduction studies have not been conducted with methoxsalen. It is also not known whether methoxsalen can cause fetal harm when administered to a pregnant woman or can affect reproduction capacity. Methoxsalen should be given to a woman with reproductive capacity only if clearly needed.

G. NURSING MOTHERS:
It is not known whether this drug is excreted in human milk. Because many drugs are excreted in human milk, either methoxsalen ingestion or nursing should be discontinued.

H. PEDIATRIC USE:
Safety in children has not been established. Potential hazards of long-term therapy include the possibilities of carcinogenicity and cataractogenicity as described in the Warnings Section as well as the probability of actinic degeneration which is also described in the Warnings Section.

ADVERSE REACTIONS

A. METHOXSALEN:
The most commonly reported side effect of methoxsalen alone is nausea, which occurs with approximately 10% of all patients. This effect may be minimized or avoided by instructing the patient to take methoxsalen with milk or food, or to divide the dose into two portions, taken approximately one-half hour apart. Other effects include nervousness, insomnia, and psychological depression.

B. COMBINED METHOXSALEN/UVA THERAPY:
1. PRURITUS: This adverse reaction occurs with approximately 10% of all patients. In most cases, pruritus can be alleviated with frequent application of bland emollients or other topical agents; severe pruritus may require systemic treatment. If pruritus is unresponsive to these measures, shield pruritic areas from further UVA exposure until the condition resolves. If intractable pruritus is generalized, UVA treatment should be discontinued until the pruritus disappears.
2. ERYTHEMA: Mild, transient erythema at 24–48 hours after PUVA therapy is an expected reaction and indicates that a therapeutic interaction between methoxsalen and UVA occurred. Any area showing moderate erythema (greater than Grade 2—See Table 1 for grades of erythema) should be shielded during subsequent UVA exposures until the erythema has resolved. Erythema greater than Grade 2 which appears within 24 hours after UVA treatment may signal a potentially severe burn. Erythema may become progressively worse over the next 24 hours, since the peak erythemal reaction characteristically occurs 48 hours or later after methoxsalen ingestion. The patient should be protected from further UVA exposures and sunlight, and should be monitored closely.
3. IMPORTANT DIFFERENCES BETWEEN PUVA ERYTHEMA AND SUNBURN: PUVA-induced inflammation differs from sunburn or UVB phototherapy in several ways. The percent transmission of UVB varies between 0% to 34% through skin whereas UVA varies between 1% to 80% transmission; thus, UVA is transmitted to a larger percent through the skin (Diffey, 1982[21]). The DNA lesions induced by PUVA are very different from UV-induced thymine dimers and may lead to a DNA crosslink. This DNA lesion may be more problematic to the cell because crosslinks are more lethal and psoralen-

DNA photoproducts may be "new" or unfamiliar substrates for DNA repair enzymes. DNA synthesis is also suppressed longer after PUVA. The time course of delayed erythema is different with PUVA and may not involve the usual mediators seen in sunburn. PUVA-induced redness may be just beginning at 24 hours, when UVB erythema has already passed its peak. The erythema dose-response curve is also steeper for PUVA. Compared to equally erythemogenic doses of UVB, the histologic alterations induced by PUVA show more dermal vessel damage and longer duration of epidermal and dermal abnormalities.

4. OTHER ADVERSE REACTIONS: Those reported include edema, dizziness, headache, malaise, depression, hypopigmentation, vesiculation and bullae formation, non-specific rash, herpes simplex, miliaria, urticaria, folliculitis, gastrointestinal disturbances, cutaneous tenderness, leg cramps, hypotension, and extension of psoriasis.

OVERDOSAGE

In the event of methoxsalen overdosage, induce emesis and keep the patient in a darkened room for at least 24 hours. Emesis is most beneficial within the first 2 to 3 hours after ingestion of methoxsalen, since maximum blood levels are reached by this time.

DRUG DOSAGE & ADMINISTRATION

> **CAUTION:** Oxsoralen-Ultra represents a new dose form of methoxsalen. This new dosage form of methoxsalen exhibits significantly greater bioavailability and earlier photosensitization onset time than previous methoxsalen dosage forms. Each patient should be evaluated by determining the minimum phototoxic dose (MPD) and phototoxic peak time after drug administration prior to onset of photochemotherapy with this dosage form. Human bioavailability studies have indicated the following drug dosage and administration directions are to be used as a guideline only.

PSORIASIS THERAPY

1. DRUG DOSAGE-INITIAL THERAPY: The methoxsalen capsules should be taken $1\frac{1}{2}$ to 2 hours before UVA exposure with some low fat food or milk according to the following table:

Patient's Weight

(kg)	(lbs)	Dose (mg)
<30	<65	10
30–50	65–100	20
51–65	101–145	30
66–80	146–175	40
81–90	176–200	50
91–115	201–250	60
>115	>250	70

2. INITIAL EXPOSURE: The initial UVA exposure energy level and corresponding time of exposure is determined by the patient's skin characteristics for sunburning and tanning as follows:

Skin Type	History	Recommended Joules/cm²
I	Always burn, never tan (patients with erythrodermic psoriasis are to be classed as Type I for determination of UVA dosage.)	0.5 J/cm²
II	Always burn, but sometimes tan	1.0 J/cm²
III	Sometimes burn, but always tan	1.5 J/cm²
IV	Never burn, always tan	2.0 J/cm²

Skin Type	Physician Examination	Joules/cm²
V*	Moderately pigmented	2.5 J/cm²
VI*	Blacks	3.0 J/cm²

(*Patients with natural pigmentation of these types should be classified into a lower skin type category if the sunburning history so indicates.)
If the MPD is done, start at $\frac{1}{2}$ MPD.
Additional drug dosage directions are as follows:
a. Weight Change: In the event that the weight of a patient changes during treatment such that he/she falls into an adjacent weight range/dose category, no change in the dose of methoxsalen is usually required. If, in the physician's opinion, however, a weight change is sufficiently great to modify the drug dose, then an adjustment in the time of exposure to UVA should be made.
b. Dose/Week: The number of doses per week of methoxsalen capsules will be determined by the patient's schedule of UVA exposures. In no case should treatments be given more often than once every other day because the full extent of phototoxic reactions may not be evident until 48 hours after each exposure.
c. Dosage Increase: Dosage may be increased by 10 mg after the fifteenth treatment under the conditions outlined under

PUVA treatment protocol, clearing phase, miscellaneous situations.

UVA RADIATION SOURCE SPECIFICATIONS & INFORMATION

A. IRRADIANCE UNIFORMITY
The following specifications should be met with the window of the detector held in a vertical plane:
1. Vertical variation: For readings taken at any point along the vertical center axis of the chamber (to within 15 cm from the top and bottom), the lowest reading should not be less than 70 percent of the highest reading.
2. Horizontal variation: Throughout any specific horizontal plane, the lowest reading must be at least 80 percent of the highest reading, excluding the peripheral 3 cm of the patient treatment space.

B. PATIENT SAFETY FEATURES:
The following safety features should be present: (1) Protection from electrical hazard: All units should be grounded and conform to applicable electrical codes. The patient or operator should not be able to touch any live electrical parts. There should be ground fault protection. (2) Protective shielding of lamps: The patient should not be able to come in contact with the bare lamps. In the event of lamp breakage, the patient should not be exposed to broken lamp components. (3) Hand rails and hand holds: Appropriate supports should be available to the patient. (4) Patient viewing window: A window which blocks UV should be provided for viewing the patient during treatment. (5) Door and latches: Patients should be able to open the door from the inside with only slight pressure to the door. (6) Non-skid floor: The floor should be of a non-skid nature. (7) Thermoregulation: Sufficient air flow should be provided for patient safety and comfort, limiting temperature within the UVA radiator cabinet to approximately less than 100°F. (8) Timer: The irradiator should be equipped with an automatic timer which terminates the exposure at the conclusion of a pre-set time interval. (9) Patient alarm device: An alarm device within the UVA irradiator chamber should be accessible to the patient for emergency activation. (10) Danger label: The unit should have a label prominently displayed which reads as follows:
DANGER—Ultraviolet Radiation—Follow your physicians instructions—Failure to use protective eyewear may result in eye injury.

C. UVA EXPOSURE DOSIMETRY MEASUREMENTS:
The maximum radiant exposure or irradiance (within $\pm$ 15 percent) of UVA (320–400 nm) delivered to the patient should be determined by using an appropriate radiometer calibrated to be read in Joules/cm² or mW/cm². In the absence of a standard measuring technique approved by the National Bureau of Standards, the system should use a detector corrected to a cosine spatial response. The use and recalibration frequency of such a radiometer for a specific UVA irradiator chamber should be specified by the manufacturer because the UVA dose (exposure) is determined by the design of the irradiator, the number of lamps, and the age of the lamps. If irradiance is measured, the radiometer reading in mW/cm² is used to calculate the exposure time in minutes to deliver the required UVA in Joules/cm² to a patient in the UVA irradiator cabinet. The equation is:

$$\text{Exposure Time (minutes)} = \frac{\text{Desired UVA Dose (J/cm}^2)}{0.06 \times \text{Irradiance (mW/cm}^2)}$$

Overexposure due to human error should be minimized by using an accurate automatic timing device, which is set by the operator and controlled by energizing and de-energizing the UVA irradiator lamp. The timing device calibration interval should be specified by the manufacturer. Safety systems should be included to minimize the possibility of delivering a UVA exposure which exceeds the prescribed dose, in the event the timer or radiometer should malfunction.

D. UVA SPECTRAL OUTPUT DISTRIBUTION:
The spectral distributions of the lamps should meet the following specifications:

Wavelength band (nanometers)	Output[1]
< 310	<1
310 to 320	1 to 3
320 to 330	4 to 8
330 to 340	11 to 17
340 to 350	18 to 25
350 to 360	19 to 28
360 to 370	15 to 23
370 to 380	8 to 12
380 to 390	3 to 7
390 to 400	1 to 3

[1] As a percentage of total irradiance between 320 and 400 nanometers.

PUVA TREATMENT PROTOCOL

INTRODUCTION:
The Oxsoralen-Ultra® Capsules reach their maximum bioavailability in $1\frac{1}{2}$ to 2 hours after ingestion.
On average, the serum level achieved with Oxsoralen-Ultra is twice that obtained with regular Oxsoralen® and reach

their peak concentration in less than $\frac{1}{2}$ the time of the regular capsules.
As a result the mean MED J/cm² for the Oxsoralen-Ultra Capsules is substantially less than that required for regular Oxsoralen Capsules (Levins et al., 1984 and private communication[1]).
Photosensitivity studies demonstrate a shorter time of peak photosensitivity of 1.5 to 2.1 hours vs. 3.9 to 4.25 hours for regular methoxsalen capsules.

A. INITIAL EXPOSURE:
The initial UVA exposures should be conducted according to the guidelines presented previously under Drug Dosage & Administration—Initial Therapy and Exposure.

B. CLEARING PHASE:
Specific recommendations for patient treatment are as follows:
1. SKIN TYPES I, II, & III. Patients with skin types I, II, and III may be treated 2 or 3 times per week. UVA exposure may be held constant or increased by up to 1.0 Joule/cm² at each treatment, according to the patient's response. If erythema occurs, however, do not increase exposure time until erythema resolves. The severity and extent of the patient's erythema may be used to determine whether the next exposure should be shortened, omitted, or maintained at the previous dosage. See Adverse Reactions section for additional information.
2. SKIN TYPES IV, V, & VI. Patients with skin types IV, V, and VI may be treated 2 or 3 times per week. UVA exposure may be held constant or increased by up to 1.5 Joules/cm² at each treatment unless erythema occurs. If erythema occurs, follow instructions outlined above in the procedures for patients with skin types I, II, and III.
3. ERYTHRODERMIC PSORIASIS. Patients with erythrodermic psoriasis should be treated with special attention because pre-existing erythema may obscure observations of possible treatment-related phototoxic erythema. These patients may be treated 2 or 3 times per week, as a Type I patient.
4. MISCELLANEOUS SITUATIONS:
a. If there is no response after a total of 10 treatments, the exposure of UVA energy may be increased by an additional 0.5-1.0 Joules/cm² above the prior incremental increases for each treatment. (Example: a patient whose exposure dose is being increased by 1.0 Joule/cm² may now have all subsequent doses increased by 1.5-2.0 Joules/cm².)
b. If there is no response, or only minimal response, after 15 treatments, the dosage of methoxsalen may be increased by 10 mg (a one-time increase in dosage). This increased dosage may be continued for the remainder of the course of treatment but should not be exceeded.
c. If a patient misses a treatment, the UVA exposure time of the next treatment should not be increased. If more than one treatment is missed, reduce the exposure by 0.5 Joule/cm² for each treatment missed.
d. If the lower extremities are not responding as well as the rest of the body and do not show erythema, cover all other body areas and give 25 percent of the present exposure dose as an additional exposure to the lower extremities. This additional exposure to the lower extremities should be terminated if erythema develops on these areas.
e. Non-responsive psoriasis: If a patient's generalized psoriasis is not responding, or if the condition appears to be worsening during treatment, the possibility of a generalized phototoxic reaction should be considered. This may be confirmed by the improvement of the condition following temporary discontinuance of this therapy for two weeks. If no improvement occurs during the interruption of treatment, this patient may be considered a treatment failure.

C. ALTERNATIVE EXPOSURE SCHEDULE:
As an alternative to increasing the UVA exposure at each treatment, the following schedule may be followed; this schedule may reduce the total number of Joules/cm² received by the patient over the entire course of therapy.
1. Incremental increases in UVA exposure for all patients may range from 0.5 to 1.5 Joules/cm², according to the patient's response to therapy.
2. Once Grade 2 clearing (see Table 2) has been reached and the patient is progressing adequately, UVA dosage is held constant. The dosage is maintained until Grade 4 clearing is reached.
3. If the rate of clearing significantly decreases, exposure dosage may be increased at each treatment (0.1-1.5 Joules/cm²) until Grade 3 clearing and a satisfactory progress rate is attained. The UVA exposure will be held constant again until Grade 4 clearing is attained. These increases may be used also if the rate of clearing significantly decreases between Grade 3 and Grade 4 response. However, the possibility of a phototoxic reaction should be considered; see Non-responsive Psoriasis, above.

Continued on next page

ICN Pharmaceuticals—Cont.

4. In summary, this schedule raises slightly the increments (Joules/cm^2) of UVA dosage, but limits these increases to those periods when the patient is not responding adequately. Otherwise, the UVA exposure is held at the lowest effective dose.

D. MAINTENANCE PHASE:

The goal of maintenance treatment is to keep the patient symptom-free as possible with the least amount of UVA exposure.

1. SCHEDULE OF EXPOSURES: When patients have achieved 95 percent clearing, or Grade 4 response (Table 2), they may be placed on the following maintenance schedules (M_1-M_4), in sequence. It is recommended that each maintenance schedule be adhered to for at least 2 treatments (unless erythema or psoriatic flare occurs, in which case see (2a) and (2b) below).

Maintenance Schedules
M_1—once/week
M_2—once/2 weeks
M_3—once/3 weeks
M_4—p.r.n. (i.e. for flares)

2. LENGTH OF EXPOSURE: The UVA exposure for the first maintenance treatment of any schedule (except M_4 as noted below) is the same as that of the patient's last treatment under the previous schedule. For skin types I–IV, however, it is recommended that the maximum UVA dosage during maintenance treatments not exceed the following:

Skin Types	Joules/cm^2/treatment
I	12
II	14
III	18
IV	22

If the patient develops erythema or new lesions of psoriasis, proceed as follows:

a. Erythema: During maintenance therapy, the patient's tan and threshold dose for erythema may gradually decrease. If maintenance treatments produce significant erythema, the exposure to UVA should be decreased by 25 percent until further treatments no longer produce erythema.

b. Psoriasis: If the patient develops new areas of psoriasis during maintenance therapy (but still is classified as having a Grade 4 response), the exposure to UVA may be increased by 0.5–1.5 Joules/cm^2 at each treatment; this is appropriate for all types of patients. These increases are continued until the psoriasis is brought under control and the patient is again clear. The exposure being administered when this clearing is reached should be used for further maintenance treatment.

3. FLARES DURING MAINTENANCE: If the patient flares during maintenance treatment (i.e., develops psoriasis on more than 5 percent of the originally involved areas of the body) his maintenance treatment schedule may be changed to the preceding maintenance or clearing schedule. The patient may be kept on his schedule until again 95 percent clear. If the original maintenance treatment schedule is unable to control the psoriasis, the schedule may be changed to a more frequent regimen. If a flare occurs less than 6 weeks after the last treatment, 25 percent of the maximum exposure received during the clearing phase, with the clearing schedule received during the clearing phase, may be used and then proceed with the clearing schedule previously followed for this patient. (At 95 percent clearing, follow regular maintenance until the optimum maintenance schedule is determined for the patient.) If more than 6 weeks have elapsed since the last treatment was given, treat patients as if they were beginning therapy insofar as exposure dosages are concerned, since their threshold for erythema may have decreased.

Table 1. Grades of Erythema

Grades	Erythema
0	No erythema
1	Minimally perceptible erythema—faint pink
2	Marked erythema but with no edema
3	Fiery erythema with edema
4	Fiery erythema with edema and blistering

Table 2. Response to Therapy

Grade	Criteria	Percent Improvement (compared to original extent of disease)
−1	Psoriasis worse	0
0	No change	0
1	Minimal improvement—slightly less scale and/or erythema	5–20
2	Definite improvement—partial flattening of all plaques—less scaling and less erythema	20–50
3	Considerable improvement—nearly complete flattening of all plaques but borders of plaques still palpable	50–95
4	Clearing; complete flattening of plaques including borders; plaques may be outlined by pigmentation	95

HOW SUPPLIED

Oxsoralen-Ultra Capsules, each containing 10 mg of methoxsalen (8-methoxypsoralen) in a soft gelatin capsule packaged in amber glass bottles are available as follows:

Unit Count	NDC Number
50	NDC 0187-0650-42

Copyright October, 1986   Printed in U.S.A.
ICN Pharmaceuticals, Inc.   March, 1987
Costa Mesa, Ca 92626
Manufactured for ICN Pharmaceuticals, Inc.

BIBLIOGRAPHY

1. Levins, P.C., Gauge, R.W., Momtaz-T.K., Parrish, J.A., and Fitzpatrick, T.B.: A New Liquid Formulation of 8-Methoxypsoralen: Bioactivity and Effect of Diet: JID, 82, No. 2, pp. 185–187 (1984) and private communication.
2. Artuc, M., Stuettgen, G. Schalla, W., Schaefer, H., and Gazith, J.: Reversible binding of 5- and 8-methoxypsoralen to human serum proteins (albumin) and to epidermis in vitro: Brit. J. Dermat. 101, pp. 669–677 (1979).
3. Mandula, B.B., Pathak, M.A., Nakayama, T., and Davidson, S.J.: Induction of mixed-function oxidases in mouse liver by psoralens., Ibid, 99, pp. 687–692 (1978).
4. Pathak, M.A., Fitzpatrick, T.B., Parrish, J.A.: PSORIASIS, Proceedings of the Second International Symposium. Edited by E.M. Farber, A.J. Cox, Yorke Medical Books, pp. 262–265 (1977).
5. Dall'Acqua, F., Marciani, S., Ciavatta, L., Rodighiero, G.: Formation on interstrand cross-linkings of the photoreactions between furocoumarins and DNA; Z Naturforsch (B), 26, pp. 561–569 (1971).
6. Cole, R.S.: Light-induced cross-linkings of DNA in the presence of a furocoumarin (psoralen), Biochem. Biophys. Acta, 217, pp. 30–39 (1970).
7. Musajo, L, Rodighiero, G., Caporale, G., Dall'Acqua, F, Marciani, S., Bordin, F., Baccichetti, F., Bevilacqua, R.: Photoreactions between Skin-Photosentizing Furocoumarins and Nucleic Acids, Sunlight and Man; Normal and Abnormal Photobiologic Responses. Edited by M.A. Pathak, LC. Harber, M. Seiji et al. University of Tokyo Press, pp. 369–387 (1974).
8. Dall'Acqua, F., Vedaldi, D., Bordin, F., and Rodighiero, G.: New studies in the interaction between 8-methoxypsoralen and DNA in vitro: JID, 73, pp. 191–197 (1979).
9. Yoshikawa, K., Mori, N., Sakakibara, S., Mizuno, N. Song, P.: Photo Conjugation of 8-methoxypsoralen with Proteins; Photochem. & Photobiol. 29, pp. 1127–1133 (1979).
10. Hakim, R.D., Griffin, A.C.: Knox, J.M.: Erythema and tumor formation in methoxsalen treated mice exposed to fluorescent light; Arch. Dermatol. 82, pp. 572–577 (1960).
11. O'Neal, M.A., Griffin, A.C.: The Effect of Oxypsoralen upon Ultraviolet Carcinogenesis in Albino Mice, Cancer Res., 17, pp. 911–916 (1957).
12. Stern, R.S., Unpublished personal communication.
13. Stern, R.S., Parrish, J.A., Zierler, S.: Skin Carcinoma in Patients with Psoriasis Treated with Topical Tar and Artificial Ultraviolet Radiation. Lancet, 1, pp. 732–735 (1980).
14. Stern, R.S., Laird, N., Melski, J. Parrish, J.A., Fitzpatrick, T.B., Bleich, H.L.: Cutaneous Squamous-Cell Carcinoma in Patients Treated with PUVA: NEJM, 310, No. 18, pp. 1156–1161 (1984).
15. Roenigk, Jr., H.H., and 12 Cooperating Investigators: Skin Cancer in the PUVA-48 Cooperative Study of Psoriasis. Program for Forty-First Annual Meeting for The Society of Investigative Dermatology, Inc., Sheraton Washington Hotel, Washington, D.C., May 12, 13, and 14, 1980). Abstracts JID, 74, No. 4, p. 250 (April, 1980).
16. Mosher, D.B., Pathak, M.A., Harris, T.J., Fitzpatrick, T.B.: Development of Cutaneous Lesions in Vitiligo During Long-Term PUVA Therapy. Program for Forty-First Annual Meeting for the Society for Investigative Dermatology, Inc., Sheraton Washington Hotel, Washington, D.C., May 12, 13, and 14, 1980. Abstracts JID, 74, No. 4, p 259 (April, 1980).
17. Cloud, T.M. Hakim, R., Griffin, A.C.: Photosensitization of the eye with methoxsalen. I. Acute effects; Arch. Ophthalmol. 64, pp. 346–352 (1960).
18. Cloud, T.M. Hakim, R., Griffin, A.C.: Photosensitization of the eye with methoxsalen. II. Chronic effects, Ibid, 66, pp. 689–694 (1961).
19. Freeman, R.G., Troll, D.: Photosensitization of the eye by 8-methoxypsoralen, JID, 53, pp. 449–453 (1969).
20. Lerman, S., Megaw, J., Willis, I.: Potential ocular complications from PUVA therapy and their prevention; JID, 74, pp. 197–199 (1980).
21. Diffey, B.L., Medical Physics Handbook 11, Ultraviolet Radiation in Medicine, Adam Hilger, Ltd., Bristol, p. 86 (1982).

Shown in Product Identification Section, page 412

PRECEF® ℞
(ceforanide for injection)

DESCRIPTION

Precef (ceforanide) is a semisynthetic broad spectrum cephalosporin antibiotic for parenteral administration. It is provided as a sterile sodium-free mixture of crystalline 7-[o-(aminomethyl) phenylacetamido]-3-[[[1-(carboxymethyl)-1H-tetrazol-5-yl]thio]methyl]-3-cephem-4-carboxylic acid and L (+) lysine. When reconstituted a solution of the lysine salt of ceforanide is formed. Solutions of Precef range in color from light yellow to amber depending on the concentration and diluent used. The pH of the solution ranges from 5.5 to 8.5. The structural formula is as shown below:

Clinical Pharmacology: Mean peak plasma concentrations of 40 and 76 mcg/ml occurred at 1 hr. after intramuscular administration of doses of 0.5 and 1.0 gram, respectively, of Precef to normal subjects. These concentrations declined to 3.9 and 6.7 mcg/ml at 12 hours. Following 30-minute intravenous infusions of 1.0 and 2.0 gram doses of Precef, respectively, the mean plasma concentrations were 125 and 240 mcg/ml, declining to 5.9 and 9.0 mcg/ml in 12 hours.

The terminal plasma half-life was 2.9 hours after intravenous and intramuscular administration. Plasma protein binding was 80% at plasma concentrations achieved after 0.5–2.0 gram doses. There was no evidence of drug accumulation and plasma pharmacokinetics did not change after twice daily administration of 0.5–2.0 grams for 9.5 days.

Precef was not metabolized prior to elimination and was primarily excreted by the kidneys. After intramuscular administration of 0.5 and 1.0 gram doses, mean peak urinary concentrations of 1250 and 2900 mcg/ml occurred within 2 hours. Urine levels were 110 and 265 mcg/ml, respectively, at 9–12 hours. Intravenous doses of 1.0 and 2.0 grams of Precef produced mean urinary concentrations of 2550 and 5130 mcg/ml, respectively, within 2 hours after administration. Urine levels were 190 and 440 mcg/ml, respectively, at 9–12 hours. Excretion kinetics and clearance rates did not change following twice daily administration of these doses for 9.5 days. Urinary excretion accounted for 78–95% of the 0.5–2.0 gram intramuscular and/or intravenous dose in 12 hours. Probenecid has no effect on serum concentrations of Precef. Precef reaches therapeutic levels in the gall bladder, myocardium, bone, skeletal muscle, and vaginal tissue. Therapeutic levels are also achieved in pericardial fluid, synovial fluid and bile.

Microbiology: The bactericidal activity of Precef results from inhibition of cell wall synthesis. Ceforanide has a high degree of stability in the presence of some **beta**-lactamases. Ceforanide is usually active against the following microorganisms in vitro.

Aerobes:

Gram-negative:

  Escherichia coli
  Klebsiella species
  Proteus mirabilis
  Providencia species (including **Providencia rettgeri,** formerly **Proteus rettgeri**)
  Citrobacter species
  Haemophilus influenzae
  Haemophilus parainfluenzae
  Enterobacter species
  Salmonella typhi
  Neisseria gonorrhoeae

Gram-positive:

  Staphylococci, including penicillinase-producing strains.
  Note: Methicillin-resistant staphylococci as well as some strains of **Staphylococcus epidermidis** are resistant.
  Streptococcus pneumoniae (Formerly **Diplococcus pneumoniae**)
  Group A and Group B streptococci
  Streptococcus viridans
  Note: Most strains of enterococci, e.g. **Streptococcus faecalis,** are resistant.

Anaerobes:
   Fusobacterium species
   Clostridium species
   Note: Most strains of **Clostridium difficile** are resistant.
   Peptococcus species
   Peptostreptococcus species
While most strains of **B. fragilis** are resistant, ceforanide demonstrates *in vitro* activity against some bacteroides species.
Note: **Pseudomonas, Acinetobacter calcoaceticus** (formerly **Mima** and **Herellea** species) and most **Serratia** strains are resistant to ceforanide.
Disc susceptibility test: Quantitative methods that require measurement of zone diameters give the most precise estimate of antibiotic susceptibility. One such procedure† has been recommended for use with discs to test susceptibility to ceforanide.
Reports from the laboratory giving results of the standard single-disc susceptibility test with a 30-mcg cefamandole disc should be interpreted according to the following criteria: Susceptible organisms produce zones of 18 mm or greater, indicating that the test organism is likely to respond to therapy.
Organisms that produce zones of 15 to 17 mm are expected to be susceptible if high dosage is used or if the infection is confined to tissues and fluids (e.g. urine) in which high antibiotic levels are attained.
Resistant organisms produce zones of 14 mm or less, indicating that other therapy should be selected.
For gram-positive isolates, the test may be performed with either the cephalosporin-class disc (30 mcg cephalothin) or the cefamandole disc (30 mcg cefamandole), and a zone of 18 mm is indicative of a ceforanide-susceptible organism. Gram-negative organisms should be tested with the cefamandole disc (using the above criteria) since ceforanide has been shown by *in vitro* tests to have activity against certain strains of **Enterobacteriaceae** found resistant when tested with the cephalosporin-class disc. Gram-negative organisms having zones of less than 18 mm around the cephalothin disc are not necessarily moderately susceptible or resistant to ceforanide.
In other susceptibility testing procedures, e.g. ICS agar dilution†† or the equivalent, a bacterial isolate may be considered susceptible if the MIC value for ceforanide is not more than 16 mcg/ml. Organisms are considered resistant to ceforanide if the MIC is greater than 32 mcg/ml. Organisms having an MIC value of 32 mcg/ml or less than 32 mcg/ml, but greater than 16 mcg/ml are expected to be susceptible if high dosage is used or if the infection is confined to tissues and fluids (e.g. urine) in which high antibiotic levels are attained.

INDICATIONS AND USAGE

Precef is indicated for the treatment of serious infections caused by susceptible strains of the designated microorganisms in the diseases listed below:
(1) Bone and Joint Infections—caused by **Staphylococcus aureus** (penicillinase and non-penicillinase producing strains).
(2) Endocarditis—caused by **Staphylococcus aureus** (penicillinase and non-penicilinase producing strains).
(3) Lower Respiratory Tract Infection—caused by **Staphylococcus aureus** (penicillinase and non-penicillinase producing strains), **Streptococcus pneumoniae** (formerly **D. pneumoniae**), **Klebsiella pneumoniae,** and **Haemophilus influenzae.**
(4) Bacterial Septicemia—caused by **Staphylococcus aureus** (penicillinase and non-penicillinase producing strains), **Streptococcus pneumoniae,** and **Escherichia coli.**
(5) Skin and Skin Structure Infections—caused by **Stephylococcus aureus** (penicillinase and non-penicillinase producing strains), **Staphylococcus epidermidis,** Group A and Group B streptococci, **Escherichia coli, Proteus mirabilis,** and **Klebsiella pneumoniae.**
(6) Urinary Tract Infections—caused by **Escherichia coli, Proteus mirabilis,** and **Klebsiella pneumoniae.**
NOTE: Injectable Penicillin G Benzathine is considered to be the drug of choice in the treatment and prevention of streptococcal infections including prophylaxis of rheumatic fever.
Specimens for bacteriologic cultures should be obtained in order to isolate and identify causative organisms and to determine their susceptibilities to ceforanide. Therapy may be instituted before results of susceptibility studies are known; however, once these results become available, the antibiotic treatment should be adjusted accordingly.
Prophylactic Use—PERIOPERATIVE PROPHYLAXIS: The preoperative prophylactic administration of Precef may prevent the growth of susceptible organisms and thereby may reduce the incidence of certain postoperative infections in patients undergoing surgical procedures which are classified as contaminated or potentially contaminated, (e.g., vaginal hysterectomy and cholecystectomy in high-risk patients such as those over 70 years of age, with acute cholecystitis, obstructive jaundice, or common duct bile stones). Effective prophylactic use of an antibiotic in surgery depends upon the time of administration. Precef should usually be administered sixty minutes before the operation to allow sufficient time to achieve an effective antibiotic concentration in the wound tissues during the procedure. Prophylactic administration is usually not required after the surgical procedure ends and should be discontinued within a 24 hour period. In the majority of surgical procedures, continuing prophylactic administration of any antibiotic does not reduce the incidence of subsequent infections but will increase the possibility of adverse reactions and the development of bacterial resistance.
The perioperative use of Precef may also be effective in surgical patients in whom infections at the operative site would present a serious risk, e.g. during prosthetic arthroplasty and open-heart surgery. Although ceforanide has been shown to be as effective as cephalothin in the prevention of infections following coronary artery bypass surgery, no placebo controlled trials have been conducted to evaluate any cephalosporin antibiotic in the prevention of infection following either coronary artery bypass surgery or prosthetic heart valve replacement. In these procedures where the occurrence of infection may be particularly devastating, the prophylactic administration of Precef may be continued for 2 days, administered every 12 hours following completion of surgery. If there are signs of infection, specimens for culture should be obtained for the identification of the causative organism so that the appropriate therapy may be instituted. (See Dosage and Administration).

CONTRAINDICATION

Precef is contraindicated in patients with known hypersensitivity to ceforanide and the cephalosporin group of antibiotics.

WARNINGS

BEFORE THERAPY WITH PRECEF IS INSTITUTED, CAREFUL INQUIRY SHOULD BE MADE TO DETERMINE WHETHER THE PATIENT HAS HAD PREVIOUS HYPERSENSITIVITY REACTIONS TO CEPHALOSPORINS, PENICILLIN, OR OTHER DRUGS. THIS PRODUCT SHOULD BE GIVEN CAUTIOUSLY TO PENICILLIN-SENSITIVE PATIENTS. ANTIBIOTICS SHOULD BE ADMINISTERED WITH CAUTION TO ANY PATIENT WHO HAS DEMONSTRATED SOME FORM OF ALLERGY, PARTICULARLY TO DRUGS. IF AN ALLERGIC REACTION TO PRECEF OCCURS, DISCONTINUE THE DRUG. SERIOUS ACUTE HYPERSENSITIVITY REACTION MAY REQUIRE EPINEPHRINE ANMINISTRATION AND OTHER EMERGENCY MEASURES.
Pseudomembranous colitis has been reported with the use of cephalosporins (and other broad spectrum antibiotics), therefore, it is important to consider its diagnosis in patients in whom diarrhea develops in association with cephalosporin use.
Treatment with broad spectrum antibiotics alters the normal flora of the colon and may permit overgrowth of clostridia. Studies indicate a toxin produced by **Clostridium difficile** is one primary cause of antibiotic-associated colitis. Cholestyramine and colestipol HCl resins have been shown to bind the toxin *in vitro.*
Mild cases of colitis may respond to drug discontinuance alone.
Moderate to severe cases should be managed with fluid, electrolyte, and protein supplementation as indicated.
When the colitis is not relieved by drug discontinuation or when it is severe, oral vancomycin is effective in treatment of the antibiotic-associated pseudomembranous colitis produced by **C. difficile.** Other causes of colitis should also be considered.

PRECAUTIONS

Although Precef rarely produces alterations in kidney function, evaluation of renal status during therapy is recommended, especially in seriously ill patients receiving the maximum dosage. The total daily dose of Precef should be reduced in patients with transient or persistent renal insufficiency (see Dosage) because high and prolonged serum antibiotic concentrations can occur in such individuals from usual dosage.
Cephalosporins should be given with caution to patients receiving concurrent treatment with potent diuretics as these regimens are suspected of adversely affecting renal function. Nephrotoxicity has been reported following concomitant administration of cephalosporins and aminoglycoside antibiotics.
Precef should be prescribed with caution in individuals with a history of gastrointestinal disease, particularly colitis.
As with other antibiotics, prolonged use of Precef may result in over-growth of non-susceptible organisms. Repeated evaluation of the patient's condition is essential. If superinfection occurs during therapy, appropriate measures should be taken.
Usage in Pregnancy—Pregnancy Category B—In a study in which rats where treated prior to mating and through pregnancy and lactation at dose levels (1600 mg/kg/day) 50 times the usual Precef dose (30 mg/kg/day), there was no evidence of imparied male or female fertility or reproductive performance. Results of teratogenicity tests in mice and rats employing doses as high as 25 times the human dose were also negative. In a peri-postnatal study, female rats treated subcutaneously with Precef at 50 times the usual human dose had a higher number of resorption sites than controls and there was a decrease in viability of the offspring. These phenomena may well have been secondary to the effects on the maternal animals of the high volume of solution injected (8 ml/kg/day), rather than representing a direct effect on the conceptus; neither was evident at lower dosage levels (e.g., 25 times human dose). There are, however, no adequate and well controlled studies in pregnant women. Because animal reproduction studies are not always predictive of human response, Precef should be used during pregnancy only if clearly needed.
Labor and Delivery—There are no data concerning the administration of Precef to women during labor or prior to delivery.
Nursing Mothers—It is not known whether Precef is excreted in human milk. Because many drugs are, caution should be exercised when Precef is administered to a nursing woman.
Pediatric Use—Safety and effectiveness of Precef in children below the age of one year have not been established. Therefore, if Precef is administered to infants, the physician should determine if the potential benefits of the product's use outweigh the possible risks of administration. Precef has been effectively used in children between the ages of 1–17 years. Certain recent cephalosporins have caused testicular changes in juvenile rats. During animal studies, Precef has not caused testicular changes in juvenile rats at a daily dose of 1000 mg/kg/day (25 × the human pediatric dose) for 31 days.

ADVERSE REACTIONS

Allergic reaction: Rash (one in 45 patients), pruritus (one in 200 patients) and eosinophilla (in about one in 12 patients) have been reported. Reactions are more likely to occur in patients with a history of hypersensitivity, particularly to penicillins.
Hematopoietic: As occurs during therapy with other cephalosporin antibiotics, therapy with Precef has been associated with transient thrombocytopenia (in about one in 5 patients). Some individuals (one in 40 patients) have developed positive direct Coombs Tests during treatment with ceforanide without clinical or laboratory evidence of hemolysis.
Gastrointestinal: Nausea (one in 270 patients), vomiting (one in 2,000 patients) and diarrhea (one in 140 patients) have been reported.
Symptoms of pseudomembranous colitis may appear during or after cephalosporin treatment.
Laboratory Changes: Transient elevation in SGOT (one in 16 patients), SGPT (one in 9 patients), and alkaline phosphatase levels (one in 27 patients) have been reported.
As with other cephalosporins, transient elevations in serum creatinine and BUN levels have been observed (in one in 9 and one in 50 patients, respectively). As may occur with intramuscular injection, the administration of Precef by this route has been associated with an elevation of CPK (in about one in 3 patients).
Local Effects: Local effects were reported in less than one percent of patients and included pain (one in 155 patients) and phlebitis (one in 140 patients).
Other reactions which have been reported in less than one percent of patients are local swelling, lethargy, confusion, headache, and hypotension.

DOSAGE AND ADMINISTRATION

Dosage: Adults—The usual dose range for Precef is 0.5 to 1.0 gram twice daily depending on the severity of the infection. Precef is administered every 12 hours by either the intramuscular or intravenous route. The route of administration should be dictated by the condition of the patient and anticipated ease of administration.
Children—Administration of 20–40 mg/kg/day in equally divided doses every 12 hours has been effective for most infections susceptible to Precef.
Perioperative Prophylactic Use—To prevent postoperative infection in contaminated or potentially contaminated surgery a 0.5 to 1 gram I.M. or I.V. dose administered 1 hour prior to the start of surgery is recommended. In cholecystectomy, a 1 gram dose is recommended.
It is important that the preoperative dose be given 1 hour prior to the start of surgery so that adequate antibiotic levels are present in the serum and tissues at the time of initial surgical incision.
In surgery where the occurrence of infection may be particularly devastating, e.g. prosthetic arthroplasty and open-heart surgery, the prophylactic administration of Precef may be continued for 2 days following completion of surgery.
Impaired Renal Function—Dosage should be determined by the degree of renal impairment, the severity of infection, the susceptibility of the causative organism, and therapeutic monitoring, If the creatinine clearance rate (Cl$_{cr}$) is 60

Continued on next page

ICN Pharmaceuticals—Cont.

ml/min/1.73m^2 or greater, the normal 12-hour dosing interval is maintained. When Cl$_{cr}$ is 20–59 ml/min/1.73m^2 a 24-hour dosing interval is recommended, and when Cl$_{cr}$ is 5–19 ml/min/1.73m^2 a 48-hour dosing interval is recommended. If Cl$_{cr}$ is less than 5 ml/min/1.73m^2, a 48–72 hour dosing interval may be used with monitoring of plasma ceforanide concentrations.

If only serum creatinine is available, creatinine clearance may be calculated from the following formula when renal function and serum creatinine levels are at steady state.

$$\text{Males: } Cl_{cr} = \frac{(140 - \text{age}) \times \text{Wt (kg)}}{72 \times \text{serum creatinine (mg/100 ml)}}$$

Females: 0.85 of the above value

NOTE: As with antibiotic therapy in general, administration of Precef should be continued for a minimum of 48 to 72 hours after the patient becomes asymptomatic or after evidence of bacterial eradication has been obtained. A minimum of 10 days of treatment is recommended in infections caused by group A beta-hemolytic streptococci in order to guard against the risk or reheumatic fever of glomerulonephritis.

Administration: Percef may be administered by either the intramuscular or the intravenous routes. Controlled clinical studies performed in normal adult volunteers and patients demonstrated that ceforanide was very well tolerated intramuscularly. In normal volunteers and patients receiving intravenous therapy, a low incidence of venous irritation was attributed to ceforanide. The intravenous route may be preferable for patients with bacterial septicemia, or other severe or life-threatening infections. These patients may be poor risks because of lowered resistance resulting from such debilitating conditions as malnutrition, trauma, surgery, diabetes, heart failure, or malignancy, particularly if shock is present or impending.

Intramuscular Injection: The 500 mg and 1 gram vials should be reconstituted with 1.7 ml and 3.2 ml, respectively, of Bacteriostatic Water for Injection, 0.9% Sodium Chloride Injection, Sterile Water for Injection, or Bacteriostatic Sodium Chloride Injection. Shake immediately. Each 1.0 ml contains 250 mg of ceforanide. The resulting solutions are stable for 48 hours at room temperature (25°C), 14 days under refrigeration (4°C) and 90 days in the frozen state (−15°C). After thawing, the solution is stable for 48 hours at room temperature. All injection should be administered deep into the muscle mass.

Intravenous Injection: The contents of the 500 mg vial should be diluted in 5 ml or more of the specified diluent; the 1 gram vial should be diluted in 10 ml or more of the specified diluent, and shaken immediately. Both may be administered slowly by direct I.V. administration over a 3 to 5 minute period.

Intravenous Solutions: At concentrations up to 10 mg/ml, Precef is stable and compatible for 48 hours at room temperature (25°C), 14 days under refrigeration (4°C) and 90 days in the frozen state (−15°C) followed by 48 hours at 25°C when thawed, in the following intravenous solutions:
Sterile Water for Injection, USP
0.9% Sodium Chloride Injection, USP
5% Dextrose Injection, USP
Lactated Ringer's Injection, USP
Lactated Ringer's and 5% Dextrose Injection
10% Dextrose Injection, USP
5% Dextrose and 0.2% Sodium Chloride Injection, USP
5% Dextrose and 0.45% Sodium Chloride Injection, USP
StrapKap® Piggyback I.V. Package: Reconstitute up to a concentration of 10 mg/ml with any of the appropriate I.V. solutions listed above.

Shake immediately upon reconstitution. The initial Precef Injection appears somewhat cloudy but will de-aerate upon brief standing to provide a clear solution. Parenteral drug products should be inspected visually for particulate matter and discoloration prior to administration, whenever solution and container permit.

HOW SUPPLIED

Precef is supplied in 500 mg vials and 500 mg piggybacks equivalent to 500 mg ceforanide and 1 gram vials and 1 gram piggybacks equivalent to 1 gram ceforanide.
NDC 0015-7351-20—500 mg vial
NDC 0015-7351-28—500 mg piggyback vial
NDC 0015-7352-20—1 gram vial
NDC 0015-7352-28—1 gram piggyback vial
For information on package sizes available, refer to the current price schedule.

† Bauer, et. al., Am. J. Clin. Path. 1966; 45:493 and Federal Register 1972 Sep. 30: 37:20525–20529.
†† Determine by the ICS agar-dilution method (Ericsson H. M., and Sherris J.C. Acta. Pathol. Microbiol. Scand. 1971 (B), Supplement No. 217 or any other method that has been shown to give equivalent results.
Manufactured by Bristol Laboratories
for ICN Pharmaceuticals, Inc.

PROSTIGMIN®   ℞
[pro-stig'min]
(neostigmine methylsulfate)
INJECTABLE

DESCRIPTION

Prostigmin (neostigmine methylsulfate) Injectable, an anticholinesterase agent, is a sterile aqueous solution intended for intramuscular, intravenous or subcutaneous administration.

Prostigmin Injectable is available in the following concentrations:

Prostigmin 1:2000 Ampuls — each ml contains 0.5 mg neostigmine methylsulfate compounded with 0.2% parabens (methyl and propyl) as preservatives and sodium hydroxide to adjust pH to approximately 5.9.

Prostigmin 1:4000 Ampuls — each ml contains 0.25 mg neostigmine methylsulfate compounded with 0.2% parabens (methyl and propyl) as preservatives and sodium hydroxide to adjust pH to approximately 5.9.

Prostigmin 1:1000 Multiple Dose Vials — each ml contains 1 mg neostigmine methylsulfate compounded with 0.45% phenol as preservative, 0.2 mg sodium acetate, and acetic acid and sodium hydroxide to adjust pH to approximately 5.9.

Prostigmin 1:2000 Multiple Dose Vials — each ml contains 0.5 mg neostigmine methylsulfate compounded with 0.45% phenol as preservative, 0.2 mg sodium acetate, and acetic acid and sodium hydroxide to adjust pH to approximately 5.9.

Chemically, neostigmine methylsulfate is (m-hydroxyphenyl)trimethylammonium methylsulfate dimethylcarbamate. It has a molecular weight of 334.39 and the following structural formula:

CLINICAL PHARMACOLOGY

Neostigmine inhibits the hydrolysis of acetylcholine by competing with acetylcholine for attachment to acetylcholinesterase at sites of cholinergic transmission. It enhances cholinergic action by facilitating the transmission of impulses across neuromuscular junctions. It also has a direct cholinomimetic effect on skeletal muscle and possibly on autonomic ganglion cells and neurons of the central nervous system. Neostigmine undergoes hydrolysis by cholinesterase and is also metabolized by microsomal enzymes in the liver. Protein binding to human serum albumin ranges from 15 to 25 percent.

Following intramuscular administration, neostigmine is rapidly absorbed and eliminated. In a study of five patients with myasthenia gravis, peak plasma levels were observed at 30 minutes, and the half-life ranged from 51 to 90 minutes. Approximately 80 percent of the drug was eliminated in urine within 24 hours; approximately 50% as the unchanged drug, and 30 percent as metabolites. Following intravenous administration, plasma half-life ranges from 47 to 60 minutes have been reported with a mean half-life of 53 minutes.

The clinical effects of neostigmine usually begin within 20 to 30 minutes after intramuscular injection and last from 2.5 to 4 hours.

INDICATIONS AND USAGE

Prostigmin is indicated for:
—the symptomatic control of myasthenia gravis when oral therapy is impractical.
—the prevention and treatment of postoperative distention and urinary retention after mechanical obstruction has been excluded.
—reversal of effects of nondepolarizing neuromuscular blocking agents (*e.g.*, tubocurarine, metocurine, gallamine, or pancuronium) after surgery.

CONTRAINDICATIONS

Prostigmin is contraindicated in patients with known hypersensitivity to the drug. It is also contraindicated in patients with peritonitis or mechanical obstruction of the intestinal or urinary tract.

WARNINGS

Prostigmin should be used with caution in patients with epilepsy, bronchial asthma, bradycardia, recent coronary occlusion, vagotonia, hyperthyroidism, cardiac arrhythmias or peptic ulcer. When large doses of Prostigmin are administered, the prior or simultaneous injection of atropine sulfate may be advisable. Separate syringes should be used for the Prostigmin and atropine. Because of the possibility of hypersensitivity in an occasional patient, atropine and antishock medication should always be readily available.

PRECAUTIONS

General: It is important to differentiate between myasthenic crisis and cholinergic crisis caused by overdosage of Prostigmin. Both conditions result in extreme muscle weakness but require radically different treatment. (See OVERDOSAGE section.)

Drug Interactions: Prostigmin does not antagonize, and may in fact prolong, the Phase I block of *depolarizing* muscle relaxants such as succinylcholine or decamethonium. Certain antibiotics, especially neomycin, streptomycin and kanamycin, have a mild but definite nondepolarizing blocking action which may accentuate neuromuscular block. These antibiotics should be used in the myasthenic patient only where definitely indicated, and then careful adjustment should be made of the anticholinesterase dosage. Local and some general anesthetics, antiarrhythmic agents and other drugs that interfere with neuromuscular transmission should be used cautiously, if at all, in patients with myasthenia gravis; the dose of Prostigmin may have to be increased accordingly.

Carcinogenesis, Mutagenesis and Impairment of Fertility: There have been no studies with Prostigmin which would permit an evaluation of its carcinogenic or mutagenic potential. Studies on the effect of Prostigmin on fertility and reproduction have not been performed.

Pregnancy:
Teratogenic Effects: Pregnancy Category C. There are no adequate or well-controlled studies of Prostigmin in either laboratory animals or in pregnant women. It is not known whether Prostigmin can cause fetal harm when administered to a pregnant woman or can affect reproductive capacity. Prostigmin should be given to a pregnant woman only if clearly needed.

Nonteratogenic Effects: Anticholinesterase drugs may cause uterine irritability and induce premature labor when given intravenously to pregnant women near term.

Nursing Mothers: It is not known whether Prostigmin is excreted in human milk. Because many drugs are excreted in human milk and because of the potential for serious adverse reactions from Prostigmin in nursing infants, a decision should be made whether to discontinue nursing or to discontinue the drug, taking into account the importance of the drug to the mother.

Pediatric Use: Safety and effectiveness in children have not been established.

ADVERSE REACTIONS

Side effects are generally due to an exaggeration of pharmacological effects of which salivation and fasciculation are the most common. Bowel cramps and diarrhea may also occur. The following additional adverse reactions have been reported following the use of either neostigmine bromide or neostigmine methylsulfate:
Allergic: Allergic reactions and anaphylaxis.
Neurologic: Dizziness, convulsions, loss of consciousness, drowsiness, headache, dysarthria, miosis and visual changes.
Cardiovascular: Cardiac arrhythmias (including bradycardia, tachycardia, A-V block and nodal rhythm) and nonspecific EKG changes have been reported, as well as cardiac arrest, syncope and hypotension. These have been predominantly noted following the use of the injectable form of Prostigmin.
Respiratory: Increased oral, pharyngeal and bronchial secretions, dyspnea, respiratory depression, respiratory arrest and bronchospasm.
Dermatologic: Rash and urticaria.
Gastrointestinal: Nausea, emesis, flatulence and increased peristalsis.
Genitourinary: Urinary frequency.
Musculoskeletal: Muscle cramps and spasms, arthralgia.
Miscellaneous: Diaphoresis, flushing and weakness.

OVERDOSAGE

Overdosage of Prostigmin can cause cholinergic crisis, which is characterized by increasing muscle weakness, and through involvement of the muscles of respiration, may result in death. Myasthenic crisis, due to an increase in the severity of the disease, is also accompanied by extreme muscle weakness and may be difficult to distinguish from cholinergic crisis on a symptomatic basis. However, such differentiation is extremely important because increases in the dose of Prostigmin or other drugs in this class, in the presence of cholinergic crisis or of a refractory or "insensitive" state, could have grave consequences. The two types of crises may be differentiated by the use of Tensilon® (edrophonium chloride) as well as by clinical judgment.

Treatment of the two conditions differs radically. Whereas the presence of *myasthenic crisis* requires more intensive anticholinesterase therapy, *cholinergic crisis* calls for the prompt withdrawal of all drugs of this type. The immediate use of atropine in cholinergic crisis is also recommended. Atropine may also be used to abolish or minimize gastrointestinal side effects or other muscarinic reactions; but such use, by masking signs of overdosage, can lead to inadvertent induction of cholinergic crisis.

The LD_{50} of neostigmine methylsulfate in mice is 0.3 ± 0.02 mg/kg intravenously, 0.54 ± 0.03 mg/kg subcutaneously, and 0.395 ± 0.025 mg/kg intramuscularly; in rats the LD_{50} is 0.315 ± 0.019 mg/kg intravenously, 0.445 ± 0.032 mg/kg subcutaneously, and 0.423 ± 0.032 mg/kg intramuscularly.

DOSAGE AND ADMINISTRATION

Symptomatic control of myasthenia gravis: One ml of the 1:2000 solution (0.5 mg) subcutaneously or intramuscularly. Subsequent doses should be based on the individual patient's response. In most patients, however, oral treatment with Prostigmin (neostigmine bromide) tablets, 15 mg each, is adequate for control of symptoms.

Prevention of postoperative distention and urinary retention: One ml of the 1:4000 solution (0.25 mg) subcutaneously or intramuscularly as soon as possible after operation; repeat every 4 to 6 hours for two or three days.

Treatment of postoperative distention: One ml of the 1:2000 solution (0.5 mg) subcutaneously or intramuscularly, as required.

Treatment of urinary retention: One ml of the 1:2000 solution (0.5 mg) subcutaneously or intramuscularly. If urination does not occur within an hour, the patient should be catheterized. After the patient has voided, or the bladder has been emptied, continue the 0.5 mg injections every three hours for at least 5 injections.

Reversal of Effects of Nondepolarizing Neuromuscular Blocking Agents: When Prostigmin is administered intravenously, it is recommended that atropine sulfate (0.6 to 1.2 mg) also be given intravenously using separate syringes. Some authorities have recommended that the atropine be injected several minutes before the Prostigmin rather than concomitantly. The usual dose is 0.5 to 2 mg Prostigmin given by *slow* intravenous injection, repeated as required. Only in exceptional cases should the total dose of Prostigmin exceed 5 mg. It is recommended that the patient be well ventilated and a patent airway maintained until complete recovery of normal respiration is assured. The optimum time for administration of the drug is during hyperventilation when the carbon dioxide level of the blood is low. It should never be administered in the presence of high concentrations of halothane or cyclopropane. In cardiac cases and severely ill patients, it is advisable to titrate the exact dose of Prostigmin required, using a peripheral nerve stimulator device. In the presence of bradycardia, the pulse rate should be increased to about 80/minute with atropine before administering Prostigmin.

Parenteral drug products should be inspected visually for particulate matter and discoloration prior to administration, whenever solution and container permit.

HOW SUPPLIED

Prostigmin 1:2000 (0.5 mg neostigmine methylsulfate/ml), 1-ml ampuls — boxes of 10 (NDC 0187-3100-20).

Prostigmin 1:4000 (0.25 mg neostigmine methylsulfate/ml), 1-ml ampuls — boxes of 10 (NDC 0187-3100-30).

Prostigmin 1:1000 (1 mg neostigmine methylsulfate/ml), 10-ml multiple dose vials — boxes of 10 (NDC 0187-3100-40).

Prostigmin 1:2000 (0.5 mg neostigmine methylsulfate/ml), 10-ml multiple dose vials — boxes of 10 (NDC 0187-3100-50).

Manufactured for ICN Pharmaceuticals, Inc.
Costa Mesa, CA 92626
by Hoffmann-La Roche Inc.
Nutley, N.J. 07110
Rev. 3/89

PROSTIGMIN® ℞

[*pro-stig'min*]
(neostigmine bromide)
TABLETS

DESCRIPTION

Prostigmin (neostigmine bromide), an anticholinesterase agent, is available for oral administration in 15-mg tablets. Each tablet also contains gelatin, lactose, corn starch, stearic acid, sugar and talc.

Chemically, neostigmine bromide is (*m*-hydroxyphenyl) trimethylammonium bromide dimethylcarbamate. It is a white, crystalline, bitter powder, soluble 1:1 in water, with a molecular weight of 303.20 and the following structural formula:

CLINICAL PHARMACOLOGY

Neostigmine inhibits the hydrolysis of acetylcholine by competing with acetylcholine for attachment to acetylcholinesterase at sites of cholinergic transmission. It enhances cholinergic action by facilitating the transmission of impulses across neuromuscular junctions. It also has a direct cholino-mimetic effect on skeletal muscle and possibly on autonomic ganglion cells and neurons of the central nervous system. Neostigmine undergoes hydrolysis by cholinesterase and is also metabolized by microsomal enzymes in the liver. Protein binding to human serum albumin ranges from 15 to 25 percent.

Neostigmine bromide is poorly absorbed from the gastrointestinal tract following oral administration. As a rule, 15 mg of neostigmine bromide orally is equivalent to 0.5 mg of neostigmine methylsulfate parenterally, due to poor absorption of the tablet from the intestinal tract. In a study in fasting myasthenic patients, the extent of absorption was estimated to be 1 to 2 percent of the ingested 30-mg single oral dose. Peak concentrations in plasma occurred 1 to 2 hours following drug ingestion, with considerable individual variations. The half-life ranged from 42 to 60 minutes with a mean half-life of 52 minutes.

INDICATIONS AND USAGE

Prostigmin is indicated for the symptomatic treatment of myasthenia gravis. Its greatest usefulness is in prolonged therapy where no difficulty in swallowing is present. In acute myasthenic crisis where difficulty in breathing and swallowing is present, the parenteral form (neostigmine methylsulfate) should be used. The patient can be transferred to the oral form as soon as it can be tolerated.

CONTRAINDICATIONS

Prostigmin is contraindicated in patients with known hypersensitivity to the drug. Because of the presence of the bromide ion, it should not be used in patients with a previous history of reaction to bromides. It is contraindicated in patients with peritonitis or mechanical obstruction of the intestinal or urinary tract.

WARNINGS

Prostigmin should be used with caution in patients with epilepsy, bronchial asthma, bradycardia, recent coronary occlusion, vagotonia, hyperthyroidism, cardiac arrhythmias or peptic ulcer. As a rule, 15 mg of neostigmine bromide orally is equivalent to 0.5 mg of neostigmine methylsulfate parenterally, due to poor absorption of the tablet from the intestinal tract. Large doses should be avoided in situations where there might be an increased absorption rate from the intestinal tract. It should be used with caution when co-administered with anticholinergic drugs, in order to avoid reduction of intestinal motility.

PRECAUTIONS

General: It is important to differentiate between myasthenic crisis and cholinergic crisis caused by overdosage of Prostigmin. Both conditions result in extreme muscle weakness but require radically different treatment. (See OVERDOSAGE section.)

Drug Interactions: Certain antibiotics, especially neomycin, streptomycin and kanamycin, have a mild but definite nondepolarizing blocking action which may accentuate neuromuscular block. These antibiotics should be used in the myasthenic patient only where definitely indicated, and then careful adjustment should be made of adjunctive anticholinesterase dosage.

Local and some general anesthetics, antiarrhythmic agents and other drugs that interfere with neuromuscular transmission should be used cautiously, if at all, in patients with myasthenia gravis; the dose of Prostigmin may have to be increased accordingly.

Carcinogenesis, Mutagenesis and Impairment of Fertility: There have been no studies with Prostigmin which would permit an evaluation of its carcinogenic or mutagenic potential. Studies on the effect of Prostigmin on fertility and reproduction have not been performed.

Pregnancy:
Teratogenic Effects: Pregnancy Category C. There are no adequate or well-controlled studies of Prostigmin in either laboratory animals or in pregnant women. It is not known whether Prostigmin can cause fetal harm when administered to a pregnant woman or can affect reproductive capacity. Prostigmin should be given to a pregnant woman only if clearly needed.

Nonteratogenic Effects: Anticholinesterase drugs may cause uterine irritability and induce premature labor when given intravenously to pregnant women near term.

Nursing Mothers: It is not known whether Prostigmin is excreted in human milk. Because many drugs are excreted in human milk and because of the potential for serious adverse reactions from Prostigmin in nursing infants, a decision should be made whether to discontinue nursing or to discontinue the drug, taking into account the importance of the drug to the mother.

Pediatric Use: Safety and effectiveness in children have not been established.

ADVERSE REACTIONS

Side effects are generally due to an exaggeration of pharmacological effects of which salivation and fasciculation are the most common. Bowel cramps and diarrhea may also occur.

The following additional adverse reactions have been reported following the use of either neostigmine bromide or neostigmine methylsulfate:

Allergic: Allergic reactions and anaphylaxis.

Neurologic: Dizziness, convulsions, loss of consciousness, drowsiness, headache, dysarthria, miosis and visual changes.

Cardiovascular: Cardiac arrhythmias (including bradycardia, tachycardia, A-V block and nodal rhythm) and nonspecific EKG changes have been reported, as well as cardiac arrest, syncope and hypotension. These have been predominantly noted following the use of the injectable form of Prostigmin.

Respiratory: Increased oral, pharyngeal and bronchial secretions, and dyspnea. Respiratory depression, respiratory arrest and bronchospasm have been reported following the use of the injectable form of Prostigmin.

Dermatologic: Rash and urticaria.

Gastrointestinal: Nausea, emesis, flatulence and increased peristalsis.

Genitourinary: Urinary frequency.

Musculoskeletal: Muscle cramps and spasms, arthralgia.

Miscellaneous: Diaphoresis, flushing and weakness.

OVERDOSAGE

Overdosage of Prostigmin can cause cholinergic crisis, which is characterized by increasing muscle weakness, and through involvement of the muscles of respiration, may result in death. Myasthenic crisis, due to an increase in the severity of the disease, is also accompanied by extreme muscle weakness and may be difficult to distinguish from cholinergic crisis on a symptomatic basis. However, such differentiation is extremely important because increases in the dose of Prostigmin or other drugs in this class, in the presence of cholinergic crisis or of a refractory or "insensitive" state, could have grave consequences. The two types of crises may be differentiated by the use of Tensilon® (edrophonium chloride) as well as by clinical judgment.

Treatment of the two conditions differs radically. Whereas the presence of *myasthenic crisis* requires more intensive anticholinesterase therapy, *cholinergic crisis* calls for the prompt withdrawal of all drugs of this type. The immediate use of atropine in cholinergic crisis is also recommended. Atropine may also be used to abolish or minimize gastrointestinal side effects or other muscarinic reactions; but such use, by masking signs of overdosage, can lead to inadvertent induction of cholinergic crisis.

The LD_{50} of neostigmine methylsulfate in mice is 0.3 ± 0.02 mg/kg intravenously, 0.54 ± 0.03 mg/kg subcutaneously, and 0.395 ± 0.025 mg/kg intramuscularly; in rats the LD_{50} is 0.315 ± 0.019 mg/kg intravenously, 0.445 ± 0.032 mg/kg subcutaneously, and 0.423 ± 0.032 mg/kg intramuscularly.

DOSAGE AND ADMINISTRATION

The onset of action of Prostigmin given orally is slower than when given parenterally, but the duration of action is longer and the intensity of action more uniform. Dosage requirements for optimal results vary from 15 mg to 375 mg per day. In some instances it may be necessary to exceed these dosages, but the possibility of cholinergic crisis must be recognized. The average dose is 10 tablets (150 mg) administered over a 24-hour period. The interval between doses is of paramount importance. The dosage schedule should be adjusted for each patient and changed as the need arises. Frequently, therapy is required day and night. Larger portions of the total daily dose may be given at times when the patient is more prone to fatigue (afternoon, mealtimes, etc.). The patient should be encouraged to keep a daily record of his or her condition to assist the physician in determining an optimal therapeutic regimen.

HOW SUPPLIED

Scored, white tablets containing 15 mg neostigmine bromide — bottles of 100 (NDC 0187-3100-10). Imprint on tablets: (front) PROSTIGMIN; (back) ICN.

Manufactured for ICN Pharmaceuticals, Inc.
Costa Mesa, CA 92626
by Hoffmann-La Roche Inc.
Nutley, N.J. 07110
Rev. 3/89

SOLAQUIN FORTE® 4% Cream ℞

[*sōl'a-kwin" for'tā*]
(HYDROQUINONE USP, 4%)
Skin Bleaching Cream with Sunscreens

CAUTION: FEDERAL (U.S.A.) LAW PROHIBITS DISPENSING WITHOUT PRESCRIPTION.
FOR EXTERNAL USE ONLY.

DESCRIPTION

Each gram of Solaquin Forte contains 40 mg hydroquinone, 50 mg ethyl dihydroxypropyl-p-aminobenzoate, 30 mg dioxybenzone USP and 20 mg oxybenzone USP in a vanishing

Continued on next page

ICN Pharmaceuticals—Cont.

cream base of purified water, glyceryl monostearate, octyldodecyl stearoyl stearate, glyceryl dilaurate, quaternium-26, coceth-6, stearyl alcohol, diethylaminoethyl stearate, dimethicone, polysorbate-80, lactic acid, ascorbic acid, hydroxyethylcellulose, quaternium-14, myristylkonium chloride, disodium EDTA, and sodium metabisulfite.

CLINICAL PHARMACOLOGY

Topical application of hydroquinone produces a reversible depigmentation of the skin by inhibition of the enzymatic oxidation of tyrosine to 3, 4-dihydroxyphenylalanine (dopa) and suppression of other melanocyte metabolic processes. Exposure to sunlight or ultraviolet light will cause repigmentation which may be prevented by the broad spectrum sunscreen agents contained in Solaquin Forte.

INDICATIONS AND USAGE

Solaquin Forte 4% Cream is indicated for the gradual bleaching of hyperpigmented skin conditions such as chloasma, melasma, freckles, senile lentigines, and other unwanted areas of melanin hyperpigmentation.

CONTRAINDICATIONS

Prior history of sensitivity or allergic reaction to this product or any of its ingredients. The safety of topical hydroquinone use during pregnancy or in children (12 years and under) has not been established.

WARNINGS

A. CAUTION: Hydroquinone is a skin bleaching agent which may produce unwanted cosmetic effects if not used as directed. The physician should be familiar with the contents of this insert before prescribing or dispensing this medication.

B. Test for skin sensitivity before using Solaquin Forte 4% Cream by applying a small amount to an unbroken patch of skin and check in 24 hours. Minor redness is not a contraindication, but where there is itching or vesicle formation or excessive inflammatory response further treatment is not advised. Close patient supervision is recommended. Contact with the eyes should be avoided. If no bleaching or lightening effect is noted after 2 months of treatment use, Solaquin Forte 4% Cream should be discontinued. Solaquin Forte 4% Cream is formulated for use as a skin bleaching agent and should not be used for the prevention of sunburn.

C. Sunscreen use is an essential aspect of hydroquinone therapy because even minimal sunlight exposure sustains melanocytic activity. The sunscreens in Solaquin Forte 4% Cream provide the necessary sun protection during skin bleaching therapy. After clearing and during maintenance therapy, sun exposure should be avoided on bleached skin by application of a sunscreen or sunblock agent or protective clothing to prevent repigmentation.

D. Keep this and all medication out of the reach of children. In case of accidental ingestion, call a physician or a poison control center immediately.

E. Warning: Contains sodium metabisulfite, a sulfite that may cause serious allergic type reactions (e.g. hives, itching, wheezing, anaphylaxis, severe asthma attack) in certain susceptible persons.

PRECAUTIONS

SEE WARNINGS.

A. Pregnancy Category C. Animal reproduction studies have not been conducted with topical hydroquinone. It is also not known whether hydroquinone can cause fetal harm when used topically on a pregnant woman or affect reproductive capacity. It is not known to what degree, if any, topical hydroquinone is absorbed systemically. Topical hydroquinone should be used in pregnant women only when clearly indicated.

B. Nursing mothers. It is not known whether topical hydroquinone is absorbed or excreted in human milk. Caution is advised when topical hydroquinone is used by a nursing mother.

C. Pediatric usage. Safety and effectiveness in children below the age of 12 years have not been established.

ADVERSE REACTIONS

No systemic adverse reactions have been reported. Occasional hypersensitivity (localized contact dermatitis) may occur in which case the medication should be discontinued and the physician notified immediately.

OVERDOSAGE

There have been no systemic reactions from the use of topical hydroquinone in Solaquin Forte. However, treatment should be limited to relatively small areas of the body at one time since some patients experience a transient skin reddening and a mild burning sensation which does not preclude treatment.

DRUG DOSAGE AND ADMINISTRATION

Solaquin Forte 4% Cream should be applied to the affected area and rubbed in well twice daily or as directed by a physician. There is no recommended dosage for children under 12 years of age except under the advice and supervision of a physician.

HOW SUPPLIED

SOLAQUIN FORTE 4% Cream is available as follows:

Size	NDC Number
0.5 ounce tube (15 grams)	0187-0396-35
1.0 ounce tube (30 grams)	0187-0396-31

Available without prescription for maintenance therapy: Solaquin (2% Hydroquinone) in 1 ounce tubes (NDC 0187-0372-31).
Solaquin Forte 4% Cream should be stored at room temperature (15–30°C) (59–86°F).

SOLAQUIN FORTE® 4% GEL   ℞
[sōl'a-kwĭn for'tā]
(Hydroquinone USP, 4%)
Skin Bleaching Gel with Sunscreens

CAUTION: FEDERAL (U.S.A.) LAW PROHIBITS DISPENSING WITHOUT A PRESCRIPTION.
FOR EXTERNAL USE ONLY

DESCRIPTION

Each gram of Solaquin Forte 4% Gel contains 40 mg of Hydroquinone, 50 mg Ethyl Dihydroxypropyl-p-aminobenzoate and 30 mg Dioxybenzone in a hydroalcoholic base of alcohol, purified water, propylene glycol, tetrahydroxypropyl ethylenediamine, carbomer 940, disodium EDTA and sodium metabisulfite.

CLINICAL PHARMACOLOGY

Topical application of hydroquinone produces a reversible depigmentation of the skin by inhibition of the enzymatic oxidation of tyrosine to 3,4-dihydroxyphenylalanine (dopa) and suppression of other melanocyte metabolic processes. Exposure to sunlight or ultraviolet light will cause repigmentation which may be prevented by the broad spectrum sunscreen agents contained in Solaquin Forte 4% Gel.

INDICATIONS AND USAGE

Solaquin Forte 4% Gel is indicated for the gradual bleaching of hyperpigmented skin conditions such as chloasma, melasma, freckles, senile lentigines and other unwanted areas of melanin hyperpigmentation.

CONTRAINDICATIONS

Prior history of sensitivity or allergic reaction to this product or any of its ingredients. The safety of topical hydroquinone use during pregnancy or in children (12 years and under) has not been established.

WARNINGS

A. CAUTION: Hydroquinone is a skin bleaching agent which may produce unwanted cosmetic effects if not used as directed. The physician should be familiar with the contents of this insert before prescribing or dispensing this medication.

B. Test for skin sensitivity before using Solaquin Forte 4% Gel by applying a small amount to an unbroken patch of skin and check in 24 hours. Minor redness is not a contraindication, but where there is itching or vesicle formation or excessive inflammatory response further treatment is not advised. Close patient supervision is recommended. Contact with the eyes should be avoided. If no bleaching or lightening effect is noted after 2 months of treatment use, Solaquin Forte 4% Gel should be discontinued. Solaquin Forte 4% Gel is formulated for use as a skin bleaching agent and should not be used for the prevention of sunburn.

C. Sunscreen use is an essential aspect of hydroquinone therapy because even minimal sunlight sustains melanocytic activity. The sunscreens in Solaquin Forte 4% Gel provide the necessary sun protection during skin bleaching therapy. After clearing and during maintenance therapy, sun exposure should be avoided on bleached skin by application of a sunscreen or sunblock agent or protective clothing to prevent repigmentation.

D. Keep this and all medication out of the reach of children. In case of accidental ingestion, call a physician or a poison control center immediately.

E. Warning: Contains sodium metabisulfite, a sulfite that may cause serious allergic type reactions (e.g. hives, itching, wheezing, anaphylaxis) in certain susceptible persons.

PRECAUTIONS

SEE WARNINGS

A. Pregnancy Category C. Animal reproduction studies have not been conducted with topical hydroquinone. It is also not known whether hydroquinone can cause fetal harm when used topically on a pregnant woman or affect reproductive capacity. It is not known to what degree, if

any, topical hydroquinone is absorbed systemically. Topical hydroquinone should be used in pregnant women only when clearly indicated.

B. Nursing mothers. It is not known whether topical hydroquinone is absorbed or excreted in human milk. Caution is advised when topical hydroquinone is used by a nursing mother.

C. Pediatric usage. Safety and effectiveness in children below the age of 12 years have not been established.

ADVERSE REACTIONS

No systemic adverse reactions have been reported. Occasional hypersensitivity (localized contact dermatitis) may occur in which case the medication should be discontinued and the physician notified immediately.

OVERDOSAGE

There have been no systemic reactions from the use of topical hydroquinone in Solaquin Forte 4% Gel. However, treatment should be limited to relatively small areas of the body at one time since some patients experience a transient skin reddening and a mild burning sensation which does not preclude treatment.

DRUG DOSAGE AND ADMINISTRATION

Solaquin Forte 4% Gel should be applied to the affected area and rubbed in well twice daily or as directed by a physician. There is no recommended dosage for children under 12 years of age except under the advice and supervision of a physician.

HOW SUPPLIED

SOLAQUIN FORTE 4% Gel is available as follows:

Size	NDC Number
0.5 ounce tube (15 grams)	0187-0523-35
1.0 ounce tube (30 grams)	0187-0523-31

Solaquin Forte 4% Gel should be stored at room temperature (15–30°C) (59–86°F).

TENSILON®   ℞
[ten'sil-on]
(edrophonium chloride)
Injectable Solution
ampuls • vials

DESCRIPTION

Tensilon is a short and rapid-acting cholinergic drug. Chemically, edrophonium chloride is ethyl (m- hydroxyphenyl)-dimethylammonium chloride.
10-ml vials: Each ml contains, in a sterile solution, 10 mg edrophonium chloride compounded with 0.45% phenol and 0.2% sodium sulfite as preservatives, buffered with sodium citrate and citric acid, and pH adjusted to approximately 5.4.
1-ml ampuls: Each ml contains, in a sterile solution, 10 mg edrophonium chloride compounded with 0.2% sodium sulfite, buffered with sodium citrate and citric acid, and pH adjusted to approximately 5.4.

ACTIONS

Tensilon is an anticholinesterase drug. Its pharmacological action is due primarily to the inhibition or inactivation of acetylcholinesterase at sites of cholinergic transmission. Its effect is manifest within 30 to 60 seconds after injection and lasts an average of 10 minutes.

INDICATIONS

Tensilon is recommended for the differential diagnosis of myasthenia gravis and as an adjunct in the evaluation of treatment requirements in this disease. It may also be used for evaluating emergency treatment in myasthenic crises. Because of its brief duration of action, it is not recommended for maintenance therapy in myasthenia gravis.
Tensilon is also useful whenever a curare antagonist is needed to reverse the neuromuscular block produced by curare, tubocurarine, gallamine triethiodide or dimethyl-tubocurarine. It is *not* effective against decamethonium bromide and succinylcholine chloride. It may be used adjunctively in the treatment of respiratory depression caused by curare overdosage.

CONTRAINDICATIONS

Known hypersensitivity to anticholinesterase agents; intestinal and urinary obstructions of mechanical type.

WARNINGS

Whenever anticholinesterase drugs are used for testing, a syringe containing 1 mg of atropine sulfate should be immediately available to be given in aliquots intravenously to counteract severe cholinergic reactions which may occur in the hypersensitive individual, whether he is normal or myasthenic. Tensilon should be used with caution in patients with bronchial asthma or cardiac dysrhythmias. The transient bradycardia which sometimes occurs can be relieved by atropine sulfate. Isolated instances of cardiac and respiratory arrest following administration of Tensilon have been reported. It is postulated that these are vagotonic effects. Tensilon solution contains sodium sulfite, a sulfite that may cause allergic-type reactions, including anaphylactic symptoms and life-threatening or less severe asthmatic episodes in certain susceptible people. The overall prevalence of sulfite sensitivity in the general population is unknown and probably low. Sulfite sensitivity is seen more frequently in asthmatic than in nonasthmatic people.

Usage in Pregnancy: The safety of Tensilon during pregnancy or lactation in humans has not been established. Therefore, use of Tensilon in women who may become pregnant requires weighing the drug's potential benefits against its possible hazards to mother and child.

PRECAUTIONS

Patients may develop "anticholinesterase insensitivity" for brief or prolonged periods. During these periods the patients should be carefully monitored and may need respiratory assistance. Dosages of anticholinesterase drugs should be reduced or withheld until patients again become sensitive to them.

ADVERSE REACTIONS

Careful observation should be made for severe cholinergic reactions in the hyperreactive individual. The myasthenic patient in crisis who is being tested with Tensilon should be observed for bradycardia or cardiac standstill and cholinergic reactions if an overdose is given. The following reactions common to anticholinesterase agents may occur, although not all of these reactions have been reported with the administration of Tensilon, probably because of its short duration of action and limited indications: **Eye:** Increased lacrimation, pupillary constriction, spasm of accommodation, diplopia, conjunctival hyperemia. **CNS:** Convulsions, dysarthria, dysphonia, dysphagia. **Respiratory:** Increased tracheobronchial secretions, laryngospasm, bronchiolar constriction, paralysis of muscles of respiration, central respiratory paralysis. **Cardiac:** Arrhythmias (especially bradycardia), fall in cardiac output leading to hypotension. **G.I.:** Increased salivary, gastric and intestinal secretion, nausea, vomiting, increased peristalsis, diarrhea, abdominal cramps. **Skeletal Muscle:** Weakness, fasciculations. **Miscellaneous:** Increased urinary frequency and incontinence, diaphoresis.

DOSAGE AND ADMINISTRATION

Tensilon Test in the Differential Diagnosis of Myasthenia Gravis:[1-8]

Intravenous Dosage (Adults): A tuberculin syringe containing 1 ml (10 mg) of Tensilon is prepared with an intravenous needle, and 0.2 ml (2 mg) is injected intravenously within 15 to 30 seconds. The needle is left *in situ. Only* if no reaction occurs after 45 seconds is the remaining 0.8 ml (8 mg) injected. If a cholinergic reaction (muscarinic side effects, skeletal muscle fasciculations and increased muscle weakness) occurs after injection of 0.2 ml (2 mg), the test is discontinued and atropine sulfate 0.4 mg to 0.5 mg is administered intravenously. After one-half hour the test may be repeated.

Intramuscular Dosage (Adults): In adults with inaccessible veins, dosage for intramuscular injection is 1 ml (10 mg) of Tensilon. Subjects who demonstrate hyperreactivity to this injection (cholinergic reaction), should be retested after one-half hour with 0.2 ml (2 mg) of Tensilon intramuscularly to rule out false-negative reactions.

Dosage (Children): The intravenous testing dose of Tensilon in children weighing up to 75 lbs is 0.1 ml (1 mg); above this weight, the dose is 0.2 ml (2 mg). If there is no response after 45 seconds, it may be titrated up to 0.5 ml (5 mg) in children under 75 lbs, given in increments of 0.1 ml (1 mg) every 30 to 45 seconds and up to 1 ml (10 mg) in heavier children. In infants, the recommended dose is 0.05 ml (0.5 mg). Because of technical difficulty with intravenous injection in children, the intramuscular route may be used. In children weighing up to 75 lbs, 0.2 ml (2 mg) is injected intramuscularly. In children weighing more than 75 lbs, 0.5 ml (5 mg) is injected intramuscularly. All signs which would appear with the intravenous test appear with the intramuscular test except that there is a delay of two to ten minutes before a reaction is noted.

Tensilon Test for Evaluation of Treatment Requirements in Myasthenia Gravis: The recommended dose is 0.1 ml to 0.2 ml (1 mg to 2 mg) of Tensilon, administered intravenously one hour after oral intake of the drug being used in treatment.[1-5] Response will be myasthenic in the undertreated patient, adequate in the controlled patient, and cholinergic in the overtreated patient. Responses to Tensilon in myasthenic and nonmyasthenic individuals are summarized in the accompanying chart:[2]
[See table above.]

Tensilon Test in Crisis: The term *crisis* is applied to the myasthenic whenever severe respiratory distress with objective ventilatory inadequacy occurs and the response to medication is not predictable. This state may be secondary to a sudden increase in severity of myasthenia gravis (myasthenic crisis), or to overtreatment with anticholinesterase drugs (cholinergic crisis).

When a patient is apneic, controlled ventilation must be secured immediately in order to avoid cardiac arrest and irreversible central nervous system damage. No attempt is made to test with Tensilon until respiratory exchange is adequate. *Dosage used at this time is most important:* If the pa-

tient is cholinergic, Tensilon will cause increased oropharyngeal secretions and further weakness in the muscles of respiration. If the crisis is myasthenic, the test clearly improves respiration and the patient can be treated with longer-acting intravenous anticholinesterase medication. When the test is performed, there should not be more than 0.2 ml (2 mg) Tensilon in the syringe. An intravenous dose of 0.1 ml (1 mg) is given initially. The patient's heart action is carefully observed. If, after an interval of one minute, this dose does not further impair the patient, the remaining 0.1 ml (1 mg) can be injected. If no clear improvement of respiration occurs after 0.2 ml (2 mg) dose, it is usually wisest to discontinue all anticholinesterase drug therapy and secure controlled ventilation by tracheostomy with assisted respiration.[5]

For Use as a Curare Antagonist: Tensilon should be administered by intravenous injection in 1 ml (10 mg) doses given slowly over a period of 30 to 45 seconds so that the onset of cholinergic reaction can be detected. This dosage may be repeated whenever necessary. The maximal dose for any one patient should be 4 ml (40 mg). Because of its brief effect, Tensilon should not be given prior to the administration of curare, tubocurarine, gallamine triethiodide or dimethyltubocurarine; it should be used at the time when its effect is needed. When given to counteract curare overdosage, the effect of each dose on the respiration should be carefully observed before it is repeated, and assisted ventilation should always be employed.

DRUG INTERACTIONS

Care should be given when administering this drug to patients with symptoms of myasthenic weakness who are also on anticholinesterase drugs. Since symptoms of anticholinesterase overdose (cholinergic crisis) may mimic underdosage (myasthenic weakness), their condition may be worsened by the use of this drug. (See OVERDOSAGE section for treatment.)

OVERDOSAGE

With drugs of this type, muscarine-like symptoms (nausea, vomiting, diarrhea, sweating, increased bronchial and salivary secretions and bradycardia) often appear with overdosage (cholinergic crisis). An important complication that can arise is obstruction of the airway by bronchial secretions. These may be managed with suction (especially if tracheostomy has been performed) and by the use of atropine. Many experts have advocated a wide range of dosages of atropine *(for Tensilon, see atropine dosage below),* but if there are copious secretions, up to 1.2 mg intravenously may be given initially and repeated every 20 minutes until secretions are controlled. Signs of atropine overdosage such as dry mouth, flush and tachycardia should be avoided as tenacious secretions and bronchial plugs may form. A total dose of atropine of 5 to 10 mg or even more may be required. The following steps should be taken in the management of overdosage of Tensilon:

1. Adequate respiratory exchange should be maintained by assuring an open airway, and the use of assisted respiration augmented by oxygen.
2. Cardiac function should be monitored until complete stabilization has been achieved.
3. Atropine sulfate in doses of 0.4 to 0.5 mg should be administered intravenously. This may be repeated every 3 to 10 minutes. Because of the short duration of action of Tensilon the total dose required will seldom exceed 2 mg.
4. Pralidoxime chloride (a cholinesterase reactivator) may be given intravenously at the rate of 50 to 100 mg per minute; usually the total dose does not exceed 1000 mg. Extreme caution should be exercised in the use of pralidoxime chloride when the cholinergic symptoms are induced by double-bond phosphorous anticholinesterase drugs.[9]
5. If convulsions or shock is present, appropriate measures should be instituted.

HOW SUPPLIED

Multiple Dose Vials, 10 ml, boxes of 10 (NDC 0187-3200-20).
Ampuls, 1 ml, boxes of 10 (NDC 0187-3200-10).

	Myasthenic*	Adequate†	Cholinergic‡
Muscle Strength (ptosis, diplopia, dysphonia, dysphagia, dysarthria, respiration, limb strength)	Increased	No change	Decreased
Fasciculations (orbicularis oculi, facial muscles, limb muscles)	Absent	Present or absent	Present or absent
Side reactions (lacrimation, diaphoresis, salivation, abdominal cramps, nausea, vomiting, diarrhea)	Absent	Minimal	Severe

* Myasthenic Response—occurs in untreated myasthenics and may serve to establish diagnosis; in patients under treatment, indicates that therapy is inadequate.
† Adequate Response—observed in treated patients when therapy is stabilized; a typical response in normal individuals. In addition to this response in nonmyasthenics, the phenomenon of forced lid closure is often observed in psychoneurotics.[1]
‡ Cholinergic Response—seen in myasthenics who have been overtreated with anticholinesterase drugs.

REFERENCES

1. Osserman, K.E. and Kaplan, L.I., *J.A.M.A.,* 150: 265, 1952.
2. Osserman, K.E., Kaplan, L.I. and Besson, G., *J. Mt. Sinai Hosp.,* 20: 165, 1953.
3. Osserman, K.E. and Kaplan, L.I., *Arch. Neurol. & Psychiat.,* 70: 385, 1953.
4. Osserman, K.E. and Teng, P., *J.A.M.A.,* 160: 153, 1956.
5. Osserman, K.E. and Genkins, G., *Ann. N.Y. Acad. Sci.,* 135: 312, 1966.
6. Tether, J.E., Second International Symposium Proceedings, Myasthenia Gravis, 1961, p. 444.
7. Tether, J.E., in H.F. Conn: *Current Therapy 1960,* Philadelphia, W. B. Saunders Company, p. 551.
8. Tether, J.E., in H.F. Conn: *Current Therapy 1965,* Philadelphia, W. B. Saunders Company, p. 556.
9. Grob, D. and Johns, R.J., *J.A.M.A.,* 166: 1855, 1958.

Manufactured for ICN Pharmaceuticals, Inc.
Costa Mesa, CA 92626
by Hoffman-La Roche Inc.
Nutley, NJ 07110
Rev. 3/89

TESTRED® ℞
Methyltestosterone Capsules, USP 10 mg

DESCRIPTION

The androgens are steroids that develop and maintain primary and secondary male sex characteristics. Androgens are derivatives of cyclopentanoperhydrophenanthrene. Endogenous androgens are C-19 steroids with a side chain at C-17, and with two angular methyl groups. Testosterone is the primary endogenous androgen. In their active form, all drugs in the class have a 17-beta-hydroxy group. 17-alpha alkylation (methyltestosterone) increases the pharmacologic activity per unit weight compared to testosterone when given orally. Methyltestosterone, a synthetic derivative of testosterone, is an androgenic preparation given by the oral route in a capsule form. Each capsule contains 10 mg of USP methyltestosterone, which has the following formula:

$C_{20}H_{30}O_2$ M.W. 302.46 (CAS-58-18-4) 17β-hydroxy-17-methylandrost-4-en-3-one

Methyltestosterone occurs as white or creamy white crystals or powder, which is soluble in various organic solvents but is practically insoluble in water.

CLINICAL PHARMACOLOGY

Endogenous androgens are responsible for the normal growth and development of the male sex organs and for maintenance of secondary sex characteristics. These effects include the growth and maturation of prostate, seminal vesicles, penis, and scrotum; the development of male hair distribution, such as beard, pubic, chest, and axillary hair; laryngeal enlargement, vocal chord thickening, alterations in body musculature and fat distribution. Drugs in this class also cause retention of nitrogen, sodium, potassium, phosphorus, and decreased urinary excretion of calcium. Androgens have been reported to increase protein anabolism and decrease protein catabolism. Nitrogen balance is improved only when there is sufficient intake of calories and protein. Androgens are responsible for the growth spurt of adolescence and for the eventual termination of linear growth which is brought about by fusion of the epiphyseal growth centers. In children, exogenous androgens accelerate linear growth rates, but may cause a disproportionate advancement in bone maturation. Use over long periods may result in fusion of the epiphyseal growth centers and termination of growth process. Androgens have been reported to stimu-

Continued on next page

ICN Pharmaceuticals—Cont.

late the production of red blood cells by enhancing the production of erythropoietic stimulating factor.

During exogenous administration of androgens, endogenous testosterone release is inhibited through feedback inhibition of pituitary luteinizing hormone (LH). At large doses of exogenous androgens, spermatogenesis may also be suppressed through feedback inhibition of pituitary follicle stimulating hormone (FSH).

There is a lack of substantial evidence that androgens are effective in fractures, surgery, convalescence and functional uterine bleeding.

Pharmacokinetics

Testosterone given orally is metabolized by the gut and 44 percent is cleared by the liver in the first pass. Oral doses as high as 400 mg per day are needed to achieve clinically effective blood levels for full replacement therapy. The synthetic androgen methyltestosterone is less extensively metabolized by the liver and has a longer half-life. It is more suitable than testosterone for oral administration.

Testosterone in plasma is 98 percent bound to a specific testosterone-estradiol binding globulin, and about 2 percent is free. Generally, the amount of this sex-hormone binding globulin in the plasma will determine the distribution of testosterone between free and bound forms, and the free testosterone concentration will determine its half-life.

About 90 percent of a dose of testosterone is excreted in the urine as glucuronic and sulfuric acid conjugates of testosterone and its metabolites; about 6 percent of a dose is excreted in the feces, mostly in the unconjugated form. Inactivation of testosterone occurs primarily in the liver. Testosterone is metabolized to various 17-keto steroids through two different pathways. There are considerable variations of the half-life of testosterone as reported in the literature, ranging from 10 to 100 minutes.

In many tissues the activity of testosterone appears to depend on reduction to dihydrotestosterone, which binds to cytosol receptor proteins. The steroid-receptor complex is transported to the nucleus where it initiates transcription events and cellular changes related to androgen action.

INDICATIONS AND USAGE

1. Males

Androgens are indicated for replacement therapy in conditions associated with a deficiency or absence of endogenous testosterone;

  a. Primary hypogonadism (congenital or acquired)—testicular failure due to cryptorchidism, bilateral torsion, orchitis, vanishing testis syndrome or orchidectomy.

  b. Hypogonadotropic hypogonadism (congenital or acquired)—idiopathic gonadotropin or LHRH deficiency, or pituitary-hypothalamic injury from tumors, trauma or radiation.

    If the above conditions occur prior to puberty, androgen therapy will be needed during the adolescent years for development of secondary sexual characteristics. Prolonged androgen treatment will be required to maintain sexual characteristics in these and other males who develop testosterone deficiency after puberty.

  c. Androgens may be used to stimulate puberty in carefully selected males with clearly delayed puberty. These patients usually have a familial pattern of delayed puberty that is not secondary to a pathological disorder; puberty is expected to occur spontaneously at a relatively late date. Brief treatment with conservative doses may occasionally be justified in these patients if they do not respond to psychological support. The potential adverse effect on bone maturation should be discussed with the patient and parents prior to androgen adminstration. An X-ray of the hand and wrist to determine bone age should be obtained every 6 months to assess the effect of treatment on the epiphyseal centers (see WARNINGS).

2. Females

Androgens may be used secondarily in women with advancing inoperable metastatic (skeletal) mammary cancer who are 1 to 5 years postmenopausal. Primary goals of therapy in these women include ablation of the ovaries. Other methods of counteracting estrogen activity are adrenalectomy, hypophysectomy, and/or antiestrogen therapy. This treatment has also been used in premenopausal women with breast cancer who have benefited from oophorectomy and are considered to have a hormone-responsive tumor. Judgment concerning androgen therapy should be made by an oncologist with expertise in this field.

Methyltestosterone has been used for the management of postpartum breast pain and engorgement.

CONTRAINDICATIONS

Androgens are contraindicated in men with carcinomas of the breast or with known or suspected carcinomas of the prostate, and in women who are or may become pregnant. When administered to pregnant women, androgens cause

virilization of the external genitalia of the female fetus. This virilization includes clitoromegaly, abnormal vaginal development, and fusion of genital folds to form a scrotal-like structure. The degree of masculinization is related to the amount of drug given and the age of the fetus, and is most likely to occur in the female fetus when the drugs are given in the first trimester. If the patient becomes pregnant while taking these drugs, she should be apprised of the potential hazard to the fetus.

WARNINGS

In patients with breast cancer, androgen therapy may cause hypercalcemia by stimulating osteolysis. In this case, the drug should be discontinued.

Prolonged use of high doses of androgens has been associated with the development of peliosis hepatis and hepatic neoplasms including hepatocellular carcinoma. (See PRECAUTIONS-Carcinogenesis). Peliosis hepatis can be a life-threatening or fatal complication.

Cholestatic hepatitis and jaundice occur with 17-alpha-alkylandrogens at a relatively low dose. If cholestatic hepatitis with jaundice appears or if liver function tests become abnormal, the androgen should be discontinued and the etiology should be determined. Drug-induced jaundice is reversible when the medication is discontinued.

Geriatric patients treated with androgens may be at an increased risk for the development of prostatic hypertrophy and prostatic carcinoma.

Edema with or without congestive heart failure may be a serious complication in patients with preexisting cardiac, renal, or hepatic disease. In addition to discontinuation of the drug, diuretic therapy may be required.

Gynecomastia frequently develops and occasionally persists in patients being treated for hypogonadism. Androgen therapy should be used cautiously in healthy males with delayed puberty. The effect on bone maturation should be monitored by assessing bone age of the wrist and hand every 6 months. In children, androgen treatment may accelerate bone maturation without producing compensatory gain in linear growth. This adverse effect may result in compromised adult stature. The younger the child the greater the risk of compromising final mature height.

PRECAUTIONS

General

Women should be observed for signs of virilization (deepening of the voice, hirsutism, acne, clitoromegaly and menstrual irregularities). Discontinuation of drug therapy at the time of evidence of mild virilism is necessary to prevent irreversible virilization. Such virilization is usual following androgen use at high doses. A decision may be made by the patient and the physician that some virilization will be tolerated during treatment for breast carcinoma.

Information for the Patient

The physician should instruct patients to report any of the following side effects of androgens:

Adult or Adolescent Males:	Too frequent or persistent erections of the penis. Any male adolescent patient receiving androgens for delayed puberty should have bone development checked every six months.
Women:	Hoarseness, acne, changes in menstrual periods, or more hair on the face.
All Patients:	Any nausea, vomiting, changes in skin color or ankle swelling.

Laboratory Tests

1. Women with disseminated breast carcinoma should have frequent determination of urine and serum calcium levels during the course of androgen therapy. (See WARNINGS).
2. Because of the hepatotoxicity associated with the use of 17-alpha-alkylated androgens, liver function tests should be obtained periodically.
3. Periodic (every 6 months) x-ray examinations of bone age should be made during treatment of prepubertal males to determine the rate of bone maturation and the effects of androgen therapy on the epiphyseal centers.
4. Hemoglobin and hematocrit should be checked periodically for polycythemia in patients who are receiving high doses of androgens.

Drug Interactions

1. **Anticoagulants:** C-17 substituted derivatives of testosterone, such as methandrostenolone, have been reported to decrease the anticoagulant requirements of patients receiving oral anticoagulants. Patients receiving oral anticoagulant therapy require close monitoring, especially when androgens are started or stopped.
2. **Oxyphenbutazone:** Concurrent administration of oxyphenbutazone and androgens may result in elevated serum levels of oxyphenbutazone.
3. **Insulin:** In diabetic patients the metabolic effects of androgens may decrease blood glucose and insulin requirements.

Drug/Laboratory Test Interferences

Androgens may decrease levels of thyroxine-binding globulin, resulting in decreased total T4 serum levels and increased resin uptake of T3 and T4. Free thyroid hormone levels remain unchanged, however, and there is no clinical evidence of thyroid dysfunction.

Carcinogenesis

Animal Data

Testosterone has been tested by subcutaneous injection and implantation in mice and rats. The implant induced cervical-uterine tumors in mice, which metastasized in some cases. There is suggestive evidence that injection of testosterone into some strains of female mice increases their susceptibility to hepatoma. Testosterone is also known to increase the number of tumors and decrease the degree of differentiation of chemically induced carcinomas of the liver in rats.

Human Data

There are rare reports of hepatocellular carcinoma in patients receiving long-term therapy with androgens in high doses. Withdrawal of the drugs did not lead to regression of the tumors in all cases.

Geriatric patients treated with androgens may be at an increased risk for the development of prostatic hypertrophy and prostatic carcinoma.

Pregnancy

Teratogenic effects. Pregnancy Category X (See CONTRAINDICATIONS).

Nursing Mothers

It is not known whether androgens are excreted in human milk. Because many drugs are excreted in human milk and because of the potential for serious adverse reactions in nursing infants from androgens, a decision should be made whether to discontinue nursing or to discontinue the drug, taking into account the importance of the drug to the mother.

Pediatric Use

Androgen therapy should be used very cautiously in children and only by specialists who are aware of the adverse effects on bone maturation. Skeletal maturation must be monitored every six months by an x-ray of hand and wrist (See INDICATIONS AND USAGE and WARNINGS).

ADVERSE REACTIONS

Endocrine and Urogenital

Female: The most common side effects of androgen therapy are amenorrhea and other menstrual irregularities, inhibition of gonadotropin secretion, and virilization, including deepening of the voice and clitoral enlargement. The latter usually is not reversible after androgens are discontinued. When administered to a pregnant woman androgens cause virilization of external genitalia of the female fetus.

Male: Gynecomastia, and excessive frequency and duration of penile erections. Oligospermia may occur at high dosages (see CLINICAL PHARMACOLOGY).

Skin and appendages: Hirsutism, male pattern of baldness, and acne.

Fluid and Electrolyte Disturbances: Retention of sodium, chloride, water, potassium, calcium, and inorganic phosphates.

Gastrointestinal: Nausea, cholestatic jaundice, alterations in liver function tests, rarely hepatocellular neoplasms and peliosis hepatis (see WARNINGS).

Hematologic: Suppression of clotting factors II, V, VII, and X, bleeding in patients on concomitant anticoagulant therapy, and polycythemia.

Nervous System: Increased or decreased libido, headache, anxiety, depression, and generalized paresthesia.

Metabolic: Increased serum cholesterol.

Miscellaneous: Rarely anaphylactoid reactions.

OVERDOSAGE

There have been no reports of acute overdosage with the androgens.

DOSAGE AND ADMINISTRATION

Methyltestosterone capsules are administered orally. The suggested dosage for androgens varies depending on the age, sex, and diagnosis of the individual patient. Dosage is adjusted according to the patient's response and the appearance of adverse reactions. Replacement therapy in androgen-deficient males is 10 to 50 mg of methyltestosterone daily. Various dosage regimens have been used to induce pubertal changes in hypogonadal males; some experts have advocated lower dosages initially, gradually increasing the dose as puberty progresses, with or without a decrease to maintenance levels. Other experts emphasize that higher dosages are needed to induce pubertal changes and lower dosages can be used for maintenance after puberty. The chronological and skeletal ages must be taken into consideration, both in determining the initial dose and in adjusting the dose.

Doses used in delayed puberty generally are in the range of that given above, and for a limited duration, for example, 4 to 6 months.

Women with metastatic breast carcinoma must be followed closely because androgen therapy occasionally appears to accelerate the disease. Thus, many experts prefer to use the shorter acting androgen preparations rather than those with prolonged activity for treating breast carcinoma. The dosage of methyltestosterone for androgen therapy in breast carcinoma in females is from 50–200 mg daily.

Suggested dosages of oral methyltestosterone for use in the prevention of postpartum breast pain and engorgement is 80 mg daily for 3 to 5 days after delivery.

HOW SUPPLIED

Methyltestosterone capsules USP 10 mg are red capsules imprinted "ICN 0901" on both sections. They are available in bottles of 100.

CAUTION: Federal (U.S.A.) law prohibits dispensing without prescription.

Revision June 1989

Shown in Product Identification Section, page 412

TRISORALEN® TABLETS   ℞

[trī 'sore "a-len]

(Trioxsalen USP, 5 mg)

To facilitate repigmentation in vitiligo, increase tolerance to solar exposure and enhance pigmentation.

Caution: *THIS IS A POTENT DRUG.*

CAUTION

Federal (U.S.A.) law prohibits dispensing without prescription.

DESCRIPTION

Trisoralen Tablets 5 mg.

TRISORALEN (trioxsalen) is the first synthetic psoralen compound made available to the medical profession. It possesses greater activity than Methoxsalen, yet the LD 50 of (trioxsalen) is six times that of Methoxsalen.

Contains color additives including FD&C Yellow No. 5 (Tartrazine).

ACTIONS

Pigment formation with TRISORALEN.

The normal pigmentation of the skin is due to melanin which is produced in the cytoplasm of the melanocytes located in the basal layers of the epidermis at its junction with the dermis. Melanin is formed by the oxidation of tyrosine to DOPA (Dihydroxyphenylalanine) with tyrosinase as catalyst. This enzymatic reaction, however, must be activated by radiant energy in the form of ultraviolet light, preferably between 2900 and 3800 angstroms (black light).

The exact mechanism of the action of psoralens in the process of melanogenesis is not known. One group of investigators feel that the psoralens have a specific effect on the epidermis or, more specifically, on the melanocytes. Another group feels that the primary response to the psoralens is an inflammatory one and that the process of melanogenesis is secondary.

INDICATIONS

TRISORALEN taken approximately two hours before measured periods of exposure to ultraviolet facilitates:

1. Repigmentation of idiopathic vitiligo. Repigmentation, not equally reversible in every patient, will vary in completeness, time of onset, and duration. The rate of completeness of pigmentation with respect to locations of lesions, occurs more rapidly on fleshy regions, such as the face, abdomen, and buttocks, and less rapidly over bony areas such as the dorsum of the hands and feet. Repigmentation may begin after a few weeks; however, significant results may take as long as six to nine months, and repigmentation, at the optimum level, may, in some cases, require maintenance dosage to retain the new pigment. If follicular repigmentation is not apparent after three months of daily treatment, treatment should be discontinued as a failure.

2. Increasing tolerance to sunlight. In blond persons and those with fair complexions who suffer painful reactions when exposed to sunlight, TRISORALEN aids in increasing resistance to solar damage. Certain persons who are allergic to sunlight or exhibit sun sensitivity may be benefited by the protective action of TRISORALEN. In albinism, TRISORALEN will increase the tolerance of the skin to sunlight, although no pigment is formed. This protective action seems to be related to the thickening of the horny layer and retention of melanin which produces a thickened melanized stratum corneum and formation of a stratum lucidum.

3. Enhancing pigmentation. The use of TRISORALEN accelerates pigmentation only when the administration of the drug is followed by exposure of the skin to sunlight or ultraviolet irradiation. The increase in pigmentation is not immediate but occurs gradually within a few days of repeated exposure and may become equivalent in a degree to that achieved by a full summer of sun exposure. Since sufficient pigment will have been formed within two weeks of continuous therapy, the use of TRISORALEN should not be continued beyond this period. Pigmentation can be maintained by periodic exposure to sunlight.

CONTRAINDICATIONS

In those diseases associated with photosensitivity, such as porphyria, acute lupus erythematosus, or leukoderma of infectious origin. To date, the safety of this drug in young persons (12 and under), has not been established and is, therefore contraindicated. No preparation with any photosensitizing capacity, internal or external should be used concomitantly with TRISORALEN therapy.

WARNINGS

TRISORALEN IS A POTENT DRUG.

Read entire brochure before prescribing or dispensing this medication. The dosage of this medication should not be increased.

The dosage of TRISORALEN and exposure time should not be increased. Overdosage and/or overexposure may result in serious burning and blistering. When used to increase tolerance to sunlight or accelerate tanning, TRISORALEN total dosage should not exceed 28 tablets, taken in daily single doses of two tablets on a continuous or interrupted regimen. To prevent harmful effects, the physician should carefully instruct the patient to adhere to the prescribed dosage schedule and procedure.

PRECAUTIONS

Accidental Overdosage:

If an overdose of TRISORALEN or ultraviolet light has been taken, emesis should be encouraged. The individual should be kept in a darkened room for eight hours or until cutaneous reactions subside. The treatment for severe reactions resulting from overdosage or overexposure should follow accepted procedures for treatment of severe burns. There have not been any clinical reports or tests to verify that more severe reactions may result from the concomitant ingestion of furocoumarin-containing food while on TRISORALEN therapy; but the physician should warn the patient that taking limes, figs, parsley, parsnips, mustard, carrots and celery, might be dangerous.

This product contains FD&C Yellow No. 5 (Tartrazine) as a color additive, which may cause allergic-type reactions (including bronchial asthma) in certain susceptible individuals. Although the overall incidence of FD&C Yellow No. 5 (Tartrazine) sensitivity is low, it is frequently seen in patients who also have aspirin hypersensitivity.

ADVERSE REACTIONS AND SIDE EFFECTS

Severe burns can result from excessive sunlight or sun lamp ultraviolet exposure.

Occasionally, there may occur gastric discomfort; to minimize this gastric effect, the tablets may be taken with milk or after a meal. Some patients who are unable to tolerate 10 mg will tolerate 5 mg. This dosage produces the same therapeutic effect but more slowly.

DOSAGE

(Adults and children over 12 years of age)

VITILIGO: Two tablets daily, taken two to four hours before measured periods of ultraviolet exposure or fluorescent black light. (See suggested sun exposure guide.)

To increase tolerance to sunlight and/or enhance pigmentation: Two tablets daily, taken two hours before measured periods of exposure to sun or ultraviolet irradiation. Not to be continued for longer than 14 days. The dosage should NOT be increased, as severe burning may occur. (See suggested sun exposure guide.)

SUGGESTED SUN EXPOSURE GUIDE

The exposure time to sunlight should be limited according to the following plan:

| | Basic Skin Color | |
	Light	Medium
Initial Exposure	15 min.	20 min.
Second Exposure	20 min.	25 min.
Third Exposure	25 min.	30 min.
Fourth Exposure	30 min.	35 min.
Subsequent Exposure:	Gradually increase exposure based on erythema and tenderness.	

Sunglasses should be worn during exposure and the lips protected with a light-screening lipstick.

SUN-LAMP EXPOSURE: Should be initiated according to directions of the sun-lamp manufacturer.

HOW SUPPLIED

TRISORALEN Tablets 5 mg in bottles of 28 (NDC 0187-0303-28) and 100 (NDC 0187-0303-01).

Military—TRIOXSALEN Tablets 5 mg stock # 6505-00-560-7022.

Trisoralen should be stored at room temperature (15–30°C) (59–86°F).

Shown in Product Identification Section, page 412

VIRAZOLE®   ℞

[vira 'zahl ']

(Ribavirin)

lyophilized for aerosol administration

> **WARNING:**
> **RIBAVIRIN AEROSOL SHOULD NOT BE USED FOR INFANTS REQUIRING ASSISTED VENTILATION BECAUSE PRECIPITATION OF THE DRUG IN THE RESPIRATORY EQUIPMENT MAY INTERFERE WITH SAFE AND EFFECTIVE VENTILATION OF THE PATIENT.** Conditions for safe use with a ventilator are still in development.
> Deterioration of respiratory function has been associated with ribavirin use in infants, and in adults with chronic obstructive lung disease or asthma. Respiratory function should be carefully monitored during treatment. If initiation of ribavirin aerosol treatment appears to produce sudden deterioration of respiratory function, treatment should be stopped and re-instituted only with extreme caution and continuous monitoring. Although ribavirin is not indicated in adults, the physician should be aware that it is teratogenic in animals (see CONTRAINDICATIONS).

DESCRIPTION

Virazole® (ribavirin) Aerosol, an antiviral drug, is a sterile, lyophilized powder to be reconstituted for aerosol administration. Each 100 ml glass vial contains 6 grams of ribavirin, and when reconstituted to the recommended volume of 300 ml with sterile water for injection or sterile water for inhalation (no preservatives added), will contain 20 mg/ml ribavirin, pH approximately 5.5. Aerosolization is to be carried out in a SPAG-2 nebulizer only.

Ribavirin is 1-beta-D-ribofuranosyl-1,2,4-triazole-3-carboxamide, with the following structural formula:

Ribavirin, a synthetic nucleoside, is a stable, white, crystalline compound with a maximum solubility in water of 142 mg/ml at 25°C and with only a slight solubility in ethanol. The empirical formula is $C_8H_{12}N_4O_5$ and the molecular weight is 244.2 Daltons.

CLINICAL PHARMACOLOGY

Antiviral effects: Ribavirin has antiviral inhibitory activity *in vitro* against respiratory syncytial virus,[1] influenza virus, and herpes simplex virus. Ribavirin is also active against respiratory syncytial virus (RSV) in experimentally infected cotton rats.[2]

In cell cultures, the inhibitory activity of ribavirin for RSV is selective. The mechanism of action is unknown. Reversal of the *in vitro* antiviral activity by guanosine or xanthosine suggests ribavirin may act as an analogue of these cellular metabolites.

Immunologic effects: Neutralizing antibody responses to RSV were decreased in ribavirin treated compared to placebo treated infants.[3] The clinical significance of this observation is unknown. In rats, ribavirin resulted in lymphoid atrophy of thymus, spleen, and lymph nodes. Humoral immunity was reduced in guinea pigs and ferrets. Cellular immunity was also mildly depressed in animal studies.

Microbiology: Several clinical isolates of RSV were evaluated for ribavirin susceptibility by plaque reduction in tissue culture. Plaques were reduced 85–98% by 16μg/ml; however, plaque reduction varies with the test system. The clinical significance of these data is unknown.

Pharmacokinetics: Assay for ribavirin in human materials is by a radioimmunoassay which detects ribavirin and at least one metabolite.

Ribavirin administered by aerosol is absorbed systemically. Four pediatric patients inhaling ribavirin aerosol administered by face mask for 2.5 hours each day for 3 days had plasma concentrations ranging from 0.44 to 1.55 μM, with a mean concentration of 0.76 μM. The plasma half-life was reported to be 9.5 hours. Three pediatric patients inhaling ribavirin aerosol administered by face mask or mist tent for 20 hours each day for 5 days had plasma concentrations ranging from 1.5 to 14.3 μM, with a mean concentration of 6.8 μM.

It is likely that the concentration of ribavirin in respiratory tract secretions is much higher than plasma concentrations in view of the route of administration.

Continued on next page

ICN Pharmaceuticals—Cont.

The bioavailability of ribavirin aerosol is unknown and may depend on the mode of aerosol delivery. After aerosol treatment, peak plasma concentrations are less than the concentration that reduced RSV plaque formation in tissue culture by 85 to 98%. After aerosol treatment, respiratory tract secretions are likely to contain ribavirin in concentrations many fold higher than those required to reduce plaque formation. However, RSV is an intracellular virus and serum concentrations may better reflect intracellular concentrations in the respiratory tract than respiratory secretion concentrations.

In man, rats, and rhesus monkeys, accumulation of ribavirin and/or metabolites in the red blood cells has been noted, plateauing in red cells in man in about 4 days and gradually declining with an apparent half-life of 40 days. The extent of accumulation of ribavirin following inhalation therapy is not well defined.

INDICATIONS AND USAGE

Ribavirin aerosol is indicated in the treatment of carefully selected hospitalized infants and young children with severe lower respiratory tract infections due to respiratory syncytial virus (RSV). In two placebo controlled trials in infants hospitalized with RSV lower respiratory tract infection, ribavirin aerosol treatment had a therapeutic effect, as judged by the reduction by treatment day 3 of severity of clinical manifestations of disease.[3,4] Virus titers in respiratory secretions were also significantly reduced with ribavirin in one of these studies.[4]

Only severe RSV lower respiratory tract infection is to be treated with ribavirin aerosol. The vast majority of infants and children with RSV infection have no lower respiratory tract disease or have disease that is mild, self-limited, and does not require hospitalization or antiviral treatment. Many children with mild lower respiratory tract involvement will require shorter hospitalization than would be required for a full course of ribavirin aerosol (3 to 7 days) and should not be treated with the drug. Thus the decision to treat with ribavirin aerosol should be based on the severity of the RSV infection.

The presence of an underlying condition such as prematurity or cardiopulmonary disease may increase the severity of the infection and its risk to the patient. High risk infants and young children with these underlying conditions may benefit from ribavirin treatment, although efficacy has been evaluated in only a small number of such patients.

Ribavirin aerosol treatment must be accompanied by and does not replace standard supportive respiratory and fluid management for infants and children with severe respiratory tract infection.

Diagnosis: RSV infection should be documented by a rapid diagnostic method such as demonstration of viral antigen in respiratory tract secretions by immunofluorescence[3,4] or ELISA[5] before or during the first 24 hours of treatment. Ribavirin aerosol is indicated only for lower respiratory tract infection due to RSV. Treatment may be initiated while awaiting rapid diagnostic test results. However, treatment should not be continued without documentation of RSV infection.

CONTRAINDICATIONS

Ribavirin is contraindicated in women or girls who are or may become pregnant during exposure to the drug. Ribavirin may cause fetal harm and respiratory syncytial virus infection is self-limited in this population. Ribavirin is not completely cleared from human blood even four weeks after administration. Although there are no pertinent human data, ribavirin has been found to be teratogenic and/or embryolethal in nearly all species in which it has been tested. Teratogenicity was evident after a single oral dose of 2.5 mg/kg in the hamster and after daily oral doses of 10 mg/kg in the rat. Malformations of skull, palate, eye, jaw, skeleton, and gastrointestinal tract were noted in animal studies. Survival of fetuses and offspring was reduced. The drug causes embryolethality in the rabbit at daily oral dose levels as low as 1 mg/kg.

WARNINGS

Ribavirin administered by aerosol produced cardiac lesions in mice and rats after 30 and 36 mg/kg, respectively, for 4 weeks, and after oral administration in monkeys at 120 and rats at 154 to 200 mg/kg for 1 to 6 months. Ribavirin aerosol administered to developing ferrets at 60 mg/kg for 10 or 30 days resulted in inflammatory and possibly emphysematous changes in the lungs. Proliferative changes were seen at 131 mg/kg for 30 days. The significance of these findings to human administration is unknown.

Ribavirin lyophilized in 6 gram vials is intended for use as an aerosol only.

PRECAUTIONS

General: Patients with lower respiratory tract infection due to respiratory syncytial virus require optimum monitoring and attention to respiratory and fluid status.

Drug Interactions: Interactions of ribavirin with other drugs such as digoxin, bronchodilators, other antiviral agents, antibiotics, or anti-metabolites has not been evaluated. Interference by ribavirin with laboratory tests has not been evaluated.

Carcinogenesis, mutagenesis, impairment of fertility: Ribavirin induces cell transformation in an *in vitro* mammalian system (Balb/C 3T3 cell line). However, *in vivo* carcinogenicity studies are incomplete. Results thus far, though inconclusive, suggest that chronic feeding of ribavirin to rats at dose levels in the range of 16–60 mg/kg body weight can induce benign mammary, pancreatic, pituitary and adrenal tumors. Ribavirin is mutagenic to mammalian (L5178Y) cells in culture. Results of microbial mutagenicity assays and a dominant lethal assay (mouse) were negative.

Ribavirin causes testicular lesions (tubular atrophy) in adult rats at oral dose levels as low as 16 mg/kg/day (lower doses not tested), but fertility of ribavirin-treated animals (male or female) has not been adequately investigated.

Pregnancy: Teratogenic Effects: Pregnancy Category X. See "Contraindications" section.

Nursing Mothers: Use of ribavirin aerosol in nursing mothers is not indicated because RSV infection is self-limited in this population. Ribavirin is toxic to lactating animals and their offspring. It is not known whether the drug is excreted in human milk.

ADVERSE REACTIONS

Approximately 200 patients have been treated with ribavirin aerosol in controlled or uncontrolled clinical studies.

Pulmonary function significantly deteriorated during ribavirin aerosol treatment in six of six adults with chronic obstructive lung disease and in four of six asthmatic adults. Dyspnea and chest soreness were also reported in the latter group. Minor abnormalities in pulmonary function were also seen in healthy adult volunteers.

Several serious adverse events occurred in severely ill infants with life-threatening underlying diseases, many of whom required assisted ventilation. The role of ribavirin aerosol in these events is indeterminate. The following events were associated with ribavirin use:

Pulmonary: Worsening of respiratory status, bacterial pneumonia, pneumothorax, apnea, and ventilator dependence.

Cardiovascular: Cardiac arrest, hypotension, and digitalis toxicity.

There were 7 deaths during or shortly after treatment with ribavirin aerosol. No death was attributed to ribavirin aerosol by the investigators.

Some subjects requiring assisted ventilation have experienced serious difficulties, which may jeopardize adequate ventilation and gas exchange. Precipitation of drug within the ventilatory apparatus, including the endotracheal tube, has resulted in increased positive end expiratory pressure and increased positive inspiratory pressure. Accumulation of fluid in tubing ("rain out") has also been noted.

Although anemia has not been reported with use of the aerosol, it occurs frequently with oral and intravenous ribavirin, and most infants treated with the aerosol have not been evaluated 1 to 2 weeks post-treatment when anemia is likely to occur. Reticulocytosis has been reported with aerosol use. Rash and conjunctivitis have been associated with the use of ribavirin aerosol.

Overdosage: No overdosage with ribavirin by aerosol administration has been reported in the human. The LD$_{50}$ in mice is 2 gm orally. Hypoactivity and gastrointestinal symptoms occurred. In man, ribavirin is sequestered in red blood cells for weeks after dosing.

DOSAGE AND ADMINISTRATION

Before use, read thoroughly the Viratek Small Particle Aerosol Generator (SPAG) Model SPAG-2 Operator's Manual for small particle aerosol generator operating instructions.

Treatment was effective when instituted within the first 3 days of respiratory syncytial virus lower respiratory tract infection.[3] Treatment early in the course of severe lower respiratory tract infection may be necessary to achieve efficacy.

Treatment is carried out for 12–18 hours per day for at least 3 and no more than 7 days, and is part of a total treatment program. The aerosol is delivered to an infant oxygen hood from the SPAG-2 aerosol generator. Administration by face mask or oxygen tent may be necessary if a hood cannot be employed (see SPAG-2 manual). However, the volume of distribution and condensation area are larger in a tent and efficacy of this method of administering the drug has been evaluated in only a small number of patients. Ribavirin aerosol is not to be administered with any other aerosol generating device or together with other aerosolized medications. Ribavirin aerosol should not be used for patients requiring simultaneous assisted ventilation (see Boxed Warnings).

Virazole is supplied as 6 grams of lyophilized drug per 100 ml vial for aerosol administration only. By sterile technique, solubilize drug with sterile USP water for injection or inhalation in the 100 ml vial. Transfer to the clean, sterilized 500 ml wide-mouth polysulfone reservoir (SPAG-2 Reservoir)

and further dilute to a final volume of 300 ml with sterile USP water for injection or inhalation. The final concentration should be 20 mg/ml. **Important:** This water should not have had any antimicrobial agent or other substance added. The solution should be inspected visually for particulate matter and discoloration prior to administration. Solutions that have been placed in the SPAG-2 unit should be discarded at least every 24 hours and when the liquid level is low before adding newly reconstituted solutions.

Using the recommended drug concentration of 20 mg/ml ribavirin as the starting solution in the drug reservoir of the SPAG unit, the average aerosol concentration for a 12 hour period would be 190 micrograms/liter (0.19 mg/l) of air.

HOW SUPPLIED

Virazole (ribavirin) Aerosol is supplied in 100 ml glass vials with 6 grams of sterile, lyophilized drug which is to be reconstituted with 300 ml sterile water for injection or sterile water for inhalation (no preservatives added) and administered only by a small particle aerosol generator (SPAG-2). Vials containing the lyophilized drug powder should be stored in a dry place at 15–25°C (59–78°F). Reconstituted solutions may be stored, under sterile conditions, at room temperature (20–30°C, 68–86°F) for 24 hours. Solutions which have been placed in the SPAG-2 unit should be discarded at least every 24 hours.

REFERENCES

1. Hruska JF, Bernstein JM, Douglas Jr., RG, and Hall CB. Effects of ribavirin on respiratory syncytial virus in vitro. *Antimicrob Agents Chemother* 17:770–775, 1, 1980.
2. Hruska JF, Morrow PE, Suffin SC, and Douglas Jr., RG. *In vivo* inhibition of respiratory syncytial virus by ribavirin. *Antimicrob Agents Chemother* 21:125–130, 1982.
3. Taber LH, Knight V, Gilbert BE, McClung HW et al. Ribavirin aerosol treatment of bronchiolitis associated with respiratory tract infection in infants. *Pediatrics* 72:613–618, 1983.
4. Hall CB, McBride JT, Walsh EE, Bell DM et al. Aerosolized ribavirin treatment of infants with respiratory syncytial viral infection. *N Engl J Med* 308:1443–7, 1983.
5. Hendry RM, McIntosh K, Fahnestock ML, and Pierik LT. Enzyme-linked immunosorbent assay for detection of respiratory syncytial virus infection. *J Clin Microbiol* 16:329–33, 1982.

Jan 1986

Inwood Laboratories
Subsidiary of Forest Laboratories
300 PROSPECT STREET
INWOOD, NY 11696

PRODUCT Generic Name Colors(s)	IDENTIFICATION CODE (Front/Back*)
CARBAMAZEPINE Tablets, USP, 200mg ℞ White	IL 3587/Blank
INDOMETHACIN E.R. Capsules, USP, 40mg ℞ Lavender & Clear	IL 3607/Blank
ISOSORBIDE DINITRATE E.R. Tablets, USP, 40mg ℞ Peach	IL 3549/Blank
PROPRANOLOL HYDROCHLORIDE E.R. Capsules, USP, 60mg Opaque Brown/Clear	IL 3609&Blank
PROPRANOLOL HYDROCHLORIDE E.R. Capsules, USP, 80mg Opaque Blue/Clear	IL 3610&Blank
PROPRANOLOL HYDROCHLORIDE E.R. Capsules, USP, 120mg Opaque Blue/Clear	IL 3611&Blank
PROPRANOLOL HYDROCHLORIDE E.R. Capsules, USP, 160mg Opaque Blue/Clear	IL 3612&Blank

*Front/Back for tablets or left and right side for capsules

THEOCHRON™   ℞
(theophylline, anhydrous)
Controlled Release Tablets

PRODUCT OVERVIEW

KEY FACTS

Theochron is a controlled release theophylline product. Available in three strengths, each tablet contains 100 mg, 200 mg, or 300 mg of anhydrous theophylline.

MAJOR USES

Theochron, a bronchodilator, is used to relieve the symptoms of asthma and the reversible bronchospasm that accompanies chronic bronchitis and emphysema. It may also be used to prevent such symptoms.

SAFETY INFORMATION

Contraindicated in patients who are allergic to any tablet ingredient. This product is not an appropriate treatment for acute symptoms of asthma and reversible bronchospasm. Toxicity may develop when serum theophylline concentration rises above 20 mcg/ml. Patients with reduced theophylline plasma clearance may experience increased serum levels and subsequent toxicity after taking usual doses. Theochron must not be chewed or crushed.

PRESCRIBING INFORMATION

THEOCHRON™   ℞
(theophylline, anhydrous)
Controlled Release Tablets

DESCRIPTION

Theophylline is a bronchodilator structurally classified as a xanthine derivative. It occurs as a white, odorless, crystalline powder having a bitter taste. Theophylline anhydrous has the chemical name, 1H-Purine-2, 6-dione, 3,7-dihydro-1,3-dimethyl-, and is represented by the following structural formula:

Theochron™ is available as Controlled Release Tablets intended for oral administration, which allows a 12-hour dosing interval for a majority of patients and a 24-hour dosing interval for selected patients (See **DOSAGE AND ADMINISTRATION** section for description of appropriate patient population). Theochron™ contains no color additives and is available in three strengths: 100 mg, 200 mg and 300 mg of theophylline anhydrous.
Theochron™ Controlled Release Tablets contain the following inactive ingredients: Colloidal silicon dioxide, hydroxypropyl methylcellulose, magnesium stearate and stearic acid.

CLINICAL PHARMACOLOGY

Theophylline directly relaxes the smooth muscle of the bronchial airways and pulmonary blood vessels, thus acting mainly as a bronchodilator and smooth muscle relaxant. It has also been demonstrated that aminophylline has a potent effect on diaphragmatic contractility in normal persons and may then be capable of reducing fatigability and thereby improve contractility in patients with chronic obstructive airways disease. The exact mode of action remains unsettled. Although theophylline does cause inhibition of phosphodiesterase with a resultant increase in intracellular cyclic AMP, other agents similarly inhibit the enzyme producing a rise of cyclic AMP but are unassociated with any demonstrable bronchodilation. Other mechanisms proposed include an effect on translocation of intracellular calcium; prostaglandin antagonism; stimulation of catecholamines endogenously; inhibition of cyclic guanosine monophosphate metabolism and adenosine receptor antagonism.
In vitro, theophylline has been shown to act synergistically with beta agonists and there are now available data which demonstrate an additive effect *in vivo* with combined use. Apparently, no development of tolerance occurs with chronic use of theophylline.
Pharmacokinetics: The half life of theophylline is influenced by a number of known variables. It may be prolonged in chronic alcoholics, particularly those with liver disease (cirrhosis or alcoholic liver disease), in patients with congestive heart failure, and in those taking certain other drugs (see **PRECAUTIONS, Drug Interactions**). Newborns and neonates have extremely slow clearance rates compared to older infants and children, i.e., those over 1 year. Older children have rapid clearance rates while most non-smoking adults have clearance rates between these two extremes. In premature neonates the decreased clearance is related to oxidative pathways that have yet to be established.

THEOPHYLLINE ELIMINATION CHARACTERISTICS

	Range	Half-life (in hours) Mean
Children	1–9	3.7
Adults	3–15	7.7

In cigarette smokers (1–2 packs/day) the mean half-life is 4–5 hours, much shorter than in non-smokers. The increase in clearance associated with smoking is presumably due to stimulation of the hepatic metabolic pathway by components of cigarette smoke. The duration of this effect after cessation of smoking is unknown but may require 6 months to 2 years before the rate approaches that of the non-smoker.

Pharmacokinetic Studies: A single dose three way crossover study was conducted in 18 normal subjects. Subjects were fasted for 10 to 12 hours before and for 4 additional hours after dosing. All subjects received a single 300 mg tablet, two 200 mg tablets or three 100 mg tablets with intervening washout periods. Mean peak theophylline serum levels for the 100 mg, 200 mg (normalized to an equivalent 300 mg dose) and 300 mg tablets were 3.8 plus or minus 0.9 mcg/mL, 3.9 plus or minus 1.4 mcg/mL and 3.4 plus or minus 0.9 mcg/mL, respectively. The peak serum level varied from subject to subject, occurring from 3 to 12 hours after dosing. However 80% of the subjects had serum levels of at least 75% of the maximum value between 5 and 8 hours after dosing. Therefore, blood samples taken between 5 and 8 hours should reference the peak serum level for most subjects.
A multiple dose, five day study was conducted with 18 normal subjects given 300 mg twice daily. For this group, theophylline half-lives after dosing with a liquid preparation were determined to be between 5.5 and 11.0 hours (mean 7.7 plus or minus 1.6 hours). On the fifth day, after steady state had been established, the AM dose was administered after a twelve hour fast which continued for 4 hours after dosing. Mean Cmax and Cmin levels were determined to be 8.3 plus or minus 1.4 mcg/mL and 5.3 plus or minus 1.3 mcg/mL, respectively, while the average percent fluctuation [(Cmax $-$Cmin/Cmin $\times$ 100)] was 62.9% $\pm$ 27.8%. The bioavailablility compared to an immediate release product was 88.6%.
Theochron™ 300 mg Controlled Release Tablets, given as a single 300 mg dose at 7 AM following the ingestion of a high fat meal (64 g fat; 1112 calories) to 16 healthy subjects resulted in a mean Cmax of 4.6 $\pm$ 1.4 mcg/mL and a mean Tmax of 8.2 $\pm$ 3.2 hours.
Theochron™ 300 mg Controlled Release Tablets were given to 17 healthy subjects under a multiple dose schedule either as 600 mg or 900 mg, once-a-day for seven days at 7 AM immediately following ingestion of a high fat meal. This regimen resulted in a mean Cmax of 16.9 $\pm$ 2.3 mcg/mL, a mean Cmin of 5.8 $\pm$ 1.8 mcg/mL, and an average percent fluctuation [(Cmax-Cmin/Cmin) $\times$ 100)] of 209.5% $\pm$ 82.9%.
Theochron™ 200 mg Controlled Release Tablets were given to 16 healthy subjects as a single 200 mg dose at 7 AM after a 10-hour overnight fast. This regimen resulted in a mean Cmax of 2.9 $\pm$ 0.9 mcg/mL and a mean Tmax of 6.6 $\pm$ 2.7 hours.
Theochron™ 100 mg Controlled Release Tablets were given to 16 healthy subjects as a single 100 mg dose at 7 AM after a 10-hour overnight fast. This regimen resulted in a mean Cmax of 1.7 $\pm$ 0.3 mcg/mL and a mean Tmax of 6.3 $\pm$ 1.4 hours.

INDICATIONS AND USAGE

For relief and/or prevention of symptoms of asthma and reversible bronchospasm associated with chronic bronchitis and emphysema.

CONTRAINDICATIONS

This product is contraindicated in individuals who have shown hypersensitivity to its components. It is also contraindicated in patients with active peptic ulcer disease, and in individuals with underlying seizure disorders (unless receiving appropriate anticonvulsant medication).

WARNINGS

Serum levels above 20 mcg/mL are rarely found after appropriate administration of the recommended doses. However, in individuals in whom theophylline plasma clearance is reduced *for any reason,* even conventional doses may result in increased serum levels and potential toxicity. Reduced theophylline clearance has been documented in the following readily identifiable groups: 1) patients with impaired renal or liver function; 2) patients over 55 years of age, particularly males and those with chronic lung disease; 3) those with cardiac failure from any cause; 4) patients with sustained high fever; 5) neonates and infants under 1 year of age; and 6) those patients taking certain drugs (see **PRECAUTIONS, Drug Interactions**). Frequently, such patients have markedly prolonged theophylline serum levels following discontinuation of the drug.
Reduction of dosage and laboratory monitoring is especially appropriate in the above individuals.
Serious side effects such as ventricular arrhythmias, convulsions or even death may appear as the first sign of toxicity without any previous warning. Less serious signs of theophylline toxicity (i.e., nausea and restlessness) may occur frequently when initiating therapy, but are usually transient; when such signs are persistent during maintenance therapy, they are often associated with serum concentrations above 20 mcg/mL.
Stately differently; *serious toxicity is not reliably preceded by less severe side effects.* A serum concentration measurement is the only reliable method of predicting potentially life-threatening toxicity.
Many patients who require theophylline exhibit tachycardia due to their underlying disease process so that the cause/effect relationship to elevated serum theophylline concentrations may not be appreciated.

Theophylline products may cause dysrhythmia and/or worsen pre-existing arrhythmias and any significant change in rate and/or rhythm warrants monitoring and further investigation.
Studies in laboratory animals (minipigs, rodents, and dogs) recorded the occurrence of cardiac arrhythmias and sudden death (with histological evidence of myocardial necrosis) when beta-agonists and methylxanthines were administered concurrently. The significance of these findings when applied to humans is currently unknown.

PRECAUTIONS

General: On the average, theophylline half-life is shorter in cigarette and marijuana smokers than in non-smokers, but smokers can have half-lives as long as non-smokers. Theochron™ Controlled Release Tablets should not be administered concurrently with other xanthine medications. Use with caution in patients with severe cardiac disease, severe hypoxemia, hypertension, hyperthyroidism, acute myocardial injury, cor pulmonale, congestive heart failure, liver disease, in the elderly, (especially males) and in neonates. In particular, great caution should be used in giving Theochron™ Controlled Release Tablets to patients with congestive heart failure. Frequently, such patients have markedly prolonged theophylline serum levels with theophylline persisting in serum for long periods following discontinuation of the drug. Individuals who are rapid metabolizers of theophylline such as the young, smokers and some non-smoking adults, may not be suitable candidates for once-daily dosing. These individuals will generally need to be dosed at 12-hour or sometimes 8-hour intervals. Such patients may exhibit symptoms of bronchospasm near the end of a dosing interval, or may have wider peak to trough differences than desired. Theophylline preparations should be used cautiously in patients with history of peptic ulcer, since they may occasionally act as a local irritant to the G.I. tract; gastrointestinal symptoms, however, are more commonly centrally mediated and associated with serum drug concentrations over 20 mcg/mL.
Information for Patients: The importance of taking only the prescribed dose and time interval between doses should be reinforced. Theochron™ Controlled Release Tablets should not be chewed or crushed. When dosing Theochron™ on a once daily (q24h) basis, tablets should be taken whole and not split. The patient should alert the physician if symptoms should occur repeatedly, especially near the end of a dosing interval.
Laboratory Test: Serum levels should be monitored periodically to determine the theophylline level associated with observed clinical response and as the method of predicting toxicity. For such measurements, the serum sample should be obtained at the time of peak concentration 5 to 8 hours (see **CLINICAL PHARMACOLOGY:** *Pharmacokinetic Studies*). It is important that the patient will not have missed or taken additional doses during the previous 48 hours and that dosing intervals will have been reasonably equally spaced. DOSAGE ADJUSTMENT BASED ON SERUM THEOPHYLLINE MEASUREMENTS WHEN THESE INSTRUCTIONS HAVE NOT BEEN FOLLOWED MAY RESULT IN RECOMMENDATIONS THAT PRESENT RISK OF TOXICITY TO THE PATIENT.
Drug Interactions:
Drug-Drug: Toxic synergism with ephedrine has been documented and may occur with some other sympathomimetic bronchodilators. In addition, the following drug interactions have been demonstrated:
Theophylline with:

Allopurinol (high-dose)	Increased serum theophylline levels
Cimetidine	Increased serum theophylline levels
Erythromycin, Troleandomycin	Increased serum theophylline levels
Lithium Carbonate	Increased renal excretion of lithium
Oral Contraceptives	Increased serum theophylline levels
Phenytoin	Decreased theophylline and phenytoin serum levels
Ciprofloxacin	Increased serum theophylline levels
Rifampin	Decreased serum theophylline levels

Drug—Food: There is information available from studies in which Theochron™ was administered either fasting or non-fasting (see **CLINICAL PHARMACOLOGY**, Pharmacokinetics). Administration of Theochron™ with a high-fat meal (such as 64 g fat; 1112 calories) does not result in a significantly different rate or extent of absorption of theophylline, when compared to administration of Theochron™ in the fasting state.
Drug—Laboratory Tests Interactions: Currently available analytical methods, including high pressure liquid chroma-

Continued on next page

Inwood—Cont.

tography and immunoassay techniques, for measuring serum theophylline levels are specific. Metabolites and other drugs generally do not affect the results. Other new analytic methods are also now in use. The physician should be aware of the laboratory method used and whether other drugs will interfere with the assay for theophylline.

Carcinogenesis, Mutagenesis, and Impairment of Fertility: Long-term carcnogenicity studies have not been performed with theophylline.

Chromosome-breaking activity was detected in human cell cultures at concentrations of theophylline up to 50 times the therapeutic serum concentration in humans. Theophylline was not mutagenic in the dominant lethal assay in male mice given theophylline intraperitoneally in doses up to 30 times the maximum daily human oral dose.

Studies to determine the effect on fertility have not been performed with theophylline.

Pregnancy: Category C—Animal reproduction studies have not been conducted with theophylline. It is not known whether theophylline can cause fetal harm when administered to a pregnant woman or can affect reproduction capacity. Xanthines should be given to a pregnant woman only if clearly needed.

Nursing Mothers: Theophylline is distributed into breast milk and may cause irritability or other signs of toxicity in nursing infants. Because of the potential for serious adverse reactions in nursing infants from theophylline, a decision should be made whether to discontinue nursing or to discontinue the drug, taking into account the importance of the drug to the mother.

Pediatric Use: Safety and effectiveness of Theochron™ administered:

A. Every 24 hours in children under 12 years of age, have not been established.

B. Every 12 hours in children under 6 years of age, have not been established.

ADVERSE REACTIONS

The following adverse reactions have been observed, but there has not been enough systematic collection of data to support an estimate of their frequency. The most consistent adverse reactions are usually due to overdosage.

1. *Gastrointestinal:* nausea, vomiting, epigastric pain, hematemesis, diarrhea.
2. *Central nervous system:* headaches, irritability, restlessness, insomnia, reflex hyperexcitability, muscle twitching, clonic and tonic generalized convulsions.
3. *Cardiovascular:* palpitation, tachycardia, extrasystoles, flushing hypotension, circulatory failure, ventricular arrhythmias.
4. *Respiratory:* tachypnea.
5. *Renal:* potentiation of diuresis.
6. *Others:* hyperglycemia and inappropriate ADH syndrome, rash.

OVERDOSAGE

Management: It is suggested that the management principles (consistent with the clinical status of the patient when first seen) outlined below be instituted and that simultaneous contact with a Regional Poison Control Center be established in this way both updated information and individualization regarding required therapy may be provided.

1. When potential oral overdose is established and seizure has not occurred:
a) If patient is alert and seen within the early hours after ingestion, induction of emesis may be of value. Gastric lavage has been demonstrated to be of no value in influencing outcome in patients who present more than 1 hour after ingestion.
b) Administer a cathartic. Sorbitol solution is reported to be of value.
c) Administer repeated doses of activated charcoal and monitor theophylline serum levels.
d) Prophylactic administration of phenobarbital has been shown to increase the seizure threshold in laboratory animals, and administration of this drug can be considered.
2. If patient presents with a seizure:
a) Establish an airway.
b) Administer oxygen.
c) Treat the seizure with intravenous diazepam, 0.1 to 0.3 mg/kg up to 10 mg. If seizures cannot be controlled, the use of general anesthesia should be considered.
d) Monitor vital signs, maintain blood pressure and provide adequate hydration.
3. If post seizure coma is present:
a) Maintain airway and oxygenation.
b) If a result of oral medication, follow above recommendations to prevent absorption of the drug, but intubation and lavage will have to be performed instead of inducing emesis, and the cathartic and charcoal will need to be introduced via a large bore gastric lavage tube.
c) Continue to provide full supportive care and adequate hydration until the drug is metabolized. In general, drug

metabolism is sufficiently rapid so as not to warrant dialysis. If repeated, oral activated charcoal is ineffective (as noted by stable or rising serum levels) and charcoal hemoperfusion may be indicated.

DOSAGE AND ADMINISTRATION

Theochron™ Controlled Release Tablets:
Administration of Theochron™ with a high-fat meal does not result in a significantly different rate or extent of absorption of theophylline, when compared to administration of Theochron™ in the fasting state.

Effective use of theophylline (i.e., the concentration of drug in the serum associated with optimal benefit and minimal risk of toxicity) is considered to occur when the theophylline concentration is maintained from 10 to 20 mcg/mL. The early studies from which these levels were derived were carried out in patients immediately or shortly after recovery from acute exacerbations of their disease (some hospitalized with status asthmaticus).

Although the 20 mcg/mL level remains appropriate as a critical value (above which toxicity is more likely to occur) for safety purposes, additional data are now available which indicate that the serum theophylline concentrations required to produce maximum physiologic benefit may, in fact, fluctuate with the degree of bronchospasm present and are variable. Therefore, the physician should individualize the range appropriate to the patient's requirements, based on both symptomatic response and improvement in pulmonary function. It should be stressed that serum theophylline concentrations maintained at the upper level of the 10 to 20 mcg/mL range may be associated with potential toxicity when factors known to reduce theophylline clearance are operative. (See **WARNINGS**.)

If it is not possible to obtain serum level determinations, restriction of the daily dose (in otherwise healthy adults) to not greater than 13 mg/kg/day, to a maximum of 900 mg, in divided doses will result in relatively few patients exceeding serum levels of 20 mcg/mL and the resultant greater risk of toxicity.

Caution should be excercised for younger children who cannot complain of minor side effects. Older adults, those with cor pulmonale, congestive heart failure, and/or liver disease may have unusually low dosage requirements and thus may experience toxicity at the maximal dosage recommended below.

Theophylline does not distribute into fatty tissue. Dosage should be calculated on the basis of lean (ideal) body weight where mg/kg doses are presented.

Theochron™ tablets (controlled release) are recommended for chronic or long term management and prevention of symptoms, and not for use in treating acute symptoms of asthma and reversible bronchospasm.

Dosage Guidelines Dosage guidelines are approximations only and the wide range of theophylline clearance between individuals (particularly those with concomitant disease) makes indiscriminate usage hazardous.

I. Acute Symptoms:
Theochron™ Controlled Release Tablets are not intended for patients experiencing an acute episode of bronchospasm (associated with asthma, chronic bronchitis, or emphysema). Such patients require rapid relief of symptoms and should be treated with an immediate-release or intravenous theophylline preparation (or other bronchodilators) and not with controlled release products.

II. Chronic Therapy:
A. Initiating Therapy:
It is recommended that the appropriate dosage be established using an immediate-release preparation. A dosage form which allows small incremental doses is desirable for initiating therapy. A liquid preparation should be considered for children to permit easier and more accurate dosage adjustment. Slow clinical titration is generally preferred to help assure acceptance and safety of the medication and to allow the patient to develop tolerance to transient caffeine-like side effects. Then, if the total 24-hour dose can be given by use of the available strengths of this product, the patient can usually be switched to Theochron™ giving one-half of the daily dose at 12-hour intervals or one-third the daily dose at 8-hour intervals. Patients who metabolize theophylline rapidly; such as the young, smokers and some non-smoking adults, are the most likely candidates for dosing at 8-hour intervals. Such patients can generally be identifed as having trough serum concentrations lower than desired or repeatedly exhibiting symptoms near the end of a dosing interval.
Alternatively, therapy can be initiated with Theochron™ since it is available in dosage forms/strengths which permit titration and adjustment of dosage as outlined in the following dosing guidelines. It is recommended that for *children under 25 kg* proper dosage be established with a liquid preparation to permit titration in small increments.
THE AVERAGE INITIAL ADULT AND CHILDRENS (over 25 kg) DOSE IS ONE THEOCHRON™ 200 mg TABLET q12h.

B. Titration and Adjustment and Chronic Maintenance:
If the desired response is not achieved with the above AVERAGE INITIAL DOSE recommendations, there are no adverse reactions and the serum theophylline level cannot be measured, dosage adjustment should proceed by increasing the dose in approximately 25% increments at three day intervals. Following each adjustment, if the clinical response is satisfactory, then that dosage level should be maintained. DOSAGE increases may be made in this manner up to the following.

III. Maximum dose of Theophylline Where the Serum Concentration is not Measured:
WARNING: DO NOT ATTEMPT TO MAINTAIN ANY DOSE THAT IS NOT TOLERATED.
Not to exceed the following: (or 900 mg, whichever is less)

Age 6–9 years	24 mg/kg/day
Age 9–12 years	20 mg/kg/day
Age 12–16 years	18 mg/kg/day
Age 16 years and older	13 mg/kg/day

If an increased dose is not tolerated because of headaches or stomach upset/nausea, vomiting, diarrhea, etc.) decrease dose to previous tolerated level. Do not exceed the above recommended doses unless serum theophylline levels can be measured.

It is important that no patient be maintained on any dosage that is not tolerated. In instructing patients to increase dosage according to the schedule above, they should be instructed not to take a subsequent dose if apparent side effects occur and to resume therapy at a lower dose once adverse effects have disappeared.

IV. Measurement of Serum Theophylline Concentrations During Chronic Therapy:
If the above maximum doses are to be maintained or exceeded, serum theophylline measurement is essential. (see **PRECAUTIONS, Laboratory Tests,** for guidance.)

V. Final Adjustment of Dosage:
Dosage adjustment after serum theophylline measurement:

If serum theophylline is:		Directions:
Within desired range		Maintain dosage if tolerated.
Too high	20 to 25 mcg/mL	Decrease doses by about 10% and recheck serum level after 3 days.
	25 to 30 mcg/mL	Skip the next dose and decrease subsequent doses by about 25%. Recheck serum level after 3 days.
	Over 30 mcg/mL	Skip the next 2 doses and decrease subsequent doses by 50%. Recheck serum level after 3 days.
Too low		Increase dose by 25% at 3 day intervals until either the desired serum concentration and/or clinical response is achieved. The total daily dose may need to be administered at more frequent intervals if symptoms occur repeatedly at the end of a dosing interval.

The serum concentration may be rechecked at appropriate intervals, but at least at the end of any adjustment period. When the patient's condition is otherwise clinically stable and none of the recognized factors which alter elimination are present, measurement of serum levels need be repeated only every 6 to 12 months.
DOSAGE ADJUSTMENT BASED ON SERUM THEOPHYLLINE CONCENTRATION MEASUREMENTS WHEN THESE INSTRUCTIONS HAVE NOT BEEN FOLLOWED MAY RESULT IN RECOMMENDATIONS THAT PRESENT RISK OF TOXICITY TO THE PATIENT.

Once-Daily Dosing:
The slow absorption rate of this preparation may allow once-daily administration in adult non-smokers with appropriate total body clearance and other patients with low dosage requirements. Once-daily dosing should be considered only after the patient has been gradually and satisfactorily titrated to therapeutic levels with q12h dosing. Once-daily dosing should be based on twice the q12h dose and should be initiated at the end of the last q12h dosing interval. The trough concentration (Cmin) obtained following conversion to once-daily dosing may be lower (especially in high clearance patients) and the peak concentration (Cmax) may be higher (especially in low clearance patients) than that obtained with q12h dosing. If symptoms recur, or signs of toxicity appear during the once-daily dosing interval, dosing on the q12h basis should be reinstituted.
It is essential that serum theophylline concentrations be monitored before and after transfer to once-daily dosing.
Food and posture, along with changes associated with circadian rhythm, may influence the rate of absorption and/or clearance rates of theophylline from controlled-release dosage forms administered at night. The exact relationship of these and other factors to nighttime serum concentrations

and the clinical significance of such findings require additional study. Therefore, it is not recommended that Theochron™, when used as a once-a-day product, be administered at night. Theochron™ when used as a once-a-day product must be taken whole and not broken.

HOW SUPPLIED

Theochron™ (Theophylline Anhydrous) is available as 100 mg, 200 mg, and 300 mg controlled release tablets having the following identification characteristics:
Theochron™ controlled release 300 mg—capsule shaped, white, scored tablets, imprint IL/3581.
Available in bottles of 100 (NDC 0258-3581-01), 500 (NDC 0258-3581-05), and 1000 (NDC 0258-3581-10).
Theochron™ controlled release 200 mg—oval concave, white, scored tablets, imprint IL/3583.
Available in bottles of 100 (NDC 0258-3583-01), 500 (NDC 0258-3583-05), and 1000 (NDC 0258-3583-10).
Theochron™ controlled release 100 mg—round concave, white, scored tablets, imprint IL/3584.
Available in bottles of 100 (NDC 0258-3584-01), 500 (NDC 0258-3584-05), and 1000 (NDC 0258-3584-10).

STORAGE

Store at controlled room temperature 15°–30°C (59°–86°F). Dispense in tight containers.

CAUTION

Federal law prohibits dispensing without prescription.
Manufactured by
Inwood Laboratories, Inc.
Inwood, New York, 11696
Subsidiary of FOREST LABORATORIES, INC.
Rev. 5/89   MG #3407
(01)
Shown in Product Identification Section, page 410

Jacobus Pharmaceutical Co., Inc.
**37 CLEVELAND LANE
P.O. BOX 5290
PRINCETON, NJ 08540**

DAPSONE USP ℞
[*dap'sōne*]
25 mg. & 100 mg.

PRODUCT OVERVIEW

KEY FACTS
Dapsone is a sulfone for the primary treatment of Dermatitis herpetiformis and an antibacterial drug for susceptible cases of leprosy.

MAJOR USES
Dapsone is used to control the dermatologic symptoms of Dermatitis herpetiformis. Dapsone is used alone or in combination with other anti-leprosy drugs for leprosy.

SAFETY INFORMATION
Dapsone is contraindicated in patients with Dapsone hypersensitivity. Complete blood counts and laboratory monitoring should be done frequently. See labeling.

PRODUCT INFORMATION

DAPSONE USP ℞
[*dap'sōne*]
25 mg. & 100 mg.

DESCRIPTION
Dapsone-USP, 4–4' diaminodiphenylsulfone (DDS) is a primary treatment for Dermatitis herpetiformis. It is an antibacterial drug for susceptible cases of leprosy. It is a white, odorless crystalline powder, practically insoluble in water and insoluble in fixed and vegetable oils.
Inactive Ingredients: Colloidal silicon dioxide, magnesium stearate, microcrystalline cellulose, and corn starch. Dapsone is issued on prescription in tablets of 25 and 100 mg. for oral use.

$$NH_2 - \text{(ring)} - SO_2 - \text{(ring)} - NH_2$$

CLINICAL PHARMACOLOGY
Actions: The mechanism of action in Dermatitis herpetiformis has not been established. By the kinetic method in mice, Dapsone is bactericidal as well as bacteriostatic against *Mycobacterium leprae*.
Absorption and Excretion: Dapsone, when given orally, is rapidly and almost completely absorbed. About 85 percent of the daily intake is recoverable from the urine mainly in the form of water-soluble metabolites. Excretion of the drug is slow and a constant blood level can be maintained with the usual dosage.

Blood Levels: Detected a few minutes after ingestion, the drug reaches peak concentration in 4–8 hours. Daily administration for at least eight days is necessary to achieve a plateau level. With doses of 200 mg. daily, this level averaged 2.3 µg/ml with a range of 0.1–7.0 µg/ml. The half-life in the plasma in different individuals varies from ten hours to fifty hours and averages twenty-eight hours. Repeat tests in the same individual are constant. Daily administration (50–100 mg.) in leprosy patients will provide blood levels in excess of the usual minimum inhibitory concentration even for patients with a short Dapsone half-life.

INDICATIONS AND USAGE
Dermatitis herpetiformis (D.H.) All forms of leprosy except for cases of proven Dapsone resistance.

CONTRAINDICATION
Hypersensitivity to Dapsone and/or its derivatives.

WARNINGS
The patient should be warned to respond to the presence of clinical signs such as sore throat, fever, pallor, purpura or jaundice. Deaths associated with the administration of Dapsone have been reported from agranulocytosis, aplastic anemia and other blood dyscrasias. Complete blood counts should be done frequently in patients receiving Dapsone. The FDA Dermatology Advisory Committee recommended that, when feasible counts should be done weekly for the first month, monthly for six months and semi-annually thereafter. If a significant reduction in leucocytes, platelets or hemopoiesis is noted, Dapsone should be discontinued and the patient followed intensively. Folic acid antagonists have similar effects and may increase the incidence of hematologic reactions; if co-administered with Dapsone the patient should be monitored more frequently. Patients on weekly Pyrimethamine and Dapsone have developed agranulocytosis during the second and third month of therapy.
Severe anemia should be treated prior to initiation of therapy and hemoglobin monitored. Hemolysis and methemoglobin may be poorly tolerated by patients with severe cardio-pulmonary disease.
Carcinogenesis, mutagenesis: Dapsone has been found carcinogenic (sarcomagenic) for male rats and female mice causing mesenchymal tumors in the spleen and peritoneum, and thyroid carcinoma in female rats. Dapsone is not mutagenic with or without microsomal activation in *S. typhimurium* tester strains 1535, 1537, 1538, 98, or 100.
Cutaneous reactions, especially bullous, include exfoliative dermatitis and are probably one of the most serious, though rare, complications of sulfone therapy. They are directly due to drug sensitization. Such reactions include toxic erythema, erythema multiforme, toxic epidermal necrolysis, morbilliform and scarlatiniform reactions, urticaria and erythema nodosum. If new or toxic dermatologic reactions occur, sulfone therapy must be promptly discontinued and appropriate therapy instituted.
Leprosy reactional states, including cutaneous, are not hypersensitivity reactions to Dapsone and do not require discontinuation. See special section.

PRECAUTIONS
General: Hemolysis and Heinz body formation may be exaggerated in individuals with a glucose-6-phosphate dehydrogenase (G6PD) deficiency, or methemoglobin reductase deficiency, or hemoglobin M. This reaction is frequently dose-related. Dapsone should be given with caution to these patients or if the patient is exposed to other agents or conditions such as infection or diabetic ketosis capable of producing hemolysis. Drugs or chemicals which have produced significant hemolysis in G6PD or methemoglobin reductase deficient patients include Dapsone, sulfanilamide, nitrite, aniline, phenylhydrazine, napthalene, niridazole, nitrofurantoin and 8-amino-antimalarials such as primaquine.
Toxic hepatitis and cholestatic jaundice have been reported early in therapy. Hyperbilirubinemia may occur more often in G6PD deficient patients. When feasible, baseline and subsequent monitoring of liver function is recommended. If abnormal, Dapsone should be discontinued until the source of the abnormality is established.
Drug Interactions: Rifampin lowers Dapsone levels 7 to 10-fold by accelerating plasma clearance; in leprosy this reduction has not required a change in dosage.
Folic acid antagonists such as pyrimethamine may increase the likelihood of hematologic reactions.
Pregnancy Category C: Animal reproduction studies have not been conducted with Dapsone. Extensive, but uncontrolled experience and two published surveys on the use of Dapsone in pregnant women have not shown that Dapsone increases the risk of fetal abnormalities if administered during all trimesters of pregnancy or can affect reproduction capacity. Because of the lack of animal studies or controlled human experience, Dapsone should be given to a pregnant woman only if clearly needed. In general, for leprosy, USPHS at Carville recommends maintenance of Dapsone. Dapsone has been important for the management of some pregnant D.H. patients.

Nursing Mothers: Dapsone is excreted in breast milk in substantial amounts. Hemolytic reactions can occur in neonates. See section on hemolysis. Because of the potential for tumorgenicity shown for Dapsone in animal studies a decision should be made whether to discontinue nursing or discontinue the drug taking into account the importance of the drug to the mother.
Pediatric Use: Children are treated on the same schedule as adults but with correspondingly smaller doses. Dapsone is generally not considered to have an effect on the later growth, development and functional development of the child.

ADVERSE REACTIONS
In addition to the warnings listed above, the following syndromes and serious reactions have been reported in patients on Dapsone.
Hematologic Effects: Dose-related hemolysis is the most common adverse effect and is seen in patients with or without G6PD deficiency. Almost all patients demonstrate the interrelated changes of a loss of 1–2g of HB, an increase in the reticulocytes (2–12%), a shortened red cell life span and a rise in methemoglobin. G6PD deficient patients have greater responses.
Nervous System Effects: Peripheral neuropathy is a definite but unusual complication of Dapsone therapy in non-leprosy patients. Motor loss is predominent. If muscle weakness appears, Dapsone should be withdrawn. Recovery on withdrawal is usually substantially complete. The mechanism of recovery is reportedly by axonal regeneration. Some recovered patients have tolerated retreatment at reduced dosage. In leprosy this complication may be difficult to distinguish from a leprosy reactional state.
Body As A Whole: In addition to the warnings and adverse effects reported above, additional adverse reactions include: nausea, vomiting, abdominal pains, vertigo, blurred vision, tinnitus, insomnia, fever, headache, psychosis, phototoxicity, tachycardia, albuminuria, the nephrotic syndrome, hypoalbuminemia without proteinuria, renal papillary necrosis, male infertility, drug-induced Lupus erythematosus and an infectious mononucleosis-like syndrome. In general, with the exception of the complications of severe anoxia from overdosage (retinal and optic nerve damage, etc.) these adverse reactions have regressed off drug.

OVERDOSAGE
Nausea, vomiting, hyperexcitability can appear a few minutes up to 24 hours after ingestion of an overdose. Methemoglobin induced depression, convulsions and severe cyanosis requires prompt treatment. In normal and methemoglobin reductase deficient patients, methylene blue, 1–2 mg/kg of body weight, given slowly intravenously is the treatment of choice. The effect is complete in 30 minutes, but may have to be repeated if methemoglobin reaccumulates. For non-emergencies, if treatment is needed, methylene blue may be given orally in doses of 3–5 mg/kg every 4–6 hours.
Methylene blue reduction depends on G6PD and should not be given to fully expressed G6PD deficient patients.

DOSAGE AND ADMINISTRATION
Dermatitis herpetiformis: The dosage should be individually titrated starting in adults with 50 mg. daily and correspondingly smaller doses in children. If full control is not achieved within the range of 50–300 mg. daily, higher doses may be tried. Dosage should be reduced to a minimum maintenance level as soon as possible. In responsive patients there is a prompt reduction in pruritus followed by clearance of skin lesions. There is no effect on the gastro-intestinal component of the disease.
Dapsone levels are influenced by acetylation rates. Patients with high acetylation rates, or who are receiving treatment affecting acetylation may require an adjustment in dosage. A strict gluten free diet is an option for the patient to elect, permitting many to reduce or eliminate the need for Dapsone; the average time for dosage reduction is 8 months with a range of 4 months to 2½ years and for dosage elimination 29 months with a range of 6 months to 9 years.
Leprosy: In order to reduce secondary Dapsone resistance, the WHO Expert Committee on Leprosy and the USPHS at Carville, LA, recommend that Dapsone should be commenced in combination with one or more anti-leprosy drugs. In the multi-drug program Dapsone should be maintained at the full dosage of 100 mg. daily without interruption (with correspondingly smaller doses for children) and provided to all patients who have sensitive organisms with new or recrudescent disease or who have not yet completed a two year course of Dapsone monotherapy. For advice and other drugs, the USPHS at Carville, LA, (504-642-7771) should be contacted. Before using other drugs consult appropriate product labeling.
In bacteriologically negative tuberculoid and indeterminate disease, the recommendation is the coadministration of Dapsone 100 mg. daily with six months of Rifampin 600 mg. daily. Under WHO, daily Rifampin may be replaced by 600 mg. Rifampin monthly, if supervised. The Dapsone is contin-

Continued on next page

Jacobus—Cont.

ued until all signs of clinical activity are controlled—usually after an additional six months. Then Dapsone should be continued for an additional three years for tuberculoid and indeterminate patients and for five years for borderline tuberculoid patients.

In lepromatous and borderline lepromatous patients, the recommendation is the coadministration of Dapsone 100 mg. daily with two years of Rifampin 600 mg. daily. Under WHO, daily Rifampin may be replaced by 600 mg. Rifampin monthly, if supervised. One may elect the concurrent administration of a third anti-leprosy drug, usually either Clofazamine 50–100mg. daily or Ethionamide 250–500 mg. daily. Dapsone 100 mg. daily is continued 3–10 years until all signs of clinical activity are controlled with skin scrapings and biopsies negative for one year. Dapsone should then be continued for an additional 10 years for borderline patients and for life for lepromatous patients.

Secondary Dapsone resistance should be suspected whenever a lepromatous or borderline lepromatous patient receiving Dapsone treatment relapses clinically and bacteriologically, solid staining bacilli being found in the smears taken from the new active lesions. If such cases show no response to regular and supervised Dapsone therapy within three to six months or good compliance for the past 3–6 months can be assured, Dapsone resistance should be considered confirmed clinically. Determination of drug sensitivity using the mouse footpad method is recommended and, after prior arrangement, is available without charge from the USPHS, Carville, LA. Patients with proven Dapsone resistance should be treated with other drugs.

Leprosy Reactional States: Abrupt changes in clinical activity occur in leprosy with any effective treatment and are known as reactional states. The majority can be classified into two groups.

The "Reversal" reaction (Type 1) may occur in borderline or tuberculoid leprosy patients often soon after chemotherapy is started. The mechanism is presumed to result from a reduction in the antigenic load: the patient is able to mount an enhanced delayed hypersensitivity response to residual infection leading to swelling ("Reversal") of existing skin and nerve lesions. If severe, or if neuritis is present, large doses of steroids should always be used. If severe, the patient should be hospitalized. In general anti-leprosy treatment is continued and therapy to suppress the reaction is indicated such as analgesics, steroids, or surgical decompression of swollen nerve trunks. USPHS at Carville, LA should be contacted for advice in management.

Erythema nodosum leprosum (ENL) (lepromatous lepra reaction) (Type 2 reaction) occurs mainly in lepromatous patients and small numbers of borderline patients. Approximately 50% of treated patients show this reaction in the first year. The principal clinical features are fever and tender erythematous skin nodules sometimes associated with malaise, neuritis, orchitis, albuminuria, joint swelling, iritis, epistaxis or depression. Skin lesions can become pustular and/or ulcerate. Histologically there is a vasculitis with an intense polymorphonuclear infiltrate. Elevated circulating immune complexes are considered to be the mechanism of the reaction. If severe, patients should be hospitalized. In general, anti-leprosy treatment is continued. Analgesics, steroids, and other agents available from USPHS, Carville, LA, are used to suppress the reaction.

HOW SUPPLIED

Rx: Dapsone 25 mg, round white scored tablet, debossed "25" above and "102" below the score and on the obverse "Jacobus" in light and child-resistant bottles, of 100, NDC 49938-102-01.

Dapsone 100 mg, round white scored tablet, debossed "100" above and "101" below the score and on the obverse "Jacobus" in light and child-resistant bottles of 100, NDC 49938-101-01.

Store at controlled room temperature, (59–86°F).
Protect from light.
CAUTION: Federal law prohibits dispensing without prescription.
Dispense this product in a well-closed child-resistant container.

JACOBUS PHARMACEUTICAL CO., INC.
P.O. Box 5290
Princeton, NJ 08540
7E APRIL, 1988

Products are cross-indexed by
generic and chemical names in the
YELLOW SECTION

Jamol Laboratories Inc.
13 ACKERMAN AVENUE
EMERSON, NEW JERSEY 07630

PONARIS
Nasal Mucosal Emollient

COMPOSITION
Essential oils of cajeput, eucalyptus, and peppermint in a specially prepared iodized cottonseed oil. (Total Iodine 0.6%) Assimilable hence NON-lipoid potential.

INDICATIONS AND USES
Nasal emollient, for relief of nasal congestion due to colds, nasal irritations, atrophic rhinitis, (dry inflamed nasal passages), nasal mucosal encrustations and allergy manifestations.
Also nasal intubations and sterile gauze impregnated for epistaxis packing.

ADMINISTRATION AND DOSAGE
3 to 4 drops in each nostril 3 to 4 times daily. May be used in a compressed air nebulizer or a DeVilbiss nebulizer No. 33 or 40.
Childrens Dosage: As directed by physician.

HOW SUPPLIED
One ounce bottle with dropper.

Janssen Pharmaceutica Inc.
40 KINGSBRIDGE ROAD
PISCATAWAY, NJ 08854

ALFENTA®   ℂ ℞
[ăl-fĕn´tä]
(alfentanil hydrochloride)
Injection

CAUTION: Federal Law Prohibits Dispensing Without Prescription

DESCRIPTION
ALFENTA (alfentanil hydrochloride) Injection is an opioid analgesic chemically designated as N-[1-[2-(4-ethyl-4, 5-dihydro-5-oxo-1H-tetrazol-1-yl) ethyl] -4-(methoxymethyl)-4-piperidinyl]-N-phenylpropanamide monohydrochloride (1:1) with a molecular weight of 452.98.

ALFENTA is a sterile, non-pyrogenic, preservative free aqueous solution containing alfentanil hydrochloride equivalent to 500 μg per ml of alfentanil base for intravenous injection. The solution, which contains sodium chloride for isotonicity, has a pH range of 4.0–6.0.

CLINICAL PHARMACOLOGY
ALFENTA (alfentanil hydrochloride) is an opioid analgesic with a rapid onset of action.

At doses of 8–40 μg/kg for surgical procedures lasting up to 30 minutes, ALFENTA provides analgesic protection against hemodynamic responses to surgical stress with recovery times generally comparable to those seen with equipotent fentanyl dosages. For longer procedures, doses of up to 75 μg/kg attenuate hemodynamic responses to laryngoscopy, intubation and incision, with recovery time comparable to fentanyl. At doses of 50–75 μg/kg followed by a continuous infusion of 0.5–3.0 μg/kg/min, ALFENTA attenuates the catecholamine response with more rapid recovery and reduced need for postoperative analgesics as compared to patients administered enflurane. High intrasubject and intersubject variability in the pharmacokinetic disposition of ALFENTA has been reported.

The pharmacokinetics of ALFENTA as determined in 11 patients given single bolus injections of 50 or 125 μg/kg, can be described as a three-compartment model; distribution half-life ranged from 0.4–3.1 minutes; redistribution half-life ranged from 4.6–21.6 minutes; and terminal elimination half-life ranged from 64.1–129.3 minutes (as compared to a terminal elimination half-life of approximately 219 minutes for fentanyl and approximately 164 minutes for sufentanil). Linear kinetics have been described only with plasma concentrations up to 1000 ng/ml. Repeated or continuous administration of ALFENTA produces increasing plasma concentration and an accumulation of the drug, particularly in patients with reduced plasma clearance. The liver is the major site of biotransformation.

ALFENTA has an apparent volume of distribution of 0.6–1.0 L/kg, which is approximately one-fourth that of fentanyl, with a plasma clearance range of 1.7–17.6 ml/kg/min as compared to approximately 12.6 ml/kg/min for fentanyl.

Approximately 81% of the administered dose is excreted within 24 hours and only 0.2% of the dose is eliminated as unchanged drug; urinary excretion is the major route of elimination of metabolites. Plasma protein binding of ALFENTA is approximately 92%.

In one study involving 15 patients administered ALFENTA with nitrous oxide/oxygen, a narrow range of plasma ALFENTA concentrations, approximately 310–340 ng/ml, was shown to provide adequate anesthesia for intra-abdominal surgery, while lower concentrations, approximately 190 ng/ml, blocked responses to skin closure. Plasma concentrations between 100–200 ng/ml provided adequate anesthesia for superficial surgery.

ALFENTA has an immediate onset of action. At dosages of approximately 105 μg/kg, ALFENTA produces hypnosis as determined by EEG patterns; an anesthetic ED_{90} of 182 μg/kg for ALFENTA in unpremedicated patients has been determined, based upon the ability to block response to placement of a nasopharyngeal airway. Based on clinical trials, induction dosage requirements range from 130–245 μg/kg. For procedures lasting 30–60 minutes, loading dosages of up to 50 μg/kg produce the hemodynamic responses to endotracheal intubation and skin incision comparable to those from fentanyl. A pre-intubation loading dose of 50–75 μg/kg prior to a continuous infusion attenuates the response to laryngoscopy, intubation and incision. Subsequent administration of ALFENTA infusion administered at a rate of 0.5–3.0 μg/kg/min with nitrous oxide/oxygen attenuates sympathetic responses to surgical stress with more rapid recovery than enflurane.

Requirements for volatile inhalation anesthetics were reduced by thirty to fifty percent during the first 60 minutes of maintenance in patients administered anesthetic doses (above 130 μg/kg) of ALFENTA as compared to patients given doses of 4–5 mg/kg thiopental for anesthetic induction. At anesthetic induction dosages, ALFENTA provides a deep level of anesthesia during the first hour of anesthetic maintenance and provides attenuation of the hemodynamic response during intubation and incision.

Following an anesthetic induction dose of ALFENTA, requirements for ALFENTA infusion are reduced by 30 to 50% for the first hour of maintenance.

Patients with compromised liver function and those over 65 years of age have been found to have reduced plasma clearance and extended terminal elimination for ALFENTA, which may prolong postoperative recovery.

Bradycardia may be seen in patients administered ALFENTA. The incidence and degree of bradycardia may be more pronounced when ALFENTA is administered in conjunction with non-vagolytic neuromuscular blocking agents or in the absence of anticholinergic agents such as atropine. Administration of intravenous diazepam immediately prior to or following high doses of ALFENTA has been shown to produce decreases in blood pressure that may be secondary to vasodilation; recovery may also be prolonged.

Patients administered doses up to 200 μg/kg of ALFENTA have shown no significant increase in histamine levels and no clinical evidence of histamine release.

Skeletal muscle rigidity is related to the dose and speed of administration of ALFENTA. Muscular rigidity will occur with an immediate onset following anesthetic induction dosages. Preventative measures (see WARNINGS) may reduce the rate and severity.

The duration and degree of respiratory depression and increased airway resistance usually increase with dose, but have also been observed at lower doses. Although higher doses may produce apnea and a longer duration of respiratory depression, apnea may also occur at low doses.

INDICATIONS AND USAGE
ALFENTA (alfentanil hydrochloride) is indicated:
     as an analgesic adjunct given in incremental doses in the maintenance of anesthesia with barbiturate/nitrous oxide/oxygen.
     as an analgesic administered by continuous infusion with nitrous oxide/oxygen in the maintenance of general anesthesia.
     as a primary anesthetic agent for the induction of anesthesia in patients undergoing general surgery in which endotracheal intubation and mechanical ventilation are required.
SEE DOSAGE CHART FOR MORE COMPLETE INFORMATION ON THE USE OF ALFENTA.

CONTRAINDICATIONS
ALFENTA (alfentanil hydrochloride) is contraindicated in patients with known hypersensitivity to the drug.

WARNINGS
ALFENTA SHOULD BE ADMINISTERED ONLY BY PERSONS SPECIFICALLY TRAINED IN THE USE OF INTRAVENOUS AND GENERAL ANESTHETIC AGENTS AND IN THE MANAGEMENT OF RESPIRATORY EFFECTS OF POTENT OPIOIDS.
AN OPIOID ANTAGONIST, RESUSCITATIVE AND INTUBATION EQUIPMENT AND OXYGEN SHOULD BE READILY AVAILABLE.
BECAUSE OF THE POSSIBILITY OF DELAYED RESPIRATORY DEPRESSION, MONITORING OF THE PATIENT MUST CONTINUE WELL AFTER SURGERY.

ALFENTA (alfentanil hydrochloride) administered in initial dosages up to 20 μg/kg may cause skeletal muscle rigidity, particularly of the truncal muscles. The incidence and severity of muscle rigidity is usually dose-related. Administration of ALFENTA at anesthetic induction dosages (above 130 μg/kg) will consistently produce muscular rigidity with an immediate onset. The onset of muscular rigidity occurs earlier than with other opioids. ALFENTA may produce muscular rigidity that involves all skeletal muscles, including those of the neck and extremities. The incidence may be reduced by: 1) routine methods of administration of neuromuscular blocking agents for balanced opioid anesthesia; 2) administration of up to ¼ of the full paralyzing dose of a neuromuscular blocking agent just prior to administration of ALFENTA at dosages up to 130 μg/kg; following loss of consciousness, a full paralyzing dose of a neuromuscular blocking agent should be administered; or 3) simultaneous administration of ALFENTA and a full paralyzing dose of a neuromuscular blocking agent when ALFENTA is used in rapidly administered anesthetic dosages (above 130 μg/kg).

The neuromuscular blocking agent used should be appropriate for the patient's cardiovascular status. Adequate facilities should be available for postoperative monitoring and ventilation of patients administered ALFENTA. It is essential that these facilities be fully equipped to handle all degrees of respiratory depression.

PRECAUTIONS
DELAYED RESPIRATORY DEPRESSION, RESPIRATORY ARREST, BRADYCARDIA, ASYSTOLE, ARRHYTHMIAS AND HYPOTENSION HAVE ALSO BEEN REPORTED. THEREFORE, VITAL SIGNS MUST BE MONITORED CONTINUOUSLY.

General: The initial dose of ALFENTA (alfentanil hydrochloride) should be appropriately reduced in elderly and debilitated patients. The effect of the initial dose should be considered in determining supplemental doses. In obese patients (more than 20% above ideal total body weight), the dosage of ALFENTA should be determined on the basis of lean body weight.

In one clinical trial, the dose of ALFENTA required to produce anesthesia, as determined by appearance of delta waves in EEG, was 40% lower in geriatric patients than that needed in healthy young patients.

In patients with compromised liver function and in geriatric patients, the plasma clearance of ALFENTA may be reduced and postoperative recovery may be prolonged.

Induction doses of ALFENTA should be administered slowly (over three minutes). Administration may produce loss of vascular tone and hypotension. Consideration should be given to fluid replacement prior to induction.

Diazepam administered immediately prior to or in conjunction with high doses of ALFENTA may produce vasodilation, hypotension and result in delayed recovery.

Bradycardia produced by ALFENTA may be treated with atropine. Severe bradycardia and asystole have been successfully treated with atropine and conventional resuscitative methods.

The hemodynamic effects of a particular muscle relaxant and the degree of skeletal muscle relaxation required should be considered in the selection of a neuromuscular blocking agent.

Following an anesthetic induction dose of ALFENTA, requirements for volatile inhalation anesthetics or ALFENTA infusion are reduced by 30 to 50% for the first hour of maintenance.

Administration of ALFENTA infusion should be discontinued at least 10–15 minutes prior to the end of surgery.

Respiratory depression caused by opioid analgesics can be reversed by opioid antagonists such as naloxone. Because the duration of respiratory depression produced by ALFENTA may last longer than the duration of the opioid antagonist action, appropriate surveillance should be maintained. As with all potent opioids, profound analgesia is accompanied by respiratory depression and diminished sensitivity to CO_2 stimulation which may persist into or recur in the postoperative period. Intraoperative hyperventilation may further alter postoperative response to CO_2. Appropriate postoperative monitoring should be employed, particularly after infusions and large doses of ALFENTA, to ensure that adequate spontaneous breathing is established and maintained in the absence of stimulation prior to discharging the patient from the recovery area.

Head Injuries: ALFENTA may obscure the clinical course of patients with head injuries.

Impaired Respiration: ALFENTA should be used with caution in patients with pulmonary disease, decreased respiratory reserve or potentially compromised respiration. In such patients, opioids may additionally decrease respiratory drive and increase airway resistance. During anesthesia, this can be managed by assisted or controlled respiration.

Impaired Hepatic or Renal Fuction: In patients with liver or kidney dysfunction, ALFENTA should be administered with caution due to the importance of these organs in the metabolism and excretion of ALFENTA.

	ALFENTA (N = 785) %	Fentanyl (N = 243) %	Thiopental Sodium (N = 66) %	Enflurane (N = 55) %	Halothane (N = 18) %	Saline Placebo* (N = 18) %
Gastrointestinal						
Nausea	28	44	14	5	0	22
Vomiting	18	31	11	9	13	17
Cardiovascular						
Bradycardia	14	7	8	0	0	0
Tachycardia	12	12	39	36	31	11
Hypotension	10	8	7	7	0	0
Hypertension	18	13	30	20	6	0
Arrhythmia	2	2	5	4	6	0
Musculoskeletal						
Chest Wall Rigidity	17	12	0	0	0	0
Skeletal Muscle Movements	6	2	6	2	0	0
Respiratory						
Apnea	7	0	0	0	0	0
Postoperative Respiratory Depression	2	2	0	0	0	0
CNS						
Dizziness	3	5	0	0	0	0
Sleepiness/ Postoperative Sedation	2	8	2	0	0	6
Blurred Vision	2	2	0	0	0	0

* From two clinical trials, one involving supplemented balanced barbiturate/nitrous oxide anesthesia and one in healthy volunteers who did not undergo surgery.

Drug Interactions: Both the magnitude and duration of central nervous system and cardiovascular effects may be enhanced when ALFENTA is administered in combination with other CNS depressants such as barbiturates, tranquilizers, opioids, or inhalation general anesthetics. Postoperative respiratory depression may be enhanced or prolonged by these agents. In such cases of combined treatment, the dose of one or both agents should be reduced. Limited clinical experience indicates that requirements for volatile inhalation anesthetics are reduced by 30 to 50% for the first sixty (60) minutes following ALFENTA induction.

The concomitant use of erythromycin with ALFENTA can significantly inhibit ALFENTA clearance and may increase the risk of prolonged or delayed respiratory depression.

Perioperative administration of drugs affecting hepatic blood flow or enzyme function may reduce plasma clearance and prolong recovery.

Carcinogenesis, Mutagenesis and Impairment of Fertility: No long-term animal studies of ALFENTA have been performed to evaluate carcinogenic potential. The micronucleus test in female rats and the dominant lethal test in female and male mice revealed that single intravenous doses of ALFENTA as high as 20 mg/kg (approximately 40 times the upper human dose) produced no structural chromosome mutations or induction of dominant lethal mutations. The Ames *Salmonella typhimurium* metabolic activating test also revealed no mutagenic activity.

Pregnancy Category C: ALFENTA has been shown to have an embryocidal effect in rats and rabbits when given in doses 2.5 times the upper human dose for a period of 10 days to over 30 days. These effects could have been due to maternal toxicity (decreased food consumption with increased mortality) following prolonged administration of the drug.

No evidence of teratogenic effects has been observed after administration of ALFENTA in rats or rabbits.

There are no adequate and well-controlled studies in pregnant women. ALFENTA should be used during pregnancy only if the potential benefit justifies the potential risk to the fetus.

Labor and Delivery: There are insufficient data to support the use of ALFENTA in labor and delivery. Placental transfer of the drug has been reported; therefore, use in labor and delivery is not recommended.

Nursing Mothers: In one study of nine women undergoing post-partum tubal ligation, significant levels of ALFENTA were detected in colostrum four hours after adminstration of 60 μg/kg of ALFENTA, with no detectable levels present after 28 hours. Caution should be exercised when ALFENTA is administered to a nursing woman.

Pediatric Use: Adequate data to support the use of ALFENTA in children under 12 years of age are not presently available.

ADVERSE REACTIONS
The most common adverse reactions, respiratory depression and skeletal muscle rigidity, are extensions of known pharmacological effects of opioids. See CLINICAL PHARMACOLOGY, WARNINGS and PRECAUTIONS on the management of respiratory depression and skeletal muscle rigidity.

Delayed respiratory depression, respiratory arrest, bradycardia, asystole, arrhythmias and hypotension have also been reported.

The reported incidences of adverse reactions listed in the following table are derived from controlled and open clinical trials involving 1183 patients, of whom 785 received ALFENTA. The controlled trials involved treatment comparisons with fentanyl, thiopental sodium, enflurane, saline placebo and halothane. Incidences are based on disturbing and nondisturbing adverse reactions reported. The comparative incidence of certain side effects is influenced by the type of use, e.g., chest wall rigidity has a higher reported incidence in clinical trials of alfentanil induction, and by the type of surgery, e.g., nausea and vomiting have a higher incidence in patients undergoing gynecologic surgery.
[See table above].

In addition, other adverse reactions less frequently reported (1% or less) were:

Laryngospasm, bronchospasm, postoperative confusion, headache, shivering, postoperative euphoria, hypercarbia, pain on injection, urticaria, and itching.

Some degree of skeletal muscle rigidity should be expected with induction doses of ALFENTA.

DRUG ABUSE AND DEPENDENCE
ALFENTA (alfentanil hydrochloride) is a Schedule II controlled drug substance that can produce drug dependence of the morphine type and therefore has the potential for being abused.

OVERDOSAGE
Overdosage would be manifested by extension of the pharmacological actions of ALFENTA (alfentanil hydrochloride) (see CLINICAL PHARMACOLOGY) as with other potent opioid analgesics. No experience of overdosage with ALFENTA was reported during clinical trials. The intravenous LD_{50} of ALFENTA is 43.0–50.9 mg/kg in rats, 72.2–73.6 mg/kg in mice, 71.8–81.9 mg/kg in guinea pigs and 59.5–87.5 mg/kg in dogs. Intravenous administration of an opioid antagonist such as naloxone should be employed as a specific antidote to manage respiratory depression.

The duration of respiratory depression following overdosage with ALFENTA may be longer than the duration of action of the opioid antagonist. Administration of an opioid antagonist should not preclude immediate establishment of a patent airway, administration of oxygen, and assisted or controlled ventilation as indicated for hypoventilation or apnea. If respiratory depression is associated with muscular rigidity, a neuromuscular blocking agent may be required to facilitate assisted or controlled ventilation. Intravenous fluids and vasoactive agents may be required to manage hemodynamic instability.

DOSAGE AND ADMINISTRATION
The dosage of ALFENTA (alfentanil hydrochloride) should be individualized in each patient according to body weight, physical status, underlying pathological condition, use of other drugs, and type and duration of surgical procedure and anesthesia. In obese patients (more than 20% above ideal total body weight), the dosage of ALFENTA should be deter-

Continued on next page

Janssen—Cont.

mined on the basis of lean body weight. The dose of AL-FENTA should be reduced in elderly or debilitated patients (see PRECAUTIONS).

Vital signs should be monitored routinely.

See Dosage Chart for the use of ALFENTA: 1) by incremental injection as an analgesic adjunct to anesthesia with barbiturate/nitrous oxide/oxygen for short surgical procedures (expected duration of less than one hour); 2) by continuous infusion as a maintenance analgesic with nitrous oxide/oxygen for general surgical procedures; and 3) by intravenous injection in anesthetic doses for the induction of anesthesia for general surgical procedures with a minimum expected duration of 45 minutes.

Usage in Children: Clinical data to support the use of AL-FENTA in patients under 12 years of age are not presently available. Therefore, such use is not recommended.

Premedication: The selection of preanesthetic medications should be based upon the needs of the individual patient.

Neuromuscular Blocking Agents: The neuromuscular blocking agent selected should be compatible with the patient's condition, taking into account the hemodynamic effects of a particular muscle relaxant and the degree of skeletal muscle relaxation required (see CLINICAL PHARMACOLOGY, WARNINGS and PRECAUTIONS sections).

In patients administered anesthetic (induction) dosages of ALFENTA, it is essential that qualified personnel and adequate facilities are available for the management of intraoperative and postoperative respiratory depression.

Also see WARNINGS and PRECAUTIONS sections.

For purposes of administering small volumes of ALFENTA accurately, the use of a tuberculin syringe or equivalent is recommended.

The physical and chemical compatibility of ALFENTA have been demonstrated in solution with normal saline, 5% dextrose in normal saline, 5% dextrose in water and Lactated Ringers. Clinical studies of ALFENTA infusion have been conducted with ALFENTA diluted to a concentration range of 25 μg/ml to 80 μg/ml.

As an example of the preparation of ALFENTA for infusion, 20 ml of ALFENTA added to 230 ml of diluent provides a 40 μg/ml solution of ALFENTA.

Parenteral drug products should be inspected visually for particulate matter and discoloration prior to administration, whenever solution and container permit.

[See table below].

INFUSION DOSAGE

Continuous Infusion: 0.5–3.0 μg/kg/min administered with nitrous oxide/oxygen in patients undergoing general surgery. Following an anesthetic induction dose of ALFENTA, infusion rate requirements are reduced by 30–50% for the first hour of maintenance.

Changes in vital signs that indicate a response to surgical stress or lightening of anesthesia may be controlled by increasing the rate up to a maximum of 4.0 μg/kg/min and/or administration of bolus doses of 7 μg/kg. If changes are not controlled after three bolus doses given over a five minute period, a barbiturate, vasodilator, and/or inhalation agent should be used.

DOSAGE RANGE CHART

Indication	Approximate Duration of Anesthesia	Induction Period (Initial Dose)	Maintenance Period (Increments/ Infusion)	Total Dose	Effects
Incremental Injection	≤ 30 mins	8–20 μg/kg	3–5 μg/kg or 0.5–1 μg/kg/min	8–40 μg/kg	Spontaneously breathing or assisted ventilation when required.
Incremental Injection	30–60 mins	20–50 μg/kg	5–15 μg/kg	up to 75 μg/kg	Assisted or controlled ventilation required. Attenuation of response to laryngoscopy and intubation.
Continuous Infusion See Guidelines Below	> 45 mins	50–75 μg/kg	0.5–3.0 μg/kg/min Average Infusion Rate 1–1.5 μg/kg/min	dependent on duration of procedure	Assisted or controlled ventilation required. Some attenuation of response to intubation and incision, with intraoperative stability.
Anesthetic Induction	> 45 mins	130–245 μg/kg	0.5 to 1.5 μg/kg/min or general anesthetic	dependent on duration of procedure	Assisted or controlled ventilation required. Administer slowly (over three minutes). Concentration of inhalation agents reduced by 30–50% for initial hour.

Infusion rates should always be adjusted downward in the absence of these signs until there is some response to surgical stimulation.

Rather than an increase in infusion rate, 7 μg/kg bolus doses of ALFENTA or a potent inhalation agent should be administered in response to signs of lightening of anesthesia within the last 15 minutes of surgery. Administration of ALFENTA infusion should be discontinued at least 10–15 minutes prior to the end of surgery.

HOW SUPPLIED

Each ml of ALFENTA (alfentanil hydrochloride) Injection for intravenous use contains alfentanil hydrochloride equivalent to 500 μg of alfentanil base. ALFENTA Injection is available as:

NDC 50458-060-02, 2 ml ampoules in packages of 10
NDC 50458-060-05, 5 ml ampoules in packages of 10
NDC 50458-060-10, 10 ml ampoules in packages of 5
NDC 50458-060-20, 20 ml ampoules in packages of 5
Protect from light. Store at room temperature 15°–30°C (59°–86°F).
U.S. Patent No. 4,167,574
March, 1987, April 1988
JANSSEN PHARMACEUTICA Inc.
Piscataway, N.J. 08854
Shown in Product Identification Section, page 412

HISMANAL®   ℞
[his 'ma-nal]
(astemizole) Tablets

DESCRIPTION

HISMANAL® (astemizole) is a histamine H$_1$-receptor antagonist available in scored white tablets for oral use. Each tablet contains 10 mg of astemizole and, as inactive ingredients: lactose, cornstarch, microcrystalline cellulose, pregelatinized starch, povidone K90, magnesium stearate, colloidal silicon dioxide, and sodium lauryl sulfate. Astemizole is chemically designated as 1-[(4-fluorophenyl)-methyl]-N-[1-2-(4-methoxyphenyl)ethyl]-4-piperidinyl]-1H-benzimidazol-2-amine, with a molecular weight of 458.58. The empirical formula is $C_{28}H_{31}FN_4O$.

Astemizole is a white to slightly off-white powder; it is insoluble in water, slightly soluble in ethanol and soluble in chloroform and methanol.

CLINICAL PHARMACOLOGY

HISMANAL is a long-acting, selective histamine H$_1$-receptor antagonist. Receptor binding studies in animals demonstrated that at pharmacological doses, HISMANAL occupies peripheral H$_1$-receptors but does not reach H$_1$-receptors in the brain. Whole body autoradiographic studies in rats, radiolabel tissue distribution studies in dogs and radioligand binding studies of guinea pig brain H$_1$-receptors have shown that HISMANAL does not readily cross the blood-brain barrier. Screening studies in rats at effective antihistaminic doses showed no anticholinergic effects. Studies in humans using the recommended dosage regimens have not been performed to determine whether HISMANAL is associated with a different frequency of anticholinergic effects than therapeutic doses of other antihistamines.

The absorption of HISMANAL is reduced by 60% when taken with meals. In single oral dose studies, HISMANAL was rapidly absorbed from the gastrointestinal tract; peak plasma concentrations of unchanged HISMANAL were reached within one hour. Due to extensive first pass metabolism and significant tissue distribution, plasma concentrations of unchanged drug were low. Elimination of unchanged HISMANAL occurred with a half-life of approximately one day. Elimination of HISMANAL plus hydroxylated metabolites, considered together to represent the pharmacologically active fraction in plasma, was biphasic with half-lives of 20 hours for the distribution phase and 7–11 days for the elimination phase. The pharmacokinetics of HISMANAL plus hydroxylated metabolites are dose proportional following single doses of 10 to 30 mg.

Following chronic administration, steady state plasma concentrations of HISMANAL plus hydroxylated metabolites (mainly desmethylastemizole) were reached within four to eight weeks; HISMANAL plus hydroxylated metabolites decayed biphasically with an initial half-life of 7–9 days, with plasma concentrations being reduced by 75% within this phase, and with a terminal half-life of about 19 days. The initial phase ($t_{1/2}$ = 7–9 days) appears to determine the time to reach steady state plasma concentrations of HISMANAL plus hydroxylated metabolites. Steady state plasma concentrations of unchanged HISMANAL were reached by 6 days (with a range of 6–9 days); unchanged HISMANAL was eliminated from plasma with a half-life of approximately 2 days (with a range of 1–2.5 days).

Excretion and metabolism studies with ^{14}C-labeled HISMANAL in volunteers demonstrated that the drug is almost completely metabolized in the liver and primarily excreted in the feces.

Interpatient variability in pharmacokinetic parameters may be greater in patients with liver disease as compared to normal subjects.

The in-vitro plasma protein binding of unchanged HISMANAL (100 ng/ml) was 96.7% with 2.3% being found as free drug in the plasma water. In human blood with an astemizole concentration of 100 ng/ml, 61.5% of astemizole was bound to the plasma proteins, with 36.2% being distributed to the blood cell fraction. The concentration of astemizole found in the blood was the same as that found in the plasma fraction of the blood. Binding studies for the astemizole metabolite(s) which achieve much higher concentrations than astemizole under chronic dosing conditions have not been conducted.

INDICATIONS AND USAGE

HISMANAL tablets are indicated for the relief of symptoms associated with seasonal allergic rhinitis and chronic idiopathic urticaria. Clinical trials have not been conducted to show whether HISMANAL is effective for short courses of therapy.

CONTRAINDICATIONS

HISMANAL is contraindicated in patients with known hypersensitivity to astemizole or any of the inactive ingredients.

PRECAUTIONS

General: Caution should be given to potential anticholinergic (drying) effects in patients with lower airway diseases, including asthma.

Caution should be used in patients with cirrhosis or other liver diseases (See Clinical Pharmacology section).

HISMANAL does not appear to be dialyzable.

Caution should also be used when treating patients with renal impairment.

Information for Patients: Patients taking HISMANAL should receive the following information and instructions. Antihistamines are prescribed to reduce allergic symptoms. Patients should be questioned about pregnancy or lactation before starting HISMANAL therapy, since the drug should be used in pregnancy or lactation only if the potential benefit justifies the potential risk to fetus or baby (see Pregnancy subsection). Patients should be instructed 1) to take HISMANAL only as needed, 2) not to exceed the prescribed dose, and 3) to take HISMANAL on an empty stomach, e.g., at least 2 hours after a meal. No additional food should be taken for at least 1 hour post-dosing. Patients should also be instructed to store this medication in a tightly closed container in a cool, dry place, away from heat or direct sunlight, and away from children.

Carcinogenesis, Mutagenesis, Impairment of Fertility: Carcinogenic potential has not been revealed in rats given 260× the recommended human dose of astemizole for 24 months, or in mice given 400× the recommended human dose for 18 months. Micronucleus, dominant lethal, sister chromatid exchange and Ames tests of astemizole have not revealed mutagenic activity.

Impairment of fertility was not observed in male or female rats given 200× the recommended human dose.

Pregnancy: Pregnancy Category C: Teratogenic effects were not observed in rats administered 200× the recommended human dose or in rabbits given 200× the recommended human dose. Maternal toxicity was seen in rabbits administered 200× the recommended human dose. Embryocidal effects accompanied by maternal toxicity were observed at $100\times$ the recommended human dose in rats. Embryotoxicity or maternal toxicity was not observed in rats or rabbits administered $50\times$ the recommended human dose. There are no adequate and well controlled studies in pregnant women. HISMANAL should be used during pregnancy only if the potential benefit justifies the potential risk to the fetus. Metabolites may remain in the body for as long as 4 months after the end of dosing, calculated on the basis of 6 times the terminal half-life (See Clinical Pharmacology section).

Nursing Mothers: It is not known whether this drug is excreted in human milk. Because certain drugs are known to be excreted in human milk, caution should be exercised when HISMANAL is administered to a nursing woman. HISMANAL is excreted in the milk of dogs.

Pediatric Use: Safety and efficacy in children under 12 years of age has not been demonstrated.

ADVERSE REACTIONS

The reported incidences of adverse reactions listed in the following table are derived from controlled clinical studies in adults. In these studies the usual maintenance dose of HISMANAL® (astemizole) was 10 mg once daily.
[See table right].

Adverse reaction information has been obtained from more than 7500 patients in all clinical trials. Weight gain has been reported in 3.6% of astemizole treated patients involved in controlled studies, with an average treatment duration of 53 days. In 46 of the 59 patients for whom actual weight gain data was available, the average weight gain was 3.2 kg. Less frequently occurring adverse experiences reported in clinical trials or spontaneously from marketing experience with HISMANAL include: angioedema, bronchospasm, depression, edema, epistaxis, myalgia, palpitation, photosensitivity, pruritus, and rash.

Marketing experiences include isolated cases of convulsions. A causal relationship with HISMANAL has not been established.

OVERDOSAGE

In the event of overdosage, supportive measures including gastric lavage and emesis should be employed. Cases of overdose have been reported from foreign marketing experience. Although overdoses of up to 500 mg have been reported with no ill effects, cases of serious ventricular arrhythmias, including Torsades de pointes, following overdoses of greater than 200 mg have been reported. Patients should be carefully observed and ECG monitoring is recommended in cases of suspected overdose. An appropriate antiarrhythmic treatment may be needed. HISMANAL does not appear to be dialyzable.

Care should be taken not to exceed dosing recommended in the DOSAGE AND ADMINISTRATION section.

Oral LD_{50} values for HISMANAL were 2052 mg/kg in mice and 3154 mg/kg in rats. In neonatal rats, the oral LD_{50} was 905 mg/kg in males and 1235 mg/kg in females.

DOSAGE AND ADMINISTRATION

The recommended maintenance dosage for adults and children 12 years of age and older is 10 mg (1 tablet) once daily. HISMANAL pharmacokinetics are dose proportional following single doses of 10 to 30 mg. To reduce the time to steady state concentration, a single dose of 30 mg (three 10 mg tablets) may be administered on the first day, 20 mg (two 10 mg tablets) on the second day of therapy, followed by the recommended 10 mg daily dose.

HISMANAL should be taken on an empty stomach, e.g., at least two hours after a meal. There should be no additional food intake for at least one hour post-dosing.

HOW SUPPLIED

HISMANAL is available as white, scored tablets containing 10 mg of astemizole debossed "JANSSEN" and on the reverse side debossed "AST"/$_{10}$.
NDC 50458-510-01
(10 × 10 blister)
NDC 50458-510-10
(100 tablets)
Store tablets at room temperature (59°–86°F) (15°–30°C). Protect from moisture.
U.S. Patent 4,219,559
December 1988
JANSSEN PHARMACEUTICA INC.
Piscataway, New Jersey 08854
Shown in Product Identification Section, page 412

IMODIUM®   ℞
(loperamide HCl) Capsules

DESCRIPTION

IMODIUM (loperamide hydrochloride), 4-(p-chlorophenyl)-4-hydroxy-N, N-dimethyl-α,α-diphenyl-1-piperidinebutyramide monohydrochloride, is a synthetic antidiarrheal for oral use.

IMODIUM is available in 2 mg capsules.
The inactive ingredients are:
Lactose, magnesium stearate, starch, and talc.
IMODIUM capsules contain F D & C Yellow No. 6.

CLINICAL PHARMACOLOGY

In vitro and animal studies show that IMODIUM acts by slowing intestinal motility and by affecting water and electrolyte movement through the bowel. IMODIUM inhibits peristaltic activity by a direct effect on the circular and longitudinal muscles of the intestinal wall.

In man, IMODIUM prolongs the transit time of the intestinal contents. It reduces the daily fecal volume, increases the viscosity and bulk density, and diminishes the loss of fluid and electrolytes. Tolerance to the antidiarrheal effect has not been observed.

Clinical studies have indicated that the apparent elimination half-life of loperamide in man is 10.8 hours with a range of 9.1–14.4 hours. Plasma levels of unchanged drug remain below 2 nanograms per ml after the intake of a 2 mg capsule of IMODIUM. Plasma levels are highest approximately five hours after administration of the capsule and 2.5 hours after the liquid. The peak plasma levels of loperamide were similar for both formulations. Of the total excreted in urine and feces, most of the administered drug was excreted in feces. In those patients in whom biochemical and hematological parameters were monitored during clinical trials, no trends toward abnormality during IMODIUM therapy were noted. Similarly, urinalyses, EKG and clinical ophthalmological examinations did not show trends toward abnormality.

INDICATIONS AND USAGE

IMODIUM is indicated for the control and symptomatic relief of acute nonspecific diarrhea and of chronic diarrhea associated with inflammatory bowel disease. IMODIUM is also indicated for reducing the volume of discharge from ileostomies.

CONTRAINDICATIONS

IMODIUM is contraindicated in patients with known hypersensitivity to the drug and in those in whom constipation must be avoided.

WARNINGS

IMODIUM should not be used in the case of acute dysentery, which is characterized by blood in stools and elevated temperatures.

Fluid and electrolyte depletion may occur in patients who have diarrhea. The use of IMODIUM does not preclude the administration of appropriate fluid and electrolyte therapy. In some patients with acute ulcerative colitis, and in pseudomembranous colitis associated with broad-spectrum antibiotics, agents which inhibit intestinal motility or delay intestinal transit time have been reported to induce toxic megacolon. IMODIUM therapy should be discontinued promptly if abdominal distention occurs or if other untoward symptoms develop in patients with acute ulcerative colitis.

IMODIUM should be used with special caution in young children because of the greater variability of response in this age group. Dehydration, particularly in younger children, may further influence the variability of response to IMODIUM.

PRECAUTIONS

General: In acute diarrhea, if clinical improvement is not observed in 48 hours, the administration of IMODIUM should be discontinued.

Patients with hepatic dysfunction should be monitored closely for signs of CNS toxicity because of the apparent large first pass biotransformation.

Information for Patients: Patients should be advised to check with their physician if their diarrhea doesn't stop after a few days or if they develop a fever.

Drug Interactions: There was no evidence in clinical trials of drug interactions with concurrent medications.

Carcinogenesis, mutagenesis, impairment of fertility: In an 18-month rat study with doses up to 133 times the maximum human dose (on a mg/kg basis), there was no evidence of carcinogenesis. Mutagenicity studies were not conducted. Reproduction studies in rats indicated that high doses (150–200 times the human dose) could cause marked female infertility and reduced male fertility.

Pregnancy
Teratogenic Effects
Pregnancy Category B: Reproduction studies in rats and rabbits have revealed no evidence of impaired fertility or harm to the fetus at doses up to 30 times the human dose. Higher doses impaired the survival of mothers and nursing young. The studies offered no evidence of teratogenic activity. There are, however, no adequate and well controlled studies in pregnant women. Because animal reproduction studies are not always predictive of human response, this drug should be used during pregnancy only if clearly needed.

Nursing Mothers: It is not known whether this drug is excreted in human milk. Because many drugs are excreted in human milk, caution should be exercised when IMODIUM is administered to a nursing woman.

Pediatric Use: See the "Warnings" Section for information on the greater variability of response in this age group. In case of accidental overdosage of IMODIUM by children, see "Overdosage" Section for suggested treatment.

ADVERSE REACTIONS

The adverse effects reported during clinical investigations of IMODIUM are difficult to distinguish from symptoms associated with the diarrheal syndrome. Adverse experiences recorded during clinical studies with IMODIUM were generally of a minor and self-limiting nature. They were more commonly observed during the treatment of chronic diarrhea.

The following patient complaints have been reported and are listed in decreasing order of frequency with the exception of hypersensitivity reactions which is listed first since it may be the most serious.

- Hypersensitivity reactions (including skin rash) have been reported with IMODIUM use.
- Abdominal pain, distention or discomfort
- Nausea and vomiting
- Constipation
- Tiredness
- Drowsiness or dizziness
- Dry mouth

DRUG ABUSE AND DEPENDENCE

Abuse: A specific clinical study designed to assess the abuse potential of loperamide at high doses resulted in a finding of extremely low abuse potential. Additionally, after years of extensive use there has been no evidence of abuse or dependence.

Continued on next page

	Percent of Patients Reporting		
	Controlled Studies*		
ADVERSE EVENT	Hismanal (N=1630) %	Placebo (N=1109) %	Classical** (N=304) %
Central Nervous System			
Drowsiness	7.1	6.4	22.0
Headache	6.7	9.2	3.3
Fatigue	4.2	1.6	11.8
Appetite increase	3.9	1.4	0.0
Weight increase	3.6	0.7	1.0
Nervousness	2.1	1.2	0.3
Dizzy	2.0	1.8	1.0
Gastrointestinal System			
Nausea	2.5	2.9	1.3
Diarrhea	1.8	2.0	0.7
Abdominal pain	1.4	1.2	0.7
Eye, Ear, Nose, and Throat			
Mouth dry	5.2	3.8	7.9
Pharyngitis	1.7	2.3	0.3
Conjunctivitis	1.2	1.2	0.7
Other			
Arthralgia	1.2	1.6	0.0

*Duration of treatment in Controlled Studies ranged from 7 to 182 Days
**Classical Drugs: Clemastine (N=137); Chlorpheniramine (N=100); Pheniramine Maleate (N=47); d-Chlorpheniramine (N=20)

Janssen—Cont.

Dependence: Physical dependence to IMODIUM in humans has not been observed. However, studies in morphine-dependent monkeys demonstrated that loperamide hydrochloride at doses above those recommended for humans prevented signs of morphine withdrawal. However, in humans, the naloxone challenge pupil test, which when positive indicates opiate-like effects, performed after a single high dose, or after more than two years of therapeutic use of IMODIUM, was negative. Orally administered IMODIUM (loperamide formulated with magnesium stearate) is both highly insoluble and penetrates the CNS poorly.

OVERDOSAGE

Animal pharmacological and toxicological data indicate that overdosage in man may result in constipation, CNS depression and gastrointestinal irritation. Clinical trials have demonstrated that a slurry of activated charcoal administered promptly after ingestion of loperamide hydrochloride can reduce the amount of drug which is absorbed into the systemic circulation by as much as ninefold. If vomiting occurs spontaneously upon ingestion, a slurry of 100 gms of activated charcoal should be administered orally as soon as fluids can be retained.

If vomiting has not occurred, gastric lavage should be performed followed by administration of 100 gms of the activated charcoal slurry through the gastric tube. In the event of overdosage, patients should be monitored for signs of CNS depression for at least 24 hours. Children may be more sensitive to central nervous system effects than adults. If CNS depression is observed, naloxone may be administered. If responsive to naloxone, vital signs must be monitored carefully for recurrence of symptoms of drug overdose for at least 24 hours after the last dose of naloxone.

In view of the prolonged action of loperamide and the short duration (one to three hours) of naloxone, the patient must be monitored closely and treated repeatedly with naloxone as indicated. Since relatively little drug is excreted in the urine, forced diuresis is not expected to be effective for IMODIUM overdosage.

In clinical trials an adult who took three 20 mg doses within a 24 hour period was nauseated after the second dose and vomited after the third dose. In studies designed to examine the potential for side effects, intentional ingestion of up to 60 mg of loperamide hydrochloride in a single dose to healthy subjects resulted in no significant adverse effects.

DOSAGE AND ADMINISTRATION

(1 capsule = 2 mg.)

Acute Diarrhea

Adults: The recommended initial dose is 4 mg (two capsules) followed by 2 mg (one capsule) after each unformed stool. Daily dosage should not exceed 16 mg (eight capsules). Clinical improvement is usually observed within 48 hours.

Children: IMODIUM use is not recommended for children under 2 years of age. In children 2 to 5 years of age (20 kg or less), the non-prescription liquid formulation (IMODIUM A-D 1 mg/5 ml) should be used; for ages 6 to 12, either IMODIUM Capsules or IMODIUM A-D Liquid may be used. For children 2 to 12 years of age, the following schedule for capsules or liquid will usually fulfill initial dosage requirements:

Recommended First Day Dosage Schedule

Two to five years:	1 mg t.i.d.	
(13 to 20 kg)	(3 mg daily dose)	
Six to eight years:	2 mg b.i.d.	
(20 to 30 kg)	(4 mg daily dose)	
Eight to twelve years:	2 mg t.i.d.	
(greater than 30 kg)	(6 mg daily dose)	

Recommended Subsequent Daily Dosage

Following the first treatment day, it is recommended that subsequent IMODIUM doses (1 mg/10 kg body weight) be administered only after a loose stool. Total daily dosage should not exceed recommended dosages for the first day.

Chronic Diarrhea

Children: Although IMODIUM has been studied in a limited number of children with chronic diarrhea, the therapeutic dose for the treatment of chronic diarrhea in a pediatric population has not been established.

Adults: The recommended initial dose is 4 mg (two capsules) followed by 2 mg (one capsule) after each unformed stool until diarrhea is controlled, after which the dosage of IMODIUM should be reduced to meet individual requirements. When the optimal daily dosage has been established, this amount may then be administered as a single dose or in divided doses.

The average daily maintenance dosage in clinical trials was 4 to 8 mg (two to four capsules). A dosage of 16 mg (eight capsules) was rarely exceeded. If clinical improvement is not observed after treatment with 16 mg per day for at least 10 days, symptoms are unlikely to be controlled by further administration. IMODIUM administration may be continued if diarrhea cannot be adequately controlled with diet or specific treatment.

HOW SUPPLIED

Capsules—each capsule contains 2 mg of loperamide hydrochloride. The capsules have a light green body and a dark green cap with "JANSSEN" imprinted on one segment and "IMODIUM" on the other segment. IMODIUM capsules are supplied in bottles of 100 and 500 and in blister packs of 10 × 10 capsules.
NDC 50458-400-01
(10 × 10 capsules—blister)
NDC 50458-400-10
(100 capsules)
NDC 50458-400-50
(500 capsules)
Protect from light. Store at room temperature 15°–30°C (59°–86°F)
Revised March 1988, May 1988
CAUTION: FEDERAL LAW PROHIBITS DISPENSING WITHOUT A PRESCRIPTION
JANSSEN PHARMACEUTICA INC.
Piscataway
New Jersey 08854
Printed in USA
U.S. Patent 3,714,159
Shown in Product Identification Section, page 412

INAPSINE®   ℞
[ĭn-ăp-sēn]
(droperidol) Injection
FOR INTRAVENOUS OR INTRAMUSCULAR USE ONLY

DESCRIPTION

INAPSINE (droperidol) is a neuroleptic (tranquilizer) agent available in ampoules and vials. Each milliliter contains 2.5 mg. of droperidol in an aqueous solution adjusted to pH 3.4 ± 0.4 with lactic acid. INAPSINE in 10 ml multidose vials also contains 1.8 mg of methylparaben and 0.2 mg propylparaben. Droperidol is chemically identified as 1-(1-[3-(p-fluorobenzoyl) propyl]-1,2,3,6-tetrahydro-4-pyridyl)-2-benzimidazolinone with a molecular weight of 379.43.
INAPSINE is a sterile, non-pyrogenic aqueous solution for intravenous or intramuscular injection.

CLINICAL PHARMACOLOGY

INAPSINE (droperidol) produces marked tranquilization and sedation. It allays apprehension and provides a state of mental detachment and indifference while maintaining a state of reflex alertness.

INAPSINE produces an antiemetic effect as evidenced by the antagonism of apomorphine in dogs. It lowers the incidence of nausea and vomiting during surgical procedures and provides antiemetic protection in the postoperative period.

INAPSINE potentiates other CNS depressants. It produces mild alpha-adrenergic blockade, peripheral vascular dilatation and reduction of the pressor effect of epinephrine. It can produce hypotension and decreased peripheral vascular resistance and may decrease pulmonary arterial pressure (particularly if it is abnormally high). It may reduce the incidence of epinephrine-induced arrhythmias, but it does not prevent other cardiac arrhythmias.

The onset of action of single intramuscular and intravenous doses is from three to ten minutes following administration, although the peak effect may not be apparent for up to thirty minutes. The duration of the tranquilizing and sedative effects generally is two to four hours, although alteration of alertness may persist for as long as twelve hours.

INDICATIONS AND USAGE

INAPSINE (droperidol) is indicated:
* to produce tranquilization and to reduce the incidence of nausea and vomiting in surgical and diagnostic procedures.
* for premedication, induction, and as an adjunct in the maintenance of general and regional anesthesia.
* in neuroleptanalgesia in which INAPSINE is given concurrently with an opioid analgesic, such as SUBLIMAZE (fentanyl citrate) Injection, to aid in producing tranquility and decreasing anxiety and pain.

CONTRAINDICATIONS

INAPSINE (droperidol) is contraindicated in patients with known hypersensitivity to the drug.

WARNINGS

FLUIDS AND OTHER COUNTERMEASURES TO MANAGE HYPOTENSION SHOULD BE READILY AVAILABLE.
As with other CNS depressant drugs, patients who have received INAPSINE (droperidol) should have appropriate surveillance.
It is recommended that opioids, when required, initially be used in reduced doses.

PRECAUTIONS

General: The initial dose of INAPSINE (droperidol) should be appropriately reduced in elderly, debilitated and other poor-risk patients. The effect of the initial dose should be considered in determining incremental doses.

Certain forms of conduction anesthesia, such as spinal anesthesia and some peridural anesthetics, can alter respiration by blocking intercostal nerves and can cause peripheral vasodilatation and hypotension because of sympathetic blockade. Through other mechanisms (see CLINICAL PHARMACOLOGY), INAPSINE can also alter circulation. Therefore, when INAPSINE is used to supplement these forms of anesthesia, the anesthetist should be familiar with the physiological alterations involved, and be prepared to manage them in the patients elected for these forms of anesthesia.

If hypotension occurs, the possibility of hypovolemia should be considered and managed with appropriate parenteral fluid therapy. Repositioning the patient to improve venous return to the heart should be considered when operative conditions permit. It should be noted that in spinal and peridural anesthesia, tilting the patient into a head-down position may result in a higher level of anesthesia than is desirable, as well as impair venous return to the heart. Care should be exercised in moving and positioning of patients because of a possibility of orthostatic hypotension. If volume expansion with fluids plus these other countermeasures do not correct the hypotension, then the administration of pressor agents other than epinephrine should be considered. Epinephrine may paradoxically decrease the blood pressure in patients treated with INAPSINE due to the alpha-adrenergic blocking action of INAPSINE.

Since INAPSINE may decrease pulmonary arterial pressure, this fact should be considered by those who conduct diagnostic or surgical procedures where interpretation of pulmonary arterial pressure measurements might determine final management of the patient.

Vital signs should be monitored routinely.

When the EEG is used for postoperative monitoring, it may be found that the EEG pattern returns to normal slowly.

Impaired Hepatic or Renal Function: INAPSINE should be administered with caution to patients with liver and kidney dysfunction because of the importance of these organs in the metabolism and excretion of drugs.

Drug Interactions: Other CNS depressant drugs (e.g. barbiturates, tranquilizers, opioids and general anesthetics) have additive or potentiating effects with INAPSINE. When patients have received such drugs, the dose of INAPSINE required will be less than usual. Following the administration of INAPSINE, the dose of other CNS depressant drugs should be reduced.

Carcinogenesis, Mutagenesis, Impairment of Fertility: No carcinogenicity studies have been carried out with INAPSINE. The micronucleus test in female rats revealed no mutagenic effects in single oral doses as high as 160 mg/kg. An oral study in rats (Segment I) revealed no impairment of fertility in either male or females at 0.63, 2.5 and 10 mg/kg doses (approximately 2, 9 and 36 times maximum recommended human iv/im dosage).

Pregnancy—Category C: INAPSINE administered intravenously has been shown to cause a slight increase in mortality of the newborn rat at 4.4 times the upper human dose. At 44 times the upper human dose, mortality rate was comparable to that for control animals. Following intramuscular administration, increased mortality of the offspring at 1.8 times the upper human dose is attributed to CNS depression in the dams who neglected to remove placentae from their offspring. INAPSINE has not been shown to be teratogenic in animals. There are no adequate and well-controlled studies in pregnant women. INAPSINE should be used during pregnancy only if the potential benefit justifies the potential risk to the fetus.

Labor and Delivery: There are insufficient data to support the use of INAPSINE in labor and delivery. Therefore, such use is not recommended.

Nursing Mothers: It is not known whether INAPSINE is excreted in human milk. Because many drugs are excreted in human milk, caution should be exercised when INAPSINE is administered to a nursing mother.

Pediatric Use: The safety of INAPSINE in children younger than two years of age has not been established.

ADVERSE REACTIONS

The most common adverse reactions reported to occur with INAPSINE (droperidol) are mild to moderate hypotension and tachycardia, but these effects usually subside without treatment. If hypotension occurs and is severe or persists, the possibility of hypovolemia should be considered and managed with appropriate parenteral fluid therapy. Postoperative drowsiness is also frequently reported.

Extrapyramidal symptoms (dystonia, akathisia, and oculogyric crisis) have been observed following administration of INAPSINE. Restlessness, hyperactivity and anxiety which can be either the result of inadequate dosage of INAPSINE or a part of the symptom complex of akathisia may occur. When extrapyramidal symptoms occur, they can usually be controlled with antiparkinson agents.

Other adverse reactions that have been reported are dizziness, chills and/or shivering, laryngospasm, bronchospasm and postoperative hallucinatory episodes (sometimes associated with transient periods of mental depression).

Elevated blood pressure, with or without pre-existing hypertension, has been reported following administration of INAPSINE combined with SUBLIMAZE (fentanyl citrate) or other parenteral analgesics. This might be due to unexplained alterations in sympathetic activity following large doses; however, it is also frequently attributed to anesthetic or surgical stimulation during light anesthesia.

OVERDOSAGE

Manifestations: The manifestations of INAPSINE (droperidol) overdosage are an extension of its pharmacologic actions.

Treatment: In the presence of hypoventilation or apnea, oxygen should be administered and respiration should be assisted or controlled as indicated. A patent airway must be maintained; an oropharyngeal airway or endotracheal tube might be indicated. The patient should be carefully observed for 24 hours; body warmth and adequate fluid intake should be maintained. If hypotension occurs and is severe or persists, the possibility of hypovolemia should be considered and managed with appropriate parenteral fluid therapy. (See PRECAUTIONS).

The intravenous LD_{50} of INAPSINE is 20–43 mg/kg in mice; 30 mg/kg in rats; 25 mg/kg in dogs and 11–13 mg/kg in rabbits. The intramuscular LD_{50} of INAPSINE is 195 mg/kg in mice; 104–110 mg/kg in rats; 97 mg/kg in rabbits and 200 mg/kg in guinea pigs.

DOSAGE AND ADMINISTRATION

Dosage should be individualized. Some of the factors to be considered in determining the dose are age, body weight, physical status, underlying pathological condition, use of other drugs, type of anesthesia to be used and the surgical procedure involved.

Vital signs should be monitored routinely.

Usual Adult Dosage

I.   **Premedication**—(to be appropriately modified in the elderly, debilitated and those who have received other depressant drugs) 2.5 to 10 mg (1 to 4 ml) may be administered intramuscularly 30 to 60 minutes preoperatively.

II. **Adjunct to General Anesthesia—**
Induction—2.5 mg (1 ml) per 20 to 25 pounds may be administered (usually intravenously) along with an analgesic and/or general anesthetic. Smaller doses may be adequate. The total amount of INAPSINE (droperidol) administered should be titrated to obtain the desired effect based on the individual patient's response.
Maintenance—1.25 to 2.5 mg (0.5 to 1 ml) usually intravenously.

III. *Use without a general anesthetic in diagnostic procedures*—Administer the usual I.M. premedication 2.5 to 10 mg (1 to 4 ml) 30 to 60 minutes before the procedure. Additional 1.25 to 2.5 mg (0.5 to 1 ml) amounts of INAPSINE may be administered, usually intravenously.
NOTE: When INAPSINE is used in certain procedures, such as bronchoscopy, appropriate topical anesthesia is still necessary.

IV. *Adjunct to regional anesthesia*—2.5 to 5 mg (1 to 2 ml) may be administered intramuscularly or slowly intravenously when additional sedation is required.

Usual Children's Dosage

For children two to 12 years of age, a reduced dose as low as 1.0 to 1.5 mg (0.4 to 0.6 ml) per 20 to 25 pounds is recommended for premedication or for induction of anesthesia.

See WARNINGS and PRECAUTIONS for use of INAPSINE with other CNS depressants and in patients with altered response.

Parenteral drug products should be inspected visually for particulate matter and discoloration prior to administration, whenever solution and container permit. If such abnormalities are observed, the drug should not be administered.

HOW SUPPLIED

INAPSINE (droperidol) Injection is available as:

NDC 50458-010-01, 2.5 mg/ml, 1 ml ampoules in packages of 10

NDC 50458-010-02, 2.5 mg/ml, 2 ml ampoules in packages of 10

NDC 50458-010-05, 2.5 mg/ml, 5 ml ampoules in packages of 10

NDC 50458-010-10, 2.5 mg/ml, 10 ml multiple-dose vials in packages of 10.

PROTECT FROM LIGHT. STORE AT ROOM TEMPERATURE 15°C–30°C (59°F–86°F).

Manufactured by TAYLOR PHARMACAL CO. for JANSSEN PHARMACEUTICA INC.
Piscataway, NJ 08854
U.S. Patent No. 3,161,645
Revised July 1986, November 1986

Shown in Product Identification Section, page 412

INNOVAR® INJECTION   Ⓒ Ⅱ ℞

[ĭn 'nō-vär]
(fentanyl citrate/droperidol) FOR INTRAVENOUS OR INTRAMUSCULAR USE ONLY

> The two components of INNOVAR Injection, fentanyl citrate and droperidol, have different pharmacologic actions. Before administering INNOVAR Injection, the user should become familiar with the special properties of each drug, particularly the widely differing durations of action.

DESCRIPTION

INNOVAR is a potent opioid analgesic (fentanyl citrate) and a neuroleptic (tranquilizer) agent (droperidol). Each milliliter contains (in a 1:50 ratio) fentanyl citrate equivalent to 50 µg of fentanyl base and 2.5 mg of droperidol in a solution adjusted to pH 3.5 ± 0.3 with lactic acid.

The chemical names and molecular weights of the two components of INNOVAR are: Fentanyl citrate N- (1-phenethyl-4-piperidyl) propionanilide citrate (1:1). Molecular weight: 528.60

Droperidol   1-[1-[3-(p-fluorobenzoyl)propyl]   -1,2,3,6-tetrahydro-4-pyridyl]-2- benzimidazolinone. Molecular weight: 379.43

INNOVAR is a sterile, preservative free aqueous solution for intravenous or intramuscular injection.

CLINICAL PHARMACOLOGY

INNOVAR (fentanyl citrate/droperidol) is a combination drug containing an opioid analgesic, fentanyl citrate, and a neuroleptic (major tranquilizer), droperidol. The combined effect, sometimes referred to as neuroleptanalgesia, is characterized by general quiescence, reduced motor activity, and profound analgesia; complete loss of consciousness usually does not occur from use of INNOVAR Injection alone. The incidence of early postoperative pain and emesis may be reduced.

A. Fentanyl citrate is an opioid analgesic. A dose of 100 µg (0.1 mg) (2.0 ml), is approximately equivalent in analgesic activity to 10 mg of morphine or 75 mg of meperidine. The principal actions of therapeutic value are analgesia and sedation. Alterations in respiratory rate and alveolar ventilation, associated with opioid analgesics, may last longer than the analgesic effect. As the dose of opioid is increased, the decrease in pulmonary exchange becomes greater. Large doses may produce apnea. Fentanyl citrate appears to have less emetic activity than either morphine or meperidine. Histamine assays and skin wheal testing in man indicate that clinically significant histamine release rarely occurs with fentanyl citrate. Assays in man show no clinically significant histamine release in dosages up to 50 µg/kg (0.05 mg/kg) (1 ml/kg). The pharmacokinetics of fentanyl citrate can be described as a three-compartment model, with a distribution time of 1.7 minutes, redistribution of 13 minutes and a terminal elimination half-life of 219 minutes. The volume of distribution for fentanyl citrate is 4 L/kg.

Fentanyl citrate plasma protein binding capacity increases with increasing ionization of the drug. Alterations in pH may affect its distribution between plasma and the central nervous system. It accumulates in skeletal muscle and fat, and is released slowly into the blood. Fentanyl citrate, which is primarily transformed in the liver, demonstrates a high first pass clearance and releases approximately 75% of an intravenous dose in urine, mostly as metabolites with less than 10% representing the unchanged drug. Approximately 9% of the dose is recovered in the feces, primarily as metabolites. The onset of action of fentanyl citrate is almost immediate when the drug is given intravenously; however, the maximal analgesic and respiratory depressant effect may not be noted for several minutes. The usual duration of action of the analgesic effect is 30 to 60 minutes after a single intravenous dose of up to 100 µg (0.1 mg) (2.0 ml). Following intramuscular administration, the onset of action is from seven to eight minutes, and the duration of action is one to two hours. As with longer acting opioid analgesics, the duration of the respiratory depressant effect of fentanyl citrate may be longer than the analgesic effect. The following observations have been reported concerning altered respiratory response to CO_2 stimulation following administration of fentanyl citrate to man:

1. DIMINISHED SENSITIVITY TO CO_2 STIMULATION MAY PERSIST LONGER THAN DEPRESSION OF RESPIRATORY RATE. [Altered sensitivity to CO_2 stimulation has been demonstrated for up to four hours following a single dose of 600 µg (0.6 mg) (12 ml) fentanyl citrate to healthy volunteers.] Fentanyl citrate frequently slows the respiratory rate, duration and degree of respiratory depression being dose related.

2. The peak respiratory depressant effect of a single intravenous dose of fentanyl citrate is noted 5 to 15 mi-

---

nutes following injection. See also WARNINGS and PRECAUTIONS concerning respiratory depression.

B. Droperidol produces marked tranquilization and sedation. Droperidol allays apprehension and provides a state of mental detachment and indifference while maintaining a state of reflex alertness.

Droperidol also produces an antiemetic effect as evidenced by the antagonism of apomorphine in dogs. It lowers the incidence of nausea and vomiting during surgical procedures and provides antiemetic protection in the postoperative period.

Droperidol potentiates other CNS depressants. It produces mild alpha-adrenergic blockade, peripheral vascular dilatation and reduction of the pressor effect of epinephrine. It can produce hypotension and decreased peripheral vascular resistance and may decrease pulmonary arterial pressure (particularly if it is abnormally high). It may reduce the incidence of epinephrine-induced arrhythmias, but does not prevent other cardiac arrhythmias.

The onset of action of single intramuscular and intravenous doses of droperidol is from three to ten minutes following administration, although the peak effect may not be apparent for up to thirty minutes. The duration of the tranquilizing and sedative effects generally is two to four hours, although alteration of consciousness may persist for as long as twelve hours. This is in contrast to the much shorter duration of fentanyl citrate.

INDICATIONS AND USAGE

INNOVAR (fentanyl citrate/droperidol) is indicated to produce tranquilization and analgesia for surgical and diagnostic procedures. It may be used as an anesthetic premedication, as an adjunct to the induction of anesthesia, and as an adjunct in the maintenance of general and regional anesthesia. If the supplementation of analgesia is necessary, SUBLIMAZE (fentanyl citrate) alone rather than the combination drug, INNOVAR, should usually be used, see DOSAGE AND ADMINISTRATION section.

CONTRAINDICATIONS

INNOVAR (fentanyl citrate/droperidol) is contraindicated in patients with known hypersensitivity to either component.

WARNINGS

INNOVAR (fentanyl citrate/droperidol) SHOULD BE ADMINISTERED ONLY BY PERSONS SPECIFICALLY TRAINED IN THE USE OF INTRAVENOUS ANESTHETICS AND MANAGEMENT OF THE RESPIRATORY EFFECTS OF POTENT OPIOIDS.

AN OPIOID ANTAGONIST, RESUSCITATIVE AND INTUBATION EQUIPMENT AND OXYGEN SHOULD BE READILY AVAILABLE.

See also discussion of opioid antagonists in PRECAUTIONS and OVERDOSAGE sections.

FLUIDS AND OTHER COUNTERMEASURES TO MANAGE HYPOTENSION SHOULD ALSO BE AVAILABLE.

The respiratory depressant effect of opioids persists longer than the measured analgesic effect. When used with INNOVAR, the total dose of all opioid analgesics administered should be considered by the practitioner before ordering opioid analgesics during recovery from anesthesia. It is recommended that opioids, when required, be used in reduced doses initially, as low as $\frac{1}{4}$ to $\frac{1}{3}$ those usually recommended.

INNOVAR may cause muscle rigidity, particularly involving the muscles of respiration. This effect is due to the fentanyl citrate component and is related to the dose and speed of injection. Its incidence can be reduced by the use of slow intravenous injection. Once the effect occurs, it is managed by the use of assisted or controlled respiration and, if necessary, by a neuromuscular blocking agent compatible with the patient's condition.

Head Injuries and Increased Intracranial Pressure: INNOVAR should be used with caution in patients who may be particularly susceptible to respiratory depression such as comatose patients who may have a head injury or brain tumor. In addition, INNOVAR may obscure the clinical course of patients with head injury.

PRECAUTIONS

General: The initial dose of INNOVAR (fentanyl citrate/droperidol) should be appropriately reduced in elderly, debilitated and other poor-risk patients. The effect of the initial dose should be considered in determining incremental doses. Certain forms of conduction anesthesia, such as spinal anesthesia and some peridural anesthetics, can alter respiration by blocking intercostal nerves and can cause peripheral vasodilation and hypotension because of sympathetic blockade. Through other mechanisms (see CLINICAL PHARMACOLOGY) fentanyl citrate and droperidol can also depress respiration and blood pressure. Therefore, when INNOVAR is used to supplement these forms of anesthesia, the anesthetist should be familiar with the physiological alterations

Continued on next page

Janssen—Cont.

involved, and be prepared to manage them in the patients selected for these forms of anesthesia.

The droperidol component of INNOVAR may decrease pulmonary arterial pressure. This fact should be considered by those who conduct diagnostic or surgical procedures where interpretation of pulmonary arterial pressure measurements might determine final management of the patient. Vital signs should be monitored routinely.

When the EEG is used for postoperative monitoring, it may be found that the EEG pattern returns to normal slowly.

Hypotension: If hypotension occurs, the possibility of hypovolemia should be considered and managed with appropriate parenteral fluid therapy. Repositioning the patient to improve venous return to the heart should be considered when operative conditions permit. It should be noted that in spinal and peridural anesthesia, tilting the patient into a head down position may result in a higher level of anesthesia than is desirable, as well as impair venous return to the heart. Care should be exercised in the moving and positioning of patients because of a possibility of orthostatic hypotension. If volume expansion with fluids plus these other countermeasures do not correct the hypotension, then the administration of pressor agents other than epinephrine should be considered. Epinephrine may paradoxically decrease the blood pressure in patients treated with INNOVAR due to the alpha-adrenergic blocking action of droperidol.

Impaired Respiration: INNOVAR and SUBLIMAZE (fentanyl citrate) should be used with caution in patients with chronic obstructive pulmonary disease, patients with decreased respiratory reserve and others with potentially compromised ventilation. In such patients opioids may additionally decrease respiratory drive and increase airway resistance. During anesthesia, this can be managed by assisted or controlled respiration. Respiratory depression caused by opioid analgesics can be reversed by opioid antagonists. Appropriate surveillance should be maintained because the duration of respiratory depression of doses of fentanyl citrate (as SUBLIMAZE (fentanyl citrate) or INNOVAR) employed during anesthesia may be longer than the duration of the opioid antagonist action. Consult individual prescribing information (levallorphan, nalorphine and naloxone) before employing opioid antagonists.

Impaired Hepatic or Renal Function: INNOVAR should be administered with caution to patients with liver and kidney dysfunction because of the importance of these organs in the metabolism and excretion of drugs.

Cardiovascular Effects: The fentanyl citrate component may produce bradycardia, which may be treated with atropine. INNOVAR should be used with caution in patients with cardiac bradyarrhythmias.

Drug Interactions: Other CNS depressant drugs (e.g. barbiturates, tranquilizers, opioids and general anesthetics) have additive or potentiating effects with INNOVAR. When patients have received such drugs, the dose of INNOVAR required will be less than usual. Following the administration of INNOVAR, the dose of other CNS depressant drugs should be reduced.

Carcinogenesis, Mutagenesis, Impairment of Fertility: No carcinogenicity studies have been conducted with INNOVAR or its components, SUBLIMAZE and INAPSINE. A subcutaneous study of INNOVAR in female rats revealed no impairment of fertility at doses 9 times the upper human dose. An intravenous study revealed no effects on fertility at 2 times the upper human dose (highest dosage level tested).

Pregnancy — Category C: INNOVAR had no embryotoxic effects in rats at intravenous doses approximately 2 times the upper human dose. A subcutaneous study of INNOVAR in female rats showed increased fetal resorptions at 18 times the upper human dose. No teratogenic effects were revealed at 36 times the upper human dose. In rabbits, increased resorptions and decreased litter size were found at intravenous doses approximately 2 times the upper human dose. Maternal mortality occurred at 7 times the upper human dose.

INNOVAR has not been shown to be teratogenic in animals. There are no adequate and well-controlled studies in pregnant women. INNOVAR should be used during pregnancy only if the potential benefit justifies the potential risk to the fetus.

Labor and Delivery: There are insufficient data to support the use of INNOVAR in labor and delivery. Therefore, such use is not recommended.

Nursing Mothers: It is not known whether fentanyl citrate or droperidol are excreted in human milk. Because many drugs are excreted in human milk, caution should be exercised when INNOVAR is administered to a nursing woman.

Pediatric Use: The safety and efficacy of INNOVAR in children under two years of age has not been established.

ADVERSE REACTIONS

The most common serious adverse reactions reported to occur with INNOVAR (fentanyl citrate/droperidol) are respiratory depression, apnea, muscular rigidity and hypoten-

sion; if these remain untreated, respiratory arrest, circulatory depression or cardiac arrest could occur.

Extrapyramidal symptoms (dystonia, akathisia and oculogyric crisis) have been observed following administration of INNOVAR. Restlessness, hyperactivity and anxiety which can be either the result of inadequate tranquilization or part of the symptom complex of akathisia may occur. When extrapyramidal symptoms occur, they can usually be controlled with anti-Parkinson agents.

Elevated blood pressure, with and without pre-existing hypertension, has been reported following administration of INNOVAR. This might be due to unexplained alterations of sympathetic activity following large doses; however, it is also frequently attributed to anesthetic or surgical stimulation during light anesthesia.

Postoperative drowsiness is also frequently reported.

Other adverse reactions that have been reported are dizziness, chills and/or shivering, twitching, blurred vision, laryngospasm, bronchospasm, bradycardia, tachycardia, nausea and emesis, diaphoresis, emergence delirium, and postoperative hallucinatory episodes (sometimes associated with transient periods of mental depression).

DRUG ABUSE AND DEPENDENCE

The fentanyl citrate component of INNOVAR (fentanyl citrate/droperidol) is a Schedule II opioid that can produce drug dependence of the morphine type and, therefore, has the potential for being abused.

OVERDOSAGE

MANIFESTATIONS: The manifestations of INNOVAR (fentanyl citrate/droperidol) overdosage are an extension of its pharmacologic actions.

TREATMENT: In the presence of hypoventilation or apnea, oxygen should be administered and respiration should be assisted or controlled as indicated. A patent airway must be maintained; an oropharyngeal airway or endotracheal tube might be indicated. If depressed respiration is associated with muscular rigidity, an intravenous neuromuscular blocking agent might be required to facilitate assisted or controlled respiration. The patient should be carefully observed for 24 hours; body warmth and adequate fluid intake should be maintained. If hypotension occurs and is severe or persists, the possibility of hypovolemia should be considered and managed with appropriate parenteral fluid therapy (See PRECAUTIONS). A specific opioid antagonist such as nalorphine, levallorphan or naloxone should be available for use as indicated to manage respiratory depression caused by the opioid component fentanyl citrate. This does not preclude the use of more immediate countermeasures. The duration of respiratory depression following overdosage of fentanyl citrate may be longer than the duration of opioid antagonist action. Consult the package inserts of the individual opioid antagonists for details about use.

The LD_{50} values after intravenous administration were 4.1–5.27 mg/kg for the rat and the rabbit and 17 mg/kg or more for the mouse and the dog. After intramuscular administration LD_{50} determinations were 6.7–14.5 mg/kg for the rabbit and 75 mg/kg for the mouse.

DOSAGE AND ADMINISTRATION

Dosage should be individualized. Some of the factors to be considered in determining dose are age, body weight, physical status, underlying pathological condition, use of other drugs, the type of anesthesia to be used and the surgical procedure involved.

Vital signs should be monitored routinely.

Most patients who have received INNOVAR (fentanyl citrate/droperidol) do not require opioid analgesics during the immediate postoperative period. It is recommended that opioid analgesics, when required, be used initially in reduced doses, as low as $1/4$ to $1/3$ those usually recommended.

USUAL ADULT DOSAGE:

I. **Premedication**—(to be appropriately modified in the elderly, debilitated and those who have received other depressant drugs)—0.5 to 2.0 ml may be administered **intramuscularly** 45 to 60 minutes prior to surgery with or without atropine.

II. **Adjunct to General Anesthesia**—
Induction—1 ml per 20 to 25 pounds of body weight may be slowly administered intravenously. Smaller doses may be adequate.
The total amount of INNOVAR administered should be carefully titrated to obtain the desired effect based on the individual patient's response.
There are several methods of administration of INNOVAR Injection for induction of anesthesia.

A. Intravenous injection—To allow for the variable needs of patients INNOVAR may be administered intravenously in fractional parts of the calculated dose. With the onset of somnolence, the general anesthetic may be administered.

B. Intravenous drip—10 ml of INNOVAR are added to 250 ml of 5% dextrose in water and the drip given rapidly until the onset of somnolence. At that time,

the drip may be either slowed or stopped and the general anesthetic administered.

Maintenance—INNOVAR is not indicated as the sole agent for the maintenance of surgical anesthesia. It is customarily used in combination with other measures such as nitrous oxide-oxygen, other inhalation anesthetics and/or topical or regional anesthesia.

To prevent the possibility of excessive accumulation of the relatively long-acting droperidol component, SUBLIMAZE (fentanyl citrate) alone should be used in increments of 25 to 50 µg (0.025 to 0.05 mg) (0.5 to 1.0 ml) for the maintenance of analgesia in patients initially given INNOVAR as an adjunct to general anesthesia. (See SUBLIMAZE (fentanyl citrate) package insert for additional prescribing information.) However, in prolonged operations, additional 0.5 to 1.0 ml amounts of INNOVAR may be administered with caution intravenously if changes in the patient's condition indicate lightening of tranquilization and analgesia.

III. **Use Without a General Anesthetic in Diagnostic Procedures**—Administer the usual intramuscular premedication (0.5 to 2.0 ml) 45 to 60 minutes before the procedure. To prevent the possibility of excessive accumulation of the relatively long-acting droperidol component, SUBLIMAZE (fentanyl citrate) alone should be used in increments of 25 to 50 µg (0.025 to 0.05 mg) (0.5 to 1.0 ml) for the maintenance of analgesia in patients initially given INNOVAR Injection. See SUBLIMAZE (fentanyl citrate) package insert for additional information. However, in prolonged operations, additional 0.5 to 1.0 ml amounts of INNOVAR may be administered with caution intravenously if changes in the patient's condition indicate lightening of tranquilization and analgesia. Note: When INNOVAR is used in certain procedures such as bronchoscopy, appropriate topical anesthesia is still necessary.

IV. **Adjunct to Regional Anesthesia**—1 to 2 ml may be administered intramuscularly or slowly intravenously when additional sedation and analgesia are required.

USUAL CHILDREN'S DOSAGE:

For premedication and as an adjunct to general anesthesia in children over 2 years of age (see PRECAUTIONS):

I. **Premedication**—0.25 ml per 20 lbs. body weight administered **intramuscularly** 45 to 60 minutes prior to surgery with or without atropine.

II. **Adjunct to General Anesthesia**—The total combined dose for induction and maintenance averages 0.5 ml per 20 lbs. body weight. Following induction with INNOVAR Injection, SUBLIMAZE (fentanyl citrate) alone in a dose of $1/4$ to $1/3$ that recommended in the adult dosage section should usually be used when indicated to avoid the possibility of excessive accumulation of droperidol. However, in prolonged operations, additional increments of INNOVAR may be administered with caution when changes in the patient's condition indicate lightening of tranquilization and analgesia.

See WARNINGS and PRECAUTIONS for use of INNOVAR with other CNS depressants, and in patients with altered response.

Parenteral drug products should be inspected visually for particulate matter and discoloration prior to administration, whenever solution and container permit. If such abnormalities are observed, the drug should not be administered.

HOW SUPPLIED

INNOVAR (fentanyl citrate/droperidol) Injection is available as:
NDC 50458-020-02, 2 ml ampoules in packages of 10
NDC 50458-020-05, 5 ml ampoules in packages of 10
containing fentanyl citrate equivalent to 50 µg/ml of fentanyl base and 2.5 mg/ml of droperidol.
(FOR INTRAVENOUS USE BY HOSPITAL PERSONNEL SPECIFICALLY TRAINED IN THE USE OF OPIOID ANALGESICS.)
PROTECT FROM LIGHT. STORE AT ROOM TEMPERATURE 15°–30°C (59°–86°F).
JANSSEN PHARMACEUTICA INC.
Piscataway, NJ 08854
U.S. Patent No. 3,141,823
Revised December 1986, January 1988
Shown in Product Identification Section, page 412

MONISTAT i.v.™   ℞
[mŏn-ĭ-stăt]
(miconazole)
10 mg/ml sterile solution

FOR INTRAVENOUS INFUSION

DESCRIPTION

MONISTAT i.v. (miconazole), 1-2-(2,4-dichlorophenyl)-2-[(2,4-dichlorophenyl) methoxyl] ethyl -1H-imidazole, is a synthetic antifungal agent supplied as a sterile solution for intravenous infusion. Each ml of this solution contains 10 mg of miconazole with 0.115 ml PEG 40 castor oil, 1.0 mg lactic acid USP, 0.5 mg methylparaben USP, 0.05 mg propylparaben USP in water for injection. Miconazole i.v. is a clear, colorless to slightly yellow solution having a pH of 3.7 to 5.7.

CLINICAL PHARMACOLOGY

MONISTAT i.v. is rapidly metabolized in the liver and about 14% to 22% of the administered dose is excreted in the urine, mainly as inactive metabolites. The pharmacokinetic profile fits a three compartment open model with the following biologic half life: 0.4, 2.1, and 24.1 hours for each phase respectively. The pharmacokinetic profile of MONISTAT i.v. is unaltered in patients with renal insufficiency, including those patients on hemodialysis. The in vitro antifungal activity of MONISTAT i.v. is very broad. Clinical efficacy has been demonstrated in patients with the following species of fungi: *Coccidioides immitis, Candida albicans, Cryptococcus neoformans, Pseudoallescheria boydii (Petriellidium boydii; Allescheria boydii),* and *Paracoccidioides brasiliensis.*

Recommended doses of MONISTAT i.v. produce serum concentrations of drug which exceed the in vitro minimum inhibitory concentration (MIC) values listed below.

Median Minimal Inhibitory Concentrations of Miconazole in mcg/ml

Clinical Isolates	Median	Range
Coccidioides immitis	0.4	0.1–1.6
Candida albicans	0.2	0.1–0.8
Cryptococcus neoformans	0.8	0.4–1.3
Paracoccidioides brasiliensis	0.24	0.16–0.31
Pseudoallescheria boydii (Petriellidium boydii)	1.0	0.16–10

Doses above 9 mg/kg of MONISTAT i.v. produce peak blood levels above 1 mcg/ml in most cases. The drug penetrates into joints.

INDICATIONS AND USAGE

MONISTAT i.v. is indicated for the treatment of the following severe systemic fungal infections, based on data derived from open clinical trials: coccidioidomycosis (N=52*), candidiasis (N=151), cryptococcosis (N=13), pseudoallescheriosis (petriellidiosis; allescheriosis) (N=12), paracoccidioidomycosis (N=12), and for the treatment of chronic mucocutaneous candidiasis (N=16).

*Represents treatment courses, as some patients were treated more than once.

However, in the treatment of fungal meningitis and *Candida* urinary bladder infections an intravenous infusion alone is inadequate. It must be supplemented with intrathecal administration or bladder irrigation. Appropriate diagnostic procedures should be performed and MIC's should be measured to determine if the organism is susceptible to MONISTAT®.

MONISTAT i.v. should only be used to treat severe systemic fungal diseases.

CONTRAINDICATIONS

MONISTAT i.v. is contraindicated in those patients who have shown hypersensitivity to it, or to its components.

WARNINGS

There have been several reports of cardiorespiratory arrest and/or anaphylaxis in patients receiving MONISTAT i.v. Excessively rapid administration of the drug may have been responsible in some cases. Rapid injection of undiluted MONISTAT i.v. may produce transient tachycardia or dysrhythmia. (See DOSAGE AND ADMINISTRATION.)

MONISTAT i.v. should only be used to treat severe systemic fungal diseases.

PRECAUTIONS

General: Before a treatment course of MONISTAT i.v. is started, the physician should ascertain insofar as possible that the patient is not hypersensitive to the drug product. MONISTAT i.v. should be given by intravenous infusion. The treatment should be started under stringent conditions of hospitalization but subsequently may be administered to suitable patients under ambulatory conditions with close clinical monitoring. It is recommended that an initial dose of 200 mg be administered with the physician in attendance. It is also recommended that clinical laboratory monitoring including hemoglobin, hematocrit, electrolytes and lipids be performed.

It should be borne in mind that systemic fungal mycoses may be complications of chronic underlying conditions which in themselves may require appropriate measures.

Since *Pseudoallescheria boydii* is difficult to distinguish histologically from species of Aspergillus, it is strongly recommended that cultures be planted.

Drug Interactions: Drugs containing cremophor type vehicles are known to cause electrophoretic abnormalities of the lipoprotein; for example, the values and/or patterns may be altered. These effects are reversible upon discontinuation of treatment but are usually not an indication that treatment should be discontinued.

Interaction with oral and i.v. anticoagulant drugs, resulting in an enhancement of the anticoagulant effect, may occur. However, this has only been reported with oral (coumadin)

Organism	Dosage Range*	Duration of Successful Therapy (weeks)
Candidiasis	600 to 1800 mg per day	1 to > 20
Cryptococcosis	1200 to 2400 mg per day	3 to > 12
Coccidioidomycosis	1800 to 3600 mg per day	3 to > 20
Pseudoallescheriosis (Petriellidiosis; Allecheriosis)	600 to 3000 mg per day	5 to > 20
Paracoccidioidomycosis	200 to 1200 mg per day	2 to > 16

* May be divided over 3 infusions

administration. In cases of simultaneous treatment with MONISTAT i.v. and anticoagulant drugs, the anticoagulant effect should be carefully titrated since reductions of the anticoagulant doses may be indicated.

Interactions between oral miconazole and oral hypoglycemic agents leading to severe hypoglycemia have been reported. Since concomitant administration of rifampin and ketoconazole (an imidazole) reduces the blood levels of the latter, the concurrent administration of MONISTAT i.v. (an imidazole) and rifampin should be avoided.

Ketoconazole (an imidazole) increases the blood level of cyclosporine; therefore, there is the possibility of a similar drug interaction involving cyclosporine and MONISTAT i.v. (an imidazole). Blood levels of cyclosporine should be monitored if the two drugs must be given concurrently.

Concomitant administration of miconazole with CNS-active drugs such as carbamazepine or phenytoin may alter the metabolism of one or both of the drugs. Therefore, consideration should be given to the advisability of monitoring plasma levels of these drugs. It is not known whether miconazole may affect the metabolism of other CNS-active drugs.

Pregnancy Category C: Reproduction studies using MONISTAT i.v. (miconazole) were performed in rats and rabbits. At intravenous doses of 40 mg/kg in the rat and 20 mg/kg in the rabbit, no evidence of impaired fertility or harm to the fetus appeared. There are no adequate and well-controlled studies using MONISTAT i.v. in pregnant women. MONISTAT i.v. should be given to a pregnant woman only if clearly needed.

Pediatric Use: The safety of miconazole i.v. in children under one year has not been extensively studied. However, reports in the literature describe the treatment of 21 neonates for periods ranging from 1 to 56 days at doses ranging from 3 to 50 mg/kg per day in 3 or 4 divided doses. No unanticipated adverse events occurred in children who received these doses. The majority of use was a daily dose in the 15 to 30 mg/kg range. Seven of the eleven evaluable children recovered or improved.

ADVERSE REACTIONS

Adverse reactions which have been observed with MONISTAT i.v. therapy include phlebitis, pruritus, rash, nausea, vomiting, febrile reactions, drowsiness, diarrhea, anorexia and flushes. In the U.S. studies, 29% of 209 patients studied had phlebitis, 21% pruritus, 18% nausea, 10% fever and chills, 9% rash, and 7% emesis. Transient decreases in hematocrit and serum sodium values have been observed following infusion of MONISTAT i.v.

In rare cases, anaphylaxis has occurred.

Thrombocytopenia has also been reported. No serious renal or hepatic toxicity has been reported. If pruritus and skin rashes are severe, discontinuation of treatment may be necessary. Nausea and vomiting can be lessened with antihistaminic or antiemetic drugs given prior to MONISTAT i.v. infusion, or by reducing the dose, slowing the rate of infusion, or avoiding administration with foods.

Aggregation of erythrocytes or rouleau formation on blood smears has been reported. Hyperlipemia has occurred in patients and is reported to be due to the vehicle, Cremophor EL (PEG 40 castor oil).

DOSAGE AND ADMINISTRATION

Dosage

Adults: Doses may vary from 200 to 1200 mg per infusion depending on severity of infection and sensitivity of the organism. The following daily doses, which may be divided over 3 infusions, are recommended:

[See table above].

Repeated courses may be necessitated by relapse or reinfection.

Children:

Children under one year: Total daily doses of 15 to 30 mg/kg have been used (See Pediatric Use.).

Children 1 to 12 years: Total daily doses of 20 to 40 mg/kg have generally been adequate.

However, a dose of 15 mg/kg body weight per infusion should not be exceeded.

Administration

For daily doses of up to 2400 mg, MONISTAT i.v. should be diluted in at least 200 ml of diluent per ampoule and should be administered at a rate of approximately 2 hours per ampoule. For daily doses higher than 2400 mg adjust the rate of

infusion and the diluent in terms of patient tolerability (see WARNINGS).

It is recommended that 0.9% Sodium Chloride Injection be used as the diluent to minimize the possibility of transient hyponatremia following an infusion of MONISTAT i.v. Alternatively, if clinically indicated, 5% Dextrose Injection may be used.

Generally, treatment should be continued until all clinical and laboratory tests no longer indicate that active fungal infection is present. Inadequate periods of treatment may yield poor response and lead to early recurrence of clinical symptoms. The dosing intervals and sites and the duration of treatment vary from patient to patient and depend on the causative organism.

Other Modes of Administration

Intrathecal: Administration of the undiluted injectable solution of MONISTAT i.v. by the various intrathecal routes (20 mg per dose) is indicated as an adjunct to intravenous treatment in fungal meningitis. Succeeding intrathecal injections may be alternated between lumbar, cervical, and cisternal punctures every 3 to 7 days. Bladder instillation: 200 mg of miconazole in a diluted solution is indicated in the treatment of *Candida* of the urinary bladder.

HOW SUPPLIED

MONISTAT i.v. is supplied in 20 ml (200 mg) ampoules. Store at controlled room temperatures. (15° to 30° C/59° to 86°F)

NDC 50458-200-20
U.S. Patent No. 3,717,655; 3,839,574
Rev. Oct. 1984, Nov. 1988
Janssen Pharmaceutica
Piscataway, NJ 08854
©J.P. 1979

Shown in Product Identification Section, page 412

NIZORAL®   ℞
[nī'zōr-ăl]
(ketoconazole) 2% Cream

DESCRIPTION

NIZORAL® (ketoconazole) 2% Cream contains the broad-spectrum synthetic antifungal agent, ketoconazole 2%, formulated in an aqueous cream vehicle consisting of propylene glycol, stearyl and cetyl alcohols, sorbitan monostearate, polysorbate 60, isopropyl myristate, sodium sulfite anhydrous, polysorbate 80 and purified water.

Ketoconazole is *cis*-1-acetyl-4-[4-[[2-(2,4-dichlorophenyl)-2-(1*H*-imidazol-1- ylmethyl) -1, 3- dioxolan -4- yl] methoxy] phenyl]piperazine.

CLINICAL PHARMACOLOGY

When NIZORAL® (ketoconazole) 2% Cream was applied dermally to intact or abraded skin of Beagle dogs for 28 consecutive days at a dose of 80 mg, there were no detectable plasma levels using an assay method having a lower detection limit of 2 ng/ml.

After a single topical application to the chest, back and arms of normal volunteers, systemic absorption of ketoconazole was not detected at the 5 ng/ml level in blood over a 72-hour period.

Two dermal irritancy studies, a human sensitization test, a phototoxicity study and a photoallergy study conducted in 38 male and 62 female volunteers showed no contact sensitization of the delayed hypersensitivity type, no irritation, no phototoxicity and no photoallergenic potential due to NIZORAL® (ketoconazole) 2% Cream.

Microbiology: Ketoconazole is a broad spectrum synthetic antifungal agent which inhibits the *in vitro* growth of the following common dermatophytes and yeasts by altering the permeability of the cell membrane: dermatophytes: *Trichophyton rubrum, T. mentagrophytes, T. tonsurans, Microsporum canis, M. audouini, M. gypseum* and *Epidermophyton floccosum;* yeasts: *Candida albicans, Malassezia ovale (Pityrosporum ovale)* and *C. tropicalis;* and the organism responsible for tinea versicolor, *Malassezia furfur (Pityrosporum orbiculare)*. Only those organisms listed in the INDICATIONS AND USAGE Section have been proven to be clinically affected. Development of resistance to ketoconazole has not been reported.

Continued on next page

Janssen—Cont.

Mode of Action: *In vitro* studies suggest that ketoconazole impairs the synthesis of ergosterol, which is a vital component of fungal cell membranes. It is postulated that the therapeutic effect of ketoconazole in seborrheic dermatitis is due to the reduction of M. ovale, but this has not been proven.

INDICATIONS AND USAGE

NIZORAL® (ketoconazole) 2% Cream is indicated for the topical treatment of tinea corporis and tinea cruris caused by *Trichophyton rubrum, T. mentagrophytes* and *Epidermophyton floccosum;* in the treatment of tinea (pityriasis) versicolor caused by *Malassezia furfur (Pityrosporum orbiculare);* in the treatment of cutaneous candidiasis caused by *Candida spp.* and in the treatment of seborrheic dermatitis.
*Efficacy for this organism in this organ system was studied in fewer than ten infections.

CONTRAINDICATIONS

NIZORAL® (ketoconazole) 2% Cream is contraindicated in persons who have shown hypersensitivity to the active or excipient ingredients of this formulation.

WARNINGS

NIZORAL® (ketoconazole) 2% Cream is not for ophthalmic use.
NIZORAL® (ketoconazole) 2% Cream contains sodium sulfite anhydrous, a sulfite that may cause allergic-type reactions including anaphylactic symptoms and life-threatening or less severe asthmatic episodes in certain susceptible people. The overall prevalence of sulfite sensitivity in the general population is unknown and probably low. Sulfite sensitivity is seen more frequently in asthmatic than in nonasthmatic people.

PRECAUTIONS

General: If a reaction suggesting sensitivity or chemical irritation should occur, use of the medication should be discontinued. Hepatitis (1:10,000 reported incidence) and, at high doses, lowered testosterone and ACTH induced corticosteroid serum levels have been seen with orally administered ketoconazole; these effects have not been seen with topical ketoconazole.
Carcinogenesis, Mutagenesis, Impairment of Fertility: A long-term feeding study in Swiss Albino mice and in Wistar rats showed no evidence of oncogenic activity. The dominant lethal mutation test in male and female mice revealed that single oral doses of ketoconazole as high as 80 mg/kg produced no mutation in any stage of germ cell development. The Ames' *Salmonella* microsomal activator assay was also negative.
Pregnancy: Teratogenic effects: Pregnancy Category C: Ketoconazole has been shown to be teratogenic (syndactylia and oligodactylia) in the rat when given orally in the diet at 80 mg/kg/day, (10 times the maximum recommended human oral dose). However, these effects may be related to maternal toxicity, which was seen at this and higher dose levels.
There are no adequate and well-controlled studies in pregnant women. Ketoconazole should be used during pregnancy only if the potential benefit justifies the potential risk to the fetus.
Nursing Mothers: It is not known whether NIZORAL® (ketoconazole) 2% Cream administered topically could result in sufficient systemic absorption to produce detectable quantities in breast milk. Nevertheless, a decision should be made whether to discontinue nursing or discontinue the drug, taking into account the importance of the drug to the mother.
Pediatric Use: Safety and effectiveness in children have not been established.

ADVERSE REACTIONS

During clinical trials 45 (5.0%) of 905 patients treated with NIZORAL® (ketoconazole) 2% Cream and 5 (2.4%) of 208 patients treated with placebo reported side effects consisting mainly of severe irritation, pruritus and stinging. One of the patients treated with NIZORAL Cream developed a painful allergic reaction.

DOSAGE AND ADMINISTRATION

Cutaneous candidiasis, tinea corporis, tinea cruris, and *tinea (pityriasis) versicolor:*
It is recommended that NIZORAL® (ketoconazole) 2% Cream be applied once daily to cover the affected and immediate surrounding area. Clinical improvement may be seen fairly soon after treatment is begun; however, candidal infections and tinea cruris and corporis should be treated for two weeks in order to reduce the possibility of recurrence. Patients with tinea versicolor usually require two weeks of treatment.
Seborrheic dermatitis: NIZORAL® (ketoconazole) 2% Cream should be applied to the affected area twice daily for four weeks or until clinical clearing. If a patient shows no clinical improvement after the treatment period, the diagnosis should be redetermined.

HOW SUPPLIED

NIZORAL® (ketoconazole) 2% Cream is supplied in 15 (NDC 50458-221-15), 30 (NDC 50458-221-30) and 60 (NDC 50458-221-60) gm tubes.
Rev. Nov. 1987, Feb. 1988
U.S. Patent No. 4,335,125
Manufactured by:
ALTANA, INC.
Melville, N.Y. 11747
Distributed by:
JANSSEN PHARMACEUTICA INC.
Piscataway, N.J. 08854
Shown in Product Identification Section, page 412

NIZORAL®   ℞
[nĭ´zōr-ăl]
(ketoconazole)
Tablets

> **WARNING:** Ketoconazole has been associated with hepatic toxicity, including some fatalities. Patients receiving this drug should be informed by the physician of the risk and should be closely monitored. See WARNINGS and PRECAUTIONS sections.

DESCRIPTION

NIZORAL® (ketoconazole) is a synthetic broad-spectrum antifungal agent available in scored white tablets, each containing 200 mg ketoconazole base for oral administration. Inactive ingredients are colloidal silicon dioxide, corn starch, lactose, magnesium stearate, microcrystalline cellulose, and povidone. Ketoconazole is cis-1-acetyl-4-[4-[[2-(2, 4-dichlorophenyl) -2- (1H-imidazol-1-ylmethyl)-1,3-dioxolan-4-yl] methoxyl]phenyl]piperazine.
Ketoconazole is a white to slightly beige, odorless powder, soluble in acids, with a molecular weight of 531.44.

CLINICAL PHARMACOLOGY

Mean peak plasma levels of approximately 3.5µg/ml are reached within 1 to 2 hours, following oral administration of a single 200 mg dose taken with a meal. Subsequent plasma elimination is biphasic with a half life of 2 hours during the first 10 hours and 8 hours thereafter. Following absorption from the gastrointestinal tract, NIZORAL (ketoconazole) is converted into several inactive metabolites. The major identified metabolic pathways are oxidation and degradation of the imidazole and piperazine rings, oxidative O-dealkylation and aromatic hydroxylation. About 13% of the dose is excreted in the urine, of which 2 to 4% is unchanged drug. The major route of excretion is through the bile into the intestinal tract. *In vitro*, the plasma protein binding is about 99%, mainly to the albumin fraction. Only a negligible proportion of NIZORAL reaches the cerebral-spinal fluid. NIZORAL is a weak dibasic agent and thus requires acidity for dissolution and absorption.
NIZORAL is active against clinical infections with *Blastomyces dermatitidis, Candida spp., Coccidioides immitis, Histoplasma capsulatum, Paracoccidioides brasiliensis,* and *Phialophora spp.* It is also active against *Trichophyton spp., Epidermophyton spp.,* and *Microsporum spp.* NIZORAL is active *in vitro* against a variety of fungi and yeast. In animal models, activity has been demonstrated against *Candida spp., Blastomyces dermatitidis, Histoplasma capsulatum, Malassezia furfur, Coccidioides immitis,* and *Cryptococcus neoformans.*
Mode of Action: In vitro studies suggest that NIZORAL impairs the synthesis of ergosterol, which is a vital component of fungal cell membranes.

INDICATIONS AND USAGE

NIZORAL (ketoconazole) is indicated for the treatment of the following systemic fungal infections: candidiasis, chronic mucocutaneous candidiasis, oral thrush, candiduria, blastomycosis, coccidioidomycosis, histoplasmosis, chromomycosis, and paracoccidioidomycosis. NIZORAL should not be used for fungal meningitis because it penetrates poorly into the cerebral-spinal fluid.
NIZORAL is also indicated for the treatment of patients with severe recalcitrant cutaneous dermatophyte infections who have not responded to topical therapy or oral griseofulvin, or who are unable to take griseofulvin.

CONTRAINDICATIONS

NIZORAL is contraindicated in patients who have shown hypersensitivity to the drug.

WARNINGS

Hepatotoxicity, primarily of the hepatocellular type, has been associated with the use of NIZORAL (ketoconazole), including some fatalities. The reported incidence of hepatotoxicity has been about 1:10,000 exposed patients, but this probably represents some degree of under-reporting, as is the case for most reported adverse reactions to drugs. The median duration of ketoconazole therapy in patients who devel- oped symptomatic hepatotoxicity was about 28 days, although the range extended to as low as 3 days. The hepatic injury has usually, but not always, been reversible upon discontinuation of NIZORAL (ketoconazole) treatment. Several cases of hepatitis have been reported in children.
Prompt recognition of liver injury is essential. Liver function tests (such as SGGT, alkaline phosphatase, SGPT, SGOT and bilirubin) should be measured before starting treatment and at frequent intervals during treatment. Patients receiving ketoconazole concurrently with other potentially hepatotoxic drugs should be carefully monitored, particularly those patients requiring prolonged therapy or those who have had a history of liver disease.
Most of the reported cases of hepatic toxicity have to date been in patients treated for onychomycosis. Of 180 patients worldwide developing idiosyncratic liver dysfunction during ketoconazole therapy, 61.3% had onychomycosis and 16.8% had chronic recalcitrant dermatophytoses.
Transient minor elevations in liver enzymes have occurred during ketoconazole treatment. The drug should be discontinued if these persist, if the abnormalities worsen, or if the abnormalities become accompanied by symptoms of possible liver injury.
In rare cases anaphylaxis has been reported after the first dose. Several cases of hypersensitivity reactions including urticaria have also been reported.
In European clinical trials involving 350 patients with metastatic prostatic cancer, eleven deaths were reported within two weeks of starting treatment with high doses of ketoconazole (1200 mg/day). It is not possible to ascertain from the information available whether death was related to ketoconazole therapy in these patients with serious underlying disease. However, high doses of ketoconazole are known to suppress adrenal corticosteroid secretion.
In female rats treated three to six months with ketoconazole at dose levels of 80 mg/kg and higher, increased fragility of long bones, in some cases leading to fracture, was seen. The maximum "no-effect" dose level in these studies was 20 mg/kg (2.5 times the maximum recommended human dose). The mechanism responsible for this phenomenon is obscure. Limited studies in dogs failed to demonstrate such an effect on the metacarpals and ribs.

PRECAUTIONS

General: NIZORAL (ketoconazole) has been demonstrated to lower serum testosterone. Once therapy with NIZORAL has been discontinued, serum testosterone levels return to baseline values. Testosterone levels are impaired with doses of 800 mg per day and abolished by 1600 mg per day. NIZORAL also decreases ACTH induced corticosteroid serum levels at similar high doses. The recommended dose of 200 mg–400 mg daily should be followed closely.
In four subjects with drug-induced achlorhydria, a marked reduction in NIZORAL (ketoconazole) absorption was observed. NIZORAL requires acidity for dissolution. If concomitant antacids, anticholinergics, and H₂-blockers are needed, they should be given at least two hours after NIZORAL administration. In cases of achlorhydria, the patients should be instructed to dissolve each tablet in 4 ml aqueous solution of 0.2 N HCl. For ingesting the resulting mixture, they should use a drinking straw so as to avoid contact with the teeth. This administration should be followed with a cup of tap water.
Information for patients: Patients should be instructed to report any signs and symptoms which may suggest liver dysfunction so that appropriate biochemical testing can be done. Such signs and symptoms may include unusual fatigue, anorexia, nausea and/or vomiting, jaundice, dark urine or pale stools (see WARNINGS).
Drug interactions: Imidazole compounds like ketoconazole may enhance the anticoagulant effect of coumarin-like drugs. In simultaneous treatment with imidazole drugs and coumarin drugs, the anticoagulant effect should be carefully titrated and monitored.
Concomitant administration of rifampin with ketoconazole reduces the blood levels of the latter. INH (Isoniazid) is also reported to affect ketoconazole concentrations adversely. These drugs should not be given concomitantly.
Ketoconazole increases the blood level of cyclosporin A. Blood levels of cyclosporin A should be monitored if the two drugs are given concomitantly.
Concomitant administration of ketoconazole with phenytoin may alter the metabolism of one or both of the drugs. It is suggested to monitor both ketoconazole and phenytoin.
Because severe hypoglycemia has been reported in patients concomitantly receiving oral miconazole (an imidazole) and oral hypoglycemic agents, such a potential interaction involving the latter agents when used concomitantly with ketoconazole (an imidazole) can not be ruled out.
Carcinogenesis, Mutagenesis, Impairment of Fertility: The dominant lethal mutation test in male and female mice revealed that single oral doses of NIZORAL (ketoconazole) as high as 80 mg/kg produced no mutation in any stage of germ cell development. The *Ames Salmonella* microsomal activator assay was also negative. A long term feeding study in

Swiss Albino mice and in Wistar rats showed no evidence of oncogenic activity.

Pregnancy: Teratogenic effects: *Pregnancy Category C.* NIZORAL (ketoconazole) has been shown to be teratogenic (syndactylia and oligodactylia) in the rat when given in the diet at 80 mg/kg/day, (10 times the maximum recommended human dose). However, these effects may be related to maternal toxicity, evidence of which also was seen at this and higher dose levels.

There are no adequate and well controlled studies in pregnant women. NIZORAL should be used during pregnancy only if the potential benefit justifies the potential risk to the fetus.

Nonteratogenic effects: NIZORAL has also been found to be embryotoxic in the rat when given in the diet at doses higher than 80 mg/kg during the first trimester of gestation.

In addition, dystocia (difficult labor) was noted in rats administered NIZORAL during the third trimester of gestation. This occurred when NIZORAL was administered at doses higher than 10 mg/kg (higher than 1.25 times the maximum human dose).

It is likely that both the malformations and the embryotoxicity resulting from the administration of NIZORAL (ketoconazole) during gestation are a reflection of the particular sensitivity of the female rat to this drug. For example, the oral LD_{50} of NIZORAL given by gavage to the female rat is 166 mg/kg whereas in the male rat the oral LD_{50} is 287 mg/kg.

Nursing Mothers: Since NIZORAL is probably excreted in the milk, mothers who are under treatment should not breast feed.

Pediatric Use: NIZORAL has not been systematically studied in children of any age, and essentially no information is available on children under 2 years. NIZORAL should not be used in pediatric patients unless the potential benefit outweighs the risks.

ADVERSE REACTIONS

In rare cases anaphylaxis has been reported after the first dose. Several cases of hypersensitivity reactions including urticaria have also been reported. However, the most frequent adverse reactions were nausea and/or vomiting in approximately 3%, abdominal pain in 1.2%, pruritus in 1.5%, and the following in less than 1% of the patients: headache, dizziness, somnolence, fever and chills, photophobia, diarrhea, gynecomastia, impotence, thrombocytopenia, leukopenia, hemolytic anemia, and bulging fontanelles. Oligospermia has been reported in investigational studies with the drug at dosages above those currently approved. Although oligospermia has not been reported at dosages up to 400 mg daily, sperm counts have been obtained infrequently in patients treated with these dosages. Most of these reactions were mild and transient and rarely required discontinuation of NIZORAL (ketoconazole). In contrast, the rare occurrences of hepatic dysfunction require special attention (see WARNINGS).

Neuropsychiatric disturbances, including suicidal tendencies and severe depression have occurred rarely in patients using NIZORAL.

OVERDOSAGE

In the event of accidental overdosage, supportive measures, including gastric lavage with sodium bicarbonate, should be employed.

DOSAGE AND ADMINISTRATION

Adults: The recommended starting dose of NIZORAL is a single daily administration of 200 mg (one tablet). In very serious infections or if clinical responsiveness is insufficient within the expected time, the dose of NIZORAL may be increased to 400 mg (two tablets) once daily.

Children: In small numbers of children over 2 years of age, a single daily dose of 3.3 to 6.6 mg/kg has been used. NIZORAL (ketoconazole) has not been studied in children under 2 years of age.

There should be laboratory as well as clinical documentation of infection prior to starting ketoconazole therapy. Treatment should be continued until tests indicate that active fungal infection has subsided. Inadequate periods of treatment may yield poor response and lead to early recurrence of clinical symptoms. Minimum treatment for candidiasis is one or two weeks. Patients with chronic mucocutaneous candidiasis usually require maintenance therapy. Minimum treatment for the other indicated systemic mycoses is six months.

Minimum treatment for recalcitrant dermatophyte infections is four weeks in cases involving glabrous skin. Palmar and plantar infections may respond more slowly. Apparent cures may subsequently recur after discontinuation of therapy in some cases.

HOW SUPPLIED

NIZORAL (ketoconazole) is available as white, scored tablets containing 200 mg of ketoconazole debossed "JANSSEN" and on the reverse side debossed "NIZORAL". They are supplied in bottles of 100 tablets (NDC 50458-220-10) and in blister packs of 10 × 10 tablets (NDC 50458-220-01).

Store at room temperature 15°–30°C (59°–86°F).
U.S. Patent 4,335,125
Rev. Aug 1988, March 1989
Janssen Pharmaceutica Inc.
Piscataway, New Jersey 08854
USA

Shown in Product Identification Section, page 412

SUBLIMAZE®   ℂ ℞

[sa ′blĭ-māz]
(fentanyl citrate) Injection
CAUTION: Federal Law Prohibits Dispensing Without Prescription

DESCRIPTION

SUBLIMAZE (fentanyl citrate) is a potent narcotic analgesic. Each milliliter of solution contains fentanyl citrate equivalent to 50 μg of fentanyl base, adjusted to pH 4.0 –7.5 with sodium hydroxide. SUBLIMAZE is chemically identified as N-(1-phenethyl-4-piperidyl) propionanilide citrate (1:1) with a molecular weight of 528.60. The empirical formula is $C_{22}H_{28}N_2O.C_6H_8O_7$.

SUBLIMAZE is a sterile, non-pyrogenic, preservative free aqueous solution for intravenous or intramuscular injection.

CLINICAL PHARMACOLOGY

SUBLIMAZE (fentanyl citrate) is a narcotic analgesic. A dose of 100 μg (0.1 mg) (2.0 ml) is approximately equivalent in analgesic activity to 10 mg of morphine or 75 mg of meperidine. The principal actions of therapeutic value are analgesia and sedation. Alterations in respiratory rate and alveolar ventilation, associated with narcotic analgesics, may last longer than the analgesic effect. As the dose of narcotic is increased, the decrease in pulmonary exchange becomes greater. Large doses may produce apnea. SUBLIMAZE appears to have less emetic activity than either morphine or meperidine. Histamine assays and skin wheal testing in man indicate that clinically significant histamine release rarely occurs with SUBLIMAZE. Recent assays in man show no clinically significant histamine release in dosages up to 50 μg/kg (0.05 mg/kg) (1 ml/kg). SUBLIMAZE preserves cardiac stability, and blunts stress-related hormonal changes at higher doses.

The pharmacokinetics of SUBLIMAZE can be described as a three-compartment model, with a distribution time of 1.7 minutes, redistribution of 13 minutes and a terminal elimination half life of 219 minutes. The volume of distribution for SUBLIMAZE is 4 L/kg.

SUBLIMAZE plasma protein binding capacity increases with increasing ionization of the drug. Alterations in pH may affect its distribution between plasma and the central nervous system. It accumulates in skeletal muscle and fat, and is released slowly into the blood. SUBLIMAZE, which is primarily transformed in the liver, demonstrates a high first pass clearance and releases approximately 75% of an intravenous dose in urine, mostly as metabolites with less than 10% representing the unchanged drug. Approximately 9% of the dose is recovered in the feces, primarily as metabolites. The onset of action of SUBLIMAZE is almost immediate when the drug is given intravenously; however, the maximal analgesic and respiratory depressant effect may not be noted for several minutes. The usual duration of action of the analgesic effect is 30 to 60 minutes after a single intravenous dose of up to 100 μg (0.1 mg) (2.0 ml). Following intramuscular administration, the onset of action is from seven to eight minutes, and the duration of action is one to two hours. As with longer acting narcotic analgesics, the duration of the respiratory depressant effect of SUBLIMAZE may be longer than the analgesic effect. The following observations have been reported concerning altered respiratory response to CO_2 stimulation following administration of SUBLIMAZE to man.

1. DIMINISHED SENSITIVITY TO CO_2 STIMULATION MAY PERSIST LONGER THAN DEPRESSION OF RESPIRATORY RATE. (Altered sensitivity to CO_2 stimulation has been demonstrated for up to four hours following a single dose of 600 μg (0.6 mg) (12 ml) SUBLIMAZE to healthy volunteers.) SUBLIMAZE frequently slows the respiratory rate, duration and degree of respiratory depression being dose related.
2. The peak respiratory depressant effect of a single intravenous dose of SUBLIMAZE is noted 5 to 15 minutes following injection. See also WARNINGS and PRECAUTIONS concerning respiratory depression.

INDICATIONS AND USAGE

SUBLIMAZE (fentanyl citrate) is indicated:
—for analgesic action of short duration during the anesthetic periods, premedication, induction and maintenance, and in the immediate postoperative period (recovery room) as the need arises.
—for use as a narcotic analgesic supplement in general or regional anesthesia.
—for administration with a neuroleptic such as INAPSINE® (droperidol) Injection as an anesthetic premedica-

tion, for the induction of anesthesia and as an adjunct in the maintenance of general and regional anesthesia.
—for use as an anesthetic agent with oxygen in selected high risk patients, such as those undergoing open heart surgery or certain complicated neurological or orthopedic procedures.

CONTRAINDICATIONS

SUBLIMAZE (fentanyl citrate) is contraindicated in patients with known intolerance to the drug.

WARNINGS

SUBLIMAZE (fentanyl citrate) SHOULD BE ADMINISTERED ONLY BY PERSONS SPECIFICALLY TRAINED IN THE USE OF INTRAVENOUS ANESTHETICS AND MANAGEMENT OF THE RESPIRATORY EFFECTS OF POTENT OPIOIDS.

AN OPIOID ANTAGONIST, RESUSCITATIVE AND INTUBATION EQUIPMENT AND OXYGEN SHOULD BE READILY AVAILABLE.

See also discussion of narcotic antagonists in PRECAUTIONS and OVERDOSAGE.

If SUBLIMAZE is administered with a tranquilizer such as INAPSINE (droperidol), the user should become familiar with the special properties of each drug, particularly the widely differing duration of action. In addition, when such a combination is used, fluids and other countermeasures to manage hypotension should be available.

As with other potent narcotics, the respiratory depressant effect of SUBLIMAZE may persist longer than the measured analgesic effect. The total dose of all narcotic analgesics administered should be considered by the practitioner before ordering narcotic analgesics during recovery from anesthesia. It is recommended that narcotics, when required, should be used in reduced doses initially, as low as $1/4$ to $1/3$ those usually recommended.

SUBLIMAZE may cause muscle rigidity, particularly involving the muscles of respiration. This rigidity has been reported to occur or recur infrequently in the extended postoperative period usually following high dose administration. In addition, skeletal muscle movements of various groups in the extremities, neck and external eye have been reported during induction of anesthesia with fentanyl; these reported movements have, on rare occasions, been strong enough to pose patient management problems. This effect is related to the dose and speed of injection and its incidence can be reduced by: 1) administration of up to $1/4$ of the full paralyzing dose of a non-depolarizing neuromuscular blocking agent just prior to administration of SUBLIMAZE; 2) administration of a full paralyzing dose of a neuromuscular blocking agent following loss of eyelash reflex when SUBLIMAZE is used in anesthetic doses titrated by slow intravenous infusion; or, 3) simultaneous administration of SUBLIMAZE and a full paralyzing dose of a neuromuscular blocking agent when SUBLIMAZE is used in rapidly administered anesthetic dosages. The neuromuscular blocking agent used should be compatible with the patient's cardiovascular status.

Adequate facilities should be available for postoperative monitoring and ventilation of patients administered anesthetic doses of SUBLIMAZE. Where moderate or high doses are used (above 10 μg/kg), there must be adequate facilities for postoperative observation, and ventilation if necessary, of patients who have received SUBLIMAZE. It is essential that these facilities be fully equipped to handle all degrees of respiratory depression.

SUBLIMAZE may also produce other signs and symptoms characteristic of narcotic analgesics including euphoria, miosis, bradycardia and bronchoconstriction.

Severe and unpredictable potentiation by MAO inhibitors has been reported for other narcotic analgesics. Although this has not been reported for fentanyl, there are insufficient data to establish that this does not occur with fentanyl. Therefore, when fentanyl is administered to patients who have received MAO inhibitors within 14 days, appropriate monitoring and ready availability of vasodilators and beta-blockers for the treatment of hypertension is indicated.

Head Injuries and Increased Intracranial Pressure—SUBLIMAZE should be used with caution in patients who may be particularly susceptible to respiratory depression, such as comatose patients who may have a head injury or brain tumor. In addition, SUBLIMAZE may obscure the clinical course of patients with head injury.

PRECAUTIONS

General: The initial dose of SUBLIMAZE (fentanyl citrate) should be appropriately reduced in elderly and debilitated patients. The effect of the initial dose should be considered in determining incremental doses.

Nitrous oxide has been reported to produce cardiovascular depression when given with higher doses of SUBLIMAZE. Certain forms of conduction anesthesia, such as spinal anesthesia and some peridural anesthetics, can alter respiration by blocking intercostal nerves. Through other mechanisms (see CLINICAL PHARMACOLOGY) SUBLIMAZE can also

Continued on next page

Janssen—Cont.

SUBLIMAZE® DOSAGE RANGE CHART

TOTAL DOSAGE

Low Dose—2 μg/kg (0.002 mg/kg) (0.04 ml/kg) SUBLIMAZE. SUBLIMAZE in small doses is most useful for minor, but painful, surgical procedures. In addition to the analgesia during surgery, SUBLIMAZE may also provide some pain relief in the immediate postoperative period.

Moderate Dose—2–20 μg/kg (0.002–0.02 mg/kg) (0.04 –0.4 ml/kg) SUBLIMAZE. Where surgery becomes more major, a larger dose is required. With this dose, in addition to adequate analgesia, one would expect to see some abolition of the stress response. However, respiratory depression will be such that artificial ventilation during anesthesia is necessary and careful observation of ventilation postoperatively is essential.

High Dose—20–50 μg/kg (0.02 –0.05 mg/kg) (0.4–1 ml/kg) SUBLIMAZE. During open heart surgery and certain more complicated neurosurgical and orthopedic procedures where surgery is more prolonged, and in the opinion of the anesthesiologist, the stress response to surgery would be detrimental to the well being of the patient, dosages of 20–50 μg/kg (0.02–0.05 mg) (0.4–1 ml) of SUBLIMAZE with nitrous oxide/oxygen have been shown to attenuate the stress response as defined by increased levels of circulating growth hormone, catecholamine, ADH and prolactin. When dosages in this range have been used during surgery, postoperative ventilation and observation are essential due to extended post operative respiratory depression. The main objective of this technique would be to produce "stress free" anesthesia.

SUBLIMAZE® DOSAGE RANGE CHART

MAINTENANCE DOSE

Low Dose—2 μg/kg (0.002 mg/kg) (0.04 ml/kg) SUBLIMAZE.

Additional dosages of SUBLIMAZE are infrequently needed in these minor procedures.

Moderate Dose—2–20 μg/kg (0.002–0.02 mg/kg) (0.04–0.4 ml/kg) SUBLIMAZE.

25 to 100 μg (0.025 to 0.1 mg) (0.5 to 2.0 ml) may be administered intravenously or intramuscularly when movement and/or changes in vital signs indicate surgical stress or lightening of analgesia.

High Dose—20–50 μg/kg (0.02–0.05 mg/kg) (0.4–1.0 ml/kg) SUBLIMAZE.

Maintenance dosage (ranging from 25 μg (0.025 mg) (0.5 ml) to one half the initial loading dose) will be dictated by the changes in vital signs which indicate stress and lightening of analgesia. However, the additional dosage selected must be individualized especially if the anticipated remaining operative time is short.

alter respiration. Therefore, when SUBLIMAZE is used to supplement these forms of anesthesia, the anesthetist should be familiar with the physiological alterations involved, and be prepared to manage them in the patients selected for these forms of anesthesia.

When a tranquilizer such as INAPSINE (droperidol) is used with SUBLIMAZE, pulmonary arterial pressure may be decreased. This fact should be considered by those who conduct diagnostic and surgical procedures where interpretation of pulmonary arterial pressure measurements might determine final management of the patient. When high dose or anesthetic dosages of SUBLIMAZE are employed, even relatively small dosages of diazepam may cause cardiovascular depression.

When SUBLIMAZE is used with a tranquilizer such as INAPSINE (droperidol), hypotension can occur. If it occurs, the possibility of hypovolemia should also be considered and managed with appropriate parenteral fluid therapy. Repositioning the patient to improve venous return to the heart should be considered when operative conditions permit. Care should be exercised in moving and positioning of patients because of the possibility of orthostatic hypotension. If volume expansion with fluids plus other countermeasures do not correct hypotension, the administration of pressor agents other than epinephrine should be considered. Because of the alpha-adrenergic blocking action of INAPSINE (droperidol), epinephrine may paradoxically decrease the blood pressure in patients treated with INAPSINE (droperidol).

Elevated blood pressure, with and without pre-existing hypertension, has been reported following administration of SUBLIMAZE combined with INAPSINE (droperidol). This might be due to unexplained alterations in sympathetic activity following large doses; however, it is also frequently attributed to anesthetic and surgical stimulation during light anesthesia.

When INAPSINE (droperidol) is used with SUBLIMAZE and the EEG is used for postoperative monitoring, it may be found that the EEG pattern returns to normal slowly.

Vital signs should be monitored routinely.

Respiratory depression caused by opioid analgesics can be reversed by opioid antagonists such as naloxone. Because the duration of respiratory depression produced by SUB-LIMAZE may last longer than the duration of the opioid antagonist action, appropriate surveillance should be maintained. As with all potent opioids, profound analgesia is accompanied by respiratory depression and diminished sensitivity to CO_2 stimulation which may persist into or recur in the postoperative period. Respiratory depression secondary to chest wall rigidity has been reported in the post-operative period. Intraoperative hyperventilation may further alter postoperative response to CO_2. Appropriate postoperative monitoring should be employed to ensure that adequate spontaneous breathing is established and maintained in the absence of stimulation prior to discharging the patient from the recovery area.

Impaired Respiration: SUBLIMAZE should be used with caution in patients with chronic obstructive pulmonary disease, patients with decreased respiratory reserve, and others with potentially compromised respiration. In such patients, narcotics may additionally decrease respiratory drive and increase airway resistance. During anesthesia, this can be managed by assisted or controlled respiration.

Impaired Hepatic or Renal Function: SUBLIMAZE should be administered with caution to patients with liver and kidney dysfunction because of the importance of these organs in the metabolism and excretion of drugs.

Cardiovascular Effects: SUBLIMAZE may produce bradycardia, which may be treated with atropine. SUBLIMAZE should be used with caution in patients with cardiac bradyarrhythmias.

Drug Interactions: Other CNS depressant drugs (e.g. barbiturates, tranquilizers, narcotics and general anesthetics) will have additive or potentiating effects with SUBLIMAZE. When patients have received such drugs, the dose of SUBLIMAZE required will be less than usual. Following the administration of SUBLIMAZE, the dose of other CNS depressant drugs should be reduced.

Carcinogenesis, Mutagenesis, Impairment of Fertility: No carcinogenicity or mutagenicity studies have been conducted with SUBLIMAZE. Reproduction studies in rats revealed a significant decrease in the pregnancy rate of all experimental groups. This decrease was most pronounced in the high dosed group (1.25 mg/kg—12.5X human dose) in which one of twenty animals became pregnant.

Pregnancy—Category C: SUBLIMAZE has been shown to impair fertility and to have an embryocidal effect in rats when given in doses 0.3 times the upper human dose for a period of 12 days. No evidence of teratogenic effects have been observed after administration of SUBLIMAZE to rats. There are no adequate and well-controlled studies in pregnant women. SUBLIMAZE should be used during pregnancy only if the potential benefit justifies the potential risk to the fetus.

Labor and Delivery: There are insufficient data to support the use of SUBLIMAZE in labor and delivery. Therefore, such use is not recommended.

Nursing Mothers: It is not known whether this drug is excreted in human milk. Because many drugs are excreted in human milk, caution should be exercised when SUBLIMAZE is administered to a nursing woman.

Pediatric Use: The safety and efficacy of SUBLIMAZE in children under two years of age has not been established. Rare cases of unexplained clinically significant methemoglobinemia have been reported in premature neonates undergoing emergency anesthesia and surgery which included combined use of fentanyl, pancuronium and atropine. A direct cause and effect relationship between the combined use of these drugs and the reported cases of methemoglobinemia has not been established.

ADVERSE REACTIONS

As with other narcotic analgesics, the most common serious adverse reactions reported to occur with SUBLIMAZE (fentanyl citrate) are respiratory depression, apnea, rigidity, and bradycardia; if these remain untreated, respiratory arrest, circulatory depression or cardiac arrest could occur. Other adverse reactions that have been reported are hypertension, hypotension, dizziness, blurred vision, nausea, emesis, laryngospasm, and diaphoresis.

It has been reported that secondary rebound respiratory depression may occasionally occur postoperatively. Patients should be monitored for this possibility and appropriate countermeasures taken as necessary.

When a tranquilizer such as INAPSINE (droperidol) is used with SUBLIMAZE, the following adverse reactions can occur: chills and/or shivering, restlessness, and postoperative hallucinatory episodes (sometimes associated with transient periods of mental depression); extrapyramidal symptoms (dystonia, akathisia, and oculogyric crisis) have been observed up to 24 hours postoperatively. When they occur, extrapyramidal symptoms can usually be controlled with antiparkinson agents. Postoperative drowsiness is also frequently reported following the use of INAPSINE (droperidol).

DRUG ABUSE AND DEPENDENCE

SUBLIMAZE (fentanyl citrate) is a Schedule II controlled drug substance that can produce drug dependence of the morphine type and therefore has the potential for being abused.

OVERDOSAGE

Manifestations: The manifestations of SUBLIMAZE (fentanyl citrate) overdosage are an extension of its pharmacologic actions (see CLINICAL PHARMACOLOGY) as with other opioid analgesics. The intravenous LD_{50} of SUBLIMAZE is 3 mg/kg in rats, 1 mg/kg in cats, 14 mg/kg in dogs and 0.03 mg/kg in monkeys.

Treatment: In the presence of hypoventilation or apnea, oxygen should be administered and respiration should be assisted or controlled as indicated. A patent airway must be maintained; an oropharyngeal airway or endotracheal tube might be indicated. If depressed respiration is associated with muscular rigidity, an intravenous neuromuscular blocking agent might be required to facilitate assisted or controlled respiration. The patient should be carefully observed for 24 hours; body warmth and adequate fluid intake should be maintained. If hypotension occurs and is severe or persists, the possibility of hypovolemia should be considered and managed with appropriate parenteral fluid therapy. A specific narcotic antagonist such as nalorphine, levallorphan or naloxone should be available for use as indicated to manage respiratory depression. This does not preclude the use of more immediate countermeasures. The duration of respiratory depression following overdosage of SUBLIMAZE may be longer than the duration of narcotic antagonist action. Consult the package insert of the individual narcotic antagonists for details about use.

DOSAGE AND ADMINISTRATION

$$50 \ \mu g = 0.05 \ mg = 1 \ ml$$

Dosage should be individualized. Some of the factors to be considered in determining the dose are age, body weight, physical status, underlying pathological condition, use of other drugs, type of anesthesia to be used and the surgical procedure involved. Dosage should be reduced in elderly or debilitated patients (see PRECAUTIONS).

Vital signs should be monitored routinely.

I. Premedication—Premedication (to be appropriately modified in the elderly, debilitated and those who have received other depressant drugs)—50 to 100 μg (0.05 to 0.1 mg) (1 to 2 ml) may be administered intramuscularly 30 to 60 minutes prior to surgery.

II. Adjunct to General Anesthesia—See Dosage Range Chart

III. Adjunct to Regional Anesthesia—50 to 100 μg (0.05 to 0.1 mg) (1 to 2 ml) may be administered intramuscularly or slowly intravenously, over one to two minutes, when additional analgesia is required.

IV. Postoperatively (recovery room)—50 to 100 μg (0.05 to 0.1 mg) (1 to 2 ml) may be administered intramuscularly for the control of pain, tachypnea and emergence delirium. The dose may be repeated in one to two hours as needed.

Usage in Children: For induction and maintenance in children 2 to 12 years of age, a reduced dose as low as 2 to 3 μg/kg is recommended.

[See table on preceding page].

As a General Anesthetic

When attenuation of the responses to surgical stress is especially important, doses of 50 to 100 μg/kg (0.05 to 0.1 mg/kg) (1 to 2 ml/kg) may be administered with oxygen and a muscle relaxant. This technique has been reported to provide anesthesia without the use of additional anesthetic agents. In certain cases, doses up to 150 μg/kg (0.15 mg/kg) (3 ml/kg) may be necessary to produce this anesthetic effect. It has been used for open heart surgery and certain other major surgical procedures in patients for whom protection of the myocardium from excess oxygen demand is particularly indicated, and for certain complicated neurological and orthopedic procedures.

As noted above, it is essential that qualified pesonnel and adequate facilities be available for the management of respiratory depression.

See WARNINGS and PRECAUTIONS for use of SUBLIMAZE (fentanyl citrate) with other CNS depressants, and in patients with altered response.

Parenteral drug products should be inspected visually for particulate matter and discoloration prior to administration, whenever solution and container permit.

HOW SUPPLIED

SUBLIMAZE (fentanyl citrate) Injection is available as:

NDC 50458-030-02 50 μg/ml of fentanyl base, 2 ml ampoules in packages of 10

NDC 50458-030-05 50 μg/ml of fentanyl base, 5 ml ampoules in packages of 10

NDC 50458-030-10 50 μg/ml of fentanyl base, 10 ml ampoules in packages of 5

NDC 50458-030-20 50 μg/ml of fentanyl base, 20 ml ampoules in packages of 5

PROTECT FROM LIGHT. STORE AT ROOM TEMPERATURE 15°C–30°C (59°F–86°F).

JANSSEN PHARMACEUTICA INC.

Piscataway, NJ 08854

U.S. Patent No. 3,164,600

Revised February 1987, March 1989

Shown in Product Identification Section, page 412

SUFENTA®   Ⓒ ℞

[su-fĕn 'ta]

(sufentanil citrate)

Injection

CAUTION: Federal Law Prohibits Dispensing Without Prescription

DESCRIPTION

SUFENTA® (sufentanil citrate) is a potent opioid analgesic chemically designated as N-[4-(methoxymethyl)-1-[2-(2-thienyl) ethyl] -4- piperidinyl]-N-phenylpropanamide 2-hydroxy-1,2,3-propanetricarboxylate (1:1) with a molecular weight of 578.68.

SUFENTA is a sterile, preservative free, aqueous solution containing sufentanil citrate equivalent to 50 μg per ml of sufentanil base for intravenous injection. The solution has a pH range of 3.5–6.0.

CLINICAL PHARMACOLOGY

SUFENTA is an opioid analgesic. When used in balanced general anesthesia, SUFENTA has been reported to be as much as 10 times as potent as fentanyl. When administered as a primary anesthetic agent with 100% oxygen, SUFENTA is approximately 5 to 7 times as potent as fentanyl. (See dosage chart for more complete information on the use of SUFENTA). At doses of up to 8 μg/kg, SUFENTA provides profound analgesia; at doses ≥ 8 μg/kg, SUFENTA produces a deep level of anesthesia. SUFENTA produces a dose related attenuation of catecholamine release, particularly norepinephrine.

The pharmacokinetics of SUFENTA can be described as a three-compartment model, with a distribution time of 1.4 minutes, redistribution of 17.1 minutes and an elimination half-life of 164 minutes. The liver and small intestine are the major sites of biotransformation. Approximately 80% of the administered dose is excreted within 24 hours and only 2% of the dose is eliminated as unchanged drug. Plasma protein binding of SUFENTA is approximately 92.5%.

SUFENTA has an immediate onset of action, with relatively limited accumulation. Rapid elimination from tissue storage sites allows for relatively more rapid recovery as compared with equipotent dosages of fentanyl. At dosages of

SUFENTA of 1–2 μg/kg, recovery times are comparable to those observed with fentanyl; at dosages of > 2–6 μg/kg, recovery times are comparable to enflurane, isoflurane and fentanyl. Within the anesthetic dosage range of 8–30 μg/kg of SUFENTA, recovery times are more rapid compared to equipotent fentanyl dosages.

At dosages of ≥ 8 μg/kg, SUFENTA produces hypnosis and anesthesia without the use of additional anesthetic agents. A deep level of anesthesia is maintained at these dosages, as demonstrated by EEG patterns. Dosages of up to 25 μg/kg attenuate the sympathetic response to surgical stress. The catecholamine response, particularly norepinephrine, is further attenuated at doses of SUFENTA of 25–30 μg/kg, with hemodynamic stability and preservation of favorable myocardial oxygen balance.

The vagolytic effects of pancuronium may produce a dose dependent elevation in heart rate during SUFENTA-oxygen anesthesia. The vagolytic effect of pancuronium may be reduced in patients administered nitrous oxide with SUFENTA. The use of moderate doses of pancuronium or of a less vagolytic neuromuscular blocking agent may be used to maintain a stable lower heart rate and blood pressure during SUFENTA-oxygen anesthesia.

Preliminary data suggest that in patients administered high doses of SUFENTA, initial dosage requirements for neuromuscular blocking agents are generally lower as compared to patients given fentanyl or halothane, and comparable to patients given enflurane.

Bradycardia is infrequently seen in patients administered SUFENTA-oxygen anesthesia. The use of nitrous oxide with high doses of SUFENTA may decrease mean arterial pressure, heart rate and cardiac output.

Assays of histamine in patients administered SUFENTA have shown no elevation in plasma histamine levels and no indication of histamine release.

SUFENTA at 20 μg/kg has been shown to provide more adequate reduction in intracranial volume than equivalent doses of fentanyl, based upon requirements for furosemide and anesthesia supplementation in one study of patients undergoing craniotomy. During carotid endarterectomy, SUFENTA-nitrous oxide/oxygen produced reductions in cerebral blood flow comparable to those of enflurane-nitrous oxide/oxygen. During cardiovascular surgery, SUFENTA-oxygen produced EEG patterns similar to fentanyl-oxygen; these EEG changes were judged to be compatible with adequate general anesthesia.

The intraoperative use of SUFENTA at anesthetic dosages maintains cardiac output, with a slight reduction in systemic vascular resistance during the initial postoperative period. The incidence of postoperative hypertension, need for vasoactive agents and requirements for postoperative analgesics are generally reduced in patients administered moderate or high doses of SUFENTA as compared to patients given inhalation agents.

Skeletal muscle rigidity is related to the dose and speed of

administration of SUFENTA. This muscular rigidity may occur unless preventative measures are taken (see WARNINGS).

Decreased respiratory drive and increased airway resistance occur with SUFENTA. The duration and degree of respiratory depression are dose related when SUFENTA is used at sub-anesthetic dosages. At high doses, a pronounced decrease in pulmonary exchange and apnea may be produced.

INDICATIONS AND USAGE

SUFENTA (sufentanil citrate) is indicated:

as an analgesic adjunct in the maintenance of balanced general anesthesia.

as a primary anesthetic agent for the induction and maintenance of anesthesia with 100% oxygen in patients undergoing major surgical procedures, such as cardiovascular surgery or neurosurgical procedures in the sitting position, to provide favorable myocardial and cerebral oxygen balance or when extended postoperative ventilation is anticipated.

SEE DOSAGE CHART FOR MORE COMPLETE INFORMATION ON THE USE OF SUFENTA.

CONTRAINDICATIONS

SUFENTA is contraindicated in patients with known hypersensitivity to the drug.

WARNINGS

SUFENTA should be administered only by persons specifically trained in the use of intravenous anesthetics and management of the respiratory effects of potent opioids.

An opioid antagonist, resuscitative and intubation equipment and oxygen should be readily available.

SUFENTA may cause skeletal muscle rigidity, particularly of the truncal muscles. The incidence and severity of muscle rigidity is dose related. Administration of SUFENTA may produce muscular rigidity with a more rapid onset than that seen with fentanyl. SUFENTA may produce muscular rigidity that involves the skeletal muscles of the neck and extremities. As with fentanyl, muscular rigidity has been reported to occur or recur infrequently in the extended post-operative period. The incidence can be reduced by: 1) administration of up to ¼ of the full paralyzing dose of a non-depolarizing neuromuscular blocking agent just prior to administration of SUFENTA at dosages of up to 8 μg/kg, 2) administration of a full paralyzing dose of a neuromuscular blocking agent following loss of consciousness when SUFENTA is used in anesthetic dosages (above 8 μg/kg) titrated by slow intravenous infusion, or, 3) simultaneous administration of SUFENTA and a full paralyzing dose of a neuromuscular blocking agent when SUFENTA is used in rapidly administered anesthetic dosages (above 8 μg/kg).

The neuromuscular blocking agent used should be compatible with the patient's cardiovascular status. Adequate facilities should be available for postoperative monitoring and ventilation of patients administered SUFENTA. It is essential that these facilities be fully equipped to handle all degrees of respiratory depression.

PRECAUTIONS

General: The initial dose of SUFENTA should be appropriately reduced in elderly and debilitated patients. The effect of the initial dose should be considered in determining supplemental doses.

Vital signs should be monitored routinely.

Nitrous oxide may produce cardiovascular depression when given with high doses of SUFENTA (see CLINICAL PHARMACOLOGY).

The hemodynamic effects of a particular muscle relaxant and the degree of skeletal muscle relaxation required should be considered in the selection of a neuromuscular blocking agent.

High doses of pancuronium may produce increases in heart rate during SUFENTA-oxygen anesthesia. Bradycardia has been reported infrequently with SUFENTA-oxygen anesthesia and has been responsive to atropine.

Respiratory depression caused by opioid analgesics can be reversed by opioid antagonists such as naloxone. Because the duration of respiratory depression produced by SUFENTA may last longer than the duration of the opioid antagonist action, appropriate surveillance should be maintained. As with all potent opioids, profound analgesia is accompanied by respiratory depression and diminished sensitivity to CO_2 stimulation which may persist into or recur in the postoperative period. Appropriate postoperative monitoring should be employed to ensure that adequate spontaneous breathing is established and maintained prior to discharging the patient from the recovery area.

Interaction with Other Central Nervous System Depressants: Both the magnitude and duration of central nervous system and cardiovascular effects may be enhanced when SUFENTA is administered to patients receiving barbiturates, tranquilizers, other opioids, general anesthetics or other CNS depressants. In such cases of combined treatment, the dose of one or both agents should be reduced.

Continued on next page

Janssen—Cont.

Head Injuries: SUFENTA may obscure the clinical course of patients with head injuries.

Impaired Respiration: SUFENTA should be used with caution in patients with pulmonary disease, decreased respiratory reserve or potentially compromised respiration. In such patients, opioids may additionally decrease respiratory drive and increase airway resistance. During anesthesia, this can be managed by assisted or controlled respiration.

Impaired Hepatic or Renal Function: In patients with liver or kidney dysfunction, SUFENTA should be administered with caution due to the importance of these organs in the metabolism and excretion of SUFENTA.

Carcinogenesis, Mutagenesis and Impairment of Fertility: No long-term animal studies of SUFENTA have been performed to evaluate carcinogenic potential. The micronucleus test in female rats revealed that single intravenous doses of SUFENTA as high as 80 μg/kg (approximately 2.5 times the upper human dose) produced no structural chromosome mutations. The Ames *Salmonella typhimurium* metabolic activating test also revealed no mutagenic activity. See ANIMAL TOXICOLOGY for reproduction studies in rats and rabbits.

Pregnancy Category C: SUFENTA has been shown to have an embryocidal effect in rats and rabbits when given in doses 2.5 times the upper human dose for a period of 10 days to over 30 days. These effects were most probably due to maternal toxicity (decreased food consumption with increased mortality) following prolonged administration of the drug. No evidence of teratogenic effects have been observed after administration of SUFENTA in rats or rabbits. There are no adequate and well-controlled studies in pregnant women. SUFENTA should be used during pregnancy only if the potential benefit justifies the potential risk to the fetus.

Labor and Delivery: There are insufficient data to support the use of SUFENTA in labor and delivery. Therefore, such use is not recommended.

Nursing Mothers: It is not known whether this drug is excreted in human milk. Because many drugs are excreted in human milk, caution should be exercised when SUFENTA is administered to a nursing woman.

Pediatric Use: The safety and efficacy of SUFENTA in children under two years of age undergoing cardiovascular surgery has been documented in a limited number of cases.

Animal Toxicology: The intravenous LD_{50} of SUFENTA is 16.8 to 18.0 mg/kg in mice, 11.8 to 13.0 mg/kg in guinea pigs and 10.1 to 19.5 mg/kg in dogs. Reproduction studies performed in rats and rabbits given doses of up to 2.5 times the upper human dose for a period of 10 to over 30 days revealed high maternal mortality rates due to decreased food consumption and anoxia, which preclude any meaningful interpretation of the results.

ADVERSE REACTIONS

The most common adverse reactions of opioids are respiratory depression and skeletal muscle rigidity. See CLINICAL PHARMACOLOGY, WARNINGS and PRECAUTIONS on the management of respiratory depression and skeletal muscle rigidity.

The most frequent adverse reactions in clinical trials involving 320 patients administered SUFENTA were: hypotension (7%), hypertension (3%), chest wall rigidity (3%) and bradycardia (3%).

Other adverse reactions with a reported incidence of less than 1% were:

Cardiovascular: tachycardia, arrhythmia
Gastrointestinal: nausea, vomiting
Respiratory: apnea, postoperative respiratory depression, bronchospasm
Dermatological: itching, erythema
Central Nervous System: chills
Miscellaneous: intraoperative muscle movement

DRUG ABUSE AND DEPENDENCE

SUFENTA (sufentanil citrate) is a Schedule II controlled drug substance that can produce drug dependence of the morphine type and therefore has the potential for being abused.

OVERDOSAGE

Overdosage would be manifested by an extension of the pharmacological actions of SUFENTA (see CLINICAL PHARMACOLOGY) as with other potent opioid analgesics. However, no experiences of overdosage with SUFENTA have been established during clinical trials. The intravenous LD_{50} of SUFENTA in male rats is 9.34 to 12.5 mg/kg (see ANIMAL TOXICOLOGY for LD_{50}s in other species). Intravenous administration of an opioid antagonist such as naloxone should be employed as a specific antidote to manage respiratory depression. The duration of respiratory depression following overdosage with SUFENTA may be longer than the duration of action of the opioid antagonist. Administration of an opioid antagonist should not preclude more immediate countermeasures. In the event of overdosage, oxygen should be administered and ventilation assisted or controlled as indicated for hypoventilation or apnea. A patent airway must be maintained, and a nasopharyngeal airway or endotracheal tube may be indicated. If depressed respiration is associated with muscular rigidity, a neuromuscular blocking agent may be required to facilitate assisted or controlled respiration. Intravenous fluids and vasopressors for the treatment of hypotension and other supportive measures may be employed.

DOSAGE AND ADMINISTRATION

The dosage of SUFENTA should be individualized in each case according to body weight, physical status, underlying pathological condition, use of other drugs, and type of surgical procedure and anesthesia. In obese patients (more than 20% above ideal total body weight), the dosage of SUFENTA should be determined on the basis of lean body weight. Dosage should be reduced in elderly and debilitated patients (see PRECAUTIONS).

Vital signs should be monitored routinely.

See dosage range chart for the use of SUFENTA by intravenous injection 1) in doses of up to 8 μg/kg as an analgesic adjunct to general anesthesia, and 2) in doses ≥ 8 μg/kg as a primary anesthetic agent for induction and maintenance of anesthesia with 100% oxygen.

Usage in Children: For induction and maintenance of anesthesia in children less than 12 years of age undergoing cardiovascular surgery, an anesthetic dose of 10–25 μg/kg administered with 100% oxygen is generally recommended. Supplemental dosages of up to 25–50 μg are recommended for maintenance, based on response to initial dose and as determined by changes in vital signs indicating surgical stress or lightening of anesthesia.

Premedication: The selection of preanesthetic medications should be based upon the needs of the individual patient.

Neuromuscular Blocking Agents: The neuromuscular blocking agent selected should be compatible with the patient's condition, taking into account the hemodynamic effects of a particular muscle relaxant and the degree of skeletal muscle relaxation required (see CLINICAL PHARMACOLOGY, WARNINGS and PRECAUTIONS).

[See table above].

In patients administered high (anesthetic) doses of SUFENTA, it is essential that qualified personnel and adequate facilities are available for the management of postoperative respiratory depression.

Also see WARNINGS and PRECAUTIONS sections.

For purposes of administering small volumes of SUFENTA accurately, the use of a tuberculin syringe or equivalent is recommended.

Parenteral drug products should be inspected visually for particulate matter and discoloration prior to administration, whenever solution and container permit.

HOW SUPPLIED

SUFENTA (sufentanil citrate) Injection for intravenous use is available as:

NDC 50458-050-01   50 μg/ml sufentanil base, 1 ml ampoules in packages of 10
NDC 50458-050-02   50 μg/ml sufentanil base, 2 ml ampoules in packages of 10
NDC 50458-050-05   50 μg/ml sufentanil base, 5 ml ampoules in packages of 10

Protect from light. Store at room temperature 15°–30°C (59°–86°F).

U.S. Patent No. 3,998,834
October 1986, March 1987

Shown in Product Identification Section, page 412

VERMOX®   ℞
[vĕr′mŏx]
(mebendazole)
Chewable Tablets

DESCRIPTION

VERMOX® (mebendazole) is a (synthetic) broad-spectrum anthelmintic available as chewable tablets, each containing 100 mg of mebendazole. Inactive ingredients are: colloidal silicon dioxide, corn starch, hydrogenated vegetable oil, magnesium stearate, microcrystalline cellulose, sodium lauryl sulfate, sodium saccharin, sodium starch glycolate, talc, tetrarome orange, and FD&C yellow No. 6.

Mebendazole is methyl 5-benzoylbenzimidazole-2-carbamate.

Mebendazole is a white to slightly yellow powder with a molecular weight of 295.29. It is less than 0.05% soluble in water, dilute mineral acid solutions, alcohol, ether and chloroform, but is soluble in formic acid.

CLINICAL PHARMACOLOGY

Following administration of 100 mg twice daily for three consecutive days, plasma levels of VERMOX® and its primary metabolite, the 2-amine, do not exceed 0.03 μg/ml and 0.09 μg/ml, respectively. All metabolites are devoid of ant-

---

SUFENTA®   ADULT DOSAGE RANGE CHART

TOTAL DOSAGE	MAINTENANCE DOSAGE
ADMINISTRATION WITH NITROUS OXIDE/OXYGEN FOR SURGICAL PROCEDURES LASTING UP TO EIGHT HOURS: ● **TOTAL DOSAGE REQUIREMENTS OF 1 μG/KG/HR OR LESS ARE RECOMMENDED**	
1–2 μg/kg: Expected duration of anesthesia 1–2 hours. Approximately 75% or more of total SUFENTA dosage may be administered prior to intubation. Administered with nitrous oxide/oxygen in patients undergoing general surgery in which endotracheal intubation and mechanical ventilation are required.	**10–25 μg (0.2–0.5 ml):** as needed when movement and/or changes in vital signs indicate surgical stress or lightening of analgesia. Supplemental dosages should be individualized and adjusted to remaining operative time anticipated.
2–8 μg/kg: Expected duration of anesthesia 2–8 hours. Approximately 50 to 75% of total SUFENTA dosage may be administered prior to intubation. Administered with nitrous oxide/oxygen in patients undergoing more complicated major surgical procedures. At dosages in this range, SUFENTA has been shown to provide some attenuation of sympathetic reflex activity in response to surgical stimuli, provide hemodynamic stability, and provide relatively rapid recovery.	**10–50 μg (0.2–1 ml):** as determined by changes in vital signs that indicate stress or lightening of analgesia. Supplemental dosages should be individualized, and adjusted to the remaining operative time anticipated.
ADMINISTRATION WITH 100% OXYGEN	
8–30 μg/kg: (anesthetic doses) administered with 100% oxygen and a muscle relaxant. SUFENTA has been found to produce sleep at dosages ≥ 8 μg/kg and to maintain a deep level of anesthesia without the use of additional anesthetic agents. At dosages in this range of up to 25 μg/kg, catecholamine release is attenuated. Dosages of 25–30 μg/kg have been shown to block sympathetic responses including catecholamine release. High doses are indicated in patients undergoing major surgical procedures, such as cardiovascular surgery and neurosurgery in the sitting position with maintenance of favorable myocardial and cerebral oxygen balance. Postoperative mechanical ventilation and observation are essential at these dosages due to extended postoperative respiratory depression.	**25–50 μg (0.5–1 ml):** as determined by changes in vital signs that indicate stress and lightening of anesthesia.

helmintic activity. In man, approximately 2% of administered VERMOX® is excreted in urine and the remainder in the feces as unchanged drug or a primary metabolite.

Mode of Action: VERMOX® inhibits the formation of the worms' microtubules and causes the worms' glucose depletion.

INDICATIONS AND USAGE

VERMOX® is indicated for the treatment of *Enterobius vermicularis* (pinworm), *Trichuris trichiura* (whipworm), *Ascaris lumbricoides* (common roundworm), *Ancylostoma duodenale* (common hookworm), *Necator americanus* (American hookworm) in single or mixed infections.

Efficacy varies as a function of such factors as pre-existing diarrhea and gastrointestinal transit time, degree of infection, and helminth strains. Efficacy rates derived from various studies are shown in the table below:

[See table above right].

CONTRAINDICATIONS

VERMOX® is contraindicated in persons who have shown hypersensitivity to the drug.

WARNINGS

There is no evidence that VERMOX®, even at high doses, is effective for hydatid disease.

PRECAUTIONS

Information for Patients: Patients should be informed of the potential risk to the fetus in women taking VERMOX® during pregnancy, especially during the first trimester (see Use in Pregnancy).

Patients should also be informed that cleanliness is important to prevent reinfection and transmission of the infection.

Carcinogenesis, Mutagenesis: In carcinogenicity tests of VERMOX® in mice and rats, no carcinogenic effects were seen at doses as high as 40 mg/kg given daily over two years. Dominant lethal mutation tests in mice showed no mutagenicity at single doses as high as 640 mg/kg. Neither the spermatocyte test, the F_1 translocation test, nor the Ames test indicated mutagenic properties.

Impairment of Fertility: Doses up to 40 mg/kg in mice, given to males for 60 days and to females for 14 days prior to gestation, had no effect upon fetuses and offspring, though there was slight maternal toxicity.

Use in Pregnancy: Pregnancy Category C. VERMOX® has shown embryotoxic and teratogenic activity in pregnant rats at single oral doses as low as 10 mg/kg. In view of these findings the use of VERMOX® is not recommended in pregnant women. In humans, a post-marketing survey has been done of a limited number of women who inadvertently had consumed VERMOX® during the first trimester of pregnancy. The incidence of spontaneous abortion and malformation did not exceed that in the general population. In 170 deliveries on term, no teratogenic risk of VERMOX® was identified. During pregnancy, especially during the first trimester, VERMOX® should be used only if the potential benefit justifies the potential risk to the fetus.

Nursing Mothers: It is not known whether VERMOX® is excreted in human milk. Because many drugs are excreted in human milk, caution should be exercised when VERMOX® is administered to a nursing woman.

Pediatric Use: The drug has not been extensively studied in children under two years; therefore, in the treatment of children under two years the relative benefit/risk should be considered.

ADVERSE REACTIONS

Transient symptoms of abdominal pain and diarrhea have occurred in cases of massive infection and expulsion of worms.

OVERDOSAGE

In the event of accidental overdosage gastrointestinal complaints lasting up to a few hours may occur. Vomiting and purging should be induced.

DOSAGE AND ADMINISTRATION

The same dosage schedule applies to children and adults. The tablet may be chewed, swallowed, or crushed and mixed with food.

[See table below].

If the patient is not cured three weeks after treatment, a second course of treatment is advised. No special procedures, such as fasting or purging, are required.

Vermox®	Pinworm (enterobiasis)	Whipworm (trichuriasis)	Common Roundworm (ascariasis)	Hookworm
Cure rates mean	95%	68%	98%	96%
Egg reduction mean	—	93%	99%	99%

HOW SUPPLIED

VERMOX® is available as chewable tablets, each containing 100 mg of mebendazole, and is supplied in boxes of thirty-six tablets.

Store at room temperature 15°–30°C (59°–86°F).

NDC 50458-110-30 (36 tablets-blister)

JANSSEN PHARMACEUTICA INC.

Piscataway, NJ 08854

Rev. Sept 1986, Sept 1988

U.S. Patent 3,657,267

Shown in Product Identification Section, page 412

Johnson & Johnson Patient Care, Inc.
410 GEORGE STREET
NEW BRUNSWICK, NJ 08901-2023

DEBRISAN®
[deb'ri-san]
wound cleaning beads and paste.
Draws Exudate from Wet Ulcers and Wounds

DESCRIPTION

DEBRISAN® consists of spherical hydrophilic beads of dextranomer, 0.1–0.3mm in diameter; the paste is a mixture of the beads and polyethylene glycol. The beads are composed of a three dimensional network of macromolecular chains of cross-linked dextran which is large enough to allow substances with a molecular weight of less than 1000 to enter freely. Substances with a molecular weight of 1000–5000 enter the beads less freely, while those with a molecular weight greater than 5000 remain in the interspaces between the beads.

Characteristics: Because of its hydrophilic properties, each gram of DEBRISAN® beads absorbs approximately 4 ml. of fluid. The beads swell to approximately four times their original size. This swelling causes significant suction forces and capillary action in the spaces between the beads. This action is continuous as long as unsaturated beads or paste is in proximity to the ulcer or wound.

When DEBRISAN® beads or paste are applied to the surface of wet ulcers or wounds suction forces begin removing various exudates and particles that tend to impede tissue repair. For example, low molecular weight components of wound exudates are drawn up within the DEBRISAN® beads while higher molecular weight components, such as plasma proteins, and fibrinogen are found between the swollen beads. Removal of these latter components, particularly fibrin and fibrinogen, retards eschar formation. Additionally, there is *in vitro* evidence that the suction forces created by the beads remove bacteria and inflammatory exudates from the surface of the wound.

The use of DEBRISAN® beads or paste to remove exudates continuously from the surface of the wound results in a concomitant reduction of inflammation and edema.

INDICATIONS

DEBRISAN® beads and paste are indicated for use in cleaning wet ulcers and wounds such as venous stasis ulcers, decubitus ulcers, and infected traumatic and surgical wounds. DEBRISAN® beads are also indicated for use in cleaning infected burns.

PRECAUTIONS

To minimize the possibility of cross-contamination, contents of a DEBRISAN® bead container should be limited to use in one patient.

When treating cratered decubitus ulcers, do not pack the wounds tightly. Allow for expansion of the beads. Do not use

DEBRISAN® beads or paste in deep fistulas, sinus tracts, or any body cavity where complete removal is not assured.

Once the DEBRISAN® is saturated it should be removed. This avoids encrustation which makes removal more difficult. All DEBRISAN® must be removed before any surgical procedure to close the wound (ie graft or flap).

Wounds may appear larger during the first few days of treatment due to the reduction of edema.

DEBRISAN® beads and paste are not effective in cleaning dry wounds.

Not all wounds require treatment with DEBRISAN® to complete healing. When the wound is no longer wet and a healthy granulation base has been established, the application of DEBRISAN® beads or paste should be discontinued. Treatment of the underlying condition (venous or arterial flow, pressure, etc.) should be addressed, in addition to using DEBRISAN® beads or paste.

ADVERSE REACTIONS

Upon application and/or removal of DEBRISAN® beads, transitory pain, bleeding, blistering and erythema have been reported in isolated cases.

DIRECTIONS FOR USE

Applying DEBRISAN®

Debride and wash the area in the usual manner. **DEBRISAN® beads and paste are not enzymes and will not debride.** Leave the area moist since this facilitates the action of DEBRISAN®

Apply DEBRISAN® beads or paste to at least $\frac{1}{4}$ inch (6mm) thickness. At least $\frac{1}{4}$ inch thickness is required to achieve desired suction effects.

Apply a dressing. Close all four sides.

Use of paste

A paste mixture of DEBRISAN® beads may be used for application on irregular body surfaces or hard to reach areas. Three methods of application are possible:

1. DEBRISAN® may be purchased in a convenient, premixed paste form.
2. A paste mixture may be prepared by carefully pouring a small amount of glycerin on a dry dressing large enough to cover the wound and adding a sufficient amount of DEBRISAN® beads to make a layer at least $\frac{1}{4}$ inch thick.

3. Or, DEBRISAN® beads (3 parts) may be mixed with glycerin (1 part) in a receptacle and applied directly to the wound with a spatula. Do not mix with any substance other than glycerin.

In any case, dress the wound in the usual manner. Use fresh paste for each application. Do not reuse.

Removing DEBRISAN®

When DEBRISAN® beads or paste become saturated, a color change will be noted indicating that they should be removed. Removal should be as complete as possible and is best achieved by irrigation. Occasionally vigorous irrigation,

---

		Vermox®			

	Pinworm (enterobiasis)	Whipworm (trichuriasis)	Common Roundworm (ascariasis)	Hookworm
Dose	1 tablet, once	1 tablet morning and evening for 3 consecutive days.	1 tablet morning and evening for 3 consecutive days.	1 tablet morning and evening for 3 consecutive days.

Continued on next page

Johnson & Johnson—Cont.

soaking, or whirlpool may be required to remove patches of DEBRISAN® that adhere to the wound.

Reapply DEBRISAN® beads or paste every 12 hours, or more frequently if necessary. Reduce the number of applications as the exudate diminishes.

When to Discontinue:
When the area is free of exudate and edema.
When a healthy granulation base is present.
The patient should consult the physician if the condition worsens or persists beyond the expected length of treatment (normally 14–21 days).

HOW SUPPLIED
DEBRISAN® beads are supplied sterile, in containers of 25 or 60 grams each and 4 gram packets in boxes of 7 or 14. DEBRISAN® paste is also available in a pre-mixed sterile form, in 10 gram foil packets, six per box.
Store in a dry place below 85°F.
Avoid contact with eyes.
For external use only.
Spilling beads or paste onto the floor will result in a slippery surface.
Materials Available: Free samples and clinical literature available to physicians. Call 800-526-JJPC.
MANUFACTURED IN SWEDEN FOR
JOHNSON & JOHNSON PATIENT CARE, INC.
NEW BRUNSWICK, NEW JERSEY 08901-2023
© **JOHNSON & JOHNSON PATIENT CARE, INC., 1989**

INSTAT™   ℞
[in'stat]
collagen absorbable
hemostat

DESCRIPTION
INSTAT Collagen Absorbable Hemostat is a purified and lyophilized bovine dermal collagen. The material, prepared as a sponge-like pad, is lightly crosslinked, sterile, non-pyrogenic, and absorbable. Hemostatic activity, which is an inherent property of collagen, is largely dependent on the basic helical structure of this protein. The helical structure of native collagen is preserved during the manufacture of IN-STAT. When collagen comes into contact with blood, platelets aggregate on the collagen and release coagulation factors which, together with plasma factors result in the formation of fibrin, and finally in the formation of a clot.

INDICATIONS
INSTAT Collagen Absorbable Hemostat is indicated in surgical procedures (other than in neurosurgical, and ophthalmological surgery) for use as an adjunct to hemostasis when control of bleeding by ligature or other conventional methods is ineffective or impractical.

CONTRAINDICATIONS
INSTAT Collagen Absorbable Hemostat should not be used in the closure of skin incisions as it may interfere with the healing of skin edges. This interference is due to simple mechanical interposition of dry collagen and not due to any intrinsic interference with wound healing. It has been reported with another absorbable collagen hemostat that, in filling porosities of cancellous bone, collagen may reduce the bonding strength of methylmethacrylate. Therefore, IN-STAT should not be applied on bone surfaces to which prosthetic materials are to be attached with methylmethacrylate adhesives.

WARNINGS
INSTAT Collagen Absorbable Hemostat is inactivated by autoclaving. It should not be resterilized. As with any foreign substance, use in contaminated wounds may enhance infection.
INSTAT should not be used in instances of pumping arterial hemorrhage.
INSTAT should not be used where blood or other fluids have pooled or in cases where the point of hemorrhage is submerged. INSTAT will not act as a tampon or plug in a bleed-

ing site nor will it close off an area of blood collecting behind a tampon.
Only the amount of INSTAT necessary to provide hemostasis should be used. The long-term effects of leaving **in situ** are unknown. Opened, unused INSTAT should be discarded because it cannot be resterilized.

PRECAUTIONS
As with other hemostatic agents, it is not recommended that INSTAT Collagen Absorbable Hemostat be left in an infected or contaminated space, nor is it recommended for use in persons known to be sensitive to materials of bovine origin. When placed into cavities or closed spaces, care should be exercised to avoid overpacking INSTAT as it may absorb fluid and expand and press against neighboring structures. In urological procedures, INSTAT should not be left in the renal pelvis or ureters to eliminate the potential focci for calculus formation.
Safety of this product has not been established in children and pregnant women; therefore, INSTAT should only be used when benefit to risk clearly warrants its use.
INSTAT is not intended to be used to treat systemic coagulation disorders.

ADVERSE REACTIONS
INSTAT Collagen Absorbable Hemostat is a collagen product. Although several types of post-operative complications were observed in INSTAT treated patients, none were attributed to INSTAT except one case of fibrotic reaction where INSTAT involvement could not be ruled out. Adverse reactions reported for other collagen hemostats include hematoma, potentiation of infection, wound dehiscence, inflammation and edema. Other reported adverse reactions that may be related to the use of collagen hemostats include adhesion formation, allergic reaction, foreign body reaction and subgaleal seroma (in a single case). The use of microfibrillar collagen in dental extraction sockets has been reported to increase the incidence of alveolalgia. The possibility that all of the above reactions may occur with INSTAT cannot be excluded.

ADMINISTRATION
INSTAT Collagen Absorbable Hemostat is applied directly to the bleeding surface with pressure. INSTAT can be cut to size. The amount needed and the period of time necessary to apply pressure will vary with the type and amount of bleeding to be controlled. Hemostasis time depends upon the type of surgery and degree of pretreatment bleeding. It usually occurred between 2 to 5 minutes with INSTAT.
INSTAT maintains its integrity in the presence of blood and is not dispersed when wet. It is easily removed from the site following hemostasis. It is most effective when used dry.
INSTAT may be left **in situ** whenever necessary. However, the surgeon, at his discretion, should remove any excess of INSTAT prior to wound closure. Animal implant studies have demonstrated that absorption and tissue reaction to INSTAT are similar to those observed with another absorbable collagen hemostatic agent. In these studies, on visual examination, most of INSTAT was found to be absorbed in 8 to 10 weeks after implantation.

CLINICAL STUDIES
The safety, effectiveness and handling characteristics of INSTAT Collagen Absorbable Hemostat were evaluated in a variety of surgical procedures. The median time to hemostasis for INSTAT was 3 minutes. Passive Hemagglutination Assay (PHA) and Enzyme-Linked Immunoabsorbent Assay (ELISA) methods have been used to evaluate the immunologic potential for INSTAT to produce antibodies in patients. These assays revealed mild elevation of antibody titers in both INSTAT treated patients and patients treated with a collagen control hemostat, confirming that INSTAT, like other collagen hemostats, is a weak antigen.

HOW SUPPLIED
INSTAT Collagen Absorbable Hemostat is supplied in a sponge-like form in peelable plastic envelopes in the following sizes:
1 in. × 2 in. (2.5 cm × 5.1 cm)
3 in. × 4 in. (7.6 cm × 10.2 cm)
The sterility of the product is guaranteed unless the individual envelope is damaged or opened.

STORAGE
Store at controlled room temperature 15°–30°C (59°–86°F).

CAUTION
Federal law restricts this device to sale, distribution, and use by or on the order of a physician.

MATERIALS AVAILABLE
Free samples and clinical literature available to physicians, Call 800-526-JJPC.
JOHNSON & JOHNSON PATIENT CARE, INC.
NEW BRUNSWICK, NEW JERSEY 08901-2023
© **JOHNSON & JOHNSON PATIENT CARE, INC., 1989**

SURGICEL® and SURGICEL   ℞
NU-KNIT™ Absorbable Hemostat
[ser'ji-sel]
(oxidized regenerated cellulose)

For surgical use
(For dental application of this product, reference should be made to the package insert for dental use.)

DESCRIPTION
SURGICEL Absorbable Hemostat is a sterile absorbable knitted fabric prepared by the controlled oxidation of regenerated cellulose. The fabric is white with a pale yellow cast and has a faint, caramel-like aroma. It is strong and can be sutured or cut without fraying. It is stable and can be stored at controlled room temperature. A slight discoloration may occur with age, but this does not affect performance.

ACTIONS
The mechanism of action whereby SURGICEL Absorbable Hemostat accelerates clotting is not completely understood, but it appears to be a physical effect rather than any alteration of the normal physiologic clotting mechanism. After SURGICEL has been saturated with blood, it swells into a brownish or black gelatinous mass which aids in the formation of a clot, thereby serving as a hemostatic adjunct in the control of local hemorrhage. When used properly in minimal amounts, SURGICEL is absorbed from the sites of implantation with practically no tissue reaction. Absorption depends upon several factors including the amount used, degree of saturation with blood, and the tissue bed.
In addition to its local hemostatic properties, SURGICEL Absorbable Hemostat is bactericidal **in vitro** against a wide range of gram positive and gram negative organisms including aerobes and anaerobes. SURGICEL is bactericidal **in vitro** against strains of species including those of:
Staphylococcus aureus
Staphylococcus epidermidis
Micrococcus luteus
Streptococcus pyogenes Group A
Streptococcus pyogenes Group B
Bacillus subtilis
Proteus vulgaris
Corynebacterium xerosis
Mycobacterium phlei
Clostridium tetani
Streptococcus salivarius
Branhamella catarrhalis
Escherichia coli
Klebsiella aerogenes
Lactobacillus sp.
Salmonella enteritidis
Shigella dysenteriae
Serratia marscescens
Clostridium perfringens
Bacteroides fragilis
Enterococcus
Enterobacter cloacae
Pseudomonas aeruginosa
Pseudomonas stutzeri
Proteus mirabilis
Studies conducted in animals show that SURGICEL in contrast to other hemostatic agents does not tend to enhance experimental infection. (1–4)

INDICATIONS
SURGICEL Absorbable Hemostat (oxidized regenerated cellulose) is used adjunctively in surgical procedures to assist in the control of capillary, venous, and small arterial hemorrhage when ligation or other conventional methods of control are impractical or ineffective.

CONTRAINDICATIONS
Although packing or wadding sometimes is medically necessary, SURGICEL Absorbable Hemostat should not be used in this manner unless it is to be removed after hemostasis is achieved. (See WARNINGS and PRECAUTIONS)
SURGICEL should not be used for implantation in bone defects, such as fractures, since there is a possibility of interference with callus formation and a theoretical chance of cyst formation.
When SUGICEL is used to help achieve hemostasis in, around, or in proximity to foromina in bone, areas of bony confine, the spinal cord, or the optic nerve and chiasm, it must always be removed once hemostasis is achieved since it will swell and could exert unwanted pressure.
SURGICEL should not be used to control hemorrhage from large arteries.
SURGICEL should not be used on non-hemorrhagic serous oozing surfaces, since body fluids other than whole blood, such as serum, do not react with SURGICEL to produce satisfactory hemostatic effect.
SURGICEL is not indicated for use as an absorbable adhesion barrier.

CONTRAINDICATIONS

THROMBOGEN is contraindicated in persons known to be sensitive to any of its components and/or to material of bovine origin.

WARNING

Because of its action in the clotting mechanism, THROMBOGEN must not be injected or otherwise allowed to enter large blood vessels. Extensive intravascular clotting and even death may result. THROMBOGEN is an antigenic substance and has caused sensitivity and allergic reactions when injected into animals.

PRECAUTIONS

General—Consult the Absorbable Gelatin Sponge, USP product labeling for complete information for use prior to utilizing the thrombin-saturated sponge procedure.

Pregnancy—Category C—Animal reproduction studies have not been conducted with Thrombin, Topical USP (Bovine origin). It is also not known whether Thrombin, Topical USP (Bovine origin) can cause fetal harm when administered to a pregnant woman or can affect reproduction capacity. Thrombin, Topical USP (Bovine origin) should be given to a pregnant woman only if clearly indicated.

Pediatric Use—Safety and effectiveness in children have not been established.

ADVERSE REACTIONS

Allergic reactions may be encountered in persons known to be sensitive to bovine materials.

DOSAGE AND ADMINISTRATION

Solutions of THROMBOGEN may be prepared in sterile distilled water or isotonic saline. The intended use determines the strength of the solution to prepare. For general use in plastic surgery, dental extractions, skin grafting, neurosurgery, etc. solutions containing approximately 100 units per ml are frequently used. For this, 10 ml of diluent added to the 1000 unit package is suitable. Where bleeding is profuse, as from abraded surfaces of liver and spleen, concentrations as high as 1000 to 2000 units per ml may be required. Intermediate strengths to suit the needs of the case may be prepared by selecting the proper strength package and dissolving the contents in an appropriate volume of diluent. In many situations, it may be advantageous to use THROMBOGEN in dry form on oozing surfaces.

Caution: Solutions should be used immediately upon reconstitution. However, the solution may be refrigerated at 2–8°C for up to three hours.

The following techniques are suggested for the topical application of THROMBOGEN.

1. The recipient surface should be sponged (not wiped) free of blood BEFORE THROMBOGEN IS APPLIED.
2. A spray may be used or the surface may be flooded using a sterile syringe and small gauge needle. The most effective hemostasis results when the THROMBOGEN mixes freely with the blood as soon as it reaches the surface.
3. In instances where a concentration of approximately 1,000 units per ml is desired, the contents of the vial of sterile isotonic saline diluent may be easily transferred into the vial of THROMBOGEN with a sterile syringe or a sterile transfer needle. If the transfer needle method is utilized, transfer the diluent as follows:
   (a) Flip plastic cover off of diluent vial.
   (b) Remove clear plastic cover from the transfer needle by twisting to break the seal.
   (c) Insert the exposed needle into the diluent.
   (d) Flip the plastic cover up on the THROMBOGEN vial and tear counterclockwise to remove the aluminum seal.
   (e) Remove the pink plastic cap from the transfer needle exposing the needle.
   (f) Invert the vial of diluent and insert the exposed needle into the THROMBOGEN vial.
   (g) Allow the vacuum to draw the complete contents of the diluent vial into the THROMBOGEN vial.

IMPORTANT
Insert needle in DILUENT first

4. In instances where THROMBOGEN in dry form is needed, the vial is opened by removing the metal ring by flipping up the metal tab and tearing counterclockwise. The rubber-diaphragm cap may be easily removed and the dried THROMBOGEN is then broken up into a powder by means of a sterile glass rod or other suitable sterile instrument.
5. Sponging of treated surfaces should be avoided in order that the clot remain securely in place.

THROMBOGEN may be used in conjunction with Absorbable Gelatin Sponge, USP as follows:

1. Prepare THROMBOGEN solution of the desired strength.
2. Immerse sponge strips of the desired size in the THROMBOGEN solution. Knead the sponge strips vigorously with moistened fingers to remove trapped air, thereby facilitating saturation of the sponge.
3. Apply saturated sponge to the bleeding area. Hold in place for 10 to 15 seconds with a pledget of cotton or a small gauze pad.

HOW SUPPLIED

THROMBOGEN is supplied as:

NDC 0137-0019-10	Package contains one 1,000 unit vial of THROMBIN, TOPICAL USP THROMBOGEN
NDC 0137-0019-11	Package contains one 5,000 unit vial of THROMBIN, TOPICAL USP THROMBOGEN with one 5 ml vial of isotonic saline diluent and a transfer needle
NDC 0137-0019-12	Package contains one 10,000 unit vial of THROMBIN, TOPICAL USP THROMBOGEN with one 10 ml vial of isotonic saline diluent and a transfer needle
NDC 0137-0019-13	Package contains one 20,000 unit vial of THROMBIN, TOPICAL USP THROMBOGEN with one 20 ml vial of isotonic saline diluent and a transfer needle

STORAGE

Store at normal, controlled room temperature.

Manufactured by:
GENTRAC INC.
MIDDLETON, WI 53562
Distributed by:
JOHNSON & JOHNSON PATIENT CARE, INC.
NEW BRUNSWICK, NEW JERSEY 08901-2023
© **JOHNSON & JOHNSON PATIENT CARE, INC. 1989**
For further information call 1-800-526-JJPC

Johnson & Johnson Professional Diagnostics Inc.
ROUTE 202
RARITAN, NEW JERSEY 08869

MICRhoGAM™   ℞

[mike'ro-gam]
Rho (D) Immune Globulin (Human)
For Intramuscular Injection Only

Micro-Dose for use *only* after spontaneous or induced abortion or termination of ectopic pregnancy up to and including 12 weeks' gestation.

DESCRIPTION

MICRhoGAM Rho(D) Immune Globulin (Human) is a sterile solution containing IgG anti-Rho(D) for use in preventing Rh immunization in Rh negative individuals exposed to Rh positive red blood cells. A single dose of MICRhoGAM contains sufficient anti-Rho(D) (approximately 50 µg)† to suppress the immune response to 2.5 ml (or less) of Rh positive red blood cells.

All plasma used in the preparation of MICRhoGAM was tested for hepatitis B surface antigen (HBsAg) by a licensed third generation test and found to be nonreactive. All donors are carefully screened to eliminate those in high risk groups for disease transmission. Fractionation of the plasma is done by a modification of the cold alcohol procedure. Human immune globulins prepared by cold alcohol fractionation have not been reported to transmit hepatitis or other infectious diseases. Glycine (15 mg/ml) is included in the final product as a stabilizer. The final product contains 5% ± 1% globulin, 2.9 mg/ml sodium chloride, 0.01% polysorbate 80 and 0.003% thimerosal (mercury derivations).

This product is for intramuscular injection only.

† A full dose of Rho(D) Immune Globulin (Human) has traditionally been referred to as a "300 µg" dose and this usage is employed here for convenience in terminology. *It should not be construed as the actual anti-D content.* Each full dose of Rho(D) Immune Globulin (Human) must contain at least as much anti-D as 1 milliliter of the U.S. Reference Rho(D) Immune Globulin (Human). Studies performed at the Food and Drug Administration have shown that the U.S. Reference contains 820 international units (IU) of anti-D per milliliter. When the conversion factor determined for the International (WHO) Reference Preparation is used, 820 IU per milliliter is equivalent to 164 µg per milliliter of anti-D. MICRhoGAM contains approximately one-sixth the amount of anti-D contained in the full dose.

CLINICAL PHARMACOLOGY

MICRhoGAM acts by suppressing the immune response of Rh negative women to Rh positive red blood cells. The risk of immunization is related to the number of Rh positive red cells received. The risk was found to be 3% when 0.1 ml of fetal red blood cells is present in the mother and 65% when 5 ml is present. In the first 12 weeks of gestation the total volume of red blood cells in the fetus is estimated at less than 2.5 ml.

Clinical studies demonstrated that administration of MICRhoGAM within three (3) hours following abortion was 100% effective in preventing Rh immunization. Studies in male volunteers showed MICRhoGAM to be effective when given as long as 72 hours after the infusion of Rh positive red cells. A lesser degree of protection is afforded if the antibody is administered beyond this time period.

INDICATIONS AND USAGE

MICRhoGAM is indicated for an Rh negative woman following spontaneous or induced abortion or termination of ectopic pregnancy up to and including 12 weeks' gestation, unless the father is conclusively shown to be Rh negative.

CONTRAINDICATIONS

MICRhoGAM must not be used for genetic amniocentesis at 15 to 18 weeks' gestation or antepartum prophylaxis at 28 weeks' gestation. RhoGAM™ Rho(D) Immune Globulin (Human) is recommended for any indication beyond 12 weeks' gestation.

Individuals known to have had an anaphylactic or severe systemic reaction to human globulin should not receive MICRhoGAM or any other Rho(D) Immune Globulin (Human).

WARNINGS

Do not inject intravenously.

PRECAUTIONS

Pregnancy Category C—Animal reproduction studies have not been conducted with MICRhoGAM. It is also not known whether Rho(D) Immune Globulin (Human) can cause fetal harm when administered to a pregnant woman or can affect reproduction capacity. Rho(D) Immune Globulin (Human) should be given to a pregnant woman only if clearly needed.

ADVERSE REACTIONS

Systemic reactions associated with administration of MICRhoGAM are extremely rare. Discomfort at the site of injection has been reported and a small number of women have noted a slight elevation in temperature.

DOSAGE AND ADMINISTRATION

Parenteral drug products should be inspected visually for particulate matter and discoloration prior to administration, whenever solution and container permit.

A single dose (approximately 50 µg)† of MICRhoGAM will completely suppress the immune response to 2.5 ml of Rh positive red blood cells (packed cells, not whole blood). Administer a single dose of MICRhoGAM intramuscularly as soon as possible after termination of a pregnancy up to and including 12 weeks' gestation. At or beyond 13 weeks' gestation it is recommended that a single dose of RhoGAM Rho(D) Immune Globulin (Human) (approximately 300 µg)† be given instead of MICRhoGAM.

Since there is no lot number and expiration date on the prefilled syringes, they should not be removed from the protective pouch until immediately before use.

† See footnote under Description.

HOW SUPPLIED

- 5 prefilled single-dose syringes of MICRhoGAM (Product code 783810)
- package insert
- 5 control forms
- 5 patient identification cards

STORAGE

Store at 2° to 8°C. DO NOT FREEZE.

RhoGAM™   ℞

[ro'gam]
Rho (D) Immune Globulin (Human)
For Intramuscular Injection Only

DESCRIPTION

RhoGAM Rho(D) Immune Globulin (Human) is a sterile solution containing IgG anti-Rho(D) for use in preventing Rh immunization in Rh negative individuals exposed to Rh positive red blood cells. Each single dose of RhoGAM contains sufficient anti-Rho(D) (approximately 300 µg)† to suppress

Continued on next page

1098

Johnson & Johnson Diag.—Cont.

the immune response to 15 ml (or less) of Rh positive red blood cells.

All plasma used in the preparation of RhoGAM was tested for hepatitis B surface antigen (HBsAg) by a licensed third generation test and found to be nonreactive. All donors are carefully screened to eliminate those in high risk groups for disease transmission. Fractionation of the plasma is done by a modification of the cold alcohol procedure. Human immune globulins prepared by cold alcohol fractionation have not been reported to transmit hepatitis or other infectious diseases. Glycine (15 mg/ml) is included in the final product as a stabilizer. The final product contains 5% ± 1% globulin, 2.9 mg/ml sodium chloride, 0.01% polysorbate 80 and 0.003% thimerosal (mercury derivative).

This product is for intramuscular injection only.

† A full dose of Rh_o(D) Immune Globulin (Human) has traditionally been referred to as a "300 μg" dose and this usage is employed here for convenience in terminology. *It should not be construed as the actual anti-D content.* Each full dose of Rh_o(D) Immune Globulin (Human) must contain at least as much anti-D as 1 milliliter of the U.S. Reference Rh_o(D) Immune Globulin (Human). Studies performed at the Food and Drug Administration have shown that the U.S. Reference contains 820 international units (IU) of anti-D per milliliter. When the conversion factor determined for the International (WHO) Reference Preparation is used, 820 IU per milliliter is equivalent to 164 μg per milliliter of anti-D.

CLINICAL PHARMACOLOGY

RhoGAM acts by suppressing the immune response of Rh negative individuals to Rh positive red blood cells. The risk of immunization is related to the number of Rh positive red blood cells received and the route of introduction.

The obstetrical patient may be exposed to red blood cells from her Rh positive fetus during the normal course of pregnancy as a consequence of abdominal trauma, amniocentesis, abortion, or full-term delivery. Clinical studies proved that the incidence of Rh immunization as a result of pregnancy was reduced to 1% to 2% when RhoGAM was given within 72 hours following delivery, compared with 12% to 13% incidence in untreated women. Further studies in which patients received two doses of Rh immune globulin, one at 28 to 32 weeks of gestation and another after delivery if the baby was Rh positive, showed this regimen reduced the risk of immunization to less than 0.1%.

An Rh negative individual who receives a transfusion of one unit of Rh positive whole blood or Rh positive red blood cells has about an 80% likelihood of producing anti-Rh_o(D).

Protection from Rh immunization has been accomplished by administering the appropriate number of single doses of RhoGAM as described under Dosage and Administration.

INDICATIONS AND USAGE

Pregnancy and Other Obstetric Conditions—RhoGAM is indicated whenever it is known or suspected that fetal red cells have entered the circulation of an Rh negative mother unless the fetus or the father can be shown conclusively to be Rh negative. Small fetal-maternal hemorrhages that could cause the mother to produce anti-Rh_o(D) have been reported in association with abortion, amniocentesis, full-term delivery and in the normal course of pregnancy.

Transfusion—RhoGAM is indicated for any Rh negative female of childbearing age who receives Rh positive red blood cells or whole blood, or components such as platelets or granulocytes prepared from Rh positive blood.

CONTRAINDICATIONS

Individuals known to have had an anaphylactic or severe systemic reaction to human globulin should not receive RhoGAM or any other Rh_o(D) Immune Globulin (Human).

WARNINGS

Do not inject intravenously.
Do not inject infant.

PRECAUTIONS

The presence of passively acquired anti-Rh_o(D) in the maternal serum may cause a positive antibody screening test subsequent to administration of Rh_o(D) Immune Globulin (Human). This does not preclude further antepartum or postpartum prophylaxis.

Some babies born of women given Rh_o(D) Immune Globulin (Human) antepartum have weakly positive direct antiglobulin tests at birth.

Late in pregnancy or following delivery there may be sufficient fetal red blood cells in the maternal circulation to cause a positive result if one tests for the Rh_o(D) variant known as D^u. When there is any doubt as to the patient's Rh type, RhoGAM should be administered.

Pregnancy Category C—Animal reproduction studies have not been conducted with RhoGAM. It is also not known whether Rh_o(D) Immune Globulin (Human) can cause fetal harm when administered to a pregnant woman or can affect reproduction capacity. Rh_o(D) Immune Globulin (Human)

should be given to a pregnant woman only if clearly needed. However, use of Rh antibody during the third trimester in full doses of antibody has been reported to produce no evidence of hemolysis in the infant.

ADVERSE REACTIONS

Systemic reactions associated with administration of RhoGAM are extremely rare. Discomfort at the site of injection has been reported and a small number of women have noted a slight elevation in temperature.

About one-quarter of a group of 22 individuals who were given multiple doses of RhoGAM to treat mismatched transfusions noted fever, myalgia and lethargy. Bilirubin levels of 0.4 to 6.8 mg/dl were observed in some of the treated individuals and one had splenomegaly.

DOSAGE AND ADMINISTRATION

Parenteral drug products should be inspected visually for particulate matter and discoloration prior to administration, whenever solution and container permit.

A single dose (approximately 300 μg)† is contained in each prefilled syringe of RhoGAM. This is the usual dose for the indications associated with pregnancy unless there is clinical or laboratory evidence of a fetal-maternal hemorrhage in excess of 15 ml of Rh positive red blood cells. The indications and recommended dosage for RhoGAM are summarized in the following table.

Indications and Recommended Dosage

Indication	Dose (approximately)
Threatened abortion at any stage of gestation with continuation of pregnancy	300 μg†
Abortion or termination of ectopic pregnancy at or beyond 13 weeks' gestation**	300 μg
Genetic amniocentesis at 15 to 18 weeks' gestation	300 μg
Abdominal trauma in second or third trimester	300 μg
Third trimester amniocentesis	300 μg
Antepartum prophylaxis at 26 to 28 weeks' gestation††	300 μg
Postpartum (if newborn Rh positive)	300 μg

†See footnote under Description

**If abortion or termination of ectopic pregnancy occurs up to and including 12 weeks' gestation, a single dose of MICRhoGAM™ Rh_o(D) Immune Globulin (Human) (approximately 50 μg)† may be used instead of RhoGAM.

††If antepartum prophylaxis is indicated, it is essential that the mother receive a postpartum dose if the infant is Rh positive.

If abdominal trauma, amniocentesis, abortion, or other adverse event requires the administration of RhoGAM at 13 to 18 weeks of gestation, another dose should be given at 26 to 28 weeks. To maintain protection throughout pregnancy, the level of passively acquired anti-Rh_o(D) should not be allowed to fall below the level required to prevent an immune response to Rh positive red cells. The half-life of IgG is 23 to 26 days. In any case, a dose of RhoGAM should be given within 72 hours after delivery if the baby is Rh positive. If delivery occurs within three weeks after the last dose, the postpartum dose may be withheld unless there is a fetal-maternal hemorrhage in excess of 15 ml of Rh positive red blood cells.

Whenever there is a fetal-maternal hemorrhage in excess of 15 ml of Rh positive red blood cells, multiple doses of RhoGAM are required. Based on the blood volume of the fetus at different stages of gestation, a fetal-maternal hemorrhage of this magnitude is unlikely prior to the last trimester of pregnancy. Patients who may need multiple doses of RhoGAM can be identified by a screening test based on rosetting. If the test is positive, the volume of the fetal-maternal hemorrhage should be determined by using an approved laboratory assay and a single dose of RhoGAM administered for every 15 ml of fetal red blood cells. If the dose calculation results in a fraction, administer the next number of prefilled syringes of RhoGAM.

Multiple doses of RhoGAM are usual for indications associated with transfusion. For every 15 ml of Rh positive red blood cells transfused, whether as red blood cells, in whole blood or in components such as platelets or granulocytes prepared from Rh positive blood, the patient should receive a single dose of RhoGAM.

Administer RhoGAM intramuscularly. Do not inject intravenously. The contents of prefilled syringes may be given at one time into different sites, or at different times, as long as the total dose is administered within three days after delivery or receipt of Rh positive red cells.

Since there is no lot number and expiration date on the prefilled syringes, they should not be removed from the protective pouch until immediately before use.

HOW SUPPLIED

RhoGAM is supplied in packages containing:
—5 prefilled single-dose syringes of RhoGAM (Product code 782610) CPT 90742

—package insert
—suggested office protocol
—5 injection records
—5 patient information booklets
—5 patient identification cards
—5 labels for patients' charts
and
—25 prefilled single-dose syringes of RhoGAM (Product code 782650) CPT 90742
—package insert
—suggested office protocol
—25 injection records
—25 patient information booklets
—25 patient identification cards
—25 labels for patients' charts

STORAGE
Store at 2° to 8°C. DO NOT FREEZE.

Jones Medical Industries, Inc.
11710 LACKLAND INDUSTRIAL DRIVE
ST. LOUIS, MO 63146

LIQUI–CHAR™ UNIT–DOSE ANTIDOTE   OTC

DESCRIPTION
Each bottle contains Activated Charcoal, U.S.P. in liquid base.

HOW SUPPLIED

LIQUI-CHAR 12.5™	12.5 grams-2 ounce (60 ml) (NDC-52604-8001-2)
LIQUI-CHAR 25™	25 grams-4 ounce (120 ml) (NDC-52604-8001-4)
LIQUI-CHAR 30™	30 grams-4 ounce (120 ml) (NDC-52604-8003-4)
LIQUI-CHAR 50™	50 grams-8 ounce (240 ml) (NDC-52604-8001-8)

NICO–400® CAPSULE   OTC

DESCRIPTION
Each capsule contains:
nicotinic acid (niacin)..................................400 mg
  (equivalent to 20 times the R.D.A. for adults)

HOW SUPPLIED
Bottle of 100   (NDC-52604-1575-1)

THEREVAC PLUS™ MINI ENEMA   OTC

DESCRIPTION
Each yellow, 4ml, soft-gelatin ampul contains:
docusate sodium ....283 mg
glycerine ....275 mg
benzocaine..20 mg
medicinal soft soap
base of polyethylene glycol

HOW SUPPLIED
Bottle of 50   (NDC 52604-8315-5)

THEREVAC SB   OTC

Same as Theravac Plus, except without benzocaine.

HOW SUPPLIED
Bottle of 30   (NDC-52604-8317-3)

THYROID STRONG™ TABLETS   ℞

DESCRIPTION
THYROID STRONG™ tablets are available in the following labeled strengths. It should be noted that the potency shown is 1 ½ times the activity of the equivalent potency of thyroid, U.S.P.

HOW SUPPLIED
In potencies from ½ to 3 grains, bottles of 100.

Products are cross-indexed by
generic and chemical names
in the
YELLOW SECTION

KabiVitrum, Inc.

Pharmaceutical Division
160 INDUSTRIAL DRIVE
FRANKLIN, OH 45005

Nutritional Products Division
P.O. BOX 597
CLAYTON, NC 27520

PHARMACEUTICAL PRODUCTS

CYKLOKAPRON®
R
[sĭklō-kap′ron]
(Tranexamic acid)
Tablets and Injection

DESCRIPTION
Each tablet contains 500 mg of tranexamic acid.
Each ml of the sterile solution for intravenous injection contains 100 mg tranexamic acid and Water for Injection to 1 mL.

FORMULATION
Chemical Name: trans-4-(aminomethyl)cyclohexanecarboxylic acid.
Structural Formula:

$$H_2N-CH_2-CH \overset{CH_2-CH_2}{\underset{CH_2-CH_2}{\diagdown}} CH-COOH$$

Empirical Formula: $C_8H_{15}NO_2$ Molecular Weight: 157.2
Tranexamic acid is a white crystalline powder. Inert ingredients in the tablets are microcrystalline cellulose, talc, magnesium stearate, silicon dioxide and povidone. The aqueous solution for injection has a pH of 6.5–7.5

HOW SUPPLIED
Tablets 500 mg (flat, white, round with bevelled edges, arcs above and below the letters CY): 100 tablets.
Ampoules 100 mg/mL, 10 × 10 mL
TABLETS   NDC 0601-0114-00
AMPOULES   NDC 0601-0114-08

KABIKINASE®
R
[kah′be-ki″nas]
(Streptokinase)

DESCRIPTION
KABIKINASE (streptokinase) is a purified preparation of a bacterial protein elaborated by group C B-hemolytic streptococci. It is supplied as a water soluble white lyophilized powder for intravenous infusion following reconstitution and dilution. KABIKINASE (streptokinase) contains 11.0 mg Sodium I-Glutamate and 13 mg Albumin Human per 100,000 IU of streptokinase as stabilizers.

HOW SUPPLIED
KABIKINASE (streptokinase) is supplied as a lyophilized powder in 5 ml vials containing 250,000, 600,000, or 750,000 IU per vial of purified streptokinase or in a 10 ml vial containing 1,500,000 IU per vial of purified streptokinase, and shipped in cartons containing 10 vials.
In each vial there is a 10% overfill above that stated on the label. Each vial also contains 11.0 mg of Sodium I-Glutamate per 100,000 IU of streptokinase and 13 mg of Albumin Human per 100,000 IU of streptokinase as stabilizers.
250,000 IU NDC 0601-0110-59
600,000 IU NDC 0601-0110-67
750,000 IU NDC 0601-0119-35
1,500,000 IU NDC 0601-0110-75

NUTRITION PRODUCTS

Product	National Drug Code

Aminess® 5.2%—essential amino acids injection with histidine primarily for intravenous nutrition of renal failure patients.
    size   400 mL   0601-0479-27
Aminess™ Tablets—essential amino acid tablets containing 690 mg of essential amino acids plus histidine per tablet. Order Code 561–75

Intralipid® 10%—a soybean oil emulsion for intravenous use

size	50 mL	0601-0490-12
	100 mL	0601-0490-10
	250 mL	0601-0490-13
	500 mL	0601-0490-15

Intralipid® 20%—a soybean oil emulsion for intravenous use

size	50 mL	0601-1490-22
	100 mL	0601-1490-20
	250 mL	0601-1490-23
	500 mL	0601-1490-25

Novamine™ 11.4%—an amino acid injection for intravenous nutrition

size	100 mL	0388-0489-02
	250 mL	0338-0489-03
	500 mL	0338-0489-04

Novamine™ 15%—an amino acid injection for intravenous nutrition

size	500 mL	0601-0480-27
	1000 mL	0601-0480-30

R-Gene® 10—10% arginine hydrochloride injection, USP.
Order Code 436-24

Kenwood Laboratories
a division of
BRADLEY PHARMACEUTICALS, INC.
383 ROUTE 46 WEST
FAIRFIELD, NJ 07006-2402

APATATE® Liquid/Tablets

COMPOSITION
Each teaspoonful (5 cc) or tablet contains: thiamine, 15 mg; cyanocobalamin, 25 mcg; pyridoxine, 0.5 mg.

HOW SUPPLIED
Liquid	Bottles of 4 fl. oz.	NDC 0482-0130-13
	Bottles of 8 fl. oz.	NDC 0482-0130-14
Tablets	Bottles of 50	NDC 0482-0135-18

GLUTOFAC® Tablets

COMPOSITION
Each tablet contains: ascorbic acid, 300 mg; thiamine hydrochloride, 15 mg; riboflavin, 10 mg; niacinamide, 50 mg; pyridoxine hydrochloride, 50 mg; pantothenic acid, 20 mg; zinc, elemental, 18 mg; magnesium, elemental, 133 mg; selenium, 25 mcg; GTF chromium (Glucose Tolerance Factor), 25 mcg—in a base of 200 mg rice bran containing B-complex vitamins. In addition to label content, GLUTOFAC Tablets contain the following elements in trace amounts, manganese, potassium, iron, copper and phosphorus. FREE OF SUGAR, STARCH AND YEAST.

HOW SUPPLIED
Bottles of 90   NDC 0482-0154-90

I•L•X® B₁₂ Elixir
Crystalline

COMPOSITION
Each three (3) teaspoonfuls (15 cc) contains: elemental iron (from iron ammonium citrate, brown), 102 mg; liver fraction 1, 98 mg; thiamine hydrochloride, 5 mg; riboflavin, 2 mg; nicotinamide, 10 mg; vitamin B_{12} crystalline, 10 mcg; alcohol 8% by volume.

HOW SUPPLIED
Bottles of 12 fl. oz.   NDC 0482-0106-15

I•L•X® B₁₂ Tablets
Crystalline

COMPOSITION
Each tablet contains: elemental iron (from ferrous gluconate 324 mg), 37 mg; liver (dessicated), 130 mg; ascorbic acid, 120 mg; thiamine hydrochloride, 2 mg; riboflavin, 2 mg; niacinamide, 20 mg; vitamin B_{12} crystalline, 12 mcg.

HOW SUPPLIED
Bottles of 100   NDC 0482-0110-23

IPSATOL® Expectorant Syrup

COMPOSITION
Each teaspoon (5 ml) contains 0.24 mg ipecac alkaloids as the fluidglycerite and 22 mg ammonium chloride in a pleasantly flavored tolu balsam syrup.

HOW SUPPLIED
Bottles of 4 fl. oz.   NDC 0482-0650-04

IRCON® Tablets

COMPOSITION
Each tablet contains ferrous fumarate, 200 mg.

HOW SUPPLIED
Bottles of 100   NDC 0482-0628-01

IRCON®–FA Tablets

COMPOSITION
Each tablet contains ferrous fumarate, 250 mg and folic acid, 0.8 mg.

HOW SUPPLIED
Bottles of 100   NDC 0482-0932-01

NITROGLYN® Sustained Release Capsules
R

COMPOSITION
Each sustained release capsule contains nitroglycerin in one of three available dosage forms; 2.5 mg; 6.5 mg; 9 mg. The capsules are not sublingual or chewable.

HOW SUPPLIED
Bottles of 100
2.5 mg	NDC 0482-1025-01
6.5 mg	NDC 0482-1065-01
9 mg	NDC 0482-1090-01

For full prescribing information, please see package insert.

TYZINE®
R
Nasal Solution/Nasal Spray/Pediatric Nasal Drops

DESCRIPTION
TYZINE Nasal Solution and TYZINE Nasal Spray contain a solution of 0.1% tetrahydrozoline HCl in water with sodium chloride, sodium citrate, edetate disodium, and benzalkonium chloride, with adjusted pH. TYZINE Pediatric Nasal Drops contain a solution of 0.05% tetrahydrozoline HCl in water with sodium chloride, sodium citrate, edetate disodium and benzalkonium chloride, with adjusted pH.

HOW SUPPLIED
Nasal Solution: Bottle of 30 ml (1 fl. oz.) with dropper
     NDC 0482-4760-30
Nasal Spray: Spray bottle of 15 ml (½ fl. oz.)
     NDC 0482-4760-15
Pediatric Nasal Drops: Bottle of 15 ml (½ fl. oz.) with dropper NDC 0482-4770-15
For full prescribing information, please see package insert.

The following are additional KENWOOD LABORATORIES products for which literature is available upon request:

Product Name	How Supplied
BONACAL® PLUS Tablets (Prenatal formulation containing fat- and water-soluble vitamins, iron and minerals)	Bottles of 100
I•L•X® Elixir (High-potency hematinic; formulated with iron, liver and vitamins)	12 oz. bottles
KENWOOD THERAPEUTIC LIQUID (Non-alcoholic, sugar-free nutritional formulation of nine fat- and water-soluble vitamins and five minerals)	12 oz. bottles
POSTERISAN® Hemorrhoidal Ointment	25 gm. tubes
Hemorrhoidal Suppositories	Boxes of 10 and 20

IDENTIFICATION PROBLEM?
Consult PDR's
Product Identification Section
where you'll find over 1700
products pictured actual size
and in full color.

Key Pharmaceuticals, Inc.
GALLOPING HILL ROAD
KENILWORTH, NJ 07033

GENAPAX®
(gentian violet) tampons

℞

DESCRIPTION
Each **GENAPAX®** (gentian violet) tampon contains 5 mg of gentian violet, a topical antifungal, on the anterior portion of a conventional vaginal tampon. The empirical formula of gentian violet is ($C_{25}H_{30}ClN_3$) and has the chemical name n-(4-bis(4-(dimethylamino)phenyl)methylene-2, 5-cyclohexadien-1-ylidene)-N-methylmethanaminium chloride.

CLINICAL PHARMACOLOGY
GENAPAX provides a simple and effective mode of administration of gentian violet in the treatment of monilial vaginitis and eliminates the messiness associated with gentian violet solutions. **GENAPAX** tampons: 1) separate the walls of the vagina; 2) convey soluble medication to the cervix and to the surface of the vaginal vault; 3) keep medication in prolonged contact with vaginal mucosa; 4) provide for the absorption of exudates; and 5) serve as a mechanical barrier to prevent leakage. The mechanism of antifungal action of gentian violet is not known. No information is available on the systemic absorption of gentian violet following topical application.

INDICATIONS AND USAGE
GENEPAX is indicated in the treatment of vaginal infections caused by *Candida albicans*. The diagnosis should be confirmed by KOH smears and/or cultures. Other pathogens associated with vaginitis (*Trichomonis* and *Haemophilus vaginalis* [Gardnerella]) should be ruled out by appropriate methods.

CONTRAINDICATIONS
Patients known to be hypersensitive to gentian violet.

WARNINGS
Although topical gentian violet is usually well tolerated, the drug may cause irritation or sensitivity reactions. Discoloration of the skin may occur when gentian violet is applied to granulation tissue; therefore, the drug should not be used on ulcerative lesions.
Tampons are associated with Toxic Shock Syndrome (TSS). TSS is a rare but serious disease that may cause death. Please refer to Patient Package Insert for more information concerning TSS.

PRECAUTIONS
Do not use in the presence of extensive excoriation or ulceration. Patients should be advised to refrain from coitus during treatment.
Carcinogenesis, mutagenesis, and impairment of fertility: Long-term animal studies have not been performed to evaluate the carcinogenic potential, mutagenic potential, or the effect of gentian violet on fertility.
Pregnancy
Category C—Animal reproduction studies have not been conducted with gentian violet. It is not known whether gentian violet can cause fetal harm when administered to a pregnant woman or can affect reproductive capacity. Therefore, gentian violet is not recommended for use in pregnant women.
Nursing Mothers
Studies have not been performed to evaluate breast milk excretion, so caution should be exercised when **GENAPAX** is administered to a nursing woman.

DOSAGE AND ADMINISTRATION
Patients should be instructed to insert a **GENAPAX** tampon intravaginally for 3 to 4 hours, once or twice daily, for a period of 12 days. In resistant cases, use an additional **GENAPAX** overnight. **GENAPAX** tampons should be inserted in the same manner as the usual tampons utilized for menstrual hygiene. Treatment should be continued through menstruation. If infection persists, a second course of treatment may be required.

HOW SUPPLIED
GENAPAX (gentian violet) tampons are available in boxes of 12 tampons, each individually sealed. Store at 15–30°C (59–86°F).

NDC 0085-0587-12   0686
                                                    I004613
Key Pharmaceuticals, Inc.
Copyright © 1987, Kenilworth, New Jersey 07033 USA

K-DUR®
[*kay-dur*]
Microburst Release System®
(potassium chloride, USP)
Extended Release Tablets

℞

DESCRIPTION
K-DUR® 20 is an immediately dispersing extended release oral dosage form of potassium chloride containing 1500 mg of microencapsulated potassium chloride USP equivalent to 20 mEq of potassium in a tablet.
K-DUR® 10 is an immediately dispersing extended release oral dosage form of potassium chloride containing 750 mg of microencapsulated potassium chloride USP equivalent to 10 mEq of potassium in a tablet.
These formulations are intended to slow the release of potassium so that the likelihood of a high localized concentration of potassium chloride within the gastrointestinal tract is reduced.
K-DUR is an electrolyte replenisher. The chemical name of the active ingredient is potassium chloride, and the structural formula is KCl. Potassium chloride USP occurs as a white, granular powder or as colorless crystals. It is odorless and has a saline taste. Its solutions are neutral to litmus. It is freely soluble in water and insoluble in alcohol.
K-DUR is a tablet formulation (not enteric coated or wax matrix) containing individually microencapsulated potassium chloride crystals which disperse upon tablet disintegration. In simulated gastric fluid at 37°C and in the absence of outside agitation, K-DUR begins disintegrating into microencapsulated crystals within seconds and completely disintegrates within one minute. The microencapsulated crystals are formulated to provide an extended release of potassium chloride.
Inactive Ingredients: Crospovidone, Ethylcellulose, Hydroxypropyl Cellulose, Magnesium Stearate, and Microcrystalline Cellulose.

CLINICAL PHARMACOLOGY
Potassium ion is the principal intracellular cation of most body tissues. Potassium ions participate in a number of essential physiological processes including the maintenance of intracellular tonicity, the transmission of nerve impulses, the contraction of cardiac, skeletal and smooth muscle and the maintenance of normal renal function. The intracellular concentration of potassium is approximately 150 to 160 mEq per liter. The normal adult plasma concentration is 3.5 to 5 mEq per liter. An active ion transport system maintains this gradient across the plasma membrane.
Potassium is a normal dietary constituent and under steady state conditions the amount of potassium absorbed from the gastrointestinal tract is equal to the amount excreted in the urine. The usual dietary intake of potassium is 50 to 100 mEq per day. Potassium depletion will occur whenever the rate of potassium loss through renal excretion and/or loss from the gastrointestinal tract exceeds the rate of potassium intake. Such depletion usually develops slowly as a consequence of therapy with diuretics, primary or secondary hyperaldosteronism, diabetic ketoacidosis, or inadequate replacement of potassium in patients on prolonged parenteral nutrition. Depletion can develop rapidly with severe diarrhea, especially if associated with vomiting.
Potassium depletion due to these causes is usually accompanied by a concomitant loss of chloride and is manifested by hypokalemia and metabolic alkalosis. Potassium depletion may produce weakness, fatigue, disturbances of cardiac rhythm (primarily ectopic beats), prominent U-waves in the electrocardiogram, and in advanced cases, flaccid paralysis and/or impaired ability to concentrate urine.
If potassium depletion associated with metabolic alkalosis cannot be managed by correcting the fundamental cause of the deficiency, e.g., where the patient requires long term diuretic therapy, supplemental potassium in the form of high potassium food or potassium chloride may be able to restore normal potassium levels. In rare circumstances (e.g., patients with renal tubular acidosis) potassium depletion may be associated with metabolic acidosis and hyperchloremia. In such patients potassium replacement should be accomplished with potassium salts other than the chloride, such as potassium bicarbonate, potassium citrate, potassium acetate, or potassium gluconate.

INDICATIONS AND USAGE
BECAUSE OF REPORTS OF INTESTINAL AND GASTRIC ULCERATION AND BLEEDING WITH CONTROLLED RELEASE POTASSIUM CHLORIDE PREPARATIONS, THESE DRUGS SHOULD BE RESERVED FOR THOSE PATIENTS WHO CANNOT TOLERATE OR REFUSE TO TAKE LIQUID OR EFFERVESCENT POTASSIUM PREPARATIONS OR FOR PATIENTS IN WHOM THERE IS A PROBLEM OF COMPLIANCE WITH THESE PREPARATIONS.
1. For the treatment of patients with hypokalemia with or without metabolic alkalosis, in digitalis intoxication and in patients with hypokalemic familial periodic paralysis.
   If hypokalemia is the result of diuretic therapy, consider-

ation should be given to the use of a lower dose of diuretic, which may be sufficient without leading to hypokalemia.
2. For the prevention of hypokalemia in patients who would be at particular risk if hypokalemia were to develop, e.g., digitalized patients or patients with significant cardiac arrhythmias.
3. The use of potassium salts in patients receiving diuretics for uncomplicated essential hypertension is often unnecessary when such patients have a normal dietary pattern and when low doses of the diuretic are used. Serum potassium should be checked periodically, however, and if hypokalemia occurs, dietary supplementation with potassium-containing foods may be adequate to control milder cases. In more severe cases, and if dose adjustment of the diuretic is ineffective or unwarranted, supplementation with potassium salts may be indicated.

CONTRAINDICATIONS
Potassium supplements are contraindicated in patients with hyperkalemia since a further increase in serum potassium concentration in such patients can produce cardiac arrest. Hyperkalemia may complicate any of the following conditions: chronic renal failure, systemic acidosis such as diabetic acidosis, acute dehydration, extensive tissue breakdown as in severe burns, adrenal insufficiency, or the administration of a potassium-sparing diuretic (e.g., spironolactone, triamterene, amiloride) (see **OVERDOSAGE**).
Controlled release formulations of potassium chloride have produced esophageal ulceration in certain cardiac patients with esophageal compression due to enlarged left atrium. Potassium supplementation, when indicated in such patients, should be given as a liquid preparation or as an aqueous (water) suspension of K-DUR (see **PRECAUTIONS; Information for Patients**, and **DOSAGE AND ADMINISTRATION** sections).
All solid oral dosage forms of potassium chloride are contraindicated in any patient in whom there is structural, pathological (e.g., diabetic gastroparesis) or pharmacologic (use of anticholinergic agents or other agents with anticholinergic properties at sufficient doses to exert anticholinergic effects) cause for arrest or delay in tablet passage through the gastrointestinal tract.

WARNINGS
Hyperkalemia (see **OVERDOSAGE**) In patients with impaired mechanisms for excreting potassium, the administration of potassium salts can produce hyperkalemia and cardiac arrest. This occurs most commonly in patients given potassium by the intravenous route but may also occur in patients given potassium orally. Potentially fatal hyperkalemia can develop rapidly and be asymptomatic. The use of potassium salts in patients with chronic renal disease, or any other condition which impairs potassium excretion, requires particularly careful monitoring of the serum potassium concentration and appropriate dosage adjustment.
Interaction with Potassium Sparing Diuretics— Hypokalemia should not be treated by the concomitant administration of potassium salts and a potassium-sparing diuretic (e.g., spironolactone, triamterene or amiloride) since the simultaneous administration of these agents can produce severe hyperkalemia.
Interaction with Angiotensin Converting Enzyme Inhibitors —Angiotensin converting enzyme (ACE) inhibitors (e.g., captopril, enalapril) will produce some potassium retention by inhibiting aldosterone production. Potassium supplements should be given to patients receiving ACE inhibitors only with close monitoring.
Gastrointestinal Lesions—Solid oral dosage forms of potassium chloride can produce ulcerative and/or stenotic lesions of the gastrointestinal tract. Based on spontaneous adverse reaction reports, enteric coated preparations of potassium chloride are associated with an increased frequency of small bowel lesions (40–50 per 100,000 patient years) compared to sustained release wax matrix formulations (less than one per 100,000 patient years). Because of the lack of extensive marketing experience with microencapsulated products, a comparison between such products and wax matrix or enteric coated products is not available. K-DUR is a tablet formulated to provide a controlled rate of release of microencapsulated potassium chloride and thus to minimize the possibility of a high local concetration of potassium near the gastrointestinal wall.
Prospective trials have been conducted in normal human volunteers in which the upper gastrointestinal tract was evaluated by endoscopic inspection before and after one week of solid oral potassium chloride therapy. The ability of this model to predict events occurring in usual clinical practice is unknown. Trials which approximated usual clinical practice did not reveal any clear differences between the wax matrix and microencapsulated dosage forms. In contrast, there was a higher incidence of gastric and duodenal lesions in subjectss receiving a high dose of a wax matrix controlled release formulation under conditions which did not resemble usual or recommended clinical practice (i.e., 96 mEq per day in divided doses of potassium chloride administered to fasted patients, in the presence of an anticholinergic drug to delay

gastric emptying). The upper gastrointestinal lesions observed by endoscopy were asymptomatic and were not accompanied by evidence of bleeding (Hemoccult testing). The relevance of these findings to the usual conditions (i.e., nonfasting, no anticholinergic agent, smaller doses) under which controlled release potassium chloride products are used is uncertain; epidemiologic studies have not identified an elevated risk, compared to microencapsulated products, for upper gastrointestinal lesions in patients receiving wax matrix formulations. K-DUR should be discontinued immediately and the possibility of ulceration, obstruction or perforation considered if severe vomiting, abdominal pain, distention, or gastrointestinal bleeding occurs.

Metabolic Acidosis—Hypokalemia in patients with metabolic acidosis should be treated with an alkalinizing potassium salt such as potassium bicarbonate, potassium citrate, potassium acetate, or potassium gluconate.

PRECAUTIONS

GENERAL: The diagnosis of potassium depletion is ordinarily made by demonstrating hypokalemia in a patient with a clinical history suggesting some cause for potassium depletion. In interpreting the serum potassium level, the physician should bear in mind that acute alkalosis per se can produce hypokalemia in the absence of a deficit in total body potassium while acute acidosis per se can increase the serum potassium concentration into the normal range even in the presence of a reduced total body potassium. The treatment of potassium depletion, particularly in the presence of cardiac disease, renal disease, or acidosis requires careful attention to acid-base balance and appropriate monitoring of serum electrolytes, the electrocardiogram, and the clinical status of the patient.

Information for Pateints: Physicians should consider reminding the patient of the following:

To take each dose with meals and with a full glass of water or other liquid.

To take each dose without crushing, chewing, or sucking the tablets. If those patients are having difficulty swallowing whole tablets, they may try one of the following alternate methods of administration:

a. Break the tablet in half, and take each half separately with a glass of water.

b. Prepare an aqueous (water) suspension as follows:

1. Place the whole tablet in approximately one-half glass of water (4 fluid ounces).
2. Allow 2–3 minutes for the tablet to disintegrate.
3. Stir for about half a minute after the tablet has disintegrated.
4. Drink the entire contents of the glass immediately.
5. Then, add another small quantity of water, stir, and drink immediately.

Aqueous suspension of K-DUR tablets that is not taken immediately should be discarded. The use of other liquids for suspending K-DUR tablets is not recommended.

To take this medicine following the frequency and amount prescribed by the physician. This is especially important if the patient is also taking diuretics and/or digitalis preparations.

To check with the physician at once if tarry stools or other evidence of gastrointestinal bleeding is noticed.

Laboratory Tests: When blood is drawn for analysis of plasma potassium it is important to recognize that artifactual elevations can occur after improper venipuncture technique or as a result of in-vitro hemolysis of the sample.

Drug Interactions: Potassium-sparing diuretics, angiotensin converting enzyme inhibitors (see **WARNINGS**).

Carcinogenesis, Mutagenesis, Impairment of Fertility: Carcinogenicity, mutagenicity and fertility studies in animals have not been performed. Potassium is a normal dietary constituent.

Pregnancy Category C: Animal reproduction studies have not been conducted with K-DUR. It is unlikely that potassium supplementation that does not lead to hyperkalemia would have an adverse effect on the fetus or would affect reproductive capacity.

Nursing Mothers: The normal potassium ion content of human milk is about 13 mEq per liter. Since oral potassium becomes part of the body potassium pool, so long as body potassium is not excessive, the contribution of potassium chloride supplementation should have little or no effect on the level in human milk.

Pediatric Use: Safety and effectiveness in children have not been established.

ADVERSE REACTIONS

One of the most severe adverse effects is hyperkalemia (see CONTRAINDICATIONS, WARNINGS, and OVERDOSAGE). There have also been reports of upper and lower gastrointestinal conditions including obstruction, bleeding, ulceration, and perforation (see CONTRAINDICATIONS and WARNINGS).

The most common adverse reactions to oral potassium salts are nausea, vomiting, flatulence, abdominal discomfort, and diarrhea. These symptoms are due to irritation of the gastrointestinal tract and are best managed by diluting the prepa-

ration further, taking the dose with meals or reducing the amount taken at one time.

OVERDOSAGE

The administration of oral potassium salts to persons with normal excretory mechanisms for potassium rarely causes serious hyperkalemia. However, if excretory mechanisms are impaired or if potassium is administered too rapidly intravenously, potentially fatal hyperkalemia can result (see CONTRAINDICATIONS and WARNINGS). It is important to recognize that hyperkalemia is usually asymptomatic and may be manifested only by an increased serum potassium concentration (6.5–8.0 mEq/L) and characteristic electrocardiographic changes (peaking of T-waves, loss of P-waves, depression of S-T segment, and prolongation of the QT-interval). Late manifestations include muscle-paralysis and cardiovascular collapse from cardiac arrest. (9–12 mEq/L).

Treatment measures for hyperkalemia include the following:

1. Elimination of foods and medications containing potassium and of any agents with potassium-sparing properties.
2. Intravenous administration of 300 to 500 mL/hr of 10% dextrose solution containing 10–20 units of crystalline insulin per 1,000 mL.
3. Correction of acidosis, if present, with intravenous sodium bicarbonate.
4. Use of exchange resins, hemodialysis, or peritoneal dialysis.

In treating hyperkalemia, it should be recalled that in patients who have been stabilized on digitalis, too rapid a lowering of the serum potassium concentration can produce digitalis toxicity.

DOSAGE AND ADMINISTRATION

The usual dietary intake of potassium by the average adult is 50 to 100 mEq per day. Potassium depletion sufficient to cause hypokalemia usually requires the loss of 200 or more mEq of potassium from the total body store.

Dosage must be adjusted to the individual needs of each patient. The dose for the prevention of hypokalemia is typically in the range of 20 mEq per day. Doses of 40–100 mEq per day or more are used for the treatment of potassium depletion. Dosage should be divided if more than 20mEq per day is given such that no more than 20 mEq is given in a single dose.

Each K-DUR 20 tablet provides 20 mEq of potassium chloride.

Each K-DUR 10 tablet provides 10 mEq of potassium chloride.

K-DUR tablets should be taken with meals and with a glass of water or other liquid. This product should not be taken on an empty stomach because of its potential for gastric irritation (see **WARNINGS**).

Patients having difficulty swallowing whole tablets may try one of the following alternate methods of administration:

a. Break the tablet in half, and take each half separately with a glass of water.

b. Prepare an aqueous (water) suspension as follows:

1. Place the whole tablet in approximately one-half glass of water (4 fluid ounces).
2. Allow 2–3 minutes for the tablet to disintegrate.
3. Stir for about half a minute after the tablet has disintegrated.
4. Drink the entire contents of the glass immediately.
5. Then, add another small quantity of water, stir, and drink immediately.

Aqueous suspension of K-DUR tablets that is not taken immediately should be discarded. The use of other liquids for suspending K-DUR tablets is not recommended.

CAUTION

Federal law prohibits dispensing without prescription.

HOW SUPPLIED

K-DUR 20 mEq Extended Release Tablets are available in bottles of 100 (NDC 0085-0787-01); bottles of 1000 (NDC 0085-0787-10) and boxes of 100 for unit dose dispensing (NDC 0085-0787-81). K-DUR 20 mEq tablets are white, oblong, imprinted K-DUR 20 and scored for flexibility of dosing.

K-DUR 10 mEq Extended Release Tablets are available in bottles of 100 (NDC 0085-0263-01) and boxes of 100 for unit dose dispensing (NDC 0085-0263-81). K-DUR 10 mEq tablets are white, oblong, imprinted K-DUR 10.

STORAGE CONDITIONS

Keep tightly closed. Store at controlled room temperature 15–30°C (59–86°F).

Rev. 4/89

Copyright © 1986, 1989
Key Pharmaceuticals, Inc.
Kenilworth, NJ 07033 USA
All rights reserved.

Shown in Product Identification Section, page 412

NITRO–DUR® ℞

[ni'tra-dur]

(nitroglycerin)

Transdermal Infusion System

DESCRIPTION

Nitroglycerin is 1,2,3-propanetriol trinitrate, an organic nitrate whose structural formula is:

$$H_2CONO_2$$
$$HCONO_2$$
$$H_2CONO_2$$

and whose molecular weight is 227.09. The organic nitrates are vasodilators, active on both arteries and veins.

The NITRO-DUR (nitroglycerin) transdermal infusion system is a flat unit designed to provide continuous controlled release of nitroglycerin through intact skin. The rate of release of nitroglycerin is linearly dependent upon the area of the applied system; each cm^2 of applied system delivers approximately 0.02 mg of nitroglycerin per hour. Thus, the 5-, 10-, 15-, 20-, and 30-cm^2 systems deliver approximately 0.1, 0.2, 0.3, 0.4 and 0.6 mg of nitroglycerin per hour, respectively.

The remainder of the nitroglycerin in each system serves as a reservoir and is not delivered in normal use.

After 12 hours, for example, each system has delivered approximately 6% of its original content of nitroglycerin.

The NITRO-DUR transdermal system contains nitroglycerin in acrylic-based polymer adhesives with a resinous cross-linking agent to provide a continuous source of active ingredient. Each unit is sealed in a paper polyethylene-foil pouch.

Cross section of the system:

Impermeable Backing

Nitroglycerin/Adhesive

CLINICAL PHARMACOLOGY

The principal pharmacological action of nitroglycerin is relaxation of vascular smooth muscle and consequent dilatation of peripheral arteries and veins, especially the latter. Dilatation of the veins promotes peripheral pooling of blood and decreases venous return to the heart, thereby reducing left ventricular end-diastolic pressure and pulmonary capillary wedge pressure (preload). Arteriolar relaxation reduces systemic vascular resistance, systolic arterial pressure, and mean arterial pressure (afterload). Dilatation of the coronary arteries also occurs. The relative importance of preload reduction, afterload reduction, and coronary dilatation remains undefined.

Dosing regimens for most chronically used drugs are designed to provide plasma concentrations that are continuously greater than a minimally effective concentration. This strategy is inappropriate for organic nitrates. Several well-controlled clinical trials have used exercise testing to assess the anti-anginal efficacy of continuously-delivered nitrates. In the large majority of these trials, active agents were indistinguishable from placebo after 24 hours (or less) of continuous therapy. Attempts to overcome nitrate tolerance by dose escalation, even to doses far in excess of those used acutely, have consistently failed. Only after nitrates had been absent from the body for several hours was their anti-anginal efficacy restored.

Pharmacokinetics: The volume of distribution of nitroglycerin is about 3 L/kg, and nitroglycerin is cleared from this volume at extremely rapid rates, with a resulting serum half-life of about 3 minutes. The observed clearance rates (close to 1 L/kg/min) greatly exceed hepatic blood flow; known sites of extrahepatic metabolism include red blood cells and vascular walls.

The first products in the metabolism of nitroglycerin are inorganic nitrate and the 1,2- and 1,3-dinitroglycerols. The dinitrates are less effective vasodilators than nitroglycerin, but they are longer-lived in the serum, and their net contribution to the overall effect of chronic nitroglycerin regimens is not known. The dinitrates are further metabolized to (nonvasoactive) mononitrates and, ultimately, to glycerol and carbon dioxide.

To avoid development of tolerance to nitroglycerin, drug-free intervals of 10–12 hours are known to be sufficient; shorter intervals have not been well studied. In one well-controlled clinical trial, subjects receiving nitroglycerin appeared to exhibit a rebound or withdrawal effect, so that their exercise tolerance at the end of the daily drug-free interval was *less* than that exhibited by the parallel group receiving placebo.

In the healthy volunteers, steady-state plasma concentrations of nitroglycerin are reached by about 2 hours after ap-

Continued on next page

Key—Cont.

plication of a patch and are maintained for the duration of wearing the system (observations have been limited to 24 hours). Upon removal of the patch, the plasma concentration declines with a half-life of about an hour.

Clinical trials: Regimens in which nitroglycerin patches were worn for 12 hours daily have been studied in well-controlled trials up to 4 weeks in duration. Starting about 2 hours after application and continuing until 10–12 hours after application, patches that deliver at least 0.4 mg of nitroglycerin per hour have consistently demonstrated greater anti-anginal activity than placebo. Lower-dose patches have not been as well studied, but in one large, well-controlled trial in which higher-dose patches were also studied, patches delivering 0.2 mg/hr had significantly *less* anti-anginal activity than placebo.

It is reasonable to believe that the rate of nitroglycerin absorption from patches may vary with the site of application, but this relationship has not been adequately studied.

The onset of action of transdermal nitroglycerin is not sufficiently rapid for this product to be useful in aborting an acute anginal episode.

INDICATIONS AND USAGE

This drug product has been conditionally approved by the FDA for the prevention of angina pectoris due to coronary artery disease. Tolerance to the antianginal effects of nitrates (measured by exercise stress testing) has been shown to be a major factor limiting efficacy when transdermal nitrates are used continuously for longer than 12 hours each day. The development of tolerance can be altered (prevented or attenuated) by use of a noncontinuous (intermittent) dosing schedule with a nitrate-free interval of 10–12 hours.

Controlled clinical trial data suggest that the intermittent use of nitrates is associated with decreased exercise tolerance, in comparison to placebo, during the last part of the nitrate-free interval; the clinical relevance of this observation is unknown, but the possibility of increased frequency or severity of angina during the nitrate-free interval should be considered. Further investigations of the tolerance phenomenon and best regimen are ongoing. A final evaluation of the effectiveness of the product will be announced by the FDA.

CONTRAINDICATIONS

Allergic reactions to organic nitrates are extremely rare, but they do occur. Nitroglycerin is contraindicated in patients who are allergic to it. Allergy to the adhesives used in nitroglycerin patches has also been reported, and it similarly constitutes a contraindication to the use of this product.

WARNINGS

The benefits of transdermal nitroglycerin in patients with acute myocardial infarction or congestive heart failure have not been established. If one elects to use nitroglycerin in these conditions, careful clinical or hemodynamic monitoring must be used to avoid the hazards of hypotension and tachycardia.

A cardiovertor/defibrillator should not be discharged through a paddle electrode that overlies a NITRO-DUR patch. The arcing that may be seen in this situation is harmless in itself, but it may be associated with local current concentration that can cause damage to the paddles and burns to the patient.

PRECAUTIONS

General: Severe hypotension, particularly with upright posture, may occur with even small doses of nitroglycerin. This drug should therefore be used with caution in patients who may be volume depleted or who, for whatever reason, are already hypotensive. Hypotension induced by nitroglycerin may be accompanied by paradoxical bradycardia and increased angina pectoris.

Nitrate therapy may aggravate the angina caused by hypertrophic cardiomyopathy.

As tolerance to other forms of nitroglycerin develops, the effects of sublingual nitroglycerin on exercise tolerance, although still observable, is somewhat blunted.

In industrial workers who have had long-term exposure to unknown (presumably high) doses of organic nitrates, tolerance clearly occurs. Chest pain, acute myocardial infarction, and even sudden death have occurred during temporary withdrawal of nitrates from these workers, demonstrating the existence of true physical dependence.

Some clinical trials in angina patients have provided nitroglycerin for about 12 continuous hours of every 24-hour day. During the nitrate-free intervals in some of these trials, anginal attacks have been more easily provoked than before treatment, and patients have demonstrated hemodynamic rebound and *decreased* exercise tolerance. The importance of these observations to the routine, clinical use of transdermal nitroglycerin is not known.

Information for Patients: Daily headaches sometimes accompany treatment with nitroglycerin. In patients who get these headaches, the headaches are a marker of the activity of the drug. Patients should resist the temptation to avoid headaches by altering the schedule of their treatment with nitroglycerin, since loss of headache is likely to be associated with simultaneous loss of antianginal efficacy.

Treatment with nitroglycerin may be associated with lightheadedness on standing, especially just after rising from a recumbent or seated position. This effect may be more frequent in patients who have also consumed alcohol.

After normal use, there is enough residual nitroglycerin in discarded patches that they are a potential hazard to children and pets.

A patient leaflet is supplied with the systems.

Drug Interactions: The vasodilating effects of nitroglycerin may be additive with those of other vasodilators. Alcohol, in particular, has been found to exhibit additive effects of this variety.

Marked symptomatic orthostatic hypotension has been reported when calcium channel blockers and organic nitrates were used in combination. Dose adjustments of either class of agents may be necessary.

Carcinogenesis, Mutagenesis, Impairment of Fertility: No long-term animal studies have examined the carcinogenic or mutagenic potential of nitroglycerin. Nitroglycerin's effect upon reproductive capacity is similarly unknown.

Pregnancy Category C: Animal reproduction studies have not been conducted with nitroglycerin. It is also not known whether nitroglycerin can cause fetal harm when administered to a pregnant woman or whether it can affect reproductive capacity. Nitroglycerin should be given to a pregnant woman only if clearly needed.

Nursing Mothers: It is not known whether nitroglycerin is excreted in human milk. Because many drugs are excreted in human milk, caution should be exercised when nitroglycerin is administered to a nursing woman.

Pediatric Use: Safety and effectiveness in children have not been established.

ADVERSE REACTIONS

Adverse reactions to nitroglycerin are generally dose-related, and almost all of these reactions are the result of nitroglycerin's activity as a vasodilator. Headache, which may be severe, is the most commonly reported side effect. Headache may be recurrent with each daily dose, especially at higher doses. Transient episodes of lightheadedness, occasionally related to blood pressure changes, may also occur. Hypotension occurs infrequently, but in some patients it may be severe enough to warrant discontinuation of therapy. Syncope, crescendo angina, and rebound hypertension have been reported but are uncommon.

Extremely rarely, ordinary doses of organic nitrates have caused methemoglobinemia in normal-seeming patients. Methemoglobinemia is so infrequent at these doses that further discussion of its diagnosis and treatment is deferred (see **OVERDOSAGE**).

Application-site irritation may occur but is rarely severe.

In two placebo-controlled trials of intermittent therapy with nitroglycerin patches at 0.2 to 0.8 mg/hr, the most frequent adverse reactions among 307 subjects were as follows:

	placebo	patch
headache	18%	63%
lightheadedness	4%	6%
hypotension, and/or syncope	0%	4%
increased angina	2%	2%

OVERDOSAGE

Hemodynamic Effects: The ill effects of nitroglycerin overdose are generally the results of nitroglycerin's capacity to induce vasodilatation, venous pooling, reduced cardiac output, and hypotension. These hemodynamic changes may have protean manifestations, including increased intracranial pressure, with any or all of persistent throbbing headache, confusion, and moderate fever; vertigo; palpitations; visual disturbances; nausea and vomting (possibly with colic and even bloody diarrhea); syncope (especially in the upright posture); air hunger and dyspnea, later followed by reduced ventilatory effort, diaphoresis, with the skin either flushed or cold and clammy; heart block and bradycardia; paralysis; coma; seizures; and death.

Laboratory determinations of serum levels of nitroglycerin and its metabolites are not widely available, and such determinations have, in any event, no established role in the management of nitroglycerin overdose.

No data are available to suggest physiological maneuvers (e.g., maneuvers to change the pH of the urine) that might accelerate elimination of nitroglycerin and its active metabolites. Similarly, it is not known which—if any—of these substances can usefully be removed from the body by hemodialysis.

No specific antagonist to the vasodilator effects of nitroglycerin is known, and no intervention has been subject to controlled study as a therapy of nitroglycerin overdose. Because the hypotension associated with nitroglycerin overdose is the result of venodilatation and arterial hypovolemia, prudent therapy in this situation should be directed toward increase in central fluid volume. Passive elevation of the patient's legs may be sufficient, but intravenous infusion of normal saline or similar fluid may also be necessary.

The use of epinephrine or other arterial vasoconstrictors in this setting is likely to do more harm than good.

In patients with renal disease or congestive heart failure, therapy resulting in central volume expansion is not without

Nitro-Dur System Rated Release In Vivo*	Total Nitroglycerin Content	System Size	Package Size
0.1 mg/hr	20 mg	5 cm²	Unit Dose 30 (NDC 0085-3305-30) Hospital Unit Dose 100 (NDC 0085-3305-01) Institutional Package 30 (NDC 0085-3305-35) Institutional Package 100 (NDC 0085-3305-10)
0.2 mg/hr	40 mg	10 cm²	Unit Dose 30 (NDC 0085-3310-30) Hospital Unit Dose 100 (NDC 0085-3310-01) Institutional Package 30 (NDC 0085-3310-35) Institutional Package 100 (NDC 0085-3310-10)
0.3 mg/hr	60 mg	15 cm²	Unit Dose 30 (NDC 0085-3315-30) Hospital Unit Dose 100 (NDC 0085-3315-01) Institutional Package 30 (NDC 0085-3315-35) Institutional Package 100 (NDC 0085-3315-10)
0.4 mg/hr	80 mg	20 cm²	Unit Dose 30 (NDC 0085-3320-30) Hospital Unit Dose 100 (NDC 0085-3320-01) Institutional Package 30 (NDC 0085-3320-35) Institutional Package 100 (NDC 0085-3320-10)
0.6 mg/hr	120 mg	30 cm²	Unit Dose 30 (NDC 0085-3330-30) Hospital Unit Dose 100 (NDC 0085-3330-01) Institutional Package 30 (NDC 0085-3330-35) Institutional Package 100 (NDC 0085-3330-10)

* Release rates were formerly described in terms of drug delivered per 24 hours. In these terms, the supplied NITRO-DUR Systems would be rated at 2.5 mg/24 hours (0.1 mg/hour), 5 mg/24 hours (0.2 mg/hour), 7.5 mg/24 hours (0.3 mg/hour), 10 mg/24 hours (0.4 mg/hour), and 15 mg/24 hours (0.6 mg/hour).

hazard. Treatment of nitroglycerin overdose in these patients may be subtle and difficult, and invasive monitoring may be required.

Methemoglobinemia: Nitrate ions liberated during metabolism of nitroglycerin can oxidize hemoglobin into methemoglobin. Even in patients totally without cytochrome b_5 reductase activity, however, and even assuming that the nitrate moieties of nitroglycerin are quantitatively applied to oxidation of hemoglobin, about 1 mg/kg of nitroglycerin should be required before any of these patients manifests clinically significant ($\geq 10\%$) methemoglobinemia. In patients with normal reductase function, significant production of methemoglobin should require even larger doses of nitroglycerin. In one study in which 36 patients received 2–4 weeks of continuous nitroglycerin therapy at 3.1 to 4.4 mg/hr, the average methemoglobin level measured was 0.2%; this was comparable to that observed in parallel patients who received placebo.

Notwithstanding these observations, there are case reports of significant methemoglobinemia in association with moderate overdoses of organic nitrates. None of the affected patients had been thought to be unusually susceptible.

Methemoglobin levels are available from most clinical laboratories. The diagnosis should be suspected in patients who exhibit signs of impaired oxygen delivery despite adequate cardiac output and adequate arterial pO_2. Classically, methemoglobinemic blood is described as chocolate brown, without color change on exposure to air.

When methemoglobinemia is diagnosed, the treatment of choice is methylene blue, 1–2 mg/kg intravenously.

DOSAGE AND ADMINISTRATION

The suggested starting dose is between 0.2 mg/hr*, and 0.4 mg/hr*. Doses between 0.4 mg/hr* and 0.8 mg/hr* have shown continued effectiveness for 10–12 hours daily for at least one month (the longest period studied) of intermittent administration. Although the minimum nitrate-free interval has not been defined, data show that a nitrate-free interval of 10–12 hours is sufficient (see **CLINICAL PHARMACOLOGY**). Thus, an appropriate dosing schedule for nitroglycerin patches would include a daily patch-on period of 12–14 hours and a daily patch-off period of 10–12 hours.

Although some well controlled clinical trials using exercise tolerance testing have shown maintenance of effectiveness when patches are worn continuously, the large majority of such controlled trials have shown the development of tolerance (i.e., complete loss of effect) within the first 24 hours after therapy was initiated. Dose adjustment even to levels much higher than generally used, did not restore efficacy.

* Release rates were formerly described in terms of drug delivered per 24 hours. In these terms, the supplied NITRO-DUR systems would be rated at 2.5 mg/24 hours (0.1 mg/hour), 5 mg/24 hours (0.2 mg/hour), 7.5 mg/24 hours (0.3 mg/hour), 10 mg/24 hours (0.4 mg/hour), and 15 mg/24 hours (0.6 mg/hour).

HOW SUPPLIED

[See table on preceding page.]

CAUTION: Federal Law prohibits dispensing without prescription.

Key Pharmaceuticals, Inc.
Kenilworth, NJ 07033 USA
Revised 8/89
Copyright © 1987, 1989 Key Pharmaceuticals, Inc.
All Rights Reserved.

Shown in Product Identification Section, page 412

QUINORA® ℞
[*kwin-ō-ra*]
(quinidine sulfate tablets, USP)

DESCRIPTION

Quinidine sulfate occurs as minute needlelike white crystals (frequently cohering in masses) or fine white powder. It is odorless, has a very bitter taste, and darkens on exposure to light. It is slightly soluble in water, soluble in alcohol and in chloroform, and insoluble in ether.

Quinidine sulfate is the sulfate salt of quinidine (cinchonan-ς-ol, 6'-methoxy-,(9S)-sulfate (2:1) dihydrate), a diastereomer of quinine sulfate. The structural formula is as follows:
[See Chemical Formula at top of next column.]

Each Quinora 300 mg tablet contains 300 mg quinidine sulfate (equivalent to 249 mg of quinidine base).

CLINICAL PHARMACOLOGY

The action of quinidine in preventing aberrant cardiac rhythms of atrial and ventricular origin resides in its ability to (a) depress excitability of cardiac muscle, (b) slow the rate of spontaneous rhythm, (c) decrease vagal tone, and (d) prolong conduction and effective refractory period. Besides

M.W. = 782.95

these direct effects, quinidine exerts some indirect activity on the heart through an anticholinergic action. Large oral doses may reduce the arterial pressure by means of peripheral vasodilation. Hypotension of a serious degree is more likely with the parenteral use of the drug.

Quinidine is rapidly absorbed from the gastrointestinal tract. The peak concentrations in serum are attained in 60 to 90 minutes and activity persists 6 to 8 hours or more. Quinidine is metabolized in the liver and excreted by the kidney. Ten to 50% of quinidine is excreted in the urine as unchanged drug within 24 hours.

Serum levels of quinidine can be measured. Values vary according to the assay employed. Traditionally, plasma concentrations for effective use of quinidine have been reported to range from 2–7 mcg/mL and levels of 8 mcg/mL or greater are associated with toxicity. This information is based upon less specific analytic methods which quantitate metabolites as well as intact quinidine. However, plasma quinidine concentrations will be lower using more specific assays. Therefore, clinicians requesting serum quinidine determinations should be aware of the method of analysis. There is a wide individual variation in response to quinidine therapy. In all cases, the physician should carefully consider patient response and evidence of toxicity along with blood levels in determining optimal quinidine therapy.

INDICATIONS AND USAGE

Quinidine sulfate is indicated in the treatment of:
1. Premature atrial and ventricular contractions
2. Paroxysmal atrial tachycardia
3. Paroxysmal atrioventricular (A-V) junctional rhythm
4. Atrial flutter
5. Paroxysmal atrial fibrillation
6. Established atrial fibrillation when therapy is appropriate
7. Paroxysmal ventricular tachycardia when not associated with complete heart block
8. Maintenance therapy after electrical conversion of atrial fibrillation and/or flutter.

CONTRAINDICATIONS

Hypersensitivity or idiosyncrasy to the drug, digitalis intoxication manifested by A-V conduction disorders, complete A-V block with an A-V nodal or idioventricular pacemaker, left bundle branch block or other severe intraventricular conduction defects with marked QRS widening. Ectopic impulses and abnormal rhythms due to escape mechanisms. Also, myasthenia gravis.

WARNINGS

In the treatment of atrial flutter, reversion to sinus rhythm may be preceded by a progressive reduction in the degree of A-V block to a 1:1 ratio, which results in extremely rapid ventricular rate. This possible hazard may be reduced by digitalization prior to administration of quinidine.

In susceptible individuals, such as those with marginally compensated cardiovascular disease, quinidine may produce clinically important depression of cardiac function manifested by hypotension, bradycardia, or heartblock. Quinidine therapy should be carefully monitored in such individuals. Evidence of quinidine cardiotoxicity (excessive prolongation of Q-T interval, widening of QRS complex, and ventricular tachyarrhythmias) mandates immediate discontinuation of the drug and subsequent close clinical and electrocardiographic monitoring of the patient.

Quinidine should be used with extreme caution when there is incomplete A-V block, since complete block and asystole may result. The drug may cause unpredictable abnormalities of rhythm in digitalized hearts, and it should be used with special caution in the presence of digitalis intoxication. The cardiotoxic effect of quinidine is increased by hyperkalemia and decreased by hypokalemia.

Patients taking quinidine occasionally have syncopal episodes which usually result from ventricular tachycardia or fibrillation. This syndrome has not been shown to be related to dose or serum levels. Syncopal episodes frequently terminate spontaneously or in response to treatment, but sometimes are fatal.

Recent reports have described increased, potentially toxic, digoxin serum levels when quinidine is administered concurrently. When concurrent use is necessary, reduction of digoxin dosage may have to be considered, its serum concentration should be monitored and the patient observed closely for digitalis intoxication.

Caution should be used when quinidine is administered concurrently with coumarin anticoagulants. The combination may reduce prothrombin levels and cause bleeding. Quinidine should be used with caution in patients exhibiting renal, cardiac or hepatic insufficiency because of potential accumulation of quinidine in serum leading to toxicity.

Cases of hepatotoxicity, including granulomatous hepatitis, due to quinidine hypersensitivity have been reported. Unexplained fever and/or elevation of hepatic enzymes, particularly in the early stages of therapy, warrant consideration of possible hepatotoxicity. Monitoring liver function during the first 4–8 weeks should be considered. Cessation of quinidine in these cases usually results in the disappearance of toxicity.

PRECAUTIONS

General

A preliminary test dose of a single tablet of quinidine sulfate may be administered to determine if the patient has an idiosyncrasy to quinidine. Hypersensitivity to quinidine, although rare, should constantly be considered, especially during the first weeks of therapy. Hospitalization for close clinical observation, electrocardiographic monitoring, and possible determination of serum quinidine levels is indicated when large doses are used, or with patients who present an increased risk.

Drug Interactions

Drug	Effect
Quinidine with:	
Anticholinergics	Additive vagolytic effect
Cholinergics	Antagonism of cholinergic effects
Carbonic anhydrase inhibitors, sodium bicarbonate, thiazide diuretics	Alkalination of urine resulting in decreased excretion of quinidine
Coumarin anticoagulants	Reduction of clotting factor concentrations (see **WARNINGS**)
Tubocurarine, succinylcholine, decamethonium and pancuronium	Potentiation of neuromuscular blockage
Phenothiazines and reserpine	Additive cardiac depressive effects
Hepatic enzyme-inducing drugs (phenobarbital, phenytoin, rifampin)	Decreased plasma half-life of quinidine
Digoxin	Increased serum concentrations of digoxin (see **WARNINGS**)
Amiodarone	Increased serum concentration of quinidine
Cimetidine	Prolonged quinidine half-life and an inrease in serum quinidine level
Ranitidine	Premature ventricular contractions and/or bigeminy
Verapamil	Increased quinidine half-life and an increase in serum quinidine level; potential hypotensive reactions
Nifedipine	Decreased serum concentrations of quinidine

Laboratory Tests

Continuous electrocardiographic monitoring and determination of serum quinidine levels are indicated when large doses (more than 2 g/day) are used.

Periodic blood counts and liver and kidney function tests should be performed during long-term therapy; the drug should be discontinued if blood dyscrasias or evidence of hepatic or renal dysfunction occurs.

Carcinogenesis, Mutagenesis and Impairment of Fertility

Studies in animals have not been performed to evaluate the carcinogenic potential of quinidine.

Usage in Pregnancy

Teratogenic Effects: Pregnancy Category C. Animal reproduction studies have not been conducted with quinidine. There are no adequate and well-controlled studies in pregnant women. Quinidine should be given to a pregnant woman only if clearly needed.

Nonteratogenic Effects: Like quinine, quinidine has been reported to have oxytocic properties. The significance of this property in the clinical setting has not been established.

Labor and Delivery

There is no known use of quinidine sulfate in labor and delivery. However, quinidine has been reported to have oxytocic properties. The significance of this property in the clinical setting has not been established.

Continued on next page

Key—Cont.

Nursing Mothers
Caution should be exercised when quinidine is administered to a nursing mother due to passage of the drug into breast milk.

Pediatric Use
There are no adequate and well-controlled studies establishing the safety and effectiveness of quinidine sulfate in children.

ADVERSE REACTIONS
Symptoms of cinchonism, such as ringing in ears, loss of hearing, dizziness, lightheadedness, headache, nausea, and/or disturbed vision may appear in sensitive patients after a single dose of the drug. The most frequently encountered side effects to quinidine are gastrointestinal.

Gastrointestinal: Nausea, vomiting, abdominal pain, diarrhea, anorexia, granulomatous hepatitis (which may be preceded by fever), esophagitis.

Cardiovascular: Ventricular extrasystoles occurring at a rate of one or more every 6 normal beats; widening of the QRS complex and prolonged Q-T interval; complete A-V block; ventricular tachycardia and fibrillation; ventricular flutter; torsade de pointes; arterial embolism; hypotension, syncope.

Central Nervous System: Headache, vertigo, apprehension, excitement, confusion, delirium, dementia, ataxia, depression.

Ophthalmologic and Otologic: Disturbed hearing (tinnitus, decreased auditory acuity), disturbed vision (mydriasis, blurred vision, disturbed color perception, photophobia, diplopia, night blindness, scotomata), optic neuritis, reduced visual field.

Dermatologic: Cutaneous flushing with intense pruritus, photosensitivity, urticaria, rash, eczema, exfoliative eruptions, psoriasis, abnormalities of pigmentation.

Hypersensitivity: Angioedema, acute asthmatic episode, vascular collapse, respiratory arrest, hepatotoxicity, granulomatous hepatitis (see **WARNINGS**), purpura, vasculitis.

Hematologic: Thrombocytopenia, thrombocytopenic purpura, agranulocytosis, acute hemolytic anemia, hypoprothrombinemia, leukocytosis, shift to left in WBC differential, neutropenia.

Immunologic: Systemic lupus erythematosus, lupus nephritis.

Miscellaneous: Fever, increase in serum skeletal muscle creatine phosphokinase, arthralgia, myalgia.

OVERDOSAGE
Symptoms: Overdosage of quinidine can lead to accelerated idioventricular rhythm, morphologic appearance of QRS complexes, prolonged Q-T intervals, intermittent sinus capture beats, paroxysms of tachycardia, ventricular arrhythmias, hypotension, oliguria, respiratory depression, pulmonary edema, acidosis, seizures, and coma.

Treatment: Early treatment to empty the stomach using syrup of ipecac and/or gastric lavage is recommended. Administration of activated charcoal may reduce absorption. Other general supportive measures should be employed as indicated by patient response in severe cases, circulation should be stabilized and measurements of pulmonary capillary wedge pressure should be performed to assure adequate left ventricular filling pressure. Electrolyte and blood gas abnormalities should be corrected. In quinidine-induced vasodilation, catecholamines and other alpha-adrenergic agonists may be tried. Arrhythmias may be treated with lidocaine, pacing, and cardioversion. Administration of sodium lactate reportedly reduces the cardiotoxicity of quinidine; however sodium lactate is contraindicated in the presence of alkalosis as increased urinary pH can lead to an increase in the renal tubular absorption of quinidine. Acidification of the urine may enhance the urinary excretion of quinidine.

DOSAGE AND ADMINISTRATION
A preliminary test dose of a single tablet of quinidine sulfate should be administered to determine whether the patient has an idiosyncrasy to it. Continuous electrocardiographic monitoring is recommended in all cases in which quinidine is used in large doses.

Usual Adult Dose
Premature Atrial and Ventricular Contractions: 200 to 300 mg, 3 or 4 times daily.

Paroxysmal Supraventricular Tachycardias: 400 to 600 mg, every 2 to 3 hours until the paroxysm is terminated.

Atrial Flutter: Quinidine should be administered after digitalization for this indication. Dosage is to be individualized.

Conversion of Atrial Fibrillation: Various schedules of quinidine administration have been in clinical use. A widely used technique is to give 200 mg of quinidine sulfate orally every 2 or 3 hours for 5 to 8 doses, with subsequent daily increases of the individual dose until sinus rhythm is restored or toxic effects occur. The total daily dose should not exceed 3 to 4 grams in any regimen. Prior to quinidine administration, the ventricular rate and congestive heart failure (if

present) should be brought under control by digitalis therapy.

Usual Maintenance Therapy: 200 to 300 mg, 3 or 4 times daily.

Although most patients may be maintained in normal rhythm on a dosage of 200 to 300 mg of quinidine sulfate every 6 to 8 hours, other patients may require larger doses or more frequent administration than the usually recommended schedule. Such increased dosage should be instituted only after careful clinical and laboratory evaluation of the patient, including monitoring of serum quinidine levels and, if possible, serial electrocardiograms.

Gastrointestinal disturbances, if they occur, may be minimized by administering the drug with food.

HOW SUPPLIED
QUINORA Tablets (300 mg): round, convex, white to off-white, unscored, tablet debossed QUINORA 300 on one side; bottles of 100 (NDC 0085-0073-01).

Storage Conditions
Tablets must be dispensed in tight, light-resistant containers as defined in the USP. Tablets must be stored at controlled room temperature between 15° and 30°C (59° and 86°F).

Caution: Federal law prohibits dispensing without prescription.

Key Pharmaceuticals, Inc.
Kenilworth, NJ 07033 USA
            Revised 10/88
Copyright © 1988, Key Pharmaceuticals, Inc.
All rights reserved.

THEO-DUR®   ℞
[thē-a-dur]
theophylline (anhydrous)
Sustained Action Tablets

DESCRIPTION
THEO-DUR® Sustained Action Tablets contain anhydrous theophylline, a bronchodilator, in a sustained release formulation which allows a 12-hour dosing interval for a majority of patients and a 24-hour dosing interval for selected patients (see DOSAGE AND ADMINISTRATION section for description of appropriate patient populations). THEO-DUR contains no color additives and is available in three strengths: 100 mg, 200 mg and 300 mg and 450 mg.

Theophylline is 1H-Purine-2, 6-dione, 3, 7-dihydro-1, 3-dimethyl.

Anhydrous theophylline is a white, odorless, crystalline powder having a bitter taste.

CLINICAL PHARMACOLOGY
Theophylline directly relaxes the smooth muscle of the bronchial airways and pulmonary blood vessels, thus acting mainly as a bronchodilator and smooth muscle relaxant. The drug also produces other actions typical of the xanthine derivatives: coronary vasodilator, cardiac stimulant, diuretic, cerebral stimulant, and skeletal muscle stimulant. The actions of theophylline may be mediated through inhibition of phosphodiesterase and a resultant increase in intracellular cyclic AMP.

In vitro theophylline has been shown to act synergistically with beta agonists that increase intracellular cyclic AMP through the stimulation of adenyl cyclase, but synergism has not been demonstrated in patient studies. More data are needed to determine if theophylline and beta agonists have a clinically important additive effect *in vivo*. Apparently, no development of tolerance occurs with chronic use of theophylline.

PHARMACOKINETICS
The half-life of theophylline is influenced by a number of known variables. It is prolonged in patients suffering from chronic alcoholism, impaired hepatic or renal function, congestive heart failure, and in patients receiving macrolide antibiotics and cimetidine. Older adults (over age 55) and patients with chronic obstructive pulmonary disease, with or without cor pulmonale, may also have much slower clearance rates. For such patients, the theophylline half-life may exceed 24 hours.

Newborns and neonates have extremely slow clearance rates compared to older infants (over 6 months) and children, and may also have a theophylline half-life of over 24 hours. High fever for prolonged periods may also reduce the rate of theophylline elimination.

THEOPHYLLINE ELIMINATION CHARACTERISTICS

Theophylline Clearance Rates (mean ± S.D.)	Half-life Average (mean ± S.D.)
Children (over 6 months of age)	
1.45 ± 0.58 ml/kg/min	3.7 ± 1.1 hrs.
Adult non-smokers uncomplicated asthma	
0.65 ± 0.19 ml/kg/min	8.7 ± 2.2 hrs.

The half-life of theophylline in smokers (1 to 2 packs/day) averages 4–5 hours, much shorter than the half-life in non-smokers which averages 7–9 hours. The increase in theophylline clearance caused by smoking is probably the result of induction of drug-metabolizing enzymes that do not readily normalize after cessation of smoking. It appears that between 3 months and 2 years may be necessary for normalization of the effect of smoking on theophylline pharmacokinetics.

THEO-DUR (100, 200 and 300 mg and 450 mg) Sustained Action Tablets:
In single dose studies with 18 normal fasting subjects, THEO-DUR, at 8 mg/kg body weight (300–700 mg/dose), produced mean peak theophylline plasma levels of 7.5 ± 1.9 mcg/ml at 9.2 ± 1.9 hours following administration. In multiple dose, steady-state, 3 and 5 day studies with 12 normal subjects, THEO-DUR administered at 8mg/kg (300–600 mg/dose) twice daily, achieved an average peak-trough difference of 4 mcg/ml. The Cmax and Cmin were 13.9 ± 6.9 and 9.9 ± 6.0, respectively. The mean % fluctuation ± S.D. of the plasma concentration at steady-state [% fluctuation = 100 (Cmax—Cmin)/Cmin] was 54.2 ± 45.7%. These pharmacokinetic parameters were measured under fasting conditions.

THEO-DUR (200 and 300 mg and 450 mg) Sustained Action Tablets:
In a multiple dose (300–500 mg BID), steady-state, 5 day study involving 14 normal, nonfasting, subjects with theophylline half-lives between 5.8 and 12.3 hours (mean 8.0 ± 1.8 hours), THEO-DUR, dosed twice daily, produced mean Cmax and Cmin levels of 12.2 ± 2.0 and 10.2 ± 1.6 mcg/ml, respectively, over the a.m. dosing interval and Cmax and Cmin of 11.6 ± 1.6 and 8.7 ± 1.8 mcg/ml, respectively, over the p.m. dosing interval. The mean % fluctuation ± S.D. over the a.m. dosing interval was 30.4 ± 12.9% and 33.7 ± 13.1% over the p.m. dosing interval. In the same subjects, THEO-DUR given once daily, in the morning, in doses ranging from 600–1000 mg (same daily dose as for BID, above) produced a mean Cmax and Cmin of 14.4 ± 2.2 and 5.5 ± 2.0, respectively and a mean % fluctuation ± S.D. of 195.8 ± 106.0%. Average peak-trough differences over 24 hours were 8.9 ± 1.3 and 3.7 ± 1.2 mcg/ml when THEO-DUR was given once or twice daily, respectively. In both the twice daily and once daily dosing regimens, THEO-DUR exhibited complete bioavailability when compared to an immediate release product.

THEO-DUR (200 and 300 mg and 450 mg) Sustained Action Tablets:
In a single-dose bioavailability study in eleven subjects, 1000 mg of THEO-DUR was administered under fasting conditions and immediately following a moderately high fat content (37g) breakfast of approximately 1000 Calories. The rate and extent of absorption of theophylline from THEO-DUR administered in fasting and fed conditions was similar.

INDICATIONS
THEO-DUR is indicated for relief and/or prevention of symptoms of asthma and for reversible bronchospasm associated with chronic bronchitis and emphysema.

CONTRAINDICATIONS
THEO-DUR is contraindicated in individuals who have shown hypersensitivity to theophylline or any of the tablet components.

WARNINGS
Status asthmaticus should be considered a medical emergency and is defined as that degree of bronchospasm which is not rapidly responsive to usual doses of conventional bronchodilators. Optimal therapy for such patients frequently requires both *additional medication,* parenterally administered, and *close monitoring,* preferably in an intensive care setting.

Although increasing the dose of theophylline may bring about relief, such treatment may be associated with toxicity. The likelihood of such toxicity developing increases significantly when the serum theophylline concentration exceeds 20 mcg/ml. Therefore, determination of serum theophylline levels is recommended to assure maximal benefit without excessive risk.

Serum levels above 20 mcg/ml are rarely found after appropriate administration of the recommended doses. However, in individuals in whom theophylline plasma clearance is reduced *for any reason,* even conventional doses may result in increased serum levels and potential toxicity. Reduced theophylline clearance has been documented in the following readily identifiable groups: 1) patients with impaired renal or liver function; 2) patients over 55 years of age, particularly males and those with chronic lung disease; 3) those with cardiac failure from any cause; 4) neonates; and 5) those patients taking certain drugs (macrolide antibiotics and cimetidine). Decreased clearance of theophylline may be associated with either influenza immunization or active infection with influenza.

Reduction of dosage and laboratory monitoring is especially appropriate in the above individuals.

Less serious signs of theophylline toxicity, i.e. nausea and restlessness, may appear in up to 50% of patients. Unfortunately, however, serious side effects such as ventricular arrhythmias, convulsions or even death may appear as the first sign of toxicity without any previous warning. Stated differently; *serious toxicity is not reliably preceded by less severe side effects.*

Many patients who require theophylline may exhibit tachycardia due to their underlying disease process so that the cause/effect relationship to elevated serum theophylline concentrations may not be appreciated.

Theophylline products may cause dysrhythmia and/or worsen pre-existing arrhythmias and any significant change in rate and/or rhythm warrants monitoring and further investigation.

The occurrence of arrhythmias and sudden death (with histological evidence of necrosis of the myocardium) has been recorded in laboratory animals (minipigs, rodents and dogs) when theophylline and beta agonists were administered concomitantly, although not when either was administered alone. The significance of these findings when applied to human usage is currently unknown.

PRECAUTIONS

THEO-DUR TABLETS SHOULD NOT BE CHEWED OR CRUSHED.

General: Theophylline half-life is shorter in smokers than in non-smokers. Therefore, smokers may require larger or more frequent doses. Morphine and curare should be used with caution in patients with airway obstruction as they may suppress respiration and stimulate histamine release. Alternative drugs should be used when possible. Theophylline should not be administered concurrently with other xanthine medications. Use with caution in patients with severe cardiac disease, severe hypoxemia, hypertension, hyperthyroidism, acute myocardial injury, cor pulmonale, congestive heart failure, liver disease, in the elderly (especially males) and in neonates. In particular, great caution should be used in giving theophylline to patients with congestive heart failure. Frequently, such patients have markedly prolonged theophylline serum levels with theophylline persisting in serum for long periods following discontinuation of the drug. Individuals who are rapid metabolizers of theophylline, such as the young, smokers, and some non-smoking adults, may not be suitable candidates for once-daily dosing. These individuals will generally need to be dosed at 12 hourly or sometimes 8 hourly intervals. Such patients may exhibit symptoms of bronchospasm near the end of a dosing interval, or may have wider peak-to-trough differences than desired.

Use theophylline cautiously in patients with history of peptic ulcer. Theophylline may occasionally act as a local irritant to the G.I. tract although gastrointestinal symptoms are more commonly centrally mediated and associated with serum drug concentrations over 20 mcg/ml.

Information for Patients: The physician should reinforce the importance of taking only the prescribed dose and time interval between doses. THEO-DUR tablets should not be chewed or crushed. When dosing THEO-DUR on a once daily (q24h) basis, tablets should be taken whole and not split. As with any controlled-release theophylline product, the patient should alert the physician if symptoms occur repeatedly, especially near the end of the dosing interval.

Drug Interactions:

Drug—Drug:

Toxic synergism with ephedrine has been documented and may occur with some other sympathomimetic bronchodilators. In addition, the following drug interactions have been demonstrated:

Drug	Effect
Theophylline with Lithium Carbonate	Increased excretion of Lithium Carbonate
Theophylline with Propranolol	Antagonism of Propranolol effect
Theophylline with Cimetidine	Increased theophylline blood levels
Theophylline with troleandomycin, erythromycin	Increased theophylline blood levels

Drug—Food:

THEO-DUR 100 mg Sustained Action Tablets have not been adequately studied to determine whether their bioavailability is altered when given with food. Available data suggest that drug administration at the time of food ingestion may infuence the absorption characteristics of theophylline controlled-release products resulting in serum values different from those found after administration in the fasting state. A drug-food effect, if any, would likely have its greatest clinical significance when high theophylline serum levels are being maintained and/or when large single doses (greater than 13 mg/kg or 900 mg) of a controlled-release theophylline product are given.

THEO-DUR (200 and 300 mg and 450 mg) Sustained Action Tablets: The rate and extent of absorption of theophylline from THEO-DUR 200 and 300 mg and 450 mg tablets when administered fasting or immediately after a moderately high fat content breakfast is similar (see CLINICAL PHARMACOLOGY, Pharmacokinetics).

Drug-Laboratory Test Interactions: When plasma levels of theophylline are measured by spectrophotometric methods, coffee, tea, cola beverages, chocolate, and acetaminophen contribute falsely high values.

Carcinogenesis, Mutagenesis, and Impairment of Fertility: Long-term animal studies have not been performed to evaluate the carcinogenic potential, mutagenic potential, or the effect on fertility of xanthine compounds.

Pregnancy: Category C-Animal reproduction studies have not been conducted with theophylline. It is not known whether theophylline can cause fetal harm when administered to a pregnant woman or can affect reproduction capacity. Xanthines should be given to a pregnant woman only if clearly needed.

Nursing Mothers: It has been reported that theophylline distributes readily into breast milk and may cause adverse effects in the infant. Caution must be used if prescribing xanthine to a mother who is nursing, taking into account the risk-benefit of this therapy.

Pediatric Use: Safety and effectiveness of THEO-DUR administered:

1. Every 24 hours in children under 12 years of age, have not been established.
2. Every 12 hours in children under 6 years of age, have not been established.

ADVERSE REACTIONS

The most consistent adverse reactions are usually due to overdose and are:

1. *Gastrointestinal:* nausea, vomiting, epigastric pain, hematemesis, diarrhea.
2. *Central nervous system:* headaches, irritability, restlessness, insomnia, reflex hyperexcitability, muscle twitching, clonic and tonic generalized convulsions.
3. *Cardiovascular:* palpitation, tachycardia, extrasystoles, flushing, hypotension, circulatory failure, ventricular arrhythmias.
4. *Respiratory:* tachypnea.
5. *Renal:* albuminuria, increased excretion of renal tubular and red blood cells, potentiation of diuresis.
6. *Others:* rash, hyperglycemia and inappropriate ADH syndrome.

OVERDOSAGE

Management:

If potential oral overdose is established and seizure has not occurred:

A. Induce vomiting.
B. Administer a cathartic (this is particularly important if sustained-release preparations have been taken).
C. Administer activated charcoal.

If patient is having a seizure:

A. Establish an airway.
B. Administer oxygen.
C. Treat the seizure with intravenous diazepam, 0.1 to 0.3 mg/kg up to 10 mg.
D. Monitor vital signs, maintain blood pressure and provide adequate hydration.

Post Seizure Coma:

A. Maintain airway and oxygenation.
B. If a result of oral medication, follow above recommendations to prevent absorption of the drug, but intubation and lavage will have to be performed instead of inducing emesis, and the cathartic and charcoal will need to be introduced via a large bore gastric lavage tube.
C. Continue to provide full supportive care and adequate hydration while waiting for drug to be metabolized. In general, the drug is metabolized sufficiently rapid so as not to warrant consideration of dialysis; however, if serum levels exceed 50 mcg/ml, charcoal hemoperfusion may be indicated.

DOSAGE AND ADMINISTRATION

THEO-DUR (200, 300mg and 450 mg) Sustained Action Tablets: The rate and extent of absorption of theophylline from THEO-DUR 200, 300 and 450 mg tablets when administered fasting or immediately after a moderately high fat content breakfast is similar (see CLINICAL PHARMACOLOGY, Pharmacokinetics).

THEO-DUR 100 mg Sustained Action Tablets have not been adequately studied for their bioavailability when administered with food (see PRECAUTIONS, Drug-Food Interactions).

For most patients, *effective use* of theophylline, i.e. associated with optimal likelihood of benefit combined with minimal risk of toxicity, is considered to occur when serum levels are maintained between 10 and 20 mcg/ml. Levels above 20 mcg/ml may produce toxicity, and in a small number of patients, toxicity may even be seen with serum levels between 15-20 mcg/ml, particularly during initiation of therapy.

There is considerable variation from patient to patient in the dosage required to achieve and maintain therapeutic and safe levels, primarily due to variable rates of elimination. Therefore, it is essential that not only must dosage be individualized, but titration and monitoring of serum levels be utilized where available. When serum concentration cannot be obtained, restriction of dosage to the amounts and intervals recommended in the guidelines listed below becomes essential. Dosage should be calculated on the basis of lean (ideal) body weight where mg/kg doses are presented. Theophylline does not distribute into fatty tissue.

As a practical consideration, it is not always possible to obtain serum level determinations. Under such conditions, restriction of the daily dose (in otherwise healthy adults) to not greater than 13 mg/kg/day or up to 900 mg (of anhydrous theophylline) will result in relatively few patients exceeding serum levels of 20 mcg/ml and the resultant risk of toxicity. THEO-DUR is not intended for patients experiencing an acute episode of bronchospasm (associated with asthma, chronic bronchitis, or emphysema). Such patients require *rapid* relief of symptoms and should be treated with an immediate-release or intravenous theophylline preparation (or other bronchodilators) and not with controlled release products.

Dosage Guidelines:

WARNING: DO NOT ATTEMPT TO MAINTAIN ANY DOSE THAT IS NOT TOLERATED.

Dosage guidelines are approximations only, and the wide range of clearance of theophylline among individuals (particularly those with concomitant disease) makes indiscriminate usage hazardous. It is recommended that dosing be considered in two stages: initiation of therapy with THEO-DUR, and titration, adjustment, and chronic maintenance.

Initiation of therapy:

It is recommended that the appropriate dosage be established using an immediate-release preparation. Slow clinical titration is generally preferred to help assure acceptance and safety of the medication and to allow the patient to develop tolerance to the transient caffeine-like side effects. Then, if the total 24 hour dose can be given by use of the available strengths of this product, the patient can usually be switched to THEO-DUR giving one-half of the daily dose at 12 hour intervals. However, certain patients, such as the young, smokers and some non-smoking adults are likely to metabolize theophylline rapidly and require dosing at 8 hour intervals. Such patients can generally be identified as having trough serum concentrations lower than desired or repeatedly exhibiting symptoms near the end of a dosing interval.

Alternatively, therapy can be initiated with THEO-DUR since it is available in dosage forms/strengths which permit titration and adjustment of dosage as outlined in the following dosing guidelines. It is recommended that for children under 25 kg, proper dosage be established with a liquid preparation to permit titration in small increments.

THE AVERAGE INITIAL ADULT AND CHILDREN'S (over 25 kg) DOSE IS ONE THEO-DUR 200 mg TABLET q12h.

Titration, Adjustment and Chronic Maintenance:

If the desired response is not achieved with the above AVERAGE INITIAL DOSE recommendations, there are no adverse reactions and the serum theophylline level cannot be measured, dosage adjustment should proceed by increasing the dose in approximately 25% increments at three day intervals. Following each adjustment, if the clinical reponse is satisfactory, then that dosage level should be maintained. Dosage increases may be made in this manner up to the following:

MAXIMUM DOSE WITHOUT MEASUREMENT OF SERUM CONCENTRATION

	Dose Per Interval
Children (25–35 kg)	250 mg q12h
Adults and Children (35–70 kg)	300 mg q12h
Adults (over 70 kg)	450 mg q12h

If an increased dose is not tolerated because of headaches or stomach upset (nausea, vomiting, diarrhea, etc.), decrease dose to previous tolerated level. Do not exceed the above recommended doses unless serum theophylline levels can be measured.

If serum theophylline levels can be measured and the concentration is between 10 and 20 mcg/ml, maintain dose if tolerated. CHECK SERUM CONCENTRATION AT APPROXIMATELY 8 HOURS AFTER A DOSE WHEN NONE HAVE BEEN MISSED OR ADDED FOR AT LEAST 3 DAYS. RECHECK SERUM THEOPHYLLINE CONCENTRATION AT 6 TO 12 MONTH INTERVALS. THIS INTER-

Continued on next page

Key—Cont.

VAL MAY NEED TO BE MORE FREQUENT IN SOME INDIVIDUALS.

Take the following action if the measured serum theophylline concentration is too high.

20 to 25 mcg/ml—Decrease dose by about 10% and serum theophylline levels should be rechecked after 3 days.*

25 to 30 mcg/ml—Skip next dose and decrease subsequent doses by 25% and serum theophylline levels should be rechecked after 3 days.

Over 30 mcg/ml—Skip next 2 doses and decrease subsequent doses by 50% and serum theophylline levels should be rechecked after 3 days.

Take the following action if the measured serum theophylline concentration is too low. 7.5 to 10 mcg/ml—Increase dose by 25%.**

5 to 7.5 mcg/ml—Increase dose by 25% RECHECK SERUM THEOPHYLLINE FOR GUIDANCE IN FURTHER DOSAGE ADJUSTMENT.

*Finer adjustments in dosage may be needed for some patients.

** Dividing the daily dosage into 3 doses administered at 8 hour intervals may be indicated if symptoms occur repeatedly at the end of a dosing interval.

DOSAGE ADJUSTMENT BASED ON SERUM THEOPHYLLINE CONCENTRATION MEASUREMENTS WHEN THESE INSTRUCTIONS HAVE NOT BEEN FOLLOWED MAY RESULT IN RECOMMENDATIONS THAT PRESENT RISK OF TOXICITY TO THE PATIENT.

Once-Daily Dosing:

The slow absorption rate of this preparation may allow once-daily administration in adult non-smokers with appropriate total body clearance and patients with low dosage requirements. Once-daily dosing should be considered only after the patient has been gradually and satisfactorily titrated to therapeutic levels with q12h dosing. Once-daily dosing should be based on twice the q12h dose and should be initiated at the end of the last q12h dosing interval. The trough concentration (Cmin) obtained following conversion to once-daily dosing may be lower (especially in high clearance patients) and the peak concentration (Cmax) may be higher (especially in low clearance patients) than that obtained with q12h dosing. If symptoms recur, or signs of toxicity appear during the once-daily dosing interval, dosing on the q12h basis should be reinstituted.

It is essential that serum theophylline concentrations be monitored before and after transfer to once-daily dosing.

Food and posture, along with changes associated with circadian rhythm, may influence the rate of absorption and/or clearance rates of theophylline from controlled-release dosage forms administered at night. The exact relationship of these and other factors to nighttime serum concentrations and the clinical significance of such findings require additional study. Therefore, it is not recommended that THEO-DUR, when used as a once-a-day product, be administered at night.

THEO-DUR, when used as a once-a-day product, must be taken whole and not broken.

Caution should be exercised for younger children who cannot complain of minor side effects. Older adults, those with cor pulmonale, congestive heart failure, and/or liver disease may have unusually low dosage requirements and thus may experience toxicity at the maximal dosage recommended above.

It is important that no patient be maintained on any dosage that is not tolerated. In instructing patients to increase dosage according to the schedule above, they should be instructed not to take a subsequent dose if apparent side effects occur and to resume therapy at a lower dose once adverse effects have disappeared.

HOW SUPPLIED

THEO-DUR 100 mg, 200 mg and 300 mg Sustained Action Tablets are available in bottles of 100, 500, 1000 and 5000, and in unit dose packages of 100.

THEO-DUR 450 mg Sustained Action Tablet are available in bottles of 100, and unit dose packages of 100.

100 mg tablet: NDC 0085-0487: round, white to off-white, debossed THEO-DUR 100 on one side and scored on the other side.

200 mg tablet: NDC 0085-0933: oval, white to off-white, debossed THEO-DUR 200 on one side and scored on the other side.

300 mg tablet: NDC 0085-0584: capsule shaped, white to off-white debossed THEO-DUR 300 on one side and scored on the other side.

450 mg tablet: NDC 0085-0806: oval white to off-white scored debossed Theo-DUR 450 on one side

STORAGE CONDITIONS

Keep tightly closed. Store at controlled room temperature 15–30°C (59–86°F).

CAUTION

Federal law prohibits dispensing without prescription.
Revised 2/87

Shown in Product Identification Section, page 412

THEO–DUR® SPRINKLE   ℞
[thē-a-dur]
theophylline (anhydrous)
Sustained Action Capsules

DESCRIPTION

THEO-DUR® SPRINKLE Sustained Action Capsules contain 50 mg, 75 mg, 125 mg or 200 mg theophylline anhydrous in the form of long acting, microencapsulated beads within a hard gelatin capsule and are intended for oral administration.

The theophylline has been microencapsulated in a proprietary coating of polymers to mask the bitter taste associated with the drug, while providing a prolonged effect. The entire contents of a THEO-DUR SPRINKLE capsule is intended to be sprinkled on a small amount of soft food immediately prior to ingestion, or may be swallowed whole. SUBDIVIDING THE CONTENTS OF A CAPSULE IS NOT RECOMMENDED. Each capsule is oversized to allow ease of opening.

Theophylline is a bronchodilator and is a member of the xanthine class of chemical compounds related to both theobromine and caffeine. Theophylline is a white, odorless, crystalline powder having a bitter taste. Theophylline is 3.7-dihydro-1,3-dimethyl-1h-purine-2,6-dione.

CLINICAL PHARMACOLOGY

Theophylline directly relaxes the smooth muscle of the bronchial airways and pulmonary blood vessels, thus acting mainly as a bronchodilator and smooth muscle relaxant. The drug also produces other actions typical of the xanthine derivatives: cardiac stimulation, coronary vasodilation, stimulation of skeletal muscles, cerebral stimulation, and diuresis. The actions of theophylline may be mediated through inhibition of phosphodiesterase and a resultant increase in intracellular cyclic AMP.

In vitro theophylline has been shown to act synergistically with beta agonists that increase intracellular cyclic AMP through the stimulation of adenyl cyclase, but synergism has not been demonstrated in patient studies. More data are needed to determine if theophylline and beta agonists have a clinically important additive effect *in vivo* . Apparently, no development of tolerance occurs with chronic use of theophylline.

Pharmacokinetics: The half-life of theophylline is influenced by a number of known variables. It is prolonged in patients suffering from chronic alcoholism, impaired hepatic or renal function, congestive heart failure, and in patients receiving macrolide antibiotics and cimetidine. Older adults (over age 55) and patients with chronic obstructive pulmonary disease, with or without cor pulmonale, may also have much slower clearance rates. For such patients, the theophylline half-life may exceed 24 hours.

Newborns and neonates have extremely slow clearance rates compared to older infants (over 6 months) and children, and may also have a theophylline half-life of over 24 hours. High fever for prolonged periods may also reduce the rate of theophylline elimination.

THEOPHYLLINE ELIMINATION CHARACTERISTICS

Theophylline Clearance Rates (mean±S.D.)	Half-Life Average (mean±S.D.)
Children (over 6 months of age)	
1.45±0.58 ml/kg/min	3.7±1.1 hrs
Adult non-smokers uncomplicated asthma	
0.65±0.19 ml/kg/min	8.7±2.2 hrs

The half-life of theophylline in smokers (1 to 2 packs/day) averages 4–5 hours, much shorter than the half-life in non-smokers which averages 7–9 hours. The increase in theophylline clearance caused by smoking is probably the result of induction of drug-metabolizing enzymes that do not readily normalize after cessation of smoking. It appears that between 3 months and 2 years may be necessary for normalization of the effect of smoking on theophylline pharmacokinetics.

In two separate single dose studies utilizing different subjects, the following bioavailability parameters were observed. THEO-DUR SPRINKLE administered in a 500 mg dose as pellets on applesauce to 6 healthy adults produced mean peak theophylline serum levels of 9.03 ±2.59 mcg/ml at 8.67 ±1.03 hours following administration. Administration of two lots of THEO-DUR SPRINKLE as intact capsules in a 600 mg dose to 6 healthy adults produced mean peak

theophylline serum levels of 9.08 ±1.30 mcg/ml and 7.60 ±0.95 mcg/ml at 8.33 ±1.50 and 8.67 ±3.01 hours after administration respectively. In these studies THEO-DUR SPRINKLE exhibited complete bioavailability when compared to an immediate release product. In both of these studies, the subjects fasted for 10 hours prior to dosing and for 4 hours after dosing.

In a multiple dose, two-way, crossover study with 18 healthy, normal adults, the bioavailability from THEO-DUR SPRINKLE administered as intact capsules was evaluated using THEO-DUR Sustained Action Tablets as the reference product. Fifteen subjects received 400 mg at 7:00 AM and 7:00 PM while three subjects received 200 mg because of low theophylline clearance. All meals and snacks were provided to the subjects during the course of this study, with breakfast at 9:00 AM, lunch at 12:30 PM a snack at 3:00 PM, and dinner at 9:00 PM. THEO-DUR SPRINKLE produced mean Cmax and Cmin levels of 10.4 ±2.6 and 6.9 ±1.8 mcg/ml as compared to a Cmax and Cmin of 10.5 ±2.8 and 7.5 ±2.7 mcg/ml for THEO-DUR tablets. The mean percent fluctuation normalized to Css was 38.8 ±8.5% for THEO-DUR SPRINKLE and 33.4 ±9.7% for THEO-DUR tablets [100(Cmax-Cmin)/Css where Css = AUC_{0-12}/dosing interval]. The mean percent fluctuation when normalized to Cmin was 51.9 ±15.4% for THEO-DUR SPRINKLE and 43.9 ±17.4% for THEO-DUR tablets [% fluctuation = 100 (Cmax-Cmin)/Cmin]. The average peak-trough differences over 12 hours for THEO-DUR SPRINKLE and THEO-DUR tablets were 3.5 ±1.2 and 3.0 ±0.7 mcg/ml respectively. The AUC for THEO-DUR SPRINKLE was 108.4 ±26.0 while that for THEO-DUR tablets was 112.1 ±32.5 mcg-hr/ml. In a separate study, THEO-DUR exhibited complete bioavailability when compared to an immediate release product. This would suggest that bioavailability from THEO-DUR SPRINKLE was complete and not statistically different from that of the THEO-DUR tablets.

INDICATIONS AND USE

For relief and/or prevention of symptoms of asthma and for reversible bronchospasm associated with chronic bronchitis and emphysema.

CONTRAINDICATIONS

THEO-DUR SPRINKLE is contraindicated in individuals who have shown hypersensitivity to theophylline or any of the capsule components.

WARNINGS

Status asthmaticus should be considered a medical emergency and is defined as that degree of bronchospasm which is not rapidly responsive to usual doses of conventional bronchodilators. Optimal therapy for such patients frequently requires both *additional medication*, parenterally administered, and *close monitoring*, preferably in an intensive care setting. Although increasing the dose of theophylline may bring about relief, such treatment may be associated with toxicity. The likelihood of such toxicity developing increases significantly when the serum theophylline concentration exceeds 20 mcg/ml. Therefore, determination of serum theophylline levels is recommended to assure maximal benefit without excessive risk.

Serum levels above 20 mcg/ml are rarely found after appropriate administration of the recommended doses. However, in individuals in whom theophylline plasma clearance is reduced for any reason, even conventional doses may result in increased serum levels and potential toxicity. Reduced theophylline clearance has been documented in the following readily identifiable groups: 1) patients with impaired renal or liver function; 2) patients over 55 years of age, particularly males and those with chronic lung disease; 3) those with cardiac failure from any cause; 4) neonates; and 5) those patients taking certain drugs (macrolide antibiotics and cimetidine). Decreased clearance of theophylline may be associated with either influenza immunization or active infection with influenza.

Reduction of dosage and laboratory monitoring is especially appropriate in the above individuals.

Less serious signs of theophylline toxicity (i.e., nausea and restlessness) may occur frequently when initiating therapy, but are usually transient; when such signs are persistent during maintenance therapy, they are often associated with serum concentrations above 20 mcg/ml.

Unfortunately, however, serious side effects such as ventricular arrhythmias, convulsions or even death may appear as the first sign of toxicity without any previous warning. *Stated differently; serious toxicity is not reliably preceded by less severe side effects.*

Many patients who require theophylline may exhibit tachycardia due to their underlying disease process so that the cause/effect relationship to elevated serum theophylline concentrations may not be appreciated.

Theophylline products may cause dysrhythmia and/or worsen pre-existing arrhythmias and any significant change in rate and/or rhythm warrants monitoring and futher investigation.

The occurrence of arrhythmias and sudden death (with histological evidence of necrosis of the myocardium) has been recorded in laboratory animals (minipigs, rodents and dogs) when theophylline and beta agonists were administered concomitantly, although not when either was administered alone. The significance of these findings when applied to human usage is currently unknown.

PRECAUTIONS
THE CONTENTS OF THE THEO-DUR SPRINKLE CAPSULE SHOULD NOT BE CHEWED OR CRUSHED.

General: Mean half-life in smokers is shorter than non-smokers. Therefore, smokers may require larger or more frequent doses of theophylline. Morphine and curare should be used with caution in patients with airway obstruction as they may suppress respiration and stimulate histamine release. Alternative drugs should be used when possible. Theophylline should not be administered concurrently with other xanthine preparations. Use with caution in patients with severe cardiac disease, severe hypoxemia, hypertension, hyperthyroidism, acute myocardial injury, cor pulmonale, congestive heart failure, alcoholism, liver disease and in the elderly, especially males, and in neonates. Great caution should be used in giving theophylline to patients with congestive heart failure. Frequently, such patients have shown markedly prolonged theophylline blood levels with theophylline persisting in serum for long periods following discontinuation of the drug. Use theophylline cautiously in patients with a history of peptic ulcer. Theophylline may occasionally act as a local gastrointestinal irritant although G.I. symptoms are more commonly centrally mediated and associated with serum drug concentrations over 20 mcg/ml.

Information for Patients: The physician should reinforce the importance of taking only the prescribed dose at the prescribed time intervals. The patient should alert the physician if symptoms occur repeatedly, especially near the end of a dosing interval.

When prescribing administration by the sprinkle method, details of the proper technique should be explained to the patient (see DOSAGE AND ADMINISTRATION Sprinkling Contents on Food).

Patients should be informed of the need to take this drug in the fasting state, and that drug administration should be one hour before, or two hours after meals (see PRECAUTIONS, Drug-Food Interactions and DOSAGE AND ADMINISTRATION).

Drug Interactions:
Drug-Drug: Toxic synergism with ephedrine has been documented and may occur with some other sympathomimetic bronchodilators. In addition, the following drug interactions have been demonstrated.

Drug	Effect
Theophylline with Lithium Carbonate	Increased excretion of Lithium Carbonate
Theophylline with Propranolol	Increased theophylline serum concentrations Antagonism of Propranolol effect
Theophylline with troleandomycin or erythromycin	Increased theophylline serum concentrations
Theophylline with Cimetidine	Increased theophylline serum concentrations

Drug-Food: THEO-DUR SPRINKLE has not been adequately studied to determine the extent of alteration of bioavailability when it is given with food as compared to the fasting state.

However, there is data to indicate that drug administration at the time of food ingestion will result in significantly lower peak serum concentrations and reduced extent of absorption (bioavailability).

The influence of the type and amount of food as well as the time interval between drug and food, on performance of THEO-DUR SPRINKLE is under study.

Drug/Laboratory Test Interactions: When plasma levels of theophylline are measured by spectrophotometric methods, coffee, tea, cola beverages, chocolate, and acetaminophen contribute falsely high values.

Carcinogenesis, Mutagenesis, and Impairment of Fertility: Long-term animal studies have not been performed to evaluate the carcinogenic potential, mutagenic potential, or the effect on fertility of xanthine compounds.

Pregnancy: Pregnancy Category C: Animal reproduction studies have not been conducted with theophylline. It is not known whether theophylline can cause fetal harm when administered to a pregnant woman or can affect reproduction capacity. Theophylline should be give to a pregnant woman only if clearly needed.

Nursing Mothers: It has been reported that theophylline distributes readily into breast milk and may cause adverse effects in the infant. Caution must be used if prescribing xanthines to a mother who is nursing, taking into account the risk-benefit of this therapy.

Pediatric Use: Safety and effectiveness in children under 6 years of age have not been established with this product.

ADVERSE REACTIONS
The most consistent adverse reactions are usually due to overdose and are:

Gastrointestinal: nausea, vomiting, epigastric pain, hematemesis, diarrhea.

Central nervous system: headaches, irritability, restlessness, insomnia, reflex hyperexcitability, muscle twitching, clonic and tonic generalized convulsions.

Cardiovascular: palpitation, tachycardia, extrasystoles, flushing, hypotension, circulatory failure, ventricular arrhythmias.

Respiratory: tachypnea.

Renal: albuminuria, increased excretion of renal tubular cells and red blood cells, potentiation of diuresis.

Other: hyperglycemia and inappropriate ADH syndrome and rash.

OVERDOSAGE
Management:
A. If potential oral overdose is established and seizure has not occurred:
  1. Induce vomiting.
  2. Administer a cathartic (this is particulary important if sustained-released preparations have been taken).
  3. Administer activated charcoal.
  4. Monitor vital signs, maintain blood pressure and provide adequate hydration.
B. If patient is having a seizure:
  1. Establish an airway.
  2. Administer oxygen.
  3. Treat the seiure with intravenous diazepam, 0.1 to 0.3 mg/kg up to a total dose of 10 mg.
  4. Monitor vital signs, maintain blood pressure and provide adequate hydration.
C. Post Seizure Coma:
  1. Maintain airway and oxygenation.
  2. If a result of oral medication, follow above recommendations to prevent absorption of the drug, but intubation and lavage will have to be performed instead of inducing emesis, and the cathartic and charcoal will need to be introduced via a large bore gastric lavage tube.
  3. Continue to provide full supportive care and adequate hydration while waiting for drug to be metabolized. In general, the drug is metabolized sufficiently rapidly so as to not warrant consideration of dialysis. However, if serum levels exceed 50 mcg/ml, charcoal hemoperfusion may be indicated.

DOSAGE AND ADMINISTRATION
There is data to indicate that administration of THEO-DUR SPRINKLE at the time of food ingestion will result in significantly lower peak serum concentrations and reduced extent of absorption (bioavailability).

Therefore, the patient should be instructed to take this medication at least one hour before or two hours after a meal (See PRECAUTIONS, Drug-Food Interactions).

For most patients, effective use of theophylline, i.e. associated with optimal likelihood of benefit combined with minimal risk of toxicity, is considered to occur when serum levels are maintained between 10 and 20 mcg/ml. Levels above 20 mcg/ml may produce toxicity and in a small number of patients, toxicity may even be seen with serum levels between 15–20 mcg/ml, particularly during initation of therapy.

There is considerable variation from patient to patient in the dosage required to achieve and maintain therapeutic and safe levels, primarily due to variable rates of elimination. Therefore, it is essential that not only must dosage be individualized but titration and monitoring of serum levels be utilized where available. When serum concentrations cannot be obtained, restriction of dosage to the amounts and intervals recommended in the guidelines listed below becomes essential. Dosage should be calculated on the basis of lean (ideal) body weight where mg/kg doses are presented. Theophylline does not distribute into fatty tissue.

As a practical consideration, it is not always possible to obtain serum level determinations. Under such conditions, restriction of the daily dose (in otherwise healthy adults) to not greater than 13 mg/kg/day of anhydrous theophylline in divided doses will result in relatively few patients exceeding serum levels of 20 mcg/ml and the resultant risk of toxicity.

Sprinkling Contents on Food: *THEO-DUR SPRINKLE may be administered by carefully opening the capsule and sprinkling the beaded contents on a spoonful of soft food such as applesauce or pudding. The soft food should be swallowed immediately without chewing and followed with a glass of cool water or juice to ensure complete swallowing of the beads. It is recommended that the food used should not be hot and should be soft enough to be swallowed without chewing. Any bead/food mixture should be used immediately and not stored for future use. The small amount of food (one spoonful) used to administer the dose will not alter the bioavailability of THEO-DUR SPRINKLE, however, the dosing should be at least one hour before or two hours after a meal. SUBDIVIDING THE CONTENTS OF A CAPSULE IS NOT RECOMMENDED.*

Dosage Guidelines: Because administration of Theo-Dur Sprinkle at the time of food ingestion has been shown to result in significantly lower peak serum concentrations and reduced extent of absorption (bioavailability), patients should be instructed to take this medication at least one hour before or two hours after a meal (See PRECAUTIONS, Drug-Food Interactions).

Taking THEO-DUR SPRINKLE at 12 hour intervals under the above restrictive recommendations in regard to food ingestion may be difficult for the patient to follow. Under such circumstances, consideration should be given to prescribing this drug every 8 hours (giving one third of the 24 hour dosage requirement with each dose), if this regimen would more easily permit dosing under fasting conditions.

I. Acute Symptoms: THEO-DUR SPRINKLE is not intended for patients experiencing an acute episode of bronchospasm (associated with asthma, chronic bronchitis, or emphysema). Such patients require rapid relief of symptoms and should be treated with an immediate-release or intravenous theophylline preparation (or other bronchodilators) and not with controlled release products.

II. Chronic Therapy:
A. Initating Therapy with an Immediate-Release Product: It is recommended that the appropriate dosage be established using an immediate-release preparation. Children weighing less than 25 kg should have their daily dosage requirements established with a liquid preparation to permit small dosage increments. Slow clinical titration is generally preferred to help assure acceptance and safety of the medication, and to allow the patient to develop tolerance to transient caffeine-like side effects. Then, if the total 24 hour dose can be given by use of the sustained release product, the patient can usually be switched to THEO-DUR SPRINKLE giving one-half of the daily dose at 12 hour intervals. Patients who metabolize theophylline rapidly such as the young, smokers, and some non-smoking adults are the most likely candidates for dosing at 8-hour intervals. Such patients can generally be identified as having trough serum concentrations lower than desired or repeatedly exhibiting symptoms near the end of a dosing interval.

B. Initating Therapy with THEO-DUR SPRINKLE: Alternatively, therapy can be initiated with THEO-DUR SPRINKLE since they are available in dosage strengths which permit titration and adjustments of dosage in adults and older children:

Initial Dose	16 mg/kg/24 hours or 400 mg/24 hours (whichever is less) of anhydrous theophylline in 2 divided doses 12-hour intervals.
Increasing Dose	The above dosage may be increased in approximately 25 percent increments at 3-day intervals so long as the drug is tolerated; until clinical reponse is satisfactory or the maximum dose as indicated in section III (below) is reached. The serum concentration may be checked at these intervals, but at a minimum, should be determined at the end of this adjustment period.

III. Maintenance Dose of Theophylline where the Serum Concentration is not Measured:
WARNING: DO NOT ATTEMPT TO MAINTAIN ANY DOSE THAT IS NOT TOLERATED.
Not to exceed the following:

Age			Dose per 12 hours
Age	6–9 years	24mg/kg/day	12.0 mg/kg
Age	9–12 years	20mg/kg/day	10.0 mg/kg
Age	12–16 years	18 mg/kg/day	9.0 mg/kg
Age	Over 16 years	13 mg/kg/day or 900 mg	6.5 mg/kg
(WHICHEVER IS LESS)			

IV. Measurement of Serum Theophylline Concentrations During Chronic Therapy: If the above maximum doses are to be maintained or exceeded, serum theophylline measurement is recommended. The serum sample should be obtained at the time of peak absorption: 1 to 2 hours after administration for immediate-release products and 5 to 10 hours after dosing for THEO-DUR SPRINKLE. It is important that the patient will have missed no doses during the previous 48 hours and that the dosing intervals will have been reasonably typical with no added doses during that period of time. DOSAGE ADJUSTMENT BASED ON SERUM THEOPHYLLINE CONCENTRATION MEASUREMENTS WHEN THESE INSTRUCTIONS HAVE NOT BEEN FOLLOWED MAY RESULT IN RECOMMENDATIONS THAT PRESENT RISK OF TOXICITY TO THE PATIENT.

V. Final Adjustment of Dosage (see Table 1)
Table 1—Dosage adjustment after serum theophylline measurement

Continued on next page

Key—Cont.

If serum theophylline is:		Directions:
Within normal Limits	10 to 20 mcg/ml	Maintain dosage if tolerated. Recheck serum theophylline concentration at 6- to 12-month intervals*
Too high	20 to 25 mcg/ml	Decrease doses by about 10%. Recheck serum theophylline concentration at 6- to 12-month intervals*
	25 to 30 mcg/ml	Skip next dose and decrease subsequent doses by about 25%.
	over 30 mcg/ml	Skip next 2 doses and decrease subsequent doses by 50%. Recheck serum theophylline.
Too low	7.5 to 10 mcg/ml	Increase dose by about 25%.** Recheck serum theophylline concentration at 6- to 12-month intervals.*
	5 to 7.5 mcg/ml	Increase dose by about 25% to the nearest dose increment and recheck serum theophylline for guidance in further dosage adjustment (another increase will probably be needed, but this provides a safety check).

*Finer adjustments in dosage may be needed for some patients.

**The total daily dose may need to be administered at more frequent intervals if symptoms occur repeatedly at the end of a dosing interval.

From the Journal of Respiratory Diseases 2(7):16.1981. Caution should be exercised for younger children who cannot complain of minor side effects. Those with cor pulmonale, congestive heart failure, and/or liver disease may have unusually low dosage requirements and thus may experience toxicity at the maximal dosage recommended above. It is important that no patient be maintained on any dosage that is not tolerated. In instructing patients to increase dosage according to the schedule above, they should be instructed not to take a subsequent dose if apparent side effects occur and to resume therapy at a lower dose once adverse effects have disappeared.

HOW SUPPLIED

THEO-DUR SPRINKLE 50, 75, 125 and 200 mg Sustained Action Capsules are available in bottles of 100.

50 mg capsule: NDC 0085-0928: white opaque capsule body with clear cap embossed in black, THIS END UP THEO-DUR® SPRINKLE 50 mg

75 mg capsule: NDC 0085-0875: white opaque capsule body with clear cap embossed in green, THIS END UP THEO-DUR® SPRINKLE 75 mg

125 mg capsule: NDC 0085-0381: white opaque capsule body with clear cap embossed in red, THIS END UP THEO-DUR® SPRINKLE 125 mg

200 mg capsule: NDC 0085-0620: white opaque capsule body with clear cap embossed in blue, THIS END UP THEO-DUR® SPRINKLE 200 mg

STORAGE CONDITIONS

Keep tightly closed. Store at controlled room temperature 15–30°C (59–86°F).

CAUTION

Federal law prohibits dispensing without prescription.

Keep this and all medications out of the reach of children.

Rev. 3/87

KEY PHARMACEUTICALS, INC.

Copyright © 1987, Kenilworth, New Jersey 07033 USA
All rights reserved

Shown in Product Identification Section, page 412

Knoll Pharmaceuticals
A Unit of BASF K&F Corporation
WHIPPANY, NJ 07981

BASF Group

AKINETON® TABLETS AND AMPULES ℞
[ā-kĭn 'ĕ-ton]
biperiden hydrochloride and biperiden lactate

DESCRIPTION

Each AKINETON® Tablet for oral administration contains 2 mg biperiden hydrochloride. Other ingredients may include corn syrup, lactose, magnesium stearate, potato starch and talc. Each 1 mL AKINETON Ampule for intramuscular or intravenous administration contains 5 mg biperiden lactate in an aqueous 1.4 percent sodium lactate solution. No added preservative. AKINETON is an anticholinergic agent. Biperiden is α-5-Norbornen-2-yl-α-phenyl-1-piperidinepropanol. It is a white, crystalline, odorless powder, slightly soluble in water and alcohol. It is stable in air at normal temperatures. Biperiden may be represented by the following structural formula:

CLINICAL PHARMACOLOGY

AKINETON is a weak peripheral anticholinergic agent. It has, therefore, some antisecretory, antispasmodic and mydriatic effects. In addition, AKINETON possesses nicotinolytic activity. Parkinsonism is thought to result from an imbalance between the excitatory (cholinergic) and inhibitory (dopaminergic) systems in the corpus striatum. The mechanism of action of centrally active anticholinergic drugs such as AKINETON is considered to relate to competitive antagonism of acetylcholine at cholinergic receptors in the corpus striatum, which then restores the balance.

The parenteral form of AKINETON is an effective and reliable agent for the treatment of acute episodes of extrapyramidal disturbances sometimes seen during treatment with neuroleptic agents. Akathisia, akinesia, dyskinetic tremors, rigor, oculogyric crisis, spasmodic torticollis, and profuse sweating are markedly reduced or eliminated. With parenteral AKINETON, these drug-induced disturbances are rapidly brought under control. Subsequently, this can usually be maintained with oral doses which may be given with tranquilizer therapy in psychotic and other conditions requiring an uninterrupted therapeutic program.

Pharmacokinetics and Metabolism: Only limited pharmacokinetic studies of biperiden in humans are available The serum concentration at 1 to 1.5 hours following a single, 4 mg oral dose was 4–5 ng/mL. Plasma levels (0.1–0.2 ng/mL) could be determined up to 48 hours after dosing. Six hours after an oral dose of 250 mg/kg in rats, 87% of the drug had been absorbed. The metabolism of AKINETON is also incompletely understood, but does involve hydroxylation. In normal volunteers a single 10 mg intravenous dose of biperiden seemed to cause a transient rise in plasma cortisol and prolactin. No change in GH, LH, FSH, or TSH levels were seen. Biperiden lactate (10 mg/mL) was not irritating to the tissue of rabbits when injected intramuscularly (1.0 mL) into the sacrospinalis muscles and intradermally (0.25 mL) and subcutaneously (0.5 mL) into the shaved abdominal skin.

INDICATIONS AND USAGE

- As an adjunct in the therapy of all forms of parkinsonism (idiopathic, postencephalitic, arteriosclerotic)
- Control of extrapyramidal disorders secondary to neuroleptic drug therapy (e.g., phenothiazines)

CONTRAINDICATIONS

1) Hypersensitivity to biperiden 2) Narrow angle glaucoma 3) Bowel obstruction 4) Megacolon

WARNINGS

Isolated instances of mental confusion, euphoria, agitation and disturbed behavior have been reported in susceptible patients. Also, the central anticholinergic syndrome can occur as an adverse reaction to properly prescribed anticholinergic medication, although it is more frequently due to overdosage. It may also result from concomitant administration of an anticholinergic agent and a drug that has secondary anticholinergic actions (see Drug Interactions and Overdosage sections). Caution should be observed in patients with manifest glaucoma, though no prohibitive rise in intraocular pressure has been noted following either oral or parenteral administration. Patients with prostatism, epilepsy or cardiac arrhythmia should be given this drug with caution.

Occasionally, drowsiness may occur, and patients who drive a car or operate any other potentially dangerous machinery should be warned of this possibility. As with other drugs acting on the central nervous system, the consumption of alcohol should be avoided during AKINETON therapy.

PRECAUTIONS

Drug Interactions: The central anticholinergic syndrome can occur when anticholinergic agents such as AKINETON are administered concomitantly with drugs that have secondary anticholinergic actions, e.g., certain narcotic analgesics such as meperidine, the phenothiazines and other antipsychotics, tricyclic antidepressants, certain antiarrhythmics such as the quinidine salts, and antihistamines. See Overdosage section for signs and symptoms of the central anticholinergic syndrome, and for treatment.

Pregnancy: Pregnancy Category C. Animal reproduction studies have not been conducted with AKINETON. It is also not known whether AKINETON can cause fetal harm when administered to a pregnant woman or can affect reproduction capacity. AKINETON should be given to a pregnant woman only if clearly needed.

Nursing Mothers: It is not known whether this drug is excreted in human milk. Because many drugs are excreted in human milk, caution should be exercised when AKINETON is administered to a nursing woman.

Pediatric Use: Safety and effectiveness in children have not been established.

ADVERSE REACTIONS

Atropine-like side effects such as dry mouth; blurred vision; drowsiness; euphoria or disorientation; urinary retention; postural hypotension; constipation; agitation; disturbed behavior may be seen. There usually are no significant changes in blood pressure or heart rate in patients who have been given the parenteral form of AKINETON. Mild transient postural hypotension and bradycardia may occur. These side effects can be minimized or avoided by slow intravenous administration. No local tissue reactions have been reported following intramuscular injection. If gastric irritation occurs following oral administration, it can be avoided by administering the drug during or after meals.

The central anticholinergic syndrome can occur as an adverse reaction to properly prescribed anticholinergic medication. See Overdosage section for signs and symptoms of the central anticholinergic syndrome, and for treatment.

OVERDOSAGE

Signs and Symptoms: Overdosage with AKINETON produces typical central symptoms of atropine intoxication (the central anticholinergic syndrome). Correct diagnosis depends upon recognition of the peripheral signs of parasympathetic blockade including dilated and sluggish pupils; warm, dry skin; facial flushing; decreased secretions of the mouth, pharynx, nose, and bronchi; foul-smelling breath; elevated temperature; tachycardia; cardiac arrhythmias, decreased bowel sounds, and urinary retention. Neuropsychiatric signs such as delirium, disorientation, anxiety, hallucinations, illusions, confusion, incoherence, agitation, hyperactivity, ataxia, loss of memory, paranoia, combativeness, and seizures may be present. The condition can progress to stupor, coma, paralysis, and cardiac and respiratory arrest and death.

Treatment: Treatment of acute overdose revolves around symptomatic and supportive therapy. If AKINETON was administered orally, gastric lavage or other measures to limit absorption should be instituted. A small dose of diazepam or a short acting barbiturate may be administered if CNS excitation is observed. Phenothiazines are contraindicated because the toxicity may be intensified due to their antimuscarinic action, causing coma. Respiratory support, artificial respiration or vasopressor agents may be necessary. Hyperpyrexia must be reversed, fluid volume replaced and acid-base balance maintained. Urinary catheterization may be necessary.

Routine use of physostigmine for overdose is controversial. Delirium, hallucinations, coma, and supraventricular tachycardia (not ventricular tachycardias or conduction defects) seem to respond. If indicated, 1 mg (half this amount for children or the elderly) may be given intramuscularly or by slow intravenous infusion. If there is no response within 20 minutes, an additional 1 mg dose may be given; this may be repeated until a total of 4 mg has been administered, a reversal of the toxic effects occur or excessive cholinergic signs are seen. Frequent monitoring of clinical signs should be done. Since physostigmine is rapidly destroyed, additional injections may be required every one or two hours to maintain control. The relapse intervals tend to lengthen as the toxic anticholinergic agent is metabolized, so the patient should be carefully observed for 8 to 12 hours following the last relapse.

Toxicity in Animals: The LD$_{50}$ of biperiden in the white mouse is 545 mg/kg orally, 195 mg/kg subcutaneously, and 56 mg/kg intravenously. The acute oral toxicity (LD$_{50}$) in rats is 750 mg/kg. The intraperitoneal toxicity (LD$_{50}$) of biperiden lactate in rats was 270 mg/kg and the intravenous toxicity (LD$_{50}$) in dogs is 222 mg/kg. In dogs under general anesthesia, respiratory arrest occurred at 33 mg/kg (intravenous) and circulatory standstill at 45 mg/kg (intravenous). The oral LD_{50} in dogs was 340 mg/kg. Chronic toxicity studies in both rat and dog have been reported.

DOSAGE AND ADMINISTRATION

Drug-Induced Extrapyramidal Symptoms:
Parenteral: The average adult dose is 2 mg intramuscularly or intravenously. May be repeated every half-hour until there is resolution of symptoms, but not more than four consecutive doses should be given in a 24-hour period.
Note: Parenteral drug products should be inspected visually for particulate matter and discoloration prior to administration, whenever solution and container permit.
Oral: One tablet one to three times daily.
Parkinson's Disease: Oral: The usual beginning dose is one tablet three or four times daily. The dosage should be individualized with the dose titrated upward to a maximum of 8 tablets (16 mg) per 24 hours.

HOW SUPPLIED

AKINETON Tablets, 2 mg each, white, embossed on one face with a triangle, bisected on the reverse and imprinted with the number "11."
Bottles of 100—NDC #0044-0120-02.
Bottles of 1000—NDC #0044-0120-04.
Shown in Product Identification Section, page 413
AKINETON Ampules, 1 mL each containing 5 mg biperiden lactate per mL.
Boxes of 10—NDC #0044-0110-01.
Storage: All dosage forms of AKINETON should be stored at 59°–86°F (15°–30°C).
Dispense in tight, light-resistant container as defined in USP.
MR 1987/5427
Revised June, 1987   5427

COLLAGENASE SANTYL® Ointment ℞
[săn'tĭl]
(collagenase)

DESCRIPTION

SANTYL® OINTMENT is a sterile enzymatic debriding ointment which contains 250 collagenase units per gram of white petrolatum USP. The enzyme collagenase is derived from the fermentation by *Clostridium histolyticum*. It possesses the unique ability to digest native and denatured collagen in necrotic tissue.

CLINICAL PHARMACOLOGY

Since collagen accounts for 75% of the dry weight of skin tissue, the ability of collagenase to digest collagen in the physiological pH range and temperature makes it particularly effective in the removal of detritus.[1] Collagenase thus contributes towards the formation of granulation tissue and subsequent epithelization of dermal ulcers and severely burned areas.[2,3,4,5,6] Collagen in healthy tissue or in newly formed granulation tissue is not attacked.[2,3,4,5,6,7,8]

INDICATIONS

Santyl Ointment is indicated for debriding chronic dermal ulcers[2,3,4,5,6,8,9,10,11,12,13,14,15,16,17,18] and severely burned areas.[3,4,5,7,16,19,20,21]

CONTRAINDICATIONS

Santyl Ointment is contraindicated in patients who have shown local or systemic hypersensitivity to collagenase.

PRECAUTIONS

The optimal pH range of collagenase is 6 to 8. Higher or lower pH conditions will decrease the enzyme's activity and appropriate precautions should be taken. The enzymatic activity is also adversely affected by detergents, hexachlorophene and heavy metal ions such as mercury and silver which are used in some antiseptics. When it is suspected such materials have been used, the site should be carefully cleansed by repeated washings with normal saline before Santyl Ointment is applied. Soaks containing metal ions or acidic solutions such as Burow's solution should be avoided because of the metal ion and low pH. Cleansing materials such as hydrogen peroxide, Dakin's solution, and sterile saline are compatible with Santyl Ointment.
Debilitated patients should be closely monitored for systemic bacterial infections because of the theoretical possibility that debriding enzymes may increase the risk of bacteremia. A slight transient erythema has been noted occasionally in the surrounding tissue, particularly when Santyl Ointment was not confined to the lesion. Therefore, the ointment should be applied carefully within the area of the lesion.

ADVERSE REACTIONS

No allergic sensitivity or toxic reactions have been noted in the recorded clinical investigations. However, one case of systemic manifestations of hypersensitivity to collagenase in a patient treated for more than one year with a combination of collagenase and cortisone has been reported to us.

OVERDOSAGE

Action of the enzyme may be stopped, should this be desired, by the application of Burow's solution USP (pH 3.6–4.4) to the lesion.

DOSAGE AND ADMINISTRATION

Santyl Ointment should be applied once daily (or more frequently if the dressing becomes soiled, as from incontinence) in the following manner:

(1) Prior to application the lesion should be cleansed of debris and digested material by gently rubbing with a gauze pad saturated with hydrogen peroxide or Dakin's solution followed by sterile normal saline.

(2) Whenever infection is present it is desirable to use an appropriate topical antibiotic powder. The antibiotic should be applied to the lesion prior to the application of Santyl Ointment. Should the infection not respond, therapy with Santyl Ointment should be discontinued until remission of the infection.

(3) Santyl Ointment should be applied directly to deep lesions with a wooden tongue depressor or spatula. For shallow lesions, Santyl Ointment may be applied to a sterile gauze pad which is then applied to the wound and properly secured.

(4) Crosshatching thick eschar with a #10 blade allows collagenase more surface contact with necrotic debris. It is also desirable to remove, with forceps and scissors, as much loosened detritus as can be done readily.

(5) All excess ointment should be removed each time dressing is changed.

(6) Use of Santyl Ointment should be terminated when debridement of necrotic tissue is complete and granulation tissue is well established.

HOW SUPPLIED

Santyl Ointment contains 250 units of collagenase enzyme per gram of white petrolatum USP. The potency assay of undenatured collagenase is based on the digestion of undenatured collagen (from bovine Achilles tendon) at pH 7.2 and 37°C for 24 hours. The number of peptide bonds cleaved are measured by reaction with ninhydrin. Amino groups released by a trypsin digestion control are subtracted. One net collagenase unit will solubilize ninhydrin reactive material equivalent to 4 micromoles of leucine.

REFERENCES

1— Mandl, I., Adv. Enzymol. 23:163, 1961.
2— Boxer, A.M., Gottesman, N., Bernstein, H., & Mandl, I., Geriatrics 24:75, 1969.
3— Mazurek, I., Med. Welt 22:150, 1971.
4— Zimmerman, W.E., in "Collagenase," I. Mandl, ed., Gordon & Breach, Science Publishers, New York, 1971, p. 131, p. 185.
5— Vetra, H., & Whittaker, D., Geriatrics 30:53, 1975.
6— Rao, D.B., Sane, P.G., & Georgiev, E.L., J. Am. Geriatrics Soc. 23:22, 1975.
7— Vrabec, R., Moserova, J., Konickova, Z., Behounkova, E., & Blaha, J., J. Hyg. Epidemiol. Microbiol. Immunol. 18:496, 1974.
8— Lippmann, H.I., Arch. Phys. Med. Rehabil. 54:588,1973.
9— German, F.M., in "Collagenase," I. Mandl, ed. Gordon & Breach, Science Publishers,New York,1971, p. 165.
10— Haimovici, H. & Strauch, B., in "Collagenase," I. Mandl, ed., Gordon & Breach, Science Publishers, New York, 1971, p. 177.
11— Lee, L.K., & Ambrus, J.L., Geriatrics 30:91, 1975.
12— Locke, R.K., & Heifitz, N.M., J. Am. Pod. Assoc. 65:242, 1975.
13— Varma, A.O., Bugatch, E., & German, F.M., Surg. Gynecol. Obstet. 136:281, 1973.
14— Barrett, D., Jr., & Klibanski, A., Am. J. Nurs. 73:849, 1973.
15— Bardfeld, L.A., J. Pod. Ed. 1:41, 1970.
16— Blum, G., Schweiz. Rundschau Med. Praxis 62:820, 1973. Abstr. in Dermatology Digest, Feb. 1974, p. 36.
17— Zaruba, F., Lettl, A., Brozkova, L., Skrdlantova, H., & Krs, V., J. Hyg. Epidemiol. Microbiol. Immunol. 18:499, 1974.
18— Altman, M.I., Goldstein, L., Horowitz, S., J. Am. Pod. Assoc. 68:11, 1978.
19— Rehn, V.J., Med. Klin. 58:799, 1963.
20— Krauss, H., Koslowski, L., & Zimmermann, W.E., Langenbecks Arch. Klin. Chir. 303:23, 1963.
21— Gruenagel, H.H., Med. Klin. 58:442, 1963.
Manufactured by
ADVANCE BIOFACTURES CORP.
35 Wilbur Street
Lynbrook, New York 11563
Distributed by
Knoll Pharmaceuticals
A Unit of BASF K & F Corporation
30 North Jefferson Road
Whippany, New Jersey 07981
Revised: November, 1987   6103
Shown in Product Identification Section, page 413

DILAUDID® ℂ ℞
[dĭ"law'dĭd]
(hydromorphone hydrochloride)

DESCRIPTION

DILAUDID (hydromorphone hydrochloride) (**WARNING:** May be habit forming), a hydrogenated ketone of morphine, is a narcotic analgesic. It is available in:
Ampules (for parenteral administration) containing: 1 mg, 2 mg, and 4 mg hydromorphone hydrochloride per mL with 0.2% sodium citrate, 0.2% citric acid solution. DILAUDID ampules are sterile.
Multiple Dose Vials (for parenteral administration) containing 20 mL of solution. Each mL contains 2 mg hydromorphone hydrochloride and 0.5 mg edetate disodium with 1.8 mg methylparaben and 0.2 mg propylparaben as preservatives. Sodium hydroxide or hydrochloric acid is used for pH adjustment. DILAUDID multiple dose vials are sterile.
Color Coded Tablets (for oral administration) containing:
    1 mg hydromorphone hydrochloride (green tablet) and FD&C blue #1 Lake dye, D&C yellow #10 Lake dye, lactose, and magnesium stearate.
    2 mg hydromorphone hydrochloride (orange tablet) and FD&C yellow #6 Lake dye, D&C yellow #10 Lake dye, lactose, and magnesium stearate.
    3 mg hydromorphone hydrochloride (pink tablet) and D&C red #30 Lake dye, lactose, and magnesium stearate.
    4 mg hydromorphone hydrochloride (yellow tablet) and D&C yellow #10 Lake dye, lactose, and magnesium stearate.
Suppositories (for rectal administration) containing 3 mg hydromorphone hydrochloride in a cocoa butter base with silicon dioxide.
Powder (for prescription compounding) containing hydromorphone hydrochloride.
The structural formula of DILAUDID (hydromorphone hydrochloride) is:

CLINICAL PHARMACOLOGY

DILAUDID is a narcotic analgesic; its principal therapeutic effect is relief of pain. The precise mechanism of action of DILAUDID and other opiates is not known, although it is believed to relate to the existence of opiate receptors in the central nervous system. There is no intrinsic limit to the analgesic effect of DILAUDID; like morphine, adequate doses will relieve even the most severe pain. Clinically, however, dosage limitations are imposed by the adverse effects, primarily respiratory depression, nausea, and vomiting, which can result from high doses.
DILAUDID has diverse additional actions. It may produce drowsiness, changes in mood and mental clouding, depress the respiratory center and the cough center, stimulate the vomiting center, produce pinpoint constriction of the pupil, enhance parasympathetic activity, elevate cerebrospinal fluid pressure, increase biliary pressure, produce transient hyperglycemia.
Generally, the analgesic action of parenterally administered DILAUDID is apparent within 15 minutes and usually remains in effect for more than five hours. The onset of action of oral DILAUDID is somewhat slower, with measurable analgesia occurring within 30 minutes.
In human plasma the half-life of a DILAUDID 4 mg tablet is 2.6 hours. In a random crossover study in six subjects, 4 mg of *oral* DILAUDID produced a mean concentration/time curve similar to that of 2 mg DILAUDID I.V., after the first hours.

INDICATIONS AND USAGE

DILAUDID is indicated for the relief of moderate to severe pain such as that due to:
    Surgery
    Cancer
    Trauma (soft tissue & bone)
    Biliary Colic
    Myocardial Infarction
    Burns
    Renal Colic

Continued on next page

Knoll—Cont.

CONTRAINDICATIONS

DILAUDID is contraindicated in patients with a known hypersensitivity to hydromorphone; in the presence of an intracranial lesion associated with increased intracranial pressure; and whenever ventilatory function is depressed (chronic obstructive pulmonary disease, cor pulmonale, emphysema, kyphoscoliosis, status asthmaticus).

WARNINGS

Respiratory Depression: DILAUDID produces dose-related respiratory depression by acting directly on brain stem respiratory centers. DILAUDID also affects centers that control respiratory rhythm, and may produce irregular and periodic breathing.

Head Injury and Increased Intracranial Pressure: The respiratory depressant effects of narcotics and their capacity to elevate cerebrospinal fluid pressure may be markedly exaggerated in the presence of head injury, other intracranial lesions or a preexisting increase in intracranial pressure. Furthermore, narcotics produce effects which may obscure the clinical course of patients with head injuries.

Acute Abdominal Conditions: The administration of narcotics may obscure the diagnosis or clinical course of patients with acute abdominal conditions.

PRECAUTIONS

Special Risk Patients: DILAUDID should be used with caution in elderly or debilitated patients and those with impaired renal or hepatic function, hypothyroidism, Addison's disease, prostatic hypertrophy or urethral stricture. As with any narcotic analgesic agent, the usual precautions should be observed and the possibility of respiratory depression should be kept in mind.

Cough Reflex: DILAUDID suppresses the cough reflex; as with all narcotics, caution should be exercised when DILAUDID is used postoperatively and in patients with pulmonary disease.

Usage in Ambulatory Patients: Narcotics may impair the mental and/or physical abilities required for the performance of potentially hazardous tasks such as driving a car or operating machinery; patients should be cautioned accordingly.

Drug Interactions: Patients receiving other narcotic analgesics, general anesthetics, phenothiazines, tranquilizers, sedative-hypnotics, tricyclic antidepressants or other CNS depressants (including alcohol) concomitantly with DILAUDID may exhibit an additive CNS depression. When such combined therapy is contemplated, the dose of one or both agents should be reduced.

Parenteral Administration: The parenteral form of DILAUDID may be given intravenously, but the injection should be given very slowly. Rapid intravenous injection of narcotic analgesics increases the possibility of side effects such as hypotension and respiratory depression.

Pregnancy: Pregnancy Category C. DILAUDID has been shown to be teratogenic in hamsters when given in doses 600 times the human dose. There are no adequate and well-controlled studies in pregnant women. DILAUDID should be used during pregnancy only if the potential benefit justifies the potential risk to the fetus.

Nonteratogenic effects: Babies born to mothers who have been taking opioids regularly prior to delivery will be physically dependent. The withdrawal signs include irritability and excessive crying, tremors, hyperactive reflexes, increased respiratory rate, increased stools, sneezing, yawning, vomiting, and fever. The intensity of the syndrome does not always correlate with the duration of maternal opioid use or dose. There is no consensus on the best method of managing withdrawal. Chlorpromazine 0.7 to 1.0 mg/kg q6h, phenobarbital 2 mg/kg q6h, and paregoric 2 to 4 drops/kg q4h, have been used to treat withdrawal symptoms in infants. The duration of therapy is 4 to 28 days, with the dosages decreased as tolerated.

Labor and Delivery: As with all narcotics, administration of DILAUDID to the mother shortly before delivery may result in some degree of respiratory depression in the newborn, especially if higher doses are used.

Nursing Mothers: It is not known whether this drug is excreted in human milk. Because many drugs are excreted in human milk and because of the potential for serious adverse reactions in nursing infants from DILAUDID, a decision should be made whether to discontinue nursing or to discontinue the drug, taking into account the importance of the drug to the mother.

Pediatric Use: Safety and effectiveness in children have not been established.

ADVERSE REACTIONS

Central Nervous System: Sedation, drowsiness, mental clouding, lethargy, impairment of mental and physical performance, anxiety, fear, dysphoria, dizziness, psychic dependence, mood changes.

Gastrointestinal System: Nausea and vomiting occur infrequently; they are more frequent in ambulatory than in recumbent patients. The antiemetic phenothiazines are useful in suppressing these effects; however, some phenothiazine derivatives seem to be antianalgesic and to increase the amount of narcotic required to produce pain relief, while other phenothiazines reduce the amount of narcotic required to produce a given level of analgesia. Prolonged administration of DILAUDID may produce constipation. Opiate agonist-induced increase in intraluminal pressure may endanger surgical anastomosis.

Cardiovascular System: Circulatory depression, peripheral circulatory collapse and cardiac arrest have occurred after rapid intravenous injection. Orthostatic hypotension and fainting may occur if a patient stands up suddenly after receiving an injection of DILAUDID.

Genitourinary System: Ureteral spasm, spasm of vesical sphincters and urinary retention have been reported.

Respiratory Depression: DILAUDID produces dose-related respiratory depression by acting directly on brain stem respiratory centers. DILAUDID also affects centers that control respiratory rhythm, and may produce irregular and periodic breathing. If significant respiratory depression occurs, it may be antagonized by the use of naloxone hydrochloride. The usual adult dose of 0.4 to 0.8 mg given *intramuscularly* or *intravenously,* promptly reverses the effects of morphine-like opioid agonists such as DILAUDID. In patients who are physically dependent, small doses of naloxone may be sufficient not only to antagonize respiratory depression, but also to precipitate withdrawal phenomena. The dose of naloxone should therefore be adjusted accordingly in such patients. Since the duration of action of DILAUDID may exceed that of the antagonist, the patient should be kept under continued surveillance; repeated doses of the antagonist may be required to maintain adequate respiration. Apply other supportive measures when indicated.

DRUG ABUSE AND DEPENDENCE

DILAUDID is a Schedule Ⓒ narcotic. Psychic dependence, physical dependence, and tolerance may develop upon repeated administration of narcotics; therefore, DILAUDID should be prescribed and administered with caution. However, psychic dependence is unlikely to develop when DILAUDID is used for a short time for the treatment of pain. Physical dependence, the condition in which continued administration of the drug is required to prevent the appearance of a withdrawal syndrome, usually assumes clinically significant proportions only after several weeks of continued narcotic use, although some mild degree of physical dependence may develop after a few days of narcotic therapy. Tolerance, in which increasingly large doses are required in order to produce the same degree of analgesia, is manifested initially by a shortened duration of analgesic effect, and subsequently by decreases in the intensity of analgesia. The rate of development of tolerance varies among patients.

OVERDOSAGE

Signs and Symptoms: Serious overdosage with DILAUDID is characterized by respiratory depression (a decrease in respiratory rate and/or tidal volume, Cheyne-Stokes respiration, cyanosis), extreme somnolence progressing to stupor or coma, skeletal muscle flaccidity, cold and clammy skin, and sometimes bradycardia and hypotension. In severe overdosage, particularly by the intravenous route, apnea, circulatory collapse, cardiac arrest, and death may occur.

Treatment: Primary attention should be given to the reestablishment of adequate respiratory exchange through provision of a patent airway and institution of assisted or controlled ventilation. The narcotic antagonist naloxone hydrochloride is a specific antidote against respiratory depression which may result from overdosage or unusual sensitivity to narcotics, including DILAUDID. Therefore, naloxone hydrochloride should be administered as described under *Adverse Reactions* (see *Respiratory Depression*) in conjunction with ventilatory assistance.

Since the duration of action of DILAUDID may exceed that of the antagonist, the patient should be kept under continued surveillance; repeated doses of the antagonist may be required to maintain adequate respiration. An antagonist should not be administered in the absence of clinically significant respiratory or cardiovascular depression. Oxygen, intravenous fluids, vasopressors, and other supportive measures should be employed as indicated.

In cases of overdosage with oral DILAUDID, gastric lavage or induced emesis may be useful in removing unabsorbed drug from conscious patients.

DOSAGE AND ADMINISTRATION

Parenteral: The usual starting dose is 1–2 mg *subcutaneously* or *intramuscularly* every 4 to 6 hours as necessary for pain control. The dose should be adjusted according to the severity of pain, as well as the patient's underlying disease, age, and size. Patients with terminal cancer may be tolerant to narcotic analgesics and may, therefore, require higher doses for adequate pain relief. Intravenous or subcutaneous administration is usually not painful. Should intravenous administration be necessary, the injection should be given

slowly, over at least 2 to 3 minutes, depending on the dose. A gradual increase in dose may be required if analgesia is inadequate, tolerance occurs, or if pain severity increases. The first sign of tolerance is usually a reduced duration of effect.

NOTE: Parenteral drug products should be inspected visually for particulate matter and discoloration prior to administration, whenever solution and container permit. A slight yellowish discoloration may develop in DILAUDID ampules and multiple dose vials. No loss of potency has been demonstrated.

Oral: The usual oral dose is 2 mg every 4 to 6 hours as necessary. The dose must be individually adjusted according to severity of pain, patient response and patient size. More severe pain may require 4 mg or more every 4 to 6 hours. If the pain increases in severity, analgesia is not adequate or tolerance occurs, a gradual increase in dosage may be required. If pain is exceedingly severe, or if prompt response is desired, parenteral DILAUDID should be used initially in adequate amounts to control the pain.

Rectal: DILAUDID suppositories (3 mg) may provide longer duration of relief which could obviate additional medication during the sleeping hours. The usual adult dose is one (1) suppository inserted rectally every 6 to 8 hours or as directed by physician.

HOW SUPPLIED

Ampules: (One mL sterile solution for parenteral administration)
1 mg/mL ampules—Boxes of 10—
NDC# 0044-1011-01.
2 mg/mL ampules—Boxes of 10—
NDC# 0044-1012-01.
Boxes of 25—NDC# 0044-1012-09.
4 mg/mL ampules—Boxes of 10—
NDC# 0044-1014-01.

Multiple Dose Vials: (20 mL sterile solution for parenteral administration)
2 mg/mL—20 mL multiple dose vials
NDC# 0044-1062-05.

Oral Color Coded Tablets: (NOT FOR INJECTION)
1 mg tablet (green)—Bottles of 100—
NDC# 0044-1021-02.
2 mg tablet (orange)—Bottles of 100—
NDC# 0044-1022-02.
Unit Dose of 100 (4 × 25)—
NDC# 0044-1022-45
Bottles of 500—NDC# 0044-1022-03.
3 mg tablet (pink)—Bottles of 100—
NDC# 0044-1023-02.
4 mg tablet (yellow)—Bottles of 100—
NDC# 0044-1024-02.
Unit Dose of 100 (4 × 25)—
NDC# 0044-1024-45
Bottles of 500—NDC# 0044-1024-03.

Rectal Suppositories: 3 mg suppositories—
Boxes of 6—NDC# 0044-1053-01.

Powder: For prescription compounding.
15 grain vial—NDC# 0044-1040-01.

Storage: Parenteral and oral dosage forms of DILAUDID should be stored at 59°–86°F (15°–30°C).

Protect from light. DILAUDID suppositories should be stored in a refrigerator.

A Schedule Ⓒ Narcotic.   6690

DEA order form required.

MR 1987/6690

Revised January 1987

Shown in Product Identification Section, page 413

DILAUDID® COUGH SYRUP   Ⓒ ℞

[dī"law'dĭd]

(hydromorphone hydrochloride)

DESCRIPTION

Each 5 mL (1 teaspoonful) contains 1 mg DILAUDID (hydromorphone HCl) (WARNING: May be habit forming) and 100 mg guaifenesin in a peach-flavored syrup containing 5% alcohol. DILAUDID is a hydrogenated ketone of morphine; it is a narcotic analgesic and antitussive.

The structural formula of DILAUDID (hydromorphone hydrochloride) is:

CLINICAL PHARMACOLOGY

DILAUDID (hydromorphone HCl) is a centrally acting narcotic antitussive which acts directly on the cough reflex center.

DILAUDID is also a narcotic analgesic; its principal therapeutic effect is relief of pain. The precise mechanism of action of DILAUDID and other opiates is not known, although it is believed to relate to the existence of opiate receptors in the central nervous system. There is no intrinsic limit to the analgesic effect of DILAUDID; like morphine, adequate doses will relieve even the most severe pain. Clinically, however, dosage limitations are imposed by the adverse effects, primarily respiratory depression, nausea, and vomiting, which can result from high doses.

DILAUDID has diverse additional actions. It produces drowsiness, changes in mood and mental clouding, depresses the respiratory center and the cough center, stimulates the vomiting center, produces pinpoint constriction of the pupil, enhances parasympathetic activity, elevates cerebrospinal fluid pressure, increases biliary pressure, produces transient hyperglycemia.

Generally, the analgesic action of parenterally administered DILAUDID is apparent within 15 minutes and usually remains in effect for more than five hours. The onset of action of oral DILAUDID is somewhat slower, with measurable analgesia occurring within 30 minutes.

Radioimmunoassay techniques have recently been developed for the analysis of DILAUDID in human plasma. In humans the half-life of a DILAUDID 4 mg tablet is 2.6 hours. In a random crossover study in six subjects, 4 mg of oral DILAUDID produced a mean concentration/time curve similar to that of 2 mg DILAUDID I.V., after the first hour.

Guaifenesin (glyceryl guaiacolate) reduces the viscosity of secretions, thereby increasing the efficiency of the cough reflex and of ciliary action in removing accumulated secretions from the trachea and bronchi. Unlike many other expectorants, guaifenesin rarely causes gastric irritation.

INDICATIONS AND USAGE

DILAUDID Cough Syrup is indicated for the control of persistent, exhausting cough or dry, non-productive cough.

CONTRAINDICATIONS

DILAUDID Cough Syrup is contraindicated in patients known to have a hypersensitivity to hydromorphone; in the presence of an intracranial lesion associated with increased intracranial pressure; and whenever ventilatory function is depressed (chronic obstructive pulmonary disease, cor pulmonale, emphysema, kyphoscoliosis, status asthmaticus).

WARNINGS

Respiratory Depression: DILAUDID produces dose-related respiratory depression by acting directly on brain stem respiratory centers. DILAUDID also affects centers that control respiratory rhythm and may produce irregular and periodic breathing.

Head Injury and Increased Intracranial Pressure: The respiratory depressant effects of narcotics and their capacity to elevate cerebrospinal fluid pressure may be markedly exaggerated in the presence of head injury, other intracranial lesions or a preexisting increase in intracranial pressure. Furthermore, narcotics produce adverse effects which may obscure the clinical course of patients with head injuries.

Acute Abdominal Conditions: The administration of narcotics may obscure the diagnosis or clinical course of patients with acute abdominal conditions.

PRECAUTIONS

Special Risk Patients: DILAUDID Cough Syrup should be used with caution in elderly or debilitated patients and those with impaired renal or hepatic function, hypothyroidism, Addison's disease, prostatic hypertrophy or urethral stricture. As with any narcotic analgesic agent, the usual precautions should be observed and the possibility of respiratory depression should be kept in mind.

Cough Reflex: DILAUDID Cough Syrup suppresses the cough reflex; as with all narcotics, caution should be exercised when DILAUDID Cough Syrup is used postoperatively and in patients with pulmonary disease.

Usage in Ambulatory Patients: Narcotics may impair the mental and/or physical abilities required for the performance of potentially hazardous tasks such as driving a car or operating machinery; patients should be cautioned accordingly.

Drug Interactions: Patients receiving other narcotic analgesics, general anesthetics, phenothiazines, tranquilizers, sedative-hypnotics, tricyclic antidepressants or other CNS depressants (including alcohol) concomitantly with DILAUDID Cough Syrup may exhibit an additive CNS depression. When such combined therapy is contemplated, the dose of one or both agents should be reduced.

Usage in Pregnancy: Pregnancy Category C. DILAUDID has been shown to be teratogenic in hamsters when given in doses 600 times the human dose. There are no adequate and well-controlled studies in pregnant women. DILAUDID Cough Syrup should be used during pregnancy only if the potential benefit justifies the potential risk to the fetus.

Nonteratogenic effects: Babies born to mothers who have been taking opioids regularly prior to delivery will be physically dependent. The withdrawal signs include irritability and excessive crying, tremors, hyperactive reflexes, in-

creased respiratory rate, increased stools, sneezing, yawning, vomiting, and fever. The intensity of the syndrome does not always correlate with the duration of maternal opioid use or dose. There is no consensus on the best method of managing withdrawal. Chlorpromazine 0.7 to 1.0 mg/kg q6h, phenobarbital 2 mg/kg q6h, and paregoric 2 to 4 drops/kg q4h, have been used to treat withdrawal symptoms in infants. The duration of therapy is 4 to 28 days, with the dosage decreased as tolerated.

Labor and Delivery: As with all narcotics, administration of DILAUDID Cough Syrup to the mother shortly before delivery may result in some degree of respiratory depression in the newborn, especially if higher doses are used.

Nursing Mothers: It is not known whether this drug is excreted in human milk. Because many drugs are excreted in human milk and because of the potential for serious adverse reactions in nursing infants from DILAUDID Cough Syrup, a decision should be made whether to discontinue nursing or to discontinue the drug, taking into account the importance of the drug to the mother.

Pediatric Use: Safety and effectiveness in children have not been established.

FD&C Yellow No. 5: DILAUDID Cough Syrup contains FD&C Yellow No. 5 (tartrazine) dye which may cause allergic-type reactions (including bronchial asthma) in certain susceptible individuals. Although the overall incidence of FD&C Yellow No. 5 (tartrazine) dye sensitivity in the general population is low, it is frequently seen in patients who also have aspirin hypersensitivity.

ADVERSE REACTIONS

Central Nervous System: Sedation, drowsiness, mental clouding, lethargy, impairment of mental and physical performance, anxiety, fear, dysphoria, dizziness, psychic dependence, mood changes.

Gastrointestinal System: Nausea and vomiting occur more frequently in ambulatory than in recumbent patients. The antiemetic phenothiazines are useful in suppressing these effects. Prolonged administration of DILAUDID may produce constipation. Opiate agonist-induced increase in intraluminal pressure may endanger surgical anastomosis.

Genitourinary System: Ureteral spasm, spasm of vesical sphincters and urinary retention have been reported.

Respiratory Depression: DILAUDID produces dose-related respiratory depression by acting on brain stem respiratory centers. DILAUDID also affects centers that control respiratory rhythm, and may produce irregular and periodic breathing. If significant respiratory depression occurs, it may be antagonized by the use of naloxone hydrochloride. The usual adult dose of 0.4 to 0.8 mg given intramuscularly or intravenously, promptly reverses the effects of morphine-like opioid agonists such as DILAUDID. In patients who are physically dependent, small doses of naloxone may be sufficient not only to antagonize respiratory depression, but also to precipitate withdrawal phenomena. The dose of naloxone should therefore be adjusted accordingly in such patients. Since the duration of action of DILAUDID may exceed that of the antagonist, the patient should be kept under continued surveillance; repeated doses of the antagonist may be required to maintain adequate respiration. Apply other supportive measures when indicated.

DRUG ABUSE AND DEPENDENCE

DILAUDID is a Schedule Ⅱ narcotic. Psychic dependence, physical dependence, and tolerance may develop upon repeated administration of narcotics; therefore, DILAUDID should be prescribed and administered with caution. However, psychic dependence is unlikely to develop when DILAUDID Cough Syrup is used for a short time as indicated. Physical dependence, the condition in which continued administration of the drug is required to prevent the appearance of a withdrawal syndrome, usually assumes clinically significant proportions only after several weeks of continued narcotic use, although some mild degree of physical dependence may develop after few days of narcotic therapy.

OVERDOSAGE

Signs and Symptoms: Serious overdosage with DILAUDID is characterized by respiratory depression (a decrease in respiratory rate and/or tidal volume, Cheyne-Stokes respiration, cyanosis), extreme somnolence progressing to stupor or coma, skeletal muscle flaccidity, cold and clammy skin, and sometimes bradycardia and hypotension. In severe overdosage particularly by the intravenous route, apnea, circulatory collapse, cardiac arrest and death may occur.

Treatment: Primary attention should be given to the reestablishment of adequate respiratory exchange through provision of a patent airway and the institution of assisted or controlled ventilation. The narcotic antagonist naloxone hydrochloride is a specific antidote against respiratory depression which may result from overdosage or unusual sensitivity to narcotics, including DILAUDID. Therefore, naloxone hydrochloride should be administered as described under ADVERSE REACTIONS (see Respiratory Depression) in conjunction with ventilatory assistance.

Since the duration of action of Dilaudid may exceed that of the antagonist, the patient should be kept under continued

surveillance; repeated doses of the antagonist may be required to maintain adequate respiration. An antagonist should not be administered in the absence of clinically significant respiratory or cardiovascular depression. Oxygen, intravenous fluids, vasopressors and other supportive measures should be employed as indicated.

In cases of overdosage with oral DILAUDID, gastric lavage or induced emesis may be useful in removing unabsorbed drug from conscious patients.

DOSAGE AND ADMINISTRATION

The usual adult dose of DILAUDID Cough Syrup is one teaspoonful (5 mL) every 3 to 4 hours.

HOW SUPPLIED

Bottles of 1 pint (473 mL)—NDC #0044-1080-01.
Storage: Store at 59°–86°F (15°–30°C).
A Schedule Ⅱ Narcotic.
DEA order form required.
Revised September 1986   8074

DILAUDID–HP® INJECTION   Ⅱ ℞
[dī"law 'dĭd]
10 mg/mL
(hydromorphone hydrochloride)

PRODUCT OVERVIEW

KEY FACTS

Dilaudid-HP is a narcotic analgesic, containing 10 mg of hydromophone per ml; it is administered by subcutaneous and intramuscular injection. Because of its highly concentrated solution, a smaller injection volume can be used than with other parenteral narcotic formulations, thereby avoiding the discomfort associated with the intramuscular or subcutaneous injection of an unusually large volume of solution.

MAJOR USE

This high-potency hydromorphone formulation is used to relieve moderate-to severe pain in narcotic-tolerant patients who require abnormally high doses of narcotic analgesics for adequate pain relief. Usually these are patients who have already been treated with other narcotic analgesics.

SAFETY INFORMATION

Is contraindicated in: patients who are not already receiving large amounts of parenteral narcotics, patients with known hypersensitivity to the drug, patients with respiratory depression in the absence of resuscitative equipment, patients with status asthmaticus, and for use in obstetrical analgesia. Similar to other narcotic analgesics, the major adverse reactions include respiratory depression and apnea, and, to a lesser extent, circulatory depression, respiratory arrest, shock and cardiac arrest.

PRESCRIBING INFORMATION

DILAUDID–HP® INJECTION   Ⅱ ℞
[dī"law 'dĭd]
10 mg/mL
(hydromorphone hydrochloride)

WARNING

DILAUDID-HP® (HIGH POTENCY) IS A HIGHLY CONCENTRATED SOLUTION OF HYDROMORPHONE INTENDED FOR USE IN NARCOTIC-TOLERANT PATIENTS. DO NOT CONFUSE DILAUDID-HP WITH STANDARD PARENTERAL FORMULATIONS OF DILAUDID OR OTHER NARCOTICS. OVERDOSE AND DEATH COULD RESULT.

DESCRIPTION

DILAUDID (hydromorphone hydrochloride) (WARNING: May be habit forming), a hydrogenated ketone of morphine, is a narcotic analgesic, *HIGH POTENCY* DILAUDID is available in AMBER ampules for subcutaneous (SC) or intramuscular (IM) administration. Each 1 mL of sterile solution contains 10 mg hydromorphone hydrochloride with 0.2% sodium citrate, 0.2% citric acid solution.

The structural formula of DILAUDID (hydromorphone hydrochloride) is:

CLINICAL PHARMACOLOGY

Many of the effects described below are common to the class of narcotic analgesics. In some instances, data may not exist to demonstrate that DILAUDID-HP possesses similar or different effects than those observed with other narcotic analgesics. However, in the absence of data to the contrary,

Continued on next page

Knoll—Cont.

it is assumed that DILAUDID-HP would possess these effects.

Central Nervous System: Narcotic analgesics have multiple actions but exert their primary effects on the central nervous system and organs containing smooth muscle. The principal actions of therapeutic value are analgesia and sedation. A significant feature of the analgesia is that it occurs without loss of consciousness. Narcotic analgesics also suppress the cough reflex and cause respiratory depression, mood changes, mental clouding, euphoria, dysphoria, nausea, vomiting and electroencephalographic changes. The precise mode of analgesic action of narcotic analgesics is unknown. However, specific CNS opiate receptors have been identified. Narcotics are believed to express their pharmacological effects by combining with these receptors.

Narcotics depress the cough reflex by direct effect on the cough center in the medulla.

Narcotics produce respiratory depression by direct effect on brain stem respiratory centers. The mechanism of respiratory depression also involves a reduction in the responsiveness of the brain stem respiratory centers to increases in carbon dioxide tension.

Narcotics cause miosis. Pinpoint pupils are a common sign of narcotic overdose but are not pathognomonic (e.g., pontine lesions of hemorrhagic or ischemic origin may produce similar findings) and marked mydriasis occurs when asphyxia intervenes.

Gastrointestinal Tract and Other Smooth Muscle: Gastric, biliary and pancreatic secretions are decreased by narcotics. Narcotics cause a reduction in motility associated with an increase in tone in the antrum portion of the stomach and duodenum. Digestion of food in the small intestine is delayed and propulsive contractions are decreased. Propulsive peristaltic waves in the colon are decreased, and tone may be increased to the point of spasm. The end result is constipation. Narcotics can cause a marked increase in biliary tract pressure as a result of spasm of the sphincter of Oddi.

Cardiovascular System: Certain narcotics produce peripheral vasodilation which may result in orthostatic hypotension. Release of histamine may occur with narcotics and may contribute to narcotic-induced hypotension. Other manifestations of histamine release and/or peripheral vasodilation may include pruritus, flushing, and red eyes.

Effects on the myocardium after i.v. administration of narcotics are not significant in normal persons, vary with different narcotic analgesic agents and vary with the hemodynamic state of the patient, state of hydration and sympathetic drive.

Pharmacokinetics: In normal human volunteers hydromorphone is metabolized primarily in the liver. It is excreted primarily as the glucuronidated conjugate, with small amounts of parent drug and minor amounts of 6-hydroxy reduction metabolites.

Following intravenous administration of DILAUDID to normal volunteers, the mean half-life of elimination was 2.64 +/− 0.88 hours. The mean volume of distribution was 91.5 liters, suggesting extensive tissue uptake. DILAUDID is rapidly removed from the blood stream and distributed to skeletal muscle, kidneys, liver, intestinal tract, lungs, spleen and brain. DILAUDID also crosses the placental membranes.

In terms of area under the analgesic time-effect curve, hydromorphone is approximately 8 times more potent than morphine (i.e., 1.3 mg of hydromorphone produces analgesia equal to that produced by 10 mg of morphine). After intramuscular administration, hydromorphone has a slightly more rapid onset and slightly shorter duration of action than morphine. The duration of DILAUDID analgesia in the nontolerant patient with usual doses may be up to 4–5 hours. However, in tolerant subjects, duration will vary substantially depending on tolerance and dose. Dose should be adjusted so that 3–4 hours of pain relief may be achieved.

INDICATIONS AND USAGE

DILAUDID-HP is indicated for the relief of moderate to severe pain in narcotic tolerant patients who require larger than usual doses of narcotics to provide adequate pain relief. Because DILAUDID-HP contains 10 mg of hydromorphone per mL, a smaller injection volume can be used than with other parenteral narcotic formulations. Discomfort associated with the intramuscular or subcutaneous injection of an unusually large volume of solution can therefore be avoided.

Contraindications: DILAUDID-HP is contraindicated in: patients who are not already receiving large amounts of parenteral narcotics, patients with known hypersensitivity to the drug, patients with respiratory depression in the absence of resuscitative equipment, and in patients with status asthmaticus. DILAUDID-HP is also contraindicated for use in obstetrical analgesia.

Warnings—Drug Dependence: DILAUDID-HP can produce drug dependence of the morphine type and therefore has the potential for being abused. Psychic dependence,

physical dependence and tolerance may develop upon repeated administration of DILAUDID-HP, and it should be prescribed and administered with the same degree of caution appropriate for the use of morphine. Since DILAUDID-HP is indicated for use in patients who are already tolerant to and hence physically dependent on narcotics, abrupt discontinuance in the administration of DILAUDID-HP is likely to result in a withdrawal syndrome. (See ***Drug Abuse and Dependence***).

Infants born to mothers physically dependent on DILAUDID-HP will also be physically dependent and may exhibit respiratory difficulties and withdrawal symptoms (see ***Drug Abuse and Dependence***).

Impaired Respiration: Respiratory depression is the chief hazard of DILAUDID-HP. Respiratory depression occurs most frequently in the elderly, in the debilitated, and in those suffering from conditions accompanied by hypoxia or hypercapnia when even moderate therapeutic doses may dangerously decrease pulmonary ventilation.

DILAUDID-HP should be used with extreme caution in patients with chronic obstructive pulmonary disease or cor pulmonale, patients having a substantially decreased respiratory reserve, hypoxia, hypercapnia, or preexisting respiratory depression. In such patients even usual therapeutic doses of narcotic analgesics may decrease respiratory drive while simultaneously increasing airway resistance to the point of apnea.

Head Injury and Increased Intracranial Pressure: The respiratory depressant effects of DILAUDID-HP with carbon dioxide retention and secondary elevation of cerebrospinal fluid pressure may be markedly exaggerated in the presence of head injury, other intracranial lesions, or preexisting increase in intracranial pressure. Narcotic analgesics including DILAUDID-HP may produce effects which can obscure the clinical course and neurologic signs of further increase in pressure in patients with head injuries.

Hypotensive Effect: Narcotic analgesics, including DILAUDID-HP, may cause severe hypotension in an individual whose ability to maintain his blood pressure has already been compromised by a depleted blood volume, or a concurrent administration of drugs such as phenothiazines or general anesthetics (see also ***Precautions—Drug Interactions***). DILAUDID-HP may produce orthostatic hypotension in ambulatory patients.

DILAUDID-HP should be administered with caution to patients in circulatory shock, since vasodilation produced by the drug may further reduce cardiac output and blood pressure.

PRECAUTIONS

General: Because of its high concentration, the delivery of precise doses of DILAUDID-HP may be difficult if low doses of hydromorphone are required. Therefore, DILAUDID-HP should be used only if the amount of hydromorphone required can be delivered accurately with this formulation.

In general, narcotics should be given with caution and the initial dose should be reduced in the elderly or debilitated and those with severe impairment of hepatic, pulmonary or renal function; myxedema or hypothyroidism; adrenocortical insufficiency (e.g., Addison's Disease); CNS depression or coma; toxic psychoses; prostatic hypertrophy or urethral stricture; gallbladder disease; acute alcoholism; delirium tremens; or kyphoscoliosis.

In the case of DILAUDID-HP, however, the patient is presumed to be receiving a narcotic to which he or she exhibits tolerance and the initial dose of DILAUDID-HP selected should be estimated based on the relative potency of hydromorphone and the narcotic previously used by the patient. See (***Dosage and Administration*** section.

The administration of narcotic analgesics including DILAUDID-HP may obscure the diagnosis or clinical course in patients with acute abdominal conditions and may aggravate preexisting convulsions in patients with convulsive disorders.

Narcotic analgesics including DILAUDID-HP should also be used with caution in patients about to undergo surgery of the biliary tract since it may cause spasm of the sphincter of Oddi.

Drug Interactions: The concomitant use of other central nervous system depressants including sedatives or hypnotics, general anesthetics, phenothiazines, tranquilizers and alcohol may produce additive depressant effects. Respiratory depression, hypotension and profound sedation or coma may occur. When such combined therapy is contemplated, the dose of one or both agents should be reduced. Narcotic analgesics, including DILAUDID-HP, may enhance the action of neuromuscular blocking agents and produce an increased degree of respiratory depression.

Pregnancy—Category C:

Human: Adequate animal studies on reproduction have not been performed to determine whether hydromorphone affects fertility in males or females. There are no well-controlled studies in women. Reports based on marketing experience do not identify any specific teratogenic risks following routine (short-term) clinical use. Although there is no clearly defined risk, such reports do not exclude the possibility of

infrequent or subtle damage to the human fetus. DILAUDID-HP should be used in pregnant women only when clearly needed (see ***Labor and Delivery*** and ***Drug Abuse and Dependence***).

Animal: Literature reports of hydromorphone hydrochloride administration to pregnant Syrian hamsters show that DILAUDID is teratogenic at a dose of 20 mg/kg which is 600 times the human dose. A maximal teratogenic effect (50% of fetuses affected) in the Syrian hamster was observed at a dose of 125 mg/kg.

Labor and Delivery: DILAUDID-HP is contraindicated in Labor and Delivery (see ***Contraindications*** section).

Nursing Mothers: Low levels of narcotic analgesics have been detected in human milk. As a general rule, nursing should not be undertaken while a patient is receiving DILAUDID-HP since it, and other drugs in this class, may be excreted in the milk.

Pediatric Use: Safety and effectiveness in children have not been established.

ADVERSE REACTIONS

The adverse effects of DILAUDID-HP are similar to those of other narcotic analgesics, and represent established pharmacological effects of the drug class. The major hazards include respiratory depression and apnea. To a lesser degree, circulatory depression, respiratory arrest, shock and cardiac arrest have occurred.

The most frequently observed adverse effects are lightheadedness, dizziness, sedation, nausea, vomiting, and sweating. These effects seem to be more prominent in ambulatory patients and in those not experiencing severe pain. Some adverse reactions in ambulatory patients may be alleviated if the patient lies down.

Less Frequently Observed With Narcotic Analgesics:

General and CNS: Dysphoria, euphoria, weakness, headache, agitation, tremor, uncoordinated muscle movements, alterations of mood (nervousness, apprehension, depression, floating feelings, dreams), muscle rigidity, paresthesia, muscle tremor, blurred vision, nystagmus, diplopia and miosis, transient hallucinations* and disorientation, visual disturbances, insomnia and increased intracranial pressure may occur.

* Hallucinations, although unusual with pure agonist narcotics, have been observed in one patient following both a 6 mg and a 4 mg DILAUDID-HP dose. However, the patient was receiving several concomitant medications during the second episode and a causal relationship cannot be established.

Cardiovascular: Flushing of the face, chills, tachycardia, bradycardia, palpitation, faintness, syncope, hypotension and hypertension have been reported.

Respiratory: Bronchospasm and laryngospasm have been known to occur.

Gastrointestinal: Dry mouth, constipation, biliary tract spasm, anorexia, diarrhea, cramps and taste alterations have been reported.

Genitourinary: Urinary retention or hesitancy, and antidiuretic effects have been reported.

Dermatologic: Pruritis, urticaria, other skin rashes, wheal and flare over the vein with intravenous injection, and diaphoresis have been reported with narcotic analgesics.

Other: In clinical trials, neither local tissue irritation nor induration was observed at the site of subcutaneous injection of DILAUDID-HP; pain at the injection site was rarely observed. However, local irritation and induration have been seen following parenteral injection of other narcotic drug products.

DRUG ABUSE AND DEPENDENCE

Narcotic analgesics may cause psychological and physical dependence (see ***Warnings***). Physical dependence results in withdrawal symptoms in patients who abruptly discontinue the drug. Withdrawal symptoms also may be precipitated in the patient with physical dependence by the administration of a drug with narcotic antagonist activity, e.g., naloxone (see also ***Overdosage***). Physical dependence usually does not occur to a clinically significant degree until after several weeks of continued narcotic usage. Tolerance, in which increasingly large doses are required in order to produce the same degree of analgesia, is initially manifested by a shortened duration of analgesic effect, and subsequently, by decreases in the intensity of analgesia. In chronic pain patients, and in narcotic-tolerant cancer patients, the dose of DILAUDID-HP should be guided by the degree of tolerance manifested.

In chronic pain patients in whom narcotic analgesics including DILAUDID-HP are abruptly discontinued, a severe abstinence syndrome should be anticipated. This may be similar to the abstinence syndrome noted in patients who withdraw from heroin. The latter abstinence syndrome may be characterized by restlessness, lacrimation, rhinorrhea, yawning, perspiration, gooseflesh, restless sleep or "yen" and mydriasis during the first 24 hours. These symptoms may increase in severity and over the next 72 hours may be accompanied by increasing irritability, anxiety, weakness, twitching and spasms of muscles, kicking movements, severe backache, abdominal and leg pains, abdominal and muscle cramps, hot and cold flashes, insomnia, nausea, anorexia, vomiting, intestinal spasm, diarrhea, coryza and repetitive sneezing, increase in body temperature, blood pressure, respiratory rate and heart rate.

Because of excessive loss of fluids through sweating, or vomiting and diarrhea, there is usually marked weight loss, dehydration, ketosis, and disturbances in acid-base balance. Cardiovascular collapse can occur. Without treatment most observable symptoms disappear in 5–14 days; however, there appears to be a phase of secondary or chronic abstinence which may last for 2–6 months characterized by insomnia, irritability, muscular aches, and autonomic instability.

In the treatment of physical dependence on DILAUDID-HP, the patient may be detoxified by gradual reduction of the dosage, although this is unlikely to be necessary in the terminal cancer patient. If abstinence symptoms become severe, the patient may be given methadone. Temporary administration of tranquilizers and sedatives may aid in reducing patient anxiety. Gastrointestinal disturbances or dehydration should be treated accordingly.

OVERDOSAGE

Serious overdosage with DILAUDID-HP is characterized by respiratory depression, somnolence progressing to stupor or coma, skeletal muscle flaccidity, cold and clammy skin, constricted pupils, and sometimes bradycardia and hypotension. In serious overdosage, particularly following intravenous injection, apnea, circulatory collapse, cardiac arrest and death may occur.

In the treatment of overdosage primary attention should be given to the reestablishment of adequate respiratory exchange through provision of a patent airway and institution of assisted or controlled ventilation.

NARCOTIC-TOLERANT PATIENT: Since tolerance to the respiratory and CNS depressant effects of narcotics develops concomitantly with tolerance to their analgesic effects, serious respiratory depression due to an acute overdose is unlikely to be seen in narcotic-tolerant patients receiving DILAUDID-HP for chronic pain.

NOTE: In such an individual who is physically dependent on narcotics, administration of the usual dose of the antagonist will precipitate an acute withdrawal syndrome. The severity will depend on the degree of physical dependence and the dose of the antagonist administered. Use of a narcotic antagonist in such a person should be avoided. If necessary to treat serious respiratory depression in the physically-dependent patient, the antagonist should be administered with extreme care and by titration with smaller than usual doses of the antagonist.

NON-TOLERANT PATIENT: The narcotic antagonist, naloxone, is a specific antidote against respiratory depression which may result from overdosage, or unusual sensitivity to DILAUDID-HP. A dose of naloxone (usually 0.4 to 2.0 mg) should be administered intravenously, if possible, simultaneously with respiratory resuscitation. The dose can be repeated in 3 minutes. Naloxone should not be administered in the absence of clinically significant respiratory or circulatory depression. Naloxone should be administered cautiously to persons who are known, or suspected to be physically dependent on DILAUDID-HP. In such cases, an abrupt or complete reversal of narcotic effects may precipitate an acute abstinence syndrome.

Since the duration of action of DILAUDID may exceed that of the antagonist, the patient should be kept under continued surveillance; repeated doses of the antagonist may be required to maintain adequate respiration. Apply other supportive measures when indicated.

Supportive measures (including oxygen, vasopressors) should be employed in the management of circulatory shock and pulmonary edema accompanying overdose as indicated. Cardiac arrest or arrhythmias may require cardiac massage or defibrillation.

DOSAGE AND ADMINISTRATION

Parenteral: **DILAUDID-HP SHOULD BE GIVEN ONLY TO PATIENTS WHO ARE ALREADY RECEIVING LARGE DOSES OF NARCOTICS.** DILAUDID-HP is indicated for relief of moderate-to-severe pain in narcotic-tolerant patients. Thus, these patients will already have been treated with other narcotic analgesics. If the patient is being changed from regular DILAUDID to DILAUDID-HP, similar doses should be used, depending on the patient's clinical response to the drug. If DILAUDID-HP is substituted for a different narcotic analgesic, the following equivalency table should be used as a guide to determine the appropriate starting dose of DILAUDID-HP (hydromorphone hydrochloride). [See table above right].

In open clinical trials with DILAUDID-HP in patients with terminal cancer, doses ranged from 1–14 mg subcutaneously or intramuscularly; one patient received 30 mg subcutaneously on two occasions. In these trials, both subcutaneous and intramuscular injections of DILAUDID-HP were well-tolerated, with minimal pain and/or burning at the injection site. Mild erythema was rarely noted after intramuscular injection. There was no induration after either intramuscu-

STRONG ANALGESICS AND STRUCTURALLY RELATED DRUGS USED IN THE TREATMENT OF CANCER PAIN*

Nonproprietary (Trade) Names	Dose, mg Equianalgesic to 10 mg of IM Morphine†	Duration Compared With Morphine
Morphine sulfate	10	Same
Papaveretum (Pantopon)	20	Same
Hydromorphone hydrochloride (DILAUDID)	1.3	Slightly shorter
Oxymorphone hydrochloride (Numorphan)	1.1	Slightly shorter
Nalbuphine hydrochloride (Nubain)	12	Same
Heroin, diamorphine hydrochloride (NA in U.S.)	4–5	Slightly shorter
Levorphanol tartrate (Levo-Dromoran)	2.3	Same
Butorphanol tartrate (Stadol)	1.5–2.5	Same
Pentazocine lactate or hydrochloride (Talwin)	60	Shorter
Meperidine, pethidine hydrochloride (Demerol)	80	Shorter
Methadone hydrochloride (Dolophine)	10	Same

* from Beaver WT
Management of cancer pain with parenteral medication J. Am. Med. Assoc. 244:2653–2657 (1980)
† (in terms of the area under the analgesic time-effect curve.)

lar or subcutaneous administration of DILAUDID-HP. Subcutaneous injections of DILAUDID-HP were particularly well accepted when administered with a short, 30-gauge needle.

Experience with administration of DILAUDID-HP by the intravenous route is limited. Should intravenous administration be necessary, the injection should be given slowly, over at least 2 to 3 minutes. The intravenous route is usually painless.

A gradual increase in dose may be required if analgesia is inadequate, tolerance occurs, or if pain severity increases. The first sign of tolerance is usually a reduced duration of effect.

NOTE: Parenteral drug products should be inspected visually for particulate matter and discoloration prior to administration, whenever solution and container permit. A slight yellowish discoloration may develop in DILAUDID-HP ampules. No loss of potency has been demonstrated. Dilaudid injection is physically compatible and chemically stable for at least 24 hours at 25°C protected from light in most common large volume parenteral solutions.

HOW SUPPLIED

DILAUDID-HP *amber* ampules contain 10 mg hydromorphone hydrochloride per mL with 0.2% sodium citrate and 0.2% citric acid solution. No added preservative.
NOTE: DILAUDID-HP ampules are *amber* in color and marked with a distinctive identification band.

HIGH POTENCY
10 mg/mL—Box of 10 ampules
        NDC 0044 1017-10
*50 mg/5 mL—Box of 10 ampules
        NDC 0044 1017-25
* FOR USE IN THE PREPARATION OF LARGE VOLUME PARENTERAL SOLUTIONS

STORAGE

Parenteral forms of DILAUDID should be stored at 59°–86°F, (15–30°C). Protect from light.
DEA Order Form Required
A Schedule ⓒ Narcotic.
September 1986   6687
Shown in Product Identification Section, page 413

ISOPTIN®   ℞
[ĭ-sŏp″tĭn]
(verapamil hydrochloride)
Intravenous Injection

DESCRIPTION

ISOPTIN® (verapamil hydrochloride) is a calcium antagonist or slow channel inhibitor. ISOPTIN is available in 5 mg/2 mL and 10 mg/4 mL ampules, 5 mg/2 mL and 10 mg/4 mL single dose vials (for intravenous administration). Each 1 mL of solution contains 2.5 mg verapamil HCl and 8.5 mg sodium chloride in water for injection. Hydrochloric acid is used for pH adjustment. The pH of the solution is between 4.1 and 6.0. Protect contents from light. ISOPTIN ampules, and vials are sterile.

The structural formula of verapamil HCl is given below:

$C_{27}H_{38}N_2O_4 \cdot HCl$ M.W. = 491.08
Benzeneacetonitrile, α-[3-[[2-(3,4-dimethoxyphenyl) ethyl] methylamino]propyl] - 3,4-dimethoxy-α-(1-methylethyl) hydrochloride
Verapamil HCl is an almost white, crystalline powder, practically free of odor, with a bitter taste. It is soluble in water, chloroform and methanol. Verapamil HCl is not chemically related to other antiarrhythmic drugs.

CLINICAL PHARMACOLOGY

Mechanism of Action: ISOPTIN (verapamil HCl) inhibits the calcium ion (and possibly sodium ion) influx through slow channels into conductile and contractile myocardial cells and vascular smooth muscle cells. The antiarrhythmic effect of ISOPTIN appears to be due to its effect on the slow channel in cells of the cardiac conduction system. The vasodilatory effect of ISOPTIN appears to be due to its effect on blockade of calcium channels as well as α-receptors.

In the isolated rabbit heart, concentrations of ISOPTIN that markedly affect SA nodal fibers or fibers in the upper and middle regions of the AV node, have very little effect on fibers in the lower AV node (NH region) and no effect on atrial action potentials or His bundle fibers.

Electrical activity in the SA and AV nodes depends, to a large degree, upon calcium influx through the slow channel. By inhibiting this influx, ISOPTIN slows AV conduction and prolongs the effective refractory period within the AV node in a rate-related manner. This effect results in a reduction of the ventricular rate in patients with atrial flutter and/or atrial fibrillation and a rapid ventricular response.

By interrupting reentry at the AV node, ISOPTIN can restore normal sinus rhythm in patients with paroxysmal supraventricular tachycardias (PSVT), including PSVT associated with Wolff-Parkinson-White syndrome.

ISOPTIN does not induce peripheral arterial spasm.

ISOPTIN has a local anesthetic action that is 1.6 times that of procaine on an equimolar basis. It is not known whether this action is important at the doses used in man.

ISOPTIN does not alter total serum calcium levels.

Hemodynamics: ISOPTIN (verapamil HCl) reduces afterload and myocardial contractility. The commonly used intravenous doses of 5–10 mg ISOPTIN produce transient, usually asymptomatic, reduction in normal systemic arterial pressure, systemic vascular resistance and contractility; left ventricular filling pressure is slightly increased. In most patients, including those with organic cardiac disease, the negative inotropic action of ISOPTIN is countered by reduction of afterload, and cardiac index is usually not reduced. However, in patients with moderately severe to severe cardiac dysfunction (pulmonary wedge pressure above 20 mm Hg, ejection fraction less than 30%), acute worsening of heart failure may be seen. Peak therapeutic effects occur within 3 to 5 minutes after a bolus injection.

Pharmacokinetics: Intravenously administered ISOPTIN (verapamil HCl) has been shown to be rapidly metabolized. Following intravenous infusion in man, verapamil is elimi-

Continued on next page

Knoll—Cont.

nated biexponentially, with a rapid early distribution phase (half-life about 4 minutes) and a slower terminal elimination phase (half-life 2–5 hours). In healthy men, orally administered ISOPTIN undergoes extensive metabolism in the liver; 12 metabolites having been identified, most in only trace amounts. The major metabolites have been identified as various N- and O-dealkylated products of ISOPTIN. Approximately 70% of an administered dose is excreted in the urine and 16% or more in the feces within 5 days. About 3–4% is excreted as unchanged drug.

Aging may affect the pharmacokinetics of verapamil given to hypertensive patients. Elimination half-life may be prolonged in the elderly.

INDICATIONS AND USAGE

ISOPTIN (verapamil HCl) is indicated for the following:
- Rapid conversion to sinus rhythm of paroxysmal supraventricular tachycardias, including those associated with accessory bypass tracts (Wolff-Parkinson-White [W-P-W] and Lown-Ganong-Levine [L-G-L] syndromes). When clinically advisable, appropriate vagal maneuvers (e.g. Valsalva maneuver) should be attempted prior to ISOPTIN administration.
- Temporary control of rapid ventricular rate in atrial flutter or atrial fibrillation **except** when the atrial flutter and/or atrial fibrillation are associated with accessory bypass tracts (Wolff-Parkinson-White [W-P-W] and Lown-Ganong-Levine [L-G-L] syndromes).

In controlled studies in the United States, about 60% of patients with supraventricular tachycardia converted to normal sinus rhythm within 10 minutes after intravenous ISOPTIN. Uncontrolled studies reported in the world literature describe a conversion rate of about 80%. About 70% of patients with atrial flutter and/or fibrillation with a fast ventricular rate respond with a decrease in ventricular rate of at least 20%. Conversion of atrial flutter or fibrillation to sinus rhythm is uncommon (about 10%) after ISOPTIN and may reflect the spontaneous conversion rate, since the conversion rate after placebo was similar. Slowing of the ventricular rate in patients with atrial fibrillation/flutter lasts 30–60 minutes after a single injection.

Because a small fraction (< 1.0%) of patients treated with ISOPTIN respond with life-threatening adverse responses (rapid ventricular rate in atrial flutter/fibrillation and an accessory bypass tract, marked hypotension, or extreme bradycardia/asystole—see Contraindications and Warnings), the initial use of intravenous ISOPTIN should, if possible, be in a treatment setting with monitoring and resuscitation facilities, including DC-cardioversion capability (see Suggested Treatment of Acute Cardiovascular Adverse Reactions). As familiarity with the patient's response is gained, use in an office setting may be acceptable. Cardioversion has been used safely and effectively after intravenous ISOPTIN.

CONTRAINDICATIONS

ISOPTIN (verapamil HCl) is contraindicated in:
1. Severe hypotension or cardiogenic shock
2. Second- or third-degree AV block (except in patients with a functioning artificial ventricular pacemaker)
3. Sick sinus syndrome (except in patients with a functioning artificial ventricular pacemaker)
4. Severe congestive heart failure (unless secondary to a supraventricular tachycardia amenable to verapamil therapy)
5. Patients receiving **intravenous** beta adrenergic blocking drugs (e.g., propranolol). **Intravenous** verapamil and **intravenous** beta adrenergic blocking drugs should not be administered in close proximity to each other (within a few hours), since both may have a depressant effect on myocardial contractility and AV conduction.
6. Patients with atrial flutter or atrial fibrillation and an accessory bypass tract (e.g. Wolff-Parkinson-White, Lown-Ganong-Levine syndromes) are at risk to develop ventricular tachyarrhythmia including ventricular fibrillation if verapamil is administered. Therefore the use of verapamil in these patients is contraindicated.
7. Ventricular Tachycardia. Administration of intravenous verapamil to patients with wide-complex ventricular tachycardia (QRS ≥ 0.12 sec) can result in marked hemodynamic deterioration and ventricular fibrillation. Proper pre-therapy diagnosis and differentiation from wide complex supraventricular tachycardia is imperative in the emergency room setting.
8. Known hypersensitivity to verapamil hydrochloride.

WARNINGS

ISOPTIN SHOULD BE GIVEN AS A SLOW INTRAVENOUS INJECTION OVER AT LEAST A TWO MINUTE PERIOD OF TIME. (See Dosage and Administration)

Hypotension: Intravenous ISOPTIN (verapamil HCl) often produces a decrease in blood pressure below baseline levels that is usually transient and asymptomatic but may result in dizziness. Systolic pressure less than 90 mm Hg and/or dia-

stolic pressure less than 60 mm Hg was seen in 5–10% of patients in controlled U.S. trials in supraventricular tachycardia and in about 10% of the patients with atrial flutter/fibrillation. The incidence of symptomatic hypotension observed in studies conducted in the U.S. was approximately 1.5%. Three of the five symptomatic patients required intravenous pharmacologic treatment (levarterenol bitartrate, metaraminol bitartrate, or 10% calcium gluconate). All recovered without sequelae.

Extreme Bradycardia/Asystole: ISOPTIN (verapamil HCl) affects the AV and SA nodes and rarely may produce second- or third-degree AV block, bradycardia and, in extreme cases, asystole. This is more likely to occur in patients with a sick sinus syndrome (SA nodal disease), which is more common in older patients. Bradycardia associated with sick sinus syndrome was reported in 0.3% of the patients treated in controlled double-blind trials in the United States. The total incidence of bradycardia (ventricular rate less than 60 beats/min) was 1.2% in these studies. Asystole in patients other than those with sick sinus syndrome is usually of short duration (few seconds or less), with spontaneous return to AV nodal or normal sinus rhythm. If this does not occur promptly, appropriate treatment should be initiated immediately. (See Adverse Reactions and Treatment of Adverse Reactions.)

Heart Failure: When heart failure is not severe or rate related, it should be controlled with digitalis glycosides and diuretics, as appropriate, before ISOPTIN is used. In patients with moderately severe to severe cardiac dysfunction (pulmonary wedge pressure above 20 mm Hg, ejection fraction less than 30%), acute worsening of heart failure may be seen.

Concomitant Antiarrhythmic Therapy:

Digitalis: Intravenous verapamil has been used concomitantly with digitalis preparations without the occurrence of serious adverse effects. However, since both drugs slow AV conduction, patients should be monitored for AV block or excessive bradycardia.

Procainamide: Intravenous verapamil has been administered to a small number of patients receiving oral procainamide without the occurrence of serious adverse effects.

Quinidine: Intravenous verapamil has been administered to a small number of patients receiving oral Quinidine without the occurrence of serious adverse effects. However, three patients have been described in whom the combination resulted in an exaggerated hypotensive response presumably from the combined ability of both drugs to antagonize the effects of catecholamines on α-adrenergic receptors. Caution should therefore be used when employing this combination of drugs.

Beta Adrenergic Blocking Drugs: Intravenous verapamil has been administered to patients receiving oral beta blockers without the development of serious adverse effects. However, since both drugs may depress myocardial contractility or AV conduction, the possibility of detrimental interactions should be considered. The concomitant administration of **intravenous** beta blockers and **intravenous** verapamil has resulted in serious adverse reactions (see Contraindications), especially in patients with severe cardiomyopathy, congestive heart failure or recent myocardial infarction.

Disopyramide: Until data on possible interactions between verapamil and all forms of disopyramide phosphate are obtained, disopyramide should not be administered within 48 hours before or 24 hours after verapamil administration.

Flecainide: A study in healthy volunteers showed that the concomitant administration of flecainide and verapamil have additive effects on myocardial contractility, AV conduction, and repolarization. Concomitant therapy with flecainide and verapamil may result in additive negative inotropic effect and prolongation of atrioventricular conduction.

Heart Block: ISOPTIN (verapamil HCl) prolongs AV conduction time. While high degree AV block has not been observed in controlled clinical trials in the U.S., a low percentage (less than 0.5%) has been reported in the world literature. Development of second- or third-degree AV block or unifascicular, bifascicular or trifascicular bundle branch block requires reduction in subsequent doses or discontinuation of verapamil and institution of appropriate therapy, if needed. (See Treatment of Acute Cardiovascular Adverse Reactions.)

Hepatic and Renal Failure: Significant hepatic and renal failure should not increase the effects of a single intravenous dose of ISOPTIN (verapamil HCl) but may prolong its duration. Repeated injections of intravenous ISOPTIN in such patients may lead to accumulation and an excessive pharmacologic effect of the drug. There is no experience to guide use of multiple doses in such patients and this generally should be avoided. If repeated injections are essential, blood pressure and PR interval should be closely monitored and smaller repeat doses should be utilized. Verapamil cannot be removed by hemodialysis.

Premature Ventricular Contractions: During conversion to normal sinus rhythm, or marked reduction in ventricular rate, a few benign complexes of unusual appearance (some-

times resembling premature ventricular contractions) may be seen after treatment with ISOPTIN (verapamil HCl). Similar complexes are seen during spontaneous conversion of supraventricular tachycardias, after DC-cardioversion and other pharmacologic therapy. These complexes appear to have no clinical significance.

Duchenne's Muscular Dystrophy: Intravenous ISOPTIN (verapamil HCl) can precipitate respiratory muscle failure in these patients and should, therefore, be used with caution.

Increased Intracranial Pressure: Intravenous ISOPTIN (verapamil HCl) has been seen to increase intracranial pressure in patients with supratentorial tumors at the time of anesthesia induction. Caution should be taken and appropriate monitoring performed.

PRECAUTIONS

Drug Interactions: (See Warnings: Concomitant Antiarrhythmic Therapy) Intravenous ISOPTIN (verapamil HCl) has been used concomitantly with other cardioactive drugs (especially digitalis) without evidence of serious negative drug interactions. In rare instances, when patients with severe cardiomyopathy, congestive heart failure or recent myocardial infarction were given **intravenous** beta-adrenergic blocking agents or disopyramide concomitantly with intravenous verapamil, serious adverse effects have occurred. Concomitant use of ISOPTIN with α-adrenergic blockers may result in an exaggerated hypotensive response. Such an effect was observed in one study following the concomitant administrtation of verapamil and prazosin. As verapamil is highly bound to plasma proteins, it should be administered with caution to patients receiving other highly protein bound drugs.

Other

Cimetidine: The interaction between cimetidine and chronically administered verapamil has not been studied. Variable results on clearance have been obtained in acute studies of healthy volunteers; clearance of verapamil was either reduced or unchanged.

Lithium: Pharmacokinetic and pharmacodynamic interactions between oral verapamil and lithium have been reported. The former may result in a lowering of serum lithium levels in patients receiving chronic stable oral lithium therapy. The latter may result in an increased sensitivity to the effects of lithium. Patients receiving both drugs must be monitored carefully.

Carbamazepine: Verapamil therapy may increase carbamazepine concentrations during combined therapy. This may produce carbamazepine side effects such as diplopia, headache, ataxia, or dizziness.

Rifampin: Therapy with rifampin may markedly reduce oral verapamil bioavailability.

Phenobarbital: Phenobarbital therapy may increase verapamil clearance.

Cyclosporin: Verapamil therapy may increase serum levels of cyclosporin.

Inhalation Anesthetics: Animal experiments have shown that inhalation anesthetics depress cardiovascular activity by decreasing the inward movement of calcium ions. When used concomitantly, inhalation anesthetics and calcium antagonists, such as verapamil, should be titrated carefully to avoid excessive cardiovascular depression.

Neuromuscular Blocking Agents: Clinical data and animal studies suggested that verapamil may potentiate the activity of neuromuscular blocking agents (curare-like and depolarizing). It may be necessary to decrease the dose of verapamil and/or the dose of neuromuscular blocking agent when the drugs are used concomitantly.

Dantrolene: Two animal studies suggest concomitant use of intravenous verapamil and intravenous dantrolene sodium may result in cardiovascular collapse. There has been one report of hyperkalemia and myocardial depression following the coadministration of oral verapamil and intravenous dantrolene.

Pregnancy: Pregnancy Category C. Reproduction studies have been performed in rabbits and rats at oral verapamil doses up to 1.5 (15 mg/kg/day) and 6 (60 mg/kg/day) times the human oral daily dose, respectively, and have revealed no evidence of teratogenicity. In the rat, however, this multiple of the human dose was embryocidal and retarded fetal growth and development, probably because of adverse maternal effects reflected in reduced weight gains of the dams. This oral dose has also been shown to cause hypotension in rats. There are no adequate and well-controlled studies in pregnant women. Because animal reproduction studies are not always predictive of human response, this drug should be used during pregnancy only if clearly needed.

Labor and Delivery: There have been few controlled studies to determine whether the use of verapamil during labor or delivery has immediate or delayed adverse effects on the fetus, or whether it prolongs the duration of labor or increases the need for forceps delivery or other obstetric intervention. Such adverse experiences have not been reported in the literature, despite a long history of use of intravenous ISOPTIN in Europe in the treatment of cardiac side effects of beta-adrenergic agonist agents used to treat premature labor.

Nursing Mothers: ISOPTIN crosses the placental barrier and can be detected in umbilical vein blood at delivery. Also, ISOPTIN is excreted in human milk. Because of the potential for adverse reactions in nursing infants from verapamil, nursing should be discontinued while verapamil is administered.

Pediatrics: Controlled studies with verapamil have not been conducted in pediatric patients, but uncontrolled experience with intravenous administration in more than 250 patients, about half under 12 months of age and about 25% newborn, indicates that results of treatment are similar to those in adults. However, in rare instances, severe hemodynamic side effects have occurred following the intravenous administration of verapamil in neonates and infants. Caution should therefore be used when administering verapamil to this group of pediatric patients.

The most commonly used single doses in patients up to 12 months of age have ranged from 0.1 to 0.2 mg/kg of body weight, while in patients aged 1 to 15 years, the most commonly used single doses ranged from 0.1 to 0.3 mg/kg of body weight. Most of the patients received the lower dose of 0.1 mg/kg once but, in some cases, the dose was repeated once or twice every 10 to 30 minutes.

ADVERSE REACTIONS

The following reactions were reported with intravenous ISOPTIN (verapamil HCl) use in controlled U.S. clinical trials involving 324 patients:

Cardiovascular: Symptomatic hypotension (1.5%); bradycardia (1.2%); severe tachycardia (1.0%). The worldwide experience in open clinical trials in more than 7,900 patients was similar.

Central Nervous System Effects: Dizziness (1.2%); headache (1.2%). Occasional cases of seizures during verapamil injection have been reported.

Gastrointestinal: Nausea (0.9%); abdominal discomfort (0.6%).

In rare cases of hypersensitive patients, broncho/laryngeal spasm accompanied by itch and urticaria have been reported.

The following reactions were reported in a few patients: emotional depression, rotary nystagmus, sleepiness, vertigo, muscle fatigue, diaphoresis or respiratory failure.

[See table above right].

OVERDOSAGE

Treatment of overdosage should be supportive and individualized. Beta-adrenergic stimulation and/or parenteral administration of calcium solutions may increase calcium ion flux across the slow channel, and have been effectively used in treatment of deliberate overdosage with oral ISOPTIN (verapamil HCL). Verapamil cannot be removed by hemodialysis. Clinically significant hypotensive reactions or high degree AV block should be treated with vasopressor agents or cardiac pacing, respectively. Asystole should be handled by the usual measures including isoproterenol hydrochloride, other vasopressor agents or cardiopulmonary resuscitation. (See Treatment of Cardiovascular Adverse Reactions.)

DOSAGE AND ADMINISTRATION

(For Intravenous Use Only): ISOPTIN SHOULD BE GIVEN AS A SLOW INTRAVENOUS INJECTION OVER AT LEAST A TWO MINUTE PERIOD OF TIME UNDER CONTINUOUS ELECTROCARDIOGRAPHIC AND BLOOD PRESSURE MONITORING.

The recommended intravenous doses of ISOPTIN are as follows:

ADULT: Initial dose: 5–10 mg (0.075–0.15 mg/kg body weight) given as an intravenous bolus over at least 2 minutes.

Repeat dose: 10 mg (0.15 mg/kg body weight) 30 minutes after the first dose if the initial response is not adequate. An optimal interval for subsequent I.V. doses has not been determined, and should be individualized for each patient.

Older Patients: The dose should be administered over at least 3 minutes to minimize the risk of untoward drug effects.

PEDIATRIC: Initial dose:

0–1 year: 0.1–0.2 mg/kg body weight (usual single dose range 0.75–2 mg) should be administered as an intravenous bolus over at least 2 minutes **under continuous ECG monitoring.**

1–15 years: 0.1–0.3 mg/kg body weight (usual single dose range 2–5 mg) should be administered as an intravenous bolus over at least 2 minutes. **Do not exceed 5 mg.**

Repeat dose:

0–1 year: 0.1–0.2 mg/kg body weight (usual single dose range 0.75–2 mg) 30 minutes after the first dose if the initial response is not adequate **(under continuous ECG monitoring).** An optimal interval for subsequent I.V. doses has not been determined, and should be individualized for each patient.

1–15 years: 0.1–0.3 mg/kg body weight (usual single dose range 2–5 mg) 30 minutes after the first dose if the initial response is not adequate. **Do not exceed 10 mg as a single dose.** An optimal interval for subsequent I.V. doses has not

Suggested Treatment of Acute Cardiovascular Adverse Reactions*

The frequency of these adverse reactions was quite low and experience with their treatment has been limited.

Adverse Reaction	Proven Effective Treatment	Supportive Treatment
1. Symptomatic hypotension requiring treatment	Calcium chloride (IV) Levarterenol bitartrate (IV) Metaraminol bitartrate (IV) Isoproterenol HCl (IV) Dopamine (IV)	Intravenous fluids Trendelenburg position
2. Bradycardia, AV block, Asystole	Isoproterenol HCl (IV) Calcium chloride (IV) Cardiac pacing Levarterenol bitartrate (IV) Atropine (IV)	Intravenous fluids (slow drip)
3. Rapid ventricular rate (due to antegrade conduction in flutter/fibrillation with W-P-W or L-G-L syndromes)	DC-cardioversion (high energy may be required) Procainamide (IV) Lidocaine (IV)	Intravenous fluids (slow drip)

* Actual treatment and dosage should depend on the severity of the clinical situation and the judgment and experience of the treating physician.

been determined, and should be individualized for each patient.

NOTE

Parenteral drug products should be inspected visually for particulate matter and discoloration prior to administration, whenever solution and container permit. ISOPTIN is physically compatible and chemically stable for at least 24 hours at 25°C protected from light in most common large volume parenteral solutions. Admixing ISOPTIN with albumin, amphotericin B, hydralazine HCl and trimethoprim with sulfamethoxazole should be avoided. ISOPTIN will precipitate in any solution with a pH above 6.0.

HOW SUPPLIED

Each 1 mL of sterile solution contains 2.5 mg verapamil HCl and 8.5 mg sodium chloride. pH adjusted with hydrochloric acid.

5 mg/2 mL ampule—Individual unit carton—NDC 0044-1815-01

Space saver pack of 10 ampules—NDC 0044-1815-05

5 mg/2 mL vial—Single dose. No preservative. Individual unit carton—NDC 0044-1816-21

10 mg/4 mL ampule—Individual unit carton—NDC 0044-1815-11

Space saver pack of 10 ampules—NDC 0044-1815-15

10 mg/4 mL vial—Single dose. No preservative. Individual unit carton—NDC 0044-1816-41

Storage: 59°–86°F (15°–30°C). Protect from light.

MR 1988/1207

RE-5/lso 1207A/1-17-89

Revised January, 1989

Printed in U.S.A.

Shown in Product Identification Section, page 413

ISOPTIN®   ℞

[ī-sŏp"tĭn]

(verapamil hydrochloride)

Oral Tablets

DESCRIPTION

ISOPTIN (verapamil hydrochloride) is a calcium ion influx inhibitor (slow channel blocker or calcium ion antagonist). ISOPTIN is available for oral administration as round, scored, film-coated tablets containing 40 mg, 80 mg or 120 mg of verapamil hydrochloride.

The structural formula of verapamil HCl is given below:

$$C_{27}H_{38}N_2O_4 \cdot HCl \qquad M.W. = 491.08$$

Benzeneacetonitrile,

α-[3-[[2-(3,4-dimethoxyphenyl) ethyl] methylamino] propyl]-3,4-dimethoxy-α-(1-methylethyl) hydrochloride

Verapamil HCl is an almost white, crystalline powder, practically free of odor, with a bitter taste. It is soluble in water, chloroform and methanol. Verapamil HCl is not chemically related to other cardioactive drugs.

In addition to verapamil HCl, ISOPTIN tablets may contain: colloidal silicon dioxide, corn starch, dibasic calcium phosphate, lactose, gelatin, microcrystalline cellulose, sodium carboxymethylcellulose, talc, and magnesium stearate. The film coating used for ISOPTIN 40mg, 80mg and 120mg tablets contains hydroxypropyl methylcellulose, polyethylene glycol, propylene glycol, titanium dioxide and polysorbate 80. ISOPTIN 80mg tablets also contain D&C yellow #10

Lake dye. The ISOPTIN 40mg tablet contains FD&C blue #2 Aluminum Lake dye.

CLINICAL PHARMACOLOGY

ISOPTIN is a calcium ion influx inhibitor (slow channel blocker or calcium ion antagonist) that exerts its pharmacologic effects by modulating the influx of ionic calcium across the cell membrane of the arterial smooth muscle as well as in conductile and contractile myocardial cells.

Mechanism of Action

Angina

The precise mechanism of action of ISOPTIN as an antianginal agent remains to be fully determined, but includes the following two mechanisms:

1. **Relaxation and prevention of coronary artery spasm**
   ISOPTIN dilates the main coronary arteries and coronary arterioles, both in normal and ischemic regions, and is a potent inhibitor of coronary artery spasm, whether spontaneous or ergonovine-induced. This property increases myocardial oxygen delivery in patients with coronary artery spasm, and is responsible for the effectiveness of ISOPTIN in vasospastic (Prinzmetal's or variant) as well as unstable angina at rest. Whether this effect plays any role in classical effort angina is not clear, but studies of exercise tolerance have not shown an increase in the maximum exercise rate-pressure product, a widely accepted measure of oxygen utilization. This suggests that, in general, relief of spasm or dilation of coronary arteries is not an important factor in classical angina.

2. **Reduction of oxygen utilization**
   ISOPTIN regularly reduces the total peripheral resistance (afterload) against which the heart works both at rest and at a given level of exercise by dilating peripheral arterioles. This unloading of the heart reduces myocardial energy consumption and oxygen requirements and probably accounts for the effectiveness of ISOPTIN in chronic stable effort angina.

Arrhythmia

Electrical activity through the AV node depends, to a significant degree, upon calcium influx through the slow channel. By decreasing the influx of calcium, ISOPTIN prolongs the effective refractory period within the AV node and slows AV conduction in a rate-related manner. This property accounts for the ability of ISOPTIN to slow the ventricular rate in patients with chronic atrial flutter or atrial fibrillation. Normal sinus rhythm is usually not affected, but in patients with sick sinus syndrome, ISOPTIN may interfere with sinus node impulse generation and may induce sinus arrest, or sinoatrial block. Atrioventricular block can occur in patients without preexisting conduction defects (see WARNINGS). ISOPTIN decreases the frequency of episodes of paroxysmal supraventricular tachycardia.

ISOPTIN does not alter the normal atrial action potential or intraventricular conduction time, but in depressed atrial fibers it decreases amplitude, velocity of depolarization and conduction velocity. ISOPTIN may shorten the antegrade effective refractory period of accessory bypass tracts. Acceleration of ventricular rate and/or ventricular fibrillation has been reported in patients with atrial flutter or atrial fibrillation and a coexisting accessory AV pathway following administration of verapamil (see WARNINGS).

ISOPTIN has a local anesthetic action that is 1.6 times that of procaine on an equimolar basis. It is not known whether this action is important at the doses used in man.

Continued on next page

Knoll—Cont.

Essential Hypertension

ISOPTIN exerts antihypertensive effects by decreasing systemic vascular resistance usually without orthostatic decreases in blood pressure or reflex tachycardia; bradycardia (rate less than 50 beats/min) is uncommon (1.4%). During isometric or dynamic exercise ISOPTIN does not alter systolic cardiac function in patients with normal ventricular function.

ISOPTIN does not alter total serum calcium levels. However, one report suggested that calcium levels above the normal range may alter the therapeutic effect of ISOPTIN.

Pharmacokinetics and Metabolism: More than 90% of the orally administered dose of ISOPTIN is absorbed. Because of rapid biotransformation of verapamil during its first pass through the portal circulation, bioavailability ranges from 20% to 35%. Peak plasma concentrations are reached between 1 and 2 hours after oral administration. Chronic oral administration of 120 mg of ISOPTIN every 6 hours resulted in plasma levels of verapamil ranging from 125 to 400 ng/mL with higher values reported occasionally. A nonlinear correlation between the verapamil dose administered and verapamil plasma levels does exist.

In early dose titration with verapamil a relationship exists between verapamil plasma concentrations and the prolongation of the PR interval. However, during chronic administration this relationship may disappear. The mean elimination half-life in single dose studies ranged from 2.8 to 7.4 hours. In these same studies, after repetitive dosing, the half-life increased to a range from 4.5 to 12.0 hours (after less than 10 consecutive doses given 6 hours apart). Half-life of verapamil may increase during titration. Aging may affect the pharmacokinetics of verapamil. Elimination half-life may be prolonged in the elderly.

In healthy men, orally administered ISOPTIN undergoes extensive metabolism in the liver. Twelve metabolites have been identified in plasma; all except norverapamil are present in trace amounts only. Norverapamil can reach steady-state plasma concentrations approximately equal to those of verapamil itself. The cardiovascular activity of norverapamil appears to be approximately 20% that of verapamil. Approximately 70% of an administered dose is excreted as metabolites in the urine and 16% or more in the feces within 5 days. About 3% to 4% is excreted in the urine as unchanged drug. Approximately 90% is bound to plasma proteins. In patients with hepatic insufficiency, metabolism is delayed and elimination half-life prolonged up to 14 to 16 hours (see PRECAUTIONS); the volume of distribution is increased and plasma clearance reduced to about 30% of normal. Verapamil clearance values suggest that patients with liver dysfunction may attain therapeutic verapamil plasma concentrations with one-third of the oral daily dose required for patients with normal liver function.

After four weeks of oral dosing (120 mg q.i.d.), verapamil and norverapamil levels were noted in the cerebral spinal fluid with estimated partition coefficient of 0.06 for verapamil and 0.04 for norverapamil.

Hemodynamics and Myocardial Metabolism: ISOPTIN reduces afterload and myocardial contractility. Improved left ventricular diastolic function in patients with IHSS and those with coronary heart disease has also been observed with ISOPTIN therapy. In most patients, including those with organic cardiac disease, the negative inotropic action of ISOPTIN is countered by reduction of afterload and cardiac index is usually not reduced. However, in patients with severe left ventricular dysfunction (e.g., pulmonary wedge pressure above 20 mmHg or ejection fraction lower than 30%), or in patients on beta-adrenergic blocking agents or other cardiodepressant drugs, deterioration of ventricular function may occur (see DRUG INTERACTIONS).

Pulmonary Function: ISOPTIN does not induce bronchoconstriction and hence, does not impair ventilatory function.

INDICATIONS AND USAGE

ISOPTIN tablets are indicated for the treatment of the following:

Angina
1. Angina at rest including:
   - Vasospastic (Prinzmetal's, variant) angina
   - Unstable (crescendo, pre-infarction) angina
2. Chronic stable angina (classic effort-associated angina)

Arrhythmias
1. In association with digitalis, for the control of ventricular rate at rest and during stress in patients with chronic atrial flutter and/or atrial fibrillation (see WARNINGS: Accessory Bypass Tract)
2. Prophylaxis of repetitive paroxysmal supraventricular tachycardia

Essential Hypertension

CONTRAINDICATIONS

Verapamil HCl tablets are contraindicated in:
1. Severe left ventricular dysfunction (see WARNINGS)
2. Hypotension (systolic pressure less than 90 mmHg) or cardiogenic shock
3. Sick sinus syndrome (except in patients with a functioning artificial ventricular pacemaker)
4. Second- or third-degree AV block (except in patients with a functioning artificial ventricular pacemaker)
5. Patients with atrial flutter or atrial fibrillation and an accessory bypass tract (e.g., Wolff-Parkinson-White, Lown-Ganong-Levine syndromes) (see Warnings)
6. Patients with known hypersensitivity to verapamil hydrochloride

WARNINGS

Heart Failure: Verapamil has a negative inotropic effect which, in most patients, is compensated by its afterload reduction (decreased systemic vascular resistance) properties without a net impairment of ventricular performance. In clinical experience with 4,954 patients, 87 (1.8%) developed congestive heart failure or pulmonary edema. Verapamil should be avoided in patients with severe left ventricular dysfunction (e.g., ejection fraction less than 30%) or moderate to severe symptoms of cardiac failure and in patients with any degree of ventricular dysfunction if they are receiving a beta adrenergic blocker (see DRUG INTERACTIONS). Patients with milder ventricular dysfunction should, if possible, be controlled with optimum doses of digitalis and/or diuretics before verapamil treatment (Note interactions with digoxin under: PRECAUTIONS).

Hypotension: Occasionally, the pharmacologic action of verapamil may produce a decrease in blood pressure below normal levels which may result in dizziness or symptomatic hypotension. The incidence of hypotension observed in 4,954 patients enrolled in clinical trials was 2.5%. In hypertensive patients, decreases in blood pressure below normal are unusual. Tilt table testing (60 degrees) was not able to induce orthostatic hypotension.

Elevated Liver Enzymes: Elevations of transaminases with and without concomitant elevations in alkaline phosphatase and bilirubin have been reported. Such elevations have sometimes been transient and may disappear even with continued verapamil treatment. Several cases of hepatocellular injury related to verapamil have been proven by rechallenge; half of these cases had clinical symptoms (malaise, fever, and/or right upper quadrant pain) in addition to elevations of SGOT, SGPT and alkaline phosphatase. Periodic monitoring of liver function in patients receiving verapamil is therefore prudent.

Accessory Bypass Tract (Wolff-Parkinson-White or Lown-Ganong-Levine): Some patients with paroxysmal and/or chronic atrial fibrillation or atrial flutter and a coexisting accessory AV pathway have developed increased antegrade conduction across the accessory pathway bypassing the AV node, producing a very rapid ventricular response or ventricular fibrillation after receiving intravenous verapamil (or digitalis). Although a risk of this occurring with oral verapamil has not been established, such patients receiving oral verapamil may be at risk and its use in these patients is contraindicated (see CONTRAINDICATIONS).

Treatment is usually DC-cardioversion. Cardioversion has been used safely and effectively after oral ISOPTIN.

Atrioventricular Block: The effect of verapamil on AV conduction and the SA node may cause asymptomatic first-degree AV block and transient bradycardia, sometimes accompanied by nodal escape rhythms. PR interval prolongation is correlated with verapamil plasma concentrations, especially during the early titration phase of therapy. Higher degrees of AV block, however, were infrequently (0.8%) observed. Marked first-degree block or progressive development to second- or third-degree AV block requires a reduction in dosage or, in rare instances, discontinuation of verapamil HCl and institution of appropriate therapy depending upon the clinical situation.

Patients with Hypertrophic Cardiomyopathy (IHSS): In 120 patients with hypertrophic cardiomyopathy (most of them refractory or intolerant to propranolol) who received therapy with verapamil at doses up to 720 mg/day, a variety of serious adverse effects were seen. Three patients died in pulmonary edema; all had severe left ventricular outflow obstruction and a past history of left ventricular dysfunction. Eight other patients had pulmonary edema and/or severe hypotension; abnormally high (greater than 20 mmHg) pulmonary wedge pressure and a marked left ventricular outflow obstruction were present in most of these patients. Concomitant administration of quinidine (See DRUG INTERACTIONS) preceded the severe hypotension in 3 of the 8 patients (2 of whom developed pulmonary edema). Sinus bradycardia occurred in 11% of the patients, second-degree AV block in 4% and sinus arrest in 2%. It must be appreciated that this group of patients had a serious disease with a high mortality rate. Most adverse effects responded well to dose reduction and only rarely did verapamil have to be discontinued.

PRECAUTIONS

General

Use in Patients with Impaired Hepatic Function: Since verapamil is highly metabolized by the liver, it should be administered cautiously to patients with impaired hepatic function. Severe liver dysfunction prolongs the elimination half-life of verapamil to about 14 to 16 hours; hence, approximately 30% of the dose given to patients with normal liver function should be administered to these patients. Careful monitoring for abnormal prolongation of the PR interval or other signs of excessive pharmacologic effects (See OVERDOSAGE) should be carried out.

Use in Patients with Attenuated (decreased) Neuromuscular Transmission: It has been reported that verapamil decreases neuromuscular transmission in patients with Duchenne's muscular dystrophy, and that verapamil prolongs recovery from the neuromuscular blocking agent vecuronium. It may be necessary to decrease the dosage of verapamil when it is administered to patients with attenuated neuromuscular transmission.

Use in Patients with Impaired Renal Function: About 70% of an administered dose of verapamil is excreted as metabolites in the urine. Verapamil is not removed by hemodialysis. Until further data are available, verapamil should be administered cautiously to patients with impaired renal function. These patients should be carefully monitored for abnormal prolongation of the PR interval or other signs of overdosage (see OVERDOSAGE).

Drug Interactions

Beta Blockers: Controlled studies in small numbers of patients suggest that the concomitant use of ISOPTIN and oral beta-adrenergic blocking agents may be beneficial in certain patients with chronic stable angina or hypertension, but available information is not sufficient to predict with confidence the effects of concurrent treatment in patients with left ventricular dysfunction or cardiac conduction abnormalities. Concomitant therapy with beta-adrenergic blockers and verapamil may result in additive negative effects on heart rate, atrioventricular conduction and/or cardiac contractility.

In one study involving 15 patients treated with high doses of propranolol (median dose: 480 mg/day, range 160 to 1280 mg/day) for severe angina, with preserved left ventricular function (ejection fraction greater than 35%), the hemodynamic effects of additional therapy with verapamil HCl were assessed using invasive methods. The addition of verapamil to high-dose beta blockers induced modest negative inotropic and chronotropic effects which were not severe enough to limit short-term (48 hours) combination therapy in this study. These modest cardiodepressant effects persisted for greater than 6, but less than 30 hours after abrupt withdrawal of beta blockers and were closely related to plasma levels of propranolol. The primary verapamil/beta-blocker interaction in this study appeared to be hemodynamic rather than electrophysiologic.

In other studies, verapamil did not generally induce significant negative inotropic, chronotropic, or dromotropic effects in patients with preserved left ventricular function receiving low or moderate doses of propranolol (less than or equal to 320 mg/day); in some patients, however, combined therapy did produce such effects. Therefore, if combined therapy is used, close surveillance of clinical status should be carried out. Combined therapy should usually be avoided in patients with atrioventricular conduction abnormalities and those with depressed left ventricular function.

Asymptomatic bradycardia (36 beats/min) with a wandering atrial pacemaker has been observed in a patient receiving concomitant timolol (a beta-adrenergic blocker) eyedrops and oral verapamil.

A decrease in metoprolol clearance has been observed when verapamil and metoprolol were administered together. A similar effect has not been seen when verapamil and atenolol were given together.

Digitalis: Clinical use of verapamil in digitalized patients has shown the combination to be well tolerated if digoxin doses are properly adjusted. However, chronic verapamil treatment can increase serum digoxin levels by 50% to 75% during the first week of therapy, and this can result in digitalis toxicity. In patients with hepatic cirrhosis the influence of verapamil on digoxin kinetics is magnified. Verapamil may reduce total body clearance and extrarenal clearance of digitoxin by 27% and 29%, respectively. Maintenance and digitalization doses should be reduced when verapamil is administered, and the patient should be reassessed to avoid over- or underdigitalization. Whenever overdigitalization is suspected, the daily dose of digitalis should be reduced or temporarily discontinued. Upon discontinuation of ISOPTIN (verapamil HCl), the patient should be reassessed to avoid underdigitalization.

Antihypertensive Agents: Verapamil administered concomitantly with oral antihypertensive agents (e.g., vasodilators, angiotensin-converting enzyme inhibitors, diuretics, beta blockers) will usually have an additive effect on lowering blood pressure. Patients receiving these combinations should be appropriately monitored. Concomitant use of agents that attenuate alpha-adrenergic function with verapamil may result in a reduction in blood pressure that is excessive in some patients. Such an effect was observed in one study following the concomitant administration of verapamil and prazosin.

Antiarrhythmic Agents

Disopyramide: Until data on possible interactions between verapamil and disopyramide are obtained, disopyramide should not be administered within 48 hours before or 24 hours after verapamil administration.

Flecainide: A study in healthy volunteers showed that the concomitant administration of flecainide and verapamil may have additive effects on myocardial contractility, AV conduction, and repolarization. The clinical significance of these findings is not known.

Quinidine: In a small number of patients with hypertrophic cardiomyopathy (IHSS), concomitant use of verapamil and quinidine resulted in significant hypotension. Until further data are obtained, combined therapy of verapamil and quinidine in patients with hypertrophic cardiomyopathy should probably be avoided.

The electrophysiological effects of quinidine and verapamil on AV conduction were studied in 8 patients. Verapamil significantly counteracted the effects of quinidine on AV conduction. There has been a report of increased quinidine levels during verapamil therapy.

Other

Nitrates: Verapamil has been given concomitantly with short- and long-acting nitrates without any undesirable drug interactions. The pharmacologic profile of both drugs and the clinical experience suggest beneficial interactions.

Cimetidine: The interaction between cimetidine and chronically administered verapamil has not been studied. Variable results on clearance have been obtained in acute studies of healthy volunteers; clearance of verapamil was either reduced or unchanged.

Lithium: Pharmacokinetic and pharmacodynamic interactions between oral verapamil and lithium have been reported. The former may result in a lowering of serum lithium levels in patients receiving chronic stable oral lithium therapy. The latter may result in an increased sensitivity to the effects of lithium. Patients receiving both drugs must be monitored carefully.

Carbamazepine: Verapamil therapy may increase carbamazepine concentrations during combined therapy. This may produce carbamazepine side effects such as diplopia, headache, ataxia, or dizziness.

Rifampin: Therapy with rifampin may markedly reduce oral verapamil bioavailability.

Phenobarbital: Phenobarbital therapy may increase verapamil clearance.

Cyclosporin: Verapamil therapy may increase serum levels of cyclosporin.

Inhalation Anesthetics: Animal experiments have shown that inhalation anesthetics depress cardiovascular activity by decreasing the inward movement of calcium ions. When used concomitantly, inhalation anesthetics and calcium antagonists, such as verapamil, should each be titrated carefully to avoid excessive cardiovascular depression.

Neuromuscular Blocking Agents: Clinical data and animal studies suggest that verapamil may potentiate the activity of neuromuscular blocking agents (curare-like and depolarizing). It may be necessary to decrease the dose of verapamil and/or the dose of the neuromuscular blocking agent when the drugs are used concomitantly.

Carcinogenesis, Mutagenesis, Impairment of Fertility: An 18-month toxicity study in rats, at a low multiple (6 fold) of the maximum recommended human dose, and not the maximum tolerated dose, did not suggest a tumorigenic potential. There was no evidence of a carcinogenic potential of verapamil administered in the diet of rats for two years at doses of 10, 35 and 120 mg/kg per day or approximately 1x, 3.5x and 12x, respectively, the maximum recommended human daily dose (480 mg per day or 9.6 mg/kg/day).

Verapamil was not mutagenic in the Ames test in 5 test strains at 3 mg per plate, with or without metabolic activation.

Studies in female rats at daily dietary doses up to 5.5 times (55 mg/kg/day) the maximum recommended human dose did not show impaired fertility. Effects on male fertility have not been determined.

Pregnancy: Pregnancy Category C. Reproduction studies have been performed in rabbits and rats at oral doses up to 1.5 (15 mg/kg/day) and 6 (60 mg/kg/day) times the human oral daily dose, respectively, and have revealed no evidence of teratogenicity. In the rat, however, this multiple of the human dose was embryocidal and retarded fetal growth and development, probably because of adverse maternal effects reflected in the reduced weight gains of the dams. This oral dose has also been shown to cause hypotension in rats. There are no adequate and well-controlled studies in pregnant women. Because animal reproduction studies are not always predictive of human response, this drug should be used during pregnancy only if clearly needed.

Verapamil crosses the placental barrier and can be detected in umbilical vein blood at delivery.

Labor and Delivery: It is not known whether the use of verapamil during labor or delivery has immediate or delayed adverse effects on the fetus, or whether it prolongs the duration of labor or increases the need for forceps delivery or other obstetric intervention. Such adverse experiences have not been reported in the literature, despite a long history of use of verapamil in Europe in the treatment of cardiac side effects of beta-adrenergic agonist agents used to treat premature labor.

Nursing Mothers: Verapamil is excreted in human milk. Because of the potential for adverse reactions in nursing infants from verapamil, nursing should be discontinued while verapamil is administered.

Pediatric Use: Safety and efficacy of ISOPTIN in children below the age of 18 years have not been established.

Animal Pharmacology and/or Animal Toxicology: In chronic animal toxicology studies verapamil caused lenticular and/or suture line changes at 30 mg/kg/day or greater and frank cataracts at 62.5 mg/kg/day or greater in the beagle dog but not the rat. Development of cataracts due to verapamil has not been reported in man.

ADVERSE REACTIONS

Serious adverse reactions are uncommon when ISOPTIN therapy is initiated with upward dose titration within the recommended single and total daily dose. See WARNINGS for discussion of heart failure, hypotension, elevated liver enzymes, AV block and rapid ventricular response. The following reactions to orally administered verapamil occurred at rates greater than 1.0% or occurred at lower rates but appeared clearly drug-related in clinical trials in 4,954 patients.

Constipation	7.3%	Fatigue	1.7%
Dizziness	3.3%	Dyspnea	1.4%
Nausea	2.7%	Bradycardia (HR < 50/min)	1.4%
Hypotension	2.5%	AV block— total 1°, 2°, 3°	1.2%
Headache	2.2%	2° and 3°	0.8%
Edema	1.9%	Rash	1.2%
CHF, Pulmonary		Flushing	0.6%
Edema	1.8%		

Elevated Liver Enzymes (see WARNINGS)

In clinical trials related to the control of ventricular response in digitalized patients who had atrial fibrillation or flutter, ventricular rate below 50 at rest occurred in 15% of patients and asymptomatic hypotension occurred in 5% of patients.

The following reactions, reported in 1.0% or less of patients, occurred under conditions (open trials, marketing experience) where a causal relationship is uncertain; they are listed to alert the physician to a possible relationship:

Cardiovascular: angina pectoris, atrioventricular dissociation, chest pain, claudication, myocardial infarction, palpitations, purpura (vasculitis), syncope.

Digestive System: diarrhea, dry mouth, gastrointestinal distress, gingival hyperplasia.

Hemic and Lymphatic: ecchymosis or bruising.

Nervous System: cerebrovascular accident, confusion, equilibrium disorders, insomnia, muscle cramps, paresthesia, psychotic symptoms, shakiness, somnolence.

Skin: arthralgia and rash, exanthema, hair loss, hyperkeratosis, maculae, sweating, urticaria, Stevens-Johnson syndrome, erythema multiforme.

Special Senses: blurred vision.

Urogenital: gynecomastia, increased urination, spotty menstruation, impotence.

Treatment of Acute Cardiovascular Adverse Reactions: The frequency of cardiovascular adverse reactions which require therapy is rare; hence, experience with their treatment is limited. Whenever severe hypotension or complete AV block occur following oral administration of verapamil, the appropriate emergency measures should be applied immediately, e.g., intravenously administered norepinephrine bitartrate, atropine sulfate, isoproterenol HCl (all in the usual doses), or calcium gluconate (10% solution). In patients with hypertrophic cardiomyopathy (IHSS), alpha-adrenergic agents (phenylephrine HCl, metaraminol bitartrate or methoxamine HCl) should be used to maintain blood pressure, and isoproterenol and norepinephrine should be avoided. If further support is necessary, dopamine HCl or dobutamine HCl may be administered. Actual treatment and dosage should depend on the severity and the clinical situation and the judgment and experience of the treating physician.

OVERDOSAGE

Treatment of overdosage should be supportive. Beta-adrenergic stimulation or parenteral administration of calcium solutions may increase calcium ion flux across the slow channel, and have been used effectively in treatment of deliberate overdosage with verapamil. Verapamil cannot be removed by hemodialysis. Clinically significant hypotensive reactions or fixed high degree AV block should be treated with vasopressor agents or cardiac pacing, respectively. Asystole should be handled by the usual measures including cardiopulmonary resuscitation.

DOSAGE AND ADMINISTRATION

The dose of verapamil must be individualized by titration. ISOPTIN is available in 40 mg, 80 mg, and 120 mg tablets. The usefulness and safety of dosages exceeding 480 mg/day have not been established; therefore, this daily dosage should not be exceeded. Since the half-life of verapamil increases during chronic dosing, maximum response may be delayed.

Angina: Clinical trials show that the usual dose is 80 mg to 120 mg three times a day. However, 40 mg three times a day may be warranted in patients who may have an increased response to verapamil (e.g., decreased hepatic function, elderly, etc.). Upward titration should be based on therapeutic efficacy and safety evaluated approximately eight hours after dosing. Dosage may be increased at daily (e.g., patients with unstable angina) or weekly intervals until optimum clinical response is obtained.

Arrhythmias: The dosage in digitalized patients with chronic atrial fibrillation (see PRECAUTIONS) ranges from 240 to 320 mg per day in divided (t.i.d. or q.i.d.) doses. The dosage for prophylaxis of PSVT (non-digitalized patients) ranges from 240 to 480 mg in divided (t.i.d. or q.i.d.) doses. In general, maximum effects for any given dosage will be apparent during the first 48 hours of therapy.

Essential Hypertension: Dose should be individualized by titration. The usual initial monotherapy dose in clinical trials was 80 mg three times a day (240 mg). Daily dosages of 360 and 480 mg have been used but there is no evidence that doses beyond 360 mg provide added effect. Consideration should be given to beginning titration at 40 mg, three times per day in patients who might respond to lower doses, such as the elderly or people of small stature. The antihypertensive effects of ISOPTIN are evident within the first week of therapy. Upward titration should be based on therapeutic efficacy, assessed at the end of the dosing interval.

HOW SUPPLIED

ISOPTIN (verapamil HCl) tablets are supplied as round, scored, film-coated tablets containing either 40mg, 80 mg or 120 mg of verapamil hydrochloride. The 80mg and 120mg tablets are embossed with "ISOPTIN 80" or "ISOPTIN 120" on one side and "Knoll" on the reverse side. The 40mg tablet is embossed on one side with the number "40" surrounded by the Knoll triangle.

40mg (lt. blue)—
  Bottle of 100—NDC #0044-1821-02
  Hospital Unit Dose (100 tablets-
  Strips of 10)—NDC #0044-1821-10
80 mg (yellow)—
  Bottle of 100—NDC #0044-1822-02
  Bottle of 500—NDC #0044-1822-05
  Bottle of 1000—NDC #0044-1822-04
  Hospital Unit Dose (100 tablets-
  Strips of 10)—NDC #0044-1822-10
120 mg (white)—
  Bottle of 100—NDC #0044-1823-02
  Bottle of 500—NDC #0044-1823-05
  Bottle of 1000—NDC #0044-1823-04
  Hospital Unit Dose (100 tablets-
  Strips of 10)—NDC #0044-1823-10

Storage: 59° to 86°F (15° to 30°C).
Dispense in a tight, light-resistant container as defined in the USP.
MR 1988/ 2636
Revised March 1988   2636
Shown in Product Identification Section, page 413

ISOPTIN® SR   ℞
[ī-sŏp"tin]
(verapamil HCl)

DESCRIPTION

ISOPTIN SR (verapamil hydrochloride) is a calcium ion influx inhibitor (slow channel blocker or calcium ion antagonist). ISOPTIN SR is available for oral administration as light green, capsule shaped, scored, film-coated tablets containing 240 mg verapamil hydrochloride. The tablets are designed for sustained release of the drug in the gastrointestinal tract; sustained release characteristics are not altered when the tablet is divided in half.

The structural formula of verapamil HCl is given below:

CH_3O CN CH_3 OCH_3
CH_3O —⬡— $C(CH_2)_3$ NCH_2CH_2 —⬡— $OCH_3 \cdot HCl$
     $CH(CH_3)_2$

$C_{27}H_{38}N_2O_4 \cdot HCl$ M.W. = 491.08

Benzeneacetonitrile,
α[[3-[[2-(3,4-dimethoxyphenyl) ethyl]
methylamino]
propyl]-3,4-dimethoxy-α-(1-methylethyl) hydrochloride
Verapamil HCl is an almost white, crystalline powder, practically free of odor, with a bitter taste. It is soluble in water,

Continued on next page

Knoll—Cont.

chloroform and methanol. Verapamil HCl is not chemically related to other cardioactive drugs.

In addition to verapamil HCl, the ISOPTIN SR tablet contains the following ingredients: alginate, hydroxypropyl methylcellulose, magnesium stearate, microcrystalline cellulose, polyethylene glycol, polyvinyl pyrrolidone, talc, titanium dioxide, D&C yellow #10 Lake dye, and FD&C blue #2 Lake dye.

CLINICAL PHARMACOLOGY

ISOPTIN is a calcium ion influx inhibitor (slow channel blocker or calcium ion antagonist) which exerts its pharmacologic effects by modulating the influx of ionic calcium across the cell membrane of the arterial smooth muscle as well as in conductile and contractile myocardial cells.

Mechanism of Action
Essential Hypertension

ISOPTIN exerts antihypertensive effects by decreasing systemic vascular resistance, usually without orthostatic decreases in blood pressure or reflex tachycardia; bradycardia (rate less than 50 beats/min) is uncommon (1.4%). During isometric or dynamic exercise ISOPTIN does not alter systolic cardiac function in patients with normal ventricular function.

ISOPTIN does not alter total serum calcium levels. However, one report suggested that calcium levels above the normal range may alter the therapeutic effect of ISOPTIN.

Other Pharmacological Actions of ISOPTIN include the Following

ISOPTIN (verapamil HCl) dilates the main coronary arteries and coronary arterioles, both in normal and ischemic regions, and is a potent inhibitor of coronary artery spasm, whether spontaneous or ergonovine-induced. This property increases myocardial oxygen delivery in patients with coronary artery spasm, and is responsible for the effectiveness of ISOPTIN in vasospastic (Prinzmetal's or variant) as well as unstable angina at rest. Whether this effect plays any role in classical effort angina is not clear, but studies of exercise tolerance have not shown an increase in the maximum exercise rate-pressure product, a widely accepted measure of oxygen utilization. This suggests that, in general, relief of spasm or dilation of coronary arteries is not an important factor in classical angina.

ISOPTIN regularly reduces the total systemic resistance (afterload) against which the heart works both at rest and at a given level of exercise by dilating peripheral arterioles. Electrical activity through the AV node depends, to a significant degree, upon calcium influx through the slow channel. By decreasing the influx of calcium, ISOPTIN prolongs the effective refractory period within the AV node and slows AV conduction in a rate-related manner.

Normal sinus rhythm is usually not affected, but in patients with sick sinus syndrome, ISOPTIN may interfere with sinus node impulse generation and may induce sinus arrest or sinoatrial block. Atrioventricular block can occur in patients without preexisting conduction defects (see WARNINGS). ISOPTIN does not alter the normal atrial action potential or intraventricular conduction time, but depresses amplitude, velocity of depolarization and conduction in depressed atrial fibers. ISOPTIN may shorten the antegrade effective refractory period of accessory bypass tracts. Acceleration of ventricular rate and/or ventricular fibrillation has been reported in patients with atrial flutter or atrial fibrillation and a coexisting accessory AV pathway following administration of verapamil (see WARNINGS).

ISOPTIN has a local anesthetic action that is 1.6 times that of procaine on an equimolar basis. It is not known whether this action is important at the doses used in man.

Pharmacokinetics and Metabolism: With the immediate release formulation, more than 90% of the orally administered dose of ISOPTIN is absorbed. Because of rapid biotransformation of verapamil during its first pass through the portal circulation, bioavailability ranges from 20% to 35%. Peak plasma concentrations are reached between 1 and 2 hours after oral administration. Chronic oral administration of 120 mg of ISOPTIN every 6 hours resulted in plasma levels of verapamil ranging from 125 to 400 ng/mL with higher values reported occasionally. A nonlinear correlation between the verapamil dose administered and verapamil plasma levels does exist.

In early dose titration with verapamil a relationship exists between verapamil plasma concentrations and the prolongation of the PR interval. However, during chronic administration this relationship may disappear. The mean elimination half-life in single dose studies ranged from 2.8 to 7.4 hours. In these same studies, after repetitive dosing, the half-life increased to a range from 4.5 to 12.0 hours (after less than 10 consecutive doses given 6 hours apart). Half-life of verapamil may increase during titration.

Aging may affect the pharmacokinetics of verapamil. Elimination half-life may be prolonged in the elderly.

In multiple dose studies under fasting conditions the bioavailability measured by AUC of ISOPTIN SR was similar to ISOPTIN immediate release; rates of absorption were, of course, different. In a randomized, single-dose, crossover study using healthy volunteers, administration of 240 mg ISOPTIN SR with food produced peak plasma verapamil concentrations of 79 ng/mL, time to peak plasma verapamil concentration of 7.71 hours, and AUC (0-24 hr) of 841 ng.hr/mL. When ISOPTIN SR was administered to fasting subjects, peak plasma verapamil concentration was 164 ng/mL; time to peak plasma verapamil concentration was 5.21 hours; and AUC (0-24 hr) was 1,478 ng.hr/mL. Similar results were demonstrated for plasma norverapamil. Food thus produces decreased bioavailability (AUC) but a narrower peak to through ratio. Good correlation of dose and response is not available, but controlled studies of ISOPTIN SR have shown effectiveness of doses similar to the effective doses of ISOPTIN (immediate release). In hypertensive patients, plasma verapamil levels are not related to antihypertensive efficacy at the dosages usually administered (240 to 480 mg/day).

In healthy man, orally administered ISOPTIN undergoes extensive metabolism in the liver. Twelve metabolites have been identified in plasma; all except norverapamil are present in trace amounts only. Norverapamil can reach steady-state plasma concentrations approximately equal to those of verapamil itself. The cardiovascular activity of norverapamil appears to be approximately 20% that of verapamil. Approximately 70% of an administered dose is excreted as metabolites in the urine and 16% or more in the feces within 5 days. About 3% to 4% is excreted in the urine as unchanged drug. Approximately 90% is bound to plasma proteins. In patients with hepatic insufficiency, metabolism of immediate release verapamil is delayed and elimination half-life prolonged up to 14 to 16 hours (see PRECAUTIONS); the volume of distribution is increased and plasma clearance reduced to about 30% of normal. Verapamil clearance values suggest that patients with liver dysfunction may attain therapeutic verapamil plasma concentrations with one-third of the oral daily dose required for patients with normal liver function.

After four weeks of oral dosing (120 mg q.i.d.), verapamil and norverapamil levels were noted in the cerebral spinal fluid with estimated partition coefficient of 0.06 for verapamil and 0.04 for norverapamil.

Hemodynamics and Myocardial Metabolism: ISOPTIN reduces afterload and myocardial contractility. Improved left ventricular diastolic function in patients with IHSS and those with coronary heart disease has also been observed with ISOPTIN therapy. In most patients, including those with organic cardiac disease, the negative inotropic action of ISOPTIN is countered by reduction of afterload and cardiac index is usually not reduced. In patients with severe left ventricular dysfunction however, (e.g., pulmonary wedge pressure above 20 mmHg or ejection fraction lower than 30%), or in patients on beta-adrenergic blocking agents or other cardiodepressant drugs, deterioration of ventricular function may occur (see DRUG INTERACTIONS).

Pulmonary Function: ISOPTIN does not induce bronchoconstriction and hence, does not impair ventilatory function.

INDICATIONS AND USAGE

ISOPTIN SR (verapamil HCl) is indicated for the management of essential hypertension.

CONTRAINDICATIONS

Verapamil HCl is contraindicated in:
1. Severe left ventricular dysfunction (see WARNINGS).
2. Hypotension (less than 90 mmHg systolic pressure) or cardiogenic shock.
3. Sick sinus syndrome (except in patients with a functioning artificial ventricular pacemaker).
4. Second- or third-degree AV block (except in patients with a functioning artificial ventricular pacemaker).
5. Patients with atrial flutter or atrial fibrillation and an accessory bypass tract (e.g., Wolff-Parkinson-White, Lown-Ganong-Levine syndromes). (see WARNINGS).
6. Patients with known hypersensitivity to verapamil hydrochloride.

WARNINGS

Heart Failure: Verapamil has a negative inotropic effect which, in most patients, is compensated by its afterload reduction (decreased systemic vascular resistance) properties without a net impairment of ventricular performance. In clinical experience with 4,954 patients, 87 (1.8%) developed congestive heart failure or pulmonary edema. Verapamil should be avoided in patients with severe left ventricular dysfunction (e.g., ejection fraction less than 30%, pulmonary wedge pressure above 20 mm Hg, or severe symptoms of cardiac failure) and in patients with any degree of ventricular dysfunction if they are receiving a beta adrenergic blocker (see DRUG INTERACTIONS). Patients with milder ventricular dysfunction should, if possible, be controlled with optimum doses of digitalis and/or diuretics before verapamil treatment (*Note interactions with digoxin under: PRECAUTIONS*).

Hypotension: Occasionally, the pharmacologic action of verapamil may produce a decrease in blood pressure below normal levels which may result in dizziness or symptomatic hypotension. The incidence of hypotension observed in 4,954 patients enrolled in clinical trials was 2.5%. In hypertensive patients, decreases in blood pressure below normal are unusual. Tilt table testing (60 degrees) was not able to induce orthostatic hypotension.

Elevated Liver Enzymes: Elevations of transaminases with and without concomitant elevations in alkaline phosphatase and bilirubin have been reported. Such elevations have sometimes been transient and may disappear even in the face of continued verapamil treatment. Several cases of hepatocellular injury related to verapamil have been proven by rechallenge; half of these had clinical symptoms (malaise, fever, and/or right upper quadrant pain) in addition to elevations of SGOT, SGPT and alkaline phosphatase. Periodic monitoring of liver function in patients receiving verapamil is therefore prudent.

Accessory Bypass Tract (Wolff-Parkinson-White or Lown-Ganong-Levine): Some patients with paroxysmal and/or chronic atrial fibrillation or atrial flutter and a coexisting accessory AV pathway have developed increased antegrade conduction across the accessory pathway bypassing the AV node, producing a very rapid ventricular response or ventricular fibrillation after receiving intravenous verapamil (or digitalis). Although a risk of this occurring with oral verapamil has not been established, such patients receiving oral verapamil may be at risk and its use in these patients is contraindicated (see CONTRAINDICATIONS).

Treatment is usually DC-cardioversion. Cardioversion has been used safely and effectively after oral ISOPTIN.

Atrioventricular Block: The effect of verapamil on AV conduction and the SA node may lead to asymptomtic first-degree AV block and transient bradycardia, sometimes accompanied by nodal escape rhythms. PR interval prolongation is correlated with verapamil plasma concentrations, especially during the early titration phases of therapy. Higher degrees of AV block, however, were infrequently (0.8%) observed. Marked first-degree block or progressive development to second- or third-degree AV block requires a reduction in dosage or, in rare instances, discontinuation of verapamil HCl and institution of appropriate therapy depending upon the clinical situation.

Patients with Hypertrophic Cardiomyopathy (IHSS): In 120 patients with hypertrophic cardiomyopathy (most of them refractory or intolerant to propranolol) who received therapy with verapamil at doses up to 720 mg/day, a variety of serious adverse effects were seen. Three patients died in pulmonary edema; all had severe left ventricular outflow obstruction and a past history of left ventricular dysfunction. Eight other patients had pulmonary edema and/or severe hypotension; abnormally high (over 20 mmHg) capillary wedge pressure and a marked left ventricular outflow obstruction were present in most of these patients. Concomitant administration of quinidine (see DRUG INTERACTIONS) preceded the severe hypotension in 3 of the 8 patients (2 of whom developed pulmonary edema). Sinus bradycardia occurred in 11% of the patients, second-degree AV block in 4% and sinus arrest in 2%. It must be appreciated that this group of patients had a serious disease with a high mortality rate. Most adverse effects responded well to dose reduction and only rarely did verapamil have to be discontinued.

PRECAUTIONS
General

Use in Patients with Impaired Hepatic Function: Since verapamil is highly metabolized by the liver, it should be administered cautiously to patients with impaired hepatic function. Severe liver dysfunction prolongs the elimination half-life of immediate release verapamil to about 14 to 16 hours; hence, approximately 30% of the dose given to patients with normal liver function should be administered to these patients. Careful monitoring for abnormal prolongation of the PR interval or other signs of excessive pharmacologic effects (see OVERDOSAGE) should be carried out.

Use in Patients with Attenuated (Decreased) Neuromuscular Transmission: It has been reported that verapamil decreases neuromuscular transmission in patients with Duchenne's muscular dystrophy, and that verapamil prolongs recovery from the neuromuscular blocking agent vecuronium. It may be necessary to decrease the dosage of verapamil when it is administered to patients with attenuated neuromuscular transmission.

Use in Patients with Impaired Renal Function: About 70% of an administered dose of verapamil is excreted as metabolites in the urine. Verapamil is not removed by hemodialysis. Until further data are available, verapamil should be administered cautiously to patients with impaired renal function. These patients should be carefully monitored for abnormal prolongation of the PR interval or other signs of overdosage (see OVERDOSAGE).

Drug Interactions

Beta Blockers: Concomitant therapy with beta-adrenergic blockers and verapamil may result in additive negative effects on heart rate, atrioventricular conduction, and/or cardiac contractility. The combination of sustained-release verapamil and beta-adrenergic blocking agents has not been studied. However, there have been reports of excessive bradycardia and AV block, including complete heart block, when the combination has been used for the treatment of hypertension. For hypertensive patients, the risks of combined therapy may outweigh the potential benefits. The combination should be used only with caution and close monitoring.

Asymptomatic bradycardia (36 beats/min) with a wandering atrial pacemaker has been observed in a patient receiving concomitant timolol (a beta-adrenergic blocker) eyedrops and oral verapamil.

A decrease in metoprolol clearance has been observed when verapamil and metoprolol were administered together. A similar effect has not been seen when verapamil and atenolol are given together.

Digitalis: Clinical use of verapamil in digitalized patients has shown the combination to be well tolerated if digoxin doses are properly adjusted. Chronic verapamil treatment can increase serum digoxin levels by 50 to 75% during the first week of therapy, and this can result in digitalis toxicity. In patients with hepatic cirrhosis the influence of verapamil on digoxin kinetics is magnified. Verapamil may reduce total body clearance and extrarenal clearance of digitoxin by 27% and 29%, respectively. Maintenance digitalis doses should be reduced when verapamil is administered, and the patient should be carefully monitored to avoid over- or underdigitalization. Whenever overdigitalization is suspected, the daily dose of digitalis should be reduced or temporarily discontinued. Upon discontinuation of ISOPTIN (verapamil HCl), the patient should be reassessed to avoid underdigitalization.

Antihypertensive Agents: Verapamil administered concomitantly with oral antihypertensive agents (e.g., vasodilators, angiotensin-converting enzyme inhibitors, diuretics, beta blockers) will usually have an additive effect on lowering blood pressure. Patients receiving these combinations should be appropriately monitored. Concomitant use of agents that attenuate alpha-adrenergic function with verapamil may result in a reduction in blood pressure that is excessive in some patients. Such an effect was observed in one study following the concomitant administration of verapamil and prazosin.

Antiarrhythmic Agents

Disopyramide: Until data on possible interactions between verapamil and disopyramide phosphate are obtained, disopyramide should not be administered within 48 hours before or 24 hours after verapamil administration.

Flecainide: A study in healthy volunteers showed that the concomitant administration of flecainide and verapamil may have additive effects on myocardial contractility, AV conduction, and repolarization. Concomitant therapy with flecainide and verapamil may result in additive negative inotropic effect and prolongation of atrioventricular conduction.

Quinidine: In a small number of patients with hypertrophic cardiomyopathy (IHSS), concomitant use of verapamil and quinidine resulted in significant hypotension. Until further data are obtained, combined therapy of verapamil and quinidine in patients with hypertrophic cardiomyopathy should probably be avoided.

The electrophysiological effects of quinidine and verapamil on AV conduction were studied in 8 patients. Verapamil significantly counteracted the effects of quinidine on AV conduction. There has been a report of increased quinidine levels during verapamil therapy.

Nitrates: Verapamil has been given concomitantly with short- and long-acting nitrates without any undesirable drug interactions. The pharmacologic profile of both drugs and the clinical experience suggest beneficial interactions.

Other

Cimetidine: The interaction between cimetidine and chronically administered verapamil has not been studied. Variable results on clearance have been obtained in acute studies of healthy volunteers; clearance of verapamil was either reduced or unchanged.

Lithium: Pharmacokinetic and pharmacodynamic interactions between oral verapamil and lithium have been reported. The former may result in a lowering of serum lithium levels in patients receiving chronic stable oral lithium therapy. The latter may result in an increased sensitivity to the effects of lithium. Patients receiving both drugs must be monitored carefully.

Carbamazepine: Verapamil therapy may increase carbamazepine concentrations during combined therapy. This may produce carbamazepine side effects such as diplopia, headache, ataxia, or dizziness.

Rifampin: Therapy with rifampin may markedly reduce oral verapamil bioavailability.

Phenobarbital: Phenobarbital therapy may increase verapamil clearance.

Cyclosporin: Verapamil therapy may increase serum levels of cyclosporin.

Inhalation Anesthetics: Animal experiments have shown that inhalation anesthetics depress cardiovascular activity by decreasing the inward movement of calcium ions. When used concomitantly, inhalation anesthetics and calcium an-

tagonists, such as verapamil, should be titrated carefully to avoid excessive cardiovascular depression.

Neuromuscular Blocking Agents: Clinical data and animal studies suggest that verapamil may potentiate the activity of neuromuscular blocking agents (curare-like and depolarizing). It may be necessary to decrease the dose of verapamil and/or the dose of the neuromuscular blocking agent when the drugs are used concomitantly.

Carcinogenesis, Mutagenesis, Impairment of Fertility: An 18-month toxicity study in rats, at a low multiple (6 fold) of the maximum recommended human dose, and not the maximum tolerated dose, did not suggest a tumorigenic potential. There was no evidence of a carcinogenic potential of verapamil administered in the diet of rats for two years at doses of 10, 35, and 120 mg/kg per day or approximately 1x, 3.5x, and 12x, respectively, the maximum recommended human daily dose (480 mg per day or 9.6 mg/kg/day).

Verapamil was not mutagenic in the Ames test in 5 test strains at 3 mg per plate, with or without metabolic activation.

Studies in female rats at daily dietary doses up to 5.5 times (55 mg/kg/day) the maximum recommended human dose did not show impaired fertility. Effects on male fertility have not been determined.

Pregnancy: Pregnancy Category C. Reproduction studies have been peformed in rabbits and rats at oral doses up to 1.5 (15 mg/kg/day) and 6 (60 mg/kg/day) times the human oral daily dose, respectively, and have revealed no evidence of teratogenicity. In the rat, however, this multiple of the human dose was embryocidal and retarded fetal growth and development, probably because of adverse maternal effects reflected in the reduced weight gains of the dams. This oral dose has also been shown to cause hypotension in rats. There are no adequate and well-controlled studies in pregnant women. Because animal reproduction studies are not always predictive of human response, this drug should be used during pregnancy only if clearly needed. ISOPTIN (verapamil HCl) crosses the placental barrier and can be detected in umbilical vein blood at delivery.

Labor and Delivery: It is not known whether the use of verapamil during labor or delivery has immediate or delayed adverse effects on the fetus, or whether it prolongs the duration of labor or increases the need for forceps delivery or other obstetric intervention. Such adverse experiences have not been reported in the literature, despite a long history of use of ISOPTIN in Europe in the treatment of cardiac side effects of beta-adrenergic agonist agents used to treat premature labor.

Nursing Mothers: ISOPTIN is excreted in human milk. Because of the potential for adverse reactions in nursing infants from verapamil, nursing should be discontinued while verapamil is administered.

Pediatric Use: Safety and efficacy of ISOPTIN in children below the age of 18 years have not been established.

Animal Pharmacology and/or Animal Toxicology: In chronic animal toxicology studies verapamil caused lenticular and/or suture line changes at 30 mg/kg/day or greater and frank cataracts at 62.5 mg/kg/day or greater in the beagle dog but not the rat. Development of cataracts due to verapamil has not been reported in man.

ADVERSE REACTIONS

Serious adverse reactions are uncommon when ISOPTIN (verapamil HCl) therapy is initiated with upward dose titration within the recommended single and total daily dose. See WARNINGS for discussion of heart failure, hypotension, elevated liver enzymes, AV block, and rapid ventricular response. The following reactions to orally administered ISOPTIN occurred at rates greater than 1.0% or occurred at lower rates but appeared clearly drug-related in clinical trials in 4,954 patients.

Constipation	7.3%	Fatigue	1.7%
Dizziness	3.3%	Dyspnea	1.4%
Nausea	2.7%	Bradycardia (HR <50/min)	1.4%
Hypotension	2.5%	AV Block—total 1°, 2°, 3°	1.2%
Headache	2.2%	2° and 3°	0.8%
Edema	1.9%	Rash	1.2%
CHF/	1.8%	Flushing	0.6%
Pulmonary Edema			

Elevated Liver Enzymes (see WARNINGS)

In clinical trials related to the control of ventricular response in digitalized patients who had atrial fibrillation or atrial flutter, ventricular rates below 50/min at rest occurred in 15% of patients and asymptomatic hypotension occurred in 5% of patients.

The following reactions, reported in 1.0% or less of patients, occurred under conditions (open trials, marketing experience) where a causal relationship is uncertain; they are listed to alert the physician to a possible relationship:

Cardiovascular: angina pectoris, atrioventricular dissociation, chest pain, claudication, myocardial infarction, palpitations, purpura (vasculitis), syncope.

Digestive System: diarrhea, dry mouth, gastrointestinal distress, gingival hyperplasia.

Hemic and Lymphatic: ecchymosis or bruising.

Nervous System: cerebrovascular accident, confusion, equilibrium disorders, insomnia, muscle cramps, paresthesia, psychotic symptoms, shakiness, somnolence.

Skin: arthralgia and rash, exanthema, hair loss, hyperkeratosis, maculae, sweating, urticaria, Stevens-Johnson syndrome, erythema multiforme.

Special Senses: blurred vision.

Urogenital: gynecomastia, impotence, increased urination, spotty menstruation.

Treatment of Acute Cardiovascular Adverse Reactions: The frequency of cardiovascular adverse reactions which require therapy is rare; hence, experience with their treatment is limited. Whenever severe hypotension or complete AV block occur following oral administration of verapamil, the appropriate emergency measures should be applied immediately, e.g., intravenously administered isoproterenol HCl, levarterenol bitartrate, atropine (all in the usual doses), or calcium gluconate (10% solution). In patients with hypertrophic cardiomyopathy (IHSS), alpha-adrenergic agents (phenylephrine, metaraminol bitartrate or methoxamine) should be used to maintain blood pressure, and isoproterenol and levarterenol should be avoided. If further support is necessary, inotropic agents (dopamine or dobutamine) may be administered. Actual treatment and dosage should depend on the severity and the clinical situation and the judgment and experience of the treating physician.

OVERDOSAGE

Treatment of overdosage should be supportive. Beta-adrenergic stimulation or parenteral administration of calcium solutions may increase calcium ion flux across the slow channel, and have been used effectively in treatment of deliberate overdosage with verapamil. Verapamil cannot be removed by hemodialysis. Clinically significant hypotensive reactions or high degree AV block should be treated with vasopressor agents or cardiac pacing, respectively. Asystole should be handled by the usual measures including cardiopulmonary resuscitation.

DOSAGE AND ADMINISTRATION

Essential Hypertension

The dose of ISOPTIN SR should be individualized by titration and the drug should be administered with food. The usual daily dose of sustained release verapamil, ISOPTIN SR, in clinical trials has been 240 mg given by mouth once daily in the morning. However, initial doses of 120 mg (½ tablet) a day may be warranted in patients who may have an increased response to verapamil (e.g., elderly, small people etc.). Upward titration should be based on therapeutic efficacy and safety evaluated approximately 24 hours after dosing. The antihypertensive effects of ISOPTIN SR are evident within the first week of therapy.

If adequate response is not obtained, the dose may be titrated upward in the following manner:
a) 240 mg (1 tablet) each morning,
b) 240 mg (1 tablet) each morning plus 120 mg (½ tablet) each evening,
c) 240 mg (1 tablet) every twelve hours.

When switching from immediate release ISOPTIN to ISOPTIN SR the total daily dose in milligrams may remain the same.

HOW SUPPLIED

ISOPTIN® SR tablets are supplied as light green, capsule shaped, scored, film-coated tablets containing 240 mg of verapamil hydrochloride. The tablet is embossed with a double Knoll triangle on one side and "ISOPTIN SR" on the other side.

Bottle of 30-NDC #0044-1826-93
Bottle of 100—NDC # 0044-1826-02
Hospital Unit Dose (100 Tablets-Strips of 10)—NDC # 0044-1826-10
Storage: 59° to 86°F (15° to 30°C).
Protect from light and moisture
Dispense in a tight, light-resistant container as defined in the USP.

Knoll Pharmaceuticals
A Unit of BASF K&F Corporation
30 North Jefferson Road
Whippany, New Jersey 07981
BASF Group
MR 1987/2624
RE-1/IsoSR2628C/12-18-87
Revised November 1987
Printed in U.S.A.

Shown in Product Identification Section, page 413

QUADRINAL™ Tablets ℞
[kwă'drĭ-nawl]

DESCRIPTION

Each QUADRINAL™ Tablet contains ephedrine hydrochloride 24 mg; phenobarbital 24 mg [Warning: May be habit

Continued on next page

Knoll—Cont.

forming]; theophylline calcium salicylate 130 mg (equivalent to 65 mg anhydrous theophylline); potassium iodide 320 mg. Other ingredients include magnesium stearate, potato starch, sodium thiosulfate and talc.

QUADRINAL contains two bronchodilators, theophylline and ephedrine. Phenobarbital serves as a mild sedative to help counteract central nervous system stimulation which may be caused by ephedrine. Wheezing and coughing are relieved by improved bronchodilation while the expectorant action of potassium iodide helps to remove secretions from the bronchial tree. Dyspnea is thus relieved or prevented and acute episodes of bronchospasm are often eliminated with consequent lessening of apprehension and distress.

CLINICAL PHARMACOLOGY
Theophylline directly relaxes the smooth muscle of the bronchial airways and pulmonary blood vessels, thus acting mainly as a bronchodilator, pulmonary vasodilator and smooth muscle relaxant. It also possesses other actions typical of the xanthine derivatives: coronary vasodilator, diuretic, and cardiac, cerebral, and skeletal muscle stimulant. The actions of theophylline may be mediated through inhibition of phosphodiesterase and a resultant increase in intracellular cyclic AMP which could mediate smooth muscle relaxation.

In vitro, theophylline has been shown to react synergistically with beta agonists (such as isoproterenol) that increase intracellular cyclic AMP through the stimulation of adenyl cyclase, but synergism has not been demonstrated in clinical studies and more data are needed to determine if theophylline and beta agonists have clinically important additive effects *in vivo*.

Apparently, tolerance does not develop with chronic use of theophylline.

The half-life is shortened with cigarette smoking. The half-life of theophylline in smokers (1 to 2 packs/day) averaged 4 to 5 hours in various studies, much shorter than the 7 to 9 hour half-life in nonsmokers. The increase in theophylline clearance caused by smoking is probably the result of induction of drug-metabolizing enzymes that do not readily normalize after cessation of smoking. It appears that between 3 months and 2 years may be necessary for normalization of the effect of smoking on theophylline pharmacokinetics.

The half-life is prolonged in alcoholism, reduced hepatic or renal function, congestive heart failure, and in patients receiving cimetidine or antibiotics such as troleandomycin (TAO, Cyclamycin), erythromycin, lincomycin and clindamycin. High fever for prolonged periods may decrease theophylline elimination.

Newborn infants have extremely slow clearances with half-lives exceeding 24 hours. These approach those seen for older children after about 3-6 months.

Older adults with chronic obstructive pulmonary disease, patients with cor pulmonale or other causes of heart failure, and patients with liver pathology may have much lower clearances with half-lives that may exceed 24 hours.

Theophylline Elimination Characteristics

	Theophylline Clearance Rates (mean ± S.D.)	Half-life Average (mean ± S.D.)
Children (over 6 months of age)	$1.45 \pm .58$ mL/kg/min	3.7 ± 1.1 hours
Adult non-smokers with uncomplicated asthma	$0.65 \pm .19$ mL/kg/min	8.7 ± 2.2 hours

INDICATIONS
For chronic respiratory disease in which tenacious mucus and bronchospasm are dominant symptoms, such as bronchial asthma, chronic bronchitis and pulmonary emphysema.

CONTRAINDICATIONS
Use of QUADRINAL is contraindicated in patients with enlarged thyroid or goiter or with known sensitivity to theophylline, potassium iodide, ephedrine or sympathomimetics, or barbiturates.

The iodide in QUADRINAL can cause fetal harm when administered to a pregnant woman. Development of goiter has been reported in infants whose mothers received iodide-containing medications during pregnancy. A few neonatal deaths resulting from tracheal obstruction due to congenital goiters have been reported. Use of barbiturates during pregnancy may cause physical dependence with resulting withdrawal symptoms in the neonate; may cause birth defects; may be associated with neonatal hemorrhage due to reduction in levels of vitamin K-dependent clotting factors in the neonate; may cause respiratory depression in the neonate.

QUADRINAL is contraindicated in women who are or may become pregnant. If this drug is used during pregnancy, or if the patient becomes pregnant while taking this drug, the patient should be apprised of the potential hazard to the fetus.

WARNINGS
QUADRINAL contains thiosulfate, a sulfite that may cause allergic-type reactions including anaphylactic symptoms and life-threatening or less severe asthmatic episodes in certain susceptible people. The overall prevalence of sulfite sensitivity in the general population is unknown and probably low. Sulfite sensitivity is seen more frequently in asthmatic than non-asthmatic people.

QUADRINAL contains theophylline calcium salicylate. Salicylates have been reported to be associated with the development of Reye's syndrome in children and teenagers with chicken pox or flu.

Excessive theophylline doses may be associated with toxicity; determination of serum theophylline levels is recommended to assure maximal benefit without excessive risk. Incidence of toxicity increases at serum levels greater than 20 mcg/mL. Because of the theophylline content of QUADRINAL, it is unlikely that toxic levels of theophylline would be reached unless a serious overdosage occurs.

Morphine, curare, and stilbamidine should be used with caution in patients with airflow obstruction since they stimulate histamine release and can induce asthmatic attacks. They may also suppress respiration leading to respiratory failure. Alternative drugs should be chosen whenever possible.

There is an excellent correlation between clinical manifestations of toxicity and high blood levels of theophylline resulting from conventional doses in patients with lowered body plasma clearances (due to transient cardiac decompensation), patients with liver dysfunction or chronic obstructive lung disease, and patients who are older than 55 years of age, particularly males. In about 50% of patients, nausea and restlessness precede more severe manifestations of toxicity. In other patients, ventricular arrhythmias or seizures may be the first signs of toxicity. These more serious side effects are more likely to occur after intravenous administration of theophylline. Many patients who have high theophylline serum levels exhibit a tachycardia, and theophylline may worsen preexisting arrhythmias.

PRECAUTIONS
Mean half-life in smokers is shorter than in nonsmokers; therefore, smokers may require larger doses of theophylline. QUADRINAL, like all theophylline products, should not be administered concurrently with other xanthine medications. Use with caution in patients with severe cardiac disease, severe hypoxemia, hypertension, hyperthyroidism, acute myocardial injury, cor pulmonale, congestive heart failure, liver disease, peptic ulcer and in the elderly (especially males) and in neonates. Great caution should be used especially in giving theophylline to patients in congestive heart failure; such patients have shown markedly prolonged theophylline blood level curves with theophylline persisting in serum for long periods following discontinuation of the drug. Theophylline may occasionally act as a local irritant to the G.I. tract although gastrointestinal symptoms are more commonly central in origin and associated with serum concentrations over 20 mcg/mL.

Ephedrine-containing medications should be used with caution in patients with cardiovascular disease, diabetes mellitus, predisposition to glaucoma, hypertension, hyperthyroidism, or prostatic hypertrophy.

Potassium iodide may aggravate acne in adolescents and adults.

Phenobarbital should be used with caution in patients with a history of drug abuse or dependence, impaired renal or hepatic function, hyperkinesis, uncontrolled pain, or history of porphyria.

Usage in Pregnancy: Pregnancy Category X. See "Contraindications" section.

Nursing Mothers: Because of the potential for serious adverse reactions in nursing infants from the potassium iodide, ephedrine and phenobarbital in QUADRINAL, a decision should be made whether to discontinue nursing or to discontinue the drug, taking into account the importance of the drug to the mother.

Pediatric Use: QUADRINAL is indicated for use in children on a short term basis. Chronic use should be reserved for patients in whom other expectorants have not been effective. If QUADRINAL is used chronically in children, the patient should be observed for signs of thyroid enlargement and worsening of acne.

Geriatric Patients: Geriatric patients may be more sensitive to the effects of ephedrine.

ADVERSE REACTIONS
The most frequent adverse reactions to theophylline are usually due to overdose (serum levels in excess of 20 mcg/mL) and are: nausea, vomiting, epigastric pain, hematemesis, diarrhea, headaches, irritability, restlessness, insomnia, reflex hyperexcitability, muscle twitching, clonic and tonic generalized convulsions, palpitations, tachycardia, extra systoles, flushing, hypotension, circulatory failure, ventricular arrhythmias, tachypnea, albuminuria, increased excretion of renal tubular cells and red blood cells, potentiation of diuresis, hyperglycemia and inappropriate ADH syndrome.

Thyroid adenoma, goiter and myxedema are possible side effects of potassium iodide.

Hypersensitivity to iodides may be manifested by angioneurotic edema, cutaneous and mucosal hemorrhages, and symptoms resembling serum sickness, such as fever, arthralgia, lymph node enlargement and eosinophilia.

Chronic ingestion of iodides may result in chronic iodide poisoning, or iodism. Initial symptoms include an unpleasant brassy taste, burning in the mouth and throat, soreness

Drug	Effect
Aminophylline with lithium carbonate	Increased excretion of lithium carbonate
Potassium iodide with lithium	Increased hypothyroid and goiterogenic effects
Aminophylline with propranolol	Antagonism of propranolol effect
Theophylline with furosemide	Increased diuresis
Theophylline with hexamethonium	Decreased hexamethonium induced chronotropic effect
Theophylline with reserpine	Reserpine-induced tachycardia
Theophylline with chlordiazepoxide	Chlordiazepoxide-induced fatty acid mobilization
Theophylline with troleandomycin (TAO, Cyclamycin), erythromycin, lincomycin, clindamycin	Increased theophylline plasma levels
Theophylline with phenytoin	Decreased phenytoin levels
Theophylline with cimetidine	Increased theophylline blood levels
Ephedrine with digitalis glycosides or anesthetics	May cause cardiac arrhythmias
Ephedrine with ergonovine, methylergonovine or oxytocin	Hypertension
Ephedrine with guanethidine	Decreased hypotensive effect
Ephedrine with MAO inhibitors	Potentiation of pressor effect of ephedrine
Ephedrine with reserpine	Decreased pressor effect of ephedrine
Ephedrine with other sympathomimetics	Increased effects of either medication
Ephedrine with tricyclic antidepressants	May antagonize the pressor action of ephedrine
Phenobarbital with alcohol, general anesthetics, other CNS depressants, or MAO inhibitors	Increased effects of either medication
Phenobarbital with oral anticoagulants	Decreased anticoagulant effects
Phenobarbital with corticosteroids, digitalis, digitoxin, doxycycline, tricyclic antidepressants, griseofulvin or phenytoin	Decreased effects of these drugs

of the teeth and gums, increased salivation, coryza, sneezing, irritation of the eyes with swelling of the eyelids, headache, cough, skin lesions, diarrhea, gastric irritation, anorexia, fever and depression. The symptoms of iodism disappear spontaneously within a few days after stopping the administration of iodide. Therefore, treatment consists of stopping QUADRINAL therapy and providing supportive measures as indicated by the symptoms. Abundant fluid and sodium chloride intake may hasten iodide elimination. In severe cases, the use of mannitol to establish an osmotic diuresis may be appropriate. Potassium iodide may produce hyperkalemia and, if ingested chronically, may lead to goiter.

Adverse reactions to ephedrine include nervousness, restlessness, trouble in sleeping, irregular heartbeat, difficult or painful urination, dizziness or light-headedness, headache, loss of appetite, nausea or vomiting, trembling, troubled breathing, unusual increase in sweating, unusual paleness, feeling of warmth, and weakness. Tolerance to ephedrine may develop with prolonged or excessive use.

Adverse reactions to phenobarbital include mental confusion or depression, shortness of breath or troubled breathing, skin rash, hives, swelling of eyelids, face or lips, wheezing or tightness in chest, sore throat and fever, unusual bleeding or bruising, unusual excitement, tiredness or weakness, unusually slow heartbeat, yellowing of eyes or skin.

DRUG INTERACTIONS

Toxic synergism of theophylline with ephedrine has been documented and may occur with some other sympathomimetic bronchodilators.
[See table on preceding page].

OVERDOSAGE

A. If potential overdose is established and seizure has not occurred and patient is conscious:
  1) Induce vomiting.
  2) Administer a cathartic.
  3) Administer activated charcoal.
B. If patient is having a seizure:
  1) Establish an airway.
  2) Administer O_2.
  3) Treat the seizure with intravenous diazepam, 0.1 to 0.3 mg/kg up to 10 mg.
  4) Monitor vital signs, maintain blood pressure and provide adequate hydration.
C. Post-seizure coma:
  1) Maintain airway and oxygenation.
  2) Following above recommendations to prevent absorption of drug, but intubation and lavage will have to be performed instead of inducing emesis, and introduce the cathartic and charcoal via a large bore gastric lavage tube.
  3) Continue to provide full supportive care and adequate hydration while waiting for drug to be metabolized. In general, the drug is metabolized sufficiently rapidly so as not to require dialysis.

DOSAGE AND ADMINISTRATION

When rapidly absorbed products such as uncoated tablets with rapid dissolution are used, dosing to maintain "around the clock" blood levels generally requires administration every 6 hours in children; dosing intervals up to 8 hours may be satisfactory for adults because of their slower elimination rate.

Pulmonary function measurements before and after a period of treatment permit an objective assessment of response to QUADRINAL.

Usual dose:

Adults—One tablet 3 or 4 times daily; if needed, an additional one tablet upon retiring for nighttime relief. In severe attacks, the usual dose may be increased by one half.
Children 6 to 12 years—one half tablet three times daily.
Children under 6 years—dose is proportionately less.

HOW SUPPLIED

QUADRINAL Tablets— white, round, bi-convex tablets, engraved with a triangle on one side, bisected on the other side and imprinted with the number "14".
Bottles of 100—NDC #0044-4520-02.

STORAGE

Store at 59°–86°F (15°–30°C).
Dispense in tight, light-resistant container as defined in USP.
MR 1987/8448
Revised May, 1987   8449
Shown in Product Identification Section, page 413

VICODIN® TABLETS   Ⓒ Ⅲ ℞
[vī′kō-dĭn]

DESCRIPTION

Each VICODIN® tablet contains:
Hydrocodone Bitartrate .... 5 mg
  (WARNING: May be habit forming.)
Acetaminophen .... 500 mg
Other ingredients include colloidal silicon dioxide, corn starch, croscarmellose sodium Type A, dibasic calcium phosphate, magnesium stearate, microcrystalline cellulose, povidone, stearic acid and sodium metabisulfite.

Hydrocodone bitartrate is an opioid analgesic and antitussive and occurs as fine, white crystals or as a crystalline powder. It is affected by light. The chemical name is 4,5α-epoxy-3-methoxy-17-methylmorphinan-6-one tartrate (1:1) hydrate (2:5).
Its structure is as follows:

$$C_{18}H_{21}NO_3 \cdot C_4H_6O_6 \cdot 2\tfrac{1}{2}H_2O \qquad\qquad \text{M.W. 494.50}$$

Acetaminophen, 4′-hydroxyacetanilide, is a non-opiate, non-salicylate analgesic and antipyretic which occurs as a white, odorless, crystalline powder possessing a slightly bitter taste. Its structure is as follows:

$$C_8H_9NO_2 \qquad\qquad \text{M.W. 151.16}$$

CLINICAL PHARMACOLOGY

Hydrocodone is a semisynthetic narcotic analgesic and antitussive with multiple actions qualitatively similar to those of codeine. Most of these involve the central nervous system and smooth muscle. The precise mechanism of action of hydrocodone and other opiates is not known, although it is believed to relate to the existence of opiate receptors in the central nervous system. In addition to analgesia, narcotics may produce drowsiness, changes in mood and mental clouding.

Radioimmunoassay techniques have recently been developed for the analysis of hydrocodone in human plasma. After a 10 mg oral dose of hydrocodone bitartrate, a mean peak serum drug level of 23.6 ng/mL and an elimination half-life of 3.8 hours were found.

The analgesic action of acetaminophen involves peripheral and central influences, but the specific mechanism is as yet undetermined. Antipyretic activity is mediated through hypothalamic heat regulating centers. Acetaminophen inhibits prostaglandin synthetase. Therapeutic doses of acetaminophen have negligible effects on the cardiovascular or respiratory systems; however, toxic doses may cause circulatory failure and rapid, shallow breathing. Acetaminophen is rapidly and almost completely absorbed from the gastrointestinal tract, producing maximum serum concentrations within 30 minutes to one hour. The plasma half-life in adults and children ranges from 0.90 hours to 3.25 hours with an average of approximately 2 hours. The drug distributes uniformly in most body fluids and is approximately 25% protein bound. Acetaminophen is conjugated in the liver, with less than 3% of the dose excreted unchanged in 24 hours. The primary metabolic pathway is conjugation to sulfate and glucuronide by-products. A minor oxidative pathway forms cysteine and mercapturic acid. These compounds are subsequently excreted by the kidneys into the urine.

INDICATIONS AND USAGE

For the relief of moderate to moderately severe pain.

CONTRAINDICATIONS

Hypersensitivity to acetaminophen or hydrocodone.

WARNINGS

Allergic-Type Reaction: VICODIN Tablets contain sodium metabisulfite, a sulfite that may cause allergic-type reactions including anaphylactic symptoms and life-threatening or less severe asthmatic episodes in certain susceptible people. The overall prevalence of sulfite sensitivity in the general population is unknown and probably low. Sulfite sensitivity is seen more frequently in asthmatic than non-asthmatic people.

Respiratory Depression: At high doses or in sensitive patients, hydrocodone may produce dose-related respiratory depression by acting directly on brain stem respiratory centers. Hydrocodone also affects centers that control respiratory rhythm, and may produce irregular and periodic breathing.

Head Injury and Increased Intracranial Pressure: The respiratory depressant effects of narcotics and their capacity to elevate cerebrospinal fluid pressure may be markedly exaggerated in the presence of head injury, other intracranial lesions or a preexisting increase in intracranial pressure. Furthermore, narcotics produce adverse reactions which may obscure the clinical course of patients with head injuries.

Acute Abdominal Conditions: The administration of narcotics may obscure the diagnosis or clinical course of patients with acute abdominal conditions.

PRECAUTIONS

Special Risk Patients: As with any narcotic analgesic agent, VICODIN Tablets should be used with caution in elderly or debilitated patients and those with severe impairment of hepatic or renal function, hypothyroidism, Addison's disease, prostatic hypertrophy or urethral stricture. The usual precautions should be observed and the possibility of respiratory depression should be kept in mind.

Information for Patients: VICODIN Tablets, like all narcotics, may impair the mental and/or physical abilities required for the performance of potentially hazardous tasks such as driving a car or operating machinery; patients should be cautioned accordingly.

Cough Reflex: Hydrocodone suppresses the cough reflex; as with all narcotics, caution should be exercised when VICODIN Tablets are used postoperatively and in patients with pulmonary disease.

Drug Interactions: Patients receiving other narcotic analgesics, antipsychotics, antianxiety agents, or other CNS depressants (including alcohol) concomitantly with VICODIN Tablets may exhibit an additive CNS depression. When combined therapy is contemplated, the dose of one or both agents should be reduced.

The use of MAO inhibitors or tricyclic antidepressants with hydrocodone preparations may increase the effect of either the antidepressant or hydrocodone.

The concurrent use of anticholinergics with hydrocodone may produce paralytic ileus.

Usage in Pregnancy:

Teratogenic Effects: Pregnancy Category C. Hydrocodone has been shown to be teratogenic in hamsters when given in doses 700 times the human dose. There are no adequate and well-controlled studies in pregnant women. VICODIN Tablets should be used during pregnancy only if the potential benefit justifies the potential risk to the fetus.

Nonteratogenic Effects: Babies born to mothers who have been taking opioids regularly prior to delivery will be physically dependent. The withdrawal signs include irritability and excessive crying, tremors, hyperactive reflexes, increased respiratory rate, increased stools, sneezing, yawning, vomiting, and fever. The intensity of the syndrome does not always correlate with the duration of maternal opioid use or dose. There is no consensus on the best method of managing withdrawal. Chlorpromazine 0.7 to 1.0 mg/kg q6h, and paregoric 2 to 4 drops/kg q4h, have been used to treat withdrawal symptoms in infants. The duration of therapy is 4 to 28 days, with the dosage decreased as tolerated.

Labor and Delivery: As with all narcotics, administration of VICODIN Tablets to the mother shortly before delivery may result in some degree of respiratory depression in the newborn, especially if higher doses are used.

Nursing Mothers: It is not known whether this drug is excreted in human milk. Because many drugs are excreted in human milk and because of the potential for serious adverse reactions in nursing infants from VICODIN Tablets, a decision should be made whether to discontinue nursing or to discontinue the drug, taking into account the importance of the drug to the mother.

Pediatric Use: Safety and effectiveness in children have not been established.

ADVERSE REACTIONS

The most frequently observed adverse reactions include lightheadedness, dizziness, sedation, nausea and vomiting. These effects seem to be more prominent in ambulatory than in nonambulatory patients and some of these adverse reactions may be alleviated if the patient lies down.
Other adverse reactions include:

Central Nervous System: Drowsiness, mental clouding, lethargy, impairment of mental and physical performance, anxiety, fear, dysphoria, dizziness, psychic dependence, mood changes.

Gastrointestinal System: The antiemetic phenothiazines are useful in suppressing the nausea and vomiting which may occur (see above) however, some phenothiazine derivatives seem to be antianalgesic and to increase the amount of narcotic required to produce pain relief, while other phenothiazines reduce the amount of narcotic required to produce a given level of analgesia. Prolonged administration of VICODIN Tablets may produce constipation.

Genitourinary System: Ureteral spasm, spasm of vesical sphincters and urinary retention have been reported.

Respiratory Depression: Hydrocodone bitartrate may produce dose-related respiratory depression by acting directly on brain stem respiratory centers. Hydrocodone also affects centers that controls respiratory rhythm, and may produce

Continued on next page

Knoll—Cont.

irregular and periodic breathing. If significant respiratory depression occurs, it may be antagonized by the use of naloxone hydrochloride. Apply other supportive measures when indicated.

DRUG ABUSE AND DEPENDENCE

VICODIN Tablets are subject to the Federal Controlled Substances Act (Schedule ⓒ).

Psychic dependence, physical dependence, and tolerance may develop upon repeated administration of narcotics; therefore, VICODIN Tablets should be prescribed and administered with caution. However, psychic dependence is unlikely to develop when VICODIN Tablets are used for a short time for the treatment of pain.

Physical dependence, the condition in which continued administration of the drug is required to prevent the appearance of a withdrawal syndrome, assumes clinically significant proportions only after several weeks of continued narcotic use, although some mild degree of physical dependence may develop after a few days of narcotic therapy. Tolerance, in which increasingly large doses are required in order to produce the same degree of analgesia, is manifested initially by a shortened duration of analgesic effect, and subsequently by decreases in the intensity of analgesia. The rate of development of tolerance varies among patients.

OVERDOSAGE

Acetaminophen:

Signs and Symptoms: In acute acetaminophen overdosage, dose-dependent, potentially fatal hepatic necrosis is the most serious adverse effect. Renal tubular necrosis, hypoglycemic coma, and thrombocytopenia may also occur.

In adults, hepatic toxicity has rarely been reported with acute overdoses of less than 10 grams and fatalities with less than 15 grams. Importantly, young children seem to be more resistant than adults to the hepatotoxic effect of an acetaminophen overdosage. Despite this, the measures outlined below should be initiated in any adult or child suspected of having ingested an acetaminophen overdose.

Early symptoms following a potentially hepatotoxic overdose may include: nausea, vomiting, diaphoresis and general malaise. Clinical and laboratory evidence of hepatic toxicity may not be apparent until 48 to 72 hours post-ingestion.

Treatment: The stomach should be emptied promptly by lavage or by induction of emesis with syrup of ipecac. Patients' estimates of the quantity of a drug ingested are notoriously unreliable. Therefore, if an acetaminophen overdose is suspected, a serum acetaminophen assay should be obtained as early as possible, but no sooner than four hours following ingestion. Liver function studies should be obtained initially and repeated at 24-hours intervals.

The antidote, N-acetylcysteine, should be administered as early as possible, preferably within 16 hours of the overdose ingestion for optimal results, but in any case, within 24 hours. Following recovery, there are no residual, structural or functional hepatic abnormalities.

Hydrocodone:

Signs and Symptoms: Serious overdose with hydrocodone is characterized by respiratory depression (a decrease in respiratory rate and/or tidal volume, Cheyne-Stokes respiration, cyanosis), extreme somnolence progressing to stupor or coma, skeletal muscle flaccidity, cold and clammy skin, and sometimes bradycardia and hypotension. In severe overdosage, apnea, circulatory collapse, cardiac arrest and death may occur.

Treatment: Primary attention should be given to the reestablishment of adequate respiratory exchange through provision of a patent airway and the institution of assisted or controlled ventilation. The narcotic antagonist naloxone is a specific antidote against respiratory depression which may result from overdosage or unusual sensitivity to narcotics, including hydrocodone. Therefore, an appropriate dose of naloxone hydrochloride (see package insert) should be administered, preferably by the intravenous route, and simultaneously with efforts at respiratory resuscitation. Since the duration of action of hydrocodone may exceed that of the antagonist, the patient should be kept under continued surveillance and repeated doses of the antagonist should be administered as needed to maintain adequate respiration.

An antagonist should not be administered in the absence of clinically significant respiratory or cardiovascular depression. Oxygen, intravenous fluids, vasopressors and other supportive measures should be employed as indicated.

Gastric emptying may be useful in removing unabsorbed drug.

DOSAGE AND ADMINISTRATION

Dosage should be adjusted according to the severity of the pain and the response of the patient. However, it should be kept in mind that tolerance to hydrocodone can develop with continued use and the incidence of untoward effects is dose related.

The usual adult dosage is one or two tablets every four to six hours as needed for pain. The total 24 hour dose should not exceed 8 tablets.

HOW SUPPLIED

White, capsule shaped tablet bisected on one side and imprinted with "VICODIN" on the other side.

Bottles of 100—NDC #0044-0727-02.
Bottles of 500—NDC #0044-0727-03.
Hospital Unit Dose Package—100 tablets (4×25 tablets)—NDC #0044-0727-41.

Storage: Store at controlled room temperature 15°–30°C (59°–86°F).

Dispense in a tight, light-resistant container as defined in the USP.

A Schedule ⓒ Narcotic.
MR 1987/5809
Revised February, 1988   5828
Shown in Product Identification Section, page 413

VICODIN ES® TABLETS   ⓒ ℞

DESCRIPTION

Each VICODIN ES® tablet contains:
Hydrocodone Bitartrate   7.5 mg
(**WARNING:** May be habit forming.)
Acetaminophen   750 mg
Other ingredients include colloidal silicon dioxide, corn starch, croscarmellose sodium, Type A magnesium stearate, povidone, stearic acid, and sodium metabisulfite.

Hydrocodone bitartrate is an opioid analgesic and antitussive and occurs as fine, white crystals or as a crystalline powder. It is affected by light. The chemical name is: 4,5α-epoxy-3-methoxy-17-methylmorphinan-6-one tartrate (1:1) hydrate (2:5). Its structure is as follows:

$$C_{18}H_{21}NO_3 \cdot C_4H_6O_6 \cdot 2\tfrac{1}{2}H_2O \qquad\qquad \text{M.W. } 494.50$$

Acetaminophen, 4'-hydroxyacetanilide, is a non-opiate, non-salicylate analgesic and antipyretic which occurs as a white, odorless crystalline powder possessing a slightly bitter taste. Its structure is as follows:

$$C_8H_9NO_2 \qquad\qquad \text{M.W. } 151.16$$

CLINICAL PHARMACOLOGY

Hydrocodone is a semisynthetic narcotic analgesic and antitussive with multiple actions qualitatively similar to those of codeine. Most of these involve the central nervous system and smooth muscle. The precise mechanism of action of hydrocodone and other opiates is not known, although it is believed to relate to the existence of opiate receptors in the central nervous system. In addition to analgesia, narcotics may produce drowsiness, changes in mood and mental clouding.

Radioimmunoassay techniques have recently been developed for the analysis of hydrocodone in human plasma. After a 10 mg oral dose of hydrocodone bitartrate, a mean peak serum drug level of 23.6 ng/mL and an elimination half-life of 3.8 hours were found.

The analgesic action of acetaminophen involves peripheral and central influences, but the specific mechanism is as yet undetermined. Antipyretic activity is mediated through hypothalmic heat regulating centers. Acetaminophen inhibits prostaglandin synthetase. Therapeutic doses of acetaminophen have negligible effects on the cardiovascular or respiratory systems; however, toxic doses may cause circulatory failure and rapid, shallow breathing. Acetaminophen is rapidly and almost completely absorbed from the gastrointestinal tract, producing maximum serum concentrations within 30 minutes to one hour. The plasma half-life in adults and children ranges from 0.90 hours to 3.25 hours with an average of approximately 2 hours. The drug distributes uniformly in most body fluids and is approximately 25% protein bound. Acetaminophen is conjugated in the liver, with less than 3% of the dose excreted unchanged in 24 hours. The primary metabolic pathway is conjugation to sulfate and glucuronide by-products. A minor oxidative pathway forms

cysteine and mercapturic acid. These compounds are subsequently excreted by the kidneys into the urine.

INDICATIONS AND USAGE

For the relief of moderate to moderately severe pain.

CONTRAINDICATIONS

Hypersensitivity to acetaminophen or hydrocodone.

WARNINGS

VICODIN ES Tablets contain sodium metabisulfite, a sulfite that may cause allergic-type reactions including anaphylactic symptoms and life-threatening or less severe asthmatic episodes in certain susceptible people. The overall prevalence of sulfite sensitivity in the general population is unknown and probably low. Sulfite sensitivity is seen more frequently in asthmatic than non-asthmatic people.

Respiratory Depression: At high doses or in sensitive patients, hydrocodone may produce dose-related respiratory depression by acting directly on the brain stem respiratory center. Hydrocodone also affects the center that controls respiratory rhythm, and may produce irregular and periodic breathing.

Head Injury and Increased Intracranial Pressure: The respiratory depressant effects of narcotics and their capacity to elevate cerebrospinal fluid pressure may be markedly exaggerated in the presence of head injury, other intracranial lesions or a preexisting increase in intracranial pressure. Furthermore, narcotics produce adverse reactions which may obscure the clinical course of patients with head injuries.

Acute Abdominal Conditions: The administration of narcotics may obscure the diagnosis or clinical course of patients with acute abdominal conditions.

PRECAUTIONS

Special Risk Patients: As with any narcotic analgesic agent, VICODIN ES Tablets should be used with caution in elderly or debilitated patients and those with severe impairment of hepatic or renal function, hypothyroidism, Addison's disease, prostatic hypertrophy or urethral stricture. The usual precautions should be observed and the possibility of respiratory depression should be kept in mind.

Information for Patients: VICODIN ES Tablets, like all narcotics, may impair the mental and/or physical abilities required for the performance of potentially hazardous tasks such as driving a car or operating machinery; patients should be cautioned accordingly.

Cough Reflex: Hydrocodone suppresses the cough reflex; as with all narcotics, caution should be exercised when VICODIN ES Tablets are used postoperatively and in patients with pulmonary disease.

Drug Interactions: Patients receiving other narcotic analgesics, antipsychotics, antianxiety agents, or other CNS depressants (including alcohol) concomitantly with VICODIN ES Tablets may exhibit an additive CNS depression. When combined therapy is contemplated, the dose of one or both agents should be reduced.

The use of MAO inhibitors or tricyclic antidepressants with hydrocodone preparations may increase the effect of either the antidepressant or hydrocodone.

The concurrent use of anticholinergics with hydrocodone may produce paralytic ileus.

Usage in Pregnancy:

Teratogenic Effects: Pregnancy Category C. Hydrocodone has been shown to be teratogenic in hamsters when given in doses 700 times the human dose. There are no adequate and well-controlled studies in pregnant women. VICODIN ES Tablets should be used during pregnancy only if the potential benefit justifies the potential risk to the fetus.

Nonteratogenic Effects: Babies born to mothers who have been taking opioids regularly prior to delivery will be physically dependent. The withdrawal signs include irritability and excessive crying, tremors, hyperactive reflexes, increased respiratory rate, increased stools, sneezing, yawning, vomiting, and fever. The intensity of the syndrome does not always correlate with the duration of maternal opioid use or dose. There is no consensus on the best method of managing withdrawal. Chlorpromazine 0.7 to 1 mg/kg q6h, and paregoric 2 to 4 drops/kg q4h, have been used to treat withdrawal symptoms in infants. The duration of therapy is 4 to 28 days, with the dosage decreased as tolerated.

Labor and Delivery: As with all narcotics, administration of VICODIN ES Tablets to the mother shortly before delivery may result in some degree of respiratory depression in the newborn, especially if higher doses are used.

Nursing Mothers: It is not known whether this drug is excreted in human milk. Because many drugs are excreted in human milk and because of the potential for serious adverse reactions in nursing infants from VICODIN ES Tablets, a decision should be made whether to discontinue nursing or to discontinue the drug, taking into account the importance of the drug to the mother.

Pediatric Use: Safety and effectiveness in children have not been established.

ADVERSE REACTIONS

The most frequently observed adverse reactions include lightheadedness, dizziness, sedation, nausea and vomiting. These effects seem to be more prominent in ambulatory than in nonambulatory patients and some of these adverse reactions may be alleviated if the patient lies down.

Other adverse reactions include:

Central Nervous System: Drowsiness, mental clouding, lethargy, impairment of mental and physical performance, anxiety, fear, dysphoria, psychic dependence, mood changes.

Gastrointestinal System: The antiemetic phenothiazines are useful in suppressing the nausea and vomiting which may occur (see above); however, some phenothiazine derivatives seem to be antianalgesic and to increase the amount of narcotic required to produce pain relief, while other phenothiazines reduce the amount of narcotic required to produce a given level of analgesia. Prolonged administration of VICODIN ES Tablets may produce constipation.

Genitourinary System: Ureteral spasm, spasm of vesical sphincters and urinary retention have been reported.

Respiratory Depression: Hydrocodone bitartrate may produce dose-related respiratory depression by acting directly on the brain stem respiratory center. Hydrocodone also affects the center that controls respiratory rhythm, and may produce irregular and periodic breathing. If significant respiratory depression occurs, it may be antagonized by the use of naloxone hydrochloride. Apply other supportive measures when indicated.

DRUG ABUSE AND DEPENDENCE

VICODIN ES Tablets are subject to the Federal Controlled Substance Act (Schedule Ⅲ).

Psychic dependence, physical dependence, and tolerance may develop upon repeated administration of narcotics; therefore, VICODIN ES Tablets should be prescribed and administered with caution. However, psychic dependence is unlikely to develop when VICODIN ES Tablets are used for a short time for the treatment of pain.

Physical dependence, the condition in which continued administration of the drug is required to prevent the appearance of a withdrawal syndrome, assumes clinically significant proportions only after several weeks of continued narcotic use, although some mild degree of physical dependence may develop after a few days of narcotic therapy. Tolerance, in which increasingly large doses are required in order to produce the same degree of analgesia, is manifested initially by a shortened duration of analgesic effect, and subsequently by decreases in the intensity of analgesia. The rate of development of tolerance varies among patients.

OVERDOSAGE

Acetaminophen:

Signs and Symptoms: In acute acetaminophen overdosage, dose-dependent, potentially fatal hepatic necrosis is the most serious adverse effect. Renal tubular necrosis, hypoglycemic coma, and thrombocytopenia may also occur.

In adults, hepatic toxicity has rarely been reported with acute overdoses of less than 10 grams and fatalities with less than 15 grams. Importantly, young children seem to be more resistant than adults to the hepatotoxic effect of an acetaminophen overdose. Despite this, the measures outlined below should be initiated in any adult or child suspected of having ingested an acetaminophen overdose.

Early symptoms following a potentially hepatotoxic overdose may include nausea, vomiting, diaphoresis and general malaise. Clinical and laboratory evidence of hepatic toxicity may not be apparent until 48 to 72 hours post-ingestion.

Treatment: The stomach should be emptied promptly by lavage or by induction of emesis with syrup of ipecac. Patients' estimates of the quantity of a drug ingested are notoriously unreliable. Therefore, if an acetaminophen overdose is suspected, a serum acetaminophen assay should be obtained as early as possible, but no sooner than four hours following ingestion. Liver function studies should be obtained initially and repeated at 24-hour intervals.

The antidote, N-acetylcysteine, should be administered as early as possible, preferably within 16 hours of the overdose ingestion for optimal results, but in any case, within 24 hours. Following recovery, there are no residual, structural or functional hepatic abnormalities.

Hydrocodone:

Signs and Symptoms: Serious overdose with hydrocodone is characterized by respiratory depression (a decrease in respiratory rate and/or tidal volume, Cheyne-Stokes respiration, cyanosis), extreme somnolence progressing to stupor or coma, skeletal muscle flaccidity, cold and clammy skin, and sometimes bradycardia and hypotension. In severe overdosage, apnea, circulatory collapse, cardiac arrest and death may occur.

Treatment: Primary attention should be given to the reestablishment of adequate respiratory exchange through provision of a patent airway and the institution of assisted or controlled ventilation. The narcotic antagonist naloxone is a specific antidote against respiratory depression which may result from overdosage or unusual sensitivity to narcotics, including hydrocodone. Therefore, an appropriate dose of naloxone hydrochloride (see package insert) should be administered, preferably by the intravenous route, and simultaneously with efforts at respiratory resuscitation. Since the duration of action of hydrocodone may exceed that of the antagonist, the patient should be kept under continued surveillance and repeated doses of the antagonist should be administered as needed to maintain adequate respiration.

An antagonist should not be administered in the absence of clinically significant respiratory or cardiovascular depression. Oxygen, intravenous fluids, vasopressors and other supportive measures should be employed as indicated.

Gastric emptying may be useful in removing unabsorbed drug.

DOSAGE AND ADMINISTRATION

Dosage should be adjusted according to the severity of the pain and the response of the patient. However, it should be kept in mind that tolerance to hydrocodone can develop with continued use and that the incidence of untoward effects is dose related.

The usual adult dosage is one tablet every four to six hours as needed for pain. The total 24 hour dose should not exceed 5 tablets.

HOW SUPPLIED

White, oval-shaped, faceted edged tablet bisected on one side and imprinted with "VICODIN ES" on the other side. Bottles of 100—NDC #0044-0728-02.

Hospital Unit Dose Package—100 tablets (4×25 tablets)—NDC #0044-0728-41.

Storage: Store at controlled room temperature 15°–30°C (59°–86°F).

Dispense in a tight, light-resistant container as defined in the USP.

A Schedule Ⅲ Narcotic.

MR 1987/5811

RE-3/VicES5832/3-21-88

Revised March, 1988

Knoll Pharmaceuticals

A Unit of BASF K&F Corporation

30 North Jefferson Road

Whippany, New Jersey 07981

BASF Group

Shown in Product Identification Section, page 413

EDUCATIONAL MATERIAL

Continuing Education Booklets

"Calcium in Cardiac Metabolism" (3 credits)
  Home Study Module - Pharmacists
"Cardiac Arrhythmias" (2 credits)
  Home Study Module - Pharmacists
"Treatment of Cardiac Arrhythmias" (3 credits)
  Home Study Module - Pharmacists
"Angina Pectoris" (2 credits)
  Home Study Module - Pharmacists
"Management of Angina Pectoris" (3 credits)
  Home Study Module - Pharmacists
"Management of Essential Hypertension" (3 credits)
  Home Study Module - Pharmacists

Kramer Laboratories, Inc.
8778 S.W. 8TH STREET
MIAMI, FL 33174

CHARCOAL PLUS
Antiflatulent/Antidiarrheal

DESCRIPTION

Each two-phase tablet contains simethicone, 80 mg., in the layer for immediate release in the stomach and activated charcoal, 400 mg. USP, in an enteric-coated core for release in the small intestine.

INDICATIONS

For the relief of the symptoms of gas distress. CHARCOAL PLUS has a two-fold action on the painful symptoms of gas distress: simethicone acts in the stomach to neutralize and prevent the formation of gas pockets and provides for the relief of the pain and pressure symptoms of excess gas; activated charcoal is an adsorbent, detoxicant and soothing agent which provides for the relief of the symptoms of intestinal gas, diarrhea, and gastrointestinal distress associated with indigestion.

DIRECTIONS

One tablet, four times daily, after meals and at bedtime. May also be taken as needed, up to 6 tablets daily, or as directed by a physician.

WARNING

Keep this and all medications out of the reach of children.

HOW SUPPLIED

Dark brown, round tablets in boxes of 60 tablets. (NDC 55505-105-13)

FUNGI-NAIL®
[fun 'gi-nāl]
Tincture

DESCRIPTION

Resorcinol 1%; Salicylic Acid 2%; Parachlorometaxylenol 2%; Benzocaine 0.5%; Acetic Acid 2.5%; Propylene glycol, Hydroxypropylmethyl Cellulose, Alcohol 50%.

INDICATIONS

For topical treatment of ringworm infections of the nails tinea unguium (onychomycosis), and other fungus and bacterial infections of the skin.

PRECAUTIONS

Avoid contact with eyes and mucous membranes. Do not use on broken skin or irritated areas.

DOSAGE AND ADMINISTRATION

Apply to affected nails and other affected areas of the skin twice daily.

HOW SUPPLIED

1 oz. bottle with brush applicator. (NDC 55505-103-26)

YOHIMEX™ Tablets   ℞
[yō-him 'eks]

DESCRIPTION

Each tablet for oral administration contains yohimbine hydrochloride, 5.4 mg. (1/12 grain). Yohimbine is an indoalkylamine alkaloid with chemical similarity to reserpine. It is the principal alkaloid of the bark of the West African Corynanthe yohimbe tree and is also found in Rauwolfia Serpentina (L) Benth.

ACTIONS

Yohimbine is primarily an alpha-2 adrenergic blocker, which blocks presynaptic alpha-2-adrenoreceptors.

PHARMACOLOGY: Its peripheral autonomic nervous system effect is to increase parasympathetic (cholinergic) and decrease sympathetic (adrenergic) activity. In male sexual performance, erection is linked to cholinergic activity which theoretically results in increased penile blood inflow, decreased penile blood outflow or both, causing erectile stimulation without increasing sexual desire. Yohimbine exerts a stimulating action on mood and may increase anxiety. Such actions are not adequately studied, although they appear to require high doses. Yohimbine has a mild antidiuretic action, probably via stimulation of hypothalmic centers and release of posterior pituitary hormone. Its action on peripheral blood vessels resembles that of reserpine, though it is weaker and of short duration. The drug reportedly exerts no significant influence on cardiac stimulation and other effects mediated by beta-adrenergic receptors.

INDICATIONS

Sympatholytic and mydriatic agent. Impotence has been successfully treated with yohimbine in male patients with vascular or diabetic origins and psychogenic origins (18 mg./day). Urologists have used yohimbine experimentally for the treatment and the diagnostic classification of certain types of male erectile impotence.

CONTRAINDICATIONS

In patients with renal disease; hypersensitivity to any component.

WARNINGS

Not for use in geriatric patients, psychiatric patients or cardio-renal patients with a history of gastric or duodenal ulcer. Generally not for use in females.

USAGE IN PREGNANCY: Do not use during pregnancy.
USAGE IN CHILDREN: Do not use in children.

DRUG INTERACTIONS

Do not use yohimbine with antidepressants and other mood-modifying drugs.

ADVERSE REACTIONS

CNS: Yohimbine readily penetrates the CNS and produces a complex pattern of responses in doses lower than those required to produce peripheral alpha-adrenergic blockade. These include: antidiuresis and central excitation including elevated blood pressure and heart rate, increased motor activity, nervousness, irritability and tremor. Dizziness, headache and skin flushing have been reported.

Continued on next page

Kramer—Cont.

OVERDOSAGE
Daily doses of 20–30 mg. may produce increases in heart rate and blood pressure, piloerection and rhinorrhea. More severe symptoms may include paresthesias, incoordination, tremulousness and a dissociative state with higher doses.

DOSAGE AND ADMINISTRATION
USUAL ADULT DOSE: One tablet taken 3 times daily. If side effects occur, the dosage is to be reduced to ½ tablet 3 times a day followed by gradual increase to 1 tablet 3 times a day. The therapy reported is not more than 10 weeks.

HOW SUPPLIED
Pink, round tablets in bottles of 100 tablets (NDC 55505-100-15)

Kremers Urban Company
See SCHWARZ PHARMA

Lactaid Inc.
P.O. BOX 111
PLEASANTVILLE, NJ 08232-0111

LACTAID®
[lăkt 'ād]
Lactaid Drops
and
Lactaid Caplets
(lactase enzyme)

PRODUCT OVERVIEW
KEY FACTS
Lactaid® lactase enzyme hydrolyzes lactose into digestible sugars: glucose and galactose. Lactaid Drops are added to milk for *in vitro* treatment; Lactaid Caplets are taken orally for *in vivo* hydrolysis.

MAJOR USES
Lactaid lactase enzyme (liquid and caplets) have proven to be clinically effective for lactose intolerant people when consuming milk and/or dairy foods, by permitting consumption of lactose-containing foods without gas, cramps, bloating and/or diarrhea.

SAFETY INFORMATION
Lactaid enzyme should be discontinued in anyone who develops hypersensitivity to the enzyme.

PRESCRIBING INFORMATION
LACTAID®
[lăkt 'ād]
Lactaid Drops
and
Lactaid Caplets
(lactase enzyme)

DESCRIPTION
Drops: Each 5 drop dosage contains not less than 1250 NLU (Neutral Lactase Units) of Beta-D-galactosidase derived from *Kluyveromyces lactis* yeast. The enzyme is in a liquid carrier of glycerol (50%), water (30%), and inert yeast dry matter (20%). 5 drops hydrolyze approximately 70% of the lactose in 1 quart of milk at refrigerator temperature, @ 43°F (6°C) in 24 hours, or will do the same in 2 hours @ 85°F (30°C). Additional time and/or enzyme required for 100% lactose conversion. 1 U.S. quart of milk will contain approximately 50 gm lactose prior to lactose hydrolysis and will contain 15 gm or less, after 70% conversion.

ACTION
Hydrolysis converts the lactose into its simple sugar components: glucose and galactose.

INDICATIONS
Lactase insufficiency in the patient, suspected from g.i. disturbances after consumption of milk or milk-content products: e.g., bloat, distension, flatulence, diarrhea; or identified by a lactose tolerance test.

USAGE
Added to milk. 5–15 drops per quart of milk depending on level of lactose conversion desired.

OTHER USES
In vivo activity has been demonstrated, indicating usage in tube feedings and other lactose-content solid and liquid foods, with addition at time of consumption.

HOW SUPPLIED
Lactase enzyme in a stable liquid form, in sales units of 12, 30 and 75 one-quart dosages at 5 drops per dose.

CAPLETS: Each caplet contains not less than 3000 FCC lactase units of Beta-D-Galactosidase from *Aspergillus oryzae*. One to two caplets taken with a meal will normally handle a lactose challenge equal to 1 glass of milk. In severe cases, 3 caplets may be required.

TOXICITY
None.

DRUG INTERACTIONS
None. Both liquid and tablets are classified as food, not drugs.

WARNINGS
Should hypersensitivity occur, discontinue use.

PRECAUTIONS
Diabetics should be aware that the milk sugar will now be metabolized available and must be taken into account (17.5 gm glucose and 17.5 gm galactose per quart @ 70% hydrolysis). No reports received of any diabetics' reactions. Galactosemics may not have milk in any form, lactase enzyme modified or not.

ADVERSE REACTIONS
The most frequently reported adverse reactions to Lactaid lactase caplets are gastrointestinal in nature, sometimes mimicking the symptoms of lactose intolerance. No reactions of any kind observed from Lactaid liquid drops. Total reactions to caplets estimated at under 0.1 (¹/₁₀)% of users.

HOW SUPPLIED
In bottles of 100, bottles of 12 and boxes of 25-2 caplet "take along" packets.

OTHER LACTOSE REDUCED PRODUCTS
In most areas of the U.S.: Fresh lactose reduced lowfat milk from dairies, ready to drink, sold in food markets. Lactose hydrolysis level: 70%. If desired, further conversion of the dairy-treated milk can be done at home or institution with the Lactaid liquid enzyme. Also in some areas: Lactaid lactose reduced cottage cheese and American process cheese. Any person or institution unable to locate Lactaid enzyme locally can order direct from Lactaid Inc. retail or wholesale. Samples and full product information to doctors, institutions and nutritionists on request.
Call toll-free 1-800-257-8650.
Shown in Product Identification Section, page 413

EDUCATIONAL MATERIAL

Brochures
Patient brochure—"Why Lactaid? The Problem with Milk and the Answer"
Professional brochure—"Lactaid Specially Digestible Milk and Dairy Products as Part of a Nutritional Program"
Samples
Dispensing samples of Lactaid Caplets and Lactaid Drops.
PATIENT STARTER KITS
Contains patient brochure, 12 Lactaid Caplets and Lactaid Drops for treating 4 quarts of milk.
All literature, samples and patient starter kits are available free to physicians and dietitians.

Lakeside Pharmaceuticals
Division of Merrell Dow Pharmaceuticals Inc.
CINCINNATI, OH 45242-9553

BENTYL®   ℞
[bĕn 'til]
(dicyclomine hydrochloride USP)
Tablets, Capsules, Syrup, Injection

CAUTION: Federal law prohibits dispensing without prescription.

DESCRIPTION
Bentyl is an antispasmodic and anticholinergic (antimuscarinic) agent available in the following forms:
1. Bentyl capsules for oral use contain 10 mg dicyclomine hydrochloride USP. Bentyl 10 mg capsules also contain inactive ingredients: calcium sulfate, corn starch, FD&C Blue No. 1, FD&C Red No. 3, gelatin, lactose, magnesium stearate, pregelatinized corn starch, and titanium dioxide.
2. Bentyl tablets for oral use contain 20 mg dicyclomine hydrochloride USP. Bentyl 20 mg tablets also contain inactive ingredients: acacia, dibasic calcium phosphate, corn starch, FD&C Blue No. 1, lactose, magnesium stearate, pregelatinized corn starch, and sucrose.
3. Bentyl syrup for oral use contains 10 mg dicyclomine hydrochloride USP in each 5 mL (1 teaspoonful). Bentyl syrup also contains inactive ingredients: citric acid, D&C Red No. 33, FD&C Blue No. 1, FD&C Red No. 40, FD&C

Yellow No. 6, flavors, glucose, methylparaben, propylene glycol, propylparaben, saccharin sodium, and water.
4. Bentyl Injection is a sterile, aqueous solution for intramuscular injection (NOT FOR INTRAVENOUS USE).
Ampul—2 mL—Each mL contains 10 mg dicyclomine hydrochloride USP in sterile water for injection, made isotonic with sodium chloride.
Vial—10 mL—Each mL contains 10 mg dicyclomine hydrochloride USP in sterile water for injection, made isotonic with sodium chloride. A preservative containing 0.5% chlorobutanol hydrous (chloral derivative) has been added.
The aqueous vehicle, Water for Injection, meets the USP requirements of the Pyrogen Test.
Chemically, Bentyl (dicyclomine hydrochloride) is [bicyclohexyl]-1-carboxylic acid, 2-(diethylamino)ethyl ester, hydrochloride with the chemical structure:

Dicyclomine hydrochloride occurs as a fine, white, crystalline, practically odorless powder with a bitter taste. It is soluble in water, freely soluble in alcohol and chloroform, and very slightly soluble in ether.

CLINICAL PHARMACOLOGY
Dicyclomine relieves smooth muscle spasm of the gastrointestinal tract. Animal studies indicate that this action is achieved via a dual mechanism: (1) a specific anticholinergic effect (antimuscarinic) at the acetylcholine-receptor sites with approximately ⅛ the milligram potency of atropine (*in vitro*, guinea pig ileum); and (2) a direct effect upon smooth muscle (musculotropic) as evidenced by dicyclomine's antagonism of bradykinin- and histamine-induced spasms of the isolated guinea pig ileum. Atropine did not affect responses to these two agonists. *In vivo* studies in cats and dogs showed dicyclomine to be equally potent against acetylcholine (ACh)- or barium chloride (BaCl$_2$)-induced intestinal spasm while atropine was at least 200 times more potent against effects of ACh than BaCl$_2$. Tests for mydriatic effects in mice showed that dicyclomine was approximately ¹/₅₀₀ as potent as atropine: antisialogogue tests in rabbits showed dicyclomine to be ¹/₃₀₀ as potent as atropine.
In man, dicyclomine is rapidly absorbed after oral administration, reaching peak values within 60–90 minutes. The principal route of elimination is via the urine (79.5% of the dose). Excretion also occurs in the feces, but to a lesser extent (8.4%). Mean half-life of plasma elimination in one study was determined to be approximately 1.8 hours when plasma concentrations were measured for 9 hours after a single dose. In subsequent studies, plasma concentrations were followed for up to 24 hours after a single dose, showing a secondary phase of elimination with a somewhat longer half-life. Mean volume of distribution for a 20 mg oral dose is approximately 3.65 L/kg suggesting extensive distribution in tissues.
In controlled clinical trials involving over 100 patients who received drug, 82% of patients treated for functional bowel-/irritable bowel syndrome with dicyclomine hydrochloride at initial doses of 160 mg daily (40 mg q.i.d.) demonstrated a favorable clinical response compared with 55% treated with placebo. (P < .05). In these trials, most of the side effects were typically anticholinergic in nature (see table) and were reported by 61% of the patients.

Side Effect	Dicyclomine Hydrochloride (40 mg q.i.d.) %	Placebo %
Dry Mouth	33	5
Dizziness	29	2
Blurred Vision	27	2
Nausea	14	6
Light-headedness	11	3
Drowsiness	9	1
Weakness	7	1
Nervousness	6	2

Nine percent (9%) of patients were discontinued from the drug because of one or more of these side effects (compared with 2% in the placebo group). In 41% of the patients with side effects, side effects disappeared or were tolerated at the 160 mg daily dose without reduction. A dose reduction from 160 mg daily to an average daily dose of 90 mg was required in 46% of the patients with side effects who then continued to experience a favorable clinical response; their side effects either disappeared or were tolerated. (See **ADVERSE RE-ACTIONS.**)

INDICATIONS AND USAGE

For the treatment of functional bowel/irritable bowel syndrome.

CONTRAINDICATIONS

1. Obstructive uropathy
2. Obstructive disease of the gastrointestinal tract
3. Severe ulcerative colitis (see PRECAUTIONS)
4. Reflux esophagitis
5. Unstable cardiovascular status in acute hemorrhage
6. Glaucoma
7. Myasthenia gravis
8. Evidence of prior hypersensitivity to dicyclomine hydrochloride or other ingredients of these formulations
9. Infants less than 6 months of age (See WARNINGS and PRECAUTIONS: *Information for Patients.*)

WARNINGS

In the presence of a high environmental temperature, heat prostration can occur with drug use (fever and heat stroke due to decreased sweating). If symptoms occur, the drug should be discontinued and supportive measures instituted.

Diarrhea may be an early symptom of incomplete intestinal obstruction, especially in patients with ileostomy or colostomy. In this instance, treatment with this drug would be inappropriate and possibly harmful.

Bentyl may produce drowsiness or blurred vision. The patient should be warned not to engage in activities requiring mental alertness, such as operating a motor vehicle or other machinery or performing hazardous work while taking this drug.

Psychosis has been reported in sensitive individuals given anticholinergic drugs. CNS signs and symptoms include confusion, disorientation, short-term memory loss, hallucinations, dysarthria, ataxia, coma, euphoria, decreased anxiety, fatigue, insomnia, agitation and mannerisms, and inappropriate affect. These CNS signs and symptoms usually resolve within 12 to 24 hours after discontinuation of the drug.

There are reports that administration of dicyclomine hydrochloride syrup to infants has been followed by serious respiratory symptoms (dyspnea, shortness of breath, breathlessness, respiratory collapse, apnea, asphyxia), seizures, syncope, pulse rate fluctuations, muscular hypotonia, and coma. Death has been reported. No causal relationship between these effects observed in infants and dicyclomine administration has been established. BENTYL IS CONTRAINDICATED IN INFANTS LESS THAN 6 MONTHS OF AGE. (See CONTRAINDICATIONS and PRECAUTIONS.)

Safety and efficacy of dicyclomine hydrochloride in children have not been established.

PRECAUTIONS

General

Use with caution in patients with:
1. Autonomic neuropathy
2. Hepatic or renal disease
3. Ulcerative colitis—large doses may suppress intestinal motility to the point of producing a paralytic ileus and the use of this drug may precipitate or aggravate the serious complication of toxic megacolon (see CONTRAINDICATIONS)
4. Hyperthyroidism
5. Hypertension
6. Coronary heart disease
7. Congestive heart failure
8. Cardiac tachyarrhythmia
9. Hiatal hernia (see CONTRAINDICATIONS: reflux esophagitis)
10. Known or suspected prostatic hypertrophy.

Investigate any tachycardia before administration of dicyclomine hydrochloride, since it may increase the heart rate.

With overdosage, a curare-like action may occur (i.e., neuromuscular blockade leading to muscular weakness and possible paralysis).

Information For Patients

Bentyl may produce drowsiness or blurred vision. The patient should be warned not to engage in activities requiring mental alertness, such as operating a motor vehicle or other machinery or to perform hazardous work while taking this drug.

Bentyl is contraindicated in infants less than 6 months of age. (See CONTRAINDICATIONS and WARNINGS.)

In the presence of a high environmental temperature, heat prostration can occur with drug use (fever and heat stroke due to decreased sweating). If symptoms occur, the drug should be discontinued and a physician contacted.

Drug Interactions

The following agents may increase certain actions or side effects of anticholinergic drugs: amantadine, antiarrhythmic agents of class I (e.g., quinidine), antihistamines, antipsychotic agents (e.g., phenothiazines), benzodiazepines, MAO inhibitors, narcotic analgesics (e.g., meperidine), nitrates and nitrites, sympathomimetic agents, tricyclic antidepressants, and other drugs having anticholinergic activity.

Anticholinergics antagonize the effects of antiglaucoma agents. Anticholinergic drugs in the presence of increased intraocular pressure may be hazardous when taken concurrently with agents such as corticosteroids. (See also CONTRAINDICATIONS.)

Anticholinergic agents may affect gastrointestinal absorption of various drugs, such as slowly dissolving dosage forms of digoxin; increased serum digoxin concentrations may result. Anticholinergic drugs may antagonize the effects of drugs that alter gastrointestinal motility, such as metoclopramide. Because antacids may interfere with the absorption of anticholinergic agents, simultaneous use of these drugs should be avoided.

The inhibiting effects of anticholinergic drugs on gastric hydrochloric acid secretion are antagonized by agents used to treat achlorhydria and those used to test gastric secretion.

Carcinogenesis, Mutagenesis, Inpairment of Fertility

There are no known human data on long-term potential for carcinogenicity or mutagenicity.

Long-term studies in animals to determine carcinogenic potential are not known to have been conducted.

In studies in rats at doses of up to 100 mg/kg/day, Bentyl produced no deleterious effects on breeding, conception, or parturition.

Pregnancy

Tetatogenic Effects

Pregnancy Category B

Reproduction studies have been performed in rats and rabbits at doses up to 33 times the maximum recommended human dose based on 160 mg/day (3 mg/kg) and have revealed no evidence of impaired fertility or harm to the fetus due to dicyclomine. Epidemiologic studies in pregnant women with products containing dicyclomine hydrochloride (at doses up to 40 mg/day) have not shown that dicyclomine increases the risk of fetal abnormalities if administered during the first trimester of pregnancy. There are, however, no adequate and well-controlled studies in pregnant women at the recommended doses (80–160 mg/day). Because animal reproduction studies are not always predictive of human response, Bentyl as indicated for functional bowel/irritable bowel syndrome should be used during pregnancy only if clearly needed.

Nursing Mothers

It is not known whether dicyclomine hydrochloride is excreted in human milk. Because many drugs are excreted in human milk, caution should be exercised when Bentyl is administered to a nursing woman. (See PRECAUTIONS: *Pediatric Use* and ADVERSE REACTIONS.)

Pediatric Use (See CONTRAINDICATIONS and WARNINGS.) BENTYL IS CONTRAINDICATED IN INFANTS LESS THAN 6 MONTHS OF AGE.

Safety and effectiveness in children have not been established.

ADVERSE REACTIONS

Controlled clinical trials have provided frequency information for reported adverse effects of dicyclomine hydrochloride listed in a decreasing order of frequency. (See CLINICAL PHARMACOLOGY.)

Not all of the following adverse reactions have been reported with dicyclomine hydrochloride. Adverse reactions are included here that have been reported for pharmacologically similar drugs with anticholinergic/antispasmodic action.

Gastrointestinal: dry mouth, nausea, vomiting, constipation, bloated feeling, abdominal pain, taste loss, anorexia

Central Nervous System: dizziness, light-headedness, tingling, headache, drowsiness, weakness, nervousness, numbness, mental confusion and/or excitement (especially in elderly persons), dyskinesia, lethargy, syncope, speech disturbance, insomnia

Ophthalmologic: blurred vision, diplopia, mydriasis, cycloplegia, increased ocular tension

Dermatologic/Allergic: rash, urticaria, itching, and other dermal manifestations; severe allergic reaction or drug idiosyncrases including anaphylaxis

Genitourinary: urinary hesitancy, urinary retention

Cardiovascular: tachycardia, palpitations

Respiratory: Dyspnea, apnea, asphyxia (see WARNINGS)

Other: decreased sweating, nasal stuffiness or congestion, sneezing, throat congestion, impotence, suppression of lactation (see PRECAUTIONS: *Nursing Mothers*)

With the injectable form, there may be a temporary sensation of light-headedness. Some local irritation and focal coagulation necrosis may occur following the I.M. injection of the drug.

DRUG ABUSE AND DEPENDENCE

Tolerance, abuse, or dependence with Bentyl has not been reported.

OVERDOSAGE

Signs and Symptoms

The signs and symptoms of overdosage are headache; nausea; vomiting; blurred vision; dilated pupils; hot, dry skin; dizziness; dryness of the mouth; difficulty in swallowing; and CNS stimulation. A curare-like action may occur (i.e., neuro-

muscular blockade leading to muscular weakness and possible paralysis).

Oral LD$_{50}$

The acute oral LD$_{50}$ of the drug is 625 mg/kg in mice.

Minimum Human Lethal Dose/Maximum Human Dose Recorded

The amount of drug in a single dose that is ordinarily associated with symptoms of overdosage or that is likely to be life threatening, has not been defined. The maximum human oral dose recorded was 600 mg by mouth in a 10-month-old child and approximately 1500 mg in an adult, each of whom survived.

In three of the infants who died following administration of dicyclomine hydrochloride (see WARNINGS), the blood concentrations of drug were 200, 220, and 505 ng/mL, respectively.

Dialysis

It is not known if Bentyl is dialyzable.

Treatment

Treatment should consist of gastric lavage, emetics, and activated charcoal. Sedatives (e.g., short-acting barbiturates, benzodiazepines) may be used for management of overt signs of excitement. If indicated, an appropriate parenteral cholinergic agent may be used as an antidote.

DOSAGE AND ADMINISTRATION

DOSAGE MUST BE ADJUSTED TO INDIVIDUAL PATIENT NEEDS. (See CLINICAL PHARMACOLOGY.)

Adults—Oral

The only oral dose clearly shown to be effective is 160 mg per day (in 4 equally divided doses). Since this dose is associated with a significant incidence of side effects, it is prudent to begin with 80 mg per day (in 4 equally divided doses). Depending upon the patient's response during the first week of therapy, the dose should be increased to 160 mg per day unless side effects limit dosage escalation.

If efficacy is not achieved within 2 weeks or side effects require doses below 80 mg per day, the drug should be discontinued. Documented safety data are not available for doses above 80 mg daily for periods longer than 2 weeks.

Adults—Intramuscular injection

NOT FOR INTRAVENOUS USE.

The intramuscular dosage form is to be used temporarily when the patient cannot take oral medication. Intramuscular injection is about twice as bioavailable as oral dosage forms; consequently, the recommended intramuscular dose is 80 mg daily (in 4 equally divided doses).

Oral dicyclomine hydrochloride should be started as soon as possible and the intramuscular form should not be used for periods longer than 1 or 2 days.

ASPIRATE THE SYRINGE BEFORE INJECTING TO AVOID INTRAVASCULAR INJECTION, SINCE THROMBOSIS MAY OCCUR IF THE DRUG IS INADVERTENTLY INJECTED INTRAVASCULARLY. Parenteral drug products should be inspected visually for particulate matter and discoloration prior to administration, whenever solution and container permit.

HOW SUPPLIED

10 mg blue capsules, imprinted BENTYL 10
  NDC 0068-0120-41: unit dose dispenser of 100
  NDC 0068-0120-61: bottles of 100
  NDC 0068-0120-65: bottles of 500
Store at room temperature, preferably below 86°F (30°C).
20 mg compressed, light blue, round tablets, debossed BENTYL 20
  NDC 0068-0123-41: unit dose dispenser of 100
  NDC 0068-0123-61: bottles of 100
  NDC 0068-0123-65: bottles of 500
  NDC 0068-0123-71: bottles of 1000
To prevent fading, avoid exposure to direct sunlight. Store at room temperature, preferably below 86°F (30°C).
10 mg/5mL pink syrup
  NDC 0068-0125-16: 16 ounce bottle
Store at room temperature, preferably below 86°F (30°C).
Protect from excessive heat.
10 mg/mL injection (for intramuscular use only, NOT FOR INTRAVENOUS USE)
  NDC 0068-0810-61: 10 mL multiple dose vials
Store at room temperature, preferably below 86°F (30°C).
Protect from freezing.
  NDC 0068-0809-23: boxes of five 2 mL ampuls
Store at room temperature, preferably below 86°F (30°C).
Protect from freezing.

Product Information as of February, 1989

Injectable dosage forms manufactured by
CONNAUGHT LABORATORIES, INC.
Swiftwater, Pennsylvania 18370 or
TAYLOR PHARMACAL COMPANY
Decatur, Illinois 62525 for

Continued on next page

Lakeside—Cont.

LAKESIDE PHARMACEUTICALS
Division of Merrell Dow Pharmaceuticals Inc.
Cincinnati, Ohio 45215, U.S.A.
Shown in Product Identification Section, page 413

BRICANYL® ℞
[brĭk'ă-nĭl]
(terbutaline sulfate USP)
Subcutaneous Injection

CAUTION: Federal law prohibits dispensing without prescription.

DESCRIPTION
Bricanyl (terbutaline sulfate USP) Subcutaneous Injection is a sterile isotonic solution. Each mL of solution contains 1 mg terbutaline sulfate (equivalent to 0.82 mg free base) and 8.9 mg sodium chloride in water for injection. Hydrochloric acid is used to adjust pH to 3–5.
Terbutaline sulfate (5-[2-[(1,1-dimethylethyl)amino]-1-hydroxyethyl]-1,3-benzenediol sulfate) is a β-adrenergic agonist bronchodilator having the chemical structure:

$$\left[\text{HO} \underset{\text{HO}}{\bigcirc} \text{CHCH}_2\text{NHC(CH}_3)_3 \atop \text{OH} \right]_2 \cdot \text{H}_2\text{SO}_4$$

CLINICAL PHARMACOLOGY
Bricanyl is a β-adrenergic receptor agonist which has been shown by *in vitro* and *in vivo* pharmacologic studies in animals to exert a preferential effect on β_2-adrenergic receptors, such as those located in bronchial smooth muscle. However, controlled clinical studies of patients who were administered the drug have not revealed a preferential β_2-adrenergic effect.
It has been postulated that β-adrenergic agonists produce many of their pharmacologic effects by activation of adenyl cyclase, the enzyme which catalyzes the conversion of adenosine triphosphate to cyclic adenosine monophosphate.
Bricanyl Injection has been shown in controlled clinical studies to relieve acute bronchospasm in acute and chronic obstructive pulmonary disease, resulting in a clinically significant increase in pulmonary flow rates, e.g., an increase of 15% or greater in FEV_1 in some patients. Following administration of 0.25 mg by subcutaneous injection, a measurable change in flow rate is usually observed within five minutes, and a clinically significant increase in FEV_1 occurs by 15 minutes following the injection. The maximum effect usually occurs within 30–60 minutes and clinically significant bronchodilator activity has been observed to persist for 90 minutes to four hours in most patients. The duration of clinically significant improvement is comparable to that found with equimilligram doses of epinephrine.
Subcutaneously administered Bricanyl shows peak plasma concentrations 15–30 minutes after injection (0.5 mg dose, mean peak plasma level 7.6 μg/L). Approximately one-third is metabolized (inactive), the majority of the dose being excreted in urine unchanged. A half-life of 3–4 hours has been reported.
Terbutaline crosses the placenta. After single dose IV administration of terbutaline to 22 women in late pregnancy who were delivered by elective Caesarean section due to clinical reasons, umbilical blood levels of terbutaline were found to range from 11 to 48% of the maternal blood levels.
Recent studies in laboratory animals (minipigs, rodents, and dogs) recorded the occurrence of cardiac arrhythmias and sudden death (with histologic evidence of myocardial necrosis) when β agonists and methylxanthines were administered concurrently. The significance of these findings when applied to humans is currently unknown.

INDICATIONS AND USAGE
Bricanyl is indicated as a bronchodilator for the relief of reversible bronchospasm in patients with obstructive airway diseases such as asthma, bronchitis and emphysema.

CONTRAINDICATIONS
Bricanyl is contraindicated in patients with a history of hypersensitivity to any of its components or sympathomimetic amines.

WARNINGS
Usage in Labor and Delivery: Bricanyl is not indicated and should not be used for the management of preterm labor. Serious adverse reactions have been reported following administration of terbutaline sulfate to women in labor. These reports have included transient hypokalemia, pulmonary edema (sometimes after delivery) and hypoglycemia in the mother and/or the neonatal child. Maternal death has been reported with terbutaline sulfate and other drugs of this class.

There have been rare reports of seizures occurring in patients receiving terbutaline, which do not recur when the drug is discontinued and have not been explained on any other basis.

PRECAUTIONS
General
Terbutaline sulfate is a sympathomimetic amine and as such should be used with caution in patients with cardiovascular disorders (including arrhythmias, coronary insufficiency and hypertension), in patients with hyperthyroidism or diabetes mellitus, history of seizures, or in patients who are unusually responsive to sympathomimetic amines. Age-related differences in the hemodynamic response to β-adrenergic receptor stimulation have been reported.
Patients susceptible to hypokalemia should be monitored because transient early falls in serum potassium levels have been reported with β agonists.
Immediate hypersensitivity reactions and exacerbation of bronchospasm have been reported after terbutaline administration.
Preparation of Other Dosage Forms: Use of the subcutaneous injection for preparation of other dosage forms, e.g., IV infusion, is not appropriate. Sterility, stability, and accurate dosing cannot be assured if the ampuls are not used in accordance with information in DOSAGE AND ADMINISTRATION.
Large doses of intravenous terbutaline sulfate have been reported to aggravate preexisting diabetes and ketoacidosis.
Information for Patients
Patients should be advised regarding the potential adverse reactions associated with Bricanyl.
Drug Interactions
Other sympathomimetic bronchodilators or epinephrine should not be used concomitantly with terbutaline sulfate since their combined effect on the cardiovascular system may be deleterious to the patient.
Terbutaline sulfate should be administered with caution in patients being treated with monoamine oxidase (MAO) inhibitors or tricyclic antidepressants, since the action of terbutaline sulfate on the vascular system may be potentiated.
β-adrenergic receptor blocking agents not only block the pulmonary effect of terbutaline but may produce severe asthmatic attacks in asthmatic patients. Therefore, patients requiring treatment for both bronchospastic disease and hypertension should be treated with medication other than β-adrenergic blocking agents for hypertension.
Carcinogenesis, Mutagenesis, Impairment of Fertility
A two-year, oral carcinogenesis bioassay of terbutaline sulfate (50, 500, 1000, and 2000 mg/kg, corresponding to 5,000, 50,000, 100,000, and 200,000 times the recommended daily adult subcutaneous dose, respectively) in the Sprague-Dawley rat revealed drug-related changes in the female genital system. Females showed dose-related increases in leiomyomas of the mesovarium: 3 (5%) at 50 mg/kg, 17 (28%) at 500 mg/kg, 21 (35%) at 1000 mg/kg, and 23 (38%) at 2000 mg/kg, which were significant at the three highest levels. None occurred in female controls. The incidence of ovarian cysts was significantly elevated at all dose levels except at 2000 mg/kg and hyperplasia of the mesovarium was increased significantly at 500 and 2000 mg/kg. A 21-month oral study of terbutaline sulfate (5, 50 and 200 mg/kg, corresponding to 500, 5,000 and 20,000 times the recommended daily adult subcutaneous dose, respectively) in the mouse revealed no evidence of carcinogenicity.
Studies of terbutaline sulfate have not been conducted to determine mutagenic potential.
An oral reproduction study of terbutaline sulfate up to 50 mg/kg (corresponding to 5,000 times the human subcutaneous dose) in the rat revealed no adverse effects on fertility.
Pregnancy
Teratogenic Effects
Pregnancy Category B: Reproduction studies in mice (up to 1.1 mg/kg subcutaneously, corresponding to 110 times the human subcutaneous dose) and in rats and rabbits (up to 50 mg/kg orally, corresponding to 5,000 times the human subcutaneous dose) have revealed no evidence of impaired fertility or harm to the fetus due to terbutaline. There are, however, no adequate and well-controlled studies in pregnant women. Because animal reproduction studies are not always predictive of human response, this drug should be used during pregnancy only if clearly needed.
Labor and Delivery
Usage in Labor and Delivery: The safe use of Bricanyl for the management of preterm labor or for other uses during labor and delivery has not been established and the drug should not be used. (See WARNINGS.)
Nursing Mothers
Terbutaline is excreted in breast milk. Caution should be exercised when Bricanyl is administered to a nursing woman.
Pediatric Use
Safety and effectiveness in children below the age of 12 have not been established.

ADVERSE REACTIONS
The adverse reactions of terbutaline sulfate are similar to those of other sympathomimetic agents.
The most commonly observed side effects are tremor and nervousness. These occur more frequently at doses in excess of 0.25 mg. Other commonly reported reactions include increased heart rate, palpitations and dizziness. Other reported reactions include headache, drowsiness, vomiting, nausea, sweating, and muscle cramps. These reactions are generally transient and usually do not require treatment.

OVERDOSAGE
Overdosage information is limited. Excessive adrenergic-receptor stimulation may augment the signs and symptoms listed under ADVERSE REACTIONS and may be accompanied by other adrenergic effects.
Signs and symptoms of overdosage may include the following—
CARDIOVASCULAR: tachycardia of varying degrees, transient arrhythmias, and extrasystoles. A significant drop in blood pressure may occur due to peripheral vasodilation.
NEUROMUSCULAR: tremors of varying degrees, nervousness, drowsiness, muscle cramps, headache, and sweating.
GASTROINTESTINAL: nausea and vomiting.
ENDOCRINE: varying degrees of hyperglycemia and rise in insulin levels which could be followed by rebound hypoglycemia. Hypokalemia in the early stages may occur. The duration of these signs and symptoms will be dependent on the degree of overdosage.
In the case of terbutaline overdosage, the patient should be treated symptomatically for sympathomimetic overdosage with careful consideration to the appropriateness of any chosen therapy and possible effect on the patient's underlying disease state. (See also WARNINGS.)
Studies in mice, rats, rabbits, and dogs have established the LD_{50} of terbutaline to be 1–9 g/kg orally and 0.3–1.6 g/kg subcutaneously.
It is not known whether terbutaline is dialyzable.

DOSAGE AND ADMINISTRATION
Parenteral drug products should be inspected visually for particulate matter and discoloration prior to administration, whenever solution and container permit.
The usual subcutaneous dose of Bricanyl is 0.25 mg (0.25 mL, $1/4$ ampul contents) injected into the lateral deltoid area. If significant clinical improvement does not occur by 15–30 minutes, a second dose of 0.25 mg may be administered. A total dose of 0.5 mg should not be exceeded within a four-hour period. If a patient fails to respond to a second 0.25 mg (0.25 mL) dose within 15–30 minutes, other therapeutic measures should be considered.

HOW SUPPLIED
Each 2 mL size ampul contains 1 mL of solution (1 mg terbutaline sulfate). Note: 0.25 mL of solution will provide the usual clinical dose of 0.25 mg.
NDC 0068-0702-20: package of 10 ampuls
Solutions of terbutaline sulfate are sensitive to excessive heat and light. Ampuls should, therefore, be stored at controlled room temperature 15°–30°C (59°–86°F) in their original carton to provide protection from light until dispensed. Solutions should not be used if discolored.
Product Information as of August, 1987
Manufactured by
Astra Pharmaceutical Products, Inc.
Westborough, Mass. 01581 for
LAKESIDE PHARMACEUTICALS
Division of Merrell Dow Pharmaceuticals Inc.
Cincinnati, Ohio 45215, U.S.A.
Shown in Product Identification Section, page 413

BRICANYL® ℞
[brĭk'ă-nĭl]
(terbutaline sulfate USP)
Tablets

CAUTION: Federal law prohibits dispensing without prescription.

DESCRIPTION
Bricanyl (terbutaline sulfate USP) Tablets for oral administration contain 2.5 mg or 5 mg of terbutaline sulfate (equivalent to 2.05 and 4.1 mg free base, respectively). Both the 2.5 and 5 mg tablets contain the following inactive ingredients: corn starch (or pregelatinized corn starch), lactose, magnesium stearate, microcrystalline cellulose, and povidone.
Terbutaline sulfate (5-[2-[(1,1-dimethylethyl)amino]-1-hydroxyethyl]-1,3-benzenediol sulfate) is a β-adrenergic agonist bronchodilator having the chemical structure:

$$\left[\text{HO} \underset{\text{HO}}{\bigcirc} \text{CHCH}_2\text{NHC(CH}_3)_3 \atop \text{OH} \right]_2 \cdot \text{H}_2\text{SO}_4$$

CLINICAL PHARMACOLOGY

Bricanyl is a β-adrenergic receptor agonist which has been shown by *in vitro* and *in vivo* pharmacologic studies in animals to exert a preferential effect on β_2-adrenergic receptors, such as those located in bronchial smooth muscle. However, controlled clinical studies on patients who were administered the drug have not revealed a preferential β_2-adrenergic effect.

It has been postulated that β-adrenergic agonists produce many of their pharmacologic effects by activation of adenyl cyclase, the enzyme which catalyzes the conversion of adenosine triphosphate to cyclic adenosine monophosphate.

Bricanyl Tablets have been shown in controlled clinical studies to relieve bronchospasm in chronic obstructive pulmonary disease such as asthma, chronic bronchitis and emphysema. This action was manifested by a clinically significant increase in pulmonary function as demonstrated by an increase of 15% or greater in FEV_1 in some patients. A measurable change in pulmonary function usually occurs within 30 minutes following oral administration. The maximum effect usually occurs within 120–180 minutes. There is a clinically significant decrease in airway and pulmonary resistance which persists for at least 4 hours or longer in most patients. Significant bronchodilator action as measured by various pulmonary function determinations (airway resistance, MMEFR, PEFR) has been demonstrated in studies for periods up to 8 hours in many patients.

Clinical studies have evaluated the effectiveness of oral Bricanyl for periods up to 12 months and the drug continued to produce significant improvement of pulmonary function throughout the period of treatment.

Orally administered terbutaline sulfate is 30–70% absorbed in the GI tract (food reduces bioavailability by one third). Sixty percent of the absorbed oral dose is metabolized via first pass conjugation in the gut wall and liver. There are no known active metabolites. After single oral doses, peak concentrations are found 30 minutes to 5 hours after administration. Each mg of orally administered terbutaline sulfate (in fasting adults) produces an average peak serum concentration of approximately 1 μg/L. Terbutaline has a half-life of 3–4 hours and is excreted in the urine.

Terbutaline crosses the placenta. After single dose IV administration of terbutaline to 22 women in late pregnancy who were delivered by elective Caesarean section due to clinical reasons, umbilical blood levels of terbutaline were found to range from 11 to 48% of the maternal blood levels.

Recent studies in laboratory animals (minipigs, rodents, and dogs) recorded the occurrence of cardiac arrhythmias and sudden death (with histologic evidence of myocardial necrosis) when β agonist and methylxanthines were administered concurrently. The significance of these findings when applied to humans is currently unknown.

INDICATIONS AND USAGE

Bricanyl is indicated as a bronchodilator for the relief of reversible bronchospasm in patients with obstructive airway diseases such as asthma, bronchitis and emphysema.

CONTRAINDICATIONS

Bricanyl is contraindicated in patients with a history of hypersensitivity to any of its components or sympathomimetic amines.

WARNINGS

Usage in Labor and Delivery: Bricanyl is not indicated and should not be used for the management of preterm labor. Serious adverse reactions have been reported following administration of terbutaline sulfate to women in labor. These reports have included transient hypokalemia, pulmonary edema (sometimes after delivery) and hypoglycemia in the mother and/or neonatal child. Maternal death has been reported with terbutaline sulfate and other drugs of this class. There have been rare reports of seizures occurring in patients receiving terbutaline, which do not recur when the drug is discontinued and have not been explained on any other basis.

PRECAUTIONS

General

Terbutaline sulfate is a sympathomimetic amine and as such should be used with caution in patients with cardiovascular disorders (including arrhythmias, coronary insufficiency, and hypertension), in patients with hyperthyroidism or diabetes mellitus, history of seizures, or in patients who are unusually responsive to sympathomimetic amines. Age-related differences in the hemodynamic response to β-adrenergic receptor stimulation have been reported.

Patients susceptible to hypokalemia should be monitored because transient early falls in serum potassium levels have been reported with β agonists.

Large doses of intravenous terbutaline sulfate have been reported to aggravate preexisting diabetes and ketoacidosis. The relevance of this observation to the use of Bricanyl Tablets is unknown.

Immediate hypersensitivity reactions and exacerbation of bronchospasm have been reported after terbutaline administration.

Information for Patients

The patient should be advised regarding the potential adverse reactions associated with Bricanyl and that: (1) the action of Bricanyl Tablets may last up to 8 hours and, therefore should not be used more frequently than recommended. (2) the number or frequency of doses should not be increased without medical consultation, (3) medical consultation should be sought promptly if symptoms get worse, and (4) other medicines should not be used while taking Bricanyl without consulting the physician.

Drug Interactions

Other sympathomimetic bronchodilators or epinephrine should not be used concomitantly with terbutaline sulfate, since their combined effect on the cardiovascular system may be deleterious to the patient. This recommendation does not preclude the judicious use of an aerosol bronchodilator of the adrenergic stimulant type in patients receiving Bricanyl Tablets. Such concomitant use, however, should be individualized and not given on a routine basis. If regular coadministration is required, alternative therapy should be considered. Terbutaline sulfate should be administered with caution in patients being treated with monoamine oxidase (MAO) inhibitors or tricyclic antidepressants, since the action of terbutaline sulfate on the vascular system may be potentiated. β-adrenergic receptor blocking agents not only block the pulmonary effect of terbutaline but may produce severe asthmatic attacks in asthmatic patients. Therefore, patients requiring treatment for both bronchospastic disease and hypertension should be treated with medication other than β-adrenergic blocking agents for their hypertension.

Carcinogenesis, Mutagenesis, Impairment of Fertility

A two-year, oral carcinogenesis bioassay of terbutaline sulfate (50, 500, 1000 and 2000 mg/kg, corresponding to 167, 1667, 3333, and 6667 times the recommended daily adult oral dose, respectively) in the Sprague-Dawley rat revealed drug-related changes in the female genital system. Females showed dose-related increases in leiomyomas of the mesovarium: 3 (5%) at 50 mg/kg, 17 (28%) at 500 mg/kg, 21 (35%) at 1000 mg/kg, and 23 (38%) at 2000 mg/kg, which were significant at the three highest levels. None occurred in female controls. The incidence of ovarian cysts was significantly elevated at all dose levels except at 2000 mg/kg and hyperplasia of the mesovarium was increased significantly at 500 and 2000 mg/kg. A 21-month oral study of terbutaline sulfate (5, 50 and 200 mg/kg, corresponding to 17, 167 and 667 times the recommended daily adult oral dose, respectively) in the mouse revealed no evidence of carcinogenicity.

Studies of terbutaline sulfate have not been conducted to determine mutagenic potential.

An oral reproduction study of terbutaline sulfate up to 50 mg/kg (corresponding to 167 times the human oral dose) in the rat revealed no adverse effects on fertility.

Pregnancy

Teratogenic Effects

Pregnancy Category B: Reproduction studies in mice (up to 1.1 mg/kg subcutaneously, corresponding to 4 times the human oral dose) and in rats and rabbits (up to 50 mg/kg orally, corresponding to 167 times the human oral dose) have revealed no evidence of impaired fertility or harm to the fetus due to terbutaline. There are, however, no adequate and well-controlled studies in pregnant women. Because animal reproduction studies are not always predictive of human response, this drug should be used during pregnancy only if clearly needed.

Labor and Delivery

Usage in Labor and Delivery: The safe use of Bricanyl for mangement of preterm labor or for other uses during labor and delivery has not been established and the drug should not be used. (See WARNINGS.)

Nursing Mothers

Terbutaline is excreted in breast milk. Caution should be exercised when Bricanyl is administered to a nursing woman.

Pediatric Use

Safety and effectiveness in children below the age of 12 have not been established.

ADVERSE REACTIONS

The adverse reactions of terbutaline sulfate are similar to those of other sympathomimetic agents.

The most commonly observed side effects are tremor and nervousness. The frequency of these side effects appear to diminish with continued therapy. Other commonly reported reactions include increased heart rate, palpitations and dizziness. Other reported reactions include headache, drowsiness, vomiting, nausea, sweating, and muscle cramps. These reactions are generally transient and usually do not require treatment.

OVERDOSAGE

Overdosage information is limited. Excessive adrenergic-receptor stimulation may augment the signs and symptoms listed under ADVERSE REACTIONS and may be accompanied by other adrenergic effects.

Signs and symptoms of overdosage may include the following—*CARDIOVASCULAR:* tachycardia of varying degrees, transient arrhythmias, and extrasystoles. A significant drop in blood pressure may occur due to peripheral vasodilation.

NEUROMUSCULAR: tremors of varying degrees, nervousness, drowsiness, muscle cramps, headache, and sweating.

GASTROINTESTINAL: nausea and vomiting.

ENDOCRINE: varying degrees of hyperglycemia and rise in insulin levels which could be followed by rebound hypoglycemia. Hypokalemia in the early stages may occur. The duration of these signs and symptoms will be dependent on the degree of overdosage.

Treat the alert patient who has taken excessive oral medication by emptying the stomach by means of induced emesis, followed by gastric lavage. In the unconscious patient, secure the airway with a cuffed endotracheal tube before beginning lavage (do not induce emesis). Instillation of activated charcoal slurry may help reduce absorption of terbutaline sulfate. Maintain adequate respiratory exchange. Provide cardiac and respiratory support as needed. Continue observation until symptom-free. Careful consideration should be given to the appropriateness of any chosen therapy and possible effect on the patient's underlying disease state. (See also WARNINGS.)

Studies in mice, rats, rabbits, and dogs have established the LD_{50} of terbutaline to be 1–9 g/kg orally and 0.3–1.6 g/kg subcutaneously.

It is not known whether terbutaline is dialyzable.

DOSAGE AND ADMINISTRATION

ADULTS: Usual dose is 5 mg three times daily. Dosing may be initiated at 2.5 mg three or four times daily and titrated upward depending on clinical response. A total dose of 15 mg in a 24-hour period should not be exceeded.

CHILDREN (12–15 yrs): 2.5 mg three times daily.

If a previously effective dosage regimen fails to provide the usual relief, medical advice should be sought immediately as this is often a sign of seriously worsening asthma which would require reassessment of therapy.

HOW SUPPLIED

2.5 mg tablets (*round*, white, debossed "BRICANYL 2½''):

    NDC 0068-0725-61: Bottle of 100

    NDC 0068-0725-71: Bottle of 1000

5.0 mg tablets (*square*, white, scored, debossed "BRICANYL 5''):

    NDC 0068-0750-61: Bottle of 100

    NDC 0068-0750-71: Bottle of 1000

Store at controlled room temperature (59°–86°F) (15°–30°C).

Product Information as of August, 1987

CEPACOL® Mouthwash/Gargle

[sēp'ă-cŏl]

(See PDR For Nonprescription Drugs)

CEPACOL® Throat Lozenges

[sēp'ă-cŏl]

(See PDR For Nonprescription Drugs)

CEPACOL® Anesthetic Lozenges (Troches)

[sēp'ă-cŏl]

(See PDR For Nonprescription Drugs)

CEPASTAT® Lozenges

[sēp'ă-stăt]

(See PDR For Nonprescription Drugs)

Cherry Flavor

CEPASTAT® Sore Throat Lozenges

[sēp'ă-stăt]

(See PDR For Nonprescription Drugs)

NICORETTE®   ℞

[nĭk'ō-rĕt'']

(nicotine polacrilex)

CAUTION

Federal law prohibits dispensing without prescription.

DESCRIPTION

Nicorette (nicotine polacrilex) contains nicotine bound to an ion exchange resin in a sugar-free flavored chewing gum base. Nicotine is absorbed through the buccal mucosa when Nicorette is chewed. Each piece of Nicorette contains nico-

Continued on next page

Information on Lakeside Pharmaceuticals products is based on labeling in effect in June, 1989.

Lakeside—Cont.

tine polacrilex equivalent to 2 mg nicotine and also contains flavors, glycerin, gum base, sodium bicarbonate, sodium carbonate, and sorbitol. Nicorette is to be used as an adjunct to smoking cessation programs. The chemical name for nicotine is (S)-3-(1-methyl-2-pyrrolidinyl)pyridine.

CLINICAL PHARMACOLOGY

Nicotine is an agonist at nicotinic receptors in the peripheral and central nervous systems. In man, as in animals, nicotine has been shown to produce both behavioral stimulation and depression.

Nicotine's effects are generally dose-dependent, and extremely high doses (achievable through parenteral, rectal, and perhaps percutaneous routes), can produce toxic symptoms, i.e., delirium. These effects can occur in nicotine-tolerant individuals. In nonsmokers, CNS-mediated symptoms of hiccups, nausea, and emesis are commonly associated with the use of even small doses of inhaled smoke or chewed Nicorette gum. However, in smokers these symptoms occur only with much larger doses.

Nicotine has actions at the sympathetic ganglia and on the chemoreceptors of the aorta and carotid bodies. Nicotine also affects the adrenal medulla, with the attendant release of catecholamines. The overall effect on the cardiovascular system leads to acceleration of the heart, peripheral vasoconstriction, and elevation of blood pressure with an attendant increase in the work of the heart. Nicotine may induce vasospasm and cardiac arrhythmias. Tolerance does not develop to the catecholamine-releasing effects of nicotine.

Results of cardiovascular studies comparing Nicorette with cigarettes document that each source of nicotine produces similar dose-dependent effects on cardiovascular performance (see *Biopharmaceutics and Pharmacokinetics* section). However, if Nicorette gum (2 mg/piece) is used by smokers at a rate not exceeding one piece per hour, the cardiovascular effects produced do not differ from those seen with placebo. Reinforcement of cigarette smoking behavior is considered to have both psychologic (or learned) and pharmacologic components. Buffered nicotine-containing gum is designed to provide an alternative source of nicotine for nicotine-dependent individuals acutely withdrawing from tobacco smoking.

Biopharmaceutics and Pharmacokinetics

The nicotine in Nicorette is bound to an ion exchange resin and is released only during chewing; nicotine will not be released in significant amounts if the gum is swallowed. The blood level of nicotine obtained with Nicorette will depend upon the vigor, rapidity, and duration of chewing.

In studies comparing the nicotine blood level achieved with Nicorette to that achieved with smoking, it was found that the trough level of nicotine obtained by smoking one cigarette per hour is approximately twice that of chewing one 2 mg Nicorette per hour.

The pronounced early peak in nicotine blood levels seen with the inhalation of cigarette smoke is not observed with the chewing of Nicorette. Swallowing Nicorette does not produce clinically significant blood levels of nicotine. Nicotine is metabolized mainly by the liver, but may also be metabolized to a lesser extent by the kidney and the lung. The principal metabolites are cotinine and nicotine-1'-N-oxide. Both nicotine and its metabolites are excreted through the kidneys with about 10 to 20% of absorbed nicotine excreted unchanged in the urine. Excretion of nicotine is increased in acid urine and by high urine output. The metabolism of nicotine absorbed buccally from Nicorette is qualitatively similar to the metabolism observed when nicotine is absorbed through inhalation of cigarette smoke.

INDICATION AND USAGE

Nicorette is indicated as a temporary aid to the cigarette smoker seeking to give up his or her smoking habit while participating in a behavioral modification program under medical or dental supervision.

The efficacy of Nicorette as an aid to smoking cessation was demonstrated in clinical studies which showed that Nicorette gum, in comparison to control chewing gums, increased the likelihood of smoking cessation among participants in behavioral modification programs. As used in the context of this labeling, behavioral modification refers to supervised programs of education, counselling and psychologic support. The efficacy of Nicorette use without concomitant participation in a behavioral modification program has not been established.

In general, smokers who have a high 'physical' type of nicotine dependence are most likely to benefit from the use of Nicorette. The following subject characteristics are correlated with a 'physical' type of nicotine dependence: (1) smoke more than 15 cigarettes per day, (2) prefer brands of cigarettes with nicotine levels of greater than 0.9 mg/cigarette, (3) usually inhale the smoke frequently and deeply, (4) find the first cigarette in the morning the hardest to give up, (5) find the first cigarette in the morning the hardest to give up, (6) smoke more frequently during the morning than the rest of the day, (7) find it difficult to refrain from smoking in places

where it is forbidden, or (8) smoke even when they are so ill they are confined to bed most of the day.

The benefits of Nicorette use beyond three months have not been demonstrated.

CONTRAINDICATIONS

Nicorette is contraindicated in non-smokers.

Nicorette is contraindicated in patients during the immediate post-myocardial infarction period, patients with life-threatening arrhythmias, and patients with severe or worsening angina pectoris. (See WARNINGS.)

Also, Nicorette is contraindicated in patients with active temporomandibular joint disease.

Current medical opinion indicates that nicotine in any form may be harmful to an unborn child. Nicorette and cigarettes both contain nicotine.

Nicorette may cause fetal harm when administered to a pregnant woman.

Use of cigarettes or Nicorette during the last trimester has been associated with a decrease in fetal breathing movements. These effects may be the result of decreased placental perfusion caused by nicotine. Rare reports of miscarriages have been received, and a relationship to drug therapy as a contributing factor cannot be excluded. Studies in pregnant rhesus monkeys have shown that maternal nicotine administration produced acidosis, hypoxia and hypercarbia in the fetus.

Nicotine has been shown to be teratogenic in mice treated subcutaneously with 25 mg/kg, which is approximately 300 times the human buccal dose. Studies in rats and monkeys have not demonstrated a teratogenic effect of nicotine in doses which would occur during cigarette smoking.

Nicorette is therefore contraindicated in women who are or may become pregnant, and female patients should be advised to take adequate precautions to avoid becoming pregnant. The physician may wish to consider a pregnancy test before instituting therapy with Nicorette. If this drug is used during pregnancy, or if the patient becomes pregnant while taking this drug, the patient should be apprised of the potential hazard to the fetus.

WARNINGS

The risks of nicotine in patients with certain cardiovascular and endocrine diseases should be carefully weighed against the benefits of including Nicorette in a smoking cessation program in these patients. Specifically, patients with coronary heart disease (history of myocardial infarction and/or angina pectoris), serious cardiac arrhythmias, or vasospastic diseases (Buerger's disease, Prinzmetal variant angina) should be carefully screened and evaluated before Nicorette is prescribed. Occasional reports of tachyarrhythmias occurring in association with the use of Nicorette have been reported; therefore, if an increase in cardiovascular symptoms occurs with the use of Nicorette, it should be discontinued. As the action of nicotine on the adrenal medulla (release of catecholamines) does not appear to be affected by tolerance, Nicorette should be used with caution in patients with hyperthyroidism, pheochromocytoma or insulin-dependent diabetes. Cigarette smoking is felt to play a perpetuating role in hypertension and peptic ulcer disease. Therefore, Nicorette should be used in patients with systemic hypertension or peptic ulcer (active or inactive) only when the benefits of including Nicorette in a smoking cessation program outweigh the risks.

PRECAUTIONS

Nicorette should be used with caution in patients with oral or pharyngeal inflammation and in patients with a history of esophagitis or peptic ulcer.

The dosage form of Nicorette dictates that it be used with caution in patients whose dental problems might be exacerbated by chewing gum. In such patients prior dental evaluation may be advisable.

Nicorette is sugar-free and has been formulated to minimize stickiness. As with other gums, however, the degree to which Nicorette may stick to dentures, dental caps or partial bridges may depend on the materials from which they are made and other factors such as amount of saliva produced, possible interaction with denture adhesives, denture cleaning compounds, dryness of mouth due to other causes and salivary constituents. Should an excessive degree of stickiness to dental work occur, there is the possibility that as with other gums, Nicorette may damage dental work; if this should occur, the patient should discontinue its use and consult a physician or dentist.

The sustained use of Nicorette by ex-smokers is not to be encouraged because the chronic consumption of nicotine is toxic and addicting. The physician must, however, weigh the relative risks of a possible return to smoking versus continued, long-term use of the gum.

Information for Patients

The patient instruction sheet is attached at the end of the professional labeling text. It is intended for detachment by the pharmacist and inclusion in the package of Nicorette dispensed to the patient. It contains important selected information on patient selection, risks and adverse effects and instructions on how to use Nicorette properly.

Drug Interactions

Smoking cessation, with or without nicotine substitutes, may alter response to concomitant medication in ex-smokers. Smoking is considered to increase metabolism and thus lower blood levels of drugs such as phenacetin, caffeine, theophylline, imipramine and pentazocine, through enzyme induction. Cessation of smoking may result in increased levels of these drugs. Absorption of glutethimide may be decreased, and the "first pass" metabolism of propoxyphene may be decreased by smoking cessation. Other reported effects of smoking, which do not involve enzyme induction, include reduced diuretic effects of furosemide and decreased cardiac output, and increased blood pressure with propranolol, which may also relate to the hormonal effects of nicotine. Smoking cessation may reverse these actions.

Both smoking and nicotine can increase circulating cortisol and catecholamines. Therapy with adrenergic agonists or with adrenergic blockers may need to be adjusted according to changes in nicotine therapy or smoking status.

Carcinogenesis, Mutagenesis, Impairment of Fertility

Nicotine was not mutagenic in the Ames *Salmonella* test. Literature reports indicate that nicotine is neither an initiator nor a tumor-promoter in mice. There is inconclusive evidence to suggest that cotinine, an oxidized metabolite of nicotine, may be carcinogenic in rats. Cotinine was not mutagenic in the Ames *Salmonella* test.

Studies have shown a decrease of litter size in rats treated with nicotine during the time of fertilization.

Pregnancy

Pregnancy Category X. (See CONTRAINDICATIONS.)

Nursing Mothers

Nicotine passes freely into the breast milk. Because of the potential for serious adverse reactions in nursing infants from nicotine, a decision should be made whether to discontinue nursing or to discontinue the drug, taking into account the importance of the drug to the mother.

Pediatric Use

Safety and effectiveness in children and adolescents who smoke have not been evaluated.

ADVERSE REACTIONS

Adverse reactions reported in association with the use of Nicorette include both local effects and systemic effects representing the pharmacologic action of nicotine. Rare reports of an apparent severe allergic reaction have been received.

Local side effects

Mechanical effects of gum chewing include traumatic injury to oral mucosa or teeth, jaw ache, and eructation secondary to air swallowing. These side effects may be minimized by modifying chewing technique. Oral mucosal changes such as stomatitis, glossitis, gingivitis, pharyngitis, and aphthous ulcers, in addition to changes in taste perception, can occur during smoking cessation efforts with or without the use of Nicorette.

Systemic side effects

Although the systemic effects seen in trials were generally similar, the reported frequency of adverse drug effects was highly variable, as illustrated by the variation observed in adverse event incidences estimated from the results of two well controlled studies (one performed in the United States, and the other in England) designed to evaluate the safety and efficacy of Nicorette. (See table, below.) Given this variability, the table can be used only as an indication of the relative frequency of adverse events reported in representative clinical trials. It can not predict expected incidences of these effects during the course of usual medical practice.

[See table on next page].

The only potentially serious systemic adverse effect observed among the 152 patients evaluated in the controlled clinical trials used to support the efficacy of Nicorette was cardiac irritability: a patient displayed what may have been nicotine-induced, but reversible, atrial fibrillation. Cardiac irritability is a well known consequence of cigarette smoking. A 46-year-old male patient participating in a clinical trial of Nicorette was reported to have developed nicotine intoxication requiring his hospitalization. After 4 days, he was discharged, fully recovered. He died suddenly one month later. Nicorette was not used during this one-month interval. The relationship of the patient's death to his prior treatment is undetermined.

Since the marketing of Nicorette in the U.S., reports of several other deaths and reports including myocardial infarction, congestive heart failure, cerebrovascular accident and cardiac arrest have been received. A cause and effect relationship between these reports and the use of Nicorette has not been established.

In addition to the reported effects listed above, the following events have been reported: *CARDIOVASCULAR*—edema, flushing, hypertension, palpitations, tachyarrhythmias, tachycardia; *CNS*—confusion, convulsions, depression, euphoria, numbness, paresthesia, syncope, tinnitus, weakness; *DERMATOLOGIC*—erythema, itching, rash, urticaria; *GASTROINTESTINAL*—alteration of liver function tests, constipation, diarrhea; *RESPIRATORY*—breathing difficulty, cough, hoarseness, sneezing, wheezing; *OTHER*—dry mouth, systemic nicotine intoxication.

Rare reports of miscarriages have been received, and a relationship to drug therapy as a contributing factor cannot be excluded.

DRUG ABUSE AND DEPENDENCE

Dependence on the use of Nicorette gum has been reported. Such dependence may result from transference to Nicorette of tobacco-based nicotine dependence. The use of the Nicorette beyond three months has not been demonstrated to increase the smoking cessation rate. Use beyond 3 months should be discouraged. To minimize the risk of dependence, after 3 months' usage, patients should be encouraged to gradually withdraw over the next 3 months or stop gum usage altogether. (See DOSAGE AND ADMINISTRATION.) In patients who have used the gum for longer periods, gradual withdrawal should be instituted. (See PRECAUTIONS.)

OVERDOSAGE

Overdosage could occur if many pieces were chewed simultaneously or in rapid succession. Risk of poisoning by swallowing the gum is small because absorption in the absence of chewing is slow and incomplete. The consequences of overdose will most likely be minimized by the early nausea and vomiting known to occur with excessive nicotine intake. However, toxic systemic effects may occur. Should an overdose occur, the symptoms would be those of acute nicotine poisoning. Symptoms and signs include nausea, salivation, abdominal pain, vomiting, diarrhea, cold sweat, headache, dizziness, disturbed hearing and vision, mental confusion and marked weakness. Faintness and prostration will likely ensue and hypotension may occur; breathing is difficult; the pulse may be rapid, weak and irregular; circulatory collapse may be followed by terminal convulsions. Death may result within a few minutes from respiratory failure caused by paralysis of the muscles of respiration.

The oral LD_{50} for nicotine in rodents varies with species but is in excess of 24 mg/kg. Death in rodents was due to respiratory paralysis. The oral minimum lethal dose of nicotine in dogs is greater than 5 mg/kg. The oral minimum lethal dose for nicotine in human adults is 40–60 mg.

Under no circumstances should Nicorette be used in children.

TREATMENT OF OVERDOSAGE

In view of the lack of actual experience in the treatment of Nicorette overdose, the procedures recommended are those that have been suggested for the treatment of acute nicotine poisoning.

If emesis has not occurred, it should be induced with ipecac syrup in conscious patients. A saline cathartic will speed gastrointestinal passage of the gum. In unconscious patients with a secure airway, gastric lavage with a wide-bore tube followed by suspension of activated charcoal will aid in nicotine removal. Mechanical ventilation for respiratory paralysis may be necessary in severe nicotine poisoning. Hypotension and/or cardiovascular collapse may occur and should be treated vigorously.

DOSAGE AND ADMINISTRATION

Nicorette is an adjunct to smoking cessation programs (see INDICATION AND USAGE), and dosage should be individualized. A patient who is a candidate for Nicorette therapy must desire to stop smoking and should be instructed to *stop smoking immediately*. The patient should be given an instruction sheet on Nicorette gum chewing, and be allowed to read the instruction sheet and ask any questions. The patient should arrange for follow-up visits at intervals not greater than one month. At follow-up visits the patient's progress in smoking cessation should be determined and continued usage of Nicorette reassessed; successful abstainers at three months should stop using gum or gradually withdraw from gum usage. Patients who chew gum beyond a 3-month period should be considered as possibly using Nicorette as a substitute source of nicotine for their nicotine dependence. (See DRUG ABUSE AND DEPENDENCE.)

At the initial office or group visit, patients should be instructed to chew one piece of gum whenever they have the urge to smoke. Each piece should be chewed slowly and intermittently for about 30 minutes. The aim of this chewing is to promote even, slow, buccal absorption of the nicotine released from the buffered gum. Chewing quickly can release the nicotine too rapidly, leading to effects similar to oversmoking; e.g., nausea, hiccups or irritation of the throat.

As the nature of adverse effects experienced by an individual patient will be primarily related to the balance between the degree of nicotine tolerance and the rate and degree of absorption of nicotine from the gum, it is important for the patient to learn to chew the gum slowly and to self-titrate the nicotine dose, in order to minimize side effects. (SEE PATIENT INSTRUCTION SHEET AT END OF PRODUCT LABELING.)

Most patients require approximately 10 to 12 pieces of gum per day during the first month of treatment. Patients should be instructed not to exceed 30 Nicorette pieces per day. Patients should be assessed after one month of treatment to determine smoking status, and the use of Nicorette as an adjunct should be reevaluated. Gradual withdrawal from

Treatment Emergent
Symptom Incidence for the 2 mg Gum

	U.S.		British	
	Drug	Placebo	Drug	Placebo
Number of Subjects Reporting	94	95	58	58
Percent of Subjects Reporting				
Autonomic				
Excess Salivation	2.1	0.0		
CNS				
Insomnia	1.1	1.1		
Dizziness/Light-headedness	2.1	2.1	19.0	13.8
Irritable/Fussy	1.1	1.1		
Headache	1.1	5.3	24.1	29.3
Gastrointestinal				
Nonspecific GI Distress	9.6	6.3		
Eructation	6.4	1.1		
Indigestion			41.4	20.7
Nausea/Vomiting	18.1	4.2	31.0	15.5
Reactions Referable to Mouth, Throat, Jaw, or Teeth				
Mouth or Throat Soreness	37.2	31.6	56.9	53.4
Jaw Muscle Ache	18.1	9.5	44.8	44.8
Others				
Anorexia	1.1	1.1		
Hiccups	14.9	0.0	22.4	3.4

Nicorette should be initiated after 3 months' usage and completed by 6 months. The use of Nicorette beyond 6 months is not recommended.

Gradual Reduction Procedures

With Nicorette, as with cigarette smoking, the abrupt cessation of nicotine may result in withdrawal symptoms which may lead to a return to smoking. Therefore, Nicorette dosing should be gradually reduced. The suggested procedures for a gradual reduction of Nicorette include, but are not limited to, the following:

1. decrease the total number of pieces of Nicorette used per day by one or more pieces every 4 to 7 days,
2. decrease the chewing time with each piece of Nicorette from the normal 30 minutes to 10 or 15 minutes for 4 to 7 days then gradually decrease the total number of pieces used per day, while continuing the 10 or 15 minute chewing time,
3. substitute one or more pieces of sugarless gum for an equal number of pieces of Nicorette. The number of pieces of sugarless gum substituted for Nicorette should be increased every 4 to 7 days.

Combination or modification of the above procedures may be adjusted to the individual patient. Nicorette dosing may be stopped when usage has been reduced to one or two pieces per day.

Most patients in Nicorette assisted programs who resumed smoking have done so within six months of treatment. If necessary, a separate course of Nicorette may be prescribed at a later time for patients who continue or resume smoking.

HOW SUPPLIED

Nicorette is available in 2 mg (beige) square chewing pieces, packaged in child-resistant blister strips of 12 chewing pieces per strip with 8 strips per box.

Each chewing piece contains nicotine polacrilex equivalent to 2 mg nicotine.

Boxes of 96 chewing pieces, 2 mg (NDC 0068-0045-55). Store at room temperature, below 86°F (30°C). Protect from light.

Product Information as of September, 1988
Manufactured by Aktiebolaget Leo, Helsingborg, Sweden for
LAKESIDE PHARMACEUTICALS
Division of Merrell Dow Pharmaceuticals Inc.
Cincinnati, Ohio 45215, U.S.A.

NICORETTE®
(nicotine polacrilex)

INSTRUCTIONS FOR USE

You must read these instructions carefully before using Nicorette. While this pamphlet contains important information about Nicorette, it does not contain all information about the drug. If you have questions on the use of Nicorette, you should consult your physician.

WARNING TO FEMALE PATIENTS: NICORETTE CONTAINS NICOTINE WHICH MAY CAUSE FETAL HARM WHEN ADMINISTERED TO A PREGNANT WOMAN. DO NOT TAKE NICORETTE IF YOU ARE PREGNANT OR NURSING. TAKE PRECAUTIONS TO AVOID PREGNANCY WHILE USING NICORETTE, BUT IF YOU SUSPECT YOU ARE PREGNANT, STOP MEDICATION AND TELL YOUR DOCTOR AT ONCE.

THIS DRUG HAS BEEN PRESCRIBED FOR YOU BY YOUR PHYSICIAN. DO NOT LET ANYONE ELSE USE IT. KEEP THIS AND ALL OTHER DRUGS OUT OF THE REACH OF CHILDREN.

1. Starting now you must give up smoking completely. Gradually cutting down your tobacco consumption will not work. The continued use of cigarettes while using Nicorette gum will markedly decrease your chances of becoming a non-smoker and will increase the likelihood of adverse effects.
2. Your physician has prescribed Nicorette as part of a program to help you stop smoking.
3. Whenever you feel that you want to smoke, put *one* piece of gum into your mouth.
4. When you chew the gum properly, nicotine is slowly released and is absorbed through the lining of your mouth.
5. Chew the gum *very slowly* until you sense a peppery taste or feel a slight tingling in your mouth. (This is *usually* after about 15 chews—the number of chews is not the same for all people.) Because of its nicotine content, the gum does not taste like ordinary chewing gum.
6. As soon as you taste the gum, or feel the tingling, stop chewing and "park" the Nicorette between the cheek and gums.
7. After the taste or tingling is almost gone (about one minute), chew *slowly* again until the taste or tingling returns. Then stop chewing and "park" the gum again, using a different location in the mouth.
8. This procedure (repeated chewing and parking) should release most of the nicotine from each Nicorette in approximately 30 minutes.
9. Most people find that 10 to 12 pieces per day of 2 mg Nicorette are enough to control their urge to smoke. Depending on your needs, you can adjust the rate of chewing and the time between pieces. Not more than 30 pieces of 2 mg gum should be chewed in any one day.
10. **WARNING:** If you chew the gum too fast or too vigorously, you may get effects like people get when they inhale a cigarette for the first time, or when they smoke too fast. These effects include light-headedness, nausea and vomiting, throat and mouth irritation, hiccups, and stomach upset. Most of these side effects are controlled by chewing more slowly. See instructions above. Some other effects sometimes seen—particularly during the first few days of using gum—include mouth ulcers, jaw muscle ache, headaches, heart palpitations, and more than the usual amount of saliva in the mouth. In addition, the mechanical effects of gum chewing (any gum) include traumatic injury to oral mucosa or teeth, jaw ache and belching from swallowing air. These side effects may be minimized by proper chewing technique (see steps 5 through 8 above). *There are other side effects which have been infrequently reported with the use of Nicorette. Your physician can answer questions you may have as to possible side effects. Report any disturbing symptoms to your doctor.*
11. If you accidentally swallow a piece of gum, you ordinarily should not experience adverse effects. However, if you do experience adverse effects, call your doctor. Overdosage could occur if many pieces are chewed simultaneously or in rapid succession. IN CASE OF ACCIDENTAL OVERDOSE OR IF A CHILD CHEWS OR SWALLOWS ONE OR MORE PIECES OF THE GUM, YOU

Continued on next page

Information on Lakeside Pharmaceuticals products is based on labeling in effect in June, 1989.

Lakeside—Cont.

SHOULD CONTACT YOUR PHYSICIAN OR LOCAL POISON CONTROL CENTER IMMEDIATELY.

12. As your urge to smoke fades, gradually reduce the number of pieces of gum you chew each day. This may be possible within 2 to 3 months. WARNING: DEPENDENCE ON THE USE OF NICORETTE GUM HAS BEEN REPORTED. SUCH DEPENDENCE MAY OCCUR WHEN PATIENTS WHO ARE DEPENDENT ON THE NICOTINE IN TOBACCO TRANSFER THAT DEPENDENCE TO THE NICOTINE IN NICORETTE GUM. Unless your physician tells you otherwise, stop using the gum when your craving is satisfied with 1 or 2 pieces a day, and do not use the gum for more than 6 months.

13. Remember to carry the gum with you at all times in case you feel the sudden urge to smoke again. DO NOT FORGET THAT ONE CIGARETTE IS ENOUGH TO START YOU ON THE SMOKING HABIT AGAIN.

PLEASE NOTE

Nicorette is sugar-free and has been formulated to minimize stickiness. As with other gums, however, the degree to which Nicorette may stick to your dentures, dental caps or partial bridges may depend on the materials from which they are made and other factors. Should an excessive degree of stickiness to your dental work occur, there is the possibility that as with other gums, Nicorette may damage dental work, and you should discontinue its use and consult your physician or dentist.

To remove the gum, tear off single unit.　　Peel off backing starting at corner with loose edge.　　Push gum through foil.

Store at room temperature, below 86°F (30°C). Remember, the trunk and glove compartments of your car can reach temperatures much higher than this in the summer. Also, you should protect the gum from light.

NOVAFED® Capsules ℞
[nō'vă-fĕd]
(pseudoephedrine hydrochloride)
Controlled-Release Decongestant

CAUTION: Federal law prohibits dispensing without prescription.

DESCRIPTION

Each Novafed capsule contains 120 mg of pseudoephedrine hydrochloride in specially formulated pellets designed to provide continuous therapeutic effect for 12 hours. About one-half of the active ingredient is released soon after administration and the rest slowly over the remaining time period. Each capsule also contains as inactive ingredients: corn starch, FD&C Blue No. 1, FD&C Red No. 3, FD&C Yellow No. 6, gelatin, sucrose, titanium dioxide, and other ingredients.

ACTIONS

Pseudoephedrine (a sympathomimetic) is an orally effective nasal decongestant with peripheral effects similar to epinephrine and central effects similar to, but less intense than, amphetamines. It has the potential for excitatory side effects. At the recommended oral dosage, it has little or no pressor effect in normotensive adults. Patients have not been reported to experience the rebound congestion sometimes experienced with frequent, repeated use of topical decongestants.

INDICATIONS

Relief of nasal congestion or eustachian tube congestion. May be given concomitantly with analgesics, antihistamines, expectorants and antibiotics.

CONTRAINDICATIONS

Patients with severe hypertension, severe coronary artery disease, and patients on MAO inhibitor therapy. Also contraindicated in patients with hypersensitivity or idiosyncrasy to sympathomimetic amines which may be manifested by insomnia, dizziness, weakness, tremor or arrhythmias.
Children under 12: Should not be used by children under 12 years.
Nursing Mothers: Contraindicated because of the higher than usual risk for infants from sympathomimetic amines.

WARNINGS

Use judiciously and sparingly in patients with hypertension, diabetes mellitus, ischemic heart disease, increased intraocular pressure, hyperthyroidism, or prostatic hypertrophy. See, however, Contraindications. Sympathomimetics may produce central nervous stimulation with convulsions or cardiovascular collapse with accompanying hypotension.

Do not exceed recommended dosage.
Use in Pregnancy: Safety in pregnancy has not been established.
Use in Elderly: The elderly (60 years and older) are more likely to have adverse reactions to sympathomimetics. Overdosage of sympathomimetics in the elderly may cause hallucinations, convulsions, CNS depression, and death. Safe use of a short-acting sympathomimetic should be demonstrated in the individual elderly patient before considering the use of a sustained-action formulation.

PRECAUTIONS

Patients with diabetes, hypertension, cardiovascular disease and hyper-reactivity to ephedrine.

ADVERSE REACTIONS

Hyper-reactive individuals may display ephedrine-like reactions such as tachycardia, palpitations, headache, dizziness or nausea. Sympathomimetics have been associated with certain untoward reactions including fear, anxiety, tenseness, restlessness, tremor, weakness, pallor, respiratory difficulty, dysuria, insomnia, hallucinations, convulsions, CNS depression, arrhythmias, and cardiovascular collapse with hypotension.

DRUG INTERACTIONS

MAO inhibitors and beta adrenergic blockers increase the effects of pseudoephedrine. Sympathomimetics may reduce the antihypertensive effects of methyldopa, mecamylamine, reserpine and veratrum alkaloids.

DOSAGE AND ADMINISTRATION

One capsule every 12 hours. Do not give to children under 12 years of age.

HOW SUPPLIED

Brown and orange colored hard gelatin capsules with the identification code ___ or NOVAFED. Bottle of 100 capsules (NDC 0068-0104-61).
Product Information as of May, 1986
Manufactured by KV Pharmaceutical Company
St. Louis, Mo. 63144 for
LAKESIDE PHARMACEUTICALS
Division of Merrell Dow Pharmaceuticals Inc.
Cincinnati, Ohio 45215, U.S.A.
Shown in Product Identification Section, page 413

NOVAFED® A Capsules ℞
[nō'vă-fĕd]
Controlled-Release
Decongestant plus Antihistamine

CAUTION: Federal law prohibits dispensing without prescription.

DESCRIPTION

Each Novafed A capsule for oral use contains 120 mg pseudoephedrine hydrochloride and 8 mg chlorpheniramine maleate. The specially formulated pellets in each capsule are designed to provide continuous therapeutic effect for 12 hours. About one-half of the active ingredients is released soon after administration and the remainder is released slowly over the remaining time period. Each capsule also contains as inactive ingredients: calcium stearate, corn starch, FD&C Blue No. 1, FD&C Red No. 3, FD&C Yellow No. 6, gelatin, pharmaceutical glaze, povidone, sucrose, talc, titanium dioxide, and other ingredients.
Pseudoephedrine hydrochloride is a nasal decongestant. Chemically it is α-[1-(methylamino) ethyl]-[S-(R*, R*)]-benzenemethanol hydrochloride with the following structure:

Chlorpheniramine maleate is an antihistamine. Chemically it is γ-(4-chlorophenyl)-N,N-dimethyl-2-pyridinepropanamine with the following structure:

CLINICAL PHARMACOLOGY

Pseudoephedrine is an orally active sympathomimetic amine and exerts a decongestant action on the nasal mucosa. Pseudoephedrine produces peripheral effects similar to those of ephedrine and central effects similar to, but less intense than amphetamines. It has the potential for excitatory side effects. At the recommended oral dosages it has little or no pressor effect in normotensive adults. The serum half-life (T 1/2) of pseudoephedrine is approximately 4 to 6

hours. T 1/2 is decreased with increased excretion of drug at urine pH lower than 6 and may be increased with decreased excretion at urine pH higher than 8.
Chlorpheniramine is an antihistaminic that possesses anticholinergic and sedative effects. It is considered one of the most effective and least toxic of the histamine antagonists. Chlorpheniramine is an H_1 receptor antagonist. It antagonizes many of the pharmacologic actions of histamine. It prevents released histamine from dilating capillaries and causing edema of the respiratory mucosa. Chlorpheniramine has a duration of action of 4 to 6 hours in clinical studies. Its half-life in serum, however, is 12 to 16 hours.

INDICATIONS AND USAGE

Relief of nasal congestion and eustachian tube congestion associated with the common cold, sinusitis and acute upper respiratory infections. It is also indicated for perennial and seasonal allergic rhinitis, vasomotor rhinitis, allergic conjunctivitis due to inhalant allergens and foods and for mild, uncomplicated allergic skin manifestations of urticaria and angioedema. Decongestants in combination with antihistamines have been used for many years to relieve eustachian tube congestion associated with acute eustachian salpingitis, aerotitis media, acute otitis media and serous otitis media. May be given concomitant with analgesics and antibiotics.

CONTRAINDICATIONS

Patients with severe hypertension, severe coronary artery disease, and in patients on MAO inhibitor therapy. Antihistamines are contraindicated in patients with narrow-angle glaucoma, urinary retention, peptic ulcer, during an asthmatic attack, and in patients receiving MAO inhibitors.
Hypersensitivity: Contraindicated in patients with hypersensitivity or idiosyncrasy to sympathomimetic amines or phenanthrene derivatives.
Nursing Mothers: Contraindicated because of the higher than usual risk for infants from sympathomimetic amines.

WARNINGS

Sympathomimetic amines should be used judiciously and sparingly in patients with hypertension, diabetes mellitus, ischemic heart disease, increased intraocular pressure, hyperthyroidism, or prostatic hypertrophy (see CONTRAINDICATIONS). Sympathomimetics may produce CNS stimulation and convulsions or cardiovascular collapse with accompanying hypotension.
Chlorpheniramine maleate has an atropine-like action and should be used with caution in patients with increased intraocular pressure, cardiovascular disease, hypertension or in patients with a history of bronchial asthma (see CONTRAINDICATIONS). Do not exceed recommended dose.
Use in Elderly: The elderly (60 years and older) are more likely to have adverse reactions to sympathomimetics. Overdosage of sympathomimetics in this age group may cause hallucinations, convulsions, CNS depression and death.

PRECAUTIONS

General: Should be used with caution in patients with diabetes, hypertension, cardiovascular disease and hyperreactivity to ephedrine. The antihistaminic may cause drowsiness and ambulatory patients who operate machinery or motor vehicles should be cautioned accordingly.
Information for Patients: Antihistamines may impair mental and physical abilities required for the performance of potentially hazardous tasks, such as driving a vehicle or operating machinery and mental alertness in children.
Drug Interactions: MAO inhibitors and beta adrenergic blockers increase the effect of sympathomimetics. Sympathomimetics may reduce the antihypertensive effects of methyldopa, mecamylamine, reserpine and veratrum alkaloids. Concomitant use of antihistamines with alcohol, tricyclic antidepressants, barbiturates and other CNS depressants may have an additive effect.
Pregnancy Category C: Animal reproduction studies have not been conducted with Novafed A capsules. It is also not known whether Novafed A capsules can cause fetal harm when administered to a pregnant woman or can affect reproduction capacity. Novafed A capsules may be given to a pregnant woman only if clearly needed.
Nursing Mothers: Pseudoephedrine is contraindicated in nursing mothers because of the higher than usual risk for infants from sympathomimetic amines.

ADVERSE REACTIONS

Hyperreactive individuals may display ephedrine-like reactions such as tachycardia, palpitations, headache, dizziness, or nausea. Patients sensitive to antihistamines may experience mild sedation. Sympathomimetic drugs have been associated with certain untoward reactions including fear, anxiety, tenseness, restlessness, tremor, weakness, pallor, respiratory difficulty, dysuria, insomnia, hallucinations, convulsions, CNS depression, arrhythmias, and cardiovascular collapse with hypotension.
Possible side effects of antihistamines are drowsiness, restlessness, dizziness, weakness, dry mouth, anorexia, nausea, headache, nervousness, blurring of vision, heartburn, dysuria and very rarely dermatitis. Patient idiosyncrasy to ad-

renergic agents may be manifested by insomnia, dizziness, weakness, tremor or arrhythmias.

OVERDOSAGE

Acute overdosage with Novafed A capsules may produce clinical signs of CNS stimulation and variable cardiovascular effects. Pressor amines should be used with great caution in the presence of pseudoephedrine. Patients with signs of stimulation should be treated conservatively.

DOSAGE AND ADMINISTRATION

One capsule every 12 hours. Do not give to children under 12 years of age.

HOW SUPPLIED

Novafed A is supplied in red and orange-colored hard gelatin capsules monogrammed with the Dow diamond followed by the number 106 or NOVAFED A, in bottles of 100 capsules (NDC 0068-0106-61).

Product Information as of April, 1986
Manufactured by KV Pharmaceutical Company
St. Louis, Mo. 63144 for
LAKESIDE PHARMACEUTICALS
Division of Merrell Dow Pharmaceuticals Inc.
Cincinnati, Ohio 45215, U.S.A.
Shown in Product Identification Section, page 413

NOVAHISTINE® DH ©
[nō"vă-hĭs'tēn]
Antitussive-Decongestant-Antihistamine

DESCRIPTION

Each 5 ml teaspoonful contains Codeine Phosphate, 10 mg (Warning: may be habit forming), Pseudoephedrine Hydrochloride, 30 mg, Chlorpheniramine Maleate, 2 mg. Also contains: Alcohol, 5%, FD&C Blue No. 1, FD&C Red No. 40, Flavors, Glycerin, Hydrochloric Acid, Invert Sugar, Saccharin Sodium, Sodium Chloride, Sorbitol, and Water.

ACTIONS

Antitussive, decongestant and antihistaminic actions. Codeine, at the recommended dose, causes suppression of the cough reflex by a direct effect on the cough center in the medulla of the brain. Codeine has antitussive, mild analgesic and sedative effects.
Pseudoephedrine hydrochloride, an orally effective nasal decongestant, is a sympathomimetic amine with peripheral effects similar to epinephrine and central effects similar to, but less intense than, amphetamines. Therefore, it has the potential for excitatory side effects. Pseudoephedrine at the recommended oral dosage has little or no pressor effect in normotensive adults. Patients taking pseudoephedrine orally have not been reported to experience the rebound congestion sometimes experienced with frequent, repeated use of topical decongestants. Pseudoephedrine is not known to produce drowsiness.
Chlorpheniramine possesses antihistaminic, mild anticholinergic and sedative effects. It antagonizes many of the pharmacologic actions of histamine. It prevents released histamine from dilating capillaries and causing edema of the respiratory mucosa.

INDICATIONS

For the temporary relief of cough associated with minor throat and bronchial irritation or nasal congestion due to the common cold, sinusitis, and hay fever (allergic rhinitis).
A minimum dosage of codeine is provided for the symptomatic relief of nonproductive cough. Decongestants have been used to relieve eustachian salpingitis, aerotitis, otitis, and serous otitis media. Chlorpheniramine maleate provides temporary relief from runny nose, sneezing, itching of nose or throat, and itchy and watery eyes as may occur in hay fever (allergic rhinitis).
May be used as supportive therapy for acute otitis media and relief of mild otalgia.
May be given concomitantly, when indicated, with analgesics and antibiotics.

CONTRAINDICATIONS

Patients with severe hypertension, severe coronary artery disease, and in patients on MAO inhibitor therapy.
Nursing Mothers: Pseudoephedrine is contraindicated in nursing mothers because of the higher than usual risk for infants from sympathomimetic amines.
Hypersensitivity: This drug is contraindicated in patients with hypersensitivity or idiosyncrasy to its ingredients. Patient idiosyncrasy to adrenergic agents may be manifested by insomnia, dizziness, weakness, tremor or arrhythmias.

WARNINGS

Codeine should be prescribed and administered with the same degree of caution as all oral medications containing a narcotic analgesic. Codeine appears in the milk of nursing mothers.
If sympathomimetic amines are used in patients with hypertension, diabetes mellitus, ischemic heart disease, hyperthyroidism, increased intraocular pressure or prostatic hypertrophy, judicious caution should be exercised. See, however,

Contraindications. Sympathomimetics may produce CNS stimulation with convulsions or cardiovascular collapse with accompanying hypotension. Do not exceed recommended dosage.
The elderly (60 years and older) are more likely to have adverse reactions to sympathomimetics. Safety for use during pregnancy has not been established.
Antihistamines may cause excitability, especially in children.

PRECAUTIONS

If cough persists for more than one week, tends to recur or is accompanied by fever, rash or headache, discontinue treatment. Other medications containing a narcotic analgesic, phenothiazines, tranquilizers, sedatives, hypnotics and other CNS depressants, including alcohol, may have an additive CNS depressant effect when used concomitantly. The dose should be reduced when such combined therapy is contemplated.
Caution should be exercised if used in patients with high blood pressure, heart disease, asthma, emphysema, diabetes, thyroid disease and hyperreactivity to ephedrine.
The antihistamine may cause drowsiness, and ambulatory patients who operate machinery or motor vehicles should be cautioned accordingly.

ADVERSE REACTIONS

Nausea, vomiting, constipation, dizziness, sedation, palpitations or pruritus may occur. More frequent or higher than recommended dosage may cause respiratory depression, especially in patients with respiratory disease associated with carbon dioxide retention.
Drugs containing sympathomimetic amines have been associated with certain untoward reactions including fear, anxiety, tenseness, restlessness, tremor, weakness, pallor, respiratory difficulty, dysuria, insomnia, hallucinations, convulsions, CNS depression, arrhythmias and cardiovascular collapse with hypotension.
Patients sensitive to antihistamine drugs may experience mild sedation. Other side effects from antihistamines may include dry mouth, dizziness, weakness, anorexia, nausea, vomiting, headache, nervousness, polyuria, heartburn, diplopia, dysuria, and very rarely, dermatitis.

DRUG INTERACTIONS

Codeine may potentiate the effects of other narcotics, general anesthetics, tranquilizers, sedatives and hypnotics, tricyclic antidepressants, MAO inhibitors, alcohol and other CNS depressants.
Beta adrenergic blockers and MAO inhibitors potentiate the sympathomimetic effects of pseudoephedrine. Sympathomimetics may reduce the antihypertensive effects of methyldopa, mecamylamine, reserpine and veratrum alkaloids.
Antihistamines have been shown to enhance one or more of the effects of alcohol, tricyclic antidepressants, barbiturates and other CNS depressants.

DOSAGE

Adults, 2 teaspoonfuls; children 50–90 lbs, ½ to 1 teaspoonful; 25–50 lbs, ¼ to ½ teaspoonful. Repeat every 4 to 6 hours. May be given to children under 2 at the discretion of the physician. *Do not exceed 4 doses in a 24-hour period.*
Product label dosage is as follows: Adults and children 12 years and older, 2 teaspoonfuls every 4 to 6 hours. Children 6 to under 12 years, 1 teaspoonful every 4 to 6 hours. Do not exceed 4 doses in 24 hours. For children under 6 years, give only as directed by a physician.

HOW SUPPLIED

In 4 fluid ounce bottles (NDC 0068-1027-04), and pints (NDC 0068-1027-16).
Product Information as of May, 1986
Shown in Product Identification Section, page 413

NOVAHISTINE® DMX
[nō"vă-hĭs'tēn]
Antitussive-Decongestant-Expectorant
Liquid

(See PDR For Nonprescription Drugs)

NOVAHISTINE® ELIXIR
[nō"vă-hĭs'tēn]
Decongestant—Antihistaminic

(See PDR For Nonprescription Drugs)

NOVAHISTINE® EXPECTORANT ©
[nō"vă-hĭs'tēn]
Antitussive-Decongestant-Expectorant

DESCRIPTION

Each 5 ml teaspoonful contains Codeine Phosphate, 10 mg (Warning: may be habit forming), Pseudoephedrine Hydrochloride, 30 mg, Guaifenesin (glyceryl guaiacolate), 100 mg. Also contains: Alcohol, 7.5%, D&C Yellow No. 10, FD&C

Blue No. 1, FD&C Red No. 40, Flavors, Glycerin, Hydrochloric Acid, Invert Sugar, Saccharin Sodium, Sodium Chloride, Sodium Gluconate, Sorbitol, and Water.

ACTIONS

Expectorant, antitussive and decongestant actions. Codeine, at the recommended dose, causes suppression of the cough reflex by a direct effect on the cough center in the medulla of the brain. Codeine has antitussive and mild analgesic and sedative effects.
Pseudoephedrine hydrochloride, an orally effective nasal decongestant, is a sympathomimetic amine with peripheral effects similar to epinephrine and central effects similar to, but less intense than, amphetamines. Therefore, it has the potential for excitatory side effects. Pseudoephedrine at the recommended oral dosage has little or no pressor effect in normotensive adults. Patients taking pseudoephedrine orally have not been reported to experience the rebound congestion sometimes experienced with frequent, repeated use of topical decongestants. Pseudoephedrine is not known to produce drowsiness.
Guaifenesin helps drainage of bronchial tubes by thinning the mucus, and facilitates expectoration by loosening phlegm and bronchial secretions.

INDICATIONS

For loosening tenacious pulmonary secretions associated with cough and respiratory congestion.
A minimum dosage of codeine phosphate is provided for the symptomatic relief of nonproductive cough. Decongestants have been used to relieve eustachian tube congestion associated with acute eustachian salpingitis, aerotitis, otitis and serous otitis media. Guaifenesin helps loosen phlegm (sputum) and bronchial secretions.
May be used as supportive therapy for acute otitis media and relief of mild otalgia.
May be given concomitantly, when indicated, with analgesics and antibiotics.

CONTRAINDICATIONS

Patients with severe hypertension, severe coronary artery disease, and in patients on MAO inhibitor therapy.
Nursing Mothers: Pseudoephedrine is contraindicated in nursing mothers because of the higher than usual risk for infants from sympathomimetic amines.
Hypersensitivity: This drug is contraindicated in patients with hypersensitivity or idiosyncrasy to its ingredients. Patient idiosyncrasy to adrenergic agents may be manifested by insomnia, dizziness, weakness, tremor or arrhythmias.

WARNINGS

Codeine should be prescribed and administered with the same degree of caution as all oral medications containing a narcotic analgesic. Codeine appears in the milk of nursing mothers.
If sympathomimetic amines are used in patients with hypertension, diabetes mellitus, ischemic heart disease, hyperthyroidism, increased intraocular pressure and prostatic hypertrophy, judicious caution should be exercised. See, however, Contraindications. Sympathomimetics may produce CNS stimulation with convulsions or cardiovascular collapse with accompanying hypotension. Do not exceed recommended dosage.
The elderly (60 years and older) are more likely to have adverse reactions to sympathomimetics. Safety for use during pregnancy has not been established.

PRECAUTIONS

If cough persists for more than one week, tends to recur or is accompanied by fever, rash or headache, discontinue treatment.
Other medications containing a narcotic analgesic, phenothiazines, tranquilizers, sedatives, hypnotics, and other CNS depressants, including alcohol, may have an additive CNS depressant effect when used concomitantly. The dose should be reduced when such combined therapy is contemplated.
Caution should be exercised if used in patients with high blood pressure, heart disease, asthma, emphysema, diabetes, thyroid disease and hyperreactivity to ephedrine.

ADVERSE REACTIONS

Nausea, vomiting, constipation, dizziness, sedation, palpitations, or pruritus may occur. More frequent or higher than recommended dosage may cause respiratory depression, especially in patients with respiratory disease associated with carbon dioxide retention.
Drugs containing sympathomimetic amines have been associated with certain untoward reactions including fear, anxiety, tenseness, restlessness, tremor, weakness, pallor, respiratory difficulty, dysuria, insomnia, hallucinations, convulsions, CNS depression, arrhythmias and cardiovascular collapse with hypotension.

Continued on next page

Lakeside—Cont.

Note: Guaifenesin interferes with the colorimetric determination of 5-hydroxyindoleacetic acid (5-HIAA) and vanillylmandelic acid (VMA).

DRUG INTERACTIONS

Codeine may potentiate the effects of other narcotics, general anesthetics, tranquilizers, sedatives and hypnotics, tricyclic antidepressants, MAO inhibitors, alcohol and other CNS depressants.

Beta adrenergic blockers and MAO inhibitors potentiate the sympathomimetic effects of pseudoephedrine. Sympathomimetics may reduce the antihypertensive effects of methyldopa, mecamylamine, reserpine and veratrum alkaloids.

DOSAGE

Adults, 2 teaspoonfuls; children 50–90 lbs, $\frac{1}{2}$ to 1 teaspoonful; 25–50 lbs, $\frac{1}{4}$ to $\frac{1}{2}$ teaspoonful. Repeat every 4 to 6 hours. May be given to children under 2 at the discretion of the physician. *Do not exceed 4 doses in a 24-hour period.* Product label dosage is as follows: Adults and children 12 years and older, 2 teaspoonfuls every 4 to 6 hours. Children 6 to under 12 years, 1 teaspoonful every 4 to 6 hours. Do not exceed 4 doses in 24 hours. For children under 6 years, give only as directed by a physician.

HOW SUPPLIED

As a liquid in 4 fluid ounce bottles (NDC 0068-1028-04) and pints (NDC 0068-1028-16).

Product Information as of May, 1986
Shown in Product Identification Section, page 413

SINGLET®
[sĭn 'glĕt]
Long-Acting Tablets
Decongestant-Antihistamine-Analgesic

(See PDR For Nonprescription Drugs)

TENUATE®   Ⓒ   ℞
[tĕn 'ū-āt]
(diethylpropion hydrochloride USP)
TENUATE DOSPAN®   Ⓒ   ℞
(diethylpropion hydrochloride USP)
controlled-release
75 mg tablets

CAUTION: Federal law prohibits dispensing without prescription.

DESCRIPTION

Tenuate is available for oral administration in immediate-release tablets containing 25 mg diethylpropion hydrochloride and in controlled-release tablets containing 75 mg diethylpropion hydrochloride. The inactive ingredients in each immediate-release tablet are: corn starch, lactose, magnesium stearate, pregelatinized corn starch, talc, and tartaric acid. The inactive ingredients in each controlled-release tablet are: carbomer 934P, mannitol, povidone, tartaric acid, zinc stearate. Diethylpropion hydrochloride is a sympathomimetic agent. The chemical name for diethylpropion hydrochloride is 1-phenyl-2-diethylamino-1-propanone hydrochloride.

Its chemical structure is:

$$CH_3CHC \cdots \text{(phenyl ring)} \qquad \cdot HCl$$
$$\underset{N(C_2H_5)_2}{\overset{O}{\|}}$$

In Tenuate Dospan tablets, diethylpropion hydrochloride is dispersed in a hydrophilic matrix. On exposure to water, the diethylpropion hydrochloride is released at a relatively uniform rate as a result of slow hydration of the matrix. The result is controlled release of the anorectic agent.

CLINICAL PHARMACOLOGY

Diethylpropion hydrochloride is a sympathomimetic amine with some pharmacologic activity similar to that of the prototype drugs of this class used in obesity, the amphetamines. Actions include some central nervous system stimulation and elevation of blood pressure. Tolerance has been demonstrated with all drugs of this class in which these phenomena have been looked for.

Drugs of this class used in obesity are commonly known as "anorectics" or "anorexigenics." It has not been established, however, that the action of such drugs in treating obesity is primarily one of appetite suppression. For example, other central nervous system actions or metabolic effects may be involved.

Adult obese subjects instructed in dietary management and treated with "anorectic" drugs lose more weight on the average than those treated with placebo and diet, as determined in relatively short-term clinical trials.

The magnitude of increased weight loss of drug-treated patients over placebo-treated patients averages some fraction of a pound a week. However, individual weight loss may vary substantially from patient to patient. The rate of weight loss is greatest in the first weeks of therapy for both drug and placebo subjects and tends to decrease in succeeding weeks. The possible origins of the increased weight loss due to the various drug effects are not established. The amount of weight loss associated with the use of an "anorectic" drug varies from trial to trial, and the increased weight loss appears to be related in part to variables other than the drug prescribed, such as the physician/investigator relationship, the population treated, and the diet prescribed. Studies do not permit conclusions as to the relative importance of the drug and non-drug factors on weight loss.

The natural history of obesity is measured in years, whereas most studies cited are restricted to a few weeks duration; thus, the total impact of drug-induced weight loss over that of diet alone is unknown.

Diethylpropion is rapidly absorbed from the GI tract after oral administration and is extensively metabolized through a complex pathway of biotransformation involving N-dealkylation and reduction. Many of these metabolites are biologically active and may participate in the therapeutic action of Tenuate or Tenuate Dospan. Due to the varying lipid solubilities of these metabolites, their circulating levels are affected by urinary pH. Diethylpropion and/or its active metabolites are believed to cross the blood-brain barrier and the placenta.

Diethylpropion and its metabolites are excreted mainly by the kidney. It has been reported that between 75–106% of the dose is recovered in the urine within 48 hours after dosing. Using a phosphorescence assay that is specific for basic compounds containing a benzoyl group, the plasma half-life of the aminoketone metabolites is estimated to be between 4 to 6 hours.

The controlled-release characteristics of Tenuate Dospan have been demonstrated by studies in humans in which plasma levels of diethylpropion-related materials were measured by phosphorescence analysis. Plasma levels obtained with the 75 mg Dospan formulation administered once daily indicated a more gradual release than the immediate-release formulation (three 25 mg tablets given in a single dose). Tenuate Dospan has not been shown superior in effectiveness to the same dosage of the immediate-release formulation (one 25 mg tablet three times daily). After administration of a single dose of Tenuate Dospan (one 75 mg controlled-release tablet) or diethylpropion hydrochloride solution (75 mg dose) in a crossover study using normal human subjects, the amount of parent compound and its active metabolites recovered in the urine within 48 hours for the two dosage forms were not statistically different.

INDICATIONS AND USAGE

Tenuate and Tenuate Dospan are indicated in the management of exogenous obesity as a short-term adjunct (a few weeks) in a regimen of weight reduction based on caloric restriction. The usefulness of agents of this class (see CLINICAL PHARMACOLOGY) should be measured against possible risk factors inherent in their use such as those described below.

CONTRAINDICATIONS

Advanced arteriosclerosis, hyperthyroidism, known hypersensitivity, or idiosyncrasy to the sympathomimetic amines, glaucoma, severe hypertension. (See PRECAUTIONS.) Agitated states.

Patients with a history of drug abuse.

During or within 14 days following the administration of monoamine oxidase inhibitors, hypertensive crises may result.

WARNINGS

If tolerance develops, the recommended dose should not be exceeded in an attempt to increase the effect; rather, the drug should be discontinued. Tenuate or Tenuate Dospan may impair the ability of the patient to engage in potentially hazardous activities such as operating machinery or driving a motor vehicle; the patient should therefore be cautioned accordingly.

When central nervous system active agents are used, consideration must always be given to the possibility of adverse interactions with alcohol.

PRECAUTIONS
General

Caution is to be exercised in prescribing Tenuate or Tenuate Dospan for patients with hypertension or with symptomatic cardiovascular disease, including arrhythmias. Tenuate or Tenuate Dospan should not be administered to patients with severe hypertension.

Reports suggest that diethylpropion hydrochloride may increase convulsions in some epileptics. Therefore, epileptics receiving Tenuate of Tenuate Dospan should be carefully monitored. Titration of dose or discontinuance of Tenuate or Tenuate Dospan may be necessary.

The least amount feasible should be prescribed or dispensed at one time in order to minimize the possibility of overdosage.

Information for Patient

The patient should be cautioned about concomitant use of alcohol or other CNS-active drugs and Tenuate or Tenuate Dospan. (See WARNINGS.) The patient should be advised to observe caution when driving or engaging in any potentially hazardous activity.

Laboratory Tests

None

Drug Interactions

Antidiabetic drug requirements (i.e., insulin) may be altered. Concurrent use with general anesthetics may result in arrhythmias. The pressor effects of diethylpropion and those of other drugs may be additive when the drugs are used concomitantly; conversely, diethylpropion may interfere with antihypertensive drugs (i.e., guanethidine, α-methyldopa). Concurrent use of phenothiazines may antagonize the anorectic effect of dietylpropion.

CARCINOGENESIS, MUTAGENESIS, AND IMPAIRMENT OF FERTILITY

No long-term studies have been done to evaluate diethylpropion hydrochloride for carcinogenicity. Mutagenicity studies have not been conducted. Animal reproduction studies revealed no evidence of impairment of fertility (see Pregnancy).

Pregnancy

TERATOGENIC EFFECTS: PREGNANCY CATEGORY B

Reproduction studies have been performed in rats at doses up to 9 times the human dose and have revealed no evidence of impaired fertility or harm to the fetus due to diethylpropion hydrochloride. There are, however, no adequate and well-controlled studies in pregnant women. Because animal reproduction studies are not always predictive of human response, this drug should be used during pregnancy only if clearly needed.

NON-TERATOGENIC EFFECTS

Abuse with diethylpropion hydrochloride during pregnancy may result in withdrawal symptoms in the human neonate.

NURSING MOTHERS

Since diethylpropion hydrochloride and/or its metabolites have been shown to be excreted in human milk, caution should be exercised when Tenuate or Tenuate Dospan is administered to a nursing woman.

PEDIATRIC USE

Since safety and effectiveness in children below the age of 12 have not been established, Tenuate or Tenuate Dospan is *not* recommended for use in children under 12 years of age.

ADVERSE REACTIONS

Cardiovascular: Precordial pain, arrhythmia, ECG changes, tachycardia, elevation of blood pressure, palpitation.

Central Nervous System: In a few epileptics an increase in convulsive episodes has been reported; rarely psychotic episodes at recommended doses; dyskinesia, blurred vision, overstimulation, nervousness, restlessness, dizziness, jitteriness, insomnia, anxiety, euphoria, depression, dysphoria, tremor, mydriasis, drowsiness, malaise, headache.

Gastrointestinal: Vomiting, diarrhea, abdominal discomfort, dryness of the mouth, unpleasant taste, nausea, constipation, other gastrointestinal disturbances.

Allergic: Urticaria, rash, ecchymosis, erythema.

Endocrine: Impotence, changes in libido, gynecomastia, menstrual upset.

Hematopoietic System: Bone marrow depression, agranulocytosis, leukopenia.

Miscellaneous: A variety of miscellaneous adverse reactions has been reported by physicians. These include complaints such as dysuria, dyspnea, hair loss, muscle pain, increased sweating, and polyuria.

DRUG ABUSE AND DEPENDENCE

Tenuate and Tenuate Dospan are schedule IV controlled substances. Diethylpropion hydrochloride has some chemical and pharmacologic similarities to the amphetamines and other related stimulant drugs that have been extensively abused. There have been reports of subjects becoming psychologically dependent on diethylpropion. The possibility of abuse should be kept in mind when evaluating the desirability of including a drug as part of a weight reduction program. Abuse of amphetamines and related drugs may be associated with varying degrees of psychologic dependence and social dysfunction which, in the case of certain drugs, may be severe. There are reports of patients who have increased the dosage to many times that recommended. Abrupt cessation following prolonged high dosage administration results in extreme fatigue and mental depression; changes are also noted on the sleep EEG. Manifestations of chronic intoxication with anorectic drugs include severe dermatoses, marked insomnia, irritability, hyperactivity, and personality changes. The most severe manifestation of chronic intoxication is psychosis, often clinically indistinguishable from schizophrenia.

OVERDOSAGE

Manifestations of acute overdosage include restlessness, tremor, hyperreflexia, rapid respiration, confusion, assaultiveness, hallucinations, panic states.

Fatigue and depression usually follow the central stimulation.

Cardiovascular effects include arrhythmias, hypertension or hypotension and circulatory collapse. Gastrointestinal symptoms include nausea, vomiting, diarrhea, and abdominal cramps. Overdosage of pharmacologically similar compounds has resulted in convulsions, coma and death.

The reported oral LD_{50} for mice is 600 mg/kg, for rats is 250 mg/kg and for dogs is 225 mg/kg.

Management of acute diethylpropion hydrochloride intoxication is largely symptomatic and includes lavage and sedation with a barbiturate. Experience with hemodialysis or peritoneal dialysis is inadequate to permit recommendation in this regard. Intravenous phentolamine (Regitine®) has been suggested on pharmacologic grounds for possible acute, severe hypertension, if this complicates Tenuate or Tenuate Dospan overdosage.

DOSAGE AND ADMINISTRATION

Tenuate (diethylpropion hydrochloride) immediate-release:
One immediate-release 25 mg tablet three times daily, one hour before meals, and in midevening if desired to overcome night hunger.

Tenuate Dospan (diethylpropion hydrochloride) controlled-release:
One controlled-release 75 mg tablet daily, swallowed whole, in midmorning.

HOW SUPPLIED

NDC 0068-0697-61
25 mg immediate-release tablets in bottles of 100
Each white, round tablet is debossed TENUATE 25 or MERRELL 697
Keep tightly closed, store at room temperature, preferably below 86°F.
Protect from excessive heat.
NDC 0068-0698-61
75 mg controlled-release tablets in bottles of 100
NDC 0068-0698-62
75 mg controlled-release tablets in bottles of 250
Each white, capsule-shaped tablet is debossed TENUATE 75 or MERRELL 698

Keep tightly closed. Store at room temperature, below 86°F.
Product Information as of January, 1985
Shown in Product Identification Section, page 413

Information on Lakeside Pharmaceuticals products is based on labeling in effect in June, 1989.

Lannett Company, Inc.
9000 STATE ROAD
PHILADELPHIA, PA 19136

ACNEDERM™ LOTION

(See PDR For Nonprescription Drugs)

CODALAN™   ℂ ℞

COMPOSITION

Each tablet contains: Codeine Phosphate* 8 mg. in No. 1; 15 mg. in No. 2; 30 mg. in No. 3; Acetaminophen 500 mg., and caffeine 30 mg.
*Warning: May be habit-forming.

HOW SUPPLIED

No. 1 orange color, No. 2 white color, No. 3 green color; all strengths in bottles of 100, 500 and 1000.

LITERATURE AVAILABLE

Complete Data Card.

DISONATE™ Capsules, Liquid and Syrup
(dioctyl sodium sulfosuccinate)

COMPOSITION

Docusate Sodium, U.S.P. (Dioctyl sodium sulfosuccinate), an effective stool-softener.

HOW SUPPLIED

Capsules of 100 mg., and 240 mg. Bottles of 100, 500 and 1000 capsules. Solution, 10 mg/cc Pint Bottle. Syrup, 20 mg/5 cc Pint and Gallon Bottle.

LITERATURE AVAILABLE

Yes.

LANIAZID SYRUP™   ℞
(Isoniazid Syrup, USP)

Each 5 mL (teaspoonful) contains:
Isoniazid, USP, 50 mg in a raspberry flavored base containing Sorbitol Solution.

HOW SUPPLIED

16 fl. oz. bottles

LITERATURE AVAILABLE

MAGNATRIL™ SUSPENSION AND TABLETS

(See PDR For Nonprescription Drugs)

QUINALAN™
(Sustained release tablets of Quinidine Gluconate)

Each tablet contains:
324 mgs. of Quinidine Gluconate in a specifically designed base for sustained release of the drug in the gastrointestinal tract.

HOW SUPPLIED

In white to yellowish white convex tablets, each containing 324 mg. of Quinidine Gluconate, and with a single score on one side and the letter "Q" on the other.
In bottles of 100, 250, and 500 tablets.

LITERATURE AVAILABLE

Laser, Inc.
2000 N. MAIN ST.
P.O. BOX 905
CROWN POINT, IN 46307

DALLERGY® SYRUP, TABLETS, CAPSULES   ℞

Each 5 ml. of syrup contains: chlorpheniramine maleate 2 mg., phenylephrine hydrochloride 10 mg., methscopolamine nitrate 0.625 mg. Each tablet contains: chlorpheniramine maleate 4 mg., phenylephrine hydrochloride 10 mg., methscopolamine nitrate 1.25 mg. Each sustained-release capsule contains: chlorpheniramine maleate 8 mg., phenylephrine hydrochloride 20 mg., methscopolamine nitrate 2.5 mg.

DALLERGY® –JR. CAPSULES   ℞

Each Sustained-Release Capsule contains: Brompheniramine Maleate, 6 mg., Pseudoephedrine Hydrochloride 60 mg.

DONATUSSIN DC SYRUP   ℂ ℞

Each 5 ml. contains: hydrocodone bitartrate 2.5 mg. (WARNING: May be habit forming), phenylephrine hydrochloride 7.5 mg., guaifenesin 50 mg. Red syrup.

DONATUSSIN DROPS   ℞

Each ml. contains: chlorpheniramine maleate 1 mg., phenylephrine hydrochloride 2 mg., guaifenesin 20 mg.

LACTOCAL–F TABLETS   ℞

Multivitamin, Multimineral supplement for pregnant or lactating women. White coated dye free tablet.

RESPAIRE®–SR CAPSULES 60 & 120   ℞

Each Sustained-Release RESPAIRE-60 SR Capsule contains pseudoephedrine hydrochloride 60 mg. and guaifenesin 200 mg. Each Sustained-Release RESPAIRE-120 SR Capsule contains pseudoephrine hydrochloride 120 mg. and guaifenesin 250 mg.

THEOSPAN® –SR CAPSULES   ℞
(theophylline anhydrous, 130 mg. & 260 mg.)

Each sustained-release THEOSPAN-SR Capsule 130 mg. contains theophylline anhydrous 130 mg. Each sustained-release THEOSPAN-SR Capsule 260 mg. contains theophylline anhydrous 260 mg.

THEOSTAT® 80 SYRUP   ℞
(theophylline anhydrous)

Each 15 ml. contains theophylline anhydrous 80 mg., alcohol 1%. Dye-free cherry-vanilla flavor.

TRIMSTAT® TABLETS   ℂ ℞
(phendimetrazine tartrate)

Each orange tablet contains: phendimetrazine tartrate 35 mg., embossed Laser, 35 .

IDENTIFICATION PROBLEM?
Consult PDR's
Product Identification Section
where you'll find over 1700
products pictured actual size
and in full color.

Continued on next page

Lederle Laboratories
A Division of American Cyanamid Co.
ONE CYANAMID PLAZA
WAYNE, NJ 07470

Lederle Parenterals, Inc.
CAROLINA, PUERTO RICO 00630

Lederle Piperacillin, Inc.
CAROLINA, PUERTO RICO 00630

LEDERLE PRODUCTS

The following list of Lederle products includes the alphanumeric LEDERMARK® codes which provide quick and positive identification of Lederle capsules and tablets:

PRODUCT IDENTITY CODE NO.	PRODUCT
A10	AMICAR® Tabs., 500mg
—	AMICAR® IV, 250mg/mL
—	AMICAR® Syrup, 25%
—	ARISTOCORT® Cream, LP, 0.025%
—	ARISTOCORT® Cream, R, 0.1%
—	ARISTOCORT® Cream, HP, 0.5%
—	ARISTOCORT® Forte Parenteral, 40mg/mL
—	ARISTOCORT® Intralesional, 25mg/mL
—	ARISTOCORT® Ointment, R, 0.1%
—	ARISTOCORT® Ointment, HP, 0.5%
—	ARISTOCORT A® Cream 0.025%
—	ARISTOCORT A® Cream 0.1%
—	ARISTOCORT A® Cream 0.5%
—	ARISTOCORT A® Ointment 0.1%
—	ARISTOSPAN® Intralesional 5mg/mL
—	ARISTOSPAN® Parenteral 20mg/mL
A 9	ARTANE® SEQUELS®, 5mg
A11	ARTANE® Tabs., 2mg
A12	ARTANE® Tabs., 5mg
—	ARTANE® Elixir, 2mg/5mL
A13	ASENDIN® Tabs., 25mg
A15	ASENDIN® Tabs., 50mg
A17	ASENDIN® Tabs., 100mg
A18	ASENDIN® Tabs., 150mg
—	AUREOMYCIN® Ointment 3%, 30mg/g
—	AUREOMYCIN® Ointment (Ophthalmic) 1%, 10mg/g
C600	CALTRATE® 600 Tabs.
C40	CALTRATE® 600—Vit. D Tabs.
C45	CALTRATE® 600—Iron Tabs.
C360	CALTRATE® Jr. Tabs.
C1	CENTRUM® Tabs.
C2	CENTRUM, JR.® +Iron Tabs.
C39	CENTRUM, JR.® Extra C Tabs.
C60	CENTRUM, JR.® + Extra Calcium Tabs.
—	Cholera Vaccine (India Strains) 1mL vial
—	CYCLOCORT® Cream 0.1%
—	CYCLOCORT® Lotion 0.1%
—	CYCLOCORT® Ointment 0.1%
D 9	DECLOMYCIN® Caps., 150mg
D11	DECLOMYCIN® Tabs., 150mg
D12	DECLOMYCIN® Tabs., 300mg
D 1	DIAMOX® Tabs., 125mg
D 2	DIAMOX® Tabs., 250mg
D 3	DIAMOX® SEQUELS® 500mg
—	DIAMOX® PARENTERAL, 500mg
—	Diphtheria & Tetanus Toxoids Adsorbed PUROGENATED®
—	Diphtheria & Tetanus Toxoids & Pertussis Vaccine Adsorbed TRI-IMMUNOL®
F 2	FERRO-SEQUELS®
F66	FIBERCON® Tabs., 625mg
F4	FILIBON® Tabs.
F5	FILIBON® F.A. Tabs.
F6	FILIBON® FORTE Tabs
—	FLU-IMUNE™ Influenza virus vaccine
—	GEVRABON® vitamin-mineral supplement 16 fl. oz.
G 1	GEVRAL® Tabs.
G 2	GEVRAL® T Tabs.
—	GEVRAL® PROTEIN ½ pound can
H 1	HYDROMOX® Tabs., 50mg
H 2	HYDROMOX® R Tabs.
—	INCREMIN® w/Iron Syrup 4 fl. oz.
—	INCREMIN® w/Iron Syrup 16 fl. oz.
L 6	LEDERPLEX® Caps.
—	LEDERPLEX® Liquid 12 fl. oz.

C33	Leucovorin Calcium Tabs., 5mg
C12	Leucovorin Calcium Tabs., 10mg
C35	Leucovorin Calcium Tabs., 15mg
—	Leucovorin Calcium Injection, USP, 3mg/mL
—	Leucovorin Calcium IM, 50mg vial, 100mg vial
—	LEVOPROME® IM 20mg/mL
L 1	LOXITANE® Caps., 5mg
L 2	LOXITANE® Caps., 10mg
L 3	LOXITANE® Caps., 25mg
L 4	LOXITANE® Caps., 50mg
—	LOXITANE® IM 50mg base/mL
—	LOXITANE® C Oral Concentrate 25mg/mL
M40	MATERNA® Tabs.
M 8	MAXZIDE® Tabs., 75/50mg
M 9	MAXZIDE®-25MG Tabs., 37.5/25mg
M 1	Methotrexate Tabs., 2.5 mg
—	Methotrexate Sodium Parenteral, 5mg, 20mg, 50mg, 100mg, 250mg, 1g
—	Methotrexate LPF® Sodium Parenteral 50mg, 100mg, 200mg, 250mg
M 2	MINOCIN® Caps., 50mg
M 3	MINOCIN® Tabs., 50mg
M 4	MINOCIN® Caps., 100mg
M 5	MINOCIN® Tabs., 100mg
—	MINOCIN® IV 100mg vial
—	MINOCIN® Oral Suspension 50mg/5mL
M 6	MYAMBUTOL® Tabs., 100mg
M 7	MYAMBUTOL® Tabs., 400mg
—	NEOLOID® emulsified Castor oil 4 fl. oz.
N 1	NEPTAZANE® Tabs., 50mg
N 2	NEPTAZANE® Tabs., 25mg
—	NOVANTRONE® 20mg/mL, 10mL vial
—	NOVANTRONE® 25mg/mL, 12.5mL vial
—	NOVANTRONE® 30mg/mL, 15mL vial
—	ORIMUNE® Poliovirus vaccine live oral trivalent
P 4	PATHILON® Tabs., 25mg
P 8	PERITINIC® Tabs.
—	PIPRACIL® 2gm
—	PIPRACIL® 3gm
—	PIPRACIL® 4gm
—	PIPRACIL® 40gm
—	PNU-IMUNE® 23 Pneumococcal vaccine Polyvalent
P 9	PRONEMIA® Caps.
M 1	RHEUMATREX® Tabs. 2.5mg
S 5	STRESSCAPS®
S 1	STRESSTABS®
S 2	STRESSTABS® w/Iron
S 3	STRESSTABS® w/Zinc
—	SUPRAX® Tablets, 200 mg
—	SUPRAX® Tablets, 400 mg
—	SUPRAX® Powder for oral suspension
—	Tetanus Toxoid Adsorbed PUROGENATED®
—	Tetanus Toxoid PUROGENATED®
—	Tetanus & Diphtheria Toxoids, Adsorbed PUROGENATED®
—	Thiotepa Parenteral 15 mg/vial
T1	TriHEMIC® 600 Tabs.
—	TRI-IMMUNOL® diphtheria and tetanus toxoids and pertussis vaccine, adsorbed
—	Tuberculin, OLD, TINE TEST®
—	Tuberculin Purified Protein Derivative TINE TEST (PPD)
—	ZINCON®

PRODUCT IDENTITY CODE NO.	STANDARD PRODUCTS
—	Acetaminophen Liquid, 160mg/5mL
A19	Acetaminophen Tablets, USP, 500mg
A20	Acetaminophen Capsules, USP, 500mg
A21	Acetaminophen Tablets, USP, 325mg
A23	Acetaminophen w/Codeine Tablets, 30mg
A39	Acetaminophen w/Codeine Tablets, 60mg
—	ACHROMYCIN® IM, 250mg
—	ACHROMYCIN® IV, 250mg
—	ACHROMYCIN® IV, 500mg
—	ACHROMYCIN® Ointment 3%
—	ACHROMYCIN® Ophthalmic Ointment 1%, 10mg/gm.
—	ACHROMYCIN® Ophthalmic Suspension 1%
A3	ACHROMYCIN® V Caps., 250mg
A5	ACHROMYCIN® V Caps., 500mg
—	ACHROMYCIN® V Oral Suspension 125mg/5mL
A43	Allopurinol Tablets, 100mg
A44	Allopurinol Tablets, 300mg
A14	Amiloride HCl/HCTZ Tablets, USP, 5mg/50mg
A24	Amitriptyline HCl Tablets, USP, 10mg
A25	Amitriptyline HCl Tablets, USP, 25mg
A26	Amitriptyline HCl Tablets, USP, 50mg
A27	Amitriptyline HCl Tablets, USP, 75mg

A28	Amitriptyline HCl Tablets, USP, 100mg
A33	Amoxicillin Capsules, USP, 250mg
A34	Amoxicillin Capsules, USP, 500mg
—	Amoxicillin for Oral Suspension, USP, 125mg/5mL
—	Amoxicillin for Oral Suspension, USP, 250mg/5mL
A31	Ampicillin Trihydrate Capsules, USP, 250mg
A32	Ampicillin Trihydrate Capsules, USP, 500mg
—	Ampicillin Trihydrate for Oral Suspension, USP, 125mg/5mL
—	Ampicillin Trihydrate for Oral Suspension, USP, 250mg/5mL
—	ARISTOCORT® Syrup, 2mg/5mL
A 1	ARISTOCORT® Tabs., 1mg
A 2	ARISTOCORT® Tabs., 2mg
A 8	ARISTOCORT® Tabs., 8mg
A 4	ARISTOCORT® Tabs., 4mg
A 4	ARISTO-PAK® Tabs., 4mg
B10	Benztropine Mesylate Tablets, USP, 1mg
B11	Benztropine Mesylate Tablets, USP, 2mg
C66	Carbamazepine Tablets, USP, 200mg
C64	Cephalexin Capsules, USP, 250mg
C65	Cephalexin Capsules, USP, 500mg
C81	Cephalexin Tablets, USP, 250mg
C82	Cephalexin Tablets, USP, 500mg
—	Cephalexin for Oral Suspension, USP, 125mg/5mL
—	Cephalexin for Oral Suspension, USP, 250mg/5mL
C61	Cephradine Capsules, USP, 250mg
C62	Cephradine Capsules, USP, 500mg
C67	Chlordiazepoxide and Amitriptyline HCl Tablets, USP, 5mg/12.5mg
C68	Chlordiazepoxide and Amitriptyline HCl Tablets, USP, 10mg/25mg
C16	Chlorpheniramine Maleate Tablets, USP, 4mg
C18	Chlorpheniramine Maleate T.D. Capsules, 12mg
—	Chlorpromazine HCl Liquid Concentrate 100mg/mL
C37	Chlorpropamide Tablets, USP, 100mg
C38	Chlorpropamide Tablets, USP, 250mg
C 7	Chlorthalidone Tablets, USP, 25mg
C15	Chlorthalidone Tablets, USP, 50mg
—	Clindamycin Phosphate Injection, USP, 150mg/mL, 2mL vial
—	Clindamycin Phosphate Injection, USP, 150mg/mL, 4mL vial
—	Clindamycin Phosphate Injection, USP, 150mg/mL, 6mL vial
C42	Clonidine HCl Tablets, USP, 0.1mg
C43	Clonidine HCl Tablets, USP, 0.2mg
C44	Clonidine HCl Tablets, USP, 0.3mg
C55	Clorazepate Dipotassium Capsules, USP, 3.75mg
C56	Clorazepate Dipotassium Capsules, USP, 7.5mg
C57	Clorazepate Dipotassium Capsules, USP, 15mg
C69	Clorazepate Dipotassium Tablets, USP, 3.75mg
C70	Clorazepate Dipotassium Tablets, USP, 7.5mg
C71	Clorazepate Dipotassium Tablets, USP, 15mg
C30	Cloxacillin Sodium Capsules, USP, 250mg
C31	Cloxacillin Sodium Capsules, USP, 500mg
—	Diazepam Injection, USP, 5mg/mL, 2mL vial
—	Diazepam Injection, USP, 5mg/mL, 10mL vial
—	Diazepam Injection, USP, 5mg/mL, 2mL ampule
—	Diazepam Injection, USP, 5mg/mL, 2mL disposable syringe
D51	Diazepam Tablets, USP, 2mg
D52	Diazepam Tablets, USP, 5mg
D53	Diazepam Tablets, USP, 10mg
D16	Dicloxacillin Sodium Capsules, USP, 250mg
D17	Dicloxacillin Sodium Capsules, USP, 500mg
D23	Dicyclomine HCl Capsules, USP, 10mg
D24	Dicyclomine HCl Tablets, USP, 20mg
D18	Dilvalproex Sodium Enteric-Coated Tablets, 125mg
D19	Dilvalproex Sodium Enteric-Coated Tablets, 250mg
D20	Dilvalproex Sodium Enteric-Coated Tablets, 500mg
—	Diphenhydramine HCl Cough Syrup, 12.5mg/5mL
—	Diphenhydramine HCl Elixir, USP, 12.5mg/5mL
D31	Diphenoxylate HCl 2.5mg and Atropine Sulfate 0.025mg Tablets, USP
D44	Dipyridamole Tablets, 25mg
D45	Dipyridamole Tablets, 50mg
D46	Dipyridamole Tablets, 75mg
D62	Disopyramide Phosphate Capsules, 100mg

D43	Disopyramide Phosphate Capsules, USP, 150mg
D32	Docusate Sodium, (DSS) Capsules, USP, 100mg
D33	Docusate Sodium, (DSS) Capsules, USP, 250mg
D34	Docusate Sodium, (DSS), 100 mg USP w/Casanthrol 30 mg, Capsules
—	Docusate Sodium (DSS) Syrup, USP, 20mg/5mL
—	Docusate Sodium (DSS) 60mg/15mL, w/Casanthranol, 30mg/15mL syrup
D36	DOLENE® Propoxyphene HCl Capsules, USP, 65mg
D35	DOLENE® AP-65 Propoxyphene HCl w/Acetaminophen Tablets, USP
D50	Doxepin HCl Capsules, USP, 10mg
D47	Doxepin HCl Capsules, USP, 25mg
D48	Doxepin HCl Capsules, USP, 50mg
D49	Doxepin HCl Capsules, USP, 75mg
D54	Doxepin HCl Capsules, USP, 100mg
D55	Doxepin HCl Capsules, USP, 150mg
D22	Doxycycline Hyclate Capsules, USP, 50mg
D25	Doxycycline Hyclate Capsules, USP, 100mg
D41	Doxycycline Hyclate Tablets, USP, 100mg
E 3	Ergoloid Mesylates Oral Tablets, 1mg
—	Erythromycin Estolate for Oral Suspension, USP, 125mg/5mL
—	Erythromycin Estolate for Oral Suspension, USP, 250mg/5mL
E10	Erythromycin Ethylsuccinate Tablets, USP 400mg
—	Erythromycin Ethylsuccinate for Oral Suspension, USP, 200mg/5mL
—	Erythromycin Ethylsuccinate for Oral Suspension, USP, 400mg/5mL
—	Erythromycin Ethylsuccinale/Sulfisoxazole Acetyl for Oral Suspension, 200mg/5mL
—	Sterile Erythromycin Lactobionate for Injection, USP, 500 mg/10mL
—	Sterile Erythromycin Lactobionate for Injection, USP, 500 mg/100mL
—	Sterile Erythromycin Lactobionate for Injection, USP, 1000mg/100mL
E 2	Erythromycin Stearate Tablets, USP, 250mg
E 5	Erythromycin Stearate Tablets, USP, 500mg
F22	Fenoprofen Calcium Tablets, USP, 600mg
F21	Ferrous Gluconate Iron Supplement Tablets, USP, 300mg
—	Ferrous Sulfate Elixir, 220mg/5mL
F20	Ferrous Sulfate Tablets, USP, 300mg
F15	Flurazepam HCl Capsules, USP, 15mg
F30	Flurazepam HCl Capsules, USP, 30mg
F 1	FOLVITE® Tabs., 1mg
—	FOLVITE® Solution, 5mg/mL
F11	Furosemide Tablets, USP, 20mg
F12	Furosemide Tablets, USP, 40mg
F13	Furosemide Tablets, USP, 80mg
—	Guaifenesin Syrup, USP, 100mg/5mL
—	Guaifenesin, 100mg, w/D-Methorphan Hydrobromide Syrup, 15mg/5mL
—	Haloperidol Oral Solution, USP, 2mg/mL
H25	Haloperidol Tablets, USP, 0.5mg
H26	Haloperidol Tablets, USP, 1mg
H27	Haloperidol Tablets, USP, 2mg
H28	Haloperidol Tablets, USP, 5mg
H29	Haloperidol Tablets, USP, 10mg
H11	Hydralazine HCl Tablets, USP, 25mg
H12	Hydralazine HCl Tablets, USP, 50mg
H14	Hydrochlorothiazide Tablets, USP, 25mg
H15	Hydrochlorothiazide Tablets, USP, 50mg
H17	Hydroxyzine HCl Tablets, 10mg
H18	Hydroxyzine HCl Tablets, USP, 25mg
I27	Aches-N-Pain™, Ibuprofen, USP, 200mg
I28	Ibuprofen Tablets, USP, 400mg
I29	Ibuprofen Tablets, USP, 600mg
I30	Ibuprofen Tablets, USP, 800mg
I11	Imipramine HCl Tablets, USP, 10mg
I12	Imipramine HCl Tablets, USP, 25mg
I13	Imipramine HCl Tablets, USP, 50mg
I19	Indomethacin Capsules, USP, 25mg
I20	Indomethacin Capsules, USP, 50mg
I15	Isosorbide Dinitrate Tablets, oral, 5mg
I24	Isosorbide Dinitrate Tablets, oral, 20mg
I23	Isosorbide Dinitrate SA Tablets, 40mg
—	LEDERCILLIN® VK, for Oral Solution, 125mg/5mL
—	LEDERCILLIN® VK, for Oral Solution, 250mg/5mL
L10	LEDERCILLIN® VK, Tablets, USP, 250mg
L 9	LEDERCILLIN® VK, Tablets, USP, 500mg
L11	Levothyroxine Sodium Tablets, USP, 0.1mg
L12	Levothyroxine Sodium Tablets, USP, 0.2mg
L13	Levothyroxine Sodium Tablets, USP, 0.3mg
L30	Lorazepam Tablets, 0.5mg

L31	Lorazepam Tablets, 1mg
L32	Lorazepam Tablets, 2mg
M12	Meclizine HCl Tablets, USP, 12.5mg
M13	Meclizine HCl Tablets, USP, 25mg
M41	Meclofenamate Sodium Capsules, USP, 50mg
M42	Meclofenamate Sodium Capsules, USP, 100mg
M35	Medroxyprogesterone Acetate Tablets, 10mg
—	Methenamine Mandelate Suspension Forte, 500mg/5mL
M19	Methocarbamol Tablets, USP, 500mg
M20	Methocarbamol Tablets, USP, 750mg
M25	Methyclothiazide Tablets, 5mg
M21	Methyldopa Tablets, USP, 125mg
M22	Methyldopa Tablets, USP, 250mg
M23	Methyldopa Tablets, USP, 500mg
M36	Methyldopa and Hydrochlorothiazide Tablets, USP, 250mg/15mg
M37	Methyldopa and Hydrochlorothiazide Tablets, USP, 250mg/25mg
M28	Metoclopramide Tablets, 10mg
M26	Metronidazole Tablets, USP, 250mg
M27	Metronidazole Tablets, USP, 500mg
N10	Neomycin Sulfate Tablets, USP, 500mg
N 5	NILSTAT® Oral Tabs.
N 6	NILSTAT® Vaginal Tabs.
—	NILSTAT® Oral Suspension, 100,000 units/mL
—	NILSTAT® Powder, USP
—	NILSTAT® Topical Cream, 100,000 units/g
—	NILSTAT® Topical Ointment, 100,000 units/g
N8	Nitrofurantoin Macrocrystals Capsules, 50 mg
N9	Nitrofurantoin Macrocrystals Capsules, 100 mg
N20	Nitroglycerin S.R. Capsules, 2.5mg
N21	Nitroglycerin S.R. Capsules, 6.5mg
N22	Nitroglycerin S.R. Capsules, 9mg
P11	Papaverine HCl T.R. Capsules, 150mg
P13	Papaverine HCl Tablets, USP, 100mg
P72	Perphenazine and Amitriptyline HCl Tablets, USP, 2mg/10mg
P73	Perphenazine and Amitriptyline HCl Tablets, USP, 2mg/25mg
P74	Perphenazine and Amitriptyline HCl Tablets, USP, 4mg/10mg
P75	Perphenazine and Amitriptyline HCl Tablets, USP, 4mg/25mg
P76	Perphenazine and Amitriptyline HCl Tablets, USP, 4mg/50mg
P21	Phenobarbital Tablets, USP, 30mg (½ gr)
P53	Extended Phenytoin Sodium Caps., USP, 100mg
K7	Potassium Chloride Extended Release Tablets, USP, 8m Eg
—	Potassium Chloride Liquid 10%
—	Potassium Chloride Liquid Concentrate 20%
P69	Prazosin HCl Capsules, 1mg
P70	Prazosin HCl Capsules, 2mg
P71	Prazosin HCl Capsules, 5mg
P24	Prednisone Tablets, USP, 5mg
P25	Probenecid Tablets, USP, 500mg
P26	Probenecid w/Colchicine Tablets, 500mg/0.5mg
P29	Procainamide HCl Capsules, USP, 250mg
P30	Procainamide HCl Capsules, USP, 375mg
P31	Procainamide HCl Capsules, USP, 500mg
P48	Procainamide HCl S.R. Tablets, 250mg
P49	Procainamide HCl S.R. Tablets, 500mg
P50	Procainamide HCl S.R. Tablets, 750mg
—	Promethazine HCl Syrup, Plain, 6.25mg/5mL
—	Promethazine HCl Syrup w/Codeine, 10mg/5mL
—	Promethazine HCl Syrup VC w/Codeine, 10mg/5mL
—	Promethazine HCl Syrup VC, Plain
P35	Propoxyphene HCl USP, 65mg Acetaminophen USP, 650 mg Tablets
P36	Propoxyphene HCl Capsules, USP, 65mg
P39	Propoxyphene Napsylate with Acetaminophen Tablets, USP, 100mg/650mg
P44	Propranolol HCl Tablets, USP, 10mg
P45	Propranolol HCl Tablets, USP, 20mg
P46	Propranolol HCl Tablets, USP, 40mg
P65	Propranolol HCl Tablets, USP, 60mg
P47	Propranolol HCl Tablets, USP, 80mg
P33	Propylthiouracil Tablets, USP, 50mg
—	Pseudoephedrine HCl Syrup, USP, 30mg/5mL
P35	Pseudoephedrine HCl Tablets, USP, 30mg
P34	Pseudoephedrine HCl Tablets, USP, 60mg
P36	Pyrazinamide Tablets, 500mg
Q13	Quinidine Gluconate SR Tablets, 324mg
Q11	Quinidine Sulfate Tablets, USP, 200mg
Q15	Quinine Sulfate Capsules, USP, 325mg
H22	Reserpine 0.1mg, Hydrochlorothiazide 15mg and Hydralazine HCl 25mg Combination Tablets USP

S13	Spironolactone Tablets, USP, 25mg
S12	Spironolactone w/Hydrochlorothiazide Tablets, 25mg/25mg
—	Sulfamethoxazole and Trimethoprim Pediatric Suspension, USP, 200mg/40mg per 5 mL
T13	Sulfamethoxazole and Trimethoprim Tablets, USP, 400mg/80mg
T16	Sulfamethoxazole and Trimethoprim Tablets, USP, 800mg/160mg
S14	Sulfasalazine Tablets, USP, 0.5g
T32	Temazepam Capsules, 15mg
T33	Temazepam Capsules, 30mg
T34	Theophylline Controlled Release Tablets, 100mg
T35	Theophylline Controlled Release Tablets, 200mg
T36	Theophylline Controlled Release Tablets, 300mg
T10	Thioridazine HCl Tablets, USP, 10mg
T25	Thioridazine HCl Tablets, USP, 25mg
T27	Thioridazine HCl Tablets, USP, 50mg
T28	Thioridazine HCl Tablets, USP, 100mg
T6	Timolol Maleate Tablets, USP, 5mg
T7	Timolol Maleate Tablets, USP, 10mg
T8	Timolol Maleate Tablets, USP, 20mg
—	Tobramycin Sulfate Injection, USP, 40mg/mL
T19	Tolazamide Tablets, USP, 100mg
T20	Tolazamide Tablets, USP, 250mg
T22	Tolazamide Tablets, USP, 500mg
T17	Tolbutamide Tablets, USP, 500mg
T29	Trazodone HCl Tablets, 50mg
T30	Trazodone HCl Tablets, 100mg
T31	Trazodone HCl Tablets, 150mg
—	Triprolidine HCl with Pseudoephedrine HCl Syrup 1.25mg/30mg per 5mL
T23	Triprolidine HCl with Pseudoephedrine HCl Tablets, USP, 2.5mg/60mg
—	VANCOLED® sterile vancomycin HCl, USP, 500mg vial
—	VANCOLED® sterile vancomycin HCl, USP, 1g vial
—	VANCOLED® sterile vancomycin HCl, USP, 2g vial
—	VANCOLED® sterile vancomycin HCl, USP, 5g vial
V4	Verapamil HCl Tablets, 80mg
V5	Verapamil HCl Tablets, 120mg

ACHROMYCIN®   ℞
[a-krō-mī-cin]
Sterile Tetracycline Hydrochloride, Intramuscular/Intravenous

ACHROMYCIN is an antibiotic isolated from *Streptomyces aureofaciens*. Chemically it is the hydrochloride of 4-dimethylamino-1, 4, 4a, 5, 5a, 6, 11, 12a-octahydro-3, 6, 10, 12, 12a-pentahydroxy -6- methyl-1, 11-dioxo -2-naphthacenecarboxamide.

ACTIONS
The tetracyclines are primarily bacteriostatic and are thought to exert their antimicrobial effect by the inhibition of protein synthesis. Tetracyclines are active against a wide range of gram-negative and gram-positive organisms.
The drugs in the tetracycline class have closely similar antimicrobial spectra, and cross-resistance among them is common. Microorganisms may be considered susceptible if the MIC (minimum inhibitory concentration) is not more than 4 mcg/mL and intermediate if the MIC is 4 to 12.5 mcg/mL. Susceptibility plate testing: A tetracycline disc may be used to determine microbial susceptibility to drugs in the tetracycline class. If the Kirby-Bauer method of disc susceptibility testing is used, a 30 mcg tetracycline disc should give a zone of at least 19 mm when tested against a tetracycline-susceptible bacterial strain.
Tetracyclines are readily absorbed and are bound to plasma proteins in varying degrees. They are concentrated by the liver in the bile and excreted in the urine and feces at high concentrations and in a biologically active form.

INDICATIONS
ACHROMYCIN is indicated in infections caused by the following microorganisms:
Rickettsiae: (Rocky Mountain spotted fever, typhus fever and the typhus group, Q fever, rickettsialpox and tick fevers).

Continued on next page

Information on Lederle products listed on these pages is the full prescribing information from product literature or package inserts effective in August, 1989. Information concerning all Lederle products may be obtained from the Professional Services Department, Lederle Laboratories, Pearl River, New York, 10965.

Lederle—Cont.

Mycoplasma pneumoniae (PPLO, Eaton Agent).

Agents of psittacosis and ornithosis.

Agents of lymphogranuloma venereum and granuloma inguinale.

The spirochetal agent of relapsing fever (*Borrelia recurrentis*).

The following gram-negative microorganisms:

Haemophilus ducreyi (chancroid),

Yersinia pestis and *Francisella tularensis*, formerly *Pasteurella pestis* and *Pasteurella tularensis*,

Bartonella bacilliformis,

Bacteroides species,

Vibrio comma and *Vibrio fetus*

Brucella species (in conjunction with streptomycin).

Because many strains of the following groups of microorganisms have been shown to be resistant to tetracyclines, culture and susceptibility testing are recommended.

Tetracycline is indicated for treatment of infections caused by the following gram-negative microorganisms, when bacteriologic testing indicates appropriate susceptibility to the drug:

Escherichia coli,

Enterobacter aerogenes (formerly *Aerobacter aerogenes*),

Shigella species,

Mima species and *Herellea* species,

Haemophilus influenzae (respiratory infections),

Klebsiella species (respiratory and urinary infections).

Tetracycline is indicated for treatment of infections caused by the following gram-positive microorganisms when bacteriologic testing indicates appropriate susceptibility to the drug:

Streptococcus species:

Up to 44% of strains of *Streptococcus pyogenes* and 74% of *Streptococcus faecalis* have been found to be resistant to tetracycline drugs. Therefore, tetracyclines should not be used for streptococcal disease unless the organism has been demonstrated to be sensitive.

For upper respiratory infections due to Group A beta-hemolytic streptococci, penicillin is the usual drug of choice, including prophylaxis of rheumatic fever.

Streptococcus pneumoniae,

Staphylococcus aureus, skin and soft tissue infections.

Tetracyclines are not the drugs of choice in the treatment of any type of staphylococcal infection.

When penicillin is contraindicated, tetracyclines are alternative drugs in the treatment of infections due to:

Neisseria gonorrhoeae and *Neisseria meningitidis*,

Treponema pallidum and *Treponema pertenue* (syphillis and yaws),

Listeria monocytogenes,

Clostridium species,

Bacillus anthracis,

Fusobacterium fusiforme (Vincent's infection),

Actinomyces species.

In acute intestinal amebiasis, the tetracyclines may be a useful adjunct to amebicides. ACHROMYCIN *sterile tetracycline HCl* is indicated in the treatment of trachoma, although the infectious agent is not always eliminated, as judged by immunofluorescence.

Inclusion conjunctivitis may be treated with oral tetracyclines or with a combination of oral and topical agents.

CONTRAINDICATIONS

This drug is contraindicated in persons who have shown hypersensitivity to any of the tetracyclines.

WARNINGS

In the presence of renal dysfunction, particularly in pregnancy, intravenous tetracycline therapy in daily doses exceeding 2 grams has been associated with deaths through liver failure.

When the need for intensive treatment outweighs its potential dangers (mostly during pregnancy or in individuals with known or suspected renal or liver impairment), it is advisable to perform renal and liver function tests before and during therapy. Also tetracycline serum concentrations should be followed.

If renal impairment exists, even usual oral or parenteral doses may lead to excessive systemic accumulation of the drug and possible liver toxicity. Under such conditions, lower than usual total doses are indicated, and if therapy is prolonged, serum level determinations of the drug may be advisable. This hazard is of particular importance in the parenteral administration of tetracyclines to pregnant or postpartum patients with pyelonephritis. When used under these circumstances, the blood level should not exceed 15 micrograms/mL and liver function tests should be made at frequent intervals. Other potentially hepatotoxic drugs should not be prescribed concomitantly.

THE USE OF DRUGS OF THE TETRACYCLINE CLASS DURING TOOTH DEVELOPMENT (LAST HALF OF PREGNANCY, INFANCY AND CHILDHOOD TO THE AGE OF 8 YEARS) MAY CAUSE PERMANENT DISCOL-

ORATION OF THE TEETH (YELLOW-GRAY-BROWN). This adverse reaction is more common during long-term use of the drugs but has been observed following repeated short-term courses. Enamel hypoplasia has also been reported. TETRACYCLINES, THEREFORE, SHOULD NOT BE USED IN THIS AGE GROUP UNLESS OTHER DRUGS ARE NOT LIKELY TO BE EFFECTIVE OR ARE CONTRAINDICATED.

Photosensitivity manifested by an exaggerated sunburn reaction has been observed in some individuals taking tetracyclines. Patients apt to be exposed to direct sunlight or ultraviolet light should be advised that this reaction can occur with tetracycline drugs, and treatment should be discontinued at the first evidence of skin erythema.

The antianabolic action of the tetracyclines may cause an increase in BUN. While this is not a problem in those with normal renal function, in patients with significantly impaired function, higher serum levels of tetracycline may lead to azotemia, hyperphosphatemia, and acidosis.

Usage In Pregnancy (See above **WARNINGS** about use during tooth development.) Results of animal studies indicate that tetracyclines cross the placenta, are found in fetal tissues and can have toxic effects on the developing fetus (often related to retardation of skeletal development). Evidence of embryotoxicity has also been noted in animals treated early in pregnancy.

Usage in newborns, infants, and children (See above **WARNINGS** about use during tooth development.)

All tetracyclines form a stable calcium complex in any bone-forming tissue. A decrease in the fibula growth rate has been observed in prematures given oral tetracycline in doses of 25 mg/kg every six hours. This reaction was shown to be reversible when the drug was discontinued.

Tetracyclines are present in the milk of lactating women who are taking a drug in this class.

PRECAUTIONS

General: Pseudotumor cerebri (benign intracranial hypertension) in adults has been associated with the use of tetracyclines. The usual clinical manifestations are headache and blurred vision. Bulging fontanels have been associated with the use of tetracyclines in infants. While both of these conditions and related symptoms usually resolve soon after discontinuation of the tetracycline, the possibility for permanent sequelae exists.

As with other antibiotic preparations, use of this drug may result in overgrowth of nonsusceptible organisms, including fungi. If superinfection occurs, the antibiotic should be discontinued and appropriate therapy should be instituted.

In venereal diseases when coexistent syphilis is suspected, darkfield examination should be done before treatment is started and the blood serology repeated monthly for at least 4 months.

In long-term therapy, periodic laboratory evaluation of organ systems, including hematopoietic, renal and hepatic studies should be performed.

All infections due to Group A beta hemolytic streptococci should be treated for at least ten days.

Drug Interactions: Because the tetracyclines have been shown to depress plasma prothrombin activity, patients who are on anticoagulant therapy may require downward adjustment of their anticoagulant dosage.

Since bacteriostatic drugs may interfere with the bactericidal action of penicillin, it is advisable to avoid giving tetracycline in conjunction with penicillin.

Concurrent use of tetracycline may render oral contraceptives less effective. Breakthrough bleeding has been reported.

ADVERSE REACTIONS

Local irritation may be present after intramuscular injection. The injection should be deep, with care taken not to injure the sciatic nerve nor inject intravascularly.

Gastrointestinal: Anorexia, nausea, vomiting, diarrhea, glossitis, dysphagia, enterocolitis, and inflammatory lesions (with monilial overgrowth) in the anogenital region. Hepatic toxicity has been reported rarely. These reactions have been caused by both the oral and parenteral administration of tetracyclines.

Skin: Maculopapular and erythematous rashes. Exfoliative dermatitis has been reported but is uncommon. Photosensitivity is discussed above. (See **WARNINGS**.)

Renal toxicity: Rise in BUN has been reported and is apparently dose related. (See **WARNINGS**.)

Hypersensitivity reactions: Urticaria, angioneurotic edema, anaphylaxis, anaphylactoid purpura, pericarditis and exacerbation of systemic lupus erythematosus.

Blood: Hemolytic anemia, thrombocytopenia, neutropenia and eosinophilia have been reported.

CNS: Pseudotumor cerebri (benign intracranial hypertension) in adults and bulging fontanels in infants (See **PRECAUTIONS—General**).

Other: When given over prolonged periods, tetracyclines have been reported to produce brown-black microscopic discoloration of thyroid glands. No abnormalities of thyroid function studies are known to occur.

PREPARATION OF SOLUTION

Intravenous

Vials of ACHROMYCIN *sterile tetracycline hydrochloride*, intravenous should be initially reconstituted by adding 5 mL of Sterile Water for Injection to 250 mg vial and 10 mL of Sterile Water for Injection to the 500 mg vial, and then further diluted prior to administration to at least 100 mL (up to 1000 mL) with any of the following diluents:

Ringer's Injection, USP

Sodium Chloride Injection, USP

Dextrose Injection, USP

  (5% Dextrose in Sterile Water for Injection, USP)

Dextrose and Sodium Chloride Injection, USP (5% in Sodium Chloride Injection, USP)

Lactated Ringer's Injection, USP

Protein Hydrolysate Injection, Low Sodium, USP 5%,

  5% with Dextrose 5%,

  5% with Invert Sugar 10%

The initial reconstituted solutions are stable at room temperature for 12 hours without significant loss of potency. The final dilution for administration should be administered immediately.

Note: The use of solutions containing calcium should be avoided as these tend to form precipitates (especially in neutral to alkaline solution) and, therefore, should not be used unless necessary. However, Ringer's Injection, USP and Lactated Ringer's Injection, USP can be used with caution since the calcium ion content in these diluents does not normally precipitate tetracycline in an acid media.

Intramuscular

Add 2 mL of Sterile Water for Injection USP (or Sodium Chloride Injection USP) to the 100 mg or 250 mg vial. The resulting solution may be stored at room temperature and should not be used after 24 hours.

DOSAGE AND ADMINISTRATION

Intravenous administration:

Note: Rapid administration is to be avoided. Parenteral therapy is indicated only when oral therapy is not adequate or tolerated. Oral therapy should be instituted as soon as possible. If intravenous therapy is given over prolonged periods of time, thrombophlebitis may result.

Adults: The usual adult dose: 250 to 500 mg every 12 hours and should not exceed 500 mg every six hours. The drug may be dissolved and then diluted in 100–1,000 mL of Dextrose 5 percent in water, Isotonic Sodium Chloride Solution or Ringer's Solution, but not in other solutions containing calcium (a precipitate may form).

For children above eight years of age: The usual dose: 12mg/kg/day, divided into 2 doses, but from 10 to 20 mg/kg/day may be given, depending on the severity of the infection.

Gonorrhea patients sensitive to penicillin may be treated with tetracycline administered as an initial oral dose of 1.5 grams followed by 0.5 grams every 6 hours for 4 days, a total dosage of 9 grams. Intravenous therapy should be reserved for situations in which oral therapy is not feasible. In patients with renal impairment: (see **WARNINGS**).

Total dosage should be decreased by reduction of recommended individual doses and/or by extending time intervals between doses.

Intramuscular Administration: Adults: The usual daily dose is 250 mg administered once every 24 hours or 300 mg given in divided doses at 8- to 12-hour intervals.

For children above eight years of age: 15–25 mg/kg body weight up to a maximum of 250 mg per single daily injection. Dosage may be divided and given at 8- to 12-hour intervals.

Gonorrhea patients sensitive to penicillin may be treated with tetracycline administered as an initial oral dose of 1.5 grams followed by 0.5 grams every six hours for four days to a total dosage of 9 grams. Intramuscular therapy should be reserved for situations in which oral therapy is not feasible. In patients with renal impairment: (see **WARNINGS**).

Total dosage should be decreased by reduction of recommended individual doses and/or by extending time intervals between doses.

The intramuscular administration of ACHROMYCIN *sterile tetracycline hydrochloride* produces lower blood levels than oral administration in the recommended dosages. Patients placed on intramuscular tetracyclines should be changed to the oral dosage form as soon as possible. If rapid, high blood levels are needed, ACHROMYCIN should be administered intravenously.

ACHROMYCIN *sterile tetracycline hydrochloride* Intramuscular should be injected deeply into a large muscle mass such as the gluteal region. Inadvertent injection into the subcutaneous or fat layers may cause pain and induration, which can be relieved by applying an ice pack.

HOW SUPPLIED

Intravenous:

Sterile Tetracycline Hydrochloride 250 mg with 625 mg ascorbic acid/vial Product Number NDC 0005-5352-95

Sterile Tetracycline Hydrochloride 500 mg with 1250 mg ascorbic acid/vial Product Number NDC 0005-4771-96

Lederle—Cont.

1.5 grams followed by 0.5 gram every 6 hours for 4 days to a total dosage of 9 grams.

Uncomplicated urethral, endocervical, or rectal infection in adults caused by *Chlamydia trachomatis:* 500 mg, by mouth, 4 times a day for at least 7 days.[1]

HOW SUPPLIED

ACHROMYCIN V *tetracycline HCl* oral dosage forms are available as follows:

CAPSULES

500 mg - Two-piece, hard shell, elongated, opaque capsules with a blue cap and a yellow body, printed with Lederle over A5 on one half and Lederle over 500 mg on the other in gray ink, supplied as follows:

NDC 0005-4875-23—Bottle of 100
NDC 0005-4875-34—Bottle of 1,000
NDC 0005-4875-59—Unit of Issue 12 × 20s
NDC 0005-4875-60—Unit Dose 10 × 10s

250 mg - Two-piece, hard shell, opaque capsules with a blue cap and yellow body, printed with Lederle over A3 on one half and Lederle over 250 mg on the other in gray ink, are supplied as follows:

NDC 0005-4880-23—Bottles of 100
NDC 0005-4880-34—Bottles of 1,000
NDC 0005-4880-59—Unit of Issue 12 × 20s
NDC 0005-4880-60—Unit Dose 10 × 10s
NDC 0005-4880-61—Unit of Issue 12 × 40s
NDC 0005-4880-63—Unit of Issue 12 × 28s
NDC 0005-4880-65—Unit of Issue 12 × 100s

Store at Controlled Room Temperature 15–30°C (59–86°F).
Shown in Product Identification Section, page 413

ORAL SUSPENSION

Tetracycline equivalent to 125 mg tetracycline HCl per teaspoonful (5 mL). Preserved with Methylparaben 0.12% and Propylparaben 0.03%, cherry-flavored, is supplied as follows:

NDC 0005-5410-65—Bottle of 16 fl oz (473 mL)
Store at Controlled Room Temperature 15–30°C (59–86°F).
DO NOT FREEZE.

Reference: 1. CDC Sexually Transmitted Diseases Treatment Guidelines 1982.

Military Depots:
NSN 6505-01-059-8997–250 mg.—40s
NSN 6505-00-655-8355–250 mg.—100s
NSN 6505-00-963-4924–250 mg.—1000s
LEDERLE LABORATORIES DIVISION
American Cyanamid Company,
Pearl River, N.Y. 10965   Rev. 2/89
                                24474

ACHROMYCIN®
tetracycline

is also supplied in a number of other dosage forms and combinations for special purposes (for details of indications, dosage, administration and precautions, see circular in package).

ACHROMYCIN®   ℞
tetracycline HCl
Ophthalmic Ointment, USP, 1% (sterile)

⅛ oz. tube NDC 0005-3501-51.
(see PDR for Ophthalmology)

ACHROMYCIN®
tetracycline HCl
3% Ointment
(For topical use)—

½ oz. tube—NDC 0005-4796-56
1 oz. tube—NDC 0005-4796-55
℞ not required

AMICAR®   ℞
[ă-mĭ-car]
Aminocaproic Acid
Intravenous, Syrup, and Tablets, USP

DESCRIPTION

AMICAR is 6-amino-hexanoic acid which acts as an effective inhibitor of fibrinolysis.

The chemical structure is $NH_2CH_2(CH_2)_3CH_2COOH$
$C_6H_{13}NO_2$ MW 131.17

AMICAR Intravenous contains 250 mg/mL Aminocaproic Acid, Benzyl Alcohol, 0.9% and Water for Injection, qs 100%. Hydrochloric acid may be added during manufacture to adjust pH to approximately 6.8.

AMICAR Syrup, 25%, contains 250 mg/mL of Aminocaproic Acid and the following inactive ingredients: Citric Acid, Flavorings, Potassium Sorbate, Preservatives, Sodium Saccharin and Sorbitol.

Each AMICAR Tablet contains 500 mg of Aminocaproic Acid and the following inactive ingredients: Magnesium Stearate, Stearic Acid and Povidone.

ACTIONS

The beneficial fibrinolysis-inhibitory effects of AMICAR appear to be principally via inhibition of plasminogen activator substances and, to a lesser degree, through antiplasmin activity. The drug is absorbed rapidly following oral administration. Whether administered by the oral or intravenous route, a major portion of the compound is recovered unmetabolized in the urine. The renal clearance of AMICAR is high (about 75% of the creatinine clearance). Thus the drug is excreted rapidly. After prolonged administration, AMICAR distributes throughout both the extravascular and intravascular compartments of the body and readily penetrates human red blood and other tissue cells.

INDICATIONS

AMICAR is useful in enhancing hemostasis when fibrinolysis contributes to bleeding. In life-threatening situations, fresh whole blood transfusions, fibrinogen infusions, and other emergency measures may be required.

Fibrinolytic bleeding may frequently be associated with *surgical complications* following heart surgery (with or without cardiac bypass procedures) and portacaval shunt; *hematological disorders* such as aplastic anemia, *abruptio placentae, hepatic cirrhosis, neoplastic disease* such as carcinoma of the prostate, lung, stomach, and cervix.

Urinary fibrinolysis, usually a normal physiological phenomenon, may frequently be associated with life-threatening complications following severe trauma, anoxia and shock. Symptomatic of such complications is *surgical hematuria* (following prostatectomy and nephrectomy) or *nonsurgical hematuria* (accompanying polycystic or neoplastic diseases of the genitourinary system). (See WARNINGS.)

CONTRAINDICATIONS

AMICAR should not be used when there is evidence of an active intravascular clotting process.

When there is uncertainty as to whether the cause of bleeding is primary fibrinolysis or disseminated intravascular coagulation (DIC), this distinction must be made before administering AMICAR.

The following tests can be applied to differentiate the two conditions:

• Platelet count is usually decreased in DIC but normal in primary fibrinolysis.

• Protamine Paracoagulation test is positive in DIC; a precipitate forms when protamine sulphate is dropped into citrated plasma. The test is negative in the presence of primary fibrinolysis.

• The euglobulin clot lysis test is abnormal in primary fibrinolysis, but normal in DIC.

AMICAR must not be used in the presence of DIC without concomitant heparin.

WARNINGS

Safe use of AMICAR *aminocaproic acid* has not been established with respect to adverse effects upon fetal development. Therefore, it should not be used in women of childbearing potential and particularly during early pregnancy, unless in the judgement of the physician the potential benefits outweigh the possible hazards. Antifertility effects, consistent with the drug's antifibrinolytic activity, have been suggested in some rodent studies.

In patients with upper urinary tract bleeding, AMICAR administration has been known to cause intrarenal obstruction in the form of glomerular capillary thrombosis, or clots in the renal pelvis and ureters. For this reason, AMICAR should not be used in hematuria of upper urinary tract origin, unless the possible benefits outweigh the risk.

PRECAUTIONS

AMICAR has a very specific action in that it inhibits both plasminogen activator substances and, to a lesser degree, plasmin activity. The drug should NOT be administered without a definite diagnosis, and/or laboratory findings indicative of hyperfibrinolysis (hyperplasminemia).*

*Stefanini, M. and Dameshek, W.: The Hemorrhagic Disorders, Ed. 2, New York, Grune and Stratton, pp. 510–514, 1962.

The use of AMICAR should be accompanied by tests designed to determine the amount of fibrinolysis present. There are presently available (a) general tests, such as those for the determination of the lysis of a clot of blood or plasma and (b) more specific tests for the study of various phases of fibrinolytic mechanisms. These latter tests include both semiquantitative and quantitative techniques for the determination of profibrinolysin, fibrinolysin, and antifibrinolysin.

Animal experiments indicate particular caution should be taken in administering AMICAR to patients with cardiac, hepatic or renal diseases.

Demonstrable animal pathology in some cases has shown endocardial hemorrhages and myocardial fat degeneration. Rarely, skeletal muscle weakness with necrosis of muscle fibers has been reported clinically. The possibility of cardiac muscle damage should be considered also when skeletal my-

opathy occurs. CPK levels should be monitored in patients on long-term therapy. AMICAR administration should be stopped if a rise in CPK is noted.

The use of this drug should thus be restricted to patients in whom the benefit expected would outweigh the potential hazard. Physicians are cautioned in the use of this product because of animal data showing rat teratogenicity and kidney concretions.

Rapid intravenous administration of the drug should be avoided since this may induce hypotension, bradycardia, and/or arrhythmia.

One case of *cardiac* and *hepatic lesions* observed in man has been reported. The patient received 2 grams of aminocaproic acid every 6 hours for a total dose of 26 grams. Death was due to continued cerebrovascular hemorrhage. Necrotic changes in the heart and liver were noted at autopsy.

Fibrinolysis is a normal process, presumably active at all times to ensure the fluidity of blood. Inhibition of fibrinolysis by aminocaproic acid *may* theoretically result in clotting or thrombosis. However, there is no definite evidence that administration of aminocaproic acid has been responsible for the few reported cases of *intravascular clotting* which followed this treatment. Rather, it appears that such intravascular clotting was most likely due to the patient's preexisting clinical condition, eg, the presence of DIC.

It has been postulated that *extravascular clots* formed *in vivo* may not undergo spontaneous lysis as do normal clots.

Reports have appeared in the literature of an increased incidence of certain neurological deficits, such as hydrocephalus, cerebral ischemia, or cerebral vasospasm, associated with the use of fibrinolytic agents in the treatment of subarachnoid hemorrhage. All of these events have also been described as part of the natural course of SAH, or as a consequence of diagnostic procedures such as angiography. Drug relatedness remains unclear.

Drug/Laboratory Test Interactions: Prolongation of the template bleeding time has been reported during continuous intravenous infusion of AMICAR; however, platelet function studies in these patients have not demonstrated any significant platelet dysfunction. The clinical significance of this observation is unknown.

ADVERSE REACTIONS

Occasionally nausea, cramps, diarrhea, hypotension, dizziness, tinnitus, malaise, conjunctival suffusion, nasal stuffiness, headache, myopathy, and skin rash have been reported as results of the administration of aminocaproic acid. The myopathy may be accompanied with general weakness, fatigue, and elevated serum enzymes. Rarely, rhabdomyolysis with myoglobinuria and renal failure may occur. Only rarely has it been necessary to discontinue or reduce medication because of one or more of these effects.

There have also been some reports of dry ejaculation during the period of AMICAR *aminocaproic acid* treatment. These have been reported to date only in hemophilia patients who received the drug after undergoing dental surgical procedures. However, this symptom resolved in all patients within 24 to 48 hours of completion of therapy.

Two cases of convulsions occurring following intravenous administration of AMICAR have been reported. However, definite associations between the seizures and the drug have not been established.

Thrombophlebitis, a possibility with all intravenous therapy, should be guarded against by strict attention to the proper insertion of the needle and the fixing of its position.

DOSAGE AND ADMINISTRATION

Initial Therapy: An initial priming dose of 5 grams of AMICAR administered either orally or intravenously followed by 1.0 to 1.25 gram doses at hourly intervals thereafter should achieve and sustain plasma levels of 0.130 mg/mL of the drug. This is the concentration apparently necessary for the inhibition of fibrinolysis. Administration of more than 30 grams in any 24-hour period is not recommended.

Intravenous: AMICAR Intravenous is administered by infusion, utilizing the usual compatible intravenous vehicles (eg, Sterile Water for Injection, physiologic saline, 5% dextrose or Ringer's Solution). RAPID INJECTION OF AMICAR INTRAVENOUS UNDILUTED INTO A VEIN IS NOT RECOMMENDED.

For the treatment of *acute* bleeding syndromes due to elevated fibrinolytic activity, it is suggested that 16 to 20 mL (4 to 5 grams) of AMICAR *aminocaproic acid* Intravenous in 250 mL of diluent be administered by infusion during the first hour of treatment, followed by a continuing infusion at the rate of 4 mL (1 gram) per hour in 50 mL of diluent. This method of treatment would ordinarily be continued for about 8 hours or until the bleeding situation has been controlled.

Oral Therapy: If the patient is able to take medication by mouth, an identical dosage regimen may be followed by administering AMICAR Tablets or 25% Syrup as follows: For the treatment of *acute* bleeding syndromes due to elevated fibrinolytic activity, it is suggested that 10 tablets (5 grams) or 4 teaspoonfuls of syrup (5 grams) of AMICAR be administered during the first hour of treatment, followed by a continuing rate of 2 tablets (1 gram) or 1 teaspoonful of syrup

(1.25 grams) per hour. This method of treatment would ordinarily be continued for about 8 hours or until the bleeding situation has been controlled.

HOW SUPPLIED

AMICAR *Intravenous:* Each 20 mL vial contains 5 grams of aminocaproic acid (250 mg per mL) as an aqueous solution, with 0.9% benzyl alcohol as a preservative. The pH is adjusted to approx. 6.8 with hydrochloric acid. 20 mL vials, Product No. NDC 0205-4668-37.

Each 96 mL vial contains 24 grams of aminocaproic acid (250 mg per mL) as an aqueous solution, with 0.9% benzyl alcohol as a preservative. The pH is adjusted to approx. 6.8 with hydrochloric acid. 96 mL vials, Product No. NDC 0205-4668-73.

Store at Controlled Room Temperature 15–30°C (59–86°F).
LEDERLE PARENTERALS, INC.

Carolina, Puerto Rico 00630

AMICAR *25% Syrup:* Each mL of raspberry flavored syrup contains 250 mg of aminocaproic acid. 16 Fl. Oz. Bottle, Product No. NDC 0005-4667-65.

AMICAR *Tablets:* Each round, white tablet, engraved with LL on one side and scored on the other with A to the left of the score and 10 on the right, contains 500 mg of aminocaproic acid. Bottle of 100, Product No. NDC 0005-4665-23.

Store at Controlled Room Temperature 15–30°C (59–86°F).

Military Depot:
NSN 6505-01-147-9535—500 Tablets mg (100s)
LEDERLE LABORATORIES DIVISION
American Cyanamid Company
Pearl River, N.Y. 10965   Rev. 9/88
                                       24558

Shown in Product Identification Section, page 413

ARISTOCORT®   ℞
[*a-ris-tō-cort*]
triamcinolone
TABLETS
ARISTOCORT®
triamcinolone diacetate
SYRUP

DESCRIPTION
ARISTOCORT is a synthetic adrenocorticosteroid. The tablets contain 1, 2, 4, or 8 mg triamcinolone, 9-Fluoro-11β,16α,17,21-tetrahydroxypregna-1,4-diene-3,20-dione. Syrup contains triamcinolone diacetate which is 9-Fluoro-11β,16α,17,21-tetrahydroxypregna-1,4-diene-3,20-dione 16,21-diacetate. It is readily absorbed from the gastrointestinal tract.

INACTIVE INGREDIENTS
ARISTOCORT tablets contain the following inactive ingredients: Cornstarch, Dibasic Calcium Phosphate, Docusate Sodium, Lactose, Magnesium Stearate, Microcrystalline Cellulose, Red 30, Sodium Benzoate, Sodium Starch Glycolate and Yellow 10.

Syrup contains Flavoring, Kaolin, Magnesium Aluminum Silicate, Methylparaben, Monobasic Sodium Phosphate, Propylparaben, Red 33, Red 40, Sodium Phosphate, Sucrose, Water.

ACTION
ARISTOCORT is primarily glucocorticoid in action and has potent anti-inflammatory, hormonal, and metabolic effects common to cortisone-like drugs. It is essentially devoid of mineralocorticoid activity when administered in therapeutic doses, causing little or no sodium retention, with potassium excretion minimal or absent. The body's immune responses to diverse stimuli are also modified by its action.

INDICATIONS
1. Endocrine Disorders:
Primary or secondary adrenocortical insufficiency (hydrocortisone or cortisone is the first choice; synthetic analogs may be used in conjunction with mineralocorticoids where applicable; in infancy mineralocorticoid supplementation is of particular importance).
Congenital adrenal hyperplasia.
Nonsuppurative thyroiditis.
Hypercalcemia associated with cancer.
2. Rheumatic Disorders:
As adjunctive therapy for short-term administration (to tide the patient over an acute episode or exacerbation) in:
Psoriatic arthritis.
Rheumatoid arthritis, including juvenile rheumatoid arthritis (selected cases may require low-dose maintenance therapy).
Ankylosing spondylitis.
Acute and subacute bursitis.
Acute nonspecific tenosynovitis.
Acute gouty arthritis.
Posttraumatic osteoarthritis.
Synovitis of osteoarthritis.
Epicondylitis.

3. Collagen Diseases:
During an exacerbation or as maintenance therapy in selected cases of—
Systemic lupus erythematosus.
Acute rheumatic carditis.
4. Dermatologic Diseases:
Pemphigus.
Bullous dermatitis herpetiformis.
Severe erythema multiforme (Stevens-Johnson syndrome).
Exfoliative dermatitis.
Mycosis fungoides.
Severe psoriasis.
Severe seborrheic dermatitis.
5. Allergic States:
Control of severe or incapacitating allergic conditions intractable to adequate trials of conventional treatment:
Seasonal or perennial allergic rhinitis.
Bronchial asthma.
Contact dermatitis.
Atopic dermatitis.
Serum sickness.
Drug hypersensitivity reactions.
6. Ophthalmic Diseases:
Severe acute and chronic allergic and inflammatory processes involving the eye and its adnexa such as—
Allergic conjunctivitis.
Keratitis.
Allergic corneal marginal ulcers.
Herpes zoster ophthalmicus.
Iritis and iridocyclitis.
Chorioretinitis.
Anterior segment inflammation.
Diffuse posterior uveitis and choroiditis.
Optic neuritis.
Sympathetic ophthalmia.
7. Respiratory Diseases:
Symptomatic sarcoidosis.
Loeffler's syndrome not manageable by other means.
Berylliosis.
Fulminating or disseminated pulmonary tuberculosis when used concurrently with appropriate antituberculous chemotherapy.
Aspiration pneumonitis.
8. Hematologic Disorders:
Idiopathic thrombocytopenic purpura in adults.
Secondary thrombocytopenia in adults.
Acquired (autoimmune) hemolytic anemia.
Erythroblastopenia (RBC anemia).
Congenital (erythroid) hypoplastic anemia.
9. Neoplastic Diseases:
For palliative management of:
Leukemias and lymphomas in adults.
Acute leukemia of childhood.
10. Edematous States:
To induce a diuresis or remission of proteinuria in the nephrotic syndrome, without uremia, of the idiopathic type or that due to lupus erythematosus.
11. Gastrointestinal Diseases:
To tide the patient over a critical period of the disease in:
Ulcerative colitis.
Regional enteritis.
12. Nervous System:
Acute exacerbations of multiple sclerosis.
13. Miscellaneous:
Tuberculous meningitis with subarachnoid block or impending block when used concurrently with appropriate antituberculous chemotherapy.
Trichinosis with neurologic or myocardial involvement.

CONTRAINDICATIONS
Systemic fungal infections.
Sensitivity to the drug or any of its components.

WARNINGS
In patients on corticosteroid therapy subjected to unusual stress, increased dosage of rapidly acting corticosteroids before, during, and after the stressful situation is indicated.
Corticosteroids may mask some signs of infection, and new infections may appear during their use. There may be decreased resistance and inability to localize infection when corticosteroids are used.
Prolonged use of corticosteroids may produce posterior subcapsular cataracts, glaucoma with possible damage to the optic nerves, and may enhance the establishment of secondary ocular infections due to fungi or viruses.
Usage in pregnancy: Since adequate human reproduction studies have not been done with corticosteroids, the use of these drugs in pregnancy, nursing mothers or women of childbearing potential requires that the possible benefits of the drug be weighed against the potential hazards to the mother and embryo or fetus. Infants born of mothers who have received substantial doses of corticosteroids during pregnancy should be carefully observed for signs of hypoadrenalism.

Average and large doses of hydrocortisone or cortisone can cause elevation of blood pressure, salt and water retention, and increased excretion of potassium. These effects are less likely to occur with ARISTOCORT *triamcinolone* except when used in large doses. Dietary salt restriction and potassium supplementation may be necessary. All corticosteroids increase calcium excretion.

While on Corticosteroid Therapy Patients Should Not Be Vaccinated Against Smallpox. Other Immunization Procedures Should Not Be Undertaken in Patients Who Are on Corticosteroids, Especially on High Doses, Because of Possible Hazards of Neurological Complications and a Lack of Antibody Response.

The use of triamcinolone in active tuberculosis should be restricted to those cases of fulminating or disseminated tuberculosis in which the corticosteroid is used for the management of the disease in conjunction with an appropriate antituberculous regimen.

If corticosteroids are indicated in patients with latent tuberculosis or tuberculin reactivity, close observation is necessary as reactivation of the disease may occur. During prolonged corticosteroid therapy, these patients should receive chemoprophylaxis.

PRECAUTIONS
Drug-induced secondary adrenocortical insufficiency may be minimized by gradual reduction of dosage. This type of relative insufficiency may persist for months after discontinuation of therapy; therefore, in any situation of stress occurring during that period, hormone therapy should be reinstituted. Since mineralocorticoid secretion may be impaired, salt and/or a mineralocorticoid should be administered concurrently.

There is an enhanced effect of corticosteroids on patients with hypothyroidism and in those with cirrhosis.

Corticosteroids should be used cautiously in patients with ocular herpes simplex because of possible corneal perforation.

The lowest possible dose of corticosteroid should be used to control the condition under treatment, and when reduction in dosage is possible, the reduction should be gradual.

Psychic derangements may appear when corticosteroids are used, ranging from euphoria, insomnia, mood swings, personality changes, and severe depression to frank psychotic manifestations. Also, existing emotional instability or psychotic tendencies may be aggravated by corticosteroids.

Aspirin should be used cautiously in conjunction with corticosteroids in hypoprothrombinemia.

Steroids should be used with caution in nonspecific ulcerative colitis if there is a probability of impending perforation, abscess or other pyogenic infection, diverticulitis, fresh intestinal anastomoses, active or latent peptic ulcer, renal insufficiency, hypertension, osteoporosis, and myasthenia gravis.

Growth and development of infants and children on prolonged corticosteroid therapy should be carefully observed.

Although controlled clinical trials have shown corticosteroids to be effective in speeding the resolution of acute exacerbations of multiple sclerosis, they do not show that they affect the ultimate outcome or natural history of the disease. The studies do show that relatively high doses of corticosteroids are necessary to demonstrate a significant effect. (See **DOSAGE AND ADMINISTRATION**.)

Since complications of treatment with glucocorticoid are dependent on the size of the dose and the duration of treatment, a risk/benefit decision must be made in each individual case as to dose and duration of treatment and as to whether daily or intermittent therapy should be used.

ADVERSE REACTIONS
Fluid and Electrolyte Disturbances:
Sodium retention.
Fluid retention.
Congestive heart failure in susceptible patients.
Potassium loss.
Hypokalemic alkalosis.
Hypertension.
Musculoskeletal:
Muscle weakness.
Steroid myopathy.
Loss of muscle mass.
Osteoporosis.
Vertebral compression fractures.
Aseptic necrosis of femoral and humeral heads.

Continued on next page

Lederle—Cont.

Pathologic fracture of long bones.

Gastrointestinal:

Peptic ulcer with possible subsequent perforation and hemorrhage.

Pancreatitis.

Abdominal distention.

Ulcerative esophagitis.

Dermatologic:

Impaired wound healing.

Thin fragile skin.

Petechiae and ecchymoses.

Facial erythema.

Increased sweating.

May suppress reactions to skin tests.

Neurological:

Convulsions.

Increased intracranial pressure with papilledema (pseudotumor cerebri) usually after treatment.

Vertigo.

Headache.

Endocrine:

Menstrual irregularities.

Development of cushingoid state.

Suppression of growth in children.

Secondary adrenocortical and pituitary unresponsiveness, particularly in times of stress, as in trauma, surgery or illness.

Decreased carbohydrate tolerance.

Manifestations of latent diabetes mellitus.

Increased requirements for insulin or oral hypoglycemic agents in diabetics.

Ophthalmic:

Posterior subcapsular cataracts.

Increased intraocular pressure.

Glaucoma.

Exophthalmos.

Metabolic:

Negative nitrogen balance due to protein catabolism.

Hypersensitivity Reactions:

Anaphylactoid reactions have been reported, rarely, with products of this class.

DOSAGE AND ADMINISTRATION

General Principles:

1. The initial dosage of ARISTOCORT *triamcinolone* may vary from 4 mg to 48 mg per day depending on the specific disease entity being treated. In situations of less severity lower doses will generally suffice while in selected patients higher initial doses may be required. The initial dosage should be maintained or adjusted until a satisfactory response is noted. If after a reasonable period of time there is a lack of satisfactory clinical response, the drug should be discontinued and the patient transferred to another appropriate therapy. IT SHOULD BE EMPHASIZED THAT DOSAGE REQUIREMENTS ARE VARIABLE AND MUST BE INDIVIDUALIZED ON THE BASIS OF THE DISEASE UNDER TREATMENT AND THE RESPONSE OF THE PATIENT. After a favorable response is noted, the proper maintenance dosage should be determined by decreasing the initial drug dosage in small increments at appropriate time intervals until the lowest dosage is reached which will maintain an adequate clinical response. It should be kept in mind that constant monitoring is needed in regard to drug dosage. Included in the situations which may make dosage adjustments necessary are changes in clinical status secondary to remissions or exacerbations in the disease process, the patient's individual drug responsiveness, and the effect of patient exposure to stressful situations not directly related to the disease entity under treatment; in this latter situation it may be necessary to increase the dosage of ARISTOCORT for a period of time consistent with the patient's condition. If after long-term therapy the drug is to be stopped, it is recommended that it be withdrawn gradually rather than abruptly.

2. Dosage should be individualized according to the severity of the disease and the response of the patient. For infants and children, the recommended dosage should be governed by the same considerations rather than by strict adherence to the ratio indicated by age or body weight.

3. Hormone therapy is an adjunct to, and not a replacement for, conventional therapy.

4. The severity, prognosis and expected duration of the disease, and the reaction of the patient to medication are primary factors in determining dosage.

5. If a period of spontaneous remission occurs in a chronic condition, treatment should be discontinued.

6. Blood pressure, body weight, routine laboratory studies, including two-hour postprandial blood glucose and serum potassium, and a chest x-ray should be obtained at regular intervals during prolonged therapy. Upper GI x-rays are desirable in patients with known or suspected peptic ulcer disease.

7. Suppression of autogenous pituitary function, a common effect of exogenous corticosteroid administration, may be reduced, modified or minimized by revision of dose schedules. The time of maximum corticoid effect is from midnight to 8 a.m. and minimal during the intervening hours. Use of a single daily dose at or about 8 a.m. will be effective in most conditions, will lower corticoid overload and will cause the least interference with the diurnal system of endogenous secretion and hypothalamopituitary-adrenal function; alternate-day dosage in some conditions and intermittent administration in certain severe disorders requiring long-term and/or high dose maintenance levels have proven both clinically effective and less likely to produce adverse reactions.

The maximum daily morning dose not associated with lasting adrenocorticoid suppression is 8 mg.

8. *Alternate-Day Therapy.* After the conventional dose has been established, some patients may be maintained on alternate-day therapy. It has been shown that the activity of the adrenal cortex varies throughout the day, being greatest from about midnight to 8 a.m. Exogenous corticoid suppresses this activity least when given at the time of maximum activity. A 48-hour interval appears to be necessary since shorter intervals are accompanied by adrenal suppression similar to that of conventional daily divided doses. Therefore, with the alternate-day dose plan, a total 48-hour requirement is given every other day at 8 a.m. As with other regimens, the minimum effective dose level should be sought.

9.* *Intermittent-Type Therapy.* An additional modification of corticosteroid usage has been recommended and used for treatment of disorders often requiring long-term administration of medium or high dose range. It is generally recommended that treatment be initiated with a single calculated dose of ARISTOCORT *triamcinolone* given once daily and continued daily until clinical response is adequate or appropriate. The time of maximum corticoid effect is from midnight to 8 a.m. and minimal during the intervening hours. Therefore, dosage beginning at or after 8 a.m. will offer good effect and lower corticoid overload. Thereafter, the patient is maintained on a calculated single daily dose given each morning for 3–4 consecutive days, followed by a "rest period" of 3 days, during which no corticosteroid is administered. This schedule is continued for as long as therapeutically indicated.

*For syrup only.

Specific Dosage Recommendations:

1. *Endocrine Disorders:* Wide variation in dosage requirements for the endocrine disorders such as *congenital adrenal hyperplasia, nonsuppurative thyroiditis,* and *hypercalcemia* associated with *cancer* precludes specific recommendation except for *adrenocortical insufficiency* where the dose is usually 4–12 mg daily in addition to mineralocorticoid therapy.

2. *Rheumatic Disorders: Rheumatoid arthritis; acute gouty arthritis; ankylosing spondylitis;* and *selected cases of psoriatic arthritis;* in *acute* and *subacute bursitis;* and in *acute nonspecific tenosynovitis.* The initial suppressive dose of ARISTOCORT in these conditions ranges from 8 to 16 mg per day, although the occasional patient may require higher doses. Patients may show an early or a delayed effect, characterized by a reduction in the inflammatory reaction and in joint swelling, together with alleviation of pain and stiffness, resulting in an increased range of motion of the affected joints or tissues. Maintenance doses are adjusted to keep symptoms at a level tolerable to the patient. Rapid reduction of the steroid or its abrupt discontinuance may result in recurrence or even exacerbation of signs and symptoms. Short-term administration is desirable as a rule. ARISTOCORT *triamcinolone* is ordinarily administered as a single morning dose, daily or on alternate days, depending on the need of the patient. Occasional patients may secure more effective relief on divided daily doses, either 2 to 4 times daily.

3. *Collagen Diseases: Systemic Lupus Erythematosus* The initial dose is usually 20 to 32 mg daily continued until the desired response is obtained, when reduced maintenance levels are sought. Patients with more severe symptoms may require higher initial doses, 48 mg or more daily, and higher maintenance doses. Although some patients with systemic lupus erythematosus appear to have spontaneous remissions or to tolerate the disorder in its milder forms for prolonged periods of time, adjustment of dosage scheduling to reduce adverse suppression of the pituitary-adrenal axis may be useful.

For Syrup: Intermittent higher doses may be given daily for three or four successive days followed by a rest period of several days; this regimen being repeated each week. *Acute Rheumatic Carditis.* In severely ill patients with carditis, pericardial effusion and/or congestive heart failure, corticosteroid therapy is effective in the control of the acute and severe inflammatory changes and may be lifesaving. Initial doses of ARISTOCORT may be from 20 to 60 mg daily, and clinical response is usually rapid and the drug can then be reduced. Maintenance therapy should be continued for at least 6 to 8 weeks and is seldom required beyond a period of 3 months. Corticosteroid therapy does not preclude conventional treatment, including antibiotics and salicylization.

4. *Dermatological Disorders: Pemphigus; bullous dermatitis herpetiformis, severe erythema multiforme* (Stevens-Johnson syndrome); *exfoliative dermatitis;* and *mycosis fungoides.* The initial dose is 8 to 16 mg daily. In these conditions, as well as in certain allergic dermatoses, *alternate-day* administration has been found effective and apparently less likely to produce adverse side effects.

Severe psoriasis: ARISTOCORT may produce reduction or remission of the disabling skin manifestations following initial doses of 8 to 16 mg daily. The period of maintenance is dependent on the clinical response. Corticosteroid reduction or discontinuation of therapy should be attempted with caution since relapse may occur and may appear in a more aggravated form, the so-called "rebound phenomenon."

5. *Allergic States:* ARISTOCORT *triamcinolone* is administered in doses of 8 to 12 mg daily in acute seasonal or perennial *allergic rhinitis.* Intractable cases may require high initial and maintenance doses. In *bronchial asthma,* 8 to 16 mg daily are usually effective. The usual therapeutic measures for control of bronchial asthma should be carried out in addition to ARISTOCORT therapy. In both allergic rhinitis and bronchial asthma, therapy is directed at alleviation of acute distress and chronic long-term use of corticosteroids is neither desirable nor often essential. Some patients may be maintained on alternate-day therapy. In such conditions as *contact dermatitis* and *atopic dermatitis,* topical therapy may be supplemented with short courses of ARISTOCORT by mouth in doses of 8 to 16 mg daily. In severely ill patients with *serum sickness,* epinephrine may be the drug of choice for immediate therapy, often supplemented by antihistamines.

ARISTOCORT is frequently useful as adjunctive treatment in such cases, with the dosage determined by the severity of the disorder, the speed with which therapeutic response is desired and the response of the patient to initial therapy.

6. *Ophthalmological Diseases: Allergic conjunctivitis; keratitis; allergic corneal marginal ulcers, iritis* and *iridocyclitis; chorioretinitis; anterior segment inflammation; diffuse posterior uveitis* and *choroiditis; optic neuritis* and *sympathetic ophthalmia.* Initial doses range from 12 to 40 mg daily depending on the severity of the condition, the nature and degree of involvement of ocular structure, but response is usually rapid and therapy of short-term duration.

7. *Respiratory Diseases: Symptomatic sarcoidosis; Loeffler's Syndrome; berylliosis;* and in certain cases of *fulminating* or *disseminated pulmonary tuberculosis* when concurrently accompanied by appropriate antituberculous chemotherapy. Initial doses are usually in the range of 16 to 48 mg daily.

8. *Hematologic Disorders: Idiopathic* and secondary *thrombocytopenia in adults, acquired* (autoimmune) *hemolytic anemia; erythroblastopenia* (RBC anemia); *congenital* (erythroid) *hypoplastic anemia.* ARISTOCORT is used to produce a remission of symptoms and may, in some instances, produce an apparent regression of abnormal cellular blood elements to normal states, temporary or permanent. The recommended dose varies between 16 and 60 mg daily, with reduction after adequate clinical response.

9. *Neoplastic Diseases: Acute leukemia in childhood.* The usual dose of ARISTOCORT is 1 mg per kilogram of body weight daily, although as much as 2 mg per kilogram may be necessary. Initial response is usually seen within 6 to 21 days and continued from 4 to 6 weeks. *Acute leukemia* and *lymphoma in adults.* The usual dose of ARISTOCORT *triamcinolone* is 16 to 40 mg daily, although it may be necessary to give as much as 100 mg daily in leukemia. ARISTOCORT therapy in these neoplasias is only palliative and not curative. Other therapeutic and supportive measures must be used when appropriate.

10. *Edematous States: Nephrotic Syndrome:* ARISTOCORT may be used to induce a diuresis or remission of proteinuria in the *nephrotic syndrome,* without uremia, of the idiopathic type or that due to *lupus erythematosus.* The average dose is 16 to 20 mg (up to 48 mg) daily until diuresis occurs. The diuresis may be massive and usually occurs by the 14th day, but occasionally may be delayed. After diuresis begins it is advisable to continue treatment until maximal or complete chemical and clinical remission occurs, at which time the dosage should be reduced gradually and then discontinued. In less severe cases maintenance dosages of as little as 4 mg daily may be adequate. Alternatively and when maintenance therapy may be prolonged, ARISTOCORT may be administered on alternate-day dose schedules.

11. *Miscellaneous: Tuberculous meningitis:* ARISTOCORT may be useful when accompanied by appropriate antituberculous therapy when there is subarachnoid block or impending block. The average dosage is 32 to 48 mg daily in either single or divided doses.

[See table on top next page].

HOW SUPPLIED

ARISTOCORT *triamcinolone* Tablets are supplied as follows:

1 mg—oblong, flat, scored, yellow tablet engraved with LL on one side and A1 on the other.

	Anti-inflammatory Relative Potency		Frequently Used Tablet Strength (mg)		Tablet × Potency Equivalent Value
Hydrocortisone	1	×	20	=	20
Prednisolone	4	×	5	=	20
ARISTOCORT triamcinolone	5	×	4	=	20
Dexamethasone	25	×	0.75	=	18.75

NDC 0005-4409-18—bottles of 50

2 mg—oblong, flat, scored, pink tablet engraved with LL on one side and A2 on the other.

NDC 0005-4405-23—bottles of 100

4 mg—oblong, flat, scored, white tablet engraved with LL on one side and A4 on the other.

NDC 0005-4406-13—bottles of 30

NDC 0005-4406-23—bottles of 100

NDC 0005-4406-07—ARISTO-PAK® *triamcinolone* 16s (for 6 days therapy)

8 mg—oblong, flat, scored, yellow tablet engraved with LL on one side and A8 on the other.

NDC 0005-4444-18—bottles of 50

ARISTOCORT Triamcinolone Diacetate Syrup contains 2 mg/5 mL of triamcinolone diacetate in a cherry-flavored base, supplied as follows:

NDC 0005-4421-58—4 fl oz bottle

Store at Controlled Room Temperature 15–30° C (59–86° F).

LEDERLE LABORATORIES DIVISION
American Cyanamid Company,
Pearl River, N.Y. 10965   Rev. 7/85–5/87
       17015, 21051

Tablets and Aristo-Pak 4 mg shown in Product Identification Section, page 414

ARISTOCORT®   ℞

[*a-ris-tō-cort*]

triamcinolone acetonide

Topical Products

[See table below].

The topical corticosteroids constitute a class of primarily synthetic steroids used as anti-inflammatory and antipruritic agents.

CLINICAL PHARMACOLOGY

Topical corticosteroids share anti-inflammatory, antipruritic, and vasoconstrictive actions.

The mechanism of anti-inflammatory activity of the topical corticosteroids is unclear. Various laboratory methods, including vasoconstrictor assays, are used to compare and predict potencies and/or clinical efficacies of the topical corticosteroids. There is some evidence to suggest that a recognizable correlation exists between vasoconstrictor potency and therapeutic efficacy in man.

PHARMACOKINETICS

The extent of percutaneous absorption of topical corticosteroids is determined by many factors including the vehicle, the integrity of the epidermal barrier, and the use of occlusive dressings.

Topical corticosteroids can be absorbed from normal intact skin. Inflammation and/or other disease processes in the skin increase percutaneous absorption. Occlusive dressings substantially increase the percutaneous absorption of topical corticosteroids. Thus, occlusive dressings may be a valuable therapeutic adjunct for treatment of resistant dermatoses. (See **DOSAGE AND ADMINISTRATION**.)

Once absorbed through the skin, topical corticosteroids are handled through pharmacokinetic pathways similar to systemically administered corticosteroids. Corticosteroids are bound to plasma proteins in varying degrees. Corticosteroids are metabolized primarily in the liver and are then excreted by the kidneys. Some of the topical corticosteroids and their metabolites are also excreted into the bile.

INDICATIONS AND USAGE

Topical corticosteroids are indicated for the relief of the inflammatory and pruritic manifestations of corticosteroid-responsive dermatoses.

CONTRAINDICATIONS

Topical corticosteroids are contraindicated in those patients with a history of hypersensitivity to any of the components of the preparation.

PRECAUTIONS

General: Systemic absorption of topical corticosteroids has produced reversible hypothalamic-pituitary-adrenal (HPA) axis suppression, manifestations of Cushing's syndrome, hyperglycemia, and glucosuria in some patients.

Conditions which augment systemic absorption include the application of the more potent steroids, use over large surface areas, prolonged use, and the addition of occlusive dressings.

Therefore, patients receiving a large dose of a potent topical steroid applied to a large surface area or under an occlusive dressing should be evaluated periodically for evidence of HPA axis suppression by using the urinary free cortisol and ACTH stimulation tests. If HPA axis suppression is noted, an attempt should be made to withdraw the drug, to reduce the frequency of application, or to substitute a less potent steroid.

Recovery of HPA axis function is generally prompt and complete upon discontinuation of the drug. Infrequently, signs and symptoms of steroid withdrawal may occur, requiring supplemental systemic corticosteroids.

Children may absorb proportionally larger amounts of topical corticosteroids and thus be more susceptible to systemic toxicity. (See **PRECAUTIONS-Pediatric Use**.)

If irritation develops, topical corticosteroids should be discontinued and appropriate therapy instituted.

In the presence of dermatological infections, the use of an appropriate antifungal or antibacterial agent should be instituted. If a favorable response does not occur promptly, the corticosteroid should be discontinued until the infection has been adequately controlled.

Information for the Patient: Patients using topical corticosteroids should receive the following information and instructions:

1. This medication is to be used as directed by the physician. It is for external use only. Avoid contact with the eyes.
2. Patients should be advised not to use this medication for any disorder other than for which it was prescribed.
3. The treated skin area should not be bandaged or otherwise covered or wrapped as to be occlusive unless directed by the physician.
4. Patients should report any signs of local adverse reactions especially under occlusive dressing.
5. Parents of pediatric patients should be advised not to use tight-fitting diapers or plastic pants on a child being treated in the diaper area since these garments may constitute occlusive dressings.

Laboratory Tests: The following tests may be helpful in evaluating the HPA axis suppression:

Urinary free cortisol test

ACTH stimulation test

Carcinogenesis, Mutagenesis, and Impairment of Fertility: Long-term animal studies have not been performed to evaluate the carcinogenic potential or the effect on fertility of topical corticosteroids.

Studies to determine mutagenicity with prednisolone and hydrocortisone have revealed negative results.

Pregnancy Category C: Corticosteroids are generally teratogenic in laboratory animals when administered systemically at relatively low dosage levels. The more potent corticosteroids have been shown to be teratogenic after dermal application in laboratory animals. There are no adequate and well-controlled studies in pregnant women on teratogenic effects from topically applied corticosteroids. Therefore, topical corticosteroids should be used during pregnancy only if the potential benefit justifies the potential risk to the fetus. Drugs of this class should not be used extensively on pregnant patients, in large amounts, or for prolonged periods of time.

Nursing Mothers: It is not known whether topical administration of corticosteroids could result in sufficient systemic absorption to produce detectable quantities in breast milk. Systemically administered corticosteroids are secreted into breast milk in quantities *not* likely to have a deleterious effect on the infant. Nevertheless, caution should be exercised when topical corticosteroids are administered to a nursing woman.

Pediatric Use: *Pediatric patients may demonstrate greater susceptibility to topical corticosteroid-induced HPA axis suppression and Cushing's syndrome than mature patients because of a larger skin surface area to body weight ratio.*

Hypothalamic-pituitary-adrenal (HPA) axis suppression, Cushing's syndrome, and intracranial hypertension have been reported in children receiving topical corticosteroids. Manifestations of adrenal suppression in children include linear growth retardation, delayed weight gain, low plasma cortisol levels, and absence of response to ACTH stimulation. Manifestations of intracranial hypertension include bulging fontanelles, headaches, and bilateral papilledema.

Administration of topical corticosteroids to children should be limited to the least amount compatible with an effective therapeutic regimen. Chronic corticosteroid therapy may interfere with the growth and development of children.

ADVERSE REACTIONS

The following local adverse reactions are reported infrequently with topical corticosteroids, but may occur more frequently with the use of occlusive dressings. These reactions are listed in an approximate decreasing order of occurrence:

Burning	Perioral dermatitis
Itching	Allergic contact dermatitis
Irritation	Maceration of the skin
Dryness	Secondary infection
Folliculitis	Skin atrophy
Hypertrichosis	Striae
Acneiform eruptions	Miliaria
Hypopigmentation	

OVERDOSAGE

Topically applied corticosteroids can be absorbed in sufficient amounts to produce systemic effects (See **PRECAUTIONS**).

HOW SUPPLIED

Cream 0.025% (0.25 mg/g)

15 g tubes—   NDC 0005-5130-09

60 g tubes—   NDC 0005-5130-40

5.25 lb jars—   NDC 0005-5130-54

ARISTOCORT Triamcinolone Acetonide TOPICAL PRODUCTS

	Cream 0.025%	Cream 0.1%	Cream 0.5%	Ointment 0.1%	0.5%
Each gram contains Triamcinolone Acetonide	0.25 mg	1 mg	5 mg	1 mg	5 mg
Preservatives:					
Sorbic Acid	0.1%	0.1%	0.1%		
Potassium Sorbate	0.1%	0.1%	0.1%		
Inactive Ingredients:	Mono- and Diglycerides, Squalane, Polysorbate 80, Cetyl Esters Wax, Stearyl Alcohol, Tenox II (butylated hydroxyanisole, propyl gallate, citric acid, propylene glycol), Sorbitol Solution, Sorbic Acid 0.1%, and Potassium Sorbate 0.1%.			White Petrolatum	

Chemical name: Triamcinolone acetonide is pregna-1,4-diene-3,20-dione,9-fluoro-11,21-dihydroxy-16,17-[(1-methylethylidene)bis(oxy)]-,(11β,16α)-.

Dosage and Administration	Apply to the affected areas as a thin film three to four times daily. Occlusive dressings may be used for the management of psoriasis or recalcitrant conditions. If an infection develops, the use of occlusive dressings should be discontinued and appropriate antimicrobial therapy instituted.

Continued on next page

Information on Lederle products listed on these pages is the full prescribing information from product literature or package inserts effective in August, 1989. Information concerning all Lederle products may be obtained from the Professional Services Department, Lederle Laboratories, Pearl River, New York, 10965.

Lederle—Cont.

Cream 0.1%
15 g tubes— NDC 0005-5131-09
60 g tubes— NDC 0005-5131-40
240 g jars— NDC 0005-5131-57
5.25 lb jars— NDC 0005-5131-54
Cream 0.5% (5 mg/g)
15 g tubes— NDC 0005-5132-09
240 g jars— NDC 0005-5132-57
Ointment 0.1% (1 mg/g)
15 g tubes— NDC 0005-5175-09
60 g tubes— NDC 0005-5175-40
240 g jars— NDC 0005-5175-57
5 lb jars— NDC 0005-5175-70
Ointment 0.5% (5 mg/g)
15 g tubes— NDC 0005-5178-09
240 g jars— NDC 0005-5178-57
Store at Controlled Room Temperature 15–30° C (59–86°F)
Do Not Freeze.
LEDERLE LABORATORIES DIVISION
American Cyanamid Company,
Pearl River, N.Y. 10965   Rev. 1/88
21996
Shown in Product Identification Section, page 413

Suspensions
ARISTOCORT®
[a-ris-tō-cort]
Sterile triamcinolone diacetate
Forte parenteral 40 mg/mL
Intralesional 25 mg/mL
NOT FOR INTRAVENOUS USE

DESCRIPTION
FORTE PARENTERAL:
A sterile suspension of 40 mg/mL of triamcinolone diacetate (micronized) suspended in a vehicle consisting of:
Polysorbate 80 NF 0.20%
Polyethylene Glycol 3350 NF 3%
Sodium Chloride.........................0.85%
Benzyl Alcohol.........................0.90%
Water for Injection q.s...................100%
Hydrochloric acid and/or sodium hydroxide may be used during manufacture to adjust pH of suspension to approximately 6.
This preparation is a slightly soluble suspension suitable for parenteral administration through a 24-gauge needle (or larger), but NOT suitable for intravenous use. It may be administered by the intramuscular, intra-articular, or intrasynovial routes, depending upon the situation. The response to each glucocorticoid varies considerably with each type of disease indication and each corticosteroid prescribed. Irreversible clumping occurs when product is frozen.
Chemically triamcinolone diacetate is Pregna-1,4-diene-3,20-dione,16,21-bis(acetyloxy)-9-fluoro-11,17-dihydroxy-,(11β,16α)- or 9-Fluoro-11β,16α,17,21-tetrahydroxypregna-1,4-diene-3,20-dione 16,21-diacetate.

ACTION
FORTE PARENTERAL:
ARISTOCORT is primarily glucocorticoid in action and has potent anti-inflammatory, hormonal and metabolic effects common to cortisone-like drugs. It is essentially devoid of mineralocorticoid activity when administered in therapeutic doses, causing little or no sodium retention, with potassium excretion minimal or absent. The body's immune responses to diverse stimuli are also modified by its action.

INDICATIONS
FORTE PARENTERAL:
Where oral therapy is not feasible or temporarily desirable in the judgment of the physician, sterile triamcinolone diacetate suspension, 40 mg/mL, is indicated for intramuscular use as follows:
1. Endocrine disorders.
   Primary or secondary adrenocortical insufficiency (hydrocortisone or cortisone is the drug of choice; synthetic analogs may be used in conjunction with mineralocorticoids where applicable; in infancy, mineralocorticoid supplementation is of particular importance). Preoperatively and in the event of serious trauma or illness, in patients with known adrenal insufficiency or when adrenocortical reserve is doubtful.
   Congenital adrenal hyperplasia.
   Nonsuppurative thyroiditis.
   Hypercalcemia associated with cancer.
2. Rheumatic disorders. As adjunctive therapy for short-term administration (to tide the patient over an acute episode or exacerbation) in:
   Posttraumatic osteoarthritis.
   Synovitis of osteoarthritis.
   Rheumatoid arthritis, including juvenile rheumatoid arthritis (selected cases may require low-dose maintenance therapy).

Acute and subacute bursitis.
Epicondylitis.
Acute nonspecific tenosynovitis.
Acute gouty arthritis.
Psoriatic arthritis.
Ankylosing spondylitis.
3. Collagen diseases. During an exacerbation or as maintenance therapy in selected cases of:
   Systemic lupus erythematosus.
   Acute rheumatic carditis.
4. Dermatologic diseases. Pemphigus.
   Severe erythema multiforme (Stevens-Johnson syndrome).
   Exfoliative dermatitis.
   Bullous dermatitis herpetiformis.
   Severe seborrheic dermatitis.
   Severe psoriasis.
   Mycosis fungoides.
5. Allergic states. Control of severe or incapacitating allergic conditions intractable to adequate trials of conventional treatment in:
   Bronchial asthma.
   Contact dermatitis.
   Atopic dermatitis.
   Serum sickness.
   Seasonal or perennial allergic rhinitis.
   Drug hypersensitivity reactions.
   Urticarial transfusion reactions.
   Acute noninfectious laryngeal edema (epinephrine is the drug of first choice).
6. Ophthalmic diseases. Severe acute and chronic allergic and inflammatory processes involving the eye, such as:
   Herpes zoster ophthalmicus.
   Iritis, iridocyclitis.
   Chorioretinitis.
   Diffuse posterior uveitis and choroiditis.
   Optic neuritis.
   Sympathetic ophthalmia.
   Allergic conjunctivitis.
   Allergic corneal marginal ulcers.
   Keratitis.
7. Gastrointestinal disease. To tide the patient over a critical period of disease in:
   Ulcerative colitis - (Systemic therapy).
   Regional enteritis - (Systemic therapy).
8. Respiratory diseases.
   Symptomatic sarcoidosis.
   Berylliosis.
   Fulminating or disseminated pulmonary tuberculosis when used concurrently with appropriate antituberculous chemotherapy.
   Loeffler's syndrome not manageable by other means.
   Aspiration pneumonitis.
9. Hematologic disorders.
   Acquired (autoimmune) hemolytic anemia.
   Secondary thrombocytopenia in adults.
   Erythroblastopenia (RBC anemia).
   Congenital (erythroid) hypoplastic anemia.
10. Neoplastic diseases. For palliative management of:
    Leukemias and lymphomas in adults.
    Acute leukemia of childhood.
11. Edematous state. To induce diuresis or remission of proteinuria in the nephrotic syndrome, without uremia, of the idiopathic type or that due to lupus erythematosus.
12. Nervous System.
    Acute exacerbations of multiple sclerosis.
13. Miscellaneous. Tuberculous meningitis with subarachnoid block or impending block when used concurrently with appropriate antituberculous chemotherapy.
    Trichinosis with neurologic or myocardial involvement.

ARISTOCORT *triamcinolone diacetate* FORTE 40 mg/mL is indicated for intra-articular or soft tissue use as follows:
As adjunctive therapy for short-term administration (to tide the patient over an acute episode or exacerbation) in:
Synovitis of osteoarthritis.
Rheumatoid arthritis.
Acute and subacute bursitis.
Acute gouty arthritis.
Epicondylitis.
Acute nonspecific tenosynovitis.
Posttraumatic osteoarthritis.
ARISTOCORT FORTE is indicated for intralesional use as follows:
Keloids.
Localized hypertrophic, infiltrated, inflammatory lesion of: Lichen planus, psoriatic plaques, granuloma annulare and lichen simplex chronicus (neurodermatitis).
Discoid lupus erythematosus.
Necrobiosis lipoidica diabeticorum.
Alopecia areata.
It may also be useful in cystic tumors of an aponeurosis or tendon (ganglia).

DESCRIPTION
INTRALESIONAL:
ARISTOCORT *triamcinolone diacetate* possesses glucocorticoid properties while being essentially devoid of mineralocorticoid activity thus causing little or no sodium retention. Supplied as a sterile suspension of 25 mg/mL micronized triamcinolone diacetate in the following vehicle:
Polysorbate 80 NF 0.20%
Polyethylene Glycol 3350 NF 3%
Sodium Chloride................0.85%
Benzyl Alcohol................0.90%
Water for Injection q.s...........100%
Hydrochloric acid and/or sodium hydroxide may be used during manufacture to adjust pH of suspension to approximately 6.
Chemically triamcinolone diacetate is Pregna - 1, 4 - diene - 3, 20 - dione, 16, 21 - bis(acetyloxy) - 9 - fluoro - 11, 17-dihydroxy-,(11β, 16α)- or 9-Fluoro-11β, 16α, 17, 21-tetrahydroxypregna-1, 4-diene-3,20-dione 16,21-diacetate. Molecular weight is 478.51.

ACTIONS
INTRALESIONAL:
Naturally occurring glucocorticoids (hydrocortisone), which also have salt-retaining properties, are used as replacement therapy in adrenocortical deficiency states. Their synthetic analogs are primarily used for their potent anti-inflammatory effects in disorders of many organ systems.
Glucocorticoids cause profound and varied metabolic effects. In addition, they modify the body's immune responses to diverse stimuli.

INDICATIONS
INTRALESIONAL:
ARISTOCORT *triamcinolone diacetate* Intralesional is indicated by the intralesional route for:
Keloids
Localized hypertrophic, infiltrated, inflammatory lesion of:
lichen planus, psoriatic plaques, granuloma annulare and lichen simplex chronicus (neurodermatitis).
Discoid lupus erythematosus.
Necrobiosis lipoidica diabeticorum.
Alopecia areata.
It may also be useful in cystic tumors of an aponeurosis or tendon (ganglia).
When used intra-articularly it is also indicated for:
Adjunctive therapy for short-term administration (to tide the patient over an acute episode or exacerbation) in:
Synovitis of osteoarthritis.
Rheumatoid arthritis.
Acute and subacute bursitis.
Acute gouty arthritis.
Epicondylitis.
Acute nonspecific tenosynovitis.
Posttraumatic osteoarthritis.

CONTRAINDICATIONS
FORTE PARENTERAL AND INTRALESIONAL:
Systemic fungal infections.

WARNINGS
In patients on corticosteroid therapy subjected to any unusual stress, increased dosage of rapidly acting corticosteroids before, during, and after the stressful situation is indicated.
Corticosteroids may mask some signs of infection, and new infections may appear during their use. There may be decreased resistance and inability to localize infection when corticosteroids are used.
Prolonged use of corticosteroids may produce posterior subcapsular cataracts, glaucoma with possible damage to the optic nerves and may enhance the establishment of secondary ocular infections due to fungi or viruses.
Usage in Pregnancy
Since adequate human reproduction studies have not been done with corticosteroids, the use of these drugs in pregnancy, nursing mothers, or women of childbearing potential requires that the possible benefits of the drug be weighed against the potential hazards to the mother and embryo or fetus. Infants born of mothers who have received substantial doses of corticosteroids during pregnancy should be carefully observed for signs of hypoadrenalism.
Average and large doses of cortisone or hydrocortisone can cause elevation of blood pressure, salt and water retention, and increased excretion of potassium. These effects are less likely to occur with the synthetic derivatives except when used in large doses. Dietary salt restriction and potassium supplementation may be necessary. All corticosteroids increase calcium excretion.
While on Corticosteroid Therapy Patients Should Not Be Vaccinated Against Smallpox. Other Immunization Procedures Should Not Be Undertaken in Patients Who Are on Corticosteroids, Especially in High Doses, Because of Possible Hazards of Neurological Complications and Lack of Antibody Response.

The use of ARISTOCORT *triamcinolone diacetate* in active tuberculosis should be restricted to those cases of fulminating or disseminated tuberculosis in which the corticosteroid is used for the management of the disease in conjunction with appropriate antituberculous regimen.

If corticosteroids are indicated in patients with latent tuberculosis or tuberculin reactivity, close observation is necessary as reactivation of the disease may occur. During prolonged corticosteroid therapy, these patients should receive chemoprophylaxis.

Because rare instances of anaphylactoid reactions have occurred in patients receiving parenteral corticosteroid therapy, appropriate precautionary measures should be taken prior to administration, especially when the patient has a history of allergy to any drug.

Postinjection flare (following intra-articular use) and Charcot-like arthropathy have been associated with parenteral corticosteroid therapy.

Intralesional or sublesional injection of excessive dosage whether by single or multiple injection into any given area may cause cutaneous or subcutaneous atrophy.

PRECAUTIONS

FORTE PARENTERAL AND INTRALESIONAL:

Drug-induced secondary adrenocortical insufficiency may be minimized by gradual reduction of dosage. This type of relative insufficiency may persist for months after discontinuation of therapy; therefore, in any situation of stress occurring during that period, hormone therapy should be reinstituted. Since mineralocorticoid secretion may be impaired, salt and/or a mineralocorticoid should be administered concurrently.

There is an enhanced effect of corticosteroids in patients with hypothyroidism and in those with cirrhosis.

Corticosteroids should be used cautiously in patients with ocular herpes simplex for fear of corneal perforation.

The lowest possible dose of corticosteroid should be used to control the condition under treatment, and when reduction in dosage is possible, the reduction must be gradual.

Psychic derangements may appear when corticosteroids are used, ranging from euphoria, insomnia, mood swings, personality changes, and severe depression to frank psychotic manifestations. Also, existing emotional instability or psychotic tendencies may be aggravated by corticosteroids.

Aspirin should be used cautiously in conjunction with corticosteroids in hypoprothrombinemia.

Steroids should be used with caution in nonspecific ulcerative colitis, if there is a probability of impending perforation, abscess or other pyogenic infection, also in diverticulitis, fresh intestinal anastomoses, active or latent peptic ulcer, renal insufficiency, hypertension, osteoporosis, and myasthenia gravis.

Growth and development of infants and children on prolonged corticosteroid therapy should be carefully followed. The following additional precautions apply for parenteral corticosteroids.

Intra-articular injection of a corticosteroid may produce systemic as well as local effects.

Appropriate examination of any joint fluid present is necessary to exclude a septic process.

A marked increase in pain accompanied by local swelling, further restriction of joint motion, fever, and malaise are suggestive of septic arthritis. If this complication occurs and the diagnosis of sepsis is confirmed, appropriate antimicrobial therapy should be instituted.

Local injection of a steroid into a previously infected joint is to be avoided.

Corticosteroid should not be injected into unstable joints.

The slower rate of absorption by intramuscular administration should be recognized.

Atrophy at the site of injection has been reported.

Routine laboratory studies, such as urinalysis, two-hour postprandial blood sugar, determination of blood pressure and body weight, and a chest X-ray should be made at regular intervals during prolonged therapy. Upper GI X-rays are desirable in patients with an ulcer history or significant dyspepsia.

FORTE PARENTERAL:

Accidental injection into soft tissue during intra-articular administration decreases local effectiveness in the joint and, by increasing rate of absorption, may produce systemic effects.

Although controlled clinical trials have shown corticosteroids to be effective in speeding the resolution of acute exacerbations of multiple sclerosis they do not show that they affect the ultimate outcome or natural history of the disease. The studies do show that relatively high doses of corticosteroids are necessary to demonstrate a significant effect. (See **DOSAGE AND ADMINISTRATION**.)

Since complications of treatment with glucocorticoid are dependent on the size of the dose and the duration of treatment, a risk/benefit decision must be made in each individual case as to dose and duration of treatment and as to whether daily or intermittent therapy should be used.

ADVERSE REACTIONS

Fluid and electrolyte disturbances:
 Sodium retention.
 Fluid retention.
 Congestive heart failure in susceptible patients.
 Potassium loss.
 Hypokalemic alkalosis.
 Hypertension.
Musculoskeletal:
 Muscle weakness.
 Steroid myopathy.
 Loss of muscle mass.
 Osteoporosis.
 Vertebral compression fractures.
 Aseptic necrosis of femoral and humeral heads.
 Pathologic fracture of long bones.
Gastrointestinal:
 Peptic ulcer with possible subsequent perforation and hemorrhage.
 Pancreatitis.
 Abdominal distention.
 Ulcerative esophagitis.
Dermatologic:
 Impaired wound healing.
 Thin fragile skin.
 Petechiae and ecchymoses.
 Facial erythema.
 Increased sweating.
 May suppress reactions to skin tests.
Neurological:
 Convulsions.
 Increased intracranial pressure with papilledema (pseudotumor cerebri) usually after treatment.
 Vertigo.
 Headache.
Endocrine:
 Menstrual irregularities.
 Development of cushingoid state.
 Suppression of growth in children.
 Secondary adrenocortical and pituitary unresponsiveness, particularly in times of stress, as in trauma, surgery, or illness.
 Decreased carbohydrate tolerance.
 Manifestations of latent diabetes mellitus.
 Increased requirements for insulin or oral hypoglycemic agents in diabetics.
Ophthalmic:
 Posterior subcapsular cataracts.
 Increased intraocular pressure.
 Glaucoma.
 Exophthalmos.
Metabolic:
 Negative nitrogen balance due to protein catabolism.
The following additional adverse reactions are related to parenteral and intralesional corticosteroid therapy:
 Rare instances of blindness associated with intralesional therapy around the face and head.
 Hyperpigmentation or hypopigmentation.
 Subcutaneous and cutaneous atrophy.
 Sterile abscess.
Anaphylactoid reactions have been reported rarely with products of this class.

DOSAGE AND ADMINISTRATION

General: The initial dosage of ARISTOCORT *triamcinolone diacetate* may vary from 3 to 48 mg per day depending on the specific disease entity being treated. In situations of less severity, lower doses will generally suffice while in selected patients higher initial doses may be required. Usually the parenteral dosage ranges are one-third to one-half the oral dose given every 12 hours. However, in certain overwhelming, acute, life-threatening situations, administration in dosages exceeding the usual dosages may be justified and may be in multiples of the oral dosages.

The initial dosage should be maintained or adjusted until a satisfactory response is noted. If after a reasonable period of time there is a lack of satisfactory clinical response, ARISTOCORT should be discontinued and the patient transferred to other appropriate therapy. It Should Be Emphasized That Dosage Requirements Are Variable and Must Be Individualized on the Basis of the Disease Under Treatment and the Response of the Patient. After a favorable response is noted, the proper maintenance dosage should be determined by decreasing the initial drug dosage in small increments at appropriate time intervals until the lowest dosage which will maintain an adequate clinical response is reached. It should be kept in mind that constant monitoring is needed in regard to drug dosage. Included in the situations which may make dosage adjustments necessary are changes in clinical status secondary to remissions or exacerbations in the disease process, the patient's individual drug responsiveness, and the effect of patient exposure to stressful situations not directly related to the disease entity under treatment; in this latter situation, it may be necessary to increase the dosage of ARISTOCORT for a period of time consistent with the patient's condition. If after long-term therapy the drug is to be stopped, it is recommended that it be withdrawn gradually rather than abruptly.

For intra-articular, intralesional and soft tissue use, a lesser initial dosage range of triamcinolone diacetate may produce the desired effect when the drug is administered to provide a localized concentration. The site of the injection and the volume of the injection should be carefully considered when triamcinolone diacetate is administered for this purpose.

Specific: FORTE PARENTERAL: ARISTOCORT FORTE Parenteral is sterile *triamcinolone diacetate* (40 mg/mL) suspended in a suitable vehicle. The full-strength suspension may be employed. If preferred, the suspension may be diluted with normal saline or water. The diluent may also be prepared by mixing equal parts of normal saline and 1% procaine hydrochloride or other similar local anesthetics. The use of diluents containing preservatives such as methylparaben, propylparaben, phenol, etc, must be avoided as these preparations tend to cause flocculation of the steroid. These dilutions retain full potency for at least one week. Topical ethyl chloride spray may be used locally prior to injection.

Since this product has been designed for ease of administration, a small bore needle (not smaller than 24 gauge) may be used.

Intramuscular: Although ARISTOCORT FORTE Parenteral may be administered intramuscularly for initial therapy, most physicians prefer to adjust the dose orally until adequate control is attained. Intramuscular administration provides a sustained or depot action which can be used to supplement or replace initial oral therapy. With intramuscular therapy, greater supervision of the amount of steroid used is made possible in the patient who is inconsistent in following an oral dosage schedule. In maintenance therapy, the patient-to-patient response is not uniform and, therefore, the dose must be individualized for optimal control.

Although triamcinolone diacetate may possess greater anti-inflammatory potency than many glucocorticoids, this is only dose-related since side effects, such as osteoporosis, peptic ulcer, etc, related to glucocorticoid activity, have not been diminished.

The average dose is 40 mg (1 mL) administered intramuscularly once a week for conditions in which anti-inflammatory action is desired.

In general, a single parenteral dose 4 to 7 times the oral daily dose may be expected to control the patient from 4 to 7 days up to 3 to 4 weeks. Dosage should be adjusted to the point where adequate but not necessarily complete relief of symptoms is obtained.

Intra-Articular and Intrasynovial: The usual dose varies from 5 to 40 mg. The average for the knee, for example, is 25 mg. The duration of effect varies from one week to 2 months. However, acutely inflamed joints may require more frequent injections.

A lesser initial dosage range of triamcinolone diacetate may produce the desired effect when the drug is administered to provide a localized concentration. The site of the injection and the volume of the injection should be carefully considered when triamcinolone diacetate is administered for this purpose.

A specific dose depends largely on the size of the joint. Strict surgical asepsis is mandatory. The physician should be familiar with anatomical relationships as described in standard text books. ARISTOCORT FORTE *triamcinolone diacetate* Parenteral may be used in any accessible joint except the intervertebrals. In general, intrasynovial therapy is suggested under the following circumstances:

1. When systemic steroid therapy is contraindicated because of side effects such as peptic ulcer.
2. When it is desirable to secure relief in one or two specific joints.
3. When good systemic maintenance fails to control flare-ups in a few joints and it is desirable to secure relief without increasing oral therapy.

Such treatment should not be considered to constitute a cure; for although this method will ameliorate the joint symptoms, it does not preclude the need for the conventional measures usually employed.

It is suggested that infiltration of the soft tissue by local anesthetic precede intra-articular injection. A 24-gauge or larger needle on a dry syringe may be inserted into the joint and excess fluid aspirated. For the first few hours following injection, there may be local discomfort in the joint but this is usually followed rapidly by effective relief of pain and improvement in local function.

Continued on next page

Information on Lederle products listed on these pages is the full prescribing information from product literature or package inserts effective in August, 1989. Information concerning all Lederle products may be obtained from the Professional Services Department, Lederle Laboratories, Pearl River, New York, 10965.

Lederle—Cont.

	Anti-inflammatory Relative Potency		Frequently Used Tablet Strength (mg)		Tablet × Potency Equivalent Value
Hydrocortisone	1	×	20	=	20
Prednisolone	4	×	5	=	20
ARISTOCORT triamcinolone	5	×	4	=	20
Dexamethasone	25	×	0.75	=	18.75

INTRALESIONAL

When ARISTOCORT Intralesional is administered by injection, strict aseptic technique is mandatory. Full strength suspensions may be employed, or if preferred, the suspension may be diluted, either to a 1:1 or 1:10 concentration, thus obtaining a working concentration of 12.5 mg/mL or approximately 2.5 mg/mL respectively. Normal (isotonic) saline solution alone or equal parts of normal (isotonic) saline solution and 1% procaine or other local anesthetics may be used as diluents. These dilutions usually retain full potency for at least one week. Topical ethyl chloride spray may be used as a local anesthetic. The use of diluents containing preservatives such as methylparaben, propylparaben, phenol, etc, must be avoided as these preparations tend to cause flocculations of the steroid.

Since this product has been designed for ease of administration, a small bore needle (not smaller than 24 gauge) may be used.

Intralesional or Sublesional: For small lesions, injection is usually well tolerated and a local anesthetic is not necessary. The location and type of lesion will determine the route of injection: intralesional, sublesional, intradermal, subdermal, intracutaneous, or subcutaneous. The size of the lesion will determine: the total amount of drug needed, the concentration used, and the number and pattern of injection sites utilized (eg, from a total of 5 mg ARISTOCORT Intralesional in a 2 mL volume divided over several locations in small lesions, ranging up to 48 mg total ARISTOCORT Intralesional for large psoriatic plaques). Avoid injecting too superficially. In general, no more than 12.5 mg per injection site should be used. An average of 25 mg is the usual limit for any one lesion. Large areas require multiple injections with smaller doses per injection. For a majority of conditions, sublesional injection directly through the lesion into the deep dermal tissue is suggested. In cases where it is difficult to inject intradermally, the suspension may be introduced subcutaneously, as superficially as possible.

Two or three injections at one to two week intervals may suffice as an average course of treatment for many conditions. Within 5-7 days after initial injection involution of the lesion can usually be seen, with pronounced clearing towards normal tissue after 12-14 days. Multiple injections of small amounts of equal strength may be convenient in alopecia areata and in psoriasis where there are large or confluent lesions. This is best accomplished by a series of fan-like injections ½ to 1 inch apart.

Alopecia areata and totalis require an average dose of 25 mg to 30 mg in a concentration of 10 mg/ml subcutaneously 1 to 2 times a week, to stimulate hair regrowth. Results may be expected in 3 to 6 weeks on this dosage, and hair growth may last 3-6 months after initial injection. No more than 0.5 mL should be given in any one site, because excessive deposition may produce local skin atrophy. Continued periodic local injections may be necessary to maintain response and continued hair growth. Use of more dilute solutions diminishes the incidence and degree of local atrophy in the injection site.

In keloids and similar dense scars injections are usually made directly into the lesion.

Injections may be repeated as required, but probably a total of no more than 75 mg of ARISTOCORT *triamcinolone diacetate* a week should be given to any one patient. The need for repeated injections is best determined by clinical response. Remissions may be expected to last from a few weeks up to 11 months.

Intra-articular or Intrasynovial: Strict surgical asepsis is mandatory. The physician should be familiar with anatomical relationships as described in standard text books. A recent paper details the anatomy and the technical approach in arthrocentesis.

It is usually recommended that infiltration by local anesthetic of the soft tissue precede intra-articular injection. A 22-gauge or larger needle on a dry syringe should be inserted into the joint and excess fluid if present should be aspirated. The specific dose depends primarily on the size of the joint. The usual dose varies from 5 mg to 40 mg with the average for the knee being 25 mg. Smaller joints as in the fingers require 2 mg to 5 mg. The duration of effect varies from one week to two months. However, acutely inflamed joints may require more frequent injections. Accidental injection into

soft tissue is usually not harmful but decreases the local effectiveness. Injection into subcutaneous lipoid tissue may produce "pseudoatrophy" with a persistent depression of the overlying dermis, lasting several weeks or months.

Administration and dosage of ARISTOCORT Intralesional *triamcinolone diacetate* must be individualized according to the nature, severity and chronicity of the disease or disorder treated, and should be undertaken with a view of the patient's entire clinical condition. Corticosteroid therapy is considered an adjunct to and not usually a replacement for conventional therapy. Therapy with ARISTOCORT Intralesional, as with all steroids, is of the suppressive type, related to its anti-inflammatory effect. The dose should be regulated during therapy according to the degree of therapeutic response, and should be reduced gradually to maintenance levels, whereby the patient obtains adequate or acceptable control of symptoms. When such control occurs, consideration should be given to gradual decrease in dosage and eventual cessation of therapy. Remission of symptoms may be due to therapy or may be spontaneous and a therapeutic test of gradual withdrawal of steroid treatment is usually indicated.

HOW SUPPLIED

Forte Parenteral: (40 mg/mL): 1 mL Vial—NDC 0205-4450-24 5 mL Vial—NDC 0205-4450-31.
Intralesional: (25 mg/mL) sterile suspension, Not For Intravenous Use: 5 ml Vial—NDC 0205-4422-31.
Store at Controlled Room Temperature 15°–30°C (59°–86°F).
LEDERLE PARENTERALS INC.
Carolina, Puerto Rico 00630   Rev. 3/88
21781,
21783

Shown in Product Identification Section, page 414

ARISTOCORT A® ℞
[a-ris-tō-cort]
Triamcinolone Acetonide Topical Cream with AQUATAIN™ hydrophilic base

ARISTOCORT A® ℞
Triamcinolone Acetonide Topical Ointment with propylene glycol

PRODUCT OVERVIEW

KEY FACTS

ARISTOCORT A is a topical corticosteroid containing Triamcinolone Acetonide in strengths of 0.025%, 0.1%, and 0.5%. Aristocort A is formulated both in a self-occluding ointment and in the patented AQUATAIN™ hydrophilic base that contains no parabens, lanolin, or propylene glycol.

MAJOR USES

ARISTOCORT A is indicated for the relief of the inflammatory and pruritic manifestations of corticosteroid-responsive dermatoses.

SAFETY INFORMATION

ARISTOCORT A may be prescribed without a two-week restriction. The possibility of systemic effects may increase with use over large surface areas, prolonged use, and the addition of occlusive dressings. The most common adverse effects are burning, itching, irritation, and dryness. ARISTOCORT A is not for ophthalmic use.

PRESCRIBING INFORMATION

ARISTOCORT A® ℞
[a-ris-tō-cort]
Triamcinolone Acetonide Topical Cream with AQUATAIN™ hydrophilic base

ARISTOCORT A® ℞
Triamcinolone Acetonide Topical Ointment with propylene glycol

DESCRIPTION

Each gram of 0.025% Topical Cream contains 0.25 mg of the highly active steroid, Triamcinolone Acetonide (a derivative of triamcinolone); each gram of 0.1% Topical Cream contains 1 mg Triamcinolone Acetonide; each gram of 0.5% Topical Cream contains 5 mg of Triamcinolone Acetonide; all in AQUATAIN™, a specially formulated cream base composed of emulsifying wax NF, isopropyl palmitate, glycerin USP, sorbitol solution USP, lactic acid, 2% benzyl alcohol, and purified water. AQUATAIN is non-staining, water-washable, paraben-free, spermaceti-free, and has a light texture and consistency.

Each gram of 0.1% Topical Ointment contains 1 mg Triamcinolone Acetonide in a specially formulated ointment base composed of emulsifying wax NF, white petrolatum, and propylene glycol, Tenox II (butylated hydroxyanisole, propyl gallate, citric acid, propylene glycol) and lactic acid.

Triamcinolone acetonide is (11β, 16α)-9-fluoro-11,21-dihydroxy-16,17-[(1-methylethylidene)bis(oxy)]pregna-1,4-diene-3,20-dione.

The topical corticosteroids constitute a class of primarily synthetic steroids used as anti-inflammatory and antipruritic agents.

CLINICAL PHARMACOLOGY

Topical corticosteroids share anti-inflammatory, anti-pruritic and vasoconstrictive actions.

The mechanism of anti-inflammatory activity of the topical corticosteroids is unclear. Various laboratory methods, including vasoconstrictor assays, are used to compare and predict potencies and/or clinical efficacies of the topical corticosteroids. There is some evidence to suggest that a recognizable correlation exists between vasoconstrictor potency and therapeutic efficacy in man.

Pharmacokinetics: The extent of percutaneous absorption of topical corticosteroids is determined by many factors including the vehicle, the integrity of the epidermal barrier, and the use of occlusive dressings.

Topical corticosteroids can be absorbed from normal intact skin. Inflammation and/or other disease processes in the skin increase percutaneous absorption. Occlusive dressings substantially increase the percutaneous absorption of topical corticosteroids. Thus, occlusive dressings may be a valuable therapeutic adjunct for treatment of resistant dermatoses. (See **DOSAGE AND ADMINISTRATION**).

Once absorbed through the skin, topical corticosteroids are handled through pharmacokinetic pathways similar to systemically administered corticosteroids. Corticosteroids are bound to plasma proteins in varying degrees.

Corticosteroids are metabolized primarily in the liver and are then excreted by the kidneys. Some of the topical corticosteroids and their metabolites are also excreted into the bile.

INDICATIONS AND USAGE

Topical corticosteroids are indicated for the relief of the inflammatory and pruritic manifestations of corticosteroid-responsive dermatoses.

CONTRAINDICATIONS

Topical corticosteroids are contraindicated in those patients with a history of hypersensitivity to any of the components of the preparation.

PRECAUTIONS

General: Systemic absorption of topical corticosteroids has produced reversible hypothalamic-pituitary-adrenal (HPA) axis suppression, manifestations of Cushing's syndrome, hyperglycemia, and glucosuria in some patients.

Conditions which augment systemic absorption include the application of the more potent steroids, use over large surface areas, prolonged use, and the addition of occlusive dressings.

Therefore, patients receiving a large dose of a potent topical steroid applied to a large surface area or under an occlusive dressing should be evaluated periodically for evidence of HPA axis suppression by using the urinary free cortisol and ACTH stimulation tests. If HPA axis suppression is noted, an attempt should be made to withdraw the drug, to reduce the frequency of application, or to substitute a less potent steroid.

Recovery of HPA axis function is generally prompt and complete upon discontinuation of the drug. Infrequently, signs and symptoms of steroid withdrawal may occur, requiring supplemental systemic corticosteroids.

Children may absorb proportionally larger amounts of topical corticosteroids and thus be more susceptible to systemic toxicity. (See **PRECAUTIONS—Pediatric Use.**)

If irritation develops, topical corticosteroids should be discontinued and appropriate therapy instituted.

In the presence of dermatological infections, the use of an appropriate antifungal or antibacterial agent should be instituted. If a favorable response does not occur promptly, the corticosteroid should be discontinued until the infection has been adequately controlled.

Information for the Patient: Patients using topical corticosteroids should receive the following information and instructions:

1. This medication is to be used as directed by the physician. It is for external use only. Avoid contact with the eyes.
2. Patients should be advised not to use this medication for any disorder other than for which it was prescribed.
3. The treated skin area should not be bandaged or otherwise covered or wrapped as to be occlusive unless directed by the physician.
4. Patients should report any signs of local adverse reactions especially under occlusive dressing.
5. Parents of pediatric patients should be advised not to use tight-fitting diapers or plastic pants on a child being treated in the diaper area, as these garments may constitute occlusive dressings.

Laboratory Tests: The following tests may be helpful in evaluating the HPA axis suppression:
Urinary free cortisol test
ACTH stimulation test

Carcinogenesis, Mutagenesis, and Impairment of Fertility: Long-term animal studies have not been performed to evaluate the carcinogenic potential or the effect on fertility of topical corticosteroids.

Studies to determine mutagenicity with prednisolone and hydrocortisone have revealed negative results.

Lederle—Cont.

and body weight, and a chest x-ray should be made at regular intervals during prolonged therapy. Upper GI x-rays are desirable in patients with an ulcer history or significant dyspepsia.

ADVERSE REACTIONS

Fluid and electrolyte disturbances:
Sodium retention.
Fluid retention.
Congestive heart failure in susceptible patients.
Potassium loss.
Hypokalemic alkalosis.
Hypertension.

Musculoskeletal:
Muscle weakness.
Steroid myopathy.
Loss of muscle mass.
Osteoporosis.
Vertebral compression fractures.
Aseptic necrosis of femoral and humeral heads.
Pathologic fracture of long bones.

Gastrointestinal:
Peptic ulcer with possible subsequent perforation and hemorrhage.
Pancreatitis.
Abdominal distention.
Ulcerative esophagitis.

Dermatologic:
Impaired wound healing.
Thin fragile skin.
Petechiae and ecchymoses.
Facial erythema.
Increased sweating.
May suppress reactions to skin tests.

Neurological:
Convulsions.
Increased intracranial pressure with papilledema (pseudotumor cerebri) usually after treatment.
Vertigo.
Headache.

Endocrine:
Menstrual irregularities.
Development of Cushingoid state.
Suppression of growth in children.
Secondary adrenocortical and pituitary unresponsiveness, particularly in times of stress, as in trauma, surgery, or illness.
Decreased carbohydrate tolerance.
Manifestations of latent diabetes mellitus.
Increased requirements for insulin or oral hypoglycemic agents in diabetics.

Ophthalmic:
Posterior subcapsular cataracts.
Increased intraocular pressure.
Glaucoma.
Exophthalmos.

Metabolic:
Negative nitrogen balance due to protein catabolism.
The following additional adverse reactions are related to parenteral and intralesional corticosteroid therapy:
Rare instances of blindness associated with intralesional therapy around the orbit or intranasally.
Hyperpigmentation or hypopigmentation.
Subcutaneous and cutaneous atrophy.
Sterile abscess.
Anaphylactoid reactions have been reported rarely with products of this class.

DOSAGE AND ADMINISTRATION

General: The initial dosage of ARISTOSPAN *sterile triamcinolone hexacetonide suspension* may vary from 2 to 48 mg per day depending on the specific disease entity being treated. In situations of less severity, lower doses will generally suffice while in selected patients higher initial doses may be required. Usually the parenteral dosage ranges are one-third to one-half the oral dose given every 12 hours. However, in certain overwhelming, acute, life-threatening situations, administration in dosages exceeding the usual dosages may be justified and may be in multiples of the oral dosages.
The initial dosage should be maintained or adjusted until a satisfactory response is noted. If after a reasonable period of time there is a lack of satisfactory clinical response, ARISTOSPAN should be discontinued and the patient transferred to other appropriate therapy. It Should Be Emphasized That Dosage Requirements Are Variable and Must Be Individualized on the Basis of the Disease Under Treatment and the Response of the Patient. After a favorable response is noted, the proper maintenance dosage should be determined by decreasing the initial drug dosage in small increments at appropriate time intervals until the lowest dosage which will maintain an adequate clinical response is reached. It should be kept in mind that constant monitoring

is needed in regard to drug dosage. Included in the situations which may make dosage adjustments necessary are changes in clinical status secondary to remissions or exacerbations in the disease process, the patient's individual drug responsiveness, and the effect of patient exposure to stressful situations not directly related to the disease entity under treatment; in this latter situation it may be necessary to increase the dosage of ARISTOSPAN for a period of time consistent with the patient's condition. If after long-term therapy the drug is to be stopped, it is recommended that it be withdrawn gradually rather than abruptly.

Directions for Use: Strict aseptic administration technique is mandatory. Topical ethyl chloride spray may be used locally before injection.
The syringe should be gently agitated to achieve uniform suspension before use. Since this product has been designed for ease of administration, a small bore needle (not smaller than 24 gauge) may be used.

Dilution: *Intralesional:* ARISTOSPAN suspension may be diluted, if desired, with Dextrose and Sodium Chloride Injection USP, (5% and 10% Dextrose), Sodium Chloride Injection USP, or Sterile Water for Injection USP.
The optimum dilution, ie, 1:1, 1:2, 1:4, should be determined by the nature of the lesion, its size, the depth of injection, the volume needed, and location of the lesion. In general, more superficial injections should be performed with greater dilution. Certain conditions, such as keloids, require a less dilute suspension such as 5 mg/mL, with variation in dose and dilution as dictated by the condition of the individual patient. Subsequent dosage, dilution, and frequency of injections are best judged by the clinical response.
The suspension may also be mixed with 1% or 2% Lidocaine Hydrochloride, using the formulations which do not contain parabens. Similar local anesthetics may also be used. Diluents containing methylparaben, propylparaben, phenol, etc. should be avoided since these compounds may cause flocculation of the steroid. These dilutions will retain full potency for one week, but care should be exercised to avoid contamination of the vial's contents and the dilutions should be discarded after 7 days.

Intralesional or Sublesional: Average Dose—Up to 0.5 mg per square inch of affected skin injected intralesionally or sublesionally. The frequency of subsequent injections is best determined by the clinical response. If desired, the vial may be diluted as indicated under **Directions for Use.**
A lesser initial dosage range of ARISTOSPAN *triamcinolone hexacetonide* may produce the desired effect when the drug is administered to provide a localized concentration. The site of the injection and the volume of the injection should be carefully considered when ARISTOSPAN is administered for this purpose.

Dilution: *Intra-articular:* ARISTOSPAN suspension may be mixed with 1% or 2% Lidocaine Hydrochloride, using the formulations which do not contain parabens. Similar local anesthetics may also be used. Diluents containing methylparaben, propylparaben, phenol, etc, should be avoided since these compounds may cause flocculation of the steroid. These dilutions will retain full potency for one week, but care should be exercised to avoid contamination.

Intra-articular
Average dose—2 to 20 mg (0.1 mL to 1.0 mL.)
The dose depends on the size of the joint to be injected, the degree of inflammation, and the amount of fluid present. In general, large joints (such as knee, hip, shoulder) require 10 to 20 mg. For small joints (such as interphalangeal, metacarpophalangeal), 2 to 6 mg may be employed. When the amount of synovial fluid is increased, aspiration may be performed before administering ARISTOSPAN. Subsequent dosage and frequency of injections can best be judged by clinical response.
The usual frequency of injection into a single joint is every three or four weeks, and injection more frequently than that is generally not advisable. To avoid possible joint destruction from repeated use of intra-articular corticosteroids, injection should be as infrequent as possible, consistent with adequate patient care. Attention should be paid to avoiding deposition of drug along the needle path which might produce atrophy.

HOW SUPPLIED

Intralesional: 5 mL (in a 12.5 mL size vial)—NDC 0205-4502-31
Intra-articular 20 mg/mL: 1 mL vial—NDC 0205-4505-24; 5 mL vial—NDC 0205-4505-31.
Color Code Violet Cap
Store at Controlled Room Temperature 15–30°C (59–86°F).
DO NOT FREEZE
Military Depot: NSN-6505-00-148-6985, 5 mL vial Intra-articular
LEDERLE PARENTERALS INC.
Carolina, Puerto Rico 00630   Rev. 12/88
                             25002

Shown in Product Identification Section, page 414

ARTANE®   ℞

[*ar-tāne*]
trihexyphenidyl HCl
Tablets, Elixir, and SEQUELS®
Sustained Release Capsules

DESCRIPTION

ARTANE is a synthetic antispasmodic drug available in the following forms:
TABLETS: Containing 2 mg and 5 mg ARTANE, each strength also containing as inactive ingredients Corn Starch, Dibasic Calcium Phosphate, Magnesium Stearate and Modified Starch.
ELIXIR: Containing 2 mg/5 mL ARTANE in a clear, colorless, lime-mint flavored preparation, also containing as inactive ingredients Alcohol, Citric Acid, Flavorings, Methylparaben, Propylparaben, Sodium Chloride and Sorbitol.
SEQUELS: Containing 5 mg ARTANE as Sustained Release soft shell capsules, also containing as inactive ingredients Beeswax, Benzoin Gum, Blue 1, Colloidal Silicon Dioxide, Dibasic Calcium Phosphate, Ethyl Cellulose, Ethyl Vanillin, Gelatin, Glycerin, Glyceryl Stearate, Magnesium Stearate, Methylparaben, Mineral Oil, Nonpareil Seeds, Propylene Glycol, Propylparaben, Sucrose, Talc and Terpene Resin.

ACTIONS

ARTANE is the substituted piperidine salt, 3-(1-piperidyl)-1-phenyl-cyclohexyl-1-propanol hydrochloride, which exerts a direct inhibitory effect upon the parasympathetic nervous system. It also has a relaxing effect on smooth musculature; exerted both directly upon the muscle tissue itself and indirectly through an inhibitory effect upon the parasympathetic nervous system. Its therapeutic properties are similar to those of atropine, although undesirable side effects are ordinarily less frequent and severe than with the latter.

INDICATIONS

This drug is indicated as an adjunct in the treatment of all forms of parkinsonism (postencephalitic, arteriosclerotic, and idiopathic). It is often useful as adjuvant therapy when treating these forms of parkinsonism with levodopa. Additionally, it is indicated for the control of extrapyramidal disorders caused by central nervous system drugs such as the dibenzoxazepines, phenothiazines, thioxanthenes, and butyrophenones.
SEQUELS—For maintenance therapy after patients have been stabilized on trihexyphenidyl hydrochloride in conventional dosage forms (tablets or elixir).

WARNING

Patients to be treated with ARTANE should have a gonioscope evaluation and close monitoring of intraocular pressures at regular periodic intervals.

PRECAUTIONS

Although trihexyphenidyl HCl is not contraindicated for patients with cardiac, liver, or kidney disorders, or with hypertension, such patients should be maintained under close observation.
Since the use of trihexyphenidyl HCl may in some cases continue indefinitely and since it has atropine-like properties, patients should be subjected to constant and careful long-term observation to avoid allergic and other untoward reactions. Inasmuch as trihexyphenidyl HCl possesses some parasympatholytic activity, it should be used with caution in patients with glaucoma, obstructive disease of the gastrointestinal or genitourinary tracts, and in elderly males with possible prostatic hypertrophy. Geriatric patients, particularly over the age of 60, frequently develop increased sensitivity to the actions of drugs of this type, and hence, require strict dosage regulation. Incipient glaucoma may be precipitated by parasympatholytic drugs such as trihexyphenidyl HCl.
Tardive dyskinesia may appear in some patients on long-term therapy with antipsychotic drugs or may occur after therapy with these drugs has been discontinued. Antiparkinsonism agents do not alleviate the symptoms of tardive dyskinesia, and in some instances may aggravate them. However, parkinsonism and tardive dyskinesia often coexist in patients receiving chronic neuroleptic treatment, and anticholinergic therapy with ARTANE may relieve some of these parkinsonism symptoms.

ADVERSE REACTIONS

Minor side effects, such as dryness of the mouth, blurring of vision, dizziness, mild nausea or nervousness, will be experienced by 30 to 50 percent of all patients. These sensations, however, are much less troublesome with ARTANE *trihexyphenidyl HCl* than with belladonna alkaloids and are usually less disturbing than unalleviated parkinsonism. Such reactions tend to become less pronounced, and even to disappear, as treatment continues. Even before these reactions have remitted spontaneously, they may often be controlled by careful adjustment of dosage form, amount of drug, or interval between doses.

Isolated instances of suppurative parotitis secondary to excessive dryness of the mouth, skin rashes, dilatation of the colon, paralytic ileus, and certain psychiatric manifestations such as delusions and hallucinations, plus one doubtful case of paranoia, all of which may occur with any of the atropine-like drugs, have been reported rarely with ARTANE.

Patients with arteriosclerosis or with a history of idiosyncrasy to other drugs may exhibit reactions of mental confusion, agitation, disturbed behavior, or nausea and vomiting. Such patients should be allowed to develop a tolerance through the initial administration of a small dose and gradual increase in dose until an effective level is reached. If a severe reaction should occur, administration of the drug should be discontinued for a few days and then resumed at a lower dosage. Psychiatric disturbances can result from indiscriminate use (leading to overdosage) to sustain continued euphoria.

Potential side effects associated with the use of any atropine-like drugs include constipation, drowsiness, urinary hesitancy or retention, tachycardia, dilation of the pupil, increased intraocular tension, weakness, vomiting, and headache.

The occurrence of angle-closure glaucoma due to long-term treatment with trihexyphenidyl hydrochloride has been reported.

DOSAGE AND ADMINISTRATION

Dosage should be individualized. The initial dose should be low and then increased gradually, especially in patients over 60 years of age. Whether ARTANE may best be given before or after meals should be determined by the way the patient reacts. Postencephalitic patients, who are usually more prone to excessive salivation, may prefer to take it after meals and may, in addition, require small amounts of atropine which, under such circumstances, is sometimes an effective adjuvant. If ARTANE *trihexyphenidyl HCl* tends to dry the mouth excessively, it may be better to take it before meals, unless it causes nausea. If taken after meals, the thirst sometimes induced can be allayed by mint candies, chewing gum or water.

ARTANE in Idiopathic Parkinsonism: As initial therapy for parkinsonism, 1 mg of ARTANE in tablet or elixir form may be administered the first day. The dose may then be increased by 2 mg increments at intervals of three to five days, until a total of 6 to 10 mg is given daily. The total daily dose will depend upon what is found to be the optimal level. Many patients derive maximum benefit from this daily total of 6 to 10 mg, but some patients, chiefly those in the postencephalitic group, may require a total daily dose of 12 to 15 mg.

ARTANE in Drug-Induced Parkinsonism: The size and frequency of dose of ARTANE needed to control extrapyramidal reactions to commonly employed tranquilizers, notably the phenothiazines, thioxanthenes, and butyrophenones, must be determined empirically. The total daily dosage usually ranges between 5 and 15 mg although, in some cases, these reactions have been satisfactorily controlled on as little as 1 mg daily. It may be advisable to commence therapy with a single 1 mg dose. If the extrapyramidal manifestations are not controlled in a few hours, the subsequent doses may be progressively increased until satisfactory control is achieved. Satisfactory control may sometimes be more rapidly achieved by temporarily reducing the dosage of the tranquilizer on instituting ARTANE therapy and then adjusting dosage of both drugs until the desired ataractic effect is retained without onset of extrapyramidal reactions.

It is sometimes possible to maintain the patient on a reduced ARTANE dosage after the reactions have remained under control for several days. Instances have been reported in which these reactions have remained in remission for long periods after ARTANE therapy was discontinued.

Concomitant Use of ARTANE with Levodopa: When ARTANE is used concomitantly with levodopa, the usual dose of each may need to be reduced. Careful adjustment is necessary, depending on side effects and degree of symptom control. ARTANE dosage of 3 to 6 mg daily, in divided doses, is usually adequate.

Concomitant Use of ARTANE with Other Parasympathetic Inhibitors: ARTANE may be substituted, in whole or in part, for other parasympathetic inhibitors. The usual technique is partial substitution initially, with progressive reduction in the other medication as the dose of trihexyphenidyl HCl is increased.

ARTANE TABLETS and ELIXIR—The total daily intake of ARTANE tablets or elixir is tolerated best if divided into 3 doses and taken at mealtimes. High doses (> 10 mg daily) may be divided into 4 parts, with 3 doses administered at mealtimes and the fourth at bedtime.

ARTANE SEQUELS—Because of the relatively high dosage in each controlled release capsule, this dosage form should not be used for initial therapy. After patients are stabilized on trihexyphenidyl HCl in conventional dosage forms (tablet or elixir), for convenience of administration they may be switched to the controlled release capsule on a milligram per milligram total daily dose basis, as a single dose after breakfast or in two divided doses 12 hours apart. Most patients will be adequately maintained on the controlled re-

lease form, but some may develop an exacerbation of parkinsonism and have to be returned to the conventional form.

HOW SUPPLIED

ARTANE *trihexyphenidyl HCl* is available as follows:
TABLETS: 2 mg—round, flat, scored, white tablets; engraved ARTANE above 2 on one side and LL above A11 below the score on the other side, are supplied as follows:

    NDC 0005-4434-23—Bottle of 100
    NDC 0005-4434-34—Bottle of 1000
    NDC 0005-4434-60—Unit Dose 10 × 10s

5 mg—round, flat, scored, white tablets; engraved ARTANE above 5 on one side and LL above A12 below the score on the other side, are supplied as follows:

    NDC 0005-4436-23—Bottle of 100
    NDC 0005-4436-60—Unit Dose 10 × 10s

Store at Controlled Room Temperature 15–30°C (59–86°F).
ELIXIR: 2 mg/5 mL—NDC 0005-4440-65—Bottle of 16 fl oz.
Store at Controlled Room Temperature 15–30°C (59–86°F).
DO NOT FREEZE.
SEQUELS SUSTAINED RELEASE CAPSULES: 5 mg—soft shell, oval shaped, clear blue, printed A9L, are supplied as follows:

    NDC 0005-4438-32—Unit-of-Issue 60s with CRC

Store at Controlled Room Temperature 15–30°C (59–86°F).
LEDERLE LABORATORIES DIVISION
American Cyanamid Company,
Pearl River, NY 10965   Rev. 6/89
                                25464

Shown in Product Identification Section, page 414

ASENDIN®   ℞
[a-sen-din]
amoxapine tablets

DESCRIPTION

ASENDIN is an antidepressant of the dibenzoxazepine class, chemically distinct from the dibenzazepines, dibenzocycloheptenes, and dibenzoxepines.
It is designated chemically as 2-chloro-11-(1-piperazinyl) dibenz-$[b,f][1,4]$oxazepine. The molecular weight is 313.8. The empirical formula is $C_{17}H_{16}CIN_3O$.
ASENDIN is supplied for oral administration as 25 mg, 50 mg, 100 mg, and 150 mg tablets.
Inactive Ingredients: All tablets contain Corn Starch, Dibasic Calcium Phosphate, Magnesium Stearate, Pregelatinized Starch and Stearic Acid. Additionally, the 50 and 150 mg tablets contain FD&C Yellow No. 6* and the 100 mg tablet contains Blue 2.
* Contain FD&C Yellow No. 6 (Sunset Yellow) as a color additive.

CLINICAL PHARMACOLOGY

ASENDIN is an antidepressant with a mild sedative component to its action. The mechanism of its clinical action in man is not well understood. In animals, amoxapine reduced the uptake of norepinephrine and serotonin and blocked the response of dopamine receptors to dopamine. Amoxapine is not a monoamine oxidase inhibitor.
ASENDIN is absorbed rapidly and reaches peak blood levels approximately 90 minutes after ingestion. It is almost completely metabolized. The main route of excretion is the kidney. *In vitro* tests show that amoxapine binding to human serum is approximately 90%.
In man, amoxapine serum concentration declines with a half-life of eight hours. However, the major metabolite, 8-hydroxyamoxapine, has a biologic half-life of 30 hours. Metabolites are excreted in the urine in conjugated form as glucuronides.
Clinical studies have demonstrated that ASENDIN has a more rapid onset of action than either amitriptyline or imipramine. The initial clinical effect may occur within four to seven days and occurs within two weeks in over 80% of responders.

INDICATIONS AND USAGE

ASENDIN is indicated for the relief of symptoms of depression in patients with neurotic or reactive depressive disorders as well as endogenous and psychotic depressions. It is indicated for depression accompanied by anxiety or agitation.

CONTRAINDICATIONS

ASENDIN is contraindicated in patients who have shown prior hypersensitivity to dibenzoxazepine compounds. It should not be given concomitantly with monoamine oxidase inhibitors. Hyperpyretic crises, severe convulsions, and deaths have occurred in patients receiving tricyclic antidepressants and monoamine oxidase inhibitors simultaneously. When it is desired to replace a monoamine oxidase inhibitor with ASENDIN, a minimum of 14 days should be allowed to elapse after the former is discontinued. ASENDIN should then be initiated cautiously with gradual increase in dosage until optimum response is achieved. The drug is not

recommended for use during the acute recovery phase following myocardial infarction.

WARNINGS

Tardive Dyskinesia: Tardive dyskinesia, a syndrome consisting of potentially irreversible, involuntary, dyskinetic movements may develop in patients treated with neuroleptic (ie, antipsychotic) drugs. (Amoxapine is not an antipsychotic, but it has substantive neuroleptic activity.) Although the prevalence of the syndrome appears to be highest among the elderly, especially elderly women, it is impossible to rely upon prevalence estimates to predict, at the inception of neuroleptic treatment, which patients are likely to develop the syndrome. Whether neuroleptic drug products differ in their potential to cause tardive dyskinesia is unknown.

Both the risk of developing the syndrome and the likelihood that it will become irreversible are believed to increase as the duration of treatment and the total cumulative dose of neuroleptic drugs administered to the patient increase. However, the syndrome can develop, although much less commonly, after relatively brief treatment periods at low doses.

There is no known treatment for established cases of tardive dyskinesia, although the syndrome may remit, partially or completely, if neuroleptic treatment is withdrawn. Neuroleptic treatment itself, however, may suppress (or partially suppress) the signs and symptoms of the syndrome and thereby may possibly mask the underlying disease process. The effect that symptomatic suppression has upon the long-term course of the syndrome is unknown.

Given these considerations, neuroleptics should be prescribed in a manner that is most likely to minimize the occurrence of tardive dyskinesia. Chronic neuroleptic treatment should generally be reserved for patients who suffer from a chronic illness that, 1) is known to respond to neuroleptic drugs, and, 2) for whom alternative, equally effective, but potentially less harmful treatments are *not* available or appropriate. In patients who do require chronic treatment, the smallest dose and the shortest duration of treatment producing a satisfactory clinical response should be sought. The need for continued treatment should be reassessed periodically.

If signs and symptoms of tardive dyskinesia appear in a patient on neuroleptics, drug discontinuation should be considered. However, some patients may require treatment despite the presence of the syndrome.

(For further information about the description of tardive dyskinesia and its clinical detection, please refer to the sections on **Information for the Patient** and **ADVERSE REACTIONS**.)

Neuroleptic Malignant Syndrome (NMS): A potentially fatal symptom complex sometimes referred to as Neuroleptic Malignant Syndrome (NMS) has been reported in association with antipsychotic drugs and with amoxapine. Clinical manifestations of NMS are hyperpyrexia, muscle rigidity, altered mental status and evidence of autonomic instability (irregular pulse or blood pressure, tachycardia, diaphoresis, and cardiac dysrhythmias).

The diagnostic evaluation of patients with this syndrome is complicated. In arriving at a diagnosis, it is important to identify cases where the clinical presentation includes both serious medical illness (eg, pneumonia, systemic infection, etc.) and untreated or inadequately treated extrapyramidal signs and symptoms (EPS). Other important considerations in the differential diagnosis include central anticholinergic toxicity, heat stroke, drug fever, and primary central nervous system (CNS) pathology.

The management of NMS should include 1) immediate discontinuation of antipsychotic drugs and other drugs not essential to concurrent therapy, 2) intensive symptomatic treatment and medical monitoring, and 3) treatment of any concomitant serious medical problems for which specific treatments are available. There is no general agreement about specific pharmacological treatment regimens for uncomplicated NMS.

If a patient requires antipsychotic drug treatment after recovery from NMS, the potential reintroduction of drug therapy should be carefully considered. The patient should be carefully monitored since recurrences of NMS have been reported.

ASENDIN *amoxapine* should be used with caution in patients with a history of urinary retention, angle-closure glaucoma, or increased intraocular pressure. Patients with cardiovascular disorders should be watched closely. Tricyclic antidepressant drugs, particularly when given in high doses, can induce sinus tachycardia, changes in conduction time, and

Continued on next page

Lederle—Cont.

arrhythmias. Myocardial infarction and stroke have been reported with drugs of this class.

Extreme caution should be used in treating patients with a history of convulsive disorder or those with overt or latent seizure disorders.

PRECAUTIONS

General: In prescribing the drug, it should be borne in mind that the possibility of suicide is inherent in any severe depression, and persists until a significant remission occurs; the drug should be dispensed in the smallest suitable amount. Manic depressive patients may experience a shift to the manic phase. Schizophrenic patients may develop increased symptoms of psychosis; patients with paranoid symptomatology may have an exaggeration of such symptoms. This may require reduction of dosage or the addition of a major tranquilizer to the therapeutic regimen. Antidepressant drugs can cause skin rashes and/or "drug fever" in susceptible individuals. These allergic reactions may, in rare cases, be severe. They are more likely to occur during the first few days of treatment, but may also occur later. ASENDIN should be discontinued if rash and/or fever develop. Amoxapine possesses a degree of dopamine-blocking activity which may cause extrapyramidal symptoms in <1% of patients. Rarely, symptoms indicative of tardive dyskinesia have been reported.

Information for the Patient: Given the likelihood that some patients exposed chronically to neuroleptics will develop tardive dyskinesia, it is advised that all patients in whom chronic use is contemplated be given, if possible, full information about this risk. The decision to inform patients and/or their guardians must obviously take into account the clinical circumstances and the competency of the patient to understand the information provided.

Patients should be warned of the possibility of drowsiness that may impair performance of potentially hazardous tasks such as driving an automobile or operating machinery.

Drug Interactions: See CONTRAINDICATIONS about concurrent usage of tricyclic antidepressants and monoamine oxidase inhibitors. Paralytic ileus may occur in patients taking tricyclic antidepressants in combination with anticholinergic drugs. ASENDIN may enhance the response to alcohol and the effects of barbiturates and other CNS depressants. Serum levels of several tricyclic antidepressants have been reported to be significantly increased when cimetidine is administered concurrently. Although such an interaction has not been reported to date with ASENDIN, specific interaction studies have not been done, and the possibility should be considered.

Therapeutic Interactions: Concurrent administration with electroshock therapy may increase the hazards associated with such therapy.

Carcinogenesis, Impairment of Fertility: In a 21-month toxicity study at three dose levels in rats, pancreatic islet cell hyperplasia occurred with slightly increased incidence at doses 5–10 times the human dose. Pancreatic adenocarcinoma was detected in low incidence in the mid-dose group only, and may possibly have resulted from endocrine-mediated organ hyperfunction. The significance of these findings to man is not known.

Treatment of male rats with 5–10 times the human dose resulted in a slight decrease in the number of fertile matings. Female rats receiving oral doses within the therapeutic range displayed a reversible increase in estrous cycle length. **Pregnancy:** *Pregnancy Category C:* Studies performed in mice, rats, and rabbits have demonstrated no evidence of teratogenic effect due to ASENDIN. Embryotoxicity was seen in rats and rabbits given oral doses approximating the human dose. Fetotoxic effects (intrauterine death, stillbirth, decreased birth weight) were seen in animals studied at oral doses 3–10 times the human dose. Decreased postnatal survival (between days 0–4) was demonstrated in the offspring of rats at 5–10 times the human dose. There are no adequate and well-controlled studies in pregnant women. ASENDIN *amoxapine* should be used during pregnancy only if the potential benefit justifies the potential risk to the fetus.

Nursing Mothers: ASENDIN, like many other systemic drugs, is excreted in human milk. Because effects of the drug on infants are unknown, caution should be exercised when ASENDIN is administered to nursing women.

Pediatric Use: Safety and effectiveness in children below the age of 16 have not been established.

ADVERSE REACTIONS

Adverse reactions reported in controlled studies in the United States are categorized with respect to incidence below. Following this is a listing of reactions known to occur with other antidepressant drugs of this class but not reported to date with ASENDIN.

INCIDENCE GREATER THAN 1%

The most frequent types of adverse reactions occurring with ASENDIN in controlled clinical trials were sedative and anticholinergic: these included drowsiness (14%), dry mouth (14%), constipation (12%), and blurred vision (7%).

Less frequently reported reactions are:

CNS and Neuromuscular: anxiety, insomnia, restlessness, nervousness, palpitations, tremors, confusion, excitement, nightmares, ataxia, alterations in EEG patterns.

Allergic: edema, skin rash.

Endocrine: elevation of prolactin levels.

Gastrointestinal: nausea.

Other: dizziness, headache, fatigue, weakness, excessive appetite, increased perspiration.

INCIDENCE LESS THAN 1%

Anticholinergic: disturbances of accommodation, mydriasis, delayed micturition, urinary retention, nasal stuffiness.

Cardiovascular: hypotension, hypertension, syncope, tachycardia.

Allergic: drug fever, urticaria, photosensitization, pruritus, rarely vasculitis, hepatitis.

CNS and Neuromuscular: tingling, paresthesias of the extremities, tinnitus, disorientation, seizures, hypomania, numbness, incoordination, disturbed concentration, hyperthermia, extrapyramidal symptoms, including, rarely, tardive dyskinesia. Neuroleptic malignant syndrome has been reported. (See **WARNINGS.**)

Hematologic: leukopenia, agranulocytosis.

Gastrointestinal: epigastric distress, vomiting, flatulence, abdominal pain, peculiar taste, diarrhea.

Endocrine: increased or decreased libido, impotence, menstrual irregularity, breast enlargement and galactorrhea in the female, syndrome of inappropriate antidiuretic hormone secretion.

Other: lacrimation, weight gain or loss, altered liver function, painful ejaculation.

DRUG RELATIONSHIP UNKNOWN

The following reactions have been reported very rarely, and occurred under uncontrolled circumstances where a drug relationship was difficult to assess. These observations are listed to serve as alerting information to physicians.

Anticholinergic: paralytic ileus.

Cardiovascular: atrial arrhythmias (including atrial fibrillation), myocardial infarction, stroke, heart block.

CNS and Neuromuscular: hallucinations.

Hematologic: thrombocytopenia, eosinophilia, purpura, petechiae.

Gastrointestinal: parotid swelling.

Endocrine: change in blood glucose levels.

Other: pancreatitis, hepatitis, jaundice, urinary frequency, testicular swelling, anorexia, alopecia.

ADDITIONAL ADVERSE REACTIONS

The following reactions have been reported with other antidepressant drugs, but not with ASENDIN *amoxapine*.

Anticholinergic: sublingual adenitis, dilation of the urinary tract.

CNS and Neuromuscular: delusions.

Gastrointestinal: stomatitis, black tongue.

Endocrine: gynecomastia.

OVERDOSAGE

Signs and Symptoms: Toxic manifestations of ASENDIN overdosage differ significantly from those of other tricyclic antidepressants. Serious cardiovascular effects are seldom if ever observed. However, CNS effects—particularly grand mal convulsions—occur frequently, and treatment should be directed primarily toward prevention or control of seizures. Status epilepticus may develop and constitutes a neurologic emergency. Coma and acidosis are other serious complications of substantial ASENDIN overdosage in some cases. Renal failure may develop two to five days after toxic overdosage in patients who may appear otherwise recovered. Acute tubular necrosis with rhabdomyolysis and myoglobinuria is the most common renal complication in such cases. This reaction probably occurs in less than 5% of overdose cases, and typically in those who have experienced multiple seizures.

Treatment: Treatment of ASENDIN overdosage should be symptomatic and supportive, but with special attention to prevention or control of seizures. If the patient is conscious, induced emesis followed by gastric lavage with appropriate precautions to prevent pulmonary aspiration should be accomplished as soon as possible. Following lavage, activated charcoal may be administered to reduce absorption, and repeated administrations may facilitate drug elimination. An adequate airway should be established in comatose patients and assisted ventilation instituted if necessary. Seizures may respond to standard anticonvulsant therapy such as intravenous diazepam and/or phenytoin. The value of physostigmine appears less certain. Status epilepticus, should it develop, requires vigorous treatment such as that described by Delgado-Escueta et al (*N Engl J Med* 1982; 306:1337-1340).

Convulsions, when they occur, typically begin within 12 hours after ingestion. Because seizures may occur precipitously in some overdosage patients who appear otherwise relatively asymptomatic, the treating physician may wish to consider prophylactic administration of anticonvulsant medication during this period.

Treatment of renal impairment, should it occur, is the same as that for nondrug-induced renal dysfunction.

Serious cardiovascular effects are remarkably rare following ASENDIN *amoxapine* overdosage, and the ECG typically remains within normal limits except for sinus tachycardia. Hence, prolongation of the QRS interval beyond 100 milliseconds within the first 24 hours is *not* a useful guide to the severity of overdosage with this drug.

Fatalities and, rarely, neurologic sequelae have resulted from prolonged status epilepticus in ASENDIN overdosage patients. While the lethal dose appears higher than that of other tricyclic antidepressants (80% of lethal ASENDIN overdosages have involved ingestion of 3 grams or more), many factors other than amount ingested are important in assessing probability of survival. These include age and physical condition of the patient, concomitant ingestion of other drugs, and especially the interval between drug ingestion and initiation of emergency treatment.

DOSAGE AND ADMINISTRATION

Effective dosage of ASENDIN may vary from one patient to another. Usual effective dosage is 200 to 300 mg daily. Three weeks constitutes an adequate period of trial providing dosage has reached 300 mg daily (or lower level of tolerance) for at least two weeks. If no response is seen at 300 mg, dosage may be increased, depending upon tolerance, up to 400 mg daily. Hospitalized patients who have been refractory to antidepressant therapy and who have no history of convulsive seizures may have dosage raised cautiously up to 600 mg daily in divided doses.

ASENDIN may be given in a single daily dose, not to exceed 300 mg, preferably at bedtime. If the total daily dosage exceeds 300 mg, it should be given in divided doses.

Initial Dosage for Adults: Usual starting dosage is 50 mg two or three times daily. Depending upon tolerance, dosage may be increased to 100 mg two or three times daily by the end of the first week. (Initial dosage of 300 mg daily may be given, but notable sedation may occur in some patients during the first few days of therapy at this level.) Increases above 300 mg daily should be made only if 300 mg daily has been ineffective during a trial period of at least two weeks. When effective dosage is established, the drug may be given in a single dose (not to exceed 300 mg) at bedtime.

Elderly Patients: In general, lower dosages are recommended for these patients. Recommended starting dosage of ASENDIN is 25 mg two or three times daily. If no intolerance is observed, dosage may be increased by the end of the first week to 50 mg two or three times daily. Although 100–150 mg daily may be adequate for many elderly patients, some may require higher dosage. Careful increases up to 300 mg daily are indicated in such cases.

Once an effective dosage is established, ASENDIN may conveniently be given in a single bedtime dose, not to exceed 300 mg.

Maintenance: Recommended maintenance dosage of ASENDIN is the lowest dose that will maintain remission. If symptoms reappear, dosage should be increased to the earlier level until they are controlled.

For maintenance therapy at dosages of 300 mg or less, a single dose at bedtime is recommended.

HOW SUPPLIED

ASENDIN *amoxapine* Tablets are supplied as follows:

25 mg—White, heptagon-shaped tablets, engraved on one side with LL above 25 and with A13 on the other scored side.

Product No. NDC 0005-5389-23—Bottle of 100

50 mg—Orange, heptagon-shaped tablets, engraved on one side with LL above 50 and with A15 on the other scored side.

Product No. NDC 0005-5390-23—Bottle of 100
Product No. NDC 0005-5390-31—Bottle of 500
Product No. NDC 0005-5390-60—10 ×10 Unit Dose

100 mg—Blue, heptagon-shaped tablets, engraved on one side with LL above 100 and with A17 on the other scored side.

Product No. NDC 0005-5391-23—Bottle of 100
Product No. NDC 0005-5391-60—10×10 Unit Dose

150 mg—Peach, heptagon-shaped tablets, engraved on one side with LL above 150 and with A18 on the other scored side.

Product No. NDC 0005-5392-38—Bottle of 30 with CRC

Store at Controlled Room Temperature 15–30° C (59–86° F).

Military and VA Depot:

NSN 6505-01-111-3195 50 mg—(100s)
NSN 6505-01-111-3194 100mg—(100s)

LEDERLE LABORATORIES DIVISION
American Cyanamid Company,
Pearl River, NY 10965   Rev. 11/87
                                        28824

Shown in Product Identification Section, page 414

CALTRATE® 600
[căl-trāt]
High potency calcium supplement

DESCRIPTION
Each CALTRATE 600 tablet provides 1500 mg calcium carbonate, which provides 600 mg elemental calcium, 60% of the US Recommended Daily Allowance (US RDA) of calcium. *Inactive ingredients:* Croscarmellose Sodium, Hydroxypropyl Methylcellulose, Magnesium Stearate, Microcrystalline Cellulose, PVPP, Sodium Lauryl Sulfate, Titanium Dioxide, and other ingredients.

INDICATIONS
To supplement diets deficient in calcium.

RECOMMENDED INTAKE
One or two tablets daily or as directed by the physician.

WARNING
Keep out of the reach of children.

HOW SUPPLIED
Film-coated tablets, Bottle of 60—NDC 0005-5510-19
Store at Room Temperature.

Rev. 3/89
24192

Shown in Product Identification Section, page 414

CALTRATE® 600 + Vitamin D
[căl-trāt]
High potency calcium supplement with Vitamin D

DESCRIPTION
Each CALTRATE 600 + Vitamin D provides:

	Adults—US RDA %
1500 mg calcium carbonate which provides 600 mg elemental calcium	60%
Vitamin D, 125 IU	31%

Inactive ingredients: Blue 2, Croscarmellose Sodium, Hydroxypropyl Methylcellulose, Magnesium Stearate, Microcrystalline Cellulose, Povidone, PVPP, Red 40, Sodium Lauryl Sulfate, Titanium Dioxide and Yellow 6.

INDICATIONS
To supplement diets deficient in calcium. Vitamin D aids calcium absorption.

RECOMMENDED INTAKE
Minimum dosage one tablet daily; two or more if directed by the physician.

WARNING
Keep out of the reach of children.

HOW SUPPLIED
Film-coated tablets, Bottle of 60—NDC 0005-5509-19
Store at Room Temperature.

Rev. 6/89
22841

Shown in Product Identification Section, page 414

CALTRATE® 600 + Iron & Vitamin D
[căl-trāt]
High potency calcium supplement with Iron and Vitamin D

DESCRIPTION
Each CALTRATE 600 + Iron and Vitamin D tablet provides:

	Adults—US RDA
1500 mg calcium carbonate, which provides 600 mg elemental calcium	60%
18 mg elemental Iron in the Optisorb® Time Release System (as ferrous fumarate)	100%
Vitamin D, 125 IU	31%

Inactive ingredients: Diethyl Phthalate, Ethylcellulose, Hydroxypropyl Cellulose, Magnesium Stearate, Microcrystalline Cellulose, Pharmaceutical Glaze, Povidone, Red 40, Silica Gel, Sodium Lauryl Sulfate, Sodium Starch Glycolate, Stearic Acid, Talc, Titanium Dioxide, and other ingredients.

INDICATIONS
Pure calcium and time-release iron for diets deficient in both minerals, plus Vitamin D to aid in calcium absorption.

RECOMMENDED INTAKE
One or two tablets daily or as directed by the physician.

WARNING
Keep out of the reach of children.

HOW SUPPLIED
Film coated tablets, Bottles of 60—NDC-0005-5523-19
Store at Room Temperature.

(9/86)

Shown in Product Identification Section, page 414

CALTRATE®, JR.
[căl-trāt]
Calcium Supplement for Children

DESCRIPTION
Each chewable, orange-flavored CALTRATE, JR. contains the following daily requirements:

	Children 4+—% US RDA
750 mg calcium carbonate which provides 300 mg elemental calcium	30%
Vitamin D - 60 I.U.	15%

Inactive Ingredients: Dextrose, dl-Alpha Tocopheryl, Gelatin, Magnesium Stearate, Malto Dextrin, Mannitol, Orange Flavor, Silica Gel, Sorbitol, Stearic Acid, Sucrose, Yellow 6 and other ingredients.

INDICATIONS
To supplement children's diets deficient in calcium.

RECOMMENDED INTAKE
One to two tablets daily or as directed by a physician.

WARNING
Keep out of the reach of children.

HOW SUPPLIED
Chewable tablets. Bottles of 60—NDC 0005-5516–19.
Store at Room Temperature.

Rev. 12/87
18053

Shown in Product Identification Section, page 414

Advanced Formula CENTRUM®
[sĕn-trŭm]
High Potency
Multivitamin-Multimineral Formula

(See PDR For Nonprescription Drugs)

Children's Chewable CENTRUM, JR.®
[sĕn-trŭm]
Vitamin/Mineral Formula + Iron

(See PDR For Nonprescription Drugs)

Advanced Formula Children's Chewable CENTRUM, JR.®
[sĕn-trŭm]
Vitamin/Mineral Formula + Extra C

(See PDR For Nonprescription Drugs)

Children's Chewable CENTRUM, JR.®
[sĕn-trŭm]
Vitamin/Mineral Formula + Extra Calcium

(See PDR For Nonprescription Drugs)

CYCLOCORT®   ℞
Amcinonide
Topical Lotion 0.1%
Topical Cream 0.1%
with AQUATAIN™ hydrophilic base
Topical Ointment 0.1%

PRODUCT OVERVIEW
KEY FACTS
CYCLOCORT is a potent topical corticosteroid containing 0.1% Amcinonide in three distinct bases. CYCLOCORT Cream and Lotion are formulated with the patented AQUATAIN™ hydrophilic base for enhanced penetration without lanolin, parabens, or propylene glycol. CYCLOCORT ointment is a specially formulated base with Tenox II which contains propylene glycol.

MAJOR USES
CYCLOCORT is indicated for the relief of the inflammatory and pruritic manifestations of corticosteroid-responsive dermatoses.

SAFETY INFORMATION
CYCLOCORT may be prescribed without a two-week restriction. The possibility of systemic effects of potent corticosteroids may increase with use over large surface areas, prolonged use, and the addition of occlusive dressings. The most common adverse effects are burning, itching, irritation, and dryness. CYCLOCORT is not for ophthalmic use.

PRESCRIBING INFORMATION

CYCLOCORT®   ℞
Amcinonide
Topical Lotion 0.1%
Topical Cream 0.1%
with AQUATAIN™ hydrophilic base
Topical Ointment 0.1%

DESCRIPTION
The topical corticosteroids constitute a class of primarily synthetic steroids used as anti-inflammatory and antipruritic agents.
TOPICAL LOTION 0.1%
Each gram of CYCLOCORT *amcinonide* topical Lotion contains 1 mg of the active steroid amcinonide in AQUATAIN,* a white, smooth, homogeneous, opaque emulsion composed of Benzyl Alcohol 1% (wt/wt) as preservative, Emulsifying Wax, Glycerin, Isopropyl Palmitate, Lactic Acid, Purified Water, and Sorbitol Solution. In addition, contains Polyethylene Glycol 400.
Sodium hydroxide may be used to adjust pH to approximately 4.4 during manufacture.
TOPICAL CREAM 0.1%
Each gram of CYCLOCORT topical Cream contains 1 mg of the active steroid amcinonide in AQUATAIN,* a white, smooth, homogeneous, opaque emulsion composed of Benzyl Alcohol 2% (wt/wt) as preservative, Emulsifying Wax, Glycerin, Isopropyl Palmitate, Lactic Acid, Purified Water and Sorbitol Solution.
* AQUATAIN is nonstaining, water-washable, paraben-free, spermaceti-free and has a light texture and consistency.
TOPICAL OINTMENT 0.1%
Each gram of CYCLOCORT *amcinonide* topical Ointment contains 1 mg of the active steroid amcinonide in a specially formulated base composed of Benzyl Alcohol 2% (wt/wt) as preservative, White Petrolatum, Emulsifying Wax and Tenox II (Butylated Hydroxyanisole, Propyl Gallate, Citric Acid, Propylene Glycol).
Chemically amcinonide is: Pregna-1,4-diene-3,20-dione, 21-(acetyloxy)-16, 17-[cyclopentylidenebis(oxy)]-9-fluoro-11-hydroxy-, $(11\beta, 16\alpha)$.

CLINICAL PHARMACOLOGY
Topical corticosteroids have anti-inflammatory, antipruritic and vasconstrictive actions.
The mechanism of anti-inflammatory activity of the topical corticosteroids is unclear. Various laboratory methods, including vasoconstrictor assays, are used to compare and predict potencies and/or clinical efficacies of the topical corticosteroids. There is some evidence to suggest that a recognizable correlation exists between vasoconstrictor potency and therapeutic efficacy in man.
Pharmacokinetics: The extent of percutaneous absorption of topical corticosteroids is determined by many factors including the vehicle, the integrity of the epidermal barrier, and the use of occlusive dressings.
Topical corticosteroids can be absorbed from normal intact skin. Inflammatory and/or other disease processes in the skin increase percutaneous absorption. Occlusive dressings substantially increase the percutaneous absorption of topical corticosteroids (see **DOSAGE AND ADMINISTRATION**).
Once absorbed through the skin, topical corticosteroids are handled through pharmacokinetic pathways similar to systemically administered corticosteroids. Corticosteroids are bound to plasma proteins in varying degrees.
Corticosteroids are metabolized primarily in the liver and are then excreted by the kidneys. Some of the topical corticosteroids and their metabolites are also excreted into the bile.

INDICATIONS AND USAGE
Topical corticosteroids are indicated for the relief of the inflammatory and pruritic manifestations of corticosteroid-responsive dermatoses.

CONTRAINDICATIONS
Topical corticosteroids are contraindicated in those patients with a history of hypersensitivity to any of the components of the preparation.

PRECAUTIONS
General: Systemic absorption of topical corticosteroids has produced reversible hypothalamic-pituitary-adrenal (HPA) axis suppression, manifestations of Cushing's syndrome, hyperglycemia, and glucosuria in some patients.

Continued on next page

Lederle—Cont.

Conditions which augment systemic absorption include the application of the more potent steroids, use over large surface areas, prolonged use, and the addition of occlusive dressings.

Therefore, patients receiving a large dose of a potent topical steroid applied to a large surface area or under an occlusive dressing should be evaluated periodically for evidence of HPA axis suppression by using the urinary free cortisol and ACTH stimulation tests. If HPA axis suppression is noted, an attempt should be made to withdraw the drug, to reduce the frequency of application, or to substitute a less potent steroid.

Recovery of HPA axis function is generally prompt and complete upon discontinuation of the drug. Infrequently, signs and symptoms of steroid withdrawal may occur, requiring supplemental systemic corticosteroids.

Children may absorb proportionally larger amounts of topical corticosteroids and thus be more susceptible to system toxicity. (See PRECAUTIONS—Pediatric Use.)

If irritation develops, topical corticosteroids should be discontinued and appropriate therapy instituted.

In the presence of dermatological infections, the use of an appropriate antifungal or antibacterial agent should be instituted. If a favorable response does not occur promptly, the corticosteroid should be discontinued until the infection has been adequately controlled.

The products are not for ophthalmic use.

Information for the Patient: Patients using topical corticosteroids should receive the following information and instructions:

1. This medication is to be used as directed by the physician. It is for external use only. Avoid contact with the eyes.
2. Patients should be advised not to use this medication for any disorder other than for which it was prescribed.
3. The treated skin area should not be bandaged or otherwise covered or wrapped as to be occlusive unless directed by the physician.
4. Patients should report any signs of local adverse reactions especially under occlusive dressings.
5. Parents of pediatric patients should be advised not to use tight-fitting diapers or plastic pants on a child being treated in the diaper area, as these garmets may constitute occlusive dressings.

Laboratory Tests: The following tests may be helpful in evaluating the HPA axis suppression:
Urinary free cortisol test
ACTH stimulation test

Carcinogenesis, Mutagenesis, and Impairment of Fertility: Long-term animal studies have not been performed to evaluate the carcinogenic potential of topical corticosteroids or their effect on fertility.

Studies to determine mutagenicity with prednisolone and hydrocortisone have revealed negative results.

Pregnancy Category C: Corticosteroids are generally teratogenic in laboratory animals when administered systemically at relatively low dosage levels. The more potent corticosteroids have been shown to be teratogenic after dermal application in laboratory animals. There are no adequate and well-controlled studies in pregnant women on teratogenic effects from topically applied corticosteroids. Therefore, topical corticosteroids should be used during pregnancy only if the potential benefit justifies the potential risk to the fetus. Drugs of this class should not be used extensively on pregnant patients, in large amounts, or for prolonged periods of time.

Nursing Mothers: It is not known whether topical administration of corticosteroids could result in sufficient systemic absorption to produce detectable quantities in breast milk. Systemically administered corticosteroids are secreted into breast milk in quantities not likely to have a deleterious effect on the infant. Nevertheless, a decision should be made whether to discontinue nursing or to discontinue the drug, taking into account the importance of the drug to the mother.

Pediatric Use: *Pediatric patients may demonstrate greater susceptibility to topical corticosteroid-induced HPA axis suppression and Cushing's syndrome than mature patients because of a higher ratio of skin surface area to body weight.*

Hypothalamic-pituitary-adrenal (HPA) axis suppression, Cushing's syndrome, and intracranial hypertension have been reported in children receiving topical corticosteroids. Manifestations of adrenal suppression in children include linear growth retardation, delayed weight gain, low plasma cortisol levels, and absence of response to ACTH stimulation. Manifestations of intracranial hypertension include bulging fontanelles, headaches, and bilateral papilledema.

Administration of topical corticosteroids to children should be limited to the least amount compatible with an effective therapeutic regimen. Chronic corticosteroid therapy may interfere with the growth and development of children.

ADVERSE REACTIONS

In the clinical trials with CYCLOCORT *amcinonide* Lotion, the investigators reported a 4.7% incidence of side effects. In a weekly acceptability evaluation, approximately 20% of the patients treated with CYCLOCORT Lotion or placebo reported itching, stinging, soreness or burning at one or more of the visits.

The following local adverse reactions are reported infrequently with topical corticosteroids, but may occur more frequently with the use of occlusive dressings. These reactions are listed in an approximate decreasing order of occurrence: burning, itching, irritation, dryness, folliculitis, hypertrichosis, acneiform eruptions, hypopigmentation, perioral dermatitis, allergic contact dermatitis, maceration of the skin, secondary infection, skin atrophy, striae, miliaria.

OVERDOSAGE

Topically applied corticosteroids can be absorbed in sufficient amounts to produce systemic effects (see **PRECAUTIONS**).

DOSAGE AND ADMINISTRATION

Topical corticosteroids are generally applied to the affected area as a thin film from two to three times daily, depending on the severity of the condition.

The lotion may be applied topically to the specified lesions, particularly to those in hairy areas, two times per day. The lotion should be rubbed into the affected area completely, and the area should be protected from washing, clothing, rubbing, etc. until the lotion has dried.

Occlusive dressings may be used for the management of psoriasis or recalcitrant conditions.

If an infection develops, the use of occlusive dressings should be discontinued and appropriate antimicrobial therapy instituted.

HOW SUPPLIED

CYCLOCORT *amcinonide* topical Lotion 0.1% (1 mg/g) with AQUATAIN hydrophilic base is available as follows:
NDC 0005-9363-37—20 mL (19.6 g) bottle
NDC 0005-9363-41—60 mL (58.8 g) bottle

CYCLOCORT topical Cream 0.1% (1 mg/g) with AQUATAIN hydrophilic base is available as follows:
NDC 0005-9183-09—15 gram tube
NDC 0005-9183-32—30 gram tube
NDC 0005-9183-40—60 gram tube

CYCLOCORT topical Ointment 0.1% (1 mg/g) is available as follows:
NDC 0005-9345-09—15 gram tube
NDC 0005-9345-32—30 gram tube
NDC 0005-9345-40—60 gram tube
Store at Controlled Room Temperature 15°–30°C (59°–86°F).

DO NOT FREEZE.

CYCLOCORT Amcinonide Topical Cream 0.1% with AQUATAIN hydrophilic base
Military Depot:
NSN 6505-01-139-5001—15 g tube
Military and VA Depots:
NSN 6505-01-093-7968—60 g tube
CYCLOCORT Amcinonide Topical Ointment 0.1%
NSN 6505-01-150-3824—60 g tube
LEDERLE LABORATORIES DIVISION
American Cyanamid Company, Pearl River, NY 10965
Rev. 2/89
24587

Shown in Product Identification Section, page 414

DECLOMYCIN® ℞
[dĕk-lō-mī-sĭn]
Demeclocycline Hydrochloride
For Oral Use

DESCRIPTION

DECLOMYCIN is an antibiotic isolated from a mutant strain of *Streptomyces aureofaciens*. Chemically it is [4S-(4α,4aα,5aα,6β,12aα)]-7-Chloro-4-dimethylamino)-1,4,4a,5,5a,6,11,12a-octahydro-3,6,10,12,12a-pentahydroxy-1,11-dioxo-2-naphthacenecarboxamide monohydrochloride.

DECLOMYCIN contains the following inactive ingredients: Capsules: Benzoin Gum, Blue 1, Colloidal Silicon Dioxide, Corn Starch, Ethyl Vanillin, Gelatin, Glycerin, Methylparaben, Propenyl Guaethol, Propylene Glycol, Propylparaben, Red 33, Red 40, Terpene Resin, Titanium Dioxide, Yellow 6 and other ingredients.

Tablets: Alginic Acid, Corn Starch, Ethylcellulose, Hydroxypropyl Methylcellulose, Magnesium Stearate, Red 7, Sorbitol, Titanium Dioxide, Yellow 10 and other ingredients. May also contain Sodium Lauryl Sulfate.

CLINICAL PHARMACOLOGY

The tetracyclines are primarily bacteriostatic and are thought to exert their antimicrobial effect by the inhibition of protein synthesis. Tetracyclines are active against a wide range of gram-negative and gram-positive organisms.

The drugs in the tetracycline class have closely similar antimicrobial spectra, and cross-resistance among them is common. Microorganisms may be considered susceptible if the MIC (minimum inhibitory concentration) is not more than 4 mcg/mL and intermediate if the MIC is 4 to 12.5 mcg/mL. Susceptibility plate testing: A tetracycline disc may be used to determine microbial susceptibility to drugs in the tetracycline class. If the Kirby-Bauer method of disc susceptibility testing is used, a 30 mcg tetracycline disc should give a zone of at least 19 mm when tested against a tetracycline-susceptible bacterial strain.

Tetracyclines are readily absorbed and are bound to plasma proteins in varying degrees. They are concentrated by the liver in the bile and excreted in the urine and feces at high concentrations and in a biologically active form.

INDICATIONS AND USAGE

DECLOMYCIN is indicated in infections caused by the following microorganisms:
Rickettsiae: (Rocky Mountain spotted fever, typhus fever and the typhus group, Q fever, rickettsialpox, tick fevers).
Mycoplasma pneumoniae (PPLO, Eaton agent).
Agents of psittacosis and ornithosis.
Agents of lymphogranuloma venereum and granuloma inguinale.
The spirochetal agent of relapsing fever (*Borrelia recurrentis*).
The following gram-negative microorganisms:
Haemophilus ducreyi (chancroid),
Yersinia pestis and *Francisella tularensis*, formerly *Pasteurella pestis* and *Pasteurella tularensis*,
Bartonella bacilliformis,
Bacteroides species,
Vibrio comma and *Vibrio fetus*.
Brucella species (in conjunction with streptomycin).
Because many strains of the following groups of microorganisms have been shown to be resistant to tetracyclines, culture and susceptibility testing are recommended.
Demeclocycline is indicated for treatment of infections caused by the following gram-negative microorganisms, when bacteriologic testing indicates appropriate susceptibility to the drug:
Escherichia coli,
Enterobacter aerogenes (formerly *Aerobacter aerogenes*),
Shigella species,
Mima species and *Herellea* species,
Haemophilus influenzae (respiratory infections),
Klebsiella species (respiratory and urinary infections).
DECLOMYCIN *demeclocycline hydrochloride* is indicated for treatment of infections caused by the following gram-positive microorganisms when bacteriologic testing indicates appropriate susceptibility to the drug:
Streptococcus species:
Up to 44% of strains of *Streptococcus pyogenes* and 74% of *Streptococcus faecalis* have been found to be resistant to tetracycline drugs. Therefore, tetracyclines should not be used for streptococcal disease unless the organism has been demonstrated to be sensitive.
For upper respiratory infections due to Group A beta-hemolytic streptococci, penicillin is the usual drug of choice, including prophylaxis of rheumatic fever.
Streptococcus pneumoniae,
Staphylococcus aureus, skin and soft tissue infections. Tetracyclines are not the drugs of choice in the treatment of any type of staphylococcal infection.
When penicillin is contraindicated, tetracyclines are alternative drugs in the treatment of infections due to:
Neisseria gonorrhoeae,
Treponema pallidum and *Treponema pertenue* (syphilis and yaws),
Listeria monocytogenes,
Clostridium species,
Bacillus anthracis,
Fusobacterium fusiforme (Vincent's infection),
Actinomyces species.
In acute intestinal amebiasis, the tetracyclines may be a useful adjunct to amebicides.
DECLOMYCIN is indicated in the treatment of trachoma, although the infectious agent is not always eliminated, as judged by immunofluorescence.
Inclusion conjunctivitis may be treated with oral tetracyclines or with a combination of oral and topical agents.

CONTRAINDICATIONS

This drug is contraindicated in persons who have shown hypersensitivity to any of the tetracyclines.

WARNINGS

THE USE OF DRUGS OF THE TETRACYCLINE CLASS DURING TOOTH DEVELOPMENT (LAST HALF OF PREGNANCY, INFANCY, AND CHILDHOOD TO THE AGE OF 8 YEARS) MAY CAUSE PERMANENT DISCOLORATION OF THE TEETH (YELLOW-GRAY-BROWN).

This adverse reaction is more common during long-term use of the drugs but has been observed following repeated short-term courses. Enamel hypoplasia has also been reported.

TETRACYCLINE DRUGS, THEREFORE, SHOULD NOT BE USED IN THIS AGE GROUP UNLESS OTHER DRUGS ARE NOT LIKELY TO BE EFFECTIVE OR ARE CONTRAINDICATED.

If renal impairment exists, even usual oral or parenteral doses may lead to excessive systemic accumulation of the drug and possible liver toxicity. Under such conditions, lower than usual total doses are indicated and, if therapy is prolonged, serum level determinations of the drug may be advisable.

Phototoxic reactions can occur in individuals taking demeclocycline, and are characterized by severe burns of exposed surfaces resulting from direct exposure of patients to sunlight during therapy with moderate or large doses of demeclocycline. Patients apt to be exposed to direct sunlight or ultraviolet light should be advised that this reaction can occur, and treatment should be discontinued at the first evidence of skin erythema.

The anti-anabolic action of the tetracyclines may cause an increase in BUN. While this is not a problem in those with normal renal function, in patients with significantly impaired function, higher serum levels of tetracycline may lead to azotemia, hyperphosphatemia, and acidosis.

Administration of DECLOMYCIN *demeclocycline hydrochloride* has resulted in appearance of the diabetes insipidus syndrome (polyuria, polydipsia and weakness) in some patients on long-term therapy. The syndrome has been shown to be nephrogenic, dose-dependent, and reversible on discontinuance of therapy.

Usage in pregnancy (See above **WARNINGS** about use during tooth development). Results of animal studies indicate that tetracyclines cross the placenta, are found in fetal tissues and can have toxic effects on the developing fetus (often related to retardation of skeletal development). Evidence of embryotoxicity has also been noted in animals treated early in pregnancy.

Usage in newborns, infants, and children (See above **WARNINGS** about use during tooth development).

All tetracyclines form a stable calcium complex in any bone forming tissue. A decrease in the fibula growth rate has been observed in prematures given oral tetracycline in doses of 25 mg/kg every 6 hours. This reaction was shown to be reversible when the drug was discontinued.

Tetracyclines are present in the milk of lactating women who are taking a drug in this class.

PRECAUTIONS

General: Pseudotumor cerebri (benign intracranial hypertension) in adults has been associated with the use of tetracyclines. The usual clinical manifestations are headache and blurred vision. Bulging fontanels have been associated with the use of tetracyclines in infants. While both of these conditions and related symptoms usually resolve soon after discontinuation of the tetracycline, the possibility for permanent sequelae exists.

As with other antibiotic preparations, use of this drug may result in overgrowth of nonsusceptible organisms, including fungi. If superinfection occurs, the antibiotic should be discontinued and appropriate therapy should be instituted.

In venereal diseases when coexistent syphilis is suspected, darkfield examination should be done before treatment is started and the blood serology repeated monthly for at least 4 months.

In long-term therapy, periodic laboratory evaluation of organ systems, including hematopoietic, renal and hepatic studies should be performed.

All infections due to Group A beta-hemolytic streptococci should be treated for at least ten days.

Interpretation of Bacteriologic Studies: Following a course of therapy, persistence for several days in both urine and blood of bacterio-suppressive levels of demeclocycline may interfere with culture studies. These levels should not be considered therapeutic.

DRUG INTERACTIONS

Because the tetracyclines have been shown to depress plasma prothrombin activity, patients who are on anticoagulant therapy may require downward adjustment of their anticoagulant dosage.

Since bacteriostatic drugs may interfere with the bactericidal action of penicillin, it is advisable to avoid giving demeclocycline in conjunction with penicillin.

Concurrent use of tetracycline may render oral contraceptives less effective. Breakthrough bleeding has been reported.

ADVERSE REACTIONS

Gastrointestinal: Anorexia, nausea, vomiting, diarrhea, glossitis, dysphagia, enterocolitis, and inflammatory lesions (with monilial overgrowth) in the anogenital region. Hepatic toxicity has been reported rarely. These reactions have been caused by both the oral and parenteral administration of tetracyclines.

Skin: Maculopapular and erythematous rashes. Exfoliative dermatitis has been reported but is uncommon. Photosensitivity is discussed above. (See **WARNINGS**.)

Renal toxicity: Rise in BUN has been reported and is apparently dose related. Nephrogenic diabetes insipidus. (See **WARNINGS**.)

Hypersensitivity Reactions: Urticaria, angioneurotic edema, anaphylaxis, anaphylactoid purpura, pericarditis, and exacerbation of systemic lupus erythematosus.

Blood: Hemolytic anemia, thrombocytopenia, neutropenia, and eosinophilia have been reported.

CNS: Pseudotumor cerebri (benign intracranial hypertension) in adults and bulging fontanels in infants (See **PRECAUTIONS—General**).

Other: When given over prolonged periods, tetracyclines have been reported to produce brown-black microscopic discoloration of thyroid glands. No abnormalities of thyroid function studies are known to occur.

DOSAGE AND ADMINISTRATION

Therapy should be continued for at least 24 to 48 hours after symptoms and fever have subsided.

Concomitant therapy: Antacids containing aluminum, calcium, or magnesium impair absorption and should not be given to patients taking oral tetracycline.

Foods and some dairy products also interfere with absorption. Oral forms of tetracycline should be given one hour before or two hours after meals.

In patients with renal impairment: (See **WARNINGS**.) Total dosage should be decreased by reduction of recommended individual doses and/or by extending time intervals between doses.

In the treatment of streptococcal infections, a therapeutic dose of demeclocycline should be administered for at least 10 days.

Adults: Usual daily dose—Four divided doses of 150 mg each or two divided doses of 300 mg each.

For children over eight years of age: Usual daily dose, 3–6 mg per pound body weight per day, depending upon the severity of the disease, divided into two to four doses.

Gonorrhea patients sensitive to penicillin may be treated with demeclocycline administered as an initial oral dose of 600 mg followed by 300 mg every 12 hours for four days to a total of 3 grams.

HOW SUPPLIED

DECLOMYCIN *demeclocycline hydrochloride* Capsules, 150 mg are two-tone, coral colored, soft gelatin capsules, printed with LL followed by D9 on the light side in blue ink, supplied as follows: NDC 0005-9208-23—Bottle of 100

DECLOMYCIN Tablets, 150 mg are round, convex, red, film coated tablets, engraved with LL on one side and D11 on the other, supplied as follows:

NDC 0005-9218-23—Bottle of 100

DECLOMYCIN Tablets, 300 mg are round, convex, red, film coated tablets, engraved with LL on one side and D12 on the other, supplied as follows:

NDC 0005-9270-29—Bottle of 48

Store at Controlled Room Temperature 15–30°C (59–86°F).

LEDERLE LABORATORIES DIVISION

American Cyanamid Company

Pearl River, N.Y. 10965   Rev. 2/89

23995

Shown in Product Identification Section, page 414

DIAMOX® ℞

[dīa-mŏx]

Acetazolamide

SEQUELS® Sustained-Release

Capsules 500 mg

(See PDR For Ophthalmology)

Shown in Product Identification Section, page 414

DIAMOX® ℞

[di'ah-moks]

Acetazolamide Tablets and

DIAMOX Sterile Acetazolamide Sodium

Parenteral

(See PDR For Ophthalmology)

Shown in Product Identification Section, page 414

DIPHTHERIA AND TETANUS ℞

TOXOIDS ADSORBED PUROGENATED®

Aluminum Phosphate-Adsorbed

For Pediatric Use

DESCRIPTION

Diphtheria and Tetanus Toxoids Adsorbed, aluminum phosphate—adsorbed PUROGENATED® is a sterile combination of refined diphtheria and tetanus toxoids for intramuscular use only. After shaking, the vaccine is a homogeneous white suspension.

The diphtheria and tetanus toxins are produced according to the method of Mueller and Miller[1,2] and are detoxified by use of formaldehyde. The toxoids are refined by the Pillemer alcohol fractionation method[3] and are diluted with a solution containing sodium phosphate monobasic, sodium phosphate dibasic, aluminum phosphate, glycine and thimerosal (mercury derivative) as a preservative. The final concentration of thimerosal in the combined vaccine is 1:10,000. The aluminum content of the final product does not exceed 0.80 mg per 0.5 ml dose.

Each 0.5 ml dose is formulated to contain 12.5 Lf units of diphtheria toxoid, and 5 Lf units of tetanus toxoid.

CLINICAL PHARMACOLOGY

Diphtheria is primarily a localized and generalized intoxication caused by diphtheria toxin, an extracellular protein metabolite of toxinogenic strains of *Corynebacterium diphtheriae*. While the incidence of diphtheria in the U.S. has decreased from over 200,000 cases reported in 1921 before the general use of diphtheria toxoid, to only 15 cases reported from 1980 through 1983, the ratio of fatalities to attack rate has remained constant at about 5% to 10%.[4] The highest case fatality rates are in the very young and the elderly.

Following adequate immunization with diphtheria toxoid, which induces antitoxin, it is thought that protection lasts for at least 10 years.[4] This significantly reduces both the risk of developing diphtheria and the severity of clinical illness. It does not, however, eliminate carriage of *C diphtheriae* in the pharynx or on the skin.[4]

Tetanus is an intoxication manifested primarily by neuromuscular dysfunction, caused by a potent exotoxin elaborated by *Clostridium tetani*. The incidence of tetanus in the U.S. has dropped dramatically with the routine use of tetanus toxoid, remaining relatively constant over the last decade at about 90 cases reported annually.[4] Spores of *C tetani* are ubiquitous, and there is essentially no natural immunity to tetanus toxin. Thus, universal primary immunization with tetanus toxoid, and subsequent maintenance of adequate antitoxin levels by means of timed boosters, is necessary to protect all age groups.[4,6] Tetanus toxoid is a highly effective antigen, and a completed primary series generally induces protective levels of serum antitoxin that persists for at least 10 years.[4]

INDICATIONS AND USAGE

Diphtheria and Tetanus Toxoids Adsorbed is indicated for active immunization of infants and children from 2 months of age up to their seventh birthday both for routine protection and as a preventive measure against diphtheria and tetanus, in circumstances in which the use of a combined triple vaccine containing pertussis antigen is contraindicated.[4,5]

Tetanus or diphtheria infection may not confer immunity; therefore, initiation or completion of active immunization is indicated at the time of recovery from these infections.[4]

CONTRAINDICATIONS

HYPERSENSITIVITY TO ANY COMPONENT OF THE VACCINE, INCLUDING THIMEROSAL, A MERCURY DERIVATIVE, IS A CONTRAINDICATION.

THE OCCURRENCE OF ANY NEUROLOGICAL SYMPTOMS OR SIGNS FOLLOWING ADMINISTRATION OF THIS PRODUCT IS A CONTRAINDICATION TO FURTHER USE.

IMMUNIZATION SHOULD BE DEFERRED DURING THE COURSE OF ANY FEBRILE ILLNESS OR ACUTE INFECTION. A MINOR AFEBRILE ILLNESS SUCH AS A MILD UPPER RESPIRATORY INFECTION IS NOT USUALLY REASON TO DEFER IMMUNIZATION.[4,5]

The clinical judgment of the attending physician should prevail at all times.

Routine immunization should be deferred during an outbreak of poliomyelitis, providing the patient has not sustained an injury that increases the risk of tetanus and providing an outbreak of diphtheria does not occur simultaneously.

WARNINGS

THIS PRODUCT IS NOT RECOMMENDED FOR IMMUNIZING PERSONS ON OR AFTER THEIR SEVENTH BIRTHDAY. For individuals 7 years of age or older, Tetanus and Diphtheria Toxoids Adsorbed For Adult Use (Td) should be used instead of Diphtheria and Tetanus Toxoids Adsorbed For Pediatric Use (DT). The concentration of diphtheria toxoid in preparations intended for use in persons 7 years of age or older is lower than that of the pediatric formulation; a lower dosage of diphtheria toxoid is recommended for persons 7 years of age or older because adverse reactions to the diphtheria component are thought to be related to both dose and age.[4]

Continued on next page

Lederle—Cont.

THE OCCURRENCE OF A NEUROLOGICAL OR SEVERE HYPERSENSITIVITY REACTION FOLLOWING A PREVIOUS DOSE IS A CONTRAINDICATION TO FURTHER USE OF THIS PRODUCT.[4]

DT should not be given to infants or children with thrombocytopenia or any coagulation disorder that would contraindicate intramuscular injection unless the potential benefits clearly outweigh the risk of administration.

Patients with impaired immune responsiveness, whether due to the use of immunosuppressive therapy (including irradiation, corticosteroids, antimetabolites, alkylating agents, and cytotoxic agents), a genetic defect, human immunodeficiency virus (HIV) infection, or other causes, may have a reduced antibody response to active immunization procedures.[4,5,6] Deferral of administration of DT may be considered in individuals receiving immunosuppressive therapy.[4,5] Other groups should generally receive this vaccine according to the usual recommended schedule.[4-7]

Special care should be taken to prevent injection into a blood vessel.

PRECAUTIONS

General:

1. THIS PRODUCT SHOULD BE USED FOR THE AGE GROUP BETWEEN 2 MONTHS AND THE SEVENTH BIRTHDAY.
2. PRIOR TO ADMINISTRATION OF ANY DOSE OF DT, THE PARENT OR GUARDIAN SHOULD BE ASKED ABOUT THE RECENT HEALTH STATUS OF THE INFANT OR CHILD TO BE IMMUNIZED IN ORDER TO DETERMINE THE EXISTENCE OF ANY CONTRAINDICATION TO IMMUNIZATION WITH DT (SEE **CONTRAINDICATIONS, WARNINGS**).
3. WHEN AN INFANT OR CHILD RETURNS FOR THE NEXT DOSE IN A SERIES, THE PARENT OR GUARDIAN SHOULD BE QUESTIONED CONCERNING OCCURRENCE OF ANY SYMPTOM AND/OR SIGN OF AN ADVERSE REACTION AFTER THE PREVIOUS DOSE (SEE **CONTRAINDICATIONS, ADVERSE REACTIONS**).
4. BEFORE THE INJECTION OF ANY BIOLOGICAL, THE PHYSICIAN SHOULD TAKE ALL PRECAUTIONS KNOWN FOR PREVENTION OF ALLERGIC OR ANY OTHER SIDE REACTIONS. This should include: a review of the patient's history regarding possible sensitivity; the ready availability of epinephrine 1:1,000 and other appropriate agents used for control of immediate allergic reactions; and a knowledge of the recent literature pertaining to use of the biological concerned, including the nature of side effects and adverse reactions that may follow its use.
5. A separate sterile syringe and needle or a sterile disposable unit should be used for each individual patient to prevent transmission of hepatitis or other infectious agents from one person to another.
6. Shake vigorously before withdrawing each dose to resuspend the contents of the vial.
7. NATIONAL CHILDHOOD VACCINE INJURY ACT OF 1986 (AS AMENDED IN 1987)
   This Act requires that the manufacturer and lot number of the vaccine administered be recorded by the health care provider in the vaccine recipient's permanent medical record, along with the date of administration of the vaccine and the name, address and title of the person administering the vaccine.
   The Act further requires the health care provider to report to a health department or to the FDA the occurrence following immunization of any event set forth in the Vaccine Injury Table including: anaphylaxis or anaphylactic shock within 24 hours, encephalopathy or encephalitis within 7 days, residual seizure disorder, any acute complication or sequelae (including death) of above events, or any event that would contraindicate further doses of vaccine, according to this package insert.[8]

Information for the Patient: PRIOR TO THE ADMINISTRATION OF THIS VACCINE, HEALTH CARE PERSONNEL SHOULD INFORM THE PARENT, GUARDIAN, OR OTHER RESPONSIBLE ADULT OF THE BENEFITS AND RISKS TO THE CHILD OF VACCINATION AGAINST DIPHTHERIA AND TETANUS.

Use in Pregnancy: This product is not recommended for administration to females of child-bearing age.

ADVERSE REACTIONS

Local reactions, manifested by varying degrees of erythema, induration, and tenderness, may occur after administration of DT.[9,10] Such local reactions are usually self-limited and require no therapy. Nodule,[11] sterile abscess formation, or subcutaneous atrophy may occur at the site of injection. Systemic symptoms, including drowsiness, fretfulness, vomiting, anorexia, and persistent crying have been described following DT immunization.[9,10]

In one study, fever ≥ 38°C (100.4°F) was reported in 9.3% of DT recipients, and fever ≥ 39°C (102.2°F) was reported in 0.7% of recipients.[9]

Pallor, coldness, and hyporesponsiveness has been reported in a child receiving a DT vaccine.[10]

NEUROLOGICAL COMPLICATIONS,[12] SUCH AS CONVULSIONS,[13] ENCEPHALOPATHY,[13,14] AND VARIOUS MONO- AND POLYNEUROPATHIES,[14-20] INCLUDING GUILLAIN-BARRE SYNDROME,[21,22] HAVE BEEN REPORTED FOLLOWING ADMINISTRATION OF PREPARATIONS CONTAINING DIPHTHERIA AND/OR TETANUS ANTIGENS.

URTICARIA, ERYTHEMA MULTIFORME OR OTHER RASH, ARTHRALGIAS[13] AND, MORE RARELY, A SEVERE ANAPHYLACTIC REACTION (IE, URTICARIA WITH SWELLING OF THE MOUTH, DIFFICULTY BREATHING, HYPOTENSION, OR SHOCK) HAVE BEEN REPORTED FOLLOWING ADMINISTRATION OF PREPARATIONS CONTAINING DIPHTHERIA, AND/OR TETANUS ANTIGENS.

DOSAGE AND ADMINISTRATION

For Intramuscular Use Only: Shake vigorously before withdrawing each dose to resuspend the contents of the vial. Parenteral drug products should be inspected visually for particulate matter and discoloration prior to administration. (See **DESCRIPTION**.)

The vaccine should be injected intramuscularly, preferably into the midlateral muscles of the thigh or deltoid, with care to avoid major peripheral nerve trunks.

Before injection, the skin at the injection site should be cleansed and prepared with a suitable germicide.

After insertion of the needle, aspirate to help avoid inadvertent injection into a blood vessel.

This combined preparation against both diphtheria and tetanus is designed particularly to meet the need of children less than 7 years of age for whom the use of a combined triple vaccine containing pertussis antigen is contraindicated.

It is recommended that active immunization against diphtheria and tetanus be started at 2 months of age.

Unimmunized infants and children less than 1 year of age for whom vaccine containing pertussis antigen is contraindicated should receive three doses of 0.5 ml each of DT at 4 to 8 week intervals, followed by a fourth (reinforcing) dose of 0.5 ml, 6 to 12 months after the third dose, for the primary series.

Unimmunized children 1 year of age or older for whom vaccine containing pertussis antigen is contraindicated should receive two doses of 0.5 ml each of DT, 4 to 8 weeks apart, followed by a third (reinforcing) dose 6 to 12 months later, for the primary series.

If after beginning a DTP series, further doses of vaccine containing pertussis antigen become contraindicated, DT should be substituted for each of the remaining doses.[4,5]

The reinforcing dose is an integral part of the primary immunizing series.

Interruption of the recommended schedule with a delay between doses does not interfere with the final immunity achieved, nor does it necessitate starting the series over again, regardless of the length of time elapsed between doses.[4,5]

A booster dose of 0.5 ml is indicated at age 4 to 6 years, preferably prior to entrance into kindergarten or elementary school. However, if the last dose of the primary immunizing series was administered after the fourth birthday, a booster prior to school entry is not considered necessary.[4,5]

For either primary or booster immunization against tetanus and diphtheria of individuals 7 years of age and older, the use of Tetanus and Diphtheria Toxoids Adsorbed For Adult Use is recommended.[4,5]

Diphtheria Prophylaxis for Case Contacts: All case contacts, household and others, who have previously received fewer than three doses of diphtheria toxoid should receive an immediate dose of an appropriate diphtheria toxoid-containing preparation and should complete the series according to schedule. Case contacts who previously received three or more doses, but who have not received a dose of a preparation containing diphtheria toxoid within the previous five years, should receive a dose of a diphtheria toxoid-containing preparation appropriate for their age. This combined preparation against both diphtheria and tetanus is designed particularly to meet the need of children less than 7 years of age for whom the use of a combined triple vaccine containing pertussis antigen is contraindicated.

Tetanus Prophylaxis in Wound Management: For routine wound management of children under 7 years of age who are not completely immunized, DT should be used instead of single-antigen tetanus toxoid (if pertussis antigen is contraindicated or individual circumstances are such that potential febrile reactions following DTP might confound the management of the patient).[4] Completion of primary vaccination thereafter should be ensured.

For tetanus-prone wounds in children who have had fewer than three, or an unknown number of immunizations with a tetanus-toxoid containing product, passive immunization with human Tetanus-Immune Globulin (TIG) is also recom-

mended.[4] A separate syringe and site of injection should be used.

HOW SUPPLIED

1858-31 5.0 ml vial

STORAGE

DO NOT FREEZE. STORE REFRIGERATED, AWAY FROM FREEZER COMPARTMENT, AT 2°C to 8°C (36°F to 46°F).

REFERENCES

1. Mueller JH, Miller PA: Production of diphtheria toxin of high potency (100Lf) on a reproducible medium. *J Immunol* 1941;40:21–32.
2. Mueller JH, Miller PA: Factors influencing the production of tetanal toxin. *J Immunol* 1947;56:143–147.
3. Pillemer L, Grossberg DB, Wittler RG: The immunochemistry of toxins and toxoids. II. The preparation and immunological evaluation of purified tetanal toxoid. *J Immunol* 1946;54:213–224.
4. Recommendation of the Immunization Practices Advisory Committee (ACIP): Diphtheria, tetanus and pertussis: Guidelines for vaccine prophylaxis and other preventive measures. *MMWR* 1985;34:405–426.
5. American Academy of Pediatrics: Report of the Committee on Infectious Diseases, ed 20. Elk Grove Village, IL, American Academy of Pediatrics, 1986.
6. Recommendation of the ACIP: Immunization of children infected with Human T-Lymphotrophic Virus Type III/Lymphadenopathy associated virus. *MMWR* 1986;35(38):595–606.
7. Immunization of children infected with Human Immunodeficiency Virus—Supplementary ACIP statement *MMWR* 1988;37(12):181–183.
8. National Childhood Vaccine Injury Act: Requirements for permanent vaccination records and for reporting of selected events after vaccination. *MMWR* 1988;37(13):197–200.
9. Cody C, et al: Nature and rates of adverse reactions associated with DTP and DT immunizations in infants and children. *Pediatrics* 1981;68:650–660.
10. Feery BJ: Incidence and type of reactions to triple antigen (DTP) and DT (CDT) vaccines. *Med Jour of Australia* 1982;2:511–515.
11. Fawcett HA, Smith NP: Injection-site granuloma due to aluminum. *Arch Dermatol* 1984;120:1318–1322.
12. Rutledge SL, Snead OC: Neurological complications of immunizations. *J Pediatr* 1986;109:917–924.
13. Adverse Events Following Immunization. *MMWR* 1985;34(3):43–47.
14. Schlenska GK: Unusual neurological complications following tetanus toxoid administration. *J Neurol* 1977;215:299–302.
15. Blumstein GI, Kreithen H: Peripheral neuropathy following tetanus toxoid administration. *JAMA* 1966;198:1030–1031.
16. Reinstein L, Pargament JM, Goodman JS: Peripheral neuropathy after multiple tetanus toxoid injections. *Arch Phys Med Rehabil* 1982;63:332–334.
17. Tsairis P, Duck PJ, Mulder DW: Natural history of brachial plexus neuropathy. *Arch Neurol* 1972;27:109–117.
18. Quast U, Hennessen W, Widmark RM: Mono- and polyneuritis after tetanus vaccination. *Devel Bio Stand* 1979;43:25–32.
19. Holliday PL, Bauer RB: Polyradiculoneuritis secondary to immunization with tetanus and diphtheria toxoids. *Arch Neurol* 1983;40:56–57.
20. Fenichel GM: Neurological complications of tetanus toxoid. *Arch Neurol* 1983;40:390.
21. Pollard JD, Selby G: Relapsing neuropathy due to tetanus toxoid. *J Neurol Sci* 1978;37:113–125.
22. Newton N, Janati A: Guillain-Barre syndrome after vaccination with purified tetanus toxoid. *S Med J* 1987;80:1053–1054.

LEDERLE LABORATORIES DIVISION
American Cyanamid Company,
Pearl River, NY 10965

Rev. 5/88
23590

FERRO—SEQUELS®

[fĕrrō-sē-quls]
High potency, time-release iron supplement

DESCRIPTION

Each FERRO-SEQUELS tablet contains 150 mg of ferrous fumarate, equivalent to approximately 50 mg of elemental iron and 100 mg of docusate sodium (DSS). FERRO-SEQUELS is a high potency iron supplement that employs a time release system to deliver iron slowly to maximize absorption, and to reduce the irritation associated with iron tablets.

Inactive Ingredients: Blue 1, Colloidal Silicon Dioxide, Corn Starch, Diethyl Phthalate, Ethycellulose, Hydroxypropyl Cellulose, Magnesium Stearate, Microcrystalline Cellulose,

Pharmaceutical Glaze, Povidone, Sodium Benzoate, Talc, Titanium Dioxide, Yellow 10 and other ingredients.

INDICATIONS

For the treatment of simple iron deficiency and iron deficiency anemia.

RECOMMENDED INTAKE

One tablet, once or twice daily, or as prescribed by the physician.

WARNING

As with any drug, if you are pregnant or nursing a baby, seek the advice of a health professional before using this product. Keep this and all medications out of the reach of children. In case of accidental overdose, seek professional assistance or contact a Poison Control Center immediately.

HOW SUPPLIED

Box of 30 tablets, NDC 0005-5267-68
Bottle of 30 tablets, NDC 0005-5267-13
Bottle of 100 tablets, NDC 0005-5267-23
Unit Dose Package 10-10s, NDC 0005-5267-60
Bottles of 1,000 tablets, NDC 0005-4612-34
Store at Controlled Room Temperature 15–30°C (59–86°F).
LEDERLE LABORATORIES DIVISION
American Cyanamid Company,
Pearl River, N.Y. 10965
MADE IN USA   9/87
                       21560

Shown in Product Identification Section, page 414

FIBERCON®

[fi-ber-con]
Calcium polycarbophil
Bulk-forming fiber laxative
Concentrated fiber laxative

DESCRIPTION

Each FIBERCON tablet contains 625 mg calcium polycarbophil equivalent to 500 mg polycarbophil. FIBERCON promotes normal function of the bowel by increasing bulk volume and water content of the stool. Contains no chemical stimulants and is non-habit forming.
Inactive Ingredients: Magnesium Stearate, Microcrystalline Cellulose, Silica Gel, Stearic Acid and other ingredients.

INDICATIONS

For the relief of constipation or irregularity. May be used in the treatment of bowel disorders other than constipation when recommended by a physician. This product generally produces a bowel movement in 12 to 72 hours.

RECOMMENDED INTAKE

Adults and children 12 years and older: swallow 2 tablets one to four times a day. Children 6 to 12 years: swallow 1 tablet one to three times a day. Children under 6 years: consult a physician.
A full glass (8 fl. oz.) of liquid should be taken with each dose. See package insert for additional information.

WARNING

If you have noticed a sudden change in bowel habits that persists over a period of 2 weeks, consult a physician before using a laxative. If the recommended use of this product for 1 week has no effect, discontinue use and consult a physician. Do not use laxative products when abdominal pain, nausea or vomiting is present except under the direction of a physician. Discontinue use and consult a physician if rectal bleeding occurs after use of any laxative product.
Interaction Precaution: Contains calcium. Take this product at least one hour before or two hours after taking an oral dose of a prescription antibiotic containing any form of tetracycline. Keep this and all medicines out of the reach of children.

HOW SUPPLIED

Film coated tablets, scored, engraved LL and F66.
Package of 36 tablets, NDC 0005-2500-02
Package of 60 tablets, NDC 0005-2500-86
Package of 90 tablets, NDC 0005-2500-33
Bottle of 500 tablets, NDC 0005-2500-31
Unit Dose Pkg, NDC 0005-2500-28
Store at Controlled Room Temperature 15–30° C (59–86° F).
Protect contents from moisture.   Rev. 3/88
LEDERLE LABORATORIES DIVISION
American Cyanamid Company
Pearl River, N.Y. 10965

Shown in Product Identification Section, page 414

INFLUENZA VIRUS VACCINE
FLU-IMUNE™*
Purified Surface Antigen Vaccine, Trivalent, Types A and B
1989–1990 Formula

DESCRIPTION

Influenza Virus Vaccine, FLU-IMUNE, Types A and B (Surface Antigen) is a sterile parenteral for intramuscular use only. The vaccine is a slightly opalescent liquid.
FLU-IMUNE is prepared from the extraembryonic fluid of embryonated chicken eggs inoculated with a specific type of influenza virus suspension containing neomycin and polymyxin. The fluid containing the virus is harvested and clarified by centrifugation and filtration prior to inactivation with betapropiolactone. The inactivated virus is concentrated and purified by zonal centrifugation. The surface antigens, hemagglutinin and neuraminidase, are obtained from the influenza virus particle by further centrifugation in the presence of Triton®† N101, a process which removes most of the internal proteins. The Triton® N101 is removed from the surface antigen preparation, and the antigens are suspended in 0.01M phosphate buffered saline. The hemagglutinin content is standardized according to current US Public Health Service requirements. Each dose (0.5 mL) contains the recommended ratio of not less than 15 mcg of hemagglutinin of each strain similar to: A/Taiwan/1/86 (H1N1), A/Shanghai/11/87 (H3N2), and B/Yamagata/16/88. Thimerosal (mercury derivative) 0.01% is added as a preservative. Polymyxin, neomycin, and betapropiolactone cannot be detected in the final product by current assay procedures. This vaccine is produced and filled by Evans Medical Limited: labeled, packaged, and released by Lederle Laboratories under a divided manufacturing arrangement.

CLINICAL PHARMACOLOGY

Influenza A viruses are classified into subtypes on the basis of two surface antigens: hemagglutinin (H) and neuraminidase (N). Three subtypes of hemagglutinin (H1, H2 and H3) and two subtypes of neuraminidase (N1, N2) are recognized among influenza A viruses that have caused widespread human disease.
Immunity to these antigens, especially the hemagglutinin, reduces the likelihood of infection and lessens the severity of the disease if infection occurs. However, over time, there may be enough antigenic variation (antigenic drift) within the same subtype that infection or immunization with one strain may not induce immunity to distantly related strains of the same subtype. Although infuenza B viruses have shown more antigenic stability than influenza A viruses, antigenic variation does occur. For these reasons major epidemics of respiratory disease caused by new variants of influenza continue to occur. The antigenic characteristics of current strains provide the basis for selecting the virus strains included in each year's vaccine.[1]
Typical influenza illness is characterized by abrupt onset of fever, sore throat, and nonproductive cough. Unlike many other common respiratory infections, influenza can cause extreme malaise lasting several days. More severe illness can result if influenza virus invades the lungs (primary viral pneumonia) or if secondary bacterial pneumonia occurs. High attack rates of acute illness during influenza epidemics usually result in dramatic increases in visits to physicians' offices, walk-in clinics, and emergency rooms by persons of all ages and in increases in hospitalization for management of lower respiratory tract complications.
Elderly persons and persons with underlying health problems are at increased risk of complications from influenza infection. Such high-risk persons are more likely than the general population to require hospitalization if infected. One recent study showed that, during major epidemics, hospitalization rates for high-risk adults increased two to fivefold, depending on age group. Previously healthy children and young adults may also require hospitalization for influenza-related complications, but the relative increase in their hospitalization rates is less than the increase for high-risk groups.[1]
An increase in mortality further indicates the impact of influenza epidemics. Increased mortality results from not only pneumonia, but also cardiopulmonary or other chronic diseases that can be exacerbated by influenza infection. Ten thousand or more excess deaths were documented in each of 19 different epidemics from 1957 to 1986. More than 40,000 excess deaths occurred in each of several recent epidemics. Approximately 80% to 90% of the excess deaths attributed to pneumonia and influenza were among persons 65 years of age and older. However, influenza-associated deaths also occur among children and previously healthy adults less than 65 years of age during major epidemics.[1]
Because the proportion of elderly persons in the United States population is increasing and because age and its associated chronic diseases are risk factors for severe influenza illness, the toll from influenza can be expected to increase unless control measures are used more vigorously. The number of younger persons at high risk for infection-related complications is also increasing for various reasons, including

the success of neonatal intensive care units, improved management of diseases such as cystic fibrosis, better survival rates for organ-transplant recipients, and the spread of human immunodeficiency virus (HIV) infections.[1]
Field studies have demonstrated that influenza vaccines give between 70% and 80% protection when the vaccine strain and infecting strain are related. Lower levels of protection occur when the infecting virus is antigenically different from the vaccine virus.[2]
Based upon epidemiological studies of circulating influenza virus strains, the Public Health Service has recommended that the 1989–1990 vaccine will be trivalent and contain 15 mcg of hemagglutinin of each strain similar to: A/Taiwan/1/86 (H1N1), A/Shanghai/11/87 (H3N2), and B/Yamagata/16/88 per 0.5 mL dose.

INDICATIONS AND USAGE

Influenza Virus Vaccine FLU-IMUNE, Types A and B (Surface Antigen) is indicated for immunization against influenza viruses containing antigens related to those in the vaccine.
Influenza vaccine is strongly recommended for persons 6 months of age or older who, by virtue of age or underlying medical condition, are at increased risk of complications from influenza, for their medical-care providers or household contacts, and for other persons wishing to reduce their chances of acquiring influenza. Guidelines for the use of vaccine among different segments of the population are given below.
Although the current Influenza Virus Vaccine often contains one or more antigens used in previous years, immunity declines in the year following immunization.[1] Therefore, a history of immunization in any previous year with a vaccine containing one or more antigens included in the current vaccine does not preclude the need to be reimmunized for the 1989–1990 influenza season.
TARGET GROUPS FOR SPECIAL IMMUNIZATION PROGRAMS:
To maximize protection of high-risk persons, both the persons at risk and their close contacts should be targeted for organized vaccination programs.
Groups at increased medical risk of influenza-related complications.
1. Adults and children with chronic disorders of the pulmonary or cardiovascular systems, including children with asthma.[1]
2. Residents of nursing homes and other chronic-care facilities housing patients of any age with chronic medical conditions.[1]
3. Persons 65 years of age or older, regardless of health status.[1]
4. Adults and children who have required regular medical follow-up or hospitalization during the preceding year because of chronic metabolic diseases (including diabetes mellitus), renal dysfunction, hemoglobinopathies, or immunosuppression.[1]
5. Children and teenagers (6 months through 18 years of age) who are receiving long-term aspirin therapy and, therefore, may be at risk of developing Reye syndrome following influenza infection.[1]
Groups potentially capable of transmitting influenza to high-risk persons.
Individuals attending high-risk persons can transmit influenza infections to them while they are incubating infection, undergoing subclinical infection, or working despite the existence of symptoms. Some high-risk persons [eg, the elderly, transplant recipients, or persons with acquired immunodeficiency syndrome (AIDS)] can have relatively low antibody responses to influenza vaccine. Efforts to protect them against influenza may be improved by reducing the chances that their care providers may expose them to influenza. Therefore, the following groups should be immunized:[1]
1. Physicians, nurses, and other personnel in both hospital and outpatient care settings who have extensive contact with high-risk patients in all age groups, including infants.[1]
2. Providers of care to high-risk persons in the home setting (eg, visiting nurses, volunteer workers).[1]
3. Household members of high-risk persons, including children, whether or not they provide care.[1]
IMMUNIZATION OF OTHER GROUPS:
General Population. Physicians should administer influenza vaccine to any person who wishes to reduce his/her chances of acquiring influenza infection. Persons providing essential community services and students or other healthy individuals in institutional settings may be considered for

Continued on next page

Lederle—Cont.

immunization to minimize disruption of routine activities during severe outbreaks.

Pregnant Women: Influenza-associated excess mortality among pregnant women has not been documented, except in the largest pandemics of 1918–1919 and 1957–1958. However, the Immunization Practices Advisory Committee (ACIP) of the US Public Health Service recommends that pregnant women who have other medical conditions that increase their risk for complications from influenza should be immunized, as the vaccine is considered safe for pregnant women.[1] Administering the vaccine after the first trimester is a reasonable precaution to minimize any concern over the theoretical possibility of teratogenicity. However, it may be undesirable to delay immunization of pregnant women with high-risk conditions who will still be in the first trimester of pregnancy when the influenza season begins.[1]

The clinical judgment of the attending physician should prevail at all times (see PRECAUTIONS, Use in Pregnancy).

Persons Infected with Human Immunodeficiency Virus (HIV): Because influenza may result in serious illness and complications in some HIV infected persons, immunization is a prudent precaution.[1]

Foreign Travelers: Increasingly, the elderly and persons with high-risk medical conditions are embarking on international travel. Influenza can occur throughout the year in the tropics; the season of greatest influenza activity in the southern hemisphere is April–September. Because of the short incubation period for influenza, exposure to the virus during travel will often result in clinical illness that begins during travel, an inconvenient or potentially dangerous situation, especially for those at increased risk for complications. Persons preparing to travel to the tropics at any time of year or to the southern hemisphere during April–September should review their immunization histories. If not immunized the previous fall/winter, they should be considered for influenza immunization prior to travel. The most current available vaccine should be used. High-risk persons given the previous season's vaccine prior to travel should be reimmunized in the fall/winter with current vaccine.

TIMING OF IMMUNIZATION: Influenza vaccine may be offered to high-risk persons presenting for routine care or hospitalization beginning in September but *not* until new vaccine is available. Except in years of pandemic influenza (eg, 1957 and 1968), high levels of influenza activity have not occurred in the contiguous 48 states before December. Therefore, November is the optimal time for organized immunization campaigns in chronic-care facilities, worksites, and other places where high-risk persons are routinely accessible. In facilities such as nursing homes, it is particularly important to avoid administering vaccine too far in advance of the influenza season because antibodies can begin to decline within a few months. Immunization may be undertaken in September or October (as soon as the current vaccine is available): 1) in regions that have experienced earlier than normal epidemic activity; and 2) for persons who should be immunized and who received medical check-ups or treatment during September or October and thus may not be seen in November. In addition, hospitalized high-risk adults and children who are discharged from September through March should be immunized as part of the discharge procedure.[1] Children under 13 years of age who have not been immunized previously require two doses with at least one month between doses. The second dose should be given before December, if possible. Vaccine can be given to both children and adults up to the time influenza virus activity is documented in a region, and even thereafter, which may be as late as April in some areas.

CONTRAINDICATIONS

INFLUENZA VIRUS FOR THE PREPARATION OF INFLUENZA VIRUS VACCINE IS PROPAGATED IN EGGS. THUS, THIS VACCINE SHOULD NOT BE ADMINISTERED TO ANYONE WITH A HISTORY OF HYPERSENSITIVITY (ALLERGY) TO CHICKEN EGGS, CHICKEN, CHICKEN FEATHERS, OR CHICKEN DANDER. THE VACCINE IS ALSO CONTRAINDICATED IN INDIVIDUALS HYPERSENSITIVE TO ANY COMPONENT OF THE VACCINE INCLUDING THIMEROSAL (A MERCURY DERIVATIVE) (SEE **ADVERSE REACTIONS**). EPINEPHRINE INJECTION (1:1000) MUST BE IMMEDIATELY AVAILABLE SHOULD AN ACUTE ANAPHYLACTIC REACTION OCCUR DUE TO ANY COMPONENT OF THE VACCINE.

IMMUNIZATION SHOULD BE DELAYED IN PERSONS WITH AN ACTIVE NEUROLOGICAL DISORDER CHARACTERIZED BY CHANGING NEUROLOGICAL FINDINGS, BUT SHOULD BE CONSIDERED WHEN THE DISEASE PROCESS HAS BEEN STABILIZED.

THE OCCURRENCE OF ANY NEUROLOGICAL SYMPTOMS OR SIGNS FOLLOWING ADMINISTRATION OF THIS PRODUCT IS A CONTRAINDICATION TO FURTHER USE.

THE VACCINE SHOULD NOT BE ADMINISTERED TO PERSONS WITH ACUTE FEBRILE ILLNESSES UNTIL THEIR TEMPORARY SYMPTOMS AND/OR SIGNS HAVE ABATED.

The clinical judgment of the attending physician should prevail at all times.

WARNINGS

THIS PRODUCT SHOULD NOT BE ADMINISTERED TO CHILDREN YOUNGER THAN 6 MONTHS OF AGE.

THE OCCURRENCE OF A NEUROLOGICAL OR SEVERE HYPERSENSITIVITY REACTION FOLLOWING PREVIOUS IMMUNIZATION WITH INFLUENZA VIRUS VACCINE IS A CONTRAINDICATION TO FURTHER USE OF THIS PRODUCT.

Influenza Virus Vaccine should not be given to individuals with thrombocytopenia or any coagulation disorder that would contraindicate intramuscular injection unless, in the judgment of the physician, the potential benefits clearly outweigh the risk of administration.

Patients with impaired immune responsiveness, whether due to the use of immunosuppressive therapy (including irradiation, corticosteroids, antimetabolites, alkylating agents, and cytotoxic agents), a genetic defect, human immunodeficiency virus (HIV) infection, or other causes, may have a reduced antibody response to active immunization procedures.

Since the likelihood of febrile convulsions from any cause is greater in children between 6 and 35 months, special care should be taken in weighing the relative risks and benefits of immunization in this age group.

Influenza virus antigens change significantly from time to time. Influenza Virus Vaccine is not effective against all possible strains of influenza virus. Protection is afforded to most people only against those strains of virus from which the vaccine is prepared, or against closely related strains. Infuenza Virus Vaccine often contains one or more antigens used in previous years. However, immunity declines during the year following immunization. Therefore, reimmunization on a yearly basis is necessary to provide optimal protection for the current season.

As with any vaccine, immunization with Influenza Virus Vaccine may not result in seroconversion of all individuals given the vaccine.

Special care should be taken to prevent injection into a blood vessel.

PRECAUTIONS

General:

1. PRIOR TO ADMINISTRATION OF ANY DOSE OF INFLUENZA VIRUS VACCINE, THE PARENT, GUARDIAN, OR ADULT PATIENT SHOULD BE ASKED ABOUT THE RECENT HEALTH STATUS, MEDICAL AND IMMUNIZATION HISTORY OF THE PATIENT TO BE IMMUNIZED IN ORDER TO DETERMINE THE EXISTENCE OF ANY CONTRAINDICATION TO IMMUNIZATION WITH INFLUENZA VIRUS VACCINE (SEE CONTRAINDICATIONS, WARNINGS).

2. BEFORE ADMINISTRATION OF ANY BIOLOGICAL, THE PHYSICIAN SHOULD TAKE ALL PRECAUTIONS KNOWN FOR PREVENTION OF ALLERGIC OR ANY OTHER SIDE REACTIONS. This should include: a review of the patient's history regarding possible sensitivity, the ready availability of epinephrine 1:1,000 and other appropriate agents used for control of immediate allergic reactions, and a knowledge of the recent literature pertaining to use of the biological concerned, including the nature of side effects and adverse reactions that may follow its use.

3. A separate sterile syringe and needle or a sterile disposable unit should be used for each individual patient to prevent transmission of hepatitis or other infectious agents from one person to another.

Information for the Patient: PRIOR TO ADMINISTRATION OF THIS VACCINE, HEALTH CARE PERSONNEL SHOULD INFORM THE PATIENT, GUARDIAN, OR ADULT PATIENT OF THE BENEFITS AND RISKS OF IMMUNIZATION AGAINST INFLUENZA.

Drug Interactions: Influenza immunization can inhibit the clearance of warfarin and theophylline. Most clinical studies have failed to show any adverse effects attributable to these drugs in patients receiving influenza vaccine.[1]

Use in Pregnancy: *Pregnancy Category C.* Animal reproduction studies have not been conducted with Influenza Virus Vaccine. It is also not known whether Influenza Virus Vaccine can cause fetal harm when administered to a pregnant woman or can affect reproductive capacity. Influenza Virus Vaccine should therefore be given to a pregnant woman ONLY if clearly indicated.

See INDICATIONS AND USAGE, Pregnant Women.

The clinical judgment of the attending physician should prevail at all times.

ADVERSE REACTIONS

Because influenza vaccine contains only noninfectious purified viral proteins, it cannot cause influenza. Occasional cases of respiratory disease following immunization represent coincidental illnesses unrelated to influenza immunization.[1]

Local Symptoms: Slight tenderness, redness, or induration at the site of injection lasting for 1 or 2 days may occur in less than one third of recipients.[1]

Systemic Symptoms: Fever, malaise, myalgia, and other systemic symptoms occur infrequently and most often affect persons who have had no exposure to the influenza virus antigens in the vaccine (eg, young children). These reactions begin 6 to 12 hours after immunization and can persist for 1 or 2 days.[1]

Immediate, presumably allergic, reactions such as hives, angioedema, allergic asthma, or systemic anaphylaxis occur rarely after influenza immunization. These reactions probably result from hypersensitivity to some vaccine component —most likely residual egg protein. Although current influenza vaccines contain only a small quantity of egg protein, they are presumed capable of inducing immediate hypersensitivity reactions in persons with severe egg allergy, and such persons should not be given influenza vaccine. This includes persons who develop hives, have swelling of the lips or tongue, or experience acute respiratory distress or collapse after eating eggs. Persons with a documented immunoglobulin E (IgE)-mediated hypersensitivity to eggs, including those who have experienced occupational asthma or other allergic responses from occupational exposure to egg protein, may also be at increased risk of reactions from influenza vaccine[1] (see CONTRAINDICATIONS).

Unlike the 1976 swine influenza vaccine, subsequent vaccines that have been prepared from other virus strains have not been associated with an increased frequency of Guillain-Barre syndrome (GBS).[3,4,5] Nevertheless, candidates for Influenza Virus Vaccine should be made aware of the benefits and possible risks of administration, including GBS.[1]

Other neurological disorders, including encephalopathies not defined as GBS, have been temporarily associated with influenza immunization, but no causal link has been established.[6,7]

DOSAGE AND ADMINISTRATION

For Intramuscular Use Only: Shake well before withdrawing each dose. DO NOT INJECT INTRAVENOUSLY.

Parenteral drug products should be inspected visually for particulate matter and discoloration prior to administration (see DESCRIPTION).

Remaining 1988–1989 influenza vaccine should not be used.

Although Influenza Virus Vaccine often contains one or more antigens used in previous years, immunity declines during the year following immunization. Therefore, a history of immunization in any previous year with a vaccine containing one or more antigens included in the current vaccine does NOT preclude the need for reimmunization for the 1989–1990 influenza season in order to provide optimal protection.

See INDICATIONS AND USAGE section for information regarding the optimal time of administration of this vaccine. During the past decade, data on influenza vaccine immunogenicity and side effects have generally been obtained when vaccine has been administered intramuscularly. Because there has been no adequate evaluation of recent influenza vaccines administered by other routes, the imtramuscular route should be used. Adults and older children should be immunized in the deltoid muscle, and infants and young children in the anterolateral aspect of the thigh.

Before injection, the skin over the site to be injected should be cleansed with a suitable germicide. After insertion of the needle, aspirate to help avoid inadvertent injection into a blood vessel.

Age Group	Dose	No. of Doses (See below for details)
6 to 35 months	0.25 mL	1 or 2 Doses
3 to 12 years	0.5 mL	1 or 2 Doses
13 years and older	0.5 mL	1 Dose

Two doses are recommended for children under 13 years of age who are receiving influenza vaccine for the first time. With the two-dose regimen, allow four weeks or more between doses.

It is recommended that only a subvirion vaccine, such as Influenza Virus Vaccine FLU-IMUNE, Types A and B (Surface Antigen), be administered to children under 13 years of age because of lower potential for causing febrile reactions.[1]

Simultaneous Administration with Other Vaccines: The target groups for influenza and pneumococcal vaccination overlap considerably. Both vaccines can be given at the same time at different sites without increasing side effects. However, influenza vaccine is given annually, *while it is currently recommended that, with few exceptions, pneumococcal vaccine be given only once.* Detailed immunization records should be provided to each patient to record the date when pneumococcal vaccine was administered.[1]

The American Academy of Pediatrics recommends that influenza vaccine should not be administered within 3 days of immunization with a pertussis-containing vaccine.[2]

HOW SUPPLIED

NDC 0005 2060-31 5.0 mL vial

STORAGE

DO NOT FREEZE. STORE REFRIGERATED, AWAY FROM FREEZER COMPARTMENT, AT 2°C to 8°C (36°F to 46°F).

REFERENCES

1. Recommendations of the Immunization Practices Advisory Committee (ACIP). Prevention and control of influenza: Part 1, Vaccines. *MMWR* 1989; 38(17) 297-311.
2. American Academy of Pediatrics: *Report of the Committee on Infectious Diseases*, ed. 21. Elk Grove Village, IL, American Academy of Pediatrics, 1988.
3. Schonberger, L, et al.: Guillain-Barre syndrome: Its epidemiology and associations with influenza vaccination. *Ann Neurol* 1981; 9 (Suppl. 31).
4. Hurwitz E, et al.: Guillain-Barre syndrome and the 1978-1979 influenza vaccine. *N Eng J Med* 1981; 304:1557-1561.
5. Kaplan J, et al.: Guillain-Barre syndrome in the United States, 1979-1980 and 1980-1981. Lack of association with influenza vaccination. *JAMA* 1982; 248:689-700.
6. Center for Disease Control: December 1986; Adverse events following immunization: Report No. 2, 1982-1984.
7. Retailliou H, et al.: Illness after influenza vaccination reported through a nation-wide surveillance system, 1976-1977. *Am J Epidemiol* 1980; 111:270-278.
†Triton® is a registered Trademark of Rohm & Haas Corp.

IMPORTANT INFORMATION FOR GROUP IMMUNIZATION PROGRAMS: If this vaccine is to be used in an immunization program sponsored by any organizations WHERE A TRADITIONAL PHYSICIAN/PATIENT RELATIONSHIP DOES NOT EXIST, each recipient (or legal guardian) must be made aware of the benefits and risks of immunization. These are summarized in the current labeling, and informed consent should be obtained from the recipient (or legal guardian) before immunization. PLEASE CONTACT YOUR LOCAL LEDERLE REPRESENTATIVE for copies of the CDC Important Information About Influenza and Influenza Consent Form.

*Trademark of Lederle Laboratories
Manufactured by:
EVANS MEDICAL LIMITED
Langhurst, Horsham
West Sussex RH12 4QD, England
and
LEDERLE LABORATORIES DIVISION
American Cyanamid Company
Pearl River, NY 10965

Rev. 6/89
22862

GEVRABON®

[jĕv-ra-bŏn]
Vitamin-Mineral Supplement

(See PDR For Nonprescription Drugs)

GEVRAL®

[jĕv-ral]
Multivitamin and Multimineral Supplement Tablets

(See PDR For Nonprescription Drugs)

GEVRAL® T

[jĕv-ral]
High Potency
Multivitamin and Multimineral Supplement Tablets

(See PDR For Nonprescription Drugs)

HYDROMOX®   ℞

[hū-drō-mŏx]
quinethazone
Tablets

DESCRIPTION

Chemistry: HYDROMOX is a quinazoline derivative, in which a cyclic carbamyl group replaces the cyclic sulfamyl group present in the thiazide derivatives.
Quinethazone is 7 - chloro - 2 - ethyl - 1, 2, 3, 4-tetrahydro-4-oxo-6-quinazolinesulfonamide.
HYDROMOX tablets contain the following inactive ingredients: Corn Starch, Dibasic Calcium Phosphate, Magnesium Stearate, Modified Food Starch.

ACTIONS

HYDROMOX produces urinary excretion of sodium and chloride in approximately equivalent amounts (saluresis), while potassium is excreted to a much lesser degree. The saluretic effect of HYDROMOX is rapid and relatively prolonged, beginning within 2 hours after administration,

reaching a peak at 6 hours, and lasting for 18 to 24 hours. While HYDROMOX is chemically different, it is pharmacologically genetic to the benzothiadiazine group of drugs. The dominant action of quinethazone is to increase the renal excretion of sodium and chloride and an accompanying volume of water. This results from inhibition of the tubular mechanism of electrolyte reabsorption. The renal effect is virtually independent of alterations in acid-base balance. HYDROMOX, like other drugs in this class, inhibits the proximal reabsorption of sodium and chloride. The excretion of potassium results from increased potassium secretion by the distal tubule where potassium is exchanged for sodium. HYDROMOX may exert its antihypertensive effect by diuresis and sodium loss and/or on vascular function to reduce peripheral resistance.

INDICATIONS

HYDROMOX, a nonmercurial oral diuretic agent, is indicated as adjunctive therapy in edema associated with congestive heart failure, hepatic cirrhosis and corticosteroid and estrogen therapy.
HYDROMOX has also been found useful in edema due to various forms of renal dysfunction such as: nephrotic syndrome; acute glomerulonephritis; and chronic renal failure.
HYDROMOX is indicated in the management of hypertension either as the sole therapeutic agent or to enhance the effectiveness of other antihypertensive drugs in the more severe forms of hypertension.
Usage in Pregnancy: The routine use of diuretics in an otherwise healthy woman is inappropriate and exposes mother and fetus to unnecessary hazard. Diuretics do not prevent development of toxemia of pregnancy, and there is no satisfactory evidence that they are useful in the treatment of developed toxemia.
Edema during pregnancy may arise from pathological causes or from the physiologic and mechanical consequences of pregnancy. Diuretics are indicated in pregnancy when edema is due to pathologic causes, just as they are in the absence of pregnancy (however, see **WARNINGS**, below). Dependent edema in pregnancy, resulting from restriction of venous return by the expanded uterus, is properly treated through elevation of the lower extremities and use of support hose; use of diuretics to lower intravascular volume in this case is illogical and unnecessary. There is hypervolemia during normal pregnancy which is harmful to neither the fetus nor the mother (in the absence of cardiovascular disease), but which is associated with edema, including generalized edema, in the majority of pregnant women. If this edema produces discomfort, increased recumbency will often provide relief. In rare instances, this edema may cause extreme discomfort which is not relieved by rest. In these cases, a short course of diuretics may provide relief and may be appropriate.

CONTRAINDICATIONS

A. Anuria.
B. Hypersensitivity to this or other sulfonamide derived drugs.

WARNINGS

Diuretics should be used with caution in severe renal disease. In patients with renal disease, diuretics may precipitate azotemia. Cumulative effects of the drug may develop in patients with impaired renal function.
Diuretics should be used with caution in patients with impaired hepatic function or progressive liver disease, since minor alterations of fluid and electrolyte balance may precipitate hepatic coma.
Quinethazone may add to or potentiate the action of other antihypertensive drugs. Potentiation occurs with ganglionic or peripheral adrenergic blocking drugs.
Sensitivity reactions may occur in patients with a history of allergy or bronchial asthma.
The possibility of exacerbation or activation of systemic lupus erythematosus has been reported.
Usage in Pregnancy: HYDROMOX *quinethazone* crosses the placental barrier and appears in cord blood. The use of quinethazone in pregnant women requires that the anticipated benefit be weighed against possible hazards to the fetus. These hazards include fetal or neonatal jaundice, thrombocytopenia, and possible other adverse reactions which have occurred in the adult.
Nursing Mothers: HYDROMOX appears in breast milk. If use of the drug is deemed essential, the patient should stop nursing.

PRECAUTIONS

(1) HYDROMOX should be used with caution in patients with impaired hepatic function or progressive liver disease, since minor alterations of fluid and electrolyte balance may precipitate hepatic coma.
(2) Whereas electrolyte abnormalities are often present in such conditions as heart failure and cirrhosis as a result of underlying disease process, they may also be aggravated or may be produced independently by any potent diuretic affecting electrolyte excretion. Caution is especially important during prolonged or intensive therapy and when salt intake is restricted or during concomitant use of steroids or ACTH.

Hypokalemia attributable to HYDROMOX therapy has been mild and infrequent, and other electrolyte abnormalities have been rare.
The possibility of potassium depletion and its toxic sequelae must be kept in mind, particularly in cirrhotics and patients receiving digitalis. As a preventive measure the use of foods rich in potassium, such as orange juice, or supplements of potassium chloride may be desirable.
(3) In patients with impaired renal function, azotemia and-/or excessive drug accumulation may develop.
(4) As with other potent diuretics, when HYDROMOX is added to a regimen that includes ganglionic-blocking agents, the dosage of these latter preparations should be reduced to avoid a sudden drop in blood pressure. Reduction of dosage is also necessary when one or more of these antihypertensive agents is added to an established HYDROMOX regimen.
(5) As with the thiazide diuretics, increases of serum uric acid may occur but precipitation of gout has been rare.
(6) A decreased glucose tolerance as evidenced by hyperglycemia and glycosuria thus aggravating or provoking diabetes mellitus has occurred.
(7) HYDROMOX *quinethazone* may decrease arterial responsiveness to norepinephrine and therefore should be withdrawn 48 hours before elective surgery. If emergency surgery is indicated, preanesthetic and anesthetic agents should be administered in reduced dosage. Quinethazone may also increase the responsiveness to tubocurarine. The antihypertensive effects of the drug may be enhanced in the postsympathectomy patient.
(8) Sensitivity reactions may be more likely to occur in patients with a history of allergy or bronchial asthma.
(9) The possibility of exacerbation or activation of systemic lupus erythematosus has been suggested for sulfonamide derived drugs.

ADVERSE REACTIONS

The following adverse reactions have been reported with the diuretic drugs, some of which may be expected to occur with quinethazone:
A. *Gastrointestinal System Reactions:* 1. anorexia, 2. gastric irritation, 3. nausea, 4. vomiting, 5. cramping, 6. diarrhea, 7. constipation, 8. jaundice (intrahepatic cholestatic jaundice), 9. pancreatitis, 10. hyperglycemia, 11. glycosuria.
B. *Central Nervous System Reactions:* 1. dizziness, 2. vertigo, 3. paresthesias, 4. headache, 5. xanthopsia.
C. *Hematologic Reactions:* 1. leukopenia, 2. thrombocytopenia, 3. agranulocytosis, 4. aplastic anemia.
D. *Dermatologic—Hypersensitivity Reactions:* 1. purpura, 2. photosensitivity, 3. rash, 4. urticaria, 5. necrotizing angiitis (vasculitis) (cutaneous vasculitis).
E. *Cardiovascular Reactions:* 1. orthostatic hypotension may occur and may be potentiated by alcohol, barbiturates or narcotics.
F. *Miscellaneous:* 1. muscle spasm, 2. weakness, 3. restlessness.
Whenever adverse reactions are moderate or severe, thiazide dosage should be reduced or therapy withdrawn.

DOSAGE AND ADMINISTRATION

Average Adult Dosage: One or two 50 mg tablets, orally, once a day. Because of its relatively prolonged duration of activity, a single daily dose is generally sufficient. Occasionally, 1 tablet (50 mg) is administered twice a day. Infrequently, a total daily dose of 3 to 4 tablets (150 to 200 mg) may be necessary. The dosage employed depends upon the severity of the condition being treated and the responsiveness of the patient, and often must be adjusted at the beginning or during the course of therapy. When HYDROMOX is used in combination with other antihypertensive agents, the dosage of each drug may often be reduced because of potentiation. (See under **PRECAUTIONS** concerning the necessity for dosage adjustment when one or more of these drugs is added to an already established therapeutic regime.)

HOW SUPPLIED

HYDROMOX *quinethazone* Tablets, are round, white, flat-faced, scored, beveled, engraved with H above and 1 below the score on one side and LL on the other side, supplied as follows:
NDC 0005-4458-23—Bottle of 100
Store at Controlled Room Temperature 15–30° C (59–86° F).
LEDERLE LABORATORIES DIVISION
American Cyanamid Company
Pearl River, N.Y. 10965   Rev. 12/85
17404

Shown in Product Identification Section, page 414

Continued on next page

Lederle—Cont.

HYDROMOX® R ℞
[hī-drō-mŏx]
Quinethazone-Reserpine
TABLETS

WARNINGS

> This fixed combination drug is not indicated for initial therapy of hypertension. Hypertension requires therapy titrated to the individual patient. If the fixed combination represents the dosage so determined, its use may be more convenient in patient management. The treatment of hypertension is not static, but must be reevaluated as conditions in each patient warrant.

DESCRIPTION

HYDROMOX R tablets each contain 50 mg quinethazone and 0.125 mg reserpine. Quinethazone is a nonmercurial oral diuretic agent, effective in the treatment of edema and hypertension. It is chemically distinct from the benzothiadiazine series of compounds. Reserpine, an antihypertensive agent, has been combined with quinethazone in a dosage form designed to be useful in the treatment of hypertension with or without edema.

Chemistry: Quinethazone is a quinazoline derivative, in which a carbamyl group replaces the cyclic sulfamyl group present in the thiazide derivatives.
Quinethazone has the following chemical name: 7-Chloro-2-ethyl-1,2,3,4-tetrahydro-4-oxo-6-quinazoline-sulfonamide. Reserpine has the following chemical name: 3β, 16β, 17α, 18β, 20α)-11,17-Dimethoxy-18-[(3,4,5-trimethoxybenzoyl) oxy]-yohimban-16-carboxylic acid methyl ester.
HYDROMOX R also contains the following inactive ingredients: Corn Starch, Dibasic Calcium Phosphate, Magnesium Stearate, Methylcellulose, Yellow 10.

ACTIONS

HYDROMOX produces urinary excretion of sodium and chloride in approximately equivalent amounts (saluresis), while potassium is excreted to a much lesser degree. The saluretic effect of HYDROMOX is rapid and relatively prolonged, beginning within two hours after administration, reaching a peak at six hours, and lasting for 18 to 24 hours. While quinethazone is chemically different from the benzothiadiazine group of drugs, its pharmacologic effects are similar to those elicited by benzothiadiazine derivatives.
The dominant action of quinethazone is to increase the renal excretion of sodium and chloride and an accompanying volume of water. This results from inhibition of the tubular mechanism of electrolyte reabsorption. The renal effect is virtually independent of alterations in acid-base balance. Quinethazone, like other drugs in its class, inhibits the proximal reabsorption of sodium and chloride. The excretion of potassium results from increased potassium secretion by the distal tubule where potassium is exchanged for sodium.
Quinethazone may exert its antihypertensive effect by diuresis and sodium loss and/or on vascular function to reduce peripheral resistance.
Reserpine is an antihypertensive agent which produces a mild type of sedation that is tranquilizing rather than hypnotic. The most prominent actions of reserpine are upon the cardiovascular and central nervous systems. In clinical hypertension, reserpine produces a gradual and moderate fall in both systolic and diastolic blood pressures after oral administration for several days to 2-3 weeks. Its effects persist about 3-4 weeks after medication is withdrawn. With an increase in dose, a prolongation of hypotensive effect, rather than an intensification of blood pressure fall, tends to occur. The doses employed in the therapy of hypertension are smaller than those used in psychiatric disorders.
The dosage form combining quinethazone with reserpine is designed to provide effective antihypertensive action in patients who have failed to show satisfactory response to the use of quinethazone or reserpine alone. This combination of quinethazone and reserpine frequently permits use of a lower dosage of each agent and hence tends to produce the desired antihypertensive effect while eliminating, or at least minimizing, adverse reactions. Blood pressure reductions averaging about –30/–15 have been demonstrated within the first 2 weeks of treatment. Continuation of therapy beyond 2 weeks may be expected to produce further *small* drops in blood pressure. The enhanced reduction in blood pressure produced by quinethazone with reserpine appears to be an additive rather than a potentiating effect.

INDICATIONS

HYDROMOX R *quinethazone-reserpine* is indicated in the management of hypertension (see box **WARNINGS**) either as the sole therapeutic agent or to enhance the effectiveness of other antihypertensive drugs in the more severe forms of hypertension.
Usage in Pregnancy: The routine use of diuretics in an otherwise healthy woman is inappropriate and exposes mother and fetus to unnecessary hazard. Diuretics do not prevent development of toxemia of pregnancy, and there is no satisfactory evidence that they are useful in the treatment of developed toxemia.
Edema during pregnancy may arise from pathological causes or from the physiologic and mechanical consequences of pregnancy. Diuretics are indicated in pregnancy when edema is due to pathologic causes, just as they are in the absence of pregnancy (however, see **WARNINGS**, below). Dependent edema in pregnancy, resulting from restriction of venous return by the expanded uterus, is properly treated through elevation of the lower extremities and use of support hose; use of diuretics to lower intravascular volume in this case is illogical and unnecessary. There is hypervolemia during normal pregnancy which is harmful to neither the fetus nor the mother (in the absence of cardiovascular disease), but which is associated with edema, including generalized edema, in the majority of pregnant women. If this edema produces discomfort, increased recumbency will often provide relief. In rare instances, this edema may cause extreme discomfort which is not relieved by rest. In these cases, a short course of diuretics may provide relief and may be appropriate.

CONTRAINDICATIONS

A. Anuria.
B. Hypersensitivity to this or other sulfonamide-derived drugs.
C. Progressively impaired renal function. Since reserpine may increase gastric secretion and motility, its use alone or in combination requires caution and is sometimes contraindicated in patients with a history of peptic or duodenal ulcer or other gastrointestinal disorders.
D. HYDROMOX R *quinethazone-reserpine* should not be administered to patients with severe hepatic dysfunction. The use of the drug should be avoided in patients with a history of mental depression or psychosis. HYDROMOX R should not be used by patients who are known to be hypersensitive to either agent.
E. History of mental depression.

WARNINGS

Diuretics should be used with caution in severe renal disease. In patients with renal disease, diuretics may precipitate azotemia.
Cumulative effects of the drug may develop in patients with impaired renal function.
Diuretics should be used with caution in patients with impaired hepatic function or progressive liver disease, since minor alterations of fluid and electrolyte balance may precipitate hepatic coma.
HYDROMOX R may add to or potentiate the action of other antihypertensive drugs. Potentiation occurs with ganglionic or peripheral adrenergic blocking drugs.
Sensitivity reactions may occur in patients with a history of allergy or bronchial asthma.
The possibility of exacerbation or activation of systemic lupus erythematosus has been reported with sulfonamide-derived drugs.
Reserpine may cause mental depression. Recognition of depression may be difficult because this condition may often be disguised by somatic complaints (Masked Depression). The drug should be discontinued at first signs of depression such as despondency, early morning insomnia, loss of appetite, impotence, or self-deprecation. Drug-induced depression may persist for several months after drug withdrawal and may be severe enough to result in suicide.
Usage in Pregnancy: HYDROMOX R crosses the placental barrier and appears in cord blood. The use of HYDROMOX R in pregnant women requires that the anticipated benefit be weighed against possible hazards to the fetus. These hazards include fetal or neonatal jaundice, thrombocytopenia, and possibly other adverse reactions which have occurred in the adult.
Nursing Mothers: HYDROMOX R appears in breast milk. If use of the drug is deemed essential, the patient should stop nursing.
Reserpine has been reported to cause central nervous system depression of the newborn infant when given to the mother in the immediate antepartum period.
HYDROMOX R should be discontinued promptly if any symptoms of mental depression occur with the use of the drug.

PRECAUTIONS

Quinethazone:
(1) Quinethazone should be used with caution in patients with impaired hepatic function or progressive liver disease, since minor alterations of fluid and electrolyte balance may precipitate hepatic coma.
(2) Whereas electrolyte abnormalities are often present in such conditions as heart failure and cirrhosis as a result of underlying disease process, they may also be aggravated or may be produced independently by any potent diuretic affecting electrolyte excretion. Caution is especially important during prolonged or intensive therapy and when salt intake is restricted or during concomitant use of steroids or ACTH. Hypokalemia attributable to HYDROMOX *quinethazone* therapy has been mild and infrequent, and other electrolyte abnormalities have been rare.
The possibility of potassium depletion and its toxic sequelae must be kept in mind, particularly in cirrhotics and patients receiving digitalis. As a preventive measure the use of foods rich in potassium, such as orange juice, or supplements of potassium chloride may be desirable.
(3) In patients with impaired renal function, azotemia and/or excessive drug accumulation may develop.
(4) As with other potent diuretics, when HYDROMOX is added to a regimen that includes ganglionic-blocking agents, the dosage of these latter preparations should be reduced to avoid a sudden drop in blood pressure. Reduction of dosage is also necessary when one or more of these antihypertensive agents is added to an established HYDROMOX regimen.
(5) As with the thiazide diuretics, increases of serum uric acid may occur but precipitation of gout has been rare.
(6) A decreased glucose tolerance as evidenced by hyperglycemia and glycosuria thus aggravating or provoking diabetes mellitus has occurred.
(7) Quinethazone may decrease arterial responsiveness to norepinephrine and therefore should be withdrawn 48 hours before elective surgery. If emergency surgery is indicated, preanesthetic and anesthetic agents should be administered in reduced dosage. Quinethazone may also increase the responsiveness to tubocurarine. The antihypertensive effects of the drug may be enhanced in the post-sympathectomy patient.
(8) Sensitivity reactions may be more likely to occur in patients with a history of allergy or bronchial asthma.
(9) The possibility of exacerbation or activation of systemic lupus erythematosus has been suggested for sulfonamide-derived drugs.
Reserpine: Reserpine may precipitate biliary colic in patients with gallstones, or bronchial asthma in susceptible patients. Reserpine preparations should be used with caution in patients with a history of peptic ulcer, ulcerative colitis, and other gastrointestinal disorders. It may cause severe depression and suicidal risk and may produce pseudoparkinsonism (a paralysis agitans-like syndrome).
Administration of reserpine should be discontinued 2 weeks or more before electroconvulsant therapy if possible to preclude severe, even fatal, reactions.
Reserpine may cause cardiotoxic effects, eg, premature ventricular contractions and other arrhythmias, possible sensitization to digitalis (which might be further complicated by any hypokalemic effects of quinethazone), fluid retention, and congestive failure.
Animal tumorigenicity: Rodent studies have shown that reserpine is an animal tumorigen, causing an increased incidence of mammary fibroadenomas in female mice, malignant tumors of the seminal vesicles in male mice, and malignant adrenal medullary tumors in male rats. These findings arose in 2-year studies in which the drug was administered in the feed at concentrations of 5 and 10 ppm—about 100 to 300 times the usual human dose. The breast neoplasms are thought to be related to reserpine's prolactin-elevating effect. Several other prolactin-elevating drugs have also been associated with an increased incidence of mammary neoplasia in rodents.
The extent to which these findings indicate a risk to humans is uncertain. Tissue culture experiments show that about one-third of human breast tumors are prolactin-dependent *in vitro*, a factor of considerable importance if the use of the drug is contemplated in a patient with previously detected breast cancer. The possibility of an increased risk of breast cancer in reserpine users has been studied extensively; however, no firm conclusion has emerged. Although a few epidemiologic studies have suggested a slightly increased risk (less than twofold in all studies except one) in women who have used reserpine, other studies of generally similar design have not confirmed this. Epidemiologic studies conducted using other drugs (neuroleptic agents) that, like reserpine, increase prolactin levels, and therefore would be considered rodent mammary carcinogens, have not shown an association between chronic administration of the drug and human mammary tumorigenesis. While long-term clinical observation has not suggested such an association, the available evidence is considered too limited to be conclusive at this time. An association of reserpine intake with pheochromocytoma or tumors of the seminal vesicles has not been explored.

ADVERSE REACTIONS

The following adverse reactions have been reported with the diuretic drugs some of which may be expected to occur with quinethazone:

A. Gastrointestinal System Reactions
1. anorexia
2. gastric irritation
3. nausea
4. vomiting
5. cramping
6. diarrhea
7. constipation
8. jaundice (intrahepatic cholestatic jaundice)
9. pancreatitis
10. hyperglycemia
11. glycosuria
B. Central Nervous System Reactions
1. dizziness
2. vertigo
3. paresthesias
4. headache
5. xanthopsia
C. Hematologic Reactions
1. leukopenia
2. thrombocytopenia
3. agranulocytosis
4. aplastic anemia
D. Dermatologic—Hypersensitivity Reactions
1. purpura
2. photosensitivity
3. rash
4. urticaria
5. necrotizing angiitis (vasculitis) (cutaneous vasculitis)
E. Cardiovascular Reactions
1. orthostatic hypotension may occur and may be potentiated by alcohol, barbiturates, or narcotics
F. Miscellaneous
1. muscle spasm
2. weakness
3. restlessness

Reserpine:
With reserpine, nasal congestion, weight gain, and diarrhea are the most frequently noted side effects. The drug may reactivate old peptic ulcers because it increases hydrochloric acid secretion by the stomach. More serious reactions are excessive drowsiness, fatigue, weakness, insomnia, nightmares, excitement, irrational behavior, and incipient parkinsonism. Sodium retention edema may occur when reserpine is used.
Whenever adverse reactions are moderate or severe, thiazide dosage should be reduced or therapy withdrawn.

DOSAGE AND ADMINISTRATION
Dosage: As determined by individual titration (see boxed **WARNINGS**).
Average (or Maintenance) Adult Dosage: 1 to 2 HYDROMOX R tablets (50 mg quinethazone with 0.125 mg reserpine to 100 mg quinethazone with 0.25 mg reserpine) administered orally, once a day.
Because of the relatively prolonged effect of HYDROMOX R, a single daily dose is usually sufficient. Occasionally 1 tablet is administered twice a day but ordinarily medication is administered only in the morning to avoid the inconvenience of nocturia.
For doses of quinethazone greater than 100 mg, the combination product is not appropriate because its use would lead to an excessive dose of reserpine.
When HYDROMOX R tablets are used in combination with other antihypertensive drugs, the dosage of each drug may often be reduced because of potentiation. (See under **PRECAUTIONS** concerning the necessity for dosage adjustment when one or more of these drugs is added to an already established therapeutic regimen.)

HOW SUPPLIED
HYDROMOX R *quinethazone-reserpine* tablets, each containing 50 mg quinethazone and 0.125 mg reserpine, are round, yellow, scored tablets, engraved with LL on one side and H above and 2 below the score on the other side, supplied as follows:
NDC 0005-4457-23—Bottle of 100
Store at Controlled Room Temperature 15–30° C (59–86° F).
LEDERLE LABORATORIES DIVISION
American Cyanamid Company,
Pearl River, N.Y. 10965
         Rev. 7/88
            23569
Shown in Product Identification Section, page 414

INCREMIN®
[*ĭn-cre-mĭn*]
WITH IRON SYRUP
(Vitamins B_1, B_6, B_{12}-Lysine-Iron)
Dietary Supplement
For the prevention of iron deficiency anemia in children and adults.

(See PDR For Nonprescription Drugs)

LEDERPLEX®
[*lĕder-plĕx*]
Dietary Supplement of B-Complex Vitamins
Capsules—Liquid

(See PDR For Nonprescription Drugs)

LEUCOVORIN CALCIUM INJECTION ℞
LEUCOVORIN CALCIUM FOR INJECTION ℞
[*lu-cō-vor-ĭn căl-sēē-um*]

DESCRIPTION
Leucovorin is one of several active, chemically reduced derivatives of folic acid. It is useful as an antidote to drugs which act as folic acid antagonists. Also known as folinic acid, Citrovorum factor, or 5-formyl-5,6,7,8-tetrahydrofolic acid, this compound has the chemical designation of L-Glutamic acid, N-[4-[[(2-amino-5-formyl-1, 4, 5, 6, 7, 8-hexahydro-4-oxo-6-pteridinyl)-methyl]amino]benzoyl]-, calcium salt (1:1). The formula weight is 511.51.
Leucovorin Calcium Injection: Leucovorin Calcium Injection is indicated for intravenous or intramuscular administration and is supplied as a sterile solution in 1 mL ampules. Each ampule contains 3 mg of leucovorin with benzyl alcohol 0.9% w/v as a preservative. The inactive ingredient is sodium chloride 0.56% w/v. Sodium hydroxide and/or hydrochloric acid are used to adjust the pH to approximately 7.7 during manufacture. There is 0.004 mEq of calcium per mg of leucovorin.
Leucovorin Calcium for Injection: Leucovorin Calcium for Injection is indicated for intravenous or intramuscular administration and is supplied as a sterile cryodesiccated powder. The 50, 100, and 350 mg vials are preservative free. The inactive ingredient is sodium chloride 40 mg/vial for the 50 mg vial, 80 mg/vial for the 100 mg vial, and 140 mg/vial for the 350 mg vial. Sodium hydroxide and/or hydrochloric acid are used to adjust the pH to approximately 8.1 during manufacture. There is 0.004 mEq of calcium per mg of leucovorin in each dosage form.

CLINICAL PHARMACOLOGY
Leucovorin is a mixture of the diastereoisomers of the 5-formyl derivative of tetrahydrofolic acid. The biologically active compound of the mixture is the (-)-L-isomer, known as Citrovorum factor or (-)-folinic acid. Leucovorin does not require reduction by the enzyme dihydrofolate reductase in order to participate in reactions utilizing folates as a source of "one-carbon" moieties. Following oral administration, leucovorin is rapidly absorbed and enters the general body pool of reduced folates.
The pharmacokinetics after intravenous, intramuscular, and oral administration of a 25 mg dose of leucovorin were studied in male volunteers. After intravenous administration, serum total reduced folates (as measured by *Lactobacillus casei* assay) reached a mean peak of 1259 ng/mL (range 897–1625). The mean time to peak was 10 minutes. This initial rise in total reduced folates was primarily due to the parent compound 5-formyl-THF (measured by *Streptococcus faecalis* assay) which rose to 1206 ng/mL at 10 minutes. A sharp drop in parent compound followed and coincided with the appearance of the metabolite (also active) 5-methyl-THF which became the predominant circulating form of the drug. The mean peak of 5-methyl-THF was 258 ng/mL and occurred at 1.3 hours. The terminal half-life for total reduced folates was 6.2 hours.
After intramuscular injection, the mean peak of serum total reduced folates was 436 ng/mL (range 240–725) and occurred at 52 minutes. Similar to IV administration, the initial sharp rise was due to the parent compound. The mean peak of 5-formyl-THF was 360 ng/mL and occurred at 28 minutes. The level of the metabolite 5-methyl-THF increased subsequently over time until at 1.5 hours it represented 50% of the circulating total folates. The mean peak of 5-methyl-THF was 226 ng/mL at 2.8 hours. The terminal half-life of total reduced folates was 6.2 hours. There was no difference of statistical significance between IM and IV administration in the AUC for total reduced folates, 5-formyl-THF, or 5-methyl-THF.

INDICATIONS AND USAGE
Leucovorin Calcium rescue is indicated after high-dose methotrexate therapy in osteosarcoma. Leucovorin Calcium is also indicated to diminish the toxicity and counteract the effects of impaired methotrexate elimination and of inadvertent overdosages of folic acid antagonists. Leucovorin Calcium Injection is indicated in the treatment of megaloblastic anemias due to folic acid deficiency when oral therapy is not feasible.

CONTRAINDICATIONS
Leucovorin is improper therapy for pernicious anemia and other megaloblastic anemias secondary to the lack of vitamin B_{12}. A hematologic remission may occur while neurologic manifestations continue to progress.

WARNINGS
In the treatment of accidental overdosages of folic acid antagonists, leucovorin should be administered as promptly as possible. As the time interval between antifolate administration [eg, methotrexate (MTX)] and leucovorin rescue increases, leucovorin's effectiveness in counteracting toxicity decreases.
Monitoring of the serum MTX concentration is essential in determining the optimal dose and duration of treatment with leucovorin.
Delayed MTX excretion may be caused by a third space fluid accumulation (ie, ascites, pleural effusion), renal insufficiency, or inadequate hydration. Under such circumstances, higher doses of leucovorin or prolonged administration may be indicated. Doses higher than those recommended for oral use must be given intravenously.
Because of the benzyl alcohol contained in the 1 mL ampule and in the recommended diluent for Leucovorin Calcium for Injection, doses greater than 10 mg/m² of either formulation are not recommended. If greater doses are required (see **DOSAGE AND ADMINISTRATION**), Leucovorin Calcium for Injection should be reconstituted with Sterile Water for Injection, USP, and used immediately.
Because of the Ca^{++} content of the leucovorin solution, no more than 16 mL (160 mg of leucovorin) should be injected intravenously per minute.
Leucovorin may enhance the toxicity of fluorouracil. Deaths from severe enterocolitis, diarrhea, and dehydration have been reported in elderly patients receiving leucovorin and fluorouracil.[1] Concomitant granulocytopenia and fever were present in some but not all of the patients.

PRECAUTIONS
General: Parenteral administration is preferable to oral dosing if there is a possibility that the patient may vomit or not absorb the leucovorin. Leucovorin has no effect on other established toxicities of MTX such as the nephrotoxicity resulting from drug and/or metabolite precipitation in the kidney.
Drug Interactions: Folic acid in large amounts may counteract the antiepileptic effect of phenobarbital, phenytoin, and primidone, and increase the frequency of seizures in susceptible children.
Preliminary animal and human studies have shown that small quantities of systemically administered leucovorin enter the CSF primarily as 5-methyltetrahydrofolate and, in humans, remain 1–3 orders of magnitude lower than the usual methotrexate concentrations following intrathecal administration. However, high doses of leucovorin may reduce the efficacy of intrathecally administered methotrexate.
Leucovorin may enhance the toxicity of fluorouracil (see **WARNINGS**).
Pregnancy: Teratogenic Effects: *Pregnancy Category C.* Animal reproduction studies have not been conducted with leucovorin. It is also not known whether leucovorin can cause fetal harm when administered to a pregnant woman or can affect reproduction capacity. Leucovorin should be given to a pregnant woman only if clearly needed.
Nursing Mothers: It is not known whether this drug is excreted in human milk. Because many drugs are excreted in human milk, caution should be exercised when leucovorin is administered to a nursing mother.
Pediatric Use: See **Drug Interactions.**

ADVERSE REACTIONS
Allergic sensitization has been reported following both oral and parenteral administration of folic acid.

OVERDOSAGE
Excessive amounts of leucovorin may nullify the chemotherapeutic effect of folic acid antagonists.

DOSAGE AND ADMINISTRATION
Leucovorin Rescue After High-Dose Methotrexate Therapy: The recommendations for leucovorin rescue are based on a methotrexate dose of 12–15 grams/m² administered by intravenous infusion over 4 hours (see methotrexate package insert for full Prescribing Information).[2] Leucovorin rescue at a dose of 15 mg (approximately 10 mg/m²) every 6 hours for 10 doses starts 24 hours after the beginning of the methotrexate infusion. In the presence of gastrointestinal toxicity, nausea or vomiting, leucovorin should be administered parenterally.
Serum creatinine and methotrexate levels should be determined at least once daily. Leucovorin administration, hydration, and urinary alkalinization (pH of 7.0 or greater) should

Continued on next page

Lederle—Cont.

be continued until the methotrexate level is below 5×10^{-8}M (0.05 micromolar). The leucovorin dose should be adjusted or leucovorin rescue extended based on the following guidelines:

[See table below].

Patients who experience delayed early methotrexate elimination are likely to develop reversible renal failure. In addition to appropriate leucovorin therapy, these patients require continuing hydration and urinary alkalinization, and close monitoring of fluid and electrolyte status, until the serum methotrexate level has fallen to below 0.05 micromolar and the renal failure has resolved.

Some patients will have abnormalities in methotrexate elimination or renal function following methotrexate administration, which are significant but less severe than the abnormalities described in the table above. These abnormalities may or may not be associated with significant clinical toxicity. If significant clinical toxicity is observed, leucovorin rescue should be extended for an additional 24 hours (total of 14 doses over 84 hours) in subsequent courses of therapy. The possibility that the patient is taking other medications which interact with methotrexate (eg, medications which may interfere with methotrexate elimination or binding to serum albumin) should always be reconsidered when laboratory abnormalities or clinical toxicities are observed.

Impaired Methotrexate Elimination or Inadvertent Overdosage: Leucovorin rescue should begin as soon as possible after an inadvertent overdosage and within 24 hours of methotrexate administration when there is delayed excretion (see **WARNINGS**). Leucovorin 10 mg/m^2 should be administered IV, IM, or PO every 6 hours until the serum methotrexate level is less than 10^{-8} M. In the presence of gastrointestinal toxicity, nausea, or vomiting, leucovorin should be administered parenterally.

Serum creatinine and methotrexate levels should be determined at 24-hour intervals. If the 24-hour serum creatinine has increased 50% over baseline or if the 24-hour methotrexate level is greater than 5×10^{-6} M or the 48-hour level is greater than 9×10^{-7} M, the dose of leucovorin should be increased to 100 mg/m^2 IV every 3 hours until the methotrexate level is less than 10^{-8} M.

Hydration (3 L/d) and urinary alkalinization with NaHCO$_3$ should be employed concomitantly. The bicarbonate dose should be adjusted to maintain the urine pH at 7.0 or greater.

Megaloblastic Anemia Due to Folic Acid Deficiency: Up to 1 mg daily. There is no evidence that doses greater than 1 mg/day have greater efficacy than those of 1 mg; additionally, loss of folate in urine becomes roughly logarithmic as the amount administered exceeds 1 mg. Each 1 mL ampule of Leucovorin Calcium Injection contains 3 mg of leucovorin with benzyl alcohol 0.9% w/v as a preservative.

Each 50 and 100 mg vial of Leucovorin Calcium for Injection when reconstituted with 5 and 10 mL, respectively, of sterile diluent yields a leucovorin concentration of 10 mg per mL. Each 350 mg vial of Leucovorin Calcium for Injection when reconstituted with 17 mL of sterile diluent yields a leucovorin concentration of 20 mg leucovorin per mL. Contains no preservative. Reconstitute with Bacteriostatic Water for Injection, USP, which contains benzyl alcohol, or with Sterile Water for Injection, USP. When reconstituted with Bacteriostatic Water for Injection, USP, the resulting solution must be used within seven days. If the product is reconstituted with Sterile Water for Injection, USP, it must be used immediately.

Because of the benzyl alcohol contained in the 1 mL ampule and in Bacteriostatic Water for Injection, USP, doses greater than 10 mg/m^2 of either formulation are not recommended. If greater doses are required, Leucovorin Calcium for Injection should be reconstituted with Sterile Water for Injection, USP, and used immediately. Because of the Ca^{++} content of the leucovorin solution, no more than 16 mL (160 mg of leucovorin) should be injected intravenously per minute. Parenteral drug products should be inspected visually for particulate matter and discoloration prior to administration, whenever solution and container permit.

HOW SUPPLIED

Leucovorin Calcium Injection
Product Number NDC 0205-4004-51—6–1 mL (3 mg/mL) ampules
Store at Controlled Room Temperature 15°–30°C (59°–86°F). Protect From Light.

Leucovorin Calcium for Injection
Product Number NDC 0205-5330-92—50 mg vial of cryodesiccated powder
Product Number NDC 0205-5330-19—50 mg vial of cryodesiccated powder—box of 25
Product Number NDC 0205-4646-94—100 mg vial of cryodesiccated powder
Product Number NDC 0205-4645-77—350 mg vial of cryodesiccated powder

Military and VA Depots:
Product Number NSN 6505-01-054-7008—50 mg vial for IM use
Store at Controlled Room Temperature 15°–30°C (59°–86°F). Protect From Light.

REFERENCES
1. Grem JL, Shoemaker DD, Petrelli NJ, Douglas HO: "Severe and Fatal Toxic Effects Observed in Treatment with High- and Low-Dose Leucovorin Plus 5-Fluorouracil for Colorectal Carcinoma."*Cancer Treat Rep* 71:1122, 1987.
2. Link MP, Goorin AH, Miser AW, et al: "The Effect of Adjuvant Chemotherapy on Relapse-Free Survival in Patients with Osteosarcoma of the Extremity."*N Engl J Med* 314:1600–1606, 1986.

LEDERLE PHARMACEUTICALS, INC.
Carolina, Puerto Rico 00630

Rev. 7/89
25602

Shown in Product Identification Section, page 414

LEUCOVORIN CALCIUM TABLETS   ℞
[lu-có-vor-ĭn căl-sēē-um]

DESCRIPTION
Leucovorin is one of several active, chemically reduced derivatives of folic acid. It is useful as an antidote to drugs which act as folic acid antagonists. Also known as folinic acid, Citrovorum factor, or 5-formyl-5,6,7,8-tetrahydrofolic acid, this compound has the chemical designation of L-Glutamic acid, N-[4-[[(2-amino-5-formyl-1,4,5,6,7,8-hexahydro-4-oxo-6=pteridinyl)methyl] amino] benzoyl]-, calcium salt (1:1). The formula weight is 511.51.

Leucovorin Calcium Tablets, 5 mg, contain 5 mg of leucovorin (equivalent to 5.40 mg of anhydrous leucovorin calcium) and the following inactive ingredients: Corn Starch, Dibasic Calcium Phosphate, Magnesium Stearate, and Pregelatinized Starch.

Leucovorin Calcium Tablets, 10 mg, contain 10 mg of leucovorin (equivalent to 10.80 mg of anhydrous leucovorin calcium) and the following inactive ingredients: Lactose, Magnesium Stearate, Microcrystalline Cellulose, Pregelatinized Starch, and Sodium Starch Glycolate.

Leucovorin Calcium Tablets, 15 mg, contain 15 mg of leucovorin (equivalent to 16.20 mg of anhydrous leucovorin calcium) and the following inactive ingredients: Lactose, Magnesium Stearate, Microcrystalline Cellulose, Pregelatinized Starch, and Sodium Starch Glycolate.

Leucovorin Calcium Tablets are indicated for oral administration only.

CLINICAL PHARMACOLOGY
Leucovorin is a mixture of the diastereoisomers of the 5-formyl derivative of tetrahydrofolic acid. The biologically active component of the mixture is the (-)-L-isomer, known as Citrovorum factor, or (-)-folinic acid. Leucovorin does not require reduction by the enzyme dihydrofolate reductase in order to participate in reactions utilizing folates as a source of "one-carbon" moieties. Following oral administration, leucovorin is rapidly absorbed and enters the general body pool of reduced folates.

The increase in plasma and serum reduced folate activity (determined microbiologically with *Lactobacillus casei*) seen after oral administration of leucovorin is predominantly due to 5-methyltetrahydrofolate.

Following a 20 mg dose of leucovorin calcium, the mean maximum serum total reduced folate concentrations were:
Tablet   364±12.1 ng/mL at 2.0±0.07 hours
Oral Solution   375±12.8 ng/mL at 2.1±0.11 hours
Parenteral   355±17.2 ng/mL at 0.96±0.10 hours
The half-life of plasma 5-formyltetrahydrofolate was 1.5±0.08 hours and that of the 5-methyltetrahydrofolate was 3.0±0.09 hours.

Oral tablets produced equivalent bioavailability (8% difference) when compared to the parenteral administration. The parenteral solution also provided equal bioavailability to the tablets when administered orally (2% difference). Oral absorption of leucovorin is saturable at doses above 25 mg. The apparent bioavailability of leucovorin was 97% for 25 mg, 75% for 50 mg, and 37% for 100 mg.

INDICATIONS
Leucovorin calcium rescue is indicated after high-dose methotrexate therapy in osteosarcoma. Leucovorin is also indicated to diminish the toxicity and counteract the effects of impaired methotrexate elimination and of inadvertent overdosages of folic acid antagonists.

CONTRAINDICATIONS
Leucovorin is improper therapy for pernicious anemia and other megaloblastic anemias secondary to the lack of vitamin B$_{12}$. A hematologic remission may occur while neurologic manifestations remain progressive.

WARNINGS
In the treatment of accidental overdosages of folic acid antagonists, leucovorin should be administered as promptly as possible. As the time interval between antifolate administration [eg, methotrexate (MTX)]and leucovorin rescue increases, leucovorin's effectiveness in counteracting hematologic toxicity diminshes.

Monitoring of serum MTX concentration is essential in determining the optimal dose and duration of treatment with leucovorin.

Delayed MTX excretion may be caused by a third-space fluid accumulation (ie, ascites, pleural effusion), renal insuffi-

GUIDELINES FOR LEUCOVORIN DOSAGE AND ADMINISTRATION

Clinical Situation	Laboratory Findings	Leucovorin Dosage and Duration
Normal Methotrexate Elimination	Serum methotrexate level approximately 10 micromolar at 24 hours after administration, 1 micromolar at 48 hours, and less than 0.2 micromolar at 72 hours.	15mg PO, IM, or IV q6h for 60 hours (10 doses starting at 24 hours after start of methotrexate infusion).
Delayed Late Methotrexate Elimination	Serum methotrexate level remaining above 0.2 micromolar at 72 hours, and more than 0.05 micromolar at 96 hours after administration.	Continue 15mg PO, IM, or IV q6h, until methotrexate level is less than 0.05 micromolar.
Delayed Early Methotrexate Elimination and/or Evidence of Acute Renal Injury	Serum methotrexate level of 50 micromolar or more at 24 hours, or 5 micromolar or more at 48 hours after administration, OR; a 100% or greater increase in serum creatinine level at 24 hours after methotrexate administration (eg an increase from 0.5 mg/dL to a level of 1 mg/dL or more).	150 mg IV q3h, until methotrexate level is less than 1 micromolar; then 15 mg IV q3h, until methotrexate level is less than 0.05 micromolar.

ciency, or inadequate hydration. Under such circumstances, higher doses of leucovorin or prolonged administration may be indicated. Doses higher than those recommended for oral use must be given intravenously.

Leucovorin may enhance the toxicity of fluorouracil. Deaths from severe enterocolitis, diarrhea, and dehydration have been reported in elderly patients receiving weekly leucovorin and fluorouracil.[1] Concomitant granulocytopenia and fever were present in some but not all of the patients.

PRECAUTIONS

General: Parenteral administration is preferable to oral dosing if there is a possibility that the patient may vomit or not absorb the leucovorin. Leucovorin has no effect on other established toxicities of MTX such as the nephrotoxicity resulting from drug and/or metabolite precipitation in the kidney.

Drug Interactions: Folic acid in large amounts may counteract the antiepileptic effect of phenobarbital, phenytoin, and primidone, and increase the frequency of seizures in susceptible children.

Preliminary animal and human studies have shown that small quantities of systemically administered leucovorin enter the CSF primarily as 5-methyltetrahydrofolate and, in humans, remain 1–3 orders of magnitude lower than the usual methotrexate concentrations following intrathecal administration. However, high doses of leucovorin may reduce the efficacy of intrathecally administered methotrexate.

Leucovorin may enhance the toxicity of fluorouracil (see **WARNINGS**).

Pregnancy: *Teratogenic Effects:* Pregnancy Category C. Animal reproduction studies have not been conducted with leucovorin. It is also not known whether leucovorin can cause fetal harm when administered to a pregnant woman or can affect reproduction capacity. Leucovorin should be given to a pregnant woman only if clearly needed.

Nursing Mothers: It is not known whether this drug is excreted in human milk. Because many drugs are excreted in human milk, caution should be exercised when leucovorin is administered to a nursing mother.

Pediatric Use: See **Drug Interactions.**

ADVERSE REACTIONS

Allergic sensitization has been reported following both oral and parenteral administration of folic acid.

OVERDOSAGE

Excessive amounts of leucovorin may nullify the chemotherapeutic effect of folic acid antagonists.

DOSAGE AND ADMINISTRATION

Leucovorin Calcium Tablets are intended for oral administration. Beause absorption is saturable, oral administration of doses greater than 25 mg is not recommended.

Leucovorin Rescue after High-Dose Methotrexate Therapy: The recommendations for leucovorin rescue are based on a methotrexate dose of 12–15 grams/m^2 administered by intravenous infusion over 4 hours (see methotrexate package insert for full Prescribing Information).[2] Leucovorin rescue at a dose of 15 mg (approximately 10 mg/m^2) every 6 hours for 10 doses starts 24 hours after the beginning of the methotrexate infusion. In the presence of gastrointestinal toxicity, nausea or vomiting, leucovorin should be administered parenterally.

Serum creatinine and methotrexate levels should be determined at least once daily. Leucovorin administration, hydration and urinary alkalinization (pH of 7.0 or greater) should be continued until the methotrexate level is below 5×10^{-8} M (0.05 micromolar). The leucovorin dose should be adjusted or leucovorin rescue extended based on the following guidelines:

[See table above right].

Patients who experience delayed early methotrexate elimination are likely to develop reversible renal failure. In addition to appropriate leucovorin therapy, these patients require continuing hydration and urinary alkalinization, and close monitoring of fluid and electrolyte status, until the serum methotrexate level has fallen to below 0.05 micromolar and the renal failure has resolved.

Some patients will have abnormalities in methotrexate elimination or renal function following methotrexate administration, which are significant but less severe than the abnormalities described in the table above. These abnormalities may or may not be associated with significant clinical toxicity. If significant clinical toxicity is observed, leucovorin rescue should be extended for an additional 24 hours (total of 14 doses over 84 hours) in subsequent courses of therapy. The possibility that the patient is taking other medications which interact with methotrexate [eg, medications which may interfere with methotrexate elimination or binding to serum (albumin)] should always be reconsidered when laboratory abnormalities or clinical toxicities are observed.

Impaired Methotrexate Elimination or Inadvertent Overdosage: The same dosage and administration guidelines may be used. However, leucovorin administration should

GUIDELINES FOR LEUCOVORIN DOSAGE AND ADMINISTRATION

Clinical Situation	Laboratory Findings	Leucovorin Dosage and Duration
Normal Methotrexate Elimination	Serum methotrexate level approximately 10 micromolar at 24 hours after administration, 1 micromolar at 48 hours, and less than 0.2 micromolar at 72 hours.	15 mg PO, IM, or IV q 6 hours for 60 hours (10 doses starting at 24 hours after start of methotrexate infusion)
Delayed Late Methotrexate Elimination	Serum methotrexate level remaining above 0.2 micromolar at 72 hours, and more than 0.05 micromolar at 96 hours after administration.	Continue 15 mg PO, IM, or IV q 6 hours, until methotrexate level is less than 0.05 micromolar
Delayed Early Methotrexate Elimination and/or Evidence of Acute Renal Injury	Serum methotrexate level of 50 micromolar or more at 24 hours, or 5 micromolar or more at 48 hours after administration, OR; a 100% or greater increase in serum creatinine level at 24 hours after methotrexate (eg, an increase from 0.5 mg/dL to a level of 1 mg/dL or more).	150 mg IV q 3 hours, until methotrexate level is less than 1 micromolar; then 15 mg IV q 3 hours until methotrexate level is less than 0.05 micromolar.

begin as soon as possible after an inadvertent overdosage is recognized.

HOW SUPPLIED

Leucovorin Calcium Tablets, 5 mg are round, convex, yellowish-white, engraved LL above 5 on one side, scored in half on the other side and engraved C above the score and 33 below, each containing 5 mg of leucovorin as the calcium salt, supplied as follows:

NDC 0005-4536-83—Bottle of 30 with CRC
NDC 0005-4536-23—Bottle of 100
NDC 0005-4536-40—Unit Dose 10 × 5s

Leucovorin Calcium Tablets, 10 mg are square with rounded corners, convex, yellowish-white, engraved LL above 10 on one side and scored in half on the other side with C above the score and 12 below, containing 10 mg of leucovorin as the calcium salt, supplied as follows:

NDC 0005-4525-83—Bottle of 12 with CRC
NDC 0005-4525-90—Bottle of 24 with CRC
NDC 0005-4525-64—Unit Dose 5 × 10s

Leucovorin Calcium Tablets, 15 mg are oval, convex, yellowish-white, engraved LL on left and 15 on right on one side, scored in half on the other side and engraved C to the left of the score and 35 to the right, each containing 15 mg of leucovorin as the calcium salt, supplied as follows:

NDC 0005-4501-83—Bottle of 12 with CRC
NDC 0005-4501-90—Bottle of 24 with CRC
NDC 0005-4501-64—Unit Dose 5 × 10s

Store at Controlled Room Temperature 15°–30°C (59°–86°F). Protect From Light.

REFERENCES

1. Grem JL, Shoemaker DD, Petrelli NJ, Douglas HO, "Severe and Fatal Toxic Effects Observed in Treatment with High- and Low-Dose Leucovorin Plus 5-Fluorouracil for Colorectal Carcinoma," *Cancer Treat Rep* 71:1122, 1987.
2. Link MP, Goorin AM, Miser AW, et al: "The Effect of Adjuvant Chemotherapy on Relapse-Free Survival in Patients with Osteosarcoma of The Extremity." *N Engl J Med* 314:1600–1606, 1986.

LEDERLE LABORATORIES DIVISION
American Cyanamid Company, Pearl River, NY 10965

Rev. 5/89
25439

Shown in Product Identification Section, page 414

LOXITANE® ℞
[*lŏks-ĭ-tāne*]
Loxapine Succinate
Capsules
LOXITANE® C ℞
Loxapine Hydrochloride
Oral Concentrate
For Oral Use
LOXITANE® IM ℞
Loxapine Hydrochloride
For Intramuscular Use Only

DESCRIPTION

LOXITANE, a dibenzoxazepine compound, represents a new subclass of tricyclic antipsychotic agent, chemically distinct from the thioxanthenes, butyrophenones, and phenothiazines. Chemically, it is 2-chloro-11-(4-methyl-1-piperazinyl)-dibenz[*b,f*][1,4]oxazepine. It is present in capsules as the succinate salt, and in the concentrate and parenteral primarily as the hydrochloride salt.

CAPSULES
Each capsule contains loxapine succinate equivalent to 5, 10, 25 or 50 mg of loxapine base and the following inactive ingredients: Blue 1, Gelatin, Lactose, Magnesium Stearate, Titanium Dioxide, and Yellow 10. Additionally, the 5 mg capsule contains Red 33, the 10 mg capsule contains Red 28 and Red 33 and the 25 mg capsule contains Yellow 6.

ORAL CONCENTRATE
Each mL contains loxapine hydrochloride equivalent to 25 mg of loxapine base and propylene glycol as an inactive ingredient.
Hydrochloric acid and, if necessary, sodium hydroxide are used to adjust pH to approx. 5.8 during manufacture.

INTRAMUSCULAR (Sterile)
Not for Intravenous Use—Each mL contains loxapine hydrochloride equivalent to 50 mg of loxapine base. Inactive Ingredients: Polysorbate 80 NF 5% w/v, Propylene Glycol 70% v/v, and Water for Injection qs ad 100% v.

Continued on next page

Lederle—Cont.

Hydrochloric acid and, if necessary, sodium hydroxide are used to adjust pH to approx. 5.8 during manufacture.

CLINICAL PHARMACOLOGY

Pharmacodynamics: Pharmacologically, loxapine is a tranquilizer for which the exact mode of action has not been established. However, changes in the level of excitability of subcortical inhibitory areas have been observed in several animal species in association with such manifestations of tranquilization as calming effects and suppression of aggressive behavior.

In normal human volunteers, signs of sedation were seen within 20 to 30 minutes after administration, were most pronounced within 1½ to three hours, and lasted through 12 hours. Similar timing of primary pharmacologic effects was seen in animals.

Absorption, Distribution, Metabolism, and Excretion: After administration of LOXITANE as an oral solution, systemic bioavailability of the parent drug was only about one third that after an equivalent intramuscular dose (25 mg base) in male volunteers. C_{max} for the parent drug was similar for the IM and oral administrations, whereas T_{max} was significantly longer for the IM administration than the oral administration (approximately 5 vs one hour). The lower systemic availability of the parent drug after oral administration as compared to the IM administration may be due to first pass metabolism of the oral form. This is supported by the finding that two metabolites found in serum (8-hydroxyloxapine and 8-hydroxydesmethylloxapine) were formed to a lesser extent after IM administration of loxapine as compared to oral administration.

The apparent half-life of loxapine after oral and IM administration is approximately four hours (range, one–14 hours) and 12 hours (range, eight—23 hours) respectively. The extended half-life for the IM administration as compared to the oral administration may be explained by prolonged absorption of loxapine from the muscle during the concurrent elimination process.

Loxapine is extensively metabolized, and urinary recovery over 48 hours resulted in recoveries of approximately 30% and 40% of an IM and orally administered loxapine dose as five metabolites.

INDICATIONS

LOXITANE is indicated for the management of the manifestations of psychotic disorders. The antipsychotic efficacy of LOXITANE *loxapine* was established in clinical studies which enrolled newly hospitalized and chronically hospitalized acutely ill schizophrenic patients as subjects.

CONTRAINDICATIONS

LOXITANE is contraindicated in comatose or severe drug-induced depressed states (alcohol, barbiturates, narcotics, etc).

LOXITANE is contraindicated in individuals with known hypersensitivity to dibenzoxazepines.

WARNINGS

Tardive Dyskinesia: Tardive dyskinesia, a syndrome consisting of potentially irreversible, involuntary, dyskinetic movements, may develop in patients treated with neuroleptic (antipsychotic) drugs. Although the prevalence of the syndrome appears to be highest among the elderly, especially elderly women, it is impossible to rely upon prevalence estimates to predict, at the inception of neuroleptic treatment, which patients are likely to develop the syndrome. Whether neuroleptic drug products differ in their potential to cause tardive dyskinesia is unknown.

Both the risk of developing the syndrome and the likelihood that it will become irreversible are believed to increase as the duration of treatment and the total cumulative dose of neuroleptic drugs administered to the patient increase. However, the syndrome can develop, although much less commonly, after relatively brief treatment periods at low doses. There is no known treatment for established cases of tardive dyskinesia, although the syndrome may remit, partially or completely, if neuroleptic treatment is withdrawn. Neuroleptic treatment, itself, however, may suppress (or partially suppress) the signs and symptoms of the syndrome, and thereby may possibly mask the underlying disease process. The effect that symptomatic suppression has upon the long-term course of the syndrome is unknown.

Given these considerations, neuroleptics should be prescribed in a manner that is most likely to minimize the occurrence of tardive dyskinesia. Chronic neuroleptic treatment should generally be reserved for patients who suffer from a chronic illness that (1) is known to respond to neuroleptic drugs, and (2) for whom alternative, equally effective, but potentially less harmful treatments are *not* available or appropriate. In patients who do require chronic treatment, the smallest dose and the shortest duration of treatment producing a satisfactory clinical response should be sought. The need for continued treatment should be reassessed periodically.

If signs and symptoms of tardive dyskinesia appear in a patient on neuroleptics, drug discontinuation should be considered. However, some patients may require treatment despite the presence of the syndrome. (See **ADVERSE REACTIONS** and **Information for Patients** sections.)

Neuroleptic Malignant Syndrome (NMS): A potentially fatal symptom complex sometimes referred to as Neuroleptic Malignant Syndrome (NMS) has been reported in association with antipsychotic drugs. Clinical manifestations of NMS are hyperpyrexia, muscle rigidity, altered mental status and evidence of autonomic instability (irregular pulse or blood pressure, tachycardia, diaphoresis, and cardiac dysrhythmias).

The diagnostic evaluation of patients with this syndrome is complicated. In arriving at a diagnosis, it is important to identify cases where the clinical presentation includes both serious medical illness (eg, pneumonia, systemic infection, etc) and untreated or inadequately treated extrapyramidal signs and symptoms (EPS). Other important considerations in the differential diagnosis include central anticholinergic toxicity, heat stroke, drug fever and primary central nervous system (CNS) pathology.

The management of NMS should include: (1) immediate discontinuation of antipsychotic drugs and other drugs not essential to concurrent therapy, (2) intensive symptomatic treatment and medical monitoring, and (3) treatment of any concomitant serious medical problems for which specific treatments are available. There is no general agreement about specific pharmacological treatment regimens for uncomplicated NMS.

If a patient requires antipsychotic drug treatment after recovery from NMS, the potential reintroduction of drug therapy should be carefully considered. The patient should be carefully monitored, since recurrences of NMS have been reported.

LOXITANE, like other tranquilizers, may impair mental and/or physical abilities, especially during the first few days of therapy. Therefore, ambulatory patients should be warned about activities requiring alertness (eg, operating vehicles or machinery) and about concomitant use of alcohol and other CNS depressants.

LOXITANE has not been evaluated for the management of behavioral complications in patients with mental retardation, and therefore, it cannot be recommended.

PRECAUTIONS

General: LOXITANE *loxapine* should be used with extreme caution in patients with a history of convulsive disorders since it lowers the convulsive threshold. Seizures have been reported in patients receiving LOXITANE at antipsychotic dose levels, and may occur in epileptic patients even with maintenance of routine anticonvulsant drug therapy.

LOXITANE has an antiemetic effect in animals. Since this effect may also occur in man, LOXITANE may mask signs of overdosage of toxic drugs and may obscure conditions such as intestinal obstruction and brain tumor.

LOXITANE should be used with caution in patients with cardiovascular disease. Increased pulse rates have been reported in the majority of patients receiving antipsychotic doses; transient hypotension has been reported. In the presence of severe hypotension requiring vasopressor therapy, the preferred drugs may be norepinephrine and angiotensin. Usual doses of epinephrine may be ineffective because of inhibition of its vasopressor effect by LOXITANE.

The possiblity of ocular toxicity from loxapine cannot be excluded at this time. Therefore, careful observation should be made for pigmentary retinopathy and lenticular pigmentation, since these have been observed in some patients receiving certain other antipsychotic drugs for prolonged periods.

Because of possible anticholinergic action, the drug should be used cautiously in patients with glaucoma or a tendency to urinary retention, particularly with concomitant administration of anticholinergic-type antiparkinson medication.

Experience to date indicates the possibility of a slightly higher incidence of extrapyramidal effects following intramuscular administration than normally anticipated with oral formulations. The increase may be attributable to higher plasma levels following intramuscular injection.

Neuroleptic drugs elevate prolactin levels; the elevation persists during chronic administration. Tissue culture experiments indicate that approximately one third of human breast cancers are prolactin-dependent *in vitro*, a factor of potential importance if the prescription of these drugs is contemplated in a patient with a previously detected breast cancer. Although disturbances such as galactorrhea, amenorrhea, gynecomastia, and impotence have been reported, the clinical significance of elevated serum prolactin levels is unknown for most patients. An increase in mammary neoplasms has been found in rodents after chronic administration of neuroleptic drugs. Neither clinical studies nor epidemiologic studies conducted to date, however, have shown an association between chronic administration of these drugs and mammary tumorigenesis; the available evidence is considered too limited to be conclusive at this time.

Information for Patients: Given the likelihood that some patients exposed chronically to neuroleptics will develop tardive dyskinesia, it is advised that all patients in whom chronic use is contemplated be given, if possible, full information about this risk. The decision to inform patients and/or their guardians must obviously take into account the clinical circumstances and the competency of the patient to understand the information provided.

Usage in Pregnancy: Safe use of LOXITANE *loxapine* during pregnancy or lactation has not been established; therefore, its use in pregnancy, in nursing mothers, or in women of childbearing potential requires that the benefits of treatment be weighed against the possible risks to mother and child. No embryotoxicity or teratogenicity was observed in studies in rats, rabbits, or dogs although, with the exception of one rabbit study, the highest dosage was only two times the maximum recommended human dose and in some studies it was below this dose. Perinatal studies have shown renal papillary abnormalities in offspring of rats treated from midpregnancy with doses of 0.6 and 1.8 mg/kg, doses which approximate the usual human dose but which are considerably below the maximum recommended human dose.

Nursing Mothers: The extent of the excretion of LOXITANE or its metabolites in human milk is not known. However, LOXITANE and its metabolites have been shown to be transported into the milk of lactating dogs. LOXITANE administration to nursing women should be avoided if clinically possible.

Usage in Children: Studies have not been performed in children; therefore, this drug is not recommended for use in children below the age of 16.

ADVERSE REACTIONS

CNS Effects: Manifestations of adverse effects on the central nervous system, other than extrapyramidal effects, have been seen infrequently. Drowsiness, usually mild, may occur at the beginning of therapy or when dosage is increased. It usually subsides with continued LOXITANE therapy. The incidence of sedation has been less than that of certain aliphatic phenothiazines and slightly more than the piperazine phenothiazines. Dizziness, faintness, staggering gait, shuffling gait, muscle twitching, weakness, insomnia, agitation, tension, seizures, akinesia, slurred speech, numbness and confusional states have been reported. Neuroleptic malignant syndrome (NMS) has been reported (see **WARNINGS**).

Extrapyramidal Reactions: Neuromuscular (extrapyramidal) reactions during the administration of LOXITANE *loxapine* have been reported frequently, often during the first few days of treatment. In most patients, these reactions involved parkinsonian-like symptoms such as tremor, rigidity, excessive salivation, and masked facies. Akathisia (motor restlessness) also has been reported relatively frequently. These symptoms are usually not severe and can be controlled by reduction of LOXITANE dosage or by administration of antiparkinson drugs in usual doses. Dystonic and dyskinetic reactions have occurred less frequently, but may be more severe. Dystonias include spasms of muscles of the neck and face, tongue protrusion, and oculogyric movement. Dyskinetic reactions have been described in the form of choreoathetoid movements. These reactions sometimes require reduction or temporary withdrawal of loxapine dosage in addition to appropriate counteractive drugs.

Persistent Tardive Dyskinesia: As with all antipsychotic agents, tardive dyskinesia may appear in some patients on long-term therapy or may appear after drug therapy has been discontinued. The risk appears to be greater in elderly patients on high-dose therapy, especially females. The symptoms are persistent and in some patients appear to be irreversible. The syndrome is characterized by rhythmical involuntary movement of the tongue, face, mouth, or jaw (eg, protrusion of tongue, puffing of cheeks, puckering of mouth, chewing movements). Sometimes these may be accompanied by involuntary movements of extremities.

There is no known effective treatment for tardive dyskinesia; antiparkinson agents usually do not alleviate the symptoms of this syndrome. It is suggested that all antipsychotic agents be discontinued if these symptoms appear. Should it be necessary to reinstitute treatment, or increase the dosage of the agent, or switch to a different antipsychotic agent, the syndrome may be masked. It has been suggested that fine vermicular movements of the tongue may be an early sign of the syndrome, and if the medication is stopped at that time the syndrome may not develop.

Cardiovascular Effects: Tachycardia, hypotension, hypertension, orthostatic hypotension, lightheadedness, and syncope have been reported.

A few cases of ECG changes similar to those seen with phenothiazines have been reported. It is not known whether these were related to LOXITANE *loxapine* administration.

Hematologic: Rarely, agranulocytosis, thrombocytopenia, leukopenia.

Skin: Dermatitis, edema (puffiness of face), pruritus, rash, alopecia and seborrhea have been reported with loxapine.

Anticholinergic Effects: Dry mouth, nasal congestion, constipation, blurred vision, urinary retention and paralytic ileus have occurred.

Gastrointestinal: Nausea and vomiting have been reported in some patients. Hepatocellular injury (ie, SGOT/SGPT elevation) has been reported in association with loxapine administration and rarely, jaundice and/or hepatitis questionably related to LOXITANE treatment.

Other Adverse Reactions: Weight gain, weight loss, dyspnea, ptosis, hyperpyrexia, flushed facies, headache, paresthesia, and polydipsia have been reported in some patients. Rarely, galactorrhea, amenorrhea, gynecomastia and menstrual irregularity of uncertain etiology have been reported.

DOSAGE AND ADMINISTRATION

LOXITANE is administered, usually in divided doses, two to four times a day. Daily dosage (in terms of base equivalents) should be adjusted to the individual patient's needs as assessed by the severity of symptoms and previous history of response to antipsychotic drugs.

Oral Administration: Initial dosage of 10 mg twice daily is recommended, although in severely disturbed patients initial dosage up to a total of 50 mg daily may be desirable. Dosage should then be increased fairly rapidly over the first seven to ten days until there is effective control of psychotic symptoms. The usual therapeutic and maintenance range is 60 to 100 mg daily. However, as with other antipsychotic drugs, some patients respond to lower dosage and others require higher dosage for optimal benefit. Daily dosage higher than 250 mg daily is not recommended.

LOXITANE C Oral Concentrate should be mixed with orange or grapefruit juice shortly before administration. Use only the enclosed calibrated (10 mg, 15 mg, 25 mg, 50 mg) dropper for dosage.

Maintenance Therapy: For maintenance therapy, dosage should be reduced to the lowest level compatible with symptom control; many patients have been maintained satisfactorily at dosages in the range of 20 to 60 mg daily.

Intramuscular Administration: LOXITANE IM is utilized for prompt symptomatic control in the acutely agitated patient and in patients whose symptoms render oral medication temporarily impractical. During clinical trial there were only rare reports of significant local tissue reaction. LOXITANE IM is administered by intramuscular (not intravenous) injection in doses of 12.5 mg (1/4 mL) to 50 mg (1 mL) at intervals of four to six hours or longer, both dose and interval depending on patient response. Many patients have responded satisfactorily to twice-daily dosage. As described above for oral administration, attention is directed to the necessity for dosage adjustment on an individual basis over the early days of loxapine administration.

Once the desired symptomatic control is achieved and the patient is able to take medication orally, loxapine should be administered in capsule or oral concentrate form. Usually this should occur within five days.

OVERDOSAGE

Signs and symptoms of overdosage will depend on the amount ingested and individual patient tolerance. As would be expected from the pharmacologic actions of the drug, the clinical findings may range from mild depression of the CNS and cardiovascular systems to profound hypotension, respiratory depression, and unconsciousness. The possibility of occurrence of extrapyramidal symptoms and/or convulsive seizures should be kept in mind. Renal failure following loxapine overdosage has also been reported.

The treatment of overdosage is essentially symptomatic and supportive. Early gastric lavage and extended dialysis might be expected to be beneficial. Centrally acting emetics may have little effect because of the antiemetic action of loxapine. In addition, emesis should be avoided because of the possibility of aspiration of vomitus. Avoid analeptics, such as pentylenetetrazol, which may cause convulsions. Severe hypotension might be expected to respond to the administration of levarterenol or phenylephrine. EPINEPHRINE SHOULD NOT BE USED SINCE ITS USE IN A PATIENT WITH PARTIAL ADRENERGIC BLOCKADE MAY FURTHER LOWER THE BLOOD PRESSURE. Severe extrapyramidal reactions should be treated with anticholinergic antiparkinson agents or diphenhydramine hydrochloride, and anticonvulsant therapy should be initiated as indicated. Additional measures include oxygen and intravenous fluids.

HOW SUPPLIED

LOXITANE *loxapine succinate* capsules are available in the following base equivalent strengths:

5 mg—Hard shell, opaque, dark green capsules, printed with Lederle over L1 on one half and 5 mg on the other, are supplied as follows:
NDC 0005-5359-23—Bottle of 100
NDC 0005-5359-60—Unit Dose 10 ×10

10 mg—Hard shell, opaque, with yellow body and a dark green cap, printed with Lederle over L2 on one half and 10 mg on the other, are supplied as follows:
NDC 0005-5360-23—Bottle of 100
NDC 0005-5360-34—Bottle of 1000
NDC 0005-5360-60—Unit Dose 10 × 10

25 mg—Hard shell, opaque, with a light green body and a dark green cap, printed with Lederle over L3 on one half and 25 mg on the other, are supplied as follows:

NDC 0005-5361-23—Bottle of 100
NDC 0005-5361-34—Bottle of 1000
NDC 0005-5361-60—Unit Dose 10 × 10

50 mg—Hard shell, opaque, with a blue body and a dark green cap, printed with Lederle over L4 on one half and 50 mg on the other, are supplied as follows:
NDC 0005-5362-23—Bottle of 100
NDC 0005-5362-34—Bottle of 1000
NDC 0005-5362-60—Unit Dose 10 × 10

Store at Controlled Room Temperature 15–30° C (59–86° F).

LOXITANE C *loxapine hydrochloride* Oral Concentrate is supplied as follows:
NDC 0005-5387-58—4 Fl oz (120 mL) with calibrated dropper. Each mL contains loxapine HCl equivalent to 25 mg of loxapine base.

Store at Controlled Room Temperature 15–30° C (59–86° F). DO NOT FREEZE.

LOXITANE loxapine succinate Capsules
VA Depot:
NSN 6505-01-048-3719—25 mg (1000s)
NSN 6505-01-048-3718—50 mg (1000s)
LOXITANE C loxapine hydrochloride Oral Concentrate For Oral Use
VA Depot:
NSN 6505-01-026-0101—25 mg/mL (4 oz)
LEDERLE LABORATORIES DIVISION
American Cyanamid Company
Pearl River, NY 10965
LOXITANE IM for Intramuscular use only is supplied as follows:
NDC 0205-5385-55—sterile 10—1 mL ampuls
NDC 0205-5385-34—10 mL multidose vial
Each mL contains loxapine HCl equivalent to 50 mg of loxapine base.
Keep package closed to protect from light. Intensification of the straw color to a light amber will not alter potency or therapeutic efficacy; if noticeably discolored, ampul or vial should not be used.
Store at Controlled Room Temperature 15–30° C (59–86° F). DO NOT FREEZE.
LEDERLE PARENTERALS, INC.
Carolina, Puerto Rico 00630
Rev. 2/88
21971

Shown in Product Identification Section, page 414

MATERNA® ℞
[*ma-ter-na*]
Enhanced Formula
Prenatal Vitamin and
Mineral Tablets

Each tablet contains:		For Pregnant or Lactating Women Percentage of U.S. Recommended Daily Allowance (U.S. RDA)
Vitamin A (as Acetate)	5,000 I.U.	(62.5%)
Vitamin D	400 I.U.	(100%)
Vitamin E (as *dl*-Alpha Tocopheryl Acetate)	30 I.U.	(100%)
Vitamin C (Ascorbic Acid)	100 mg	(167%)
Folic Acid	1 mg	(125%)
Vitamin B_1 (as Thiamine Mononitrate)	3 mg	(224%)
Vitamin B_2 (as Riboflavin)	3.4 mg	(170%)
Vitamin B_6 (as Pyridoxine Hydrochloride)	10 mg	(400%)
Niacinamide	20 mg	(100%)
Vitamin B_{12} (Cyanocobalamin)	12 mcg	(150%)
Biotin	30 mcg	(10%)
Pantothenic Acid (as Calcium Pantothenate)	10 mg	(100%)
Calcium (as Calcium Carbonate)	250 mg	(19%)
Iodine (as Potassium Iodide)	150 mcg	(100%)
Iron (as Ferrous Fumarate)	60 mg	(333%)
Magnesium (as Magnesium Oxide)	25 mg	(6%)
Copper (as Cupric Oxide)	2 mg	(100%)
Zinc (as Zinc Oxide)	25 mg	(167%)
Chromium (as Chromium Chloride)	25 mcg*	
Molybdenum (as Sodium Molybdate)	25 mcg*	
Manganese (as Manganese Sulfate)	5 mg*	

*Recognized as essential in human nutrition, but no U.S. RDA established.

Inactive Ingredients: Gelatin, Hydrolyzed Protein, Hydroxypropyl Methylcellulose, Lactose, Magnesium Stearate, Methylparaben, Modified Food Starch, Mono- and Di-glycerides, Polacrilin, Potassium Sorbate, Povidone, Propylparaben, Silica Gel, Sodium Benzoate, Sodium Lauryl Sulfate, Sodium Starch Glycolate, Sorbic Acid, Stearic Acid, Sucrose, Titanium Dioxide.

Contains no Color or Dyes from Artificial Sources.
CAUTION: Federal law prohibits dispensing without prescription.
RECOMMENDED INTAKE: 1 daily with or without food or as prescribed by physician.
WARNING: Keep out of the reach of children.
Notice: Contact with moisture may produce surface discoloration or erosion of the tablet.
PRECAUTION: Folic Acid may obscure pernicious anemia in that the peripheral blood picture may revert to normal while neurological manifestations remain progressive. Allergic sensitization has been reported following both oral and parenteral administration of Folic Acid.
Store at Controlled Room Temperature 15°–30°C (59°–86°F).
HOW SUPPLIED: Bottles of 100.
NDC 0005-5560-23
PATENTED Made in U.S.A.
U.S. Pat. No. 4,431,634
©1986
LEDERLE LABORATORIES DIVISION
American Cyanamid Company, Pearl River, N.Y. 10965
Rev. 6/87
18697

Shown in Product Identification Section, page 414

MAXZIDE® and MAXZIDE®-25 MG Tablets ℞
Triamterene/Hydrochlorothiazide

PRODUCT OVERVIEW

KEY FACTS

MAXZIDE is a potassium-sparing diuretic, antihypertensive product. MAXZIDE delivers optimally bioavailable doses of both hydrochlorothiazide and triamterene in an optimal ratio of HCTZ to TMT for potassium-sparing action.

MAJOR USES

This fixed combination drug is indicated for the following: (1) the treatment of hypertension or edema in patients who develop hypokalemia on hydrochlorothiazide alone; (2) those patients who require a thiazide diuretic and in whom the development of hypokalemia cannot be risked.

MAXZIDE may be used alone or in combination with other antihypertensive drugs such as beta blockers. Since MAXZIDE may enhance the actions of these drugs, dosage adjustments may be necessary.

Use caution when used concomitantly with ACE inhibitors due to the possibility of hyperkalemia. (See **SAFETY INFORMATION**).

SAFETY INFORMATION

MAXZIDE should not be used in the presence of elevated serum potassium levels (greater than or equal to 5.5 mEg/L). Hyperkalemia is more likely to occur in patients with renal impairment, diabetes (even without evidence of renal impairment); and elderly or severely ill patients. Since uncorrected hyperkalemia may be fatal, serum potassium levels must be monitored at frequent intervals, especially in patients first receiving MAXZIDE, when dosages are changed, or with any illness that may influence renal function. Avoid potassium-conserving therapy in severely ill patients in whom respiratory or metabolic acidosis may occur. Acidosis may be associated with rapid elevations in serum potassium levels. If MAXZIDE is employed, frequent evaluation of acid balance and serum electrolytes are necessary. (See full Prescribing Information). If hyperkalemia develops, discontinue drug and substitute a thiazide alone. MAXZIDE should not be given to patients receiving other potassium-conserving agents, potassium containing salt substitutes, or potassium-enriched diets. Because of the potassium-sparing properties of angiotensin-converting enzymes (ACE) inhibitors, use MAXZIDE cautiously, if at all, with these agents.

PRESCRIBING INFORMATION

MAXZIDE® and MAXZIDE®-25 MG Tablets ℞
Triamterene/Hydrochlorothiazide

DESCRIPTION

MAXZIDE combines triamterene, a potassium-conserving diuretic, with the natriuretic agent, hydrochlorothiazide. Each MAXZIDE tablet contains triamterene, USP, 75 mg and hydrochlorothiazide, USP, 50 mg.
Each MAXZIDE-25 MG tablet contains triamterene, USP, 37.5 mg and hydrochlorothiazide, USP, 25 mg.

Continued on next page

Lederle—Cont.

MAXZIDE and MAXZIDE–25 MG tablets for oral administration contain the following inactive ingredients: Colloidal Silicon Dioxide, Croscarmellose Sodium, Magnesium Stearate, Microcrystalline Cellulose, Powdered Cellulose, Sodium Lauryl Sulfate, and D&C Yellow #10. MAXZIDE–25 MG tablets also contain FD&C Blue #1.

Triamterene is 2,4,7-triamino-6-phenylpteridine. Triamterene is practically insoluble in water, benzene, chloroform, ether and dilute alkali hydroxides. It is soluble in formic acid and sparingly soluble in methoxyethanol. Triamterene is very slightly soluble in acetic acid, alcohol and dilute mineral acids. Its molecular weight is 253.27.

Hydrochlorothiazide is 6-chloro-3,4-dihydro-$2H$-1,2,4, benzothiadiazine-7-sulfonamide 1, 1-dioxide. Hydrochlorothiazide is slightly soluble in water and freely soluble in sodium hydroxide solution, n-butylamine and dimethylformamide. It is sparingly soluble in methanol and insoluble in ether, chloroform and dilute mineral acids. Its molecular weight is 297.73.

CLINICAL PHARMACOLOGY

MAXZIDE is a diuretic, antihypertensive drug product, principally due to its hydrochlorothiazide component; the triamterene component of MAXZIDE reduces the excessive potassium loss which may occur with hydrochlorothiazide use.

Hydrochlorothiazide: Hydrochlorothiazide is a diuretic and antihypertensive agent. It blocks the renal tubular absorption of sodium and chloride ions. This natriuresis and diuresis is accompanied by a secondary loss of potassium and bicarbonate. Onset of hydrochlorothiazide's diuretic effect occurs within two hours and the peak action takes place in four hours. Diuretic activity persists for approximately six to twelve hours.

The exact mechanism of hydrochlorothiazide's antihypertensive action is not known although it may relate to the excretion and redistribution of body sodium. Hydrochlorothiazide does not affect normal blood pressure.

Following oral administration, peak hydrochlorothiazide plasma levels are attained in approximately two hours. It is excreted rapidly and unchanged in the urine.

Well-controlled studies have demonstrated that doses of hydrochlorothiazide as low as 25 mg given once daily are effective in treating hypertension, but the dose response has not been clearly established.

Triamterene: Triamterene is a potassium-conserving (antikaliuretic) diuretic with relatively weak natriuretic properties. It exerts its diuretic effect on the distal renal tubule to inhibit the reabsorption of sodium in exchange for potassium and hydrogen. With this action, triamterene increases sodium excretion and reduces the excessive loss of potassium and hydrogen associated with hydrochlorothiazide. Triamterene is not a competitive antagonist of the mineralocorticoids and its potassium-conserving effect is observed in patients with Addison's disease, ie, without aldosterone. Triamterene's onset and duration of activity is similar to hydrochlorothiazide. No predictable antihypertensive effect has been demonstrated with triamterene.

Triamterene is rapidly absorbed following oral administration. Peak plasma levels are achieved within one hour after dosing. Triamterene is primarily metabolized to the sulfate conjugate of hydroxytriamterene. Both the plasma and urine levels of this metabolite greatly exceed triamterene levels.

The amount of triamterene added to 50 mg of hydrochlorothiazide in MAXZIDE tablets was determined from steady-state dose response evaluations in which various doses of liquid preparations of triamterene were administered to hypertensive persons who developed hypokalemia with hydrochlorothiazide (50 mg/day). Daily doses of 75 mg triamterene produced maximal increases in serum potassium levels. Doses exceeding 75 mg daily provided no additional elevations in serum potassium levels. The amount of triamterene added to the 25 mg of hydrochlorothiazide in MAXZIDE-25 MG tablets was also determined from steady-state dose response evaluations in which various doses of liquid preparations of triamterene were administered to hypertensive persons who developed hypokalemia with hydrochlorothiazide (25 mg/day). Daily doses of 37.5 mg triamterene produced maximal increases in serum potassium levels. Doses exceeding 37.5 mg daily produced no additional elevations in serum potassium levels. The potassium-sparing properties of triamterene were also evaluated in hypokalemic patients receiving 50 mg hydrochlorothiazide as two divided doses. Triamterene given twice daily restored serum potassium levels towards normal in a dose-related fashion. The largest increase in this study was observed with a total daily dose of 100 mg, the largest dose tested. However, the combination of triamterene and hydrochlorothiazide given twice daily in this trial appeared to produce an increased frequency of elevation in serum BUN and creatinine levels. Ordinarily, triamterene does not entirely reverse the kaliuretic effect of hydrochlorothiazide and some patients

may remain hypokalemic while receiving triamterene and hydrochlorothiazide. In some individuals, however, it may induce hyperkalemia (see **WARNINGS**).

The triamterene and hydrochlorothiazide components of MAXZIDE and MAXZIDE-25 MG are well absorbed and are bioequivalent to liquid preparations of the individual components administered orally. Food does not influence the absorption of triamterene or hydrochlorothiazide from MAXZIDE or MAXZIDE-25 MG tablets. The hydrochlorothiazide component of MAXZIDE is bioequivalent to single-entity hydrochlorothiazide tablet formulations.

INDICATIONS AND USAGE

This fixed combination drug is not indicated for the initial therapy of edema or hypertension except in individuals in whom the development of hypokalemia cannot be risked.

1. MAXZIDE *triamterene/hydrochlorothiazide* is indicated for the treatment of hypertension or edema in patients who develop hypokalemia on hydrochlorothiazide alone.
2. MAXZIDE is also indicated for those patients who require a thiazide diuretic and in whom the development of hypokalemia cannot be risked (eg, patients on concomitant digitalis preparations, or with a history of cardiac arrhythmias, etc.).

MAXZIDE may be used alone or in combination with other antihypertensive drugs such as beta-blockers. Since MAXZIDE may enhance the actions of these drugs, dosage adjustments may be necessary.

Usage in Pregnancy: The routine use of diuretics in an otherwise healthy woman is inappropriate and exposes mother and fetus to unnecessary hazard. Diuretics do not prevent development of toxemia of pregnancy, and there is no satisfactory evidence that they are useful in the treatment of developed toxemia.

Edema during pregnancy may arise from pathological causes or from the physiologic and mechanical consequences of pregnancy. Thiazides are indicated in pregnancy when edema is due to pathologic causes, just as they are in absence of pregnancy. Dependent edema in pregnancy, resulting from restriction of venous return by the expanded uterus, is properly treated through elevation of the lower extremities and use of support hose; use of diuretics to lower intravascular volume in this case is illogical and unnecessary. There is hypervolemia during normal pregnancy which is harmful to neither the fetus nor the mother (in the absence of cardiovascular disease), but which is associated with edema, including generalized edema, in the majority of pregnant women. If this edema produces discomfort, increased recumbency will often provide relief. In rare instances, this edema may cause extreme discomfort which is not relieved by rest. In these cases, a short course of diuretics may provide relief and may be appropriate.

CONTRAINDICATIONS

Hyperkalemia: MAXZIDE *triamterene/hydrochlorothiazide* should not be used in the presence of elevated serum potassium levels (greater than or equal to 5.5 mEq/liter). If hyperkalemia develops, this drug should be discontinued and a thiazide alone should be substituted.

Antikaliuretic Therapy or Potassium Supplementation: MAXZIDE should not be given to patients receiving other potassium-conserving agents such as spironolactone, amiloride HCl or other formulations containing triamterene. Concomitant potassium supplementation in the form of medication, potassium-containing salt substitute or potassium-enriched diets should also not be used.

Impaired Renal Function: MAXZIDE is contraindicated in patients with anuria, acute and chronic renal insufficiency or significant renal impairment.

Hypersensitivity: MAXZIDE should not be used in patients who are hypersensitive to triamterene or hydrochlorothiazide or other sulfonamide-derived drugs.

WARNINGS

Hyperkalemia. Abnormal elevation of serum potassium levels (greater than or equal to 5.5 mEq/liter) can occur with all potassium-conserving diuretic combinations, including MAXZIDE. Hyperkalemia is more likely to occur in patients with renal impairment, diabetes (even without evidence of renal impairment), or elderly or severely ill patients. Since uncorrected hyperkalemia may be fatal, serum potassium levels must be monitored at frequent intervals especially in patients first receiving MAXZIDE, when dosages are changed or with any illnesses that may influence renal function.

If hyperkalemia is suspected (warning signs include paresthesias, muscular weakness, fatigue, flaccid paralysis of the extremities, bradycardia, and shock) an electrocardiogram (ECG) should be obtained. However, it is important to monitor serum potassium levels because mild hyperkalemia may not be associated with ECG changes.

If hyperkalemia is present, MAXZIDE should be discontinued immediately and a thiazide alone should be substituted. If the serum potassium exceeds 6.5 mEq/liter, more vigorous

therapy is required. The clinical situation dictates the procedures to be employed. These include the intravenous administration of calcium chloride solution, sodium bicarbonate solution and/or the oral or parenteral administration of glucose with a rapid-acting insulin preparation. Cationic exchange resins such as sodium polystyrene sulfonate may be orally or rectally administered. Persistent hyperkalemia may require dialysis.

The development of hyperkalemia associated with potassium-sparing diuretics is accentuated in the presence of renal impairment (see **CONTRAINDICATIONS**). Patients with mild renal functional impairment should not receive this drug without frequent and continuing monitoring of serum electrolytes. Cumulative drug effects may be observed in patients with impaired renal function. The renal clearances of hydrochlorothiazide and the pharmacologically active metabolite of triamterene, the sulfate ester of hydroxytriamterene, have been shown to be reduced and the plasma levels increased following MAXZIDE *triamterene/hydrochlorothiazide* administration to elderly patients and patients with impaired renal function.

Hyperkalemia has been reported in diabetic patients with the use of potassium-conserving agents even in the absence of apparent renal impairment. Accordingly, MAXZIDE should be avoided in diabetic patients. If it is employed, serum electrolytes must be frequently monitored.

Because of the potassium-sparing properties of angiotensin-converting enzyme (ACE) inhibitors, MAXZIDE should be used cautiously, if at all, with these agents (see **PRECAUTIONS, Drug Interactions**).

Metabolic or Respiratory Acidosis: Potassium-conserving therapy should also be avoided in severely ill patients in whom respiratory or metabolic acidosis may occur. Acidosis may be associated with rapid elevations in serum potassium levels. If MAXZIDE is employed, frequent evaluations of acid/base balance and serum electrolytes are necessary.

PRECAUTIONS

General: Electrolyte Imbalance and BUN Increases: Patients receiving MAXZIDE should be carefully monitored for fluid or electrolyte imbalances, ie, hyponatremia, hypochloremic alkalosis, hypokalemia, and hypomagnesemia. Determination of serum electrolytes to detect possible electrolyte imbalance should be performed at appropriate intervals. Serum and urine electrolyte determinations are especially important and should be frequently performed when the patient is vomiting or receiving parenteral fluids. Warning signs or symptoms of fluid and electrolyte imbalance include: dryness of mouth, thirst, weakness, lethargy, drowsiness, restlessness, muscle pains or cramps, muscular fatigue, hypotension, oliguria, tachycardia and gastrointestinal disturbances such as nausea and vomiting.

Any chloride deficit during thiazide therapy is generally mild and usually does not require any specific treatment except under extraordinary circumstances (as in liver disease or renal disease). Dilutional hyponatremia may occur in edematous patients in hot weather; appropriate therapy is water restriction, rather than administration of salt, except in rare instances when the hyponatremia is life threatening. In actual salt depletion, appropriate replacement is the therapy of choice.

Hypokalemia may develop with thiazide therapy, especially with brisk diuresis, when severe cirrhosis is present, or during concomitant use of corticosteroids, ACTH, amphotericin B or after prolonged thiazide therapy. However, hypokalemia of this type is usually prevented by the triamterene component of MAXZIDE.

Interference with adequate oral electrolyte intake will also contribute to hypokalemia. Hypokalemia can sensitize or exaggerate the response of the heart to the toxic effects of digitalis (eg, increased ventricular irritability).

MAXZIDE *triamterene/hydrochlorothiazide* may produce an elevated blood urea nitrogen level (BUN), creatinine level or both. This is probably not the result of renal toxicity but is secondary to a reversible reduction of the glomerular filtration rate or a depletion of the intravascular fluid volume. Elevations in BUN and creatinine levels may be more frequent in patients receiving divided dose diuretic therapy. Periodic BUN and creatinine determinations should be made especially in elderly patients, patients with suspected or confirmed hepatic disease or renal insufficiencies. If azotemia increases, MAXZIDE should be discontinued.

Hepatic Coma: MAXZIDE should be used with caution in patients with impaired hepatic function or progressive liver disease, since minor alterations of fluid and electrolyte balance may precipitate hepatic coma.

Renal Stones: Triamterene has been reported in renal stones in association with other calculus components. MAXZIDE should be used with caution in patients with histories of renal lithiasis.

Folic Acid Deficiency: Triamterene is a weak folic acid antagonist and may contribute to the appearance of megaloblastosis in instances where folic acid stores are decreased. In such patients, periodic blood evaluations are recommended.

Hyperuricemia: Hyperuricemia may occur or acute gout may be precipitated in certain patients receiving thiazide therapy.

Metabolic and Endocrine Effects: The thiazides may decrease serum PBI levels without signs of thyroid disturbance.

Calcium excretion is decreased by thiazides. Pathological changes in the parathyroid gland with hypercalcemia and hypophosphatemia have been observed in a few patients on prolonged thiazide therapy. The common complications of hyperparathyroidism such as renal lithiasis, bone resorption, and peptic ulceration have not been seen. Thiazides should be discontinued before carrying out tests for parathyroid function.

Insulin requirements in diabetic patients may be increased, decreased or unchanged. Diabetes mellitus which has been latent may become manifest during thiazide administration.

Hypersensitivity: Sensitivity reactions to thiazides may occur in patients with or without a history of allergy or bronchial asthma.

Possible exacerbation or activation of systemic lupus erythematosus by thiazides has been reported.

Drug Interactions: Thiazides may add to or potentiate the action of other antihypertensive drugs.

The thiazides may decrease arterial responsiveness to norepinephrine. This diminution is not sufficient to preclude effectiveness of the pressor agent for therapeutic use. Thiazides have also been shown to increase responsiveness to tubocurarine.

Lithium generally should not be given with diuretics because they reduce its renal clearance and add a high risk of lithium toxicity. Refer to the package insert on lithium before use of such concomitant therapy.

Acute renal failure has been reported in a few patients receiving indomethacin and formulations containing triamterene and hydrochlorothiazide. Caution is therefore advised when administering nonsteroidal anti-inflammatory agents with MAXZIDE *triamterene/hydrochlorothiazide.*

Potassium-sparing agents should be used very cautiously, if at all, in conjunction with angiotensin-converting enzyme (ACE) inhibitors due to a greatly increased risk of hyperkalemia. Serum potassium should be monitored frequently.

Drug/Laboratory Test Interactions: Triamterene and quinidine have similar fluorescence spectra; thus MAXZIDE may interfere with the measurement of quinidine.

Pregnancy Category C: The safe use of MAXZIDE in pregnancy has not been established. Animal reproduction studies have not been conducted with MAXZIDE. It is also not known if MAXZIDE can cause fetal harm when administered to a pregnant woman or can affect reproductive capacity. Thiazides cross the placental barrier and appear in cord blood. The use of thiazides in pregnant women requires that the anticipated benefit be weighed against possible hazards to the fetus. These hazards include fetal or neonatal jaundice, thrombocytopenia, pancreatitis, and possibly other adverse reactions which have occurred in the adult. MAXZIDE should be given to a pregnant woman only if clearly needed.

Nursing Mothers: Thiazides appear in breast milk. If the use of MAXZIDE is deemed essential, the patient should stop nursing.

Pediatric Use: The safety and effectiveness of MAXZIDE in children have not been established.

ADVERSE REACTIONS

Side effects observed in association with the use of MAXZIDE or other triamterene/hydrochlorothiazide combination products include drowsiness and fatigue, insomnia, muscle cramps and weakness, headache, nausea, appetite disturbance, vomiting, diarrhea, constipation, urine discoloration, dizziness, decreased sexual performance, tachycardia, shortness of breath and chest pain, dry mouth, depression and anxiety. Rare incidents of acute interstitial nephritis and acute renal failure have been reported. Other adverse reactions which have been reported with the individual active drugs include:

Hydrochlorothiazide: *Gastrointestinal:* anorexia, gastric irritation, cramping, jaundice (intrahepatic cholestatic jaundice), pancreatitis, sialadenitis.
Central Nervous System: vertigo, paresthesias, xanthopsia.
Hematologic: leukopenia, agranulocytosis, thrombocytopenia, aplastic anemia, hemolytic anemia, megaloblastosis.
Cardiovascular: orthostatic hypotension (may be aggravated by alcohol, barbiturates, or narcotics).
Hypersensitivity: anaphylaxis, purpura, photosensitivity, rash, urticaria, necrotizing angiitis (vasculitis, cutaneous vasculitis), fever, respiratory distress including pneumonitis.
Other: hyperglycemia, glycosuria, hyperuricemia, restlessness, transient blurred vision.
Triamterene: *Hypersensitivity:* anaphylaxis, photosensitivity and rash.
Other: Triamterene has been reported in renal stones in association with other calculus materials. Triamterene has been associated with blood dyscrasias.
Whenever adverse reactions are moderate to severe, therapy should be reduced or withdrawn.

OVERDOSAGE

No specific data are available regarding MAXZIDE *triamterene/hydrochlorothiazide* overdosage in humans and no specific antidote is available.

Fluid and electrolyte imbalances are the most important concern. Excessive doses of the triamterene component may elicit hyperkalemia, dehydration, nausea, vomiting and weakness and possibly hypotension. Overdosing with hydrochlorothiazide has been associated with hypokalemia, hypochloremia, hyponatremia, dehydration, lethargy (may progress to coma) and gastrointestinal irritation. Treatment is symptomatic and supportive. Therapy with MAXZIDE should be discontinued. Induce emesis or institute gastric lavage. Monitor serum electrolyte levels and fluid balance. Institute supportive measures as required to maintain hydration, electrolyte balance, respiratory, cardiovascular and renal function.

DOSAGE AND ADMINISTRATION

The usual dose of MAXZIDE-25 MG is one or two tablets daily, given as a single dose, with appropriate monitoring of serum potassium (see **WARNINGS**). The usual dose of MAXZIDE is one tablet daily, with appropriate monitoring of serum potassium (see **WARNINGS**). There is no experience with the use of more than one MAXZIDE tablet daily or more than two MAXZIDE-25 MG tablets daily. Clinical experience with the administration of two MAXZIDE-25 MG tablets daily in divided doses (rather than as a single dose) suggests an increased risk of electrolyte imbalance and renal dysfunction.

Patients receiving 50 mg of hydrochlorothiazide who become hypokalemic may be transferred to MAXZIDE directly. Patients receiving 25 mg hydrochlorothiazide who become hypokalemic may be transferred to MAXZIDE-25 MG 37.5 mg triamterene/25 mg hydrochlorothiazide directly.

In patients requiring hydrochlorothiazide therapy and in whom hypokalemia cannot be risked, therapy may be initiated with MAXZIDE-25 MG. If an optimal blood pressure response is not obtained with MAXZIDE-25 MG, the dose should be increased to two MAXZIDE-25 MG tablets daily as a single dose, or one MAXZIDE tablet daily. If blood pressure still is not controlled, another antihypertensive agent may be added (see **PRECAUTIONS, Drug Interactions**).

Clinical studies have shown that patients taking less bioavailable formulations of triamterene and hydrochlorothiazide (totaling 75-100 mg hydrochlorothiazide and 150-200 mg triamterene) may be safely changed to one MAXZIDE tablet per day. Patients receiving less bioavailable formulations of triamterene and hydrochlorothiazide in daily doses of 25-50 mg hydrochlorothiazide and 50-100 mg triamterene may be safely changed to one MAXZIDE-25 MG tablet daily. All patients changed from less bioavailable formulations to MAXZIDE should be monitored clinically and for serum potassium after the transfer.

HOW SUPPLIED

MAXZIDE *triamterene/hydrochlorothiazide* tablets are bow-tie-shaped, flat-faced beveled, light yellow tablets, engraved with MAXZIDE on one side and scored on the other with LL on the left and M8 on the right of the score. Each tablet contains 75 mg of triamterene, USP and 50 mg of hydrochlorothiazide, USP. They are supplied as follows:

    NDC 0005-4460-43—Bottle of 100 with CRC
    NDC 0005-4460-31—Bottle of 500
    NDC 0005-4460-60—Unit Dose 10 × 10

MAXZIDE-25 MG tablets are bowtie-shaped, flat-faced beveled, light green tablets, engraved with MAXZIDE on one side and scored on the other with LL on the left and M9 on the right of the score. Each tablet contains 37.5 mg of triamterene, USP and 25 mg hydrochlorothiazide, USP. They are supplied as follows:

    NDC 0005-4464-43—Bottle of 100 with CRC
    NDC 0005-4464-60—Unit Dose 10 × 10

    Store at Controlled Room Temperature 15–30°C (59–86°F).
Protect From Light.
Dispense in a tight, light-resistant, child-resistant container.
MAXZIDE Triamterene 75 mg/Hydrochlorothiazide 50 mg VA Depot:
NSN 6505-01-196-5403—Unit Dose (10 × 10s)
NSN 6505-01-223-8008—(30s)
Manufactured for
LEDERLE LABORATORIES DIVISION
American Cyanamid Company, Pearl River, NY 10965
by
MYLAN PHARMACEUTICALS, INC.
Morgantown, West Virginia 26505

          Rev. 8/88
          22348
Shown in Product Identification Section, page 415

METHOTREXATE Tablets   ℞
METHOTREXATE Sodium   ℞
METHOTREXATE LPF® Sodium Parenteral   ℞

WARNINGS
METHOTREXATE SHOULD BE USED ONLY BY PHYSICIANS WHOSE KNOWLEDGE AND EXPERIENCE INCLUDES THE USE OF ANTIMETABOLITE THERAPY.
THE USE OF METHOTREXATE HIGH-DOSE REGIMENS RECOMMENDED FOR OSTEOSARCOMA REQUIRES METICULOUS CARE (see **DOSAGE AND ADMINISTRATION**). HIGH-DOSAGE REGIMENS FOR OTHER NEOPLASTIC DISEASES ARE INVESTIGATIONAL AND A THERAPEUTIC ADVANTAGE HAS NOT BEEN ESTABLISHED.
BECAUSE OF THE POSSIBILITY OF SERIOUS TOXIC REACTIONS, THE PATIENT SHOULD BE INFORMED BY THE PHYSICIAN OF THE RISKS INVOLVED AND SHOULD BE UNDER A PHYSICIAN'S CONSTANT SUPERVISION.
DEATHS HAVE BEEN REPORTED WITH THE USE OF METHOTREXATE IN THE TREATMENT OF MALIGNANCY, PSORIASIS, AND RHEUMATOID ARTHRITIS.
IN THE TREATMENT OF PSORIASIS OR RHEUMATOID ARTHRITIS, METHOTREXATE USE SHOULD BE RESTRICTED TO PATIENTS WITH SEVERE, RECALCITRANT, DISABLING DISEASE, WHICH IS NOT ADEQUATELY RESPONSIVE TO OTHER FORMS OF THERAPY, AND ONLY WHEN THE DIAGNOSIS HAS BEEN ESTABLISHED AND AFTER APPROPRIATE CONSULTATION.
1. Methotrexate has been reported to cause fetal death and/or congenital anomalies. Therefore, it is not recommended for women of childbearing potential unless there is clear medical evidence that the benefits can be expected to outweigh the considered risks. Pregnant patients with psoriasis or rheumatoid arthritis should not receive methotrexate. (See **CONTRAINDICATIONS.**)
2. Periodic monitoring for toxicity, including CBC with differential and platelet counts, and liver and renal function tests is a mandatory part of methotrexate therapy. Periodic liver biopsies may be indicated in some situations. Patients at increased risk for impaired methotrexate elimination (eg, renal dysfunction, pleural effusions, or ascites) should be monitored more frequently. (See **PRECAUTIONS.**)
3. Methotrexate causes hepatotoxicity, fibrosis and cirrhosis, but generally only after prolonged use. Acutely, liver enzyme elevations are frequently seen; these are usually transient and asymptomatic, and also do not appear predictive of subsequent hepatic disease. Liver biopsy after sustained use often shows histologic changes, and fibrosis and cirrhosis have been reported; these latter lesions often are not preceded by symptoms or abnormal liver function tests. (See **PRECAUTIONS.**)
4. Methotrexate-induced lung disease is a potentially dangerous lesion, which may occur acutely at any time during therapy and which has been reported at doses as low as 7.5 mg/week. It is not always fully reversible. Pulmonary symptoms (especially a dry, nonproductive cough) may require interruption of treatment and careful investigation.
5. Methotrexate may produce marked bone marrow depression, with resultant anemia, leukopenia, and/or thrombocytopenia.
6. Diarrhea and ulcerative stomatitis require interruption of therapy; otherwise, hemorrhagic enteritis and death from intestinal perforation may occur.
7. Methotrexate therapy in patients with impaired renal function should be undertaken with extreme caution, and at reduced dosages, because renal dysfunction will prolong methotrexate elimination.
8. Unexpectedly severe (sometimes fatal) marrow suppression and gastrointestinal toxicity have been reported with concomitant administration of methotrexate (usually in high dosage) along with some nonsteroidal anti-inflammatory drugs (NSAIDs). (See **PRECAUTIONS, Drug Interactions.**)

Continued on next page

Lederle—Cont.

METHOTREXATE FORMULATIONS AND DILUENTS CONTAINING PRESERVATIVES MUST NOT BE USED FOR INTRATHECAL OR HIGH-DOSE METHOTREXATE THERAPY.

DESCRIPTION

Methotrexate (formerly Amethopterin) is an antimetabolite used in the treatment of certain neoplastic diseases, severe psoriasis, and adult rheumatoid arthritis. Chemically methotrexate is N-[4-[[(2,4-diamino-6-pteridinyl)-methyl]methylamino]benzoyl]-L-glutamic acid. Methotrexate Tablets for oral administration are available in bottles of 100 and in a packaging system designated as the RHEUMATREX® Methotrexate Dose Pack for therapy with a weekly dosing schedule of 5 mg, 7.5 mg, 10 mg, 12.5 mg, and 15 mg. Methotrexate tablets contain an amount of methotrexate sodium equivalent to 2.5 mg of methotrexate and the following inactive ingredients: Lactose, Magnesium Stearate and Pregelatinized Starch. May also contain Corn Starch.

Methotrexate Sodium Parenteral products are sterile and may be given by the intramuscular, intravenous, intra-arterial or intrathecal route. (see **DOSAGE AND ADMINISTRATION.**) However, the preservative formulation contains Benzyl Alcohol and must not be used for intrathecal or high-dose therapy.

Methotrexate Sodium Parenteral Isotonic Liquid Preservative Protected is available in 25 mg/mL, 2 mL (50 mg) and 10 mL (250 mg) vials.

Each 25 mg/mL, 2 mL and 10 mL vial contains methotrexate sodium equivalent to 50 mg and 250 mg methotrexate respectively, 0.90% w/v of Benzyl Alcohol as a preservative, and the following inactive ingredients: Sodium Chloride 0.260% w/v and Water for Injection qs ad 100% v. Sodium Hydroxide and, if necessary, Hydrochloric Acid are added to adjust the pH to approximately 8.5. Each 25 mg/mL, 2 mL vial contains methotrexate sodium equivalent to 50 mg methotrexate, 0.90% w/v of Benzyl Alcohol as a preservative, and the following inactive ingredients: Sodium Chloride 0.260% w/v and Water for Injection qs ad 100% v. Sodium Hydroxide and, if necessary, Hydrochloric Acid are added to adjust the pH to approximately 8.5.

Methotrexate LPF® Sodium Parenteral Isotonic Liquid, Preservative Free, for single use only, is available in 25 mg/mL, 2 mL (50 mg), 4 mL (100 mg), 8 mL (200 mg) and 10 mL (250 mg) vials.

Each 25 mg/mL, 2 mL, 4 mL, 8 mL and 10 mL vial contains methotrexate sodium equivalent to 50 mg, 100 mg, 200 mg, and 250 mg methotrexate respectively, and the following inactive ingredients: Sodium Chloride 0.490% w/v and Water for Injection qs ad 100% v. Sodium Hydroxide and, if necessary, Hydrochloric Acid are added to adjust the pH to approximately 8.5. The 2 mL, 4 mL, 8 mL and 10 mL solutions contain approximately 0.43 mEq, 0.86 mEq, 1.72 mEq and 2.15 mEq of Sodium per vial, respectively and are isotonic solutions.

Methotrexate Sodium Parenteral, Freeze Dried, Preservative Free, Low Sodium, for single use only, is available in 20 mg, 50 mg and 1 gram vials.

Each low sodium 20 mg, 50 mg and 1 g vial of cryodesiccated powder contains methotrexate sodium equivalent to 20 mg, 50 mg an 1 g methotrexate respectively. Contains no preservative. Sodium Hydroxide and, if necessary, Hydrochloric Acid are added during manufacture to adjust the pH. The 20 mg vial contains approximately 0.14 mEq of Sodium; the 50 mg vial contains approximately 0.33 mEq of Sodium, and the 1 g vial contains approximately 7 mEq Sodium.

CLINICAL PHARMACOLOGY

Methotrexate inhibits dihydrofolic acid reductase. Dihydrofolates must be reduced to tetrahydrofolates by this enzyme before they can be utilized as carriers of one-carbon groups in the synthesis of purine nucleotides and thymidylate. Therefore, methotrexate interferes with DNA synthesis, repair, and cellular replication. Actively proliferating tissues such as malignant cells, bone marrow, fetal cells, buccal and intestinal mucosa, and cells of the urinary bladder are in general more sensitive to this effect of methotrexate. When cellular proliferation in malignant tissues is greater than in most normal tissues, methotrexate may impair malignant growth without irreversible damage to normal tissues.

The mechanism of action in rheumatoid arthritis is unknown; it may affect immune function. Two reports describe *in vitro* methotrexate inhibition of DNA precursor uptake by stimulated mononuclear cells, and another describes, in animal polyarthritis, partial correction by methotrexate of spleen cell hyporesponsiveness and suppressed IL 2 production. Other laboratories, however, have been unable to demonstrate similar effects. Clarification of methotrexate's effect on immune activity and its relation to rheumatoid immunopathogenesis await further studies.

In patients with rheumatoid arthritis, effects of methotrexate on articular swelling and tenderness can be seen as early as 3 to 6 weeks. Although methotrexate clearly ameliorates symptoms of inflammation (pain, swelling, stiffness), there is no evidence that it induces remission of rheumatoid arthritis nor has a beneficial effect been demonstrated on bone erosions and other radiologic changes which result in impaired joint use, functional disability, and deformity.

Most studies of methotrexate in patients with rheumatoid arthritis are relatively short term (3 to 6 months). Limited data from long-term studies indicate that an initial clinical improvement is maintained for at least two years with continued therapy.

In psoriasis, the rate of production of epithelial cells in the skin is greatly increased over normal skin. This differential in proliferation rates is the basis for the use of methotrexate to control the psoriatic process.

Methotrexate in high doses, followed by leucovorin rescue, is used as a part of the treatment of patients with nonmetastatic osteosarcoma. The original rationale for high-dose methotrexate therapy was based on the concept of selective rescue of normal tissues by leucovorin. More recent evidence suggests that high-dose methotrexate may also overcome methotrexate resistance caused by impaired active transport, decreased affinity of dihydrofolic acid reductase for methotrexate, increased levels of dihydrofolic acid reductase resulting from gene amplification, or decreased polyglutamation of methotrexate. The actual mechanism of action is unknown.

Two Pediatric Oncology Group studies (one randomized and one nonrandomized) demonstrated a significant improvement in relapse-free survival in patients with nonmetastatic osteosarcoma, when high-dose methotrexate with leucovorin rescue was used in combination with other chemotherapeutic agents following surgical resection of the primary tumor. These studies were not designed to demonstrate the specific contribution of high-dose methotrexate/leucovorin rescue therapy to the efficacy of the combination. However, a contribution can be inferred from the reports of objective responses to this therapy in patients with metastatic osteosarcoma, and from reports of extensive tumor necrosis following preoperative administration of this therapy to patients with nonmetastatic osteosarcoma.

Pharmacokinetics: *Absorption:* In adults, oral absorption appears to be dose dependent. Peak serum levels are reached within one to two hours. At doses of 30 mg/m^2 or less, methotrexate is generally well absorbed with a mean bioavailability of about 60%. The absorption of doses greater than 80 mg/m^2 is significantly less, possibly due to a saturation effect.

In leukemic children, oral absorption has been reported to vary widely (23% to 95%). A twentyfold difference between highest and lowest peak levels (Cmax: 0.11 to 2.3 micromolar after a 20 mg/m^2 dose) has been reported. Significant interindividual variability has also been noted in time to peak concentration (Tmax: 0.67 to 4h after a 15 mg/m^2 dose) and fraction of dose absorbed. Food has been shown to delay absorption and reduce peak concentration.

Methotrexate is generally completely absorbed from parenteral routes of injection. After intramuscular injection, peak serum concentrations occur in 30 to 60 minutes.

Distribution: After intravenous administration, the initial volume of distribution is approximately 0.18 L/kg (18% of body weight) and steady-state volume of distribution is approximately 0.4 to 0.8 L/kg (40% to 80% of body weight). Methotrexate competes with reduced folates for active transport across cell membranes by means of a single carrier-mediated active transport process. At serum concentrations greater than 100 micromolar, passive diffusion becomes a major pathway by which effective intracellular concentrations can be achieved. Methotrexate in serum is approximately 50% protein bound. Laboratory studies demonstrate that it may be displaced from plasma albumin by various compounds including sulfonamides, salicylates, tetracyclines, chloramphenicol, and phenytoin.

Methotrexate does not penetrate the blood-cerebrospinal fluid barrier in therapeutic amounts when given orally or parenterally. High CSF concentrations of the drug may be attained by intrathecal administration.

In dogs, synovial fluid concentrations after oral dosing were higher in inflamed than uninflamed joints. Although salicylates did not interfere with this penetration, prior prednisone treatment reduced penetration into inflamed joints to the level of normal joints.

Metabolism: After absorption, methotrexate undergoes hepatic and intracellular metabolism to polyglutamated forms which can be converted back to methotrexate by hydrolase enzymes. These polyglutamates act as inhibitors of dihydrofolate reductase and thymidylate synthetase. Small amounts of methotrexate polyglutamates may remain in tissues for extended periods. The retention and prolonged drug action of these active metabolites vary among different cells, tissues and tumors. A small amount of metabolism to 7-hydroxymethotrexate may occur at doses commonly prescribed. Accumulation of this metabolite may become significant at the high doses used in osteogenic sarcoma. The aqueous solubility of 7-hydroxymethotrexate is three- to fivefold lower than the parent compound. Methotrexate is partially metabolized by intestinal flora after oral administration.

Half-Life: The terminal half-life reported for methotrexate is approximately three to ten hours for patients receiving treatment for psoriasis, or rheumatoid arthritis or low-dose antineoplastic therapy (less than 30 mg/m^2). For patients receiving high doses of methotrexate, the terminal half-life is eight to 15 hours.

Excretion: Renal excretion is the primary route of elimination and is dependent upon dosage and route of administration. With IV administration, 80% to 90% of the administered dose is excreted unchanged in the urine within 24 hours. There is limited biliary excretion amounting to 10% or less of the administered dose. Enterohepatic recirculation of methotrexate has been proposed.

Renal excretion occurs by glomerular filtration and active tubular secretion. Nonlinear elimination due to saturation of renal tubular reabsorption has been observed in psoriatic patients at doses between 7.5 and 30 mg. Impaired renal function, as well as concurrent use of drugs such as weak organic acids that also undergo tubular secretion, can markedly increase methotrexate serum levels. Excellent correlation has been reported between methotrexate clearance and endogenous creatinine clearance.

Methotrexate clearance rates vary widely and are generally decreased at higher doses. Delayed drug clearance has been identified as one of the major factors responsible for methotrexate toxicity. It has been postulated that the toxicity of methotrexate for normal tissues is more dependent upon the duration of exposure to the drug rather than the peak level achieved. When a patient has delayed drug elimination due to compromised renal function, a third-space effusion, or other causes, methotrexate serum concentrations may remain elevated for prolonged periods.

The potential for toxicity from high-dose regimens or delayed excretion is reduced by the administration of leucovorin calcium during the final phase of methotrexate plasma elimination. Pharmacokinetic monitoring of methotrexate serum concentrations may help identify those patients at high risk for methotrexate toxicity and aid in proper adjustment of leucovorin dosing. Guidelines for monitoring serum methotrexate levels, and for adjustment of leucovorin dosing to reduce the risk of methotrexate toxicity, are provided below in **DOSAGE AND ADMINISTRATION.**

Methotrexate has been detected in human breast milk. The highest breast milk to plasma concentration ratio reached was 0.08:1.

INDICATIONS AND USAGE

Neoplastic Diseases: Methotrexate is indicated in the treatment of gestational choriocarcinoma, chorioadenoma destruens, and hydatidiform mole.

In acute lymphocytic leukemia, methotrexate is indicated in the prophylaxis of meningeal leukemia and is used in maintenance therapy in combination with other chemotherapeutic agents. Methotrexate is also indicated in the treatment of meningeal leukemia.

Methotrexate is used alone or in combination with other anticancer agents in the treatment of breast cancer, epidermoid cancers of the head and neck, advanced mycosis fungoides, and lung cancer, particularly squamous cell and small cell types. Methotrexate is also used in combination with other chemotherapeutic agents in the treatment of advanced stage non-Hodgkin's lymphomas.

Methotrexate in high doses followed by leucovorin rescue in combination with other chemotherapeutic agents is effective in prolonging relapse-free survival in patients with nonmetastatic osteosarcoma who have undergone surgical resection or amputation for the primary tumor.

Psoriasis: Methotrexate is indicated in the symptomatic control of severe, recalcitrant, disabling psoriasis that is not adequately responsive to other forms of therapy, *but only when the diagnosis has been established, as by biopsy and/or after dermatologic consultation.* It is important to ensure that a psoriasis "flare" is not due to an undiagnosed concomitant disease affecting immune responses.

Rheumatoid Arthritis: Methotrexate is indicated in the management of selected adults with severe, active, classical or definite rheumatoid arthritis (ARA criteria) who have had an insufficient therapeutic response to, or are intolerant of, an adequate trial of first-line therapy including full dose NSAIDs and usually a trial of at least one or more disease-modifying antirheumatic drugs.

Aspirin, nonsteroidal anti-inflammatory agents, and/or low-dose steroids may be continued, although the possibility of increased toxicity with concomitant use of NSAIDs including salicylates has not been fully explored (see **PRECAUTIONS, Drug Interactions**). Steroids may be reduced gradually in patients who respond to methotrexate. Combined use of methotrexate with gold, penicillamine, hydroxychloroquine, sulfasalazine, or cytotoxic agents, has not been studied and may increase the incidence of adverse effects. Rest and physiotherapy as indicated should be continued.

CONTRAINDICATIONS

Methotrexate can cause fetal death or teratogenic effects when administered to a pregnant woman. Methotrexate is contraindicated in pregnant patients with psoriasis or rheumatoid arthritis and should be used in the treatment of neoplastic diseases only when the potential benefit outweighs the risk to the fetus. Women of childbearing potential should not be started on methotrexate unitl pregnancy is excluded and should be fully counseled on the serious risk to the fetus (see **PRECAUTIONS**) should they become pregnant while undergoing treatment. Pregnancy should be avoided if either partner is receiving methotrexate; during and for a minimum of three months after therapy for male patients, and during and for at least one ovulatory cycle after therapy for female patients. (See Boxed **WARNINGS**.)

Because of the potential for serious adverse reactions from methotrexate in breast fed infants, it is contraindicated in nursing mothers.

Patients with psoriasis or rheumatoid arthritis with alcoholism, alcoholic liver disease, or other chronic liver disease should not receive methotrexate.

Patients with psoriasis or rheumatoid arthritis who have overt or laboratory evidence of immunodeficiency syndromes should not receive methotrexate.

Patients with psoriasis or rheumatoid arthritis who have preexisting blood dyscrasias, such as bone marrow hypoplasia, leukopenia, thrombocytopenia, or significant anemia, should not receive methotrexate.

Patients with a known hypersensitivity to methotrexate should not receive the drug.

WARNINGS—SEE BOXED WARNINGS.

PRECAUTIONS

General: Methotrexate has the potential for serious toxicity (see Boxed **WARNINGS**). Toxic effects may be related in frequency and severity to dose or frequency of administration but have been seen at all doses. Because they can occur at any time during therapy, it is necessary to follow patients on methotrexate closely. Most adverse reactions are reversible if detected early. When such reactions do occur, the drug should be reduced in dosage or discontinued and appropriate corrective measures should be taken. If necessary, this could include the use of leucovorin calcium (see **OVERDOSAGE**). If methotrexate therapy is reinstituted, it should be carried out with caution, with adequate consideration of further need for the drug, and with increased alertness as to possible recurrence of toxicity.

The clinical pharmacology of methotrexate has not been well studied in older individuals. Due to diminished hepatic and renal function as well as decreased folate stores in this population, relatively low doses should be considered, and these patients should be closely monitored for early signs of toxicity.

Information for Patients: Patients should be informed of the early signs and symptoms of toxicity, of the need to see their physician promptly if they occur, and the need for close follow-up, including periodic laboratory tests to monitor toxicity.

Both the physician and pharmacist should emphasize to the patient that the recommended dose is taken weekly in rheumatoid arthritis and psoriasis, and that mistaken daily use of the recommended dose has led to fatal toxicity. Patients should be encouraged to read the Patient Instructions sheet within the Dose Pack. Prescriptions should not be written or refilled on a PRN basis.

Patients should be informed of the potential benefit and risk in the use of methotrexate. The risk of effects on reproduction should be discussed with both male and female patients taking methotrexate.

Laboratory Tests: Patients undergoing methotrexate therapy should be closely monitored so that toxic effects are detected promptly. Baseline assessment should include a complete blood count with differential and platelet counts, hepatic enzymes, renal function tests, and a chest X-ray. During therapy of rheumatoid arthritis and psoriasis, monitoring of these parameters is recommended: hematology at least monthly, and liver and renal function every 1 to 3 months. More frequent monitoring is usually indicated during antineoplastic therapy. *During initial or changing doses*, or during periods of increased risk of elevated methotrexate blood levels (eg, dehydration), more frequent monitoring may also be indicated.

A relationship between abnormal liver function tests and fibrosis or cirrhosis of the liver has not been established. Transient liver function test abnormalities are observed frequently after methotrexate administration and are usually not cause for modification of methotrexate therapy. Persistent liver function test abnormalities just prior to dosing and/or depression of serum albumin may be indicators of serious liver toxicity and require evaluation.

Pulmonary function tests may be useful if methotrexate-induced lung disease is suspected, especially if baseline measurements are available.

Drug Interactions: Nonsteroidal anti-inflammatory drugs should not be administered prior to or concomitantly with the high doses of methotrexate used in the treatment of osteosarcoma. Concomitant administration of some NSAIDs with high-dose methotrexate therapy has been reported to elevate and prolong serum methotrexate levels, resulting in deaths from severe hematologic and gastrointestinal toxicity.

Caution should be used when NSAIDs and salicylates are administered concomitantly with lower doses of methotrexate. These drugs have been reported to reduce the tubular secretion of methotrexate in an animal model and may enhance its toxicity.

Despite the potential interactions, studies of methotrexate in patients with rheumatoid arthritis have usually included concurrent use of dosage regimens of NSAIDs, without apparent problems. It should be appreciated however, that the doses used in rheumatoid arthritis (7.5 to 15 mg/week) are somewhat lower than those used in psoriasis and that larger doses could lead to unexpected toxicity.

Methotrexate is partially bound to serum albumin, and toxicity may be increased because of displacement by certain drugs, such as salicylates, phenylbutazone, phenytoin, and sulfonamides. Renal tubular transport is also diminished by probenecid; use of methotrexate with this drug should be carefully monitored.

In the treatment of patients with osteosarcoma, caution must be exercised if high-dose methotrexate is administered in combination with a potentially nephrotoxic chemotherapeutic agent (eg, cisplatin).

Oral antibiotics such as tetracycline, chloramphenicol, and nonabsorbable broad-spectrum antibiotics, may decrease intestinal absorption of methotrexate or interfere with the enterohepatic circulation by inhibiting bowel flora and suppressing metabolism of the drug by bacteria.

Vitamin preparations containing folic acid or its derivatives may decrease responses to systemically administered methotrexate. Preliminary animal and human studies have shown that small quantities of intravenously administered leucovorin enter the CSF primarily as 5-methyltetrahydrofolate and, in humans, remain 1–3 orders of magnitude lower than the usual methotrexate concentrations following intrathecal administration. However, high doses of leucovorin may reduce the efficacy of intrathecally administered methotrexate.

Folate deficiency states may increase methotrexate toxicity. Trimethoprim/sulfamethoxazole has been reported rarely to increase bone marrow suppression in patients receiving methotrexate, probably by an additive antifolate effect.

Carcinogenesis, Mutagenesis, and Impairment of Fertility: No controlled human data exist regarding the risk of neoplasia with methotrexate. Methotrexate has been evaluated in a number of animal studies for carcinogenic potential with inconclusive results. Although, there is evidence that methotrexate causes chromosomal damage to animal somatic cells and human bone marrow cells, the clinical significance remains uncertain. Assessment of the carcinogenic potential of methotrexate is complicated by conflicting evidence of an increased risk of certain tumors in rheumatoid arthritis. Benefit should be weighed against this potential risk before using methotrexate alone or in combination with other drugs, especially in children or young adults. Methotrexate causes embryotoxicity, abortion, and fetal defects in humans. It has also been reported to cause impairment of fertility, oligospermia and menstrual dysfunction in humans, during and for a short period after cessation of therapy.

Pregnancy: Psoriasis and rheumatoid arthritis: Methotrexate is in Pregnancy Category X. See **CONTRAINDICATIONS**.

Nursing Mothers: See **CONTRAINDICATIONS**.

Pediatric Use: Safety and effectiveness in children have not been established, other than in cancer chemotherapy.

Organ System Toxicity: Gastrointestinal: If vomiting, diarrhea, or stomatitis occur, which may result in dehydration, methotrexate should be discontinued until recovery occurs. Methotrexate should be used with extreme caution in the presence of peptic ulcer disease or ulcerative colitis.

Hematologic: Methotrexate can suppress hematopoiesis and cause anemia, leukopenia, and/or thrombocytopenia. In patients with malignancy and preexisting hematopoietic impairment, the drug should be used with caution, if at all. In controlled clinical trials in rheumatoid arthritis (n = 128), leukopenia (WBC < 3000/mm^3) was seen in 2 patients, thrombocytopenia (platelets < 100,000/mm^3) in 6 patients, and pancytopenia in 2 patients.

In psoriasis and rheumatoid arthritis, methotrexate should be stopped immediately if there is a significant drop in blood counts. In the treatment of neoplastic diseases, methotrexate should be continued only if the potential benefit warrants the risk of severe myelosuppression. Patients with profound granulocytopenia and fever should be evaluated immediately and usually require parenteral broad-spectrum antibiotic therapy.

Hepatic: Methotrexate has the potential for acute (elevated transaminases) and chronic (fibrosis and cirrhosis) hepatotoxicity. Chronic toxicity is potentially fatal; it generally has occurred after prolonged use (generally two years or more) and after a total dose of at least 1.5 grams. In studies in psoriatic patients, hepatotoxicity appeared to be a function of total cumulative dose and appeared to be enhanced by alcoholism, obesity, diabetes, and advanced age. An accurate incidence rate has not been determined; the rate of progression and reversibility of lesions is not known. Special caution is indicated in the presence of preexisting liver damage or impaired hepatic function.

Liver function tests, including serum albumin, should be performed periodically prior to dosing but are often normal in the face of developing fibrosis or cirrhosis. These lesions may be detectable only by biopsy.

In psoriasis, the usual recommendation is to obtain a liver biopsy at a total cumulative dose of 1.5 grams. Moderate fibrosis or any cirrhosis normally leads to discontinuation of the drug; mild fibrosis normally suggests a repeat biopsy in 6 months. Milder histologic findings, such as fatty change and low grade portal inflammation, are relatively common pretherapy. Although these mild changes are usually not a reason to avoid or discontinue methotrexate therapy, the drug should be used with caution.

Clinical experience with liver disease in rheumatoid arthritis is limited, but the same risk factors should be anticipated. Liver function tests are also usually not reliable predictors of histological changes in this population.

When to perform a liver biopsy in rheumatoid arthritis patients has not been established, either in terms of cumulative methotrexate dose or duration of therapy. There is a combined reported experience in 217 rheumatoid arthritis patients with liver biopsies both before and during treatment (after a cumulative dose of at least 1500 mg) and in 714 patients with a biopsy only during treatment. There are 64 (7%) cases of fibrosis and 1 (0.1%) case of cirrhosis. Of the 64 cases of fibrosis, 60 were deemed mild. The reticulin stain is more sensitive for early fibrosis and its use may increase these figures. It is unknown whether even longer use will increase these risks.

Infection or Immunologic States: Methotrexate should be used with extreme caution in the presence of active infection, and is usually contraindicated in patients with overt or laboratory evidence of immunodeficiency syndromes. Immunization may be ineffective when given during methotrexate therapy. Immunization with live virus vaccines is generally not recommended. There have been reports of disseminated vaccinia infections after smallpox immunization in patients receiving methotrexate therapy. Hypogammaglobulinemia has been reported rarely.

Neurologic: There have been reports of leukoencephalopathy following intravenous administration of methotrexate to patients who have had craniospinal irradiation. Chronic leukoencephalopathy has also been reported in patients with osteosarcoma who received repeated doses of high-dose methotrexate with leucovorin rescue even without cranial irradiation. Discontinuation of methotrexate does not always result in complete recovery.

A transient acute neurologic syndrome has been observed in patients treated with high dosage regimens. Manifestations of this neurologic disorder may include behavioral abnormalities, focal sensorimotor signs, and abnormal reflexes. The exact cause is unknown.

After the intrathecal use of methotrexate, the central nervous system toxicity which may occur can be classified as follows: chemical arachnoiditis manifested by such symptoms as headache, back pain, nuchal rigidity, and fever; paresis, usually transient, manifested by paraplegia associated with involvement with one or more spinal nerve roots; leukoencephalopathy manifested by confusion, irritability, somnolence, ataxia, dementia, and occasionally major convulsions.

Pulmonary: Pulmonary symptoms (especially a dry, nonproductive cough) or a nonspecific pneumonitis occurring during methotrexate therapy may be indicative of a potentially dangerous lesion and require interruption of treatment and careful investigation. Although clinically variable, the typical patient with methotrexate-induced lung disease presents with fever, cough, dyspnea, hypoxemia, and an infiltrate on chest X-ray; infection needs to be excluded. This lesion can occur at all dosages.

Renal: High doses of methotrexate used in the treatment of osteosarcoma may cause renal damage leading to acute renal failure. Nephrotoxicity is due primarily to the precipitation of methotrexate and 7-hydroxymethotrexate in the renal tubules. Close attention to renal function including adequate hydration, urine alkalinization and measurement of serum methotrexate and creatinine levels are essential for safe administration.

Continued on next page

Information on Lederle products listed on these pages is the full prescribing information from product literature or package inserts effective in August, 1989. Information concerning all Lederle products may be obtained from the Professional Services Department, Lederle Laboratories, Pearl River, New York, 10965.

Lederle—Cont.

Other precautions: Methotrexate should be used with extreme caution in the presence of debility.

Methotrexate exits slowly from third-space compartments (eg, pleural effusions or ascites). This results in a prolonged terminal plasma half-life and unexpected toxicity. In patients with significant third-space accumulations, it is advisable to evacuate the fluid before treatment and to monitor plasma methotrexate levels.

Lesions of psoriasis may be aggravated by concomitant exposure to ultraviolet radiation. Radiation dermatitis and sunburn may be "recalled" by the use of methotrexate.

ADVERSE REACTIONS

IN GENERAL, THE INCIDENCE AND SEVERITY OF ACUTE SIDE EFFECTS ARE RELATED TO DOSE AND FREQUENCY OF ADMINISTRATION. THE MOST SERIOUS REACTIONS ARE DISCUSSED ABOVE UNDER ORGAN SYSTEM TOXICITY IN THE PRECAUTION SECTION. THAT SECTION SHOULD ALSO BE CONSULTED WHEN LOOKING FOR INFORMATION ABOUT ADVERSE REACTIONS WITH METHOTREXATE.

The most frequently reported adverse reactions include ulcerative stomatitis, leukopenia, nausea, and abdominal distress. Other frequently reported adverse effects are malaise, undue fatigue, chills and fever, dizziness, and decreased resistance to infection.

Other adverse reactions that have been reported with methotrexate are listed below by organ system. In the oncology setting, concomitant treatment and the underlying disease make specific attribution of a reaction to methotrexate difficult.

Alimentary System: Gingivitis, pharyngitis, stomatitis, anorexia, nausea, vomiting, diarrhea, hematemesis, melena, gastrointestinal ulceration and bleeding, enteritis.

Central Nervous System: Headaches, drowsiness, blurred vision. Aphasia, hemiparesis, paresis, and convulsions have also occurred following administration of methotrexate.

Pulmonary System: Interstitial pneumonitis deaths have been reported, and chronic interstitial obstructive pulmonary disease has occasionally occurred.

Skin: Erythematous rashes, pruritus, urticaria, photosensitivity, pigmentary changes, alopecia, ecchymosis, telangiectasia, acne, furunculosis.

Urogenital System: Severe nephropathy or renal failure, azotemia, cystitis, hematuria; defective oogenesis or spermatogenesis, transient oligospermia, menstrual dysfunction and vaginal discharge; infertility, abortion, fetal defects.

Other rarer reactions related to or attributed to the use of methotrexate such as arthralgia/myalgia, diabetes, osteoporosis and sudden death. A few cases of anaphylactoid reactions have been reported.

Adverse Reactions in Double-Blind Rheumatoid Arthritis Studies: The approximate incidences of methotrexate-attributed (ie, placebo rate subtracted) adverse reactions in 12-to 18-week double-blind studies of patients (n = 128) with rheumatoid arthritis treated with low-dose oral (7.5–15 mg/week) pulse methotrexate, are listed below. Virtually all of these patients were on concomitant nonsteroidal anti-inflammatory medication and some were also taking low dosages of corticosteroids.

Incidence greater than 10%: Elevated liver function tests 15%, nausea/vomiting 10%.

Incidence 3% to 10%: Stomatitis, thrombocytopenia, (platelet count less than 100,000/mm³).

Incidence 1% to 3%: Rash/pruritus/dermatitis, diarrhea, alopecia, leukopenia (WBC <3000/mm³), pancytopenia, dizziness.

No pulmonary toxicity was seen in these two trials. Thus, the incidence is probably less than 2.5% (95% C.L.). Hepatic histology was not examined in these short-term studies (see PRECAUTIONS).

Other less common reactions included decreased hematocrit, headache, upper respiratory infection, anorexia, arthralgias, chest pain, coughing, dysuria, eye discomfort, epistaxis, fever, infection, sweating, tinnitus, and vaginal discharge.

Adverse Reactions in Psoriasis: There are no recent placebo-controlled trials in patients with psoriasis. There are two literature reports (Roenigk, 1969 and Nyfors, 1978) describing large series (n = 204, 248) of psoriasis patients treated with methotrexate. Dosages ranged up to 25 mg per week, and treatment was administered for up to four years. With the exception of alopecia, photosensitivity, and "burning of skin lesions" (each 3% to 10%), the adverse reaction rates in these reports were very similar to those in the rheumatoid arthritis studies.

OVERDOSAGE

Leucovorin is indicated to diminish the toxicity and counteract the effect of inadvertently administered overdosages of methotrexate. Leucovorin administration should begin as promptly as possible. As the time interval between methotrexate administration and leucovorin initiation increases, the effectiveness of leucovorin in counteracting toxicity de-creases. Monitoring of the serum methotrexate concentration is essential in determining the optimal dose and duration of treatment with leucovorin.

In cases of massive overdosage, hydration and urinary alkalinization may be necessary to prevent the precipitation of methotrexate and/or its metabolites in the renal tubules. Neither hemodialysis nor peritoneal dialysis has been shown to improve methotrexate elimination.

DOSAGE AND ADMINISTRATION

Neoplastic Diseases: Oral administration in tablet form is often preferred when low doses are being administered since absorption is rapid and effective serum levels are obtained. Methotrexate sodium parenteral may be given by the intramuscular, intravenous, intra-arterial or intrathecal route. However, the preserved formulation contains Benzyl Alcohol and must not be used for intrathecal or high-dose therapy.

Choriocarcinoma and similar trophoblastic diseases: Methotrexate is administered orally or intramuscularly in doses of 15 to 30 mg daily for a five-day course. Such courses are usually repeated for 3 to 5 times as required, with rest periods of one or more weeks interposed between courses, until any manifesting toxic symptoms subside. The effectiveness of therapy is ordinarily evaluated by 24-hour quantitative analysis of urinary chorionic gonadotropin (hCG), which should return to normal or less than 50 IU/24h usually after the third or fourth course and usually be followed by a complete resolution of measurable lesions in 4 to 6 weeks. One to two courses of methotrexate after normalization of hCG is usually recommended. Before each course of the drug careful clinical assessment is essential. Cyclic combination therapy of methotrexate with other antitumor drugs has been reported as being usual.

Since hydatidiform mole may precede choriocarcinoma, prophylactic chemotherapy with methotrexate has been recommended.

Chorioadenoma destruens is considered to be an invasive form of hydatidiform mole. Methotrexate is administered in these disease states in doses similar to those recommended for choriocarcinoma.

Leukemia: Acute lymphoblastic leukemia in children and young adolescents is the most responsive to present day chemotherapy. In young adults and older patients, clinical remission is more difficult to obtain and early relapse is more common.

Methotrexate alone or in combination with steroids was used initially for induction of remission in acute lymphoblastic leukemias. More recently corticosteroid therapy, in combination with other antileukemic drugs or in cyclic combinations with methotrexate included, has appeared to produce rapid and effective remissions. When used for induction, methotrexate in doses of 3.3 mg/m² in combination with 60 mg/m² of prednisone, given daily, produced remissions in 50% of patients treated, usually within a period of 4 to 6 weeks. Methotrexate in combination with other agents appears to be the drug of choice for securing maintenance of drug-induced remissions. When remission is achieved and supportive care has produced general clinical improvement, maintenance therapy is initiated, as follows: Methotrexate is administered 2 times weekly either by mouth or intramuscularly in total weekly doses of 30 mg/m². It has also been given in doses of 2.5 mg/kg intravenously every 14 days. If and when relapse does occur, reinduction of remission can again usually be obtained by repeating the initial induction regimen.

A variety of combination chemotherapy regimens have been used for both induction and maintenance therapy in acute lymphoblastic leukemia. The physician should be familiar with the new advances in antileukemic therapy.

Meningeal leukemia: In the treatment or prophylaxis of meningeal leukemia, methotrexate must be administered intrathecally. Preservative-free methotrexate is diluted to a concentration of 1 mg/mL in an appropriate sterile, preservative-free medium such as 0.9% Sodium Chloride Injection, USP.

The cerebrospinal fluid volume is dependent on age and not on body surface area. The CSF is at 40% of the adult volume at birth and reaches the adult volume in several years.

Intrathecal methotrexate administration at a dose of 12 mg/m² (maximum 15 mg) has been reported to result in low CSF methotrexate concentrations and reduced efficacy in children and high concentrations and neurotoxicity in adults. The following dosage regimen is based on age instead of body surface area:

Age (years)	Dose (mg)
<1	6
1	8
2	10
3 or older	12

In one study in patients under the age of 40, this dosage regimen appeared to result in more consistent CSF methotrexate concentrations and less neurotoxicity. Another study in chil-dren with acute lymphocytic leukemia compared this regimen to a dose of 12 mg/m² (maximum 15 mg). A significant reduction in the rate of CNS relapse was observed in the group whose dose was based on age.

Because the CSF volume and turnover may decrease with age, a dose reduction may be indicated in elderly patients. For the treatment of meningeal leukemia, intrathecal methotrexate may be given at intervals of 2 to 5 days. However, administration at intervals of less than 1 week may result in increased subacute toxicity. Methotrexate is administered until the cell count of the cerebrospinal fluid returns to normal. At this point one additional dose is advisable. For prophylaxis against meningeal leukemia, the dosage is the same as for treatment except for the intervals of administration. On this subject, it is advisable for the physician to consult the medical literature.

Untoward side effects may occur with any given intrathecal injection and are commonly neurological in character. Large doses may cause convulsions. Methotrexate given by the intrathecal route appears significantly in the systemic circulation and may cause systemic methotrexate toxicity. Therefore, systemic antileukemic therapy with the drug should be appropriately adjusted, reduced, or discontinued. Focal leukemic involvement of the central nervous system may not respond to intrathecal chemotherapy and is best treated with radiotherapy.

Lymphomas: In Burkitt's Tumor, Stages I–II, methotrexate has produced prolonged remissions in some cases. Recommended dosage is 10 to 25 mg/day orally for 4 to 8 days. In stage III, methotrexate is commonly given concomitantly with other antitumor agents. Treatment in all stages usually consists of several courses of the drug interposed with 7- to 10-day rest periods. Lymphosarcomas in Stage III may respond to combined drug therapy with methotrexate given in doses of 0.625 to 2.5 mg/kg daily.

Mycosis fungoides: Therapy with methotrexate appears to produce clinical remissions in one half of the cases treated. Dosage is usually 2.5 to 10 mg daily by mouth for weeks or months. Dose levels of drug and adjustment of dose regimen by reduction or cessation of drug are guided by patient response and hematologic monitoring. Methotrexate has also been given intramuscularly in doses of 50 mg once weekly or 25 mg 2 times weekly.

Osteosarcoma: An effective adjuvant chemotherapy regimen requires the administration of several cytotoxic chemotherapeutic agents. In addition to high-dose methotrexate with leucovorin rescue, these agents may include doxorubicin, cisplatin, and the combination of bleomycin, cyclophosphamide and dactinomycin (BCD) in the doses and schedule shown in the table below. The starting dose for high-dose methotrexate treatment is 12 grams/m². If this dose is not sufficient to produce a peak serum methotrexate concentration of 1,000 micromolar (10^{-3} mol/L) at the end of the methotrexate infusion, the dose may be escalated to 15 grams/m² in subsequent treatments. If the patient is vomiting or is unable to tolerate oral medication, leucovorin is given IV or IM at the same dose and schedule.

[See table on next page].

When these higher doses of methotrexate are to be administered, the following safety guidelines should be closely observed.

GUIDELINES FOR METHOTREXATE THERAPY WITH LEUCOVORIN RESCUE

1. Administration of methotrexate should be delayed until recovery if:
   - the WBC count is <1500/microliter
   - the neutrophil count is <200/microliter
   - the platelet count is <75,000/microliter
   - the serum bilirubin level is >1.2 mg/dL
   - the SGPT level is >450 U
   - mucositis is present, until there is evidence of healing
   - persistent pleural effusion is present; this should be drained dry prior to infusion.

2. Adequate renal function must be documented.
   a. Serum creatinine must be normal, and creatinine clearance must be greater than 60 mL/min, before initiation of therapy.
   b. Serum creatinine must be measured prior to each subsequent course of therapy. If serum creatinine has increased by 50% or more compared to a prior value, the creatinine clearance must be measured and documented to be greater than 60 mL/min (even if the serum creatinine is still within the normal range).

3. Patients must be well hydrated, and must be treated with sodium bicarbonate for urinary alkalinization.
   a. Administer 1,000 mL/m² of intravenous fluid over 6 hours prior to initiation of the methotrexate infusion. Continue hydration at 125 mL/m²/hr (3 liters/m²/day) during the methotrexate infusion, and for 2 days after the infusion has been completed.
   b. Alkalinize urine to maintain pH above 7.0 during methotrexate infusion and leucovorin calcium therapy. This can be accomplished by the administration of sodium bicarbonate orally or by incorporation into a separate intravenous solution.

4. Repeat serum creatinine and serum methotrexate 24 hours after starting methotrexate and at least once daily until the methotrexate level is below 5×10^{-8} mol/L (0.05 micromolar).

5. The table below provides guidelines for leucovorin calcium dosage based upon serum methotrexate levels. (See table below.‡)

Patients who experience delayed early methotrexate elimination are likely to develop nonreversible oliguric renal failure. In addition to appropriate leucovorin therapy, these patients require continuing hydration and urinary alkalinization, and close monitoring of fluid and electrolyte status, until the serum methotrexate level has fallen to below 0.05 micromolar and the renal failure has resolved.

6. Some patients will have abnormalities in methotrexate elimination, or abnormalities in renal function following methotrexate administration, which are significant but less severe than the abnormalities described in the table below. These abnormalities may or may not be associated with significant clinical toxicity. If significant clinical toxicity is observed, leucovorin rescue should be extended for an additional 24 hours (total 14 doses over 84 hours) in subsequent courses of therapy. The possibility that the patient is taking other medications which interact with methotrexate (eg, medications which may interfere with methotrexate binding to serum albumin, or elimination) should always be reconsidered when laboratory abnormalities or clinical toxicities are observed.

Psoriasis and Rheumatoid Arthritis: *The patient should be fully informed of the risks involved and should be under constant supervision of the physician.* (See **Information for Patients** under **PRECAUTIONS**.) Assessment of hematologic, hepatic, renal, and pulmonary function should be made by history, physical examination, and laboratory tests before beginning, periodically during, and before reinstituting methotrexate therapy (see **PRECAUTIONS**). Appropriate steps should be taken to avoid conception during methotrexate therapy. (See **PRECAUTIONS** and **CONTRAINDICATIONS**.)

Weekly therapy may be instituted with the RHEUMATREX® Methotrexate 2.5 mg Tablet Dose Packs which are designed to provide doses over a range of 5 mg to 15 mg administered as a single weekly dose. The dose packs are not recommended for administration of methotrexate in weekly doses greater than 15 mg. All schedules should be continually tailored to the individual patient. An initial test dose may be given prior to the regular dosing schedule to detect any extreme sensitivity to adverse effects (See **ADVERSE REACTIONS**). Maximal myelosuppression usually occurs in seven to ten days.

Psoriasis: Recommended Starting Dose Schedules
1. Weekly single oral, IM or IV dose schedule: 10 to 25 mg per week until adequate response is achieved.
2. Divided oral dose schedule: 2.5 mg at 12-hour intervals for three doses.

Dosages in each schedule may be gradually adjusted to achieve optimal clinical response; 30 mg/week should not ordinarily be exceeded.

Once optimal clinical response has been achieved, each dosage schedule should be reduced to the lowest possible amount of drug and to the longest possible rest period. The use of methotrexate may permit the return to conventional topical therapy, which should be encouraged.

Rheumatoid Arthritis: Recommended Starting Dosage Schedules
1. Single oral doses of 7.5 mg once weekly.

Drug*	Dose*	Treatment Week After Surgery
Methotrexate	12g/m² IV as 4 hour infusion (starting dose)	4, 5, 6, 7, 11, 12, 15, 16, 29, 30, 44, 45
Leucovorin	15 mg orally every six hours for 10 doses starting at 24 hours after start of methotrexate infusion.	
Doxorubicin† as a single drug	30 mg/m²/day IV × 3 days	8, 17
Doxorubicin†	50 mg/m² IV	20, 23, 33, 36
Cisplatin†	100 mg/m² IV	20, 23, 33, 36
Bleomycin†	15 units/m² IV × 2 days	2, 13, 26, 39, 42
Cyclophosphamide†	600 mg/m² IV × 2 days	2, 13, 26, 39, 42
Dactinomycin†	0.6 mg/m² IV × 2 days	2, 13, 26, 39, 42

* Link MP, Goorin AM, Miser AW, et al: The effect of adjuvant chemotherapy on relapse-free survival in patients with osteosarcoma of the extremity. *N Engl J Med* 1986; 314(no.25):1600–1606.
† See each respective package insert for full prescribing information. Dosage modifications may be necessary because of drug-induced toxicity.

2. Divided oral dosages of 2.5 mg at 12-hour intervals for 3 doses given as a course once weekly.

Dosages in each schedule may be adjusted gradually to achieve an optimal response, but not ordinarily to exceed a total weekly dose of 20 mg. Limited experience shows a significant increase in the incidence and severity of serious toxic reactions, especially bone marrow suppression, at doses greater than 20 mg/wk.

Once response has been achieved, each schedule should be reduced, if possible, to the lowest possible effective dose.

Therapeutic response usually begins within 3 to 6 weeks and the patient may continue to improve for another 12 weeks or more.

The optimal duration of therapy is unknown. Limited data available from long-term studies indicate that the initial clinical improvement is maintained for at least two years with continued therapy. When methotrexate is discontinued, the arthritis usually worsens within 3 to 6 weeks.

HANDLING AND DISPOSAL
Procedures for proper handling and disposal of anticancer drugs should be considered. Several guidelines on this subject have been published.[1-6] There is no general agreement that all of the procedures recommended in the guidelines are necessary or appropriate.

RECONSTITUTION OF LOW SODIUM CRYO-DESICCATED POWDERS
Reconstitute immediately prior to use.

Methotrexate parenteral should be reconstituted with an appropriate sterile, preservative-free medium such as 5% Dextrose Solution, USP, or Sodium Chloride Injection, USP. Reconstitute the 20 mg and 50 mg vials to a concentration no greater than 25 mg/mL. **The 1 gram vial should be reconstituted with 19.4 mL to a concentration of 50 mg/mL.**

When high doses of methotrexate are administered by IV infusion, the total dose is diluted in 5% Dextrose Solution. For intrathecal injection, reconstitute to a concentration of 1 mg/mL with an appropriate sterile, preservative-free medium such as Sodium Chloride Injection, USP.

DILUTION INSTRUCTIONS FOR LIQUID METHOTREXATE SODIUM PARENTERAL PRODUCTS
Methotrexate Sodium Parenteral, Preserved: If desired, the solution may be further diluted with a compatible medium such as Sodium Chloride Injection, USP. Storage for 24 hours at a temperature of 21° to 25° C results in a product which is within 90% of label potency.

Methotrexate LPF® Sodium Parenteral, Isotonic, Preservative-Free, for Single Use Only: If desired, the solution may be further diluted immediately prior to use with an appropriate sterile, preservative-free medium such as 5% Dextrose Solution, USP or Sodium Chloride Injection, USP.

HOW SUPPLIED
Parenterals:
Methotrexate Sodium Parenteral Freeze-Dried, Preservative-Free Low Sodium for Single Use Only
NDC 0205-4654-90 (Dark Blue Cap)—20 mg vial
NDC 0205-9337-92 (Violet Cap)—50 mg vial
NDC 0205-4653-02 (Red Cap)—1 gram vial

Military Depot:
NSN 6505-01-125-6505—25 mg/mL—8 mL vial
Methotrexate LPF® Sodium Parenteral Isotonic Liquid Preservative-Free, for Single Use Only
NDC 0205-5325-26 (Brown Cap)—50 mg (25 mg/mL)—2 mL vials
NDC 0205-5326-18 (Light Blue Cap)—100 mg (25 mg/mL)—4 mL vials
NDC 0205-5327-30 (Orange Cap)—200 mg (25 mg/mL)—8 mL vials
NDC 0205-5337-34 (Violet Cap)—250 mg (25 mg/mL)—10 mL vials
NDC 0205-5337-98 (Violet Cap)—250 mg (25 mg/mL)—10 mL vials—25 vials per box
Methotrexate Sodium Parenteral Isotonic Liquid Preservative Protected
NDC 0205-4556-26 (Red Cap)—50 mg (25 mg/mL)—2 mL vials
NDC 0205-5338-34 (Brown Cap)—250 mg (25 mg/mL)—10 mL vials
Store at Controlled Room Temperature 15°–30°C (59°–86° F). Protect From Light.
LEDERLE PARENTERALS, INC.
Carolina, Puerto Rico 00630

Oral: Description: Methotrexate tablets contain an amount of methotrexate sodium equivalent to 2.5 mg of methotrexate and are round, convex, yellow tablets, engraved with LL on one side, scored in half on the other side, and engraved with M above the score, and 1 below.
NDC 0005-4507-23—Bottle of 100
NDC 0005-4507-04—RHEUMATREX® Methotrexate 2.5 mg Tablet Dose Pack: 4 cards each containing two 2.5 mg tablets, ie, 5 mg per week.
NDC 0005-4507-05—RHEUMATREX® Methotrexate 2.5 mg Tablet Dose Pack: 4 cards each containing three 2.5 mg tablets, ie, 7.5 mg per week.
NDC 0005-4507-07—RHEUMATREX® Methotrexate 2.5 mg Tablet Dose Pack: 4 cards each containing four 2.5 mg tablets, ie, 10 mg per week.
NDC 0005-4507-09—RHEUMATREX® Methotrexate 2.5 mg Tablet Dose Pack: 4 cards each containing five 2.5 mg tablets, ie, 12.5 mg per week.

Continued on next page

Information on Lederle products listed on these pages is the full prescribing information from product literature or package inserts effective in August, 1989. Information concerning all Lederle products may be obtained from the Professional Services Department, Lederle Laboratories, Pearl River, New York, 10965.

‡LEUCOVORIN RESCUE SCHEDULES FOLLOWING TREATMENT WITH HIGHER DOSES OF METHOTREXATE

Clinical Situation	Laboratory Findings	Leucovorin Dosage and Duration
Normal Methotrexate Elimination	Serum methotrexate level approximately 10 micromolar at 24 hours after administration, 1 micromolar at 48 hours, and less than 0.2 micromolar at 72 hours.	15 mg PO, IM or IV q6h for 60h (10 doses starting at 24h after start of methotrexate infusion).
Delayed Late Methotrexate Elimination	Serum methotrexate level remaining above 0.2 micromolar at 72 hours, and more than 0.05 micromolar at 96 hours after administration.	Continue 15 mg PO, IM or IV q6h, until methotrexate level is less than 0.05 micromolar.
Delayed Early Methotrexate Elimination and/or Evidence of Acute Renal Injury	Serum methotrexate level of 50 micromolar or more at 24 hours, or 5 micromolar or more at 48 hours after administration, OR; a 100% or greater increase in serum creatinine level at 24 hours after methotrexate administration (eg, an increase from 0.5 mg/dL to a level of 1.0 mg/dL or more).	150 mg IV q3h, until methotrexate level is less than 1 micromolar; then 15 mg IV q3h, until methotrexate level is less than 0.05 micromolar.

Lederle—Cont.

NDC 0005-4507-91—RHEUMATREX® Methotrexate 2.5 mg Tablet Dose Pack: 4 cards each containing six 2.5 mg tablets, ie, 15 mg per week.
Military Depot:
NSN 6505-00-963-5353—Bottle of 100
Store at Controlled Room Temperature 15°–30° C (59°–86° F). Protect From Light.
LEDERLE LABORATORIES DIVISION
American Cyanamid Company, Pearl River, NY 10965
Rev. 6/89
21516

REFERENCES

1. Recommendations for the Safe Handling of Parenteral Antineoplastic Drugs. NIH Publication No. 83-2621. For sale by the Superintendent of Documents, U.S. Government Printing Office, Washington, D.C. 20402.
2. AMA Council Report. Guidelines for Handling Parenteral Antineoplastics. *JAMA*, March 15, 1985.
3. National Study Commission on Cytotoxic Exposure—Recommendations for Handling Cytotoxic Agents. Available from Louis P. Jeffrey, Sc. D., Director of Pharmacy Services, Rhode Island Hospital, 593 Eddy Street, Providence, Rhode Island 02902.
4. Clinical Oncological Society of Australia: Guidelines and recommendations for safe handling of antineoplastic agents. *Med J Australia* 1983; 1:426–428.
5. Jones, R.B., et al. Safe handling of chemotherapeutic agents: A report from the Mount Sinai Medical Center. *CA: A Cancer Journal for Clinicians* Sept/Oct, 1983; 258–263.
6. American Society of Hospital Pharmacists technical assistance bulletin on handling cytotoxic drugs in hospitals. *Am J Hosp Pharm* 1985; 42:131–137.

Shown in Product Identification Section, page 415

MINOCIN®

[mĭ-nŏ-sĭn]
Sterile
minocycline hydrochloride
Intravenous
100 mg/Vial

DESCRIPTION

MINOCIN, a semisynthetic derivative of tetracycline, is named [4S-(4α, 4aα, 5aα, 12aα)]-4,7-bis(dimethylamino) - 1,4,4a,5,5a,6,11,12a-octahydro-3,10,12,12a-tetrahydroxy-1, 11-dioxo-2-naphthacenecarboxamide monohydrochloride. Each vial, dried by cryodesiccation, contains sterile minocycline HCl equivalent to 100 mg minocycline. When reconstituted with 5 mL of Sterile Water For Injection, the pH ranges from 2.0 to 2.8.

ACTIONS

Microbiology: The tetracyclines are primarily bacteriostatic and are thought to exert their antimicrobial effect by the inhibition of protein synthesis. Minocycline HCl is a tetracycline with antibacterial activity comparable to other tetracyclines with activity against a wide range of gram-negative and gram-positive organisms.
Tube dilution testing: Microorganisms may be considered susceptible (likely to respond to minocycline therapy) if the minimum inhibitory concentration (MIC) is not more than 4 mcg/mL. Microorganisms may be considered intermediate (harboring partial resistance) if the MIC is 4 to 12.5 mcg/mL and resistant (not likely to respond to minocycline therapy) if the MIC is greater than 12.5 mcg/mL.
Susceptibility plate testing: If the Kirby-Bauer method of susceptibility testing (using a 30 mcg tetracycline disc) gives a zone of 18 mm or greater, the bacterial strain is considered to be susceptible to any tetracycline. Minocycline shows moderate *in vitro* activity against certain strains of staphylococci which have been found resistant to other tetracyclines. For such strains, minocycline susceptibility powder may be used for additional susceptibility testing.
Human Pharmacology: Following a single dose of 200 mg, administered intravenously to 10 healthy male volunteers, serum levels ranged from 2.52 to 6.63 mcg/mL (average 4.18); after 12 hours they ranged from 0.82 to 2.64 mcg/mL (average 1.38). In a group of 5 healthy male volunteers, serum levels of 1.4 to 1.8 mcg/mL were maintained at 12 and 24 hours with dosages of 100 mg every 12 hours for three days. When given 200 mg once daily for three days, the serum levels had fallen to approximately 1 mcg/mL at 24 hours. The serum half-life following IV doses of 100 mg every 12 hours or 200 mg once daily did not differ significantly and ranged from 15 to 23 hours. The serum half-life following a single 200 mg oral dose in 12 essentially normal volunteers ranged from 11 to 17 hours, in 7 patients with hepatic dysfunction ranged from 11 to 16 hours, and in 5 patients with renal dysfunction from 18 to 69 hours.
Intravenously administered minocycline appears similar to oral doses in excretion. The urinary and fecal recovery of oral minocycline when administered to 12 normal volunteers is one-half to one-third that of other tetracyclines.

INDICATIONS

MINOCIN *minocycline HCl* is indicated in infections caused by the following microorganisms:
Rickettsiae: (Rocky Mountain spotted fever, typhus fever and the typhus group, Q fever, rickettsialpox, tick fevers).
Mycoplasma pneumoniae (PPLO, Eaton agent).
Agents of psittacosis and ornithosis.
Agents of lymphogranuloma venereum and granuloma inguinale. The spirochetal agent of relapsing fever (*Borrelia recurrentis*).
The following gram-negative microorganisms:
Haemophilus ducreyi (chancroid), *Yersinia pestis* and *Francisella tularensis*, formerly *Pasteurella pestis* and *Pasteurella tularensis*, *Bartonella bacilliformis*, *Bacteroides* species, *Vibrio comma* and *Vibrio fetus*, *Brucella* species (in conjunction with streptomycin).
Because many strains of the following groups of microorganisms have been shown to be resistant to tetracyclines, culture and susceptibility testing are recommended.
MINOCIN is indicated for treatment of infections caused by the following gram-negative microorganisms, when bacteriologic testing indicates appropriate susceptibility to the drug:
Escherichia coli, Enterobacter aerogenes (formerly *Aerobacter aerogenes*), *Shigella* species, *Mima* species and *Herellea* species, *Haemophilus influenzae* (respiratory infections), *Klebsiella* species (respiratory and urinary infections).
MINOCIN is indicated for treatment of infections caused by the following gram-positive microorganisms when bacteriologic testing indicates appropriate susceptibility to the drug:
Streptococcus species: Up to 44% of strains of *Streptococcus pyogenes* and 74% of *Streptococcus faecalis* have been found to be resistant to tetracycline drugs. Therefore, tetracyclines should not be used for streptococcal disease unless the organism has been demonstrated to be sensitive.
For upper respiratory infections due to Group A beta-hemolytic streptococci, penicillin is the usual drug of choice, including prophylaxis of rheumatic fever.
Streptococcus pneumoniae, Staphylococcus aureus, skin and soft tissue infections.
Tetracyclines are not the drugs of choice in the treatment of any type of staphylococcal infection.
When penicillin is contraindicated, tetracyclines are alternative drugs in the treatment of infections due to:
Neisseria gonorrhoeae, and *Neisseria meningitidis*, *Treponema pallidum* and *Treponema pertenue* (syphilis and yaws), *Listeria monocytogenes*, *Clostridium* species, *Bacillus anthracis*, *Fusobacterium fusiforme* (Vincent's infection), *Actinomyces* species.
In acute intestinal amebiasis, the tetracyclines may be a useful adjunct to amebicides.
MINOCIN is indicated in the treatment of trachoma, although the infectious agent is not always eliminated, as judged by immunofluorescence.
Inclusion conjunctivitis may be treated with oral tetracyclines or with a combination of oral and topical agents.

CONTRAINDICATIONS

This drug is contraindicated in persons who have shown hypersensitivity to any of the tetracyclines.

WARNINGS

In the presence of renal dysfunction, particularly in pregnancy, intravenous tetracycline therapy in daily doses exceeding 2 g has been associated with deaths through liver failure.
When the need for intensive treatment outweighs its potential dangers (mostly during pregnancy or in individuals with known or suspected renal or liver impairment), it is advisable to perform renal and liver function tests before and during therapy. Also, tetracycline serum concentrations should be followed.
If renal impairment exists, even usual oral or parenteral doses may lead to excessive systemic accumulation of the drug and possible liver toxicity. Under such conditions, lower than usual total doses are indicated, and if therapy is prolonged, serum level determinations of the drug may be advisable. This hazard is of particular importance in the parenteral administration of tetracyclines to pregnant or postpartum patients with pyelonephritis. When used under these circumstances, the blood level should not exceed 15 mcg/mL and liver function tests should be made at frequent intervals. Other potentially hepatotoxic drugs should not be prescribed concomitantly.
THE USE OF TETRACYCLINES DURING TOOTH DEVELOPMENT (LAST HALF OF PREGNANCY, INFANCY, AND CHILDHOOD TO THE AGE OF 8 YEARS) MAY CAUSE PERMANENT DISCOLORATION OF THE TEETH (YELLOW-GRAY-BROWN). This adverse reaction is more common during long-term use of the drugs but has been observed following repeated short-term courses. Enamel hypoplasia has also been reported. TETRACYCLINES, THEREFORE, SHOULD NOT BE USED IN THIS AGE GROUP UNLESS OTHER DRUGS ARE NOT LIKELY TO BE EFFECTIVE OR ARE CONTRAINDICATED.
Photosensitivity manifested by an exaggerated sunburn reaction has been observed in some individuals taking tetracyclines. Patients apt to be exposed to direct sunlight or ultraviolet light should be advised that this reaction can occur with tetracycline drugs, and treatment should be discontinued at the first evidence of skin erythema. Studies to date indicate that photosensitivity is rarely reported with MINOCIN *minocycline HCl*.
The anti-anabolic action of the tetracyclines may cause an increase in BUN. While this is not a problem in those with normal renal function, in patients with significantly impaired function, higher serum levels of tetracycline may lead to azotemia, hyperphosphatemia, and acidosis.
CNS side effects including lightheadedness, dizziness or vertigo have been reported. Patients who experience these symptoms should be cautioned about driving vehicles or using hazardous machinery while on minocycline therapy. These symptoms may disappear during therapy and usually disappear rapidly when the drug is discontinued.
Usage in Pregnancy: (See above **WARNINGS** about use during tooth development.)
Results of animal studies indicate that tetracyclines cross the placenta, are found in fetal tissues and can have toxic effects on the developing fetus (often related to retardation of skeletal development). Evidence of embryotoxicity has also been noted in animals treated early in pregnancy.
The safety of MINOCIN for use during pregnancy has not been established.
Usage in Newborns, Infants, and Children: (See above **WARNINGS** about use during tooth development.)
All tetracyclines form a stable calcium complex in any bone-forming tissue. A decrease in the fibula growth rate has been observed in prematures given oral tetracycline in doses of 25 mg/kg every six hours. This reaction was shown to be reversible when the drug was discontinued.
Tetracyclines are present in the milk of lactating women who are taking a drug in this class.

PRECAUTIONS

General: Pseudotumor cerebri (benign intracranial hypertension) in adults has been associated with the use of tetracyclines. The usual clinical manifestations are headache and blurred vision. Bulging fontanels have been associated with the use of tetracyclines in infants. While both of these conditions and related symptoms usually resolve soon after discontinuation of the tetracycline, the possibility for permanent sequelae exists.
As with other antibiotic preparations, use of this drug may result in overgrowth of nonsusceptible organisms, including fungi. If superinfection occurs, the antibiotic should be discontinued and appropriate therapy should be instituted.
In venereal diseases when coexistent syphilis is suspected, darkfield examination should be done before treatment is started and the blood serology repeated monthly for at least four months.
In long-term therapy, periodic laboratory evaluation of organ systems, including hematopoietic, renal, and hepatic studies should be performed.
All infections due to Group A beta-hemolytic streptococci should be treated for at least ten days.
Drug Interactions: Because tetracyclines have been shown to depress plasma prothrombin activity, patients who are on anticoagulant therapy may require downward adjustment of their anticoagulant dosage.
Since bacteriostatic drugs may interfere with the bactericidal action of penicillin, it is advisable to avoid giving tetracycline in conjunction with penicillin.
Concurrent use of tetracyclines may render oral contraceptives less effective. Breakthrough bleeding has been reported.

ADVERSE REACTIONS

Gastrointestinal: Anorexia, nausea, vomiting, diarrhea, glossitis, dysphagia, enterocolitis, inflammatory lesions (with monilial overgrowth) in the anogenital region, and increases in liver enzymes and, rarely, hepatitis. These reactions have been caused by both the oral and parenteral administration of tetracyclines.
Skin: Maculopapular and erythematous rashes.
Exfoliative dermatitis has been reported but is uncommon. Erythema multiforme and rarely Stevens-Johnson syndrome have been reported. Photosensitivity is discussed above. (see **WARNINGS**.)
Pigmentation of the skin and mucous membranes has been reported.
Tooth discoloration has been reported, rarely, in adults.
Renal Toxicity: Rise in BUN has been reported and is apparently dose related (see **WARNINGS**).

Hypersensitivity Reactions: Urticaria, angioneurotic edema, polyarthralgia, anaphylaxis, anaphylactoid purpura, pericarditis, exacerbation of systemic lupus erythematosus and, rarely, pulmonary infiltrates with eosinophilia.

Blood: Hemolytic anemia, thrombocytopenia, neutropenia, and eosinophilia have been reported.

CNS: (see **WARNINGS.**) Pseudotumor cerebri (benign intracranial hypertension) in adults and bulging fontanels in infants (see **PRECAUTIONS—General**).

Other: When given over prolonged periods, tetracyclines have been reported to produce brown-black microscopic discoloration of thyroid glands. No abnormalities of thyroid function studies are known to occur.

DOSAGE AND ADMINISTRATION

Note: Rapid administration is to be avoided. Parenteral therapy is indicated only when oral therapy is not adequate or tolerated. Oral therapy should be instituted as soon as possible. If intravenous therapy is given over prolonged periods of time, thrombophlebitis may result.

Adults: Usual adult dose: 200 mg followed by 100 mg every 12 hours and should not exceed 400 mg in 24 hours. The drug should be initially dissolved and then further diluted to 500 mL–1,000 mL with either Sodium Chloride Injection USP, Dextrose Injection USP, Dextrose and Sodium Chloride Injection USP, Ringer's Injection USP, or Lactated Ringer's Injection USP but not in other solutions containing calcium (a precipitate may form).

The reconstituted solutions are stable at room temperature for 24 hours without significant loss of potency. Any unused portions must be discarded after that period. The final dilution for administration should be administered immediately.

For children above 8 years of age: Usual pediatric dosage: 4 mg/kg followed by 2 mg/kg every 12 hours.

In patients with renal impairment: (see **WARNINGS**). Total dosage should be decreased by reduction of recommended individual doses and/or by extending time intervals between doses.

HOW SUPPLIED

MINOCIN *monocycline HCl* Intravenous is supplied as 100 mg vials of sterile cryodesiccated powder
Product No. NDC 0205-5305-94
Store at Controlled Room Temperature 15–30°C (59–86°F).
Military Depot: Intravenous NSN 6505-00-149-0574
LEDERLE PARENTERALS, INC.
Carolina, Puerto Rico 00630   Rev. 2/89
                                                              24140
Shown in Product Identification Section, page 415

MINOCIN®   ℞
[mĭ-nō-sĭn]
Minocycline Hydrochloride
for Oral Use

PRODUCT OVERVIEW

KEY FACTS

Tablets, Capsules, Oral Solution
MINOCIN is a long acting, semisynthetic derivative of tetracycline. MINOCIN is indicated for treatment of infections caused by gram-negative and gram-positive microorganisms when bacteriologic testing indicates appropriate susceptibility to the drug. (See full Prescribing Information.) Highly lipophilic MINOCIN achieves high concentrations in body tissue and fluids. MINOCIN is unaffected by β-lactamase enzymes. Bid dosing encourages patient compliance.

MAJOR USES

MINOCIN is indicated for the treatment of single or mixed upper and lower respiratory infections due to susceptible aerobes and anerobes, skin and soft tissue infections, STD due to Chlamydia or *Ureaplasma urealyticum*, STD due to *Neisseria gonorrhoeae* in women, uncomplicated gonococcal urethritis in men due to *Neisseria gonorrhoeae*, and as adjunctive therapy in severe acne.

SAFETY INFORMATION

MINOCIN is contraindicated in persons who have shown hypersensitivity to any of the tetracyclines. Adverse reactions most frequently observed in clinical trials were nausea (8.9%) and dizziness/lightheadedness (6.8%).
Photosensitivity is rarely reported. For more information on adverse reactions, see full Prescribing Information.

PRESCRIBING INFORMATION

MINOCIN®   ℞
[mĭ-nō-sĭn]
Minocycline Hydrochloride
for Oral Use

DESCRIPTION

MINOCIN, a semisynthetic derivative of tetracycline, is named [4S-(4α,4aα,5aα,12aα)]-4,7-bis(dimethylamino)-1,4,4a,5,5a,6,11,12a-octahydro-3,10,12,12a-tetrahydroxy-1,11-dioxo-2-naphthacenecarboxamide monohydrochloride.

MINOCIN Capsules contain minocycline HCl equivalent to 50 or 100 mg minocycline and the following inactive ingredients: Corn Starch, Magnesium Stearate, Titanium Dioxide and Yellow 6. Additionally, the 100 mg capsules contain Blue 1 and Red 28.

MINOCIN Oral Suspension contains minocycline HCl equivalent to 50 mg of minocycline per 5 mL (10 mg/mL) and the following inactive ingredients: Alcohol, Butylparaben, Calcium Hydroxide, Cellulose, Decaglyceryl Tetraoleate, Edetate Calcium Disodium, Glycol, Guar Gum, Polysorbate 80, Propylparaben, Propylene Glycol, Sodium Saccharin, Sodium Sulfite (see **WARNINGS**) and Sorbitol.

MINOCIN Tablets contain minocycline HCl equivalent to 50 or 100 mg minocycline and the following inactive ingredients: Lactose, Microcrystalline Cellulose, Magnesium Stearate, Povidone, Sodium Lauryl Sulfate, Sodium Starch Glycolate, Sorbitol, Stearic Acid, Titanium Dioxide, Yellow 6, Yellow 10, and other ingredients.

ACTIONS

Microbiology: The tetracyclines are primarily bacteriostatic and are thought to exert their antimicrobial effect by the inhibition of protein synthesis. Minocycline HCl is a tetracycline with antibacterial activity comparable to other tetracyclines with activity against a wide range of gram-negative and gram-positive organisms.

Tube dilution testing: Microorganisms may be considered susceptible (likely to respond to minocycline therapy) if the minimum inhibitory concentration (MIC) is not more than 4 mcg/mL. Microorganisms may be considered intermediate (harboring partial resistance) if the MIC is 4 to 12.5 mcg/mL and resistant (not likely to respond to minocycline therapy) if the MIC is greater than 12.5 mcg/mL.

Susceptibility plate testing: If the Kirby-Bauer method of susceptibility testing (using a 30 mcg tetracycline disc) gives a zone of 18 mm or greater, the bacterial strain is considered to be susceptible to any tetracycline. Minocycline shows moderate *in vitro* activity against certain strains of staphylococci which have been found resistant to other tetracyclines. For such strains minocycline susceptibility powder may be used for additional susceptibility testing.

Human Pharmacology: Following a single dose of two 100 mg of minocycline HCl capsules administered to ten normal adult volunteers, serum levels ranged from 0.74 to 4.45 mcg/mL in one hour (average 2.24); after 12 hours, they ranged from 0.34 to 2.36 mcg/mL (average 1.25). The serum half-life following a single 200 mg dose in 12 essentially normal volunteers ranged from 11 to 17 hours, in 7 patients with hepatic dysfunction it ranged from 11 to 16 hours, and in 5 patients with renal dysfunction, from 18 to 69 hours. The urinary and fecal recovery of minocycline when administered to 12 normal volunteers is one-half to one-third that of other tetracyclines.

INDICATIONS

MINOCIN *minocycline HCl* is indicated in infections caused by the following microorganisms:

Rickettsiae: (Rocky Mountain spotted fever, typhus fever and the typhus group, Q fever, rickettsialpox, tick fevers).

Mycoplasma pneumoniae (PPLO, Eaton agent).

Agents of psittacosis and ornithosis.

Agents of lymphogranuloma venereum and granuloma inguinale. The spirochetal agent of relapsing fever (*Borrelia recurrentis*).

The following gram-negative microorganisms:
Haemophilus ducreyi (chancroid), *Yersinia pestis* and *Francisella tularensis* formerly *Pasteurella pestis* and *Pasteurella tularensis*, *Bartonella bacilliformis*, *Bacteroides* species, *Vibrio comma* and *Vibrio fetus*, *Brucella* species (in conjunction with streptomycin).

Because many strains of the following groups of microorganisms have been shown to be resistant to tetracyclines, culture and susceptibility testing are recommended.

MINOCIN is indicated for treatment of infections caused by the following gram-negative microorganisms when bacteriologic testing indicates appropriate susceptibility to the drug:
Escherichia coli, *Enterobacter aerogenes* (formerly *Aerobacter aerogenes*), *Shigella* species, *Acinetobacter calcoaceticus* (formerly *Herellea*, *Mima*), *Haemophilus influenzae* (respiratory infections), *Klebsiella* species (respiratory and urinary infections).

MINOCIN is indicated for treatment of infections caused by the following gram-positive microorganisms when bacteriologic testing indicates appropriate susceptibility to the drug:
Streptococcus species: Up to 44% of strains of *Streptococcus pyogenes* and 74% of *Streptococcus faecalis* have been found to be resistant to tetracycline drugs.

Therefore, tetracyclines should not be used for streptococcal disease unless the organism has been demonstrated to be sensitive.

For upper respiratory infections due to Group A beta-hemolytic streptococci, penicillin is the usual drug of choice, including prophylaxis of rheumatic fever.

Streptococcus pneumoniae, *Staphylococcus aureus*, skin and soft tissue infections.

Tetracyclines are not the drugs of choice in the treatment of any type of staphylococcal infection.

MINOCIN is indicated for the treatment of uncomplicated gonococcal urethritis in men due to *Neisseria gonorrhoeae*. When penicillin is contraindicated, tetracyclines are alternative drugs in the treatment of infections due to:
Neisseria gonorrhoeae (in women), *Treponema pallidum* and *Treponema pertenue* (syphilis and yaws), *Listeria monocytogenes*, *Clostridium* species, *Bacillus anthracis*, *Fusobacterium fusiforme* (Vincent's infection), *Actinomyces* species.

In acute intestinal amebiasis, the tetracyclines may be a useful adjunct to amebicides.

In severe acne, the tetracyclines may be useful adjunctive therapy.

MINOCIN is indicated in the treatment of trachoma, although the infectious agent is not always eliminated, as judged by immunofluorescence.

MINOCIN *minocycline HCl is indicated for the treatment of uncomplicated urethral, endocervical or rectal infections in adults caused by Chlamydia trachomatis or Ureaplasma urealyticum*.[1]

Inclusion conjunctivitis may be treated with oral tetracyclines or with a combination of oral and topical agents.

MINOCIN is indicated in the treatment of asymptomatic carriers of *Neisseria meningitidis* to eliminate meningococci from the nasopharynx.

In order to preserve the usefulness of MINOCIN in the treatment of asymptomatic meningococcal carriers, diagnostic laboratory procedures, including serotyping and susceptibility testing, should be performed to establish the carrier state and the correct treatment. It is recommended that the drug be reserved for situations in which the risk of meningococcal meningitis is high.

Minocycline by oral administration is not indicated for the treatment of meningococcal infection.

Although no controlled clinical efficacy studies have been conducted, limited clinical data show that oral minocycline hydrochloride has been used successfully in the treatment of infections caused by Mycobacterium marinum.

CONTRAINDICATIONS

This drug is contraindicated in persons who have shown hypersensitivity to any of the tetracyclines.

WARNINGS

THE USE OF DRUGS OF THE TETRACYCLINE CLASS DURING TOOTH DEVELOPMENT (LAST HALF OF PREGNANCY, INFANCY, AND CHILDHOOD TO THE AGE OF 8 YEARS) MAY CAUSE PERMANENT DISCOLORATION OF THE TEETH (YELLOW-GRAY-BROWN). This adverse reaction is more common during long-term use of the drugs but has been observed following repeated short-term courses. Enamel hypoplasia has also been reported. TETRACYCLINE DRUGS, THEREFORE, SHOULD NOT BE USED IN THIS AGE GROUP UNLESS OTHER DRUGS ARE NOT LIKELY TO BE EFFECTIVE OR ARE CONTRAINDICATED.

If renal impairment exists, even usual oral or parenteral doses may lead to excessive systemic accumulations of the drug and possible liver toxicity. Under such conditions, lower-than-usual total doses are indicated, and if therapy is prolonged, serum level determinations of the drug may be advisable.

Photosensitivity manifested by an exaggerated sunburn reaction has been observed in some individuals taking tetracyclines. Patients apt to be exposed to direct sunlight or ultraviolet light should be advised that this reaction can occur with tetracycline drugs, and treatment should be discontinued at the first evidence of skin erythema. Studies to date indicate that photosensitivity is rarely reported with MINOCIN *minocycline HCl*.

The anti-anabolic action of the tetracyclines may cause an increase in BUN. While this is not a problem in those with normal renal function, in patients with significantly impaired function, higher serum levels of tetracycline may lead to azotemia, hyperphosphatemia, and acidosis.

CNS side effects including lightheadedness, dizziness, or vertigo have been reported. Patients who experience these symptoms should be cautioned about driving vehicles or using hazardous machinery while on minocycline therapy. These symptoms may disappear during therapy and usually disappear rapidly when the drug is discontinued.

MINOCIN Oral Suspension contains sodium sulfite, a sulfite that may cause allergic-type reactions including anaphylactic symptoms and life-threatening or less severe asthmatic

Continued on next page

Lederle—Cont.

episodes in certain susceptible people. The overall prevalence of sulfite sensitivity in the general population is unknown and probably low. Sulfite sensitivity is seen more frequently in asthmatic than in nonasthmatic people.

Usage in pregnancy: (See above WARNINGS about use during tooth development.) Results of animal studies indicate that tetracyclines cross the placenta, are found in fetal tissues, and can have toxic effects on the developing fetus (often related to retardation of skeletal development). Evidence of embryotoxicity has also been noted in animals treated early in pregnancy.

The safety of minocycline HCl for use during pregnancy has not been established.

Usage in newborns, infants, and children: (See above WARNINGS about use during tooth development.)

All tetracyclines form a stable calcium complex in any bone-forming tissue. A decrease in the fibula growth rate has been observed in prematures given oral tetracycline in doses of 25 mg/kg every six hours. This reaction was shown to be reversible when the drug was discontinued.

Tetracyclines are present in the milk of lactating women who are taking a drug in this class.

PRECAUTIONS

General: Pseudotumor cerebri (benign intracranial hypertension) in adults has been associated with the use of tetracyclines. The usual clinical manifestations are headache and blurred vision. Bulging fontanels have been associated with the use of tetracyclines in infants. While both of these conditions and related symptoms usually resolve soon after discontinuation of the tetracycline, the possibility for permanent sequelae exists.

As with other antibiotic preparations, use of this drug may result in overgrowth of nonsusceptible organisms, including fungi. If superinfection occurs, the antibiotic should be discontinued and appropriate therapy should be instituted.

In venereal diseases when coexistent syphilis is suspected, darkfield examination should be done before treatment is started and the blood serology repeated monthly for at least 4 months.

In long-term therapy, periodic laboratory evaluation of organ systems, including hematopoietic, renal, and hepatic studies should be performed.

All infections due to Group A beta-hemolytic streptococci should be treated for at least ten days.

Drug Interactions: Because tetracyclines have been shown to depress plasma prothrombin activity, patients who are on anticoagulant therapy may require downward adjustment of their anticoagulant dosage.

Since bacteriostatic drugs may interfere with the bactericidal action of penicillin, it is advisable to avoid giving tetracycline in conjunction with penicillin.

Concurrent use of tetracyclines may render oral contraceptives less effective. Breakthrough bleeding has been reported.

ADVERSE REACTIONS

Gastrointestinal: Anorexia, nausea, vomiting, diarrhea, glossitis, dysphagia, enterocolitis, inflammatory lesions (with monilial overgrowth) in the anogenital region, and increases in liver enzymes, rarely, hepatitis. These reactions have been caused by both the oral and parenteral administration of tetracyclines.

Skin: Maculopapular and erythematous rashes. Exfoliative dermatitis has been reported but is uncommon. Erythema multiforme and rarely Stevens-Johnson syndrome have been reported. Photosensitivity is discussed above (see WARNINGS). Pigmentation of the skin and mucous membranes has been reported. Tooth discoloration has been reported rarely in adults.

Renal toxicity: Rise in BUN has been reported and is apparently dose related (see WARNINGS).

Hypersensitivity Reactions: Urticaria, angioneurotic edema, polyarthralgia, anaphylaxis, anaphylactoid purpura, pericarditis, exacerbation of systemic lupus erythematosus and, rarely, pulmonary infiltrates with eosinophilia.

Blood: Hemolytic anemia, thrombocytopenia, neutropenia, and eosinophilia have been reported.

CNS: (see WARNINGS.) Pseudotumor cerebri (benign intracranial hypertension) in adults and bulging fontanels in infants (see PRECAUTIONS—General).

Other: When given over prolonged periods, tetracyclines have been reported to produce brown-black microscopic discoloration of thyroid glands. No abnormalities of thyroid function studies are known to occur.

DOSAGE AND ADMINISTRATION

Therapy should be continued for at least 24 to 48 hours after symptoms and fever have subsided.

Concomitant therapy: Antacids containing aluminum, calcium, or magnesium impair absorption and should not be given to patients taking oral tetracycline.

Studies to date have indicated that the absorption of MINOCIN is not notably influenced by foods and dairy products.

In patients with renal impairment: (See WARNINGS.) Total dosage should be decreased by reduction of recommended individual doses and/or extending time intervals between doses.

In the treatment of streptococcal infections, a therapeutic dosage of tetracycline should be administered for at least ten days.

ADULTS: The usual dosage of MINOCIN *minocycline HCl* is 200 mg initially followed by 100 mg every 12 hours. Alternatively, if more frequent doses are preferred, two or four 50 mg capsules or tablets may be given initially, followed by one 50 mg capsule or tablet four times daily.

For children above 8 years of age: The usual dosage of MINOCIN is 4 mg/kg initially followed by 2 mg/kg every 12 hours.

For treatment of syphilis, the usual dosage of MINOCIN should be administered over a period of 10 to 15 days. Close follow-up, including laboratory tests, is recommended.

Gonorrhea patients sensitive to penicillin may be treated with MINOCIN, administered as 200 mg initially, followed by 100 mg every 12 hours for a minimum of four days, with post-therapy cultures within 2 to 3 days.

In the treatment of meningococcal carrier state recommended dosage is 100 mg every 12 hours for five days.

Mycobacterium marinum infections: Although optimal doses have not been established, 100 mg twice a day for 6 to 8 weeks have been used successfully in a limited number of cases.

Uncomplicated urethral, endocervical, or rectal infection in adults caused by *Chlamydia trachomatis* or *Ureaplasma urealyticum:* 100 mg, by mouth, 2 times a day for at least seven days.[1]

In the treatment of uncomplicated gonococcal urethritis in men, 100 mg twice a day orally for five days is recommended.

HOW SUPPLIED

CAPSULES

MINOCIN equivalent to 100 mg minocycline.
Hardshell orange and purple with Lederle over M4 printed on one half and MINOCIN over 100 mg on the other.

NDC 0005-5301-18 Bottle of 50s
Military Depot: NSN 6505-00-003-5112
NDC 0005-5301-23 Bottle of 100s
VA Depot: NSN 6505-01-108-9040
NDC 0005-5301-60 Unit Dose (strips) 10×10s
Military Depot: NSN 6505-01-153-3577

MINOCIN equivalent to 50 mg minocycline.
Hardshell orange with Lederle over M2 printed on one half and MINOCIN over 50 mg on the other.

NDC 0005-5300-23 Bottle of 100s
Military and VA Depots: NSN 6505-01-015-4147
NDC 0005-5300-60 Unit Dose (strips) 10×10s
Store at Controlled Room Temperature 15°-30° C (59°-86° F).

ORAL SUSPENSION

MINOCIN Oral Suspension contains minocycline hydrochloride equivalent to 50 mg minocycline per teaspoonful (5 mL). Preserved with propylparaben 0.10% and butylparaben 0.06% with Alcohol USP 5% v/v, Custard-flavored.

NDC 0005-5313-56 Bottle 2 fl oz (60 mL)
Store at Controlled Room Temperature 15°-30° C (59°-86° F)
DO NOT FREEZE.

TABLETS

MINOCIN equivalent to 100 mg minocycline. Round, convex, orange film-coated tablet engraved with M over bisect and 5 under bisect on one side of the tablet and LL on the other.

NDC 0005-9376-18 Bottle of 50s

MINOCIN equivalent to 50 mg minocycline. Round, convex, orange film-coated tablet engraved with M3 on one side and LL on the other.

NDC 0005-9375-23 Bottle of 100s
Store at Controlled Room Temperature 15-30° C (59-86° F).

ANIMAL PHARMACOLOGY AND TOXICOLOGY

MINOCIN *minocycline HCl* has been found to produce high blood concentrations following oral dosage to various animal species and to be extensively distributed to all tissues examined in ^{14}C-labeled drug studies in dogs. MINOCIN has been found experimentally to produce discoloration of the thyroid glands. This finding has been observed in rats and dogs. Changes in thyroid function have also been found in these animal species. However, no change in thyroid function has been observed in humans.

Reference: 1. CDC Sexually Transmitted Diseases Treatment Guidelines 1982.

LEDERLE LABORATORIES DIVISION
American Cyanamid Company,
Pearl River, NY 10965   Rev. 2/89
                       23996

Shown in Product Identification Section, page 415

MYAMBUTOL®   ℞
[mī-am-bū-tōl]
ethambutol hydrochloride
Tablets

DESCRIPTION

MYAMBUTOL is an oral chemotherapeutic agent which is specifically effective against actively growing microorganisms of the genus *Mycobacterium*, including *M tuberculosis*. MYAMBUTOL 100 mg and 400 mg tablets contain the following inactive ingredients: Gelatin, Hydroxypropyl Methylcellulose, Magnesium Stearate, Sodium Lauryl Sulfate, Sorbitol, Stearic Acid, Sucrose, Titanium Dioxide and other ingredients.

ACTION

MYAMBUTOL, following a single oral dose of 25 mg/kg of body weight, attains a peak of 2 to 5 micrograms/mL in serum 2 to 4 hours after administration. When the drug is administered daily for longer periods of time at this dose, serum levels are similar. The serum level of MYAMBUTOL falls to undetectable levels by 24 hours after the last dose except in some patients with abnormal renal function. The intracellular concentrations of erythrocytes reach peak values approximately twice those of plasma and maintain this ratio throughout the 24 hours.

During the 24-hour period following oral administration of MYAMBUTOL, approximately 50% of the initial dose is excreted unchanged in the urine, while an additional 8% to 15% appears in the form of metabolites. The main path of metabolism appears to be an initial oxidation of the alcohol to an aldehydic intermediate, followed by conversion to a dicarboxylic acid. From 20% to 22% of the initial dose is excreted in the feces as unchanged drug. No drug accumulation has been observed with consecutive single daily doses of 25 mg/kg in patients with normal kidney function, although marked accumulation has been demonstrated in patients with renal insufficiency.

MYAMBUTOL diffuses into actively growing *mycobacterium* cells such as tubercle bacilli. MYAMBUTOL appears to inhibit the synthesis of one or more metabolites, thus causing impairment of cell metabolism, arrest of multiplication, and cell death. No cross resistance with other available antimycobacterial agents has been demonstrated.

MYAMBUTOL has been shown to be effective against strains of *Mycobacterium tuberculosis* but does not seem to be active against fungi, viruses, or other bacteria. *Mycobacterium tuberculosis* strains previously unexposed to MYAMBUTOL have been uniformLy sensitive to concentrations of 8 or less micrograms/mL, depending on the nature of the culture media. When MYAMBUTOL has been used alone for treatment of tuberculosis, tubercle bacilli from these patients have developed resistance to MYAMBUTOL by *in vitro* susceptibility tests; the development of resistance has been unpredictable and appears to occur in a step-like manner. No cross resistance between MYAMBUTOL and other antituberculous drugs has been reported. MYAMBUTOL has reduced the incidence of the emergence of mycobacterial resistance to isoniazid when both drugs have been used concurrently.

An agar diffusion microbiologic assay, based upon inhibition of *Mycobacterium smegmatis* (ATCC 607) may be used to determine concentrations of MYAMBUTOL in serum and urine. This technique has not been published, but further information can be obtained upon inquiry to Lederle Laboratories.

ANIMAL PHARMACOLOGY

Toxicological studies in dogs on high prolonged doses produced evidence of myocardial damage and failure, and depigmentation of the tapetum lucidum of the eyes, the significance of which is not known. Degenerative changes in the central nervous system, apparently not dose-related, have also been noted in dogs receiving ethambutol hydrochloride over a prolonged period.

In the rhesus monkey, neurological signs appeared after treatment with high doses given daily over a period of several months. These were correlated with specific serum levels of ethambutol hydrochloride and with definite neuro-anatomical changes in the central nervous system. Focal interstitial carditis was also noted in monkeys which received ethambutol hydrochloride in high doses for a prolonged period.

When pregnant mice or rabbits were treated with high doses of ethambutol hydrochloride, fetal mortality was slightly but not significantly (P > 0.05) increased. Female rats treated with ethambutol hydrochloride displayed slight but insignificant (P > 0.05) decreases in fertility and litter size.

In fetuses born of mice treated with high doses of MYAMBUTOL during pregnancy, a low incidence of cleft palate, exencephaly and abnormality of the vertebral column were observed. Minor abnormalities of the cervical vertebra were seen in the newborn of rats treated with high doses of MYAMBUTOL during pregnancy. Rabbits receiving high doses of MYAMBUTOL during pregnancy gave birth to two fetuses with monophthalmia, one with a shortened right

Initial Snellen Reading	Reading Indicating Significant Decrease	Significant Number of Lines	Decrease Number of Points
20/13	20/25	3	12
20/15	20/25	2	10
20/20	20/30	2	10
20/25	20/40	2	15
20/30	20/50	2	20
20/40	20/70	2	30
20/50	20/70	1	20

forearm accompanied by bilateral wrist-joint contracture and one with harelip and cleft palate.

INDICATIONS

MYAMBUTOL *ethambutol hydrochloride* is indicated for the treatment of pulmonary tuberculosis. It should not be used as the sole antituberculous drug, but should be used in conjunction with at least one other antituberculous drug. Selection of the companion drug should be based on clinical experience, considerations of comparative safety and appropriate *in vitro* susceptibility studies. In patients who have not received previous antituberculous therapy, ie, initial treatment, the most frequently used regimens have been the following:

MYAMBUTOL plus isoniazid
MYAMBUTOL plus isoniazid plus streptomycin.

In patients who have received previous antituberculous therapy, mycobacterial resistance to other drugs used in initial therapy is frequent. Consequently, in such retreatment patients, MYAMBUTOL should be combined with at least one of the second line drugs not previously administered to the patient and to which bacterial susceptibility has been indicated by appropriate *in vitro* studies. Antituberculous drugs used with MYAMBUTOL have included cycloserine, ethionamide, pyrazinamide, viomycin and other drugs. Isoniazid, aminosalicylic acid, and streptomycin have also been used in multiple drug regimens. Alternating drug regimens have also been utilized.

CONTRAINDICATIONS

MYAMBUTOL *ethambutol hydrochloride* is contraindicated in patients who are known to be hypersensitive to this drug. It is also contraindicated in patients with known optic neuritis unless clinical judgment determines that it may be used.

PRECAUTIONS

The effects of combinations of MYAMBUTOL with other antituberculous drugs on the fetus is not known. While administration of this drug to pregnant human patients has produced no detectable effect upon the fetus, the possible teratogenic potential in women capable of bearing children should be weighed carefully against the benefits of therapy. There are published reports of five women who received the drug during pregnancy without apparent adverse effect upon the fetus.

MYAMBUTOL is not recommended for use in children under thirteen years of age since safe conditions for use have not been established.

Patients with decreased renal function need the dosage reduced as determined by serum levels of MYAMBUTOL, since the main path of excretion of this drug is by the kidneys.

Because this drug may have adverse effects on vision, physical examination should include ophthalmoscopy, finger perimetry and testing of color discrimination. In patients with visual defects such as cataracts, recurrent inflammatory conditions of the eye, optic neuritis, and diabetic retinopathy, the evaluation of changes in visual acuity is more difficult, and care should be taken to be sure the variations in vision are not due to the underlying disease conditions. In such patients, consideration should be given to relationship between benefits expected and possible visual deterioration since evaluation of visual changes is difficult. (For recommended procedures, see next paragraphs under ADVERSE REACTIONS.)

As with any potent drug, periodic assessment of organ system functions, including renal, hepatic, and hematopoietic, should be made during long-term therapy.

ADVERSE REACTIONS

MYAMBUTOL may produce decreases in visual acuity which appear to be due to optic neuritis and to be related to dose and duration of treatment. The effects are generally reversible when administration of the drug is discontinued promptly. In rare cases recovery may be delayed for up to one year or more and the effect may possibly be irreversible in these cases.

Patients should be advised to report promptly to their physician any change of visual acuity.

The change in visual acuity may be unilateral or bilateral and hence *each eye must be tested separately and both eyes tested together*. Testing of visual acuity should be performed before beginning MYAMBUTOL therapy and periodically during drug administration, except that it should be done monthly when a patient is on a dosage of more than 15 mg per kilogram per day. Snellen eye charts are recommended for testing of visual acuity. Studies have shown that there are definite fluctuations of one or two lines of the Snellen chart in the visual acuity of many tuberculous patients *not* receiving MYAMBUTOL *ethambutol hydrochloride*.

The following table may be useful in interpreting possible changes in visual acuity attributable to MYAMBUTOL. [See table above].

In general, changes in visual acuity less than those indicated under "Significant Number of Lines" and "Decrease-Number of Points," may be due to chance variation, limitations of the testing method or physiologic variability. Conversely, changes in visual acuity equaling or exceeding those under "Significant Number of Lines" and "Decrease-Number of Points" indicate need for retesting and careful evaluation of the patient's visual status. If careful evaluation confirms the magnitude of visual change and fails to reveal another cause, MYAMBUTOL should be discontinued and the patient reevaluated at frequent intervals. Progressive decreases in visual acuity during therapy must be considered to be due to MYAMBUTOL *ethambutol hydrochloride*.

If corrective glasses are used prior to treatment, these must be worn during visual acuity testing. During 1 to 2 years of therapy, a refractive error may develop which must be corrected in order to obtain accurate test results. Testing the visual acuity through a pinhole eliminates refractive error. Patients developing visual abnormality during MYAMBUTOL treatment may show subjective visual symptoms before, or simultaneously with, the demonstration of decreases in visual acuity, and all patients receiving MYAMBUTOL should be questioned periodically about blurred vision and other subjective eye symptoms.

Recovery of visual acuity generally occurs over a period of weeks to months after the drug has been discontinued. Patients have then received MYAMBUTOL again without recurrence of loss of visual acuity.

Other adverse reactions reported include: anaphylactoid reactions, dermatitis pruritus and joint pain; anorexia, nausea, vomiting, gastrointestinal upset, abdominal pain; fever, malaise, headache, and dizziness; mental confusion, disorientation and possible hallucinations. Numbness and tingling of the extremities due to peripheral neuritis have been reported infrequently.

Elevated serum uric acid levels occur and precipitation of acute gout has been reported. Transient impairment of liver function as indicated by abnormal liver function tests is not an unusual finding. Since MYAMBUTOL is recommended for therapy in conjunction with one or more other antituberculous drugs, these changes may be related to the concurrent therapy.

DOSAGE AND ADMINISTRATION

MYAMBUTOL should not be used alone, in initial treatment or in retreatment. MYAMBUTOL should be administered on a once every 24-hour basis only. Absorption is not significantly altered by administration with food. Therapy, in general, should be continued until bacteriological conversion has become permanent and maximal clinical improvement has occurred.

MYAMBUTOL is not recommended for use in children under thirteen years of age since safe conditions for use have not been established.

Initial Treatment: In patients who have not received previous antituberculous therapy, administer MYAMBUTOL 15 mg per kilogram (7 mg per pound) of body weight, as a single oral dose once every 24 hours. In the more recent studies, isoniazid has been administered concurrently in a single, daily, oral dose.

Retreatment: In patients who have received previous antituberculous therapy, administer MYAMBUTOL 25 mg per kilogram (11 mg per pound) of body weight, as a single oral dose once every 24 hours. Concurrently administer at least one other antituberculous drug to which the organisms have been demonstrated to be susceptible by appropriate *in vitro* tests. Suitable drugs usually consist of those not previously used in the treatment of the patient. After 60 days of MYAMBUTOL administration, decrease the dose to 15 mg per kilogram (7 mg per pound) of body weight, and administer as a single oral dose once every 24 hours.

During the period when a patient is on a daily dose of 25 mg/kg, monthly eye examinations are advised.

See Table for easy selection of proper weight-dose tablet(s).

Weight-Dose Table
15 mg/kg (7 mg/lb) Schedule

Weight Range Pounds	Kilograms	Daily Dose In mg
Under 85 lbs	Under 37 kg	500
85–94.5	37–43	600
95–109.5	43–50	700
110–124.5	50–57	800
125–139.5	57–64	900
140–154.5	64–71	1000
155–169.5	71–79	1100
170–184.5	79–84	1200
185–199.5	84–90	1300
200–214.5	90–97	1400
215 and Over	Over 97	1500

25 mg/kg (11 mg/lb) Schedule

Under 85 lbs	Under 38 kg	900
85–92.5	38–42	1000
93–101.5	42–45.5	1100
102–109.5	45.5–50	1200
110–118.5	50–54	1300
119–128.5	54–58	1400
129–136.5	58–62	1500
137–146.5	62–67	1600
147–155.5	67–71	1700
156–164.5	71–75	1800
165–173.5	75–79	1900
174–182.5	79–83	2000
183–191.5	83–87	2100
192–199.5	87–91	2200
200–209.5	91–95	2300
210–218.5	95–99	2400
219 and Over	Over 99	2500

HOW SUPPLIED

MYAMBUTOL *ethambutol hydrochloride* Tablets 100 mg round, convex, white, coated tablets engraved M6 on one side and LL on the other, are supplied as follows:

NDC 0005-5015-23 - Bottle of 100
NDC 0005-5015-34 Bottle of 1000

400 mg - round, convex, white, scored, film-coated tablets engraved with LL on one side and M to the left and 7 to the right of the score on the other side, are supplied as follows:

NDC 0005-5084-62 Unit-of-Issue 100s with CRC
NDC 0005-5084-34 Bottle of 1000
NDC 0005-5084-60 - Unit Dose 10 × 10s

Store at Controlled Room Temperature 15–30°C (59–86°F).

Military Depot:
Tablets, 100 mg NSN 6505-00-403-7645, 100s
Tablets 400 mg NSN 6505-00-812-2579, 100s
VA Depot: Tablets, 400 mg NSN 6505-00-812-2543, 1000s
LEDERLE LABORATORIES DIVISION
American Cyanamid Company,
Pearl River, NY 10965   Rev. 6/87
21225

Shown in Product Identification Section, page 415

NEOLOID®

[*nēo-loid*]
Emulsified Castor Oil
For the treatment of isolated bouts of constipation
Peppermint Flavored - Shake Well

CONTAINS

Castor Oil USP 36.4% (w/w) with 0.1% (w/w) Sodium Benzoate and 0.2% (w/w) Potassium Sorbate added as preservatives, emulsifying and flavoring agents in water. Also contains the following inactive ingredients: Citric Acid, Glyceryl Monostearate, Polysorbate 80, Propylene Glycol, Sodium Alginate, Sodium Saccharin, Stearic Acid, Tenox II. NEOLOID is an emulsion with an exceptionally bland, pleasant taste.

DOSAGE

Infants ½ to 1½ teaspoonfuls; children, adjust between infant and adult dose. Average adult dose, 2 to 4 tablespoonfuls, or as prescribed by the physician. Not to be used when abdominal pain, nausea, vomiting, or other symptoms of appendicitis are present. Frequent or continued use of this preparation may result in dependence on laxatives. Do not use during pregnancy except on a physician's advice. Keep this and all drugs out of the reach of children.

WARNING

As with any drug, if you are pregnant or nursing a baby, seek the advice of a health professional before using this product.

Continued on next page

Information on Lederle products listed on these pages is the full prescribing information from product literature or package inserts effective in August, 1989. Information concerning all Lederle products may be obtained from the Professional Services Department, Lederle Laboratories, Pearl River, New York, 10965.

Lederle—Cont.

In case of accidental overdose, seek professional assistance or contact a Poison Control Center immediately.
Store at Room Temperature.
DO NOT FREEZE
NET 4 Fl. Oz. (118 mL) NDC 0005-5442-58.
LEDERLE LABORATORIES DIVISION
American Cyanamid Company
Pearl River, N.Y. 10965   Rev. 8/85
      16838

NEPTAZANE® ℞
[nĕp-ta-zāne]
methazolamide
Tablets

(See PDR For Ophthalmology)
Shown in Product Identification Section, page 415

NOVANTRONE® ℞
[nō-văn-trōne]
Mitoxantrone Hydrochloride Concentrate for Injection

PRODUCT OVERVIEW

KEY FACTS
NOVANTRONE is a synthetic antineoplastic anthracenedione for intravenous use. The precise mechanism of action by which NOVANTRONE exerts its tumoricidal effect has not been fully defined. It is believed to be associated with the inhibition of nucleic acid synthesis, resulting in cell death. Several studies have demonstrated that NOVANTRONE inhibits both RNA and DNA synthesis.

MAJOR USES
NOVANTRONE, in combination with other approved drugs, is indicated for initial therapy of acute nonlymphocytic leukemia (ANLL) in adults, including myelogenous, promelocytic, monocytic, and erythroid acute leukemias.

SAFETY INFORMATION
NOVANTRONE is intended for intravenous use only. The nonvesicant properties of NOVANTRONE minimize the likelihood of severe local reaction. When NOVANTRONE is used as indicated for leukemia, severe myelosuppression will occur as expected. It is, therefore, recommended that NOVANTRONE be administered by physicians experienced in the chemotherapy of this disease. Therapy with NOVANTRONE should be accompanied by close and frequent monitoring of hematologic and chemical laboratory parameters, as well as frequent patient observation.

PRESCRIBING INFORMATION

NOVANTRONE® ℞
[nō-văn-trōne]
Mitoxantrone Hydrochloride Concentrate for Injection

DESCRIPTION
NOVANTRONE is a synthetic antineoplastic anthracenedione for intravenous use. Its molecular formula is $C_{22}H_{28}N_4O_6 \cdot 2HCl$ and its molecular weight is 517.4. It is supplied as a concentrate which **MUST BE DILUTED PRIOR TO INJECTION.** The concentrate is a sterile, dark blue aqueous solution containing mitoxantrone hydrochloride equivalent to 2 mg/mL mitoxantrone free base, with sodium chloride (0.80% w/v), sodium acetate (0.005% w/v), and acetic acid (0.046% w/v) as inactive ingredients. The solution has a pH of 3.0 to 4.5 and contains 0.14 mEq of sodium per mL. The product does not contain preservatives. Its chemical name is: 1,4-Dihydroxy-5, 8-bis [[2-[(2-hydroxyethyl) amino] ethyl] amino-9, 10-anthracenedione dihydrochloride.

CLINICAL PHARMACOLOGY
Athough its mechanism of action is not fully elucidated, NOVANTRONE is a DNA-reactive agent. It has a cytocidal effect on both proliferating and nonproliferating cultured human cells, suggesting lack of cell cycle phase specificity. Pharmacokinetic studies have not been performed in humans receiving multiple daily doses. Pharmacokinetic studies in adult patients following a single intravenous administration of NOVANTRONE have demonstrated multi-exponential plasma clearance. Distribution to tissues is rapid and extensive. Distribution to the brain, spinal cord, eye, and spinal fluid in the monkey is low. The apparent steady-state volume of distribution exceeds $1000L/M^2$. Elimination of drug is slow with an apparent mean terminal plasma half-life of 5.8 days (range 2.3–13.0). The half-life in tissues may be longer. Multiple intravenous doses in dogs daily for five days resulted in significant accumulation in plasma and tissue. The extent of accumulation was fourfold. NOVANTRONE is 78% bound to plasma proteins in the observed concentration range of 26–455 ng/mL. This binding is independent of concentration and was not affected by the presence of diphenylhydantoin, doxorubicin, methotrexate, prednisone, prednisolone, heparin, or acetylsalicylic acid.

NOVANTRONE is excreted via the renal and hepatobiliary systems. Renal excretion is limited; only 6%–11% of the dose is recovered in the urine within five days after drug administration. Of the material recovered in the urine, 65% is unchanged drug; the remaining 35% is comprised primarily of two inactive metabolites and their glucuronide conjugates. The metabolites are mono- and dicarboxylic acid derivatives. Hepatobiliary elimination of drug appears to be of greater significance with as much as 25% of the dose recovered in the feces within five days of intravenous dosing. No significant difference in the pharmacokinetics of NOVANTRONE was observed in seven patients with moderately impaired liver function (serum bilirubin 1.3–3.4 mg/dL) as compared with 16 patients without hepatic dysfunction. Results of pharmacokinetic studies on four patients with severe hepatic dysfunction (bilirubin greater than 3.4 mg/dL) suggest that these patients have a lower total body clearance and a larger Area under Curve than other patients at a comparable NOVANTRONE dose.

In two large randomized multicenter trials, remission induction therapy for ANLL with NOVANTRONE *mitoxantrone* HCl 12 mg/M^2 daily for three days as a ten-minute intravenous infusion and cytosine arabinoside 100 mg/M^2 for seven days given as a continous 24-hour infusion was compared with daunorubicin 45 mg/M^2 daily by intravenous infusion for three days plus the same dose and schedule of cytosine arabinoside used with NOVANTRONE. Patients who had an incomplete antileukemic response received a second induction course in which NOVANTRONE or daunorubicin was given for two days and cytosine arabinoside for five days using the same daily dosage schedule. Response rates and median survival information for both the US and international multicenter trials are given in the following table:

Trial	% Complete Response (CR)		Median Time to CR (days)		Median Survival (days)	
	NOV	DAUN	NOV	DAUN	NOV	DAUN
US	63 (62/98)	53 (54/102)	35	42	312	237
Foreign	50 (56/112)	51 (62/123)	36	42	192	230

NOV = NOVANTRONE + Cytosine arabinoside
DAUN = Daunorubicin + Cytosine arabinoside
In these studies, two consolidation courses were administered to complete responders on each arm. Consolidation therapy consisted of the same drug and daily dosage used for remission induction, but only five days of cytosine arabinoside and two days of NOVANTRONE *mitoxantrone* HCL or daunorubicin were given. The first consolidation course was administered 6 weeks after the start of the final induction course if the patient achieved a complete remission. The second consolidation course was generally administered 4 weeks later. Full hematologic recovery was necessary for patients to receive consolidation therapy. For the US trial, median granulocyte nadirs for patients receiving NOVANTRONE + cytosine arabinoside for consolidation courses 1 and 2 were 10/mm^3 for both courses, and for those patients receiving daunorubicin + cytosine arabinoside were 170/mm^3 and 260/mm^3, respectively. Median platelet nadirs for patients who received NOVANTRONE + cytosine arabinoside for consolidation courses 1 and 2 were 17,000/mm^3 and 14,000/mm^3, respectively, and were 33,000/mm^3 and 22,000/mm^3 in courses 1 and 2 for those patients who received daunorubicin + cytosine arabinoside. The benefit of consolidation therapy in ANLL patients who achieve a complete remission remains controversial. However, in the only well-controlled prospective, randomized multicenter trials with NOVANTRONE in ANLL, consolidation therapy was given to all patients who achieved a complete remission. During consolidation in the US study, two myelosuppression-related deaths occurred on the NOVANTRONE arm and one on the daunorubicin arm. However, in the foreign study there were eight deaths on the NOVANTRONE arm during consolidation which were related to the myelosuppression and none on the daunorubicin arm where less myelosuppression occurred.

INDICATIONS AND USAGE
NOVANTRONE in combination with other approved drug(s) is indicated in the initial therapy of acute nonlymphocytic leukemia (ANLL) in adults. This category includes myelogenous, promyelocytic, monocytic, and erythroid acute leukemias.

CONTRAINDICATIONS
NOVANTRONE is contraindicated in patients who have demonstrated prior hypersensitivity to it.

WARNINGS
WHEN NOVANTRONE IS USED IN DOSES INDICATED FOR THE TREATMENT OF LEUKEMIA, SEVERE MYELOSUPPRESSION WILL OCCUR. THEREFORE, IT IS RECOMMENDED THAT NOVANTRONE BE ADMINISTERED ONLY BY PHYSICIANS EXPERIENCED IN THE CHEMOTHERAPY OF THIS DISEASE. LABORATORY AND SUPPORTIVE SERVICES MUST BE AVAILABLE FOR HEMATOLOGIC AND CHEMISTRY MONITORING AND ADJUNCTIVE THERAPIES, INCLUDING ANTIBIOTICS: BLOOD AND BLOOD PRODUCTS MUST BE AVAILABLE TO SUPPORT PATIENTS DURING THE EXPECTED PERIOD OF MEDULLARY HYPOPLASIA AND SEVERE MYELOSUPPRESSION. PARTICULAR CARE SHOULD BE GIVEN TO ASSURING FULL HEMATOLOGIC RECOVERY BEFORE UNDERTAKING CONSOLIDATION THERAPY (IF THIS TREATMENT IS USED) AND PATIENTS SHOULD BE MONITORED CLOSELY DURING THIS PHASE.

Patients with preexisting myelosuppression as the result of prior drug therapy should not receive NOVANTRONE unless it is felt that the possible benefit from such treatment warrants the risk of further medullary suppression. Because of the possible danger of cardiac effects in patients previously treated with daunorubicin or doxorubicin, the benefit-to-risk ratio of NOVANTRONE therapy in such patients should be determined before starting therapy.

The safety of NOVANTRONE in patients with hepatic insufficiency is not established. (See CLINICAL PHARMACOLOGY.)

Cardiac Effects: *General:* Functional cardiac changes including congestive heart failure and decreases in left ventricular ejection fraction (LVEF) occur with NOVANTRONE. Cardiac toxicity may be more common in patients with prior treatment with anthracyclines, prior mediastinal radiotherapy, or with preexisting cardiovascular disease. Such patients should have regular cardiac monitoring of LVEF from the initiation of therapy. In investigational trials of intermittent single doses in other tumor types, patients who received up to the cumulative dose of 140 mg/M^2 had a cumulative 2.6% probability of clinical congestive heart failure. The overall cumulative probability rate of moderate or serious decreases in LVEF at this dose was 13% in comparative trials.

Leukemia: Acute CHF may occasionally occur in patients treated with NOVANTRONE for ANLL. In first-line comparative trials of NOVANTRONE + cytosine arabinoside *vs* daunorubicin + cytosine arabinoside in adult patients with previously untreated ANLL, therapy was associated with congestive heart failure in 6.5% of patients on each arm. A causal relationship between drug therapy and cardiac effects is difficult to establish in this setting since myocardial function is frequently depressed by the anemia, fever and infection, and hemorrhage, which often accompany the underlying disease.

Pregnancy Category D: NOVANTRONE *mitoxantrone* HCl may cause fetal harm when administered to a pregnant woman. In treated rats, low fetal birth weight and retarded development of the fetal kidney were seen in greater frequency. In rabbits an increased incidence of premature delivery was observed. NOVANTRONE was not teratogenic in rabbits. There are no adequate and well-controlled studies in pregnant women. If this drug is used during pregnancy, or if the patient becomes pregnant while taking this drug, the patient should be apprised of the potential hazard to the fetus. Women of childbearing potential should be advised to avoid becoming pregnant.

Safety for use by routes other than intravenous administration has not been established.

PRECAUTIONS
General: Therapy with NOVANTRONE should be accompanied by close and frequent monitoring of hematologic and chemical laboratory parameters, as well as frequent patient observation.

Hyperuricemia may occur as a result of rapid lysis of tumor cells by NOVANTRONE. Serum uric acid levels should be monitored and hypouricemic therapy instituted prior to the initiation of antileukemic therapy.

Systemic infections should be treated concomitantly with or just prior to commencing therapy with NOVANTRONE.

Information for Patients: NOVANTRONE may impart a blue-green color to the urine for 24 hours after administration, and patients should be advised to expect this during therapy. Bluish discoloration of the sclera may also occur. Patients should be advised of the signs and symptoms of myelosuppression.

Laboratory Tests: Serial complete blood counts and liver function tests are necessary for appropriate dose adjustments. (See **DOSAGE AND ADMINISTRATION** section.)

Carcinogenesis, Mutagenesis: NOVANTRONE *mitoxantrone* HCL can result in chromosomal aberrations in animals and it is mutagenic in bacterial systems. NOVANTRONE caused DNA damage and sister chromatid exchanges *in vitro.*

Pregnancy Category D: (See WARNINGS section.)

Nursing Mothers: It is not known whether NOVANTRONE is excreted in human milk. Because of the potential for serious adverse reactions in infants from NOVANTRONE, breast feeding should be discontinued before starting treatment.

Pediatric Use: Safety and effectiveness in children have not been established.

ADVERSE REACTIONS

NOVANTRONE has been studied in approximately 600 patients with acute nonlymphocytic leukemia. The table below represents the adverse reaction experience in the large US comparative study of NOVANTRONE + cytosine arabinoside vs daunorubicin + cytosine arabinoside. Experience in the large foreign study was similar. A much wider experience in a variety of other tumor types revealed no additional important reactions other than cardiomyopathy (See **WARNINGS.**) It should be appreciated that the listed adverse reaction categories include overlapping clinical symptoms related to the same condition, eg, dyspnea, cough, and pneumonia. In addition, the listed adverse reactions cannot all necessarily be attributed to chemotherapy as it is often impossible to distinguish effects of the drug and effects of the underlying disease. It is clear, however, that the combination of NOVANTRONE + cytosine arabinoside was responsible for nausea and vomiting, alopecia, mucositis/stomatitis, and myelosuppression.

The following table summarizes adverse reactions occurring in patients treated with NOVANTRONE + cytosine arabinoside in comparison with those who received daunorubicin + cytosine arabinoside for therapy of ANLL in a large, multicenter, randomized prospective US trial. Adverse reactions are presented as major categories and selected examples of clinically significant subcategories.

[See table right].

Allergic Reaction: Hypotension, urticaria, dyspnea, and rashes have been reported occasionally.

Cutaneous: Phlebitis has been reported infrequently at the site of infusion. There have been rare reports of tissue necrosis following extravasation.

Hematologic: Myelosuppression is rapid in onset and is consistent with the requirement to produce significant marrow hypoplasia in order to achieve a response. The incidences of infection and bleeding seen in the US trial are consistent with those reported for other standard induction regimens.

Gastrointestinal: Nausea and vomiting occurred acutely in most patients, but were generally mild to moderate and could be controlled through the use of antiemetics. Stomatitis/mucositis occurs within one week of therapy.

Cardiovascular: Congestive heart failure, tachycardia, EKG changes including arrhythmias, chest pain, and asymptomatic decreases in left ventricular ejection fraction have occurred (See **WARNINGS.**)

OVERDOSAGE

There is no known specific antidote for NOVANTRONE mitoxantrone HCL. Accidental overdoses have been reported. Four patients receiving 140–180 mg/M^2 as a single bolus injection died as a result of severe leukopenia with infection. Hematologic support and antimicrobial therapy may be required during prolonged periods of medullary hypoplasia. Although patients with severe renal failure have not been studied, NOVANTRONE is extensively tissue bound and it is unlikely that the therapeutic effect or toxicity would be mitigated by peritoneal or hemodialysis.

DOSAGE AND ADMINISTRATION

(See **WARNINGS.**)

NOVANTRONE SOLUTION MUST BE DILUTED PRIOR TO USE.

Combination Initial Therapy for ANLL in Adults: For induction, the recommended dosage is 12 mg/M^2 of NOVANTRONE daily on days 1–3 given as an intravenous infusion, and 100 mg/M^2 cytosine arabinoside for seven days given as a continuous 24-hour infusion on days 1–7.

Most complete remissions will occur following the initial course of induction therapy. In the event of an incomplete antileukemic response, a second induction course may be given. NOVANTRONE should be given for two days and cytosine arabinoside for five days using the same daily dosage levels.

If severe or life-threatening nonhematologic toxicity is observed during the first induction course, the second induction course should be withheld until toxicity clears.

Consolidation therapy which was used in two large, randomized multicenter trials consisted of NOVANTRONE 12 mg/M^2 given by intravenous infusion daily for days one and two, and cytosine arabinoside 100 mg/M^2 for five days given as a continuous 24-hour infusion on days 1–5. The first course was given approximately 6 weeks after the final induction course; the second was generally administered 4 weeks after the first. Severe myelosuppression occurred. (See CLINICAL PHARMACOLOGY Section.)

NOVANTRONE solution should be diluted to at least 50 mL with either 0.9% Sodium Chloride Injection (USP) or 5% Dextrose Injection (USP). This solution should be introduced into the tubing as a freely running intravenous infusion of 0.9% Sodium Chloride Injection (USP) or 5% Dextrose Injection (USP) over a period of not less than three minutes. Unused infusion solutions should de discarded in an appropriate fashion. If extravasation occurs, the administration

	ALL INDUCTION (percentage of pts entering induction)		ALL CONSOLIDATION (percentage of pts entering consolidation)	
	NOV N=102	DAUN N=102	NOV N=55	DAUN N=49
Cardiovascular	26	28	11	24
CHF	5	6	0	0
Arrhythmias	3	3	4	4
Bleeding	37	41	20	6
GI	16	12	2	2
Petechiae/Ecchymoses	7	9	11	2
Gastrointestinal	88	85	58	51
Nausea/Vomiting	72	67	31	31
Diarrhea	47	47	18	8
Abdominal Pain	15	9	9	4
Mucositis/Stomatitis	29	33	18	8
Hepatic	10	11	14	2
Jaundice	3	8	7	0
Infections	66	73	60	43
UTI	7	2	7	2
Pneumonia	9	7	9	0
Sepsis	34	36	31	18
Fungal Infections	15	13	9	6
Renal Failure	8	6	0	2
Fever	78	71	24	18
Alopecia	37	40	22	16
Pulmonary	43	43	24	14
Cough	13	9	9	2
Dyspnea	18	20	6	0
CNS	30	30	34	35
Seizures	4	4	2	8
Headache	10	9	13	8
Eye	7	6	2	4
Conjunctivitis	5	1	0	0

should be stopped immediately and restarted in another vein. The nonvesicant properties of NOVANTRONE minimize the possibility of severe local reactions following extravasation. However, care should be taken to avoid extravasation at the infusion site and to avoid contact of NOVANTRONE with the skin, mucous membranes, or eyes. Skin accidentally exposed to NOVANTRONE should be rinsed copiously with warm water and if the eyes are involved, standard irrigation techniques should be used immediately. The use of goggles, gloves, and protective gowns is recommended during preparation and administration of the drug. Spills on equipment and environmental surfaces may be cleaned using an aqueous solution of calcium hypochlorite (5.5 parts calcium hypochlorite in 13 parts by weight of water for each 1 part of NOVANTRONE). Absorb the solution with gauze or towels and dispose of these in a safe manner. Appropriate safety equipment such as goggles and gloves should be worn while working with calcium hypochlorite.

NOVANTRONE should not be mixed in the same infusion as heparin since a precipitate may form. Because specific compatibility data are not available, it is recommended that NOVANTRONE not be mixed in the same infusion with other drugs.

Procedures for proper handling and disposal of anticancer drugs should be considered. Several guidelines on this subject have been published.[1–6] There is no general agreement that all of the procedures recommended in the guidelines are necessary or appropriate.

REFERENCES

1. Recommendations for the Safe Handling of Parenteral Antineoplastic Drugs. NIH Publication No. 83-2621. For sale by the Superintendent of Documents, U.S. Government Printing Office, Washington, D.C. 20402.
2. AMA Council Report. Guidelines for Handling Parenteral Antineoplastics. *JAMA*, March 15, 1985.
3. National Study Commission on Cytotoxic Exposure—Recommendations for Handling Cytotoxic Agents. Available from Louis P. Jeffrey, Sc. D., Director of Pharmacy Services, Rhode Island Hospital, 593 Eddy Street, Providence, Rhode Island 02902.
4. Clinical Oncological Society of Australia: Guidelines and recommendations for safe handling of antineoplastic agents. *Med J Australia* 1:426–428 1983.
5. Jones R.B., et al. Safe handling of chemotherapeutic agents: A report from the Mount Sinai Medical Center. *Ca—A Cancer Journal for Clinicians* Sept/Oct, 258–263 1983.
6. American Society of Hospital Pharmacists: Technical assistance bulletin on handling cytotoxic drugs in hospitals. *Am J Hosp Pharm* 42:131–137 1985.

NOVANTRONE may be further diluted into Dextrose 5% in Water, Normal Saline or Dextrose 5% with Normal Saline and used immediately. DO NOT FREEZE.

Parenteral drug products should be inspected visually for particulate matter and discoloration prior to administration whenever solution and container permit.

HOW SUPPLIED

NOVANTRONE mitoxantrone HCl concentrate for injection is a sterile aqueous solution at a concentration equivalent to 2 mg mitoxantrone free base per mL and is supplied in vials for single dose use as follows:

  NDC 0005-9393-34—10 mL/vial (20 mg)
  NDC 0005-9393-72—12.5 mL/vial (25 mg)
  NDC 0005-9393-36—15 mL/vial (30 mg)

NOVANTRONE is stable for two years from time of manufacture.

NOVANTRONE should be stored at Controlled Room Temperature 15–30°C (59–86°F). DO NOT FREEZE.

Rev. 2/88
22251

Manufactured by
LEDERLE LABORATORIES
Gosport, Hampshire, England
Distributed by
LEDERLE LABORATORIES DIVISION
American Cyanamid Company
Pearl River, NY 10965

Shown in Product Identification Section, page 415

OCCUCOAT™
2% Hydroxypropylmethylcellulose

(See PDR For Ophthalmology)

ORIMUNE®   ℞
[or-ĭ-mune]
POLIOVIRUS VACCINE
LIVE ORAL TRIVALENT
0.5 mL Dose Contains Sorbitol
SABIN STRAINS TYPES 1, 2 and 3
FOR ORAL ADMINISTRATION—NOT
FOR INJECTION

DESCRIPTION

Manufacture and Composition: *Poliovirus vaccine live oral trivalent* ORIMUNE is a mixture of three types of attenuated polioviruses which have been propagated in monkey kidney cell culture. The cells are grown in the presence of Eagle's Basal Medium consisting of Earle's Balanced Salt Solution containing amino acids, antibiotics and calf serum. After cell growth, the medium is removed and replaced with fresh medium containing the inoculating virus but no calf serum. The

Continued on next page

Lederle—Cont.

final vaccine is diluted with a modified cell culture maintenance medium containing sorbitol. Each dose (0.5 mL) contains less than 25 micrograms of each of the antibiotics, streptomycin and neomycin.

The potency is expressed in terms of the amount of virus contained in the recommended dose as tissue culture infective doses ($TCID_{50}$). The human dose of vaccine containing all three virus types shall be constituted to have infectivity titers in the final container material of $10^{5.4}$ to $10^{6.4}$ for Type 1, $10^{4.5}$ to $10^{5.5}$ for Type 2, and $10^{5.2}$ to $10^{6.2}$ for Type 3.[1]

CLINICAL PHARMACOLOGY

Administration of attenuated, live oral poliovirus vaccine (OPV) simulates natural infection, inducing active mucosal and systemic immunity without producing untoward symptoms of disease. For optimal mucosal immunity to occur, it is necessary for the virus to multiply in the intestinal tract. A primary series of trivalent vaccine is designed to produce an antibody response to poliovirus Types 1, 2, and 3. This response is comparable to the immunity induced by the natural disease. The antibodies thus formed help protect the individual against clinical poliomyelitis infection by any of the three types of poliovirus. Multiple doses of OPV in the primary series are not administered as boosters, but to insure that immunity to all three types of poliovirus has been achieved.[2] When used in the prescribed manner for immunization, type specific neutralizing antibodies will be induced in 90% or more of susceptibles.

INDICATIONS AND USAGE

This vaccine is indicated for use in the prevention of poliomyelitis caused by poliovirus Types 1, 2, and 3.

Infants starting at 6 to 12 weeks of age, all unimmunized children and adolescents up to age 18 are the usual candidates for routine prophylaxis.

The Immunization Practices Advisory Committee (ACIP) of the Public Health Service states that trivalent oral poliovirus vaccine (OPV) and inactivated poliovirus vaccine (IPV) are both effective in preventing poliomyelitis.

The choice of OPV as the preferred poliovirus vaccine for primary administration to children in the United States has been made by the ACIP, the Committee on Infectious Diseases of the American Academy of Pediatrics, and a special expert committee of the Institute of Medicine, National Academy of Science.[2,3,4] OPV is preferred because it induces intestinal immunity, is simple to administer, is well accepted by patients, results in immunization of some contacts of vaccinated persons, and has a record of having essentially eliminated disease associated with wild poliovirus in this country.[3] OPV is also recommended for control of epidemic poliomyelitis.[2,3]

Past history of clinical poliomyelitis or prior vaccination with IPV in otherwise healthy individuals does not preclude the administration of OPV when otherwise indicated.

Serologic evidence indicates that measles and rubella vaccines or combinations (measles-mumps-rubella vaccine) given simultaneously with trivalent oral poliovirus vaccine can be expected to give adequate antibody response.[5]

Routine poliomyelitis immunization for adults residing in the continental United States is not necessary because of extreme unlikelihood of exposure. However, primary immunization with IPV is recommended whenever feasible for those unimmunized adults subject to *increased risk* of exposure, as by travel to or contact with epidemic or endemic areas and for those employed in hospitals, medical laboratories, clinics, or sanitation facilities. If less than 4 weeks are available before protection is needed, a single dose of TOPV is recommended, with the remaining doses of vaccine given later if the person remains at increased risk. Immunization with IPV may be indicated for unimmunized parents and those in other special situations where, in the judgment of the attending physician, protection may be needed.[3] (See CONTRAINDICATIONS and ADVERSE REACTIONS.)

Community Programs: Poliovirus vaccine live oral trivalent ORIMUNE has been recommended for epidemic control. Within an epidemic area, OPV should be provided for all persons over 6 weeks of age who have not been completely immunized or whose immunization status is unknown, with the exceptions noted under immunodeficiency.[2,3] (See CONTRAINDICATIONS.)

In certain tropical endemic areas, where poliomyelitis has been increasing in recent years, the physician may wish to administer OPV to the infant at birth. Because successful immunization is less likely in newborn infants, a complete series of OPV should follow the neonatal dose beginning when the infants are 2 months old.[2] If the physician chooses to immunize the infant at birth, it may be wise to wait until the child is three days old, and it may be prudent to recommend abstention from breastfeeding for two to three hours before and after oral vaccination to permit the establishment of the vaccine viruses in the gut.[6]

CONTRAINDICATIONS

Under no circumstances should this vaccine be administered parenterally.

Administration of the vaccine should be postponed or avoided in those experiencing any acute illness and in those with any advanced debilitated condition or persistent vomiting or diarrhea.

Other viruses (including poliovirus and other enterovirus) may interfere with the desired response to this vaccine, since their presence in the intestinal tract may interfere with the replication of the attenuated strains of poliovirus in the vaccine.

ORIMUNE **must not** be administered to patients with immune deficiency diseases such as combined immunodeficiency, hypogammaglobulinemia and agammaglobulinemia. Further, *Poliovirus vaccine live oral trivalent* ORIMUNE **must not** be administered to patients with altered immune states, such as those occurring in thymic abnormalities, leukemia, lymphoma, or generalized malignancy or by lowered resistance from therapy with corticosteroids, alkylating drugs, antimetabolites, or radiation. Because vaccine viruses are excreted by the vaccinee, and may spread to contacts, ORIMUNE should not be used in families with immunodeficient members.[2]

Recipients of the vaccine should avoid close household-type contact with all persons with altered immune status for at least 6 to 8 weeks.

Because of the possibility of immunodeficiency in other children born to a family in which there has been one such case, OPV should not be given to a member of a household in which there is a family history of immunodeficiency until the immune status of the intended recipient and other children in the family is determined to be normal.

IPV is preferred for immunizing all persons in the above described circumstances regarding immunodeficiency.

WARNINGS

Under no circumstances should this vaccine be administered parenterally.

Administration of the vaccine should be postponed or avoided in those experiencing any acute illness and in those with any advanced debilitated condition or persistent vomiting or diarrhea.

Other viruses (including poliovirus and other enterovirus) may interfere with the desired response to this vaccine, since their presence in the intestinal tract may interfere with the replication of the attenuated strains of poliovirus in the vaccine.

PRECAUTIONS

Preliminary data indicate that Immune Globulin (Human) (IG) does not appear to interfere with immunization with OPV.[7] However, until more data are available, it would seem prudent not to administer OPV shortly after Immune Globulin (IG) unless such a procedure is unavoidable, for example, with unexpected travel to or contact with epidemic or endemic areas. If OPV is given with or shortly after IG, the dose probably should be repeated after three months if immunization is still indicated.[8]

The vaccine is not effective in modifying or preventing cases of existing and/or incubating poliomyelitis.

National Childhood Vaccine Injury Act of 1986 (as amended in 1987): This Act requires that the manufacturer and lot number of the vaccine administered be recorded by the health care provider in the vaccine recipient's permanent record, along with the date of administration of the vaccine and the name, address, and title of the person administering the vaccine.

The Act further requires the health care provider to report to a health department or to the FDA the occurrence following immunization of any event set forth in the Vaccine Injury Table including: paralytic poliomyelitis—in a nonimmunodeficient recipient within 30 days of vaccination,—in an immunodeficient recipient within 6 months of vaccination; any vaccine-associated community case of paralytic poliomyelitis; or any acute complication or sequela (including death) of above events.[9]

Use in Pregnancy: Pregnancy Category C: Animal reproduction studies have not been conducted with *poliovirus vaccine live oral trivalent.* It is also not known whether OPV can cause fetal harm when administered to a pregnant woman or can affect reproduction capacity.

Although there is no convincing evidence documenting adverse effects of either OPV or IPV on the developing fetus or pregnant women, it is prudent on theoretical grounds to avoid vaccinating pregnant women. However, if immediate protection against poliomyelitis is needed, OPV is recommended.[3] (See CONTRAINDICATIONS and ADVERSE REACTIONS.)

ADVERSE REACTIONS

Paralytic disease following the ingestion of live poliovirus vaccines has been, on rare occasion, reported in individuals receiving the vaccine, and in persons who were in close contact with vaccinees.[2,3,4,10,11,12,13,14] The vaccine viruses are shed in the vaccinee's stools for at least six to eight weeks as well as via the pharyngeal route. Most reports of paralytic disease following ingestion of the vaccine or contact with a recent vaccinee are based on epidemiological analysis and temporal association between vaccination or contact and the onset of symptoms. Most authorities believe that a causal relationship exists.[2,11,14,15,16]

Prior to administration of the vaccine, the attending physician should warn or specifically direct personnel acting under his authority to convey the warnings to the vaccinee, parent, guardian, or other responsible person of the possibility of vaccine-associated paralysis, particularly to the recipient, susceptible family members, and other close personal contacts.[3]

The Centers for Disease Control report that during the years 1973 through 1984 approximately 274.1 million OPV doses were distributed in the United States. During this same period, 105 vaccine-associated cases were reported (1 case per 2.6 million doses distributed). Of these 105 cases, 35 occurred in vaccine recipients (1 case per 7.8 million doses distributed), 50 occurred in household and nonhousehold contacts of vaccines (1 case per 5.5 million doses distributed), 14 occurred in immunodeficient recipients or contacts, and 6 occurred in persons with no history of vaccine exposure, from whom vaccine-like viruses were isolated.[14]

Thirty-three (94%) of the receipient cases, 41 (82%) of the contact cases, and 5 (36%) of the immune deficient cases were associated with the recipient's first dose of OPV. Because most cases of vaccine-associated paralysis have occurred in association with the first dose, the CDC has estimated the likelihood of paralysis in association with first *v* subsequent doses of OPV, using the number of births during 1973–1984 to estimate the number of first doses distributed, and subtracting this from the total distribution to estimate the number of subsequent doses distributed. This method estimates a frequency of paralysis for recipients of 1 case per 1.2 million first doses *v* 1 case per 116.5 million subsequent doses; for contacts one case per 1 million first doses *v* 25.9 million subsequent doses; with an overall frequency of 1 case per 520,000 first doses *v* 1 case per 12.3 million subsequent doses.[14]

Other methods of estimating the likelihood of paralysis in association with OPV have been described. Because the number of susceptible vaccine recipients or contacts of recipients is not known, the true risk of vaccine-associated poliomyelitis is impossible to determine precisely.[14]

When the attenuated vaccine strains are to be introduced into a household with adults who have not been adequately vaccinated or whose immune status cannot be determined, the risk of vaccine-associated paralysis can be reduced by giving these adults three doses of IPV a month apart before the children receive *poliovirus vaccine live oral trivalent* ORIMUNE.[3] The children may receive the first dose of ORIMUNE at the same visit that the adult receives the third dose of IPV. The CDC reports that no paralytic reactions to IPV are known to have occurred since the 1955 cluster of poliomyelitis cases caused by vaccine that contained live polioviruses that had escaped inactivation.[3]

The ACIP states: "Because of the overriding importance of ensuring prompt and complete immunization of the child and the extreme rarity of OPV-associated disease in contacts, the Committee recommends the administration of OPV to a child regardless of the poliovirus-vaccine status of adult household contacts. This is the usual practice in the United States. The responsible adult should be informed of the small risk involved. An acceptable alternative, if there is a strong assurance that ultimate, full immunization of the child will not be jeopardized or unduly delayed, is to immunize adults according to the schedule outlined above before giving OPV to the child."[3]

The ACIP has concluded that "Oral polio vaccine remains the vaccine of choice for primary immunization of children."[3]

DOSAGE AND ADMINISTRATION

ORIMUNE is to be administered *orally, under the supervision of a physician. Under no circumstances should this vaccine be administered parenterally.* For convenience, the vaccine is supplied in a disposable pipette containing a single dose of 0.5 mL. The vaccine can be administered directly or mixed with distilled water, tap water free of chlorine, simple syrup NF, or milk. Alternatively, it may be adsorbed on any one of a number of foods such as bread, cake, or cube sugar. Breast feeding does not interfere with successful immunization.[3]

Initial Administration (Primary Series)

Infants: The primary series is three doses. The ACIP and the American Academy of Pediatrics recommends that the three-dose immunization series be started at 6 to 12 weeks of age, commonly with the first DTP inoculation at 2 months of age. The second dose should be given not less than 6 and preferably 8 weeks later, commonly at 4 months of age. The third dose is an integral part of the primary immunization and should be administered 8 to 12 months after the second dose, commonly at 18 months of age. An optional dose of OPV may be given at 6 months of age in areas where poliomyelitis is endemic.[2,3]

Older Children and Adolescents (up to age 18): Two doses, given not less than 6 and preferably 8 weeks apart and the third dose 6 to 12 months after the second dose.[2,3]

Adults: See INDICATIONS and ADVERSE REACTIONS. Where *Poliovirus vaccine live oral trivalent* ORIMUNE is given to unimmunized adults, the dosage is as indicated for children and adolescents.

Booster Doses: *School Entrance:* On entering elementary school, all children who have completed the primary series should be given a single follow-up dose of trivalent oral poliovirus vaccine.[2,3] All others should complete the primary series. The fourth supplemental dose is not required in those who received the third primary dose on or after their fourth birthday.[3] The ACIP does not recommend routine booster doses of vaccine on the basis of current information, beyond that given at the time of entering school.[3] It has been shown that over 95% of children studied five years after full immunization with oral poliovirus vaccine had protective antibodies to all three types of poliovirus.[17]

Increased Risk: If an individual who has completed a primary series is subjected to a substantially increased risk by virtue of contact, travel, or occupation, a single dose of OPV has been suggested.[3]

STORAGE

To maintain potency, it is necessary to store this vaccine at a temperature which will maintain ice continuously in a solid state. This vaccine may remain fluid at temperatures above −14°C (+7°F) because of its sorbitol content. If frozen, the vaccine must be completely thawed prior to use. A container of vaccine that has been frozen and then is thawed may be carried through a maximum of 10 freeze-thaw cycles, provided the temperature does not exceed 8°C (46°F) during the periods of thaw, and provided the total cumulative duration of thaw does not exceed 24 hours. If the 24-hour period is exceeded, the vaccine then must be used within 30 days, during which time it must be stored at a temperature between 2°-8°C (36°-46°F).

Color Change: This vaccine contains phenol red as a pH indicator. The usual color of the vaccine is pink, although some containers of vaccine, shipped or stored in dry ice, may exhibit a yellow coloration due to the very low temperature or possible absorption of carbon dioxide. The color of the vaccine prior to use (red-pink-yellow) has no effect on the virus or efficacy of the vaccine.

DISCLAIMER OF REPRESENTATIONS AND WARRANTIES

This vaccine has been produced and tested in accordance with the regulations of the United States Food and Drug Administration for the production of Poliovirus vaccine live oral trivalent. The manufacturer makes no representation or warranty, expressed or implied, with respect to the merchantability or fitness for use of this vaccine other than that the vaccine has been produced in accordance with the standards for its production prescribed by the United States Food and Drug Administration and applicable thereto at the time of its release by the manufacturer. While the use of this preparation and other measures described herein are consistent with accepted standards of medical practice, their use as described cannot be expected necessarily to assure a specific result.

DIRECTIONS FOR USE: Pull off the protective cap and squeeze to expel contents.

HOW SUPPLIED

2084-08-10 (0.5 mL) DISPETTES®
2084-12-50 (0.5 mL) DISPETTES

Military Depot: NSN 6505-01-185-8848, 50 × 1 dose Dispettes

REFERENCES

1. *Code of Federal Regulations.* 21 CFR 630.17[c] p 97 (revised Apr 1985).
2. Report of the Committee on the Control of Infectious Diseases. *Amer Acad of Pediatr* 1982; 19:207–211.
3. Recommendations of the Public Health Service Immunization Practices Advisory Committee [ACIP]. *MMWR* 1982; 31:22–34.
4. Nightingale EO: Recommendations for a national policy on poliomyelitis vaccination. *N Engl J Med* 1977; 297:249–253.
5. Recommendations of ACIP Simultaneous Administration of Certain Live Virus Vaccines. *MMWR* 1972; 21:403.
6. Welsh JH, et al: Anti-infective properties of breast milk. *J Pediatr* 1979; 94:1–9.
7. Melnick JL: Advantages and disadvantages of killed and live poliomyelitis vaccines. *Bull WHO* 1978; 56:21–38.
8. Immunization Practices Advisory Committee [ACIP], general recommendations on immunization. *MMWR* 1980; 29:76–83.
9. National Childhood Injury Act: Requirements for Permanent Vaccination Records and for Reporting Selected Events after Vaccination. *MMWR* 37[13]:197–200 [April 8] 1988.
10. Henderson DA, et al. Paralytic disease associated with oral polio vaccines. *JAMA* 1964; 190:41–48.
11. Morse LJ, et al. Vaccine-acquired paralytic poliomyelitis in an unvaccinated mother. *JAMA* 1966; 197: 1034–1035.
12. Swanson PD, et al. Poliomyelitis associated with type 2 virus. *JAMA* 1967; 201:771–773.
13. Balduzzi P, et al. Paralytic poliomyelitis in a contact of a vaccinated child. *New Engl J Med* 1967; 276:796–797.
14. Nkowane BM, Wassilak, SGF, Orenstein, WA et al: Vaccine-associated Paralytic Poliomyelitis. United States: 1973 through 1984. *JAMA* 1987 257[10]: 1335–1340.
15. Center for Disease Control: *Neurotropic Diseases Surveillance Annual Poliomyelitis Summary 1971.* [March 1973].
16. Evidence on the Safety and Efficacy of Live Poliomyelitis Vaccines Currently in Use with Special Reference to Type 3 Poliovirus. *Bull WHO* 40[6]:925–945, 1969.
17. Krugman, RD, et al: Antibody persistence after primary immunization with trivalent oral poliovirus vaccine. *Pediatrics* 1977:60:80–82.

LEDERLE LABORATORIES DIVISION
American Cyanamid Company
Pearl River, NY 10965   Rev. 10/88
24370

PERITINIC

[perĭ-tĭn-ĭk]
Hematinic with Vitamins and Fecal Softener Tablets (Film Coated)

DESCRIPTION

In the prevention of nutritional anemias, certain vitamin deficiencies and iron-deficiency anemias.
Each tablet contains:

Elemental Iron	100 mg	
(as Ferrous Fumarate)		
Docusate Sodium USP	100 mg	
(DSS) (to counteract the constipating effect of iron)		
Vitamin B₁	7.5 mg	(7½ MDR)
(as Thiamine Mononitrate)		
Vitamin B₂	7.5 mg	(6¼ MDR)
(Riboflavin)		
Vitamin B₆	7.5 mg	
(Pyridoxine Hydrochloride)		
Vitamin B₁₂	50 mcg	
(Cyanocobalamin)		
Vitamin C	200 mg	(6⅔ MDR)
(Ascorbic Acid)		
Niacinamide	30 mg	(3 MDR)
Folic Acid	0.05 mg	
Pantothenic Acid	15 mg	
(as D-Pantothenyl Alcohol)		

MDR—Adult Minimum Daily Requirement

Inactive Ingredients: Alginic Acid, Amberlite Resin, Blue 2, Ethyl Cellulose, Hydroxypropyl Methylcellulose, Lactose, Magnesium Stearate, Modified Food Starch, Povidone, Red 40, Silica Gel, Titanium Dioxide, Yellow 6, and other ingredients.

RECOMMENDED INTAKE

Adults, 1 or 2 tablets daily.

WARNING

As with any drug, if you are pregnant or nursing a baby, seek the advice of a health professional before using this product. Keep out of the reach of children.
In case of accidental overdose, seek professional assistance or contact a Poison Control Center immediately.

HOW SUPPLIED

Embossed LL and P8
NDC 0005-5124-19—Bottles of 60
LEDERLE LABORATORIES DIVISION
American Cyanamid Company,
Pearl River, N.Y. 10965   Rev. 5/87
18649

PIPRACIL®   ℞

[pĭp-ra-sĭl]
sterile piperacillin sodium
For Intravenous and Intramuscular Use

PRODUCT OVERVIEW

KEY FACTS

PIPRACIL is a semisynthetic broad-spectrum penicillin antibiotic for parenteral administration. PIPRACIL is bactericidal against a wide range of gram-negative and gram-positive pathogens, including aerobic and anaerobic strains. PIPRACIL has demonstrated excellent activity against *Pseudomonas aeruginosa*, with little development of resistance. It is particularly useful for treating mixed infections and for presumptive therapy prior to identifying the causative organisms.

MAJOR USES

PIPRACIL has been proven effective for treatment of serious infections, including bacteremia, caused by susceptible strains of microorganisms. (See full Prescribing Information.) PIPRACIL may be administered as a single drug in some situations where two antibiotics might otherwise be employed. It has also been used successfully with aminoglycosides. Before initiating therapy, obtain cultures for susceptibility testing; once results are known, adjust therapy, if necessary.

SAFETY INFORMATION

PIPRACIL is contraindicated in patients with a history of hypersensitivity reaction to any of the penicillins and/or cephalosporins. While PIPRACIL possesses the characteristic low toxicity of the penicillin group of antibiotics, periodic assessment of organ system functions, including renal, hepatic, and hematopoietic, is advisable during prolonged therapy.

PRESCRIBING INFORMATION

PIPRACIL®   ℞

[pĭp-ra-sĭl]
sterile piperacillin sodium
For Intravenous and Intramuscular Use

DESCRIPTION

PIPRACIL is a semisynthetic broad-spectrum penicillin for parenteral use derived from D (-) α-aminobenzylpenicillin. The chemical name of piperacillin sodium is [2S-[2α,5α,6β(S*)]]-6-[[[[(4-ethyl-2,3-dioxo-1-piperazinyl)carbonyl]amino] phenylacetyl] amino] -3, 3- dimethyl-7 -oxo-4-thia-1-azabicyclo[3.2.0]heptane-2-carboxylic acid, monosodium salt.

PIPRACIL is a white to off-white hygroscopic cryodesiccated crystalline powder which is readily soluble in water and gives a colorless to pale-yellow solution. The pH of the aqueous solution is 5.5 to 7.5. One g contains 1.85 mEq (42.5 mg) of sodium (Na⁺).

CLINICAL PHARMACOLOGY

Intravenous Administration: In healthy adult volunteers, mean serum levels immediately after a two- to three-minute intravenous injection of 2, 4, or 6 g were 305, 412, and 775 mcg/mL. Serum levels lack dose proportionality. [See table on next page].
A 30-minute infusion of 6 g every 6 h gave, on the fourth day, a mean peak serum concentration of 420 mcg/mL.

Intramuscular Administration: PIPRACIL is rapidly absorbed after intramuscular injection. In healthy volunteers, the mean peak serum concentration occurs approximately 30 minutes after a single dose of 2 g and is about 36 mcg/mL. The oral administration of 1 g probenecid before injection produces an increase in piperacillin peak serum level of about 30%. The area under the curve (AUC) is increased by approximately 60%.

General: PIPRACIL is not absorbed when given orally. Peak serum concentrations are attained approximately 30 minutes after intramuscular injections and immediately after completion of intravenous injection or infusion. The serum half-life in healthy volunteers ranges from 36 minutes to one hour and 12 minutes. The mean elimination half-life of PIPRACIL in healthy adult volunteers is 54 minutes following administration of 2 g and 63 minutes following 6 g. As with other penicillins, PIPRACIL is eliminated primarily by glomerular filtration and tubular secretion; it is excreted rapidly as unchanged drug in high concentrations in the urine. Approximately 60% to 80% of the administered dose is excreted in the urine in the first 24 hours. Piperacillin urine concentrations, determined by microbioassay, were as high as 14,100 mcg/mL following a 6 g intravenous dose and 8,500 mcg/mL following a 4 g intravenous dose. These urine drug concentrations remained well above 1,000 mcg/mL throughout the dosing interval. The elimination half-life is increased twofold in mild-to-moderate renal impairment and fivefold to sixfold in severe impairment.

PIPRACIL binding to human serum proteins is 16%. The drug is widely distributed in human tissues and body fluids, including bone, prostate, and heart, and reaches high concentrations in bile. After a 4 gram bolus, maximum biliary concentrations averaged 3,205 mcg/mL. It penetrates into the cerebrospinal fluid in the presence of inflamed meninges. Because PIPRACIL is excreted by the biliary route as well as by the renal route, it can be used safely in appropriate dosage (see DOSAGE AND ADMINISTRATION) in

Continued on next page

Information on Lederle products listed on these pages is the full prescribing information from product literature or package inserts effective in August, 1989. Information concerning all Lederle products may be obtained from the Professional Services Department, Lederle Laboratories, Pearl River, New York, 10965.

Lederle—Cont.

patients with severely restricted kidney function, and can be used effectively in treatment of hepatobiliary infections.

Microbiology: PIPRACIL *sterile piperacillin sodium* is an antibiotic which exerts its bactericidal activity by inhibiting both septum and cell wall synthesis. It is active against a variety of gram-positive and gram-negative aerobic and anaerobic bacteria. *In vitro*, piperacillin is active against most strains of clinical isolates of the following microorganisms:

Aerobic and facultatively anaerobic organisms

Gram-negative bacteria

Escherichia coli
Proteus mirabilis
Proteus vulgaris
Morganella morganii (formerly *Proteus morganii*)
Providencia rettgeri (formerly *Proteus rettgeri*)
Serratia species including *S marcescens* and *S liquefaciens*
Klebsiella pneumoniae
Klebsiella species
Enterobacter species including *E aerogenes* and *E cloacae*
Citrobacter species including *C freundii* and *C diversus*
Salmonella species*
Shigella species*
Pseudomonas aeruginosa
Pseudomonas species including *P cepacia,* *P maltophilia,* and *P fluorescens*
Acinetobacter species (formerly *Mima-Herellea*)
Haemophilus influenzae (non-β-lactamase-producing strains)
Neisseria gonorrhoeae
Neisseria meningitidis
Moraxella species*
Yersinia species* (formerly *Pasteurella*)

Gram-positive bacteria

Group D streptococci including
    Enterococci (*Streptococcus faecalis, S faecium*)
    Non-enterococci*
β-hemolytic streptococci including
    Group A *Streptococcus* (*S pyogenes*)
    Group B *Streptococcus* (*S agalactiae*)
Streptococcus pneumoniae
Streptococcus viridans
Staphylococcus aureus (non-penicillinase-producing)*
Staphylococcus epidermidis (non-penicillinase-producing)*

Anaerobic bacteria

Actinomyces species*
Bacteroides species including
    B fragilis group (*B fragilis, B vulgatus*)
    Non-*B fragilis* group (*B melaninogenicus*)
    B asaccharolyticus
Clostridium species including
    C perfringens and *C difficile**
Eubacterium species
Fusobacterium species including
    F nucleatum and *F necrophorum*
Peptococcus species
Peptostreptococcus species
Veillonella species

*Piperacillin has been shown to be active *in vitro* against these organisms; however, clinical efficacy has not yet been established.

In vitro, PIPRACIL *sterile piperacillin sodium* is inactivated by staphylococcal β-lactamases and β-lactamases produced by gram-negative bacteria. However, it is active against β-lactamase-producing gonococci.

Many strains of gram-negative organisms resistant to certain antibiotics have been found to be susceptible to PIPRACIL.

PIPRACIL has excellent activity against gram-positive organisms, including enterococci (*S faecalis*). It is active against obligate anaerobes such as *Bacteroides* species and

also against *C difficile* (which has been associated with pseudomembranous colitis).

Piperacillin is active against many gram-negative bacteria including *Enterobacteriaceae, Klebsiella, Serratia, Pseudomonas, E coli, Proteus,* and *Citrobacter,* and, in addition, it is active against anaerobes and enterococci.

In vitro tests show piperacillin to act synergistically with aminoglycoside antibiotics against most isolates of *P aeruginosa.*

Susceptibility Testing: The use of a 100 mcg piperacillin antibiotic disk with susceptibility test methods which measure zone diameter gives an accurate estimation of susceptibility of organisms to PIPRACIL. The following standard procedure† has been recommended for use with disks for testing antimicrobials.

†NCCLS Approved Standard; M2-A2 (Formerly ASM-2) Performance Standards for Antimicrobic Disk Susceptibility Tests, Second Edition, available from the National Committee of Clinical Laboratory Standards.

With this type of procedure, a report of "susceptible" from the laboratory indicates that the infecting organism is likely to respond to therapy. A report of "intermediate susceptibility" suggests that the organism would be susceptible if high dosage is used or if the infection is confined to tissue and fluids (eg, urine) in which high antibiotic levels are obtained. A report of "resistant" indicates that the infecting organism is not likely to respond to therapy. With the piperacillin disk, a zone of 18 mm or greater indicates susceptibility, zone sizes of 14 mm or less indicate resistance, and zone sizes of 15 to 17 mm indicate intermediate susceptibility.

Haemophilus and *Neisseria* species which give zones of ≥ 29 mm are susceptible; resistant strains give zones of ≤ 28 mm. The above interpretive criteria are based on the use of the standardized procedure. Antibiotic susceptibility testing requires carefully prescribed procedures. Susceptibility tests are biased to a considerable degree when different methods are used.

The standardized procedure requires the use of control organisms. The 100 mcg piperacillin disk should give zone diameters between 24 and 30 mm for *E coli* ATCC No. 25922 and between 25 and 33 mm for *Pseudomonas aeruginosa* ATCC No. 27853.

Dilution methods such as those described in the International Collaborative Study‡ have been used to determine susceptibility of organisms to PIPRACIL *sterile piperacillin sodium.*

‡*Acta Pathol Microbiol Scand* [B] 1971; (suppl) 217.

Enterobacteriaceae, Pseudomonas species and *Acinetobacter* sp are considered susceptible if the minimal inhibitory concentration (MIC) of piperacillin is no greater than 64 mcg/mL and are considered resistant if the MIC is greater than 128 mcg/mL.

Haemophilus and *Neisseria* species are considered susceptible if the MIC of piperacillin is ≤ to 1 mcg/mL.

When anaerobic organisms are isolated from infection sites, it is recommended that other tests such as the modified Broth-Disk Method§ be used to determine the antibiotic susceptibility of these slowly growing organisms.

§ Wilkins TD, Thiel T: *Antimicrob Agents Chemother* 1973; 3:350–356.

INDICATIONS AND USAGE

Therapeutic: PIPRACIL is indicated for the treatment of serious infections caused by susceptible strains of the designated organisms in the conditions as listed below.

Intra-abdominal Infections including hepatobiliary and surgical infections caused by *E coli, P aeruginosa,* enterococci, *Clostridium* sp, anaerobic cocci, and *Bacteroides* sp, including *B fragilis.*

Urinary Tract Infections caused by *E coli, Klebsiella* sp, *P aeruginosa, Proteus* sp, including *P mirabilis,* and enterococci.

Gynecologic Infections including endometritis, pelvic inflammatory disease, pelvic cellulitis caused by *Bacteroides* sp including *B fragilis,* anaerobic cocci, *Neisseria gonorrhoeae,* and enterococci (*S faecalis*).

Septicemia including bacteremia caused by *E coli, Klebsiella* sp, *Enterobacter* sp, *Serratia* sp, *P mirabilis, S pneumoniae,* enterococci, *P aeruginosa, Bacteroides* sp, and anaerobic cocci.

Lower Respiratory Tract Infections caused by *E coli, Klebsiella* sp, *Enterobacter* sp, *Pseudomonas aeruginosa, Serratia* sp, *H influenzae, Bacteroides* sp, and anaerobic cocci. Although improvement has been noted in patients with cystic fibrosis, lasting bacterial eradication may not necessarily be achieved.

Skin and Skin Structure Infections caused by *E coli, Klebsiella* sp, *Serratia* sp, *Acinetobacter* sp, *Enterobacter* sp, *Pseudomonas aeruginosa,* indole-positive *Proteus* sp, *Proteus mirabilis, Bacteroides* sp, including *B fragilis,* anaerobic cocci, and enterococci.

Bone and Joint Infections caused by *P aeruginosa,* enterococci, *Bacteroides* sp, and anaerobic cocci.

Gonococcal Infections: PIPRACIL has been effective in the treatment of uncomplicated gonococcal urethritis.

PIPRACIL *sterile piperacillin sodium* has also been shown to be clinically effective for the treatment of infections at various sites caused by *Streptococcus* species including Group A β-hemolytic *Streptococcus* and *S pneumoniae;* however, infections caused by these organisms are ordinarily treated with more narrow spectrum penicillins. Because of its broad spectrum of bactericidal activity against gram-positive and gram-negative aerobic and anaerobic bacteria, PIPRACIL is particularly useful for the treatment of mixed infections and presumptive therapy prior to the identification of the causative organisms.

Also, PIPRACIL may be administered as single drug therapy in some situations where normally two antibiotics might be employed.

Piperacillin has been successfully used with aminoglycosides, especially in patients with impaired host defenses. Both drugs should be used in full therapeutic doses.

Appropriate cultures should be made for susceptibility testing before initiating therapy and therapy adjusted, if appropriate, once the results are known.

Prophylaxis: PIPRACIL is indicated for prophylactic use in surgery including intra-abdominal (gastrointestinal and biliary) procedures, vaginal hysterectomy, abdominal hysterectomy, and cesarean section. Effective prophylactic use depends on the time of administration, and PIPRACIL should be given one-half to one hour before the operation so that effective levels can be achieved in the site prior to the procedure.

The prophylactic use of piperacillin should be stopped within 24 hours, since continuing administration of any antibiotic increases the possibility of adverse reactions, but in the majority of surgical procedures, does not reduce the incidence of subsequent infections. If there are signs of infection, specimens for culture should be obtained for identification of the causative organism so that appropriate therapy can be instituted.

CONTRAINDICATIONS

A history of allergic reactions to any of the penicillins and/or cephalosporins.

WARNINGS

Serious and occasionally fatal hypersensitivity (anaphylactic) reactions have been reported in patients receiving therapy with penicillins. These reactions are more apt to occur in persons with a history of sensitivity to multiple allergens. There have been reports of patients with a history of penicillin hypersensitivity who have experienced severe hypersensitivity reactions when treated with a cephalosporin. Before initiating therapy with PIPRACIL, careful inquiry should be

PIPERACILLIN SERUM LEVELS IN ADULTS (mcg/mL) AFTER A TWO- TO THREE-MINUTE IV INJECTION

DOSE	0	10 min	20 min	30 min	1 h	1.5 h	2 h	3 h	4 h	6 h	8 h
2	305 (159–615)	202 (164–225)	156 (52–165)	67 (41–88)	40 (25–57)	24 (18–31)	20 (14–24)	8 (3–11)	3 (2–4)	2 (<0.6–3)	—
4	412 (389–484)	344 (315–379)	295 (269–330)	117 (98–138)	93 (78–110)	60 (50–67)	36 (26–51)	20 (17–24)	8 (7–11)	4 (3.7–4.1)	0.9 (0.7–1)
6	775 (695–849)	609 (530–670)	563 (492–630)	325 (292–363)	208 (180–239)	138 (115–175)	90 (71–113)	38 (29–53)	33 (25–44)	8 (3–19)	3.2 (<2–6)

PIPERACILLIN SERUM LEVELS IN ADULTS (mcg/mL) AFTER A 30-MINUTE IV INFUSION

DOSE	0	5 min	10 min	15 min	30 min	45 min	1 h	1.5 h	2 h	4 h	6 h	7.5 h
4	244 (155–298)	215 (169–247)	186 (140–209)	177 (142–213)	141 (122–156)	146 (110–265)	105 (85–133)	72 (53–105)	53 (36–69)	15 (6–24)	4 (1–9)	2 (0.5–3)
6	353 (324–371)	298 (242–339)	298 (232–331)	272 (219–314)	229 (185–249)	180 (144–209)	149 (117–171)	104 (89–113)	73 (66–94)	22 (12–39)	16 (5–49)	—

made concerning previous hypersensitivity reactions to penicillins, cephalosporins, and other allergens. If an allergic reaction occurs during therapy with PIPRACIL, the antibiotic should be discontinued. The usual agents (antihistamines, pressor amines, and corticosteroids) should be readily available. SERIOUS ANAPHYLACTOID REACTIONS REQUIRE IMMEDIATE EMERGENCY TREATMENT WITH EPINEPHRINE. OXYGEN AND INTRAVENOUS CORTICOSTEROIDS AND AIRWAY MANAGEMENT INCLUDING INTUBATION SHOULD ALSO BE ADMINISTERED AS NECESSARY.

PRECAUTIONS

General: While piperacillin possesses the characteristic low toxicity of the penicillin group of antibiotics, periodic assessment of organ system functions, including renal, hepatic, and hematopoietic, during prolonged therapy is advisable. Bleeding manifestations have occurred in some patients receiving β-lactam antibiotics, including piperacillin. These reactions have sometimes been associated with abnormalities of coagulation tests such as clotting time, platelet aggregation and prothrombin time and are more likely to occur in patients with renal failure.

If bleeding manifestations occur, the antibiotic should be discontinued and appropriate therapy instituted.

The possibility of the emergence of resistant organisms which might cause superinfections should be kept in mind, particularly during prolonged treatment. If this occurs, appropriate measures should be taken.

As with other penicillins, patients may experience neuromuscular excitability or convulsions if higher than recommended doses are given intravenously.

PIPRACIL *sterile piperacillin sodium* is a monosodium salt containing 1.85 mEq of Na⁺ per g. This should be considered when treating patients requiring restricted salt intake. Periodic electrolyte determinations should be made in patients with low potassium reserves, and the possibility of hypokalemia should be kept in mind with patients who have potentially low potassium reserves and who are receiving cytotoxic therapy or diuretics.

Antimicrobials used in high doses for short periods to treat gonorrhea may mask or delay the symptoms of incubating syphilis. Therefore, prior to treatment, patients with gonorrhea should also be evaluated for syphilis. Specimens for darkfield examination should be obtained from patients with any suspected primary lesion, and serologic tests should be performed. In all cases where concomitant syphilis is suspected, monthly serological tests should be made for a minimum of 4 months.

As with other semisynthetic penicillins, PIPRACIL therapy has been associated with an increased incidence of fever and rash in cystic fibrosis patients.

Drug Interactions: The mixing of piperacillin with an aminoglycoside *in vitro* can result in substantial inactivation of the aminoglycosides.

Pregnancy: *Pregnancy Category B:* Although reproduction studies in mice and rats performed at doses up to 4 times the human dose have shown no evidence of impaired fertility or harm to the fetus, safety of PIPRACIL use in pregnant women has not been determined by adequate and well-controlled studies. Because animal reproduction studies are not always predictive of human response, this drug should be used during pregnancy only if clearly needed. It has been found to cross the placenta in rats.

Nursing Mothers: Caution should be exercised when PIPRACIL *sterile piperacillin sodium* is administered to nursing mothers. It is excreted in low concentrations in milk.

Pediatric Use: Dosages for children under the age of 12 have not been established. The safety of PIPRACIL in neonates is not known. In dog neonates, dilated renal tubules and peri-tubular hyalinization occurred following administration of PIPRACIL.

ADVERSE EFFECTS

PIPRACIL is generally well tolerated. The most common adverse reactions have been local in nature, following intravenous or intramuscular injection. The following adverse reactions may occur.

Local Reactions: In clinical trials thrombophlebitis was noted in 4% of patients. Pain, erythema, and/or induration at the injection site occurred in 2% of patients. Less frequent reactions including ecchymosis, deep vein thrombosis and hematomas have also occurred.

Gastrointestinal: Diarrhea and loose stools were noted in 2% of patients. Other less frequent reactions included vomiting, nausea, increases in liver enzymes, (LDH, SGOT, SGPT), hyperbilirubinemia, cholestatic hepatitis, bloody diarrhea and, rarely, pseudomembranous colitis.

Hypersensitivity Reactions: Anaphylactoid Reactions, see WARNINGS.

Rash was noted in 1% of patients. Other less frequent findings included pruritus, vesicular eruptions, positive Coombs tests.

Other dermatologic manifestations such as erythema multiforme and Stevens-Johnson syndrome have been reported rarely.

Renal: Elevations of creatinine or BUN, and, rarely, interstitial nephritis.

Central Nervous System: Headache, dizziness, fatigue.

Hemic and Lymphatic: Reversible leukopenia, neutropenia, thrombocytopenia, and/or eosinophilia have been reported. As with other β-lactam antibiotics, reversible leukopenia (neutropenia) is more apt to occur in patients receiving prolonged therapy at high dosages or in association with drugs known to cause this reaction.

Serum Electrolytes: Individuals with liver disease or individuals receiving cytotoxic therapy or diuretics were reported rarely to demonstrate a decrease in serum potassium concentrations with high doses of piperacillin.

Skeletal: Rarely, prolonged muscle relaxation.

Other: Superinfection, including candidiasis. Hemorrhagic manifestations.

DOSAGE AND ADMINISTRATION

PIPRACIL may be administered by the intramuscular route (see Note) or intravenously or given in a three to five minute intravenous injection. The usual dosage of PIPRACIL for serious infections is 3- to 4-g given every four to six hours as a 20- to 30-minute infusion. For serious infections, the intravenous route should be used.

PIPRACIL should not be mixed with an aminoglycoside in a syringe or infusion bottle since this can result in inactivation of the aminoglycoside.

The maximum daily dose for adults is usually 24 g/day, although higher doses have been used.

Intramuscular injections (See Note) should be limited to 2 g per injection site. This route of administration has been used primarily in the treatment of patients with uncomplicated gonorrhea and urinary tract infections.

NOTE: THE ADD-Vantage VIAL IS <u>NOT</u> FOR IM USE.

DOSAGE RECOMMENDATIONS

Type of Infection	Usual Total Daily Dose
Serious infections such as septicemia, nosocomial pneumonia, intra-abdominal infections, aerobic and anaerobic gynecologic infections, and skin and soft tissue infections	12–18 g/d IV (200–300 mg/kg/d) in divided doses every 4 to 6 h
Complicated urinary tract infections	8–16 g/d IV (125–200 mg/kg/d) in divided doses every 6 to 8 h
Uncomplicated urinary tract infections and most community-acquired pneumonia	6–8 g/d IM or IV (100–125 mg/kg/d) in divided doses every 6 to 12 h
Uncomplicated gonorrhea infections	2 g IM″ as a one-time dose

″ One gram of probenecid given orally one-half hour prior to injection.

The average duration of PIPRACIL *sterile piperacillin sodium* treatment is from seven to ten days, except in the treatment of gynecologic infections, in which it is from three to ten days; the duration should be guided by the patient's clinical and bacteriological progress. For most acute infections, treatment should be continued for at least 48 to 72 hours after the patient becomes asymptomatic. Antibiotic therapy for Group A β-hemolytic streptococcal infections should be maintained for at least ten days to reduce the risk of rheumatic fever or glomerulonephritis.

When PIPRACIL is given concurrently with aminoglycosides, both drugs should be used in full therapeutic doses.

Renal Impairment

Dosage in Renal Impairment

Creatinine Clearance mL/min	Urinary Tract Infection (uncomplicated)	Urinary Tract Infection (complicated)	Serious Systemic Infection
>40	No dosage adjustment necessary		
20–40	No dosage adjustment necessary	9g/day 3g every 8 h	12g/day 4g every 8 h
<20	6g/day 3g every 12 h	6g/day 3g every 12 h	8g/day 4g every 12 h

For patients on hemodialysis, the maximum daily dose is 6 g/day (2 g every 8 h). In addition, because hemodialysis

removes 30%–50% of piperacillin in 4 hours, 1 g additional dose should be administered following each dialysis period. For patients with renal failure and hepatic insufficiency, measurement of serum levels of PIPRACIL *sterile piperacillin sodium* will provide additional guidance for adjusting dosage.

Prophylaxis: When possible, PIPRACIL should be administered as a 20–30 minute infusion just prior to anaesthesia. Administration while the patient is awake will facilitate identification of possible adverse reactions during drug infusion.

INDICATION	1st Dose	2nd Dose	3rd Dose
Intra-abdominal Surgery	2g IV just prior to surgery	2g during surgery	2g every 6 h postop for no more than 24 h
Vaginal Hysterectomy	2g IV just prior to surgery	2g 6 h after 1st dose	2g 12 h after 1st dose
Cesarean Section	2g IV after cord is clamped	2g 4 h after 1st dose	2g 8 h after 1st dose
Abdominal Hysterectomy	2g IV just prior to surgery	2g on return to recovery room	2g after 6 h

Infants and Children: Dosages in infants and children under 12 years of age have not been established.

PRODUCT RECONSTITUTION/DOSAGE PREPARATION

Conventional Vials:
Diluents for Reconstitution
  Sterile Water for Injection
  Bacteriostatic£ Water for Injection
  Sodium Chloride Injection
  Bacteriostatic£ Sodium Chloride Injection
  Dextrose 5% in Water
  Dextrose 5% and 0.9% Sodium Chloride
  #Lidocaine HCl 0.5%–1% (without epinephrine)

£ Either Parabens or Benzyl Alcohol
For Intramuscular Use Only. Lidocaine is contraindicated in patients with a known history of hypersensitivity to local anesthetics of the amide type.

Conventional Vials:
Intravenous Solutions
  Dextrose 5% in Water
  0.9% Sodium Chloride
  Dextrose 5% and 0.9% Sodium Chloride
  Lactated Ringer's Injection
  Dextran 6% in 0.9% Sodium Chloride
Intravenous Admixtures
  Normal Saline [+ KCl 40 mEq]
  5% Dextrose in Water [+ KCl 40 mEq]
  5% Dextrose/Normal Saline [+ KCl 40 mEq]
  Ringer's Injection [+ KCl 40 mEq]
  Lactated Ringer's Injection [+ KCl 40 mEq]
ADD-Vantage Vials:**
ADD-Vantage System Admixtures
  Dextrose 5% in Water (50 or 100 mL)
  0.9% Sodium Chloride (50 or 100 mL)
** (ADD-Vantage is the registered trademark of Abbott Laboratories)

INTRAVENOUS ADMINISTRATION:

Reconstitution Directions for Conventional Vials: Reconstitute each gram of PIPRACIL *sterile piperacillin sodium* with at least 5 mL of a suitable diluent (except Lidocaine HCl 0.5% to 1% without epinephrine) listed above. Shake well until dissolved. Reconstituted solution may be further diluted to the desired volume (eg, 50 or 100 mL) in the above listed intravenous solutions and admixtures.

Reconstitution Directions for ADD-Vantage Vials: See Instruction Sheet provided in box.

Reconstitution Directions for PHARMACY BULK VIAL: Reconstitute the 40 g vial with 172 mL of a suitable diluent (except Lidocaine HCl 0.5%–1% without epinephrine) listed above to achieve a concentration of 1 g per 5 mL.

Directions for Administration: *Intermittent IV Infusion* —Infuse diluted solution over period of about 30 minutes.

Continued on next page

Information on Lederle products listed on these pages is the full prescribing information from product literature or package inserts effective in August, 1989. Information concerning all Lederle products may be obtained from the Professional Services Department, Lederle Laboratories, Pearl River, New York, 10965.

Lederle—Cont.

During infusion it is desirable to discontinue the primary intravenous solution.

Intravenous Injection (Bolus) — Reconstituted solution should be injected slowly over a three- to five-minute period to help avoid vein irritation.

INTRAMUSCULAR ADMINISTRATION (CONVENTIONAL VIALS ONLY)

Reconstitution Directions: Reconstitute each gram of PIPRACIL with 2 mL of a suitable diluent listed above to achieve a concentration of 1 g per 2.5 mL. Shake well until dissolved.

Directions for Administration: When indicated by clinical and bacteriological findings, intramuscular administration of 6 to 8 g daily of PIPRACIL, in divided doses, may be utilized for initiation of therapy. In addition, intramuscular administration of the drug may be considered for maintenance therapy after clinical and bacteriologic improvement has been obtained with intravenous piperacillin sodium treatment. Intramuscular administration should not exceed 2 g per injection at any one site.

The preferred site is the upper outer quadrant of the buttock (ie, gluteus maximus).

The deltoid area should be used only if well-developed, and then only with caution to avoid radial nerve injury. Intramuscular injections should not be made into the lower or mid-third of the upper arm.

STABILITY OF PIPRACIL FOLLOWING RECONSTITUTION:

PIPRACIL is stable in both glass and plastic containers when reconstituted with recommended diluents and when diluted with the intravenous solutions and intravenous admixtures indicated above.

Extensive stability studies have demonstrated chemical stability (potency, pH, and clarity) through 24 hours at room temperature, up to one week refrigerated, and up to one month frozen (−10° to −20°C). (Note: The 40 g Pharmacy Bulk Vial should not be frozen after reconstitution.) Appropriate consideration of aseptic technique and individual hospital policy, however, may recommend discarding unused portions after storage for 48 hours under refrigeration and discarding after 24 hours storage at room temperature.

ADD-Vantage System:

Stability studies with the ad-mixed ADD-Vantage system have demonstrated chemical stability (potency, pH and clarity) through 24 hours at room temperature. (Note: The ad-mixed ADD-Vantage should not be refrigerated or frozen after reconstitution.)

Additional stability data available upon request.

HOW SUPPLIED

PIPRACIL *sterile piperacillin sodium* is available in vials containing sterile freeze-dried piperacillin sodium powder equivalent to two, three, four, and 40 g of piperacillin. One g of piperacillin (as a monosodium salt) contains 1.85mEq (42.5 mg) of sodium.

Product Numbers:
2 gram/Vial—10 per box—NDC 0206-3879-16
3 gram/Vial—10 per box—NDC 0206-3882-55
4 gram/Vial—10 per box—NDC 0206-3880-25
2 gram infusion Bottle—10 per box—NDC 0206-3879-47
3 gram infusion Bottle—10 per box—NDC 0206-3882-65
4 gram infusion Bottle—10 per box—NDC 0206-3880-66
2 gram ADD-Vantage Vial—10 per box—NDC 0206-3879-27
3 gram ADD-Vantage Vial—10 per box—NDC 0206-3882-28
4 gram ADD-Vantage Vial—10 per box—NDC 0206-3380-29
40 gram Pharmacy Bulk Vial—NDC 0206-3877-60
This product should be stored at controlled room temperature 15–30°C (59–86°F).

Military and VA depots:
NSN 6505-01-148-5040—2 g vial (10s)
NSN 6505-01-280-2317—3 g vial (10s)
NSN 6505-01-137-0039—3 g infusion bottle (10s)
NSN 6505-01-280-2318—4 g vial (10s)
LEDERLE PIPERACILLIN, INC.

Carolina, Puerto Rico 00630   Rev. 7/88
                                   24378

Shown in Product Indentification Section, page 415

PNU-IMUNE® 23   ℞
[new-ĭ-mune]
Pneumococcal Vaccine,
Polyvalent

DESCRIPTION

Pneumococcal Vaccine Polyvalent, PNU-IMUNE 23 is a sterile liquid vaccine for intramuscular or subcutaneous use, consisting of a mixture of purified capsular polysaccharides from 23 pneumococcal types: [See table below].

It is indicated for immunization against infections caused by the 23 most prevalent types of pneumococci responsible for approximately 90% of serious pneumococcal disease in the United States and the rest of the world.[1-5] Each of the pneumococcal polysaccharide types is produced separately by Lederle Laboratories to give a high degree of purity. After an individual pneumococcal type is grown, the polysaccharide is separated from the cell and purified by a series of steps including ethanol fractionation. The resultant 23 purified polysaccharides are combined in amounts to give 25 micrograms of each type per dose (0.5 mL) in the final vaccine. Thimerosal (a mercury derivative) at a final concentration of 0.01% is added as a preservative.

CLINICAL PHARMACOLOGY

Pneumococci are the etiologic agents for a significant number of the pneumonias occurring throughout the world. The emergence of strains of pneumococci with increased resistance to one or more of the common antibiotics[4] and recent isolations of pneumococci with multiple-antibiotic resistance[6] emphasize the importance of vaccine prophylaxis against pneumococcal disease.

Based on projections from limited observations in the United States, it has been estimated that 150,000 to 570,000 cases of pneumococcal pneumonia may occur annually. The overall case fatality rate ranges from 5%–7%.[2] As many as 60% of all deaths among patients with pneumococcal bacteremia treated with penicillin or tetracycline occur within five days of onset of the illness.[6] Thus vaccination offers an effective means for further reducing the mortality and morbidity of this disease. Populations at high risk are the elderly,[7-8] individuals with immune deficiencies, asplenics and patients with splenic deficiencies including sickle cell anemia and other severe hemoglobinopathies, alcoholics and patients with the following diseases: chronic respiratory illness, the nephrotic syndrome, multiple myeloma, Hodgkin's disease and cirrhosis.[2] Antibiotics have only been partially effective in reducing the mortality of pneumococcal pneumonia. The pneumococcus is also a major infectious agent in meningitis[9] and otitis media. Other illnesses caused by pneumococci include sinus infection, arthritis and conjunctivitis. The annual incidence of pneumococcal meningitis is approximately 1.5 to 2.5 per 100,000 population. One-half of the cases occur in children in whom the fatality rate is about 40%.[1,8]

The polysaccharide capsules of pneumococci endow these organisms with resistance to the phagocytic action of polymorphonuclear leukocytes and monocytes. The opsonin activity of type-specific antibody facilitates their destruction in the body by complement-mediated activities.

The protection induced by the vaccine is of long duration but its extent is not yet known. Elevated antibody levels have been shown to persist for at least 5 years after immunization with other pneumococcal vaccines.[10] Children under 2 years of age do not respond adequately to some of the important polysaccharide types.[12] PNU-IMUNE 23 *pneumococcal vaccine, polyvalent* has not been studied in children under 2 years of age. Recipients of polyvalent vaccines acquired less nasopharyngeal carriage of pneumococcal types included in the vaccine.[2,11]

A repeat (booster) injection of pneumococcal vaccine *should not be given* to previously vaccinated subjects regardless of the time interval from the previous injection. Available data indicate that revaccination may result in more frequent and severe local reactions at the site of injection, especially in persons who have retained high antibody titers. Such adverse reactions have occurred with booster doses given after long intervals from the initial vaccination. There is also evidence that booster doses do not result in increased antibody titers.[2]

In clinical studies with PNU-IMUNE 23, more than 90% of all adults showed a twofold or greater increase in geometric mean antibody titer for each vaccine capsular type.[13]

Patients over the age of 2 years with anatomical or functional asplenia and otherwise intact lymphoid function responded to PNU-IMUNE 23 and other comparable pneumococcal vaccines with a serological conversion comparable to that observed in healthy individuals of the same age.[14]

Polyvalent pneumococcal vaccines, from other sources, were shown to be effective in preventing pneumococcal disease. Controlled field trials in South Africa involving 12,000 gold miners have shown a 6-valent and a 13-valent pneumococcal vaccine to be 78.5% effective in preventing type-specific pneumococcal pneumonia and 82.3% effective in preventing pneumococcal bacteremia with the types in the vaccine.[15] In a preliminary study of an 8-valent polysaccharide vaccine in a group consisting of 77 patients with sickle cell disease and 19 asplenic persons, there were no pneumococcal infections

in the immunized patients within two years of immunization. There were eight cases of pneumococcal infection in 106 unimmunized, age-matched patients with sickle cell disease. Antibody response of the asplenic patients was comparable to normal controls.[16]

In a study carried out by Austrian, et al,[15] with 13-valent pneumococcal vaccines prepared for the National Institute of Allergy and Infectious Disease, the reduction in pneumonias caused by the capsular types in the vaccines was 79%. Reduction in type-specific pneumococcal bacteremia was 82%.

In a double-blind study of a 14-valent pneumococcal vaccine carried out in Papua, New Guinea, pneumococcal infection was less in the vaccinated group by 84%. Mortality from pneumonia was less by 44%.[17]

Pneumococcal polysaccharide vaccine was found to significantly reduce clinical cases of pneumococcal otitis media in a six-month post vaccination period of observation. In a controlled study there were 455 children ages two to six years with a history of prior episodes of otitis media. Two hundred seventy-four of these patients received 14-valent pneumococcal vaccine. Overall, there was a 73% reduction in frequency of cases caused by serotypes in the pneumococcal vaccine, other than type 6 for which no protection was found. These Finnish otitis studies revealed a marked fall-off of protective efficacy later than six months after immunization.[18]

INDICATIONS AND USAGE

PNU-IMUNE 23 *pneumococcal vaccine, polyvalent* is indicated for immunization against pneumococcal disease caused by those pneumococcal types included in the vaccine. Use in preventing pneumococcal otitis media. Children two years or older who, in the judgment of the physician, are clearly in need of protection due to a risk of developing otitis media. (See CLINICAL PHARMACOLOGY for clinical data.)

Use in Selected Individuals: Persons over 2 years of age as follows: (1) who have anatomical asplenia or who have splenic dysfunction due to sickle cell disease or other causes; (2) persons with chronic illnesses in which there is an increased risk of pneumococcal disease, such as diabetes mellitus, functional impairment of cardiorespiratory, hepatic and renal systems; (3) persons 50 years of age or older, and (4) patients about to undergo immunosuppressive therapy.[2] It is reasonable to assume that patients on immunosuppressive therapy are at increased risk of pneumococcal disease. When possible, vaccination should be given at least ten days and preferably more than 14 days prior to initiation of such immunosuppressive therapy. Impairment of antibody response in Hodgkin's disease patients receiving radiotherapy, chemotherapy or both, was demonstrated.[20]

Use in Communities: Persons over 2 years of age as follows: (1) closed groups such as those in residential schools, nursing homes and other institutions; (2) groups epidemiologically at risk in the community when there is a generalized outbreak in the population due to a single pneumococcal type included in the vaccine, and (3) patients at high risk of influenza complications, particularly pneumonia.[11]

Simultaneous administration of pneumococcal polysaccharide vaccine and whole-virus influenza vaccine has been found to give satisfactory antibody response without increasing the incidence of side effects. Although not yet studied, simultaneous administration of the pneumococcal vaccine and split-virus influenza vaccine may also be expected to yield satisfactory results.[2,19]

CONTRAINDICATIONS

Children below 2 years of age: While pneumococcal polysaccharide vaccines have been shown to be highly immunogenic and effective in adults, their usefulness in children is still being evaluated. Although some pneumococcal polysaccharides have been reported to be immunogenic from the age of 3 months (particularly serotype 3), serum antibody responses to most of the polysaccharides present in the 14-valent vaccine have been shown to be poor in children under 2 years of age.[22]

Hypersensitivity: Known hypersensitivity to any component of the vaccine including hypersensitivity to thimerosal. Remedial measures for anaphylactoid reactions, including epinephrine injection (1:1000), must be available for immediate use.

Patients on Immunosuppressive Therapy: Immunization of patients should not be attempted less than ten days prior to or during treatment with immunosuppressive drugs or irradiation. Administration of vaccine to patients on such therapy for Hodgkin's disease resulted in reduction of preexisting antibody levels.[20]

Previously vaccinated subjects: The use of PNU-IMUNE 23 *pneumococcal vaccine, polyvalent* is contraindicated in persons who have been immunized with any polyvalent pneumococcal vaccine.

WARNINGS

PNU-IMUNE 23 is not an effective agent for prophylaxis against pneumococcal disease caused by types not present in the vaccine. The vaccine may not be effective in patients undergoing treatment causing therapeutic suppression of the immune-response system.

Nomenclature	Pneumococcal Types																						
Danish	1	2	3	4	5	6B	7F	8	9N	9V	10A	11A	12F	14	15B	17F	18C	19A	19F	20	22F	23F	33F
U.S.	1	2	3	4	5	26	51	8	9	68	34	43	12	14	54	17	56	57	19	20	22	23	70

Patients who have received extensive chemotherapy and/or splenectomy for the treatment of Hodgkin's disease have been shown to have an impaired serum antibody response to pneumococcal vaccine.[20]

A repeat (booster) injection of pneumococcal vaccine *should not be given* to previously vaccinated subjects regardless of the time interval from the previous injection. Available data indicate that revaccination may result in more frequent and severe local reactions at the site of injection, especially in persons who have retained high antibody titers. Such adverse reactions have occurred with booster doses given after long intervals from the initial vaccination. There is also evidence that booster doses do not result in increased antibody titers.[2]

Intradermal administration may cause severe local reactions.

PRECAUTIONS

General: The vaccine should be injected subcutaneously or intramuscularly. *Do not inject intravenously.*

In the presence of any febrile respiratory illness or other active infection, the vaccine should not be used.

The parenteral administration of any biological product should be surrounded by every known precaution for the prevention and arrest of allergic and other untoward reactions. (See **CONTRAINDICATIONS.**)

When administering this vaccine, a separate heat-sterilized syringe and needle or a new disposable equivalent should be used for each patient to prevent transmission of hepatitis B (homologous serum hepatitis) or other infectious agents.

Patients who have had episodes of pneumococcal pneumonia or other pneumococcal infection may have high levels of preexisting pneumococcal antibodies which may result in increased reactions to PNU-IMUNE 23, mostly local, but occasionally systemic.[21] Caution should be exercised if such patients are considered for vaccination with PNU-IMUNE 23.

Pregnancy Category C: Animal reproduction studies have not been conducted with PNU-IMUNE 23. It is also not known whether PNU-IMUNE 23 can cause fetal harm when administered to a pregnant woman or can affect reproduction capacity. PNU-IMUNE 23 is not recommended for use in pregnant women.

It is not known whether the drug is excreted in human milk. Because many drugs are excreted in human milk, caution should be exercised when PNU-IMUNE 23 *pneumococcal vaccine, polyvalent* is administered to a nursing woman.

Pediatric Use. PNU-IMUNE 23 has not been studied in children under 2 years of age. While pneumococcal polysaccharide vaccines have been shown to be highly immunogenic and effective in adults, their usefulness in children is still being evaluated. Although some pneumococcal polysaccharides have been reported to be immunogenic from the age of three months (particularly serotype 3), serum antibody responses to most of the polysaccharides present in the 14-valent vaccine have been shown to be poor in children under two years of age.[22]

ADVERSE REACTIONS

PNU-IMUNE 23 is associated with a relatively low incidence of adverse reactions. The adverse reactivity observed in clinical studies was not serious and of short duration.

In a study of 32 individuals who received PNU-IMUNE 23, 23 (72%) experienced a local reaction characterized by local soreness at the injection site within three days after vaccination.

Low grade fever (less than 100°F) and mild myalgia occur occasionally with PNU-IMUNE 23 and are usually confined to the 24-hour period following vaccination. Rash and arthralgia have been reported rarely.

Although rare, fever over 102° and marked local swelling has been reported with pneumococcal polysaccharide vaccine.

Patients with otherwise stabilized idiopathic thrombocytopenic purpura have, on rare occasions, experienced a relapse in their thrombocytopenia, occurring two to 14 days after vaccination, and lasting up to 2 weeks.[23]

Reactions of greater severity, or extent are unusual. Rarely, anaphylactoid reactions have been reported.

A repeat (booster) injection of pneumococcal vaccine *should not be given* to previously vaccinated subjects regardless of the time interval from the previous injection. Available data indicate that revaccination may result in more frequent and severe local reactions at the site of injection, especially in persons who have retained high antibody titers. Such adverse reactions have occurred with booster doses given after long intervals from the initial vaccination. There is also evidence that booster doses do not result in increased antibody titers.[2]

Temporal association of neurological disorders have been reported following parenteral injections of biological products.

DOSAGE AND ADMINISTRATION

Do not inject intravenously. The immunization schedule consists of a single 0.5 mL dose given subcutaneously or intramuscularly.

Parenteral drug products should be inspected visually for particulate matter and discoloration prior to administration, whenever solution and container permit.

PNU-IMUNE 23 *must not* be administered to persons who have been immunized previously with any polyvalent pneumococcal vaccine.

A repeat (booster) injection of pneumococcal vaccine *should not be given* to previously vaccinated subjects regardless of the time interval from the previous injection. Available data indicate that revaccination may result in more frequent and severe local reactions at the site of injection, especially in persons who have retained high antibody titers. Such adverse reactions have occurred with booster doses given after long intervals from the initial vaccination. There is also evidence that booster doses do not result in increased antibody titers.[2]

Directions for Use of the LEDERJECT® Disposable Syringe:
1. Twist the plunger rod clockwise to be sure that rod is secure to rubber plunger base.
2. Hold needle shield in place with index finger and thumb of one hand while with the other thumb exert light pressure on plunger rod until the plunger base has been freed and demonstrates slight movement when pressure is applied.
3. Grasp the rubber needle shield at its base; twist and pull to remove.
4. Pull back plunger rod slowly and carefully to insure smooth plunger operation.
5. Expel the air bubble.

Storage and Use: Store syringes and unopened or opened vials at 2°–8°C (35°–46°F).

The vaccine is used directly as supplied. No dilution or reconstitution is necessary. Thimerosal (a mercury derivative) is present in the vaccine as a preservative at a final concentration of 0.01%. Discard unused vials beyond expiration date.

HOW SUPPLIED

PNU-IMUNE *pneumococcal vaccine, polyvalent* 23 is supplied as follows:

    NDC 0005-2309-31 5 dose vial, for use with syringe only.
    NDC 0005-2309-33 5 × One dose LEDERJECT Disposable Syringes.

References:
1. Austrian, R "Surveillance of Pneumococcal Infection for Field Trials of Polyvalent Vaccines." Annual Contract Prog. Report to the Nat. Inst. of Allerg. and Inf. Dis. (1975) Updated to Dec. 1977, personal communication.
2. Recommendation of the Immunization Practices Advisory Committee, Morb. Mort. Weekly Report 30 (33):410–419 August 28, 1981.
3. Lund, E "Distribution of Pneumococcal Types at Different Times and Different Areas" in *Bayer Symposium III. Bacterial Infections.* "Changes in Their Causative Agents, Trends and Possible Basis." M Finland, W Marget and K Bartman (eds.) Berlin, Springer-Verlag:49, (1971).
4. Mufson, MA, Kruss, DM, Wasil, RE and Metzger, WI "Capsular Types and Outcome of Bacteremic Pneumococcal Disease in the Antibiotic Era." Arch. Int. Med., 134:505, (1974).
5. Robbins, JB, Austrian, R, Lee, CJ, Rastogi, SC, Schiffman, G, Henrichsen, J, Mäkelä, PH, Broome, CV, Facklam, RR, Tiesjema, RH, and Parke, JC, Jr. "Consideration for Formulating the Second Generation Pneumococcal Capsule Polysaccharide Vaccine with Emphasis on the Cross-Reactive Types Within Groups." J. Infec. Dis. 148(6):1136–1159, 1983.
6. Epidemiologic Notes and Reports, Multiple-Antibiotic Resistance of Pneumococci—South Africa Morb. Mort. Weekly Report 26 (35):285–286 September 2, 1977.
7. Austrian, R, and Gold, J "Pneumococcal Bacteremia with Especial Reference to Bacteremic Pneumococcal Pneumonia." Ann. Int. Med., 60:759, (1964).
8. Valenti, WM, Jenzer, M and Bently, W "Type-Specific Pneumococcal Respiratory Disease in the Elderly and Chronically Ill." Am. Rev. Resp. Dis., 117:233, (1978).
9. Fraser, DW, Geil, CC, and Feldman, RA "Meningitis in Bernalillo County, New Mexico. A Comparison with Three Other American Populations." Am. J. Epidemiol., 100:29, (1974).
10. Mufson, MA, Krause, HE and Schiffman, G "Long Term Persistence of Antibody Following Immunization with Pneumococcal Polysaccharide Vaccine" Proc. Soc. Exptl. Biol. & Med. 173(2):270–275, 1983.
11. Mufson, MA and Krause, HE "Role of Antibody in Prevention of Acquisition of Pneumococcal Carriage Among Vaccinees." Clin. Res., 24:577A, (1976).
12. Report of the Committee on Infectious Diseases. Pneumococcal Infections. Amer. Acad. of Ped. 19th Edition: 205–206, 1982.
13. Data on File, Lederle Laboratories.
14. Sullivan, JL, Ochs, HD, Schiffman, G, Hammerschlag, MR, Miser, J, Vichinsky, E, and Wedgwood, RJ "Immune Response After Splenectomy." Lancet, 178, (1978).
15. Austrian, R, Douglas, RM, Schiffman, G, Coetzee, AM, Koornhof, HJ, Hayden-Smith, S and Reid, RDW "Prevention of Pneumococcal Pneumonia by Vaccination." Trans. Asc. Am. Physicians, 89:184, (1976).
16. Amman, AJ, Addiego, K, Wara, DW, Lubin, B, Smith, WB and Mentzer, WC "Polyvalent Pneumococcal-Polysaccharide Immunization of Patients with Sickle-Cell Anemia and Patients with Splenectomy." New Eng. J. Med., 297:897, (1977).
17. Riley, ID, Andrews, M, Howard, R, Tarr, PI, Pfeiffer, M, Challands, P and Jennison, G "Immunization with Polyvalent Pneumococcal Vaccine." Lancet, 1338, (1977).
18. Makela, PH, Sibakov, M, Herva, E, Henrichsen, J, Luotonen, J, Timonen, M, Lienonen, M, Koskela, M, Pukander, J, Pontynen, S, Gronroos, P, Karma, P Pneumococcal Vaccine and Otitis Media. Lancet 547-551, 1980.
19. DeStefano, F, Goodman, RA, Noble, GR, McClary, GD, Smith, SJ and Broome, CV "Simultaneous Administration of Influenza and Pneumococcal Vaccines" JAMA 247:2551–2554, (1982).
20. Siber, GR, Weitzman, SA, Aisenberg, AC, Weinstein, HJ, and Schiffman, G "Impaired Antibody Response to Pneumococcal Vaccine After Treatment for Hodgkin's Disease." New Eng. J. Med., 299:442, (1978).
21. Pönkä, A and Leinonen, M "Adverse Reactions to Polyvalent Pneumococcal Vaccine." Scand. J. Infect. Dis., 14:67–71, (1982).
22. Douglas, RM, Paton, JC, Duncan, SJ, and Hansman, DJ "Antibody Response to Pneumococcal Vaccination in Children Younger than Five Years of Age." J. Infec. Dis., (1):13-137, (1983).
23. Kelton, JG "Vaccination-Associated Relapse of Immune Thrombocytopenia." J. Am. Med. Assoc., 245(4):369-371, (1981).

LEDERLE LABORATORIES DIVISION
American Cyanamid Company,
Pearl River, NY 10965   Rev. 11/85
                                                  17541

RHEUMATREX® Dose Pack   ℞
Methotrexate 2.5 mg. Tablets

PRODUCT OVERVIEW

KEY FACTS

RHEUMATREX is a folic acid antagonist given orally in second-line therapy for adult rheumatoid arthritis. While it has not been shown to modify the disease process, RHEUMATREX reduces articular swelling and tenderness and ameliorates signs and symptoms of inflammation (pain, swelling, stiffness). Clinical improvement may begin as early as three to six weeks and is maintained with continued therapy.

Tablets are supplied in a Dose Pack in weekly doses of 5 mg, 7.5 mg, 10 mg, 12.5 mg, and 15 mg.

MAJOR USES

RHEUMATREX is used in the treatment of selected adults with active, rheumatoid arthritis (ARA Criteria).

SAFETY INFORMATION

There is a potential for severe toxic reactions. Physicians should monitor patients closely. Patients should be informed of early signs of toxicity plus the need to see their physicians promptly if these signs occur, and of the need for regular follow-up, including periodic lab tests. Physician and pharmacist should emphasize that the recommended dose is taken weekly and that mistaken daily use has led to fatal toxicity. (See box **Warnings, Precautions,** and **Adverse Reactions** sections in full Prescribing Information for Methotrexate).

PRESCRIBING INFORMATION

Please see page 1163 for full Prescribing Information for Methotrexate.

Shown in Product Identification Section, page 415

STRESSCAPS®
[strĕs-caps]
Stress Formula B + C Vitamins
(See PDR For Nonprescription Drugs)

Continued on next page

Lederle—Cont.

STRESSTABS® Advanced Formula
[strĕs-tabs]
High Potency
Stress Formula Vitamins

(See PDR For Nonprescription Drugs)

STRESSTABS® with IRON,
[strĕs-tabs]
Advanced Formula
High Potency
Stress Formula Vitamins

(See PDR For Nonprescription Drugs)

STRESSTABS® with ZINC,
[strĕs-tabs]
Advanced Formula
High Potency
Stress Formula Vitamins

(See PDR For Nonprescription Drugs)

SUPRAX®　　　　　　　　　　　　　　　℞
Cefixime
ORAL

PRODUCT OVERVIEW

KEY FACTS
SUPRAX is a semisynthetic, third-generation cephalosporin antibiotic for oral administration. The bactericidal action of SUPRAX results from inhibition of cell-well synthesis. SUPRAX is highly beta-lactamase stable and, as a result, many organisms resistant to penicillins and some cephalosporins, due to the presence of beta-lactamases, may be susceptible to SUPRAX.
SUPRAX has been shown to be active against most strains of gram-negative and gram-positive organisms, both *in vitro* and in clinical studies. (See full **Prescribing Information**.) The serum half-life of SUPRAX averages 3.0 to 4.0 hours, but may range up to 9 hours in some normal volunteers.

MAJOR USES
SUPRAX is indicated for the treatment of the following infections caused by susceptible strains of the designated microorganisms; Otitis media caused by *Haemophilus influenzae* (beta-lactamase positive and negative strains), *Branhamella catarrhalis* (most of which are beta-lactamase positive), and *Streptococcus pyogenes* (see **CLINICAL STUDIES** section of full Prescribing Information for information on *Streptococcus pneumoniae*); pharyngitis and tonsillitis caused by *S pyogenes*; acute bronchitis, caused by *S pneumoniae* and *H influenzae* (beta-lactamase positive and negative strains); uncomplicated urinary tract infections caused by *Escherichia coli* and *Proteus mirabilis*.

SAFETY INFORMATION
SUPRAX is contraindicated in patients with known allergy to the cephalosporin group of antibiotics. In patients with renal impairment, dosage adjustment is necessary. Prescribe with caution in patients with a history of gastrointestinal disease, particularly colitis.

PRESCRIBING INFORMATION

SUPRAX®　　　　　　　　　　　　　　　℞
Cefixime
ORAL

DESCRIPTION
SUPRAX is a semisynthetic, cephalosporin antibiotic for oral administration. Chemically, it is [6R-[6α, 7β(Z)]]-7-[[(2-amino-4-thiazolyl)[(carboxymethoxy)imino]acetyl]amino]-3-ethenyl-8-oxo-5-thia -1- azabicyclo [4.2.0] oct-2-ene-2-carboxylic acid. Molecular weight = 507.50 as the trihydrate.
SUPRAX is available in scored 200 mg and 400 mg film-coated tablets and in a powder for oral suspension which, when reconstituted, provides 100 mg/5 mL.
Inactive ingredients contained in the 200 mg and 400 mg tablets are: dibasic calcium phosphate, hydroxypropyl methylcellulose 2910, light mineral oil, magnesium stearate, microcrystalline cellulose, pregelatinized starch, sodium lauryl sulfate, and titanium dioxide. The powder for oral suspension is strawberry flavored and contains sodium benzoate, sucrose, and xanthan gum.

CLINICAL PHARMACOLOGY
SUPRAX *cefixime*, given orally, is about 40%–50% absorbed whether administered with or without food; however, time to maximal absorption is increased approximately 0.8 hours when administered with food. A single 200 mg tablet of SUPRAX produces an average peak serum concentration of approximately 2 mcg/mL (range 1 to 4 mcg/mL); a single 400 mg tablet produces an average peak concentration of approximately 3.7 mcg/mL (range 1.3 to 7.7 mcg/mL). The oral suspension produces average peak concentrations approximately 25%–50% higher than the tablets. Two hundred mg and 400 mg doses of oral suspension produce average peak concentrations of 3 mcg/mL (range 1 to 4.5 mcg/mL) and 4.6 mcg/mL (range 1.9 to 7.7 mcg/mL), respectively. The area under the time versus concentration curve is greater by approximately 10%–25% with the oral suspension than with the tablet after doses of 100 mg to 400 mg. This increased absorption should be taken into consideration if the oral suspension is to be substituted for the tablet. Because of the lack of bioequivalence, tablets should not be substituted for oral suspension in the treatment of otitis media. (See **DOSAGE AND ADMINISTRATION**.)
Peak serum concentrations occur between 2 and 6 hours following oral administration of a single 200 mg tablet, a single 400 mg tablet, or 400 mg of suspension of SUPRAX. Peak serum concentrations occur between 2 and 5 hours following a single administration of 200 mg of suspension.

TABLE
Serum Levels of Cefixime After Administration of Tablets (mcg/mL)

DOSE	1h	2h	4h	6h	8h	12h	24h
100 mg	0.3	0.8	1.0	0.7	0.4	0.2	0.02
200 mg	0.7	1.4	2.0	1.5	1.0	0.4	0.03
400 mg	1.2	2.5	3.5	2.7	1.7	0.6	0.04

Serum Levels of Cefixime After Administration of Oral Suspension (mcg/mL)

DOSE	1h	2h	4h	6h	8h	12h	24h
100 mg	0.7	1.1	1.3	0.9	0.6	0.2	0.02
200 mg	1.2	2.1	2.8	2.0	1.3	0.5	0.07
400 mg	1.8	3.3	4.4	3.3	2.2	0.8	0.07

Approximately 50% of the absorbed dose is excreted unchanged in the urine in 24 hours. In animal studies, it was noted that cefixime is also excreted in the bile in excess of 10% of the administered dose. Serum protein binding is concentration-independent with a bound fraction of approximately 65%. In a multiple dose study conducted with a research formulation which is less bioavailable than the tablet or suspension, there was little accumulation of drug in serum or urine after dosing for 14 days.
The serum half-life of cefixime in healthy subjects is independent of dosage form and averages 3.0–4.0 hours but may range up to 9 hours in some normal volunteers. Average AUCs at steady state in elderly patients are approximately 40% higher than average AUCs in other healthy adults.
In subjects with moderate impairment of renal function (20 to 40 mL/min creatinine clearance), the average serum half-life of cefixime is prolonged to 6.4 hours. In severe renal impairment (5 to 20 mL/min creatinine clearance), the half-life increased to an average of 11.5 hours. The drug is not cleared significantly from the blood by hemodialysis or peritoneal dialysis. However, a study indicated that with doses of 400 mg, patients undergoing hemodialysis have similar blood profiles as subjects with creatinine clearances of 21–60 mL/min. There is no evidence of metabolism of cefixime *in vivo*.
Adequate data on CSF levels of cefixime are not available.
Microbiology: As with other cephalosporins, bactericidal action of SUPRAX *cefixime* results from inhibition of cell-wall synthesis. SUPRAX is highly stable in the presence of beta-lactamase enzymes. As a result, many organisms resistant to penicillins and some cephalosporins, due to the presence of beta-lactamases, may be susceptible to cefixime. SUPRAX has been shown to be active against most strains of the following organisms both *in vitro* and in clinical infections (see **INDICATIONS and USAGE**):
Gram-positive Organisms
Streptococcus pneumoniae
Streptococcus pyogenes
Gram-negative Organisms
Haemophilus influenzae (beta-lactamase positive and negative strains)
Moraxella (Branhamella) catarrhalis (most of which are beta-lactamase positive)
Escherichia coli
Proteus mirabilis
SUPRAX has been shown to be active *in vitro* against most strains of the following organisms; however, clinical efficacy has not been established.
Gram-positive Organisms
Streptococcus agalactiae
Gram-negative Organisms
Neisseria gonorrhoeae (beta-lactamase positive and negative strains)
Haemophilus parainfluenzae (beta-lactamase positive and negative strains)
Proteus vulgaris
Klebsiella pneumoniae
Klebsiella oxytoca
Pasteurella multocida
Providencia species
Salmonella species
Shigella species
Citrobacter amalonaticus
Citrobacter diversus
Serratia marcescens
Note: *Pseudomonas* species, strains of group D streptococci (including enterococci), *Listeria monocytogenes*, most strains of staphylococci (including methicillin-resistant strains) and most strains of *Enterobacter* are resistant to SUPRAX. In addition, most strains of *Bacteroides fragilis* and clostridia are resistant to SUPRAX.

SUSCEPTIBILITY TESTING
Susceptibility Tests: *Diffusion Techniques:* Quantitative methods that require measurement of zone diameters give an estimate of antibiotic susceptibility. One such procedure[1-3] has been recommended for use with disks to test susceptibility to cefixime. Interpretation involves correlation of the diameters obtained in the disk test with minimum inhibitory concentration (MIC) for cefixime.
Reports from the laboratory giving results of the standard single-disk susceptibility test with a 5 mcg cefixime disk should be interpreted according to the following criteria:

Zone diameter (mm)	Interpretation
≥ 19	(S) Susceptible
16–18	(MS) Moderately Susceptible
≤ 15	(R) Resistant

A report of "Susceptible" indicates that the pathogen is likely to be inhibited by generally achievable blood levels. A report of "Moderately Susceptible" indicates that inhibitory concentrations of the antibiotic may well be achieved if high dosage is used or if the infection is confined to tissues and fluids (eg, urine) in which high antibiotic levels are attained. A report of "Resistant" indicates that achievable concentrations of the antibiotic are unlikely to be inhibitory and other therapy should be selected.
Standardized procedures require the use of laboratory control organisms. The 5 mcg disk should give the following zone diameter:

Organism	Zone diameter (mm)
E coli ATCC 25922	23–27

The class disk for cephalosporin susceptibility testing (the cephalothin disk) is not appropriate because of spectrum differences with cefixime. The 5 mcg cefixime disk should be used for all *in vitro* testing of isolates.
Dilution Techniques: In other susceptibility testing procedures, eg, ICS agar dilution or equivalent, a bacterial isolate may be considered susceptible if the MIC value for cefixime is 1 mcg/mL or less. Organisms are considered resistant to cefixime if the MIC is equal to or greater than 4 mcg/mL. Organisms having an MIC of 2 mcg/mL are moderately susceptible.
As with standard diffusion methods, dilution procedures require the use of laboratory control organisms. Standard cefixime powder should give MIC values in the range of 0.25–1 mcg/mL for *E coli* ATCC 25922 and in the range of 8–32 mcg/mL for *S aureus* ATCC 29213.

INDICATIONS AND USAGE
SUPRAX *cefixime* is indicated in the treatment of the following infections when caused by susceptible strains of the designated microorganisms:
Uncomplicated Urinary Tract Infections caused by *Escherichia coli* and *Proteus mirabilis*.
Otitis Media caused by *Haemophilus influenzae* (beta-lactamase positive and negative strains), *Moraxella (Branhamella) catarrhalis*, (most of which are beta-lactamase positive) and *Streptococcus pyogenes*.*
Note: For information on otitis media caused by *Streptococcus pneumoniae*, see **CLINICAL STUDIES** section.
Pharyngitis and Tonsillitis, caused by *Streptococcus pyogenes*.
Note: Penicillin is the usual drug of choice in the treatment of *Streptococcus pyogenes* infections, including the prophylaxis of rheumatic fever. SUPRAX *cefixime* is generally effective in the eradication of *Streptococcus pyogenes* from the nasopharynx; however, data establishing the efficacy of SUPRAX in the subsequent prevention of rheumatic fever are not available.
Acute Bronchitis and Acute Exacerbations of Chronic Bronchitis, caused by *Streptococcus pneumoniae* and *Haemophilus influenzae* (beta-lactamase positive and negative strains). Appropriate cultures and susceptibility studies should be performed to determine the causative organism and its susceptibility to SUPRAX; however, therapy may be started

while awaiting the results of these studies. Therapy should be adjusted, if necessary, once these results are known.
*Efficacy for this organism in this organ system was studied in fewer than 10 infections.

CLINICAL STUDIES

In clinical trials of otitis media in nearly 400 children between the ages of 6 months to 10 years, *Streptococcus pneumoniae* was isolated from 47% of the patients, *Haemophilus influenzae* from 34%, *Moraxella (Branhamella) catarrhalis* from 15% and *Streptococcus pyogenes* from 4%.

The overall response rate of *Streptococcus pneumoniae* to cefixime was approximately 10% lower and that of *Haemophilus influenzae* or *Moraxella (Branhamella) catarrhalis* approximately 7% higher (12% when beta-lactamase positive strains of *H influenzae* are included) than the response rates of these organisms to the active control drugs.

In these studies, patients were randomized and treated with either cefixime at dose regimens of 4 mg/kg BID or 8 mg/kg QD, or with a standard antibiotic regimen. Sixty-nine to 70% of the patients in each group had resolution of signs and symptoms of otitis media when evaluated two to four weeks posttreatment, but persistent effusion was found in 15% of the patients. When evaluated at the completion of therapy, 17% of patients receiving cefixime and 14% of patients receiving effective comparative drugs (18% including those patients who had *Haemophilus influenzae* resistant to the control drug and who received the control antibiotic) were considered to be treatment failures. By the two- to four-week follow-up, a total of 30%–31% of patients had evidence of either treatment failure or recurrent disease.
[See table above].

CONTRAINDICATIONS

SUPRAX *cefixime* is contraindicated in patients with known allergy to the cephalosporin group of antibiotics.

WARNINGS

BEFORE THERAPY WITH SUPRAX IS INSTITUTED, CAREFUL INQUIRY SHOULD BE MADE TO DETERMINE WHETHER THE PATIENT HAS HAD PREVIOUS HYPERSENSITIVITY REACTIONS TO CEPHALOSPORINS, PENICILLINS, OR OTHER DRUGS. IF THIS PRODUCT IS TO BE GIVEN TO PENICILLIN-SENSITIVE PATIENTS, CAUTION SHOULD BE EXERCISED BECAUSE CROSS HYPERSENSITIVITY AMONG BETA-LACTAM ANTIBIOTICS HAS BEEN CLEARLY DOCUMENTED AND MAY OCCUR IN UP TO 10% OF PATIENTS WITH A HISTORY OF PENICILLIN ALLERGY. IF AN ALLERGIC REACTION TO SUPRAX OCCURS, DISCONTINUE THE DRUG. SERIOUS ACUTE HYPERSENSITIVITY REACTIONS MAY REQUIRE TREATMENT WITH EPINEPHRINE AND OTHER EMERGENCY MEASURES, INCLUDING OXYGEN, INTRAVENOUS FLUIDS, INTRAVENOUS ANTIHISTAMINES, CORTICOSTEROIDS, PRESSOR AMINES AND AIRWAY MANAGEMENT, AS CLINICALLY INDICATED.

Antibiotics, including SUPRAX, should be administered cautiously to any patient who has demonstrated some form of allergy, particularly to drugs.

Treatment with broad-spectrum antibiotics, including SUPRAX, alters the normal flora of the colon and may permit overgrowth of clostridia. Studies indicate that a toxin produced by *Clostridium difficile* is a primary cause of severe antibiotic-associated diarrhea including pseudomembranous colitis. Pseudomembranous colitis has been reported with the use of SUPRAX *cefixime* and other broad-spectrum antibiotics (including macrolides, semisynthetic penicillins, and cephalosporins); therefore, it is important to consider this diagnosis in patients who develop diarrhea in association with the use of antibiotics. Symptoms of pseudomembranous colitis may occur during or after antibiotic treatment and may range in severity from mild to life threatening. Mild cases of pseudomembranous colitis usually respond to drug discontinuation alone. In moderate-to-severe cases, management should include fluids, electrolytes, and protein supplementation. If the colitis does not improve after the drug has been discontinued, or if the symptoms are severe, oral vancomycin is the drug of choice for antibiotic-associated pseudomembranous colitis produced by *C difficile*. Other causes of colitis should be excluded.

PRECAUTIONS

General: The possibility of the emergence of resistant organisms which might result in overgrowth should be kept in mind, particularly during prolonged treatment. In such use, careful observation of the patient is essential. If superinfection occurs during therapy, appropriate measures should be taken.

The dose of SUPRAX should be adjusted in patients with renal impairment as well as those undergoing continuous ambulatory peritoneal dialysis (CAPD) and hemodialysis (HD). Patients on dialysis should be monitored carefully. (See **DOSAGE AND ADMINISTRATION**).

SUPRAX should be prescribed with caution in individuals with a history of gastrointestinal disease, particularly colitis.

Drug Interactions: No significant drug interactions have been reported to date.

Bacteriological Outcome of Otitis Media at Two- to Four-Weeks Posttherapy
Based on Repeat Middle Ear Fluid Culture or
Extrapolation from Clinical Outcome

Organism	Cefixime[a] 4 mg/kg BID		Cefixime[a] 8 mg/kg QD		Control[a] drugs	
Streptococcus pneumoniae	48/70	(69%)	18/22	(82%)	82/100	(82%)
Haemophilus influenzae beta-lactamase negative	24/34	(71%)	13/17	(76%)	23/34	(68%)
Haemophilus influenzae beta-lactamase positive	17/22	(77%)	9/12	(75%)	1/1[b]	
Moraxella (Branhamella) catarrhalis	26/31	(84%)	5/5		18/24	(75%)
Streptococcus pyogenes	5/5		3/3		6/7	
All Isolates	120/162	(74%)	48/59	(81%)	130/166	(78%)

[a] Number eradicated/number isolated.
[b] An additional 20 beta-lactamase positive strains of *Haemophilus influenzae* were isolated, but were excluded from this analysis because they were resistant to the control antibiotic. In nineteen of these, the clinical course could be assessed and a favorable outcome occurred in 10. When these cases are included in the overall bacteriological evaluation of therapy with the control drugs, 140/185 (76%) of pathogens were considered to be eradicated.

Drug/Laboratory Test Interactions: A false-positive reaction for ketones in the urine may occur with tests using nitroprusside but not with those using nitroferricyanide.

The administration of SUPRAX may result in a false-positive reaction for glucose in the urine using Clinitest®**, Benedict's solution, or Fehling's solution. It is recommended that glucose tests based on enzymatic glucose oxidase reactions (such as Clinistix®** or Tes-Tape®**) be used.

A false-positive direct Coombs test has been reported during treatment with other cephalosporin antibiotics; therefore, it should be recognized that a positive Coombs test may be due to the drug.

Carcinogenesis, Mutagenesis, Impairment of Fertility: Lifetime studies in animals to evaluate carcinogenic potential have not been conducted. SUPRAX did not cause point mutations in bacteria or mammalian cells, DNA damage, or chromosome damage *in vitro* and did not exhibit clastogenic potential *in vivo* in the mouse micronucleus test. In rats, fertility and reproductive performance were not affected by cefixime at doses up to 125 times the adult therapeutic dose.

Usage in Pregnancy: *Pregnancy Category B:* Reproduction studies have been performed in mice and rats at doses up to 400 times the human dose and have revealed no evidence of harm to the fetus due to SUPRAX. There are no adequate and well-controlled studies in pregnant women. Because animal reproduction studies are not always predictive of human response, this drug should be used during pregnancy only if clearly needed.

Labor and Delivery: SUPRAX *cefixime* has not been studied for use during labor and delivery. Treatment should only be given if clearly needed.

Nursing Mothers: It is not known whether SUPRAX is excreted in human milk. Consideration should be given to discontinuing nursing temporarily during treatment with this drug.

Pediatric Use: Safety and effectiveness of SUPRAX in children aged less than six months old have not been established. The incidence of gastrointestinal adverse reactions, including diarrhea and loose stools, in the pediatric patients receiving the suspension, was comparable to the incidence seen in adult patients receiving tablets.

ADVERSE REACTIONS

Most of the adverse reactions observed in clinical trials were of a mild and transient nature. Five percent (5%) of patients in the U.S. trials discontinued therapy because of drug-related adverse reactions. The most commonly seen adverse reactions in U.S. trials of the tablet formulation were gastrointestinal events, which were reported in 30% of adult patients on either the BID or the QD regimen. Clinically mild gastrointestinal side effects occurred in 20% of all patients, moderate events occurred in 9% of all patients, and severe adverse reactions occurred in 2% of all patients. Individual event rates included diarrhea 16%, loose or frequent stools 6%, abdominal pain 3%, nausea 7%, dyspepsia 3%, and flatulence 4%. The incidence of gastrointestinal adverse reactions, including diarrhea and loose stools, in pediatric patients receiving the suspension was comparable to the incidence seen in adult patients receiving tablets.

These symptoms usually responded to symptomatic therapy or ceased when SUPRAX was discontinued.

Several patients developed severe diarrhea and/or documented pseudomembranous colitis, and a few required hospitalization.

The following adverse reactions have been reported following the use of SUPRAX. Incidence rates were less than 1 in 50 (less than 2%), except as noted above for gastrointestinal events.

Gastrointestinal: (SEE ABOVE): Diarrhea, loose stools, abdominal pain, dyspepsia, nausea, and vomiting. Several cases of documented pseudomembranous colitis were identified during the studies. The onset of pseudomembranous colitis symptoms may occur during or after therapy.

Hypersensitivity Reactions: Skin rashes, urticaria, drug fever, and pruritus.

Hepatic: Transient elevations in SGPT, SGOT, and alkaline phosphatase.

Renal: Transient elevations in BUN or creatinine.

Central Nervous System: Headaches or dizziness.

Hemic and Lymphatic Systems: Transient thrombocytopenia, leukopenia, and eosinophilia. Prolongation in prothrombin time was seen rarely.

Other: Genital pruritus, vaginitis, candidiasis.

In addition to the adverse reactions listed above which have been observed in patients treated with SUPRAX, the following adverse reactions and altered laboratory tests have been reported for cephalosporin-class antibiotics:

Adverse Reactions: Allergic reactions including anaphylaxis, Stevens-Johnson syndrome, erythema multiforme, toxic epidermal necrolysis, superinfection, renal dysfunction, toxic nephropathy, hepatic dysfunction including cholestasis, aplastic anemia, hemolytic anemia, hemorrhage.

Several cephalosporins have been implicated in triggering seizures, particularly in patients with renal impairment when the dosage was not reduced (see DOSAGE AND ADMINISTRATION and OVERDOSAGE). If seizures associated with drug therapy occur, the drug should be discontinued. Anticonvulsant therapy can be given if clinically indicated.

Abnormal Laboratory Tests: Positive direct Coombs test, elevated bilirubin, elevated LDH, pancytopenia, neutropenia, agranulocytosis.

OVERDOSAGE

Gastric lavage may be indicated; otherwise, no specific antidote exists. Cefixime is not removed in significant quantities from the circulation by hemodialysis or peritoneal dialysis. Adverse reactions in small numbers of healthy adult volunteers receiving single doses up to 2 g of SUPRAX *cefixime* did not differ from the profile seen in patients treated at the recommended doses.

DOSAGE AND ADMINISTRATION

Adults: The recommended dose of SUPRAX *cefixime* is 400 mg daily. This may be given as a 400 mg tablet daily or as a 200 mg tablet every 12 hours.

Children: The recommended dose is 8 mg/kg/day of the suspension. This may be administered as a single daily dose or may be given in two divided doses, as 4 mg/kg every 12 hours.

Children weighing more than 50 kg or older than 12 years should be treated with the recommended adult dose.

Otitis media should be treated with the suspension. Clinical studies of otitis media were conducted with the suspension, and the suspension results in higher peak blood levels than the tablet when administered at the same dose. Therefore, the tablet should not be substituted for the suspension in the

Continued on next page

Lederle—Cont.

PEDIATRIC DOSAGE CHART

WEIGHT kg	DOSE/DAY mg	DOSE/DAY tsp of suspension	DOSE/DAY mL
6	48	0.5	2.4
12.5	100	1.0	5.0
19	152	1.5	7.6
25	200	2.0	10.0
35	280	3.0	14.0

treatment of otitis media (see **CLINICAL PHARMACOLOGY**).

Efficacy and safety in infants aged less than six months have not been established.

In the treatment of infections due to *S pyogenes*, a therapeutic dosage of SUPRAX should be administered for at least 10 days.

Renal Impairment: SUPRAX may be administered in the presence of impaired renal function. Normal dose and schedule may be employed in patients with creatinine clearances of 60 mL/min or greater. Patients whose clearance is between 21 and 60 mL/min or patients who are on renal hemodialysis may be given 75% of the standard dosage at the standard dosing interval (ie, 300 mg daily). Patients whose clearance is < 20 mL/min, or patients who are on continuous ambulatory peritoneal dialysis may be given half the standard dosage at the standard dosing interval (ie, 200 mg daily). Neither hemodialysis nor peritoneal dialysis remove significant amounts of drug from the body.

Reconstitution Directions for Oral Suspension

Bottle Size	Reconstitution Directions
100 mL	Suspend in a total of 66 mL water. Method: Add 33 mL of water to the contents in the bottle, invert and shake to wet powder. Then add a further 33 mL water and shake to suspend.
50 mL	Suspend in a total of 33 mL water. Method: Add 17 mL of water to the contents in the bottle, invert and shake to wet powder. Then add a further 16 mL water and shake to suspend. A calibrated dropper for dose administration is included.

After mixing, the suspension may be kept for 14 days at room temperature without significant loss of potency. DO NOT REFRIGERATE. Keep tightly closed. Shake well before using. Discard unused portion after 14 days.

HOW SUPPLIED

SUPRAX *cefixime* Tablets, 200 mg are convex, rectangular, white, film-coated tablets with rounded corners and beveled edges and a divided break line on each side, engraved with SUPRAX across one side and LL to the left and 200 to the right on the other side, supplied as follows:
NDC 0005-3899-23—Bottle of 100
Store at Controlled Room Temperature 15°–30°C (59°–86°F).
SUPRAX Tablets, 400 mg are convex, rectangular, white, film-coated tablets with rounded corners and beveled edges and a divided break line on each side, engraved with SUPRAX across one side and LL to the left and 400 to the right on the other side, supplied as follows:
NDC 0005-3897-18—Bottle of 50
NDC 0005-3897-23—Bottle of 100
Store at Controlled Room Temperature 15°–30°C (59°–86°F).
SUPRAX Powder for Oral Suspension is an off-white to cream-colored powder which when reconstituted as directed contains cefixime 100 mg/5 mL, supplied as follows:
NDC 0005-3898-40—50 mL Bottle
NDC 0005-3898-46—100 mL Bottle
Prior to Reconstitution: Store at Controlled Room Temperature 15°–30°C (59°–86°F).

REFERENCES

1. Bauer AW, Kirby WMM, Sherris JC, et al: Antibiotic susceptibility testing by a standard single disk method. *Am J Clin Pathol* 1966; 45: 493.
2. National Committee for Clinical Laboratory Standards, Approved Standard: Performance Standards for Antimicrobial Disk Susceptibility Tests (M2-A3), December 1984.
3. Standardized disk susceptibility test. Federal Register 1974; 39 (May 30): 19182–19184.
**Clinitest® and Clinistix® are registered trademarks of Ames Division, Miles Laboratories, Inc. Tes-Tape® is a registered trademark of Eli Lilly and Company.

Manufactured for
LEDERLE LABORATORIES DIVISION
American Cyanamid Company, Pearl River, NY 10965
By
BIOCRAFT LABORATORIES, INC.
Elmwood Park, NJ 07407
Under License of
Fujisawa Pharmaceutical Co., Ltd.
Osaka, Japan

Rev. 4/89
28780

Shown in Product Identification Section, page 415

TETANUS AND DIPHTHERIA TOXOIDS ADSORBED PUROGENATED®   ℞
For Adult Use
Aluminum Phosphate-Adsorbed

DESCRIPTION

Tetanus and Diphtheria Toxoids Adsorbed, For Adult Use, aluminum phosphate—adsorbed PUROGENATED® is a sterile combination of refined tetanus and diphtheria toxoids for intramuscular use only. After shaking, the vaccine is a homogeneous white suspension.

The tetanus and diphtheria toxins are produced according to the method of Mueller and Miller,[1,2] and are detoxified by use of formaldehyde. The toxoids are refined by the Pillemer alcohol fractionation method[3] and are diluted with a solution containing sodium phosphate monobasic, sodium phosphate dibasic, aluminum phosphate, glycine and thimerosal (mercury derivative) as a preservative. The final concentration of thimerosal in the combined vaccine is 1:10,000. The aluminum content of the final product does not exceed 0.80 mg per 0.5 ml dose.

Each 0.5 ml dose is formulated to contain 5 Lf units of tetanus toxoid and 2 Lf units of diphtheria toxoid.

CLINICAL PHARMACOLOGY

Tetanus is an intoxication manifested primarily by neuromuscular dysfunction, caused by a potent exotoxin elaborated by *Clostridium tetani*. The incidence of tetanus in the U.S. has dropped dramatically with the routine use of tetanus toxoid, remaining relatively constant over the last decade at about 90 cases reported annually.[4] Spores of *C tetani* are ubiquitous, and there is essentially no natural immunity to tetanus toxin. Thus, universal primary immunization with tetanus toxoid, and subsequent maintenance of adequate antitoxin levels by means of timed boosters, is necessary to protect all age groups.[4] Tetanus toxoid is a highly effective antigen, and a completed primary series generally induces protective levels of serum antitoxin that persist for at least 10 years.[4]

Diphtheria is primarily a localized and generalized intoxication caused by diphtheria toxin, an extracellular protein metabolite of toxinogenic strains of *Corynebacterium diphtheriae*. While the incidence of diphtheria in the U.S. has decreased from over 200,000 cases reported in 1921 before the general use of diphtheria toxoid, to only 15 cases reported from 1980 through 1983, the ratio of fatalities to attack rate has remained constant at about 5% to 10%.[4] The highest case fatality rates are in the very young and the elderly.

Following adequate immunization with diphtheria toxoid, which induces antitoxin, it is thought that protection lasts for at least 10 years.[4] This significantly reduces both the risk of developing diphtheria and the severity of clinical illness. It does not, however, eliminate carriage of *C diphtheriae* in the pharynx or on the skin.[4]

INDICATIONS AND USAGE

Tetanus and Diphtheria Toxoids adsorbed PUROGENATED (Td) For Adult Use, is indicated for active immunization against tetanus and diphtheria in adults and children 7 years of age and older.[4,5]

The Immunization Practices Advisory Committee (ACIP) of the U.S. Public Health Service recommends the use of the combined toxoids vaccine rather than single component vaccines for both primary and booster injections, including active tetanus immunization in wound management.[4]

Persons recovering from tetanus or diphtheria: Tetanus or diphtheria infection may not confer immunity; therefore, initiation or completion of active immunization is indicated at the time of recovery from these infections.[4]

Neonatal tetanus prevention: There is no evidence that tetanus and diphtheria toxoids are teratogenic. A previously unimmunized pregnant woman, who may deliver her child under nonhygienic circumstances and/or surroundings, should receive two properly spaced doses of Td before delivery, preferably during the last two trimesters. Incompletely immunized pregnant women should complete the three-dose series. Those immunized more than 10 years previously should have a booster dose.[4] (See also pregnancy information under **PRECAUTIONS**.)

CONTRAINDICATIONS

HYPERSENSITIVITY TO ANY COMPONENT OF THE VACCINE, INCLUDING THIMEROSAL, A MERCURY DERIVATIVE, IS A CONTRAINDICATION.
THE OCCURRENCE OF ANY NEUROLOGICAL SYMPTOMS OR SIGNS FOLLOWING ADMINISTRATION OF THIS PRODUCT IS A CONTRAINDICATION TO FURTHER USE.
IMMUNIZATION SHOULD BE DEFERRED DURING THE COURSE OF ANY FEBRILE ILLNESS OR ACUTE INFECTION. A MINOR AFEBRILE ILLNESS SUCH AS A MILD UPPER RESPIRATORY INFECTION IS NOT USUALLY REASON TO DEFER IMMUNIZATION.[4]
The clinical judgment of the attending physician should prevail at all times.
Routine immunization should be deferred during an outbreak of poliomyelitis, providing the patient has not sustained an injury that increases the risk of tetanus and providing an outbreak of diphtheria does not occur simultaneously.

WARNINGS

THIS PRODUCT IS NOT RECOMMENDED FOR IMMUNIZING PERSONS LESS THAN 7 YEARS OF AGE. The concentration of diphtheria toxoid in preparations intended for use in persons 7 years of age or older is lower than that of the pediatric formulation (Diphtheria and Tetanus Toxoids Adsorbed, for pediatric use, [DT]): a lower dosage of diphtheria toxoid is recommended for persons 7 years of age or older because adverse reactions to the diphtheria component are thought to be related to both dose and age.[4]
THE OCCURRENCE OF A NEUROLOGICAL OR SEVERE HYPERSENSITIVITY REACTION FOLLOWING A PREVIOUS DOSE IS A CONTRAINDICATION TO FURTHER USE OF THIS PRODUCT.[4]
THE ADMINISTRATION OF BOOSTER DOSES MORE FREQUENTLY THAN RECOMMENDED (see **DOSAGE AND ADMINISTRATION**) MAY BE ASSOCIATED WITH INCREASED INCIDENCE AND SEVERITY OF REACTIONS.[4]
Persons who experience Arthus-type hypersensitivity reactions or temperature greater than 39.4°C (103°F), after a previous dose of tetanus toxoid usually have very high serum tetanus antitoxin levels and should not be given even emergency doses of Td more frequently than every 10 years, even if they have a wound that is neither clean nor minor.[4]
If a contraindication to using tetanus toxoid-containing preparations exists in a person who has not completed a primary immunizing course of tetanus toxoid, and other than a clean, minor wound is sustained, only passive immunization should be given using human Tetanus Immune Globulin (TIG).[4]
Td should not be given to individuals with thrombocytopenia or any coagulation disorder that would contraindicate intramuscular injection unless the potential benefits clearly outweigh the risk of administration.
Patients with impaired immune responsiveness, whether due to the use of immunosuppressive therapy (including irradiation, corticosteroids, antimetabolites, alkylating agents, and cytotoxic agents), a genetic defect, human immunodeficiency virus (HIV) infection, or other causes, may have a reduced antibody response to active immunization procedures.[4–6] Deferral of administration of vaccine may be considered in individuals receiving immunosuppressive therapy.[4,5]
Special care should be taken to prevent injection into a blood vessel.

PRECAUTIONS

General:

1. **THIS PRODUCT SHOULD BE USED FOR INDIVIDUALS 7 YEARS OF AGE OR OLDER.**
2. PRIOR TO ADMINISTRATION OF ANY DOSE OF Td, THE PARENT, GUARDIAN, OR ADULT PATIENT SHOULD BE ASKED ABOUT THE RECENT HEALTH STATUS AND IMMUNIZATION HISTORY OF THE PATIENT TO BE IMMUNIZED IN ORDER TO DETERMINE THE EXISTENCE OF ANY CONTRAINDICATION TO IMMUNIZATION WITH Td (SEE **CONTRAINDICATIONS, WARNINGS**).
3. WHEN THE PATIENT RETURNS FOR THE NEXT DOSE IN A SERIES, THE PARENT, GUARDIAN, OR ADULT PATIENT SHOULD BE QUESTIONED CONCERNING OCCURRENCE OF ANY SYMPTOM AND/OR SIGN OF AN ADVERSE REACTION AFTER THE PREVIOUS DOSE (SEE **CONTRAINDICATIONS, ADVERSE REACTIONS**).
4. BEFORE THE INJECTION OF ANY BIOLOGICAL, THE PHYSICIAN SHOULD TAKE ALL PRECAUTIONS KNOWN FOR PREVENTION OF ALLERGIC OR ANY OTHER SIDE REACTIONS. This should include: a review of the patient's history regarding possible sensitivity; the ready availability of epinephrine 1:1,000 and other appropriate agents used for control of immediate allergic reactions; and a knowledge of the recent literature pertaining

to use of the biological concerned, including the nature of side effects and adverse reactions that may follow its use.

5. A separate sterile syringe and needle or a sterile disposable unit should be used for each individual patient to prevent transmission of hepatitis or other infectious agents from one person to another.

6. Shake vigorously before withdrawing each dose to resuspend the contents of the vial or vial.

7. NATIONAL CHILDHOOD VACCINE INJURY ACT OF 1986 (AS AMENDED IN 1987)

This Act requires that the manufacturer and lot number of the vaccine administered be recorded by the health care provider in the vaccine recipient's permanent medical record, along with the date of administration of the vaccine and the name, address and title of the person administering the vaccine.

The Act further requires the health care provider to report to a health department or to the FDA the occurrence following immunization of any event set forth in the Vaccine Injury Table including: anaphylaxis or anaphylactic shock within 24 hours, encephalopathy or encephalitis within 7 days, residual seizure disorder, any acute complication or sequelae (including death) of above events, or any event that would contraindicate further doses of vaccine, according to this package insert.[7]

Information for the Patient: PRIOR TO THE ADMINISTRATION OF THIS VACCINE, HEALTH CARE PERSONNEL SHOULD INFORM THE PARENT, GUARDIAN, OR ADULT PATIENT OF THE BENEFITS AND RISKS OF VACCINATION AGAINST TETANUS AND DIPHTHERIA.

Use in Pregnancy: *Pregnancy Category C:* Animal reproductive studies have not been conducted with this product. There is no evidence that tetanus and diphtheria toxoids are teratogenic. Td should be given to inadequately immunized pregnant women because it affords protection against neonatal tetanus.[8] Waiting until the second trimester is a reasonable precaution to minimize any theoretical concern.[4] Maintenance of adequate immunization by routine boosters in nonpregnant women of childbearing age (see **DOSAGE AND ADMINISTRATION**) can obviate the need to vaccinate women during pregnancy.

ADVERSE REACTIONS

Local reactions, such as erythema, induration, and tenderness, are common after the administration of Td.[9,10,11,12] Such local reactions are usually self-limited and require no therapy. Nodule,[13] sterile abscess formation, or subcutaneous atrophy may occur at the site of injection. Systemic reactions, such as fever, chills, myalgias, and headaches also may occur.[9,10,11,12]

Arthus-type hypersensitivity reactions, or high fever, may occur in persons who have very high serum antitoxin antibodies due to overly frequent injections of toxoid (see **WARNINGS**).

NEUROLOGICAL COMPLICATIONS,[14] SUCH AS CONVULSIONS,[15] ENCEPHALOPATHY,[15,16] AND VARIOUS MONO- AND POLYNEUROPATHIES,[16-22] INCLUDING GUILLAIN-BARRE SYNDROME,[23,24] HAVE BEEN REPORTED FOLLOWING ADMINISTRATION OF PREPARATIONS CONTAINING TETANUS AND/OR DIPHTHERIA ANTIGENS.

URTICARIA, ERYTHEMA MULTIFORME OR OTHER RASH, ARTHRALGIAS[15] AND, MORE RARELY, A SEVERE ANAPHYLACTIC REACTION (I.E., URTICARIA WITH SWELLING OF THE MOUTH, DIFFICULTY BREATHING, HYPOTENSION, OR SHOCK) HAVE BEEN REPORTED FOLLOWING ADMINISTRATION OF PREPARATIONS CONTAINING TETANUS AND/OR DIPHTHERIA ANTIGENS.

DOSAGE AND ADMINISTRATION

For Intramuscular Use Only: Shake vigorously before withdrawing each dose to resuspend the contents of the vial or syringe.

Parenteral drug products should be inspected visually for particulate matter and discoloration prior to administration. (See **DESCRIPTION**.)

The vaccine should be injected intramuscularly, preferably into the deltoid muscle, with care to avoid major peripheral nerve trunks. Before injection, the skin at the injection site should be cleansed and prepared with a suitable germicide. After insertion of the needle, aspirate to help avoid inadvertent injection into a blood vessel.

The primary immunizing course for unimmunized individuals 7 years of age or older consists of two doses of 0.5 ml each, 4 to 8 weeks apart, followed by a third (reinforcing) dose of 0.5 ml 6 to 12 months after the second dose. The reinforcing dose is an integral part of the primary immunizing course.[4] Interruption of the recommended schedule with a delay between doses does not interfere with the final immunity achieved, nor does it necessitate starting the series over again, regardless of the length of time elapsed between doses.[4]

A booster dose of 0.5 ml of Td is given 10 years after completion of primary immunization and every 10 years thereafter.

If a dose is given sooner than 10 years, as part of wound management or on exposure to diphtheria, the next booster is not needed for 10 years thereafter. MORE FREQUENT BOOSTER DOSES ARE NOT INDICATED AND MAY BE ASSOCIATED WITH INCREASED INCIDENCE AND SEVERITY OF REACTIONS.[4] (See **WARNINGS**.)

Diphtheria Prophylaxis for Case Contacts: All case contacts, household and others, who have previously received fewer than three doses of diphtheria toxoid, should receive an immediate dose of an appropriate diphtheria toxoid-containing preparation and should complete the series according to schedule. Case contacts who previously received three or more doses, but who have not received a dose of a preparation containing diphtheria toxoid within the previous five years, should receive a booster dose of a diphtheria toxoid-containing preparation appropriate for their age.[4] Td is an appropriate preparation in these circumstances for persons 7 years of age or older.

Tetanus Prophylaxis in Wound Management: The need for active immunization with a tetanus toxoid-containing preparation, with or without passive immunization with human Tetanus Immune Globulin (TIG) depends on both the condition of the wound and the patient's immunization history. Tetanus has rarely occurred among persons with a documented primary series of tetanus toxoid injections. A thorough attempt must be made to determine whether a patient has completed primary immunization.[4]

Individuals who have completed primary immunization against tetanus, and who sustain wounds which are minor and uncontaminated, should receive a booster dose of a tetanus-toxoid preparation only if they have not received tetanus toxoid within the preceding 10 years. For other wounds, a booster is appropriate if the patient has not received tetanus toxoid within the preceding 5 years. Antitoxin antibodies develop rapidly in persons who have previously received at least two doses of tetanus toxoid.[4]

Individuals who have not completed primary immunization against tetanus, or whose immunization history is unknown or uncertain, should be immunized with a tetanus toxoid-containing product. Completion of primary immunization thereafter should be ensured. In addition, if these individuals have sustained a tetanus-prone wound, the use of human Tetanus Immune Globulin (TIG) is recommended. A separate syringe and site of administration should be used.[4]

Summary guide to tetanus prophylaxis in routine wound management[4•]

History of tetanus toxoid (doses)	Clean, minor wounds		All other wounds†	
	Td	TIG	Td	TIG
Unknown <three	Yes	No	Yes	Yes
≥three‡	No§	No	No″	No

* Important details are in the text.

† Such as, but not limited to, wounds contaminated with dirt, feces, soil, saliva, etc.; puncture wounds; avulsions; and wounds resulting from missiles, crushing, burns and frostbite.

‡ If only three doses of **fluid** toxoid have been received, a fourth dose of toxoid, preferably an adsorbed toxoid, should be given.

§ Yes, if more than 10 years since last dose.

″ Yes, if more than 5 years since last dose. (More frequent boosters are not needed and can accentuate side effects.)

Td is the preferred preparation for active tetanus immunization in wound management of patients 7 years of age or older. This is to enhance diphtheria protection, since a large proportion of adults are susceptible. Thus, by taking advantage of acute health care visits for wound management, some patients can be protected who otherwise would remain susceptible.[4]

HOW SUPPLIED

1875-31 5.0 ml vial
1875-47 10 (0.5 ml) LEDERJECT® disposable syringe. For directions on use of LEDERJECT® disposable syringe, please see package insert accompanying product.

STORAGE

DO NOT FREEZE. STORE REFRIGERATED, AWAY FROM FREEZER COMPARTMENT, AT 2°C to 8°C (36°F to 46°F).

REFERENCES

1. Mueller JH, Miller PA: Factors influencing the production of tetanal toxin. *J Immunol* 1947;56:143–147.
2. Mueller JH, Miller PA: Production of diphtheria toxin of high potency (100Lf) on a reproducible medium. *J Immunol* 1941;40:21–32.
3. Pillemer L, Grossberg DB, Wittler RG: The immunochemistry of toxins and toxoids. II. The preparation and immunological evaluation of purified tetanal toxoid. *J Immunol* 1946;54:213–224.
4. Recommendation of the Immunization Practices Advisory Committee (ACIP): Diphtheria, tetanus and pertus-

sis: Guidelines for vaccine prophylaxis and other preventive measures. *MMWR* 1985;34:405–426.
5. Committee on Immunization, Council of Medical Societies American College of Physicians: Guide for Adult Immunization, 1st Edition 1985; Philadelphia, PA.
6. Recommendation of the ACIP: Immunization of children infected with Human T-Lymphotrophic Virus Type III/Lymphadenopathy associated virus. *MMWR* 1986;35(38):595–606.
7. National Childhood Vaccine Injury Act: Requirements for permanent vaccination records and for reporting of selected events after vaccination. *MMWR* 1988;37(13):197–200.
8. Recommendations of the ACIP: General recommendations on immunization. *MMWR* 1983;32(1):1–17.
9. Deacon SP, et al: A comparative clinical study of adsorbed tetanus vaccine and adult-type tetanus-diphtheria vaccine. *J Hyg (Cambridge)* 1982;89:513–519.
10. Macko MB, Powell CE: Comparison of the morbidity of tetanus toxoid boosters with tetanus-diphtheria toxoid boosters. *Ann Emerg Med* 1985;14:(1):33–35.
11. Myers MG, et al: Primary immunization with tetanus and diphtheria toxoids. *JAMA* 1982;248:(19):2478–2480.
12. Sisk CW, et al: Reactions to tetanus-diphtheria toxoid (adult). *Arch Environ Health* 1965;11:34–36.
13. Fawcett HA, Smith NP: Injection-site granuloma due to aluminum. *Arch Dermatol* 1984;120:1318–1322.
14. Rutledge SL, Snead OC: Neurological complications of immunizations. *J Pediatr* 1986;109:917–924.
15. Adverse Events Following Immunization. *MMWR* 1985;34(3):43–47.
16. Schlenska GK: Unusual neurological complications following tetanus toxoid administration. *J Neurol* 1977;215:299–302.
17. Blumstein GI, Kreithen H: Peripheral neuropathy following tetanus toxoid administration. *JAMA* 1966;198:1030–1031.
18. Reinstein L, Pargament JM, Goodman JS: Peripheral neuropathy after multiple tetanus toxoid injections. *Arch Phys Med Rehabil* 1982;63:332–334.
19. Tsairis P, Duck PJ, Mulder DW: Natural history of brachial plexus neuropathy. *Arch Neurol* 1972;27:109–117.
20. Quast U, Hennessen W, Widmark RM: Mono- and polyneuritis after tetanus vaccination. *Devel Bio Stand* 1979;43:25–32.
21. Holliday PL, Bauer RB: Polyradiculoneuritis secondary to immunization with tetanus and diphtheria toxoids. *Arch Neurol* 1983;40:56–67.
22. Fenichel GM: Neurological complications of tetanus toxoid. *Arch Neurol* 1983;40:390.
23. Pollard JD, Selby G: Relapsing neuropathy due to tetanus toxoid. *J Neurol Sci* 1978;37:113–125.
24. Newton N, Janati A: Guillain-Barre syndrome after vaccination with purified tetanus toxoid. *S Med J* 1987;80:1053–1054.

LEDERLE LABORATORIES DIVISION
American Cyanamid Company,
Pearl River, NY 10965

Rev. 5/88
23591

TETANUS TOXOID ADSORBED PUROGENATED®   ℞
Tetanus Toxoid Aluminum Phosphate Adsorbed

DESCRIPTION

Tetanus Toxoid Adsorbed, aluminum phosphate—adsorbed, PUROGENATED® is a sterile preparation of refined tetanus toxoid for intramuscular use only. After shaking, the product is a homogeneous white suspension.

The tetanus toxin is produced according to the method of Mueller and Miller[1] and is detoxified by use of formaldehyde. The toxoid is refined by the Pillemer alcohol fractionation method[2] and is diluted with a solution containing sodium phosphate dibasic, sodium phosphate monobasic, glycine, sodium chloride and thimerosal (mercury derivative) in a final concentration of 1:10,000 as a preservative and aluminum phosphate as adjuvant. The aluminum content does not exceed 0.80 mg per 0.5 mL dose.

Each 0.5 mL dose is formulated to contain 5 Lf units of tetanus toxoid.

CLINICAL PHARMACOLOGY

Tetanus is an intoxication manifested primarily by neuromuscular dysfunction, caused by a potent exotoxin elabo-

Continued on next page

Lederle—Cont.

rated by *Clostridium tetani*. The incidence of tetanus in the U.S. has dropped dramatically with the routine use of tetanus toxoid, remaining relatively constant over the last decade at about 90 cases reported annually.[3] Spores of *C tetani* are ubiquitous, and there is essentially no natural immunity to tetanus toxin. Thus, universal primary immunization with tetanus toxoid, and subsequent maintenance of adequate antitoxin levels by means of timed boosters, is necessary to protect all age groups.[3] Tetanus toxoid is a highly effective antigen, and a completed primary series generally induces protective levels of serum antitoxin that persist for at least 10 years.[3]

INDICATIONS AND USAGE

Tetanus Toxoid Adsorbed is indicated for active immunization against tetanus in adults and children 2 months of age or older.

Immunization of persons 7 years of age or older may be accomplished by the use of Tetanus and Diphtheria Toxoids Adsorbed, for Adult Use, (Td), Tetanus Toxoid Adsorbed, or Tetanus Toxoid Fluid. The Immunization Practices Advisory Committee (ACIP) of the U.S. Public Health Service recommends the use of the combined toxoids vaccine rather than single component vaccines for both primary and booster injections, including active tetanus immunization in wound management.[3] Individuals for whom the use of a vaccine containing diphtheria toxoid is contraindicated should receive a single-component tetanus toxoid-containing vaccine. Immunization of infants and children 2 months of age up to the seventh birthday is usually accomplished by the use of Diphtheria and Tetanus Toxoids and Pertussis Vaccine Adsorbed (DTP) or Diphtheria and Tetanus Toxoids Adsorbed, for pediatric use (DT). Tetanus Toxoid Adsorbed may be used for immunizing infants and children for whom the use of a vaccine containing diphtheria toxoid and pertussis antigen is contraindicated.

Comparative tests have shown that the adsorbed toxoids are superior to the fluid toxoids in antibody titers produced and in the durability of protection achieved. The promptness of antibody response to booster doses of either fluid or adsorbed toxoid is not sufficiently different to be of clinical importance. When Tetanus Immune Globulin (TIG) is to be administered at the same visit as tetanus toxoid, the adsorbed toxoid should be used. [3,4]

Persons recovering from tetanus: Tetanus infection may not confer immunity; therefore, initiation or completion of active immunization is indicated at the time of recovery from this infection.[3]

Neonatal tetanus prevention: There is no evidence that tetanus toxoid is teratogenic. A previously unimmunized pregnant woman, who may deliver her child under nonhygienic circumstances and/or surroundings, should receive two properly spaced doses of a tetanus toxoid-containing preparation before delivery, preferably during the last two trimesters. Incompletely immunized pregnant women should complete the three-dose series. Those immunized more than 10 years previously should have a booster dose.[3] (See also pregnancy information under **PRECAUTIONS**).

CONTRAINDICATIONS

HYPERSENSITIVITY TO ANY COMPONENT OF THE VACCINE, INCLUDING THIMEROSAL, A MERCURY DERIVATIVE, IS A CONTRAINDICATION.
THE OCCURRENCE OF ANY TYPE OF NEUROLOGICAL SYMPTOMS OR SIGNS FOLLOWING ADMINISTRATION OF THIS PRODUCT IS A CONTRAINDICATION TO FURTHER USE.
IMMUNIZATION SHOULD BE DEFERRED DURING THE COURSE OF ANY FEBRILE ILLNESS OR ACUTE INFECTION. A MINOR AFEBRILE ILLNESS SUCH AS A MILD UPPER RESPIRATORY INFECTION IS NOT USUALLY REASON TO DEFER IMMUNIZATION.[3]
The clinical judgment of the attending physician should prevail at all times.
Routine immunization should be deferred during an outbreak of poliomyelitis, providing the patient has not sustained an injury that increases the risk of tetanus.

WARNINGS

THE OCCURRENCE OF A NEUROLOGICAL OR SEVERE HYPERSENSITIVITY REACTION FOLLOWING A PREVIOUS DOSE IS A CONTRAINDICATION TO FURTHER USE OF THIS PRODUCT.[3]
THE ADMINISTRATION OF BOOSTER DOSES MORE FREQUENTLY THAN RECOMMENDED (See **DOSAGE AND ADMINISTRATION**) MAY BE ASSOCIATED WITH INCREASED INCIDENCE AND SEVERITY OF REACTIONS.[3]
Persons who experience Arthus-type hypersensitivity reactions or temperature greater than 39.4°C (103°F), after a previous dose of tetanus toxoid usually have very high serum tetanus antitoxin levels and should not be given even emergency doses of tetanus toxoid more frequently than every 10

years, even if they have a wound that is neither clean nor minor.[3]
If a contraindication to using tetanus toxoids exists in a person who has not completed a primary immunizing course of tetanus toxoid, and other than a clean, minor wound is sustained, only passive immunization should be given using human Tetanus Immune Globulin (TIG).[3]
Tetanus Toxoid Adsorbed should not be given to individuals with thrombocytopenia or any coagulation disorder that would contraindicate intramuscular injection, unless the potential benefit clearly outweighs the risk of administration.
Patients with impaired immune responsiveness, whether due to the use of immunosuppressive therapy (including irradiation, corticosteroids, antimetabolites, alkylating agents, and cytotoxic agents), a genetic defect, human immunodeficiency virus (HIV) infection, or other causes, may have a reduced antibody response to active immunization procedures.[3–5] Deferral of administration of vaccine may be considered in individuals receiving immunosuppressive therapy.[3,4]
Special care should be taken to prevent injection into a blood vessel.

PRECAUTIONS

General:

1. PRIOR TO ADMINISTRATION OF ANY DOSE OF VACCINE THE PARENT, GUARDIAN, OR ADULT PATIENT SHOULD BE ASKED ABOUT THE RECENT HEALTH STATUS AND IMMUNIZATION HISTORY OF THE PATIENT TO BE IMMUNIZED IN ORDER TO DETERMINE THE EXISTENCE OF ANY CONTRAINDICATION TO IMMUNIZATION (SEE **CONTRAINDICATIONS, WARNINGS**).
2. WHEN THE PATIENT RETURNS FOR THE NEXT DOSE IN A SERIES, THE PARENT, GUARDIAN, OR ADULT PATIENT SHOULD BE QUESTIONED CONCERNING OCCURRENCE OF ANY SYMPTOM AND/OR SIGN OF AN ADVERSE REACTION AFTER THE PREVIOUS DOSE (SEE **CONTRAINDICATIONS, ADVERSE REACTIONS**).
3. BEFORE THE INJECTION OF ANY BIOLOGICAL, THE PHYSICIAN SHOULD TAKE ALL PRECAUTIONS KNOWN FOR PREVENTION OF ALLERGIC OR ANY OTHER SIDE REACTIONS. This should include: a review of the patient's history regarding possible sensitivity; the ready availability of epinephrine 1:1,000 and other appropriate agents used for control of immediate allergic reactions; and a knowledge of the recent literature pertaining to use of the biological concerned, including the nature of side effects and adverse reactions that may follow its use.
4. A separate sterile syringe and needle or a sterile disposable unit should be used for each individual patient to prevent transmission of hepatitis or other infectious agents from one person to another.
5. Shake vigorously before withdrawing each dose to resuspend the contents of the vial.
6. NATIONAL CHILDHOOD VACCINE INJURY ACT OF 1986 (AS AMENDED IN 1987)
This Act requires that the manufacturer and lot number of the vaccine administered be recorded by the health care provider in the vaccine recipient's permanent record, along with the date of administration of the vaccine and the name, address and title of the person administering the vaccine.
The Act further requires the health care provider to report to a health department or to the FDA the occurrence following immunization of any event set forth in the Vaccine Injury Table including: anaphylaxis or anaphylactic shock within 24 hours, encephalopathy or encephalitis within 7 days, residual seizure disorder, any acute complication or sequelae (including death) of above events, or any event that would contraindicate further doses of vaccine, according to this package insert.[6]

Information for the Patient: PRIOR TO ADMINISTRATION OF THIS VACCINE, HEALTH CARE PERSONNEL SHOULD INFORM THE PARENT, GUARDIAN, OR ADULT PATIENT OF THE BENEFITS AND RISKS OF VACCINATION AGAINST TETANUS.

Use in Pregnancy: *Pregnancy Category C:* Animal reproductive studies have not been conducted with this product. There is no evidence that tetanus toxoid is teratogenic. An appropriate tetanus-toxoid containing preparation (usually Td) should be given to inadequately immunized pregnant women because it affords protection against neonatal tetanus.[7] Waiting until the second trimester is a reasonable precaution to minimize any theoretical concern.[4] Maintenance of adequate immunization by routine boosters in non-pregnant women of child-bearing age (see **DOSAGE AND ADMINISTRATION**) can obviate the need to vaccinate women during pregnancy.

ADVERSE REACTIONS

Local reactions, such as erythema, induration, and tenderness, are common after the administration of tetanus toxoid.[8,9,10] Such local reactions are usually self-limiting and

require no therapy. Nodule,[11] sterile abscess formation, or subcutaneous atrophy may occur at the site of injection. Systemic reactions, such as fever, chills, myalgia, and headaches also may occur.[8,9,10]
Arthus-type hypersensitivity reactions, or high fever, may occur in persons who have very high serum antitoxin antibodies due to overly frequent injections of toxoid.[3] (See **WARNINGS.**)
NEUROLOGICAL COMPLICATIONS,[12] SUCH AS CONVULSIONS,[13] ENCEPHALOPATHY,[13,14] AND VARIOUS MONO- AND POLYNEUROPATHIES,[14–20] INCLUDING GUILLAIN-BARRE SYNDROME,[21,22] HAVE BEEN REPORTED FOLLOWING ADMINISTRATION OF PREPARATIONS CONTAINING TETANUS ANTIGENS.
URTICARIA, ERYTHEMA MULTIFORME OR OTHER RASH, ARTHRALGIAS[13] AND, MORE RARELY, A SEVERE ANAPHYLACTIC REACTION (I.E., URTICARIA WITH SWELLING OF THE MOUTH, DIFFICULTY BREATHING, HYPOTENSION, OR SHOCK) HAVE BEEN REPORTED FOLLOWING ADMINISTRATION OF PREPARATIONS CONTAINING TETANUS ANTIGEN.

DOSAGE AND ADMINISTRATION

For Intramuscular Use Only: Shake vigorously before withdrawing each dose to resuspend the contents of the vial or syringe.
Parenteral drug products should be inspected visually for particulate matter and discoloration prior to administration. (See **DESCRIPTION.**)
Preferred injection sites for intramuscular injection include the anterolateral aspect of the upper thigh and the deltoid area of the upper arm. Care should be taken to avoid major peripheral nerve trunks.
Before injection, the skin at the injection site should be cleansed and prepared with a suitable germicide.
After insertion of the needle, aspirate to help avoid inadvertent injection into a blood vessel.
The primary immunizing course for unimmunized individuals one year of age or older consists of **two** doses of 0.5 mL each, 4 to 8 weeks apart, followed by a **third** (reinforcing) dose of 0.5 mL, 6 to 12 months after the second dose. The reinforcing dose is an integral part of the primary immunizing course.
If, after beginning combined immunization against diphtheria, tetanus, and pertussis, further doses of vaccine containing pertussis and diphtheria antigens become contraindicated, Tetanus Toxoid Adsorbed may be substituted for each of the remaining doses.
When immunization with Tetanus Toxoid Adsorbed is begun in the first year of life, the primary series consists of **three** doses of 0.5 mL each, 4 to 8 weeks apart, followed by a **fourth** (reinforcing) dose of 0.5 mL, 6 to 12 months after the third dose.
Interruption of the recommended schedule with a delay between doses does not interfere with the final immunity achieved with Tetanus Toxoid Adsorbed. There is no need to start the series over again, regardless of the length of time elapsed between doses.[3]
Booster Doses: A single injection of 0.5 mL of Tetanus Toxoid Adsorbed is given 10 years after completion of primary immunization and every 10 years thereafter. If a dose is given sooner as part of wound management, the next booster is not needed for 10 years thereafter. MORE FREQUENT BOOSTER DOSES ARE NOT INDICATED AND MAY BE ASSOCIATED WITH INCREASED INCIDENCE AND SEVERITY OF REACTIONS.[3]
Tetanus Prophylaxis in Wound Management: The need for active immunization with a tetanus toxoid-containing preparation, with or without passive immunization with human Tetanus Immune Globulin (TIG) depends on both the condition of the wound and the patient's immunization history. Tetanus has rarely occurred among persons with a documented primary series of toxoid injections. A thorough attempt must be made to determine whether a patient has completed primary immunization.[3]
Individuals who have completed primary immunization against tetanus, and who sustain wounds which are minor and uncontaminated, should receive a booster dose of a tetanus toxoid-containing preparation (see **INDICATIONS AND USAGE**) only if they have not received tetanus toxoid within the preceding 10 years. For other wounds, a booster is appropriate if the patient has not received tetanus toxoid within the preceding 5 years. Antitoxin antibodies develop rapidly in persons who have previously received at least two doses of tetanus toxoid.[3]
Individuals who have not completed primary immunization against tetanus, or whose immunization history is unknown or uncertain, should be immunized with a tetanus toxoid-containing product (see **INDICATIONS AND USAGE**). Completion of primary immunization thereafter should be ensured. In addition, if these individuals have sustained a tetanus-prone wound, the use of human Tetanus Immune Globulin (TIG) is recommended. A separate syringe and site of administration should be used. When TIG is to be administered at the same visit as tetanus toxoid, an adsorbed tetanus toxoid-containing preparation should be used.[3]

SUMMARY GUIDE TO TETANUS PROPHYLAXIS IN ROUTINE WOUND MANAGEMENT[3]*

History of tetanus toxoid (doses)	Clean, minor wounds		All other wounds†	
	Td‡	TIG	Td‡	TIG
Unknown or < three	Yes	No	Yes	Yes
≥ three§	No″	No	No£	No

* Important details are in the text.

† Such as, but not limited to, wounds contaminated with dirt, feces, soil, saliva, etc.; puncture wounds; avulsions; and wounds resulting from missiles, crushing, burns and frostbite.

‡ For children under 7 years old DPT (DT, if pertussis vaccine is contraindicated) is preferred to tetanus toxoid alone. For persons 7 years and older, Td is preferred to tetanus toxoid alone.

§ If only three doses of **fluid** toxoid have been received, a fourth dose of toxoid, preferably an adsorbed toxoid, should be given.

″ Yes, if more than 10 years since last dose.

£ Yes, if more than 5 years since last dose. (More frequent boosters are not needed and can accentuate side effects.)

In order to enhance diphtheria protection in the population, the ACIP recommends Tetanus and Diphtheria Toxoid For Adult Use as the preferred preparation for active tetanus immunization in wound management of patients 7 years of age or older.[3]

HOW SUPPLIED

NDC 0005-1938-31   5.0 mL vial

NDC 0005-1938-47   10×0.5 mL LEDERJECT® disposable syringe. For directions on use of LEDERJECT® disposable syringe, please see package insert accompanying product.

STORAGE

DO NOT FREEZE. STORE REFRIGERATED, AWAY FROM FREEZER COMPARTMENT, AT 2°C to 8°C (36°F to 46°F).

REFERENCES

1. Mueller JH, Miller PA: Factors influencing the production of tetanal toxin. *J Immunol* 1947;56:143–147.
2. Pillemer L, Grossberg DB, Wittler RG: The immunochemistry of toxins and toxoids. II. The preparation and immunological evaluation of purified tetanal toxoid. *J Immunol* 1946;54:213–224.
3. Recommendation of the Immunization Practices Advisory Committee (ACIP): Diphtheria, tetanus and pertussis: Guidelines for vaccine prophylaxis and other preventive measures. *MMWR* 1985;34:405–426.
4. Committee on Immunization, Council of Medical Societies American College of Physicians: Guide for Adult Immunization, Philadelphia, 1985.
5. Recommendation of the ACIP: Immunization of children infected with Human T-Lymphotrophic Virus Type III/Lymphadenopathy associated virus. *MMWR* 1986;35(38):595–606.
6. National Childhood Vaccine Injury Act: Requirements for permanent vaccination records and for reporting of selected events after vaccination. *MMWR* 1988;37(13):197–200.
7. Recommendations of the ACIP: General recommendations on immunization. *MMWR* 1983;32(1):1–17.
8. Macko MB, Powell CE: Comparison of the morbidity of tetanus toxoid boosters with tetanus-diphtheria toxoid boosters. *Ann Emerg Med* 1985;14:(1):33–35.
9. Deacon SP, et al: A comparative clinical study of adsorbed tetanus vaccine and adult-type tetanus-diphtheria vaccine. *J Hyg (Cambridge)* 1982;89:513–519.
10. Jacobs RL, et al: Adverse reactions to tetanus toxoid. *JAMA* 1982: 247;(1):40–42.
11. Fawcett HA, Smith N: Injection-site granuloma due to aluminum. *Arch Dermatol* 1984;120:1318–1322.
12. Rutledge SL, Snead OC: Neurological complications of immunizations. *J Pediatr* 1986;109:917–924.
13. Adverse Events Following Immunization. *MMWR* 1985;34(3):43–47.
14. Schlenska GK: Unusual neurological complications following tetanus toxoid administration. *J Neurol* 1977;215:299–302.
15. Blumstein GI, Kreithen H: Peripheral neuropathy following tetanus toxoid administration. *JAMA* 1966;198:1030–1031.
16. Reinstein L, Pargament JM, Goodman JS: Peripheral neuropathy after multiple tetanus toxoid injections. *Arch Phys Med Rehabil* 1982;63:332–334.
17. Tsairis P, Duck PJ, Mulder DW: Natural history of brachial plexus neuropathy. *Arch Neurol* 1972;27:109–117.
18. Quast U, Hennessen W, Widmark RM: Mono- and polyneuritis after tetanus vaccination. *Devel Bio Stand* 1979;43:25–32.
19. Holliday PL, Bauer RB: Polyradiculoneuritis secondary to immunization with tetanus and diphtheria toxoids. *Arch Neurol* 1983;40:56–57.
20. Fenichel GM: Neurological complications of tetanus toxoid. *Arch Neurol* 1983;40:390.
21. Pollard JD, Selby G: Relapsing neuropathy due to tetanus toxoid. *J Neurol Sci* 1978;37:113–125.
22. Newton N, Janati A: Guillain-Barre syndrome after vaccination with purified tetanus toxoid. *S Med J* 1987;80:1053–1054.

LEDERLE LABORATORIES DIVISION
American Cyanamid Company,
Pearl River, NY 10965

Rev. 5/88
23588

TETANUS TOXOID PUROGENATED®   ℞
Tetanus Toxoid Fluid

DESCRIPTION

Tetanus Toxoid PUROGENATED® Tetanus Toxoid Fluid is a sterile preparation of refined tetanus toxoid for intramuscular or subcutaneous use. The product is a clear, practically colorless liquid.

The tetanus toxin is produced according to the method of Mueller and Miller[1] and is detoxified by use of formaldehyde. The toxoid is refined by the Pillemer alcohol fractionation method[2] and is diluted with a solution containing sodium phosphate dibasic and glycine. Thimerosal (mercury derivative) is present in a final concentration of 1:10,000 as a preservative.

Each 0.5 mL dose is formulated to contain 5 Lf units of tetanus toxoid.

CLINICAL PHARMACOLOGY

Tetanus is an intoxication manifested primarily by neuromuscular dysfunction, caused by a potent exotoxin elaborated by *Clostridium tetani*. The incidence of tetanus in the U.S. has dropped dramatically with the routine use of tetanus toxoid, remaining relatively constant over the last decade at about 90 cases reported annually.[3] Spores of *C tetani* are ubiquitous and there is essentially no natural immunity to tetanus toxin. Thus, universal primary immunization with tetanus toxoid, and subsequent maintenance of adequate antitoxin levels by means of timed boosters, is necessary to protect all age groups.[3]

Tetanus toxoid is a highly effective antigen, and a completed primary series generally induces protective levels of serum antitoxin that persist for at least 10 years.[3]

INDICATIONS AND USAGE

Tetanus Toxoid Fluid is indicated for active immunization against tetanus in adults and children 2 months of age or older. While either Tetanus Toxoid Adsorbed or Tetanus Toxoid Fluid can be used for active immunization of individuals against tetanus, the adsorbed preparation is preferred.[3] Immunization of persons 7 years of age or older may be accomplished by the use of Tetanus and Diphtheria Toxoids Adsorbed, for Adult Use (Td), Tetanus Toxoid Adsorbed, or Tetanus Toxoid Fluid. The Immunization Practices Advisory Committee (ACIP) of the U.S. Public Health Service recommends the use of the combined toxoids vaccine rather than single component vaccines for both primary and booster injections, including active tetanus immunization in wound management.[3] Individuals for whom the use of a vaccine containing diphtheria toxoid is contraindicated should receive a single-component tetanus toxoid-containing vaccine. Immunization of infants and children 2 months of age up to the seventh birthday is usually accomplished by the use of Diphtheria and Tetanus Toxoids and Pertussis Vaccine Adsorbed (DTP) or Diphtheria and Tetanus Toxoids Adsorbed, for pediatric use (DT). A single-component tetanus toxoid-containing vaccine may be used for immunizing infants and children for whom the use of a vaccine containing diphtheria toxoid and pertussis antigen is contraindicated.

Comparative tests have shown that the adsorbed toxoids are superior to the fluid toxoids in antibody titers produced and in the durability of protection achieved. The promptness of antibody response to booster doses of either fluid or adsorbed toxoid is not sufficiently different to be of clinical importance. When Tetanus Immune Globulin (TIG) is to be administered at the same visit as tetanus toxoid, the adsorbed toxoid should be used.[3,4]

Persons recovering from tetanus: Tetanus infection may not confer immunity; therefore, initiation or completion of active immunization is indicated at the time of recovery from this infection.[3]

Neonatal tetanus prevention: There is no evidence that tetanus toxoid is teratogenic. A previously unimmunized pregnant woman who may deliver her child under nonhygienic circumstances and/or surroundings should receive two properly spaced doses of a tetanus toxoid-containing preparation before delivery, preferably during the last two trimesters. Incompletely immunized pregnant women should complete the three-dose series. Those immunized more than 10 years previously should have a booster dose.[3] (See also pregnancy information under **PRECAUTIONS**.)

CONTRAINDICATIONS

HYPERSENSITIVITY TO ANY COMPONENT OF THE VACCINE, INCLUDING THIMEROSAL, A MERCURY DERIVATIVE, IS A CONTRAINDICATION.

THE OCCURRENCE OF ANY TYPE OF NEUROLOGICAL SYMPTOMS OR SIGNS FOLLOWING ADMINISTRATION OF THIS PRODUCT IS A CONTRAINDICATION TO FURTHER USE.

IMMUNIZATION SHOULD BE DEFERRED DURING THE COURSE OF ANY FEBRILE ILLNESS OR ACUTE INFECTION. A MINOR AFEBRILE ILLNESS SUCH AS A MILD UPPER RESPIRATORY INFECTION IS NOT USUALLY REASON TO DEFER IMMUNIZATION.[3]

The clinical judgment of the attending physician should prevail at all times.

Routine immunization should be deferred during an outbreak of poliomyelitis, providing the patient has not sustained an injury that increases the risk of tetanus.

WARNINGS

THE OCCURRENCE OF A NEUROLOGICAL OR SEVERE HYPERSENSITIVITY REACTION FOLLOWING A PREVIOUS DOSE IS A CONTRAINDICATION TO FURTHER USE OF THIS PRODUCT.[3]

THE ADMINISTRATION OF BOOSTER DOSES MORE FREQUENTLY THAN RECOMMENDED (see **DOSAGE AND ADMINISTRATION**) MAY BE ASSOCIATED WITH INCREASED INCIDENCE AND SEVERITY OF REACTIONS.[3]

Persons who experience Arthus-type hypersensitivity reactions or temperature greater than 39.4°C (103°F), after a previous dose of tetanus toxoid usually have very high serum tetanus antitoxin levels and should not be given even emergency doses of tetanus toxoid more frequently than every 10 years, even if they have a wound that is neither clean nor minor.[3]

If a contraindication to using tetanus toxoid exists in a person who has not completed a primary immunizing course of tetanus toxoid, and other than a clean, minor wound is sustained, only passive immunization should be given using human Tetanus Immune Globulin (TIG).[3]

Tetanus Toxoid Fluid should not be administered with Tetanus Immune Globulin (TIG). In this situation the adsorbed preparation should be used.[4]

Tetanus Toxoid Fluid should not be given by intramuscular injection to individuals with thrombocytopenia or any coagulation disorder that would contraindicate intramuscular injection, unless the potential benefit clearly outweighs the risk of administration.

Patients with impaired immune responsiveness, whether due to the use of immunosuppressive therapy (including irradiation, corticosteroids, antimetabolites, alkylating agents, and cytotoxic agents), a genetic defect, human immunodeficiency virus (HIV) infection, or other causes, may have a reduced antibody response to active immunization procedures.[3–5] Deferral of administration of vaccine may be considered in individuals receiving immunosuppressive therapy.[3,4]

Special care should be taken to prevent injection into a blood vessel.

PRECAUTIONS

General:

1. PRIOR TO ADMINISTRATION OF ANY DOSE OF VACCINE THE PARENT, GUARDIAN, OR ADULT PATIENT SHOULD BE ASKED ABOUT THE RECENT HEALTH STATUS AND IMMUNIZATION HISTORY OF THE PATIENT TO BE IMMUNIZED IN ORDER TO DETERMINE THE EXISTENCE OF ANY CONTRAINDICATIONS TO IMMUNIZATION (SEE **CONTRAINDICATIONS, WARNINGS**).
2. WHEN THE PATIENT RETURNS FOR THE NEXT DOSE IN A SERIES, THE PARENT, GUARDIAN, OR ADULT PATIENT SHOULD BE QUESTIONED CONCERNING OCCURRENCE OF ANY SYMPTOM AND/OR SIGN OF AN ADVERSE REACTION AFTER THE PREVIOUS DOSE (SEE **CONTRAINDICATIONS, ADVERSE REACTIONS**).
3. BEFORE THE INJECTION OF ANY BIOLOGICAL, THE PHYSICIAN SHOULD TAKE ALL PRECAUTIONS KNOWN FOR PREVENTION OF ALLERGIC OR ANY OTHER SIDE REACTIONS. This should include: a review of the patient's history regarding possible sensitivity; the ready availability of epinephrine 1:1,000 and other appro-

Continued on next page

Lederle—Cont.

priate agents used for control of immediate allergic reactions; and a knowledge of the recent literature pertaining to use of the biological concerned, including the nature of side effects and adverse reactions that may follow its use.

4. A separate sterile syringe and needle or a sterile disposable unit should be used for each individual patient to prevent transmission of hepatitis or other infectious agents from one person to another.

5. NATIONAL CHILDHOOD VACCINE INJURY ACT OF 1986 (AS AMENDED IN 1987)

This Act requires that the manufacturer and lot number of the vaccine administered be recorded by the health care provider in the vaccine recipient's permanent record, along with the date of administration of the vaccine and the name, address and title of the person administering the vaccine.

The Act further requires the health care provider to report to a health department or to the FDA the occurrence following immunization of any event set forth in the Vaccine Injury Table including: anaphylaxis or anaphylactic shock within 24 hours, encephalopathy or encephalitis within 7 days, residual seizure disorder, any acute complication or sequelae (including death) of above events, or any event that would contraindicate further doses of vaccine, according to this package insert.[6]

Information for the Patient: PRIOR TO THE ADMINISTRATION OF THIS VACCINE, HEALTH CARE PERSONNEL SHOULD INFORM THE PARENT, GUARDIAN, OR ADULT PATIENT OF THE BENEFITS AND RISKS OF VACCINATION AGAINST TETANUS.

Use in Pregnancy: *Pregnancy Category C:* Animal reproductive studies have not been conducted with this product. There is no evidence that tetanus toxoid is teratogenic. An appropriate tetanus-toxoid containing preparation (usually Td) should be given to inadequately immunized women because it affords protection against neonatal tetanus.[7] Waiting until the second trimester is a reasonable precaution to minimize any theoretical concern.[4] Maintenance of adequate immunization by routine boosters in non-pregnant women of childbearing age (see **DOSAGE AND ADMINISTRATION**) can obviate the need to vaccinate women during pregnancy.

ADVERSE REACTIONS

Local reactions, such as erythema, induration, and tenderness, are common after the administration of tetanus toxoid.[8,9,10] Such local reactions are usually self-limited and require no therapy. Nodule, sterile abscess formation, or subcutaneous atrophy may occur at the site of injection. Systemic reactions, such as fever, chills, myalgia, and headaches also may occur.[8,9,10]

Arthus-type hypersensitivity reactions, or high fever, may occur in persons who have very high serum antitoxin antibodies due to overly frequent injections of toxoid.[3] (See **WARNINGS.**)

NEUROLOGICAL COMPLICATIONS,[11] SUCH AS CONVULSIONS,[12] ENCEPHALOPATHY,[12,13] AND VARIOUS MONO- AND POLYNEUROPATHIES,[13–19] INCLUDING GUILLAIN-BARRE SYNDROME,[20,21] HAVE BEEN REPORTED FOLLOWING ADMINISTRATION OF PREPARATIONS CONTAINING TETANUS ANTIGEN.

URTICARIA, ERYTHEMA MULTIFORME OR OTHER RASH, ARTHRALGIAS[12] AND, MORE RARELY, A SEVERE ANAPHYLACTIC REACTION (I.E., URTICARIA WITH SWELLING OF THE MOUTH, DIFFICULTY BREATHING, HYPOTENSION OR SHOCK) HAVE BEEN REPORTED FOLLOWING ADMINISTRATION OF PREPARATIONS CONTAINING TETANUS ANTIGEN.

DOSAGE AND ADMINISTRATION

For Intramuscular or Subcutaneous Use Only: Parenteral drug products should be inspected visually for particulate matter and discoloration prior to administration. (See **DESCRIPTION.**)

Preferred injection sites for intramuscular or subcutaneous injection include the anterolateral aspect of the upper thigh and the deltoid area of the upper arm. Care should be taken to avoid major peripheral nerve trunks.

Before injection, the skin at the injection site should be cleansed and prepared with a suitable germicide.

After insertion of the needle, aspirate to help avoid inadvertent injection into a blood vessel.

The primary immunizing course for unimmunized individuals 2 months of age or older consists of three doses of 0.5 mL each, 4 to 8 weeks apart, followed by a fourth (reinforcing) dose of 0.5 mL, 6 to 12 months after the third dose. The reinforcing dose is an integral part of the primary immunizing course.

If, after beginning combined immunization against diphtheria, tetanus, and pertussis, further doses of vaccine containing pertussis and diphtheria antigens become contraindicated, a single-component tetanus toxoid-containing vaccine may be substituted for each of the remaining doses.

Interruption of the recommended schedule with a delay between doses does not interfere with the final immunity achieved with Tetanus Toxoid Fluid. There is no need to start the series over again, regardless of the length of time elapsed between doses.[3]

Booster Doses: A single injection of 0.5 mL of Tetanus Toxoid Fluid is given 10 years after completion of primary immunization and every 10 years thereafter. If a dose is given sooner as part of wound management, the next booster is not needed for 10 years thereafter. MORE FREQUENT BOOSTER DOSES ARE NOT INDICATED AND MAY BE ASSOCIATED WITH INCREASED INCIDENCE AND SEVERITY OF REACTIONS.[3]

Tetanus Prophylaxis in Wound Management: The need for active immunization with a tetanus toxoid-containing preparation, with or without passive immunization with human Tetanus Immune Globulin (TIG) depends on both the condition of the wound and the patient's immunization history. Tetanus has rarely occurred among persons with a documented primary series of toxoid injections. A thorough attempt must be made to determine whether a patient has completed primary immunization.[3]

Individuals who have completed primary immunization against tetanus, and who sustain wounds which are minor and uncontaminated, should receive a booster dose of the appropriate tetanus toxoid-containing preparation (see **INDICATIONS AND USAGE**) only if they have not received tetanus toxoid within the preceding 10 years. For other wounds, a booster is appropriate if the patient has not received tetanus toxoid within the preceding 5 years. Antitoxin antibodies develop rapidly in persons who have previously received at least two doses of tetanus toxoid.[3]

Individuals who have not completed primary immunization against tetanus, or whose immunization history is unknown or uncertain, should be immunized with the appropriate tetanus toxoid-containing product (see **INDICATIONS AND USAGE**). Completion of primary immunization thereafter should be ensured. In addition, if these individuals have sustained a tetanus-prone wound, the use of human Tetanus Immune Globulin (TIG) is recommended. A separate syringe and site of administration should be used. When TIG is to be administered at the same visit as tetanus toxoid, an adsorbed tetanus toxoid-containing preparation should be used.[3]

Summary Guide to Tetanus Prophylaxis in Routine Wound Management[3*]

History of tetanus toxoid (doses)	Clean, minor wounds		All other wounds†	
	Td‡	TIG	Td‡	TIG
Unknown or <three	Yes	No	Yes	Yes
≥three§	No″	No	No£	No

* Important details are in the text.

† Such as, but not limited to, wounds contaminated with dirt, feces, soil, saliva, etc.; puncture wounds; avulsions; and wounds resulting from missiles, crushing, burns and frostbite.

‡ For children under 7 years old DTP (DT, if pertussis vaccine is contraindicated) is preferred to tetanus toxoid alone. For persons 7 years and older, Td is preferred to tetanus toxoid alone.

§ If only three doses of **fluid** toxoid have been received, a fourth dose of toxoid, preferably an adsorbed toxoid, should be given.

″ Yes, if more than 10 years since last dose.

£ Yes, if more than 5 years since last dose. (More frequent boosters are not needed and can accentuate side effects.)

In order to enhance diphtheria protection in the population, the ACIP recommends Tetanus and Diphtheria Toxoids For Adult Use as the preferred preparation for active tetanus immunization in wound management of patients 7 years of age or older.[3]

HOW SUPPLIED

NDC 0005-1942-33   7.5 mL vial

NDC 0005-1942-47   10×0.5 mL; LEDERJECT® disposable syringe. For directions on use of LEDERJECT disposable syringe, please see package insert accompanying product.

STORAGE

DO NOT FREEZE. STORE REFRIGERATED, AWAY FROM FREEZER COMPARTMENT, AT 2°C to 8°C (36°F to 46°F).

REFERENCES

1. Mueller JH, Miller PA: Factors influencing the production of tetanal toxin. *J Immunol* 1947;56:143–147.
2. Pillemer L, Grossberg DB, Wittler RG: The immunochemistry of toxins and toxoids. II. The preparation and immunological evaluation of purified tetanal toxoid. *J Immunol* 1946;54:213–224.
3. Recommendation of the Immunization Practices Advisory Committee (ACIP): Diphtheria, tetanus and pertussis: Guidelines for vaccine prophylaxis and other preventive measures. *MMWR* 1985;34:405–426.
4. Committee on Immunization, Council of Medical Societies, American College of Physicians: Guide for Adult Immunization, 1st Edition 1985; Philadelphia, PA.
5. Recommendation of the ACIP: Immunization of children infected with Human T-Lymphotrophic Virus Type III/Lymphadenopathy associated virus. *MMWR* 1986;35(38):595–606.
6. National Childhood Vaccine Injury Act: Requirements for permanent vaccination records and for reporting of selected events after vaccination. *MMWR* 1988;37(13):197–200.
7. Recommendations of the ACIP: General recommendations on immunization. *MMWR* 1983;32(1):1–17.
8. Macko MB, Powell CE: Comparison of the morbidity of tetanus toxoid boosters with tetanus-diphtheria toxoid boosters. *Ann Emerg Med* 1985;14(1):33–35.
9. Deacon SP, et al: A comparative clinical study of adsorbed tetanus vaccine and adult-type tetanus-diphtheria vaccine. *J Hyg (Cambridge)* 1982;89:513–519.
10. Jacobs RL, et al: Adverse reactions to tetanus toxoid *JAMA*, 1982; 247(1):40–42.
11. Rutledge SL, Snead OC: Neurological complications of immunizations. *J Pediatr* 1986;109:917–924.
12. Adverse Events Following Immunization. *MMWR* 1985;34(3):43–47.
13. Schlenska GK: Unusual neurological complications following tetanus toxoid administration. *J Neurol* 1977;215:299–302.
14. Blumstein GI, Kreithen H: Peripheral neuropathy following tetanus toxoid administration. *JAMA* 1966;198:1030–1031.
15. Reinstein L, Pargament JM, Goodman JS: Peripheral neuropathy after multiple tetanus toxoid injections. *Arch Phys Med Rehabil* 1982;63:332–334.
16. Tsairis P, Duck PJ, Mulder DW: Natural history of brachial plexus neuropathy. *Arch Neurol* 1972;27:109–117.
17. Quast U, Hennessen W, Widmark RM: Mono- and polyneuritis after tetanus vaccination. *Devel Bio Stand* 1979;43:25–32.
18. Holliday PL, Bauer RB: Polyradiculoneuritis secondary to immunization with tetanus and diphtheria toxoids. *Arch Neurol* 1983;40:56–57.
19. Fenichel GM: Neurological complications of tetanus toxoid. *Arch Neurol* 1983;40:390.
20. Pollard JD, Selby G: Relapsing neuropathy due to tetanus toxoid. *J Neurol Sci* 1978;37:113–125.
21. Newton N, Janati A: Guillain-Barre syndrome after vaccination with purified tetanus toxoid. *S Med J* 1987;80:1053–1054.

LEDERLE LABORATORIES DIVISION
American Cyanamid Company,
Pearl River, NY 10965

Rev. 5/88
23589

THIOTEPA   ℞

[*thī″o-tĕpa*]
Parenteral
Sterile
15 mg Vial

THIOTEPA *Lederle* **is a polyfunctional alkylating agent used in the chemotherapy of certain neoplastic diseases.**

DESCRIPTION

Thiotepa is an ethylenimine-type compound, 1,1′,1″-phosphinothioylidynetris-aziridine available in powder form in vials which contain a sterile mixture of 15 mg Thiotepa, 80 mg NaCl, and 50 mg NaHCO₃. Thiotepa has also been known as TESPA and TSPA and is not the same as TEPA. Thiotepa is stable in alkaline medium and unstable in acid medium. When reconstituted with Sterile Water for Injection, the resulting solution has a pH of approximately 7.6.

ACTION

Thiotepa is a cytotoxic agent of the polyfunctional alkylating type (more than one reactive ethylenimine group) related chemically and pharmacologically to nitrogen mustard. Its radiomimetic action is believed to occur through the release of ethylenimine radicals which, like irradiation, disrupt the bonds of DNA. One of the principal bond disruptions is initiated by alkylation of guanine at the N-7 position, which severs the linkage between the purine base and the sugar and liberates alkylated guanines.

On the basis of tissue concentration studies, it is reported that Thiotepa has no differential affinity for neoplasms. Most of the drug appears to be excreted unchanged in the urine.

INDICATIONS

Thiotepa has been tried with varying results in the palliation of a wide variety of neoplastic diseases. However, the most consistent results have been seen in the following tumors:

1. Adenocarcinoma of the breast.
2. Adenocarcinoma of the ovary.
3. For controlling intracavitary effusions secondary to diffuse or localized neoplastic disease of various serosal cavities.
4. For the treatment of superficial papillary carcinoma of the urinary bladder.

While now largely superseded by other treatments, Thiotepa has been effective against other lymphomas, such as lymphosarcoma and Hodgkin's disease.

CONTRAINDICATIONS

Therapy is probably contraindicated in cases of existing hepatic, renal, or bone marrow damage. However, if the need overweighs the risk in such patients, Thiotepa may be used in low dosage, and accompanied by hepatic, renal, and hemopoietic function tests.

Thiotepa is contraindicated in patients with a known hypersensitivity (allergy) to this preparation.

WARNINGS

The administration of Thiotepa to pregnant women is not recommended except in cases where the benefit to be gained outweighs the risk of teratogenicity involved.

Thiotepa is highly toxic to the hematopoietic system. A rapidly falling white blood cell or platelet count indicates the necessity for discontinuing or reducing the dosage of Thiotepa. Weekly blood and platelet counts are recommended during therapy and for at least three weeks after therapy has been discontinued.

Thiotepa is a polyfunctional alkylating agent, capable of cross-linking the DNA within a cell and changing its nature. The replication of the cell is, therefore, altered, and Thiotepa may be described as mutagenic. An *in vitro* study has shown that it causes chromosomal aberrations of the chromatid type and that the frequency of induced aberrations increases with the age of the subject.

Like all alkylating agents, Thiotepa is carcinogenic. Carcinogenicity is shown most clearly in mouse studies, but there is strong circumstantial evidence of carcinogenicity in man.

PRECAUTIONS

The serious complication of excessive Thiotepa therapy, or sensitivity to the effects of Thiotepa, is bone marrow depression. If proper precautions are not observed, Thiotepa may cause leukopenia, thrombocytopenia, and anemia. Death from septicemia and hemorrhage has occurred as a direct result of hematopoietic depression by Thiotepa.

It is not advisable to combine, simultaneously or sequentially, cancer chemotherapeutic agents or a cancer chemotherapeutic agent and a therapeutic modality having the same mechanism of action. Therefore, Thiotepa combined with other alkylating agents such as nitrogen mustard or cyclophosphamide or Thiotepa combined with irradiation would serve to intensify toxicity rather than to enhance therapeutic response. If these agents must follow each other, it is important that recovery from the first agent, as indicated by white blood cell count, be complete before therapy with the second agent is instituted.

The most reliable guide to Thiotepa toxicity is the white blood cell count. If this falls to 3000 or less, the dose should be discontinued. Another good index of Thiotepa toxicity is the platelet count; if this falls to 150,000, therapy should be discontinued. Red blood cell count is a less accurate indicator of Thiotepa toxicity.

Other drugs which are known to produce bone marrow depression should be avoided.

There is no known antidote for overdosage with Thiotepa. Transfusions of whole blood or platelets or leukocytes have proved beneficial to the patient in combating hematopoietic toxicity.

ADVERSE REACTIONS

Apart from its effect on the blood-forming elements, Thiotepa may cause other adverse reactions. These include pain at the site of injection, nausea, vomiting, anorexia, dizziness, headache, amenorrhea, and interference with spermatogenesis.

Febrile reaction and weeping from a subcutaneous lesion may occur as the result of breakdown of tumor tissue.

Allergic reactions are rare, but hives and skin rash have been noted occasionally. One case of alopecia has been reported. In addition, a patient who has received Thiotepa and other anticancer agents experienced prolonged apnea after succinylcholine was administered prior to surgery. It was theorized that this was caused by decrease of pseudocholinesterase activity caused by the anticancer drugs.

There have been rare reports of chemical cystitis or hemorrhagic cystitis following intravesical, but not parenteral administration of Thiotepa.

DOSAGE

Parenteral routes of administration are most reliable since absorption of Thiotepa from the gastrointestinal tract is variable.

Since Thiotepa is nonvesicant, intravenous doses may be given directly and rapidly without need for slow drip or large volumes of diluent. Some physicians prefer to give Thiotepa directly into the tumor mass. This may be effected transrectally, transvaginally, or intracerebrally. The technique is discussed in the appropriate section which follows. For the control of malignant effusions, Thiotepa is instilled directly into the cavity involved.

Dosage must be carefully individualized. A slow response to Thiotepa may be deceptive and may occasion unwarranted frequency of administration with subsequent signs of toxicity. After maximum benefit is obtained by initial therapy, it is necessary to continue patient on maintenance therapy (1 to 4 week intervals). In order to continue optimal effect, maintenance doses should be no more frequent than weekly in order to preserve correlation between dose and blood counts.

Initial and Maintenance Doses: Initially the higher dose in the given range is commonly administered. The maintenance dose should be adjusted weekly on the basis of pretreatment control blood counts and subsequent blood counts.

Intravenous Administration: Thiotepa may be given by rapid intravenous administration in doses of 0.3–0.4 mg/kg. Doses should be given at 1 to 4 week intervals.

For conversion of mg/kg of body weight to mg/M^2 of body surface or the reverse, a ratio of 1:30 is given as a guideline. The conversion factor varies between 1:20 and 1:40 depending on age and body build.

Intratumor Administration: Thiotepa in initial doses of 0.6–0.8 mg/kg may be injected directly into a tumor by means of a 22-gauge needle. A small amount of local anesthetic is injected first; then the syringe is removed and the Thiotepa solution is injected through the same needle. The drug is diluted in Sterile Water for Injection, 10 mg per 1 mL. Maintenance doses at one to four week intervals range from 0.07 mg/kg to 0.8 mg/kg depending on the condition of the patient.

Intracavitary Administration: The dosage recommended is 0.6–0.8 mg/kg. Administration is usually effected through the same tubing which is used to remove the fluid from the cavity involved.

Intravesical Administration: Patients with papillary carcinoma of the bladder are dehydrated for 8 to 12 hours prior to treatment. Then 60 mg of Thiotepa in 30–60 mL of Sterile Water for Injection is instilled into the bladder by catheter. For maximum effect, the solution should be retained for two hours. If the patient finds it impossible to retain 60 mL for two hours, the dose may be given in a volume of 30 mL. If desired, the patient may be positioned every 15 minutes for maximum area contact. The usual course of treatment is once a week for 4 weeks. The course may be repeated if necessary, but second and third courses must be given with caution since bone marrow depression may be increased. Deaths have occurred after intravesical administration, caused by bone marrow depression from systemically absorbed drug.

Preparation of Solution: The powder should be reconstituted preferably in Sterile Water for Injection. The amount of diluent most often used is 1.5 mL. resulting in a drug concentration of 5 mg in each 0.5 mL of solution. Larger volumes are usually employed for intracavitary use, intravenous drip, or perfusion therapy. The 1.5 mL reconstituted preparation may be added to larger volumes of other diluents: Sodium Chloride Injection USP, Dextrose Injection USP, Dextrose and Sodium Chloride Injection USP, Ringer's Injection USP, or Lactated Ringer's Injection USP. Reconstituted solutions should be clear to slightly opaque but solutions that are grossly opaque or precipitated should not be used.

Since the original powder form contains 15 mg Thiotepa, 80 mg NaCl, and 50 mg NaHCO₃, the addition of Sterile Water for Injection produces an isotonic solution. The addition of other diluents may result in hypertonic solutions, which may cause mild to moderate discomfort on injection.

For local use into single or multiple sites, Thiotepa may be mixed with procaine HCl 2%, epinephrine HCl 1:1000, or both.

Procedures for proper handling and disposal of anti-cancer drugs should be considered. Several guidelines on this subject have been published.[1–6] There is no general agreement that all of the procedures recommended in the guidelines are necessary or appropriate.

HOW SUPPLIED

15 mg vials, sterile, for parenteral use—NDC 0005-4650-91. Whether in its original powder form or in reconstituted solution, Thiotepa must be stored in the refrigertor at 2–8° C. (35–46° F.) Reconstituted solutions may be kept for 5 days in a refrigerator without substantial loss of potency.

MILITARY DEPOT:

15 mg vial
NSN 6505-01-047-3872

REFERENCES

1. Recommendations for the Safe Handling of Parenteral Antineoplastic Drugs. NIH Publication No. 83-2621. For sale by the Superintendent of Documents, U.S. Government Printing Office, Washington, D.C. 20402.
2. AMA Council Report. Guidelines for Handling Parenteral Antineoplastics. *JAMA*, March 15, 1985.
3. National Study Commission on Cytotoxic Exposure—Recommendations for Handling Cytotoxic Agents. Available from Louis P. Jeffrey, Sc. D., Director of Pharmacy Services, Rhode Island Hospital, 593 Eddy Street, Providence, Rhode Island 02902.
4. Clinical Oncological Society of Australia: Guidelines and recommendations for safe handling of antineoplastic agents. *Med J Australia* 1:426–428, 1983.
5. Jones, R.B., et al. Safe handling of chemotherapeutic agents: A report from the Mount Sinai Medical Center. *Ca—A Cancer Journal for Clinicians* Sept/Oct, 258–263, 1983.
6. American Society of Hospital Pharmacists technical assistance bulletin on handling cytotoxic drugs in hospitals. *Am J Hosp Pharm* 42:131–137, 1985.

LEDERLE LABORATORIES DIVISION
American Cyanamid Company
Pearl River, N.Y. 10965   Rev. 3/87
18452

Shown in Product Identification Section, page 415

TRI-IMMUNOL®   ℞
Diphtheria and Tetanus Toxoids and Pertussis Vaccine Adsorbed

DESCRIPTION

Diphtheria and Tetanus Toxoids and Pertussis Vaccine Adsorbed, (DTP), TRI-IMMUNOL, is a sterile combination of PUROGENATED® Diphtheria Toxoid aluminum phosphate-adsorbed, PUROGENATED Tetanus Toxoid aluminum phosphate-adsorbed, and Pertussis Vaccine for intramuscular use only. After shaking, the vaccine is a homogeneous white suspension.

The diphtheria and tetanus toxins are produced according to the method of Mueller and Miller[1,2] and are detoxified by use of formaldehyde. The toxoids are refined by the Pillemer alcohol fractionation method[3] and are diluted with a solution containing sodium phosphate monobasic, sodium phosphate dibasic, glycine, and thimerosal (mercury derivative) as a preservative. Pertussis Vaccine is prepared by growing Phase I *Bordetella pertussis* in a modified Cohen-Wheeler broth containing acid hydrolysate of casein. The *B pertussis* culture is harvested, inactivated, and then suspended in a solution containing potassium phosphate monobasic, sodium phosphate dibasic, aluminum phosphate, sodium chloride, and thimerosal as a preservative and is then combined with the refined Diphtheria and Tetanus Toxoids in physiological saline diluent containing thimerosal as a preservative. The final concentration of thimerosal (mercury derivative) in the combined vaccine is 1:10,000. The aluminum content of the final product does not exceed 0.80 mg per 0.5 mL dose.

Each 0.5 mL dose is formulated to contain 12.5 Lf of diphtheria toxoid, and 5 Lf of tetanus toxoid. The total human immunizing dose (the first three 0.5 mL doses given) contains an estimate of 12 units of pertussis vaccine. Each component of the vaccine—diphtheria, tetanus and pertussis—meets the required potency standards.

The primary immunization against diphtheria, tetanus, and pertussis consists of four 0.5 mL doses when administered as recommended.[4,5]

CLINICAL PHARMACOLOGY

Simultaneous immunization against diphtheria, tetanus, and pertussis during infancy and childhood has been a routine practice in the United States since the late 1940s. It has played a major role in markedly reducing the incidence of cases and deaths from each of these diseases.

Diphtheria is primarily a localized and generalized intoxication caused by diphtheria toxin, an extracellular protein metabolite of toxinogenic strains of *Corynebacterium diphtheriae*. While the incidence of diphtheria in the U.S. has decreased from over 200,000 cases reported in 1921, before the general use of diphtheria toxoid, to only 15 cases reported from 1980 to 1983,[4] the ratio of fatalities to attack rate has remained constant at about 5% to 10%. The highest case fatality rates are in the very young and in the elderly. Following adequate immunization with diphtheria toxoid, which induces antitoxin, it is thought that protection lasts for at least ten years.[4] This significantly reduces both the risk of developing diphtheria and the severity of clinical illness. It does not, however, eliminate carriage of *C diphtheria* in the pharynx or on the skin.[4]

Tetanus is an intoxication manifested primarily by neuromuscular dysfunction caused by a potent exotoxin elabo-

Continued on next page

Lederle—Cont.

rated by *Clostridium tetani*. The incidence of tetanus in the U.S. has dropped dramatically with the routine use of tetanus toxoid, remaining relatively constant over the last decade at about 90 cases reported annually. Spores of *C tetani* are ubiquitous, and there is essentially no natural immunity to tetanus toxin. Thus, universal primary immunization with tetanus toxoid with subsequent maintenance of adequate antitoxin levels, by means of timed boosters, is necessary to protect all age groups.[4] Tetanus toxoid is a highly effective antigen and a completed primary series generally induces protective levels of serum antitoxin that persist for at least 10 years.[4]

Pertussis is a disease of the respiratory tract caused by *B pertussis*. This Gram-negative coccobacillus produces a variety of active components including endotoxin and a number of other substances that have been defined primarily on the basis of their biological activity in animals, such as lymphocytosis, leukocytosis, sensitivity to histamine, changes in glucose and/or insulin levels, possible neurological effects and adjuvant activity.[6] The role of each of the different components in either the pathogenesis of, or immunity to, pertussis is not well understood.

Pertussis is a highly communicable disease which has an attack rate in unimmunized populations of over 90%.[4] Since pertussis vaccine has come into widespread use, the number of reported cases and associated mortality in the U.S. has declined from about 120,000 cases and 1,100 deaths in 1950,[7] to an annual average of about 2,000 cases and 10 fatalities over the last 10 years.[4] Accurate data do not exist, as bacteriological confirmation of pertussis can be obtained in less than half of the suspected cases. Most reported illnesses from *B pertussis* occur in infants and young children; two thirds of reported deaths occur in children less than one year old. Older children and adults, in whom classic signs are often absent, may go undiagnosed and serve as reservoirs of disease.[4]

Evidence of the efficacy of pertussis vaccine can be provided by the recent British experience, where a reduction in the number of immunized individuals from 79% in 1973, to 31% in 1978 resulted in an epidemic of 102,500 pertussis cases and 36 deaths between late 1977 and 1980, and 1,440 cases per week reported during the winter of 1981 to 1982. A similar situation occurred in Japan.[7]

Because the severity of pertussis decreases with age, and the vaccine may cause side effects and adverse reactions, routine pertussis immunization is not recommended for persons 7 years of age or older.[4]

INDICATIONS AND USAGE

Diphtheria and Tetanus Toxoids and Pertussis Vaccine Adsorbed TRI-IMMUNOL is indicated for active immunization of infants and children from 2 months of age up to their seventh birthday against diphtheria, tetanus, and pertussis.[4,5] Children who have recovered from culture-confirmed pertussis need not receive further doses of a vaccine containing pertussis.[4]

CONTRAINDICATIONS

HYPERSENSITIVITY TO ANY COMPONENT OF THE VACCINE, INCLUDING THIMEROSAL, A MERCURY DERIVATIVE, IS A CONTRAINDICATION.

IMMUNIZATION SHOULD BE DEFERRED DURING THE COURSE OF ANY FEBRILE ILLNESS OR ACUTE INFECTION. A MINOR AFEBRILE ILLNESS SUCH AS A MILD UPPER RESPIRATORY INFECTION IS NOT USUALLY REASON TO DEFER IMMUNIZATION.[4,5]

THE OCCURRENCE OF ANY TYPE OF NEUROLOGICAL SYMPTOMS OR SIGNS, INCLUDING ONE OR MORE CONVULSIONS (SEIZURES) FOLLOWING ADMINISTRATION OF THIS PRODUCT IS A CONTRAINDICATION TO FURTHER USE. USE OF THIS PRODUCT IS ALSO CONTRAINDICATED IF THE CHILD HAS A PERSONAL HISTORY OF SEIZURES (SEE FOLLOWING DISCUSSION FOR INFORMATION REGARDING CHILDREN WITH A FAMILY HISTORY OF SEIZURES). THE PRESENCE OF ANY EVOLVING OR CHANGING DISORDER AFFECTING THE CENTRAL NERVOUS SYSTEM IS A CONTRAINDICATION TO ADMINISTRATION OF DTP REGARDLESS OF WHETHER THE SUSPECTED NEUROLOGICAL DISORDER IS ASSOCIATED WITH OCCURRENCE OF SEIZURE ACTIVITY OF ANY TYPE.

STUDIES HAVE INDICATED THAT A PERSONAL OR FAMILY HISTORY OF SEIZURES IS ASSOCIATED WITH INCREASED FREQUENCY OF SEIZURES FOLLOWING PERTUSSIS IMMUNIZATION.[8,9,10]

Personal History: THE IMMUNIZATION PRACTICES ADVISORY COMMITTEE (ACIP) OF THE U.S. PUBLIC HEALTH SERVICE STATES: "THE PRESENCE OF A NEUROLOGIC CONDITION CHARACTERIZED BY CHANGING DEVELOPMENTAL OR NEUROLOGIC FINDINGS, REGARDLESS OF WHETHER A DEFINITIVE DIAGNOSIS HAS BEEN MADE, IS ... CONSIDERED A CONTRAINDICATION TO RECEIPT OF PERTUSSIS VAC-

CINE, BECAUSE ADMINISTRATION OF DTP MAY COINCIDE WITH OR POSSIBLY EVEN AGGRAVATE MANIFESTATIONS OF THE DISEASE. SUCH DISORDERS INCLUDE UNCONTROLLED EPILEPSY, INFANTILE SPASMS, AND PROGRESSIVE ENCEPHALOPATHY."[4]

THE IMMUNIZATION PRACTICES ADVISORY COMMITTEE (ACIP) AND THE AMERICAN ACADEMY OF PEDIATRICS (AAP) RECOGNIZE CERTAIN CIRCUMSTANCES IN WHICH CHILDREN WITH STABLE CENTRAL NERVOUS SYSTEM DISORDERS, INCLUDING WELL-CONTROLLED SEIZURES OR SATISFACTORILY EXPLAINED SINGLE SEIZURES, MAY RECEIVE PERTUSSIS VACCINE. THE DECISION TO ADMINISTER VACCINE TO SUCH CHILDREN MUST BE MADE BY THE PHYSICIAN ON AN INDIVIDUAL BASIS, WITH CONSIDERATION OF ALL RELEVANT FACTORS, TO ALLOW AN ACCURATE ASSESSMENT OF RISKS AND BENEFITS FOR THAT INDIVIDUAL. THE PHYSICIAN SHOULD REVIEW THE FULL TEXT OF THE ACIP AND AAP GUIDELINES PRIOR TO CONSIDERING VACCINATION FOR SUCH CHILDREN.[4,5,8] THE PARENT OR GUARDIAN SHOULD BE ADVISED OF THE INCREASED RISK INVOLVED.

Family History: *THE ACIP AND AAP DO NOT CONSIDER A FAMILY HISTORY OF SEIZURES TO BE A CONTRAINDICATION TO PERTUSSIS VACCINE.[4,5] DESPITE THE INCREASED RISK OF SEIZURES IN THESE INDIVIDUALS. THE DECISION TO ADMINISTER VACCINE TO SUCH CHILDREN MUST BE MADE BY THE PHYSICIAN ON AN INDIVIDUAL BASIS, WITH CONSIDERATION OF ALL RELEVANT FACTORS, TO ALLOW AN ACCURATE ASSESSMENT OF RISKS AND BENEFITS FOR THAT INDIVIDUAL. THE PARENT OR GUARDIAN SHOULD BE ADVISED OF THE INCREASED RISK INVOLVED.*

THE ACIP STATES: "THERE ARE NO DATA ON WHETHER THE PROPHYLACTIC USE OF ANTIPYRETICS CAN DECREASE THE RISK OF FEBRILE CONVULSIONS. HOWEVER, PRELIMINARY DATA SUGGEST THAT ACETAMINOPHEN... WILL REDUCE THE INCIDENCE OF POSTVACCINATION FEVER. THUS, IT IS REASONABLE TO CONSIDER ADMINISTERING... ACETAMINOPHEN AT AGE-APPROPRIATE DOSES AT THE TIME OF VACCINATION AND EVERY 4 TO 6 HOURS FOR 48 TO 72 HOURS TO CHILDREN AT HIGHER RISK FOR SEIZURES THAN THE GENERAL POPULATION."[8]

Adverse Events Following Previous Immunization: THE ACIP AND AAP CONSIDER THE OCCURRENCE OF ANY OF THE FOLLOWING EVENTS AFTER VACCINATION WITH PERTUSSIS-CONTAINING VACCINE TO BE AN ABSOLUTE CONTRAINDICATION TO FURTHER PERTUSSIS VACCINATION:

1. ALLERGIC HYPERSENSITIVITY TO ANY COMPONENT OF THE VACCINE
2. FEVER OF 40.5°C (105°F) OR GREATER WITHIN 48 HOURS
3. COLLAPSE OR SHOCK-LIKE STATE (HYPOTONIC-HYPORESPONSIVE EPISODE) WITHIN 48 HOURS
4. PERSISTING, INCONSOLABLE CRYING LASTING THREE HOURS OR MORE, OR AN UNUSUAL HIGH-PITCHED CRY OCCURRING WITHIN 48 HOURS
5. CONVULSION(S) WITH OR WITHOUT FEVER OCCURRING WITHIN THREE DAYS. (For convulsions occurring beyond three days, see discussion in **CONTRAINDICATIONS** section and in references 4 and 5 concerning children with a personal history of convulsions.)
6. ENCEPHALOPATHY OCCURRING WITHIN SEVEN DAYS; THIS INCLUDES SEVERE ALTERATIONS IN CONSCIOUSNESS WITH GENERALIZED OR FOCAL NEUROLOGIC SIGNS.[4,5]

The clinical judgment of the attending physician should prevail at all times.

Routine immunization should be deferred during an outbreak of poliomyelitis, providing the patient has not sustained an injury that increases the risk of tetanus and providing an outbreak of diphtheria or pertussis does not occur simultaneously.

WARNINGS

THIS PRODUCT IS NOT RECOMMENDED FOR IMMUNIZING PERSONS ON OR AFTER THEIR SEVENTH BIRTHDAY. DO NOT ATTEMPT IMMUNIZATION IF THE CHILD HAS OR IS SUSPECTED TO HAVE AN EVOLVING NEUROLOGICAL DISORDER. STUDIES HAVE INDICATED THAT A PERSONAL OR FAMILY HISTORY OF SEIZURES IS ASSOCIATED WITH INCREASED FREQUENCY OF SEIZURES FOLLOWING PERTUSSIS IMMUNIZATION.[8,9,10] (SEE DISCUSSION IN **CONTRAINDICATIONS** SECTION.)

SHOULD ANY SYMPTOMATOLOGY RELATED TO NEUROLOGICAL DISORDERS DEVELOP FOLLOWING ADMINISTRATION, DO NOT ATTEMPT FURTHER ADMINISTRATION OF PERTUSSIS VACCINE. THE OCCURRENCE OF ENCEPHALOPATHY (INCLUDING SEVERE ALTERATIONS IN CONSCIOUSNESS WITH GENERALIZED OR FOCAL NEUROLOGICAL SIGNS), CONVUL-

SION, PERSISTING INCONSOLABLE CRYING FOR THREE OR MORE HOURS DURATION, AN UNUSUAL HIGH-PITCHED CRY, COLLAPSE OR SHOCK-LIKE STATE, FEVER OF 40.5°C (105°F) OR GREATER, AND ALLERGIC REACTIONS AFTER ADMINISTRATION ARE CONTRAINDICATIONS FOR ANY FURTHER USE OF PERTUSSIS-CONTAINING VACCINE. (SEE **CONTRAINDICATIONS** SECTION.)

If a contraindication to pertussis is found, the infant or child should be given Diphtheria and Tetanus Toxoids, Adsorbed, for pediatric use (DT) instead of DTP.

Unimmunized children less than 1 year of age should receive three doses of DT at 4 to 8 week intervals, followed by a fourth dose 6 to 12 months after the third dose, for the primary series. **Unimmunized children 1 year of age or older** should receive two doses of DT 4 to 8 weeks apart, followed by a third dose 6 to 12 months after the second dose for the primary series. If, after beginning a DTP series, further doses of vaccine containing pertussis antigen become contraindicated, DT should be substituted for each of the remaining doses.[4,5]

PARTIAL DOSES OF DTP VACCINE SHOULD NOT BE GIVEN.[4,5] Neither the efficacy of such practice in reducing the frequency of associated serious adverse events, nor the resulting protection against disease has been determined. The occurrence of sudden-infant-death syndrome (SIDS) has been reported following administration of DTP.[11,12,13] However, a large case-control study in the U.S. revealed no causal relationship between receipt of DTP vaccine and SIDS.[14] Onset of infantile spasms has occurred in infants who have recently received DTP or DT. Analysis of data from the National Childhood Encephalopathy Study on children with infantile spasms showed that receipt of DTP or DT was not causally related to infantile spasms.[15] The incidence of onset of infantile spasms increases at 3–9 months of age, the time period in which the second and third doses of DTP are generally given. Therefore, some cases of infantile spasms can be expected to be related by chance alone to recent receipt of DTP.[4]

DTP should not be given to infants or children with thrombocytopenia or any coagulation disorder that would contraindicate intramuscular injection unless the potential benefit clearly outweighs the risk of administration.

Patients with impaired immune responsiveness, whether due to the use of immunosuppressive therapy (including irradiation, corticosteroids, antimetabolites, alkylating agents, and cytotoxic agents), a genetic defect, human immunodeficiency virus (HIV) infection, or other causes may have a reduced antibody response to active immunization procedures.[4,5,16] Deferral of administration of vaccine may be considered in individuals receiving immunosuppressive therapy.[4,5] Other groups should receive this vaccine according to the usual recommended schedule.[4,5,16,17]

Special care should be taken to prevent injection into a blood vessel.

PRECAUTIONS

General

1. THIS PRODUCT SHOULD BE USED FOR THE AGE GROUP BETWEEN 2 MONTHS AND THE 7TH BIRTHDAY.
2. PRIOR TO ADMINISTRATION OF ANY DOSE OF DTP, THE PARENT OR GUARDIAN SHOULD BE ASKED ABOUT THE PERSONAL AND FAMILY HISTORY AND THE RECENT HEALTH STATUS OF THE INFANT OR CHILD TO BE IMMUNIZED IN ORDER TO DETERMINE THE EXISTENCE OF ANY CONTRAINDICATION TO IMMUNIZATION WITH DTP AND TO ALLOW AN ACCURATE ASSESSMENT OF BENEFITS AND RISKS. (SEE **CONTRAINDICATIONS; WARNINGS.**)
3. WHEN AN INFANT OR CHILD RETURNS FOR THE NEXT DOSE IN THE SERIES, THE PARENT OR GUARDIAN SHOULD BE QUESTIONED CONCERNING OCCURRENCE OF ANY SYMPTOM AND/OR SIGNS OF AN ADVERSE REACTION AFTER THE PREVIOUS DOSE (SEE **CONTRAINDICATIONS, ADVERSE REACTIONS.**)
4. BEFORE THE INJECTION OF ANY BIOLOGICAL, THE PHYSICIAN SHOULD TAKE ALL PRECAUTIONS KNOWN FOR PREVENTION OF ALLERGIC OR ANY OTHER SIDE REACTIONS. This should include: a review of the patient's history regarding possible sensitivity; the ready availability of epinephrine 1:1,000 and other appropriate agents used for control of immediate allergic reactions; and a knowledge of the recent literature pertaining to use of the biological concerned, including the nature of side effects and adverse reactions that may follow its use.
5. *Since this product contains both a bacterial suspension and an adjuvant, shake vigorously before withdrawing each dose from multiple dose vials.*
6. A separate sterile syringe and needle or a sterile disposable unit should be used for each individual patient to prevent transmission of hepatitis or other infectious agents from one person to another.

7. NATIONAL CHILDHOOD VACCINE INJURY ACT OF 1986 (AS AMENDED IN 1987). This Act requires that the manufacturer and lot number of the vaccine administered be recorded by the health care provider in the vaccine recipient's permanent medical record, along with the date of administration of the vaccine and the name, address and title of the person administering the vaccine.

The Act further requires the health care provider to report to a health department or to the FDA the occurrence following immunization of any event set forth in the Vaccine Injury Table including: anaphylaxis or anaphylactic shock within 24 hours, encephalopathy or encephalitis within 7 days, shock-collapse or hypotonic-hyporesponsive collapse within 7 days, residual seizure disorder, any acute complication or sequelae (including death) of above events, or any event that would contraindicate further doses of vaccine, according to this package insert.[18]

Information for Patient: PRIOR TO ADMINISTRATION OF THIS VACCINE, HEALTH CARE PERSONNEL SHOULD INFORM THE PARENT, GUARDIAN, OR OTHER RESPONSIBLE ADULT OF THE BENEFITS AND RISKS TO THE CHILD OF DTP VACCINE, GUIDANCE SHOULD BE PROVIDED ON MEASURES TO BE TAKEN SHOULD ADVERSE EVENTS OCCUR, EG, ANTIPYRETIC MEASURES FOR ELEVATED TEMPERATURES.

ADVERSE REACTIONS

Local reactions are common after administration of DTP, occurring in 35% to 50% of recipients[19] and are manifested by varying degrees of erythema, induration and tenderness which may occasionally be severe. Such local reactions are usually self-limited and require no therapy. A nodule may be palpable at the injection site for a few weeks. Sterile abscess formation,[20] or subcutaneous atrophy at the site of injection has been reported. Cervical lymphadenopathy has been reported following DTP injections into the arm.[21]

Temperature elevations, fretfulness, drowsiness, vomiting, and anorexia frequently follow DTP administration.[19,22,23] Approximately 50% of DTP recipients will develop temperature elevations > 38°C (100.4°F) after one or more doses of the series; approximately 6% > 39°C (102.2°F);[20] and approximately 0.3% ≥ 40.5°C (105°F).[4] Some data suggest that febrile reactions are more likely to occur in those who have experienced such responses after prior doses.[22]

SIGNIFICANT REACTIONS ATTRIBUTED TO THE PERTUSSIS VACCINE COMPONENT HAVE BEEN: HIGH FEVER OF 40.5°C (105°F), A TRANSIENT SHOCK-LIKE EPISODE, EXCESSIVE SCREAMING (PERSISTING CRYING OR SCREAMING FOR THREE OR MORE HOURS DURATION), AN UNUSUAL HIGH-PITCHED CRY AND CONVULSIONS.

ENCEPHALOPATHY HAS BEEN REPORTED FOLLOWING PERTUSSIS VACCINATION; ONE STUDY SUGGESTS THE INCIDENCE OF ENCEPHALOPATHY OCCURRING WITHIN SEVEN DAYS OF VACCINATION MAY BE 1 PER 140,000 DOSES, WITH ENCEPHALOPATHY RESULTING IN DEATH OR PERMANENT DAMAGE TO THE CENTRAL NERVOUS SYSTEM ESTIMATED TO OCCUR IN 1 PER 330,000 DOSES.[24] (SEE CONTRAINDICATIONS AND WARNINGS.)

THE INCIDENCE OF CONVULSION OR TRANSIENT SHOCK-LIKE EPISODE OCCURRING WITHIN 48 HOURS OF VACCINATION HAS BEEN ESTIMATED TO BE 1 PER 1,750 DOSES.[19]

BULGING FONTANEL[25,26,27] HAS BEEN REPORTED AFTER DTP IMMUNIZATION, ALTHOUGH NO CAUSE AND EFFECT RELATIONSHIP HAS BEEN ESTABLISHED.

CARDIAC EFFECTS[28,29,30] AND RESPIRATORY DIFFICULTIES, INCLUDING APNEA HAVE BEEN REPORTED RARELY.

PERTUSSIS VACCINE HAS BEEN ASSOCIATED WITH A GREATER PROPORTION OF ADVERSE REACTIONS THAN MANY OTHER CHILDHOOD IMMUNIZATIONS.[31] SHOULD SYMPTOMATOLOGY REFERABLE TO THE CENTRAL NERVOUS SYSTEM DEVELOP WITHIN SEVEN DAYS FOLLOWING ADMINISTRATION, FURTHER IMMUNIZATION WITH THIS PRODUCT IS CONTRAINDICATED. (SEE CONTRAINDICATIONS.) NEUROLOGICAL COMPLICATIONS,[32] SUCH AS CONVULSIONS,[19,31] ENCEPHALOPATHY,[24,33] AND VARIOUS MONO- AND POLYNEUROPATHIES,[32–39] INCLUDING GUILLAIN-BARRE SYNDROME,[40,41] HAVE BEEN REPORTED FOLLOWING ADMINISTRATION OF PREPARATIONS CONTAINING DIPHTHERIA, TETANUS AND/OR PERTUSSIS ANTIGENS.

URTICARIA, ERYTHEMA MULTIFORME OR OTHER RASH, ARTHRALGIAS[31] AND RARELY, A SEVERE ANAPHYLACTIC REACTION (IE, URTICARIA WITH SWELLING OF THE MOUTH, DIFFICULTY BREATHING, HYPOTENSION OR SHOCK) HAVE BEEN REPORTED FOLLOWING ADMINISTRATION OF PREPARATIONS CONTAINING DIPHTHERIA, TETANUS, AND/OR PERTUSSIS ANTIGENS.

DOSAGE AND ADMINISTRATION

For Intramuscular Use Only: *Shake vigorously before withdrawing each dose from the multiple dose vials.*

Parenteral drug products should be inspected visually for particulate matter and discoloration prior to administration. (See **DESCRIPTION**.)

The vaccine should be injected intramuscularly, preferably into the midlateral muscles of the thigh or deltoid, with care to avoid major peripheral nerve trunks.

Before injection, the skin at the injection site should be cleansed and prepared with a suitable germicide.

After insertion of the needle, aspirate to help avoid inadvertent injection into a blood vessel.

The primary immunizing course for infants and children from 2 months of age up to their seventh birthday consists of three doses of 0.5 mL each at 4 to 8 week intervals, followed by a fourth dose of 0.5 mL 6 to 12 months after the third dose.[4,5]

If a contraindication to the pertussis component occurs, Diphtheria and Tetanus Toxoids, Adsorbed for pediatric use (DT) should be substituted for the remaining doses, according to the schedule discussed under **WARNINGS**.

The simultaneous administration of DTP, oral poliovirus vaccine (OPV), and/or measles-mumps-rubella vaccine (MMR) has resulted in seroconversion rates and rates of side effects similar to those observed when the vaccines are administered separately.[34] Therefore, if there is any doubt that a vaccine recipient will return for further vaccine doses, the ACIP and AAP recommend that these three vaccines may be given simultaneously (at separate sites) if appropriate for the age and previous vaccination status of the recipient.[5,42]

Premature infants may be immunized with DTP at the usual chronological age.[5]

Interruption of the recommended schedule with a delay between doses does not interfere with the final immunity achieved; nor does it necessitate starting the series over again, regardless of the length of time elapsed between doses.[4,5]

A booster dose of 0.5 mL is indicated at age 4 to 6 years, preferably prior to entrance into kindergarten or elementary school. (Substitute DT when contraindication to pertussis-containing vaccine exists.) (See **CONTRAINDICATIONS** and **WARNINGS** sections.) However, if the fourth dose of the basic immunizing series was administered after the fourth birthday a booster prior to school entry is not considered necessary.[4]

For either primary or booster immunization against tetanus and diphtheria of individuals 7 years of age and older, the use of Tetanus and Diphtheria Toxoids Adsorbed For Adult Use is recommended.[4,5]

HOW SUPPLIED

NDC 0005-1948-33   7.5 mL vial

STORAGE

DO NOT FREEZE. STORE REFRIGERATED, AWAY FROM FREEZER COMPARTMENT, AT 2°C TO 8°C (36°F TO 46°F).

REFERENCES

1. Mueller JH, Miller PA: Production of diphtheria toxin of high potency (100Lf) on a reproducible medium. *J Immunol* 1941;40:21–32.
2. Mueller JH, Miller PA: Factors influencing the production of tetanal toxin. *J Immunol* 1947;56:143–147.
3. Pillemer L, Grossberg DB, Wittler RG: The immunochemistry of toxins and toxoids. II. The preparation and immunological evaluation of purified tetanal toxoid. *J Immunol* 1946;54:213–224.
4. Diphtheria, tetanus and pertussis: Guidelines for vaccine prophylaxis and other preventive measures—recommendation of the Immunization Practices Advisory Committee (ACIP), *MMWR* 1985;34(27):405–426.
5. American Academy of Pediatrics: Report of the Committee on Infectious Diseases, ed 20. Elk Grove Village, IL, American Academy of Pediatrics, 1986.
6. Manclark CR, Cowell JL: Pertussis Vaccine, in Germanier R. (ed): Bacterial Vaccines. New York, Academic Press Inc., 1984;69–106.
7. Reported incidence of notifiable diseases in the United States. *MMWR* 1970;19(53):44.
8. Pertussis immunization: family history of convulsions and use of antipyretics—supplementary ACIP statement. *MMWR* 1987;36(18):281–282.
9. Stetler HC, et al: History of convulsions and use of pertussis vaccine. *J Pediatr* 1985;107(2):175–179.
10. Hirtz DG, et al: Seizures following childhood immunizations. *J Pediatr* 1983;102(1):14–18.
11. Bernier R, et al: Diphtheria-tetanus toxoids, pertussis vaccination and sudden infant deaths in Tennessee. *J Pediatr* 1982;101:419–421.
12. Baraff L, et al: Possible temporal association between diphtheria-tetanus toxoid, pertussis vaccination and sudden infant death syndrome. *Pediatr Inf Dis* 1983;2:7–11.
13. Walker AM, et al: Diphtheria-tetanus-pertussis immunization and sudden infant death syndrome. *AJPH* 1987;77(8):945–951.
14. Hoffman HJ, et al: Diphtheria-tetanus-pertussis immunization and sudden infant death; results of the National Institute of Child Health and Human Development cooperative study of sudden infant death syndrome risk factors. *Pediatrics* 1987;79(4):598–611.
15. Bellman MH, et al: Infantile spasms and pertussis immunization. *Lancet* 1983;1:1031–1034.
16. Recommendation of the ACIP: Immunization of children infected with Human T-Lymphotrophic Virus Type III/Lymphadenopathy-associated virus. *MMWR* 1986;35(38):595–606.
17. Immunization of children infected with Human Immunodeficiency Virus—Supplementary ACIP statement. *MMWR* 1988;37(12):181–183.
18. National Childhood Vaccine Injury Act: Requirements for permanent vaccination records and for reporting of selected events after vaccination. *MMWR* 1988; 37(13):197–200.
19. Cody C, et al: Nature and rates of adverse reactions associated with DTP and DT immunizations in infants and children. *Pediatrics* 1981;68:650–660.
20. Bernier R, et al: Abscesses complicating DTP vaccination. *Am J Dis Child* 1981;135:826–828.
21. Omokoku B, Castells S: Post-DPT inoculation-caused lymphadenitis in children. *NY State J Med* 1981;81:1667–1668.
22. Baraff L, et al: DTP-associated reactions: An analysis by injection site, manufacturer, prior reactions and dose. *Pediatrics* 1984;73:31–36.
23. Barkin R, Pichichero M: Diphtheria-pertussis-tetanus vaccine: Reactogenicity of commercial products. *Pediatrics* 1979;63:256–260.
24. Miller DL, et al: Pertussis vaccine and whooping cough as risk factors in acute neurological illness and death in young children. *Dev Biol Stand* 1985;61:389–394.
25. Mathur et al: Bulging fontanel following triple vaccine (letter). *Indian Pediatrics* 1981;18(6):417–418.
26. Shendurnikar et al: Bulging fontanel following DTP vaccine (letter). *Indian Pediatrics* 1986;23(11):960.
27. Jacob et al: Increased intracranial pressure after diphtheria, tetanus, and pertussis immunization. *Am J Dis Child* 1979;133:217–218.
28. Leung A: Congenital heart disease and DTP vaccination. *Can Med Assoc J* 1984;131:541.
29. Park JM, et al: Paroxysmal supraventricular tachycardia precipitated by pertussis vaccine. *Pediatrics* 1983;102(6):883–885.
30. Amsel SG, et al: Myocarditis after triple immunization. *Arch Dis Child* 1986;61:403–404.
31. Adverse events following immunization. *MMWR* 1985;34:43–47.
32. Rutledge SL, Snead OC: Neurologic complications of immunizations. *J Pediatr* 1986;109:917–924.
33. Schlenska GK: Unusual neurological complications following tetanus toxoid administration. *J Neurol* 1977;215:299–302.
34. Blumstein GI, Kreithen H: Peripheral neuropathy following tetanus toxoid administration. *JAMA* 1966;198:1030–1031.
35. Reinstein L, Pargament JM, Goodman JS: Peripheral neuropathy after multiple tetanus toxoid injections. *Arch Phys Med Rehabil* 1982;63:332–334.
36. Tsairis P, Duck PJ, Mulder DW: Natural history of brachial plexus neuropathy. *Arch Neurol* 1972;27:109–117.
37. Quast U, Hennessen W, Widmark RM: Mono- and polyneuritis after tetanus vaccination. *Devel Bio Stand* 1979;43:25–32.
38. Holliday PL, Bauer RB: Polyradiculoneuritis secondary to immunization with tetanus and diphtheria toxoids. *Arch Neurol* 1983;40:56–67.
39. Fenichel GM: Neurological complications of tetanus toxoid. *Arch Neurol* 1983;40:390.
40. Pollard JD, Selby G: Relapsing neuropathy due to tetanus toxoid. *J Neurol Sci* 1978;37:113–125.
41. Newton N, Janati A: Guillain-Barre syndrome after vaccination with purified tetanus toxoid. *S Med J* 1987;80:1053–1054.

Continued on next page

Lederle—Cont.

42. Recommendation of the ACIP: New recommended schedule for active immunization of normal infants and children. *MMWR* 1986;35(37):577–579.

LEDERLE LABORATORIES DIVISION
American Cyanamid Company,
Pearl River, NY 10965

Rev. 5/88
23587

ZINCON® Pyrithione Zinc 1%
[*zink 'on*]
Dandruff Shampoo

(See PDR For Nonprescription Drugs)

EDUCATIONAL MATERIAL

Films
Product: ASENDIN® *amoxapine*
Film Titles
Antidepressant Therapy—Why Aren't We Content?
Raymond Anton, MD—Major Depressive Disorders With Psychotic Features
Product: LOXITANE® *loxapine*
Film Titles
New Techniques in the Diagnosis and Treatment Evaluation of Schizophrenia
Neuroleptic Side Effects: Medicolegal Aspects
Today's Clinical Perceptions of a Chemically Distinct Neuroleptic Rapid Rehabilitation of the Schizophrenic Patient
Free Samples available for ASENDIN and LOXITANE.
Call: 800-L-E-D-E-R-L-E—between the hours of 8:30 am and 4:30 pm

Brochures
Product: FiberCon® Bulk-Forming Fiber Laxative
Patient Information Brochure
For consumer information on *Digestive Regularity*, write to:
Lederle Promotional Center
Bradley Corporate Park
2200 Bradley Hill Road
Blauvelt, NY 10913

Slide Lecture Kits
Product: MAXZIDE® *75 triamterene/50 mg hydrochlorothiazide*
Practical Considerations in Hypertension
Electrolytes in Cardiovascular Disease: Focus on Magnesium
Free Samples available for MAXZIDE
Call: 800-L-E-D-E-R-L-E—between the hours of 8:30 am and 4:30 pm

---

Leeming Division
Pfizer, Inc.
100 JEFFERSON ROAD
PARSIPPANY, NJ 07054

BEN–GAY® **EXTERNAL**
[*ben-gā'*]
ANALGESIC PRODUCTS

(See PDR For Nonprescription Drugs)

BONINE®
(Meclizine hydrochloride)
Chewable Tablets

ACTIONS
BONINE is an antihistamine which shows marked protective activity against nebulized histamine and lethal doses of intravenously injected histamine in guinea pigs. It has a marked effect in blocking the vasodepressor response to histamine, but only a slight blocking action against acetylcholine. Its activity is relatively weak in inhibiting the spasmogenic action of histamine on isolated guinea pig ileum.

INDICATIONS
BONINE is effective in the management of nausea, vomiting and dizziness associated with motion sickness.

CONTRAINDICATIONS
Asthma, glaucoma, emphysema, chronic pulmonary disease, shortness of breath, difficulty in breathing, or difficulty in urination due to enlargement of the prostate gland unless directed by a doctor.

WARNINGS
May cause drowsiness; alcohol, sedatives and tranquilizers may increase the drowsiness effect. Avoid alcoholic beverages while taking this product. Do not take this product if you are taking sedatives or tranquilizers without first con-

sulting your doctor. Do not drive or operate dangerous machinery while taking this medication.
Usage in Children:
Clinical studies establishing safety and effectiveness in children have not been done; therefore, usage is not recommended in children under 12 years of age.
Usage in Pregnancy:
As with any drug, if you are pregnant or nursing a baby, seek advice of a health care professional before taking this product.

ADVERSE REACTIONS
Drowsiness, dry mouth, and on rare occasions, blurred vision have been reported.

DOSAGE AND ADMINISTRATION
For motion sickness 1 or 2 tablets of BONINE should be taken one hour prior to embarkation. Thereafter, the dose may be repeated every 24 hours for the duration of the journey.

HOW SUPPLIED
BONINE (meclizine HCl) is available in convenient packets of 8 chewable tablets of 25 mg. meclizine HCl.

INACTIVE INGREDIENTS
Cornstarch, FD&C Red #40, Lactose, Magnesium Stearate, Purified Siliceous Earth, Raspberry Flavor, Sodium Saccharin, Talc.

DESITIN® **OINTMENT**
[*des "i-tin '*]

(See PDR For Nonprescription Drugs)

RHEABAN® Maximum Strength
TABLETS
[*rē 'ăban*]
(attapulgite)

(See PDR For Nonprescription Drugs)

RID® Spray
Lice Control Spray

PRODUCT OVERVIEW
KEY FACTS
Rid Lice Control Spray is a pediculicide spray for controlling lice and louse eggs on inanimate objects, to help prevent reinfestation. It contains a highly active synthetic pyrethroid that kills lice and their eggs on inanimate objects.

MAJOR USES
Rid Lice Control Spray effectively kills lice and louse eggs on garments, bedding, furniture and other inanimate objects that cannot be either laundered or dry cleaned.

SAFETY INFORMATION
Rid Lice Control Spray is intended for use on inanimate objects only; it is not for use on humans or animals. It is harmful if swallowed. It should not be sprayed in the eyes or on the skin and should not be inhaled. The product should be used only in well ventilated areas; room(s) should be vacated after treatment and ventilated before reoccupying.

PRESCRIBING INFORMATION
RID® Spray
Lice Control Spray

THIS PRODUCT IS NOT FOR USE ON HUMANS OR ANIMALS

ACTIVE INGREDIENT
(5-Benzyl-3-Furyl) methyl 2, 2-dimethyl-3-(2-methylpropenyl) cyclopropanecarboxylate

	0.500%
Related Compounds	0.068%
Aromatic petroleum hydrocarbons	0.664%
Inert Ingredients	98.768%
	100.000%

ACTIONS
A highly active synthetic pyrethroid for the control of lice and louse eggs on garments, bedding, furniture and other inanimate objects.

WARNINGS
Avoid contamination of feed and foodstuffs. Cover or remove fishbowls. HARMFUL IF SWALLOWED. This product is not for use on humans or animals. If lice infestations should occur on humans, consult either your physician or pharmacist for a product for use on humans.

PHYSICAL AND CHEMICAL HAZARDS
Contents under pressure. Do not use or store near heat or open flame. Do not puncture or incinerate container. Exposure to temperatures above 130° F may cause bursting.

CAUTION: Avoid spraying in eyes. Avoid breathing spray mist. Use only in well ventilated areas. Avoid contact with skin. In case of contact wash immediately with soap and water. Vacate room after treatment and ventilate before reoccupying.
Statement of Practical Treatment:
If inhaled: Remove affected person to fresh air. Apply artificial respiration if indicated.
If in eyes: Flush with plenty of water. Contact physician if irritation persists.
If on skin: Wash affected areas immediately with soap and water.

DIRECTION FOR USE
It is a violation of Federal law to use this product in a manner inconsistent with its labeling.
Shake well before each use. Remove protective cap. Aim spray opening away from person. Push button to spray.
To kill lice and louse eggs: Spray in an inconspicuous area to test for possible staining or discoloration. Inspect again after drying, then proceed to spray entire area to be treated. Hold container upright with nozzle away from you. Depress valve and spray from a distance of 8 to 10 inches.
Spray each square foot for 3 seconds. Spray only those garments, parts of bedding, including mattresses and furniture that cannot be either laundered or dry cleaned.
Allow all sprayed articles to dry thoroughly before use. Repeat treatment as necessary.
Buyer assumes all risks of use, storage or handling of this material not in strict accordance with direction given herewith.

DISPOSAL OF CONTAINER
Wrap container and dispose of in trash. Do not incinerate.

HOW SUPPLIED
5 ounce aerosol can.
Also available in combination with RID® Lice Treatment Kit as the RID® Lice Elimination System.

RID®
Lice Treatment Kit

PRODUCT OVERVIEW
KEY FACTS
The Rid Lice Treatment Kit contains a liquid pediculicide effective against head, body, and pubic lice and their eggs. The active ingredients in Rid are pyrethrins, which attack the louse's nervous system and piperonyl butoxide, a synergist. Rid rinses out completely after treatment and its active ingredients are poorly absorbed through the skin. Rid works faster than other OTC pediculicides. Each Rid Lice Treatment Kit package also contains an exclusive nit removal comb that removes all nits.

MAJOR USES
Rid has proved to be clinically effective in treating infestations of head lice, body lice, and pubic (crab) lice and their eggs.

SAFETY INFORMATION
Rid should be used with caution by ragweed sensitized persons. It is intended for external use only and is harmful if swallowed. It should not be inhaled or allowed to come in contact with the eyes or mucous membranes. Contamination of feed or foodstuffs should be avoided.

PRESCRIBING INFORMATION
RID®
Lice Treatment Kit
DESCRIPTION
Rid contains a liquid pediculicide whose active ingredients are: pyrethrins 0.3% and piperonyl butoxide, technical 3.00%, equivalent to 2.4% (butylcarbityl) (6-propylpiperonyl) ether and to 0.6% related compounds. Also contains petroleum distillate 1.20% and benzyl alcohol 2.4%. Inert ingredients 93.1%.

ACTIONS
RID kills head lice (Pediculus humanus capitis), body lice (Pediculus humanus humanus), and pubic or crab lice (Phthirus pubis), and their eggs.
The pyrethrins act as a contact poison and affect the parasite's nervous system, resulting in paralysis and death. The efficacy of the pyrethrins is enhanced by the synergist, piperonyl butoxide. Rid rinses out completely after treatment and is not designed to leave long-acting residues. The active ingredients in RID are poorly absorbed through the skin. Of the relatively minor amounts that are absorbed, they are rapidly metabolized to water-soluble compounds and eliminated from the body without ill effects. RID works faster than other OTC pediculicides.

INDICATIONS
RID is indicated for the treatment of infestations of head lice, body lice and pubic (crab) lice and their eggs.

WARNING

RID should be used with caution by ragweed sensitized persons.

PRECAUTIONS

This product is for external use only. It is harmful if swallowed. It should not be inhaled. It should be kept out of the eyes and contact with mucous membranes should be avoided. If accidental contact with eyes occurs, flush immediately with water. In case of infection or skin irritation, discontinue use and consult a physician. Consult a physician if infestation of eyebrows or eyelashes occurs. Avoid contamination of feed or foodstuffs.

STORAGE AND DISPOSAL

Do not store below 32°F (0°C). Do not reuse empty container. Wrap in several layers of newspaper and discard in trash.

DOSAGE AND ADMINISTRATION

(1) Shake well. Apply undiluted RID to dry hair and scalp or to any other infested area until entirely wet. Do not use on eyelashes or eyebrows. (2) Allow RID to remain on area for 10 minutes but no longer. (3) Wash thoroughly with warm water and soap or shampoo. (4) Dead lice and eggs should be removed with special nit comb provided. (5) Repeat treatment in 7 to 10 days to kill any newly hatched lice. Do not exceed two consecutive applications within 24 hours.

Since lice infestations are spread by contact, each family member should be examined carefully. If infested, he or she should be treated promptly to avoid spread or reinfestation of previously treated individuals. Contaminated clothing and other articles, such as hats, etc., should be dry cleaned, boiled or otherwise treated until decontaminated to prevent reinfestation or spread.

HOW SUPPLIED

In 2, 4 and 8 fl. oz. plastic bottles. Exclusive nit removal comb that removes all the nits and patient instruction booklet (English and Spanish) are included in each package of RID. Also available in combination with RID Lice Control Spray as the RID Lice Elimination System.

UNISOM DUAL RELIEF®   OTC
[yu 'na-som]
Nighttime Sleep Aid and Pain Reliever

PRODUCT OVERVIEW

KEY FACTS

Unisom Dual Relief (diphenhydramine sleep aid/acetaminophen pain relief formula) is a product with a dual antihistamine sleep aid/analgesic action to utilize the sedative effects of an antihistamine and relieve mild to moderate pain that may disturb normal sleep patterns. If patients have difficulty in falling asleep but are not experiencing pain at the same time, regular Unisom Sleep Aid which contains doxylamine succinate is indicated.

MAJOR USES

One Unisom Dual Relief is indicated 30 minutes before retiring to help reduce difficulty in falling asleep while relieving accompanying minor aches and pains, such as headache, muscle aches or menstrual discomfort.

SAFETY INFORMATION

Unisom Dual Relief is contraindicated in patients with asthma, glaucoma, or enlargement of the prostate, or in pregnancy or in nursing mothers. Excessive dosing may lead to liver damage. Product is intended for patients 12 years and older. Caution should be used if taken when alcohol is being consumed. Concurrent use with other medication must be done with caution due to anticholinergic properties of antihistamines.

PRESCRIBING INFORMATION

UNISOM DUAL RELIEF®
[yu 'na-som]
Nighttime Sleep Aid and Pain Reliver

DESCRIPTION

Unisom Dual Relief® is a pale blue, capsule-shaped, coated tablet.

ACTIVE INGREDIENTS

650 mg. acetaminophen and 50 mg. diphenhydramine HCl per tablet.

INDICATIONS

Unisom Dual Relief (diphenhydramine sleep aid formula) is indicated to help reduce difficulty in falling asleep while relieving accompanying minor aches and pains such as headache, muscle ache or menstrual discomfort. If there is difficulty in falling asleep, but pain is not being experienced at the same time, regular Unisom sleep aid is indicated which contains doxylamine succinate as its active ingredient.

ADMINISTRATION AND DOSAGE

One tablet 30 minutes before retiring. Take once daily or as directed by a physician.

CONTRAINDICATIONS

DO NOT TAKE THIS PRODUCT IF YOU HAVE ASTHMA, GLAUCOMA OR ENLARGEMENT OF THE PROSTATE GLAND EXCEPT UNDER THE ADVICE AND SUPERVISION OF A PHYSICIAN. Do not take this product if pregnant or nursing a baby.

Do not take this product for treatment of arthritis except under the advice and supervision of a physician.

WARNINGS

Do not exceed recommended dosage because severe liver damage may occur. If symptoms persist continuously for more than ten days, consult your physician. Insomnia may be a symptom of serious underlying medical illness. Take this product with caution if alcohol is being consumed. For adults only. Do not give to children under 12 years of age. Keep this and all medications out of reach of children. IN CASE OF ACCIDENTAL OVERDOSE SEEK PROFESSIONAL ADVICE OR CONTACT A POISON CONTROL CENTER IMMEDIATELY.

CAUTION

This product contains an antihistamine and will cause drowsiness. It should be used only at bedtime.

DRUG INTERACTION

Monoamine oxidase (MAO) inhibitors prolong and intensify the anticholinergic effects of antihistamines. The CNS depressant effect is heightened by alcohol and other CNS depressant drugs.

ATTENTION

Use only if tablet blister seals are unbroken. Child resistant packaging.

HOW SUPPLIED

Boxes of 8 and 16 tablets in child resistant blisters.

INACTIVE INGREDIENTS

Corn starch, FD&C Blue #1, FD&C Blue #2, hydroxypropyl methylcellulose, magnesium stearate, polyethylene glycol, polysorbate 80, polyvinylpyrrolidone, stearic acid, titanium dioxide.

UNISOM®   OTC
[yu 'na-som]
Nighttime Sleep Aid
(doxylamine succinate)

PRODUCT OVERVIEW

KEY FACTS

Unisom is an ethanolamine antihistamine (doxylamine) which characteristically shows a high incidence of sedation. It produces a reduced latency to end of wakefulness and early onset of sleep.

MAJOR USES

Unisom has been shown to be clinically effective as a sleep aid when 1 tablet is given 30 minutes before retiring.

SAFETY INFORMATION

Unisom is contraindicated in pregnancy and nursing mothers. It is also contraindicated in patients with asthma, glaucoma, and enlargement of the prostate. Caution should be used if taken when alcohol is being consumed. Caution is also indicated when taken concurrently with other medications due to the anticholinergic properties of antihistamines.

PRESCRIBING INFORMATION

UNISOM®   OTC
[yu 'na-som]
Nighttime Sleep Aid
(doxylamine succinate)

DESCRIPTION

Pale blue oval scored tablets containing 25 mg. of doxylamine succinate, 2-(α-(2-dimethylaminoethoxy)α-methylbenzyl) pyridine succinate.

ACTION AND USES

Doxylamine succinate is an antihistamine of the ethanolamine class, which characteristically shows a high incidence of sedation. In a comparative clinical study of over 20 antihistamines on more than 3000 subjects, doxylamine succinate 25 mg. was one of the three most sedating antihistamines, producing a significantly reduced latency to end of wakefulness and comparing favorably with established hypnotic drugs such as secobarbital and pentobarbital in sedation activity. It was chosen as the antihistamine, based on dosage, causing the earliest onset of sleep. In another clinical study, doxylamine succinate 25 mg. scored better than secobarbital 100 mg. as a nighttime hypnotic. Two additional, identical clinical studies, involving a total of 121 subjects demonstrated that doxylamine succinate 25 mg. reduced the sleep latency period by a third, compared to placebo. Duration of sleep was 26.6% longer with doxylamine succinate, and the quality of sleep was rated higher with the drug than with placebo. An EEG study on 6 subjects confirmed the re-

sults of these studies. In yet another study, no statistically significant difference was found between doxylamine succinate and flurazepam in the average time required for 200 patients with mild to moderate insomnia to fall asleep over 5 nights following a nightly dose of doxylamine succinate 25 mg. or flurazepam 30 mg., nor was any statistically significant difference found in the total time the 200 patients slept. Patients on doxylamine succinate awoke an average of 1.2 times per night while those on flurazepam awoke an average of 0.9 times per night. In either case the patients awoke rested the following morning. On a rating scale of 1 to 5, doxylamine succinate was given a 3.0, flurazepam a 3.4 by patients rating the degree of restfulness provided by their medication (5 represents "very well rested"). Although statistically significant, the difference between doxylamine succinate 25 mg. and flurazepam 30 mg. in the number of awakenings and degree of restfulness are clinically insignificant.

ADMINISTRATION AND DOSAGE

One tablet 30 minutes before retiring. Not for children under 12 years of age.

SIDE EFFECTS

Occasional anticholinergic effects may be seen.

PRECAUTIONS

Unisom® should be taken only at bedtime.

CONTRAINDICATIONS

Asthma, glaucoma, enlargement of the prostate gland. This product should not be taken by pregnant women or those who are nursing a baby.

WARNINGS

Should be taken with caution if alcohol is being consumed. Product should not be taken if patient is concurrently on any other drug, without prior consultation with physician. Should not be taken for longer than two weeks unless approved by physician.

HOW SUPPLIED

Boxes of 8, 16, 32 or 48 tablets.

INACTIVE INGREDIENTS

Dibasic Calcium Phosphate, FD&C Blue #1 Aluminum Lake, Magnesium Stearate, Microcrystalline Cellulose, Sodium Starch Glycolate.

VISINE®
Tetrahydrozoline Hydrochloride
Redness Reliever Eye Drops

(See PDR For Nondescription Drugs)

VISINE a.c.®
Astringent/Redness Reliever Eye
Drops

(See PDR For Nonprescription Drugs)

VISINE EXTRA®
Redness Reliever/Lubricant Eye
Drops

(See PDR For Nonprescription Drugs)

WART–OFF™
Liquid

ACTIVE INGREDIENT

Salicylic Acid, U.S.P., 17%, in Flexible Collodion, U.S.P.

INACTIVE INGREDIENTS

Alcohol, 18.1%, Camphor, Castor Oil, Ether, 47.7%, Lactic Acid, Pyroxylin.

INDICATIONS

Removal of Warts

WARNINGS

Keep this and all medications out of reach of children to avoid accidental poisoning.

Flammable—Do not use near fire or flame. For external use only. In case of accidental ingestion, contact a physician or a Poison Control Center immediately. Do not use near eyes or on mucous membranes. Diabetics or other people with impaired circulation should not use Wart-Off™. Do not use on moles, birthmarks or unusual warts with hair growing from them. If wart persists, see your physician. If pain should develop, consult your physician. **Do not apply to surrounding skin.**

DOSAGE AND ADMINISTRATION

Instructions For Use: Read warning and enclosed instructional brochure. Do not apply to surrounding skin. Make sure that surrounding skin is protected from accidental ap-

Continued on next page

Leeming—Cont.

plication. Apply Wart-Off™ to warts only. Before applying, soak affected area in hot water for several minutes. If any tissue has loosened, remove by rubbing surface of wart gently with cleaning brush enclosed in Wart-Off™ package. Dry thoroughly. Warts are contagious, so don't share your towel. Apply once or twice daily. Using pinpoint applicator attached to cap, apply one drop at a time until entire wart is covered. Lightly cover with small adhesive bandage. Replace cap tightly. This treatment may be used daily for three to four weeks if necessary.

HOW SUPPLIED

0.5 fluid ounce bottle with special pinpoint plastic applicator, cleaning brush and instructional brochure.

Legere Pharmaceuticals
7326 EAST EVANS ROAD
SCOTTSDALE, AZ 85260

Product Number	Product Name	
1038	ACE + Z Tablets	OTC
	Vitamin A	5000 I.U.
	Vitamin C	1000 mg.
	Vitamin E (Succinate)	50 I.U.
	Magnesium (oxide)	100 mg.
	Zinc Sulfate	100 mg.
1066	ACETACO Tablets	℞ CIII
	Acetaminophen	300 mg.
	Codeine Phosphate	30 mg.
043	ADENOSINE 10 ml.	℞
	Adenosine Monophosphate	25 mg.
046	ALLERDRYL 50 10 ml.	℞
	Diphenhydramine HCL.	50 mg.
008	ALLERPHEN 100 10 ml.	℞
	Chlorpheniramine Maleate	100 mg.
1128	AMFED TD Capsules	OTC
	Phenylpropanolamine	75 mg.
805	AQUAMED 10 ml.	℞
	Furosemide	10 mg.
1140	AQUAMED TABLETS	℞
	Furosemide	40 mg.
005	B COMPLEX 100 30 ml.	℞
	Thiamine HCl	100 mg.
	Riboflavin	2 mg.
	Pyridoxine HCl	2 mg.
	Panthenol	2 mg.
	Niacinamide	100 mg.
095	B-S-P 5 ml.	℞
	Betamethasone Sodium Phosphate	4 mg.
060	CAL IM 100 ml.	℞
	Calcium Glycerophosphate	10 mg.
	Calcium Levulinate	15 mg.
052	CEE 250 30 ml.	℞
	Sodium Ascorbate	250 mg.
086	CEE-500 50 ml.	℞
	Ascorbic Acid	500 mg.
1073	CEE-1000 T.D. Tablets	OTC
	Ascorbic Acid	1000 mg.
057	CHORIONIC GONADOTROPIN 10 ml.	℞
	Chorionic Gonadotropin	10,000 I.U.
055	CINALONE 40 5 ml.	℞
	Triamcinolone Diacetate	40 mg.
101	CINONIDE 40 5 ml.	℞
	Triamcinolone Acetonide	40 mg.
004	COBOLIN-M 30 ml.	℞
	Cyanocobalamin	1000 mcg.
299	CYLOMINE 10 ml	℞
	Dicyclomine HCl	10 mg.
078	DEPO-COBOLIN 10 ml.	℞
	Hydroxocobalamin 1000 mcg.	
062	DEPO-PREDATE 80 5 ml.	℞
	Methylprednisolone Acetate	80 mg.
121	DEPO-PREDATE 40 10 ml.	℞
	Methylprednisolone Acetate	40 mg.
010	DEXASONE 4 5 ml.	℞
	Dexamethasone Phosphate	4 mg.
011	DEXASONE LA 5 ml.	℞
	Dexamethasone Acetate	8 mg.
113	DEXASONE 10 10 ml.	℞
	Dexamethasone Sodium Phosphate	10 mg.
1058	DEXOL T.D. Tablets	OTC
	Pantothenic Acid	1000 mg.
107	DEXOL 250 10 ml.	℞
	Dexpanthenol	250 mg.

1111	DI-ATRO Tablets		℞ CV
	Diphenoxylate HCl	2.5 mg.	
	Atropine Sulfate	0.025 mg.	
1003	DICAL Gelcaps	OTC	
	Vitamin D	333 I.U.	
	Calcium Phosphate	75 mg.	
	Calcium Gluconate	14 mg.	
	Phosphorous	58 mg.	
1130	DIEUTRIM Capsules	OTC	
	Phenylpropanolamine HCl	75 mg.	
	Benzocaine	9 mg.	
	Carboxymethylcellulose	75 mg.	
015	E-CYPIONATE 10 ml.		℞
	Estradiol Cypionate	5 mg.	
080	EDTA 20 ml.		℞
	Edetate Disodium	150 mg.	
019	ESTRONE 10 ml.		℞
	Estrone	2 mg.	
1074	FUMARCEE Tablets	OTC	
	Ferrous Fumarate	200 mg.	
	Ascorbic Acid	300 mg.	
1002	HYDROCHLOR 50		℞
	Hydrochlorothiazide	50 mg.	
114	KABOLIN 2 ml.		℞
	Nandrolone Decanoate	50 mg.	
026	LIDOCAINE 1% 50 ml.		℞
	Lidocaine Hydrochloride	10 mg.	
027	LIDOCAINE 2%		℞
	Lidocaine Hydrochloride	20 mg.	
1129	LIPO B-C Tablets	OTC	
	Lipotropics		
	B Complex with Vitamin C		
059	LIVOLEX 30 ml.		℞
	Liver Vitamins and Iron		
1057	MEGAPLEX Tablets	OTC	
	Multi-Vitamin		
117	MENAVAL 20 10 ml.		℞
	Estradiol Valerate	20 mg.	
023	MENAVAL 40 10 ml.		℞
	Estradiol Valerate	40 mg.	
064	MYOTROL 10 ml.		℞
	Orphenadrine Citrate	30 mg.	
018	NATURAL ESTROGENIC SUBSTANCE 10 ml.		℞
	Estrone Suspension	2 mg.	
049	NEUCALM 50 10 ml.		℞
	Hydroxyzine HCl	50 mg.	
1063	O. B. THERA Tablets	OTC	
	Pre-natal Vitamins		
1022	PHENAZINE Tablets and Capsules		℞ CIII
	Phendimetrazine Tartrate	35 mg.	
031	PREDATE 50 10 ml.		℞
	Prednisolone Acetate Suspension	50 mg.	
032	PREDATE S 10 ml.		℞
	Prednisolone Sodium Phosphate	20 mg.	
033	PREDATE TBA 10 ml.		℞
	Prednisolone Tebutate Suspension	20 mg.	
1064	PREVENZYME Tablets	OTC	
	Pancreatin	600 mg.	
	Pepsin	225 mg.	
	Amylase	15 mg.	
	Diastase	150 mg.	
	Papain	150 mg.	
	Glutamic Acid HCL	30 mg.	
	Betaine HCL	30 mg.	
602	PROBAHIST		℞
	Brompheniramine maleate	10 mg.	
1132	PROBAHIST Capsules		℞
	Pseudoephedrine	120 mg.	
	Chlorpheniramine	8 mg.	
1150	PROBASIN-LA Capulets		℞
	Phenylpropanolamine HCl	75 mg.	
	Guaifenesin	400 mg.	
088	PRODROX 250 5 ml.		℞
	Hydroxyprogesterone Caproate	250 mg.	
081	PROGESTERONE 50 10 ml.		℞
	Progesterone	50 mg.	
034	PROMET 50 10 ml.		℞
	Promethazine Hydrochloride	50 mg.	
1133	PT 105 Capsules		℞ CIII
	Phendimetrazine	105 mg.	
073	RODEX 30 ml.		℞
	Pyridoxine HCl	100 mg.	
1037	RODEX T.D. Capsules	OTC	
	Pyridoxine	150 mg.	
035	SOLATE 30 ml.		℞
	Sodium Thiosalicylate	50 mg.	
1095	SPASGESIC		℞
	Chlorzoxazone	250 mg.	
	Acetaminophen	300 mg.	

054	STEMETIC 20 ml.		℞
	Trimethobenzamide HCl	100 mg.	
039	T-CYPIONATE 10 ml.		℞
	Testosterone Cypionate	200 mg.	
051	T-E CYPIONATE 10 ml.		℞
	Testosterone Cypionate	50 mg.	
	Estradiol Cypionate	2 mg.	
1025	TERAMINE Capsules		℞ CIV
	Phentermine HCl	30 mg.	
050	TESTAVAL 90/4 10 ml.		℞
	Testosterone Enanthate	90 mg.	
	Estradiol Valerate	4 mg.	
030	TESTOSTERONE SUSPENSION 10 ml.		℞
	Testosterone 100 Aqueous	100 mg.	
1044	VITABESE Capsules	OTC	
	Multi-Vitamins		

Lehn & Fink
Division of Sterling Drug Inc.
Personal Products Division
225 SUMMIT AVENUE
MONTVALE, NJ 07645

DIAPARENE®

[See table on next page].

DIAPARENE® BABY POWDER

DESCRIPTION

Powder comprised of corn starch, magnesium carbonate, methylbenzethonium chloride 0.055% and fragrance.

ACTION AND USES

Diaparene Baby Powder has a corn starch base for high absorbency to help keep baby's skin dry and for soothing diaper rash, prickly heat and chafing.

ADMINISTRATION AND DOSAGE

Apply liberally to baby's skin after bath and with each diaper change.

HOW SUPPLIED

Available in 4 oz, 9 oz, 14 oz containers.

DIAPARENE® SUPERS BABY WASH CLOTHS

DESCRIPTION

Wash cloths are impregnated with a cleansing solution containing water, SD alcohol-40, propylene glycol, PEG/60, lanolin, sodium nonoxynol-9-phosphate, sorbic acid, citric acid, disodium phosphate, oleth-20, and fragrance.

ACTION AND USES

Diaparene Baby Wash Cloths contain lanolin and a mild cleansing solution to clean and condition baby's skin.

ADMINISTRATION AND DOSAGE

Wipe baby's skin with solution-impregnated wash cloths as required.

HOW SUPPLIED

Available in canisters of 70 and 150 wash cloths.

Lemmon Company
P.O. BOX 630
SELLERSVILLE, PA 18960

Additional LEMMON Products:

Acetaminophen and Codeine Phosphate Tablets CIII
Alphaderm Cream (Hydrocortisone)
Amantadine HCl Capsules
Amitriptyline HCl Tablets
Amoxicillin Capsules
Betamethasone Dipropionate Cream, Lotion and Ointment
Beta-Val Cream, Lotion and Ointment (Betamethasone Valerate)
Carbamazepine Tablets
Cefadroxil Capsules and Tablets
Cefazolin Sodium Sterile Injection
Cephalexin Capsules and Suspension
Cephradine Capsules
Chlorpropamide Tablets
Chlorzoxazone Tablets
Clindamycin Phosphate Injection

	Diaparene® **Medicated Cream**	**Diaparene®** **Peri-Anal®** **Medicated Ointment**	**Diaparene®** **Cradol®**
DESCRIPTION	Special lotion formula to soothe and protect baby's skin.	Ointment that soothes and helps heal diaper rash, helps protect against wetness and irritation.	Medicated lotion scalp treatment for "cradle cap" developed by babies.
	Contains: Methylbenzethonium Chloride 0.1% (w/w) Also contains: Dibasic Sodium Phosphate, Fragrance, Glycerin, Mineral Oil, Parabens, Polysorbate 60, Purified Water, Sorbitan Monostearate, Stearyl Alcohol, White Petrolatum.	Contains: Cod Liver Oil (vitamins A & D), Zine Oxide, Methylbenzethonium Chloride 0.1% (w/w) Also contains: Calcium Caseinate, Fragrance, Lanolin, Lanolin Alcohol, Mineral Oil, Starch, Paraffin, White Petrolatum, Yellow Wax.	Contains: Methylbenzethonium Chloride 0.07%. Also contains: Anhydrous Lanolin, Fragrance, Glyceryl Stearate, Lanolin, Lanolin Alcohol, Light Mineral Oil, Mineral Oil, Parabens, Paraffin, PEG-6 Stearate, Purified Water, Stearamidoethyl Diethylamine, Yellow Wax.
ACTION AND USES	Nonstaining cream formula soothes and protects diaper area, knees, elbows— anywhere baby's skin needs comfort.	The antibacterial action of methylbenzethonium chloride combats ammonia-forming bacteria that can cause diaper rash and odor. Provides a water repellent shield to keep out wetness, and to protect skin from irritating urine, stool and perspiration.	Gently softens and separates crust and scales from the scalp. Helps prevent and treat local infection.
ADMINISTRATION AND DOSAGE	Directions: Apply anywhere skin chafing or irritation may develop. Use liberally, taking care to include skin folds where moisture collects.	Directions: At the first sign of redness or diaper rash, apply liberally to diaper area three times daily as needed. To help prevent diaper rash, apply to diaper area after each diaper change. Especially important at bedtime, or anytime that exposure to wet diapers may be prolonged. For minor skin irritations, apply a thin layer, using a gauze dressing if necessary.	Directions for "cradle cap" and scalp infection: Massage into wet or dry scalp 3 times daily for 3 days. Do not wash off or shampoo between applications. After 3 days, shampoo with mild soap and use a fine comb or scalp brush to gently brush away crusts and scales from baby's scalp. To prevent reoccurrence: Massage into wet or dry scalp 3 times weekly.
HOW SUPPLIED	NDC 12843-246-21 1 ounce tube NDC 12843-246-22 2 ounce tube NDC 12843-246-24 4 ounce tube	NDC 12843-236-10 1 ounce tube NDC 12843-236-20 2 ounce tube NDC 12843-236-40 4 ounce tube	NDC 12843-070-21 3 ounce bottle

Clonidine HCl Tablets
Cotrim Tablets, I.V. Infusion and Pediatric Suspension (Sulfamethoxazole and Trimethoprim)
Desipramine HCl Tablets
Diazepam Injection Ⓒ
Diphenhydramine HCl Capsules
Doxycycline Hyclate Capsules and Tablets
Epitol Tablets (Carbamazepine)
Fenoprofen Calcium Capsules and Tablets
Fluocinonide Cream, Gel and Topical Solution
Fluocinonide Cream (Emulsified Base)
Haloperidol Oral Solution, Injection and Tablets
Hydrocortisone Cream
Ibuprofen Tablets
Indomethacin Capsules
Indomethacin SR Capsules
Isoxsuprine HCl Tablets
Lorazepam Tablets Ⓒ
Meclofenamate Sodium Capsules
Metoclopramide HCl Tablets
Metronidazole Tablets
Myco-Triacet II Cream and Ointment (Nystatin & Triamcinolone Acetonide)
Neothylline Tablets (Dyphylline)
Neothylline GG Tablets (Dyphylline and Guaifenesin)
Nystatin Cream, Oral Tablets, Oral Suspension and Vaginal Tablets
Otocort Sterile Ear Solution and Suspension

Perphenazine Tablets
Perphenazine and Amitriptyline HCl Tablets
Propacet -100 Tablets Ⓒ (Propoxyphene Napsylate and Acetaminophen)
Propoxyphene Compound 65 Capsules Ⓒ (Propoxyphene HCl, Aspirin, Caffeine)
Propoxyphene HCl Capsules Ⓒ
Propoxyphene HCl and Acetaminophen Tablets Ⓒ
Propoxyphene Napsylate and Acetaminophen Tablets (Pink) Ⓒ
Propranolol HCl Extended Release Capsules
Racet Cream (Iodochlorhydroxyquin, Hydrocortisone)
Rhinex D-Lay Tablets (Acetaminophen, Salicylamide, Phenylpropanolamine HCl, Chlorpheniramine Maleate)
Rhus Tox Antigen Poison Ivy Extract
Sofarin Tablets (Warfarin Sodium)
Statobex Tablets Ⓒ (Phendimetrazine Tartrate)
Sulfanilamide Vaginal Cream 15%
Tetracycline HCl Capsules
Thiothixene HCl Oral Solution
Trazodone HCl Tablets
Triacet Cream (Triamcinolone Acetonide)
Triamterene and Hydrochlorothiazide Capsules 50 mg/25 mg
Triamterene and Hydrochlorothiazide Tablets 75 mg/50 mg
Vagilia Triple Sulfa Vaginal Cream (Sulfathiazole, Sulfacetamide, Sulfabenzamide)

ADIPEX-P®

       Ⓒ Ⱦ

[ă′dĭ-pĕx]

(phentermine hydrochloride 37.5 mg)

DESCRIPTION

Phentermine Hydrochloride has the chemical name of α, α-dimethylphene-thylamine hydrochloride. The structural formula is as follows.

$C_{10}H_{15}N \cdot HCl$ M.W. 185.7

Phentermine hydrochloride is a white, odorless, hygroscopic, crystalline powder which is soluble in water and lower alcohols, slightly soluble in chloroform and insoluble in ether. ADIPEX-P, an anorectic agent for oral administration, is available as a capsule or tablet containing 37.5 mg of phentermine hydrochloride (equivalent to 30mg of phentermine base).

ADIPEX-P capsules contain the inactive ingredients Corn Starch, Gelatin, Lactose, Magnesium Stearate, and Coloring. ADIPEX-P Tablets contain the inactive ingredients Acacia, Confectioner's Sugar, Corn Starch, Lactose, Magnesium Stearate, Stearic Acid, and Coloring.

CLINICAL PHARMACOLOGY

Phentermine hydrochloride is a sympathomimetic amine with pharmacologic activity similar to the prototype drugs of this class used in obesity, the amphetamines. Actions include central nervous system stimulation and elevation of blood pressure. Tachyphylaxis and tolerance have been demonstrated with all drugs of this class in which these phenomena have been looked for.

Drugs of this class used in obesity are commonly known as "anorectics" or "anorexigenics". It has not been established, however, that the action of such drugs in treating obesity is primarily one of appetite suppression. Other central nervous system actions, or metabolic effects, may be involved, for example.

Adult obese subjects instructed in dietary management and treated with "anorectic" drugs, lose more weight on the average than those treated with placebo and diet, as determined in relatively short-term clinical trials.

The magnitude of increased weight loss of drug-treated patients over placebo-treated patients is only a fraction of a pound a week. The rate of weight loss is greatest in the first weeks of therapy for both drug and placebo subjects and tends to decrease in succeeding weeks. The possible origins of the increased weight loss due to the various drug effects are not established. The amount of weight loss associated with the use of "anorectic" drugs varies from trial to trial, and the increased weight loss appears to be related in part to variables other than the drug prescribed, such as the physician-investigator, the population treated, and the diet prescribed. Studies do not permit conclusions as to the relative importance of the drug and non-drug factors on weight loss.

The natural history of obesity is measured in years, whereas the studies cited are restricted to a few weeks duration; thus, the total impact of drug-induced weight loss over that of diet alone must be considered clinically limited.

INDICATIONS AND USAGE

ADIPEX-P® (phentermine hydrochloride) is indicated in the management of exogenous obesity as a short term adjunct (a few weeks) in a regimen of weight reduction based on caloric restriction.

The limited usefulness of agents of this class (see CLINICAL PHARMACOLOGY) should be measured against possible risk factors inherent in their use such as those described below.

CONTRAINDICATIONS

Advanced arteriosclerosis, symptomatic cardiovascular disease, moderate to severe hypertension, hyperthyroidism, known hypersensitivity or idiosyncrasy to the sympathomimetic amines, glaucoma.

Agitated states.

Patients with a history of drug abuse.

During or within 14 days following the administration of monoamine oxidase inhibitors (hypertensive crisis may result).

WARNINGS

Tolerance to the anorectic effect usually develops within a few weeks. When this occurs, the recommended dose should not be exceeded in an attempt to increase the effect; rather, the drug should be discontinued.

Phentermine hydrochloride may impair the ability of the patient to engage in potentially hazardous activities such as operating machinery or driving a motor vehicle; the patient should therefore be cautioned accordingly.

Usage in Pregnancy: Safe use in pregancy has not been established. Use of phentermine hydrochloride by women

Continued on next page

Lemmon—Cont.

who are or may become pregnant, and those in the first trimester of pregnancy, requires that the potential benefit be weighed against the possible hazard to mother and infant.

Usage in Children: Phentermine hydrochloride is not recommended for use in children under 12 years of age.

Usage with Alcohol: Concomitant use of alcohol with phentermine hydrochloride may result in an adverse drug interaction.

PRECAUTIONS

Caution is to be exercised in prescribing phentermine hydrochloride for patients with even mild hypertension.

Insulin requirements in diabetes mellitus may be altered in association with the use of phentermine hydrochloride and the concomitant dietary regimen.

Phentermine hydrochloride may decrease the hypotensive effect of guanethidine.

The least amount feasible should be prescribed or dispensed at one time in order to minimize the possibility of overdosage.

ADVERSE REACTIONS

Cardiovascular: Palpitation, tachycardia, elevation of blood pressure.

Central Nervous System: Overstimulation, restlessness, dizziness, insomnia, euphoria, dysphoria, tremor, headache, rarely psychotic episodes at recommended doses.

Gastrointestinal: Dryness of the mouth, unpleasant taste, diarrhea, constipation, other gastrointestinal disturbances.

Allergic: Urticaria.

Endocrine: Impotence, changes in libido.

DRUG ABUSE AND DEPENDENCE

Phentermine hydrochloride is a Scheduled IV controlled substance. Phentermine hydrochloride is related chemically and pharmacologically to the amphetamines. Amphetamines and related stimulant drugs have been extensively abused, and the possibility of abuse of phentermine hydrochloride should be kept in mind when evaluating the desirability of including a drug as part of a weight reduction program. Abuse of amphetamines and related drugs may be associated with intense psychological dependence and severe social dysfunction. There are reports of patients who have increased the dosage to many times that recommended. Abrupt cessation following prolonged high dosage administration results in extreme fatigue and mental depression; changes are also noted in the sleep EEG. Manifestations of chronic intoxication with anorectic drugs include severe dermatoses, marked insomnia, irritability, hyperactivity, and personality changes. The most severe manifestation of chronic intoxications is psychosis, often clinically indistinguishable from schizophrenia.

OVERDOSAGE

Manifestations of acute overdosage with phentermine hydrochloride include restlessness, tremor, hyperreflexia, rapid respiration, confusion, assaultiveness, hallucinations, panic states.

Fatigue and depression usually follow the central stimulation.

Cardiovascular effects include arrhythmias, hypertension or hypotension and circulatory collapse. Gastrointestinal symptoms include nausea, vomiting, diarrhea, and abdominal cramps. Fatal poisoning usually terminates in convulsions and coma.

Management of acute phentermine hydrochloride intoxication is largely symptomatic and includes lavage and sedation with a barbiturate. Experience with hemodialysis or peritoneal dialysis is inadequate to permit recommendation in this regard. Acidification of the urine increases phentermine excretion. Intravenous phentolamine has been suggested for possible acute, severe hypertension, if this complicates phentermine hydrochloride overdosage.

DOSAGE AND ADMINISTRATION

Dosage should be individualized to obtain an adequate response with the lowest effective dose.

The usual adult dose is one capsule or tablet (37.5 mg) daily, administered before breakfast or 1-2 hours after breakfast. For tablets, the dosage may be adjusted to the patient's need. For some patients $\frac{1}{2}$ tablet (18.75 mg) daily may be adequate, while in some cases it may be desirable to give $\frac{1}{2}$ tablet (18.75 mg) two times a day.

Late evening medication should be avoided because of the possibility of resulting insomnia.

Phentermine hydrochloride is NOT recommended for use in children under 12 years of age.

HOW SUPPLIED

Available in tablets and capsules containing 37.5 mg phentermine hydrochloride (equivalent to 30 mg phentermine base). Each blue and white, oblong, scored tablet is imprinted with "LEMMON"/"9"-"9". The #3 capsule has an opaque white body and an opaque light blue cap. Each capsule is imprinted with "ADIPEX-P"-"37.5" on the cap and two blue stripes on the body.

Tablets are packaged in bottles of 100 (NDC 0093-0009-01); 400 (NDC 0093-0009-26); and 1000 (NDC 0093-0009-10). Capsules are packaged in bottles of 100 (NDC 0093-0019-01); and 400 (NDC 0093-0019-26).

Shown in Product Identification Section, page 415

ORAP™   ℞
(Pimozide)
Tablets

DESCRIPTION

ORAP (pimozide) is an orally active antipsychotic agent of the diphenyl-butylpiperidine series. The structural formula of pimozide, 1-(1-(4,4- bis(4-fluorophenyl)-butyl)-4-piperidinyl)-1,3-dihydro-2H-benzimidazol-2-one is:

The solubility of pimozide in water is less than 0.01 mg/ml; it is slightly soluble in most organic solvents.

Each white ORAP tablet contains 2 mg of pimozide and the following inactive ingredients: calcium stearate, cellulose, lactose and corn starch.

CLINICAL PHARMACOLOGY

Pharmacodynamic Actions

ORAP (pimozide) is an orally active antipsychotic drug product which shares with other antipsychotics the ability to blockade dopaminergic receptors on neurons in the central nervous system. Although its exact mode of action has not been established, the ability of pimozide to suppress motor and phonic tics in Tourette's Disorder is thought to be a function of its dopaminergic blocking activity. However, receptor blockade is often accompanied by a series of secondary alterations in central dopamine metabolism and function which may contribute to both pimozide's therapeutic and untoward effects. In addition, pimozide, in common with other antipsychotic drugs, has various effects on other central nervous system receptor systems which are not fully characterized.

Metabolism and Pharmacokinetics

More than 50% of a dose of pimozide is absorbed after oral administration. Based on the pharmacokinetic and metabolic profile, pimozide appears to undergo significant first pass metabolism. Peak serum levels occur generally six to eight hours (range 4–12 hours) after dosing. Pimozide is extensively metabolized, primarily by N-dealkylation in the liver. Two major metabolites have been identified, 1-(4-piperidyl)-2-benzimidazolinone and 4,4-bis(4-fluorophenyl) butyric acid. The antipsychotic activity of these metabolites is undetermined. The major route of elimination of pimozide and its metabolites is through the kidney.

The mean serum elimination half-life of pimozide in schizophrenic patients was approximately 55 hours. There was a 13-fold interindividual difference in the area under the serum pimozide level-time curve and an equivalent degree of variation in peak serum levels among patients studied. The significance of this is unclear since there are few correlations between plasma levels and clinical findings.

Effects of food, disease or concomitant medication upon the absorption, distribution, metabolism and elimination of pimozide are not known.

INDICATIONS AND USAGE

ORAP (pimozide) is indicated for the suppression of motor and phonic tics in patients with Tourette's Disorder who have failed to respond satisfactorily to standard treatment. ORAP is not intended as a treatment of first choice nor is it intended for the treatment for tics that are merely annoying or cosmetically troublesome. ORAP should be reserved for use in Tourette's Disorder patients whose development and/or daily life function is severely compromised by the presence of motor and phonic tics.

Evidence supporting approval of pimozide for use in Tourette's Disorder was obtained in two controlled clinical investigations which enrolled patients between the ages of 8 and 53 years. Most subjects in the two trials were 12 or older.

CONTRAINDICATIONS

1. ORAP (pimozide) is contraindicated in the treatment of simple tics or tics other than those associated with Tourette's Disorder.

2. ORAP should not be used in patients taking drugs that may, themselves, cause motor and phonic tics (e.g., pemoline, methylphenidate and amphetamines) until such patients have been withdrawn from these drugs to determine whether or not the drugs, rather than Tourette's Disorder, are responsible for the tics.

3. Because ORAP prolongs the QT interval of the electrocardiogram it is contraindicated in patients with congenital long QT syndrome, patients with a history of cardiac arrhythmias, or patients taking other drugs which prolong the QT interval of the electrocardiogram (see DRUG INTERACTIONS).

4. ORAP is contraindicated in patients with severe toxic central nervous system depression or comatose states from any cause.

5. ORAP is contraindicated in patients with hypersensitivity to it. As it is not known whether cross-sensitivity exists among the antipsychotics, pimozide should be used with appropriate caution in patients who have demonstrated hypersensitivity to other antipsychotic drugs.

WARNINGS

The use of ORAP (pimozide) in the treatment of Tourette's Disorder involves different risk/benefit considerations than when antipsychotic drugs are used to treat other conditions. Consequently, a decision to use ORAP should take into consideration the following (see also PRECAUTIONS—Information for Patients).

Tardive Dyskinesia

A syndrome consisting of potentially irreversible, involuntary, dyskinetic movements may develop in patients treated with antipsychotic drugs. Although the prevalence of the syndrome appears to be highest among the elderly, especially elderly women, it is impossible to rely upon prevalence estimates to predict, at the inception of antipsychotic treatment, which patients are likely to develop the syndrome. Whether antipsychotic drug products differ in their potential to cause tardive dyskinesia is unknown.

Both the risk of developing tardive dyskinesia and the likelihood that it will become irreversible are believed to increase as the duration of treatment and the total cumulative dose of antipsychotic drugs administered to the patient increase. However, the syndrome can develop, although much less commonly, after relatively brief treatment periods at low doses.

There is no known treatment for established cases of tardive dyskinesia, although the syndrome may remit, partially or completely, if antipsychotic treatment is withdrawn. Antipsychotic treatment, itself, however, may suppress (or partially suppress) the signs and symptoms of the syndrome and thereby may possibly mask the underlying process. The effect that symptomatic suppression has upon the long-term course of the syndrome is unknown.

Given these considerations, antipsychotic drugs should be prescribed in a manner that is most likely to minimize the occurrence of tardive dyskinesia. Chronic antipsychotic treatment should generally be reserved for patients who suffer from a chronic illness that, 1) is known to respond to antipsychotic drugs, and 2) for whom alternative, equally effective, but potentially less harmful treatments are not available or appropriate. In patients who do require chronic treatment, the smallest dose and the shortest duration of treatment producing a satisfactory clinical response should be sought. The need for continued treatment should be reassessed periodically.

If signs and symptoms of tardive dyskinesia appear in a patient on antipsychotics, drug discontinuation should be considered. However, some patients may require treatment despite the presence of the syndrome.

(For further information about the description of tardive dyskinesia and its clinical detection, please refer to ADVERSE REACTIONS and PRECAUTIONS—Information for Patients).

Neuroleptic Malignant Syndrome (NMS)

A potentially fatal symptom complex sometimes referred to as Neuroleptic Malignant Syndrome (NMS) has been reported in association with antipsychotic drugs. Clinical manifestations of NMS are hyperpyrexia, muscle rigidity, altered mental status (including catatonic signs) and evidence of autonomic instability (irregular pulse or blood pressure, tachycardia, diaphoresis, and cardiac dysrhythmias). Additional signs may include elevated creatine phosphokinase, myoglobinuria (rhabdomyolysis) and acute renal failure.

The diagnostic evaluation of patients with this syndrome is complicated. In arriving at a diagnosis, it is important to identify cases where the clinical presentation includes both serious medical illness (e.g., pneumonia, systemic infection, etc.) and untreated or inadequately treated extrapyramidal signs and symptoms (EPS). Other important considerations in the differential diagnosis include central anticholinergic toxicity, heat stroke, drug fever and primary central nervous system (CNS) pathology.

The management of NMS should include 1) immediate discontinuation of antipsychotic drugs and other drugs not essential to concurrent therapy, 2) intensive symptomatic treatment and medical monitoring, and 3) treatment of any concomitant serious medical problems for which specific treatments are available. There is no general agreement about specific pharmacological treatment regimens for uncomplicated NMS.

If a patient requires antipsychotic drug treatment after recovery from NMS, the potential reintroduction of drug therapy should be carefully considered. The patient should be carefully monitored, since recurrences of NMS have been reported.

Hyperpyrexia, not associated with the above symptom complex, has been reported with other antipsychotic drugs.

Other

Sudden, unexpected deaths have occurred in experimental studies of conditions other than Tourette's Disorder. These deaths occurred while patients were receiving dosages in the range of 1 mg per kg. One possible mechanism for such deaths is prolongation of the QT interval predisposing patients to ventricular arrhythmia. An electrocardiogram should be performed before ORAP treatment is initiated and periodically thereafter, especially during the period of dose adjustment.

ORAP may have a tumorigenic potential. Based on studies conducted in mice, it is known that pimozide can produce a dose related increase in pituitary tumors. The full significance of this finding is not known, but should be taken into consideration in the physician's and patient's decisions to use this drug product. This finding should be given special consideration when the patient is young and chronic use of pimozide is anticipated. (see PRECAUTIONS—Carcinogenesis, Mutagenesis. Impairment of Fertility).

PRECAUTIONS

General

ORAP (pimozide) may impair the mental and/or physical abilities required for the performance of potentially hazardous tasks, such as driving a car or operating machinery, especially during the first few days of treatment.

ORAP produces anticholinergic side effects and should be used with caution in individuals whose conditions may be aggravated by anticholinergic activity.

ORAP should be administered cautiously to patients with impairment of liver or kidney function, because it is metabolized by the liver and excreted by the kidneys.

Antipsychotics should be administered with caution to patients receiving anticonvulsant medication, with a history of seizures, or with EEG abnormalities, because they may lower the convulsive threshold. If indicated, adequate anticonvulsant therapy should be maintained concomitantly.

Information for Patients

Treatment with ORAP exposes the patient to serious risks. A decision to use ORAP chronically in Tourette's Disorder is one that deserves full consideration by the patient (or patient's family) as well as by the treating physician. Because the goal of treatment is symptomatic improvement, the patient's view of the need for treatment and assessment of response are critical in evaluating the impact of therapy and weighing its benefits against the risks. Since the physician is the primary source of information about the use of a drug in any disease, it is recommended that the following information be discussed with patients and/or their families.

ORAP is intended only for use in patients with Tourette's Disorder whose symptoms are severe and who cannot tolerate, or who do not respond to HALDOL® (haloperidol).

Given the likelihood that a proportion of patients exposed chronically to antipsychotics will develop tardive dyskinesia, it is advised that all patients in whom chronic use is contemplated be given, if possible, full information about this risk. The decision to inform patients and/or their guardians must obviously take into account the clinical circumstances and the competency of the patient to understand the information provided.

There is *very* little information available on the use of ORAP in children under 12 years of age.

The information available on ORAP from foreign marketing experience and from U.S. clinical trials indicate that ORAP has a side effect profile similar to that of other antipsychotic drugs. Patients should be informed that all types of side effects associated with the use of antipsychotics may be associated with the use of ORAP.

In addition, sudden, unexpected deaths have occurred in patients taking high doses of ORAP for conditions other than Tourette's Disorder. These deaths may have been the result of an effect of ORAP upon the heart. Therefore, patients should be instructed not to exceed the prescribed dose of ORAP and they should realize the need for the initial ECG and for follow-up ECGs during treatment.

Also, pimozide, at a dose about 15 times that given humans, caused an increase in the number of benign tumors of the pituitary gland in female mice. It is not possible to say how important this is. Similar tumors were not seen in rats given pimozide, nor at lower doses in mice, which is reassuring. However, any such finding must be considered to suggest a possible risk of long term use of the drug.

Laboratory Tests

An ECG should be done at baseline and periodically thereafter throughout the period of dose adjustment. Any indication of prolongation of the QT, interval beyond an absolute limit of 0.47 seconds (children) or 0.52 seconds (adults), or more than 25% above the patient's original baseline should be considered a basis for stopping further dose increase (see CONTRAINDICATIONS) and considering a lower dose. Since hypokalemia has been associated with ventricular arrhythmias, potassium insufficiency, secondary to diuretics, diarrhea, or other cause, should be corrected before

ORAP therapy is initiated and normal potassium maintained during therapy.

Drug Interactions

Because ORAP prolongs the QT interval of the electrocardiogram, an additive effect on QT interval would be anticipated if administered with other drugs, such as phenothiazines, tricyclic antidepressants or antiarrhythmic agents, which prolong the QT interval. Such concomitant administration should not be undertaken (see CONTRAINDICATIONS). ORAP may be capable of potentiating CNS depressants, including analgesics, sedatives, anxiolytics, and alcohol.

Carcinogenesis, Mutagenesis, Impairment of Fertility

Carcinogenesis studies were conducted in mice and rats. In mice, pimozide causes a dose-related increase in pituitary and mammary tumors.

When mice were treated for up to 18 months with pimozide, pituitary gland changes developed in females only. These changes were characterized as hyperplasia at doses approximating the human dose and adenoma at doses about fifteen times the maximum recommended human dose on a mg per kg basis. The mechanism for the induction of pituitary tumors in mice is not known.

Mammary gland tumors in female mice were also increased, but these tumors are expected in rodents treated with antipsychotic drugs which elevate prolactin levels. Chronic administration of an antipsychotic also causes elevated prolactin levels in humans. Tissue culture experiments indicate that approximately one-third of human breast cancers are prolactin-dependent *in vitro*, a factor of potential importance if the prescription of these drugs is contemplated in a patient with a previously detected breast cancer. Although disturbances such as galactorrhea, amenorrhea, gynecomastia, and impotence have been reported with antipsychotic drugs, the clinical significance of elevated serum prolactin levels is unknown for most patients. Neither clinical studies nor epidemiologic studies conducted to date have shown an association between chronic administration of these drugs and mammary tumorigenesis. The available evidence, however, is considered too limited to be conclusive at this time.

In a 24 month carcinogenicity study in rats, animals received up to 50 times the maximum recommended human dose. No increased incidence of overall tumors or tumors at any site was observed in either sex. Because of the limited number of animals surviving this study, the meaning of these results is unclear.

Pimozide did not have mutagenic activity in the Ames test with four bacterial test strains, in the mouse dominant lethal test or in the micronucleus test in rats.

Reproduction studies in animals were not adequate to assess all aspects of fertility. Nevertheless, female rats administered pimozide had prolonged estrus cycles, an effect also produced by other antipsychotic drugs.

Pregnancy

Category C. Reproduction studies performed in rats and rabbits at oral doses up to 8 times the maximum human dose did not reveal evidence of teratogenicity. In the rat, however, this multiple of the human dose resulted in decreased pregnancies and in the retarded development of fetuses. These effects are thought to be due to an inhibition or delay in implantation which is also observed in rodents administered other antipsychotic drugs. In the rabbit, maternal toxicity, mortality, decreased weight gain, and embryotoxicity including increased resorptions were dose related. Because animal reproduction studies are not always predictive of human response, pimozide should be given to a pregnant woman only if the potential benefits of treatment clearly outweigh the potential risks.

Labor and Delivery

This drug has no recognized use in labor or delivery.

Nursing Mothers

It is not known whether pimozide is excreted in human milk. Because many drugs are excreted in human milk and because of the potential for tumorigenicity and unknown cardiovascular effects in the infant, a decision should be made whether to discontinue nursing or to discontinue the drug, taking into account the importance of the drug to the mother.

Pediatric Use

Although Tourette's Disorder most often has its onset between the ages of 2 and 15 years, information on the use and efficacy of ORAP in patients less than 12 years of age is limited. Because its use and safety have not been evaluated in other childhood disorders, ORAP is not recommended for use in any condition other than Tourette's Disorder.

ADVERSE REACTIONS

General

Extrapyramidal reactions: Neuromuscular (extrapyramidal) reactions during the administration of ORAP (pimozide) have been reported frequently, often during the first few days of treatment. In most patients, these reactions involved Parkinson-like symptoms which, when first observed, were usually mild to moderately severe and usually reversible. Other types of neuromuscular reactions (motor restlessness, dystonia, akathisia, hyperreflexia, opisthotonos, oculogyric crises) have been reported far less frequently. Severe extra-

pyramidal reactions have been reported to occur at relatively low doses. Generally the occurrence and severity of most extrapyramidal symptoms are dose related since they occur at relatively high doses and have been shown to disappear or become less severe when the dose is reduced. Administration of antiparkinson drugs such as benztropine mesylate or trihexyphenidyl hydrochloride may be required for control of such reactions. It should be noted that persistent extrapyramidal reactions have been reported and that the drug may have to be discontinued in such cases.

Withdrawal Emergent Neurological Signs: Generally, patients receiving short term therapy experience no problems with abrupt discontinuation of antipsychotic drugs. However, some patients on maintenance treatment experience transient dyskinetic signs after abrupt withdrawal. In certain of these cases the dyskinetic movements are indistinguishable from the syndrome described below under "Tardive Dyskinesia" except for duration. It is not known whether gradual withdrawal of antipsychotic drugs will reduce the rate of occurrence of withdrawal emergent neurological signs but until further evidence becomes available, it seems reasonable to gradually withdraw use of ORAP.

Tardive Dyskinesia: ORAP may be associated with persistent dyskinesias. Tardive dyskinesia, a syndrome consisting of potentially irreversible, involuntary, dyskinetic movements, may appear in some patients on long-term therapy or may occur after drug therapy has been discontinued. The risk appears to be greater in elderly patients on high-dose therapy, especially females. The symptoms are persistent and in some patients appear irreversible. The syndrome is characterized by rhythmical involuntary movements of tongue, face, mouth or jaw (e.g., protrusion of tongue, puffing of cheeks, puckering of mouth, chewing movements). Sometimes these may be accompanied by involuntary movements of extremities and the trunk.

There is no known effective treatment for tardive dyskinesia; antiparkinson agents usually do not alleviate the symptoms of this syndrome. It is suggested that all antipsychotic agents be discontinued if these symptoms appear. Should it be necessary to reinstitute treatment, or increase the dosage of the agent, or switch to a different antipsychotic agent, this syndrome may be masked.

It has been reported that fine vermicular movement of the tongue may be an early sign of tardive dyskinesia and if the medication is stopped at that time the syndrome may not develop.

Electrocardiographic Changes: Electrocardiographic changes have been observed in clinical trials of ORAP In Tourette's Disorder and schizophrenia. These have included prolongation of the QT interval, flattening, notching and inversion of the T wave and the appearance of U waves. Sudden, unexpected deaths and grand mal seizure have occurred at doses above 20 mg/day.

Neuroleptic Malignant Syndrome: Neuroleptic malignant syndrome (NMS) has been reported with ORAP. (See WARNINGS for further information concerning NMS.)

Hyperpyrexia: Hyperpyrexia has been reported with other antipsychotic drugs.

Clinical Trials

The following adverse reaction tabulation was derived from 20 patients in a 6 week long placebo controlled clinical trial of ORAP in Tourette's Disorder.

Body System/ Adverse Reaction	Pimozide (N = 20)	Placebo N = 20
Body as a Whole		
Headache	1	2
Gastrointestinal		
Dry mouth	5	1
Diarrhea	1	0
Nausea	0	2
Vomiting	0	1
Constipation	4	2
Eructations	0	1
Thirsty	1	0
Appetite increase	1	0
Endocrine		
Menstrual disorder	0	1
Breast secretions	0	1
Musculoskeletal		
Muscle cramps	0	1
Muscle tightness	3	0
Stooped posture	2	0
CNS		
Drowsiness	7	3
Sedation	14	5
Insomnia	2	2
Dizziness	0	1
Akathisia	8	0
Rigidity	2	0
Speech disorder	2	0
Handwriting change	1	0
Akinesia	8	0

Continued on next page

Lemmon—Cont.

Psychiatric

Depression	2	3
Excitement	0	1
Nervous	1	0
Adverse behavior effect	5	0

Special Senses

Visual disturbance	4	0
Taste change	1	0
Sensitivity of eyes to light	1	0
Decreased accommodation	4	1
Spots before eyes	0	1

Urogenital

Impotence	3	0

Because clinical investigational experience with ORAP in Tourette's Disorder is limited, uncommon adverse reactions may not have been detected. The physician should consider that other adverse reactions associated with antipsychotics may occur.

Other Adverse Reactions
In addition to the adverse reactions listed above, those listed below have been reported in U.S. clinical trials of ORAP in conditions other than Tourette's Disorder.
Body as a Whole: Asthenia, chest pain, periorbital edema
Cardiovascular/Respiratory: Postural hypotension, hypotension, hypertension, tachycardia, palpitations
Gastrointestinal: Increased salivation, nausea, vomiting, anorexis, GI distress
Endocrine: Loss of libido
Metabolic/Nutritional: Weight gain, weight loss
Central Nervous System: Dizziness, tremor, parkinsonism, fainting, dyskinesia
Psychiatric: Excitement
Skin: Rash, sweating, skin irritation
Special Senses: Blurred vision, cataracts
Urogenital: Nocturia, urinary frequency

OVERDOSAGE
In general, the signs and symptoms of overdosage with ORAP (pimozide) would be an exaggeration of known pharmacologic effects and adverse reactions, the most prominent of which would be: 1) electrocardiographic abnormalities, 2) severe extrapyramidal reactions, 3) hypotension, 4) a comatose state with respiratory depression.
In the event of overdosage, gastric lavage, establishment of a patent airway and, if necessary, mechanically-assisted respiration are advised. Electrocardiographic monitoring should commence immediately and continue until the ECG parameters are within the normal range. Hypotension and circlatory collapse may be counteracted by use of intravenous fluids, plasma, or concentrated albumin, and vasopressor agents such as metaraminol, phenylephrine and norepinephrine. Epinephrine should not be used. In case of severe extrapyramidal reactions, antiparkinson medication should be administered. Because of the long half-life of pimozide, patients who take an overdose should be observed for at least 4 days. As with all drugs, the physician should consider contacting a poison control center for additional information on the treatment of overdose.

DOSAGE AND ADMINISTRATION
Reliable dose response data for the effects of ORAP (pimozide) on tic manifestations in Tourette's Disorder patients below the age of twelve are not available. Consequently, the suppression of tics by ORAP requires a slow and gradual introduction of the drug. The patient's dose should be carefully adjusted to a point where the suppression of tics and the relief afforded by the drug is balanced against the untoward side effects of the drug.
An ECG should be done at baseline and periodically thereafter especially during the period of dose adjustment (see WARNINGS and PRECAUTIONS-Laboratory Tests).
In general, treatment with ORAP should be initiated with a dose of 1 to 2 mg a day in divided doses. The dose may be increased thereafter every other day. Most patients are maintained at less than 0.2 mg/kg per day, or 10 mg/day, whichever is less. Doses greater than 0.2 mg/kg/day or 10 mg/day are not recommended.
Periodic attempts should be made to reduce the dosage of ORAP to see whether or not tics persist at the level and extent first identified. In attempts to reduce the dosage of ORAP, consideration should be given to the possibility that increases of tic intensity and frequency may represent a transient, withdrawal related phenomenon rather than a return of disease symptoms. Specifically, one to two weeks should be allowed to elapse before one concludes that an increase in tic manifestations is a function of the underlying disease syndrome rather than a response to drug withdrawal. A gradual withdrawal is recommended in any case.

ANIMAL PHARMACOLOGY
A chronic study in dogs indicated that pimozide caused gingival hyperplasia when administered for several months at about 5 times the maximum recommended human dose. This condition was reversible after withdrawal. This condition has not been observed following chronic administration of ORAP to man.

HOW SUPPLIED
ORAP™ (pimozide) 2 mg tablets, white, scored, imprinted "LEMMON" and "ORAP 2"—NDC 0093-0187-01, bottles of 100.
Dispense in tight, light-resistant containers as defined in the official compendium.
Shown in Product Identification Section, page 415

Lexis Pharmaceuticals, Inc.
100 CONGRESS AVENUE
SUITE 400
AUSTIN, TX 78701-4042

NDC #	PRODUCT	
3521/3528	**N.E.E. 1/35**™ (norethindrone 1 mg and ethinyl estradiol 35 mcg tablets USP)	℞
0521/0528	**N.E.E. .5/35**™ (norethindrone .5 mg and ethinyl estradiol 35 mcg tablets USP)	℞
5021/5028	**N.E.E. 1/50**™ (norethindrone 1 mg and ethinyl estradiol 50 mcg tablets USP)	℞
1021/1028	**N.E.E. 10/11**™	℞
7777	**Furonatal FA**™ **prenatal vitamin tablets**	℞

Vitamin A (as Acetate)	8000 IU
Vitamin C (as Ascorbic Acid)	90 mg
Thiamine (as Thiamine Mononitrate Vitamin B$_1$)	2.55 mg
Riboflavin	3 mg
Niacinamide	20 mg
Calcium (as Calcium Carbonate)	0.2 mg
Iron (as Ferrous Fumarate)	65 mg
Vitamin D$_2$	400 IU
E (as dl-Alpha Tocopheryl Acetate)	30 IU
Vitamin B$_6$ (as Pyridoxine Hydrochloride)	10 mg
Folic Acid	1 mg
Vitamin B$_{12}$ (Cyanocobalamin)	12 mcg
Iodine (as Potassium Iodide)	150 mcg
Magnesium (as Magnesium Oxide)	100 mg
Zinc (as Zinc Oxide)	25 mg

NDC #	PRODUCT	
3603	**Histamic**™ **capsules** (Phenylpropanolamine HCl 50 mg, Phenylephrine HCl 25 mg, Phenyltoloxamine Citrate 30 mg, Chlorpheniramine Maleate 12 mg)	℞
3002	**Span FF**® **ferrous fumarate capsules** 325 mg, (equivalent to 106 mg elemental iron))	OTC

Eli Lilly and Company
LILLY CORPORATE CENTER
INDIANAPOLIS, IN 46285

LEGEND

ADD-Vantage®—*Vials and Diluent Containers, Abbott*
Aspirol®—*Inhalant in an Ampoule, Lilly*
CP—*Convenience Pak, Lilly*
Disket®—*Dispersible Tablet, Lilly*
Enseal®—*Enteric-Release Tablet, Lilly*
Faspak®—*Flexible Plastic Bag, Lilly*
Gelseal®—*Filled Elastic Capsule, Lilly*
Identi-Code®—*Formula Identification Code, Lilly*
Identi-Dose®—*Unit Dose Medication, Lilly*
Pulvule®—*Filled Gelatin Capsule, Lilly*
Redi Vial®—*Dual Compartment Vial, Lilly*
℞Pak—*Prescription Package, Lilly*
Solvet®—*Soluble Tablet, Lilly*
Traypak™—*Multivial Carton, Lilly*

IDENTI-CODE® **Index**
(formula Identification code, Lilly)
Provides Positive Product Identification
A letter-number symbol, a 4-digit number, the name of the product, the strength of the product, or a combination of these appears on each Lilly capsule and most tablets and on each label of pediatric liquids, powders for oral suspension, and suppositories. The letter/number or 4-digit number identifies the product.

Identi-Code®	Product Name

A01-A33 (Enseals®**)**

A01	**Ammonium Chloride**	Composition (Each Enseal®): Ammonium Chloride, USP, 7½ grs (486 mg)
A02	**Ferrous Sulfate**	Composition (Each Enseal®): Ferrous Sulfate, USP, 5 grs (324 mg) (equiv. to 65 mg elemental iron), Red
A04	**Pancreatin**	Composition (Each Enseal®): Pancreatin, Triple Strength, equivalent to 1 g Pancreatin, USP
A05	**Potassium Chloride**	Composition (Each Enseal®): Potassium chloride, 300 mg
A06	**Potassium Iodide**	Composition (Each Enseal®): Potassium Iodide, USP, 300 mg
A09	**Sodium Chloride**	Composition (Each Enseal®): Sodium Chloride, USP, 15½ grs (1.004 g)
A10	**Sodium Salicylate**	Composition (Each Enseal®): Sodium Salicylate, USP, 5 grs (324 mg)
A11	**Sodium Salicylate**	Composition (Each Enseal®): Sodium Salicylate, USP, 10 grs (648 mg)
A14	**Thyroid**	Composition (Each Enseal®): Thyroid, USP, 30 mg
A15	**Thyroid**	Composition (Each Enseal®): Thyroid, USP, 60 mg
A22	**Diethylstilbestrol**	Composition (Each Enseal®): Diethylstilbestrol, USP, 1 mg
A25	**A.S.A.**®	Composition (Each Enseal®): Aspirin, USP, 5 grs (324 mg)
A26	**Ox Bile Extract**	Composition (Each Enseal®): Ox bile extract, 5 grs (324 mg)
A31	**Potassium Chloride**	Composition (Each Enseal®): Potassium chloride, 1 g
A32	**A.S.A.**®	Composition (Each Enseal®): Aspirin, USP, 10 grs (648 mg)
A33	**Diethylstilbestrol**	Composition (Each Enseal®): Diethylstilbestrol, USP, 5 mg

C06-C71 (Coated Tablets)

C06	**Cascara**	Composition (Each Coated Tablet): Cascara, USP, 5 grs (324 mg)

C13 Ferrous Sulfate
Composition (Each Coated Tablet): Ferrous Sulfate, USP, 5 grs (324 mg) (equiv. to 65 mg elemental iron)

C27 V-Cillin K®
Composition (Each Coated Tablet): Penicillin V Potassium, USP, 125 mg

C29 V-Cillin K®
Composition (Each Coated Tablet): Penicillin V Potassium, USP, 250 mg

C36 Quinine Sulfate
Composition (Each Coated Tablet): Quinine Sulfate, USP, 5 grs (324 mg)

C46 V-Cillin K®
Composition (Each Coated Tablet): Penicillin V Potassium, USP, 500 mg

C47 Hepicebrin®
Composition (Each Coated Tablet): Vitamin A acetate, 5000 IU (1.5 mg); vitamin D (as ergocalciferol), 400 IU (10 mcg); ascorbic acid (vitamin C), 75 mg; thiamine mononitrate (vitamin B₁), 2 mg; riboflavin (vitamin B₂), 3 mg; niacinamide, 20 mg (USP)

C51 Darvocet-N® 50
Composition (Each Coated Tablet): Propoxyphene napsylate, 50 mg; acetaminophen, 325 mg (USP)

C53 Darvon-N®
Composition (Each Coated Tablet): Propoxyphene Napsylate, USP, 100 mg

C54 Darvon-N® with A.S.A.®
Composition (Each Coated Tablet): Propoxyphene napsylate, 100 mg; aspirin, 325 mg (USP)

C63 Darvocet-N® 100
Composition (Each Coated Tablet): Propoxyphene napsylate, 100 mg; acetaminophen, 650 mg (USP)

C71 Multicebrin®
Composition (Each Coated Tablet): Thiamine (vitamin B₁), 3 mg; riboflavin (vitamin B₂), 3 mg; pyridoxine (vitamin B₆), 1.2 mg; pantothenic acid, 5 mg; niacinamide, 25 mg; vitamin B₁₂ (activity equivalent), 3 mcg; ascorbic acid (vitamin C), 75 mg; dl-alpha tocopheryl acetate (vitamin E), 6.6 IU (6.6 mg); vitamin A, 10,000 IU (3 mg); vitamin D, 400 IU (10 mcg)

F03-H72 (Pulvules®)

F03 Zentinic®
Composition (Each Pulvule®): Iron, elemental (as ferrous fumarate), 100 mg; folic acid, 0.05 mg; thiamine mononitrate (vitamin B₁), 7.5 mg; riboflavin (vitamin B₂), 7.5 mg; pyridoxine hydrochloride (vitamin B₆), 7.5 mg; vitamin B₁₂ (activity equivalent), 50 mcg; pantothenic acid (as calcium pantothenate), 15 mg; niacinamide, 30 mg; ascorbic acid (vitamin C), 200 mg

F04 Seromycin®
Composition (Each Pulvule®): Cycloserine, USP, 250 mg

F11 A.S.A.®
Composition (Each Pulvule®): Aspirin, USP, 5 grs (324 mg), Clear

F14 Ephedrine and Amytal®
Composition (Each Pulvule®): Ephedrine sulfate, 25 mg; amobarbital, 50 mg

F15 Lextron®
Composition (Each Pulvule®): Liver-stomach concentrate (as intrinsic powder), 50 mg; iron, elemental (as iron and ammonium citrates green), 30 mg; vitamin B₁₂ (activity equivalent), 2 mcg; thiamine hydrochloride (vitamin B₁), 1 mg; riboflavin (vitamin B₂), 0.25 mg; with other factors of vitamin B complex present in the liver-stomach concentrate

F16 Lextron® Ferrous
Composition (Each Pulvule®): Liver-stomach concentrate (as intrinsic powder), 50 mg; iron, elemental (as ferrous sulfate), 35 mg; vitamin B₁₂ (activity equivalent), 2 mcg; thiamine hydrochloride (vitamin B₁), 1 mg; riboflavin (vitamin B₂), 0.25 mg; with other factors of vitamin B complex present in the liver-stomach concentrate

F19 Extralin®
Composition (Each Pulvule®): Liver-stomach concentrate (as intrinsic powder), 50 mg

F23 Amytal® Sodium
Composition (Each Pulvule®): Amobarbital Sodium, USP, 65 mg

F24 Ephedrine Sulfate
Composition (Each Pulvule®): Ephedrine Sulfate, USP, 25 mg

F25 Ephedrine Sulfate
Composition (Each Pulvule®): Ephedrine Sulfate, USP, 50 mg

F26 Quinine Sulfate
Composition (Each Pulvule®): Quinine Sulfate, USP, 2 grs (130 mg)

F27 Quinine Sulfate
Composition (Each Pulvule®): Quinine Sulfate, USP, 3 grs (194 mg)

F29 Quinine Sulfate
Composition (Each Pulvule®): Quinine Sulfate, USP, 5 grs (324 mg)

F31 Acidulin®
Composition (Each Pulvule®): Glutamic acid hydrochloride, 340 mg

F33 Amytal® Sodium
Composition (Each Pulvule®): Amobarbital Sodium, USP, 200 mg

F34 Carbarsone
Composition (Each Pulvule®): Carbarsone, USP, 250 mg

F36 Copavin®
Composition (Each Pulvule®): Codeine sulfate, 15 mg; papaverine hydrochloride, 15 mg

F39 Quinidine Sulfate
Composition (Each Pulvule®): Quinidine Sulfate, USP, 200 mg

F40 Seconal® Sodium
Composition (Each Pulvule®): Secobarbital Sodium, USP, 100 mg

F41 Bilron®
Composition (Each Pulvule®): Iron bile salts, 300 mg

F42 Seconal® Sodium
Composition (Each Pulvule®): Secobarbital Sodium, USP, 50 mg

F43 Vitamin B Complex (Betalin® Compound)
Composition (Each Pulvule®): Thiamine (vitamin B₁), 1 mg; riboflavin (vitamin B₂), 2 mg; pyridoxine (vitamin B₆), 0.4 mg; pantothenic acid, 3.333 mg; niacinamide, 10 mg; vitamin B₁₂ (activity equivalent), 1 mcg

F44 Ferrous Gluconate
Composition (Each Pulvule®): Ferrous Gluconate, USP, 5 grs (324 mg)

F52 Dibasic Calcium Phosphate with Vitamin D
Composition (Each Pulvule®): Dibasic calcium phosphate, anhydrous, equivalent to 500 mg of dibasic calcium phosphate dihydrate; vitamin D synthetic, 33 IU (0.825 mcg)

F56 Calcium Gluconate with Vitamin D
Composition (Each Pulvule®): Calcium gluconate, 325 mg; vitamin D synthetic, 0.825 mcg

F61 Bilron®
Composition (Each Pulvule®): Iron bile salts, 150 mg

F64 Tuinal®
Composition (Each Pulvule®): Secobarbital sodium, 25 mg; amobarbital sodium, 25 mg (USP)

F65 Tuinal®
Composition (Each Pulvule®): Secobarbital sodium, 50 mg; amobarbital sodium, 50 mg (USP)

F66 Tuinal®
Composition (Each Pulvule®): Secobarbital sodium, 100 mg; amobarbital sodium, 100 mg (USP)

F72 Seconal® Sodium
Composition (Each Pulvule®): Secobarbital Sodium, USP, 30 mg

F74 Tycopan®
Composition: Three Pulvules® contain thiamine mononitrate (vitamin B₁), 10 mg; riboflavin (vitamin B₂), 8 mg; pyridoxine hydrochloride (vitamin B₆), 10 mg; pantothenic acid (as calcium pantothenate), 60 mg; niacinamide, 60 mg; vitamin B₁₂ (activity equivalent), 15 mcg; ascorbic acid (vitamin C), 200 mg; dl-alpha tocopheryl acetate (vitamin E), 22 IU (22 mg); biotin, 0.16 mg; folic acid, 0.45 mg; aminobenzoic acid, 33 mg; inositol, 160 mg; choline (as choline bitartrate), 160 mg; lipoic acid, 0.3 mg; vitamin A synthetic, 20,000 IU (6 mg); vitamin D synthetic, 1000 IU (25 mg)

F96 Reticulex®
Composition (Each Pulvule®): Liver-stomach concentrate (as intrinsic powder), 222 mg; vitamin B₁₂ (activity equivalent), 10 mcg; iron, elemental (as ferrous sulfate), 75 mg; ascorbic acid (vitamin C), 50 mg; folic acid, 0.3 mg

H02 Darvon®
Composition (Each Pulvule®): Propoxyphene Hydrochloride, USP, 32 mg

H03 Darvon®
Composition (Each Pulvule®): Propoxyphene Hydrochloride, USP, 65 mg

H04 Darvon® with A.S.A.®
Composition (Each Pulvule®): Propoxyphene hydrochloride, 65 mg; aspirin, 325 mg

H10 En-Cebrin® F
Composition (Each Pulvule®): Vitamin A synthetic, 4000 IU (1.2 mg); thiamine mononitrate (vitamin B₁), 3 mg; riboflavin (vitamin B₂), 2 mg; niacinamide, 10 mg; pyridoxine hydrochloride (vitamin B₆), 2 mg; folic acid, 1 mg; vitamin B₁₂ (activity equivalent), 5 mcg; pantothenic acid (as calcium pantothenate), 5 mg; ascorbic acid (vitamin C), 50 mg; vitamin D synthetic, 400 IU (10 mcg); calcium (as the carbonate), 250 mg; iron (as ferrous fumarate), 30 mg; iodine (as potassium iodide), 0.15 mg; copper (as the sulfate), 1 mg; magnesium (as the hydroxide), 5 mg; manganese (as the glycerophosphate), 1 mg; zinc (as the chloride), 1.5 mg

H12 En-Cebrin®
Composition (Each Pulvule®): Vitamin A, 4000 IU (1.2 mg); thiamine mononitrate (vitamin B₁), 3 mg; riboflavin (vitamin B₂), 2 mg; niacinamide, 10 mg; pyridoxine (vitamin B₆), 1.7 mg; vitamin B₁₂ (activity equivalent), 5 mcg; pantothenic acid, 5 mg; ascorbic acid (vitamin C), 50 mg; vitamin D, 400 IU (10 mcg); calcium (as the carbonate), 250 mg; iron (as ferrous fumarate), 30 mg; iodine (as potassium iodide), 0.15 mg; copper (as the sulfate), 1 mg; magnesium (as the hydroxide), 5 mg; manganese (as the glycerophosphate), 1 mg; zinc (as the chloride), 1.5 mg

H17 Aventyl® HCl
Composition (Each Pulvule®): Nortriptyline Hydrochloride, USP, 10 mg (equiv. to base)

H19 Aventyl® HCl
Composition (Each Pulvule®): Nortriptyline Hydrochloride, USP, 25 mg (equiv. to base)

H72 Theracebrin®
Composition (Each Pulvule®): Thiamine (as the mononitrate) (vitamin B₁), 15 mg; riboflavin (vitamin B₂), 10 mg; pyridoxine (as the hydrochloride) (vitamin B₆), 2.5 mg; pantothenic acid (as d-calcium pantothenate), 20 mg; niacinamide, 150 mg; vitamin B₁₂ (activity equivalent), 10 mcg; ascorbic acid (vitamin C), 150 mg; dl-alpha tocopheryl acetate (vitamin E), 18.5 IU (18.5 mg); vitamin A synthetic, 25,000 IU (7.5 mg); vitamin D synthetic, 1500 IU (37.5 mcg)

3061 Ceclor®
Composition (Each Pulvule®): Cefaclor, USP, 250 mg

3062 Ceclor®
Composition (Each Pulvule®): Cefaclor, USP, 500 mg

3075 Histadyl® and A.S.A.®
Composition (Each Pulvule®): Chlorpheniramine maleate, 4 mg; aspirin, 325 mg

3101 Cesamet®
Composition (Each Pulvule®): Nabilone, 1 mg

3110 Darvon® Compound
Composition (Each Pulvule®): Propoxyphene hydrochloride, 32 mg; aspirin, 389 mg; caffeine, 32.4 mg

3111 Darvon® Compound-65
Composition (Each Pulvule®): Propoxyphene hydrochloride, 65 mg; aspirin, 389 mg; caffeine, 32.4 mg

3113 A.S.A.® and Codeine Compound, No. 3
Composition (Each Pulvule®): Codeine phosphate, 30 mg; aspirin, 380 mg; caffeine, 30 mg

3125 Vancocin®
Composition (Each Pulvule®): Vancomycin hydrochloride, 125 mg

3126 Vancocin®
Composition (Each Pulvule®): Vancomycin hydrochloride, 250 mg

3144 Axid®
Composition (Each Pulvule®): Nizatidine, 150 mg

3145 Axid®
Composition (Each Pulvule®): Nizatidine, 300 mg

Continued on next page

* Identi-Code® symbol.

Lilly—Cont.

J02-J96 (Compressed Tablets)

J02 **Atropine Sulfate**
Composition (Each Compressed Tablet): Atropine Sulfate, USP, 0.4 mg

J03 **Belladonna Extract**
Composition (Each Compressed Tablet): Belladonna Extract, USP, 15 mg (¼ gr) (total alkaloids, 0.187 mg)

J05 **Citrated Caffeine**
Composition (Each Compressed Tablet): Citrated caffeine, 1 gr (64.8 mg)

J09 **Codeine Sulfate**
Composition (Each Compressed Tablet): Codeine Sulfate, USP, 15 mg

J10 **Codeine Sulfate**
Composition (Each Compressed Tablet): Codeine Sulfate, USP, 30 mg

J11 **Codeine Sulfate**
Composition (Each Compressed Tablet): Codeine Sulfate, USP, 60 mg

J13 **Colchicine**
Composition (Each Compressed Tablet): Colchicine, USP, 0.6 mg

J20 **Quinidine Sulfate**
Composition (Each Compressed Tablet): Quinidine Sulfate, USP, 200 mg

J23 **Soda Mint**
Composition (Each Compressed Tablet): Sodium bicarbonate, 5 grs; oil peppermint

J24 **Sodium Bicarbonate**
Composition (Each Compressed Tablet): Sodium Bicarbonate, USP, 5 grs (324 mg)

J25 **Thyroid**
Composition (Each Compressed Tablet): Thyroid, USP, 60 mg

J26 **Thyroid**
Composition (Each Compressed Tablet): Thyroid, USP, 120 mg

J29 **Thyroid**
Composition (Each Compressed Tablet): Thyroid, USP, 30 mg

J31 **Phenobarbital**
Composition (Each Compressed Tablet): Phenobarbital, USP, 15 mg

J32 **Phenobarbital**
Composition (Each Compressed Tablet): Phenobarbital, USP, 30 mg

J33 **Phenobarbital**
Composition (Each Compressed Tablet): Phenobarbital, USP, 100 mg

J36 **Ergotrate® Maleate**
Composition (Each Compressed Tablet): Ergonovine Maleate, USP, 0.2 mg

J37 **Phenobarbital**
Composition (Each Compressed Tablet): Phenobarbital, USP, 60 mg

J41 **Niacin**
Composition (Each Compressed Tablet): Niacin, USP, 20 mg

J42 **Niacin**
Composition (Each Compressed Tablet): Niacin, USP, 100 mg

J43 **Niacin**
Composition (Each Compressed Tablet): Niacin, USP, 50 mg

J45 **Pyridoxine Hydrochloride (Hexa-Betalin®)**
Composition (Each Compressed Tablet): Pyridoxine Hydrochloride, USP, 25 mg

J46 **Niacinamide**
Composition (Each Compressed Tablet): Niacinamide, USP, 50 mg

J47 **Riboflavin**
Composition (Each Compressed Tablet): Riboflavin, USP, 5 mg

J52 **Diethylstilbestrol**
Composition (Each Compressed Tablet): Diethylstilbestrol, USP, 1 mg

J54 **Diethylstilbestrol**
Composition (Each Compressed Tablet): Diethylstilbestrol, USP, 5 mg

J60 **Crystodigin®**
Composition (Each Compressed Tablet): Digitoxin, USP, 0.1 mg

J61 **Papaverine Hydrochloride**
Composition (Each Compressed Tablet): Papaverine Hydrochloride, USP, 30 mg

J62 **Papaverine Hydrochloride**
Composition (Each Compressed Tablet): Papaverine Hydrochloride, USP, 60 mg

J63 **Riboflavin**
Composition (Each Compressed Tablet): Riboflavin, USP, 10 mg

J64 **Dolophine® Hydrochloride**
Composition (Each Compressed Tablet): Methadone Hydrochloride, USP, 5 mg

J69 **Propylthiouracil**
Composition (Each Compressed Tablet): Propylthiouracil, USP, 50 mg

J72 **Dolophine® Hydrochloride**
Composition (Each Compressed Tablet): Methadone Hydrochloride, USP, 10 mg

J73 **Methyltestosterone**
Composition (Each Compressed Tablet): Methyltestosterone, USP, 10 mg

J74 **Methyltestosterone**
Composition (Each Compressed Tablet): Methyltestosterone, USP, 25 mg

J75 **Crystodigin®**
Composition (Each Compressed Tablet): Digitoxin, USP, 0.05 mg

J76 **Crystodigin®**
Composition (Each Compressed Tablet): Digitoxin, USP, 0.15 mg

J94 **Tapazole®**
Composition (Each Compressed Tablet): Methimazole, USP, 5 mg

J95 **Tapazole®**
Composition (Each Compressed Tablet): Methimazole, USP, 10 mg

J96 **Tylosterone®**
Composition (Each Compressed Tablet): Diethylstilbestrol, 0.25 mg; methyltestosterone, 5 mg

S11 (Suppositories)

S11 **Seconal® Sodium**
Composition (Each Suppository): Secobarbital sodium, 200 mg

T01-U56 (Compressed Tablets)

T01 **Zentron® Chewable**
Composition (Each Compressed Tablet): Iron, elemental (as ferrous fumarate), 20 mg; thiamine mononitrate (vitamin B_1), 1 mg; riboflavin (vitamin B_2), 1 mg; pyridoxine hydrochloride (vitamin B_6), 1 mg; cyanocobalamin (vitamin B_{12} crystalline), 5 mcg; pantothenic acid (as panthenol), 1 mg; niacinamide, 5 mg; ascorbic acid (vitamin C), 100 mg

T05 **A.S.A.®**
Composition (Each Compressed Tablet): Aspirin, USP, 5 grs (324 mg)

T13 **Calcium Lactate**
Composition (Each Compressed Tablet): Calcium Lactate, USP, 5 grs (324 mg)

T14 **Calcium Lactate**
Composition (Each Compressed Tablet): Calcium Lactate, USP, 10 grs (648 mg)

T23 **Sodium Chloride**
Composition (Each Compressed Tablet): Sodium Chloride, USP, 2.25 g

T24 **Sodium Chloride**
Composition (Each Compressed Tablet): Sodium Chloride, USP, 1 g

T26 **Pancreatin**
Composition (Each Compressed Tablet): Pancreatin, Single Strength, equivalent to 325 mg Pancreatin, USP

T29 **Sodium Bicarbonate**
Composition (Each Compressed Tablet): Sodium Bicarbonate, USP, 10 grs (648 mg)

T32 **Amytal®**
Composition (Each Compressed Tablet): Amobarbital, USP, 100 mg

T35 **Calcium Carbonate**
Composition (Each Compressed Tablet): Calcium Carbonate, USP, Aromatic, 10 grs (648 mg)

T36 **Calcium Gluconate**
Composition (Each Compressed Tablet): Calcium Gluconate, USP, 1 g

T37 **Amytal®**
Composition (Each Compressed Tablet): Amobarbital, USP, 50 mg

T39 **Calcium Gluconate**
Composition (Each Compressed Tablet): Calcium Gluconate, USP, 7½ grs (486 mg)

T44 **Calcium Gluconate with Vitamin D**
Composition (Each Compressed Tablet): Calcium gluconate, 1 g; vitamin D synthetic, 1.65 mcg

T45 **Vitamin C (Cevalin®)**
Composition (Each Compressed Tablet): Ascorbic Acid, USP, 100 mg

T46 **Sulfapyridine**
Composition (Each Compressed Tablet): Sulfapyridine, USP, 0.5 g

T52 **Thiamine Hydrochloride (Betalin® S)**
Composition (Each Compressed Tablet): Thiamine Hydrochloride, USP, 10 mg

T53 **Niacinamide**
Composition (Each Compressed Tablet): Niacinamide, USP, 100 mg

T54 **Sulfadiazine**
Composition (Each Compressed Tablet): Sulfadiazine, USP, 0.5 g

T55 **Papaverine Hydrochloride**
Composition (Each Compressed Tablet): Papaverine Hydrochloride, USP, 100 mg

T56 **Amytal®**
Composition (Each Compressed Tablet): Amobarbital, USP, 30 mg

T59 **Thiamine Hydrochloride (Betalin® S)**
Composition (Each Compressed Tablet): Thiamine Hydrochloride, USP, 25 mg

T60 **Vitamin C (Cevalin®)**
Composition (Each Compressed Tablet): Ascorbic Acid, USP, 250 mg

T61 **Dibasic Calcium Phosphate**
Composition (Each Compressed Tablet): Dibasic calcium phosphate, anhydrous, equivalent to 7½ grs (486 mg) of dibasic calcium phosphate dihydrate (USP)

T62 **Thiamine Hydrochloride (Betalin® S)**
Composition (Each Compressed Tablet): Thiamine Hydrochloride, USP, 50 mg

T63 **Thiamine Hydrochloride (Betalin® S)**
Composition (Each Compressed Tablet): Thiamine Hydrochloride, USP, 100 mg

T67 **Vitamin C (Cevalin®)**
Composition (Each Compressed Tablet): Ascorbic Acid, USP, 500 mg

T72 **Pyridoxine Hydrochloride (Hexa-Betalin®)**
Composition (Each Compressed Tablet): Pyridoxine Hydrochloride, USP, 50 mg

T73 **Papaverine Hydrochloride**
Composition (Each Compressed Tablet): Papaverine Hydrochloride, USP, 200 mg

T75 **Neotrizine®**
Composition (Each Compressed Tablet): Sulfadiazine, 167 mg; sulfamerazine, 167 mg sulfamethazine, 167 mg (USP)

T93 **Isoniazid**
Composition (Each Compressed Tablet): Isoniazid, USP, 100 mg

T96 **Neomycin Sulfate**
Composition (Each Compressed Tablet): Neomycin Sulfate, USP, 500 mg (equiv. to 350 mg base)

T99 **Haldrone®**
Composition (Each Compressed Tablet): Paramethasone Acetate, USP, 1 mg

U01 **Haldrone®**
Composition (Each Compressed Tablet): Paramethasone Acetate, USP, 2 mg

U03 **Dymelor®**
Composition (Each Compressed Tablet): Acetohexamide, USP, 250 mg

U07 **Dymelor®**
Composition (Each Compressed Tablet): Acetohexamide, USP, 500 mg

U09 **Anhydron®**
Composition (Each Compressed Tablet): Cyclothiazide, USP, 2 mg

U23 **Isoniazid**
Composition (Each Compressed Tablet): Isoniazid, USP, 300 mg

U29 **Reserpine (Sandril®)**
Composition (Each Compressed Tablet): Reserpine, USP, 0.25 mg

U53 **Methadone Hydrochloride**
Composition (Each Disket®): Methadone Hydrochloride, USP, 40 mg

U56 **Folic Acid**
Composition (Each Compressed Tablet): Folic Acid, USP, 1 mg

4067 **A.S.A.® and Codeine Compound, No. 3**
Composition (Each Compressed Tablet): Codeine phosphate, 30 mg; aspirin, 80 mg; caffeine, 30 mg

4131 **Permax®**
Composition (Each Compressed Tablet): Pergolide mesylate, 0.05 mg

4133 **Permax®**
Composition (Each Compressed Tablet): Pergolide mesylate, 0.25 mg

4135 **Permax®**
Composition (Each Compressed Tablet): Pergolide mesylate, 1 mg

W07-W16 (Miscellaneous)

W07   **V-Cillin K®, for Oral Solution**
Composition (When Mixed as Directed): Each 5 ml contain penicillin V potassium equivalent to penicillin V, 125 mg (USP).

W16   **V-Cillin K®, for Oral Solution**
Composition (When Mixed as Directed): Each 5 ml contain penicillin V potassium equivalent to penicillin V, 250 mg (USP).

5057   **Ceclor®, for Oral Suspension**
Composition (When Mixed as Directed): Each 5 ml contain cefaclor, 125 mg (USP).

5058   **Ceclor®, for Oral Suspension**
Composition (When Mixed as Directed): Each 5 ml contain cefaclor, 250 mg (USP).

UNIT-DOSE PACKAGING

Identi-Dose® (unit dose medication, Lilly)
Reverse-Numbered Package
Closed-circuit control of medication from pharmacy to nurse to patient and return. Simplifies counting and dispensing whether in single-unit or prescription-size quantities. Fits into any dispensing system for ready identification and legibility, better inventory control, protection from contamination, easier handling and recording under Medicare, prevention of drug loss through pilferage or spilling, better control of Federal Controlled Substances, and less chance of medication errors.

The following products are available through normal channels of supply:

Identi-Dose® (ID100)
Pulvules®
No.

ℭ 240	Seconal® Sodium, 100 mg
ℭ 365	Darvon®, 65 mg
ℭ 369	Darvon® Compound-65
387	Aventyl® HCl, 10 mg
389	Aventyl® HCl, 25 mg
3061	Ceclor®, 250 mg
3062	Ceclor®, 500 mg

Tablets
No.

100	Multicebrin®
186	A.S.A.®, 5 grs
1125	Quinidine Sulfate, USP, 200 mg
ℭ 1544	Phenobarbital, USP, 15 mg
ℭ 1545	Phenobarbital, USP, 30 mg
1572	Ergotrate® Maleate, 0.2 mg
1803	Neomycin Sulfate, USP, 500 mg
1842	Dymelor®, 250 mg
1843	Dymelor®, 500 mg, Yellow
ℭ 1883	Darvon-N®, 100 mg
ℭ 1890	Darvocet-N® 50
ℭ 1893	Darvocet-N® 100

Reverse-Numbered Package (RN500)
Pulvules®
No.

ℭ 365	Darvon®, 65 mg

Tablets
No.

ℭ 1893	Darvocet-N® 100

Single-Cut Identi-Dose® (ID500)
Tablets
No.

ℭ 1893	Darvocet-N® 100

ℭ, ℭ, ℭ Federal Controlled Substances.

AXID®   ℞
[ake′sid]
(nizatidine capsules)
PULVULES®

DESCRIPTION

Axid® (Nizatidine, Lilly) is a histamine H_2-receptor antagonist. Chemically, it is N-[2-[[[2-[(dimethylamino)methyl]-4-thiazolyl]methyl]thio]-ethyl]-N′-methyl-2-nitro-1,1-ethenediamine.
The structural formula is as follows:

Nizatidine

Nizatidine has the empirical formula $C_{12}H_{21}N_5O_2S_2$ representing a molecular weight of 331.46. It is an off-white to buff crystalline solid that is soluble in water. Each Pulvule®

(capsule) contains for oral administration gelatin, pregelatinized starch, silicone, starch, titanium dioxide, yellow iron oxide, 150 mg or 300 mg of nizatidine, and other inactive ingredients. The 150-mg Pulvule also contains magnesium stearate, and the 300-mg Pulvule also contains carboxymethylcellulose sodium, povidone, red iron oxide, and talc.

CLINICAL PHARMACOLOGY

Axid® (Nizatidine, Lilly) is a competitive, reversible inhibitor of histamine at the histamine H_2 receptors, particularly those in the gastric parietal cells.
Antisecretory Activity—1. Effects on Acid Secretion: Axid significantly inhibited nocturnal gastric acid secretion for up to 12 hours. Axid also significantly inhibited gastric acid secretion stimulated by food, caffeine, betazole, and pentagastrin (Table 1).

Table 1
Effect of Oral Axid on Gastric Acid Secretion

	Time After Dose (h)	% Inhibition of Gastric Acid Output by Dose (mg)				
		20–50	75	100	150	300
Nocturnal	Up to 10	57		73		90
Betazole	Up to 3		93		100	99
Pentagastrin	Up to 6		25		64	67
Meal	Up to 4	41	64		98	97
Caffeine	Up to 3		73		85	96

2. Effects on Other Gastrointestinal Secretions—Pepsin: Oral administration of 75 to 300 mg of Axid did not affect pepsin activity in gastric secretions. Total pepsin output was reduced in proportion to the reduced volume of gastric secretions.
Intrinsic Factor: Oral administration of 75 to 300 mg of Axid increased betazole-stimulated secretion of intrinsic factor.
Serum Gastrin: Axid had no effect on basal serum gastrin. No rebound of gastrin secretion was observed when food was ingested 12 hours after administration of Axid.
3. Other Pharmacologic Actions—
a. Hormones: Axid was not shown to affect the serum concentrations of gonadotropins, prolactin, growth hormone, antidiuretic hormone, cortisol, triiodothyronine, thyroxin, testosterone, 5α-dihydrotestosterone, androstenedione, or estradiol.
b. Axid had no demonstrable antiandrogenic action.
4. Pharmacokinetics—The absolute oral bioavailability of nizatidine exceeds 90%. Peak plasma concentrations (700 to 1,800 µg/L for a 150-mg dose and 1,400 to 3,600 µg/L for a 300-mg dose) occur from 0.5 to 3 hours following the dose. A concentration of 1,000 µg/L is equivalent to 3 µmol/L; a dose of 300 mg is equivalent to 905 µmoles. Plasma concentrations 12 hours after administration are less than 10 µg/L. The elimination half-life is 1 to 2 hours, plasma clearance is 40 to 60 L/h, and the volume of distribution is 0.8 to 1.5 L/kg. Because of the short half-life and rapid clearance of nizatidine, accumulation of the drug would not be expected in individuals with normal renal function who take either 300 mg once daily at bedtime or 150 mg twice daily. Axid exhibits dose proportionality over the recommended dose range.
The oral bioavailability of nizatidine is unaffected by concomitant ingestion of propantheline. Antacids consisting of aluminum and magnesium hydroxides with simethicone decrease the absorption of nizatidine by about 10%. With food the AUC and C_{max} increase by approximately 10%.
In humans, less than 7% of an oral dose is metabolized as N2-monodesmethylnizatidine, an H_2-receptor antagonist, which is the principal metabolite excreted in the urine. Other likely metabolites are the N2-oxide (less than 5% of the dose) and the S-oxide (less than 6% of the dose).
More than 90% of an oral dose of nizatidine is excreted in the urine within 12 hours. About 60% of an oral dose is excreted as unchanged drug. Renal clearance is about 500 mL/min,

Table 2
Healing Response of Ulcers to Axid® (Nizatidine, Lilly)

	Axid				Placebo	
	300 mg h.s.		150 mg b.i.d.			
	Number Entered	Healed/ Evaluable	Number Entered	Healed/ Evaluable	Number Entered	Healed/ Evaluable
STUDY 1						
Week 2			276	93/265 (35%)*	279	55/260 (21%)
Week 4				198/259 (76%)*		95/243 (39%)
STUDY 2						
Week 2	108	24/103 (23%)*	106	27/101 (27%)*	101	9/93 (10%)
Week 4		65/97 (67%)*		66/97 (68%)*		24/84 (29%)
STUDY 3						
Week 2	92	22/90 (24%)†			98	13/92 (14%)
Week 4		52/85 (61%)*				29/88 (33%)
Week 8		68/83 (82%)*				39/79 (49%)

* $P < 0.01$ as compared with placebo.
† $P < 0.05$ as compared with placebo.

which indicates excretion by active tubular secretion. Less than 6% of an administered dose is eliminated in the feces. Moderate to severe renal impairment significantly prolongs the half-life and decreases the clearance of nizatidine. In individuals who are functionally anephric, the half-life is 3.5 to 11 hours, and the plasma clearance is 7 to 14 L/h. To avoid accumulation of the drug in individuals with clinically significant renal impairment, the amount and/or frequency of doses of Axid should be reduced in proportion to the severity of dysfunction (see Dosage and Administration).
Approximately 35% of nizatidine is bound to plasma protein, mainly to $α_1$-acid glycoprotein. Warfarin, diazepam, acetaminophen, propantheline, phenobarbital, and propranolol did not affect plasma protein binding of nizatidine in vitro.
Clinical Trials—1. Active Duodenal Ulcer: In multicenter, double-blind, placebo-controlled studies in the United States, endoscopically diagnosed duodenal ulcers healed more rapidly following administration of Axid, 300 mg h.s. or 150 mg b.i.d., than with placebo (Table 2). Lower doses, such as 100 mg h.s., had slightly lower effectiveness.
[See table above.]
2. Maintenance of Healed Duodenal Ulcer:
Treatment with a reduced dose of Axid has been shown to be effective as maintenance therapy following healing of active duodenal ulcers. In multicenter, double-blind, placebo-controlled studies, 150 mg of Axid taken at bedtime resulted in a significantly lower incidence of duodenal ulcer recurrence in patients treated for up to 1 year (Table 3).

Table 3
Percentage of Ulcers Recurring by 3, 6, and 12 Months in
Double-Blind Studies Conducted in the United States

Month	Axid, 150 mg h.s.	Placebo
3	13% (28/208)*	40% (82/204)
6	24% (45/188)*	57% (106/187)
12	34% (57/166)*	64% (112/175)

* $P < 0.001$ as compared with placebo.

INDICATIONS AND USAGE

Axid® (Nizatidine, Lilly) is indicated for up to 8 weeks for the treatment of active duodenal ulcer. In most patients, the ulcer will heal within 4 weeks.
Axid is indicated for maintenance therapy for duodenal ulcer patients, at a reduced dosage of 150 mg h.s. after healing of an active duodenal ulcer. The consequences of continuous therapy with Axid for longer than 1 year are not known.

CONTRAINDICATION

Axid® (Nizatidine, Lilly) is contraindicated in patients with known hypersensitivity to the drug and should be used with caution in patients with hypersensitivity to other H_2-receptor antagonists.

PRECAUTIONS

General—1. Symptomatic response to nizatidine therapy does not preclude the presence of gastric malignancy.
2. Because nizatidine is excreted primarily by the kidney, dosage should be reduced in patients with moderate to severe renal insufficiency (see Dosage and Administration).
3. Pharmacokinetic studies in patients with hepatorenal syndrome have not been done. Part of the dose of nizatidine is metabolized in the liver. In patients with normal renal function and uncomplicated hepatic dysfunction, the disposition of nizatidine is similar to that in normal subjects.
Laboratory Tests—False-positive tests for urobilinogen with Multistix® may occur during therapy with nizatidine.
Drug Interactions—No interactions have been observed between Axid® (Nizatidine, Lilly) and theophylline, chlordiazepoxide, lorazepam, lidocaine, phenytoin, and warfarin. Axid does not inhibit the cytochrome P-450-linked drug-me-

Continued on next page

---

* Identi-Code® symbol.

Lilly—Cont.

tabolizing enzyme system; therefore, drug interactions mediated by inhibition of hepatic metabolism are not expected to occur. In patients given very high doses (3,900 mg) of aspirin daily, increases in serum salicylate levels were seen when nizatidine, 150 mg b.i.d., was administered concurrently.

Carcinogenesis, Mutagenesis, Impairment of Fertility—A 2-year oral carcinogenicity study in rats with doses as high as 500 mg/kg/day (about 80 times the recommended daily therapeutic dose) showed no evidence of a carcinogenic effect. There was a dose-related increase in the density of enterochromaffin-like (ECL) cells in the gastric oxyntic mucosa. In a 2-year study in mice, there was no evidence of a carcinogenic effect in male mice, although hyperplastic nodules of the liver were increased in the high-dose males as compared with placebo. Female mice given the high dose of Axid (2,000 mg/kg/day, about 330 times the human dose) showed marginally statistically significant increases in hepatic carcinoma and hepatic nodular hyperplasia with no numerical increase seen in any of the other dose groups. The rate of hepatic carcinoma in the high-dose animals was within the historical control limits seen for the strain of mice used. The female mice were given a dose larger than the maximum tolerated dose, as indicated by excessive (30%) weight decrement as compared with concurrent controls and evidence of mild liver injury (transaminase elevations). The occurrence of a marginal finding at high dose only in animals given an excessive and somewhat hepatotoxic dose, with no evidence of a carcinogenic effect in rats, male mice, and female mice (given up to 360 mg/kg/day, about 60 times the human dose), and a negative mutagenicity battery is not considered evidence of a carcinogenic potential for Axid.

Axid was not mutagenic in a battery of tests performed to evaluate its potential genetic toxicity, including bacterial mutation tests, unscheduled DNA synthesis, sister chromatid exchange, the mouse lymphoma assay, chromosome aberration tests, and a micronucleus test.

In a 2-generation, perinatal and postnatal fertility study in rats, doses of nizatidine up to 650 mg/kg/day produced no adverse effects on the reproductive performance of parental animals or their progeny.

Pregnancy—Teratogenic Effects—Pregnancy Category C—Oral reproduction studies in rats at doses up to 300 times the human dose and in Dutch Belted rabbits at doses up to 55 times the human dose revealed no evidence of impaired fertility or teratogenic effect; but, at a dose equivalent to 300 times the human dose, treated rabbits had abortions, decreased number of live fetuses, and depressed fetal weights. On intravenous administration to pregnant New Zealand White rabbits, nizatidine at 20 mg/kg produced cardiac enlargement, coarctation of the aortic arch, and cutaneous edema in 1 fetus, and at 50 mg/kg it produced ventricular anomaly, distended abdomen, spina bifida, hydrocephaly, and enlarged heart in 1 fetus. There are, however, no adequate and well-controlled studies in pregnant women. It is also not known whether nizatidine can cause fetal harm when administered to a pregnant woman or can affect reproduction capacity. Nizatidine should be used during pregnancy only if the potential benefit justifies the potential risk to the fetus.

Nursing Mothers—Studies conducted in lactating women have shown that 0.1% of the administered oral dose of nizatidine is secreted in human milk in proportion to plasma concentrations. Because of the growth depression in pups reared by lactating rats treated with nizatidine, a decision should be made whether to discontinue nursing or discontinue the drug, taking into account the importance of the drug to the mother.

Pediatric Use—Safety and effectiveness in children have not been established.

Use in Elderly Patients—Ulcer healing rates in elderly patients are similar to those in younger age groups. The incidence rates of adverse events and laboratory test abnormalities are also similar to those seen in other age groups. Age alone may not be an important factor in the disposition of nizatidine. Elderly patients may have reduced renal function (*see* Dosage and Administration).

ADVERSE REACTIONS

Clinical trials of nizatidine included almost 5,000 patients given nizatidine in studies of varying durations. Domestic placebo-controlled trials included over 1,900 patients given nizatidine and over 1,300 given placebo. Among the more common adverse events in the domestic placebo-controlled trials, sweating (1% vs 0.2%), urticaria (0.5% vs <0.01%), and somnolence (2.4% vs 1.3%) were significantly more common in the nizatidine group. A variety of less common events were also reported; it was not possible to determine whether these were caused by nizatidine.

Hepatic—Hepatocellular injury, evidenced by elevated liver enzyme tests (SGOT [AST], SGPT [ALT], or alkaline phosphatase), occurred in some patients and was possibly or probably related to nizatidine. In some cases there was marked elevation of SGOT/SGPT enzymes (greater than 500 IU/L)

and in a single instance SGPT was greater than 2,000 IU/L. The overall rate of occurrences of elevated liver enzymes and elevations to 3 times the upper limit of normal, however, did not significantly differ from the rate of liver enzyme abnormalities in placebo-treated patients. All abnormalities were reversible after discontinuation of Axid® (Nizatidine, Lilly).

Cardiovascular—In clinical pharmacology studies, short episodes of asymptomatic ventricular tachycardia occurred in 2 individuals administered Axid and in 3 untreated subjects.

CNS—Rare cases of reversible mental confusion have been reported.

Endocrine—Clinical pharmacology studies and controlled clinical trials showed no evidence of antiandrogenic activity due to Axid. Impotence and decreased libido were reported with equal frequency by patients who received Axid and by those given placebo. Rare reports of gynecomastia occurred.

Hematologic—Fatal thrombocytopenia was reported in a patient who was treated with Axid and another H_2-receptor antagonist. On previous occasions, this patient had experienced thrombocytopenia while taking other drugs. Rare cases of thrombocytopenic purpura have been reported.

Integumental—Sweating and urticaria were reported significantly more frequently in nizatidine- than in placebo-treated patients. Rash and exfoliative dermatitis were also reported.

Hypersensitivity—As with other H_2-receptor antagonists, rare cases of anaphylaxis following administration of nizatidine have been reported. Because cross-sensitivity in this class of compounds has been observed, H_2-receptor antagonists should not be administered to individuals with a history of previous hypersensitivity to these agents. Rare episodes of hypersensitivity reactions (eg, bronchospasm, laryngeal edema, rash, and eosinophilia) have been reported.

Other—Hyperuricemia unassociated with gout or nephrolithiasis was reported. Eosinophilia, fever, and nausea related to nizatidine administration have been reported.

OVERDOSAGE

Overdoses of Axid® (Nizatidine, Lilly) have been reported rarely. The following is provided to serve as a guide should such an overdose be encountered.

Signs and Symptoms—There is little clinical experience with overdosage of Axid in humans. Test animals that received large doses of nizatidine have exhibited cholinergic-type effects, including lacrimation, salivation, emesis, miosis, and diarrhea. Single oral doses of 800 mg/kg in dogs and of 1,200 mg/kg in monkeys were not lethal. Intravenous median lethal doses in the rat and mouse were 301 mg/kg and 232 mg/kg respectively.

Treatment—To obtain up-to-date information about the treatment of overdose, a good resource is your certified Regional Poison Control Center. Telephone numbers of certified poison control centers are listed in the *Physicians' Desk Reference (PDR)*. In managing overdosage, consider the possibility of multiple drug overdoses, interaction among drugs, and unusual drug kinetics in your patient.

If overdosage occurs, use of activated charcoal, emesis, or lavage should be considered along with clinical monitoring and supportive therapy. Renal dialysis for 4 to 6 hours increased plasma clearance by approximately 84%.

DOSAGE AND ADMINISTRATION

Active Duodenal Ulcer—The recommended oral dosage for adults is 300 mg once daily at bedtime. An alternative dosage regimen is 150 mg twice daily.

Maintenance of Healed Duodenal Ulcer—The recommended oral dosage for adults is 150 mg once daily at bedtime.

Dosage Adjustment for Patients With Moderate to Severe Renal Insufficiency—The dose for patients with renal dysfunction should be reduced as follows:

Active Duodenal Ulcer

Ccr	Dose
20–50 mL/min	150 mg daily
<20 mL/min	150 mg every other day

Maintenance Therapy

Ccr	Dose
20–50 mL/min	150 mg every other day
<20 mL/min	150 mg every 3 days

Some elderly patients may have creatinine clearances of less than 50 mL/min, and, based on pharmacokinetic data in patients with renal impairment, the dose for such patients should be reduced accordingly. The clinical effects of this dosage reduction in patients with renal failure have not been evaluated.

HOW SUPPLIED

℞Pulvules*:
150 mg, pale yellow and dark yellow (No. 3144)—(CP†-30s)
  NDC 0002-3144-85; (Rx Pak‡ of 60) NDC 0002-3144-60

300 mg, pale yellow and peach (No. 3145)—(CP-30s) NDC 0002-3145-85; (Rx Pak of 30) NDC 0002-3145-30

* Pulvules® (filled gelatin capsules, Lilly)
† CP (convenience pak)
‡Rx Pak (prescription package, Lilly)
Store at controlled room temperature, 59° to 86°F (15° to 30°C).

[032389]

Shown in Product Identification Section, page 415

BREVITAL® SODIUM　　　　　　　　℞
[*brĕv'ĭ-tăl sō'dĭ-ŭm*]
(methohexital sodium)
For Injection, USP
For Intravenous Use

> **WARNING**
> This drug should be administered by persons qualified in the use of intravenous anesthetics. Cardiac life support equipment must be immediately available during use of methohexital.

DESCRIPTION

Brevital® Sodium (Methohexital Sodium for Injection, USP, Lilly) is 2,4,6 (1H,3H,5H)-Pyrimidinetrione, 1-methyl-5-(1-methyl-2-pentynyl)-5-(2-propenyl)-(±)-, monosodium salt.

Methohexital sodium for injection is a freeze-dried, sterile, nonpyrogenic mixture of methohexital sodium and anhydrous sodium carbonate added as a buffer, which is prepared from an aqueous solution of methohexital, sodium hydroxide, and sodium carbonate. It contains not less than 90% and not more than 110% of the labeled amount of $C_{14}H_{17}N_2NaO_3$. This mixture is ordinarily intended to be reconstituted so as to contain 1% methohexital sodium in Sterile Water for Injection for direct intravenous injection or 0.2% methohexital sodium in 5% dextrose injection (or 0.9% sodium chloride injection) for administration by continuous intravenous drip. The pH of the 1% solution is between 10 and 11; the pH of the 0.2% solution in 5% dextrose is between 9.5 and 10.5

Methohexital sodium is a rapid, ultrashort-acting barbiturate anesthetic. It occurs as a white, crystalline powder that is freely soluble in water.

CLINICAL PHARMACOLOGY

Compared with thiamylal and thiopental, methohexital is at least twice as potent on a weight basis, and its duration of action is only about half as long. Although the metabolic fate of methohexital in the body is not clear, the drug does not appear to concentrate in fat depots to the extent that other barbiturate anesthetics do. Thus, cumulative effects are fewer and recovery is more rapid with methohexital than with thiobarbiturates. In experimental animals, the drug cannot be detected in the blood 24 hours after administration.

Methohexital differs chemically from the established barbiturate anesthetics in that it contains no sulfur. Little analgesia is conferred by barbiturates; their use in the presence of pain may result in excitation.

Intravenous administration of methohexital results in rapid uptake by the brain (within 30 seconds) and rapid induction of sleep. With single doses, the rate of redistribution determines duration of pharmacologic effect. Metabolism occurs in the liver through demethylation and oxidation. Side-chain oxidation is the most important biotransformation involved in terminatin of biologic activity. Excretion occurs via the kidneys through glomerular filtration.

INDICATIONS AND USAGE

Brevital® Sodium (Methohexital Sodium for Injection, USP, Lilly) can be used as follows:

1. For intravenous induction of anesthesia prior to the use of other general anesthetic agents.
2. For intravenous induction of anesthesia and as an adjunct to subpotent inhalational anesthetic agents (such as nitrous oxide in oxygen) for short surgical procedures; Brevital Sodium may be given by infusion or intermittent injection.
3. For use along with other parental agents, usually narcotic analgesics, to supplement subpotent inhalational anesthetic agents (such as nitrous oxide in oxygen) for longer surgical procedures.
4. As intravenous anesthesia for short surgical, diagnostic, or therapeutic procedures associated with minimal painful stimuli (*see* Precautions).
5. As an agent for inducing a hypnotic state.

CONTRAINDICATIONS

Brevital® Sodium (Methohexital Sodium for Injection, USP, Lilly) is contraindicated in patients in whom general anesthesia is contraindicated, in those with latent or manifest porphyria, or in patients with a known hypersensitivity to barbiturates.

WARNINGS

See boxed Warning.

AS WITH ALL POTENT ANESTHETIC AGENTS AND ADJUNCTS, THIS DRUG SHOULD BE ADMINISTERED ONLY BY THOSE TRAINED IN THE ADMINISTRATION OF GENERAL ANESTHESIA, THE MAINTENANCE OF A PATENT AIRWAY AND VENTILATION, AND THE MANAGEMENT OF CARDIOVASCULAR DEPRESSION ENCOUNTERED DURING ANESTHESIA AND SURGERY.

Because the liver is involved in demethylation and oxidation of methohexital and because barbiturates may enhance preexisting circulatory depression, severe hepatic dysfunction, severe cardiovascular instability, or a shock-like condition may be reason for selecting another induction agent. Psychomotor seizures may be elicited in susceptible individuals.

Prolonged administration may result in cumulative effects, including extended somnolence, protracted unconsciousness, and respiratory and cardiovascular depression. Respiratory depression in the presence of an impaired airway may lead to hypoxia, cardiac arrest, and death.

The CNS-depressant effect of Brevital® Sodium (Methohexital Sodium for Injection, USP, Lilly) may be additive with that of other CNS depressants, including ethyl alcohol and propylene glycol.

DANGER OF INTRA-ARTERIAL INJECTION—Unintended intra-arterial injection of barbiturate solutions may be followed by the production of platelet aggregates and thrombosis, starting in arterioles distal to the site of injection. The resulting necrosis may lead to gangrene, which may require amputation. The first sign in conscious patients may be a complaint of fiery burning that roughly follows the distribution path of the injected artery; if noted, the injection should be stopped immediately and the situation reevaluated. Transient blanching may or may not be noted very early; blotchy cyanosis and dark discoloration may then be the first sign in anesthetized patients. There is no established treatment other than prevention. The following should be considered prior to injection.

1. The extent of injury is related to concentration. Concentrations of 1% methohexital will usually suffice; higher concentrations should ordinarily be avoided.
2. Check the infusion to ensure that the catheter is in the lumen of a vein before injection. Injection through a running intravenous infusion may enhance the possibility of detecting arterial placement; however, it should be remembered that the characteristic bright-red color of arterial blood is often altered by contact with drugs. The possibility of aberrant arteries should always be considered.

Postinjury arterial injection of vasodilators and/or arterial infusion of parenteral fluids are generally regarded to be of no value in altering outcome. Animal experiments and published individual case reports concerned with a variety of arteriolar irritants, including barbiturates, suggest that one or more of the following may be of benefit in reducing the area of necrosis:

1. Arterial injection of heparin at the site of injury, followed by systemic anticoagulation.
2. Sympathetic blockade (or brachial plexus blockade in the arm).
3. Intra-arterial glucocorticoid injection at the site of injury, followed by systemic steroids.
4. A recent case report (nonbarbiturate injury) suggests that intra-arterial urokinase may promote fibrinolysis, even if administered late in treatment.

If extravasation is noted during injection of methohexital, the injection should be discontinued until the situation is remedied. Local irritation may result from extravasation; subcutaneous swelling may also serve as a sign of arterial or periarterial placement of the catheter.

PRECAUTIONS

General—Maintenance of a patent airway and adequacy of ventilation must be ensured during induction and maintenance of anesthesia with methohexital sodium solution. Laryngospasm is common during induction with all barbiturates and may be due to a combination of secretions and accentuated reflexes following induction or may result from painful stimuli during light anesthesia. Transient apnea may be noted during induction, which may impair pulmonary ventilation; the duration of apnea may be longer than that produced by other barbiturate anesthetics. Cardiorespiratory arrest may occur. Intravenous administration of Brevital® Sodium (Methohexital Sodium for Injection, USP, Lilly) is often associated with hiccups, coughing, and/or muscle twitching, which may also impair pulmonary ventilation.

Following induction, temporary hypotension and tachycardia may occur.

Recovery from methohexital anesthesia is rapid and smooth. The incidence of postoperative nausea and vomiting is low if the drug is administered to fasting patients. Postanesthetic shivering has occurred in a few instances.

The usual precautions taken with any barbiturate anesthetic should be observed with Brevital Sodium. The drug

Preparation of Solutions of Brevital® Sodium (Methohexital Sodium for Injection, USP)

Preparation of Solution—FOLLOW DILUTING INSTRUCTIONS EXACTLY.
Diluents—DO NOT USE DILUENTS CONTAINING BACTERIOSTATS.
Sterile Water for Injection is the preferred diluent.
Dextrose Injection (5%) or Sodium Chloride Injection (0.9%) may be used.
(Brevital Sodium is not compatible with Lactated Ringer's Injection.)
Dilution Instructions—For a 1% solution (10 mg/mL), contents of vials should be diluted as follows:
  Vials No. 660 (500 mg)—add 50 mL of diluent
  Vials No. 760 (500 mg)—add 50 mL of accompanying diluent
  Vials No. 664 (2.5 g)—add 250 mL of diluent
  Vials No. 662 (5 g)—add 500 mL of diluent

Vial No.	Amount of Diluent to Be Added to the Vial	For 1% Solution Dilute to
663 (2.5 g)	15 mL	250 mL
659 (5 g)	30 mL	500 mL

When the first dilution is made with Vials No. 663 or No. 659, the solution in the vial will be yellow. When further diluted to make a 1% solution, it must be *clear and colorless* or should not be used.

should be used with caution in patients with asthma, obstructive pulmonary disease, severe hypertension or hypotension, myocardial disease, congestive heart failure, severe anemia, or extreme obesity.

Methohexital sodium should be used with extreme caution in patients in status asthmaticus.

Caution should be exercised in debilitated patients or in those with impaired function of respiratory, circulatory, renal, hepatic, or endocrine systems.

Information for Patients—When appropriate, patients should be instructed as to the hazards of drowsiness that may follow use of Brevital® Sodium (Methohexital Sodium for Injection, USP, Lilly). Outpatients should be released in the company of another individual, and no skilled activities, such as operating machinery or driving a motor vehicle, should be engaged in for 8 to 12 hours.

Laboratory Tests—BSP and liver function studies may be influenced by administration of a single dose of barbiturates.

Drug Interactions—Barbiturates may influence the absorption and elimination of other concomitantly used drugs, such as diphenylhydantoin, halothane, anticoagulants, corticosteroids, ethyl alcohol, and propylene glycol-containing solutions.

Carcinogenesis, Mutagenesis, Impairment of Fertility—Studies of Brevital Sodium in animals to evaluate the carcinogenic and mutagenic potential or the effect on fertility have not been conducted.

Usage in Pregnancy—Pregnancy Category B—Reproduction studies have been performed in rabbits and rats at doses up to 4 and 7 times the human dose respectively and have revealed no evidence of impaired fertility or harm to the fetus due to methohexital sodium. There are, however, no adequate and well-controlled studies in pregnant women. Because animal reproduction studies are not always predictive of human response, this drug should be used during pregnancy only if clearly needed.

Labor and Delivery—Brevital Sodium has been used in cesarean section delivery but, because of its solubility and lack of protein binding, it readily and rapidly traverses the placenta.

Nursing Mothers—Caution should be exercised when Brevital Sodium is administered to a nursing woman.

Usage in Children—Safety and effectiveness in children have not been established.

ADVERSE REACTIONS

Side effects associated with Brevital® Sodium (Methohexital Sodium for Injection, USP, Lilly) are extensions of pharmacologic effects and include:

Cardiovascular—Circulatory depression, thrombophlebitis, hypotension, peripheral vascular collapse, and convulsions in association with cardiorespiratory arrest

Respiratory—Respiratory depression (including apnea), cardiorespiratory arrest, laryngospasm, bronchospasm, hiccups, and dyspnea

Neurologic—Skeletal muscle hyperactivity (twitching), injury to nerves adjacent to injection site, and seizures

Psychiatric—Emergence delirium, restlessness, and anxiety may occur, especially in the presence of postoperative pain

Gastrointestinal—Nausea, emesis, and abdominal pain

Allergic—Erythema, pruritus, and urticaria

Other—Other adverse reactions include pain at injection site, salivation, headache, and rhinitis

DRUG ABUSE AND DEPENDENCE

Controlled Substance—Brevital® Sodium (Methohexital Sodium for Injection, USP, Lilly) is a Schedule IV drug. Brevital Sodium may be habit-forming.

OVERDOSAGE

Signs and Symptoms—The onset of toxicity following an overdose of intravenously administered methohexital will be within seconds of the infusion. If methohexital is administered rectally or is ingested, the onset of toxicity may be delayed. The manifestations of an ultrashort-acting barbitu-

rate in overdose include central nervous system depression, respiratory depression, hypotension, loss of peripheral vascular resistance, and muscular hyperactivity ranging from twitching to convulsive-like movements. Other findings may include convulsions and allergic reactions. An acute allergic reaction to methohexital may include erythema, pruritus, urticaria, rhinitis, dyspnea, hypotension, anxiety, abdominal pain, and peripheral vascular collapse. Following massive exposure to any barbiturate, pulmonary edema, circulatory collapse with loss of peripheral vascular tone, and cardiac arrest may occur.

Treatment—To obtain up-to-date information about the treatment of overdose, a good resource is your certified Regional Poison Control Center. Telephone numbers of certified poison control centers are listed in the *Physicians' Desk Reference (PDR)*. In managing overdosage, consider the possibility of multiple drug overdoses, interaction among drugs, and unusual drug kinetics in your patient.

Establish an airway and ensure oxygenation and ventilation. Resuscitative measures should be initiated promptly. For hypotension, intravenous fluids should be administered and the patient's legs raised. If desirable increase in blood pressure is not obtained, vasopressor and/or inotropic drugs may be used as dictated by the clinical situation.

For convulsions, diazepam intravenously and phenytoin may be required. If the seizures are refractory to diazepam and phenytoin, general anesthesia and paralysis with a neuromuscular blocking agent may be necessary.

Protect the patient's airway and support ventilation and perfusion. Meticulously monitor and maintain, within acceptable limits, the patient's vital signs, blood gases, serum electrolytes, etc. Absorption of drugs from the gastrointestinal tract may be decreased by giving activated charcoal, which, in many cases, is more effective than emesis or lavage; consider charcoal instead of or in addition to gastric emptying. Repeated doses of charcoal over time may hasten elimination of some drugs that have been absorbed. Safeguard the patient's airway when employing gastric emptying or charcoal.

DOSAGE AND ADMINISTRATION

Preanesthetic medication is generally advisable. Brevital® Sodium (Methohexital Sodium for Injection, USP, Lilly) may be used with any of the recognized preanesthetic medications, but the phenothiazines are less satisfactory than the combination of an opiate and a belladonna derivative. Facilities for assisting respiration and administering oxygen are necessary adjuncts for intravenous anesthesia. Since cardiorespiratory arrest may occur, patients should be observed carefully during and after the use of Brevital Sodium. Resuscitative equipment (ie, intubation and cardioversion equipment, oxygen, suction, and a secure intravenous line) and personnel qualified in its use must be immediately available.

[See table above].

For continuous drip anesthesia, prepare a 0.2% solution by adding 500 mg of Brevital Sodium to 250 mL of diluent. For this dilution, either 5% glucose solution or isotonic (0.9%) sodium chloride solution is recommended instead of distilled water in order to avoid extreme hypotonicity.

Administration—Brevital® Sodium (Methohexital Sodium for Injection, USP, Lilly) is administered intravenously in a concentration of no higher than 1%. Higher concentrations markedly increase the incidence of muscular movements and irregularities in respiration and blood pressure. Dosage is highly individualized; the drug should be administered only by those completely familiar with its quantitative differences from other barbiturate anesthetics.

Continued on next page

* Identi-Code® symbol.

Lilly—Cont.

Brevital Sodium may be dissolved in Sterile Water for Injection, 5% Dextrose Injection, or Sodium Chloride Injection. For induction of anesthesia, a 1% solution is administered at a rate of about 1 mL/5 seconds. Gaseous anesthetics and/or skeletal muscle relaxants may be administered concomitantly. The dose required for induction may range from 50 to 120 mg or more but averages about 70 mg. The induction dose usually provides anesthesia for 5 to 7 minutes.

The usual dosage in adults ranges from 1 to 1.5 mg/kg. Data on dosage requirements in children are not available.

Maintenance of anesthesia may be accomplished by intermittent injections of the 1% solution or, more easily, by continuous intravenous drip of a 0.2% solution. Intermittent injections of about 20 to 40 mg (2 to 4 mL of a 1% solution) may be given as required, usually every 4 to 7 minutes. For continuous drip, the average rate of administration is about 3 mL of a 0.2% solution/minute (1 drop/second). The rate of flow must be individualized for each patient. For longer surgical procedures, gradual reduction in the rate of administration is recommended (see discussion of prolonged administration in Warnings). Other parenteral agents, usually narcotic analgesics, are ordinarily employed along with Brevital Sodium during longer procedures.

Parenteral drug products should be inspected visually for particulate matter and discoloration prior to administration, whenever solution and container permit.

COMPATIBILITY INFORMATION

Solutions of Brevital® Sodium (Methohexital Sodium for Injection, USP, Lilly) should not be mixed in the same syringe or administered simultaneously during intravenous infusion through the same needle with acid solutions, such as atropine sulfate, Metubine® Iodide (Metocurine Iodide Injection, USP, Lilly), and succinylcholine chloride. Alteration of pH may cause free barbituric acid to be precipitated. Solubility of the soluble sodium salts of barbiturates, including Brevital Sodium, is maintained only at a relatively high (basic) pH.

Because of numerous requests from anesthesiologists for information regarding the chemical compatibility of these mixtures, the following chart contains information obtained from compatibility studies in which a 1% solution of Brevital Sodium was mixed with therapeutic amounts of agents whose solutions have a low (acid) pH.

[See table below].

Solutions of Brevital Sodium are incompatible with silicone and should not be allowed to come in contact with rubber stoppers or parts of disposable syringes that have been treated with silicone.

HOW SUPPLIED

Storage—Brevital Sodium is stable in Sterile Water for Injection at room temperature 77°F (25°C or below) for at least *6 weeks.* Solutions may be stored and used as long as they remain clear and colorless. Five percent Dextrose Injection or isotonic (0.9%) Sodium Chloride Injection may be used as diluents, but the resulting solutions are not stable for much more than *24 hours.*

The vials may be stored at room temperature, 77°F (25°C or below). The expiration period for the vials is 2 years.

(C) *Vials* Brevital® Sodium (Methohexital Sodium for Injection, USP)* are supplied as follows:

500 mg (with 30 mg anhydrous sodium carbonate), 50-mL size, multiple dose (No. 660)—(1s) NDC 0002-1446-01; (25s) NDC 0002-1446-25

500 mg (with 30 mg anhydrous sodium carbonate), 50-mL size, multiple dose, with one 50-mL vial Sterile Water for Injection (No. 760)—(1s) NDC 0002-1465-01

2.5 g (with 150 mg anhydrous sodium carbonate) (No. 663)—(1s) NDC 0002-1448-01; (25s), NDC 0002-1448-25

2.5 g (with 150 mg anhydrous sodium carbonate), 250-mL size, multiple dose (No. 664)—(1s) NDC 0002-1449-01; (25s) NDC 0002-1449-25

5 g (with 300 mg anhydrous sodium carbonate) (No. 659)—(1s) NDC 0002-1445-01

5 g (with 300 mg anhydrous sodium carbonate), 500-mL size, multiple dose (No. 662)—(1s) NDC 0002-1447-01; (25s) NDC 0002-1447-25

* In crystalline form.

[102388]

CAPASTAT® SULFATE   ℞
[kăp 'a-stăt sŭl 'făt]
(capreomycin sulfate)
Sterile, USP
Not for Pediatric Use

Warnings
The use of Capastat® Sulfate (Sterile Capreomycin Sulfate, USP, Lilly) in patients with renal insufficiency or preexisting auditory impairment must be undertaken with great caution, and the risk of additional 8th-nerve impairment or renal injury should be weighed against the benefits to be derived from therapy.
Refer to animal pharmacology section for additional information.
Since other parenteral antituberculosis agents (streptomycin, viomycin) also have similar and sometimes irreversible toxic effects, particularly on 8th-cranial-nerve and renal function, simultaneous administration of these agents with Capastat Sulfate is not recommended. Use with nonantituberculosis drugs (polymyxin A sulfate, colistin sulfate, amikacin, gentamicin, tobramycin, vancomycin, kanamycin, and neomycin) having ototoxic or nephrotoxic potential should be undertaken only with great caution.
Usage in Pregnancy—The safety of the use of Capastat Sulfate in pregnancy has not been determined.
Pediatric Usage—Safety of the use of Capastat Sulfate in infants and children has not been established.

DESCRIPTION

Capastat® Sulfate (Sterile Capreomycin Sulfate, USP, Lilly) is a polypeptide antibiotic isolated from *Streptomyces capreolus.* It is a complex of 4 microbiologically active components, which have been characterized in part; however, complete structural determination of all the components has not been established.

Capreomycin is supplied as the disulfate salt and is soluble in water. In complete solution, it is almost colorless.

Each vial contains the equivalent of 1 g capreomycin activity.

CLINICAL PHARMACOLOGY

Human Pharmacology—Capreomycin is not absorbed in significant quantities from the gastrointestinal tract and must be administered parenterally. In 2 studies of 10 patients each, peak serum concentrations following 1 g of capreomycin given intramuscularly were achieved 1 to 2 hours after administration, and average peak levels reached were 28 and 32 mg/L, respectively (range, 20 to 47 mg/L). Low serum concentrations were present at 24 hours. However, 1 g of capreomycin daily for 30 days or more produced no significant accumulation in subjects with normal renal function. Two patients with marked reduction of renal function had high serum concentrations 24 hours after administration of the drug. When a 1-g dose of capreomycin was given intramuscularly to normal volunteers, 52% was excreted in the urine within 12 hours.

Paper chromatographic studies indicated that capreomycin is excreted essentially unaltered. Urine concentrations averaged 1.68 mg/mL (average urine volume, 228 mL) during the 6 hours following a 1-g dose.

Microbiology—Capreomycin is active against human strains of *Mycobacterium tuberculosis.*

Susceptibility Tests—The susceptibility of strains of *M tuberculosis* in vitro varies with the media and techniques employed. In general, the minimum inhibitory concentrations for *M tuberculosis* are lowest in liquid media that are free of egg protein (7H10 or Dubos) and range from 1 to 5 mg/L

when the indirect method is used. Comparable inhibitory concentrations are obtained when 7H10 agar is used for direct susceptibility testing. When indirect susceptibility tests are performed on standard tube slants with 7H10 media, susceptible strains are inhibited by 10 to 25 mg/L. Egg-containing media, such as Löwenstein-Jensen or ATS, require concentrations of 25 to 50 mg/L to inhibit susceptible strains.

Cross-Resistance—Frequent cross-resistance occurs between capreomycin and viomycin. Varying degrees of cross-resistance between capreomycin and kanamycin and neomycin have been reported. No cross-resistance has been observed between capreomycin and isoniazid, aminosalicylic acid, cycloserine, streptomycin, ethionamide, or ethambutol.

INDICATIONS AND USAGE

Capastat® Sulfate (Sterile Capreomycin Sulfate, USP, Lilly), which is to be used concomitantly with other appropriate antituberculosis agents, is indicated in pulmonary infections caused by capreomycin-susceptible strains of *M tuberculosis* when the primary agents (isoniazid, rifampin, ethambutol, aminosalicylic acid, and streptomycin) have been ineffective or cannot be used because of toxicity or the presence of resistant tubercle bacilli.

Susceptibility studies should be performed to determine the presence of a capreomycin-susceptible strain of *M tuberculosis.*

CONTRAINDICATION

Capastat® Sulfate (Sterile Capreomycin Sulfate, USP, Lilly) is contraindicated in those patients who are hypersensitive to it.

PRECAUTIONS

General—Audiometric measurements and assessment of vestibular function should be performed prior to initiation of therapy with capreomycin and at regular intervals during treatment.

Renal injury, with tubular necrosis, elevation of the blood urea nitrogen (BUN) or serum creatinine, and abnormal urinary sediment, has been noted. Slight elevation of the BUN and serum creatinine has been observed in a significant number of patients receiving prolonged therapy. The appearance of casts, red cells, and white cells in the urine has been noted in a high percentage of these cases. Elevation of the BUN above 30 mg/100 mL or any other evidence of decreasing renal function with or without a rise in BUN levels calls for careful evaluation of the patient, and the dosage should be reduced or the drug completely withdrawn. The clinical significance of abnormal urine sediment and slight elevation in the BUN (or serum creatinine) observed during long-term therapy with Capastat® Sulfate (Sterile Capreomycin Sulfate, USP, Lilly) has not been established.

The peripheral neuromuscular blocking action that has been attributed to other polypeptide antibiotics (colistin sulfate, polymyxin A sulfate, paromomycin, and viomycin) and to aminoglycoside antibiotics (streptomycin, dihydrostreptomycin, neomycin, and kanamycin) has been studied with Capastat Sulfate. A partial neuromuscular blockade was demonstrated after large intravenous doses of Capastat Sulfate. This action was enhanced by ether anesthesia (as has been reported for neomycin) and was antagonized by neostigmine.

Caution should be exercised in the administration of antibiotics, including Capastat Sulfate, to any patient who has demonstrated some form of allergy, particularly to drugs.

Laboratory Tests—Regular tests of renal function should be made throughout the period of treatment, and reduced dosage should be employed in patients with known or suspected renal impairment.

Renal function studies should be made both before therapy with Capastat Sulfate is started and on a weekly basis during treatment.

Since hypokalemia may occur during therapy, serum potassium levels should be determined frequently.

Drug Interactions—For neuromuscular blocking action of this drug, see Precautions, General.

Carcinogenesis, Mutagenesis, Impairment of Fertility—Studies have not been performed to determine potential for carcinogenicity, mutagenicity, or impairment of fertility.

Usage in Pregnancy—Pregnancy Category C—Capastat Sulfate has been shown to be teratogenic in rats when given in does 3½ times the human dose. There are no adequate and well-controlled studies in pregnant women. Capastat Sulfate should be used during pregnancy only if the potential benefit justifies the potential risk to the fetus (see boxed Warnings and Animal Pharmacology).

Nursing Mothers—It is not known whether this drug is excreted in human milk. Because many drugs are excreted in human milk, caution should be exercised when Capastat Sulfate is administered to a nursing woman.

Pediatric Use—Safety and effectiveness in children have not been established (see boxed Warnings).

ADVERSE REACTIONS

Nephrotoxicity—In 36% of 722 patients treated with Capastat® Sulfate (Sterile Capreomycin Sulfate, USP, Lilly),

---

Compatibility of Brevital® Sodium (Methohexital Sodium for Injection, USP) with Solutions Having a Low pH

Active Ingredient	Potency per mL	Volume Used	Physical Change			
			Immediate	15 min	30 min	1 h
BREVITAL SODIUM	10 mg	10 mL		CONTROL		
Atropine sulfate	1/150 gr	1 mL	None	Haze		
Atropine sulfate	1/100 gr	1 mL	None	Ppt	Ppt	
Succinylcholine chloride	0.5 mg	4 mL	None	None	Haze	
Succinylcholine chloride	1 mg	4 mL	None	None	Haze	
Metocurine iodide	0.5 mg	4 mL	None	None	Ppt	
Metocurine iodide	1 mg	4 mL	None	None	Ppt	
Scopolamine hydrobromide	1/120 gr	1 mL	None	None	None	Haze
Tubocurarine chloride	3 mg	4 mL	None	Haze		

elevation of the BUN above 20 mg/100 mL has been observed. In many instances, there was also depression of PSP excretion and abnormal urine sediment. In 10% of this series, the BUN elevation exceeded 30 mg/100 mL.

Toxic nephritis was reported in 1 patient with tuberculosis and portal cirrhosis who was treated with Capastat Sulfate (1 g) and aminosalicylic acid daily for 1 month. This patient developed renal insufficiency and oliguria and died. Autopsy showed subsiding acute tubular necrosis.

Electrolyte disturbances resembling Bartter's syndrome have been reported in 1 patient.

Ototoxicity—Subclinical auditory loss was noted in approximately 11% of 722 patients undergoing treatment with Capastat Sulfate. This was a 5- to 10-decibel loss in the 4,000 to 8,000-CPS range. Clinically apparent hearing loss occurred in 3% of the 722 subjects. Some audiometric changes were reversible. Other cases with permanent loss were not progressive following withdrawal of Capastat Sulfate. Tinnitus and vertigo have occurred.

Liver—Serial tests of liver function have demonstrated a decrease in BSP excretion without change in SGOT or SGPT in the presence of preexisting liver disease. Abnormal results in liver function tests have occurred in many persons receiving Capastat Sulfate in combination with other antituberculosis agents that also are known to cause changes in hepatic function. The role of Capastat Sulfate in producing these abnormalities is not clear; however, periodic determinations of liver function are recommended.

Blood—Leukocytosis and leukopenia have been observed. The majority of patients treated have had eosinophilia exceeding 5% while receiving daily injections of Capastat Sulfate. This has subsided with reduction of the dosage of Capastat Sulfate to 2 or 3 g weekly.

Pain and induration at the injection sites have been observed. Excessive bleeding at the injection site has been reported. Sterile abscesses have been noted. Rare cases of thrombocytopenia have been reported.

Hypersensitivity—Urticaria and maculopapular skin rashes associated in some cases with febrile reactions have been reported when Capastat Sulfate and other antituberculosis drugs were given concomitantly.

OVERDOSAGE

Signs and Symptoms—Nephrotoxicity following the parenteral administration of Capastat® Sulfate (Sterile Capreomycin Sulfate, USP, Lilly) is most closely related to the area under the curve of the serum concentration versus time graph. The elderly patient, patients with abnormal renal function or dehydration, and patients receiving other nephrotoxic drugs are at much greater risk for developing acute tubular necrosis.

Damage to the auditory and vestibular divisions of the 8th cranial nerve has been associated with Capastat Sulfate given to patients with abnormal renal function or dehydration, or to those receiving medications with additive auditory toxicities. These patients often experience dizziness, tinnitus, vertigo, and a loss of high-tone acuity.

Neuromuscular blockage or respiratory paralysis may occur following rapid intravenous administration.

If capreomycin is ingested, toxicity would be unlikely because it is poorly absorbed (less then 1%) from an intact gastrointestinal system.

Hypokalemia, hypocalcemia, hypomagnesemia, and an electrolyte disturbance resembling Bartter's syndrome have been reported to occur in patients with capreomycin toxicity.

Treatment—To obtain up-to-date information about the treatment of overdose, a good resource is your certified Regional Poison Control Center. Telephone numbers of certified poison control centers are listed in the *Physician's Desk Reference (PDR)*. In managing overdosage, consider the possibility of multiple drug overdoses, interaction among drugs, and unusual drug kinetics in your patient.

Protect the patient's airway and support ventilation and perfusion. Meticulously monitor and maintain, within acceptable limits, the patient's vital signs, blood gases, serum electrolytes, etc. Absorption of drugs from the gastrointestinal tract may be decreased by giving acitivated charcoal, which, in many cases, is more effective than emesis or lavage; consider charcoal instead of or in addition to gastric emptying. Repeated doses of charcoal over time may hasten elimination of some drugs that have been absorbed. Safeguard the patient's airway when employing gastric emptying or charcoal.

Patients who have received an overdose of capreomycin and have normal renal function should be carefully hydrated to maintain a urine output of 3 to 5 mL/kg/h. Fluid balance, electrolytes, and creatinine clearance should be carefully monitored.

Hemodialysis may be effectively used to remove capreomycin in patients with significant renal disease.

DOSAGE AND ADMINISTRATION

Capastat® Sulfate (Sterile Capreomycin Sulfate, USP, Lilly) should be dissolved in 2 mL of 0.9% Sodium Chloride Injection or Sterile Water for Injection. Two to 3 minutes should be allowed for complete solution. For administration of a 1-g dose, the entire contents of the vial should be given. For dosages lower than 1 g, the accompanying dilution table may be used.
[See table above].

DILUTION TABLE FOR CAPASTAT® SULFATE (Sterile Capreomycin Sulfate, USP)

Diluent Added to 1-g Vial	Volume of Capastat Sulfate Solution	Concentration* (Approx.)
2.15 mL	2.85 mL	350 mg/mL
2.63 mL	3.33 mL	300 mg/mL
3.3 mL	4 mL	250 mg/mL
4.3 mL	5 mL	200 mg/mL

*Stated in terms of mg of capreomycin activity.

The solution may acquire a pale straw color and darken with time, but this is not associated with loss of potency or the development of toxicity. After reconstitution, solutions of Capastat Sulfate may be stored for 48 hours at room temperature and up to 14 days under refrigeration.

Capastat Sulfate should be given by deep intramuscular injection into a large muscle mass, since superficial injections may be associated with increased pain and the development of sterile abscesses.

Capreomycin is always administered in combination with at least 1 other antituberculosis agent to which the patient's strain of tubercle bacilli is susceptible. The usual dose is 1 g daily (not to exceed 20 mg/kg/day) given intramuscularly for 60 to 120 days, followed by 1 g intramuscularly 2 or 3 times weekly. (*Note*—Therapy for tuberculosis should be maintained for 12 to 24 months. If facilities for administering injectable medication are not available, a change to appropriate oral therapy is indicated on the patient's release from the hospital.)

Patients with reduced renal function should have dosage reduction based on creatinine clearance using the guidelines included in Table 1. These dosages are designed to achieve a mean steady-state capreomycin level of 10 mg/L.
[See table below].

ANIMAL PHARMACOLOGY

In addition to renal and 8th-cranial-nerve toxicity demonstrated in animal toxicology studies, 2 dogs have developed cataracts while on doses of 62 mg/kg and 100 mg/kg for prolonged periods.

In teratology studies, a low incidence of "wavy ribs" was noted in litters of female rats treated with daily doses of 50 mg/kg or more of capreomycin.

HOW SUPPLIED

(℞) Vials No. 718, *Capastat® Sulfate (Sterile Capreomycin Sulfate, USP)*, equivalent to 1 g capreomycin activity, 10-mL size, rubber-stoppered (Dry Powder), in singles (NDC 0002-1485-01) (10 per carton).

[110988]

CECLOR® ℞
[sē'klôr]
(cefaclor)
USP

DESCRIPTION

Ceclor® (Cefaclor, USP, Lilly) is a semisynthetic cephalosporin antibiotic for oral administration. It is chemically designated as 3-chloro-7-D-(2-phenylglycinamido)-3-cephem-4-carboxylic acid.

Each Pulvule® contains cefaclor monohydrate equivalent to 250 mg or 500 mg cefaclor. The Pulvules also contain cornstarch, FD&C Blue No. 1, FD&C Red No. 3, gelatin, magnesium stearate, silicone, titanium dioxide, and other inactive ingredients. The 500-mg Pulvule also contains iron oxide. After mixing, each 5 mL of Ceclor for Oral Suspension will contain cefaclor monohydrate equivalent to 125 mg, 187 mg, 250 mg, or 375 mg cefaclor. The suspensions also contain cellulose, cornstarch, FD&C Red No. 40, flavors, silicone, sodium lauryl sulfate, sucrose, and xanthan gum.

CLINICAL PHARMACOLOGY

Cefaclor is well absorbed after oral administration to fasting subjects. Total absorption is the same whether the drug is given with or without food; however, when it is taken with food, the peak concentration achieved is 50% to 75% of that observed when the drug is administered to fasting subjects and generally appears from three-fourths to 1 hour later. Following administration of 250-mg, 500-mg, and 1-g doses to fasting subjects, average peak serum levels of approximately 7, 13, and 23 mg/L respectively were obtained within 30 to 60 minutes. Approximately 60% to 85% of the drug is excreted unchanged in the urine within 8 hours, the greater portion being excreted within the first 2 hours. During this 8-hour period, peak urine concentrations following the 250-mg, 500-mg, and 1-g doses were approximately 600, 900, and 1,900 mg/L respectively. The serum half-life in normal subjects is 0.6 to 0.9 hour. In patients with reduced renal function, the serum half-life of cefaclor is slightly prolonged. In those with complete absence of renal function, the biologic half-life of the intact molecule is 2.3 to 2.8 hours. Excretion pathways in patients with markedly impaired renal function have not been determined. Hemodialysis shortens the half-life by 25% to 30%.

Microbiology—In vitro tests demonstrate that the bactericidal action of the cephalosporins results from inhibition of cell-wall synthesis. Cefaclor is active in vitro against most strains of clinical insolates of the following organisms:

Staphylococci, including coagulase-positive, coagulase-negative, and penicillinase-producing strains (when tested by in vitro methods), exhibit cross-resistance between cefaclor and methicillin

Streptococcus pyogenes (group A β-hemolytic streptococci)

S. pneumoniae (formerly *Diplococcus pneumoniae*)

Moraxella (Branhamella) catarrhalis

Haemophilus influenzae, including β-lactamase-producing ampicillin-resistant strains

Escherichia coli

Proteus mirabilis

Klebsiella

Citrobacter diversus

Neisseria gonorrhoeae

Propionibacteria acnes and *Bacteroides* sp (excluding *Bacteroides fragilis*)

Peptococci

Peptostreptococci

Note: *Pseudomonas* species, *Acinetobacter calcoaceticus* (formerly *Mima* sp and *Herellea* sp), and most strains of enterococci (*Enterococcus faecalis* [formerly *Streptococcus faecalis*], group D streptococci), *Enterobacter* sp, indole-positive *Proteus*, and *Serratia* sp are resistant to cefaclor. When tested by in vitro methods, staphylococci exhibit cross-resistance between cefaclor and methicillin-type antibiotics.

Table 1. Dose estimates, by renal function, to attain a mean steady-state serum capreomycin concentration of 10 mg/L

CrCl mL/min	Capreomycin Clearance L/kg/h $\times 10^{-2}$	Half-life Hours	Dose[a], mg/kg, for the following dosing intervals (hours)		
			24	48	72
0	0.54	55.5	1.29	2.58	3.87
10	1.01	29.4	2.43	4.87	7.30
20	1.49	20.0	3.58	7.16	10.7
30	1.97	15.1	4.72	9.45	14.2
40	2.45	12.2	5.87	11.7	
50	2.92	10.2	7.01	14.0	
60	3.40	8.8	8.16		
80	4.35	6.8	10.4[b]		
100	5.31	5.6	12.7[b]		
110	5.78	5.2	13.9[b]		

a—For renal patients, initial maintenance dose estimates are given for optional dosing intervals; longer dosing intervals are expected to provide greater peak and lower trough serum capreomycin levels than shorter dosing intervals.
b—The usual dose for patients with *normal* renal function is 1,000 mg daily, not to exceed 20 mg/kg/day, for 60 to 120 days, then 1,000 mg 2 to 3 times weekly.

Continued on next page

* Identi-Code® symbol.

Lilly—Cont.

Disk Susceptibility Tests —Quantitative methods that require measurement of zone diameters give the most precise estimates of antibiotic susceptibility. One such procedure[1] has been recommended for use with disks for testing susceptibility to cephalothin. The currently accepted zone diameter interpretive criteria for the cephalothin disk are appropriate for determining bacterial susceptibility to cefaclor. With this procedure, a report from the laboratory of "resistant" indicates that the infecting organism is not likely to respond to therapy. A report of "intermediate susceptibility" suggests that the organism would be susceptible if the infection is confined to tissues and fluids (eg, urine) in which high antibiotic levels can be obtained or if high dosage is used.

INDICATIONS AND USAGE

Ceclor® (Cefaclor, USP, Lilly) is indicated in the treatment of the following infections when caused by susceptible strains of the designated microorganisms:

Otitis media caused by *S pneumoniae (D pneumoniae), H influenzae,* staphylococci, and *S pyogenes* (group A β-hemolytic streptococci)

Lower respiratory infections, including pneumonia, caused by *S pneumoniae (D pneumoniae), H influenzae,* and *S pyogenes* (group A β-hemolytic streptococci)

Upper respiratory infections, including pharyngitis and tonsillitis, caused by *S pyogenes* (group A β-hemolytic streptococci)

Note: Penicillin is the usual drug of choice in the treatment and prevention of streptococcal infections, including the prophylaxis of rheumatic fever. Ceclor is generally effective in the eradication of streptococci from the nasopharynx; however, substantial data establishing the efficacy of Ceclor in the subsequent prevention of rheumatic fever are not available at present.

Urinary tract infections, including pyelonephritis and cystitis, caused by *E coli, P mirabilis, Klebsiella* sp, and coagulase-negative staphylococci

Skin and skin-structure infections caused by *Staphylococcus aureus* and *S pyogenes* (group A β-hemolytic streptococci)

Appropriate culture and susceptibility studies should be performed to determine susceptibility of the causative organism to Ceclor.

CONTRAINDICATION

Ceclor® (Cefaclor, USP, Lilly) is contraindicated in patients with known allergy to the cephalosporin group of antibiotics.

WARNINGS

IN PENICILLIN-SENSITIVE PATIENTS, CEPHALOSPORIN ANTIBIOTICS SHOULD BE ADMINISTERED CAUTIOUSLY. THERE IS CLINICAL AND LABORATORY EVIDENCE OF PARTIAL CROSS-ALLERGENICITY OF THE PENICILLINS AND THE CEPHALOSPORINS, AND THERE ARE INSTANCES IN WHICH PATIENTS HAVE HAD REACTIONS, INCLUDING ANAPHYLAXIS, TO BOTH DRUG CLASSES.

Antibiotics, including Ceclor® (Cefaclor, USP, Lilly), should be administered cautiously to any patient who has demonstrated some form of allergy, particularly to drugs.

Pseudomembranous colitis has been reported with virtually all broad-spectrum antibiotics (including macrolides, semisynthetic penicillins, and cephalosporins); therefore, it is important to consider its diagnosis in patients who develop diarrhea in association with the use of antibiotics. Such colitis may range in severity from mild to life-threatening.

Treatment with broad-spectrum antibiotics alters the normal flora of the colon and may permit overgrowth of clostridia. Studies indicate that a toxin produced by *Clostridium difficile* is one primary cause of antibiotic-associated colitis. Mild cases of pseudomembranous colitis usually respond to drug discontinuance alone. In moderate to severe cases, management should include sigmoidoscopy, appropriate bacteriologic studies, and fluid, electrolyte, and protein supplementation. When the colitis does not improve after the drug has been discontinued, or when it is severe, oral vancomycin is the drug of choice for antibiotic-associated pseudomembranous colitis produced by *C difficile.* Other causes of colitis should be ruled out.

PRECAUTIONS

General —If an allergic reaction to Ceclor® (Cefaclor, USP, Lilly) occurs, the drug should be discontinued, and, if necessary, the patient should be treated with appropriate agents, eg, pressor amines, antihistamines, or corticosteroids.

Prolonged use of Ceclor may result in the overgrowth of nonsusceptible organisms. Careful observation of the patient is essential. If superinfection occurs during therapy, appropriate measures should be taken.

Positive direct Coombs' tests have been reported during treatment with the cephalosporin antibiotics. In hematologic studies or in transfusion cross-matching procedures when antiglobulin tests are performed on the minor side or in Coombs' testing of newborns whose mothers have received cephalosporin antibiotics before parturition, it should be recognized that a positive Coombs' test may be due to the drug.

Ceclor should be administered with caution in the presence of markedly impaired renal function. Since the half-life of cefaclor in anuria is 2.3 to 2.8 hours, dosage adjustments for patients with moderate or severe renal impairment are usually not required. Clinical experience with cefaclor under such conditions is limited; therefore, careful clinical observation and laboratory studies should be made.

As a result of administration of Ceclor, a false-positive reaction for glucose in the urine may occur. This has been observed with Benedict's and Fehling's solutions and also with Clinitest® tablets but not with Tes-Tape® (Glucose Enzymatic Test Strip, USP, Lilly).

Broad-spectrum antibiotics should be prescribed with caution in individuals with a history of gastrointestinal disease, particularly colitis.

Usage in Pregnancy —*Pregnancy Category B* —Reproduction studies have been performed in mice and rats at doses up to 12 times the human dose and in ferrets given 3 times the maximum human dose and have revealed no evidence of impaired fertility or harm to the fetus due to Ceclor. There are, however, no adequate and well-controlled studies in pregnant women. Because animal reproduction studies are not always predictive of human response, this drug should be used during pregnancy only if clearly needed.

Nursing Mothers —Small amounts of Ceclor have been detected in mother's milk following administration of single 500-mg doses. Average levels were 0.18, 0.20, 0.21, and 0.16 mg/L at 2, 3, 4, and 5 hours respectively. Trace amounts were detected at 1 hour. The effect on nursing infants is not known. Caution should be exercised when Ceclor is administered to a nursing woman.

Usage in Children —Safety and effectiveness of this product for use in infants less than 1 month of age have not been established.

ADVERSE REACTIONS

Adverse effects considered related to therapy with Ceclor® (Cefaclor, USP, Lilly) are listed below:

Hypersensitivity reactions have been reported in about 1.5% of patients and include morbilliform eruptions (1 in 100). Pruritus, urticaria, and positive Coombs' tests each occur in less than 1 in 200 patients. Cases of **serum-sickness-like** reactions have been reported with the use of Ceclor. These are characterized by findings of erythema multiforme, rashes, and other skin manifestations accompanied by arthritis/arthralgia, with or without fever, and differ from classic serum sickness in that there is infrequently associated lymphadenopathy and proteinuria, no circulating immune complexes, and no evidence to date of sequelae of the reaction. While further investigation is ongoing, **serum-sickness-like** reactions appear to be due to hypersensitivity and more often occur during or following a second (or subsequent) course of therapy with Ceclor. Such reactions have been reported more frequently in children than in adults with an overall occurrence ranging from 1 in 200 (0.5%) in one focused trial to 2 in 8,346 (0.024%) in overall clinical trials (with an incidence in children in clinical trials of 0.055%) to 1 in 38,000 (0.003%) in spontaneous event reports. Signs and symptoms usually occur a few days after initiation of therapy and subside within a few days after cessation of therapy; occasionally these reactions have resulted in hospitalization, usually of short duration (median hospitalization = two to three days, based on postmarketing surveillance studies). In those requiring hospitalization, the symptoms have ranged from mild to severe at the time of admission with more of the severe reactions occurring in children. Antihistamines and glucocorticoids appear to enhance resolution of the signs and symptoms. No serious sequelae have been reported.

More severe hypersensitivity reactions, including Stevens-Johnson syndrome, toxic epidermal neocrolysis, and anaphylaxis, have been reported rarely. Anaphylaxis may be more common in patients with a history of penicillin allergy.

Gastrointestinal symptoms occur in about 2.5% of patients and include diarrhea (1 in 70).

Symptoms of pseudomembranous colitis may appear either during or after antibiotic treatment. Nausea and vomiting have been reported rarely. As with some penicillins and some other cephalosporins, transient hepatitis and cholestatic jaundice have been reported rarely.

Other effects considered related to therapy included eosinophilia (1 in 50 patients), genital pruritus or vaginitis (less than 1 in 100 patients), and rarely, thrombocytopenia, or reversible interstitial nephritis.

Causal Relationship Uncertain —*CNS* —Rarely, reversible hyperactivity, nervousness, insomnia, confusion, hypertonia, dizziness, and somnolence have been reported.

Transitory abnormalities in clinical laboratory test results have been reported. Although they were of uncertain etiology, they are listed below to serve as alerting information for the physician.

Hepatic —Slight elevations of SGOT, SGPT, or alkaline phosphatase values (1 in 40).

Hematopoietic —Transient lymphocytosis, leukopenia, and rarely, reversible neutropenia of possible clinical significance, as has also been reported with other β-lactam antibiotics.

Renal —Slight elevations in BUN or serum creatinine (less than 1 in 500) or abnormal urinalysis (less than 1 in 200).

OVERDOSAGE

Signs and Symptoms —The toxic symptoms following an overdose of cefaclor may include nausea, vomiting, epigastric distress, and diarrhea. The severity of the epigastric distress and the diarrhea are dose related. If other symptoms are present, it is probable that they are secondary to an underlying disease state, an allergic reaction, or the effects of other intoxication.

Treatment —To obtain up-to-date information about the treatment of overdose, a good resource is your certified Regional Poison Control Center. Telephone numbers of certified poison control centers are listed in the *Physicians' Desk Reference* (PDR). In managing overdosage, consider the possibility of multiple drug overdoses, interaction among drugs, and unusual drug kinetics in your patient.

Unless 5 times the normal dose of cefaclor has been ingested, gastrointestinal decontamination will not be necessary.

Protect the patients's airway and support ventilation and perfusion. Meticulously monitor and maintain, within acceptable limits, the patient's vital signs, blood gases, serum electrolytes, etc. Absorption of drugs from the gastrointestinal tract may be decreased by giving activated charcoal, which, in many cases, is more effective than emesis or lavage; consider charcoal instead of or in addition to gastric emptying. Repeated doses of charcoal over time may hasten elimination of some drugs that have been absorbed. Safeguard the patient's airway when employing gastric emptying or charcoal.

Forced diuresis, peritoneal dialysis, hemodialysis, or charcoal hemoperfusion have not been established as beneficial for an overdose of cefaclor.

DOSAGE AND ADMINISTRATION

Ceclor® (Cefaclor, USP, Lilly) is administered orally.

Adults —The usual adult dosage is 250 mg every 8 hours. For more severe infections (such as pneumonia) or those caused by less susceptible organisms, doses may be doubled.

Children —The usual recommended daily dosage for children is 20 mg/kg/day in divided doses every 8 hours. In more serious infections, otitis media, and infections caused by less susceptible organisms, 40 mg/kg/day are recommended, with a maximum dosage of 1 g/day.

	Ceclor Suspension 20 mg/kg/day	
Child's Weight	125 mg/5 mL	250 mg/5 mL
9 kg	½ tsp t.i.d.	
18 kg	1 tsp t.i.d.	½ tsp t.i.d.
	40 mg/kg/day	
9 kg	1 tsp t.i.d.	½ tsp t.i.d.
18 kg		1 tsp t.i.d.

B.I.D. Treatment Option —For the treatment of otitis media and pharyngitis, the total daily dosage may be divided and administered every 12 hours.

	Ceclor Suspension 20 mg/kg/day (Pharyngitis)	
Child's Weight	187 mg/5 mL	375 mg/5 mL
9 kg	½ tsp b.i.d.	
18 kg	1 tsp b.i.d.	½ tsp b.i.d.
	40 mg/kg/day (Otitis Media)	
9 kg	1 tsp b.i.d.	½ tsp b.i.d.
18 kg		1 tsp b.i.d.

Ceclor may be administered in the presence of impaired renal function. Under such a condition, the dosage usually is unchanged (*see* Precautions).

In the treatment of β-hemolytic streptococcal infections, a therapeutic dosage of Ceclor should be administered for at least 10 days.

HOW SUPPLIED

(℞) Pulvules:

250 mg, purple and white (No. 3061)—RxPak* of 15) NDC 0002-3061-15; (100s) NDC 0002-3061-02; (ID†100) NDC 0002-3061-33

500 mg, purple and gray (No. 3062)—(RxPak of 15) NDC 0002-3062-15; (100s) NDC 0002-3062-02; (ID100) NDC 0002-3062-33

(℞) For Oral Suspension:

125 mg/5 mL, strawberry flavor (M-5057‡)—(75-mL size) NDC 0002-5057-18; (150-mL size) NDC 0002-5057-68

187 mg/5 mL, strawberry flavor (M-5130‡)—(50-mL size) NDC 0002-5130-87; (100-mL size) NDC 0002-5130-48

250 mg/5 mL, strawberry flavor (M-5058‡)—(75-mL size) NDC 0002-5058-18; (150-mL size) NDC 0002-5058-68

375 mg/5 mL, strawberry flavor (M-5132‡)—(50 mL size) NDC 0002-5132-87; (100-mL size) NDC 0002-5132-48

* All RxPaks (prescription packages, Lilly) have safety closures.
† Identi-Dose® (unit dose medication, Lilly)
‡ After mixing, store in a refrigerator. Shake well before using. Keep tightly closed. The mixture may be kept for 14 days without significant loss of potentcy. Discard unused portion after 14 days.

Store at controlled room temperature, 59° to 86°F (15° to 30°C).

M-5057—150 mL—6505-01-141-9488
M-5058—75 mL—6505-01-152-3607
M-5058—150 mL—6505-01-141-9489
Pulvules® No. 3061—100's—6505-01-150-2101
Shown in Product Identification Section, page 415

———
1. *Am J Clin Pathol* 1966;45:493; *Federal Register* 1974;39:19182–19184.

[052689]

CEFACLOR, *see* Ceclor® (Cefaclor, USP, Lilly).

CEFAMANDOLE NAFATE, *see* Mandol® (Cefamandole Nafate, USP, Lilly).

CEFAZOLIN SODIUM, *see* Kefzol® (Cefazolin Sodium, USP, Lilly).

CEFTAZIDIME, *see* Tazidime® (Ceftazidime, USP, Lilly).

CEFUROXIME SODIUM, *see* Kefurox® (Cefuroxime Sodium, USP, Lilly).

CESAMET®
[*sĕs ʹá-mĕt*]
(nabilone)
PULVULES®

C II

DESCRIPTION

Cesamet® (Nabilone, Lilly) is a synthetic cannabinoid for oral administration. Nabilone as a raw material occurs as a white, polymorphic crystalline powder. In aqueous media, the solubility of nabilone is less than 0.5 mg/L, with pH values ranging from 1.2 to 7.0.

Chemically, nabilone is (±)-*trans*-3-(1,1-dimethylheptyl)-6,6a,7,8,10,10a-hexahydro-1-hydroxy-6-6-dimethyl-9H-dibenzo[b,d]pyran-9-one and has the empirical formula $C_{24}H_{36}O_3$. It has a molecular weight of 372.55.

Each Pulvule Cesamet contains 1 mg nabilone. The Pulvules also contain F D & C Blue No. 2, gelatin, iron oxides, povidone, cornstarch, titanium dioxide, and other inactive ingredients.

CLINICAL PHARMACOLOGY

Nontherapeutic Effects —Cesamet® (Nabilone, Lilly), a synthetic cannabinoid, is highly abusable and has the potential to produce psychologic dependence. Cesamet has complex effects on the central nervous system. Its effects on the mental state (ie, "inner mental life") are similar to those of cannabis. Subjects given Cesamet may experience changes in mood (euphoria, detachment, depression, anxiety, panic, paranoia, etc), decrements in cognitive performance and memory, a decreased ability to control drives and impulses, and alterations in the experience of reality (eg, distortions in the perception of objects and the sense of time, hallucinations, etc). These phenomena appear to be more common when larger doses of Cesamet are administered; however, a full-blown picture of psychosis (psychotic organic brain syndrome) may occur in patients receiving doses within the lower portion of the therapeutic range.

Data on the chronic use of Cesamet are not available; experience with cannabis suggests that chronic use of cannabinoids may be associated with a variety of untoward effects on motivation, cognition, judgment, etc, but whether these phenomena reflect the underlying character of individuals chronically abusing cannabis or are a result of the use of cannabis is not known.

The simultaneous use of Cesamet and alcohol or barbiturates may produce additive depressive effects on central nervous system function. Possible changes in mood and other adverse behavioral effects may occur in patients receiving Cesamet. Patients should remain under supervision of a responsible adult while using Cesamet.

Cesamet has central nervous system activity. It produces relaxation, drowsiness, and euphoria in the recommended dosage range. Tolerance to these effects develops rapidly and is readily reversible.

In addition to effects on the mental state, Cesamet has several systemic actions; most prominent are dry mouth and hypotension. Cesamet has been observed to elevate supine and standing heart rates and to cause supine and orthostatic hypotension. In clinical studies, oral administration of 2 mg

of Cesamet did produce some decrease in airway resistance in normal controls but had no effect in patients with asthma. No other nontherapeutic effects of clinical significance due to Cesamet have been reported.

Metabolism and Pharmacokinetics —Following oral administration of Pulvules Cesamet, peak plasma concentrations occur within about 2 hours. Precise information concerning the relative accumulation of nabilone and its "active" metabolites following repeated administration is not available. Available evidence suggests, however, that one or more of the metabolites has a terminal elimination half-life that exceeds that of nabilone. Consequently, in repeated use, the metabolites may accumulate at concentrations in excess of the parent drug.

The extent to which nabilone undergoes presystemic clearance (first-pass effect) is unknown. Metabolism of nabilone, however, is extensive, and several metabolites have been identified. The relative activities of the metabolites and the parent drug have not been established. Following oral administration of a 2-mg dose of radiolabeled nabilone, peak serum concentration of approximately 10 ng/mL of nabilone are achieved. The plasma half-life ($T^{1/2}$) values for nabilone and total radioactivity of identified and unidentified metabolites are about 2 and 35 hours, respectively. Dose proportionality for the parent drug and its metabolites has not been determined. The effects of age, hepatic dysfunction, and renal insufficiency on the metabolism and elimination of nabilone have not been determined.

When Cesamet is administered orally or intravenously, the drug and its metabolites are eliminated mainly in the feces (approximately 65%) and to a lesser extent in the urine (approximately 20%). It appears that the major excretory pathway is the biliary system.

INDICATIONS AND USAGE

Pulvules Cesamet® (Nabilone, Lilly) are indicated for the treatment of the nausea and vomiting associated with cancer chemotherapy in patients who have failed to respond adequately to conventional antiemetic treatments. This restriction is required because a substantial proportion of any group of patients treated with Cesamet can be expected to experience disturbing psychotomimetic reactions not observed with other antiemetic agents.

Because of its potential to alter the mental state, Cesamet is intended for use in circumstances that permit close supervision of the patient by a responsible individual.

Cesamet is highly abusable and controlled as nabilone under Schedule II of the Controlled Substances Act. Prescriptions for Cesamet should be limited to the amount necessary for a single cycle of chemotherapy (ie, a few days).

Evidence supporting the efficacy of Cesamet in the treatment of nausea and vomiting induced by cancer chemotherapy was obtained from both active-controlled (prochlorperazine) and placebo-controlled trials. Persuasive evidence was obtained in subjects being treated with a wide variety of chemotherapy regimens, including low-dose cisplatin (20 mg/m²).

CONTRAINDICATIONS

Cesamet® (Nabilone, Lilly) is contraindicated in patients whose nausea and vomiting arises from any cause other than cancer chemotherapy.

Cesamet is contraindicated in any patient known to be hypersensitive to it.

WARNINGS

Because of its profound effects on mental status, patients should be warned not to drive, operate complex machinery, or engage in any activity requiring sound judgment and unimpaired coordination while receiving treatment with Cesamet® (Nabilone, Lilly). The effects of Cesamet may persist for a variable and unpredictable period of time following its oral administration. Adverse psychiatric reactions can persist for 48 to 72 hours following cessation of treatment. Because of individual variation in response and tolerance to the effects of Cesamet, the physician should determine on clinical grounds the period of patient supervision required. Patients receiving Cesamet should be closely observed, if possible, within an inpatient setting. This is especially important during the treatment of naive patients. However, even patients experienced with Cesamet or cannabis may have serious untoward responses not predicted by prior uneventful exposures. Because a psychotic patient is a potential danger to himself/herself and/or others, any patient who has a psychotic experience with Cesamet should be closely observed in an appropriate setting until his/her mental state returns to normal. The patient should not be given additional doses of Cesamet until he/she has been examined and the circumstances evaluated by a physician. If the clinical situation warrants it, a lower dose of Cesamet may be administered under very close supervision. The patient should be counseled about the experience and should share in the decision about further use of Cesamet.

Cesamet should not be taken with alcohol, sedatives, hypnotics, or other psychotomimetic substances.

PRECAUTIONS

General —Since Cesamet® (Nabilone, Lilly) can elevate supine and standing heart rates and cause postural hypotension, it should be used with caution in the elderly and in patients with hypertension or heart disease.

Cesamet should also be used with caution in patients with current or previous psychiatric disorders, (including manic-depressive illness and schizophrenia), because the symptoms of these disease states may be unmasked by the use of cannabinoids.

Cesamet should be used with caution in individuals receiving other psychoactive drugs.

Information for Patients —Persons taking Cesamet should be alerted to the potential for additive central nervous system depression resulting from simultaneous use of Cesamet and alcohol or barbiturates. This combination should be avoided. Operation of machinery or a motor vehicle should be avoided during therapy with Cesamet. Patients using Cesamet should be made aware of possible changes in mood and other adverse behavioral effects of the drug so as to avoid panic in the event of such manifestations. Patients should remain under supervision of a responsible adult while using Cesamet.

Drug Interactions —Potential interactions between Cesamet, 2 mg, and diazepam, 5 mg; sodium secobarbital, 100 mg; alcohol, 45 mL (absolute laboratory alcohol); or codeine, 65 mg, were evaluated in 15 subjects. Only a single combination was utilized at any one time. The subjects were evaluated according to physiologic (ie, heart rate and blood pressure), psychometric, psychomotor, and subjective parameters. In this study, as expected, the depressant effects of the combinations were additive. Psychomotor function was particularly impaired with concurrent use of diazepam. Caution must be used when administering nabilone in combination with any CNS depressant.

Carcinogenesis, Mutagenesis, Impairment of Fertility —Carcinogenicity studies have not been performed with Cesamet. The influence of Cesamet on fertility and reproduction at doses of 150 and 40 times the maximum recommended human dose was evaluated in rats and rabbits, respectively. In these studies there was no evidence of teratogenicity due to Cesamet. In high-dose groups, however, Cesamet produced a decrease in pregnancy rate.

Pregnancy —*Pregnancy Category B.* Reproduction studies performed in rats at 150 times the human dose and in rabbits at 40 times the human dose revealed a dose-related reduction in litter size, an increase in the incidence of fetal resorptions, and an increase in the incidence of stillborn pups. These effects appear related to the dose-dependent reduction in maternal food intake and gain in body weight induced by Cesamet. At 150 times the maximum recommended human dose, Cesamet produced a reduction in neonatal survival that may be related to reduced milk production by mothers. Cesamet is known to have an inhibitory effect on prolactin release, which could contribute to the observed reduction in milk production. Hypothermia was also reported in the offspring of high-dose groups of female rats, which may have also contributed to reduced neonatal survival. There are no adequate and well-controlled studies in pregnant women. Because animal reproduction studies are not always predictive of human response, this drug should be used during pregnancy only if clearly needed.

Nursing Mothers —It is not known whether this drug is excreted in breast milk. Because many drugs are excreted in breast milk, it is recommended that Cesamet not be given to nursing mothers.

Pediatric Use —Safety and effectiveness have not been established in patients younger than 18 years of age.

ADVERSE REACTIONS

Commonly Encountered Reactions —During controlled clinical trials of Cesamet® (Nabilone, Lilly), virtually all patients experienced at least one adverse reaction. The most commonly encountered events were drowsiness, vertigo, dry mouth, euphoria (high), ataxia, headache, and concentration difficulties.

Comparative Incidence of Reactions —Accurate estimates of the incidence of adverse events associated with the use of any drug are difficult to obtain. Estimates are influenced by drug dose, detection technique, setting, physician judgments, etc. Consequently, the accompanying tables are presented solely to indicate the relative frequency of adverse events reported in representative controlled clinical studies conducted to evaluate the safety and efficacy of Cesamet under relatively similar conditions of use. The figures cited cannot be used to predict precisely the incidence of untoward events in the usual course of medical practice, in which patient characteristics and other factors may differ from those that prevailed in the clinical trials. Also, these incidence figures cannot be compared with those obtained from other clinical studies

Continued on next page

* Identi-Code® symbol.

Lilly—Cont.

involving related drug products because each group of drug trials is conducted under a different set of conditions. Finally, it is important to emphasize that these tabulations do not reflect the relative severity and/or clinical importance of the adverse events. A better perspective on the serious adverse events associated with the use of Cesamet is provided in the WARNINGS and PRECAUTIONS sections.

The accompanying tables list in order of decreasing frequency the adverse reactions encountered by a substantial proportion of patients treated with Cesamet participating in representative controlled clinical trials.

[See table below].

Adverse Reactions by Body System —The following list of adverse events is organized by decreasing frequency within body systems for patients treated with Cesamet® (Nabilone, Lilly) in controlled clinical trials. All events are listed regardless of causality assessment.

Blood and Hematopoietic —Anemia

Cardiovascular —Orthostatic hypotension, hypotension, tachycardia, syncope, palpitation, flushing, hypertension, arrhythmia, and cerebral vascular accident.

Eye and Ear —Vision disturbance, ear tightness, eye irritation, eye dryness, equilibrium dysfunction, tinnitus, eye disorder, amblyopia, eye swelling, eyelid diseases, pupil dilation, photophobia, and visual field defect.

Gastrointestinal —Dry mouth, nausea, anorexia, vomiting, diarrhea, abdominal pain, constipation, aphthous ulcer, mouth irritation, gastritis, and dyspepsia.

Genitourinary —Increased urination, decreased urination, hot flashes, urinary retention, and frequency of micturition.

Infection —Bacterial infection

Metabolic and Endocrine —Thirst

Musculoskeletal —Muscle pain, back pain, neck pain, joint pain, and unspecified pain.

Nervous System —Drowsiness, vertigo, ataxia, decreased concentration, sedation, hallucinations, paresthesia, tremor, memory disturbance, perception disturbance, convulsions, dystonia, numbness, and akathisia.

Psychiatric —Euphoria (high), sleep disturbance, depression, confusion, disorientation, anxiety, depersonalization syndrome, speech disorder, abnormal dreams, insomnia, mood swings, inebriated feeling, toxic psychosis, paranoia, apathy, thought disorder, withdrawal, panic disorder, phobic neurosis, emotional disorder, and hyperactivity.

Respiratory —Dyspnea, pharyngitis, nasal congestion, sinus headache, thick tongue, dry throat, dry nose, wheezing, nosebleed, cough, voice change, and chest pain.

Skin and Appendages —Anhidrosis, photosensitivity, pruritus, rash, and allergic reactions.

Miscellaneous and Ill-Defined Conditions —Headache, fatigue, lightheadedness, coordination disturbance, asthesia, dysphoria, dizziness, taste change, excessive appetite, chills, excessive sweating, nervousness, malaise, postural dizziness, twitch, irritability, fever, inhibited walking, unconsciousness, hypotonia, and impaired urination.

Spontaneously Reported Adverse Reactions —Cesamet has been marketed internationally since 1982. The following adverse reactions listed in order of decreasing frequency by body system have been reported since Cesamet has been marketed. All events are listed regardless of causality assessment.

Blood and Hematopoietic —Leukopenia

Cardiovascular —Hypotension and tachycardia

Eye and Ear —Visual disturbances

Gastrointestinal —Dry mouth, nausea, vomiting, and constipation

Nervous System —Hallucinations, CNS depression, CNS stimulation, ataxia, stupor, vertigo, convulsion, and circumoral paresthesia

Psychiatric —Somnolence, confusion, euphoria, depression, dysphoria, depersonalization, anxiety, psychosis, and emotional lability

Miscellaneous and Ill-Defined Conditions —Dizziness, headache, insomnia, abnormal thinking, chest pain, lack of effect, and face edema

DRUG ABUSE AND DEPENDENCE

Controlled Substance —Cesamet® (Nabilone, Lilly), a synthetic cannabinoid closely related to dronabinol (formerly known as delta-9-THC), is a highly abusable substance. Cesamet is controlled under Schedule II of the Controlled Substances Act. Prescriptions for Cesamet should be limited to the amount necessary for a single cycle of chemotherapy (ie, a few days).

It is not known what proportion of individuals exposed chronically to Cesamet or cannabinoids will develop either psychologic or physical dependence. Long-term use of these compounds has, however, been associated with disorders of motivation, judgment, and cognition. It is not clear, though, whether this is a manifestation of the underlying personalities of chronic users of this class of drugs or whether these drugs are directly responsible for these effects. An abstinence syndrome has been reported following discontinuation of high doses of dronabinol (200 mg/day). The acute phase was characterized by psychic distress, insomnia, and signs of autonomic hyperactivity (sweating, rhinorrhea, loose stools, hiccups). A protracted abstinence phase may have occurred as subjects reported sleep disturbances for several weeks after dronabinol discontinuation.

Abuse —Cesamet may produce subjective side effects that may be interpreted as a euphoria or marijuana-like "high" at therapeutic doses. Cesamet was shown to be qualitatively and quantitatively similar to dronabinol in the production of cannabis-like effects, thus demonstrating that Cesamet has a high potential for abuse.

Preclinical studies peformed in both dogs and monkeys demonstrated that Cesamet was cannabinoid-like. As with dronabinol, tolerance develops rapidly to the pharmacologic effects in both the dog and the monkey. Cross-tolerance between Cesamet and dronabinol was demonstrated in the monkey.

Dependence —The physical dependence capability of Cesamet is unknown at this time. Patients who participated in clinical trials of up to 5 days' duration evidenced no withdrawal symptoms on cessation of dosing.

OVERDOSAGE

Signs and symptoms of overdosage are an extension of the psychotomimetic and physiologic effects of Cesamet® (Nabilone, Lilly).

Treatment —To obtain up-to-date information about the treatment of overdose, a good resource is your certified Regional Poison Control Center. Telephone numbers of certified poison control centers are listed in the *Physicians' Desk Reference (PDR)*. In managing overdosage, consider the possibility of multiple drug overdoses, interaction among drugs, and unusual drug kinetics in your patient.

Overdosage may be considered to have occurred, even at prescribed dosages, if disturbing psychiatric symptoms are present. In these cases, the patient should be observed in a quiet environment and supportive measures, including reassurance, should be used. Subsequent doses should be withheld until patients have returned to their baseline mental status; routine dosing may then be resumed if clinically indicated. In such instances, a lower initiating dose is suggested. In controlled clinical trials, alterations in mental status related to the use of Cesamet resolved within 72 hours without specific medical therapy.

In overdose settings, attention should be paid to vital signs, since both hypertension and hypotension have been known to occur; tachycardia and orthostatic hypotension were most commonly reported.

No cases of overdosage with more than 10 mg/day of nabilone were reported during clinical trials. Signs and symptoms that would be expected to occur in large overdose situations are psychotic episodes, including hallucinations, anxiety reactions, respiratory depression, and coma.

If psychotic episodes occur, the patient should be managed conservatively, if possible. For moderate psychotic episodes and anxiety reactions, verbal support and comforting may be sufficient. In more severe cases, antipsychotic drugs may be useful; however, the utility of antipsychotic drugs in cannabinoid psychosis has not been systematically evaluated. Support for their use is drawn from limited experience using antipsychotic agents to manage cannabis overdoses. Because of the potential for drug-drug interactions (eg, additive CNS-depressant effects due to nabilone and chlorpromazine), such patients should be closely monitored.

Protect the patient's airway and support ventilation and perfusion. Meticulously monitor and maintain, within acceptable limits, the patient's vital signs, blood gases, serum electrolytes, etc. Absorption of drugs from the gastrointestinal tract may be decreased by giving activated charcoal, which, in many cases, is more effective than emesis or lavage; consider charcoal instead of or in addition to gastric emptying. Repeated doses of charcoal over time may hasten elimination of some drugs that have been absorbed. Safeguard the patient's airway when employing gastric emptying or charcoal.

The use of forced diuresis, peritoneal dialysis, hemodialysis, charcoal hemoperfusion, or cholestyramine has not been reported. In the presence of normal renal function, most of a dose of nabilone is eliminated through the biliary system. Treatment for respiratory depression and comatose state consists in symptomatic and supportive therapy. Particular attention should be paid to the occurrence of hypothermia. If the patient becomes hypotensive, consider fluids, inotropes, and/or vasopressors.

The estimated oral LD_{50} in female mice is between 1,000 and 2,000 mg/kg; in the female rat, it is greater than 2,000 mg/kg. *See* Clinical Pharmacology.

DOSAGE AND ADMINISTRATION

The usual adult dosage is 1 or 2 mg b.i.d. On the day of chemotherapy, the initial dose should be given 1 to 3 hours before the oncolytic agent is administered. To minimize side effects, it is recommended that the lower starting dose be used and that the dose be increased as necessary. A dose of 1 or 2 mg the night before may be useful. The maximum recommended daily dose is 6 mg given in divided doses t.i.d. Cesamet® (Nabilone, Lilly) may be administered 2 or 3 times daily during the entire course of each cycle of chemotherapy and, if needed, for 48 hours after the last dose of each cycle of chemotherapy.

ANIMAL PHARMACOLOGY AND/OR ANIMAL TOXICOLOGY

Monkeys treated with Cesamet® (Nabilone, Lilly) at doses as high as 2 mg/kg/day for a year experienced no significant adverse events. This result contrasts with the findings in a planned 1-year dog study that was prematurely terminated because of deaths associated with convulsions in dogs receiving as little as 0.5 mg/kg/day. The earliest deaths, however, occurred at 104 days in dogs receiving 1 mg/kg/day. The unusual vulnerability of the dog to Cesamet is not understood; it is hypothesized, however, that the explanation lies in the fact that the dog differs from other species in its metabolism of Cesamet.

TABLE 1
INCIDENCE OF ADVERSE REACTIONS IN PLACEBO-CONTROLLED STUDIES

Adverse Event	Nabilone (Cesamet) (n = 132)		Placebo (n = 119)	
	Patients	Percent	Patients	Percent
Vertigo	69	52	3	3
Drowsiness	69	52	6	5
Dry Mouth	47	36	2	2
Ataxia	19	14	0	0
Euphoria	14	11	1	1
Sleep Disturbance	14	11	1	1
Dysphoria	12	9	0	0
Headache	8	6	0	0
Nausea	5	4	0	0
Disorientation	3	2	0	0
Depersonalization	2	2	1	1

TABLE 2
INCIDENCE OF ADVERSE REACTIONS IN ACTIVE-CONTROLLED STUDIES

Adverse Event	Nabilone (Cesamet) (n = 250)		Prochlorperazine (n = 232)	
	Patients	Percent	Patients	Percent
Drowsiness	165	66	108	47
Vertigo/Dizziness	147	59	53	23
Euphoria	95	38	12	5
Dry Mouth	54	22	11	5
Depression	35	14	37	16
Ataxia	32	13	4	2
Visual Disturbance	32	13	9	4
Concentration Difficulties	31	12	3	1
Hypotension	20	8	3	1
Asthenia	19	8	10	4
Anorexia	19	8	22	9
Headache	18	7	14	6
Sedation	7	3	2	1
Increased Appetite	6	2	2	1

HOW SUPPLIED

(©) Pulvules (blue and white):
1 mg (No. 3101) (ID20*), NDC 0002-3101-42

*Identi-Dose® (unit dose medication, Lilly).

[080388]

CRYSTODIGIN® R

[krĭs-tō-dĭj'ĭn]
(digitoxin)
Tablets, USP

DESCRIPTION

Crystodigin® (Digitoxin Tablets, USP, Lilly) is a crystalline-pure single cardiac glycoside obtained from *Digitalis purpurea* and is identical in pharmacologic action with whole-leaf digitalis.

Digitoxin is the most slowly excreted of all digitalis compounds (excretion time is 14 to 21 days). It is most useful in patients with impaired renal function, since excretion and metabolism are independent of renal function.

Crystodigin is noted for its uniform potency, complete absorption, and lack of gastrointestinal irritation. It permits accurate dosage adjustments to produce maximum therapeutic effect smoothly and dependably.

Crystodigin, for oral administration, is available in tablets containing 0.1 mg crystalline digitoxin.

The tablets also contain cornstarch, lactose, magnesium stearate, povidone, and FD&C Red No. 40.

Digitoxin is a cardiotonic glycoside. The chemical name is card-20 (22) - enolide,3-[(O -2,6-dideoxy-β- D -ribo -hexopyranosyl-(1 → 4)-O -2,6 - dideoxy-β- D - ribo -hexopyranosyl-(1 → 4) -2,6- dideoxy- β-D-ribo- hexopyranosyl) oxy]-14-hydroxy,(3β,5β)-. The empirical formula of digitoxin is $C_{41}H_{64}O_{13}$.

CLINICAL PHARMACOLOGY

The cellular basis for the inotropic effects of digitalis is probably enhancement of excitation-contraction coupling, that process by which chemical energy is converted into mechanical energy when triggered by membrane depolarization. Most evidence relates this process to the entry of calcium ions into the cell during depolarization of the membrane and/or to the release of calcium from intracellular binding sites on the sarcoplasmic reticulum. The free calcium ion mediates the interaction of actin and myosin, resulting in contraction.

The amount of glycoside absorbed depends largely on its polarity, which is a function of the net electronic charge on the molecule. The more nonpolar or lipid soluble, the better is the absorption, because of the greater permeability of lipid membrane of the intestinal mucosa for lipid-soluble substances. The nonpolar, lipophilic digitoxin is completely absorbed. Other glycosides are not as well absorbed.

Nonpolar digitoxin is over 90% bound to tissue proteins. The firm binding of digitoxin to protein is responsible for its long half-life (7 to 9 days).

Digitoxin differs from other commonly used glycosides not only in its firm binding to protein but also because it is metabolized in the liver, with the only active metabolite being digoxin, which represents only a small fraction of the total metabolites. All other metabolites are inert and are probably excreted as such in the urine. The portion of digitoxin that is not metabolized is excreted in the bile to the intestines and recycled to the liver until it is completely metabolized. The portion of digitoxin that is bound to protein is in equilibrium with free digitoxin in the serum. Thus, as more and more of the free digitoxin is metabolized after a single dose, there is proportionately less bound digitoxin.

INDICATIONS AND USAGE

Crystodigin® (Digitoxin Tablets, USP, Lilly) is indicated in the treatment of heart failure, atrial flutter, atrial fibrillation, and supraventricular tachycardia.

CONTRAINDICATIONS

If the indications are carefully observed, there are few contraindications to digitalis therapy except toxic response or idiosyncrasy to digitalis, ventricular tachycardia, beriberi heart disease, and some instances of the hypersensitive carotid sinus syndrome.

Patients already taking digitalis preparations must not be given the rapid digitalizing dose of Crystodigin® (Digitoxin Tablets, USP, Lilly) or parenteral calcium.

WARNINGS

Many of the arrhythmias for which digitalis is advised are identical with those reflecting digitalis intoxication. When the possibility of digitalis intoxication cannot be excluded, cardiac glycosides should be withheld temporarily if the clinical situation permits.

The patient with congestive heart failure may complain of nausea and vomiting. Since these symptoms may also be associated with digitalis intoxication, a clinical determination of their cause must be attempted before further administration of the drug.

Cases of idiopathic hypertrophic subaortic stenosis must be managed with extreme care. Unless cardiac failure is severe, it is doubtful whether digitalis should be employed.

NOTE: Digitalis glycosides are an important cause of accidental poisoning in children.

PRECAUTIONS

General —When the risk of digitalis intoxication is great, the use of a short-acting, rapidly eliminated glycoside, such as digoxin, is advisable. Although intoxication cannot always be prevented by the selection of one glycoside over another, certain glycosides may be preferred in patients who have fixed disabilities (eg, liver impairment, drug intolerance). However, digitoxin can be used in patients with impaired renal function.

Special care must be exercised in elderly patients receiving digitalis, because their body mass tends to be small and renal clearance is likely to be reduced. Frequent electrocardiographic monitoring is important in these patients. In addition, digitalis must be used cautiously in the presence of active heart disease, such as acute myocardial infarction or acute myocarditis. In patients with acute or unstable chronic atrial fibrillation, digitalis may not normalize the ventricular rate even when the serum concentration exceeds the usual therapeutic level. Although these patients may be less sensitive to the toxic effects of digitalis than are patients with normal sinus rhythm, dosage should not be increased to potentially toxic levels.

Hypokalemia predisposes to digitalis toxicity, and even a moderate decrease in the concentration of serum potassium can precipitate serious arrhythmias.

Impaired liver function may necessitate reduction in dosage of any digitalis preparation, including digitoxin.

Sensitive radioimmunoassay techniques have been developed for measuring serum levels of digitoxin, and these procedures can be instituted in almost any hospital. Serum levels must, however, be evaluated in conjunction with clinical history and the results of the electrocardiogram and other laboratory tests. A therapeutic serum level for one patient may be excessive or inadequate for another patient.

Drug Interactions —The synthesis of microsomal enzymes that metabolize digitoxin in the liver is subject to stimulation by a number of drugs, such as antihistamines, anticonvulsants, barbiturates, oral hypoglycemic agents, and others.

When digitoxin is the glycoside used for digitalis maintenance, drugs that are liver-microsomal-enzyme inducers should not be used at the same time. Phenobarbital, phenylbutazone, and diphenylhydantoin will increase the rate of metabolism of digitoxin. In patients receiving 60 mg of phenobarbital 3 times a day for 12 weeks, the steady-state concentration of digitoxin in plasma fell approximately 50% when the drugs were administered concurrently and returned to previous levels when phenobarbital was discontinued.

When drugs that increase the rate of metabolism of digitoxin in the liver are discontinued, toxicity may occur.

Hypokalemia is most frequently encountered in patients receiving concomitant diuretic therapy, because the most widely used and most effective diuretics (ie, thiazides and furosemide) increase the urinary loss of potassium. Prescribing a potassium-sparing agent (spironolactone or triamterene) together with the potassium-wasting diuretic is a reliable means for maintaining the serum potassium level. Alternatively, potassium chloride supplements may be prescribed.

Mineralocorticoids (eg, prednisone) and, rarely, certain antibiotics (eg, amphotericin B) may also cause increased excretion of potassium.

Usage in Pregnancy —*Pregnancy Category C* —Animal reproduction studies have not been conducted with Crystodigin® (Digitoxin Tablets, USP, Lilly). It is also not known whether this drug can cause fetal harm when administered to a pregnant woman or can affect reproduction capacity. Crystodigin should be given to a pregnant woman only if clearly needed.

Labor and Delivery —No information is available concerning the use of Crystodigin in labor and delivery.

Nursing Mothers —It is not known whether this drug is excreted in human milk. Because many drugs are excreted in human milk, caution should be exercised when Crystodigin is administered to a nursing woman.

ADVERSE REACTIONS

Anorexia, nausea, and vomiting have been reported. These effects are central in origin, but following large oral doses, there is also a local emetic action. Abdominal discomfort or pain and diarrhea may also occur.

OVERDOSAGE

Signs and Symptoms —Symptoms may include alterations in mental status, nausea, vomiting, bradycardia, visual disturbances, heart block, and all known cardiac arrhythmias. Hyperkalemia may be present following acute overdose, whereas hypokalemia is associated with chronic overdose. Peak toxic effects following acute overdose may be delayed up to 12 hours.

Older patients, particularly those with coronary insufficiency, are more susceptible to dysrhythmias. Ventricular fibrillation is the most common cause of death from digitalis poisoning. There is insufficient information to accurately determine the minimum toxic or lethal dose in humans. Death from ventricular fibrillation was reported 24 hours after admission in a patient with a plasma concentration of 124 ng/mL shortly before death.

Treatment —To obtain up-to-date information about the treatment of overdose, a good resource is your certified Regional Poison Control Center. Telephone numbers of certified poison control centers are listed in the *Physicians' Desk Reference (PDR)*. In managing overdosage, consider the possibility of multiple drug overdoses, interaction among drugs, and unusual drug kinetics in your patient.

Continuous ECG monitoring is necessary. For any suspected digitoxin-induced dysrhythmia, discontinue the drug. Monitor potassium and digitoxin concentrations. Severe hyperkalemia may require administration of sodium bicarbonate, glucose, and regular insulin.

Protect the patient's airway and support ventilation and perfusion. Meticulously monitor and maintain, within acceptable limits, the patient's vital signs, blood gases, serum electrolytes, etc. Absorption of drugs from the gastrointestinal tract may be decreased by giving activated charcoal, which, in many cases, is more effective than emesis or lavage; consider charcoal instead of or in addition to gastric emptying. Repeated doses of charcoal over time may hasten elimination of some drugs that have been absorbed. Safeguard the patient's airway when employing gastric emptying or charcoal.

Atropine or a pacemaker may be used for bradycardia and heart block. Phenytoin (15 mg/kg), at a rate not to exceed 50 mg/min, may be useful for treating ventricular dysrhythmias and to improve atrioventricular conduction. Lidocaine may also be used, but impaired AV conduction may require a pacemaker. Consider use of digitalis-specific Fab fragments.

Forced diuresis, peritoneal dialysis, hemodialysis, or charcoal hemoperfusion have not been established as beneficial for an overdose of Crystodigin® (Digitoxin Tablets, USP, Lilly).

DOSAGE AND ADMINISTRATION

Adults: Slow Digitalization —0.2 mg twice daily for a period of 4 days, followed by maintenance dosage.

Rapid Digitalization —Preferably 0.6 mg initially, followed by 0.4 mg and then 0.2 mg at intervals of 4 to 6 hours.

Maintenance Dosage —Ranges from 0.05 to 0.3 mg daily, the most common dose being 0.15 mg daily.

After the neonatal period, the dose is as follows:
Under 1 year of age—0.045 mg/kg
1 to 2 years of age—0.04 mg/kg
Over 2 years of age—0.03 mg/kg (0.75 mg/m²)

The total dose should be divided into 3, 4, or more portions, with 6 hours or more between doses.

For a maintenance dose, the patient should be given one-tenth of the digitalizing dose.

HOW SUPPLIED

(R) Tablets (scored)
0.05 mg. orange (No. 1736)—(100s) NDC 0002-1075-02
0.1 mg, pink (No. 1703)—(100s) NDC 0002-1060-02; (500s) NDC 0002-1060-03

Protect from light. Store at controlled room temperature, 59° to 86°F (15° to 30°C). [072688]

Shown in Product Identification Section, page 415

CYCLOSERINE, *see* Seromycin® (Cycloserine, USP, Lilly).

DARVOCET-N® 50 ©

[där'vō-sĕt ĕn]
and
DARVOCET-N® 100

(propoxyphene napsylate and acetaminophen)
USP

DARVON-N®

[där'vŏn ĕn]
(propoxyphene napsylate)
USP

DARVON-N® WITH A.S.A.®

[där'vŏn ĕn with ā'ĕs-ā]
(propoxyphene napsylate and aspirin)
USP

DESCRIPTION

Darvon-N® (Propoxyphene Napsylate, USP) is an odorless, white crystalline solid with a bitter taste. It is very slightly

Continued on next page

* Identi-Code® symbol.

Lilly—Cont.

soluble in water and soluble in methanol, ethanol, chloroform, and acetone. Chemically, it is α-(+)- 4- (Dimethylamino) -3 - methyl - 1, 2 - diphenyl - 2 - butanol Propionate (ester) 2-Naphthalene-sulfonate (salt) Hydrate.

Propoxyphene napsylate differs from propoxyphene hydrochloride in that it allows more stable liquid dosage forms and tablet formulations. Because of differences in molecular weight, a dose of 100 mg of propoxyphene napsylate is required to supply an amount of propoxyphene equivalent to that present in 65 mg of propoxyphene hydrochloride.

Each tablet of Darvocet-N 50 contains 50 mg propoxyphene napsylate and 325 mg acetaminophen.

Each tablet of Darvocet-N 100 contains 100 mg propoxyphene napsylate and 650 mg acetaminophen.

Tablets Darvocet-N 50 and Darvocet-N 100 also contain amberlite, cellulose, cornstarch, F D & C Yellow No. 6, magnesium stearate, stearic acid, titanium dioxide, and other inactive ingredients.

Each tablet of Darvon-N contains 100 mg propoxyphene napsylate. The tablets also contain cellulose, cornstarch, iron oxides, lactose, magnesium stearate, silicon dioxide, stearic acid, and titanium dioxide.

Each 5 mL of Suspension Darvon-N contain 50 mg propoxyphene napsylate. The suspension also contains butylparaben, D&C Yellow No. 10, FD&C Yellow No. 6, flavors, glucose, hydroxypropyl methylcellulose, methylparaben, propylparaben, saccharin, silicone, sodium-2-naphthalene sulfonate, and sucrose.

Each tablet of Darvon-N with A.S.A. contains 100 mg propoxyphene napsylate and 325 mg aspirin. Each tablet also contains cellulose, FD&C Yellow No. 6, silicon dioxide, starch, stearic acid, titanium dioxide, yellow iron oxide, and other inactive ingredients.

CLINICAL PHARMACOLOGY

Propoxyphene is a centrally acting narcotic analgesic agent. Equimolar doses of propoxyphene hydrochloride or napsylate provide similar plasma concentrations. Following administration of 65, 130, or 195 mg of propoxyphene hydrochloride, the bioavailability of propoxyphene is equivalent to that of 100, 200, or 300 mg respectively of propoxyphene napsylate. Peak plasma concentrations of propoxyphene are reached in 2 to 2 ½ hours. After a 100-mg oral dose of propoxyphene napsylate, peak plasma levels of 0.05 to 0.1 mg/L are achieved. As shown in Figure 1, the napsylate salt tends to be absorbed more slowly than the hydrochloride. At or near therapeutic doses, this difference is small when compared with that among subjects and among doses. (See Figure 1)

Figure 1. Mean plasma concentrations of propoxyphene in 8 human subjects following oral administration of 65 and 130 mg of the hydrochloride salt and 100 and 200 mg of the napsylate salt and in 7 given 195 mg of the hydrochloride and 300 mg of the napsylate salt

Because of this several hundredfold difference in solubility, the absorption rate of very large doses of the napsylate salt is significantly lower than that of equimolar doses of the hydrochloride.

Repeated doses of propoxyphene at 6-hour intervals lead to increasing plasma concentrations, with a plateau after the ninth dose at 48 hours.

Propoxyphene is metabolized in the liver to yield norpropoxyphene. Propoxyphene has a half-life of 6 to 12 hours, whereas that of norpropoxyphene is 30 to 36 hours.

Norpropoxyphene has substantially less central-nervous-system-depressant effect than propoxyphene but a greater local anesthetic effect, which is similar to that of amitriptyline and antiarrhythmic agents, such as lidocaine and quinidine.

In animal studies in which propoxyphene and norpropoxyphene were continuously infused in large amounts, intracardiac conduction time (PR and QRS intervals) was prolonged. Any intracardiac conduction delay attributable to high concentrations of norpropoxyphene may be of relatively long duration.

ACTIONS

Propoxyphene is a mild narcotic analgesic structurally related to methadone. The potency of propoxyphene napsylate is from two-thirds to equal that of codeine.

Darvocet-N 50 and Darvocet-N 100 provide the analgesic activity of propoxyphene napsylate and the antipyretic-analgesic activity of acetaminophen.

The combination of propoxyphene and acetaminophen produces greater analgesia than that produced by either propoxyphene or acetaminophen administered alone.

The combination of propoxyphene with aspirin produces greater analgesia than that produced by either drug administered alone.

INDICATIONS

Darvocet-N 50, Darvocet-N 100, and Darvon-N with A.S.A. are indicated for the relief of mild to moderate pain, either when pain is present alone or when it is accompanied by fever.

Darvon-N® (propoxyphene napsylate, Lilly) is indicated for the relief of mild to moderate pain.

CONTRAINDICATIONS

Hypersensitivity to propoxyphene, acetaminophen, or aspirin.

WARNINGS

- Do not prescribe propoxyphene for patients who are suicidal or addiction-prone.
- Prescribe propoxyphene with caution for patients taking tranquilizers or antidepressant drugs and patients who use alcohol in excess.
- Tell your patients not to exceed the recommended dose and to limit their intake of alcohol.

Propoxyphene products in excessive doses, either alone or in combination with other CNS depressants, including alcohol, are a major cause of drug-related deaths. Fatalities within the first hour of overdosage are not uncommon. In a survey of deaths due to overdosage conducted in 1975, in approximately 20% of the fatal cases, death occurred within the first hour (5% occurred within 15 minutes). Propoxyphene should not be taken in doses higher than those recommended by the physician. The judicious prescribing of propoxyphene is essential to the safe use of this drug. With patients who are depressed or suicidal, consideration should be given to the use of non-narcotic analgesics. Patients should be cautioned about the concomitant use of propoxyphene products and alcohol because of potentially serious CNS-additive effects of these agents. Because of its added depressant effects, propoxyphene should be prescribed with caution for those patients whose medical condition requires the concomitant administration of sedatives, tranquilizers, muscle relaxants, antidepressants, or other CNS-depressant drugs. Patients should be advised of the additive depressant effects of these combinations.

Many of the propoxyphene-related deaths have occurred in patients with previous histories of emotional disturbances or suicidal ideation or attempts as well as histories of misuse of tranquilizers, alcohol, and other CNS-active drugs. Some deaths have occurred as a consequence of the accidental ingestion of excessive quantities of propoxyphene alone or in combination with other drugs. Patients taking propoxyphene should be warned not to exceed the dosage recommended by the physician.

Drug Dependence —Propoxyphene, when taken in higher-than-recommended doses over long periods of time, can produce drug dependence characterized by psychic dependence and, less frequently, physical dependence and tolerance. Propoxyphene will only partially suppress the withdrawal syndrome in individuals physically dependent on morphine or other narcotics. The abuse liability of propoxyphene is qualitatively similar to that of codeine although quantita-

tively less, and propoxyphene should be prescribed with the same degree of caution appropriate to the use of codeine.

Usage in Ambulatory Patients —Propoxyphene may impair the mental and/or physical abilities required for the performance of potentially hazardous tasks, such as driving a car or operating machinery. The patient should be cautioned accordingly.

Warning —Reye syndrome is a rare but serious disease which can follow flu or chickenpox in children and teenagers. Although the cause of Reye syndrome is unknown, some reports claim aspirin (or salicylates) may increase the risk of developing this disease.

PRECAUTIONS

General —Propoxyphene should be administered with caution to patients with hepatic or renal impairment, since higher serum concentrations or delayed elimination may occur.

Salicylates should be used with extreme caution in the presence of peptic ulcer or coagulation abnormalities.

Drug Interactions —The CNS-depressant effect of propoxyphene is additive with that of other CNS depressants, including alcohol.

As is the case with many medicinal agents, propoxyphene may slow the metabolism of a concomitantly administered drug. Should this occur, the higher serum concentrations of that drug may result in increased phamacologic or adverse effects of that drug. Such occurrences have been reported when propoxyphene was administered to patients on antidepressants, anticonvulsants, or warfarinlike drugs.

Salicylates may enhance the effect of anticoagulants and inhibit the uricosuric effect of uricosuric agents.

Usage in Pregnancy —Safe use in pregnancy has not been established relative to possible adverse effects on fetal development. Instances of withdrawal symptoms in the neonate have been reported following usage during pregnancy. Therefore, propoxyphene should not be used in pregnant women unless, in the judgment of the physician, the potential benefits outweigh the possible hazards.

Usage in Nursing Mothers —Low levels of propoxyphene have been detected in human milk. In postpartum studies involving nursing mothers who were given propoxyphene, no adverse effects were noted in infants receiving mother's milk.

Usage in Children —Propoxyphene is not recommended for use in children, because documented clinical experience has been insufficient to establish safety and a suitable dosage regimen in the pediatric age group.

Usage in the Elderly —The rate of propoxyphene metabolism may be reduced in some patients. Increased dosing interval should be considered.

A Patient Information Sheet is available for these products. See text following "How Supplied" section below.

ADVERSE REACTIONS

In a survey conducted in hospitalized patients, less than 1% of patients taking propoxyphene hydrochloride at recommended doses experienced side effects. The most frequently reported have been dizziness, sedation, nausea, and vomiting. Some of these adverse reactions may be alleviated if the patient lies down.

Other adverse reactions include constipation, abdominal pain, skin rashes, lightheadedness, headache, weakness, euphoria, dysphoria, hallucinations, and minor visual disturbances.

Liver dysfunction has been reported in association with both active components of Darvocet-N 50 and Darvocet-N 100.

Propoxyphene therapy has been associated with abnormal liver function tests and, more rarely, with instances of reversible jaundice. Hepatic necrosis may result from acute overdoses of acetaminophen (*see* Management of Overdosage). In chronic ethanol abusers, this has been reported rarely with short-term use of acetaminophen doses of 2.5 to 10 g/day. Fatalities have occurred.

Renal papillary necrosis may result from chronic acetaminophen use, particularly when the dosage is greater than recommended and when combined with aspirin.

Subacute painful myopathy has occurred following chronic propoxyphene overdosage.

DOSAGE AND ADMINISTRATION

These products are given orally. The usual dose of Darvocet-N 50 or Darvocet-N 100 is 100 mg propoxyphene napsylate and 650 mg acetaminophen every 4 hours as needed for pain. The usual dose of Darvon-N® (propoxyphene napsylate, Lilly) is 100 mg every 4 hours as needed for pain.

The usual dose of Darvon-N with A.S.A. is 100 mg propoxyphene napsylate and 325 mg aspirin every 4 hours as needed for pain.

The maximum recommended dose of propoxyphene napsylate is 600 mg/day.

Consideration should be given to a reduced total daily dosage in patients with hepatic or renal impairment.

MANAGEMENT OF OVERDOSAGE

In all cases of suspected overdosage, call your regional Poison Control Center to obtain the most up-to-date information about the treatment of overdose. This recommendation is made because, in general, information regarding the treatment of overdosage may change more rapidly than do package inserts.

Initial consideration should be given to the management of the CNS effects of propoxyphene overdosage. Resuscitative measures should be initiated promptly.

Symptoms of Propoxyphene Overdosage —The manifestations of acute overdosage with propoxyphene are those of narcotic overdosage. The patient is usually somnolent but may be stuporous or comatose and convulsing. Respiratory depression is characteristic. The ventilatory rate and/or tidal volume is decreased, which results in cyanosis and hypoxia. Pupils, initially pinpoint, may become dilated as hypoxia increases. Cheyne-Stokes respiration and apnea may occur. Blood pressure and heart rate are usually normal initially, but blood pressure falls and cardiac performance deteriorates, which ultimately results in pulmonary edema and circulatory collapse, unless the respiratory depression is corrected and adequate ventilation is restored promptly. Cardiac arrhythmias and conduction delay may be present. A combined respiratory-metabolic acidosis occurs owing to retained CO_2 (hypercapnea) and to lactic acid formed during anaerobic glycolysis. Acidosis may be severe if large amounts of salicylates have also been ingested. Death may occur.

Treatment of Propoxyphene Overdosage — Attention should be directed first to establishing a patent airway and to restoring ventilation. Mechanically assisted ventilation, with or without oxygen, may be required, and positive pressure respiration may be desirable if pulmonary edema is present. The narcotic antagonist naloxone will markedly reduce the degree of respiratory depression, and 0.4 to 2 mg should be administered promptly, preferably intravenously. If the desired degree of counteraction with improvement in respiratory functions is not obtained, naloxone should be repeated at 2 to 3-minute intervals. The duration of action of the antagonist may be brief. If no response is observed after 10 mg of naloxone have been administered, the diagnosis of propoxyphene toxicity should be questioned. Naloxone may also be administered by continuous intravenous infusion.

Treatment of Propoxyphene Overdosage in Children —The usual inital dose of naloxone in children is 0.01 mg/kg body weight given intravenously. If this dose does not result in the desired degree of clinical improvement, a subsequent increased dose of 0.1 mg/kg body weight may be administered. If an IV route of administration is not available, naloxone may be administered IM or subcutaneously in divided doses. If necessary, naloxone can be diluted with Sterile Water for Injection.

Blood gases, pH, and electrolytes should be monitored in order that acidosis and any electrolyte disturbance present may be corrected promptly. Acidosis, hypoxia, and generalized CNS depression predispose to the development of cardiac arrhythmias. Ventricular fibrillation or cardiac arrest may occur and necessitate the full complement of cardiopulmonary resuscitation (CPR) measures. Respiratory acidosis rapidly subsides as ventilation is restored and hypercapnea eliminated, but lactic acidosis may require intravenous bicarbonate for prompt correction.

Electrocardiographic monitoring is essential. Prompt correction of hypoxia, acidosis, and electrolyte disturbance (when present) will help prevent these cardiac complications and will increase the effectiveness of agents administered to restore normal cardiac function.

In addition to the use of a narcotic antagonist, the patient may require careful titration with an anticonvulsant to control convulsions. Analeptic drugs (for example, caffeine or amphetamine) should not be used because of their tendency to precipitate convulsions.

General supportive measures, in addition to oxygen, include, when necessary, intravenous fluids, vasopressor-inotropic compounds, and, when infection is likely, anti-infective agents. Gastric lavage may be useful, and activated charcoal can adsorb a significant amount of ingested propoxyphene. Dialysis is of little value in poisoning due to propoxyphene. Efforts should be made to determine whether other agents, such as alcohol, barbiturates, tranquilizers, or other CNS depressants, were also ingested, since these increase CNS depression as well as cause specific toxic effects.

Symptoms of Acetaminophen Overdosage — Shortly after oral ingestion of an overdose of acetaminophen and for the next 24 hours, anorexia, nausea, vomiting, diaphoresis, general malaise, and abdominal pain have been noted. The patient may then present no symptoms, but evidence of liver dysfunction may be apparent up to 72 hours after ingestion, with elevated serum transaminase and lactic dehydrogenase levels, an increase in serum bilirubin concentrations, and a prolonged prothrombin time. Death from hepatic failure may result 3 to 7 days after overdosage.

Acute renal failure may accompany the hepatic dysfunction and has been noted in patients who do not exhibit signs of fulminant hepatic failure. Typically, renal impairment is more apparent 6 to 9 days after ingestion of the overdose.

Treatment of Acetaminophen Overdosage —Acetaminophen in massive overdosage may cause hepatic toxicity in some

patients. *In all cases of suspected overdose, immediately call your regional poison center or the Rocky Mountain Poison Center's toll-free number* (800-525-6115) *for assistance in diagnosis and for directions in the use of N-acetylcysteine as an antidote.*

In adults, hepatic toxicity has rarely been reported with acute overdoses of less than 10 g and fatalities with less than 15 g. Importantly, young children seem to be more resistant than adults to the hepatotoxic effect of an acetaminophen overdose. Despite this, the measures outlined below should be initiated in any adult or child suspected of having ingested an acetaminophen overdose.

Because clinical and laboratory evidence of hepatic toxicity may not be apparent until 48 to 72 hours postingestion, liver function studies should be obtained initially and repeated at 24-hour intervals.

Consider emptying the stomach promptly by lavage or by induction of emesis with syrup of ipecac. Patients' estimates of the quantity of a drug ingested are notoriously unreliable. Therefore, if an acetaminophen overdose is suspected, a serum acetaminophen assay should be obtained as early as possible, but no sooner than 4 hours following ingestion. The antidote, N-acetylcysteine, should be administered as early as possible, and within 16 hours of the overdose ingestion for optimal results. Following recovery, there are no residual, structural, or functional hepatic abnormalities.

Symptoms of Salicylate Overdosage —Such symptoms include central nausea and vomiting, tinnitus and deafness, vertigo and headaches, mental dullness and confusion, diaphoresis, rapid pulse, and increased respiration and respiratory alkalosis.

Treatment of Salicylate Overdosage —When Darvon-N with A.S.A. has been ingested, the clinical picture may be complicated by salicylism.

The treatment of acute salicylate intoxication includes minimizing drug absorption, promoting elimination through the kidneys, and correcting metabolic derangements affecting body temperature, hydration, acid-base balance, and electrolyte balance. The technique to be employed for eliminating salicylate from the bloodstream depends on the degree of drug intoxication.

If the patient is seen within 4 hours of ingestion, the stomach should be emptied by inducing vomiting or by gastric lavage as soon as possible.

The nomogram of Done is a useful prognostic guide in which the expected severity of salicylate intoxication is based on serum salicylate levels and the time interval between ingestion and taking the blood sample.

Exchange transfusion is most feasible for a small infant. Intermittent peritoneal dialysis is useful for cases of moderate severity in adults. Intravenous fluids alkalinized by the addition of sodium bicarbonate or potassium citrate are helpful. Hemodialysis with the artificial kidney is the most effective means of removing salicylate and is indicated for the very severe cases of salicylate intoxication.

ANIMAL TOXICOLOGY

The acute lethal doses of the hydrochloride and napsylate salts of propoxyphene were determined in 4 species. The results shown in Figure 2 indicate that, on a molar basis, the napsylate salt is less toxic than the hydrochloride. This may be due to the relative insolubility and retarded absorption of propoxyphene napsylate

Figure 2. Acute oral toxicity of propoxyphene

Species	LD_{50} (mg/kg) $\pm$ SE	
	LD_{50} (mmole/kg)	
	Propoxyphene Hydrochloride	Propoxyphene Napsylate
Mouse	282 ± 39	915 ± 163
	0.75	1.62
Rat	230 ± 44	647 ± 95
	0.61	1.14
Rabbit	ca. 82	>183
	0.22	>0.32
Dog	ca. 100	>183
	0.27	>0.32

Some indication of the relative insolubility and retarded absorption of propoxyphene napsylate was obtained by measuring plasma propoxyphene levels in 2 groups of 4 dogs following oral administration of equimolar doses of the 2 salts. As shown in Figure 3, the peak plasma concentration observed with propoxyphene hydrochloride was much higher than that obtained after administration of the napsylate salt.

Figure 3. Plasma propoxyphene concentrations in dogs following large doses of the hydrochloride and napsylate salts

Although none of the animals in this experiment died, 3 of the 4 dogs given propoxyphene hydrochloride exhibited convulsive seizures during the time interval corresponding to the peak plasma levels. The 4 animals receiving the napsylate salt were mildly ataxic but not acutely ill.

HOW SUPPLIED

(℞) Tablets:
Darvocet-N 50, dark orange (No. 1890)—(RxPak* of 100) NDC 0002-0351-02; (ID†100) NDC 0002-0351-33; (500s) NDC 0002-0351-03
Darvocet-N 100, dark orange (No. 1893)—(RxPak* of 100) NDC 0002-0363-02; (ID100) NDC 0002-0363-33; (500s) NDC 0002-0363-03; (ID500) NDC 0002-0363-43; (RN‡500) NDC 0002-0363-46

* All RxPaks (prescription packages, Lilly) have safety closures.
† Identi-Dose® (unit dose medication, Lilly).
‡ Reverse-numbered package.
Store at controlled room temperature, 59° to 86°F (15° to 30°C).
(℞) Tablets Darvon-N, 100 mg, buff (No. 1883)—(RxPak* of 100) NDC 0002-0353-02; (ID†100) NDC 0002-0353-33; (500s) NDC 0002-0353-03
(℞) Darvon-N, Suspension, ‡ 50 mg/5 mL (No. M-135)—(16 fl oz) NDC 0002-2371-05

* All RxPaks (prescription packages, Lilly) have safety closures.
† Identi-Dose® (unit dose medication, Lilly).
‡ Shake well before using. Avoid frezing. Keep tightly closed.
Store at controlled room temperature, 59° to 86°F (15° to 30°C).
(℞) Tablets Darvon-N with A.S.A., orange (No. 1884)—(RxPak* of 100) NDC 0002-0354-02; (500s) NDC 0002-0354-03
Store at controlled room temperature, 59° to 86°F (15° to 30°C).

* All RxPaks (prescription packages, Lilly) have safety closures.

Shown in Product Identification Section, page 415
The following information, including illustrations of dosage forms and the maximum daily dosage of each, is available to patients receiving Darvon products.

Patient Information Sheet
YOUR PRESCRIPTION FOR A DARVON® (PROPOXYPHENE) PRODUCT ℞
Summary: Products containing Darvon are used to relieve pain.
LIMIT YOUR INTAKE OF ALCOHOL WHILE TAKING THIS DRUG. Make sure your doctor knows that you are taking tranquilizers, sleep aids, antidepressants, antihistamines, or any other drugs that make you sleepy. Combining propoxyphene with alcohol or these drugs in excessive doses is dangerous.
Use care while driving a car or using machines until you see how the drug affects you, because propoxyphene can make you sleepy. Do not take more of the drug than your doctor prescribed. Dependence has occurred when patients have taken propoxyphene for a long period of time at doses greater than recommended.
The rest of this leaflet gives you more information about propoxyphene. Please read it and keep it for future use.
Uses of Darvon: Products containing Darvon are used for the relief of mild to moderate pain. Products that contain Darvon plus aspirin or acetaminophen are prescribed for the relief of pain or pain associated with fever.
Before Taking Darvon: Make sure your doctor knows if you have ever had an allergic reaction to propoxyphene, aspirin, or acetaminophen. Some forms of propoxyphene products

Continued on next page

Lilly—Cont.

contain aspirin to help relieve the pain. Your doctor should be advised if you have a history of ulcers or if you are taking an anticoagulant ("blood thinner"). The aspirin may irritate the stomach lining and may cause bleeding, particularly if an ulcer is present. Also, bleeding may occur if you are taking an anticoagulant. In a small group of people, aspirin may cause an asthma attack. If you are one of these people, be sure your drug does not contain aspirin.

The effect of propoxyphene in children under 12 has not been studied. Therefore, use of the drug in this age group is not recommended.

Also, due to the possible association between aspirin and Reye syndrome, those propoxyphene products containing aspirin should not be given to children, including teenagers, with chickenpox or flu unless prescribed by a physician. The following propoxyphene products contain aspirin:

Darvon® with A.S.A.® (Propoxyphene Hydrochloride and Aspirin, Lilly)

Darvon® Compound and Darvon® Compound-65 (Propoxyphene Hydrochloride, Aspirin, and Caffeine, USP, Lilly)

Darvon-N® with A.S.A.® (Propoxyphene Napsylate and Aspirin, USP, Lilly)

How to Take Darvon: Follow your doctor's directions exactly. Do not increase the amount you take without your doctor's approval. If you miss a dose of the drug, do not take twice as much the next time.

Pregnancy: Do not take propoxyphene during pregnancy unless your doctor knows you are pregnant and specifically recommends its use. Cases of temporary dependence in the newborn have occurred when the mother has taken propoxyphene consistently in the weeks before delivery. As a general principle, no drug should be taken during pregnancy unless it is clearly necessary.

General Cautions: Heavy use of alcohol with propoxyphene is hazardous and may lead to overdosage symptoms (see "Overdose" below). THEREFORE, LIMIT YOUR INTAKE OF ALCOHOL WHILE TAKING PROPOXYPHENE.

Combinations of excessive doses of propoxyphene, alcohol, and tranquilizers are dangerous. Make sure your doctor knows you are taking tranquilizers, sleep aids, antidepressant drugs, antihistamines, or any other drugs that make you sleepy. The use of these drugs with propoxyphene increases their sedative effects and may lead to overdosage symptoms, including death (see "Overdose" below).

Propoxyphene may cause drowsiness or impair your mental and/or physical abilities; therefore, use caution when driving a vehicle or operating dangerous machinery. DO NOT perform any hazardous task until you have seen your response to this drug.

Propoxyphene may increase the concentration in the body of medications such as anticoagulants ("blood thinners"), antidepressants, or drugs used for epilepsy. The result may be excessive or adverse effects of these medications. Make sure your doctor knows if you are taking any of these medications.

Dependence: You can become dependent on propoxyphene if you take it in higher than recommended doses over a long period of time. Dependence is a feeling of need for the drug and a feeling that you cannot perform normally without it.

Overdose: An overdose of Darvon, alone or in combination with other drugs, including alcohol, may cause weakness, difficulty in breathing, confusion, anxiety, and more severe drowsiness and dizziness. Extreme overdosage may lead to unconsciousness and death.

If the propoxyphene product contains acetaminophen, the overdosage symptoms include nausea, vomiting, lack of appetite, and abdominal pain. Liver damage may occur.

When the propoxyphene product contains aspirin, symptoms of taking too much of the drug are headache, dizziness, ringing in the ears, difficulty in hearing, dim vision, confusion, drowsiness, sweating, thirst, rapid breathing, nausea, vomiting, and, occasionally, diarrhea.

In any suspected overdosage situation, contact your doctor or nearest hospital emergency room. GET EMERGENCY HELP IMMEDIATELY.

KEEP THIS DRUG AND ALL DRUGS OUT OF THE REACH OF CHILDREN.

Possible Side Effects: When propoxyphene is taken as directed, side effects are infrequent. Among those reported are drowsiness, dizziness, nausea, and vomiting. If these effects occur, it may help if you lie down and rest.

Less frequently reported side effects are constipation, abdominal pain, skin rashes, lightheadedness, headache, weakness, hallucinations, minor visual disturbances, and feelings of elation or discomfort.

If side effects occur and concern you, contact your doctor.

Other Information: The safe and effective use of propoxyphene depends on your taking it exactly as directed. This drug has been prescribed specifically for you and your present condition. Do not give this drug to others who may have similar symptoms. Do not use it for any other reason.

If you would like more information about propoxyphene, ask your doctor or pharmacist. They have a more technical leaflet (professional labeling) you may read.

Prescription Vial Sticker

Tell your doctor if you are taking tranquilizers, antidepressant drugs, or sleep aids. LIMIT alcohol use with Darvon-N® (propoxyphene napsylate) and Darvon® (propoxyphene hydrochloride) products.

[111688]

DARVON® ℞
[där′von]
(propoxyphene hydrochloride)
Capsules, USP

DARVON® COMPOUND and
[där′vŏn kŏm′pound]
DARVON® COMPOUND–65
(propoxyphene hydrochloride, aspirin, and caffeine)

DARVON® WITH A.S.A®
[där′vŏn with ā′ĕs-ā]
(propoxyphene hydrochloride and aspirin)

DESCRIPTION

Darvon® (Propoxyphene Hydrochloride, USP, Lilly) is an odorless, white crystalline powder with a bitter taste. It is freely soluble in water. Chemically, it is α-(+)-4-(Dimethylamino)-3-methyl- 1,2-diphenyl-2-butanol Propionate Hydrochloride.

Each Pulvule® Darvon contains 32 or 65 mg propoxyphene hydrochloride. Each Pulvule also contains D & C Red No. 33, F D & C Yellow No. 6, gelatin, magnesium stearate, silicone, starch, titanium dioxide, and other inactive ingredients.

	Pulvules No. 368 Darvon Compound	Pulvules No. 369 Darvon Compound-65
32 mg	Darvon	65 mg
389 mg	A.S.A.®	389 mg
	(Aspirin, USP, Lilly)	
32.4 mg	Caffeine	32.4 mg

Pulvules Darvon Compound and Darvon Compound-65 also contain FD&C Yellow No. 6, gelatin, glutamic acid hydrochloride, iron oxide, kaolin, silicone, titanium dioxide, and other inactive ingredients. Darvon Compound also contains D&C Red No. 33. Darvon Compound-65 also contains FD&C Red No. 3.

Each Pulvule Darvon with A.S.A. contains 65 mg propoxyphene hydrochloride and 325 mg aspirin. Each Pulvule also contains D&C Red No. 33, FD&C Red No. 3, FD&C Yellow No. 6, gelatin, glutamic acid hydrochloride, silicone, starch, titanium dioxide, and other inactive ingredients.

CLINICAL PHARMACOLOGY

Propoxyphene is a centrally acting narcotic analgesic agent. Equimolar doses of propoxyphene hydrochloride or napsylate provide similar plasma concentrations. Following administration of 65, 130, or 195 mg of propoxyphene hydrochloride, the bioavailability of propoxyphene is equivalent to that of 100, 200, or 300 mg respectively of propoxyphene napsylate. Peak plasma concentrations of propoxyphene are reached in 2 to 2 ½ hours. After a 65-mg oral dose of propoxyphene hydrochloride, peak plasma levels of 0.05 to 0.1 mg/L are achieved.

Repeated doses of propoxyphene at 6-hour intervals lead to increasing plasma concentrations, with a plateau after the ninth dose at 48 hours.

Propoxyphene is metabolized in the liver to yield norpropoxyphene. Propoxyphene has a half-life of 6 to 12 hours, whereas that of norpropoxyphene is 30 to 36 hours.

Norpropoxyphene has substantially less central-nervous-system-depressant effect than propoxyphene but a greater local anesthetic effect, which is similar to that of amitriptyline and antiarrhythmic agents, such as lidocaine and quinidine.

In animal studies in which propoxyphene and norpropoxyphene were continuously infused in large amounts, intracardiac conduction time (PR and QRS intervals) was prolonged. Any intracardiac conduction delay attributable to high concentrations of norpropoxyphene may be of relatively long duration.

ACTIONS

Propoxyphene is a mild narcotic analgesic structurally related to methadone. The potency of propoxyphene hydrochloride is from two-thirds to equal that of codeine.

The combination of propoxyphene with a mixture of aspirin and caffeine produces greater analgesia than that produced by either propoxyphene or aspirin and caffeine administered alone.

INDICATIONS

Darvon® (propoxyphene hydrochloride, Lilly) is indicated for the relief of mild to moderate pain.

Darvon Compound, Darvon Compound-65, and Darvon with A.S.A. are indicated for the relief of mild to moderate pain, either when pain is present alone or when it is accompanied by fever.

CONTRAINDICATION

Hypersensitivity to propoxyphene, aspirin, or caffeine.

WARNINGS: *See under Darvocet-N®.*

PRECAUTIONS: *See under Darvocet-N®.*

ADVERSE REACTIONS: *See under Darvocet-N®.*

DOSAGE AND ADMINISTRATION

These products are given orally. The usual dosage of Darvon® (propoxyphene hydrochloride, Lilly) is 65 mg every 4 hours as needed for pain.

The usual dosage of Darvon Compound and Darvon Compound-65 is 32 or 65 mg propoxyphene hydrochloride, 389 mg aspirin, and 32.4 mg caffeine every 4 hours as needed for pain.

The usual dosage of Darvon with A.S.A. is 65 mg propoxyphene hydrochloride and 325 mg aspirin every 4 hours as needed for pain.

The maximum recommended dose of propoxyphene hydrochloride is 390 mg/day.

Consideration should be given to a reduced total daily dosage in patients with hepatic or renal impairment.

MANAGEMENT OF OVERDOSAGE

In all cases of suspected overdosage, call your regional Poison Control Center to obtain the most up-to-date information about the treatment of overdose. This recommendation is made because, in general, information regarding the treatment of overdosage may change more rapidly than do package inserts.

Initial consideration should be given to the management of the CNS effects of propoxyphene overdosage. Resuscitative measures should be initiated promptly.

Symptoms of Propoxyphene Overdosage —See under Darvocet-N®.

Treatment of Propoxyphene Overdosage —See under Darvocet-N®.

Treatment of Propoxyphene Overdosage in Children —See under Darvocet-N®.

Symptoms of Salicylate Overdosage —See under Darvocet-N®.

Treatment of Salicylate Overdosage —When Darvon Compound, Darvon Compound-65, or Darvon with A.S.A. has been ingested, the clinical picture may be complicated by salicylism.

See also under Darvocet-N®.

HOW SUPPLIED

(℞) Pulvules:
32 mg, pink (No. 364)—(RxPak* of 100) NDC 0002-0802-02; (500s) NDC 0002-0802-03
65 mg, pink (No. 365)—(RxPak of 100) NDC 0002-0803-03; (ID100) NDC 0002-0803-33; (500s) NDC 0002-0803-03; (RN‡500) NDC 0002-0803-46

* All RxPaks (prescription packages, Lilly) have safety closures.
† Identi-Dose® (unit dose medication, Lilly).
‡ Reverse-numbered package.
Store at controlled room temperature, 59° to 86°F (15° to 30°C).

(℞) Pulvules:
Darvon Compound, pink and gray (No. 368)—(RxPak* of 100) NDC 0002-3110-02; (500s) NDC 0002-3110-03
Darvon Compound-65, red and gray (No. 369)—(RxPak of 100) NDC 0002-3111-02; (ID†100) NDC 0002-3111-33; (500s) NDC 0002-3111-03

* All RxPaks (prescription packages, Lilly) have safety closures.
† Identi-Dose® (unit dose medication, Lilly).
Store at controlled room temperature, 59° to 86°F (15° to 30°C).
(℞) Pulvules Darvon with A.S.A., red and pink (No. 366)—(RxPak* of 100) NDC 0002-0804-02

* All RxPaks (prescription packages, Lilly) have safety closures.
Store at controlled room temperature, 59° to 86°F (15° to 30°C).

Shown in Product Identification Section, page 415
Patient information, including illustrations of dosage forms and the maximum daily dosage of each, is available to patients receiving Darvon (propoxyphene) products.
See under Darvocet-N®.

[102888]

DIETHYLSTILBESTROL   ℞
[dī-eth′il-stil-bĕs′trōl]
USP

---

1. USE OF ESTROGENS HAS BEEN REPORTED TO INCREASE THE RISK OF ENDOMETRIAL CARCINOMA

Three independent case-control studies have reported an increased risk of endometrial cancer in postmenopausal women exposed to exogenous estrogens for more than 1 year. This risk was independent of other known risk factors for endometrial cancer. These studies are further supported by the finding that, since 1969, the incidence rate of endometrial cancer has increased sharply in 8 different areas of the United States which have population-based cancer reporting systems.

The 3 case-control studies reported that the risk of endometrial cancer in estrogen users was about 4.5 to 13.9 times greater than in nonusers. The risk appears to depend on both the duration of treatment and the dose of estrogen. In view of these findings, the lowest dose that will control symptoms should be utilized when estrogens are used for the treatment of menopausal symptoms, and medication should be discontinued as soon as possible. When prolonged treatment is medically indicated, a reassessment should be made on at least a semiannual basis to determine the need for continued therapy. Although the evidence must be considered preliminary, one study suggests that cyclic administration of low doses of estrogen may carry less risk than does continuous administration; it therefore appears prudent to utilize such a regimen.

Close clinical surveillance of all women taking estrogens is important. In all cases of undiagnosed persistent or recurring abnormal vaginal bleeding, adequate diagnostic measures should be undertaken to rule out malignancy.

At present, there is no evidence that "natural" estrogens are more or less hazardous than "synthetic" estrogens at equivalent estrogenic doses.

2. ESTROGENS SHOULD NOT BE USED DURING PREGNANCY

The use of female sex hormones, both estrogens and progestogens, during early pregnancy may affect the offspring. It has been reported that females exposed *in utero* to diethylstilbestrol, a nonsteroidal estrogen, may have an increased risk of developing later in life a rare form of vaginal or cervical cancer. This risk has been estimated to be 0.14 to 1.4 per 1,000 exposures. Furthermore, from 30% to 90% of such exposed women have been found to have vaginal adenosis and epithelial changes of the vagina and cervix. Although these changes are histologically benign, it is not known whether they are precursors of malignancy. Even though similar data are not available with the use of other estrogens, it cannot be presumed that they would not induce similar changes.

Several reports suggest that there is an association between intrauterine exposure to female sex hormones and congenital anomalies, including congenital heart defects and limb-reduction defects. One case-control study estimated a 4.7-fold increased risk of limb-reduction defects in infants exposed *in utero* to sex hormones (oral contraceptives, hormone withdrawal tests for pregnancy, or attempted treatment for threatened abortion). Some of these exposures were very short and involved only a few days of treatment. The data suggest that the risk of limb-reduction defects in exposed fetuses is somewhat less than 1 per 1,000.

In the past, female sex hormones have been used during pregnancy in an attempt to treat threatened or habitual abortion; however, their efficacy was never conclusively proved or disproved.

If diethylstilbestrol is administered during pregnancy, or if the patient becomes pregnant while taking this drug, she should be apprised of the potential risks to the fetus and of the advisability of pregnancy continuation.

THIS DRUG PRODUCT SHOULD NOT BE USED AS A POSTCOITAL CONTRACEPTIVE

DESCRIPTION

Diethylstilbestrol is a crystalline synthetic estrogenic substance capable of producing all the pharmacologic and therapeutic responses attributed to natural estrogens. Diethylstilbestrol may be administered orally (in the form of Enseals® [enteric-release tablets, Lilly] and tablets). Chemically, diethylstilbestrol is α,α′-diethyl-4,4′-stilbenediol.

The Enseals contain cornstarch, FD&C Blue No. 2, FD&C Red No. 3, FD&C Yellow No. 6, lactose, magnesium stearate, sucrose, talc, titanium dioxide, and other inactive ingredients.

The tablets contain cornstarch, lactose, magnesium stearate, and talc.

INDICATIONS

Diethylstilbestrol is indicated in the treatment of:

1. Breast cancer (for palliation only) in appropriately selected women and men with metastatic disease
2. Prostatic carcinoma—palliative therapy of advanced disease

DIETHYLSTILBESTROL SHOULD NOT BE USED FOR ANY PURPOSE DURING PREGNANCY. ITS USE MAY CAUSE SEVERE HARM TO THE FETUS (SEE BOXED WARNING).

CONTRAINDICATIONS

Estrogens should not be used in women (or men) with any of the following conditions:

1. Known or suspected cancer of the breast, except in appropriately selected patients being treated for metastatic disease
2. Known or suspected estrogen-dependent neoplasia
3. Known or suspected pregnancy (see boxed warning)
4. Undiagnosed abnormal genital bleeding
5. Active thrombophlebitis or thromboembolic disorders
6. A past history of thrombophlebitis, thrombosis, or thromboembolic disorders associated with previous use of estrogen (except when used in treatment of breast or prostatic malignancy)

WARNINGS

1. *Induction of Malignant Neoplasms* —In certain animal species, long-term continuous administration of natural and synthetic estrogens increases the frequency of carcinomas of the breast, cervix, vagina, kidney, and liver. There are now reports that prolonged use of estrogens increases the risk of carcinoma of the endometrium in humans (see boxed warning).

At the present time, there is no satisfactory evidence that administration of estrogens to postmenopausal women increases the risk of cancer of the breast. This possibility, however, has been raised by a recent long-term follow-up of one physician's practice. Because of the animal data, there is a need for caution in prescribing estrogens for women with a family history of breast cancer or for women who have breast nodules, fibrocystic disease, or abnormal mammograms.

2. *Gallbladder Disease* —A recent study reported a 2-to-3-fold increase in the risk of gallbladder disease occurring in women receiving postmenopausal estrogen therapy, similar to the twofold increased risk previously noted in women using oral contraceptives. In the case of oral contraceptives, this increased risk appeared after 2 years of use.

3. *Effects Similar to Those Caused by Estrogen-Progestogen Oral Contraceptives* —There are several serious adverse effects associated with the use of oral contraceptives; however, most of these adverse effects have not as yet been documented as consequences of postmenopausal estrogen therapy. This may reflect the comparatively low doses of estrogen used in postmenopausal women. It would be expected that these adverse effects are more likely to occur following administration of the larger doses of estrogen used for treating prostatic or breast cancer. It has, in fact, been shown that there is an increased risk of thrombosis with the administration of estrogens for prostatic cancer in men and for postpartum breast engorgement in women.

  a. *Thromboembolic Disease* —It is now well established that women taking oral contraceptives run an increased risk of various thromboembolic and thrombotic vascular diseases, such as thrombophlebitis, pulmonary embolism, stroke, and myocardial infarction. Cases of retinal thrombosis, mesenteric thrombosis, and optic neuritis have been reported in users of oral contraceptives. There is evidence that the risk of several of these adverse reactions is related to the dose of the drug. An increased risk of postsurgical thromboembolic complications has also been reported in users of oral contraceptives. If feasible, estrogen therapy should be discontinued at least 4 weeks before surgery that may be associated with an increased risk of thromboembolism or that may require periods of prolonged immobilization.

Although an increased rate of thromboembolic and thrombotic disease has not been noted in postmenopausal users of estrogen, this does not rule out the possibility that such an increase may be present or that it exists in subgroups of women who have underlying risk factors or who are receiving relatively large doses of estrogens. Therefore, estrogens should not be used in persons with active thrombophlebitis or thromboembolic disorders, nor should they be used (except in treatment of malignancy) in persons with a history of such disorders associated with estrogen therapy. Estrogens should be administered cautiously to patients with cerebral vascular or coronary artery disease and only when such therapy is clearly needed.

In a large prospective clinical trial in men, large doses of estrogen (5 mg of conjugated estrogens per day), comparable to those used to treat cancer of the prostate and breast, have been shown to increase the risk of nonfatal myocardial infarction, pulmonary embolism, and thrombophlebitis. When such large doses of estrogen are used, any of the thromboembolic and thrombotic adverse effects associated with the use of oral contraceptives should be considered a clear risk.

  b. *Hepatic Adenoma* —Benign hepatic adenomas appear to be associated with the use of oral contraceptives. Although these adenomas are benign and rare, they may rupture and may cause death by intra-abdominal hemorrhage. Such lesions have not yet been reported in association with the administration of other estrogen or progestogen preparations, but they should be considered when abdominal pain and tenderness, abdominal mass, or hypovolemic shock occurs in persons receiving estrogen therapy. Hepatocellular carcinoma has also been reported in women taking estrogen-containing oral contraceptives. The relationship of this malignancy to such drugs is not known at this time.

  c. *Elevated Blood Pressure* —Increased blood pressure is not uncommon in women taking oral contraceptives. There is now one report that this may occur with use of estrogens in the menopause, and blood pressure should be monitored during estrogen therapy, especially if high doses are used.

  d. *Glucose Tolerance* —A decrease in glucose tolerance has been observed in a significant percentage of patients on estrogen-containing oral contraceptives. For this reason, diabetic patients should be carefully observed while receiving estrogen.

4. *Hypercalcemia* —Administration of estrogens may lead to severe hypercalcemia in patients with breast cancer and bone metastases. If this occurs, the drug should be stopped and appropriate measures taken to reduce the serum calcium level.

PRECAUTIONS

General —1. A complete medical and family history should be taken prior to initiation of any estrogen therapy. In the pretreatment and periodic physical examinations, special consideration should be given to blood pressure, breasts, abdomen, and pelvic organs, and a Papanicolaou smear should be performed. As a general rule, estrogen should not be prescribed for over a year without another physical examination.

2. Fluid retention—Because estrogens may cause some degree of fluid retention, conditions which might be influenced by this factor, such as epilepsy, migraine, and cardiac or renal dysfunction, require careful observation.

3. Certain patients may develop undesirable manifestations of excessive estrogenic stimulation, such as abnormal or excessive uterine bleeding, mastodynia, etc.

4. Oral contraceptives appear to be associated with an increased incidence of mental depression. Although it is not clear whether this is due to the estrogenic or progestogenic component of the contraceptive agent, patients with a history of depression should be carefully observed.

5. Preexisting uterine leiomyomata may increase in size with administration of estrogens.

6. The pathologist should be advised of estrogen therapy when relevant specimens are submitted.

7. Patients with a past history of jaundice during pregnancy run an increased risk of recurrence of jaundice while receiving estrogen-containing oral contraceptive therapy. If jaundice develops in any patient receiving estrogen, the medication should be discontinued while the cause is investigated.

8. Estrogens may be poorly metabolized in patients with impaired liver function, and they should therefore be administered with caution in such patients.

9. Because estrogens influence the metabolism of calcium and phosphorus, they should be used with caution in patients with metabolic bone diseases associated with hypercalcemia or in patients with renal insufficiency.

10. Because of the effects of estrogens on epiphyseal closure, they should be used judiciously in young patients in whom bone growth is not complete.

11. Certain endocrine and liver function tests may be affected by estrogen-containing oral contraceptives. The following similar changes may be expected with larger doses of estrogen:

  a. Increased sulfobromophthalein retention
  b. Increased prothrombin and factors VII, VIII, IX, and X; decreased antithrombin 3; increased norepinephrine-induced platelet aggregability
  c. Increased thyroid-binding globulin (TBG) leading to increased circulating total thyroid hormone, as measured by PBI, T^4 by column, or T^4 by radioimmunoassay. Free T^3 resin uptake is decreased, reflecting the elevated TBG; free T^4 concentration is unaltered
  d. Impaired glucose tolerance
  e. Decreased pregnanediol excretion
  f. Reduced response to metyrapone test
  g. Reduced serum folate concentration
  h. Increased serum triglyceride and phospholipid concentration

Information for the Patient —See text of Patient Package Insert.

Continued on next page

---

* Identi-Code® symbol.

Lilly—Cont.

Pregnancy Category X—See Contraindications and boxed warning.

Nursing Mothers—As a general principle, any drug should be administered to nursing mothers only when clearly necessary, since many drugs are excreted in human milk.

ADVERSE REACTIONS

(*See* Warnings regarding induction of neoplasia, adverse effects on the fetus, increased incidence of gallbladder disease, and adverse effects similar to those of oral contraceptives, including thromboembolism.) The following additional adverse reactions have been reported with estrogenic therapy, including oral contraceptives:

1. *Genitourinary System*
   Breakthrough bleeding, spotting, change in menstrual flow
   Dysmenorrhea
   Premenstrual-like syndrome
   Amenorrhea during and after treatment
   Increase in size of uterine fibromyomata
   Vaginal candidiasis
   Change in cervical eversion and in degree of cervical secretion
   Cystitis-like syndrome
2. *Breasts*
   Tenderness, enlargement, secretion
3. *Gastrointestinal*
   Nausea, vomiting
   Abdominal cramps, bloating
   Cholestatic jaundice
4. *Skin*
   Chloasma or melasma which may persist when drug is discontinued
   Erythema multiforme
   Erythema nodosum
   Hemorrhagic eruption
   Loss of scalp hair
   Hirsutism
5. *Eyes*
   Steepening of corneal curvature
   Intolerance to contact lenses
6. *CNS*
   Headache, migraine, dizziness
   Mental depression
   Chorea
7. *Miscellaneous*
   Increase or decrease in weight
   Reduced carbohydrate tolerance
   Aggravation of porphyria
   Edema
   Changes in libido

OVERDOSAGE

Signs and Symptoms—Symptoms of acute overdose include anorexia, nausea, vomiting, abdominal cramps, and diarrhea. Withdrawal vaginal bleeding may follow large doses. Chronic toxicity may include salt and water retention, edema, headache, vertigo, leg cramps, gynecomastia, chloasma, and porphyria cutanea tarda. Polydipsia, polyuria, fatigue, and an abnormal glucose tolerance may occur in some patients with preclinical diabetes mellitus.

No information is available on the following: LD_{50}, concentration of diethylstilbestrol in biologic fluids associated with toxicity and/or death, the amount of drug in a single dose usually associated with symptoms of overdosage, or the amount of diethylstilbestrol in a single dose likely to be life-threatening.

Treatment—Chronic diethylstilbestrol toxicity should be treated by discontinuing all estrogenic medications and providing supportive care for any symptoms that may be present.

To obtain up-to-date information about the treatment of overdose, a good resource is your certified Regional Poison Control Center. Telephone numbers of certified poison control centers are listed in the *Physicians' Desk Reference (PDR)*. In managing overdosage, consider the possibility of multiple drug overdoses, interaction among drugs, and unusual drug kinetics in your patient.

In treating acute overdose, protect the patient's airway and support ventilation and perfusion. Meticulously monitor and maintain, within acceptable limits, the patient's vital signs, blood gases, serum electrolytes, etc. Absorption of drugs from the gastrointestinal tract may be decreased by giving activated charcoal, which, in many cases, is more effective than emesis or lavage; consider charcoal instead of or in addition to gastric emptying. Repeated doses of charcoal over time may hasten elimination of some drugs that have been absorbed. Safeguard the patient's airway when employing gastric emptying or charcoal.

Forced diuresis, peritoneal dialysis, hemodialysis, or charcoal hemoperfusion have not been established as beneficial for an overdose of diethylstilbestrol.

DOSAGE AND ADMINISTRATION

Given Chronically:
   Inoperable progressing prostatic cancer
      1 to 3 mg daily initially, increased in advanced cases; the dosage may later be reduced to an average of 1 mg daily.
   Inoperable progressing breast cancer in appropriately selected men and postmenopausal women (*see* Indications)
      15 mg daily
Patients with an intact uterus should be closely monitored for signs of endometrial cancer, and appropriate diagnostic measures should be taken to rule out malignancy in the event of persistent or recurring abnormal vaginal bleeding.

HOW SUPPLIED

(℞) Diethylstilbestrol, USP, is supplied in the following forms:

Enseals:
1 mg (No. 49)—(100s) NDC 0002-0122-02; (1,000s) NDC 0002-0122-04
5 mg (No. 85)—(100s) NDC 0002-0133-02
Tablets:
1 mg (No. 1649)—(100s) NDC 0002-1052-02; (1,000s) NDC 0002-1052-04
5 mg (No. 1685)—(100s) NDC 0002-1054-02   [083188]

DOBUTREX® SOLUTION   ℞
[dō′bū-trĕks]
(dobutamine hydrochloride)
Injection

DESCRIPTION

Dobutrex® Solution (Dobutamine Hydrochloride Injection, Lilly) is (±)-4-[2-[[3-(p-hydroxyphenyl)-1-methylpropyl]amino]-ethyl]-pyrocatechol hydrochloride. It is a synthetic catecholamine.
Molecular Formula:$C_{18}H_{23}NO_3 \cdot HCl$
Molecular Weight: 337.85
The clinical formulation is supplied in a sterile form for intravenous use only. Each mL contains 12.5 mg dobutamine, 0.24 mg sodium bisulfite (added during manufacture), and water for injection, q.s. Hydrochloric acid and/or sodium hydroxide may have been added during manufacture to adjust the pH.

CLINICAL PHARMACOLOGY

Dobutrex® Solution (Dobutamine Hydrochloride Injection, Lilly) is a direct-acting inotropic agent whose primary activity results from stimulation of the β receptors of the heart while producing comparatively mild chronotropic, hypertensive, arrhythmogenic, and vasodilative effects. It does not cause the release of endogenous norepinephrine, as does dopamine. In animal studies, dobutamine produces less increase in heart rate and less decrease in peripheral vascular resistance for a given inotropic effect than does isoproterenol.

In patients with depressed cardiac function, both dobutamine and isoproterenol increase the cardiac output to a similar degree. In the case of dobutamine, this increase is usually not accompanied by marked increases in heart rate (although tachycardia is occasionally observed), and the cardiac stroke volume is usually increased. In contrast, isoproterenol increases the cardiac index primarily by increasing the heart rate while stroke volume changes little or declines.

Facilitation of atrioventricular conduction has been observed in human electrophysiologic studies and in patients with atrial fibrillation.

Systemic vascular resistance is usually decreased with administration of dobutamine. Occasionally, minimum vasoconstriction has been observed.

Most clinical experience with dobutamine is short-term—not more than several hours in duration. In the limited number of patients who were studied for 24, 48, and 72 hours, a persistent increase in cardiac output occurred in some, whereas output returned toward baseline values in others.

The onset of action of Dobutrex Solution is within 1 to 2 minutes; however, as much as 10 minutes may be required to obtain the peak effect of a particular infusion rate.

The plasma half-life of dobutamine in humans is 2 minutes. The principal routes of metabolism are methylation of the catechol and conjugation. In human urine, the major excretion products are the conjugates of dobutamine and 3-O-methyl dobutamine. The 3-O-methyl derivative of dobutamine is inactive.

Alteration of synaptic concentrations of catecholamines with either reserpine or tricyclic antidepressants does not alter the actions of dobutamine in animals, which indicates that the actions of dobutamine are not dependent on presynaptic mechanisms.

INDICATIONS AND USAGE

Dobutrex® Solution (Dobutamine Hydrochloride Injection, Lilly) is indicated when parenteral therapy is necessary for inotropic support in the <u>short-term</u> treatment of adults with

---

cardiac decompensation due to depressed contractility resulting either from organic heart disease or from cardiac surgical procedures.

In patients who have atrial fibrillation with rapid ventricular response, a digitalis preparation should be used prior to institution of therapy with Dobutrex Solution.

CONTRAINDICATION

Dobutrex® Solution (Dobutamine Hydrochloride Injection, Lilly) is contraindicated in patients with idiopathic hypertrophic subaortic stenosis and in patients who have shown previous manifestations of hypersensitivity to Dobutrex Solution.

WARNINGS

1. *Increase in Heart Rate or Blood Pressure*—Dobutrex® Solution (Dobutamine Hydrochloride Injection, Lilly) may cause a marked increase in heart rate or blood pressure, especially systolic pressure. Approximately 10% of patients in clinical studies have had rate increases of 30 beats/minute or more, and about 7.5% have had a 50-mm Hg or greater increase in systolic pressure. Usually, reduction of dosage promptly reverses these effects. Because dobutamine facilitates atrioventricular conduction, patients with atrial fibrillation are at risk of developing rapid ventricular response. Patients with preexisting hypertension appear to face an increased risk of developing an exaggerated pressor response.

2. *Ectopic Activity*—Dobutrex may precipitate or exacerbate ventricular ectopic activity, but it rarely has caused ventricular tachycardia.

3. *Hypersensitivity*—Reactions suggestive of hypersensitivity associated with administration of Dobutrex Solution, including skin rash, fever, eosinophilia, and bronchospasm, have been reported occasionally.

4. Dobutrex Solution contains sodium bisulfite, a sulfite that may cause allergic-type reactions, including anaphylactic symptoms and life-threatening or less severe asthmatic episodes, in certain susceptible people. The overall prevalence of sulfite sensitivity in the general population is unknown and probably low. Sulfite sensitivity is seen more frequently in asthmatic than in nonasthmatic people.

PRECAUTIONS

1. During the administration of Dobutrex® Solution (Dobutamine Hydrochloride Injection, Lilly), as with any adrenergic agent, ECG and blood pressure should be continuously monitored. In addition, pulmonary wedge pressure and cardiac output should be monitored whenever possible to aid in the safe and effective infusion of Dobutrex Solution.

2. Hypovolemia should be corrected with suitable volume expanders before treatment with Dobutrex Solution is instituted.

3. Animal studies indicate that dobutamine may be ineffective if the patient has recently received a β-blocking drug. In such a case, the peripheral vascular resistance may increase.

4. No improvement may be observed in the presence of marked mechanical obstruction, such as severe valvular aortic stenosis.

Usage Following Acute Myocardial Infarction—Clinical experience with Dobutrex Solution following myocardial infarction has been insufficient to establish the safety of the drug for this use. There is concern that any agent which increases contractile force and heart rate may increase the size of an infarction by intensifying ischemia, but it is not known whether dobutamine does so.

Usage in Pregnancy—Reproduction studies performed in rats and rabbits have revealed no evidence of impaired fertility, harm to the fetus, or teratogenic effects due to dobutamine. However, the drug has not been administered to pregnant women and should be used only when the expected benefits clearly outweigh the potential risks to the fetus.

Pediatric Use—The safety and effectiveness of Dobutrex Solution for use in children have not been studied.

Drug Interactions—There was no evidence of drug interactions in clinical studies in which Dobutrex Solution was administered concurrently with other drugs, including digitalis preparations, furosemide, spironolactone, lidocaine, glyceryl trinitrate, isosorbide dinitrate, morphine, atropine, heparin, protamine, potassium chloride, folic acid, and acetaminophen. Preliminary studies indicate that the concomitant use of dobutamine and nitroprusside results in a higher cardiac output and, usually, a lower pulmonary wedge pressure than when either drug is used alone.

ADVERSE REACTIONS

Increased Heart Rate, Blood Pressure, and Ventricular Ectopic Activity—A 10 to 20-mm increase in systolic blood pressure and an increase in heart rate of 5 to 15 beats/minute have been noted in most patients (*see* Warnings regarding exaggerated chronotropic and pressor effects). Approximately 5% of patients have had increased premature ventricular beats during infusions. These effects are dose related.

Hypotension—Precipitous decreases in blood pressure have occasionally been described in association with dobutamine therapy. Decreasing the dose or discontinuing the infusion typically results in rapid return of blood pressure to baseline values.

Reactions at Sites of Intravenous Infusion—Phlebitis has occasionally been reported. Local inflammatory changes have been described following inadvertent infiltration.

Miscellaneous Uncommon Effects—The following adverse effects have been reported in 1% to 3% of patients: nausea, headache, anginal pain, nonspecific chest pain, palpitations, and shortness of breath.

No abnormal laboratory values attributable to Dobutrex® Solution (Dobutamine Hydrochloride Injection, Lilly) have been observed.

Longer-Term Safety—Infusions of up to 72 hours have revealed no adverse effects other than those seen with shorter infusions.

OVERDOSAGE

Overdoses of dobutamine have been reported rarely. The following is provided to serve as a guide if such an overdose is encountered.

Signs and Symptoms—Toxicity from dobutamine hydrochloride is usually due to excessive cardiac β-receptor stimulation. The duration of action of dobutamine hydrochloride is generally short ($T_{1/2}$= 2 minutes) because it is rapidly metabolized by catechol-O-methyltransferase. The symptoms of toxicity may include anorexia, nausea, vomiting, tremor, anxiety, palpitations, headache, shortness of breath, and anginal and nonspecific chest pain. The positive inotropic and chronotropic effects of dobutamine on the myocardium may cause hypertension, tachyarrhythmias, myocardial ischemia, and ventricular fibrillation. Hypotension may result from vasodilation.

If the product is ingested, unpredictable absorption may occur from the mouth and the gastrointestinal tract.

Treatment—To obtain up-to-date information about the treatment of overdose, a good resource is your certified Regional Poison Control Center. Telephone numbers of certified poison control centers are listed in the *Physicians' Desk Reference (PDR)*. In managing overdosage, consider the possibility of multiple drug overdoses, interaction among drugs, and unusual drug kinetics in your patient.

The initial actions to be taken in a dobutamine hydrochloride overdose are discontinuing administration, establishing an airway, and ensuring oxygenation and ventilation. Resuscitative measures should be initiated promptly. Severe ventricular tachyarrhythmias may be successfully treated with propranolol or lidocaine. Hypertension usually responds to a reduction in dose or discontinuation of therapy.

Protect the patient's airway and support ventilation and perfusion. If needed, meticulously monitor and maintain, within acceptable limits, the patient's vital signs, blood gases, serum electrolytes, etc. Absorption of drugs from the gastrointestinal tract may be decreased by giving activated charcoal, which, in many cases, is more effective than emesis or lavage; consider charcoal instead of or in addition to gastric emptying. Repeated doses of charcoal over time may hasten elimination of some drugs that have been absorbed. Safeguard the patient's airway when employing gastric emptying or charcoal.

Forced diuresis, peritoneal dialysis, hemodialysis, or charcoal hemoperfusion have not been established as beneficial for an overdose of dobutamine hydrochloride.

DOSAGE AND ADMINISTRATION

Note—Do not add Dobutrex® Solution (Dobutamine Hydrochloride Injection, Lilly) to 5% Sodium Bicarbonate Injection or to any other strongly alkaline solutions. Dobutrex Solution should not be used in conjunction with other agents or diluents containing both sodium bisulfite and ethanol.

Reconstitution and Stability—At the time of administration, Dobutrex Solution must be further diluted in an IV container to at least a 50 mL solution using one of the following intravenous solutions as a diluent: 5% Dextrose Injection, 5% Dextrose and 0.45% Sodium Chloride Injection, 5% Dextrose and 0.9% Sodium Chloride Injection, 10% Dextrose Injection, Isolyte® M with 5% Dextrose Injection, Lactated Ringer's Injection, 5% Dextrose in Lactated Ringer's Injection, Normosol®-M in D5-W, 20% Osmitrol® in Water for Injection, 0.9% Sodium Chloride Injection, or Sodium Lactate Injection. Intravenous solutions should be used within 24 hours.

Solutions containing Dobutrex Solution may exhibit a pink color that, if present, will increase with time. This color change is due to slight oxidation of the drug, but there is no significant loss of potency during the reconstituted time periods stated above.

Recommended Dosage—The rate of infusion needed to increase cardiac output usually ranges from 2.5 to 10 μg/kg/min (see table). On rare occasions, infusion rates up to 40 μg/kg/min have been required to obtain the desired effect.

[See table above].

The rate of administration and the duration of therapy should be adjusted according to the patient's response, as determined by heart rate, presence of ectopic activity, blood pressure, urine flow, and, whenever possible, measurement

---

Dobutrex® Solution (Dobutamine Hydrochloride Injection, Lilly)—Rates of Infusion for Concentrations of 250, 500, and 1,000 mg/L

Drug Delivery Rate (μg/kg/min)	Infusion Delivery Rate		
	250 mg/mL* (mL/kg/min)	500 mg/L† (mL/kg/min)	1,000 mg/L‡ (mL/kg/min)
2.5	0.01	0.005	0.0025
5	0.02	0.01	0.005
7.5	0.03	0.015	0.0075
10	0.04	0.02	0.01
12.5	0.05	0.025	0.0125
15	0.06	0.03	0.015

*250 mg/L of diluent
†500 mg/L or 250 mg/500 mL of diluent
‡1,000 mg/L or 250 mg/250 mL of diluent

of central venous or pulmonary wedge pressure and cardiac output.

Concentrations up to 5,000 mg/L have been administered to humans (250 mg/50 mL). The final volume administered should be determined by the fluid requirements of the patient.

HOW SUPPLIED

(℞) Vials:
250 mg,*20-mL size (No. 7175)—(1s) NDC 0002-7175-01; (Traypak† of 10) NDC 0002-7175-10

* Equivalent to dobutamine.
† Traypak™(multivial carton, Lilly)
Store at controlled room temperature, 59° to 86°F (15° to 30°C).

[120288]

DOLOPHINE® HYDROCHLORIDE   Ⅽ
[dō′lō-fēn hī-drō-klō′rīd]
(methadone hydrochloride)
Injection, USP

AMPOULES AND VIALS

> **CONDITIONS FOR DISTRIBUTION AND USE OF METHADONE PRODUCTS:**
> Code of Federal Regulations,
> Title 21, Sec. 291.505
>
> METHADONE PRODUCTS, WHEN USED FOR THE TREATMENT OF NARCOTIC ADDICTION IN DETOXIFICATION OR MAINTENANCE PROGRAMS, SHALL BE DISPENSED ONLY BY APPROVED HOSPITAL PHARMACIES, APPROVED COMMUNITY PHARMACIES, AND MAINTENANCE PROGRAMS APPROVED BY THE FOOD AND DRUG ADMINISTRATION AND THE DESIGNATED STATE AUTHORITY.
> APPROVED MAINTENANCE PROGRAMS SHALL DISPENSE AND USE METHADONE IN ORAL FORM ONLY AND ACCORDING TO THE TREATMENT REQUIREMENTS STIPULATED IN THE FEDERAL METHADONE REGULATIONS (21 CFR 291.505). FAILURE TO ABIDE BY THE REQUIREMENTS IN THESE REGULATIONS MAY RESULT IN CRIMINAL PROSECUTION, SEIZURE OF THE DRUG SUPPLY, REVOCATION OF THE PROGRAM APPROVAL, AND INJUNCTION PRECLUDING OPERATION OF THE PROGRAM.
> A METHADONE PRODUCT, WHEN USED AS AN ANALGESIC, MAY BE DISPENSED IN ANY LICENSED PHARMACY.

DESCRIPTION

Dolophine® Hydrochloride (Methadone Hydrochloride, USP, Lilly) (4,4- diphenyl-6-dimethylamino-heptanone-3 hydrochloride) is a white crystalline material which is water soluble.

Each mL contains methadone hydrochloride, 10 mg, and sodium chloride, 0.9%. Sodium hydroxide and/or hydrochloric acid may have been added during manufacture to adjust the pH. The 20-mL vials also contain chlorobutanol (chloroform derivative), 0.5%, as a preservative.

ACTIONS

Methadone hydrochloride is a synthetic narcotic analgesic with multiple actions quantitatively similar to those of morphine, the most prominent of which involve the central nervous system and organs composed of smooth muscle. The principal actions of therapeutic value are analgesia and sedation and detoxification or temporary maintenance in narcotic addiction. The methadone abstinence syndrome, although qualitatively similar to that of morphine, differs in that the onset is slower, the course is more prolonged, and the symptoms are less severe.

A parenteral dose of 8 to 10 mg of methadone is approximately equivalent in analgesic effect to 10 mg of morphine. With single-dose administration, the onset and duration of analgesic action of the 2 drugs are similar.

When administered orally, methadone is approximately one-half as potent as when given parenterally. Oral administration results in a delay of the onset, a lowering of the peak, and an increase in the duration of analgesic effect.

INDICATIONS

(See boxed Note.)
For relief of severe pain.
For detoxification treatment of narcotic addiction.
For temporary maintenance treatment of narcotic addiction.

> **NOTE**
> If methadone is administered for treatment of heroin dependence for more than 3 weeks, the procedure passes from treatment of the acute withdrawal syndrome (detoxification) to maintenance therapy. Maintenance treatment is permitted to be undertaken only by approved methadone programs. This does not preclude the maintenance treatment of an addict who is hospitalized for medical conditions other than addiction and who requires temporary maintenance during the critical period of his stay or whose enrollment has been verified in a program approved for maintenance treatment with methadone.

CONTRAINDICATION

Hypersensitivity to methadone.

WARNINGS

Methadone hydrochloride, a narcotic, is a Schedule II controlled substance under the Federal Controlled Substances Act. Appropriate security measures should be taken to safeguard stocks of methadone against diversion.

DRUG DEPENDENCE—METHADONE CAN PRODUCE DEPENDENCE OF THE MORPHINE TYPE AND, THEREFORE, HAS THE POTENTIAL FOR BEING ABUSED. PSYCHIC DEPENDENCE, PHYSICAL DEPENDENCE, AND TOLERANCE MAY DEVELOP ON REPEATED ADMINISTRATION OF METHADONE, AND IT SHOULD BE PRESCRIBED AND ADMINISTERED WITH THE SAME DEGREE OF CAUTION APPROPRIATE TO THE USE OF MORPHINE.

Interaction With Other Central-Nervous-System Depressants—Methadone should be used with caution and in reduced dosage in patients who are concurrently receiving other narcotic analgesics, general anesthetics, phenothiazines, other tranquilizers, sedative-hypnotics, tricyclic antidepressants, and other CNS depressants (including alcohol). Respiratory depression, hypotension, and profound sedation or coma may result.

Anxiety—Since methadone, as used by tolerant subjects at a constant maintenance dosage, is not a tranquilizer, patients who are maintained on this drug will react to life problems and stresses with the same symptoms of anxiety as do other individuals. The physician should not confuse such symptoms with those of narcotic abstinence and should not attempt to treat anxiety by increasing the dosage of methadone. The action of methadone in maintenance treatment is limited to the control of narcotic symptoms and is ineffective for relief of general anxiety.

Head Injury and Increased Intracranial Pressure—The respiratory depressant effects of methadone and its capacity to elevate cerebrospinal-fluid pressure may be markedly exaggerated in the presence of increased intracranial pressure. Furthermore, narcotics produce side effects that may obscure the clinical course of patients with head injuries. In

Continued on next page

* Identi-Code® symbol.

Lilly—Cont.

such patients, methadone must be used with caution and only if it is deemed essential.

Asthma and Other Respiratory Conditions— Methadone should be used with caution in patients having an acute asthmatic attack, in those with chronic obstructive pulmonary disease or cor pulmonale, and in individuals with a substantially decreased respiratory reserve, preexisting respiratory depression, hypoxia, or hypercapnia. In such patients, even usual therapeutic doses of narcotics may decrease respiratory drive while simultaneously increasing airway resistance to the point of apnea.

Hypotensive Effect—The administration of methadone may result in severe hypotension in an individual whose ability to maintain normal blood pressure has already been compromised by a depleted blood volume or concurrent administration of such drugs as the phenothiazines or certain anesthetics.

Use in Ambulatory Patients—Methadone may impair the mental and/or physical abilities required for the performance of potentially hazardous tasks, such as driving a car or operating machinery. The patient should be cautioned accordingly.

Methadone, like other narcotics, may produce orthostatic hypotension in ambulatory patients.

Use in Pregnancy—Safe use in pregnancy has not been established in relation to possible adverse effects on fetal development. Therefore, methadone should not be used in pregnant women unless, in the judgment of the physician, the potential benefits outweigh the possible hazards.

Methadone is not recommended for obstetric analgesia because its long duration of action increases the probability of respiratory depression in the newborn.

Use in Children—Methadone is not recommended for use as an analgesic in children, since documented clinical experience has been insufficient to establish a suitable dosage regimen for the pediatric age group.

PRECAUTIONS

Interaction with Pentazocine—**Patients who are addicted to heroin or who are on the methadone maintenance program may experience withdrawal symptoms when given pentazocine.**

Interaction with Rifampin—The concurrent administration of rifampin may possibly reduce the blood concentration of methadone to a degree sufficient to produce withdrawal symptoms. The mechanism by which rifampin may decrease blood concentrations of methadone is not fully understood, although enhanced microsomal drug-metabolized enzymes may influence drug disposition.

Acute Abdominal Conditions—The administration of methadone or other narcotics may obscure the diagnosis or clinical course in patients with acute abdominal conditions.

Interaction with Monoamine Oxidase (MAO) Inhibitors—Therapeutic doses of meperidine have precipitated severe reactions in patients concurrently receiving monoamine oxidase inhibitors or those who have received such agents within 14 days. Similar reactions thus far have not been reported with methadone; but if the use of methadone is necessary in such patients, a sensitivity test should be performed in which repeated small incremental doses are administered over the course of several hours while the patient's condition and vital signs are under careful observation.

Special-Risk Patients—Methadone should be given with caution and the initial dose should be reduced in certain patients, such as the elderly or debilitated and those with severe impairment of hepatic or renal function, hypothyroidism, Addison's disease, prostatic hypertrophy, or urethral stricture.

ADVERSE REACTIONS

THE MAJOR HAZARDS OF METHADONE, AS OF OTHER NARCOTIC ANALGESICS, ARE RESPIRATORY DEPRESSION AND, TO A LESSER DEGREE, CIRCULATORY DEPRESSION. RESPIRATORY ARREST, SHOCK, AND CARDIAC ARREST HAVE OCCURRED.

The most frequently observed adverse reactions include lightheadedness, dizziness, sedation, nausea, vomiting, and sweating. These effects seem to be more prominent in ambulatory patients and in those who are not suffering severe pain. In such individuals, lower doses are advisable. Some adverse reactions may be alleviated in the ambulatory patient if he/she lies down.

Other adverse reactions include the following:

Central Nervous System—Euphoria, dysphoria, weakness, headache, insomnia, agitation, disorientation, and visual disturbances.

Gastrointestinal—Dry mouth, anorexia, constipation, and biliary tract spasm.

Cardiovascular—Flushing of the face, bradycardia, palpitation, faintness, and syncope.

Genitourinary—Urinary retention or hesitancy, antidiuretic effect, and reduced libido and/or potency.

Allergic—Pruritus, urticaria, other skin rashes, edema, and, rarely, hemorrhagic urticaria.

Hematologic—Reversible thrombocytopenia has been described in a narcotics addict with chronic hepatitis.

In addition, pain at injection site; local tissue irritation and induration following subcutaneous injection, particularly when repeated.

OVERDOSAGE

Signs and Symptoms—Methadone is an opioid and produces effects similar to those of morphine. Symptoms of overdose begin within seconds after intravenous administration and within minutes of nasal, oral, or rectal administration. Prominent symptoms are miosis, respiratory depression, somnolence, coma, cool clammy skin, skeletal muscle flaccidity that may progress to hypotension, apnea, bradycardia, and death. Noncardiac pulmonary edema may occur and monitoring of heart filling pressures may be helpful.

Treatment—To obtain up-to-date information about the treatment of overdose, a good resource is your certified Regional Poison Control Center. Telephone numbers of certified poison control centers are listed in the *Physicians' Desk Reference (PDR)*. In managing overdosage, consider the possibility of multiple drug overdoses, interaction among drugs, and unusual drug kinetics in your patient.

Initial management of opioid overdose should include establishment of a secure airway and support ventilation and perfusion. Naloxone may be given to antagonize opioid effects, but the airway must be secured as vomiting may ensue. **The duration of methadone effect is much longer (36 to 48 hours) than the duration of naloxone effect (1 to 3 hours) and repeated doses (or continuous intravenous infusion) of naloxone may be required.**

If the patient has chronically abused opioids, administration of naloxone may precipitate a withdrawal syndrome that may include yawning, tearing, restlessness, sweating, dilated pupils, piloerection, vomiting, diarrhea, and abdominal cramps. If these symptoms develop, they should abate quickly as the effects of naloxone dissipate.

If methadone has been taken by mouth, protect the patient's airway and support ventilation and perfusion. Meticulously monitor and maintain, within acceptable limits, the patient's vital signs, blood gases, serum electrolytes, etc. Absorption of drugs from the gastrointestinal tract may be decreased by giving activated charcoal, which, in many cases, is more effective than emesis or lavage; consider charcoal instead of or in addition to gastric emptying. Repeated doses of charcoal over time may hasten elimination of some drugs that have been absorbed. Safeguard the patient's airway when employing gastric emptying or charcoal.

Forced diuresis, pertoneal dialysis, hemodialysis, or charcoal hemoperfusion have not been established as beneficial for an overdose of methadone.

NOTE: IN AN INDIVIDUAL PHYSICALLY DEPENDENT ON NARCOTICS, THE ADMINISTRATION OF THE USUAL DOSE OF A NARCOTIC ANTAGONIST WILL PRECIPITATE AN ACUTE WITHDRAWAL SYNDROME. THE SEVERITY OF THIS SYNDROME WILL DEPEND ON THE DEGREE OF PHYSICAL DEPENDENCE AND THE DOSE OF THE ANTAGONIST ADMINISTERED. THE USE OF A NARCOTIC ANTAGONIST IN SUCH A PERSON SHOULD BE AVOIDED IF POSSIBLE. IF IT MUST BE USED TO TREAT SERIOUS RESPIRATORY DEPRESSION IN THE PHYSICALLY DEPENDENT PATIENT, THE ANTAGONIST SHOULD BE ADMINISTERED WITH EXTREME CARE AND BY TITRATION WITH SMALLER THAN USUAL DOSES OF THE ANTAGONIST.

DOSAGE AND ADMINISTRATION

For Relief of Pain—Dosage should be adjusted according to the severity of the pain and the response of the patient. Occasionally, it may be necessary to exceed the usual dosage recommended in cases of exceptionally severe pain or in those patients who have become tolerant to the analgesic effect of narcotics.

Although subcutaneous administration is suitable for occasional use, intramuscular injection is preferred when repeated doses are required.

The usual adult dosage is 2.5 to 10 mg intramuscularly or subcutaneously every 3 or 4 hours as necessary.

For Detoxification Treatment—THE DRUG SHALL BE ADMINISTERED DAILY UNDER CLOSE SUPERVISION AS FOLLOWS:

A detoxification treatment course shall not exceed 21 days and may not be repeated earlier than 4 weeks after completion of the preceding course.

The oral form of administration is preferred. However, if the patient is unable to ingest oral medication, he may be started on the parenteral form initially.

In detoxification, the patient may receive methadone when there are significant symptoms of withdrawal. The dosage schedules indicated below are recommended but could be varied in accordance with clinical judgment. Initially, a single dose of 15 to 20 mg of methadone will often be sufficient to suppress withdrawal symptoms. Additional methadone may be provided if withdrawal symptoms are not suppressed or if symptoms reappear. When patients are physically dependent on high doses, it may be necessary to exceed these levels. Forty mg/day in single or divided doses will usually constitute an adequate stabilizing dosage level. Stabilization can be continued for 2 to 3 days, and then the amount of methadone normally will be gradually decreased. The rate at which methadone is decreased will be determined separately for each patient. The dose of methadone can be decreased on a daily basis or at 2-day intervals, but the amount of intake shall always be sufficient to keep withdrawal symptoms at a tolerable level. In hospitalized patients, a daily reduction of 20% of the total daily dose may be tolerated and may cause little discomfort. In ambulatory patients, a somewhat slower schedule may be needed. If methadone is administered for more than 3 weeks, the procedure is considered to have progressed from detoxification or treatment of the acute withdrawal syndrome to maintenance treatment, even though the goal and intent may be eventual total withdrawal.

HOW SUPPLIED

(℃) Ampoules:
10 mg, 1 mL(No. 456)—(12s) NDC 0002-1687-12; (100s) NDC 0002-1687-02
(℃) Multiple-Dose Vials:
10 mg/mL, 20 mL (No. 435)—(1s) NDC 0002-1682-01; (25s) NDC 0002-1682-25
Store at controlled room temperature, 59° to 86°F (15° to 30°C).

[080288]

DOLOPHINE® HYDROCHLORIDE   (℃)
[dō'lō-fĕn hī-drō-klō'rĭd]
(methadone hydrochloride)
Tablets, USP

CONDITIONS FOR DISTRIBUTION AND USE OF METHADONE PRODUCTS: *See under* Ampoules Dolophine Hydrochloride.

DESCRIPTION, ACTIONS, INDICATIONS, and CONTRAINDICATIONS
See under Ampoules Dolophine Hydrochloride.

Each tablet contains 5 mg (No. 1712) or 10 mg (No. 1730) methadone hydrochloride. They also contain cellulose, cornstarch, lactose, magnesium stearate, sucrose, and talc. The 10-mg tablet also contains acacia.

WARNINGS

Tablets Dolophine® Hydrochloride (Methadone Hydrochloride, USP, Lilly) are for oral administration only and *must not* be used for injection. It is recommended that Tablets Dolophine Hydrochloride, if dispensed, be packaged in child-resistant containers and kept out of the reach of children to prevent accidental ingestion.

See also under Ampoules Dolophine Hydrochloride.

PRECAUTIONS and ADVERSE REACTIONS
See under Ampoules Dolophine Hydrochloride.

OVERDOSAGE
See under Ampoules Dolophine Hydrochloride.

DOSAGE AND ADMINISTRATION
For Relief of Pain—Dosage should be adjusted according to the severity of the pain and the response of the patient. Occasionally it may be necessary to exceed the usual dosage recommended in cases of exceptionally severe pain or in those patients who have become tolerant to the analgesic effect of narcotics.

The usual adult dosage is 2.5 to 10 mg every 3 or 4 hours as necessary.

See also under Ampoules Dolophine Hydrochloride.

If the patient cannot ingest methadone orally, parenteral administration may be substituted.

HOW SUPPLIED

(℃) Tablets:
5 mg (No. 1712)—(100s) NDC 0002-1064-092
10 mg (No. 1730)—(100s) NDC 0002-1072-02
Store at controlled room temperature, 59° to 86°F (15° to 30°C).

[080288]

FLUOXETINE HYDROCHLORIDE, *see* Prozac®
(Fluoxetine Hydrochloride, Dista).

GLUCAGON FOR INJECTION   ℞

[glōō′ka-gŏn]
USP

DESCRIPTION

Glucagon, manufactured by Eli Lilly and Company, is extracted from beef and pork pancreas.

Chemically unrelated to insulin, glucagon is a single-chain polypeptide containing 29 amino acid residues and having a molecular weight of 3,483.

The empirical formula is $C_{153}H_{225}N_{43}O_{49}S$. The structure of glucagon is shown below.

His-Ser-Gln-Gly-Thr-Phe-Thr-Ser-Asp-Tyr-Ser-Lys-Tyr-Leu-Asp-Ser-
1 2 3 4 5 6 7 8 9 10 11 12 13 14 15 16
Arg-Arg-Ala-Gln-Asp-Phe-Val-Gln-Trp-Leu-Met-Asn-Thr 4a
17 18 19 20 21 22 23 24 25 26 27 28 29

Crystalline glucagon is a white powder containing less than 0.05% zinc. It is relatively insoluble in water but is soluble at a pH of less than 3 or more than 9.5. Glucagon is stable in lyophilized form at room temperatures. Glucagon should be used immediately after reconstitution. It may be kept at 41°F (5°C) for up to 48 hours, if necessary.

Vials No. 666, Glucagon for Injection, USP, contain 1 unit (1 mg) of glucagon as the hydrochloride with 49 mg of lactose. (Vials No. 667, Diluting Solution for Glucagon for Injection, USP, 1 mL, contain glycerin, 1.6%, with 0.2% phenol added as a preservative. Sodium hydroxide and/or hydrochloric acid may have been added during manufacture to adjust the pH.)

Vials No. 668, Glucagon for Injection, USP, contain 10 units (10 mg) of glucagon as the hydrochloride with 140 mg of lactose. (Vials No. 669, Diluting Solution for Glucagon for Injection, USP, 10 mL, contain glycerin, 1.6%, with 0.2% phenol added as a preservative. Sodium hydroxide and/or hydrochloric acid may have been added during manufacture to adjust the pH.) Glucagon should be used immediately after reconstitution. It may be kept at 41°F (5°C) for up to 48 hours, if necessary.

If glucagon is to be given at doses higher than 2 mg, it should be reconstituted with Sterile Water for Injection instead of the diluting solution supplied and used immediately.

CLINICAL PHARMACOLOGY

Glucagon causes an increase in blood glucose concentration and is used in the treatment of hypoglycemic states. It is effective in small doses, and no evidence of toxicity has been reported with its use. Glucagon acts only on liver glycogen, converting it to glucose.

Parenteral administration of glucagon produces relaxation of the smooth muscle of the stomach, duodenum, small bowel, and colon.

The half-life of glucagon in plasma is approximately 3 to 6 minutes, which is similar to that of insulin.

INDICATIONS AND USAGE

For the treatment of hypoglycemia: Glucagon is useful in counteracting severe hypoglycemic reactions in diabetic patients or during insulin shock therapy in psychiatric patients. Glucagon is helpful in hypoglycemia only if liver glycogen is available. It is of little or no help in states of starvation, adrenal insufficiency, or chronic hypoglycemia.

The patient with type I diabetes does not have as great a response in blood glucose levels as does the type II stable patient. Therefore, supplementary carbohydrate should be given as soon as possible, to the child or adolescent patient especially.

For use as a diagnostic aid: Glucagon is indicated as a diagnostic aid in the radiologic examination of the stomach, duodenum, small bowel, and colon when a hypotonic state would be advantageous.

Glucagon is as effective for this examination as are the anticholinergic drugs, but it has fewer side effects. When glucagon is administered concomitantly with an anticholinergic agent, the response is not significantly greater than when either drug is used alone. However, the addition of the anticholinergic agent results in increased side effects.

CONTRAINDICATION

Glucagon is contraindicated in patients with known hypersensitivity and in patients with pheochromocytoma.

WARNINGS

Glucagon should be administered cautiously to patients with a history suggestive of insulinoma and/or pheochromocytoma. In patients with insulinoma, intravenous administration of glucagon will produce an initial increase in blood glucose but, because of its insulin-releasing effect, may cause the insulinoma to release its insulin and thus, may subsequently cause hypoglycemia. A patient developing symptoms of hypoglycemia after a dose of glucagon should be given glucose orally, intravenously, or by gavage, whichever is more appropriate.

Exogenous glucagon also stimulates the release of catecholamines. In the presence of pheochromocytoma, glucagon can cause the tumor to release catecholamines, which results in a sudden and marked increase in blood pressure. If a patient suddenly develops a marked increase in blood pressure, 5 to 10 mg of phentolamine mesylate may be administered intravenously in an attempt to control the blood pressure.

Generalized allergic reactions, including urticaria, respiratory distress, and hypotension, have been reported in patients who received glucagon injection.

PRECAUTIONS

General —In the treatment of hypoglycemic shock with glucagon, liver glycogen must be available. Glucose by the intravenous route or by gavage should be considered in the hypoglycemic patient.

Laboratory Tests —Blood glucose determinations may be obtained to follow the patient in hypoglycemic shock until he or she is asymptomatic.

Carcinogenesis, Mutagenesis, Impairment of Fertility —Glucagon is administered in 1 or 2 doses to patients in hypoglycemic shock or for diagnostic radiology. The drug has a half-life of approximately 3 to 6 minutes. Because glucagon is usually given in a single dose and has a very short half-life, no studies have been done regarding carcinogenesis.

Reproduction studies have been performed in rats at doses up to 2 mg/kg b.i.d. (or 90 to 120 times the human dose) and have revealed no evidence of impaired fertility.

Usage in Pregnancy —*Pregnancy Category B* —Reproduction studies have been performed in rats at doses up to 2 mg/kg b.i.d., or 90 to 120 times the human dose, and have revealed no evidence of harm to the fetus due to glucagon. There are, however, no adequate and well-controlled studies in pregnant women. Because animal reproduction studies are not always predictive of human response, this drug should be used during pregnancy only if clearly needed.

Nursing Mothers —It is not known whether this drug is excreted in human milk. Because many drugs are excreted in human milk, caution should be exercised when glucagon is administered to a nursing woman. The plasma half-life of glucagon is approximately 3 to 6 minutes. If the drug is excreted in human milk during this short period, it will be handled like any other polypeptide, ie, it will be hydrolyzed and absorbed. Glucagon is not active when taken orally because it is destroyed in the gastrointestinal tract before it is absorbed.

ADVERSE REACTIONS

Glucagon is relatively free of adverse reactions except for occasional nausea and vomiting, which may also occur with hypoglycemia. Generalized allergic reactions have been reported (see Warnings).

OVERDOSAGE

Signs and Symptoms —There have been no reported cases of human overdosage of glucagon. Glucagon is generally well tolerated. If overdosage occurred, it would not be expected to cause consequential toxicity, but would be expected to be associated with nausea, vomiting, gastric hypotonicity, and diarrhea.

The administration of intravenous glucagon has been shown to have a positive inotropic and chronotropic effect. A transient increment in both blood pressure and pulse rate may occur following the administration of glucagon. Those patients taking β-blockers might be expected to have a greater increment in both pulse and blood pressure. This increase will be transient because of glucagon's short half-life. The increase in blood pressure and pulse rate may require therapy in patients with pheochromocytoma, insulinomas, or coronary artery disease.

When glucagon was given in large doses to cardiac patients, investigators reported a positive inotropic effect. These investigators administered glucagon in doses of 0.5 to 16 mg/hour by continuous infusion for periods of 5 to 166 hours. Total doses ranged from 25 to 996 mg, and a 21-month child received approximately 8.25 mg in 165 hours. Side effects included nausea, vomiting, and decreasing serum potassium. The serum potassium could be maintained within normal limits with supplemental potassium.

The oral median lethal dose for glucagon in mice is approximately 300 mg/kg.

Because of glucagon's polypeptide structure, it would be rapidly destroyed in the gastrointestinal tract if it were to be accidentally ingested.

Treatment —To obtain up-to-date information about the treatment of overdose, a good resource is your certified Regional Poison Control Center. Telephone numbers of certified poison control centers are listed in the *Physicians' Desk Reference (PDR)*. In managing overdosage, consider the possibility of multiple drug overdoses, interaction among drugs, and unusual drug kinetics in your patient.

In view of the extremely short half-life of glucagon and its prompt destruction and excretion, the treatment of overdosage is symptomatic, primarily for nausea, vomiting, and possible hypokalemia.

If the patient develops a dramatic increase in blood pressure, 5 mg to 10 mg of phentolamine has been shown to be effecitve in lowering blood pressure for the short time that control would be needed.

Forced diuresis, peritoneal dialysis, hemodialysis, or charcoal hemoperfusion have not been established as beneficial for an overdose of glucagon; however, it would be extremely unlikely that one of these procedures would even be indicated.

DOSAGE AND ADMINISTRATION

For the treatment of hypoglycemia: The diluent is provided for use only in the preparation of glucagon for *intermittent* parenteral injection and for no other use.

If glucagon is to be given at doses higher than 2 mg, it should be reconstituted with Sterile Water for Injection instead of the diluting solution supplied and used immediately.

Directions for Use of Glucagon —1. Dissolve the lyophilized glucagon in the accompanying solvent.

2. Glucagon should not be used at concentrations greater than 1 unit/mL.

3. Glucagon solutions should not be used unless they are clear and of a water-like consistency.

4. Give 0.5 to 1 unit of glucagon by subcutaneous, intramuscular, or intravenous injection.

5. The patient will usually awaken in 5 to 20 minutes. If the response is delayed, there is no contraindication to the administration of 1 or 2 additional doses of glucagon; however, in view of the deleterious effects of cerebral hypoglycemia and depending on the duration and depth of coma, the use of parenteral glucose *must* be considered by the physician.

6. Intravenous glucose *must* be given if the patient fails to respond to glucagon.

7. When the patient responds, give supplemental carbohydrate to restore the liver glycogen and prevent secondary hypoglycemia.

General Management of Hypoglycemia —The following are helpful measures in the prevention of hypoglycemic reactions due to insulin:

1. Reasonable uniformity from day to day with regard to diet, insulin, and exercise.

2. Careful adjustment of the insulin program so that the type (or types) of insulin, dose, and time (or times) of administration are suited to the individual patient.

3. Frequent testing of the blood or urine so that a change in insulin requirements can be foreseen.

4. Routine carrying of sugar, candy, or other readily absorbable carbohydrate by the patient so that it may be taken at the first warning of an oncoming reaction.

If the patient is unaware of the symptoms of hypoglycemia, he/she may lapse into insulin shock; therefore, the physician should instruct the patient in this regard when feasible.

It is important that the patient be aroused as quickly as possible, for prolonged hypoglycemic reactions may result in cortical damage. Glucagon or intravenous glucose will awaken the patient sufficiently so that oral carbohydrates may be taken.

Instructions to the Family —Instructions describing the method of using this preparation are included in the literature that accompanies the patient's package. It is advisable for the patient and family members to become familiar with the technique of preparing Glucagon for Injection before an emergency arises. Patient instructions include the use of 0.5 unit for small children if recommended by the physician.

CAUTION—Although glucagon may be used for the treatment of hypoglycemia by the patient during an emergency, the physician must still be notified when hypoglycemic reactions occur so that the dose of insulin may be adjusted more accurately.

Insulin Shock Therapy —Dissolve the lyophilized glucagon in the accompanying diluting solution.

After 1 hour of coma, inject 0.5 to 1 unit of glucagon by the subcutaneous, intramuscular, or intravenous route. Larger doses may be employed if desired.

Glucagon should not be used at concentrations greater than 1 unit/mL.

The patient will usually awaken in 10 to 25 minutes. If no response occurs within the desired interval, the dose may be repeated. Upon awakening, the patient should be fed orally as soon as possible and the usual dietary regimen followed. In a very deep state of coma, such as Stage IV or Stage V of Himwich, intravenous glucose should be given in addition to glucagon for a more immediate response. Glucagon and glucose may be used together without decreasing the efficacy of glucose administration.

For use as a diagnostic aid: Dissolve the lyophilized glucagon in the accompanying diluting solution.

Glucagon should not be used at concentrations greater than 1 unit/mL.

The doses in the accompanying chart may be administered for relaxation of the stomach, duodenum, and small bowel, depending on the time of onset of action and the duration of effect required for the examination. Since the stomach is less

Continued on next page

Lilly—Cont.

sensitive to the effect of glucagon, ½ unit IV or 2 units IM are recommended.
[See table below].
For examination of the colon, it is recommended that a 2-unit dose (2 mg) be administered intramuscularly approximately 10 minutes prior to initiation of the procedure. Relaxation of the colon and reduction of discomfort to the patient will allow the radiologist to perform a more satisfactory examination.

HOW SUPPLIED

Glucagon is supplied in lyophilized form with accompanying diluting solution.
(℞) Vials:
1 unit (1 mg)—(No. 666), with 1-mL vial of diluting solution (1s) NDC 0002-1450-01
10 units (10 mg)—(No. 668), multiple dose, with 10-mL vial of diluting solution (1s) NDC 00902-1451-01
Prior to reconstitution, the vials may be stored at controlled room temperature, 59° to 86°F (15° to 30°C).
Glucagon should be used immediately after reconstitution. It may be kept at 41°F (5°C) for up to 48 hours, if necessary. Glucagon solutions should not be used unless they are clear and of a water-like consistency.
If glucagon is to be given at doses higher than 2 mg, it should be reconstituted with Sterile Water for Injection instead of the diluting solution supplied and used immediately.
Also available:
Glucagon Emergency Kit for Diabetic Insulin Reaction (M-8030)—(1s) NDC 0002-8030-01. This emergency kit contains 1 vial of Glucagon for Injection, USP, 1 Unit (1 mg)—(No. 7286) NDC 0002-7286-01; and 1 Hyporet® of Diluting Solution for Glucagon for Injection. USP, 1 mL (No. 7287).

Hyporet® (disposable syringe, Lilly)

[120288]

HUMATROPE®
[hū′ma-trōp]
(somatropin (rDNA origin) for injection)

℞

DESCRIPTION

Humatrope® (Somatropin, rDNA Origin, for Injection, Lilly) is a polypeptide hormone of recombinant DNA origin. Humatrope has 191 amino acid residues and a molecular weight of about 22,125 daltons. The amino acid sequence of the product is identical to that of human growth hormone of pituitary origin. Humatrope is synthesized in a strain of *Escherichia coli* that has been modified by the addition of the gene for human growth hormone.
Humatrope is a sterile, white, lyophilized powder intended for intramuscular administration after reconstitution. Each vial of Humatrope contains 5 mg somatropin (approximately 13 IU or 225 picomoles); 25 mg mannitol; 5 mg glycine; and 1.13 mg dibasic sodium phosphate. Phosphoric acid and/or sodium hydroxide may have been added at the time of manufacture to adjust the pH. Each vial is supplied in a combination package with an accompanying 5-mL vial of diluting solution. Each vial contains water for injection as the diluent with 0.3% m-cresol as a preservative and 1.7% glycerin, both added at the time of manufacture.
Humatrope is a highly purified preparation. The 1.7% glycerin content makes the reconstituted product nearly isotonic at a concentration of 2 mg of Humatrope/mL Diluent. Reconstituted solutions have a pH of approximatey 7.5.

CLINICAL PHARMACOLOGY

Linear Growth —Humatrope® (Somatropin, rDNA Origin, for Injection, Lilly) stimulates linear growth in children who lack adequate normal endogenous growth hormone. In vitro, preclinical, and clinical tests have demonstrated that Humatrope is therapeutically equivalent to human growth hormone of pituitary origin and achieves equivalent pharmacokinetic profiles in normal adults. Treatment of growth hormone-deficient children with Humatrope produces increased growth rate and IGF-1 (Insulin-like Growth Factor/Somatomedin-C) concentrations that are similar to those seen after therapy with human growth hormone of pituitary origin.

In addition, the following actions have been demonstrated for Humatrope and/or human growth hormone of pituitary origin.
A. Tissue Growth —1. Skeletal Growth: Humatrope stimulates skeletal growth in patients with growth hormone deficiency. The measurable increase in body length after administration of either Humatrope or human growth hormone of pituitary origin results from an effect on the growth plates of long bones. Concentrations of IGF-1, which may play a role in skeletal growth, are low in the serum of growth hormone-deficient children but increase during treatment with Humatrope. Elevations in mean serum alkaline phosphatase concentrations are also seen. 2. Cell Growth: It has been shown that there are fewer skeletal muscle cells in short-statured children who lack endogenous growth hormone as compared with normal children. Treatment with human growth hormone of pituitary origin results in an increase in both the number and size of muscle cells.
B. Protein Metabolism —Linear growth is facilitated in part by increased cellular protein synthesis. Nitrogen retention, as demonstrated by decreased urinary nitrogen excretion and serum urea nitrogen, follows the initiation of therapy with human growth hormone of pituitary origin. Treatment with Humatrope results in a similar decrease in serum urea nitrogen.
C. Carbohydrate Metabolism —Children with hypopituitarism sometimes experience fasting hypoglycemia that is improved by treatment with Humatrope. Large doses of human growth hormone may impair glucose tolerance.
D. Lipid Metabolism —In growth hormone-deficient patients, administration of human growth hormone of pituitary origin has resulted in lipid mobilization, reduction in body fat stores, and increased plasma fatty acids.
E. Mineral Metabolism —Retention of sodium, potassium, and phosphorus is induced by human growth hormone of pituitary origin. Serum concentrations of inorganic phosphate increased in patients with growth hormone deficiency after therapy with Humatrope or human growth hormone of pituitary origin. Serum calcium is not significantly altered in patients with either human growth hormone of pituitary origin or Humatrope.

INDICATION AND USAGE

Humatrope® (Somatropin, rDNA Origin, for Injection, Lilly) is indicated only for the long-term treatment of children who have growth failure due to an inadequate secretion of normal endogenous growth hormone.

CONTRAINDICATIONS

Humatrope® (Somatropin, rDNA Origin, for Injection, Lilly) should not be used in subjects with closed epiphyses. Humatrope should not be used when there is any evidence of activity of a tumor. Intracranial lesions must be inactive and antitumor therapy complete prior to the institution of therapy. Humatrope should be discontinued if there is evidence of tumor growth.
Humatrope should not be reconstituted with the supplied Diluent for Humatrope by patients with a known sensitivity to either m-cresol or glycerin.

WARNING

If sensitivity to the diluent should occur, the vials may be reconstituted with Sterile Water for Injection, USP. When Humatrope® (Somatropin, rDNA Origin, for Injection, Lilly) is reconstituted in this manner, (1) use only one reconstituted dose per vial, (2) refrigerate the solution (36° to 46°F [2° to 8°C]) if it is not used immediately after reconstitution, (3) use the reconstituted dose within 24 hours, and (4) discard the unused portion.

PRECAUTIONS

Therapy with Humatrope® (Somatropin, rDNA Origin, for Injection, Lilly) should be directed by physicians who are experienced in the diagnosis and management of patients with growth hormone deficiency.
Patients with growth hormone deficiency secondary to an intracranial lesion should be examined frequently for progression or recurrence of the underlying disease process.
Because human growth hormone may induce a state of insulin resistance, patients should be observed for evidence of glucose intolerance.
Excessive glucocorticoid therapy will inhibit the growth-promoting effect of human growth hormone. Patients with coexisting ACTH deficiency should have their glucocorticoid

replacement dose carefully adjusted to avoid an inhibitory effect on growth.
Hypothyroidism may develop during treatment with human growth hormone, and inadequate treatment of hypothyroidism may prevent optimal response to human growth hormone. Therefore, patients should have periodic thyroid function tests and be treated with thyroid hormone when indicated.
Patients with endocrine disorders, including growth hormone deficiency, may develop slipped capital epiphyses more frequently. Any child with the onset of a limp during growth hormone therapy should be evaluated.

ADVERSE REACTIONS

Approximately 2% of 481 naive and previously treated clinical trial patients treated with Humatrope® (Somatropin, rDNA Origin, for Injection, Lilly) have developed antibodies to growth hormone, as demonstrated by a binding capacity determination threshold ≥ 0.02 mg/L. Nevertheless, even these patients experienced increases in linear growth and other salutary effects of Humatrope and did not have any unusual adverse events. Although growth-limiting antibodies have been observed with other growth hormone preparations (including products of pituitary origin), antibodies in patients treated with Humatrope have not limited growth. The long-term implications of antibody development are uncertain at this time.
Of the 232 naive and previously treated clinical trial patients receiving Humatrope for 6 months or more, 4.7% had serum binding of radiolabeled growth hormone in excess of twice the binding observed in control sera when the serum samples were assayed at a tenfold dilution. Among these patients were 160 naive patients of whom 6.9% had positive serum binding. In comparison, 74.5% of 106 naive patients treated for 6 months or more with Lilly somatrem in a similar clinical trial, had serum binding of radiolabeled growth hormone of at least twice the binding observed in control sera.
In addition to an evaluation of compliance with the treatment program and of thyroid status, testing for antibodies to human growth hormone should be carried out in any patient who fails to respond to therapy.
In clinical studies in which high doses of Humatrope were administered to healthy adult volunteers, the following events have occurred infrequently: headache, localized muscle pain, weakness, mild hyperglycemia, and glucosuria. In studies with growth hormone-deficient children, injection site pain was reported infrequently. A mild and transient edema, which appeared in 2.5% of patients, was observed early during the course of treatment.
Leukemia has been reported in a small number of children who have been treated with growth hormone, including growth hormone of pituitary origin and recombinant somatrem and somatropin. The relationship, if any, between leukemia and growth hormone therapy is uncertain.

OVERDOSAGE

The recommended dosage is up to 0.06 mg/kg (0.16 IU/kg) of body weight 3 times per week. Acute overdosage could lead initially to hypoglycemia and subsequently to hyperglycemia. Long-term overdosage could result in signs and symptoms of acromegaly consistent with the known effects of excess human growth hormone.

DOSAGE AND ADMINISTRATION

A dosage of up to 0.06 mg/kg (0.16 IU/kg) of body weight administered 3 times per week by intramuscular injection is recommended. The dosage and administration schedule for Humatrope® (Somatropin, rDNA Origin, for Injection, Lilly) should be individualized for each patient.
Each 5-mg vial of Humatrope should be reconstituted with 1.5 to 5 mL of Diluent for Humatrope. The diluent should be injected into the vial of Humatrope by aiming the stream of liquid against the glass wall. Following reconstitution, the vial should be swirled with a GENTLE rotary motion until the contents are completely dissolved. DO NOT SHAKE. The resulting solution should be clear, without particulate matter. If the solution is cloudy or contains particulate matter, the contents MUST NOT be injected.
Before and after injection, the septum of the vial should be wiped with rubbing alcohol or an alcoholic antiseptic solution to prevent contamination of the contents by repeated needle insertions. Sterile disposable syringes and needles should be used for administration of Humatrope. The volume of the syringe should be small enough so that the prescribed dose can be withdrawn from the vial with reasonable accuracy. The needle should be of sufficient length (usually 1 inch or more) to ensure that the injection reaches the muscle layer.

STABILITY AND STORAGE

Before Reconstitution —Vials of Humatrope® (Somatropin, rDNA Origin, for Injection, Lilly) as well as the Diluent for Humatrope are stable when refrigerated (36° to 46°F [2° to 8°C]). Avoid freezing Diluent for Humatrope. Expiration dates are stated on the labels.
After Reconstitution —Vials of Humatrope are stable for up to 14 days when reconstituted with Diluent for Humatrope

Dosage of Glucagon as a Diagnostic Aid

Dose	Route of Administration	Time of Onset of Action	Approximate Duration of Effect
¼–½ unit (0.25–0.5 mg)	IV	1 minute	9–17 minutes
1 unit (1 mg)*	IM	8–10 minutes	12–27 minutes
2 units (2 mg)*	IV	1 minute	22–25 minutes
2 units (2 mg)*	IM	4–7 minutes	21–32 minutes

*Administration of 2-unit doses produces a higher incidence of nausea and vomiting than do lower doses.

and stored in a refrigerator at 36° to 46°F (2° to 8°C). Avoid freezing the reconstituted Vial of Humatrope.

HOW SUPPLIED

(R) Vials:

5 mg (No. 7335) (6s), NDC 0002-7335-16, and 5-mL vial of Diluent for Humatrope (No. 7336)

[120888]

HUMULIN® 70/30   OTC
(70% Human Insulin Isophane Suspension and 30% Human Insulin Injection [Recombinant DNA origin])

INFORMATION TO THE PATIENT
WARNINGS
THIS LILLY HUMAN INSULIN PRODUCT DIFFERS FROM ANIMAL-SOURCE INSULINS, BECAUSE IT IS STRUCTURALLY IDENTICAL TO THE INSULIN PRODUCED BY YOUR BODY'S PANCREAS AND BECAUSE OF ITS UNIQUE MANUFACTURING PROCESS.

ANY CHANGE OF INSULIN SHOULD BE MADE CAUTIOUSLY AND ONLY UNDER MEDICAL SUPERVISION. CHANGES IN REFINEMENT, PURITY, STRENGTH, BRAND (MANUFACTURER), TYPE (REGULAR, NPH, LENTE®, ETC), AND/OR METHOD OF MANUFACTURE (RECOMBINANT DNA VERSUS ANIMAL-SOURCE INSULIN) MAY RESULT IN THE NEED FOR A CHANGE IN DOSAGE.

SOME PATIENTS TAKING HUMULIN® (HUMAN INSULIN, RECOMBINANT DNA ORIGIN, LILLY) WILL REQUIRE A CHANGE IN DOSAGE FROM THAT USED WITH ANIMAL-SOURCE INSULINS. IF AN ADJUSTMENT IS NEEDED, IT MAY OCCUR WITH THE FIRST DOSE OR OVER A PERIOD OF SEVERAL WEEKS.

INSULIN AND DIABETES

Your doctor has explained that you have diabetes. You have learned that the treatment of your diabetes requires injections of insulin.

Insulin is a hormone produced by the pancreas, a large gland that lies near the stomach. This hormone is necessary for the body's correct use of food, especially sugar. Diabetes occurs when the pancreas does not make enough insulin to meet your body's needs.

To control your diabetes, your doctor has prescribed injections of insulin to keep your blood sugar at a nearly normal level and to keep your urine as free of sugar as possible. Each case of diabetes is different. Your doctor has told you which insulin to use, how much, and when and how often to inject it. This schedule has been individualized for you. Proper control of your diabetes requires close and constant cooperation with your doctor.

In spite of diabetes, you can lead an active, healthy, and useful life if you eat a balanced diet daily, exercise regularly, and take your insulin injections exactly as prescribed by your doctor.

You have been instructed to test your urine and/or your blood regularly for sugar. If your urine tests consistently show the presence of sugar or your blood tests consistently show above-normal sugar levels, your diabetes is not properly controlled and you must let your doctor know.

USE THE PROPER TYPE OF INSULIN

This insulin, manufactured by Eli Lilly and Company, has the trademark Humulin and is available in 6 formulations—Regular, NPH, Lente, Buffered Regular, Ultralente, and 70/30. These products can be identified by the large letter or numbers that appear on the carton and vial (bottle) label following the name Humulin: Humulin R (Regular), Humulin N (NPH), Humulin L (Lente), Humulin BR (Buffered Regular), Humulin U (Ultralente) or Humulin 70/30 (70% Human Insulin Isophane Suspension [NPH]/30% Human Insulin Injection [buffered regular]).

These types of insulin differ mainly in the time they require to take effect and in the length of time their action lasts. Your doctor has prescribed the type of insulin that he/she believes is best for you. DO NOT USE ANY OTHER INSULIN EXCEPT ON HIS/HER ADVICE AND DIRECTION.

If your physician has directed you to take Humulin, when you receive your insulin from the pharmacy, always check to see that:

1. The name Humulin appears on the carton and bottle label and is followed by the proper letter designation and name for the insulin formulation: R-Regular; N-NPH; L-Lente; BR-Buffered Regular; Humulin U-Ultralente; 70/30-70% Human Insulin Isophane Suspension/30% Human Insulin Injection.
2. The carton and bottle label are correct for your type of insulin.
3. The human insulin is of recombinant DNA origin.
4. The insulin strength is U-100.
5. The expiration date on the package will allow you to use the insulin before that date.

70/30 HUMAN INSULIN

Humulin® 70/30 (Human Insulin Isophane Suspension and Human Insulin Injection, Recombinant DNA Origin, Lilly)

is synthesized in a non-disease producing special laboratory strain of *Escherichia coli* bacteria that has been genetically altered by the addition of the human gene for insulin production. Humulin 70/30 is a mixture of 70% Human Insulin Isophane Suspension and 30% Human Insulin Injection. It is an intermediate-acting insulin with a more rapid onset of action than NPH alone. Humulin 70/30 has a peak ranging between 2 and 12 hours. The duration of activity may last up to 24 hours following injection. Humulin 70/30 is for subcutaneous use only.

Humulin 70/30 should look uniformly cloudy or milky. If the insulin substance (the cloudy material) settles at the bottom of the bottle, the bottle must be rotated or carefully shaken before the injection so that the contents are uniformly mixed (see instructions under Preparing the Dose). Do not use a vial of Humulin 70/30 if a deposit of solid particles remains on the bottom or wall of the vial or if there are clumps floating in the insulin after the bottle has been rotated or carefully shaken. Also, the insulin should not be used if it is clear and remains clear after the bottle is rotated or carefully shaken.

STORAGE

Insulin should be stored in a cold place, preferably in a refrigerator, but not in the freezing compartment. Do not let it freeze or leave it in direct sunlight. If refrigeration is not possible, the bottle of insulin that you are currently using can be kept unrefrigerated as long as it is kept as cool as possible and away from heat and sunlight. Do not use a bottle of insulin after the expiration date stamped on the label.

USE THE CORRECT SYRINGE

Doses of insulin are measured in units. The number of units in each milliliter (mL) is clearly stated on the package. It is important to use a syringe which is marked for an insulin preparation with 100 units per mL. Failure to use the proper syringe can lead to a mistake in dosage, and you may receive too little or too much insulin. This can cause serious problems for you, ranging from a blood sugar level that is too low or too high, to coma (unconsciousness) or, rarely, death.

IMPORTANT: TO HELP AVOID CONTAMINATION AND POSSIBLE INFECTION, FOLLOW THESE INSTRUCTIONS EXACTLY.

DISPOSABLE SYRINGES

Disposable syringes and needles require no sterilization; they should be used only once and then discarded.

STERILIZING AND ASSEMBLING REUSABLE SYRINGES

Your reusable syringe and needle must be sterilized before each injection—follow the package directions supplied with your syringe. Boiling, as described below, is the best method of sterilizing.

1. Put syringe, plunger, and needle in strainer, place in saucepan, and cover with water. Boil for 5 minutes.
2. Remove articles from water. When they have cooled, insert plunger into barrel and fasten needle to syringe with a slight twist.
3. Push plunger in and out several times until water is completely removed. (If the syringe, plunger, and needle cannot be boiled, as when you are traveling, they may be sterilized by immersion for at least 5 minutes in Isopropyl Alcohol, 91%. Do not use bathing, rubbing, or medicated alcohol for this sterilization. If the syringe is sterilized with alcohol, it must be absolutely dry before use.)

PREPARING THE DOSE

1. Wash your hands.
2. Roll or carefully shake the insulin bottle several times to mix the insulin. Be sure it is completely mixed. Flip off the colored protective cap on the bottle, but do not remove the rubber stopper.
3. Wipe top of bottle with alcohol swab.
4. Draw air into the syringe by pulling back on the plunger. The amount of air should be equal to your insulin dose.
5. Remove the needle cover. Put the needle through rubber top of insulin bottle.
6. Push plunger in. The air injected into the bottle will allow insulin to be easily withdrawn into syringe.
7. Turn bottle and syringe upside down in 1 hand. Be sure tip of needle is in insulin. Your other hand will be free to move the plunger. Draw back on plunger slowly to draw the correct dose of insulin into syringe.
8. Check for air bubbles. The air is harmless, but too large an air bubble will reduce the insulin dose. To remove air bubbles, push insulin back into the bottle and measure your correct dose of insulin.
9. Double-check your dose. Remove needle from bottle. Cover needle with guard or lay syringe down so that needle does not touch anything.

INJECTING THE DOSE

1. Cleanse the skin where the injection is to be made.
2. With 1 hand, stabilize the skin by spreading it or pinching up a large area of skin.
3. Pick up syringe with other hand, and hold it as you would a pencil. Insert needle straight into the skin (90° angle). After the needle is in, pull back the plunger very slightly.

If blood comes into the syringe, the needle has entered a blood vessel. Remove the needle and put it in at another location. If blood does not appear in the syringe, push the plunger in slowly as far as it will go.

4. To inject the insulin, push plunger all the way down, using less than 5 seconds to inject the dose.
5. Hold alcohol swab near the needle and pull needle straight out of skin. Press alcohol swab over injection site for several seconds.
6. Use disposable syringe only once to ensure sterility of syringe and needle and accuracy of dose. Destroy syringes as directed.
7. To avoid tissue damage, always change the site for each injection.

WARNINGS—SEE ADDITIONAL WARNINGS ABOVE

Humulin 70/30 is a fixed mixture of human insulins consisting of 70% Human Insulin Isophane Suspension and 30% Human Insulin Injection. Humulin 70/30 should be used only if your physician has prescribed insulins mixed in a ratio of 70% NPH and 30% Regular. You should not attempt to change the ratio of this product by adding additional NPH or Regular insulin to this vial. If Humulin N and Humulin R mixtures are prescribed in a different proportion, the individual insulins should be mixed in the amounts recommended by your physician.

USAGE IN PREGNANCY

Pregnancy may make managing your diabetes more difficult. If you are pregnant or nursing a baby, consult your physician, pharmacist, or nurse-educator when using this product.

INSULIN REACTION AND SHOCK

Insulin reaction (too little sugar in the blood, also called "hypoglycemia") can be brought about by:

1. Taking too much insulin
2. Missing or delaying meals
3. Exercising or working too hard just before a meal
4. An infection or illness (especially with diarrhea or vomiting)
5. A change in the body's need for insulin

The first symptoms of insulin reaction usually come on suddenly and may include fatigue, nervousness or "shakiness," headache, rapid heartbeat, nausea, and a cold sweat.

A few patients who experienced hypoglycemic reactions after being transferred to Humulin have reported that these early warning symptoms were less pronounced than they were with animal-source insulin.

Eating sugar or a sugar-sweetened product will often correct the condition and prevent more serious symptoms.

If the reaction becomes more severe, breathing will be shallow and the skin pale. Severe hypoglicemia can result in confusion, loss of consciousness, or convulsions. Contact a doctor at once if you develop any of these symptoms.

DIABETIC ACIDOSIS AND COMA

Diabetic acidosis may develop if your body has too little insulin. (This is the opposite of insulin reaction, which is the result of too much insulin in the blood.) Diabetic acidosis may be brought on if you omit your insulin or take less than the doctor has prescribed, eat significantly more than your diet calls for, or develop a fever or infection. With acidosis, urine tests show a large amount of sugar and acetone.

The first symptoms of diabetic acidosis usually come on gradually, over a period of hours or days, and include a drowsy feeling, flushed face, thirst, and loss of appetite. Heavy breathing and a rapid pulse are more severe symptoms. It is important that you notify your doctor immediately, because diabetic coma (unconsciousness) can follow.

ALLERGY TO INSULIN

Patients occasionally experience redness, swelling, and itching at the site of injection of insulin. This condition, called "local allergy", usually clears up in a few days to a few weeks. If you have local reactions, contact your doctor, who may recommend a change in the type or species of insulin. Less common, but potentially more serious, is generalized allergy to insulin, which may cause rash over the whole body, shortness of breath, wheezing, reduction in blood pressure, fast pulse, or sweating. Severe cases of generalized allergy may be life-threatening. If you think you are having a generalized allergic reaction to insulin, notify a physician immediately. Your doctor may recommend skin testing—injecting small doses of other insulins into the skin—in order to select the best insulin for you to use. Patients who have had severe generalized allergic reactions to insulin should be skin-tested with each new preparation to be used before treatment with that preparation is started.

IMPORTANT NOTES

1. Never change from the insulin that has been prescribed for you to another insulin without instructions from your

Continued on next page

* Identi-Code® symbol.

Lilly—Cont.

doctor. Changing the type, strength, species, or manufacturer of insulin can cause problems with your diabetes.

2. Your doctor will tell you what to do if you miss a dose of insulin or miss a meal because of illness. Always keep an extra supply of insulin, as well as spare syringe and needle, on hand. If you miss a meal, use a substitute of sugar, sugar-sweetened candy, fruit juice, or sugar-sweetened beverage according to your doctor's instructions.

3. If you become ill from any cause, especially with nausea and vomiting, your insulin requirements may change. Test your urine and/or blood and notify your doctor at once.

4. Consult your doctor if you notice anything unusual or have doubts about your condition or your use of insulin.

5. Always wear diabetic identification so that appropriate treatment can be given if complications occur away from home.

6. Understand how to manage your diabetes so that your life can be active and healthy.

DIABETES FORECAST is a national magazine designed especially for patients with diabetes and their families and is available on subcription from the American Diabetes Association, National Service Center, 1660 Duke Street, Alexandria, Virginia 22314.

Another publication, **DIABETES COUNTDOWN,** is available from the Juvenile Diabetes Foundation, 60 Madison Avenue, New York, New York 10010.　　　[051689]

HUMULIN® BR　　　OTC
[hū'mŭ-lĭn bē är]
Buffered Regular
(insulin human injection, USP
[recombinant DNA origin])
FOR EXTERNAL INSULIN PUMPS ONLY

WARNINGS
**FOR USE ONLY IN EXTERNAL INSULIN PUMPS.
DO NOT MIX WITH OTHER INSULIN PRODUCTS.
HUMULIN BR SHOULD NOT BE MIXED WITH OTHER INSULINS BECAUSE THE BUFFERING INGREDIENT COULD INTERACT WITH OTHER INSULINS AND CHANGE THEIR ACTIVITY. THIS COULD LEAD TO AN UNDESIRED EFFECT ON BLOOD SUGAR, SUCH AS HYPOGLYCEMIA (LOW BLOOD SUGAR).
HUMULIN BR HAS BEEN TESTED ONLY IN CARDIAC PACEMAKERS, INC, SERIES 9100 AND 9200 INFUSION DEVICES. PATIENTS PARTICIPATING IN THE STUDY CHANGED THE INSULIN IN THE RESERVOIR (SYRINGE) EVERY 24 HOURS.
THIS LILLY HUMAN INSULIN PRODUCT DIFFERS FROM ANIMAL-SOURCE INSULINS BECAUSE IT IS STRUCTURALLY IDENTICAL TO THE INSULIN PRODUCED BY YOUR BODY'S PANCREAS, AND BECAUSE OF ITS UNIQUE MANUFACTURING PROCESS.
ANY CHANGE OF INSULIN SHOULD BE MADE CAUTIOUSLY AND ONLY UNDER MEDICAL SUPERVISION. CHANGES IN REFINEMENT, PURITY, STRENGTH, BRAND (MANUFACTURER), TYPE (REGULAR, NPH, LENTE®, ETC), SPECIES (BEEF, PORK, BEEF-PORK, HUMAN), AND /OR METHOD OF MANUFACTURE (RECOMBINANT DNA VERSUS ANIMAL-SOURCE INSULIN) MAY RESULT IN THE NEED FOR A CHANGE IN DOSAGE.
SOME PATIENTS TAKING HUMULIN® (HUMAN INSULIN, RECOMBINANT DNA ORIGIN, LILLY) MAY REQUIRE A CHANGE IN DOSAGE FROM THAT USED WITH ANIMAL-SOURCE INSULINS. IF AN ADJUSTMENT IS NEEDED, IT MAY OCCUR WITH THE FIRST DOSE OR OVER A PERIOD OF SEVERAL WEEKS.
INFORMATION FOR THE PATIENT:**
See under Humulin® L.
Always check the carton and the bottle label for the name and letter designation of the insulin you receive from your pharmacy to make sure it is the same as that your doctor has prescribed.

BUFFERED REGULAR HUMAN INSULIN
Humulin is synthesized in a non-disease-producing special laboratory strain of *Escherichia coli* bacteria that has been genetically altered by the addition of the human gene for insulin production. Humulin® BR (Buffered Regular Insulin Human Injection, USP [Recombinant DNA Origin], Lilly) consists of zinc-insulin crystals dissolved in a clear fluid containing disodium phosphate buffer. Humulin BR has the same rapid effect and relatively short duration of activity (6 to 8 hours) as that of regular insulin.

Always check the appearance of a bottle of insulin before withdrawing a dose. Humulin BR is a clear and colorless liquid with a water-like appearance and consistency. Do not use it if it appears cloudy, thickened, or slightly colored or if solid particles are visible. A bottle that appears cloudy, thickened, or slightly colored or contains solid particles should be returned to the place of purchase for exchange.

If you note anything unusual in the appearance of your insulin or notice your insulin requirements changing markedly, check the appearance of the bottle you are using and consult your doctor.

In some individuals who use insulin infusion pumps, the catheters tend to become clogged with insulin crystals. The phosphate buffer in this preparation may prevent this type of blockage. During menses, there may still be a tendency toward insulin-related catheter obstruction. This may be treated by changing catheter sets more frequently or by minimizing direct contact of the catheter with the skin.

USE THE CORRECT SYRINGE/RESERVOIR FOR THE PUMP THAT YOU ARE USING
Doses of insulin are measured in units. The number of units in each milliliter (mL) is clearly stated on the package. It is important to follow the instructions from the manufacturer of the pump that you are using regarding loading the syringe or reservoir. Failure to do so can lead to a mistake in dosage, and you may receive too little or too much insulin. This can cause serious problems for you, such as a blood sugar level that is too low or too high.　　　[042688]

HUMULIN® L　　　OTC
[hū'-mŭ-lĭn ĕl]
Lente (human insulin [recombinant DNA origin]
zinc suspension)
INFORMATION FOR THE PATIENT
WARNINGS
**THIS LILLY HUMAN INSULIN PRODUCT DIFFERS FROM ANIMAL-SOURCE INSULINS BECAUSE IT IS STRUCTURALLY IDENTICAL TO THE INSULIN PRODUCED BY YOUR BODY'S PANCREAS AND BECAUSE OF ITS UNIQUE MANUFACTURING PROCESS.
ANY CHANGE OF INSULIN SHOULD BE MADE CAUTIOUSLY AND ONLY UNDER MEDICAL SUPERVISION. CHANGES IN REFINEMENT, PURITY, STRENGTH, BRAND (MANUFACTURER), TYPE (REGULAR, NPH, LENTE®, ETC), SPECIES (BEEF, PORK, BEEF-PORK, HUMAN), AND /OR METHOD OF MANUFACTURE (RECOMBINANT DNA VERSUS ANIMAL-SOURCE INSULIN) MAY RESULT IN THE NEED FOR A CHANGE IN DOSAGE.
SOME PATIENTS TAKING HUMULIN® (HUMAN INSULIN, RECOMBINANT DNA ORIGIN, LILLY) MAY REQUIRE A CHANGE IN DOSAGE FROM THAT USED WITH ANIMAL-SOURCE INSULINS. IF AN ADJUSTMENT IS NEEDED, IT MAY OCCUR WITH THE FIRST DOSE OR OVER A PERIOD OF SEVERAL WEEKS.**

INSULIN AND DIABETES
Your doctor has explained that you have diabetes. You have learned that the treatment of your diabetes requires injections of insulin.

Insulin is a hormone produced by the pancreas, a large gland that lies near the stomach. This hormone is necessary for the body's correct use of food, especially sugar. Diabetes occurs when the pancreas does not make enough insulin to meet your body's needs.

To control your diabetes, your doctor has prescribed injections of insulin to keep your blood sugar at a nearly normal level and to keep your urine as free of sugar as possible. Each case of diabetes is different. You doctor has told you which insulin to use, how much, and when and how often to inject it. This schedule has been individualized for you. Proper control of your diabetes requires close and constant cooperation with your doctor.

In spite of diabetes, you can lead an active, healthy, and useful life if you eat a balanced diet daily, exercise regularly, and take your insulin injections exactly as prescribed by your doctor.

You have been instructed to test your blood and/or your urine regularly for sugar. If your blood tests consistently show above-normal sugar levels or your urine tests consistently show the presence of sugar, your diabetes is not properly controlled and you must let your doctor know.

If you become ill from any cause, especially with nausea and vomiting, your insulin requirements may change. Test your urine and/or blood and notify your doctor at once.

Always keep an extra supply of insulin as well as spare syringe and needle on hand. Always wear diabetic identification so that appropriate treatment can be given if complications occur away from home.

USE THE PROPER TYPE OF INSULIN
This insulin, manufactured by Eli Lilly and Company, has the trademark Humulin and is available in 5 formulations—Regular, Buffered Regular, NPH, Lente, and Ultralente®. These products can be identified by a large letter(s) that appears on the carton and vial (bottle) label following the name Humulin: Humulin R (Regular), Humulin BR (Buffered Regular), Humulin N (NPH), Humulin L (Lente), or Humulin U (Ultralente).

These types of insulin differ mainly in the time they require to take effect and in the length of time their action lasts. Your doctor has prescribed the type of insulin that he/she believes is best for you. **DO NOT USE ANY OTHER INSULIN EXCEPT ON HIS/HER ADVICE AND DIRECTION.**

Always check the carton and the bottle label for the name and letter designation of the insulin you receive from your pharmacy to make sure it is the same as that your doctor has prescribed.　　[See below].

LENTE HUMAN INSULIN
Humulin is synthesized in a non-disease-producing special laboratory strain of *Escherichia coli* bacteria that has been genetically altered by the addition of the human gene for insulin production. Humulin® L (Lente Human Insulin [Recombinant DNA Origin] Zinc Suspension, Lilly) is a suspension of zinc-insulin crystals providing a different duration of action than that of regular insulin. The result is an intermediate-acting insulin with a slower onset of action and a longer duration of activity (up to 24 hours) than that of regular insulin.

Always examine the appearance of a bottle of insulin before withdrawing each dose. A bottle of Humulin L must be rotated or carefully shaken before each injection so that the contents are uniformly mixed. Humulin L should look uniformly cloudy or milky after mixing. Do not use if the insulin substance (the white material) remains at the bottom of the bottle after mixing, leaving a clear liquid above (Figure 1). Do not use a bottle of Humulin L if there are clumps floating in the insulin after mixing (Figure 2). A bottle that remains clear or has clumps floating in the insulin after mixing should be returned to the place of purchase for exchange.

If you note anything unusual in the appearance of your insulin or notice your insulin requirements changing markedly, check the appearance of the bottle you are using and consult your doctor.

EXPIRATION DATE

EXPIRATION DATE

BRAND NAME

SPECIES

CONCENTRATION

INTERNATIONAL SYMBOL

TYPE

U-100

PA 6350 AMP

Fig. 1.—Do not use if the insulin material remains at the bottom of the bottle after mixing.

Fig. 2.—Do not use if clumps are floating in the insulin after mixing.

STORAGE

Insulin should be stored in a cold place, preferably in a refrigerator, but not in the freezing compartment. Do not let it freeze or leave it in direct sunlight. If refrigeration is not possible, the bottle of insulin which you are currently using can be kept unrefrigerated as long as it is kept as cool as possible and away from heat and sunlight. Do not use a bottle of insulin after the expiration date stamped on the label.

USE THE CORRECT SYRINGE

Doses of insulin are measured in **units**. The number of units in each milliliter (mL) is clearly stated on the package. It is important to use a syringe which is marked for an insulin preparation with 100 units per mL. Failure to use the proper syringe can lead to a mistake in dosage, and you may receive too little or too much insulin. This can cause serious problems for you, such as a blood sugar level that is too low or too high.

IMPORTANT: TO HELP AVOID CONTAMINATION AND POSSIBLE INFECTION, FOLLOW THESE INSTRUCTIONS EXACTLY.

DISPOSABLE SYRINGES

Disposable syringes and needles require no sterilization; they should be used only once and then discarded.

STERILIZING AND ASSEMBLING REUSABLE SYRINGES

Your reusable syringe and needle must be sterilized before each injection—**follow the package directions supplied with your syringe.** Boiling, as described below, is the best method of sterilizing.

1. Put syringe, plunger, and needle in strainer, place in saucepan, and cover with water. Boil for 5 minutes.
2. Remove articles from water. When they have cooled, insert plunger into barrel, and fasten needle to syringe with a slight twist.
3. Push plunger in and out several times until water is completely removed.
   (If the syringe, plunger, and needle cannot be boiled, as when you are traveling, they may be sterilized by immersion for at least 5 minutes in Isopropyl Alcohol, 91%. Do not use bathing, rubbing, or medicated alcohol for this sterilization. If the syringe is sterilized with alcohol, it must be absolutely dry before use.)

PREPARING THE DOSE

1. Wash your hands.
2. Roll or carefully shake the insulin bottle several times to mix the insulin. Be sure it is completely mixed. Flip off the colored protective cap on the bottle, but **do not** remove the rubber stopper.

3. Wipe top of bottle with alcohol swab.

4. Draw air into the syringe by pulling back on the plunger. The amount of air should be equal to your insulin dose.

5. Remove the needle cover. Put the needle through rubber top of insulin bottle.

6. Push plunger in. The air injected into the bottle will allow insulin to be easily withdrawn into syringe.

7. Turn bottle and syringe upside down in one hand. Be sure tip of needle is in insulin. Your other hand will be free to move the plunger. Draw back on plunger slowly to draw the correct dose of insulin into syringe.

8. Check for air bubbles. The air is harmless, but too large an air bubble will reduce the insulin dose. To remove air bubbles, push insulin back into the bottle and measure your correct dose of insulin.

9. Double check your dose. Remove needle from bottle. Cover needle with guard or lay syringe down so that needle does not touch anything.

INJECTING THE DOSE

1. Cleanse the skin where the injection is to be made.

2. With one hand, stabilize the skin by spreading it or pinching up a large area of skin.

3. Pick up syringe with other hand, and hold it as you would a pencil. Insert needle straight into the skin (90° angle). After the needle is in, pull back the plunger very slightly. If blood comes into the syringe, the needle has entered a blood vessel. Remove the needle and put it at another location. If blood does not appear in the syringe, push the plunger in slowly as far as it will go.

4. To inject the insulin, push plunger all the way down, using less than 5 seconds to inject the dose.

5. Hold alcohol swab near the needle and pull needle straight out of skin. Press alcohol swab over injection site for several seconds.

6. Use disposable syringe only once to ensure sterility of syringe and needle and accuracy of dose. Destroy syringes as directed.

7. To avoid tissue damage, always change the site for each injection.

WARNINGS—SEE ADDITIONAL WARNINGS ABOVE

Patients who have been directed by their doctors to mix 2 types of insulin should be aware that insulin hypodermic syringes of different manufacturers may vary in the amount of space between the bottom line and the needle. Because of this, do not change:

1. The order of mixing that the doctor has prescribed or
2. The model and brand of syringe or needle without first consulting your physician.

The mixing should be done immediately prior to injection. Failure to heed this warning could result in a dosage error.

Continued on next page

* Identi-Code® symbol.

Lilly—Cont.

USAGE IN PREGNANCY

Pregnancy may make managing your diabetes more difficult. If you are pregnant or nursing a baby, consult your doctor, pharmacist, or diabetes-educator when using this product.

INSULIN REACTION AND SHOCK

Insulin reaction (too little sugar in the blood, also called "hypoglycemia") can be brought about by:
1. Taking too much insulin
2. Missing or delaying meals
3. Exercising or working too hard just before a meal
4. An infection or illness (especially with diarrhea or vomiting)
5. A change in the body's need for insulin

The first symptoms of insulin reaction usually come on suddenly and may include fatigue, nervousness or "shakiness," headache, rapid heartbeat, nausea, and a cold sweat.

A few patients who experienced hypoglycemic reactions after being transferred to Humulin have reported that these early warning symptoms were less pronounced than they were with animal-source insulin.

Eating sugar or a sugar-sweetened product will often correct the condition and prevent more serious symptoms.

If the reaction becomes more severe, breathing will be shallow and the skin pale. If uncorrected, loss of consciousness, coma, or death can result. Therefore, it is important that you obtain medical assistance immediately.

DIABETIC ACIDOSIS AND COMA

Diabetic acidosis may develop if your body has too little insulin. (This is the opposite of insulin reaction, which is the result of too much insulin in the blood.) Diabetic acidosis may be brought on if you omit your insulin or take less than the doctor has prescribed, eat significantly more than your diet calls for, or develop a fever or infection. With acidosis, urine tests show a large amount of sugar and acetone.

The first symptoms of diabetic acidosis usually come on gradually, over a period of hours or days, and include a drowsy feeling, flushed face, thirst, and loss of appetite. Heavy breathing and a rapid pulse are more severe symptoms. If uncorrected, loss of consciousness, coma, or death can result. Therefore, it is important that you obtain medical assistance immediately.

ALLERGY TO INSULIN

Patients occasionally experience redness, swelling, and itching at the site of injection of insulin. This condition, called local allergy, usually clears up in a few days to a few weeks. If you have local reactions, contact your doctor, who may recommend a change in the type or species source of insulin. Less common, but potentially more serious, is generalized allergy to insulin, which may cause rash over the whole body, shortness of breath, wheezing, reduction in blood pressure, fast pulse, or sweating. Severe cases of generalized allergy may be life-threatening. If you think you are having a generalized allergic reaction to insulin, notify a doctor immediately. Your doctor may recommend skin testing, that is, injecting small doses of other insulins into the skin, in order to select the best insulin for you to use. Patients who have had severe generalized allergic reactions to insulin should be skin tested with each new preparation to be used before starting treatment with that preparation.

PUBLICATIONS

DIABETES FORECAST is a national magazine designed especially for patients with diabetes and their families and is available on subscription from the American Diabetes Association, National Service Center, 1660 Duke Street, Alexandria, Virginia 22314.

Another publication, **DIABETES COUNTDOWN,** is available from the Juvenile Diabetes Foundation, 60 Madison Avenue, New York, New York 10010.

[042688]

HUMULIN® N   OTC
[hū 'mŭ-lĭn ĕn]
NPH
(human insulin [recombinant DNA origin]
isophane suspension)

INFORMATION FOR THE PATIENT: *See under* Humulin® L.
Always check the carton and the bottle label for the name and letter designation of the insulin you receive from your pharmacy to make sure it is the same as that your doctor has prescribed.

NPH HUMAN INSULIN

Humulin is synthesized in a non-disease-producing special laboratory strain of *Escherichia coli* bacteria which has been genetically altered by the addition of the human gene for insulin production. Humulin® N (NPH Human Insulin, Recombinant DNA Origin, Isophane Suspension, Lilly) is a modification of a solution of zinc-insulin crystals providing a different duration of action than that of regular insulin. The result is an intermediate-acting insulin with a slower onset of action and a longer duration of activity (slightly less than 24 hours) that that of regular insulin.

Always examine the appearance of a bottle of insulin before withdrawing each dose. A bottle of Humulin N must be rotated or carefully shaken before each injection so that the contents are uniformly mixed. Humulin N should look uniformly cloudy or milky after mixing. Do not use if the insulin substance (the white material) remains at the bottom of the bottle after mixing. Do not use a bottle of Humulin N if there are clumps floating in the insulin after mixing (Figure 1). Do not use a bottle of Humulin N if solid white particles stick to the bottom or wall of the bottle, giving it a frosted appearance (Figure 2). A bottle that appears frosted should be returned to the place of purchase for exchange.

If you note anything unusual in the appearance of your insulin or notice your insulin requirements changing markedly, check the appearance of the bottle you are using and consult your doctor.

[042688]

Fig. 1.—Do not use if clumps are floating in the insulin after mixing.

Fig. 2.—Do not use if particles on the bottom or wall give the bottle a frosted appearance.

HUMULIN® R   OTC
[hū 'mŭ-lĭn är]
Regular
(insulin human injection, USP [recombinant DNA origin])

INFORMATION FOR THE PATIENT: *See under* Humulin® L.
Always check the carton and the bottle label for the name and letter designation of the insulin you receive from your pharmacy to make sure it is the same as that your doctor has prescribed.

NEUTRAL REGULAR HUMAN INSULIN

Humulin is synthesized in a non-disease-producing special laboratory strain of *Escherichia coli* bacteria that has been genetically altered by the addition of the human gene for insulin production. Humulin® R (Regular Insulin Human Injection, USP [Recombinant DNA Origin], Lilly) consists of zinc-insulin crystals dissolved in a clear fluid. Humulin R has had nothing added to change the speed or length of its action. It takes effect rapidly and has a relatively short duration of activity (6 to 8 hours) as compared with other insulins. Always check the appearance of a bottle of insulin before withdrawing a dose. Humulin R is a clear and colorless liquid with a water-like appearance and consistency. Do not use Humulin R if it appears cloudy, thickened, or slightly colored or if solid particles are visible. A bottle that appears cloudy, thickened, or slightly colored or contains solid particles should be returned to the place of purchase for exchange.

If you note anything unusual in the appearance of your insulin or notice your insulin requirements changing markedly, check the appearance of the bottle you are using and consult your doctor.

PREPARING THE DOSE

See under Humulin® L, *except:* Do not roll or shake the insulin bottle.

[042688]

HUMULIN® U   OTC
[hū '-mŭ-lĭn ū]
Ultralente
(human Insulin [recombinant DNA origin]
extended zinc suspension)

INFORMATION FOR THE PATIENT: *See under* Humulin® L.
Always check the carton and the bottle label for the name and letter designation of the insulin you receive from your pharmacy to make sure it is the same as that your doctor has prescribed.

ULTRALENTE HUMAN INSULIN

Humulin is synthesized in a non-disease-producing special laboratory strain of *Escherichia coli* bacteria that has been genetically altered by the addition of the human gene for insulin. Humulin® U (Ultralente Human Insulin [Recombinant DNA Origin] Extended Zinc Suspension, Lilly) is a suspension of zinc-insulin crystals that has a slower onset and a longer and less intense duration of activity than that of regular insulin or the intermediate-acting insulins (NPH and Lente). The time course of action of any insulin may vary considerably in different individuals or at different times in the same individual. As with all insulin preparations, the duration of action of Humulin U is somewhat dose dependent (24 to 28 hours following administration of 0.5 U/kg (0.25 U/lb).

Always examine the appearance of a bottle of insulin before withdrawing each dose. A bottle of Humulin U must be rotated or carefully shaken before each injection so that the contents are uniformly mixed. Humulin U should look uniformly cloudy or milky after mixing. Do not use if the insulin substance (the white material) remains at the bottom of the bottle after mixing, leaving a clear liquid above (Figure 1). Do not use a bottle of Humulin U if there are clumps floating in the insulin after mixing (Figure 2). A bottle that remains clear or has clumps floating in the insulin after mixing should be returned to the place of purchase for exchange.

If you note anything unusual in the appearance of your insulin or notice your insulin requirements changing markedly, check the appearance of the bottle you are using and consult your doctor.

WARNINGS—SEE ADDITIONAL WARNINGS UNDER HUMULIN L

Unless directed by their doctors, patients should not mix Humulin U with other insulins and should not change the model and brand of syringe or needle. When regular insulin is mixed with Humulin U, the quick effect of the regular insulin is lost.

After the dose is prepared, the injection should be made promptly to avoid clogging the needle.

[042688]

ILETIN® (INSULIN, LILLY)—   OTC
[ĭ 'lĕ-tĭn]
REGULAR AND MODIFIED
INSULIN PRODUCTS

All of the insulins listed below are prepared from a mixture of insulin crystals extracted from beef and pork pancreas, except for Regular (Concentrated) Iletin® II (purified pork insulin injection, Lilly), U-500, which is prepared from pork insulin only. Regular Iletin® II (purified insulin injection, Lilly), Lente® Iletin® II (purified insulin zinc suspension, Lilly),

NPH Iletin® II (isophane purified insulin suspension, Lilly), and Protamine, Zinc & Iletin® II (protamine zinc purified insulin suspension, Lilly) made solely from beef or pork source are available in U-100 strength only. When insulin is prepared from a single animal source, the species is indicated on the vial label and on the package.

REGULAR ILETIN® I
[rĕg´ū-lĕr ĭ´lĕ-tĭn wŭn]
(Beef-Pork)
(insulin injection)
USP

INFORMATION FOR THE PATIENT

WARNINGS
ANY CHANGE OF INSULIN SHOULD BE MADE CAUTIOUSLY AND ONLY UNDER MEDICAL SUPERVISION. CHANGES IN REFINEMENT, PURITY, STRENGTH (U-40, U-100), BRAND (MANUFACTURER), TYPE (LENTE®, NPH, REGULAR, ETC.), AND SPECIES SOURCE (BEEF, PORK, BEEF-PORK, OR HUMAN) MAY RESULT IN THE NEED FOR A CHANGE IN DOSAGE.
SOME PATIENTS TAKING THIS BEEF-PORK INSULIN WILL REQUIRE SUCH A CHANGE IN DOSAGE. IF AN ADJUSTMENT IS NEEDED, IT MAY OCCUR WITH THE FIRST DOSE OR OVER A PERIOD OF SEVERAL WEEKS.

INSULIN AND DIABETES
Your doctor has explained that you have diabetes. You have learned that the treatment of your diabetes requires injections of insulin.
Insulin is a hormone produced by the pancreas, a large gland that lies near the stomach. This hormone is necessary for the body's correct use of food, especially sugar. Diabetes occurs when the pancreas does not make enough insulin to meet the body's needs.
To control your diabetes, your doctor has prescribed injections of insulin to keep your blood sugar at a nearly normal level and to keep your urine as free of sugar as possible. Each case of diabetes is different. Your doctor has told you which insulin to use, how much, and when and how often to inject it. This schedule has been individualized for you. Proper control of your diabetes requires close and constant cooperation with your doctor.
In spite of diabetes, you can lead an active, healthy, and useful life if you eat a balanced diet daily, exercise regularly, and take your insulin injections exactly as prescribed by your doctor.
You have been instructed to test your urine and/or blood regularly for sugar. If your urine tests consistently show the presence of sugar or your blood tests consistently show above-normal sugar levels, your diabetes is not properly controlled and you must let your doctor know.

USE THE PROPER TYPE OF INSULIN
This insulin, manufactured by Eli Lilly and Company, has the trademark Iletin® I (insulin, Lilly) and is available in various types—Regular, NPH, Protamine Zinc, Lente, Semilente®, and Ultralente®.
These types of insulin differ mainly in the time they require to take effect and in the length of time their action lasts. Your doctor has prescribed the type of insulin that he/she believes is best for you. **Do not use any other type of insulin except on his/her advice and direction.**

REGULAR BEEF-PORK INSULIN
Regular Iletin I, consisting of zinc-insulin crystals dissolved in a clear fluid, is obtained from beef and pork pancreas. Regular beef-pork insulin is "unmodified" (that is, nothing has been added to change the speed or length of its action). It takes effect rapidly and has a relatively short duration of activity (six to eight hours) as compared with other insulins. Regular beef-pork insulin should be clear and colorless. Do not use it if it is cloudy, unusually viscous, precipitated, or even slightly colored.

STORAGE
Insulin should be stored in a cold place, preferably in a refrigerator, but not in the freezing compartment. Do not let it freeze or leave it in direct sunlight. If refrigeration is not possible, the bottle of insulin which you are currently using can be kept unrefrigerated as long as it is kept as cool as possible and away from heat and sunlight. Do not use a bottle of insulin after the expiration date stamped on the label.

USE THE CORRECT SYRINGE
Doses of insulin are measured in **units.** The number of units in each cubic centimeter (cc) is clearly stated on the package. Two strengths are available for some types of insulin: U-40 (40 units per cc) and U-100 (100 units per cc). It is important that you understand the markings on your syringe, because the volume of insulin you inject depends on the strength, that is, the number of units per cc. For this reason, you should always use a syringe marked for the strength of insulin you are injecting. Failure to use the proper syringe can lead to a mistake in dosage, and you may receive too little or too much insulin. This can cause serious problems for you,

ranging from a blood sugar that is too low or too high to coma (unconsciousness) or, rarely, death.
IMPORTANT: TO HELP AVOID CONTAMINATION AND POSSIBLE INFECTION, FOLLOW THESE INSTRUCTIONS EXACTLY.

DISPOSABLE SYRINGES
Disposable syringes and needles require no sterilization; they should be used only once and then discarded.

STERILIZING AND ASSEMBLING REUSABLE SYRINGES
Your reusable syringe and needle must be sterilized before each injection—**follow the package directions supplied with your syringe.** Boiling, as described below, is the best method of sterilizing.
1. Put syringe, plunger, and needle in strainer, place in saucepan, and cover with water. Boil for 5 minutes.
2. Remove articles from water. When they have cooled, insert plunger into barrel, and fasten needle to syringe with a slight twist.
3. Push plunger in and out several times until water is completely removed. (If the syringe, plunger, and needle cannot be boiled, as when you are traveling, they may be sterilized by immersion for at least 5 minutes in Isopropyl Alcohol, 91%. Do not use bathing, rubbing, or medicated alcohol for this sterilization. If the syringe is sterilized with alcohol, it must be absolutely dry before use.)

PREPARING THE DOSE
1. Wash your hands.
2. Flip off the colored protective cap on the bottle, but **do not** remove rubber stopper.
3. Wipe top of bottle with alcohol swab.
4. Draw air into the syringe by pulling back on the plunger. The amount of air should be equal to your insulin dose.
5. Remove the needle cover. Put the needle through rubber top of insulin bottle.
6. Push plunger in. The air injected into the bottle will allow insulin to be easily withdrawn into syringe.
7. Turn bottle and syringe upside down in one hand. Be sure tip of needle is in insulin. Your other hand will be free to move the plunger. Draw back on plunger slowly to draw the correct dose of insulin into syringe.
8. Check for air bubbles. The air is harmless, but too large an air bubble will reduce the insulin dose. To remove air bubbles, push insulin back into the bottle and measure your correct dose of insulin.
9. Double check your dose. Remove needle from bottle. Cover needle with guard or lay syringe down so that needle does not touch anything.

INJECTING THE DOSE
1. Clean the skin where the injection is to be made.
2. With one hand, stabilize the skin by spreading it or pinching up a large area of skin.
3. Pick up syringe with other hand, and hold it as you would a pencil. Insert needle straight into the skin (90° angle). After the needle is in, pull back the plunger very slightly. If blood comes into the syringe, the needle has entered a blood vessel. Remove the needle and put it in at another location. If blood does not appear in the syringe, push the plunger in slowly as far as it will go.
4. To inject the insulin, push plunger all the way down, using less than 5 seconds to inject the dose.
5. Hold alcohol swab near the needle and pull needle straight out of skin. Press alcohol swab over injection site for several seconds.
6. Use disposable syringe only once to insure sterility of syringe and needle and accuracy of dose. Destroy syringes as directed.
7. To avoid tissue damage, always change the site for each injection.

WARNINGS—SEE ADDITIONAL WARNINGS ABOVE
Patients who have been directed by their physicians to mix 2 types of insulin should be aware that insulin hypodermic syringes of different manufacturers may vary in the amount of space between the bottom line and the needle.
Because of this, do not change:
1. The order of mixing that the physician has prescribed or
2. The model and brand of syringe or needle without first consulting your physician.
The mixing should be done immediately prior to injection. Failure to heed this warning could result in a dosage error.

USAGE IN PREGNANCY
Pregnancy may make managing your diabetes more difficult. If you are pregnant or nursing a baby, consult your physician, pharmacist, or nurse-educator when using this product.

INSULIN REACTION AND SHOCK
Insulin reaction (too little sugar in the blood, also called "hy-

poglycemia") can be brought about by:
1. Taking too much insulin
2. Missing or delaying meals
3. Exercising or working too hard just before a meal
4. An infection or illness (especially with diarrhea or vomiting)
5. A change in the body's need for insulin
The first symptoms of insulin reaction usually come on suddenly and may include fatigue, nervousness or "shakiness," headache, rapid heartbeat, nausea, and a cold sweat. Eating sugar or a sugar-sweetened product will often correct the condition and prevent more serious symptoms. If the reaction becomes more severe, breathing will be shallow and the skin pale. Contact your doctor at once if you develop any of these symptoms.

DIABETIC ACIDOSIS AND COMA
Diabetic acidosis may develop if your body has too little insulin. (This is the opposite of insulin reaction, which is the result of too much insulin in the blood.) Diabetic acidosis may be brought on if you omit your insulin or take less than the doctor has prescribed, eat significantly more than your diet calls for, or develop a fever or infection. With acidosis, urine tests show a large amount of sugar and acetone.
The first symptoms of diabetic acidosis usually come on gradually, over a period of hours or days, and include a drowsy feeling, flushed face, thirst, and loss of appetite. Heavy breathing and a rapid pulse are more severe symptoms. It is important that you notify your doctor immediately, because diabetic coma (unconsciousness) can follow.

ALLERGY TO INSULIN
Patients occasionally experience redness, swelling, and itching at the site of injection of insulin. This condition, called local allergy, usually clears up in a few days to a few weeks. If you have local reactions, contact your physician, who may recommend a change in the type or species source of insulin. Less common, but potentially more serious, is generalized allergy to insulin, which may cause rash over the whole body, shortness of breath, wheezing, reduction in blood pressure, fast pulse, or sweating. Severe cases of generalized allergy may be life-threatening. If you think you are having a generalized allergic reaction to insulin, notify a physician immediately. Your doctor may recommend skin testing, injecting small doses of other insulins into the skin, in order to select the best insulin for you to use. Patients who have had severe generalized allergic reactions to insulin should be skin tested with each new preparation to be used before starting treatment with that preparation.

IMPORTANT NOTES
1. Never change from the insulin that has been prescribed for you to another insulin without instructions from your doctor. Changing the type, strength, species, or manufacturer of insulin can cause problems with your diabetes.
2. Your doctor will tell you what to do if you miss a dose of insulin or miss a meal because of illness. Always keep an extra supply of insulin, as well as spare syringe and needle, on hand. If you miss a meal, use a substitute of sugar, sugar-sweetened candy, fruit juice, or sugar-sweetened beverage according to your doctor's instructions.
3. If you become ill from any cause, especially with nausea and vomiting, your insulin requirement may change. Test your urine and /or blood and notify your doctor at once.
4. Consult your doctor if you notice anything unusual or have doubts about your condition or your use of insulin.
5. Always wear diabetic identification so that appropriate treatment can be given if complications occur away from home.
6. Understand how to manage your diabetes so that your life can be active and healthy.

HOW SUPPLIED
Regular Iletin ® I (Insulin Injection, USP) (Beef-Pork) is supplied in rubber-stoppered vials as follows:
CP-240, U-40, 40 units/cc, 10 cc (400 units) (NDC 0002-8240-01).
CP-210, U-100, 100 units/cc, 10 cc (1000 units) (NDC 0002-8210-01). The above products are supplied 10 per carton. *Refrigerate. Avoid freezing.*

[021787]

Continued on next page

* Identi-Code® symbol.

Lilly—Cont.

REGULAR (CONCENTRATED) ILETIN® II, U-500   ℞
[rĕg-ū-lĕr ī'lĕ-tĭn]
(insulin injection, USP, purified pork)

WARNINGS
ANY CHANGE OF INSULIN SHOULD BE MADE CAUTIOUSLY AND ONLY UNDER MEDICAL SUPERVISION. CHANGES IN PURITY, STRENGTH (U-40, U-100), BRAND (MANUFACTURER), TYPE (LENTE®, NPH, REGULAR, ETC.), AND/OR SPECIES SOURCE (BEEF, PORK, BEEF-PORK, OR HUMAN) MAY RESULT IN THE NEED FOR A CHANGE IN DOSAGE. SEE BELOW.
IT IS NOT POSSIBLE TO IDENTIFY WHICH PATIENTS WILL REQUIRE A REDUCTION IN DOSE TO AVOID HYPOGLYCEMIA WHEN USING THIS INSULIN. HOWEVER, IT IS KNOWN THAT A SMALL NUMBER OF PATIENTS MAY REQUIRE A SIGNIFICANT CHANGE. ADJUSTMENT MAY BE NEEDED WITH THE FIRST DOSE OR OCCUR OVER A PERIOD OF SEVERAL WEEKS. BE AWARE OF THE POSSIBILITY OF SYMPTOMS OF EITHER HYPOGLYCEMIA OR HYPERGLYCEMIA.
This insulin is prepared from pork pancreas only. The dose of pork insulin for patients with insulin resistance due to antibodies to beef insulin may be only a fraction of that of beef insulin.
This insulin preparation contains 500 units of insulin in each milliliter. Extreme caution must be observed in the measurement of dosage because inadvertent overdose may result in irreversible insulin shock. Serious consequences may result if it is used other than under constant medical supervision.

DESCRIPTION
This Lilly pork insulin product differs from previous pork insulin preparations because it has undergone additional steps of chromatographic purification.
Regular (Concentrated) Iletin® II (insulin injection, USP, purified pork, Lilly), U-500, is an aqueous solution made from the antidiabetic principle of pork pancreas as stated on the label. Each milliliter contains 500 units of regular (unmodified) insulin and approximately 1.6% glycerin (w/v), with approximately 0.25% m-cresol (w/v) as a preservative. Sodium hydroxide and hydrochloric acid are added during manufacture to adjust the *p*H. All preparations of Iletin® II (insulin purified pork, Lilly) are made from zinc-insulin crystals.

CLINICAL PHARMACOLOGY
Adequate insulin dosage permits the diabetic patient to utilize carbohydrates and fats in a comparatively satisfactory manner. Regardless of concentration, the action of insulin is basically the same: to enable carbohydrate metabolism to occur and thus to prevent the production of ketone bodies by the liver. Although, under usual circumstances, diabetes can be controlled with doses in the vicinity of 40 to 60 units or less, an occasional patient develops such resistance or becomes so unresponsive to the effect of insulin that daily doses of several hundred, or even several thousand, units are required. Patients who require doses in excess of 300 to 500 units daily usually have impaired receptor function.
Occasionally, a cause of the insulin resistance can be found (such as hemochromatosis, cirrhosis of the liver, some complicating disease of the endocrine glands other than the pancreas, allergy, or infection), but in other cases, no cause of the high insulin requirement can be determined.
Iletin II, U-500, is unmodified by any agent that might prolong its action; however, clinical experience has shown that it frequently has a time action similar to a repository insulin preparation and that a single dose may show activity over a 24-hour period. This effect has been credited to the high concentration of the preparation.

INDICATIONS AND USAGE
Iletin® II (insulin injection, purified pork, Lilly), U-500, is especially useful for the treatment of diabetic patients with marked insulin resistance (daily requirements more than 200 units), since a large dose may be administered subcutaneously in a reasonable volume.

CONTRAINDICATIONS
Patients with a history of systemic allergic reactions to pork or mixed beef/pork insulin should not receive the insulin formulation unless they have been successfully desensitized.

PRECAUTIONS
General—Every patient exhibiting insulin resistance who requires Iletin® II (insulin injection, purified pork, Lilly), U-500, for control of diabetes should be under close observation until dosage is established. The response will vary among patients. Some can be controlled with a single dose daily; others may require 2 or 3 injections per day. Most patients will show a "tolerance" to insulin, so that minor varia-

tions in dosage can occur without the development of untoward symptoms of insulin shock.
Insulin resistance is frequently self-limited; after several weeks or months during which high dosage is required, responsiveness to the pharmacologic effect of insulin may be regained and dosage can be reduced.
Patients with immunologic insulin resistance to beef insulin (this diagnosis is usually confirmed by the finding of increased serum antibody titers) may require an immediate dosage reduction of 20 to 50% when treated with pork insulin.
Information for Patients—Patients should be instructed regarding their dosage and should be reminded that this formulation requires the administration of a smaller volume of solution than is the case with less concentrated formulations.
Laboratory Tests—Blood and urine glucose, glycohemoglobin, and urine ketones should be monitored frequently.
Drug Interactions—The concurrent use of oral hypoglycemic agents with Iletin II, U-500, is not recommended since there are no data to support such use.
Pregnancy—Teratogenic Effects—No reproduction studies have been conducted in animals, and there are no adequate and well-controlled studies in pregnant women. It would be anticipated that the benefits of this insulin preparation would outweigh any risk to the developing fetus.
Nonteratogenic Effects—Insulin does not cross the placenta as does glucose.
Labor and Delivery—Careful monitoring of the patient is required, since the insulin requirement may decrease following delivery.
Nursing Mothers—It is not known whether insulin is excreted in significant amounts in human milk. Because many drugs are excreted in human milk, caution should be exercised when Iletin II, U-500, is administered to a nursing woman.
Pediatric Use—There are no special precautions relating to the use of this insulin formulation in the pediatric age group.

ADVERSE REACTIONS
As with other insulin preparations, hypoglycemic reactions may be associated with the administration of Iletin® II (insulin injection, purified pork, Lilly), U-500. However, deep secondary hypoglycemic reactions may develop 18 to 24 hours after the original injection of Iletin II, U-500. Consequently, patients should be carefully observed, and prompt treatment of such reactions should be initiated with glucagon injections and/or with glucose by intravenous injection or gavage.

ALLERGIC REACTIONS
Erythema, swelling, or pruritus may occur at injection sites. Such localized allergic manifestations usually resolve within a few days to a few weeks.
Less common, but potentially more serious, is systemic allergy to insulin, which may cause generalized urticaria, dyspnea, or wheezing, which may progress to anaphylaxis. If a severe allergic reaction occurs, the drug should be discontinued and the patient treated with the usual agents (eg, epinephrine, antihistamines, or corticosteroids). Patients who have experienced severe systemic allergic reactions to insulin (eg, generalized urticaria, angioedema, anaphylaxis) should be skin-tested with each new preparation to be used before starting therapy with that preparation. Desensitization procedures may permit resumption of insulin administration.

DOSAGE AND ADMINISTRATION
Iletin® II (insulin injection, purified pork, Lilly), U-500, can be administered by both the subcutaneous and the intramuscular routes. It is inadvisable to inject Iletin II, U-500, intravenously because of the possible development of allergic or anaphylactoid reactions.
It is recommended that a tuberculin type of syringe be utilized for the measurement of dosage. Variations in dosage are frequently possible in the insulin-resistant patient, since the individual is unresponsive to the pharmacologic effect of the insulin. Nevertheless, accuracy of measurement is to be encouraged because of the potential danger of the preparation.

HOW SUPPLIED
Insulin should be kept in a cold place, preferably in a refrigerator, but must not be frozen.
Do not inject insulin that is not water-clear. Discoloration, turbidity, or unusual viscosity indicates deterioration or contamination.
Use of a package of insulin should not be started after the expiration date stamped on it.
(℞) Vials, U-500, 500 units/cc, 20 cc (No. CP-2500) (1's), NDC 0002-8500-01

[013186]

LENTE® ILETIN® I   OTC
[lĕn-ta ī-lĕ-tĭn]
(Beef-Pork)
(insulin zinc suspension)
USP

SEMILENTE® ILETIN® I
[sĕm'ĭ-lĕn'ta ī'lĕ-tĭn]
(Beef-Pork)
(prompt insulin zinc suspension)
USP

ULTRALENTE® ILETIN® I
[ŭl'tra-lĕn'ta ī'lĕ-tĭn]
(Beef-Pork)
(extended insulin zinc suspension)
USP

INFORMATION FOR THE PATIENT
WARNINGS, Insulin and Diabetes, and Use of Proper Type of Insulin: *See under* Regular Iletin® I.

LENTE BEEF-PORK INSULIN
Lente beef-pork insulin is obtained from beef and pork pancreas. Insulin has been combined with zinc to form small crystals. Lente beef-pork insulin has an intermediate time of activity. Its action starts more slowly than does that of regular beef-pork insulin and lasts somewhat longer (slightly over 24 hours).
Lente beef-pork insulin should look uniformly cloudy or milky. If the insulin substance (the cloudy material) settles at the bottom of the vial, the vial must be rotated or carefully shaken before the injection so that the contents are uniformly mixed (see instructions under Preparing the Dose). Do not use a vial of insulin if you see lumps that float or stick to the sides. Also, the insulin should not be used if it is clear and remains clear after the vial is rotated or shaken.

SEMILENTE BEEF-PORK INSULIN
Semilente beef-pork insulin comes from beef and pork pancreas. Insulin has been combined with zinc to form small crystals. Semilente beef-pork insulin has a short period of activity. Its action starts nearly as rapidly as that of regular insulin and lasts slightly longer (approximately 12 to 16 hours). This type of insulin will shorten the action time of Lente insulin (an intermediate-acting form) when they are mixed.
Semilente beef-pork insulin should look uniformly cloudy or milky. If the insulin substance (the cloudy material) settles at the bottom of the vial, the vial must be rotated or carefully shaken before the injection so that the contents are uniformly mixed (see instructions under Preparing the Dose). Do not use a vial of insulin if you see lumps that float or stick to the sides. Also, the insulin should not be used if it is clear and remains clear after the vial is rotated or shaken.

ULTRALENTE BEEF-PORK INSULIN
Ultralente beef-pork insulin comes from beef and pork pancreas. Insulin has been combined with zinc to form small crystals. Ultralente beef-pork insulin takes effect very gradually and, in comparison with regular insulin, has a long period of activity (more than 36 hours). This type of insulin will lengthen the action time of Lente insulin (an intermediate-acting form) when they are mixed.
Ultralente beef-pork insulin should look uniformly cloudy or milky. If the insulin substance (the cloudy material) settles at the bottom of the vial, the vial must be rotated or carefully shaken before the injection so that the contents are uniformly mixed (see instructions under Preparing the Dose). Do not use a vial of insulin if you see lumps that float or stick to the sides. Also, the insulin should not be used if it is clear and remains clear after the vial is rotated or shaken.
Storage, Use the Correct Syringe, Disposable Syringes, and Sterilizing and Assembling Reusable Syringes: *See under* Regular Iletin® I.

PREPARING THE DOSE
1. Wash your hands.
2. Roll or carefully shake the insulin bottle several times to mix the insulin. Be sure it is completely mixed. Flip off the colored protective cap on the bottle, but **do not** remove the rubber stopper. *See also under* Regular Iletin® I.
Injecting the Dose, Warnings, Usage in Pregnancy, Insulin Reaction and Shock, Diabetic Acidosis and Coma, Allergy to Insulin, and **Important Notes:** *See under* Regular Iletin® I.

HOW SUPPLIED
Lente® Iletin® I (Insulin Zinc Suspension, USP) is supplied in rubber-stoppered vials as follows:
CP-440, U-40, 40 units/cc, 10 cc (400 units) (NDC 0002-8440-01).
CP-410, U-100, 100 units/cc, 10 cc (1000 units) (NDC 0002-8410-01).
Semilente® Iletin® I (Prompt Insulin Zinc Suspension, USP) is supplied in rubber-stoppered vials as follows:
CP-540, U-40, 40 units/cc, 10 cc (400 units) (NDC 0002-8540-01).

CP-510, U-100, 100 units/cc, 10 cc (1000 units) (NDC 0002-8510-01).

Ultralente ® Iletin ® I (Extended Insulin Zinc Suspension, USP) is supplied in rubber-stoppered vials as follows:
CP-640, U-40, 40 units/cc, 10 cc (400 units) (NDC 0002-8640-01).
CP-610, U-100, 100 units/cc, 10 cc (1000 units) (NDC 0002-8610-01).
The above products are supplied 10/carton. *Refrigerate. Avoid freezing.*

[021787]

NPH ILETIN® I   OTC
[ĕn'pē-āch ī'lĕ-tĭn]
(Beef-Pork)
(isophane insulin suspension)
USP

INFORMATION FOR THE PATIENT
WARNINGS, Insulin and Diabetes, and Use of Proper Type of Insulin: *See under* Regular Iletin® I.

NPH BEEF-PORK INSULIN
NPH beef-pork insulin is obtained from beef and pork pancreas. Insulin has been combined with protamine and zinc so that its action is similar to that of a mixture of Regular and Protamine Zinc insulins. The result is an intermediate-acting insulin with a slower speed of action than Regular insulin and a shorter time of activity than Protamine Zinc insulin. The effect of NPH beef-pork insulin lasts slightly more than 24 hours.

NPH beef-pork insulin should look uniformly cloudy or milky. If the insulin substance (the cloudy material) settles at the bottom of the vial, the vial must be rotated or carefully shaken before the injection so that the contents are uniformly mixed (see instructions under Preparing the Dose). Do not use a vial of insulin if you see lumps that float or stick to the sides. Also, the insulin should not be used if it is clear and remains clear after the vial is rotated or shaken.

Storage, Use the Correct Syringe, Disposable Syringes, and Sterilizing and Assembling Reusable Syringes: *See under* Regular Iletin® I.
Preparing the Dose: *See under* Lente® Iletin® I and Regular Iletin® I.
Injecting the Dose, Warnings, Usage in Pregnancy, Insulin Reaction and Shock, Diabetic Acidosis and Coma, Allergy to Insulin, and Important Notes: *See under* Regular Iletin® I.

HOW SUPPLIED
NPH Iletin ® I (Isophane Insulin Suspension, USP) is supplied in rubber-stoppered vials as follows:
CP-340, U-40, 40 units/cc, 10 cc (400 units) (NDC 0002-8340-01).
CP-310, U-100, 100 units/cc, 10 cc (1000 units) (NDC 0002-8310-01).
The above products are supplied 10/carton. *Refrigerate. Avoid freezing.*

[021787]

PROTAMINE, ZINC & ILETIN® I   OTC
[prō'ta-mĕn zĭngk ănd ī'lĕ-tĭn]
(Beef-Pork)
(protamine zinc insulin suspension)
USP

INFORMATION FOR THE PATIENT
WARNINGS, Insulin and Diabetes, and Use of Proper Type of Insulin: *See under* Regular Iletin® I.

PROTAMINE ZINC BEEF-PORK INSULIN
Protamine zinc beef-pork insulin is obtained from beef and pork pancreas. Protamine and zinc have been added to lengthen the time of action. Protamine zinc beef-pork insulin takes effect gradually and, in comparison with regular beef-pork insulin, has a long period of activity (well over 24 hours).

Protamine zinc beef-pork insulin should look uniformly cloudy or milky. If the insulin substance (the cloudy material) settles at the bottom of the vial, the vial must be rotated or carefully shaken before the injection so that the contents are uniformly mixed (see instructions under Preparing the Dose). Do not use a vial of insulin if you see lumps that float or stick to the sides. Also, the insulin should not be used if it is clear and remains clear after the vial is rotated or shaken.

Storage, Use the Correct Syringe, Disposable Syringes, and Sterilizing and Assembling Reusable Syringes: - *See under* Regular Iletin® I.
Preparing the Dose: *See under* Lente® Iletin® I and Regular Iletin® I.
Injecting the Dose, Warnings, Usage in Pregnancy, Insulin Reaction and Shock, Diabetic Acidosis and Coma, Allergy to Insulin, and **Important Notes:** *See under* Regular Iletin® I.

HOW SUPPLIED
Protamine, Zinc & Iletin® I (Protamine Zinc Insulin Suspension, USP) is supplied in rubber-stoppered vials as follows:
CP-140, U-40, 40 units/cc, 10 cc (400 units) (NDC 0002-8140-01).
CP-110, U-100, 100 units/cc, 10 cc (1000 units) (NDC 0002-8110-01).
The above products are supplied 10/carton. *Refrigerate. Avoid freezing.*

[021787]

KEFUROX®   ℞
[kĕf'yū-rŏeks]
(sterile cefuroxime sodium)
USP

DESCRIPTION
Kefurox® (Sterile Cefuroxime Sodium, USP, Lilly) is a semisynthetic, broad-spectrum cephalosporin antibiotic for parenteral administration. It has the chemical formula (6R,7R)-7-[2-(2-Furyl) glyoxylamido]-3-(hydroxymethyl)-8-oxo-5-thia-1-azabicyclo [4.2.0] oct-2-ene-2-carboxylic acid (Z)-mono(0-methyloxime) carbamate (ester), monosodium salt (USAN). Kefurox contains approximately 54.2 mg (2.4 mEq) of sodium per gram of cefuroxime activity. Solutions of Kefurox range from light yellow to amber, depending on the concentration and diluent used. The pH of freshly reconstituted solutions usually ranges from 6.0 to 8.5.

CLINICAL PHARMACOLOGY
After intramuscular injection of a 750-mg dose of cefuroxime to normal volunteers, the mean peak serum concentration was 27 mg/L. The peak occurred at approximately 45 minutes (range 15–60 minutes). Following intravenous doses of 750 mg and 1.5 g, serum concentrations were approximately 50 mg/L and 100 mg/L, respectively, at 15 minutes. Therapeutic serum concentrations of approximately 2 mg/L or more were maintained for 5.3 hours and 8 hours or more, respectively. There was no evidence of accumulation of cefuroxime in the serum following intravenous administration of 1.5-g doses every 8 hours to normal volunteers. The serum half-life after either intramuscular or intravenous injections is approximately 80 minutes.

Approximately 89% of a dose of cefuroxime is excreted by the kidneys over an 8-hour period, resulting in high urinary concentrations.

Following the intramuscular administration of a 750-mg single dose, urinary concentrations averaged 1,300 mg/L during the first 8 hours. Intravenous doses of 750 mg and 1.5 g produced urinary levels averaging 1,150 mg/L and 2,500 mg/L, respectively, during the first 8-hour period.

The concomitant oral administration of probenecid with cefuroxime slows tubular secretion, decreases renal clearance by approximately 40%, increases the peak serum level by approximately 30%, and increases the serum half-life by approximately 30%. Kefurox® (Sterile Cefuroxime Sodium, USP, Lilly) is detectable in therapeutic concentrations in pleural fluid, joint fluid, bile, sputum, bone, cerebrospinal fluid (in patients with meningitis), and aqueous humor. Cefuroxime is approximately 50% bound to serum protein.

Microbiology—Cefuroxime has in vitro activity against a wide range of gram-positive and gram-negative organisms, and it is highly stable in the presence of β-lactamases of certain gram-negative bacteria. The bactericidal action of cefuroxime results from inhibition of cell-wall synthesis.
Cefuroxime is usually active against the following organisms in vitro.

Gram-Negative—Haemophilus influenzae (including ampicillin-resistant strains), *Haemophilus parainfluenzae, Neisseria gonorrhoeae* (including penicillinase- and non-penicillinase-producing strains), *Neisseria meningitidis, Escherichia coli, Klebsiella* sp (including *Klebsiella* pneumoniae), Enterobacter sp, *Citrobacter* sp, *Salmonella* sp, *Shigella* sp, *Proteus mirabilis, Proteus inconstans* (formerly *Providencia),* *Providencia rettgeri* (formerly *Proteus rettgeri), Morganella morganii* (formerly *Proteus morganii).*
Some strains of *M morganii, Enterobacter cloacae,* and *Citrobacter* sp have been shown by in vitro tests to be resistant to cefuroxime and other cephalosporins.
Gram-Positive—Staphyloccus aureus (including penicillinase- and non-penicillinase-producing strains), *Staphylococcus epidermidis, Streptococcus pyogenes* (and other streptococci), *Streptococcus pneumoniae* (formerly *Diplococcus pneumoniae*).
Certain strains of enterococci, eg, *Enterococcus faecalis* (formerly *Streptococcus faecalis*), are resistant.
Anaerobic Organisms —Gram-positive and gram-negative cocci (including *Peptococcus* and *Peptostreptococcus* sp), gram-positive bacilli (including *Clostridium* sp), gram-negative bacilli (including *Bacteroides* and *Fusobacterium* sp). Most strains of *Bacteroides fragilis* are resistant.
Pseudomonas and *Campylobacter* sp, *Acinetobacter calcoaceticus* (formerly *Mima* and *Herellea* sp), and most strains of *Serratia* and *Proteus vulgaris* are resistant to cephalosporins. Methicillin-resistant staphylococci, *Clostridium difficile,* and *Listeria monocytogenes* are resistant to cefuroxime.
Susceptibility Tests —Diffusion Techniques—Quantitative methods that require measurement of zone diameters give the most precise estimates of antibiotic susceptibility. One such procedure[1] has been recommended for use with disks to test susceptibility to cefuroxime. Interpretation involves correlation of the diameters obtained in the disk test with minimum inhibitory concentration (MIC) values for cefuroxime.
Reports from the laboratory giving results of the standardized single-disk susceptibility test[1] using a 30- µg cefuroxime disk should be interpreted according to the following criteria:

1. Bauer AW, Kirby WMM, Sherris JC, Turck M: Antibiotic susceptibility testing by a standardized single disk method. *Am J Clin Pathol* 1966; 45:493. Standardized disk susceptibility test. *Federal Register* 1974; 39:19182–19184. National Committee for Clinical Laboratory Standards, Approved Standard: ASM-2 Performance Standards for Antimicrobial Disk Susceptibility Tests,—Third Edition, December, 1984.

Susceptible organisms produce zones of 18 mm or greater, indicating that the tested organism is likely to respond to therapy.
Organisms that produce zones of 15 to 17 mm are expected to be susceptible if high dosage is used or if the infection is confined to tissues and fluids (eg, urine), in which high antibiotic levels are attained.
Resistant organisms produce zones of 14 mm or less, indicating that other therapy should be selected.
For gram-positive isolates, the test may be performed with either the cephalosporin-class disk (30 µg cephalothin) or the cefuroxime disk (30 µg cefuroxime) and a zone of 18 mm or greater indicates a cefuroxime-susceptible organism.
Gram-negative organisms should be tested with the cefuroxime disk (using the above criteria), since cefuroxime has been shown by in vitro tests to have activity against certain strains of *Enterobacteriaceae* found resistant when tested with the cephalosporin-class disk. Gram-negative organisms having zones of less than 18 mm around the cephalothin disk are not necessarily of intermediate susceptibility or resistant to cefuroxime. The cefuroxime disk should not be used for testing susceptibility to other cephalosporins.
Standardized procedures require the use of laboratory control organisms. The 30-µg cefuroxime disk should give zone diameters between 27 and 35 mm for *S. aureus* ATCC 25923. For *E coli* ATCC 25922, the zone diameters should be between 20 and 26 mm.
Dilution Techniques —A bacterial isolate may be considered susceptible if the MIC value for cefuroxime is not more than 16 mg/L. Organisms are considered resistant if the MIC is greater than 32 mg/L.
As with standard diffusion methods, dilution procedures require the use of laboratory control organisms. Standard cefuroxime powder should give MIC values in the range of 0.5 mg/L and 2 mg/L for *S aureus* ATCC 25923. For *E coli* ATCC 25922, the MIC range should be between 2 mg/L and 8 mg/L.

INDICATIONS AND USAGE
Kefurox® (Sterile Cefuroxime Sodium, USP, Lilly) is indicated for the treatment of infections caused by susceptible strains of the designated microorganisms in the diseases listed below:
Lower Respiratory Infections, including pneumonia caused by *S pneumoniae* (formerly *Diplococcus pneumoniae*), *H influenzae* (including ampicillin-resistant strains), *Klebsiella* sp, *S aureus* (penicillinase- and non-penicillinase producing), *S pyogenes,* and *E coli.*
Urinary Tract Infections caused by *E coli* and *Klebsiella* sp.
Skin and Skin-Structure Infections caused by *S aureus* (penicillinase- and non-penicillinase-producing), *S pyogenes, E coli, Klebsiella* sp, and *Enterobacter* sp.
Septicemia caused by *S aureus* (penicillinase-and non-penicillinase-producing), *S pneumoniae, E coli, H influenzae* (including ampicillin-resistant strains), and *Klebsiella* sp.
Meningitis caused by *S pneumoniae, H influenzae* (including ampicillin-resistant strains), *N meningitidis,* and *S aureus* (penicillinase- and non-penicillinase-producing).
Gonorrhea—Uncomplicated and disseminated gonococcal infections due to *N gonorrhoeae* (penicillinase- and non-penicillinase-producing strains) in both males and females.
Bone and Joint Infections —Caused by *S aureus* (including penicillinase- and non-penicillinase-producing strains).
Clinical microbiologic studies in skin and skin-structure infections frequently reveal the growth of susceptible strains of both aerobic and anaerobic organisms. Kefurox has been used successfully in these mixed infections in which several organisms have been isolated. Appropriate cultures and sus-

Continued on next page

* Identi-Code® symbol.

Lilly—Cont.

ceptibility studies should be performed to determine the susceptibility of the causative organisms to Kefurox. Therapy may be started while awaiting the results of these studies; however, once these results become available, the antibiotic treatment should be adjusted accordingly. In certain cases of confirmed or suspected gram-positive or gram-negative sepsis or in patients with other serious infections in which the causative organism has not been identified, Kefurox may be used concomitantly with an aminoglycoside (*see* Precautions). The recommended doses of both antibiotics may be given depending on the severity of the infection and the patient's condition.

Prevention: The preoperative prophylactic administration of Kefurox® (Sterile Cefuroxime Sodium, USP, Lilly) may prevent the growth of susceptible disease-causing bacteria and, thereby, may reduce the incidence of certain postoperative infections in patients undergoing surgical procedures (eg, vaginal hysterectomy) that are classified as clean-contaminated or potentially contaminated procedures. Effective prophylactic use of antibiotics in surgery depends on the time of administration. Kefurox should usually be given ½ to 1 hour before the operation to allow sufficient time to achieve effective antibiotic concentrations in the wound tissues during the procedure. The dose should be repeated intraoperatively if the surgical procedure is lengthy. Prophylactic administration is usually not required after the surgical procedure ends and should be stopped within 24 hours. In the majority of surgical procedures, continuing prophylactic administration of any antibiotic does not reduce the incidence of subsequent infections but will increase the possibility of adverse reactions and the development of bacterial resistance. The perioperative use of Kefurox has also been effective during open heart surgery for surgical patients in whom infections at the operative site would present a serious risk. For these patients, it is recommended that therapy with Kefurox be continued for at least 48 hours after the surgical procedure ends. If an infection is present, specimens for culture should be obtained for the identification of the causative organism and appropriate antimicrobial therapy should be instituted.

CONTRAINDICATIONS

Kefurox® (Sterile Cefuroxime Sodium, USP, Lilly) is contraindicated in patients with known allergy to the cephalosporin group of antibiotics.

WARNINGS

BEFORE THERAPY WITH KEFUROX® (STERILE CEFUROXIME SODIUM, USP, LILLY) IS INSTITUTED, CAREFUL INQUIRY SHOULD BE MADE TO DETERMINE WHETHER THE PATIENT HAS HAD PREVIOUS HYPERSENSITIVITY REACTIONS TO CEPHALOSPORINS, PENICILLINS, OR OTHER DRUGS. THIS PRODUCT SHOULD BE GIVEN CAUTIOUSLY TO PENICILLIN-SENSITIVE PATIENTS. ANTIBIOTICS SHOULD BE ADMINISTERED WITH CAUTION TO ANY PATIENT WHO HAS DEMONSTRATED SOME FORM OF ALLERGY, PARTICULARLY TO DRUGS. IF AN ALLERGIC REACTION TO KEFUROX OCCURS, DISCONTINUE THE DRUG. SERIOUS ACUTE HYPERSENSITIVITY REACTIONS MAY REQUIRE EPINEPHRINE AND OTHER EMERGENCY MEASURES.

Pseudomembranous colitis has been reported with the use of cephalosporins (and other broad-spectrum antibiotics); therefore, it is important to consider its daignosis in patients who develop diarrhea in association with antibiotic use.

Treatment with broad-spectrum antibiotics alters normal flora of the colon and may permit overgrowth of clostridia. Studies indicate a toxin produced by *C difficile* is one primary cause of antibiotic-associated colitis. Cholestyramine and colestipol resins have been shown to bind the toxin in vitro.

Mild cases of colitis may respond to drug discontinuance alone. Moderate to severe cases should be managed with fluid, electrolyte, and protein supplementation as indicated. When the colitis is not relieved by drug discontinuance or when it is severe, oral vancomycin is the treatment of choice for antibiotic-associated pseudomembranous colitis produced by *C difficile*. Other causes of colitis should also be considered.

PRECAUTIONS

Although Kefurox® (Sterile Cefuroxime Sodium, USP, Lilly) rarely produces alterations in kidney function, evaluation of renal status during therapy is recommended, especially in seriously ill patients receiving the maximum doses. Cephalosporins should be given with caution to patients receiving concurrent treatment with potent diuretics, as these regimens are suspected of adversely affecting renal function. The total daily dose of Kefurox should be reduced in patients with transient or persistent renal insufficiency (*see* Dosage), because high and prolonged serum antibiotic concentrations can occur in such individuals from usual doses.

As with other antibiotics, prolonged use of Kefurox may result in overgrowth of nonsusceptible organisms. Careful observation of the patient is essential. If superinfection does occur during therapy, appropriate measures should be taken.

Broad-spectrum antibiotics should be prescribed with caution in individuals with a history of gastrointestinal disease, particularly colitis.

Nephrotoxicity has been reported following concomitant administration of aminoglycoside antibiotics and cephalosporins.

Interference with Laboratory Tests —A false-positive reaction for glucose in the urine may occur with copper reduction tests (Benedict's or Fehling's solution or with Clinitest® tablets), but not with enzyme-based tests for glycosuria (eg, Tes-Tape®). A false-negative reaction may occur in the ferricyanide test for blood glucose.

Cefuroxime does not interfere with the assay of serum and urine creatinine by the the alkaline picrate method.

Carcinogenesis, Mutagenesis, and Impairment of Fertility —Although no long-term studies in animals have been performed to evaluate carcinogenic potential, no mutagenic potential of cefuroxime was found in standard laboratory tests.

Reproductive studies revealed no impairment of fertility in animals.

*Usage in Pregnancy—Pregnancy Category B —*Reproduction studies have been performed in mice and rabbits at doses up to 60 times the human dose and have revealed no evidence of impaired fertility or harm to the fetus due to cefuroxime. There are, however, no adequate, well-controlled studies in pregnant women. Because animal reproduction studies are not always predictive of human response, this drug should be used during pregnancy only if clearly needed.

Nursing Mothers —Since Kefurox is excreted in human milk, caution should be exercised when Kefurox is administered to a nursing woman.

Pediatric Use —Safety and effectiveness in children below the age of 3 months have not been established. Accumulation of other members of the cephalosporin class in newborn infants (with resulting prolongation of drug half-life) has been reported.

ADVERSE REACTIONS

Kefurox® (Sterile Cefuroxime Sodium, USP, Lilly) is generally well tolerated. The most common adverse effects have been local reactions following intravenous administration. Other adverse reactions have been encountered only rarely.

Local Reactions —Thrombophlebitis has occurred with intravenous administration in 1 in 60 patients.

Gastrointestinal —Gastrointestinal symptoms occurred in 1 in 150 patients and included diarrhea (1 in 220 patients) and nausea (1 in 440 patients). Symptoms of pseudomembranous colitis can appear during or after antibiotic treatment.

Hypersensitivity Reactions —Hypersensitivity reactions have been reported in less than 1% of the patients treated with Kefurox and include rash (1 in 125). Pruritus and urticaria and positive Coombs' test each occurred in less than 1 in 250 patients, and, as with other cephalosporins, cases of anaphylaxis have occurred rarely.

Blood —A decrease in hemoglobin and hematocrit has been observed in 1 in 10 patients and transient eosinophilia in 1 in 14 patients. Less common reactions seen were transient neutropenia (less than 1 in 100 patients) and leukopenia (1 in 750 patients). A similar pattern and incidence were seen with other cephalosporins used in controlled studies.

Hepatic —Transient rise in SGOT and SGPT (1 in 25 patients), alkaline phosphatase (1 in 50 patients), LDH (1 in 75 patients), and bilirubin (1 in 500 patients) levels has been noted.

Kidney —Elevations in serum creatinine and/or blood urea nitrogen and a decreased creatinine clearance have been observed, but their relationship to cefuroxime is unknown.

OVERDOSAGE

Signs and Symptoms —Experience with overdose of cefuroxime sodium in humans is limited. The administration of inappropriately large doses of parenteral cephalosporins may cause seizures, particularly in patients with renal failure where accumulation is likely to occur.

The oral LD_{50} in the adult mouse was > 10 g/kg, representing 83 times the routine maximum adult dose. In animals, doses up to 5 g/kg produced no tissue toxicity. With chronic doses greater than 5 g/kg, tubular necrosis was seen in animals.

Treatment —To obtain up-to-date information about the treatment of overdose, a good resource is your certified Regional Poison Control Center. Telephone numbers of certified poison control centers are listed in the *Physicians' Desk Reference (PDR)*. In managing overdosage, consider the possibility of multiple drug overdoses, interaction among drugs, and unusual drug kinetics in your patient.

Protect the patient's airway and support ventilation and perfusion. Meticulously monitor and maintain, within acceptable limits, the patient's vital signs, blood gases, serum electrolytes, etc. If the patient develops convulsions, the drug

should be promptly discontinued; anticonvulsant therapy may be administered if clinically indicated. The use of hemodialysis in the treatment of cefuroxime overdose has not been established.

DOSAGE AND ADMINISTRATION

Adults—The usual adult dosage range for Kefurox® (Sterile Cefuroxime Sodium, USP, Lilly) is 750 mg to 1.5 g every 8 hours, usually for 5 to 10 days. In uncomplicated urinary tract infections, skin and skin-structure infections, disseminated gonococcal infections, and uncomplicated pneumonia, a 750-mg dose every 8 hours is recommended. In severe or complicated infections, a 1.5-g dose every 8 hours is recommended.

In bone and joint infections, a dosage of 1.5 g every 8 hours is recommended. In clinical trials, surgical intervention was performed, when indicated, as an adjunct to therapy with Kefurox. A course of oral antibiotic therapy was administered when appropriate following the completion of parenteral administration of Kefurox.

In life-threatening infections or infections due to less susceptible organisms, 1.5 g every 6 hours may be required. In bacterial meningitis, the dose should not exceed 3.0 g every 8 hours. The recommended dose for uncomplicated gonococcal infection is 1.5 g intramuscularly, given as a single dose at two different sites together with 1.0 g of oral probenecid. For preventive use for clean-contaminated or potentially contaminated surgical procedures, a 1.5-g dose administered intravenously just prior to surgery (approximately ½ to 1 hour before the initial incision) is recommended. Thereafter, give 750 mg intravenously or intramuscularly every 8 hours when the procedure is prolonged.

For preventive use during open heart surgery, a 1.5-g dose administered intravenously at the induction of anesthesia and every 12 hours thereafter for a total of 6.0 g is recommended.

Impaired Renal Function —When renal function is impaired, a reduced dosage must be employed. Dosage should be determined by the degree of renal impairment and the susceptibility of the causative organism (see Table 1).

TABLE 1: Dosage of Kefurox® (Sterile Cefuroxime Sodium, USP) in Adults With Reduced Renal Function

Creatinine Clearance (mL/min.)	Dose	Frequency
> 20	750 mg–1.5 g	Every 8 hours
10–20	750 mg	Every 12 hours
< 10	750 mg	Every 24 hours*

*Since Kefurox is dialyzable, patients on hemodialysis should be given a further dose at the end of the dialysis.

When only serum creatinine is available, the following formula (based on sex, weight, and age of the patient) may be used to convert this value into creatinine clearance. The serum creatinine should represent a steady state of renal function.

Male:
$$\frac{\text{Weight (kg)} \times (140 - \text{age})}{72 \times \text{serum creatinine (mg/100 dL)}}$$

Females: 0.9 × above value

Note: As with antibiotic therapy in general, administration of Kefurox should be continued for a minimum of 48 to 72 hours after the patient becomes asymptomatic or after evidence of bacterial eradication has been obtained; a minimum of 10 days of treatment is recommended in infections caused by *Streptococcus pyogenes* in order to guard against the risk of rheumatic fever or glomerulonephritis; frequent bacteriologic and clinical appraisal is necessary during therapy of chronic urinary tract infection and may be required for several months after therapy has been completed; persistent infections may require treatment for several weeks; and doses smaller than those indicated above should not be used. In staphylococcal and other infections involving a collection of pus, surgical drainage should be carried out when indicated.

Infants and Children Above 3 Months of Age —Administration of 50 to 100 mg/kg/day in equally divided doses every 6 to 8 hours has been successful for most infections susceptible to cefuroxime. The higher dose of 100 mg/kg/day (not to exceed the maximum adult dose) should be used for the more severe or serious infections.

In cases of bacterial meningitis, larger doses of Kefurox are recommended, initially 200 to 240 mg/kg/day intravenously in divided doses every 6 to 8 hours.

In children with renal insufficiency, the frequency of dosage should be modified consistent with the recommendations for adults.

Preparation of Solution and Suspension —The directions for preparing Kefurox for both intravenous and intramuscular use are summarized in Table 2.   [See table next page]

For Intramuscular Use —Each 750-mg/10 mL vial of Kefurox should be reconstituted with 3.6 mL of Sterile Water for Injection. Shake gently to disperse and withdraw 3.6 mL of the resulting suspension for injection.

For Intravenous Use—Each 750-mg/10 mL vial should be reconstituted with 9.0 mL of Sterile Water for Injection. Withdraw 8.0 mL of the resulting solution for injection. Each 1.5-g/20 mL vial should be reconstituted with 14.0 mL of Sterile Water for Injection and the solution completely withdrawn for injection.

For infusion, each 750-mg or 1.5-g dose should be reconstituted with 50 to 100 mL of Sterile Water for Injection, 5% Dextrose Injection, 0.9% Sodium Chloride Injection, or any of the solutions listed under the Intravenous portion of the Compatibility and Stability section. If Sterile Water for Injection is used as the diluent, reconstitute with approximately 20 mL/g to avoid a hypotonic solution.

[See table right].

Administration—After reconstitution, Kefurox® (Sterile Cefuroxime Sodium, USP, Lilly) may be given intravenously or by deep intramuscular injection into a large muscle mass (such as the gluteus or lateral part of the thigh). Prior to injecting intramuscularly, aspiration is necessary to avoid inadvertent injection into a blood vessel.

Intravenous Administration—The intravenous route may be preferable for patients with bacterial septicemia or other severe or life-threatening infections or for patients who may be poor risks because of lowered resistance, particularly if shock is present or impending.

For Direct Intermittent Intravenous Administration—Slowly inject the solution into a vein over a period of 3 to 5 minutes or give it through the tubing system by which the patient is also receiving other intravenous solutions.

For Intermittent Intravenous Infusion with a Y-Type Administration Set—Dosing can be accomplished through the tubing system by which the patient may be receiving other intravenous solutions. However, during infusion of the solution containing Kefurox, it is advisable to discontinue administration of any other solutions at the same site temporarily.

For Continuous Intravenous Infusion—A solution of Kefurox may be added to an intravenous bottle containing 1 of the following fluids:

0.9% Sodium Chloride Injection, 5% Dextrose Injection, 10% Dextrose Injection, 5% Dextrose and 0.9% Sodium Chloride Injection, 5% Dextrose and 0.45% Sodium Chloride Injection, or M/6 Sodium Lactate Injection

Solutions of Kefurox, like those of most β-lactam antibiotics, should not be added to solutions of aminglycoside antibiotics because of potential interaction.

However, if concurrent therapy with Kefurox and an aminoglycoside is indicated, each of these antibiotics can be administered separately to the same patient.

Compatibility and Stability—Intramuscular—When reconstituted as directed with Sterile Water for Injection, suspensions of Kefurox® (Sterile Cefuroxime Sodium, USP, Lilly) for intramuscular injection maintain satisfactory potency for 24 hours at room temperature and for 48 hours under refrigeration (5℃).

After the periods mentioned above, any unused suspensions should be discarded.

Intravenous—When the 750-mg and 1.5-g vials are reconstituted as directed with Sterile Water for Injection, the solutions of Kefurox for intravenous administration maintain satisfactory potency for 24 hours at room temperature and for 48 hours under refrigeration (5℃). More dilute solutions, such as 750 mg or 1.5 g plus 50 to 100 mL of Sterile Water for Injection, 5% Dextrose Injection, or 0.9% Sodium Chloride Injection, maintain satisfactory potency for 24 hours at room temperature and for 7 days under refrigeration.

These solutions may be further diluted to concentrations of between 1 mg/mL and 30 mg/mL in the following solutions and will lose not more than 10% activity for 24 hour at room temperature or for at least 7 days under refrigeration: 0.9% Sodium Chloride Injection, M/6 Sodium Lactate Injection, Ringer's Injection USP, Lactated Ringer's Injection USP, 5% Dextrose and 0.9% Sodium Chloride Injection, 5% Dextrose Injection, 5% Dextrose and 0.45% Sodium Chloride Injection, 5% Dextrose and 0.225% Sodium Chloride Injection, 10% Dextrose Injection, and 10% Invert Sugar in Water for Injection.

Unused solutions should be discarded after the time periods mentioned above.

Kefurox has also been found compatible for 24 hours at room temperature when admixed in intravenous infusion with: Heparin (10 and 50 units/mL) in 0.9% Sodium Chloride Injection, and Potassium Chloride (10 and 40 mEq/L) in 0.9% Sodium Chloride Injection.

Note: Parenteral drug products should be inspected visually for particulate matter and discoloration prior to administration whenever solution and container permit.

As with other cephalosporins, however, cefuroxime powder as well as solutions and suspensions tend to darken, depending on storage conditions, without adversely affecting product potency.

Protect from light. Prior to reconstitution, store at controlled room temperature, 59° to 86°F (15° to 30℃).

TABLE 2
Preparation of Solution and Suspension
(Glass Vials, ADD-Vantage®, and Faspak)

Strength	Amount of Diluent to Be Added (mL)		Volume to Be Withdrawn (mL)	Approximate Concentration (mg/mL)
750 mg/10 mL vial	3.6	(IM)	3.6*	200
750 mg/10 mL vial	9	(IV)	8	100
1.5 g/20 mL vial	14	(IV)	Total	100
750 mg/100 mL bottle	50	(IV)	—	15
750 mg/100 mL bottle	100	(IV)	—	7.5
1.5 g/100 mL bottle	50	(IV)	—	30
1.5 g/100 mL bottle	100	(IV)	—	15
750 mg/Faspak	50	(IV)	—	15
750 mg/Faspak	100	(IV)	—	7.5
1.5 g/Faspak	50	(IV)	—	30
1.5 g/Faspak	100	(IV)	—	15
750 mg/ADD-Vantage†	50	(IV)	—	15
750 mg/ADD-Vantage†	100	(IV)	—	7.5
1.5 g/ADD-Vantage†	50	(IV)	—	30
1.5 g/ADD-Vantage†	100	(IV)	—	15

* KEFUROX® (Sterile Cefuroxime Sodium, USP, Lilly) is a suspension at IM concentrations.
† Instructions for use of the ADD-Vantage Vials are enclosed in the package.

HOW SUPPLIED
(℞) Vials:
750 mg,* 10-mL size (No. 7271)—(Traypak† of 25) NDC 0002-7271-25
1.5 g,* 20-mL size (No. 7272)—(Traypak of 10) NDC 0002-7272-10
750 mg,* 100-mL size (No. 7273)—(Traypak of 10) NDC 0002-7273-10
1.5 g,* 100-mL size (No. 7274)—(Traypak of 10) NDC 0002-7274-10
(℞) Faspak‡:
750 mg (No. 7276)—(24s) NDC 0002-7276-24
1.5 g (No. 7277)—(24s) NDC 0002-7277-24
(℞) ADD-Vantage§ Vials:
750 mg,* (No. 7278)—(Tray pak of 25) NDC 0002-7278-25
1.5 g,* (No. 7279)—(Traypak of 10) NDC 0002-7279-10
The above ADD-Vantage Vials are to be used with Abbott Laboratories' ADD-Vantage Antibiotic Diluent Container. Instructions for use of the ADD-Vantage Vials are enclosed in the package.
Also available:
(℞) Pharmacy Bulk Package;
7.5 g,* 100-mL size (No. 7275)—(Traypak of 6) NDC 0002-7275-16

---

* Equivalent to cefuroxime.
† Traypak™ (multivial carton, Lilly)
‡ Faspak® (flexible plastic bag, Lilly)
§ ADD-Vantage® (vials and diluent containers, Abbott).
[070688]

KEFZOL®   ℞
[kĕf'zōl]
(cefazolin sodium)
Sterile, USP

DESCRIPTION
Kefzol® (cefazolin sodium, Lilly) is a semisynthetic cephalosporin for parenteral administration. It is the sodium salt of 3- [[(5-methyl-1,3,4-thiadiazol-2-yl)-thio]methyl] -7- [2 - (1H-tetrazol-1-yl)acetamido] -3- cephem-4-carboxylic acid. The sodium content is 48.3 mg/g of cefazolin sodium. In addition to cefazolin sodium, the Faspak® (flexible plastic bag, Lilly) and the ADD-Vantage® System vial also contain 0.04% polysorbate 80.
The molecular formula is $C_{14}H_{14}N_8O_4S_3$ (sodium salt). The molecular weight is 476.5.
The pH of the reconstituted solution is between 4.5 and 6.

CLINICAL PHARMACOLOGY
Human Pharmacology—Table 1 demonstrates the blood levels and duration of cefazolin following intramuscular administration.

TABLE 1. SERUM CONCENTRATIONS AFTER INTRAMUSCULAR ADMINISTRATION

Dose	Serum Concentrations (µg/mL)					
	½ h	1 h	2 h	4 h	6 h	8 h
250 mg	15.5	17	13	5.1	2.5	
500 mg	36.2	36.8	37.9	15.5	6.3	3
1 g*	60.1	63.8	54.3	29.3	13.2	7.1

*Average of 2 studies

Clinical pharmacology studies in patients hospitalized with infections indicate that cefazolin produces mean peak serum levels approximately equivalent to those seen in normal volunteers.

In a study (using normal volunteers) of constant intravenous infusion with dosages of 3.5 mg/kg for 1 hour (approximately 250 mg) and 1.5 mg/kg the next 2 hours (approximately 100 mg), cefazolin produced a steady serum level at the third hour of approximately 28 µg/mL. Table 2 shows the average serum concentrations after IV injection of a single 1-g dose; average half-life was 1.4 hours.

TABLE 2. SERUM CONCENTRATIONS AFTER 1-G INTRAVENOUS DOSE

Serum Concentrations (µg/mL)					
5 min	15 min	30 min	1 h	2 h	4 h
188.4	135.8	106.8	73.7	45.6	16.5

Controlled studies on adult normal volunteers receiving 1 g 4 times a day for 10 days, monitoring CBC, SGOT, SGPT, bilirubin, alkaline phosphatase, BUN, creatinine, and urinalysis, indicated no clinically significant changes attributed to cefazolin.

Cefazolin is excreted unchanged in the urine, primarily by glomerular filtration and, to a lesser degree, by tubular secretion. Following intramuscular injection of 500 mg, 56% to 89% of the administered dose is recovered within 6 hours and 80% to nearly 100% in 24 hours. Cefazolin achieves peak urine concentrations greater than 1,000 µg/mL and 4,000 µg/mL, respectively, following 500-mg and 1-g intramuscular doses.

In patients undergoing peritoneal dialysis (2 L/h), mean serum levels of cefazolin were approximately 10 and 30 µg/mL after 24 hours' instillation of a dialyzing solution containing 50 mg/L and 150 mg/L, respectively. Mean peak levels were 29 µg/mL (range 13-44 µg/mL) with 50 mg/L (3 patients), and 72 µg/mL (range 26-142 µg/mL) with 150 mg/L (6 patients). Intraperitoneal administration of cefazolin is usually well tolerated.

When cefazolin is administered to patients with unobstructed biliary tracts, high concentrations well over serum levels occur in the gallbladder tissue and bile. In the presence of obstruction, however, concentration of the antibiotic is considerably lower in bile than in serum.

Cefazolin readily crosses an inflamed synovial membrane, and the concentration of the antibiotic achieved in the joint space is comparable to levels measured in the serum.

Cefazolin readily crosses the placental barrier into the cord blood and amniotic fluid. It is present in very low concentrations in the milk of nursing mothers.

Microbiology—In vitro tests demonstrate that the bactericidal action of cephalosporins results from inhibition of cellwall synthesis. Kefzol® (cefazolin sodium, Lilly) is active against the following organisms in vitro and in clinical infections.

Staphylococcus aureus (including penicillinase-producing strains)
Staphylococcus epidermidis

Continued on next page

* Identi-Code® symbol.

Lilly—Cont.

Methicillin-resistant staphylococci are uniformly resistant to cefazolin.

Group A β-hemolytic streptococci and other strains of streptococci (many strains of enterococci are resistant)
Streptococcus (Diplococcus) pneumoniae
Escherichia coli
Proteus mirabilis
Klebsiella sp
Enterobacter aerogenes
Haemophilus influenzae

Most strains of indole-positive *Proteus* (*P vulgaris*), *Enterobacter cloacae*, *Morganella morganii*, and *Providencia rettgeri* are resistant. *Serratia, Pseudomonas,* and *Acinetobacter calcoaceticus* (formerly *Mima* and *Herellea* sp) are almost uniformly resistant to cefazolin.

Disk Susceptibility Tests—Quantitative methods that require measurement of zone diameters give the most precise estimates of antibiotic susceptibility. One such procedure* has been recommended for use with disks for testing susceptibility to cefazolin. With this procedure, a report from the laboratory of "susceptible" indicates that the infecting organism is likely to respond to therapy. A report of "resistant" indicates that the infecting organism is not likely to respond to therapy. A report of "intermediate susceptibility" suggests that the organism would be susceptible if high dosage is used or if the infection were confined to tissues and fluids (eg, urine) in which high antibiotic levels are attained.
*National Committee for Clinical Laboratory Standards (NCCLS), 1984. Performance Standards for Antimicrobial Disk Susceptibility Tests, Approved Standard, M2-A3, NCCLS, Villanova, PA 19085.

For gram-positive isolates, a zone of 18 mm is indicative of a cefazolin-susceptible organism when tested with either the cephalosporin-class disk (30 μg cephalothin) or the cefazolin disk (30 μg cefazolin).
Gram-negative organisms should be tested with the cefazolin disk (using the above criteria), because cefazolin has been shown by in vitro tests to have activity against certain strains of *Enterobacteriaceae* found resistant when tested with the cephalothin disk. Gram-negative organisms having zones of less than 18 mm around the cephalothin disk may be susceptible to cefazolin.
The cefazolin disk should not be used for testing susceptibility to other cephalosporins.
Dilution Techniques—A bacterial isolate may be considered susceptible if the minimum inhibitory concentration (MIC) for cefazolin is not more than 16 μg/mL. Organisms are considered resistant if the MIC is equal to or greater than 64 μg/mL.

INDICATIONS AND USAGE

Kefzol® (cefazolin sodium, Lilly) is indicated in the treatment of the following serious infections due to susceptible organisms:
Respiratory tract infections due to *S pneumoniae, Klebsiella* sp, *H influenzae, S aureus* (including penicillinase-producing strains), and group A β-hemolytic streptococci
Injectable penicillin G benzathine is considered to be the drug of choice in the treatment and prevention of streptococcal infections, including the prophylaxis of rheumatic fever. Kefzol is effective in the eradication of streptococci from the nasopharynx; however, data establishing the efficacy of Kefzol in the subsequent prevention of rheumatic fever are not available at present.
Genitourinary tract infections due to *E coli, P mirabilis, Klebsiella* sp, and some strains of *Enterobacter* and enterococci
Skin and skin-structure infections due to *S aureus* (including penicillinase-producing strains) and group A β-hemolytic streptococci and other strains of streptococci
Biliary tract infections due to *E coli*, various strains of streptococci, *P mirabilis, Klebsiella* sp, and *S aureus*
Bone and joint infections due to *S aureus*
Septicemia due to *S pneumoniae, S aureus* (penicillin-susceptible and penicillin-resistant), *P mirabilis, E coli,* and *Klebsiella* sp
Endocarditis due to *S aureus* (penicillin-susceptible and penicillin-resistant) and group A β-hemolytic streptococci

Appropriate culture and susceptibility studies should be performed to determine susceptibility of the causative organism to Kefzol.
Perioperative Prophylaxis—The prophylactic administration of Kefzol preoperatively, intraoperatively, and postoperatively may reduce the incidence of certain postoperative infections in patients undergoing surgical procedures that are classified as contaminated or potentially contaminated (eg, vaginal hysterectomy or cholecystectomy in high-risk patients such as those over 70 years of age, with acute cholecystitis, obstructive jaundice, or common-bile-duct stones). The perioperative use of Kefzol also may be effective in surgical patients in whom infection at the operative site would present a serious risk (eg, during open-heart surgery and prosthetic arthroplasty).
The prophylactic administration of Kefzol should usually be discontinued within a 24-hour period after the surgical procedure. In surgery in which the occurrence of infection may be particularly devastating (eg, open-heart surgery and prosthetic arthroplasty), the prophylactic administration of Kefzol may be continued for 3 to 5 days following the completion of surgery. If there are signs of infection, specimens for culture should be obtained for the identification of the causative organism so that appropriate therapy may be instituted. (*See* DOSAGE AND ADMINISTRATION.)

CONTRAINDICATION

Kefzol® (cefazolin sodium, Lilly) is contraindicated in patients with known allergy to the cephalosporin group of antibiotics.

WARNINGS

BEFORE CEFAZOLIN THERAPY IS INSTITUTED, CAREFUL INQUIRY SHOULD BE MADE CONCERNING PREVIOUS HYPERSENSITIVITY REACTIONS TO CEPHALOSPORINS AND PENICILLIN. CEPHALOSPORIN C DERIVATIVES SHOULD BE GIVEN CAUTIOUSLY TO PENICILLIN-SENSITIVE PATIENTS.
SERIOUS ACUTE HYPERSENSITIVITY REACTIONS MAY REQUIRE EPINEPHRINE AND OTHER EMERGENCY MEASURES.
There is some clinical and laboratory evidence of partial cross-allergenicity of the penicillins and the cephalosporins. Patients have been reported to have had severe reactions (including anaphylaxis) to both drugs.
Antibiotics, including Kefzol® (cefazolin sodium, Lilly), should be administered cautiously to any patient who has demonstrated some form of allergy, particularly to drugs. Pseudomembranous colitis has been reported with virtually all broad-spectrum antibiotics (including macrolides, semisynthetic penicillins, and cephalosporins); therefore, it is important to consider its diagnosis in patients who develop diarrhea in association with the use of antibiotics. Such colitis may range in severity from mild to life-threatening.
Treatment with broad-spectrum antibiotics alters the normal flora of the colon and may permit overgrowth of clostridia. Studies indicate that a toxin produced by *Clostridium difficile* is one primary cause of antibiotic-associated colitis. Mild cases of pseudomembranous colitis usually respond to drug discontinuance alone. In moderate to severe cases, management should include sigmoidoscopy, appropriate bacteriologic studies, and fluid, electrolyte, and protein supplementation. When the colitis does not improve after the drug has been discontinued, or when it is severe, oral vancomycin is the drug of choice for antibiotic-associated pseudomembranous colitis produced by *C difficile*. Other causes of colitis should be ruled out.
Usage in Infants—Safety for use in prematures and infants under 1 month of age has not been established.

PRECAUTIONS

General—If an allergic reaction to Kefzol® (cefazolin sodium, Lilly) occurs, the drug should be discontinued and the patient treated with the usual agents (eg, epinephrine or other pressor amines, antihistamines, or corticosteroids).
Prolonged use of Kefzol may result in the overgrowth of nonsusceptible organisms. Careful clinical observation of the patient is essential. If superinfection occurs during therapy, appropriate measures should be taken.
When Kefzol is administered to patients with low urinary output because of impaired renal function, lower daily dosage is required (see dosage instructions).
Drug Interactions—Probenecid may decrease renal tubular secretion of cephalosporins when used concurrently, which

results in increased and more prolonged cephalosporin blood levels.
Drug/Laboratory Test Interactions—A false-positive reaction for glucose in the urine may occur with Benedict's solution, Fehling's solution, or Clinitest® tablets but not with enzyme-based tests, such as Clinistix® and Tes-Tape® (Glucose Enzymatic Test Strip, USP, Lilly).
Positive direct and indirect antiglobulin (Coombs') tests have occurred; these may also occur in neonates whose mothers received cephalosporins before delivery.
Broad-spectrum antibiotics should be prescribed with caution in individuals with a history of gastrointestinal disease, particularly colitis.
Carcinogenesis, Mutagenesis—Mutagenicity studies and long-term studies in animals to determine the carcinogenic potential of cefazolin have not been performed.
Usage in Pregnancy—Pregnancy Category B—Reproduction studies have been performed in rats given doses of 500 mg or 1 g of cefazolin/kg and have revealed no evidence of impaired fertility or harm to the fetus due to Kefzol. There are, however, no adequate and well-controlled studies in pregnant women. Because animal reproduction studies are not always predictive of human response, this drug should be used during pregnancy only if clearly needed.
Labor and Delivery—When cefazolin has been administered prior to cesarean section, drug levels in cord blood have been approximately one-fourth to one-third of maternal drug levels. The drug appears to have no adverse effect on the fetus.
Nursing Mothers—Cefazolin is present in very low concentrations in the milk of nursing mothers. Caution should be exercised when cefazolin is administered to a nursing woman.

ADVERSE REACTIONS

The following reactions have been reported:
Hypersensitivity—Drug fever, skin rash, vulvar pruritus, eosinophilia, and anaphylaxis have occurred.
Blood—Neutropenia, leukopenia, thrombocythemia, and positive direct and indirect Coombs' tests have occurred.
Renal—Transient rise in BUN levels has been observed without clinical evidence of renal impairment.
Hepatic—Transient rise in SGOT, SGPT, and alkaline phosphatase levels has been observed rarely. As with some penicillins and some other cephalosporins, transient hepatitis and cholestatic jaundice have been reported rarely.
Gastrointestinal—Symptoms of pseudomembranous colitis may appear either during or after antibiotic treatment. Nausea and vomiting have been reported rarely. Anorexia, diarrhea, and oral candidiasis (oral thrush) have been reported.
Other—Pain on intramuscular injection, sometimes with induration, has occurred infrequently. Phlebitis at the site of injection has been noted. Other reactions have included genital and anal pruritus, genital moniliasis, and vaginitis.

OVERDOSAGE

The administration of inappropriately large doses of parenteral cephalosporins may cause seizures, particularly in patients with renal impairment. Dosage reduction is necessary when renal function is impaired (*see* Dosage and Administration). If seizures occur, the drug should be promptly discontinued; anticonvulsant therapy may be administered if clinically indicated. Hemodialysis may be considered in cases of overwhelming overdosage.

DOSAGE AND ADMINISTRATION

Kefzol® (cefazolin sodium, Lilly) may be administered intramuscularly or intravenously after reconstitution.
Intramuscular Administration—Reconstitute with 0.9% Sodium Chloride Injection, Sterile Water for Injection, or Bacteriostatic Water for Injection according to Table 3. Shake well until dissolved. Kefzol should be injected into a large muscle mass. Pain on injection is infrequent with Kefzol.
[See table below].
Intravenous Administration—Kefzol® (cefazolin sodium, Lilly) may be administered by intravenous injection or by continuous or intermittent infusion. Total daily dosages are the same as with intramuscular injection.
Intermittent intravenous infusion: Kefzol can be administered along with primary intravenous fluid management programs in a volume control set or in a separate, secondary IV bottle. Reconstituted 500 mg or 1 g of Kefzol may be diluted in 50 to 100 mL of 1 of the following intravenous solutions: 0.9% Sodium Chloride Injection, 5% or 10% Dextrose Injection, 5% Dextrose in Lactated Ringer's Injection, 5% Dextrose and 0.9% Sodium Chloride Injection (also may be used with 5% Dextrose and 0.45% or 0.2% Sodium Chloride Injection), Lactated Ringer's Injection, 5% or 10% Invert Sugar in Sterile Water for Injection, Ringer's Injection, Normosol®-M in D5-W, Ionosol® B with Dextrose 5%, or Plasma-Lyte® with 5% Dextrose.
ADD-Vantage Vials of Kefzol are to be reconstituted *only* with 0.9% Sodium Chloride Injection or 5% Dextrose Injection in the 50-mL or 100-mL Flexible Diluent Containers.
Intravenous injection (Administer solution directly into vein or though tubing): Dilute the reconstituted 500 mg or 1 g of Kefzol in a minimum of 10 mL of Sterile Water for Injection.

TABLE 3. DILUTION TABLE FOR KEFZOL® (CEFAZOLIN SODIUM)

Vial Size	Diluent to Be Added	Approximate Available Volume	Approximate Average Concentration
250 mg	2 mL	2 mL	125 mg/mL
500 mg	2 mL	2.2 mL	225 mg/mL
1 g*	2.5 mL	3 mL	330 mg/mL

* The 1-g vial should be reconstituted only with Sterile Water for Injection or Bacteriostatic Water for Injection.

Inject solution slowly over 3 to 5 minutes. (NOTE: ADD-VANTAGE VIALS ARE NOT TO BE USED IN THIS MANNER.)

Direct intravenous injection: Dilute the reconstituted 500 mg or 1 g of Kefzol in a minimum of 10 mL of Sterile Water for Injection. Inject solution slowly over 3 to 5 minutes. It may be administered directly into a vein or through the tubing for a patient receiving the above parenteral fluids.
Dosage—The usual adult dosages are given in Table 4.

TABLE 4. USUAL ADULT DOSAGE OF KEFZOL® (CEFAZOLIN SODIUM)

Type of Infection	Dose	Frequency
Pneumococcal pneumonia	500 mg	q12h
Mild infections caused by susceptible gram-positive cocci	250 to 500 mg	q8h
Acute uncomplicated urinary tract infections	1 g	q12h
Moderate to severe infections	500 mg to 1 g	q6 to 8h
Severe, life-threatening infections (eg, endo-carditis, septicemia)*	1 g to 1.5 g	q6h

* In rare instances, doses up to 12 g of cefazolin per day have been used.

Dosage Adjustment for Patients with Reduced Renal Function—Kefzol may be used in patients with reduced renal function with the following dosage adjustments: Patients with a creatinine clearance of 55 mL/min or greater or a serum creatinine of 1.5 mg % or less can be given full doses. Patients with creatinine clearance rates of 35 to 54 mL/min or serum creatinine of 1.6 to 3.0 mg % can also be given full doses, but dosage should be restricted to at least 8-hour intervals. Patients with creatinine clearance rates of 11 to 34 mL/min or serum creatinine of 3.1 to 4.5 mg % should be given one-half the usual dose every 12 hours. Patients with creatinine clearance rates of 10 mL/min or less or serum creatinine of 4.6 mg % or greater should be given one-half the usual dose every 18 to 24 hours. All reduced dosage recommendations apply after an initial loading dose appropriate to the severity of the infection. Patients undergoing peritoneal dialysis: See *Human Pharmacology.*
Perioperative Prophylactic Use—To prevent postoperative infection in contaminated or potentially contaminated surgery, the recommended doses are as follows:

a. 1 g IV or IM administered one-half to 1 hour prior to the start of surgery.
b. For lengthy operative procedures (eg, 2 hours or more), 0.5 to 1 g IV or IM during surgery (administration modified according to the duration of the operative procedure).
c. 0.5 to 1 g IV or IM every 6 to 8 hours for 24 hours postoperatively.

It is important that (1) the preoperative dose be given just (one-half to 1 hour) prior to the start of surgery so that adequate antibiotic levels are present in the serum and tissues at the time of the initial surgical incision and (2) Kefzol be administered, if necessary, at appropriate intervals during surgery to provide sufficient levels of the antibiotic at the anticipated moments of greatest exposure to infective organisms.
In surgery in which the occurrence of infection may be particularly devastating (eg, open-heart surgery and prosthetic arthroplasty), the prophylactic administration of Kefzol may be continued for 3 to 5 days following the completion of surgery.
In children, a total daily dosage of 25 to 50 mg/kg (approximately 10 to 20 mg/lb) of body weight, divided into 3 or 4 equal doses, is effective for most mild to moderately severe infections (Table 5). Total daily dosage may be increased to 100 mg/kg (45 mg/lb) of body weight for severe infections.
In children with mild to moderate renal impairment (creatinine clearance of 70 to 40 mL/min), 60% of the normal daily dose given in divided doses every 12 hours should be sufficient. In children with moderate impairment (creatinine clearance of 40 to 20 mL/min), 25% of the normal daily dose given in divided doses every 12 hours should be sufficient. In children with severe impairment (creatinine clearance of 20 to 5 mL/min), 10% of the normal daily dose given every 24 hours should be adequate. All dosage recommendations apply after an initial loading dose.

TABLE 5. PEDIATRIC DOSAGE GUIDE FOR KEFZOL® (CEFAZOLIN SODIUM)

Weight		25 mg/kg/Day Divided into 3 Doses		25 mg/kg/Day Divided into 4 Doses	
			Vol. (mL) Needed with Dilution of 125		Vol. (mL) Needed with Dilution of 125
lb	kg	Approximate Single Dose (mg q8h)	mg/mL	Approximate Single Dose (mg q6h)	mg/mL
10	4.5	40 mg	0.35 mL	30 mg	0.25 mL
20	9	75 mg	0.6 mL	55 mg	0.45 mL
30	13.6	115 mg	0.9 mL	85 mg	0.7 mL
40	18.1	150 mg	1.2 mL	115 mg	0.9 mL
50	22.7	190 mg	1.5 mL	140 mg	1.1 mL

Weight		50 mg/kg/Day Divided into 3 Doses		50 mg/kg/Day Divided into 4 Doses	
			Vol. (mL) Needed with Dilution of 225		Vol. (mL) Needed with Dilution of 225
lb	kg	Approximate Single Dose (mg q8h)	mg/mL	Approximate Single Dose (mg q6h)	mg/mL
10	4.5	75 mg	0.35 mL	55 mg	0.25 mL
20	9	150 mg	0.7 mL	110 mg	0.5 mL
30	13.6	225 mg	1 mL	170 mg	0.75 mL
40	18.1	300 mg	1.35 mL	225 mg	1 mL
50	22.7	375 mg	1.7 mL	285 mg	1.25 mL

Since safety for use in premature infants and in infants under 1 month of age has not been established, the use of Kefzol in these patients is not recommended.

STABILITY

In those situations in which the drug and diluent have been mixed, but not immediately administered to the patient, the admixture may be sorted under the following conditions:
Vials, Redi Vials, and Faspak Containers—Reconstituted Kefzol® (cefazolin sodium, Lilly) diluted in Sterile Water for Injection, 5% Dextrose Injection, 0.9% Sodium Chloride Injection, or Bacteristatic Water for Injection is stable for 24 hours at room temperature and for 10 days if stored under refrigeration.
Solutions of Kefzol in Sterile Water for Injection, 5% Dextrose Injection, or 0.9% Sodium Chloride Injection that are frozen immediately after reconstitution in the original vials or Faspak containers are stable for as long as 12 weeks when stored at −20°C Once thawed, these solutions are stable for 24 hours at room temperature or for 10 days if stored under refrigeration. If the product is warmed, care should be taken to avoid heating it after the thawing is complete. Once thawed, the solution should not be refrozen.
Secondary Diluents—Solutions of Kefzol for infusion in 10% Dextrose Injection, 5% Dextrose in Lactated Ringer's Injection, 5% Dextrose and 0.9% Sodium Chloride Injection (also may be used with 5% Dextrose and 0.45% or 0.2% Sodium Chloride Injection), Lactated Ringer's Injection, 5% or 10% Invert Sugar in Sterile Water for Injection, Ringer's Injection, Normosol®-M in D5-W, Ionosol®-B with Dextrose 5%, or Plasma-Lyte with 5% Dextrose should be used within 24 hours after dilution when stored at room temperature or within 96 hours if stored under refrigeration. (DO NOT FREEZE KEFZOL DILUTED WITH THE ABOVE DILUENTS.)
ADD-Vantage Vials—Only 0.9% Sodium Chloride Injection and 5% Dextrose Injection in the 50-mL or 100-mL Flexible Diluent Containers are approved for reconstituting ADD-Vantage Kefzol. Ordinarily, ADD-Vantage vials should be reconstituted only when it is certain that the patient is ready to receive the drug. However, reconstituted Kefzol diluted in 5% Dextrose Injection and 0.9% Sodium Chloride Injection is stable of 24 hours at room temperature. (DO NOT REFRIGERATE OR FREEZE KEFZOL IN ADD-VANTAGE VIALS.)
Directions for Dispensing, Pharmacy Bulk Package—Not for direct infusion. Pharmacy bulk package is for use in the Hospital Pharmacy Admixture Service only in a suitable work area, such as under a laminar flow hood. Entry into the vial must be made with a sterile transfer set or other sterile dispensing device, and contents dispensed as aliquots using aseptic technique. Use of a syringe and needle is not recommended as it may cause leakage. (*See* Dosage and Administration section above.) AFTER ENTRY USE ENTIRE CONTENTS OF VIAL PROMPTLY. ANY UNUSED PORTION

MUST BE DISCARDED WITHIN 24 HOURS AFTER INITIAL ENTRY.

HOW SUPPLIED

(℞) *Vials Kefzol® (Sterile Cefazolin Sodium, USP)*, rubber-stoppered (Dry Powder): *No. 766*, 250 mg,* 10-mL size (NDC 0002-1496-01), in singles (10/carton); *No. 767*, 500 mg,* and *No. 768*, 1 g,* 10-mL size, in singles (NDC 0002-1497-01 and NDC 0002-1498-01) (10/carton) and in Traypak™ (multivial carton, Lilly) of 25 (NDC 0002-1497-25 and NDC 0002-1498-25); *No. 7018*, † 500 mg* (NDC 0002-7018-10), and *No. 7011*, † 1 g* (NDC 0002-7011-10), 100-mL size, in Traypak of 10; *No. 7014*, 10 g,* 100-mL size, in Traypak of 6 (NDC 0002-7014-16); *No. 7021*, 20 g, 100-mL size, in Traypak of 6 (0002-7021-16).
(℞) *Redi Vial® (dual compartment vial, Lilly) Kefzol® (Sterile Cefazolin Sodium, USP): No. 7082*, 500 mg,* and *No. 7083*, 1 g,* in singles (NDC 0002-7082-01 and NDC 0002-7083-01) (10/carton) and in Traypak of 10 (NDC 0002-7082-10 and NDC 0002-7083-10).
(℞) *Faspak® (flexible plastic bag, Lilly) Kefzol® (Sterile Cefazolin Sodium, USP), No. 7201*, 500 mg,* and *No. 7202*, 1 g,* in Faspak of 96 (NDC 0002-7201-74 and NDC 0002-7202-74).
(℞) *ADD-Vantage® (vials and diluent containers, Abbott) Vials: No. 7265*, 500 mg,* in Traypak of 25 (NDC 0002-7265-25); *No. 7266*, 1 g,*Traypak of 25 (NDC 0002-7266-25).
The above ADD-Vantage Vials are to be used only with Abbott Laboratories' Diluent Containers.
Instructions for use of the ADD-Vantage Vials are enclosed in the package.

*Equivalent to cefazolin.
†For IV use.

[111687]

LENTE® ILETIN® I
[lĕn'tā' ī lĕ-tĭn]
(insulin zinc suspension, Lilly), *see under* Iletin® (insulin, Lilly).

MANDOL®   ℞
[măn'dōl]
(cefamandole nafate)
For Injection
USP

DESCRIPTION

Mandol® (cefamandole nafate, Lilly) is a semisynthetic broad-spectrum cephalosporin antibiotic for parenteral administration. It is the sodium salt of 7-D-mandelamido-3-[[(1-methyl-1H-tetrazol-5-yl) -thio]methyl] -3-cephem-4-carboxylic acid, formate (ester). Mandol also contains 63 mg sodium carbonate/g of cefamandole activity. The total sodium content is approximately 77 mg (3.3 mEq sodium ion) per g of cefamandole activity. After addition of diluent, cefamandole nafate rapidly hydrolyzes to cefamandole, and both compounds have microbiologic activity in vivo. Solutions of Mandol range from light yellow to amber, depending on concentration and diluent used. The pH of freshly reconstituted solutions usually ranges from 6.0 to 8.5.

CLINICAL PHARMACOLOGY

After intramuscular administration of a 500-mg dose of cefamandole to normal volunteers, the mean peak serum concentration was 13 μg/mL. After a 1-g dose, the mean peak concentration was 25 μg/mL. These peaks occurred at 30 to 120 minutes. Following intravenous doses of 1, 2, and 3 g, serum concentrations were 139, 240, and 533 μg/mL, respectively, at 10 minutes. These concentrations declined to 0.8, 2.2, and 2.9 μg/mL at 4 hours. Intravenous administration of 4-g doses every 6 hours produced no evidence of accumulation in the serum. The half-life after an intravenous dose is 32 minutes; after intramuscular administration, the half-life is 60 minutes.
Sixty-five to 85% of cefamandole is excreted by the kidneys over an 8-hour period, resulting in high urinary concentrations. Following intramuscular doses of 500 mg and 1 g, urinary concentrations averaged 254 and 1,357 μg/mL, respectively. Intravenous doses of 1 and 2 g produced urinary levels averaging 750 and 1,380 μg/mL respectively. Probenecid slows tubular excretion and doubles the peak serum level and the duration of measurable serum concentrations.
The antibiotic reaches therapeutic levels in pleural and joint fluids and in bile and bone.
Microbiology—The bactericidal action of cefamandole results from inhibition of cell-wall synthesis. Cephalosporins have in vitro activity against a wide range of gram-positive and gram-negative organisms. Cefamandole is usually active

Continued on next page

* Identi-Code® symbol.

Lilly—Cont.

against the following organisms in vitro and in clinical infections:

Gram-positive

Staphylococcus aureus, including penicillinase- and non-penicillinase-producing strains

S epidermidis

β-hemolytic and other streptococci (Most strains of enterococci, eg, *Streptococcus faecalis,* are resistant.)

S pneumoniae (formerly *Diplococcus pneumoniae*)

Gram-negative

Escherichia coli

Klebsiella sp

Enterobacter sp (Initially susceptible organisms occasionally may become resistant during therapy.)

Haemophilus influenzae

Proteus mirabilis

P rettgeri

P morganii

P vulgaris (Some strains of *P vulgaris* have been shown by in vitro tests to be resistant to cefamandole and other cephalosporins.)

Anaerobic organisms

Gram-positive and gram-negative cocci (including *Peptococcus* and *Peptostreptococcus* sp)

Gram-positive bacilli (including *Clostridium* sp)

Gram-negative bacilli (including *Bacteroides* and *Fusobacterium* sp). Most strains of *Bacteroides fragilis* are resistant.

Pseudomonas, Acinetobacter calcoaceticus (formerly *Mima* and *Herellea* sp), and most *Serratia* strains are resistant to cephalosporins. Cefamandole is resistant to degradation by β-lactamases from certain members of the *Enterobacteriaceae.*

Susceptibility Tests —Quantitative methods that require measurement of zone diameters give the most precise estimates of antibiotic susceptibility. One such procedure[1] has been recommended for use with disks to test susceptibility to cefamandole. Interpretation involves correlation of the diameters obtained in the disk test with minimum inhibitory concentration (MIC) values for cefamandole.

Reports from the laboratory giving results of the standardized single-disk susceptibility test[1] using a 30-μg cefamandole disk should be interpreted according to the following criteria:

Susceptible organisms produce zones of 18 mm or greater, indicating that the tested organism is likely to respond to therapy.

Organisms of intermediate susceptibility produce zones of 15 to 17 mm, indicating that the tested organism would be susceptible if high dosage is used or if the infection is confined to tissues and fluids (eg, urine), in which high antibiotic levels are attained.

Resistant organisms produce zones of 14 mm or less, indicating that other therapy should be selected.

For gram-positive isolates, the test may be performed with either the cephalosporin-class disk (30 μg cephalothin) or the cefamandole disk (30 μg cefamandole), and a zone of 18 mm is indicative of a cefamandole-susceptible organism.

Gram-negative organisms should be tested with the cefamandole disk (using the above criteria), since cefamandole has been shown by in vitro tests to have activity against certain strains of *Enterobacteriaceae* found resistant when tested with the cephalosporin-class disk. Gram-negative organisms having zones of less than 18 mm around the cephalothin disk are not necessarily of intermediate susceptibility or resistant to cefamandole.

The cefamandole disk should not be used for testing susceptibility to other cephalosporins.

A bacterial isolate may be considered susceptible if the MIC value for cefamandole[2] is not more than 16 μg/mL. Organisms are considered resistant if the MIC is greater than 32 μg/mL.

INDICATIONS AND USAGE

Mandol® (cefamandole nafate, Lilly) is indicated for the treatment of serious infections caused by susceptible strains of the designated microorganisms in the diseases listed below:

Lower respiratory infections, including pneumonia caused by *S pneumoniae (D pneumoniae), H influenzae, Klebsiella* sp, *S aureus* (penicillinase- and non-penicillinase-producing), β-hemolytic streptococci, and *P. mirabilis*

Urinary tract infections caused by *E coli, Proteus* sp (both indole-negative and indole-positive), *Enterobacter* sp, *Klebsiella* sp, group D streptococci (Note: Most enterococci, eg, *S faecalis,* are resistant), and *S epidermidis*

Peritonitis caused by *E coli* and *Enterobacter* sp

Septicemia caused by *E coli, S aureus* (penicillinase- and non-penicillinase-producing), *S pneumoniae, S pyogenes* (group A β-hemolytic streptococci), *H influenzae,* and *Klebsiella* sp

Skin and skin-structure infections caused by *S aureus* (penicillinase- and non-penicillinase-producing), *S. pyog-*

enes (group A β-hemolytic streptococci), *H influenzae, E coli, Enterobacter* sp, and *P mirabilis*

Bone and joint infections caused by *S aureus* (penicillinase- and non-penicillinase-producing)

Clinical microbiologic studies in nongonococcal pelvic inflammatory disease in females, lower respiratory infections, and skin infections frequently reveal the growth of susceptible strains of both aerobic and anaerobic organisms. Mandol has been used successfully in these infections in which several organisms have been isolated. Most strains of *B fragilis* are resistant in vitro; however, infections caused by susceptible strains have been treated successfully.

Specimens for bacteriologic cultures should be obtained in order to isolate and identify causative organisms and to determine their susceptibilities to cefamandole. Therapy may be instituted before results of susceptibility studies are known; however, once these results become available, the antibiotic treatment should be adjusted accordingly.

In certain cases of confirmed or suspected gram-positive or gram-negative sepsis or in patients with other serious infections in which the causative organism has not been identified, Mandol may be used concomitantly with an aminoglycoside (*see* PRECAUTIONS). The recommended doses of both antibiotics may be given, depending on the severity of the infection and the patient's condition. The renal function of the patient should be carefully monitored, especially if higher dosages of the antibiotics are to be administered.

Antibiotic therapy of β-hemolytic streptococcal infections should continue for at least 10 days.

Preventive Therapy —The administration of Mandol preoperatively, intraoperatively, and postoperatively may reduce the incidence of certain postoperative infections in patients undergoing surgical procedures that are classified as contaminated or potentially contaminated (eg, gastrointestinal surgery, cesarean section, vaginal hysterectomy, or cholecystectomy in high-risk patients such as those with acute cholecystitis, obstructive jaundice, or common-bile-duct stones).

In major surgery in which the risk of postoperative infection is low but serious (cardiovascular surgery, neurosurgery, or prosthetic arthroplasty), Mandol may be effective in preventing such infections.

The perioperative use of Mandol should be discontinued after 24 hours; however, in prosthetic arthroplasty, it is recommended that administration be continued for 72 hours. If signs of infection occur, specimens for culture should be obtained for identification of the causative organism so that appropriate antibiotic therapy may be instituted.

CONTRAINDICATION

Mandol® (cefamandole nafate, Lilly) is contraindicated in patients with known allergy to the cephalosporin group of antibiotics.

WARNINGS

BEFORE THERAPY WITH MANDOL® (cefamandole nafate, Lilly) IS INSTITUTED, CAREFUL INQUIRY SHOULD BE MADE TO DETERMINE WHETHER THE PATIENT HAS HAD PREVIOUS HYPERSENSITIVITY REACTIONS TO CEPHALOSPORINS, PENICILLINS, OR OTHER DRUGS. THIS PRODUCT SHOULD BE GIVEN CAUTIOUSLY TO PENICILLIN-SENSITIVE PATIENTS. ANTIBIOTICS SHOULD BE ADMINISTERED WITH CAUTION TO ANY PATIENT WHO HAS DEMONSTRATED SOME FORM OF ALLERGY, PARTICULARLY TO DRUGS. SERIOUS ACUTE HYPERSENSITIVITY REACTIONS MAY REQUIRE EPINEPHRINE AND OTHER EMERGENCY MEASURES.

In newborn infants, accumulation of other cephalosporin-class antibiotics (with resulting prolongation of drug half-life) has been reported.

Pseudomembranous colitis has been reported with virtually all broad-spectrum antibiotics (including macrolides, semisynthetic penicillins, and cephalosporins); therefore, it is important to consider its diagnosis in patients who develop diarrhea in association with the use of antibiotics. Such colitis may range in severity from mild to life-threatening.

Treatment with broad-spectrum antibiotics alters the normal flora of the colon and may permit overgrowth of clostridia. Studies indicate that a toxin produced by *Clostridium difficile* is one primary cause of antibiotic-associated colitis.

Mild cases of pseudomembranous colitis usually respond to drug discontinuance alone. In moderate to severe cases, management should include sigmoidoscopy, appropriate bacteriologic studies, and fluid, electrolyte, and protein supplementation. When the colitis does not improve after the drug has been discontinued, or when it is severe, oral vancomycin is the drug of choice for antibiotic-associated pseudomembranous colitis produced by *C difficile.* Other causes of colitis should be ruled out.

PRECAUTIONS

General —Although Mandol® (cefamandole nafate, Lilly) rarely produces alteration in kidney function, evaluation of renal status is recommended, especially in seriously ill patients receiving maximum doses.

Prolonged use of Mandol may result in the overgrowth of nonsusceptible organisms. Careful observation of the patient

is essential. If superinfection occurs during therapy, appropriate measures should be taken.

Nephrotoxicity has been reported following concomitant administration of aminoglycoside antibiotics and cephalosporins.

A false-positive reaction for glucose in the urine may occur with Benedict's or Fehling's solution or with Clinitest® tablets but not with Tes-Tape® (Glucose Enzymatic Test Strip, USP, Lilly). There may be a false-positive test for proteinuria with acid and denaturization-precipitation tests.

As with other broad-spectrum antibiotics, hypoprothrombinemia, with or without bleeding, has been reported rarely, but it has been promptly reversed by administration of vitamin K. Such episodes usually have occurred in elderly, debilitated, or otherwise compromised patients with deficient stores of vitamin K. Treatment of such individuals with antibiotics possessing significant gram-negative and/or anaerobic activity is thought to alter the number and/or type of intestinal bacterial flora, with consequent reduction in synthesis of vitamin K. Prophylactic administration of vitamin K may be indicated in such patients, especially when intestinal sterilization and surgical procedures are performed.

In a few patients receiving Mandol, nausea, vomiting, and vasomotor instability with hypotension and peripheral vasodilatation occurred following the ingestion of ethanol. Cefamandole inhibits the enzyme acetaldehyde dehydrogenase in laboratory animals. This causes accumulation of acetaldehyde when ethanol is administered concomitantly. Broad-spectrum antibiotics should be prescribed with caution in individuals with a history of gastrointestinal disease, particularly colitis.

Carcinogenesis, Mutagenesis, Impairment of Fertility —Certain β-lactam antibiotics containing the N-methylthiotetrazole side chain have been reported to cause delayed maturity of the testicular germinal epithelium when given to neonatal rats during initial spermatogenic development (6 to 36 days of age). In animals that were treated from 6 to 36 days of age with 1,000 mg/kg/day of cefamandole (approximately 5 times the maximum clinical dose), the delayed maturity was pronounced and was associated with decreased testicular weights and a reduced number of germinal cells in the leading waves of spermatogenic development. The effect was slight in rats given 50 or 100 mg/kg/day. Some animals that were given 1,000 mg/kg/day during days 6 to 36 were infertile after becoming sexually mature. No adverse effects have been observed in rats exposed in utero, in neonatal rats (4 days of age or younger) treated prior to the initiation of spermatogenesis, or in older rats (more than 36 days of age) after exposure for up to 6 months. The significance to man of these findings in rats is unknown because of differences in the time of initiation of spermatogenesis, rate of spermatogenic development, and duration of puberty.

Usage in Pregnancy —*Pregnancy Category B* —Reproduction studies have been performed in rats given doses of 500 or 1,000 mg/kg/day and have revealed no evidence of impaired fertility or harm to the fetus due to Mandol. There are, however, no adequate and well-controlled studies in pregnant women. Because animal reproduction studies are not always predictive of human response, this drug should be used during pregnancy only if clearly needed.

Nursing Mothers —Caution should be exercised when Mandol is administered to a nursing woman.

Usage in Infancy —Mandol has been effectively used in this age group, but all laboratory parameters have not been extensively studied in infants between 1 and 6 months of age; safety of this product has not been established in prematures and infants under 1 month of age. Therefore, if Mandol is administered to infants, the physician should determine whether the potential benefits outweigh the possible risks involved.

ADVERSE REACTIONS

Gastrointestinal —Symptoms of pseudomembranous colitis may appear either during or after antibiotic treatment. Nausea and vomiting have been reported rarely. As with some penicillins and some other cephalosporins, transient hepatitis and cholestatic jaundice have been reported rarely.

Hypersensitivity —Anaphylaxis, maculopapular rash, urticaria, eosinophilia, and drug fever have been reported. These reactions are more likely to occur in patients with a history of allergy, particularly to penicillin.

Blood —Thrombocytopenia has been reported rarely. Neutropenia has been reported, especially in long courses of treatment. Some individuals have developed positive direct Coombs' tests during treatment with the cephalosporin antibiotics.

Liver —Transient rise in SGOT, SGPT, and alkaline phosphatase levels has been noted.

Kidney —Decreased creatinine clearance has been reported in patients with prior renal impairment. As with some other cephalosporins, transitory elevations of BUN have occasionally been observed with Mandol® (cefamandole nafate, Lilly); their frequency increases in patients over 50 years of age. In some of these cases, there was also a mild increase in serum creatinine.

Local Reactions—Pain on intramuscular injection is infrequent. Thrombophlebitis occurs rarely.

OVERDOSAGE

The administration of inappropriately large doses of parenteral cephalosporins may cause seizures, particularly in patients with renal impairment. Dosage reduction is necessary when renal function is impaired (*see* Dosage and Administration). If seizures occur, the drug should be promptly discontinued; anticonvulsant therapy may be administered if clinically indicated. Hemodialysis may be considered in cases of overwhelming overdosage.

DOSAGE AND ADMINISTRATION

Dosage—Adults: The usual dosage range for cefamandole is 500 mg to 1 g every 4 to 8 hours.

In infections of skin structures and in uncomplicated pneumonia, a dosage of 500 mg every 6 hours is adequate.

In uncomplicated urinary tract infections, a dosage of 500 mg every 8 hours is sufficient. In more serious urinary tract infections, a dosage of 1 g every 8 hours may be needed.

In severe infections, 1-g doses may be given at 4 to 6-hour intervals.

In life-threatening infections or infections due to less susceptible organisms, doses up to 2 g every 4 hours (ie, 12 g/day) may be needed.

Infants and Children: Administration of 50 to 100 mg/kg/day in equally divided doses every 4 to 8 hours has been effective for most infections susceptible to Mandol® (cefamandole nafate, Lilly). This may be increased to a total daily dose of 150 mg/kg (not to exceed the maximum adult dose) for severe infections. (*See* Warnings and Precautions for this age group.)

Note: As with antibiotic therapy in general, administration of Mandol should be continued for a minimum of 48 to 72 hours after the patient becomes asymptomatic or after evidence of bacterial eradication has been obtained; a minimum of 10 days of treatment is recommended in infections caused by group A β-hemolytic streptococci in order to guard against the risk of rheumatic fever or glomerulonephritis; frequent bacteriologic and clinical appraisal is necessary during therapy of chronic urinary tract infection and may be required for several months after therapy has been completed; persistent infections may require treatment for several weeks; and doses smaller than those indicated above should not be used.

For perioperative use of Mandol, the following dosages are recommended:

Adults—1 or 2 g intravenously or intramuscularly one-half to 1 hour prior to the surgical incision followed by 1 or 2 g every 6 hours for 24 to 48 hours.

Children (3 months of age and older)—50 to 100 mg/kg/day in equally divided doses by the routes and schedule designated above.

Note: In patients undergoing prosthetic arthroplasty, administration is recommended for as long as 72 hours.

In patients undergoing cesarean section, the initial dose may be administered just prior to surgery or immediately after the cord has been clamped.

Impaired Renal Function—When renal function is impaired, a reduced dosage must be employed and the serum levels closely monitored. After an initial dose of 1 to 2 g (depending on the severity of infection), a maintenance dosage schedule should be followed (see chart). Continued dosage should be determined by degree of renal impairment, severity of infection, and susceptibility of the causative organism. [See table above.]

When only serum creatinine is available, the following formula (based on sex, weight, and age of the patient) may be used to convert this value into creatinine clearance. The serum creatinine should represent a steady state of renal function.

Males: $\dfrac{\text{Weight (kg)} \times (140 - \text{age})}{72 \times \text{serum creatinine}}$

Females: $0.9 \times$ above value

Modes of Administration—Mandol® (cefamandole nafate, Lilly) may be given intravenously or by deep intramuscular injection into a large muscle mass (such as the gluteus or lateral part of the thigh) to minimize pain.

Intramuscular Administration—Each g of Mandol should be diluted with 3 mL of one of the following diluents: Sterile Water for Injection, Bacteriostatic Water for Injection, 0.9% Sodium Chloride Injection, or Bacteriostatic Sodium Chloride Injection. Shake well until dissolved.

Intravenous Administration—The intravenous route may be preferable for patients with bacterial septicemia, localized parenchymal abscesses (such as intra-abdominal abscess), peritonitis, or other severe or life-threatening infections when they may be poor risks because of lowered resistance. In those with normal renal function, the intravenous dosage for such infections is 3 to 12 g of Mandol daily. In conditions such as bacterial septicemia, 6 to 12 g/day may be given initially by the intravenous route for several days, and dosage

MANDOL® (CEFAMANDOLE NAFATE)—MAINTENANCE DOSAGE GUIDE FOR PATIENTS WITH RENAL IMPAIRMENT

Creatinine Clearance (mL/min/1.73 m²)	Renal Function	Life-Threatening Infections— Maximum Dosage	Less Severe Infections
>80	Normal	2 g q4h	1–2 g q6h
80–50	Mild Impairment	1.5 g q4h OR 2 g q6h	0.75–1.5 g q6h
50–25	Moderate Impairment	1.5 g q6h OR 2 g q8h	0.75–1.5 g q8h
25–10	Severe Impairment	1 g q6h OR 1.25 g q8h	0.5–1 g q8h
10–2	Marked Impairment	0.67 g q8h OR 1 g q12h	0.5–0.75 g q12h
<2	None	0.5 g q8h OR 0.75 g q12h	0.25–0.5 g q12h

may then be gradually reduced according to clinical response and laboratory findings.

If combination therapy with Mandol and an aminoglycoside is indicated, each of these antibiotics should be administered in different sites. *Do not mix an aminoglycoside with Mandol in the same intravenous fluid container.*

A SOLUTION OF 1 G OF MANDOL IN 22 ML OF STERILE WATER FOR INJECTION IS ISOTONIC.

The choice of saline, dextrose, or electrolyte solution and the volume to be employed are dictated by fluid and electrolyte management.

For direct intermittent intravenous administration, each g of cefamandole should be reconstituted with 10 mL of Sterile Water for Injection, 5% Dextrose Injection, or 0.9% Sodium Chloride Injection. Slowly inject the solution into the vein over a period of 3 to 5 minutes, or give it through the tubing of an administration set while the patient is also receiving one of the following intravenous fluids: 0.9% Sodium Chloride Injection; 5% Dextrose Injection; 10% Dextrose Injection; 5% Dextrose and 0.9% Sodium Chloride Injection; 5% Dextrose and 0.45% Sodium Chloride Injection; 5% Dextrose and 0.2% Sodium Chloride Injection; or Sodium Lactate Injection (M/6).

Intermittent intravenous infusion with a Y-type administration set or volume control set can also be accomplished while any of the above-mentioned intravenous fluids are being infused. However, during infusion of the solution containing Mandol® (cefamandole nafate, Lilly), it is desirable to discontinue the other solution. When this technique is employed, careful attention should be paid to the volume of the solution containing Mandol so that the calculated dose will be infused. When a Y-tube hookup is used, 100 mL of the appropriate diluent should be added to the 1 or 2-g piggyback (100-mL) vial. If Sterile Water for Injection is used as the diluent, reconstitute with approximately 20 mL/g to avoid a hypotonic solution.

For continuous intravenous infusion, each g of cefamandole should be diluted with 10 mL of Sterile Water for Injection. An appropriate quantity of the resulting solution may be added to an IV bottle containing one of the following fluids: 0.9% Sodium Chloride Injection; 5% Dextrose Injection; 10% Dextrose Injection; 5% Dextrose and 0.9% Sodium Chloride Injection; 5% Dextrose and 0.45% Sodium Chloride Injection; 5% Dextrose and 0.2% Sodium Chloride Injection; or Sodium Lactate Injection (M/6).

STABILITY

Reconstituted Mandol® (cefamandole nafate, Lilly) is stable for 24 hours at room temperature (25°C) and for 96 hours if stored under refrigeration (5°C). *During storage at room temperature, carbon dioxide develops inside the vial after reconstitution. This pressure may be dissipated prior to withdrawal of the vial contents, or it may be used to aid withdrawal if the vial is inverted over the syringe needle and the contents are allowed to flow into the syringe.*

Solutions of Mandol in Sterile Water for Injection, 5% Dextrose Injection, or 0.9% Sodium Chloride Injection that are frozen immediately after reconstitution in Faspak containers and the conventional vials in which the drugs are supplied are stable for 6 months when stored at −20°C. **If the product is warmed (to a maximum of 37°C), care should be taken to avoid heating it after the thawing is complete. Once thawed, the solution should not be refrozen.**

HOW SUPPLIED

(℞) *Vials* Mandol ® *(Cefamandole Nafate for Injection, USP)*, rubber-stoppered (Dry Powder): No. 7060, 500 mg*

(NDC 0002-7060-25), and *No.* 7061, 1 g* (NDC 0002-7061-25), 10-mL size, in Traypak™ (multivial carton, Lilly) of 25; *No.* 7068, 1 g,* 100-mL size (NDC 0002-7068-10), No. 7064, 2 g,* 20-mL size (NDC 0002-7064-10), and *No.* 7069, 2 g,* 100-mL size (NDC 0002-7069-10), in Traypak of 10; No. 7072, 10 g,* 100-mL size (NDC 0002-7072-16), in Traypak of 6.

(℞) *Faspak ® (flexible plastic bag, Lilly) Mandol ® (Cefamandole Nafate for Injection, USP):* No. 7208, 1 g* (NDC 0002-7208-74), and *No.* 7209, 2 g* (NDC 0002-7209-74), in Faspak of 96.

(℞) *ADD-Vantage® (vials and diluent containers, Abbott)* Vials: No. 7268, 1 g,* in Traypak of 25 (NDC 0002-7268-25); No. 7269, 2 g,* in Traypak of 10 (NDC 0002-7269-10).

The above ADD-Vantage® Vials are to be used only with Abbott Laboratories' Add-Vantage Diluent Containers. Instructions for use of the ADD-Vantage Vials are enclosed in the package.

*Equivalent to cefamandole activity.

[013087]

1. Bauer, A. W., Kirby, W. M. M., Sherris, J. C., and Turck, M.: Antibiotic Susceptibility Testing by a Standardized Single Disk Method, Am. J. Clin. Pathol., 45:493, 1966; Standardized Disc Susceptibility Test, Federal Register, 39:19182-19184, 1974. National Committee for Clinical Laboratory Standards. Approved Standard: ASM-2, Performance Standards for Antimicrobial Disc Susceptibility Tests, July, 1975.
2. Determined by the ICS agar-dilution method (Ericsson, H. M., and Sherris, J. C.: Acta Pathol. Microbiol. Scand. [B], Supplement No. 217, 1971) or any other method that has been shown to give equivalent results.

METHADONE HYDROCHLORIDE   Ⓒ

[mĕth 'ă-dōn hī-drō- klō-rĭd]

DISKETS® (dispersible tablets, Lilly)
Tablets, USP
(*See also* **Dolophine® Hydrochloride)**

CONDITIONS FOR DISTRIBUTION
AND USE OF METHADONE
PRODUCTS:

Code of Federal Regulations,
Title 21, Sec. 291.505

METHADONE PRODUCTS, WHEN USED FOR THE TREATMENT OF NARCOTIC ADDICTION IN DETOXIFICATION OR MAINTENANCE PROGRAMS, SHALL BE DISPENSED ONLY BY APPROVED HOSPITAL PHARMACIES, APPROVED COMMUNITY PHARMACIES, AND MAINTENANCE PROGRAMS APPROVED BY THE FOOD AND DRUG ADMINISTRATION AND THE DESIGNATED STATE AUTHORITY.

APPROVED MAINTENANCE PROGRAMS SHALL DISPENSE AND USE METHADONE IN ORAL FORM ONLY AND ACCORDING TO THE TREATMENT RE-

Continued on next page

* Identi-Code® symbol.

Lilly—Cont.

QUIREMENTS STIPULATED IN THE FEDERAL METHADONE REGULATIONS (21 CFR 291.505). FAILURE TO ABIDE BY THE REQUIREMENTS IN THESE REGULATIONS MAY RESULT IN CRIMINAL PROSECUTION, SEIZURE OF THE DRUG SUPPLY, REVOCATION OF THE PROGRAM APPROVAL, AND INJUNCTION PRECLUDING OPERATION OF THE PROGRAM.

DESCRIPTION

Methadone Hydrochloride, USP (4,4-diphenyl -6-dimethylamino - heptanone-3 hydrochloride), is a white crystalline material which is water soluble. However, the Disket preparation of methadone hydrochloride has been specially formulated with insoluble excipients to deter the use of this drug by injection.

Each Disket contains 40 mg methadone hydrochloride. Each tablet also contains cellulose, FD&C Yellow No. 6, flavors, magnesium stearate, potassium phosphate, silicon dioxide, starch, and stearic acid.

ACTIONS

Methadone hydrochloride is a synthetic narcotic analgesic with multiple actions quantitatively similar to those of morphine, the most prominent of which involve the central nervous system and organs composed of smooth muscle. The principal actions of therapeutic value are analgesia and sedation and detoxification or maintenance in narcotic addiction. The methadone abstinence syndrome, although qualitatively similar to that of morphine, differs in that the onset is slower, the course is more prolonged, and the symptoms are less severe.

When administered orally, methadone is approximately one-half as potent as when given parenterally. Oral administration results in a delay of the onset, a lowering of the peak, and an increase in the duration of analgesic effect.

INDICATIONS

1. Detoxification treatment of narcotic addiction (heroin or other morphine-like drugs).
2. Maintenance treatment of narcotic addiction (heroin or other morphine-like drugs), in conjunction with appropriate social and medical services.

NOTE

If methadone is administered for treatment of heroin dependence for more than 3 weeks, the procedure passes from treatment of the acute withdrawal syndrome (detoxification) to maintenance therapy. Maintenance treatment is permitted to be undertaken only by approved methadone programs. This does not preclude the maintenance treatment of an addict who is hospitalized for medical conditions other than addiction and who requires temporary maintenance during the critical period of his/her stay or whose enrollment has been verified in a program which has approval for maintenance treatment with methadone.

CONTRAINDICATION

Hypersensitivity to methadone.

WARNINGS

Diskets Methadone Hydrochloride are for oral administration only. This preparation contains insoluble excipients and therefore *must not* be injected. It is recommended that Diskets Methadone Hydrochloride, if dispensed, be packaged in child-resistant containers to prevent accidental ingestion.

Methadone hydrochloride, a narcotic, is a Schedule II controlled substance under the Federal Controlled Substances Act. Appropriate security measures should be taken to safeguard stocks of methadone against diversion.

DRUG DEPENDENCE—**METHADONE CAN PRODUCE DRUG DEPENDENCE OF THE MORPHINE TYPE AND, THEREFORE, HAS THE POTENTIAL FOR BEING ABUSED. PSYCHIC DEPENDENCE, PHYSICAL DEPENDENCE, AND TOLERANCE MAY DEVELOP ON REPEATED ADMINISTRATION OF METHADONE, AND IT SHOULD BE PRESCRIBED AND ADMINISTERED WITH THE SAME DEGREE OF CAUTION APPROPRIATE TO THE USE OF MORPHINE.**

Interaction with Other Central-Nervous-System Depressants —Methadone should be used with caution and in reduced dosage in patients who are concurrently receiving other narcotic analgesics, general anesthetics, phenothiazines, other tranquilizers, sedative-hypnotics, tricyclic antidepressants, and other CNS depressants (including alcohol). Respiratory depression, hypotension, and profound sedation or coma may result.

Anxiety—Since methadone, as used by tolerant subjects at a constant maintenance dosage, is not a tranquilizer, patients who are maintained on this drug will react to life problems and stresses with the same symptoms of anxiety as do other individuals. The physician should not confuse such symptoms with those of narcotic abstinence and should not attempt to treat anxiety by increasing the dosage of methadone. The action of methadone in maintenance treatment is limited to the control of narcotic symptoms and is ineffective for relief of general anxiety.

Head Injury and Increased Intracranial Pressure —The respiratory depressant effects of methadone and its capacity to elevate cerebrospinal-fluid pressure may be markedly exaggerated in the presence of increased intracranial pressure. Furthermore, narcotics produce side effects that may obscure the clinical course of patients with head injuries. In such patients, methadone must be used with caution and only if it is deemed essential.

Asthma and Other Respiratory Conditions —Methadone should be used with caution in patients having an acute asthmatic attack, in those with chronic obstructive pulmonary disease or cor pulmonale, and in individuals with a substantially decreased respiratory reserve, preexisting respiratory depression, hypoxia, or hypercapnia. In such patients, even usual therapeutic doses of narcotics may decrease respiratory drive while simultaneously increasing airway resistance to the point of apnea.

Hypotensive Effect —The administration of methadone may result in severe hypotension in an individual whose ability to maintain his blood pressure has already been compromised by a depleted blood volume or concurrent administration of such drugs as the phenothiazines or certain anesthetics.

Use in Ambulatory Patients —Methadone may impair the mental and/or physical abilities required for the performance of potentially hazardous tasks, such as driving a car or operating machinery. The patient should be cautioned accordingly.

Methadone, like other narcotics, may produce orthostatic hypotension in ambulatory patients.

Use in Pregnancy —Safe use in pregnancy has not been established in relation to possible adverse effects on fetal development. Therefore, methadone should not be used in pregnant women unless, in the judgment of the physician, the potential benefits outweigh the possible hazards.

PRECAUTIONS

Interaction With Pentazocine— **Patients who are addicted to heroin or who are on the methadone maintenance program may experience withdrawal symptoms when given pentazocine.**

Interaction With Rifampin —The concurrent administration of rifampin may possibly reduce the blood concentration of methadone to a degree sufficient to produce withdrawal symptoms. The mechanism by which rifampin may decrease blood concentrations of methadone is not fully understood, although enhanced microsomal drug-metabolized enzymes may influence drug disposition.

Acute Abdominal Conditions —The administration of methadone or other narcotics may obscure the diagnosis or clinical course in patients with acute abdominal conditions.

Interaction with Monoamine Oxidase (MAO) Inhibitors— Therapeutic doses of meperidine have precipitated severe reactions in patients concurrently receiving monoamine oxidase inhibitors or those who have received such agents within 14 days. Similar reactions thus far have not been reported with methadone; but if the use of methadone is necessary in such patients, a sensitivity test should be performed in which repeated small incremental doses are administered over the course of several hours while the patient's condition and vital signs are under careful observation.

Special-Risk Patients —Methadone should be given with caution and the initial dose should be reduced in certain patients, such as the elderly or debilitated and those with severe impairment of hepatic or renal function, hypothyroidism, Addison's disease, prostatic hypertrophy, or urethral stricture.

ADVERSE REACTIONS

Heroin Withdrawal —During the induction phase of methadone maintenance treatment, patients are being withdrawn from heroin and may therefore show typical withdrawal symptoms, which should be differentiated from methadone-induced side effects. They may exhibit some or all of the following symptoms associated with acute withdrawal from heroin or other opiates: lacrimation, rhinorrhea, sneezing, yawning, excessive perspiration, gooseflesh, fever, chilliness alternating with flushing, restlessness, irritability, "sleepy yen," weakness, anxiety, depression, dilated pupils, tremors, tachycardia, abdominal cramps, body aches, involuntary twitching and kicking movements, anorexia, nausea, vomiting, diarrhea, intestinal spasms, and weight loss.

Initial Administration —Initially, the dosage of methadone should be carefully titrated to the individual. Induction too rapid for the patient's sensitivity is more likely to produce the following effects.

THE MAJOR HAZARDS OF METHADONE, AS OF OTHER NARCOTIC ANALGESICS, ARE RESPIRATORY DEPRESSION AND, TO A LESSER DEGREE, CIRCULATORY DEPRESSION. RESPIRATORY ARREST, SHOCK, AND CARDIAC ARREST HAVE OCCURRED.

The most frequently observed adverse reactions include lightheadedness, dizziness, sedation, nausea, vomiting, and sweating. These effects seem to be more prominent in ambulatory patients and in those who are not suffering severe pain. In such individuals, lower doses are advisable. Some adverse reactions may be alleviated if the patient lies down.

Other adverse reactions include the following:

Central Nervous System —Euphoria, dysphoria, weakness, headache, insomnia, agitation, disorientation, and visual disturbances.

Gastrointestinal —Dry mouth, anorexia, constipation, and biliary tract spasm.

Cardiovascular —Flushing of the face, bradycardia, palpitation, faintness, and syncope.

Genitourinary —Urinary retention or hesitancy, antidiuretic effect, and reduced libido and/or potency.

Allergic —Pruritus, urticaria, other skin rashes, edema, and, rarely, hemorrhagic urticaria.

Hematologic —Reversible thrombocytopenia has been described in a narcotics addict with chronic hepatitis.

Maintenance on a Stabilized Dose —During prolonged administration of methadone, as in a methadone maintenance treatment program, there is a gradual, yet progressive, disappearance of side effects over a period of several weeks. However, constipation and sweating often persist.

OVERDOSAGE

Signs and Symptoms —Methadone is an opioid and produces effects similar to those of morphine. Symptoms of overdose begin within seconds after intravenous administration and within minutes of nasal, oral, or rectal administration. Prominent symptoms are miosis, respiratory depression, somnolence, coma, cool clammy skin, skeletal muscle flaccidity that may progress to hypotension, apnea, bradycardia, and death. Noncardiac pulmonary edema may occur and monitoring of heart filling pressures may be helpful.

Treatment —To obtain up-to-date information about the treatment of overdose, a good resource is your certified Regional Poison Control Center. Telephone numbers of certified poison control centers are listed in the *Physicians' Desk Reference (PDR)*. In managing overdosage, consider the possibility of multiple drug overdoses, interaction among drugs, and unusual drug kinetics in your patient.

Initial management of opioid overdose should include establishment of a secure airway and support of ventilation and perfusion. Naloxone may be given to antagonize opioid effects, but the airway must be secured as vomiting may ensue. **The duration of methadone effect is much longer (36 to 48 hours) than the duration of naloxone effect (1 to 3 hours), and repeated doses (or continuous intravenous infusion) of naloxone may be required.**

If the patient has chronically abused opioids, administration of naloxone may precipitate a withdrawal syndrome that may include yawning, tearing, restlessness, sweating, dilated pupils, piloerection, vomiting, diarrhea, and abdominal cramps. If these symptoms develop, they should abate quickly as the effects of naloxone dissipate.

If methadone has been taken by mouth, protect the patient's airway and support ventilation and perfusion. Meticulously monitor and maintain, within acceptable limits, the patient's vital signs, blood gases, serum electrolytes, etc. Absorption of drugs from the gastrointestinal tract may be decreased by giving activated charcoal, which, in many cases, is more effective than emesis or lavage; consider charcoal instead of or in addition to gastric emptying. Repeated doses of charcoal over time may hasten elimination of some drugs that have been absorbed. Safeguard the patient's airway when employing gastric emptying or charcoal.

Forced diuresis, peritoneal dialysis, hemodialysis, or charcoal hemoperfusion have not been established as beneficial for an overdose of methadone.

NOTE IN AN INDIVIDUAL PHYSICALLY DEPENDENT ON NARCOTICS, THE ADMINISTRATION OF THE USUAL DOSE OF A NARCOTIC ANTAGONIST WILL PRECIPITATE AN ACUTE WITHDRAWAL SYNDROME. THE SEVERITY OF THIS SYNDROME WILL DEPEND ON THE DEGREE OF PHYSICAL DEPENDENCE AND THE DOSE OF THE ANTAGONIST ADMINISTERED. THE USE OF A NARCOTIC ANTAGONIST IN SUCH A PERSON SHOULD BE AVOIDED IF POSSIBLE. IF IT MUST BE USED TO TREAT SERIOUS RESPIRATORY DEPRESSION IN THE PHYSICALLY DEPENDENT PATIENT, THE ANTAGONIST SHOULD BE ADMINISTERED WITH EXTREME CARE AND BY TITRATION WITH SMALLER THAN USUAL DOSES OF THE ANTAGONIST.

DOSAGE AND ADMINISTRATION

For Detoxification Treatment—THE DRUG SHALL BE ADMINISTERED DAILY UNDER CLOSE SUPERVISION AS FOLLOWS:

A detoxification treatment course shall not exceed 21 days and may not be repeated earlier than 4 weeks after completion of the preceding course.

In detoxification, the patient may receive methadone when there are significant symptoms of withdrawal. The dosage schedules indicated below are recommended but could be varied in accordance with clinical judgment. Initially, a single oral dose of 15 to 20 mg of methadone will often be sufficient to suppress withdrawal symptoms. Additional methadone may be provided if withdrawal symptoms are not suppressed or if symptoms reappear. When patients are physically dependent on high doses, it may be necessary to exceed these levels. Forty mg/day in single or divided doses will usually constitute an adequate stabilizing dosage level. Stabilization can be continued for 2 to 3 days, and then the amount of methadone normally will be gradually decreased. The rate at which methadone is decreased will be determined separately for each patient. The dose of methadone can be decreased on a daily basis or at 2-day intervals, but the amount of intake shall always be sufficient to keep withdrawal symptoms at a tolerable level. In hospitalized patients, a daily reduction of 20% of the total daily dose may be tolerated and may cause little discomfort. In ambulatory patients, a somewhat slower schedule may be needed. If methadone is administered for more than 3 weeks, the procedure is considered to have progressed from detoxification or treatment of the acute withdrawal syndrome to maintenance treatment, even though the goal and intent may be eventual total withdrawal.

For Maintenance Treatment—In maintenance treatment, the initial dosage of methadone should control the abstinence symptoms that follow withdrawal of narcotic drugs but should not be so great as to cause sedation, respiratory depression, or other effects of acute intoxication. It is important that the initial dosage be adjusted on an individual basis to the narcotic tolerance of the new patient. If such a patient has been a heavy user of heroin up to the day of admission, he may be given 20 mg 4 to 8 hours later or 40 mg in a single oral dose. If he enters treatment with little or no narcotic tolerance (eg, if he has recently been released from jail or other confinement), the initial dosage may be one-half these quantities. When there is any doubt, the smaller dose should be used initially. The patient should then be kept under observation, and, if symptoms of abstinence are distressing, additional 10-mg doses may be administered as needed. Subsequently, the dosage should be adjusted individually, as tolerated and required, up to a level of 120 mg daily. The patient will initially ingest the drug under observation daily, or at least 6 days a week, for the first 3 months. After demonstrating satisfactory adherence to the program regulations for at least 3 months, the patient may be permitted to reduce to 3 times weekly the occasions when he must ingest the drug under observation. He shall receive no more than a 2-day take-home supply. With continuing adherence to the program's requirements for at least 2 years, he may then be permitted twice-weekly visits to the program for drug ingestion under observation, with a 3-day take-home supply. A daily dose of 120 mg or more shall be justified in the medical record. Prior approval from state authority and the Food and Drug Administration is required for any dose above 120 mg administered at the clinic and for any dose above 100 mg to be taken at home. A regular review of dosage level should be made by the responsible physician, with careful consideration given to reduction of dosage as indicated on an individual basis. A new dosage level is only a test level until stability is achieved.

Special Considerations for a Pregnant Patient—Caution shall be taken in the maintenance treatment of pregnant patients. Dosage levels shall be kept as low as possible if continued methadone treatment is deemed necessary. It is the responsibility of the program sponsor to assure that each female patient be fully informed concerning the possible risks to a pregnant woman or her unborn child from the use of methadone.

Special Limitations —
Treatment of Patients under Age 18

1. The safety and effectiveness of methadone for use in the treatment of adolescents have not been proved by adequate clinical study. Special procedures are therefore necessary to assure that patients under age 16 will not be admitted to a program and that patients between 16 and 18 years of age will be admitted to maintenance treatment only under limited conditions.

2. Patients between 16 and 18 years of age who were enrolled and under treatment in approved programs on December 15, 1972, may continue in maintenance treatment. No new patients between 16 and 18 years of age may be admitted to a maintenance treatment program after March 15, 1973, unless a parent, legal guardian, or responsible adult designated by the state authority completes and signs Form FD 2635, "Consent for Methadone Treatment."

Methadone treatment of new patients between the ages of 16 and 18 years will be permitted after December 15, 1972, only with a documented history of 2 or more unsuccessful attempts at detoxification and a documented history of dependence on heroin or other morphine-like drugs beginning 2 years or more prior to application for treatment. No patient under age 16 may be continued or started on methadone treatment after December 15, 1972, but these patients may be detoxified and retained in the program in a drug-free state for follow-up and aftercare.

3. Patients under age 18 who are not placed on maintenance treatment may be detoxified. Detoxification may not exceed 3 weeks. A repeat episode of detoxification may not be initiated until 4 weeks after the completion of the previous detoxification.

HOW SUPPLIED

(Ⓒ) Diskets*:
　　40 mg (peach-colored, cross-scored) (No. 1)—(100s) NDC 0002-2153-02
Store at controlled room temperature, 59° to 86°C (15° to 30°F).

* Diskets® (dispersible tablets, Lilly)

[080288]

Shown in Product Identification Section, page 415

METUBINE® IODIDE　　　　℞
[mĕ-tū́ˈbēn ī-ō-dīd]
(metocurine iodide)
Injection, USP

THIS DRUG SHOULD BE ADMINISTERED ONLY BY ADEQUATELY TRAINED INDIVIDUALS WHO ARE FAMILIAR WITH ITS ACTIONS, CHARACTERISTICS, AND HAZARDS.

DESCRIPTION

Metubine® Iodide (Metocurine Iodide Injection, USP, Lilly) is a nondepolarizing muscle relaxant and is presented as a sterile isotonic solution for intravenous injection.

Each ml contains 2 mg metocurine iodide and sodium chloride, 0.9%, with 0.5% phenol as a preservative. Sodium carbonate and/or hydrochloric acid may have been added during manufacture to adjust the pH in the range of 4 to 4.3. The empirical formula is $C_{40}H_{48}I_2N_2O_6$, and the molecular weight is 906.64.

CLINICAL PHARMACOLOGY

Metubine® Iodide (Metocurine Iodide Injection, USP, Lilly) is a methyl analogue of tubocurarine which produces nondepolarizing (competitive) neuromuscular blockade at the myoneural junction. Recent animal studies suggest that Metubine Iodide does not produce the autonomic ganglionic blockade seen with other nondepolarizing muscle relaxants. Recent clinical findings suggest that Metubine Iodide reaches the neuromuscular junction more rapidly than does tubocurarine. After intravenous injection, there is rapid onset (1 to 4 minutes) of muscle relaxation with maximum twitch inhibition (96%) in 1.5 to 10 minutes. The maximum effect lasts 35 to 60 minutes. The time for recovery to 50% of control twitch response is in excess of 3 hours.

Following bolus injection of 0.05 mg/kg, the mean terminal half-life of Metubine Iodide was 3.6 hours (217 minutes). Approximately 50% of the dose was excreted as unchanged drug in the urine over 48 hours, and 2% was excreted unchanged in the bile. Approximately 35% is protein bound, mainly to the beta and gamma globulins.

The use of repeated doses may be accompanied by a cumulative effect. The duration of action and degree of muscle relaxation may be altered by dehydration, body temperature changes, hypocalcemia, excess magnesium, or acid-base imbalance. Concurrently administered general anesthetics, certain antibiotics, and neuromuscular disease may potentiate the neuromuscular blocking action of Metubine Iodide. Histamine release with Metubine Iodide occurs less frequently than with *d*-tubocurarine and is related to dosage and rapidity of administration. Effects on the cardiovascular system (eg, changes in pulse rate, hypotension) are less than those reported with equipotent doses of *d*-tubocurarine and gallamine.

Because the main excretory pathway for Metubine Iodide is through the kidneys, severe renal disease or conditions associated with poor renal perfusion (shock states) may result in prolonged neuromuscular blockade.

Following intravenous injection in the mother, placental transfer of Metubine Iodide occurs rapidly, and, after 6 minutes, the fetal plasma concentration is approximately one-tenth the maternal level.

INDICATIONS AND USAGE

Metubine® Iodide (Metocurine Iodide Injection, USP, Lilly) is indicated as an adjunct to anesthesia to induce skeletal-muscle relaxation. It may be employed to reduce the intensity of muscle contractions in pharmacologically or electrically induced convulsions. It may also be employed to facilitate the management of patients undergoing mechanical ventilation.

CONTRAINDICATIONS

Metubine® Iodide (Metocurine Iodide Injection, USP, Lilly) is contraindicated in those persons with known hypersensitivity to the drug or to its iodide content.

WARNINGS

METUBINE® IODIDE (METOCURINE IODIDE INJECTION, USP, LILLY) SHOULD BE ADMINISTERED IN CAREFULLY ADJUSTED DOSES BY OR UNDER THE SUPERVISION OF EXPERIENCED CLINICIANS WHO ARE FAMILIAR WITH THE COMPLICATIONS WHICH MAY OCCUR WITH THE USE OF THIS DRUG. Metubine Iodide should not be administered unless facilities for intubation, artificial ventilation, oxygen therapy, and reversal agents are immediately available. The clinician must be prepared to assist or control respiration.

Metubine Iodide should be used with extreme caution in patients with myasthenia gravis. In such patients, a peripheral nerve stimulator may be valuable in assessing the effects of administration.

PRECAUTIONS

*General —*Metubine® Iodide (Metocurine Iodide Injection, USP, Lilly) should be used with caution in patients with poor renal perfusion or severe renal disease (*see* Clinical Pharmacology).

Rapid administration of large doses of Metubine Iodide may produce changes in blood pressure or heart rate or signs of histamine release.

Metubine Iodide has no effect on consciousness, pain threshold, or cerebration; therefore, it should be used with adequate anesthesia.

*Drug Interactions —*Synergistic or antagonistic effects may result when depolarizing and nondepolarizing muscle relaxants are administered simultaneously or sequentially.

Parenteral administration of high doses of certain antibiotics may intensify or resemble the neuroblocking action of muscle relaxants. These include neomycin, streptomycin, bacitracin, kanamycin, gentamicin, dihydrostreptomycin, polymyxin B, colistin, sodium colistimethate, and tetracyclines. If muscle relaxants and antibiotics must be administered simultaneously, the patient should be observed closely for any unexpected prolongation of respiratory depression. Certain general anesthetics have a synergistic action with neuromuscular blocking agents. Diethyl ether, halothane, and isoflurane potentiate the neuromuscular blocking action of other nondepolarizing agents and may be presumed to do so with Metubine Iodide.

Administration of quinidine shortly after recovery may produce recurrent paralysis.

The effect of diazepam on neuromuscular blockade by Metubine Iodide is not clear. Until more information is available, patients should be carefully monitored for unexpected drug response and prolongation of action.

The use of magnesium sulfate in preeclamptic patients potentiates the effects of both depolarizing and nondepolarizing muscle relaxants.

*Usage in Pregnancy —Pregnancy Category C —*Intrauterine growth retardation and limb deformities resembling clubfoot were produced by *d*-tubocurarine chloride and succinylcholine chloride when administered to the rat fetus between the 16th and 19th days of gestation or when injected in chick embryos from the 5th to the 15th day of incubation. When *d*-tubocurarine was injected intramuscularly into the interscapular region of the fetuses on the 16th to the 19th day of gestation, the incidence of growth retardation and limb deformity ranged from 21 to 23% and 7 to 8% respectively. There are no adequate and well-controlled studies of Metubine Iodide in pregnant women. Metubine Iodide should be used during pregnancy only if the potential benefit justifies the risk to the fetus.

*Labor and Delivery —*It is not known whether the use of muscle relaxants during labor or delivery has immediate or delayed adverse effects on the fetus, prolongs the duration of labor, or increases the likelihood that forceps delivery, obstetric intervention, or resuscitation of the newborn will be necessary.

*Nursing Mothers —*It is not known whether Metubine Iodide is excreted in human milk. Because many drugs are excreted in human milk, caution should be exercised when Metubine Iodide is administered to a nursing woman.

*Usage in Children —*A clinical study has shown that Metubine Iodide is twice as potent as *d*-tubocurarine in children, but the rate of recovery is the same. There may be a slight increase in heart rate, but no change occurs in blood pressure or ECG. Doses calculated on the basis of body weight or body surface area may be applicable when the advantages of nondepolarizing neuromuscular blockade are desired.

Continued on next page

• **Identi-Code® symbol.**

Lilly—Cont.

ADVERSE REACTIONS

The most frequently noted adverse reaction is prolongation of the drug's pharmacologic action. Neuromuscular effects may range from skeletal-muscle weakness to a profound relaxation that produces respiratory insufficiency or apnea. Possible adverse reactions include allergic or hypersensitivity reactions to the drug or its iodide content and histamine release when large doses are administered rapidly. Signs of histamine release include erythema, edema, flushing, tachycardia, arterial hypotension, bronchospasm, and circulatory collapse.

Prolonged apnea and respiratory depression have occurred following the use of muscle relaxants. Many physiologic factors, drug interactions, and individual sensitivities may contribute to the development of respiratory paralysis (*see* Clinical Pharmacology *and* Precautions).

OVERDOSAGE

An overdose of Metubine® Iodide (Metocurine Iodide Injection, USP, Lilly) may result in prolonged apnea, cardiovascular collapse, and sudden release of histamine.

Massive doses of metocurarine are not reversible by the antagonists edrophonium or neostigmine and atropine.

Overdosage may be avoided by the careful monitoring of response by means of a peripheral nerve stimulator.

The primary treatment for residual neuromuscular blockade with respiratory paralysis or inadequate ventilation is maintenance of the patient's airway and manual or mechanical ventilation.

Accompanying derangements of blood pressure, electrolyte imbalance, or circulating blood volume should be determined and corrected by appropriate fluid and electrolyte therapy.

Residual neuromuscular blockade following surgery may be reversed by the use of anticholinesterase inhibitors such as neostigmine or pyridostigmine bromide and atropine. Prescribing information should be consulted for the appropriate drug selection based on dosage and desired duration of action.

DOSAGE AND ADMINISTRATION

Metubine® Iodide (Metocurine Iodide Injection, USP, Lilly) should be administered intravenously as a sustained injection over a period of 30 to 60 seconds. INTRAMUSCULAR ADMINISTRATION OF METUBINE IODIDE IS NOT RECOMMENDED. Care must be taken to avoid overdosage. The use of a peripheral nerve stimulator to monitor response will minimize the risk of overdosage. The type of anesthetic used and nature of the surgical procedure will influence the amount of Metubine Iodide required. Doses of 0.2 to 0.4 mg/kg have been found satisfactory for endotracheal intubation. Relaxation following the initial dose may be expected to be effective for periods of 25 to 90 minutes, with an average of approximately 60 minutes. Supplemental administration may be made as indicated to provide needed surgical relaxation. Supplemental doses average 0.5 to 1 mg. The use of strong anesthetics that potentiate the effect of neuromuscular blocking drugs such as halothane, diethyl ether, isoflurane, or enflurane reduces the requirement for Metubine Iodide. Incremental doses should be reduced by approximately one-third to one-half.

Recommended Doses for Use During Electroshock Therapy — Doses required for satisfactory relaxation range from 1.75 to 5.5 mg. When the patient is treated for the first time, the drug is administered slowly by the intravenous route as a sustained injection until a head-drop response ensues. After dosage has been established, subsequent injections are completed in 15 to 50 seconds. The average dose ranges from 2 to 3 mg.

Drug Incompatibilities — Metubine Iodide is unstable in alkaline solutions. When it is combined with barbiturate solutions, precipitation may occur. Solutions of barbiturates, meperidine, and morphine sulfate should not be administered from the same syringe.

Parenteral drug products should be inspected visually for particulate matter and discoloration prior to administration, whenever solution and container permit.

HOW SUPPLIED

(℞) Multiple-Dose Vials:

2 mg/mL, 20 mL (No. 586) (1s), NDC 0002-1421-01

Store at controlled room temperature, 59° to 86°F (15° to 30°C).

Metubine Iodide is a clear, colorless solution.

[022387]

NEBCIN®   ℞
[nĕb'sĭn]
(tobramycin sulfate)
Injection, USP

<table>
<tr><td>

WARNINGS

Patients treated with Nebcin® (Tobramycin Sulfate Injection, USP, Lilly) and other aminoglycosides should be under close clinical observation, because these drugs have an inherent potential for causing ototoxicity and nephrotoxicity.

Neurotoxicity, manifested as both auditory and vestibular ototoxicity, can occur. The auditory changes are irreversible, are usually bilateral, and may be partial or total. Eighth-nerve impairment and nephrotoxicity may develop, primarily in patients having preexisting renal damage and in those with normal renal function to whom aminoglycosides are administered for longer periods or in higher doses than those recommended. Other manifestations of neurotoxicity may include numbness, skin tingling, muscle twitching, and convulsions. The risk of aminoglycoside-induced hearing loss increases with the degree of exposure to either high peak or high trough serum concentrations. Patients who develop cochlear damage may not have symptoms during therapy to warn them of eighth-nerve toxicity, and partial or total irreversible bilateral deafness may continue to develop after the drug has been discontinued. Rarely, nephrotoxicity may not become manifest until the first few days after cessation of therapy. Aminoglycoside-induced nephrotoxicity usually is reversible.

Renal and eighth-nerve function should be closely monitored in patients with known or suspected renal impairment and also in those whose renal function is initially normal but who develop signs of renal dysfunction during therapy. Peak and trough serum concentrations of aminoglycosides should be monitored periodically during therapy to assure adequate levels and to avoid potentially toxic levels. Prolonged serum concentrations above 12 mg/L should be avoided. Rising trough levels (above 2 mg/L) may indicate tissue accumulation. Such accumulation, excessive peak concentrations, advanced age, and cumulative dose may contribute to ototoxicity and nephrotoxicity (*see* Precautions). Urine should be examined for decreased specific gravity and increased excretion of protein, cells, and casts. Blood urea nitrogen, serum creatinine, and creatinine clearance should be measured periodically. When feasible, it is recommended that serial audiograms be obtained in patients old enough to be tested, particularly high-risk patients. Evidence of impairment of renal, vestibular, or auditory function requires discontinuation of the drug or dosage adjustment.

Nebcin should be used with caution in premature and neonatal infants because of their renal immaturity and the resulting prolongation of serum half-life of the drug. Concurrent and sequential use of other neurotoxic and/or nephrotoxic antibiotics, particularly other aminoglycosides (eg, amikacin, streptomycin, neomycin, kanamycin, gentamicin, and paromomycin), cephaloridine, viomycin, polymyxin B, colistin, cisplatin, and vancomycin, should be avoided. Other factors that may increase patient risk are advanced age and dehydration. Aminoglycosides should not be given concurrently with potent diuretics, such as ethacrynic acid and furosemide. Some diuretics themselves cause ototoxicity, and intravenously administered diuretics enhance aminoglycoside toxicity by altering antibiotic concentrations in serum and tissue.

Aminoglycosides can cause fetal harm when administered to a pregnant woman (*see* Precautions).

</td></tr>
</table>

DESCRIPTION

Tobramycin sulfate, a water-soluble antibiotic of the aminoglycoside group, is derived from the actinomycete *Streptomyces tenebrarius.* Nebcin® (Tobramycin Sulfate, USP, Lilly), Injection, is a clear and colorless sterile aqueous solution for parenteral administration.

Each mL also contains phenol as a preservative (5 mg, multiple-dose vials; 1.25 mg, ADD-Vantage® vials), sodium bisulfite (3.2 mg, multiple-dose vials; 1.6 mg, ADD-Vantage vials), 0.1 mg edetate disodium, and water for injection, qs. Sulfuric acid and/or sodium hydroxide may have been added to adjust the pH. Tobramycin is 4-0-[2,6-diamino-2, 3, 6-trideoxy-α-D-glucopyranosyl]-6-   0- [3-amino -3-   deoxy-α-D-glucopyranosyl] -2- deoxystreptamine.

CLINICAL PHARMACOLOGY

Tobramycin is rapidly absorbed following intramuscular administration. Peak serum concentrations of tobramycin occur between 30 and 90 minutes after intramuscular administration. Following an intramuscular dose of 1 mg/kg of

---

body weight, maximum serum concentrations reach about 4 mg/L, and measurable levels persist for as long as 8 hours. Therapeutic serum levels are generally considered to range from 4 to 6 mg/L. When Nebcin® (Tobramycin Sulfate, USP, Lilly) is administered by intravenous infusion over a 1-hour period, the serum concentrations are similar to those obtained by intramuscular administration. Nebcin is poorly absorbed from the gastrointestinal tract.

In patients with normal renal function, except neonates, Nebcin administered every 8 hours does not accumulate in the serum. However, in those with reduced renal function and in neonates, the serum concentration of the antibiotic is usually higher and can be measured for longer periods of time than in normal adults. Dosage for such patients must, therefore, be adjusted accordingly (*see* Dosage and Administration).

Following parenteral administration, little, if any, metabolic transformation occurs, and tobramycin is eliminated almost exclusively by glomerular filtration. Renal clearance is similar to that of endogenous creatinine. Ultrafiltration studies demonstrate that practically no serum protein binding occurs. In patients with normal renal function, up to 84% of the dose is recoverable from the urine in 8 hours and up to 93% in 24 hours.

Peak urine concentrations ranging from 75 to 100 mg/L have been observed following the intramuscular injection of a single dose of 1 mg/kg. After several days of treatment, the amount of tobramycin excreted in the urine approaches the daily dose administered. When renal function is impaired, excretion of Nebcin is slowed, and accumulation of the drug may cause toxic blood levels.

The serum half-life in normal individuals is 2 hours. An inverse relationship exists between serum half-life and creatinine clearance, and the dosage schedule should be adjusted according to the degree of renal impairment (*see* Dosage and Administration). In patients undergoing dialysis, 25% to 70% of the administered dose may be removed, depending on the duration and type of dialysis.

Tobramycin can be detected in tissues and body fluids after parenteral administration. Concentrations in bile and stools ordinarily have been low, which suggests minimum biliary excretion. Tobramycin has appeared in low concentration in the cerebrospinal fluid following parenteral administration, and concentrations are dependent on dose, rate of penetration, and degree of meningeal inflammation. It has also been found in sputum, peritoneal fluid, synovial fluid, and abscess fluids, and it crosses the placental membranes. Concentrations in the renal cortex are several times higher than the usual serum levels.

Probenecid does not affect the renal tubular transport of tobramycin.

Microbiology —In vitro tests demonstrate that tobramycin is bactericidal and that it acts by inhibiting the synthesis of protein in bacterial cells.

Tobramycin is usually active against most strains of the following organisms in vitro and in clinical infections:

> *Pseudomonas aeruginosa*
> *Proteus* species (indole-positive and indole-negative), including *Proteus mirabilis, Morganella morganii, Providencia rettgeri* (formerly *Proteus rettgeri*), and *Proteus vulgaris*
> *Escherichia coli*
> *Klebsiella-Enterobacter-Serratia* group
> *Citrobacter* sp
> *Providencia* sp
> Staphylococci, including *Staphylococcus aureus* (coagulase-positive and coagulase-negative)

Aminoglycosides have a low order of activity against most gram-positive organisms, including *Streptococcus pyogenes, Streptococcus pneumoniae,* and enterococci.

Although most strains of group D streptococci demonstrate in vitro resistance, some strains in this group are susceptible. In vitro studies have shown that an aminoglycoside combined with an antibiotic that interferes with cell-wall synthesis affects some group D streptococcal strains synergistically. The combination of penicillin G and tobramycin results in a synergistic bactericidal effect in vitro against certain strains of *Enterococcus faecalis* (formerly *Streptococcus faecalis*). However, this combination is not synergistic against other closely related organisms, eg, *Enterococcus faecium* (formerly *Streptococcus faecium*). Speciation of group D streptococci alone cannot be used to predict susceptibility. Susceptibility testing and tests for antibiotic synergism are emphasized.

Cross-resistance between aminoglycosides occurs and depends largely on inactivation by bacterial enzymes.

Susceptibility Tests —If the FDA Standardized Disc Test method (formerly the Bauer-Kirby-Sherris-Turck method) of disk susceptibility testing is used, a disk containing 10 µg tobramycin should give a zone of at least 15 mm when tested against a tobramycin-susceptible bacterial strain, a zone of 13 to 14 mm against strains of intermediate susceptibility, and a zone of 12 mm or less against resistant organisms. The minimum inhibitory concentration correlates are ≤4 mg/L for susceptibility and ≥ 8 mg/L for resistance.

INDICATIONS AND USAGE

Nebcin® (Tobramycin Sulfate, USP, Lilly) is indicated for the treatment of serious bacterial infections caused by susceptible strains of the designated microorganisms in the diseases listed below:

Septicemia in the neonate, child, and adult caused by *P aeruginosa*, *E coli*, and *Klebsiella* sp

Lower respiratory tract infections caused by *P aeruginosa*, *Klebsiella* sp, *Enterobacter* sp, *Serratia* sp, *E coli*, and *S aureus* (penicillinase- and non-penicillinase-producing strains)

Serious central-nervous-system infections (meningitis) caused by susceptible organisms

Intra-abdominal infections, including peritonitis, caused by *E coli*, *Klebsiella* sp, and *Enterobacter* sp

Skin, bone, and skin-structure infections caused by *P aeruginosa*, *Proteus* sp, *E coli*, *Klebsiella* sp, *Enterobacter* sp, and *S aureus*

Complicated and recurrent urinary tract infections caused by *P aeruginosa*, *Proteus* sp (indole-positive and indole-negative), *E coli*, *Klebsiella* sp, *Enterobacter* sp, *Serratia* sp, *S aureus*, *Providencia* sp, and *Citrobacter* sp

Aminoglycosides, including Nebcin, are not indicated in uncomplicated initial episodes of urinary tract infections unless the causative organisms are not susceptible to antibiotics having less potential toxicity. Nebcin may be considered in serious staphylococcal infections when penicillin or other potentially less toxic drugs are contraindicated and when bacterial susceptibility testing and clinical judgment indicate its use.

Bacterial cultures should be obtained prior to and during treatment to isolate and identify etiologic organisms and to test their susceptibility to tobramycin. If susceptibility tests show that the causative organisms are resistant to tobramycin, other appropriate therapy should be instituted. In patients in whom a serious life-threatening gram-negative infection is suspected, including those in whom concurrent therapy with a penicillin or cephalosporin and an aminoglycoside may be indicated, treatment with Nebcin may be initiated before the results of susceptibility studies are obtained. The decision to continue therapy with Nebcin should be based on the results of susceptibility studies, the severity of the infection, and the important additional concepts discussed in the WARNINGS box above.

CONTRAINDICATIONS

A hypersensitivity to any aminoglycoside is a contraindication to the use of tobramycin. A history of hypersensitivity or serious toxic reactions to aminoglycosides may also contraindicate the use of any other aminoglycoside because of the known cross-sensitivity of patients to drugs in this class.

WARNINGS

See WARNINGS box above.

Nebcin® (Tobramycin Sulfate, USP, Lilly) contains sodium bissulfite, a sulfite that may cause allergic-type reactions, including anaphylactic symptoms and life-threatening or less severe asthmatic episodes, in certain susceptible people. The overall prevalence of sulfite sensitivity in the general population is unknown and probably low. Sulfite sensitivity is seen more frequently in asthmatic than in nonasthmatic people.

PRECAUTIONS

Serum and urine specimens for examination should be collected during therapy, as recommended in the WARNINGS box. Serum calcium, magnesium, and sodium should be monitored.

Peak and trough serum levels should be measured periodically during therapy. Prolonged concentrations above 12 mg/L should be avoided. Rising trough levels (above 2 mg/L) may indicate tissue accumulation. Such accumulation, advanced age, and cumulative dosage may contribute to ototoxicity and nephrotoxicity. It is particularly important to monitor serum levels closely in patients with known renal impairment.

A useful guideline would be to perform serum-level assays after 2 or 3 doses, so that the dosage could be adjusted if necessary, and also at 3 to 4-day intervals during therapy. In the event of changing renal function, more frequent serum levels should be obtained and the dosage or dosage interval adjusted according to the guidelines provided in the Dosage and Administration section.

In order to measure the peak level, a serum sample should be drawn about 30 minutes following intravenous infusion or 1 hour after an intramuscular injection. Trough levels are measured by obtaining serum samples at 8 hours or just prior to the next dose of Nebcin®(Tobramycin Sulfate, USP, Lilly). These suggested time intervals are intended only as guidelines and may vary according to institutional practices. It is important, however, that there be consistency within the individual patient program unless computerized pharmacokinetic dosing programs are available in the institution. These serum-level assays may be especially useful for monitoring the treatment of severely ill patients with changing renal function or of those infected with less sensitive organisms or those receiving maximum dosage.

Neuromuscular blockade and respiratory paralysis have been reported in cats receiving very high doses of tobramycin (40 mg/kg). The possibility that prolonged or secondary apnea may occur should be considered if tobramycin is administered to anesthetized patients who are also receiving neuromuscular blocking agents, such as succinylcholine, tubocurarine, or decamethonium, or to patients receiving massive transfusions of citrated blood. If neuromuscular blockade occurs, it may be reversed by the administration of calcium salts.

Cross-allergenicity among aminoglycosides has been demonstrated.

In patients with extensive burns, altered pharmacokinetics may result in reduced serum concentrations of aminoglycosides. In such patients treated with Nebcin, measurement of serum concentration is especially recommended as a basis for determination of appropriate dosage.

Elderly patients may have reduced renal function that may not be evident in the results of routine screening tests, such an BUN or serum creatinine. A creatinine clearance determination may be more useful. Monitoring of renal function during treatment with aminoglycosides is particularly important in such patients.

An increased incidence of nephrotoxicity has been reported following concomitant administration of aminoglycoside antibiotics and cephalosporins.

Aminoglycosides should be used with caution in patients with muscular disorders, such as myasthenia gravis or parkinsonism, since these drugs may aggravate muscle weakness because of their potential curare-like effect on neuromuscular function.

Aminoglycosides may be absorbed in significant quantities from body surfaces after local irrigation or application and may cause neurotoxicity and nephrotoxicity.

See WARNINGS box regarding concurrent use of potent diuretics and concurrent and sequential use of other neurotoxic or nephrotoxic drugs.

The inactivation of tobramycin and other aminoglycosides by β-lactam-type antibiotics (penicillins or cephalosporins) has been demonstrated in vitro and in patients with severe renal impairment. Such inactivation has not been found in patients with normal renal function who have been given the drugs by separate routes of administration.

Therapy with tobramycin may result in overgrowth of nonsusceptible organisms. If overgrowth of nonsusceptible organisms occurs, appropriate therapy should be initiated.

Pregnancy Category D—Aminoglycosides can cause fetal harm when administered to a pregnant woman. Aminoglycoside antibiotics cross the placenta, and there have been several reports of total irreversible bilateral congenital deafness in children whose mothers received streptomycin during pregnancy. Serious side effects to mother, fetus, or newborn have not been reported in the treatment of pregnant women with other aminoglycosides. If tobramycin is used during pregnancy or if the patient becomes pregnant while taking tobramycin, she should be apprised of the potential hazard to the fetus.

Usage in Children—See Indications and Usage *and* Dosage and Administration.

ADVERSE REACTIONS

Neurotoxicity—Adverse effects on both the vestibular and auditory branches of the eighth nerve have been noted, especially in patients receiving high doses or prolonged therapy, in those given previous courses of therapy with an ototoxin, and in cases of dehydration. Symptoms include dizziness, vertigo, tinnitus, roaring in the ears, and hearing loss. Hearing loss is usually irreversible and is manifested initially by diminution of high-tone acuity. Tobramycin and gentamicin sulfates closely parallel each other in regard to ototoxic potential.

Nephrotoxicity—Renal function changes, as shown by rising BUN, NPN, and serum creatinine and by oliguria, cylindruria, and increased proteinuria, have been reported, especially in patients with a history of renal impairment who are treated for longer periods or with higher doses than those recommended. Adverse renal effects can occur in patients with initially normal renal function.

Clinical studies and studies in experimental animals have been conducted to compare the nephrotoxic potential of tobramycin and gentamicin. In some of the clinical studies and in the animal studies, tobramycin caused nephrotoxicity significantly less frequently than gentamicin. In some other clinical studies, no significant difference in the incidence of nephrotoxicity between tobramycin and gentamicin was found.

Other reported adverse reactions possibly related to Nebcin® (Tobramycin Sulfate, USP, Lilly) include anemia, granulocytopenia, and thrombocytopenia; and fever, rash, itching, urticaria, nausea, vomiting, diarrhea, headache, lethargy, pain at the injection site, mental confusion, and disorientation. Laboratory abnormalities possibly related to Nebcin include increased serum transaminases (SGOT, SGPT); increased serum LDH and bilirubin; decreased serum calcium, magnesium, sodium, and potassium; and leukopenia, leukocytosis, and eosinophilia.

OVERDOSAGE

Signs and Symptoms—The severity of the signs and symptoms following a tobramycin overdose are dependent on the dose administered, the patient's renal function, state of hydration, and age and whether or not other medications with similar toxicities are being administered concurrently. Toxicity may occur in adults given more than 5 mg/kg/day, children given more than 7.5 mg/kg/day, or patients with reduced renal function whose dose has not been appropriately adjusted.

Nephrotoxicity following the parenteral administration of an aminoglycoside is most closely related to the area under the curve of the serum concentration versus time graph. Nephrotoxicity is more likely if nadir blood concentrations fail to fall below 2 mg/L and is also proportional to the average blood concentration. Patients who are elderly, who have abnormal renal function, are receiving other nephrotoxic drugs, or are volume depleted are at greater risk for developing acute tubular necrosis. Auditory and vestibular toxicity has been associated with aminoglycoside overdose in patients with abnormal renal function, dehydrated patients, or in patients receiving medications with additive auditory toxicities. These patients often experience dizziness, tinnitus, vertigo, and a loss of high-tone acuity.

Neuromuscular blockade or respiratory paralysis may occur following rapid intravenous administration of many aminoglycosides. This has also been reported in cats given extremely large doses of tobramycin (40 mg/kg). Neuromuscular blockade and respiratory failure may occur more commonly in patients with myasthenia gravis or Parkinson's disease. Prolonged respiratory paralysis may occur more commonly in patients with myasthenia gravis or Parkinson's disease. Prolonged respiratory paralysis may also occur in patients receiving decamethonium, tubocurarine, or succinylcholine.

If tobramycin were ingested, toxicity would be unlikely because aminoglycosides are poorly absorbed (less than 1%) from an intact gastrointestinal tract.

Treatment—To obtain up-to-date information about the treatment of overdose, a good resource is your certified Regional Poison Control Center. Telephone numbers of certified poison control centers are listed in the *Physicians' Desk Reference (PDR)*. In managing overdosage, consider the possibility of multiple drug overdoses, interaction among drugs, and unusual drug kinetics in your patient.

The initial intervention in a tobramycin overdose is to establish an airway and ensure oxygenation and ventilation. Resuscitative measures should be initiated promptly if respiratory paralysis occurs.

Patients that have received an overdose of tobramycin and have normal renal function should be carefully hydrated to maintain a urine output of 3 to 5 mL/kg/hr. Fluid balance, creatinine clearance, and tobramycin plasma levels should be carefully monitored until the serum tobramycin level falls below 2 mg/L.

Patients in whom the elimination half-life is greater than 2 hours or whose renal function is abnormal may require more aggressive therapy. In such patients, hemodialysis may be beneficial.

DOSAGE AND ADMINISTRATION

Nebcin® (Tobramycin Sulfate, USP, Lilly) may be given intramuscularly or intravenously. ADD-Vantage vials are not for intramuscular administration. Recommended dosages are the same for both routes. The patient's pretreatment body weight should be obtained for calculation of correct dosage. It is desirable to measure both peak and trough serum concentrations (see WARNINGS box *and* Precautions).

Administration for Patients With Normal Renal Function—*Adults With Serious Infections:* 3 mg/kg/day in 3 equal doses every 8 hours (see Table 1).

Adults with Life-Threatening Infections: Up to 5 mg/kg/day may be administered in 3 or 4 equal doses (see Table 1). The dosage should be reduced to 3 mg/kg/day as soon as clinically indicated. To prevent increased toxicity due to excessive blood levels, dosage should not exceed 5 mg/kg/day unless serum levels are monitored (see Warnings box *and* Precautions).

[See table on next page.]

Children: 6 to 7.5 mg/kg/day in 3 or 4 equally divided doses (2 to 2.5 mg/kg every 8 hours or 1.5 to 1.89 mg/kg every 6 hours).

Premature or Full-Term Neonates 1 Week of Age or Less: Up to 4 mg/kg/day may be administered in 2 equal doses every 12 hours.

It is desirable to limit treatment to a short term. The usual duration of treatment is 7 to 10 days. A longer course of therapy may be necessary in difficult and complicated infections. In such cases, monitoring of renal, auditory, and vestibular

Continued on next page

* Identi-Code® symbol.

Lilly—Cont.

functions is advised, because neurotoxicity is more likely to occur when treatment is extended longer than 10 days.

Administration for Patients With Impaired Renal Function —Whenever possible, serum tobramycin concentrations should be monitored during therapy.

Following a loading dose of 1 mg/kg, subsequent dosage in these patients must be adjusted, either with reduced doses administered at 8-hour intervals or with normal doses given at prolonged intervals. Either of these methods can be used when serum levels of tobramycin cannot be measured directly. They are based on either the creatinine clearance level or the serum creatinine level of the patient, because these values correlate with the half-life of tobramycin. The dosage schedule derived from either method should be used in conjunction with careful clinical and laboratory observations of the patient and should be modified as necessary. Neither method should be used when dialysis is being performed.

Reduced dosage at 8-hour intervals: When the creatinine clearance rate is 70 mL or less per minute or when the serum creatinine value is known, the amount of the reduced dose can be determined by multiplying the normal dose from Table 1 by the percent of normal dose from the accompanying nomogram.

REDUCED DOSAGE NOMOGRAM*
Creatinine Clearance (mL/min/1.73m²)

Serum Creatinine
(mg/100 mL)
*Scales have been adjusted to
facilitate dosage calculations.

An alternate rough guide for determining reduced dosage at 8-hour intervals (for patients whose steady-state serum creatinine values are known) is to divide the normally recommended dose by the patient's serum creatinine.

Normal dosage at prolonged intervals: If the creatinine clearance rate is not available and the patient's condition is stable, a dosage frequency *in hours* for the dosage given in

Table 1 can be determined by multiplying the patient's serum creatinine by 6.

Dosage in Obese Patients —The appropriate dose may be calculated by using the patient's estimated lean body weight plus 40% of the excess as the basic weight on which to figure mg/kg.

Intramuscular Administration —Nebcin may be administered by withdrawing the appropriate dose directly from a vial or by using a prefilled Hyporet®. ADD-Vantage vials are not for intramuscular administration.

Intravenous Administration—For intravenous administration, the usual volume of diluent (0.9% Sodium Chloride Injection or 5% Dextrose Injection) is 50 to 100 mL for adult doses. For children, the volume of diluent should be proportionately less than for adults. The diluted solution usually should be infused over a period of 20 to 60 minutes. Infusion periods of less than 20 minutes are not recommended, because peak serum levels may exceed 12 mg/L (*see* WARNINGS box).

Use of ADD-Vantage Nebcin Vials —ADD-Vantage Nebcin vials are not intended for multiple use and should not be used with a syringe in the conventional way. These products are intended for use only with Abbott ADD-Vantage diluent containers and in those instances in which the physician's order specified 60-mg or 80-mg doses. Use within 24 hours after activation.

Nebcin® (Tobramycin Sulfate, USP, Lilly) should not be physically premixed with other drugs but should be administered separately according to the recommended dose and route.

HOW SUPPLIED
(℞) Multiple-Dose Vials:
  80 mg*/2 mL, 2 mL (No. 781)—(1s) NDC 0002-1499-01; (Traypak† of 25) NDC 0002-1499-25
  Pediatric, 20 mg*/2 mL (No. 782)—(1s) NDC 0002-0501-01
  1.2 g*/30 mL (Pharmacy Bulk Package) (No. 7090)—(Traypak of 6) NDC 0002-7090-16
(℞) Hyporets®,‡ each scored with a 10-mg (0.25-mL) fractional dose scale:
  60 mg*/1.5 mL, 1.5 mL (No. 55)—(24s) NDC 0002-0509-24
  80 mg*/2 mL, 2 mL (No. 42)—(24s) NDC 0002-0503-24
(℞) ADD-Vantage§ Vials
  60 mg*/6 mL, 6 mL (No. 7293)—(Traypak of 25) NDC 0002-7293-25
  80 mg*/8 mL, 8 mL (No. 7294)—(Traypak of 25) NDC 0002-7294-25
The above ADD-Vantage vials are to be used only with Abbott Laboratories' diluent containers.
Instructions for the use of ADD-Vantage vials are enclosed in the package.

* equivalent to tobramycin
† Traypack™ (multivial carton, Lilly)
‡ Hyporet® (disposable syringe, Lilly)
§ ADD-Vantage® Vials (vials and diluent containers, Abbott)

[020588]

NEBCIN®   ℞
[něb´sin]
(tobramycin sulfate)
Sterile

PHARMACY BULK PACKAGE—NOT FOR DIRECT INFUSION

WARNINGS
See *under* Nebcin, Injection, USP.

DESCRIPTION
Tobramycin sulfate, a water-soluble antibiotic of the aminoglycoside group, is derived from the actinomycete *Streptomyces tenebrarius*. Nebcin® (Tobramycin Sulfate Injection, USP, Lilly), Sterile, is supplied as a sterile dry powder and is intended for reconstitution with 30 ml of Sterile Water for Injection, USP. Sulfuric acid and/or sodium hydroxide may have been added during manufacture to adjust the pH. Each vial contains 1,200 mg of tobramycin activity. After dilution, the solution will contain 40 mg of tobramycin per mL. The product contains no preservative or sodium bisulfite. *See also under* Nebcin, Injection, USP.
The pharmacy bulk package of Nebcin is a sterile preparation for parenteral use that contains multiple single doses. It is intended for use in a pharmacy admixture program. Package use is restricted to the preparation of admixtures for intravenous infusion or to the filling of empty sterile syringes for intravenous injections for patients with individualized dosing requirements.

CLINICAL PHARMACOLOGY, INDICATIONS AND USAGE, CONTRAINDICATIONS, PRECAUTIONS, ADVERSE REACTIONS, and OVERDOSAGE
See *under* Nebcin, Injection, USP.

WARNINGS
See Warnings box under Nebcin, Injection, USP.

DOSAGE AND ADMINISTRATION
The patient's pretreatment body weight should be obtained for calculation of correct dosage. It is desirable to measure both peak and trough serum concentrations (*see* Warnings box *and* Precautions *under* Nebcin, Injection, USP).
Administration for Patients With Normal Renal Function —Adults With Serious Infections: 3 mg/kg/day in 3 equal doses every 8 hours (*see* Table 1 under Nebcin, Injection, USP).
Adults With Life-Threatening Infections: Up to 5 mg/kg/day may be administered in 3 or 4 equal doses (*see* Table 1). The dosage should be reduced to 3 mg/kg/day as soon as clinically indicated. To prevent increased toxicity due to excessive blood levels, dosage should not exceed 5 mg/kg/day unless serum levels are monitored (*see* Warnings box *and* Precautions under Nebcin, Injection, USP).
Children: 6 to 7.5 mg/kg/day in 3 or 4 equally divided doses (2 to 2.5 mg/kg every 8 hours or 1.5 to 1.89 mg/kg every 6 hours).
Premature or Full-Term Neonates 1 Week of Age or Less: Up to 4 mg/kg/day may be administered in 2 equal doses every 12 hours.
It is desirable to limit treatment to a short term. The usual duration of treatment is 7 to 10 days. A longer course of therapy may be necessary in difficult and complicated infections. In such cases, monitoring of renal, auditory, and vestibular functions is advised, because neurotoxicity is more likely to occur when treatment is extended longer than 10 days.
Administration for Patients With Impaired Renal Function —Whenever possible, serum tobramycin concentrations should be monitored during therapy.
Following a loading dose of 1 mg/kg, subsequent dosage in these patients must be adjusted, either with reduced doses administered at 8-hour intervals or with normal doses given at prolonged intervals. Both of these methods can be used when serum levels of tobramycin cannot be measured directly. They are based on either the creatinine clearance level or the serum creatinine level of the patient, because these values correlate with the half-life of tobramycin. The dosage schedules derived from either method should be used in conjunction with careful clinical and laboratory observations of the patient and should be modified as necessary. Neither method should be used when dialysis is being performed.
Reduced dosage at 8-hour intervals: When the creatinine clearance rate is 70 mL or less per minute or when the serum creatinine value is known, the amount of the reduced dose can be determined by multiplying the normal dose from Table 1 by the percent of normal dose from the nomogram *under* Nebcin, Injection, USP.
An alternate rough guide for determining reduced dosage at 8-hour intervals (for patients whose steady-state serum creatinine values are known) is to divide the normally recommended dose by the patient's serum creatinine.
Normal dosage at prolonged intervals: If the creatinine clearance rate is not available and the patient's condition is

TABLE 1. DOSAGE SCHEDULE GUIDE FOR NEBCIN® (TOBRAMYCIN SULFATE, USP) IN ADULTS WITH NORMAL RENAL FUNCTION
(Dosage at 8-Hour Intervals)

For Patient Weighing kg	lb	Usual Dose for Serious Infections 1 mg/kg q8h (Total, 3 mg/kg/day) mg/dose q8h	mL/dose*		Maximum Dose for Life-Threatening Infections (Reduce as soon as possible) 1.66 mg/kg q8h (Total, 5 mg/kg/day) mg/dose q8h	mL/dose*	
120	264	120 mg	3	mL	200 mg	5	mL
115	253	115 mg	2.9	mL	191 mg	4.75	mL
110	242	110 mg	2.75	mL	183 mg	4.5	mL
105	231	105 mg	2.6	mL	175 mg	4.4	mL
100	220	100 mg	2.5	mL	166 mg	4.2	mL
95	209	95 mg	2.4	mL	158 mg	4	mL
90	198	90 mg	2.25	mL	150 mg	3.75	mL
85	187	85 mg	2.1	mL	141 mg	3.5	mL
80	176	80 mg	2	mL	133 mg	3.3	mL
75	165	75 mg	1.9	mL	125 mg	3.1	mL
70	154	70 mg	1.75	mL	116 mg	2.9	mL
65	143	65 mg	1.6	mL	108 mg	2.7	mL
60	132	60 mg	1.5	mL	100 mg	2.5	mL
55	121	55 mg	1.4	mL	91 mg	2.25	mL
50	110	50 mg	1.25	mL	83 mg	2.1	mL
45	99	45 mg	1.1	mL	75 mg	1.9	mL
40	88	40 mg	1	mL	66 mg	1.6	mL

*Applicable to all product forms except Nebcin, Pediatric, Injection (*see* How Supplied).

stable, a dosage frequency *in hours* for the dosage given in Table 1 can be determined by multiplying the patient's serum creatinine by 6.

Dosage in Obese Patients —The appropriate dose may be calculated by using the patient's estimated lean body weight plus 40% of the excess as the basic weight on which to figure mg/kg.

Intravenous Administration —For intravenous administration, the usual volume of diluent (0.9% Sodium Chloride Injection or 5% Dextrose Injection) is 50 to 100 mL for adult doses. For children, the volume of diluent should be proportionately less than for adults. The diluted solution usually should be infused over a period of 20 to 60 minutes. Infusion periods of less than 20 minutes are not recommended, because peak serum levels may exceed 12 mg/L (*see* WARNINGS box).

Nebcin® (Sterile Tobramycin Sulfate, USP, Lilly) should not be physically premixed with other drugs but should be administered separately according to the recommended dose and route.

PREPARATION AND STORAGE

Directions for Proper Use of Pharmacy Bulk Package —Not for direct infusion. The pharmacy bulk package is for use in the Hospital Pharmacy Admixture Service and only in a suitable work area, such as a laminar flow hood. Using aseptic technique, the closure may be penetrated only 1 time after reconstitution using a suitable sterile transfer device or dispensing set, which allows measured dispensing of the contents. Use of a syringe and needle is not recommended as it may cause leakage. After entry, entire contents of bulk vial should be dispensed within 24 hours.

Nebcin, Sterile, is supplied as a dry powder. The contents of the vial (No. 7040) should be diluted with 30 mL of Sterile Water for Injection, USP, to provide a solution containing 40 mg of tobramycin per mL. Prior to reconstitution, the vial should be stored at controlled room temperature, 59° to 86°F (15° to 30°C). After reconstitution, the solution should be kept in a refrigerator and used within 96 hours. If kept at room temperature, the solution must be used within 24 hours.

HOW SUPPLIED

(℞) Pharmacy Bulk Vial:
    1.2 g* (Dry Powder) (40-mL size) (No. 7040)—(Traypak† of 6) NDC 0002-7040-16

Also Available:
(℞) Pharmacy Liquid Bulk Package:
    1.2 g*/30 mL, 30 mL (No. 7090)—(Traypak of 6) NDC 0002-7090-16

---

* Equivalent to tobramycin
†Traypak™ (multivial carton, Lilly)

[092088]

ONCOVIN®   ℞

[ŏn′kō-vĭn]
(vincristine sulfate injection)
Solution

DESCRIPTION

Oncovin® (Vincristine Sulfate, USP, Lilly) is the salt of an alkaloid obtained from a common flowering herb, the periwinkle plant (*Vinca rosea* Linn.). Originally known as leurocristine, it has also been referred to as LCR and VCR. The empirical formula for vincristine sulfate is $C_{46}H_{56}N_4O_{10} \cdot H_2SO_4$.

Vincristine sulfate is a white to slightly yellow, amorphous powder. It is soluble in methanol, freely soluble in water, but only slightly soluble in 95% ethanol. In 98% ethanol, vincristine sulfate has an ultraviolet spectrum with maxima at 221 nm ($E + 47,100$).

Each mL contains vincristine sulfate, 1 mg (1.08 μmoL); mannitol, 100 mg; methylparaben, 1.3 mg; propylparaben, 0.2 mg; and water for injection, qs. Acetic acid and sodium acetate have been added for pH control. The pH of Oncovin Solution ranges from 3.5 to 5.5. This product is a sterile solution for cancer/oncolytic use.

This preparation is for intravenous use only. It should be administered by individuals experienced in the administration of Oncovin. The intrathecal administration of Oncovin results in death. Syringes containing this product should be labeled "ONCOVIN FOR INTRAVENOUS USE ONLY."

Caution —It is extremely important that the intravenous needle or catheter be properly positioned before any vincristine is injected. Leakage into surrounding tissue during intravenous administration of Oncovin may cause considerable irritation. If extravasation occurs, the injection should be discontinued immediately, and any remaining portion of the dose should then be introduced into another vein. Local injection of hyaluronidase and the application of moderate heat to the area of leakage help disperse the drug and are thought to minimize discomfort and the possibility of cellulitis.

CLINICAL PHARMACOLOGY

The mechanisms of action of Oncovin® (Vincristine Sulfate, USP, Lilly) remain under investigation. Treatment of neo-

plastic cells in vitro with Oncovin causes mitotic arrest. The antineoplastic effects of vinca alkaloids are related to interference with intracellular tubulin function.

Central-nervous-system leukemia has been reported in patients undergoing otherwise successful therapy with Oncovin. This suggests that Oncovin does not penetrate well into the cerebrospinal fluid.

Pharmacokinetic studies in patients with cancer have shown a triphasic serum decay pattern following rapid intravenous injection. The initial, middle, and terminal half-lives are 5 minutes, 2.3 hours, and 85 hours respectively; however, the range of the terminal half-life in humans is from 19 to 155 hours. The liver is the major excretory organ in humans and animals; about 80% of an injected dose of Oncovin appears in the feces and 10% to 20% can be found in the urine. Within 15 to 30 minutes after injection, over 90% of the drug is distributed from the blood into tissue, where it remains tightly, but not irreversibly, bound.

Current principles of cancer chemotherapy involve the simultaneous use of several agents. Generally, each agent used has a unique toxicity and mechanism of action so that therapeutic enhancement occurs without additive toxicity. It is rarely possible to achieve equally good results with single-agent methods of treatment. Thus, Oncovin is often chosen as part of polychemotherapy because of lack of significant bone-marrow suppression (at recommended doses) and of unique clinical toxicity (neuropathy). *See* Dosage and Administration for possible increased toxicity when used in combination therapy.

INDICATIONS AND USAGE

Oncovin® (Vincristine Sulfate, USP, Lilly) is indicated in acute leukemia.

Oncovin has also been shown to be useful in combination with other oncolytic agents in Hodgkin's disease, non-Hodgkin's malignant lymphomas (lymphocytic, mixed-cell, histiocytic, undifferentiated, nodular, and difuse types), rhabdomyosarcoma, neuroblastoma, and Wilms' tumor.

CONTRAINDICATIONS

Patients with the demyelinating form of Charcot-Marie-Tooth syndrome should not be given Oncovin® (Vincristine Sulfate, USP, Lilly). Careful attention should be given to those conditions listed under Warnings *and* Precautions.

WARNINGS

> *This preparation is for intravenous use only. It should be administered by individuals experienced in the administration of Oncovin® (Vincristine Sulfate, USP, Lilly). The intrathecal administration of Oncovin results in death. Syringes containing this product should be labeled "ONCOVIN FOR INTRAVENOUS USE ONLY."*

Pregnancy Category D —Oncovin can cause fetal harm when administered to a pregnant woman. When pregnant mice and hamsters were given doses of Oncovin that caused the resorption of 23% to 85% of fetuses, fetal malformations were produced in those that survived. Five monkeys were given single doses of Oncovin between days 27 and 34 of their pregnancies; 3 of the fetuses were normal at term, and 2 viable fetuses had grossly evident malformations at term. In several animal species, Oncovin can induce teratogenesis as well as embryo death at doses that are nontoxic to the pregnant animal. There are no adequate and well-controlled studies in pregnant women. If this drug is used during pregnancy or if the patient becomes pregnant while receiving this drug, she should be apprised of the potential hazard to the fetus. Women of childbearing potential should be advised to avoid becoming pregnant.

PRECAUTIONS

General —Acute uric acid nephropathy, which may occur after the administration of oncolytic agents, has also been reported with Oncovin® (Vincristine Sulfate, USP, Lilly). In the presence of leukopenia or a complicating infection, administration of the next dose of Oncovin warrants careful consideration.

If central-nervous-system leukemia is diagnosed, additional agents may be required, because Oncovin does not appear to cross the blood-brain barrier in adequate amounts.

Particular attention should be given to dosage and neurologic side effects if Oncovin is administered to patients with preexisting neuromuscular disease and when other drugs with neurotoxic potential are also being used.

Acute shortness of breath and severe bronchospasm have been reported following the administration of vinca alkaloids. These reactions have been encountered most frequently when the vinca alkaloid was used in combination with mitomycin-C and may require aggressive treatment, particularly when there is preexisting pulmonary dysfunction. The onset of these reactions may occur minutes to several hours after the vinca is injected and may occur up to 2 weeks following the dose of mitomycin.

Care must be taken to avoid contamination of the eye with concentrations of Oncovin used clinically. If accidental contamination occurs, severe irritation (or, if the drug was deliv-

ered under pressure, even corneal ulceration) may result. The eye should be washed immediately and thoroughly.

Laboratory Tests —Since dose-limiting clinical toxicity is manifested as neurotoxicity, clinical evaluation (eg, history, physical examination) is necessary to detect the need for dosage modification. Following administration of Oncovin, some individuals may have a fall in the white-blood-cell count or platelet count, particularly when previous therapy or the disease itself has reduced bone-marrow function. Therefore, a complete blood count should be done before administration of each dose. Acute elevation of serum uric acid may also occur during induction of remission in acute leukemia; thus, such levels should be determined frequently during the first 3 to 4 weeks of treatment or appropriate measures taken to prevent uric acid nephropathy. The laboratory performing these tests should be consulted for its range of normal values.

Carcinogenesis, Mutagenesis, Impairment of Fertility —Neither in vivo nor in vitro laboratory tests have conclusively demonstrated the mutagenicity of this product. Fertility following treatment with Oncovin alone for malignant disease has not been studied in humans. Clinical reports of both male and female patients who received multiple-agent chemotherapy that included Oncovin indicate that azoospermia and amenorrhea can occur in postpubertal patients. Recovery occurred many months after completion of chemotherapy in some, but not all, patients. When the same treatment is administered to prepubertal patients, permanent azoospermia and amenorrhea are much less likely.

Patients who received Oncovin chemotherapy in combination with anticancer drugs known to be carcinogenic have developed second malignancies. The contributing role of Oncovin in this development has not been determined. No evidence of carcinogenicity was found following intraperitoneal administration of Oncovin in rats and mice, although this study was limited.

Usage in Pregnancy —*Pregnancy Category D* —See Warnings.

Nursing Mothers —It is not known whether this drug is excreted in human milk. Because many drugs are excreted in human milk and because of the potential for serious adverse reactions due to Oncovin in nursing infants, a decision should be made either to discontinue nursing or the drug, taking into account the importance of the drug to the mother.

ADVERSE REACTIONS

Prior to the use of this drug, patients and/or their parents/ guardian should be advised of the possibility of untoward symptoms.

In general, adverse reactions are reversible and are related to dosage. The most common adverse reaction is hair loss; the most troublesome adverse reactions are neuromuscular in origin.

When single weekly doses of the drug are employed, the adverse reactions of leukopenia, neuritic pain, and constipation occur but are usually of short duration (ie, less than 7 days). When the dosage is reduced, these reactions may lessen or disappear. The severity of such reactions seems to increase when the calculated amount of drug is given in divided doses. Other adverse reactions, such as hair loss, sensory loss, paresthesia, difficulty in walking, slapping gait, loss of deep-tendon reflexes, and muscle wasting, may persist for at least as long as therapy is continued. Generalized sensorimotor dysfunction may become progressively more severe with continued treatment. Although most such symptoms usually disappear by about the sixth week after discontinuance of treatment, some neuromuscular difficulties may persist for prolonged periods in some patients. Regrowth of hair may occur while maintenance therapy continues.

The following adverse reactions have been reported:

Hypersensitivity —Rare cases of allergic-type reactions, such as anaphylaxis, rash, and edema, that are temporally related to vincristine therapy have been reported in patients receiving vincristine as a part of multidrug chemotherapy regimens.

Gastrointestinal —Constipation, abdominal cramps, weight loss, nausea, vomiting, oral ulceration, diarrhea, paralytic ileus, intestinal necrosis and/or perforation, and anorexia have occurred. Constipation may take the form of upper-colon impaction, and, on physical examination, the rectum may be empty. Colicky abdominal pain coupled with an empty rectum may mislead the physician. A flat film of the abdomen is useful in demonstrating this condition. All cases have responded to high enemas and laxatives. A routine prophylactic regimen against constipation is recommended for all patients receiving Oncovin® (Vincristine Sulfate, USP, Lilly).

Paralytic ileus (which mimics the "surgical abdomen") may occur, particularly in young children. The ileus will reverse itself with temporary discontinuance of Oncovin and with symptomatic care.

Continued on next page

---

* Identi-Code® symbol.

Lilly—Cont.

Genitourinary—Polyuria, dysuria, and urinary retention due to bladder atony have occurred. Other drugs known to cause urinary retention (particularly in the elderly) should, if possible, be discontinued for the first few days following administration of Oncovin.

Cardiovascular—Hypertension and hypotension have occurred. Chemotherapy combinations that have included vincristine sulfate, when given to patients previously treated with mediastinal radiation, have been associated with coronary artery disease and myocardial infarction. Causality has not been established.

Neurologic—Frequently there is a sequence to the development of neuromuscular side effects. Initially, only sensory impairment and paresthesia may be encountered. With continued treatment, neuritic pain and, later, motor difficulties may occur. There have been no reports made of any agent that can reverse the neuromuscular manifestations that may accompany therapy with Oncovin.

Loss of deep-tendon reflexes, foot drop, ataxia, and paralysis have been reported with continued administration. Cranial nerve manifestations, including isolated paresis and/or paralysis of muscles controlled by cranial motor nerves, may occur in the absence of motor impairment elsewhere; extraocular and laryngeal muscles are most commonly involved. Jaw pain, pharyngeal pain, parotid gland pain, bone pain, back pain, limb pain, and myalgias have been reported; pain in these areas may be severe. Convulsions, frequently with hypertension, have been reported in a few patients receiving Oncovin. Several instances of convulsions followed by coma have been reported in children. Transient cortical blindness and optic atrophy with blindness have been reported.

Pulmonary—See Precautions.

Endocrine—Rare occurrences of a syndrome attributable to inappropriate antidiuretic hormone secretion have been observed in patients treated with Oncovin. This syndrome is characterized by high urinary sodium excretion in the presence of hyponatremia; renal or adrenal disease, hypotension, dehydration, azotemia, and clinical edema are absent. With fluid deprivation, improvement occurs in the hyponatremia and in the renal loss of sodium.

Hematologic—Oncovin does not appear to have any constant or significant effect on platelets or red blood cells. Serious bone-marrow depression is usually not a major dose-limiting event. However, anemia, leukopenia, and thrombocytopenia have been reported. Thrombocytopenia, if present when therapy with Oncovin is begun, may actually improve before the appearance of marrow remission.

Skin—Alopecia and rash have been reported.

Other—Fever and headache have occurred.

OVERDOSAGE

Side effects following the use of Oncovin® (Vincristine Sulfate, USP, Lilly) are dose related. In children under 13 years of age, death has occurred following doses of Oncovin that were 10 times those recommended for therapy. Severe symptoms may occur in this patient group following dosages of 3 to 4 mg/m^2. Adults can be expected to experience severe symptoms after single doses of 3 mg/m^2 or more (see Adverse Reactions). Therefore, following administration of doses higher than those recommended, patients can be expected to experience exaggerated side effects. Supportive care should include the following (1) prevention of side effects resulting from the syndrome of inappropriate antidiuretic hormone secretion (preventive treatment would include restriction of fluid intake and perhaps the administration of a diuretic affecting the function of Henle's loop and the distal tubule); (2) administration of anticonvulsants; (3) use of enemas or cathartics to prevent ileus (in some instances, decompression of the gastrointestinal tract may be necessary); (4) monitoring the cardiovascular system; and (5) determining daily blood counts for guidance in transfusion requirements.

Folinic acid has been observed to have a protective effect in normal mice that were administered lethal doses of Oncovin (*Cancer Res* 1963, 23:1390). Isolated case reports suggest that folinic acid may be helpful in treating humans who have received an overdose of Oncovin. It is suggested that 100 mg of folinic acid be administered intravenously every 3 hours for 24 hours and then every 6 hours for at least 48 hours. Theoretically (based on pharmacokinetic data), tissue levels of Oncovin can be expected to remain significantly elevated for at least 72 hours. Treatment with folinic acid does not eliminate the need for the above-mentioned supportive measures.

Most of an intravenous dose of Oncovin is excreted into the bile after rapid tissue binding (see Clinical Pharmacology). Because only very small amounts of the drug appear in dialysate, hemodialysis is not likely to be helpful in cases of overdosage. An increase in the severity of side effects may be experienced by patients with liver disease that is severe enough to decrease biliary excretion.

Enhanced fecal excretion of parenterally administered vincristine has been demonstrated in dogs pretreated with cho-

lestyramine. There are no published clinical data on the use of cholestyramine as an antidote in humans.

There are no published clinical data on the consequences of oral ingestion of vincristine. Should oral ingestion occur, the stomach should be evacuated. Evacuation should be followed by oral administration of activated charcoal and a cathartic.

DOSAGE AND ADMINISTRATION

This preparation is for intravenous use only (see Warnings). Neurotoxicity appears to be dose related. Extreme care must be used in calculating and administering the dose of Oncovin® (Vincristine Sulfate, USP, Lilly), since overdosage may have a very serious or fatal outcome.

The concentration of vincristine contained in all vials and Hyporets® of Oncovin is 1 mg/mL. Do not add extra fluid to the vial prior to removal of the dose. Withdraw the solution of Oncovin into an accurate dry syringe, measuring the dose carefully. Do not add extra fluid to the vial in an attempt to empty it completely.

Caution—It is extremely important that the intravenous needle or catheter be properly positioned before any vincristine is injected. Leakage into surrounding tissue during intravenous administration of Oncovin may cause considerable irritation. If extravasation occurs, the injection should be discontinued immediately, and any remaining portion of the dose should then be introduced into another vein. Local injection of hyaluronidase and the application of moderate heat to the area of leakage will help disperse the drug and may minimize discomfort and the possibility of cellulitis.

Oncovin must be administered via an intact, free-flowing intravenous needle or catheter. Care should be taken that there is no leakage or swelling occurring during administration (see Caution statement *under* Description).

The solution may be injected either directly into a vein or into the tubing of a running intravenous infusion. *See* Drug Interactions below. Injection of Oncovin should be accomplished within 1 minute.

The drug is administered intravenously *at weekly intervals*. The usual dose of Oncovin for children is 2mg/m^2. For children weighing 10 kg or less, the starting dose should be 0.05 mg/kg, administered once a week. The usual dose of Oncovin for adults is 1.4 mg/m^2. A 50% reduction in the dose of Oncovin is recommended for patients having a direct serum bilirubin value above 3 mg/100 mL.

Oncovin should not be given to patients while they are receiving radiation therapy through ports that include the liver. When Oncovin is used in combination with L-asparaginase, Oncovin should be given 12 to 24 hours before administration of the enzyme in order to minimize toxicity; administering L-asparaginase before Oncovin may reduce hepatic clearance of Oncovin.

Drug Interactions—Oncovin should not be diluted in solutions that raise or lower the pH outside the range of 3.5 to 5.5. It should not be mixed with anything other than normal saline or glucose in water.

Whenever solution and container permit, parenteral drug products should be inspected visually for particulate matter and discoloration prior to administration.

Procedures for proper handling and disposal of anticancer drugs should be considered. Several guidelines on this subject have been published. There is no general agreement that all of the procedures recommended in the guidelines are necessary or appropriate.

See package insert for references.

HOW SUPPLIED

(℞) Multiple-Dose Vials:
1 mg/1 mL, 1 mL (No. 7194) (1s), NDC 0002-7194-01
2 mg/2 mL, 2 mL (No. 7195) (1s), NDC 0002-7195-01
5 mg/5 mL, 5 mL (No. 7196) (1s), NDC 0002-7196-01
(℞) Hyporets® (disposable syringes, Lilly), each marked with a 0.1-mg (0.1-mL) fractional dose scale:
1 mg/1 mL, 1 mL (No. 7198) (3s), NDC 0002-7198-09
2 mg/2 mL, 2 mL (No. 7199) (3s), NDC 0002-7199-09
This product should be refrigerated.

[101488]

PERMAX®   ℞
[pĕr 'măks]
(pergolide mesylate)

DESCRIPTION

Permax® (Pergolide Mesylate, Lilly) is a dopamine receptor agonist at both D_1 and D_2 receptor sites. Pergolide mesylate is chemically designated as 8β-[(Methylthio)methyl]-6-propylergoline monomethanesulfonate; the structural formula is as follows:
[See Chemical Formula at top of next column].
The formula weight of the base is 314.5; 1 mg of base corresponds to 3.18 μmol.
Permax is provided for oral administration in tablets containing 0.05, 0.25, and 1 mg pergolide as the base. They also contain carboxymethylcellulose sodium, iron oxide, lactose, magnesium stearate, and povidone. The 0.25 mg tablet also contains F D & C Blue No. 1.

CLINICAL PHARMACOLOGY

Pharmacodynamic Information—Pergolide mesylate is a potent dopamine receptor agonist. Pergolide is 10 to 1,000 times more potent than bromocriptine on a milligram per milligram basis in various in vitro and in vivo test systems. Pergolide mesylate inhibits the secretion of prolactin in humans; it causes a transient rise in serum concentrations of growth hormone and a decrease in serum concentrations of luteinizing hormone. In Parkinson's disease, pergolide mesylate is believed to exert its therapeutic effect by directly stimulating postsynaptic dopamine receptors in the nigrostriatal system.

Pharmacokinetic Information (Absorption, Distribution, Metabolism, and Elimination)—Information on oral systemic bioavailability of pergolide mesylate is unavailable because of the lack of a sufficiently sensitive assay to detect the drug after the administration of single doses. However, following oral administration of ^{14}C radiolabeled pergolide mesylate, approximately 55% of the administered radioactivity can be recovered from the urine and 5% from expired CO_2, suggesting that a significant fraction is absorbed. Nothing can be concluded about the extent of presystemic clearance, if any. Data on postabsorption distribution of pergolide are unavailable.

At least 10 metabolites have been detected, including N-despropylpergolide, pergolide sulfoxide, and pergolide sulfone. Pergolide sulfoxide and pergolide sulfone are dopamine agonists in animals. The other detected metabolites have not been identified, and it is not known whether any other metabolites are active pharmacologically.

The major route of excretion is via the kidney.

Pergolide is approximately 90% bound to plasma proteins. This extent of protein binding may be important to consider when pergolide mesylate is coadministered with other drugs known to affect protein binding.

INDICATIONS AND USAGE

Permax is indicated as adjunctive treatment to levodopa/carbidopa in the management of the signs and symptoms of Parkinson's disease.

Evidence to support the efficacy of pergolide mesylate as an antiparkinsonian adjunct was obtained in a multicenter study enrolling 376 patients with mild to moderate Parkinson's disease who were intolerant to *l*-dopa/carbidopa as manifested by moderate to severe dyskinesia and/or on-off phenomena. On average, the sample of patients evaluated had been on *l*-dopa/carbidopa for 3.9 years (range, 2 days to 16.8 years). The administration of pergolide mesylate permitted a 5% to 30% reduction in the daily dose of *l*-dopa. On average these patients treated with pergolide mesylate maintained an equivalent or better clinical status than they exhibited at baseline.

CONTRAINDICATIONS

Pergolide mesylate is contraindicated in patients who are hypersensitive to this drug or other ergot derivatives.

WARNINGS

Symptomatic Hypotension—In clinical trials, approximately 10% of patients taking pergolide mesylate with *l*-dopa vs. 7% taking placebo with *l*-dopa experienced symptomatic orthostatic and/or sustained hypotension, especially during initial treatment. With gradual dosage titration, tolerance to the hypotension usually develops. It is, therefore, important to warn patients of the risk, to begin therapy with low doses, and to increase the dosage in carefully adjusted increments over a period of 3 to 4 weeks (see Dosage and Administration).

Hallucinosis—In controlled trials, pergolide mesylate with *l*-dopa caused hallucinosis in about 14% of patients as opposed to 3% taking placebo with *l*-dopa. This was of sufficient severity to cause discontinuation of treatment in about 3% of those enrolled; tolerance to this untoward effect was not observed.

Fatalities—In the placebo-controlled trial, 2 of 187 patients treated with placebo died as compared with 1 of 189 patients treated with pergolide mesylate. Of the 2,299 patients treated with pergolide mesylate in premarketing studies evaluated as of October 1988, 143 died while on the drug or shortly after discontinuing the drug. The patient population under evaluation was elderly, ill, and at high risk for death. It seems unlikely that pergolide mesylate played any role in these deaths, but the possibility that pergolide shortens survival of patients cannot be excluded with absolute certainty. In particular, a case-by-case review of the clinical course of the patients who died failed to disclose any unique set of signs, symptoms, or laboratory results that would suggest that treatment with pergolide caused their deaths. Sixty-eight percent (68%) of the patients who died were 65 years of age or over. No death (other than a suicide) occurred within the first month of treatment; most of the patients who died had been on pergolide for years. A relative frequency of the causes of death by organ system are: Pulmonary failure/ Pneumonia, 35%; Cardiovascular, 30%; Cancer, 11%; Unknown, 8.4%; Infection, 3.5%; Extrapyramidal syndrome, 3.5%; Stroke, 2.1%; Dysphagia, 2.1%; Injury, 1.4%; Suicide, 1.4%; Dehydration, 0.7%; Glomerulonephritis, 0.7%.

PRECAUTIONS

General —Caution should be exercised when administering pergolide mesylate to patients prone to cardiac dysrhythmias.

In a study comparing pergolide mesylate and placebo, patients taking pergolide mesylate were found to have significantly more episodes of atrial premature contractions (APCs) and sinus tachycardia.

The use of pergolide mesylate in patients on *l*-dopa may cause and/or exacerbate preexisting states of confusion and hallucinations (*see* Warnings).

The administration of pergolide mesylate to patients receiving *l*-dopa may cause and/or exacerbate preexisting dyskinesia.

Information for Patients —Patients and their families should be informed of the common adverse consequences of the use of pergolide mesylate (*see* Adverse Reactions) and the risk of hypotension (*see* Warnings).

Patients should be advised to notify their physician if they become pregnant or intend to become pregnant during therapy.

Patients should be advised to notify their physician if they are breast-feeding an infant.

Laboratory Tests —No specific laboratory tests are deemed essential for the management of patients on Permax® (Pergolide Mesylate, Lilly). Periodic routine evaluation of all patients, however, is appropriate.

Drug Interactions —Dopamine antagonists, such as the neuroleptics (phenothiazines, butyrophenones, thioxanthines) or metoclopramide, ordinarily should not be administered concurrently with Permax (a dopamine agonist); these agents may diminish the effectiveness of Permax.

Because pergolide mesylate is approximately 90% associated with plasma proteins, caution should be exercised if pergolide mesylate is coadministered with other drugs known to affect protein binding.

Carcinogenesis, Mutagenesis, and Impairment of Fertility —A 2-year carcinogenicity study was conducted in mice using dietary levels of pergolide mesylate equivalent to oral doses of 0.6, 3.7, and 36.4 mg/kg/day in males and 0.6, 4.4, and 40.8 mg/kg/day in females. A 2-year study in rats was conducted using dietary levels equivalent to oral doses of 0.04, 0.18, and 0.88 mg/kg/day in males and 0.05, 0.28, and 1.42 mg/kg/day in females. The highest doses tested in the mice and rats were approximately 340 and 12 times the maximum human oral dose administered in controlled clinical trials (6 mg/day equivalent to 0.12 mg/kg/day).

A low incidence of uterine neoplasms occurred in both rats and mice. Endometrial adenomas and carcinomas were observed in rats. Endometrial sarcomas were observed in mice. The occurrence of these neoplasms is probably attributable to the high estrogen/progesterone ratio which would occur in rodents as a result of the prolactin-inhibiting action of pergolide mesylate. The endocrine mechanisms believed to be involved in the rodents are not present in humans. However, even though there is no known correlation between uterine malignancies occurring in pergolide-treated rodents and human risk, there are no human data to substantiate this conclusion.

Pergolide mesylate was evaluated for mutagenic potential in a battery of tests that included an Ames bacterial mutation assay, a DNA repair assay in cultured rat hepatocytes, a point-mutation assay in cultured L5178Y cells, and a determination of chromosome alteration in bone marrow cells of Chinese hamsters. A weak mutagenic response was noted in the in vitro mammalian cell-point-mutation assay using L5178Y cells only after metabolic activation with rat liver microsomes. No mutagenic effects were obtained in the 2 other in vitro assays and in the in vivo assay. The relevance of these findings to humans is unknown.

A fertility study in male and female mice showed the fertility was maintained at 0.6 and 1.7 mg/kg/day but decreased at 5.6 mg/kg/day. Prolactin has been reported to be involved in stimulating and maintaining progesterone levels required for implantation in mice, and, therefore, the impaired fertility at high dose may occur because of depressed prolactin levels.

Usage in Pregnancy —Pregnancy Category B —Reproduction studies were conducted in mice at doses of 5, 16, and 45 mg/kg/day and in rabbits at doses of 2, 6, and 16 mg/kg/day. The highest doses tested in mice and rabbits were 375 and 133 times the 6 mg/day maximum human dose administered in controlled clinical trials. In these studies, there was no evidence of harm to the fetus due to pergolide mesylate.

There are, however, no adequate and well-controlled studies in pregnant women. Among women who received pergolide mesylate for endocrine disorders in premarketing studies,

Incidence of Treatment-Emergent Adverse Experiences in the Placebo-Controlled Clinical Trial

Percentage of Patients Reporting Events

Body System/ Adverse Event*	Pergolide Mesylate N = 189	Placebo N = 187
Body as a Whole		
Pain	7.0	2.1
Abdominal pain	5.8	2.1
Injury, accident	5.8	7.0
Headache	5.3	6.4
Asthenia	4.2	4.8
Chest pain	3.7	2.1
Flu syndrome	3.2	2.1
Neck pain	2.7	1.6
Back pain	1.6	2.1
Surgical procedure	1.6	<1
Chills	1.1	0
Face edema	1.1	0
Infection	1.1	0
Cardiovascular		
Postural hypotension	9.0	7.0
Vasodilatation	3.2	<1
Palpitation	2.1	<1
Hypotension	2.1	<1
Syncope	2.1	1.1
Hypertension	1.6	1.1
Arrhythmia	1.1	<1
Myocardial infarction	1.1	<1
Digestive		
Nausea	24.3	12.8
Constipation	10.6	5.9
Diarrhea	6.4	2.7
Dyspepsia	6.4	2.1
Anorexia	4.8	2.7
Dry mouth	3.7	<1
Vomiting	2.7	1.6
Hemic and Lymphatic		
Anemia	1.1	<1
Metabolic and Nutritional		
Peripheral edema	7.4	4.3
Edema	1.6	0
Weight gain	1.6	0
Musculoskeletal		
Arthralgia	1.6	2.1
Bursitis	1.6	<1
Myalgia	1.1	<1
Twitching	1.1	0
Nervous System		
Dyskinesia	62.4	24.6
Dizziness	19.1	13.9
Hallucinations	13.8	3.2
Dystonia	11.6	8.0
Confusion	11.1	9.6
Somnolence	10.1	3.7
Insomnia	7.9	3.2
Anxiety	6.4	4.3
Tremor	4.2	7.5
Depression	3.2	5.4
Abnormal dreams	2.7	4.3
Personality disorder	2.1	<1
Psychosis	2.1	0
Abnormal gait	1.6	1.6
Akathisia	1.6	0
Extrapyramidol syndrome	1.6	1.1
Incoordination	1.6	<1
Paresthesia	1.6	3.2
Akinesia	1.1	1.1
Hypertonia	1.1	0
Neuralgia	1.1	<1
Speech disorder	1.1	1.6
Respiratory System		
Rhinitis	12.2	5.4
Dyspnea	4.8	1.1
Epistaxis	1.6	<1
Hiccup	1.1	0
Skin and Appendages		
Rash	3.2	2.1
Sweating	2.1	2.7
Special Senses		
Abnormal vision	5.8	5.4
Diplopia	2.1	0
Taste perversion	1.6	0
Eye disorder	1.1	0
Urogenital System		
Urinary frequency	2.7	6.4
Urinary tract infection	2.7	3.7
Hematuria	1.1	<1

*Events reported by at least 1% of patients receiving pergolide mesylate are included.

Continued on next page

* Identi-Code® symbol.

Lilly—Cont.

there were 33 pregnancies that resulted in healthy babies and 4 pregnancies that resulted in congential abnormalities (2 major, 2 minor); a causal relationship has not been established. Because human data are limited and because animal reproduction studies are not always predictive of human response, this drug should be used during pregnancy only if clearly needed.

Nursing Mothers —It is not known whether this drug is excreted in human milk. The pharmacologic action of pergolide mesylate suggests that it may interfere with lactation. Because many drugs are excreted in human milk and because of the potential for serious adverse reactions to pergolide mesylate in nursing infants, a decision should be made whether to discontinue nursing or to discontinue the drug, taking into account the importance of the drug to the mother.

Pediatric Use —Safety and effectiveness in children have not been established.

ADVERSE REACTIONS

Commonly Observed —In premarketing clinical trials, the most commonly observed adverse events associated with use of pergolide mesylate which were not seen at an equivalent incidence among placebo-treated patients were: nervous system complaints, including dyskinesia, hallucinations, somnolence, insomnia; digestive complaints, including nausea, constipation, diarrhea, dyspepsia; and respiratory system complaints, including rhinitis.

Associated With Discontinuation of Treatment —Twenty-seven percent (27%) of approximately 1,200 patients receiving pergolide mesylate for treatment of Parkinson's disease in premarketing clinical trials in the US and Canada discontinued treatment due to adverse reactions. The events most commonly causing discontinuation were related to the nervous system (15.5%), primarily hallucinations (7.8%) and confusion (1.8%).

Fatalities —See Warnings.

Incidence in Controlled Clinical Trials —The table that follows enumerates adverse events that occurred at a frequency of 1% or more among patients taking pergolide mesylate who participated in the premarketing controlled clinical trials comparing pergolide mesylate with placebo. In a double-blind, controlled study of 6 months' duration, patients with Parkinson's disease were continued on *l*-dopa/carbidopa and were randomly assigned to receive either pergolide mesylate or placebo as additional therapy.

The prescriber should be aware that these figures cannot be used to predict the incidence of side effects in the course of usual medical practice where patient characteristics and other factors differ from those which prevailed in the clinical trials. Similarly, the cited frequencies cannot be compared with figures obtained from other clinical investigations involving different treatments, uses, and investigators. The cited figures, however, do provide the prescribing physician with some basis for estimating the relative contribution of drug and nondrug factors to the side-effect incidence rate in the population studied.

[See table on preceding page].

Events Observed During the Premarketing Evaluation of Permax® (Pergolide Mesylate, Lilly) — This section reports event frequencies evaluated as of October 1988 for adverse events occurring in a group of approximately 1,800 patients who took multiple doses of pergolide mesylate. The conditions and duration of exposure to pergolide mesylate varied greatly, involving well-controlled studies as well as experience in open and uncontrolled clinical settings. In the absence of appropriate controls in some of the studies, a causal relationship between these events and treatment with pergolide mesylate cannot be determined.

The following enumeration by organ system describes events in terms of their relative frequency of reporting in the data base. Events of major clinical importance are also described in the Warnings and Precautions sections.

The following definitions of frequency are used: frequent adverse events are defined as those occurring in at least 1/100 patients; infrequent adverse events are those occurring in 1/100 to 1/1,000 patients; rare events are those occurring in fewer than 1/1,000 patients.

Body as a Whole—*Frequent:* headache, asthenia, accidental injury, abdominal pain, chest pain, back pain, flu syndrome, neck pain, fever; *Infrequent:* facial edema, chills, enlarged abdomen, malaise, neoplasm, hernia, pelvic pain, sepsis, cellulitis, moniliasis, abscess, jaw pain, hypothermia; *Rare:* acute abdominal syndrome, LE syndrome

Cardiovascular System—*Frequent:* postural hypotension, syncope, hypertension, palpitations, vasodilatations, congestive heart failure; *Infrequent:* myocardial infarction, tachycardia, heart arrest, abnormal electrocardiogram, angina pectoris, thrombophlebitis, bradycardia, ventricular extrasystoles, cerebrovascular accident, ventricular tachycar-

dia, cerebral ischemia, atrial fibrillation, varicose vein, pulmonary embolus, AV block, shock; *Rare:* vasculitis, pulmonary hypertension, pericarditis, migraine, heart block, cerebral hemorrhage

Digestive System—*Frequent:* nausea, vomiting, dyspepsia, diarrhea, constipation, dry mouth, dysphagia; *Infrequent:* flatulence, abnormal liver function tests, increased appetite, salivary bland enlargement, thirst, gastroenteritis, gastritis, periodontal abscess, intestinal obstruction, nausea and vomiting, gingivitis, esophagitis, cholelithiasis, tooth caries, hepatitis, stomach ulcer, melena, hepatomegaly, hematemesis, eructation; *Rare:* sialadenitis, peptic ulcer, pancreatitis, jaundice, glossitis, fecal incontinence, duodenitis, colitis, cholecystitis, aphthous stomatitis, esophageal ulcer

Endocrine System—*Infrequent:* hypothyroidism, adenoma, diabetes mellitus, ADH inappropriate; *Rare:* endocrine disorder, thyroid adenoma

Hemic and Lymphatic System—*Frequent:* anemia; *Infrequent:* leukopenia, lymphadenopathy, leukocytosis, thrombocytopenia, petechia, megaloblastic anemia, cyanosis; *Rare:* purpura, lymphocytosis, eosinophilia, thrombocythemia, acute lymphoblastic leukemia, polycythemia, splenomegaly

Metabolic and Nutritional System—*Frequent:* peripheral edema, weight loss, weight gain; *Infrequent:* dehydration, hypokalemia, hypoglycemia, iron deficiency anemia, hyperglycemia, gout, hypercholesteremia; *Rare:* electrolyte imbalance, cachexia, acidosis, hyperuricemia

Musculoskeletal System—*Frequent:* twitching, myalgia, arthralgia; *Infrequent:* bone pain, tenosynovitis, myositis, bone sarcoma, arthritis; *Rare:* osteoporosis, muscle atrophy, osteomyelitis

Nervous System—*Frequent:* dyskinesia, dizziness, hallucinations, confusion, somnolence, insomnia, dystonia, paresthesia, depression, anxiety, tremor, akinesia, extrapyramidal syndrome, abnormal gait, abnormal dreams, incoordination, psychosis, personality disorder, nervousness, choreoathetosis, amnesia, paranoid reaction, abnormal thinking; *Infrequent:* akathisia, neuropathy, neuralgia, hypertonia, delusions, convulsion, libido increased, euphoria, emotional lability, libido decreased, vertigo, myoclonus, coma, apathy, paralysis, neurosis, hyperkinesia, ataxia, acute brain syndrome, torticollis, meningitis, manic reaction, hypokinesia, hostility, agitation, hypotonia; *Rare:* stupor, neuritis, intracranial hypertension, hemiplegia, facial paralysis, brain edema, myelitis

Respiratory System—*Frequent:* rhinitis, dyspnea, pneumonia, pharyngitis, cough increased; *Infrequent:* epistaxis, hiccup, sinusitis, bronchitis, voice alteration, hemoptysis, asthma, lung edema, pleural effusion, laryngitis, emphysema, apnea, hyperventilation; *Rare:* pneumothorax, lung fibrosis, larynx edema, hypoxia, hypoventilation, hemothorax, carcinoma of lung

Skin and Appendages System—*Frequent:* sweating, rash; *Infrequent:* skin discoloration, pruritus, acne, skin ulcer, alopecia, dry skin, skin carcinoma, seborrhea, hirsutism, herpes simplex, eczema, fungal dermatitis, herpes zoster; *Rare:* vesiculobullous rash, subcutaneous nodule, skin nodule, skin benign neoplasm, lichenoid dermatitis

Special Senses System—*Frequent:* diplopia; *Infrequent:* otitis media, conjunctivitis, tinnitus, deafness, taste perversion, ear pain, eye pain, glaucoma, eye hemorrhage, photophobia, visual field defect; *Rare:* blindness, cataract, retinal detachment, retinal vascular disorder

Urogenital System—*Frequent:* urinary tract infection, urinary frequency, urinary incontinence, hematuria, dysmenorrhea; *Infrequent:* dysuria, breast pain, menorrhagia, impotence, cystitis, urinary retention, abortion, vaginal hemorrhage, vaginitis, priapism, kidney calculus, fibrocystic breast, lactation, uterine hemorrhage, urolithiasis, salpingitis, pyuria, metrorrhagia, menopause, kidney failure, breast carcinoma, cervical carcinoma; *Rare:* amenorrhea, bladder carcinoma, breast engorgement, epididymitis, hypogonadism, leukorrhea, nephrosis, pyelonephritis, urethral pain, uricaciduria, withdrawal bleeding

OVERDOSAGE

There is no clinical experience with massive overdosage. The largest overdose involved a young hospitalized adult patient who was not being treated with pergolide mesylate but who intentionally took 60 mg of pergolide mesylate. He experienced vomiting, hypotension, and agitation. Another patient receiving a daily dosage of 7 mg of pergolide mesylate, unintentionally took 19 mg/day for 3 days, after which his vital signs were normal but he experienced severe hallucinations. Within 36 hours of resumption of the prescribed dosage level, the hallucinations stopped. One patient unintentionally took 14 mg/day for 23 days instead of her prescribed 1.4 mg/day dosage. She experienced severe involuntary movements and tingling in her arms and legs. Another patient who inadvertently received 7 mg instead of the prescribed 0.7 mg experienced palpitations, hypotension, and ventricular extrasystoles. The highest total daily dose (prescribed for several patients with refractory Parkinson's disease) has exceeded 30 mg.

Symptoms —Animal studies indicate that the manifestations of overdosage in man might include nausea, vomiting, convulsions, decreased blood pressure, and CNS stimulation. The oral median lethal doses in mice and rats were 54 and 15 mg/kg respectively.

Treatment —To obtain up-to-date information about the treatment of overdose, a good resource is your certified Regional Poison Control Center. Telephone numbers of certified poison control centers are listed in the *Physicians' Desk Reference (PDR)*. In managing overdosage, consider the possibility of multiple drug overdoses, interaction among drugs, ·and unusual drug kinetics in your patient.

Management of overdosage may require supportive measures to maintain arterial blood pressure. Cardiac function should be monitored; an antiarrhythmic agent may be necessary. If signs of CNS stimulation are present, a phenothiazine or other butyrophenone neuroleptic agent may be indicated; the efficacy of such drugs in reversing the effects of overdose has not been assessed.

Protect the patient's airway and support ventilation and perfusion. Meticulously monitor and maintain, within acceptable limits, the patient's vital signs, blood gases, serum electrolytes, etc. Absorption of drugs from the gastrointestinal tract may be decreased by giving activated charcoal, which, in many cases, is more effective than emesis or lavage; consider charcoal instead of or in addition to gastric emptying. Repeated doses of charcoal over time may hasten elimination of some drugs that have been absorbed. Safeguard the patient's airway when employing gastric emptying or charcoal.

There is no experience with dialysis or hemoperfusion, and these procedures are unlikely to be of benefit.

DOSAGE AND ADMINISTRATION

Administration of Permax® (Pergolide Mesylate, Lilly) should be initiated with a daily dosage of 0.05 mg for the first 2 days. The dosage should then be gradually increased by 0.1 or 0.15 mg/day every third day over the next 12 days of therapy. The dosage may then be increased by 0.25 mg/day every third day until an optimal therapeutic dosage is achieved. Permax is usually administered in divided doses 3 times per day. During dosage titration, the dosage of concurrent *l*-dopa/carbidopa may be cautiously decreased.

In clinical studies, the mean therapeutic daily dosage of Permax was 3 mg/day. The average concurrent daily dosage of *l*-dopa/carbidopa (expressed as *l*-dopa) was approximately 650 mg/day. The efficacy of Permax at doses above 5 mg/day has not been systematically evaluated.

HOW SUPPLIED

(℞) *Permax®* (Pergolide Mesylate, Lilly)

Tablets (scored):
0.05 mg, ivory (No. 4131)—(RxPak* of 30) NDC 0002-4131-30
0.25 mg, green (No. 4133)—(RxPak of 30) NDC 0002-4133-30;
(RxPak of 100) NDC 0002-4133-02
1 mg, pink (No. 4135)—(RxPak of 100) NDC 0002-4135-02

* All RxPaks (prescription packages, Lilly) have safety closures.
Store at controlled room temperature, 59° to 86°F (15° to 30°C).

[012089]

Shown in Product Identification Section, page 415

PROTAMINE SULFATE   ℞
[prō'ta-mĕn sŭl'fāt]
Injection, USP

DESCRIPTION

Protamines are simple proteins of low molecular weight that are rich in arginine and strongly basic. They occur in the sperm of salmon and certain other species of fish.

Protamine sulfate occurs as fine white or off-white amorphous or crystalline powder. It is sparingly soluble in water. The pH is between 6.0 and 7.5. The cationic hydrogenated protamine at a pH of 6.8 to 7.1 reacts with anionic heparin at a pH of 5.0 to 7.5 to form an inactive complex.

Protamine Sulfate Injection, USP, is a sterile, isotonic solution of protamine sulfate. It acts as a heparin antagonist. It is also a weak anticoagulant.

Each 5-mL ampoule of Protamine Sulfate Injection contains protamine sulfate equivalent to 50 mg of activity, and each 25-mL vial contains protamine sulfate equivalent to 250 mg of activity. Both products also contain 0.9% sodium chloride. Sodium phosphate and/or sulfuric acid may have been added during manufacture to adjust the pH. Contains no preservative.

Protamine sulfate is administered intravenously.

CLINICAL PHARMACOLOGY

When administered alone, protamine has an anticoagulant effect. However, when it is given in the presence of heparin (which is strongly acidic), a stable salt is formed and the anticoagulant activity of both drugs is lost.

Protamine sulfate has a rapid onset of action. Neutralization of heparin occurs within 5 minutes after intravenous administration of an appropriate dose of protamine sulfate. Although the metabolic fate of the heparin-protamine complex has not been elucidated, it has been postulated that protamine sulfate in the heparin-protamine complex may be partially metabolized or may be attacked by fibrinolysin, thus freeing heparin.

INDICATIONS AND USAGE
Protamine sulfate is indicated in the treatment of heparin overdosage.

CONTRAINDICATION
Protamine sulfate is contraindicated in patients who have shown previous intolerance to the drug.

WARNINGS
Hyperheparinemia or bleeding has been reported in experimental animals and in some patients 30 minutes to 18 hours after cardiac surgery (under cardiopulmonary bypass) in spite of complete neutralization of heparin by adequate doses of protamine sulfate at the end of the operation. It is important to keep the patient under close observation after cardiac surgery. Additional doses of protamine sulfate should be administered if indicated by coagulation studies, such as the heparin titration test with protamine and the determination of plasma thrombin time.

Too-rapid administration of protamine sulfate can cause severe hypotensive and anaphylactoid reactions (see Dosage and Administration and Warnings**). Facilities to treat shock should be available.**

PRECAUTIONS
General—**Because of the anticoagulant effect of protamine, it is unwise to give more than 100 mg over a short period unless a larger dose is clearly needed.**
Patients with a history of allergy to fish may develop hypersensitivity reactions to protamine, although to date no relationship has been established between allergic reactions to protamine and fish allergy.
Previous exposure to protamine through use of protamine-containing insulins or during heparin neutralization may predispose susceptible individuals to the development of untoward reactions from the subsequent use of this drug. Reports of the presence of antiprotamine antibodies in the serums of infertile or vasectomized men suggest that some of these individuals may react to use of protamine sulfate.
Drug Interactions—Protamine sulfate has been shown to be incompatible with certain antibiotics, including several of the cephalosporins and penicillins (see Dosage and Administration).
Carcinogenesis, Mutagenesis, Impairment of Fertility—Studies have not been performed to determine potential for carcinogenicity, mutagenicity, or impairment of fertility.
Usage in Pregnancy—Pregnancy Category C—Animal reproduction studies have not been conducted with protamine sulfate. It is also not known whether protamine sulfate can cause fetal harm when administered to a pregnant woman or can affect reproduction capacity. Protamine sulfate should be given to a pregnant woman only if clearly needed.
Nursing Mothers—It is not known whether this drug is excreted in human milk. Because many drugs are excreted in human milk, caution should be exercised when protamine sulfate is administered to a nursing woman.
Usage in Children—Safety and effectiveness in children have not been established.

ADVERSE REACTIONS
Intravenous injections of protamine may cause a sudden fall in blood pressure, bradycardia, pulmonary hypertension, dyspnea, or transitory flushing and a feeling of warmth. There have been reports of anaphylaxis that resulted in respiratory embarrassment (see Warnings and Precautions). Other reported adverse reactions include systemic hypertension, nausea, vomiting, and lassitude. Back pain has been reported rarely in conscious patients undergoing such procedures as cardiac catheterization.
Because fatal reactions often resembling anaphylaxis have been reported after administration of protamine sulfate, the drug should be given only when resuscitation techniques and treatment of anaphylactoid shock are readily available.

OVERDOSAGE
Signs and Symptoms—Overdose of protamine sulfate may cause bleeding. Protamine has a weak anticoagulant effect due to an interaction with platelets and with many proteins including fibrinogen. This effect should be distinguished from the rebound anticoagulation that may occur 30 minutes to 18 hours following the reversal of heparin with protamine.
Rapid administration of protamine is more likely to result in bradycardia, dyspnea, a sensation of warmth, flushing, and severe hypotension. Hypertension has also occurred.
The LD_{50} of protamine sulfate is 100 mg/kg in mice. Serum concentrations of protamine sulfate are not clinically useful. Information is not available on the amount of drug in a single dose that is associated with overdosage or is likely to be life-threatening.

Treatment—To obtain up-to-date information about the treatment of overdose, a good resource is your certified Regional Poison Control Center. Telephone numbers of certified poison control centers are listed in the Physicians' Desk Reference (PDR). In managing overdosage, consider the possibility of multiple drug overdoses, interaction among drugs, and unusual drug kinetics in your patient.
Replace blood loss with blood transfusions or fresh frozen plasma.
If the patient is hypotensive, consider fluids, epinephrine, dobutamine, or dopamine.

DOSAGE AND ADMINISTRATION
Each mg of protamine sulfate neutralizes approximately 90 USP units of heparin activity derived from lung tissue or about 115 USP units of heparin activity derived from intestinal mucosa.
Protamine Sulfate Injection should be given by very slow intravenous injection over a 10-minute period in doses not to exceed 50 mg (see Warnings).
Protamine sulfate is intended for injection without further dilution; however, if further dilution is desired, D5-W or normal saline may be used. Diluted solutions should not be stored since they contain no preservative.
Protamine sulfate should not be mixed with other drugs without knowledge of their compatibility, because protamine sulfate has been shown to be incompatible with certain antibiotics, including several of the cephalosporins and penicillins.
Because heparin disappears rapidly from the circulation, the dose of protamine sulfate required also decreases rapidly with the time elapsed following intravenous injection of heparin. For example, if the protamine sulfate is administered 30 minutes after the heparin, one-half the usual dose may be sufficient.
The dosage of protamine sulfate should be guided by blood coagulation studies (see Warnings).
Parenteral drug products should be inspected visually for particulate matter and discoloration prior to administration whenever solution and container permit.

HOW SUPPLIED
(℞) Ampoules:
    5 mL (No. 473)—(6s) NDC 0002-1691-16; (25s) NDC 0002-1691-25
(℞) Vials:
    25 mL (No. 735)—(1s) NDC 0002-1462-01
Ampoules and vials should be stored in the refrigerator and kept above freezing and below 50°F.
CAUTION—The total dose of protamine sulfate contained in Vials No. 735 (250 mg of activity in 25 mL) is 5 times greater than that in Ampoules No. 473 (50 mg of activity in 5 mL).
The large-size vials (No. 735) are designed for antiheparin treatment only when large doses of heparin have been given during surgery and are to be neutralized by large doses of protamine sulfate after surgical procedures.

[052488]

REGULAR ILETIN® I
[rĕg ʹū-lĕr ī ʹlĕ-tĭn]
(insulin injection, Lilly), see under Iletin® (insulin, Lilly).

SEMILENTE® ILETIN® I
[sĕm ʹĭ-lĕn ʹtā ī ʹlĕ-tĭn]
(prompt insulin zinc suspension, Lilly), see under Iletin® (insulin, Lilly).

SEROMYCIN®   ℞
[sĕr-ō-mī ʹsĭn]
(cycloserine)
Capsules, USP

DESCRIPTION
Seromycin® (Cycloserine Capsules, USP, Lilly), 3-isoxazolidinone, 4-amino-, (R)-, is a broad-spectrum antibiotic that is produced by a strain of Streptomyces orchidaceus and has also been synthesized. Cycloserine is a white powder that is soluble in water and stable in alkaline solution. It is rapidly destroyed at a neutral or acid pH.
Cycloserine has a pH between 5.5 and 6.5 in a solution containing 100 mg/mL. The molecular weight of cycloserine is 102.09, and it has an empirical formula of $C_3H_6N_2O_2$.
Each Pulvule® contains cycloserine, 250 mg (2.45 mmoL); D & C Yellow No. 10, F D & C Blue No. 1, F D & C Red No. 3, F D & C Yellow No. 6, gelatin, iron oxide, mineral oil, talc, titanium dioxide, and other inactive ingredients.

CLINICAL PHARMACOLOGY
After oral administration, cycloserine is readily absorbed from the gastrointestinal tract, with peak blood levels occurring in 4 to 8 hours. Blood levels of 25 to 30 mg/L can generally be maintained with the usual dosage of 250 mg twice a day, although the relationship of plasma levels to dosage is not always consistent. Concentrations in the cerebrospinal fluid, pleural fluid, fetal blood, and mother's milk approach those found in the serum. Detectable amounts are found in ascitic fluid, bile, sputum, amniotic fluid, and lung and lymph tissues. Approximately 65% of a single dose of cycloserine can be recovered in the urine within 72 hours after oral administration. The remaining 35% is apparently metabolized to unknown substances. The maximum excretion rate occurs 2 to 6 hours after administration, with 50% of the drug eliminated in 12 hours.
Microbiology—Cycloserine inhibits cell-wall synthesis in susceptible strains of gram-positive and gram-negative bacteria and in Mycobacterium tuberculosis.
Susceptibility Tests—Cycloserine clinical laboratory standard powder is available for both direct and indirect methods[1] of determining the susceptibility of strains of mycobacteria. Cycloserine MICs for susceptible strains are 25 mg/L or lower.

INDICATIONS AND USAGE
Seromycin® (Cycloserine Capsules, USP, Lilly) is indicated in the treatment of active pulmonary and extrapulmonary tuberculosis (including renal disease) when the organisms are susceptible to this drug when treatment with the primary medications (streptomycin, isoniazid, rifampin, and ethambutol) has proved inadequate. Like all antituberculosis drugs, Seromycin should be administered in conjunction with other effective chemotherapy and not as the sole therapeutic agent.
Seromycin may be effective in the treatment of acute urinary tract infections caused by susceptible strains of gram-positive and gram-negative bacteria, especially Enterobacter sp and Escherichia coli. It is generally no more and is usually less effective than other antimicrobial agents in the treatment of urinary tract infections caused by bacteria other than mycobacteria. Use of Seromycin in these infections should be considered only when the more conventional therapy has failed and when the organism has been demonstrated to be susceptible to the drug.

CONTRAINDICATIONS
Administration is contraindicated in patients with any of the following:
    Hypersensitivity to cycloserine
    Epilepsy
    Depression, severe anxiety, or psychosis
    Severe renal insufficiency
    Excessive concurrent use of alcoholic beverages

WARNINGS
Administration of Seromycin® (Cycloserine Capsules, USP, Lilly) should be discontinued or the dosage reduced if the patient develops allergic dermatitis or symptoms of CNS toxicity, such as convulsions, psychosis, somnolence, depression, confusion, hyperreflexia, headache, tremor, vertigo, paresis, or dysarthria.
The toxicity of Seromycin is closely related to excessive blood levels (above 30 mg/L), as determined by high dosage or inadequate renal clearance. The ratio of toxic dose to effective dose in tuberculosis is small.
The risk of convulsions is increased in chronic alcoholics. Patients should be monitored by hematologic, renal excretion, blood level, and liver function studies.

PRECAUTIONS
General—Before treatment with Seromycin® (Cycloserine Capsules, USP, Lilly) is initiated, cultures should be taken and the organism's susceptibility to the drug should be established. In tuberculous infections, the organism's susceptibility to the other antituberculosis agents in the regimen should also be demonstrated.
Anticonvulsant drugs or sedatives may be effective in controlling symptoms of CNS toxicity, such as convulsions, anxiety, and tremor. Patients receiving more than 500 mg of Seromycin daily should be closely observed for such symptoms. The value of pyridoxine in preventing CNS toxicity from cycloserine has not been proved.
Administration of Seromycin and other antituberculosis drugs has been associated in a few instances with vitamin B_{12} and/or folic acid deficiency, megaloblastic anemia, and sideroblastic anemia. If evidence of anemia develops during treatment, appropriate studies and therapy should be instituted.
Laboratory Tests—Blood levels should be determined at least weekly for patients with reduced renal function, for individuals receiving a daily dosage of more than 500 mg, and for those showing signs and symptoms suggestive of toxicity. The dosage should be adjusted to keep the blood level below 30 mg/L.

Continued on next page

• Identi-Code® symbol.

Lilly—Cont.

Drug Interactions—Concurrent administration of ethionamide has been reported to potentiate neurotoxic side effects.

Alcohol and Seromycin are "incompatible," especially during a regimen calling for large doses of the latter. Alcohol increases the possibility and risk of epileptic episodes.

Concurrent administration of isoniazid may result in increased incidence of CNS effects, such as dizziness or drowsiness. Dosage adjustments may be necessary and patients should be monitored closely for signs of CNS toxicity.

Carcinogenesis, Mutagenicity, and Impairment of Fertility—Studies have not been performed to determine potential for carcinogenicity, mutagenicity, or impairment of fertility.

Pregnancy Category C—Animal reproduction studies have not been conducted with Seromycin. It is also not known whether Seromycin can cause fetal harm when administered to a pregnant woman or can affect reproduction capacity. Seromycin should be given to a pregnant woman only if clearly needed.

Nursing Mothers—Because of the potential for serious adverse reactions in nursing infants from Seromycin, a decision should be made whether to discontinue nursing or to discontinue the drug, taking into account the importance of the drug to the mother.

Usage in Children—Safety and dosage have not been established for pediatric use.

ADVERSE REACTIONS

Most adverse reactions occurring during therapy with Seromycin® (Cycloserine Capsules, USP, Lilly) involve the nervous system or are manifestations of drug hypersensitivity. The following side effects have been observed in patients receiving Seromycin:

Nervous system symptoms (which appear to be related to higher dosages of the drug, ie, more than 500 mg daily)
  Convulsions
  Drowsiness and somnolence
  Headache
  Tremor
  Dysarthria
  Vertigo
  Confusion and disorientation with loss of memory
  Psychoses, possibly with suicidal tendencies
    Character changes
    Hyperirritability
    Aggression
  Paresis
  Hyperreflexia
  Paresthesias
  Major and minor (localized)
    clonic seizures
  Coma
Cardiovascular
  Sudden development of congestive heart failure in patients receiving 1 to 1.5 g of Seromycin daily has been reported.
Allergy (apparently not related to dosage)
Skin rash
Miscellaneous
  Elevated serum transaminase, especially in patients with preexisting liver disease

OVERDOSAGE

Signs and Symptoms—Acute toxicity from cycloserine can occur if more than 1 g is ingested by an adult. Chronic toxicity from cycloserine is dose related and can occur if more than 500 mg is administered daily. Patients with renal impairment will accumulate cycloserine and may develop toxicity if the dosing regimen is not modified. Patients with severe renal impairment should not receive the drug. The central nervous system is the most common organ system involved with toxicity. Toxic effects may include headache, vertigo, confusion, drowsiness, hyperirritability, paresthesias, dysarthria, and psychosis. Following larger ingestions, paresis, convulsions, and coma often occur. Ethyl alcohol may increase the risk of seizures in patients receiving cycloserine.

The oral median lethal dose in mice is 5,290 mg/kg.

Treatment—To obtain up-to-date information about the treatment of overdose, a good resource is your certified Regional Poison Control Center. Telephone numbers of certified poison control centers are listed in the *Physicians' Desk Reference (PDR)*. In managing overdosage, consider the possibility of multiple drug overdoses, interaction among drugs, and unusual drug kinetics in your patient.

Overdoses of cycloserine have been reported rarely. The following is provided to serve as a guide should such an overdose be encountered.

Protect the patient's airway and support ventilation and perfusion. Meticulously monitor and maintain, within acceptable limits, the patient's vital signs, blood gases, serum electrolytes, etc. Absorption of drugs from the gastrointestinal tract may be decreased by giving activated charcoal,

which, in many cases, is more effective than emesis or lavage; consider charcoal instead of or in addition to gastric emptying. Repeated doses of charcoal over time may hasten elimination of some drugs that have been absorbed. Safeguard the patient's airway when employing gastric emptying or charcoal.

In adults, many of the neurotoxic effects of cycloserine can be both treated and prevented with the administration of 200 to 300 mg of pyridoxine daily.

The use of hemodialysis has been shown to remove cycloserine from the bloodstream. This procedure should be reserved for patients with life-threatening toxicity that is unresponsive to less invasive therapy.

DOSAGE AND ADMINISTRATION

Seromycin® (Cycloserine Capsules, USP, Lilly) is effective orally and is currently administered only by this route. The usual dosage is 500 mg to 1 g daily in divided doses monitored by blood levels.[2] The initial adult dosage most frequently given is 250 mg twice daily at 12-hour intervals for the first 2 weeks. A daily dosage of 1 g should not be exceeded.

References

1. Kubica GP, Dye WE: Laboratory methods for clinical and public health—mycobacteriology. US Department of Health, Education and Welfare, Public Health Service, 1967, pp. 47–55, 66–70.
2. Jones LR: Colorimetric determination of cycloserine, a new antibiotic. *Anal Chem* 1956; 28:39.

HOW SUPPLIED

(R) Pulvules, 250 mg (No. 12)—(40s) NDC 0002-0604-40
Store at controlled room temperature, 59° to 86°F (15° to 30°C).

[032289]

TAZIDIME®   R

[tă 'zĭ-dēm]
(ceftazidime)
for injection
USP

DESCRIPTION

Tazidime® (Ceftazidime, USP, Lilly) is a semisynthetic, broad-spectrum β-lactam antibiotic for parenteral administration. It is the pentahydrate of pyridinium, 1-[[7-[[(2-amino-4-thiazolyl) [(1-carboxy-1-methylethoxy) imino] acetyl]-amino]-2-carboxy -8- oxo-5-thia -1-azabicyclo[4.2.0] oct-2-en-3-yl]methyl]-, hydroxide, inner salt, [6R-[6α,7β(Z)]]. Tazidime is a sterile, dry powder. Tazidime also contains 118 mg sodium carbonate/g of ceftazidime activity. The total sodium content of the mixture is approximately 54 mg (2.3 mEq)/g of ceftazidime activity. Solutions of Tazidime range from light yellow to amber, depending on the diluent and concentration. The pH of freshly reconstituted solutions usually ranges from 5.0 to 8.0.

CLINICAL PHARMACOLOGY

After intravenous administration of a 500-mg or a 1-g dose of ceftazidime over 5 minutes to normal adult male volunteers, mean peak serum concentrations were 45 mg/L and 90 mg/L, respectively. Following intravenous infusion of 500-mg, 1-g, and 2-g doses of ceftazidime over 20 to 30 minutes to normal adult male volunteers, mean peak serum concentrations of 42, 69, and 170 mg/L, respectively, were achieved. The average serum concentrations following intravenous infusion of 500-mg, 1-g, and 2-g doses to these volunteers over an 8-hour period are given in Table 1.

Table 1. Ceftazidime Concentration in Serum

Ceftazidime Dosage IV	Serum Concentrations (mg/L)				
	½ h	1 h	2 h	4 h	8 h
500 mg	42	25	12	6	2
1 g	60	39	23	11	3
2 g	129	75	42	13	5

The absorption and elimination of ceftazidime were directly proportional to the size of the dose. Following intravenous administration, the half-life was approximately 1.9 hours. Less than 10% of ceftazidime was protein bound. The degree of protein binding was independent of concentration. Following multiple intravenous doses of 1 g and 2 g every 8 hours for 10 days, there was no evidence of accumulation of ceftazidime in the serum in individuals with normal renal function.

Following intramuscular administration of 500-mg and 1-g doses of ceftazidime to normal adult volunteers, the mean peak serum concentrations at approximately 1 hour were 17 mg/L and 39 mg/L, respectively. Serum concentrations remained above 4 mg/L for 6 and 8 hours after the intramuscular administration of 500-mg and 1-g doses, respectively. The half-life of ceftazidime in these volunteers was approximately 2 hours.

The presence of hepatic dysfunction had no effect on the pharmacokinetics of ceftazidime in individuals who received 2 g intravenously every 8 hours for 5 days. Therefore, dosage adjustment is not required for patients with hepatic dysfunction, unless renal function is impaired.

Approximately 80% to 90% of an intramuscular or intravenous dose of ceftazidime is excreted unchanged by the kidneys over a 24-hour period. After the intravenous administration of a single 500-mg or 1-g dose, approximately 50% of the dose appeared in the urine in the first 2 hours. An additional 20% was excreted 2 and 4 hours after administration, and approximately another 12% of the dose appeared in the urine 4 to 8 hours later. The elimination of ceftazidime by the kidneys resulted in high urinary concentrations.

The mean renal clearance of ceftazidime was approximately 100 mL/min. The calculated plasma clearance of approximately 115 mL/min indicated almost complete elimination of ceftazidime by the renal route. The administration of probenecid prior to administration of ceftazidime had no effect on the elimination kinetics of ceftazidime. This suggested that ceftazidime is eliminated by glomerular filtration and is not actively secreted by renal tubular mechanisms.

Since ceftazidime is eliminated almost solely by the kidneys, its serum half-life is significantly prolonged in patients with impaired renal function. Consequently, dosage for such patients must be adjusted (see Dosage and Administration). Therapeutic concentrations of ceftazidime are achieved in the following tissues and body fluids: [See table below].

Microbiology—In vitro tests demonstrate that ceftazidime is bactericidal, exerting its effect by inhibition of enzymes responsible for cell-wall synthesis. Ceftazidime has in vitro activity against a wide range of gram-negative organisms, including strains resistant to gentamicin and other aminoglycosides. In addition, ceftazidime has been shown to be active against gram-positive organisms. It is highly stable to most clinically important β-lactamases, plasmid or chromosomal, that are produced by gram-negative or gram-positive organisms and consequently is active against many strains resistant to ampicillin and other cephalosporins.

Ceftazidime has been shown to be active against the following organisms both in vitro and in clinical infections:

Gram-Negative—*Pseudomonas* sp (including *Pseudomonas aeruginosa*); *Klebsiella* sp (including *Klebsiella pneumoniae*); *Proteus mirabilis*; *Proteus vulgaris*; *Escherichia coli*; *Enterobacter* sp (including *Enterobacter cloacae* and *En-*

Table 2: Ceftazidime Concentrations in Tissues and Body Fluids

Tissue or Fluid	Dose/ Route	No. of Patients	Time of Sample Post-Dose	Average Tissue or Fluid Level (mg/L)
Urine	500 mg IM	6	0–2 h	2,100.0
	2 g IV	6	0–2 h	12,000.0
Bile	2 g IV	3	90 min	36.4
Synovial fluid	2 g IV	13	2 h	25.6
Peritoneal fluid	2 g IV	8	2 h	48.6
Sputum	1 g IV	8	1 h	9.0
Cerebrospinal fluid	2 g q8h IV	5	120 min	9.8
(inflamed meninges)	2 g q8h IV	6	180 min	9.4
Aqueous humor	2 g IV	13	1–3 h	11.0
Blister fluid	1 g IV	7	2–3 h	19.7
Lymphatic fluid	1 g IV	7	2–3 h	23.4
Bone	2 g IV	8	0.67 h	31.1
Heart muscle	2 g IV	35	30–280 min	12.7
Skin	2 g IV	22	30–180 min	6.6
Skeletal muscle	2 g IV	35	30–280 min	9.4
Myometrium	2 g IV	31	1–2 h	18.7

terobacter aerogenes); Citrobacter sp (including Citrobacter freundii and Citrobacter diversus); Serratia sp; Haemophilus influenzae, including ampicillin-resistant strains; and Neisseria meningitidis.

Gram-Positive —Staphylococcus aureus, including penicillinase- and non-penicillinase-producing strains; Streptococcus pyogenes (group A β-hemolytic streptococci); Streptococcus agalactiae (group B streptococci); and Streptococcus pneumoniae.

Anaerobic Organisms —Bacteroides sp (NOTE: most strains of Bacteroides fragilis are resistant).

Although clinical efficacy has not been established, ceftazidime has also been shown to demonstrate in vitro activity against the following microorganisms:

Staphylococcus epidermidis; Morganella morganii (formerly Proteus morganii); Providencia sp (including Providencia rettgeri, formerly Proteus rettgeri); Acinetobacter sp; Salmonella sp; Clostridium sp (not including Clostridium difficile); Peptococcus sp; Peptostreptococcus sp; Neisseria gonorrhoeae; Haemophilus parainfluenzae; Yersinia enterocolitica; and Shigella sp.

Ceftazidime and the aminoglycosides have been shown to be synergistic in vitro against some strains of P aeruginosa and the Enterobacteriaceae. Ceftazidime and carbenicillin have also been shown to be synergistic in vitro against P aeruginosa.

Ceftazidime is not active in vitro against methicillin-resistant staphylococci; Enterococcus faecalis (formerly Streptococcus faecalis) and many other enterococci; Listeria monocytogenes; Campylobacter sp; or C difficile.

Susceptibility Tests —Quantitative methods that require measurement of zone diameters give the most precise estimates of antibiotic susceptibility. One such procedure[1-3] has been recommended for use with disks to test susceptibility to ceftazidime.

Reports from the laboratory giving results of the standardized single-disk susceptibility test using a 30-µg ceftazidime disk should be interpreted according to the following criteria:

Susceptible organisms produce zones of 18 mm or greater, indicating that the tested organism is likely to respond to therapy.

Organisms of intermediate susceptibility produce zones of 15 to 17 mm, indicating that the tested organism would be susceptible if high dosage is used or if the infection is confined to tissues and fluids (eg, urine) in which high antibiotic levels are attained.

Resistant organisms produce zones of ≤14 mm, indicating that other therapy should be selected.

Organisms should be tested with the ceftazidime disk, because ceftazidime has been shown by in vitro tests to have activity against certain strains found to be resistant when tested with other β-lactam disks.

Standardized procedures require the use of laboratory control organisms. The 30-µg ceftazidime disk should give zone diameters between 25 mm and 32 mm for E coli ATCC 25922, between 22 mm and 29 mm for P aeruginosa ATCC 27853, and between 16 mm and 20 mm for S aureus ATCC 25923.

In other susceptibility testing procedures (eg, ICS agar dilution or its equivalent), a bacterial isolate may be considered susceptible if the MIC value for ceftazidime is not >16 mg/L. Organisms are considered resistant if the MIC is ≥64 mg/L. Organisms having an MIC value of <64 mg/L but >16 mg/L are expected to be susceptible if high dosage is used or if the infection is confined to tissues and fluids (eg, urine) in which high antibiotic levels are attained.

As with standard diffusion methods, dilution procedures require the use of laboratory control organisms. Standard ceftazidime powder should give MIC values of 4 mg/L to 16 mg/L for S aureus ATCC 25923, 0.125 mg/L to 0.5 mg/L for E coli ATCC 25922, and 0.5 mg/L to 2 mg/L for P aeruginosa ATCC 27853.

INDICATIONS AND USAGE

Tazidime® (Ceftazidime, USP, Lilly) is indicated for the treatment of infections caused by susceptible strains of the designated organisms in the diseases listed below:

Lower respiratory tract infections, including pneumonia, caused by P aeruginosa and other Pseudomonas sp; H influenzae (including ampicillin-resistant strains); Klebsiella sp; Enterobacter sp; P mirabilis; E coli; Serratia sp; Citrobacter sp; S pneumoniae; and S aureus (methicillin-susceptible strains)

Skin and skin-structure infections caused by P aeruginosa; Klebsiella sp; E coli; Proteus sp (including P mirabilis and indole-positive Proteus); Enterobacter sp; Serratia sp; S aureus (methicillin-susceptible strains); and S pyogenes (group A β-hemolytic streptococci)

Urinary tract infections, both complicated and uncomplicated, caused by P aeruginosa; Enterobacter sp; Proteus sp (including P mirabilis and indole-positive Proteus); Klebsiella sp; and E coli

Bacterial septicemia caused by P aeruginosa; Klebsiella sp; H influenzae; E coli; Serratia sp; S pneumoniae; and S aureus (methicillin-susceptible strains)

Bone and joint infections caused by P aeruginosa; Klebsiella sp; Enterobacter sp; and S aureus (methicillin-susceptible strains)

Gynecologic infections, including endometritis, pelvic cellulitis, and other infections of the female genital tract, caused by E coli

Intra-abdominal infections, including peritonitis, caused by E coli, Klebsiella sp, and S aureus (methicillin-susceptible strains) and polymicrobial infections caused by aerobic and anaerobic organisms and Bacteroides sp (NOTE: Most strains of B. fragilis are resistant)

Central-nervous-system infections, including meningitis, caused by H influenzae and Neisseria meningitidis. Tazidime has also been used successfully in a limited number of cases of menigitis due to P aeruginosa and S pneumoniae

Specimens for bacteriologic cultures should be obtained prior to therapy in order to isolate and identify causative organisms and to determine their susceptibilities to ceftazidime. Therapy may be instituted before results of susceptibility studies are known; however, once these results become available, the antibiotic treatment should be adjusted accordingly.

Tazidime may be used alone in cases of confirmed or suspected sepsis. Tazidime has been used successfully as empiric therapy in clinical trial cases involving concomitant therapies with other antibiotics.

Tazidime may also be used concomitantly with other antibiotics, such as aminoglycosides, vancomycin, and clindamycin, in severe and life-threatening infections and in the immunocompromised patient. When such concomitant treatment is appropriate, prescribing information in the labeling for the other antibiotics should be followed. The dose depends on the severity of the infection and the patient's condition.

CONTRAINDICATIONS

Tazidime® (Ceftazidime, USP, Lilly) is contraindicated in patients who have shown hypersensitivity to ceftazidime or the cephalosporin group of antibiotics.

WARNINGS

BEFORE THERAPY WITH TAZIDIME® (Ceftazidime, USP, Lilly) IS INSTITUTED, CAREFUL INQUIRY SHOULD BE MADE TO DETERMINE WHETHER THE PATIENT HAS HAD PREVIOUS HYPERSENSITIVITY REACTIONS TO CEFTAZIDIME, CEPHALOSPORINS, PENICILLINS, OR OTHER DRUGS. ANTIBIOTICS SHOULD BE ADMINISTERED WITH CAUTION TO ANY PATIENT WHO HAS DEMONSTRATED SOME FORM OF ALLERGY, PARTICULARLY TO DRUGS. THIS PRODUCT SHOULD BE GIVEN WITH CAUTION TO PATIENTS WITH TYPE 1 HYPERSENSITIVITY REACTIONS TO PENICILLIN. IF AN ALLERGIC REACTION TO TAZIDIME OCCURS, DISCONTINUE TREATMENT WITH THE DRUG. SERIOUS ACUTE HYPERSENSITIVITY REACTIONS MAY REQUIRE EPINEPHRINE AND OTHER EMERGENCY MEASURES.

Pseudomembranous colitis has been reported with virtually all broad-spectrum antibiotics (including macrolides, semisynthetic penicillins, and cephalosporins); therefore, it is important to consider its diagnosis in patients who develop diarrhea in association with the use of antibiotics.

Treatment with broad-spectrum antibiotics alters normal flora of the colon and may permit overgrowth of clostridia. Studies indicate a toxin produced by C difficile is a primary cause of antibiotic-associated colitis.

Mild cases of pseudomembranous colitis responded to drug discontinuance alone. In moderate to severe cases, management should include fluid, electrolyte, and protein supplementation. When the colitis does not improve by drug discontinuance or when it is severe, oral vancomycin is the drug of choice for antibiotic-associated pseudomembranous colitis produced by C difficile. Other causes of colitis should be ruled out.

PRECAUTIONS

General —Tazidime® (Ceftazidime, USP, Lilly) has not been shown to be nephrotoxic; however, because high and prolonged serum antibiotic concentrations can occur from usual doses in patients with transient or persistent reduction of urinary output because of renal insufficiency, the total daily dosage should be reduced when ceftazidime is administered to such patients (see Dosage and Administration). In such cases, dosage should be determined by degree of renal impairment, severity of infection, and susceptibility of the causative organisms.

As with other antibiotics, prolonged use of Tazidime may result in overgrowth of nonsusceptible organisms. Repeated evaluation of the patient's condition is essential. If superinfection occurs during therapy, appropriate measures should be taken.

Tazidime should be prescribed with caution in individuals with a history of gastrointestinal disease, particularly colitis.

Drug Interactions —Nephrotoxicity has been reported following the concomitant administration of cephalosporins with aminoglycoside antibiotics or potent diuretics, such as furosemide. Renal function should be carefully monitored

because of the potential nephrotoxicity and ototoxicity of aminoglycoside antibiotics, especially if higher dosages of the aminoglycosides are to be administered or if therapy is prolonged. Nephrotoxicity and ototoxicity were not noted when Tazidime was given alone in clinical trials.

Carcinogenesis, Mutagenesis, Impairment of Fertility —Long-term studies in animals have not been performed to evaluate carcinogenic potential. However, a mouse micronucleus test and an Ames test were both negative for mutagenic effects.

Usage in Pregnancy —Pregnancy Category B —Reproduction studies have been performed in mice and rats at doses up to 40 times the human dose and have revealed no evidence of impaired fertility or harm to the fetus due to Tazidime. There are, however, no adequate and well-controlled studies in pregnant women. Because animal reproduction studies are not always predictive of human response, this drug should be used during pregnancy only if clearly needed.

Nursing Mothers —Ceftazidime is excreted in human milk in low concentrations. Caution should be exercised when Tazidime is administered to a nursing woman.

ADVERSE REACTIONS

Tazidime® (Ceftazidime, USP, Lilly) is generally well tolerated. The incidence of adverse reactions associated with the administration of Tazidime was low in clinical trials. The most common were local reactions following intravenous injection and allergic and gastrointestinal reactions. Other adverse reactions were encountered infrequently. No disulfiram-like reactions were reported. The following adverse effects during clinical trials were considered to be either related to ceftazidime therapy or of uncertain etiology:

Local effects, reported in <2% of patients, were phlebitis and inflammation at the site of injection (1 in 69 patients).

Hypersensitivity reactions, reported in 2% of patients, were pruritus, rash, and fever. Immediate hypersensitivity reactions occurred in 1 in 285 patients.

Gastrointestinal symptoms, reported in <2% of patients, were diarrhea (1 in 78), nausea (1 in 156), vomiting (1 in 500), and abdominal pain (1 in 416).

Less frequent adverse events (<1%) were candidiasis and vaginitis; central-nervous-system events included headache, dizziness, and paresthesia.

Laboratory test changes noted during clinical trials with Tazidime were transient and included eosinophilia (1 in 13), positive Coombs' test without hemolysis (1 in 23), thrombocytosis (1 in 45), and slight elevations in 1 or more of the hepatic enzymes: SGOT (1 in 16), SGPT (1 in 15), LDH (1 in 18), and alkaline phosphatase (1 in 23). As with some other cephalosporins, transient elevations of blood urea, blood urea nitrogen, and/or serum creatinine were observed occasionally. Transient leukopenia, neutropenia, thrombocytopenia, and lymphocytosis were seen very rarely.

OVERDOSAGE

Signs and Symptoms —Toxic signs and symptoms following an overdose of ceftazidime may include pain, inflammation, and phlebitis at the injection site.

The administration of inappropriately large doses of parenteral cephalosporins may cause dizziness, paresthesias, and headaches. Seizures may occur following overdosage with some cephalosporins, particularly in patients with renal impairment where accumulation is likely to occur.

Laboratory abnormalities that may occur after an overdose include elevations in creatinine, BUN, liver enzymes, and bilirubin, a positive Coombs' test, thrombocytosis, thrombocytopenia, eosinophilia, leukopenia, and prolongation of the prothrombin time.

The subcutaneous LD_{50} values in rats and mice ranged from 5.8 to 20 g/kg, and the intravenous LD_{50} values in rabbits were >2 g/kg.

Treatment —To obtain up-to-date information about the treatment of overdose, a good resource is your certified Regional Poison Control Center. Telephone numbers of certified poison control centers are listed in the Physicians' Desk Reference (PDR). In managing overdosage, consider the possibility of multiple drug overdoses, interaction among drugs, and unusual drug kinetics in your patient.

If seizures occur, the drug should be discontinued promptly; anticonvulsant therapy may be administered if clinically indicated. Protect the patient's airway and support ventilation and perfusion. Meticulously monitor and maintain, within acceptable limits, the patient's vital signs, blood gases, serum electrolytes, etc.

In cases of severe overdosage, especially in a patient with renal failure, combined hemodialysis and hemoperfusion may be considered if response to more conservative therapy fails. However, no data supporting such therapy are available.

Continued on next page

Lilly—Cont.

DOSAGE AND ADMINISTRATION

The usual adult dosage is 1 g administered intravenously or intramuscularly every 8 or 12 hours. The dosage and route of administration should be determined by the susceptibility of the causative organisms, the severity of infection, and the condition and renal function of the patient.

The guidelines for dosage of Tazidime® (Ceftazidime, USP, Lilly) are listed in Table 3. The following dosage schedule is recommended:

[See table below].

Patients with Impaired Hepatic Function —No adjustment in dosage is required for patients with hepatic dysfunction.

Patients with Impaired Renal Function —Ceftazidime is excreted by the kidneys, almost exclusively by glomerular filtration. Therefore, in patients with impaired renal function (GFR < 50 mL/min), it is recommended that the dose of Tazidime be reduced to compensate for its slower excretion. In patients with suspected renal insufficiency, an initial loading dose of 1 g of Tazidime may be given. An estimate of GFR should be made to determine the appropriate maintenance dose. The recommended dosage is presented in Table 4.

Table 4. Recommended Maintenance Dosage of Tazidime® (Ceftazidime, USP, Lilly) in Patients With Renal Insufficiency

Creatinine Clearance (mL/min)	Recommended Dose of Tazidime	Frequency
50–31	1 g	q12h
30–16	1 g	q24h
15–6	500 mg	q24h
<5	500 mg	q48h

When only serum creatinine is available, the following formula (Cockcroft's equation)[4] may be used to estimate creatinine clearance. The serum creatinine should represent a steady state of renal function:

$$\text{Males:} = \frac{\text{Weight (kg)} \times (140 - \text{age})}{72 \times \text{serum creatinine (mg/dL)}}$$

Creatinine Clearance (mL/min)

Females: $0.85 \times$ above value

In patients with severe infections who would normally receive 6 g of Tazidime daily were it not for renal insufficiency, the dose given in the above table may be increased by 50% or the dosing frequency increased appropriately. Continued dosage should be determined by therapeutic monitoring, severity of the infection, and susceptibility of the causative organism.

In children, as in adults, the creatinine clearance should be adjusted for body surface area or lean body mass and the dosing frequency should be reduced in cases of renal insufficiency.

In patients undergoing hemodialysis, a loading dose of 1 g of Tazidime is recommended, followed by 1 g after each hemodialysis period.

Tazidime can also be used in patients undergoing intraperitoneal dialysis (IPD) and continuous ambulatory peritoneal dialysis (CAPD). In such patients, a loading dose of 1 g of Tazidime may be given, followed by 500 mg every 24 hours. In addition to intravenous use, Tazidime can be incorporated in dialysis fluid at a concentration of 250 mg/2 L of dialysis fluid.

NOTE: Tazidime should generally be continued for 2 days after the signs and symptoms of infection have disappeared; however, in complicated infections, longer therapy may be required.

Administration —Tazidime® (Ceftazidime, USP, Lilly) may be given intravenously or by deep intramuscular injection into a large muscle mass (such as the upper outer quadrant of the gluteus maximus or lateral part of the thigh).

Intramuscular Administration —For intramuscular administration, Tazidime should be reconstituted with 1 of the following diluents: Sterile Water for Injection, Bacteriostatic Water for Injection, or 0.5% or 1.0% Lidocaine Hydrochloride Injection. Refer to Table 5.

Intravenous Administration —The IV route is preferable for patients with bacterial septicemia, bacterial meningitis, peritonitis, or other severe or life-threatening infections. It is also preferable for patients who may be poor risks because of lowered resistance resulting from such debilitating conditions as malnutrition, trauma, surgery, diabetes, heart failure, or malignancy, particularly if shock is present or impending.

For direct intermittent intravenous administration, reconstitute Tazidime with Sterile Water for Injection (see Table 5). Slowly inject the solution directly into the vein over a period of 3 to 5 minutes or give through the tubing of an administration set while the patient is also receiving 1 of the compatible intravenous fluids (see Compatibility and Stability).

For intravenous infusion, reconstitute the 1-g or 2-g piggyback (100-mL) vial with 50 or 100 mL Sterile Water for Injection or 1 of the compatible intravenous fluids listed in the Compatibility and Stability section. Alternatively, reconstitute the 500-mg, 1-g, or 2-g vial and add an appropriate quantity of the resulting solution to an IV container with 1 of the compatible intravenous fluids.

Table 5: Preparation of Solutions of Tazidime® (Ceftazidime, USP, Lilly)

	Amount of Diluent to Be Added (mL)	Approximate Available Volume (mL)	Approximate Ceftazidime Concentration (mg/mL)
Intramuscular			
500 mg, Vial No. 7230	1.5	1.8	280
1 g, Vial No. 7231	3.0	3.6	280
Intravenous			
500 mg, Vial No. 7230	5	5.3	100
1 g, Vial No. 7231	5 or 10	5.6 or 10.6	180 or 100
2 g, Vial No. 7234	10	11.2	180
Piggyback (100 mL)			
1 g, Vial No. 7238	50* or 100*	50 or 100	20 or 10
2 g, Vial No. 7239	50* or 100*	50 or 100	40 or 20

*Note: Addition should be in 2 stages (see Instructions for Reconstitution below).

Intermittent intravenous infusion with a Y-type administration set can be accomplished with compatible solutions. However, during infusion of a solution containing ceftazidime, it is desirable to discontinue the other solution.

ADD-Vantage® vials are to be used only with Abbott ADD-Vantage diluent bags according to the printed tray card instructions included in each Traypak of vials.

ADD-Vantage vials that have been joined to Abbott ADD-Vantage bags of diluent and activated to dissolve the drug are stable for 24 hours at room temperature. Joined vials which have not been activated may be used within a 14-day period; this period corresponds to that for use of Abbott ADD-Vantage containers following removal of the outer packaging (overwrap).

Freezing solutions of Tazidime in the ADD-Vantage system is not recommended.

[See table above].

When Tazidime® (Ceftazidime, USP, Lilly) is dissolved, carbon dioxide is released and a positive pressure develops. For ease of use, please follow the recommended techniques of reconstitution described below.

Solutions of Tazidime, like those of most β-lactam antibiotics, should not be added to solutions of aminoglycoside antibiotics because of potential interaction. However, if concurrent therapy with Tazidime and an aminoglycoside is indicated, each of these antibiotics should be administered in different sites.

Instructions for Reconstitution:

For 500-mg IM/IV, 1-g IM/IV, and 2-g IV vials

1. Inject the diluent and shake well to dissolve.
2. Carbon dioxide is released as the antibiotic dissolves, generating pressure within the vial. The solution will become clear within 1 to 2 minutes.
3. Invert the vial, and completely depress the syringe plunger prior to insertion.
4. Insert the needle through the vial stopper. Be sure the needle remains within the solution, and withdraw contents of the vial in the usual manner. Pressure in the vial may aid withdrawal.
5. The withdrawn solution may contain carbon dioxide bubbles which should be expelled from the syringe before injection.

For 1-g and 2-g piggyback vials

1. Inject 10 mL of the diluent and shake to dissolve.
2. Carbon dioxide is released as the antibiotic dissolves, generating pressure within the vial. The solution will become clear within 1 to 2 minutes.
3. Insert a vent needle to release pressure before adding additional diluent to the vial. Add diluent and then remove the vent needle.
4. After storage, any additional pressure that may develop in the vial prior to administration should be released.

COMPATIBILITY AND STABILITY

Intramuscular —Vials of Tazidime® (Ceftazidime, USP, Lilly), when reconstituted as directed with Sterile Water for Injection, Bacteriostatic Water for Injection, or 0.5% or 1% Lidocaine Hydrochloride Injection, maintain satisfactory potency for 24 hours at room temperature or for 10 days under refrigeration. Solutions in Sterile Water for Injection that are frozen immediately after reconstitution in the original container are stable for 3 months when stored at −20°C. Once thawed, solutions should not be refrozen. Thawed solutions may be stored for up to 24 hours at room temperature or for 4 days in a refrigerator.

Intravenous —Vials of Tazidime, when reconstituted as directed with Sterile Water for Injection, maintain satisfactory potency for 24 hours at room temperature or for 10 days under refrigeration. Solutions in Sterile Water for Injection in the original container or in 0.9% Sodium Chloride Injection or 5% Dextrose Injection in PVC small-volume containers that are frozen immediately after reconstitution are stable for 3 months when stored at −20°C. When it is necessary to warm a large volume of the frozen product (to a maximum

Table 3: Recommended Dosage Schedule for Ceftazidime

	Dose	Frequency
Adults		
Usual recommended dose	**1 g IV or IM**	**q8 or 12h**
Uncomplicated urinary tract infections	250 mg IV or IM	q12h
Bone and joint infections	2 g IV	q12h
Complicated urinary tract infections	500 mg IV or IM	q8 or 12h
Uncomplicated pneumonia; mild skin and skin-structure infections	500 mg–1 g IV or IM	q8h
Serious gynecologic and intra-abdominal infections	2 g IV	q8h
Meningitis	2 g IV	q8h
Very severe life-threatening infections, especially in immunocompromised patients	2 g IV	q8h
Pseudomonal lung infections in patients with cystic fibrosis with normal renal function*	30–50 mg/kg IV to a maximum of 6 g/day	q8h
Neonates (0 to 4 weeks)	30 mg/kg IV	q12h
Infants and Children (1 month to 12 years of age)	30–50 mg/kg IV to a maximum of 6 g/day†	q8h

* Although clinical improvement has been shown, bacteriologic cures cannot be expected in patients with chronic respiratory disease and cystic fibrosis.

† The higher dose should be reserved for immunocompromised children or children with cystic fibrosis or meningitis.

of 40°C), care should be taken to avoid heating it after thawing is complete. Once thawed, solutions should not be refrozen. Thawed solutions may be stored for up to 24 hours at room temperature or for 4 days in a refrigerator.

Tazidime is compatible with the more commonly used intravenous infusion fluids. Solutions at concentrations from 1 mg/mL to 40 mg/mL in the following infusion fluids may be stored for up to 24 hours at room temperature or for 10 days if refrigerated: 0.9% Sodium Chloride Injection; M/6 Sodium Lactate Injection; Ringer's Injection, USP; Lactated Ringer's Injection, USP; 5% Dextrose Injection; 5% Dextrose and 0.225% Sodium Chloride Injection; 5% Dextrose and 0.45% Sodium Chloride Injection; 5% Dextrose and 0.9% Sodium Chloride Injection; 10% Dextrose Injection; 10% Invert Sugar in Water for Injection; and Normosol®-M in 5% Dextrose Injection.

When diluted with Abbott's ADD-Vantage diluents, 0.9% Sodium Chloride Injection and 5% Dextrose Injection, ADD-Vantage Tazidime may be stored for up to 24 hours at room temperature.

Tazidime is less stable in Sodium Bicarbonate Injection than in other intravenous fluids. Sodium Bicarbonate Injection is not recommended as a diluent. Solutions of Tazidime in 5% Dextrose or 0.9% Sodium Chloride Injection are stable for at least 6 hours at room temperature in plastic tubing, drip chambers, and volume control devices of common intravenous infusion sets.

At a concentration of 4 mg/mL, Tazidime has been found to be compatible for 24 hours at room temperature or for 10 days under refrigeration in 0.9% Sodium Chloride Injection or 5% Dextrose Injection when admixed with cefuroxime sodium, 3 mg/mL; heparin, 10 units/mL or 50 units/mL; or potassium chloride, 10 mEq/L or 40 mEq/L.

Note: Parenteral drug products should be inspected visually for particulate matter whenever solution and container permit.

Tazidime powder and solutions will darken under certain storage conditions. However, product potency is not adversely affected if proper storage conditions and periods are observed.

HOW SUPPLIED

(℞) Vials (Dry Powder):

500 mg,* 10-mL size (No. 7230)—(Traypak† of 25) NDC 0002-7230-25

1 g,* 20-mL size (No. 7231)—(Traypak of 25) NDC 0002-7231-25

1 g,* 100-mL size (No. 7238)—(Traypak of 10) NDC 0002-7238-10

2 g,* 50-mL size (No. 7234)—(Traypak of 10) NDC 0002-7234-10

2 g,* 100-mL size (No. 7239)—(Traypak of 10) NDC 0002-7239-10

(℞) Faspak§:

1 g* (No. 7245)—(Faspak of 24) NDC 0002-7245-24

2 g* (No. 7246)—(Faspak of 24) NDC 0002-7246-24

(℞) ADD-Vantage‡ Vials:

1 g* (No. 7290)—(Traypak of 25) NDC 0002-7290-25

2 g* (No. 7291)—(Traypak of 10) NDC 0002-7291-10

The above ADD-Vantage Vials are to be used only with Abbott Laboratories' ADD-Vantage Diluent Containers. Instructions for the use of ADD-Vantage Vials are enclosed in the package.

Also available:

Pharmacy Bulk Package:

6 g,* 100-mL size (No. 7241)—(Traypak of 6) NDC 0002-7241-16

---

*Equivalent to ceftazidime activity.

†Traypak™(multivial carton, Lilly).

‡ADD-Vantage® (vials and diluent containers, Abbott).

§Faspak® (flexible plastic bag, Lilly).

REFERENCES

1. Bauer AW, Kirby WMM, Sherris J C, et al: Antibiotic susceptibility testing by a standardized single disk method. Am J Clin Pathol 1966; 45:493.

2. National Committee for Clinical Laboratory Standards, Approved Standard: Performance standards for antimicrobial disk susceptibility tests (M2-A3), December, 1984.

3. Standardized disc susceptibility test, Federal Register 1974; 39 (May 30):19182–19184.

4. Cockcroft DW, Gault MH: Prediction of creatinine clearance from serum creatinine, Nephron 1978; 16:31–41.

[021389]

TOBRAMYCIN SULFATE, see Nebcin® (Tobramycin Sulfate Injection, USP, Lilly)

ULTRALENTE® ILETIN® I

[ŭl ′trá-lĕn ′tā ī ′lĕ-tĭn]

(extended insulin zinc suspension, Lilly), see under Iletin® (insulin, Lilly).

VANCOCIN® HCl   ℞

[văn ′kō-sĭn āch ′sē-ĕl]

(vancomycin hydrochloride)

Sterile, USP

IntraVenous

DESCRIPTION

Vancocin® HCl (Sterile Vancomycin Hydrochloride, USP, Lilly), IntraVenous, is a chromatographically purified, tricyclic glycopeptide antibiotic derived from Nocardia orientalis (formerly Streptomyces orientalis) and has the chemical formula $C_{66}H_{75}Cl_2N_9O_{24} \cdot HCl$. The molecular weight is 1,486; 500 mg of the base are equivalent to 0.34 mmol.

The vials contain sterile vancomycin hydrochloride equivalent to either 500 mg or 1 g vancomycin base. Vancomycin hydrochloride is an off-white lyophilized plug. When reconstituted in water, it forms a clear solution with a pH range of 2.5 to 4.5.

CLINICAL PHARMACOLOGY

Vancomycin is poorly absorbed after oral administration; it is given intravenously for therapy of systemic infections. Intramuscular injection is painful.

In subjects with normal kidney function, multiple intravenous dosing of 1 g of vancomycin (15 mg/kg) infused over 60 minutes produces mean plasma concentrations of approximately 63 mg/L immediately at the completion of infusion, mean plasma concentrations of approximately 23 mg/L 2 hours after infusion, and mean plasma concentrations of approximately 8 mg/L 11 hours after the end of the infusion. Multiple dosing of 500 mg infused over 30 minutes produces mean plasma concentrations of about 49 mg/L at the completion of infusion, mean plasma concentrations of about 19 mg/L 2 hours after infusion, and mean plasma concentrations of about 10 mg/L 6 hours after infusion. The plasma concentrations during multiple dosing are similar to those after a single dose.

The mean elimination half-life of vancomycin from plasma is 4 to 6 hours in subjects with normal renal function. In the first 24 hours, about 75% of an administered dose of vancomycin is excreted in urine by glomerular filtration. Mean plasma clearance is about 0.058 L/kg/h, and mean renal clearance is about 0.048 L/kg/h. Renal dysfunction slows excretion of vancomycin. In anephric patients, the average half-life of elimination is 7.5 days. The distribution coefficient is from 0.3 to 0.43 L/kg. There is no apparent metabolism of the drug. About 60% of an intraperitoneal dose of vancomycin administered during peritoneal dialysis is absorbed systemically in 6 hours. Serum concentrations of about 10 mg/L are achieved by intraperitoneal injection of 30 mg/kg of vancomycin. Vancomycin is not effectively removed by either hemodialysis or peritoneal dialysis; there have been no reports of vancomycin clearance with hemoperfusion and hemofiltration.

Total systemic and renal clearance of vancomycin may be reduced in the elderly.

Vancomycin is approximately 55% serum protein bound as measured by ultrafiltration at vancomycin serum concentrations of 10 to 100 mg/L. After IV administration of Vancocin® HCl (Sterile Vancomycin Hydrochloride, USP, Lilly), inhibitory concentrations are present in pleural, pericardial, ascitic, and synovial fluids; in urine; in peritoneal dialysis fluid; and in atrial appendage tissue. Vancocin HCl does not readily diffuse across normal meninges into the spinal fluid; but, when the meninges are inflamed, penetration into the spinal fluid occurs.

Microbiology —The bactericidal action of vancomycin results primarily from inhibition of cell-wall biosynthesis. In addition, vancomycin alters bacterial-cell-membrane permeability and RNA synthesis. There is no cross-resistance between vancomycin and other antibiotics. Vancomycin is active against staphylococci, including Staphylococcus aureus and Staphylococcus epidermidis (including heterogeneous methicillin-resistant strains); streptococci, including Streptococcus pyogenes, Streptococcus pneumoniae (including penicillin-resistant strains), Streptococcus agalactiae, the viridans group, Streptococcus bovis, and enterococci (eg, Enterococcus faecalis [formerly Streptococcus faecalis]); Clostridium difficile (eg, toxigenic strains implicated in pseudomembranous enterocolitis); and diphtheroids. Other organisms that are susceptible to vancomycin in vitro include Listeria monocytogenes, Lactobacillus species, Actinomyces species, Clostridium species, and Bacillus species.

Vancomycin is not active in vitro against gram-negative bacilli, mycobacteria, or fungi.

Synergy —The combination of vancomycin and an aminoglycoside acts synergistically in vitro against many strains of S aureus, nonenterococcal group D streptococci, enterococci, and Streptococcus species (viridans group).

Disk Susceptibility Tests —The standardized disk method described by the National Committee for Clinical Laboratory Standards has been recommended to test susceptibility to vancomycin. Results of standard susceptibility tests with a 30-μg vancomycin hydrochloride disk should be interpreted according to the following criteria: Susceptible organisms

produce zones greater than or equal to 12 mm, indicating that the test organism is likely to respond to therapy. Organisms that produce zones of 10 or 11 mm are considered to be of intermediate susceptibility. Organisms in this category are likely to respond if the infection is confined to tissues or fluids in which high antibiotic concentrations are attained. Resistant organisms produce zones of 9 mm or less, indicating that other therapy should be selected.

With a standardized dilution method, a bacterial isolate may be considered susceptible if the MIC value for vancomycin is 4 mg/L or less. Organisms are considered resistant to vancomycin if the MIC is greater than or equal to 16 mg/L. Organisms having an MIC value of less than 16 mg/L but greater than 4 mg/L are considered to be of intermediate susceptibility.[1-3]

Standardized procedures require the use of laboratory control organisms. The 30-μg vancomycin disk should give zone diameters between 15 and 19 mm for S aureus ATCC 25923. As with the standard diffusion methods, dilution procedures require the use of laboratory control organisms. Standard vancomycin powder should give MIC values in the range of 0.5 mg/L to 2.0 mg/L for S aureus ATCC 29213. For E faecalis ATCC 29212, the MIC range should be 1.0 to 4.0 mg/L.

INDICATIONS AND USAGE

Vancocin® HCl (Sterile Vancomycin Hydrochloride, USP, Lilly) is indicated for the treatment of serious or severe infections caused by susceptible strains of methicillin-resistant (β-lactam-resistant) staphylococci. It is indicated for penicillin-allergic patients, for patients who cannot receive or who have failed to respond to other drugs, including the penicillins or cephalosporins, and for infections caused by vancomycin-susceptible organisms that are resistant to other antimicrobial drugs. Vancocin HCl is indicated for initial therapy when methicillin-resistant staphylococci are suspected, but after susceptibility data are available, therapy should be adjusted accordingly.

Vancocin HCl is effective in the treatment of staphylococcal endocarditis. Its effectiveness has been documented in other infections due to staphylococci, including septicemia, bone infections, lower respiratory tract infections, and skin and skin-structure infections. When staphylococcal infections are localized and purulent, antibiotics are used as adjuncts to appropriate surgical measures.

Vancocin HCl has been reported to be effective alone or in combination with an aminoglycoside for endocarditis caused by Streptococcus viridans or S bovis. For endocarditis caused by enterococci (eg, E faecalis), Vancocin HCl has been reported to be effective only in combination with an aminoglycoside.

Vancocin HCl has been reported to be effective for the treatment of diphtheroid endocarditis. Vancocin HCl has been used successfully in combination with either rifampin, an aminoglycoside, or both in early-onset prosthetic valve endocarditis caused by S epidermidis or diphtheroids.

Specimens for bacteriologic cultures should be obtained in order to isolate and identify causative organisms and to determine their susceptibilities to Vancocin HCl.

The parenteral form of Vancocin HCl may be administered orally for treatment of antibiotic-associated pseudomembranous colitis caused by C difficile and staphylococccal enterocolitis. Parenteral administration of Vancocin HCl alone is of unproven benefit for these indications. Vancocin HCl is not effective by the oral route for other types of infection. Although no controlled clinical efficacy studies have been conducted, intravenous vancomycin has been suggested by the American Heart Association and the American Dental Association as prophylaxis against bacterial endocarditis in penicillin-allergic patients who have congenital heart disease or rheumatic or other acquired valvular heart disease when these patients undergo dental procedures or surgical procedures of the upper respiratory tract.

Note: When selecting antibiotics for the prevention of bacterial endocarditis, the physician or dentist should read the full joint statement of the American Heart Association and the American Dental Association.[4]

CONTRAINDICATION

Vancocin® HCl (Sterile Vancomycin Hydrochloride, USP, Lilly) is contraindicated in patients with known hypersensitivity to this antibiotic.

WARNINGS

Rapid bolus administration (eg, over several minutes) may be associated with exaggerated hypotension and, rarely, cardiac arrest.

Vancocin® HCl (Sterile Vancomycin Hydrochloride, USP, Lilly) should be administered in a dilute solution over a period of not less than 60 minutes to avoid rapid-infusion-related reactions. Stopping the infusion usually results in prompt cessation of these reactions.

Continued on next page

---

* Identi-Code® symbol.

Lilly—Cont.

Ototoxicity has occurred in patients receiving Vancocin HCl. It may be transient or permanent. It has been reported mostly in patients who have been given excessive doses, who have an underlying hearing loss, or who are receiving concomitant therapy with another ototoxic agent, such as an aminoglycoside. Vancomycin should be used with caution in patients with renal insufficiency because the risk of toxicity is appreciably increased by high, prolonged blood concentrations.

Dosage of Vancocin HCl must be adjusted for patients with renal dysfunction (see Precautions and Dosage and Administration).

PRECAUTIONS

General—Clinically significant serum concentrations have been reported in some patients who have taken multiple oral doses of vancomycin for active *C difficile*-induced pseudomembranous colitis.

Prolonged use of Vancocin HCl may result in the overgrowth of nonsusceptible organisms. Careful observation of the patient is essential. If superinfection occurs during therapy, appropriate measures should be taken.

In order to minimize the risk of nephotoxicity when treating patients with underlying renal dysfunction or patients receiving concomitant therapy with an aminoglycoside, serial monitoring of renal function should be performed and particular care should be taken in following appropriate dosing schedules (see Dosage and Administration).

Serial tests of auditory function may be helpful in order to minimize the risk of ototoxicity.

Reversible neutropenia has been reported in patients receiving Vancocin® HCl (Sterile Vancomycin Hydrochloride, USP, Lilly) (see Adverse Reactions). Patients who will undergo prolonged therapy with Vancocin HCl or those who are receiving concomitant drugs that may cause neutropenia should have periodic monitoring of the leukocyte count.

Vancocin HCl is irritating to tissue and must be given by a secure intravenous route of administration. Pain, tenderness, and necrosis occur with intramuscular injection of Vancocin HCl or with inadvertent extravasation. Thrombophlebitis may occur, the frequency and severity of which can be minimized by administering the drug slowly as a dilute solution (2.5 to 5 g/L) and by rotating the sites of infusion. There have been reports that the frequency of infusion-related events (including hypotension, flushing, erythema, urticaria, and pruritus) increases with the concomitant administration of anesthetic agents. Infusion-related events may be minimized by the administration of Vancocin HCl as a 60-minute infusion prior to anesthetic induction.

The safety and efficacy of vancomycin administration by the intrathecal (intralumbar or intraventricular) routes have not been assessed.

Concurrent and/or sequential systemic or topical use of other potentially neurotoxic and/or nephrotoxic drugs, such as amphotericin B, aminoglycosides, bacitracin, polymyxin B, colistin, viomycin, or cisplatin, requires careful monitoring.

Drug Interactions—Concomitant administration of vancomycin and anaesthetic agents has been associated with erythema and histamine-like flushing (see Usage in Pediatrics under Precautions and Adverse Reactions).

Usage in Pregnancy—Pregnancy Category C—Animal reproduction studies have not been conducted with Vancocin HCl. It is also not known whether Vancocin HCl can affect reproduction capacity. In a controlled clinical study, Vancocin HCl was administered to pregnant women for serious staphylococcal infections complicating intravenous drug abuse to evaluate potential ototoxic and nephrotoxic effects on the infant. Vancocin HCl was found in cord blood. No sensorineural hearing loss or nephrotoxicity attributable to Vancocin HCl was noted. One infant whose mother received Vancocin HCl in the third trimester experienced conductive hearing loss that was not attributed to the administration of Vancocin HCl. Because the number of patients treated in this study was limited and Vancocin HCl was administered only in the second and third trimesters, it is not known whether Vancocin HCl cause fetal harm. Vancocin HCl should be given to a pregnant woman only if clearly needed.

Nursing Mothers—Vancocin HCl is excreted in human milk. Caution should be exercised when Vancocin HCl is administered to a nursing woman. Because of the potential for adverse events, a decision should be made whether to discontinue nursing or to discontinue the drug, taking into account the importance of the drug to the mother.

Usage in Pediatrics—In premature neonates and young infants, it may be appropriate to confirm desired vancomycin serum concentrations. Concomitant administration of vancomycin and anesthetic agents has been associated with erythema and histamine-like flushing in children (see Adverse Reactions).

Geriatrics—The natural decrement of glomerular filtration with increasing age may lead to elevated vancomycin serum concentrations if dosage is not adjusted. Vancomycin dosage schedules should be adjusted in elderly patients (see Dosage and Administration).

ADVERSE REACTIONS

Infusion-Related Events—During or soon after rapid infusion of Vancocin® HCl (Sterile Vancomycin Hydrochloride, USP, Lilly), patients may develop anaphylactoid reactions, including hypotension, wheezing, dyspnea, urticaria, or pruritus. Rapid infusion may also cause flushing of the upper body ("red neck") or pain and muscle spasm of the chest and back. These reactions usually resolve within 20 minutes but may persist for several hours. Such events are infrequent if Vancocin HCl is given by a slow infusion over 60 minutes. In studies of normal volunteers, infusion-related events did not occur when Vancocin HCl was administered at a rate of 10 mg/min or less.

Nephrotoxicity—Rarely, renal failure, principally manifested by increased serum creatinine or BUN concentrations, especially in patients given large doses of Vancocin HCl, has been reported. Rare cases of interstitial nephritis have been reported. Most of these have occurred in patients who were given aminoglycosides concomitantly or who had preexisting kidney dysfunction. When Vancocin HCl was discontinued, azotemia resolved in most patients.

Ototoxicity—A few dozen cases of hearing loss associated with Vancocin HCl have been reported. Most of these patients had kidney dysfunction or a preexisting hearing loss or were receiving concomitant treatment with an ototoxic drug. Vertigo, dizziness, and tinnitus have been reported rarely.

Hematopoietic—Reversible neutropenia, usually starting 1 week or more after onset of therapy with Vancocin HCl or after a total dose of more than 25 g, has been reported for several dozen patients. Neutropenia appears to be promptly reversible when Vancocin HCl is discontinued. Thrombocytopenia has rarely been reported.

Phlebitis—Inflammation at the injection site has been reported.

Miscellaneous—Infrequently, patients have been reported to have had anaphylaxis, drug fever, nausea, chills, eosinophilia, rashes, including exfoliative dermatitis, Stevens-Johnson syndrome, and rare cases of vasculitis in association with administration of Vancocin HCl.

OVERDOSAGE

Supportive care is advised, with maintenance of glomerular filtration. Vancomycin is poorly removed by dialysis. Hemofiltration and hemoperfusion with polysulfone resin have been reported to result in increased vancomycin clearance.

DOSAGE AND ADMINISTRATION

A concentration of no more than 10 mg/mL is recommended. An infusion of 10 mg/min or less is associated with fewer infusion-related events (see Adverse Reactions).

Patients With Normal Renal Function

Adults—The usual daily intravenous dose is 2 g divided either as 500 mg every 6 hours or 1 g every 12 hours. Each dose should be administered over a period of at least 60 minutes. Other patient factors, such as age or obesity, may call for modification of the usual daily intravenous dose.

Children—The total daily intravenous dosage of Vancocin® HCl (Sterile Vancomycin Hydrochloride, USP, Lilly), calculated on the basis of 40 mg/kg of body weight, can be divided and incorporated into the child's 24-hour fluid requirement. Each dose should be administered over a period of at least 60 minutes.

Infants and Neonates—In neonates and young infants, the total daily intravenous dosage may be lower. In both neonates and infants, an initial dose of 15 mg/kg is suggested, followed by 10 mg/kg every 12 hours for neonates in the first week of life and every 8 hours thereafter up to the age of 1 month. Close monitoring of serum concentrations of vancomycin may be warranted in these patients.

Patients With Impaired Renal Function and Elderly Patients
Dosage adjustment must be made in patients with impaired renal function. In the elderly, dosage reductions greater than expected may be necessary because of decreased renal function. Measurement of vancomycin serum concentrations can be helpful in optimizing therapy, especially in seriously ill patients with changing renal function. Vancomycin serum concentrations can be determined by use of microbiologic assay, radioimmunoassay, fluorescence polarization immunoassay, fluorescence immunoassay, or high-pressure liquid chromatography.

If creatinine clearance can be measured or estimated accurately, the dosage for most patients with renal impairment can be calculated by using the following table. The dosage of Vancocin HCl per day in mg is about 15 times the glomerular filtration rate in mL/min:

DOSAGE TABLE FOR VANCOMYCIN
IN PATIENTS WITH IMPAIRED RENAL FUNCTION
(Adapted from Moellering et al[5])

Creatinine Clearance mL/min	Vancomycin Dose mg/24 h
100	1,545
90	1,390
80	1,235
70	1,080
60	925
50	770
40	620
30	465
20	310
10	155

The initial dose should be no less than 15 mg/kg, even in patients with mild to moderate renal insufficiency.

The table is not valid for functionally anephric patients. For such patients, an initial dose of 15 mg/kg of body weight should be given to achieve prompt therapeutic serum concentrations. The dose required to maintain stable concentrations is 1.9 mg/kg/24 h. In patients with marked renal impairment, it may be more convenient to give maintenance doses of 250 to 1,000 mg once every several days rather than administering the drug on a daily basis. In anuria, a dose of 1,000 mg every 7 to 10 days has been recommended.

When only the serum creatinine concentration is known, the following formula (based on sex, weight, and age of the patient) may be used to calculate creatinine clearance. Calculated creatinine clearances (mL/min) are only estimates. The creatinine clearance should be measured promptly.

Men:
$$\frac{\text{Weight (kg)} \times (140 - \text{age in years})}{72 \times \text{serum creatinine concentration (mg/dL)}}$$

Women: $0.85 \times$ above value

The serum creatinine must represent a steady state of renal function. Otherwise, the estimated value for creatinine clearance is not valid. Such a calculated clearance is an overestimate of actual clearance in patients with conditions: (1) characterized by decreasing renal function, such as shock, severe heart failure, or oliguria; (2) in which a normal relationship between muscle mass and total body weight is not present, such as obese patients or those with liver disease, edema, or ascites; and (3) accompanied by debilitation, malnutrition, or inactivity.

The safety and efficacy of vancomycin administration by the intrathecal (intralumbar or intraventricular) routes have not been assessed.

Intermittent infusion is the recommended method of administration.

PREPARATION AND STABILITY

At the time of use, reconstitute by adding 10 mL of Sterile Water for Injection to the 500-mg vial or 20 mL of Sterile Water for Injection to the 1-g vial of dry, sterile vancomycin powder. Vials reconstituted in this manner will give a solution of 50 mg/mL. FURTHER DILUTION IS REQUIRED. After reconstitution, the vials may be stored in a refrigerator for 14 days without significant loss of potency. Reconstituted solutions containing 500 mg of vancomycin must be diluted with at least 100 mL of diluent. Reconsitiued solutions containing 1 g must be diluted with at least 200 mL of diluent. The desired dose, diluted in this manner, should be administered by intermittent intravenous infusion over a period of at least 60 minutes.

Compatibility With Intravenous Fluids—Solutions that are diluted with 5% Dextrose Injection or 0.9% Sodium Chloride Injection may be stored in a refrigerator for 14 days without significant loss of potency. Solutions that are diluted with the following infusion fluids may be stored in a refrigerator for 96 hours:

    5% Dextrose Injection and 0.9% Sodium Chloride Injection, USP
    Lactated Ringer's Injection, USP
    Lactated Ringer's and 5% Dextrose Injection
    Normosol®-M and 5% Dextrose
    Isolyte® E
    Acetated Ringer's Injection

Vancomycin solution has a low pH and may cause physical instability of other compounds.

Prior to administration, parenteral drug products should be inspected visually for particulate matter and discoloration whenever solution or container permits.

For Oral Administration—The usual adult total daily dosage for antibiotic-associated pseudomembranous colitis caused by *C. difficile* and staphylococcal enterocolitis is 500 mg to 2 g given in 3 or 4 divided doses for 7 to 10 days. The total daily dosage in children is 40 mg/kg of body weight in 3 or 4 divided doses for 7 to 10 days. The total daily dosage should not exceed 2 g. The appropriate dose may be diluted in 1 oz of water and given to the patient to drink. Common flavoring syrups may be added to the solution to improve the taste for oral administration. The diluted solution may be administered via a nasogastric tube.

HOW SUPPLIED

(℞) Vials:

500 mg,* 10-mL size (No. 657)—(1s) NDC 0002-1444-01; (Traypak† of 10) NDC 0002-1444-10

1 g,* 20-mL size (No. 7321)—(Traypak of 10) NDC 0002-7321-10

Also available:

(℞) ADD-Vantage‡ Vials:

500 mg,* 15-mL size (No. 7297)—(Traypak of 10) NDC 0002-7297-10

1 g,* 15-mL size (No. 7298)—(Traypak of 10) NDC 0002-7298-10

(℞) Pharmacy Bulk Package:

10 g,* 100-mL size (No. 7355)—(1s) NDC 0002-7355-01

Prior to reconstitution, the vials may be stored at room temperature, 59° to 86°F (15° to 30°C).

---

*Equivalent to vancomycin.

†Traypak™ (multivial carton, Lilly).

‡ADD-Vantage® (vials and diluent containers, Abbott).

REFERENCES

1. National Committee for Clinical Laboratory Standards, 1984. Performance standards for antimicrobial disk susceptibility tests, MZ-A3, NCCLS, Villanova, PA 19805.
2. National Committee for Clinical Laboratory Standards, 1983. Methods for dilution antimicrobial susceptibility tests for bacteria that grow aerobically, M7-T, NCCLS, Villanova, PA 19805.
3. National Committee for Clinical Laboratory Standards, 1984. Reference agar dilution procedure for antimicrobial susceptibility testing of anaerobic bacteria, M11-A, NCCLS, Villanova, PA 19805.
4. Shulman ST, Amren DP, Bisno AL, et al: Prevention of bacterial endocarditis. *Circulation* 1984, 70:1123A.
5. Moellering RC, Krogstad DJ, Greenblatt DJ: Vancomycin therapy in patients with impaired renal function: A nomogram for dosage. *Ann Intern Med* 1981; 94:343.

[091288]

VANCOCIN® HCl   ℞

[văn 'kō-sĭn āch 'sē-ĕl]

(vancomycin hydrochloride)

For Oral Solution, USP

Pulvules®

Capsules, USP

This preparation for the treatment of colitis is for oral use only and is not systemically absorbed. Vancocin HCl must be given orally for treatment of staphylococcal enterocolitis and antibiotic-associated pseudomembranous colitis produced by *Clostridium difficile.* Orally administered Vancocin HCl is *not* effective for other types of infection.

Parenteral administration of Vancocin HCl is not effective for treatment of staphylococcal enterocolitis and antibiotic-associated pseudomembranous colitis produced by *Clostridium difficile.* If parenteral vancomycin therapy is desired, use Vancocin® HCl (Sterile Vancomycin Hydrochloride, USP, Lilly), IntraVenous, and consult package insert accompanying that preparation.

DESCRIPTION

Vancocin® HCl for Oral Solution (Vancomycin Hydrochloride for Oral Solution, USP, Lilly) and Pulvules® Vancocin® HCl (Vancomycin Hydrochloride Capsules, USP, Lilly), contain chromatographically purified vancomycin hydrochloride, a tricyclic glycopeptide antibiotic derived from *Nocardia orientalis* (formerly *Streptomyces orientalis*), which has the chemical formula $C_{66}H_{75}Cl_2N_9O_{24} \cdot HCl$. The molecular weight of vancomycin hydrochloride is 1,486; 500 mg of the base are equivalent to 0.34 mmol.

Vancocin HCl for Oral Solution contains vancomycin hydrochloride equivalent to 10 g or 1 g vancomycin.

Each Pulvule contains 125 mg or 250 mg of vancomycin hydrochloride. The Pulvules also contain FD&C Blue No. 2, gelatin, iron oxide, polyethylene glycol, titanium dioxide, and other inactive ingredients.

CLINICAL PHARMACOLOGY

Vancomycin is poorly absorbed after oral administration. During multiple dosing of 250 mg every 8 hours for 7 doses, fecal concentrations of vancomycin in volunteers exceeded 100 mg/kg in the majority of samples. No blood concentrations were detected, and urinary recovery did not exceed 0.76%. In anephric patients with no inflammatory bowel disease, blood concentrations of vancomycin were barely measurable (0.66 mg/L) in 2 of 5 subjects who received 2 g of Vancocin HCl for Oral Solution daily for 16 days. No measurable blood concentrations were attained in the other 3 patients. With doses of 2 g daily, very high concentrations of drug can be found in the feces (> 3,100 mg/kg) and very low concentrations (< 1 mg/L) can be found in the serum of patients with normal renal function who have pseudomembranous colitis. Orally administered vancomycin does not usually enter the systemic circulation even when inflammatory

lesions are present. After multiple-dose oral administration of vancomycin, measurable serum concentrations may infrequently occur in patients with active *C difficile* -induced pseudomembranous colitis, and, in the presence of renal impairment, the possibility of accumulation exists.

Microbiology —The bactericidal action of vancomycin results primarily from inhibition of cell-wall biosynthesis. In addition, vancomycin alters bacterial-cell-membrane permeability and RNA synthesis. There is no cross-resistence between vancomycin and other antibiotics. Vancomycin is active against *C difficile* (eg, toxigenic strains implicated in pseudomembranous enterocolitis). It is also active against staphylococci, including *Staphylococcus aureus.*

For further information, see prescribing information for Vancocin HCl, IntraVenous.

Vancomycin is not active in vitro against gram-negative bacilli, mycobacteria, or fungi.

Disk Susceptibility Tests —The standardized disk and/or dilution methods described by the National Committee for Clinical Laboratory Standards have been recommended for use to test susceptibility to vancomycin.

INDICATIONS AND USAGE

Vancocin® HCl (vancomycin hydrochloride, Lilly) is administered orally for treatment of staphylococcal enterocolitis and antibiotic-associated pseudomembranous colitis produced by *C difficile.* Parenteral administration of Vancocin HCl is not effective for the above indications; therefore, Vancocin HCl must be given orally for these indications. Orally administered Vancocin HCl is *not* effective for other types of infection.

CONTRAINDICATION

Vancocin® HCl (vancomycin hydrochloride, Lilly) is contraindicated in patients with known hypersensitivity to this antibiotic.

PRECAUTIONS

Some patients with inflammatory disorders of the intestinal mucosa may have significant systemic absorption of vancomycin and, therefore, may be at risk for the development of adverse reactions associated with the parenteral administration of vancomycin (See package insert accompanying the intravenous preparation.) The risk is greater if renal impairment is present. It should be noted that the total systemic and renal clearances of vancomycin are reduced in the elderly.

Ototoxicity has occurred in patients receiving Vancocin® HCl (vancomycin hydrochloride, Lilly). It may be transient or permanent. It has been reported mostly in patients who have been given excessive intravenous doses, who have an underlying hearing loss, or who are receiving concomitant therapy with another ototoxic agent, such as an aminoglycoside. Serial tests of auditory function may be helpful in order to minimize the risk of ototoxicity.

When patients with underlying renal dysfunction or those receiving concomitant therapy with an aminoglycoside are being treated, serial monitoring of renal function should be performed.

*Usage in Pregnancy —Pregnancy Category C —*Animal reproduction studies have not been conducted with Vancocin HCl. It is also not known whether Vancocin HCl can cause fetal harm when administered to a pregnant woman or can affect reproduction capacity. Vancocin HCl should be given to a pregnant woman only if clearly needed.

Nursing Mothers —It is not known whether this drug is excreted in human milk. Because many drugs are excreted in human milk, caution should be exercised when Vancocin HCl is administered to a nursing woman. It is unlikely that a nursing infant can absorb a significant amount of vancomycin from the normal gastrointestinal tract.

ADVERSE REACTIONS

Nephrotoxicity —A few dozen cases of increased serum creatinine or BUN concentrations in patients given intravenously administered Vancocin® HCl (vancomycin hydrochloride, Lilly) have been reported. Most of these have occurred in patients who were given aminoglycosides concomitantly or who had preexisting kidney dysfunction. When Vancocin HCl was discontinued, azotemia resolved in most patients.

Ototoxicity —A few dozen cases of hearing loss associated with intravenously administered Vancocin HCl have been reported. Most of these patients had kidney dysfunction, preexisting hearing loss, or concomitant treatment with an ototoxic drug. Vertigo, dizziness, and tinnitus have been reported rarely.

Hematopoietic —Reversible neutropenia, usually starting 1 week or more after onset of intravenous therapy with Vancocin HCl or after a total dose of more than 25 g, has been reported for several dozen patients. Neutropenia appears to be promptly reversible when Vancocin HCl is discontinued. Thrombocytopenia has rarely been reported.

Miscellaneous —Infrequently, patients have been reported to have anaphylaxis, urticaria, drug fever, chills, nausea, and rashes, including exfoliative dermatitis, in association with Vancocin HCl.

OVERDOSAGE

Supportive care is advised, with maintenance of glomerular filtration. Vancomycin is poorly removed by dialysis. Hemoperfusion with Amberlite XAD-4 resin has been reported to be of limited benefit.

DOSAGE AND ADMINISTRATION

Adults —The usual daily dosage for staphyloccus enterocolitis and antibiotic-associated pseudomembranous colitis produced by *C difficile* is 500 mg to 2 g administered orally in 3 or 4 divided doses for 7 to 10 days.

Children —The usual daily dosage is 40 mg/kg in 3 or 4 divided doses for 7 to 10 days. The total daily dosage should not exceed 2 g.

PREPARATION AND STABILITY

Vancocin® HCl (vancomycin hydrochloride, Lilly) for Oral Solution

The contents of the 10-g vial may be mixed with distilled or deionized water (115 mL) for oral administration. When mixed with 115 mL of water, each 6 mL provide approximately 500 mg of vancomycin. The contents of the 1-g vial may be mixed with distilled or deionized water (20 mL). When reconstituted with 20 mL, each 5 mL contains approximately 250 mg of vancomycin. Mix thoroughly to dissolve. These mixtures may be kept for 2 weeks in a refrigerator without significant loss of potency.

The appropriate oral solution dose may be diluted in 1 oz of water and given to the patient to drink. The diluted material may be administered via nasogastric tube. Common flavoring syrups may be added to the solution to improve the taste for oral administration.

HOW SUPPLIED

(℞) For Oral Solution:

10 g* (screw-cap bottle) (No. M-206)—(1s) NDC 0002-2372-37

1 g* (screw-cap bottle) (No. M-5105)—(Traypak† of 6) NDC 0002-5105-16

Prior to reconstitution, store at controlled room temperature, 59° to 86°F (15° to 30°C).

(℞) Pulvules.®

125 mg,* blue and brown (No. 3125)—(ID‡20) NDC 0002-3125-42

250 mg,* blue and gray (No. 3126)—(ID20) NDC 0002-3126-42

Store at controlled room temperature, 59° to 86°F (15° to 30°C).

---

*Equivalent to vancomycin.

†Traypak™ (multivial carton, Lilly).

‡Identi-Dose® (unit dose medication, Lilly).

[032688]

VANCOMYCIN HYDROCHLORIDE,

[văn 'kō-sĭn āch 'sē-ĕl]

see Vancocin® HCl (Vancomycin Hydrochloride, USP, Lilly).

VELBAN®   ℞

[vĕl 'băn]

(vinblastine sulfate)

Sterile, USP

DESCRIPTION

Velban® (Vinblastine Sulfate, USP, Lilly) is the salt of an alkaloid extracted from *Vinca rosea* Linn., a common flowering herb known as the periwinkle (more properly known as *Catharanthus roseus* G Don). Previously, the generic name was vincaleukoblastine, abbreviated VLB. It is a stathmokinetic oncolytic agent. When treated in vitro with this preparation, growing cells are arrested in metaphase.

Chemical and physical evidence indicates that Velban has the empirical formula $C_{46}H_{58}N_4O_9 \cdot H_2SO_4$ and that it is a dimeric alkaloid containing both indole and dihydroindole moieties.

Vials of Velban contain 10 mg of sterile vinblastine sulfate, in the form of a lyophilized plug, without excipients. When sodium chloride solution is added prior to injection, the pH of the resulting solution lies in the range of 3.5 to 5.

Caution—It is extremely important that the needle be properly positioned in the vein before this product is injected. If leakage into surrounding tissue should occur during intravenous administration of Velban, it may cause considerable irritation. The injection should be discontinued immediately, and any remaining portion of the dose should then be introduced into another vein. Local injection of hyaluronidase and the application of moderate heat to the area of leakage

---

Continued on next page

---

* Identi-Code® symbol.

Lilly—Cont.

help disperse the drug and are thought to minimize discomfort and the possibility of cellulitis.

This preparation is for intravenous use only. It should be administered by individuals experienced in the administration of Velban. The intrathecal administration of Velban results in death.

CLINICAL PHARMACOLOGY

Experimental data indicate that the action of Velban® (Vinblastine Sulfate, USP, Lilly) is different from that of other recognized antineoplastic agents. Tissue-culture studies suggest an interference with metabolic pathways of amino acids leading from glutamic acid to the citric acid cycle and to urea. In vivo experiments tend to confirm the in vitro results. A number of studies in vitro and in vivo have demonstrated that Velban produces a stathmokinetic effect and various atypical mitotic figures. The therapeutic responses, however, are not fully explained by the cytologic changes, since these changes are sometimes observed clinically and experimentally in the absence of any oncolytic effects.

Reversal of the antitumor effect of Velban by glutamic acid or tryptophan has been observed. In addition, glutamic acid and aspartic acid have protected mice from lethal doses of Velban. Aspartic acid was relatively ineffective in reversing the antitumor effect.

Other studies indicate that Velban has an effect on cell-energy production required for mitosis and interferes with nucleic acid synthesis.

Pharmacokinetic studies in patients with cancer have shown a triphasic serum decay pattern following rapid intravenous injection. The initial, middle, and terminal half-lives are 3.7 minutes, 1.6 hours, and 24.8 hours respectively. The volume of the central compartments is 70% of body weight, probably reflecting very rapid tissue binding to formed elements of the blood. Extensive reversible tissue binding occurs. Low body stores are present at 48 and 72 hours after injection. Since the major route of excretion may be through the biliary system, toxicity from this drug may be increased when there is hepatic excretory insufficiency. Following injection of tritiated vinblastine in the human cancer patient, 10% of the radioactivity was found in the feces and 14% in the urine; the remaining activity was not accounted for. Similar studies in dogs demonstrated that, over 9 days, 30% to 36% of radioactivity was found in the bile and 12% to 17% in the urine. A similar study in the rat demonstrated that the highest concentrations of radioactivity were found in the lung, liver, spleen, and kidney 2 hours after injection.

Hematologic Effects—Clinically, leukopenia is an expected effect of Velban® (Vinblastine Sulfate, USP, Lilly), and the level of the leukocyte count is an important guide to therapy with this drug. In general, the larger the dose employed, the more profound and longer lasting the leukopenia will be. The fact that the white-blood-cell count returns to normal levels after drug-induced leukopenia is an indication that the white-cell-producing mechanism is not permanently depressed. Usually, the white count has completely returned to normal after the virtual disappearance of white cells from the peripheral blood.

Following therapy with Velban, the nadir in white-blood-cell count may be expected to occur 5 to 10 days after the last day of drug administration. Recovery of the white blood count is fairly rapid thereafter and is usually complete within another 7 to 14 days. With the smaller doses employed for maintenance therapy, leukopenia may not be a problem. Although the thrombocyte count ordinarily is not significantly lowered by therapy with Velban, patients whose bone marrow has been recently impaired by prior therapy with radiation or with other oncolytic drugs may show thrombocytopenia (less than 200,000 platelets/mm³). When other chemotherapy or radiation has not been employed previously, thrombocyte reduction below the level of 200,000/mm³ is rarely encountered, even when Velban may be causing significant leukopenia. Rapid recovery from thrombocytopenia within a few days is the rule.

The effect of Velban upon the red-cell count and hemoglobin is usually insignificant when other therapy does not complicate the picture. It should be remembered, however, that patients with malignant disease may exhibit anemia even in the absence of any therapy.

INDICATIONS AND USAGE

Vinblastine sulfate is indicated in the palliative treatment of the following:

I. Frequently Responsive Malignancies—
    Generalized Hodgkin's disease (Stages III and IV, Ann Arbor modification of Rye staging system)
    Lymphocytic lymphoma (nodular and diffuse, poorly and well differentiated)
    Histiocytic lymphoma
    Mycosis fungoides (advanced stages)
    Advanced carcinoma of the testis
    Kaposi's sarcoma
    Letterer-Siwe disease (histiocytosis X)

II. Less Frequently Responsive Malignancies—
    Choriocarcinoma resistant to other chemotherapeutic agents
    Carcinoma of the breast, unresponsive to appropriate endocrine surgery and hormonal therapy

Current principles of chemotherapy for many types of cancer include the concurrent administration of several antineoplastic agents. For enhanced therapeutic effect without additive toxicity, agents with different dose-limiting clinical toxicities and different mechanisms of action are generally selected. Therefore, although Velban® (Vinblastine Sulfate, USP, Lilly) is effective as a single agent in the aforementioned indications, it is usually administered in combination with other antineoplastic drugs. Such combination therapy produces a greater percentage of response than does a single-agent regimen. These principles have been applied, for example, in the chemotherapy of Hodgkin's disease.

Hodgkin's Disease—Velban has been shown to be one of the most effective single agents for the treatment of Hodgkin's disease. Advanced Hodgkin's disease has also been successfully treated with several multiple-drug regimens that included Velban. Patients who had relapses after treatment with the MOPP program—mechlorethamine hydrochloride (nitrogen mustard), vincristine sulfate (Oncovin® [Vincristine Sulfate Injection, USP, Lilly]), prednisone, and procarbazine—have likewise responded to combination-drug therapy that included Velban. A protocol using cyclophosphamide in place of nitrogen mustard and Velban instead of Oncovin is an alternative therapy for previously untreated patients with advanced Hodgkin's disease.

Advanced testicular germinal-cell cancers (embryonal carcinoma, teratocarcinoma, and choriocarcinoma) are sensitive to Velban alone, but better clinical results are achieved when Velban is administered concomitantly with other antineoplastic agents. The effect of bleomycin is significantly enhanced if Velban is administered 6 to 8 hours prior to the administration of bleomycin; this schedule permits more cells to be arrested during metaphase, the stage of the cell cycle in which bleomycin is active.

CONTRAINDICATIONS

Velban® (Vinblastine Sulfate, USP, Lilly) is contraindicated in patients who have significant granulocytopenia unless this is a result of the disease being treated. It should not be used in the presence of bacterial infections. Such infections must be brought under control prior to the initiation of therapy with Velban.

WARNINGS

This product is for intravenous use only. It should be administered by individuals experienced in the administration of Velban. The intrathecal administration of Velban® (Vinblastine Sulfate, USP, Lilly) results in death.

Usage in Pregnancy—Caution is necessary with the administration of all oncolytic drugs during pregnancy. Information on the use of Velban during human pregnancy is very limited. Animal studies with Velban suggest that teratogenic effects may occur. Vinblastine sulfate can cause fetal harm when administered to a pregnant woman. Laboratory animals given this drug early in pregnancy suffer resorption of the conceptus: surviving fetuses demonstrate gross deformities. There are no adequate and well-controlled studies in pregnant women. If this drug is used during pregnancy, or if the patient becomes pregnant while receiving this drug, she should be apprised of the potential hazard to the fetus. Women of childbearing potential should be advised to avoid becoming pregnant.

Aspermia has been reported in man. Animal studies show metaphase arrest and degenerative changes in germ cells. Leukopenia (granulocytopenia) may reach dangerously low levels following administration of the higher recommended doses. It is therefore important to follow the dosage technique recommended under the Dosage and Administration section. Stomatitis and neurologic toxicity, although not common or permanent, can be disabling.

PRECAUTIONS

General—Toxicity may be enhanced in the presence of hepatic insufficiency.

If leukopenia with less than 2,000 white blood cells/mm³ occurs following a dose of Velban® (Vinblastine Sulfate, USP, Lilly), the patient should be watched carefully for evidence of infection until the white-blood-cell count has returned to a safe level.

When cachexia or ulcerated areas of the skin surface are present, there may be a more profound leukopenic response to the drug; therefore, its use should be avoided in older persons suffering from either of these conditions.

In patients with malignant-cell infiltration of the bone marrow, the leukocyte and platelet counts have sometimes fallen precipitously after moderate doses of Velban. Further use of the drug in such patients is inadvisable.

Acute shortness of breath and severe bronchospasm have been reported following the administration of vinca alkaloids. These reactions have been encountered most frequently when the vinca alkaloid was used in combination with mitomycin-C and may require aggressive treatment, particularly when there is preexisting pulmonary dysfunction. The onset may be within minutes or several hours after the vinca is injected and may occur up to 2 weeks following a dose of mitomycin.

The use of small amounts of Velban daily for long periods is not advised, even though the resulting total weekly dosage may be similar to that recommended. Little or no added therapeutic effect has been demonstrated when such regimens have been used. *Strict adherence to the recommended dosage schedule is very important.* When amounts equal to several times the recommended weekly dosage were given in 7 daily installments for long periods, convulsions, severe and permanent central-nervous-system damage, and even death occurred.

Care must be taken to avoid contamination of the eye with concentrations of Velban used clinically. If accidental contamination occurs, severe irritation (or, if the drug was delivered under pressure, even corneal ulceration) may result. The eye should be washed with water immediately and thoroughly.

It is not necessary to use preservative-containing solvents if unused portions of the remaining solutions are discarded immediately. Unused preservative-containing solutions should be refrigerated for future use.

Information for Patients—The patient should be warned to report immediately the appearance of sore throat, fever, chills, or sore mouth. Advice should be given to avoid constipation, and the patient should be made aware that alopecia may occur and that jaw pain and pain in the organs containing tumor tissue may occur. The latter is thought possibly to result from swelling of tumor tissue during its response to treatment. Scalp hair will regrow to its pretreatment extent even with continued treatment with Velban® (Vinblastine Sulfate, USP, Lilly). Nausea and vomiting, although not common, may occur. Any other serious medical event should be reported to the physician.

Laboratory Tests—Since dose-limiting clinical toxicity is the result of depression of the white-blood-cell count, it is imperative that this count be obtained just before the planned dose of Velban. Following administration of Velban, a fall in the white-blood-cell count may occur. The nadir of this fall is observed from 5 to 10 days following a dose. Recovery to pretreatment levels is usually observed from 7 to 14 days after treatment. These effects will be exaggerated when preexisting bone marrow damage is present and also with the higher recommended doses (see Dosage and Administration). The presence of this drug or its metabolites in blood or body tissues is not known to interfere with clinical laboratory tests.

Drug Interactions—Velban should not be diluted with solvents that raise or lower the pH of the resulting solution from between 3.5 and 5. Solutions should be made with either normal saline or 5% glucose in water (each with or without preservative) and should not be combined in the same container with any other chemical.

Carcinogenesis, Mutagenesis, Impairment of Fertility—Aspermia has been reported in man. Animal studies suggest that teratogenic effects may occur. See Warnings regarding impaired fertility. Animal studies have shown metaphase arrest and degenerative changes in germ cells. Amenorrhea has occurred in some patients treated with the combination consisting of an alkylating agent, procarbazine, prednisone, and Velban. Its occurrence was related to the total dose of these 4 agents used. Recovery of menses was frequent. The same combination of drugs given to male patients produced azoospermia; if spermatogenesis did return, it was not likely to do so with less than 2 years of unmaintained remission.

Mutagenicity—Tests in *Salmonella typhimurium* and with the dominant lethal assay in mice failed to demonstrate mutagenicity. Sperm abnormalities have been noted in mice. Velban has produced an increase in micronuclei formation in bone marrow cells of mice; however, since Velban inhibits mitotic spindle formation, it cannot be concluded that this is evidence of mutagenicity. Additional studies in mice demonstrated no reduction in fertility of males. Chromosomal translocations did occur in male mice. First-generation male offspring of these mice were not heterozygous translocation carriers.

In vitro tests using hamster lung cells in culture have produced chromosomal changes, including chromatid breaks and exchanges, whereas tests using another type of hamster cell failed to demonstrate mutation. Breaks and aberrations were not observed on chromosome analysis of marrow cells from patients being treated with this drug.

It is not clear from the literature how this drug affects synthesis of DNA and RNA. Some believe that there is no interference. Others believe that vinblastine interferes with nucleic acide metabolism but may not do so by direct effect but possibly as the result of biochemical disturbance in some other part of the molecular organization of the cell. No inhibition of RNA synthesis occurred in rat hepatoma cells exposed in culture to noncytotoxic levels of vinblastine. Conflicting results have been noted by others regarding interference with DNA synthesis.

Carcinogenesis—There is no currently available evidence to indicate that Velban itself has been carcinogenic in humans since the inception of its clinical use in the late 1950s. Patients treated for Hodgkin's disease have developed leukemia following radiation therapy and administration of Velban in combination with other chemotherapy, including agents known to intercalate with DNA. It is not known to what extent Velban may have contributed to the appearance of leukemia. Available data in rats and mice have failed to demonstrate clearly evidence of carcinogenesis when the animals were treated with the maximum tolerated dose and with one-half that dose for 6 months. This testing system demonstrated that other agents were clearly carcinogenic, whereas Velban was in the group of drugs causing slightly increased or the same tumor incidence as controls in one study and 1.5 to twofold increase in tumor incidence over controls in another study.

Usage in Pregnancy—Pregnancy Category D (See Warnings). Velban should be given to a pregnant woman only if clearly needed. Animal studies suggest that teratogenic effects may occur.

Pediatric Use—The dosage schedule for children is indicated under Dosage and Administration.

Nursing Mothers—It is not known whether this drug is excreted in human milk. Because many drugs are excreted in human milk and because of the potential for serious adverse reactions from Velban in nursing infants, a decision should be made whether to discontinue nursing or the drug, taking into account the importance of the drug to the mother.

ADVERSE REACTIONS

Prior to the use of the drug, patients should be advised of the possibility of untoward symptoms.

In general, the incidence of adverse reactions attending the use of Velban® (Vinblastine Sulfate, USP, Lilly) appears to be related to the size of the dose employed. With the exception of epilation, leukopenia, and neurologic side effects, adverse reactions generally have not persisted for longer than 24 hours. Neurologic side effects are not common; but when they do occur, they often last for more than 24 hours. Leukopenia, the most common adverse reaction, is usually the dose-limiting factor.

The following are manifestations which have been reported as adverse reactions, in decreasing order of frequency. The most common adverse reactions are underlined:

Hematologic—Leukopenia (granulocytopenia), anemia, thrombocytopenia (myelosuppression).

Dermatologic—Alopecia is common. A single case of light sensitivity associated with this product has been reported.

Gastrointestinal—Constipation, anorexia, nausea, vomiting, abdominal pain, ileus, vesiculation of the mouth, pharyngitis, diarrhea, hemorrhagic enterocolitis, bleeding from an old peptic ulcer, rectal bleeding.

Neurologic—Numbness of digits (paresthesias), loss of deep tendon reflexes, peripheral neuritis, mental depression, headache, convulsions.

Cardiovascular—Hypertension. Cases of unexpected myocardial infarction and cerebrovascular accidents have occurred in patients undergoing combination chemotherapy with vinblastine, bleomycin, and cisplatin. Raynaud's phenomenon has also been reported with this combination.

Pulmonary—See Precautions.

Miscellaneous—Malaise, bone pain, weakness, pain in tumor-containing tissue, dizziness, jaw pain, skin vesiculation, hypertension, Raynaud's phenomenon when patients are being treated with Velban in combination with bleomycin and cis-platinum for testicular cancer. The syndrome of inappropriate secretion of antidiuretic hormone has occurred with higher-than-recommended doses.

Nausea and vomiting usually may be controlled with ease by antiemetric agents. When epilation develops, it frequently is not total; and, in some cases, hair regrows while maintenance therapy continues.

Extravasation during intravenous injection may lead to cellulitis and phlebitis. If the amount of extravasation is great, sloughing may occur.

OVERDOSAGE

Signs and Symptoms—Side effects following the use of Velban® (Vinblastine Sulfate, USP, Lilly) are dose related. Therefore, following administration of more than the recommended dose, patients can be expected to experience these effects in an exaggerated fashion. (*See* Clinical Pharmacology, Contraindications, Warnings, Precautions, and Adverse Reactions.) There is no specific antidote. In addition, neurotoxicity similar to that with Oncovin may be observed. Since the major route of excretion may be through the biliary system, toxicity from this drug may be increased when there is hepatic insufficiency.

Treatment—To obtain up-to-date information about the treatment of overdose, a good resource is your certified Regional Poison Control Center. Telephone numbers of certified poison control centers are listed in the *Physicians' Desk Reference (PDR)*. In managing overdosage, consider the possibility of multiple drug overdoses, interaction among drugs, and unusual drug kinetics in your patient. Overdoses of Velban have been reported rarely. The following is provided to serve as a guide should such an overdose be encountered.

Supportive care should include the following: (1) prevention of side effects that result from the syndrome of inappropriate secretion of antidiuretic hormone (this would include restriction of the volume of daily fluid intake to that of the urine output plus insensible loss and perhaps the administration of a diuretic affecting the function of the loop of Henle and the distal tubule); (2) administration of an anticonvulsant; (3) prevention of ileus; (4) monitoring the cardiovascular system; and (5) determining daily blood counts for guidance in transfusion requirements and assessing the risk of infection. The major effect of excessive doses of Velban will be myelosuppression, which may be life threatening. There is no information regarding the effectiveness of dialysis nor of cholestyramine for the treatment of overdosage.

Velban in the dry state is irregularly and unpredictably absorbed from the gastrointestinal tract following oral administration. Absorption of the solution has not been studied. If vinblastine is swallowed, activated charcoal in a water slurry may be given by mouth along with a cathartic. The use of cholestyramine in this situation has not been reported. Symptoms of overdose will appear when greater-than-recommended doses are given. Any dose of Velban that results in elimination of platelets and neutrophils from blood and marrow and their precursors from marrow should be considered life threatening. The exact dose that will do this in all patients is unknown. Overdoses occurring during prolonged, consecutive-day infusions may be more toxic than the same total dose given by rapid intravenous injection. The intravenous LD$_{50}$ in mice is 10 mg/kg body weight; in rats, it is 2.9 mg/kg. The oral LD$_{50}$ in rats is 7 mg/kg.

Protect the patient's airway and support ventilation and perfusion. Meticulously monitor and maintain, within acceptable limits, the patient's vital signs, blood gases, serum electrolytes, etc. Absorption of drugs from the gastrointestinal tract may be decreased by giving activated charcoal, which, in many cases, is more effective than emesis or lavage; consider charcoal instead of or in addition to gastric emptying if the drug has been swallowed. Repeated doses of charcoal over time may hasten elimination of some drugs that have been absorbed. Safeguard the patient's airway when employing gastric emptying or charcoal.

DOSAGE AND ADMINISTRATION

Caution—**It is extremely important that the needle be properly positioned in the vein before this product is injected.**

If leakage into surrounding tissue should occur during intravenous administration of Velban® (Vinblastine Sulfate, USP, Lilly), it may cause considerable irritation. The injection should be discontinued immediately, and any remaining portion of the dose should then be introduced into another vein. Local injection of hyaluronidase and the application of moderate heat to the area of leakage help disperse the drug and are thought to minimize discomfort and the possibility of cellulitis.

There are variations in the depth of the leukopenic response that follows therapy with Velban. For this reason, it is recommended that the drug be given no more frequently than *once every 7 days*. It is wise to initiate therapy for adults by administering a single intravenous dose of 3.7 mg/m^2 of body surface area (bsa); the initial dose for children should be 2.5 mg/m^2. Thereafter, white-blood-cell counts should be made to determine the patient's sensitivity to Velban. A reduction of 50% in the dose of Velban is recommended for patients having a direct serum bilirubin value above 3 mg/mL. Since metabolism and excretion are primarily hepatic, no modification is recommended for patients with impaired renal function.

A simplified and conservative incremental approach to dosage *at weekly intervals* may be outlined as follows:

	Adults		Children	
First dose	3.7	mg/m^2 bsa	2.5	mg/m^2 bsa
Second dose	5.5	mg/m^2 bsa	3.75	mg/m^2 bsa
Third dose	7.4	mg/m^2 bsa	5.0	mg/m^2 bsa
Fourth dose	9.25	mg/m^2 bsa	6.25	mg/m^2 bsa
Fifth dose	11.1	mg/m^2 bsa	7.5	mg/m^2 bsa

The above-mentioned increases may be used until a maximum dose (not exceeding 18.5 mg/m^2 bsa for adults and 12.5 mg/m^2 bsa for children) is reached. The dose should not be increased after that dose which reduces the white-cell count to approximately 3,000 cells/mm^3. In some adults, 3.7 mg/m^2 bsa may produce this leukopenia; other adults may require more than 11.1 mg/m^2 bsa; and, very rarely, as much as 18.5 mg/m^2 bsa may be necessary. For most adult patients, however, the weekly dosage will prove to be 5.5 to 7.4 mg/m^2 bsa.

When the dose of Velban which will produce the above degree of leukopenia has been established, a dose *1 increment smaller* than this should be administered at weekly intervals for maintenance. Thus, the patient is receiving the maximum dose that does not cause leukopenia. *It should be emphasized that, even though 7 days have elapsed, the next dose*

of Velban should not be given until the white-cell count has returned to at least 4,000/mm^3. In some cases, oncolytic activity may be encountered before leukopenic effect. When this occurs, there is no need to increase the size of subsequent doses (*see* Precautions).

The duration of maintenance therapy varies according to the disease being treated and the combination of antineoplastic agents being used. There are differences of opinion regarding the duration of maintenance therapy with the same protocol for a particular disease; for example, various durations have been used with the MOPP program in treating Hodgkin's disease. Prolonged chemotherapy for maintaining remissions involves several risks, among which are life-threatening infectious diseases, sterility, and possibly the appearance of other cancers through suppression of immune surveillance.

In some disorders, survival following complete remission may not be as prolonged as that achieved with shorter periods of maintenance therapy. On the other hand, failure to provide maintenance therapy in some patients may lead to unnecessary relapse; complete remissions in patients with testicular cancer, unless maintained for at least 2 years, often result in early relapse.

To prepare a solution containing 1 mg of Velban/mL, add 10 mL of Sodium Chloride Injection (preserved with phenol or benzyl alcohol) to the 10 mg of Velban in the sterile vial. Other solutions are not recommended. The drug dissolves instantly to give a clear solution. After a solution has been made in this way and a portion of it has been removed from a vial, the remainder of the vial's contents may be stored in a refrigerator for future use for 30 days without significant loss of potency.

The dose of Velban (calculated to provide the desired amount) may be injected either into the tubing of a running intravenous infusion or directly into a vein. The latter procedure is readily adaptable to outpatient therapy. In either case, the injection may be completed in about 1 minute. If care is taken to insure that the needle is securely within the vein and that no solution containing Velban is spilled extravascularly, cellulitis and/or phlebitis will not occur. To minimize further the possibility of extravascular spillage, it is suggested that the syringe and needle be rinsed with venous blood before withdrawal of the needle. The dose should not be diluted in large volumes of diluent (ie, 100 to 250 mL) or given intravenously for prolonged periods (ranging from 30 to 60 minutes or more), since this frequently results in irritation of the vein and increases the chance of extravasation.

Because of the enhanced possibility of thrombosis, it is considered inadvisable to inject a solution of Velban® (Vinblastine Sulfate, USP, Lilly) into an extremity in which the circulation is impaired or potentially impaired by such conditions as compressing or invading neoplasm, phlebitis, or varicosity.

Parenteral drug products should be inspected visually for particulate matter and discoloration prior to administration, whenever solution and container permit.

It is not necessary to use preservative-containing solvents if unused portions of the remaining solutions are discarded immediately. Unused preservative-containing solutions should be refrigerated for future use.

Procedures for proper handling and disposal of anticancer drugs should be considered. Several guidelines on this subject have been published. There is no general agreement that all of the procedures recommended in the guidelines are necessary or appropriate.

References are available in the package insert or on request.

HOW SUPPLIED

(℞) Vials, 10 mg, 10-mL size (No. 687)—(1s) NDC 0002-1452-01.

The vials should be stored in a refrigerator (2° to 8°C, or 36° to 46°F) to assure extended stability.

[101288]

ZINC-INSULIN CRYSTALS

[ĭ'lĕ-tĭn]
see under Iletin® (insulin, Lilly).

---

* Identi-Code® symbol.

Products are cross-indexed by generic and chemical names in the **YELLOW SECTION**

Lunsco, Inc.
ROUTE 2, BOX 62
PULASKI, VA 24301

APPECON   Ⓒ Ⅲ ℞

COMPOSITION
Each sustained release capsule contains: Phendimetrazine Tartrate 105 mg.

SUPPLIED
bottles of 100

DYTUSS   ℞

COMPOSITION
Each 30cc represents: Diphenhydramine HCl. 80 mg., Alcohol 5%.

SUPPLIED
Pint

FETRIN   ℞

COMPOSITION
Each sustained-release capsule contains: Ferrous Fumarate (Equivalent to 66 mg. Elemental Iron) 200 mg., Ascorbic Acid 60 mg., Cyanocobalamin 5mcg with Intrinsic Factor

SUPPLIED
Bottles of 100.

HYCO–PAP   Ⓒ Ⅲ ℞

COMPOSITION
Each capsule contains: Hydrocodone Bitartrate 5 mg., (Warning: May be Habit Forming), Acetaminophen 500 mg.

SUPPLIED
Bottles of 100.

PACAPS   ℞

COMPOSITION
Each capsule represents: Butalbital 50 mg., Caffeine 40 mg., Acetaminophen 325 mg.

SUPPLIED
Bottles of 100.

PROTID   ℞

COMPOSITION
Each tablet represents: Acetaminophen 500 mg., Chlorpheniramine Maleate 8 mg., Phenylephrine HCl. 40 mg.

SUPPLIED
Bottles of 100.

Lyphomed, Inc.
10401 WEST TOUHY AVENUE
ROSEMONT, IL 60018-3392

NEBUPENT™   ℞
(Pentamidine Isethionate)
For Inhalation Solution

DESCRIPTION
NebuPent™ (Pentamidine Isethionate), an anti-protozoal agent, is a sterile and non-pyrogenic lyophilized product. After reconstitution with Sterile Water for Injection USP, NebuPent™ is administered by inhalation via the Respirgard® II nebulizer [Marquest, Englewood, CO] (see DOSAGE AND ADMINISTRATION).

Pentamidine isethionate, 4,4′-diamidinodiphenoxypentane di-(β-hydroxyethanesulfonate), is a white crystalline powder soluble in water and glycerin and insoluble in ether, acetone, and chloroform.

$C_{23}H_{36}N_4O_{10}S_2$ 592.68
Each vial contains 300 mg sterile pentamidine isethionate.

CLINICAL PHARMACOLOGY
Microbiology
Pentamidine isethionate, an aromatic diamidine, is known to have activity against *Pneumocystis carinii*. The mode of action is not fully understood. *In vitro* studies indicate that the drug interferes with protozoal nuclear metabolism by inhibition of DNA, RNA, phospholipid and protein synthesis.

Pharmacokinetics
In 5 AIDS patients with suspected *Pneumocystis carinii* pneumonia (PCP), the mean concentrations of pentamidine determined 18 to 24 hours after inhalation therapy were 23.2 ng/mL (range 5.1 to 43.0 ng/mL) in bronchoalveolar lavage fluid and 705 ng/mL (range, 140 to 1336 ng/mL) in sediment after administration of a 300 mg single dose via the Respirgard® II nebulizer. In 3 AIDS patients with suspected PCP, the mean concentrations of pentamidine determined 18 to 24 hours after a 4 mg/kg intravenous dose were 2.6 ng/mL (range 1.5 to 4.0 ng/mL) in bronchoalveolar lavage fluid and 9.3 ng/mL (range, 6.9 to 12.8 ng/mL) in sediment. In the patients who received aerosolized pentamidine, the peak plasma levels of pentamidine were at or below the lower limit of detection of the assay (2.3 ng/mL).

Following a single 2-hour intravenous infusion of 4 mg/kg of pentamidine isethionate to 6 AIDS patients, the mean plasma Cmax, T 1/2 and clearance were 612 ± 371 ng/mL, 6.4 ± 1.3 hr and 248 ± 91 L/hr respectively. In another study of aerosolized pentamidine in 13 AIDS patients with acute PCP who received 4 mg/kg/day administered via the Ultra Vent® jet nebulizer, peak plasma levels of pentamidine averaged 18.8 ± 11.9 ng/mL after the first dose. During the next 14 days of repeated dosing, the highest observed Cmax averaged 20.5 ± 21.2 ng/mL. In a third study, following daily administration of 600 mg of inhaled pentamidine isethionate with the Respirgard® II nebulizer for 21 days in 11 patients with acute PCP, mean plasma levels measured shortly after the 21st dose averaged 11.8 ± 10.0 ng/mL. Plasma concentrations after aerosol administration are substantially lower than those observed after a comparable intravenous dose. The extent of pentamidine accumulation and distribution following chronic inhalation therapy are not known.

In rats, intravenous administration of a 5 mg/kg dose resulted in concentrations of pentamidine in the liver and kidney that were 87.5 and 62.3-fold higher, respectively, than levels in those organs following 5 mg/kg administered as an aerosol.

No pharmacokinetic data are available following aerosol administration of pentamidine in humans with impaired hepatic or renal function.

INDICATIONS AND USAGE
NebuPent™ is indicated for the prevention of *Pneumocystis carinii* pneumonia (PCP) in high-risk, HIV-infected patients defined by one or both of the following criteria:
i. a history of one or more episodes of PCP
ii. a peripheral CD4+ (T4 helper/inducer) lymphocyte count less than or equal to 200/mm³.

These indications are based on the results of an 18-month randomized, dose-response trial in high risk HIV-infected patients and on existing epidemiological data from natural history studies.

The patient population of the controlled trial consisted of 408 patients, 237 of whom had a history of one or more episodes of PCP. The remaining patients without a history of PCP included 55 patients with Kaposi's sarcoma and 116 patients with other AIDS diagnoses, ARC or asymptomatic HIV infection. Patients were randomly assigned to receive NebuPent™ via the Respirgard® II nebulizer at one of the following three doses: 30 mg every two weeks (n=135), 150 mg every two weeks (n=134) or 300 mg every four weeks (n=139). The results of the trial demonstrated a significant protective effect (p < 0.01) against PCP with the 300 mg every four week dosage regimen compared to the 30 mg every two week dosage regimen. The 300 mg dose regimen reduced the risk of developing PCP by 50 to 70% compared to the 30 mg regimen. A total of 293 patients (72% of all patients) also received zidovudine at sometime during the trial. The analysis of the data demonstrated the efficacy of the 300 mg dose even after adjusting for the effect of zidovudine.

The results of the trial further demonstrate that the dose and frequency of dosing are important to the efficacy of NebuPent™ prophylaxis in that multiple analyses consistently demonstrated a trend toward greater efficacy with 300 mg every four weeks as compared to 150 mg every two weeks.

No dose-response was observed for reduction in overall mortality; however, mortality from PCP was low in all three dosage groups.

CONTRAINDICATIONS
NebuPent™ is contraindicated in patients with a history of an anaphylactic reaction to inhaled or parenteral pentamidine isethionate.

WARNINGS
The potential for development of acute PCP still exists in patients receiving NebuPent™ prophylaxis. Therefore, any patient with symptoms suggestive of the presence of a pulmonary infection, including but not limited to dyspnea, fever or cough, should receive a thorough medical evaluation and appropriate diagnostic tests for possible acute PCP as well as for other opportunistic and non-opportunistic pathogens. The use of NebuPent™ may alter the clinical and radiographic features of PCP and could result in an atypical presentation, including but not limited to mild disease or focal infection.

Prior to initiating NebuPent™ prophylaxis, symptomatic patients should be evaluated appropriately to exclude the presence of PCP. The recommended dose of NebuPent™ for the prevention of PCP is insufficient to treat acute PCP.

PRECAUTIONS
IMPORTANT; DO NOT MIX THE NEBUPENT™ SOLUTION WITH ANY OTHER DRUGS. DO NOT USE THE RESPIRGARD® II NEBULIZIER TO ADMINISTER A BRONCHODILATOR. (See DOSAGE AND ADMINISTRATION).
Pulmonary
Inhalation of NebuPent™ may induce bronchospasm or cough. This has been noted particularly in some patients who have a history of smoking or asthma. In clinical trials, cough and bronchospasm were the most frequently reported adverse experiences associated with NebuPent™ administration (38% and 15%, respectively, of patients receiving the 300 mg dose); however less than 1% of the doses were interrupted or terminated due to these effects. For the majority of patients, cough and bronchospasm were controlled by administration of an aerosolized bronchodilator (only 1% of patients withdrew from the study due to treatment-associated cough or bronchospasm). In patients who experience bronchospasm or cough, administration of an inhaled bronchodilator prior to giving each NebuPent™ dose may minimize recurrence of the symptoms.
General
The extent and consequence of pentamidine accumulation following chronic inhalation therapy are not known. As a result, patients receiving NebuPent™ should be closely monitored for the development of serious adverse reactions that have occurred in patients receiving parenteral pentamidine, including hypotension, hypoglycemia, hyperglycemia, hypocalcemia, anemia, thrombocytopenia, leukopenia, hepatic or renal dysfunction, ventricular tachycardia, pancreatitis and Stevens-Johnson syndrome.

Extrapulmonary infection with *P. carinii* has been reported infrequently. Most, but not all, of the cases have been reported in patients who have a history of PCP. The presence of extrapulmonary pneumocystosis should be considered when evaluating patients with unexplained signs and symptoms. Cases of acute pancreatitis have been reported in patients receiving aerosolized pentamidine. NebuPent™ should be discontinued if signs or symptoms of acute pancreatitis develop.
Drug Interactions
While specific studies on drug interactions with NebuPent™ have not been conducted, the majority of patients in clinical trials received concomitant medications, including zidovudine, with no reported interactions.
Carcinogenesis, Mutagenesis and Impairment of Fertility
No studies have been conducted to evaluate the potential of pentamidine isethionate as a carcinogen or mutagen or to determine its effects on fertility.
Pregnancy. Pregnancy Category C
Animal reproduction studies have not been conducted with NebuPent™. It is also not known whether NebuPent™ can cause fetal harm when administered to a pregnant woman or can affect reproduction capacity. NebuPent™ should be given to a pregnant woman only if clearly needed. NebuPent™ should not be given to a pregnant woman unless the potential benefits are judged to outweigh the unknown risk.
Nursing Mothers
It is not known whether NebuPent™ is excreted in human milk. Because of the potential for serious adverse reactions in nursing infants from NebuPent™, a decision should be made whether to discontinue nursing or to discontinue the drug, taking into account the importance of the drug to the mother. Because many drugs are excreted in human milk, NebuPent™ should not be given to a nursing mother unless the potential benefits are judged to outweigh the unknown risk.
Pediatric Use
The safety and effectiveness of NebuPent™ in children have not been established.

ADVERSE REACTIONS
The most frequent adverse effects attributable to NebuPent™ administration are cough and bronchospasm (reported by 38% and 15%, respectively, of patients receiving 300 mg every four weeks).

The most frequently reported adverse experiences in the controlled clinical trials in which 607 patients were treated with NebuPent™ (139 patients at 300 mg every four weeks,

232 at 150 mg every two weeks, 101 at 100 mg every two weeks and 135 at 30 mg every two weeks) using the Respirgard® II nebulizer were as follows:

53–72%	fatigue, bad (metallic) taste, shortness of breath and decreased appetite;
31–47%	dizziness and rash;
10–23%	nausea, pharyngitis, chest pain or congestion, night sweats, chills and vomiting.

In nearly all cases neither the relationship to treatment or underlying disease nor the severity of adverse experiences was recorded.

Other less frequently occurring adverse experiences (reported by greater than 1% and up to 5% of patients in two clinical trials) were pneumothorax, diarrhea, headache, anemia (generally associated with zidovudine use), myalgia, abdominal pain and edema.

From a total experience with 1130 patients adverse events reported with a frequency of 1% or less were as follows. No causal relationship to treatment has been established for these adverse events.

General: Allergic reaction and extrapulmonary pneumocystosis.

Cardiovascular: Tachycardia, hypotension, hypertension, palpitations, syncope, cerebrovascular accident, vasodilatation and vasculitis.

Metabolic: Hypoglycemia, hyperglycemia, and hypocalcemia.

Gastrointestinal: Gingivitis, dyspepsia, oral ulcer/abscess, gastritis, gastric ulcer, hypersalivation, dry mouth, splenomegaly, melena, hematochezia, esophagitis, colitis, and pancreatitis.

Hematological: Pancytopenia, neutropenia, eosinophilia and thrombocytopenia.

Hepatorenal: Hepatitis, hepatomegaly, hepatic dysfunction, renal failure, flank pain and nephritis.

Musculoskeletal: Arthralgia.

Neurological: Tremors, confusion, anxiety, memory loss, seizure, neuropathy, paresthesia, insomnia, hypesthesia, drowsiness, emotional lability, vertigo, paranoia, neuralgia, hallucination, depression and unsteady gait.

Respiratory: Rhinitis, laryngitis, laryngospasm, hyperventilation, hemoptysis, gagging, eosinophilic or interstitial pneumonitis, pleuritis, cyanosis, tachypnea, and rales.

Skin: Pruritis, erythema, dry skin, desquamation and urticaria.

Special Senses: Eye discomfort, conjunctivitis, blurred vision, blepharitis and loss of taste and smell.

Urogenital: Incontinence.

Reproductive: Miscarriage.

OVERDOSAGE

Overdosage has not been reported with NebuPent™. The symptoms and signs of overdosage are not known.

A serious overdosage, to the point of producing systemic drug levels similar to those following parenteral administration, would have the potential of producing similar types of serious systemic toxicity. (See **PRECAUTIONS**).

Available clinical pharmacology data (see **CLINICAL PHARMACOLOGY**) suggest that a dose up to 40 times the recommended NebuPent™ dosage would be required to produce systemic levels similar to a single 4 mg/kg intravenous dose.

DOSAGE AND ADMINISTRATION

IMPORTANT: NEBUPENT™ MUST BE DISSOLVED ONLY IN STERILE WATER FOR INJECTION, USP. DO NOT USE SALINE SOLUTION FOR RECONSTITUTION BECAUSE THE DRUG WILL PRECIPITATE. DO NOT MIX THE NEBUPENT™ SOLUTION WITH ANY OTHER DRUGS. DO NOT USE THE RESPIRGARD® II NEBULIZER TO ADMINISTER A BRONCHODILATOR.

Reconstitution

The contents of one vial (300 mg) must be dissolved in 6 mL Sterile Water for Injection, USP. Place the entire reconstituted contents of the vial into the Respirgard® II nebulizer reservoir for administration.

Dosage

The recommended adult dosage of NebuPent™ for the prevention of *Pneumocystis carinii* pneumonia is 300 mg once every four weeks administered via the Respirgard® II nebulizer.

The dose should be delivered until the nebulizer chamber is empty (approximately 30 to 45 minutes). The flow rate should be 5 to 7 liters per minute from a 40 to 50 pounds per square inch (PSI) air or oxygen source. Alternatively, a 40 to 50 PSI air compressor can be used with flow limited by setting the flowmeter at 5 to 7 liters per minute or by setting the pressure at 22 to 25 PSI. Low pressure (less than 20 PSI) compressors should not be used.

Stability

Freshly prepared solutions for aerosol use are recommended. After reconstitution with sterile water, the Nebupent™ solution is stable for 48 hours in the original vial at room temperature if protected from light.

HOW SUPPLIED

Product No.	NDC No.	
877-15	0469-8770-90	NebuPent™ (Pentamidine Isethionate) 300 mg lyophilized product in single dose vials individually packaged.

Store the dry product at controlled room temperature 15°-30°C (59°-86°F).

Protect the dry product and the reconstituted solution from light.

CAUTION

Federal (USA) law prohibits dispensing without prescription

Lyphomed, Inc.
Rosemont, IL 60018

45-474
June 1989

PENTAM® 300   ℞
(Sterile Pentamidine Isethionate)

DESCRIPTION

PENTAM® 300 (Sterile Pentamidine Isethionate), an antiprotozoal agent, is a nonpyrogenic, lyophilized product. After reconstitution, it should be administered by intramuscular or intravenous (IM or IV) routes. (See DOSAGE AND ADMINISTRATION).

Pentamidine isethionate is a white crystalline powder soluble in water and glycerin and insoluble in ether, acetone, and chloroform. It is chemically designated as 4,4'-diamidinodiphenoxypentane di (β-hydroxyethanesulfonate) with the following structural formula:

$C_{23}H_{36}N_4O_{10}S_2$ 592.68

Each vial contains:
Pentamidine isethionate .... 300 mg

CLINICAL PHARMACOLOGY

Pentamidine isethionate, an aromatic diamidine, is known to have activity against *Pneumocystis carinii*.

The mode of action of pentamidine is not fully understood. *In vitro* studies with mammalian tissues and the protozoan *Crithidia oncopelti* indicate that the drug interferes with nuclear metabolism producing inhibition of the synthesis of DNA, RNA, phospholipids and proteins.

Little is known about the drug's pharmacokinetics. Preliminary studies have shown that in seven patients treated with daily IM doses of pentamidine at 4 mg/kg for 10 to 12 days, plasma concentrations were between 0.3 and 0.5 mcg/ml. The levels did not appreciably change with time after injection or from day to day. Higher plasma levels were encountered in patients with an elevated BUN. The patients continued to excrete decreasing amounts of pentamidine in urine up to six to eight weeks after cessation of the treatment.

Tissue distribution has been studied in mice given a single intraperitoneal injection of pentamidine at 10 mg/kg. The concentration in the kidneys was the highest followed by that in the liver. In mice pentamidine was excreted unchanged, primarily via the kidneys with some elimination in the feces. The ratio of amounts excreted in the urine and feces (4:1) was constant over the period of study.

INDICATIONS AND USAGE

PENTAM® 300 (Sterile Pentamidine Isethionate) is indicated for the treatment of pneumonia due to *Pneumocystis carinii*.

CONTRAINDICATIONS

Once the diagnosis of *Pneumocystis carinii* pneumonia has been firmly established, there are no absolute contraindications to the use of pentamidine isethionate.

WARNINGS

Fatalities due to severe hypotension, hypoglycemia and cardiac arrhythmias have been reported in patients treated with pentamidine isethionate, both by the IM and IV routes. Severe hypotension may result after a single dose (see PRECAUTIONS). The administration of the drug should, therefore, be limited to the patients in whom *Pneumocystis carinii* has been demonstrated. Patients should be closely monitored for the development of serious adverse reactions (see PRECAUTIONS and ADVERSE REACTIONS).

PRECAUTIONS

General

Pentamidine isethionate should be used with caution in patients with hypertension, hypotension, hypoglycemia, hyperglycemia, hypocalcemia, leukopenia, thrombocytopenia, anemia, and hepatic or renal dysfunction.

Patients may develop sudden, severe hypotension after a single dose of pentamidine isethionate, whether given IV or IM. Therefore, patients receiving the drug should be lying down and the blood pressure should be monitored closely during administration of the drug and several times thereafter until the blood pressure is stable. Equipment for emergency resuscitation should be readily available. If pentamidine isethionate is administered IV, it should be infused over a period of 60 minutes.

Pentamidine isethionate-induced hypoglycemia has been associated with pancreatic islet cell necrosis and inappropriately high plasma insulin concentrations. Hyperglycemia and diabetes mellitus, with or without preceding hypoglycemia, have also occurred, sometimes several months after therapy with pentamidine isethionate. Therefore, blood glucose levels should be monitored daily during therapy with pentamidine isethionate, and several times thereafter.

Laboratory Tests

The following tests should be carried out before, during and after therapy:

a) Daily blood urea nitrogen and serum creatinine determinations.
b) Daily blood glucose determinations.
c) Complete blood count and platelet count.
d) Liver function test, including bilirubin, alkaline phosphatase, AST (SGOT), and ALT (SGPT).
e) Serum calcium determinations.
f) Electrocardiograms at regular intervals.

Carcinogensis, Mutagensis, Impairment of Fertility

No studies have been conducted to evaluate the potential of pentamidine isethionate as a carcinogen, mutagen, or cause of impaired fertility.

Pregnancy Category C

Animal reproduction studies have not be conducted with pentamidine isethionate. It is also not known whether pentamidine isethionate can cause fetal harm when administered to a pregnant woman or can affect reproduction capacity. Pentamidine isethionate should be given to a pregnant woman only if clearly needed.

ADVERSE REACTIONS

CAUTION: Fatalities due to severe hypotension, hypoglycemia and cardiac arrhythmias have been reported in patients treated with pentamidine isethionate, both by the IM and IV routes. The administration of the drug should, therefore, be limited to the patients in whom *Pneumocystis carinii* has been demonstrated.

Of 424 patients treated with pentamidine isethionate, 244 (57.5%) developed some adverse reaction. Most of the patients had the acquired immunodeficiency syndrome (AIDS). In the following table, "Severe" refers to life-threatening reactions or reactions that require immediate corrective measures and led to discontinuation of pentamidine isethionate.

Adverse Reactions	Number	%
Severe		
Leukopenia (<1000/mm³)	12	2.8
Hypoglycemia (<25 mg/dL)	10	2.4
Thrombocytopenia (<20,000/mm³)	7	1.7
Hypotension (<60 mm Hg systolic)	4	0.9
Acute renal failure (serum creatinine >6 mg/dl)	2	0.5
Hypocalcemia	1	0.2
Stevens-Johnson syndrome	1	0.2
Ventricular tachycardia	1	0.2
Total number of patients with severe effects*	37	8.7
Moderate		
Elevated serum creatinine (2.4 to 6.0 mg/dl)	98	23.1
Sterile abscess, pain, or induration at the site of IM injection	47	11.1
Elevated liver function tests	37	8.7
Leukopenia	32	7.5
Nausea, anorexia	25	5.9
Hypotension	17	4.0
Fever	15	3.5
Hypoglycemia	15	3.5
Rash	14	3.3
Bad taste in mouth	7	1.7
Confusion/hallucinations	7	1.7
Anemia	5	1.2
Neuralgia	4	0.9
Thrombocytopenia	4	0.9
Hyperkalemia	3	0.7
Phlebitis	3	0.7
Dizziness (without hypotension)	2	0.5
Other moderate adverse reactions**	5	1.2
Total number of patients with moderate adverse reactions*	207	48.8

*Patient total may not equal sum of reactions, since some patients had more than one reaction.

Continued on next page

Lyphomed—Cont.

**Each of the following moderate adverse reactions was reported in one patient: Hypocalcemia, abnormal ST segment of electrocardiogram, bronchospasm, diarrhea, and hyperglycemia.

DOSAGE AND ADMINISTRATION

Pentamidine isethionate should be administered IM or IV only. The recommended regimen for adults and children is 4 mg/kg once a day for 14 days. The benefits and risk of therapy with pentamidine isethionate for more than 14 days are not well defined.

Intramuscular Injection

The contents of one vial (300 mg) should be dissolved in 3 mL of Sterile Water for Injection, USP. The calculated daily dose should then be withdrawn and administered by deep IM injection.

Intravenous Injection

The contents of one vial should first be dissolved in 3 to 5 mL of Sterile Water for Injection, USP or 5% Dextrose Injection, USP. The calculated dose of pentamidine isethionate should then be withdrawn and diluted further in 50 to 250 ml of 5% Dextrose Injection, USP. **The diluted IV solutions containing pentamidine isethionate should be infused over a period of 60 minutes.**

Aseptic technique should be employed in preparation of all solutions. Parenteral drug products should be inspected visually for particulate matter and discoloration prior to administration.

Stability: Intravenous infusion solutions of pentamidine isethionate at 1 mg and 2.5 mg/mL prepared in 5% Dextrose Injection, USP are stable at room temperature for up to 24 hours.

HOW SUPPLIED

Product No.	NDC No.	
113-10	0469-1130-91	PENTAM® 300 (Sterile Pentamidine Isethionate) 300 mg, lyophilized product in single dose vials, packages of 10.

Store the dry product at controlled room temperature 15°–30°C (59°–86°F). Protect the dry product and reconstituted solution from light.

Discard unused portions.

CAUTION: Federal (USA) law prohibits dispensing without prescription.

Lyphomed, Inc.
Rosemont, IL 60018

45-485
Revised: January 1989

EDUCATIONAL MATERIAL

COMPLIMENTARY EDUCATIONAL AND TEACHING MATERIALS FROM LYPHOMED, INC.

Booklets, Brochures
Case Study Number 1: *Treating Pneumocystis carinii Pneumonia*, by Hetty Waskins, M.D.
Monograph: *Diagnosis and Treatment of Pulmonary Disease in AIDS*, by Richard E. Chaisson, M.D., and Philip C. Hopewell, M.D.
Symposium Summaries: *Pentamidine Isethionate Inhalation*
Free to all health care professionals.

Book
Clinical Guide to Parenteral Micronutrition
Edited by Thomas G. Baumgartner, Pharm D, M.Ed.
Free to all health care professionals

Quarterly Newsletters
Clinical Trends in Hospital Pharmacy
(ACPE Provider of Continuing Education)
Free to all health care professionals.
Problem-Solving in Office Oncology Nursing
Free to all health care professionals.

3M Riker
225-1S-07 3M CENTER
ST. PAUL, MN 55144

[See table below].

ALU-TAB® Tablets
and
ALU-CAP® Capsules

DESCRIPTION

Each green Alu-Tab "swallow" tablet contains dried aluminum hydroxide gel 600 mg. Alu-Tab tablets also contain: acetylated monoglycerides, cellulose, ethylcellulose, hydrogenated vegetable oil, hydroxypropyl cellulose, hydroxypropyl methylcellulose, magnesium stearate, polyethylene glycol, sodium starch glycolate, starch, talc, titanium dioxide, D&C yellow #10, FD&C blue #1, and FD&C yellow #6 (Sunset yellow) as color additives. Each red and green Alu-Cap capsule contains dried aluminum hydroxide gel 475 mg. Alu-Cap capsules also contain: cellulose, gelatin, polyethylene glycol, talc, titanium dioxide, FD&C red #40, D&C yellow #10, FD&C blue #1, FD&C green #3, and FD&C yellow #6 (Sunset yellow) as color additives.

ACTIONS

Antacid actions include neutralization of gastric hyperacidity and mild astringent and absorbent properties. Aluminum hydroxide dried gel increases phosphate excretion in the bowel by the formation of non-absorbable salts.*

INDICATIONS

Treatment in uncomplicated peptic ulcer and gastric hyperacidity.

PRECAUTIONS

Aluminum hydroxide is essentially a nontoxic compound. If constipation occurs, medication should be discontinued and a physician should be consulted. Aluminum hydroxide must be given with care to patients who have recently suffered massive upper gastrointestinal hemorrhage. Do not give this product to any patient presently taking a prescription antibiotic drug containing any form of tetracycline.

DIRECTIONS

Three Alu-Tab "swallow" tablets three times a day or as prescribed by physician. Three Alu-Cap capsules three times a day or as prescribed by physician.

HOW SUPPLIED

Bottles of 250 green film-coated Alu-Tab "swallow" tablets (NDC **0089-0107-25**). Bottles of 100 red and green Alu-Cap capsules (NDC **0089-0106-10**).

*Goodman, L.S., and Gilman, A.: *The Pharmacological Basis of Therapeutics*, 6th ed., Macmillan Publishing Co., Inc. New York, 1980, p. 990.

CALCIUM DISODIUM VERSENATE*   ℞
(edetate calcium disodium injection, U.S.P.)
Injection

WARNING
Edetate Calcium Disodium is capable of producing toxic and potentially fatal effects. The dosage schedule should be followed and at no time should the recommended daily dose be exceeded. In lead encephalopathy avoid rapid infusion; intramuscular route is preferred.

DESCRIPTION

Calcium Disodium Versonate injection (edetate calcium disodium injection, U.S.P.) is a sterile concentrated solution for intravenous infusion or intramuscular injection. Each 5 ml ampule contains 1000 mg of edetate calcium disodium (equivalent to 200 mg/ml) in water for injection.

CLINICAL PHARMACOLOGY

The calcium in edetate calcium disodium is readily displaced by heavy metals, such as lead, to form stable complexes. Following parenteral injection, the chelate formed is excreted in the urine, with 50 percent appearing in the first hour after administration.

INDICATIONS AND USAGE

Edetate calcium disodium is indicated for the reduction of blood levels and depot stores of lead in lead poisoning (acute and chronic) and lead encephalopathy.

CONTRAINDICATIONS

Edetate calcium disodium should not be given during periods of anuria.

WARNINGS

See box warning above.

Usage in pregnancy: The safe use of edetate calcium disodium has not been established with respect to possible adverse effects upon fetal development. Therefore, it should not be used in women of child-bearing potential and particularly during early pregnancy unless, in the judgment of the physician, the potential benefits outweigh the possible hazards.

PRECAUTIONS

Severe acute lead poisoning by itself may cause proteinuria and microscopic hematuria. Edetate calcium disodium may produce the same signs of renal damage. Routine urinalysis should be done daily during each course of therapy to determine whether the proteinuria and hematuria is improving or the evidence of renal tubular injury is getting worse. The presence of large renal epithelial cells or increasing numbers of red blood cells in the urinary sediment or greater proteinuria call for immediate stopping of edetate calcium disodium administration. Evidence of renal impairment should be looked for by periodic blood urea nitrogen determinations before and during each course of therapy. The patient should also be monitored for irregularities of cardiac rhythm.

ADVERSE REACTIONS

The principal toxic effect is renal tubular necrosis.

DOSAGE AND ADMINISTRATION

Edetate calcium disodium is equally effective whether administered intravenously, subcutaneously or intramuscularly. Because of convenience in administration and greater safety in treating symptomatic children, many physicians experienced in the treatment of lead poisoning prefer the intramuscular route which is recommended in patients with either overt or incipient lead encephalopathy. Rapid intravenous infusions may be lethal by suddenly increasing intracranial pressure in this group of patients with cerebral edema.

Note: In patients with lead encephalopathy and increased intracranial pressure, excess fluids must be avoided. In such case a 20 percent solution of edetate calcium disodium is mixed with procaine to give a final concentration of 0.5 percent of procaine in the mixture which is administered intramuscularly.

Acutely ill individuals may be dehydrated from vomiting. Since edetate calcium disodium is excreted almost exclusively in the urine, it is very important to establish urine flow by intravenous infusion before the first dose of the chelating agent is given. Once urine flow is established further intravenous fluid is restricted to basal water and electrolyte requirements. Administration of edetate calcium disodium should be stopped whenever there is cessation of urine flow in order to avoid unduly high tissue levels of the drug.

Intravenous Administration: Dilute the 5 ml. (1 gram, 20% solution) from an ampule with 250-500 ml. of Solution Isotonic Sodium Chloride, USP, or sterile 5% dextrose solution in water. In asymptomatic adults, administer this diluted solution over a period of at least one hour. Such doses may be administered twice daily for periods up to 5 days. The therapy should then be interrupted for 2 days and followed by an additional 5 days of treatment, if indicated.

In mildly affected or asymptomatic individuals the dosage of 50 mg./kg. per day should not be exceeded.

In symptomatic adults, fluids should be kept to basal levels and the time of administration increased to two hours. A second daily infusion is to be given six or more hours after the first.

Intramuscular Administration: This is the route of choice for children. The dosage should not exceed 0.5 gram per 30 pounds of body weight twice daily (total, 1.0 gram/30 lbs./day). This is equivalent to 35 mg./kg. twice daily (total, approx. 75 mg./kg./day). In mild cases a dose of 50 mg./kg. per day should not be exceeded. For young children the total daily dose may be given in divided doses every 8 or 12 hours for 3 to 5 days. A second course may be given after a rest period of 4 or more days. Procaine to produce a concentration of 0.5% should be added to minimize pain at injection site. (1 ml. of 1% procaine solution for each ml. of concentrated Calcium Disodium Versonate solution, or crystalline procaine may be used to reduce volume.)

The following Riker products are available in Military and Veterans Administration depots:

Military Depot Items	National Stock Number
Duo-Medihaler® (aerosol) w/adapter 22.5 ml.	6505-00-071-7861
Medihaler-Iso® (aerosol) w/adapter 15 ml.	6505-00-023-6481
Medihaler-Iso® (aerosol) w/adapter 22.5 ml.	6505-00-014-8486
Norflex Tablets 100's	6505-00-138-8462
Theolair™ 125 mg. Tablets 100's	6505-01-074-0490
Theolair™ 250 mg. Tablets 100's	6505-01-149-3555
Urex® Tablets 100's	6505-00-126-3207

Veterans Administration Depot Items	National Stock Number
Medihaler-Iso® (aerosol) w/adapter 22.5 ml.	6505-00-014-8486
Norflex Tablets 100's	6505-00-138-8462

Regardless of method of administration, doses larger than those recommended should not be undertaken.

Lead Encephalopathy: This condition is relatively rare in adults but is quite common in children in whom the mortality rate has been high. Recent reports by Chisolm and by Coffin et al who employed a combination of BAL and edetate calcium disodium, suggest that this may be the preferred treatment, although edetate calcium disodium alone has been used over a longer period of time. Each group administered edetate calcium disodium intramuscularly concurrently with BAL in separate deep I.M. sites. Procaine was added to the 20% solution of edetate calcium disodium to give a procaine concentration of 0.5%. In the studies of Coffin and Chisolm, 125 children with acute lead encephalopathy have been treated with this combined therapy with only one death.

HOW SUPPLIED

Calcium Disodium Versenate Injection, 5 ml. ampules containing 200 mg. of edetate calcium disodium per ml., boxes containing 6 ampules.
(NDC **0089-0510-06**).
*Registered trademark of the Dow Chemical Company

CAUTION

Federal law prohibits dispensing without prescription.

DISALCID®   ℞
(salsalate)
Tablets and Capsules

DESCRIPTION

DISALCID (salsalate) is a nonsteroidal anti-inflammatory agent for oral administration. Chemically, salsalate (salicylsalicylic acid or 2-hydroxy-benzoic acid 2-carboxyphenyl ester) is a dimer of salicylic acid.

Each round, aqua, scored film coated DISALCID tablet contains 500 mg salsalate.

Each aqua and white DISALCID capsule contains 500 mg salsalate. DISALCID capsules also contain: colloidal silicon dioxide, gelatin, magnesium stearate, starch, titanium dioxide, FD&C blue #1, and D&C yellow #10.

Each capsule-shaped aqua, scored, film coated DISALCID tablet contains 750 mg salsalate. DISALCID tablets also contain: hydroxypropyl methylcellulose, magnesium stearate, microcrystalline cellulose, polyethylene glycol, polysorbate 80, polypropylene glycol, starch, talc, titanium dioxide, FD&C blue #1, and D&C yellow #10. (See HOW SUPPLIED).

CLINICAL PHARMACOLOGY

DISALCID is insoluble in acid gastric fluids (< 0.1 mg/ml at pH 1.0), but readily soluble in the small intestine where it is partially hydrolyzed to two molecules of salicylic acid. A significant portion of the parent compound is absorbed unchanged and undergoes rapid esterase hydrolysis in the body; its half-life is about one hour. About 13% is excreted through the kidneys as a glucuronide conjugate of the parent compound, the remainder as salicylic acid and its metabolites. Thus, the amount of salicylic acid available from DISALCID is about 15% less than from aspirin, when the two drugs are administered on a salicylic acid molar equivalent basis (3.6 g salsalate/5 g aspirin). Salicylic acid biotransformation is saturated at anti-inflammatory doses of DISALCID. Such capacity-limited biotransformation results in an increase in the half-life of salicylic acid from 3.5 to 16 or more hours. Thus, dosing with DISALCID twice a day will satisfactorily maintain blood levels within the desired therapeutic range (10 to 30 mg/100 ml) throughout the 12-hour intervals. Therapeutic blood levels continue for up to 16 hours after the last dose. The parent compound does not show capacity-limited biotransformation, nor does it accumulate in the plasma on multiple dosing. Food slows the absorption of all salicylates including DISALCID.

The mode of anti-inflammatory action of DISALCID and other nonsteroidal anti-inflammatory drugs is not fully defined. Although salicylic acid (the primary metabolite of DISALCID) is a weak inhibitor of prostaglandin synthesis in vitro, DISALCID appears to selectively inhibit prostaglandin synthesis in vivo,[1] providing anti-inflammatory activity equivalent to aspirin[2] and indomethacin.[3] Unlike aspirin, DISALCID does not inhibit platelet aggregation.[4]

The usefulness of salicylic acid, the active in vivo product of DISALCID, in the treatment of arthritic disorders has been established.[5,6] In contrast to aspirin, DISALCID causes no greater fecal gastrointestinal blood loss than placebo.[7]

INDICATIONS AND USAGE

DISALCID is indicated for relief of the signs and symptoms of rheumatoid arthritis, osteoarthritis and related rheumatic disorders.

CONTRAINDICATIONS

DISALCID is contraindicated in patients hypersensitive to salsalate.

WARNINGS

Reye's Syndrome may develop in individuals who have chicken pox, influenza, or flu symptoms. Some studies suggest possible association between the development of Reye's Syndrome and the use of medicines containing salicylate or aspirin. DISALCID contains a salicylate and therefore is not recommended for use in patients with chicken pox, influenza, or flu symptoms.

PRECAUTIONS

General Precautions: Patients on treatment with DISALCID should be warned not to take other salicylates so as to avoid potentially toxic concentrations. Great care should be exercised when DISALCID is prescribed in the presence of chronic renal insufficiency or peptic ulcer disease. Protein binding of salicylic acid can be influenced by nutritional status, competitive binding of other drugs, and fluctuations in serum proteins caused by disease (rheumatoid arthritis, etc.).

Although cross reactivity, including bronchospasm, has been reported occasionally with non-acetylated salicylates, including salsalate, in aspirin-sensitive patients,[8,9] salsalate is less likely than aspirin to induce asthma in such patients.[10]

Laboratory Tests: Plasma salicylic acid concentrations should be periodically monitored during long-term treatment with DISALCID to aid maintenance of therapeutically effective levels: 10 to 30 mg/100 ml. Toxic manifestations are not usually seen until plasma concentrations exceed 30 mg/100 ml (see OVERDOSAGE). Urinary pH should also be regularly monitored: sudden acidification, as from pH 6.5 to 5.5, can double the plasma level, resulting in toxicity.

Drug Interactions: Salicylates antagonize the uricosuric action of drugs used to treat gout. ASPIRIN AND OTHER SALICYLATE DRUGS WILL BE ADDITIVE TO DISALCID AND MAY INCREASE PLASMA CONCENTRATIONS OF SALICYLIC ACID TO TOXIC LEVELS. Drugs and foods that raise urine pH will increase renal clearance and urinary excretion of salicylic acid, thus lowering plasma levels; acidifying drugs or foods will decrease urinary excretion and increase plasma levels. Salicylates given concomitantly with anticoagulant drugs may predispose to systemic bleeding. Salicylates may enhance the hypoglycemic effect of oral antidiabetic drugs of the sulfonylurea class. Salicylate competes with a number of drugs for protein binding sites, notably penicillin, thiopental, thyroxine, triiodothyronine, phenytoin, sulfinpyrazone, naproxen, warfarin, methotrexate, and possibly corticosteroids.

Drug/Laboratory Test Interactions: Salicylate competes with thyroid hormone for binding to plasma proteins, which may be reflected in a depressed plasma T_4 value in some patients; thyroid function and basal metabolism are unaffected.

Carcinogenesis: No long-term animal studies have been performed with DISALCID to evaluate its carcinogenic potential.

Use in Pregnancy: Pregnancy Category C: Salsalate and salicylic acid have been shown to be teratogenic and embryocidal in rats when given in doses 4 to 5 times the usual human dose. These effects were not observed at doses twice as great as the usual human dose. There are no adequate and well-controlled studies in pregnant women. DISALCID should be used during pregnancy only if the potential benefit justifies the potential risk to the fetus.

Labor and Delivery: There exist no adequate and well-controlled studies in pregnant women. Although adverse effects on mother or infant have not been reported with DISALCID use during labor, caution is advised when anti-inflammatory dosage is involved. However, other salicylates have been associated with prolonged gestation and labor, maternal and neonatal bleeding sequelae, potentiation of narcotic and barbiturate effects (respiratory or cardiac arrest in the mother), delivery problems and stillbirth.

Nursing Mothers: It is not known whether salsalate per se is excreted in human milk; salicylic acid, the primary metabolite of DISALCID, has been shown to appear in human milk in concentrations approximating the maternal blood level. Thus the infant of a mother on DISALCID therapy might ingest in mother's milk 30 to 80% as much salicylate per kg body weight as the mother is taking. Accordingly, caution should be exercised when DISALCID is administered to a nursing woman.

Pediatric Use: Safety and effectiveness of DISALCID use in children have not been established. (See WARNINGS section.)

ADVERSE REACTIONS

In two well-controlled clinical trials, the following reversible adverse experiences characteristic of salicylates were most commonly reported with DISALCID (n = 280 pts; listed in descending order of frequency): tinnitus, nausea, hearing impairment, rash, and vertigo. These common symptoms of salicylates, i.e., tinnitus or reversible hearing impairment, are often used as a guide to therapy.

Although cause-and-effect relationships have not been established, spontaneous reports over a ten-year period have included the following additional medically significant adverse

experiences: abdominal pain, abnormal hepatic function, anaphylactic shock, angioedema, bronchospasm, decreased creatinine clearance, diarrhea, G.I. bleeding, hepatitis, hypotension, nephritis and urticaria.

DRUG ABUSE AND DEPENDENCE

Drug abuse and dependence have not been reported with DISALCID.

OVERDOSAGE

Death has followed ingestion of 10 to 30 g of salicylates in adults, but much larger amounts have been ingested without fatal outcome.

Symptoms: The usual symptoms of salicylism—tinnitus, vertigo, headache, confusion, drowsiness, sweating, hyperventilation, vomiting and diarrhea—will occur. More severe intoxication will lead to disruption of electrolyte balance and blood pH, and hyperthermia and dehydration.

Treatment: Further absorption of DISALCID from the G.I. tract should be prevented by emesis (syrup of ipecac) and, if necessary, by gastric lavage.

Fluid and electrolyte imbalance should be corrected by the administration of appropriate I.V. therapy. Adequate renal function should be maintained. Hemodialysis or peritoneal dialysis may be required in extreme cases.

DOSAGE AND ADMINISTRATION

Adults: The usual dosage is 3000 mg daily, given in divided doses as follows: 1) two doses of two 750 mg tablets; 2) two doses of three 500 mg tablets/capsules; or 3) three doses of two 500 mg tablets/capsules. Some patients, e.g., the elderly, may require a lower dosage to achieve therapeutic blood concentrations and to avoid the more common side affects such as auditory.

Alleviation of symptoms is gradual, and full benefit may not be evident for 3 to 4 days, when plasma salicylate levels have achieved steady state. There is no evidence for development of tissue tolerance (tachyphylaxis), but salicylate therapy may induce increased activity of metabolizing liver enzymes, causing a greater rate of salicyluric acid production and excretion, with a resultant increase in dosage requirement for maintenance of therapeutic serum salicylate levels.

Children: Dosage recommendations and indications for DISALCID use in children have not been established.

HOW SUPPLIED

750 mg tablets in bottles of 100 (NDC **0089-0151-10**)
750 mg tablets in boxes of 100 in unit-dose blister strips (NDC **0089-0151-16**)
750 mg tablets in bottles of 500 (NDC **0089-0151-50**)
500 mg tablets in bottles of 100 (NDC **0089-0149-10**)
500 mg tablets in boxes of 100 in unit-dose blister strips (NDC **0089-0149-16**)
500 mg tablets in bottles of 500 (NDC **0089-0149-50**)
500 mg capsules in bottles of 100 (NDC **0089-0148-10**)
Store at controlled room temperature 15°–30°C (59°–86°F).
CAUTION: Federal law prohibits dispensing without prescription.

REFERENCES

1. Morris HG, Sherman NA, McQuain C, et al: Effects of Salsalate (Non-Acetylated) Salicylate and Aspirin (ASA) on Serum and Urine Prostaglandins in Man. Clin Pharm Therap. **33**:(2) 197, 1983.
2. April PA, Curran NJ, Ekholm, BP, et al: Multicenter Comparative Study of Salsalate (SSA) vs Aspirin (ASA) in Rheumatoid Arthritis (RA). Arthritis Rheumatism **50**(4 supplement):S93, 1987.
3. Deodhar SD, McLeod MM, Dick WC, et al: A Short-Term Comparative Trial of Salsalate and Indomethacin in Rheumatoid Arthritis. Curr. Med. Res. Opin., **5**:185–188, 1987.
4. Estes D, Kaplan K: Lack of Platelet Effect With the Aspirin Analog, Salsalate. Arthritis and Rheumatism **23**:1303–1307, 1980.
5. Dick C, Dick PH, Nuki G, et al: Effect of Anti-inflammatory Drug Therapy on Clearance of ^{133}Xe from Knee Joints of Patients with Rheumatoid Arthritis. British Med. J. **3**:278–280, 1969.
6. Dick WC, Grayson MF, Woodburn A, et al: Indices of Inflammatory Activity. Ann. of the Rheum. Dis. **29**:643–648, 1970.
7. Cohen A: Fecal Blood Loss and Plasma Salicylate Study of Salicylsalicylic Acid and Aspirin. J. Clin. Pharmacol. **19**:242–247, 1979.
8. Chudwin DS, Strub M, Golden HE, et al: Sensitivity to Non-Acetylated Salicylates in Patients with Asthma, Nasal Polyps, and Rheumatoid Arthritis, Annals of Allergy **57**:133–134, 1986.
9. Spector SL, Wangaard CH, Farr RS: Aspirin and Concomitant Idiosyncrasies in Adult Asthmatic Patients. J. Allergy Clin. Immunol. **64**:500–506, 1979.

Continued on next page

3M Riker—Cont.

10. Stevenson DD, Schrank PJ, Hougham AJ, et al: Salsalate Cross Sensitivity in Aspirin-Sensitive Asthmatics. J. Allergy Clin. Immunol. **81**:181, 1988.

DSD-15   April 1988

Shown in Product Identification Section, page 415

DUO-MEDIHALER®   ℞
(isoproterenol hydrochloride and phenylephrine bitartrate)

DESCRIPTION

Duo-Medihaler (isoproterenol hydrochloride and phenylephrine bitartrate) is an aerosol device which delivers micronized particles of isoproterenol hydrochloride and phenylephrine bitartrate. Also contains: cetylpyridinium chloride, dichlorodifluoromethane, dichlorotetrafluoroethane, sorbitan trioleate, and trichloromonofluoromethane. This drug-propellant system is contained in a hermetically sealed metal vial. Each valve actuation releases a uniform aerosolized dose of 0.16 mg. isoproterenol hydrochloride (equivalent to 0.137 mg. of isoproterenol base) and 0.24 mg. phenylephrine bitartrate (equivalent to 0.126 mg. of phenylephrine base).

HOW SUPPLIED

Duo-Medihaler with adapter (450 doses, 22.5 ml.) NDC **0089-0732-21.**
Duo-Medihaler refill vial (450 doses, 22.5 ml.) NDC **0089-0732-11.**
Duo-Medihaler with adapter (300 doses, 15 ml.) NDC **0089-0735-21.**
Duo-Medihaler refill (300 doses, 15 ml.) NDC **0089-0735-11.**

MAXAIR® Inhaler   ℞
pirbuterol acetate inhalation aerosol
Bronchodilator Aerosol
For Inhalation Only

DESCRIPTION

The active component of MAXAIR Inhaler is α^6-{[(1,1-dimethylethyl)amino]methyl}-3-hydroxy-2,6-pyridine-dimethanol monoacetate salt having the following chemical structure:

MAXAIR (pirbuterol acetate) is a white, crystalline powder, freely soluble in water, with a molecular weight of 300.3 and empirical formula of $C_{12}H_{20}N_2O_3 \cdot C_2H_4O_2$.
MAXAIR Inhaler is a metered dose aerosol unit for oral inhalation. It provides a fine-particle suspension of pirbuterol acetate in the propellant mixture of trichloromonofluoromethane and dichlorodifluoromethane, with sorbitan trioleate. Each actuation delivers from the mouthpiece pirbuterol acetate equivalent to 0.2 mg of pirbuterol with the majority of particles less than 5 microns in diameter. Each cannister provides at least 300 inhalations.

CLINICAL PHARMACOLOGY

In vitro studies and *in vivo* pharmacologic studies have demonstrated that MAXAIR has a preferential effect on beta-2 adrenergic receptors compared with isoproterenol. While it is recognized that beta-2 adrenergic receptors are the predominant receptors in bronchial smooth mucle, recent data indicate that there is a population of beta-2 receptors in the human heart, existing in a concentration between 10–50%. The precise function of these, however, is not yet established (see WARNINGS section).
The pharmacologic effects of beta adrenergic agonist drugs, including MAXAIR, are at least in part attributable to stimulation through beta adrenergic receptors of intracellular adenyl cyclase, the enzyme which catalyzes the conversion of adenosine triphosphate (ATP) to cyclic-3',5'-adenosine monophosphate (c-AMP). Increased c-AMP levels are associated with relaxation of bronchial smooth muscle and inhibition of release of mediators of immediate hypersensitivity from cells, especially from mast cells.
Bronchodilator activity of MAXAIR was manifested clinically by an improvement in various pulmonary function parameters (FEV$_1$, MMF, PEFR, airway resistance [RAW] and conductance [GA/V$_{tg}$]).
In controlled double-blind single dose clinical trials, the onset of improvement in pulmonary function occurred within 5 minutes in most patients as determined by forced expiratory volume in one second (FEV$_1$). FEV$_1$ and MMF measurements also showed that maximum improvement in pulmonary function generally occurred 30–60 minutes after one (1) or two (2) inhalations of pirbuterol (0.2–0.4 mg). The duration of action of MAXAIR is maintained for 5 hours (the time at which the last observations were made) in a substan-

tial number of patients, based on a 15% greater increase in FEV$_1$. In controlled repetitive dose studies of 12 weeks' duration, 74% of 156 patients on pirbuterol and 62% of 141 patients on metaproterenol showed a clinically significant improvement based on a 15% or greater increase in FEV$_1$ on at least half of the days. Onset and duration were equivalent to that seen in single dose studies. Continued effectiveness was demonstrated over the 12-week period in the majority (94%) of responding patients; however, chronic dosing was associated with the development of tachyphylaxis (tolerance) to the bronchodilator effect in some patients in both treatment groups.
A placebo-controlled double-blind single dose study (24 patients per treatment group), utilizing continuous Holter monitoring for 5 hours after drug administration, showed no significant difference in ectopic activity between the placebo control group and MAXAIR at the recommended dose (0.2–0.4 mg), and twice the recommended dose (0.8 mg). As with other inhaled beta adrenergic agonists, supraventricular and ventricular ectopic beats have been seen with MAXAIR (see WARNINGS).
Recent studies in laboratory animals (minipigs, rodents, and dogs) recorded the occurrence of cardiac arrhythmias and sudden death (with histologic evidence of myocardial necrosis) when beta agonists and methylxanthines were administered concurrently. The significance of these findings when applied to humans is currently unknown.

Pharmacokinetics

As expected by extrapolation from oral data, systemic blood levels of pirbuterol are below the limit of assay sensitivity (2–5 ng/ml) following inhalation of doses up to 0.8 mg (twice the maximum recommended dose). A mean of 51% of the dose is recovered in urine as pirbuterol plus its sulfate conjugate following administration by aerosol. Pirbuterol is not metabolized by catechol-O-methyltransferase. The percent of administered dose recovered as pirbuterol plus its sulfate conjugate does not change significantly over the dose range of 0.4 mg to 0.8 mg and is not significantly different from that after oral administration of pirbuterol. The plasma half-life measured after oral administration is about two hours.

INDICATIONS AND USAGE

MAXAIR Inhaler is indicated for the prevention and reversal of bronchospasm in patients with reversible bronchospasm including asthma. It may be used with or without concurrent theophylline and/or steroid therapy.

CONTRAINDICATIONS

MAXAIR is contraindicated in patients with a history of hypersensitivity to any of its ingredients.

WARNINGS

As with other beta adrenergic aerosols, MAXAIR should not be used in excess. Controlled clinical studies and other clinical experience have shown that MAXAIR like other inhaled beta adrenergic agonists can produce a significant cardiovascular effect in some patients, as measured by pulse rate, blood pressure, symptoms, and/or ECG changes. As with other beta adrenergic aerosols, the potential for paradoxical bronchospasm (which can be life threatening) should be kept in mind. If it occurs, the preparation should be discontinued immediately and alternative therapy instituted.
Fatalities have been reported in association with excessive use of inhaled sympathomimetic drugs.
The contents of MAXAIR Inhaler are under pressure. Do not puncture. Do not use or store near heat or open flame. Exposure to temperature above 120°F may cause bursting. Never throw container into fire or incinerator. Keep out of reach of children.

PRECAUTIONS

General

Since pirbuterol is a sympathomimetic amine, it should be used with caution in patients with cardiovascular disorders, including ischemic heart disease, hypertension, or cardiac arrhythmias, in patients with hyperthyroidism or diabetes mellitus, and in patients who are unusually responsive to sympathomimetic amines or who have convulsive disorders. Significant changes in systolic and diastolic blood pressure could be expected to occur in some patients after use of any beta adrenergic aerosol bronchodilator.

Information for Patients

MAXAIR effects may last up to five hours or longer. It should not be used more often than recommended and the patient should not increase the number of inhalations or frequency of use without first asking the physician. If symptoms of asthma get worse, adverse reactions occur, or the patient does not respond to the usual dose, the patient should be instructed to contact the physician immediately. The patient should be advised to see the Illustrated Directions for Use.

Drug Interactions

Other beta adrenergic aerosol bronchodilators should not be used concomitantly with MAXAIR because they may have additive effects. Beta adrenergic agonists should be administered with caution to patients being treated with monoamine oxidase inhibitors or tricyclic antidepressants, since the ac-

tion of beta adrenergic agonists on the vascular system may be potentiated.

Carcinogenesis, Mutagenesis and Impairment of Fertility

Pirbuterol hydrochloride administered in the diet to rats for 24 months and to mice for 18 months was free of carcinogenic activity at doses corresponding to 200 times the maximum human inhalation dose. In addition, the intragastric intubation of the drug at doses corresponding to 6250 times the maximum recommended human daily inhalation dose resulted in no increase in tumors in a 12-month rat study. Studies with pirbuterol revealed no evidence of mutagenesis. Reproduction studies in rats revealed no evidence of impaired fertility.

Teratogenic Effects—Pregnancy Category C

Reproduction studies have been performed in rats and rabbits by the inhalation route at doses up to 12 times (rat) and 16 times (rabbit) the maximum human inhalation dose and have revealed no significant findings. Animal reproduction studies in rats at *oral doses* up to 300 mg/kg and in rabbits at oral doses up to 100 mg/kg have shown no adverse effect on reproductive behavior, fertility, litter size, peri- and postnatal viability or fetal development. In rabbits at the highest dose level given, 300 mg/kg, abortions and fetal mortality were observed. There are no adequate and well controlled studies in pregnant women and MAXAIR should be used during pregnancy only if the potential benefit justifies the potential risk to the fetus.

Nursing Mothers

It is not known whether MAXAIR is excreted in human milk. Therefore, MAXAIR should be used during nursing only if the potential benefit justifies the possible risk to the newborn.

Pediatric Use

MAXAIR Inhaler is not recommended for patients under the age of 12 years because of insufficient clinical data to establish safety and effectiveness.

ADVERSE REACTIONS

The following rates of adverse reaction to pirbuterol are based on single and multiple dose clinical trials involving 761 patients, 400 of whom received multiple doses (mean duration of treatment was 2.5 months and maximum was 19 months).
The following were the adverse reactions reported more frequently than 1 in 100 patients:
CNS: nervousness (6.9%), tremor (6.0%), headache (2.0%), dizziness (1.2%).
Cardiovascular: palpitations (1.7%), tachycardia (1.2%).
Respiratory: cough (1.2%).
Gastrointestinal: nausea (1.7%).
The following adverse reactions occurred less frequently than 1 in 100 patients and there may be a causal relationship with pirbuterol:
CNS: depression, anxiety, confusion, insomnia, weakness, hyperkinesia, syncope.
Cardiovascular: hypotension, skipped beats, chest pain.
Gastrointestinal: dry mouth, glossitis, abdominal pain/cramps, anorexia, diarrhea, stomatitis, nausea and vomiting.
Ear, Nose and Throat: smell/taste changes, sore throat.
Dermatological: rash, pruritus.
Other: numbness in extremities, alopecia, bruising, fatigue, edema, weight gain, flushing.
Other adverse reactions were reported with a frequency of less than 1 in 100 patients but a causal relationship between pirbuterol and the reaction could not be determined: migraine, productive cough, wheezing, and dermatitis.
The following rates of adverse reactions during three-month controlled clinical trials involving 310 patients are noted. The table does not include mild reactions.

PERCENT OF PATIENTS WITH MODERATE TO SEVERE ADVERSE REACTIONS

Reaction	Pirbuterol N = 157	Metaproterenol N = 153
Central Nervous System		
tremors	1.3%	3.3%
nervousness	4.5%	2.6%
headache	1.3%	2.0%
weakness	.0%	1.3%
drowsiness	.0%	0.7%
dizziness	0.6%	.0%
Cardiovascular		
palpitations	1.3%	1.3%
tachycardia	1.3%	2.0%
Respiratory		
chest pain/tightness	1.3%	.0%
cough	.0%	0.7%
Gastrointestinal		
nausea	1.3%	2.0%
diarrhea	1.3%	0.7%
dry mouth	1.3%	1.3%
vomiting	.0%	0.7%
Dermatological		
skin reaction	.0%	0.7%
rash	.0%	1.3%

Other

bruising	0.6%	.0%
smell/taste change	0.6%	.0%
backache	.0%	0.7%
fatigue	.0%	0.7%
hoarseness	.0%	0.7%
nasal congestion	.0%	0.7%

OVERDOSAGE

The expected symptoms with overdosage are those of excessive beta-stimulation and/or any of the symptoms listed under adverse reactions, e.g., angina, hypertension or hypotension, arrhythmias, nervousness, headache, tremor, dry mouth, palpitation, nausea, dizziness, fatigue, malaise, and insomnia.

Treatment consists of discontinuation of pirbuterol together with appropriate symptomatic therapy.

The oral acute lethal dose in male and female rats and mice was greater than 2000 mg base/kg. The aerosol acute lethal dose was not determined.

DOSAGE AND ADMINISTRATION

The usual dose for adults and children 12 years and older is two inhalations (0.4 mg) repeated every 4–6 hours. One inhalation (0.2 mg) repeated every 4–6 hours may be sufficient for some patients.

A total daily dose of 12 inhalations should not be exceeded. If a previously effective dosage regimen fails to provide the usual relief, medical advice should be sought immediately as this is often a sign of seriously worsening asthma which would require reassessment of therapy.

HOW SUPPLIED

MAXAIR Inhaler is supplied in pressurized aluminum canisters. Each actuation delivers pirbuterol acetate equivalent to 0.2 mg of pirbuterol from the mouthpiece.

Vial with plastic actuator, net content weight 25.6 g, a minimum of 300 actuations (NDC **0089-0790-21**).

Refill vial only, net content weight 25.6 g, a minimum of 300 actuations (NDC **0089-0790-11**).

CAUTION

Federal law prohibits dispensing without prescription.
Store between 15° and 30°C (59° to 86°F).
PIR-2   FEBRUARY 1988
Shown in Product Identification Section, page 416

MEDIHALER-EPI®
(epinephrine bitartrate)
FOR TEMPORARY RELIEF FROM ACUTE PAROXYSMS OF BRONCHIAL ASTHMA.

FOR ORAL INHALATION THERAPY ONLY

Each inhalation delivers 0.3 mg epinephrine bitartrate equivalent to 0.16 mg of epinephrine base. Also contains: cetylpyridinium chloride, dichlorodifluoromethane, dichlorotetrafluoroethane, sorbitan trioleate, and trichloromonofluoromethane.

HOW SUPPLIED

15 ml. size: Available as a combination package (vial with oral adapter) or as a refill (vial only).

MEDIHALER ERGOTAMINE®   ℞
(ergotamine tartrate)

DESCRIPTION

Medihaler Ergotamine (ergotamine tartrate) is an aerosol device which contains a fine particle suspension of 9.0 mg. ergotamine tartrate per ml. in an inert, nontoxic aerosol vehicle. The inert ingredients are dichlorodifluoromethane, dichlorotetrafluoroethane, sorbitan trioleate, and trichloromonofluoromethane. Each depression of the valve delivers a measured dose of 0.36 mg. to the patient.

ACTION

Ergotamine exerts a constrictor action upon the cranial vessels.

INDICATIONS

As therapy to abort vascular headache, e.g., migraine, migraine variants, or so-called "histaminic cephalalgia."

CONTRAINDICATIONS

Ergotamine tartrate should not be used in the presence of coronary artery disease, peripheral vascular disease, hypertension, impaired renal or hepatic function, infectious states or malnutrition.

Ergotamine tartrate is contraindicated in patients with a history of hypersensitivity reactions.

Pregnancy: Ergotamine tartrate is contraindicated in pregnancy.

WARNINGS

Patients who are being treated with Medihaler Ergotamine should be informed adequately of the symptoms of ergotism. Close medical supervision by the physician is recommended so that he may react appropriately should signs of ergotism develop. Six inhalations per day, if continued daily, entail the risk of vasospastic complications. Avoid prolonged administration or in excess of the recommended dosage because of the danger of ergotism and gangrene.

Pediatric Patients: Since there is no experience in children who have received this drug, safety and efficacy in children have not been established.

Nursing Mothers: Whether ergotamine tartrate is excreted in mothers' milk is not known. As a general rule, nursing should not be undertaken while a patient is on a drug (since many drugs are excreted in human milk).

ADVERSE REACTIONS

Ergotamine tartrate may cause nausea and vomiting. Patients with headaches may become nauseated and drug induced distress may be difficult to evaluate.

Ergotamine in large doses raises arterial pressure, produces coronary vasoconstriction and slows the heart both by direct action and its effect on the vagus. Under this condition, ergotamine also has oxytocic and spasmolytic properties. The above conditions are seen as a consequence of overdosage and may be manifested at the dosage recommended for control of headaches.

Vasoconstrictive complications, at times of a serious nature, may occur. These include pulselessness, weakness, muscle pains and paresthesias of the extremities and precordial distress and pain. Although these effects occur most commonly with long term therapy at relatively high doses, they have also been reported with short term or normal doses. Other adverse effects include transient tachycardia or bradycardia, nausea, vomiting, localized edema and itching.

DOSAGE AND ADMINISTRATION

Adults: A single inhalation at the first sign of headache or prodrome. Repeat this procedure in 5 minutes if relief is not obtained. Space any additional inhalations at no less than 5-minute intervals. No more than 6 inhalations should be administered in any 24-hour period, and no more than 15 in a one week period.

Children: A recommended dose for children has not been determined.

Directions For Use: Before each use, remove dust cap and shake Medihaler Ergotamine.
1. Breathe out fully and place mouthpiece well into the mouth, aimed at the back of the throat.
2. As you begin to breathe in deeply, press the vial firmly down into the adapter with the index finger. This releases one dose.
3. Release pressure on vial and remove unit from mouth. Hold the breath as long as possible, then breathe out slowly.

HOW SUPPLIED

Metal vial (2.5 ml.) and adapter. Each depression of the valve delivers 0.36 mg. ergotamine tartrate. (NDC **0089-0762-21**).

CAUTION

Federal law prohibits dispensing without prescription.
Shown in Product Identification Section, page 416

MEDIHALER-ISO®   ℞
(isoproterenol sulfate)

DESCRIPTION

Medihaler-Iso (isoproterenol sulfate) is an aerosol device which contains a fine particle suspension of 2.0 mg. per ml. isoproterenol sulfate. Also contains: dichlorodifluoromethane, dichlorotetrafluoroethane, sorbitan trioleate, and trichloromonofluoromethane. Each depression of the valve delivers a measured dose of 0.08 mg. to the patient.

HOW SUPPLIED

Medihaler-Iso (isoproterenol sulfate) with oral adapter (300 doses 15 ml.) NDC **0089-0785-21**.

Medihaler-Iso (isoproterenol sulfate) refill vial only (300 doses 15 ml.) NDC **0089-0785-11**.

Medihaler-Iso (isoproterenol sulfate) with oral adapter (450 doses 22.5 ml.) NDC **0089-0782-21**.

Medihaler-Iso (isoproterenol sulfate) refill vial only (450 doses 22.5 ml.) NDC **0089-0782-11**.

MINITRAN®   ℞
(nitroglycerin)
Transdermal Delivery System

DESCRIPTION

The MINITRAN transdermal delivery system contains nitroglycerin in a hypoallergenic, medical grade, acrylate-based polymer adhesive. Components of this system are used in various medical tapes. The MINITRAN system is available in dosage strengths which deliver 2.5 mg/24 hours (3.3 cm^2), 5 mg/24 hours (6.7 cm^2), 10 mg/24 hours (13.3 cm^2), and 15 mg/24 hours (20 cm^2). These contain 9 mg, 18 mg, 36 mg, and 54 mg, respectively, and provide a range of continuous dosing levels of nitroglycerin. The rate of release of nitroglycerin is dependent upon the area of the system applied to the skin; approximately 0.75 mg nitroglycerin is released per 24 hours for every square centimeter of system area. Each patch is packaged in foil/polymer film laminate.

CLINICAL PHARMACOLOGY

When the MINITRAN system is applied to the skin, nitroglycerin is absorbed continuously through the skin into the systemic circulation. This results in active drug reaching the target organs (heart, vascular system) before deactivation by the liver. Nitroglycerin is a smooth muscle relaxant with vascular effects manifested predominately by venous dilation with pooling. The major beneficial effect of nitroglycerin in angina pectoris is a reduction in myocardial oxygen consumption secondary to vascular dilatation with resultant reduction in cardiac preload and afterload. Recent data also indicate a direct vasodilator effect of nitroglycerin on the coronary vessels.

In studies of MINITRAN in healthy volunteers, transdermal absorption of nitroglycerin was demonstrated by attainment of continuous venous plasma levels for a minimum of 24 hours. In most cases, detectable plasma levels are attained within 30 minutes, reaching steady state 2 hours after application of the system. Levels were maintained for 24 hours and diminished rapidly when the system was removed. Precise definition of "therapeutic plasma level" for nitroglycerin is not known at this time. The amount of nitroglycerin released (2.5 mg, 5 mg, 10 mg, or 15 mg per 24 hours) represents the mean release rate of nitroglycerin as determined from healthy volunteers and, hence, the amount potentially available for absorption from the skin. Absorption will vary among individuals.

INDICATIONS AND USAGE

This drug product has been conditionally approved by the FDA for the prevention and treatment of angina pectoris due to coronary artery disease. The conditional approval reflects a determination that the drug may be marketed while further investigation of its effectiveness is undertaken. A final evaluation of the effectiveness of the product will be announced by the FDA.

CONTRAINDICATIONS

Intolerance of organic nitrate drugs or marked anemia.

WARNINGS

The MINITRAN system should be used under careful clinical and/or hemodynamic monitoring in patients with acute myocardial infarction or congestive heart failure.

In terminating treatment of anginal patients, both the dosage and frequency of application must be gradually reduced over a period of 4 to 6 weeks to prevent sudden withdrawal reactions, which are characteristic of all vasodilators in the nitroglycerin class.

PRECAUTIONS

Symptoms of hypotension, such as faintness, weakness or dizziness, particularly orthostatic hypotension, may be due to overdosage. If these symptoms occur during the course of treatment, the dosage should be reduced or use of the product discontinued.

MINITRAN is not intended for use in the treatment of acute anginal attacks. For this purpose, occasional use of sublingual nitroglycerin may be necessary.

Pregnancy: Pregnancy Category C. Animal reproduction studies have not been conducted with MINITRAN. It is also not known whether MINITRAN can cause fetal harm when administered to a pregnant woman or can affect reproductive capacity. MINITRAN should be given to a pregnant woman only if clearly needed.

Nursing Mothers: It is not known whether nitroglycerin is excreted in human milk. Because many drugs are excreted in human milk, caution should be exercised when MINITRAN is administered to a nursing woman.

ADVERSE REACTIONS

Transient headache is the most common side effect, especially when higher doses of the drug are administered. Headaches should be treated with mild analgesics while continuing MINITRAN therapy. If headache persists, the MINITRAN dosage should be reduced, or use of the product discontinued.

Adverse reactions reported less frequently include hypotension, increased heart rate, faintness, flushing, dizziness, nausea, vomiting, and dermatitis. Except for dermatitis, these symptoms are attributed to the pharmacologic effects of nitroglycerin; however, they may be symptoms of overdosage. When they persist, the MINITRAN dosage should be reduced or use of the product discontinued.

DOSAGE AND ADMINISTRATION

To apply the MINITRAN system, tear (do not cut) the foil pouch open and remove the unit. With the "PEEL OFF" message on the plastic liner facing you, peel away the smaller portion of the plastic liner while holding the product in your other hand. Firmly apply the exposed adhesive surface to the

Continued on next page

3M Riker—Cont.

site of application. Gently peel away the remaining portion of the plastic liner and firmly press the entire patch against the skin to insure complete adhesion. Dispose of both portions of the plastic liner. Remove and discard the system after 24 hours. Place a new system on a different skin site. The initial starting dose is usually 5 mg/24 hours. To achieve optimum therapeutic effect in some patients, it may be necessary to titrate to a higher dosing strength.

Dosage should be titrated while monitoring clinical response, ie, blood pressure, episodes of angina and subsequent use of sublingual nitroglycerin. A 2.5 mg/24 hours dose is useful principally for increasing or decreasing the dosage gradually, though it may provide adequate therapy for some patients when used alone. The MINITRAN system may remain in place for periods of up to 24 hours as required to provide continuous levels of nitroglycerin.

The MINITRAN system may be applied to any convenient skin area; a recommended site of application is the arm or chest. A suitable area may be lightly shaved if necessary. Do not apply the MINITRAN system to the distal part of the extremities, ie, below the elbow or knee.

STORAGE CONDITIONS

Store at controlled room temperature 15°–30°C (59°–86°F). **Do not refrigerate.** Extremes of temperature and/or humidity should be avoided.

HOW SUPPLIED

[See table below].

MINITRAN transdermal delivery system, 2.5 mg/24 hours, 5 mg/24 hours, 10 mg/24 hours, and 15 mg/24 hours, is available in cartons of 33 patches.

CAUTION

Federal law prohibits dispensing without prescription.

PATIENT INFORMATION

Patient instructions for application appear on each unit dose package. Additional patient information is supplied with the systems.

NTR-2   AUGUST 1988

Shown in Product Identification Section, page 416

NORFLEX®   ℞
(orphenadrine citrate)
Tablets and Injectable

PRODUCT OVERVIEW

KEY FACTS

Norflex sustained-release tablets provide 12 hours relief from the pain of muscle spasm. Also available in injectable form, IV or IM, also given every 12 hours.

MAJOR USES

Norflex is indicated as an adjunct to rest, physical therapy, and other measures for the relief of discomfort associated with painful musculoskeletal disorders.

SAFETY INFORMATION

Contraindicated in patients with glaucoma, pyloric or duodenal obstruction, stenosing peptic ulcers, prostatic hypertrophy or obstruction of the bladder neck, cardiospasm (megaesophagus) and myasthenia gravis. Contraindicated in patients who have a previous sensitivity to the drug.

PRESCRIBING INFORMATION

NORFLEX®   ℞
(orphenadrine citrate)
Tablets and Injectable

DESCRIPTION

Orphenadrine citrate is the citrate salt of orphenadrine (2-dimethylaminoethyl 2-methylbenzhydryl ether citrate). It occurs as a white, crystalline powder having a bitter taste. It is practically odorless; sparingly soluble in water, slightly soluble in alcohol.

Each Norflex Tablet contains 100 mg orphenadrine citrate. Norflex Tablets also contain: calcium stearate, ethylcellulose, and lactose. Norflex injectable contains 60 mg of orphenadrine citrate in aqueous solution in each ampul. Norflex injectable also contains: water for injection, USP; sodium chloride; sodium bisulfite; and sodium hydroxide.

ACTIONS

The mode of therapeutic action has not been clearly identified, but may be related to its analgesic properties. Orphenadrine citrate also possesses anti-cholinergic actions.

INDICATIONS

Orphenadrine citrate is indicated as an adjunct to rest, physical therapy, and other measures for the relief of discomfort associated with acute painful musculo skeletal conditions. The mode of action of the drug has not been clearly identified, but may be related to its analgesic properties. Orphenadrine citrate does not directly relax tense skeletal muscles in man.

CONTRAINDICATIONS

Contraindicated in patients with glaucoma, pyloric or duodenal obstruction, stenosing peptic ulcers, prostatic hypertrophy or obstruction of the bladder neck, cardio-spasm (megaesophagus) and myasthenia gravis. Contraindicated in patients who have demonstrated a previous hypersensitivity to the drug.

WARNINGS

Some patients may experience transient episodes of lightheadedness, dizziness or syncope. Norflex may impair the ability of the patient to engage in potentially hazardous activities such as operating machinery or driving a motor vehicle; ambulatory patients should therefore be cautioned accordingly.

Norflex injectable contains sodium bisulfite, a sulfite that may cause allergic-type reactions including anaphylactic symptoms and life-threatening or less severe asthmatic episodes in certain susceptible people. The overall prevalence of sulfite sensitivity in the general population is unknown and probably low. Sulfite sensitivity is seen more frequently in asthmatic than nonasthmatic people.

USAGE IN PREGNANCY

Safe use of orphenadrine has not been established with respect to adverse effects upon fetal development. Therefore, Norflex should be used in women of childbearing potential and particularly during early pregnancy only when in the judgment of the physician the potential benefits outweigh the possible hazards.

USAGE IN CHILDREN

Safety and effectiveness in children have not been established; therefore, this drug is not recommended for use in the pediatric age group.

PRECAUTIONS

Confusion, anxiety and tremors have been reported in few patients receiving propoxyphene and orphenadrine concomitantly. As these symptoms may be simply due to an additive effect, reduction of dosage and/or discontinuation of one or both agents is recommended in such cases.

Orphenadrine citrate should be used with caution in patients with tachycardia, cardiac decompensation, coronary insufficiency, cardiac arrhythmias.

Safety of continuous long-term therapy with orphenadrine has not been established. Therefore, if orphenadrine is prescribed for prolonged use, periodic monitoring of blood, urine and liver function values is recommended.

ADVERSE REACTIONS

Adverse effects of orphenadrine are mainly due to the mild anticholinergic action of orphenadrine, and are usually associated with higher dosage. Dryness of the mouth is usually the first adverse effect to appear. When the daily dose is increased, possible adverse effects include: tachycardia, palpitation, urinary hesitancy or retention, blurred vision, dilatation of pupils, increased ocular tension, weakness, nausea, vomiting, headache, dizziness, constipation, drowsiness, hypersensitivity reactions, pruritus, hallucinations, agitation, tremor, gastric irritation, and rarely urticaria and other dermatoses. Infrequently, an elderly patient may experience some degree of mental confusion. These adverse reactions can usually be eliminated by reduction in dosage. Very rare cases of aplastic anemia associated with the use of orphenadrine tablets have been reported. No causal relationship has been established.

Rare instances of anaphylactic reaction have been reported associated with the intramuscular injection of Norflex injectable.

DOSAGE AND ADMINISTRATION

TABLETS:Adults—Two tablets per day; one in the morning and one in the evening.

INJECTABLE: Adults—One 2 ml. ampul (60 mg.) intravenously or intramuscularly; may be repeated every 12 hours. Relief may be maintained by 1 Norflex tablet twice daily.

HOW SUPPLIED

TABLETS: Bottles of 100 (NDC **0089-0221-10**) and 500 (NDC **0089-0221-50**). Boxes of 100 in unit dose, aluminum foil strips (NDC **0089-0221-16**). Each tablet contains 100 mg of orphenadrine citrate.

INJECTABLE: Boxes of 6 (NDC **0089-0540-06**) and 50 (NDC **0089-0540-50**) 2 ml ampuls, each ampul containing 60 mg of orphenadrine citrate in aqueous solution.

A.H.F.S. Category 12:08

CAUTION

Federal law prohibits dispensing without prescription.

Shown in Product Identification Section, page 416

NORGESIC®   ℞
and
NORGESIC® FORTE   ℞

ACTIONS

Orphenadrine citrate is a centrally acting (brain stem) compound which in animals selectively blocks facilitatory functions of the reticular formation. Orphenadrine does not produce myoneural block, nor does it affect crossed extensor reflexes. Orphenadrine prevents nicotine-induced convulsions but not those produced by strychnine.

Chronic administration of Norgesic to dogs and rats has revealed no drug-related toxicity. No blood or urine changes were observed, nor were there any macroscopic or microscopic pathological changes detected. Extensive experience with combinations containing aspirin and caffeine has established them as safe agents. The addition of orphenadrine citrate does not alter the toxicity of aspirin and caffeine. The mode of therapeutic action of orphenadrine has not been clearly identified, but may be related to its analgesic properties. Orphenadrine citrate also possesses anti-cholinergic actions.

INDICATIONS

1. Symptomatic relief of mild to moderate pain of acute musculo-skeletal disorders.
2. The orphenadrine component is indicated as an adjunct to rest, physical therapy, and other measures for the relief of discomfort associated with acute painful musculo-skeletal conditions.

The mode of action of orphenadrine has not been clearly identified, but may be related to its analgesic properties. Norgesic and Norgesic Forte do not directly relax tense skeletal muscles in man.

CONTRAINDICATIONS

Because of the mild anticholinergic effect of orphenadrine, Norgesic or Norgesic Forte should not be used in patients with glaucoma, pyloric or duodenal obstruction, achalasia, prostatic hypertrophy or obstructions at the bladder neck. Norgesic or Norgesic Forte is also contraindicated in patients with myasthenia gravis and in patients known to be sensitive to aspirin or caffeine.

The drug is contraindicated in patients who have demonstrated a previous hypersensitivity to the drug.

WARNINGS

Reye Syndrome may develop in individuals who have chicken pox, influenza, or flu symptoms. Some studies suggest possible association between the development of Reye Syndrome and the use of medicines containing salicylate or aspirin. Norgesic and Norgesic Forte contain aspirin and therefore are not recommended for use in patients with chicken pox, influenza, or flu symptoms.

Norgesic Forte may impair the ability of the patient to engage in potentially hazardous activities such as operating machinery or driving a motor vehicle; ambulatory patients should therefore be cautioned accordingly.

Aspirin should be used with extreme caution in the presence of peptic ulcers and coagulation abnormalities.

USAGE IN PREGNANCY

Since safety of the use of this preparation in pregnancy, during lactation, or in the childbearing age has not been established, use of the drug in such patients requires that the potential benefits of the drug be weighed against its possible hazard to the mother and child.

USAGE IN CHILDREN

The safe and effective use of this drug in children has not been established. Usage of this drug in children under 12 years of age is not recommended.

PRECAUTIONS

Confusion, anxiety and tremors have been reported in few patients receiving propoxyphene and orphenadrine concomitantly. As these symptoms may be simply due to an additive effect, reduction of dosage and/or discontinuation of one or both agents is recommended in such cases.

MINITRAN System Rated Release In-Vivo	System Size	Total Nitroglycerin in System	NDC Number
2.5 mg/24 hr	3.3 cm^2	9 mg	NDC-0089-0301-03
5 mg/24 hr	6.7 cm^2	18 mg	NDC-0089-0302-03
10 mg/24 hr	13.3 cm^2	36 mg	NDC-0089-0303-03
15 mg/24 hr	20.0 cm^2	54 mg	NDC-0089-0304-03

Safety of continuous long term therapy with Norgesic Forte has not been established; therefore, if Norgesic Forte is prescribed for prolonged use, periodic monitoring of blood, urine and liver function values is recommended.

ADVERSE REACTIONS

Side effects of Norgesic or Norgesic Forte are those seen with aspirin and caffeine or those usually associated with mild anticholinergic agents. These may include tachycardia, palpitation, urinary hesitancy or retention, dry mouth, blurred vision, dilatation of the pupil, increased intraocular tension, weakness, nausea, vomiting, headache, dizziness, constipation, drowsiness, and rarely, urticaria and other dermatoses. Infrequently an elderly patient may experience some degree of confusion. Mild central excitation and occasional hallucinations may be observed. These mild side effects can usually be eliminated by reduction in dosage. One case of aplastic anemia associated with the use of Norgesic has been reported. No causal relationship has been established. Rare G.I. hemorrhage due to aspirin content may be associated with the administration of Norgesic or Norgesic Forte. Some patients may experience transient episodes of light-headedness, dizziness or syncope.

DOSAGE AND ADMINISTRATION

Norgesic: Adults 1 to 2 tablets 3 to 4 times daily.
Norgesic Forte: Adults ½ to 1 tablet 3 to 4 times daily.

HOW SUPPLIED

Norgesic tablets can be identified by their three layers colored light green, white and yellow. Each round tablet contains orphenadrine citrate (2-dimethylaminoethyl 2-methylbenzhydryl ether citrate) 25 mg., aspirin 385 mg., and caffeine 30 mg.

Norgesic Forte tablets are exactly twice the strength of Norgesic. They are identified by their scored capsule shape and by their three layers colored light green, white and yellow. Each capsule shaped tablet contains orphenadrine citrate 50 mg., aspirin 770 mg., and caffeine 60 mg.

Norgesic and Norgesic Forte also contain: lactose, polyethylene glycol, povidone, starch, sucrose, zinc stearate, and D&C yellow #10, and FD&C blue #1.

Norgesic: Bottles of 100 (NDC **0089-0231-10**) and 500 tablets (NDC **0089-0231-50**); Boxes of 100 in unit dose, aluminum foil strips (NDC **0089-0231-16**).

Norgesic Forte: Bottles of 100 tablets (NDC **0089-0233-10**) and 500 tablets (NDC **0089-0233-50**); Boxes of 100 in unit dose, aluminum foil strips (NDC **0089-0233-16**)

CAUTION

Federal law prohibits dispensing without prescription.
Shown in Product Identification Section, page 416

TAMBOCOR® ℞

[tăm-ba-kŏr]
(flecainide acetate)
Oral Tablets

DESCRIPTION

TAMBOCOR® (flecainide acetate) is an antiarrhythmic drug available in tablets of 50, 100 or 150 mg for oral administration.

Flecainide acetate is benzamide, N-(2-piperidinylmethyl)-2,5-bis(2,2,2-trifluoroethoxy)-, monoacetate. The structural formula is given below.

$$CF_3CH_2O-\text{(benzene ring)}-CONHCH_2-\text{(piperidine ring, NH)} \cdot CH_3COOH$$
$$OCH_2CF_3$$

Flecainide acetate is a white crystalline substance with a pK_a of 9.3. It has a aqueous solubility of 48.4 mg/ml at 37°C. TAMBOCOR tablets also contain: croscarmellose sodium, hydrogenated vegetable oil, magnesium stearate, microcrystalline cellulose and starch.

CLINICAL PHARMACOLOGY

TAMBOCOR has local anesthetic activity and belongs to the membrane stabilizing (Class I) group of antiarrhythmic agents; it has electrophysiologic effects characteristic of the IC class of antiarrhythmics.

Electrophysiology. In man, TAMBOCOR produces a dose-related decrease in intracardiac conduction in all parts of the heart with the greatest effect on the His-Purkinje system (H-V connduction). Effects upon atrioventricular (AV) nodal conduction time and intra-atrial conduction times, although present, are less pronounced than those on ventricular conduction velocity. Significant effects on refractory periods were observed only in the ventricle. Sinus node recovery times (corrected) following pacing and spontaneous cycle lengths are somewhat increased. This latter effect may become significant in patients with sinus node dysfunction. (See Warnings.)

TAMBOCOR causes a dose-related and plasma-level related decrease in single and multiple PVCs and can suppress recurrence of ventricular tachycardia. In limited studies of patients with a history of ventricular techycardia, TAMBOCOR has been successful 30-40% of the time in fully suppressing the inducibility of arrhythmias by programmed electrical stimulation. Based on PVC suppression, it appears that plasma levels of 0.2 to 1.0 ug/ml may be needed to obtain the maximal therapeutic effect. It is more difficult to assess the dose needed to suppress serious arrhythmias, but trough plasma levels in patients successfully treated for recurrent ventricular tachycardia were between 0.2 and 1.0 ug/ml. Plasma levels above 0.7-1.0 ug/ml are associated with a higher rate of cardiac adverse experiences such as conduction defects or bradycardia. The relation of plasma levels to proarrhythmic events is not established, but dose reduction in clinical trials of patients with ventricular tachycardia appears to have led to a reduced frequency and severity of such events.

Hemodynamics. TAMBOCOR does not usually alter heart rate, although bradycardia and tachycardia have been reported occasionally.

In animals and isolated myocardium, a negative inotropic effect of flecainide has been demonstrated. Decreases in ejection fraction, consistent with a negative inotropic effect, have been observed after single administration of 200 to 250 mg of the drug in man; both increases and decreases in ejection fraction have been encountered during multidose therapy in patients at usual therapeutic dose. (See Warnings.)

Metabolism in Humans. Following oral administration, the absorption of TAMBOCOR is nearly complete. Peak plasma levels are attained at about three hours in most individuals (range, 1 to 6 hours). Flecainide does not undergo any consequential presystemic biotransformation (first-pass effect). Food or antacid do not affect absorption.

The apparent plasma half-life averages about 20 hours but is quite variable (range, 12 to 27 hours) after multiple oral doses in patients with premature ventricular contractions (PVCs). With multiple dosing, plasma levels increase because of its long half-life with steady-state levels approached in 3 to 5 days; once at steady-state, no additional (or unexpected) accumulation of drug in plasma occurs during chronic therapy. Over the usual therapeutic range, data suggest that plasma levels in an individual are approximately proportional to dose, deviating upwards from linearity only slightly (about 10 to 15% per 100 mg on average). In healthy subjects, about 30% of a single oral dose (range, 10 to 50%) is excreted in urine as unchanged drug. The two major urinary metabolites are meta-O-dealkylated flecainide (active, but about one fifth as potent) and the meta-O-dealkylated lactam of flecainide (non-active metabolite). These two metabolites (primarily conjugated) account for most of the remaining portion of the dose. Several minor metabolites (3% of the dose or less) are also found in urine; only 5% of an oral dose is excreted in feces. In patients, free (unconjuated) plasma levels of the two major metabolites are very low (less than 0.05 ug/ml).

When urinary pH is very alkaline (8 or higher), as may occur in rare conditions (e.g., renal tubular acidosis, strict vegetarian diet), flecainide elimination from plasma is much slower. The elimination of flecainide from the body depends on renal function (i.e., 10 to 50% appears in urine as unchanged drug). With increasing renal impairment, the extent of unchanged drug excretion in urine is reduced and the plasma half-life of flecainide is prolonged. Since flecainide is also extensively metabolized, there is no simple relationship between creatinine clearance and the rate of flecainide elimination from plasma. (See Dosage and Administration.)

In patients with congestive heart failure (NYHA class III), the rate of flecainide elimination from plasma (mean half-life, 19 hours) is moderately slower than for healty subjects (mean half-life, 14 hours), but similar to the rate for otherwise well patients with PVCs. The extent of unchanged drug excretion in urine is also similar. (See Dosage and Administration.)

From age 20 to 80, plasma levels are only slightly higher with advancing age; flecainide elimination from plasma is somewhat slower in elderly subjects than in younger subjects. Patients up to age 80+ have been safely treated with usual dosages.

The extent of flecainide binding to human plasma proteins is about 40% and is independent of plasma drug level over the range of 0.015 to about 3.4 ug/ml. Thus, clinically significant drug interactions based on protein binding effects would not be expected.

Hemodialysis removes only about 1% of an oral dose as unchanged flecainide.

Small increases in plasma digoxin levels are seen during coadministration of TAMBOCOR with digoxin. Small increases in both flecainide and propranolol plasma levels are seen during coadministration of these two drugs. (See Precautions, Drug Interaction.)

INDICATIONS AND USAGE

TAMBOCOR is indicated for the treatment of documented ventricular arrhythmias, such as sustained ventricular tachycardia, that in the judgment of the physician, are life-threatening. Because of the proarrhythmic effects of TAM-

BOCOR, its use should be reserved for patients in whom, in the opinion of the physician, the benefits of treatment outweigh the risks. The use of TAMBOCOR is not recommended in patients with less severe ventricular arrhythmias even if the patients are symptomatic.

Use of TAMBOCOR for the treatment of sustained ventricular tachycardia, like other antiarrhythmics, should be initiated in the hospital.

The effects of TAMBOCOR in patients with recent myocardial infarction (except as described in the WARNINGS section) and in patients with supraventricular tachycardia have not been adequately studied. As is the case for other antiarrhythmic agents, there is no evidence from controlled trials that the use of TAMBOCOR favorably affects survival or the incidence of sudden death.

CONTRAINDICATIONS

TAMBOCOR is contraindicated in patients with preexisting second- or third-degree AV block, or with right bundle branch block when associated with a left hemiblock (bifascicular block), unless a pacemaker is present to sustain the cardiac rhythm should complete heart block occur. TAMBOCOR is also contraindicated in the presence of cardiogenic shock or known hypersensitivity to the drug.

WARNINGS

> **Mortality.** TAMBOCOR was included in the National Heart Lung and Blood Institute's Cardiac Arrhythmia Suppression Trial (CAST), a long-term multi-center, randomized, doubled-blind study in patients with asymptomatic non-life-threatening arrhythmias who had a myocardial infarction more than six days, but less than two years previously. An excessive mortality or non-fatal cardiac arrest rate was seen in patients treated with TAMBOCOR compared with that seen in a carefully matched placebo-treated group. This rate was 16/315 (5.1%) for TAMBOCOR and 7/309 (2.3%) for its matched placebo. The average duration of treatment with TAMBOCOR in this study was 10 months.

The applicability of these results to other populations (e.g., those without recent infarction) is uncertain, but at present it is prudent to consider the risks of Class IC agents, coupled with the lack of any evidence of improved survival, generally unacceptable in patients without life-threatening ventricular arrhythmias, even if the patients are experiencing unpleasant, but not life-threatening, symptoms or signs.

Proarrhythmic Effects. TAMBOCOR, like other antiarrhythmic agents, can cause new or worsened arrhythmias. Such proarrhythmic effects range from an increase in frequency of PVCs to the development of more severe ventricular tachycardia, e.g., tachycardia that is more sustained or more resistant to conversion to sinus rhythm, with potentially fatal consequences. In studies of ventricular arrhythmia patients treated with TAMBOCOR, three-fourths of proarrhythmic events were new or worsened ventricular tachyarrhythmias, the remainder being increased frequency of PVCs or new supraventricular arrhythmias. It is uncertain if TAMBOCOR's risk of proarrhythmia is exaggerated in patients with chronic atrial fibrillation (CAF), high ventricular rate, and/or exercise. Wide complex tachycardia and ventricular fibrillation have been reported in two of 12 CAF patients undergoing maximal exercise tolerance testing.

In patients with complex arrhythmias, it is often difficult to distinguish a spontaneous variation in the patient's underlying rhythm disorder from drug-induced worsening, so that the following occurence rates must be considered approximations. Their frequency appears to be related to dose and to the underlying cardiac disease.

Among patients treated for *sustained* ventricular tachycardia (who frequently also had heart failure, a low ejection fraction, a history of myocardial infarction and/or an episode of cardiac arrest), the incidence of proarrhythmic events was 13% when dosage was initiated at 200 mg/day with slow upward titration, and did not exceed 300 mg/day in most patients. In early studies in patients with *sustained* ventricular tachycardia utilizing a higher initial dose (400 mg/day) the incidence of proarrhythmic events was 26%; moreover, in about 10% of the patients treated proarrhythmic events resulted in death, despite prompt medical attention. With lower initial doses, the incidence of proarrhythmic events resulting in death decreased to 0.5% of these patients. Accordingly, it is extremely important to follow the recommended dosage schedule. (See Dosage and Administration.)

The relatively high frequency of proarrhythmic events in patients with sustained ventricular tachycardia and serious underlying heart disease, and the need for careful titration and monitoring, requires that therapy of patients with sustained ventricular tachycardia be started in the hospital. Hospitalization should also be considered for other patients

Continued on next page

3M Riker—Cont.

with underlying structural heart disease. (See Dosage and Administration.)

Heart Failure. TAMBOCOR has a negative inotropic effect and may cause or worsen congestive heart failure (CHF), particularly in patients with cardiomyopathy, preexisting severe heart failure (NYHA functional class III or IV) or low ejection fractions (less than 30%). CHF developed rarely (1%) in patients who had no previous history of CHF. In ventricular arrhythmia patients with preexisting heart failure, 15% developed worsening of CHF at some time during TAMBOCOR treatment. Exacerbation of preexisting CHF occurred more commonly in studies which included patients with class III or IV failure than in studies which excluded such patients. TAMBOCOR should be used cautiously in patients who are known to have a history of congestive heart failure or myocardial dysfunction. The initial dosage in such patients should be no more than 100 mg bid (see Dosage and Administration) and patients should be monitored carefully. Close attention must be given to maintenance of cardiac function, including optimization of digitalis, diuretic, or other therapy. In cases where CHF has developed or worsened during treatment with TAMBOCOR, the time of onset has ranged from a few hours to several months after starting therapy. Some patients who develop evidence of reduced myocardial function while on TAMBOCOR can continue to TAMBOCOR with adjustment of digitalis or diuretics, others may require dosage reduction or discontinuation of TAMBOCOR. When feasible, it is recommended that plasma flecainide levels be monitored. Attempts should be made to keep trough plasma levels below 0.7 to 1.0 ug/ml.

Effects on Cardiac Conduction. TAMBOCOR slows cardiac conduction in most patients to produce dose-related increases in PR, QRS, and QT intervals.

PR interval increases on average about 25% (0.04 seconds) and as much as 118% in some patients. Approximately one-third of patients may develop new first degree AV heart block (PR interval $\geq$ 0.20 seconds). The QRS complex increases on average about 25% (0.02 seconds) and as much as 150% in some patients. Many patients develop QRS complexes with a duration of 0.12 seconds or more. In one study, 4% of patients developed new bundle branch block while on TAMBOCOR. The degree of lengthening of PR and QRS intervals does not predict either efficacy or the development of cardiac adverse effects. In clinical trials, it was unusual for PR intervals to increase to 0.30 seconds or more, or for QRS intervals to increase to 0.18 seconds or more. Thus, caution should be used when such intervals occur, and dose reductions may be considered. The QT interval widens about 8%, but most of this widening (about 60% to 90%) is due to widening of the QRS duration. The JT interval (QT minus QRS) only widens about 4% on the average. Significant JT prolongation occurs in less than 2% of patients. There have been rare cases of Torsade de Pointes-type arrhythmia associated with TAMBOCOR therapy.

Clinically significant conduction changes have been observed at these rates: sinus node dysfunction such as sinus pause, sinus arrest and symptomatic bradycardia (1.2%), second-degree AV block (0.5%) and third-degree AV block (0.4%). An attempt should be made to manage the patient on the lowest effective dose in an effort to minimize these effects. (See Dosage and Administration.) If second or third-degree AV block, or right bundle branch block associated with a left hemiblock occur, TAMBOCOR therapy should be discontinued unless a temporary or implanted ventricular pacemaker is in place to ensure an adequate ventrivcular rate.

Sick Sinus Syndrome (Bradycardia-Tachycardia Syndrome). TAMBOCOR should be used only with extreme caution in patients with sick sinus syndrome because it may cause sinus bracycardia, sinus pause, or sinus arrest.

Effects on Pacemaker Thresholds. TAMBOCOR is known to increase endocardial pacing thresholds and may suppress ventricular escape rhythms. These effects are reversible if flecainide is discontinued. It should be used with caution in patients with permanent pacemakers or temporary pacing electrodes and should not be administered to patients with existing poor thresholds or nonprogrammable pacemakers unless suitable pacing rescue is available.

The pacing threshold in patients with pacemakers should be determined prior to instituting therapy with TAMBOCOR, again after one week of administration and at regular intervals thereafter. Generally threshold changes are within the range of multiprogrammable pacemakers and, when these occur, a doubling of either voltage or pulse width is usually sufficient to regain capture.

Electrolyte Disturbances. Hypokalemia or hyperkalemia may alter the effects of Class I antiarrhythmic drugs. Preexisting hypokalemia or hyperkalemia should be corrected before administration of TAMBOCOR.

PRECAUTIONS

Drug Interactions. TAMBOCOR has been administered to patients receiving digitalis preparations or beta-adrenergic blocking agents without adverse effects. During administration of multiple oral doses of TAMBOCOR to healthy subjects stabilized on a maintenance dose of digoxin, a 13% $\pm$ 19% increase in plasma digoxin levels occurred at six hours postdose.

In a study involving healthy subjects receiving TAMBOCOR and propranolol concurrently, plasma flecainide levels were increased about 20% and propranolol levels were increased about 30% compared to control values. In this formal interaction study, TAMBOCOR and propranolol were each found to have negative inotropic effects; when the drugs were administered together, the effects were additive. The effects of concomitant administration of TAMBOCOR and propranolol on the PR interval were less than additive. In TAMBOCOR clinical trials, patients who were receiving beta blockers concurrently did not experience an increased incidence of side effects. Nevertheless, the possibility of additive negative inotropic effects of beta blockers and flecainide should be recognized.

Flecainide is not extensively bound to plasma proteins. In vitro studies with several drugs which may be administered concomitantly showed that the extent of flecainide binding to human plasma proteins is either unchanged or only slightly less. Consequently, interactions with other drugs which are highly protein bound (e.g., anticoagulants) would not be expected. TAMBOCOR has been used in a large number of patients receiving diuretics without apparent interaction. Limited data in patients receiving known enzyme inducers (phenytoin, phenobarbital, carbamazepine) indicate only a 30% increase in the rate of flecainide elimination. In healty subjects receiving cimetidine (1 gm daily) for one week, plasma flecainide levels increased by about 30% and half-life increasd by about 10%.

When amiodarone is added to flecainide therapy, plasma flecainide levels may increase two-fold or more in some patients, if flecainide dosage is not reduced. (See Dosage and Administration.)

There has been little experience with the coadministration of TAMBOCOR and either disopyramide or verapamil. Because both of these drugs have negative inotropic properties and the effects of coadministration with TAMBOCOR are unknown, neither disopyramide nor verapamil should be administered concurrently with TAMBOCOR unless, in the judgment of the physician, the benefits of this combination outweigh the risks. There has been too little experience with the coadministrator of TAMBOCOR with nifedipine or diltiazem to recommend concomitant use.

Carcinogenesis, Mutagenesis, Impairment of Fertility. Long-term studies with flecainide in rats and mice at doses up to about eight times the usual human dose of 8 mg/kg/day, (assuming patient weight of 50 kg), have not revealed any compound-related carcinogenic effects. Mutagenicity studies (Ames test, mouse lymphoma and in vivo cytogenetics) did not reveal any mutagenic effects. A rat reproduction study at doses up to 50 mg/kg/day (seven times the usual human dose) did not reveal any adverse effect on male or female fertility.

Pregnancy. Pregnancy Category C. Flecainide has been shown to have teratogenic effects (club paws, sternebrae and vertebrae abnormalities, pale hearts with contracted ventricular septum) and an embryotoxic effect (increased resorptions) in one breed of rabbit (New Zealand White) but not in another breed of rabbit (Dutch Belted) when given in doses about four times (but not three times) the usual human dose (assuming a patient weight of 50 kg). No teratogenic effects were observed in rats and mice given doses up to 50 and 80 mg/kg/day, respectively; however, delayed sternebral and vertebral ossification was observed at the high dose in rats. Because there are no adequate and well-controlled studies in pregnant women, TAMBOCOR should be used during pregnancy only if the potential benefit justifies the potential risk to the fetus.

Labor and Delivery. It is not known whether the use of TAMBOCOR during labor or delivery has immediate or delayed adverse effects on the mother or fetus, affects the duration of labor or delivery, or increases the possibility of forceps delivery or other obstetrical intervention.

Nursing Mothers. Limited data suggest that flecainide is excreted in human milk. Because of the drug's potential for serious adverse effects in nursing infants, a decision should be made whether to discontinue nursing or discontinue the drug, taking into account the importance of the drug to the mother.

Pediatric Use. The safety and effectiveness of TAMBOCOR in children less than 18 years of age have not been established.

Hepatic Impairment. Since flecainide elimination from plasma can be markedly slower in patients with significant hepatic impairment, TAMBOCOR should not be used in such patients unless the potential benefits clearly outweigh the risks. If used, frequent and early plasma level monitoring is required to guide dosage (See Plasma Level Monitoring); dosage increases should be made very cautiously when plasma levels have plateaued (after more than four days).

ADVERSE REACTIONS

In post-myocardial infarction patients with asymptomatic PVCs and non-sustained ventricular tachycardia, TAMBOCOR therapy was found to be associated with a 5.1% rate of death and non-fatal cardiac arrest, compared with a 2.3% rate in a matched placebo group. (See Warnings.)

Adverse effects reported for TAMBOCOR, described in detail in the Warnings section, were new or exacerbated ventricular arrhythmias which occurred in 7% of 1330 patients with PVCs, non-sustained or sustained ventricular tachycardia. 198 patients with sustained ventricular tachycardia experienced a 13% incidence of new or exacerbated ventricular arrhythmias when dosage was initiated at 200 mg/day with slow upward titration, and did not exceed 300 mg/day in most patients. In some patients, TAMBOCOR treatment has been associated with episodes of unresuscitatable ventricular tachycardia or ventricular filbrillation. (See Warnings.) New or worsened congestive heart failure occurred in 6.3% of 1046 patients with PVCs, non-sustained or sustained ventricular tachycardia. Of 297 patients with sustained ventricular tachycardia, 9.1% experienced new or worsened CHF. There have also been instances of second- (0.5%) or third-degree (0.4%) AV block. Patients have developed sinus bradycardia, sinus pause, or sinus arrest, about 1.2% altogether (see Warnings). The frequency of most of these serious adverse events probably increases with higher trough plasma levels, especially when these trough levels exceed 1.0 ug/ml.

There have been rare reports of isolated elevations of serum alkaline phosphatase and isolated elevations of serum transaminase levels. These elevations have been asymptomatic and no cause and effect relationship with TAMBOCOR has been established. In foreign postmarketing surveillance studies, there have been rare reports of hepatic dysfunction including reports of cholestasis and hepatic failure, and extremely rare reports of blood dyscrasias. Although no cause and effect relationship has been established, it is advisable to discontinue TAMBOCOR in patients who develop unexplained jaundice or signs of hepatic dysfunction or blood dyscrasias in order to eliminate TAMBOCOR as the possible causative agent.

Incidence figures for other adverse effects are based on a multicenter efficacy study, utilizing starting doses of 200 mg/day with gradual upward titration to 400 mg/day. Patients were treated for an average of 4.7 months, some receiving up to 22 months of therapy. In this trial, 5.4% of patients discontinued due to non-cardiac adverse effects. [See table on next page].

The following additional adverse experiences, possibly related to TAMBOCOR therapy and occurring in 1% to less than 3% of patients, have been reported in acute and chronic studies: Body as a Whole—malaise, fever; Cardiovascular—tachycardia, sinus pause or arrest; Gastrointestinal—vomiting, diarrhea, dyspepsia, anorexia; Skin—rash; Visual—diplopia; Nervous System—hypoesthesia, paresthesia, paresis, ataxia, flushing, increased sweating, vertigo, syncope, somnolence, tinnitus; Psychiatric—anxiety, insomnia, depression.

The following additional adverse experiences, possibly related to TAMBOCOR, have been reported in less than 1% of patients: Body as a Whole—swollen lips, tongue and mouth; arthralgia, bronchospasm, myalgia; Cardiovascular—angina pectoris, second-degree and third-degree AV block, bradycardia, hypertension, hypotension; Gastrointestinal—flatulence; Urinary System—polyuria, urinary retention; Hematologic—leukopenia, thrombocytopenia; Skin—urticaria, exfoliative dermatitis, pruritis; Visual—eye pain or irritation, photophobia, nystagmus; Nervous System—twitching, weakness, change in taste, dry mouth, convulsions, impotence, speech disorder, stupor; Psychiatric—amnesia, confusion, decreased libido, depersonalization, euphoria, morbid dreams, apathy.

OVERDOSAGE

No specific antidote has been identified for the treatment of TAMBOCOR overdosage. Animal studies suggest that the following events might occur with overdosage: lengthening of the PR interval; increase in the QRS duration, QT interval and amplitude of the T-wave; a reduction in myocardial rate and contractility; conduction disturbances; hypotension; and death from respiratory failure or asystole. Treatment of overdosage should be supportive and may include the following: removal of unabsorbed drug from the gastrointestinal tract, administration of inotropic agents or cardiac stimulants such a dopamine, dobutamine or isoproterenol; mechanically assisted respiration; circulatory assists such as intra-aortic balloon pumping; and transvenous pacing in the event of conduction block. Because of the long plasma half-life of flecainide (12 to 27 hours in patients receiving usual doses), and the possibility of markedly non-linear elimination kinetics at very high doses, these supportive treatments may need to be continued for extended periods of time. Hemodialysis is not an effective means of removing flecainide from the body. Since flecainide elimination is much slower when urine is very alkaline (ph 8 or higher), theoretically, acidification of urine to promote drug excretion may be beneficial in overdose cases with very alkaline urine. There is no evidence that acidification from normal urinary pH increases excretion.

DOSAGE AND ADMINISTRATION

For patients with sustained ventricular tachycardia, no matter what their cardiac status, TAMBOCOR, like other antiarrhythmics, should be initiated in-hospital with rhythm monitoring. (See Warnings).

Flecainide has a long half-life (12 to 27 hours in patients). Steady-state plasma levels, in patients with normal renal and hepatic function, may not be achieved until the patient has received 3 to 5 days of therapy at a given dose. Therefore, increases in dosage should be made no more frequently than once every four days, since during the first 2 to 3 days of therapy the optimal effect of a given dose may not be achieved. The recommended starting dose is 100 mg every 12 hours. This dose may be increased in increments of 50 mg bid every four days until efficacy is achieved. Most patients with sustained ventricular tachycardia do not require more than 150 mg every 12 hours (300 mg/day), and the maximum dose is 400 mg/day.

Use of higher initial doses and more rapid dosage adjustments have resulted in an increased incidence of proarrhythmic events and congestive heart failure, particularly during the first few days of dosing (see Warnings). Therefore, a loading dose is not recommended.

Intravenous lidocaine has been used occasionally with TAMBOCOR while awaiting the therapeutic effect of TAMBOCOR. No adverse drug interactions were apparent. However, no formal studies have been performed to demonstrate the usefulness of this regimen.

An occasional patient not adequately controlled by (or intolerant to) a dose given at 12-hour intervals may be dosed at eight-hour intervals.

Once adequate control of the arrhythmia has been achieved, it may be possible in some patients to reduce the dose as necessary to minimize side effects or effects on conduction. In such patients, efficacy at the lower dose should be evaluated. TAMBOCOR should be used cautiously in patients with a history of congestive heart failure or myocardial dysfunction (see Warnings).

In patients with severe renal impairment (creatinine clearance of 35 ml/min/1.73 square meters or less), the initial dosage should be 100 mg once daily (or 50 mg bid); when used in such patients, frequent plasma level monitoring is required to guide dosage adjustments (See Plasma Level Monitoring). In patients with less severe renal disease, the initial dosage should be 100 mg every 12 hours; plasma level monitoring may also be useful in these patients during dosage adjustment. In both groups of patients, dosage increases should be made very cautiously when plasma levels have plateaued (after more than four days), observing the patient closely for signs of adverse cardiac effects or other toxicity. It should be borne in mind that in these patients it may take longer than four days before a new steady-state plasma level is reached following a dosage change.

Based on theoretical considerations, rather than experimental data, the following suggestion is made: when transferring patients from another antiarrhythmic drug to TAMBOCOR allow at least two to four plasma half-lives to elapse for the drug being discontinued before starting TAMBOCOR at the usual dosage. In patients where withdrawal of a previous antiarrhythmic agent is likely to produce life-threatening arrhythmias, the physician should consider hospitalizing the patient.

When flecainide is given in the presence of amiodarone, reduce the usual flecainide dose by 50% and monitor the patient closely for adverse effects. Plasma level monitoring is strongly recommended to guide dosage with such combination therapy·

Plasma Level Monitoring: The large majority of patients successfully treated with TAMBOCOR were found to have trough plasma levels between 0.2 and 1.0 ug/ml. The probability of adverse experiences, especially cardiac, may increase with higher trough plasma levels, especially when these exceed 1.0 ug/ml. Periodic monitoring of trough plasma levels may be useful in patient management. Plasma level monitoring is required in patients with severe renal failure or severe hepatic disease, such elimination of flecainide from plasma may be markedly slower. Monitoring of plasma levels is strongly recommended in patients on concurrent amiodarone therapy and may also be helpful in patients with congestive heart failure and in patients with moderate renal disease.

HOW SUPPLIED

All tablets are embossed with RIKER on one side and TR 50, TR 100 or TR 150 on the other side.

Tambocor, 50 mg per white, round tablet, is available in
 Bottles of 100—NDC #0089-0305-10.
 Boxes of 100 in unit dose blister strips—NDC #0089-0305-16.

Table 1
Most Common Non-Cardiac Adverse Effects in Patients Treated with TAMBOCOR in the Multicenter Study

Adverse Effect	Incidence in All 429 Patients at Any Dose	Incidence By Dose During Upward Titration		
		200 mg/Day (N=426)	300 mg/Day (N=293)	400 mg/Day (N=100)
Dizziness*	18.9%	11.0%	10.6%	13.0%
Visual Disturbance+	15.9%	5.4%	12.3%	18.0%
Dyspnea	10.3%	5.2%	7.5%	4.0%
Headache	9.6%	4.5%	6.1%	9.0%
Nausea	8.9%	4.9%	4.8%	6.0%
Fatigue	7.7%	4.5%	4.4%	3.0%
Palpitation	6.1%	3.5%	2.4%	7.0%
Chest Pain	5.4%	3.1%	3.8%	1.0%
Asthenia	4.9%	2.6%	2.0%	4.0%
Tremor	4.7%	2.4%	3.4%	2.0%
Constipation	4.4%	2.8%	2.1%	1.0%
Edema	3.5%	1.9%	1.4%	2.0%
Abdominal pain	3.3%	1.9%	2.4%	1.0%

* Dizziness includes reports of dizziness, lightheadedness, faintness, unsteadiness, near syncope, etc.
+Visual disturbance includes reports of blurred vision, difficulty in focusing, spots before eyes, etc.

Tambocor, 100 mg per white, round, scored tablet, is available in
 Bottles of 100—NDC #0089-0307-10.
 Boxes of 100 in unit dose blister strips—NDC #0089-0307-16.
Tambocor, 150 mg per white, oval, scored tablet, is available in
 Bottles of 100—NDC #0089-0314-10.
Store at controlled room temperature 15°–30°C (59°–86°F) in a tight, light resistant container.
CAUTION: Federal law prohibits dispensing without prescription.
Manufactured by
3M Riker
3M Health Care
Northridge, CA 91324

TEPANIL® ℞
(diethylpropion hydrochloride, U.S.P.)
TEPANIL® TEN-TAB® ℞
(diethylpropion hydrochloride U.S.P.)
sustained-release tablets

DESCRIPTION

Diethylpropion hydrochloride, a sympathomimetic agent, is 1-phenyl-2-diethylamino-1-propanone hydrochloride. Tepanil tablets also contain: magnesium stearate, mannitol, starch, talc, and tartaric acid.

In Tepanil Ten-Tab tablets, diethylpropion hydrochloride is dispersed in a hydrophilic matrix. On exposure to water the diethylpropion hydrochloride is released at a relatively uniform rate as a result of slow hydration of the matrix. The result is sustained-release of the drug. Tepanil Ten-Tab tablets also contain : carbomer, mannitol, povidone, tartaric acid, and zinc stearate.

HOW SUPPLIED

Tepanil 25 mg.: bottles of 100 (NDC **0089-0351-10**) white tablets, Tepanil Ten-Tab 75 mg.: bottles of 30 (NDC **0089-0353-03**), 100 (NDC **0089-0353-10**), and 250 (NDC **0089-0353-25**) white tablets.

Shown in Product Identification Section, page 416

THEOLAIR™ ℞
(theophylline)
TABLETS
THEOLAIR™ ℞
(theophylline)
LIQUID
THEOLAIR™–SR ℞
(theophylline)
TABLETS

DESCRIPTION

THEOLAIR Tablets contain 125 mg or 250 mg anhydrous theophylline. Theolair tablets also contain: colloidal silicon dioxide, lactose, magnesium stearate, and pregelatinized starch.
THEOLAIR Liquid contains 80 mg theophylline per 15 ml (tablespoonful) in a nonalcoholic solution. Theolair liquid also contains: flavor, methyl & propyl parabens, purified water, sorbitol, and sucrose.
THEOLAIR-SR Tablets contain 200 mg, 250 mg, 300 mg or 500 mg anhydrous theophylline, in a sustained-release formulation. Theolair-SR tablets also contain: cellulose acetate phthalate, lactose, and magnesium stearate.

HOW SUPPLIED

THEOLAIR Tablets:
 125 mg tablets—Bottles of 100 (NDC 0089-0342-10). Each round, white, scored tablet imprinted with "RIKER" on one side and "342" on the other.

 250 mg tablets—Bottles of 100 (NDC **0089-0344-10**). Each capsule-shaped, white, scored tablet imprinted with "RIKER" on one side and "THEOLAIR 250" on the other.
 STORE BELOW 30° C (86° F).
THEOLAIR Liquid:
 1 pint bottles (NDC 0089-0960-16)
 STORE BETWEEN 15–30° C (59–86° F).
THEOLAIR-SR Tablets:
 200 mg sustained-release tablets—Bottles of 100 (NDC **0089-0341-10**) and 1,000 (NDC 0089-0341-80). Each round white, scored tablet imprinted with "RIKER" on one side and "SR 200" on the other.
 250 mg sustained-release tablets—Bottles of 100 (NDC **0089-0345-10**) and 250 (NDC **0089-0345-25**). Each round, white, scored tablet imprinted with "RIKER" on one side and "SR 250" on the other.
 300 mg sustained-release tablets—Bottles of 100 (NDC **0089-0343-10**) and 1,000 (NDC 0089-0343-80). Each oval white, scored tablet imprinted with "RIKER" on one side and "SR 300" on the other.
 500 mg sustained-release tablets—Bottles of 100 (NDC **0089-0347-10**) and 250 (NDC **0089-0347-25**). Each capsule-shaped, white, scored tablet imprinted on one side with "RIKER" and "SR 500" on the other.
 STORE AT CONTROLLED ROOM TEMPERATURE 15°–30° C (59°–86° F).
Shown in Product Identification Section, page 416

UREX® ℞
(methenamine hippurate)

DESCRIPTION

Urex (methenamine hippurate) is the hippuric acid salt of methenamine (hexamethylenetetramine). Urex tablets also contain: magnesium stearate, povidone, and saccharin sodium.

HOW SUPPLIED

One gram scored, white tablets, bottles of 100 (NDC **0089-0371-10**) and 500 (NDC **0089-0371-50**).

EDUCATIONAL MATERIAL

Books, Booklets, Brochures
Exercises for better care of the back, neck, knee and shoulder. Back exercises feature the "Williams Exercises," Free to physicians for distribution to their patients and available through local 3M Riker representatives.
Films, Slides, Videos
Videotapes of current interests are available for viewing and may be obtained through your local 3M Riker representatives.
Samples
Patient starter packets are available by mail and through your local 3M Riker representative.

Products are cross-indexed by
generic and chemical names in the
YELLOW SECTION

MDR Fitness Corp.
5207 N.W. 163RD STREET
MIAMI, FL 33014

MDR
Fitness Tabs for Men and Women

DESCRIPTION
Formulated by M.D.'s to provide an improved absorption capability of nutrients needed for health with an A.M. and P.M. dosage. More micronutrients are required for energy producing reactions in the A.M. when activity is greater.

Each Fitness Tab Contains:	MEN		WOMEN	
Vitamin A (Fish Oil)	5000	IU	5000	IU
Vitamin E (d-alpha tocopherol succinate with other mixed tocopherols)	40	IU	60	IU
Vitamin D-3 (Colecalciferol)	400	IU	400	IU
Vitamin C (Ascorbic Acid)	250	mg	200	mg
Vitamin B1 (Thiamine Mononitrate)	6	mg	6	mg
Vitamin B2 (Riboflavin)	6	mg	6	mg
Niacinamide	40	mg	40	mg
Vitamin B6	6	mg	8	mg
Folic Acid	400	mcg	400	mcg
Vitamin B12	6	mcg	6	mcg
Pantothenic Acid	20	mg	20	mg
Biotin	200	mcg	200	mcg
Calcium (Carbonate)	510	mg	535	mg
Magnesium (Oxide)	200	mg	200	mg
Iron (Fumarate)	10	mg	20	mg
Zinc (Sulfate)	20	mg	20	mg
Manganese (Sulfate)	5	mg	5	mg
Selenium (Nutrition 21)	40	mcg	40	mcg
Chromium	100	mcg	100	mcg
Copper (Sulfate)	0.5	mg	0.5	mg
Garlic (odorless)	100	mg	100	mg

Free of sugar, starches, and coloring additives.

DIRECTIONS
With breakfast or lunch, take one "AM" Fitness Tab. After dinner, take one "PM" Fitness Tab.

HOW SUPPLIED
Bottles of 60 Fitness Tabs.

M.D.R. HIGH PERFORMANCE TABS

DESCRIPTION
An additional two tablet per day supplement to be taken with the M.D.R. FITNESS TABS.
Ideally suited for persons whose nutritional requirements may be increased by illness, smoking or an increase in physical and athletic activity.

DIRECTIONS
Take one tablet after breakfast or lunch and one tablet after dinner. Two tablets per day.

HOW SUPPLIED
Bottles of 120 HIGH PERFORMANCE TABS.
CALL 1-800-MDR TABS, 1-800-837-8227 OR (305) 624-4466 FOR INFORMATION.

Macsil, Inc.
1326 FRANKFORD AVENUE
PHILADELPHIA, PA 19125

BALMEX® BABY POWDER

(See PDR For Nonprescription Drugs)

BALMEX® EMOLLIENT LOTION

(See PDR For Nonprescription Drugs)

BALMEX® OINTMENT

(See PDR For Nonprescription Drugs)

Products are
listed alphabetically
in the
PINK SECTION.

Marion Laboratories, Inc.
MARION PARK DRIVE
KANSAS CITY, MO 64137

PRODUCT IDENTIFICATION
NUMERICAL SUMMARY
SOLID ORAL DOSAGE FORMS

Marion Laboratories, Inc.
Kansas City, MO 64137
To provide quick and positive identification of Marion Laboratories prescription drug products, we have imprinted an identifying number and the name MARION on the following tablets or capsules.

1375   DITROPAN® Tablets (oxybutynin chloride)
1550   NITRO-BID® Capsules, 2.5 mg (nitroglycerin)*
1551   NITRO-BID® Capsules, 6.5 mg (nitroglycerin)†
1553   NITRO-BID® Capsules, 9 mg (nitroglycerin)**
1555   PAVABID® Capsules, 150 mg (papaverine hydrochloride)‡
1771   CARDIZEM® Tablets, 30 mg (diltiazem hydrochloride)
1772   CARDIZEM® Tablets, 60 mg (diltiazem hydrochloride)

CARAFATE® Tablets, 1 gm (sucralfate) is identified by the brand name CARAFATE embossed on one side and 1712 bracketed by C's imprinted on the reverse side.
CARDIZEM® Tablets, 90 mg (diltiazem hydrochloride) is imprinted with the brand name CARDIZEM on one side and 90 mg on the reverse side.
CARDIZEM® Tablets, 120 mg (diltiazem hydrochloride) is imprinted with the brand name CARDIZEM on one side and 120 mg on the reverse side.
CARDIZEM® SR Capsules, 60 mg (diltiazem hydrochloride) is imprinted with the Cardizem logo on one end and Cardizem SR 60 mg on the other.
CARDIZEM® SR Capsules, 90 mg (diltiazem hydrochloride) is imprinted with the Cardizem logo on one end and Cardizem SR 90 mg on the other.
CARDIZEM® SR Capsules, 120 mg (diltiazem hydrochloride) is imprinted with the Cardizem logo on one end and Cardizem SR 120 mg on the other.
PAVABID® HP Capsulets, 300 mg (papaverine hydrochloride) is identified by the name MARION on one side and PAVABID HP on the reverse side.
* NITRO-BID® Capsules, 2.5 mg (nitroglycerin) also bear the brand name NITRO-BID 2.5.
† NITRO-BID® Capsules, 6.5 mg (nitroglycerin) also bear the brand name NITRO-BID 6.5.
** NITRO-BID® Capsules, 9 mg (nitroglycerin) also bear the brand name NITRO-BID 9.
‡ PAVABID Capsules, 150 mg (papaverine hydrochloride) also bear the brand name PAVABID.

CARAFATE® Tablets   ℞
[kar′af-āt]
(sucralfate) 1 gm

DESCRIPTION
CARAFATE® (sucralfate) is α-D-Glucopyranoside, β-D-fructofuranosyl-, octakis-(hydrogen sulfate), aluminum complex.

$$R = SO_3[Al_2(OH)_5 \cdot (H_2O)_2]$$

Tablets for oral administration contain 1 gm of sucralfate. Also contain: D&C Red #30 Lake, FD&C Blue #1 Lake, magnesium stearate, microcrystalline cellulose, and starch. Therapeutic category: antiulcer

CLINICAL PHARMACOLOGY
Sucralfate is only minimally absorbed from the gastrointestinal tract. The small amounts of the sulfated disaccharide that are absorbed are excreted primarily in the urine.
Although the mechanism of sucralfate's ability to accelerate healing of duodenal ulcers remains to be fully defined, it is known that it exerts its effect through a local, rather than systemic, action. The following observations also appear pertinent:
1. Studies in human subjects and with animal models of ulcer disease have shown that sucralfate forms an ulcer-adherent complex with proteinaceous exudate at the ulcer site.
2. In vitro, a sucralfate-albumin film provides a barrier to diffusion of hydrogen ions.
3. In human subjects, sucralfate given in doses recommended for ulcer therapy inhibits pepsin activity in gastric juice by 32%.
4. In vitro, sucralfate adsorbs bile salts.
These observations suggest that sucralfate's antiulcer activity is the result of formation of an ulcer-adherent complex that covers the ulcer site and protects it against further attack by acid, pepsin, and bile salts. Sucralfate has negligible acid-neutralizing capacity, and its antiulcer effects cannot be attributed to neutralization of gastric acid.

CLINICAL TRIALS
Over 600 patients have participated in well-controlled clinical trials worldwide. Multicenter trials conducted in the United States, both of them placebo-controlled studies with endoscopic evaluation at 2 and 4 weeks, showed:

STUDY 1

Treatment Groups	Ulcer Healing/No. Patients	
	2 wk	4 wk (Overall)
Sucralfate	37/105 (35.2%)	82/109 (75.2%)
Placebo	26/106 (24.5%)	68/107 (63.6%)

STUDY 2

Treatment Groups	Ulcer Healing/No. Patients	
	2 wk	4 wk (Overall)
Sucralfate	8/24 (33%)	22/24 (92%)
Placebo	4/31 (13%)	18/31 (58%)

The sucralfate-placebo differences were statistically significant in both studies at 4 weeks but not at 2 weeks. The poorer result in the first study may have occurred because sucralfate was given two hours after meals and at bedtime rather than one hour before meals and at bedtime, the regimen used in international studies and in the second United States study. In addition, in the first study liquid antacid was utilized as needed, whereas in the second study antacid tablets were used.

INDICATIONS AND USAGE
CARAFATE (sucralfate) is indicated in the short-term (up to 8 weeks) treatment of duodenal ulcer.
Antacids may be prescribed as needed for relief of pain.

CONTRAINDICATIONS
There are no known contraindications to the use of sucralfate.

PRECAUTIONS
Duodenal ulcer is a chronic, recurrent disease. While short-term treatment with sucralfate can result in complete healing of the ulcer, a successful course of treatment with sucralfate should not be expected to alter the post-healing frequency or severity of duodenal ulceration.
Drug Interactions: Animal studies have shown that simultaneous administration of CARAFATE (sucralfate) with tetracycline, phenytoin, or digoxin will result in a statistically significant reduction in the bioavailability of these agents. The bioavailability of these agents may be restored simply by separating the administration of these agents from that of CARAFATE by two hours. This interaction appears to be nonsystemic in origin, presumably resulting from these agents being bound by CARAFATE in the gastrointestinal tract. The clinical significance of these animal studies is yet to be defined. However, because of the potential of CARAFATE to alter the absorption of some drugs from the gastrointestinal tract, the separate administration of CARAFATE from that of other agents should be considered when alterations in bioavailability are felt to be critical for concomitantly administered drugs.
Carcinogenesis, Mutagenesis, Impairment of Fertility: Chronic oral toxicity studies of 24 months' duration were conducted in mice and rats at doses up to 1 gm/kg (12 times the human dose). There was no evidence of drug-related tumorigenicity. A reproduction study in rats at doses up to 38 times the human dose did not reveal any indication of fertility impairment. Mutagenicity studies were not conducted.
Pregnancy: Teratogenic effects. Pregnancy Category B. Teratogenicity studies have been performed in mice, rats, and rabbits at doses up to 50 times the human dose and have revealed no evidence of harm to the fetus due to sucralfate. There are, however, no adequate and well-controlled studies in pregnant women. Because animal reproduction studies are not always predictive of human response, this drug should be used during pregnancy only if clearly needed.
Nursing Mothers: It is not known whether this drug is excreted in human milk. Because many drugs are excreted in human milk, caution should be exercised when sucralfate is administered to a nursing woman.
Pediatric Use: Safety and effectiveness in children have not been established.

ADVERSE REACTIONS
Adverse reactions to sucralfate in clinical trials were minor and only rarely led to discontinuation of the drug. In studies

involving over 2,500 patients treated with sucralfate, adverse effects were reported in 121 (4.7%).

Constipation was the most frequent complaint (2.2%). Other adverse effects, reported in no more than one of every 350 patients, were diarrhea, nausea, gastric discomfort, indigestion, dry mouth, rash, pruritus, back pain, dizziness, sleepiness, and vertigo.

OVERDOSAGE

There is no experience in humans with overdosage. Acute oral toxicity studies in animals, however, using doses up to 12 gm/kg body weight, could not find a lethal dose. Risks associated with overdosage should, therefore, be minimal.

DOSAGE AND ADMINISTRATION

The recommended adult oral dosage for duodenal ulcer is 1 gm four times a day on an empty stomach.

Antacids may be prescribed as needed for relief of pain but should not be taken within one-half hour before or after sucralfate.

While healing with sucralfate may occur during the first week or two, treatment should be continued for 4 to 8 weeks unless healing has been demonstrated by x-ray or endoscopic examination.

HOW SUPPLIED

CARAFATE (sucralfate) 1-gm tablets are supplied in bottles of 100 (NDC 0088-1712-47) and 500 (NDC 0088-1712-55) and in Unit Dose Identification Paks of 100 (NDC 0088-1712-49). Light pink scored oblong tablets are embossed with CARAFATE on one side and 1712 bracketed by C's on the other.

Issued 3/88

Shown in Product Identification Section, page 416

CARDIZEM® Tablets ℞
[kar'diz-em]
(diltiazem HCl)
30 mg, 60 mg, 90 mg, and 120 mg

DESCRIPTION

CARDIZEM® (diltiazem hydrochloride) is a calcium ion influx inhibitor (slow channel blocker or calcium antagonist). Chemically, diltiazem hydrochloride is 1,5-Benzothiazepin-4(5H)one,3-(acetyloxy)-5-[2-(dimethylamino) ethyl]-2,3-dihydro-2-(4-methoxyphenyl)-, monohydrochloride,(+)-cis-.

Diltiazem hydrochloride is a white to off-white crystalline powder with a bitter taste. It is soluble in water, methanol, and chloroform. It has a molecular weight of 450.98. Each tablet of CARDIZEM contains 30 mg, 60 mg, 90 mg, or 120 mg diltiazem hydrochloride.

Also contains: D&C Yellow #10, FD&C Yellow #6 (60 mg and 120 mg), or FD&C Blue #1 (30 mg and 90 mg), hydroxypropylcellulose, hydroxypropyl methylcellulose, lactose, magnesium stearate, methylparaben, polyethylene glycol, talc, and other ingredients.

For oral administration.

CLINICAL PHARMACOLOGY

The therapeutic benefits achieved with CARDIZEM are believed to be related to its ability to inhibit the influx of calcium ions during membrane depolarization of cardiac and vascular smooth muscle.

Mechanisms of Action. Although precise mechanisms of its antianginal actions are still being delineated, CARDIZEM is believed to act in the following ways:

1. Angina Due to Coronary Artery Spasm: CARDIZEM has been shown to be a potent dilator of coronary arteries both epicardial and subendocardial. Spontaneous and ergonovine-induced coronary artery spasm are inhibited by CARDIZEM.
2. Exertional Angina: CARDIZEM has been shown to produce increases in exercise tolerance, probably due to its ability to reduce myocardial oxygen demand. This is accomplished via reductions in heart rate and systemic blood pressure at submaximal and maximal exercise work loads.

In animal models, diltiazem interferes with the slow inward (depolarizing) current in excitable tissue. It causes excitation-contraction uncoupling in various myocardial tissues without changes in the configuration of the action potential. Diltiazem produces relaxation of coronary vascular smooth muscle and dilation of both large and small coronary arteries at drug levels which cause little or no negative inotropic effect. The resultant increases in coronary blood flow (epicardial and subendocardial) occur in ischemic and nonischemic models and are accompanied by dose-dependent decreases in systemic blood pressure and decreases in peripheral resistance.

Hemodynamic and Electrophysiologic Effects. Like other calcium antagonists, diltiazem decreases sinoatrial and atrioventricular conduction in isolated tissues and has a negative inotropic effect in isolated preparations. In the intact animal, prolongation of the AH interval can be seen at higher doses.

In man, diltiazem prevents spontaneous and ergonovine-provoked coronary artery spasm. It causes a decrease in pe-

ripheral vascular resistance and a modest fall in blood pressure and, in exercise tolerance studies in patients with ischemic heart disease, reduces the heart rate-blood pressure product for any given work load. Studies to date, primarily in patients with good ventricular function, have not revealed evidence of a negative inotropic effect; cardiac output, ejection fraction, and left ventricular end diastolic pressure have not been affected. There are as yet few data on the interaction of diltiazem and beta-blockers. Resting heart rate is usually unchanged or slightly reduced by diltiazem.

Intravenous diltiazem in doses of 20 mg prolongs AH conduction time and AV node functional and effective refractory periods approximately 20%. In a study involving single oral doses of 300 mg of CARDIZEM in six normal volunteers, the average maximum PR prolongation was 14% with no instances of greater than first-degree AV block. Diltiazem-associated prolongation of the AH interval is not more pronounced in patients with first-degree heart block. In patients with sick sinus syndrome, diltiazem significantly prolongs sinus cycle length (up to 50% in some cases).

Chronic oral administration of CARDIZEM in doses of up to 240 mg/day has resulted in small increases in PR interval, but has not usually produced abnormal prolongation.

Pharmacokinetics and Metabolism. Diltiazem is absorbed from the tablet formulation to about 80% of a reference capsule and is subject to an extensive first-pass effect, giving an absolute bioavailability (compared to intravenous dosing) of about 40%. CARDIZEM undergoes extensive hepatic metabolism in which 2% to 4% of the unchanged drug appears in the urine. In vitro binding studies show CARDIZEM is 70% to 80% bound to plasma proteins. Competitive ligand binding studies have also shown CARDIZEM binding is not altered by therapeutic concentrations of digoxin, hydrochlorothiazide, phenylbutazone, propranolol, salicylic acid, or warfarin. Single oral doses of 30 to 120 mg of CARDIZEM result in detectable plasma levels within 30 to 60 minutes and peak plasma levels two to three hours after drug administration. The plasma elimination half-life following single or multiple drug administration is approximately 3.5 hours. Desacetyl diltiazem is also present in the plasma at levels of 10% to 20% of the parent drug and is 25% to 50% as potent as a coronary vasodilator as diltiazem. Therapeutic blood levels of CARDIZEM appear to be in the range of 50–200 ng/mL. There is a departure from dose-linearity when single doses above 60 mg are given; a 120-mg dose gave blood levels three times that of the 60-mg dose. There is no information about the effect of renal or hepatic impairment on excretion or metabolism of diltiazem.

INDICATIONS AND USAGE

1. **Angina Pectoris Due to Coronary Artery Spasm.** CARDIZEM is indicated in the treatment of angina pectoris due to coronary artery spasm. CARDIZEM has been shown effective in the treatment of spontaneous coronary artery spasm presenting as Prinzmetal's variant angina (resting angina with ST-segment elevation occurring during attacks).
2. **Chronic Stable Angina (Classic Effort-Associated Angina).** CARDIZEM is indicated in the management of chronic stable angina in patients who cannot tolerate therapy with beta-blockers and/or nitrates or who remain symptomatic despite adequate doses of these agents. CARDIZEM has been effective in short-term controlled trials in reducing angina frequency and increasing exercise tolerance but confirmation of sustained effectiveness is incomplete.

There are few controlled studies of the effectiveness of the concomitant use of diltiazem and beta-blockers or of the safety of this combination in patients with impaired ventricular function or conduction abnormalities.

CONTRAINDICATIONS

CARDIZEM is contraindicated in (1) patients with sick sinus syndrome except in the presence of a functioning ventricular pacemaker, (2) patients with second- or third-degree AV block except in the presence of a functioning ventricular pacemaker, (3) patients with hypotension (less than 90 mm Hg systolic), (4) patients who have demonstrated hypersensitivity to the drug, and (5) patients with acute myocardial infarction and pulmonary congestion documented by x-ray on admission.

WARNINGS

1. **Cardiac Conduction.** CARDIZEM prolongs AV node refractory periods without significantly prolonging sinus node recovery time, except in patients with sick sinus syndrome. This effect may rarely result in abnormally slow heart rates (particularly in patients with sick sinus syndrome) or second- or third-degree AV block (six of 1,243 patients for 0.48%). Concomitant use of diltiazem with beta-blockers or digitalis may result in additive effects on cardiac conduction. A patient with Prinzmetal's angina developed periods of asystole (2 to 5 seconds) after a single dose of 60 mg of diltiazem.
2. **Congestive Heart Failure.** Although diltiazem has a negative inotropic effect in isolated animal tissue preparations, hemodynamic studies in humans with normal ventricular

function have not shown a reduction in cardiac index nor consistent negative effects on contractility (dp/dt). Experience with the use of CARDIZEM alone or in combination with beta-blockers in patients with impaired ventricular function is very limited. Caution should be exercised when using the drug in such patients.

3. **Hypotension.** Decreases in blood pressure associated with CARDIZEM therapy may occasionally result in symptomatic hypotension.
4. **Acute Hepatic Injury.** In rare instances, significant elevations in enzymes such as alkaline phosphatase, LDH, SGOT, SGPT, and other phenomena consistent with acute hepatic injury have been noted. These reactions have been reversible upon discontinuation of drug therapy. The relationship to CARDIZEM is uncertain in most cases, but probable in some. (See PRECAUTIONS.)

PRECAUTIONS

General. CARDIZEM (diltiazem hydrochloride) is extensively metabolized by the liver and excreted by the kidneys and in bile. As with any drug given over prolonged periods, laboratory parameters should be monitored at regular intervals. The drug should be used with caution in patients with impaired renal or hepatic function. In subacute and chronic dog and rat studies designed to produce toxicity, high doses of diltiazem were associated with hepatic damage. In special subacute hepatic studies, oral doses of 125 mg/kg and higher in rats were associated with histological changes in the liver which were reversible when the drug was discontinued. In dogs, doses of 20 mg/kg were also associated with hepatic changes; however, these changes were reversible with continued dosing.

Dermatological events (see ADVERSE REACTIONS section) may be transient and may disappear despite continued use of CARDIZEM. However, skin eruptions progressing to erythema multiforme and/or exfoliative dermatitis have also been infrequently reported. Should a dermatologic reaction persist, the drug should be discontinued.

Drug Interaction. Due to the potential for additive effects, caution and careful titration are warranted in patients receiving CARDIZEM concomitantly with any agents known to affect cardiac contractility and/or conduction. (See WARNINGS.)

Pharmacologic studies indicate that there may be additive effects in prolonging AV conduction when using beta-blockers or digitalis concomitantly with CARDIZEM. (See WARNINGS.)

As with all drugs, care should be exercised when treating patients with multiple medications. CARDIZEM undergoes biotransformation by cytochrome P-450 mixed function oxidase. Coadministration of CARDIZEM with other agents which follow the same route of biotransformation may result in the competitive inhibition of metabolism. Dosages of similarly metabolized drugs, particularly those of low therapeutic ratio or in patients with renal and/or hepatic impairment, may require adjustment when starting or stopping concomitantly administered CARDIZEM to maintain optimum therapeutic blood levels.

Beta-blockers: Controlled and uncontrolled domestic studies suggest that concomitant use of CARDIZEM and beta-blockers or digitalis is usually well tolerated. Available data are not sufficient, however, to predict the effects of concomitant treatment, particularly in patients with left ventricular dysfunction or cardiac conduction abnormalities.

Administration of CARDIZEM (diltiazem hydrochloride) concomitantly with propranolol in five normal volunteers resulted in increased propranolol levels in all subjects and bioavailability of propranolol was increased approximately 50%. If combination therapy is initiated or withdrawn in conjunction with propranolol, an adjustment in the propranolol dose may be warranted. (See WARNINGS.)

Cimetidine: A study in six healthy volunteers has shown a significant increase in peak diltiazem plasma levels (58%) and area-under-the-curve (53%) after a 1-week course of cimetidine at 1,200 mg per day and diltiazem 60 mg per day. Ranitidine produced smaller, nonsignificant increases. The effect may be mediated by cimetidine's known inhibition of hepatic cytochrome P-450, the enzyme system probably responsible for the first-pass metabolism of diltiazem. Patients currently receiving diltiazem therapy should be carefully monitored for a change in pharmacological effect when initiating and discontinuing therapy with cimetidine. An adjustment in the diltiazem dose may be warranted.

Digitalis: Administration of CARDIZEM with digoxin in 24 healthy male subjects increased plasma digoxin concentrations approximately 20%. Another investigator found no increase in digoxin levels in 12 patients with coronary artery disease. Since there have been conflicting results regarding the effect of digoxin levels, it is recommended that digoxin levels be monitored when initiating, adjusting, and discontinuing CARDIZEM therapy to avoid possible over- or underdigitalization. (See WARNINGS.)

Anesthetics: The depression of cardiac contractility, conductivity, and automaticity as well as the vascular dilation

Continued on next page

Marion—Cont.

associated with anesthetics may be potentiated by calcium channel blockers. When used concomitantly, anesthetics and calcium blockers should be titrated carefully.

Carcinogenesis, Mutagenesis, Impairment of Fertility. A 24-month study in rats and a 21-month study in mice showed no evidence of carcinogenicity. There was also no mutagenic response in in vitro bacterial tests. No intrinsic effect on fertility was observed in rats.

Pregnancy. Category C. Reproduction studies have been conducted in mice, rats, and rabbits. Administration of doses ranging from five to ten times greater (on a mg/kg basis) than the daily recommended therapeutic dose has resulted in embryo and fetal lethality. These doses, in some studies, have been reported to cause skeletal abnormalities. In the perinatal/postnatal studies, there was some reduction in early individual pup weights and survival rates. There was an increased incidence of stillbirths at doses of 20 times the human dose or greater.

There are no well-controlled studies in pregnant women; therefore, use CARDIZEM in pregnant women only if the potential benefit justifies the potential risk to the fetus.

Nursing Mothers. Diltiazem is excreted in human milk. One report suggests that concentrations in breast milk may approximate serum levels. If use of CARDIZEM is deemed essential, an alternative method of infant feeding should be instituted.

Pediatric Use. Safety and effectiveness in children have not been established.

ADVERSE REACTIONS

Serious adverse reactions have been rare in studies carried out to date, but it should be recognized that patients with impaired ventricular function and cardiac conduction abnormalities have usually been excluded.

In domestic placebo-controlled trials, the incidence of adverse reactions reported during CARDIZEM therapy was not greater than that reported during placebo therapy.

The following represent occurrences observed in clinical studies which can be at least reasonably associated with the pharmacology of calcium influx inhibition. In many cases, the relationship to CARDIZEM has not been established. The most common occurrences as well as their frequency of presentation are: edema (2.4%), headache (2.1%), nausea (1.9%), dizziness (1.5%), rash (1.3%), asthenia (1.2%). In addition, the following events were reported infrequently (less than 1%):

Cardiovascular: Angina, arrhythmia, AV block (first degree), AV block (second or third degree—see conduction warning), bradycardia, congestive heart failure, flushing, hypotension, palpitations, syncope.

Nervous System: Amnesia, depression, gait abnormality, hallucinations, insomnia, nervousness, paresthesia, personality change, somnolence, tinnitus, tremor.

Gastrointestinal: Anorexia, constipation, diarrhea, dysgeusia, dyspepsia, mild elevations of alkaline phosphatase, SGOT, SGPT, and LDH (see hepatic warnings), vomiting, weight increase.

Dermatologic: Petechiae, pruritus, photosensitivity, urticaria.

Other: Amblyopia, CPK elevation, dyspnea, epistaxis, eye irritation, hyperglycemia, nasal congestion, nocturia, osteoarticular pain, polyuria, sexual difficulties.

The following postmarketing events have been reported infrequently in patients receiving CARDIZEM: alopecia, gingival hyperplasia, erythema multiforme, and leukopenia. However, a definitive cause and effect between these events and CARDIZEM therapy is yet to be established.

OVERDOSAGE OR EXAGGERATED RESPONSE

Overdosage experience with oral diltiazem has been limited. Single oral doses of 300 mg of CARDIZEM have been well tolerated by healthy volunteers. In the event of overdosage or exaggerated response, appropriate supportive measures should be employed in addition to gastric lavage. The following measures may be considered:

Bradycardia: Administer atropine (0.60 to 1.0 mg). If there is no response to vagal blockade, administer isoproterenol cautiously.

High-Degree AV Block: Treat as for bradycardia above. Fixed high-degree AV block should be treated with cardiac pacing.

Cardiac Failure: Administer inotropic agents (isoproterenol, dopamine, or dobutamine) and diuretics.

Hypotension: Vasopressors (eg, dopamine or levarterenol bitartrate).

Actual treatment and dosage should depend on the severity of the clinical situation and the judgment and experience of the treating physician.

The oral LD$_{50}$'s in mice and rats range from 415 to 740 mg/kg and from 560 to 810 mg/kg, respectively. The intravenous LD$_{50}$'s in these species were 60 and 38 mg/kg, respectively. The oral LD$_{50}$ in dogs is considered to be in excess of 50 mg/kg, while lethality was seen in monkeys at 360 mg/kg.

The toxic dose in man is not known. Due to extensive metabolism, blood levels after a standard dose of diltiazem can vary over tenfold, limiting the usefulness of blood levels in overdose cases. Overdoses with as much as 10.8 gm of oral diltiazem have been survived following appropriate supportive care.

DOSAGE AND ADMINISTRATION

Exertional Angina Pectoris Due to Atherosclerotic Coronary Artery Disease or Angina Pectoris at Rest Due to Coronary Artery Spasm. Dosage must be adjusted to each patient's needs. Starting with 30 mg four times daily, before meals and at bedtime, dosage should be increased gradually (given in divided doses three or four times daily) at one- to two-day intervals until optimum response is obtained. Although individual patients may respond to any dosage level, the average optimum dosage range appears to be 180 to 360 mg/day. There are no available data concerning dosage requirements in patients with impaired renal or hepatic function. If the drug must be used in such patients, titration should be carried out with particular caution.

Concomitant Use With Other Cardiovascular Agents.
1. **Sublingual NTG** may be taken as required to abort acute anginal attacks during CARDIZEM (diltiazem hydrochloride) therapy.
2. **Prophylactic Nitrate Therapy**—CARDIZEM may be safely coadministered with short- and long-acting nitrates, but there have been no controlled studies to evaluate the antianginal effectiveness of this combination.
3. **Beta-blockers.** (See WARNINGS and PRECAUTIONS.)

HOW SUPPLIED

CARDIZEM 30-mg tablets are supplied in bottles of 100 (NDC 0088-1771-47) and in Unit Dose Identification Paks of 100 (NDC 0088-1771-49). Each green tablet is engraved with MARION on one side and 1771 engraved on the other.
CARDIZEM 60-mg scored tablets are supplied in bottles of 100 (NDC 0088-1772-47) and in Unit Dose Identification Paks of 100 (NDC 0088-1772-49). Each yellow tablet is engraved with MARION on one side and 1772 on the other.
CARDIZEM 90-mg scored tablets are supplied in bottles of 100 (NDC 0088-1791-47) and in Unit Dose Identification Paks of 100 (NDC 0088-1791-49). Each green oblong tablet is engraved with CARDIZEM on one side and 90 mg on the other.
CARDIZEM 120-mg scored tablets are supplied in bottles of 100 (NDC 0088-1792-47) and in Unit Dose Identification Paks of 100 (NDC 0088-1792-49). Each yellow oblong tablet is engraved with CARDIZEM on one side and 120 mg on the other.

Store at controlled room temperature 59–86°F (15–30°C).

           Issued 11/88

Shown in Product Identification Section, page 416

CARDIZEM® SR   ℞
[kar'diz-em]
(diltiazem hydrochloride)
Sustained Release Capsules

DESCRIPTION

CARDIZEM® (diltiazem hydrochloride) is a calcium ion influx inhibitor (slow channel blocker or calcium antagonist). Chemically, diltiazem hydrochloride is 1,5-Benzothiazepin-4(5H)one,3-(acetyloxy)-5-[2-(dimethylamino) ethyl]-2,3-dihydro-2-(4-methoxyphenyl)-, monohydrochloride,(+) -cis-.
Diltiazem hydrochloride is a white to off-white crystalline powder with a bitter taste. It is soluble in water, methanol, and chloroform. It has a molecular weight of 450.98. Each CARDIZEM SR capsule contains either 60 mg, 90 mg, or 120 mg diltiazem hydrochloride.
Also contains: fumaric acid, povidone, starch, sucrose, talc, and other ingredients.
For oral administration.

CLINICAL PHARMACOLOGY

The therapeutic effects of CARDIZEM are believed to be related to its ability to inhibit the influx of calcium ions during membrane depolarization of cardiac and vascular smooth muscle.

Mechanisms of Action. CARDIZEM SR produces its antihypertensive effect primarily by relaxation of vascular smooth muscle and the resultant decrease in peripheral vascular resistance. The magnitude of blood pressure reduction is related to the degree of hypertension; thus hypertensive individuals experience an antihypertensive effect, whereas there is only a modest fall in blood pressure in normotensives.

Hemodynamic and Electrophysiologic Effects. Like other calcium antagonists, diltiazem decreases sinoatrial and atrioventricular conduction in isolated tissues and has a negative inotropic effect in isolated preparations. In the intact animal, prolongation of the AH interval can be seen at higher doses.
In man, diltiazem prevents spontaneous and ergonovine-provoked coronary artery spasm. It causes a decrease in peripheral vascular resistance and a modest fall in blood pres-

sure in normotensive individuals and, in exercise tolerance studies in patients with ischemic heart disease, reduces the heart rate-blood pressure product for any given work load. Studies to date, primarily in patients with good ventricular function, have not revealed evidence of a negative inotropic effect; cardiac output, ejection fraction, and left ventricular end diastolic pressure have not been affected. Increased heart failure has, however, been reported in occasional patients with preexisting impairment of ventricular function. There are as yet few data on the interaction of diltiazem and beta-blockers in patients with poor ventricular function. Resting heart rate is usually slightly reduced by diltiazem. CARDIZEM SR produces antihypertensive effects both in the supine and standing positions. Postural hypotension is infrequently noted upon suddenly assuming an upright position. No reflex tachycardia is associated with the chronic antihypertensive effects. CARDIZEM SR decreases vascular resistance, increases cardiac output (by increasing stroke volume), and produces a slight decrease or no change in heart rate. During dynamic exercise, increases in diastolic pressure are inhibited while maximum achievable systolic pressure is usually reduced. Heart rate at maximum exercise does not change or is slightly reduced. Chronic therapy with CARDIZEM produces no change or an increase in plasma catecholamines. No increased activity of the renin-angiotensin-aldosterone axis has been observed. CARDIZEM SR antagonizes the renal and peripheral effects of angiotensin II. Hypertensive animal models respond to diltiazem with reductions in blood pressure and increased urinary output and natriuresis without a change in urinary sodium/potassium ratio.
Intravenous diltiazem in doses of 20 mg prolongs AH conduction time and AV node functional and effective refractory periods approximately 20%. In a study involving single oral doses of 300 mg of CARDIZEM in six normal volunteers, the average maximum PR prolongation was 14% with no instances of greater than first-degree AV block. Diltiazem-associated prolongation of the AH interval is not more pronounced in patients with first-degree heart block. In patients with sick sinus syndrome, diltiazem significantly prolongs sinus cycle length (up to 50% in some cases).
Chronic oral administration of CARDIZEM in doses of up to 360 mg/day has resulted in small increases in PR interval, and on occasion produces abnormal prolongation. (See WARNINGS.)

Pharmacokinetics and Metabolism. Diltiazem is well absorbed from the gastrointestinal tract and is subject to an extensive first-pass effect, giving an absolute bioavailability (compared to intravenous administration) of about 40%. CARDIZEM undergoes extensive metabolism in which 2% to 4% of the unchanged drug appears in the urine. In vitro binding studies show CARDIZEM is 70% to 80% bound to plasma proteins. Competitive in vitro ligand binding studies have also shown CARDIZEM binding is not altered by therapeutic concentrations of digoxin, hydrochlorothiazide, phenylbutazone, propranolol, salicylic acid, or warfarin. The plasma elimination half-life following single or multiple drug administration is approximately 3.0 to 4.5 hours. Desacetyl diltiazem is also present in the plasma at levels of 10% to 20% of the parent drug and is 25% to 50% as potent a coronary vasodilator as diltiazem. Minimum therapeutic plasma levels of CARDIZEM appear to be in the range of 50–200 ng/mL. There is a departure from linearity when dose strengths are increased; the half-life is slightly increased with dose. A study that compared patients with normal hepatic function to patients with cirrhosis found an increase in half-life and a 69% increase in bioavailability in the hepatically impaired patients. A single study in patients with severely impaired renal function showed no difference in the pharmacokinetic profile of diltiazem compared to patients with normal renal function.

Cardizem SR Capsules. Diltiazem is absorbed from the capsule formulation to about 92% of a reference solution at steady-state. A single 120-mg dose of the capsule results in detectable plasma levels within two to three hours and peak plasma levels at six to 11 hours. The apparent elimination half-life after single or multiple dosing is five to seven hours. A departure from linearity similar to that observed with the CARDIZEM tablet is observed. As the dose of CARDIZEM SR capsules is increased from a daily dose of 120 mg (60 mg bid) to 240 mg (120 mg bid) daily, there is an increase in bioavailability of 2.6 times. When the dose is increased from 240 mg to 360 mg daily there is an increase in bioavailability of 1.8 times. The average plasma levels of the capsule dosed twice daily at steady-state are equivalent to the tablet dosed four times daily when the same total daily dose is administered.

INDICATIONS AND USAGE

CARDIZEM SR is indicated for the treatment of hypertension. It may be used alone or in combination with other antihypertensive medications, such as diuretics.

CONTRAINDICATIONS

CARDIZEM is contraindicated in (1) patients with sick sinus syndrome except in the presence of a functioning ventricular pacemaker, (2) patients with second- or third-degree AV block except in the presence of a functioning ventricular pacemaker, (3) patients with hypotension (less than 90 mm Hg systolic), (4) patients who have demonstrated hypersensitivity to the drug, and (5) patients with acute myocardial infarction and pulmonary congestion documented by x-ray on admission.

WARNINGS

1. **Cardiac Conduction.** CARDIZEM prolongs AV node refractory periods without significantly prolonging sinus node recovery time, except in patients with sick sinus syndrome. This effect may rarely result in abnormally slow heart rates (particularly in patients with sick sinus syndrome) or second- or third-degree AV block (nine of 2,111 patients or 0.43%). Concomitant use of diltiazem with beta-blockers or digitalis may result in additive effects on cardiac conduction. A patient with Prinzmetal's angina developed periods of asystole (2 to 5 seconds) after a single dose of 60 mg of diltiazem.

2. **Congestive Heart Failure.** Although diltiazem has a negative inotropic effect in isolated animal tissue preparations, hemodynamic studies in humans with normal ventricular function have not shown a reduction in cardiac index nor consistent negative effects on contractility (dp/dt). An acute study of oral diltiazem in patients with impaired ventricular function (ejection fraction 24%±6%) showed improvement in indices of ventricular function without significant decrease in contractile function (dp/dt). Experience with the use of CARDIZEM (diltiazem hydrochloride) in combination with beta-blockers in patients with impaired ventricular function is limited. Caution should be exercised when using this combination.

3. **Hypotension.** Decreases in blood pressure associated with CARDIZEM therapy may occasionally result in symptomatic hypotension.

4. **Acute Hepatic Injury.** Mild elevations of transaminases with and without concomitant elevation in alkaline phosphatase and bilirubin have been observed in clinical studies. Such elevations were usually transient and frequently resolved even with continued diltiazem treatment. In rare instances, significant elevations in enzymes such as alkaline phosphatase, LDH, SGOT, SGPT, and other phenomena consistent with acute hepatic injury have been noted. These reactions tended to occur early after therapy initiation (1 to 8 weeks) and have been reversible upon discontinuation of drug therapy. The relationship to CARDIZEM is uncertain in some cases, but probable in some. (See PRECAUTIONS.)

PRECAUTIONS

General. CARDIZEM (diltiazem hydrochloride) is extensively metabolized by the liver and excreted by the kidneys and in bile. As with any drug given over prolonged periods, laboratory parameters should be monitored at regular intervals. The drug should be used with caution in patients with impaired renal or hepatic function. In subacute and chronic dog and rat studies designed to produce toxicity, high doses of diltiazem were associated with hepatic damage. In special subacute hepatic studies, oral doses of 125 mg/kg and higher in rats were associated with histological changes in the liver which were reversible when the drug was discontinued. In dogs, doses of 20 mg/kg were also associated with hepatic changes; however, these changes were reversible with continued dosing.

Dermatological events (see ADVERSE REACTIONS section) may be transient and may disappear despite continued use of CARDIZEM. However, skin eruptions progressing to erythema multiforme and/or exfoliative dermatitis have also been infrequently reported. Should a dermatologic reaction persist, the drug should be discontinued.

Drug Interaction. Due to the potential for additive effects, caution and careful titration are warranted in patients receiving CARDIZEM concomitantly with any agents known to affect cardiac contractility and/or conduction. (See WARNINGS.) Pharmacologic studies indicate that there may be additive effects in prolonging AV conduction when using beta-blockers or digitalis concomitantly with CARDIZEM. (See WARNINGS.)

As with all drugs, care should be exercised when treating patients with multiple medications. CARDIZEM undergoes biotransformation by cytochrome P-450 mixed function oxidase. Coadministration of CARDIZEM with other agents which follow the same route of biotransformation may result in the competitive inhibition of metabolism. Dosages of similarly metabolized drugs, particularly those of low therapeutic ratio or in patients with renal and/or hepatic impairment, may require adjustment when starting or stopping concomitantly administered CARDIZEM to maintain optimum therapeutic blood levels.

Beta-blockers: Controlled and uncontrolled domestic studies suggest that concomitant use of CARDIZEM and beta-blockers or digitalis is usually well tolerated, but available data are not sufficient to predict the effects of concomitant treatment in patients with left ventricular dysfunction or cardiac conduction abnormalities.

Administration of CARDIZEM (diltiazem hydrochloride) concomitantly with propranolol in five normal volunteers resulted in increased propranolol levels in all subjects and bioavailability of propranolol was increased approximately 50%. If combination therapy is initiated or withdrawn in conjunction with propranolol, an adjustment in the propranolol dose may be warranted. (See WARNINGS.)

Cimetidine: A study in six healthy volunteers has shown a significant increase in peak diltiazem plasma levels (58%) and area-under-the-curve (53%) after a 1-week course of cimetidine at 1,200 mg per day and diltiazem 60 mg per day. Ranitidine produced smaller, nonsignificant increases. The effect may be mediated by cimetidine's known inhibition of hepatic cytochrome P-450, the enzyme system probably responsible for the first-pass metabolism of diltiazem. Patients currently receiving diltiazem therapy should be carefully monitored for a change in pharmacological effect when initiating and discontinuing therapy with cimetidine. An adjustment in the diltiazem dose may be warranted.

Digitalis: Administration of CARDIZEM with digoxin in 24 healthy male subjects increased plasma digoxin concentrations approximately 20%. Another investigator found no increase in digoxin levels in 12 patients with coronary artery disease. Since there have been conflicting results regarding the effect of digoxin levels, it is recommended that digoxin levels be monitored when initiating, adjusting, and discontinuing CARDIZEM therapy to avoid possible over- or under-digitalization. (See WARNINGS.)

Anesthetics: The depression of cardiac contractility, conductivity, and automaticity as well as the vascular dilation associated with anesthetics may be potentiated by calcium channel blockers. When used concomitantly, anesthetics and calcium blockers should be titrated carefully.

Carcinogenesis, Mutagenesis, Impairment of Fertility. A 24-month study in rats and a 21-month study in mice showed no evidence of carcinogenicity. There was also no mutagenic response in in vitro bacterial tests. No intrinsic effect on fertility was observed in rats.

Pregnancy. Category C. Reproduction studies have been conducted in mice, rats, and rabbits. Administration of doses ranging from five to ten times greater (on a mg/kg basis) than the daily recommended therapeutic dose has resulted in embryo and fetal lethality. These doses, in some studies, have been reported to cause skeletal abnormalities. In the perinatal/postnatal studies, there was some reduction in early individual pup weights and survival rates. There was an increased incidence of stillbirths at doses of 20 times the human dose or greater.

There are no well-controlled studies in pregnant women; therefore, use CARDIZEM in pregnant women only if the potential benefit justifies the potential risk to the fetus.

Nursing Mothers. Diltiazem is excreted in human milk. One report suggests that concentrations in breast milk may approximate serum levels. If use of CARDIZEM is deemed essential, an alternative method of infant feeding should be instituted.

Pediatric Use. Safety and effectiveness in children have not been established.

ADVERSE REACTIONS

Serious adverse reactions have been rare in studies carried out to date, but it should be recognized that patients with impaired ventricular function and cardiac conduction abnormalities have usually been excluded from these studies.

The adverse events described below represent events observed in clinical studies of hypertensive patients receiving either CARDIZEM Tablets or CARDIZEM SR Capsules as well as experiences observed in studies of angina and during marketing. The most common events in hypertension studies are shown in a table with rates in placebo patients shown for comparison. Less common events are listed by body system; these include any adverse reactions seen in angina studies that were not observed in hypertension studies. In all hypertensive patients studied (over 900), the most common adverse events were edema (9%), headache (8%), dizziness (6%), asthenia (5%), sinus bradycardia (3%), flushing (3%), and 1° AV block (3%). Only edema and perhaps bradycardia and dizziness were dose related. The most common events observed in clinical studies (over 2,100 patients) of angina patients and hypertensive patients receiving CARDIZEM Tablets or CARDIZEM SR Capsules were (ie, greater than 1%) edema (5.4%), headache (4.5%), dizziness (3.4%), asthenia (2.8%), first-degree AV block (1.8%), flushing (1.7%), nausea (1.6%), bradycardia (1.5%), and rash (1.5%).

DOUBLE BLIND PLACEBO CONTROLLED HYPERTENSION TRIALS

Adverse	Diltiazem N=315 # pts (%)	Placebo N=211 # pts (%)
headache	38 (12%)	17 (8%)
AV block first degree	24 (7.6%)	4 (1.9%)
dizziness	22 (7%)	6 (2.8%)
edema	19 (6%)	2 (0.9%)
bradycardia	19 (6%)	3 (1.4%)
ECG abnormality	13 (4.1%)	3 (1.4%)
asthenia	10 (3.2%)	1 (0.5%)
constipation	5 (1.6%)	2 (0.9%)
dyspepsia	4 (1.3%)	1 (0.5%)
nausea	4 (1.3%)	2 (0.9%)
palpitations	4 (1.3%)	2 (0.9%)
polyuria	4 (1.3%)	2 (0.9%)
somnolence	4 (1.3%)	—
alk phos increase	3 (1%)	1 (0.5%)
hypotension	3 (1%)	1 (0.5%)
insomnia	3 (1%)	1 (0.5%)
rash	3 (1%)	1 (0.5%)
AV block second degree	2 (0.6%)	—

In addition, the following events were reported infrequently (less than 1%) or have been observed in angina trials. In many cases, the relation to drug is uncertain.

Cardiovascular: Angina, arrhythmia, bundle branch block, tachycardia, ventricular extrasystoles, congestive heart failure, syncope.

Nervous System: Amnesia, depression, gait abnormality, hallucinations, nervousness, paresthesia, personality change, tinnitus, tremor, abnormal dreams.

Gastrointestinal: Anorexia, diarrhea, dysgeusia, mild elevations of SGOT, SGPT, and LDH (see hepatic warnings), vomiting, weight increase, thirst.

Dermatological: Petechiae, pruritus, photosensitivity, urticaria.

Other: Amblyopia, CPK increase, dyspnea, epistaxis, eye irritation, hyperglycemia, erythema multiforme, sexual difficulties, nasal congestion, nocturia, osteoarticular pain, impotence, dry mouth.

The following postmarketing events have been reported infrequently in patients receiving CARDIZEM: alopecia, gingival hyperplasia, erythema multiforme, and leukopenia. Definitive cause and effect relationship between these events and CARDIZEM therapy cannot yet be established.

OVERDOSAGE OR EXAGGERATED RESPONSE

Overdosage experience with oral diltiazem has been limited. Single oral doses of 300 mg of CARDIZEM have been well tolerated by healthy volunteers. In the event of overdosage or exaggerated response, appropriate supportive measures should be employed in addition to gastric lavage. The following measures may be considered:

Bradycardia: Administer atropine (0.60 to 1.0 mg). If there is no response to vagal blockade, administer isoproterenol cautiously.

High-Degree AV Block: Treat as for bradycardia above. Fixed high-degree AV block should be treated with cardiac pacing.

Cardiac Failure: Administer inotropic agents (isoproterenol, dopamine, or dobutamine) and diuretics.

Hypotension: Vasopressors (eg, dopamine or levarterenol bitartrate).

Actual treatment and dosage should depend on the severity of the clinical situation and the judgment and experience of the treating physician.

The oral LD$_{50}$'s in mice and rats range from 415 to 740 mg/kg and from 560 to 810 mg/kg, respectively. The intravenous LD$_{50}$'s in these species were 60 and 38 mg/kg, respectively. The oral LD$_{50}$ in dogs is considered to be in excess of 50 mg/kg, while lethality was seen in monkeys at 360 mg/kg. The toxic dose in man is not known. Due to extensive metabolism, blood levels after a standard dose of diltiazem can vary

Continued on next page

Marion—Cont.

over tenfold, limiting the usefulness of blood levels in overdose cases. Overdoses with as much as 10.8 gm of oral diltiazem have been survived following appropriate supportive care.

DOSAGE AND ADMINISTRATION

Dosages must be adjusted to each patient's needs, starting with 60 to 120 mg twice daily. Maximum antihypertensive effect is usually observed by 14 days of chronic therapy; therefore, dosage adjustments should be scheduled accordingly. Although individual patients may respond to lower doses, the usual optimum dosage range in clinical trials was 240 to 360 mg/day.

CARDIZEM SR has an additive antihypertensive effect when used with other antihypertensive agents. Therefore, the dosage of CARDIZEM SR or the concomitant antihypertensives may need to be adjusted when adding one to the other. See WARNINGS and PRECAUTIONS regarding use with beta-blockers.

HOW SUPPLIED

[See table below].

Issued 1/89

Shown in Product Identification Section, page 416

DEBROX® Drops   OTC
[de 'brox]

DESCRIPTION

Carbamide peroxide 6.5%. Also contains citric acid, glycerin, propylene glycol, sodium stannate, water, and other ingredients.

ACTIONS

DEBROX®, used as directed, cleanses the ear with sustained microfoam. DEBROX Drops foam on contact with earwax due to the release of oxygen.

INDICATIONS

DEBROX Drops provide a safe, nonirritating method of softening and removing earwax.

FDA APPROVED USES

For occasional use as an aid to soften, loosen, and remove excessive earwax.

DIRECTIONS

FOR USE IN THE EAR ONLY. Adults and children over 12 years of age: tilt head sideways and place 5 to 10 drops into ear. Tip of applicator should not enter ear canal. Keep drops in ear for several minutes by keeping head tilted or placing cotton in the ear. Use twice daily for up to four days if needed, or as directed by a doctor. Any wax remaining after treatment may be removed by gently flushing the ear with warm water, using a soft rubber bulb ear syringe. Children under 12 years of age: consult a doctor.

WARNINGS

Do not use if you have ear drainage or discharge, ear pain, irritation, or rash in the ear or are dizzy; consult a doctor. Do not use if you have an injury or perforation (hole) of the eardrum or after ear surgery unless directed by a doctor. Do not use for more than four days; if excessive earwax remains after use of this product, consult a doctor. Avoid contact with the eyes.

CAUTIONS

Avoid exposing bottle to excessive heat and direct sunlight. Keep color tip on bottle when not in use. AVOID CONTACT WITH EYES. KEEP THIS AND ALL DRUGS OUT OF THE REACH OF CHILDREN. IN CASE OF ACCIDENTAL INGESTION, SEEK PROFESSIONAL ASSISTANCE OR CONTACT A POISON CONTROL CENTER IMMEDIATELY.

HOW SUPPLIED

DEBROX Drops are available in ½- or 1-fl-oz plastic squeeze bottles with applicator spouts.

Issued 12/86

Shown in Product Identification Section, page 416

DITROPAN® Tablets and Syrup   ℞
[di 'tro-pan]
(oxybutynin chloride)

DESCRIPTION

Each scored biconvex, engraved blue DITROPAN® Tablet contains 5 mg of oxybutynin chloride. Each 5 mL of DITROPAN® Syrup contains 5 mg of oxybutynin chloride. Chemically, oxybutynin chloride is d,l (racemic) 4-diethylamino-2-butynyl phenylcyclohexylglycolate hydrochloride. The empirical formula of oxybutynin chloride is $C_{22}H_{31}NO_3 \cdot HCl$.

Oxybutynin chloride is a white crystalline solid with a molecular weight of 393.9. It is readily soluble in water and acids, but relatively insoluble in alkalis.

DITROPAN® Tablets
Also contains: calcium stearate, FD&C Blue #1 Lake, lactose, and microcrystalline cellulose.

DITROPAN® Syrup
Also contains: citric acid, FD&C Green #3, glycerin, methylparaben, flavor, sodium citrate, sorbitol, sucrose, and water.

DITROPAN® Tablets and Syrup are for oral administration.

Therapeutic Category: Antispasmodic, anticholinergic.

CLINICAL PHARMACOLOGY

DITROPAN® (oxybutynin chloride) exerts direct antispasmodic effect on smooth muscle and inhibits the muscarinic action of acetylcholine on smooth muscle. DITROPAN exhibits only one fifth of the anticholinergic activity of atropine on the rabbit detrusor muscle, but four to ten times the antispasmodic activity. No blocking effects occur at skeletal neuromuscular junctions or autonomic ganglia (antinicotinic effects).

DITROPAN relaxes bladder smooth muscle. In patients with conditions characterized by involuntary bladder contractions, cystometric studies have demonstrated that DITROPAN increases bladder (vesical) capacity, diminishes the frequency of uninhibited contractions of the detrusor muscle, and delays the initial desire to void. DITROPAN thus decreases urgency and the frequency of both incontinent episodes and voluntary urination.

DITROPAN was well tolerated in patients administered the drug in controlled studies of 30 days' duration and in uncontrolled studies in which some of the patients received the drug for 2 years. Pharmacokinetic information is not currently available.

INDICATIONS AND USAGE

DITROPAN is indicated for the relief of symptoms of bladder instability associated with voiding in patients with uninhibited neurogenic or reflex neurogenic bladder (ie, urgency, frequency, urinary leakage, urge incontinence, dysuria).

CONTRAINDICATIONS

DITROPAN® (oxybutynin chloride) is contraindicated in patients with increased intraocular pressure (ie, glaucoma) associated with angle closure, since anticholinergic drugs may aggravate this condition.

It is also contraindicated in partial or complete obstruction of the gastrointestinal tract, paralytic ileus, intestinal atony of the elderly or debilitated patient, megacolon, toxic megacolon complicating ulcerative colitis, severe colitis, and myasthenia gravis. It is contraindicated in patients with ob-

structive uropathy and in patients with unstable cardiovascular status in acute hemorrhage.

DITROPAN is contraindicated in patients who have demonstrated hypersensitivity to the product.

WARNINGS

DITROPAN® (oxybutynin chloride), when administered in the presence of high environmental temperature, can cause heat prostration (fever and heat stroke due to decreased sweating).

Diarrhea may be an early symptom of incomplete intestinal obstruction, especially in patients with ileostomy or colostomy. In this instance treatment with DITROPAN would be inappropriate and possibly harmful.

DITROPAN may produce drowsiness or blurred vision. The patient should be cautioned regarding activities requiring mental alertness such as operating a motor vehicle or other machinery or performing hazardous work while taking this drug.

Alcohol or other sedative drugs may enhance the drowsiness caused by DITROPAN.

PRECAUTIONS

DITROPAN® (oxybutynin chloride) should be used with caution in the elderly and in all patients with autonomic neuropathy, hepatic or renal disease. DITROPAN may aggravate the symptoms of hyperthyroidism, coronary heart disease, congestive heart failure, cardiac arrhythmias, hiatal hernia, tachycardia, hypertension, and prostatic hypertrophy. Administration of DITROPAN® (oxybutynin chloride) to patients with ulcerative colitis may suppress intestinal motility to the point of producing a paralytic ileus and precipitate or aggravate toxic megacolon, a serious complication of the disease.

CARCINOGENESIS, MUTAGENESIS, IMPAIRMENT OF FERTILITY. A 24-month study in rats at dosages up to approximately 400 times the recommended human dosage showed no evidence of carcinogenicity.

DITROPAN showed no increase of mutagenic activity when tested in *Schizosaccharomyces pompholiciformis, Saccharomyces cerevisiae* and *Salmonella typhimurium* test systems. Reproduction studies in the hamster, rabbit, rat, and mouse have shown no definite evidence of impaired fertility.

PREGNANCY: Category B. Reproduction studies in the hamster, rabbit, rat, and mouse have shown no definite evidence of impaired fertility or harm to the animal fetus. The safety of DITROPAN administered to women who are or who may become pregnant has not been established. Therefore, DITROPAN should not be given to pregnant women unless, in the judgment of the physician, the probable clinical benefits outweigh the possible hazards.

NURSING MOTHERS. It is not known whether this drug is excreted in human milk. Because many drugs are excreted in human milk, caution should be exercised when DITROPAN is administered to a nursing woman.

PEDIATRIC USE. The safety and efficacy of DITROPAN administration have been demonstrated for children 5 years of age and older (see DOSAGE AND ADMINISTRATION). However, as there is insufficient clinical data for children under age 5, DITROPAN is not recommended for this age group.

ADVERSE REACTIONS

Following administration of DITROPAN® (oxybutynin chloride), the symptoms that can be associated with the use of other anticholinergic drugs may occur:

Cardiovascular: Palpitations, tachycardia, vasodilatation.
Dermatologic: Decreased sweating, rash.
Gastrointestinal/Genitourinary: Constipation, decreased gastrointestinal motility, dry mouth, nausea, urinary hesitance and retention.
Nervous System: Asthenia, dizziness, drowsiness, hallucinations, insomnia, restlessness.
Ophthalmic: Amblyopia, cycloplegia, decreased lacrimation, mydriasis.
Other: Impotence, suppression of lactation.

OVERDOSAGE

The symptoms of overdosage with DITROPAN® (oxybutynin chloride) may be any of those seen with other anticholinergic agents. Symptoms may include signs of central nervous system excitation (eg, restlessness, tremor, irritability, convulsions, delirium, hallucinations), flushing, fever, nausea, vomiting, tachycardia, hypotension or hypertension, respiratory failure, paralysis, and coma.

In the event of an overdose or exaggerated response, treatment should be symptomatic and supportive. Maintain respiration and induce emesis or perform gastric lavage (emesis is contraindicated in precomatose, convulsive, or psychotic state). Activated charcoal may be administered as well as a cathartic. Physostigmine may be considered to reverse symptoms of anticholinergic intoxication. Hyperpyrexia may be treated symptomatically with ice bags or other cold applications and alcohol sponges.

CARDIZEM® SR
(diltiazem hydrochloride)
Sustained Release Capsules

Strength	Quantity	NDC Number	Description
60 mg	100 btl 100 UDIP®	0088-1777-47 0088-1777-49	Ivory/brown capsule imprinted with CARDIZEM logo on one end and CARDIZEM SR 60 mg on the other
90 mg	100 btl 100 UDIP®	0088-1778-47 0088-1778-49	Gold/brown capsule imprinted with CARDIZEM logo on one end and CARDIZEM SR 90 mg on the other
120 mg	100 btl 100 UDIP®	0088-1779-47 0088-1779-49	Caramel/brown capsule imprinted with CARDIZEM logo on one end and CARDIZEM SR 120 mg on the other

Storage Conditions: Store at controlled room temperature 59–86°F (15–30°C).

DOSAGE AND ADMINISTRATION

Tablets

Adults: The usual dose is one 5-mg tablet two to three times a day. The maximum recommended dose is one 5-mg tablet four times a day.

Children over 5 years of age: The usual dose is one 5-mg tablet two times a day. The maximum recommended dose is one 5-mg tablet three times a day.

Syrup

Adults: The usual dose is one teaspoon (5 mg/5 mL) syrup two to three times a day. The maximum recommended dose is one teaspoon (5 mg/5 mL) syrup four times a day.

Children over 5 years of age: The usual dose is one teaspoon (5 mg/5 mL) two times a day. The maximum recommended dose is one teaspoon (5 mg/5 mL) three times a day.

HOW SUPPLIED

DITROPAN® (oxybutynin chloride) Tablets are supplied in bottles of 100 tablets (NDC 0088-1375-47) and 1,000 tablets (NDC 0088-1375-58) and in Unit Dose Identification Paks of 100 tablets (NDC 0088-1375-49).

Blue scored tablets (5 mg) are engraved with MARION on one side and 1375 on the other side.

DITROPAN® Syrup (5 mg/5 mL) is supplied in bottles of 16 fluid ounces (473 mL) (NDC 0088-1373-18).

Pharmacist: Dispense in tight, light-resistant container as defined in the USP.

Store at controlled room temperature (59°–86° F).

Issued 3/88

Shown in Product Identification Section, page 416

A III Color Wound Care Product
ENVICLUSIVE™
[ĕn-vĭ-clū 'sĭv]
Semi-occlusive adhesive film dressing

DIRECTIONS FOR USE

1. Clean application site and surrounding skin and thoroughly dry surface of intact skin.
2. Apply sterile dressing and/or wound care product to the application site.
3. Measure and cut the required length of ENVICLUSIVE™.
4. Peel off the film backing and apply, ensuring that the ENVICLUSIVE™ is firmly secured to dry, healthy skin around the application site.

Directions for Use With ENVISAN™ Paste

1. Preparation. Debride the necrotic areas mechanically. Clean the wound with a swab soaked in normal saline. Leave wound bed moist.

2. Lay ENVINET™ fine mesh dressing over wound. Place a fine mesh dressing over the bed of the wound, leaving an overlap of about 12 mm (½ in), and moisten with saline. Make sure sensitive skin around the wound is covered.

3. Spread ENVISAN™ Paste into wound. Remove ENVISAN™ Paste from packet and spread onto the mesh dressing to a depth of at least 6 mm (¼ in) covering the wound

4. Select ENVICLUSIVE™ semi-occlusive film. Measure and cut the required length of ENVICLUSIVE™ to a size at least 12 mm (½ in) larger than the mesh dressing.

5–6. Secure the dressing. Peel off backing and cover dressing and ENVISAN™ Paste with ENVICLUSIVE™, ensuring that it is firmly secured to dry, healthy skin around the wound.

7. Remove discolored dressing. Remove the dressing complete with ENVISAN™ Paste when it becomes discolored (usually after 12 to 24 hours). If necessary, syringe carefully with saline to assist removal.

8. Renewal. Clean the wound with a swab soaked in normal saline. Leave the wound bed moist. Renew the dressing as required.

For external use only.
Please see package insert for ENVISAN™ Paste and ENVISAN™ Pads.
Mfd in Sweden for
Marion Laboratories, Inc.

Issued 10/87

A III Color Wound Care Product
ENVINET™ Nylon Net for ENVISAN™ Treatment
[ĕn 'vĭ-nĕt]

1. Preparation. Debride the necrotic areas mechanically. Clean the wound with a swab soaked in normal saline. Leave wound bed moist.

2. Lay ENVINET™ fine mesh dressing over wound. Place a fine mesh dressing over the bed of the wound, leaving an overlap of about 12 mm (½ in), and moisten with saline. Make sure sensitive skin around the wound is covered.

3. Spread ENVISAN™ Paste into wound. Remove ENVISAN™ Paste from packet and spread onto the mesh dressing to a depth of at least 6 mm (¼ in) covering the wound area.

4. Select ENVICLUSIVE™ semi-occlusive film. Measure and cut the required length of ENVICLUSIVE™ to a size at least 12 mm (½ in) larger than the mesh dressing.

5–6. Secure the dressing. Peel off backing and cover dressing and ENVISAN™ Paste with ENVICLUSIVE™, ensuring that it is firmly secured to dry, healthy skin around the wound.

7. Remove discolored dressing. Remove the dressing complete with ENVISAN™ Paste when it becomes discolored (usually after 12 to 24 hours). If necessary, syringe carefully with saline to assist removal.

8. Renewal. Clean the wound with a swab soaked in normal saline. Leave the wound bed moist. Renew the dressing as required.

Please see package insert for ENVISAN™ Paste.
Mfd in Sweden for
Marion Laboratories, Inc.

Issued 10/87

A III Color Wound Care Product
ENVISAN™ Wound Cleaning Pad
[ĕn 'vĭ-san]
(dextranomer, polyethylene glycol 3,000, polyethylene glycol 600, water qs)

PRODUCT INFORMATION

DESCRIPTION

ENVISAN™ Wound Cleaning Pad consists of spherical hydrophilic beads of dextranomer, 0.1 to 0.3 mm in diameter, polyethylene glycol 3,000, polyethylene glycol 600, and water qs enclosed in a polyamide net bag.

The beads are composed of a three-dimensional network of macromolecular chains of cross-linked dextran which is large enough to allow substances with a molecular weight of less than 1,000 to enter freely. Substances with a molecular

Continued on next page

Marion—Cont.

weight of 1,000–5,000 enter the beads less freely, while those with a molecular weight greater than 5,000 remain in the interspaces between the beads.

CHARACTERISTICS

Because of its hydrophilic properties, each gram of dextranomer beads absorbs approximately 4 mL of fluid. The beads swell to approximately four times their original size. This swelling causes significant suction forces and capillary action in the spaces between the beads. This action is continuous as long as the unsaturated beads are in proximity to the ulcer or wound.

When ENVISAN™ Wound Cleaning Pad is applied to the surface of wet ulcers or wet wounds, suction forces begin removing various exudates and particles that tend to impede tissue repair. For example, low molecular weight components of wound exudates are drawn up within the beads while higher molecular weight components, such as plasma proteins and fibrinogen, are found between the swollen beads. Removal of these latter components, particularly fibrin and fibrinogen, retards eschar formation. Additionally, there is in vitro evidence that the suction forces created by the beads remove bacteria and inflammatory exudates from the surface of the wound.

The use of ENVISAN™ Wound Cleaning Pad to remove exudates continuously from the surface of the wound results in a concomitant reduction of inflammation and edema and thus provides an environment conducive to the normal healing process.

INDICATIONS

ENVISAN™ Wound Cleaning Pad is indicated for use in cleaning wet ulcers and wet wounds such as venous stasis ulcers, pressure (decubitus) ulcers, infected traumatic and surgical wounds, and infected burns.

PRECAUTIONS

When treating cratered pressure ulcers, fistulas, or wounds with narrow openings, do not pack the wound tightly. Allow for expansion of the pad. Do not use in cases where complete removal of the pad cannot be assured.

Once the ENVISAN™ Wound Cleaning Pad is saturated, it should be removed since it will no longer be effective and the potential for encrustation can be reduced.

The pad must be removed prior to any surgical procedure to close the wound.

Avoid contact with the eyes.

Wounds may appear larger during the first few days of treatment due to the reduction of edema.

ENVISAN™ Wound Cleaning Pad is not effective in cleaning nonsecreting wounds.

Not all wounds require treatment to complete healing. When the wound is no longer exuding and a healthy granulation base has been established, the use of ENVISAN™ Wound Cleaning Pad should be discontinued. At this point the natural healing process usually leads to complete closure of the wound.

Treatment of the underlying condition (venous or arterial flow, pressure, etc) should proceed concurrently with the use of the pad.

ADVERSE REACTIONS

Transitory pain, bleeding, blistering, edema, and erythema have occasionally been reported in isolated cases.

INSTRUCTIONS FOR USE

Application

Debride and clean the wound in the usual manner. Leave the wound moist since this facilitates the action of the ENVISAN™ Wound Cleaning Pad.

ENVISAN™ Wound Cleaning Pad is not an enzyme and will not debride a wound.

Remove the pad from the packet and apply to the wound. Press lightly to ensure contact with the wound surface. Cover with ENVICLUSIVE™ semi-occlusive film, allowing sufficient room for expansion of the beads.

Use a fresh pad or pads for each application.

Removal

Remove the ENVISAN™ Wound Cleaning Pad when it becomes saturated.

Gentle irrigation may be required to aid in removal.

Reapplication

Initially reapply fresh ENVISAN™ Wound Cleaning Pad every 12 to 24 hours.

Thereafter, the time interval for reapplication should be adjusted to accommodate the amount of exudate present. Reduce the number of applications as the amount of exudate diminishes.

Discontinuation

Use of ENVISAN™ Wound Cleaning Pad should be discontinued when the wound is free of exudate and edema and a healthy granulation base has been established.

The physician should be consulted if the patient's condition worsens or persists beyond the expected treatment period.

HOW SUPPLIED

Each ENVISAN™ Wound Cleaning Pad (double absorbent pad, 1.8 in × 1.2 in) is supplied sterile and contains 3 g (0.11 oz) ENVISAN™ Wound Cleaning Paste. Each double absorbent pad is individually packaged. Available in cartons of six sterile packets.

For use with ENVICLUSIVE™ semi-occlusive film dressing.

Store at 59° to 86°F (15° to 30°C)

For external use only

Avoid contact with the eyes

Mfd in Sweden for

Marion Laboratories, Inc.

Issued 10/87

A III Color Wound Care Product
ENVISAN™ Wound Cleaning Paste

[ĕn 'vĭ-san]

(dextranomer, polyethylene
glycol 600, water qs)

PRODUCT INFORMATION

DESCRIPTION

ENVISAN™ Paste consists of spherical hydrophilic beads of dextranomer, 0.1 to 0.3 mm in diameter, polyethylene glycol 600, and water qs.

The beads are composed of a three-dimensional network of macromolecular chains of cross-linked dextran which is large enough to allow substances with a molecular weight of less than 1,000 to enter freely. Substances with a molecular weight of 1,000 to 5,000 enter the beads less freely, while those with a molecular weight greater than 5,000 remain in the interspaces between the beads.

CHARACTERISTICS

Because of its hydrophilic properties, each gram of dextranomer beads absorbs approximately 4 mL of fluid. The beads swell to approximately four times their original size. This swelling causes significant suction forces and capillary action in the spaces between the beads. This action is continuous as long as the unsaturated beads are in proximity to the ulcer or wound.

When ENVISAN™ Paste is applied to the surface of wet ulcers or wet wounds, suction forces begin removing various exudates and particles that tend to impede tissue repair. For example, low molecular weight components of wound exudates are drawn up within the beads while higher molecular weight components, such as plasma proteins and fibrinogen, are found between the swollen beads. Removal of these latter components, particularly fibrin and fibrinogen, retards eschar formation. Additionally, there is in vitro evidence that the suction forces created by the beads remove bacteria and inflammatory exudates from the surface of the wound.

The use of ENVISAN™ Paste to remove exudates continuously from the surface of the wound results in a concomitant reduction of inflammation and edema and thus provides an environment conducive to the normal healing process.

INDICATIONS

ENVISAN™ Paste is indicated for use in cleaning wet ulcers and wet wounds such as venous stasis ulcers, pressure (decubitus) ulcers, infected traumatic and surgical wounds, and infected burns.

PRECAUTIONS

When treating cratered pressure ulcers, fistulas, or wounds with narrow openings, do not pack the wound tightly. Allow for expansion of the paste. Do not use in cases where complete removal of the paste cannot be assured.

Once the ENVISAN™ Paste is saturated, it should be removed since it will no longer be effective and the potential for encrustation can be reduced.

The paste must be removed prior to any surgical procedure to close the wound.

Avoid contact with the eyes.

Wounds may appear larger during the first few days of treatment due to the reduction of edema.

ENVISAN™ Paste is not effective in cleaning nonsecreting wounds.

Not all wounds require treatment to complete healing. When the wound is no longer exuding and a healthy granulation base has been established, the use of ENVISAN™ Paste should be discontinued. At this point the natural healing process usually leads to complete closure of the wound.

Treatment of the underlying condition (venous or arterial flow, pressure, etc) should proceed concurrently with the use of the paste.

ADVERSE REACTIONS

Transitory pain, bleeding, blistering, edema, and erythema have occasionally been reported in isolated cases.

INSTRUCTIONS FOR USE (See diagram.)

Application

Debride and clean the wound in the usual manner. Leave the wound moist since this facilitates the action of the ENVISAN™ Paste.

ENVISAN™ Paste is not an enzyme and will not debride a wound.

Line the wound with ENVINET™ nylon net.

Remove the paste from the packet and apply to ENVINET™ lining the wound.

Press lightly to ensure contact with the wound surface.

Cover with ENVICLUSIVE™ semi-occlusive film, allowing sufficient room for expansion of the beads.

Use fresh paste for each application.

Removal

Remove the ENVISAN™ Paste when it becomes saturated. Gentle irrigation may be required to aid in removal.

Reapplication

Initially reapply fresh ENVISAN™ Paste every 12 to 24 hours.

Thereafter, the time interval for reapplication should be adjusted to accommodate the amount of exudate present. Reduce the number of applications as the amount of exudate diminishes.

Discontinuation

Use of ENVISAN™ Paste should be discontinued when the wound is free of exudate and edema and a healthy granulation base has been established.

The physician should be consulted if the patient's condition worsens or persists beyond the expected treatment period.

HOW SUPPLIED

ENVISAN™ Paste is supplied sterile in a 10g (0.35oz) packet. Available in cartons of six sterile packets.

For use with ENVINET™ nylon net and ENVICLUSIVE™ semi-occlusive film dressing.

Store at 59°–86°F (15°–30°C)

For external use only

Avoid contact with the eyes

ENVISAN™ PASTE—Directions for Use

1. Preparation. Debride the necrotic areas mechanically. Clean the wound with a swab soaked in normal saline. Leave wound bed moist.

2. Lay ENVINET™ fine mesh dressing over wound. Place a fine mesh dressing over the bed of the wound, leaving an overlap of about 12 mm (½ in), and moisten with saline. Make sure sensitive skin around the wound is covered.

3. Spread ENVISAN™ Paste into wound. Remove ENVISAN™ Paste from packet and spread onto the mesh dressing to a depth of at least 6 mm (¼ in) covering the wound area.

4. Select ENVICLUSIVE™ semi-occlusive film. Measure and cut the required length of ENVICLUSIVE™ to a size at least 12 mm (½ in) larger than the mesh dressing.

5–6. Secure the dressing. Peel off backing and cover dressing and ENVISAN™ Paste with ENVICLUSIVE™, ensuring that it is firmly secured to dry, healthy skin around the wound.

7. Remove discolored dressing. Remove the dressing complete with ENVISAN™ Paste when it becomes discolored (usually after 12 to 24 hours). If necessary, syringe carefully with saline to assist removal.

8. Renewal. Clean the wound with a swab soaked in normal saline. Leave the wound bed moist. Renew the dressing as required.

Please see package insert for ENVISAN™ Paste.
Mfd in Sweden for
Marion Laboratories, Inc.

Issued 10/87

GAVISCON® Antacid Tablets   OTC
[gav ′is-kon]

COMPOSITION
Each chewable tablet contains the following active ingredients:
Aluminum hydroxide dried gel .... 80 mg
Magnesium trisilicate .... 20 mg
and the following inactive ingredients: alginic acid, calcium stearate, flavor, sodium bicarbonate, starch (may contain cornstarch), and sucrose.

INDICATIONS
GAVISCON is specifically formulated for the temporary relief of heartburn (acid indigestion) due to acid reflux. GAVISCON is not indicated for the treatment of peptic ulcers.

DIRECTIONS
Chew 2 to 4 tablets four times a day or as directed by a physician. Tablets should be taken after meals and at bedtime or as needed. For best results follow by a half glass of water or other liquid. Do not swallow whole.

WARNINGS
Do not take more than 16 tablets in a 24-hour period or 16 tablets daily for more than 2 weeks, except under the advice and supervision of a physician. Do not use this product except under the advice and supervision of a physician if you are on a sodium-restricted diet. Each GAVISCON Tablet contains approximately 0.8 mEq sodium.

DRUG INTERACTION PRECAUTIONS
Do not take this product if you are presently taking a prescription antibiotic drug containing any form of tetracycline. Store at a controlled room temperature in a dry place.

Keep this and all drugs out of the reach of children.
In case of accidental overdose, seek professional assistance or contact a poison control center immediately.

HOW SUPPLIED
Available in bottles of 100 tablets and in foil-wrapped 2s in boxes of 30 tablets.

Issued 2/87

Shown in Product Identification Section, page 416

GAVISCON® EXTRA STRENGTH   OTC
RELIEF FORMULA Antacid Tablets
[găv ′ĭs-kŏn]

COMPOSITION
Each chewable tablet contains the following active ingredients:
Aluminum hydroxide ....160 mg
Magnesium carbonate ....105 mg
and the following inactive ingredients: alginic acid, calcium stearate, flavor, mannitol, sodium bicarbonate, stearic acid, and sucrose.

DIRECTIONS
Chew 2 to 4 tablets four times a day or as directed by a physician. Tablets should be taken after meals and at bedtime or as needed. For best results follow by a half glass of water or other liquid. DO NOT SWALLOW WHOLE.

> **FDA APPROVED USES**
> For the relief of heartburn, sour stomach, and/or acid indigestion, and upset stomach associated with heartburn, sour stomach, and/or acid indigestion.

WARNINGS
Do not take more than 16 tablets in a 24-hour period or 16 tablets daily for more than 2 weeks, except under the advice and supervision of a physician. Do not use this product except under the advice and supervision of a physician if you are on a sodium-restricted diet. Each tablet contains approximately 1.3 mEq sodium.

DRUG INTERACTION PRECAUTIONS
Do not take this product if you are presently taking a prescription antibiotic drug containing any form of tetracycline. Store at a controlled room temperature in a dry place.
Keep this and all drugs out of the reach of children.
In case of accidental overdose, seek professional assistance or contact a poison control center immediately.

HOW SUPPLIED
Available in bottles of 100 tablets.

Issued 4/87

Shown in Product Identification Section, page 416

GAVISCON® EXTRA STRENGTH   OTC
RELIEF FORMULA
Liquid Antacid
[găv ′ĭs-kŏn]

COMPOSITION
Each 2 teaspoonfuls (10 mL) contains the following active ingredients:
Aluminum hydroxide ....508 mg
Magnesium carbonate ....475 mg
And the following inactive ingredients: butylparaben, edetate disodium, flavor, glycerin, propylparaben, saccharin sodium, simethicone emulsion, sodium alginate, sorbitol solution, water, and xanthan gum.

> **FDA APPROVED USES**
> For the relief of heartburn, sour stomach and/or acid indigestion, and upset stomach associated with heartburn, sour stomach and/or acid indigestion.

DIRECTIONS
SHAKE WELL BEFORE USING. Take 2 to 4 teaspoonfuls four times a day or as directed by a physician. GAVISCON Extra Strength Relief Formula Liquid should be taken after meals and at bedtime, followed by half a glass of water. Dispense product only by spoon or other measuring device.

WARNINGS
Except under the advice and supervision of a physician, do not take more than 16 teaspoonfuls in a 24-hour period or 16 teaspoonfuls daily for more than 2 weeks. May have laxative effect. Do not use this product if you have a kidney disease; do not use this product if you are on a sodium-restricted diet. Each teaspoonful contains approximately 0.9 mEq sodium.

DRUG INTERACTION PRECAUTIONS
Do not take this product if you are presently taking a prescription antibiotic drug containing any form of tetracycline.

Keep tightly closed. Avoid freezing. Store at a controlled room temperature.
Keep this and all drugs out of the reach of children.
In case of accidental overdose, seek professional assistance or contact a poison control center immediately.

HOW SUPPLIED
Available in 12 fl oz (355 mL) bottles.

Issued 2/89

Shown in Product Identification Section, page 416

GAVISCON® Liquid Antacid   OTC
[gav ′is-kon]

COMPOSITION
Each tablespoonful (15 ml) contains the following active ingredients:
Aluminum hydroxide .... 95 mg
Magnesium carbonate .... 412 mg
And the following inactive ingredients: D&C Yellow #10, edetate disodium, FD&C Blue #1, flavor, glycerin, paraben preservatives, saccharin sodium, sodium alginate, sorbitol solution, water, and xanthan gum.

> **FDA APPROVED USES**
> For the relief of heartburn, sour stomach and/or acid indigestion, and upset stomach associated with heartburn, sour stomach and/or acid indigestion.

DIRECTIONS
Shake well before using. Take 1 or 2 tablespoonfuls four times a day or as directed by a physician. GAVISCON Liquid should be taken after meals and at bedtime, followed by half a glass of water.
Dispense product only by spoon or other measuring device.

WARNINGS
Except under the advice and supervision of a physician, do not take more than 8 tablespoonfuls in a 24-hour period or 8 tablespoonfuls daily for more than 2 weeks. May have laxative effect. Do not use this product if you have a kidney disease; do not use this product if you are on a sodium-restricted diet. Each tablespoonful of GAVISCON Liquid contains approximately 1.7 mEq sodium.

DRUG INTERACTION PRECAUTIONS
Do not take this product if you are presently taking a prescription antibiotic drug containing any form of tetracycline. Keep tightly closed. Avoid freezing. Store at a controlled room temperature.
Keep this and all drugs out of the reach of children.
In case of accidental overdose, seek professional assistance or contact a poison control center immediately.

HOW SUPPLIED
Bottles of 12 fluid ounces (355 ml) and 6 fluid ounces (177 ml).

Issued 2/87

Shown in Product Identification Section, page 416

GLY-OXIDE® Liquid   OTC
[gli ′ok-sīd]

DESCRIPTION
GLY-OXIDE® Liquid contains carbamide peroxide 10%. Also contains citric acid, flavor, glycerin, propylene glycol, sodium stannate, water, and other ingredients.

ACTIONS
GLY-OXIDE® Liquid has an oxygen-rich formula that works to relieve the pain of canker sores by cleaning and debriding damaged tissue so natural healing can occur.

ADMINISTRATION
Do not dilute. Apply directly from bottle. Replace color tip on bottle when not in use.

INDICATIONS
For local treatment and hygienic prevention of minor oral inflammation such as canker sores, denture irritation, and postdental procedure irritation, place several drops on affected area four times daily, after meals and at bedtime, or as directed by a dentist or physician; expectorate after two to three minutes. Or place 10 drops onto tongue, mix with saliva, swish for several minutes, and expectorate.
As an adjunct to oral hygiene (orthodontics, dental appliances) after regular brushing, swish 10 or more drops vigorously. Continue for two to three minutes; expectorate.
When normal oral hygiene is inadequate or impossible (total care geriatrics, etc), swish 10 or more drops vigorously after meals and expectorate.

PRECAUTIONS
Severe or persistent oral inflammation, denture irritation, or gingivitus may be serious. If these conditions or unex-

Continued on next page

Marion—Cont.

pected side effects occur, consult a dentist or physician immediately.

Avoid contact with eyes. Protect from heat and direct light. Keep this and all drugs out of the reach of children. In case of accidental overdose, seek professional assistance or contact a poison control center immediately.

HOW SUPPLIED

GLY-OXIDE® Liquid is available in ½-fl-oz and 2-fl-oz non-spill, plastic squeeze bottles with applicator spouts.

Issued 2/86

Shown in Product Identification Section, page 416

NITRO–BID® Plateau CAPS®   ℞
[ni'tro-bid]
(nitroglycerin) 2.5 mg, 6.5 mg, 9 mg

DESCRIPTION

Each NITRO-BID® Controlled-Release Capsule contains:
2.5 mg nitroglycerin: Light purple and clear capsule with white beads; identification imprint MARION/1550.
6.5 mg nitroglycerin: Dark blue and yellow capsule with white beads; identification imprint MARION/1551.
9 mg nitroglycerin: Green and yellow capsule with white beads; identification imprint MARION/1553.
Also contains: calcium stearate, lactose, silica gel, starch, sucrose, talc, and other ingredients.

ACTION

The mechanism of action of nitroglycerin in the relief of angina pectoris is not as yet known. However, its main pharmacologic action is to relax smooth muscle, principally in the smaller blood vessels, thus dilating arterioles and capillaries, especially in the coronary circulation. In therapeutic doses, nitroglycerin is thought to increase the blood supply to the myocardium which may, in turn, relieve myocardial ischemia, the possible functional basis for the pain of angina pectoris. The sublingual administration of nitroglycerin is normally rapid and transient, but nitroglycerin in controlled-release NITRO-BID® 2.5, NITRO-BID® 6.5, and NITRO-BID® 9 produces a prolonged action.

INDICATIONS

Based on a review of this drug and a related drug by the National Academy of Sciences-National Research Council and/or other information, FDA has classified the indications as follows:
"Possibly" effective:
For the management, prophylaxis, or treatment of anginal attacks.
Final classification of the less-than-effective indications requires further investigation.

CONTRAINDICATIONS

Acute or recent myocardial infarction, severe anemia, closed-angle glaucoma, postural hypotension, increased intracranial pressure, and idiosyncrasy to the drug.

WARNINGS

Capsules must be swallowed. FOR ORAL, NOT SUBLINGUAL, USE. NITRO-BID® 2.5, NITRO-BID® 6.5, and NITRO-BID® 9 Controlled-Release Capsules are not intended for immediate relief of anginal attacks.

PRECAUTIONS

Intraocular pressure may be increased; therefore, caution is required in administering to patients with glaucoma. Tolerance to this drug and cross-tolerance to other organic nitrites and nitrates may occur. If blurring of vision, dryness of mouth, or lack of benefit occurs, the drug should be discontinued.

ADVERSE REACTIONS

Severe and persistent headaches, cutaneous flushing, dizziness, and weakness. Occasionally, drug rash or exfoliative dermatitis and nausea and vomiting may occur; these responses may disappear with a decrease in dosage. Adverse effects are enhanced by ingestion of alcohol, which appears to increase absorption from the gastrointestinal tract.

DOSAGE AND ADMINISTRATION

Administer the smallest effective dose two or three times daily at 8- to 12-hour intervals, unless clinical response suggests a different regimen. Patient should be titrated to anginal relief or hemodynamic response. Hemodynamic response can be measured by drop in systolic blood pressure. Discontinue if not effective.

HOW SUPPLIED

NITRO-BID® (nitroglycerin) 2.5, 6.5, and 9 Controlled-Release Capsules are available in 60- and 100-count bottles.

CAUTION

Federal law prohibits dispensing without prescription.

STORAGE

Store at a controlled room temperature. Dispense only in the original unopened container.

Issued 9/85

Shown in Product Identification Section, page 416

NITRO–BID® IV   ℞
[ni'tro-bid]
(nitroglycerin)
FOR INTRAVENOUS USE ONLY

NOT FOR DIRECT INTRAVENOUS INJECTION. NITRO-BID IV MUST BE DILUTED IN DEXTROSE (5%) INJECTION, USP OR SODIUM CHLORIDE (0.9%) INJECTION, USP BEFORE INTRAVENOUS ADMINISTRATION. THE ADMINISTRATION SET USED FOR INFUSION MAY AFFECT THE AMOUNT OF NITRO-BID IV DELIVERED TO THE PATIENT. (SEE **WARNINGS** AND **DOSAGE AND ADMINISTRATION** SECTIONS.)
CAUTION: SEVERAL PREPARATIONS OF NITRO-GLYCERIN FOR INJECTION ARE AVAILABLE. THEY DIFFER IN CONCENTRATION AND/OR VOLUME PER VIAL. WHEN SWITCHING FROM ONE PRODUCT TO ANOTHER, ATTENTION MUST BE PAID TO THE DILUTION AND DOSAGE AND ADMINISTRATION INSTRUCTIONS.

DESCRIPTION

NITRO-BID IV (nitroglycerin) is a clear, practically colorless additive solution for intravenous infusion after dilution. Each milliliter contains 5 mg nitroglycerin and 45 mg propylene glycol dissolved in 70% ethanol.
The solution is sterile, nonpyrogenic, and nonexplosive. NITRO-BID IV, an organic nitrate, is a vasodilator. The chemical name for nitroglycerin is 1,2,3 propanetriol trinitrate.

CLINICAL PHARMACOLOGY

Relaxation of vascular smooth muscle is the principal pharmacologic action of NITRO-BID IV (nitroglycerin). Although venous effects predominate, nitroglycerin produces, in a dose-related manner, dilation of both arterial and venous beds. Dilation of the postcapillary vessels, including large veins, promotes peripheral pooling of blood and decreases venous return to the heart, reducing left ventricular end-diastolic pressure (preload). Arteriolar relaxation reduces systemic vascular resistance and arterial pressure (afterload). Myocardial oxygen consumption or demand (as measured by the pressure-rate product, tension-time index, and stroke-work index) is decreased by both the arterial and venous effects of nitroglycerin, and a more favorable supply-demand ratio can be achieved.

Therapeutic doses of intravenous nitroglycerin reduce systolic, diastolic, and mean arterial blood pressures. Effective coronary perfusion pressure is usually maintained, but can be compromised if blood pressure falls excessively or increased heart rate decreases diastolic filling time.

Elevated central venous and pulmonary capillary wedge pressures, pulmonary vascular resistance, and systemic vascular resistance are also reduced by nitroglycerin therapy. Heart rate is usually slightly increased, presumably a reflex response to the fall in blood pressure. Cardiac index may be increased, decreased, or unchanged. Patients with elevated left ventricular filling pressure and systemic vascular resistance values in conjunction with a depressed cardiac index are likely to experience an improvement in cardiac index. On the other hand, when filling pressures and cardiac index are normal, cardiac index may be slightly reduced by intravenous nitroglycerin.

Nitroglycerin is widely distributed in the body with an apparent volume of distribution of approximately 200 liters in adult male subjects, and is rapidly metabolized to dinitrates and mononitrates, with a short half-life, estimated at one to four minutes. This results in a low plasma concentration after intravenous infusion. At plasma concentrations of between 50 and 100 ng/ml, the binding of nitroglycerin to plasma proteins is approximately 60%, while that of 1,2 dinitroglycerin and 1,3 dinitroglycerin is 60% and 30%, respectively. The activity and half-life of the dinitroglycerins are not well characterized. The mononitrate is not active.

INDICATIONS AND USAGE

NITRO-BID IV (nitroglycerin) is indicated for:
1. **Control of blood pressure in perioperative hypertension,** ie, hypertension associated with surgical procedures, especially cardiovascular procedures, such as the hypertension seen during intratracheal intubation, anesthesia, skin incision, sternotomy, cardiac bypass, and in the immediate postsurgical period.
2. **Congestive heart failure associated with acute myocardial infarction.**
3. **Treatment of angina pectoris** in patients who have not responded to recommended doses of organic nitrates and/or a beta-blocker.
4. **Production of controlled hypotension during surgical procedures.**

CONTRAINDICATIONS

NITRO-BID IV (nitroglycerin) should not be administered to individuals with:
1. A known hypersensitivity to nitroglycerin or a known idiosyncratic reaction to organic nitrates.
2. Hypotension or uncorrected hypovolemia, as the use of NITRO-BID IV in such states could produce severe hypotension or shock.
3. Increased intracranial pressure (eg, head trauma or cerebral hemorrhage).
4. Inadequate cerebral circulation, constrictive pericarditis, and pericardial tamponade.

WARNINGS

1. Nitroglycerin readily migrates into many plastics. To avoid absorption of nitroglycerin into plastic parenteral solution containers, the dilution and storage of nitroglycerin for intravenous infusion should be made only in glass parenteral solution bottles.
2. Some filters also absorb nitroglycerin; they should be avoided.
3. Forty percent to 80% of the total amount of nitroglycerin in the final diluted solution for infusion is absorbed by the polyvinyl chloride (PVC) tubing of the intravenous administration sets currently in general use. The higher rates of absorption occur when flow rates are low, nitroglycerin concentrations are high, and tubing is long. Although the rate of loss is highest during the early phase of administration (when flow rates are lowest), the loss is neither constant nor self-limiting; consequently, no simple calculation or correction can be performed to convert the theoretical infusion rate (based on the concentration of the infusion solution) to the actual delivery rate. Because of this problem, Marion Laboratories recommends the use of the least absorptive infusion tubing available for infusions of NITRO-BID IV. DOSING INSTRUCTIONS MUST BE FOLLOWED WITH CARE. IT SHOULD BE NOTED THAT WHEN THESE INFUSION SETS ARE USED, THE CALCULATED DOSE WILL BE DELIVERED TO THE PATIENT DEPENDENT UPON THE LOSS OF NITROGLYCERIN DUE TO ABSORPTIVE TUBING. NOTE THAT THE DOSAGES COMMONLY USED IN PUBLISHED STUDIES UTILIZED GENERAL-USE PVC TUBING, AND RECOMMENDED DOSES BASED ON THIS EXPERIENCE ARE TOO HIGH IF NEW, LESS ABSORPTIVE INFUSION TUBING IS USED.
4. PROTECT FROM LIGHT UNTIL READY FOR USE.
5. NITRO-BID IV VIALS ARE INTENDED FOR SINGLE-DOSE ONLY. PROPERLY DISCARD ANY UNUSED PORTION.

PRECAUTIONS

NITRO-BID IV (nitroglycerin) should be used with caution in patients who have severe hepatic or renal disease.

Excessive hypotension, especially for prolonged periods of time, must be avoided because of possible deleterious effects on the brain, heart, liver, and kidney from poor perfusion and the attendant risk of ischemia, thrombosis, and altered function of these organs. Patients with normal or low pulmonary capillary wedge pressure are especially sensitive to the hypotensive effects of NITRO-BID IV. If pulmonary capillary wedge pressure is being monitored, it will be noted that a fall in wedge pressure precedes the onset of arterial hypotension, and the pulmonary capillary wedge pressure is thus a useful guide to safe titration of the drug.

Carcinogenesis, Mutagenesis, Impairment of Fertility: No long-term studies in animals were performed to evaluate carcinogenic potential of NITRO-BID IV (nitroglycerin).
Pregnancy: Category C. Animal reproduction studies have not been conducted with NITRO-BID IV. It is also not known whether NITRO-BID IV can cause fetal harm when administered to a pregnant woman or can affect reproduction capacity. NITRO-BID IV should be given to a pregnant woman only if clearly needed.
Nursing Mothers: It is not known whether nitroglycerin is excreted in human milk. Because many drugs are excreted in human milk, caution should be exercised when NITRO-BID IV is administered to a nursing woman.
Pediatric Use: The safety and effectiveness of NITRO-BID IV in children have not been established.
NITRO-BID IV contains alcohol and propylene glycol; safety for intracoronary injection has not been shown.

ADVERSE REACTIONS

The most frequent adverse reaction in patients treated with nitroglycerin is headache, which occurs in approximately 2% of patients. Other adverse reactions occurring in less than 1% of patients are the following: tachycardia, nausea, vomiting, apprehension, restlessness, muscle twitching, retrosternal discomfort, palpitations, dizziness, and abdominal pain. Paradoxical bradycardia and increased angina pectoris may accompany nitroglycerin-induced hypotension. The following additional adverse reactions have been reported with the oral and/or topical use of nitroglycerin: cutaneous flushing, weakness, and occasionally, drug rash or exfoliative dermatitis.

OVERDOSAGE

Accidental overdosage of nitroglycerin may result in severe hypotension and reflex tachycardia which can be treated by elevating the legs and decreasing or temporarily terminating the infusion until the patient's condition stabilizes. Since the duration of the hemodynamic effects following nitroglycerin administration is quite short, additional corrective measures are usually not required. However, if further therapy is indicated, administration of an intravenous alpha-adrenergic agonist (eg, methoxamine or phenylephrine) should be considered.

DOSAGE AND ADMINISTRATION

NOT FOR DIRECT INTRAVENOUS INJECTION.

NITRO-BID IV (NITROGLYCERIN) IS A CONCENTRATED, POTENT DRUG WHICH MUST BE DILUTED IN DEXTROSE (5%) INJECTION, USP OR SODIUM CHLORIDE (0.9%) INJECTION, USP PRIOR TO ITS INFUSION. NITRO-BID IV SHOULD NOT BE ADMIXED WITH OTHER DRUGS.

Dilution: It is important to consider the fluid requirements of the patient as well as the expected duration of infusion in selecting the appropriate dilution of NITRO-BID IV. [See table right].

Dosage: Dosage is affected by the type of infusion set used (see **WARNINGS**). Although the usual starting adult dose range reported in clinical studies was 25 mcg/min or more, those studies used PVC TUBING. **The use of nonabsorbing tubing will result in the need to use reduced doses.**

The dosage for NITRO-BID IV (nitroglycerin) infusion should initially be 5 mcg/min delivered through an infusion pump capable of exact and constant delivery of the drug. Subsequent titration must be adjusted to the clinical situation, with dose increments becoming more cautious as partial response is seen. Initial titration should be in 5-mcg/min increments, with increases every three to five minutes until some response is noted. If no response is seen at 20 mcg/min, increments of 10 and later 20 mcg/min can be used. Once a partial blood pressure response is observed, the dose increase should be reduced and the interval between increments should be lengthened. Patients with normal or low left ventricular filling pressure or pulmonary capillary wedge pressure (eg, angina patients without other complications) may be hypersensitive to the effects of NITRO-BID IV and may respond fully to doses as small as 5 mcg/min. These patients require especially careful titration and monitoring.

There is no fixed optimum dose of NITRO-BID IV. Due to variations in the responsiveness of individual patients to the drug, each patient must be titrated to the desired level of hemodynamic function. Therefore, continuous monitoring of physiologic parameters (eg, blood pressure, heart rate, and pulmonary capillary wedge pressure) MUST BE PERFORMED to achieve the correct dose. Adequate systemic blood pressure and coronary perfusion pressure must be maintained.

HOW SUPPLIED

NITRO-BID® IV is supplied in boxes of ten 1-ml vials (NDC 0088-1800-31), each vial containing 5 mg of nitroglycerin (5 mg/ml); ten 5-ml vials (NDC 0088-1800-32), each vial containing 25 mg nitroglycerin (5 mg/ml); and five 10-ml vials (NDC 0088-1800-33), each vial containing 50 mg nitroglycerin (5 mg/ml).

Mfd by Taylor Pharmacal Co., Decatur, IL 62525 for Marion Laboratories, Inc.

Issued 3/85

NITRO-BID® Ointment
[ni'tro-bid]
(nitroglycerin 2%)

℞

DESCRIPTION

Nitroglycerin, an organic nitrate, is a vasodilator which has effects on both arteries and veins. The chemical name for nitroglycerin is 1,2,3-Propanetriol, trinitrate. The compound has a molecular weight of 227.09.

NITRO-BID® Ointment contains 2% nitroglycerin ointment and lactose in a lanolin and white petrolatum base. Each inch, as squeezed from the tube, contains approximately 15 mg nitroglycerin.

CLINICAL PHARMACOLOGY

The principal pharmacological action of nitroglycerin is relaxation of vascular smooth muscle, producing a vasodilator effect on both peripheral arteries and veins with more prominent effects on the latter. Dilation of the post-capillary vessels, including large veins, promotes peripheral pooling of blood and decreases venous return to the heart, thereby reducing left ventricular end-diastolic pressure (preload). Arteriolar relaxation reduces systemic vascular resistance and arterial pressure (afterload).

NITRO-BID® IV Administration Table

Each 1-ml vial = 5 mg nitroglycerin
Each 5-ml vial = 25 mg nitroglycerin
Each 10-ml vial = 50 mg nitroglycerin

Mixing Instructions	1 ml in 100 ml 5 ml in 500 ml 10 ml in 1000 ml	1 ml in 50 ml 5 ml in 250 ml 10 ml in 500 ml 20 ml in 1000 ml	2 ml in 50 ml 10 ml in 250 ml 20 ml in 500 ml 40 ml in 1000 ml	FLOW RATE milliliters/hour microdrops/minute
Concentration	50 mcg/ml	100 mcg/ml	200 mcg/ml	
Dosage	mcg/min	mcg/min	mcg/min	microdrops/min
	2.5	5	10	3
	5	10	20	6
	10	20	40	12
	20	40	80	24
	40	80	160	48
	60	120	240	72
	80	160	320	96

The mechanism by which nitroglycerin relieves angina pectoris is not fully understood. Myocardial oxygen consumption or demand (as measured by the pressure-rate product, tension-time index, and stroke work index) for a given level of external exercise is decreased by both the arterial and venous effects of nitroglycerin and, presumably, a more favorable supply-demand ratio is achieved. While the large epicardial coronary arteries are also dilated by nitroglycerin, the extent to which this action contributes to relief of exertional angina is unclear.

Nitroglycerin is rapidly metabolized, principally by a liver reductase to form glycerol nitrate metabolites and inorganic nitrate. Two active major metabolites, the 1, 2 and 1, 3 dinitroglycerols, the products of hydrolysis, appear to be less potent than nitroglycerin as vasodilators but have longer plasma half-lives.

The dinitrates are further metabolized to mononitrates (biologically inactive with respect to cardiovascular effects) and ultimately glycerol and carbon dioxide. There is extensive first-pass deactivation by the liver of nitroglycerin following gastrointestinal absorption.

Adequate studies defining the pharmacokinetics of NITRO-BID have not been reported. The clinical relevance of nitroglycerin blood levels has not been established, since therapeutic levels of the drug and metabolites have not been defined. In general, it appears that blood levels are proportional to surface covered, but they are also related to location (chest placement gives higher levels than extremities) and to the thickness of the applied paste. Duration of effect would be expected to depend on the total amount of nitroglycerin (thickness of paste) per unit of surface area, but this has not been well studied.

Therapeutic doses of nitroglycerin have been shown to reduce systolic and mean arterial blood pressures, especially when the patient assumes upright posture, for as long as seven hours after a single application. Nitroglycerin ointment reduces abnormally elevated left ventricular end-diastolic pressure (LVEDP), a hemodynamic concomitant of acute episodes of angina pectoris. The onset of hemodynamic effects of nitroglycerin ointment is not sufficiently rapid to be of use in aborting an acute episode of angina pectoris.

INDICATIONS AND USAGE

NITRO-BID is indicated for the treatment and prevention of angina pectoris due to coronary artery disease. Controlled clinical trials have demonstrated that this form of nitroglycerin is effective in improving exercise tolerance in patients with exertional angina pectoris. Double-blind, placebo-controlled trials have shown significant improvement in exercise time until chest pain for up to six hours after single application of various doses of nitroglycerin ointment (mean doses ranged from 5 to 36 mg) to a 36-inch^2 area of trunk.

CONTRAINDICATIONS

Nitroglycerin is contraindicated in patients who have shown purported hypersensitivity or idiosyncrasy to it or other nitrates or nitrites.

WARNINGS

The benefits of nitroglycerin ointment during the early days of acute myocardial infarction have not been established. If one elects to use organic nitrates in early infarction, careful assessment and hemodynamic monitoring should be used because of the potential deleterious effects of hypotension.

PRECAUTIONS

General. Severe hypotensive response, particularly with upright posture, may occur even with small doses of nitroglycerin. The drug therefore should be used with caution in patients who may have volume depletion from diuretic therapy or in patients who have low systolic blood pressure (eg, below 90 mm Hg). Paradoxical bradycardia and increased angina pectoris may accompany nitroglycerin-induced hypotension.

Nitrate therapy may aggravate the angina caused by hypertrophic cardiomyopathy.

Tolerance to this drug and cross-tolerance to other nitrates and nitrites may occur. Tolerance to the vascular and antianginal effects of nitrates has been demonstrated in clinical trials, in experience through occupational exposure, and in isolated tissue experiments. The importance of tolerance to the appropriate use of nitroglycerin ointment in the management of patients with angina pectoris has not been determined. In controlled clinical trials in angina pectoris patients, sustained therapy with some nitrate preparations has resulted in significantly less improvement and a shorter duration of improvement in exercise time than had been seen when therapy was initiated. Sustained improvement in exercise tolerance has been reported in patients with angina pectoris who applied nitroglycerin ointment three times daily for 8 to 12 weeks in open studies, but there have been no controlled clinical studies involving exercise testing that have examined the efficacy of repetitive doses of NITRO-BID for the long-term treatment of angina pectoris.

In industrial workers continuously exposed to nitroglycerin, tolerance clearly occurs. Moreover, physical dependence also occurs since chest pain, acute myocardial infarction, and even sudden death have occurred during temporary withdrawal of nitroglycerin from the workers. In clinical trials in angina patients, there are reports of anginal attacks being more easily provoked and of rebound in the hemodynamic effects soon after nitrate withdrawal. The relative importance of these observations to the routine, clinical use of nitroglycerin is not known, but it seems prudent to gradually withdraw patients from nitroglycerin when the therapy is being terminated, rather than stopping the drug abruptly.

Drug Interactions. Alcohol may enhance sensitivity to the hypotensive effects of nitrates.

Nitroglycerin acts directly on vascular muscle. Therefore, any other agent that directly or indirectly acts on vascular smooth muscle may have decreased or increased effect depending upon the agent.

Marked symptomatic orthostatic hypotension has been reported when calcium channel blockers and organic nitrates were used in combination. Dose adjustments of either class of agents may be necessary.

Carcinogenesis, Mutagenesis, Impairment of Fertility. No long-term studies in animals have been performed to evaluate carcinogenic potential of NITRO-BID; neither has its mutagenic potential been studied. It is also not known whether nitroglycerin can affect reproduction capacity.

Pregnancy. Pregnancy Category C. Animal reproduction studies have not been conducted with NITRO-BID. It is also not known whether nitroglycerin can cause fetal harm when administered to a pregnant woman. Nitroglycerin should be given to a pregnant woman only if clearly needed.

Nursing Mothers. It is not known whether nitroglycerin is excreted in human milk. Because many drugs are excreted in human milk, caution should be exercised when NITRO-BID is administered to a nursing woman.

Pediatric Use. Safety and effectiveness in children have not been established.

ADVERSE REACTIONS

Adverse reactions to NITRO-BID, particularly headache and hypotension, are generally dose-related. In clinical trials at various doses of nitroglycerin, the following adverse effects have been observed.

Headache, which may be severe and persistent, is the most commonly reported side effect of nitroglycerin, with an incidence in the order of 50% in some studies. Cutaneous vasodilation with flushing may occur. Transient episodes of dizziness and weakness, as well as other signs of cerebral ischemia associated with postural hypotension may occasionally develop. An occasional individual may exhibit marked sensitivity to the hypotensive effects of nitrates and severe responses (nausea, vomiting, weakness, restlessness, pallor, perspiration, and collapse) may occur even with therapeutic doses of nitrates. Drug rash and/or exfoliative dermatitis have been reported in patients receiving nitrate therapy. Nausea and vomiting can occur, but appear to be uncommon.

Continued on next page

Marion—Cont.

OVERDOSAGE

Signs and Symptoms. Nitrate overdosage may result in: severe hypotension, persistent throbbing headache, vertigo, palpitation, visual disturbance, flushing and perspiring skin (later becoming cold and cyanotic), nausea and vomiting (possibly with colic and even bloody diarrhea), syncope (especially in the upright posture), methemoglobinemia with cyanosis and anorexia, initial hyperpnea, dyspnea and slow breathing, slow pulse (dicrotic and intermittent), heart block, increased intracranial pressure with cerebral symptoms of confusion and moderate fever, paralysis and coma followed by clonic convulsions and possibly death due to circulatory collapse.

Treatment of Overdosage. Keep the patient recumbent in a shock position and comfortably warm. Wipe the skin clean of the nitroglycerin ointment. Passive movement of the extremities may aid venous return. Administer oxygen and artificial ventilation if necessary. If methemoglobinemia is present, administration of methylene blue (1% solution), 1 to 2 mg/kg intravenously, may be required.

Methemoglobin. Case reports of clinically significant methemoglobinemia are rare at conventional doses of organic nitrates. The formation of methemoglobin is dose-related and in the case of genetic abnormalities of hemoglobin that favor methemoglobin formation, even conventional doses of organic nitrates could produce harmful concentrations of methemoglobin.

WARNINGS

Epinehprine is ineffective in reversing the severe hypotensive events associated with overdose. It and related compounds are contraindicated in this situation.

DOSAGE AND ADMINISTRATION

When applying the ointment, place the dose-determining applicator supplied with the package printed-side down and squeeze the necessary amount of ointment from the tube onto the applicator. Then place the applicator with the ointment-side down onto the desired area of skin, usually the chest or back. Several studies suggest that absorption of nitroglycerin through the skin varies with the site of application of the drug. Application of the drug to the skin of the chest is reported to give higher blood levels of nitroglycerin and greater hemodynamic effects than application to the extremities.

The amount of nitroglycerin entering the circulation varies directly with the size of skin area exposed to the drug and the amount of ointment applied. Although in major clinical trials the dose of nitroglycerin was often applied to a 6×6-inch (150×150-mm) area of skin, in clinical practice the dose is usually applied to a smaller area. The ointment should be applied in a thin, uniform layer and the dose-to-area ratio kept reasonably constant. For example: 1 inch on a 2×3-inch area; 2 inches on a 3×4-inch area; 3 inches on a 4×5-inch area. When doubling the dose, the surface area over which the ointment is placed should also be doubled.

As with all nitrates, clinical studies suggest that clinical response is variable. A suggested starting dose for NITRO-BID is ½ inch (7.5 mg) applied to a 1×3-inch area every eight hours. Response to treatment should be assessed over the next several days. If angina occurs while the ointment is in place, the dose should be increased, for example, to 1 inch on a 2×3-inch area. NITRO-BID should be titrated upward until a dose effective in controlling angina is determined or until side effects limit the dose. If angina occurs after the ointment has been in place for several hours, the frequency of dosing should be increased (eg, every six hours). Administer the smallest effective dose three to four times daily, unless clinical response suggests a different regimen. At initiation of therapy or change in dosage, blood pressure (patient standing) should be monitored. Controlled trials have been carried out for up to seven hours after dosing, therefore, it is not known whether the drug is effective in prevention of exertional angina beyond seven hours after dosing. The effectiveness of repetitive applications of nitroglycerin ointment for the chronic management of angina pectoris has not been established.

NITRO-BID is not intended for immediate relief of anginal attacks.

HOW SUPPLIED

NITRO-BID® Ointment (nitroglycerin 2%) is available in 20-gm (NDC 0088-1552-20) and 60-gm (NDC 0088-1552-60) tubes and in Unit Dose Identification Paks of 100 1-gm foil pouches (NDC 0088-1552-49).

Issued 10/86

OS-CAL® 250+D Tablets   OTC
[ahs'kal]
calcium supplement with vitamin D

Each Tablet Contains:
625 mg of calcium carbonate from oyster shell, an organic calcium source.
Elemental calcium .... 250 mg
Vitamin D .... 125 USP Units
Ingredients: Oyster shell powder, corn syrup solids, talc, cornstarch, hydroxypropyl methylcellulose, calcium stearate, polysorbate 80, titanium dioxide, methyl propyl paraben, polyethylene glycol, pharmaceutical glaze, vitamin D, polyvinylpyrrolidone, carnauba wax, D&C Yellow #10, acetylated monoglyceride, edetate disodium, FD&C Blue #1, simethicone emulsion, and edible gray ink.

INDICATIONS

OS-CAL® 250+D Tablets provide a source of calcium when it is desired to increase the dietary intake of this mineral. OS-CAL 250+D also contains vitamin D to aid in the absorption of calcium.

DIRECTIONS

Take one tablet three times a day with meals, or as recommended by your physician.
Three tablets provide:

	Quantity	% U.S. RDA* for Adults
Calcium	750 mg	75%
Vitamin D	375 units	94%

*Percent U.S. Recommended Daily Allowance.
Store at room temperature.
Keep out of reach of children.

HOW SUPPLIED

Bottles of 100, 240, 500, and 1,000 tablets.

Issued 10/87

Shown in Product Identification Section, page 416

OS-CAL® 500 Chewable Tablets   OTC
[ahs'kal]
calcium supplement

Each Tablet Contains:
1,250 mg of calcium carbonate.
Elemental calcium .... 500 mg
Ingredients: Calcium carbonate, dextrose monohydrate, maltodextrin, microcrystalline cellulose, magnesium stearate, Bavarian cream flavor, sodium chloride, and coconut cream flavor.

INDICATIONS

OS-CAL 500 Chewable Tablets provide a source of calcium when it is desired, or recommended by a physician, to increase the dietary intake of this mineral.

DIRECTIONS

One tablet two to three times a day with meals, or as recommended by your physician.
Two tablets provide: 1,000 mg calcium, 100% of U.S. RDA for adults and children 12 or more years of age.
Three tablets provide: 1,500 mg calcium, 115% of U.S. RDA for pregnant and lactating women.
Store at room temperature.
Keep out of reach of children.

HOW SUPPLIED

OS-CAL® 500 Chewable Tablets are available in bottles of 60 tablets.

Issued 10/87

Shown in Product Identification Section, page 416

OS-CAL® 500 Tablets   OTC
[ahs'kal]
calcium supplement

Each tablet contains:
1,250 mg of calcium carbonate from oyster shell, an organic calcium source.
Elemental calcium .... 500 mg
Ingredients: Oyster shell powder, corn syrup solids, talc, hydroxypropyl methylcellulose, cornstarch, sodium starch glycolate, calcium stearate, polysorbate 80, pharmaceutical glaze, titanium dioxide, methyl propyl paraben, polyethylene glycol, polyvinylpyrrolidone, carnauba wax, D&C Yellow #10, acetylated monoglyceride, edetate disodium, FD&C Blue #1, and simethicone emulsion.

INDICATIONS

OS-CAL 500 Tablets provide a source of calcium when it is desired or recommended by a physician to increase the dietary intake of this mineral.

DIRECTIONS

Take one tablet two to three times a day with meals, or as recommended by your physician.

Two tablets daily provide:

	Quantity	%U.S. RDA†
Calcium	1,000 mg	100%*
		77%**

Three tablets daily provide:

	Quantity	%U.S. RDA†
Calcium	1,500 mg	150%*
		115%**

†Percent U.S. Recommended Daily Allowance.
*For adults and children 12 or more years of age.
**For pregnant and lactating women.
Store at room temperature.
Keep out of reach of children.

HOW SUPPLIED

Bottles of 60 and 120 tablets.

Issued 10/87

Shown in Product Identification Section, page 416

OS-CAL® 500+D Tablets   OTC
[ahs'kal]
calcium supplement with vitamin D

EACH TABLET CONTAINS

1,250 mg of calcium carbonate from oyster shell, an organic calcium source.
Elemental calcium..500 mg
Vitamin D..125 USP Units

INGREDIENTS

Oyster shell powder, corn syrup solids, talc, hydroxypropyl methylcellulose, cornstarch, sodium starch glycolate, calcium stearate, polysorbate 80, pharmaceutical glaze, titanium dioxide, methyl propyl paraben, polyethylene glycol, polyvinylpyrrolidone, vitamin D, carnauba wax, D&C Yellow #10, acetylated monoglyceride, edetate disodium, FD&C Blue #1, and simethicone emulsion.

DIRECTIONS

One tablet two or three times a day with meals, or as recommended by your physician.
Two tablets provide: 1,000 mg calcium, 100% of U.S. RDA for adults and children 12 or more years of age and 64% of vitamin D.
Three tablets provide: 1,500 mg calcium, 115% of U.S. RDA for pregnant and lactating women and 94% of vitamin D.
Store at room temperature.
Keep out of reach of children.

HOW SUPPLIED

OS-CAL® 500+D is available in bottles of 60 tablets.

Issued 10/87

Shown in Product Identification Section, page 416

OS-CAL® FORTIFIED Tablets   OTC
[ahs'kal for 'te-fid]
multivitamin and mineral supplement
New name—Formerly marketed as Os-Cal Forte

Each tablet contains:

Vitamin A (palmitate)	1668 USP Units
Vitamin D	125 USP Units
Thiamine mononitrate (vitamin B₁)	1.7 mg
Riboflavin (vitamin B₂)	1.7 mg
Pyridoxine hydrochloride (vitamin B₆)	2.0 mg
Ascorbic acid (vitamin C)	50 mg
dl-alpha-locopherol acetate (vitamin E)	0.8 IU
Niacinamide	15 mg
Calcium (from oyster shell)	250 mg
Iron (as ferrous fumarate)	5 mg
Magnesium (as oxide)	1.6 mg
Manganese (as sulfate)	0.3 mg
Zinc (as sulfate)	0.5 mg

Ingredients: Oyster shell powder, ascorbic acid, corn syrup solids, niacinamide, D&C Yellow #10 Aluminum Lake, ferrous fumarate, calcium stearate, FD&C Blue #1 Aluminum Lake, cornstarch, vitamin A palmitate, polysorbate 80, magnesium oxide, pyridoxine, thiamine, riboflavin, vitamin E, pharmaceutical glaze, methyl paraben, zinc sulfate, manganese sulfate, propylparaben, povidone, vitamin D, hydroxypropyl methylcellulose, carnauba wax, titanium dioxide, ethylcellulose, and acetylated monoglyceride.

INDICATION

Multivitamin and mineral supplement.

DIRECTIONS

One tablet three times a day with meals or as recommended by your physician.

THREE TABLETS PROVIDE

VITAMIN/MINERAL	% RDA
Vitamin A	100.0%
Vitamin C	250.0%
Thiamine (vitamin B₁)	340.0%

Riboflavin (vitamin B$_2$)	300.0%
Vitamin B$_6$	300.0%
Niacin	225.0%
Vitamin D	93.8%
Vitamin E	8.0%
Iron (elemental)	83.3%
Calcium (elemental)	75.0%
Magnesium	1.2%

Store at room temperature.
Keep out of the reach of children. In case of accidental overdose, seek professional assistance or contact a poison control center immediately.

HOW SUPPLIED
Bottles of 100 tablets.

Issued 6/89

Shown in Product Identification Section, page 416

OS-CAL® PLUS Tablets   OTC
[ahs 'kal]
multivitamin and multimineral supplement

Each Tablet Contains:

Elemental calcium (from oyster shell)	250 mg
Vitamin D	125 USP Units
Vitamin A (palmitate)	1666 USP Units
Vitamin C (ascorbic acid)	33 mg
Vitamin B$_2$ (riboflavin)	0.66 mg
Vitamin B$_1$ (thiamine mononitrate)	0.5 mg
Vitamin B$_6$ (pyridoxine HCl)	0.5 mg
Niacinamide	3.33 mg
Iron (as ferrous fumarate)	16.6 mg
Zinc (as the sulfate)	0.75 mg
Manganese (as the sulfate)	0.75 mg

Ingredients: Oyster shell powder, corn syrup solids, ferrous fumarate, ascorbic acid, calcium stearate, cornstarch, hydroxypropyl methylcellulose, polysorbate 80, titanium dioxide, vitamin A palmitate, niacinamide, ethylcellulose, manganese sulfate, methylpropyl paraben, zinc sulfate, pharmaceutical glaze, acetylated monoglyceride, riboflavin, thiamine mononitrate, pyridoxine hydrochloride, povidone, vitamin D, carnauba wax, and D&C Red #33.

INDICATIONS
As a multivitamin and multimineral supplement.

DOSAGE
One (1) tablet three times a day before meals or as directed by a physician. For children under 4 years of age, consult a physician.
Store at room temperature.
Keep out of the reach of children. In case of accidental overdose, seek professional assistance or contact a poison control center immediately.

HOW SUPPLIED
Bottles of 100 tablets.

Issued 5/87

Shown in Product Identification Section, page 416

PAVABID® Plateau CAPS®   ℞
[pav 'uh-bid]
(papaverine hydrochloride) 150 mg

COMPOSITION
Each capsule contains:
Papaverine hydrochloride .... 150 mg
in a specially prepared base to provide prolonged activity.
Also contains: calcium stearate, starch, stearic acid, sucrose, talc, and other ingredients.

ACTION AND USES
The main actions of papaverine are exerted on cardiac and smooth muscle. Like quinidine, papaverine acts directly on the heart muscle to depress conduction and prolong the refractory period. Papaverine relaxes various smooth muscles. This relaxation may be prominent if spasm exists. The muscle cell is not paralyzed by papaverine and still responds to drugs and other stimuli causing contraction. The antispasmodic effect is a direct one, and unrelated to muscle innervation. Papaverine is practically devoid of effects on the central nervous system.
Papaverine relaxes the smooth musculature of the larger blood vessels, especially coronary, systemic peripheral, and pulmonary arteries. Perhaps by its direct vasodilating action on cerebral blood vessels, papaverine increases cerebral blood flow and decreases cerebral vascular resistance in normal subjects; oxygen consumption is unaltered. These effects may explain the benefit reported from the drug in cerebral vascular encephalopathy.
The direct actions of papaverine on the heart to depress conduction and irritability and to prolong the refractory period of the myocardium provide the basis for its clinical trial in abrogating atrial and ventricular premature systoles and ominous ventricular arrhythmias. The coronary vasodilator action could be an additional factor of therapeutic value

when such rhythms are secondary to insufficiency or occlusion of the coronary arteries.
In patients with acute coronary thrombosis, the occurrence of ventricular rhythms is serious and requires measures designed to decrease myocardial irritability. Papaverine may have advantages over quinidine, used for a similar purpose, in that it may be given in an emergency by the intravenous route, does not depress myocardial contraction or cause cinchonism, and produces coronary vasodilation.

INDICATIONS
For the relief of cerebral and peripheral ischemia associated with arterial spasm and myocardial ischemia complicated by arrhythmias.

PRECAUTIONS
Use with caution in patients with glaucoma. Hepatic hypersensitivity has been reported with gastrointestinal symptoms, jaundice, eosinophilia, and altered liver function tests. Discontinue medication if these occur.

ADVERSE REACTIONS
Although occurring rarely, the reported side effects of papaverine include nausea, abdominal distress, anorexia, constipation, malaise, drowsiness, vertigo, sweating, headache, diarrhea, and skin rash.

DOSAGE AND ADMINISTRATION
One capsule every 12 hours. In difficult cases administration may be increased to one capsule every 8 hours, or two capsules every 12 hours.

HOW SUPPLIED
PAVABID® (papaverine hydrochloride) Capsules are available in bottles of 100, 250, 1000 and in Unit Dose Identification Paks of 100 capsules. Capsules are imprinted with MARION/1555.

CAUTION
Federal law prohibits dispensing without prescription.

Issued 11/85

Shown in Product Identification Section, page 416

PAVABID® HP Capsulets   ℞
[pav 'uh-bid]
(papaverine hydrochloride) 300 mg

COMPOSITION
Each capsulet contains:
Papaverine hydrochloride .... 300 mg
Also contains: calcium stearate, FD&C yellow #6, FD&C yellow #6 lake, lactose, microcrystalline cellulose, starch, and other ingredients.

ACTION AND USES
The main actions of papaverine are exerted on cardiac and smooth muscle. Like quinidine, papaverine acts directly on the heart muscle to depress conduction and prolong the refractory period. Papaverine relaxes various smooth muscles. This relaxation may be prominent if spasm exists. The muscle cell is not paralyzed by papaverine, and still responds to drugs and other stimuli causing contraction. The antispasmodic effect is a direct one, and unrelated to muscle innervation. Papaverine is practically devoid of effects on the central nervous system.
Papaverine relaxes the smooth musculature of the larger blood vessels, especially coronary, systemic peripheral, and pulmonary arteries. Perhaps by its direct vasodilating action on cerebral blood vessels, papaverine increases cerebral blood flow and decreases cerebral vascular resistance in normal subjects; oxygen consumption is unaltered. These effects may explain the benefit reported from the drug in cerebral vascular encephalopathy.
The direct actions of papaverine on the heart to depress conduction and irritability and to prolong the refractory period of the myocardium provide the basis for its clinical trial in abrogating atrial and ventricular premature systoles and ominous ventricular arrhythmias. The coronary vasodilator action could be an additional factor of therapeutic value when such rhythms are secondary to insufficiency or occlusion of the coronary arteries.
In patients with acute coronary thrombosis, the occurrence of ventricular rhythms is serious and requires measures designed to decrease myocardial irritability. Papaverine may have advantages over quinidine, used for a similar purpose, in that it may be given in an emergency by the intravenous route, does not depress myocardial contraction or cause cinchonism, and produces coronary vasodilation.

INDICATIONS
For the relief of cerebral and peripheral ischemia associated with arterial spasm and myocardial ischemia complicated by arrhythmias.

PRECAUTIONS
Use with caution in patients with glaucoma. Hepatic hypersensitivity has been reported with gastrointestinal symptoms, jaundice, eosinophilia, and altered liver function tests. Discontinue medication if these occur.

ADVERSE REACTIONS
Although occurring rarely, the reported side effects of papaverine include nausea, abdominal distress, anorexia, constipation, malaise, drowsiness, vertigo, sweating, headache, diarrhea, and skin rash.

DOSAGE AND ADMINISTRATION
Dosage should be started at 150 mg (one-half capsulet) two to three times daily and titrated upward to the desired level. The 300-mg capsulet breaks into two separate half capsulets. To break: place capsulet on a hard surface with the embossed MARION M facing up, press down on the embossed M.

HOW SUPPLIED
PAVABID® (papaverine hydrochloride) HP Capsulets are available in 60-count bottles. Each light orange capsulet is embossed with a raised M stamped MARION on one side and PAVABID HP on the other side.

CAUTION
Federal law prohibits dispensing without prescription.

Issued 11/85

Shown in Product Identification Section, page 416

SILVADENE® Cream 1%   ℞
[sil 'vuh-dĕn]
(silver sulfadiazine)

DESCRIPTION
SILVADENE Cream 1% is a soft, white, water-miscible cream containing the antimicrobial agent silver sulfadiazine in micronized form.
Each gram of SILVADENE Cream 1% contains 10 mg of micronized silver sulfadiazine. The cream vehicle consists of white petrolatum, stearyl alcohol, isopropyl myristate, sorbitan monooleate, polyoxyl 40 stearate, propylene glycol, and water, with methylparaben 0.3% as a preservative.

CLINICAL PHARMACOLOGY
SILVADENE Cream 1% (silver sulfadiazine) spreads easily and can be washed off readily with water.
Silver sulfadiazine has broad antimicrobial activity. It is bactericidal for many gram-negative and gram-positive bacteria as well as being effective against yeast. Results from in vitro testing are listed below.
Sufficient data have been obtained to demonstrate that silver sulfadiazine will inhibit bacteria that are resistant to other antimicrobial agents and that the compound is superior to sulfadiazine.

Number of Sensitive Strains/Total Strains Tested
Concentration of Silver Sulfadiazine

Genus & Species	50 µg/ml	100 µg/ml
Pseudomonas aeruginosa	130/130	130/130
Pseudomonas maltophilia	7/7	7/7
Enterobacter species	48/50	50/50
Enterobacter cloacae	24/24	24/24
Klebsiella	53/54	54/54
Escherichia coli	63/63	63/63
Serratia	27/28	28/28
Proteus mirabilis	53/53	53/53
Proteus morganii	10/10	10/10
Proteus rettgeri	2/2	2/2
Proteus vulgaris	2/2	2/2
Providencia	1/1	1/1
Citrobacter	10/10	10/10
Herellea	8/9	9/9
Mima	2/2	2/2
Staphylococcus aureus	100/101	101/101
Staphylococcus epidermidis	51/51	51/51
β-Hemolytic *Streptococcus*	4/4	4/4
Enterococcus (group D *Streptococcus*)	52/53	53/53
Corynebacterium diphtheriae	2/2	2/2
Clostridium perfringens	0/2	2/2
Candida albicans	43/50	50/50

Studies utilizing radioactive micronized silver sulfadiazine, electron microscopy, and biochemical techniques have revealed that the mechanism of action of silver sulfadiazine on bacteria differs from silver nitrate and sodium sulfadiazine. SILVADENE Cream 1% (silver sulfadiazine) acts only on the cell membrane and cell wall to produce its bactericidal effect.

INDICATIONS AND USAGE
SILVADENE Cream 1% (silver sulfadiazine) is a topical antimicrobial drug indicated as an adjunct for the prevention and treatment of wound sepsis in patients with second- and third-degree burns.

Continued on next page

Marion—Cont.

CONTRAINDICATIONS

Because sulfonamide therapy is known to increase the possibility of kernicterus, SILVADENE Cream 1% should not be used at term pregnancy, on premature infants, or on newborn infants during the first 2 months of life.

WARNINGS

GENERAL. SILVADENE Cream 1% should be administered with great caution to patients with history of hypersensitivity to SILVADENE Cream 1%. There is potential cross-sensitivity between SILVADENE Cream 1% and other sulfonamides. If allergic reactions attributable to treatment with SILVADENE Cream 1% occur, discontinuation of SILVADENE Cream 1% must be considered.

Fungal proliferation in and below the eschar may occur. However, the incidence of clinically reported fungal superinfection is low.

PRECAUTIONS

GENERAL. If hepatic and renal functions become impaired and elimination of drug decreases, accumulation may occur and discontinuation of SILVADENE Cream 1% (silver sulfadiazine) should be weighed against the therapeutic benefit being achieved.

In considering the use of topical proteolytic enzymes in conjunction with SILVADENE Cream 1%, the possibility should be noted that silver may inactivate such enzymes. The use of SILVADENE Cream 1% in some cases of glucose-6-phosphate dehydrogenase-deficient individuals may be hazardous as hemolysis may occur.

LABORATORY TESTS. In the treatment of burn wounds involving extensive areas of the body, the serum sulfa concentrations may approach adult therapeutic levels (8 to 12 mg%). Therefore, in these patients it would be advisable to monitor serum sulfa concentrations. Renal function should be carefully monitored and the urine should be checked for sulfa crystals. Absorption of the propylene glycol vehicle has been reported to affect serum osmolality, which may affect the interpretation of laboratory tests.

CARCINOGENESIS, MUTAGENESIS, IMPAIRMENT OF FERTILITY. Long-term dermal toxicity studies of 24 months' duration in rats and 18 months in mice with concentrations of silver sulfadiazine three to ten times the concentration in SILVADENE Cream 1% revealed no evidence of carcinogenicity.

PREGNANCY CATEGORY B. A reproductive study has been performed in rabbits at concentrations of silver sulfadiazine three to ten times the concentration in SILVADENE Cream 1%. The results of this study showed no harmful effect on the fetus. There are, however, no adequate and well-controlled studies in pregnant women. Because animal reproduction studies are not always predictive of human response, this drug should be used during pregnancy only if clearly needed.

NURSING MOTHERS. It is not known whether SILVADENE Cream 1% is excreted in human milk. However, sulfonamides are known to be excreted in human milk. Since all sulfonamide derivatives are known to increase the possibility of kernicterus, caution should be exercised when SILVADENE Cream 1% is administered to a nursing woman.

ADVERSE REACTIONS

In the original clinical trials, an aggregate of 2,297 patients were treated with SILVADENE Cream 1% and reported 59 drug related reactions (2.5%). These included burning sensation (2.2%), rash (0.2%), itching (0.1%), and one report of interstitial nephritis.

In postmarketing experience with SILVADENE Cream 1%, there have been additional reports of infrequently occurring events. These include skin necrosis, erythema multiforme, and leukopenia. The propylene glycol vehicle has also been reported to cause hyperosmolality.

Skin discoloration may rarely occur in some patients. The majority of reports to date indicate that this discoloration is transient and subsides upon discontinuation of therapy. There have also been several cases of transient leukopenia reported in patients receiving silver sulfadiazine therapy. In an uncontrolled study, leukopenia (WBC < 3500) was reported to occur with a frequency of one in 20 patients.[1] However, in a placebo-controlled study in which 69 patients received silver sulfadiazine and 60 received placebo, six (10%) patients in the placebo group and five (7%) patients in the treatment group developed leukopenia[2] (WBC < 5000). The leukopenia associated with silver sulfadiazine is characterized by decreased neutrophil count with maximal white blood cell depression occurring within two to four days of initiation of therapy. Leukocyte levels usually rebound to normal levels within two to three days without discontinuation of therapy.

Absorption of silver sulfadiazine varies depending upon the percent of body surface area and the extent of the tissue damage. Although few have been reported, it is possible that any adverse reaction associated with sulfonamides may occur. Some of the reactions which have been associated with sul-

fonamides are as follows: blood dyscrasias, including agranulocytosis, aplastic anemia, thrombocytopenia, leukopenia and hemolytic anemia; dermatologic and allergic reactions, including Stevens-Johnson syndrome and exfoliative dermatitis; gastrointestinal reactions; hepatitis and hepatocellular necrosis; CNS reactions; and toxic nephrosis.

DOSAGE AND ADMINISTRATION

Prompt institution of appropriate regimens for care of the burned patient is of prime importance and includes the control of shock and pain. The burn wounds are then cleansed and debrided and SILVADENE Cream 1% (silver sulfadiazine) is applied with sterile, gloved hand. The burn areas should be covered with SILVADENE Cream 1% at all times. The cream should be applied once to twice daily to a thickness of approximately $\frac{1}{16}$ inch. Whenever necessary, the cream should be reapplied to any areas from which it has been removed by patient activity. Administration may be accomplished in minimal time because dressings are not required. However, if individual patient requirements make dressings necessary, they may be used.

When feasible, the patient should be bathed daily. This is an aid in debridement. A whirlpool bath is particularly helpful, but the patient may be bathed in bed or in a shower.

Reduction in bacterial growth after application of topical antibacterial agents has been reported to permit spontaneous healing of deep partial-thickness burns by preventing conversion of the partial thickness to full thickness by sepsis. However, reduction in bacterial colonization has caused delayed separation, in some cases necessitating escharotomy in order to prevent contracture.

Treatment with SILVADENE Cream 1% should be continued until satisfactory healing has occurred or until the burn site is ready for grafting. **The drug should not be withdrawn from the therapeutic regimen while there remains the possibility of infection except if a significant adverse reaction occurs.**

HOW SUPPLIED

SILVADENE Cream 1% (silver sulfadiazine) is available in jars containing 50 grams (NDC 0088-1050-50), 400 grams (NDC 0088-1050-72), and 1,000 grams (NDC 0088-1050-58) and tubes containing 20 grams (NDC 0088-1050-20) and 85 grams (NDC 0088-1050-85).

BIBLIOGRAPHY

1. Jarret F, Ellerbe S, Demling R: Acute leukopenia during topical burn therapy with silver sulfadiazine. *Amer J Surg* 1978;135:818–819.
2. Kiker RG, Carvajal HF, Micak RP, Larson DL: A controlled study of the effects of silver sulfadiazine on white blood cell counts in burned children. *J Trauma* 1977;17:835–836.

U.S. Patent 3,761,590   Issued 2/88

Shown in Product Identification Section, page 416

THROAT DISCS®   **OTC**
[thrōt disks]
Throat Lozenges

DESCRIPTION

Each lozenge contains sucrose, starch (may contain cornstarch), acacia, glycyrrhiza extract (licorice), gum tragacanth, anethole, linseed, cubeb oleoresin, anise oil, peppermint oil, capsicum, and mineral oil.

INDICATIONS

Effective for soothing, temporary relief of minor throat irritations from hoarseness and coughs due to colds.

PRECAUTIONS

For severe or persistent cough or sore throat, or sore throat accompanied by high fever, headache, nausea, and vomiting, consult physician promptly. Not recommended for children under 3 years of age.

DOSAGE

Allow lozenge to dissolve slowly in mouth. One or two should give the desired relief.

HOW SUPPLIED

Boxes of 60 lozenges.

Issued 5/85

Shown in Product Identification Section, page 416

Products are cross-indexed
by product classifications
in the
BLUE SECTION

Marlyn Health Care
6324 FERRIS SQUARE
SAN DIEGO, CA 92121

HEP-FORTE®
[hep-for 'tay]

DESCRIPTION

Hep Forte is a comprehensive formulation of protein, B factors and other nutritional factors which can be important as a dietary supplement for maintenance and support of normal hepatic function.

COMPOSITION

Each capsule contains:

Vitamin A (Palmitate)	1,200 I.U.
Vitamin E (d-Alpha Tocopherol)	10 I.U.
Vitamin C (Ascorbic Acid)	10 mg.
Folic Acid	0.06 mg.
Vitamin B1 (Thiamine Mononitrate)	1 mg.
Vitamin B2 (Riboflavin)	1 mg.
Niacinamide	10 mg.
Vitamin B6 (Pyridoxine HCl)	0.5 mg.
Vitamin B12 (Cobalamin)	1 mcg.
Biotin	3.3 mg.
Pantothenic Acid	2 mg.
Choline Bitartrate	21 mg.
Zinc (Zinc Sulfate)	2 mg.
Desiccated Liver	194.4 mg.
Liver Concentrate	64.8 mg.
Liver Fraction Number 2	64.8 mg.
Yeast (Dried)	64.8 mg.
dl-Methionine	10 mg.
Inositol	10 mg.

INDICATIONS

Hep Forte is a balanced formulation of vitamins, minerals, lipotropic factors, and vitamin-protein supplements. It is of value as a nutritional supplement for persons who are receiving professional treatment for alcoholism, hepatic dysfunction due to hepatotoxic drugs and liver poisons, male and female infertility due to hormonal imbalance caused by hepatic dysfunction, and for nutritional supplementation after treatment.

CONTRAINDICATIONS

There are no known contraindications to Hep Forte.

DOSAGE

Three to six capsules daily.

HOW SUPPLIED

Bottles of 100, 300 or 500 capsules.
Literature Available.

MARLYN FORMULA 50®

PRODUCT OVERVIEW

KEY FACTS

MARLYN FORMULA 50 is a combination of amino acids and B6 in a gelatin capsule which provides protein "building blocks" important to growth and development of all protein containing tissue including nails, hair and skin.

MAJOR USES

Dermatologists recommend Formula 50 not only for splitting, peeling nails but also prescribe it in conjunction with their favorite topical cream for control of nail fungus. OB-Gyn's recommend it for help in controlling excessive hair fall-out after child birth.

The recommended daily dose is six capsules daily.

SAFETY INFORMATION

There are no known contraindications or adverse reactions.

PRESCRIBING INFORMATION

MARLYN FORMULA 50®

COMPOSITION

Each capsule contains:

Amino Acids	0.3 Gm*
Vitamin B6 (pyridoxine HCl)	1.0 mg.

*Approximate analysis of the amino acids: indispensable amino acids (lysine, tryptophan, phenylalanine, methionine, threonine, leucine, isoleucine, valine), 35.30%; semi-dispensable amino acids (arginine, histidine, tyrosine, cystine, glycine), 19.18%; dispensable amino acids (glutamic acid, alanine, aspartic acid, serine, proline), 45.56%.

Amino acids: Protein "building blocks" important to growth and development of all protein containing tissue including nails, hair, and skin.

DOSAGE AND ADMINISTRATION

The recommended daily dose is 6 capsules daily.

SUPPLY

Bottles of 100, 250 and 1000 capsules.

MARLYN FORMULA 50 MEGA FORTE

PRODUCT OVERVIEW

KEY FACTS

MARLYN FORMULA 50 MEGA FORTE is a combination of amino acids and B6 in a gelatin capsule which provides protein "building blocks" important to growth and development of all protein containing tissues including nails, hair, and skin. In addition FORMULA 50 MEGA FORTE has the added advantages of Silicon, L-Cysteine and natural Mucopolysaccharides (from bovine cartilage.)

MAJOR USES

Dermatologists recommend FORMULA 50 MEGA FORTE not only for splitting, peeling nails but also prescribe it in conjunction with their favorite topical cream for control of nail fungus. OB-Gyn's recommend it for help in controlling excessive hair fall-out after child birth.
The recommended daily dose is six capsules daily.

SAFETY INFORMATION

There are no known contraindications or adverse reactions.

PRESCRIBING INFORMATION

MARLYN FORMULA 50 MEGA FORTE

Each 6 capsules contain:

Amino Acids	1980	mg
Vitamin B$_6$	6	mg
Silicon		
(from Amino Acid Chelate)	90	mg
L-Cysteine HCl	120	mg
(Natural Extract)		
Mucopolysaccharides	60	mg
(from Bovine cartilage extract)		

Approximate analysis of amino acids: indispensable amino acids: (lysine, tryptophan, phenylalanine, methionine, threonine, leucine, isoleucine, valine) 35.30%; semi-dispensable amino acids; (arginine, histidine, tyrosine, cystine, glycine, 19.18%; dispensable amino acids (glutamic acids, alanine, aspartic acid, serine, proline), 45.56%.
Amino Acids; Protein "building blocks" important to growth and development of all protein containing tissue including nails, hair, and skin.

DOSAGE AND ADMINISTRATION

The recommended daily dose is 6 capsules daily

SUPPLY

Bottles of 100, 240, 500 and 1000

PRO-HEPATONE

PRODUCT OVERVIEW

KEY FACTS

PRO-HEPATONE is an all-inclusive formulation of vitamins, hematinic factors, amino acids, lipotropic factors, and other nutritional supplements to help overcome dietary deficiencies of these nutrients.

MAJOR USES

PRO-HEPATONE is specially designed to be of help as a nutritional adjuvant for persons under professional care for the avoidance of liver problems that may result from improper diet or excesses of alcohol or drugs, and to be of assistance in some types of occasional impotence.

SAFETY INFORMATION

There are no known contraindications or adverse reactions.

PRESCRIBING INFORMATION

PRO-HEPATONE

EACH TWO CAPSULES SUPPLY:

Choline Bitartrate	100	mg
Methionine	100	mg
Inositol	100	mg
Lecithin	632	mg
Liver Concentrate	64.8	mg
Desiccated Liver	64.8	mg
Unsaturated Fatty Acid	20	mg
Vitamin E (Alpha Tocopheryl)	20	I.U.
Vitamin C (Ascorbic Acid)	20	mg
Vitamin B$_1$ (Thiamine)	5	mg
Vitamin B$_2$ (Riboflavin)	5	mg
Niacinamide (Vitamin P)	20	mg
Vitamin B$_6$ (Pyridoxine HCl)	5	mg
L-Cysteine HCl	10	mg
Gluthathione	5	mg
Desoxycholic Acid	25	mg
Thiotic Acid	5	mg
d-Calcium Pantothenate	20	mg
Vitamin B$_{12}$ (Cyanocobalamin)	64.8	mcg
L-Arginine	5	mg
L-Glutamine	10	mg
L-Aspartic Acid	10	mg

L-Ornithine	5	mg
Ferrous Fumarate	648	mcg
Glycine	100	mg
Fructose	100	mg

DOSAGE AND ADMINISTRATION

The recommended daily dose is 2–3 capsules daily.

SUPPLY

Bottles of 90, 180, 240

Mason Pharmaceuticals, Inc.

**5000 BIRCH
SUITE 6100
NEWPORT BEACH, CA 92660**

DAMASON-P   ⒸR

[dă 'mă-sŭn-p]
(Hydrocodone Bitartrate 5 mg., USP, Aspirin 224 mg., Caffeine 32 mg.)

PRODUCT OVERVIEW

KEY FACTS

Damason-P is a narcotic analgesic combining Hydrocodone Bitartrate with aspirin and caffeine. Hydrocodone exerts its narcotic effects centrally. Aspirin acts both centrally and peripherally in the relief of pain. Caffeine has been reported to be an effective adjuvant to aspirin.

MAJOR USES

Damason-P is an analgesic intended for the relief of moderate to moderately severe pain.

SAFETY INFORMATION

Damason-P is contraindicated for patients who have developed a hypersensitivity to aspirin, caffeine, or hydrocodone. The benefit/risk potential should be considered before using Damason-P in patients with head injury, head lesions, increased intracranial pressure, or abdominal conditions because of the potential of narcotic induced respiratory depression and the possibility of masking of the diagnosis or clinical course of patients.
Damason-P should be avoided in the presence of peptic ulcer and coagulation abnormalities. Use in children and teenagers is also better avoided if flu or chicken pox is suspected.

PRESCRIBING INFORMATION

DAMASON-P   ⒸR

[dă 'mă-sŭn-p]
(Hydrocodone Bitartrate 5mg, USP, Aspirin 224mg, Caffeine 32mg)

DESCRIPTION

Each pink tablet of DAMASON-P contains:

ACTIVE INGREDIENTS

Hydrocodone Bitartrate	5 mg
(Warning: May be habit forming)	
Aspirin	224 mg
Caffeine	32 mg

INACTIVE INGREDIENTS

Cellulose
Corn Starch
Stearic Acid
Color, Red #3 Lake
Narcotic analgesic tablet for oral administration.
Hydrocodone is a hydrogenated ketone of codeine available as bitartrate salt. Hydrocodone bitartrate is an opioid analgesic and antitussive and occurs as fine, white crystals or as a crystalline powder. It is affected by light.

CLINICAL PHARMACOLOGY

Hydrocodone is a semisynthetic narcotic analgesic with multiple actions similar to those of codeine. Most of these actions involve the central nervous system and smooth muscle. The precise mechanism of action of hydrocodone and other opiates is not known, although it is believed to relate to the existence of opiate receptors in the central nervous system. In addition to analgesia, narcotics may produce drowsiness, changes in mood and mental clouding. There is no history of hepatic toxicity.
Radioimmunoassay techniques have recently been developed for the analysis of hydrocodone in human plasma. After a 10 mg. oral dose of hydrocodone bitartrate, a mean peak serum drug level of 23.6 ng/ml and an elimination half-life of 3.8 hours were found. DAMASON-P also contains the nonnarcotic, anti-inflammatory, antipyretic analgesic, aspirin and caffeine.

INDICATIONS AND USAGE

For the relief of moderate to moderately severe pain.

CONTRAINDICATIONS

Hypersensitivity to aspirin, caffeine or hydrocodone.

WARNINGS

Reye Syndrome: This is a rare but serious disease which can follow flu or chicken pox in children and teenagers. While the cause of the Reye Syndrome is unknown, some reports claim aspirin (or salicylates) may increase the risk of developing this disease. Consult a doctor before use in children or teenagers with flue or chicken pox.
Acute Abdominal Conditions: The administration of narcotics may obscure the diagnosis or clinical course of patients with acute abdominal conditions.
Head Injury and Increased Intracranial Pressure: The respiratory depressant effects of narcotics and their capacity to elevate cerebrospinal fluid pressure may be markedly exaggerated in the presence of head injury, other intracranial lesions or a preexisting increase in intracranial pressure. Furthermore, narcotics produce adverse reactions which may obscure the clinical course of patients with head injuries.
Respiratory Depression: At high doses or in sensitive patients, hydrocodone may produce dose-related respiratory depression by acting directly on brain stem respiratory centers. Hydrocodone also affects centers that control respiratory rhythm, and may produce irregular and periodic breathing.
Other: Salicylates should be used with extreme caution in the presence of peptic ulcer or coagulation abnormalities.

PRECAUTIONS

Special Risk Patients: As with any narcotic analgesic agent, DAMASON-P should be used with caution in elderly or debilitated patients and those with severe impairment of hepatic or renal functions, hypothyroidism, Addison's disease, prostatic hypertrophy or urethral stricture. The usual precautions should be observed and the possibility of respiratory depression should be kept in mind.
Information for Patients: DAMASON-P, like all narcotics, may impair the mental and/or physical abilities required for the performance of potentially hazardous tasks such as driving a car or operating machinery; patients should be cautioned accordingly. DAMASON-P should be taken after meals or with a full glass of water.
Cough Reflex: Hydrocodone suppresses the cough reflex; as with all narcotics, caution should be exercised when DAMASON-P is used postoperatively and in patients with pulmonary disease.
Drug Interactions: Patients receiving other narcotic analgesics, general anesthetics, phenothiazines, other tranquilizers, sedative-hypnotics or other CNS depressants (including alcohol) concomitantly with DAMASON-P may exhibit an additive CNS depression. When such combined therapy is contemplated, the dose of one or both agents should be reduced. Aspirin may enhance the effects of anti-coagulants and inhibit the uricosuric effects of uricosuric agents.
The concurrent use of anticholinergics with hydrocodone may produce paralytic ileus.
The use of MAO inhibitors or tricyclic antidepressants with hydrocodone preparations may increase the effect of either the antidepressant or hydrocodone.
Usage In Pregnancy: "Pregnancy Category C." Hydrocodone has been shown to be teratogenic in hamsters when given in doses 700 times the human dose. There are no adequate and well-controlled studies in pregnant women. DAMASON-P should be used during pregnancy only if the potential benefit justifies the potential risk to the fetus.
Nonteratogenic Effects: Babies born to mothers who have been taking opioids regularly prior to delivery will be physically dependent. The withdrawal signs include irritability and excessive crying, tremors, hyperactive reflexes, increased respiratory rate, increased stools, sneezing, yawning, vomiting, and fever. The intensity of the syndrome does not always correlate with the duration of maternal opioid use or dose. There is no consensus on the best method of managing withdrawal.
Chlorpromazine 0.7 to 1.0 mg/kg q6h, and paregoric 2 to 4 drops/kg q4h, have been used to treat withdrawal symptoms in infants. The duration of therapy is 4 to 28 days, with the dosage decreased as tolerated.
Labor and Delivery: As with all narcotics, administration of DAMASON-P to the mother shortly before delivery may result in some degree of respiratory depression in the newborn, especially if higher doses are used.
Nursing Mothers: It is not known whether this drug is excreted in human milk. Because many drugs are excreted in human milk and because of the potential for serious adverse reactions in nursing infants from DAMASON-P, a decision should be made whether to discontinue nursing or to discontinue the drug, taking into account the importance of the drug to the mother. Hydrocodone is almost completely excreted within 72 hours.
Pediatric Use: Safety and efficacy in children have not been established.

Continued on next page

Mason—Cont.

ADVERSE REACTIONS

Central Nervous System: As with all narcotics, sedation, drowsiness, mental clouding, lethargy, impairment of mental and physical performance, anxiety, fear, dysphoria, dizziness, psychic dependence and mood changes may occur.

Gastrointestinal System: Nausea and vomiting occur infrequently; they are more frequent in ambulatory than in recumbent patients. Administration with meals may help reduce this problem. The antiemetic phenothiazines are useful in suppressing these effects; however, some phenothiazine derivatives seem to be antianalgesic and to increase the amount of narcotic required to produce a given level of analgesia. Prolonged administration of DAMASON-P may produce constipation.

Genitourinary System: Ureteral spasm, spasm of vesical sphincters and urinary retention have been reported with codeine and its derivatives.

Drug Abuse and Dependence: DAMASON-P is subject to the Federal Controlled Substance Act (Schedule III). Psychic dependence, physical dependence, and tolerance may develop upon repeated administration of narcotics; therefore, DAMASON-P Tablets should be prescribed and administered with caution. However, psychic dependence is unlikely to develop when DAMASON-P Tablets are used for a short time for the treatment of pain.

Physical dependence, the condition in which continued administration of the drug is required to prevent the appearance of a withdrawal syndrome, assumes clinically significant proportions only after several weeks of continued narcotic use, although some mild degree of physical dependence may develop after a few days of narcotic therapy. Tolerance, in which increasingly larger doses are required in order to produce the same degree of analgesia, is manifested initially by a shortened duration of analgesic effect, and subsequently by decreases in the intensity of analgesia. The rate of development of tolerance varies among patients.

OVERDOSAGE

Aspirin:

Signs and Symptoms: Respiratory alkalosis is characteristic of the early phase in intoxication with aspirin while hyperventilation is occurring, and is quickly followed by metabolic acidosis in most people with severe intoxication. This occurs more readily in children. Hypoglycemia may occur in children who have taken large overdoses. Other laboratory findings associated with aspirin intoxication include ketonuria, hyponatremia, hypokalemia, and occasionally proteinuria. A slight rise in lactic dehydrogenase and hydroxybutyric dehydrogenase may occur.

Methemoglobin and sulfhemoglobin formation are seldom clinically significant in adults but may contribute to general toxicity. When prominent, they appear as a grayish cyanosis seen most clearly in the lips and nailbeds. Definitive diagnosis is made by spectroscopic analysis of water-diluted (1:100) blood specimen, which shows an abnormal band at 630 nm for methamoglobin and at 618 nm for sulfhemoglobin.

Concentrations of aspirin in plasma above 30 mg/100 ml are associated with toxicity. The single lethal dose of aspirin in adults is probably about 25–30 gm, but is not known with certainty.

Hydrocodone:

Signs and Symptoms: Serious overdose with hydrocodone is characterized by respiratory depression (a decrease in respiratory rate and/or tidal volume, Cheyne-Stokes respiration, cyanosis), extreme somnolence progressing to stupor or coma, skeletal muscle flaccidity, cold and clammy skin, and sometimes bradycardia and hypotension. In severe overdosage, apnea, circulatory collapse, cardiac arrest and death may occur.

Treatment: Primary attention should be given to the reestablishment of adequate respiratory exchange through provision of a patent airway and the institution of assisted or controlled ventilation. The narcotic antagonist naloxone hydrochloride is a specific antidote against respiratory depression which may result from overdosage or unusual sensitivity to narcotics, including hydrocodone. Therefore, an appropriate dose of naloxone hydrochloride, 0.55 mg/kgm, should be administered intravenously, (see package insert), simultaneously with efforts at respiratory resuscitation. Since the duration of action of hydrocodone may exceed that of the antagonist, the patient should be kept under continued surveillance and repeated doses of the antagonist should be administered as needed to maintain adequate respiration. An antagonist should not be administered in the absence of clinically significant respiratory or cardiovascular depression. Oxygen, intravenous fluids, vasopressors and other supportive measures should be employed as indicated. Gastric emptying may be useful in removing unabsorbed drug.

DOSAGE AND ADMINISTRATION

Given orally, the dosage should be adjusted according to the severity of the pain and the response of the patient. How-

ever, it should be kept in mind that tolerance to hydrocodone can develop with continued use and that the incidence of untoward effects may be dose-related.

The usual dose is one tablet, orally, every six hours as needed for pain, with water or other liquids. If necessary, this dose may be repeated at four hour intervals. In cases of more severe pain, two tablets every six hours (up to 8 tablets in 24 hours) may be required.

CAUTION

Federal Law prohibits dispensing without prescription. DAMASON-P has a schedule III classification which permits prescription refill up to six months or five times on physician's specification.

HOW SUPPLIED

DAMASON-P is supplied as 7/16", round, pink mottled tablets with an "M" logo on one side and "D-P" on the other. Supplied in bottles of 100, NDC 12758-055-01, bottles of 500, NDC 12758-055-05, and in hospital packs of 100, NDC 12758-055-25.

Storage: DAMASON-P should be stored at 59°-86°F, 15°-30°C.

Manufactured by:
Anabolic Inc.
Irvine, CA 92714
Manufactured expressly for:
Mason Pharmaceuticals, Inc.
Newport Beach, CA 92660
5901A Revised May, 1989

Shown in Product Identification Section, page 416

DUOCET™   Ⓒ Ⱦ

[du "oset]
(Hydrocodone 5 mg., Acetominophen 500 mg.)

PRODUCT OVERVIEW

KEY FACTS

DuoCet is a narcotic analgesic combining Hydrocodone Bitartrate with Acetaminophen. Hydrocodone exerts its narcotic effects centrally. The analgesic action of acetaminophen involves peripheral and central influences, but the specific mechanism is as yet undetermined.

MAJOR USES

DuoCet is an analgesic intended for the relief of moderate to moderately severe pain.

SAFETY INFORMATION

DuoCet is contraindicated for patients who have developed a hypersensitivity to hydrocodone or acetaminophen.

The benefit/risk potential should be considered before using DuoCet in patients with head injury, head lesions, increased intracranial pressure, or abdominal conditions because of the potential of narcotic induced respiratory depression and the possibility of masking of the diagnosis or clinical course of patients.

PRESCRIBING INFORMATION

DUOCET™   Ⓒ Ⱦ

[du "oset]
Hydrocodone and Acetaminophen Tablets

DESCRIPTION

Each DuoCet tablet contains:
Active Ingredients:
Hydrocodone bitartrate .... 5 mg
    Warning. may be habit forming
Acetaminophen ....500 mg
Inactive Ingredients: Calcium Stearate, Microcrystalline Cellulose, Progelatinized Starch (Corn), Sodium Lauryl Sulfate, Starch (Corn), and Stearic Acid.

Narcotic analgesic tablet for oral administration.
Hydrocodone bitartrate is an opioid analgesic and antitussive and occurs as fine, white crystals or as a crystalline powder. It is affected by light. The chemical formula of hydrocodone bitartrate is: $C_{18}H_{21}NO_3 \cdot C_4H_6O_6 \cdot 2\frac{1}{2}H_2O$

Acetaminophen is a non-opiate, non-salicylate analgesic and antipyretic which occurs as a white, odorless, crystalline powder possessing a slightly bitter taste. It may be represented by the following chemical formula: $C_8H_9NO_2$

CLINICAL PHARMACOLOGY

Hydrocodone is a semisynthetic narcotic analgesic and antitussive with multiple actions qualitatively similar to those of codeine. Most of these involve the central nervous system and smooth muscle. The precise mechanism of action of hydrocodone and other opiates is not known, although it is believed to relate to the existence of opiate receptors in the central nervous system. In addition to analgesia, narcotics may produce drowsiness, changes in mood and mental clouding.

Radioimmunoassay techniques have recently been developed for the analysis of hydrocodone in human plasma. After a 10 mg. oral dose of hydrocodone bitartrate, a mean peak serum drug level of 23.6 ng/ml and an elimination half-life of 3.8 hours were found.

The analgesic action of acetaminophen involves peripheral and central influences, but the specific mechanism is as yet undetermined. Antipyretic activity is mediated through hypothalamic heat regulating centers. Acetaminophen inhibits prostaglandin synthetase. Therapeutic doses of acetaminophen have negligible effects on the cardiovascular or respiratory systems; however, toxic doses may cause circulatory failure and rapid, shallow breathing. Acetaminophen is rapidly and almost completely absorbed from the gastrointestinal tract, producing maximum serum concentrations within 30 minutes to one hour. The plasma half-life in adults and children ranges from 0.90 hours to 3.25 hours with an average of approximately 2 hours. The drug distributes uniformly in most body fluids and is approximately 25% protein bound. Acetaminophen is conjugated in the liver, with less than 3% of the dose excreted unchanged in 24 hours. The primary metabolic pathway is conjugation to sulfate and glucuronide by-products. A minor oxidative pathway forms cysteine and mercapturic acid. These compounds are subsequently excreted by the kidneys into the urine.

INDICATIONS AND USAGE

For the relief of moderate to moderately severe pain.

CONTRAINDICATIONS

Hypersensitivity to acetaminophen or hydrocodone.

WARNINGS

Respiratory Depression: At high doses or in sensitive patients, hydrocodone may produce dose-related respiratory depression by acting directly on brain stem respiratory centers. Hydrocodone also affects centers that control respiratory rhythm, and may produce irregular and periodic breathing.

Head Injury and Increased Intracranial Pressure: The respiratory depressant effects of narcotics and their capacity to elevate cerebrospinal fluid pressure may be markedly exaggerated in the presence of head injury, other intracranial lesions or a preexisting increase in intracranial pressure. Furthermore, narcotics produce adverse reactions which may obscure the clinical course of patients with head injuries.

Acute Abdominal Conditions: The administration of narcotics may obscure the diagnosis or clinical course of patients with acute abdominal conditions.

PRECAUTIONS

Special Risk Patients: As with any narcotic analgesic agent, DuoCet tablets should be used with caution in elderly or debilitated patients and those with severe impairment of hepatic or renal functions, hypothyroidism, Addison's disease, prostatic hypertrophy or urethral stricture. The usual precautions should be observed and the possibility of respiratory depression should be kept in mind.

Information for Patients: DuoCet tablets, like all narcotics, may impair the mental and/or physical abilities required for the performance of potentially hazardous tasks such as driving a car or operating machinery; patients should be cautioned accordingly.

Cough Reflex: Hydrocodone suppresses the cough reflex; as with all narcotics, caution should be exercised when DuoCet tablets are used postoperatively and in patients with pulmonary disease.

Drug Interactions: Patients receiving other narcotic analgesics, antipsychotics, antianxiety agents, or other CNS depressants (including alcohol) concomitantly with DuoCet tablets may exhibit an additive CNS depression. When combined therapy is contemplated, the dose of one or both agents should be reduced.

The use of MAO inhibitors or tricyclic antidepressants with hydrocodone preparations may increase the effect of either the antidepressant or hydrocodone.

The concurrent use of anticholinergics with hydrocodone may produce paralytic ileus.

Usage in Pregnancy: "Pregnancy Category C." Hydrocodone has been shown to be teratogenic in hamsters when given in doses 700 times the human dose. There are no adequate and well-controlled studies in pregnant women. DuoCet tablets should be used during pregnancy only if the potential benefit justifies the potential risk to the fetus.

Nonteratogenic Effects: Babies born to mothers who have been taking opioids regularly prior to delivery will be physically dependent. The withdrawal signs include irritability and excessive crying, tremors, hyperactive reflexes, increased respiratory rate, increased stools, sneezing, yawning, vomiting and fever. The intensity of the syndrome does not always correlate with the duration of maternal opioid use or dose. There is no consensus on the best method of managing withdrawal. Chlorpromazine 0.7 to 1.0 mg/kg q6h, and paregoric 2 to 4 drops/kg q4h, have been used to treat withdrawal symptoms in infants. The duration of therapy is 4 to 28 days, with the dosage decreased as tolerated.

Labor and Delivery: As with all narcotics, administration of DuoCet tablets to the mother shortly before delivery may result in some degree of respiratory depression in the newborn, especially if higher doses are used.

Nursing Mothers: It is not known whether this drug is excreted in human milk. Because many drugs are excreted in human milk and because of the potential for serious adverse reactions in nursing infants from DuoCet tablets, a decision should be made whether to discontinue nursing or to discontinue the drug, taking into account the importance of the drug to the mother.

Pediatric Use: Safety and effectiveness in children have not been established.

ADVERSE REACTIONS

The most frequently observed reactions include lightheadedness, dizziness, sedation, nausea and vomiting. These effects seem to be more prominent in ambulatory than in nonambulatory patients and some of these adverse reactions may be alleviated if the patient lies down.

Other adverse ractions include:

Central Nervous System: Drowsiness, mental clouding, lethargy, impairment of mental and physical performance, anxiety, fear, dysphoria, psychic dependence, mood changes.

Gastrointestinal System: Nausea and vomiting may occur; they are more frequent in ambulatory than in recumbent patients. The antiemetic phenothiazines are useful in suppressing these effects; however, some phenothiazine derivatives seem to be antianalgesic and to increase the amount of narcotic required to produce pain relief while other phenothiazines reduce the amount of narcotic required to produce a given level of analgesia. Prolonged administration of Duo-Cet tablets may produce constipation.

Genitourinary System: Ureteral spasm, spasm of vesical sphincters and urinary retention have been reported.

Respiratory Depression: DuoCet tablets may produce dose-related respiratory depression by acting directly on brain stem respiratory centers. Hydrocodone also affects centers that control respiratory rhythm, and may produce irregular and periodic breathing. If significant respiratory depression occurs, it may be antagonized by the use of naloxone hydrochloride (see package insert). Apply other supportive measures when indicated.

Drug Abuse and Dependence: DuoCet tablets are subject to the Federal Controlled Substance Act (Schedule CIII). Psychic dependence, physical dependence, and tolerance may develop upon repeated administration of narcotics; therefore, DuoCet tablets should be prescribed and administered with caution. However, psychic dependence is unlikely to develop when DuoCet tablets are used for a short time for the treatment of pain. Physical dependence, the condition in which continued administration of the drug is required to prevent the appearance of a withdrawal syndrome, assumes clinically significant proportions only after several weeks of continued narcotic use, although some mild degree of physical dependence may develop after a few days of narcotic therapy. Tolerance, in degree of physical dependence may develop after a few days of narcotic therapy. Tolerance, in which increasingly large doses are required in order to produce the same degree of analgesia, is manifested initially by a shortened duration of analgesic effect, and subsequently by decreases in the intensity of analgesia. The rate of development of tolerance varies among patients.

OVERDOSAGE

Hydrocodone:

Signs and Symptoms: Serious overdose with hydrocodone is characterized by respiratory depression (a decrease in respiratory rate and/or tidal volume, Cheyne-Stokes respiration, cyanosis), extreme somnolence progressing to stupor or coma, skeletal muscle flaccidity, cold and clammy skin, and sometimes bradycardia and hypotension. In severe overdosage, apnea, circulatory collapse, cardiac arrest, and death may occur.

Treatment: Primary attention should be given to the reestablishment of adequate respiratory exchange through provision of a patent airway and the institution of assisted or controlled ventilation. The narcotic antagonist naloxone is a specific antidote against respiratory depression which may result from overdosage or unusual sensitivity to narcotics, including hydrocodone. Therefore, an appropriate dose of naloxone HCl (see package insert) should be administered, preferably by the intravenous route, and simultaneously with efforts at respiratory resuscitation. Since the duration of action of hydrocodone may exceed that of the antagonist, the patient should be kept under continued surveillance and repeated doses of the antagonist should be administered as needed to maintain adequate respiration.

An antagonist should not be administered in the absence of clinically significant respiratory or cardiovascular depression. Oxygen, intravenous fluids, vasopressors and other supportive measures should be employed as indicated. Gastric emptying may be useful in removing unabsorbed drug.

Acetaminophen:

Signs and Symptoms: In acute acetaminophen overdosage, dose-dependent, potentially fatal hepatic necrosis is the most serious adverse effect. Renal tubular necrosis, hypoglycemic coma, and thrombocytopenia may also occur.

In adults, hepatic toxicity has rarely been reported with acute overdoses of less than 10 grams and fatalities with less than 15 grams. Importantly, young children seem to be more resistant than adults to the hepatotoxic effect of an acetaminophen overdose. Despite this, the measures outlined below should be initiated in any adult or child suspected of having ingested an acetaminophen overdose.

Early symptoms following a potentially hepatotoxic overdose may include: nausea, vomiting, diaphoresis and general malaise. Clinical and laboratory evidence of hepatic toxicity may not be apparent until 48 to 72 hours post-ingestion.

Treatment: The stomach should be emptied promptly by lavage or by induction of emesis with syrup of ipecac. Patients' estimates of the quantity of a drug ingested are notoriously unreliable. Therefore, if an acetaminophen overdose is suspected, a serum acetaminophen assay should be obtained as early as possible, but no sooner than four hours following ingestion. Liver function studies should be obtained initially and repeated at 24-hour intervals.

The antidote, N-acetylcysteine, should be administered as early as possible, preferably within 16 hours of the overdose ingestion for optimal results but in any case within 24 hours. Following recovery, there are no residual, structural or functional hepatic abnormalities.

DOSAGE AND ADMINISTRATION

Given orally, the dosage should be adjusted according to the severity of the pain and the response of the patient. However, tolerance to hydrocodone can develop with continued use and the incidence of untoward effects is dose related. The usual dosage is one or two tablets every four to six hours as needed for pain. The total 24-hour dose should not exceed eight tablets.

CAUTION

Federal law prohibits dispensing without prescription. DUO-CET has a schedule III classification which permits prescription refill up to six months or five times on physician's specification.

HOW SUPPLIED

DUOCET is supplied as white, bar-shaped tablets, scored on one side with DUOCET debossed on the other.

Supplied in bottles of 100, NDC 12758-067-01

Storage: DUOCET should be stored at 59°–86°F, 15°–30°C.

Manufactured by:

Pharmaceutical Basics, Inc.

Denver, CO 80223

Manufactured expressly for

Mason Pharmaceuticals, Inc.

Newport Beach, CA 92660

5915A-Revised May, 1989

Shown in Product Identification Section, page 416

Matrix Technologies, Inc.
1020 BAY AREA BLVD.
HOUSTON, TX 77058

SAAVE™

DESCRIPTION

SAAVE is an amino acid and vitamin nutritional supplement carefully formulated toward the specific brain nutritional deficiencies common in alcoholics, children of alcoholics and polydrug abusers. SAAVE is a nutritional adjunct to therapy and is nonaddictive and hypoallergenic.

COMPOSITION

Each capsule contains a combination of 460 mg DL-phenylalanine, 25 mg L-tryptophan, 25 mg L-glutamine and 3 mg of pyridoxal-5-phosphate (vitamin B6 active metabolite). No binders, yeast, sugars, dyes, or preservatives.

ACTIONS AND USES

SAAVE is recommended for use as a nutritional adjunct to therapy for alcoholics and abusers of heroin, related opiates, and other depressants. Alcohol and drug abuse and the genetic predisposition to alcoholism lead to nutritional deficiencies in amino acid based neurotransmitters, amino acids, minerals, vitamins. SAAVE is formulated to aid in correcting these deficiencies.

CONTRAINDICATIONS

SAAVE should not be used by phenylketonurics (PKU), pregnant or lactating females and persons who are hypersensitive to any of its ingredients. Children under 14 should use SAAVE only with the advice of a physician. Do not use with monoamine oxidase inhibitors (MAO).

AMOUNT AND FREQUENCY

It is recommended that persons within the first 6 months of sobriety take 6 capsules per day (preferably 2 three times per day or, alternatively, 3 two times per day) one to two hours before meals. It is recommended that those who have been sober over 6 months and adult children of alcoholics take 3–4 capsules per day. If occasional dull headaches occur, reduce

the amount taken to 3–4 capsules per day. If headaches continue, discontinue use. SAAVE should be used on a continuing daily basis as long as needed (generally over one year).

HOW SUPPLIED

SAAVE is supplied in 42 and 180 capsule bottles and in hospital unit dose packages of 100 capsules in blister packs.

TROPAMINE™

DESCRIPTION

TROPAMINE is an amino acid, mineral and vitamin combination formulated to foster the nutritional replacement of specific deficiencies common in cocaine and stimulant abusers. It is nonaddictive and hypoallergenic.

COMPOSITION

Each 6 capsules (daily intake) contain:

DL-Phenylalanine	1500 mg
L-Tyrosine	900 mg
L-Tryptophan	400 mg
L-Glutamine	300 mg
Zinc (chelate)	30 mg
Magnesium (oxide)	150 mg
Calcium (chelate)	150 mg
Thiamine (HCl)	100 mg
Riboflavin	15 mg
Niacinamide	100 mg
Pantothenic acid	90 mg
Pyridoxal-5-phosphate	20 mg
Cyanocobalamin	6 ug
Calcium ascorbate	600 mg
Folic acid	400 ug

No binders, yeast, sugars, dyes, or preservatives.

ACTIONS AND USES

Dependence on cocaine (and other nervous system stimulants) leads to nutritional deficiencies in amino acid based neurotransmitters, amino acids, minerals and vitamins. TROPAMINE is formulated to aid in correcting these deficiencies and is recommended for use as a nutritional adjunct to therapy for cocaine, amphetamine and stimulant abuse.

CONTRAINDICATIONS

TROPAMINE should not be used by phenylketonurics (PKU), pregnant or lactating females and persons who are hypersensitive to any of its ingredients. Children under 14 should use Tropamine only with the advice of a physician. Do not use with monoamine oxidase inhibitors (MAO).

AMOUNT AND FREQUENCY

The recommended daily amount is 6 capsules (preferably 2 three times per day or, alternatively, 3 two times per day) one to two hours before meals. If occasional dull headaches occur, reduce the amount taken to 3–4 capsules per day. If headaches continue, discontinue use. TROPAMINE should be used on a continuing daily basis as long as needed for nutritional supplementation. This period is generally about one year.

HOW SUPPLIED

Tropamine is supplied in 42 and 180 capsule bottles and in hospital unit dose packages of 100 capsules in blister packs.

EDUCATIONAL MATERIAL

Chart

A 24″ × 36″ chart showing the neurochemistry of alcohol addiction and recovery is available free to physicians.

IDENTIFICATION PROBLEM?
Consult PDR's
Product Identification Section
where you'll find over 1700
products pictured actual size
and in full color.

Mayrand, Inc.
P. O. BOX 8869
FOUR DUNDAS CIRCLE
GREENSBORO, NC 27419

B–A–C TABLETS ℞

DESCRIPTION
Each yellow and white tablet for oral administration contains:

Butalbital*	50 mg

*WARNING: May be habit forming.

Aspirin	650 mg
Caffeine	40 mg

HOW SUPPLIED
Available as yellow and white scored capsule-shaped tablets imprinted "M/R" in bottles of 100's, NDC #0259-1256-01.

ELDERCAPS ℞

DESCRIPTION
Each capsule contains: Vitamin A Acetate, 4000 I.U.; Vitamin D_2, 400 I.U.; Vitamin E, 25 I.U.; Ascorbic Acid, 200 mg.; Thiamine Mononitrate, 10 mg.; Riboflavin, 5 mg.; Pyridoxine HCl, 2 mg.; Niacinamide, 25 mg.; d-Calcium Pantothenate, 10 mg.; Zinc Sulfate, 110 mg.; Magnesium Sulfate, 70 mg.; Manganese Sulfate, 5 mg.; Folic Acid, 1 mg.

INDICATIONS
ELDERCAPS are indicated for the prophylaxis or treatment of vitamin and mineral deficiencies associated with restricted diets, improper food intake, and decreased absorption or utilization. ELDERCAPS are also indicated in patients with increased requirements for vitamins and minerals due to chronic disease, infection or the stress of surgery.

WARNINGS
Folic acid alone is improper therapy in the treatment of pernicious anemia and other megaloblastic anemias where vitamin B_{12} is deficient.

PRECAUTIONS
Folic acid, especially in doses above 0.1 mg. daily, may obscure pernicious anemia, that is, hematological remission may occur while neurologic manifestations remain progressive.

DOSAGE
One capsule daily or as directed by the physician.

HOW SUPPLIED
Bottles of 100 capsules.

ELDERTONIC

DESCRIPTION
Each 45 ml. contains: Thiamine HCl, 1.5 mg.; Riboflavin, 1.7 mg.; Pyridoxine HCl, 2.0 mg.; Cyanocobalamin, 6.0 mcg.; Dexpanthenol, 10.0 mg.; Niacinamide, 20.0 mg.; Zinc, 15 mg. (as zinc sulfate); Manganese, 2.0 mg. (as manganese sulfate); Magnesium (minimum content as added magnesium), 2.0 mg. (as magnesium sulfate); Alcohol, 13.5%.
In a special sherry wine base.

INDICATIONS
B-complex vitamins with minerals for nutritional supplementation.

DOSAGE
Adults: one tablespoonful three times a day with meals.

WARNING
Do not exceed recommended dosage unless directed by a physician.

USAGE IN PREGNANCY
Safe use of this product in pregnancy has not been established.

CAUTION
Keep out of the reach of children.

HOW SUPPLIED
8 fl. oz.; Pints; Gallons

MAY–VITA ELIXIR ℞

DESCRIPTION
Each 45 ml. contains: Dexpanthenol, 10 mg; Niacinamide, 40 mg.; Pyridoxine HCl (B-6), 4 mg.; Cyanocobalamin (B-12), 12 mcg.; Folic Acid, 1 mg.; Iron, 36 mg. (as polysaccharide iron complex); Zinc, 15 mg. (as zinc sulfate); Manganese, 4 mg. (as manganese sulfate); Alcohol, 13%.

INDICATIONS
For vitamin and mineral replacement therapy in deficiency states and for treatment of iron deficiency anemia and/or nutritional megaloblastic anemias due to inadequate diet.

WARNINGS
Folic acid alone is improper therapy in the treatment of pernicious anemia and other megaloblastic anemias where vitamin B_{12} is deficient.

PRECAUTIONS
Folic acid, especially in doses above 0.1 mg. daily, may obscure pernicious anemia, in that hematologic remission may occur while neurological manifestations remain progressive.

ADVERSE REACTIONS
Allergic sensitization has been reported following both oral and parenteral administration of folic acid.

USE IN PREGNANCY
Safe use of this product in pregnancy has not been established.

DOSAGE
Usual adult dosage is one tablespoonful three times daily with meals. Do not exceed recommended dosage unless directed by a physician.

HOW SUPPLIED
Pint bottles.

NU–IRON 150 CAPS
NU–IRON Elixir (polysaccharide-iron complex)
Sugar Free

DESCRIPTION
NU-IRON is a highly water soluble complex of iron and a low molecular weight polysaccharide.
Each NU-IRON 150 Capsule contains:

Iron (elemental)	150 mg.
(as Polysaccharide Iron Complex)	

Each 5 ml. of NU-IRON Elixir contains:

Iron (elemental)	100 mg.
(as Polysaccharide Iron Complex)	
Alcohol	10%

ACTION AND USES
NU-IRON is a non-ionic, easily assimilated, relatively non-toxic form of iron. Full therapeutic doses may be achieved with virtually no gastrointestinal side effects. There is no metallic aftertaste and no staining of teeth.

INDICATIONS
For treatment of uncomplicated iron deficiency anemia.

CONTRAINDICATIONS
Hemochromatosis, hemosiderosis or a known hypersensitivity to any of the ingredients.

DOSAGE
ADULTS; One or two NU-IRON 150 Caps daily, or one or two teaspoonfuls NU-IRON Elixir daily. CHILDREN; 6 to 12 years old; one teaspoonful NU-IRON Elixir daily. For younger children consult physician.

HOW SUPPLIED
NU-IRON 150 Caps in bottles of 100. NU-IRON Elixir in 8 fl. oz. bottles.

SEDAPAP TABLETS ℞

DESCRIPTION
Each white, capsule-shaped tablet for oral administration contains:

Butalbital*	50 mg

*(WARNING: May be habit forming.)

Acetaminophen	650 mg

$C_{11}H_{16}N_2O_3$　　　　　　　　　M.W. 224.25
Butalbital

$C_8H_9NO_2$　　　　　　　　　M.W. 151.16
Acetaminophen

Butalbital, 5-allyl-5-isobutylbarbituric acid, a white, odorless, crystalline powder having a slightly bitter taste, is a short to intermediate-acting barbiturate.

Acetaminophen, 4-hydroxyacetanilide, is a non-opiate, nonsalicylate analgesic and antipyretic which occurs as a white, odorless, crystalline powder possessing a slightly bitter taste.

CLINICAL PHARMACOLOGY
Pharmacologically, SEDAPAP TABLETS combine the analgesic properties of acetaminophen with the anxiolytic and muscle relaxant properties of butalbital.

INDICATIONS AND USAGE
SEDAPAP TABLETS are indicated for the relief of the symptom complex of tension (or muscle contraction) headache.

CONTRAINDICATIONS
Hypersensitivity to acetaminophen or barbiturates. Patients with porphyria.

PRECAUTIONS
General: Barbiturates should be administered with caution, if at all, to patients who are mentally depressed, have suicidal tendencies, or a history of drug abuse.
Elderly or debilitated patients may react to barbiturates with marked excitement, depression, and confusion. In some persons, barbiturates repeatedly produce excitement rather than depression.

Information For Patients: Practitioners should give the following information and instructions to patients receiving barbiturates:

A. The use of barbiturates carries with it an associated risk of psychological and/or physical dependence. The patient should be warned against increasing the dose of the drug without consulting a physician.

B. Barbiturates may impair mental and/or physical abilities required for the performance of potentially hazardous tasks (e.g., driving, operating machinery, etc.).

C. Alcohol should not be consumed while taking barbiturates. Concurrent use of the barbiturates with other CNS depressants (e.g., alcohol, narcotics, tranquilizers, and antihistamines) may result in additional CNS depressant effects.

Drug Interactions: Patients receiving narcotic analgesics, antipsychotics, antianxiety agents, or other CNS depressants (including alcohol) concomitantly with SEDAPAP TABLETS may exhibit additive CNS depressant effects.

DRUGS	EFFECT
Butalbital with coumarin coumarin anti-couglants	Decreased effect of anti-coagulant because of increased metabolism resulting from enzyme induction.
Butalbital with tricyclic anti-coagulant	Decreased blood levels of the anti-depressant.

Usage In Pregnancy: Adequate studies have not been performed in animals to determine whether this drug affects fertility in males or females, has teratogenic potential or has other adverse effects on the fetus. There are no well-controlled studies in pregnant women. Although there is no clearly defined risk, one cannot exclude the possibility of infrequent or subtle damage to the human fetus. SEDAPAP TABLETS should be used in pregnant women only when clearly needed.

Nursing Mothers: The effects of SEDAPAP TABLETS on infants of nursing mothers are not known. Barbiturates are excreted in the breast milk of nursing mothers. The serum levels in infants are believed to be insignificant with therapeutic doses.

Pediatric Use: Safety and effectiveness in children below the age of twelve have not been established.

ADVERSE REACTIONS
The most frequent adverse reactions are drowsiness and dizziness. Less frequent adverse reactions are lightheadedness and gastrointestinal disturbances including nausea, vomiting, and flatulence. Mental confusion or depression can occur due to intolerance or overdosage of butalbital.

DRUG ABUSE AND DEPENDENCE
Prolonged use of barbiturates can produce drug dependence, characterized by psychic dependence and tolerance. The abuse liability of SEDAPAP TABLETS is similar to that of other barbiturate-containing drug combinations. Caution should be exercised when prescribing medication for patients with a known propensity for taking excessive quanti-

ties of drugs, which is not uncommon in patients with chronic tension headache.

OVERDOSAGE
The toxic effects of acute overdosage of SEDAPAP TABLETS are attributable mainly to its barbiturate component, and, to a lesser extent, acetaminophen.

Barbiturate
SIGNS AND SYMPTOMS: Drowsiness, confusion, coma; respiratory depression; hypotension; shock.
TREATMENT:
Maintenance of an adequate airway, with assisted respiration and oxygen administration as necessary.
Monitoring of vital signs and fluid balance.
If the patient is conscious and has not lost the gag reflex, emesis may be induced with ipecac. Care should be taken to prevent pulmonary aspiration of vomitus. After completion of vomiting, 30 grams of activated charcoal in a glass of water may be administered.
If emesis is contraindicated, gastric lavage may be performed with a cuffed endotracheal tube in place with the patient in the facedown position. Activated charcoal may be left in the emptied stomach and a saline cathartic administered.
Fluid therapy and other standard treatment for shock, if needed.
If renal function is normal, forced diuresis may aid in the elimination of the barbiturate. Alkalinization of the urine increases renal excretion of some barbiturates, especially phenobarbital.
Although not recommended as a routine procedure, hemodialysis may be used in severe barbiturate intoxication or if the patient is anuric or in shock.

Acetaminophen
SIGNS AND SYMPTOMS: In acute acetaminophen overdosage, dose-dependent, potentially fatal hepatic necrosis is the most serious adverse effect. Renal tubular necrosis, hypoglycemic coma, and thrombocytopenia may also occur.
In adults, hepatic toxicity has rarely been reported with acute overdoses of less than 10 grams and fatalities with less than 15 grams. Importantly, young children seem to be more resistant than adults to the hepatotoxic effects of an acetaminophen overdose.
Early symptoms following a potentially hepatotoxic overdosage may include: nausea, vomiting, diaphoresis and general malaise. Clinical and laboratory evidence of hepatic toxicity may not be apparent until 48 to 72 hours post-ingestion.
TREATMENT: The stomach should be emptied promptly by lavage or by induction of emesis with syrup of ipecac. Patients' estimates of the quantity of a drug ingested are notoriously unreliable. Therefore, if an acetaminophen overdose is suspected, a serum acetaminophen assay should be obtained as early as possible, but no sooner than four hours following ingestion. Liver function studies should be obtained initially and repeated at 24-hour intervals.
The antidote, N-acetylcysteine, should be administered as early as possible, preferably within 16 hours of the overdose ingestion for optimal results, but in any case, within 24 hours. Following recovery, there are no residual, structural or functional hepatic abnormalities.

DOSAGE AND ADMINISTRATION
One tablet every four hours as needed. Do not exceed 6 tablets per day.

HOW SUPPLIED
SEDAPAP TABLETS [Butalbital 50 mg (WARNING: May be habit forming) and Acetaminophen 650 mg] are available as white, capsule-shaped tablets scored on one side with an "M" appearing on the left side of the score, and an "R" appearing on the right side of the score. In bottles of 100, NDC #0259-1278-01.

STERAPRED UNIPAK   ℞

DESCRIPTION
Each blue tablet contains:
Prednisone ....5 mg.

HOW SUPPLIED
Available in 21 tablet dispensing pack.

STERAPRED DS UNIPAK   ℞
STERAPRED DS 12 DAY UNIPAK

DESCRIPTION
Each white tablet contains:
Prednisone ....10 mg.

HOW SUPPLIED
STERAPRED DS UNIPAK available in 21 tablet dispensing pack.
STERAPRED DS 12 DAY UNIPAK available in 48 tablet dispensing pack.

McGregor
Pharmaceuticals Inc.
32580 GRAND RIVER AVENUE
FARMINGTON, MI 48024

ALL McGREGOR PRODUCTS ARE COMPLETELY DYE FREE.

Full prescribing information for all McGregor Pharmaceuticals products is available from your McGregor Pharmaceuticals representative.

Product Identification Codes
To provide quick and positive identification of McGregor Pharmaceuticals products, we have had imprinted the product identification number on our capsules. In order that you may quickly identify a product by its code number, we provide the following list of code numbers:

Product	Code Number
Rhindecon™ (Phenylpropanolamine HCl, 75 mg) Sustained Release Capsules ℞	MCG 215
Rhinolar™ (Phenylpropanolamine HCl 75 mg, Chlorpheniramine Maleate 8 mg, Methscopolamine Nitrate 2.5 mg) Sustained Release Capsule ℞	MCG 219
Rhinolar-EX™ (Phenylpropanolamine HCl 75 mg, Chlorpheniramine Maleate 8 mg) Sustained Release Capsule ℞	MCG 210
Rhinolar-EX 12™ (Phenylpropanolamine HCl 75 mg, Chlorpheniramine Maleate 12 mg) Sustained Release Capsule ℞	MCG 211

EDUCATIONAL MATERIAL

Samples: Starter samples on above products available upon request.

McNeil Consumer Products Company
Division of McNeil-PPC, Inc.
FORT WASHINGTON, PA 19034

DELSYM®   OTC
[del'sim]
(dextromethorphan polistirex)

DESCRIPTION
Each teaspoonful (5 ml) contains dextromethorphan polistirex equivalent to 30 mg dextromethorphan hydrobromide.

ACTIONS
Delsym® contains a clinically proven cough suppressant, dextromethorphan hydrobromide, to provide 12-hour relief of coughs due to minor throat and bronchial irritation.

INDICATIONS
For temporary relief of cough due to minor throat and bronchial irritation as may occur with the common cold or with inhaled irritants.

USUAL DOSAGE
Shake well before using. Adults: 2 teaspoonful every 12 hours; do not exceed 4 teaspoonsful in 24 hours. Children 6–12: 1 teaspoonful every 12 hours; do not exceed 2 teaspoonsful in 24 hours. Children 2–5: ½ teaspoonful every 12 hours: do not exceed 1 teaspoonful in 24 hours. Children under 2: Use only under the advice and supervision of a physician.
Note: Since DELSYM dextromethorphan polistirex syrup is available without prescription, the following appears on the package labels.
Warning: Do not give this product to children under 2 years except under the advice and supervision of a physician. Do not take this product for persistent or chronic cough such as occurs with smoking, asthma, or emphysema, or where cough is accompanied by excessive phlegm (mucus) unless directed by a physician.
As with any drug, if you are pregnant or nursing a baby, seek the advice of a health professional before using this product.

A persistent cough may be a sign of a serious condition. If cough persists for more than 1 week, tends to recur or is accompanied by fever, rash or persistent headache, consult a physician. Keep this and all medications out of reach of children. In case of accidental overdose, seek professional assistance or contact a Poison Control Center immediately. Do not use if carton is opened, or break-away ring is separated or missing.

OVERDOSAGE
Acute dextromethorphan overdose usually does not result in serious signs and symptoms unless a massive amount has been ingested. Signs and symptoms of a substantial overdose may include nausea and vomiting, visual disturbance, CNS disturbances, and urinary retention. Because of the sustained action of DELSYM, the onset of symptoms may be delayed, and the duration of symptoms may be prolonged.

INACTIVE INGREDIENTS
Citric Acid; Ethylcellulose; Flavor; High Fructose Corn Syrup; Methylparaben; Polyethylene Glycol 3350; Polysorbate 80; Propylene Glycol; Propylparaben; Sucrose; Tragacanth; Vegetable Oil; Purified Water; Xanthan Gum, Yellow #6 (Sunset Yellow).

HOW SUPPLIED
Orange flavored syrup in 3 fl. oz. bottles (NDC 0045-0288-03)
Shown in Product Identification Section, page 417

IMODIUM® A–D
(loperamide hydrochloride)

PRODUCT OVERVIEW
KEY FACTS
IMODIUM® A–D is a liquid antidiarrheal containing 1mg of loperamide per teaspoon. IMODIUM® A–D acts by slowing intestinal motility and by affecting water and electrolyte movement through the bowel.

MAJOR USES
IMODIUM® A–D is indicated for the control and symptomatic relief of acute nonspecific diarrhea.

SAFETY INFORMATION
No known drug interactions. Do not use if diarrhea is accompanied by high fever (greater than 101°F), or if blood is present in the stool.

PRESCRIBING INFORMATION
IMODIUM® A–D
(loperamide hydrochloride)

DESCRIPTION
Each 5 ml (teaspoon) of Imodium A-D liquid contains loperamide hydrochloride 1 mg. Imodium A-D liquid is stable, cherry flavored, and clear in color.

ACTIONS
Imodium A-D contains a clinically proven antidiarrheal medication. Loperamide HCl acts by slowing intestinal motility and by affecting water and electrolyte movement through the bowel.

INDICATION
Imodium A-D is indicated for the control and symptomatic relief of acute nonspecific diarrhea.

USUAL DOSAGE
Adults: Take four teaspoonfuls after first loose bowel movement. If needed, take two teaspoonfuls after each subsequent loose bowel movement. Do not exceed eight teaspoonfuls in any 24 hour period, unless directed by a physician.
9–11 years old (60–95 lbs.): Two teaspoonfuls after first loose bowel movement, followed by one teaspoonful after each subsequent loose bowel movement. Do not exceed six teaspoonfuls a day.
6–8 years old (48–59 lbs.): Two teaspoonfuls after first loose bowel movement, followed by one teaspoonful after each subsequent loose bowel movement. Do not exceed four teaspoonfuls a day.
Professional Dosage Schedule for children two-five years old (24–27 lbs): one teaspoon after first loose bowel movement, followed by one after each subsequent loose bowel movement. Do not exceed three teaspoonfuls a day.
Warnings: Since Imodium A-D liquid is available without a prescription, the following information appears on the package label: "WARNINGS: DO NOT USE FOR MORE THAN TWO DAYS UNLESS DIRECTED BY A PHYSICIAN. Do not use if diarrhea is accompanied by high fever (greater than 101°F), or if blood is present in the stool, or if you have had a rash or other allergic reaction to loperamide HCl. If you are taking antibiotics or have a history of liver disease, consult a physician before using this product. As with any drug, if you are pregnant or nursing a baby, seek the advice of a physician before using this product. Keep this and all drugs out of the reach of children. In case of accidental over-

Continued on next page

McNeil Consumer—Cont.

dose, seek professional assistance or contact a poison control center immediately. Store at room temperature."

OVERDOSAGE

Overdosage of loperamide HCl in man may result in constipation, CNS depression and nausea. A slurry of activated charcoal administered promptly after ingestion of loperamide hydrochloride can reduce the amount of drug which is absorbed. If vomiting occurs spontaneously upon ingestion, a slurry of 100 grams of activated charcoal should be administered orally as soon as fluids can be retained. If vomiting has not occurred, and CNS depression is evident, gastric lavage should be performed followed by administration of 100 gms of the activated charcoal slurry through the gastric tube. In the event of overdosage, patients should be monitored for signs of CNS depression for at least 24 hours. Children may be more sensitive to central nervous system effects than adults. If CNS depression is observed, naloxone may be administered. If responsive to naloxone, vital signs must be monitored carefully for recurrence of symptoms of drug overdose for at least 24 hours after the last dose of naloxone.

INACTIVE INGREDIENTS

Alcohol (5.25%), citric acid, flavors, glycerin, methylparaben, propylparaben and purified water.

HOW SUPPLIED

Cherry flavored liquid (clear) 2 fl. oz., 3 fl. oz., and 4 fl. oz. tamper resistant bottles with child resistant safety caps and special dosage cups.

BK403

Shown in Product Identification Section, page 417

MEDIPREN®   OTC
Ibuprofen Caplets and Tablets
Pain Reliever/Fever Reducer

WARNING

ASPIRIN SENSITIVE PATIENTS. Do not take this product if you have had a severe allergic reaction to aspirin (e.g., asthma, swelling, shock or hives) because even though this product contains no aspirin or salicylates, cross-reactions may occur in patients allergic to aspirin.

DESCRIPTION

Each MEDIPREN Caplet or Tablet contains ibuprofen 200 mg.

INDICATIONS

For the temporary relief of minor aches and pains associated with the common cold, headache, toothaches, muscular aches, backache, for the minor pain of arthritis, for the pain of menstrual cramps, and for reduction of fever.

USUAL DOSAGE

Adults: One Caplet or Tablet every 4 to 6 hours while symptoms persist. If pain or fever does not respond to 1 Caplet or Tablet, 2 Caplets or Tablets may be used but do not exceed 6 Caplets or Tablets in 24 hours, unless directed by a doctor. The smallest effective dose should be used. Take with food or milk if occasional and mild heartburn, upset stomach, or stomach pain occurs with use. Consult a doctor if these symptoms are more than mild or if they persist.

Children: Do not give this product to children under 12 except under the advice and supervision of a doctor.

WARNINGS

Do not take for pain for more than 10 days or for fever for more than 3 days unless directed by a doctor. If pain or fever persists or gets worse, if new symptoms occur, or if the painful area is red or swollen, consult a doctor. These could be signs of serious illness. If you are under a doctor's care for any serious condition, consult a doctor before taking this product. As with aspirin and acetaminophen, if you have any condition which requires you to take prescription drugs or if you have had any problems or serious side effects from taking any non-prescription pain reliever, do not take this product without first discussing it with your doctor. If you experience any symptoms which are unusual or seem unrelated to the condition for which you took ibuprofen, consult a doctor before taking any more of it. Although ibuprofen is indicated

for the same conditions as aspirin and acetaminophen, it should not be taken with them except under a doctor's direction. Do not combine this product with any other ibuprofen containing product. As with any drug, if you are pregnant or nursing a baby, seek the advice of a health professional before using this product. IT IS ESPECIALLY IMPORTANT NOT TO USE IBUPROFEN DURING THE LAST 3 MONTHS OF PREGNANCY UNLESS SPECIFICALLY DIRECTED TO DO SO BY A DOCTOR BECAUSE IT MAY CAUSE PROBLEMS IN THE UNBORN CHILD OR COMPLICATIONS DURING DELIVERY. Keep this and all drugs out of the reach of children.

OVERDOSAGE

In case of accidental overdose, contact a physician or poison control center.

STORAGE

Store at room temperature; avoid excessive heat 40°C (104°F).

INACTIVE INGREDIENTS

Colloidal silicon dioxide, glyceryl triacetate, hydroxypropyl methylcellulose, microcrystalline cellulose, pregelatinized starch, sodium lauryl sulfate, sodium starch glycolate, titanium dioxide, FD&C blue #1 and D&C yellow #10.

HOW SUPPLIED

Coated Caplets (colored white, imprinted "MEDIPREN")— bottles of 24's, 50's, 100's. Coated Tablets (colored white, imprinted "MEDIPREN")—bottles of 24's, 50's, 100's.

Shown in Product Identification Section, page 416

PEDIACARE® Cold Formula Liquid   OTC
PEDIACARE® Cough-Cold Formula Liquid and Chewable Tablets
PEDIACARE® Night Rest Cough-Cold Formula Liquid
PEDIACARE® Infants' Oral Decongestant Drops

PRODUCT OVERVIEW

KEY FACTS

PediaCare® Cold Relief Products are formulated specifically for relief of pediatric cold and cough symptoms. These products are formulated to allow accurate dosing by age and weight, especially when using the enclosed dropper or dosage cup.

Recommended dosage schedules for PediaCare Infants' Drops, Cold Formula, Cough-Cold Formula are the same as recommended dosage schedules for Children's TYLENOL Infants' Drops, Elixir and Chewable Tablets, respectively.

PRESCRIBING INFORMATION

PEDIACARE® Cold Formula Liquid   OTC
PEDIACARE® Cough-Cold Formula Liquid and Chewable Tablets
PEDIACARE® Nigh Rest Cough-Cold Formula Liquid
PEDIACARE® Infants' Oral Decongestant Drops

DESCRIPTION

Each 5 ml of PEDIACARE Cold Formula Liquid contains pseudoephedrine hydrochloride 15 mg and chlorpheniramine maleate 1 mg. Each 5 ml of PEDIACARE Cough-Cold Formula Liquid contains pseudoephedrine hydrochloride 15 mg, chlorpheniramine maleate 1 mg and dextromethorphan hydrobromide 5 mg. Each PEDIACARE Cough-Cold Formula Chewable Tablet contains pseudoephedrine hydrochloride 7.5 mg, chlorpheniramine maleate 0.5 mg and dextromethorphan hydrobromide 2.5 mg. Each 0.8 ml oral dropper of PEDIACARE Infants' Oral Decongestant Drops contains pseudoephedrine hydrochloride 7.5 mg. PEDIACARE Night Rest contains pseudoephedrine hydrochloride 15 mg, chlorpheniramine maleate 1 mg and dextromethorphan hydrobromide 7.5 mg per 5 ml. PEDIACARE Liquid Products and Infants' Drops are stable, cherry flavored and red in color. PEDIACARE Cough-Cold Formula Chewable Tablets are fruit flavored and pink in color.

ACTIONS

PEDIACARE Cold Products are available in four different formulas, allowing you to select the ideal cold product to temporarily relieve the patient's cold symptoms. PEDIACARE Cold Formula Liquid contains a decongestant, pseudoephedrine hydrochloride, and an antihistamine, chlorpheniramine maleate, to provide temporary relief of nasal congestion, runny nose and sneezing due to the common cold, hay

fever or other upper respiratory allergies. PEDIACARE Cough-Cold Formula Liquid and Chewable Tablets contain both of the above ingredients plus a cough suppressant, dextromethorphan hydrobromide, to provide temporary relief of nasal congestion, runny nose, sneezing and coughing due to the common cold, hay fever or other upper respiratory allergies. PEDIACARE Night Rest Cough-Cold Formula Liquid contains a decongestant, pseudoephedrine hydrochloride, an antihistamine, chlorpheniramine maleate, and a cough suppressant, dextromethorphan hydrobromide to provide temporary relief of coughs, nasal congestion, runny nose and sneezing due to the common cold. PEDIACARE Nigh Rest may be used day or night to relieve cough and cold symptoms. PEDIACARE Infants' Oral Decongestant Drops contain a decongestant, pseudoephedrine hydrochloride, to provide temporary relief of nasal congestion due to the common cold, hay fever or other upper respiratory allergies.

Professional Dosage: A calibrated dosage cup is provided for accurate dosing of the PEDIACARE Liquid formulas. A calibrated oral dropper is provided for accurate dosing of PEDIACARE Infants' Drops. All doses of PEDIACARE Cold Formula Liquid, PEDIACARE Cough-Cold Formula Liquid and Chewable Tablets and PEDIACARE Infants' Drops may be repeated every 4–6 hours, not to exceed 4 doses in 24 hours. PEDIACARE Night Rest Liquid may be repeated every 6–8 hrs, not to exceed 4 doses in 24 hours. [See table below].

Note: Since PEDIACARE cold products are available without prescription, the following information appears on the package labels: "WARNINGS: Do not use if carton is opened, or if printed plastic bottle wrap or foil inner seal is broken. Keep this and all medication out of the reach of children. In case of accidental overdosage, contact a physician or poison control center immediately."

The following information appears on the appropriate package labels:

PEDIACARE Cold Formula Liquid: "Do not exceed the recommended dosage because nervousness, dizziness or sleeplessness may occur. If symptoms do not improve within seven days or are accompanied by fever, consult a physician before continuing use. This preparation may cause drowsiness, or in some cases, excitability. Do not give this product to children who have heart disease, high blood pressure, thyroid disease, diabetes, glaucoma or asthma, or are taking a prescription drug for high blood pressure or depression, except under the advise and supervision of a physician."

"Inactive Ingredients: Benzoic acid, citric acid, flavors, glycerin, polyethylene glycol, propylene glycol, sodium benzoate, sorbitol, sucrose, purified water, Red #33, Blue #1 and Red #40.

PEDIACARE Cough-Cold Formula Liquid and Chewable Tablets: "Do not exceed the recommended dosage because nervousness, dizziness or sleeplessness may occur. A persistent cough may be a sign of a serious condition. If symptoms do not improve within seven days, tend to recur, or are accompanied by fever, rash, excessive mucus, persistent cough or headache, consult a physician before continuing use. This preparation may cause drowsiness or, in some cases, excitability. Do not give this product to children who have heart disease, high blood pressure, thyroid disease, diabetes, glaucoma or asthma, or are taking a prescription drug for high blood pressure or depression, except under the advice and supervision of a physician."

PEDIACARE Cough-Cold Formula Liquid: Inactive Ingredients: Benzoic acid, citric acid, flavors, glycerin, polyethylene glycol, propylene glycol, sodium benzoate, sorbitol, sucrose, purified water, Red #33, Blue #1 and Red #40. PEDIACARE Cough-Cold Formula Chewable Tablets also contain the warning, "Phenylketonurics: contains phenylalanine 3 mg per tablet", and the inactive ingredient listing, "Inactive Ingredients: Aspartame, cellulose, citric acid, dextrose, flavors, magnesium stearate, magnesium trisilicate, mannitol, starch, sucrose and Red #3."

PEDIACARE Night Rest Cough-Cold Formula Liquid: "Do not exceed the recommended dosage because nervousness, dizziness or sleeplessness may occur. A persistent cough may be a sign of a serious condition. If symptoms do not improve within seven days, tend to recur, or are accompanied by fever, rash, excessive mucus, persistent cough or headache, consult a physician before continuing use. This preparation may cause drowsiness or, in some cases, excitability. Do not give this product to children who have heart disease, high

Age Group	0–3 mos	4–11 mos	12–23 mos	2–3 yrs	4–5 yrs	6–8 yrs	9–10 yrs	11 yrs	Dosage
Weight (lbs)	6–11 lb	12–17 lb	18–23 lb	24–35 lb	36–47 lb	48–59 lb	60–71 lb	72–95 lb	
PEDIACARE Infants' Drops*	½ dropper (0.4 ml)	1 dropper (0.8 ml)	1½ droppers (1.2 ml)	2 droppers (1.6 ml)					q4–6h
PEDIACARE Cold Formula Liquid**				1 tsp	1½ tsp	2 tsp	2½ tsp	3 tsp	q4–6h
PEDIACARE Cough-Cold Formula Liquid**				1 tsp	1½ tsp	2 tsp	2½ tsp	3 tsp	q4–6h
Chewable Tablets**				2 tabs	3 tabs	4 tabs	5 tabs	6 tabs	q4–6h
PEDIACARE Night Rest Liquid**					2 tsp	2 tsp	2 tsp		q6–8

* administer to children under 2 years only on the advice of a physician
** administer to children under 6 years only on the advice of a physician

blood pressure, thyroid disease, diabetes, glaucoma or asthma, or are taking a prescription drug for high blood pressure or depression, except under the advice and supervision of a physician."

PEDIACARE Night Rest Cough-Cold Formula Liquid: Inactive ingredients Benzoic acid, citric acid, flavors, glycerin, polyethylene glycol, propylene glycol, sodium benzoate, sorbitol, sucrose, purified water, Red #33, blue #1 and Red #40.

PEDIACARE Infants' Oral Decongestant Drops: "Do not exceed the recommended dosage because at higher doses nervousness, dizziness or sleeplessness may occur. Do not give this product to children who have heart disease, high blood pressure, thyroid disease or diabetes unless directed by a physician. Do not give this product to children for more than seven days. If symptoms do not improve or are accompanied by fever, consult a physician. Do not give this product to children who are taking a prescription drug for high blood pressure or depression without first consulting a physician. Take by mouth only. Not for nasal use."

"Inactive Ingredients: Benzoic acid, citric acid, flavors, glycerin, polyethylene glycol, propylene glycol, purified water, sodium benzoate, sorbitol, sucrose and Red #40."

OVERDOSAGE

Acute dextromethorphan overdose usually does not result in serious signs and symptoms unless massive amounts have been ingested. Signs and symptoms of a substantial overdose may include nausea and vomiting, visual disturbances, CNS disturbances, and urinary retention. Symptoms from pseudoephedrine overdose consist most often of mild anxiety, tachycardia and/or mild hypertension. Symptoms usually appear within 4 to 8 hours of ingestion and are transient, usually requiring no treatment. Chlorpheniramine toxicity should be treated as you would an antihistamine/anticholinergic overdose and is likely to be present within a few hours after acute ingestion.

HOW SUPPLIED

PEDIACARE Liquid products (colored red)—bottles of 4 fl. oz with child-resistant safety cap and calibrated dosage cup. PEDIACARE Cough-Cold Formula Chewable Tablets (pink, scored)—bottles of 24 with child-resistant safety cap. PEDIACARE Infants' Drops (colored red)—bottles of ½ fl. oz with calibrated dropper.

Shown in Product Identification Section, page 417

MAXIMUM STRENGTH SINE-AID®   OTC
Sinus Headache Caplets and Tablets

DESCRIPTION
Each MAXIMUM STRENGTH SINE-AID® Caplet or Tablet contains acetaminophen 500 mg and pseudoephedrine hydrochloride 30 mg.

ACTIONS
MAXIMUM STRENGTH SINE-AID® Caplets and Tablets contain a clinically proven analgesic-antipyretic and a decongestant. Maximum allowable non-prescription levels of acetaminophen and pseudophedrine provide temporary relief of sinus congestion and pain. Acetaminophen is equal to aspirin in analgesic and antipyretic effectiveness and it is unlikely to produce many of the side effects associated with aspirin and aspirin-containing products. Acetaminophen produces analgesia by elevation of the pain threshold and antipyresis through action on the hypothalamic heat-regulating center. Pseudoephedrine hydrochloride is a sympathomimetic amine that promotes sinus cavity drainage by reducing nasopharyngeal mucosal congestion.

INDICATIONS
MAXIMUM STRENGTH SINE-AID® Caplets and Tablets provide effective symptomatic relief from sinus headache pain and congestion. SINE-AID® is particularly well-suited in patients with aspirin allergy, hemostatic disturbances (including anticoagulant therapy), and bleeding diatheses (e.g. hemophilia) and upper gastrointestinal disease (e.g. ulcer, gastritis, hiatus hernia).

PRECAUTIONS
If a rare sensitivity occurs, the drug should be discontinued. Although pseudoephedrine is virtually without pressor effect in normotensive patients, it should be used with caution in hypertensives.

USUAL DOSAGE
Adult dosage: Two caplets or tablets every four to six hours. Do not exceed eight caplets or tablets in any 24 hour period. **Note:** Since MAXIMUM STRENGTH SINE-AID® Caplets and Tablets are available without a prescription, the following appears on the package labels: "**WARNING:** Do not exceed the recommended dosage because at higher doses nervousness, dizziness or sleeplessness may occur. Do not administer to children under 12. If you have high blood pressure, heart disease, diabetes, thyroid disease, difficulty in urination due to enlargement of the prostate gland, or are presently taking a prescription drug for the treatment of

high blood pressure or depression, do not take except under the advice and supervision of a physician. Do not take this product for more than 7 days. If symptoms do not improve or are accompanied by high fever, consult a physician. **Do not use if carton is opened, or if printed red neck wrap or printed foil inner seal is broken. Keep this and all medication out of the reach of children. As with any drug, if you are pregnant or nursing a baby, seek the advice of a health professional before using this product. In case of accidental overdosage, contact a physician or poison control center immediately."**

OVERDOSAGE
Acetaminophen in massive overdosage may cause hepatic toxicity in some patients. In adults and adolescents, hepatic toxicity has rarely been reported following ingestion of acute overdoses of less than 10 grams. Fatalities are infrequent (less than 3–4% of untreated cases) and have rarely been reported with overdoses of less than 15 grams. In children, an acute overdosage of less than 150 mg/kg has not been associated with hepatic toxicity.

Early symptoms following a potentially hepatotoxic overdose may include: nausea, vomiting, diaphoresis and general malaise. Clinical and laboratory evidence of hepatic toxicity may not be apparent until 48 to 72 hours postingestion.

In adults and adolescents, regardless of the quantity of acetaminophen reported to have been ingested, administer MUCOMYST® acetylcysteine immediately if 24 hours or less have elapsed from the reported time of ingestion. For full prescribing information, refer to the MUCOMYST package insert. Do not await results of assays for acetaminophen level before initiating treatment with MUCOMYST acetylcysteine. The following additional procedures are recommended: The stomach should be emptied promptly by lavage or by induction of emesis with syrup of ipecac. A serum acetaminophen assay should be obtained as early as possible, but no sooner than four hours following ingestion. Liver function studies should be obtained initially and repeated at 24-hour intervals.

Serious toxicity or fatalities are extremely infrequent in children, possibly due to differences in the way they metabolize acetaminophen. In children, the maximum potential amount ingested can be more easily estimated. If more than 150 mg/kg or an unknown amount was ingested, obtain an acetaminophen plasma level. The acetaminophen plasma level should be obtained as soon as possible, but no sooner than 4 hours following the ingestion. Induce emesis using syrup of ipecac. If the plasma level is obtained and falls above the broken line on the acetaminophen overdose nomogram, the MUCOMYST acetylcysteine therapy should be initiated and continued for a full course of therapy. If acetaminophen plasma assay capability is not available, and the estimated acetaminophen ingestion exceeds 150 mg/kg, MUCOMYST acetylcysteine therapy should be initiated and continued for a full course of therapy.

For additional emergency information, call your regional poison center or call the Rocky Mountain Poison Center toll-free, (1-800-525-6115).

Symptoms from pseudoephedrine overdose consist most often of mild anxiety, tachycardia and/or mild hypertension. Symptoms usually appear within 4 to 8 hours of ingestion and are transient, usually requiring no treatment.

INACTIVE INGREDIENTS
Cellulose, hydroxypropyl methylcellulose, magnesium stearate, polyethylene glycol, sodium starch glycolate, starch, titanium dioxide, Blue #1 and Red #40.

HOW SUPPLIED
Caplets (colored white imprinted "Maximum SINE-AID")—blister pack of 24 and tamper-resistant bottles of 50. Tablets (colored white embossed "Sine-Aid")—blister package of 24 and tamper resistant bottles of 50 and 100
Shown in Product Identification Section, page 417

CHILDREN'S TYLENOL®   OTC
acetaminophen
Chewable Tablets, Elixir, Drops

DESCRIPTION
Each Children's TYLENOL Chewable Tablet contains 80 mg. acetaminophen in a fruit or grape flavored tablet. Children's TYLENOL acetaminophen Elixir is stable and alcohol free, cherry flavored is red in color grape flavored purple in color. Infants' TYLENOL Drops are stable, fruit flavored, orange in color and are alcohol free.
Children's TYLENOL Elixir: Each 5 ml. contains 160 mg. acetaminophen.
Infant's TYLENOL Drops: Each 0.8 ml. (one calibrated dropperful) contains 80 mg. acetaminophen.

ACTIONS
Acetaminophen is a clinically proven analgesic/antipyretic. Acetaminophen produces analgesia by elevation of the pain threshold and antipyresis through action on the hypothalamic heat regulating center. Acetaminophen is equal to aspirin in analgesic and antipyretic effectiveness and it is un-

likely to produce many of the side effects associated with aspirin and aspirin containing products.

INDICATIONS
Children's TYLENOL Chewable Tablets, Elixir and Drops are designed for treatment of infants and children with conditions requiring temporary relief of fever and discomfort due to colds and "flu," and of simple pain and discomfort due to teething, immunizations and tonsillectomy.

PRECAUTIONS
If a rare sensitivity reaction occurs, the drug should be stopped.

USUAL DOSAGE
All dosages may be repeated every 4 hours, but not more than 5 times daily. Administer to children under 2 years only on the advice of a physician. Children's TYLENOL Chewable Tablets: 2–3 years: two tablets. 4–5 years: three tablets, 6–8 years: four tablets. 9–10 years: five tablets. 11–12 years: six tablets.

Children's TYLENOL Elixir: (special cup for measuring dosage is provided) 4–11 months: one-half teaspoon. 12–23 months: three-quarters teaspoon. 2–3 years: one teaspoon. 4–5 years: one and one-half teaspoons. 6–8 years: 2 teaspoons. 9–10 years: two and one-half teaspoons. 11–12 years: three teaspoons.

Infants' TYLENOL Drops: 0–3 months: 0.4 ml. 4–11 months: 0.8 ml. 12–23 months: 1.2 ml. 2–3 years: 1.6 ml. 4–5 years: 2.4 ml.

Warning: Keep this and all medication out of reach of children. In case of accidental overdose, contact a physician or poison control center immediately. Consult your physician if fever persists for more than 3 days or if pain continues for more than 5 days. Store at room temperature.
NOTE: In addition to the above:
Children's TYLENOL® Drops—Do not use if printed carton overwrap or printed plastic bottle wrap is broken or missing or if carton is opened.
Children's TYLENOL Elixir—Do not use if printed carton overwrap is broken or missing or if carton is opened. Do not use if printed plastic bottle wrap or printed foil inner seal is broken. Not a USP elixir.
Children's TYLENOL Chewables—Do not use if carton is opened or if printed plastic bottle wrap or printed foil inner seal is broken. Phenylketonurics: contains phenylalanine 3mg per tablet.

OVERDOSAGE
Acetaminophen in massive overdosage may cause hepatic toxicity in some patients. In adults and adolescents, hepatic toxicity has rarely been reported following ingestion of acute overdoses of less than 10 grams. Fatalities are infrequent (less than 3–4% of untreated cases) and have rarely been reported with overdoses of less than 15 grams. In children, an acute overdosage of less than 150 mg/kg has not been associated with hepatic toxicity.

Early symptoms following a potentially hepatotoxic overdose may include: nausea, vomiting, diaphoresis and general malaise. Clinical and laboratory evidence of hepatic toxicity may not be apparent until 48 to 72 hours postingestion.

In adults and adolescents, regardless of the quantity of acetaminophen reported to have been ingested, administer MUCOMYST® acetylcysteine immediately if 24 hours or less have elapsed from the reported time of ingestion. For full prescribing information, refer to the MUCOMYST package insert. Do not await results of assays for acetaminophen level before initiating treatment with MUCOMYST acetylcysteine. The following additional procedures are recommended: The stomach should be emptied promptly by lavage or by induction of emesis with syrup of ipecac. A serum acetaminophen assay should be obtained as early as possible, but no sooner than four hours following ingestion. Liver function studies should be obtained initially and repeated at 24-hour intervals.

Serious toxicity or fatalities are extremely infrequent in children, possibly due to differences in the way they metabolize acetaminophen. In children, the maximum potential amount ingested can be more easily estimated. If more than 150 mg/kg or an unknown amount was ingested, obtain an acetaminophen plasma level. The acetaminophen plasma level should be obtained as soon as possible, but no sooner than 4 hours following the ingestion. Induce emesis using syrup of ipecac. If the plasma level is obtained and falls above the broken line on the acetaminophen overdose nomogram, the MUCOMYST acetylcysteine therapy should be initiated and continued for a full course of therapy. If acetaminophen plasma assay capability is not available, and the estimated acetaminophen ingestion exceeds 150 mg/kg, MUCOMYST acetylcysteine therapy should be initiated and continued for a full course of therapy.

For additional emergency information, call your regional poison center or call the Rocky Mountain Poison Center toll free, (1-800-525-6115).

Continued on next page

McNeil Consumer—Cont.

INACTIVE INGREDIENTS

Children's Tylenol Chewable Tablets—Aspartame, Cellulose, Citric Acid, Ethylcellulose, Flavors, Hydroxypropyl Methylcellulose, Mannitol, Starch, Magnesium Stearate, Red #7 and Blue #1 (Grape only).

Children's Tylenol Elixir—Benzoic Acid, Citric Acid, Flavors, Glycerin, Polyethylene Glycol, Propylene Glycol, Sodium Benzoate, Sorbitol, Sucrose, Purified Water, Red #40. In addition to the above ingredients cherry flavored elixir contains Red #33 and grape flavored elixir contains malic acid and Blue #1.

Infant's Tylenol Drops—Flavors, Propylene Glycol, Saccharin, Purified Water, Yellow #6.

HOW SUPPLIED

Chewable Tablets (pink colored fruit, purple colored grape, scored, imprinted "TYLENOL")—Bottles of 30 and child resistant blister packs of 48 (fruit only). Elixir (cherry colored red and grape colored purple)—bottles of 2 and 4 fl. oz. Drops (colored orange)—bottles of ½ oz. (15 ml.) with calibrated plastic dropper.

All packages listed above have child-resistant safety caps.

Shown in Product Identification Section, page 416

Junior Strength TYLENOL®   OTC
acetaminophen
Coated Caplets

DESCRIPTION

Each Junior Strength Caplet contains 160mg acetaminophen in a small, coated, capsule shaped tablet.

ACTIONS

Acetaminophen is a clinically proven analgesic/antipyretic. Acetaminophen produces analgesia by elevation of the pain threshold and antipyresis through action on the hypothalamic heat-regulating center. Acetaminophen is equal to aspirin in analgesic and antipyretic effectiveness and it is unlikely to produce many of the side effects associated with aspirin and aspirin-containing products.

INDICATIONS

Junior Strength TYLENOL Caplets are designed for easy swallowability in older children and young adults to provide fast, effective temporary relief of fever and discomfort due to colds and "flu," and pain and discomfort due to simple headaches, minor muscle aches, sprains and overexertion.

PRECAUTIONS

If a rare sensitivity reaction occurs, the drug should be stopped.

USUAL DOSAGE

All dosages shouold be taken with liquid and may be repeated every 4 hours, but not more than 5 times daily. For ages: 6–8 years: two Caplets, 9–10 years: two and one-half Caplets, 11 years: three Caplets, 12–14 years: four Caplets.

Note: Since Junior Strength TYLENOL acetaminophen Caplets are available without a prescription as an analgesic, the following appears on the package labels:

Warnings: Do not use if carton is opened or if a blister unit is broken. Keep this and all medications out of the reach of children. In case of accidental overdosage, contact a physician or poison control center immediately. Consult your physician if fever persists for more than three days or if pain continues for more than five days. As with any drugs, if you are pregnant or nursing a baby, seek the advice of a health professional before using this product. Not for children who have difficulty swallowing tablets.

OVERDOSAGE

Acetaminophen in massive overdosage may cause hepatic toxicity in some patients. In adults and adolescents, hepatic toxicity has rarely been reported following ingestion of acute overdosage of less than 10 grams. Fatalities are infrequent (less than 3–4% of untreated cases) and have rarely been reported with overdoses of less than 15 grams. In children, an acute overdosage of less than 150 mg/kg has not been associated with hepatic toxicity.

Early symptoms following a potentially hepatotoxic overdose may include: nausea, vomiting, diaphoresis and general malaise. Clinical and laboratory evidence of hepatic toxicity may not be apparent until 48 to 72 hours postingestion.

In adults and adolescents, regardless of the quantity of acetaminophen reported to have been ingested, administer MUCOMYST® acetylcysteine immediately if 24 hours or less have elapsed from the reported time of ingestion. For full prescribing information, refer to the MUCOMYST package insert. Do not await the results of assays for acetaminophen level before initiating treatment with MUCOMYST acetylcysteine. The following additional procedures are recommended: The stomach should be emptied promptly by lavage or by induction of emesis with syrup of ipecac. A serum acetaminophen assay should be obtained as early as possible, but no sooner than four hours following ingestion. Liver function studies should be obtained initially and repeated at 24-hour intervals.

Serious toxicity or fatalities are extremely infrequent in children, possibly due to differences in the way they metabolize acetaminophen. In children, the maximum potential amount ingested can be more easily estimated. If more than 150 mg/kg or an unknown amount was ingested, obtain an acetaminophen plasma level. The acetaminophen plasma level should be obtained as soon as possible, but no sooner than 4 hours following the ingestion. Induce emesis using syrup of ipecac. If the plasma level is obtained and falls above the broken line on the acetaminophen overdose nomogram, the MUCOMYST acetylcysteine therapy should be initiated and continued for a full course of therapy. If acetaminophen plasma assay capability is not available, and the estimated acetaminophen ingestion exceeds 150 mg/kg, MUCOMYST acetylcysteine therapy should be initiated and continued for a full course of therapy.

For additional emergency information, call your regional poison center or call the Rocky Mountain Poison Center toll-free, (1-800-525-6115).

INACTIVE INGREDIENTS

Cellulose, Ethylcellulose, Magnesium Stearate, Sodium Lauryl Sulfate, Sodium Starch Glycolate, Starch.

HOW SUPPLIED

Coated Caplets, (colored white, coated, scored, imprinted "TYLENOL 160"). Package of 30. All packages are safety sealed and use child resistant blister packaging.

Shown in Product Identification Section, page 416

Regular Strength
TYLENOL® acetaminophen Tablets   OTC
and Caplets

DESCRIPTION

Each Regular Strength TYLENOL Tablet or Caplet contains acetaminophen 325 mg.

ACTIONS

Acetaminophen is a clinically proven analgesic and antipyretic. Acetaminophen produces analgesia by elevation of the pain threshold and antipyresis through action on the hypothalamic heat-regulating center. Acetaminophen is equal to aspirin in analgesic and antipyretic effectiveness and it is unlikely to produce many of the side effects associated with aspirin and aspirin-containing products.

INDICATIONS

Acetaminophen acts safely and quickly to provide temporary relief from: simple headache; minor muscular aches; the minor aches and pains associated with bursitis, neuralgia, sprains, overexertion, menstrual cramps; and from the discomfort of fever due to colds and "flu." Also for temporary relief of minor aches and pains of arthritis and rheumatism. Acetaminophen is particularly well suited as an analgesic-antipyretic in the presence of aspirin allergy, hemostatic disturbances (including anticoagulant therapy), and bleeding diatheses (e.g., hemophilia) and upper gastrointestinal disease (e.g., ulcer, gastritis, hiatus hernia).

PRECAUTIONS

If a rare sensitivity reaction occurs, the drug should be discontinued.

USUAL DOSAGE

Adults: One to two tablets or caplets three or four times daily. Children (6 to 12): One-half to one tablet 3 or 4 times daily. (Junior Strength TYLENOL acetaminophen Swallowable Tablets, Chewable Tablets, Elixir and Drops are available for greater convenience in younger patients).

Note: Since TYLENOL acetaminophen tablets and caplets are available without prescription as an analgesic, the following appears on the package labels: Warning: Do not take for pain for more than 10 days (for adult) or 5 days (for children) and do not take for fever for more than 3 days unless directed by a doctor.

Do not use if printed red neck wrap or printed foil inner seal is broken. Keep this and all medications out of the reach of children. As with any drug, if you are pregnant or nursing a baby, seek the advice of a health professional before using this product. In case of accidental overdosage, contact a doctor or poison control center immediately."

OVERDOSAGE

Acetaminophen in massive overdosage may cause hepatic toxicity in some patients. In adults and adolescents, hepatic toxicity has rarely been reported following ingestion of acute overdoses of less than 10 grams. Fatalities are infrequent (less than 3–4% of untreated cases) and have rarely been reported with overdoses of less than 15 grams. In children, an acute overdosage of less than 150 mg/kg has not been associated with hepatic toxicity.

Early symptoms following a potentially hepatotoxic overdose may include: nausea, vomiting, diaphoresis and general malaise. Clinical and laboratory evidence of hepatic toxicity may not be apparent until 48 to 72 hours postingestion.

In adults and adolescents, regardless of the quantity of acetaminophen reported to have been ingested, administer MUCOMYST® acetylcysteine immediately if 24 hours or less have elapsed from the reported time of ingestion. For full prescribing information, refer to the MUCOMYST package insert. Do not await results of assays for acetaminophen level before initiating treatment with MUCOMYST acetylcysteine. The following additional procedures are recommended: The stomach should be emptied promptly by lavage or by induction of emesis with syrup of ipecac. A serum acetaminophen assay should be obtained as early as possible, but no sooner than four hours following ingestion. Liver function studies should be obtained initially and repeated at 24-hour intervals.

Serious toxicity or fatalities are extremely infrequent in children, possibly due to differences in the way they metabolize acetaminophen. In children, the maximum potential amount ingested can be more easily estimated. If more than 150 mg/kg or an unknown amount was ingested, obtain an acetaminophen plasma level. The acetaminophen plasma level should be obtained as soon as possible, but no sooner than 4 hours following the ingestion. Induce emesis using syrup of ipecac. If the plasma level is obtained and falls above the broken line on the acetaminophen overdose nomogram, the MUCOMYST acetylcysteine therapy should be initiated and continued for a full course of therapy. If acetaminophen plasma assay capability is not available, and the estimated acetaminophen ingestion exceeds 150 mg/kg, MUCOMYST acetylcysteine therapy should be initiated and continued for a full course of therapy.

For additional emergency information, call your regional poison center or call the Rocky Mountain Poison Center toll-free (1-800-525-6115).

INACTIVE INGREDIENTS

Tablets—Calcium Stearate or Magnesium Stearate, Cellulose, Docusate Sodium and Sodium Benzoate or Sodium Lauryl Sulfate, and Starch. Caplets—Cellulose, Hydroxypropyl Methylcellulose, Magnesium Stearate, Polyethylene Glycol, Sodium Starch Glycolate and Starch.

HOW SUPPLIED

Tablets (colored white, scored, imprinted "TYLENOL")—tins and vials of 12, and tamper-resistant bottles of 24, 50, 100 and 200. Caplets (colored white, "TYLENOL")—tamper-resistant bottles of 24, 50, 100. For additional pain relief, Extra-Strength TYLENOL® Tablets and Caplets, 500 mg, and Extra-Strength TYLENOL® Adult Liquid Pain Reliever are available (colored green; 1 fl. oz. = 1000 mg.)

Shown in Product Identification Section, page 416

Extra-Strength
TYLENOL® acetaminophen   OTC
Caplets, Gelcaps, Tablets

DESCRIPTION

Each Extra-Strength TYLENOL Caplet, Gelcap or Tablet contains acetaminophen 500 mg.

ACTIONS

Acetaminophen is a clinically proven analgesic and antipyretic. Acetaminophen produces analgesia by elevation of the pain threshold and antipyresis through action on the hypothalamic heat-regulating center. Acetaminophen is equal to aspirin in analgesic and antipyretic effectiveness and it is unlikely to produce many of the side effects associated with aspirin and aspirin-containing products.

INDICATIONS

For the temporary relief of minor aches, pains, headaches and fever.

PRECAUTIONS

If a rare sensitivity reaction occurs, the drug should be discontinued.

USUAL DOSAGE

Adults: Two Caplets, Gelcaps or Tablets 3 or 4 times daily. No more than a total of eight Caplets, Gelcaps or Tablets in any 24-hour period.

Note: Since Extra-Strength TYLENOL acetaminophen is available without a prescription, the following appears on the package labels: **Warning:** Do not take for more than 10 days or for fever for more than 3 days unless directed by a doctor. Severe or recurrent pain or high or continued fever may be indicative of serious illness. Under these conditions, consult a doctor.**Do not use if printed red neck wrap or printed foil inner seal is broken. Keep this and all medication out of the reach of children. As with any drug, if you are pregnant or nursing a baby, seek the advice of a health professional before using this product. In case of accidental overdosage, contact a doctor or poison control center immediately."**

OVERDOSAGE

Acetaminophen in massive overdosage may cause hepatic toxicity in some patients. In adults and adolescents, hepatic toxicity has rarely been reported following ingestion of acute overdosage of less than 10 grams. Fatalities are infrequent (less than 3-4% of untreated cases) and have rarely been reported with overdoses of less than 15 grams. In children, an acute overdosage of less than 150 mg/kg has not been associated with hepatic toxicity.

Early symptoms following a potentially hepatotoxic overdose may include: nausea, vomiting, diaphoresis and general malaise. Clinical and laboratory evidence of hepatic toxicity may not be apparent until 48 to 72 hours postingestion.

In adults and adolescents, regardless of the quantity of acetaminophen reported to have been ingested, administer MUCOMYST® acetylcysteine immediately if 24 hours or less have elapsed from the reported time of ingestion. For full prescribing information, refer to the MUCOMYST package insert. Do not await the results of assays for acetaminophen level before initiating treatment with MUCOMYST acetylcysteine. The following additional procedures are recommended: The stomach should be emptied promptly by lavage or by induction of emesis with syrup of ipecac. A serum acetaminophen assay should be obtained as early as possible, but no sooner than four hours following ingestion. Liver function studies should be obtained initially and repeated at 24-hour intervals.

Serious toxicity or fatalities are extremely infrequent in children, possibly due to differences in the way they metabolize acetaminophen. In children, the maximum potential amount ingested can be more easily estimated. If more than 150 mg/kg or an unknown amount was ingested, obtain an acetaminophen plasma level. The acetaminophen plasma level should be obtained as soon as possible, but no sooner than 4 hours following the ingestion. Induce emesis using syrup of ipecac. If the plasma level is obtained and falls above the broken line on the acetaminophen overdose nomogram, the MUCOMYST acetylcysteine therapy should be initiated and continued for a full course of therapy. If acetaminophen plasma assay capability is not available, and the estimated acetaminophen ingestion exceeds 150 mg/kg, MUCOMYST acetylcysteine therapy should be initiated and continued for a full course of therapy.

For additional emergency information, call your regional poison center or call the Rocky Mountain Poison Center toll-free, (1-800-525-6115).

INACTIVE INGREDIENTS

Tablets—Calcium Stearate or Magnesium Stearate, Cellulose, Docusate Sodium and Sodium Benzoate or Sodium Lauryl Sulfate and Starch. Caplets—Cellulose, Hydroxypropyl Methylcellulose, Magnesium Stearate, Polyethylene Glycol, Sodium Starch Glycolate, Starch and Red #40.
Gelcaps—Benzyl Alcohol, Butylparaben, Castor Oil, Cellulose, Edetate Calcium Disodium, Gelatin, Hydroxypropyl Methylcellulose, Magnesium Stearate, Methylparaben, Propylparaben, Sodium Lauryl Sulfate, Sodium Propionate, Sodium Starch Glycolate, Starch, Titanium Dioxide, Blue #1 and #2, Red #40 and Yellow #10.

HOW SUPPLIED

Tablets (colored white, imprinted "TYLENOL" and "500")—vials of 10 and tamper-resistant bottles of 30, 60, 100, and 200. Caplets (colored white, imprinted "TYLENOL 500 mg")—vials of 10 and tamper-resistant bottles of 24, 50, 100, 175, and 250's.
Gelcaps (colored yellow and red, imprinted "Tylenol 500") tamper-resistant bottles of 24, 50 and 100. For adults who prefer liquids or can't swallow solid medication, Extra-Strength TYLENOL® Adult Liquid Pain Reliever, mint flavored, is also available (colored green; 1 fl. oz. = 1000 mg.).

Shown in Product Identification Section, page 416

Extra-Strength   OTC
TYLENOL® acetaminophen
Adult Liquid Pain Reliever

DESCRIPTION

Each 15 ml. (½ fl. oz. or one tablespoonful) contains 500 mg. acetaminophen (alcohol 7%).

ACTIONS

TYLENOL acetaminophen is a clinically proven analgesic and antipyretic. Acetaminophen produces analgesia by elevation of the pain threshold and antipyresis through action on the hypothalamic heat-regulating center. Acetaminophen is equal to aspirin in analgesic & antipyretic effectiveness and it is unlikely to produce many of the side effects associated with aspirin and aspirin-containing products.

INDICATIONS

Acetaminophen provides temporary relief of minor aches, pains, headaches and fevers.

PRECAUTIONS

If a rare sensitivity reaction occurs, the drug should be discontinued.

USUAL DOSAGE

Extra-Strength TYLENOL Adult Liquid Pain Reliever is an adult preparation for those adults who prefer liquids or can't swallow solid medication. Not for use in children under 12. Measuring cup is marked for accurate dosage. Extra-Strength Dose—1 fl. oz. (30 ml or 2 tablespoonsful, 1000 mg), which is equivalent to two 500 mg Extra-Strength TYLENOL Tablets or Caplets. Take every 4–6 hours, no more than 4 doses in any 24-hour period.

Note: Since Extra-Strength TYLENOL Adult Liquid Pain Reliever is available without a prescription, the following appears on the package labels: **Warning:** Do not take for pain for more than 10 days (for adults) or 5 days (for children) and do not take for fever for more than 3 days unless directed by a doctor. Severe or recurrent pain or high or continued fever may be indicative of serious illness. Under these conditions, consult a physician. **Do not use if printed plastic overwrap or printed foil inner seal is broken. Keep this and all medication out of the reach of children. As with any drug, if you are pregnant or nursing a baby, seek the advice of a health professional before using this product. In case of accidental overdosage, contact a doctor or poison control center immediately."**

OVERDOSAGE

Acetaminophen in massive overdosage may cause hepatic toxicity in some patients. In adults and adolescents, hepatic toxicity has rarely been reported following ingestion of acute overdosage of less than 10 grams. Fatalities are infrequent (less than 3-4% of untreated cases) and have rarely been reported with overdoses of less than 15 grams. In children, an acute overdosage of less than 150 mg/kg has not been associated with hepatic toxicity.

Early symptoms following a potentially hepatotoxic overdose may include: nausea, vomiting, diaphoresis and general malaise. Clinical and laboratory evidence of hepatic toxicity may not be apparent until 48 to 72 hours postingestion.

In adults and adolescents, regardless of the quantity of acetaminophen reported to have been ingested, administer MUCOMYST® acetylcysteine immediately if 24 hours or less have elapsed from the reported time of ingestion. For full prescribing information, refer to the MUCOMYST package insert. Do not await the results of assays for acetaminophen level before initiating treatment with MUCOMYST acetylcysteine. The following additional procedures are recommended: The stomach should be emptied promptly by lavage or by induction of emesis with syrup of ipecac. A serum acetaminophen assay should be obtained as early as possible, but no sooner than four hours following ingestion. Liver function studies should be obtained initially and repeated at 24-hour intervals.

Serious toxicity or fatalities are extremely infrequent in children, possibly due to differences in the way they metabolize acetaminophen. In children, the maximum potential amount ingested can be more easily estimated. If more than 150 mg/kg or an unknown amount was ingested, obtain an acetaminophen plasma level. The acetaminophen plasma level should be obtained as soon as possible, but no sooner than 4 hours following the ingestion. Induce emesis using syrup of ipecac. If the plasma level is obtained and falls above the broken line on the acetaminophen overdose nomogram, the MUCOMYST acetylcysteine therapy should be initiated and continued for a full course of therapy. If acetaminophen plasma assay capability is not available, and the estimated acetaminophen ingestion exceeds 150 mg/kg, MUCOMYST acetylcysteine therapy should be initiated and continued for a full course of therapy.

For additional emergency information, call your regional poison center or call the Rocky Mountain Poison Center toll-free, (1-800-525-6115).

INACTIVE INGREDIENTS

Alcohol, Citric Acid, Flavors, Glycerin, Polyethylene Glycol, Purified Water, Sodium Benzoate, Sorbitol, Sucrose, Yellow #6 (Sunset Yellow), Yellow #10 and Blue #1.

HOW SUPPLIED

Mint-flavored liquid (colored green), 8 fl. oz. tamper-resistant bottle with child resistent safety cap and special dosage cup.

CHILDREN'S TYLENOL COLD®   OTC
Chewable Cold Tablets and Liquid Cold Formula

PRODUCT OVERVIEW

KEY FACTS

Children's Tylenol Cold® Products are formulated to relieve a child's fever, aches and pains, congestion and runny nose. The products are aspirin free and formulated for accurate dosing by age and weight.

MAJOR USES

Children's Tylenol Cold Products contain the same amount of acetaminophen as comparable Children's Tylenol Cold Products (80mg per tablet, 160mg. per 5ml) for relief of fever and pain resulting from a cold in children ages 11 and under. Additionally, Children's TYLENOL Cold Products contain pseudoephedrine hydrochloride (7.5mg per tablet, 15mg per 5ml) for treatment of nasal congestion and chlorpheniramine maleate (0.5mg per tablet, 1mg per 5ml) for treatment of runny noses and sneezing.

PRESCRIBING INFORMATION

CHILDREN'S TYLENOL COLD®   OTC
Chewable Cold Tablets and Liquid Cold Formula

DESCRIPTION

Each Children's Tylenol Cold Chewable Grape-Flavored Tablet contains acetaminophen 80 mg, chlorpheniramine maleate 0.5 mg and pseudoephedrine hydrochloride 7.5 mg. Children's Tylenol Cold Liquid Formula is grape flavored, and contains no alcohol. Each teaspoon (5 ml) contains acetaminophen 160 mg, chlorpheniramine maleate 1 mg, and pseudoephedrine hydrochloride 15 mg.

ACTIONS

Children's Tylenol Cold Chewable Tablets and Liquid combine the analgesic-antipyretic acetaminophen with the decongestant pseudoephedrine hydrochloride and the antihistamine chlorpheniramine maleate to help relieve nasal congestion, dry runny noses and prevent sneezing as well as to relieve the fever, aches, pains and general discomfort associated with colds and upper respiratory infections.

Acetaminophen is equal to aspirin in analgesic and antipyretic effectiveness and it is unlikely to produce the side effects often associated with aspirin or aspirin-containing products.

INDICATIONS

Provides fast, effective temporary relief of nasal congestion, runny nose, sneezing, minor aches and pains, headaches and fever due to the common cold, hay fever or other upper respiratory allergies.

USUAL DOSAGE

Administer to children under 6 years only on the advice of a physician. Children's Tylenol Cold Chewable Tablets: 2–5 years—2 tablets, 6–11 years—4 tablets. Children's Tylenol Cold Liquid Formula: 2–5 years—1 teaspoonful; 6–11 years—2 teaspoonsful. Measuring cup is provided and marked for accurate dosing.

Doses may be repeated every 4-6 hours as needed, not to exceed 4 doses in 24 hours.

Note: Since Children's Tylenol Cold Chewable Tablets and Liquid Formula are available without prescription, the following information appears on the package labels. The Warnings are identical for the two dosage forms except the Liquid Cold Formula does not contain the phenylketonurics statement since the product does not contain aspartame.

Warning: Do not use if carton is opened, or if printed plastic bottle wrap or printed foil inner seal is broken. **Keep this and all medication out of the reach of children. In case of accidental overdosage, contact a physician or poison control center immediately. Phenylketonurics: contains phenylalanine, 4 mg per tablet.** Do not exceed the recommended dosage because nervousness, dizziness or sleeplessness may occur. If fever persists for more than three days, or if symptoms do not improve or new ones occur within five days or are accompanied by high fever, consult a physician before continuing use. This preparation may cause drowsiness, or in some cases, excitability. Do not give this product to children who have heart disease, high blood pressure, thyroid disease, diabetes, glaucoma or asthma or are taking a prescription drug for high blood pressure or depression, except under the advice and supervision of a physician.

OVERDOSAGE

Acetaminophen in massive overdosage may cause hepatic toxicity in some patients. In adults and adolescents, hepatic toxicity has rarely been reported following ingestion of acute overdosage of less than 10 grams. Fatalities are infrequent (less than 3-4% of untreated cases) and have rarely been reported with overdoses of less than 15 grams. In children, an acute overdosage of less than 150 mg/kg has not been associated with hepatic toxicity.

Early symptoms following a potentially hepatotoxic overdose may include: nausea, vomiting, diaphoresis and general malaise. Clinical and laboratory evidence of hepatic toxicity may not be apparent until 48 to 72 hours postingestion.

In adults and adolescents, regardless of the quantity of acetaminophen reported to have been ingested, administer MUCOMYST® acetylcysteine immediately if 24 hours or less have elapsed from the reported time of ingestion. For

Continued on next page

McNeil Consumer—Cont.

full prescribing information, refer to the MUCOMYST package insert. Do not await the results of assays for acetaminophen level before initiating treatment with MUCOMYST acetylcysteine. The following additional procedures are recommended: The stomach should be emptied promptly by lavage or by induction of emesis with syrup of ipecac. A serum acetaminophen assay should be obtained as early as possible, but no sooner than four hours following ingestion. Liver function studies should be obtained initially and repeated at 24-hour intervals.

Serious toxicity or fatalities are extremely infrequent in children, possibly due to differences in the way they metabolize acetaminophen. In children, the maximum potential amount ingested can be more easily estimated. If more than 150 mg/kg or an unknown amount was ingested, obtain an acetaminophen plasma level. The acetaminophen plasma level should be obtained as soon as possible, but no sooner than 4 hours following the ingestion. Induce emesis using syrup of ipecac. If the plasma level is obtained and falls above the broken line on the acetaminophen overdose nomogram, the MUCOMYST acetylcysteine therapy should be initiated and continued for a full course of therapy. If acetaminophen plasma assay capability is not available, and the estimated acetaminophen ingestion exceeds 150 mg/kg, MUCOMYST acetylcysteine therapy should be initiated and continued for a full course of therapy.

For additional emergency information, call your regional poison center or call the Rocky Mountain Poison Center toll-free, (1-800-525-6115).

Chlorpheniramine toxicity should be treated as you would an antihistamine/anticholinergic overdose and is likely to be present within a few hours after acute ingestion.

Pseudoephedrine may produce central nervous system stimulation and sympathomimetic effects on the cardiovascular system which are likely to be manifested within a few hours following ingestion.

INACTIVE INGREDIENTS

Chewable Tablets—Aspartame, citric acid, ethylcellulose, flavors, magnesium stearate, mannitol, microcrystalline cellulose, pregelatinized starch, sucrose, Blue #1 and Red #7.

Liquid—Benzoic acid, citric acid, flavors, glycerin, malic acid, polyethylene glycol, propylene glycol, sodium benzoate, sorbitol, sucrose, purified water, Blue #1 and Red #40.

HOW SUPPLIED

Chewable Tablets (colored purple, scored, imprinted "Tylenol Cold") on one side and "TC" on opposite side—bottles of 24. Cold Formula—bottles (colored purple) of 4 fl. oz.

Shown in Product Identification Section, page 417

TYLENOL® Cold Medication   OTC
Liquid

DESCRIPTION

Each 30 ml (1 fl. oz.) contains acetaminophen 650 mg., chlorpheniramine maleate 4 mg., pseudoephedrine hydrochloride 60 mg., and dextromethorphan hydrobromide 30 mg. (alcohol 7%).

ACTIONS

TYLENOL Cold Medication Liquid contains a clinically proven analgesic-antipyretic, decongestant, cough suppressant and antihistamine. Acetaminophen produces analgesia by elevation of the pain threshold and antipyresis through action on the hypothalamic heat-regulating center. Acetaminophen component is equal to aspirin in analgesic and antipyretic effectiveness and it is unlikely to produce many of the side effects associated with aspirin and aspirin-containing products. Pseudoephedrine hydrochloride is a sympathomimetic amine which provides temporary relief of nasal congestion. Dextromethorphan is a cough suppressant which provides temporary relief of coughs due to minor throat irritations that may occur with the common cold. Chlorpheniramine is an antihistamine which helps provide temporary relief of runny nose, sneezing and watery and itchy eyes.

INDICATIONS

TYLENOL Cold Medication Liquid provides effective temporary relief of runny nose, sneezing, watery and itchy eyes, nasal congestion, coughing, and aches, pains and fevers due to a cold or "flu".

PRECAUTIONS

If a rare sensitivity reaction occurs, the drug should be stopped. Although pseudoephedrine is virtually without pressor effect in normotensive patients, it should be used with caution in hypertensives.

USUAL DOSAGE

Measuring cup is provided and marked for accurate dosing. Adults: 1 fluid ounce (2 tbsp.) every 6 hours as needed, not to exceed 4 doses in 24 hours. Children (6–12 yrs): ½ the

adult dose (1 tbsp.) as indicated on the measuring cup provided, not to exceed 4 doses in 24 hours for 5 days.

Note: Since TYLENOL Cold Medication Liquid is available without a prescription, the following appears on the package label: "WARNING: Do not administer to children under 6 or exceed the recommended dosage because nervousness, dizziness or sleeplessness may occur. May cause excitability especially in children. A persistent cough may be a sign of a serious condition. If fever persists for more than three days, or if symptoms do not improve or new ones occur within five days or are accompanied by high fever, rash, excessive mucus, persistent cough or headache, consult a physician before continuing use. This preparation may cause drowsiness; alcohol may increase the drowsiness effect. Avoid alcoholic beverages when taking this product. Use caution when driving a motor vehicle or operating machinery. Do not take this product if you have heart disease, high blood pressure, thyroid disease, diabetes, asthma, glaucoma, emphysema, chronic pulmonary disease, shortness of breath, difficulty in breathing, or difficulty in urination due to enlargement of the prostate gland or are taking a prescription drug for high blood pressure or depression, unless directed by a doctor. Do not use if carton is opened, or if printed plastic overwrap or printed foil inner seal is broken. Keep this and all medication out of the reach of children. As with any drug, if you are pregnant or nursing a baby, seek the advice of a health professional before using this product. In case of accidental overdosage, contact a physician or poison control center immediately."

OVERDOSAGE

Acetaminophen in massive overdosage may cause hepatic toxicity in some patients. In adults and adolescents, hepatic toxicity has rarely been reported following ingestion of acute overdosage of less than 10 grams. Fatalities are infrequent (less than 3–4% of untreated cases) and have rarely been reported with overdoses of less than 15 grams. In children, an acute overdosage of less than 150 mg/kg has not been associated with hepatic toxicity.

Early symptoms following a potentially hepatotoxic overdose may include: nausea, vomiting, diaphoresis and general malaise. Clinical and laboratory evidence of hepatic toxicity may not be apparent until 48 to 72 hours postingestion.

In adults and adolescents, regardless of the quantity of acetaminophen reported to have been ingested, administer MUCOMYST® acetylcysteine immediately if 24 hours or less have elapsed from the reported time of ingestion. For full prescribing information, refer to the MUCOMYST package insert. Do not await results of assays for acetaminophen level before initiating treatment with MUCOMYST acetylcysteine. The following additional procedures are recommended: The stomach should be emptied promptly by lavage or by induction of emesis with syrup of ipecac. A serum acetaminophen assay should be obtained as early as possible, but no sooner than four hours following ingestion. Liver function studies should be obtained initially and repeated at 24-hour intervals.

Serious toxicity or fatalities are extremely infrequent in children, possibly due to differences in the way they metabolize acetaminophen. In children, the maximum potential amount ingested can be more easily estimated. If more than 150 mg/kg or an unknown amount was ingested, obtain an acetaminophen plasma level. The acetaminophen plasma level should be obtained as soon as possible, but no sooner than 4 hours following the ingestion. Induce emesis using syrup of ipecac. If the plasma level is obtained and falls above the broken line on the acetaminophen overdose nomogram, the MUCOMYST acetylcysteine therapy should be initiated and continued for a full course of therapy. If acetaminophen plasma assay capability is not available, and the estimated acetaminophen ingestion exceeds 150 mg/kg, MUCOMYST acetylcysteine therapy should be initiated and continued for a full course of therapy.

For additional emergency information, call your regional poison center or call the Rocky Mountain Poison Center toll-free, (1-800-525-6115).

Chlorpheniramine toxicity should be treated as you would an antihistamine/anticholinergic overdose and is likely to be present within a few hours after acute ingestion.

Symptoms from pseudoephedrine overdose consist most often of mild anxiety, tachycardia and/or mild hypertension. Symptoms usually appear within 4 to 8 hours of ingestion and are transient, usually requiring no treatment.

Acute dextromethorphan overdose usually does not result in serious signs and symptoms unless massive amounts have been ingested. Signs and symptoms of a substantial overdose may include nausea and vomiting, visual disturbances, CNS disturbances, and urinary retention.

INACTIVE INGREDIENTS

Alcohol (7%), Citric Acid, Flavors, Glycerin, Liquid Polyethylene Glycol, Saccharin, Sodium Benzoate, Sorbitol, Sucrose, Purified Water, Yellow #6 (sunset yellow) and Blue #1.

HOW SUPPLIED

Cherry/mint mentholated flavored (colored amber) in 5 oz. bottles with child-resistant safety cap, special dosage cup

graded in ounces and tablespoons, and tamper-resistant packaging.

Shown in Product Identification Section, page 417

TYLENOL® Cold Medication   OTC
Tablets and Caplets

DESCRIPTION

Each TYLENOL Cold Tablet or Caplet contains acetaminophen 325 mg., chlorpheniramine maleate 2 mg., pseudoephedrine hydrochloride 30 mg. and dextromethorphan hydrobromide 15 mg.

ACTIONS

TYLENOL Cold Medication Tablets and Caplets contain a clinically proven analgesic-antipyretic, decongestant, cough suppressant and antihistamine. Acetaminophen produces analgesia by elevation of the pain threshold and antipyresis through action on the hypothalamic heat-regulating center. Acetaminophen is equal to aspirin in analgesic and antipyretic effectiveness and it is unlikely to produce many of the side effects associated with aspirin and aspirin-containing products. Pseudoephedrine hydrochloride is a sympathomimetic amine which provides temporary relief of nasal congestion. Dextromethorphan is a cough suppressant which provides temporary relief of coughs due to minor throat irritations that may occur with the common cold. Chlorpheniramine is an antihistamine which helps provide temporary relief of runny nose, sneezing and watery and itchy eyes.

INDICATIONS

TYLENOL Cold Medication provides effective temporary relief of runny nose, sneezing, watery and itchy eyes, nasal congestion, coughing, and aches, pains and fever due to a cold or "flu".

PRECAUTIONS

If a rare sensitivity reaction occurs, the drug should be stopped. Although pseudoephedrine is virtually without pressor effect in normotensive patients, it should be used with caution in hypertensives.

USUAL DOSAGE

Adults: Two tablets or caplets every 6 hours, not to exceed 8 tablets or caplets in 24 hours. Children (6–12 years): One caplet or tablet every 6 hours, not to exceed 4 tablets or caplets in 24 hours for 5 days.

Note: Since TYLENOL Cold Medication Tablets and Caplets are available without prescription, the following appears on the package label: "WARNING: Do not administer to children under 6 or exceed the recommended dosage because nervousness, dizziness or sleeplessness may occur. May cause excitability especially in children. A persistent cough may be a sign of a serious condition. If fever persists for more than three days, or if symptoms do not improve or new ones occur within five days or are accompanied by high fever, rash, excessive mucus, persistent cough or headache, consult a physician before continuing use. This preparation may cause drowsiness; alcohol may increase the drowsiness effect. Avoid alcoholic beverages when taking this product. Use caution when driving a motor vehicle or operating machinery. Do not take this product if you have heart disease, high blood pressure, thyroid disease, diabetes, asthma, glaucoma, emphysema, chronic pulmonary disease, shortness of breath, difficulty in breathing, or difficulty in urination due to enlargement of the prostate gland or are taking a prescription drug for high blood pressure or depression, unless directed by a doctor. Do not use if carton is opened, or if printed green neck wrap or printed foil inner seal is broken. Keep this and all medication out of the reach of children. As with any drug, if you are pregnant or nursing a baby, seek the advice of a health professional before using this product. In case of accidental overdosage, contact a physician or poison control center immediately."

OVERDOSAGE

Acetaminophen in massive overdosage may cause hepatic toxicity in some patients. In adults and adolescents, hepatic toxicity has rarely been reported following ingestion of acute overdosage of less than 10 grams. Fatalities are infrequent (less than 3–4% of untreated cases) and have rarely been reported with overdoses of less than 15 grams. In children, an acute overdosage of less than 150 mg/kg has not been associated with hepatic toxicity.

Early symptoms following a potentially hepatotoxic overdose may include: nausea, vomiting, diaphoresis and general malaise. Clinical and laboratory evidence of hepatic toxicity may not be apparent until 48 to 72 hours postingestion.

In adults and adolescents, regardless of the quantity of acetaminophen reported to have been ingested, administer MUCOMYST® acetylcysteine immediately if 24 hours or less have elapsed from the reported time of ingestion. For full prescribing information, refer to the MUCOMYST package insert. Do not await results of assays for acetaminophen level before initiating treatment with MUCOMYST acetylcysteine. The following additional procedures are recommended: The stomach should be emptied promptly by lavage or by induction of emesis with syrup of ipecac. A serum acetaminophen assay should be obtained as early as possible, but no sooner than four hours following ingestion. Liver function studies should be obtained initially and repeated at 24-hour intervals.

Serious toxicity or fatalities are extremely infrequent in children, possibly due to differences in the way they metabolize acetaminophen. In children, the maximum potential amount ingested can be more easily estimated. If more than 150 mg/kg or an unknown amount was ingested, obtain an acetaminophen plasma level. The acetaminophen plasma level should be obtained as soon as possible, but no sooner than 4 hours following the ingestion. Induce emesis using syrup of ipecac. If the plasma level is obtained and falls above the broken line on the acetaminophen overdose nomogram, the MUCOMYST acetylcysteine therapy should be initiated and continued for a full course of therapy. If acetaminophen plasma assay capability is not available, and the estimated acetaminophen ingestion exceeds 150 mg/kg, MUCOMYST acetylcysteine therapy should be initiated and continued for a full course of therapy.

For additional emergency information, call your regional poison center or call the Rocky Mountain Poison Center toll-free, (1-800-525-6115).

Chlorpheniramine toxicity should be treated as you would an antihistamine/anticholinergic overdose and is likely to be present within a few hours after acute ingestion.

Symptoms from pseudoephedrine overdose consist most often of mild anxiety, tachycardia and/or mild hypertension. Symptoms usually appear within 4 to 8 hours of ingestion and are transient, usually requiring no treatment.

Acute dextromethorphan overdose usually does not result in serious signs and symptoms unless massive amounts have been ingested. Signs and symptoms of a substantial overdose may include nausea and vomiting, visual disturbances, CNS disturbances, and urinary retention.

INACTIVE INGREDIENTS

Tablets: Cellulose, Starch, Magnesium Stearate, Yellow #6 and Yellow #10. Caplets: Cellulose, Glyceryl, Triacetate, Hydroxypropyl, Methylcellulose, Magnesium Stearate, Sodium Starch Glycolate, Starch, Titanium Dioxide, Blue #1 and Yellow #6 & #10.

HOW SUPPLIED

Tablets (colored yellow, imprinted "TYLENOL Cold")—blister packs of 24 and tamper-resistant bottles of 50. Caplets (light yellow, imprinted "TYLENOL Cold")—blister packs of 24 and tamper-resistant bottles of 50.

Shown in Product Identification Section, page 417

TYLENOL® Cold Medication   OTC
No Drowsiness Formula
Caplets

DESCRIPTION

Each TYLENOL Cold Medication No Drowsiness Formula Caplet contains acetaminophen 325 mg., pseudoephedrine hydrochloride 30 mg. and dextromethorphan hydrobromide 15 mg.

ACTIONS

TYLENOL Cold Medication No Drowsiness Formula Caplets contain a clinically proven analgesic-antipyretic, decongestant and cough suppressant. Acetaminophen produces analgesia by elevation of the pain threshold and antipyresis through action on the hypothalamic heat-regulating center. Acetaminophen is equal to aspirin in analgesic and antipyretic effectiveness and it is unlikely to produce many of the side effects associated with aspirin and aspirin-containing products. Pseudoephedrine hydrochloride is a sympathomimetic amine which provides temporary relief of nasal congestion. Dextromethorphan is a cough suppressant which provides temporary relief of coughs due to minor throat irritations that may occur with the common cold.

INDICATIONS

TYLENOL Cold Medication No Drowsiness Formula provides effective temporary relief of the nasal congestion, coughing, and aches, pains and fever due to a cold or "flu".

PRECAUTIONS

If a rare sensitivity reaction occurs, the drug should be stopped. Although pseudoephedrine is virtually without pressor effect in normotensive patients, it should be used with caution in hypertensives.

USUAL DOSAGE

Adults: Two caplets every 6 hours, not to exceed 8 caplets in 24 hours. Children (6–12 years): One caplet every 6 hours, not to exceed 4 tablets or caplets in 24 hours for 5 days.

Note: Since TYLENOL Cold Medication No Drowsiness Formula Caplets are available without prescription, the following appears on the package label: "WARNING: Do not administer to children under 6 or exceed the recommended dosage because nervousness, dizziness or sleeplessness may occur. May cause excitability especially in children. A persistent cough may be a sign of a serious condition. If fever persists for more than three days, or if symptoms do not im-

---

prove or new ones occur within five days or are accompanied by fever, rash, excessive mucus, persistent cough or headache, consult a physician before continuing use. Avoid alcoholic beverages when taking this product. Use caution when driving a motor vehicle or operating machinery. Do not take this product if you have heart disease, high blood pressure, thyroid disease, diabetes, asthma, glaucoma, emphysema, chronic pulmonary disease, shortness of breath, difficulty in breathing, or difficulty in urination due to enlargement of the prostate gland or are taking a prescription drug for high blood pressure or depression, unless directed by a doctor. Do not use if carton is opened, or if printed green neck wrap or printed foil inner seal is broken. Keep this and all medication out of the reach of children. As with any drug, if you are pregnant or nursing a baby, seek the advice of a health professional before using this product. In case of accidental overdosage, contact a physician or poison control center immediately."

OVERDOSAGE

Acetaminophen in massive overdosage may cause hepatic toxicity in some patients. In adults and adolescents, hepatic toxicity has rarely been reported following ingestion of acute overdosage of less than 10 grams. Fatalities are infrequent (less than 3–4% of untreated cases) and have rarely been reported with overdoses of less than 15 grams. In children, an acute overdosage of less than 150 mg/kg has not been associated with hepatic toxicity.

Early symptoms following a potentially hepatotoxic overdose may include: nausea, vomiting, diaphoresis and general malaise. Clinical and laboratory evidence of hepatic toxicity may not be apparent until 48 to 72 hours postingestion.

In adults and adolescents, regardless of the quantity of acetaminophen reported to have been ingested, administer MUCOMYST® acetylcysteine immediately if 24 hours or less have elapsed from the reported time of ingestion. For full prescribing information, refer to the MUCOMYST package insert. Do not await results of assays for acetaminophen level before initiating treatment with MUCOMYST acetylcysteine. The following additional procedures are recommended: The stomach should be emptied promptly by lavage or by induction of emesis with syrup of ipecac. A serum acetaminophen assay should be obtained as early as possible, but no sooner than four hours following ingestion. Liver function studies should be obtained initially and repeated at 24-hour intervals.

Serious toxicity or fatalities are extremely infrequent in children, possibly due to differences in the way they metabolize acetaminophen. In children, the maximum potential amount ingested can be more easily estimated. If more than 150 mg/kg or an unknown amount was ingested, obtain an acetaminophen plasma level. The acetaminophen plasma level should be obtained as soon as possible, but no sooner than 4 hours following the ingestion. Induce emesis using syrup of ipecac. If the plasma level is obtained and falls above the broken line on the acetaminophen overdose nomogram, the MUCOMYST acetylcysteine therapy should be initiated and continued for a full course of therapy. If acetaminophen plasma assay capability is not available, and the estimated acetaminophen ingestion exceeds 150 mg/kg, MUCOMYST acetylcysteine therapy should be initiated and continued for a full course of therapy.

For additional emergency information, call your regional poison center or call the Rocky Mountain Poison Center toll-free, (1-800-525-6115).

Symptoms from pseudoephedrine overdose consist most often of mild anxiety, tachycardia and/or mild hypertension. Symptoms usually appear within 4 to 8 hours of ingestion and are transient, usually requiring no treatment.

Acute dextromethorphan overdose usually does not result in serious signs and symptoms unless massive amounts have been ingested. Signs and symptoms of a substantial overdose may include nausea and vomiting, visual disturbances, CNS disturbances, and urinary retention.

INACTIVE INGREDIENTS

Cellulose, Glyceryl, Triacetate, Hydroxypropyl Methylcellulose, Magnesium Stearate, Sodium Starch Glycolate, Starch, Titanium Dioxide, Blue #1 and Yellow #10.

HOW SUPPLIED

Caplets (colored white, imprinted TYLENOL "cold")—blister packs of 24 and tamper-resistant bottles of 50.

Shown in Product Identification Section, page 417

Maximum-Strength   OTC
TYLENOL® Allergy Sinus Medication Caplets

DESCRIPTION

Each TYLENOL® Allergy Sinus Caplet contains acetaminophen 500 mg, chlorpheniramine maleate 2 mg, and pseudoephedrine hydrochloride 30 mg.

ACTIONS

TYLENOL® Allergy Sinus Caplets contain a clinically proven analgesic-antipyretic, decongestant, and antihistamine. Acetaminophen produces analgesia by elevation of the pain threshold and antipyresis through action on the hypothalamic heat-regulating center. Acetaminophen is equal to aspirin in analgesic and antipyretic effectiveness, and it is unlikely to produce many of the side effects associated with aspirin and aspirin-containing products. Pseudoephedrine hydrochloride is a sympathomimetic amine which provides temporary relief of nasal congestion. Chlorpheniramine is an antihistamine which helps provide temporary relief of runny nose, sneezing and watery and itchy eyes.

INDICATIONS

TYLENOL® Allergy Sinus provides effective temporary relief of these upper respiratory allergy, hayfever and sinusitis symptoms: sneezing, itchy, watery eyes, runny nose, itching of the nose or throat, nasal and sinus congestion and sinus pain and headaches.

PRECAUTIONS

If a rare sensitivity reaction occurs, the drug should be stopped. Although pseudoephedrine is virtually without pressor effect in normotensive patients, it should be used with caution in hypertensives.

USUAL DOSAGE

Adults: Two caplets every 6 hours, not to exceed 8 caplets in 24 hours.

NOTE: Since TYLENOL® Allergy Sinus Caplets are available without a prescription, the following appears on the package label: "WARNING: Do not administer to children under 12 or exceed the recommended dosage because nervousness, dizziness, or sleeplessness may occur. May cause excitability, especially in children. This preparation may cause drowsiness; alcohol may increase the drowsiness effect. Avoid alcoholic beverages when taking this product. Use caution when driving a motor vehicle or operating machinery. Do not take this product if you have heart disease, high blood pressure, thyroid disease, diabetes, asthma, glaucoma, emphysema, chronic pulmonary disease, shortness of breath, difficulty in breathing or difficulty in urination due to enlargement of prostate gland unless directed by a doctor. Do not take this product for more than 7 days. If symptoms do not improve or are accompanied by a high fever, consult a physician." **DO NOT USE IF CARTON IS OPEN OR IF A BLISTER UNIT IS BROKEN. KEEP THIS AND ALL MEDICATION OUT OF THE REACH OF CHILDREN. AS WITH ANY DRUG, IF YOU ARE PREGNANT OR NURSING A BABY, SEEK THE ADVICE OF A HEALTH PROFESSIONAL BEFORE USING THIS PRODUCT. IN THE CASE OF ACCIDENTAL OVERDOSE, CONTACT A PHYSICIAN OR POISON CONTROL CENTER IMMEDIATELY.**

DRUG INTERACTION PRECAUTION: Do not take this product if you are presently taking a prescription drug for high blood pressure or depression without first consulting your doctor.

OVERDOSAGE

Acetaminophen in massive overdosage may cause hepatic toxicity in some patients. In adults and adolescents, hepatic toxicity has rarely been reported following ingestion of acute overdosage of less than 10 grams. Fatalities are infrequent (less than 3–4% of untreated cases) and have rarely been reported with overdoses of less than 15 grams. In children, an acute overdosage of less than 150 mg/kg has not been associated with hepatic toxicity.

Early symptoms following a potentially hepatotoxic overdose may include: nausea, vomiting, diaphoresis and general malaise. Clinical and laboratory evidence of hepatic toxicity may not be apparent until 48 to 72 hours postingestion. In adults and adolescents, regardless of the quantity of acetaminophen reported to have been ingested, administer MUCOMYST® acetylcysteine immediately if 24 hours or less have elapsed from the reported time of ingestion. For full prescribing information, refer to the MUCOMYST package insert. Do not await results of assays for acetaminophen level before initiating treatment with MUCOMYST acetylcysteine. The following additional procedures are recommended: The stomach should be emptied promptly by lavage or by induction of emesis with syrup of ipecac. A serum acetaminophen assay should be obtained as early as possible, but no sooner than four hours following ingestion. Liver function studies should be obtained initially and repeated at 24-hour intervals.

Several toxicity or fatalities are extremely infrequent in children, possibly due to differences in the way they metabolize acetaminophen. In children, the maximum potential amount ingested can be easily estimated. If more than 150 mg/kg or an unknown amount was ingested, obtain an acetaminophen plasma level. The acetaminophen plasma level should be obtained as soon as possible, but no sooner than 4 hours following ingestion. Induce emesis using syrup of ipecac. If the plasma level is obtained and falls above the broken line on the acetaminophen overdose nomogram, the MUCOMYST acetylcysteine therapy should be initiated and continued for a full course of therapy. If acetaminophen plasma assay capability is not available, and the estimated acetami-

Continued on next page

McNeil Consumer—Cont.

nophen ingestion exceeds 150 mg/kg, MUCOMYST acetyl-cysteine therapy should be initiated and continued for a full course of therapy.

For additional emergency information, call your regional poison center or call the Rocky Mountain Poison Control Center toll-free, (1-800-525-6115).

Chlorpheniramine toxicity should be treated as you would an antihistamine/anticholinergic overdose and is likely to be present within a few hours after acute ingestion.

Symptoms from pseudoephedrine overdose consist most often of mild anxiety, tachycardia and/or hypertension. Symptoms usually appear within 4 to 8 hours of ingestion and are transient, usually requiring no treatment.

INACTIVE INGREDIENTS

cellulose, hydroxypropyl cellulose, hydroxypropyl methylcellulose, magnesium stearate, polyethylene glycol, sodium starch glycolate, starch, titanium dioxide, blue #1, yellow #6, yellow #10.

HOW SUPPLIED

Caplets: (dark · yellow, imprinted "TYLENOL Allergy Sinus")—Blister packs of 24 and tamper-resistant bottles of 50.

Shown in Product Identification Section, page 417

Maximum-Strength
TYLENOL® Sinus Medication   OTC
Tablets and Caplets

DESCRIPTION

Each Maximum-Strength TYLENOL® Sinus Medication tablet or caplet contains acetaminophen 500 mg and pseudo-ephedrine hydrochloride 30 mg.

ACTIONS

TYLENOL Sinus Medication contains a clinically proven analgesic-antipyretic and a decongestant. Maximum allowable non-prescription levels of acetaminophen and pseudo-ephedrine provide temporary relief of sinus headache and congestion. Acetaminophen is equal to aspirin in analgesic and antipyretic effectiveness and it is unlikely to produce many of the side effects associated with aspirin and aspirin-containing products.

Acetaminophen produces analgesia by elevation of the pain threshold and antipyresis through action on the hypothalamic heat-regulating center. Pseudoephedrine hydrochloride is a sympathomimetic amine which promotes sinus cavity drainage by reducing nasopharyngeal mucosal congestion.

INDICATIONS

Maximum-Strength TYLENOL Sinus Medication provides effective symptomatic relief from sinus headache pain and congestion. Maximum-Strength TYLENOL Sinus Medication is particularly well-suited in patients with aspirin allergy, hemostatic disturbances (including anticoagulant therapy), and bleeding diatheses (e.g. hemophilia) and upper gastrointestinal disease (e.g. ulcer, gastritis, hiatus hernia).

PRECAUTIONS

If a rare sensitivity occurs, the drug should be discontinued. Although pseudoephedrine is virtually without pressor effect in normotensive patients, it should be used with caution in hypertensives.

USUAL DOSAGE

Adult dosage: Two tablets or caplets every four to six hours. Do not exceed eight tablets or caplets in any 24 hour period. **Note:** Since TYLENOL Sinus Medication tablets and caplets are available without a prescription, the following appears on the package labels: "WARNING: Do not exceed the recommended dosage because at higher doses nervousness, dizziness, or sleeplessness may occur. Do not administer to children under 12. If you have high blood pressure, heart disease, diabetes, thyroid disease, difficulty in urination due to enlargement of the prostate gland, or are presently taking a prescription drug for the treatment of high blood pressure or depression, do not take except under the advice and supervision of a physician. Do not take this product for more than 7 days. If symptoms do not improve or are accompanied by high fever, consult a physician. **Do not use if carton is opened or if printed green neck wrap or printed foil inner seal is broken. Keep this and all medication out of the reach of children. As with any drug, if you are pregnant or nursing a baby, seek the advice of a health professional before using this product. In case of accidental overdosage, contact a physician or poison control center immediately.**

OVERDOSAGE

Acetaminophen in massive overdosage may cause hepatic toxicity in some patients. In adults and adolescents, hepatic toxicity has rarely been reported following ingestion of acute overdosage of less than 10 grams. Fatalities are infrequent (less than 3–4% of untreated cases) and have rarely been reported with overdoses of less than 15 grams. In children,

---

an acute overdosage of less than 150 mg/kg has not been associated with hepatic toxicity.

Early symptoms following a potentially hepatotoxic overdose may include: nausea, vomiting, diaphoresis and general malaise. Clinical and laboratory evidence of hepatic toxicity may not be apparent until 48 to 72 hours postingestion.

In adults and adolescents, regardless of the quantity of acetaminophen reported to have been ingested, administer MUCOMYST® acetylcysteine immediately if 24 hours or less have elapsed from the reported time of ingestion. For full prescribing information, refer to the MUCOMYST package insert. Do not await the results of assays for acetaminophen level before initiating treatment with MUCOMYST acetylcysteine. The following additional procedures are recommended: The stomach should be emptied promptly by lavage or by induction of emesis with syrup of ipecac. A serum acetaminophen assay should be obtained as early as possible, but no sooner than four hours following ingestion. Liver function studies should be obtained initially and repeated at 24-hour intervals.

Serious toxicity or fatalities are extremely infrequent in children, possibly due to differences in the way they metabolize acetaminophen. In children, the maximum potential amount ingested can be more easily estimated. If more than 150 mg/kg or an unknown amount was ingested, obtain an acetaminophen plasma level. The acetaminophen plasma level should be obtained as soon as possible, but no sooner than 4 hours following the ingestion. Induce emesis using syrup of ipecac. If the plasma level is obtained and falls above the broken line on the acetaminophen overdose nomogram, the MUCOMYST acetylcysteine therapy should be initiated and continued for a full course of therapy. If acetaminophen plasma assay capability is not available, and the estimated acetaminophen ingestion exceeds 150 mg/kg, MUCOMYST acetylcysteine therapy should be initiated and continued for a full course of therapy.

For additional emergency information, call your regional poison center or call the Rocky Mountain Poison Center toll-free, (1-800-525-6115).

Symptoms from pseudoephedrine overdose consist most often of mild anxiety, tachycardia and/or mild hypertension. Symptoms usually appear within 4 to 8 hours of ingestion and are transient, usually requiring no treatment.

INACTIVE INGREDIENTS

Caplets—Cellulose, Hydroxypropyl Methylcellulose, Magnesium Stearate, Polysorbate 80, Sodium Starch Glycolate, Starch, Titanium Dioxide, Blue #1, Red #40 and Yellow #10. Tablets—Cellulose, Magnesium Stearate, Sodium Lauryl Sulfate, Starch, Yellow #6 (Sunset Yellow), Yellow #10 and Blue #1.

HOW SUPPLIED

Tablets (colored light green, imprinted "Maximum-Strength TYLENOL Sinus")—tamper-resistant bottles of 24 and 50. Caplets (light green coating, printed "TYLENOL Sinus" in dark green) tamper resistant bottles of 24 and 50.

Shown in Product Identification Section, page 417

McNeil Pharmaceutical
McNEILAB, INC.
SPRING HOUSE, PA 19477

HALDOL® brand of haloperidol   ℞
[*hal 'dawl*]
Tablets/Concentrate/Injection
  ½ mg (1000's):
NSN 6505-01-153-3213
  1 mg (1000's):
NSN 6505-01-003-2415
  2 mg (1000's):
NSN 6505-00-876-7239
  5 mg (100's)
NSN 6505-01-153-3049
  5 mg (1000's):
NSN 6505-01-003-2416
  10 mg (100's):
NSN 6505-01-037-3145
  10 mg (1000's):
NSN 6505-01-003-2417
  20 mg (100's):
NSN 6505-01-134-8386
  Concentrate 4 oz:
NSN 6505-01-003-5341
  Concentrate 8 oz:
NSN 6505-01-259-2566
  Injection 1 mL:
NSN 6505-00-268-8530

DESCRIPTION

Haloperidol is the first of the butyrophenone series of major tranquilizers. The chemical designation is 4-[4-(p-chloro-

---

phenyl)-4- hydroxy-piperidino]-4'-fluorobutyrophenone and it has the following structural formula:

HALDOL haloperidol dosage forms include: tablets (½, 1*, 2, 5*, 10* and 20 mg); a concentrate with 2 mg per mL haloperidol (as the lactate); and a sterile parenteral form for intramuscular injection. The injection provides 5 mg haloperidol (as the lactate) with 1.8 mg methylparaben and 0.2 mg propylparaben per mL, and lactic acid for pH adjustment between 3.0–3.6.

Inactive ingredients: tablets—calcium phosphate, calcium stearate, corn starch, natural flavor—1 mg contains FD&C * Yellow No. 5*; 2 mg contains D&C Red No. 33 and FD&C Blue No. 2; 5 mg contains FD&C Blue No. 1 and FD&C Yellow No. 5*; 10 mg contains FD&C Blue No. 1 and FD&C Yellow No. 5*; and 20 mg contains FD&C Red No. 40; concentrate—lactic acid and methylparaben.

* See Precautions

ACTIONS

The precise mechanism of action has not been clearly established.

INDICATIONS

HALDOL haloperidol is indicated for use in the management of manifestations of psychotic disorders.

HALDOL is indicated for the control of tics and vocal utterances of Tourette's Disorder in children and adults.

HALDOL is effective for the treatment of severe behavior problems in children of combative, explosive hyperexcitability (which cannot be accounted for by immediate provocation). HALDOL is also effective in the short-term treatment of hyperactive children who show excessive motor activity with accompanying conduct disorders consisting of some or all of the following symptoms: impulsivity, difficulty sustaining attention, aggressivity, mood lability and poor frustration tolerance. HALDOL should be reserved for these two groups of children only after failure to respond to psychotherapy or medications other than antipsychotics.

CONTRAINDICATIONS

HALDOL haloperidol is contraindicated in severe toxic central nervous system depression or comatose states from any cause and in individuals who are hypersensitive to this drug or have Parkinson's disease.

WARNINGS

Tardive Dyskinesia—A syndrome consisting of potentially irreversible, involuntary, dyskinetic movements may develop in patients treated with antipsychotic drugs. Although the prevalence of the syndrome appears to be highest among the elderly, especially elderly women, it is impossible to rely upon prevalence estimates to predict, at the inception of antipsychotic treatment, which patients are likely to develop the syndrome. Whether antipsychotic drug products differ in their potential to cause tardive dyskinesia is unknown.

Both the risk of developing the syndrome and the likelihood that it will become irreversible are believed to increase as the duration of treatment and the total cumulative dose of antipsychotic drugs administered to the patient increase. However, the syndrome can develop, although much less commonly, after relatively brief treatment periods at low doses.

There is no known treatment for established cases of tardive dyskinesia, although the syndrome may remit, partially or completely, if antipsychotic treatment is withdrawn. Antipsychotic treatment, itself, however, may suppress (or partially suppress) the signs and symptoms of the syndrome and thereby may possibly mask the underlying process. The effect that symptomatic suppression has upon the long-term course of the syndrome is unknown.

Given these considerations, antipsychotic drugs should be prescribed in a manner that is most likely to minimize the occurrence of tardive dyskinesia. Chronic antipsychotic treatment should generally be reserved for patients who suffer from a chronic illness that, 1) is known to respond to antipsychotic drugs, and, 2) for whom alternative, equally effective, but potentially less harmful treatments are not available or appropriate. In patients who do require chronic treatment, the smallest dose and the shortest duration of treatment producing a satisfactory clinical response should be sought. The need for continued treatment should be reassessed periodically.

If signs and symptoms of tardive dyskinesia appear in a patient on antipsychotics, drug discontinuation should be considered. However, some patients may require treatment despite the presence of the syndrome. (For further information about the description of tardive dyskinesia and its clinical detection, please refer to ADVERSE REACTIONS.)

Neuroleptic Malignant Syndrome (NMS)—A potentially fatal symptom complex sometimes referred to as Neuroleptic Malignant Syndrome (NMS) has been reported in association with antipsychotic drugs. Clinical manifestations of NMS are hyperpyrexia, muscle rigidity, altered mental status (including catatonic signs) and evidence of autonomic instability (irregular pulse or blood pressure, tachycardia, diaphoresis, and cardiac dysrhythmias). Additional signs may include elevated creatine phosphokinase, myoglobinuria (rhabdomyolysis) and acute renal failure.

The diagnostic evaluation of patients with this syndrome is complicated. In arriving at a diagnosis, it is important to identify cases where the clinical presentation includes both serious medical illness (e.g., pneumonia, systemic infection, etc.) and untreated or inadequately treated extrapyramidal signs and symptoms (EPS). Other important considerations in the differential diagnosis include central anticholinergic toxicity, heat stroke, drug fever and primary central nervous system (CNS) pathology.

The management of NMS should include 1) immediate discontinuation of antipsychotic drugs and other drugs not essential to concurrent therapy, 2) intensive symptomatic treatment and medical monitoring, and 3) treatment of any concomitant serious medical problems for which specific treatments are available. There is no general agreement about specific pharmacological treatment regimens for uncomplicated NMS.

If a patient requires antipsychotic drug treatment after recovery from NMS, the potential reintroduction of drug therapy should be carefully considered. The patient should be carefully monitored, since recurrences of NMS have been reported.

Hyperpyrexia and heat stroke, not associated with the above symptom complex, have also been reported with HALDOL.

Usage in Pregnancy—Rodents given 2 to 20 times the usual maximum human dose of haloperidol by oral or parenteral routes showed an increase in incidence of resorption, reduced fertility, delayed delivery and pup mortality. No teratogenic effect has been reported in rats, rabbits or dogs at dosages within this range, but cleft palate has been observed in mice given 15 times the usual maximum human dose. Cleft palate in mice appears to be a non-specific response to stress or nutritional imbalance as well as to a variety of drugs, and there is no evidence to relate this phenomenon to predictable human risk for most of these agents.

There are no well controlled studies with HALDOL haloperidol in pregnant women. There are reports, however, of cases of limb malformations observed following maternal use of HALDOL along with other drugs which have suspected teratogenic potential during the first trimester of pregnancy. Causal relationships were not established in these cases. Since such experience does not exclude the possibility of fetal damage due to HALDOL, this drug should be used during pregnancy or in women likely to become pregnant only if the benefit clearly justifies a potential risk to the fetus. Infants should not be nursed during drug treatment.

Combined Use of HALDOL and Lithium—An encephalopathic syndrome (characterized by weakness, lethargy, fever, tremulousness and confusion, extrapyramidal symptoms, leukocytosis, elevated serum enzymes, BUN, and FBS) followed by irreversible brain damage has occurred in a few patients treated with lithium plus HALDOL. A causal relationship between these events and the concomitant administration of lithium and HALDOL has not been established; however, patients receiving such combined therapy should be monitored closely for early evidence of neurological toxicity and treatment discontinued promptly if such signs appear.

General—A number of cases of bronchopneumonia, some fatal, have followed the use of antipsychotic drugs, including HALDOL. It has been postulated that lethargy and decreased sensation of thirst due to central inhibition may lead to dehydration, hemoconcentration and reduced pulmonary ventilation. Therefore, if the above signs and symptoms appear, especially in the elderly, the physician should institute remedial therapy promptly.

Although not reported with HALDOL, decreased serum cholesterol and/or cutaneous and ocular changes have been reported in patients receiving chemically-related drugs.

HALDOL may impair the mental and/or physical abilities required for the performance of hazardous tasks such as operating machinery or driving a motor vehicle. The ambulatory patient should be warned accordingly.

The use of alcohol with this drug should be avoided due to possible additive effects and hypotension.

PRECAUTIONS

HALDOL haloperidol should be administered cautiously to patients:

— with severe cardiovascular disorders, because of the possibility of transient hypotension and/or precipitation of anginal pain. Should hypotension occur and a vasopressor be required, epinephrine should not be used since HALDOL may block its vasopressor activity and paradoxical further lowering of the blood pressure may oc-

cur. Instead, metaraminol, phenylephrine or norepinephrine should be used.

— receiving anticonvulsant medications, with a history of seizures or EEG abnormalities, because HALDOL may lower the convulsive threshold. If indicated, adequate anticonvulsant therapy should be concomitantly maintained.

— with known allergies, or with a history of allergic reactions to drugs.

— receiving anticoagulants, since an isolated instance of interference occurred with the effects of one anticoagulant (phenindione).

If concomitant antiparkinson medication is required, it may have to be continued after HALDOL is discontinued because of the difference in excretion rates. If both are discontinued simultaneously, extrapyramidal symptoms may occur. The physician should keep in mind the possible increase in intraocular pressure when anticholinergic drugs, including antiparkinson agents, are administered concomitantly with HALDOL.

As with other antipsychotic agents, it should be noted that HALDOL may be capable of potentiating CNS depressants such as anesthetics, opiates, and alcohol.

When HALDOL is used to control mania in cyclic disorders, there may be a rapid mood swing to depression.

Severe neurotoxicity (rigidity, inability to walk or talk) may occur in patients with thyrotoxicosis who are also receiving antipsychotic medication, including HALDOL.

Carcinogenicity studies using oral haloperidol were conducted in Wistar rats (dosed at up to 5 mg/kg daily for 24 months) and in Albino Swiss mice (dosed at up to 5 mg/kg daily for 18 months). In the rat study survival was less than optimal in all dose groups, reducing the number of rats at risk for developing tumors. However, although a relatively greater number of rats survived to the end of the study in high dose male and female groups, these animals did not have a greater incidence of tumors than control animals. Therefore, although not optimal, this study does suggest the absence of a haloperidol related increase in the incidence of neoplasia in rats at doses up to 20 times the usual daily human dose for chronic or resistant patients.

In female mice at 5 and 20 times the highest initial daily dose for chronic or resistant patients, there was a statistically significant increase in mammary gland neoplasia and total tumor incidence; at 20 times the same daily dose there was a statistically significant increase in pituitary gland neoplasia. In male mice, no statistically significant differences in incidences of total tumors or specific tumor types were noted.

Antipsychotic drugs elevate prolactin levels; the elevation persists during chronic administration. Tissue culture experiments indicate that approximately one-third of human breast cancers are prolactin dependent *in vitro*, a factor of potential importance if the prescription of these drugs is contemplated in a patient with a previously detected breast cancer. Although disturbances such as galactorrhea, amenorrhea, gynecomastia, and impotence have been reported, the clinical significance of elevated serum prolactin levels is unknown for most patients. An increase in mammary neoplasms has been found in rodents after chronic administration of antipsychotic drugs. Neither clinical studies nor epidemiologic studies conducted to date, however, have shown an association between chronic administration of these drugs and mammary tumorigenesis; the available evidence is considered too limited to be conclusive at this time.

FD&C Yellow No. 5 (tartrazine) may cause allergic-type reactions (including bronchial asthma) in certain susceptible individuals. Although the overall incidence of FD&C Yellow No. 5 (tartrazine) sensitivity in the general population is low, it is frequently seen in patients who also have aspirin hypersensitivity.

ADVERSE REACTIONS

CNS Effects:

Extrapyramidal Reactions—Neuromuscular (extrapyramidal) reactions during the administration of HALDOL haloperidol have been reported frequently, often during the first few days of treatment. In most patients, these reactions involved Parkinson-like symptoms which, when first observed, were usually mild to moderately severe and usually reversible. Other types of neuromuscular reactions (motor restlessness, dystonia, akathisia, hyperreflexia, opisthotonos, oculogyric crises) have been reported far less frequently, but were often more severe. Severe extrapyramidal reactions have been reported to occur at relatively low doses. Generally the occurrence and severity of most extrapyramidal symptoms are dose related since they occur at relatively high doses and have been shown to disappear or become less severe when the dose is reduced. Administration of antiparkinson drugs such as benztropine mesylate U.S.P. or trihexyphenidyl hydrochloride U.S.P. may be required for control of such reactions. It should be noted that persistent extrapyramidal reactions have been reported and that the drug may have to be discontinued in such cases.

Withdrawal Emergent Neurological Signs— Generally, patients receiving short term therapy experience no problems with abrupt discontinuation of antipsychotic drugs. How-

ever, some patients on maintenance treatment experience transient dyskinetic signs after abrupt withdrawal. In certain of these cases the dyskinetic movements are indistinguishable from the syndrome described below under "Tardive Dyskinesia" except for duration. It is not known whether gradual withdrawal of antipsychotic drugs will reduce the rate of occurrence of withdrawal emergent neurological signs but until further evidence becomes available, it seems reasonable to gradually withdraw use of HALDOL.

Tardive Dyskinesia—As with all antipsychotic agents HALDOL has been associated with persistent dyskinesias. Tardive dyskinesia, a syndrome consisting of potentially irreversible, involuntary, dyskinetic movements, may appear in some patients on long-term therapy or may occur after drug therapy has been discontinued. The risk appears to be greater in elderly patients on high-dose therapy, especially females. The symptoms are persistent and in some patients appear irreversible. The syndrome is characterized by rhythmical involuntary movements of tongue, face, mouth or jaw (e.g., protrusion of tongue, puffing of cheeks, puckering of mouth, chewing movements). Sometimes these may be accompanied by involuntary movements of extremities and the trunk.

There is no known effective treatment for tardive dyskinesia; antiparkinson agents usually do not alleviate the symptoms of this syndrome. It is suggested that all antipsychotic agents be discontinued if these symptoms appear. Should it be necessary to reinstitute treatment, or increase the dosage of the agent, or switch to a different antipsychotic agent, this syndrome may be masked.

It has been reported that fine vermicular movement of the tongue may be an early sign of tardive dyskinesia and if the medication is stopped at that time the full syndrome may not develop.

Tardive Dystonia—Tardive dystonia, not associated with the above syndrome, has also been reported. Tardive dystonia is characterized by delayed onset of choreic or dystonic movements, is often persistent, and has the potential of becoming irreversible.

Other CNS Effects—Insomnia, restlessness, anxiety, euphoria, agitation, drowsiness, depression, lethargy, headache, confusion, vertigo, grand mal seizures, exacerbation of psychotic symptoms including hallucinations, and catatonic-like behavorial states which may be responsive to drug withdrawal and/or treatment with anticholinergic drugs.

Body as a Whole: Neuroleptic malignant syndrome (NMS), hyperpyrexia and heat stroke have been reported with HALDOL. (See WARNINGS for further information concerning NMS.)

Cardiovascular Effects: Tachycardia, hypotension, hypertension and ECG changes.

Hematologic Effects: Reports have appeared citing the occurrence of mild and usually transient leukopenia and leukocytosis, minimal decreases in red blood cell counts, anemia, or a tendency toward lymphomonocytosis. Agranulocytosis has rarely been reported to have occurred with the use of HALDOL, and then only in association with other medication.

Liver Effects: Impaired liver function and/or jaundice have been reported.

Dermatologic Reactions: Maculopapular and acneiform skin reactions and isolated cases of photosensitivity and loss of hair.

Endocrine Disorders: Lactation, breast engorgement, mastalgia, menstrual irregularities, gynecomastia, impotence, increased libido, hyperglycemia, hypoglycemia and hyponatremia.

Gastrointestinal Effects: Anorexia, constipation, diarrhea, hypersalivation, dyspepsia, nausea and vomiting.

Autonomic Reactions: Dry mouth, blurred vision, urinary retention, diaphoresis and priapism.

Respiratory Effects: Laryngospasm, bronchospasm and increased depth of respiration.

Special Senses: Cataracts, retinopathy and visual disturbances.

Other: Cases of sudden and unexpected death have been reported in association with the administration of HALDOL. The nature of the evidence makes it impossible to determine definitively what role, if any, HALDOL played in the outcome of the reported cases. The possibility that HALDOL caused death cannot, of course, be excluded, but it is to be kept in mind that sudden and unexpected death may occur in psychotic patients when they go untreated or when they are treated with other antipsychotic drugs.

OVERDOSAGE

Manifestations—In general, the symptoms of overdosage would be an exaggeration of known pharmacologic effects and adverse reactions, the most prominent of which would

Continued on next page

Information on McNeil Pharmaceutical Products is based on labeling in effect in August, 1989.

McNeil Pharm.—Cont.

be: 1) severe extrapyramidal reactions, 2) hypotension, or 3) sedation. The patient would appear comatose with respiratory depression and hypotension which could be severe enough to produce a shock-like state. The extrapyramidal reaction would be manifest by muscular weakness or rigidity and a generalized or localized tremor as demonstrated by the akinetic or agitans types respectively. With accidental overdosage, hypertension rather than hypotension occurred in a two-year old child.

Treatment—Gastric lavage or induction of emesis should be carried out immediately followed by administration of activated charcoal. Since there is no specific antidote, treatment is primarily supportive. A patent airway must be established by use of an oropharyngeal airway or endotracheal tube or, in prolonged cases of coma, by tracheostomy. Respiratory depression may be counteracted by artificial respiration and mechanical respirators. Hypotension and circulatory collapse may be counteracted by use of intravenous fluids, plasma, or concentrated albumin, and vasopressor agents such as metaraminol, phenylephrine and norepinephrine. Epinephrine should not be used. In case of severe extrapyramidal reactions, antiparkinson medication should be administered.

DOSAGE AND ADMINISTRATION

There is considerable variation from patient to patient in the amount of medication required for treatment. As with all antipsychotic drugs, dosage should be individualized according to the needs and response of each patient. Dosage adjustments, either upward or downward, should be carried out as rapidly as practicable to achieve optimum therapeutic control.

To determine the initial dosage, consideration should be given to the patient's age, severity of illness, previous response to other antipsychotic drugs, and any concomitant medication or disease state. Children, debilitated or geriatric patients, as well as those with a history of adverse reactions to antipsychotic drugs, may require less HALDOL haloperidol. The optimal response in such patients is usually obtained with more gradual dosage adjustments and at lower dosage levels, as recommended below.

Clinical experience suggests the following recommendations:

Oral Administration
Initial Dosage Range
Adults

Moderate Symptomatology	0.5 mg to 2.0 mg b.i.d. or t.i.d.
Severe Symptomatology	3.0 mg to 5.0 mg b.i.d. or t.i.d.

To achieve prompt control, higher doses may be required in some cases.

Geriatric or Debilitated Patients	0.5 mg to 2.0 mg b.i.d. or t.i.d.
Chronic or Resistant Patients	3.0 mg to 5.0 mg b.i.d. or t.i.d.

Patients who remain severely disturbed or inadequately controlled may require dosage adjustment. Daily dosages up to 100 mg may be necessary in some cases to achieve an optimal response. Infrequently, HALDOL has been used in doses above 100 mg for severely resistant patients; however, the limited clinical usage has not demonstrated the safety of prolonged administration of such doses.

Children
The following recommendations apply to children between the ages of 3 and 12 years (weight range 15 to 40 kg). HALDOL is not intended for children under 3 years old. Therapy should begin at the lowest dose possible (0.5 mg per day). If required, the dose should be increased by an increment of 0.5 mg at 5 to 7 day intervals until the desired therapeutic effect is obtained. (See chart below).

The total dose may be divided, to be given b.i.d. or t.i.d.

Psychotic Disorders	0.05 mg/kg/day to 0.15 mg/kg/day
Non-Psychotic Behavior Disorders and Tourette's Disorder	0.05 mg/kg/day to 0.075 mg/kg/day

Severely disturbed psychotic children may require higher doses.
In severely disturbed, non-psychotic children or in hyperactive children with accompanying conduct disorders, who have failed to respond to psychotherapy or medications other than antipsychotics, it should be noted that since these behaviors may be short-lived, short-term administration of HALDOL may suffice. There is no evidence establishing a maximum effective dosage. There is little evidence that behavior improvement is further enhanced in dosages beyond 6 mg per day.

Maintenance Dosage
Upon achieving a satisfactory therapeutic response, dosage should then be gradually reduced to the lowest effective maintenance level.

Intramuscular Administration
Adults
Parenteral medication, administered intramuscularly in doses of 2 to 5 mg, is utilized for prompt control of the acutely agitated patient with moderately severe to very severe symptoms. Depending on the response of the patient, subsequent doses may be given, administered as often as every hour, although 4 to 8 hour intervals may be satisfactory.

Controlled trials to establish the safety and effectiveness of intramuscular administration in children have not been conducted.

Parenteral drug products should be inspected visually for particulate matter and discoloration prior to administration, whenever solution and container permit.

Switchover Procedure
The oral form should supplant the injectable as soon as practicable. In the absence of bioavailability studies establishing bioequivalence between these two dosage forms the following guidelines for dosage are suggested. For an initial approximation of the total daily dose required, the parenteral dose administered in the preceeding 24 hours may be used. Since this dose is only an initial estimate, it is recommended that careful monitoring of clinical signs and symptoms, including clinical efficacy, sedation, and adverse effects, be carried out periodically for the first several days following the initiation of switchover. In this way, dosage adjustments, either upward or downward, can be quickly accomplished. Depending on the patient's clinical status, the first oral dose should be given within 12–24 hours following the last parenteral dose.

HOW SUPPLIED

HALDOL* brand of haloperidol Tablets Scored, Imprinted "McNEIL" and "HALDOL"
[See table below].
HALDOL® brand of haloperidol Concentrate 2 mg per mL (as the lactate) Colorless, Odorless, and Tasteless Solution—NDC 0045-0250, bottles of 15 mL, 120 mL and 240 mL.

HALDOL® brand of haloperidol Injection 5 mg per mL (as the lactate)—NDC 0045-0255, units of 10 × 1 mL ampuls, 10 mL multiple-dose vial and units of 10 × 1 mL disposable Prefilled Syringe.

Dispense HALDOL haloperidol tablets and concentrate in a tight, light-resistant container as defined in the official compendium.

Revised 6/3/87

Shown in Product Identification Section, page 417

HALDOL® Decanoate ℞
[hal 'dawl dek "ah-nō 'āt]
(haloperidol) Decanoate Injection

PRODUCT OVERVIEW

KEY FACTS

HALDOL Decanoate is a long-acting injectable form of HALDOL. The basic effects of HALDOL Decanoate are those of HALDOL, with the exception of duration of action. HAL-

DOL Decanoate reaches peak plasma concentration about six days after administration, with an apparent half-life of about three weeks. The recommended interval between doses is four weeks.

MAJOR USES

HALDOL Decanoate is intended for use in the management of patients requiring prolonged parenteral antipsychotic therapy.

SAFETY INFORMATION

See complete safety information provided below.

PRESCRIBING INFORMATION

HALDOL® Decanoate ℞
[hal 'dawl dek "ah-nō 'āt]
(haloperidol) Decanoate Injection
NSN 6505-01-241-8602—1 mL Ampul
NSN 6505-01-293-5628—5 mL Vial

DESCRIPTION

HALDOL® (haloperidol) Decanoate is the decanoate ester of the butyrophenone, HALDOL haloperidol. It has a markedly extended duration of effect. It is available in sterile form for intramuscular injection. The structural formula of haloperidol decanoate, 4-(4-chlorophenyl)-1-[4-(4-fluorophenyl)-4-oxobutyl]-4 piperidinyl decanoate, is:

Haloperidol decanoate is almost insoluble in water (0.01 mg/mL), but is soluble in most organic solvents. Each mL contains 50 mg haloperidol (present as haloperidol decanoate 70.52 mg) in a sesame oil vehicle, with 1.2% (w/v) benzyl alcohol as a preservative.

CLINICAL PHARMACOLOGY

HALDOL (haloperidol) Decanoate is a long-acting form of HALDOL. The basic effects of HALDOL Decanoate are no different from those of HALDOL with the exception of duration of action. Haloperidol blocks the effects of dopamine and increases its turnover rate; however, the precise mechansim of action is unknown.

Administration of haloperidol decanoate in sesame oil results in slow and sustained release of haloperidol. The plasma concentrations of haloperidol gradually rise, reaching a peak at about 6 days after the injection, and falling thereafter, with an apparent half-life of about 3 weeks. Steady state plasma concentrations are achieved after the third or fourth dose. The relationship between dose of haloperidol decanoate and plasma haloperidol concentration is roughly linear for doses below 450 mg. It should be noted, however, that the pharmacokinetics of haloperidol decanoate following intramuscular injections can be quite variable between subjects.

INDICATIONS AND USAGE

HALDOL Decanoate is a long-acting parenteral antipsychotic drug intended for use in the management of patients requiring prolonged parenteral antipsychotic therapy (e.g., patients with chronic schizophrenia).

CONTRAINDICATIONS

Since the pharmacologic and clinical actions of HALDOL (haloperidol) Decanoate are attributed to HALDOL as the active medication, Contraindications, Warnings, and additional information are those of HALDOL, modified only to reflect the prolonged action.

HALDOL is contraindicated in severe toxic central nervous system depression or comatose states from any cause and in individuals who are hypersensitive to this drug or have Parkinson's disease.

WARNINGS

Tardive Dyskinesia—A syndrome consisting of potentially irreversible, involuntary, dyskinetic movements may develop in patients treated with antipsychotic drugs. Although the prevalence of the syndrome appears to be highest among the elderly, especially elderly women, it is impossible to rely upon prevalence estimates to predict, at the inception of antipsychotic treatment, which patients are likely to develop the syndrome. Whether antipsychotic drug products differ in their potential to cause tardive dyskinesia is unknown.

Both the risk of developing tardive dyskinesia and the likelihood that it will become irreversible are believed to increase as the duration of treatment and the total cumulative dose of antipsychotic drugs administered to the patient increase. However, the syndrome can develop, although much less commonly, after relatively brief treatment periods at low doses.

There is no known treatment for established cases of tardive dyskinesia, although the syndrome may remit, partially or

		Bottles Containing		Unit Dose Blister Pack		
		100	1000	10 × 10	31 × 32	10 × 32
½mg, white	NDC 0045-0240	x	x	x	x	
1mg, yellow	NDC 0045-0241	x	x	x	x	
2mg, pink	NDC 0045-0242	x	x	x	x	
5mg, green	NDC 0045-0245	x	x	x	x	
10mg, aqua	NDC 0045-0246	x		x	x	
20mg, salmon	NDC 0045-0248	x		x		x

completely, if antipsychotic treatment is withdrawn. Antipsychotic treatment, itself, however, may suppress (or partially suppress) the signs and symptoms of the syndrome and thereby may possibly mask the underlying process. The effect that symptomatic suppression has upon the long-term course of the syndrome is unknown.

Given these considerations, antipsychotic drugs should be prescribed in a manner that is most likely to minimize the occurrence of tardive dyskinesia. Chronic antipsychotic treatment should generally be reserved for patients who suffer from a chronic illness that 1) is known to respond to antipsychotic drugs, and 2) for whom alternative, equally effective, but potentially less harmful treatments are **not** available or appropriate. In patients who do require chronic treatment, the smallest dose and the shortest duration of treatment producing a satisfactory clinical response should be sought. The need for continued treatment should be reassessed periodically.

If signs and symptoms of tardive dyskinesia appear in a patient on antipsychotics, drug discontinuation should be considered. However, some patients may require treatment despite the presence of the syndrome. (For further information about the description of tardive dyskinesia and its clinical detection, please refer to ADVERSE REACTIONS.)

Neuroleptic Malignant Syndrome (NMS)—A potentially fatal symptom complex sometimes referred to as Neuroleptic Malignant Syndrome (NMS) has been reported in association with antipsychotic drugs. Clinical manifestations of NMS are hyperpyrexia, muscle rigidity, altered mental status (including catatonic signs) and evidence of autonomic instability (irregular pulse or blood pressure, tachycardia, diaphoresis, and cardiac dysrhythmias). Additional signs may include elevated creatine phosphokinase, myoglobinuria (rhabdomyolysis) and acute renal failure.

The diagnostic evaluation of patients with this syndrome is complicated. In arriving at a diagnosis, it is important to identify cases where the clinical presentation includes both serious medical illness (e.g., pneumonia, systemic infection, etc.) and untreated or inadequately treated extrapyramidal signs and symptoms (EPS). Other important considerations in the differential diagnosis include central anticholinergic toxicity, heat stroke, drug fever and primary central nervous system (CNS) pathology.

The management of NMS should include 1) immediate discontinuation of antipsychotic drugs and other drugs not essential to concurrent therapy, 2) intensive symptomatic treatment and medical monitoring, and 3) treatment of any concomitant serious medical problems for which specific treatments are available. There is no general agreement about specific pharmacological treatment regimens for uncomplicated NMS.

If a patient requires antipsychotic drug treatment after recovery from NMS, the potential reintroduction of drug therapy should be carefully considered. The patient should be carefully monitored, since recurrences of NMS have been reported.

Hyperpyrexia and heat stroke, not associated with the above symptom complex, have also been reported with HALDOL.

General—A number of cases of bronchopneumonia, some fatal, have followed the use of antipsychotic drugs, including HALDOL (haloperidol). It has been postulated that lethargy and decreased sensation of thirst due to central inhibition may lead to dehydration, hemoconcentration and reduced pulmonary ventilation. Therefore, if the above signs and symptoms appear, especially in the elderly, the physician should institute remedial therapy promptly.

Although not reported with HALDOL, decreased serum cholesterol and/or cutaneous and ocular changes have been reported in patients receiving chemically-related drugs.

PRECAUTIONS

HALDOL (haloperidol) Decanoate should be administered cautiously to patients:

—with severe cardiovascular disorders, because of the possibility of transient hypotension and/or precipitation of anginal pain. Should hypotension occur and a vasopressor be required, epinephrine should not be used since HALDOL may block its vasopressor activity, and paradoxical further lowering of the blood pressure may occur. Instead, metaraminol, phenylephrine or norepinephrine should be used.

—receiving anticonvulsant medications, with a history of seizures, or with EEG abnormalities, because HALDOL may lower the convulsive threshold. If indicated, adequate anticonvulsant therapy should be concomitantly maintained.

—with known allergies, or with a history of allergic reactions to drugs.

—receiving anticoagulants, since an isolated instance of interference occurred with the effects of one anticoagulant (phenindione).

If concomitant antiparkinson medication is required, it may have to be continued after HALDOL Decanoate is discontinued because of the prolonged action of HALDOL Decanoate. If both drugs are discontinued simultaneously, extrapyramidal symptoms may occur. The physician should keep in mind

the possible increase in intraocular pressure when anticholinergic drugs, including antiparkinson agents, are administered concomitantly with HALDOL Decanoate.

In patients with thyrotoxicosis who are also receiving antipsychotic medication, including HALDOL Decanoate, severe neurotoxicity (rigidity, inability to walk or talk) may occur.

When HALDOL is used to control mania in bipolar disorders, there may be a rapid mood swing to depression.

Information for Patients: HALDOL Decanoate may impair the mental and/or physical abilities required for the performance of hazardous tasks such as operating machinery or driving a motor vehicle. The ambulatory patient should be warned accordingly.

The use of alcohol with this drug should be avoided due to possible additive effects and hypotension.

Drug Interactions: An encephalopathic syndrome (characterized by weakness, lethargy, fever, tremulousness and confusion, extrapyramidal symptoms, leukocytosis, elevated serum enzymes, BUN, and FBS) followed by irreversible brain damage has occurred in a few patients treated with lithium plus HALDOL. A causal relationship between these events and the concomitant administration of lithium and HALDOL has not been established; however, patients receiving such combined therapy should be monitored closely for early evidence of neurological toxicity and treatment discontinued promptly if such signs appear.

As with other antipsychotic agents, it should be noted that HALDOL may be capable of potentiating CNS depressants such as anesthetics, opiates, and alcohol.

Carcinogenesis, Mutagenesis, and Impairment of Fertility: No mutagenic potential of haloperidol decanoate was found in the Ames Salmonella microsomal activation assay.

Carcinogenicity studies using oral haloperidol were conducted in Wistar rats (dosed at up to 5 mg/kg daily for 24 months) and in Albino Swiss mice (dosed at up to 5 mg/kg daily for 18 months). In the rat study survival was less than optimal in all dose groups, reducing the number of rats at risk for developing tumors. However, although a relatively greater number of rats survived to the end of the study in high dose male and female groups, these animals did not have a greater incidence of tumors than control animals. Therefore, although not optimal, this study does suggest the absence of a haloperidol related increase in the incidence of neoplasia in rats at doses up to 20 times the usual daily human dose for chronic or resistant patients.

In female mice at 5 and 20 times the highest initial daily dose for chronic or resistant patients, there was a statistically significant increase in mammary gland neoplasia and total tumor incidence; at 20 times the same daily dose there was a statistically significant increase in pituitary gland neoplasia. In male mice, no statistically significant differences in incidences of total tumors or specific tumor types were noted.

Antipsychotic drugs elevate prolactin levels; the elevation persists during chronic administration. Tissue culture experiments indicate that approximately one-third of human breast cancers are prolactin dependent *in vitro*, a factor of potential importance if the prescription of these drugs is contemplated in a patient with a previously detected breast cancer. Although disturbances such as galactorrhea, amenorrhea, gynecomastia, and impotence have been reported, the clinical significance of elevated serum prolactin levels is unknown for most patients.

An increase in mammary neoplasms has been found in rodents after chronic administration of antipsychotic drugs. Neither clinical studies nor epidemiologic studies conducted to date, however, have shown an association between chronic administration of these drugs and mammary tumorigenesis; the available evidence is considered too limited to be conclusive at this time.

Usage in Pregnancy: Pregnancy Category C. Rodents given up to 3 times the usual maximum human dose of haloperidol decanoate showed an increase in incidence of resorption, fetal mortality, and pup mortality. No fetal abnormalities were observed.

Cleft palate has been observed in mice given oral haloperidol at 15 times the usual maximum human dose. Cleft palate in mice appears to be a non-specific response to stress or nutritional imbalance as well as to a variety of drugs, and there is no evidence to relate this phenomenon to predictable human risk for most of these agents.

There are no adequate and well-controlled studies in pregnant women. There are reports, however, of cases of limb malformations observed following maternal use of HALDOL along with other drugs which have suspected teratogenic potential during the first trimester of pregnancy. Causal relationships were not established with these cases. Since such experience does not exclude the possibility of fetal damage due to HALDOL, HALDOL Decanoate should be used during pregnancy or in women likely to become pregnant only if the benefit clearly justifies a potential risk to the fetus.

Nursing Mothers: Since haloperidol is excreted in human breast milk, infants should not be nursed during drug treatment with HALDOL Decanoate.

Pediatric Use: Safety and effectiveness of HALDOL Decanoate in children have not been established.

ADVERSE REACTIONS

Adverse reactions following the administration of HALDOL (haloperidol) Decanoate are those of HALDOL. Since vast experience has accumulated with HALDOL, the adverse reactions are reported for that compound as well as for HALDOL Decanoate. As with all injectable medications, local tissue reactions have been reported with HALDOL Decanoate.

CNS Effects: *Extrapyramidal Reactions*—Neuromuscular (extrapyramidal) reactions during the administration of HALDOL have been reported frequently, often during the first few days of treatment. These have also been reported with HALDOL Decanoate. In most patients, these reactions involved Parkinson-like symptoms which, when first observed, were usually mild to moderately severe and usually reversible. Other types of neuromuscular reactions (motor restlessness, dystonia, akathisia, hyperreflexia, opisthotonos, oculogyric crises) have been reported far less frequently, but were often more severe. Severe extrapyramidal reactions have been reported to occur at relatively low doses. Generally the occurrence and severity of most extrapyramidal symptoms are dose-related since they occur at relatively high doses and have been shown to disappear or become less severe when the dose is reduced. Administration of antiparkinson drugs such as benztropine mesylate U.S.P. or trihexyphenidyl hydrochloride U.S.P. may be required for control of such reactions. It should be noted that persistent extrapyramidal reactions have been reported and that the drug may have to be discontinued in such cases.

Withdrawal Emergent Neurological Signs—Generally, patients receiving short term therapy experience no problems with abrupt discontinuation of antipsychotic drugs. However, some patients on maintenance treatment experience transient dyskinetic signs after abrupt withdrawal. In certain of these cases the dyskinetic movements are indistinguishable from the syndrome described below under "Tardive Dyskinesia" except for duration. Although the long acting properties of HALDOL Decanoate provide gradual withdrawal, it is not known whether gradual withdrawal of antipsychotic drugs will reduce the rate of occurrence of withdrawal emergent neurological signs.

Tardive Dyskinesia—As with all antipsychotic agents HALDOL has been associated with persistent dyskinesias. Tardive dyskinesia, a syndrome consisting of potentially irreversible, involuntary, dyskinetic movements, may appear in some patients on long-term therapy with HALDOL Decanoate or may occur after drug therapy has been discontinued. The risk appears to be greater in elderly patients on high-dose therapy, especially females. The symptoms are persistent and in some patients appear irreversible. The syndrome is characterized by rhythmical involuntary movements of tongue, face, mouth, or jaw (e.g., protrusion of tongue, puffing of cheeks, puckering of mouth, chewing movements). Sometimes these may be accompanied by involuntary movements of extremities and the trunk.

There is no known effective treatment for tardive dyskinesia; antiparkinson agents usually do not alleviate the symptoms of this syndrome. It is suggested that all antipsychotic agents be discontinued if these symptoms appear. Should it be necessary to reinstitute treatment, or increase the dosage of the agent, or switch to a different antipsychotic agent, this syndrome may be masked.

It has been reported that fine vermicular movement of the tongue may be an early sign of tardive dyskinesia and if the medication is stopped at that time the full syndrome may not develop.

Tardive Dystonia—Tardive dystonia, not associated with the above syndrome, has also been reported. Tardive dystonia is characterized by delayed onset of choreic or dystonic movements, is often persistent, and has the potential of becoming irreversible.

Other CNS effects—Insomnia, restlessness, anxiety, euphoria, agitation, drowsiness, depression, lethargy, headache, confusion, vertigo, grand mal seizures, exacerbation of psychotic symptoms including hallucinations, and catatonic-like behavioral states which may be responsive to drug withdrawal and/or treatment with anticholinergic drugs.

Body as a Whole: Neuroleptic malignant syndrome (NMS), hyperpyrexia and heat stroke have been reported with HALDOL. (See WARNINGS for further information concerning NMS.)

Cardiovascular Effects: Tachycardia, hypotension, hypertension and ECG changes.

Hematologic Effects: Reports have appeared citing the occurrence of mild and usually transient leukopenia and leukocytosis, minimal decreases in red blood cell counts, anemia, or a tendency toward lymphomonocytosis. Agranu-

Continued on next page

Information on McNeil Pharmaceutical Products is based on labeling in effect in August, 1989.

McNeil Pharm.—Cont.

locytosis has rarely been reported to have occurred with the use of HALDOL, and then only in association with other medication.

Liver Effects: Impaired liver function and/or jaundice have been reported.

Dermatologic Reactions: Maculopapular and acneiform skin reactions and isolated cases of photosensitivity and loss of hair.

Endocrine Disorders: Lactation, breast engorgement, mastalgia, menstrual irregularities, gynecomastia, impotence, increased libido, hyperglycemia, hypoglycemia and hyponatremia.

Gastrointestinal Effects: Anorexia, constipation, diarrhea, hypersalivation, dyspepsia, nausea and vomiting.

Autonomic Reactions: Dry mouth, blurred vision, urinary retention, diaphoresis and priapism.

Respiratory Effects: Laryngospasm, bronchospasm and increased depth of respiration.

Special Senses: Cataracts, retinopathy and visual disturbances.

Other: Cases of sudden and unexpected death have been reported in association with the administration of HALDOL. The nature of the evidence makes it impossible to determine definitively what role if any, HALDOL played in the outcome of the reported cases. The possibility that HALDOL caused death cannot, of course, be excluded, but it is to be kept in mind that sudden and unexpected death may occur in psychotic patients when they go untreated or when they are treated with other antipsychotic drugs.

OVERDOSAGE

While overdosage is less likely to occur with a parenteral than with an oral medication, information pertaining to HALDOL (haloperidol) is presented, modified only to reflect the extended duration of action of HALDOL Decanoate.

Manifestations—In general, the symptoms of overdosage would be an exaggeration of known pharmacologic effects and adverse reactions, the most prominent of which would be: 1) severe extrapyramidal reactions, 2) hypotension, or 3) sedation. The patient would appear comatose with respiratory depression and hypotension which could be severe enough to produce a shock-like state. The extrapyramidal reactions would be manifested by muscular weakness or rigidity and a generalized or localized tremor, as demonstrated by the akinetic or agitans types, respectively. With accidental overdosage, hypertension rather than hypotension occurred in a two-year old child.

Treatment—Since there is no specific antidote, treatment is primarily supportive. A patent airway must be established by use of an oropharyngeal airway or endotracheal tube or, in prolonged cases of coma, by tracheostomy. Respiratory depression may be counteracted by artificial respiration and mechanical respirators. Hypotension and circulatory collapse may be counteracted by use of intravenous fluids, plasma, or concentrated albumin, and vasopressor agents such as metaraminol, phenylephrine and norepinephrine. Epinephrine should not be used. In case of severe extrapyramidal reactions, antiparkinson medication should be administered, and should be continued for several weeks, and then withdrawn gradually as extrapyramidal symptoms may emerge.

DOSAGE AND ADMINISTRATION

HALDOL (haloperidol) Decanoate should be administered by deep intramuscular injection. A 21 gauge needle is recommended. The maximum volume per injection site should not exceed 3 mL. The recommended interval between doses is 4 weeks. DO NOT ADMINISTER INTRAVENOUSLY.

Parenteral drug products should be inspected visually for particulate matter and discoloration prior to administration, whenever solution and container permit.

HALDOL Decanoate is intended for use in chronic psychotic patients who require prolonged parenteral antipsychotic therapy. These patients should be previously stabilized on antipsychotic medication before considering a conversion to HALDOL Decanoate. Furthermore, it is recommended that patients being considered for HALDOL Decanoate therapy have been treated with, and tolerate well, short-acting HALDOL in order to exclude the possibility of an unexpected adverse sensitivity to haloperidol. Close clinical supervision is required during the initial period of dose adjustment in order to minimize the risk of overdosage or reappearance of psychotic symptoms before the next injection. During dose adjustment or episodes of exacerbation of psychotic symptoms, HALDOL Decanoate therapy can be supplemented with short-acting forms of haloperidol.

The dose of HALDOL Decanoate should be expressed in terms of its haloperidol content. The starting dose of HALDOL Decanoate should be based on the patient's clinical history, physical condition, and response to previous antipsychotic therapy. The preferred approach to determining the minimum effective dose is to begin with lower initial doses and to adjust the dose upward as needed. For patients previ-

ously maintained on low doses of antipsychotics (e.g. up to the equivalent of 10 mg/day oral haloperidol), it is recommended that the initial dose of HALDOL Decanoate be 10–15 times the previous daily dose in oral haloperidol equivalents; limited clinical experience suggests that lower initial doses may be adequate. The initial dose of HALDOL Decanoate should not exceed 100 mg, regardless of previous antipsychotic dose requirements. HALDOL Decanoate has been effectively administered at monthly intervals in several clinical studies. However, variation in patient response may dictate a need for adjustment of the dosing interval as well as the dose.

Lower initial doses and more gradual adjustment are recommended for elderly or debilitated patients.

Clinical experience with HALDOL Decanoate at doses greater than 300 mg per month has been limited.

HOW SUPPLIED

HALDOL® (haloperidol) Decanoate contains 50 mg haloperidol as 70.5 mg per mL haloperidol decanoate for IM use only. NDC 0045-0253, 10×1 mL ampuls, 3 × 1 mL ampuls and 5 mL multiple-dose vials.

Store at controlled room temperature (15°–30°C, 59°–86°F). Do not refrigerate or freeze.

Protect from light.

Revised 2/15/89

Shown in Product Identification Section, page 417

PANCREASE®   ℞
[pan'kre-ace]
(pancrelipase) Capsules
Enteric Coated Microspheres
NSN 6505-01-095-4174—100's
NSN 6505-01-077-2780—250's

DESCRIPTION

PANCREASE pancrelipase is a white, dye-free, orally administered capsule containing enteric coated microspheres of porcine pancreatic enzyme concentrate, predominately steapsin (pancreatic lipase), amylase and protease. Each capsule contains no less than:

Lipase	4,000 U.S.P. Units
Amylase	20,000 U.S.P. Units
Protease	25,000 U.S.P. Units

Inactive ingredients include cellulose acetate phthalate, diethyl phthalate, gelatin, povidone, sodium starch glycollate, corn starch, sugar, talc and titanium dioxide.

CLINICAL PHARMACOLOGY

PANCREASE pancrelipase capsules resist gastric inactivation and deliver predictable, high levels of biologically active enzymes into the duodenum. The enzymes catalyze the hydrolysis of fats into glycerol and fatty acids, protein into proteoses and derived substances, and starch into dextrins and sugars. PANCREASE capsules are effective in controlling steatorrhea and its consequences at low daily dosage levels.

INDICATIONS AND USAGE

PANCREASE pancrelipase capsules are indicated for patients with exocrine pancreatic enzyme deficiency as in but not limited to:

* cystic fibrosis
* chronic pancreatitis
* post-pancreatectomy
* post-gastrointestinal bypass surgery (e.g. Billroth II gastroenterostomy)
* ductal obstruction from neoplasm (e.g. of the pancreas or common bile duct).

CONTRAINDICATIONS

PANCREASE pancrelipase capsules are contraindicated in patients known to be hypersensitive to pork protein.

WARNINGS

Should hypersensitivity occur, discontinue medication and treat symptomatically.

PRECAUTIONS

TO PROTECT ENTERIC COATING, MICROSPHERES SHOULD NOT BE CRUSHED OR CHEWED.

Where swallowing of capsules is difficult, they may be opened and the microspheres shaken onto a small quantity of a soft food (e.g. applesauce, gelatin, etc.), which does not require chewing, and swallowed immediately. Contact of the microspheres with foods having a pH greater than 5.5 can dissolve the protective enteric shell.

Pregnancy Category C. Diethyl phthalate, an enteric coating component of PANCREASE pancrelipase capsules has been shown with high intraperitoneal dosing to be tetratogenic in rats. However, when this coating was administered orally to rats up to 100 times the human dose, no teratogenic or embryocidal effects were observed. There were no adequate and well-controlled studies in pregnant women. PANCREASE capsules should be used in pregnancy only if the potential benefit justifies the potential risk to the fetus.

ADVERSE REACTIONS

The most frequently reported adverse reactions to PANCREASE pancrelipase capsules are gastrointestinal in nature. Less frequently, allergic-type reactions have also been observed. Extremely high doses of exogenous pancreatic enzymes have been associated with hyperuricosuria and hyperuricemia.

DOSAGE AND ADMINISTRATION

Usual dosage: One or two capsules during each meal and one capsule with snacks. Occasionally a third capsule with meals may be required depending upon individual requirements for control of steatorrhea.

HOW SUPPLIED

PANCREASE® pancrelipase capsules (white, dye-free, imprinted "McNeil" and "Pancrease") in bottles of:

100	NDC 0045-0095-60
250	NDC 0045-0095-69

Keep bottle tightly closed. Store at controlled room temperature (15°–30°C, 59°–86°F), in a dry place. Do not refrigerate.

4/18/85

Shown in Product Identification Section, page 417

PANCREASE® MT   ℞
[pan'kre-ace MT]
(pancrelipase) Capsules
Enteric Coated Microtablets

PRODUCT OVERVIEW

KEY FACTS

Microtablet formulation allows for higher enzyme concentrations and smaller capsule size than the original PANCREASE capsules—more enzymatic activity per gram of protein. Enteric coating protects against gastric deactivation and allows delivery of predictable, high levels of biologically active enzymes into the duodenum. Available in three convenient capsule strengths for increased dosage flexibility.

MAJOR USES

PANCREASE MT capsules are indicated for patients with exocrine pancreatic enzyme deficiency.

SAFETY INFORMATION

See complete safety information provided below.

PRESCRIBING INFORMATION

PANCREASE® MT   ℞
[pan'kre-ace MT]
(pancrelipase) Capsules
Enteric Coated Microtablets

DESCRIPTION

PANCREASE MT pancrelipase capsules are orally administered capsules containing enteric coated microtablets of porcine pancreatic enzyme concentrate, predominately steapsin (pancreatic lipase), amylase and protease.

Each PANCREASE MT 4 capsule contains:

Lipase	4,000 U.S.P. Units
Amylase	12,000 U.S.P. Units
Protease	12,000 U.S.P. Units

Each PANCREASE MT 10 capsule contains:

Lipase	10,000 U.S.P. Units
Amylase	30,000 U.S.P. Units
Protease	30,000 U.S.P. Units

Each PANCREASE MT 16 capsule contains:

Lipase	16,000 U.S.P. Units
Amylase	48,000 U.S.P. Units
Protease	48,000 U.S.P. Units

Inactive ingredients: benzyl alcohol, cellulose, crospovidone, gelatin, iron oxide, magnesium stearate, methacrylic acid copolymer, methylparaben, polydimethylsiloxane, propylparaben, sodium lauryl sulfate, silicon dioxide, talc, titanium dioxide, triethylcitrate, wax and other trace ingredients.

CLINICAL PHARMACOLOGY

PANCREASE MT pancrelipase capsules resist gastric inactivation and deliver predictable, high levels of biologically active enzymes into the duodenum. The enzymes catalyze the hydrolysis of fats into glycerol and fatty acids, protein into proteoses and derived substances, and starch into dextrins and sugars. PANCREASE MT capsules are effective in controlling steatorrhea and its consequences.

INDICATIONS AND USAGE

PANCREASE MT pancrelipase capsules are indicated for patients with exocrine pancreatic enzyme deficiency such as:

* cystic fibrosis
* chronic pancreatitis
* post-pancreatectomy
* post-gastrointestinal bypass surgery (e.g. Billroth II gastroenterostomy)
* ductal obstruction from neoplasm (e.g. of the pancreas or common bile duct).

CONTRAINDICATIONS

PANCREASE MT pancrelipase capsules are contraindicated in patients known to be hypersensitive to pork protein. PANCREASE MT capsules are contraindicated in patients with acute pancreatitis or with acute exacerbations of chronic pancreatic diseases.

WARNINGS

Should hypersensitivity occur, discontinue medication and treat symptomatically.

PRECAUTIONS

General

TO PROTECT ENTERIC COATING, MICROTABLETS SHOULD NOT BE CRUSHED OR CHEWED. Where swallowing of capsules is difficult, they may be opened and the microtablets shaken onto a small quantity of a soft food (e.g. applesauce, gelatin, etc.), which does not require chewing, and swallowed immediately. Contact of the microtablets with foods having a pH greater than 6.0 can dissolve the protective enteric shell.

Pregnancy Category C. Animal reproduction studies have not been conducted with PANCREASE MT pancrelipase capsules. It is also not known whether PANCREASE MT can cause fetal harm when administered to a pregnant woman or can affect reproduction capacity. PANCREASE MT should be given to a pregnant woman only if clearly needed.

ADVERSE REACTIONS

The most frequently reported adverse reactions to pancrelipase-containing products are gastrointestinal in nature. Less frequently, allergic-type reactions have also been observed. Extremely high doses of exogenous pancreatic enzymes have been associated with hyperuricosuria and hyperuricemia when the preparations given were pancrelipase in powdered or capsule form, or pancreatin in tablet form.

DOSAGE AND ADMINISTRATION

Dosage should be adjusted according to the severity of the exocrine pancreatic enzyme deficiency. The number of capsules or capsule strength given with meals and/or snacks should be estimated by assessing which dose minimizes steatorrhea and maintains good nutritional status.

In some patients with pancreatic enzyme deficiency, satisfactory responses have been achieved with dosages (expressed in U.S.P. units of lipase) similar to the ones stated below. However, dosages should be adjusted according to the response of the patient.

Children 7 to 12 years: 4,000 to 12,000 units (more if necessary) with each meal and with snacks.

Children 1 to 6 years: 4,000 to 8,000 units with each meal and 4,000 units with snacks.

Children under 1 year: Dosage for children under 6 months of age has not been established. Children 6 months to 1 year have responded to 2,000 units of lipase per meal.

The assessment of the end points in children is aided by charting growth curves.

Adults: 4,000 to 16,000 units (more if necessary) with each meal and with snacks.

HOW SUPPLIED

PANCREASE® MT 4 pancrelipase capsules (yellow and clear, imprinted "McNEIL" and "PANCREASE MT 4") in bottles of 100—NDC 0045-0341-60.

PANCREASE® MT 10 pancrelipase capsules (pink and clear imprinted "McNEIL" and "PANCREASE MT 10") in bottles of 100—NDC 0045-0342-60.

PACREASE® MT 16 pancrelipase capsules (salmon and clear, imprinted "McNEIL" and "PANCREASE MT 16") in bottles of 100—NDC 0045-0343-60.

Keep bottle tightly closed. Store at controlled room temperature (15°–30°C, 59°–86°F), in a dry place. Do not refrigerate. Dispense in tight container as defined in the official compendium.

Microtablets manufactured by Nordmark Pharmaceutical, Uetersen, W. Germany.

Revised 4/20/88

Shown in Product Identification Section, page 417

PARAFLEX® (chlorzoxazone) Tablets   ℞
[par'a-flex]

DESCRIPTION

Each tablet contains chlorzoxazone* 250 mg.
*5-chlorobenzoxazolinone
Inactive ingredients: calcium phosphate, calcium stearate, corn starch, wheat gluten, FD&C Red No. 3 and FD&C Yellow No. 6.

ACTIONS

Chlorzoxazone is a centrally-acting agent for painful musculoskeletal conditions. Data available from animal experiments as well as human study indicate that chlorzoxazone acts primarily at the level of the spinal cord and subcortical areas of the brain where it inhibits multisynaptic reflex arcs involved in producing and maintaining skeletal muscle spasm of varied etiology. The clinical result is a reduction of the skeletal muscle spasm with relief of pain and increased mobility of the involved muscles. Blood levels of chlorzoxazone can be detected in people during the first 30 minutes and peak levels may be reached, in the majority of subjects, in about 1 to 2 hours after oral administration of PARAFLEX. Chlorzoxazone is rapidly metabolized and is excreted in the urine, primarily in a conjugated form as the glucuronide. Less than one percent of a dose of chlorzoxazone is excreted unchanged in the urine in 24 hours.

INDICATIONS

PARAFLEX chlorzoxazone is indicated as an adjunct to rest, physical therapy, and other measures for the relief of discomfort associated with acute, painful musculoskeletal conditions. The mode of action of this drug has not been clearly identified, but may be related to its sedative properties. Chlorzoxazone does not directly relax tense skeletal muscles in man.

CONTRAINDICATIONS

PARAFLEX chlorzoxazone is contraindicated in patients with known intolerance to the drug.

WARNINGS

The concomitant use of alcohol or other central nervous system depressants may have an additive effect.
Usage in Pregnancy: The safe use of PARAFLEX chlorzoxazone has not been established with respect to the possible adverse effects upon fetal development. Therefore, it should be used in women of childbearing potential only when, in the judgment of the physician, the potential benefits outweigh the possible risks.

PRECAUTIONS

PARAFLEX chlorzoxazone should be used with caution in patients with known allergies or with a history of allergic reactions to drugs. If a sensitivity reaction occurs such as urticaria, redness, or itching of the skin, the drug should be stopped.
If any symptoms suggestive of liver dysfunction are observed, the drug should be discontinued.

ADVERSE REACTIONS

After more than twenty-six years of extensive clinical use of PARAFLEX chlorzoxazone and other chlorzoxazone-containing products in an estimated thirty-two million patients, it is apparent that the drug is well tolerated and seldom produces undesirable side effects. Occasional patients may develop gastrointestinal disturbances. It is possible in rare instances that PARAFLEX chlorzoxazone may have been associated with gastrointestinal bleeding. Drowsiness, dizziness, lightheadedness, malaise, or overstimulation may be noted by an occasional patient. Rarely, allergic-type skin rashes, petechiae, or ecchymoses may develop during treatment. Angioneurotic edema or anaphylactic reactions are extremely rare. There is no evidence that the drug will cause renal damage. Rarely, a patient may note discoloration of the urine resulting from a phenolic metabolite of chlorzoxazone. This finding is of no known clinical significance.

Approximately thirty-six patients have been reported in whom the administration of PARAFLEX chlorzoxazone or other chlorzoxazone-containing products was suspected as being the cause of liver damage. In one case, the jaundice was subsequently considered to be due to a carcinoma of the head of the pancreas rather than to the drug. In a second case, there was no jaundice but an elevated alkaline phosphatase and BSP retention. In this patient there was a malignancy with bony and liver metastases. The role of the drug was difficult to determine. A third and fourth case had cholelithiasis. Diagnosis in a fifth case was submassive hepatic necrosis possibly due to abusive use of the drug for approximately one year. The remaining cases had a clinical picture compatible with either a viral hepatitis or a drug-induced hepatitis. In all these latter cases the drug was stopped, and, with one exception, the patients recovered. It is not possible to state that the hepatitis in these patients was or was not drug-induced.

DOSAGE AND ADMINISTRATION

Usual Adult Dosage: One tablet (250 mg) three or four times daily. Initial dosage for *painful musculoskeletal conditions* should be two tablets (500 mg) three or four times daily. If adequate response is not obtained with this dose, it may be increased to three tablets (750 mg) three or four times daily. As improvement occurs dosage can usually be reduced.

Usual Child's Dosage: One-half to two tablets (125 mg to 500 mg) three or four times daily given according to age and weight. The tablets may be crushed and mixed with food or a suitable vehicle for administration to children.

OVERDOSAGE

Symptoms: Initially, gastrointestinal disturbances such as nausea, vomiting, or diarrhea together with drowsiness, dizziness, lightheadedness or headache may occur. Early in the course there may be malaise or sluggishness followed by marked loss of muscle tone, making voluntary movement impossible. The deep tendon reflexes may be decreased or absent. The sensorium remains intact, and there is no peripheral loss of sensation. Respiratory depression may occur with rapid, irregular respiration and intercostal and substernal retraction. The blood pressure is lowered, but shock has not been observed.
Treatment: Gastric lavage or induction of emesis should be carried out, followed by administration of activated charcoal. Thereafter, treatment is entirely supportive. If respirations are depressed, oxygen and artificial respiration should be employed and a patent airway assured by use of an oropharyngeal airway or endotracheal tube. Hypotension may be counteracted by use of dextran, plasma, concentrated albumin or a vasopressor agent such as norepinephrine. Cholinergic drugs or analeptic drugs are of no value and should not be used.

HOW SUPPLIED

PARAFLEX® (chlorzoxazone) 250 mg tablets (colored orange, scored, imprinted "PARAFLEX" "McNeil") —bottles of 100 NDC 0045-0317-60.
Dispense in tight container as defined in the official compendium.

9/17/86

PARAFON FORTE™ DSC   ℞
[par'a-fahn for'ta]
(chlorzoxazone) Caplets 500 mg
NSN 6505-01-264-4453—100's

DESCRIPTION

Each caplet contains:
Chlorzoxazone* .... 500 mg
Inactive ingredients: FD&C Blue No. 1, microcrystalline cellulose, docusate sodium, lactose (hydrous), magnesium stearate, sodium benzoate, sodium starch glycolate, pregelatinized corn starch, D&C Yellow No. 10.
* 5-chlorobenzoxazolinone

ACTIONS

Chlorzoxazone is a centrally-acting agent for painful musculoskeletal conditions. Data available from animal experiments as well as human study indicate that chlorzoxazone acts primarily at the level of the spinal cord and subcortical areas of the brain where it inhibits multisynaptic reflex arcs involved in producing and maintaining skeletal muscle spasm of varied etiology. The clinical result is a reduction of the skeletal muscle spasm with relief of pain and increased mobility of the involved muscles. Blood levels of chlorzoxazone can be detected in people during the first 30 minutes and peak levels may be reached, in the majority of the subjects, in about 1 to 2 hours after oral administration of chlorzoxazone. Chlorzoxazone is rapidly metabolized and is excreted in the urine, primarily in a conjugated form as the glucuronide. Less than one percent of a dose of chlorzoxazone is excreted unchanged in the urine in 24 hours.

INDICATIONS

PARAFON FORTE DSC chlorzoxazone is indicated as an adjunct to rest, physical therapy, and other measures for the relief of discomfort associated with acute, painful musculoskeletal conditions. The mode of action of this drug has not been clearly identified, but may be related to its sedative properties. Chlorzoxazone does not directly relax tense skeletal muscles in man.

CONTRAINDICATIONS

PARAFON FORTE DSC chlorzoxazone is contraindicated in patients with known intolerance to the drug.

WARNINGS

The concomitant use of alcohol or other central nervous system depressants may have an additive effect.
Usage in Pregnancy: The safe use of PARAFON FORTE DSC chlorzoxazone has not been established with respect to the possible adverse effects upon fetal development. Therefore, it should be used in women of childbearing potential only when, in the judgment of the physician, the potential benefits outweigh the possible risks.

PRECAUTIONS

PARAFON FORTE DSC chlorzoxazone should be used with caution in patients with known allergies or with a history of allergic reactions to drugs. If a sensitivity reaction occurs such as urticaria, redness, or itching of the skin, the drug should be stopped.
If any signs or symptoms suggestive of liver dysfunction are observed, the drug should be discontinued.

ADVERSE REACTIONS

After more than twenty-six years of extensive clinical use of chlorzoxazone-containing products in an estimated thirty-two million patients, it is apparent that the drug is well tolerated and seldom produces undesirable side effects. Occasional patients may develop gastrointestinal disturbances. It

Continued on next page

Information on McNeil Pharmaceutical Products is based on labeling in effect in August, 1989.

McNeil Pharm.—Cont.

is possible in rare instances that chlorzoxazone may have been associated with gastrointestinal bleeding. Drowsiness, dizziness, lightheadedness, malaise, or overstimulation may be noted by an occasional patient. Rarely, allergic-type skin rashes, petechiae, or ecchymoses may develop during treatment. Angioneurotic edema or anaphylactic reactions are extremely rare. There is no evidence that the drug will cause renal damage. Rarely, a patient may note discoloration of the urine resulting from a phenolic metabolite of chlorzoxazone. This finding is of no known clinical significance.

Approximately thirty-six patients have been reported in whom the administration of chlorzoxazone-containing products was suspected as being the cause of liver damage. In one case, the jaundice was subsequently considered to be due to a carcinoma of the head of the pancreas rather than to the drug. In a second case, there was no jaundice but an elevated alkaline phosphatase and BSP retention. In this patient there was a malignancy with bony and liver metastases. The role of the drug was difficult to determine. A third and fourth case had cholelithiasis. Diagnosis in a fifth case was submassive hepatic necrosis possibly due to abusive use of the drug for approximately one year. The remaining cases had a clinical picture compatible with either a viral hepatitis or a drug-induced hepatitis. In all these latter cases, the drug was stopped, and, with one exception, the patients recovered. It is not possible to state that the hepatitis in these patients was or was not drug-induced.

DOSAGE AND ADMINISTRATION

Usual Adult Dosage: One caplet three or four times daily. If adquate reponse is not obtained with this dose, it may be increased to 1½ caplets (750 mg) three or four times daily. As improvement occurs dosage can usually be reduced.

OVERDOSE

Symptoms: Initially, gastrointestinal disturbances such as nausea, vomiting, or diarrhea together with drowsiness, dizziness, lightheadedness or headache may occur. Early in the course there may be malaise or sluggishness followed by marked loss of muscle tone, making voluntary movement impossible. The deep tendon reflexes may be decreased or absent. The sensorium remains intact, and there is no peripheral loss of sensation. Respiratory depression may occur with rapid, irregular respiration and intercostal and substernal retraction. The blood pressure is lowered, but shock has not been observed.

Treatment: Gastric lavage or induction of emesis should be carried out, followed by administration of activated charcoal. Thereafter, treatment is entirely supportive. If respirations are depressed, oxygen and artificial respiration should be employed and a patent airway assured by use of an oropharyngeal airway or endotracheal tube. Hypotension may be counteracted by use of dextran, plasma, concentrated albumin or a vasopressor agent such as norepinephrine. Cholinergic drugs or analeptic drugs are of no value and should not be used.

HOW SUPPLIED

PARAFON FORTE™ DSC (chlorzoxazone) 500 mg caplets, (capsule shaped tablet, colored light green, imprinted "PARAFON FORTE DSC" and "McNEIL", scored).
NDC 0045-0325, bottles of 100, 500 and unit dose 100's. Dispense in a tight container as defined in the official compendium.
Store at room temperature.

Revised 12/20/88
Shown in Product Identification Section, page 417

TOLECTIN® 600 (tolmetin sodium) ℞
[*to-lek 'tin*]
  600 mg Tablets
TOLECTIN® DS (tolmetin sodium)
  400 mg Capsules
TOLECTIN® 200 (tolmetin sodium)
  200 mg Tablets

PRODUCT OVERVIEW

KEY FACTS

TOLECTIN is rapidly and almost completely absorbed with peak plasma levels being reached within 30–60 minutes. A therapeutic response to TOLECTIN can be expected in a few days to a week. TOLECTIN displays a biphasic elimination from the plasma consisting of a rapid phase with a half-life of one to 2 hours followed by a slower phase with a half-life of about 5 hours. Essentially all of the dose is recovered in the urine in 24 hours.

MAJOR USES

TOLECTIN is indicated for the relief of signs and symptoms of rheumatoid arthritis, osteoarthritis and juvenile rheumatoid arthritis.

SAFETY INFORMATION
See complete safety information provided below.

PRESCRIBING INFORMATION

TOLECTIN® 600 (tolmetin sodium) ℞
[*to-lek 'tin*]
  600 mg Tablets
TOLECTIN® DS (tolmetin sodium)
  400 mg Capsules
  NSN 6505-01-091-9624—100's
TOLECTIN® 200 (tolmetin sodium)
  200 mg Tablets
  NSN 6505-01-038-7460—100's

DESCRIPTION

TOLECTIN 200 (tolmetin sodium) tablets for oral administration contain tolmetin sodium as the dihydrate in an amount equivalent to 200 mg of tolmetin (scored for 100 mg). Each tablet contains 18 mg (0.784 mEq) of sodium and the following inactive ingredients: cellulose, magnesium sterate, silicon dioxide, corn starch and talc.

TOLECTIN DS (tolmetin sodium) capsules for oral administration contain tolmetin sodium as the dihydrate in an amount equivalent to 400 mg of tolmetin. Each capsule contains 36 mg (1.568 mEq) of sodium and the following inactive ingredients: gelatin, magnesium stearate, corn starch, talc, FD&C Red No. 3, FD&C Yellow No. 6 and titanium dioxide.

TOLECTIN 600 (tolmetin sodium) tablets for oral administration contain tolmetin sodium as the dihydrate in an amount equivalent to 600 mg of tolmetin. Each tablet contains 54 mg (2.35 mEq) of sodium and the following inactive ingredients: cellulose, silicon dioxide, crospovidone, hydroxypropyl methyl cellulose, magnesium stearate, polyethylene glycol, corn starch, titanium dioxide, FD&C Yellow No. 6 and D&C Yellow No. 10.

The pKa of tolmetin is 3.5 and tolmetin sodium is freely soluble in water.
Tolmetin sodium is a nonsteroidal anti-inflammatory agent. The structural formula is:

Sodium 1-methyl-5-(4-methylbenzoyl)-1*H*-pyrrole-2-acetate dihydrate.

CLINICAL PHARMACOLOGY

Studies in animals have shown TOLECTIN (tolmetin sodium) to possess anti-inflammatory, analgesic and antipyretic activity. In the rat, TOLECTIN prevents the development of experimentally induced polyarthritis and also decreases established inflammation.

The mode of action of TOLECTIN is not known. However, studies in laboratory animals and man have demonstrated that the anti-inflammatory action of TOLECTIN is *not* due to pituitary-adrenal stimulation. TOLECTIN inhibits prostaglandin synthetase *in vitro* and lowers the plasma level of prostaglandin E in man. This reduction in prostaglandin synthesis may be responsible for the anti-inflammatory action. TOLECTIN does not appear to alter the course of the underlying disease in man.

In patients with rheumatoid arthritis and in normal volunteers, tolmetin sodium is rapidly and almost completely absorbed with peak plasma levels being reached within 30–60 minutes after an oral therapeutic dose. In controlled studies, the time to reach peak tolmetin plasma concentration is approximately 20 minutes longer following administration of a 600 mg tablet, compared to an equivalent dose given as 200 mg tablets. The clinical meaningfulness of this finding, if any, is unknown. Tolmetin displays a biphasic elimination from the plasma consisting of a rapid phase with a half-life of one to 2 hours followed by a slower phase with a half-life of about 5 hours. Peak plasma levels of approximately 40 µg/mL are obtained with a 400 mg oral dose. Essentially all of the administered dose is recovered in the urine in 24 hours either as an inactive oxidative metabolite or as conjugates of tolmetin. An 18-day multiple dose study demonstrated no accumulation of tolmetin when compared with a single dose.

In two fecal blood loss studies of 4 to 6 days duration involving 15 subjects each, TOLECTIN did not induce an increase in blood loss over that observed during a 4-day drug-free control period. In the same studies, aspirin produced a greater blood loss than occurred during the drug-free control period, and a greater blood loss than occurred during the TOLECTIN treatment period. In one of the two studies, indomethacin produced a greater fecal blood loss than occurred during the drug free control period; in the second study, indomethacin did not induce a significant increase in blood loss.

TOLECTIN is effectve in treating both the acute flares and in the long term management of the symptoms of rheumatoid arthritis, osteoarthritis and juvenile rheumatoid arthritis.

In patients with either rheumatoid arthritis or osteoarthritis, TOLECTIN is as effective as aspirin and indomethacin in controlling disease activity, but the frequency of the milder gastrointestinal adverse effects and tinnitus was less than in aspirin-treated patients, and the incidence of central nervous system adverse effects was less than in indomethacin-treated patients.

In patients with juvenile rheumatoid arthritis, TOLECTIN is as effective as aspirin in controlling disease activity, with a similar incidence of adverse reactions. Mean SGOT values, initially elevated in patients on previous aspirin therapy, remained elevated in the aspirin group and decreased in the TOLECTIN group.

TOLECTIN has produced additional therapeutic benefit when added to a regimen of gold salts and, to a lesser extent, with corticosteroids. TOLECTIN should not be used in conjunction with salicylates since greater benefit from the combination is not likely, but the potential for adverse reactions is increased.

INDICATIONS AND USAGE

TOLECTIN (tolmetin sodium) is indicated for the relief of signs and symptoms of rheumatoid arthritis and osteoarthritis. TOLECTIN is indicated in the treatment of acute flares and the long-term management of the chronic disease.

TOLECTIN is also indicated for treatment of juvenile rheumatoid arthritis. The safety and effectiveness of TOLECTIN have not been established in children under 2 years of age (see PRECAUTIONS—Pediatric Use and DOSAGE AND ADMINISTRATION).

CONTRAINDICATIONS

Anaphylactoid reactions have been reported with TOLECTIN as with other nonsteroidal anti-inflammatory drugs. Because of the possibility of cross-sensitivity to other nonsteroidal anti-inflammatory drugs, particularly zomepirac sodium, anaphylactoid reactions may be more likely to occur in patients who have exhibited allergic reactions to these compounds. For this reason, TOLECTIN should not be given to patients in whom aspirin and other nonsteroidal anti-inflammatory drugs induce symptoms of asthma, rhinitis, urticaria and other symptoms of allergic or anaphylactoid reactions. Patients experiencing anaphylactoid reactions on TOLECTIN should be treated with conventional therapy, such as epinephrine, antihistamines and/or steroids.

WARNINGS

Risk of GI Ulceration, Bleeding and Perforation with NSAID Therapy:

Serious gastrointestinal toxicity such as bleeding, ulceration, and perforation, can occur at any time, with or without symptoms, in patients treated chronically with NSAID (Nonsteroidal Anti-Inflammatory Drug) therapy. Although minor upper gastrointestinal problems, such as dyspepsia, are common, usually developng early in therapy, physicians should remain alert for ulceration and bleeding in patients treated chronically with NSAID's even in the absence of previous GI tract symptoms. In patients observed in clinical trials of several months to two years duration, symptomatic upper GI ulcers, gross bleeding or perforation appear to occur in approximately 1% of patients treated for 3–6 months, and in about 2–4% of patients treated for one year. Physicians should inform patients about the signs and/or symptoms of serious GI toxicity and what steps to take if they occur.

Studies to date have not identified any subset of patients not at risk of developing peptic ulceration and bleeding. Except for a prior history of serious GI events and other risk factors known to be associated with peptic ulcer disease, such as alcoholism, smoking, etc., no risk factor (e.g., age, sex) have been associated with increased risk. Elderly or debilitated patients seem to tolerate ulceration or bleeding less well than other individuals and most spontaneous reports of fatal GI events are in this population. Studies to date are inconclusive concerning the relative risk of various NSAID's in causing such reactions. High doses of any NSAID probably carry a greater risk of these reactions, although controlled clinical trials showing this do not exist in most cases. In considering the use of relatively large doses (within the recommended dosage range), sufficient benefit should be anticipated to offset the potential increased risk of GI toxicity.

PRECAUTIONS

General

Because of ocular changes observed in animals and reports of adverse eye findings with nonsteroidal anti-inflammatory agents, it is recommended that patients who develop visual disturbances during treatment with TOLECTIN have ophthalmologic evaluations.

As with other nonsteroidal anti-inflammatory drugs, long-term administration of tolmetin to animals has resulted in renal papillary necrosis and other abnormal renal pathology. In humans, there have been reports of acute interstitial nephritis with hematuria, proteinuria, and occasionally nephrotic syndrome.

A second form of renal toxicity has been seen in patients with prerenal conditions leading to a reduction in renal blood flow or blood volume, where the renal prostaglandins have a supportive role in the maintenance of renal perfusion. In these patients administration of an NSAID may cause a dose dependent reduction in prostaglandin formation and may precipitate overt renal decompensation. Patients at greatest risk of this reaction are those with heart failure, liver dysfunction, those taking diuretics, and the elderly. Discontinuation of NSAID therapy is typically followed by recovery to the pretreatment state.

Since TOLECTIN and its metabolites are eliminated primarily by the kidneys, patients with impaired renal function should be closely monitored, and it should be anticipated that they will require lower doses.

TOLECTIN prolongs bleeding time. Patients who may be adversely affected by prolongation of bleeding time should be carefully observed when TOLECTIN is administered.

In patients receiving concomitant TOLECTIN-steroid therapy, any reduction in steroid dosage should be gradual to avoid the possible complications of sudden steroid withdrawal.

Peripheral edema has been reported in some patients receiving TOLECTIN therapy. Therefore, as with other nonsteroidal anti-inflammatory drugs, TOLECTIN should be used with caution in patients with compromised cardiac function, hypertension, or other conditions predisposing to fluid retention.

The antipyretic and anti-inflammatory activities of the drug may reduce fever and inflammation, thus diminishing their utility as diagnostic signs in detecting complications of presumed non-infectious, non-inflammatory painful conditions. As with other nonsteroidal anti-inflammatory drugs, borderline elevations of one or more liver tests may occur in up to 15% of patients. These abnormalities may progress, may remain essentially unchanged, or may be transient with continued therapy. The SGPT (ALT) test is probably the most sensitive indicator of liver dysfunction. Meaningful (3 times the upper limit of normal) elevations of SGPT or SGOT (AST) occurred in controlled clinical trials in less than 1% of patients. A patient with symptoms and/or signs suggesting liver dysfunction, or in whom an abnormal liver test has occurred, should be evaluated for evidence of the development of more severe hepatic reaction while on therapy with TOLECTIN. Severe hepatic reactions, including jaundice and fatal hepatitis, have been reported with TOLECTIN as with other nonsteroidal anti-inflammatory drugs. Although such reactions are rare, if abnormal liver tests persist or worsen, if clinical signs and symptoms consistent with liver disease develop, or if systemic manifestations occur (e.g. eosinophilia, rash, etc.), TOLECTIN should be discontinued.

Carcinogenesis, Mutagenesis, Impairment of Fertility
Tolmetin sodium did not possess any carcinogenic liability in the following long-term studies: a 24-month study in rats at doses as high as 75 mg/kg/day, and an 18-month study in mice at doses as high as 50 mg/kg/day.

No mutagenic potential of tolmetin sodium was found in the Ames Salmonella-Microsomal Activation Test.

Reproductive studies revealed no impairment of fertility in animals. Effects on parturition have been shown, however, as with other prostaglandin inhibitors. This information is detailed in the Pregnancy section below.

Pregnancy
Pregnancy Category C. Reproduction studies in rats and rabbits at doses up to 50 mg/kg (1.5 times the maximum clinical dose based on a body weight of 60 kg) revealed no evidence of teratogenesis or impaired fertility due to TOLECTIN. However, TOLECTIN is an inhibitor of prostaglandin synthetase. Drugs in this class have known effects on the fetal cardiovascular system which may cause constriction of the ductus arteriosus *in utero* during the third trimester of pregnancy, which may result in persistent pulmonary hypertension of the newborn.

There are no adequate and well-controlled studies in pregnant women. TOLECTIN should be used during pregnancy only if the potential benefit justifies the potential risk to the fetus.

Non-Teratogenic Effects
Prostaglandin inhibitors have also been shown to increase the incidence of dystocia and delayed parturition in animals.

Nursing Mothers
TOLECTIN has been shown to be secreted in human milk. Because of the possible adverse effects of prostaglandin inhibiting drugs on neonates, use in nursing mothers should be avoided.

Pediatric Use
The safety and effectiveness of TOLECTIN in children under 2 years of age have not been established.

Drug Interactions
The *in vitro* binding of warfarin to human plasma proteins is unaffected by tolmetin, and tolmetin does not alter the prothrombin time of normal volunteers. However, increased prothrombin time and bleeding have been reported in patients on concomitant TOLECTIN and warfarin therapy. Therefore, caution should be exercised when administering TOLECTIN to patients on anticoagulants.

In adult diabetic patients under treatment with either sulfonylureas or insulin there is no change in the clinical effects of either TOLECTIN or the hypoglycemic agents.

Caution should be used if TOLECTIN is administered concomitantly with methotrexate. TOLECTIN and other nonsteroidal anti-inflammatory drugs have been reported to reduce the tubular secretion of methotrexate in an animal model, possibly enhancing the toxicity of methotrexate.

Laboratory Tests
Because serious GI tract ulceration and bleeding can occur without warning symptoms, physicians should follow chronically treated patients for the signs and symptoms of ulceration and bleeding and should inform them of the importance of this follow-up (see Warnings—Risk of GI Ulceration, Bleeding and Perforation with NSAID Therapy).

Drug/Laboratory Test Interaction
The metabolites of tolmetin sodium in urine have been found to give positive tests for proteinuria using tests which rely on acid precipitation as their endpoint (e.g. sulfosalicylic acid). No interference is seen in the tests for proteinuria using dye-impregnated commercially available reagent strips (e.g. Albustix®, Uristix®, etc.).

Drug-Food Interaction
In a controlled single dose study, administration of TOLECTIN with milk had no effect on peak plasma tolmetin concentrations, but decreased total tolmetin bioavailability by 16%. When TOLECTIN was taken immediately after a meal, peak plasma tolmetin concentrations were reduced by 50% while total bioavailability was again decreased by 16%.

Information for Patients
TOLECTIN, like other drugs of its class, is not free of side effects. The side effects of these drugs can cause discomfort and, rarely, there are more serious side effects, such as gastrointestinal bleeding, which may result in hospitalization and even fatal outcomes.

NSAID's (Nonsteroidal Anti-Inflammatory Drugs) are often essential agents in the management of arthritis, but they also may be commonly employed for conditions which are less serious.

Physicians may wish to discuss with their patients the potential risks (see Warnings, Precautions, and Adverse Reactions sections) and likely benefits of NSAID treatment, particularly when the drugs are used for less serious conditions where treatment without NSAID's may represent an acceptable alternative to both the patient and physician.

ADVERSE REACTIONS
The adverse reactions which have been observed in clinical trials encompass observations in about 4370 patients treated with TOLECTIN (tolmetin sodium), over 800 of whom have undergone at least one year of therapy. These adverse reactions, reported below by body system, are among those typical of nonsteroidal anti-inflammatory drugs and, as expected, gastrointestinal complaints were most frequent. In clinical trials with TOLECTIN, about 10% of patients dropped out because of adverse reactions, mostly gastrointestinal in nature.

Incidence Greater Than 1%
The following adverse reactions which occurred more frequently than 1 in 100 were reported in controlled clinical trials.

Gastrointestinal: Nausea (11%), dyspepsia,* gastrointestinal distress,* abdominal pain,* diarrhea,* flatulence,* vomiting,* constipation, gastritis, and peptic ulcer. Forty percent of the ulcer patients had a prior history of peptic ulcer disease and/or were receiving concomitant anti-inflammatory drugs including corticosteroids, which are known to produce peptic ulceration.

Body as a Whole: Headache,* asthenia,* chest pain
Cardiovascular: Elevated blood pressure,* edema*
Central Nervous System: Dizziness,* drowsiness, depression
Metabolic/Nutritional: Weight gain,* weight loss*
Dermatologic: Skin irritation
Special Senses: Tinnitus, visual disturbance
Hematologic: Small and transient decreases in hemoglobin and hematocrit not associated with gastrointestinal bleeding have occurred. These are similar to changes reported with other nonsteroidal anti-inflammatory drugs.
Urogenital: Elevated BUN, urinary tract infection
* Reactions occurring in 3% to 9% of patients treated with TOLECTIN. Reactions occurring in fewer than 3% of the patients are unmarked.

Incidence Less Than 1%
(Causal Relationship Probable)
The following adverse reactions were reported less frequently than 1 in 100 in controlled clinical trials or were reported since marketing. The probability exists that there is a causal relationship between TOLECTIN and these adverse reactions.

Gastrointestinal: Gastrointestinal bleeding with or without evidence of peptic ulcer, glossitis, stomatitis, hepatitis, liver function abnormalities
Body as a Whole: Anaphylactoid reactions, fever, lymphadenopathy, serum sickness
Hematologic: Hemolytic anemia, thrombocytopenia, granulocytopenia, agranulocytosis

Cardiovascular: Congestive heart failure in patients with marginal cardiac function
Dermatologic: Urticaria, purpura, erythema multiforme, toxic epidermal necrolysis
Urogenital: Hematuria, proteinuria, dysuria, renal failure

Incidence Less Than 1%
(Causal Relationship Unknown)
Other adverse reactions were reported less frequently than 1 in 100 in controlled clinical trials or were reported since marketing, but a causal relationship between TOLECTIN and the reaction could not be determined. These rarely reported reactions are being listed as alerting information for the physician since the possibility of a causal relationship cannot be excluded.

Body as Whole: Epistaxis
Special Senses: Optic neuropathy, retinal and macular changes

MANAGEMENT OF OVERDOSAGE
In the event of overdosage, the stomach should be emptied by inducing vomiting or by gastric lavage followed by the administration of activated charcoal.

DOSAGE AND ADMINISTRATION
In adults with rheumatoid arthritis or osteoarthritis, the recommended starting dose is 400 mg three times daily (1200 mg daily), preferably including a dose on arising and a dose at bedtime. To achieve optimal therapeutic effect the dose should be adjusted according to the patient's response after one to two weeks. Control is usually achieved at doses of 600–1800 mg daily in divided doses (generally t.i.d.). Doses larger than 1800 mg/kg have not been studied and are not recommended.

The recommended starting dose for children (2 years and older) is 20 mg/kg/day in divided doses (t.i.d. or q.i.d.). When control has been achieved, the usual dose ranges from 15 to 30 mg/kg/day. Doses higher than 30 mg/kg/day have not been studied and, therefore, are not recommended.

A therapeutic response to TOLECTIN (tolmetin sodium) can be expected in a few days to a week. Progressive improvement can be anticipated during succeeding weeks of therapy. If gastrointestinal symptoms occur, TOLECTIN can be administered with antacids other than sodium bicarbonate. TOLECTIN bioavailability and pharmacokinetics are not significantly affected by acute or chronic administration of magnesium and aluminum hydroxides; however, bioavailability is affected by food or milk (see PRECAUTIONS—Drug-Food Interaction).

HOW SUPPLIED
TOLECTIN® 200 (tolmetin sodium) tablets 200 mg (white, scored, imprinted "TOLECTIN," "200" and "McNEIL"), NDC 0045-0412, bottles of 100.
TOLECTIN® DS (tolmetin sodium) capsules 400 mg (colored orange opaque, with contrasting parallel bands, imprinted "TOLECTIN DS" and "McNEIL"), NDC 0045-0414, bottles of 100, 500 and unit dose of 100's.
TOLECTIN® 600 (tolmetin sodium) tablets 600 mg (colored orange, film coated, imprinted "TOLECTIN 600" and "McNEIL"), NDC 0045-0416, bottles of 100.
Dispense in tight, light-resistant container as defined in the official compendium.
Store at controlled room temperature (15°–30°C, 59°–86°F). Protect from light.

Revised 5/12/89

Shown in Product Identification Section, page 417

TYLENOL® with Codeine ℞
[ti'len-awl co'dēn]
(acetaminophen and codeine phosphate tablets and elixir)
Tablets ⑪ and Elixir ⓒ
No. 3-NSN 6505-00-400-2054—100's
No. 3-NSN 6505-00-147-8347—500's
No. 3-NSN 6505-00-372-3032—1000's
Elixir-NSN 6505-01-035-1963—Pints

DESCRIPTION
Each tablet contains:

No. 1 Codeine Phosphate*	7.5 mg
Acetaminophen	300 mg
No. 2 Codeine Phosphate*	15 mg
Acetaminophen	300 mg
No. 3 Codeine Phosphate*	30 mg
Acetaminophen	300 mg
No. 4 Codeine Phosphate*	60 mg
Acetaminophen	300 mg

Each 5 mL of elixir contains:

Codeine Phosphate*	12 mg
Acetaminophen	120 mg
Alcohol 7%	

*Warning —May be habit forming.

Continued on next page

Information on McNeil Pharmaceutical Products is based on labeling in effect in August, 1989.

McNeil Pharm.—Cont.

Inactive ingredients: tablets—powdered cellulose, magnesium stearate, sodium metabisulfite†; elixir—alcohol, citric acid, propylene glycol, sodium benzoate, saccharin sodium, sucrose, natural and artificial flavors, FD&C Yellow No. 6.

Acetaminophen, 4'-hydroxyacetanilide, is a nonopiate, nonsalicylate analgesic and antipyretic which occurs as a white, odorless, crystalline powder, possessing a slightly bitter taste. Its structure is as follows:

$C_8H_9NO_2$ M.W. 151.16

Codeine is an alkaloid, obtained from opium or prepared from morphine by methylation. Codeine phosphate occurs as fine, white, needle-shaped crystals, or white, crystalline powder. It is affected by light. Its chemical name is: 7,8-didehydro-4,5α-epoxy-3-methoxy-17-methyl-morphinan-6α-ol phosphate (1:1) (salt) hemihydrate. Its structure is as follows:

$C_{18}H_{21}NO_3 \cdot H_3PO_4 \cdot \frac{1}{2} H_2O$
M.W. 406.37
†See WARNINGS

CLINICAL PHARMACOLOGY

TYLENOL with Codeine (acetaminophen and codeine phosphate tablets and elixir) combines the analgesic effects of a centrally acting analgesic, codeine, with a peripherally acting analgesic, acetaminophen. Both ingredients are well absorbed orally. The plasma elimination half-life ranges from 1 to 4 hours for acetaminophen, and from 2.5 to 3 hours for codeine.

Codeine retains at least one-half of its analgesic activity when administered orally. A reduced first-pass metabolism of codeine by the liver accounts for the greater oral efficacy of codeine when compared to most other morphine-like narcotics. Following absorption, codeine is metabolized by the liver and metabolic products are excreted in the urine. Approximately 10 percent of the administered codeine is demethylated to morphine, which may account for its analgesic activity.

Acetaminophen is distributed throughout most tissues of the body. Acetaminophen is metabolized primarily in the liver. Little unchanged drug is excreted in the urine, but most metabolic products appear in the urine within 24 hours.

INDICATIONS AND USAGE

TYLENOL with Codeine tablets (acetaminophen and codeine phosphate tablets) are indicated for the relief of mild to moderately severe pain.
TYLENOL with Codeine elixir (acetaminophen and codeine phosphate elixir) is indicated for the relief of mild to moderate pain.

CONTRAINDICATIONS

TYLENOL with Codeine tablets or elixir (acetaminophen and codeine phosphate tablets and elixir) should not be administered to patients who have previously exhibited hypersensitivity to any component.

WARNINGS

TYLENOL with Codeine tablets (acetaminophen and codeine phosphate tablets) contain sodium metabisulfite, a sulfite that may cause allergic-type reactions including anaphylactic symptoms and life-threatening or less severe asthmatic episodes in certain susceptible people. The overall prevalence of sulfite sensitivity in the general population is unknown and probably low. Sulfite sensitivity is seen more frequently in asthmatic than in nonasthmatic people.

PRECAUTIONS
General
Head Injury and Increased Intracranial Pressure: The respiratory depressant effects of narcotics and their capacity to elevate cerebrospinal fluid pressure may be markedly exaggerated in the presence of head injury, other intracranial lesions or a pre-existing increase in intracranial pressure. Furthermore, narcotics produce adverse reactions which may obscure the clinical course of patients with head injuries.

Acute Abdominal Conditions: The administration of this product or other narcotics may obscure the diagnosis or clinical course of patients with acute abdominal conditions.
Special Risk Patients: This drug should be given with caution to certain patients such as the elderly or debilitated, and those with severe impairment of hepatic or renal function, hypothyroidism, Addison's disease, and prostatic hypertrophy or urethral stricture.
Information for Patients
Codeine may impair the mental and/or physical abilities required for the performance of potentially hazardous tasks such as driving a car or operating machinery. The patient using this drug should be cautioned accordingly.
The patient should understand the single-dose and 24 hour dose limits, and the time interval between doses.
Drug Interactions
Patients receiving other narcotic analgesics, antipsychotics, anti-anxiety agents, or other CNS depressants (including alcohol) concomitantly with this drug may exhibit an additive CNS depression. When such combined therapy is contemplated, the dose of one or both agents should be reduced.
The use of MAO inhibitors or tricyclic antidepressants with codeine preparations may increase the effect of either the antidepressant or codeine.
The concurrent use of anticholinergics with codeine may produce paralytic ileus.
Carcinogenesis, Mutagenesis, Impairment of Fertility
No long-term studies in animals have been performed with acetaminophen or codeine to determine carcinogenic potential or effects on fertility.
Acetaminophen and codeine have been found to have no mutagenic potential using the Ames Salmonella-Microsomal Activation test, the Basc test on Drosophila germ cells, and the Micronucleus test on mouse bone marrow.
Pregnancy
Teratogenic Effects: Pregnancy Category C.
Codeine: A study in rats and rabbits reported no teratogenic effect of codeine administered during the period of organogenesis in doses ranging from 5 to 120 mg/kg. In the rat, doses at the 120 mg/kg level, in the toxic range for the adult animal, were associated with an increase in embryo resorption at the time of implantation. In another study a single 100 mg/kg dose of codeine administered to pregnant mice reportedly resulted in delayed ossification in the offspring.

There are no studies in humans, and the significance of these findings to humans, if any, is not known.
TYLENOL with Codeine (acetaminophen and codeine phosphate tablets and elixir) should be used during pregnancy only if the potential benefit justifies the potential risk to the fetus.
Nonteratogenic Effects:
Dependence has been reported in newborns whose mothers took opiates regularly during pregnancy. Withdrawal signs include irritability, excessive crying, tremors, hyperreflexia, fever, vomiting, and diarrhea. Signs usually appear during the first few days of life.
Labor and Delivery
Narcotic analgesics cross the placental barrier. The closer to delivery and the larger the dose used, the greater the possibility of respiratory depression in the newborn. Narcotic analgesics should be avoided during labor if delivery of a premature infant is anticipated. If the mother has received narcotic analgesics during labor, newborn infants should be observed closely for signs of respiratory depression. Resuscitation may be required (see OVERDOSAGE). The effect of codeine, if any, on the later growth, development, and functional maturation of the child is unknown.
Nursing Mothers
Some studies, but not others, have reported detectable amounts of codeine in breast milk. The levels are probably not clinically significant after usual therapeutic dosage. The possibility of clinically important amounts being excreted in breast milk in individuals abusing codeine should be considered.
Pediatric Use
Safe dosage of TYLENOL with Codeine elixir (acetaminophen and codeine phosphate elixir) has not been established in children below the age of three years.

ADVERSE REACTIONS
The most frequently observed adverse reactions include lightheadedness, dizziness, sedation, shortness of breath, nausea and vomiting. These effects seem to be more prominent in ambulatory than in non-ambulatory patients, and some of these adverse reactions may be alleviated if the patient lies down. Other adverse reactions include allergic reactions, euphoria, dysphoria, constipation, abdominal pain, and pruritus.
At higher doses codeine has most of the disadvantages of morphine including respiratory depression.

DRUG ABUSE AND DEPENDENCE
TYLENOL with Codeine tablets (acetaminophen and codeine phosphate tablets) are Schedule III controlled substances.

TYLENOL with Codeine elixir (acetaminophen and codeine phosphate elixir) is a Schedule V controlled substance.
Codeine can produce drug dependence of the morphine type, and therefore has the potential for being abused. Psychic dependence, physical dependence and tolerance may develop upon repeated adminstration of this drug, and it should be prescribed and administered with the same degree of caution appropriate to the use of other oral narcotic-containing medications.

OVERDOSAGE
Acetaminophen
Signs and Symptoms: In acute acetaminophen overdosage, dose-dependent, potentially fatal hepatic necrosis is the most serious adverse effect. Renal tubular necrosis, hypoglycemic coma and thrombocytopenia may also occur.
In adults, hepatic toxicity has rarely been reported with acute overdoses of less than 10 grams and fatalities with less than 15 grams. Importantly, young children seem to be more resistant than adults to the hepatotoxic effect of an acetaminophen overdose. Despite this, the measures outlined below should be initiated in any adult or child suspected of having ingested an acetaminophen overdose.
Early symptoms following a potentially hepatotoxic overdose may include: nausea, vomiting, diaphoresis and general malaise. Clinical and laboratory evidence of hepatic toxicity may not be apparent until 48 to 72 hours post-ingestion.
Treatment: The stomach should be emptied promptly by lavage or by induction of emesis with syrup of ipecac. Patients' estimates of the quantity of a drug ingested are notoriously unreliable. Therefore, if an acetaminophen overdose is suspected, a serum acetaminophen assay should be obtained as early as possible, but no sooner than four hours following ingestion. Liver function studies should be obtained initially and repeated at 24 hour intervals.
The antidote, N-acetylcysteine, should be administered as early as possible, and within 16 hours of the overdose ingestion for optimal results, but in any case, within 24 hours. Following recovery, there are no residual, structural or functional hepatic abnormalities.
Codeine
Signs and Symptoms: Serious overdose with codeine is characterized by respiratory depression (a decrease in respiratory rate and/or tidal volume, Cheyne-Stokes respiration, cyanosis), extreme somnolence progressing to stupor or coma, skeletal muscle flaccidity, cold and clammy skin, and sometimes bradycardia and hypotension. In severe overdosage, apnea, circulatory collapse, cardiac arrest and death may occur.
Treatment: Primary attention should be given to the reestablishment of adequate respiratory exchange through provision of a patent airway and the institution of assisted or controlled ventilation. The narcotic antagonist naloxone is a specific antidote against respiratory depression which may result from overdosage or unusual sensitivity to narcotics, including codeine. Therefore, an appropriate dose of naloxone hydrochloride (see package insert) should be administered, preferably by the intravenous route, and simultaneously with efforts at respiratory resuscitation. Since the duration of action of codeine may exceed that of the antagonist, the patient should be kept under continued surveillance and repeated doses of the antagonist should be administered as needed to maintain adequate respiration.
An antagonist should not be administered in the absence of clinically significant respiratory or cardiovascular depression. Oxygen, intravenous fluids, vasopressors and other supportive measures should be employed as indicated.
Gastric emptying may be useful in removing unabsorbed drug.

DOSAGE AND ADMINISTRATION
Dosage should be adjusted according to severity of pain and response of the patient.
It should be kept in mind, however, that tolerance to codeine can develop with continued use and that the incidence of untoward effects is dose related. Adult doses of codeine higher than 60 mg fail to give commensurate relief of pain but merely prolong analgesia and are associated with an appreciably increased incidence of undesirable side effects. Equivalently high doses in children would have similar effects.
The usual adult dosage for tablets is:

	Single Doses (Range)	Maximum 24 Hour Dose
Codeine Phosphate	15 mg–60mg	360 mg
Acetaminophen	300mg–1000mg	4000mg

Doses may be repeated up to every 4 hours.
The prescriber must determine the number of tablets per dose, and the maximum number of tablets per 24 hours, based upon the above dosage guidance. This information should be conveyed in the prescription.
For children, the dose of codeine phosphate is 0.5 mg/kg.
TYLENOL with Codeine elixir (acetaminophen and codeine phosphate elixir) contains 120 mg of acetaminophen and 12 mg of codeine phosphate/5 mL and is given orally.

The usual doses are:

Children (7 to 12 years): 10 mL (2 teaspoonfuls) 3 or 4 times daily. *(3 to 6 years):* 5 mL (1 teaspoonful) 3 or 4 times daily. *(under 3 years):* safe dosage has not been established.
Adults: 15 mL (1 tablespoonful) every 4 hours as needed.

HOW SUPPLIED
TYLENOL with Codeine tablets (acetaminophen and codeine phosphate tablets): (round, white, imprinted "McNEIL", "TYLENOL CODEINE" and either "1", "2", "3", "4"): No. 1—NDC 0045-0510, bottles of 100; No. 2—NDC 0045-0511, bottles of 100 and 500; No. 3—NDC 0045-0513, bottles of 100, 500, and 1000; and No. 4—NDC 0045-0515, bottles of 100 and 500. No. 2, No. 3, and No. 4 also available in unit doses (20 × 25).
TYLENOL with Codeine elixir (acetaminophen and codeine phosphate elixir) contains 120 mg acetaminophen and 12 mg codeine phosphate/5 mL (colored amber, cherry flavored)—NDC 0045-0508, bottles of 1 pint, unit dose cup (10 × 5 mL) and unit dose cup (10 × 15 mL).
Dispense in tight, light-resistant container as defined in the official compendium.

Revised 8/31/88
Shown in Product Identification Section, page 417

TYLOX® Capsules
[*ti'lox*]
(oxycodone and acetaminophen capsules USP)
NSN 6505-01-210-4450-100's
NSN 6505-01-211-6803-Unit Dose (100's)

DESCRIPTION
Each capsule of TYLOX (oxycodone and acetaminophen capsules USP) contains:

Oxycodone Hydrochloride USP .... 5 mg*
  Warning —May be habit forming.
Acetaminophen USP .... 500 mg
Inactive ingredients: docusate sodium, gelatin, magnesium stearate, sodium benzoate, sodium metabisulfite†, corn starch, FD&C Blue No. 1, FD&C Red No. 3, FD&C Red No. 40, and titanium dioxide.
Acetaminophen occurs as a white, odorless crystalline powder, possessing a slightly bitter taste.
The oxycodone component is 14-hydroxydihydrocodeinone, a white, odorless crystalline powder having a saline, bitter taste. It is derived from the opium alkaloid thebaine, and may be represented by the following structural formula:

*5 mg oxycodone hydrochloride is equivalent to 4.4815 mg oxycodone
†See Warnings

CLINICAL PHARMACOLOGY
The principal ingredient, oxycodone, is a semisynthetic narcotic analgesic with multiple actions qualitatively similar to those of morphine; the most prominent of these involve the central nervous system and organs composed of smooth muscle. The principal actions of therapeutic value of the oxycodone in TYLOX (oxycodone and acetaminophen capsules) are analgesia and sedation.
Oxycodone is similar to codeine and methadone in that it retains at least one-half of its analgesic activity when administered orally.
Acetaminophen is a non-opiate, non-salicylate analgesic and antipyretic.

INDICATIONS AND USAGE
TYLOX (oxycodone and acetaminophen capsules) are indicated for the relief of moderate to moderately severe pain.

CONTRAINDICATIONS
TYLOX (oxycodone and acetaminophen capsules) should not be administered to patients who are hypersensitive to any component.

WARNINGS
Contains sodium metabisulfite, a sulfite that may cause allergic-type reactions including anaphylactic symptoms and life-threatening or less severe asthmatic episodes in certain susceptible people. The overall prevalence of sulfite sensitivity in the general population is unknown and probably low. Sulfite sensitivity is seen more frequently in asthmatic than in nonasthmatic people.
Drug Dependence
Oxycodone can produce drug dependence of the morphine type and, therefore, has the potential for being abused. Psychic dependence, physical dependence and tolerance may develop upon repeated administration of TYLOX (oxycodone

and acetaminophen capsules), and it should be prescribed and administered with the same degree of caution appropriate to the use of other oral narcotic-containing medications. Like other narcotic-containing medications, TYLOX is subject to the Federal Control Substances Act (Schedule II).

PRECAUTIONS
General
Head Injury and Increased Intracranial Pressure: The respiratory depressant effects of narcotics and their capacity to elevate cerebrospinal fluid pressure may be markedly exaggerated in the presence of head injury, other intracranial lesions, or a pre-existing increase in intracranial pressure. Furthermore, narcotics produce adverse reactions which may obscure the clinical course of patients with head injuries.
Acute Abdominal Conditions: The administration of TYLOX (oxycodone and acetaminophen capsules) or other narcotics may obscure the diagnosis or clinical course in patients with acute abdominal conditions.
Special Risk Patients: TYLOX capsules should be given with caution to certain patients such as the elderly or debilitated, and those with severe impairment of hepatic or renal function, hypothyroidism, Addison's disease, and prostatic hypertrophy or urethral stricture.
Information for Patients
Oxycodone may impair the mental and/or physical abilities required for the performance of potentially hazardous tasks such as driving a car or operating machinery. The patient using TYLOX should be cautioned accordingly.
Drug Interactions
Patients receiving other narcotic analgesics, general anesthetics, phenothiazines, other tranquilizers, sedative-hypnotics or other CNS depressants (including alcohol) concomitantly with TYLOX may exhibit an additive CNS depression. When such combined therapy is contemplated, the dose of one or both agents should be reduced.
The use of MAO inhibitors or tricyclic antidepressants with oxycodone preparations may increase the effect of either the antidepressant or oxycodone.
The concurrent use of anticholinergics with narcotics may produce paralytic ileus.
Usage in Pregnancy
Pregnancy Category C. Animal reproductive studies have not been conducted with TYLOX. It is also not known whether TYLOX can cause fetal harm when administered to a pregnant woman or can affect reproductive capacity. TYLOX should not be given to a pregnant woman unless in the judgment of the physician, the potential benefits outweigh the possible hazards.
Nonteratogenic Effects: Use of narcotics during pregnancy may produce physical dependence in the neonate.
Labor and Delivery
As with all narcotics, administration of TYLOX to the mother shortly before delivery may result in some degree of respiratory depression in the newborn and the mother, especially if higher doses are used.
Nursing Mothers
It is not known whether the components of TYLOX are excreted in human milk. Because many drugs are excreted in human milk, caution should be exercised when TYLOX is administered to a nursing woman.
Pediatric Use
Safety and effectiveness in children have not been established.

ADVERSE REACTIONS
The most frequently observed adverse reactions include lightheadedness, dizziness, sedation, nausea, and vomiting. These effects seem to be more prominent in ambulatory than in non-ambulatory patients, and some of these adverse reactions may be alleviated if the patient lies down.
Other adverse reactions include allergic reactions, euphoria, dysphoria, constipation, skin rash, and pruritus.
At higher doses oxycodone has most of the disadvantages of morphine including respiratory depression.

OVERDOSAGE
Acetaminophen
Signs and Symptoms: In acute acetaminophen overdosage, dose-dependent potentially fatal hepatic necrosis is the most serious adverse effect. Renal tubular necrosis and hypoglycemic coma and thrombocytopenia may also occur.
In adults, hepatic toxicity has rarely been reported with acute overdoses of less than 10 grams and fatalities with less than 15 grams. Importantly, young children seem to be more resistant than adults to the hepatotoxic effect of an acetaminophen overdose. Despite this, the measures outlined below should be initiated in any adult or child suspected of having ingested an acetaminophen overdose.
Early symptoms following a potentially hepatotoxic overdose may include: nausea, vomiting, diaphoresis, and general malaise. Clinical and laboratory evidence of hepatic toxicity may not be apparent until 48 to 72 hours post-ingestion.
Treatment: The stomach should be emptied promptly by lavage or by induction of emesis with syrup of ipecac. Pa-

tients' estimates of the quantity of a drug ingested are notoriously unreliable. Therefore, if an acetaminophen overdose is suspected, a serum acetaminophen assay should be obtained as early as possible, but no sooner than four hours following ingestion. Liver function studies should be obtained initially and repeated at 24-hour intervals.
The antidote, N-acetylcysteine, should be administered as early as possible, and within 16 hours of the overdose ingestion for optimal results. Following recovery, there are no residual, structural, or functional hepatic abnormalities.
Oxycodone
Signs and symptoms: Serious overdose with oxycodone is characterized by respiratory depression (a decrease in respiratory rate and/or tidal volume, Cheyne-Stokes respiration, cyanosis), extreme somnolence progressing to stupor or coma, skeletal muscle flaccidity, cold and clammy skin, and sometimes bradycardia and hypotension. In severe overdosage, apnea, circulatory collapse, cardiac arrest, and death may occur.
Treatment: Primary attention should be given to the reestablishment of adequate respiratory exchange through provision of a patent airway and the institution of assisted or controlled ventilation. The narcotic antagonist naloxone hydrochloride is a specific antidote against respiratory depression which may result from overdosage or unusual sensitivity to narcotics, including oxycodone. Therefore, an appropriate dose of naloxone hydrochloride (usual initial adult dose 0.4 mg to 2 mg) should be administered preferably by the intravenous route and simultaneously with efforts at respiratory resuscitation (see package insert). Since the duration of action of oxycodone may exceed that of the antagonist, the patient should be kept under continued surveillance, and repeated doses of the antagonist should be administered as needed to maintain adequate respiration.
An antagonist should not be administered in the absence of clinically significant respiratory or cardiovascular depression. Oxygen, intravenous fluids, vasopressors and other supportive measures should be employed as indicated.
Gastric emptying may be useful in removing unabsorbed drug.

DOSAGE AND ADMINISTRATION
Dosage should be adjusted according to the severity of the pain and the response of the patient. However, it should be kept in mind that tolerance to oxycodone can develop with continued use and that the incidence of untoward effects is dose related. This product is inappropriate even in high doses for severe or intractable pain.
TYLOX (oxycodone and acetaminophen capsules) are given orally. The usual adult dose is one TYLOX capsule every 6 hours as needed for pain.

HOW SUPPLIED
TYLOX (oxycodone and acetaminophen capsules USP): (colored red, imprinted "TYLOX" "McNEIL") NDC 0045-0526—bottles of 100 and unit dose 100's.
Dispense in tight, light-resistant container as defined in the official compendium.

Revised 7/25/88
Shown in Product Identification Section, page 417

EDUCATIONAL MATERIAL

Haldol® (haloperidol) Decanoate
"Haldol® Films Available" Brochure
Available free to physicians and pharmacists through McNeil representatives.

Pancrease® (pancrelipase) and **Pancrease**® MT
"Tree of Life" film and brochure—film available in ½" videotape.
"The Adventures of Mr. Enzyme" Nutritional Video
Target 100%—Growth and Nutrition brochure—for CF patients and families.
CF Foundation's Patient and Family Education video and workbook.
Available free to physicians and pharmacists through McNeil representatives.

Parafon Forte™ DSC (chlorzoxazone)
"Remedial Exercises for Low Back Pain" (English & Spanish)
"Remedial Exercises for Cervical Sprain" (English & Spanish)
Both are available free to physicians and pharmacists through McNeil representatives.

Continued on next page

Information on McNeil Pharmaceutical Products is based on labeling in effect in August, 1989.

McNeil Pharm.—Cont.

Tolectin® (tolmetin sodium)
"Six Steps to Control Your Arthritis Symptoms" (English & Spanish)
Health Assessment Questionaire (English and Spanish)
Available free to physicians and pharmacists through McNeil representatives.

Mead Johnson Laboratories
A Bristol-Myers Company
2400 W. LLOYD EXPRESSWAY
EVANSVILLE, INDIANA 47721-0001

IDENTIFICATION MARKINGS
SOLID ORAL DOSE FORMS
[See table below].

ESTRACE®   ℞
[es'trās]
(estradiol)

Tablets, 1 mg, bottles of 100
NSN 6505-01-281-4829 (M)

WARNING
1. ESTROGENS HAVE BEEN REPORTED TO IN-CREASE THE RISK OF ENDOMETRIAL CARCINOMA.
Three independent case control studies have shown an increased risk of endometrial cancer in postmenopausal women exposed to exogenous estrogens for prolonged periods.[1-3] This risk was independent of the other known risk factors for endometrial cancer. These studies are further supported by the finding that incidence rates of endometrial cancer have increased sharply since 1969 in eight different areas of the United States with population based cancer reporting systems, an increase which may be related to the rapidly expanding use of estrogens during the last decade.[4]
The three case control studies reported that the risk of endometrial cancer in estrogen users was about 4.5 to 13.9 times greater than in nonusers. The risk appears to depend on both duration of treatment[1] and on estrogen dose.[3] In view of these findings, when estrogens are used for the treatment of menopausal symptoms, the lowest dose that will control symptoms should be utilized and medication should be discontinued as soon as possible. When prolonged treatment is medically indicated, the patient should be reassessed on at least a semiannual basis to determine the need for continued therapy. Although the evidence must be considered preliminary, one study suggests that cyclic administration of low doses of estrogen may carry less risk than continuous administration;[3] it therefore appears prudent to utilize such a regimen.
Close clinical surveillance of all women taking estrogens is important. In all cases of undiagnosed persistent or recurring abnormal vaginal bleeding, adequate diagnostic measures should be undertaken to rule out malignancy.
There is no evidence at present that "natural" estrogens are more or less hazardous than "synthetic" estrogens at equiestrogenic doses.
2. ESTROGENS SHOULD NOT BE USED DURING PREGNANCY.
The use of female sex hormones, both estrogens and progestogens, during early pregnancy may seriously damage the offspring. It has been shown that females exposed *in utero* to diethylstilbestrol, a nonsteroidal estrogen, have an increased risk of developing in later life a form of vaginal or cervical cancer that is ordinarily extremely rare.[5,6] This risk has been estimated as not greater than 4 per 1,000 exposures.[7] Furthermore, a high percentage of such exposed women (from 30 to 90 percent) have been found to have vaginal adenosis,[8-12] epithelial changes of the vagina and cervix. Although these changes are histologically benign, it is not known whether they are precursors of malignancy. Although similar data are not available with the use of other estrogens, it cannot be presumed they would not induce similar changes.
Several reports suggest an association between intrauterine exposure to female sex hormones and congenital anomalies, including congenital heart defects and

limb reduction defects.[13-16] One case control study[16] estimated a 4.7-fold increased risk of limb reduction defects in infants exposed *in utero* to sex hormones (oral contraceptives, hormone withdrawal tests for pregnancy, or attempted treatment for threatened abortion). Some of these exposures were very short and involved only a few days of treatment. The data suggest that the risk of limb reduction defects in exposed fetuses is somewhat less than 1 per 1,000.
In the past, female sex hormones have been used during pregnancy in an attempt to treat threatened or habitual abortion. There is considerable evidence that estrogens are ineffective for these indications, and there is no evidence from well-controlled studies that progestogens are effective for these uses.
If Estrace is used during pregnancy, or if the patient becomes pregnant while taking this drug, she should be apprised of the potential risks to the fetus and the advisability of pregnancy continuation.

DESCRIPTION
Estrace oral tablets contain 1 or 2 mg of micronized estradiol. Estradiol (17β-estradiol) is a white, crystalline solid, chemically described as estra-1,3,5(10)-triene-3,17β-diol. Estrace oral tablets provide estrogen replacement therapy. The structural formula is:

Estrace Tablets, 1 mg, contain the following active ingredients: acacia, D&C Red No. 27 (aluminum lake), dibasic calcium phosphate, FD&C Blue No. 1 (aluminum lake), lactose, magnesium stearate, colloidal silicon dioxide, starch (corn), and talc.
Estrace Tablets, 2 mg, contain the following inactive ingredients: acacia, dibasic calcium phosphate, FD&C Blue No. 1 (aluminum lake), FD&C Yellow No. 5 (tartrazine) (aluminum lake), lactose, magnesium stearate, colloidal silicon dioxide, starch (corn), and talc.
Clinical Pharmacology
17β-Estradiol is the most potent physiologic estrogen and, in fact, is the major estrogenic hormone secreted by the human. Estradiol in Estrace has been micronized and demonstrated to be rapidly and effectively absorbed from the gastrointestinal tract.[17]

INDICATIONS
Estrace affords effective treatment of:
1. Moderate to severe vasomotor symptoms associated with the menopause. (There is no evidence that estrogens are effective for nervous symptoms or depression which might occur during menopause, and they should not be used to treat these conditions.)
2. Atrophic vaginitis.
3. Kraurosis vulvae.
4. Female hypogonadism.
5. Female castration.
6. Primary ovarian failure.
7. Breast cancer (for palliation only) in appropriately selected women and men with metastatic disease.
8. Prostatic carcinoma—palliative therapy of advanced disease.
9. The lowest effective dose appropriate for the specific indication should be utilized. Studies of the addition of a progestogen for seven or more days of a cycle of estrogen administration have reported a lowered incidence of endometrial hyperplasia. Morphological and biochemical studies of endometrium suggest that 10 to 13 days of progestogen are needed to provide maximal maturation of the endometrium and to eliminate any hyperplastic changes. Whether this will provide protection from endometrial carcinoma has not been clearly established. There are possible additional risks which may be associated with the inclusion of progestogen in estrogen replacement regimens. The potential risks include adverse effects on carbohydrate and lipid metabolism. The choice of progestogen and dosage may be important in minimizing these adverse effects.
ESTRACE HAS NOT BEEN SHOWN TO BE EFFECTIVE FOR ANY PURPOSE DURING PREGNANCY AND ITS USE MAY CAUSE SEVERE HARM TO THE FETUS (SEE BOXED WARNING).

CONTRAINDICATIONS
Estrogens should not be used in women (or men) with any of the following conditions:
1. Known or suspected cancer of the breast except in appropriately selected patients being treated for metastatic disease.
2. Known or suspected estrogen-dependent neoplasia.
3. Known or suspected pregnancy (See Boxed Warning).
4. Undiagnosed abnormal genital bleeding.
5. Active thrombophlebitis or thromboembolic disorders.
6. A past history of thrombophlebitis, thrombosis, or thromboembolic disorders associated with previous estrogen use (except when used in treatment of breast or prostatic malignancy).

WARNINGS
1. Induction of malignant neoplasms. Long-term continuous administration of natural and synthetic estrogens in certain animal species increases the frequency of carcinomas of the breast, cervix, vagina, and liver. There is now evidence that estrogens increase the risk of carcinoma of the endometrium in humans. (See Boxed Warning).
At the present time there is no satisfactory evidence that estrogens given to postmenopausal women increase the risk of cancer of the breast,[18] although a recent long-term follow-up of a single physician's practice has raised this possibility.[19] Because of the animal data there is a need for caution in prescribing estrogens for women with a strong family history of breast cancer or who have breast nodules, fibrocystic disease, or abnormal mammograms.
2. Gallbladder disease. A recent study has reported a 2- to 3-fold increase in the risk of surgically confirmed gallbladder disease in women receiving postmenopausal estrogens,[18] similar to the 2-fold increase previously noted in users of oral contraceptives.[20,20a] In the case of oral contraceptives, the increased risk appeared after two years of use.[34]
3. Effects similar to those caused by estrogen-progestogen oral contraceptives. There are several serious adverse effects of oral contraceptives, most of which have not, up to now, been documented as consequences of postmenopausal estrogen therapy. This may reflect the comparatively low doses of estrogen used in postmenopausal women. It would be expected that the larger doses of estrogen used to treat prostatic or breast cancer or postpartum breast engorgement are more likely to result in these adverse effects; and, in fact, it has been shown that there is an increased risk of thrombosis in men receiving estrogens for prostatic cancer and women for postpartum breast engorgement.[21-24]
a. Thromboembolic disease. It is now well established that users of oral contraceptives have an increased risk of various thromboembolic and thrombotic vascular diseases, such as thrombophlebitis, pulmonary embolism, stroke, and myocardial infarction.[25-32] Cases of retinal thrombosis, mesenteric thrombosis, and optic neuritis have been reported in oral contraceptive users. There is evidence that the risk of several of these adverse reactions is related to the dose of the drug.[33,34] An increased risk of postsurgery thromboembolic complications has also been reported in users of oral contraceptives.[35,36] If feasible, estrogen should be discontinued at least 4 weeks before surgery of the type associated with an increased risk of thromboembolism, or during periods of prolonged immobilization.
While an increased rate of thromboembolic and thrombotic disease in postmenopausal users of estrogens has not been found,[19,37] this does not rule out the possibility that such an increase may be present or that subgroups of women who have underlying risk factors or who are receiving relatively large doses of estrogens may have increased risk. Therefore, estrogens should not be used in persons with active thrombophlebitis or thromboembolic disorders, and they should not be used (except in treatment of malignancy) in persons with a history of such disorders in association with estrogen use. They should be used with caution in patients with cerebral vascular or coronary artery disease and only for those in whom estrogens are clearly needed.
Large doses of estrogen (5 mg conjugated estrogens per day), comparable to those used to treat cancer of the prostate and breast, have been shown in a large prospective clinical trial in men[38] to increase the risk of nonfatal myocardial infarction, pulmonary embolism and thrombophlebitis. When estrogen doses of this size are used, any of the thromboembolic and thrombotic adverse effects associated with oral contraceptive use should be considered a clear risk.
b. Hepatic adenoma. Hepatic adenomas appear to be associated with the use of oral contraceptives.[39-41] Although rare, these may rupture and may cause death through intraabdominal hemorrhage. Such lesions have not yet been reported in association with other estrogen or progestogen preparations but should be considered in estrogen users having abdominal pain and tenderness, abdominal mass, or hypovolemic shock. Hepatocellular carcinoma has also been reported in women taking estrogen-containing oral contraceptives.[40] The relationship of this malignancy to these drugs is not known at this time.

Product	Strengths	Capsules	Tablets One Side
Estrace® (estradiol)	1 mg		MJ755
Estrace® (estradiol)	2 mg		MJ756

c. **Elevated blood pressure.** Increased blood pressure is not uncommon in women using oral contraceptives. There is now a report that this may occur with use of estrogens in the menopause[42] and blood pressure should be monitored with estrogen use, especially if high doses are used.

d. **Glucose tolerance.** A worsening of glucose tolerance has been observed in a significant percentage of patients on estrogen-containing oral contraceptives. For this reason, diabetic patients should be carefully observed while receiving estrogen.

4. **Hypercalcemia.** Administration of estrogens may lead to severe hypercalcemia in patients with breast cancer and bone metastases. If this occurs, the drug should be stopped and appropriate measures taken to reduce the serum calcium level.

PRECAUTIONS

A. General Precautions.

1. A complete medical and family history should be taken prior to the initiation of any estrogen therapy. The pretreatment and periodic physical examinations should include special reference to blood pressure, breasts, abdomen, and pelvic organs, and should include a Papanicolaou smear. As a general rule, estrogen should not be prescribed for longer than one year without another physical examination being performed.

2. Fluid retention—Because estrogens may cause some degree of fluid retention, conditions which might be influenced by this factor such as epilepsy, migraine, and cardiac or renal dysfunction, require careful observation.

3. Certain patients may develop undesirable manifestations of excessive estrogenic stimulation, such as abnormal or excessive uterine bleeding, mastodynia, etc.

4. Oral contraceptives appear to be associated with an increased incidence of mental depression. Although it is not clear whether this is due to the estrogenic or progestogenic component of the contraceptive, patients with a history of depression should be carefully observed.

5. Preexisting uterine leiomyomata may increase in size during estrogen use.

6. The pathologist should be advised of estrogen therapy when relevant specimens are submitted.

7. Patients with a past history of jaundice during pregnancy have an increased risk of recurrence of jaundice while receiving estrogen-containing oral contraceptive therapy. If jaundice develops in any patient receiving estrogen, the medication should be discontinued while the cause is investigated.

8. Estrogens may be poorly metabolized in patients with impaired liver function and they should be administered with caution in such patients.

9. Because estrogens influence the metabolism of calcium and phosphorus, they should be used with caution in patients with metabolic bone diseases that are associated with hypercalcemia or in patients with renal insufficiency.

10. Because of the effects of estrogens on epiphyseal closure, they should be used judiciously in young patients in whom bone growth is not complete.

11. Certain endocrine and liver function tests may be affected by estrogen-containing oral contraceptives. The following similar changes may be expected with larger doses of estrogen:

  a. Increased sulfobromophthalein retention.

  b. Increased prothrombin and factors VII, VIII, IX, and X; decreased antithrombin 3; increased norepinephrine-induced platelet aggregability.

  c. Increased thyroid binding globulin (TBG) leading to increased circulating total thyroid hormone, as measured by PBI, T4 by column, or T4 by radioimmunoassay. Free T3 resin uptake is decreased, reflecting the elevated TBG; free T4 concentration is unaltered.

  d. Impaired glucose tolerance.

  e. Decreased pregnanediol excretion.

  f. Reduced response to metyrapone test.

  g. Reduced serum folate concentration.

  h. Increased serum triglyceride and phospholipid concentration.

B. Information for the Patient. See text of Patient Package Insert.

C. Pregnancy Category X. See Contraindications and Boxed Warning.

D. Nursing Mothers. As a general principle, the administration of any drug to nursing mothers should be done only when clearly necessary since many drugs are excreted in human milk.

Estrace 2 mg tablets contain FD&C Yellow No. 5 (tartrazine) which may cause allergic-type reactions (including bronchial asthma) in certain susceptible individuals. Although the overall incidence of FD&C Yellow No. 5 (tartrazine) sensitivity in the general population is low, it is frequently seen in patients who also have aspirin hypersensitivity.

ADVERSE REACTIONS

(See Warnings regarding induction of neoplasia, adverse effects on the fetus, increased incidence of gallbladder disease, and adverse effects similar to those of oral contraceptives, including thromboembolism.) The following additional adverse reactions have been reported with estrogenic therapy, including oral contraceptives:

Genitourinary system. Breakthrough bleeding, spotting, change in menstrual flow. Dysmenorrhea. Premenstrual-like syndrome. Amenorrhea during and after treatment. Increase in size of uterine fibromyomata. Vaginal candidiasis. Change in cervical eversion and in degree of cervical secretion. Cystitis-like syndrome.

Breast. Tenderness, enlargement, secretion.

Gastrointestinal. Nausea, vomiting. Abdominal cramps, bloating. Cholestatic jaundice.

Skin. Chloasma or melasma which may persist when drug is discontinued. Erythema multiforme. Erythema nodosum. Hemorrhagic eruption. Loss of scalp hair. Hirsutism.

Eyes. Steepening of corneal curvature. Intolerance to contact lenses.

CNS. Headache, migraine, dizziness. Mental depression. Chorea.

Miscellaneous. Increase or decrease in weight. Reduced carbohydrate tolerance. Aggravation of porphyria. Edema. Changes in libido.

OVERDOSAGE

Numerous reports of ingestion of large doses of estrogen-containing oral contraceptives by young children indicate that serious ill effects do not occur. Overdosage of estrogen may cause nausea, and withdrawal bleeding may occur in females.

DOSAGE AND ADMINISTRATION

1. **Given cyclically for short-term use only:**

For treatment of moderate to severe *vasomotor* symptoms, atrophic vaginitis, or kraurosis vulvae associated with the menopause. The lowest dose that will control symptoms should be chosen and medication should be discontinued as promptly as possible. Administration should be cyclic (eg, 3 weeks on and 1 week off). Attempts to discontinue or taper medication should be made at 3 to 6 month intervals. The usual initial dosage range is 1 or 2 mg daily of micronized estradiol adjusted as necessary to control presenting symptoms. The minimal effective dose for maintenance therapy should be determined by titration.

2. **Given cyclically:**

Female hypogonadism.

Female castration.

Primary ovarian failure.

Treatment is usually initiated with a dose of 1 or 2 mg daily of micronized estradiol, adjusted as necessary to control presenting symptoms; the minimal effective dose for maintenance therapy should be determined by titration.

3. **Given chronically:**

Inoperable progressing prostatic cancer—Suggested dosage is 1 to 2 mg three times daily. The effectiveness of therapy can be judged by phosphatase determinations as well as by symptomatic improvement of the patient.

Inoperable progressing breast cancer in appropriately selected men and postmenopausal women (see INDICATIONS)—Suggested dosage is 10 mg three times daily for a period of at least three months.

Treated patients with an intact uterus should be monitored closely for signs of endometrial cancer and appropriate diagnostic measures should be taken to rule out malignancy in the event of persistent or recurring abnormal vaginal bleeding.

HOW SUPPLIED

Estrace 1 mg; lavender scored tablets

NDC 0087-0755-01	Bottles of 100
NDC 0087-0755-44	Cartons of 3 Compacts of 25

Estrace 2 mg; turquoise scored tablets

NDC 0087-0756-01	Bottles of 100
NDC 0087-0756-44	Cartons of 3 Compacts of 25

PATIENT LABELING

WHAT YOU SHOULD KNOW ABOUT ESTROGENS

Estrogens are female hormones produced principally by the ovaries. The ovaries make several different kinds of estrogens. In addition, scientists have been able to make a variety of synthetic estrogens. As far as we know, all these estrogens have the same properties and, therefore, much the same usefulness, side effects, and risks. This leaflet is intended to help you understand what estrogens are used for, the risks involved in their use, and how to use them as safely as possible.

This leaflet includes important information about Estrace® (estradiol) and estrogens in general, but not all the information. If you want to know more you can ask your doctor or pharmacist to let you read the professional package insert.

USES OF ESTROGEN

Estrogens are prescribed by doctors for a number of purposes, including:

1. To provide estrogen during a period of adjustment when a woman's ovaries no longer produce it, in order to prevent certain uncomfortable symptoms of estrogen deficiency. (All women normally experience a decrease in the production of estrogens, generally between 45–55; this is called the menopause.)

2. To prevent symptoms of estrogen deficiency when a woman's ovaries have been removed surgically before the natural menopause.

3. To prevent pregnancy. (Some estrogens are given along with a progestogen, another female hormone; these combinations are called oral contraceptives or birth control pills. They will not be discussed in this leaflet.) However, Estrace is not intended for this use.

4. To treat certain cancers in women and men.

5. To prevent painful swelling of the breasts after pregnancy in women who choose not to nurse their babies.

THERE IS NO PROPER USE OF ESTROGENS IN A PREGNANT WOMAN.

ESTROGENS IN THE MENOPAUSE

In the natural course of their lives, all women eventually experience a decrease in estrogen production. This usually occurs between ages 45 and 55 but may occur earlier or later. Sometimes the ovaries may need to be removed before natural menopause by an operation, producing a "surgical menopause."

When the amount of estrogen in the blood begins to decrease, many women may develop typical symptoms: feelings of warmth in the face, neck, and chest or sudden intense episodes of heat and sweating throughout the body (called "hot flashes" or "hot flushes"). These symptoms are sometimes very uncomfortable. A few women eventually develop changes in the vagina (called "atrophic vaginitis") which cause discomfort, especially during and after intercourse. Estrogens can be prescribed to treat these symptoms of the menopause. It is estimated that considerably more than half of all women undergoing the menopause have only mild symptoms or no symptoms at all and therefore do not need estrogens. Other women may need estrogens for a few months, while their bodies adjust to lower estrogen levels. Sometimes the need will be for periods longer than six months. In an attempt to avoid over-stimulation of the uterus (womb), estrogens are usually given cyclically during each month of use, that is, three weeks of pills followed by one week without pills.

Sometimes women experience nervous symptoms or depression during menopause. There is no evidence that estrogens are effective for such symptoms and they should not be used to treat them, although other treatment may be needed.

You may have heard that taking estrogens for long periods (years) after the menopause will keep your skin soft and supple and keep you feeling young. There is no evidence that this is so, however, and such long-term treatment carries additional risks.

ESTROGENS TO PREVENT SWELLING OF THE BREASTS AFTER PREGNANCY

If you do not breast-feed your baby after delivery, your breasts may fill up with milk and become painful and engorged. This usually begins about three to four days after delivery and may last for a few days to up to a week or more. Sometimes the discomfort is severe, but usually it is not and can be controlled by pain-relieving drugs such as aspirin and by binding the breasts up tightly. Estrogens can sometimes be used successfully to try to prevent the breasts from filling up. While this treatment is sometimes successful, in many cases the breasts fill up to some degree in spite of treatment. The dose of estrogens needed to prevent pain and swelling of the breasts is much larger than the dose needed to treat symptoms of the menopause and this may increase your chances of developing blood clots in the legs or lungs or other parts of the body (see below, 4. Abnormal Blood Clotting). Therefore, it is important that you discuss the benefits and the risks of estrogen use with your doctor, before using estrogen, if you have decided not to breast-feed your baby.

THE DANGERS OF ESTROGENS

1. **Cancer of the uterus.** If estrogens are used in the postmenopausal period for more than a year, there is an increased risk of **cancer of the endometrium** (uterine lining). Women taking estrogens have roughly 5 to 15 times as great a chance of getting this cancer as women who take no estrogens. To put this another way, while a postmenopausal woman not taking estrogens has one chance in 1,000 each year of getting cancer of the uterus, a woman taking estrogens has 5 to 15 chances in 1,000 each year. For this reason **it is important to take estrogens only when you really need them.**

The risk of this cancer is greater the longer estrogens are used and also seems to be greater when larger doses are taken. For this reason **it is important to take the lowest dose of estrogen that will control symptoms and to take it only as long as it is needed.** If estrogens are needed for longer periods of time, your doctor will want to reevaluate your need for estrogens at least every six months.

Women using estrogens should report any irregular vaginal bleeding to their doctors; such bleeding may be of no importance, but it can be an early warning of cancer of the uterus.

Continued on next page

Mead Johnson Labs.—Cont.

If you have undiagnosed vaginal bleeding, you should not use estrogens until a diagnosis is made and you are certain there is no cancer of the uterus. If you have had your uterus completely removed (total hysterectomy), there is no danger of developing cancer of the uterus.

2. **Other possible cancers.** Estrogens can cause development of other tumors in animals, such as tumors of the breast, cervix, vagina, or liver, when given for a long time. At present, there is no satisfactory evidence that women using estrogens in the menopause have an increased risk of such tumors, but there is no way yet to be sure they do not; and one study raises the possibility that use of estrogens in the menopause may increase the risk of breast cancer many years later. This is a further reason to use estrogens only when clearly needed. While you are taking estrogens, it is important that you go to your doctor at least once a year for a physical examination. Also, if members of your family have had breast cancer or if you have breast nodules or abnormal mammograms (breast x-rays), your doctor may wish to carry out more frequent examinations.

3. **Gallbladder disease.** Women who use estrogens after menopause are two or three times more likely to develop gallbladder disease needing surgery than women who do not use estrogens. Birth control pills have a similar effect.

4. **Abnormal blood clotting.** Oral contraceptives increase the risk of blood clotting in various parts of the body. This can occur in different parts of the circulatory system causing thrombophlebitis (clot in the legs or pelvis), retinal thrombosis or optic neuritis (clots affecting vision, including blindness), mesenteric thrombosis (clots in the intestinal blood vessels), stroke (clot in the brain), heart attack (clot in a vessel of the heart) or a pulmonary embolism (clot which eventually lodges in the lungs). These can be fatal.

At this time use of estrogens in the menopause is not known to cause increased blood clotting, this has not been fully studied and there could still prove to be such a risk. It is recommended that if you have had clotting in the legs or lungs or a heart attack or stroke while you were using estrogens or birth control pills, you should not use estrogens (unless they are being used to treat cancer of the breast or prostate). If you have had a stroke or heart attack or if you have angina pectoris, estrogens should be used with great caution and only if clearly needed (for example, if you have severe symptoms of the menopause).

The larger doses of estrogen used to prevent swelling of the breasts after pregnancy have been reported to cause abnormal blood clotting as indicated above.

SPECIAL WARNING ABOUT PREGNANCY

You should not receive estrogen if you are pregnant. If this should occur, there is a greater than usual chance that the developing child will be born with a birth defect, although the possibility remains fairly small. A female child may have an increased risk of developing cancer of the vagina or cervix later in life (in the teens or twenties). Every possible effort should be made to avoid exposure to estrogens during pregnancy. If exposure occurs, see your doctor.

OTHER EFFECTS OF ESTROGENS

In addition to the serious known risks of estrogens described above, estrogens have the following side effects and potential risks which, if occurring, should be discussed promptly with your doctor.

1. **Nausea and vomiting.** The most common side effect of estrogen therapy is nausea. Vomiting is less common.

2. **Effects on breasts.** Estrogens may cause breast tenderness or enlargement and may cause the breasts to secrete a liquid.

3. **Effects on the uterus.** Estrogens may cause benign fibroid tumors of the uterus to get larger. Some women will have menstrual bleeding when estrogens are stopped. But if the bleeding occurs on days you are still taking estrogens, you should report this to your doctor.

4. **Effects on liver.** Women taking oral contraceptives develop on rare occasions a tumor of the liver which can rupture, bleed into the abdomen, and cause death. So far, these tumors have not been reported in women using estrogens in the menopause, but you should report any swelling or unusual pain or tenderness in the abdomen to your doctor immediately.

Women with a past history of jaundice (yellowing of the skin and white parts of the eyes) may get jaundice again during estrogen use. If this occurs, stop taking estrogens and see your doctor.

5. **Other effects.** Estrogens may cause excess fluid to be retained in the body. This may make some conditions worse, such as epilepsy, migraine, heart disease, or kidney disease. Mental depression or high blood pressure may occur. A spotty darkening of the skin, particularly of the face, is possible and may persist.

SUMMARY

Estrogens have important uses, and they may have serious risks as well. You must decide, with your doctor, whether the risks are acceptable to you in view of the benefits of treatment. Except where your doctor has prescribed estrogens for use in special cases of cancer of the breast or prostate, you should not use estrogens if you have cancer of the breast or uterus, are pregnant, have undiagnosed abnormal vaginal bleeding, clotting in the legs or lungs or have had a stroke, heart attack or angina, or clotting in the legs or lungs in the past while you were taking estrogens.

You can use estrogens as safely as possible by understanding that your doctor will require regular physical examinations while you are taking them and will try to discontinue the drug as soon as possible and use the smallest dose possible. Be alert for signs of trouble including:

1. Abnormal bleeding from the vagina.
2. Pains in the calves or chest or sudden shortness of breath, or coughing blood (indicating possible clots in the legs, heart, or lungs).
3. Severe headache, dizziness, faintness, or changes in vision (indicating possible developing clots in the brain or eye).
4. Breast lumps (you should ask your doctor how to examine your own breasts).
5. Jaundice (yellowing of the skin).
6. Mental depression.

Based on his or her assessment of your medical needs, your doctor has prescribed this drug for you. Do not give the drug to anyone else.

REFERENCES

1. Ziel HK, Finkel WD: Increased risk of endometrial carcinoma among users of conjugated estrogens. New Eng J Med 293:1167–1170, 1975. **2.** Smith DC, Prentice R, Thompson DJ, Herrmann WL: Association of exogenous estrogen and endometrial carcinoma. New Eng J Med 293:1164–1167, 1975. **3.** Mack TM, Pike MC, Henderson BE, et al: Estrogens and endometrial cancer in a retirement community. New Eng J Med 294:1262–1267, 1976. **4.** Weiss NS, Szekely DR, Austin DF: Increasing incidence of endometrial cancer in the United States. New Eng J Med 294:1259–1262, 1976. **5.** Herbst AL, Ulfelder H, Poskanzer DC: Adenocarcinoma of vagina. New Eng J Med 284:878–881, 1971. **6.** Greenwald P, Barlow J, Nasca P, Burnett W: Vaginal cancer after maternal treatment with synthetic estrogens. New Eng J Med 285:390–392, 1971. **7.** Lanier A, Noller K, Decker D, et al: Cancer and stilbestrol. A follow-up of 1719 persons exposed to estrogens in utero and born 1943–1959. Mayo Clin Proceedings 48:793–799, 1973. **8.** Herbst A, Kurman R, Scully R: Vaginal and cervical abnormalities after exposure to stilbestrol in utero. Obstet and Gynec 40:287–298, 1972. **9.** Herbst A, Robboy S, Macdonald G, Scully R: The effects of local progesterone on stilbestrol-associated vaginal adenosis. Am J Obstet Gynec 118:607–615, 1974. **10.** Herbst A, Poskanzer D, Robboy S, et al: Prenatal exposure to stilbestrol, a prospective comparison of exposed female offspring with unexposed controls. New Eng J Med 292:334–339, 1975. **11.** Stafl A, Mattingly R, Foley D, Fetherston W: Clinical diagnosis of vaginal adenosis. Obstet Gynec 43:118–128, 1974. **12.** Sherman AI, Goldrath M, Berlin A, et al: Cervical-vaginal adenosis after in utero exposure to synthetic estrogens. Obstet Gynec 44:531–545, 1974. **13.** Gal I, Kirman B, Stern J: Hormone pregnancy tests and congenital malformation. Nature 216:83, 1967. **14.** Levy EP, Cohen A, Fraser FC: Hormone treatment during pregnancy and congenital heart defects. Lancet 1:611, 1973. **15.** Nora J, Nora A: Birth defects and oral contraceptives. Lancet 1:941–942, 1973. **16.** Janerich DT, Piper JM, Glebatis DM: Oral contraceptives and congenital limb-reduction defects. New Eng J Med 291:697–700, 1974. **17.** Yen SSC, Martin PL, Burnier AM, et al: Circulating estradiol, estrone and gonadotropin levels following the administration of orally active 17β-estradiol in postmenopausal women. J Clin Endocrinol Metab 40:518–521, 1975. **18.** Boston Collaborative Drug Surveillance Program: Surgically confirmed gallbladder disease, venous thromboembolism and breast tumors in relation to post-menopausal estrogen therapy. New Eng J Med 290:15–19, 1974. **19.** Hoover R, Gray LA Sr, Cole P, MacMahon B: Menopausal estrogens and breast cancer. New Eng J Med 295:15–19, 1974. **20.** Boston Collaborative Drug Surveillance Program: Oral contraceptives and venous thromboembolic disease, surgically confirmed gallbladder disease, and breast tumors. Lancet 1:1399–1404, 1973. **20a.** Royal College of General Practitioners: Oral Contraceptives and Health. New York, Pitman Corp, 1974. **21.** Daniel DG, Campbell H, Turnbull AC: Puerperal thromboembolism and suppression of lactation. Lancet 2:287–289, 1967. **22.** The Veterans Administration Cooperative Urological Research Group: Carcinoma of the prostate: treatment comparisons. J Urol 98:516–522, 1967. **23.** Bailar JC: Thromboembolism and oestrogen therapy. Lancet 2:560, 1967. **24.** Blackard C, Doe R, Mellinger G, Byar D: Incidence of cardiovascular disease and death in patients receiving diethylstilbestrol for carcinoma of the prostate. Cancer 26:249–256, 1970. **25.** Royal College of General Practitioners: Oral contraception and thromboembolic disease. J Roy Coll Gen Pract 13:267–279, 1967. **26.** Inman WHW, Vessey MP: Investigation of deaths from pulmonary, coronary, and cerebral thrombosis and embolism in women of child-bearing age. Brit M J 2:193–199, 1968. **27.** Vessey MP, Doll R: Investigation of relation between use of oral contraceptives and thromboembolic disease. A further report. Brit M J 2:651–657, 1969. **28.** Sartwell PE, Masi AT, Arthes FG, et al: Thromboembolism and oral contraceptives: an epidemiological case control study. Am J Epidemiol 90:365–380, 1969. **29.** Collaborative Group for the Study of Stroke in Young Women: Oral contraception and increased risk of cerebral ischemia or thrombosis. New Eng J Med 288:871–878, 1973. **30.** Collaborative Group for the Study of Stroke in Young Women: Oral contraceptives and stroke in young women: Associated risk factors. JAMA 231:718–722, 1975. **31.** Mann JI, Inman WHW: Oral contraceptives and death from myocardial infarction. Brit M J 2:245–248, 1975. **32.** Mann JI, Vessey MP, Thorogood M, Doll R: Myocardial infarction in young women with special reference to oral contraceptive practice. Brit M J 2:241–245, 1975. **33.** Inman WHW, Vessey VP, Westerholm B, Engelund A: Thromboembolic disease and the steroidal content of oral contraceptives. Brit M J 2:203–209, 1970. **34.** Stolley PD, Tonascia JA, Tockman MS, et al: Thrombosis with low-estrogen oral contraceptives. Am J Epidemiol 102:197–208, 1975. **35.** Vessey MP, Doll R, Fairbairn AS, Glober G:Post-operative thromboembolism and the use of the oral contraceptives. Brit M J 3:123–126, 1970. **36.** Greene GR, Sartwell PE: Oral contraceptive use in patients with thromboembolism following surgery, trauma or infection. Am J Pub Health 62:680–685, 1972. **37.** Rosenberg L, Armstrong MB, Jick H: Myocardial infarction and estrogen therapy in postmenopausal women. New Eng J Med 294:1256–1259, 1976. **38.** Coronary Drug Project Research Group: The coronary drug project: initial findings leading to modifications of its research protocol. JAMA 214:1303–1313, 1970. **39.** Baum J, Holtz F, Bookstein JJ, Klein EW: Possible association between benign hepatomas and oral contraceptives. Lancet 2:926–928, 1973. **40.** Mays ET, Christopherson WM, Mahr MM, Williams HC: Hepatic changes in young women ingesting contraceptive steroids, hepatic hemorrhage and primary hepatic tumors. JAMA 235:730–732, 1976. **41.** Edmondson HA, Henderson B, Benton B: Liver cell adenomas associated with the use of oral contraceptives. New Eng J Med 294:470–472, 1976. **42.** Pfeffer RI, Van Den Noort S: Estrogen use and stroke risk in postmenopausal women. Am J Epidemiol 103:445–456, 1976.

Shown in Product Identification Section, page 417

Shown in Product Identification Section, page 417

ESTRACE®   ℞

[ĕs 'trāce]

(Estradiol Vaginal Cream 0.01%)

WARNING

1. ESTROGENS HAVE BEEN REPORTED TO INCREASE THE RISK OF ENDOMETRIAL CARCINOMA. Three independent case control studies have shown an increased risk of endometrial cancer in postmenopausal women exposed to exogenous estrogens for prolonged periods.[1–3] This risk was independent of the other known risk factors for endometrial cancer. These studies are further supported by the finding that incidence rates of endometrial cancer have increased sharply since 1969 in eight different areas of the United States with population-based cancer reporting systems, an increase which may be related to the rapidly expanding use of estrogens during the last decade.[4]

The three case control studies reported that the risk of endometrial cancer in estrogen users was about 4.5 to 13.9 times greater than in nonusers. The risk appears to depend on both duration of treatment[1] and on estrogen dose.[3] In view of these findings, when estrogens are used for the treatment of menopausal symptoms, the lowest dose that will control symptoms should be utilized and medication should be discontinued as soon as possible. When prolonged treatment is medically indicated, the patient should be reassessed on at least a semiannual basis to determine the need for continued therapy. Although the evidence must be considered preliminary, one study suggests that cyclic administration of low doses of estrogen may carry less risk than continuous administration,[3] it therefore appears prudent to utilize such a regimen.

Close clinical surveillance of all women taking estrogens is important. In all cases of undiagnosed persistent or recurring abnormal vaginal bleeding, adequate diagnostic measures should be undertaken to rule out malignancy.

There is no evidence at present that "natural" estrogens are more or less hazardous than "synthetic" estrogens at equiestrogenic doses.

2. ESTROGENS SHOULD NOT BE USED DURING PREGNANCY.

The use of female sex hormones, both estrogens and progestogens, during early pregnancy may seriously damage the offspring. It has been shown that females exposed in utero to diethylstilbestrol, a nonsteroidal estrogen, have an increased risk of developing in later life a form of vaginal or cervical cancer that is ordinarily extremely rare.[5,6] This risk has been estimated as not greater than 4 per 1,000 exposures.[7] Furthermore, a high percentage of such exposed women (from 30 to 90 percent) have been found to have vaginal adenosis,[8–12] epithelial changes of the vagina and cervix. Although these changes are histologically benign, it is not known whether they are precursors of malignancy. Although similar data are not available with the use of other estrogens, it cannot be presumed they would not induce similar changes.

Several reports suggest an association between intrauterine exposure to female sex hormones and congenital anomalies, including congenital heart defects and limb reduction defects.[13–16] One case control study[16] estimated a 4.7-fold increased risk of limb reduction defects in infants exposed *in utero* to sex hormones (oral contraceptives, hormone withdrawal tests for pregnancy, or attempted treatment for threatened abortion). Some of these exposures were very short and involved only a few days of treatment. The data suggest that the risk of limb reduction defects in exposed fetuses is somewhat less than 1 per 1,000.

In the past, female sex hormones have been used during pregnancy in an attempt to treat threatened or habitual abortion. There is considerable evidence that estrogens are ineffective for these indications, and there is no evidence from well-controlled studies that progestogens are effective for these uses.

If Estrace is used during pregnancy, or if the patient becomes pregnant while taking this drug, she should be apprised of the potential risks to the fetus and the advisability of pregnancy continuation.

DESCRIPTION

Each gram of Estrace (17β-estradiol) Vaginal Cream contains 0.1 mg 17β-estradiol in a nonliquefying base containing purified water, propylene glycol, stearyl alcohol, white ceresin wax, glyceryl monostearate, hydroxypropyl methylcellulose, 2208 4000 cps, sodium lauryl sulfate, methylparaben, edetate disodium and tertiary-butylhydroquinone. Estradiol is chemically described as estra-1, 3, 5(10)-triene-3, 17β-diol. The structural formula is:

CLINICAL PHARMACOLOGY

Estrogens are important in the development and maintenance of the female reproductive system and secondary sex characteristics. They promote growth and development of the vagina, uterus, and fallopian tubes, and enlargement of the breasts. Indirectly, they contribute to the shaping of the skeleton, maintenance of tone and elasticity or urogenital structures, changes in the epiphyses of the long bones that allow for the pubertal growth spurt and its termination, growth of axillary and pubic hair, and pigmentation of the nipples and genitals. Decline of estrogenic activity at the end of the menstrual cycle can bring on menstruation, although the cessation of progesterone secretion is the most important factor in the mature ovulatory cycle. However, in the preovulatory or nonovulatory cycle, estrogen is the primary determinant in the onset of menstruation. Estrogens also affect the release of pituitary gonadotropins.

Micronized 17β-estradiol achieves its pharmacologic effect in estrogen-responsive target tissues via anabolic stimulus at the cellular level. Micronized 17β-estradiol in Estrace Vaginal Cream is readily absorbed from mucosal surfaces.

In responsive tissues (female genital organs, breasts, hypothalamus, pituitary) estrogens enter the cell and are transported into the nucleus. As a result of estrogen action, specific RNA and protein synthesis occurs.

Metabolism and inactivation occur primarily in the liver. Some estrogens are excreted into the bile; however, they are reabsorbed from the intestine and returned to the liver through the portal venous system. Water-soluble estrogen conjugates are strongly acidic and are ionized in body fluids, which favor excretion through the kidneys since tubular reabsorption is minimal.

INDICATIONS

Estrace Vaginal Cream is indicated in the treatment of atrophic vaginitis and kraurosis vulvae.

The lowest effective dose appropriate for the specific indication should be utilized. Studies of the addition of a progestogen for seven or more days of a cycle of estrogen administration have reported a lowered incidence of endometrial hyperplasia. Morphological and biochemical studies of endometrium suggest that 10 to 13 days of progestogen are needed to provide maximal maturation of the endometrium and to eliminate any hyperplastic changes. Whether this will pro-

vide protection from endometrial carcinoma has not been clearly established. There are possible additional risks which may be associated with the inclusion of progestogen in estrogen replacement regimens. The potential risks include adverse effects on carbohydrate and lipid metabolism. The choice of progestogen and dosage may be important in minimizing these adverse effects.

ESTRACE HAS NOT BEEN SHOWN TO BE EFFECTIVE FOR ANY PURPOSE DURING PREGNANCY AND ITS USE MAY CAUSE SEVERE HARM TO THE FETUS (SEE BOXED WARNING).

CONTRAINDICATIONS

Estrogens should not be used in women (or men) with any of the following conditions:

1. Known or suspected cancer of the breast, except in appropriately selected patients being treated for metastatic disease.
2. Known or suspected estrogen-dependent neoplasia.
3. Known or suspected pregnancy (See Boxed Warning).
4. Undiagnosed abnormal genital bleeding.
5. Active thrombophlebitis or thromboembolic disorders.
6. A past history of thrombophlebitis, thrombosis or thromboembolic disorders associated with previous estrogen use (except when used in treatment of breast or prostatic malignancy).

WARNINGS

1. **Induction of malignant neoplasms.** Long-term continuous administration of natural and synthetic estrogens in certain animal species increases the frequency of carcinomas of the breast, cervix, vagina, and liver. There is now evidence that estrogens increase the risk of carcinoma of the endometrium in humans. (See Boxed Warning).

At the present time there is no satisfactory evidence that estrogens given to postmenopausal women increase the risk of cancer of the breast,[17] although a recent long-term follow-up of a single physician's practice has raised this possibility.[18] Because of the animal data there is a need for caution in prescribing estrogens for women with a strong family history of breast cancer or who have breast nodules, fibrocystic disease, or abnormal mammograms.

2. **Gallbladder disease.** A recent study has reported a 2- to 3-fold increase in the risk of surgically confirmed gallbladder disease in women receiving postmenopausal estrogens,[17] similar to the 2-fold increase previously noted in users of oral contraceptives.[19,24a]

3. **Effects similar to those caused by estrogen-progestogen oral contraceptives.** There are several serious adverse effects of oral contraceptives, most of which have not, up to now, been documented as consequences of postmenopausal estrogen therapy. This may reflect the comparatively low doses of estrogen used in postmenopausal women. It would be expected that the larger doses of estrogen used to treat prostatic or breast cancer or postpartum breast engorgement are more likely to result in these adverse effects; and, in fact, it has been shown that there is an increased risk of thrombosis in men receiving estrogens for prostatic cancer and women for postpartum breast engorgement.[20–23]

a. **Thromboembolic disease.** It is now well established that users of oral contraceptives have an increased risk of various thromboembolic and thrombotic vascular diseases, such as thrombophlebitis, pulmonary embolism, stroke, and myocardial infarction.[24–31] Cases of retinal thrombosis, mesenteric thrombosis, and optic neuritis have been reported in oral contraceptive users. There is evidence that the risk of several of these adverse reactions is related to the dose of the drug.[32,33] An increased risk of postsurgery thromboembolic complications has also been reported in users of oral contraceptives.[34,35] If feasible, estrogen should be discontinued at least 4 weeks before surgery of the type associated with an increased risk of thromboembolism, or during periods of prolonged immobilization.

While an increased rate of thromboembolic and thrombotic disease in postmenopausal users of estrogens has not been found,[17–36] this does not rule out the possibility that such an increase may be present or that subgroups of women who have underlying risk factors or who are receiving relatively large doses of estrogens may have increased risk. Therefore, estrogens should not be used in persons with active thrombophlebitis or thromboembolic disorders, and they should not be used (except in treatment of malignancy) in persons with a history of such disorders in association with estrogen use. They should be used with caution in patients with cerebral vascular or coronary artery disease and only for those in whom estrogens are clearly needed.

Large doses of estrogen (5 mg conjugated estrogens per day), comparable to those used to treat cancer of the prostate and breast, have been shown in a large prospective clinical trial in men[37] to increase the risk of nonfatal myocardial infarction, pulmonary embolism and thrombophlebitis. When estrogen doses of this size are used, any of the thromboembolic and thrombotic adverse effects associated

with oral contraceptive use should be considered a clear risk.

b. **Hepatic adenoma.** Hepatic adenomas appear to be associated with the use of oral contraceptives.[38–40] Although rare, these may rupture and may cause death through intraabdominal hemorrhage. Such lesions have not yet been reported in association with other estrogen or progestogen preparations but should be considered in estrogen users having abdominal pain and tenderness, abdominal mass, or hypovolemic shock. Hepatocellular carcinoma has also been reported in women taking estrogen-containing oral contraceptives.[39] The relationship of this malignancy to these drugs is not known at this time.

c. **Elevated blood pressure.** Increased blood pressure is not uncommon in women using oral contraceptives. There is now a report that this may occur with use of estrogens in the menopause[41] and blood pressure should be monitored with estrogen use, especially if high doses are used.

d. **Glucose tolerance.** A worsening of glucose tolerance has been observed in a significant percentage of patients on estrogen-containing oral contraceptives. For this reason, diabetic patients should be carefully observed while receiving estrogen.

4. **Hypercalcemia.** Administration of estrogens may lead to severe hypercalcemia in patients with breast cancer and bone metastases. If this occurs, the drug should be stopped and appropriate measures taken to reduce the serum calcium level.

PRECAUTIONS

A. General Precautions.

1. A complete medical and family history should be taken prior to the initiation of any estrogen therapy. The pretreatment and periodic physical examinations should include special reference to blood pressure, breasts, abdomen, and pelvic organs, and should include a Papanicolaou smear. As a general rule, estrogen should not be prescribed for longer than one year without another physical examination being performed.

2. Fluid retention — Because estrogens may cause some degree of fluid retention, conditions which might be influenced by this factor such as epilepsy, migraine, and cardiac or renal dysfunction, require careful observation.

3. Certain patients may develop undesirable manifestations of excessive estrogenic stimulation, such as abnormal or excessive uterine bleeding, mastodynia, etc.

4. Oral contraceptives appear to be associated with an increased incidence of mental depression.[24a] Although it is not clear whether this is due to the estrogenic or progestogenic component of the contraceptive, patients with a history of depression should be carefully observed.

5. Pre-existing uterine leiomyomata may increase in size during estrogen use.

6. The pathologist should be advised of estrogen therapy when relevant specimens are submitted.

7. Patients with a past history of jaundice during pregnancy have an increased risk of recurrence of jaundice while receiving estrogen-containing oral contraceptive therapy. If jaundice develops in any patient receiving estrogen, the medication should be discontinued while the cause is investigated.

8. Estrogens may be poorly metabolized in patients with impaired liver function and they should be administered with caution in such patients.

9. Because estrogens influence the metabolism of calcium and phosphorus, they should be used with caution in patients with metabolic bone diseases that are associated with hypercalcemia or in patients with renal insufficiency.

10. Because of the effects of estrogens on epiphyseal closure, they should be used judiciously in young patients in whom bone growth is not complete.

11. Certain endocrine and liver function tests may be affected by estrogen-containing oral contraceptives. The following similar changes may be expected with larger doses of estrogen:

a. Increased sulfobromophthalein retention.

b. Increased prothrombin and factors VII and VIII, IX, and X; decreased antithrombin 3; increased norepinephrine-induced platelet aggregability.

c. Increased thyroid binding globulin (TBG) leading to increased circulating total thyroid hormone, as measured by PBI, T4 by column, or T4 by radioimmunoassay, free T3 resin uptake is decreased, reflecting the elevated TBG; free T4 concentration is unaltered.

d. Impaired glucose tolerance.

e. Decreased pregnanediol excretion.

f. Reduced response to metyrapone test.

g. Reduced serum folate concentration.

h. Increased serum triglyceride and phospholipid concentration.

B. Information for the Patient. See text which appears after the physician References.

C. Pregnancy Category X. See Contraindications and Boxed Warning.

Continued on next page

Mead Johnson Labs.—Cont.

D. Nursing Mothers. As a general principle, the administration of any drug to nursing mothers should be done only when clearly necessary since many drugs are excreted in human milk.

ADVERSE REACTIONS

(See Warnings regarding induction of neoplasia, adverse effects on the fetus, increased incidence of gall bladder disease, and adverse effects similar to those of oral contraceptives, including thromboembolism.) The following additional adverse reactions have been reported with estrogenic therapy, including oral contraceptives:

Genitourinary system. Breakthrough bleeding, spotting, change in menstrual flow. Dysmenorrhea. Premenstrual-like syndrome. Amenorrhea during and after treatment. Increase in size of uterine fibromyomata. Vaginal candidiasis. Change in cervical eversion and in degree of cervical secretion. Cystitis-like syndrome.

Breast. Tenderness, enlargement, secretion.

Gastrointestinal. Nausea, vomiting. Abdominal cramps, bloating. Cholestatic jaundice.

Skin. Chloasma or melasma which may persist when drug is discontinued. Erythema multiforme. Hemorrhagic eruption. Hirsutism. Erythema nodosum. Loss of scalp hair.

Eyes. Steepening of corneal curvature. Intolerance to contact lenses.

CNS. Headache, migraine, dizziness. Mental depression. Chorea.

Miscellaneous. Increase or decrease in weight. Reduced carbohydrate tolerance. Aggravation of porphyria. Edema. Changes in libido.

OVERDOSAGE

Numerous reports of ingestion of large doses of estrogen-containing oral contraceptives by young children indicate that serious ill effects do not occur. Overdosage of estrogen may cause nausea, and withdrawal bleeding may occur in females.

DOSAGE AND ADMINISTRATION

Given cyclically for short-term use only.
For treatment of atrophic vaginitis or kraurosis vulvae.
The lowest dose that will control symptoms should be chosen and medication should be discontinued as promptly as possible. Administration should be cyclic (eg, 3 weeks on and 1 week off).
Attempts to discontinue or taper medication should be made at 3 to 6 month intervals.
Usual Dosage: The usual dosage range is 2 to 4 g (marked on the applicator) daily for one or two weeks, then gradually reduced to one half initial dosage for a similar period. A maintenance dosage of 1 g one to three times a week, may be used after restoration of the vaginal mucosa has been achieved.
Patients with an intact uterus should be monitored closely for signs of endometrial cancer and appropriate diagnostic measures should be taken to rule out malignancy in eventual persistent or recurring abnormal vaginal bleeding.

HOW SUPPLIED

Estrace (estradiol) Vaginal Cream.
NDC 0087-0754-42 42.5 g Tube with applicator.

REFERENCES

1. Ziel HK, Finkel WD: Increased risk of endometrial carcinoma among users of conjugated estrogens. New Eng J Med 293:1167–1170, 1975. **2.** Smith, DC, Prentice R, Thompson DJ, Herrmann WL: Association of exogenous estrogen and endometrial carcinoma. New Eng J Med 293:1164–1167, 1975. **3.** Mack TM, Pike MC, Henderson BE, et al: Estrogens and the endometrial cancer in a retirement community. New Eng J Med 294:1262–1267, 1976. **4.** Weiss, NS, Szekely DR, Austin DF: Increasing incidence of endometrial cancer in the United States. New Eng J Med 294:1259–1262, 1976. **5.** Herbst AL, Ulfelder H, Poskanzer DC: Adenocarcinoma of vagina. New Eng J Med 284:878–881, 1971. **6.** Greenwald P, Barlow J, Nasca P, Burnett W: Vaginal cancer after maternal treatment with synthetic estrogens. New Eng J Med 285:390–392, 1971. **7.** Lanier A, Noller K, Decker D, et al: Cancer and stilbestrol. A follow-up of 1719 persons exposed to estrogens in utero and born 1943–1959. Mayo Clin Proceedings 48:793–799, 1973. **8.** Herbst A, Kurman R, Scully R: Vaginal and cervical abnormalities after exposure to stilbestrol in utero. Obstet and Gynec 40:287–298, 1972. **9.** Herbst A, Robboy S, MacDonald G, Scully R: The effects of local progesterone on stilbestrol-associated vaginal adenosis. Am J Obstet Gynec 118:607–615, 1974. **10.** Herbst A, Poskanzer D, Robboy S, et al: Prenatal exposure to stilbestrol, a prospective comparison of exposed female offspring with unexposed controls. New Eng J Med 292:334–339, 1975. **11.** Stafl A, Mattingly R, Foley D, Fetherston W: Clinical diagnosis of vaginal adenosis. Obstet and Gynec 43:118–128, 1974. **12.** Sherman Al, Goldrath M, Berlin A, et al: Cervical-vaginal adenosis after in utero exposure to synthetic estrogens. Obstet Gynec 44:531–545, 1974. **13.** Gal I, Kirman B, Stern J: Hormone pregnancy tests and congenital malformation. Nature 216:83, 1967. **14.** Levy EP, Cohen A, Fraser FC: Hormone treatment during pregnancy and congenital heart defects. Lancet 1:611, 1973. **15.** Nora J, Nora A: Birth defects and oral contraceptives. Lancet 1:941–942, 1973. **16.** Janerich DT, Piper JM, Glebatis DM: Oral contraceptives and congenital limb-reduction defects. New Engl J Med 291:697–700, 1974. **17.** Boston Collaborative Drug Surveillance Program: Surgically confirmed gallbladder disease, venous thromboembolism and breast tumors in relation to post-menopausal estrogen therapy. New Eng J Med 290:15–19, 1974. **18.** Hoover R, Gray LA Sr, Cole P, MacMahon B: Menopausal estrogens and breast cancer. New Eng J Med 295:15–19, 1974. **19.** Boston Collaborative Drug Surveillance Program: Oral contraceptives and venous thromboembolic disease, surgically confirmed gall bladder disease, and breast tumors. Lancet 1:1399–1404, 1973. **20.** Daniel DG, Campbell H, Turnbull AC: Puerperal thromboemboism and suppression of lactation. Lancet 2:287–289, 1967. **21.** The Veterans Administration Cooperative Urological Research Group: Carcinoma of the prostate; treatment comparisons. J Urol 98:516–522, 1967. **22.** Bailar JC: Thromboembolism and oestrogen therapy. Lancet 2:560, 1967. **23.** Blackard C, Doe R, Mellinger G, Byar D: Incidence of cardiovascular disease and death in patients receiving diethylstilbestrol for carcinoma of the prostate. Cancer 26:249–256, 1970. **24.** Royal College of General Practitioners: Oral contraception and thromboembolic disease. J Roy Coll Gen Pract 13:267–279, 1967. **24a.** Royal College of General Practitioners: Oral Contraceptives and Health, New York, Pitman Corp, 1974. **25.** Inman WHW, Vessey MP: Investigation of deaths from pulmonary, coronary, and cerebral thrombosis and embolism in women of childbearing age. Brit M J 2:193–199, 1968. **26.** Vessey MP, Doll R: Investigation of relation between use of oral contraceptives and thromboembolic disease. A further report. Brit M J 2:651–657, 1969. **27.** Sartwell PE, Masi AT, Arthes FG, et al: Thromboembolism and oral contraceptives: an epidemiological case control study. Am J Epidemiol 90:365–380, 1969. **28.** Collaborative Group for the Study of Stroke in Young Women: Oral contraception and increased risk of cerebral ischemia or thrombosis. New Eng J Med 288:871–878, 1973. **29.** Collaborative Group for the Study of Stroke in Young Women: Oral contraceptives and stroke in young women: Associated risk factors. JAMA 231:718–722, 1975. **30.** Mann JI, Inman WHW: Oral contraceptives and death from myocardial infarction. Brit M J 2:245–248, 1975. **31.** Mann JI, Vessey MP, Thorogood M, Doll R: Myocardial infarction in young women with special reference to oral contraceptive practice. Brit M J 2:241–245, 1975. **32.** Inman WHW, Vessey MP, Westerholm B, Engelund A: Thromboembolic disease and the steroidal content of oral contraceptives. Brit M J 2:203–209, 1970. **33.** Stolley PD, Tonascia JA, Tockman MS, et al: Thrombosis with low-estrogen oral contraceptives. Am J Epidemiol 102:197–208, 1975. **34.** Vessey MP, Doll R, Fairbairn AS, Glober G: Post-operative thromboembolism and the use of the oral contraceptives. Brit M J 3:123–126, 1970. **35.** Greene GR, Sartwell PE: Oral contraceptive use in patients with thromboembolism following surgery, trauma or infection. Am J Pub Health 62:680–685, 1972. **36.** Rosenberg L, Armstrong MB, Jick H: Myocardial infarction and estrogen therapy in postmenopausal women. New Engl J Med 294:1256–1259, 1976. **37.** Coronary Drug Project Research Group: The coronary drug project: initial findings leading to modifications of its research protocol. JAMA 214:1303–1313, 1970. **38.** Baum J, Holtz F, Bookstein JJ, Klein EW: Possible association between benign hepatomas and oral contraceptives. Lancet 2:926–928, 1973. **39.** Mays ET, Christopherson WM, Mahr MM, Williams HC: Hepatic changes in young women ingesting contraceptive steroids, hepatic hemorrhage and primary hepatic tumors. JAMA 235:730–732, 1976. **40.** Edmondson HA, Henderson B, Benton B: Liver cell adenomas associated with the use of oral contraceptives. New Eng J Med 294:470–472, 1976. **41.** Pfeffer RI, Van Den Noort S: Estrogen use and stroke risk in postmenopausal women. Am J Epidemiol 103:445–456, 1976.

INFORMATION FOR THE PATIENT

WHAT YOU SHOULD KNOW ABOUT ESTROGENS

Estrogens are female hormones produced principally by the ovaries. The ovaries make several different kinds of estrogens. In addition, scientists have been able to make a variety of synthetic estrogens. As far as we know, all these estrogens have the same properties and, therefore, much the same usefulness, side effects, and risks. This leaflet is intended to help you understand what estrogens are used for, the risks involved in their use, and how to use them as safely as possible.

This leaflet includes important information about Estrace® (estradiol) and estrogens in general, but not all the information. If you want to know more, you can ask your doctor or pharmacist to let you read the professional package insert.

USES OF ESTROGEN

Estrogens are prescribed by doctors for a number of purposes, including:

1. To provide estrogen during a period of adjustment when a woman's ovaries no longer produce it, in order to prevent certain uncomfortable symptoms of estrogen deficiency. (All women normally experience a decrease in the production of estrogens, generally between 45–55; this is called the menopause).
2. To prevent symptoms of estrogen deficiency when a woman's ovaries have been removed surgically before the natural menopause.
3. To prevent pregnancy. (Some estrogens are given along with a progestogen, another female hormone; these combinations are called oral contraceptives or birth control pills. They will not be discussed in this leaflet.) However, Estrace is not intended for this use.
4. To treat certain cancers in women and men.
5. To prevent painful swelling of the breasts after pregnancy in women who choose not to nurse their babies.

THERE IS NO PROPER USE OF ESTROGENS IN A PREGNANT WOMAN.

ESTROGENS IN THE MENOPAUSE

In the natural course of their lives, all women eventually experience a decrease in estrogen production. This usually occurs between ages 45 and 55 but may occur earlier or later. Sometimes the ovaries may need to be removed before natural menopause by an operation, producing a "surgical menopause."

When the amount of estrogen in the blood begins to decrease, many women may develop typical symptoms: feelings of warmth in the face, neck, and chest or sudden intense episodes of heat and sweating throughout the body (called "hot flashes" or "hot flushes"). These symptoms are sometimes very uncomfortable. A few women eventually develop changes in the vagina (called "atrophic vaginitis") which cause discomfort, especially during and after intercourse. Estrogens can be prescribed to treat these symptoms of the menopause. It is estimated that considerably more than half of all women undergoing the menopause have only mild symptoms or no symptoms at all and therefore do not need estrogens. Other women may need estrogens for a few months, while their bodies adjust to lower estrogen levels. Sometimes the need will be for periods longer than six months. In an attempt to avoid over-stimulation of the uterus (womb), estrogens are usually given cyclically during each month of use, that is, three weeks of therapy followed by one week without therapy.

Sometimes women experience nervous symptoms or depression during menopause. There is no evidence that estrogens are effective for such symptoms and they should not be used to treat them, although other treatment may be needed.

You may have heard that taking estrogens for long periods (years) after the menopause will keep your skin soft and supple and keep you feeling young. There is no evidence that this is so, however, and such long-term treatment carries additional risks.

ESTROGENS TO PREVENT SWELLING OF THE BREASTS AFTER PREGNANCY

If you do not breast-feed your baby after delivery, your breasts may fill up with milk and become painful and engorged. This usually begins about three to four days after delivery and may last for a few days to up to a week or more. Sometimes the discomfort is severe, but usually it is not and can be controlled by pain-relieving drugs such as aspirin and by binding the breasts up tightly. Estrogens can sometimes be used successfully to try to prevent the breasts from filling up. While this treatment is sometimes successful, in many cases the breasts fill up to some degree in spite of treatment. The dose of estrogens needed to prevent pain and swelling of the breasts is much larger than the dose needed to treat symptoms of the menopause and this may increase your chances of developing blood clots in the legs or lungs or other parts of the body (see below, 4. **Abnormal Blood Clotting**). Therefore, it is important that you discuss the benefits and the risks of estrogen use with your doctor, before using estrogen, if you have decided not to breast-feed your baby.

THE DANGERS OF ESTROGENS

1. **Cancer of the uterus.** If estrogens are used in the postmenopausal period for more than a year, there is an increased risk of **cancer of the endometrium** (uterine lining). Women taking estrogens have roughly 5 to 15 times as great a chance of getting this cancer as women who take no estrogens. To put this another way, while a postmenopausal woman not taking estrogens has one chance in 1,000 each year of getting cancer of the uterus, a woman taking estrogens has 5 to 15 chances in 1,000 each year. For this reason **it is important to take estrogens only when you really need them.**
The risk of this cancer is greater the longer estrogens are used and also seems to be greater when larger doses are taken. For this reason **it is important to take the lowest dose of estrogen that will control symptoms and to take it only as long as it is needed.** If estrogens are needed for longer periods of time, your doctor will want to reevaluate your need for estrogens at least every six months. Women using estrogens should report any irregular vaginal bleeding to their doctors; such bleeding may be of no

importance, but it can be an early warning of cancer of the uterus. If you have undiagnosed vaginal bleeding, you should not use estrogens until a diagnosis is made and you are certain there is no cancer of the uterus.

NOTE: If you have had your uterus completely removed (total hysterectomy), there is no danger of developing cancer of the uterus.

2. **Other possible cancers.** Estrogens can cause development of other tumors in animals, such as tumors of the breast, cervix, vagina, or liver, when given for a long time. At present, there is no satisfactory evidence that women using estrogens in the menopause have an increased risk of such tumors, but there is no way yet to be sure they do not; and one study raises the possibility that use of estrogens in the menopause may increase the risk of breast cancer many years later. This is a further reason to use estrogens only when clearly needed. While you are taking estrogens, it is important that you go to your doctor at least once a year for a physical examination. Also, if members of your family have had breast cancer or if you have breast nodules or abnormal mammograms (breast x-rays), your doctor may wish to carry out more frequent examinations.

3. **Gallbladder disease.** Women who use estrogens after menopause are two or three times more likely to develop gallbladder disease needing surgery than women who do not use estrogens. Birth control pills have a similar effect.

4. **Abnormal blood clotting.** Oral contraceptives increase the risk of blood clotting in various parts of the body. This can occur in different parts of the circulatory system causing thrombophlebitis (clot in the legs or pelvis), retinal thrombosis or optic neuritis (clots affecting vision, including blindness), mesenteric thrombosis (clots in the intestinal blood vessels), stroke (clot in the brain), heart attack (clot in a vessel of the heart) or a pulmonary embolism (clot which eventually lodges in the lungs). These can be fatal.

At this time, use of estrogens in the menopause is not known to cause increased blood clotting; this has not been fully studied and there could still prove to be such a risk. It is recommended that if you have had clotting in the legs or lungs or a heart attack or stroke while you were using estrogens or birth control pills, you should not use estrogens (unless they are being used to treat cancer of the breast or prostate). If you have had a stroke or heart attack or if you have angina pectoris, estrogens should be used with great caution and only if clearly needed (for example, if you have severe symptoms of the menopause). The larger doses of estrogen used to prevent swelling of the breasts after pregnancy have been reported to cause abnormal blood clotting as indicated above.

SPECIAL WARNING ABOUT PREGNANCY

You should not receive estrogen if you are pregnant. If this should occur, there is a greater than usual chance that the developing child will be born with a birth defect, although the possibility remains fairly small. A female child may have an increased risk of developing cancer of the vagina or cervix later in life (in the teens or twenties). Every possible effort should be made to avoid exposure to estrogens during pregnancy. If exposure occurs, see your doctor.

OTHER EFFECTS OF ESTROGENS

In addition to the serious known risks of estrogens described above, estrogens have the following side effects and potential risks which, if occurring, should be discussed promptly with your doctor.

1. **Nausea and vomiting.** The most common side effect of estrogen therapy is nausea. Vomiting is less common.

2. **Effects on breasts.** Estrogens may cause breast tenderness or enlargement and may cause the breasts to secrete a liquid.

3. **Effects on the uterus.** Estrogens may cause benign fibroid tumors of the uterus to get larger. Some women will have menstrual bleeding when estrogens are stopped. But if the bleeding occurs on days you are still taking estrogens, you should report this to your doctor.

4. **Effects on liver.** Women taking oral contraceptives develop on rare occasions a tumor of the liver which can rupture, bleed into the abdomen, and cause death. So far, these tumors have not been reported in women using estrogens in the menopause, but you should report any swelling or unusual pain or tenderness in the abdomen to your doctor immediately.

Women with a past history of jaundice (yellowing of the skin and white parts of the eyes) may get jaundice again during estrogen use. If this occurs, stop taking estrogens and see your doctor.

5. **Other effects.** Estrogens may cause excess fluid to be retained in the body. This may make some conditions worse, such as epilepsy, migraine, heart disease, or kidney disease. Mental depression or high blood pressure may occur. A spotty darkening of the skin, particularly of the face, is possible and may persist.

SUMMARY

Estrogens have important uses, and they may have serious risks as well. You must decide, with your doctor, whether the risks are acceptable to you in view of the benefits of treatment. Except where your doctor has prescribed estrogens for use in special cases of cancer of the breast or prostate, you should not use estrogens if you have cancer of the breast or uterus, are pregnant, have undiagnosed abnormal vaginal bleeding, clotting in the legs or lungs or have had a stroke, heart attack or angina, or clotting in the legs or lungs in the past while you were taking estrogens.

You can use estrogens as safely as possible by understanding that your doctor will require regular physical examinations while you are taking them and will try to discontinue the drug as soon as possible and use the smallest dose possible. Be alert for signs of trouble including:

1. Abnormal bleeding from the vagina.
2. Pains in the calves or chest or sudden shortness of breath, or coughing blood (indicating possible clots in the legs, heart, or lungs).
3. Severe headache, dizziness, faintness, or changes in vision (indicating possible developing clots in the brain or eye).
4. Breast lumps (you should ask your doctor how to examine your own breasts).
5. Jaundice (yellowing of the skin).
6. Mental depression.

Your doctor has prescribed this drug for you. Do not give this drug to anyone else.

Shown in Product Identification Section, page 417

NATALINS® Tablets
[nā-tă-lins]
Multivitamin and multimineral supplement

COMPOSITION
Each Natalins tablet supplies:
Vitamins

Vitamin A, IU	5,000
Vitamin D, IU	400
Vitamin E, IU	30
Vitamin C (Ascorbic acid), mg	90
Folic acid, mg	0.8
Thiamine (Vitamin B₁), mg	1.7
Riboflavin (Vitamin B₂), mg	2
Niacin, mg	20
Vitamin B₆, mg	4
Vitamin B₁₂, μg	8

Minerals

Calcium, mg	200
Iodine, μg	150
Iron, mg	45
Magnesium, mg	100

INGREDIENTS
Calcium carbonate, magnesium hydroxide, ferrous fumarate, sodium ascorbate, povidone, dl-alpha-tocopheryl acetate, acacia, niacinamide, vitamin A acetate, hydroxypropyl methylcellulose, polacrilin potassium, magnesium stearate, pyridoxine hydrochloride, polyethylene glycol, riboflavin (color), titanium dioxide (color), hydroxypropyl cellulose, silicon dioxide, thiamine mononitrate, folic acid, vitamin D₃, calcium iodate, vitamin B₁₂.

INDICATIONS AND USAGE
Diet supplementation during pregnancy or lactation.

DOSAGE AND ADMINISTRATION
One tablet a day or as indicated.

HOW SUPPLIED
Natalins® tablets
  0087-0700-01 Bottles of 100
  0087-0700-06 Bottles of 1000
    Shown in Product Identification Section, page 417

NATALINS® RX
[nā-tă-lins]
Multivitamin and Multimineral Supplement
Tablets with 1 mg folic acid and 60 mg Iron

Natalins Rx tablets provide twelve vitamins and six minerals to supplement the diet during pregnancy or lactation with no artificial flavor or color from synthetic sources.

COMPOSITION
Each Natalins Rx tablet supplies:
Vitamins

Vitamin A, IU	5,000
Vitamin D, IU	400
Vitamin E, IU	30
Vitamin C (Ascorbic acid), mg	90
Folic acid (Folacin), mg	1
Thiamine (Vitamin B₁), mg	2.5
Riboflavin (Vitamin B₂), mg	3
Niacin, mg	20
Vitamin B₆, mg	10
Vitamin B₁₂, μg	8
Biotin, mg	0.05
Pantothenic acid, mg	15

Minerals

Calcium, mg	200
Iodine, μg	150
Iron, mg	60
Magnesium, mg	100
Copper, mg	2
Zinc, mg	15

ACTIVE INGREDIENT
Each tablet contains 1 mg folic acid.

OTHER INGREDIENTS
Acacia, biotin, calcium carbonate, calcium iodate, calcium pantothenate, cholecalciferol, colloidal silicon dioxide, cupric oxide, cyanocobalamin, ferrous fumarate, hydroxypropyl cellulose, hydroxypropyl methylcellulose 2910, magnesium hydroxide, magnesium stearate, niacinamide, polacrilin potassium, polyethylene glycol, povidone, pyridoxine hydrochloride, riboflavin, sodium ascorbate, thiamine mononitrate, titanium dioxide, dl-alpha-tocopheryl acetate, vitamin A acetate, zinc oxide.

INDICATIONS AND USAGE
Natalins Rx tablets help assure an adequate intake of the vitamins and minerals listed above.
Folic acid helps prevent the development of megaloblastic anemia during pregnancy.

CONTRAINDICATIONS
Supplemental vitamins and minerals should not be prescribed for patients with hemochromatosis or Wilson's disease.

WARNING
Keep Natalins Rx tablets out of the reach of children.

PRECAUTIONS
General—pernicious anemia should be excluded before using this product since folic acid may mask the symptoms of pernicious anemia. The calcium content should be considered before prescribing for patients with kidney stones. Do not exceed the recommended dose.

ADVERSE REACTIONS
No adverse reactions or undesirable side effects have been attributed to the use of Natalins Rx tablets.

DOSAGE AND ADMINISTRATION
One tablet daily, or as prescribed.

HOW SUPPLIED
Natalins® Rx Tablets: (Available on prescription.)
  NDC 0087-0702-01 Bottles of 100
  NDC 0087-0702-02 Bottles of 1000
    Shown in Product Identification Section, page 417

OVCON® 50   ℞
[ăv′kăn]

21 tablets of norethindrone 1 mg and ethinyl estradiol 0.05 mg. Each green tablet in the 28-day regimen contains inert ingredients.

OVCON® 35   ℞

21 tablets of norethindrone 0.4 mg and ethinyl estradiol 0.035 mg. Each green tablet in the 28-day regimen contains inert ingredients.

Oral contraceptives

DESCRIPTION
28-Day OVCON® 50 and OVCON® 35 tablets (norethindrone and ethinyl estradiol) tablets provide a continuous regimen for oral contraception derived from 21 tablets composed of norethindrone and ethinyl estradiol to be followed by 7 green tablets of inert ingredients.

21-Day OVCON 50 and OVCON 35 tablets provide a regimen for oral contraception derived from 21 tablets composed of norethindrone and ethinyl estradiol. The chemical name for norethindrone is 17-hydroxy-19-nor-17α-pregn-4-en-20-yn-3-one and for ethinyl estradiol the chemical name is 19-nor-17α-pregna-1,3,5 (10)-trien-20-yne-3, 17-diol. The structural formulas are:

NORETHINDRONE

Continued on next page

Mead Johnson Labs.—Cont.

ETHINYL ESTRADIOL

The active OVCON 50 tablets contain 1 mg norethindrone and 0.05 mg ethinyl estradiol. The active OVCON 35 tablets contain 0.4 mg norethindrone and 0.035 mg ethinyl estradiol.

The green tablets contain inert ingredients.

OVCON 50, 21-Day contains the following inactive ingredients: dibasic calcium phosphate, D&C Yellow No. 10 (aluminum lake), FD&C Yellow No. 6 (aluminum lake), lactose, magnesium stearate, povidone, and sodium starch glycolate.

OVCON 50, 28-Day contains the following inactive ingredients: acacia, dibasic calcium phosphate, D&C Yellow No. 10 (aluminum lake), FD&C Blue No. 1 (aluminum lake), FD&C Yellow No. 6 (aluminum lake), lactose, magnesium stearate, povidone, sodium starch glycolate, starch (corn), and talc.

OVCON 35, 21-Day contains the following inactive ingredients: dibasic calcium phosphate, FD&C Yellow No. 6 (aluminum lake), lactose, magnesium stearate, povidone, and sodium starch glycolate.

OVCON 35, 28-Day contains the following inactive ingredients: acacia, dibasic calcium phosphate, D&C Yellow No. 10 (aluminum lake), FD&C Blue No. 1 (aluminum lake), FD&C Yellow No. 6 (aluminum lake), lactose, magnesium stearate, povidone, sodium starch glycolate, starch (corn), and talc.

Clinical Pharmacology

Combination oral contraceptives act by suppression of gonadotropins. Although the primary mechanism of this action is inhibition of ovulation, other alterations include changes in the cervical mucus (which increase the difficulty of sperm entry into the uterus) and the endometrium (which reduce the likelihood of implantation).

INDICATIONS AND USAGE

Oral contraceptives are indicated for the prevention of pregnancy in women who elect to use this product as a method of contraception.

Oral contraceptives are highly effective. Table 1 lists the typical accidental pregnancy rates for users of combination oral contraceptives and other methods of contraception. The efficacy of these contraceptive methods, except sterilization, depends upon the reliability with which they are used. Correct and consistent use of methods can result in lower failure rates.

TABLE 1
LOWEST EXPECTED AND TYPICAL FAILURE RATES DURING THE FIRST YEAR OF CONTINUOUS USE OF A METHOD

% of Women Experiencing an Accidental Pregnancy in the First Year of Continuous Use

Method	Lowest Expected*	Typical**
(No contraception)	(89)	(89)
Oral contraceptives		
combined	0.1	N/A***
progestin only	0.5	N/A***
Diaphragm with spermicidal cream or jelly	3	18
Spermicides alone (foam, creams, jellies and vaginal suppositories)	3	21
Vaginal sponge		
nulliparous	5	18
multiparous	>8	>28
IUD (medicated)	1	6#
Condom without spermicides	2	12
Periodic abstinence (all methods)	2–10	20
Female sterilization	0.2	0.4
Male sterilization	0.1	0.15

Reproduced with permission of the Population Council from J. Trussell and K. Kost: Contraceptive failure in the United States: A critical review of the literature. Studies in Family Planning, 18 (5), September–October 1987.

* The authors' best guess of the percentage of women expected to experience an accidental pregnancy among couples who initiate a method (not necessarily for the first time) and who use it consistently and correctly during the first year if they do not stop for any other reason other than pregnancy.

** This term represents "typical" couples who initiate use of a method (not necessarily for the first time), who experience an accidental pregnancy during the first year if they do not stop for any other reason other than pregnancy.

*** N/A—Data not available

\# Combined typical rate for both medicated and non-medicated IUD. The rate for medicated IUD alone is not available.

CONTRAINDICATIONS

Oral contraceptives should not be used in women who currently have the following conditions:

· Thrombophlebitis or thromboembolic disorders
· A past history of deep vein thrombophlebitis or thromboembolic disorders
· Cerebrovascular or coronary artery disease
· Known or suspected carcinoma of the breast
· Carcinoma of the endometrium or other known or suspected estrogen-dependent neoplasia
· Undiagnosed abnormal genital bleeding
· Cholestatic jaundice of pregnancy or jaundice with prior pill use
· Hepatic adenomas or carcinomas
· Known or suspected pregnancy

WARNINGS

> Cigarette smoking increases the risk of serious cardiovascular side effects from oral contraceptive use. This risk increases with age and with heavy smoking (15 or more cigarettes per day) and is quite marked in women over 35 years of age. Women who use oral contraceptives should be strongly advised not to smoke.

The use of oral contraceptives is associated with increased risk of several serious conditions including myocardial infarction, thromboembolism, stroke, hepatic neoplasia, and gallbladder disease, although the risk of serious morbidity or mortality is very small in healthy women without underlying risk factors. The risk of morbidity and mortality increases significantly in the presence of other underlying risk factors such as hypertension, hyperlipidemias, obesity and diabetes.

Practitioners prescribing oral contraceptives should be familiar with the following information relating to these risks. The information contained in this package insert is principally based on studies carried out in patients who used oral contraceptives with higher formulations of estrogens and progestogens than those in common use today. The effect of long-term use of the oral contraceptives with lower formulations of both estrogens and progestogens remains to be determined.

Throughout this labeling, epidemiological studies reported are of two types: retrospective or case control studies and prospective or cohort studies. Case control studies provide a measure of the relative risk of a disease, namely, a *ratio* of the incidence of a disease among oral contraceptive users to that among nonusers. The relative risk does not provide information on the actual clinical occurrence of a disease. Cohort studies provide a measure of attributable risk, which is the *difference* in the incidence of disease between oral contraceptive users and nonusers. The attributable risk does provide information about the actual occurrence of a disease in the population.* For further information, the reader is referred to a text on epidemiological methods.

* Adapted from Stadel BB: Oral contraceptives and cardiovascular disease. *N Engl J Med*, 1981; 305:612–618, 672–677; with author's permission.

1. THROMBOEMBOLIC DISORDERS AND OTHER VASCULAR PROBLEMS

The physician should be alert to the earliest manifestations of thromboembolic thrombotic disorders as discussed below. Should any of these occur or be suspected the drug should be discontinued immediately.

a. Myocardial Infarction

An increased risk of myocardial infarction has been associated with oral contraceptive use. This risk is primarily in smokers or women with other underlying risk factors for coronary artery disease such as hypertension, hypercholesterolemia, morbid obesity, and diabetes. The relative risk of heart attack for current oral contraceptive users has been estimated to be two to six. The risk is very low under the age of 30.

Smoking in combination with oral contraceptive use has been shown to contribute substantially to the incidence of myocardial infarctions in women in their mid-thirties or older, with smoking accounting for the majority of excess cases. Mortality rates associated with circulatory disease have been shown to increase substantially in smokers over the age of 35 and nonsmokers over the age of 40 (Figure 1) among women who use oral contraceptives.

FIGURE 1
CIRCULATORY DISEASE MORTALITY RATES PER 100,000 WOMAN-YEARS BY AGE, SMOKING STATUS AND ORAL CONTRACEPTIVE USE

Layde PM, and Beral V: Further analyses of mortality in oral contraceptive users: Royal College of General Practitioners' oral contraceptive study. (Table 5) *Lancet* 1981; 1:541–546.

Oral contraceptives may compound the effects of well-known risk factors, such as hypertension, diabetes, hyperlipidemias, age and obesity. In particular, some progestogens are known to decrease HDL cholesterol and cause glucose intolerance, while estrogens may create a state of hyperinsulinism. Oral contraceptives have been shown to increase blood pressure among users (see section 9 in Warnings). Such increases in risk factors have been associated with an increased risk of heart disease and the risk increases with the number of risk factors present. Oral contraceptives must be used with caution in women with cardiovascular disease risk factors.

b. Thromboembolism

An increased risk of thromboembolic and thrombotic disease associated with the use of oral contraceptives is well established. Case control studies have found the relative risk of users compared to nonusers to be 3 for the first episode of superficial venous thrombosis, 4 to 11 for deep vein thrombosis or pulmonary embolism, and 1.5 to 6 for women with predisposing conditions for venous thromboembolic disease. Cohort studies have shown the relative risk to be somewhat lower, about 3 for new cases and about 4.5 for new cases requiring hospitalization. The risk of thromboembolic disease due to oral contraceptives is not related to length of use and disappears after pill use is stopped.

A two- to four-fold increase in relative risk of postoperative thromboembolic complications has been reported with the use of oral contraceptives. The relative risk of venous thrombosis in women who have predisposing conditions is twice that of women without such medical conditions. If feasible, oral contraceptives should be discontinued at least four weeks prior to and for two weeks after elective surgery of a type associated with an increase in risk of thromboembolism and during and following prolonged immobilization. Since the immediate postpartum period is also associated with an increased risk of thromboembolism, oral contraceptives should be started no earlier than four to six weeks after delivery in women who elect not to breastfeed.

c. Cerebrovascular diseases

Oral contraceptives have been shown to increase both the relative and attributable risks of cerebrovascular events (thrombotic and hemorrhagic strokes); although, in general, the risk is greatest among older (> 35 years), hypertensive women who also smoke. Hypertension was found to be a risk factor for both users and nonusers, for both types of strokes, while smoking interacted to increase the risk for hemorrhagic stroke.

In a large study, the relative risk of thrombotic strokes has been shown to range from 3 for normotensive users to 14 for users with severe hypertension. The relative risk of hemorrhagic stroke is reported to be 1.2 for nonsmokers who used oral contraceptives, 2.6 for smokers who did not use oral contraceptives, 7.6 for smokers who used oral contraceptives, 1.8 for normotensive users and 25.7 for users with severe hypertension. The attributable risk is also greater in older women.

d. Dose-related risk of vascular disease from oral contraceptives

A positive association has been observed between the amount of estrogen and progestogen in oral contraceptives and the risk of vascular disease. A decline in serum high density lipoproteins (HDL) has been reported with many progestational agents. A decline in serum high density lipoproteins has been associated with an increased incidence of ischemic heart disease. Because estrogens increase HDL cholesterol, the net effect of an oral contraceptive depends on a balance achieved between doses of estrogen and progestogen and the nature and absolute amount of progestogens used in the contraceptive. The amount of both hormones should be considered in the choice of an oral contraceptive. Minimizing exposure to estrogen and progestogen is in keeping with good principles of therapeutics. For any particular estrogen/progestogen combination, the dosage regimen prescribed should be one which contains the least amount of estrogen and progestogen that is compatible with a low failure rate and the needs of the individual patient. New acceptors of oral contraceptive agents should be started on preparations containing 0.05 mg or less of estrogen.

e. Persistence of risk

There are two studies which have shown persistence of risk of vascular disease for ever-users of oral contraceptives. In a study in the United States, the risk of developing myocardial infarction after discontinuing oral contraceptives persists for at least 9 years for women 40–49 years who had used oral contraceptives for five or more years, but this increased risk was not demonstrated in other age groups. In another study in Great Britain, the risk of developing cerebrovascular disease persisted for at least 6 years after discontinuation of oral contraceptives, although excess risk was very small. However, both studies were performed with oral contraceptive formulations containing 50 micrograms or higher of estrogens.

2. ESTIMATES OF MORTALITY FROM CONTRACEPTIVE USE

One study gathered data from a variety of sources which have estimated the mortality rate associated with different methods of contraception at different ages (Table 2). [See table right]

These estimates include the combined risk of death associated with contraceptive methods plus the risk attributable to pregnancy in the event of method failure. Each method of contraception has its specific benefits and risks. The study concluded that with the exception of oral contraceptive users 35 and older who smoke and 40 and older who do not smoke, mortality associated with all methods of birth control is low and below that associated with childbirth. However, smokers 35 and older and nonsmokers 40 and older who use oral contraceptives have an increase in mortality higher than those using other methods of birth control. These facts must be weighed in conjunction with failure rates for other methods and the risk associated with subsequent pregnancy. (See Table 1.)

3. CARCINOMA OF THE REPRODUCTIVE ORGANS

Numerous epidemiological studies have been performed on the incidence of breast, endometrial, ovarian, and cervical cancer in women using oral contraceptives. The overwhelming evidence in the literature suggests that use of oral contraceptives is not associated with an increase in the risk of developing breast cancer, regardless of the age and parity of first use or with most of the marketed brands and doses. The Cancer and Steroid Hormone (CASH) study also showed no latent effect on the risk of breast cancer for at least a decade following long-term use. A few studies have shown a slightly increased relative risk of developing breast cancer, although the methodology of these studies, which included differences in examination of users and nonusers and differences in age at start of use, has been questioned.

Some studies suggest that oral contraceptive use has been associated with an increase in the risk of cervical intraepithelial neoplasia in some populations of women. However, there continues to be controversy about the extent to which such findings may be due to differences in sexual behavior and other factors.

In spite of many studies of the relationship between oral contraceptive use and breast cancer and cervical cancers, a cause and effect relationship has not been established.

4. HEPATIC NEOPLASIA

Benign hepatic adenomas are associated with oral contraceptive use, although the occurrence is rare in the United States. Indirect calculations have estimated the attributable risk to be in the range of 3.3 cases/100,000 for users, a risk that increases after four or more years of use. Rupture of hepatic adenomas may cause death through intra-abdominal hemorrhage.

Studies from Britain have shown an increased risk of developing hepatocellular carcinoma in long-term (> 8 years) oral contraceptive users. However, these cancers are extremely rare in the U.S. and the attributable risk (the excess incidence) of liver cancers in oral contraceptive users approaches less than one per million users.

5. OCULAR LESIONS

There have been clinical case reports of retinal thrombosis associated with the use of oral contraceptives. Oral contraceptives should be discontinued if there is unexplained partial or complete loss of vision; onset of proptosis or diplopia; papilledema; or retinal vascular lesions. Appropriate diagnostic and therapeutic measures should be undertaken immediately.

6. ORAL CONTRACEPTIVE USE BEFORE OR DURING EARLY PREGNANCY:

Extensive epidemiological studies have revealed no increased risk of birth defects in women who have used oral contraceptives prior to pregnancy. Studies also do not suggest a teratogenic effect, particularly in so far as cardiac anomalies and limb reduction defects are concerned, when taken inadvertently during early pregnancy.

The administration of oral contraceptives to induce withdrawal bleeding should not be used as a test for pregnancy. Oral contraceptives should not be used during pregnancy to treat threatened or habitual abortion.

TABLE 2
ANNUAL NUMBER OF BIRTH-RELATED OR METHOD-RELATED DEATHS ASSOCIATED WITH CONTROL OF FERTILITY PER 100,000 NONSTERILE WOMEN, BY FERTILITY CONTROL METHOD ACCORDING TO AGE

Method of control and outcome	AGE					
	15–19	20–24	25–29	30–34	35–39	40–44
No fertility control methods*	7.0	7.4	9.1	14.8	25.7	28.2
Oral contraceptives nonsmoker**	0.3	0.5	0.9	1.9	13.8	31.6
Oral contraceptives smoker**	2.2	3.4	6.6	13.5	51.1	117.2
IUD**	0.8	0.8	1.0	1.0	1.4	1.4
Condom*	1.1	1.6	0.7	0.2	0.3	0.4
Diaphragm/spermicide*	1.9	1.2	1.2	1.3	2.2	2.8
Periodic abstinence*	2.5	1.6	1.6	1.7	2.9	3.6

 * Deaths are birth related
** Deaths are method related

Ory HW: Mortality associated with fertility and fertility control:1983. *Fam Plann Perspect* 1983;15:50–56.

It is recommended that for any patient who has missed two consecutive periods, pregnancy should be ruled out before continuing oral contraceptive use. If the patient has not adhered to the prescribed schedule, the possibility of pregnancy should be considered at the time of the first missed period. Oral contraceptive use should be discontinued if pregnancy is confirmed.

7. GALLBLADDER DISEASE

Earlier studies have reported an increased lifetime relative risk of gallbladder surgery in users of oral contraceptives and estrogens. More recent studies, however, have shown that the relative risk of developing gallbladder disease among oral contraceptive users may be minimal.

The recent findings of minimal risk may be related to the use of oral contraceptive formulations containing lower hormonal doses of estrogens and progestogens.

8. CARBOHYDRATE AND LIPID METABOLIC EFFECTS

Oral contraceptives have been shown to cause glucose intolerance in a significant percentage of users. Oral contraceptives containing greater than 75 micrograms of estrogens cause hyperinsulinism, while lower doses of estrogen cause less glucose intolerance. Progestogens increase insulin secretion and create insulin resistance, this effect varying with different progestational agents.

However, in the nondiabetic woman, oral contraceptives appear to have no effect on fasting blood glucose. Because of these demonstrated effects, prediabetic and diabetic women should be carefully observed while taking oral contraceptives.

A small proportion of women will have persistent hypertriglyceridemia while on the pill. As discussed earlier (see Warnings 1.a. and 1.d.), changes in serum triglycerides and lipoprotein levels have been reported in oral contraceptive users.

9. ELEVATED BLOOD PRESSURE

An increase in blood pressure has been reported in women taking oral contraceptives and this increase is more likely in older oral contraceptive users and with continued use. Data from the Royal College of General Practitioners and subsequent randomized trials have shown that the incidence of hypertension increases with increasing concentrations of progestogens.

Women with a history of hypertension or hypertension-related diseases, or renal disease should be encouraged to use another method of contraception. If women elect to use oral contraceptives, they should be monitored closely and if significant elevation of blood pressure occurs, oral contraceptives should be discontinued. For most women, elevated blood pressure will return to normal after stopping oral contraceptives, and there is no difference in the occurrence of hypertension among ever- and never-users.

10. HEADACHE

The onset or exacerbation of migraine or development of headache with a new pattern which is recurrent, persistent, or severe requires discontinuation of oral contraceptives and evaluation of the cause.

11. BLEEDING IRREGULARITIES

Breakthrough bleeding and spotting are sometimes encountered in patients on oral contraceptives, especially during the first three months of use. Nonhormonal causes should be considered and adequate diagnostic measures taken to rule out malignancy or pregnancy in the event of breakthrough bleeding, as in the case of any abnormal vaginal bleeding. If pathology has been excluded, time or a change to another formulation may solve the problem. In the event of amenorrhea, pregnancy should be ruled out.

Women with a history of oligomenorrhea or secondary amenorrhea or young women without regular cycles prior to taking oral contraceptives may again have irregular bleeding or amenorrhea after discontinuation of oral contraceptives.

PRECAUTIONS

1. PHYSICAL EXAMINATION AND FOLLOW-UP

A complete medical history and physical examination should be taken prior to the initiation or reinstitution of oral contraceptives and at least annually during use of oral contraceptives. These physical examinations should include special reference to blood pressure, breasts, abdomen and pelvic organs, including cervical cytology, and relevant laboratory tests. In case of undiagnosed, persistent, or recurrent abnormal vaginal bleeding, appropriate diagnostic measures should be conducted to rule out malignancy. Women with a strong family history of breast cancer or who have breast nodules should be monitored with particular care.

2. LIPID DISORDERS

Women who are being treated for hyperlipidemias should be followed closely if they elect to use oral contraceptives. Some progestogens may elevate LDL levels and may render the control of hyperlipidemias more difficult.

3. LIVER FUNCTION

If jaundice develops in any woman receiving such drugs, the medication should be discontinued. Steroid hormones may be poorly metabolized in patients with impaired liver function.

4. FLUID RETENTION

Oral contraceptives may cause some degree of fluid retention. They should be prescribed with caution, and only with careful monitoring, in patients with conditions which might be aggravated by fluid retention.

5. EMOTIONAL DISORDERS

Women with a history of depression should be carefully observed and the drug discontinued if depression recurs to a serious degree.

Patients becoming significantly depressed while taking oral contraceptives should stop the medication and use an alternate method of contraception in an attempt to determine whether the symptom is drug related.

6. CONTACT LENSES

Contact lens wearers who develop visual changes or changes in lens tolerance should be assessed by an ophthalmologist.

7. DRUG INTERACTIONS

Reduced efficacy and increased incidence of breakthrough bleeding and menstrual irregularities have been associated with concomitant use of rifampin. A similar association, though less marked, has been suggested with barbiturates, phenylbutazone, phenytoin sodium, and possibly with griseofulvin, ampicillin, and tetracyclines.

8. INTERACTIONS WITH LABORATORY TESTS

Certain endocrine and liver function tests and blood components may be affected by oral contraceptives:
a. Increased prothrombin and factors VII, VIII, IX, and X; decreased antithrombin 3; increased norepinephrine-induced platelet aggregability.
b. Increased thyroid-binding globulin (TBG) leading to increased circulating total thyroid hormone, as measured by protein-bound iodine (PBI), T4 by column or by radioimmunoassay. Free T3 resin uptake is decreased, reflecting the elevated TBG, free T4 concentration is unaltered.
c. Other binding proteins may be elevated in serum.
d. Sex-binding globulins are increased and result in elevated levels of total circulating sex steroids and corticoids; however, free or biologically active levels remain unchanged.
e. Triglycerides may be increased.
f. Glucose tolerance may be decreased.
g. Serum folate levels may be depressed by oral contraceptive therapy. This may be of clinical significance if a woman becomes pregnant shortly after discontinuing oral contraceptives.

Continued on next page

Mead Johnson Labs.—Cont.

9. CARCINOGENESIS
See WARNINGS section.

10. PREGNANCY
Pregnancy Category X. See CONTRAINDICATIONS and WARNINGS sections.

11. NURSING MOTHERS
Small amounts of oral contraceptive steroids have been identified in the milk of nursing mothers and a few adverse effects on the child have been reported, including jaundice and breast enlargement. In addition, oral contraceptives given in the postpartum period may interfere with lactation by decreasing the quantity and quality of breast milk. If possible, the nursing mother should be advised not to use oral contraceptives but to use other forms of contraception until she has completely weaned her child.

12. SEXUALLY-TRANSMITTED DISEASES
Oral contraceptives neither prevent nor are treatment for venereal disease. Also oral contraceptives do not protect against the acquisition of the Auto-Immune Disease Syndrome (AIDS).

13. VOMITING AND/OR DIARRHEA
Although a cause-and-effect relationship has not been clearly established, several cases of oral contraceptive failure have been reported in association with vomiting and/or diarrhea. If significant gastrointestinal disturbance occurs in any woman receiving contraceptive steroids, the use of a back-up method of contraception for the remainder of that cycle is recommended.

INFORMATION FOR THE PATIENT
See Patient Labeling Printed Below

ADVERSE REACTIONS
An increased risk of the following serious adverse reactions has been associated with the use of oral contraceptives (see Warnings section).
- Thrombophlebitis
- Arterial thromboembolism
- Pulmonary embolism
- Myocardial infarction
- Cerebral hemorrhage
- Cerebral thrombosis
- Hypertension
- Gallbladder disease
- Hepatic adenomas or benign liver tumors

There is evidence of an association between the following conditions and the use of oral contraceptives, although additional confirmatory studies are needed:
- Mesenteric thrombosis
- Retinal thrombosis

The following adverse reactions have been reported in patients receiving oral contraceptives and are believed to be drug-related:
- Nausea
- Vomiting
- Gastrointestinal symptoms (such as abdominal cramps and bloating)
- Breakthrough bleeding
- Spotting
- Change in menstrual flow
- Amenorrhea
- Temporary infertility after discontinuation of treatment
- Edema
- Melasma which may persist
- Breast changes: tenderness, enlargement, and secretion
- Change in weight (increase or decrease)
- Change in cervical ectropion and secretion
- Possible diminution in lactation when given immediately postpartum
- Cholestatic jaundice
- Migraine
- Rash (allergic)
- Mental depression
- Reduced tolerance to carbohydrates
- Vaginal candidiasis
- Change in corneal curvature (steepening)
- Intolerance to contact lenses

The following adverse reactions have been reported in users of oral contraceptives, and the association has been neither confirmed nor refuted:
- Premenstrual syndrome
- Cataracts
- Changes in appetite
- Cystitis-like syndrome
- Headache
- Nervousness
- Dizziness
- Hirsutism
- Loss of scalp hair
- Erythema multiforme
- Erythema nodosum
- Hemorrhagic eruption
- Vaginitis

- Porphyria
- Impaired renal function
- Hemolytic uremic syndrome
- Budd-Chiari syndrome
- Acne
- Changes in libido
- Colitis

OVERDOSAGE
Serious ill effects have not been reported following acute ingestion of large doses of oral contraceptives by young children. Overdosage may cause nausea, and withdrawal bleeding may occur in females.

NONCONTRACEPTIVE HEALTH BENEFITS
The following noncontraceptive health benefits related to the use of oral contraceptives are supported by epidemiological studies which largely utilized oral contraceptive formulations containing estrogen doses exceeding 0.035 mg of ethinyl estradiol or 0.05 mg of mestranol.
Effects on menses:
- Increased menstrual cycle regularity
- Decreased blood loss and decreased incidence of iron deficiency anemia
- Decreased incidence of dysmenorrhea
Effects related to inhibition of ovulation:
- Decreased incidence of functional ovarian cysts
- Decreased incidence of ectopic pregnancies
Effects from long-term use:
- Decreased incidence of fibroadenomas and fibrocystic disease of the breast
- Decreased incidence of acute pelvic inflammatory disease
- Decreased incidence of endometrial cancer
- Decreased incidence of ovarian cancer

DOSAGE AND ADMINISTRATION
To achieve maximum contraceptive effectiveness, (OVCON 35 or OVCON 50) must be taken exactly as directed and at intervals not exceeding 24 hours. For the initial cycle of OVCON 35 or OVCON 50 therapy, contraceptive efficacy should not be assumed until after the first seven consecutive days of administration. The possibility of ovulation and conception prior to initiation of medication should be considered.
In subsequent cycles where more than seven days elapse from the first day of menstruation until the first pill containing active contraceptive medication is taken, an additional method of birth control should be used until the oral contraceptive has been taken for seven consecutive days.

28-DAY REGIMEN
Sunday Start
IF THIS IS YOUR FIRST PACKAGE, start taking the yellow or peach tablets on the first Sunday after your period begins, unless your period begins on Sunday. If your period begins on Sunday, start taking the tablets that very same day.
Continue to take one tablet each day.
After the last tablet in row 3 has been taken, start taking the green tablets in row 4 the very next day (Sunday).
After the last green tablet in row 4 has been taken, start your new packet the following day (Sunday) in the manner described above.
TAKE a tablet every day, without interruption. DO NOT MISS A TABLET. Your period will usually begin while you are taking the green tablets. It may continue during the first few tablets of the next packet.
Should you begin menstrual-like bleeding at another time, or if you do not have a period at all, continue to take your one tablet daily and notify your doctor. Your doctor should be informed promptly of any unusual changes in your general health.
Day Five Start
IF THIS IS YOUR FIRST PACKAGE, count the first day of your menstrual bleeding as Day 1. Take your first yellow or peach tablet on Day 5.
CONTINUE to take one tablet daily. Take the tablets in order—first the yellow or peach, then the green ones.
TAKE a tablet every day, without interruption. DO NOT MISS A TABLET. Your period will usually begin while you are taking the green tablets. It may continue during the first few yellow or peach tablets.
Should you begin menstrual-like bleeding at another time, or if you do not have a period at all, continue to take your one tablet daily and notify your doctor. Your doctor should be informed promptly of any unusual changes in your general health.
If you miss a tablet, take it as soon as remembered. Also take the usual tablet for that day. Then resume your tablet-a-day schedule. Each missed tablet increases the possibility that the medication may not work. To reduce this possibility, use an additional method of protection until your next period. Because you are to take a tablet every day, without interruption, always have a new supply of tablets ready to take.

21-DAY REGIMEN
Sunday Start
IF THIS IS YOUR FIRST PACKAGE, start taking the yellow or peach tablets on the first Sunday after your period begins, unless your period begins on Sunday. If your period begins on Sunday, start taking the tablets that very same day.

Continue to take one tablet each day.
After the last tablet in row 3 has been taken (on a Saturday), stop for one week before starting to take the tablets in your next packet. Start your new packet on Sunday in the manner described above.
TAKE a tablet every day, without interruption. DO NOT MISS A TABLET. Your period will usually begin during your week off therapy. It may continue during the first few tablets of the next packet.
Should you begin menstrual-like bleeding at another time, or if you do not have a period at all, continue to take your one tablet daily and notify your doctor. Your doctor should be informed promptly of any unusual changes in your general health.
Day Five Start
IF THIS IS YOUR FIRST PACKAGE, count the first day of your menstrual bleeding as Day 1. Take your first yellow or peach tablet on Day 5.
CONTINUE to take one tablet daily and take the tablets in order.
AFTER you have taken the last tablet, wait seven days and then begin your next package of tablets. You should begin again on the same day of the week. Thus, three weeks on, one week off tablets.
TAKE a tablet every day, without interruption. DO NOT MISS A TABLET. Your period will usually begin within four days after you have taken your last yellow or peach tablet.
Should you begin menstrual-like bleeding at another time, or if you do not have a period at all, continue to take your tablets as directed and notify your doctor. Your doctor should be informed promptly of any unusual changes in your general health.
If you miss a tablet, take it as soon as remembered. Also take the usual tablet for that day. Them resume your tablet-a-day schedule. Each missed tablet increases the possibility that the medication may not work. To reduce this possibility, use an additional method of protection until your next period. Because you are to take a tablet every day for three weeks, without interruption, always have a new supply of tablets ready to take.
Patients should be cautioned to follow the dosage schedule strictly.
If the regimen is interrupted, an additional contraceptive method is recommended for the rest of the cycle. Should spotting or breakthrough bleeding occur, it is recommended that the patient continue medication. If bleeding is persistent or recurrent, the patient should consult her physician.
Use of oral contraceptives in the event of a missed menstrual period:
1. If the patient has not adhered to the prescribed dosage regimen, the possibility of pregnancy should be considered after the first missed period and oral contraceptives should be withheld until pregnancy has been ruled out.
2. If the patient has adhered to the prescribed regimen and misses two consecutive periods, pregnancy should be ruled out before continuing the contraceptive regimen.

HOW SUPPLIED
OVCON® 50 (norethindrone and ethinyl estradiol) is available in 21- and 28-day regimens. Each package contains 21 yellow tablets of 1.0 mg norethindrone and 0.05 mg ethinyl estradiol. Each green tablet in the 28-day regimen contains inert ingredients.
OVCON 50, 21-day
NDC 0087-0584-40   Package of 21 tablets
NDC 0087-0584-42   Carton of 6 packages
OVCON 50, 28-Day
NDC 0087-0579-40   Package of 28 tablets
NDC 0087-0579-41   Carton of 6 packages
OVCON® 35 (norethindrone and ethinyl estradiol) is available in 21- and 28-day regimens. Each package contains 21 peach tablets of 0.4 mg norethindrone and 0.035 mg ethinyl estradiol. Each green tablet in the 28-day regimen contains inert ingredients.
OVCON 35, 21-Day
NDC 0087-0583-40   Package of 21 tablets
NDC 0087-0583-42   Carton of 6 packages
OVCON 35, 28-Day
NDC 0087-0578-40   Package of 28 tablets
NDC 0087-0578-41   Carton of 6 packages
References are available upon request.

PATIENT PACKAGE INSERT
BRIEF SUMMARY
Oral contraceptives, also known as "birth control pills" or "the pill," are taken to prevent pregnancy and when taken correctly, have a failure rate of about 1% per year when used without missing any pills. The typical failure rate of large numbers of pill users is less than 3% per year when women who miss pills are included.
Oral contraceptive use is associated with certain serious diseases that can be life-threatening or may cause temporary or permanent disability. The risks associated with taking oral contraceptives increase significantly if you:

- Smoke
- Are over the age of 40
- Have high blood pressure, diabetes, high cholesterol
- Have or have had clotting disorders, heart attack, stroke, angina pectoris, cancer of the breast or sex organs, jaundice or malignant or benign liver tumors.

You should not take the pill if you suspect you are pregnant or have unexplained vaginal bleeding.

> Cigarette smoking increases the risk of serious cardiovascular side effects from oral contraceptive use. This risk increases with age and with heavy smoking (15 or more cigarettes per day) and is quite marked in women over 35 years of age. Women who use oral contraceptives are strongly advised not to smoke.

Most side effects of the pill are not serious. The most common such effects are nausea, vomiting, bleeding between menstrual periods, weight gain, breast tenderness, and difficulty wearing contact lenses. These side effects, especially nausea and vomiting, may subside within the first three months of use.

The serious side effects of the pill occur very infrequently, especially if you are in good health and are young. However, you should know that the following medical conditions have been associated with or made worse by the pill:

1. Blood clots in the legs (thrombophlebitis), lungs (pulmonary embolism), stoppage or rupture of a blood vessel in the brain (stroke), blockage of blood vessels in the heart (heart attack or angina pectoris), or other organs of the body. As mentioned above, smoking increases the risk of heart attacks and strokes and subsequent serious medical consequences.
2. Liver tumors, which may rupture and cause severe bleeding. A possible but not definite association has been found with the pill and liver cancer. However, liver cancers are extremely rare. The chance of developing liver cancer from using the pill is thus even rarer.
3. High blood pressure, although blood pressure usually returns to normal when the pill is stopped.

The symptoms associated with these serious side effects are discussed in the detailed leaflet given to you with your supply of pills. Notify your doctor or health care provider if you notice any unusual physical disturbances while taking the pill. In addition, drugs such as rifampin, as well as some anticonvulsants and some antibiotics may decrease oral contraceptive effectiveness.

Studies to date of women taking the pill have not shown an increase in the incidence of cancer of the breast or cervix. There is, however, insufficient evidence to rule out the possibility that pills may cause such cancers.

Taking the pill provides some important noncontraceptive effects. These include less painful menstruation, less menstrual blood loss and anemia, fewer pelvic infections, and fewer cancers of the ovary and the lining of the uterus.

Be sure to discuss any medical condition you may have with your health care provider. Your health care provider will take a medical and family history before prescribing oral contraceptives and will examine you. You should be reexamined at least once a year while taking oral contraceptives. The detailed patient information booklet gives you further information which you should read and discuss with your health care professional.

INSTRUCTIONS TO PATIENTS

See Detailed Package Insert.

PATIENT PACKAGE INSERT

INTRODUCTION

Any woman who considers using oral contraceptives (the birth control pill or the pill) should understand the benefits and risks of using this form of birth control.

Although the oral contraceptives have important advantages over other methods of contraception, they have certain risks that no other method has and some of these risks may continue after you have stopped using the oral contraceptive. This booklet will give you much of the information you will need to make this decision and will also help you determine if you are at risk of developing any of the serious side effects of the pill. It will tell you how to use the pill properly so that it will be as effective as possible. However, this booklet is not a replacement for a careful discussion between you and your health care professional. You should discuss the information provided in this booklet with him or her, both when you first start taking the pill and during your revisits. You should also follow your health care professional's advice with regard to regular check-ups while you are on the pill.

EFFECTIVENESS OF ORAL CONTRACEPTIVES

Oral contraceptives or "birth control pills" or "the pill" are used to prevent pregnancy and are more effective than other nonsurgical methods of birth control. The chance of becoming pregnant is less than 1% (1 pregnancy per 100 women per year of use) when the pills are used correctly and no pills are missed. Typical failure rates are actually 3% per year.

ANNUAL NUMBER OF BIRTH-RELATED OR METHOD-RELATED DEATHS ASSOCIATED WITH CONTROL OF FERTILITY PER 100,000 NONSTERILE WOMEN, BY FERTILITY CONTROL METHOD ACCORDING TO AGE

Method of control and outcome	AGE					
	15–19	20–24	25–29	30–34	35–39	40–44
No fertility control methods*	7.0	7.4	9.1	14.8	25.7	28.2
Oral contraceptives nonsmoker**	0.3	0.5	0.9	1.9	13.8	31.6
Oral contraceptives smoker**	2.2	3.4	6.6	13.5	51.1	117.2
IUD**	0.8	0.8	1.0	1.0	1.4	1.4
Condom*	1.1	1.6	0.7	0.2	0.3	0.4
Diaphragm/spermicide*	1.9	1.2	1.2	1.3	2.2	2.8
Periodic abstinence*	2.5	1.6	1.6	1.7	2.9	3.6

* Deaths are birth-related
** Deaths are method-related

The change of becoming pregnant increases with each missed pill during a menstrual cycle.

In comparison, typical accidental pregnancy rates for other nonsurgical methods of birth control during the first year of use are as follows:

IUD: 6%
Diaphragm with spermicides: 18%
Spermicides alone: 21%
Vaginal sponge: 18 to 30%
Condom alone: 12%
Periodic abstinence: 20%
No methods: 89%

WHO SHOULD NOT TAKE ORAL CONTRACEPTIVES

> Cigarette smoking increases the risk of serious cardiovascular side effects from oral contraceptive use. This risk increases with age and with heavy smoking (15 or more cigarettes per day) and is quite marked in women over 35 years of age. Women who use oral contraceptives should not smoke.

Some women should not use the pill. For example, you should not take the pill if you are pregnant or think you may be pregnant. You should also not use the pill if you have or have had any of the following conditions:

- A history of heart attack or stroke
- Blood clots in the legs (thrombophlebitis), lungs (pulmonary embolism), or eyes
- A history of blood clots in the deep veins of your legs
- Chest pain (angina pectoris)
- Known or suspected breast cancer or cancer of the lining of the uterus
- Unexplained vaginal bleeding (until a diagnosis is reached by your doctor)
- Yellowing of the whites of the eyes or of the skin (jaundice) during pregnancy or during previous use of the pill
- Liver tumor (benign or cancerous)

Tell your health care professional if you have ever had any of these conditions. Your health care professional can recommend a safer method of birth control.

OTHER CONSIDERATIONS BEFORE TAKING ORAL CONTRACEPTIVES

Tell your health care provider if you have:

- Breast nodules, fibrocystic disease of the breast, or an abnormal breast x-ray or mammogram
- Diabetes
- Elevated cholesterol or triglycerides
- High blood pressure
- Migraine or other headaches or epilepsy
- Mental depression
- Gallbladder, heart, or kidney disease
- History of scanty or irregular menstrual periods

Women with any of these conditions should be checked often by their health care professional if they choose to use oral contraceptives.

Also, be sure to inform your doctor or health care professional if you smoke or are on any medications.

RISKS OF TAKING ORAL CONTRACEPTIVES

1. Risk of developing blood clots

Blood clots and blockage of blood vessels are the most serious side effects of taking oral contraceptives. In particular, a clot in the legs can cause thrombophlebitis and a clot that travels to the lungs can cause a sudden blocking of the vessel carrying blood to the lungs. Either of these can cause death or disability. Rarely, clots occur in the blood vessels of the eye and may cause blindness, double vision, or impaired vision.

If you take oral contraceptives and need elective surgery, need to stay in bed for a prolonged illness or have recently delivered a baby, you may be at risk of developing blood clots. You should consult your doctor about stopping oral contraceptives three to four weeks before surgery and not taking oral contraceptives for two weeks after surgery or during bed rest. You should also not take oral contraceptives soon after delivery of a baby. It is advisable to wait for at least four weeks after delivery if you are not breastfeeding. If you are breastfeeding see the section on Breastfeeding in General Precautions.

2. Heart attacks and strokes

Oral contraceptives may increase the tendency to develop strokes (stoppage or rupture of blood vessels in the brain) and angina pectoris and heart attacks (blockage of blood vessels in the heart). Any of these conditions can cause death or disability.

Smoking greatly increases the possibility of suffering heart attacks and strokes. Furthermore, smoking and the use of oral contraceptives greatly increase the chances of developing and dying of heart disease.

3. Gallbladder disease

Oral contraceptive users probably have a greater risk than nonusers of having gallbladder disease, although this risk may be related to pills containing high doses of estrogens.

4. Liver tumors

In rare cases, oral contraceptives can cause benign but dangerous liver tumors. These benign liver tumors can rupture and cause fatal internal bleeding. In addition, a possible but not definite, association has been found with the pill and liver cancers in two studies, in which a few women who developed these very rare cancers were found to have used oral contraceptives for long periods. However, liver cancers in general are extremely rare and the chance of developing liver cancer from using the pill is thus even rarer.

5. Cancer of the reproductive organs

There is, at present, no confirmed evidence that oral contraceptives increase the risk of cancer of the reproductive organs and breasts in human studies. Several studies have found no overall increase in the risk of developing breast cancer. However, women who use oral contraceptives and have a strong family history of breast cancer, or who have breast nodules or abnormal mammograms should be closely followed by their doctors.

Some studies have found an increase in the incidence of cancer of the cervix in women who use oral contraceptives. However, this finding may be related to factors other than the use of oral contraceptives.

ESTIMATED RISK OF DEATH FROM A BIRTH CONTROL METHOD OR PREGNANCY

All methods of birth control and pregnancy are associated with a risk of developing certain diseases which may lead to disability or death. An estimate of the number of deaths associated with different methods of birth control and pregnancy has been calculated and is shown in the following table. [See table above].

It can be seen in the table that for women aged 15 to 39, the risk of death was highest with pregnancy (7–26 deaths per 100,000 women, depending on age). Among pill users who do not smoke, the risk of death was always lower than that associated with pregnancy for any age group, although over the age of 40, the risk increases to 32 deaths per 100,000 women, compared to 28 associated with pregnancy at that age. However, for pill users who smoke and are over the age of 35, the estimated number of deaths exceeds those for other methods of birth control. If a woman is over the age of 40 and smokes, her estimated risk of death is four times higher (117/100,000 women) than the estimated risk associated with pregnancy (28/100,000 women) in that age group.

Moreover, if you do not smoke and are under the age of 35, the possible risk of death from oral contraceptive use is extremely low when you consider the failure rate associated with other methods of contraception such as the condom or diaphragm and the resulting pregnancy-associated risk.

In the above table, the risk of death from any birth control method is less than the risk of childbirth, except for oral contraceptive users over the age of 35 who smoke and pill users over the age of 40 even if they do not smoke.

You should discuss this information with your health care professional.

Continued on next page

Mead Johnson Labs.—Cont.

WARNING SIGNALS

If any of these adverse conditions occur while you are taking oral contraceptives, call your doctor immediately:

- Sharp chest pain, coughing of blood, or sudden shortness of breath (indicating a possible clot in the lung)
- Pain in the calf (indicating a possible clot in the leg)
- Crushing chest pain or heaviness in the chest (indicating a possible heart attack)
- Sudden severe headache or vomiting, dizziness or fainting, disturbances of vision or speech, weakness, or numbness in an arm or leg (indicating a possible stroke)
- Sudden partial or complete loss of vision (indicating a possible clot in the eye)
- Breast lumps (indicating possible breast cancer or fibrocystic disease of the breast; ask your doctor or health care provider to show you how to examine your breasts)
- Severe pain or tenderness in the stomach area (indicating a possibly ruptured liver tumor)
- Difficulty in sleeping, weakness, lack of energy, fatigue, or change in mood (possibly indicating severe depression)
- Jaundice or a yellowing of the skin or eyeballs, accompanied frequently by fever, fatigue, loss of appetite, dark-colored urine, or light-colored bowel movements (indicating possible liver problems)
- Abnormal vaginal bleeding (See Side Effects of Oral Contraceptives, 1. Vaginal bleeding, below.)

SIDE EFFECTS OF ORAL CONTRACEPTIVES

In addition to the risks and more serious side effects discussed above (See Risks of Taking Oral Contraceptives, Estimated Risk of Death from a Birth Control Method or Pregnancy and Warning Signals section, above), the following may also occur:

1. Vaginal bleeding

Irregular vaginal bleeding or spotting may occur while you are taking the pills. Irregular bleeding may vary from slight staining between menstrual periods to breakthrough bleeding which is a flow much like a regular period. Irregular bleeding occurs most often during the first few months of oral contraceptive use, but may also occur after you have been taking the pill for some time. Such bleeding may be temporary and usually does not indicate any serious problems. It is important to continue taking your pills on schedule. If the bleeding occurs in more than one cycle or lasts for more than a few days, talk to your doctor or health care professional.

2. Gastrointestinal Effects

The most frequent, unpleasant side effects are nausea and vomiting, stomach cramps, bloating, and a change in appetite.

3. Contact lenses

If you wear contact lenses and notice a change in vision or an inability to wear your lenses, contact your doctor or health care professional.

4. Fluid retention

Oral contraceptives may cause edema (fluid retention) with swelling of the fingers or ankles and may raise your blood pressure. If you experience fluid retention, contact your doctor or health care professional.

5. Melasma

A spotty darkening of the skin is possible, particularly of the face.

6. Other side effects

Other side effects may include change in appetite, headache, nervousness, depression, dizziness, loss of scalp hair, rash, and vaginal infections.

If any of these side effects bother you, call your doctor or health care professional.

GENERAL PRECAUTIONS

1. Missed periods and use of oral contraceptives before or during early pregnancy

There may be times when you may not menstruate regularly after you have completed taking a cycle of pills. If you have taken your pills regularly and miss one menstrual period, continue taking your pills for the next cycle but be sure to inform your health care professional before doing so. If you have not taken the pills daily as instructed and missed a menstrual period, or if you missed two consecutive menstrual periods, you may be pregnant. Check with your health care professional immediately to determine whether you are pregnant. Do not continue to take oral contraceptives until you are sure you are not pregnant, but continue to use another method of contraception.

There is no conclusive evidence that oral contraceptive use is associated with an increase in birth defects, when taken inadvertently during early pregnancy. Previously, a few studies had reported that oral contraceptives might be associated with birth defects, but these studies have not been confirmed. Nevertheless, oral contraceptives or any other drugs should not be used during pregnancy unless clearly necessary and prescribed by your doctor. You should check with

your doctor about risks to your unborn child of any medication taken during pregnancy.

2. While breastfeeding

If you are breastfeeding, consult your doctor before starting oral contraceptives. Some of the drug will be passed on to the child in the milk. A few adverse effects on the child have been reported, including yellowing of the skin (jaundice) and breast enlargement. In addition, oral contraceptives may decrease the amount and quality of your milk. If possible, do not use oral contraceptives while breastfeeding. You should use another method of contraception since breastfeeding provides only partial protection from becoming pregnant and this partial protection decreases significantly as you breastfeed for longer periods of time. You should consider starting oral contraceptives only after you have weaned your child completely.

3. Laboratory tests

If you are scheduled for any laboratory tests, tell your doctor you are taking birth control pills. Certain blood tests may be affected by birth control pills.

4. Drug interactions

Certain drugs may interact with birth control pills to make them less effective in preventing pregnancy or cause an increase in breakthrough bleeding. Such drugs include rifampin, drugs used for epilepsy such as barbiturates (for example, phenobarbital) and phenytoin (Dilantin is one brand of this drug), phenylbutazone (Butazolidin is one brand) and possibly ampicillin and tetracyclines (several brand names). You may need to use an additional method of contraception when you take drugs which can make oral contraceptives less effective.

HOW TO TAKE ORAL CONTRACEPTIVES

1. General Instructions

You must take your pill every day according to the instructions. Oral contraceptives are most effective if taken no more than 24 hours apart. Take your pill at the same time every day so that you are less likely to forget to take it. You will then maintain an effective dose of the oral contraceptive in your body.

How To Take the Pill So That it Is Most Effective.

To achieve maximum contraceptive effectiveness, OVCON 50 or OVCON 35 must be taken correctly and at intervals not exceeding 24 hours. For the initial cycle of OVCON 35 or OVCON 50 therapy, oral contraceptive efficacy (98% or greater) should not be assumed until after the first seven consecutive days of administration. The possibility of ovulation and conception prior to initiation of medication should be considered.

In subsequent cycles where more than seven days elapse from the first day of menstruation until the first pill containing active contraceptive medication is taken, an additional method of birth control should be used until the oral contraceptive has been taken for seven consecutive days.

28-DAY REGIMEN

Sunday Start

IF THIS IS YOUR FIRST PACKAGE, start taking the yellow or peach tablets on the first Sunday after your period begins, unless your period begins on Sunday. **If your period begins on Sunday, start taking the tablets that very same day.** CONTINUE to take one tablet each day.

After the last tablet in row 3 has been taken, start taking the green tablets in row 4 the very next day (Sunday).

After the last green tablet in row 4 has been taken, **start your new packet the following day** (Sunday) in the manner described above.

TAKE a tablet every day, without interruption. DO NOT MISS A TABLET. Your period will usually begin while you are taking the green tablets. It may continue during the first few tablets of the next packet.

Should you begin menstrual-like bleeding at another time, or if you do not have a period at all, **continue to take your one tablet daily** and notify your doctor. Your doctor should be informed promptly of any unusual changes in your general health.

Day Five Start

IF THIS IS YOUR FIRST PACKAGE, count the first day of your menstrual bleeding as Day 1. Take your first yellow or peach tablet on Day 5.

CONTINUE to take one tablet daily. Take the tablets in order—first the yellow or peach, then the green ones.

TAKE a tablet every day, without interruption. DO NOT MISS A TABLET. Your period will usually begin while you are taking the green tablets. It may continue during the first few yellow or peach tablets.

Should you begin menstrual-like bleeding at another time, or if you do not have a period at all, **continue to take your one tablet daily** and notify your doctor. Your doctor should be informed promptly of any unusual changes in your general health.

If you miss a tablet, take it as soon as remembered. Also take the usual tablet for that day. Then resume your tablet-a-day schedule. Each missed tablet increases the possibility that the medication may not work. To reduce this possibility, use an additional method of protection until your next period.

Because you are to take a tablet every day, without interruption, always have a new supply of tablets ready to take.

21-DAY REGIMEN

Sunday Start

IF THIS IS YOUR FIRST PACKAGE, start taking the yellow or peach tablets on the first Sunday after your period begins, unless your period begins on Sunday. **If your period begins on Sunday, start taking the tablets that very same day.** Continue to take one tablet each day.

After the last tablet in row 3 has been taken (on a Saturday), **stop for one week** before starting to take the tablets in your next packet. Start your new packet on Sunday in the manner described above.

TAKE a tablet every day, without interruption. DO NOT MISS A TABLET. Your period will usually begin your week off therapy. It may continue during the first few tablets of the next packet.

Should you begin menstrual-like bleeding at another time, or if you do not have a period at all, **continue to take your one tablet daily** and notify your doctor. Your doctor should be informed promptly of any unusual changes in your general health.

Day Five Start

IF THIS IS YOUR FIRST PACKAGE, count the first day of your menstrual bleeding as Day 1. Take your first yellow or peach tablet on Day 5.

CONTINUE to take one tablet daily and take the tablets in order.

TAKE a tablet every day, without interruption. DO NOT MISS A TABLET. Your period will usually begin within four days after you have taken your last yellow or peach tablet.

AFTER you have taken the last tablet, wait seven days and then begin your next package of tablets. You should begin again on the same day of the week. Thus, three weeks on, one week off tablets.

Should you begin menstrual-like bleeding at another time, or if you do not have a period at all, **continue to take your tablets correctly** and notify your doctor. Your doctor will also want you to let him know promptly of any unusual changes in your general health.

If you miss a tablet, take it as soon as remembered. Also take the usual tablet for that day. Then resume your tablet-a-day schedule. Each missed tablet increases the possibility that the medication may not work. To reduce this possibility, use an additional method of protection until your next period. Because you are to take a tablet every day for three weeks, without interruption, always have a new supply of tablets ready to take.

Patients should be cautioned to follow the dosage schedule strictly. If the regimen is interrupted, an additional contraceptive method is recommended for the rest of the cycle. Should spotting or breakthrough bleeding occur, it is recommended that you continue medication. If bleeding is persistent or recurrent, consult your physician.

Use of oral contraceptives in the event of a missed menstrual period:

a. If you have not adhered to the prescribed dosage regimen, the possibility of pregnancy should be considered after the first missed period (or after 45 days from the last menstrual period if the progestogen-only oral contraceptives are used) and oral contraceptives should be withheld until pregnancy has been ruled out.

b. If you have adhered to the prescribed regimen and miss two consecutive periods, pregnancy should be ruled out before continuing the contraceptive regimen.

c. At times there may be no menstrual period after a cycle of pills. Therefore, if you miss one menstrual period but have taken the pills **exactly as you were supposed to**, continue as usual into the next cycle. If you have not taken the pills correctly and miss a menstrual period, you may be pregnant and should stop taking oral contraceptives until your doctor determines whether or not you are pregnant. Until you can get to your doctor, use another form of contraception. If two consecutive menstrual periods are missed, you should stop taking pills until it is determined whether you are pregnant.

If your doctor has scheduled you for surgery, or you need prolonged bed rest, he or she may suggest that you stop taking the pill four weeks before surgery to avoid an increased risk of blood clots. It is also advisable not to start oral contraceptives sooner than four weeks after delivery of a baby.

2. If your forget to take your pill

If you miss only one pill in a cycle, the change of becoming pregnant is small. Take the missed pill as soon as you realize that you have forgotten it. Since the risk of pregnancy increases with each additional pill you skip, it is very important that you take one pill a day.

At times there may be no menstrual period after a cycle of pills. Therefore, if you miss one menstrual period but have taken the pills **exactly as you were supposed to**, continue as usual into the next cycle. If you have not taken the pills correctly and miss a menstrual period, you may be pregnant and should stop taking oral contraceptives until your doctor determines whether or not you are pregnant. Until you can get to your doctor, use another form of contraception. If two consecutive menstrual periods are missed, you should stop taking pills until it is determined whether you are pregnant.

3. Pregnancy due to pill failure

The incidence of pill failure resulting in pregnancy is approximately one percent (ie, one pregnancy per 100 women per year) if taken every day as directed, but more typical failure rates are about 3%. If failure does occur, the risk to the fetus is minimal.

4. Pregnancy after stopping the pill

There may be some delay in becoming pregnant after you stop using oral contraceptives, especially if you had irregular menstrual cycles before you used oral contraceptives. It may be advisable to postpone conception until you begin menstruating regularly once you have stopped taking the pill and desire pregnancy.

There does not appear to be any increase in birth defects in newborn babies when pregnancy occurs soon after stopping the pill.

5. Other

a. Gastrointestinal upset

If significant vomiting and/or diarrhea occur while you are taking the pill, it is recommended that you use a back-up method of contraception during the remainder of that cycle.

b. Sexually-transmitted diseases

Oral conceptives are of no value in the treatment or prevention of venereal disease. Neither do oral contraveptives protect against infection with the AIDS virus.

c. Overdosage

Serious ill effects have not been reported following ingestion of large doses of oral contraceptives by young children. Overdosage may cause nausea and withdrawal bleeding in females. In case of overdosage, contact your poison control center, health care professional, or nearest emergency room. KEEP THIS DRUG AND ALL DRUGS OUT OF THE REACH OF CHILDREN.

d. General medical information.

Your health care professional will take a medical and family history before prescribing oral contraceptives and will examine you. You should be reexamined at least once a year. Be sure to inform your health care professional if there is a family history of any of the conditions listed previously in this leaflet. Be sure to keep all appointments with your health care professional, because this is a time to determine if there are early signs of side effects of oral contraceptive use.

Do not use the drug for any condition other than the one for which it was prescribed. This drug has been prescribed specifically for you; do not give it to others who may want birth control pills.

NONCONTRACEPTIVE EFFECTS OF ORAL CONTRACEPTIVES

In addition to preventing pregnancy, use of oral contraceptives may provide certain benefits. They are:

· Menstrual cycles may become more regular
· Blood flow during menstruation may be lighter and less iron may be lost. Therefore, anemia due to iron deficiency is less likely to occur.
· Pain or other symptoms during menstruation may be encountered less frequently
· Ectopic (tubal) pregnancy may occur less frequently
· Noncancerous cysts or lumps in the breast may occur less frequently
· Acute pelvic inflammatory disease may occur less frequently
· Oral contraceptive use may provide some protection against developing two forms of cancer: cancer of the ovaries and cancer of the lining of the uterus

If you want more information about birth control pills, ask your doctor or pharmacist. They have a more technical leaflet called the Professional Labeling, which you may wish to read.

Date of latest revision: September 1989.

Shown in Product Identification Section, page 417

Each tablet supplies:	Poly-Vi-Flor chewable tablets			Percentage of U.S. Recommended Daily Allowance	
	1.0 mg	0.5 mg	0.25 mg	Children Age 2–3 Years	Adults & Children age 4 Years or More
Vitamin A, IU	2500	2500	2500	100	50
Vitamin D, IU	400	400	400	100	100
Vitamin E, IU	15	15	15	150	50
Vitamin C, mg	60	60	60	150	100
Folic acid, mg	0.3	0.3	0.3	150	75
Thiamine, mg	1.05	1.05	1.05	150	70
Riboflavin, mg	1.2	1.2	1.2	150	70
Niacin, mg	13.5	13.5	13.5	150	68
Vitamin B_6, mg	1.05	1.05	1.05	150	53
Vitamin B_{12}, µg	4.5	4.5	4.5	150	75
Fluoride, mg	1	0.5	0.25	*	*

* U.S. Recommended Daily Allowance has not been established.

Mead Johnson Nutritionals
A Bristol-Myers Company
2400 W. LLOYD EXPRESSWAY
EVANSVILLE, INDIANA 47721-0001

CASEC® powder
[kā'sek]
Calcium caseinate
Protein supplement

(See PDR For Nonprescription Drugs)

CE–VI–SOL®
[see'vi-sahl"]
Vitamin C supplement drops

(See PDR For Nonprescription Drugs)

CRITICARE HN®
[cri'tĭ-care" hn']
Ready to Use High Nitrogen Elemental Diet

(See PDR For Nonprescription Drugs)

ENFAMIL® concentrated liquid • powder
[en'fah-mil"]
Low iron infant formula

(See PDR For Nonprescription Drugs)

ENFAMIL® with Iron
[en'fah-mil"]
concentrated liquid • powder
Iron fortified infant formula

(See PDR For Nonprescription Drugs)

ENFAMIL NURSETTE®
[en'fah-mil"]
Low iron and iron fortified infant formula

(See PDR For Nonprescription Drugs)

ENFAMIL® ready-to-use
[en'fah-mil"]
Low iron infant formula

(See PDR For Nonprescription Drugs)

ENFAMIL® with Iron ready-to-use
[en'fah-mil"]
Iron fortified infant formula

(See PDR For Nonprescription Drugs)

FER–IN–SOL®
[fair'in-sahl"]
Iron supplement
• drops
• syrup
• capsules
Ferrous sulfate, Mead Johnson

(See PDR For Nonprescription Drugs)

ISOCAL®
[ĭ'sō-cal"]
Nutritionally complete liquid diet for tube and oral feeding

(See PDR For Nonprescription Drugs)

ISOCAL® HCN
[ĭ'sō-cal"]
High calorie and nitrogen nutritionally complete liquid tube-feeding formula

(See PDR For Nonprescription Drugs)

ISOCAL® HN
[ĭ'sō-cal"]
High nitrogen nutritionally complete liquid tube-feeding formula

(See PDR For Nonprescription Drugs)

LONALAC® powder
[lōn'ah-lak"]
Low sodium, high protein beverage mix

(See PDR For Nonprescription Drugs)

LYTREN®
[lĭ'tren]
Oral electrolyte solution

(See PDR For Nonprescription Drugs)

MCT Oil
Medium chain triglycerides

(See PDR For Nonprescription Drugs)

MODUCAL® Powder
[mŏd'ū-kăl]
Dietary carbohydrate

(See PDR For Nonprescription Drugs)

NUTRAMIGEN®
[nū-tram'ĭ-jen"]
Iron fortified protein hydrolysate formula
• powder, 1 lb cans
• ready-to-feed, 4 fl oz and 8 fl oz Nursette® bottles
• ready-to-feed, 32 fl oz cans
• concentrate, 13 fl oz

(See PDR For Nonprescription Drugs)

POLY–VI–FLOR®   ℞
[pahl-ē-vī'flōr"]
• 1.0 mg
• 0.5 mg
• 0.25 mg
Multivitamin and fluoride supplement chewable tablets

DESCRIPTION
[See table above].
Active ingredient for caries prophylaxis: Fluoride as sodium fluoride.

Continued on next page

Mead Johnson Nutr.—Cont.

Other ingredients: Ascorbic acid, cholecalciferol, colloidal silicon dioxide, cyanocobalamin, dextrates, FD&C Blue No. 2 (aluminum lake), FD&C Red No. 40 (aluminum lake), FD&C Yellow No. 6 (aluminum lake), folic acid, fruit flavors (artificial), lactose, magnesium stearate, niacinamide, pyridoxine hydrochloride, riboflavin, silica gel, sodium ascorbate, sodium chloride, sucrose, thiamine mononitrate, dl-alpha-tocopheryl acetate, vitamin A acetate.

CLINICAL PHARMACOLOGY

It is well established that fluoridation of the water supply (1 ppm fluoride) during the period of tooth development leads to a significant decrease in the incidence of dental caries. Poly-Vi-Flor chewable tablets provide sodium fluoride, and ten essential vitamins in a chewable tablet. Because the tablets are chewable, they provide a *topical* as well as *systemic* source of fluoride.[1,2]

Hydroxyapatite is the principal crystal for all calcified tissue in the human body. The fluoride ion reacts with the *hydroxyapatite* in the tooth as it is formed to produce the more caries-resistant crystal, *fluorapatite*. The reaction may be expressed by the equation:[3]

$Ca_{10}(PO_4)_6(OH)_2 + 2F^- \rightarrow \quad Ca_{10}(PO_4)_6F_2 + 2OH^-$
(Hydroxyapatite)   (Fluorapatite)

Three stages of fluoride deposition in tooth enamel can be distinguished:[3]

1. Small amounts (reflecting the low levels of fluoride in tissue fluids) are incorporated into the enamel crystals while they are being formed.
2. After enamel has been laid down, fluoride deposition continues in the surface enamel. Diffusion of fluoride from the surface inward is apparently restricted.
3. After eruption, the surface enamel acquires fluoride from water, food, supplementary fluoride and smaller amounts from saliva.

INDICATIONS AND USAGE

Supplementation of the diet with ten essential vitamins. Supplementation of the diet with the fluoride for caries prophylaxis.

Poly-Vi-Flor 1.0 mg chewable tablets provide fluoride in tablet form for children over 3 years in areas where the water fluoride level is less than 0.3 ppm.[4]

Poly-Vi-Flor 0.5 mg chewable tablets provide fluoride in tablet form for children 2-3 years of age where the drinking water has a fluoride content of less than 0.3 ppm, and for children 3 years of age and above where the drinking water contains 0.3 through 0.7 ppm of fluoride.[4]

Poly-Vi-Flor 0.25 mg chewable tablets provide fluoride in tablet form for children 2-3 years of age where the drinking water contains 0.3 through 0.7 ppm of fluoride.[4]

Poly-Vi-Flor chewable tablets supply significant amounts of vitamins A, D, E, C, thiamine, riboflavin, niacin, pyridoxine, cyanocobalamin and folic acid to supplement the diet, and to help assure that nutritional deficiencies of these vitamins will not develop. Thus, in a single easy-to-use preparation, children obtain ten essential vitamins and the important mineral, fluoride.

The American Academy of Pediatrics recommends that children up to age 16, in areas where drinking water contains less than optimal levels of fluoride, receive daily fluoride supplementation.

Children using Poly-Vi-Flor chewable tablets regularly should receive semiannual dental examinations. The regular brushing of teeth and attention to good oral hygiene practices are also essential.

WARNINGS

As in the case of all medications, keep out of the reach of children.

PRECAUTIONS

The suggested dose *should not be exceeded,* since dental fluorosis may result from continued ingestion of large amounts of fluoride.

Before prescribing Vi-Flor® products:
1. determine the fluoride content of the drinking water.
2. make sure the child is not receiving significant amounts of fluoride from other medications.
3. periodically check to make sure that the child does not develop significant dental fluorosis.

The Council on Dental Therapeutics of the American Dental Association recommends that no more than 264 mg of sodium fluoride should be dispensed at one time.[5] Therefore, no more than 120 Poly-Vi-Flor 1.0 mg chewable tablets (2.2 mg sodium fluoride per tablet) should be dispensed at one time.

ADVERSE REACTIONS

Allergic rash and other idiosyncrasies have been rarely reported.

DOSAGE AND ADMINISTRATION

One tablet daily or as prescribed.

HOW SUPPLIED

Poly-Vi-Flor 1.0 mg (multivitamin and fluoride supplement) chewable tablets are available in 100- and 1000-tablet bottles.
NDC 0087-0474-02 Bottles of 100
NDC 0087-0474-03 Bottles of 1000
Poly-Vi-Flor 0.5 mg (multivitamin and fluoride supplement) chewable tablets are available in 100 tablet bottles.
NDC 0087-0468-41 Bottles of 100
Poly-Vi-Flor 0.25 mg (multivitamin and fluoride supplement) chewable tablets are available in 100-tablet bottles.
NDC 0087-0487-41 Bottles of 100

LITERATURE AVAILABLE

Yes.

REFERENCES

1. Hennon, D.K.; Stookey, G.K., and Muhler, J.C.: The Clinical Anticariogenic Effectiveness of Supplementary Fluoride-Vitamin Preparations— Results at the End of Three Years, J. Dentistry for Children 33:3–12 (Jan.) 1966.
2. Hennon, D.K.; Stookey, G.K., and Muhler, J.C.: The Clinical Anticariogenic Effectiveness of Supplementary Fluoride-Vitamin Preparations— Results at the End of Four Years, J. Dentistry for Children 34:439–443 (Nov.) 1967.
3. Brudevold, F., and McCann, H.G.: Fluoride and Caries Control—Mechanism of Action, in Nizel, A.E.: The Science of Nutrition and Its Application in Clinical Dentistry, Philadelphia, W.B. Saunders Company, 1966, pp. 331–347.
4. American Academy of Pediatrics Committee on Nutrition: Fluoride Supplementation. Pediatrics 77:758, 1986.
5. Council on Dental Therapeutics, Am Dental Assoc, Accepted Dental Therapeutics, 1977, 37th Edition, page 294.

POLY–VI–FLOR®   ℞

[pahl-ē-vī′flŏr″]
● 0.5 mg
● 0.25 mg
Multivitamin and fluoride supplement drops

DESCRIPTION

[See table below].
See INDICATIONS AND USAGE section below for use by infants and children under two years of age.
Active ingredient for caries prophylaxis: Fluoride as sodium fluoride.
Other ingredients: Ascorbic acid, caramel color, cholecalciferol, cyanocobalamin, ferrous sulfate, fruit flavor (artificial), glycerin, niacinamide, polysorbate 80, pyridoxine hydrochloride, riboflavin-5-phosphate sodium, thiamine hydrochloride, d-alpha-tocopheryl acid succinate, vitamin A palmitate, water, and other ingredients.

CLINICAL PHARMACOLOGY

For information on fluoridation see Poly-Vi-Flor chewable tablets.

INDICATIONS AND USAGE

Supplementation of the diet with nine essential vitamins. Supplementation of the diet with fluoride for caries prophylaxis.

The American Academy of Pediatrics recommends that children up to age 16, in areas where drinking water contains less than optimal levels of fluoride, receive daily fluoride supplementation.

Poly-Vi-Flor 0.5 mg (multivitamin and fluoride supplement) drops provide fluoride in drop form for children ages 2–3 years in areas where the drinking water contains less than 0.3 ppm fluoride; and for children over 3 years in areas where the drinking water contains 0.3 through 0.7 ppm of fluoride. Each 1.0 mL provides sodium fluoride (0.5 mg fluoride) plus nine essential vitamins.

Poly-Vi-Flor 0.25 mg (multivitamin and fluoride supplement) drops provide fluoride in drop form for infants and young children from birth to 2 years of age in areas where the drinking water contains less than 0.3 ppm of fluoride and for children ages 2–3 years where the drinking water contains 0.3 through 0.7 ppm of fluoride. Each 1.0 mL supplies sodium fluoride (0.25 mg fluoride) plus nine essential vitamins.

The American Academy of Pediatrics[1] and the American Dental Association[2] currently recommend that infants and children under 2 years of age, in areas where drinking water contains less than 0.3 ppm of fluoride, and children 2-3, in areas where the drinking water contains 0.3 through 0.7 ppm of fluoride, receive 0.25 mg of supplemental fluoride daily which is provided in a full dose (1 mL) of Poly-Vi-Flor® 0.25 mg drops. A half dose (0.5 mL) of Poly-Vi-Flor 0.5 mg drops could also provide a daily fluoride intake of 0.25 mg; however, this dosage reduces vitamin supplementation by half.

Poly-Vi-Flor 0.5 mg drops and 0.25 mg drops supply significant amounts of vitamins A, D, E, C, thiamine, riboflavin, niacin, pyridoxine, and cyanocobalamin to supplement the diet, and to help assure that nutritional deficiencies of these vitamins will not develop. Thus in a single easy-to-use preparation, infants and children obtain nine essential vitamins and fluoride.

A comprehensive $5\frac{1}{2}$ year series of studies of the effectiveness of Tri-Vi-Flor® and Poly-Vi-Flor® products in caries protection has been published.[3-6] Children in this continuing study lived in an area where the water supply contained only 0.05 ppm fluoride. The subjects were divided into two groups, one which used only nonfluoridated Vi-Sol® vitamin products and the other Tri-Vi-Flor and Poly-Vi-Flor vitamin-fluoride products.

The three-year interim report showed 63% fewer carious surfaces in primary teeth and 43% fewer carious surfaces in permanent teeth of the children taking Vi-Flor® vitamin-fluoride products.[3]

After four years the studies continued to support the effectiveness of Tri-Vi-Flor and Poly-Vi-Flor, showing a reduction in carious surfaces of 68% in primary teeth and 46% in permanent teeth.[4]

Results at the end of $5\frac{1}{2}$ years further confirmed the previous findings and indicated that significant reductions in dental caries are apparent with the continued use of Vi-Flor vitamin-fluoride products.[5]

WARNINGS

As in the case of all medications, keep out of the reach of children.

PRECAUTIONS

The suggested dose should not be exceeded since dental fluorosis may result from continued ingestion of large amounts of fluoride.

When prescribing Vi-Flor products:
1. determine the fluoride content of the drinking water.
2. make sure the child is not receiving significant amounts of fluoride from other medications.
3. periodically check to make sure that the child does not develop significant dental fluorosis.

Poly-Vi-Flor 0.5 mg drops and 0.25 mg drops should be dispensed in the original plastic container, since contact with glass leads to instability and precipitation. (The amount of sodium fluoride in all Poly-Vi-Flor drops is well below the maximum to be dispensed at one time according to recommendations of the American Dental Association.)

ADVERSE REACTIONS

Allergic rash and other idiosyncrasies have been rarely reported.

DOSAGE AND ADMINISTRATION

1.0 mL daily or as prescribed.
Drops may be dropped directly into mouth with 'Safti-Dropper,' or mixed with cereal, fruit juice or other food.

HOW SUPPLIED

Poly-Vi-Flor 0.5 mg (multivitamin and fluoride supplement) drops are available on prescription only in bottles of 50 mL.

	Poly-Vi-Flor drops		Percentage of U.S. Recommended Daily Allowance	
	0.5 mg	0.25 mg	Infants	Children Under 4
Each 1.0 mL supplies:				
Vitamin A, IU	1500	1500	100	60
Vitamin D, IU	400	400	100	100
Vitamin E, IU	5	5	100	50
Vitamin C, mg	35	35	100	88
Thiamine, mg	0.5	0.5	100	71
Riboflavin, mg	0.6	0.6	100	75
Niacin, mg	8	8	100	89
Vitamin B_6, mg	0.4	0.4	100	57
Vitamin B_{12}, μg	2	2	100	67
Fluoride, mg	0.5	0.25	*	*

* U.S. Recommended Daily Allowance has not been established.

NDC 0087-0472-02 Bottles of 1⅔ fl oz (50 mL)
FSN 6505-080-0967 (50 mL)
Poly-Vi-Flor 0.25 mg (multivitamin and fluoride supplement) drops are available on prescription only in bottles of 50 mL.
NDC 0087-0451-41 Bottles of 50 mL.

LITERATURE AVAILABLE
Yes.

REFERENCES
1. American Academy of Pediatrics, Committee on Nutrition: Fluoride Supplementation. Pediatrics 77:758, 1986.
2. Accepted Dental Therapeutics, Ed. 38, Chicago, American Dental Association, 1979, p. 321.
3. Hennon, D.K.; Stookey, G.K., and Muhler, J.C.: The Clinical Anticariogenic Effectiveness of Supplementary Fluoride-Vitamin Preparations— Results at the End of Three Years, J. Dentistry for Children 33:3–12 (Jan.) 1966.
4. Hennon, D.K.; Stookey, G.K., and Muhler, J.C.: The Clinical Anticariogenic Effectiveness of Supplementary Fluoride-Vitamin Preparations— Results at the End of Four Years, J. Dentistry for Children 34:439–443 (Nov.) 1967.
5. Hennon, D.K.; Stookey, G.K., and Muhler, J.C.: The Clinical Anticariogenic Effectiveness of Supplementary Fluoride-Vitamin Preparations— Results at the End of Five and a Half Years, Phar. and Ther. In Dent. 1:1, 1970.
6. Hennon, D.K.; Stookey, G.K., and Beiswanger, B.B.: Fluoride Vitamin Supplements: Effects on Dental Caries and Fluorosis when Used in Areas with Suboptimum Fluoride in the Water Supply. J. Am. Dent. Assoc. 95:965, 1977.

POLY–VI–FLOR® with Iron   ℞
[pahl-ē-vī'flōr"]
● 1.0 mg
● 0.5 mg
● 0.25 mg
Multivitamin, mineral and fluoride supplement chewable tablets

DESCRIPTION
[See table above right]
Active ingredient for caries prophylaxis: Fluoride as sodium fluoride.
Other ingredients: Ascorbic acid, cholecalciferol, colloidal silicon dioxide, cupric oxide, cyanocobalamin, dextrates, FD&C Red No. 40 (aluminum lake), ferrous fumarate, folic acid, fruit flavors (artificial), lactose, magnesium stearate, niacinamide, pyridoxine hydrochloride, riboflavin, silica gel, sodium ascorbate, sodium chloride, stearic acid, sucrose, thiamine mononitrate, dl-alpha-tocopheryl acetate, vitamin A acetate, zinc oxide.

CLINICAL PHARMACOLOGY
For information on fluoridation see Poly-Vi-Flor chewable tablets.
Poly-Vi-Flor with Iron chewable tablets provide sodium fluoride, iron, copper, zinc and ten essential vitamins in a chewable tablet. Because the tablets are chewable, they provide a *topical* as well as *systemic* source of fluoride.[1,2]

INDICATIONS AND USAGE
Supplementation of the diet with ten essential vitamins, iron, copper and zinc.
Supplementation of the diet with fluoride, for caries prophylaxis.
The American Academy of Pediatrics recommends that children up to age 16, in areas where drinking water contains less than optimal levels of fluoride, receive daily fluoride supplementation.
Poly-Vi-Flor 1.0 mg with Iron chewable tablets were developed to provide fluoride in tablet form for children over 3 years in areas where the water fluoride level is less than 0.3 ppm.[3]
Poly-Vi-Flor 0.5 mg with Iron chewable tablets provides fluoride for children 2–3 years of age where the drinking water has fluoride content of less than 0.3 ppm, and for children 3 years of age and above where the drinking water contains 0.3 through 0.7 ppm of fluoride.[3]

| | Poly-Vi-Flor w/Iron chewable tablets | | | Percentage of U.S. Recommended Daily Allowance | |
	1.0 mg	0.5 mg	0.25 mg	Children Age 2–3 Years	Adults & Children 4 Years or More
Each tablet supplies:					
Vitamin A, IU	2500	2500	2500	100	50
Vitamin D, IU	400	400	400	100	100
Vitamin E, IU	15	15	15	150	50
Vitamin C, mg	60	60	60	150	100
Folic acid, mg	0.3	0.3	0.3	150	75
Thiamine, mg	1.05	1.05	1.05	150	70
Riboflavin, mg	1.2	1.2	1.2	150	70
Niacin, mg	13.5	13.5	13.5	150	68
Vitamin B$_6$, mg	1.05	1.05	1.05	150	53
Vitamin B$_{12}$, μg	4.5	4.5	4.5	150	75
Iron, mg	12	12	12	120	67
Copper, mg	1	1	1	100	50
Zinc, mg	10	10	10	125	67
Fluoride, mg	1	0.5	0.25	*	*
*U.S. Recommended Daily Allowance has not been established.

Poly-Vi-Flor 0.25 mg with Iron chewable tablets provide fluoride in tablet form for children 2–3 years of age where the drinking water contains 0.3 through 0.7 ppm of fluoride.[3]
Poly-Vi-Flor with Iron chewable tablets supply significant amounts of vitamins A, D, E, C, thiamine, riboflavin, niacin, pyridoxine, cyanocobalamin, folic acid, iron, copper and zinc to supplement the diet, and to help assure that deficiencies of these nutrients will not develop. Thus, in a single easy-to-use preparation, children obtain ten essential vitamins, iron, copper, zinc and fluoride.
Children using Poly-Vi-Flor with Iron chewable tablets regularly should receive semiannual dental examinations. The regular brushing of teeth and attention to good oral hygiene practices are also essential.

WARNINGS
As in the case of all medications, keep out of the reach of children.

PRECAUTIONS
The suggested dose of Poly-Vi-Flor with Iron chewable tablets *should not be exceeded,* since dental fluorosis may result from continued ingestion of large amounts of fluoride.
Before prescribing Vi-Flor® products:
1. determine the fluoride content of the drinking water.
2. make sure the child is not receiving significant amounts of fluoride from other medications.
3. periodically check to make sure that the child does not develop significant dental fluorosis.

ADVERSE REACTIONS
Allergic rash and other idiosyncrasies have been rarely reported.

DOSAGE AND ADMINISTRATION
One tablet daily or as prescribed.

HOW SUPPLIED
Poly-Vi-Flor 1.0 mg with Iron (multivitamin, mineral and fluoride supplement) chewable tablets are available in 100- and 1000-tablet bottles.
NDC 0087-0476-03 Bottles of 100
NDC 0087-0476-04 Bottles of 1000
Poly-Vi-Flor 0.5 mg with Iron (multivitamin, mineral and fluoride supplement) chewable tablets are available only in 100-tablet bottles.
NDC 0087-0482-41 Bottles of 100
Poly-Vi-Flor 0.25 mg with Iron (multivitamin, mineral and fluoride supplement) chewable tablets are available in 100-tablet bottles.
NDC 0087-0488-41 Bottles of 100

LITERATURE AVAILABLE
Yes.

REFERENCES
1. Hennon, D.K.; Stookey, G.K., and Muhler, J.C.: The Clinical Anticariogenic Effectiveness of Supplementary Fluoride-Vitamin Preparations— Results at the End of Three Years, J. Dentistry for Children 33:3–12 (Jan.) 1966.
2. Hennon, D.K.; Stookey, G.K., and Muhler, J.C.: The Clinical Anticariogenic Effectiveness of Supplementary Fluoride-Vitamin Preparations— Results at the End of Four Years, J. Dentistry for Children 34:439–443 (Nov.) 1967.
3. American Academy of Pediatrics Committee on Nutrition: Fluoride Supplementation. Pediatrics 77:758, 1986.

POLY–VI–FLOR® with Iron   ℞
[pahl-ē-vī'flōr"]
● 0.5 mg
● 0.25 mg
Multivitamin, iron and fluoride supplement drops

DESCRIPTION
[See table below left]
See INDICATIONS AND USAGE section below for use by infants and children under two years of age.
Active ingredient for caries prophylaxis: Fluoride as sodium fluoride.
Other ingredients: Ascorbic acid, caramel color, cholecalciferol, ferrous sulfate, fruit flavor (artificial), glycerin, niacinamide, polysorbate 80, pyridoxine hydrochloride, riboflavin-5-phosphate sodium, thiamine hydrochloride, d-alpha-tocopheryl acid succinate, vitamin A palmitate, water, and other ingredients.

CLINICAL PHARMACOLOGY
For information on fluoridation see Poly-Vi-Flor chewable tablets.

INDICATIONS AND USAGE
Supplementation of the diet with eight essential vitamins and iron.
Supplementation of the diet with fluoride for caries prophylaxis.
The American Academy of Pediatrics recommends that children up to age 16, in areas where drinking water contains less than optimal levels of fluoride, receive daily fluoride supplementation.
Poly-Vi-Flor 0.5 mg with Iron (multivitamin, iron, and fluoride supplement) drops provide fluoride in drop form for children ages 2–3 years in areas where the drinking water contains less than 0.3 ppm fluoride; and for children over 3 years in areas where the drinking water contains 0.3 through 0.7 ppm of fluoride. Each 1.0 mL provides sodium fluoride (0.5 mg fluoride) plus eight essential vitamins and iron.
Poly-Vi-Flor 0.25 mg with Iron drops provide fluoride in drop form for infants and young children from birth to 2 years of age in areas where the drinking water contains less than 0.3 ppm of fluoride and for children ages 2-3 years in areas where the drinking water contains 0.3 through 0.7 ppm of fluoride. Each 1.0 mL supplies sodium fluoride (0.25 mg fluoride) plus eight essential vitamins and iron.
The American Academy of Pediatrics[1] and the American Dental Association[2] currently recommend that infants and children under 2 years of age, in areas where drinking water contains less than 0.3 ppm of fluoride, and children 2-3, in areas where the drinking water contains 0.3 through 0.7 ppm of fluoride, receive 0.25 mg of supplemental fluoride daily which is provided in a full dose (1 mL) of Poly-Vi-Flor® 0.25 mg with Iron drops. A half dose (0.5 mL) of Poly-Vi-Flor 0.5 mg with Iron drops could also provide a daily fluoride intake of 0.25 mg; however, this dosage reduces vitamin supplementation by half.
Poly-Vi-Flor with Iron drops supply significant amounts of vitamins A, D, E, C, thiamine, riboflavin, niacin, pyridoxine,

| | Poly-Vi-Flor w/Iron drops | | Percentage of U.S. Recommended Daily Allowance | |
	0.5 mg	0.25 mg	Infants	Children Under 4
Each 1.0 mL supplies:				
Vitamin A, IU	1500	1500	100	60
Vitamin D, IU	400	400	100	100
Vitamin E, IU	5	5	100	50
Vitamin C, mg	35	35	100	88
Thiamine, mg	0.5	0.5	100	71
Riboflavin, mg	0.6	0.6	100	75
Niacin, mg	8	8	100	89
Vitamin B$_6$, mg	0.4	0.4	100	57
Iron, mg	10	10	67	100
Fluoride, mg	0.5	0.25	*	*
*U.S. Recommended Daily Allowance has not been established.

Continued on next page

Mead Johnson Nutr.—Cont.

and ferrous sulfate to supplement the diet, and to help assure that deficiencies of these nutrients will not develop. Thus, in a single easy-to-use preparation, infants and children obtain eight essential vitamins and iron, plus fluoride. A comprehensive 5½ year series of studies of the effectiveness of Tri-Vi-Flor® and Poly-Vi-Flor® products in caries protection has been published.[3-6] Children in this continuing study lived in an area where the water supply contained only 0.05 ppm fluoride. The subjects were divided into two groups, one which used only nonfluoridated Vi-Sol® vitamin products and the other Tri-Vi-Flor and Poly-Vi-Flor vitamin-fluoride products.

The three-year interim report showed 63% fewer carious surfaces in primary teeth and 43% fewer carious surfaces in permanent teeth of the children taking Vi-Flor® vitamin-fluoride products.[3]

After four years the studies continued to support the effectiveness of Tri-Vi-Flor and Poly-Vi-Flor, showing a reduction in carious surfaces of 68% in primary teeth and 46% in permanent teeth.[4]

Results at the end of 5½ years further confirmed the previous findings and indicated that significant reductions in dental caries are apparent with the continued use of Vi-Flor vitamin-fluoride products.[5]

WARNINGS
As in the case of all medications, keep out of the reach of children.

PRECAUTIONS
The suggested dose should not be exceeded since dental fluorosis may result from continued ingestion of large amounts of fluoride.

When prescribing Vi-Flor products:
1. determine the fluoride content of the drinking water.
2. make sure the child is not receiving significant amounts of fluoride from other medications.
3. periodically check to make sure that the child does not develop significant dental fluorosis.

Poly-Vi-Flor with Iron drops should be dispensed in the original plastic container, since contact with glass leads to instability and precipitation. (The amount of sodium fluoride in the 50-mL size is well below the maximum to be dispensed at one time according to recommendations of the American Dental Association.)

ADVERSE REACTIONS
Allergic rash and other idiosyncrasies have been reported rarely.

DOSAGE AND ADMINISTRATION
1.0 mL daily or as prescribed.
May be dropped directly into mouth with 'Safti-Dropper,' or mixed with cereal, fruit juice or other foods.

HOW SUPPLIED
Poly-Vi-Flor 0.5 mg with Iron (multivitamin, fluoride and iron supplement) drops are available in bottles of 50 mL.
NDC 0087-0469-41 Bottles of 1⅔ fl oz (50 mL)
Poly-Vi-Flor 0.25 mg with Iron (multivitamin, fluoride and iron supplement) drops are available in bottles of 50 mL.
NDC 0087-0483-41 Bottles of 1⅔ fl oz (50 mL)

LITERATURE AVAILABLE
Yes.

REFERENCES
1. American Academy of Pediatrics, Committee on Nutrition: Fluoride Supplementation. Pediatrics 77:758, 1986.
2. Accepted Dental Therapeutics, Ed. 38, Chicago, American Dental Association, 1979, p. 321.
3. Hennon, D.K.; Stookey, G.K., and Muhler, J.C.: The Clinical Anticariogenic Effectiveness of Supplementary Fluoride-Vitamin Preparations— Results at the End of Three Years, J. Dentistry for Children 33:3–12 (Jan.) 1966.
4. Hennon, D.K.; Stookey, G.K., and Muhler, J.C.: The Clinical Anticariogenic Effectiveness of Supplementary Fluoride-Vitamin Preparations— Results at the End of Four Years, J. Dentistry for Children 34:439–443 (Nov.) 1967.
5. Hennon, D.K.; Stookey, G.K., and Muhler, J.C.: The Clinical Anticariogenic Effectiveness of Supplementary Fluoride-Vitamin Preparations— Results at the End of Five and a Half Years, Phar. and Ther. In Dent. 1:1, 1970.
6. Hennon, D.K.; Stookey, G.K., and Beiswanger, B.B.: Fluoride-Vitamin Supplements: Effects on Dental Caries and Fluorosis When Used in Areas With Suboptimum Fluoride in the Water Supply. J. Am. Dent. Assoc. 95:965, 1977.

POLY-VI-SOL®
[pahl-ē-vī'sahl]
Vitamins
drops ● chewable tablets

(See PDR For Nonprescription Drugs)

POLY-VI-SOL® with Iron
[pahl-ē-vī'sahl]
Chewable vitamins and minerals

(See PDR For Nonprescription Drugs)

POLY-VI-SOL® with Iron
[pahl-ē-vī'sahl]
Vitamin and iron drops

(See PDR For Nonprescription Drugs)

PORTAGEN®
[port'ă-jen]
Iron fortified nutritionally complete powder with Medium Chain Triglycerides for tube and oral feeding
U.S. Patent No. 3,450,819

(See PDR For Nonprescription Drugs)

PREGESTIMIL®
[prē-jest'ĭ-mĭl]
Iron fortified protein hydrolysate formula with medium chain triglycerides
● powder, 1 lb can

(See PDR For Nonprescription Drugs)

PROSOBEE®
[prō-sō'be]
Iron-fortified, milk-free, sucrose-free, full-year soy formula
● powder, 14 oz cans
● ready-to-feed, 4 fl oz and 8 fl oz Nursette® bottles
● ready-to-feed, 8 fl oz and 32 fl oz cans
● concentrate, 13 fl oz

(See PDR For Nonprescription Drugs)

SUSTACAL®
[sŭs'tă-cal]
● liquid (ready to use)
● powder (mix with milk or water)
● pudding (ready-to-eat)
Nutritionally complete food

(See PDR For Nonprescription Drugs)

SUSTACAL® HC
[sŭs'tă-cal' hc]
High calorie nutritionally complete food for oral and tube feeding

(See PDR for Nonprescription Drugs)

SUSTACAL® with Fiber
[sŭs'tă-cal]
Nutritionally complete food with dietary fiber

(See PDR For Nonprescription Drugs)

SUSTAGEN® powder
[sus'tă-jen]
High calorie, high protein nutritional supplement

(See PDR For Nonprescription Drugs)

TEMPRA® drops, syrup, and chewable tablets
[tem'prah]
Acetaminophen

(See PDR For Nonprescription Drugs)

TRAUMACAL®
[tră'mă-cal]
High nitrogen nutritionally complete formula for metabolically stressed patients

(See PDR For Nonprescription Drugs)

TRIND® liquid
[trĭnd]
nasal decongestant ● antihistamine

(See PDR For Nonprescription Drugs)

TRIND–DM® liquid
[trĭnd]
antitussive ● nasal decongestant ● antihistamine

(See PDR For Nonprescription Drugs)

TRI–VI–FLOR® 1.0 mg   ℞
[trī'vī-flōr]
Vitamins A, D, C and fluoride chewable tablets

DESCRIPTION
[See table below left]
Active ingredient for caries prophylaxis: Fluoride as sodium fluoride.
Other ingredients: Ascorbic acid, cholecalciferol, dextrates, FD&C Blue No. 2 (aluminum lake), FD&C Red No. 40 (aluminum lake), FD&C Yellow No. 6 (aluminum lake), fruit flavors (artificial), magnesium stearate, sodium chloride, sodium ascorbate, stearic acid, surcrose, vitamin A acetate.

CLINICAL PHARMACOLOGY
For information of fluoridation see Poly-Vi-Flor® chewable tablets.
Tri-Vi-Flor tablets provide sodium fluoride (1 mg fluoride) and three basic vitamins in a chewable tablet. Because the tablets are chewable, they provide a *topical* as well as *systemic* source of fluoride.[1,2]

INDICATIONS AND USAGE
Supplementation of the diet with vitamins A, D, and C.
Supplementation of the diet with fluoride for caries prophylaxis.
The American Academy of Pediatrics recommends that children up to age 16, in areas where drinking water contains less than optimal levels of fluoride, receive daily fluoride supplementation.
Tri-Vi-Flor 1.0 mg (vitamins A, D, C and fluoride) chewable tablets provide fluoride in tablet form for children 3 years of age and older where the drinking water contains less than 0.3 ppm of fluoride.[3]
Tri-Vi-Flor 1.0 mg chewable tablets supply vitamins A, D and C to help assure that nutritional deficiencies of these vitamins will not develop.
Tri-Vi-Flor 1.0 mg chewable tablets also provide the important mineral fluoride for caries prophylaxis. Thus in a single easy-to-use preparation, children over 3 years of age obtain three basic vitamins and the important mineral fluoride.
A study of fluoride tablets given to 121 children revealed the efficacy of sodium fluoride in tablet form. The authors concluded that the caries reduction was comparable to that previously reported for children drinking fluoridated water.[4]
A comprehensive 5½ year series of studies of the effectiveness of Tri-Vi-Flor® and Poly-Vi-Flor® products in caries protection has been published.[1,2,5] Children in this continuing study lived in an area where the water supply contained only 0.05 ppm fluoride. The subjects were divided into two groups, one which used only non-fluoridated Vi-Sol® vitamin products and the other Tri-Vi-Flor and Poly-Vi-Flor vitamin-fluoride products.
The three-year interim report showed 63% fewer carious surfaces in primary teeth and 43% fewer carious surfaces in permanent teeth of the children taking Vi-Flor® vitamin-fluoride products.[1]
After four years the studies continued to support the effectiveness of Tri-Vi-Flor and Poly-Vi-Flor, showing a reduction

Each tablet supplies:	Tri-Vi-Flor Chewable Tablets 1.0 mg	Percentage of U.S. Recommended Daily Allowance	
		Children Age 2-3 Years	Adults & Children Age 4 Years or More
Vitamin A, IU	2500	100	50
Vitamin D, IU	400	100	100
Vitamin C, mg	60	150	100
Fluoride, mg	1.0	*	*

*U.S. Recommended Daily Allowance has not been established.

in carious surfaces of 68% in primary teeth and 46% in permanent teeth.[2]

Results at the end of $5\frac{1}{2}$ years further confirmed the previous findings and indicated that significant reductions in dental caries are apparent with the continued use of Vi-Flor vitamin-fluoride products.[5]

Children using Tri-Vi-Flor 1.0 mg chewable tablets regularly should receive semiannual dental examinations. The regular brushing of teeth and attention to good oral hygiene practices are also essential.

WARNINGS

As in the case of all medications, keep out of the reach of children.

PRECAUTIONS

The suggested dose of Tri-Vi-Flor 1.0 mg chewable tablets *should not be exceeded,* since dental fluorosis may result from continued ingestion of large amounts of fluoride.

When prescribing Vi-Flor products:
1. determine the fluoride content of the drinking water.
2. make sure the child is not receiving significant amounts of fluoride from other medications.
3. periodically check to make sure that the child does not develop significant dental fluorosis.

The Council on Dental Therapeutics of the American Dental Association recommends that no more than 264 mg of sodium fluoride should be dispensed at one time.[6] Therefore, no more than 120 Tri-Vi-Flor 1.0 mg chewable tablets (2.2 mg sodium fluoride per tablet) should be dispensed at one time.

ADVERSE REACTIONS

Allergic rash and other idiosyncrasies have been rarely reported.

DOSAGE AND ADMINISTRATION

One chewable tablet daily or as prescribed.

HOW SUPPLIED

Tri-Vi-Flor 1.0 mg (vitamins A, D, C and fluoride) chewable tablets are available in 100- and 1000-tablet bottles.
NDC 0087-0477-01 Bottles of 100
NDC 0087-0477-02 Bottles of 1000

LITERATURE AVAILABLE

Yes.

REFERENCES

1. Hennon, D.K., Stookey, G.K. and Muhler, J.C.: The Clinical Anticariogenic Effectiveness of Supplementary Fluoride-Vitamin Preparations—Results at the End of Three Years. J Dent for Children 33:3–12 (Jan). 1966.
2. Hennon, D.K., Stookey, G.K. and Muhler, J.C.: The Clinical Anticariogenic Effectiveness of Supplementary Fluoride-Vitamin Preparations—Results at the End of Four Years, J Dent for Children 34:439–443 (Nov.) 1967.
3. American Academy of Pediatrics, Committee on Nutrition: Fluoride Supplementation. Pediatrics 77:758, 1986.
4. Arnold, F.A., Jr., McClure, F.J. and White, C.L.: Sodium Fluoride Tablets for Children, Dental Progress 1:12–16 (Oct.) 1960.
5. Hennon, D.K., Stookey, G.K. and Muhler, J.C.: The Clinical Anticariogenic Effectiveness of Supplementary Fluoride-Vitamin Preparations—Results at the End of Five and a Half Years, Phar. and Ther. in Dent. 1:1, 1970.
6. Council on Dental Therapeutics, Am Dental Assoc, Accepted Dental Therapeutics, 1977, 37th Edition, page 294.

TRI-VI-FLOR®   ℞

[trī′vī-flor″]
● 0.5 mg
● 0.25 mg
Vitamins A, D, C and fluoride drops

DESCRIPTION

[See table above right]
See INDICATIONS AND USAGE section below for use by infants and children under two years of age.
Active ingredient for caries prophylaxis: Fluoride as sodium fluoride.
Other ingredients: Ascorbic acid, caramel color, cholecalciferol, fruit flavor (artificial), glycerin, polysorbate 80, sodium hydroxide, vitamin A palmitate, water.

CLINICAL PHARMACOLOGY

For information on fluoridation see Poly-Vi-Flor® chewable tablets.

INDICATIONS AND USAGE

Supplementation of the diet with vitamins A, D and C.
Tri-Vi-Flor drops also provide fluoride for caries prophylaxis.
The American Academy of Pediatrics recommends that children up to age 16, in areas where drinking water contains less than optimal levels of fluoride, receive daily fluoride supplementation.
Tri-Vi-Flor 0.5 mg (vitamins A, D, C and fluoride) drops provide fluoride in drop form for children ages 2-3 years in areas where the drinking water contains less than 0.3 ppm fluo-

ride; and for children over 3 years in areas where the drinking water contains 0.3 through 0.7 ppm of fluoride. Each 1.0 mL provides sodium fluoride (0.5 mg fluoride) plus three basic vitamins.
Tri-Vi-Flor 0.25 mg (vitamins A, D, C and fluoride) drops provide fluoride in drop form for infants and young children from birth to 2 years of age in areas where the drinking water contains less than 0.3 ppm of fluoride; and for children ages 2-3 years in areas where the drinking water contains 0.3 through 0.7 ppm of fluoride. Each 1.0 mL supplies sodium fluoride (0.25 mg fluoride) plus three basic vitamins.
The American Academy of Pediatrics[1] and the American Dental Association[6] currently recommend that infants and children under 2 years of age, in areas where drinking water contains less than 0.3 ppm of fluoride, and children 2-3, in areas where the drinking water contains 0.3 through 0.7 ppm of fluoride, receive 0.25 mg of supplemental fluoride daily which is provided in a full dose (1 mL) of Tri-Vi-Flor® 0.25 mg drops. A half dose (0.5 mL) of Tri-Vi-Flor 0.5 mg drops could also provide a daily fluoride intake of 0.25 mg; however, this dosage reduces vitamin supplementation by half.
A comprehensive $5\frac{1}{2}$ year series of studies of the effectiveness of Tri-Vi-Flor® and Poly-Vi-Flor® products in caries protection has been published.[2-5] Children in this continuing study lived in an area where the water supply contained only 0.05 ppm fluoride. The subjects were divided into two groups, one which used only nonfluoridated Vi-Sol® vitamin products and the other Tri-Vi-Flor and Poly-Vi-Flor vitamin-fluoride products.
The three-year interim report showed 63% fewer carious surfaces in primary teeth and 43% fewer carious surfaces in permanent teeth of the children taking Vi-Flor® vitamin-fluoride products.[2]
After four years the studies continued to support the effectiveness of Tri-Vi-Flor and Poly-Vi-Flor, showing a reduction in carious surfaces of 68% in primary teeth and 46% in permanent teeth.[3]
Results at the end of $5\frac{1}{2}$ years further confirmed the previous findings and indicated that significant reductions in dental caries are apparent with the continued use of Vi-Flor vitamin-fluoride products.[4]

WARNINGS

As in the case of all medications, keep out of the reach of children.

PRECAUTIONS

The suggested dose should not be exceeded since dental fluorosis may result from continued ingestion of large amounts of fluoride.

When prescribing Vi-Flor products:
1. determine the fluoride content of the drinking water.
2. make sure the child is not receiving significant amounts of fluoride from other medications.
3. periodically check to make sure that the child does not develop significant dental fluorosis.

Tri-Vi-Flor drops should be dispensed in the original plastic container, since contact with glass leads to instability and precipitation. (The amount of sodium fluoride in all Tri-Vi-Flor drops is well below the maximum to be dispensed at one time acccording to recommendations of the American Dental Association.)

ADVERSE REACTIONS

Allergic rash and other idiosyncrasies have been rarely reported.

DOSAGE AND ADMINISTRATION

1.0 mL daily, or as prescribed.
May be dropped directly into mouth with 'Safti-Dropper,' or mixed with cereal, fruit juice or other food.

HOW SUPPLIED

Tri-Vi-Flor 0.5 mg (vitamins A,D,C, and fluoride) drops are available in bottles of 50 mL.
NDC 0087-0473-02 Bottles of $1\frac{2}{3}$ fl oz (50 mL)
Tri-Vi-Flor 0.25 mg (vitamins A, D, C and fluoride) drops are available in bottles of 50 mL.
NDC 0087-0452-41 Bottles of 50 mL.

LITERATURE AVAILABLE

Yes.

REFERENCES

1. American Academy of Pediatrics, Committee on Nutrition: Fluoride Supplementation. Pediatrics 77:758, 1986.

	Tri-Vi-Flor Drops		Percentage of U.S. Recommended Daily Allowance	
Each 1.0 mL supplies:	0.5 mg	0.25 mg	Infants	Children Under 4
Vitamin A, IU	1500	1500	100	60
Vitamin D, IU	400	400	100	100
Vitamin C, mg	35	35	100	88
Fluoride, mg	0.5	0.25	*	*

*U.S. Recommended Daily Allowance has not been established.

2. Hennon, D.K.; Stookey, G.K., and Muhler, J.C.: The Clinical Anticariogenic Effectiveness of Supplementary Fluoride-Vitamin Preparations— Results at the End of Three Years, J. Dentistry for Children 33:3–12 (Jan.) 1966.
3. Hennon, D.K.; Stookey, G.K., and Muhler, J.C.: The Clinical Anticariogenic Effectiveness of Supplementary Fluoride-Vitamin Preparations— Results at the End of Four Years, J. Dentistry for Children 34:439–443 (Nov.) 1967.
4. Hennon, D.K.; Stookey, G.K., and Muhler, J.C.: The Clinical Anticariogenic Effectiveness of Supplementary Fluoride-Vitamin Preparations— Results at the End of Five and a Half Years, Phar. and Ther. in Dent. 1:1, 1970.
5. Hennon, D.K.; Stookey, G.K., and Beiswanger, B.B.: Fluoride-Vitamin Supplements: Effects on Dental Caries and Fluorosis when Used in Areas with Suboptimum Fluoride in the Water Supply. J. Am. Dent. Assoc. 95:965, 1977.
6. Accepted Dental Therapeutics, Ed. 38, Chicago, American Dental Association, 1979, p. 321.

TRI-VI-FLOR® 0.25 mg with Iron   ℞

[trī′vī-flor″]
Vitamins A, D, C, iron and fluoride drops

DESCRIPTION

		Percentage of U.S. Recommended Daily Allowance	
Each 1.0 mL supplies:		Infants	Children Under 4
Vitamin A, IU	1500	100	60
Vitamin D, IU	400	100	100
Vitamin C, mg	35	100	88
Iron, mg	10	67	100
Fluoride, mg	0.25	*	*

* U.S. Recommended Daily Allowance has not been established.

Active ingredient for caries prophylaxis: Fluoride as sodium fluoride.
Other ingredients: Ascorbic acid, caramel color, cholecalciferol, ferrous sulfate, fruit flavor (artificial), glycerin, polysorbate 80, propylene glycol, sodium hydroxide, vitamin A palmitate, water, and other ingredients.

CLINICAL PHARMACOLOGY

For information on fluoridation see Poly-Vi-Flor® chewable tablets.

INDICATIONS AND USAGE

Supplementation of the diet with vitamins A, D, C and iron. Supplementation of the diet with fluoride for caries prophylaxis.
The American Academy of Pediatrics[1] recommends that children up to age 16, in areas where drinking water contains less than optimal levels of fluoride, receive daily fluoride supplementation.
Tri-Vi-Flor 0.25 mg with Iron (vitamins A, D, C, iron and fluoride) drops provide fluoride in drop form for infants and young children from birth to 2 years of age in areas where the drinking water contains less than 0.3 ppm of fluoride; and for children ages 2-3 years in areas where the drinking water contains 0.3 through 0.7 ppm of fluoride. Each 1.0 mL supplies sodium fluoride (0.25 mg fluoride) plus three basic vitamins and iron.

WARNINGS

As in the case of all medications, keep out of the reach of children.

PRECAUTIONS

The suggested dose should not be exceeded since dental fluorosis may result from continued ingestion of large amounts of fluoride.

When prescribing Vi-Flor® products:
1. determine the fluoride content of the drinking water.
2. make sure the child is not receiving significant amounts of fluoride from other medications.
3. periodically check to make sure that the child does not develop significant dental fluorosis.

Tri-Vi-Flor 0.25 mg with Iron drops should be dispensed in the original plastic container, since contact with glass leads to instability and precipitation. (The amount of sodium fluoride in the 50-mL size is well below the maximum to be dis-

Continued on next page

Mead Johnson Nutr.—Cont.

pensed at one time according to recommendations of the American Dental Association.)

ADVERSE REACTIONS

Allergic rash and other idiosyncrasies have been rarely reported.

DOSAGE AND ADMINISTRATION

1.0 mL daily, or as prescribed. May be dropped directly into mouth with 'Safti-Dropper', or mixed with cereal, fruit juice or other food.
USE FULL DOSAGE.

HOW SUPPLIED

Tri-Vi-Flor 0.25 mg with Iron (vitamins A, D, C, iron and fluoride) drops are available in bottles of 50 mL.

REFERENCES

1. American Academy of Pediatrics, Committee on Nutrition: Fluoride Supplementation. Pediatrics 77:758, 1986.

TRI-VI-SOL®
[trī'vĭ-sahl"]
Vitamins A, D and C Supplement
drops

(See PDR For Nonprescription Drugs)

TRI-VI-SOL® with Iron
[trī'vĭ-sahl"]
Vitamins A, D, C and Iron
drops

(See PDR For Nonprescription Drugs)

Mead Johnson Pharmaceuticals
A Bristol-Myers Company
2400 W. LLOYD EXPRESSWAY
EVANSVILLE, INDIANA 47721-0001

BUSPAR®   ℞
[būspăr]
(buspirone HCl)

PRODUCT OVERVIEW

KEY FACTS

BuSpar® (buspirone hydrochloride) is an antianxiety agent that is neither chemically nor pharmacologically related to the benzodiazepines, barbiturates, or other sedative/anxiolytic drugs. BuSpar is less sedating than other anxiolytics. BuSpar has shown no potential for abuse or diversion and there is no evidence that it causes either physical or psychological dependence. BuSpar is not a controlled substance.

MAJOR USES

BuSpar is clinically effective for the management of anxiety disorders or the short-term relief of symptoms of anxiety. The recommended initial dose is 5 mg three times a day, with divided doses of 20–30 mg per day commonly employed after titration in 5 mg increments.

SAFETY INFORMATION

BuSpar is contraindicated in patients hypersensitive to buspirone hydrochloride. It is recommended that BuSpar not be used concomitantly with a monoamine oxidase inhibitor. Because BuSpar will not block the withdrawal syndrome often seen with benzodiazepines and other common sedative/hypnotic drugs, it is advisable to withdraw such patients gradually from their prior treatment before starting BuSpar therapy.

PRESCRIBING INFORMATION

BUSPAR®   ℞
[būspăr]
(buspirone HCl)

DESCRIPTION

BuSpar® (buspirone hydrochloride) is an antianxiety agent that is not chemically or pharmacologically related to the benzodiazepines, barbiturates, or other sedative/anxiolytic drugs.
Buspirone hydrochloride is a white crystalline, water soluble compound with a molecular weight of 422.0. Chemically, buspirone hydrochloride is 8-[4-[4-(2-pyrimidinyl)-1-piperazinyl]butyl]-8-azaspiro[4.5]decane-7,9-dione monohydrochloride. The empirical formula $C_{21}H_{31}N_5O_2 \cdot HCl$ is represented by the following structural formula:
[See Chemical Formula at top of next column].
BuSpar is supplied for oral administration in 5 mg and 10 mg white, ovoid-rectangular, scored tablets. BuSpar tablets, 5

mg and 10 mg, contain the following inactive ingredients: colloidal silicon dioxide, lactose, magnesium stearate, microcrystalline cellulose, and sodium starch glycolate.

CLINICAL PHARMACOLOGY

The mechanism of action of buspirone is unknown. Buspirone differs from typical benzodiazepine anxiolytics in that it does not exert anticonvulsant or muscle relaxant effects. It also lacks the prominent sedative effect that is associated with more typical anxiolytics. In vitro preclinical studies have shown that buspirone has a high affinity for serotonin ($5\text{-}HT_{1A}$) receptors. Buspirone has no significant affinity for benzodiazepine receptors and does not affect GABA binding in vitro or in vivo when tested in preclinical models.
Buspirone has moderate affinity for brain D_2-dopamine receptors. Some studies do suggest that buspirone may have indirect effects on other neurotransmitter systems.
BuSpar is rapidly absorbed in man and undergoes extensive first pass metabolism. In a radiolabeled study, unchanged buspirone in the plasma accounted for only about 1% of the radioactivity in the plasma. Following oral administration, plasma concentrations of unchanged buspirone are very low and variable between subjects. Peak plasma levels of 1 to 6 ng/mL have been observed 40 to 90 minutes after single oral doses of 20 mg. The single dose bioavailability of unchanged buspirone when taken as a tablet is on the average about 90% of an equivalent dose of solution, but there is large variability.
The effects of food upon the bioavailability of BuSpar have been studied in eight subjects. They were given a 20 mg dose with and without food; the area under the plasma concentration-time curve (AUC) and peak plasma concentration (Cmax) of unchanged buspirone increased by 84% and 116% respectively, but the total amount of buspirone immunoreactive material did not change. This suggests that food may decrease the extent of presystemic clearance of buspirone, but the clinical significance of these findings is unknown.
A multiple-dose study conducted in fifteen subjects suggests that buspirone has nonlinear pharmacokinetics. Thus, dose increases and repeated dosing may lead to somewhat higher blood levels of unchanged buspirone than would be predicted from results of single dose studies.
In man, approximately 95% of buspirone is plasma protein bound, but other highly bound drugs, eg, phenytoin, propranolol, and warfarin are not displaced by buspirone from plasma protein in vitro. However, in vitro binding studies show that buspirone does displace digoxin.
Buspirone is metabolized primarily by oxidation producing several hydroxylated derivatives and a pharmacologically active metabolite, 1-pyrimidinylpiperazine (1-PP). In animal models predictive of anxiolytic potential, 1-PP has about one quarter of the activity of buspirone, but is present in up to 20-fold greater amounts. However, this is probably not important in humans: blood samples from humans chronically exposed to BuSpar do not exhibit high levels of 1-PP; mean values are approximately 3 ng/mL and the highest human blood level recorded among 108 chronically dosed patients was 17 ng/mL, less than 1/200th of 1-PP levels found in animals given large doses of buspirone without signs of toxicity.
In a single-dose study using 14C-labeled buspirone, 29% to 63% of the dose was excreted in the urine within 24 hours, primarily as metabolites; fecal excretion accounted for 18 to 38% of the dose. The average elimination half-life of unchanged buspirone after single doses of 10 to 40 mg is about 2 to 3 hours.
The pharmacokinetics of BuSpar in patients with hepatic or renal dysfunction has not been determined, nor has the effect of age. The effect of BuSpar on drug metabolism or concomitant drug disposition has not been investigated.

INDICATIONS AND USAGE

BuSpar is indicated for the management of anxiety disorders or the short-term relief of the symptoms of anxiety. Anxiety or tension associated with the stress of everyday life usually does not require treatment with an anxiolytic.
The efficacy of BuSpar has been demonstrated in controlled clinical trials of outpatients whose diagnosis roughly corresponds to Generalized Anxiety Disorder (300.02) of the American Psychiatric Association's Diagnostic and Statistical Manual, III[1] as described below:
Generalized, persistent anxiety (of at least one month continual duration), manifested by symptoms from three of the following four categories:
1. Motor tension: shakiness, jitteriness, jumpiness, trembling, tension, muscle aches, fatigability, inability to relax, eyelid twitch, furrowed brow, strained face, fidgeting, restlessness, easy startle.
2. Autonomic hyperactivity: sweating, heart pounding or racing, cold, clammy hands, dry mouth, dizziness, lightheadedness, paresthesias (tingling in hands or feet), upset

stomach, hot or cold spells, frequent urination, diarrhea, discomfort in the pit of the stomach, lump in the throat, flushing, pallor, high resting pulse, and respiration rate.
3. Apprehensive expectation: anxiety, worry, fear, rumination, and anticipation of misfortune to self or others.
4. Vigilance and scanning: hyperattentiveness resulting in distractibility, difficulty in concentrating, insomnia, feeling "on edge," irritability, impatience.
The above symptoms would not be due to another mental disorder, such as a depressive disorder or schizophrenia.
The effectiveness of BuSpar in long-term use, that is, for more than three to four weeks, has not been demonstrated in controlled trials. However, patients have been treated with BuSpar for several months without ill effect. Therefore, the physician who elects to use BuSpar for extended periods should periodically reassess the usefulness of the drug for the individual patient.

CONTRAINDICATIONS

BuSpar is contraindicated in patients hypersensitive to buspirone hydrochloride.

WARNINGS

The administration of BuSpar to a patient taking a monoamine oxidase inhibitor (MAOI) may pose a hazard. There have been reports of the occurrence of elevated blood pressure when BuSpar has been added to a regimen including an MAOI. Therefore, it is recommended that BuSpar not be used concomitantly with an MAOI.
Because BuSpar has no established antipsychotic activity, it should not be employed in lieu of appropriate antipsychotic treatment.

PRECAUTIONS

General:
Interference with cognitive and motor performance:
Studies indicate that BuSpar is less sedating than other anxiolytics and that it does not produce significant functional impairment. However, its CNS effects in any individual patient may not be predictable. Therefore, patients should be cautioned about operating an automobile or using complex machinery until they are reasonably certain that buspirone treatment does not affect them adversely.
While formal studies of the interaction of BuSpar with alcohol indicate that buspirone does not increase alcohol-induced impairment in motor and mental performance, it is prudent to avoid concomitant use of alcohol and buspirone.
Potential for withdrawal reactions in sedative/hypnotic/anxiolytic drug-dependent patients:
Because BuSpar does not exhibit cross-tolerance with benzodiazepines and other common sedative/hypnotic drugs, it will not block the withdrawal syndrome often seen with cessation of therapy with these drugs. Therefore, before starting therapy with BuSpar, it is advisable to withdraw patients gradually, especially patients who have been using a CNS-depressant drug chronically, from their prior treatment. Rebound or withdrawal symptoms may occur over varying time periods, depending in part on the type of drug, and its effective half-life of elimination.
The syndrome of withdrawal from sedative/hypnotic/anxiolytic drugs can appear as any combination of irritability, anxiety, agitation, insomnia, tremor, abdominal cramps, muscle cramps, vomiting, sweating, flu-like symptoms without fever, and occasionally, even as seizures.
Possible concerns related to buspirone's binding to dopamine receptors:
Because buspirone can bind to central dopamine receptors, a question has been raised about its potential to cause acute and chronic changes in dopamine-mediated neurological function (eg, dystonia, pseudoparkinsonism, akathisia, and tardive dyskinesia). Clinical experience in controlled trials has failed to identify any significant neuroleptic-like activity; however, a syndrome of restlessness, appearing shortly after initiation of treatment, has been reported in some small fraction of buspirone-treated patients. The syndrome may be explained in several ways. For example, buspirone may increase central noradrenergic activity; alternatively, the effect may be attributable to dopaminergic effects (ie, represent akathisia). Obviously, the question cannot be totally resolved at this point in time. Generally, long-term sequelae of any drug's use can be identified only after several years of marketing.
Information for Patients:
To assure safe and effective use of BuSpar, the following information and instructions should be given to patients:
1. Inform your physician about any medications, prescription or nonprescription, alcohol, or drugs that you are now taking or plan to take during your treatment with BuSpar.
2. Inform your physician if you are pregnant, or if you are planning to become pregnant, or if you become pregnant while you are taking BuSpar.
3. Inform your physician if you are breast-feeding an infant.
4. Until you experience how this medication affects you, do not drive a car or operate potentially dangerous machinery.

Laboratory Tests:
There are no specific laboratory tests recommended.

Drug Interactions:
Because the effects of concomitant administration of BuSpar with most other psychotropic drugs have not been studied, the concomitant use of BuSpar with other CNS-active drugs should be approached with caution. (See WARNINGS.)

There is one report suggesting that the concomitant use of Desyrel® (trazodone hydrochloride) and BuSpar may have caused 3- to 6-fold elevations on SGPT (ALT) in a few patients. In a similar study, attempting to replicate this finding, no interactive effect on hepatic transaminases was identified.

In a study in normal volunteers, concomitant administration of BuSpar and haloperidol resulted in increased serum haloperidol concentrations. The clinical significance of this finding is not clear.

In vitro, buspirone does not displace tightly bound drugs like phenytoin, propranolol, and warfarin from serum proteins. However, there has been one report of prolonged prothrombin time when buspirone was added to the regimen of a patient treated with warfarin. The patient was also chronically receiving phenytoin, phenobarbital, digoxin, and Synthroid. *In vitro*, buspirone may displace less firmly bound drugs like digoxin. The clinical significance of this property is unknown.

Drug/Laboratory Test Interactions:
Buspirone is not known to interfere with commonly employed clinical laboratory tests.

Carcinogenesis, Mutagenesis, Impairment of Fertility:
No evidence of carcinogenic potential was observed in rats during a 24-month study at approximately 133 times the maximum recommended human oral dose; or in mice, during an 18-month study at approximately 167 times the maximum recommended human oral dose.

With or without metabolic activation, buspirone did not induce point mutations in 5 strains of *Salmonella typhimurium* (Ames Test) or mouse lymphoma L5178YTK⁺ cell cultures, nor was DNA damage observed with buspirone in Wi-38 human cells. Chromosomal aberrations or abnormalities did not occur in bone marrow cells of mice given one or five daily doses of buspirone.

Pregnancy: Teratogenic effects:
Pregnancy Category B: No fertility impairment or fetal damage was observed in reproduction studies performed in rats and rabbits at buspirone doses of approximately 30 times the maximum recommended human dose. In humans, however, adequate and well-controlled studies during pregnancy have *not* been performed. Because animal reproduction studies are not always predictive of human response, this drug should be used during pregnancy only if clearly needed.

Labor and Delivery:
The effect of BuSpar on labor and delivery in women is unknown. No adverse effects were noted in reproduction studies in rats.

Nursing Mothers:
The extent of the excretion in human milk of buspirone or its metabolites is not known. In rats, however, buspirone and its metabolites are excreted in milk. BuSpar administration to nursing women should be avoided if clinically possible.

Pediatric Use:
The safety and effectiveness of BuSpar have not been determined in individuals below 18 years of age.

Use in the Elderly:
BuSpar has not been systematically evaluated in older patients; however, several hundred elderly patients have participated in clinical studies with BuSpar and no unusual adverse age-related phenomena have been identified. In 87 elderly patients for whom dosage data were available, the modal total daily dose of BuSpar was 15 mg per day, the same as that in the total sample of patients treated with BuSpar.

Use in Patients with Impaired Hepatic or Renal Function:
Since BuSpar is metabolized by the liver and excreted by the kidneys, its administration to patients with severe hepatic or renal impairment cannot be recommended.

ADVERSE REACTIONS (See also PRECAUTIONS)

Commonly Observed:
The more commonly observed untoward events associated with the use of BuSpar not seen at an equivalent incidence among placebo-treated patients include dizziness, nausea, headache, nervousness, lightheadedness, and excitement.

Associated with Discontinuation of Treatment:
One guide to the relative clinical importance of adverse events associated with BuSpar is provided by the frequency with which they caused drug discontinuation during clinical testing. Approximately ten percent of the 2200 anxious patients who participated in the BuSpar premarketing clinical efficacy trials in anxiety disorders lasting three to four weeks discontinued treatment due to an adverse event. The more common events causing discontinuation included: central nervous system disturbances (3.4%), primarily dizziness, insomnia, nervousness, drowsiness and lightheaded feeling; gastrointestinal disturbances (1.2%), primarily nausea; and miscellaneous disturbances (1.1%), primarily headache and fatigue. In addition, 3.4% of patients had multiple complaints, none of which could be characterized as primary.

Incidence in Controlled Clinical Trials:
The table that follows enumerates adverse events that occurred at a frequency of 1% or more among BuSpar patients who participated in four-week, controlled trials comparing BuSpar with placebo. The frequencies were obtained from pooled data for seventeen trials. The prescriber should be aware that these figures cannot be used to predict the incidence of side effects in the course of usual medical practice where patient characteristics and other factors differ from those which prevailed in the clinical trials. Similarly, the cited frequencies cannot be compared with figures obtained from other clinical investigations involving different treatments, uses, and investigators. Comparison of the cited figures, however, does provide the prescribing physician with some basis for estimating the relative contribution of drug and non-drug factors to the side effect incidence rate in the population studied.

TREATMENT-EMERGENT ADVERSE EXPERIENCE INCIDENCE IN PLACEBO-CONTROLLED CLINICAL TRIALS*
(Percent of Patients Reporting)

Adverse Experience	BuSpar (n=477)	Placebo (n=464)
Cardiovascular		
Tachycardia/Palpitations	1	1
CNS		
Dizziness	12	3
Drowsiness	10	9
Nervousness	5	1
Insomnia	3	3
Lightheadedness	3	—
Decreased Concentration	2	2
Excitement	2	—
Anger/Hostility	2	—
Confusion	2	—
Depression	2	2
EENT		
Blurred Vision	2	—
Gastrointestinal		
Nausea	8	5
Dry Mouth	3	4
Abdominal/Gastric Distress	2	2
Diarrhea	2	—
Constipation	1	2
Vomiting	1	2
Musculoskeletal		
Musculoskeletal Aches/Pains	1	—
Neurological		
Numbness	2	—
Paresthesia	1	—
Incoordination	1	—
Tremor	1	—
Skin		
Skin Rash	1	—
Miscellaneous		
Headache	6	3
Fatigue	4	4
Weakness	2	—
Sweating/Clamminess	1	—

* Events reported by at least 1% of BuSpar patients are included.
—Incidence less than 1%.

Other Events Observed During the Entire Premarketing Evaluation of BuSpar:
During its premarketing assessment, BuSpar was evaluated in over 3500 subjects. This section reports event frequencies for adverse events occurring in approximately 3000 subjects from this group who took multiple doses of BuSpar in the dose range for which BuSpar is being recommended (ie, the modal daily dose of BuSpar fell between 10 and 30 mg for 70% of the patients studied) and for whom safety data were systematically collected. The conditions and duration of exposure to BuSpar varied greatly, involving well-controlled studies as well as experience in open and uncontrolled clinical settings. As part of the total experience gained in clinical studies, various adverse events were reported. In the absence of appropriate controls in some of the studies, a causal relationship to BuSpar treatment cannot be determined. The list includes all undesirable events reasonably associated with the use of the drug.

The following enumeration by organ system describes events in terms of their relative frequency of reporting in this data base. Events of major clinical importance are also described in the PRECAUTIONS section.

The following definitions of frequency are used: Frequent adverse events are defined as those occurring in at least 1/100 patients. Infrequent adverse events are those occurring in 1/100 to 1/1000 patients, while rare events are those occurring in less than 1/1000 patients.

Cardiovascular:
Frequent was nonspecific chest pain; infrequent were syncope, hypotension and hypertension; rare were cerebrovascular accident, congestive heart failure, myocardial infarction, cardiomyopathy and bradycardia.

Central Nervous System:
Frequent were dream disturbances; infrequent were depersonalization, dysphoria, noise intolerance, euphoria, akathisia, fearfulness, loss of interest, dissociative reaction, hallucinations, suicidal ideation and seizures; rare were feelings of claustrophobia, cold intolerance, stupor, and slurred speech and psychosis.

EENT:
Frequent were tinnitus, sore throat and nasal congestion. Infrequent were redness and itching of the eyes, altered taste, altered smell, and conjunctivitis; rare were inner ear abnormality, eye pain, photophobia, and pressure on eyes.

Endocrine:
Rare were galactorrhea and thyroid abnormality.

Gastrointestinal:
Infrequent were flatulence, anorexia, increased appetite, salivation, irritable colon and rectal bleeding; rare was burning of the tongue.

Genitourinary:
Infrequent were urinary frequency, urinary hesitancy, menstrual irregularity and spotting, and dysuria; rare were amenorrhea, pelvic inflammatory disease, enuresis and nocturia.

Musculoskeletal:
Infrequent were muscle cramps, muscle spasms, rigid/stiff muscles, and arthralgias.

Neurological:
Infrequent were involuntary movements and slowed reaction time; rare was muscle weakness.

Respiratory:
Infrequent were hyperventilation, shortness of breath and chest congestion; rare was epistaxis.

Sexual Function:
Infrequent were decreased or increased libido; rare were delayed ejaculation and impotence.

Skin:
Infrequent were edema, pruritus, flushing, easy bruising, hair loss, dry skin, facial edema and blisters; rare were acne and thinning of nails.

Clinical Laboratory:
Infrequent were increases in hepatic aminotransferases (SGOT, SGPT); rare were eosinophilia, leukopenia and thrombocytopenia.

Miscellaneous:
Infrequent were weight gain, fever, roaring sensation in the head, weight loss and malaise; rare were alcohol abuse, bleeding disturbance, loss of voice and hiccoughs.

POSTINTRODUCTION CLINICAL EXPERIENCE
Postmarketing experience has shown an adverse experience profile similar to that given above. Voluntary reports since introduction have included rare occurrences of allergic reactions, cogwheel rigidity, dystonic reactions, ecchymosis, emotional lability, tunnel vision, and urinary retention. Because of the uncontrolled nature of these spontaneous reports, a causal relationship to BuSpar treatment has not been determined.

DRUG ABUSE AND DEPENDENCE

Controlled Substance Class:
BuSpar is not a controlled substance.

Physical and Psychological Dependence:
In human and animal studies, buspirone has shown no potential for abuse or diversion and there is no evidence that it causes tolerance, or either physical or psychological dependence. Human volunteers with a history of recreational drug or alcohol usage were studied in two double-blind clinical investigations. None of the subjects were able to distinguish between BuSpar and placebo. By contrast, subjects showed a statistically significant preference for methaqualone and diazepam. Studies in monkeys, mice, and rats have indicated that buspirone lacks potential for abuse.

Following chronic administration in the rat, abrupt withdrawal of buspirone did not result in the loss of body weight commonly observed with substances that cause physical dependency.

Although there is no direct evidence that BuSpar causes physical dependence or drug-seeking behavior, it is difficult to predict from experiments the extent to which a CNS active drug will be misused, diverted and/or abused once marketed. Consequently, physicians should carefully evaluate patients for a history of drug abuse and follow such patients closely, observing them for signs of BuSpar misuse or abuse (eg, development of tolerance, incrementation of dose, drug-seeking behavior).

OVERDOSAGE

Signs and Symptoms:
In clinical pharmacology trials, doses as high as 375 mg/day were administered to healthy male volunteers. As this dose was approached, the following symptoms were observed: nausea, vomiting, dizziness, drowsiness, miosis, and gastric distress. No deaths have been reported in humans either

Continued on next page

Mead Johnson Pharm.—Cont.

with deliberate or accidental overdosage of BuSpar. Toxicology studies of buspirone yielded the following LD_{50} values: mice, 655 mg/kg; rats, 196 mg/kg; dogs, 586 mg/kg; and monkeys, 356 mg/kg. These dosages are 160–550 times the recommended human daily dose.

Recommended Overdose Treatment:
General symptomatic and supportive measures should be used along with immediate gastric lavage. Respiration, pulse, and blood pressure should be monitored as in all cases of drug overdosage. No specific antidote is known to buspirone, and dialyzability of buspirone has not been determined.

DOSAGE AND ADMINISTRATION

The recommended initial dose is 15 mg daily (5 mg three times a day). To achieve an optimal therapeutic response, at intervals of 2 to 3 days the dosage may be increased 5 mg per day, as needed. The maximum daily dosage should not exceed 60 mg per day. In clinical trials allowing dose titration, divided doses of 20–30 mg per day were commonly employed.

HOW SUPPLIED

BuSpar® (buspirone hydrochloride)
Tablets, 5 mg and 10 mg (white, ovoid-rectangular with score, MJ logo, strength and the name BuSpar embossed) are available in bottles of 100 and 500.

NDC 0087-0818-41	Bottles of 100
5 mg tablet	
NDC 0087-0818-44	Bottles of 500
5 mg tablet	
NDC 0087-0819-41	Bottles of 100
10 mg tablet	
NDC 0087-0819-44	Bottles of 500
10 mg tablet	

U.S. Patent Nos. 3,717,634
              4,182,763
Store at room temperature. Protect from temperatures greater than 86° F (30° C). Dispense in a tight, light-resistant container.

REFERENCE

1. American Psychiatric Association, Ed.: Diagnostic and Statistical Manual of Mental Disorders—III, American Psychiatric Association, May 1980.
   Shown in Product Identification Section, page 418

COLACE®
[kō'lās]
docusate sodium, Mead Johnson
capsules • syrup • liquid (drops)

30 mL bottle   **NSN 6505-00-045-7786 (M)**

PRODUCT OVERVIEW

KEY FACTS
Colace is a stool softener. This surface-active agent helps keep stools soft for easy, natural passage. Colace is not a laxative; thus, not habit forming. It is available in three forms: capsules, 50 mg and 100 mg; syrup, 20 mg/5 mL; liquid (drops, 1% solution).

MAJOR USES
Colace is useful in constipation due to hard stools in painful anorectal conditions, in cardiac and other conditions in which maximum ease of passage is desirable to avoid difficult or painful defecation, and when peristaltic stimulants are contraindicated.

SAFETY INFORMATION
There are no known contraindications to Colace. The incidence of side effects—none of a serious nature—is exceedingly small. As with any drug, if you are pregnant or nursing a baby, seek the advice of a health professional before using this product.

PRESCRIBING INFORMATION

COLACE®
[kō'lās]
docusate sodium, Mead Johnson
capsules • syrup • liquid (drops)

DESCRIPTION
Colace (docusate sodium) is a stool softener.
Colace Capsules, 50 mg, contain the following inactive ingredients: citric acid, D&C Red No. 33, FD&C Red No. 40, non-porcine gelatin, edible ink, polyethylene glycol, propylene glycol, and purified water.
Colace Capsules, 100 mg, contain the following inactive ingredients: citric acid, D&C Red No. 33, FD&C Red No. 40, FD&C Yellow No. 6, non-porcine gelatin, edible ink, polyethylene glycol, propylene glycol, titanium dioxide, and purified water.
Colace Liquid, 1%, contains the following inactive ingredients: citric acid, D&C Red No. 33, methylparaben, polox-

amer, polyethylene glycol, propylene glycol, propylparaben, sodium citrate, vanillin, and purified water.
Colace Syrup, 20 mg/5 mL, contains the following inactive ingredients: alcohol, citric acid, D&C Red No. 33, FD&C Red No. 40, flavor (natural), menthol, methylparaben, peppermint oil, poloxamer, polyethylene glycol, propylparaben, sodium citrate, sucrose, and purified water.

ACTIONS AND USES

Colace, a surface-active agent, helps to keep stools soft for easy, natural passage. Not a laxative, thus not habit forming. Useful in constipation due to hard stools, in painful anorectal conditions, in cardiac and other conditions in which maximum ease of passage is desirable to avoid difficult or painful defecation, and when peristaltic stimulants are contraindicated. *Note:* When peristaltic stimulation is needed due to inadequate bowel motility, see Peri-Colace® (laxative and stool softener).

CONTRAINDICATIONS

There are no known contraindications to Colace.

WARNING

As with any drug, if you are pregnant or nursing a baby, seek the advice of a health professional before using this product.

SIDE EFFECTS

The incidence of side effects—none of a serious nature—is exceedingly small. Bitter taste, throat irritation, and nausea (primarily associated with the use of the syrup and liquid) are the main side effects reported. Rash has occurred.

ADMINISTRATION AND DOSAGE

Orally—Suggested daily Dosage: *Adults and older children:* 50 to 200 mg. *Children 6 to 12:* 40 to 120 mg. *Children 3 to 6:* 20 to 60 mg. *Infants and children under 3:* 10 to 40 mg. The higher doses are recommended for initial therapy. Dosage should be adjusted to individual response. The effect on stools is usually apparent one to three days after the first dose. Give Colace liquid in half a glass of milk or fruit juice or in infant formula, to mask bitter taste. *In enemas*—Add 50 to 100 mg Colace (5 to 10 mL Colace liquid) to a retention or flushing enema.

HOW SUPPLIED

Colace® capsules, 50 mg
  NDC 0087-0713-01 Bottles of 30
  NDC 0087-0713-02 Bottles of 60
  NDC 0087-0713-03 Bottles of 250
  NDC 0087-0713-05 Bottles of 1000
  NDC 0087-0713-07 Cartons of 100 single unit packs
Colace® capsules, 100 mg
  NDC 0087-0714-01 Bottles of 30
  NDC 0087-0714-02 Bottles of 60
  NDC 0087-0714-03 Bottles of 250
  NDC 0087-0714-05 Bottles of 1000
  NDC 0087-0714-07 Cartons of 100 single unit packs
Note: Colace capsules should be stored at controlled room temperature (59°–86°F or 15°–30°C)
Colace® liquid, 1% solution; 10 mg/mL (with calibrated dropper)
  NDC 0087-0717-04 Bottles of 16 fl oz
  NDC 0087-0717-02 Bottles of 30 mL.
  6505-00-045-7786 (Bottle of 30 mL) Defense
Colace® syrup, 20 mg/5-mL teaspoon; contains not more than 1% alcohol
  NDC 0087-0720-01 Bottles of 8 fl oz
  NDC 0087-0720-02 Bottles of 16 fl oz
  Shown in Product Identification Section, page 418

DESYREL®   ℞
[des'ē-rel]
(trazodone HCl)

Tablets, 150 mg, bottles of 100
       NSN 6505-01-234-4439 (M&VA)

DESCRIPTION

DESYREL (trazodone hydrochloride) is an antidepressant chemically unrelated to tricyclic, tetracyclic, or other known antidepressant agents. It is a triazolopyridine derivative designated as 2-[3-[4-(3-chlorophenyl)-1-piperazinyl] propyl]-1,2,4-triazolo[4, 3-a]pyridin-3(2$\underline{H}$)-one hydrochloride. DESYREL is a white odorless crystalline powder which is freely soluble in water. Its molecular weight is 408.3. The empirical formula is $C_{19}H_{22}ClN_5O \cdot HCl$ and the structural formula is represented as follows:

DESYREL is supplied for oral administration in 50 mg, 100 mg, 150 mg and 300 mg tablets.
DESYREL Tablets, 50 mg, contain the following inactive ingredients: dibasic calcium phosphate, castor oil, microcrystalline cellulose, ethylcellulose, FD&C Yellow No. 6 (alumi-

num lake), lactose, magnesium stearate, povidone, sodium starch glycolate, and starch (corn).
DESYREL Tablets, 100 mg, contain the following inactive ingredients: dibasic calcium phosphate, castor oil, microcrystalline cellulose, ethylcellulose, lactose, magnesium stearate, povidone, sodium starch glycolate, and starch (corn).
DESYREL Tablets, 150 mg, contain the following inactive ingredients: microcrystalline cellulose, FD&C Yellow No. 6 (aluminum lake), magnesium stearate, pregelatinized starch, and stearic acid.
DESYREL Tablets, 300 mg, contain the following inactive ingredients: microcrystalline cellulose, yellow ferric oxide, magnesium stearate, sodium starch glycolate, pregelatinized starch, and stearic acid.

CLINICAL PHARMACOLOGY

The mechanism of DESYREL's antidepressant action in man is not fully understood. In animals, DESYREL selectively inhibits serotonin uptake by brain synaptosomes and potentiates the behavioral changes induced by the serotonin precursor, 5-hydroxytryptophan. Cardiac conduction effects of DESYREL in the anesthetized dog are qualitatively dissimilar and quantitatively less pronounced than those seen with tricyclic antidepressants. DESYREL is not a monoamine oxidase inhibitor and, unlike amphetamine-type drugs, does not stimulate the central nervous system.
In man, DESYREL is well absorbed after oral administration without selective localization in any tissue. When DESYREL is taken shortly after ingestion of food, there may be an increase in the amount of drug absorbed, a decrease in maximum concentration and a lengthening in the time to maximum concentration. Peak plasma levels occur approximately one hour after dosing when DESYREL is taken on an empty stomach or two hours after dosing when taken with food. Elimination of DESYREL is biphasic, consisting of an initial phase (half-life 3–6 hours) followed by a slower phase (half-life 5–9 hours), and is unaffected by the presence or absence of food. Since the clearance of DESYREL from the body is sufficiently variable, in some patients DESYREL may accumulate in the plasma.
For those patients who responded to DESYREL, one-third of the inpatients and one-half of the outpatients had a significant therapeutic response by the end of the first week of treatment. Three-fourths of all responders demonstrated a significant therapeutic effect by the end of the second week. One-fourth of responders required 2–4 weeks for a significant therapeutic response.

INDICATIONS AND USAGE

DESYREL is indicated for the treatment of depression. The efficacy of DESYREL has been demonstrated in both inpatient and outpatient settings and for depressed patients with and without prominent anxiety. The depressive illness of patients studied corresponds to the Major Depressive Episode criteria of the American Psychiatric Association's Diagnostic and Statistical Manual, III.[a]
Major Depressive Episode implies a prominent and relatively persistent (nearly every day for at least two weeks) depressed or dysphoric mood that usually interferes with daily functioning, and includes at least four of the following eight symptoms: change in appetite, change in sleep, psychomotor agitation or retardation, loss of interest in usual activities or decrease in sexual drive, increased fatigability, feelings of guilt or worthlessness, slowed thinking or impaired concentration, and suicidal ideation or attempts.

CONTRAINDICATIONS

DESYREL is contraindicated in patients hypersensitive to DESYREL.

WARNINGS

TRAZODONE HAS BEEN ASSOCIATED WITH THE OCCURRENCE OF PRIAPISM. IN APPROXIMATELY ⅓ OF THE CASES REPORTED, SURGICAL INTERVENTION WAS REQUIRED AND, IN A PORTION OF THESE CASES, PERMANENT IMPAIRMENT OF ERECTILE FUNCTION OR IMPOTENCE RESULTED. MALE PATIENTS WITH PROLONGED OR INAPPROPRIATE ERECTIONS SHOULD IMMEDIATELY DISCONTINUE THE DRUG AND CONSULT THEIR PHYSICIAN.
If an erection should persist, promptly contact Bristol-Myers USPG Medical Services Department (812/429-5591 or 812/429-5000).
The detumescence of priapism and drug-induced penile erections by the intracavernosal injection of alpha-adrenergic stimulants such as epinephrine and metaraminol has been reported.[b-g] For one case of priapism (of some 12-24 hours' duration) in a DESYREL-treated patient in whom the intracavernosal injection of epinephrine was accomplished, prompt detumescence occurred with return of normal erectile activity.
This procedure should be performed under the supervision of a urologist or a physician familiar with the procedure and should not be initiated without urologic consultation if the priapism has persisted for more than 24 hours.
DESYREL is not recommended for use during the initial recovery phase of myocardial infarction.

Caution should be used when administering DESYREL to patients with cardiac disease, and such patients should be closely monitored, since antidepressant drugs (including DESYREL) have been associated with the occurrence of cardiac arrhythmias. Recent clinical studies in patients with pre-existing cardiac disease indicate that DESYREL may be arrhythmogenic in some patients in that population. Arrhythmias identified include isolated PVCs, ventricular couplets, and in two patients short episodes (3–4 beats) of ventricular tachycardia.

PRECAUTIONS

General: The possibility of suicide in seriously depressed patients is inherent in the illness and may persist until significant remission occurs. Therefore, prescriptions should be written for the smallest number of tablets consistent with good patient management.

Hypotension, including orthostatic hypotension and syncope, has been reported to occur in patients receiving DESYREL. Concomitant administration of antihypertensive therapy with DESYREL may require a reduction in the dose of the antihypertensive drug.

Little is known about the interaction between DESYREL and general anesthetics; therefore, prior to elective surgery, DESYREL should be discontinued for as long as clinically feasible.

As with all antidepressants, the use of DESYREL should be based on the consideration of the physician that the expected benefits of therapy outweigh potential risk factors.

Information for Patients: Because priapism has been reported to occur in patients receiving DESYREL, patients with prolonged or inappropriate penile erection should immediately discontinue the drug and consult with the physician (see WARNINGS).

Antidepressants may impair the mental and/or physical ability required for the performance of potentially hazardous tasks, such as operating an automobile or machinery; the patient should be cautioned accordingly.

DESYREL may enhance the response to alcohol, barbiturates, and other CNS depressants.

DESYREL should be given shortly after a meal or light snack. Within any individual patient, total drug absorption may be up to 20% higher when the drug is taken with food rather than on an empty stomach. The risk of dizziness/lightheadedness may increase under fasting conditions.

Laboratory Tests: Occasional low white blood cell and neutrophil counts have been noted in patients receiving DESYREL. These were not considered clinically significant and did not necessitate discontinuation of the drug; however, the drug should be discontinued in any patient whose white blood cell count or absolute neutrophil count falls below normal levels. White blood cell and differential counts are recommended for patients who develop fever and sore throat (or other signs of infection) during therapy.

Drug Interactions: Increased serum digoxin or phenytoin levels have been reported to occur in patients receiving DESYREL concurrently with either of those two drugs.

It is not known whether interactions will occur between monoamine oxidase (MAO) inhibitors and DESYREL. Due to the absence of clinical experience, if MAO inhibitors are discontinued shortly before or are to be given concomitantly with DESYREL, therapy should be initiated cautiously with gradual increase in dosage until optimum response is achieved.

Therapeutic Interactions: Concurrent administration with electroshock therapy should be avoided because of the absence of experience in this area.

There have been reports of increased and decreased prothrombin time occurring in Coumadinized patients who take DESYREL.

Carcinogenesis, Mutagenesis, Impairment of Fertility: No drug- or dose-related occurrence of carcinogenesis was evident in rats receiving DESYREL in daily oral doses up to 300 mg/kg for 18 months.

Pregnancy Category C: DESYREL has been shown to cause increased fetal resorption and other adverse effects on the fetus in two studies using the rat when given at dose levels approximately 30–50 times the proposed maximum human dose. There was also an increase in congenital anomalies in one of three rabbit studies at approximately 15–50 times the maximum human dose. There are no adequate and well-controlled studies in pregnant women. DESYREL should be used during pregnancy only if the potential benefit justifies the potential risk to the fetus.

Nursing Mothers: DESYREL and/or its metabolites have been found in the milk of lactating rats, suggesting that the drug may be secreted in human milk. Caution should be exercised when DESYREL is administered to a nursing woman.

Pediatric Use: Safety and effectiveness in children below the age of 18 have not been established.

ADVERSE REACTIONS

Because the frequency of adverse drug effects is affected by diverse factors (eg, drug dose, method of detection, physician judgment, disease under treatment, etc) a single meaningful

	Treatment-Emergent Symptom Incidence			
	Inpts.		Outpts.	
	D	P	D	P
Number of Patients	142	95	157	158
% of Patients Reporting				
Allergic				
Skin Condition/Edema	2.8	1.1	7.0	1.3
Autonomic				
Blurred Vision	6.3	4.2	14.7	3.8
Constipation	7.0	4.2	7.6	5.7
Dry Mouth	14.8	8.4	33.8	20.3
Cardiovascular				
Hypertension	2.1	1.1	1.3	*
Hypotension	7.0	1.1	3.8	0.0
Shortness of Breath	*	1.1	1.3	0.0
Syncope	2.8	2.1	4.5	1.3
Tachycardia/Palpitations	0.0	0.0	7.0	7.0
CNS				
Anger/Hostility	3.5	6.3	1.3	2.5
Confusion	4.9	0.0	5.7	7.6
Decreased Concentration	2.8	2.1	1.3	0.0
Disorientation	2.1	0.0	*	0.0
Dizziness/Lightheadedness	19.7	5.3	28.0	15.2
Drowsiness	23.9	6.3	40.8	19.6
Excitement	1.4	1.1	5.1	5.7
Fatigue	11.3	4.2	5.7	2.5
Headache	9.9	5.3	19.8	15.8
Insomnia	9.9	10.5	6.4	12.0
Impaired Memory	1.4	0.0	*	*
Nervousness	14.8	10.5	6.4	8.2
Gastrointestinal				
Abdominal/Gastric Disorder	3.5	4.2	5.7	4.4
Bad Taste in Mouth	1.4	0.0	0.0	0.0
Diarrhea	0.0	1.1	4.5	1.9
Nausea/Vomiting	9.9	1.1	12.7	9.5
Musculoskeletal				
Musculoskeletal Aches/Pains	5.6	3.2	5.1	2.5
Neurological				
Incoordination	4.9	0.0	1.9	0.0
Paresthesia	1.4	0.0	0.0	*
Tremors	2.8	1.1	5.1	3.8
Sexual Function				
Decreased Libido	*	1.1	1.3	*
Other				
Decreased Appetite	3.5	5.3	0.0	*
Eyes Red/Tired/Itching	2.8	0.0	0.0	0.0
Head Full-Heavy	2.8	0.0	0.0	0.0
Malaise	2.8	0.0	0.0	0.0
Nasal/Sinus Congestion	2.8	0.0	5.7	3.2
Nightmares/Vivid Dreams	*	1.1	5.1	5.7
Sweating/Clamminess	1.4	1.1	*	*
Tinnitus	1.4	0.0	*	*
Weight Gain	1.4	0.0	4.5	1.9
Weight Loss	*	3.2	5.7	2.5

*Incidence less than 1%.

D = DESYREL   P = Placebo

estimate of adverse event incidence is difficult to obtain. This problem is illustrated by the variation in adverse event incidence observed and reported from the inpatients and outpatients treated with DESYREL. It is impossible to determine precisely what accounts for the differences observed.

Clinical Trial Reports: The table below is presented solely to indicate the relative frequency of adverse events reported in representative controlled clinical studies conducted to evaluate the safety and efficacy of DESYREL.

The figures cited cannot be used to predict precisely the incidence of untoward events in the course of usual medical practice where patient characteristics and other factors often differ from those which prevailed in the clinical trials. These incidence figures, also, cannot be compared with those obtained from other clinical studies involving related drug products and placebo, as each group of drug trials is conducted under a different set of conditions.

[See table above].

Occasional sinus bradycardia has occurred in long-term studies.

In addition to the relatively common (ie, greater than 1%) untoward events enumerated above, the following adverse events have been reported to occur in association with the use of DESYREL in the controlled clinical studies: akathisia, allergic reaction, anemia, chest pain, delayed urine flow, early menses, flatulence, hallucinations/delusions, hematuria, hypersalivation, hypomania, impaired speech, impotence, increased appetite, increased libido, increased urinary frequency, missed periods, muscle twitches, numbness, and retrograde ejaculation.

Postintroduction Reports: Although the following adverse reactions have been reported in DESYREL users, the causal association has neither been confirmed nor refuted.

Voluntary reports received since market introduction include the following: agitation, alopecia, apnea, ataxia, breast enlargement or engorgement, diplopia, edema, extrapyramidal symptoms, grand mal seizures, hallucinations, hemolytic anemia, hyperbilirubinemia, leukonychia, jaundice, lactation, liver enzyme alterations, methemoglobinemia, nausea/vomiting (most frequently), paresthesia, priapism (See WARNINGS and PRECAUTIONS, Information for Patients; some patients have required surgical intervention), pruritus, psychosis, rash, stupor, inappropriate ADH syndrome, tardive dyskinesia, unexplained death, urinary incontinence, urinary retention, urticaria, vasodilation, vertigo, and weakness.

Cardiovascular system effects which have been reported include the following: conduction block, orthostatic hypotension and syncope, palpitations, bradycardia, atrial fibrillation, myocardial infarction, cardiac arrest, arrhythmia, and ventricular ectopic activity, including ventricular tachycardia (see WARNINGS).

OVERDOSE

Animal Oral LD$_{50}$

The oral LD$_{50}$ of the drug is 610 mg/kg in mice, 486 mg/kg in rats, and 560 mg/kg in rabbits.

Signs and Symptoms: Death from overdose has occurred in patients ingesting DESYREL and other drugs concurrently (namely, alcohol; alcohol + chloral hydrate + diazepam; amobarbital; chlordiazepoxide; or meprobamate).

The most severe reactions reported to have occurred with overdose of DESYREL alone have been priapism, respiratory arrest, seizures, and EKG changes. The reactions reported most frequently have been drowsiness and vomiting. Overdosage may cause an increase in incidence or severity of any

Continued on next page

Mead Johnson Pharm.—Cont.

of the reported adverse reactions (see ADVERSE REACTIONS).

Treatment: There is no specific antidote for DESYREL. Treatment should be symptomatic and supportive in the case of hypotension or excessive sedation. Any patient suspected of having taken an overdose should have the stomach emptied by gastric lavage. Forced diuresis may be useful in facilitating elimination of the drug.

DOSAGE AND ADMINISTRATION

The dosage should be initiated at a low level and increased gradually, noting the clinical response and any evidence of intolerance. Occurrence of drowsiness may require the administration of a major portion of the daily dose at bedtime or a reduction of dosage. DESYREL should be taken shortly after a meal or light snack. Symptomatic relief may be seen during the first week, with optimal antidepressant effects typically evident within two weeks. Twenty-five percent of those who respond to DESYREL require more than two weeks (up to four weeks) of drug administration.

Usual Adult Dosage: An initial dose of 150 mg/day in divided doses is suggested. The dose may be increased by 50 mg/day every three to four days. The maximum dose for outpatients usually should not exceed 400 mg/day in divided doses. Inpatients (ie, more severely depressed patients) may be given up to but not in excess of 600 mg/day in divided doses.

Maintenance: Dosage during prolonged maintenance therapy should be kept at the lowest effective level. Once an adequate response has been achieved, dosage may be gradually reduced, with subsequent adjustment depending on therapeutic response.

Although there has been no systematic evaluation of the efficacy of DESYREL beyond six weeks, it is generally recommended that a course of antidepressant drug treatment should be continued for several months.

HOW SUPPLIED

DESYREL® (trazodone hydrochloride)

Tablets, 50 mg—round, orange/scored, film-sealed (imprinted with DESYREL and MJ 775)

NDC 0087-0775-41	Bottles of 100
NDC 0087-0775-43	Bottles of 1000
NDC 0087-0775-42	Cartons of 100 Unit Doses

Tablets, 100 mg—round, white/scored, film-sealed (imprinted with DESYREL and MJ 776)

NDC 0087-0776-41	Bottles of 100
NDC 0087-0776-43	Bottles of 1000
NDC 0087-0776-42	Cartons of 100 Unit Doses

Tablets, 150 mg—orange, in the Dividose® tablet design (imprinted with MJ and 778 on front; "50," "50," "50" on reverse)

NDC 0087-0778-43	Bottles of 100
NDC 0087-0778-44	Bottles of 500

Tablets, 300 mg—yellow, in the Dividose® tablet design (imprinted with MJ and 796 on front; "100," "100," "100" on reverse)

NDC 0087-0796-41	Bottles of 100

U.S. Patent Nos. 4,215,104
                       4,258,027

Store at room temperature. Protect from temperatures above 104°F (40°C).

Dispense in tight, light-resistant container (USP).

REFERENCES

a. Williams JBW, Ed: Diagnostic and Statistical Manual of Mental Disorders-III, American Psychiatric Association, May 1980.

b. Brindley GS: New treatment for priapism, *Lancet* July 28, 1984, ii:220.

c. Goldstein I, et al: Pharmacologic detumescence: The alternative to surgical shunting, *J Urol* April 1986, 135(4:PEII):3-08A.

d. Brindley GS: Pilot experiments on the actions of drugs injected into the human corpus cavernosum penis, *Br J Phar* 1986, 87:495-500.

e. Padma-Nathan H, et al: Treatment of prolonged or priapistic erections following intracavernosal papaverine therapy, *Semin Urol* 1986, IV(4):236-238.

f. Lue TF, et al: Priapism: A Refined Approach to Diagnosis and Treatment, *J Urol* July 1986, 136:104-110.

g. Fabre LF, Feighner JP: Long-term therapy for depression with trazodone, *J Clin Psychiatry* January 1983, 44(1):17-21.

Shown in Product Identification Section, page 418

DURICEF®   ℞
[*dur'i-sef*]
(cefadroxil monohydrate)

Capsules, 500 mg, bottles of 100
                NSN 6505-01-096-3886 (M)

DESCRIPTION

DURICEF® (cefadroxil monohydrate) is a semisynthetic cephalosporin antibiotic intended for oral administration. It is a white to yellowish-white crystalline powder. It is soluble in water and it is acid-stable. It is chemically designated as 7-[[D-2-amino-2-(4-hydroxyphenyl) acetyl] amino]-3-methyl-8-oxo -5- thia-1-azabicyclo [4.2.0] oct-2- ene-2-carboxylic acid monohydrate. It has the following structural formula:

DURICEF® tablets, 1 g, contain the following inactive ingredients: microcrystalline cellulose and magnesium stearate.

DURICEF® for Oral Suspension contains the following inactive ingredients: FD&C Yellow No. 6, flavors (natural and artificial), polysorbate 80, sodium benzoate, sucrose, and xanthan gum.

DURICEF® capsules contain the following inactive ingredients: D&C Red No. 28, FD&C Blue No. 1, FD&C Red No. 40, gelatin, magnesium stearate, and titanium dioxide.

Clinical Pharmacology—DURICEF (cefadroxil monohydrate) is rapidly absorbed after oral administration. Following single doses of 500 and 1000 mg, average peak serum concentrations were approximately 16 and 28 μg/mL, respectively. Measurable levels were present 12 hours after administration. Over 90 percent of the drug is excreted unchanged in the urine within 24 hours. Peak urine concentrations are approximately 1800 μg/mL during the period following a single 500 mg oral dose. Increases in dosage generally produce a proportionate increase in DURICEF urinary concentration. The urine antibiotic concentration, following a 1 g dose, was maintained well above the MIC of susceptible urinary pathogens for 20 to 22 hours.

Microbiology: *In vitro* tests demonstrate that the cephalosporins are bactericidal because of their inhibition of cell-wall synthesis. DURICEF is active against the following organisms *in vitro*:

    Beta- hemolytic streptococci
    Staphylococci, including coagulase-positive,
        coagulase-negative,
        and penicillinase-producing strains
    Streptococcus (Diplococcus) pneumoniae
    Escherichia coli.
    Proteus mirabilis
    Klebsiella species
    Moraxella (Branhamella) catarrhalis

Note:—Most strains of enterococci (*Streptococcus faecalis* and *S. faecium*) are resistant to DURICEF. It is not active against most strains of *Enterobacter* species, *P. morganii*, and *P. vulgaris*, It has no activity against *Pseudomonas* sp. and *Acinetobacter calcoaceticus* (formerly *Mima* and *Herellea* sp.)

Disc Susceptibility Tests.—Quantitative methods that require measurement of zone diameters give the most precise estimates of antibiotic susceptibility. One recommended procedure (CFR Section 460.1) uses cephalosporin class disc for testing susceptibility; interpretations correlate zone diameters of this disc test with MIC values for DURICEF. With this procedure, a report from the laboratory of "resistant" indicates that the infecting organism is not likely to respond to therapy. A report of "intermediate susceptibility" suggests that the organism would be susceptible if the infection is confined to the urinary tract, as DURICEF produces high antibiotic levels in the urine.

INDICATIONS AND USAGE

DURICEF (cefadroxil monohydrate) is indicated for the treatment of the following infections when caused by susceptible strains of the designated microorganisms:

    Urinary tract infections caused by *E. coli, P. mirabilis,* and *Klebsiella* species
    Skin and skin structure infections caused by staphylococci and/or streptococci
    Pharyngitis and tonsillitis caused by Group A *beta*-hemolytic streptococci (Penicillin is the usual drug of choice in the treatment and prevention of streptococcal infections, including the prophylaxis of rheumatic fever. DURICEF is generally effective in the eradication of streptococci from the nasopharynx; however, substantial data establishing the efficacy of DURICEF in the subsequent prevention of rheumatic fever are not available at present.)

Note: Culture and susceptibility tests should be initiated prior to and during therapy. Renal function studies should be performed when indicated.

CONTRAINDICATIONS

DURICEF (cefadroxil monohydrate) is contraindicated in patients with known allergy to the cephalosporin group of antibiotics.

WARNING

IN PENICILLIN-ALLERGIC PATIENTS, CEPHALOSPORIN ANTIBIOTICS SHOULD BE USED WITH GREAT CAUTION. THERE IS CLINICAL AND LABORATORY EVIDENCE OF PARTIAL CROSS-ALLERGENICITY OF THE PENICILLINS AND THE CEPHALOSPORINS, AND THERE ARE INSTANCES OF PATIENTS WHO HAVE HAD REACTIONS TO BOTH DRUGS (INCLUDING FATAL ANAPHYLAXIS AFTER PARENTERAL USE).

Any patient who has demonstrated a history of some form of allergy, particularly to drugs, should receive antibiotics cautiously and then only when absolutely necessary. No exception should be made with regard to DURICEF (cefadroxil monohydrate).

Pseudomembranous colitis has been reported with the use of cephalosporins (and other broad-spectrum antibiotics); therefore, it is important to consider its diagnosis in patients who develop diarrhea in association with antibiotic use. Treatment with broad-spectrum antibiotics alters normal flora of the colon and may permit overgrowth of clostridia. Studies indicate a toxin produced by *Clostridium difficile* is one primary cause of antibiotic-associated colitis. Cholestyramine and colestipol resins have been shown to bind the toxin *in vitro.*

Mild cases of colitis may respond to drug discontinuance alone.

Moderate to severe cases should be managed with fluid, electrolyte and protein supplementation as indicated.

When the colitis is not relieved by drug discontinuance or when it is severe, oral vancomycin is the treatment of choice for antibiotic-associated pseudomembranous colitis produced by *C. difficile.* Other causes of colitis should also be considered.

PRECAUTIONS

Patients should be followed carefully so that any side effects or unusual manifestations of drug idiosyncrasy may be detected. If a hypersensitivity reaction occurs, the drug should be discontinued and the patient treated with the usual agents (eg, epinephrine or other pressor amines, antihistamines, or corticosteroids).

DURICEF (cefadroxil monohydrate) should be used with caution in the presence of markedly impaired renal function (creatinine clearance rate of less than 50 mL/min/1.73 m^2). (See Dosage and Administration.) In patients with known or suspected renal impairment, careful clinical observation and appropriate laboratory studies should be made prior to and during therapy.

Prolonged use of DURICEF may result in the overgrowth of nonsusceptible organisms. Careful observation of the patient is essential. If superinfection occurs during therapy, appropriate measures should be taken.

Positive direct Coombs tests have been reported during treatment with the cephalosporin antibiotics. In hematologic studies or in transfusion cross-matching procedures when antiglobulin tests are performed on the minor side or in Coombs testing of newborns whose mothers have received cephalosporin antibiotics before parturition, it should be recognized that a positive Coombs test may be due to the drug.

DURICEF should be prescribed with caution in individuals with a history of gastrointestinal disease, particularly colitis.

Carcinogenesis, Mutagenesis and Impairment of Fertility: No long-term studies have been performed to determine carcinogenic potential. No genetic toxicity tests have been performed.

Pregnancy: Pregnancy Category B: Reproduction studies have been performed in mice and rats at doses up to 11 times the human dose and have revealed no evidence of impaired fertility or harm to the fetus due to cefadroxil monohydrate. There are, however, no adequate and well-controlled studies in pregnant women. Because animal reproduction studies are not always predictive of human response, this drug should be used during pregnancy only if clearly needed.

Nursing Mothers: Caution should be exercised when cefadroxil monohydrate is administered to a nursing mother.

ADVERSE REACTIONS

Gastrointestinal—Symptoms of pseudomembranous colitis can appear during antibiotic treatment. Nausea and vomiting have been reported rarely. Diarrhea has also occurred.

Hypersensitivity—Allergies (in the form of rash, urticaria, and angioedema) have been observed. These reactions usually subsided upon discontinuation of the drug.

Other reactions have included genital pruritus, genital moniliasis, vaginitis, and moderate transient neutropenia.

DOSAGE AND ADMINISTRATION

DURICEF (cefadroxil monohydrate) is acid-stable and may be administered orally without regard to meals. Administration with food may be helpful in diminishing potential gastrointestinal complaints occasionally associated with oral cephalosporin therapy.

Adults
Urinary Tract Infections: For uncomplicated lower urinary tract infections (ie, cystitis) the usual dosage is 1 or 2 g per day in single (q.d.) or divided doses (b.i.d.).

For all other urinary tract infections the usual dosage is 2 g per day in divided doses (b.i.d.).

Skin and Skin Structure Infections: For skin and skin structure infections the usual dosage is 1 g per day in single (q.d.) or divided doses (b.i.d.).

Pharyngitis and Tonsillitis: Treatment of Group A beta-hemolytic streptococcal pharyngitis and tonsillitis—1 g per day in single (q.d.) or divided doses (b.i.d.) for 10 days.

Children
For urinary tract infections and for skin and skin structure infections, the recommended daily dosage for children is 30 mg/kg/day in divided doses every 12 hours. For pharyngitis and tonsillitis, the recommended daily dosage for children is 30 mg/kg/day in single (q.d.) or divided doses (b.i.d.). In the treatment of beta-hemolytic streptococcal infections, a therapeutic dosage of DURICEF should be administered for at least 10 days.

See chart for total daily dosage for children.

[See table above.]

In patients with renal impairment, the dosage of cefadroxil monohydrate should be adjusted according to creatinine clearance rates to prevent drug accumulation. The following schedule is suggested. In adults, the initial dose is 1000 mg of DURICEF (cefadroxil monohydrate) and the maintenance dose (based on the creatinine clearance rate [(mL/min/1.73 m²]) is 500 mg at the time intervals listed below.

Creatinine Clearances	Dosage Interval
0–10 mL/min	36 hours
10–25 mL/min	24 hours
25–50 mL/min	12 hours

Patients with creatinine clearance rates over 50 mL/min may be treated as if they were patients having normal renal function.

HOW SUPPLIED

DURICEF® (cefadroxil monohydrate) for Oral Suspension

125 mg/5 mL	50 mL size	(NDC 0087-0786-42)
	100 mL size	(NDC 0087-0786-41)
250 mg/5 mL	50 mL size	(NDC 0087-0782-42)
	100 mL size	(NDC 0087-0782-41)
500 mg/5 mL	50 mL size	(NDC 0087-0783-42)
	100 mL size	(NDC 0087-0783-41)

All with orange-pineapple flavor. Directions for mixing are included on the label. Shake well before using. Keep container tightly closed. After mixing, store in refrigerator. Discard unused portion after 14 days.

DURICEF (cefadroxil monohydrate) capsules, 500 mg, in bottles of 50 (NDC 0087-0784-46), 100 (NDC 0087-0784-42) and in 10 strips of 10 individually labeled blisters each containing 1 capsule (NDC 0087-0784-44).

DURICEF (cefadroxil monohydrate) tablets, 1 g, in bottles of 50 (NDC 0087-0785-43), 100 (NDC 0087-0785-42) and in 10 strips of 10 individually labeled blisters each containing 1 tablet (NDC 0087-0785-44).

U.S. Patent Nos. 4,160,863
              4,504,657

Shown in Product Identification Section, page 418

KLOTRIX®   ℞
[klō′trix]
(potassium chloride)
Slow-Release Tablets 10 mEq

PRODUCT OVERVIEW

KEY FACTS
Klotrix is a film-coated (not enteric-coated) tablet containing 750 mg potassium chloride (equivalent to 10 mEq) in a wax matrix. Klotrix is formulated to provide a controlled release of potassium from the matrix to minimize the likelihood of producing high localized concentrations of potassium within the gastrointestinal tract.

MAJOR USES
Klotrix is suggested for therapeutic use in patients with hypokalemia with or without metabolic alkalosis; in digitalis intoxication and in patients with hypokalemic familial periodic paralysis. It also can be used for prevention of potassium depletion when the dietary intake of potassium is inadequate.

SAFETY INFORMATION
Potassium supplements are contraindicated in patients with hyperkalemia. Because of reports of intestinal and gastric ulceration and bleeding with slow-release potassium chloride preparations, these drugs should be reserved for those

Daily Dosage of DURICEF Suspension

Child's Weight				
lbs	kg	125 mg/5 mL	250 mg/5 mL	500 mg/5mL
10	4.5	1 tsp		
20	9.1	2 tsp	1 tsp	
30	13.6	3 tsp	1½ tsp	
40	18.2	4 tsp	2 tsp	1 tsp
50	22.7	5 tsp	2½ tsp	1¼ tsp
60	27.3	6 tsp	3 tsp	1½ tsp
70 & above	31.8+	—	—	2 tsp

patients who cannot tolerate or refuse to take liquid or effervescent potassium preparations or for patients in whom there is a problem of compliance with these preparations.

PRESCRIBING INFORMATION

KLOTRIX®   ℞
[klō′trix]
(potassium chloride)
Slow-Release Tablets 10 mEq

DESCRIPTION
KLOTRIX is a solid, oral dosage form of potassium chloride containing 750 mg of potassium chloride, USP (equivalent to 10 mEq of potassium) in a film-coated wax-matrix tablet. This formulation is intended to provide a controlled release of potassium from the matrix to minimize the likelihood of producing high, localized concentrations of potassium within the gastrointestinal tract.

KLOTRIX is an electrolyte replenisher. The chemical name is potassium chloride, and the structural formula is KCl. Potassium chloride, USP, occurs as a white, granular powder or as colorless crystals. It is odorless and has a saline taste. Its solutions are neutral to litmus. It is freely soluble in water and insoluble in alcohol.

This product contains the following inactive ingredients: ethylcellulose, FD&C Yellow No. 6 (aluminum lake), glycerin, hydroxypropyl methylcellulose 2910, edible ink, magnesium stearate, povidone, colloidal silicon dioxide, stearic acid, and titanium dioxide.

CLINICAL PHARMACOLOGY
The potassium ion is the principal intracellular cation of most body tissues. Potassium ions participate in a number of essential physiological processes including the maintenance of intracellular tonicity, the transmission of nerve impulses, the contraction of cardiac, skeletal, and smooth muscle, and the maintenance of normal renal function.

The intracellular concentration of potassium is approximately 150 to 160 mEq per liter. The normal adult plasma concentration is 3.5 to 5 mEq per liter. An active ion transport system maintains this gradient across the plasma membrane.

Potassium is a normal dietary constituent and, under steady state conditions, the amount of potassium absorbed from the gastrointestinal tract is equal to the amount excreted in the urine. The usual dietary intake of potassium is 50 to 100 mEq per day.

Potassium depletion will occur whenever the rate of potassium loss through renal excretion and/or loss from the gastrointestinal tract exceeds the rate of potassium intake. Such depletion usually develops as a consequence of therapy with diuretics, primary or secondary hyperaldosteronism, diabetic ketoacidosis, or inadequate replacement of potassium in patients on prolonged parenteral nutrition. Depletion can develop rapidly with severe diarrhea, especially if associated with vomiting. Potassium depletion due to these causes is usually accompanied by a concomitant loss of chloride and is manifested by hypokalemia and metabolic alkalosis. Potassium depletion may produce weakness, fatigue, disturbances of cardiac rhythm (primarily ectopic beats), prominent U-waves in the electrocardiogram, and in advanced cases, flaccid paralysis and/or impaired ability to concentrate urine.

If potassium depletion associated with metabolic alkalosis cannot be managed by correcting the fundamental cause of the deficiency, eg, where the patient requires long-term, diuretic therapy, supplemental potassium in the form of high potassium food or potassium chloride may be able to restore normal potassium levels.

In rare circumstances (eg, patients with renal tubular acidosis) potassium depletion may be associated with metabolic acidosis and hyperchloremia. In such patients potassium replacement should be accomplished with potassium salts other than the chloride, such as potassium bicarbonate, potassium citrate, potassium acetate, or potassium gluconate.

INDICATIONS AND USAGE
BECAUSE OF REPORTS OF INTESTINAL AND GASTRIC ULCERATION AND BLEEDING WITH CONTROLLED-RELEASE POTASSIUM CHLORIDE PREPARATIONS, THESE DRUGS SHOULD BE RESERVED FOR THOSE PATIENTS WHO CANNOT TOLERATE OR REFUSE TO TAKE LIQUIDS OR EFFERVESCENT POTASSIUM PREPARATIONS OR

FOR PATIENTS IN WHOM THERE IS A PROBLEM OF COMPLIANCE WITH THESE PREPARATIONS.

1. For the treatment of patients with hypokalemia with or without metabolic alkalosis; in digitalis, intoxication; and in patients with hypokalemic familial periodic paralysis. If hypokalemia is the result of diuretic therapy, consideration should be given to the use of a lower dose of diuretic, which may be sufficient without leading to hypokalemia.
2. For prevention of hypokalemia in patients who would be at particular risk if hypokalemia were to develop, eg, digitalized patients or patients with significant cardiac arrhythmias.

The use of potassium salts in patients receiving diuretics for uncomplicated essential hypertension is often unnecessary when such patients have a normal dietary pattern and when low doses of the diuretic are used. Serum potassium should be checked periodically, however; and, if hypokalemia occurs, dietary supplementation with potassium-containing foods may be adequate to control milder cases. In more severe cases, and if dose adjustment of the diuretic is ineffective or unwarranted, supplementation with potassium salts may be indicated.

CONTRAINDICATIONS
Potassium supplements are contraindicated in patients with hyperkalemia since a further increase in serum potassium concentration in such patients can produce cardiac arrest. Hyperkalemia may complicate any of the following conditions; chronic renal failure, systemic acidosis such as diabetic acidosis, acute dehydration, extensive tissue breakdown as in severe burns, adrenal insufficiency, or the administration of a potassium-sparing diuretic (eg, spironolactone, triamterene, amiloride) (see OVERDOSAGE).

Controlled-release formulations of potassium chloride have produced esophageal ulceration in certain cardiac patients with esophageal compression due to an enlarged left atrium. Potassium supplementation, when indicated in such patients, should be given as a liquid preparation.

All solid dosage forms of potassium chloride are contraindicated in any patient in whom there is structural, pathological (eg, diabetic gastroparesis) or pharmacologic (use of anticholinergic agents or other agents with anticholinergic properties at sufficient doses to exert anticholinergic effects) cause for arrest or delay in tablet passage through the gastrointestinal tract.

WARNINGS
Hyperkalemia (see OVERDOSAGE)
In patients with impaired mechanisms for excreting potassium, the administration of potassium salts can produce hyperkalemia and cardiac arrest. This occurs most commonly in patients given potassium by the intravenous route but may also occur in patients given potassium orally. Potentially fatal hyperkalemia can develop rapidly and be asymptomatic.

The use of potassium salts in patients with chronic renal disease, or any other condition which impairs potassium excretion, requires particularly careful monitoring of the serum potassium concentration and appropriate dosage adjustment.

Interaction with Potassium-Sparing Diuretics
Hypokalemia should not be treated by the concomitant administration of potassium in salts and a potassium-sparing diuretic (eg, spironolactone, triamterene, or amiloride), since the simultaneous administration of these agents can produce severe hyperkalemia.

Interaction with Angiotensin Converting Enzyme Inhibitors
Angiotensin convertying enzyme (ACE) inhibitors (eg, captopril, enalapril) will produce some potassium retention by inhibiting aldosterone production. Potassium supplements should be given to patients receiving ACE inhibitors only with close monitoring.

Gastrointestinal Lesions
Solid oral dosage forms of potassium chloride can produce ulcerative and/or stenotic lesions of the gastrointestinal tract. Based on spontaneous adverse reaction reports, enteric-coated preparations of potassium chloride are associated with an increased frequency of small bowel lesions (40-50 per 100,000 patient-years) compared to sustained-release, wax-matrix formulations (less than one per 100,000 patient-

Continued on next page

Mead Johnson Pharm.—Cont.

years). Because of the lack of extensive marketing experience with microencapsulated products, a comparison between such products and wax-matrix or enteric-coated products is not available. KLOTRIX is a wax-matrix tablet formulated to provide a controlled rate of release of potassium chloride and thus to minimize the possibility of a high local concentration of potassium near the gastrointestinal wall. Prospective trials have been conducted in normal human volunteers in which the upper gastrointestinal tract was evaluated by endoscopic inspection before and after one week of solid oral potassium chloride therapy. The ability of this model to predict events occurring in usual clinical practice is unknown. Trials which approximated usual clinical practice did not reveal any clear differences between the wax-matrix and microencapsulated dosage forms. In contrast, there was a higher incidence of gastric and duodenal lesions in subjects receiving a high dose of wax-matrix, controlled-release formulation under conditions which did not resemble usual or recommended clinical practice (ie, 96 mEq per day in divided doses of potassium chloride administered to fasted patients, in the presence of an anticholinergic drug to delay gastric emptying). The upper gastrointestinal lesions observed by endoscopy were asymptomatic and were not accompanied by evidence of bleeding (hemoccult testing). The relevance of these findings to the usual conditions (ie, non-fasting, no anticholinergic agent, smaller doses) under which controlled-release potassium chloride products are used is uncertain; epidemiologic studies have not identified an elevated risk, compared to microencapsulated products, for upper gastrointestinal lesions in patients receiving wax-matrix formulations. KLOTRIX should be discontinued immediately and the possibility of ulceration, obstruction or perforation considered if severe vomiting, abdominal pain, distension, or gastrointestinal bleeding occurs.

Metabolic Acidosis

Hypokalemia in patients with metabolic acidosis should be treated with an alkalinizing potassium salt such as potassium bicarbonate, potassium citrate, potassium acetate, or potassium gluconate.

PRECAUTIONS

General

The diagnosis of potassium depletion is ordinarily made by demonstrating hypokalemia in a patient with a clinical history suggesting some cause for potassium depletion. In interpreting the serum potassium level, the physician should bear in mind that acute alkalosis *per se* can produce hypokalemia in the absence of a deficit in total body potassium, while acute acidosis *per se* can increase the serum potassium concentration into the normal range even in the presence of a reduced total body potassium. The treatment of potassium depletion, particularly in the presence of cardiac disease, renal disease, or acidosis, requires careful attention to acid-base balance and appropriate monitoring of serum electrolytes, the electrocardiogram, and the clinical status of the patient.

Information for Patients:

Physicians should consider reminding the patient of the following:

To take each dose with meals and with a full glass of water or other liquid.

To take this medicine following the frequency and amount prescribed by the physician. This is especially important if the patient is also taking diuretics and/or digitalis preparations.

To check with the physician if there is trouble swallowing tablets or if the tablets seem to stick in the throat.

To check with the physician at once if tarry stools or other evidence of gastrointestinal bleeding is noticed.

To take each dose without crushing, chewing, or sucking the tablets.

Laboratory Tests:

When blood is drawn for analysis of plasma potassium it is important to recognize that artifactual elevations can occur after improper venipuncture technique or as a result of *in vitro* hemolysis of the sample.

Drug Interactions:

Potassium-sparing diuretic, angiotensin converting enzyme inhibitors: see WARNINGS.

Carcinogenesis, Mutagenesis, Impairment of Fertility:

Carcinogenicity, mutagenicity, and fertility studies in animals have not been performed. Potassium is a normal dietary constituent.

Pregnancy Category C:

Animal reproduction studies have not been conducted with KLOTRIX. It is unlikely that potassium supplementation that does not lead to hyperkalemia would have an adverse effect on the fetus or would affect reproductive capacity.

Nursing Mothers:

The normal potassium ion content of human milk is about 13 mEq per liter. Since oral potassium becomes part of the body potassium pool, so long as body potassium is not excessive, the contribution of potassium chloride supplementation should have little or no effect on the level in human milk.

Pediatric Use:

Safety and effectiveness in children have not been established.

ADVERSE REACTIONS

One of the most severe adverse effects is hyperkalemia (see CONTRAINDICATIONS, WARNINGS, and OVERDOSAGE). There also have been reports of upper and lower gastrointestinal conditions including obstruction, bleeding, ulceration, and perforation (see CONTRAINDICATIONS and WARNINGS). The most common adverse reactions to oral potassium salts are nausea, vomiting, abdominal pain and discomfort, and diarrhea. These symptoms are due to irritation of the gastrointestinal tract and are best managed by diluting the preparation further, taking the dose with meals, or reducing the dose.

OVERDOSAGE

The administration of oral potassium salts to persons with normal excretory mechanisms for potassium rarely causes serious hyperkalemia. However, if excretory mechanisms are impaired or if potassium is administered too rapidly intravenously, potentially fatal hyperkalemia can result (see CONTRAINDICATIONS and WARNINGS). It is important to recognize that hyperkalemia is usually asymptomatic and may be manifested only by an increased serum potassium concentration (6.5 - 8.0 mEq/L) and characteristic electrocardiographic changes (peaking of T-waves, loss of P-wave, depression of S-T segment, and prolongation of the QT interval). Late manifestations include muscle paralysis and cardiovascular collapse from cardiac arrest (9 - 12 mEq/L).

Treatment measures for hyperkalemia include the following: (1) elimination of foods and medications containing potassium and of potassium-sparing diuretics; (2) intravenous administration of 300 to 500 mL/hr of 10% dextrose solution containing 10-20 units of insulin per 1,000 mL; (3) correction of acidosis, if present, with intravenous sodium bicarbonate; (4) use of exchange resins, hemodialysis, or peritoneal dialysis.

In treating hyperkalemia, it should be recalled that in patients who have been stabilized on digitalis, too rapid a lowering of the serum potassium concentration can produce digitalis toxicity.

DOSAGE AND ADMINISTRATION

The usual dietary intake of potassium by the average adult is 50 to 100 mEq per day. Potassium depletion sufficient to cause hypokalemia usually requires the loss of 200 or more mEq of potassium from the total body store. Dosage must be adjusted to the individual needs of each patient but is typically in the range of 20 mEq per day for the prevention of hypokalemia to 40-100 mEq per day or more for the treatment of potassium depletion. Dosage should be divided if more than 20 mEq per day is given so that no more than 20 mEq is given in a single dose.

KLOTRIX provides 10 mEq of potassium chloride.

Note: KLOTRIX slow-release tablets must be taken without crushing, chewing, or sucking tablets. KLOTRIX should be taken with meals and with a glass of water or other liquid. This product should not be taken on an empty stomach because of its potential for gastric irritation (see WARNINGS). Following release of the potassium chloride, the expended wax-matrix, which is not absorbed, may be observed in the stool.

HOW SUPPLIED

Tablets (light orange, film-coated) each containing 750 mg potassium chloride (equivalent to 10 mEq each potassium and chloride).

NDC 0087-0770-41	Bottles of 100
NDC 0087-0770-42	Bottles of 1000
NDC 0087-0770-43	Cartons of 100 individually wrapped tablets

Tablets, 10 mEq, bottles of 100 NSN 6505-01-235-2631 (M)
Tablets, 10 mEq, bottles of 1000 NSN 6505-01-235-2632 (M)
U.S. Patent No. 4,140,756
Do not store at temperatures above 86°F (30°C).

Shown in Product Identification Section, page 418

PERI–COLACE® capsules ● syrup
[*peri-kō 'lās*]
casanthranol and docusate sodium

PRODUCT OVERVIEW

KEY FACTS

Peri-Colace is a combination of the mild stimulant laxative casanthranol and the stool softener Colace® (docusate sodium). This product provides gentle peristaltic stimulation and helps to keep stools soft for easier passage. It is available in two forms: capsules and syrup.

MAJOR USES

Peri-Colace is useful in the management of chronic or temporary constipation.

SAFETY INFORMATION

Do not use Peri-Colace when abdominal pain, nausea, or vomiting are present. Frequent or prolonged use of this preparation may result in dependence on laxatives.

As with any drug, if you are pregnant or nursing a baby, seek the advice of a health professional before using this product.

PRESCRIBING INFORMATION

PERI-COLACE® capsules ● syrup
[*peri-kō 'las*]
casanthranol and docusate sodium

DESCRIPTION

Peri-Colace is a combination of the mild stimulant laxative casanthranol and the stool-softener Colace (docusate sodium). Each capsule contains 30 mg of casanthranol and 100 mg of Colace; the syrup contains 30 mg of casanthranol and 60 mg of Colace per 15-mL tablespoon (10 mg of casanthranol and 20 mg of Colace per 5-mL teaspoon) and 10% alcohol. Peri-Colace Capsules contain the following inactive ingredients: D&C Red No. 33, FD&C Red No. 40, non-porcine gelatin, edible ink, polyethylene glycol, propylene glycol, titanium dioxide, and purified water.

Peri-Colace Syrup contains the following inactive ingredients: alcohol, citric acid, flavors, methyl salicylate, methylparaben, poloxamer, polyethylene glycol, propylparaben, sodium citrate, sorbitol solution, sucrose, and purified water.

ACTION AND USES

Peri-Colace provides gentle peristaltic stimulation and helps to keep stools soft for easier passage. Bowel movement is induced gently—usually overnight or in 8 to 12 hours. Nausea, griping, abnormally loose stools, and constipation rebound are minimized. Useful in management of chronic or temporary constipation.

Note: To prevent hard stools when laxative stimulation is not needed or undesirable, see Colace (stool softener).

WARNINGS

Do not use when abdominal pain, nausea, or vomiting are present. Frequent or prolonged use of this preparation may result in dependence on laxatives.

As with any drug, if you are pregnant or nursing a baby, seek the advice of a health professional before using this product.

SIDE EFFECTS

The incidence of side effects—none of a serious nature—is exceedingly small. Nausea, abdominal cramping or discomfort, diarrhea, and rash are the main side effects reported.

ADMINISTRATION AND DOSAGE

Adults —1 or 2 capsules, or 1 or 2 tablespoons syrup at bedtime, or as indicated. In severe cases, dosage may be increased to 2 capsules or 2 tablespoons twice daily, or 3 capsules at bedtime. *Children* —1 to 3 teaspoons of syrup at bedtime, or as indicated.

OVERDOSAGE

In addition to symptomatic treatment, gastric lavage, if timely, is recommended in cases of large overdosage.

HOW SUPPLIED

Peri-Colace® Capsules
  NDC 0087-0715-01 Bottles of 30
  NDC 0087-0715-02 Bottles of 60
  NDC 0087-0715-03 Bottles of 250
  NDC 0087-0715-05 Bottles of 1000
  NDC 0087-0715-07 Cartons of 100 single unit packs
Note: Peri-Colace capsules should be stored at controlled room temperatures (59°–86°F or 15°– 30°C).
Peri-Colace® Syrup
  NDC 0087-0721-01 Bottles of 8 fl oz
  NDC 0087-0721-02 Bottles of 16 fl oz
Shown in Product Identification Section, page 418

Medical Market Specialties Inc.
P.O. BOX 150
BOONTON, NJ 07005

PROGLYCEM®   ℞
[*pro-gli 'sem*]
brand of diazoxide
CAPSULES
SUSPENSION, USP
FOR ORAL ADMINISTRATION

DESCRIPTION

Diazoxide is 7-chloro-3-methyl-2H-1,2,4-benzothiadiazine 1,1-diazoxide. It is a white powder practically insoluble to sparingly soluble in water.

CLINICAL PHARMACOLOGY

Diazoxide administered orally produces a prompt dose-related increase in blood glucose level, due primarily to an inhibition of insulin release from the pancreas and also to an extrapancreatic effect. The hyperglycemic effect begins within an hour and generally lasts no more than eight hours in the presence of normal renal function.

PROGLYCEM decreases the excretion of sodium chloride and water resulting in fluid retention which may be clinically significant.

The hypotensive effect of diazoxide on blood pressure is usually not marked with the oral preparation.

Other pharmacologic actions of PROGLYCEM include increased pulse rate, increased serum uric acid levels due to decreased excretion, increased serum levels of free fatty acids, decreased para-aminohippuric acid (PAH) clearance with no appreciable effect on glomerular filtration rate.

PROGLYCEM-induced hyperglycemia is reversed by the administration of insulin or tolbutamide. The inhibition of insulin release by PROGLYCEM is antagonized by alpha-adrenergic blocking agents.

PROGLYCEM is extensively bound (more than 90%) to serum proteins, and is excreted in the kidneys. The plasma half-life 28 ± 8.3 hours. In four children aged four and six years, the plasma half-life varied from 9.5 to 24 hours. The half-life may be prolonged following overdosage, and in patients with impaired renal function.

INDICATIONS AND USAGE

PROGLYCEM (oral diazoxide) is useful in the management of hypoglycemia due to hyperinsulinism associated with the following conditions when surgery or other therapy is unsuccessful.

ADULTS: inoperable islet cell adenoma or carcinoma, or extrapancreatic malignancy.

INFANTS AND CHILDREN: leucine sensitivity, islet cell hyperplasia, nesidioblastosis, extrapancreatic malignancy, islet cell adenoma, or adenomatosis. PROGYLCEM may be used preoperatively as a temporary measure, and postoperatively, if hypoglycemia persists.

CONTRAINDICATIONS

The use of PROGLYCEM for functional hypoglycemia is contraindicated. The drug should not be used in patients hypersensitive to diazoxide or to other thiazides unless the potential benefits outweigh the possible risks.

WARNINGS

Diazoxide may lead to significant fluid retention which in patients with a compromised cardiac reserve, may precipitate congestive heart failure. The fluid retention will respond to conventional therapy with diuretics. It should be noted that concomitently administered thiazides may potentiate the hyperglycemic and hyperuricemic actions of diazoxide.

Ketoacidosis and nonketotic hyperosmolar coma have been reported in patients treated with recommended doses of PROGLYCEM usually during intercurrent illness. Prompt recognition and treatment are essential (see OVERDOSAGE), and prolonged surveillance following the acute episode is necessary because of the long drug half-life.

Transient cataracts occur in association with hyperosmolar coma in an infant, and subsided on correction of the hyperosmolarity. Cataracts have been observed in several animals receiving daily doses of intravenous or oral diazoxide.

The development of abnormal facial features in four children treated chronically (>4 years) with PROGLYCEM for hypoglycemia hyperinsulinism in the same clinic has been reported.

PRECAUTIONS

General: Treatment with PROGLYCEM should be initiated under close clinical supervision, with careful monitoring of blood glucose and clinical response until the patient's condition has stabilized. This usually requires several days. If not effective in two to three weeks, the drug should be discontinued.

Prolonged treatment requires regular monitoring of the urine for sugar and ketones, especially under stress conditions, with prompt reporting of any abnormalities to the physician. Additionally, blood sugar levels should be monitored periodically by the physician to determine the need or dose adjustment.

In some patients, higher blood levels have been observed with the oral suspension than with the capsule formulation of PROGLYCEM. Dosage should be adjusted as necessary in individual patients if changed from one formulation to the other.

The antihypertensive effect of other drugs may be enhanced by PROGLYCEM.

DRUG INTERACTIONS

Since diazoxide is highly bound to serum proteins, it may displace other substances which are also bound to protein, such as bilirubin or coumarin and its derivatives, resulting in higher blood levels of these substances. Concomitant administration of oral diazoxide and diphenylhydantoin may result in a loss of seizure control. The concomitant administration of thiazides or other commonly used diuretics may potentiate the hyperglycemic and other hyperglycemic effects of diazoxide.

Pregnancy Category C: Reproduction studies in rats and rabbits have revealed increased fetal resorptions and delayed parturition, as well as fetal skeletal and cardiac anomalies. The drug has also been demonstrated to cross the placental barrier in animals and to cause degeneration of the fetal pancreatic beta cells. Since there are no adequate data on fetal effects of this drug when given to pregnant women, safety in pregnancy has not been established. When the use of PROGLYCEM is considered, the indications should be limited to those specified for adults and the potential benefits to the mother must be weighed against possible harmful effects to the fetus.

Non-Teratogenic Effects: Diazoxide crosses the placental barrier and appears in cord blood. When given to the mother prior to delivery of the infant, the drug may produce fetal or neonatal hyperbilirubinemia, thrombocytopenia, altered carbohydrate metabolism or possibly other side effects that have occurred in adults. Alopecia and hypertrichosis lanuginosa have occurred in infants whose mothers received oral diazoxide during the last 19 to 60 days of pregnancy.

LABOR AND DELIVERY

Since intravenous administration of the drug during labor may cause cessation of uterine contractions, and administration of oxytocic agents may be required to reinstate labor, caution is advised in administering PROGLYCEM at that time.

ADVERSE REACTIONS

Frequent and Serious: Sodium and fluid retention is most common in young infants and in adults and may precipitate congestive heart failure in patients with compromised cardiac reserve. It usually responds to diuretic therapy. INFREQUENT AND SERIOUS: Diabetic ketoacidosis and hyperosmolar non-ketotic coma may develop very rapidly (see OVERDOSAGE and WARNING).

Other Frequent Adverse Reactions: Hirsutism of the lanugo type, mainly on the forehead, back and limbs subsides on discontinuation of the drug. HYPERGLYCEMIA OR GLYCOSURIA may require reduction in dosage in order to avoid progression towards ketoacidosis or hyperosmolar coma. GASTROINTESTINAL INTOLERANCE may include anorexia, nausea, vomiting, abdominal pain, illeus, diarrhea, transient loss of taste. Tachycardia, palpitations, increased levels of serum uric acid are common. THROMBOCYTOPENIA with or without purpura may require discontinuation of the drug. Neutropenia is transient, is not associated with increased susceptibility to infection, and ordinarily does not require discontinuation of the drug. Skin rash, headache, weakness, and malaise may also occur.

Other adverse reactions which have been observed are: CARDIOVASCULAR—hypotension and transient hypertension. Chest pain has been reported rarely. HEMATOLOGIC—eosinophilia, decreased hemoglobin/hemocrit, excessive bleeding, decreased IgG. HEPATO-RENAL—increased AST, alkaline phosphatase, azotemia, decreased creatinine clearance, reversible nephrotic syndrome, decreased urinary output, hematuria, albuminuria. NEUROLOGIC—anxiety, dizziness, insomnia, polyneuritis, paresthesia, pruritus, extrapyramidal signs. OPHTHALOMOLOGIC—transient cataracts, subconjunctival hemorrhage, ring scotoma, blurred vision, diplopia, lacrimation, SKELETAL, INTEGUMENTARY—monilial dermatitis, herpes, advance in bone-age, loss of scalp hair. SYSTEMIC—fever, lymphadenopathy. OTHER—gout, acute pancreatitis, pancreatic necrosis, galactorraga, enlargement of lump in breast.

OVERDOSAGE

An overdosage of PROGLYCEM causes marked hyperglycemia which may be associated with ketoacidosis. It will respond to prompt insulin administration and restoration of fluid and electrolyte balance. Because of the drug's long half-life (approximately 30 hours), the symptoms of overdosage require prolonged surveillance for periods of up to seven days, until the blood sugar level stabilizes with the normal range. Peritoneal dialysis and hemodialysis have lowered diazoxide blood levels in two patients.

DOSAGE AND ADMINISTRATION

The dosage of PROGLYCEM must be individualized based on the severity of the hypoglycemic condition and the blood glucose level and clinical response of the patient. The dosage should be adjusted until the desired clinical and laboratory effects are produced with the least amount of the drug. Special care should be taken to assure accuracy of dosage in infants and young children.

ADULTS AND CHILDREN: The usual daily dosage is 3 to 8 mg/kg, divided into two or three equal doses every 8 to 12 hours. In certain instances, patients with refractory hypoglycemia may require higher dosages.

INFANTS AND NEWBORNS: The usual daily dosage is 8 to 15 mg/kg, divided into two or three equal doses every 8 to 12 hours.

HOW SUPPLIED

PROGLYCEM Capsules, 50 mg, half opaque orange and half clear capsules, branded in black with MMS and either product identification letters, PBA, or numbers, 830, bottle of 100 (NDC #52891-830-05).

PROGLYCEM Suspension, 50 mg/ml, a chocolate-mint flavored suspension, bottle of 30 ml (NDC #52891-426-04), with dropper calibrated to deliver 10, 20, 30, 40, and 50 mg diazoxide. Shake well before each use: Protect from light. Store in carton until contents are used. Store PROGLYCEM Capsules and Suspension between 2° C and 30° C (36° and 86° F).

Medicone Company
225 VARICK ST.
NEW YORK, NY 10014

MEDICONE® DERMA Ointment

(See PDR For Nonprescription Drugs)

MEDICONE® DERMA-HC Ointment   ℞

COMPOSITION

Each gram contains:

Hydrocortisone acetate	10.0 mg.
Benzocaine	19.8 mg.
8-Hydroxyquinoline sulfate	10.4 mg.
Ephedrine hydrochloride	1.1 mg.
Menthol	4.8 mg.
Ichthammol	9.9 mg.
Zinc oxide	135.8 mg.
Petrolatum, Lanolin, perfume	q.s.

ACTION AND USES

Offers the advantage of quick, lasting comfort during treatment of severely inflamed dermatoses by affording prompt temporary local anesthetic action, inhibiting pain, burning, itching and controlling the scratch reflex. The hydrocortisone acetate reduces inflammation and swelling, aiding the normal healing process. The non-drying base will not disintegrate or liquefy at body temperature and is not washed off by exudate, perspiration or urine. Effectively suppresses inflammation, pain, swelling, burning and itching in contact dermatitis, eczematoid dermatitis, atopic dermatitis, neurodermatitis, seborrheic dermatitis, allergic dermatitis, rhus dermatitis, pruritus ani and pruritus vulvae.

ADMINISTRATION AND DOSAGE

Apply to affected area 2 to 4 times daily. When adequate improvement is noted, reduce frequency of application or continue maintenance control with regular Medicone Derma ointment.

PRECAUTIONS

Observe the usual adrenocorticosteroid precautions. Exercise care if the patient is on other corticosteroid therapy or if infection is present or if rash or irritation develops. Do not use in the eyes.

CONTRAINDICATIONS

Do not use in the presence of tuberculosis of the skin.

HOW SUPPLIED

7 gram and 20 gram tubes.
Shown in Product Identification Section, page 418

MEDICONE® DRESSING Cream

(See PDR For Nonprescription Drugs)

MEDICONE® Rectal Ointment

(See PDR For Nonprescription Drugs)

MEDICONE® Rectal Suppositories

(See PDR For Nonprescription Drugs)
Shown in Product Identification Section, page 418

MEDICONET®
(medicated rectal wipes)

(See PDR For Nonprescription Drugs)

Products are cross-indexed by
generic and chemical names
in the
YELLOW SECTION

Merck Sharp & Dohme
DIVISION OF MERCK & CO., INC.
WEST POINT, PA 19486
Product Identification Codes

To provide quick and positive identification of Merck Sharp & Dohme products, we have imprinted a code number on tablet and capsule products. In order that you may identify a product by its code number, we have compiled below a numerical list of code numbers with their corresponding product names. We are also listing the code numbers by alphabetical listing of products as a cross reference.
The code number as it appears on tablets and capsules bears the letters MSD plus the numerical code. Decadron® (Dexamethasone, MSD) tablets 0.25 mg is identified MSD 20.

Numerical Listing

MSD Code No.	Product	Product No.
14	Vasotec® (Enalapril Maleate, MSD) Tablets 2.5 mg	3411
19	Prinivil® (Lisinopril, MSD) Tablets 5 mg	3577
20	Decadron® (Dexamethasone, MSD) Tablets 0.25 mg	7592
21	Cogentin® (Benztropine Mesylate, MSD) Tablets 0.5 mg	3297
23	Elavil® (Amitriptyline HCl, MSD) Tablets 10 mg	3287
25	Indocin® (Indomethacin, MSD) Capsules 25 mg	3316
26	Vivactil® (Protriptyline HCl, MSD) Tablets 5 mg	3313
41	Decadron® (Dexamethasone, MSD) Tablets 0.5 mg	7598
42	HydroDIURIL® (Hydrochlorothiazide, MSD) Tablets 25 mg	3263
43	Mephyton® (Phytonadione, MSD) Tablets 5 mg	7776
45	Elavil® (Amitriptyline HCl, MSD) Tablets 25 mg	3288
47	Vivactil® (Protriptyline HCl, MSD) Tablets 10 mg	3314
49	Daranide® (Dichlorphenamide, MSD) Tablets 50 mg	3256
50	Indocin® (Indomethacin, MSD) Capsules 50 mg	3317
52	Inversine® (Mecamylamine HCl, MSD) Tablets 2.5 mg	3219
53	Hydropres® 25 (Reserpine-Hydrochlorothiazide, MSD) Tablets	3265
59	Blocadren® (Timolol Maleate, MSD) Tablets 5 mg	3343
60	Cogentin® (Benztropine Mesylate, MSD) Tablets 2 mg	3172
62	Periactin® (Cyproheptadine HCl, MSD) Tablets 4 mg	3276
63	Decadron® (Dexamethasone, MSD) Tablets 0.75 mg	7601
65	Edecrin® (Ethacrynic Acid, MSD) Tablets 25 mg	3321
67	Timolide® 10-25 (Timolol Maleate-Hydrochlorothiazide, MSD) Tablets	3373
90	Edecrin® (Ethacrynic Acid, MSD) Tablets 50 mg	3322
92	Midamor® (Amiloride HCl, MSD) Tablets 5 mg	3381
95	Decadron® (Dexamethasone, MSD) Tablets 1.5 mg	7638
97	Decadron® (Dexamethasone, MSD) Tablets 4 mg	7645
102	Elavil® (Amitriptyline HCl, MSD) Tablets 50 mg	3320
105	HydroDIURIL® (Hydrochlorothiazide, MSD) Tablets 50 mg	3264
106	Prinivil® (Lisinopril, MSD) Tablets 10 mg	3578
127	Hydropres® 50 (Reserpine-Hydrochlorothiazide, MSD) Tablets	3266
135	Aldomet® (Methyldopa, MSD) Tablets 125 mg	3341
136	Blocadren® (Timolol Maleate, MSD) Tablets 10 mg	3344
140	Prinzide® 12.5 (Lisinopril-Hydrochlorothiazide, MSD) Tablets	3594
142	Prinzide® 25 (Lisinopril-Hydrochlorothiazide, MSD) Tablets	3595
147	Decadron® (Dexamethasone, MSD) Tablets 6 mg	7648
150	Indocin® (Indomethacin, MSD) Suppositories 50 mg	3354

MSD Code No.	Product	Product No.
207	Prinivil® (Lisinopril, MSD) Tablets 20 mg	3579
214	Diuril® (Chlorothiazide, MSD) Tablets 250 mg	3244
219	Cortone® (Cortisone Acetate, MSD) Tablets 25 mg	7063
230	Diupres-250® (Reserpine-Chlorothiazide, MSD) Tablets	3261
237	Prinivil® (Lisinopril, MSD) Tablets 40 mg	3580
401	Aldomet® (Methyldopa, MSD) Tablets 250 mg	3290
403	Urecholine® (Bethanechol Chloride, MSD) Tablets 5 mg	7785
405	Diupres-500® (Reserpine-Chlorothiazide, MSD) Tablets	3262
410	HydroDIURIL® (Hydrochlorothiazide, MSD) Tablets 100 mg	3340
412	Urecholine® (Bethanechol Chloride, MSD) Tablets 10 mg	7787
423	Aldoril® 15 (Methyldopa-Hydrochlorothiazide, MSD) Tablets	3294
430	Elavil® (Amitriptyline HCl, MSD) Tablets 75 mg	3348
432	Diuril® (Chlorothiazide, MSD) Tablets 500 mg	3245
435	Elavil® (Amitriptyline HCl, MSD) Tablets 100 mg	3349
437	Blocadren® (Timolol Maleate, MSD) Tablets 20 mg	3371
456	Aldoril® 25 (Methyldopa-Hydrochlorothiazide, MSD) Tablets	3295
457	Urecholine® (Bethanechol Chloride, MSD) Tablets 25 mg	7788
460	Urecholine® (Bethanechol Chloride, MSD) Tablets 50 mg	7790
501	Benemid® (Probenecid, MSD) Tablets 0.5 g	3337
516	Aldomet® (Methyldopa, MSD) Tablets 500 mg	3292
517	Triavil® 4-50 (Perphenazine-Amitriptyline HCl, MSD) Tablets	3364
602	Cuprimine® (Penicillamine, MSD) Capsules 250 mg	3299
612	Aldoclor® 150 (Methyldopa-Chlorothiazide, MSD) Tablets	3318
614	ColBENEMID® (Probenecid-Colchicine, MSD) Tablets	3283
619	Hydrocortone® (Hydrocortisone, MSD) Tablets 10 mg	7604
625	Hydrocortone® (Hydrocortisone, MSD) Tablets 20 mg	7602
634	Aldoclor® 250 (Methyldopa-Chlorothiazide, MSD) Tablets	3319
635	Cogentin® (Benztropine Mesylate, MSD) Tablets 1 mg	3334
647	Sinemet® 10-100 (Carbidopa-Levodopa, MSD) Tablets	3346
650	Sinemet® 25-100 (Carbidopa-Levodopa, MSD) Tablets	3365
654	Sinemet® 25-250 (Carbidopa-Levodopa, MSD) Tablets	3347
672	Cuprimine® (Penicillamine, MSD) Capsules 125 mg	3350
673	Elavil® (Amitriptyline HCl, MSD) Tablets 150 mg	3351
675	Dolobid® (Diflunisal, MSD) Tablets 250 mg	3390
679	Cuprid® (Trientine Hydrochloride, MSD) Capsules 250 mg	3511
690	Demser® (Metyrosine, MSD) Capsules 250 mg	3355
693	Indocin® SR (Indomethacin, MSD) 75 mg, Sustained Release, Capsules	3370
694	Aldoril® D30 (Methyldopa-Hydrochlorothiazide, MSD) Tablets	3362
697	Dolobid® (Diflunisal, MSD) Tablets 500 mg	3392
705	Noroxin® (Norfloxacin, MSD) Tablets 400 mg	3522
707	Tonocard® (Tocainide HCl, MSD) Tablets 400 mg	3409
709	Tonocard® (Tocainide HCl, MSD) Tablets 600 mg	3410
712	Vasotec® (Enalapril Maleate, MSD) Tablets 5 mg	3412
713	Vasotec® (Enalapril Maleate, MSD) Tablets 10 mg	3413
714	Vasotec® (Enalapril Maleate, MSD) Tablets 20 mg	3414
720	Vaseretic® 10–25 (Enalapril Maleate-Hydrochlorothiazide, MSD) Tablets	3418

MSD Code No.	Product	Product No.
731	Mevacor® (Lovastatin, MSD) Tablets 20 mg	3561
732	Mevacor® (Lovastatin, MSD) Tablets 40 mg	3562
907	Mintezol® (Thiabendazole, MSD) Chewable Tablets 500 mg	3332
914	Triavil® 2-10 (Perphenazine-Amitriptyline HCl, MSD) Tablets	3328
917	Moduretic® (Amiloride HCl-Hydrochlorothiazide, MSD) Tablets	3385
921	Triavil® 2-25 (Perphenazine-Amitriptyline HCl, MSD) Tablets	3311
931	Flexeril® (Cyclobenzaprine HCl, MSD) Tablets 10 mg	3358
934	Triavil® 4-10 (Perphenazine-Amitriptyline HCl, MSD) Tablets	3310
935	Aldoril® D50 (Methyldopa-Hydrochlorothiazide, MSD) Tablets	3363
941	Clinoril® (Sulindac, MSD) Tablets 150 mg	3360
942	Clinoril® (Sulindac, MSD) Tablets 200 mg	3353
946	Triavil® 4-25 (Perphenazine-Amitriptyline HCl, MSD) Tablets	3312
963	Pepcid® (Famotidine, MSD) Tablets 20 mg	3535
964	Pepcid® (Famotidine, MSD) Tablets 40 mg	3536

Alphabetical Listing

MSD Code No.	Product	Product No.
612	Aldoclor® 150 (Methyldopa-Chlorothiazide, MSD) Tablets	3318
634	Aldoclor® 250 (Methyldopa-Chlorothiazide, MSD) Tablets	3319
135	Aldomet® (Methyldopa, MSD) Tablets 125 mg	3341
401	Aldomet® (Methyldopa, MSD) Tablets 250 mg	3290
516	Aldomet® (Methyldopa, MSD) Tablets 500 mg	3292
423	Aldoril® 15 (Methyldopa-Hydrochlorothiazide, MSD) Tablets	3294
456	Aldoril® 25 (Methyldopa-Hydrochlorothiazide, MSD) Tablets	3295
694	Aldoril® D30 (Methyldopa-Hydrochlorothiazide, MSD) Tablets	3362
935	Aldoril® D50 (Methyldopa-Hydrochlorothiazide, MSD) Tablets	3363
501	Benemid® (Probenecid, MSD) Tablets 0.5 g	3337
59	Blocadren® (Timolol Maleate, MSD) Tablets 5 mg	3343
136	Blocadren® (Timolol Maleate, MSD) Tablets 10 mg	3344
437	Blocadren® (Timolol Maleate, MSD) Tablets 20 mg	3371
941	Clinoril® (Sulindac, MSD) Tablets 150 mg	3360
942	Clinoril® (Sulindac, MSD) Tablets 200 mg	3353
21	Cogentin® (Benztropine Mesylate, MSD) Tablets 0.5 mg	3297
635	Cogentin® (Benztropine Mesylate, MSD) Tablets 1 mg	3334
60	Cogentin® (Benztropine Mesylate, MSD) Tablets 2 mg	3172
614	ColBENEMID® (Probenecid-Colchicine, MSD) Tablets	3283
219	Cortone® (Cortisone Acetate, MSD) Tablets 25 mg	7063
679	Cuprid® (Trientine Hydrochloride, MSD) Capsules 250 mg	3511
672	Cuprimine® (Penicillamine, MSD) Capsules 125 mg	3350
602	Cuprimine® (Penicillamine, MSD) Capsules 250 mg	3299
49	Daranide® (Dichlorphenamide, MSD) Tablets 50 mg	3256
20	Decadron® (Dexamethasone, MSD) Tablets 0.25 mg	7592
41	Decadron® (Dexamethasone, MSD) Tablets 0.5 mg	7598
63	Decadron® (Dexamethasone, MSD) Tablets 0.75 mg	7601
95	Decadron® (Dexamethasone, MSD) Tablets 1.5 mg	7638

ALDOCLOR® Tablets ℞
(Methyldopa-Chlorothiazide, MSD), U.S.P.

WARNING

This fixed combination drug is not indicated for initial therapy of hypertension. Hypertension requires therapy titrated to the individual patient. If the fixed combination represents the dosage so determined, its use may be more convenient in patient management. The treatment of hypertension is not static, but must be re-evaluated as conditions in each patient warrant.

DESCRIPTION

ALDOCLOR® (Methyldopa-Chlorothiazide, MSD) combines two antihypertensives: methyldopa and chlorothiazide.

Methyldopa

Methyldopa is an antihypertensive and is the *L* - isomer of alpha-methyldopa. It is levo-3-(3,4-dihydroxyphenyl)2-methylalanine. Its empirical formula is $C_{10}H_{13}NO_4$, with a molecular weight of 211.22, and its structural formula is:

HO—⬡—CH_2—$\overset{CH_3}{\underset{NH_2}{C}}$—$CO_2H$ (HO—)

Methyldopa is a white to yellowish white, odorless fine powder, and is soluble in water.

Chlorothiazide

Chlorothiazide is a diuretic and antihypertensive. It is 6-chloro-2H-1, 2, 4-benzothiadiazine-7-sulfonamide 1, 1-dioxide. Its empirical formula is $C_7H_6ClN_3O_4S_2$ and its structural formula is:

[structural formula of chlorothiazide with NH_2SO_2 and Cl substituents]

It is a white, or practically white crystalline powder with a molecular weight of 295.72, which is very slightly soluble in water, but readily soluble in dilute aqueous sodium hydroxide. It is soluble in urine to the extent of about 150 mg per 100 mL at pH 7.

ALDOCLOR is supplied as tablets in two strengths for oral use:

ALDOCLOR 150, contains 250 mg of methyldopa and 150 mg of chlorothiazide.

ALDOCLOR 250, contains 250 mg of methyldopa and 250 mg of chlorothiazide.

Each tablet contains the following inactive ingredients: calcium disodium edetate, cellulose, citric acid, D&C Yellow 10, ethylcellulose, FD&C Yellow 6, gelatin, glycerin, guar gum, hydroxypropyl methylcellulose, magnesium stearate, starch, talc, and titanium dioxide. ALDOCLOR 150 also contains iron oxides. ALDOCLOR 250 also contains FD&C Blue 2.

CLINICAL PHARMACOLOGY

Methyldopa

Methyldopa is an aromatic-amino-acid decarboxylase inhibitor in animals and in man. Although the mechanism of action has yet to be conclusively demonstrated, the antihypertensive effect of methyldopa probably is due to its metabolism to alpha-methylnorepinephrine, which then lowers arterial pressure by stimulation of central inhibitory alpha-adrenergic receptors, false neurotransmission, and/or reduction of plasma renin activity. Methyldopa has been shown to cause a net reduction in the tissue concentration of serotonin, dopamine, norepinephrine, and epinephrine.

Only methyldopa, the *L*-isomer of alpha-methyldopa, has the ability to inhibit dopa decarboxylase and to deplete animal tissues of norepinephrine. In man, the antihypertensive activity appears to be due solely to the *L*-isomer. About twice the dose of the racemate (*DL*-alpha-methyldopa) is required for equal antihypertensive effect.

Methyldopa has no direct effect on cardiac function and usually does not reduce glomerular filtration rate, renal blood flow, or filtration fraction. Cardiac output usually is maintained without cardiac acceleration. In some patients the heart rate is slowed.

Normal or elevated plasma renin activity may decrease in the course of methyldopa therapy.

Methyldopa reduces both supine and standing blood pressure. It usually produces highly effective lowering of the supine pressure with infrequent symptomatic postural hypotension. Exercise hypotension and diurnal blood pressure variations rarely occur.

Chlorothiazide

The mechanism of the antihypertensive effect of thiazides is unknown. Chlorothiazide does not usually affect normal blood pressure.

Chlorothiazide affects the distal renal tubular mechanism of electrolyte reabsorption. At maximal therapeutic dosage all thiazides are approximately equal in their diuretic efficacy. Chlorothiazide increases excretion of sodium and chloride in approximately equivalent amounts. Natriuresis may be accompanied by some loss of potassium and bicarbonate.

After oral use diuresis begins within 2 hours, peaks in about 4 hours and lasts about 6 to 12 hours.

Methyldopa-Chlorothiazide

The concomitant use of methyldopa and chlorothiazide, as provided in ALDOCLOR, frequently produces a more pronounced antihypertensive response than when either compound is the sole therapeutic agent. Particularly in those cases of hypertensive vascular disease where sodium and water retention is a problem, the coadministration of these two drugs in the form of ALDOCLOR will help control the fluid imbalance.

In severe essential hypertension and in malignant hypertension, ALDOCLOR may achieve effective lowering of blood pressure with fewer side effects than occur with other compounds used for this purpose.

ALDOCLOR reduces both supine and standing blood pressure; more effective lowering of the supine pressure with less frequent symptomatic postural hypotension can be obtained with ALDOCLOR than with most other antihypertensive agents. In patients treated with ALDOCLOR, exercise hypotension and diurnal blood pressure variations rarely occur.

Pharmacokinetics and Metabolism

Methyldopa

The maximum decrease in blood pressure occurs four to six hours after oral dosage. Once an effective dosage level is attained, a smooth blood pressure response occurs in most patients in 12 to 24 hours. After withdrawal, blood pressure usually returns to pretreatment levels within 24–48 hours. Methyldopa is extensively metabolized. The known urinary metabolites are: α-methyldopa mono-0-sulfate; 3-0 methyl-α-methyldopa; 3,4,-dihydroxyphenylacetone; α-methyldopamine; 3-0-methyl-α-methyldopamine and their conjugates.

Continued on next page

Information on the Merck Sharp & Dohme products listed on these pages is the full prescribing information from product circulars in use August 31, 1989.

Merck Sharp & Dohme—Cont.

Approximately 70 percent of the drug which is absorbed is excreted in the urine as methyldopa and its mono-0-sulfate conjugate. The renal clearance is about 130 mL/min in normal subjects and is diminished in renal insufficiency. The plasma half-life of methyldopa is 105 minutes. After oral doses, excretion is essentially complete in 36 hours. Methyldopa crosses the placental barrier, appears in cord blood, and appears in breast milk.

Chlorothiazide
Chlorothiazide is not metabolized but is eliminated rapidly by the kidney. The plasma half-life is 45–120 minutes. After oral doses, 20–24 percent of the dose is excreted unchanged in the urine. Chlorothiazide crosses the placental but not the blood-brain barrier and is excreted in breast milk.

INDICATION AND USAGE

Hypertension (see box warning).
Use in Pregnancy. Routine use of diuretics during normal pregnancy is inappropriate and exposes mother and fetus to unnecessary hazard. Diuretics do not prevent development of toxemia of pregnancy and there is no satisfactory evidence that they are useful in the treatment of toxemia.
Edema during pregnancy may arise from pathologic causes or from the physiologic and mechanical consequences of pregnancy. Thiazides are indicated in pregnancy when edema is due to pathologic causes, just as they are in the absence of pregnancy (see PRECAUTIONS, *Pregnancy*). Dependent edema in pregnancy, resulting from restriction of venous return by the gravid uterus, is properly treated through elevation of the lower extremities and use of support stockings. Use of diuretics to lower intravascular volume in this instance is illogical and unnecessary. During normal pregnancy there is hypervolemia which is not harmful to the fetus or the mother in the absence of cardiovascular disease. However, it may be associated with edema, rarely generalized edema. If such edema causes discomfort, increased recumbency will often provide relief. Rarely this edema may cause extreme discomfort which is not relieved by rest. In these instances, a short course of diuretic therapy, may provide relief and be appropriate.

CONTRAINDICATIONS

Active hepatic disease, such as acute hepatitis and active cirrhosis.
If previous methyldopa therapy has been associated with liver disorders (see WARNINGS).
Anuria.
Hypersensitivity to methyldopa, or to chlorothiazide or other sulfonamide-derived drugs.

WARNINGS

Methyldopa
It is important to recognize that a positive Coombs test, hemolytic anemia, and liver disorders may occur with methyldopa therapy. The rare occurrences of hemolytic anemia or liver disorders could lead to potentially fatal complications unless properly recognized and managed. Read this section carefully to understand these reactions.
With prolonged methyldopa therapy, 10 to 20 percent of patients develop a positive direct Coombs test which usually occurs between 6 and 12 months of methyldopa therapy. Lowest incidence is at daily dosage of 1 g or less. This on rare occasions may be associated with hemolytic anemia, which could lead to potentially fatal complications. One cannot predict which patients with a positive direct Coombs test may develop hemolytic anemia.
Prior existence or development of a positive direct Coombs test is not in itself a contraindication to use of methyldopa. If a positive Coombs test develops during methyldopa therapy, the physician should determine whether hemolytic anemia exists and whether the positive Coombs test may be a problem. For example, in addition to a positive direct Coombs test there is less often a positive indirect Coombs test which may interfere with cross matching of blood.
Before treatment is started, it is desirable to do a blood count (hematocrit, hemoglobin, or red cell count) for a baseline or to establish whether there is anemia. Periodic blood counts should be done during therapy to detect hemolytic anemia. It may be useful to do a direct Coombs test before therapy and at 6 and 12 months after the start of therapy.
If Coombs-positive hemolytic anemia occurs, the cause may be methyldopa and the drug should be discontinued. Usually the anemia remits promptly. If not, corticosteroids may be given and other causes of anemia should be considered. If the hemolytic anemia is related to methyldopa, the drug should not be reinstituted.
When methyldopa causes Coombs positivity alone or with hemolytic anemia, the red cell is usually coated with gamma globulin of the IgG (gamma G) class only. The positive

Coombs test may not revert to normal until weeks to months after methyldopa is stopped.
Should the need for transfusion arise in a patient receiving methyldopa, both a direct and an indirect Coombs test should be performed. In the absence of hemolytic anemia, usually only the direct Coombs test will be positive. A positive direct Coombs test alone will not interfere with typing or cross matching. If the indirect Coombs test is also positive, problems may arise in the major cross match and the assistance of a hematologist or transfusion expert will be needed.
Occasionally, fever has occurred within the first three weeks of methyldopa therapy, associated in some cases with eosinophilia or abnormalities in one or more liver function tests, such as serum alkaline phosphatase, serum transaminases (SGOT, SGPT), bilirubin, and prothrombin time. Jaundice, with or without fever, may occur with onset usually within the first two to three months of therapy. In some patients the findings are consistent with those of cholestasis. In others the findings are consistent with hepatitis and hepatocellular injury.
Rarely fatal hepatic necrosis has been reported after use of methyldopa. These hepatic changes may represent hypersensitivity reactions. Periodic determination of hepatic function should be done particularly during the first 6 to 12 weeks of therapy or whenever an unexplained fever occurs. If fever, abnormalities in liver function tests, or jaundice appear, stop therapy with methyldopa. If caused by methyldopa, the temperature and abnormalities in liver function characteristically have reverted to normal when the drug was discontinued. Methyldopa should not be reinstituted in such patients.
Rarely, a reversible reduction of the white blood cell count with a primary effect on the granulocytes has been seen. The granulocyte count returned promptly to normal on discontinuance of the drug. Rare cases of granulocytopenia have been reported. In each instance, upon stopping the drug, the white cell count returned to normal. Reversible thrombocytopenia has occurred rarely.

Chlorothiazide
Use with caution in severe renal disease. In patients with renal disease, thiazides may precipitate azotemia. Cumulative effects of the drug may develop in patients with impaired renal function.
Thiazides should be used with caution in patients with impaired hepatic function or progressive liver disease, since minor alterations of fluid and electrolyte balance may precipitate hepatic coma.
Thiazides may add to or potentiate the action of other antihypertensive drugs.
Sensitivity reactions may occur in patients with or without a history of allergy or bronchial asthma.
The possibility of exacerbation or activation of systemic lupus erythematosus has been reported.
Lithium generally should not be given with diuretics (see PRECAUTIONS, *Drug Interactions*).

PRECAUTIONS

General
Methyldopa
Methyldopa should be used with caution in patients with a history of previous liver disease or dysfunction (see WARNINGS).
Some patients taking methyldopa experience clinical edema or weight gain which may be controlled by use of a diuretic. Methyldopa should not be continued if edema progresses or signs of heart failure appear.
Hypertension has recurred occasionally after dialysis in patients given methyldopa because the drug is removed by this procedure.
Rarely involuntary choreoathetotic movements have been observed during therapy with methyldopa in patients with severe bilateral cerebrovascular disease. Should these movements occur, stop therapy.
Chlorothiazide
All patients receiving diuretic therapy should be observed for evidence of fluid or electrolyte imbalance: namely, hyponatremia, hypochloremic alkalosis, and hypokalemia. Serum and urine electrolyte determinations are particularly important when the patient is vomiting excessively or receiving parenteral fluids. Warning signs or symptoms of fluid and electrolyte imbalance, irrespective of cause include dryness of mouth, thirst, weakness, lethargy, drowsiness, restlessness, muscle pains or cramps, muscular fatigue, hypotension, oliguria, tachycardia, and gastrointestinal disturbances such as nausea and vomiting.
Hypokalemia may develop, especially with brisk diuresis, when severe cirrhosis is present, or after prolonged therapy. Interference with adequate oral electrolyte intake will also contribute to hypokalemia. Hypokalemia may cause cardiac arrhythmia and may also sensitize or exaggerate the response of the heart to the toxic effects of digitalis (e.g., increased ventricular irritability). Hypokalemia may be avoided or treated by use of potassium sparing diuretics or

potassium supplements such as foods with a high potassium content.
Although any chloride deficit is generally mild and usually does not require specific treatment except under extraordinary circumstances (as in liver disease or renal disease), chloride replacement may be required in the treatment of metabolic alkalosis.
Dilutional hyponatremia may occur in edematous patients in hot weather; appropriate therapy is water restriction, rather than administration of salt, except in rare instances when the hyponatremia is life threatening. In actual salt depletion, appropriate replacement is the therapy of choice. Hyperuricemia may occur or acute gout may be precipitated in certain patients receiving thiazides.
In diabetic patients dosage adjustments of insulin or oral hypoglycemic agents may be required. Hyperglycemia may occur with thiazide diuretics. Thus latent diabetes mellitus may become manifest during thiazide therapy.
The antihypertensive effects of the drug may be enhanced in the postsympathectomy patient.
If progressive renal impairment becomes evident, consider withholding or discontinuing diuretic therapy.
Thiazides have been shown to increase the urinary excretion of magnesium; this may result in hypomagnesemia.
Thiazides may decrease urinary calcium excretion. Thiazides may cause intermittent and slight elevation of serum calcium in the absence of known disorders of calcium metabolism. Marked hypercalcemia may be evidence of hidden hyperparathyroidism. Thiazides should be discontinued before carrying out tests for parathyroid function.
Increases in cholesterol and triglyceride levels may be associated with thiazide diuretic therapy.

Laboratory Tests
Methyldopa
Blood count, Coombs test and liver function tests are recommended before initiating therapy and at periodic intervals (see WARNINGS).
Chlorothiazide
Periodic determination of serum electrolytes to detect possible electrolyte imbalance should be done at appropriate intervals.

Drug Interactions
Methyldopa
When methyldopa is used with other antihypertensive drugs, potentiation of antihypertensive effect may occur. Patients should be followed carefully to detect side reactions or unusual manifestations of drug idiosyncrasy.
Patients may require reduced doses of anesthetics when on methyldopa. If hypotension does occur during anesthesia, it usually can be controlled by vasopressors. The adrenergic receptors remain sensitive during treatment with methyldopa.
Chlorothiazide
When given concurrently the following drugs may interact with thiazide diuretics.
Alcohol, barbiturates, or narcotics —potentiation of orthostatic hypotension may occur.
Antidiabetic drugs (oral agents and insulin)—dosage adjustment of the antidiabetic drug may be required.
Other antihypertensive drugs —additive effect or potentiation.
Corticosteroids, ACTH —intensified electrolyte depletion, particularly hypokalemia.
Pressor amines (e.g., norepinephrine) —possible decreased response to pressor amines but not sufficient to preclude their use.
Skeletal muscle relaxants, nondepolarizing (e.g., tubocurarine) —possible increased responsiveness to the muscle relaxant.
Lithium —generally should not be given with diuretics. Diuretic agents reduce the renal clearance of lithium and add a high risk of lithium toxicity. Refer to the package insert for lithium preparations before use of such preparations with ALDOCLOR.
Non-steroidal Anti-inflammatory Drugs —In some patients, the administration of a non-steroidal anti-inflammatory agent can reduce the diuretic, natriuretic, and antihypertensive effects of loop, potassium-sparing and thiazide diuretics. Therefore, when ALDOCLOR and non-steroidal anti-inflammatory agents are used concomitantly, the patient should be observed closely to determine if the desired effect of the diuretic is obtained.

Drug/Laboratory Test Interactions
Methyldopa
Methyldopa may interfere with measurement of: urinary uric acid by the phosphotungstate method, serum creatinine by the alkaline picrate method, and SGOT by colorimetric methods. Interference with spectrophotometric methods for SGOT analysis has not been reported.
Since methyldopa causes fluorescence in urine samples at the same wave lengths as catecholamines, falsely high levels of urinary catecholamines may be reported. This will interfere with the diagnosis of pheochromocytoma. It is important to recognize this phenomenon before a patient with a possible pheochromocytoma is subjected to surgery. Methyldopa does not interfere with measurement of VMA (vanillylman-

delic acid), a test for pheochromocytoma, by those methods which convert VMA to vanillin. Methyldopa is not recommended for the treatment of patients with pheochromocytoma. Rarely, when urine is exposed to air after voiding, it may darken because of breakdown of methyldopa or its metabolites.

Chlorothiazide
Thiazides should be discontinued before carrying out tests for parathyroid function (see PRECAUTIONS, *General*).

Carcinogenesis, Mutagenesis, Impairment of Fertility
Long-term studies in animals have not been performed to evaluate the effects upon fertility, mutagenic or carcinogenic potential of the combination.

Methyldopa
Methyldopa is currently under study in the U.S. Carcinogenesis Testing Program.

Methyldopa did not have mutagenic activity *in vitro* in the Ames microbial mutagen test with or without metabolic activation.

Methyldopa given in a two-litter study in rats at approximately three to six times the usual daily dose did not impair fertility.

Chlorothiazide
Carcinogenic studies have not been done with chlorothiazide.

Chlorothiazide was not mutagenic *in vitro* in the Ames microbial test at a maximum concentration of 5 mg/plate using Strains TA98 and TA100. Chlorothiazide did not produce any significant mutagenicity in the dominant lethal assay in the mouse after 8 oral doses of 50 mg/kg or single intraperitoneal doses of 525 or 644 mg/kg, although early fetal deaths and preimplantation losses were increased beyond control values. In a test using *Aspergillus nidulans,* chlorothiazide was negative and did not induce disjunction.

Chlorothiazide had no effect on fertility in a two-litter study in rats at doses up to 60 mg/kg/day (2 times the maximum recommended human dose).

Pregnancy
Teratogenic Effects—Pregnancy Category B: Reproduction studies in the rat, at doses up to 40 mg/kg/day (3–4 times the maximum recommended human dose), did not impair fertility or cause abnormalities of the fetus due to ALDOCLOR. There are no adequate and well-controlled studies with ALDOCLOR in pregnant women. Because animal reproduction studies are not always predictive of human response, this drug should be used during pregnancy only if clearly needed. (See INDICATIONS AND USAGE)

Chlorothiazide: Thiazides cross the placental barrier and appear in cord blood.

Reproduction studies in the rabbit, the mouse and the rat at doses up to 500 mg/kg/day (25 times the maximum recommended human dose) showed no evidence of external abnormalities of the fetus due to chlorothiazide. Chlorothiazide given in a two-litter study in rats at doses up to 60 mg/kg/day (2 times the maximum recommended human dose) did not impair fertility or produce birth abnormalities in the offspring.

Methyldopa: Reproduction studies have been performed in the rabbit, the mouse, and the rat at doses up to 1000 mg/kg/day (16.6 times the maximum recommended human dose) and have revealed no evidence of impaired fertility or harm to the fetus due to methyldopa. There are, however, no adequate and well-controlled studies in pregnant women in the first trimester of pregnancy. Because animal reproduction studies are not always predictive of human response, methyldopa should be used during pregnancy only if clearly needed.

Published reports of the use of methyldopa during all trimesters indicate that if this drug is used during pregnancy the possibility of fetal harm appears remote. In five studies, three of which were controlled, involving 332 pregnant hypertensive women, treatment with methyldopa was associated with an improved fetal outcome. The majority of these women were in the third trimester when methyldopa therapy was begun.

In one study, women who had begun methyldopa treatment between weeks 16 and 20 of pregnancy gave birth to infants whose average head circumference was reduced by a small amount (34.2 ± 1.7 cm vs. 34.6 ± 1.3 cm [mean ± 1 S.D.]). Long-term follow up of 195 (97.5%) of the children born to methyldopa-treated pregnant women (including those who began treatment between weeks 16 and 20) failed to uncover any significant adverse effect on the children. At four years of age, the developmental delay commonly seen in children born to hypertensive mothers was less evident in those whose mothers were treated with methyldopa during pregnancy than those whose mothers were untreated. The children of the treated group scored consistently higher than the children of the untreated group on five major indices of intellectual and motor development. At age seven and one-half developmental scores and intelligence indices showed no significant differences in children of treated or untreated hypertensive women.

Nonteratogenic Effects: These may include fetal or neonatal jaundice, thrombocytopenia, and possibly other adverse reactions which have occurred in the adult.

Nursing Mothers
Methyldopa and thiazides appear in breast milk. Therefore, because of the potential for serious adverse reactions in nursing infants from chlorothiazide, a decision should be made whether to discontinue nursing or to discontinue the drug, taking into account the importance of the drug to the mother.

Pediatric Use
Safety and effectiveness of ALDOCLOR in children has not been established.

ADVERSE REACTIONS

The following adverse reactions have been reported and, within each category, are listed in order of decreasing severity.

Methyldopa
Sedation, usually transient, may occur during the initial period of therapy or whenever the dose is increased. Headache, asthenia, or weakness may be noted as early and transient symptoms. However, significant adverse effects due to methyldopa have been infrequent and this agent usually is well tolerated.

Cardiovascular: Aggravation of angina pectoris, congestive heart failure, prolonged carotid sinus hypersensitivity, orthostatic hypotension (decrease daily dosage), edema or weight gain, bradycardia.

Digestive: Pancreatitis, colitis, vomiting, diarrhea, sialadenitis, sore or "black" tongue, nausea, constipation, distension, flatus, dryness of mouth.

Endocrine: Hyperprolactinemia.

Hematologic: Bone marrow depression, leukopenia, granulocytopenia, thrombocytopenia, hemolytic anemia; positive tests for antinuclear antibody, LE cells, and rheumatoid factor, positive Coombs test.

Hepatic: Liver disorders including hepatitis, jaundice, abnormal liver function tests (see WARNINGS).

Hypersensitivity: Myocarditis, pericarditis, lupus-like syndrome, drug-related fever.

Nervous System/Psychiatric: Parkinsonism, Bell's palsy, decreased mental acuity, involuntary choreoathetotic movements, symptoms of cerebrovascular insufficiency, psychic disturbances including nightmares and reversible mild psychoses or depression, headache, sedation, asthenia or weakness, dizziness, lightheadedness, paresthesias.

Metabolic: Rise in BUN.

Musculoskeletal: Arthralgia, with or without joint swelling; myalgia.

Respiratory: Nasal stuffiness.

Skin: Toxic epidermal necrolysis, rash.

Urogenital: Amenorrhea, breast enlargement, gynecomastia, lactation, impotence, decreased libido.

Chlorothiazide
Body as a Whole: Weakness.

Cardiovascular: Hypotension including orthostatic hypotension (may be aggravated by alcohol, barbiturates, narcotics or antihypertensive drugs).

Digestive: Pancreatitis, jaundice (intrahepatic cholestatic jaundice), diarrhea, vomiting, sialadenitis, cramping, constipation, gastric irritation, nausea, anorexia.

Hematologic: Aplastic anemia, agranulocytosis, leukopenia, hemolytic anemia, thrombocytopenia.

Hypersensitivity: Anaphylactic reactions, necrotizing angiitis (vasculitis and cutaneous vasculitis), respiratory distress including pneumonitis and pulmonary edema, photosensitivity, fever, urticaria, rash, purpura.

Metabolic: Electrolyte imbalance (see PRECAUTIONS), hyperglycemia, glycosuria, hyperuricemia.

Musculoskeletal: Muscle spasm.

Nervous System/Psychiatric: Vertigo, paresthesias, dizziness, headache, restlessness.

Renal: Renal failure, renal dysfunction, interstitial nephritis. (See WARNINGS.)

Special Senses: Transient blurred vision, xanthopsia.

Whenever adverse reactions are moderate or severe, thiazide dosage should be reduced or therapy withdrawn.

OVERDOSAGE

Acute overdosage may produce acute hypotension with other responses attributable to brain and gastrointestinal malfunction (excessive sedation, weakness, bradycardia, dizziness, lightheadedness, constipation, distention, flatus, diarrhea, nausea, vomiting).

In the event of overdosage, symptomatic and supportive measures should be employed. When ingestion is recent, gastric lavage or emesis may reduce absorption. When ingestion has been earlier, infusions may be helpful to promote urinary excretion. Otherwise, management includes special attention to cardiac rate and output, blood volume, electrolyte imbalance, paralytic ileus, urinary function and cerebral activity.

Sympathomimetic drugs [e.g., levarterenol, epinephrine, ARAMINE® (Metaraminol Bitartrate, MSD)] may be indicated. Methyldopa is dialyzable.

The oral LD_{50} of methyldopa is greater than 1.5 g/kg in both the mouse and the rat. The oral LD_{50} of chlorothiazide is 8.5 g/kg, greater than 10 g/kg, and greater than 1 g/kg in the mouse, rat, and dog respectively.

DOSAGE AND ADMINISTRATION

Dosage: As determined by individual titration (see box warning).

The usual starting dosage is 1 tablet of ALDOCLOR 150 or 1 tablet of ALDOCLOR 250 two or three times a day in the first 48 hours. The daily dosage then may be increased or decreased, preferably at intervals of not less than two days, until an adequate response is achieved. To minimize the sedation associated with methyldopa, start dosage increases in the evening. By adjustment of dosage, morning hypotension may be prevented without sacrificing control of afternoon blood pressure.

When ALDOCLOR is given to patients on other antihypertensives, the dose of these agents many need to be adjusted to effect a smooth transition. When ALDOCLOR is given with antihypertensives other than thiazides, the initial dosage of methyldopa should be limited to 500 mg daily in divided doses.

Although occasional patients have responded to higher doses, the maximum recommended daily dosage is 3.0 g of methyldopa and 1.0 to 2.0 g of chlorothiazide. Once an effective dosage range is attained, a smooth blood pressure response occurs in most patients in 12 to 24 hours. If ALDOCLOR alone does not adequately control blood pressure, additional methyldopa may be given separately to obtain the maximum blood pressure response.

Since both components of ALDOCLOR have a relatively short duration of action, withdrawal is followed by return of hypertension usually within 48 hours. This is not complicated by an overshoot of blood pressure.

Occasionally tolerance may occur, usually between the second and third month of therapy. Increasing the dosage of either methyldopa or chlorothiazide separately or together frequently will restore effective control of blood pressure. Methyldopa is largely excreted by the kidney and patients with impaired renal function may respond to smaller doses of ALDOCLOR. Syncope in older patients may be related to an increased sensitivity and advanced arteriosclerotic vascular disease. This may be avoided by lower doses.

HOW SUPPLIED

No. 3318—Tablets ALDOCLOR 150 are beige, oval, film coated tablets coded MSD 612. Each tablet contains 250 mg of methyldopa and 150 mg of chlorothiazide. They are supplied as follows:
NDC 0006-0612-68 bottles of 100.
Shown in Product Identification Section, page 418
No. 3319—Tablets ALDOCLOR 250 are green, oval, film coated tablets coded MSD 634. Each tablet contains 250 mg of methyldopa and 250 mg of chlorothiazide. They are supplied as follows:
NDC 0006-0634-68 bottles of 100.
Shown in Product Identification Section, page 418
Storage
Keep container tightly closed. Protect from light. Store container in carton until contents have been used.
A.H.F.S. Category: 24:08
DC 7059833   Issued October 1987

ALDOMET® **Tablets**   ℞
(Methyldopa, MSD), U.S.P.

ALDOMET® **Oral Suspension**   ℞
(Methyldopa, MSD), U.S.P.

DESCRIPTION

ALDOMET® (Methyldopa, MSD) is an antihypertensive drug.

Methyldopa, the *L*-isomer of alpha-methyldopa is levo-3-(3,4 - dihydroxyphenyl) -2-methylalanine. Its empirical formula is $C_{10}H_{13}NO_4$, with a molecular weight of 211.22, and its structural formula is:

Continued on next page

Information on the Merck Sharp & Dohme products listed on these pages is the full prescribing information from product circulars in use August 31, 1989.

Merck Sharp & Dohme—Cont.

Methyldopa is a white to yellowish white, odorless fine powder, and is soluble in water.

ALDOMET is supplied as tablets, for oral use, in three strengths: 125 mg, 250 mg, or 500 mg of methyldopa per tablet. Inactive ingredients in the tablets are: calcium disodium edetate, cellulose, citric acid, colloidal silicon dioxide, D&C Yellow 10, ethylcellulose, guar gum, hydroxypropyl methylcellulose, iron oxide, magnesium stearate, propylene glycol, talc, and titanium dioxide.

Oral Suspension ALDOMET is supplied as a white to off-white preparation; each 5 mL contains 250 mg of methyldopa and alcohol 1 percent, with benzoic acid 0.1 percent and sodium bisulfite 0.2 percent added as preservatives. Inactive ingredients in the oral suspension are: artificial and natural flavors, cellulose, citric acid, confectioner's sugar, disodium edetate, glycerin, polysorbate, purified water, and sodium carboxymethylcellulose.

CLINICAL PHARMACOLOGY

ALDOMET is an aromatic-amino-acid decarboxylase inhibitor in animals and in man. Although the mechanism of action has yet to be conclusively demonstrated, the antihypertensive effect of methyldopa probably is due to its metabolism to alpha-methylnorepinephrine, which then lowers arterial pressure by stimulation of central inhibitory alpha-adrenergic receptors, false neurotransmission, and/or reduction of plasma renin activity. Methyldopa has been shown to cause a net reduction in the tissue concentration of serotonin, dopamine, norepinephrine, and epinephrine.

Only methyldopa, the *L*-isomer of alpha-methyldopa, has the ability to inhibit dopa decarboxylase and to deplete animal tissues of norepinephrine. In man the antihypertensive activity appears to be due solely to the *L*-isomer. About twice the dose of the racemate (*DL*-alpha-methyldopa) is required for equal antihypertensive effect.

Methyldopa has no direct effect on cardiac function and usually does not reduce glomerular filtration rate, renal blood flow, or filtration fraction. Cardiac output usually is maintained without cardiac acceleration. In some patients the heart rate is slowed.

Normal or elevated plasma renin activity may decrease in the course of methyldopa therapy.

ALDOMET reduces both supine and standing blood pressure. Methyldopa usually produces highly effective lowering of the supine pressure with infrequent symptomatic postural hypotension. Exercise hypotension and diurnal blood pressure variations rarely occur.

Pharmacokinetics and Metabolism

The maximum decrease in blood pressure occurs four to six hours after oral dosage. Once an effective dosage level is attained, a smooth blood pressure response occurs in most patients in 12 to 24 hours. After withdrawal, blood pressure usually returns to pretreatment levels within 24–48 hours. Methyldopa is extensively metabolized. The known urinary metabolites are: α-methyldopa mono-0-sulfate; 3-0-methyl-α-methyldopa; 3,4-dihydroxyphenylacetone; α-methyldopamine; 3-0-methyl-α-methyldopamine and their conjugates. Approximately 70% of the drug which is absorbed is excreted in the urine as methyldopa and its mono-0-sulfate conjugate. The renal clearance is about 130 mL/min in normal subjects and is diminished in renal insufficiency. The plasma half-life of methyldopa is 105 minutes. After oral doses, excretion is essentially complete in 36 hours. Methyldopa crosses the placental barrier, appears in cord blood, and appears in breast milk.

INDICATION AND USAGE

Hypertension.

CONTRAINDICATIONS

Active hepatic disease, such as acute hepatitis and active cirrhosis.

If previous methyldopa therapy has been associated with liver disorders (see WARNINGS).

Hypersensitivity to any component of these products, including sulfites contained in Oral Suspension ALDOMET (see WARNINGS). Tablets ALDOMET do <u>not</u> contain sulfites.

WARNINGS

It is important to recognize that a positive Coombs test, hemolytic anemia, and liver disorders may occur with methyldopa therapy. The rare occurrences of hemolytic anemia or liver disorders could lead to potentially fatal complications unless properly recognized and managed. Read this section carefully to understand these reactions.

With prolonged methyldopa therapy, 10 to 20 percent of patients develop a positive direct Coombs test which usually occurs between 6 and 12 months of methyldopa therapy.

Lowest incidence is at daily dosage of 1 g or less. This on rare occasions may be associated with hemolytic anemia, which could lead to potentially fatal complications. One cannot predict which patients with a positive direct Coombs test may develop hemolytic anemia.

Prior existence or development of a positive direct Coombs test is not in itself a contraindication to use of methyldopa. If a positive Coombs test develops during methyldopa therapy, the physician should determine whether hemolytic anemia exists and whether the positive Coombs test may be a problem. For example, in addition to a positive direct Coombs test there is less often a positive indirect Coombs test which may interfere with cross matching of blood.

Before treatment is started, it is desirable to do a blood count (hematocrit, hemoglobin, or red cell count) for a baseline or to establish whether there is anemia. Periodic blood counts should be done during therapy to detect hemolytic anemia. It may be useful to do a direct Coombs test before therapy and at 6 and 12 months after the start of therapy.

If Coombs-positive hemolytic anemia occurs, the cause may be methyldopa and the drug should be discontinued. Usually the anemia remits promptly. If not, corticosteroids may be given and other causes of anemia should be considered. If the hemolytic anemia is related to methyldopa, the drug should not be reinstituted.

When methyldopa causes Coombs positivity alone or with hemolytic anemia, the red cell is usually coated with gamma globulin of the IgG (gamma G) class only. The positive Coombs test may not revert to normal until weeks to months after methyldopa is stopped.

Should the need for transfusion arise in a patient receiving methyldopa, both a direct and an indirect Coombs test should be performed. In the absence of hemolytic anemia, usually only the direct Coombs test will be positive. A positive direct Coombs test alone will not interfere with typing or cross matching. If the indirect Coombs test is also positive, problems may arise in the major cross match and the assistance of a hematologist or transfusion expert will be needed.

Occasionally, fever has occurred within the first 3 weeks of methyldopa therapy, associated in some cases with eosinophilia or abnormalities in one or more liver function tests, such as serum alkaline phosphatase, serum transaminases (SGOT, SGPT), bilirubin, and prothrombin time. Jaundice, with or without fever, may occur with onset usually within the first 2 to 3 months of therapy. In some patients the findings are consistent with those of cholestasis. In others the findings are consistent with hepatitis and hepatocellular injury.

Rarely, fatal hepatic necrosis has been reported after use of methyldopa. These hepatic changes may represent hypersensitivity reactions. Periodic determinations of hepatic function should be done particularly during the first 6 to 12 weeks of therapy or whenever an unexplained fever occurs. If fever, abnormalities in liver function tests, or jaundice appear, stop therapy with methyldopa. If caused by methyldopa, the temperature and abnormalities in liver function characteristically have reverted to normal when the drug was discontinued. Methyldopa should not be reinstituted in such patients.

Rarely, a reversible reduction of the white blood cell count with a primary effect on the granulocytes has been seen. The granulocyte count returned promptly to normal on discontinuance of the drug. Rare cases of granulocytopenia have been reported. In each instance, upon stopping the drug, the white cell count returned to normal. Reversible thrombocytopenia has occurred rarely.

Oral Suspension ALDOMET (but not Tablets ALDOMET) contains sodium bisulfite, a sulfite that may cause allergic-type reactions including anaphylactic symptoms and life-threatening or less severe asthmatic episodes in certain susceptible people. The overall prevalence of sulfite sensitivity in the general population is unknown and probably low. Sulfite sensitivity is seen more frequently in asthmatic than in nonasthmatic people.

PRECAUTIONS

General

Methyldopa should be used with caution in patients with a history of previous liver disease or dysfunction (see WARNINGS).

Some patients taking methyldopa experience clinical edema or weight gain which may be controlled by use of a diuretic. Methyldopa should not be continued if edema progresses or signs of heart failure appear.

Hypertension has recurred occasionally after dialysis in patients given methyldopa because the drug is removed by this procedure.

Rarely involuntary choreoathetotic movements have been observed during therapy with methyldopa in patients with severe bilateral cerebrovascular disease. Should these movements occur, stop therapy.

Laboratory Tests

Blood count, Coombs test, and liver function tests are recommended before initiating therapy and at periodic intervals (see WARNINGS).

Drug Interactions

When methyldopa is used with other antihypertensive drugs, potentiation of antihypertensive effect may occur. Patients should be followed carefully to detect side reactions or unusual manifestations of drug idiosyncrasy.

Patients may require reduced doses of anesthetics when on methyldopa. If hypotension does occur during anesthesia, it usually can be controlled by vasopressors. The adrenergic receptors remain sensitive during treatment with methyldopa.

When methyldopa and lithium are given concomitantly the patient should be carefully monitored for symptoms of lithium toxicity. Read the circular for lithium preparations.

Drug/Laboratory Test Interactions

Methyldopa may interfere with measurement of: urinary uric acid by the phosphotungstate method, serum creatinine by the alkaline picrate method, and SGOT by colorimetric methods. Interference with spectrophotometric methods for SGOT analysis has not been reported.

Since methyldopa causes fluorescence in urine samples at the same wave lengths as catecholamines, falsely high levels of urinary catecholamines may be reported. This will interfere with the diagnosis of pheochromocytoma. It is important to recognize this phenomenon before a patient with a possible pheochromocytoma is subjected to surgery. Methyldopa does not interfere with measurement of VMA (vanillylmandelic acid), a test for pheochromocytoma, by those methods which convert VMA to vanillin. Methyldopa is not recommended for the treatment of patients with pheochromocytoma. Rarely, when urine is exposed to air after voiding, it may darken because of breakdown of methyldopa or its metabolites.

Carcinogenesis, Mutagenesis, Impairment of Fertility

Methyldopa is currently under study in the U.S. Carcinogenesis Testing Program.

Methyldopa did not have mutagenic activity *in vitro* in the Ames microbial mutagen test with or without metabolic activation.

Methyldopa given in a two-liter study in rats at approximately three to six times the usual daily dose did not impair fertility.

Pregnancy

Pregnancy Category B. Reproduction studies have been performed in the rabbit, the mouse, and the rat at doses up to 1000 mg/kg/day (16.6 times the maximum recommended human dose) and have revealed no evidence of impaired fertility or harm to the fetus due to methyldopa. There are, however, no adequate and well-controlled studies in pregnant women in the first trimester of pregnancy. Because animal reproduction studies are not always predictive of human response, ALDOMET should be used during pregnancy only if clearly needed.

Published reports of the use of methyldopa during all trimesters indicate that if this drug is used during pregnancy the possibility of fetal harm appears remote. In five studies, three of which were controlled, involving 332 pregnant hypertensive women, treatment with ALDOMET was associated with an improved fetal outcome. The majority of these women were in the third trimester when methyldopa therapy was begun.

In one study, women who had begun methyldopa treatment between weeks 16 and 20 of pregnancy gave birth to infants whose average head circumference was reduced by a small amount (34.2 $\pm$ 1.7 cm vs. 34.6 $\pm$ 1.3 cm [mean $\pm$ 1 S.D.]). Long-term follow up of 195 (97.5%) of the children born to methyldopa-treated pregnant women (including those who began treatment between weeks 16 and 20) failed to uncover any significant adverse effect on the children. At four years of age, the developmental delay commonly seen in children born to hypertensive mothers was less evident in those whose mothers were treated with methyldopa during pregnancy than those whose mothers were untreated. The children of the treated group scored consistently higher than the children of the untreated group on five major indices of intellectual and motor development. At age seven and one-half developmental scores and intelligence indices showed no significant differences in children of treated or untreated hypertensive women.

Nursing Mothers

Methyldopa appears in breast milk. Therefore, caution should be exercised when methyldopa is given to a nursing woman.

ADVERSE REACTIONS

Sedation, usually transient, may occur during the initial period of therapy or whenever the dose is increased. Headache, asthenia, or weakness may be noted as early and transient symptoms. However, significant adverse effects due to

ALDOMET have been infrequent and this agent usually is well tolerated.

The following adverse reactions have been reported and, within each category, are listed in order of decreasing severity.

Cardiovascular: Aggravation of angina pectoris, congestive heart failure, prolonged carotid sinus hypersensitivity, orthostatic hypotension (decrease daily dosage), edema or weight gain, bradycardia.

Digestive: Pancreatitis, colitis, vomiting, diarrhea, sialadenitis, sore or "black" tongue, nausea, constipation, distension, flatus, dryness of mouth.

Endocrine: Hyperprolactinemia.

Hematologic: Bone marrow depression, leukopenia, granulocytopenia, thrombocytopenia, hemolytic anemia; positive tests for antinuclear antibody, LE cells, and rheumatoid factor, positive Coombs test.

Hepatic: Liver disorders including hepatitis, jaundice, abnormal liver function tests (see WARNINGS).

Hypersensitivity: Myocarditis, pericarditis, lupus-like syndrome, drug-related fever.

Nervous System/Psychiatric: Parkinsonism, Bell's palsy, decreased mental acuity, involuntary choreoathetotic movements, symptoms of cerebrovascular insufficiency, psychic disturbances including nightmares and reversible mild psychoses or depression, headache, sedation, asthenia or weakness, dizziness, lightheadedness, paresthesias.

Metabolic: Rise in BUN.

Musculoskeletal: Arthralgia, with or without joint swelling; myalgia.

Respiratory: Nasal stuffiness.

Skin: Toxic epidermal necrolysis, rash.

Urogenital: Amenorrhea, breast enlargement, gynecomastia, lactation, impotence, decreased libido.

OVERDOSAGE

Acute overdosage may produce acute hypotension with other responses attributable to brain and gastrointestinal malfunction (excessive sedation, weakness, bradycardia, dizziness, lightheadedness, constipation, distention, flatus, diarrhea, nausea, vomiting).

In the event of overdosage, symptomatic and supportive measures should be employed. When ingestion is recent, gastric lavage or emesis may reduce absorption. When ingestion has been earlier, infusions may be helpful to promote urinary excretion. Otherwise, management includes special attention to cardiac rate and output, blood volume, electrolyte balance, paralytic ileus, urinary function and cerebral activity.

Sympathomimetic drugs [e.g., levarterenol, epinephrine, ARAMINE® (Metaraminol Bitartrate, MSD)] may be indicated. Methyldopa is dialyzable.

The oral LD$_{50}$ of methyldopa is greater than 1.5 g/kg in both the mouse and the rat.

DOSAGE AND ADMINISTRATION

ADULTS

Initiation of Therapy

The usual starting dosage of ALDOMET is 250 mg two or three times a day in the first 48 hours. The daily dosage then may be increased or decreased, preferably at intervals of not less than two days, until an adequate response is achieved. To minimize the sedation, start dosage increases in the evening. By adjustment of dosage, morning hypotension may be prevented without sacrificing control of afternoon blood pressure.

When methyldopa is given to patients on other antihypertensives, the dose of these agents may need to be adjusted to effect a smooth transition. When ALDOMET is given with antihypertensives other than thiazides, the initial dosage of ALDOMET should be limited to 500 mg daily in divided doses; when ALDOMET is added to a thiazide, the dosage of thiazide need not be changed.

Maintenance Therapy

The usual daily dosage of ALDOMET is 500 mg to 2 g in two to four doses. Although occasional patients have responded to higher doses, the maximum recommended daily dosage is 3 g. Once an effective dosage range is attained, a smooth blood pressure response occurs in most patients in 12 to 24 hours. Since methyldopa has a relatively short duration of action, withdrawal is followed by return of hypertension usually within 48 hours. This is not complicated by an overshoot of blood pressure.

Occasionally tolerance may occur, usually between the second and third month of therapy. Adding a diuretic or increasing the dosage of methyldopa frequently will restore effective control of blood pressure. A thiazide may be added at any time during methyldopa therapy and is recommended if therapy has not been started with a thiazide or if effective control of blood pressure cannot be maintained on 2 g of methyldopa daily.

Methyldopa is largely excreted by the kidney and patients with impaired renal function may respond to smaller doses.

Syncope in older patients may be related to an increased sensitivity and advanced arteriosclerotic vascular disease. This may be avoided by lower doses.

CHILDREN

Initial dosage is based on 10 mg/kg of body weight daily in two to four doses. The daily dosage then is increased or decreased until an adequate response is achieved. The maximum dosage is 65 mg/kg or 3 g daily, whichever is less.

HOW SUPPLIED

No. 3341—Tablets ALDOMET, 125 mg, are yellow, film coated, round tablets, coded MSD 135. They are supplied as follows:

NDC 0006-0135-68 bottles of 100.

Shown in Product Identification Section, page 418

No. 3290—Tablets ALDOMET, 250 mg, are yellow, film coated, round tablets, coded MSD 401. They are supplied as follows:

NDC 0006-0401-68 bottles of 100
(6505-00-890-1856, 250 mg 100's)

NDC 0006-0401-28 unit dose packages of 100
(6505-00-149-0090, 250 mg individually sealed 100's)

NDC 0006-0401-78 unit of use bottles of 100

NDC 0006-0401-82 bottles of 1000
(6505-00-931-6646, 250 mg 1000's).

Shown in Product Identification Section, page 418

No. 3292—Tablets ALDOMET, 500 mg, are yellow, film coated, round tablets, coded MSD 516. They are supplied as follows:

NDC 0006-0516-54 unit of use bottles of 60

NDC 0006-0516-68 bottles of 100

NDC 0006-0516-28 unit dose packages of 100
(6505-01-046-3616, 500 mg individually sealed 100's)

NDC 0006-0516-78 unit of use bottles of 100

NDC 0006-0516-74 bottles of 500
(6505-01-199-8339, 500 mg 500's).

Shown in Product Identification Section, page 418

No. 3382—Oral Suspension ALDOMET, 250 mg per 5 mL, is an off-white, creamy suspension with a citric orange-pineapple flavor. It is supplied as follows:

NDC 0006-3382-74 bottles of 473 mL.

Storage

Store Oral Suspension ALDOMET below 26°C (78°F) in a tight, light-resistant container. Protect from freezing.

A.H.F.S. Category: 24:08

DC 7398624　Issued May 1988

COPYRIGHT © MERCK & CO., INC., 1985

ALDOMET® Ester HCl Injection
(Methyldopate Hydrochloride, MSD), U.S.P.　　℞

DESCRIPTION

Injection ALDOMET® Ester Hydrochloride (Methyldopate Hydrochloride, MSD) is an antihypertensive agent for intravenous use, each 5 mL of which contains:

Methyldopate
hydrochloride .... 250.0 mg
Inactive ingredients:
　Citric acid anhydrous .... 25.0 mg
　Disodium edetate .... 2.5 mg
　Monothioglycerol .... 10.0 mg
Sodium hydroxide to adjust pH
Water for Injection, q.s. to .... 5.0 mL
Methylparaben 7.5 mg, propylparaben 1.0 mg, and sodium bisulfite 16.0 mg added as preservatives.

Methyldopate hydrochloride [levo-3-(3,4-dihydroxyphenyl)-2-methylalanine, ethyl ester hydrochloride] is the ethyl ester of methyldopa, supplied as the hydrochloride salt. Methyldopate hydrochloride is more soluble and stable in solution than methyldopa and is the preferred form for intravenous use.

The structural formula for methyldopate hydrochloride is:

$$HO-\underset{HO}{\bigcirc}-CH_2-\underset{\underset{NH_2 \cdot HCl}{|}}{\overset{\overset{CH_3}{|}}{C}}-CO_2C_2H_5$$

ACTIONS

ALDOMET® (Methyldopa, MSD), a unique antihypertensive, is an aromatic-amino-acid decarboxylase inhibitor in animals and in man. Although the mechanism of action has yet to be conclusively demonstrated, the antihypertensive effect of methyldopa probably is due to its metabolism to alpha-methyl-norepinephrine, which then lowers arterial pressure by stimulation of central inhibitory alpha-adrenergic receptors, false neurotransmission, and/or reduction of plasma renin activity. Methyldopa has been shown to cause a

net reduction in the tissue concentration of serotonin, dopamine, norepinephrine, and epinephrine.

Only methyldopa, the *L*-isomer of alpha-methyldopa, has the ability to inhibit dopa decarboxylase and to deplete animal tissues of norepinephrine. In man the antihypertensive activity appears to be due solely to the *L*-isomer. About twice the dose of the racemate (*DL*-alpha-methyldopa) is required for equal antihypertensive effect.

Methyldopa has no direct effect on cardiac function and usually does not reduce glomerular filtration rate, renal blood flow, or filtration fraction. Cardiac output usually is maintained without cardiac acceleration. In some patients the heart rate is slowed.

Normal or elevated plasma renin activity may decrease in the course of methyldopa therapy.

Methyldopa reduces both supine and standing blood pressure. It usually produces highly effective lowering of the supine pressure with infrequent symptomatic postural hypotension. Exercise hypotension and diurnal blood pressure variations rarely occur.

Methyldopate hydrochloride is the ethyl ester of methyldopa hydrochloride and possesses the same pharmacologic attributes.

INDICATION

Hypertension, when parenteral medication is indicated. The treatment of hypertensive crises may be initiated with Injection ALDOMET Ester Hydrochloride.

CONTRAINDICATIONS

Active hepatic disease, such as acute hepatitis and active cirrhosis.

If previous methyldopa therapy has been associated with liver disorders (see WARNINGS).

Hypersensitivity to any component of this product, including sulfites (see WARNINGS).

WARNINGS

It is important to recognize that a positive Coombs test, hemolytic anemia, and liver disorders may occur with methyldopa therapy. The rare occurrences of hemolytic anemia or liver disorders could lead to potentially fatal complications unless properly recognized and managed. Read this section carefully to understand these reactions.

With prolonged methyldopa therapy, 10 to 20 percent of patients develop a positive direct Coombs test which usually occurs between 6 and 12 months of methyldopa therapy. Lowest incidence is at daily dosage of 1 g or less. This on rare occasions may be associated with hemolytic anemia, which could lead to potentially fatal complications. One cannot predict which patients with a positive direct Coombs test may develop hemolytic anemia.

Prior existence or development of a positive direct Coombs test is not in itself a contraindication to use of methyldopa. If a positive Coombs test develops during methyldopa therapy, the physician should determine whether hemolytic anemia exists and whether the positive Coombs test may be a problem. For example, in addition to a positive direct Coombs test there is less often a positive indirect Coombs test which may interfere with cross matching of blood.

At the start of methyldopa therapy, it is desirable to do a blood count (hematocrit, hemoglobin, or red cell count) for a baseline or to establish whether there is anemia. Periodic blood counts should be done during therapy to detect hemolytic anemia. It may be useful to do a direct Coombs test before therapy and at 6 and 12 months after the start of therapy.

If Coombs-positive hemolytic anemia occurs, the cause may be methyldopa and the drug should be discontinued. Usually the anemia remits promptly. If not, corticosteroids may be given and other causes of anemia should be considered. If the hemolytic anemia is related to methyldopa, the drug should not be reinstituted.

When methyldopa causes Coombs positivity alone or with hemolytic anemia, the red cell is usually coated with gamma globulin of the IgG (gamma G) class only. The positive Coombs test may not revert to normal until weeks to months after methyldopa is stopped.

Should the need for transfusion arise in a patient receiving methyldopa, both a direct and an indirect Coombs test should be performed on his blood. In the absence of hemolytic anemia, usually only the direct Coombs test will be positive. A positive direct Coombs test alone will not interfere with typing or cross matching. If the indirect Coombs test is also positive, problems may arise in the major cross match

Continued on next page

Information on the Merck Sharp & Dohme products listed on these pages is the full prescribing information from product circulars in use August 31, 1989.

Merck Sharp & Dohme—Cont.

and the assistance of a hematologist or transfusion expert will be needed.

Occasionally, fever has occurred within the first three weeks of methyldopa therapy, associated in some cases with eosinophilia or abnormalities in one or more liver function tests, such as serum alkaline phosphatase, serum transaminases (SGOT, SGPT), bilirubin, cephalin cholesterol flocculation, prothrombin time, and bromsulphalein retention. Jaundice, with or without fever, may occur with onset usually within the first two to three months of therapy. In some patients the findings are consistent with those of cholestasis.

Rarely fatal hepatic necrosis has been reported after use of methyldopa. These hepatic changes may represent hypersensitivity reactions. Periodic determination of hepatic function should be done particularly during the first 6 to 12 weeks of therapy or whenever an unexplained fever occurs. If fever, abnormalities in liver function tests, or jaundice appear, stop therapy with methyldopa. If caused by methyldopa, the temperature and abnormalities in liver function characteristically have reverted to normal when the drug was discontinued. Methyldopa should not be reinstituted in such patients.

Rarely, a reversible reduction of the white blood cell count with a primary effect on the granulocytes has been seen. The granulocyte count returned promptly to normal on discontinuance of the drug. Rare cases of granulocytopenia have been reported. In each instance, upon stopping the drug, the white cell count returned to normal. Reversible thrombocytopenia has occurred rarely.

When methyldopa is used with other antihypertensive drugs, potentiation of antihypertensive effect may occur. Patients should be followed carefully to detect side reactions or unusual manifestations of drug idiosyncrasy.

When methyldopa and lithium are given concomitantly the patient should be carefully monitored for symptoms of lithium toxicity. Read the circular for lithium preparations.

Injection ALDOMET Ester Hydrochloride contains sodium bisulfite, a sulfite that may cause allergic-type reactions including anaphylactic symptoms and life-threatening or less severe asthmatic episodes in certain susceptible people. The overall prevalence of sulfite sensitivity in the general population is unknown and probably low. Sulfite sensitivity is seen more frequently in asthmatic than in nonasthmatic people.

Pregnancy and Nursing

Use of any drug in women who are or may become pregnant or intend to nurse requires that anticipated benefits be weighed against possible risks.

Methyldopa crosses the placental barrier, appears in cord blood, and appears in breast milk.

No unusual adverse reactions have been reported in association with the use of methyldopa during pregnancy. Though no obvious teratogenic effects have been reported, the possibility of fetal injury cannot be excluded. Also, the possibility of injury to a nursing infant cannot be excluded.

PRECAUTIONS

Methyldopa should be used with caution in patients with a history of previous liver disease or dysfunction (see WARNINGS).

Methyldopa may interfere with measurement of: urinary uric acid by the phosphotungstate method, serum creatinine by the alkaline picrate method, and SGOT by colorimetric methods. Interference with spectrophotometric methods for SGOT analysis has not been reported.

A paradoxical pressor response has been reported with intravenous administration of ALDOMET Ester Hydrochloride.

Since methyldopa causes fluorescence in urine samples at the same wave lengths as catecholamines, falsely high levels of urinary catecholamines may be reported. This will interfere with the diagnosis of pheochromocytoma. It is important to recognize this phenomenon before a patient with a possible pheochromocytoma is subjected to surgery. Methyldopa does not interfere with measurement of VMA (vanillylmandelic acid), a test for pheochromocytoma, by those methods which convert VMA to vanillin. Methyldopa is not recommended for the treatment of patients with pheochromocytoma. Rarely, when urine is exposed to air after voiding, it may darken because of breakdown of methyldopa or its metabolites.

Rarely involuntary choreoathetotic movements have been observed during therapy with methyldopa in patients with severe bilateral cerebrovascular disease. Should these movements occur, stop therapy.

Patients may require reduced doses of anesthetics when on methyldopa. If hypotension does occur during anesthesia, it usually can be controlled by vasopressors. The adrenergic receptors remain sensitive during treatment with methyldopa.

Hypertension has recurred occasionally after dialysis in patients given methyldopa because the drug is removed by this procedure.

ADVERSE REACTIONS

Sedation, usually transient, may occur during the initial period of therapy or whenever the dose is increased. Headache, asthenia, or weakness may be noted as early and transient symptoms. However, significant adverse effects due to methyldopa have been infrequent and this agent usually is well tolerated.

Nervous System/Psychiatric: Sedation, headache, asthenia or weakness, dizziness, lightheadedness, symptoms of cerebrovascular insufficiency, paresthesias, parkinsonism, Bell's palsy, decreased mental acuity, involuntary choreoathetotic movements. Psychic disturbances including nightmares and reversible mild psychoses or depression.

Cardiovascular: Bradycardia, prolonged carotid sinus hypersensitivity, aggravation of angina pectoris. Paradoxical pressor response with intravenous use. Orthostatic hypotension (decrease daily dosage). Edema (and weight gain) usually relieved by use of a diuretic. (Discontinue methyldopa if edema progresses or signs of heart failure appear.)

Digestive: Nausea, vomiting, distention, constipation, flatus, diarrhea, colitis, mild dryness of mouth, sore or "black" tongue, pancreatitis, sialadenitis.

Hepatic: Abnormal liver function tests, jaundice, liver disorders.

Hematologic: Positive Coombs test, hemolytic anemia. Bone marrow depression, leukopenia, granulocytopenia, thrombocytopenia. Positive tests for antinuclear antibody, LE cells, and rheumatoid factor.

Allergic: Drug-related fever, lupus-like syndrome, myocarditis, pericarditis.

Skin: Rash as in eczema or lichenoid eruption; toxic epidermal necrolysis.

Respiratory: Nasal stuffiness.

Metabolic: Rise in BUN.

Urogenital: Breast enlargement, gynecomastia, lactation, amenorrhea, impotence, decreased libido.

Endocrine: Hyperprolactinemia.

Musculoskeletal: Mild arthralgia, with or without joint swelling; myalgia.

DOSAGE AND ADMINISTRATION

Injection ALDOMET Ester Hydrochloride, when given intravenously in effective doses, causes a decline in blood pressure that may begin in four to six hours and last 10 to 16 hours after injection.

Add the desired dose of Injection ALDOMET Ester Hydrochloride to 100 mL of 5 percent Dextrose Injection U.S.P. Alternatively the desired dose may be given in 5% dextrose in water in a concentration of 100 mg/10 mL. Give this intravenous infusion slowly over a period of 30 to 60 minutes.

ADULTS

The usual adult dosage intravenously is 250 to 500 mg at six hour intervals as required. The maximum recommended intravenous dose is 1.0 g every six hours.

When control has been obtained, oral therapy with Tablets ALDOMET (Methyldopa, MSD) may be substituted for intravenous therapy, starting with the same dosage schedule used for the parenteral route. The effectiveness and anticipated responses are described in the circular for Tablets ALDOMET (Methyldopa, MSD).

Since methyldopa has a relatively short duration of action, withdrawal is followed by return of hypertension usually within 48 hours. This is not complicated by an overshoot of blood pressure.

Occasionally tolerance may occur, usually between the second and third month of therapy. Adding a diuretic or increasing the dosage of methyldopa frequently will restore effective control of blood pressure. A thiazide may be added at any time during methyldopa therapy and is recommended if therapy has not been started with a thiazide or if effective control of blood pressure cannot be maintained on 2.0 g of methyldopa daily.

Methyldopa is largely excreted by the kidney and patients with impaired renal function may respond to smaller doses. Syncope in older patients may be related to an increased sensitivity and advanced arteriosclerotic vascular disease. This may be avoided by lower doses.

CHILDREN

The recommended daily dosage is 20 to 40 mg/kg of body weight in divided doses every six hours. The maximum dosage is 65 mg/kg or 3.0 g daily, whichever is less. When the blood pressure is under control, continue with oral therapy using Tablets ALDOMET (Methyldopa, MSD) in the same dosage as for the parenteral route.

HOW SUPPLIED

No. 3293—Injection ALDOMET Ester Hydrochloride, 250 mg per 5 mL, is a clear, colorless solution and is supplied as follows:

NDC 0006-3293-05 in 5 mL vials
(6505-01-096-2735, 5 mL vial).

A.H.F.S. Category: 24:08
DC 7347129   Issued May 1988

ALDORIL® Tablets   ℞
(Methyldopa-Hydrochlorothiazide, MSD), U.S.P.

> **WARNING**
> This fixed combination drug is not indicated for initial therapy of hypertension. Hypertension requires therapy titrated to the individual patient. If the fixed combination represents the dosage so determined, its use may be more convenient in patient management. The treatment of hypertension is not static, but must be reevaluated as conditions in each patient warrant.

DESCRIPTION

ALDORIL® (Methyldopa-Hydrochlorothiazide, MSD) combines two antihypertensives: methyldopa and hydrochlorothiazide.

Methyldopa

Methyldopa is an antihypertensive and is the L-isomer of alphamethyldopa. It is levo-3-(3,4-dihydroxyphenyl)-2-methylalanine. Its empirical formula is $C_{10}H_{13}NO_4$, with a molecular weight of 211.22, and its structural formula is:

Methyldopa is a white to yellowish white, odorless fine powder, and is soluble in water.

Hydrochlorothiazide

Hydrochlorothiazide is a diuretic and antihypertensive. It is the 3,4-dihydro derivative of chlorthiazide. Its chemical name is 6-chloro-3,4-dihydro-$2H$-1,2,4-benzothiadiazine-7-sulfonamide 1,1-dioxide. Its empirical formula is $C_7H_8ClN_3O_4S_2$ and its structural formula is:

Hydrochlorothiazide is a white, or practically white, crystalline powder with a molecular weight of 297.72, which is slightly soluble in water, but freely soluble in sodium hydroxide solution.

ALDORIL is supplied as tablets in four strengths for oral use:

ALDORIL 15, contains 250 mg of methyldopa and 15 mg of hydrochlorothiazide.

ALDORIL 25, contains 250 mg of methyldopa and 25 mg of hydrochlorothiazide.

ALDORIL D30, contains 500 mg of methyldopa and 30 mg of hydrochlorothiazide.

ALDORIL D50, contains 500 mg of methyldopa and 50 mg of hydrochlorothiazide.

Each tablet contains the following inactive ingredients: calcium disodium edetate, calcium phosphate, cellulose, citric acid, colloidal silicon dioxide, ethylcellulose, guar gum, hydroxypropyl methylcellulose, magnesium stearate, propylene glycol, talc, and titanium dioxide. ALDORIL 15 and ALDORIL D30 also contain iron oxide and FD&C Red 3.

CLINICAL PHARMACOLOGY

Methyldopa

Methyldopa is an aromatic-amino-acid decarboxylase inhibitor in animals and in man. Although the mechanism of action has yet to be conclusively demonstrated, the antihypertensive effect of methyldopa probably is due to its metabolism to alpha-methylnorepinephrine, which then lowers arterial pressure by stimulation of central inhibitory alpha-adrenergic receptors, false neurotransmission, and/or reduction of plasma renin activity. Methyldopa has been shown to cause a net reduction in the tissue concentration of serotonin, dopamine, norepinephrine, and epinephrine.

Only methyldopa, the L-isomer of alpha-methyldopa, has the ability to inhibit dopa decarboxylase and to deplete animal tissues of norepinephrine. In man, the antihypertensive activity appears to be due solely to the L-isomer. About twice the dose of the racemate (DL-alpha-methyldopa) is required for equal antihypertensive effect.

Methyldopa has no direct effect on cardiac function and usually does not reduce glomerular filtration rate, renal blood flow, or filtration fraction. Cardiac output usually is maintained without cardiac acceleration. In some patients the heart rate is slowed.

Normal or elevated plasma renin activity may decrease in the course of methyldopa therapy.

Methyldopa reduces both supine and standing blood pressure. It usually produces highly effective lowering of the supine pressure with infrequent symptomatic postural hypotension. Exercise hypotension and diurnal blood pressure variations rarely occur.

Hydrochlorothiazide

The mechanism of the antihypertensive effect of thiazides is unknown. Hydrochlorothiazide does not usually affect normal blood pressure.

Hydrochlorothiazide affects the distal renal tubular mechanism of electrolyte reabsorption. At maximal therapeutic dosage all thiazides are approximately equal in their diuretic efficacy.

Hydrochlorothiazide increases excretion of sodium and chloride in approximately equivalent amounts. Natriuresis may be accompanied by some loss of potassium and bicarbonate. After oral use diuresis begins within 2 hours, peaks in about 4 hours and lasts about 6 to 12 hours.

Methyldopa-Hydrochlorothiazide

The concomitant use of methyldopa and hydrochlorothiazide, as provided in ALDORIL, frequently produces a more pronounced antihypertensive response than when either compound is the sole therapeutic agent. Particularly in those cases of hypertensive vascular disease where sodium and water retention is a problem, the coadministration of these two drugs in the form of ALDORIL will help control the fluid imbalance.

In severe essential hypertension and in malignant hypertension ALDORIL may achieve effective lowering of blood pressure with fewer side effects than occur with other compounds used for this purpose.

ALDORIL reduces both supine and standing blood pressure; more effective lowering of the supine pressure with less frequent symptomatic postural hypotension can be obtained with ALDORIL than with most other antihypertensive agents. In patients treated with ALDORIL, exercise hypotension and diurnal blood pressure variations rarely occur.

Pharmacokinetics and Metabolism

Methyldopa

The maximum decrease in blood pressure occurs four to six hours after oral dosage. Once an effective dosage level is attained, a smooth blood pressure response occurs in most patients in 12 to 24 hours. After withdrawal, blood pressure usually returns to pretreatment levels within 24–48 hours.

Methyldopa is extensively metabolized. The known urinary metabolites are: α-methyldopa mono-0-sulfate; 3-0-methyl-α-methyldopa; 3,4-dihydroxyphenylacetone; α-methyldopamine; 3-0-methyl-α-methyldopamine and their conjugates. Approximately 70 percent of the drug which is absorbed is excreted in the urine as methyldopa and its mono-0-sulfate conjugate. The renal clearance is about 130 mL/min in normal subjects and is diminished in renal insufficiency. The plasma half-life of methyldopa is 105 minutes. After oral doses, excretion is essentially complete in 36 hours.

Methyldopa crosses the placental barrier, appears in cord blood, and appears in breast milk.

Hydrochlorothiazide

Hydrochlorothiazide is not metabolized but is eliminated rapidly by the kidney. When plasma levels have been followed for at least 24 hours, the plasma half-life has been observed to vary between 5.6 and 14.8 hours. At least 61 percent of the oral dose is eliminated unchanged within 24 hours. Hydrochlorothiazide crosses the placental but not the blood-brain barrier and is excreted in breast milk.

INDICATION AND USAGE

Hypertension (see box warning).

Use in Pregnancy. Routine use of diuretics during normal pregnancy is inappropriate and exposes mother and fetus to unnecessary hazard. Diuretics do not prevent development of toxemia of pregnancy and there is no satisfactory evidence that they are useful in the treatment of toxemia.

Edema during pregnancy may arise from pathologic causes or from the physiologic and mechanical consequences of pregnancy. Thiazides are indicated in pregnancy when edema is due to pathologic causes, just as they are in the absence of pregnancy (see PRECAUTIONS, *Pregnancy*). Dependent edema in pregnancy, resulting from restriction of venous return by the gravid uterus, is properly treated through elevation of the lower extremities and use of support stockings. Use of diuretics to lower intravascular volume in this instance is illogical and unnecessary. During normal pregnancy there is hypervolemia which is not harmful to the fetus or the mother in the absence of cardiovascular disease. However, it may be associated with edema, rarely generalized edema. If such edema causes discomfort, increased recumbency will often provide relief. Rarely this edema may cause extreme discomfort which is not relieved by rest. In these instances, a short course of diuretic therapy may provide relief and be appropriate.

CONTRAINDICATIONS

Active hepatic disease, such as acute hepatitis and active cirrhosis.

If previous methyldopa therapy has been associated with liver disorders (see WARNINGS).

Anuria.

Hypersensitivity to methyldopa, or to hydrochlorothiazide or other sulfonamide-derived drugs.

WARNINGS

Methyldopa

It is important to recognize that a positive Coombs test, hemolytic anemia, and liver disorders may occur with methyldopa therapy. The rare occurrences of hemolytic anemia or liver disorders could lead to potentially fatal complications unless properly recognized and managed. Read this section carefully to understand these reactions.

With prolonged methyldopa therapy, 10 to 20 percent of patients develop a positive direct Coombs test which usually occurs between 6 and 12 months of methyldopa therapy. Lowest incidence is at daily dosage of 1 g or less. This on rare occasions may be associated with hemolytic anemia, which could lead to potentially fatal complications. One cannot predict which patients with a positive direct Coombs test may develop hemolytic anemia.

Prior existence or development of a positive direct Coombs test is not in itself a contraindication to use of methyldopa. If a positive Coombs test develops during methyldopa therapy, the physician should determine whether hemolytic anemia exists and whether the positive Coombs test may be a problem. For example, in addition to a positive direct Coombs test there is less often a positive indirect Coombs test which may interfere with cross matching of blood.

Before treatment is started it is desirable to do a blood count (hematocrit, hemoglobin, or red cell count) for a baseline or to establish whether there is anemia. Periodic blood counts should be done during therapy to detect hemolytic anemia. It may be useful to do a direct Coombs test before therapy and at 6 and 12 months after the start of therapy.

If Coombs-positive hemolytic anemia occurs, the cause may be methyldopa and the drug should be discontinued. Usually the anemia remits promptly. If not, corticosteroids may be given and other causes of anemia should be considered. If the hemolytic anemia is related to methyldopa, the drug should not be reinstituted.

When methyldopa causes Coombs positivity alone or with hemolytic anemia, the red cell is usually coated with gamma globulin of the IgG (gamma G) class only. The positive Coombs test may not revert to normal until weeks to months after methyldopa is stopped.

Should the need for transfusion arise in a patient receiving methyldopa, both a direct and an indirect Coombs test should be performed. In the absence of hemolytic anemia, usually only the direct Coombs test will be positive. A positive direct Coombs test alone will not interfere with typing or cross matching. If the indirect Coombs test is also positive, problems may arise in the major cross match and the assistance of a hematologist or transfusion expert will be needed.

Occasionally, fever has occurred within the first three weeks of methyldopa therapy, associated in some cases with eosinophilia or abnormalities in one or more liver function tests, such as serum alkaline phosphatase, serum transaminases (SGOT, SGPT), bilirubin, and prothrombin time. Jaundice, with or without fever, may occur with onset usually within the first two to three months of therapy. In some patients the findings are consistent with those of cholestasis. In others the findings are consistent with hepatitis and hepatocellular injury.

Rarely fatal hepatic necrosis has been reported after use of methyldopa. These hepatic changes may represent hypersensitivity reactions. Periodic determination of hepatic function should be done particularly during the first 6 to 12 weeks of therapy or whenever an unexplained fever occurs. If fever, abnormalities in liver function tests, or jaundice appear, stop therapy with methyldopa. If caused by methyldopa, the temperature and abnormalities in liver function characteristically have reverted to normal when the drug was discontinued. Methyldopa should not be reinstituted in such patients.

Rarely, a reversible reduction of the white blood cell count with a primary effect on the granulocytes has been seen. The granulocyte count returned promptly to normal on discontinuance of the drug. Rare cases of granulocytopenia have been reported. In each instance, upon stopping the drug, the white cell count returned to normal. Reversible thrombocytopenia has occurred rarely.

Hydrochlorothiazide

Use with caution in severe renal disease. In patients with renal disease, thiazides may precipitate azotemia. Cumulative effects of the drug may develop in patients with impaired renal function.

Thiazides should be used with caution in patients with impaired hepatic function or progressive liver disease, since minor alterations of fluid and electrolyte balance may precipitate hepatic coma.

Thiazides may add to or potentiate the action of other antihypertensive drugs.

Sensitivity reactions may occur in patients with or without a history of allergy or bronchial asthma.

The possibility of exacerbation or activation of systemic lupus erythematosus has been reported.

Lithium generally should not be given with diuretics (see PRECAUTIONS, *Drug Interactions*).

PRECAUTIONS

General

Methyldopa

Methyldopa should be used with caution in patients with a history of previous liver disease or dysfunction (see WARNINGS).

Some patients taking methyldopa experience clinical edema or weight gain which may be controlled by use of a diuretic. Methyldopa should not be continued if edema progresses or signs of heart failure appear.

Hypertension has recurred occasionally after dialysis in patients given methyldopa because the drug is removed by this procedure.

Rarely involuntary choreoathetotic movements have been observed during therapy with methyldopa in patients with severe bilateral cerebrovascular disease. Should these movements occur, stop therapy.

Hydrochlorothiazide

All patients receiving diuretic therapy should be observed for evidence of fluid or electrolyte imbalance: namely, hyponatremia, hypochloremic alkalosis, and hypokalemia. Serum and urine electrolyte determinations are particularly important when the patient is vomiting excessively or receiving parenteral fluids. Warning signs or symptoms of fluid and electrolyte imbalance, irrespective of cause, include dryness of mouth, thirst, weakness, lethargy, drowsiness, restlessness, muscle pains or cramps, muscular fatigue, hypotension, oliguria, tachycardia, and gastrointestinal disturbances such as nausea and vomiting.

Hypokalemia may develop, especially with brisk diuresis, when severe cirrhosis is present or after prolonged therapy. Interference with adequate oral electrolyte intake will also contribute to hypokalemia. Hypokalemia may cause cardiac arrhythmia and may also sensitize or exaggerate the response of the heart to the toxic effects of digitalis (e.g., increased ventricular irritability). Hypokalemia may be avoided or treated by use of potassium sparing diuretics or potassium supplements such as foods with a high potassium content.

Although any chloride deficit is generally mild and usually does not require specific treatment except under extraordinary circumstances (as in liver disease or renal disease), chloride replacement may be required in the treatment of metabolic alkalosis.

Dilutional hyponatremia may occur in edematous patients in hot weather; appropriate therapy is water restriction, rather than administration of salt, except in rare instances when the hyponatremia is life threatening. In actual salt depletion, appropriate replacement is the therapy of choice.

Hyperuricemia may occur or acute gout may be precipitated in certain patients receiving thiazides.

In diabetic patients dosage adjustment of insulin or oral hypoglycemic agents may be required. Hyperglycemia may occur with thiazide diuretics. Thus latent diabetes mellitus may become manifest during thiazide therapy.

The antihypertensive effects of the drug may be enhanced in the postsympathectomy patient.

If progressive renal impairment becomes evident, consider withholding or discontinuing diuretic therapy.

Thiazides have been shown to increase the urinary excretion of magnesium; this may result in hypomagnesemia.

Thiazides may decrease urinary calcium excretion. Thiazides may cause intermittent and slight elevation of serum calcium in the absence of known disorders of calcium metabolism. Marked hypercalcemia may be evidence of hidden hyperparathyroidism. Thiazides should be discontinued before carrying out tests for parathyroid function.

Increases in cholesterol and triglyceride levels may be associated with thiazide diuretic therapy.

Continued on next page

Information on the Merck Sharp & Dohme products listed on these pages is the full prescribing information from product circulars in use August 31, 1989.

Merck Sharp & Dohme—Cont.

Laboratory Tests
Methyldopa
Blood count, Coombs test and liver function test, are recommended before initiating therapy and at periodic intervals (see WARNINGS).
Hydrochlorothiazide
Periodic determination of serum electrolytes to detect possible electrolyte imbalance should be done at appropriate intervals.
Drug Interactions
Methyldopa
When methyldopa is used with other antihypertensive drugs, potentiation of antihypertensive effect may occur. Patients should be followed carefully to detect side reactions or unusual manifestations of drug idiosyncrasy.
Patients may require reduced doses of anesthetics when on methyldopa. If hypotension does occur during anesthesia, it usually can be controlled by vasopressors. The adrenergic receptors remain sensitive during treatment with methyldopa.
Hydrochlorothiazide
When given concurrently the following drugs may interact with thiazide diuretics.
Alcohol, barbiturates, or narcotics —potentiation of orthostatic hypotension may occur.
Antidiabetic drugs (oral agents and insulin) —dosage adjustment of the antidiabetic drug may be required.
Other antihypertensive drugs —additive effect or potentiation.
Corticosteroids, ACTH —intensified electrolyte depletion, particularly hypokalemia.
Pressor amines (e.g., norepinephrine) —possible decreased response to pressor amines but not sufficient to preclude their use.
Skeletal muscle relaxants, nondepolarizing (e.g., tubocurarine) —possible increased responsiveness to the muscle relaxant.
Lithium —generally should not be given with diuretics. Diuretic agents reduce the renal clearance of lithium and add a high risk of lithium toxicity. Refer to the package insert for lithium preparations before use of such preparations with ALDORIL.
Non-steroidal Anti-inflammatory Drugs —In some patients, the administration of a non-steroidal anti-inflammatory agent can reduce the diuretic, natriuretic, and antihypertensive effects of loop, potassium-sparing and thiazide diuretics. Therefore, when ALDORIL and non-steroidal anti-inflammatory agents are used concomitantly, the patient should be observed closely to determine if the desired effect of the diuretic is obtained.
Drug/Laboratory Test Interactions
Methyldopa
Methyldopa may interfere with measurement of: urinary uric acid by the phosphotungstate method, serum creatinine by the alkaline picrate method, and SGOT by colorimetric methods. Interference with spectrophotometric methods for SGOT analysis has not been reported.
Since methyldopa causes fluorescence in urine samples at the same wave lengths as catecholamines, falsely high levels of urinary catecholamines may be reported. This will interfere with the diagnosis of pheochromocytoma. It is important to recognize this phenomenon before a patient with a possible pheochromocytoma is subjected to surgery. Methyldopa does not interfere with measurement of VMA (vanillylmandelic acid), a test for pheochromocytoma, by those methods which convert VMA to vanillin. Methyldopa is not recommended for the treatment of patients with pheochromocytoma. Rarely, when urine is exposed to air after voiding, it may darken because of breakdown of methyldopa or its metabolites.
Hydrochlorothiazide
Thiazides should be discontinued before carrying out tests for parathyroid function (see PRECAUTIONS, *General*).
Carcinogenesis, Mutagenesis,
Impairment of Fertility
Long-term studies in animals have not been performed to evaluate the effects upon fertility, mutagenic or carcinogenic potential of the combination.
Methyldopa
Methyldopa is currently under study in the U.S. Carcinogenesis Testing Program.
Methyldopa did not have mutagenic activity *in vitro* in the Ames microbial mutagen test with or without metabolic activation.
Methyldopa given in a two-litter study in rats at approximately three to six times the usual daily dose did not impair fertility.
Hydrochlorothiazide
Hydrochlorothiazide is currently under study in the U.S. Carcinogenesis Testing Program.
Hydrochlorothiazide was not mutagenic *in vitro,* in the Ames microbial mutagen test at a maximum concentration of 5 mg/plate using Strains TA98 and TA100. Urine samples from patients treated with hydrochlorothiazide did not have mutagenic activity in the Ames test.
The ability of a number of drugs to induce nondisjunction and crossing over was measured using *Aspergillus nidulans.* A large number of drugs, including hydrochlorothiazide, induced nondisjunction.
Hydrochlorothiazide had no effect on fertility in a two-litter study in rats at doses 4–5.6 mg/kg/day (up to 2 times the maximum recommended human dose).
Pregnancy
Teratogenic Effects—Pregnancy Category C: Animal reproduction studies have not been conducted with ALDORIL. It is also not known whether ALDORIL can affect reproduction capacity or can cause fetal harm when given to a pregnant woman. ALDORIL should be given to a pregnant woman only if clearly needed. (See INDICATIONS AND USAGE.)
Hydrochlorothiazide: Thiazides cross the placental barrier and appear in cord blood.
Reproduction studies in the rabbit, the mouse and the rat at doses up to 100 mg/kg/day (50 times the maximum recommended human dose) showed no evidence of external abnormalities of the fetus due to hydrochlorothiazide. Hydrochlorothiazide given in a two-litter study in rats at doses of 4–5.6 mg/kg/day (approximately 1–2 times the maximum recommended human dose) did not impair fertility or produce birth abnormalities in the offspring.
Methyldopa: Reproduction studies have been performed in the rabbit, the mouse, and the rat at doses up to 1000 mg/kg/day (16.6 times the maximum recommended human dose) and have revealed no evidence of impaired fertility or harm to the fetus due to methyldopa. There are, however, no adequate and well-controlled studies in pregnant women in the first trimester of pregnancy. Because animal reproduction studies are not always predictive of human response, methyldopa should be used during pregnancy only if clearly needed.
Published reports of the use of methyldopa during all trimesters indicate that if this drug is used during pregnancy the possibility of fetal harm appears remote. In five studies, three of which were controlled, involving 332 pregnant hypertensive women, treatment with methyldopa was associated with an improved fetal outcome. The majority of these women were in the third trimester when methyldopa therapy was begun.
In one study, women who had begun methyldopa treatment between weeks 16 and 20 of pregnancy gave birth to infants whose average head circumference was reduced by a small amount (34.2 ± 1.7 cm vs. 34.6 ± 1.3 cm [mean ± 1 S.D.]). Long term follow-up of 195 (97.5%) of the children born to methyldopa-treated pregnant women (including those who began treatment between weeks 16 and 20) failed to uncover any significant adverse effect on the children. At four years of age, the developmental delay commonly seen in children born to hypertensive mothers was less evident in those whose mothers were treated with methyldopa during pregnancy than those whose mothers were untreated. The children of the treated group scored consistently higher than the children of the untreated group on five major indices of intellectual and motor development. At age 7 and one-half developmental scores and intelligence indices showed no significant differences in children of treated or untreated hypertensive women.
Nonteratogenic Effects: These may include fetal or neonatal jaundice, thrombocytopenia, and possibly other adverse reactions which have occurred in the adult.
Nursing Mothers
Methyldopa and thiazides appear in breast milk. Therefore, because of the potential for serious adverse reactions in nursing infants from hydrochlorothiazide, a decision should be made whether to discontinue nursing or to discontinue the drug, taking into account the importance of the drug to the mother.
Pediatric Use
Safety and effectiveness of ALDORIL in children has not been established.

ADVERSE REACTIONS

The following adverse reactions have been reported and, within each category, are listed in order of decreasing severity.
Methyldopa
Sedation, usually transient, may occur during the initial period of therapy or whenever the dose is increased. Headache, asthenia, or weakness may be noted as early and transient symptoms. However, significant adverse effects due to methyldopa have been infrequent and this agent usually is well tolerated.
Cardiovascular: Aggravation of angina pectoris, congestive heart failure, prolonged carotid sinus hypersensitivity, orthostatic hypotension (decrease daily dosage), edema or weight gain, bradycardia.
Digestive: Pancreatitis, colitis, vomiting, diarrhea, sialadenitis, sore or "black" tongue, nausea, constipation, distension, flatus, dryness of mouth.
Endocrine: Hyperprolactinemia.
Hematologic: Bone marrow depression, leukopenia, granulocytopenia, thrombocytopenia, hemolytic anemia; positive tests for antinuclear antibody, LE cells, and rheumatoid factor, positive Coombs test.
Hepatic: Liver disorders including hepatitis, jaundice, abnormal liver function tests (see WARNINGS).
Hypersensitivity: Myocarditis, pericarditis, lupus-like syndrome, drug-related fever.
Nervous System/Psychiatric: Parkinsonism, Bell's palsy, decreased mental acuity, involuntary choreoathetotic movements, symptoms of cerebrovascular insufficiency, psychic disturbances including nightmares and reversible mild psychoses or depression, headache, sedation, asthenia or weakness, dizziness, lightheadedness, paresthesias.
Metabolic: Rise in BUN.
Musculoskeletal: Arthralgia, with or without joint swelling; myalgia.
Respiratory: Nasal stuffiness.
Skin: Toxic epidermal necrolysis, rash.
Urogenital: Amenorrhea, breast enlargement, gynecomastia, lactation, impotence, decreased libido.
Hydrochlorothiazide
Body as a Whole: Weakness.
Cardiovascular: Hypotension including orthostatic hypotension (may be aggravated by alcohol, barbiturates, narcotics or antihypertensive drugs).
Digestive: Pancreatitis, jaundice (intrahepatic cholestatic jaundice), diarrhea, vomiting, sialadenitis, cramping, constipation, gastric irritation, nausea, anorexia.
Hematologic: Aplastic anemia, agranulocytosis, leukopenia, hemolytic anemia, thrombocytopenia.
Hypersensitivity: Anaphylactic reactions, necrotizing angiitis (vasculitis and cutaneous vasculitis), respiratory distress including pneumonitis and pulmonary edema, photosensitivity, fever, urticaria, rash, purpura.
Metabolic: Electrolyte imbalance (see PRECAUTIONS), hyperglycemia, glycosuria, hyperuricemia.
Musculoskeletal: Muscle spasm.
Nervous System/Psychiatric: Vertigo, paresthesias, dizziness, headache, restlessness.
Renal: Renal failure, renal dysfunction, interstitial nephritis. (See WARNINGS.)
Special Senses: transient blurred vision, xanthopsia.
Whenever adverse reactions are moderate or severe, thiazide dosage should be reduced or therapy withdrawn.

OVERDOSAGE

Acute overdosage may produce acute hypotension with other responses attributable to brain and gastrointestinal malfunction (excessive sedation, weakness, bradycardia, dizziness, lightheadedness, constipation, distention, flatus, diarrhea, nausea, vomiting).
In the event of overdosage, symptomatic and supportive measures should be employed. When ingestion is recent, gastric lavage or emesis may reduce absorption. When ingestion has been earlier, infusions may be helpful to promote urinary excretion. Otherwise, management includes special attention to cardiac rate and output, blood volume, electrolyte balance, paralytic ileus, urinary function and cerebral activity.
Sympathomimetic drugs [e.g., levarterenol, epinephrine, ARAMINE® (Metaraminol Bitartrate, MSD)] may be indicated. Methyldopa is dialyzable.
The oral LD_{50} of methyldopa is greater than 1.5 g/kg in both the mouse and the rat. The oral LD_{50} of hydrochlorothiazide is greater than 10 g/kg in the mouse and rat.

DOSAGE AND ADMINISTRATION

Dosage: As determined by individual titration (see box warning).
The usual dosage is 1 tablet of ALDORIL 15, ALDORIL 25, ALDORIL D30, or ALDORIL D50 two or three times a day in the first 48 hours. The daily dosage then may be increased or decreased, preferably at intervals of not less than two days, until an adequate response is achieved. To minimize the sedation associated with methyldopa, start dosage increases in the evening. By adjustment of dosage, morning hypotension may be prevented without sacrificing control of afternoon blood pressure.
When ALDORIL is given to patients on other antihypertensives, the dose of these agents may need to be adjusted to effect a smooth transition. When ALDORIL is given with antihypertensives other than thiazides, the initial dosage of methyldopa should be limited to 500 mg daily in divided doses.
Although occasional patients have responded to higher doses, the maximum recommended daily dosage is 3.0 g of methyldopa and 100 to 200 mg of hydrochlorothiazide. Once an effective dosage range is attained, a smooth blood pres-

sure response occurs in most patients in 12 to 24 hours. If ALDORIL alone does not adequately control blood pressure, additional methyldopa may be given separately to obtain the maximum blood pressure response.

Since both components of ALDORIL have a relatively short duration of action, withdrawal is followed by return of hypertension usually within 48 hours. This is not complicated by an overshoot of blood pressure.

Occasionally tolerance may occur, usually between the second and third month of therapy. Increasing the dosage of either methyldopa or hydrochlorothiazide separately or together frequently will restore effective control of blood pressure.

Methyldopa is largely excreted by the kidney and patients with impaired renal function may respond to smaller doses of ALDORIL. Syncope in older patients may be related to an increased sensitivity and advanced arteriosclerotic vascular disease. This may be avoided by lower doses.

HOW SUPPLIED

No. 3294—Tablets ALDORIL 15 are salmon, round, film coated tablets, coded MSD 423. Each tablet contains 250 mg of methyldopa and 15 mg of hydrochlorothiazide. They are supplied as follows:

NDC 0006-0423-68 bottles of 100
NDC 0006-0423-28 unit dose packages of 100
NDC 0006-0423-82 bottles of 1000.

Shown in Product Identification Section, page 418
No. 3295—Tablets ALDORIL 25 are white, round, film coated tablets, coded MSD 456. Each tablet contains 250 mg of methyldopa and 25 mg of hydrochlorothiazide. They are supplied as follows:

NDC 0006-0456-68 bottles of 100
NDC 0006-0456-28 unit dose packages of 100
NDC 0006-0456-82 bottles of 1000.

Shown in Product Identification Section, page 418
No. 3362—Tablets ALDORIL D30 are salmon, oval, film coated tablets, coded MSD 694. Each tablet contains 500 mg of methyldopa and 30 mg of hydrochlorothiazide. They are supplied as follows:

NDC 0006-0694-68 bottles of 100.

Shown in Product Identification Section, page 418
No. 3363—Tablets ALDORIL D50 are white, oval, film coated tablets, coded MSD 935. Each tablet contains 500 mg of methyldopa and 50 mg of hydrochlorothiazide. They are supplied as follows:

NDC 0006-0935-68 bottles of 100.

Shown in Product Identification Section, page 418
A.H.F.S. Category: 24:08
DC 7059640   Issued October 1987
COPYRIGHT © MERCK & CO., INC., 1986
All rights reserved

AMINOHIPPURATE SODIUM, MSD "PAH" ℞
Injection, U.S.P.

DESCRIPTION

Aminohippurate sodium,* MSD is an agent to measure effective renal plasma flow (ERPF). It is the sodium salt of para-aminohippuric acid, commonly abbreviated "PAH". It is water soluble, lipid-insoluble, and has a pKa of 3.83. The empirical formula of the anhydrous salt is $C_9H_9N_2NaO_3$ and its structural formula is:

$$H_2N\text{—}\langle\text{ring}\rangle\text{—CONHCH}_2\text{COONa}$$

It is provided as a sterile, non-preserved 20 percent aqueous solution for injection, with a pH of 6.7 to 7.6. Each 10 mL contains: Aminohippurate sodium 2 g. Inactive ingredients: Sodium hydroxide to adjust pH, water for injection, q.s.

CLINICAL PHARMACOLOGY

PAH is filtered by the glomeruli and is actively secreted by the proximal tubules. At low plasma concentrations (1.0 to 2.0 mg/100 mL), an average of 90 percent of PAH is cleared by the kidneys from the renal blood stream in a single circulation. It is ideally suited for measurement of ERPF since it has a high clearance, is essentially nontoxic at the plasma concentrations reached with recommended doses and its analytical determination is relatively simple and accurate. PAH is also used to measure the functional capacity of the renal tubular secretory mechanism or transport maximum (Tm_{PAH}). This is accomplished by elevating the plasma concentration to levels (40–60 mg/100 mL) sufficient to saturate the maximal capacity of the tubular cells to secrete PAH. Inulin clearance is generally measured during Tm_{PAH} determinations since glomerular filtration rate (GFR) must be

---
*Formerly referred to as Sodium para-Aminohippurate.

known before calculations of secretory Tm measurements can be done (See *Calculations*).

INDICATIONS AND USAGE

Estimation of effective renal plasma flow.
Measurement of the functional capacity of the renal tubular secretory mechanism.

CONTRAINDICATIONS

Hypersensitivity to this product or to its components.

PRECAUTIONS

General
Intravenous solutions must be given with caution to patients with low cardiac reserve, since a rapid increase in plasma volume can precipitate congestive heart failure.
For measurement of ERPF, small doses of PAH are used. However, in research procedures to measure Tm_{PAH}, high plasma levels are required to saturate the capacity of the tubular cells. During these procedures the intravenous administration of PAH solutions should be carried out slowly and with caution. The patient should be continuously observed for any adverse reactions.
Drug Interactions
Renal clearance measurements of PAH cannot be made with any significant accuracy in patients receiving sulfonamides, procaine, or thiazolesulfone. These compounds interfere with chemical color development essential to the analytical procedures.
Probenecid depresses tubular secretion of certain weak acids such as PAH. Therefore, patients receiving probenecid will have erroneously low ERPF and Tm_{PAH} values.
Carcinogenesis, Mutagenesis, Impairment of Fertility
Long-term studies in animals have not been done to evaluate any effects upon fertility or carcinogenic potential of PAH.
Pregnancy
Pregnancy Category C. Animal reproduction studies have not been done with PAH. It is also not known whether PAH can cause fetal harm when given to a pregnant woman or can affect reproduction capacity. PAH should be given to a pregnant woman only if clearly needed.
Nursing Mothers
It is not known whether this drug is excreted in human milk. Because many drugs are excreted in human milk, caution should be exercised when PAH is administered to a nursing woman.
Pediatric Use
Safety and effectiveness in children have not been established.

ADVERSE REACTIONS

Vasomotor disturbances, flushing, tingling, nausea, vomiting, and cramps may occur.
Patients may have a sensation of warmth or the desire to defecate or urinate during or shortly following initiation of infusion.

OVERDOSAGE

The intravenous LD_{50} in female mice is 7.22 g/kg.

DOSAGE AND ADMINISTRATION

For intravenous use only
Clearance measurements using single injection technics are generally inaccurate, particularly in the measurement of ERPF. For this reason, intravenous infusions at fixed rates are used to sustain the plasma PAH concentration at the desired level.

To measure ERPF, the concentration of PAH in the plasma should be maintained at 2 mg per 100 mL, which can be achieved with a priming dose of 6 to 10 mg/kg and an infusion dose of 10 to 24 mg/min.

As a research procedure for the measurement of Tm_{PAH}, the plasma level of PAH must be sufficient to saturate the capacity of the tubular secretory cells. Concentrations of from 40 to 60 mg per 100 mL are usually necessary.
Technical details of these tests may be found in Smith[1]; Wesson[2]; Bauer[3]; Pitts[4]; and Schnurr.[5]

Parenteral drug products should be inspected visually for particulate matter and discoloration prior to use, whenever solution and container permit. NOTE: The normal color range for this product is a colorless to yellow/brown solution. The efficacy is not affected by color changes within this range.
Calculations
Effective Renal Plasma Flow (ERPF)
The clearance of PAH, which is extracted almost completely from the plasma during its passage through the renal circu-

lation, constitutes a measure of ERPF. Hence:

$$ERPF = \frac{U_{PAH}V}{P_{PAH}}$$

Where U_{PAH} = concentration of PAH (mg/mL) in the urine
V = rate of urine excretion (mL/min), and
P_{PAH} = plasma concentration of PAH (mg/mL).

Example: U_{PAH} = 8.0 mg/mL
V = 1.5 mL/min
P_{PAH} = 0.02 mg/mL

$$ERPF = \frac{8.0 \times 1.5}{0.02} = 600 \text{ mL/min.}$$

Based on PAH clearance studies, the normal values for ERPF are:
men 675 ± 150 mL/min
women 595 ± 125 mL/min.

Maximum Tubular Secretory Mechanism (Tm_{PAH})
The quantity of PAH, secreted by the tubules (Tm_{PAH}) is given by the difference between the total rate of excretion ($U_{PAH}V$) and the quantity filtered by the glomeruli (GFR × P_{PAH}). Hence:

$$Tm_{PAH} = U_{PAH}V - (GFR \times P_{PAH} \times 0.83)$$

The factor, 0.83, corrects for that portion of PAH which is bound to plasma protein and hence is unfilterable.

Example: U_{PAH} = 9.55 mg/mL
V = 16.68 mL/min
GFR = 120 mL/min
P_{PAH} = 0.60 mg/mL
Then Tm_{PAH} = 9.55 × 16.68 − (120 × 0.60 × 0.83) = 100 mL/min.

Average normal values of Tm_{PAH} are 80–90 mg/min.
The value of the expression $U_{PAH}V$, used in calculations of ERPF and Tm_{PAH}, may be found by determining the amount of PAH in a measured volume of urine excreted within a specific period of time.

These calculations are based on a body surface area of 1.73 m^2. Corrections for variations in surface area are made by multiplying the values obtained for ERPF and Tm_{PAH} by 1.73/A, where A is the subject surface area.

HOW SUPPLIED

No. 95—Aminohippurate Sodium, 20 percent sterile solution for intravenous injection, is supplied as follows:
NDC 0006-3395-11 in 10 mL vials.
Storage
Avoid storage at temperatures below −20°C (−4°F) and above 40°C (104°F).

REFERENCES

1. Smith, H. W.: Lectures on the kidney, University Extension Division, University of Kansas, Lawrence, Kansas, 1943.
2. Wesson, L. G., Jr.: "Physiology of the Human Kidney," New York, Grune & Stratton, 1969, pp. 632–655.
3. Bauer, J. D.; Ackermann, P. G.; Toro, G.: "Brays Clinical Laboratory Methods," ed. 7, St. Louis, Mosby, 1968.
4. Pitts, R. F.: "Physiology of the Kidney and Body Fluids," ed. 2, Chicago, Year Book Medical Publishers, 1968.
5. Schnurr, E., Lahme, W., Kuppers, H.: Measurement of renal clearance of inulin and PAH in the steady state without urine collection; Clinical Nephrology, *13*(1): (26–29), 1980.

A.H.F.S. Category: 36:40
DC 7470618   Issued May 1986
COPYRIGHT © MERCK & CO., INC., 1983
All rights reserved

ANTIVENIN ℞
(Latrodectus mactans), MSD, U.S.P.
Black Widow Spider Antivenin
Equine Origin

DESCRIPTION

Antivenin (Latrodectus mactans), MSD is a sterile, non-pyrogenic preparation derived by drying a frozen solution of specific venom-neutralizing globulins obtained from the blood serum of healthy horses immunized against venom of black widow spiders (Latrodectus mactans). It is standardized by biological assay on mice, in terms of one dose of antivenin neutralizing the venom in not less than 6000 mouse LD_{50} of Latrodectus mactans. Thimerosal (mercury derivative) 1:10,000 is added as a preservative. When constituted as

Continued on next page

Merck Sharp & Dohme—Cont.

specified, it is opalescent and contains not more than 20.0 percent of solids.

Each vial contains not less than 6000 Antivenin units. One unit of Antivenin will neutralize one average mouse lethal dose of black widow spider venom when the Antivenin and the venom are injected simultaneously in mice under suitable conditions.

CLINICAL PHARMACOLOGY

The pharmacological mode of action is unknown and metabolic and pharmacokinetic data in humans are unavailable.

INDICATIONS AND USAGE

Antivenin (Latrodectus mactans), MSD is used to treat patients with symptoms due to bites by the black widow spider (Latrodectus mactans). Early use of the Antivenin is emphasized for prompt relief.

Local muscular cramps begin from 15 minutes to several hours after the bite which usually produces a sharp pain similar to that caused by puncture with a needle. The exact sequence of symptoms depends somewhat on the location of the bite. The venom acts on the myoneural junctions or on the nerve endings, causing an ascending motor paralysis or destruction of the peripheral nerve endings. The groups of muscles most frequently affected are those of the thigh, shoulder, and back. After a varying length of time, the pain becomes more severe, spreading to the abdomen, and weakness and tremor usually develop. The abdominal muscles assume a boardlike rigidity, but tenderness is slight. Respiration is thoracic. The patient is restless and anxious. Feeble pulse, cold, clammy skin, labored breathing and speech, light stupor, and delirium may occur. Convulsions also may occur, particularly in small children. The temperature may be normal or slightly elevated. Urinary retention, shock, cyanosis, nausea and vomiting, insomnia, and cold sweats also have been reported. The syndrome following the bite of the black widow spider may be confused easily with any medical or surgical condition with acute abdominal symptoms.

The symptoms of black widow spider bite increase in severity for several hours, perhaps a day, and then very slowly become less severe, gradually passing off in the course of two or three days except in fatal cases. Residual symptoms such as general weakness, tingling, nervousness, and transient muscle spasm may persist for weeks or months after recovery from the acute stage.

If possible, the patient should be hospitalized. Other additional measures giving greatest relief are prolonged warm baths and intravenous injection of 10 mL of 10 percent solution of calcium gluconate repeated as necessary to control muscle pain. Morphine also may be required to control pain. Barbiturates may be used for extreme restlessness. However, as the venom is a neurotoxin, it can cause respiratory paralysis. This must be borne in mind when considering use of morphine or a barbiturate. Adrenocorticosteroids have been used with varying degrees of success. Supportive therapy is indicated by the condition of the patient. Local treatment of the site of the bite is of no value. Nothing is gained by applying a tourniquet or by attempting to remove venom from the site of the bite by incision and suction.

In otherwise healthy individuals between the ages of 16 and 60, the use of Antivenin may be deferred and treatment with muscle relaxants may be considered.

WARNINGS

Prior to treatment with any product prepared from horse serum, a careful review of the patient's history should be taken emphasizing prior exposure to horse serum or any allergies. Serious sickness and even death could result from the use of horse serum in a sensitive patient. A skin or conjunctival test should be performed prior to administration of Antivenin.

Skin test: Inject into (not under) the skin not more than 0.02 mL of the test material (1:10 dilution of normal horse serum in physiologic saline). Evaluate result in 10 minutes. A positive reaction is an urticarial wheal surrounded by a zone of erythema. A control test using Sodium Chloride Injection facilitates interpretation of the results.

Conjunctival test: For adults instill into the conjunctival sac one drop of a 1:10 dilution of horse serum and for children one drop of 1:100 dilution. Itching of the eye and reddening of the conjunctiva indicate a positive reaction, usually within 10 minutes.

Patients should be observed for serum sickness for an average of 8 to 12 days following administration of Antivenin. *Desensitization should be attempted only when the administration of Antivenin is considered necessary to save life.* Epinephrine must be available in case of untoward reaction.

Desensitization: If the history is positive or the results of the sensitivity tests are mildly or questionably positive, Antivenin should be administered as follows to reduce the risk of an immediate severe allergic reaction:

1. In separate sterile vials or syringes prepare 1:10 or 1:100 dilutions of Antivenin in Sodium Chloride for Injection.
2. Allow at least 15 but preferably 30 minutes between injections and only proceed with the next dose if no reactions occurred following the previous dose.
3. Using a tuberculin syringe, inject subcutaneously 0.1, 0.2 and 0.5 mL of the 1:100 dilution at 15 or 30 minute intervals; repeat with the 1:10 dilution, and finally the undiluted Antivenin.
4. If there is a reaction after any of the injections, place a tourniquet proximal to the sites of injection and administer epinephrine, 1:1000 (0.3 to 1.0 mL subcutaneously, 0.05 to 0.1 mL intravenously), proximal to the tourniquet or into another extremity. Wait at least 30 minutes before giving another injection of Antivenin, the amount of which should be the same as the last one not evoking a reaction.
5. If no reaction has occurred after 0.5 mL of undiluted Antivenin has been given, it is probably safe to continue the dose at 15 minute intervals until the entire dose has been injected.

PRECAUTIONS

Carcinogenesis, Mutagenesis, Impairment of Fertility
No long term studies in animals have been performed to evaluate the potential for carcinogenesis, mutagenesis, or impairment of fertility.

Pregnancy
Pregnancy Category C. Animal reproduction studies have not been conducted with Black Widow Spider Antivenin. It is also not known whether Black Widow Spider Antivenin can cause fetal harm when administered to a pregnant woman or can affect reproduction capacity. Black Widow Spider Antivenin should be given to a pregnant woman only if clearly needed.

Nursing Mothers
It is not known whether this drug is excreted in human milk. Because many drugs are excreted in human milk, caution should be exercised when Black Widow Spider Antivenin is administered to a nursing woman.

Pediatric Use
Controlled clinical studies for safety and effectiveness in children have not been conducted; however, there have been virtually no adverse effects reported in those children who have received the product.

ADVERSE REACTIONS

Anaphylaxis and serum sickness have been reported following use of Antivenin.

DOSAGE AND ADMINISTRATION

Using a sterile syringe, remove from the accompanying vial 2.5 mL of Sterile Diluent for Antivenin and inject into the vial of Antivenin. With the needle still in the rubber stopper, shake the vial to dissolve the contents completely.

Parenteral drug products should be inspected visually for particulate matter and discoloration prior to administration, whenever solution and container permit.

The dose for adults and children is the entire contents of a restored vial (2.5 mL) of Antivenin. It may be given intramuscularly, preferably in the region of the anterolateral thigh so that a tourniquet may be applied in the event of a systemic reaction. Symptoms usually subside in 1 to 3 hours. Although one dose of Antivenin usually is adequate, a second dose may be necessary in some cases.

Antivenin also may be given intravenously in 10 to 50 mL of saline solution over a 15 minute period. It is the preferred route in severe cases, or when the patient is under 12, or in shock. One restored vial usually is enough.

HOW SUPPLIED

No. 4084—Antivenin (Latrodectus mactans), MSD equine origin is a white to grey crystalline powder, each vial containing not less than 6000 Antivenin units. Thimerosal (mercury derivative) 1:10,000 is added as preservative, **NDC** 0006-4084-00. A 2.5 mL vial of Sterile Diluent for Antivenin is included. Also supplied is a 1 mL vial of normal horse serum (1:10 dilution) for sensitivity testing. Thimerosal (mercury derivative) 1:10,000 is added as preservative.

A.H.F.S. Category: 80:04
DC 6145212　Issued March 1985

AquaMEPHYTON® Injection　　　　　　　　　　　　　　℞
(Phytonadione, MSD), U.S.P.
Aqueous Colloidal Solution of Vitamin K₁

> ### WARNING—INTRAVENOUS USE
> Severe reactions, including fatalities, have occurred during and immediately after INTRAVENOUS injection of AquaMEPHYTON® (Phytonadione, MSD), even when precautions have been taken to dilute the AquaMEPHYTON and to avoid rapid infusion. Typically these severe reactions have resembled hypersensitivity or anaphylaxis, including shock and cardiac and/or respiratory arrest. Some patients have exhibited these severe reactions on receiving AquaMEPHYTON for the first time. Therefore the INTRAVENOUS route should be restricted to those situations where other routes are not feasible and the serious risk involved is considered justified.

DESCRIPTION

Phytonadione is a vitamin, which is a clear, yellow to amber, viscous, odorless or nearly odorless liquid. It is insoluble in water, soluble in chloroform and slightly soluble in ethanol. It has a molecular weight of 450.70.

Phytonadione is 2-methyl-3-phytyl-1,4-naphthoquinone. Its empirical formula is $C_{31}H_{46}O_2$ and its structural formula is:

AquaMEPHYTON injection is a yellow, sterile, aqueous colloidal solution of vitamin K₁, with a pH of 5.0 to 7.0, available for injection by the intravenous, intramuscular, and subcutaneous routes. Each milliliter contains:
Phytonadione ....2 mg or 10 mg
Inactive ingredients:
　Polyoxyethylated fatty acid
　　derivative ....70 mg
　Dextrose ....37.5 mg
　Water for Injection, q.s. ....1 mL
Added as preservative:
　Benzyl alcohol 0.9%

CLINICAL PHARMACOLOGY

AquaMEPHYTON aqueous colloidal solution of vitamin K₁ for parenteral injection, possesses the same type and degree of activity as does naturally-occurring vitamin K, which is necessary for the production via the liver of active prothrombin (factor II), proconvertin (factor VII), plasma thromboplastin component (factor IX), and Stuart factor (factor X). The prothrombin test is sensitive to the levels of three of these four factors—II, VII, and X. The mechanism by which vitamin K promotes formation of these clotting factors in the liver is not known.

Phytonadione is readily absorbed following intramuscular administration. After absorption, phytonadione is initially concentrated in the liver, but the concentration declines rapidly. Very little vitamin K accumulates in tissues. Little is known about the metabolic fate of vitamin K. Almost no free unmetabolized vitamin K appears in bile or urine.

In normal animals and humans, phytonadione is virtually devoid of pharmacodynamic activity. However, in animals and humans deficient in vitamin K, the pharmacological action of vitamin K is related to its normal physiological function, that is, to promote the hepatic biosynthesis of vitamin K dependent clotting factors.

The action of the aqueous colloidal solution, when administered intravenously, is generally detectable within an hour or two and hemorrhage is usually controlled within 3 to 6 hours. A normal prothrombin level may often be obtained in 12 to 14 hours.

In the prophylaxis and treatment of hemorrhagic disease of the newborn, phytonadione has demonstrated a greater margin of safety than that of the water-soluble vitamin K analogues.

INDICATIONS AND USAGE

AquaMEPHYTON is indicated in the following coagulation disorders which are due to faulty formation of factors II, VII, IX and X when caused by vitamin K deficiency or interference with vitamin K activity.
AquaMEPHYTON injection is indicated in:
— anticoagulant-induced prothrombin deficiency caused by coumarin or indanedione derivatives;

— prophylaxis and therapy of hemorrhagic disease of the newborn;

— hypoprothrombinemia due to antibacterial therapy;

— hypoprothrombinemia secondary to factors limiting absorption or synthesis of vitamin K, e.g., obstructive jaundice, biliary fistula, sprue, ulcerative colitis, celiac disease, intestinal resection, cystic fibrosis of the pancreas, and regional enteritis;

— other drug-induced hypoprothrombinemia where it is definitely shown that the result is due to interference with vitamin K metabolism, e.g., salicylates.

CONTRAINDICATION

Hypersensitivity to any component of this medication.

WARNINGS

Benzyl alcohol as a preservative in Bacteriostatic Sodium Chloride Injection has been associated with toxicity in newborns. Data are unavailable on the toxicity of other preservatives in this age group. There is no evidence to suggest that the small amount of benzyl alcohol contained in AquaMEPHYTON, when used as recommended, is associated with toxicity.

An immediate coagulant effect should not be expected after administration of phytonadione. It takes a minimum of 1 to 2 hours for measurable improvement in the prothrombin time. Whole blood or component therapy may also be necessary if bleeding is severe.

Phytonadione will not counteract the anticoagulant action of heparin.

When vitamin K_1 is used to correct excessive anticoagulant-induced hypoprothrombinemia, anticoagulant therapy still being indicated, the patient is again faced with the clotting hazards existing prior to starting the anticoagulant therapy. Phytonadione is not a clotting agent, but overzealous therapy with vitamin K_1 may restore conditions which originally permitted thromboembolic phenomena. Dosage should be kept as low as possible, and prothrombin time should be checked regularly as clinical conditions indicate.

Repeated large doses of vitamin K are not warranted in liver disease if the response to initial use of the vitamin is unsatisfactory. Failure to respond to vitamin K may indicate that the condition being treated is inherently unresponsive to vitamin K.

PRECAUTIONS

Drug Interactions
Temporary resistance to prothrombin-depressing anticoagulants may result, especially when larger doses of phytonadione are used. If relatively large doses have been employed, it may be necessary when reinstituting anticoagulant therapy to use somewhat larger doses of the prothrombin-depressing anticoagulant, or to use one which acts on a different principle, such as heparin sodium.

Laboratory Tests
Prothrombin time should be checked regularly as clinical conditions indicate.

Carcinogenesis, Mutagenesis, Impairment of Fertility
Studies of carcinogenicity, mutagenesis or impairment of fertility have not been conducted with AquaMEPHYTON.

Pregnancy
Pregnancy Category C: Animal reproduction studies have not been conducted with AquaMEPHYTON. It is also not known whether AquaMEPHYTON can cause fetal harm when administered to a pregnant woman or can affect reproduction capacity. AquaMEPHYTON should be given to a pregnant woman only if clearly needed.

Nursing Mothers
It is not known whether this drug is excreted in human milk. Because many drugs are excreted in human milk, caution should be exercised when AquaMEPHYTON is administered to a nursing woman.

Pediatric Use
Hemolysis, jaundice, and hyperbilirubinemia in newborns, particularly in premature infants, may be related to the dose of AquaMEPHYTON. Therefore, the recommended dose should not be exceeded (see ADVERSE REACTIONS and DOSAGE AND ADMINISTRATION).

ADVERSE REACTIONS

Deaths have occurred after intravenous administration. (See Box Warning at beginning of circular.)

Transient "flushing sensations" and "peculiar" sensations of taste have been observed, as well as rare instances of dizziness, rapid and weak pulse, profuse sweating, brief hypotension, dyspnea, and cyanosis.

Pain, swelling, and tenderness at the injection site may occur. The possibility of allergic sensitivity, including an anaphylactoid reaction, should be kept in mind.

Rarely, after repeated injections, reactions resembling erythema perstans have been reported.

AquaMEPHYTON
Summary of Dosage Guidelines
(See circular text for details)

Newborns	Dosage
Hemorrhagic Disease of the Newborn	
Prophylaxis	0.5–1.0 mg IM within 1 hour of birth
Treatment	1.0 mg SC or IM (Higher doses may be necessary if the mother has been receiving oral anticoagulants)

Adults	Initial Dosage
Anticoagulant-Induced Prothrombin Deficiency (caused by coumarin or indanedione derivatives)	2.5 mg–10 mg or up to 25 mg (rarely 50 mg)
Hypoprothrombinemia due to other causes (Antibiotics; Salicylates or other drugs; Factors limiting absorption or synthesis)	2.5 mg–25 mg or more (rarely up to 50 mg)

Hyperbilirubinemia has been observed in the newborn following administration of phytonadione. This has occurred rarely and primarily with doses above those recommended. (See PRECAUTIONS, *Pediatric Use.*)

OVERDOSAGE

The intravenous LD_{50} of AquaMEPHYTON in the mouse is 41.5 and 52 mL/kg for the 0.2% and 1.0% concentrations respectively.

DOSAGE AND ADMINISTRATION

Whenever possible, AquaMEPHYTON should be given by the subcutaneous or intramuscular route. When intravenous administration is considered unavoidable, the drug should be injected very slowly, not exceeding 1 mg per minute.

Protect from light at all times.

Parenteral drug products should be inspected visually for particulate matter and discoloration prior to administration, whenever solution and container permit.

Directions for Dilution
AquaMEPHYTON may be diluted with 0.9% Sodium Chloride Injection, 5% Dextrose Injection, or 5% Dextrose and Sodium Chloride Injection. Benzyl alcohol as a preservative has been associated with toxicity in newborns. *Therefore, all of the above diluents should be preservative-free* (see WARNINGS). *Other diluents should not be used.* When dilutions are indicated, administration should be started immediately after mixture with the diluent, and unused portions of the dilution should be discarded, as well as unused contents of the ampul.

Prophylaxis of Hemorrhagic Disease of the Newborn
The American Academy of Pediatrics recommends that vitamin K_1 be given to the newborn. A single intramuscular dose of AquaMEPHYTON 0.5 to 1.0 mg within one hour of birth is recommended.

Treatment of Hemorrhagic Disease of the Newborn
Empiric administration of vitamin K_1 should not replace proper laboratory evaluation of the coagulation mechanism. A prompt response (shortening of the prothrombin time in 2 to 4 hours) following administration of vitamin K_1 is usually diagnostic of hemorrhagic disease of the newborn, and failure to respond indicates another diagnosis or coagulation disorder.

AquaMEPHYTON 1.0 mg should be given either subcutaneously or intramuscularly.

[See table above].

Higher doses may be necessary if the mother has been receiving oral anticoagulants.

Whole blood or component therapy may be indicated if bleeding is excessive. This therapy, however, does not correct the underlying disorder and AquaMEPHYTON should be given concurrently.

Anticoagulant-Induced Prothrombin Deficiency in Adults
To correct excessively prolonged prothrombin time caused by oral anticoagulant therapy—2.5 to 10 mg or up to 25 mg initially is recommended. In rare instances 50 mg may be required. Frequency and amount of subsequent doses should be determined by prothrombin time response or clinical condition (see WARNINGS). If in 6 to 8 hours after parenteral administration the prothrombin time has not been shortened satisfactorily, the dose should be repeated.

In the event of shock or excessive blood loss, the use of whole blood or component therapy is indicated.

Hypoprothrombinemia Due to Other Causes in Adults
A dosage of 2.5 to 25 mg or more (rarely up to 50 mg) is recommended, the amount and route of administration depending upon the severity of the condition and response obtained.

If possible, discontinuation or reduction of the dosage of drugs interfering with coagulation mechanisms (such as salicylates, antibiotics) is suggested as an alternative to administering concurrent AquaMEPHYTON. The severity of the coagulation disorder should determine whether the immediate administration of AquaMEPHYTON is required in addition to discontinuation or reduction of interfering drugs.

HOW SUPPLIED

Injection AquaMEPHYTON is a yellow, sterile, aqueous colloidal solution and is supplied in the following concentrations:
No. 7780—10 mg of vitamin K_1 per mL
NDC 0006-7780-64 boxes of 6 × 1 mL ampuls (6505-00-854-2499 10 mg 1.0 mL 6's)
NDC 0006-7780-66 boxes of 25 × 1 mL ampuls.
No. 7782—10 mg of vitamin K_1 per mL
NDC 0006-7782-30 in 2.5 mL multiple dose vials
NDC 0006-7782-03 in 5 mL multiple dose vials.
No. 7784—1 mg of vitamin K_1 per 0.5 mL
NDC 0006-7784-33 boxes of 25 × 0.5 mL ampuls (6505-00-180-6372 1 mg 0.5 mL 25's).

A.H.F.S. Category: 88:24
DC 7349814 Issued August 1986

ARAMINE® Injection ℞
(Metaraminol Bitartrate, MSD), U.S.P.

DESCRIPTION

Metaraminol bitartrate is a potent sympathomimetic amine that increases both systolic and diastolic blood pressure.

Metaraminol bitartrate is $[R\text{-}(R^*,S^*)]\text{-}\alpha\text{-}(1\text{-aminoethyl})\text{-}3\text{-}$hydroxybenzenemethanol $[R\text{-}(R^*,R^*)]\text{-}2,3\text{-dihydroxy-}$butanedioate (1:1) (salt), which is levorotatory. Its empirical formula is $C_9H_{13}NO_2 \cdot C_4H_6O_6$ and its structural formula is:

Metaraminol bitartrate is a white, crystalline powder with a molecular weight of 317.29, is freely soluble in water, slightly soluble in alcohol, and practically insoluble in chloroform and in ether.

Injection ARAMINE® (Metaraminol Bitartrate, MSD) is a sterile solution. Each mL contains:

Metaraminol bitartrate equivalent to metaraminol	10 mg
Inactive ingredients:	
Sodium chloride	4.4 mg
Water for Injection q.s. ad	1 mL

Methylparaben 0.15%, propylparaben 0.02%, and sodium bisulfite 0.2% added as preservatives.

CLINICAL PHARMACOLOGY

The pressor effect of ARAMINE begins in 1 to 2 minutes after intravenous infusion, in about 10 minutes after intra-

Continued on next page

Merck Sharp & Dohme—Cont.

muscular injection, and in 5 to 20 minutes after subcutaneous injection. The effect lasts from about 20 minutes to one hour. ARAMINE has a positive inotropic effect on the heart and a peripheral vasoconstrictor action.

Renal, coronary, and cerebral blood flow are a function of perfusion pressure and regional resistance. In patients with insufficient or failing vasoconstriction, there is additional advantage to the peripheral action of ARAMINE, but in most patients with shock, vasoconstriction is adequate and any further increase is unnecessary. Blood flow to vital organs may decrease with ARAMINE if regional resistance increases excessively.

The pressor effect of ARAMINE is decreased but not reversed by alpha-adrenergic blocking agents. Primary or secondary fall in blood pressure and tachyphylactic response to repeated use are uncommon.

INDICATIONS AND USAGE

ARAMINE is indicated for prevention and treatment of the acute hypotensive state occurring with spinal anesthesia. It is also indicated as adjunctive treatment of hypotension due to hemorrhage, reactions to medications, surgical complications, and shock associated with brain damage due to trauma or tumor.

CONTRAINDICATIONS

Use of ARAMINE with cyclopropane or halothane anesthesia should be avoided, unless clinical circumstances demand such use.

Hypersensitivity to any component of this product, including sulfites (see WARNINGS).

WARNINGS

Use of sympathomimetic amines with monoamine oxidase inhibitors or tricyclic antidepressants may result in potentiation of the pressor effect. (See PRECAUTIONS, *Drug Interactions.*)

ARAMINE contains sodium bisulfite, a sulfite that may cause allergic-type reactions including anaphylactic symptoms and life-threatening or less severe asthmatic episodes in certain susceptible people. The overall prevalence of sulfite sensitivity in the general population is unknown and probably low. Sulfite sensitivity is seen more frequently in asthmatic than in nonasthmatic people.

PRECAUTIONS

General
Caution should be used to avoid excessive blood pressure response. Rapidly induced hypertensive responses have been reported to cause acute pulmonary edema, arrhythmias, cerebral hemorrhage, or cardiac arrest.

Patients with cirrhosis should be treated with caution, with adequate restoration of electrolytes if diuresis ensues. Fatal ventricular arrhythmia was reported in one patient with Laennec's cirrhosis while receiving metaraminol bitartrate. In several instances, ventricular extrasystoles that appeared during infusion of this vasopressor subsided promptly when the rate of infusion was reduced.

With the prolonged action of ARAMINE, a cumulative effect is possible. If there is an excessive vasopressor response there may be a prolonged elevation of blood pressure even after discontinuation of therapy.

When vasopressor amines are used for long periods, the resulting vasoconstriction may prevent adequate expansion of circulating volume and may cause perpetuation of shock. There is evidence that plasma volume may be reduced in all types of shock, and that the measurement of central venous pressure is useful in assessing the adequacy of the circulating blood volume. Therefore, blood or plasma volume expanders should be used when the principal reason for hypotension or shock is decreased circulating volume.

Because of its vasoconstrictor effect ARAMINE should be given with caution in heart or thyroid disease, hypertension, or diabetes. Sympathomimetic amines may provoke a relapse in patients with a history of malaria.

Drug Interactions
ARAMINE should be used with caution in digitalized patients, since the combination of digitalis and sympathomimetic amines may cause ectopic arrhythmias.

Monoamine oxidase inhibitors or tricyclic antidepressants may potentiate the action of sympathomimetic amines. Therefore, when initiating pressor therapy in patients receiving these drugs, the initial dose should be small and given with caution. (See WARNINGS.)

Carcinogenesis, Mutagenesis,
Impairment of Fertility
Studies in animals have not been performed to evaluate the mutagenic or carcinogenic potential of ARAMINE or its potential to affect fertility.

Pregnancy
Pregnancy Category C. Animal reproduction studies have not been conducted with ARAMINE. It is not known whether ARAMINE can cause fetal harm when given to a pregnant woman or can affect reproduction capacity. ARAMINE should be given to a pregnant woman only if clearly needed.

Nursing Mothers
It is not known whether this drug is secreted in human milk. Because many drugs are secreted in human milk, caution should be exercised when ARAMINE is given to a nursing woman.

Pediatric Use
Safety and effectiveness in children have not been established.

ADVERSE REACTIONS

Sympathomimetic amines, including ARAMINE, may cause sinus or ventricular tachycardia, or other arrhythmias, especially in patients with myocardial infarction. (See PRECAUTIONS.)

In patients with a history of malaria, these compounds may provoke a relapse.

Abscess formation, tissue necrosis, or sloughing rarely may follow the use of ARAMINE. In choosing the site of injection, it is important to avoid those areas recognized as *not* suitable for use of any pressor agent and to discontinue the infusion immediately if infiltration or thrombosis occurs. Although the physician may be forced by the urgent nature of the patient's condition to choose injection sites that are not recognized as suitable, he should, when possible, use the preferred areas of injection. The larger veins of the antecubital fossa or the thigh are preferred to veins in the dorsum of the hand or ankle veins, particularly in patients with peripheral vascular disease, diabetes mellitus, Buerger's disease, or conditions with coexistent hypercoagulability.

OVERDOSAGE

Overdosage may result in severe hypertension accompanied by headache, constricting sensation in the chest, nausea, vomiting, euphoria, diaphoresis, pulmonary edema, tachycardia, bradycardia, sinus arrhythmia, atrial or ventricular arrhythmias, cerebral hemorrhage, myocardial infarction, cardiac arrest or convulsions.

Should an excessive elevation of blood pressure occur, it may be immediately relieved by a sympatholytic agent, e.g. phentolamine. An appropriate antiarrhythmic agent may also be required.

The oral LD_{50} in the rat and mouse is 240 mg/kg and 99 mg/kg, respectively.

DOSAGE AND ADMINISTRATION

ARAMINE may be given intramuscularly, subcutaneously, or intravenously, the route depending on the nature and severity of the indication.

Parenteral drug products should be inspected visually for particulate matter and discoloration prior to use, whenever solution and container permit.

Allow at least 10 minutes to elapse before increasing the dose because the maximum effect is not immediately apparent. When the vasopressor is discontinued, observe the patient carefully as the effect of the drug tapers off, so that therapy can be reinitiated promptly if the blood pressure falls too rapidly. The response to vasopressors may be poor in patients with coexistent shock and acidosis. When indicated, established methods of shock management should be used, such as blood or fluid replacement.

Intramuscular or Subcutaneous Injection (for prevention of hypotension—see INDICATIONS): The recommended dose is 2 to 10 mg (0.2 to 1 mL). As with other agents given subcutaneously, only the preferred sites of injection, as set forth in standard texts, should be used.

Intravenous Infusion (for adjunctive treatment of hypotension—see INDICATIONS): The recommended dose is 15 to 100 mg (1.5 to 10 mL) in 500 mL of Sodium Chloride Injection or 5% Dextrose Injection, adjusting the rate of infusion to maintain the blood pressure at the desired level. Higher concentrations of ARAMINE, 150 to 500 mg per 500 mL of infusion fluid, have been used.

If the patient needs more saline or dextrose solution at a rate of flow that would provide an excessive dose of the vasopressor, the recommended volume of infusion fluid (500 mL) should be increased accordingly. ARAMINE may also be added to *less* than 500 mL of infusion fluid if a smaller volume is desired.

Compatibility Information
In addition to Sodium Chloride Injection and Dextrose Injection 5%, the following infusion solutions were found physically and chemically compatible with Injection ARAMINE when 5 mL of Injection ARAMINE, 10 mg/mL (metaraminol equivalent), was added to 500 mL of infusion solution: Ringer's Injection, Lactated Ringer's Injection, Dextran 6% in Saline†, Normosol®-R pH 7.4†, and Normosol®-M in D5-W†.

When Injection ARAMINE is mixed with an infusion solution, sterile precautions should be observed. Since infusion solutions generally do not contain preservatives, mixtures should be used within 24 hours.

Direct Intravenous Injection: In severe shock, when time is of great importance, this agent should be given by direct intravenous injection. The suggested dose is 0.5 to 5 mg (0.05 to 0.5 mL), followed by an infusion of 15 to 100 mg (1.5 to 10 mL) in 500 mL of infusion fluid as described previously.

Vials may be sterilized by autoclaving or by immersion in a sterilizing solution.

HOW SUPPLIED

No. 3222X—Injection ARAMINE 1%, containing metaraminol bitartrate equivalent to 10 mg of metaraminol per mL, is a clear, colorless solution and is supplied as follows:
NDC 0006-3222-10 in 10 mL vials
(6505-00-753-9601 10 mL vial).

Storage
Protect from light. Store container in carton until contents have been used.
Avoid storage at temperatures below -20°C (-4°F) and above 40°C (104°F).

A.H.F.S. Category: 12:12
DC 7348522   Issued May 1987

ATTENUVAX®   ℞
(Measles Virus Vaccine Live, MSD), U.S.P.
(More Attenuated Enders' Strain)

DESCRIPTION

ATTENUVAX® (Measles Virus Vaccine Live, MSD) is a live virus vaccine for immunization against measles (rubeola).

ATTENUVAX is a sterile lyophilized preparation of a more attenuated line of measles virus derived from Enders' attenuated Edmonston strain. The further modification of the virus in ATTENUVAX was achieved in the Merck Institute for Therapeutic Research by multiple passage of Edmonston strain virus in cell cultures of chick embryo at low temperature.

The reconstituted vaccine is for subcutaneous administration. When reconstituted as directed, the dose for injection is 0.5 mL and contains not less than the equivalent of 1,000 $TCID_{50}$ (tissue culture infectious doses) of the U.S. Reference Measles Virus. Each dose also contains approximately 25 mcg of neomycin. The product contains no preservative. Sorbitol and hydrolized gelatin are added as stabilizers.

CLINICAL PHARMACOLOGY

ATTENUVAX produces a modified measles infection in susceptible persons. Fever and rash may appear. Extensive clinical trials have demonstrated that ATTENUVAX is highly immunogenic and generally well tolerated. A single injection of the vaccine has been shown to induce measles hemagglutination-inhibiting (HI) antibodies in 97 percent or more of susceptible persons. Vaccine-induced antibody levels have been shown to persist for at least 13 years without substantial decline. If the present pattern continues, it will provide a basis for the expectation that immunity following vaccination will be permanent. However, continued surveillance will be required to demonstrate this point.

INDICATIONS AND USAGE

ATTENUVAX is indicated for immunization against measles (rubeola) in persons 15 months of age or older. A booster is not needed. Infants who are less than 15 months of age may fail to respond to the vaccine due to presence in the circulation of residual measles antibody of maternal origin; the younger the infant, the lower the likelihood of seroconversion. In geographically isolated or other relatively inaccessible populations for whom immunization programs are logistically difficult, and in population groups in which natural measles infection may occur in a significant proportion of infants before 15 months of age, it may be desirable to give the vaccine to infants at an earlier age. Infants vaccinated under these conditions at less than 12 months of age should

†Product of Abbott Laboratories

be revaccinated after reaching 15 months of age. There is some evidence to suggest that infants immunized at less than one year of age may not develop sustained antibody levels when later reimmunized. The advantage of early protection must be weighed against the chance for failure to respond adequately on reimmunization.

According to ACIP recommendations, most persons born in 1956 or earlier are likely to have been infected naturally and generally need not be considered susceptible. All children, adolescents, and adults born after 1956 are considered susceptible and should be vaccinated, if there are no contraindications. This includes persons who may be immune to measles but who lack adequate documentation of immunity as evidenced by: (1) physician-diagnosed measles, (2) laboratory evidence of measles immunity, or (3) adequate immunization with live measles vaccine on or after the first birthday.

ATTENUVAX given immediately after exposure to natural measles may provide some protection. If, however, the vaccine is given a few days before exposure, substantial protection may be provided.

Revaccination: Children vaccinated when younger than 12 months of age should be revaccinated, particularly if vaccine was administered with immune serum globulin or measles immune globulin, a standardized globulin preparation. Based on available evidence, there is no reason to routinely revaccinate persons who were vaccinated originally when 12 months of age or older. However, persons should be revaccinated if there is evidence to suggest that initial immunization was ineffective.

Despite the risk of reactions (see ADVERSE REACTIONS), persons born since 1956 who have previously been given inactivated vaccine alone or followed by live vaccine within 3 months should be revaccinated with live vaccine to reduce the risk of the severe atypical form of natural measles that may occur.

Use with other Vaccines

Routine administration of DTP (diphtheria, tetanus, pertussis) and/or OPV (oral poliovirus vaccine) concomitantly with measles, mumps and rubella vaccines is not recommended because there are insufficient data relating to the simultaneous administration of these antigens. However, the American Academy of Pediatrics has noted that in some circumstances, particularly when the patient may not return, some practitioners prefer to administer all these antigens on a single day. If done, separate sites and syringes should be used for DTP and ATTENUVAX.

ATTENUVAX should not be given less than one month before or after administration of other virus vaccines.

CONTRAINDICATIONS

Do not give ATTENUVAX to pregnant females; the possible effects of the vaccine on fetal development are unknown at this time. If vaccination of postpubertal females is undertaken, pregnancy should be avoided for three months following vaccination (see PRECAUTIONS, *Pregnancy*).

Anaphylactoid reaction to neomycin (each dose of reconstituted vaccine contains approximately 25 mcg of neomycin). History of anaphylactoid reaction to eggs (see HYPERSENSITIVITY TO EGGS below).

Any febrile respiratory illness or other active febrile infection.

Active untreated tuberculosis.

Patients receiving immunosuppressive therapy. This contraindication does not apply to patients who are receiving corticosteroids as replacement therapy, e.g., for Addison's disease.

Individuals with blood dyscrasias, leukemia, lymphomas of any type, or other malignant neoplasms affecting the bone marrow or lymphatic systems.

Primary immunodeficiency states, including cellular immune deficiencies, hypogammaglobulinemic and dysgammaglobulinemic states.

Individuals with a family history of congenital or hereditary immunodeficiency, until the immune competence of the potential vaccine recipient is demonstrated.

HYPERSENSITIVITY TO EGGS

Live measles vaccine is produced in chick embryo cell culture. Persons with a history of anaphylactoid or other immediate reactions (e.g., hives, swelling of the mouth and throat, difficulty breathing, hypotension and shock) subsequent to egg ingestion should not be vaccinated. Evidence indicates that persons are not at increased risk if they have egg allergies that are not anaphylactoid in nature. Such persons should be vaccinated in the usual manner. There is no evidence to indicate that persons with allergies to chickens or feathers are at increased risk of reaction to the vaccine.

PRECAUTIONS
General

Adequate treatment provisions including epinephrine, should be available for immediate use should an anaphylactoid reaction occur.

Due caution should be employed in administration of measles vaccine to persons with a history of febrile convulsions, or cerebral injury, or of any other condition in which stress due to fever should be avoided. The physician should be alert to the temperature elevation which may occur following vaccination. (See ADVERSE REACTIONS).

Vaccination should be deferred for at least 3 months following blood or plasma transfusions, or administration of human immune serum globulin.

There are no reports of transmission of live attenuated measles virus from vaccinees to susceptible contacts.

It has been reported that attenuated measles virus vaccine, live, may result in a temporary depression of tuberculin skin sensitivity. Therefore, if a tuberculin test is to be done, it should be administered either before or simultaneously with ATTENUVAX.

Children under treatment for tuberculosis have not experienced exacerbation of the disease when immunized with live measles virus vaccine; no studies have been reported to date of the effect of measles virus vaccines on untreated tuberculous children.

As for any vaccine, vaccination with ATTENUVAX may not result in seroconversion in 100% of susceptible persons given the vaccine.

Pregnancy

Pregnancy Category C

Animal reproduction studies have not been conducted with ATTENUVAX. It is also not known whether ATTENUVAX can cause fetal harm when administered to a pregnant woman or can affect reproduction capacity. Therefore, the vaccine should not be administered to pregnant females; furthermore, pregnancy should be avoided for three months following vaccination (see CONTRAINDICATIONS).

Reports have indicated that contracting of natural measles during pregnancy enhances fetal risk. Increased rates of spontaneous abortion, stillbirth, congenital defects and prematurity have been observed subsequent to natural measles during pregnancy. There are no adequate studies of the attenuated (vaccine) strain of measles virus in pregnancy. However, it would be prudent to assume that the vaccine strain of virus is also capable of inducing adverse fetal effects for up to three months following vaccination.

Vaccine administration to postpubertal females entails a potential for inadvertent immunization during pregnancy. Theoretical risks involved should be weighed against the risks that measles poses to the unimmunized adolescent or adult. Advisory committees reviewing this matter have recommended vaccination of postpubertal females who are presumed to be susceptible to measles and not known to be pregnant. If a measles exposure occurs during pregnancy, one should consider the possibility of providing temporary passive immunity through the administration of immune globulin (human).

Nursing Mothers

It is not known whether measles vaccine virus is secreted in human milk. Therefore, because many drugs are excreted in human milk, caution should be exercised when ATTENUVAX is administered to a nursing woman.

ADVERSE REACTIONS

Because of the slightly acidic pH (6.2–6.6) of the vaccine, patients may complain of burning and/or stinging of short duration at the injection site.

Occasional

Moderate fever [101–102.9°F (38.3–39.4°C)] may occur during the month after vaccination. Generally, fever, rash, or both appear between the 5th and the 12th days. Rash, when it occurs, is usually minimal, but rarely may be generalized.

Less Common

High fever [over 103°F (39.4°C)].

Rare

Reactions at injection site. Allergic reactions such as wheal and flare at the injection site or urticaria have been reported.

Children developing fever may, on rare occasions, exhibit febrile convulsions.

Thrombocytopenia and purpura have occurred rarely.

Forms of optic neuritis, including retrobulbar neuritis, papillitis, and retinitis may infrequently follow viral infections, and have been reported to occur 1 to 3 weeks following inoculation with some live virus vaccines.

Experience from more than 80 million doses of all live measles vaccines given in the U.S. through 1975 indicates that significant central nervous system reactions such as encephalitis and encephalopathy, occurring within 30 days after vaccination, have been temporally associated with measles vaccine approximately once for every million doses. In no case has it been shown that reactions were actually caused by vaccine. The Center for Disease Control has pointed out that "a certain number of cases of encephalitis may be expected to occur in a large childhood population in a defined

period of time even when no vaccines are administered". However, the data suggest the possibility that some of these cases may have been caused by measles vaccines. The risk of such serious neurological disorders following live measles virus vaccine administration remains far less than that for encephalitis and encephalopathy with natural measles (one per two thousand reported cases).

There have been isolated reports of ocular palsies and Guillain-Barre syndrome occurring after immunization with vaccines containing live attenuated measles virus. The ocular palsies have occurred approximately 3–24 days following vaccination. No definite causal relationship has been established between either of these events and vaccination.

There have been reports of subacute sclerosing panencephalitis (SSPE) in children who did not have a history of natural measles but did receive measles vaccine. Some of these cases may have resulted from unrecognized measles in the first year of life or possibly from the measles vaccination. Based on estimated nationwide measles vaccine distribution, the association of SSPE cases to measles vaccination is about one case per million vaccine doses distributed. This is far less than the association with natural measles, 6–22 cases of SSPE per million cases of measles. The results of a retrospective case-controlled study conducted by the Center for Disease Control suggest that the overall effect of measles vaccine is to protect against SSPE by preventing measles with its inherent higher risk of SSPE.

Local reactions characterized by marked swelling, redness and vesiculation at the injection site of attenuated live virus measles vaccines, and systemic reactions including atypical measles, have occurred in persons who have previously received killed measles vaccine. Rarely, more severe reactions that require hospitalization, including prolonged high fevers, panniculitis, and extensive local reactions, have been reported.

DOSAGE AND ADMINISTRATION

FOR SUBCUTANEOUS ADMINISTRATION

Do not inject intravenously

The dosage of vaccine is the same for all persons. Inject the total volume of the single dose vial (about 0.5 mL) or 0.5 mL of the multiple dose vial of reconstituted vaccine subcutaneously, preferably into the outer aspect of upper arm. *Do not give immune globulin (IG) concurrently with* ATTENUVAX.

During shipment, to insure that there is no loss of potency, the vaccine must be maintained at a temperature of 10°C (50°F) or less.

Before reconstitution, store ATTENUVAX at 2–8°C (35.6–46.4°F). *Protect from light.*

CAUTION: A sterile syringe free of preservatives, antiseptics, and detergents should be used for each injection and/or reconstitution of the vaccine because these substances may inactivate the live virus vaccine. A 25 gauge, 5/8" needle is recommended.

To reconstitute, use only the diluent supplied, since it is free of preservatives or other antiviral substances which might inactivate the vaccine.

Single Dose Vial—First withdraw the entire volume of diluent into the syringe to be used for reconstitution. Inject all the diluent in the syringe into the vial of lyophilized vaccine, and agitate to mix thoroughly. Withdraw the entire contents into a syringe and inject the total volume of restored vaccine subcutaneously.

It is important to use a separate sterile syringe and needle for each individual patient to prevent transmission of hepatitis B and other infectious agents from one person to another.

10 Dose Vial (available only to government agencies/institutions)—Withdraw the entire contents (7 mL) of the diluent vial into the sterile syringe to be used for reconstitution, and introduce into the 10 dose vial of lyophilized vaccine. Agitate to ensure thorough mixing. The outer labeling suggests "For Jet Injector or Syringe Use". Use with separate sterile syringes is permitted for containers of 10 doses or less. The vaccine and diluent do not contain preservatives; therefore, the user must recognize the potential contamination hazards and exercise special precautions to protect the sterility and potency of the product. The use of aseptic techniques and proper storage prior to and after restoration of the vaccine and subsequent withdrawal of the individual doses is essential. Use 0.5 mL of the reconstituted vaccine for subcutaneous injection.

It is important to use a separate sterile syringe and needle for each individual patient to prevent transmission of hepatitis B and other infectious agents from one person to another.

Continued on next page

Merck Sharp & Dohme—Cont.

50 Dose Vial (available only to government agencies/institutions)—Withdraw the entire contents (30 mL) of diluent vial into the sterile syringe to be used for reconstitution and introduce into the 50 dose vial of lyophilized vaccine. Agitate to ensure thorough mixing. With full aseptic precautions, attach the vial to the sterilized multidose jet injector apparatus. Use 0.5 mL of the reconstituted vaccine for subcutaneous injection.

Each dose of ATTENUVAX contains not less than 1,000 $TCID_{50}$ (tissue culture infectious doses) of measles virus vaccine expressed in terms of the assigned titer of the U.S. Reference Measles Virus.

Parenteral drug products should be inspected visually for particulate matter and discoloration prior to administration. ATTENUVAX, when reconstituted, is clear yellow.

HOW SUPPLIED

No. 4709—ATTENUVAX is supplied as a single-dose vial of lyophilized vaccine, **NDC** 0006-4709-00, and a vial of diluent.
No. 4589X/4309—ATTENUVAX is supplied as follows: (1) a box of 10 single-dose vials of lyophilized vaccine (package A), **NDC** 0006-4589-00; and (2) a box of 10 vials of diluent (package B). To conserve refrigerator space, the diluent may be stored separately at room temperature.
Available only to government agencies/institutions:
No. 4614X—ATTENUVAX is supplied as one 10 dose vial of lyophilized vaccine, **NDC** 0006-4614-00, and one 7 mL vial of diluent.
No. 4591X—ATTENUVAX is supplied as one 50 dose vial of lyophilized vaccine, **NDC** 0006-4591-00, and one 30 mL vial of diluent.
Storage
It is recommended that the vaccine be used as soon as possible after reconstitution. Protect vaccine from light at all times, since such exposure may inactivate the virus. Store reconstituted vaccine in the vaccine vial in a dark place at 2–8°C (35.6–46.4°F) and discard if not used within 8 hours.

A.H.F.S. Category: 80:12
DC 7075508   Issued September 1985
COPYRIGHT © MERCK & CO., INC., 1985
All rights reserved

BENEMID® Tablets   ℞
(Probenecid, MSD), U.S.P.

DESCRIPTION

BENEMID® (Probenecid, MSD) is a uricosuric and renal tubular transport blocking agent.
Probenecid is the generic name for 4-[(dipropylamino) sulfonyl] benzoic acid (molecular weight 285.36). It has the following structural formula:

Probenecid is a white or nearly white, fine, crystalline powder. Probenecid is soluble in dilute alkali, in alcohol, in chloroform, and in acetone; it is practically insoluble in water and in dilute acids.
Each tablet contains 0.5 g probenecid and the following inactive ingredients: calcium stearate, D&C Yellow 10, gelatin, hydroxypropyl methylcellulose, iron oxide, magnesium carbonate, polyethylene glycol, starch, talc, and titanium dioxide.

ACTIONS

BENEMID is a uricosuric and renal tubular blocking agent. It inhibits the tubular reabsorption of urate, thus increasing the urinary excretion of uric acid and decreasing serum urate levels. Effective uricosuria reduces the miscible urate pool, retards urate deposition, and promotes resorption of urate deposits.
BENEMID inhibits the tubular secretion of penicillin and usually increases penicillin plasma levels by any route the antibiotic is given. A 2-fold to 4-fold elevation has been demonstrated for various penicillins.
BENEMID also has been reported to inhibit the renal transport of many other compounds including aminohippuric acid (PAH), aminosalicylic acid (PAS), indomethacin, sodium iodomethamate and related iodinated organic acids, 17-ketosteroids, pantothenic acid, phenolsulfonphthalein (PSP), sulfonamides, and sulfonylureas. See also DRUG INTERACTIONS.
BENEMID decreases both hepatic and renal excretion of sulfobromophthalein (BSP). The tubular reabsorption of phosphorus is inhibited in hypoparathyroid but not in euparathyroid individuals.

BENEMID does not influence plasma concentrations of salicylates, nor the excretion of streptomycin, chloramphenicol, chlortetracycline, oxytetracycline, or neomycin.

INDICATIONS

For treatment of the hyperuricemia associated with gout and gouty arthritis.
As an adjuvant to therapy with penicillin or with ampicillin, methicillin, oxacillin, cloxacillin, or nafcillin, for elevation and prolongation of plasma levels by whatever route the antibiotic is given.

CONTRAINDICATIONS

Hypersensitivity to this product.
Children under 2 years of age.
Not recommended in persons with known blood dyscrasias or uric acid kidney stones.
Therapy with BENEMID should not be started until an acute gouty attack has subsided.

WARNINGS

Exacerbation of gout following therapy with BENEMID may occur; in such cases colchicine or other appropriate therapy is advisable.
BENEMID increases plasma concentrations of methotrexate in both animals and humans. In animal studies, increased methotrexate toxicity has been reported. If BENEMID is given with methotrexate, the dosage of methotrexate should be reduced and serum levels may need to be monitored.
In patients on BENEMID the use of salicylates in either small or large doses is contraindicated because it antagonizes the uricosuric action of BENEMID. The biphasic action of salicylates in the renal tubules accounts for the so-called "paradoxical effect" of uricosuric agents. In patients on BENEMID who require a mild analgesic agent the use of acetaminophen rather than small doses of salicylates would be preferred.
Rarely, severe allergic reactions and anaphylaxis have been reported with the use of BENEMID. Most of these have been reported to occur within several hours after readministration following prior usage of the drug.
The appearance of hypersensitivity reactions requires cessation of therapy with BENEMID.
Use in Pregnancy: BENEMID crosses the placental barrier and appears in cord blood. The use of any drug in women of childbearing potential requires that the anticipated benefit be weighed against possible hazards.

PRECAUTIONS

General
Hematuria, renal colic, costovertebral pain, and formation of uric acid stones associated with the use of BENEMID in gouty patients may be prevented by alkalization of the urine and a liberal fluid intake (*see* DOSAGE AND ADMINISTRATION). In these cases when alkali is administered, the acid-base balance of the patient should be watched.
Use with caution in patients with a history of peptic ulcer.
BENEMID has been used in patients with some renal impairment but dosage requirements may be increased. BENEMID may not be effective in chronic renal insufficiency particularly when the glomerular filtration rate is 30 mL/minute or less. Because of its mechanism of action, BENEMID is not recommended in conjunction with a penicillin in the presence of *known* renal impairment.
A reducing substance may appear in the urine of patients receiving BENEMID. This disappears with discontinuance of therapy. Suspected glycosuria should be confirmed by using a test specific for glucose.
Drug Interactions
When BENEMID is used to elevate plasma concentrations of penicillin or other beta-lactams, or when such drugs are given to patients taking BENEMID therapeutically, high plasma concentrations of the other drug may increase the incidence of adverse reactions associated with that drug. In the case of penicillin or other beta-lactams, psychic disturbances have been reported.
The use of salicylates antagonizes the uricosuric action of BENEMID (*see* WARNINGS). The uricosuric action of BENEMID is also antagonized by pyrazinamide.
BENEMID produces an insignificant increase in free sulfonamide plasma concentrations but a significant increase in total sulfonamide plasma levels. Since BENEMID decreases the renal excretion of conjugated sulfonamides, plasma concentrations of the latter should be determined from time to time when a sulfonamide and BENEMID are coadministered for prolonged periods. BENEMID may prolong or enhance the action of oral sulfonylureas and thereby increase the risk of hypoglycemia.
It has been reported that patients receiving BENEMID require significantly less thiopental for induction of anesthesia. In addition, ketamine and thiopental anesthesia were significantly prolonged in rats receiving probenecid.

The concomitant administration of probenecid increases the mean plasma elimination half-life of a number of drugs which can lead to increased plasma concentrations. These include agents such as indomethacin, acetaminophen, naproxen, ketoprofen, meclofenamate, lorazepam, and rifampin. Although the clinical significance of this observation has not been established, a lower dosage of the drug may be required to produce a therapeutic effect, and increases in dosage of the drug in question should be made cautiously and in small increments when probenecid is being co-administered. Although specific instances of toxicity due to this potential interaction have not been observed to date physicians should be alert to this possibility.
Probenecid given concomitantly with sulindac had only a slight effect on plasma sulfide levels, while plasma levels of sulindac and sulfone were increased. Sulindac was shown to produce a modest reduction in the uricosuric action of probenecid, which probably is not significant under most circumstances.
In animals and in humans, BENEMID has been reported to increase plasma concentrations of methotrexate (*see* WARNINGS).
Falsely high readings for theophylline have been reported in an *in vitro* study, using the Schack and Waxler technic, when therapeutic concentrations of theophylline and BENEMID were added to human plasma.

ADVERSE REACTIONS

The following adverse reactions have been observed and within each category are listed in order of decreasing severity.
Central Nervous System: headache, dizziness.
Metabolic: precipitation of acute gouty arthritis.
Gastrointestinal: hepatic necrosis, vomiting, nausea, anorexia, sore gums.
Genitourinary: nephrotic syndrome, uric acid stones with or without hematuria, renal colic, costovertebral pain, urinary frequency.
Hypersensitivity: anaphylaxis, fever, urticaria, pruritus.
Hematologic: aplastic anemia, leukopenia, hemolytic anemia which in some patients could be related to genetic deficiency of glucose -6- phosphate dehydrogenase in red blood cells, anemia.
Integumentary: dermatitis, alopecia, flushing.

DOSAGE AND ADMINISTRATION

Gout
Therapy with BENEMID should not be *started* until an acute gouty attack has subsided. However, if an acute attack is precipitated *during* therapy, BENEMID may be continued without changing the dosage, and full therapeutic dosage of colchicine or other appropriate therapy should be given to control the acute attack.
The recommended adult dosage is 0.25 g (½ tablet of BENEMID) twice a day for one week, followed by 0.5 g (1 tablet) twice a day thereafter.
Some degree of renal impairment may be present in patients with gout. A daily dosage of 1 g may be adequate. However, if necessary, the daily dosage may be increased by 0.5 g increments every 4 weeks within tolerance (and usually not above 2 g per day) if symptoms of gouty arthritis are not controlled or the 24 hour uric acid excretion is not above 700 mg. As noted, BENEMID may not be effective in chronic renal insufficiency particularly when the glomerular filtration rate is 30 mL/minute or less.
Gastric intolerance may be indicative of overdosage, and may be corrected by decreasing the dosage.
As uric acid tends to crystallize out of an acid urine, a liberal fluid intake is recommended, as well as sufficient sodium bicarbonate (3 to 7.5 g daily) or potassium citrate (7.5 g daily) to maintain an alkaline urine (*see* PRECAUTIONS).
Alkalization of the urine is recommended until the serum urate level returns to normal limits and tophaceous deposits disappear, i.e., during the period when urinary excretion of uric acid is at a high level. Thereafter, alkalization of the urine and the usual restriction of purine-producing foods may be somewhat relaxed.
BENEMID should be continued at the dosage that will maintain normal serum urate levels. When acute attacks have been absent for 6 months or more and serum urate levels remain within normal limits, the daily dosage may be decreased by 0.5 g every 6 months. The maintenance dosage should not be reduced to the point where serum urate levels tend to rise.
BENEMID *and Penicillin Therapy (General)*
Adults:
The recommended dosage is 2 g (4 tablets of BENEMID) daily in divided doses. This dosage should be reduced in older patients in whom renal impairment may be present.
Children 2-14 years of age:
Initial dose: 25 mg/kg body weight (or 0.7 g/square meter body surface).

BENEMID® (Probenecid, MSD)   Penicillin Therapy (Gonorrhea)*

	Recommended Regimens**	Remarks
Uncomplicated gonococcal infection in men and women (urethral, cervical, rectal)	4.8 million units of aqueous procaine penicillin G† I.M., in at least 2 doses injected at different sites at one visit + 1 g of BENEMID (Probenecid, MSD) orally just before injections *or* 3.5 g of ampicillin† orally + 1 g of BENEMID orally given simultaneously.	Follow-up: Obtain urethral and other appropriate cultures from men, and cervical, anal, and other appropriate cultures from women, 7 to 14 days after completion of treatment. Treatment of sexual partners: Persons with known recent exposure to gonorrhea should receive same treatment as those known to have gonorrhea. Examination and treatment of male sex partners of persons with gonorrhea are essential because of high prevalence of nonsymptomatic urethral gonococcal infection in such men.
Pharyngeal gonococcal infection in men and women	4.8 million units of aqueous procaine penicillin G† I.M., in at least 2 doses injected at different sites at one visit + 1 g of BENEMID orally just before injections	Pharyngeal gonococcal infections may be more difficult to treat than anogenital gonorrhea. Posttreatment cultures are essential.
Uncomplicated gonorrhea in pregnant patients	4.8 million units of aqueous procaine penicillin G† I.M., in at least 2 doses injected at different sites at one visit *or* 3.5 g of ampicillin† orally + 1 g of BENEMID orally given simultaneously	
Acute gonococcal salpingitis	*Outpatients:* Aqueous procaine penicillin G† or ampicillin† with BENEMID as for gonorrhea in pregnancy, followed by 500 mg of ampicillin 4 times a day for 10 days *Hospitalized patients:* See details in CDC recommendations	Follow-up of patients with acute salpingitis is essential. All patients should receive repeat pelvic examinations and cultures for *Neisseria gonorrhoeae* after treatment. Examination and appropriate treatment of male sex partners are essential because of high prevalence of nonsymptomatic urethral gonorrhea in such men.
Disseminated gonococcal infection (arthritis-dermatitis syndrome)	10 million units of aqueous crystalline penicillin G† I.V. a day for 3 days or till significant clinical improvement occurs. May be followed with 500 mg of ampicillin† 4 times a day orally to complete 7 days of treatment *or* 3.5 g of ampicillin† orally with 1 g of BENEMID, followed by 500 mg of ampicillin† 4 times a day for at least 7 days	
Gonococcal infection in children	For postpubertal children and/or those weighing over 45 kg (100 lb) use the dosage regimens given above for adults Uncomplicated vulvovaginitis and urethritis: aqueous procaine penicillin G† 75,000–100,000 units/kg I.M., with BENEMID 23 mg/kg orally	See CDC recommendations for detailed information about prevention and treatment of neonatal gonococcal infection and gonococcal ophthalmia.

Note: Before treating gonococcal infections in patients with suspected primary or secondary syphilis, perform proper diagnostic procedures including darkfield examinations. If concomitant syphilis is suspected, perform monthly serological tests for at least 4 months.
*   Recommended by Venereal Disease Control Advisory Committee, Center for Disease Control, U.S. Department of Health, Education, and Welfare, Public Health Service (Morbidity and Mortality Weekly Report, Vol. *23*: 341, 342, 347, 348, Oct. 11, 1974).
**   See CDC recommendations for definition of regimens of choice, alternative regimens, treatment of hypersensitive patients, and other aspects of therapy.
†   See package circulars of manufacturers for detailed information about contraindications, warnings, precautions, and adverse reactions.

Maintenance dose: 40 mg/kg body weight (*or* 1.2 g/square meter body surface) per day, divided into 4 doses.
For children weighing more than 50 kg (110 lb) the adult dosage is recommended.
BENEMID is contraindicated in children under 2 years of age.
The PSP excretion test may be used to determine the effectiveness of BENEMID in retarding penicillin excretion and maintaining therapeutic levels. The renal clearance of PSP is reduced to about one-fifth the normal rate when dosage of BENEMID is adequate.
Penicillin Therapy (Gonorrhea)
[See table above].

HOW SUPPLIED

No. 3337—Tablets BENEMID, 0.5 g, are yellow, capsule shaped, scored, film coated tablets, coded MSD 501. They are supplied as follows:
NDC 0006-0501-68 bottles of 100
(6505-00-104-9735 100's)
NDC 0006-0501-28 unit dose packages of 100
NDC 0006-0501-82 bottles of 1000
(6505-00-181-8387 1000's).
    Shown in Product Identification Section, page 418
      A.H.F.S. Category: 40:40
      DC 7399020   Issued August 1988

BIAVAX®II   ℞
(Rubella and Mumps Virus Vaccine Live, MSD), U.S.P.

DESCRIPTION

BIAVAX® II (Rubella and Mumps Virus Vaccine Live, MSD) is a live virus vaccine for immunization against rubella (German measles) and mumps.

BIAVAX II is a sterile lyophilized preparation of the Wistar RA 27/3 strain of live attenuated rubella virus grown in human diploid cell (WI-38) culture; and the Jeryl Lynn (B level) strain of mumps virus grown in cell cultures of chick embryo. The vaccine viruses are the same as those used in the manufacture of MERUVAX® II (Rubella Virus Vaccine Live, MSD) and MUMPSVAX® (Mumps Virus Vaccine Live, MSD). The two viruses are mixed before being lyophilized. The reconstituted vaccine is for subcutaneous administration. When reconstituted as directed, the dose for injection is 0.5 mL and contains not less than the equivalent of 1,000 $TCID_{50}$ of the U.S. Reference Rubella Virus and 5,000 $TCID_{50}$ of the U.S. Reference Mumps Virus. Each dose contains approximately 25 mcg of neomycin. The product contains no preservative. Sorbitol and hydrolized gelatin are added as stabilizers.

CLINICAL PHARMACOLOGY

Clinical studies of 73 double seronegative children 12 months to 2 years of age demonstrated that BIAVAX II is highly immunogenic and generally well tolerated. In these studies, a single injection of the vaccine induced rubella hemagglutination-inhibition (HI) antibodies in 100 percent, and mumps neutralizing antibodies in 97 percent of the susceptible children.
The RA 27/3 rubella strain in BIAVAX II elicits higher immediate post-vaccination HI, complement-fixing and neutralizing antibody levels than other strains of rubella vaccine and has been shown to induce a broader profile of circulating antibodies including anti-theta and anti-iota precipitating antibodies. The RA 27/3 rubella strain immunologically simulates natural infection more closely than other rubella vaccine viruses. The increased levels and broader profile of antibodies produced by RA 27/3 strain rubella virus vaccine appear to correlate with greater resistance to

subclinical reinfection with the wild virus, and provide greater confidence for lasting immunity.
Vaccine induced antibody levels following administration of BIAVAX II have been shown to persist for at least two years without substantial decline. Antibody levels after immunization with BIAVAX (Rubella and Mumps Virus Vaccine Live, MSD), containing the HPV-77 strain of rubella, have persisted for 10.5 years without substantial decline. If the present pattern continues, it will provide a basis for the expectation that immunity following vaccination will be permanent. However, continued surveillance will be required to demonstrate this point.

INDICATIONS AND USAGE

BIAVAX II is indicated for simultaneous immunization against rubella and mumps in persons 12 months of age or older. A booster is not needed.
The vaccine is not recommended for infants younger than 12 months because they may retain maternal rubella and mumps neutralizing antibodies which may interfere with the immune response.
Previously unimmunized children of susceptible pregnant women should receive live attenuated rubella vaccine, because an immunized child will be less likely to acquire natural rubella and introduce the virus into the household.
Non-Pregnant Adolescent and Adult Females
Immunization of susceptible non-pregnant adolescent and adult females of childbearing age with live attenuated rubella virus vaccine is indicated if certain precautions are

Continued on next page

Information on the Merck Sharp & Dohme products listed on these pages is the full prescribing information from product circulars in use August 31, 1989.

Merck Sharp & Dohme—Cont.

observed (see below and PRECAUTIONS). Vaccinating susceptible postpubertal females confers individual protection against subsequently acquiring rubella infection during pregnancy, which in turn prevents infection of the fetus and consequent congenital rubella injury.

Women of childbearing age should be advised not to become pregnant for three months after vaccination and should be informed of the reasons for this precaution.*

It is recommended that rubella susceptibility be determined by serologic testing prior to immunization.** If immune, as evidenced by a specific rubella antibody titer of 1:8 or greater (hemagglutination-inhibition test), vaccination is unnecessary. Congenital malformations do occur in up to seven percent of all live births. Their chance appearance after vaccination could lead to misinterpretation of the cause, particularly if the prior rubella-immune status of vaccinees is unknown.

Postpubertal females should be informed of the frequent occurrence of generally self-limited arthralgia and/or arthritis beginning 2 to 4 weeks after vaccination (see ADVERSE REACTIONS).

Postpartum Women

It has been found convenient in many instances to vaccinate rubella-susceptible women in the immediate postpartum period. (See *Nursing Mothers*).

Revaccination: Children vaccinated when younger than 12 months of age should be revaccinated. Based on available evidence, there is no reason to routinely revaccinate persons who were vaccinated originally when 12 months of age or older. However, persons should be revaccinated if there is evidence to suggest that initial immunization was ineffective.

Use with other Vaccines

Routine administration of DTP (diphtheria, tetanus, pertussis) and/or OPV (oral poliovirus vaccine) concomitantly with measles, mumps and rubella vaccines is not recommended because there are insufficient data relating to the simultaneous administration of these antigens. However, the American Academy of Pediatrics has noted that in some circumstances, particularly when the patient may not return, some practitioners prefer to administer all these antigens on a single day. If done, separate sites and syringes should be used for DTP and BIAVAX II.

BIAVAX II should not be given less than one month before or after administration of other virus vaccines.

CONTRAINDICATIONS

Do not give BIAVAX II to pregnant females; the possible effects of the vaccine on fetal development are unknown at this time. If vaccination of postpubertal females is undertaken, pregnancy should be avoided for three months following vaccination. (See PRECAUTIONS, *Pregnancy*).

Anaphylactoid reaction to neomycin (each dose of reconstituted vaccine contains approximately 25 mcg of neomycin).

History of anaphylactoid reaction to eggs (see HYPERSENSITIVITY TO EGGS below).

Any febrile respiratory illness or other active febrile infection.

Active untreated tuberculosis.

Patients receiving immunosuppressive therapy. This contraindication does not apply to patients who are receiving corticosteroids as replacement therapy, e.g., for Addison's disease.

Individuals with blood dyscrasias, leukemia, lymphomas of any type, or other malignant neoplasms affecting the bone marrow or lymphatic systems.

Primary immunodeficiency states, including cellular immune deficiencies, hypogammaglobulinemic and dysgammaglobulinemic states.

---

* NOTE: The Immunization Practices Advisory Committee (ACIP) has recommended "In view of the importance of protecting this age group against rubella, reasonable precautions in a rubella immunization program include asking females if they are pregnant, excluding those who say they are, and explaining the theoretical risks to the others."

** NOTE: The Immunization Practices Advisory Committee (ACIP) has stated "When practical, and when reliable laboratory services are available, potential vaccinees of childbearing age can have serologic tests to determine susceptibility to rubella. . . . However, routinely performing serologic tests for all females of childbearing age to determine susceptibility so that vaccine is given only to proven susceptibles is expensive and has been ineffective in some areas. Accordingly, the ACIP believes that rubella vaccination of a woman who is not known to be pregnant and has no history of vaccination is justifiable without serologic testing."

Individuals with a family history of congenital or hereditary immunodeficiency, until the immune competence of the potential vaccine recipient is demonstrated.

HYPERSENSITIVITY TO EGGS

Live mumps vaccine is produced in chick embryo cell culture. Persons with a history of anaphylactic or other immediate reactions (e.g., hives, swelling of the mouth and throat, difficulty breathing, hypotension, or shock) subsequent to egg ingestion should not be vaccinated. Evidence indicates that persons are not at increased risk if they have egg allergies that are not anaphylactic in nature. Such persons may be vaccinated in the usual manner. There is no evidence to indicate that persons with allergies to chickens or feathers are at increased risk of reaction to the vaccine.

PRECAUTIONS

General

Adequate treatment provisions including epinephrine, should be available for immediate use should an anaphylactoid reaction occur.

Vaccination should be deferred for at least 3 months following blood or plasma transfusions, or administration of human immune serum globulin.

Excretion of small amounts of the live attenuated rubella virus from the nose and throat has occurred in the majority of susceptible individuals 7–28 days after vaccination. There is no confirmed evidence to indicate that such virus is transmitted to susceptible persons who are in contact with the vaccinated individuals. Consequently, transmission through close personal contact, while accepted as a theoretical possibility, is not regarded as a significant risk. However, transmission of the rubella vaccine virus to infants via breast milk has been documented (see *Nursing Mothers*).

There are no reports of transmission of live attenuated mumps virus from vaccinees to susceptible contacts.

It has been reported that live attenuated rubella and mumps virus vaccines given individually may result in a temporary depression of tuberculin skin sensitivity. Therefore, if a tuberculin test is to be done, it should be administered either before or simultaneously with BIAVAX II.

As for any vaccine, vaccination with BIAVAX II may not result in seroconversion in 100% of susceptible persons given the vaccine.

Pregnancy

Pregnancy Category C

Animal reproduction studies have not been conducted with BIAVAX II. It is also not known whether BIAVAX II can cause fetal harm when administered to a pregnant woman or can affect reproduction capacity. Therefore, the vaccine should not be administered to pregnant females; furthermore, pregnancy should be avoided for three months following vaccination (see CONTRAINDICATIONS).

In counseling women who are inadvertently vaccinated when pregnant or who become pregnant within 3 months of vaccination, the physician should be aware of the following: (1) In a 10 year survey involving over 700 pregnant women who received rubella vaccine within 3 months before or after conception, (of whom 189 received the Wistar RA 27/3 strain) none of the newborns had abnormalities compatible with congenital rubella syndrome; and (2) although mumps virus is capable of infecting the placenta and fetus, there is no good evidence that it causes congenital malformations in humans. Mumps vaccine virus also has been shown to infect the placenta and fetus, but the virus has not been isolated from the fetal tissues from susceptible women who were vaccinated and underwent elective abortions.

Nursing Mothers

It is not known whether mumps vaccine virus is secreted in human milk. Recent studies have shown that lactating postpartum women immunized with live attenuated rubella vaccine may secrete the virus in breast milk and transmit it to breast-fed infants. In the infants with serological evidence of rubella infection, none exhibited severe disease; however, one exhibited mild clinical illness typical of acquired rubella. Caution should be exercised when BIAVAX II is administered to a nursing woman.

ADVERSE REACTIONS

Because of the slightly acidic pH (6.2–6.6) of the vaccine, patients may complain of burning and/or stinging of short duration at the injection site.

The adverse clinical reactions associated with the use of BIAVAX II are those expected to follow administration of the monovalent vaccines given separately. These may include malaise, sore throat, headache, fever, rash, nausea, and vomiting; mild local reactions such as erythema, induration, tenderness and regional lymphadenopathy; parotitis, orchitis, nerve deafness, thrombocytopenia and purpura; allergic reactions such as wheal and flare at the injection site or urticaria; polyneuritis; and arthralgia and/or arthritis (usually transient and rarely chronic).

Moderate fever [101–102.9°F (38.3–39.4°C)] occurs occasionally, and high fever [above 103°F (39.4°C)] occurs less commonly. On rare occasions, children developing fever may exhibit febrile convulsions. Rash occurs infrequently and is usually minimal, but rarely may be generalized.

Forms of optic neuritis, including retrobulbar neuritis and papillitis may infrequently follow viral infections, and have been reported to occur 1 to 3 weeks following inoculation with some live virus vaccines.

Isolated reports of polyneuropathy including Guillain-Barré syndrome have been reported after immunization with rubella containing vaccines.

Clinical experience with live attenuated rubella and mumps virus vaccines given individually indicates that encephalitis and other nervous system reactions have occurred very rarely. These might occur also with BIAVAX II.

Arthralgia and/or arthritis (usually transient and rarely chronic), and polyneuritis are features of natural rubella and vary in frequency and severity with age and sex, being greatest in adult females and least in prepubertal children. This type of involvement as well as myalgia and paresthesia have also been reported following administration of MERUVAX II (Rubella Virus Vaccine Live, MSD).

Chronic arthritis has been associated with natural rubella infection and has been related to persistent virus and/or viral antigen isolated from body tissues. Only rarely have vaccine recipients developed chronic joint symptoms.

Following vaccination in children, reactions in joints are uncommon and generally of brief duration. In women, incidence rates for arthritis and arthralgia are generally higher than those seen in children (children: 0–3%; women: 12–20%), and the reactions tend to be more marked and of longer duration. Symptoms may persist for a matter of months or on rare occasions for years. In adolescent girls, the reactions appear to be intermediate in incidence between those seen in children and in adult women. Even in older women (35–45 years), these reactions are generally well tolerated and rarely interfere with normal activities.

DOSAGE AND ADMINISTRATION

FOR SUBCUTANEOUS ADMINISTRATION

Do not inject intravenously.

The dosage of vaccine is the same for all persons. Inject the total volume (about 0.5 mL) of reconstituted vaccine subcutaneously, preferably into the outer aspect of upper arm. *Do not give immune globulin (IG) concurrently with BIAVAX II.*

During shipment, to insure that there is no loss of potency, the vaccine must be maintained at a temperature of 10°C (50°F) or less.

Before reconstitution, store BIAVAX II at 2–8°C (35.6-46.4°F). *Protect from light.*

CAUTION: A sterile syringe free of preservatives, antiseptics, and detergents should be used for each injection of the vaccine because these substances may inactivate the live virus vaccine. A 25 gauge, ⅝″ needle is recommended.

To reconstitute, use only the diluent supplied, since it is free of preservatives or other antiviral substances which might inactivate the vaccine. First withdraw the entire volume of diluent into the syringe to be used for reconstitution. Inject all the diluent in the syringe into the vial of lyophilized vaccine, and agitate to mix thoroughly. Withdraw the entire contents into a syringe and inject the total volume of restored vaccine subcutaneously.

It is important to use a separate sterile syringe and needle for each individual patient to prevent transmission of hepatitis B virus and other infectious agents from one person to another.

Each dose of BIAVAX II contains not less than the equivalent of 1,000 TCID$_{50}$ of the U.S. Reference Rubella Virus and 5,000 TCID$_{50}$ of the U.S. Reference Mumps Virus.

Parenteral drug products should be inspected visually for particulate matter and discoloration prior to administration. BIAVAX II, when reconstituted, is clear yellow.

HOW SUPPLIED

No. 4746—BIAVAX II is supplied as a single-dose vial of lyophilized vaccine, **NDC** 0006-4746-00, and a vial of diluent. No. 4669/4309—BIAVAX II is supplied as follows: (1) a box of 10 single-dose vials of lyophilized vaccine (package A), **NDC** 0006-4669-00; and (2) a box of 10 vials of diluent (package B). To conserve refrigerator space, the diluent may be stored separately at room temperature.

Storage

It is recommended that the vaccine be used as soon as possible after reconstitution. Protect the vaccine from light at all times, since such exposure may inactivate the virus. Store reconstituted vaccine in the vaccine vial in a dark place at 2–8°C (35.6-46.4°F) and discard if not used within eight hours.

A.H.F.S. Category: 80:12

DC 7411411   Issued October 1986

BLOCADREN® Tablets   ℞
(Timolol Maleate, MSD), U.S.P.

DESCRIPTION

BLOCADREN® (Timolol Maleate, MSD) is a non-selective beta-adrenergic receptor blocking agent. The chemical name for timolol maleate is (S)-1-[(1, 1-dimethylethyl) amino] -3-[[4-(4-morpholinyl)-1, 2, 5-thiadiazol-3-yl]oxy]-2-propanol, (Z)-butenedioate (1:1) salt. It possesses an asymmetric carbon atom in its structure and is provided as the levoisomer. Its empirical formula is $C_{13}H_{24}N_4O_3S \cdot C_4H_4O_4$ and its structural formula is:

Timolol maleate has a molecular weight of 432.49. It is a white, odorless, crystalline powder which is soluble in water, methanol, and alcohol.
BLOCADREN is supplied as tablets in three strengths containing 5 mg, 10 mg or 20 mg timolol maleate for oral administration. Inactive ingredients are cellulose, FD&C Blue 2, magnesium stearate, and starch.

CLINICAL PHARMACOLOGY

BLOCADREN is a $beta_1$ and $beta_2$ (non-selective) adrenergic receptor blocking agent that does not have significant intrinsic sympathomimetic, direct myocardial depressant, or local anesthetic activity.
Pharmacodynamics
Clinical pharmacology studies have confirmed the beta-adrenergic blocking activity as shown by (1) changes in resting heart rate and response of heart rate to changes in posture; (2) inhibition of isoproterenol-induced tachycardia; (3) alteration of the response to the Valsalva maneuver and amyl nitrite administration; and (4) reduction of heart rate and blood pressure changes on exercise.
BLOCADREN decreases the positive chronotropic, positive inotropic, bronchodilator, and vasodilator responses caused by beta-adrenergic receptor agonists. The magnitude of this decreased response is proportional to the existing sympathetic tone and the concentration of BLOCADREN at receptor sites.
In normal volunteers, the reduction in heart rate response to a standard exercise was dose dependent over the test range of 0.5 to 20 mg, with a peak reduction at 2 hours of approximately 30% at higher doses.
Beta-adrenergic receptor blockade reduces cardiac output in both healthy subjects and patients with heart disease. In patients with severe impairment of myocardial function beta-adrenergic receptor blockade may inhibit the stimulatory effect of the sympathetic nervous system necessary to maintain adequate cardiac function.
Beta-adrenergic receptor blockade in the bronchi and bronchioles results in increased airway resistance from unopposed parasympathetic activity. Such an effect in patients with asthma or other bronchospastic conditions is potentially dangerous.
Clinical studies indicate that BLOCADREN at a dosage of 20–60 mg/day reduces blood pressure without causing postural hypotension in most patients with essential hypertension. Administration of BLOCADREN to patients with hypertension results initially in a decrease in cardiac output, little immediate change in blood pressure, and an increase in calculated peripheral resistance. With continued administration of BLOCADREN blood pressure decreases within a few days, cardiac output usually remains reduced, and peripheral resistance falls toward pretreatment levels. Plasma volume may decrease or remain unchanged during therapy with BLOCADREN. In the majority of patients with hypertension BLOCADREN also decreases plasma renin activity. Dosage adjustment to achieve optimal antihypertensive effect may require a few weeks. When therapy with BLOCADREN is discontinued, the blood pressure tends to return to pretreatment levels gradually. In most patients the antihypertensive activity of BLOCADREN is maintained with long-term therapy and is well tolerated.
The mechanism of the antihypertensive effects of beta-adrenergic receptor blocking agents is not established at this time. Possible mechanisms of action include reduction in cardiac output, reduction in plasma renin activity, and a central nervous system sympatholytic action.
A Norwegian multi-center, double-blind study compared the effects of timolol maleate with placebo in 1,884 patients who had survived the acute phase of a myocardial infarction. Patients with systolic blood pressure below 100 mm Hg, sick sinus syndrome and contraindications to beta blockers, including uncontrolled heart failure, second or third degree AV block and bradycardia (<50 beats per minute), were excluded from the multi-center trial. Therapy with BLOCA-DREN, begun 7 to 28 days following infarction, was shown to reduce overall mortality; this was primarily attributable to a reduction in cardiovascular mortality. BLOCADREN significantly reduced the incidence of sudden deaths (deaths occurring without symptoms or within 24 hours of the onset of symptoms), including those occurring within one hour, and particularly instantaneous deaths (those occurring without preceding symptoms). The protective effect of BLOCADREN was consistent regardless of age, sex or site of infarction. The effect was clearest in patients with a first infarction who were considered at a high risk of dying, defined as those with one or more of the following characteristics during the acute phase: transient left ventricular failure, cardiomegaly, newly appearing atrial fibrillation or flutter, systolic hypotension, or SGOT (ASAT) levels greater than four times the upper limit of normal. Therapy with BLOCADREN also reduced the incidence of non-fatal reinfarction. The mechanism of the protective effect of BLOCADREN is unknown.
Pharmacokinetics and Metabolism
BLOCADREN is rapidly and nearly completely absorbed (about 90%) following oral ingestion. Detectable plasma levels of timolol occur within one-half hour and peak plasma levels occur in about one to two hours. The drug half-life in plasma is approximately 4 hours and this is essentially unchanged in patients with moderate renal insufficiency. Timolol is partially metabolized by the liver and timolol and its metabolites are excreted by the kidney. Timolol is not extensively bound to plasma proteins; i.e., <10% by equilibrium dialysis and approximately 60% by ultrafiltration. An *in vitro* hemodialysis study, using ^{14}C timolol added to human plasma or whole blood, showed that timolol was readily dialyzed from these fluids; however, a study of patients with renal failure showed that timolol did not dialyze readily. Plasma levels following oral administration are about half those following intravenous administration indicating approximately 50% first pass metabolism. The level of beta sympathetic activity varies widely among individuals, and no simple correlation exists between the dose or plasma level of timolol maleate and its therapeutic activity. Therefore, objective clinical measurements such as reduction of heart rate and/or blood pressure should be used as guides in determining the optimal dosage for each patient.

INDICATIONS AND USAGE

Hypertension
BLOCADREN is indicated for the treatment of hypertension. It may be used alone or in combination with other antihypertensive agents, especially thiazide-type diuretics.
Myocardial Infarction
BLOCADREN is indicated in patients who have survived the acute phase of a myocardial infarction, and are clinically stable, to reduce cardiovascular mortality and the risk of reinfarction.

CONTRAINDICATIONS

BLOCADREN is contraindicated in patients with bronchial asthma or with a history of bronchial asthma, or severe chronic obstructive pulmonary disease (see WARNINGS); sinus bradycardia; second and third degree atrioventricular block; overt cardiac failure (see WARNINGS); cardiogenic shock; hypersensitivity to this product.

WARNINGS

Cardiac Failure
Sympathetic stimulation may be essential for support of the circulation in individuals with diminished myocardial contractility, and its inhibition by beta-adrenergic receptor blockade may precipitate more severe failure. Although beta blockers should be avoided in overt congestive heart failure, they can be used, if necessary, with caution in patients with a history of failure who are well-compensated, usually with digitalis and diuretics. Both digitalis and timolol maleate slow AV conduction. If cardiac failure persists, therapy with BLOCADREN should be withdrawn.
In Patients Without a History of Cardiac Failure continued depression of the myocardium with beta-blocking agents over a period of time can, in some cases, lead to cardiac failure. At the first sign or symptom of cardiac failure, patients receiving BLOCADREN should be digitalized and/or given a diuretic, and the response observed closely. If cardiac failure continues, despite adequate digitalization and diuretic therapy, BLOCADREN should be withdrawn.

Exacerbation of Ischemic Heart Disease Following Abrupt Withdrawal—Hypersensitivity to catecholamines has been observed in patients withdrawn from beta blocker therapy; exacerbation of angina and, in some cases, myocardial infarction have occurred after *abrupt* discontinuation of such therapy. When discontinuing chronically administered timolol maleate, particularly in patients with ischemic heart disease, the dosage should be gradually reduced over a period of one to two weeks and the patient should be carefully monitored. If angina markedly worsens or acute coronary insufficiency develops, timolol maleate administration should be reinstituted promptly, at least temporarily, and other measures appropriate for the management of unstable angina should be taken. Patients should be warned against interruption or discontinuation of therapy without the physician's advice. Because coronary artery disease is common and may be unrecognized, it may be prudent not to discontinue timolol maleate therapy abruptly even in patients treated only for hypertension.

Obstructive Pulmonary Disease
PATIENTS WITH CHRONIC OBSTRUCTIVE PULMONARY DISEASE (e.g., CHRONIC BRONCHITIS, EMPHYSEMA) OF MILD OR MODERATE SEVERITY, BRONCHOSPASTIC DISEASE OR A HISTORY OF BRONCHOSPASTIC DISEASE (OTHER THAN BRONCHIAL ASTHMA OR A HISTORY OF BRONCHIAL ASTHMA, IN WHICH 'BLOCADREN' IS CONTRAINDICATED, see CONTRAINDICATIONS), SHOULD IN GENERAL NOT RECEIVE BETA BLOCKERS, INCLUDING 'BLOCADREN'. However, if BLOCADREN is necessary in such patients, then the drug should be administered with caution since it may block bronchodilation produced by endogenous and exogenous catecholamine stimulation of $beta_2$ receptors.
Major Surgery
The necessity or desirability of withdrawal of beta-blocking therapy prior to major surgery is controversial. Beta-adrenergic receptor blockade impairs the ability of the heart to respond to beta-adrenergically mediated reflex stimuli. This may augment the risk of general anesthesia in surgical procedures. Some patients receiving beta-adrenergic receptor blocking agents have been subject to protracted severe hypotension during anesthesia. Difficulty in restarting and maintaining the heartbeat has also been reported. For these reasons, in patients undergoing elective surgery, some authorities recommend gradual withdrawal of beta-adrenergic receptor blocking agents.
If necessary during surgery, the effects of beta-adrenergic blocking agents may be reversed by sufficient doses of such agonists as isoproterenol, dopamine, dobutamine or levarterenol (see OVERDOSAGE).
Diabetes Mellitus
BLOCADREN should be administered with caution in patients subject to spontaneous hypoglycemia or to diabetic patients (especially those with labile diabetes) who are receiving insulin or oral hypoglycemic agents. Beta-adrenergic receptor blocking agents may mask the signs and symptoms of acute hypoglycemia.
Thyrotoxicosis
Beta-adrenergic blockade may mask certain clinical signs (e.g., tachycardia) of hyperthyroidism. Patients suspected of developing thyrotoxicosis should be managed carefully to avoid abrupt withdrawal of beta blockade which might precipitate a thyroid storm.

PRECAUTIONS

General
Impaired Hepatic or Renal Function: Since BLOCADREN is partially metabolized in the liver and excreted mainly by the kidneys, dosage reductions may be necessary when hepatic and/or renal insufficiency is present.
Dosing in the Presence of Marked Renal Failure: Although the pharmacokinetics of BLOCADREN are not greatly altered by renal impairment, marked hypotensive responses have been seen in patients with marked renal impairment undergoing dialysis after 20 mg doses. Dosing in such patients should therefore be especially cautious.
Muscle Weakness: Beta-adrenergic blockade has been reported to potentiate muscle weakness consistent with certain myasthenic symptoms (e.g., diplopia, ptosis, and generalized weakness). Timolol has been reported rarely to increase muscle weakness in some patients with myasthenia gravis or myasthenic symptoms.
Cerebrovascular Insufficiency: Because of potential effects of beta-adrenergic blocking agents relative to blood pressure and pulse, these agents should be used with caution in patients with cerebrovascular insufficiency. If signs or symptoms suggesting reduced cerebral blood flow are observed, consideration should be given to discontinuing these agents.
Drug Interactions
Close observation of the patient is recommended when BLOCADREN is administered to patients receiving catecholamine-depleting drugs such as reserpine, because of possible additive effects and the production of hypotension and

Continued on next page

Merck Sharp & Dohme—Cont.

/or marked bradycardia, which may produce vertigo, syncope, or postural hypotension.

Blunting of the antihypertensive effect of beta-adrenoceptor blocking agents by non-steroidal anti-inflammatory drugs has been reported. When using these agents concomitantly, patients should be observed carefully to confirm that the desired therapeutic effect has been obtained.

Literature reports suggest that oral calcium antagonists may be used in combination with beta-adrenergic blocking agents when heart function is normal, but should be avoided in patients with impaired cardiac function. Hypotension, AV conduction disturbances, and left ventricular failure have been reported in some patients receiving beta-adrenergic blocking agents when an oral calcium antagonist was added to the treatment regimen. Hypotension was more likely to occur if the calcium antagonist were a dihydropyridine derivative, e.g. nifedipine, while left ventricular failure and AV conduction disturbances were more likely to occur with either verapamil or diltiazem.

Intravenous calcium antagonists should be used with caution in patients receiving beta-adrenergic blocking agents. The concomitant use of beta-adrenergic blocking agents with digitalis and either diltiazem or verapamil may have additive effects in prolonging AV conduction time.

Carcinogenesis, Mutagenesis, Impairment of Fertility

In a two-year study of timolol maleate in rats, there was a statistically significant (P ≤ 0.05) increase in the incidence of adrenal pheochromocytomas in male rats administered 300 mg/kg/day (250 times* the maximum recommended human dose). Similar differences were not observed in rats administered doses equivalent to approximately 20 or 80 times* the maximum recommended human dose.

In a lifetime study in mice, there were statistically significant (P ≤ 0.05) increases in the incidence of benign and malignant pulmonary tumors and benign uterine polyps in female mice at 500 mg/kg/day (approximately 400 times* the maximum recommended human dose), but not at 5 or 50 mg/kg/day. In a subsequent supplementary study in female mice at 500 mg/kg/day, a statistically significant increase in the incidence of pulmonary tumors was observed. In the initial study in mice there was also a significant increase in mammary adenocarcinomas at the 500 mg/kg/day dose. Mammary adenocarcinomas were associated with elevations in serum prolactin which occurred in female mice administered timolol at 500 mg/kg, but not at doses of 5 or 50 mg/kg/day. An increased incidence of mammary adenocarcinomas in rodents has been associated with administration of several other therapeutic agents which elevate serum prolactin, but no correlation between serum prolactin levels and mammary tumors has been established in man. Furthermore, in adult human female subjects who received oral dosages of up to 60 mg of timolol maleate, the maximum recommended human oral dosage, there were no clinically meaningful changes in serum prolactin.

Timolol maleate was devoid of mutagenic potential when evaluated *in vivo* (mouse) in the micronucleus test and cytogenetic assay (doses up to 800 mg/kg) and *in vitro* in a neoplastic cell transformation assay (up to 100 μg/mL). In Ames tests the highest concentrations of timolol employed, 5000 or 10,000 μg/plate, were associated with statistically significant elevations (P ≤ 0.05) of revertants observed with tester strain TA100 (in seven replicate assays), but not in the remaining three strains. In the assays with tester strain TA100, no consistent dose response relationship was observed, nor did the ratio of test to control revertants reach 2. A ratio of 2 is usually considered the criterion for a positive Ames test.

Reproduction and fertility studies in rats showed no adverse effect on male or female fertility at doses up to 125 times* the maximum recommended human dose.

Pregnancy

Pregnancy Category C. Teratogenicity studies with timolol in mice and rabbits at doses up to 50 mg/kg/day (50 times the maximum recommended human dose) showed no evidence of fetal malformations. Although delayed fetal ossification was observed at this dose in rats, there were no adverse effects on postnatal development of offspring. Doses of 1000 mg/kg/day (1,000 times the maximum recommended human dose) were maternotoxic in mice and resulted in an increased number of fetal resorptions. Increased fetal resorptions were also seen in rabbits at doses of 100 times the maximum recommended human dose, in this case without apparent maternotoxicity. There are no adequate and well-controlled studies in pregnant women. BLOCADREN should be used during pregnancy only if the potential benefit justifies the potential risk to the fetus.

Nursing Mothers

Because of the potential for serious adverse reactions from timolol in nursing infants, a decision should be made whether to discontinue nursing or to discontinue the drug, taking into account the importance of the drug to the mother.

Pediatric Use

Safety and effectiveness in children have not been established.

ADVERSE REACTIONS

BLOCADREN is usually well tolerated in properly selected patients. Most adverse effects have been mild and transient. In a multicenter (12-week) clinical trial comparing timolol maleate and placebo, the following adverse reactions were reported spontaneously and considered to be causally related to timolol maleate:

	Timolol Maleate (n = 176) %	Placebo (n = 168) %
BODY AS A WHOLE		
fatigue/tiredness	3.4	0.6
headache	1.7	1.8
chest pain	0.6	0
asthenia	0.6	0
CARDIOVASCULAR		
bradycardia	9.1	0
arrhythmia	1.1	0.6
syncope	0.6	0
edema	0.6	1.2
DIGESTIVE		
dyspepsia	0.6	0.6
nausea	0.6	0
SKIN		
pruritus	1.1	0
NERVOUS SYSTEM		
dizziness	2.3	1.2
vertigo	0.6	0
paresthesia	0.6	0
PSYCHIATRIC		
decreased libido	0.6	0
RESPIRATORY		
dyspnea	1.7	0.6
bronchial spasm	0.6	0
rales	0.6	0
SPECIAL SENSES		
eye irritation	1.1	0.6
tinnitus	0.6	0

* Based on patient weight of 50 kg.

These data are representative of the incidence of adverse effects that may be observed in a properly selected hypertensive patient population, e.g., a group excluding patients with bronchospastic disease, congestive heart failure or other contraindications to beta blocker therapy. These adverse reactions can also occur in patients with coronary artery disease.

In a different population, the coronary artery disease population, studied in the Norwegian multi-center trial (see CLINICAL PHARMACOLOGY), the frequency of the principal adverse reactions and the frequency with which these resulted in discontinuation of therapy in the timolol and placebo groups were:

[See table below].

The following additional adverse effects have been reported in clinical experience with the drug: *Body as a Whole:* extremity pain, decreased exercise tolerance, weight loss, fever; *Cardiovascular:* cardiac arrest, cardiac failure, cerebrovascular accident, worsening of angina pectoris, worsening of arterial insufficiency, Raynaud's phenomenon, palpitations, vasodilatation; *Digestive:* gastrointestinal pain, hepatomegaly, vomiting, diarrhea, dyspepsia; *Hematologic:* nonthrombocytopenic purpura; *Endocrine:* hyperglycemia, hypoglycemia; *Skin:* rash, skin irritation, increased pigmentation, sweating, alopecia; *Musculoskeletal:* arthralgia; *Nervous System:* local weakness, increase in signs and symptoms of myasthenia gravis; *Psychiatric:* depression, nightmares, somnolence, insomnia, nervousness, diminished concentration, hallucinations; *Respiratory:* cough; *Special Senses:* visual disturbances, diplopia, ptosis, dry eyes; *Urogenital:* impotence, urination difficulties.

There have been reports of retroperitoneal fibrosis in patients receiving timolol maleate and in patients receiving other beta-adrenergic blocking agents. A causal relationship between this condition and therapy with beta-adrenergic blocking agents has not been established.

Potential Adverse Effects: In addition, a variety of adverse effects not observed in clinical trials with BLOCADREN, but reported with other beta-adrenergic blocking agents, should be considered potential adverse effects of BLOCADREN: *Nervous System:* Reversible mental depression progressing to catatonia; an acute reversible syndrome characterized by disorientation for time and place, short-term memory loss, emotional lability, slightly clouded sensorium, and decreased performance on neuropsychometrics; *Cardiovascular:* Intensification of AV block (see CONTRAINDICATIONS); *Digestive:* Mesenteric arterial thrombosis, ischemic colitis; *Hematologic:* Agranulocytosis, thrombocytopenic purpura; *Allergic:* Erythematous rash, fever combined with aching and sore throat, laryngospasm with respiratory distress; *Miscellaneous:* Peyronie's disease.

There have been reports of a syndrome comprising psoriasiform skin rash, conjunctivitis sicca, otitis, and sclerosing serositis attributed to the beta-adrenergic receptor blocking agent, practolol. This syndrome has not been reported with BLOCADREN.

Clinical Laboratory Test Findings: Clinically important changes in standard laboratory parameters were rarely associated with the administration of BLOCADREN. Slight increases in blood urea nitrogen, serum potassium, uric acid, and triglycerides, and slight decreases in hemoglobin, hematocrit and HDL cholesterol occurred, but were not progressive or associated with clinical manifestations. Increases in liver function tests have been reported.

OVERDOSAGE

No data are available in regard to overdosage in humans. The oral LD_{50} of the drug is 1190 and 900 mg/kg in female mice and female rats, respectively.

An *in vitro* hemodialysis study, using ^{14}C timolol added to human plasma or whole blood, showed that timolol was readily dialyzed from these fluids; however, a study of patients with renal failure showed that timolol did not dialyze readily.

The most common signs and symptoms to be expected with overdosage with a beta-adrenergic receptor blocking agent are symptomatic bradycardia, hypotension, bronchospasm, and acute cardiac failure. Therapy with BLOCADREN should be discontinued and the patient observed closely. The following additional therapeutic measures should be considered:

(1) *Gastric lavage*

(2) *Symptomatic bradycardia:* Use atropine sulfate intravenously in a dosage of 0.25 mg to 2 mg to induce vagal blockade. If bradycardia persists, intravenous isoproterenol hydrochloride should be administered cautiously. In refractory cases the use of a transvenous cardiac pacemaker may be considered.

(3) *Hypotension:* Use sympathomimetic pressor drug therapy, such as dopamine, dobutamine or levarterenol. In refractory cases the use of glucagon hydrochloride has been reported to be useful.

BLOCADREN	Adverse Reaction†		Withdrawal‡	
	Timolol (n = 945) %	Placebo (n = 939) %	Timolol (n = 945) %	Placebo (n = 939) %
Asthenia or Fatigue	5	1	<1	<1
Heart Rate <40 beats/minute	5	<1	4	<1
Cardiac Failure—Nonfatal	8	7	3	2
Hypotension	3	2	3	1
Pulmonary Edema—Nonfatal	2	<1	<1	<1
Claudication	3	3	1	<1
AV Block 2nd or 3rd degree	<1	<1	<1	<1
Sinoatrial Block	<1	<1	<1	<1
Cold Hands and Feet	8	<1	<1	0
Nausea or Digestive Disorders	8	6	1	<1
Dizziness	6	4	1	0
Bronchial Obstruction	2	<1	1	<1

† When an adverse reaction recurred in a patient, it is listed only once.
‡ Only principal reason for withdrawal in each patient is listed.
These adverse reactions can also occur in patients treated for hypertension.

(4) *Bronchospasm:* Use isoproterenol hydrochloride. Additional therapy with aminophylline may be considered.

(5) *Acute cardiac failure:* Conventional therapy with digitalis, diuretics, and oxygen should be instituted immediately. In refractory cases the use of intravenous aminophylline is suggested. This may be followed if necessary by glucagon hydrochloride which has been reported to be useful.

(6) *Heart block (second or third degree):* Use isoproterenol hydrochloride or a transvenous cardiac pacemaker.

DOSAGE AND ADMINISTRATION

Hypertension

The usual initial dosage of BLOCADREN is 10 mg twice a day, whether used alone or added to diuretic therapy. Dosage may be increased or decreased depending on heart rate and blood pressure response. The usual total maintenance dosage is 20–40 mg per day. Increases in dosage to a maximum of 60 mg per day divided into two doses may be necessary. There should be an interval of at least seven days between increases in dosages.

BLOCADREN may be used with a thiazide diuretic or with other antihypertensive agents. Patients should be observed carefully during initiation of such concomitant therapy.

Myocardial Infarction

The recommended dosage for long-term prophylactic use in patients who have survived the acute phase of a myocardial infarction is 10 mg given twice daily (see CLINICAL PHARMACOLOGY).

HOW SUPPLIED

No. 3343—Tablets BLOCADREN, 5 mg, are light blue, round, compressed tablets, with code MSD 59 on one side and BLOCADREN on the other. They are supplied as follows:
NDC 0006-0059-68 bottles of 100.
Shown in Product Identification Section, page 418
No. 3344—Tablets BLOCADREN, 10 mg, are light blue, round, scored, compressed tablets, with code MSD 136 on one side and BLOCADREN on the other. They are supplied as follows:
NDC 0006-0136-68 bottles of 100
(6505-01-132-0651, 10 mg 100's)
NDC 0006-0136-28 unit dose packages of 100.
Shown in Product Identification Section, page 418
No. 3371—Tablets BLOCADREN, 20 mg, are light blue, capsule shaped, scored, compressed tablets, with code MSD 437 on one side and BLOCADREN on the other. They are supplied as follows:
NDC 0006-0437-68 bottles of 100
(6505-01-132-0652, 20 mg 100's)
Shown in Product Identification Section, page 418
Storage
Store in a well-closed container, protected from light.
A.H.F.S. Categories: 24:04, 24:08
DC 7146624 Issued July 1987
COPYRIGHT © MERCK & CO., INC., 1985
All rights reserved

CLINORIL® Tablets   ℞
(Sulindac, MSD), U.S.P.

DESCRIPTION

Sulindac is a non-steroidal, anti-inflammatory indene derivative designated chemically as (Z)- 5-fluoro-2-methyl - 1 - [*p* - (methylsulfinyl) phenyl]methylene]-1*H*-indene-3-acetic acid. It is not a salicylate, pyrazolone or propionic acid derivative. Its empirical formula is $C_{20}H_{17}FO_3S$, with a molecular weight of 356.42. Sulindac, a yellow crystalline compound, is a weak organic acid practically insoluble in water below pH 4.5, but very soluble as the sodium salt or in buffers of pH 6 or higher.
CLINORIL® (Sulindac, MSD) is available in 150 and 200 mg tablets for oral administration. Each tablet contains the following inactive ingredients: cellulose, magnesium stearate, starch.
Following absorption, sulindac undergoes two major biotransformations—reversible reduction to the sulfide metabolite, and irreversible oxidation to the sulfone metabolite. Available evidence indicates that the biological activity resides with the sulfide metabolite.
The structural formulas of sulindac and its metabolites are:
[See Chemical Formula at top of next column].

CLINICAL PHARMACOLOGY

CLINORIL is a non-steroidal anti-inflammatory drug, also possessing analgesic and antipyretic activities. Its mode of action, like that of other non-steroidal, anti-inflammatory agents, is not known; however, its therapeutic action is not due to pituitary-adrenal stimulation. Inhibition of prostaglandin synthesis by the sulfide metabolite may be involved in the anti-inflammatory action of CLINORIL.

Sulindac is approximately 90% absorbed in man after oral administration. The peak plasma concentrations of the biologically active sulfide metabolite are achieved in about two hours when sulindac is administered in the fasting state, and in about three to four hours when sulindac is administered with food. The mean half-life of sulindac is 7.8 hours while the mean half-life of the sulfide metabolite is 16.4 hours. Sustained plasma levels of the sulfide metabolite are consistent with a prolonged anti-inflammatory action which is the rationale for a twice per day dosage schedule.
Sulindac and its sulfone metabolite undergo extensive enterohepatic circulation relative to the sulfide metabolite in animals. Studies in man have also demonstrated that recirculation of the parent drug, sulindac, and its sulfone metabolite, is more extensive than that of the active sulfide metabolite. The active sulfide metabolite accounts for less than six percent of the total intestinal exposure to sulindac and its metabolites.
The primary route of excretion in man is via the urine as both sulindac and its sulfone metabolite (free and glucuronide conjugates). Approximately 50% of the administered dose is excreted in the urine, with the conjugated sulfone metabolite accounting for the major portion. Less than 1% of the administered dose of sulindac appears in the urine as the sulfide metabolite. Approximately 25% is found in the feces, primarily as the sulfone and sulfide metabolites.
The bioavailability of sulindac, as assessed by urinary excretion, was not changed by concomitant administration of an antacid containing magnesium and aluminum hydroxides (MAALOX®, William H. Rorer, Inc.).
Because CLINORIL is excreted in the urine primarily as biologically inactive forms, it may possibly affect renal function to a lesser extent than other non-steroidal anti-inflammatory drugs, however, renal adverse experiences have been reported with CLINORIL (see ADVERSE REACTIONS). In a study of patients with chronic glomerular disease treated with therapeutic doses of CLINORIL, no effect was demonstrated on renal blood flow, glomerular filtration rate, or urinary excretion of prostaglandin E_2 and the primary metabolite of prostacyclin, 6-keto-PGF$_1\alpha$. However, in other studies in healthy volunteers and patients with liver disease, CLINORIL was found to blunt the renal responses to intravenous furosemide, i.e., the diuresis, natriuresis, increments in plasma renin activity and urinary excretion of prostaglandins. These observations may represent a differentiation of the effects of CLINORIL on renal functions based on differences in pathogenesis of the renal prostaglandin dependence associated with differing dose-response relationships of different NSAIDs to the various renal functions influenced by prostaglandins. These observations need further clarification and in the interim, sulindac should be used with caution in patients whose renal function may be impaired (see PRECAUTIONS).
In healthy men, the average fecal blood loss, measured over a two-week period during administration of 400 mg per day of CLINORIL, was similar to that for placebo, and was statistically significantly less than that resulting from 4800 mg per day of aspirin.
In controlled clinical studies CLINORIL was evaluated in the following five conditions:

1. *Osteoarthritis*
In patients with osteoarthritis of the hip and knee, the anti-inflammatory and analgesic activity of CLINORIL was demonstrated by clinical measurements that included: assessments by both patient and investigator of overall response; decrease in disease activity as assessed by both patient and investigator; improvement in ARA Functional Class; relief of night pain; improvement in overall evaluation of pain, including pain on weight bearing and pain on active and passive motion; improvement in joint mobility, range of motion, and functional activities; decreased swelling and tenderness; and decreased duration of stiffness following prolonged inactivity.
In clinical studies in which dosages were adjusted according to patient needs, CLINORIL 200 to 400 mg daily was shown to be comparable in effectiveness to aspirin 2400 to 4800 mg daily. CLINORIL was generally well tolerated, and patients on it had a lower overall incidence of total adverse effects, of milder gastrointestinal reactions, and of tinnitus than did patients on aspirin. (See ADVERSE REACTIONS.)

2. *Rheumatoid Arthritis*
In patients with rheumatoid arthritis, the anti-inflammatory and analgesic activity of CLINORIL was demonstrated by clinical measurements that included: assessments by both patient and investigator of overall response; decrease in disease activity as assessed by both patient and investigator; reduction in overall joint pain; reduction in duration and severity of morning stiffness; reduction in day and night pain; decrease in time required to walk 50 feet; decrease in general pain as measured on a visual analog scale; improvement in the Ritchie articular index; decrease in proximal interphalangeal joint size; improvement in ARA Functional Class; increase in grip strength; reduction in painful joint count and score; reduction in swollen joint count and score; and increased flexion and extension of the wrist.
In clinical studies in which dosages were adjusted according to patient needs, CLINORIL 300 to 400 mg daily was shown to be comparable in effectiveness to aspirin 3600 to 4800 mg daily. CLINORIL was generally well tolerated, and patients on it had a lower overall incidence of total adverse effects, of milder gastrointestinal reactions, and of tinnitus than did patients on aspirin. (See ADVERSE REACTIONS.)
In patients with rheumatoid arthritis, CLINORIL may be used in combination with gold salts at usual dosage levels. In clinical studies, CLINORIL added to the regimen of gold salts usually resulted in additional symptomatic relief but did not alter the course of the underlying disease.

3. *Ankylosing spondylitis*
In patients with ankylosing spondylitis, the anti-inflammatory and analgesic activity of CLINORIL was demonstrated by clinical measurements that included: assessments by both patient and investigator of overall response; decrease in disease activity as assessed by both patient and investigator; improvement in ARA Functional Class; improvement in patient and investigator evaluation of spinal pain, tenderness and/or spasm; reduction in the duration of morning stiffness; increase in the time to onset of fatigue; relief of night pain; increase in chest expansion; and increase in spinal mobility evaluated by fingers-to-floor distance, occiput to wall distance, the Schober Test, and the Wright Modification of the Schober Test. In a clinical study in which dosages were adjusted according to patient need, CLINORIL 200 to 400 mg daily was as effective as indomethacin 75 to 150 mg daily. In a second study, CLINORIL 300 to 400 mg daily was comparable in effectiveness to phenylbutazone 400 to 600 mg daily. CLINORIL was better tolerated than phenylbutazone. (See ADVERSE REACTIONS.)

4. *Acute painful shoulder (Acute subacromial bursitis/supraspinatus tendinitis)*
In patients with acute painful shoulder (acute subacromial bursitis/supraspinatus tendinitis), the anti-inflammatory and analgesic activity of CLINORIL was demonstrated by clinical measurements that included: assessments by both patient and investigator of overall response; relief of night pain, spontaneous pain, and pain on active motion; decrease in local tenderness; and improvement in range of motion measured by abduction, and internal and external rotation. In clinical studies in acute painful shoulder, CLINORIL 300 to 400 mg daily and oxyphenbutazone 400 to 600 mg daily were shown to be equally effective and well tolerated.

5. *Acute gouty arthritis*
In patients with acute gouty arthritis, the anti-inflammatory and analgesic activity of CLINORIL was demonstrated by clinical measurements that included: assessments by both the patient and investigator of overall response; relief of weight-bearing pain; relief of pain at rest and on active and passive motion; decrease in tenderness; reduction in warmth and swelling; increase in range of motion; and improvement in ability to function. In clinical studies, CLINORIL at 400 mg daily and phenylbutazone at 600 mg daily were shown to be equally effective. In these short-term studies in which reduction of dosage was permitted according to response, both drugs were equally well tolerated.

Continued on next page

Information on the Merck Sharp & Dohme products listed on these pages is the full prescribing information from product circulars in use August 31, 1989.

Merck Sharp & Dohme—Cont.

INDICATIONS AND USAGE

CLINORIL is indicated for acute or long-term use in the relief of signs and symptoms of the following:
1. Osteoarthritis
2. Rheumatoid arthritis*
3. Ankylosing spondylitis
4. Acute painful shoulder (Acute subacromial bursitis/supraspinatus tendinitis)
5. Acute gouty arthritis

---

* The safety and effectiveness of CLINORIL have not been established in rheumatoid arthritis patients who are designated in the American Rheumatism Association classification as Functional Class IV (incapacitated, largely or wholly bedridden, or confined to wheelchair; little or no self-care).

CONTRAINDICATIONS

CLINORIL should not be used in:
Patients who are hypersensitive to this product.
Patients in whom acute asthmatic attacks, urticaria, or rhinitis are precipitated by aspirin or other non-steroidal anti-inflammatory agents.

WARNINGS

Gastrointestinal Effects
Peptic ulceration and gastrointestinal bleeding have been reported in patients receiving CLINORIL. Fatalities have occurred. Gastrointestinal bleeding is associated with higher morbidity and mortality in patients acutely ill with other conditions, the elderly and patients with hemorrhagic disorders. In patients with active gastrointestinal bleeding or an active peptic ulcer, an appropriate ulcer regimen should be instituted, and the physician must weigh the benefits of therapy with CLINORIL against possible hazards, and carefully monitor the patient's progress. When CLINORIL is given to patients with a history of either upper or lower gastrointestinal tract disease, it should be given under close supervision and only after consulting the ADVERSE REACTIONS section.

Risk of GI Ulcerations, Bleeding and Perforation with NSAID Therapy
Serious gastrointestinal toxicity such as bleeding, ulceration, and perforation, can occur at any time, with or without warning symptoms, in patients treated chronically with NSAID therapy. Although minor upper gastrointestinal problems, such as dyspepsia, are common, usually developing early in therapy, physicians should remain alert for ulceration and bleeding in patients treated chronically with NSAIDs even in the absence of previous GI tract symptoms. In patients observed in clinical trials of several months to two years duration, symptomatic upper GI ulcers, gross bleeding or perforation appear to occur in approximately 1% of patients treated for 3-6 months, and in about 2-4% of patients treated for one year. Physicians should inform patients about the signs and/or symptoms of serious GI toxicity and what steps to take if they occur.
Studies to date have not identified any subset of patients not at risk of developing peptic ulceration and bleeding. Except for a prior history of serious GI events and other risk factors known to be associated with peptic ulcer disease, such as alcoholism, smoking, etc., no risk factors (e.g., age, sex) have been associated with increased risk. Elderly or debilitated patients seem to tolerate ulceration or bleeding less well than other individuals and most spontaneous reports of fatal GI events are in this population. Studies to date are inconclusive concerning the relative risk of various NSAIDs in causing such reactions. High doses of any NSAID probably carry a greater risk of these reactions, although controlled clinical trials showing this do not exist in most cases. In considering the use of relatively large doses (within the recommended dosage range), sufficient benefit should be anticipated to offset the potential increased risk of GI toxicity.

Hypersensitivity
Rarely, fever and other evidence of hypersensitivity (see ADVERSE REACTIONS) including abnormalities in one or more liver function tests and severe skin reactions have occurred during therapy with CLINORIL. Fatalities have occurred in these patients. Hepatitis, jaundice, or both, with or without fever, may occur usually within the first one to three months of therapy. Determinations of liver function should be considered whenever a patient on therapy with CLINORIL develops unexplained fever, rash or other dermatologic reactions or constitutional symptoms. If unexplained fever or other evidence of hypersensitivity occurs, therapy with CLINORIL should be discontinued. The elevated temperature and abnormalities in liver function caused by CLINORIL characteristically have reverted to normal after discontinuation of therapy. Administration of CLINORIL should not be reinstituted in such patients.

Hepatic Effects
In addition to hypersensitivity reactions involving the liver, in some patients the findings are consistent with those of cholestatic hepatitis. As with other non-steroidal anti-inflammatory drugs, borderline elevations of one or more liver tests without any other signs and symptoms may occur in up to 15% of patients. These abnormalities may progress, may remain essentially unchanged, or may be transient with continued therapy. The SGPT (ALT) test is probably the most sensitive indicator of liver dysfunction. Meaningful (3 times the upper limit of normal) elevations of SGPT or SGOT (AST) occurred in controlled clinical trials in less than 1% of patients. A patient with symptoms and/or signs suggesting liver dysfunction, or in whom an abnormal liver test has occurred, should be evaluated for evidence of the development of more severe hepatic reaction while on therapy with CLINORIL. Although such reactions as described above are rare, if abnormal liver tests persist or worsen, if clinical signs and symptoms consistent with liver disease develop, or if systemic manifestations occur (e.g. eosinophilia, rash, etc.), CLINORIL should be discontinued.
In clinical trials with CLINORIL, the use of doses of 600 mg/day has been associated with an increased incidence of mild liver test abnormalities (see DOSAGE AND ADMINISTRATION for maximum dosage recommendation).

PRECAUTIONS

General
Although CLINORIL has less effect on platelet function and bleeding time than aspirin, it is an inhibitor of platelet function; therefore, patients who may be adversely affected should be carefully observed when CLINORIL is administered.
Pancreatitis has been reported in patients receiving CLINORIL (see ADVERSE REACTIONS). Should pancreatitis be suspected, the drug should be discontinued and not restarted, supportive medical therapy instituted, and the patient monitored closely with appropriate laboratory studies (e.g., serum and urine amylase, amylase/creatinine clearance ratio, electrolytes, serum calcium, glucose, lipase, etc.). A search for other causes of pancreatitis as well as those conditions which mimic pancreatitis should be conducted.
Because of reports of adverse eye findings with non-steroidal anti-inflammatory agents, it is recommended that patients who develop eye complaints during treatment with CLINORIL have ophthalmologic studies.
In patients with poor liver function, delayed, elevated and prolonged circulating levels of the sulfide and sulfone metabolites may occur. Such patients should be monitored closely; a reduction of daily dosage may be required.
Edema has been observed in some patients taking CLINORIL. Therefore, as with other non-steroidal anti-inflammatory drugs, CLINORIL should be used with caution in patients with compromised cardiac function, hypertension, or other conditions predisposing to fluid retention.
CLINORIL may allow a reduction in dosage or the elimination of chronic corticosteroid therapy in some patients with rheumatoid arthritis. However, it is generally necessary to reduce corticosteroids gradually over several months in order to avoid an exacerbation of disease or signs and symptoms of adrenal insufficiency. Abrupt withdrawal of chronic corticosteroid treatment is generally not recommended even when patients have had a serious complication of chronic corticosteroid therapy.

Renal Effects
As with other non-steroidal anti-inflammatory drugs, long term administration of sulindac to animals has resulted in renal papillary necrosis and other abnormal renal pathology. In humans, there have been reports of acute interstitial nephritis with hematuria, proteinuria, and occasionally nephrotic syndrome.
A second form of renal toxicity has been seen in patients with prerenal and renal conditions leading to a reduction in renal blood flow or blood volume, where the renal prostaglandins have a supportive role in the maintenance of renal perfusion. In these patients administration of an NSAID may cause a dose dependent reduction in prostaglandin formation and may precipitate overt renal decompensation. CLINORIL may affect renal function less than other NSAIDs in patients with chronic glomerular renal disease (see CLINICAL PHARMACOLOGY). Until these observations are better understood and clarified, however, and because renal adverse experiences have been reported with CLINORIL (see ADVERSE REACTIONS), caution should be exercised when administering the drug to patients with conditions associated with increased risk of the effects of non-steroidal anti-inflammatory drugs on renal function, such as those with renal or hepatic dysfunction, diabetes mellitus, advanced age, extracellular volume depletion from any cause, congestive heart failure, septicemia, pyelonephritis, or concomitant use of any nephrotoxic drug. Discontinuation of NSAID therapy is typically followed by recovery to the pretreatment state.

Since CLINORIL is eliminated primarily by the kidneys, patients with significantly impaired renal function should be closely monitored; a lower daily dosage should be anticipated to avoid excessive drug accumulation.
Sulindac metabolites have been reported rarely as the major or a minor component in renal stones in association with other calculus components. CLINORIL should be used with caution in patients with a history of renal lithiasis, and they should be kept well hydrated while receiving CLINORIL.

Information for Patients
CLINORIL, like other drugs of its class, is not free of side effects. The side effects of these drugs can cause discomfort and, rarely, there are more serious side effects such as gastrointestinal bleeding, which may result in hospitalization and even fatal outcomes.
NSAIDs (Non-steroidal Anti-inflammatory Drugs) are often essential agents in the management of arthritis, but they also may be commonly employed for conditions which are less serious.
Physicians may wish to discuss with their patients the potential risks (see WARNINGS, PRECAUTIONS and ADVERSE REACTIONS) and likely benefits of NSAID treatment, particularly when the drugs are used for less serious conditions where treatment without NSAIDs may represent an acceptable alternative to both the patient and physician.

Laboratory Tests
Because serious GI tract ulceration and bleeding can occur without warning symptoms, physicians should follow chronically treated patients for the signs and symptoms of ulceration and bleeding and should inform them of the importance of this follow-up (see WARNINGS, *Risk of GI Ulcerations, Bleeding and Perforation with NSAID Therapy*).

Use in Pregnancy
CLINORIL is not recommended for use in pregnant women, since safety for use has not been established, and because of the known effect of drugs of this class on the human fetal cardiovascular system (closure of the ductus arteriosus) during the third trimester of pregnancy. In reproduction studies in the rat, a decrease in average fetal weight and an increase in numbers of dead pups were observed on the first day of the postpartum period at dosage levels of 20 and 40 mg/kg/day ($2\frac{1}{2}$ and 5 times the usual maximum daily dose in humans), although there was no adverse effect on the survival and growth during the remainder of the postpartum period. CLINORIL prolongs the duration of gestation in rats, as do other compounds of this class which also may cause dystocia and delayed parturition in pregnant animals. Visceral and skeletal malformations observed in low incidence among rabbits in some teratology studies did not occur at the same dosage levels in repeat studies, nor at a higher dosage level in the same species.

Nursing Mothers
Nursing should not be undertaken while a patient is on CLINORIL. It is not known whether sulindac is secreted in human milk; however, it is secreted in the milk of lactating rats.

Use in Children
Safety and effectiveness in children have not been established.

Drug Interactions
DMSO should not be used with sulindac. Concomitant administration has been reported to reduce the plasma levels of the active sulfide metabolite and potentially reduce efficacy. In addition, this combination has been reported to cause peripheral neuropathy.
Although sulindac and its sulfide metabolite are highly bound to protein, studies, in which CLINORIL was given at a dose of 400 mg daily, have shown no clinically significant interaction with oral anticoagulants or oral hypoglycemic agents. However, patients should be monitored carefully until it is certain that no change in their anticoagulant or hypoglycemic dosage is required. Special attention should be paid to patients taking higher doses than those recommended and to patients with renal impairment or other metabolic defects that might increase sulindac blood levels.
The concomitant administration of aspirin with sulindac significantly depressed the plasma levels of the active sulfide metabolite. A double-blind study compared the safety and efficacy of CLINORIL 300 or 400 mg daily given alone or with aspirin 2.4 g/day for the treatment of osteoarthritis. The addition of aspirin did not alter the types of clinical or laboratory adverse experiences for CLINORIL; however, the combination showed an increase in the incidence of gastrointestinal adverse experiences. Since the addition of aspirin did not have a favorable effect on the therapeutic response to CLINORIL, the combination is not recommended.
The concomitant administration of CLINORIL and diflunisal in normal volunteers resulted in lowering of the plasma levels of the active sulindac sulfide metabolite by approximately one-third.
Probenecid given concomitantly with sulindac had only a slight effect on plasma sulfide levels, while plasma levels of sulindac and sulfone were increased. Sulindac was shown to produce a modest reduction in the uricosuric action of probenecid, which probably is not significant under most circumstances.

Neither propoxyphene hydrochloride nor acetaminophen had any effect on the plasma levels of sulindac or its sulfide metabolite.

ADVERSE REACTIONS

The following adverse reactions were reported in clinical trials or have been reported since the drug was marketed. The probability exists of a causal relationship between CLINORIL and these adverse reactions. The adverse reactions which have been observed in clinical trials encompass observations in 1,865 patients, including 232 observed for at least 48 weeks.

Incidence Greater Than 1%
Gastrointestinal
The most frequent types of adverse reactions occurring with CLINORIL are gastrointestinal; these include gastrointestinal pain (10%), dyspepsia*, nausea* with or without vomiting, diarrhea*, constipation*, flatulence, anorexia and gastrointestinal cramps.
Dermatologic
Rash*, pruritus.
Central Nervous System
Dizziness*, headache*, nervousness.
Special Senses
Tinnitus.
Miscellaneous
Edema (see PRECAUTIONS).

Incidence Less Than 1 in 100
Gastrointestinal
Gastritis, gastroenteritis or colitis. Peptic ulcer and gastrointestinal bleeding have been reported. GI perforation has been reported rarely.
Liver function abnormalities; jaundice, sometimes with fever; cholestasis; hepatitis.
Pancreatitis (see PRECAUTIONS).
Ageusia; glossitis.
There have been rare reports of sulindac metabolites in common bile duct "sludge" in patients with symptoms of cholecystitis who underwent a cholecystectomy.
Dermatologic
Stomatitis, sore or dry mucous membranes, alopecia, photosensitivity.
Erythema multiforme, toxic epidermal necrolysis, Stevens-Johnson syndrome, and exfoliative dermatitis have been reported.
Cardiovascular
Congestive heart failure, especially in patients with marginal cardiac function; palpitation; hypertension.
Hematologic
Thrombocytopenia; ecchymosis; purpura; leukopenia; agranulocytosis; neutropenia; bone marrow depression, including aplastic anemia; hemolytic anemia; increased prothrombin time in patients on oral anticoagulants (see PRECAUTIONS).
Genitourinary
Urine discoloration; dysuria; vaginal bleeding; hematuria; proteinuria; crystalluria; renal impairment, including renal failure; interstitial nephritis; nephrotic syndrome.
Renal calculi containing sulindac metabolites have been observed rarely.
Metabolic
Hyperkalemia.
Musculoskeletal
Muscle weakness.
Psychiatric
Depression; psychic disturbances including acute psychosis.
Nervous System
Vertigo; insomnia; somnolence; paresthesia; convulsions; syncope; aseptic meningitis.
Special Senses
Blurred vision; visual disturbances; decreased hearing; metallic or bitter taste.
Respiratory
Epistaxis.
Hypersensitivity Reactions
Anaphylaxis; angioneurotic edema; bronchial spasm; dyspnea.
Hypersensitivity vasculitis.
A potentially fatal apparent hypersensitivity syndrome has been reported. This syndrome may include constitutional symptoms (fever, chills), cutaneous findings (rash or other dermatologic reactions—see above), conjunctivitis, involvement of major organs (changes in liver function, jaundice, pancreatitis, pneumonitis with or without pleural effusion, leukopenia, eosinophilia, disseminated intravascular coagulation, anemia, renal impairment, including renal failure), and other less specific findings (adenitis, arthralgia, arthritis, myalgia, fatigue, malaise, hypotension, chest pain, tachycardia).

* Incidence between 3% and 9%. Those reactions occurring in 1 to 3% of patients are not marked with an asterisk.

Causal Relationship Unknown
Other reactions have been reported in clinical trials or since the drug was marketed, but occurred under circumstances where a causal relationship could not be established. However, in these rarely reported events, that possibility cannot be excluded. Therefore, these observations are listed to serve as alerting information to physicians.
Cardiovascular
Arrhythmia.
Metabolic
Hyperglycemia.
Nervous System
Neuritis.
Special Senses
Disturbances of the retina and its vasculature.
Miscellaneous
Gynecomastia.

MANAGEMENT OF OVERDOSAGE

Cases of overdosage have been reported and rarely, deaths have occurred. The following signs and symptoms may be observed following overdosage: stupor, coma, diminished urine output and hypotension.
In the event of overdosage, the stomach should be emptied by inducing vomiting or by gastric lavage, and the patient carefully observed and given symptomatic and supportive treatment.
Animal studies show that absorption is decreased by the prompt administration of activated charcoal and excretion is enhanced by alkalinization of the urine.

DOSAGE AND ADMINISTRATION

CLINORIL should be administered orally twice a day with food. The maximum dosage is 400 mg per day. Dosages above 400 mg per day are not recommended.
In osteoarthritis, rheumatoid arthritis, and ankylosing spondylitis, the recommended starting dosage is 150 mg twice a day. The dosage may be lowered or raised depending on the response.
A prompt response (within one week) can be expected in about one-half of patients with osteoarthritis, ankylosing spondylitis, and rheumatoid arthritis. Others may require longer to respond.
In acute painful shoulder (acute subacromial bursitis/supraspinatus tendinitis) and acute gouty arthritis, the recommended dosage is 200 mg twice a day. After a satisfactory response has been achieved, the dosage may be reduced according to the response. In acute painful shoulder, therapy for 7–14 days is usually adequate. In acute gouty arthritis, therapy for 7 days is usually adequate.

HOW SUPPLIED

No. 3360—Tablets CLINORIL 150 mg are yellow, hexagon-shaped, compressed tablets, coded MSD 941. They are supplied as follows:
NDC 0006-0941-54 unit of use bottles of 60
NDC 0006-0941-68 in bottles of 100
(6505-01-071-5559 100's)
NDC 0006-0941-78 unit of use bottles of 100
NDC 0006-0941-28 unit dose packages of 100.
    Shown in Product Identification Section, page 418
No. 3353—Tablets CLINORIL 200 mg are yellow, hexagon-shaped, scored, compressed tablets, coded MSD 942. They are supplied as follows:
NDC 0006-0942-54 unit of use bottles of 60
NDC 0006-0942-68 in bottles of 100
(6505-01-072-3426 100's)
NDC 0006-0942-78 unit of use bottles of 100
NDC 0006-0942-28 unit dose packages of 100.
    Shown in Product Identification Section, page 418
A.H.F.S. Category: 28:08
DC 7411626   Issued January 1989
COPYRIGHT © MERCK & CO., INC., 1988
All rights reserved

COGENTIN® Tablets   ℞
(Benztropine Mesylate, MSD), U.S.P.
COGENTIN® Injection   ℞
(Benztropine Mesylate, MSD), U.S.P.

DESCRIPTION

Benztropine mesylate is a synthetic compound resulting from the combination of the active portions of atropine and diphenhydramine.
It is a crystalline white powder, very soluble in water, with the following structural formula:
[See Chemical Formula at top of next column].
COGENTIN® (Benztropine Mesylate, MSD) is supplied as tablets in three strengths (0.5 mg, 1 mg, and 2 mg per tablet), and as an injection for intravenous and intramuscular use.

Tablets COGENTIN contain 0.5, 1 or 2 mg of benztropine mesylate. Each tablet contains the following inactive ingredients: calcium phosphate, cellulose, lactose, magnesium stearate and starch.
Each milliliter of the injection contains:
Benztropine mesylate ....1.0 mg
Sodium chloride..9.0 mg
Water for injection q.s. ....1.0 mL

ACTIONS

COGENTIN possesses both anticholinergic and antihistaminic effects, although only the former have been established as therapeutically significant in the management of parkinsonism.
In the isolated guinea pig ileum, the anticholinergic activity of this drug is about equal to that of atropine; however, when administered orally to unanesthetized cats, it is only about half as active as atropine.
In laboratory animals, its antihistaminic activity and duration of action approach those of pyrilamine maleate.

INDICATIONS

For use as an adjunct in the therapy of all forms of parkinsonism.
Useful also in the control of extrapyramidal disorders (except tardive dyskinesia—see PRECAUTIONS) due to neuroleptic drugs (e.g., phenothiazines).

CONTRAINDICATIONS

Hypersensitivity to COGENTIN tablets or to any component of COGENTIN injection.
Because of its atropine-like side effects, this drug is contraindicated in children under three years of age, and should be used with caution in older children.

WARNINGS

Safe use in pregnancy has not been established.
COGENTIN may impair mental and/or physical abilities required for performance of hazardous tasks, such as operating machinery or driving a motor vehicle.
When COGENTIN is given concomitantly with phenothiazines or other drugs with anticholinergic activity, patients should be advised to report gastrointestinal complaints promptly. Paralytic ileus, sometimes fatal, has occurred in patients taking anticholinergic-type antiparkinsonism drugs, including COGENTIN, in combination with phenothiazines and/or tricyclic antidepressants.
Since COGENTIN contains structural features of atropine, it may produce anhidrosis. For this reason, it should be administered with caution during hot weather, especially when given concomitantly with other atropine-like drugs to the chronically ill, the alcoholic, those who have central nervous system disease, and those who do manual labor in a hot environment. Anhidrosis may occur more readily when some disturbance of sweating already exists. If there is evidence of anhidrosis, the possibility of hyperthermia should be considered. Dosage should be decreased at the discretion of the physician so that the ability to maintain body heat equilibrium by perspiration is not impaired. Severe anhidrosis and fatal hyperthermia have occurred.

PRECAUTIONS

Since COGENTIN has cumulative action, continued supervision is advisable. Patients with a tendency to tachycardia and patients with prostatic hypertrophy should be observed closely during treatment.
Dysuria may occur, but rarely becomes a problem. Urinary retention has been reported with COGENTIN.
The drug may cause complaints of weakness and inability to move particular muscle groups, especially in large doses. For example, if the neck has been rigid and suddenly relaxes, it may feel weak, causing some concern. In this event, dosage adjustment is required.

Continued on next page

Information on the Merck Sharp & Dohme products listed on these pages is the full prescribing information from product circulars in use August 31, 1989.

Merck Sharp & Dohme—Cont.

Mental confusion and excitement may occur with large doses, or in susceptible patients. Visual hallucinations have been reported occasionally. Furthermore, in the treatment of extrapyramidal disorders due to neuroleptic drugs (e.g., phenothiazines), in patients with mental disorders, occasionally there may be intensification of mental symptoms. In such cases, antiparkinsonian drugs can precipitate a toxic psychosis. Patients wiith mental disorders should be kept under careful observation, especially at the beginning of treatment or if dosage is increased.

Tardive dyskinesia may appear in some patients on long-term therapy with phenothiazines and related agents, or may occur after therapy with these drugs has been discontinued. Antiparkinsonism agents do not alleviate the symptoms of tardive dyskinesia, and in some instances may aggravate them. COGENTIN is not recommended for use in patients with tardive dyskinesia.

The physician should be aware of the possible occurrence of glaucoma. Although the drug does not appear to have any adverse effect on simple glaucoma, it probably should not be used in angle-closure glaucoma.

ADVERSE REACTIONS

The adverse reactions below, most of which are anticholinergic in nature, have been reported and within each category are listed in order of decreasing severity.

Cardiovascular
Tachycardia.
Digestive
Constipation, dry mouth, nausea, vomiting.
If dry mouth is so severe that there is difficulty in swallowing or speaking, or loss of appetite and weight, reduce dosage, or discontinue the drug temporarily.
Slight reduction in dosage may control nausea and still give sufficient relief of symptoms. Vomiting may be controlled by temporary discontinuation, followed by resumption at a lower dosage.
Nervous System
Toxic psychosis, including confusion, disorientation, memory impairment, visual hallucinations; exacerbation of preexisting psychotic symptoms; nervousness; depression; listlessness; numbness of fingers.
Special Senses
Blurred vision, dilated pupils.
Urogenital
Urinary retention, dysuria.
Metabolic/Immune or Skin
Occasionally, an allergic reaction, e.g., skin rash, develops. If this can not be controlled by dosage reduction, the medication should be discontinued.

DOSAGE AND ADMINISTRATION

COGENTIN tablets should be used when patients are able to take oral medication.

The injection is especially useful for psychotic patients with acute dystonic reactions or other reactions that make oral medication difficult or impossible. It is recommended also when a more rapid response is desired than can be obtained with the tablets.

Since there is no significant difference in onset of effect after intravenous or intramuscular injection, usually there is no need to use the intravenous route. The drug is quickly effective after either route, with improvement sometimes noticeable a few minutes after injection. In emergency situations, when the condition of the patient is alarming, 1 to 2 mL of the injection normally will provide quick relief. If the parkinsonian effect begins to return, the dose can be repeated. Because of cumulative action, therapy should be initiated with a low dose which is increased gradually at five or six-day intervals to the smallest amount necessary for optimal relief. Increases should be made in increments of 0.5 mg, to a maximum of 6 mg, or until optimal results are obtained without excessive adverse reactions.

Postencephalitic and
Idiopathic Parkinsonism—
The usual daily dose is 1 to 2 mg, with a range of 0.5 to 6 mg orally or parenterally.

As with any agent used in parkinsonism, dosage must be individualized according to age and weight, and the type of parkinsonism being treated. Generally, older patients and thin patients cannot tolerate large doses. Most patients with postencephalitic parkinsonism need fairly large doses and tolerate them well. Patients with a poor mental outlook are usually poor candidates for therapy.

In idiopathic parkinsonism, therapy may be initiated with a single daily dose of 0.5 to 1 mg at bedtime. In some patients, this will be adequate; in others 4 to 6 mg a day may be required.

In postencephalitic parkinsonism, therapy may be initiated in most patients with 2 mg a day in one or more doses. In

highly sensitive patients, therapy may be initiated with 0.5 mg at bedtime, and increased as necessary.

Some patients experience greatest relief by taking the entire dose at bedtime; others react more favorably to divided doses, two to four times a day. Frequently, one dose a day is sufficient, and divided doses may be unnecessary or undesirable.

The long duration of action of this drug makes it particularly suitable for bedtime medication when its effects may last throughout the night, enabling patients to turn in bed during the night more easily, and to rise in the morning.

When COGENTIN is started, do not terminate therapy with other antiparkinsonian agents abruptly. If the other agents are to be reduced or discontinued, it must be done gradually. Many patients obtain greatest relief with combination therapy.

COGENTIN may be used concomitantly with SINEMET® (Carbidopa-Levodopa, MSD), or with levodopa, in which case periodic dosage adjustment may be required in order to maintain optimum response.

Drug-Induced Extrapyramidal Disorders—In treating extrapyramidal disorders due to neuroleptic drugs (e.g., phenothiazines), the recommended dosage is 1 to 4 mg once or twice a day orally or parenterally. Dosage must be individualized according to the need of the patient. Some patients require more than recommended; others do not need as much.

In acute dystonic reactions, 1 to 2 mL of the injection usually relieves the condition quickly. After that, the tablets, 1 to 2 mg twice a day, usually prevent recurrence.

When extrapyramidal disorders develop soon after initiation of treatment with neuroleptic drugs (e.g., phenothiazines), they are likely to be transient. One to 2 mg of COGENTIN tablets two or three times a day usually provides relief within one or two days. After one or two weeks, the drug should be withdrawn to determine the continued need for it. If such disorders recur, COGENTIN can be reinstituted. Certain drug-induced extrapyramidal disorders that develop slowly may not respond to COGENTIN.

OVERDOSAGE

Manifestations—May be any of those seen in atropine poisoning or antihistamine overdosage: CNS depression, preceded or followed by stimulation; confusion; nervousness; listlessness; intensification of mental symptoms or toxic psychosis in patients with mental illness being treated with neuroleptic drugs (e.g., phenothiazines); hallucinations (especially visual); dizziness; muscle weakness; ataxia; dry mouth; mydriasis; blurred vision; palpitations; tachycardia; nausea; vomiting; dysuria; numbness of fingers; dysphagia; allergic reactions, e.g., skin rash; headache; hot, dry, flushed skin; delirium; coma; shock; convulsions; respiratory arrest; anhidrosis; hyperthermia; glaucoma; constipation.

Treatment—Physostigmine salicylate, 1 to 2 mg, SC or IV, reportedly will reverse symptoms of anticholinergic intoxication (Duvoisin, R.C.; Katz, R.: J. Amer. Med. Ass. 206:1963-1965, Nov. 25, 1968). A second injection may be given after 2 hours if required. Otherwise treatment is symptomatic and supportive. Induce emesis or perform gastric lavage (contraindicated in precomatose, convulsive, or psychotic states). Maintain respiration. A short-acting barbiturate may be used for CNS excitement, but with caution to avoid subsequent depression; supportive care for depression (avoid convulsant stimulants such as picrotoxin, pentylenetetrazol, or bemegride); artificial respiration for severe respiratory depression; a local miotic for mydriasis and cycloplegia; ice bags or other cold applications and alcohol sponges for hyperpyrexia, a vasopressor and fluids for circulatory collapse. Darken room for photophobia.

HOW SUPPLIED

No. 3297—Tablets COGENTIN, 0.5 mg, are white, round, scored, compressed tablets, coded MSD 21. They are supplied as follows:
NDC 0006-0021-68 in bottles of 100.
   Shown in Product Identification Section, page 418
No. 3334—Tablets COGENTIN, 1 mg, are white, oval shaped, scored, compressed tablets, coded MSD 635. They are supplied as follows:
NDC 0006-0635-68 in bottles of 100
NDC 0006-0635-28 unit dose packages of 100.
   Shown in Product Identification Section, page 418
No. 3172—Tablets COGENTIN, 2 mg, are white, round, scored, compressed tablets, coded MSD 60. They are supplied as follows:
NDC 0006-0060-68 in bottles of 100
(6505-01-028-8726, 2 mg 100's)
NDC 0006-0060-28 unit dose packages of 100
NDC 0006-0060-82 in bottles of 1000.
   Shown in Product Identification Section, page 418
No. 3275—Injection COGENTIN, 1 mg per mL, is a clear, colorless solution and is supplied as follows:

NDC 0006-3275-16 in boxes of 6×2 mL ampuls.
   A.H.F.S. Category: 12:08
   DC 7398216   Issued July 1985

ColBENEMID® Tablets   ℞
(Probenecid-Colchicine, MSD), U.S.P.

DESCRIPTION

ColBENEMID® (Probenecid-Colchicine, MSD) contains probenecid, which is a uricosuric agent, and colchicine, which has antigout activity, the mechanism of which is unknown.

Probenecid is the generic name for 4-[(dipropylamino) sulfonyl] benzoic acid (molecular weight 285.36). It has the following structural formula:

Probenecid is a white or nearly white, fine, crystalline powder. It is soluble in dilute alkali, in alcohol, in chloroform, and in acetone; it is practically insoluble in water and in dilute acids.

Colchicine is an alkaloid obtained from various species of Colchicum. The chemical name for colchicine is (S)-N-(5,6,7,9-tetrahydro-1,2,3,10-tetramethoxy-9-oxobenzo [a] heptalen-7-yl) acetamide (molecular weight 399.43). It has the following structural formula:

Colchicine consists of pale yellow scales or powder; it darkens on exposure to light. Colchicine is soluble in water, freely soluble in alcohol and in chloroform, and slightly soluble in ether.

Each tablet contains 0.5 g probenecid and 0.5 mg colchicine and the following inactive ingredients: calcium stearate, gelatin, magnesium carbonate, starch.

ACTIONS

Probenecid is a uricosuric and renal tubular blocking agent. It inhibits the tubular reabsorption of urate, thus increasing the urinary excretion of uric acid and decreasing serum urate levels. Effective uricosuria reduces the miscible urate pool, retards urate deposition, and promotes resorption of urate deposits.

Probenecid inhibits the tubular secretion of penicillin and usually increases penicillin plasma levels by any route the antibiotic is given. A 2-fold to 4-fold elevation has been demonstrated for various penicillins.

Probenecid also has been reported to inhibit the renal transport of many other compounds including aminohippuric acid (PAH), aminosalicylic acid (PAS), indomethacin, sodium iodomethamate and related iodinated organic acids, 17-ketosteroids, pantothenic acid, phenolsulfonphthalein (PSP), sulfonamides, and sulfonylureas. See also DRUG INTERACTIONS.

Probenecid decreases both hepatic and renal excretion of sulfobromophthalein (BSP). The tubular reabsorption of phosphorus is inhibited in hypoparathyroid but not in euparathyroid individuals.

Probenecid does not influence plasma concentrations of salicylates, nor the excretion of streptomycin, chloramphenicol, chlortetracycline, oxytetracycline, or neomycin.

The mode of action of colchicine in gout is unknown. It is not an analgesic, though it relieves pain in acute attacks of gout. It is not a uricosuric agent and will not prevent progression of gout to chronic gouty arthritis. It does have a prophylactic, suppressive effect that helps to reduce the incidence of acute attacks and to relieve the residual pain and mild discomfort that patients with gout occasionally feel.

In man and certain other animals, colchicine can produce a temporary leukopenia that is followed by leukocytosis. Colchicine has other pharmacologic actions in animals: It alters neuromuscular function, intensifies gastrointestinal activity by neurogenic stimulation, increases sensitivity to central depressants, heightens response to sympathomimetic compounds, depresses the respiratory center, constricts blood vessels, causes hypertension by central vasomotor stimulation, and lowers body temperature.

INDICATIONS

For the treatment of chronic gouty arthritis when complicated by frequent, recurrent acute attacks of gout.

CONTRAINDICATIONS

Hypersensitivity to this product or to probenecid or colchicine.

Children under 2 years of age.

Not recommended in persons with known blood dyscrasias or uric acid kidney stones.

Therapy with ColBENEMID should not be started until an acute gouty attack has subsided.

Pregnancy: Probenecid crosses the placental barrier and appears in cord blood. Colchicine can arrest cell division in animals and plants. In certain species of animal under certain conditions, colchicine has produced teratogenic effects. The possibility of such effects in humans also has been reported. Because of the colchicine component, ColBENEMID is contraindicated in pregnant patients. The use of any drug in women of childbearing potential requires that the anticipated benefit be weighed against possible hazards.

WARNINGS

Exacerbation of gout following therapy with ColBENEMID may occur; in such cases additional colchicine or other appropriate therapy is advisable.

Probenecid increases plasma concentrations of methotrexate in both animals and humans. In animal studies, increased methotrexate toxicity has been reported. If ColBENEMID is given with methotrexate, the dosage of methotrexate should be reduced and serum levels may need to be monitored.

In patients on ColBENEMID the use of salicylates in either small or large doses is contraindicated because it antagonizes the uricosuric action of probenecid. The biphasic action of salicylates in the renal tubules accounts for the so-called "paradoxical effect" of uricosuric agents. In patients on ColBENEMID who require a mild analgesic agent the use of acetaminophen rather than small doses of salicylates would be preferred.

Rarely, severe allergic reactions and anaphylaxis have been reported with the use of ColBENEMID. Most of these have been reported to occur within several hours after readministration following prior usage of the drug.

The appearance of hypersensitivity reactions requires cessation of therapy with ColBENEMID.

Colchicine has been reported to adversely affect spermatogenesis in animals. Reversible azoospermia has been reported in one patient.

PRECAUTIONS

General

Hematuria, renal colic, costovertebral pain, and formation of uric acid stones associated with the use of ColBENEMID in gouty patients may be prevented by alkalization of the urine and a liberal fluid intake (*see* DOSAGE AND ADMINISTRATION). In these cases when alkali is administered, the acid-base balance of the patient should be watched.

Use with caution in patients with a history of peptic ulcer. ColBENEMID has been used in patients with some renal impairment but dosage requirements may be increased. ColBENEMID may not be effective in chronic renal insufficiency particularly when the glomerular filtration rate is 30 mL/minute or less.

A reducing substance may appear in the urine of patients receiving probenecid. This disappears with discontinuance of therapy. Suspected glycosuria should be confirmed by using a test specific for glucose.

Adequate animal studies have not been conducted to determine the carcinogenicity potential of probenecid or this drug combination. Since colchicine is an established mutagen, its ability to act as a carcinogen must be suspected and administration of ColBENEMID should involve a weighing of the benefit-vs-risk when long-term administration is contemplated.

Drug Interactions

When probenecid is used to elevate plasma concentrations of penicillin, or other beta-lactams, or when such drugs are given to patients taking probenecid therapeutically, high plasma concentrations of the other drug may increase the incidence of adverse reactions associated with that drug. In the case of penicillin, or other beta-lactams, psychic disturbances have been reported.

The use of salicylates antagonizes the uricosuric action of probenecid (*see* WARNINGS). The uricosuric action of probenecid is also antagonized by pyrazinamide.

Probenecid produces an insignificant increase in free sulfonamide plasma concentrations but a significant increase in total sulfonamide plasma levels. Since probenecid decreases the renal excretion of conjugated sulfonamides, plasma concentrations of the latter should be determined from time to time when a sulfonamide and ColBENEMID are coadministered for prolonged periods. Probenecid may prolong or enhance the action of oral sulfonylureas and thereby increase the risk of hypoglycemia.

It has been reported that patients receiving probenecid require significantly less thiopental for induction of anesthesia. In addition, ketamine and thiopental anesthesia were significantly prolonged in rats receiving probenecid.

The concomitant administration of probenecid increases the mean plasma elimination half-life of a number of drugs which can lead to increased plasma concentrations. These include agents such as indomethacin, acetaminophen, naproxen, ketoprofen, meclofenamate, lorazepam, and rifampin. Although the clinical significance of this observation has not been established, a lower dosage of the drug may be required to produce a therapeutic effect, and increases in dosage of the drug in question should be made cautiously and in small increments when probenecid is being co-administrated. Although specific instances of toxicity due to this potential interaction have not been observed to date, physicians should be alert to this possibility.

Probenecid given concomitantly with sulindac had only a slight effect on plasma sulfide levels, while plasma levels of sulindac and sulfone were increased. Sulindac was shown to produce a modest reduction in the uricosuric action of probenecid, which probably is not significant under most circumstances.

In animals and in humans, probenecid has been reported to increase plasma concentrations of methotrexate (*see* WARNINGS).

Falsely high readings for theophylline have been reported in an *in vitro* study, using the Schack and Waxler technic, when therapeutic concentrations of theophylline and probenecid were added to human plasma.

ADVERSE REACTIONS

The following adverse reactions have been observed and within each category are listed in order of decreasing severity.

Probenecid

Central Nervous System: headache, dizziness.

Metabolic: precipitation of acute gouty arthritis.

Gastrointestinal: hepatic necrosis, vomiting, nausea, anorexia, sore gums.

Genitourinary: nephrotic syndrome, uric acid stones with or without hematuria, renal colic, costovertebral pain, urinary frequency.

Hypersensitivity: anaphylaxis, fever, urticaria, pruritus.

Hematologic: aplastic anemia, leukopenia, hemolytic anemia which in some patients could be related to genetic deficiency of glucose -6- phosphate dehydrogenase in red blood cells, anemia.

Integumentary: dermatitis, alopecia, flushing.

Colchicine

Side effects due to colchicine appear to be a function of dosage. The possibility of increased colchicine toxicity in the presence of hepatic dysfunction should be considered. The appearance of any of the following symptoms may require reduction of dosage or discontinuance of the drug.

Central Nervous System: peripheral neuritis.

Musculoskeletal: muscular weakness.

Gastrointestinal: nausea, vomiting, abdominal pain, or diarrhea may be particularly troublesome in the presence of peptic ulcer or spastic colon.

Hypersensitivity: urticaria.

Hematologic: aplastic anemia, agranulocytosis.

Integumentary: dermatitis, purpura, alopecia.

At toxic doses, colchicine may cause severe diarrhea, generalized vascular damage, and renal damage with hematuria and oliguria.

DOSAGE AND ADMINISTRATION

Therapy with ColBENEMID should not be *started* until an acute gouty attack has subsided. However, if an acute attack is precipitated *during* therapy, ColBENEMID may be continued without changing the dosage, and additional colchicine or other appropriate therapy should be given to control the acute attack.

The recommended adult dosage is 1 tablet of ColBENEMID daily for one week, followed by 1 tablet twice a day thereafter.

Some degree of renal impairment may be present in patients with gout. A daily dosage of 2 tablets may be adequate. However, if necessary, the daily dosage may be increased by 1 tablet every four weeks within tolerance (and usually not above 4 tablets per day) if symptoms of gouty arthritis are not controlled or the 24 hour uric acid excretion is not above 700 mg. As noted, probenecid may not be effective in chronic renal insufficiency particularly when the glomerular filtration rate is 30 mL/minute or less.

Gastric intolerance may be indicative of overdosage, and may be corrected by decreasing the dosage.

As uric acid tends to crystallize out of an acid urine, a liberal fluid intake is recommended, as well as sufficient sodium bicarbonate (3 to 7.5 g daily) or potassium citrate (7.5 g daily) to maintain an alkaline urine (*see* PRECAUTIONS).

Alkalization of the urine is recommended until the serum urate level returns to normal limits and tophaceous deposits disappear, i.e., during the period when urinary excretion of uric acid is at a high level. Thereafter, alkalization of the urine and the usual restriction of purine-producing foods may be somewhat relaxed.

ColBENEMID (or probenecid) should be continued at the dosage that will maintain normal serum urate levels. When acute attacks have been absent for six months or more and serum urate levels remain within normal limits, the daily dosage of ColBENEMID may be decreased by 1 tablet every six months. The maintenance dosage should not be reduced to the point where serum urate levels tend to rise.

HOW SUPPLIED

No. 3283—Tablets ColBENEMID are white to off-white, capsule-shaped, scored tablets, coded MSD 614. Each tablet contains 0.5 g of probenecid and 0.5 mg of colchicine. They are supplied as follows:

NDC 0006-0614-68 bottles of 100.

Shown in Product Identification Section, page 418

Storage

Protect from light. Store container in carton until contents have been used.

    A.H.F.S. Categories: 40:40, 92:00

    DC 7398924 Issued August 1988

CORTONE® Acetate Sterile Suspension   ℞
(Cortisone Acetate, MSD), U.S.P.

For intramuscular injection only

NOT FOR INTRAVENOUS USE

DESCRIPTION

Cortisone acetate, a synthetic adrenocortical steroid, is a white or practically white, odorless, crystalline powder. It is stable in air. It is insoluble in water. The molecular weight is 402.49. It is designated chemically as 21-(acetyloxy)-17-hydroxypregn-4-ene-3,11,20-trione. The empirical formula is $C_{23}H_{30}O_6$ and the structural formula is:

CORTONE® Acetate (Cortisone Acetate, MSD) sterile suspension is a sterile suspension of cortisone acetate in an aqueous medium (pH 5.0 to 7.0). It is supplied in two strengths, one containing 25 mg of cortisone acetate per milliliter, the other containing 50 mg per milliliter. Inactive ingredients per mL: sodium chloride, 9 mg; polysorbate 80, 4 mg; sodium carboxymethylcellulose, 5 mg; Water for Injection q.s. 1 mL. Benzyl alcohol, 9 mg, added as preservative. No attempt should be made to alter CORTONE Acetate sterile suspension. Diluting it or mixing it with other substances may affect the state of suspension or change the rate of absorption and reduce its effectiveness.

ACTIONS

CORTONE Acetate sterile suspension has a slow onset but long duration of action when compared with more soluble preparations. When daily corticosteroid therapy is required and oral therapy is not feasible, the required daily dosage may be given in a single intramuscular injection of this preparation.

Naturally occurring glucocorticoids (hydrocortisone and cortisone), which also have salt-retaining properties, are used as replacement therapy in adrenocortical deficiency states. They are also used for their potent anti-inflammatory effects in disorders of many organ systems.

Glucocorticoids cause profound and varied metabolic effects. In addition, they modify the body's immune responses to diverse stimuli.

INDICATIONS

When oral therapy is not feasible:

1. *Endocrine disorders*

Primary or secondary adrenocortical insufficiency (hydrocortisone or cortisone is the drug of choice; synthetic analogs

Continued on next page

Merck Sharp & Dohme—Cont.

may be used in conjunction with mineralocorticoids where applicable; in infancy, mineralocorticoid supplementation is of particular importance)

Acute adrenocortical insufficiency (hydrocortisone or cortisone is the drug of choice; mineralocorticoid supplementation may be necessary, particularly when synthetic analogs are used)

Preoperatively, and in the event of serious trauma or illness, in patients with known adrenal insufficiency or when adrenocortical reserve is doubtful

Shock unresponsive to conventional therapy if adrenocortical insufficiency exists or is suspected
  Congenital adrenal hyperplasia
  Nonsuppurative thyroiditis
  Hypercalcemia associated with cancer
2. *Rheumatic disorders*
As adjunctive therapy for short-term administration (to tide the patient over an acute episode or exacerbation) in:
  Post-traumatic osteoarthritis
  Synovitis of osteoarthritis
  Rheumatoid arthritis, including juvenile rheumatoid arthritis (selected cases may require low-dose maintenance therapy)
  Acute and subacute bursitis
  Epicondylitis
  Acute nonspecific tenosynovitis
  Acute gouty arthritis
  Psoriatic arthritis
  Ankylosing spondylitis
3. *Collagen diseases*
During an exacerbation or as maintenance therapy in selected cases of:
  Systemic lupus erythematosus
  Acute rheumatic carditis
  Systemic dermatomyositis (polymyositis)
4. *Dermatologic diseases*
  Pemphigus
  Severe erythema multiforme (Stevens-Johnson syndrome)
  Exfoliative dermatitis
  Bullous dermatitis herpetiformis
  Severe seborrheic dermatitis
  Severe psoriasis
  Mycosis fungoides
5. *Allergic states*
Control of severe or incapacitating allergic conditions intractable to adequate trials of conventional treatment in:
  Bronchial asthma
  Contact dermatitis
  Atopic dermatitis
  Serum sickness
  Seasonal or perennial allergic rhinitis
  Drug hypersensitivity reactions
  Urticarial transfusion reactions
  Acute noninfectious laryngeal edema (epinephrine is the drug of first choice)
6. *Ophthalmic diseases*
Severe acute and chronic allergic and inflammatory processes involving the eye, such as:
  Herpes zoster ophthalmicus
  Iritis, iridocyclitis
  Chorioretinitis
  Diffuse posterior uveitis and choroiditis
  Optic neuritis
  Sympathetic ophthalmia
  Anterior segment inflammation
  Allergic conjunctivitis
  Keratitis
  Allergic corneal marginal ulcers
7. *Gastrointestinal diseases*
To tide the patient over a critical period of the disease in:
  Ulcerative colitis (Systemic therapy)
  Regional enteritis (Systemic therapy)
8. *Respiratory diseases*
  Symptomatic sarcoidosis
  Berylliosis
  Fulminating or disseminated pulmonary tuberculosis when used concurrently with appropriate antituberculous chemotherapy
  Loeffler's syndrome not manageable by other means
  Aspiration pneumonitis
9. *Hematologic disorders*
  Acquired (autoimmune) hemolytic anemia
  Erythroblastopenia (RBC anemia)
  Congenital (erythroid) hypoplastic anemia
10. *Neoplastic diseases*
  For palliative management of:
  Leukemias and lymphomas in adults
  Acute leukemia of childhood
11. *Edematous states*
  To induce diuresis or remission of proteinuria in the nephrotic syndrome, without uremia, of the idiopathic type, or that due to lupus erythematosus

12. *Miscellaneous*
  Tuberculous meningitis with subarachnoid block or impending block when used concurrently with appropriate antituberculous chemotherapy
  Trichinosis with neurologic or myocardial involvement

CONTRAINDICATIONS

Systemic fungal infections
Hypersensitivity to any component of this product

WARNINGS

Because rare instances of anaphylactoid reactions have occurred in patients receiving parenteral corticosteroid therapy, appropriate precautionary measures should be taken prior to administration, especially when the patient has a history of allergy to any drug. Anaphylactoid and hypersensitivity reactions have been reported for Sterile Suspension CORTONE Acetate (see ADVERSE REACTIONS).

In patients on corticosteroid therapy subjected to any unusual stress, increased dosage of rapidly acting corticosteroids before, during, and after the stressful situation is indicated.

Drug-induced secondary adrenocortical insufficiency may result from too rapid withdrawal of corticosteroids and may be minimized by gradual reduction of dosage. This type of relative insufficiency may persist for months after discontinuation of therapy; therefore, in any situation of stress occurring during that period, hormone therapy should be reinstituted. If the patient is receiving steroids already, dosage may have to be increased. Since mineralocorticoid secretion may be impaired, salt and/or a mineralocorticoid should be administered concurrently.

Corticosteroids may mask some signs of infection, and new infections may appear during their use. There may be decreased resistance and inability to localize infection when corticosteroids are used. Moreover, corticosteroids may affect the nitroblue-tetrazolium test for bacterial infection and produce false negative results.

In cerebral malaria, a double-blind trial has shown that the use of corticosteroids is associated with prolongation of coma and a higher incidence of pneumonia and gastrointestinal bleeding.

Corticosteroids may activate latent amebiasis. Therefore, it is recommended that latent or active amebiasis be ruled out before initiating corticosteroid therapy in any patient who has spent time in the tropics or any patient with unexplained diarrhea.

Prolonged use of corticosteroids may produce posterior subcapsular cataracts, glaucoma with possible damage to the optic nerves, and may enhance the establishment of secondary ocular infections due to fungi or viruses.

Usage in pregnancy. Since adequate human reproduction studies have not been done with corticosteroids, use of these drugs in pregnancy or in women of childbearing potential requires that the anticipated benefits be weighed against the possible hazards to the mother and embryo or fetus. Infants born of mothers who have received substantial doses of corticosteroids during pregnancy should be carefully observed for signs of hypoadrenalism.

Corticosteroids appear in breast milk and could suppress growth, interfere with endogenous corticosteroid production, or cause other unwanted effects. Mothers taking pharmacologic doses of corticosteroids should be advised not to nurse.

Average and large doses of cortisone or hydrocortisone can cause elevation of blood pressure, salt and water retention, and increased excretion of potassium. These effects are less likely to occur with the synthetic derivatives except when used in large doses. Dietary salt restriction and potassium supplementation may be necessary. All corticosteroids increase calcium excretion.

Administration of live virus vaccines, including smallpox, is contraindicated in individuals receiving immunosuppressive doses of corticosteroids. If inactivated viral or bacterial vaccines are administered to individuals receiving immunosuppressive doses of corticosteroids, the expected serum antibody response may not be obtained.

The use of CORTONE Acetate sterile suspension in active tuberculosis should be restricted to those cases of fulminating or disseminated tuberculosis in which the corticosteroid is used for the management of the disease in conjunction with an appropriate antituberculous regimen.

If corticosteroids are indicated in patients with latent tuberculosis or tuberculin reactivity, close observation is necessary as reactivation of the disease may occur. During prolonged corticosteroid therapy, these patients should receive chemoprophylaxis.

Literature reports suggest an apparent association between use of corticosteroids and left ventricular free wall rupture after a recent myocardial infarction; therefore, therapy with corticosteroids should be used with great caution in these patients.

PRECAUTIONS

CORTONE Acetate sterile suspension, like many other steroid formulations, is sensitive to heat. Therefore, it should not be autoclaved when it is desirable to sterilize the exterior of the vial.

Following prolonged therapy, withdrawal of corticosteroids may result in symptoms of the corticosteroid withdrawal syndrome including fever, myalgia, arthralgia, and malaise. This may occur in patients even without evidence of adrenal insufficiency.

There is an enhanced effect of corticosteroids in patients with hypothyroidism and in those with cirrhosis.

Corticosteroids should be used cautiously in patients with ocular herpes simplex for fear of corneal perforation.

The lowest possible dose of corticosteroid should be used to control the condition under treatment, and when reduction in dosage is possible, the reduction must be gradual.

Psychic derangements may appear when corticosteroids are used, ranging from euphoria, insomnia, mood swings, personality changes, and severe depression to frank psychotic manifestations. Also, existing emotional instability or psychotic tendencies may be aggravated by corticosteroids.

Aspirin should be used cautiously in conjunction with corticosteroids in hypoprothrombinemia.

Steroids should be used with caution in nonspecific ulcerative colitis, if there is a probability of impending perforation, abscess, or other pyogenic infection, also in diverticulitis, fresh intestinal anastomoses, active or latent peptic ulcer, renal insufficiency, hypertension, osteoporosis, and myasthenia gravis. Signs of peritoneal irritation following gastrointestinal perforation in patients receiving large doses of corticosteroids may be minimal or absent. Fat embolism has been reported as a possible complication of hypercortisonism.

When large doses are given, some authorities advise that antacids be administered between meals to help to prevent peptic ulcer.

Growth and development of infants and children on prolonged corticosteroid therapy should be carefully followed. Steroids may increase or decrease motility and number of spermatozoa in some patients.

Phenytoin, phenobarbital, ephedrine, and rifampin may enhance the metabolic clearance of corticosteroids, resulting in decreased blood levels and lessened physiologic activity, thus requiring adjustment in corticosteroid dosage.

The prothrombin time should be checked frequently in patients who are receiving corticosteroids and coumarin anticoagulants at the same time because of reports that corticosteroids have altered the response to these anticoagulants. Studies have shown that the usual effect produced by adding corticosteroids is inhibition of response to coumarins, although there have been some conflicting reports of potentiation not substantiated by studies.

When corticosteroids are administered concomitantly with potassium-depleting diuretics, patients should be observed closely for development of hypokalemia.

Injection of a steroid into an infected site is to be avoided.

ADVERSE REACTIONS

Fluid and electrolyte disturbances
  Sodium retention
  Fluid retention
  Congestive heart failure in susceptible patients
  Potassium loss
  Hypokalemic alkalosis
  Hypertension
Musculoskeletal
  Muscle weakness
  Steroid myopathy
  Loss of muscle mass
  Osteoporosis
  Vertebral compression fractures
  Aseptic necrosis of femoral and humeral heads
  Pathologic fracture of long bones
  Tendon rupture
Gastrointestinal
  Peptic ulcer with possible subsequent perforation and hemorrhage
  Perforation of the small and large bowel, particularly in patients with inflammatory bowel disease
  Pancreatitis
  Abdominal distention
  Ulcerative esophagitis
Dermatologic
  Impaired wound healing
  Thin fragile skin
  Petechiae and ecchymoses
  Erythema
  Increased sweating
  May suppress reactions to skin tests
  Other cutaneous reactions, such as allergic dermatitis, urticaria, angioneurotic edema

Neurologic
  Convulsions
  Increased intracranial pressure with papilledema (pseudotumor cerebri) usually after treatment
  Vertigo
  Headache
  Psychic disturbances
Endocrine
  Menstrual irregularities
  Development of cushingoid state
  Suppression of growth in children
  Secondary adrenocortical and pituitary unresponsiveness, particularly in times of stress, as in trauma, surgery, or illness
  Decreased carbohydrate tolerance
  Manifestations of latent diabetes mellitus
  Increased requirements for insulin or oral hypoglycemic agents in diabetics
  Hirsutism
Ophthalmic
  Posterior subcapsular cataracts
  Increased intraocular pressure
  Glaucoma
  Exophthalmos
Metabolic
  Negative nitrogen balance due to protein catabolism
Cardiovascular
  Myocardial rupture following recent myocardial infarction (see WARNINGS).
Other
  Anaphylactoid or hypersensitivity reactions
  Thromboembolism
  Weight gain
  Increased appetite
  Nausea
  Malaise
The following *additional* adverse reactions are related to parenteral corticosteroid therapy:
  Rare instances of blindness associated with intralesional therapy around the face and head
  Hyperpigmentation or hypopigmentation
  Subcutaneous and cutaneous atrophy
  Sterile abscess

OVERDOSAGE

Reports of acute toxicity and/or death following overdosage of glucocorticoids are rare. In the event of overdosage, no specific antidote is available; treatment is supportive and symptomatic.
The intraperitoneal LD_{50} of cortisone acetate in female mice was 1405 mg/kg.

DOSAGE AND ADMINISTRATION

For intramuscular injection only
NOT FOR INTRAVENOUS USE
DOSAGE REQUIREMENTS ARE VARIABLE AND MUST BE INDIVIDUALIZED ON THE BASIS OF THE DISEASE AND THE RESPONSE OF THE PATIENT.
The initial dosage varies from 20 to 300 mg a day depending on the disease being treated. In less severe diseases doses lower than 20 mg may suffice, while in severe diseases doses higher than 300 mg may be required. The initial dosage should be maintained or adjusted until the patient's response is satisfactory. If a satisfactory clinical response does not occur after a reasonable period of time, discontinue CORTONE Acetate sterile suspension and transfer the patient to other therapy.
After a favorable initial response, the proper maintenance dosage should be determined by decreasing the initial dosage in small amounts to the lowest dosage that maintains an adequate clinical response.
Patients should be observed closely for signs that might require dosage adjustment, including changes in clinical status resulting from remissions or exacerbations of the disease, individual drug responsiveness, and the effect of stress (e.g., surgery, infection, trauma). During stress it may be necessary to increase dosage temporarily.
If the drug is to be stopped after more than a few days of treatment, it usually should be withdrawn gradually.

HOW SUPPLIED

No. 7062—Sterile Suspension CORTONE Acetate is a white, mobile suspension, each mL containing 25 mg cortisone acetate, and is supplied as follows:
NDC 0006-7062-20 in 20 mL vials.
No. 7069—Sterile Suspension CORTONE Acetate is a white, mobile suspension, each mL containing 50 mg cortisone acetate, and is supplied as follows:
NDC 0006-7069-10 in 10 mL vials.
Storage
Sensitive to heat. Do not autoclave.
Protect from freezing.

A.H.F.S. Category: 68:04
DC 7411913   Issued March 1988

CORTONE® Acetate Tablets   ℞
(Cortisone Acetate, MSD), U.S.P.

DESCRIPTION

Glucocorticoids are adrenocortical steroids, both naturally occurring and synthetic, which are readily absorbed from the gastrointestinal tract.
Cortisone acetate is a white or practically white, odorless, crystalline powder. It is stable in air. It is insoluble in water. The molecular weight is 402.49. It is designated chemically as 21-(acetyloxy)-17-hydroxypregn-4-ene-3,11,20-trione. The empirical formula is $C_{23}H_{30}O_6$ and the structural formula is:

CORTONE® Acetate (Cortisone Acetate, MSD) tablets contain 25 mg of cortisone acetate in each tablet.
Inactive ingredients are lactose, magnesium stearate, and starch.

ACTIONS

Naturally occurring glucocorticoids (hydrocortisone and cortisone), which also have salt-retaining properties, are used as replacement therapy in adrenocortical deficiency states. They are also used for their potent anti-inflammatory effects in disorders of many organ systems.
Glucocorticoids cause profound and varied metabolic effects. In addition, they modify the body's immune responses to diverse stimuli.

INDICATIONS

1. *Endocrine Disorders*
Primary or secondary adrenocortical insufficiency (hydrocortisone or cortisone is the first choice; synthetic analogs may be used in conjunction with mineralocorticoids where applicable; in infancy mineralocorticoid supplementation is of particular importance).
  Congenital adrenal hyperplasia
  Nonsuppurative thyroiditis
  Hypercalcemia associated with cancer
2. *Rheumatic Disorders*
As adjunctive therapy for short-term administration (to tide the patient over an acute episode or exacerbation) in:
  Psoriatic arthritis
  Rheumatoid arthritis, including juvenile rheumatoid arthritis (selected cases may require low-dose maintenance therapy)
  Ankylosing spondylitis
  Acute and subacute bursitis
  Acute nonspecific tenosynovitis
  Acute gouty arthritis
  Post-traumatic osteoarthritis
  Synovitis of osteoarthritis
  Epicondylitis
3. *Collagen Diseases*
During an exacerbation or as maintenance therapy in selected cases of—
  Systemic lupus erythematosus
  Acute rheumatic carditis
  Systemic dermatomyositis (polymyositis)
4. *Dermatologic Diseases*
  Pemphigus
  Bullous dermatitis herpetiformis
  Severe erythema multiforme (Stevens-Johnson syndrome)
  Exfoliative dermatitis
  Mycosis fungoides
  Severe psoriasis
  Severe seborrheic dermatitis
5. *Allergic States*
Control of severe or incapacitating allergic conditions intractable to adequate trials of conventional treatment:
  Seasonal or perennial allergic rhinitis
  Bronchial asthma
  Contact dermatitis
  Atopic dermatitis
  Serum sickness
  Drug hypersensitivity reactions

---

6. *Ophthalmic Diseases*
Severe acute and chronic allergic and inflammatory processes involving the eye and its adnexa, such as—
  Allergic conjunctivitis
  Keratitis
  Allergic corneal marginal ulcers
  Herpes zoster ophthalmicus
  Iritis and iridocyclitis
  Chorioretinitis
  Anterior segment inflammation
  Diffuse posterior uveitis and choroiditis
  Optic neuritis
  Sympathetic ophthalmia
7. *Respiratory Diseases*
  Symptomatic sarcoidosis
  Loeffler's syndrome not manageable by other means
  Berylliosis
  Fulminating or disseminated pulmonary tuberculosis when used concurrently with appropriate antituberculous chemotherapy
  Aspiration pneumonitis
8. *Hematologic Disorders*
  Idiopathic thrombocytopenic purpura in adults
  Secondary thrombocytopenia in adults
  Acquired (autoimmune) hemolytic anemia
  Erythroblastopenia (RBC anemia)
  Congenital (erythroid) hypoplastic anemia
9. *Neoplastic Diseases*
For palliative management of:
  Leukemias and lymphomas in adults
  Acute leukemia of childhood
10. *Edematous States*
To induce a diuresis or remission of proteinuria in the nephrotic syndrome, without uremia, of the idiopathic type or that due to lupus erythematosus
11. *Gastrointestinal Diseases*
To tide the patient over a critical period of the disease in:
  Ulcerative colitis
  Regional enteritis
12. *Miscellaneous*
Tuberculous meningitis with subarachnoid block or impending block when used concurrently with appropriate antituberculous chemotherapy
Trichinosis with neurologic or myocardial involvement

CONTRAINDICATIONS

Systemic fungal infections
Hypersensitivity to this product

WARNINGS

In patients on corticosteroid therapy subjected to unusual stress, increased dosage of rapidly acting corticosteroids before, during, and after the stressful situation is indicated.
Drug-induced secondary adrenocortical insufficiency may result from too rapid withdrawal of corticosteroids and may be minimized by gradual reduction of dosage. This type of relative insufficiency may persist for months after discontinuation of therapy; therefore, in any situation of stress occurring during that period, hormone therapy should be reinstituted. If the patient is receiving steroids already, dosage may have to be increased. Since mineralocorticoid secretion may be impaired, salt and/or a mineralocorticoid should be administered concurrently.
Corticosteroids may mask some signs of infection, and new infections may appear during their use. There may be decreased resistance and inability to localize infection when corticosteroids are used. Moreover, corticosteroids may affect the nitroblue-tetrazolium test for bacterial infection and produce false negative results.
In cerebral malaria, a double-blind trial has shown that the use of corticosteroids is associated with prolongation of coma and a higher incidence of pneumonia and gastrointestinal bleeding.
Corticosteroids may activate latent amebiasis. Therefore, it is recommended that latent or active amebiasis be ruled out before initiating corticosteroid therapy in any patient who has spent time in the tropics or any patient with unexplained diarrhea.
Prolonged use of corticosteroids may produce posterior subcapsular cataracts, glaucoma with possible damage to the optic nerves, and may enhance the establishment of secondary ocular infections due to fungi or viruses.
Usage in pregnancy: Since adequate human reproduction studies have not been done with corticosteroids, use of these drugs in pregnancy or in women of childbearing potential

Continued on next page

Merck Sharp & Dohme—Cont.

requires that the anticipated benefits be weighed against the possible hazards to the mother and embryo or fetus. Infants born of mothers who have received substantial doses of corticosteroids during pregnancy should be carefully observed for signs of hypoadrenalism.

Corticosteroids appear in breast milk and could suppress growth, interefere with endogenous corticosteroid production, or cause other unwanted effects. Mothers taking pharmacologic doses of corticosteroids should be advised not to nurse.

Average and large doses of hydrocortisone or cortisone can cause elevation of blood pressure, salt and water retention, and increased excretion of potassium. These effects are less likely to occur with the synthetic derivatives except when used in large doses. Dietary salt restriction and potassium supplementation may be necessary. All corticosteroids increase calcium excretion.

Administration of live virus vaccines, including smallpox, is contraindicated in individuals receiving immunosuppressive doses of corticosteroids. If inactivated viral or bacterial vaccines are administered to individuals receiving immunosuppressive doses of corticosteroids, the expected serum antibody response may not be obtained. However, immunization procedures may be undertaken in patients who are receiving corticosteroids as replacement therapy, e.g., for Addison's disease.

The use of CORTONE Acetate tablets in active tuberculosis should be restricted to those cases of fulminating or disseminated tuberculosis in which the corticosteroid is used for the management of the disease in conjunction with an appropriate antituberculous regimen.

If corticosteroids are indicated in patients with latent tuberculosis or tuberculin reactivity, close observation is necessary as reactivation of the disease may occur. During prolonged corticosteroid therapy, these patients should receive chemoprophylaxis.

Literature reports suggest an apparent association between use of corticosteroids and left ventricular free wall rupture after a recent myocardial infarction; therefore, therapy with corticosteroids should be used with great caution in these patients.

PRECAUTIONS

Following prolonged therapy, withdrawal of corticosteroids may result in symptoms of the corticosteroid withdrawal syndrome including fever, myalgia, arthralgia, and malaise. This may occur in patients even without evidence of adrenal insufficiency.

There is an enhanced effect of corticosteroids in patients with hypothyroidism and in those with cirrhosis.

Corticosteroids should be used cautiously in patients with ocular herpes simplex because of possible corneal perforation.

The lowest possible dose of corticosteroid should be used to control the condition under treatment, and when reduction in dosage is possible, the reduction should be gradual.

Psychic derangements may appear when corticosteroids are used, ranging from euphoria, insomnia, mood swings, personality changes, and severe depression, to frank psychotic manifestations. Also, existing emotional instability or psychotic tendencies may be aggravated by corticosteroids.

Aspirin should be used cautiously in conjunction with corticosteroids in hypoprothrombinemia.

Steroids should be used with caution in nonspecific ulcerative colitis, if there is a probability of impending perforation, abscess, or other pyogenic infection, diverticulitis, fresh intestinal anastomoses, active or latent peptic ulcer, renal insufficiency, hypertension, osteoporosis, and myasthenia gravis. Signs of peritoneal irritation following gastrointestinal perforation in patients receiving large doses of corticosteroids may be minimal or absent. Fat embolism has been reported as a possible complication of hypercortisonism.

When large doses are given, some authorities advise that corticosteroids be taken with meals and antacids taken between meals to help to prevent peptic ulcer.

Growth and development of infants and children on prolonged corticosteroid therapy should be carefully observed. Steroids may increase or decrease motility and number of spermatozoa in some patients.

Phenytoin, phenobarbital, ephedrine, and rifampin may enhance the metabolic clearance of corticosteroids, resulting in decreased blood levels and lessened physiologic activity, thus requiring adjustment in corticosteroid dosage.

The prothrombin time should be checked frequently in patients who are receiving corticosteroids and coumarin anticoagulants at the same time because of reports that corticosteroids have altered the response to these anticoagulants. Studies have shown that the usual effect produced by adding corticosteroids is inhibition of response to coumarins, although there have been some conflicting reports of potentiation not substantiated by studies.

When corticosteroids are administered concomitantly with potassium-depleting diuretics, patients should be observed closely for development of hypokalemia.

ADVERSE REACTIONS

Fluid and Electrolyte Disturbances
   Sodium retention
   Fluid retention
   Congestive heart failure in susceptible patients
   Potassium loss
   Hypokalemic alkalosis
   Hypertension
Musculoskeletal
   Muscle weakness
   Steroid myopathy
   Loss of muscle mass
   Osteoporosis
   Vertebral compression fractures
   Aseptic necrosis of femoral and humeral heads
   Pathologic fracture of long bones
   Tendon rupture
Gastrointestinal
   Peptic ulcer with possible perforation and hemorrhage
   Perforation of the small and large bowel, particularly in patients with inflammatory bowel disease
   Pancreatitis
   Abdominal distention
   Ulcerative esophagitis
Dermatologic
   Impaired wound healing
   Thin fragile skin
   Petechiae and ecchymoses
   Erythema
   Increased sweating
   May suppress reactions to skin tests
   Other cutaneous reactions, such as allergic dermatitis, urticaria, angioneurotic edema
Neurologic
   Convulsions
   Increased intracranial pressure with papilledema (pseudotumor cerebri), usually after treatment
   Vertigo
   Headache
   Psychic disturbances
Endocrine
   Menstrual irregularities
   Development of cushingoid state
   Suppression of growth in children
   Secondary adrenocortical and pituitary unresponsiveness, particularly in times of stress, as in trauma, surgery, or illness
   Decreased carbohydrate tolerance
   Manifestations of latent diabetes mellitus
   Increased requirements for insulin or oral hypoglycemic agents in diabetics
   Hirsutism
Ophthalmic
   Posterior subcapsular cataracts
   Increased intraocular pressure
   Glaucoma
   Exophthalmos
Metabolic
   Negative nitrogen balance due to protein catabolism
Cardiovascular
   Myocardial rupture following recent myocardial infarction (see WARNINGS).
Other
   Hypersensitivity
   Thromboembolism
   Weight gain
   Increased appetite
   Nausea
   Malaise
   Psychic disturbances

OVERDOSAGE

Reports of acute toxicity and/or death following overdosage of glucocorticoids are rare. In the event of overdosage, no specific antidote is available; treatment is supportive and symptomatic.

The intraperitoneal LD_{50} of cortisone acetate in female mice was 1405 mg/kg.

DOSAGE AND ADMINISTRATION

For oral administration
DOSAGE REQUIREMENTS ARE VARIABLE AND MUST BE INDIVIDUALIZED ON THE BASIS OF THE DISEASE AND THE RESPONSE OF THE PATIENT.
The initial dosage varies from 25 to 300 mg a day depending on the disease being treated. In less severe diseases doses lower than 25 mg may suffice, while in severe diseases doses higher than 300 mg may be required. The initial dosage

should be maintained or adjusted until the patient's response is satisfactory. If satisfactory clinical response does not occur after a reasonable period of time, discontinue CORTONE Acetate tablets and transfer the patient to other therapy.

After a favorable initial response, the proper maintenance dosage should be determined by decreasing the initial dosage in small amounts to the lowest dosage that maintains an adequate clinical response.

Patients should be observed closely for signs that might require dosage adjustment, including changes in clinical status resulting from remissions or exacerbations of the disease, individual drug responsiveness, and the effect of stress (e.g., surgery, infection, trauma). During stress it may be necessary to increase dosage temporarily.

If the drug is to be stopped after more than a few days of treatment, it usually should be withdrawn gradually.

HOW SUPPLIED

No. 7063—Tablets Cortone Acetate, 25 mg each, are white, round, scored, compressed tablets, coded MSD 219. They are supplied as follows:
NDC 0006-0219-68 in bottles of 100.
Shown in Product Identification Section, page 418
    A.H.F.S. Category: 68:04
    DC 7411828   Issued March 1988

COSMEGEN® Injection   ℞
(Dactinomycin, MSD), U.S.P.

WARNING

Dactinomycin is extremely corrosive to soft tissue. If extravasation occurs during intravenous use, severe damage to soft tissues will occur. In at least one instance, this has led to contracture of the arms.

DOSAGE

The dosage of COSMEGEN® (Dactinomycin, MSD) is calculated in micrograms (mcg). The usual adult dosage is 500 micrograms (0.5 mg) daily intravenously for a maximum of five days. The dosage for adults or children should not exceed 15 mcg/kg or 400–600 mcg/square meter of body surface daily intravenously for five days. Calculation of the dosage for obese or edematous patients should be on the basis of surface area in an effort to relate dosage to lean body mass.

DESCRIPTION

Dactinomycin is one of the actinomycins, a group of antibiotics produced by various species of *Streptomyces*. Dactinomycin is the principal component of the mixture of actinomycins produced by *Streptomyces parvullus*. Unlike other species of *Streptomyces*, this organism yields an essentially pure substance that contains only traces of similar compounds differing in the amino acid content of the peptide side chains. The empirical formula is $C_{62}H_{86}N_{12}O_{16}$ and the structural formula is:

COSMEGEN is a sterile, yellow lyophilized powder for injection by the intravenous route or by regional perfusion after reconstitution. Each vial contains 0.5 mg (500 mcg) of dactinomycin and 20.0 mg of mannitol.

CLINICAL PHARMACOLOGY

Action
Generally, the actinomycins exert an inhibitory effect on gram-positive and gram-negative bacteria and on some fungi. However, the toxic properties of the actinomycins (including dactinomycin) in relation to antibacterial activity are such as to preclude their use as antibiotics in the treatment of infectious diseases.

Because the actinomycins are cytotoxic, they have an antineoplastic effect which has been demonstrated in experimental animals with various types of tumor implant. This cytotoxic action is the basis for their use in the palliative treatment of certain types of cancer.

Pharmacokinetics and Metabolism

Results of a study in patients with malignant melanoma indicate that dactinomycin (^{3}H actinomycin D) is minimally metabolized, is concentrated in nucleated cells, and does not penetrate the blood brain barrier. Approximately 30% of the dose was recovered in urine and feces in one week. The terminal plasma half-life for radioactivity was approximately 36 hours.

INDICATIONS AND USAGE

Wilms' Tumor

The neoplasm responding most frequently to COSMEGEN is Wilms' tumor. With low doses of both dactinomycin and radiotherapy, temporary objective improvement may be as good as and may last longer than with higher doses of each given alone. In the National Wilms' Tumor study, combination therapy with dactinomycin and vincristine together with surgery and radiotherapy, was shown to have significantly improved the prognosis of patients in groups II and III. Dactinomycin and vincristine were given for a total of seven cycles, so that maintenance therapy continued for approximately 15 months.

Postoperative radiotherapy in group I patients and optimal combination chemotherapy for those in group IV are unsettled issues. About 70 percent of lung metastases have disappeared with an appropriate combination of radiation, dactinomycin and vincristine.

Rhabdomyosarcoma

Temporary regression of the tumor and beneficial subjective results have occurred with dactinomycin in rhabdomyosarcoma which, like most soft tissue sarcomas, is comparatively radio-resistant.

Several groups have reported successful use of cyclophosphamide, vincristine, dactinomycin and doxorubicin hydrochloride in various combinations. Effective combinations have included vincristine and dactinomycin; vincristine, dactinomycin and cyclophosphamide (VAC therapy) and all four drugs in sequence. At present, the most effective treatment for children with inoperable or metastatic rhabdomyosarcoma has been VAC chemotherapy. Two-thirds of these children were doing well without evidence of disease at a median time of three years after diagnosis.

Carcinoma of Testis and Uterus

The sequential use of dactinomycin and methotrexate, along with meticulous monitoring of human chorionic gonadotropin levels until normal, has resulted in survival in the majority of women with metastatic choriocarcinoma. Sequential therapy is used if there is:

1. Stability in gonadotropin titers following two successive courses of an agent.
2. Rising gonadotropin titers during treatment.
3. Severe toxicity preventing adequate therapy.

In patients with nonmetastatic choriocarcinoma, dactinomycin or methotrexate or both, have been used successfully, with or without surgery.

Dactinomycin has been beneficial as a single agent in the treatment of metastatic nonseminomatour testicular carcinoma when used in cycles of 500 mcg/day for five consecutive days, every 6–8 weeks for periods of four months or longer.

Other Neoplasms

Dactinomycin has been given intravenously or by regional perfusion, either alone or with other antineoplastic compounds or x-ray therapy, in the palliative treatment of Ewing's sarcoma and sarcoma botryoides. For nonmetastatic Ewing's sarcoma, promising results were obtained when dactinomycin (45 mcg/m^2) and cyclophosphamide (1200 mg/m^2) were given sequentially and with radiotherapy, over an 18 month period. Those with metastatic disease remain the subject of continued investigation with a more aggressive chemotherapeutic regimen employed initially.

Temporary objective improvement and relief of pain and discomfort have followed the use of dactinomycin usually in conjunction with radiotherapy for sarcoma botryoides. This palliative effect ranges from transitory inhibition of tumor growth to a considerable but temporary regression in tumor size.

COSMEGEN (Dactinomycin, MSD) and Radiation Therapy

Much evidence suggests that dactinomycin potentiates the effects of x-ray therapy. The converse also appears likely; i.e., dactinomycin may be more effective when radiation therapy also is given.

With combined dactinomycin-radiation therapy, the normal skin, as well as the buccal and pharyngeal mucosa, show early erythema. A smaller than usual x-ray dose when given with dactinomycin causes erythema and vesiculation, which progress more rapidly through the stages of tanning and desquamation. Healing may occur in four to six weeks rather than two to three months. Erythema from previous x-ray therapy may be reactivated by dactinomycin alone, even when irradiation occurred many months earlier, and especially when the interval between the two forms of therapy is brief. This potentiation of radiation effect represents a special problem when the irradiation treatment area includes the mucous membrane. When irradiation is directed toward the nasopharynx, the combination may produce severe oropharyngeal mucositis. *Severe reactions may ensue if high doses of both dactinomycin and radiation therapy are used or if the patient is particularly sensitive to such combined therapy.*

Because of this potentiating effect, dactinomycin may be tried in radio-sensitive tumors not responding to doses of x-ray therapy that can be tolerated. Objective improvement in tumor size and activity may be observed when lower, better tolerated doses of both types of therapy are employed.

COSMEGEN (Dactinomycin, MSD) and Perfusion Technic

Dactinomycin alone or with other antineoplastic agents has also been given by the isolation-perfusion technic, either as palliative treatment or as an adjunct to resection of a tumor. Some tumors considered resistant to chemotherapy and radiation therapy may respond when the drug is given by the perfusion technic. Neoplasms in which dactinomycin has been tried by this technic include various types of sarcoma, carcinoma, and adenocarcinoma.

In some instances tumors regressed, pain was relieved for variable periods, and surgery made possible. On other occasions, however, the outcome has been less favorable. Nevertheless, in selected cases, the drug by perfusion may provide more effective palliation than when given systemically.

Dactinomycin by the isolation-perfusion technic offers certain advantages, provided leakage of the drug through the general circulation into other areas of the body is minimal. By this technic the drug is in continuous contact with the tumor for the duration of treatment. The dose may be increased well over that used by the systemic route, usually without adding to the danger of toxic effects. If the agent is confined to an isolated part, it should not interfere with the patient's defense mechanism. Systemic absorption of toxic products from neoplastic tissue can be minimized by removing the perfusate when the procedure is finished.

CONTRAINDICATIONS

If dactinomycin is given at or about the time of infection with chicken pox or herpes zoster, a severe generalized disease, which may result in death, may occur.

PRECAUTIONS

General

COSMEGEN should be administered only under the supervision of a physician who is experienced in the use of cancer chemotherapeutic agents.

This drug is highly toxic and both powder and solution must be handled and administered with care. Inhalation of dust or vapors and contact with skin or mucous membranes, especially those of the eyes, must be avoided. Should accidental eye contact occur, copious irrigation with water should be instituted immediately, followed by prompt ophthalmologic consultation. Should accidental skin contact occur, the affected part must be irrigated immediately with copious amounts of water for at least 15 minutes.

As with all antineoplastic agents, dactinomycin is a toxic drug and very careful and frequent observation of the patient for adverse reactions is necessary. These reactions may involve any tissue of the body. The possibility of an anaphylactoid reaction should be borne in mind.

Increased incidence of gastrointestinal toxicity and marrow suppression has been reported when dactinomycin was given with x-ray therapy.

Particular caution is necessary when administering dactinomycin within two months of irradiation for the treatment of right-sided Wilms' tumor, since hepatomegaly and elevated SGOT levels have been noted.

Nausea and vomiting due to dactinomycin make it necessary to give this drug intermittently. It is extremely important to observe the patient daily for toxic side effects when multiple chemotherapy is employed, since a full course of therapy occasionally is not tolerated. If stomatitis, diarrhea, or severe hemopoietic depression appear during therapy, these drugs should be discontinued until the patient has recovered. Recent reports indicate an increased incidence of second primary tumors following treatment with radiation and anti-neoplastic agents, such as dactinomycin. Multi-modal therapy creates the need for careful, long-term observation of cancer survivors.

Laboratory Tests

Many abnormalities of renal, hepatic, and bone marrow function have been reported in patients with neoplastic disease and receiving dactinomycin. It is advisable to check renal, hepatic, and bone marrow functions frequently.

Drug/Laboratory Test Interactions

It has been reported that dactinomycin may interfere with bioassay procedures for the determination of antibacterial drug levels.

Carcinogenesis, Mutagenesis, Impairment of Fertility

The International Agency on Research on Cancer has judged that dactinomycin is a positive carcinogen in animals. Local sarcomas were produced in mice and rats after repeated subcutaneous or intraperitoneal injection. Mesenchymal tumors occurred in male F344 rats given intraperitoneal injections of 0.05 mg/kg, 2 to 5 times per week for 18 weeks. The first tumor appeared at 23 weeks.

Dactinomycin has been shown to be mutagenic in a number of test systems *in vitro* and *in vivo* including human fibroblasts and leucocytes, and HELA cells. DNA damage and cytogenetic effects have been demonstrated in the mouse and the rat.

Adequate fertility studies have not been reported.

Pregnancy

Pregnancy Category C. COSMEGEN has been shown to cause malformations and embryotoxicity in the rat, rabbit and hamster when given in doses of 50–100 mcg/kg intravenously (3–7 times the maximum recommended human dose). There are no adequate and well-controlled studies in pregnant women. COSMEGEN should be used during pregnancy only if the potential benefit justifies the potential risk to the fetus.

Nursing Mothers

It is not known whether this drug is excreted in human milk. Because many drugs are excreted in human milk and because of the potential for serious adverse reactions in nursing infants from COSMEGEN, a decision should be made whether to discontinue nursing or to discontinue the drug, taking into account the importance of the drug to the mother.

Pediatric Use

The greater frequency of toxic effects of dactinomycin in infants suggest that this drug should be given to infants only over the age of 6 to 12 months.

ADVERSE REACTIONS

Toxic effects (excepting nausea and vomiting) usually do not become apparent until two to four days after a course of therapy is stopped, and may not be maximal before one to two weeks have elapsed. Deaths have been reported. However, adverse reactions are usually reversible on discontinuance of therapy. They include the following:

Miscellaneous: malaise, fatigue, lethargy, fever, myalgia, proctitis, hypocalcemia.

Oral: cheilitis, dysphagia, esophagitis, ulcerative stomatitis, pharyngitis.

Gastrointestinal: anorexia, nausea, vomiting, abdominal pain, diarrhea, gastrointestinal ulceration, liver toxicity including ascites, hepatomegaly, hepatitis, and liver function test abnormalities. Nausea and vomiting, which occur early during the first few hours after administration, may be alleviated by giving antiemetics.

Hematologic: anemia, even to the point of aplastic anemia, agranulocytosis, leukopenia, thrombocytopenia, pancytopenia, reticulopenia. Platelet and white cell counts should be done *daily* to detect severe hemopoietic depression. If either count markedly decreases, the drug should be withheld to allow marrow recovery. This often takes up to three weeks.

Dermatologic: alopecia, skin eruptions, acne, flare-up of erythema or increased pigmentation of previously irradiated skin.

Soft tissues. Dactinomycin is extremely corrosive. If extravasation occurs during intravenous use, severe damage to soft tissues will occur. In at least one instance, this has led to contracture of the arms.

OVERDOSAGE

The intravenous LD$_{50}$ of COSMEGEN in the rat is 460 mcg/kg.

DOSAGE AND ADMINISTRATION

Toxic reactions due to dactinomycin are frequent and may be severe (see ADVERSE REACTIONS), thus limiting in many instances the amount that may be given. However, the severity of toxicity varies markedly and is only partly dependent on the dose employed. The drug must be given in short courses.

Continued on next page

Merck Sharp & Dohme—Cont.

Intravenous Use

The dosage of dactinomycin varies depending on the tolerance of the patient, the size and location of the neoplasm, and the use of other forms of therapy. It may be necessary to decrease the usual dosages suggested below when other chemotherapy or x-ray therapy is used concomitantly or has been used previously.

The dosage for adults or children should not exceed 15 mcg/kg or 400–600 mcg/square meter of body surface daily intravenously for five days. Calculation of the dosage for obese or edematous patients should be on the basis of surface area in an effort to relate dosage to lean body mass.

Adults: The usual adult dosage is 500 mcg (0.5 mg) daily intravenously for a maximum of five days.

Children: In children 15 mcg (0.015 mg) per kilogram of body weight is given intravenously daily for five days. An alternative schedule is a total dosage of 2500 mcg (2.5 mg) per square meter of body surface given intravenously over a one week period.

In both adults and children, a second course may be given after at least three weeks have elapsed, provided all signs of toxicity have disappeared.

Reconstitute COSMEGEN by adding 1.1 ml of **Sterile Water for Injection (without preservative)** using aseptic precautions. The resulting solution of dactinomycin will contain approximately 500 mcg or 0.5 mg per ml.

Parenteral drug products should be inspected visually for particulate matter and discoloration prior to administration, whenever solution and container permit. When reconstituted, COSMEGEN is a clear, gold-colored solution.

Once reconstituted, the solution of dactinomycin can be added to infusion solutions of Dextrose Injection 5 percent or Sodium Chloride Injection either directly or to the tubing of a running intravenous infusion.

Although reconstituted COSMEGEN is chemically stable, the product does not contain a preservative and accidental microbial contamination might result. Any unused portion should be discarded. Use of water containing preservatives (benzyl alcohol or parabens) to reconstitute COSMEGEN for injection, results in the formation of a precipitate.

Partial removal of dactinomycin from intravenous solutions by cellulose ester membrane filters used in some intravenous in-line filters has been reported.

Since dactinomycin is extremely corrosive to soft tissue, precautions for materials of this nature should be observed.

If the drug is given directly into the vein without the use of an infusion, the "two-needle technic" should be used. Reconstitute and withdraw the calculated dose from the vial with one sterile needle. Use another sterile needle for direct injection into the vein.

Discard any unused portion of the dactinomycin solution.

Isolation-Perfusion Technic

The dosage schedules and the technic itself vary from one investigator to another; the published literature, therefore, should be consulted for details. In general, the following doses are suggested:

    50 mcg (0.05 mg) per kilogram of body weight for lower extremity or pelvis.

    35 mcg (0.035 mg) per kilogram of body weight for upper extremity.

It may be advisable to use lower doses in obese patients, or when previous chemotherapy or radiation therapy has been employed.

Complications of the perfusion technic are related mainly to the amount of drug that escapes into the systemic circulation and may consist of hemopoietic depression, absorption of toxic products from massive destruction of neoplastic tissue, increased susceptibility to infection, impaired wound healing, and superficial ulceration of the gastric mucosa. Other side effects may include edema of the extremity involved, damage to soft tissues of the perfused area, and (potentially) venous thrombosis.

HOW SUPPLIED

No. 3298—Injection COSMEGEN is a lyophilized powder and is supplied as follows: **NDC** 0006-3298-22 in vials containing 0.5 mg (500 micrograms) of dactinomycin and 20.0 mg of mannitol. In the dry form the compound is an amorphous yellow powder. The solution is clear and gold-colored.

Storage

Protect from light.

Special Handling

Due to the drug's toxic and mutagenic properties, appropriate precautions including the use of appropriate safety equipment are recommended for the preparation of COSMEGEN for parenteral administration. The National Institutes of Health presently recommends that the preparation of injectable antineoplastic drugs should be performed in a Class II laminar flow biological safety cabinet and that per-

sonnel preparing drugs of this class should wear surgical gloves and a closed front surgical-type gown with knit cuffs.

A.H.F.S. Category: 10:00
DC 7496524 Issued December 1988
COPYRIGHT © MERCK & CO., INC., 1983
All rights reserved

CUPRID® Capsules   ℞
(Trientine Hydrochloride, MSD)

DESCRIPTION

Trientine hydrochloride is *N,N'*-bis (2-aminoethyl)-1,2-ethanediamine dihydrochloride. It is a white to pale yellow crystalline hygroscopic powder. It is freely soluble in water, soluble in methanol, slightly soluble in ethanol, and insoluble in chloroform and ether.

The empirical formula is $C_6H_{18}N_4 \cdot 2HCl$ with a molecular weight of 219.2. The structural formula is:

$NH_2(CH_2)_2NH(CH_2)_2NH(CH_2)_2NH_2 \cdot 2HCl$

Trientine hydrochloride is a chelating compound for removal of excess copper from the body. CUPRID® (Trientine Hydrochloride, MSD) is available as 250 mg capsules for oral administration. Capsules CUPRID contain gelatin, iron oxides, stearic acid, and titanium dioxide as inactive ingredients.

CLINICAL PHARMACOLOGY

Introduction

Wilson's disease (hepatolenticular degeneration) is an autosomal inherited metabolic defect resulting in an inability to maintain a near-zero balance of copper. Excess copper accumulates possibly because the liver lacks the mechanism to excrete free copper into the bile. Hepatocytes store excess copper but when their capacity is exceeded copper is released into the blood and is taken up into extrahepatic sites. This condition is treated with a low copper diet and the use of chelating agents that bind copper to facilitate its excretion from the body.

Clinical Summary

Forty-one patients (18 male and 23 female) between the ages of 6 and 54 with a diagnosis of Wilson's disease and who were intolerant of d-penicillamine were treated in two separate studies with trientine hydrochloride. The dosage varied from 450 to 2400 mg per day. The average dosage required to achieve an optimal clinical response varied between 1000 mg and 2000 mg per day. The mean duration of trientine hydrochloride therapy was 48.7 months (range 2–164 months). Thirty-four of the 41 patients improved, 4 had no change in clinical global response, 2 were lost to follow-up and one showed deterioration in clinical condition. One of the patients who improved while on therapy with trientine hydrochloride experienced a recurrence of the symptoms of systemic lupus erythematosus which had appeared originally during therapy with penicillamine. Therapy with trientine hydrochloride was discontinued. No other adverse reactions, except iron deficiency, were noted among any of these 41 patients.

One investigator treated 13 patients with trientine hydrochloride following their development of intolerance to d-penicillamine. Retrospectively, he compared these patients to an additional group of 12 patients with Wilson's disease who were both tolerant of and controlled with d-penicillamine therapy, but who failed to continue any copper chelation therapy. The mean age at onset of disease of the latter group was 12 years as compared to 21 years for the former group. The trientine hydrochloride group received d-penicillamine for an average of 4 years as compared to an average of 10 years for the non-treated group.

Various laboratory parameters showed changes in favor of the patients treated with trientine hydrochloride. Free and total serum copper, SGOT, and serum bilirubin all showed mean increases over baseline in the untreated group which were significantly larger than with the patients treated with trientine hydrochloride. In the 13 patients treated with trientine hydrochloride, previous symptoms and signs relating to d-penicillamine intolerance disappeared in 8 patients, improved in 4 patients, and remained unchanged in one patient. The neurological status in the trientine hydrochloride group was unchanged or improved over baseline, whereas in the untreated group, 6 patients remained unchanged and 6 worsened. Kayser-Fleischer rings improved significantly during trientine hydrochloride treatment.

The clinical outcome of the two groups also differed markedly. Of the 13 patients on therapy with trientine hydrochloride (mean duration of therapy 4.1 years; range 1 to 13 years), all were alive at the data cutoff date, and in the non-treated group (mean years with no therapy 2.7 years; range 3 months to 9 years), 9 of the 12 died of hepatic disease.

Chelating Properties

Preclinical Studies

Studies in animals have shown that trientine hydrochloride has cupriuretic activities in both normal and copper-loaded rats. In general, the effects of trientine hydrochloride on urinary copper excretion are similar to those of equimolar

doses of penicillamine, although in one study they were significantly smaller.

Human Studies

Renal clearance studies were carried out with penicillamine and trientine hydrochloride on separate occasions in selected patients treated with penicillamine for at least one year. Six-hour excretion rates of copper were determined off treatment and after a single dose of 500 mg of penicillamine or 1.2 g of trientine hydrochloride. The mean urinary excretion rates of copper were as follows:

No. of Patients	Single Dose Treatment	Basal Excretion Rate (μg Cu⁺⁺/6hr)	Test-dose Excretion Rate (μg Cu⁺⁺/6hr)
6	Trientine, 1.2 g	19	234
4	Penicillamine, 500 mg	17	320

In patients *not* previously treated with chelating agents, a similar comparison was made:

No. of Patients	Single Dose Treatment	Basal Excretion Rate (μg Cu⁺⁺/6hr)	Test-dose Excretion Rate (μg Cu⁺⁺/6hr)
8	Trientine, 1.2 g	71	1326
7	Penicillamine, 500 mg	68	1074

These results demonstrate that CUPRID is effective as a cupriuretic agent in patients with Wilson's disease although on a molar basis it appears to be less potent or less effective than penicillamine. Evidence from a radio-labelled copper study indicates that the different cupriuretic effect between these two drugs could be due to a difference in selectivity of the drugs for different copper pools within the body.

Pharmacokinetics

Data on the pharmacokinetics of trientine hydrochloride are not available. Dosage adjustment recommendations are based upon clinical use of the drug (see DOSAGE AND ADMINISTRATION).

INDICATIONS AND USAGE

CUPRID is indicated in the treatment of patients with Wilson's disease who are intolerant of penicillamine. Clinical experience with CUPRID is limited and alternate dosing regimens have not been well-characterized; all endpoints in determining an individual patient's dose have not been well defined. CUPRID and penicillamine cannot be considered interchangeable. CUPRID should be used when continued treatment with penicillamine is no longer possible because of intolerable or life endangering side effects.

Unlike penicillamine, CUPRID is not recommended in cystinuria or rheumatoid arthritis. The absence of a sulfhydryl moiety renders it incapable of binding cystine and, therefore, it is of no use in cystinuria. In 15 patients with rheumatoid arthritis, CUPRID was reported not to be effective in improving any clinical or biochemical parameter after 12 weeks of treatment.

CUPRID is not indicated for treatment of biliary cirrhosis.

CONTRAINDICATIONS

Hypersensitivity to this product.

WARNINGS

Patient experience with trientine hydrochloride is limited (see CLINICAL PHARMACOLOGY). Patients receiving CUPRID should remain under regular medical supervision throughout the period of drug administration. Patients (especially women) should be closely monitored for evidence of iron deficiency anemia.

PRECAUTIONS

General

There are no reports of hypersensitivity in patients who have been administered trientine hydrochloride for Wilson's disease. However, there have been reports of asthma, bronchitis and dermatitis occurring after prolonged environmental exposure in workers who use trientine hydrochloride as a hardener of epoxy resins. Patients should be observed closely for signs of possible hypersensitivity.

Information for Patients

Patients should be directed to take CUPRID on an empty stomach, at least one hour before meals or two hours after meals and at least one hour apart from any other drug, food, or milk. The capsules should be swallowed whole with water and should not be opened or chewed. Because of the potential for contact dermatitis, any site of exposure to the capsule contents should be washed with water promptly. For the first month of treatment, the patient should have his temperature taken nightly, and he should be asked to report any symptom such as fever or skin eruption.

Laboratory Tests

The most reliable index for monitoring treatment is the determination of free copper in the serum, which equals the difference between quantitatively determined total copper and ceruloplasmin-copper. Adequately treated patients will usually have less than 10 mcg free copper/dL of serum. Therapy may be monitored with a 24 hour urinary copper analysis periodically (i.e., every 6–12 months). Urine must be collected in copper-free glassware. Since a low copper diet should keep copper absorption down to less than one milligram a day, the patient probably will be in the desired state of negative copper balance if 0.5 to 1.0 milligram of copper is present in a 24-hour collection of urine.

Drug Interactions

In general, mineral supplements should not be given since they may block the absorption of CUPRID. However, iron deficiency may develop, especially in children and menstruating or pregnant women, or as a result of the low copper diet recommended for Wilson's disease. If necessary, iron may be given in short courses, but since iron and CUPRID each inhibit absorption of the other, two hours should elapse between administration of CUPRID and iron.

It is important that CUPRID be taken on an empty stomach, at least one hour before meals or two hours after meals and at least one hour apart from any other drug, food, or milk. This permits maximum absorption and reduces the likelihood of inactivation of the drug by metal binding in the gastrointestinal tract.

Carcinogenesis, Mutagenesis, Impairment of Fertility

Data on carcinogenesis, mutagenesis, and impairment of fertility are not available.

Pregnancy

Pregnancy Category C. Trientine hydrochloride was teratogenic in rats at doses similar to the human dose. The frequencies of both resorptions and fetal abnormalities, including hemorrhage and edema, increased while fetal copper levels decreased when trientine hydrochloride was given in the maternal diets of rats. There are no adequate and well-controlled studies in pregnant women. CUPRID should be used during pregnancy only if the potential benefit justifies the potential risk to the fetus.

Nursing Mothers

It is not known whether this drug is excreted in human milk. Because many drugs are excreted in human milk, caution should be exercised when CUPRID is administered to a nursing mother.

Pediatric Use

Controlled studies of the safety and effectiveness of CUPRID in children have not been conducted. It has been used clinically in children as young as 6 years with no reported adverse experiences.

ADVERSE REACTIONS

Clinical experience with CUPRID has been limited. The following adverse reactions have been reported in patients with Wilson's disease who were on therapy with trientine hydrochloride: iron deficiency, systemic lupus erythematosus (see CLINICAL PHARMACOLOGY).

CUPRID is not indicated for treatment of biliary cirrhosis, but in one study of 4 patients treated with trientine hydrochloride for primary biliary cirrhosis, the following adverse reactions were reported: heartburn; epigastric pain and tenderness; thickening, fissuring and flaking of the skin; hypochromic microcytic anemia; acute gastritis; aphthoid ulcers; abdominal pain; melena; anorexia; malaise; cramps; muscle pain; weakness; rhabdomyolysis. A causal relationship of these reactions to drug therapy could not be rejected or established.

OVERDOSAGE

There is a report of an adult woman who ingested 30 grams of trientine hydrochloride without apparent ill effects. No other data on overdosage are available.

DOSAGE AND ADMINISTRATION

Systemic evaluation of dose and/or interval between dose has not been done. However, on limited clinical experience, the recommended initial dose of CUPRID is 500–750 mg/day for children and 750–1250 mg/day for adults given in divided doses two, three or four times daily. This may be increased to a maximum of 2000 mg/day for adults or 1500 mg/day for children age 12 or under. The daily dose of CUPRID should be increased only when the clinical response is not adequate or the concentration of free serum copper is persistently above 20 mcg/dL. Optimal long-term maintenance dosage should be determined at 6–12 month intervals (see PRECAUTIONS, *Laboratory Tests*).

It is important that CUPRID be given on an empty stomach, at least one hour before meals or two hours after meals and at least one hour apart from any other drug, food, or milk. The capsules should be swallowed whole with water and should not be opened or chewed.

HOW SUPPLIED

No. 3511—Capsules CUPRID, 250 mg, are light brown opaque capsules and are coded MSD 679. They are supplied as follows:

NDC 0006-0679-68 in bottles of 100.

Storage

Keep container tightly closed.

Store at 2°–8°C (35.6°–46.4°F).

A.H.F.S. Category: 12:20

DC 7325102 Issued June 1986

COPYRIGHT © MERCK & CO., INC., 1985

All rights reserved

CUPRIMINE® Capsules   ℞
(Penicillamine, MSD), U.S.P.

> Physicians planning to use penicillamine should thoroughly familiarize themselves with its toxicity, special dosage considerations, and therapeutic benefits. Penicillamine should never be used casually. Each patient should remain constantly under the close supervision of the physician. Patients should be warned to report promptly any symptoms suggesting toxicity.

DESCRIPTION

Penicillamine is 3-mercapto-D-valine. It is a white or practically white, crystalline powder, freely soluble in water, slightly soluble in alcohol, and insoluble in ether, acetone, benzene, and carbon tetrachloride. Although its configuration is D, it is levorotatory as usually measured:

$$[\alpha]25° = -63° \pm 5° (C = 1, 1\underline{N} \text{ NaOH})\cdot$$
$$D$$

The empirical formula is $C_5H_{11}NO_2S$, giving it a molecular weight of 149.21. The structural formula is:

$$\underset{(CH_3)_2C-CHCOOH}{\overset{SH \ NH_2}{| \quad |}}$$

It reacts readily with formaldehyde or acetone to form a thiazolidine-carboxylic acid.

Capsules CUPRIMINE® (Penicillamine, MSD) for oral administration contain either 125 mg or 250 mg of penicillamine. Each capsule contains the following inactive ingredients: D & C Yellow 10, gelatin, lactose, magnesium stearate, and titanium dioxide. The 125 mg capsule also contains iron oxide.

CLINICAL PHARMACOLOGY

Penicillamine is a chelating agent recommended for the removal of excess copper in patients with Wilson's disease. From *in vitro* studies which indicate that one atom of copper combines with two molecules of penicillamine, it would appear that one gram of penicillamine should be followed by the excretion of about 200 milligrams of copper; however, the actual amount excreted is about one percent of this.

Penicillamine also reduces excess cystine excretion in cystinuria. This is done, at least in part, by disulfide interchange between penicillamine and cystine, resulting in formation of penicillamine-cysteine disulfide, a substance that is much more soluble than cystine and is excreted readily.

Penicillamine interferes with the formation of cross-links between tropocollagen molecules and cleaves them when newly formed.

The mechanism of action of penicillamine in rheumatoid arthritis is unknown although it appears to suppress disease activity. Unlike cytotoxic immunosuppressants, penicillamine markedly lowers IgM rheumatoid factor but produces no significant depression in absolute levels of serum immunoglobulins. Also unlike cytotoxic immunosuppressants which act on both, penicillamine *in vitro* depresses T-cell activity but not B-cell activity.

In vitro, penicillamine dissociates macroglobulins (rheumatoid factor) although the relationship of the activity to its effect in rheumatoid arthritis is not known.

In rheumatoid arthritis, the onset of therapeutic response to CUPRIMINE may not be seen for two or three months. In those patients who respond, however, the first evidence of suppression of symptoms such as pain, tenderness, and swelling is generally apparent within three months. The optimum duration of therapy has not been determined. If remissions occur, they may last from months to years, but usually require continued treatment (see DOSAGE AND ADMINISTRATION).

In all patients receiving penicillamine, it is important that CUPRIMINE be given on an empty stomach, at least one hour before meals or two hours after meals, and at least one hour apart from any other drug, food, or milk. This permits maximum absorption and reduces the likelihood of inactivation by metal binding in the gastrointestinal tract. Methodology for determining the bioavailability of penicillamine is not available; however, penicillamine is known to be a very soluble substance.

INDICATIONS

CUPRIMINE is indicated in the treatment of Wilson's disease, cystinuria, and in patients with severe, active rheumatoid arthritis who have failed to respond to an adequate trial of conventional therapy. Available evidence suggests that CUPRIMINE is not of value in ankylosing spondylitis.

Wilson's Disease—Wilson's disease (hepatolenticular degeneration) results from the interaction of an inherited defect and an abnormality in copper metabolism. The metabolic defect, which is the consequence of the autosomal inheritance of one abnormal gene from each parent, manifests itself in a greater positive copper balance than normal. As a result, copper is deposited in several organs and appears eventually to produce pathologic effects most prominently seen in the brain, where degeneration is widespread; in the liver, after fatty infiltration, inflammation, and hepatocellular damage progress to postnecrotic cirrhosis; in the kidney, where tubular and glomerular dysfunction results; and in the eye, where characteristic corneal copper deposits are known as Kayser-Fleischer rings.

Two types of patients require treatment for Wilson's disease: (1) the symptomatic, and (2) the asymptomatic in whom it can be assumed the disease will develop in the future if the patient is not treated.

Diagnosis, suspected on the basis of family or individual history, physical examination, or a low serum concentration of ceruloplasmin*, is confirmed by the demonstration of Kayser-Fleischer rings or, particularly in the asymptomatic patient, by the quantitative demonstration in a liver biopsy specimen of a concentration of copper in excess of 250 mcg/g dry weight.

Treatment has two objectives:

(1) to minimize dietary intake and absorption of copper.

(2) to promote excretion of copper deposited in tissues.

The first objective is attained by a daily diet that contains no more than one or two milligrams of copper. Such a diet should exclude, most importantly, chocolate, nuts, shellfish, mushrooms, liver, molasses, broccoli, and cereals enriched with copper, and be composed to as great an extent as possible of foods with a low copper content. Distilled or demineralized water should be used if the patient's drinking water contains more than 0.1 mg of copper per liter.

For the second objective, a copper chelating agent is used. In symptomatic patients this treatment usually produces marked neurologic improvement, fading of Kayser-Fleischer rings, and gradual amelioration of hepatic dysfunction and psychic disturbances.

Clinical experience to date suggests that life is prolonged with the above regimen.

Noticeable improvement may not occur for one to three months. Occasionally, neurologic symptoms become worse during initiation of therapy with CUPRIMINE. Despite this, the drug should not be discontinued permanently, although temporary interruption may result in clinical improvement of the neurological symptoms but it carries an increased risk of developing a sensitivity reaction upon resumption of therapy (see WARNINGS).

Treatment of asymptomatic patients has been carried out for over ten years. Symptoms and signs of the disease appear to be prevented indefinitely if daily treatment with CUPRIMINE can be continued.

Cystinuria—Cystinuria is characterized by excessive urinary excretion of the dibasic amino acids, arginine, lysine, ornithine, and cystine, and the mixed disulfide of cysteine and homocysteine. The metabolic defect that leads to cystinuria is inherited as an autosomal, recessive trait. Metabolism of the affected amino acids is influenced by at least two abnormal factors: (1) defective gastrointestinal absorption and (2) renal tubular dysfunction.

Arginine, lysine, ornithine, and cysteine are soluble substances, readily excreted. There is no apparent pathology connected with their excretion in excessive quantities.

---

*For quantitative test for serum ceruloplasmin see: Morell, A.G.; Windsor, J.; Sternlieb, I.; Scheinberg, I.H.: Measurement of the concentration of ceruloplasmin in serum by determination of its oxidase activity, in "Laboratory Diagnosis of Liver Disease", F.W. Sunderman; F.W. Sunderman, Jr. (eds.), St. Louis, Warren H. Green, Inc., 1968, pp. 193-195.

Continued on next page

Information on the Merck Sharp & Dohme products listed on these pages is the full prescribing information from product circulars in use August 31, 1989.

Merck Sharp & Dohme—Cont.

Cystine, however, is so slightly soluble at the usual range of urinary pH that it is not excreted readily, and so crystallizes and forms stones in the urinary tract. Stone formation is the only known pathology in cystinuria.

Normal daily output of cystine is 40 to 80 mg. In cystinuria, output is greatly increased and may exceed 1 g/day. At 500 to 600 mg/day, stone formation is almost certain. When it is more than 300 mg/day, treatment is indicated.

Conventional treatment is directed at keeping urinary cystine diluted enough to prevent stone formation, keeping the urine alkaline enough to dissolve as much cystine as possible, and minimizing cystine production by a diet low in methionine (the major dietary precursor of cystine). Patients must drink enough fluid to keep urine specific gravity below 1.010, take enough alkali to keep urinary pH at 7.5 to 8, and maintain a diet low in methionine. This diet is not recommended in growing children and probably is contraindicated in pregnancy because of its low protein content (see PRECAUTIONS).

When these measures are inadequate to control recurrent stone formation, CUPRIMINE may be used as additional therapy. When patients refuse to adhere to conventional treatment, CUPRIMINE may be a useful substitute. It is capable of keeping cystine excretion to near normal values, thereby hindering stone formation and the serious consequences of pyelonephritis and impaired renal function that develop in some patients.

Bartter and colleagues depict the process by which penicillamine interacts with cystine to form penicillamine-cysteine mixed disulfide as:

$$
\begin{array}{rcl}
CSSC + PS' & \rightleftharpoons & CS' + CSSP \\
PSSP + CS' & \rightleftharpoons & PS' + CSSP \\
CSSC + PSSP & \rightleftharpoons & 2\ CSSP \\
\end{array}
$$

CSSC = cystine
CS' = deprotonated cysteine
PSSP = penicillamine
PS' = deprotonated penicillamine sulfhydryl
CSSP = penicillamine-cysteine mixed disulfide

In this process, it is assumed that the deprotonated form of penicillamine, PS', is the active factor in bringing about the disulfide interchange.

Rheumatoid Arthritis—Because CUPRIMINE can cause severe adverse reactions, its use in rheumatoid arthritis should be restricted to patients who have severe, active disease and who have failed to respond to an adequate trial of conventional therapy. Even then, benefit-to-risk ratio should be carefully considered. Other measures, such as rest, physiotherapy, salicylates, and corticosteroids should be used, when indicated, in conjunction with CUPRIMINE (see PRECAUTIONS).

CONTRAINDICATIONS

Except for the treatment of Wilson's disease or certain cases of cystinuria, use of penicillamine during pregnancy is contraindicated (see PRECAUTIONS).

Although breast milk studies have not been reported in animals or humans, mothers on therapy with penicillamine should not nurse their infants.

Patients with a history of penicillamine-related aplastic anemia or agranulocytosis should not be restarted on penicillamine (see WARNINGS and ADVERSE REACTIONS). Because of its potential for causing renal damage, penicillamine should not be administered to rheumatoid arthritis patients with a history or other evidence of renal insufficiency.

WARNINGS

The use of penicillamine has been associated with fatalities due to certain diseases such as aplastic anemia, agranulocytosis, thrombocytopenia, Goodpasture's syndrome, and myasthenia gravis.

Because of the potential for serious hematological and renal adverse reactions to occur at any time, routine urinalysis, white and differential blood cell count, hemoglobin determination, and direct platelet count must be done every two weeks for at least the first six months of penicillamine therapy and monthly thereafter. Patients should be instructed to report promptly the development of signs and symptoms of granulocytopenia and/or thrombocytopenia such as fever, sore throat, chills, bruising or bleeding. The above laboratory studies should then be promptly repeated.

Leukopenia and thrombocytopenia have been reported to occur in up to five percent of patients during penicillamine therapy. Leukopenia is of the granulocytic series and may or may not be associated with an increase in eosinophils. A confirmed reduction in WBC below 3500 per cubic mL mandates discontinuance of penicillamine therapy. Thrombocytopenia may be on an idiosyncratic basis, with decreased or absent megakaryocytes in the marrow, when it is part of an aplastic anemia. In other cases the thrombocytopenia is presumably

on an immune basis since the number of megakaryocytes in the marrow has been reported to be normal or sometimes increased. The development of a platelet count below 100,000 per cubic mL, even in the absence of clinical bleeding, requires at least temporary cessation of penicillamine therapy. A progressive fall in either platelet count or WBC in three successive determinations, even though values are still within the normal range, likewise requires at least temporary cessation.

Proteinuria and/or hematuria may develop during therapy and may be warning signs of membranous glomerulopathy which can progress to a nephrotic syndrome. Close observation of these patients is essential. In some patients the proteinuria disappears with continued therapy; in others, penicillamine must be discontinued. When a patient develops proteinuria or hematuria the physician must ascertain whether it is a sign of drug-induced glomerulopathy or is unrelated to penicillamine.

Rheumatoid arthritis patients who develop moderate degrees of proteinuria may be continued cautiously on penicillamine therapy, provided that quantitative 24-hour urinary protein determinations are obtained at intervals of one to two weeks. Penicillamine dosage should not be increased under these circumstances. Proteinuria which exceeds 1 g/24 hours, or proteinuria which is progressively increasing, requires either discontinuance of the drug or a reduction in the dosage. In some patients, proteinuria has been reported to clear following reduction in dosage.

In rheumatoid arthritis patients, penicillamine should be discontinued if unexplained gross hematuria or persistent microscopic hematuria develops.

In patients with Wilson's disease or cystinuria the risks of continued penicillamine therapy in patients manifesting potentially serious urinary abnormalities must be weighed against the expected therapeutic benefits.

When penicillamine is used in cystinuria, an annual x-ray for renal stones is advised. Cystine stones form rapidly, sometimes in six months.

Up to one year or more may be required for any urinary abnormalities to disappear after penicillamine has been discontinued.

Because of rare reports of intrahepatic cholestasis and toxic hepatitis, liver function tests are recommended every six months for the duration of therapy.

Goodpasture's syndrome has occurred rarely. The development of abnormal urinary findings associated with hemoptysis and pulmonary infiltrates on x-ray requires immediate cessation of penicillamine.

Obliterative bronchiolitis has been reported rarely. The patient should be cautioned to report immediately pulmonary symptoms such as exertional dyspnea, unexplained cough or wheezing. Pulmonary function studies should be considered at that time.

Myasthenic syndrome sometimes progressing to myasthenia gravis has been reported. Ptosis and diplopia, with weakness of the extraocular muscles, are often early signs of myasthenia. In the majority of cases, symptoms of myasthenia have receded after withdrawal of penicillamine.

Most of the various forms of pemphigus have occurred during treatment with penicillamine. Pemphigus vulgaris and pemphigus foliaceus are reported most frequently, usually as a late complication of therapy. The seborrhea-like characteristics of pemphigus foliaceus may obscure an early diagnosis. When pemphigus is suspected, CUPRIMINE should be discontinued. Treatment has consisted of high doses of corticosteroids alone or, in some cases, concomitantly with an immunosuppressant. Treatment may be required for only a few weeks or months, but may need to be continued for more than a year.

Once instituted for Wilson's disease or cystinuria, treatment with penicillamine should, as a rule, be continued on a daily basis. Interruptions for even a few days have been followed by sensitivity reactions after reinstitution of therapy.

Use in Pregnancy—Penicillamine has been shown to be teratogenic in rats when given in doses 10 times higher than the highest dose recommended for human use. Skeletal defects, cleft palates and fetal toxicity (resorptions) have been reported.

There are no controlled studies on the use of penicillamine in pregnant women. Although normal outcomes have been reported, characteristic congenital cutis laxa and associated birth defects have been reported in infants born of mothers who received therapy with penicillamine during pregnancy. Penicillamine should be used in women of childbearing potential only when the expected benefits outweigh the possible hazards. Women on therapy with penicillamine who are of childbearing potential should be apprised of this risk and followed closely for early recognition of pregnancy.

Wilson's Disease—Reported experience* shows that continued treatment with penicillamine throughout pregnancy protects the mother against relapse of the Wilson's disease, and that discontinuation of penicillamine has deleterious effects on the mother.

---

*Scheinberg, I.H., Sternlieb, I.: N. Engl. J. Med. *293* : 1300-1302, Dec. 18, 1975.

If penicillamine is administered during pregnancy to patients with Wilson's disease, it is recommended that the daily dosage be limited to 1 g. If cesarean section is planned, the daily dosage should be limited to 250 mg during the last six weeks of pregnancy and postoperatively until wound healing is complete.

Cystinuria—If possible, penicillamine should not be given during pregnancy to women with cystinuria (see CONTRAINDICATIONS). There are reports of women with cystinuria on therapy with penicillamine who gave birth to infants with generalized connective tissue defects who died following abdominal surgery. If stones continue to form in these patients, the benefits of therapy to the mother must be evaluated against the risk to the fetus.

Rheumatoid Arthritis—Penicillamine should not be administered to rheumatoid arthritis patients who are pregnant (see CONTRAINDICATIONS) and should be discontinued promptly in patients in whom pregnancy is suspected or diagnosed.

There is a report that a woman with rheumatoid arthritis treated with less than one gram a day of penicillamine during pregnancy gave birth (cesarean delivery) to an infant with growth retardation, flattened face with broad nasal bridge, low set ears, short neck with loose skin folds, and unusually lax body skin.

PRECAUTIONS

Some patients may experience drug fever, a marked febrile response to penicillamine, usually in the second to third week following initiation of therapy. Drug fever may sometimes be accompanied by a macular cutaneous eruption.

In the case of drug fever in patients with Wilson's disease or cystinuria, penicillamine should be temporarily discontinued until the reaction subsides. Then penicillamine should be reinstituted with a small dose that is gradually increased until the desired dosage is attained. Systemic steroid therapy may be necessary, and is usually helpful, in such patients in whom toxic reactions develop a second or third time.

In the case of drug fever in rheumatoid arthritis patients, because other treatments are available, penicillamine should be discontinued and another therapeutic alternative tried since experience indicates that the febrile reaction will recur in a very high percentage of patients upon readministration of penicillamine.

The skin and mucous membranes should be observed for allergic reactions. Early and late rashes have occurred. Early rash occurs during the first few months of treatment and is more common. It is usually a generalized pruritic, erythematous, maculopapular or morbilliform rash and resembles the allergic rash seen with other drugs. Early rash usually disappears within days after stopping penicillamine and seldom recurs when the drug is restarted at a lower dosage. Pruritus and early rash may often be controlled by the concomitant administration of antihistamines. Less commonly, a late rash may be seen, usually after six months or more of treatment, and requires discontinuation of penicillamine. It is usually on the trunk, is accompanied by intense pruritus, and is usually unresponsive to topical corticosteroid therapy. Late rash may take weeks to disappear after penicillamine is stopped and usually recurs if the drug is restarted.

The appearance of a drug eruption accompanied by fever, arthralgia, lymphadenopathy or other allergic manifestations usually requires discontinuation of penicillamine.

Certain patients will develop a positive antinuclear antibody (ANA) test and some of these may show a lupus erythematosus-like syndrome similar to drug-induced lupus associated with other drugs. The lupus erythematosus-like syndrome is not associated with hypocomplementemia and may be present without nephropathy. The development of a positive ANA test does not mandate discontinuance of the drug; however, the physician should be alerted to the possibility that a lupus erythematosus-like syndrome may develop in the future.

Some patients may develop oral ulcerations which in some cases have the appearance of aphthous stomatitis. The stomatitis usually recurs on rechallenge but often clears on a lower dosage. Although rare, cheilosis, glossitis and gingivostomatitis have also been reported. These oral lesions are frequently dose-related and may preclude further increase in penicillamine dosage or require discontinuation of the drug.

Hypogeusia (a blunting or diminution in taste perception) has occurred in some patients. This may last two to three months or more and may develop into a total loss of taste; however, it is usually self-limited despite continued penicillamine treatment. Such taste impairment is rare in patients with Wilson's disease.

Penicillamine should not be used in patients who are receiving concurrently gold therapy, antimalarial or cytotoxic drugs, oxyphenbutazone or phenylbutazone because these drugs are also associated with similar serious hematologic and renal adverse reactions. Patients who have had gold salt therapy discontinued due to a major toxic reaction may be at greater risk of serious adverse reactions with penicillamine but not necessarily of the same type.

Patients who are allergic to penicillin may theoretically have cross-sensitivity to penicillamine. The possibility of reactions from contamination of penicillamine by trace amounts of penicillin has been eliminated now that penicillamine is being produced synthetically rather than as a degradation product of penicillin.

Because of their dietary restrictions, patients with Wilson's disease and cystinuria should be given 25 mg/day of pyridoxine during therapy, since penicillamine increases the requirement for this vitamin. Patients also may receive benefit from a multivitamin preparation, although there is no evidence that deficiency of any vitamin other than pyridoxine is associated with penicillamine. In Wilson's disease, multivitamin preparations must be copper-free.

Rheumatoid arthritis patients whose nutrition is impaired should also be given a daily supplement of pyridoxine. Mineral supplements should not be given, since they may block the response to penicillamine.

Iron deficiency may develop, especially in children and in menstruating women. In Wilson's disease, this may be a result of adding the effects of the low copper diet, which is probably also low in iron, and the penicillamine to the effects of blood loss or growth. In cystinuria, a low methionine diet may contribute to iron deficiency, since it is necessarily low in protein. If necessary, iron may be given in short courses, but a period of two hours should elapse between administration of penicillamine and iron, since orally administered iron has been shown to reduce the effects of penicillamine.

Penicillamine causes an increase in the amount of soluble collagen. In the rat this results in inhibition of normal healing and also a decrease in tensile strength of intact skin. In man this may be the cause of increased skin friability at sites especially subject to pressure or trauma, such as shoulders, elbows, knees, toes, and buttocks. Extravasations of blood may occur and may appear as purpuric areas, with external bleeding if the skin is broken, or as vesicles containing dark blood. Neither type is progressive. There is no apparent association with bleeding elsewhere in the body and no associated coagulation defect has been found. Therapy with penicillamine may be continued in the presence of these lesions. They may not recur if dosage is reduced. Other reported effects probably due to the action of penicillamine on collagen are excessive wrinkling of the skin and development of small, white papules at venipuncture and surgical sites. The effects of penicillamine on collagen and elastin make it advisable to consider a reduction in dosage to 250 mg/day, when surgery is contemplated. Reinstitution of full therapy should be delayed until wound healing is complete.

Carcinogenesis—Long-term animal carcinogenicity studies have not been done with penicillamine. There is a report that five of ten autoimmune disease-prone NZB hybrid mice developed lymphocytic leukemia after 6 months' intraperitoneal treatment with a dose of 400 mg/kg penicillamine 5 days per week.

Nursing Mothers—See CONTRAINDICATIONS.

Usage in Children—The efficacy of CUPRIMINE in juvenile rheumatoid arthritis has not been established.

ADVERSE REACTIONS

Penicillamine is a drug with a high incidence of untoward reactions, some of which are potentially fatal. Therefore, it is mandatory that patients receiving penicillamine therapy remain under close medical supervision throughout the period of drug administration (see WARNINGS and PRECAUTIONS).

Reported incidences (%) for the most commonly occurring adverse reactions in rheumatoid arthritis patients are noted, based on 17 representative clinical trials reported in the literature (1270 patients).

Allergic—Generalized pruritus, early and late rashes (5%), pemphigus (see WARNINGS), and drug eruptions which may be accompanied by fever, arthralgia, or lymphadenopathy have occurred (see WARNINGS and PRECAUTIONS). Some patients may show a lupus erythematosus-like syndrome similar to drug-induced lupus produced by other pharmacological agents (see PRECAUTIONS).

Urticaria and exfoliative dermatitis have occurred.

Thyroiditis has been reported; hypoglycemia in association with anti-insulin antibodies has been reported. These reactions are extremely rare.

Some patients may develop a migratory polyarthralgia, often with objective synovitis (see DOSAGE AND ADMINISTRATION).

Gastrointestinal—Anorexia, epigastric pain, nausea, vomiting, or occasional diarrhea may occur (17%).

Isolated cases of reactivated peptic ulcer have occurred, as have hepatic dysfunction and pancreatitis. Intrahepatic cholestasis and toxic hepatitis have been reported rarely. There have been a few reports of increased serum alkaline phosphatase, lactic dehydrogenase, and positive cephalin flocculation and thymol turbidity tests.

Some patients may report a blunting, diminution, or total loss of taste perception (12%); or may develop oral ulcerations. Although rare, cheilosis, glossitis, and gingivostomatitis have been reported (see PRECAUTIONS).

Gastrointestinal side effects are usually reversible following cessation of therapy.

Hematological—Penicillamine can cause bone marrow depression (see WARNINGS). Leukopenia (2%) and thrombocytopenia (4%) have occurred. Fatalities have been reported as a result of thrombocytopenia, agranulocytosis, aplastic anemia, and sideroblastic anemia.

Thrombotic thrombocytopenic purpura, hemolytic anemia, red cell aplasia, monocytosis, leukocytosis, eosinophilia, and thrombocytosis have also been reported.

Renal—Patients on penicillamine therapy may develop proteinuria (6%) and/or hematuria which, in some, may progress to the development of the nephrotic syndrome as a result of an immune complex membranous glomerulopathy (see WARNINGS).

Central Nervous System—Tinnitus, optic neuritis and peripheral sensory and motor neuropathies (including polyradiculoneuropathy, i.e., Guillain-Barre syndrome) have been reported. Muscular weakness may or may not occur with the peripheral neuropathies.

Neuromuscular—Myasthenia gravis (see WARNINGS).

Other—Adverse reactions that have been reported rarely include thrombophlebitis; hyperpyrexia (see PRECAUTIONS); falling hair or alopecia; lichen planus; polymyositis; dermatomyositis; mammary hyperplasia; elastosis perforans serpiginosa; toxic epidermal necrolysis; anetoderma (cutaneous macular atrophy); and Goodpasture's syndrome, a severe and ultimately fatal glomerulonephritis associated with intra-alveolar hemorrhage (see WARNINGS). Fatal renal vasculitis has also been reported. Allergic alveolitis, obliterative bronchiolitis, interstitial pneumonitis and pulmonary fibrosis have been reported in patients with severe rheumatoid arthritis, some of whom were receiving penicillamine. Bronchial asthma also has been reported.

Increased skin friability, excessive wrinkling of skin, and development of small white papules at venipuncture and surgical sites have been reported (see PRECAUTIONS).

The chelating action of the drug may cause increased excretion of other heavy metals such as zinc, mercury and lead. There have been reports associating penicillamine with leukemia. However, circumstances involved in these reports are such that a cause and effect relationship to the drug has not been established.

DOSAGE AND ADMINISTRATION

In all patients receiving penicillamine, it is important that CUPRIMINE be given on an empty stomach, at least one hour before meals or two hours after meals, and at least one hour apart from any other drug, food, or milk.

Wilson's Disease—Optimal dosage can be determined by measurement of urinary copper excretion and the determination of free copper in the serum. The urine must be collected in copper-free glassware, and should be quantitatively analyzed for copper before and soon after initiation of therapy with CUPRIMINE.

Determination of 24-hour urinary copper excretion is of greatest value in the first week of therapy with penicillamine. In the absence of any drug reaction, a dose between 0.75 and 1.5 g that results in an initial 24-hour cupriuresis of over 2 mg should be continued for about three months, by which time the most reliable method of monitoring maintenance treatment is the determination of free copper in the serum. This equals the difference between quantitatively determined total copper and ceruloplasmin-copper. Adequately treated patients will usually have less than 10 mcg free copper/dL of serum. It is seldom necessary to exceed a dosage of 2 g/day. If the patient is intolerant to therapy with CUPRIMINE, alternative treatment is trientine hydrochloride.

In patients who cannot tolerate as much as 1 g/day initially, initiating dosage with 250 mg/day, and increasing gradually to the requisite amount, gives closer control of the effects of the drug and may help to reduce the incidence of adverse reactions.

Cystinuria—It is recommended that CUPRIMINE be used along with conventional therapy. By reducing urinary cystine, it decreases crystalluria and stone formation. In some instances, it has been reported to decrease the size of, and even to dissolve, stones already formed.

The usual dosage of CUPRIMINE in the treatment of cystinuria is 2 g/day for adults, with a range of 1 to 4 g/day. For children, dosage can be based on 30 mg/kg/day. The total daily amount should be divided into four doses. If four equal doses are not feasible, give the larger portion at bedtime. If adverse reactions necessitate a reduction in dosage, it is important to retain the bedtime dose.

Initiating dosage with 250 mg/day, and increasing gradually to the requisite amount, gives closer control of the effects of the drug and may help to reduce the incidence of adverse reactions.

In addition to taking CUPRIMINE, patients should drink copiously. It is especially important to drink about a pint of fluid at bedtime and another pint once during the night when urine is more concentrated and more acid than during the day. The greater the fluid intake, the lower the required dosage of CUPRIMINE.

Dosage must be individualized to an amount that limits cystine excretion to 100–200 mg/day in those with no history of stones, and below 100 mg/day in those who have had stone formation and/or pain. Thus, in determining dosage, the inherent tubular defect, the patient's size, age, and rate of growth, and his diet and water intake all must be taken into consideration.

The standard nitroprusside cyanide test has been reported useful as a qualitative measure of the effective dose*: Add 2 mL of freshly prepared 5 percent sodium cyanide to 5 mL of a 24-hour aliquot of protein-free urine and let stand ten minutes. Add 5 drops of freshly prepared 5 percent sodium nitroprusside and mix. Cystine will turn the mixture magenta. If the result is negative, it can be assumed that cystine excretion is less than 100 mg/g creatinine.

Although penicillamine is rarely excreted unchanged, it also will turn the mixture magenta. If there is any question as to which substance is causing the reaction, a ferric chloride test can be done to eliminate doubt: Add 3 percent ferric chloride dropwise to the urine. Penicillamine will turn the urine an immediate and quickly fading blue. Cystine will not produce any change in appearance.

Rheumatoid Arthritis—The principal rule of treatment with CUPRIMINE in rheumatoid arthritis is patience. The onset of therapeutic response is typically delayed. Two or three months may be required before the first evidence of a clinical response is noted (see CLINICAL PHARMACOLOGY).

When treatment with CUPRIMINE has been interrupted because of adverse reactions or other reasons, the drug should be reintroduced cautiously by starting with a lower dosage and increasing slowly.

Initial Therapy—The currently recommended dosage regimen in rheumatoid arthritis begins with a single daily dose of 125 mg or 250 mg which is thereafter increased at one to three month intervals, by 125 mg or 250 mg/day, as patient response and tolerance indicate. If a satisfactory remission of symptoms is achieved, the dose associated with the remission should be continued (see *Maintenance Therapy*). If there is no improvement and there are no signs of potentially serious toxicity after two to three months of treatment with doses of 500–750 mg/day, increases of 250 mg/day at two to three month intervals may be continued until a satisfactory remission occurs (see *Maintenance Therapy*) or signs of toxicity develop (see WARNINGS and PRECAUTIONS). If there is no discernible improvement after three to four months of treatment with 1000 to 1500 mg of penicillamine/day, it may be assumed the patient will not respond and CUPRIMINE should be discontinued.

Maintenance Therapy—The maintenance dosage of CUPRIMINE must be individualized, and may require adjustment during the course of treatment. Many patients respond satisfactorily to a dosage within the 500–750 mg/day range. Some need less.

Changes in maintenance dosage levels may not be reflected clinically or in the erythrocyte sedimentation rate for two to three months after each dosage adjustment.

Some patients will subsequently require an increase in the maintenance dosage to achieve maximal disease suppression. In those patients who do respond, but who evidence incomplete suppression of their disease after the first six to nine months of treatment, the daily dosage of CUPRIMINE may be increased by 125 mg or 250 mg/day at three-month intervals. It is unusual in current practice to employ a dosage in excess of 1 g/day, but up to 1.5 g/day has sometimes been required.

Management of Exacerbations—During the course of treatment some patients may experience an exacerbation of disease activity following an initial good response. These may be self-limited and can subside within twelve weeks. They are usually controlled by the addition of non-steroidal anti-inflammatory drugs, and only if the patient has demonstrated a true "escape" phenomenon (as evidenced by failure of the flare to subside within this time period) should an increase in the maintenance dose ordinarily be considered.

In the rheumatoid patient, migratory polyarthralgia due to penicillamine is extremely difficult to differentiate from an exacerbation of the rheumatoid arthritis. Discontinuance or a substantial reduction in dosage of CUPRIMINE for up to

---

*Lotz, M., Potts, J.T. and Bartter, F.C.: Brit. Med. J. 2:521, Aug. 28, 1965 (in Medical Memoranda).

Continued on next page

Information on the Merck Sharp & Dohme products listed on these pages is the full prescribing information from product circulars in use August 31, 1989.

Merck Sharp & Dohme—Cont.

several weeks will usually determine which of these processes is responsible for the arthralgia.

Duration of Therapy—The optimum duration of therapy with CUPRIMINE in rheumatoid arthritis has not been determined. If the patient has been in remission for six months or more, a gradual, stepwise dosage reduction in decrements of 125 mg or 250 mg/day at approximately three month intervals may be attempted.

Concomitant Drug Therapy—CUPRIMINE should not be used in patients who are receiving gold therapy, antimalarial or cytotoxic drugs, oxyphenbutazone, or phenylbutazone (see PRECAUTIONS). Other measures, such as salicylates, other non-steroidal anti-inflammatory drugs, or systemic corticosteroids, may be continued when penicillamine is initiated. After improvement commences, analgesic and anti-inflammatory drugs may be slowly discontinued as symptoms permit. Steroid withdrawal must be done gradually, and many months of treatment with CUPRIMINE may be required before steroids can be completely eliminated.

Dosage Frequency—Based on clinical experience dosages up to 500 mg/day can be given as a single daily dose. Dosages in excess of 500 mg/day should be administered in divided doses.

HOW SUPPLIED

No. 3299—Capsules CUPRIMINE, 250 mg, are ivory-colored capsules containing a white or nearly white powder, and are coded MSD 602. They are supplied as follows:
NDC 0006-0602-68 in bottles of 100
(6505-01-049-9494, 250 mg 100's).
Shown in Product Identification Section, page 418
No. 3350—Capsules CUPRIMINE, 125 mg, are opaque yellow and gray capsules containing a white or nearly white powder, and are coded MSD 672. They are supplied as follows:
NDC 0006-0672-68 in bottles of 100.
Shown in Product Identification Section, page 418
Storage
Keep container tightly closed.
A.H.F.S. Category: 64:00
DC 7412337   Issued May 1987

DARANIDE® Tablets ℞
(Dichlorphenamide, MSD), U.S.P.

DESCRIPTION

DARANIDE® (Dichlorphenamide, MSD) is an oral carbonic anhydrase inhibitor. Dichlorphenamide, a dichlorinated benzenedisulfonamide, is known chemically as 4,5-dichloro-1,3-benzenedisulfonamide. Its empirical formula is $C_6H_6Cl_2N_2O_4S_2$ and its structural formula is:

Dichlorphenamide is a white or practically white, crystalline compound with a molecular weight of 305.16. It is very slightly soluble in water but soluble in dilute solutions of sodium carbonate and sodium hydroxide. Dilute alkaline solutions of dichlorphenamide are stable at room temperature.
DARANIDE is supplied as tablets, for oral administration, each containing 50 mg dichlorphenamide. Inactive ingredients are D&C Yellow 10, lactose, magnesium stearate, and starch.

CLINICAL PHARMACOLOGY

Carbonic anhydrase inhibitors reduce intraocular pressure by partially suppressing the secretion of aqueous humor (inflow), although the mechanism by which they do this is not fully understood. Evidence suggests that HCO_3^- ions are produced in the ciliary body by hydration of carbon dioxide under the influence of carbonic anhydrase and diffuse into the posterior chamber with Na^+ ions. The aqueous fluid contains more Na^+ and HCO_3^- ions than does plasma and consequently is hypertonic. Water is attracted to the posterior chamber by osmosis. Systemic administration of a carbonic anhydrase inhibitor has been shown to inactivate carbonic anhydrase in the ciliary body of the rabbit's eye and to reduce the high concentration of HCO_3^- ions in ocular fluids. As is the case with all carbonic anhydrase inhibitors,

DARANIDE in high doses causes some decrease in renal blood flow and glomerular filtration rate.
In man, DARANIDE begins to act within an hour and maximal effect is observed in two to four hours. The lowered intraocular tension may be maintained for approximately 6 to 12 hours.

INDICATIONS AND USAGE

For adjunctive treatment of: chronic simple (open-angle) glaucoma, secondary glaucoma, and preoperatively in acute angle-closure glaucoma where delay of surgery is desired in order to lower intraocular pressure.

CONTRAINDICATIONS

DARANIDE is contraindicated in hepatic insufficiency, renal failure, adrenocortical insufficiency, hyperchloremic acidosis, or in conditions in which serum levels of sodium or potassium are depressed. DARANIDE should not be used in patients with severe pulmonary obstruction who are unable to increase their alveolar ventilation since their acidosis may be increased.
DARANIDE is contraindicated in patients who are hypersensitive to this product.

PRECAUTIONS

General
Potassium excretion is increased by DARANIDE and hypokalemia may develop with brisk diuresis, when severe cirrhosis is present, or during concomitant use of steroids or ACTH.
Interference with adequate oral electrolyte intake will also contribute to hypokalemia. Hypokalemia can sensitize or exaggerate the response of the heart to the toxic effects of digitalis (e.g., increased ventricular irritability). Hypokalemia may be avoided or treated by use of potassium supplements such as foods with a high potassium content. DARANIDE should be used with caution in patients with respiratory acidosis.
Drug Interactions
Caution is advised in patients receiving concomitant high-dose aspirin and carbonic anhydrase inhibitors, as anorexia, tachypnea, lethargy and coma have been rarely reported due to a possible drug interaction.
Carcinogenesis, Mutagenesis, Impairment of Fertility
Long-term studies in animals have not been performed to evaluate the effects upon fertility or carcinogenic potential of DARANIDE.
Pregnancy
Pregnancy Category C. Dichlorphenamide has been shown to be teratogenic in the rat (skeletal anomalies) when given in doses 100 times the human dose. There are no adequate and well-controlled studies in pregnant women. DARANIDE should not be used in women of childbearing age or in pregnancy, especially during the first trimester, unless the potential benefits outweigh the potential risks.
Nursing Mothers
It is not known whether dichlorphenamide is excreted in human milk. Because many drugs are excreted in human milk, caution should be exercised when dichlorphenamide is administered to a nursing woman.
Pediatric Use
Safety and effectiveness in children have not been established.

ADVERSE REACTIONS

Certain side effects characteristic of carbonic anhydrase inhibitors may occur with DARANIDE, particularly with increasing doses. The most common effects include gastrointestinal disturbances (anorexia, nausea, and vomiting), drowsiness and paresthesias.
Included in the listing which follows are some adverse reactions which have not been reported with DARANIDE. However, pharmacological similarities among the carbonic anhydrase inhibitors make it advisable to consider the following reactions when diclorphenamide is administered. *Central Nervous System/Psychiatric:* ataxia, tremor, tinnitus, headache, weakness, nervousness, globus hystericus, lassitude, depression, confusion, disorientation, dizziness; *Gastrointestinal:* constipation, hepatic insufficiency; *Metabolic:* loss of weight, metabolic acidosis, electrolyte imbalance (hypokalemia, hyperchloremia), hyperuricemia; *Hypersensitivity:* skin eruptions, pruritus, fever; *Hematologic:* leukopenia, agranulocytosis, thrombocytopenia; *Genitourinary:* urinary frequency, renal colic, renal calculi, phosphaturia.

OVERDOSAGE

The oral LD_{50} of DARANIDE is 1710 and 2600 mg/kg in the mouse and rat respectively.

Symptoms of overdosage or toxicity may include drowsiness, anorexia, nausea, vomiting, dizziness, paresthesias, ataxia, tremor and tinnitus.
In the event of overdosage, induce emesis or perform gastric lavage. The electrolyte disturbance most likely to be encountered from overdosage is hyperchloremic acidosis that may respond to bicarbonate administration. Potassium supplementation may be required. The patient should be carefully observed and given supportive treatment.

DOSAGE AND ADMINISTRATION

DARANIDE is usually given in conjunction with topical ocular hypotensive agents. In acute angle-closure glaucoma, it may be used together with miotics and osmotic agents in an attempt to reduce intraocular tension rapidly. If this is not quickly relieved, surgery may be mandatory.
Dosage must be adjusted carefully to meet the requirements of the individual patient. A priming dose of 100 to 200 mg of DARANIDE (2 to 4 tablets) is suggested for adults, followed by 100 mg (2 tablets) every 12 hours until the desired response has been obtained. The recommended maintenance dosage for adults is 25 to 50 mg (½ to 1 tablet) once to three times daily.

HOW SUPPLIED

No. 3256—Tablets DARANIDE, 50 mg each, are yellow, round, scored, compressed tablets, coded MSD 49. They are supplied as follows:
NDC 0006-0049-68 bottles of 100.
Shown in Product Identification Section, page 418
A.H.F.S. Category: 52:10
DC 7412517 Issued November 1986

DECADERM® 0.1% Topical ℞
(Dexamethasone, MSD)
in ESTERGEL®
(Isopropyl Myristate Gel, MSD)

DESCRIPTION

DECADERM® (Dexamethasone, MSD) is a topical steroid preparation containing 0.1% of dexamethasone. The topical corticosteroids constitute a class of primarily synthetic steroids used as anti-inflammatory and anti-pruritic agents. Dexamethasone is 9-fluoro-11β,17,21-trihydroxy-16α-methylpregna-1,4-diene-3,20-dione.
Its empirical formula is $C_{22}H_{29}FO_5$ and its structural formula is:

Dexamethasone has a molecular weight of 392.47.
Dexamethasone is slightly soluble both in isopropyl myristate (.23 mg/ml) and in water (.11 mg/ml) at 37°C.
Each gram of DECADERM contains 1 mg dexamethasone in ESTERGEL®, a specially formulated vehicle consisting of gelled isopropyl myristate, wool alcohols B.P., refined lanolin alcohol, microcrystalline wax, anhydrous citric acid, and anhydrous sodium phosphate dibasic.
This emollient gel vehicle is anhydrous, lipophilic, hydrophilic, and moisture-retentive. The base largely disappears when rubbed on the skin.

CLINICAL PHARMACOLOGY

Topical corticosteroids share anti-inflammatory, anti-pruritic and vasoconstrictive actions.
The mechanism of anti-inflammatory activity of the topical corticosteroids is unclear. Various laboratory methods, including vasoconstrictor assays, are used to compare and predict potencies and/or clinical efficacies of the topical corticosteroids. There is some evidence to suggest that a recognizable correlation exists between vasoconstrictor potency and therapeutic efficacy in man.
Pharmacokinetics
The extent of percutaneous absorption of topical corticosteroids is determined by many factors including the vehicle, the integrity of the epidermal barrier, and the use of occlusive dressings.
Topical corticosteroids can be absorbed from normal intact skin. Inflammation and/or other disease processes in the skin increase percutaneous absorption. Occlusive dressings

substantially increase the percutaneous absorption of topical corticosteroids. Thus, occlusive dressings may be a valuable therapeutic adjunct for treatment of resistant dermatoses. (See DOSAGE AND ADMINISTRATION)

Once absorbed through the skin, topical corticosteroids are handled through pharmacokinetic pathways similar to systemically administered corticosteroids. Corticosteroids are bound to plasma proteins in varying degrees. Corticosteroids are metabolized primarily in the liver and are then excreted by the kidneys. Some of the topical corticosteroids and their metabolites are also excreted into the bile.

INDICATIONS AND USAGE

DECADERM is indicated for relief of the inflammatory and pruritic manifestations of corticosteroid-responsive dermatoses.

CONTRAINDICATIONS

Topical corticosteroids are contraindicated in those patients with a history of hypersensitivity to any of the components of the preparation.

PRECAUTIONS

General
Systemic absorption of topical corticosteroids has produced reversible hypothalamic-pituitary-adrenal (HPA) axis suppression, manifestations of Cushing's syndrome, hyperglycemia, and glycosuria in some patients.
Conditions which augment systemic absorption include the application of the more potent corticosteroids, use over large surface areas, prolonged use, and the addition of occlusive dressings.
Therefore, patients receiving a large dose of a potent topical corticosteroid applied to a large surface area or under an occlusive dressing should be evaluated periodically for evidence of HPA axis suppression by using urinary free cortisol and ACTH stimulation tests. If HPA axis suppression is noted, an attempt should be made to withdraw the drug, to reduce the frequency of application, or to substitute a less potent corticosteroid.
Recovery of HPA axis function is generally prompt and complete upon discontinuation of the drug. Infrequently, signs and symptoms of corticosteroid withdrawal may occur, requiring supplemental systemic corticosteroids.
Children may absorb proportionally larger amounts of topical corticosteroids and thus be more susceptible to systemic toxicity (See PRECAUTIONS, *Pediatric Use*).
If irritation develops, topical corticosteroids should be discontinued and appropriate therapy instituted.
In the presence of dermatological infections, the use of an appropriate antifungal or antibacterial agent should be instituted. If a favorable response does not occur promptly, the corticosteroid should be discontinued until the infection has been adequately controlled.
This product is not for ophthalmic use. However, if applied to the eyelids or skin near the eyes, the drug may enter the eyes. In patients with a history of herpes simplex keratitis, ocular exposure to corticosteroids may lead to a recurrence. Prolonged ocular exposure may cause steroid glaucoma.
Generally, occlusive dressings should not be used on weeping or exudative lesions.
If occlusive dressing therapy is used, inspect lesions between dressings for development of infection. If infection develops, the technique should be discontinued and appropriate antimicrobial therapy instituted.
When large areas of the body are covered with an occlusive dressing, thermal homeostasis may be impaired. If elevation of body temperature occurs, use of the occlusive dressing should be discontinued.

Information for the Patient
Patients using topical corticosteroids should receive the following information and instructions:
1. This medication is to be used as directed by the physician. It is for external use only. Avoid contact with the eyes.
2. Patients should be advised not to use this medication for any disorder other than that for which it was prescribed.
3. The treated skin area should not be bandaged or otherwise covered or wrapped so as to be occlusive unless directed by the physician.
4. Patients should report any signs of local adverse reactions, especially under occlusive dressing.
5. Parents of pediatric patients should be advised not to use tight-fitting diapers or plastic pants on a child being treated in the diaper area, as these garments may constitute occlusive dressings.

Laboratory Tests
The following tests may be helpful in evaluating the HPA axis suppression:
- Urinary free cortisol test
- ACTH stimulation test

Carcinogenesis, Mutagenesis, and Impairment of Fertility
Long-term animal studies have not been performed to evaluate the carcinogenic potential or the effect on fertility of topical corticosteroids.
Studies to determine mutagenicity with prednisolone and hydrocortisone have revealed negative results.

Pregnancy
Pregnancy Category C: Corticosteroids are generally teratogenic in laboratory animals when administered systemically at relatively low dosage levels. The more potent corticosteroids have been shown to be teratogenic after dermal application in laboratory animals. There are no adequate and well-controlled studies in pregnant women on teratogenic effects from topically applied corticosteroids. Therefore, topical corticosteroids should be used during pregnancy only if the potential benefit justifies the potential risk to the fetus. Drugs of this class should not be used extensively on pregnant patients, in large amounts, or for prolonged periods of time.

Nursing Mothers
It is not known whether topical administration of corticosteroids could result in sufficient systemic absorption to produce detectable quantities in breast milk. Systemically administered corticosteroids are secreted into breast milk in quantities not likely to have a deleterious effect on the infant. Nevertheless, caution should be exercised when topical corticosteroids are administered to a nursing woman.

Pediatric Use
Pediatric patients may demonstrate greater susceptibility to topical corticosteroid-induced HPA axis suppression and Cushing's syndrome than mature patients because of a larger skin surface area to body weight ratio.
Hypothalamic-pituitary-adrenal (HPA) axis suppression, Cushing's syndrome, and intracranial hypertension have been reported in children receiving topical corticosteroids. Manifestations of adrenal suppression in children include linear growth retardation, delayed weight gain, low plasma cortisol levels, and absence of response to ACTH stimulation. Manifestations of intracranial hypertension include bulging fontanelles, headaches, and bilateral papilledema.
Administration of topical corticosteroids to children should be limited to the least amount compatible with an effective therapeutic regimen. Chronic corticosteroid therapy may interfere with the growth and development of children.

ADVERSE REACTIONS

The following adverse reactions are reported infrequently with topical corticosteroids, but may occur more frequently with the use of occlusive dressings. These reactions are listed in an approximate decreasing order of occurrence:
Burning
Itching
Irritation
Dryness
Folliculitis
Hypertrichosis
Acneiform eruptions
Hypopigmentation
Perioral dermatitis
Allergic contact dermatitis
Maceration of the skin
Secondary infection
Skin atrophy
Striae
Miliaria

OVERDOSAGE

Topically applied corticosteroids can be absorbed in sufficient amounts to produce systemic effects (See PRECAUTIONS).

DOSAGE AND ADMINISTRATION

Apply to the affected area as a thin film three or four times daily.
Occlusive dressings may be used for the management of psoriasis or recalcitrant conditions.
Before using this preparation in the ear, clean the aural canal thoroughly and sponge dry. Confirm that the eardrum is intact. With a cotton-tipped applicator, apply a thin coating of the cream to the affected canal area three or four times a day.

HOW SUPPLIED

No. 7631—0.1% Topical DECADERM is pale yellow in color, and is supplied as follows:
NDC 0006-7631-24 in 30 g tubes.
    A.H.F.S. Category: 84:06
    DC 6822406   Issued April 1983

DECADRON® Elixir   ℞
(Dexamethasone, MSD), U.S.P.

DESCRIPTION

Glucocorticoids are adrenocortical steroids, both naturally occurring and synthetic, which are readily absorbed from the gastrointestinal tract.
Dexamethasone, a synthetic adrenocortical steroid, is a white to practically white, odorless, crystalline powder. It is stable in air. It is practically insoluble in water. The molecular weight is 392.47. It is designated chemically as 9-fluoro-11β,17,21-trihydroxy-16α-methylpregna -1, 4- diene-3,20-dione. The empirical formula is $C_{22}H_{29}FO_5$ and the structural formula is:

DECADRON® (Dexamethasone, MSD) elixir contains 0.5 mg of dexamethasone in each 5 mL. Benzoic acid, 0.1%, is added as a preservative. It also contains alcohol 5%. Inactive ingredients are FD&C Red 40, flavors, glycerin, purified water, and sodium saccharin.

ACTIONS

Naturally occurring glucocorticoids (hydrocortisone and cortisone), which also have salt-retaining properties, are used as replacement therapy in adrenocortical deficiency states. Their synthetic analogs, including dexamethasone, are primarily used for their potent anti-inflammatory effects in disorders of many organ systems.
Glucocorticoids cause profound and varied metabolic effects. In addition, they modify the body's immune responses to diverse stimuli.
At equipotent anti-inflammatory doses, dexamethasone almost completely lacks the sodium-retaining property of hydrocortisone and closely related derivatives of hydrocortisone.

INDICATIONS

1. *Endocrine Disorders*
   Primary or secondary adrenocortical insufficiency (hydrocortisone or cortisone is the first choice; synthetic analogs may be used in conjunction with mineralocorticoids where applicable; in infancy mineralocorticoid supplementation is of particular importance)
   Congenital adrenal hyperplasia
   Nonsuppurative thyroiditis
   Hypercalcemia associated with cancer
2. *Rheumatic Disorders*
   As adjunctive therapy for short-term administration (to tide the patient over an acute episode or exacerbation) in:
   Psoriatic arthritis
   Rheumatoid arthritis, including juvenile rheumatoid arthritis (selected cases may require low-dose maintenance therapy)
   Ankylosing spondylitis
   Acute and subacute bursitis
   Acute nonspecific tenosynovitis
   Acute gouty arthritis
   Post-traumatic osteoarthritis
   Synovitis of osteoarthritis
   Epicondylitis
3. *Collagen Diseases*
   During an exacerbation or as maintenance therapy in selected cases of—
   Systemic lupus erythematosus
   Acute rheumatic carditis
4. *Dermatologic Diseases*
   Pemphigus
   Bullous dermatitis herpetiformis
   Severe erythema multiforme (Stevens-Johnson syndrome)

Continued on next page

Merck Sharp & Dohme—Cont.

Exfoliative dermatitis
Mycosis fungoides
Severe psoriasis
Severe seborrheic dermatitis
5. *Allergic States*
Control of severe or incapacitating allergic conditions intractable to adequate trials of conventional treatment:
Seasonal or perennial allergic rhinitis
Bronchial asthma
Contact dermatitis
Atopic dermatitis
Serum sickness
Drug hypersensitivity reactions
6. *Ophthalmic Diseases*
Severe acute and chronic allergic and inflammatory processes involving the eye and its adnexa, such as—
Allergic conjunctivitis
Keratitis
Allergic corneal marginal ulcers
Herpes zoster ophthalmicus
Iritis and iridocyclitis
Chorioretinitis
Anterior segment inflammation
Diffuse posterior uveitis and choroiditis
Optic neuritis
Sympathetic ophthalmia
7. *Respiratory Diseases*
Symptomatic sarcoidosis
Loeffler's syndrome not manageable by other means
Berylliosis
Fulminating or disseminated pulmonary tuberculosis when used concurrently with appropriate antituberculous chemotherapy
Aspiration pneumonitis
8. *Hematologic Disorders*
Idiopathic thrombocytopenic purpura in adults
Secondary thrombocytopenia in adults
Acquired (autoimmune) hemolytic anemia
Erythroblastopenia (RBC anemia)
Congenital (erythroid) hypoplastic anemia
9. *Neoplastic Diseases*
For palliative management of:
Leukemias and lymphomas in adults
Acute leukemia of childhood
10. *Edematous States*
To induce a diuresis or remission of proteinuria in the nephrotic syndrome, without uremia, of the idiopathic type or that due to lupus erythematosus
11. *Gastrointestinal Diseases*
To tide the patient over a critical period of the disease in:
Ulcerative colitis
Regional enteritis
12. *Miscellaneous*
Tuberculous meningitis with subarachnoid block or impending block when used concurrently with appropriate antituberculous chemotherapy
Trichinosis with neurologic or myocardial involvement
13. *Diagnostic testing of adrenocortical hyperfunction.*

CONTRAINDICATIONS

Systemic fungal infections
Hypersensitivity to this product

WARNINGS

In patients on corticosteroid therapy subjected to unusual stress, increased dosage of rapidly acting corticosteroids before, during, and after the stressful situation is indicated.
Drug-induced secondary adrenocortical insufficiency may result from too rapid withdrawal of corticosteroids and may be minimized by gradual reduction of dosage. This type of relative insufficiency may persist for months after discontinuation of therapy; therefore, in any situation of stress occurring during that period, hormone therapy should be reinstituted. If the patient is receiving steroids already, dosage may have to be increased. Since mineralocorticoid secretion may be impaired, salt and/or a mineralocorticoid should be administered concurrently.
Corticosteroids may mask some signs of infection, and new infections may appear during their use. There may be decreased resistance and inability to localize infection when corticosteroids are used. Moreover, corticosteroids may affect the nitroblue-tetrazolium test for bacterial infection and produce false negative results.
In cerebral malaria, a double-blind trial has shown that the use of corticosteroids is associated with prolongation of coma and a higher incidence of pneumonia and gastrointestinal bleeding.
Corticosteroids may activate latent amebiasis. Therefore, it is recommended that latent or active amebiasis be ruled out before initiating corticosteroid therapy in any patient who

has spent time in the tropics or any patient with unexplained diarrhea.
Prolonged use of corticosteroids may produce posterior subcapsular cataracts, glaucoma with possible damage to the optic nerves, and may enhance the establishment of secondary ocular infections due to fungi or viruses.
Usage in pregnancy: Since adequate human reproduction studies have not been done with corticosteroids, use of these drugs in pregnancy or in women of childbearing potential requires that the anticipated benefits be weighed against the possible hazards to the mother and embryo or fetus. Infants born of mothers who have received substantial doses of corticosteroids during pregnancy should be carefully observed for signs of hypoadrenalism.
Corticosteroids appear in breast milk and could suppress growth, interfere with endogenous corticosteroid production, or cause other unwanted effects. Mothers taking pharmacologic doses of corticosteroids should be advised not to nurse.
Average and large doses of hydrocortisone or cortisone can cause elevation of blood pressure, salt and water retention, and increased excretion of potassium. These effects are less likely to occur with the synthetic derivatives except when used in large doses. Dietary salt restriction and potassium supplementation may be necessary. All corticosteroids increase calcium excretion.
Administration of live virus vaccines, including smallpox, is contraindicated in individuals receiving immunosuppressive doses of corticosteroids. If inactivated viral or bacterial vaccines are administered to individuals receiving immunosuppressive doses of corticosteroids, the expected serum antibody response may not be obtained. However, immunization procedures may be undertaken in patients who are receiving corticosteroids as replacement therapy, e.g., for Addison's disease.
The use of DECADRON elixir in active tuberculosis should be restricted to those cases of fulminating or disseminated tuberculosis in which the corticosteroid is used for the management of the disease in conjunction with an appropriate antituberculous regimen.
If corticosteroids are indicated in patients with latent tuberculosis or tuberculin reactivity, close observation is necessary as reactivation of the disease may occur. During prolonged corticosteroid therapy, these patients should receive chemoprophylaxis.
Literature reports suggest an apparent association between use of corticosteroids and left ventricular free wall rupture after a recent myocardial infarction; therefore, therapy with corticosteroids should be used with great caution in these patients.

PRECAUTIONS

Following prolonged therapy, withdrawal of corticosteroids may result in symptoms of the corticosteroid withdrawal syndrome including fever, myalgia, arthralgia, and malaise. This may occur in patients even without evidence of adrenal insufficiency.
There is an enhanced effect of corticosteroids in patients with hypothyroidism and in those with cirrhosis.
Corticosteroids should be used cautiously in patients with ocular herpes simplex because of possible corneal perforation.
The lowest possible dose of corticosteroid should be used to control the condition under treatment, and when reduction in dosage is possible, the reduction should be gradual.
Psychic derangements may appear when corticosteroids are used, ranging from euphoria, insomnia, mood swings, personality changes, and severe depression, to frank psychotic manifestations. Also, existing emotional instability or psychotic tendencies may be aggravated by corticosteroids.
Aspirin should be used cautiously in conjunction with corticosteroids in hypoprothrombinemia.
Steroids should be used with caution in nonspecific ulcerative colitis, if there is a probability of impending perforation, abscess, or other pyogenic infection, diverticulitis, fresh intestinal anastomoses, active or latent peptic ulcer, renal insufficiency, hypertension, osteoporosis, and myasthenia gravis. Signs of peritoneal irritation following gastrointestinal perforation in patients receiving large doses of corticosteroids may be minimal or absent. Fat embolism has been reported as a possible complication of hypercortisonism.
When large doses are given, some authorities advise that corticosteroids be taken with meals and antacids taken between meals to help to prevent peptic ulcer.
Growth and development of infants and children on prolonged corticosteroid therapy should be carefully observed.
Steroids may increase or decrease motility and number of spermatozoa in some patients.
Phenytoin, phenobarbital, ephedrine, and rifampin may enhance the metabolic clearance of corticosteroids, resulting in decreased blood levels and lessened physiologic activity, thus requiring adjustment in corticosteroid dosage. These interactions may interfere with dexamethasone suppression tests which should be interpreted with caution during administration of these drugs.

False-negative results in the dexamethasone suppression test (DST) in patients being treated with indomethacin have been reported. Thus, results of the DST should be interpreted with caution in these patients.
The prothrombin time should be checked frequently in patients who are receiving corticosteroids and coumarin anticoagulants at the same time because of reports that corticosteroids have altered the response to these anticoagulants. Studies have shown that the usual effect produced by adding corticosteroids is inhibition of response to coumarins, although there have been some conflicting reports of potentiation not substantiated by studies.
When corticosteroids are administered concomitantly with potassium-depleting diuretics, patients should be observed closely for development of hypokalemia.

ADVERSE REACTIONS

Fluid and Electrolyte Disturbances
Sodium retention
Fluid retention
Congestive heart failure in susceptible patients
Potassium loss
Hypokalemic alkalosis
Hypertension
Musculoskeletal
Muscle weakness
Steroid myopathy
Loss of muscle mass
Osteoporosis
Vertebral compression fractures
Aseptic necrosis of femoral and humeral heads
Pathologic fracture of long bones
Tendon rupture
Gastrointestinal
Peptic ulcer with possible perforation and hemorrhage
Perforation of the small and large bowel, particularly in patients with inflammatory bowel disease
Pancreatitis
Abdominal distention
Ulcerative esophagitis
Dermatologic
Impaired wound healing
Thin fragile skin
Petechiae and ecchymoses
Erythema
Increased sweating
May suppress reactions to skin tests
Other cutaneous reactions, such as allergic dermatitis, urticaria, angioneurotic edema
Neurologic
Convulsions
Increased intracranial pressure with papilledema (pseudotumor cerebri) usually after treatment
Vertigo
Headache
Psychic disturbances
Endocrine
Menstrual irregularities
Development of cushingoid state
Suppression of growth in children
Secondary adrenocortical and pituitary unresponsiveness, particularly in times of stress, as in trauma, surgery, or illness
Decreased carbohydrate tolerance
Manifestations of latent diabetes mellitus
Increased requirements for insulin or oral hypoglycemic agents in diabetics
Hirsutism
Ophthalmic
Posterior subcapsular cataracts
Increased intraocular pressure
Glaucoma
Exophthalmos
Metabolic
Negative nitrogen balance due to protein catabolism
Cardiovascular
Myocardial rupture following recent myocardial infarction (see WARNINGS).
Other
Hypersensitivity
Thromboembolism
Weight gain
Increased appetite
Nausea
Malaise
Hiccups

OVERDOSAGE

Reports of acute toxicity and/or death following overdosage of glucocorticoids are rare. In the event of overdosage, no specific antidote is available; treatment is supportive and symptomatic.
The oral LD_{50} of dexamethasone in female mice was 6.5 g/kg.

DOSAGE AND ADMINISTRATION

For oral administration
DOSAGE REQUIREMENTS ARE VARIABLE AND MUST BE INDIVIDUALIZED ON THE BASIS OF THE DISEASE AND THE RESPONSE OF THE PATIENT.
The initial dosage varies from 0.75 to 9 mg a day depending on the disease being treated. In less severe diseases doses lower than 0.75 mg may suffice, while in severe diseases doses higher than 9 mg may be required. The initial dosage should be maintained or adjusted until the patient's response is satisfactory. If satisfactory clinical response does not occur after a reasonable period of time, discontinue DECADRON elixir and transfer the patient to other therapy.
After a favorable initial response, the proper maintenance dosage should be determined by decreasing the initial dosage in small amounts to the lowest dosage that maintains an adequate clinical response.
Patients should be observed closely for signs that might require dosage adjustment, including changes in clinical status resulting from remissions or exacerbations of the disease, individual drug responsiveness, and the effect of stress (e.g., surgery, infection, trauma). During stress it may be necessary to increase dosage temporarily.
If the drug is to be stopped after more than a few days of treatment, it usually should be withdrawn gradually.
The following milligram equivalents facilitate changing to DECADRON from other glucocorticoids:

DECADRON	Prednisolone and Prednisone			
Methylpred-nisolone and Triamcinolone	Hydrocortisone			
Cortisone				
0.75 mg =	4 mg =	5 mg =	20 mg =	25 mg

Dexamethasone suppression tests
1. Tests for Cushing's syndrome
   Give 1.0 mg of DECADRON orally at 11:00 p.m. Blood is drawn for plasma cortisol determination at 8:00 a.m. the following morning.
   For greater accuracy, give 0.5 mg of DECADRON orally every 6 hours for 48 hours. Twenty-four hour urine collections are made for determination of 17-hydroxycorticosteroid excretion.
2. Test to distinguish Cushing's syndrome due to pituitary ACTH excess from Cushing's syndrome due to other causes
   Give 2.0 mg of DECADRON orally every 6 hours for 48 hours. Twenty-four hour urine collections are made for determination of 17-hydroxycorticosteroid excretion.

HOW SUPPLIED

No. 7622—Elixir DECADRON, 0.5 mg dexamethasone per 5 mL, is a clear, red liquid and is supplied as follows:
NDC 0006-7622-55 bottles of 100 mL with calibrated dropper assembly.
NDC 0006-7622-66 bottles of 237 mL without dropper assembly.
Storage
Store in a container which is kept tightly closed.
A.H.F.S. Category: 68:04
DC 7412726   Issued March 1988

DECADRON® Tablets
(Dexamethasone, MSD), U.S.P.   ℞

DESCRIPTION

Glucocorticoids are adrenocortical steroids, both naturally occurring and synthetic, which are readily absorbed from the gastrointestinal tract.
Dexamethasone, a synthetic adrenocortical steroid, is a white to practically white, odorless, crystalline powder. It is stable in air. It is practically insoluble in water. The molecular weight is 392.47. It is designated chemically as 9-fluoro-11β, 17, 21-trihydroxy-16α-methylpregna-1, 4-diene-3,20-dione. The empirical formula is $C_{22}H_{29}FO_5$ and the structural formula is:
[See Chemical Formula at top of next column].
DECADRON® (Dexamethasone, MSD) tablets are supplied in six potencies, 0.25 mg, 0.5 mg, 0.75 mg, 1.5 mg, 4 mg, and 6 mg. Inactive ingredients are calcium phosphate, lactose, magnesium stearate, and starch. Tablets DECADRON 0.25

mg also contain FD&C Yellow 6. Tablets DECADRON 0.5 mg also contain D&C Yellow 10 and FD&C Yellow 6. Tablets DECADRON 0.75 mg also contain FD&C Blue 1. Tablets DECADRON 1.5 mg also contain FD&C Red 40. Tablets DECADRON 6 mg also contain FD&C Blue 1 and iron oxide.

ACTIONS

Naturally occurring glucocorticoids (hydrocortisone and cortisone), which also have salt-retaining properties, are used as replacement therapy in adrenocortical deficiency states. Their synthetic analogs including dexamethasone are primarily used for their potent anti-inflammatory effects in disorders of many organ systems.
Glucocorticoids cause profound and varied metabolic effects. In addition, they modify the body's immune responses to diverse stimuli.
At equipotent anti-inflammatory doses, dexamethasone almost completely lacks the sodium-retaining property of hydrocortisone and closely related derivatives of hydrocortisone.

INDICATIONS

1. *Endocrine Disorders*
   Primary or secondary adrenocortical insufficiency (hydrocortisone or cortisone is the first choice; synthetic analogs may be used in conjunction with mineralocorticoids where applicable; in infancy mineralocorticoid supplementation is of particular importance)
   Congenital adrenal hyperplasia
   Nonsuppurative thyroiditis
   Hypercalcemia associated with cancer
2. *Rheumatic Disorders*
   As adjunctive therapy for short-term administration (to tide the patient over an acute episode or exacerbation) in:
   Psoriatic arthritis
   Rheumatoid arthritis, including juvenile rheumatoid arthritis (selected cases may require low-dose maintenance therapy)
   Ankylosing spondylitis
   Acute and subacute bursitis
   Acute nonspecific tenosynovitis
   Acute gouty arthritis
   Post-traumatic osteoarthritis
   Synovitis of osteoarthritis
   Epicondylitis
3. *Collagen Diseases*
   During an exacerbation or as maintenance therapy in selected cases of—
   Systemic lupus erythematosus
   Acute rheumatic carditis
4. *Dermatologic Diseases*
   Pemphigus
   Bullous dermatitis herpetiformis
   Severe erythema multiforme (Stevens-Johnson syndrome)
   Exfoliative dermatitis
   Mycosis fungoides
   Severe psoriasis
   Severe seborrheic dermatitis
5. *Allergic States*
   Control of severe or incapacitating allergic conditions intractable to adequate trials of conventional treatment:
   Seasonal or perennial allergic rhinitis
   Bronchial asthma
   Contact dermatitis
   Atopic dermatitis
   Serum sickness
   Drug hypersensitivity reactions
6. *Ophthalmic Diseases*
   Severe acute and chronic allergic and inflammatory processes involving the eye and its adnexa, such as—
   Allergic conjunctivitis
   Keratitis
   Allergic corneal marginal ulcers
   Herpes zoster ophthalmicus
   Iritis and iridocyclitis
   Chorioretinitis
   Anterior segment inflammation
   Diffuse posterior uveitis and choroiditis
   Optic neuritis
   Sympathetic ophthalmia
7. *Respiratory Diseases*
   Symptomatic sarcoidosis

Loeffler's syndrome not manageable by other means
Berylliosis
Fulminating or disseminated pulmonary tuberculosis when used concurrently with appropriate antituberculous chemotherapy
Aspiration pneumonitis
8. *Hematologic Disorders*
   Idiopathic thrombocytopenic purpura in adults
   Secondary thrombocytopenia in adults
   Acquired (autoimmune) hemolytic anemia
   Erythroblastopenia (RBC anemia)
   Congenital (erythroid) hypoplastic anemia
9. *Neoplastic Diseases*
   For palliative management of:
   Leukemias and lymphomas in adults
   Acute leukemia of childhood
10. *Edematous States*
    To induce a diuresis or remission of proteinuria in the nephrotic syndrome, without uremia, of the idiopathic type or that due to lupus erythematosus
11. *Gastrointestinal Diseases*
    To tide the patient over a critical period of the disease in:
    Ulcerative colitis
    Regional enteritis
12. *Cerebral Edema* associated with primary or metastatic brain tumor, craniotomy, or head injury. Use in cerebral edema is not a substitute for careful neurosurgical evaluation and definitive management such as neurosurgery or other specific therapy.
13. *Miscellaneous*
    Tuberculous meningitis with subarachnoid block or impending block when used concurrently with appropriate antituberculous chemotherapy
    Trichinosis with neurologic or myocardial involvement
14. *Diagnostic testing of adrenocortical hyperfunction.*

CONTRAINDICATIONS

Systemic fungal infections
Hypersensitivity to this drug

WARNINGS

In patients on corticosteroid therapy subjected to unusual stress, increased dosage of rapidly acting corticosteroids before, during, and after the stressful situation is indicated.
Drug-induced secondary adrenocortical insufficiency may result from too rapid withdrawal of corticosteroids and may be minimized by gradual reduction of dosage. This type of relative insufficiency may persist for months after discontinuation of therapy; therefore, in any situation of stress occurring during that period, hormone therapy should be reinstituted. If the patient is receiving steroids already, dosage may have to be increased. Since mineralocorticoid secretion may be impaired, salt and/or a mineralocorticoid should be administered concurrently.
Corticosteroids may mask some signs of infection, and new infections may appear during their use. There may be decreased resistance and inability to localize infection when corticosteroids are used. Moreover, corticosteroids may affect the nitroblue-tetrazolium test for bacterial infection and produce false negative results.
In cerebral malaria, a double-blind trial has shown that the use of corticosteroids is associated with prolongation of coma and a higher incidence of pneumonia and gastrointestinal bleeding.
Corticosteroids may activate latent amebiasis. Therefore, it is recommended that latent or active amebiasis be ruled out before initiating corticosteroid therapy in any patient who has spent time in the tropics or any patient with unexplained diarrhea.
Prolonged use of corticosteroids may produce posterior subcapsular cataracts, glaucoma with possible damage to the optic nerves, and may enhance the establishment of secondary ocular infections due to fungi or viruses.
Usage in pregnancy: Since adequate human reproduction studies have not been done with corticosteroids, use of these drugs in pregnancy or in women of childbearing potential requires that the anticipated benefits be weighed against the possible hazards to the mother and embryo or fetus. Infants born of mothers who have received substantial doses of corticosteroids during pregnancy should be carefully observed for signs of hypoadrenalism.
Corticosteroids appear in breast milk and could suppress growth, interfere with endogenous corticosteroid production, or cause other unwanted effects. Mothers taking pharmacologic doses of corticosteroids should be advised not to nurse.

Continued on next page

Information on the Merck Sharp & Dohme products listed on these pages is the full prescribing information from product circulars in use August 31, 1989.

Merck Sharp & Dohme—Cont.

Average and large doses of hydrocortisone or cortisone can cause elevation of blood pressure, salt and water retention, and increased excretion of potassium. These effects are less likely to occur with the synthetic derivatives except when used in large doses. Dietary salt restriction and potassium supplementation may be necessary. All corticosteroids increase calcium excretion.

Administration of live virus vaccines, including smallpox, is contraindicated in individuals receiving immunosuppressive doses of corticosteroids. If inactivated viral or bacterial vaccines are administered to individuals receiving immunosuppressive doses of corticosteroid the expected serum antibody response may not be obtained. However, immunization procedures may be undertaken in patients who are receiving corticosteroids as replacement therapy, e.g., for Addison's disease.

The use of DECADRON tablets in active tuberculosis should be restricted to those cases of fulminating or disseminated tuberculosis in which the corticosteroid is used for the management of the disease in conjunction with an appropriate antituberculous regimen.

If corticosteroids are indicated in patients with latent tuberculosis or tuberculin reactivity, close observation is necessary as reactivation of the disease may occur. During prolonged corticosteroid therapy, these patients should receive chemoprophylaxis.

Literature reports suggest an apparent association between use of corticosteroids and left ventricular free wall rupture after a recent myocardial infarction; therefore, therapy with corticosteroids should be used with great caution in these patients.

PRECAUTIONS

Following prolonged therapy, withdrawal of corticosteroids may result in symptoms of the corticosteroid withdrawal syndrome including fever, myalgia, arthralgia, and malaise. This may occur in patients even without evidence of adrenal insufficiency.

There is an enhanced effect of corticosteroids in patients with hypothyroidism and in those with cirrhosis.

Corticosteroids should be used cautiously in patients with ocular herpes simplex because of possible corneal perforation.

The lowest possible dose of corticosteroids should be used to control the condition under treatment, and when reduction in dosage is possible, the reduction should be gradual.

Psychic derangements may appear when corticosteroids are used, ranging from euphoria, insomnia, mood swings, personality changes, and severe depression, to frank psychotic manifestations. Also, existing emotional instability or psychotic tendencies may be aggravated by corticosteroids.

Aspirin should be used cautiously in conjunction with corticosteroids in hypoprothrombinemia.

Steroids should be used with caution in nonspecific ulcerative colitis, if there is a probability of impending perforation, abscess, or other pyogenic infection, diverticulitis, fresh intestinal anastomoses, active or latent peptic ulcer, renal insufficiency, hypertension, osteoporosis, and myasthenia gravis. Signs of peritoneal irritation following gastrointestinal perforation in patients receiving large doses of corticosteroids may be minimal or absent. Fat embolism has been reported as a possible complication of hypercortisonism.

When large doses are given, some authorities advise that corticosteroids be taken with meals and antacids taken between meals to help to prevent peptic ulcer.

Growth and development of infants and children on prolonged corticosteroid therapy should be carefully observed.

Steroids may increase or decrease motility and number of spermatozoa in some patients.

Phenytoin, phenobarbital, ephedrine, and rifampin may enhance the metabolic clearance of corticosteroids, resulting in decreased blood levels and lessened physiologic activity, thus requiring adjustment in corticosteroid dosage. These interactions may interfere with dexamethasone suppression tests which should be interpreted with caution during administration of these drugs.

False-negative results in the dexamethasone suppression test (DST) in patients being treated with indomethacin have been reported. Thus, results of the DST should be interpreted with caution in these patients.

The prothrombin time should be checked frequently in patients who are receiving corticosteroids and coumarin anticoagulants at the same time because of reports that corticosteroids have altered the response to these anticoagulants. Studies have shown that the usual effect produced by adding corticosteroids is inhibition of response to coumarins, although there have been some conflicting reports of potentiation not substantiated by studies.

When corticosteroids are administered concomitantly with potassium-depleting diuretics, patients should be observed closely for development of hypokalemia.

ADVERSE REACTIONS

Fluid and Electrolyte Disturbances
　Sodium retention
　Fluid retention
　Congestive heart failure in susceptible patients
　Potassium loss
　Hypokalemic alkalosis
　Hypertension
Musculoskeletal
　Muscle weakness
　Steroid myopathy
　Loss of muscle mass
　Osteoporosis
　Vertebral compression fractures
　Aseptic necrosis of femoral and humeral heads
　Pathologic fracture of long bones
　Tendon rupture
Gastrointestinal
　Peptic ulcer with possible perforation and hemorrhage
　Perforation of the small and large bowel, particularly in patients with inflammatory bowel disease
　Pancreatitis
　Abdominal distention
　Ulcerative esophagitis
Dermatologic
　Impaired wound healing
　Thin fragile skin
　Petechiae and ecchymoses
　Erythema
　Increased sweating
　May suppress reactions to skin tests
　Other cutaneous reactions, such as allergic dermatitis, urticaria, angioneurotic edema
Neurologic
　Convulsions
　Increased intracranial pressure with papilledema (pseudotumor cerebri) usually after treatment
　Vertigo
　Headache
　Psychic disturbances
Endocrine
　Menstrual irregularities
　Development of cushingoid state
　Suppression of growth in children
　Secondary adrenocortical and pituitary unresponsiveness, particularly in times of stress, as in trauma, surgery, or illness
　Decreased carbohydrate tolerance
　Manifestations of latent diabetes mellitus
　Increased requirements for insulin or oral hypoglycemic agents in diabetics
　Hirsutism
Ophthalmic
　Posterior subcapsular cataracts
　Increased intraocular pressure
　Glaucoma
　Exophthalmos
Metabolic
　Negative nitrogen balance due to protein catabolism
Cardiovascular
　Myocardial rupture following recent myocardial infarction (see WARNINGS).
Other
　Hypersensitivity
　Thromboembolism
　Weight gain
　Increased appetite
　Nausea
　Malaise
　Hiccups

OVERDOSAGE

Reports of acute toxicity and/or death following overdosage of glucocorticoids are rare. In the event of overdosage, no specific antidote is available; treatment is supportive and symptomatic.
The oral LD_{50} of dexamethasone in female mice was 6.5 g/kg.

DOSAGE AND ADMINISTRATION

For oral administration
DOSAGE REQUIREMENTS ARE VARIABLE AND MUST BE INDIVIDUALIZED ON THE BASIS OF THE DISEASE AND THE RESPONSE OF THE PATIENT.
The initial dosage varies from 0.75 to 9 mg a day depending on the disease being treated. In less severe diseases doses lower than 0.75 mg may suffice, while in severe diseases doses higher than 9 mg may be required. The initial dosage should be maintained or adjusted until the patient's response is satisfactory. If satisfactory clinical response does not occur after a reasonable period of time, discontinue DECADRON tablets and transfer the patient to other therapy.

After a favorable initial response, the proper maintenance dosage should be determined by decreasing the initial dosage in small amounts to the lowest dosage that maintains an adequate clinical response.

Patients should be observed closely for signs that might require dosage adjustment, including changes in clinical status resulting from remissions or exacerbations of the disease, individual drug responsiveness, and the effect of stress (e.g., surgery, infection, trauma). During stress it may be necessary to increase dosage temporarily.

If the drug is to be stopped after more than a few days of treatment, it usually should be withdrawn gradually.

The following milligram equivalents facilitate changing to DECADRON from other glucocorticoids:

DECADRON			Prednisolone and Prednisone	
	Methylprednisolone and Triamcinolone		Hydrocortisone	
				Cortisone
0.75 mg =	4 mg =	5 mg =	20 mg =	25 mg

In *acute, self-limited allergic disorders or acute exacerbations of chronic allergic disorders*, the following dosage schedule combining parenteral and oral therapy is suggested:
DECADRON® Phosphate (Dexamethasone Sodium Phosphate, MSD) injection, 4 mg per mL:
First Day
　1 or 2 mL, intramuscularly
DECADRON tablets, 0.75 mg:
Second Day
　4 tablets in two divided doses
Third Day
　4 tablets in two divided doses
Fourth Day
　2 tablets in two divided doses
Fifth Day
　1 tablet
Sixth Day
　1 tablet
Seventh Day
　No treatment
Eighth Day
　Follow-up visit
This schedule is designed to ensure adequate therapy during acute episodes, while minimizing the risk of overdosage in chronic cases.

In *cerebral edema*, DECADRON Phosphate (Dexamethasone Sodium Phosphate, MSD) injection is generally administered initially in a dosage of 10 mg intravenously followed by 4 mg every six hours intramuscularly until the symptoms of cerebral edema subside. Response is usually noted within 12 to 24 hours and dosage may be reduced after two to four days and gradually discontinued over a period of five to seven days. For palliative management of patients with recurrent or inoperable brain tumors, maintenance therapy with either DECADRON Phosphate (Dexamethasone Sodium Phosphate, MSD) injection or DECADRON tablets in a dosage of two mg two or three times daily may be effective.

Dexamethasone suppression tests
1.　Tests for Cushing's syndrome
　　Give 1.0 mg of DECADRON orally at 11:00 p.m. Blood is drawn for plasma cortisol determination at 8:00 a.m. the following morning.
　　For greater accuracy, give 0.5 mg of DECADRON orally every 6 hours for 48 hours. Twenty-four hour urine collections are made for determination of 17-hydroxycorticosteroid excretion.
2.　Test to distinguish Cushing's syndrome due to pituitary ACTH excess from Cushing's syndrome due to other causes
　　Give 2.0 mg of DECADRON orally every 6 hours for 48 hours. Twenty-four hour urine collections are made for determination of 17-hydroxycorticosteroid excretion.

HOW SUPPLIED

Tablets DECADRON are compressed, pentagonal-shaped tablets, colored to distinguish potency. They are scored and coded on one side and are available as follows:
No. 7648—6 mg, green in color and coded MSD 147.
NDC 0006-0147-50 bottles of 50
NDC 0006-0147-28 single unit packages of 100.
　Shown in Product Identification Section, page 418
No. 7645—4 mg, white in color and coded MSD 97.
NDC 0006-0097-50 bottles of 50
NDC 0006-0097-28 single unit packages of 100.

Shown in Product Identification Section, page 418
No. 7638—1.5 mg, pink in color and coded MSD 95.
NDC 0006-0095-50 bottles of 50
NDC 0006-0095-28 single unit packages of 100.
Shown in Product Identification Section, page 418
No. 7601—0.75 mg, bluish-green in color and coded MSD 63.
NDC 0006-0063-12 5-12 PAK® (package of 12)
NDC 0006-0063-68 bottles of 100
NDC 0006-0063-28 single unit packages of 100.
Shown in Product Identification Section, page 418
No. 7598—0.5 mg, yellow in color and coded MSD 41.
NDC 0006-0041-68 bottles of 100
NDC 0006-0041-28 single unit packages of 100.
Shown in Product Identification Section, page 418
No. 7592—0.25 mg, orange in color and coded MSD 20.
NDC 0006-0020-68 bottles of 100.
Shown in Product Identification Section, page 418
A.H.F.S. Category: 68:04
DC 7420544 Issued March 1988

DECADRON® Phosphate Injection ℞
(Dexamethasone Sodium Phosphate, MSD), U.S.P.

DESCRIPTION

Dexamethasone sodium phosphate, a synthetic adrenocortical steroid, is a white or slightly yellow, crystalline powder. It is freely soluble in water and is exceedingly hygroscopic. The molecular weight is 516.41. It is designated chemically as 9-fluoro-11β, 17-dihydroxy-16α-methyl-21-(phosphonooxy)pregna-1, 4-diene-3, 20-dione disodium salt. The empirical formula is $C_{22}H_{28}FNa_2O_8P$ and the structural formula is:

DECADRON® Phosphate (Dexamethasone Sodium Phosphate, MSD) injection is a sterile solution (pH 7.0 to 8.5) of dexamethasone sodium phosphate, and is supplied in two concentrations: 4 mg/mL and 24 mg/mL. The 24 mg/mL concentration offers the advantage of less volume in indications where high doses of corticosteroids by the intravenous route are needed.
Each milliliter of DECADRON Phosphate injection, 4 mg/mL, contains dexamethasone sodium phosphate equivalent to 4 mg dexamethasone phosphate or 3.33 mg dexamethasone. Inactive ingredients per mL: 8 mg creatinine, 10 mg sodium citrate, sodium hydroxide to adjust pH, and Water for Injection q.s., with 1 mg sodium bisulfite, 1.5 mg methylparaben, and 0.2 mg propylparaben added as preservatives.
Each milliliter of DECADRON Phosphate injection, 24 mg/mL, contains dexamethasone sodium phosphate equivalent to 24 mg dexamethasone phosphate or 20 mg dexamethasone. Inactive ingredients per mL: 8 mg creatinine, 10 mg sodium citrate, 0.5 mg disodium edetate, sodium hydroxide to adjust pH, and Water for Injection q.s., with 1 mg sodium bisulfite, 1.5 mg methylparaben, and 0.2 mg propylparaben added as preservatives.

ACTIONS

DECADRON Phosphate injection has a rapid onset but short duration of action when compared with less soluble preparations. Because of this, it is suitable for the treatment of acute disorders responsive to adrenocortical steroid therapy.
Naturally occurring glucocorticoids (hydrocortisone and cortisone), which also have salt-retaining properties, are used as replacement therapy in adrenocortical deficiency states. Their synthetic analogs, including dexamethasone, are primarily used for their potent anti-inflammatory effects in disorders of many organ systems.
Glucocorticoids cause profound and varied metabolic effects. In addition, they modify the body's immune responses to diverse stimuli.
At equipotent anti-inflammatory doses, dexamethasone almost completely lacks the sodium-retaining property of hydrocortisone and closely related derivatives of hydrocortisone.

INDICATIONS

A. By intravenous or intramuscular injection when oral therapy is not feasible:
1. *Endocrine disorders*
Primary or secondary adrenocortical insufficiency (hydrocortisone or cortisone is the drug of choice; synthetic analogs may be used in conjunction with mineralocorticoids where applicable; in infancy, mineralocorticoid supplementation is of particular importance)
Acute adrenocortical insufficiency (hydrocortisone or cortisone is the drug of choice; mineralocorticoid supplementation may be necessary, particularly when synthetic analogs are used)
Preoperatively, and in the event of serious trauma or illness, in patients with known adrenal insufficiency or when adrenocortical reserve is doubtful
Shock unresponsive to conventional therapy if adrenocortical insufficiency exists or is suspected
Congenital adrenal hyperplasia
Nonsuppurative thyroiditis
Hypercalcemia associated with cancer
2. *Rheumatic disorders*
As adjunctive therapy for short-term administration (to tide the patient over an acute episode or exacerbation) in:
Post-traumatic osteoarthritis
Synovitis of osteoarthritis
Rheumatoid arthritis, including juvenile rheumatoid arthritis (selected cases may require low-dose maintenance therapy)
Acute and subacute bursitis
Epicondylitis
Acute nonspecific tenosynovitis
Acute gouty arthritis
Psoriatic arthritis
Ankylosing spondylitis
3. *Collagen diseases*
During an exacerbation or as maintenance therapy in selected cases of:
Systemic lupus erythematosus
Acute rheumatic carditis
4. *Dermatologic diseases*
Pemphigus
Severe erythema multiforme (Stevens-Johnson syndrome)
Exfoliative dermatitis
Bullous dermatitis herpetiformis
Severe seborrheic dermatitis
Severe psoriasis
Mycosis fungoides
5. *Allergic states*
Control of severe or incapacitating allergic conditions intractable to adequate trials of conventional treatment in:
Bronchial asthma
Contact dermatitis
Atopic dermatitis
Serum sickness
Seasonal or perennial allergic rhinitis
Drug hypersensitivity reactions
Urticarial transfusion reactions
Acute noninfectious laryngeal edema (epinephrine is the drug of first choice)
6. *Ophthalmic diseases*
Severe acute and chronic allergic and inflammatory processes involving the eye, such as:
Herpes zoster ophthalmicus
Iritis, iridocyclitis
Chorioretinitis
Diffuse posterior uveitis and choroiditis
Optic neuritis
Sympathetic ophthalmia
Anterior segment inflammation
Allergic conjunctivitis
Keratitis
Allergic corneal marginal ulcers
7. *Gastrointestinal diseases*
To tide the patient over a critical period of the disease in:
Ulcerative colitis (Systemic therapy)
Regional enteritis (Systemic therapy)
8. *Respiratory diseases*
Symptomatic sarcoidosis
Berylliosis
Fulminating or disseminated pulmonary tuberculosis when used concurrently with appropriate antituberculous chemotherapy
Loeffler's syndrome not manageable by other means
Aspiration pneumonitis
9. *Hematologic disorders*
Acquired (autoimmune) hemolytic anemia
Idiopathic thrombocytopenic purpura in adults (I.V. only; I.M. administration is contraindicated)
Secondary thrombocytopenia in adults
Erythroblastopenia (RBC anemia)
Congenital (erythroid) hypoplastic anemia
10. *Neoplastic diseases*
For palliative management of:
Leukemias and lymphomas in adults
Acute leukemia of childhood
11. *Edematous states*
To induce diuresis or remission of proteinuria in the nephrotic syndrome, without uremia, of the idiopathic type, or that due to lupus erythematosus

12. *Miscellaneous*
Tuberculous meningitis with subarachnoid block or impending block when used concurrently with appropriate antituberculous chemotherapy
Trichinosis with neurologic or myocardial involvement
13. *Diagnostic testing of adrenocortical hyperfunction*
14. *Cerebral Edema* associated with primary or metastatic brain tumor, craniotomy, or head injury. Use in cerebral edema is not a substitute for careful neurosurgical evaluation and definitive management such as neurosurgery or other specific therapy.
B. By intra-articular or soft tissue injection:
As adjunctive therapy for short-term administration (to tide the patient over an acute episode or exacerbation) in:
Synovitis of osteoarthritis
Rheumatoid arthritis
Acute and subacute bursitis
Acute gouty arthritis
Epicondylitis
Acute nonspecific tenosynovitis
Post-traumatic osteoarthritis.
C. By intralesional injection:
Keloids
Localized hypertrophic, infiltrated, inflammatory lesions of: lichen planus, psoriatic plaques, granuloma annulare, and lichen simplex chronicus (neurodermatitis)
Discoid lupus erythematosus
Necrobiosis lipoidica diabeticorum
Alopecia areata
May also be useful in cystic tumors of an aponeurosis or tendon (ganglia).

CONTRAINDICATIONS

Systemic fungal infections. (See WARNINGS regarding amphotericin B)
Hypersensitivity to any component of this product, including sulfites (see WARNINGS).

WARNINGS

Because rare instances of anaphylactoid reactions have occurred in patients receiving parenteral corticosteroid therapy, appropriate precautionary measures should be taken prior to administration, especially when the patient has a history of allergy to any drug. Anaphylactoid and hypersensitivity reactions have been reported for Injection DECADRON Phosphate (see ADVERSE REACTIONS).
Injection DECADRON Phosphate contains sodium bisulfite, a sulfite that may cause allergic-type reactions including anaphylactic symptoms and life-threatening or less severe asthmatic episodes in certain susceptible people. The overall prevalence of sulfite sensitivity in the general population is unknown and probably low. Sulfite sensitivity is seen more frequently in asthmatic than in nonasthmatic people.
Corticosteroids may exacerbate systemic fungal infections and therefore should not be used in the presence of such infections unless they are needed to control drug reactions due to amphotericin B. Moreover, there have been cases reported in which concomitant use of amphotericin B and hydrocortisone was followed by cardiac enlargement and congestive failure.
In patients on corticosteroid therapy subjected to any unusual stress, increased dosage of rapidly acting corticosteroids before, during, and after the stressful situation is indicated.
Drug-induced secondary adrenocortical insufficiency may result from too rapid withdrawal of corticosteroids and may be minimized by gradual reduction of dosage. This type of relative insufficiency may persist for months after discontinuation of therapy; therefore, in any situation of stress occurring during that period, hormone therapy should be reinstituted. If the patient is receiving steroids already, dosage may have to be increased. Since mineralocorticoid secretion may be impaired, salt and/or a mineralocorticoid should be administered concurrently.
Corticosteroids may mask some signs of infection, and new infections may appear during their use. There may be decreased resistance and inability to localize infection when corticosteroids are used. Moreover, corticosteroids may affect the nitroblue-tetrazolium test for bacterial infection and produce false negative results.
In cerebral malaria, a double-blind trial has shown that the use of corticosteroids is associated with prolongation of coma and a higher incidence of pneumonia and gastrointestinal bleeding.
Corticosteroids may activate latent amebiasis. Therefore, it is recommended that latent or active amebiasis be ruled out

Continued on next page

Merck Sharp & Dohme—Cont.

before initiating corticosteroid therapy in any patient who has spent time in the tropics or any patient with unexplained diarrhea.

Prolonged use of corticosteroids may produce posterior subcapsular cataracts, glaucoma with possible damage to the optic nerves, and may enhance the establishment of secondary ocular infections due to fungi or viruses.

Usage in pregnancy. Since adequate human reproduction studies have not been done with corticosteroids, use of these drugs in pregnancy or in women of childbearing potential requires that the anticipated benefits be weighed against the possible hazards to the mother and embryo or fetus. Infants born of mothers who have received substantial doses of corticosteroids during pregnancy should be carefully observed for signs of hypoadrenalism.

Corticosteroids appear in breast milk and could suppress growth, interfere with endogenous corticosteroid production, or cause other unwanted effects. Mothers taking pharmacologic doses of corticosteroids should be advised not to nurse. Average and large doses of cortisone or hydrocortisone can cause elevation of blood pressure, salt and water retention, and increased excretion of potassium. These effects are less likely to occur with the synthetic derivatives except when used in large doses. Dietary salt restriction and potassium supplementation may be necessary. All corticosteroids increase calcium excretion.

Administration of live virus vaccines, including smallpox, is contraindicated in individuals receiving immunosuppressive doses of corticosteroids. If inactivated viral or bacterial vaccines are administered to individuals receiving immunosuppressive doses of corticosteroids, the expected serum antibody response may not be obtained. However, immunization procedures may be undertaken in patients who are receiving corticosteroids as replacement therapy, e.g., for Addison's disease.

The use of DECADRON Phosphate injection in active tuberculosis should be restricted to those cases of fulminating or disseminated tuberculosis in which the corticosteroid is used for the management of the disease in conjunction with an appropriate antituberculous regimen.

If corticosteroids are indicated in patients with latent tuberculosis or tuberculin reactivity, close observation is necessary as reactivation of the disease may occur. During prolonged corticosteroid therapy, these patients should receive chemoprophylaxis.

Literature reports suggest an apparent association between use of corticosteroids and left ventricular free wall rupture after a recent myocardial infarction; therefore, therapy with corticosteroids should be used with great caution in these patients.

PRECAUTIONS

This product, like many other steroid formulations, is sensitive to heat. Therefore, it should not be autoclaved when it is desirable to sterilize the exterior of the vial.

Following prolonged therapy, withdrawal of corticosteroids may result in symptoms of the corticosteroid withdrawal syndrome including fever, myalgia, arthralgia, and malaise. This may occur in patients even without evidence of adrenal insufficiency.

There is an enhanced effect of corticosteroids in patients with hypothyroidism and in those with cirrhosis.

Corticosteroids should be used cautiously in patients with ocular herpes simplex for fear of corneal perforation.

The lowest possible dose of corticosteroid should be used to control the condition under treatment, and when reduction in dosage is possible, the reduction must be gradual.

Psychic derangements may appear when corticosteroids are used, ranging from euphoria, insomnia, mood swings, personality changes, and severe depression to frank psychotic manifestations. Also, existing emotional instability or psychotic tendencies may be aggravated by corticosteroids.

Aspirin should be used cautiously in conjunction with corticosteroids in hypoprothrombinemia.

Steroids should be used with caution in nonspecific ulcerative colitis, if there is a probability of impending perforation, abscess, or other pyogenic infection, also in diverticulitis, fresh intestinal anastomoses, active or latent peptic ulcer, renal insufficiency, hypertension, osteoporosis, and myasthenia gravis. Signs of peritoneal irritation following gastrointestinal perforation in patients receiving large doses of corticosteroids may be minimal or absent. Fat embolism has been reported as a possible complication of hypercortisonism.

When large doses are given, some authorities advise that antacids be administered between meals to help to prevent peptic ulcer.

Growth and development of infants and children on prolonged corticosteroid therapy should be carefully followed.

Steroids may increase or decrease motility and number of spermatozoa in some patients.

Phenytoin, phenobarbital, ephedrine, and rifampin may enhance the metabolic clearance of corticosteroids resulting in decreased blood levels and lessened physiologic activity, thus requiring adjustment in corticosteroid dosage. These interactions may interfere with dexamethasone suppression tests which should be interpreted with caution during administration of these drugs.

False negative results in the dexamethasone suppression test (DST) in patients being treated with indomethacin have been reported. Thus, results of the DST should be interpreted with caution in these patients.

The prothrombin time should be checked frequently in patients who are receiving corticosteroids and coumarin anticoagulants at the same time because of reports that corticosteroids have altered the response to these anticoagulants. Studies have shown that the usual effect produced by adding corticosteroids is inhibition of response to coumarins, although there have been some conflicting reports of potentiation not substantiated by studies.

When corticosteroids are administered concomitantly with potassium-depleting diuretics, patients should be observed closely for development of hypokalemia.

Intra-articular injection of a corticosteroid may produce systemic as well as local effects.

Appropriate examination of any joint fluid present is necessary to exclude a septic process.

A marked increase in pain accompanied by local swelling, further restriction of joint motion, fever, and malaise is suggestive of septic arthritis. If this complication occurs and the diagnosis of sepsis is confirmed, appropriate antimicrobial therapy should be instituted.

Injection of a steroid into an infected site is to be avoided. Corticosteroids should not be injected into unstable joints.

Patients should be impressed strongly with the importance of not overusing joints in which symptomatic benefit has been obtained as long as the inflammatory process remains active.

Frequent intra-articular injection may result in damage to joint tissues.

The slower rate of absorption by intramuscular administration should be recognized.

ADVERSE REACTIONS

Fluid and electrolyte disturbances
Sodium retention
Fluid retention
Congestive heart failure in susceptible patients
Potassium loss
Hypokalemic alkalosis
Hypertension
Musculoskeletal
Muscle weakness
Steroid myopathy
Loss of muscle mass
Osteoporosis
Vertebral compression fractures
Aseptic necrosis of femoral and humeral heads
Pathologic fracture of long bones
Tendon rupture
Gastrointestinal
Peptic ulcer with possible subsequent perforation and hemorrhage
Perforation of the small and large bowel, particularly in patients with inflammatory bowel disease
Pancreatitis
Abdominal distention
Ulcerative esophagitis
Dermatologic
Impaired wound healing
Thin fragile skin
Petechiae and ecchymoses
Erythema
Increased sweating
May suppress reactions to skin tests
Burning or tingling, especially in the perineal area (after I.V. injection)
Other cutaneous reactions, such as allergic dermatitis, urticaria, angioneurotic edema
Neurologic
Convulsions
Increased intracranial pressure with papilledema (pseudotumor cerebri) usually after treatment
Vertigo
Headache
Psychic disturbances
Endocrine
Menstrual irregularities
Development of cushingoid state
Suppression of growth in children
Secondary adrenocortical and pituitary unresponsiveness, particularly in times of stress, as in trauma, surgery, or illness

Decreased carbohydrate tolerance
Manifestations of latent diabetes mellitus
Increased requirements for insulin or oral hypoglycemic agents in diabetics
Hirsutism
Ophthalmic
Posterior subcapsular cataracts
Increased intraocular pressure
Glaucoma
Exophthalmos
Metabolic
Negative nitrogen balance due to protein catabolism
Cardiovascular
Myocardial rupture following recent myocardial infarction (see WARNINGS).
Other
Anaphylactoid or hypersensitivity reactions
Thromboembolism
Weight gain
Increased appetite
Nausea
Malaise
Hiccups
The following *additional* adverse reactions are related to parenteral corticosteroid therapy:
Rare instances of blindness associated with intralesional therapy around the face and head
Hyperpigmentation or hypopigmentation
Subcutaneous and cutaneous atrophy
Sterile abscess
Postinjection flare (following intra-articular use)
Charcot-like arthropathy

OVERDOSAGE

Reports of acute toxicity and/or death following overdosage of glucocorticoids are rare. In the event of overdosage, no specific antidote is available; treatment is supportive and symptomatic.

The oral LD_{50} of dexamethasone in female mice was 6.5 g/kg. The intravenous LD_{50} of dexamethasone sodium phosphate in female mice was 794 mg/kg.

DOSAGE AND ADMINISTRATION

DECADRON Phosphate injection, 4 mg/mL—*For intravenous, intramuscular, intra-articular, intralesional, and soft tissue injection.*
DECADRON Phosphate injection, 24 mg/mL—*For intravenous injection only.*
DECADRON Phosphate injection can be given directly from the vial or the disposable syringe, or it can be added to Sodium Chloride Injection or Dextrose Injection and administered by intravenous drip.

Solutions used for intravenous administration or further dilution of this product should be preservative-free when used in the neonate, especially the premature infant.

When it is mixed with an infusion solution, sterile precautions should be observed. Since infusion solutions generally do not contain preservatives, mixtures should be used within 24 hours.

DOSAGE REQUIREMENTS ARE VARIABLE AND MUST BE INDIVIDUALIZED ON THE BASIS OF THE DISEASE AND THE RESPONSE OF THE PATIENT.

Intravenous and Intramuscular Injection
The initial dosage of DECADRON Phosphate injection varies from 0.5 to 9 mg a day depending on the disease being treated. In less severe diseases doses lower than 0.5 mg may suffice, while in severe diseases doses higher than 9 mg may be required.

The initial dosage should be maintained or adjusted until the patient's response is satisfactory. If a satisfactory clinical response does not occur after a reasonable period of time, discontinue DECADRON Phosphate injection and transfer the patient to other therapy.

After a favorable initial response, the proper maintenance dosage should be determined by decreasing the initial dosage in small amounts to the lowest dosage that maintains an adequate clinical response.

Patients should be observed closely for signs that might require dosage adjustment, including changes in clinical status resulting from remissions or exacerbations of the disease, individual drug responsiveness, and the effect of stress (e.g., surgery, infection, trauma). During stress it may be necessary to increase dosage temporarily.

If the drug is to be stopped after more than a few days of treatment, it usually should be withdrawn gradually.

When the intravenous route of administration is used, dosage usually should be the same as the oral dosage. In certain overwhelming, acute, life-threatening situations, however, administration in dosages exceeding the usual dosages may be justified and may be in multiples of the oral dosages. The slower rate of absorption by intramuscular administration should be recognized.

Shock

There is a tendency in current medical practice to use high (pharmacologic) doses of corticosteroids for the treatment of unresponsive shock. The following dosages of DECADRON phosphate injection have been suggested by various authors:

Author[*]	Dosage
Cavanagh[1]	3 mg/kg of body weight per 24 hours by constant intravenous infusion after an initial intravenous injection of 20 mg
Dietzman[2]	2 to 6 mg/kg of body weight as a single intravenous injection
Frank[3]	40 mg initially followed by repeat intravenous injection every 4 to 6 hours while shock persists
Oaks[4]	40 mg initially followed by repeat intravenous injection every 2 to 6 hours while shock persists
Schumer[5]	1 mg/kg of body weight as a single intravenous injection

Administration of high dose corticosteroid therapy should be continued only until the patient's condition has stabilized and usually not longer than 48 to 72 hours.

Although adverse reactions associated with high dose, short term corticosteroid therapy are uncommon, peptic ulceration may occur.

*1. Cavanagh, D.; Singh, K. B.: Endotoxin shock in pregnancy and abortion, in "Corticosteroids in the Treatment of Shock", Schumer, W.; Nyhus, L. M., Editors, Urbana, University of Illinois Press, 1970, pp. 86-96.
2. Dietzman, R. H.; Ersek, R. A.; Bloch, J. M.; Lillehei, R. C.: High-output, low-resistance gram-negative septic shock in man, Angiology 20: 691-700, Dec. 1969.
3. Frank, E.: Clinical observations in shock and management (In: Shields, T. F., ed.: Symposium on current concepts and management of shock), J. Maine Med. Ass. 59: 195-200, Oct. 1968.
4. Oaks, W. W.; Cohen, H. E.: Endotoxin shock in the geriatric patient, Geriat. 22: 120-130, Mar. 1967.
5. Schumer, W.; Nyhus, L. M.: Corticosteroid effect on biochemical parameters of human oligemic shock, Arch. Surg. 100: 405-408, Apr. 1970.

Cerebral Edema

DECADRON Phosphate injection is generally administered initially in a dosage of 10 mg intravenously followed by 4 mg every six hours intramuscularly until the symptoms of cerebral edema subside. Response is usually noted within 12 to 24 hours and dosage may be reduced after two to four days and gradually discontinued over a period of five to seven days. For palliative management of patients with recurrent or inoperable brain tumors, maintenance therapy with two mg two or three times a day may be effective.

Acute Allergic Disorders

In acute, self-limited allergic disorders or acute exacerbations of chronic allergic disorders, the following dosage schedule combining parenteral and oral therapy is suggested:

DECADRON Phosphate injection, 4 mg/mL: *first day*, 1 or 2 mL (4 or 8 mg), intramuscularly.

DECADRON® (Dexamethasone, MSD) tablets, 0.75 mg: *second and third days*, 4 tablets in two divided doses each day; *fourth day*, 2 tablets in two divided doses; *fifth and sixth days*, 1 tablet each day; *seventh day*, no treatment; *eighth day*, follow-up visit.

This schedule is designed to ensure adequate therapy during acute episodes, while minimizing the risk of overdosage in chronic cases.

Intra-articular, Intralesional, and Soft Tissue Injection

Intra-articular, intralesional, and soft tissue injections are generally employed when the affected joints or areas are limited to one or two sites. Dosage and frequency of injection varies depending on the condition and the site of injection. The usual dose is from 0.2 to 6 mg. The frequency usually ranges from once every three to five days to once every two to three weeks. Frequent intra-articular injection may result in damage to joint tissues.

Some of the usual single doses are:

Site of Injection	Amount of Dexamethasone Phosphate (mg)
Large Joints (e.g., Knee)	2 to 4
Small Joints (e.g., Interphalangeal, Temporomandibular)	0.8 to 1
Bursae	2 to 3
Tendon Sheaths	0.4 to 1
Soft Tissue Infiltration	2 to 6
Ganglia	1 to 2

DECADRON Phosphate injection is particularly recommended for use in conjunction with one of the less soluble, longer-acting steroids for intra-articular and soft tissue injection.

HOW SUPPLIED

No. 7628X—Injection DECADRON Phosphate, 4 mg per mL, is a clear, colorless solution, and is available in 2.5 mL disposable syringes and in 1 mL, 5 mL, and 25 mL vials as follows:

NDC 0006-7628-66, boxes of 25 × 1 mL vials
NDC 0006-7628-30, 2.5 mL single dose disposable syringe
NDC 0006-7628-03, 5 mL vial
(6505-00-963-5355, 5 mL vial)
NDC 0006-7628-25, 25 mL vial

FOR INTRAVENOUS USE ONLY:

No. 7646—Injection DECADRON Phosphate, 24 mg per mL, is a clear, colorless to light yellow solution and is available in 5 mL and 10 mL vials as follows:

NDC 0006-7646-03, 5 mL vial
NDC 0006-7646-10, 10 mL vial.

Storage
Sensitive to heat. Do not autoclave.
Protect from freezing.
Protect from light. Store container in carton until contents have been used.

A.H.F.S. Category: 68:04
DC 7347224   Issued March 1988

DECADRON® Phosphate with XYLOCAINE®   ℞
Injection, Sterile
(Dexamethasone Sodium Phosphate-Lidocaine Hydrochloride)

> **For local injection only**

NOT FOR INTRAVENOUS USE

DESCRIPTION

Dexamethasone sodium phosphate is a white or slightly yellow, crystalline powder. It is freely soluble in water and is exceedingly hygroscopic. The molecular weight is 516.41. It is designated chemically as 9-fluoro-11β, 17-dihydroxy-16α-methyl-21-(phosphonooxy)pregna-1,4-diene-3,20-dione disodium salt. The empirical formula is $C_{22}H_{28}FNa_2O_8P$ and the structural formula is:

Lidocaine hydrochloride is a white, crystalline powder that is very soluble in water and alcohol, soluble in chloroform, and insoluble in ether. The molecular weight is 288.82. It is designated chemically as 2-(diethylamino)-N-(2,6-dimethylphenyl)acetamide, monohydrochloride, monohydrate. The empirical formula is $C_{14}H_{22}N_2O \cdot HCl \cdot H_2O$ and the structural formula is:

DECADRON® Phosphate with XYLOCAINE* (Dexamethasone Sodium Phosphate-Lidocaine Hydrochloride) Injection is provided as a sterile solution (pH 6.5 to 6.9) for the convenience of physicians who prefer to treat patients with simultaneous administration of a corticosteroid and a local anesthetic.

*Registered trademark of Astra Pharmaceutical Products, Inc.

Each milliliter contains dexamethasone sodium phosphate equivalent to dexamethasone phosphate, 4 mg; and lidocaine hydrochloride, 10 mg. Inactive ingredients per mL: citric acid anhydrous, 10 mg; creatinine, 8 mg; sodium bisulfite, 0.5 mg; disodium edetate, 0.5 mg; sodium hydroxide to adjust pH; and Water for Injection, q.s., 1 mL.
Methylparaben, 1.5 mg, and propylparaben, 0.2 mg, added as preservatives.

ACTIONS

DECADRON Phosphate (Dexamethasone Sodium Phosphate, MSD) is a synthetic glucocorticoid used primarily for its potent anti-inflammatory effects in disorders of many organ systems. Glucocorticoids cause profound and varied metabolic effects. In addition, they modify the body's immune responses to diverse stimuli.

XYLOCAINE (Lidocaine Hydrochloride) is a local anesthetic with a rapid onset and moderate duration of action.

Local anesthesia appears within a few minutes after injection of DECADRON Phosphate with XYLOCAINE and lasts 45 minutes to one hour. By the time the anesthesia wears off, steroid activity usually has begun. If the anesthesia wears off before full steroid effect appears, there may be some discomfort beginning about an hour after injection and relief of pain may be delayed for a short time.

INDICATIONS

Acute and subacute bursitis
Acute and subacute nonspecific tenosynovitis

CONTRAINDICATIONS

Hypersensitivity to any component of this product, including sulfites (see WARNINGS).
Dexamethasone Sodium Phosphate
   Systemic fungal infections
Lidocaine Hydrochloride
   Patients with known history of hypersensitivity to local anesthetics of the amide type (e.g., mepivacaine, prilocaine)
   Severe shock
   Heart block

WARNINGS

Because rare instances of anaphylactoid reactions have occurred in patients receiving parenteral corticosteroid therapy, appropriate precautionary measures should be taken prior to administration, especially when the patient has a history of allergy to any drug. Anaphylactoid and hypersensitivity reactions have been reported for Injection DECADRON Phosphate with XYLOCAINE (see ADVERSE REACTIONS).

Injection DECADRON Phosphate with XYLOCAINE contains sodium bisulfite, a sulfite that may cause allergic-type reactions including anaphylactic symptoms and life-threatening or less severe asthmatic episodes in certain susceptible people. The overall prevalence of sulfite sensitivity in the general population is unknown and probably low. Sulfite sensitivity is seen more frequently in asthmatic than in nonasthmatic people.

Lidocaine Hydrochloride
RESUSCITATIVE EQUIPMENT AND DRUGS SHOULD BE IMMEDIATELY AVAILABLE WHEN ANY LOCAL ANESTHETIC IS USED.

Usage in pregnancy: The safe use of lidocaine hydrochloride has not been established with respect to adverse effects upon fetal development. Careful consideration should be given to this fact before administering this drug to women of childbearing potential, particularly during early pregnancy.

Dexamethasone Sodium Phosphate
In patients on corticosteroid therapy subjected to unusual stress, increased dosage of rapidly acting corticosteroids before, during, and after the stressful situation is indicated.

Drug-induced secondary adrenocortical insufficiency may result from too rapid withdrawal of corticosteroids and may be minimized by gradual reduction of dosage. This type of relative insufficiency may persist for months after discontinuation of therapy; therefore, in any situation of stress occurring during that period, hormone therapy should be reinstituted. If the patient is receiving steroids already, dosage may have to be increased. Since mineralocorticoid secretion may be impaired, salt and/or a mineralocorticoid should be administered concurrently.

Continued on next page

Merck Sharp & Dohme—Cont.

Corticosteroids may mask some signs of infection, and new infections may appear during their use. There may be decreased resistance and inability to localize infection when corticosteroids are used. Moreover, corticosteroids may affect the nitroblue-tetrazolium test for bacterial infection and produce false negative results.

Corticosteroids may activate latent amebiasis. Therefore, it is recommended that latent or active amebiasis be ruled out before initiating corticosteroid therapy in any patient who has spent time in the tropics or any patient with unexplained diarrhea.

Prolonged use of corticosteroids may produce posterior subcapsular cataracts, glaucoma with possible damage to the optic nerves, and may enhance the establishment of secondary ocular infections due to fungi or viruses.

Usage in pregnancy: Since adequate human reproduction studies have not been done with corticosteroids, use of these drugs in pregnancy or in women of childbearing potential requires that the anticipated benefits be weighed against the possible hazards to the mother and embryo or fetus. Infants born of mothers who have received substantial doses of corticosteroids during pregnancy should be carefully observed for signs of hypoadrenalism.

Corticosteroids appear in breast milk and could suppress growth, interfere with endogenous corticosteroid production, or cause other unwanted effects. Mothers taking pharmacologic doses of corticosteroids should be advised not to nurse.

Average and large doses of cortisone or hydrocortisone can cause elevation of blood pressure, salt and water retention, and increased excretion of potassium. These effects are less likely to occur with the synthetic derivatives except when used in large doses. Dietary salt restriction and potassium supplementation may be necessary. All corticosteroids increase calcium excretion.

Administration of live virus vaccines, including smallpox, is contraindicated in individuals receiving immunosuppressive doses of corticosteroids. If inactivated viral or bacterial vaccines are administered to individuals receiving immunosuppressive doses of corticosteroids, the expected serum antibody response may not be obtained.

If corticosteroids are indicated in patients with latent tuberculosis or tuberculin reactivity, close observation is necessary as reactivation of the disease may occur. During prolonged corticosteroid therapy, these patients should receive chemoprophylaxis.

Literature reports suggest an apparent association between use of corticosteroids and left ventricular free wall rupture after a recent myocardial infarction; therefore, therapy with corticosteroids should be used with great caution in these patients.

PRECAUTIONS

This product, like many other steroid formulations, is sensitive to heat. Therefore, it should not be autoclaved when it is desirable to sterilize the exterior of the vial.

Therapy with this preparation does not eliminate the need for conventional supportive measures. Although capable of ameliorating symptoms, and even suppressing them completely in some patients, it is not a cure. Neither the hormone nor the anesthetic has any effect on the basic cause of inflammation.

Supportive measures, such as analgesics, pertinent orthopedic procedures, heat or cold, rest, rehabilitation, and physiotherapy must be used as applicable. If physiotherapy is applied immediately following injection, it may cause severe pain.

In some patients, a single injection fully restores mobility. Patients should be strongly impressed with the importance of not overusing the affected part as long as the inflammatory process remains active.

Injection into an infected site is to be avoided.

Dexamethasone Sodium Phosphate
Following prolonged therapy, withdrawal of corticosteroids may result in symptoms of the corticosteroid withdrawal syndrome including fever, myalgia, arthralgia, and malaise. This may occur in patients even without evidence of adrenal insufficiency.

There is an enhanced effect of corticosteroids in patients with hypothyroidism and in those with cirrhosis.

Corticosteroids should be used cautiously in patients with ocular herpes simplex for fear of corneal perforation.

Psychic derangements may appear when corticosteroids are used, ranging from euphoria, insomnia, mood swings, personality changes, and severe depression to frank psychotic manifestations. Also, existing emotional instability or psychotic tendencies may be aggravated by corticosteroids.

Aspirin should be used cautiously in conjunction with corticosteroids in hypoprothrombinemia.

Steroids should be used with caution in non-specific ulcerative colitis, if there is a probability of impending perforation, abscess, or other pyogenic infection, also in diverticuli-

tis, fresh intestinal anastomoses, active or latent peptic ulcer, renal insufficiency, hypertension, osteoporosis, and myasthenia gravis. Signs of peritoneal irritation following gastrointestinal perforation in patients receiving large doses of corticosteroids may be minimal or absent. Fat embolism has been reported as a possible complication of hypercortisonism.

When large doses are given, some authorities advise that antacids be administered between meals to help to prevent peptic ulcer.

Growth and development of infants and children on prolonged corticosteroid therapy should be carefully followed. Steroids may increase or decrease motility and number of spermatozoa in some patients.

Phenytoin, phenobarbital, ephedrine, and rifampin may enhance the metabolic clearance of corticosteroids, resulting in decreased blood levels and lessened physiologic activity, thus requiring adjustment in corticosteroid dosage.

The prothrombin time should be checked frequently in patients who are receiving corticosteroids and coumarin anticoagulants at the same time because of reports that corticosteroids have altered the response to these anticoagulants. Studies have shown that the usual effect produced by adding corticosteroids is inhibition of response to coumarins, although there have been some conflicting reports of potentiation not substantiated by studies.

When corticosteroids are administered concomitantly with potassium-depleting diuretics, patients should be observed closely for development of hypokalemia.

Lidocaine Hydrochloride
The safety and effectiveness of lidocaine hydrochloride depend on proper dosage, correct technique, adequate precautions, and readiness for emergencies.

Injection of repeated doses may cause significant increases in blood levels with each repeated dose due to slow accumulation of the drug or its metabolites. Tolerance varies with the status of the patient. Debilitated, elderly patients, acutely ill patients, and children should be given reduced doses commensurate with their age and physical status. INJECTIONS SHOULD ALWAYS BE MADE SLOWLY AND WITH FREQUENT ASPIRATIONS. Aspiration is advisable since it reduces the possibility of intravascular injection, thereby keeping the incidence of side effects and anesthetic failures to a minimum. Consult standard textbooks for specific techniques and precautions for various local anesthetic procedures.

Lidocaine hydrochloride should be used with caution in persons with known drug sensitivities. Patients allergic to para-aminobenzoic acid derivatives (procaine, tetracaine, benzocaine, etc.) have not shown cross sensitivity to lidocaine hydrochloride.

Local anesthetics react with certain metals and cause the release of their respective ions which, if injected, may cause severe local irritation. Adequate precaution should be taken to avoid this type of interaction.

ADVERSE REACTIONS

Dexamethasone Sodium Phosphate
Fluid and electrolyte disturbances
  Sodium retention
  Fluid retention
  Congestive heart failure in susceptible patients
  Potassium loss
  Hypokalemic alkalosis
  Hypertension
Musculoskeletal
  Muscle weakness
  Steroid myopathy
  Loss of muscle mass
  Osteoporosis
  Vertebral compression fractures
  Aseptic necrosis of femoral and humeral heads
  Pathologic fracture of long bones
  Tendon rupture
Gastrointestinal
  Peptic ulcer with possible subsequent perforation and hemorrhage
  Perforation of the small and large bowel, particularly in patients with inflammatory bowel disease
  Pancreatitis
  Abdominal distention
  Ulcerative esophagitis
Dermatologic
  Impaired wound healing
  Thin fragile skin
  Petechiae and ecchymoses
  Erythema
  Increased sweating
  May suppress reactions to skin tests
  Other cutaneous reactions, such as allergic dermatitis, urticaria, angioneurotic edema

Neurologic
  Convulsions
  Increased intracranial pressure with papilledema (pseudotumor cerebri) usually after treatment
  Vertigo
  Headache
  Psychic disturbances
Endocrine
  Menstrual irregularities
  Development of cushingoid state
  Suppression of growth in children
  Secondary adrenocortical and pituitary unresponsiveness, particularly in times of stress, as in trauma, surgery, or illness
  Decreased carbohydrate tolerance
  Manifestations of latent diabetes mellitus
  Increased requirements for insulin or oral hypoglycemic agents in diabetics
Ophthalmic
  Posterior subcapsular cataracts
  Increased intraocular pressure
  Glaucoma
  Exophthalmos
Metabolic
  Negative nitrogen balance due to protein catabolism
Cardiovascular
Myocardial rupture following recent myocardial infarction (see WARNINGS).
Other
  Anaphylactoid or hypersensitivity reactions
  Thromboembolism
  Weight gain
  Increased appetite
  Nausea
  Malaise
  Hiccups

The following *additional* adverse reactions are related to parenteral corticosteroid therapy:
  Rare instances of blindness associated with intralesional therapy around the face and head
  Hyperpigmentation or hypopigmentation
  Subcutaneous and cutaneous atrophy
  Sterile abscess
  Charcot-like arthropathy

Lidocaine Hydrochloride
Adverse reactions may result from high plasma levels due to excessive dosage, rapid absorption or inadvertent intravascular injection, or may result from a hypersensitivity, idiosyncrasy or diminished tolerance on the part of the patient. Such reactions are systemic in nature and involve the central nervous system and/or the cardiovascular system.

CNS reactions are excitatory and/or depressant, and may be characterized by nervousness, dizziness, blurred vision, and tremors followed by drowsiness, convulsions, unconsciousness, and possibly respiratory arrest. The excitatory reactions may be very brief or may not occur at all, in which case the first manifestations of toxicity may be drowsiness merging into unconsciousness and respiratory arrest.

Cardiovascular reactions are depressant, and may be characterized by hypotension, myocardial depression, bradycardia and possibly cardiac arrest.

Treatment of a patient with toxic manifestations consists of assuring and maintaining a patent airway and supporting ventilation using oxygen and assisted or controlled respiration as required. This usually will be sufficient in the management of most reactions. Should circulatory depression occur, vasopressors, such as ephedrine or metaraminol, and intravenous fluids may be used. Should a convulsion persist despite oxygen therapy, small increments of an ultra-short acting barbiturate (thiopental or thiamylal) or a short acting barbiturate (pentobarbital or secobarbital) may be given intravenously.

Allergic reactions are characterized by cutaneous lesions, urticaria, edema or anaphylactoid reactions. The detection of sensitivity by skin testing is of doubtful value.

DOSAGE AND ADMINISTRATION

> **For local injection only**

NOT FOR INTRAVENOUS USE
DOSAGE AND FREQUENCY OF INJECTION ARE VARIABLE AND MUST BE INDIVIDUALIZED ON THE BASIS OF THE DISEASE AND THE RESPONSE OF THE PATIENT.

Injections should always be made slowly and with frequent aspiration.
The initial dose ranges from 0.1 to 0.75 mL depending on the disease being treated and the size of the area to be injected. Frequency of injection depends on symptomatic response. In some patients, acute conditions are controlled adequately by a single injection. In others, additional injections are required, usually at intervals of four to seven days. If satisfactory clinical response does not occur after a reasonable pe-

riod of time, discontinue DECADRON Phosphate with XYLOCAINE Injection and transfer the patient to other therapy.

Patients should be observed closely for signs that might require dosage adjustment, including changes in clinical status resulting from remissions or exacerbations of the disease, and individual drug responsiveness.

The usual doses are:

	Acute and Subacute Bursitis	Acute and Subacute Nonspecific Tenosynovitis
Amount of injection (mL)	0.5 to 0.75	0.1 to 0.25
Amount of dexamethasone sodium phosphate (mg)	2 to 3	0.4 to 1
Amount of lidocaine hydrochloride (mg)	5 to 7.5	1 to 2.5

DECADRON Phosphate with XYLOCAINE may be given undiluted directly from the vial, or it may be diluted with Sterile Water for Injection or Sodium Chloride Injection, using up to five parts of diluent to each part of injection. Dilutions should be used within one hour, since there is a possibility of change in pH, and this may adversely affect the stability or activity of the components.

HOW SUPPLIED

No. 7625X—Injection DECADRON Phosphate with XYLOCAINE, containing 4 mg dexamethasone phosphate equivalent and 10 mg lidocaine hydrochloride per mL, is a clear, colorless solution, and is available as follows:
NDC 0006-7625-03 in 5 mL vials.
Storage
Sensitive to heat. Do not autoclave.
Protect from freezing.
　　A.H.F.S. Categories: 68:04-72:00
　　DC 7349316　Issued March 1988

DECADRON® Phosphate ℞
(Dexamethasone Sodium Phosphate, MSD), U.S.P.
0.05% Dexamethasone Phosphate Equivalent
Sterile Ophthalmic Ointment

DESCRIPTION

Dexamethasone sodium phosphate is 9-fluoro-11β, 17-dihydroxy-16α-methyl-21-(phosphonooxy)pregna-1,4-diene-3,20-dione disodium salt. Its empirical formula is $C_{22}H_{28}FNa_2O_8P$ and its structural formula is:

Glucocorticoids are adrenocortical steroids, both naturally occurring and synthetic. Dexamethasone is a synthetic analog of naturally occurring glucocorticoids (hydrocortisone and cortisone). Dexamethasone sodium phosphate is a water soluble, inorganic ester of dexamethasone. Its molecular weight is 516.41.
Sterile Ophthalmic Ointment DECADRON® Phosphate (Dexamethasone Sodium Phosphate, MSD) is a topical steroid ointment containing dexamethasone sodium phosphate equivalent to 0.5 mg (0.05%) dexamethasone phosphate in each gram. Inactive ingredients: white petrolatum and mineral oil.
Dexamethasone sodium phosphate is an inorganic ester of dexamethasone.

CLINICAL PHARMACOLOGY

Dexamethasone sodium phosphate suppresses the inflammatory response to a variety of agents and it probably delays or slows healing. No generally accepted explanation of these steroid properties have been advanced.

INDICATIONS AND USAGE

For the treatment of the following conditions:
Steroid responsive inflammatory conditions of the palpebral and bulbar conjunctiva, cornea, and anterior segment of the globe, such as allergic conjunctivitis, acne rosacea, superficial punctate keratitis, herpes zoster keratitis, iritis, cyclitis, selected infective conjunctivitis when the inherent hazard of steroid use is accepted to obtain an advisable diminution in edema and inflammation; corneal injury from chemical or thermal burns, or penetration of foreign bodies.

CONTRAINDICATIONS

Epithelial herpes simplex keratitis (dendritic keratitis).
Acute infectious stages of vaccinia, varicella, and many other viral diseases of the cornea and conjunctiva.
Mycobacterial infection of the eye.
Fungal diseases of ocular structures.
Hypersensitivity to a component of the medication.

WARNINGS

Prolonged use may result in ocular hypertension and/or glaucoma, with damage to the optic nerve, defects in visual acuity and fields of vision, and posterior subcapsular cataract formation. Prolonged use may suppress the host response and thus increase the hazard of secondary ocular infections. In those diseases causing thinning of the cornea or sclera, perforations have been known to occur with the use of topical corticosteroids. In acute purulent conditions of the eye, corticosteroids may mask infection or enhance existing infection. If these products are used for 10 days or longer, intraocular pressure should be routinely monitored even though it may be difficult in children and uncooperative patients.
Employment of corticosteroid medication in the treatment of herpes simplex other than epithelial herpes simplex keratitis, in which it is contraindicated, requires great caution; periodic slit-lamp microscopy is essential.

PRECAUTIONS

General
The possibility of persistent fungal infections of the cornea should be considered after prolonged corticosteroid dosing.
Carcinogenesis, Mutagenesis, Impairment of Fertility
Long-term animal studies have not been performed to evaluate the carcinogenic potential or the effect on fertility of Ophthalmic Ointment DECADRON Phosphate.
Pregnancy
Pregnancy Category C. Dexamethasone has been shown to be teratogenic in mice and rabbits following topical ophthalmic application in multiples of the therapeutic dose.
In the mouse, corticosteroids produce fetal resorptions and a specific abnormality, cleft palate. In the rabbit, corticosteroids have produced fetal resorptions and multiple abnormalities involving the head, ears, limbs, palate, etc.
There are no adequate or well-controlled studies in pregnant women. Ophthalmic Ointment DECADRON Phosphate should be used during pregnancy only if the potential benefit to the mother justifies the potential risk to the embryo or fetus. Infants born of mothers who have received substantial doses of corticosteroids during pregnancy should be observed carefully for signs of hypoadrenalism.
Nursing Mothers
Topically applied steroids are absorbed systemically. Therefore, because of the potential for serious adverse reactions in nursing infants from dexamethasone sodium phosphate, a decision should be made whether to discontinue nursing or discontinue the drug, taking into account the importance of the drug to the mother.
Pediatric Use
Safety and effectiveness in children have not been established.

ADVERSE REACTIONS

Glaucoma with optic nerve damage, visual acuity and field defects, posterior subcapsular cataract formation, secondary ocular infection from pathogens including herpes simplex, perforation of the globe.
Rarely, filtering blebs have been reported when topical steroids have been used following cataract surgery.
Rarely, stinging or burning may occur.

DOSAGE AND ADMINISTRATION

The duration of treatment will vary with the type of lesion and may extend from a few days to several weeks, according to therapeutic response. Relapses, more common in chronic active lesions than in self-limited conditions, usually respond to retreatment.
Apply a thin coating of ointment three or four times a day. When a favorable response is observed, reduce the number of daily applications to two, and later to one a day as a maintenance dose if this is sufficient to control symptoms.

Ophthalmic Ointment DECADRON Phosphate is particularly convenient when an eye pad is used. It may also be the preparation of choice for patients in whom therapeutic benefit depends on prolonged contact of the active ingredients with ocular tissues.

HOW SUPPLIED

No. 7615—0.05% Sterile Ophthalmic Ointment DECADRON Phosphate is a clear unctuous ointment and is supplied as follows:
NDC 0006-7615-04 in 3.5 g tubes
(6505-00-961-5508 0.05% 3.5 g).
　　A.H.F.S. Category: 52:08
　　DC 6033127　Issued July 1986

DECADRON® Phosphate ℞
(Dexamethasone Sodium Phosphate, MSD), U.S.P.
0.1% Dexamethasone Phosphate Equivalent
Sterile Ophthalmic Solution

DESCRIPTION

Dexamethasone sodium phosphate is 9-fluoro-11β,17-dihydroxy-16α-methyl-21-(phosphonooxy)pregna-1,4-diene-3,20-dione disodium salt. Its empirical formula is $C_{22}H_{28}FNa_2O_8P$ and its structural formula is:

Glucocorticoids are adrenocortical steroids, both naturally occurring and synthetic. Dexamethasone is a synthetic analog of naturally occurring glucocorticoids (hydrocortisone and cortisone). Dexamethasone sodium phosphate is a water soluble, inorganic ester of dexamethasone. It is approximately three thousand times more soluble in water at 25℃ than hydrocortisone. Its molecular weight is 516.41.
Ophthalmic Solution DECADRON® Phosphate (Dexamethasone Sodium Phosphate, MSD) in the 5 mL OCUMETER® ophthalmic dispenser is a topical steroid solution containing dexamethasone sodium phosphate equivalent to 1 mg (0.1%) dexamethasone phosphate in each milliliter of buffered solution. Inactive ingredients: creatinine, sodium citrate, sodium borate, polysorbate 80, disodium edetate, hydrochloric acid to adjust pH, and water for injection. Sodium bisulfite 0.1%, phenylethanol 0.25% and benzalkonium chloride 0.02% added as preservatives.

CLINICAL PHARMACOLOGY

Dexamethasone sodium phosphate suppresses the inflammatory response to a variety of agents and it probably delays or slows healing. No generally accepted explanation of these steroid properties have been advanced.

INDICATIONS AND USAGE

For the treatment of the following conditions:
Ophthalmic:
Steroid responsive inflammatory conditions of the palpebral and bulbar conjunctiva, cornea, and anterior segment of the globe, such as allergic conjunctivitis, acne rosacea, superficial punctate keratitis, herpes zoster keratitis, iritis, cyclitis, selected infective conjunctivitis when the inherent hazard of steroid use is accepted to obtain an advisable diminution in edema and inflammation; corneal injury from chemical or thermal burns, or penetration of foreign bodies.
Otic:
Steroid responsive inflammatory conditions of the external auditory meatus, such as allergic otitis externa, selected purulent and nonpurulent infective otitis externa when the hazard of steroid use is accepted to obtain an advisable diminution in edema and inflammation.

Continued on next page

Merck Sharp & Dohme—Cont.

CONTRAINDICATIONS

Epithelial herpes simplex keratitis (dendritic keratitis).
Acute infectious stages of vaccinia, varicella, and many other viral diseases of the cornea and conjunctiva.
Mycobacterial infection of the eye.
Fungal diseases of ocular or auricular structures.
Hypersensitivity to any component of this product, including sulfites (see WARNINGS).
Perforation of a drum membrane.

WARNINGS

Prolonged use may result in ocular hypertension and/or glaucoma, with damage to the optic nerve, defects in visual acuity and fields of vision, and posterior subcapsular cataract formation. Prolonged use may suppress the host response and thus increase the hazard of secondary ocular infections. In those diseases causing thinning of the cornea or sclera, perforations have been known to occur with the use of topical corticosteroids. In acute purulent conditions of the eye or ear, corticosteroids may mask infection or enhance existing infection. If these products are used for 10 days or longer, intraocular pressure should be routinely monitored even though it may be difficult in children and uncooperative patients.
Employment of corticosteroid medication in the treatment of herpes simplex other than epithelial herpes simplex keratitis, in which it is contraindicated, requires great caution; periodic slit-lamp microscopy is essential.
Ophthalmic Solution DECADRON Phosphate contains sodium bisulfite, a sulfite that may cause allergic-type reactions including anaphylactic symptoms and life-threatening or less severe asthmatic episodes in certain susceptible people. The overall prevalence of sulfite sensitivity in the general population is unknown and probably low. Sulfite sensitivity is seen more frequently in asthmatic than in nonasthmatic people.

PRECAUTIONS

General
The possibility of persistent fungal infections of the cornea should be considered after prolonged corticosteroid dosing.
Carcinogenesis, Mutagenesis, Impairment of Fertility
Long-term animal studies have not been performed to evaluate the carcinogenic potential or the effect on fertility of Ophthalmic Solution DECADRON Phosphate.
Pregnancy
Pregnancy Category C. Dexamethasone has been shown to be teratogenic in mice and rabbits following topical ophthalmic application in multiples of the therapeutic dose.
In the mouse, corticosteroids produce fetal resorptions and a specific abnormality, cleft palate. In the rabbit, corticosteroids have produced fetal resorptions and multiple abnormalities involving the head, ears, limbs, palate, etc.
There are no adequate or well-controlled studies in pregnant women. Ophthalmic Solution DECADRON Phosphate should be used during pregnancy only if the potential benefit to the mother justifies the potential risk to the embryo or fetus. Infants born of mothers who have received substantial doses of corticosteroids during pregnancy should be observed carefully for signs of hypoadrenalism.
Nursing Mothers
Topically applied steroids are absorbed systemically. Therefore, because of the potential for serious adverse reactions in nursing infants from dexamethasone sodium phosphate, a decision should be made whether to discontinue nursing or discontinue the drug, taking into account the importance of the drug to the mother.
Pediatric Use
Safety and effectiveness in children have not been established.

ADVERSE REACTIONS

Glaucoma with optic nerve damage, visual acuity and field defects, posterior subcapsular cataract formation, secondary ocular infection from pathogens including herpes simplex, perforation of the globe.
Rarely, filtering blebs have been reported when topical steroids have been used following cataract surgery.
Rarely, stinging or burning may occur.

DOSAGE AND ADMINISTRATION

The duration of treatment will vary with the type of lesion and may extend from a few days to several weeks, according to therapeutic response. Relapses, more common in chronic active lesions than in self-limited conditions, usually respond to retreatment.
Eye—Instill one or two drops of solution into the conjunctival sac every hour during the day and every two hours during the night as initial therapy. When a favorable response is observed, reduce dosage to one drop every four hours. Later,

further reduction in dosage to one drop three or four times daily may suffice to control symptoms.
Ear—Clean the aural canal thoroughly and sponge dry. Instill the solution directly into the aural canal. A suggested initial dosage is three or four drops two or three times a day. When a favorable response is obtained, reduce dosage gradually and eventually discontinue.
If preferred, the aural canal may be packed with a gauze wick saturated with solution. Keep the wick moist with the preparation and remove from the ear after 12 to 24 hours. Treatment may be repeated as often as necessary at the discretion of the physician.

HOW SUPPLIED

Sterile Ophthalmic Solution DECADRON Phosphate is a clear, colorless to pale yellow solution.
No. 7643—Ophthalmic Solution DECADRON Phosphate is supplied as follows:
NDC 0006-7643-03 in 5 mL white, opaque, plastic OCUMETER ophthalmic dispenser with a controlled drop tip. (6505-00-007-4536 0.1% 5 mL).

A.H.F.S. Category: 52:08
DC 7261515 Issued February 1987

DECADRON® Phosphate   ℞
RESPIHALER®
(Dexamethasone Sodium Phosphate, MSD), U.S.P.

DESCRIPTION

RESPIHALER® DECADRON® Phosphate (Dexamethasone Sodium Phosphate, MSD) is an aerosol for oral inhalation which contains dexamethasone sodium phosphate, an inorganic ester of dexamethasone, a synthetic adrenocortical steroid with basic glucocorticoid actions and effects.
Each RESPIHALER DECADRON Phosphate contains an amount sufficient to deliver at least 170 sprays. The metering valve of the aerosol-mechanism of the RESPIHALER dispenses dexamethasone sodium phosphate equivalent to approximately 0.1 mg of dexamethasone phosphate or approximately 0.084 mg of dexamethasone with each activation. On a regimen of 12 inhalations daily, it has been determined that the patient absorbs approximately 0.4-0.6 mg of dexamethasone. The inactive ingredients are fluorochlorohydrocarbons included as propellants. Alcohol 2%.
Dexamethasone sodium phosphate, a synthetic adrenocortical steroid, is a white or slightly yellow, crystalline powder. It is freely soluble in water and is exceedingly hygroscopic. It is prepared by a special process to produce particles in the range of 0.5 to 4 microns in size. The molecular weight is 516.41. It is designated chemically as 9-fluoro-11β, 17-dihydroxy-16α-methyl-21-(phosphono-oxy)pregna-1, 4-diene-3, 20-dione disodium salt. The empirical formula is $C_{22}H_{28}FNa_2O_8P$ and the structural formula is:

ACTIONS

Because of the high water solubility of dexamethasone sodium phosphate, the aerosolized particles dissolve readily in the secretions of the bronchial and bronchiolar mucous membrane.

INDICATIONS

RESPIHALER DECADRON Phosphate is indicated for the treatment of bronchial asthma and related corticosteroid responsive bronchospastic states intractable to adequate trial of conventional therapy.

CONTRAINDICATIONS

Systemic fungal infections.
Hypersensitivity to any component of this medication.
Persistently positive cultures of the sputum for *Candida albicans*.

WARNINGS

Rare instances of laryngeal and pharyngeal fungal infections have been observed in patients using RESPIHALER DECADRON Phosphate. These have usually responded promptly to discontinuation of therapy and institution of antifungal treatment.

In patients on therapy with RESPIHALER DECADRON Phosphate subjected to unusual stress, increased dosage of rapidly acting corticosteroids before, during, and after the stressful situation is indicated.
Drug-induced secondary adrenocortical insufficiency may result from too rapid withdrawal of corticosteroids and may be minimized by gradual reduction of dosage. This type of relative insufficiency may persist for months after discontinuation of therapy; therefore, in any situation of stress occurring during that period, hormone therapy should be reinstituted. If the patient is receiving steroids already, dosage may have to be increased. Since mineralocorticoid secretion may be impaired, salt and/or a mineralocorticoid should be administered concurrently.
Dexamethasone may mask some signs of infection, and new infections may appear during its use. There may be decreased resistance and inability to localize infection when corticosteroids are used. Moreover, dexamethasone may affect the nitroblue-tetrazolium test for bacterial infection and produce false negative results.
Corticosteroids may activate latent amebiasis. Therefore, it is recommended that latent or active amebiasis be ruled out before initiating corticosteroid therapy in any patient who has spent time in the tropics or any patient with unexplained diarrhea.
Prolonged use of RESPIHALER DECADRON Phosphate may produce posterior subcapsular cataracts, glaucoma with possible damage to the optic nerves, and may enhance the establishment of secondary ocular infections due to fungi or viruses.
Usage in pregnancy: Since adequate human reproduction studies have not been done with RESPIHALER DECADRON Phosphate, use of this drug in pregnancy or in women of childbearing potential requires that the anticipated benefits be weighed against the possible hazards to the mother and embryo or fetus. Infants born of mothers who have received substantial doses of dexamethasone during pregnancy, should be carefully observed for signs of hypoadrenalism.
Dexamethasone appears in breast milk and could suppress growth, interfere with endogenous corticosteroid production, or cause other unwanted effects. Mothers taking pharmacologic doses of dexamethasone should be advised not to nurse.
Average and large doses of hydrocortisone or cortisone can cause elevation of blood pressure, salt and water retention, and increased excretion of potassium. These effects are less likely to occur with the synthetic derivatives and with RESPIHALER DECADRON Phosphate, except when used in large doses. Dietary salt restriction and potassium supplementation may be necessary. All corticosteroids increase calcium excretion.
Administration of live virus vaccines, including smallpox, is contraindicated in individuals receiving immunosuppressive doses of corticosteroids. If inactivated viral or bacterial vaccines are administered to individuals receiving immunosuppressive doses of corticosteroids, the expected serum antibody response may not be obtained.
If RESPIHALER DECADRON Phosphate is indicated in patients with latent tuberculosis or tuberculin reactivity, close observation is necessary as reactivation of the disease may occur. During prolonged therapy with RESPIHALER DECADRON Phosphate, these patients should receive chemoprophylaxis.
Literature reports suggest an apparent association between use of corticosteroids and left ventricular free wall rupture after a recent myocardial infarction; therefore, therapy with corticosteroids should be used with great caution in these patients.

PRECAUTIONS

RESPIHALER DECADRON Phosphate is *not* indicated for relief of the occasional mild and isolated attack of asthma which is readily responsive to the immediate, though short-lived, action of epinephrine, isoproterenol, aminophylline, etc. Nor should it be employed for the treatment of severe status asthmaticus where intensive measures are required. RESPIHALER DECADRON Phosphate should be considered only for the following classes of patients: patients not on corticosteroid therapy who have not responded adequately to other treatment; patients already on systemic corticosteroid therapy—in an attempt to reduce or eliminate systemic administration.
Although systemic absorption is low when RESPIHALER DECADRON Phosphate is used in the recommended dosage, adrenal suppression may occur. In addition, other systemic effects of steroid administration must be considered as a possibility.
Following prolonged therapy, withdrawal of corticosteroids may result in symptoms of the corticosteroid withdrawal syndrome including fever, myalgia, arthralgia, and malaise. This may occur in patients even without evidence of adrenal insufficiency.
There is an enhanced effect of dexamethasone in patients with hypothyroidism and in those with cirrhosis.

RESPIHALER DECADRON Phosphate should be used cautiously in patients with ocular herpes simplex for fear of corneal perforation.

The lowest possible dose of RESPIHALER DECADRON Phosphate should be used to control the condition under treatment, and when reduction in dosage is possible, the reduction must be gradual.

Psychic derangements may appear when dexamethasone is used, ranging from euphoria, insomnia, mood swings, personality changes, and severe depression, to frank psychotic manifestations. Also, existing emotional instability or psychotic tendencies may be aggravated.

Aspirin should be used cautiously in conjunction with RESPIHALER DECADRON Phosphate in hypoprothrombinemia.

RESPIHALER DECADRON Phosphate should be used with caution in nonspecific ulcerative colitis, if there is a probability of impending perforation, abscess or other pyogenic infection; also in diverticulitis; fresh intestinal anastomoses; active or latent peptic ulcer; renal insufficiency; hypertension; osteoporosis; and myasthenia gravis. Signs of peritoneal irritation following gastrointestinal perforation in patients receiving large doses of corticosteroids may be minimal or absent. Fat embolism has been reported as a possible complication of hypercortisonism.

Growth and development of infants and children on prolonged therapy with RESPIHALER DECADRON Phosphate should be carefully followed.

Dexamethasone may increase or decrease motility and number of spermatozoa in some patients.

Phenytoin, phenobarbital, ephedrine and rifampin may enhance the metabolic clearance of dexamethasone, resulting in decreased blood levels and lessened physiologic activity, thus requiring adjustment in dexamethasone dosage.

The prothrombin time should be checked frequently in patients who are receiving RESPIHALER DECADRON Phosphate and coumarin anticoagulants at the same time because of reports that corticosteroids have altered the response to these anticoagulants. Studies have shown that the usual effect produced by adding corticosteroids is inhibition of response to coumarins, although there have been some conflicting reports of potentiation, not substantiated by studies.

When RESPIHALER DECADRON Phosphate is used concomitantly with potassium-depleting diuretics, patients should be observed closely for development of hypokalemia.

Since the contents of RESPIHALER DECADRON Phosphate are under pressure, the container should not be broken, stored in extreme heat, or incinerated. It should be stored at a temperature below 120°F.

ADVERSE REACTIONS

Side effects which may occur in patients treated with RESPIHALER DECADRON Phosphate include throat irritation, hoarseness, coughing, and laryngeal and pharyngeal fungal infections.

Patients should be observed for the hormonal effects described below:

Fluid and Electrolyte Disturbances
 Sodium retention
 Fluid retention
 Congestive heart failure in susceptible patients
 Potassium loss
 Hypokalemic alkalosis
 Hypertension
Musculoskeletal
 Muscle weakness
 Steroid myopathy
 Loss of muscle mass
 Osteoporosis
 Vertebral compression fractures
 Aseptic necrosis of femoral and humeral heads
 Pathologic fracture of long bones
 Tendon rupture
Gastrointestinal
 Peptic ulcer with possible subsequent perforation and hemorrhage
 Perforation of the small and large bowel, particularly in patients with inflammatory bowel disease
 Pancreatitis
 Abdominal distention
 Ulcerative esophagitis
Dermatologic
 Impaired wound healing
 Thin fragile skin
 Petechiae and ecchymoses
 Erythema
 Increased sweating
 May suppress reactions to skin tests
 Other cutaneous reactions, such as allergic dermatitis, urticaria, angioneurotic edema

Neurologic
 Convulsions
 Increased intracranial pressure with papilledema (pseudotumor cerebri) usually after treatment
 Vertigo
 Headache
 Psychic disturbances
Endocrine
 Menstrual irregularities
 Development of cushingoid state
 Suppression of growth in children
 Secondary adrenocortical and pituitary unresponsiveness, particularly in times of stress, as in trauma, surgery, or illness
 Decreased carbohydrate tolerance
 Manifestations of latent diabetes mellitus
 Increased requirements for insulin or oral hypoglycemic agents in diabetics
Ophthalmic
 Posterior subcapsular cataracts
 Increased intraocular pressure
 Glaucoma
 Exophthalmos
Metabolic
 Negative nitrogen balance due to protein catabolism
Cardiovascular
 Myocardial rupture following recent myocardial infarction (see WARNINGS).
Other
 Hypersensitivity
 Thromboembolism
 Weight gain
 Increased appetite
 Nausea
 Malaise
 Hiccups

OVERDOSAGE

Reports of acute toxicity and/or death following overdosage of glucocorticoids are rare. In the event of overdosage, no specific antidote is available; treatment is supportive and symptomatic.

The oral LD_{50} of dexamethasone in female mice was 6.5 g/kg. The intravenous LD_{50} of dexamethasone sodium phosphate in female mice was 794 mg/kg.

DOSAGE AND ADMINISTRATION

Recommended *initial dosage:*
 Adults —3 inhalations 3 or 4 times per day.
 Children —2 inhalations 3 or 4 times per day.
Maximum dosage:
 Adults —3 inhalations *per dose;* 12 inhalations *per day.*
 Children —2 inhalations *per dose;* 8 inhalations *per day.*

When a favorable response is attained, the dose may be gradually reduced. In patients on systemic corticosteroids, it is recommended that systemic therapy be reduced or eliminated before reduction of RESPIHALER dosage is begun. Gradual reduction of systemic corticosteroid therapy must be emphasized to avoid withdrawal symptoms.

HOW SUPPLIED

No. 7626X—RESPIHALER DECADRON Phosphate, aerosol for oral inhalation, is supplied as follows: **NDC** 0006-7626-13 in a pressurized container, and includes a plastic adapter.
Storage
Store at a temperature below 49°C (120°F).
 A.H.F.S. Category: 68:04
 DC 7413016 Issued March 1988

DECADRON® Phosphate Topical Cream
(Dexamethasone Sodium Phosphate, MSD), U.S.P.   ℞
0.1% Dexamethasone Phosphate Equivalent

DESCRIPTION

DECADRON® Phosphate (Dexamethasone Sodium Phosphate, MSD) Topical Cream is a topical steroid preparation.

The topical corticosteroids constitute a class of primarily synthetic steroids used as anti-inflammatory and anti-pruritic agents.

Dexamethasone sodium phosphate is 9-fluoro-11β,17-dihydroxy-16α-methyl-21-(phosphonooxy)pregna-1,4-diene-3,20-dione disodium salt. Its empirical formula is $C_{22}H_{28}FNa_2O_8P$ and its structural formula is:
[See Chemical Formula at top of next column].
Dexamethasone sodium phosphate has a molecular weight of 516.41.

DECADRON Phosphate Topical Cream contains in each gram: dexamethasone sodium phosphate equivalent to 1 mg (0.1%) dexamethasone phosphate in a greaseless bland base. Inactive ingredients: stearyl alcohol, cetyl alcohol, mineral oil, polyoxyl 40 stearate, sorbitol solution, methyl polysilicone emulsion, creatinine, sodium citrate, disodium edetate, sodium hydroxide to adjust pH, and purified water. Methylparaben, 0.15%, and sorbic acid, 0.1% added as preservatives.

CLINICAL PHARMACOLOGY

Topical corticosteroids share anti-inflammatory, anti-pruritic and vasoconstrictive actions.

The mechanism of anti-inflammatory activity of the topical corticosteroids is unclear. Various laboratory methods, including vasoconstrictor assays, are used to compare and predict potencies and/or clinical efficacies of the topical corticosteroids. There is some evidence to suggest that a recognizable correlation exists between vasoconstrictor potency and therapeutic efficacy in man.
Pharmacokinetics
The extent of percutaneous absorption of topical corticosteroids is determined by many factors including the vehicle, the integrity of the epidermal barrier, and the use of occlusive dressings.

Topical corticosteroids can be absorbed from normal intact skin. Inflammation and/or other disease processes in the skin increase percutaneous absorption. Occlusive dressings substantially increase the percutaneous absorption of topical corticosteroids. Thus, occlusive dressings may be a valuable therapeutic adjunct for treatment of resistant dermatoses. (See DOSAGE AND ADMINISTRATION)

Once absorbed through the skin, topical corticosteroids are handled through pharmacokinetic pathways similar to systemically administered corticosteroids. Corticosteroids are bound to plasma proteins in varying degrees. Corticosteroids are metabolized primarily in the liver and are then excreted by the kidneys. Some of the topical corticosteroids and their metabolites are also excreted into the bile.

INDICATIONS AND USAGE

DECADRON Phosphate Topical Cream is indicated for relief of the inflammatory and pruritic manifestations of corticosteroid-responsive dermatoses.

CONTRAINDICATIONS

Topical corticosteroids are contraindicated in those patients with a history of hypersensitivity to any of the components of the preparation.

PRECAUTIONS

General
Systemic absorption of topical corticosteroids has produced reversible hypothalamic-pituitary-adrenal (HPA) axis suppression, manifestations of Cushing's syndrome, hyperglycemia, and glycosuria in some patients.

Conditions which augment systemic absorption include the application of the more potent corticosteroids, use over large surface areas, prolonged use, and the addition of occlusive dressings.

Therefore, patients receiving a large dose of a potent topical corticosteroid applied to a large surface area or under an occlusive dressing should be evaluated periodically for evidence of HPA axis suppression by using urinary free cortisol and ACTH stimulation tests. If HPA axis suppression is noted, an attempt should be made to withdraw the drug, to reduce the frequency of application, or to substitute a less potent corticosteroid.

Recovery of HPA axis function is generally prompt and complete upon discontinuation of the drug. Infrequently, signs and symptoms of corticosteroid withdrawal may occur, requiring supplemental systemic corticosteroids.

Continued on next page

Information on the Merck Sharp & Dohme products listed on these pages is the full prescribing information from product circulars in use August 31, 1989.

Merck Sharp & Dohme—Cont.

Children may absorb proportionally larger amounts of topical corticosteroids and thus be more susceptible to systemic toxicity (See PRECAUTIONS, *Pediatric Use*).

If irritation develops, topical corticosteroids should be discontinued and appropriate therapy instituted.

In the presence of dermatological infections, the use of an appropriate antifungal or antibacterial agent should be instituted. If a favorable response does not occur promptly, the corticosteroid should be discontinued until the infection has been adequately controlled.

This product is not for ophthalmic use. However, if applied to the eyelids or skin near the eyes, the drug may enter the eyes. In patients with a history of herpes simplex keratitis, ocular exposure to corticosteroids may lead to a recurrence. Prolonged ocular exposure may cause steroid glaucoma. Generally, occlusive dressings should not be used on weeping or exudative lesions.

If occlusive dressing therapy is used, inspect lesions between dressings for development of infection. If infection develops, the technique should be discontinued and appropriate antimicrobial therapy instituted.

When large areas of the body are covered with an occlusive dressing, thermal homeostasis may be impaired. If elevation of body temperature occurs, use of the occlusive dressing should be discontinued.

Information for the Patient
Patients using topical corticosteroids should receive the following information and instructions:

1. This medication is to be used as directed by the physician. It is for external use only. Avoid contact with the eyes.
2. Patients should be advised not to use this medication for any disorder other than that for which it was prescribed.
3. The treated skin area should not be bandaged or otherwise covered or wrapped so as to be occlusive unless directed by the physician.
4. Patients should report any signs of local adverse reactions, especially under occlusive dressing.
5. Parents of pediatric patients should be advised not to use tight-fitting diapers or plastic pants on a child being treated in the diaper area, as these garments may constitute occlusive dressings.

Laboratory Tests
The following tests may be helpful in evaluating the HPA axis suppression:
• Urinary free cortisol test
• ACTH stimulation test

Carcinogenesis, Mutagenesis, and Impairment of Fertility
Long-term animal studies have not been performed to evaluate the carcinogenic potential or the effect on fertility of topical corticosteroids.

Studies to determine mutagenicity with prednisolone and hydrocortisone have revealed negative results.

Pregnancy
Pregnancy Category C: Corticosteroids are generally teratogenic in laboratory animals when administered systemically at relatively low dosage levels. The more potent corticosteroids have been shown to be teratogenic after dermal application in laboratory animals. There are no adequate and well-controlled studies in pregnant women on teratogenic effects from topically applied corticosteroids. Therefore, topical corticosteroids should be used during pregnancy only if the potential benefit justifies the potential risk to the fetus. Drugs of this class should not be used extensively on pregnant patients, in large amounts, or for prolonged periods of time.

Nursing Mothers
It is not known whether topical administration of corticosteroids could result in sufficient systemic absorption to produce detectable quantities in breast milk. Systemically administered corticosteroids are secreted into breast milk in quantities *not* likely to have a deleterious effect on the infant. Nevertheless, caution should be exercised when topical corticosteroids are administered to a nursing woman.

Pediatric Use
Pediatric patients may demonstrate greater susceptibility to topical corticosteroid-induced HPA axis suppression and Cushing's syndrome than mature patients because of a larger skin surface area to body weight ratio.

Hypothalamic-pituitary-adrenal (HPA) axis suppression, Cushing's syndrome, and intracranial hypertension have been reported in children receiving topical corticosteroids. Manifestations of adrenal suppression in children include linear growth retardation, delayed weight gain, low plasma cortisol levels, and absence of response to ACTH stimulation. Manifestations of intracranial hypertension include bulging fontanelles, headaches, and bilateral papilledema.

Administration of topical corticosteroids to children should be limited to the least amount compatible with an effective therapeutic regimen. Chronic corticosteroid therapy may interfere with the growth and development of children.

ADVERSE REACTIONS

The following adverse reactions are reported infrequently with topical corticosteroids, but may occur more frequently with the use of occlusive dressings. These reactions are listed in an approximate decreasing order of occurrence:

Burning
Itching
Irritation
Dryness
Folliculitis
Hypertrichosis
Acneiform eruptions
Hypopigmentation
Perioral dermatitis
Allergic contact dermatitis
Maceration of the skin
Secondary infection
Skin atrophy
Striae
Miliaria

OVERDOSAGE

Topically applied corticosteroids can be absorbed in sufficient amounts to produce systemic effects (See PRECAUTIONS).

DOSAGE AND ADMINISTRATION

Apply to the affected area as a thin film three or four times daily.

Occlusive dressings may be used for the management of psoriasis or recalcitrant conditions.

Before using this preparation in the *ear*, clean the aural canal thoroughly and sponge dry. Confirm that the eardrum is intact. With a cotton-tipped applicator, apply a thin coating of the cream to the affected canal area three or four times a day.

HOW SUPPLIED

No. 7616X — 0.1% Topical Cream DECADRON Phosphate is a white cream, and is supplied as follows:
NDC 0006-7616-12 in 15 g tubes
NDC 0006-7616-24 in 30 g tubes.
A.H.F.S. Category: 84:06
DC 6005423 Issued April 1983
Copyright © MERCK & CO., INC., 1983
All rights reserved

DECADRON® Phosphate   ℞
TURBINAIRE®
(Dexamethasone Sodium Phosphate, MSD), U.S.P.

DESCRIPTION

TURBINAIRE® DECADRON® Phosphate (Dexamethasone Sodium Phosphate, MSD) is an aerosol for intranasal application. The inactive ingredients are fluorochlorohydrocarbons as propellants and alcohol 2%. One cartridge delivers an amount sufficient to ensure delivery of 170 metered sprays, each containing dexamethasone sodium phosphate equivalent to approximately 0.1 mg dexamethasone phosphate or to approximately 0.084 mg dexamethasone. Twelve sprays deliver a theoretical maximum of 1.0 mg dexamethasone.

Dexamethasone sodium phosphate, a synthetic adrenocortical steroid, is a white or slightly yellow, crystalline powder. It is freely soluble in water and is exceedingly hygroscopic. The molecular weight is 516.41. It is designated chemically as 9-fluoro-11β, 17-dihydroxy-16α-methyl-21-(phosphonooxy) pregna-1, 4-diene-3, 20-dione disodium salt. The empirical formula is $C_{22}H_{28}FNa_2O_8P$ and the structural formula is:

ACTION

Inhibition of inflammatory response to inciting agents of mechanical, chemical or immunological nature.

INDICATIONS

Allergic or inflammatory nasal conditions, and nasal polyps (excluding polyps originating within the sinuses).

CONTRAINDICATIONS

Systemic fungal infections.
Hypersensitivity to components.
Tuberculous, viral and fungal nasal conditions, ocular herpes simplex.

WARNINGS

In patients on therapy with TURBINAIRE DECADRON Phosphate subjected to unusual stress, increased dosage of rapidly acting corticosteroids before, during, and after the stressful situation is indicated.

Drug-induced secondary adrenocortical insufficiency may result from too rapid withdrawal of corticosteroids and may be minimized by gradual reduction of dosage. This type of relative insufficiency may persist for months after discontinuation of therapy; therefore, in any situation of stress occurring during that period, hormone therapy should be reinstituted. If the patient is receiving steroids already, dosage may have to be increased. Since mineralocorticoid secretion may be impaired, salt and/or a mineralocorticoid should be administered concurrently.

Dexamethasone may mask some signs of infection, and new infections may appear during its use. There may be decreased resistance and inability to localize infection when corticosteroids are used. Therefore, patients with bacterial infections should also be given appropriate antibiotic therapy if TURBINAIRE DECADRON Phosphate is used. Moreover, dexamethasone may affect the nitroblue-tetrazolium test for bacterial infection and produce false negative results.

Corticosteroids may activate latent amebiasis. Therefore, it is recommended that latent or active amebiasis be ruled out before initiating corticosteroid therapy in any patient who has spent time in the tropics or any patient with unexplained diarrhea.

Prolonged use of TURBINAIRE DECADRON Phosphate may produce posterior subcapsular cataracts, glaucoma with possible damage to the optic nerves, and may enhance the establishment of secondary ocular infections due to fungi or viruses.

Usage in pregnancy: Since adequate human reproduction studies have not been done with TURBINAIRE DECADRON Phosphate, use of this drug in pregnancy or in women of childbearing potential requires that the anticipated benefits be weighed against the possible hazards to the mother and embryo or fetus. Infants born of mothers who have received substantial doses of dexamethasone during pregnancy, should be carefully observed for signs of hypoadrenalism.

Dexamethasone appears in breast milk and could suppress growth, interfere with endogenous corticosteroid production, or cause other unwanted effects. Mothers taking pharmacologic doses of dexamethasone should be advised not to nurse.

Average and large doses of hydrocortisone or cortisone can cause elevation of blood pressure, salt and water retention, and increased excretion of potassium. These effects are less likely to occur with the synthetic derivatives and with TURBINAIRE DECADRON Phosphate, except when used in large doses. Dietary salt restriction and potassium supplementation may be necessary. All corticosteroids increase calcium excretion.

Administration of live virus vaccines, including smallpox, is contraindicated in individuals receiving immunosuppressive doses of corticosteroids. If inactivated viral or bacterial vaccines are administered to individuals receiving immunosuppressive doses of corticosteroids, the expected serum antibody response may not be obtained.

If TURBINAIRE DECADRON Phosphate is indicated in patients with latent tuberculosis or tuberculin reactivity, close observation is necessary as reactivation of the disease may occur. During prolonged therapy with TURBINAIRE DECADRON Phosphate, these patients should receive chemoprophylaxis.

Literature reports suggest an apparent association between use of corticosteroids and left ventricular free wall rupture after a recent myocardial infarction; therefore, therapy with corticosteroids should be used with great caution in these patients.

PRECAUTIONS

During local corticosteroid therapy, the possibility of pharyngeal candidiasis should be kept in mind.

Although systemic absorption is low when TURBINAIRE DECADRON Phosphate is used in the recommended dosage, adrenal suppression may occur. In addition, other systemic effects of steroid administration must be considered as a possibility.

Following prolonged therapy, withdrawal of corticosteroids may result in symptoms of the corticosteroid withdrawal syndrome including fever, myalgia, arthralgia, and malaise. This may occur in patients even without evidence of adrenal insufficiency. Replacement of systemic steroid with TUR-

BINAIRE DECADRON Phosphate should be gradual and carefully monitored by the physician.

There is an enhanced effect of dexamethasone in patients with hypothyroidism and in those with cirrhosis.

TURBINAIRE DECADRON Phosphate should be used cautiously in patients with ocular herpes simplex for fear of corneal perforation.

The lowest possible dose of TURBINAIRE DECADRON Phosphate should be used to control the condition under treatment, and when reduction in dosage is possible, the reduction must be gradual. If beneficial effect is not evident within 7 days after initiation of therapy, the patient should be re-evaluated.

Psychic derangements may appear when dexamethasone is used, ranging from euphoria, insomnia, mood swings, personality changes, and severe depression, to frank psychotic manifestations. Also, existing emotional instability or psychotic tendencies may be aggravated.

Aspirin should be used cautiously in conjunction with TURBINAIRE DECADRON Phosphate in hypoprothrombinemia.

TURBINAIRE DECADRON Phosphate should be used with caution in patients with nonspecific ulcerative colitis, if there is a probability of impending perforation, abscess or other pyogenic infection; also in diverticulitis; fresh intestinal anastomoses; active or latent peptic ulcer; renal insufficiency; hypertension; osteoporosis; and myasthenia gravis. Signs of peritoneal irritation following gastrointestinal perforation in patients receiving large doses of corticosteroids may be minimal or absent. Fat embolism has been reported as a possible complication of hypercortisonism.

Because clinical studies have not been done, the use of this product in children under the age of 6 years is not recommended. Growth and development of children 6 years of age or older on prolonged therapy with TURBINAIRE DECADRON Phosphate should be carefully followed.

Dexamethasone may increase or decrease motility and number of spermatozoa in some patients.

Phenytoin, phenobarbital, ephedrine and rifampin may enhance the metabolic clearance of dexamethasone, resulting in decreased blood levels and lessened physiologic activity, thus requiring adjustment in dexamethasone dosage.

The prothrombin time should be checked frequently in patients who are receiving TURBINAIRE DECADRON Phosphate and coumarin anticoagulants at the same time because of reports that corticosteroids have altered the response to these anticoagulants. Studies have shown that the usual effect produced by adding corticosteroids is inhibition of response to coumarins, although there have been some conflicting reports of potentiation, not substantiated by studies.

When TURBINAIRE DECADRON Phosphate is used concomitantly with potassium-depleting diuretics, patients should be observed closely for development of hypokalemia. Since the contents of TURBINAIRE DECADRON Phosphate are under pressure, the container should not be broken, stored in extreme heat, or incinerated. It should be stored at a temperature below 120°F.

ADVERSE REACTIONS

Nasal irritation and dryness are the most common adverse reactions. The following have been reported: headache, light-headedness, urticaria, nausea, epistaxis, rebound congestion, bronchial asthma, perforation of the nasal septum, and anosmia. Signs of adrenal hypercorticism may occur in some patients, especially with overdosage.

Systemic effects from therapy with TURBINAIRE DECADRON Phosphate are less likely to occur than with oral or parenteral corticosteroid therapy because of a lower total dose administered. Nevertheless, patients should be observed for the hormonal effects described below because of absorption of dexamethasone from the nasal mucosa.

Fluid and Electrolyte Disturbances
  Sodium retention
  Fluid retention
  Congestive heart failure in susceptible patients
  Potassium loss
  Hypokalemic alkalosis
  Hypertension
Musculoskeletal
  Muscle weakness
  Steroid myopathy
  Loss of muscle mass
  Osteoporosis
  Vertebral compression fractures
  Aseptic necrosis of femoral and humeral heads
  Pathologic fracture of long bones
  Tendon rupture
Gastrointestinal
  Peptic ulcer with possible subsequent perforation and hemorrhage
  Perforation of the small and large bowel, particularly in patients with inflammatory bowel disease

  Pancreatitis
  Abdominal distention
  Ulcerative esophagitis
Dermatologic
  Impaired wound healing
  Thin fragile skin
  Petechiae and ecchymoses
  Erythema
  Increased sweating
  May suppress reactions to skin tests
  Other cutaneous reactions, such as allergic dermatitis, urticaria, angioneurotic edema.
Neurologic
  Convulsions
  Increased intracranial pressure with papilledema (pseudotumor cerebri) usually after treatment
  Vertigo
  Headache
  Psychic disturbances
Endocrine
  Menstrual irregularities
  Development of cushingoid state
  Suppression of growth in children
  Secondary adrenocortical and pituitary unresponsiveness, particularly in times of stress, as in trauma, surgery, or illness
  Decreased carbohydrate tolerance
  Manifestations of latent diabetes mellitus
  Increased requirements for insulin or oral hypoglycemic agents in diabetics
Ophthalmic
  Posterior subcapsular cataracts
  Increased intraocular pressure
  Glaucoma
  Exophthalmos
Metabolic
  Negative nitrogen balance due to protein catabolism
Cardiovascular
  Myocardial rupture following recent myocardial infarction (see WARNINGS).
Other
  Hypersensitivity
  Thromboembolism
  Weight gain
  Increased appetite
  Nausea
  Malaise
  Hiccups

OVERDOSAGE

Reports of acute toxicity and/or death following overdosage of glucocorticoids are rare. In the event of overdosage, no specific antidote is available; treatment is supportive and symptomatic.

The oral LD_{50} of dexamethasone in female mice was 6.5 g/kg. The intravenous LD_{50} of dexamethasone sodium phosphate in female mice was 794 mg/kg.

DOSAGE AND ADMINISTRATION

DO NOT EXCEED THE RECOMMENDED DOSAGE.
The usual initial dosage of TURBINAIRE DECADRON Phosphate is:
  Adults—2 sprays in each nostril 2 or 3 times a day.
  Children (6 to 12 years of age)—1 or 2 sprays in each nostril 2 times a day depending on age.
See accompanying instructions on the proper use of TURBINAIRE.

When improvement occurs the dosage should be gradually reduced. Some patients will be symptom-free on one spray in each nostril 2 times a day. The maximum daily dosage for adults is 12 sprays, and for children, 8 sprays. Therapy should be discontinued as soon as feasible. It may be reinstituted if recurrence of symptoms occurs.

HOW SUPPLIED

No. 7634—TURBINAIRE DECADRON Phosphate, aerosol for intranasal application, is supplied as follows: **NDC** 0006-7634-13 in a pressurized container and includes a plastic adapter (6505-00-885-6302, 12.6 Grams, 170 Metered Doses).
No. 7642—Refill unit for TURBINAIRE DECADRON Phosphate aerosol for intranasal application is supplied as follows: **NDC** 0006-7642-13 in a pressurized container.
Storage
Store at a temperature below 49°C (120°F).
     A.H.F.S. Category: 52:08
DC 7413122   Issued March 1988

DECADRON-LA® Sterile Suspension   ℞
(Dexamethasone Acetate, MSD), U.S.P.

NOT FOR INTRAVENOUS USE

DESCRIPTION

Dexamethasone acetate, a synthetic adrenocortical steroid, is a white to practically white, odorless powder. It is a practically insoluble ester of dexamethasone. The structural formula is:

Dexamethasone acetate is present in DECADRON-LA® (Dexamethasone Acetate, MSD) sterile suspension as the monohydrate, with the empirical formula, $C_{24}H_{31}FO_6 \cdot H_2O$, and molecular weight, 452.52. Dexamethasone acetate is designated chemically as 21-(acetyloxy)-9-fluoro-11β,17-dihydroxy-16α-methylpregna-1,4-diene-3,20-dione.

DECADRON-LA sterile suspension is a sterile white suspension (pH 5.0 to 7.5) that settles on standing, but is easily resuspended by mild shaking.

Each milliliter contains dexamethasone acetate equivalent to 8 mg dexamethasone. Inactive ingredients per mL: 6.67 mg sodium chloride; 5 mg creatinine; 0.5 mg disodium edetate; 5 mg sodium carboxymethylcellulose; 0.75 mg polysorbate 80; sodium hydroxide to adjust pH; and Water for Injection, q.s. 1 mL, with 9 mg benzyl alcohol, and 1 mg sodium bisulfite added as preservatives.

ACTIONS

DECADRON-LA sterile suspension is a long-acting, repository adrenocorticosteroid preparation with a prompt onset of action. It is suitable for intramuscular or local injection, but not when an immediate effect of short duration is desired. Naturally occurring glucocorticoids (hydrocortisone and cortisone), which also have salt-retaining properties, are used as replacement therapy in adrenocortical deficiency states. Their synthetic analogs, including dexamethasone, are primarily used for their potent anti-inflammatory effects in disorders of many organ systems.

Glucocorticoids cause profound and varied metabolic effects. In addition, they modify the body's immune responses to diverse stimuli.

At equipotent anti-inflammatory doses, dexamethasone almost completely lacks the sodium-retaining property of hydrocortisone.

INDICATIONS

A. By intramuscular injection when oral therapy is not feasible:
1. *Endocrine disorders*
Congenital adrenal hyperplasia
Nonsuppurative thyroiditis
Hypercalcemia associated with cancer
2. *Rheumatic disorders*
As adjunctive therapy for short-term administration (to tide the patient over an acute episode or exacerbation) in:
Post-traumatic osteoarthritis
Synovitis of osteoarthritis
Rheumatoid arthritis, including juvenile rheumatoid arthritis (selected cases may require low-dose maintenance therapy)
Acute and subacute bursitis
Epicondylitis
Acute nonspecific tenosynovitis
Acute gouty arthritis
Psoriatic arthritis
Ankylosing spondylitis
3. *Collagen diseases*
During an exacerbation or as maintenance therapy in selected cases of:
Systemic lupus erythematosus
Acute rheumatic carditis
4. *Dermatologic diseases*
Pemphigus
Severe erythema multiforme (Stevens-Johnson syndrome)
Exfoliative dermatitis
Bullous dermatitis herpetiformis

Continued on next page

Merck Sharp & Dohme—Cont.

Severe seborrheic dermatitis
Severe psoriasis
Mycosis fungoides

5. *Allergic states*
Control of severe or incapacitating allergic conditions intractable to adequate trials of conventional treatment in:
Bronchial asthma
Contact dermatitis
Atopic dermatitis
Serum sickness
Seasonal or perennial allergic rhinitis
Drug hypersensitivity reactions
Urticarial transfusion reactions

6. *Ophthalmic diseases*
Severe acute and chronic allergic and inflammatory processes involving the eye, such as:
Herpes zoster ophthalmicus
Iritis, Iridocyclitis
Chorioretinitis
Diffuse posterior uveitis and choroiditis
Optic neuritis
Sympathetic ophthalmia
Anterior segment inflammation
Allergic conjunctivitis
Keratitis
Allergic corneal marginal ulcers

7. *Gastrointestinal diseases*
To tide the patient over a critical period of the disease in:
Ulcerative colitis (Systemic therapy)
Regional enteritis (Systemic therapy)

8. *Respiratory diseases*
Symptomatic sarcoidosis
Berylliosis
Loeffler's syndrome not manageable by other means
Aspiration pneumonitis

9. *Hematologic disorders*
Acquired (autoimmune) hemolytic anemia
Secondary thrombocytopenia in adults
Erythroblastopenia (RBC anemia)
Congenital (erythroid) hypoplastic anemia

10. *Neoplastic diseases*
For palliative management of:
Leukemias and lymphomas in adults
Acute leukemia of childhood

11. *Edematous states*
To induce diuresis or remission of proteinuria in the nephrotic syndrome, without uremia, of the idiopathic type, or that due to lupus erythematosus

12. *Miscellaneous*
Trichinosis with neurologic or myocardial involvement.

B. By intra-articular or soft tissue injection as adjunctive therapy for short-term administration (to tide the patient over an acute episode or exacerbation) in:
Synovitis of osteoarthritis
Rheumatoid arthritis
Acute and subacute bursitis
Acute gouty arthritis
Epicondylitis
Acute nonspecific tenosynovitis
Post-traumatic osteoarthritis

C. By intralesional injection in:
Keloids
Localized hypertrophic, infiltrated, inflammatory lesions of: lichen planus, psoriatic plaques, granuloma annulare, and lichen simplex chronicus (neurodermatitis)
Discoid lupus erythematosus
Necrobiosis lipoidica diabeticorum
Alopecia areata
May also be useful in cystic tumors of an aponeurosis or tendon (ganglia).

CONTRAINDICATIONS

Systemic fungal infections
Hypersensitivity to any component of this product, including sulfites (see WARNINGS).

WARNINGS

DO NOT INJECT INTRAVENOUSLY

Because rare instances of anaphylactoid reactions have occurred in patients receiving parenteral corticosteroid therapy, appropriate precautionary measures should be taken prior to administration, especially when the patient has a history of allergy to any drug. Anaphylactoid and hypersensitivity reactions have been reported for Sterile Suspension DECADRON-LA (see ADVERSE REACTIONS).

Sterile Suspension DECADRON-LA contains sodium bisulfite, a sulfite that may cause allergic-type reactions including anaphylactic symptoms and life-threatening or less severe asthmatic episodes in certain susceptible people. The overall prevalence of sulfite sensitivity in the general population is unknown and probably low. Sulfite sensitivity is seen more frequently in asthmatic than in nonasthmatic people.

In patients on corticosteroid therapy subjected to any unusual stress, increased dosage of rapidly acting corticosteroids before, during, and after the stressful situation is indicated.

Drug-induced secondary adrenocortical insufficiency may result from too rapid withdrawal of corticosteroids and may be minimized by gradual reduction of dosage. This type of relative insufficiency may persist for months after discontinuation of therapy; therefore, in any situation of stress occurring during that period, hormone therapy should be reinstituted. If the patient is receiving steroids already, dosage may have to be increased. Since mineralocorticoid secretion may be impaired, salt and/or a mineralocorticoid should be administered concurrently.

Corticosteroids may mask some signs of infection, and new infections may appear during their use. There may be decreased resistance and inability to localize infection when corticosteroids are used. Moreover, corticosteroids may affect the nitroblue-tetrazolium test for bacterial infection and produce false negative results.

In cerebral malaria, a double-blind trial has shown that the use of corticosteroids is associated with prolongation of coma and a higher incidence of pneumonia and gastrointestinal bleeding.

Corticosteroids may activate latent amebiasis. Therefore, it is recommended that latent or active amebiasis be ruled out before initiating corticosteroid therapy in any patient who has spent time in the tropics or any patient with unexplained diarrhea.

Prolonged use of corticosteroids may produce posterior subcapsular cataracts, glaucoma with possible damage to the optic nerves, and may enhance the establishment of secondary ocular infections due to fungi or viruses.

Usage in pregnancy. Since adequate human reproduction studies have not been done with corticosteroids, use of these drugs in pregnancy or in women of childbearing potential requires that the anticipated benefits be weighed against the possible hazards to the mother and embryo or fetus. Infants born of mothers who have received substantial doses of corticosteroids during pregnancy should be carefully observed for signs of hypoadrenalism.

Corticosteroids appear in breast milk and could suppress growth, interfere with endogenous corticosteroid production, or cause other unwanted effects. Mothers taking pharmacologic doses of corticosteroids should be advised not to nurse.

Average and large doses of cortisone or hydrocortisone can cause elevation of blood pressure, salt and water retention, and increased excretion of potassium. These effects are less likely to occur with the synthetic derivatives except when used in large doses. Dietary salt restriction and potassium supplementation may be necessary. All corticosteroids increase calcium excretion.

Administration of live virus vaccines, including smallpox, is contraindicated in individuals receiving immunosuppressive doses of corticosteroids. If inactivated viral or bacterial vaccines are administered to individuals receiving immunosuppressive doses of corticosteroids, the expected serum antibody response may not be obtained.

If corticosteroids are indicated in patients with latent tuberculosis or tuberculin reactivity, close observation is necessary as reactivation of the disease may occur. During prolonged corticosteroid therapy, these patients should receive chemoprophylaxis.

Repository adrenocorticosteroid preparations may cause atrophy at the site of injection. To minimize the likelihood and/or severity of atrophy, do not inject subcutaneously, avoid injection into the deltoid muscle, and avoid repeated intramuscular injections into the same site if possible.

Dosage in children under 12 has not been established.

Literature reports suggest an apparent association between use of corticosteroids and left ventricular free wall rupture after a recent myocardial infarction; therefore, therapy with corticosteroids should be used with great caution in these patients.

PRECAUTIONS

DECADRON-LA sterile suspension is not recommended as initial therapy in acute, life-threatening situations.

This product, like many other steroid formulations, is sensitive to heat. Therefore, it should not be autoclaved when it is desirable to sterilize the exterior of the vial.

Following prolonged therapy, withdrawal of corticosteroids may result in symptoms of the corticosteroid withdrawal syndrome including fever, myalgia, arthralgia, and malaise. This may occur in patients even without evidence of adrenal insufficiency.

There is an enhanced effect of corticosteroids in patients with hypothyroidism and in those with cirrhosis.

Corticosteroids should be used cautiously in patients with ocular herpes simplex for fear of corneal perforation.

Psychic derangements may appear when corticosteroids are used, ranging from euphoria, insomnia, mood swings, personality changes, and severe depression to frank psychotic manifestations. Also, existing emotional instability or psychotic tendencies may be aggravated by corticosteroids.

Aspirin should be used cautiously in conjunction with corticosteroids in hypoprothrombinemia.

Steroids should be used with caution in nonspecific ulcerative colitis, if there is a probability of impending perforation, abscess, or other pyogenic infection, also in diverticulitis, fresh intestinal anastomoses, active or latent peptic ulcer, renal insufficiency, hypertension, osteoporosis, and myasthenia gravis. Signs of peritoneal irritation following gastrointestinal perforation in patients receiving large doses of corticosteroids may be minimal or absent. Fat embolism has been reported as a possible complication of hypercortisonism.

When large doses are given, some authorities advise that antacids be administered between meals to help to prevent peptic ulcer.

Growth and development of infants and children on prolonged corticosteroid therapy should be carefully followed.

Steroids may increase or decrease motility and number of spermatozoa in some patients.

Phenytoin, phenobarbital, ephedrine, and rifampin may enhance the metabolic clearance of corticosteroids, resulting in decreased blood levels and lessened physiologic activity, thus requiring adjustment in corticosteroid dosage.

The prothrombin time should be checked frequently in patients who are receiving corticosteroids and coumarin anticoagulants at the same time because of reports that corticosteroids have altered the response to these anticoagulants. Studies have shown that the usual effect produced by adding corticosteroids is inhibition of response to coumarins, although there have been some conflicting reports of potentiation not substantiated by studies.

When corticosteroids are administered concomitantly with potassium-depleting diuretics, patients should be observed closely for development of hypokalemia.

Intra-articular injection of a corticosteroid may produce systemic as well as local effects.

Appropriate examination of any joint fluid present is necessary to exclude a septic process.

A marked increase in pain accompanied by local swelling, further restriction of joint motion, fever, and malaise is suggestive of septic arthritis. If this complication occurs and the diagnosis of sepsis is confirmed, appropriate antimicrobial therapy should be instituted.

Injection of a steroid into an infected site is to be avoided. Corticosteroids should not be injected into unstable joints.

Patients should be impressed strongly with the importance of not overusing joints in which symptomatic benefit has been obtained as long as the inflammatory process remains active.

Frequent intra-articular injection may result in damage to joint tissues.

ADVERSE REACTIONS

Fluid and electrolyte disturbances
Sodium retention
Fluid retention
Congestive heart failure in susceptible patients
Potassium loss
Hypokalemic alkalosis
Hypertension
Musculoskeletal
Muscle weakness
Steroid myopathy
Loss of muscle mass
Osteoporosis
Vertebral compression fractures
Aseptic necrosis of femoral and humeral heads
Pathologic fracture of long bones
Tendon rupture
Gastrointestinal
Peptic ulcer with possible subsequent perforation and hemorrhage
Perforation of the small and large bowel, particularly in patients with inflammatory bowel disease
Pancreatitis
Abdominal distention
Ulcerative esophagitis
Dermatologic
Impaired wound healing
Thin fragile skin
Petechiae and ecchymoses
Erythema
Increased sweating
May suppress reactions to skin tests
Other cutaneous reactions, such as allergic dermatitis, urticaria, angioneurotic edema

Neurologic
Convulsions
Increased intracranial pressure with papilledema (pseudotumor cerebri) usually after treatment
Vertigo
Headache
Psychic disturbances
Endocrine
Menstrual irregularities
Development of cushingoid state
Suppression of growth in children
Secondary adrenocortical and pituitary unresponsiveness, particularly in times of stress, as in trauma, surgery, or illness
Decreased carbohydrate tolerance
Manifestations of latent diabetes mellitus
Increased requirements for insulin or oral hypoglycemic agents in diabetics
Hirsutism
Ophthalmic
Posterior subcapsular cataracts
Increased intraocular pressure
Glaucoma
Exophthalmos
Metabolic
Negative nitrogen balance due to protein catabolism
Cardiovascular
Myocardial rupture following recent myocardial infarction (see WARNINGS).
Other
Anaphylactoid or hypersensitivity reactions
Thromboembolism
Weight gain
Increased appetite
Nausea
Malaise
The following *additional* adverse reactions are related to parenteral corticosteroid therapy:
Rare instances of blindness associated with intralesional therapy around the face and head
Hyperpigmentation or hypopigmentation
Subcutaneous and cutaneous atrophy
Sterile abscess
Postinjection flare (following intra-articular use)
Charcot-like arthropathy
Scarring
Induration
Inflammation
Paresthesia
Delayed pain or soreness
Muscle twitching, ataxia, hiccups, and nystagmus have been reported in low incidence after injection of DECADRON-LA sterile suspension.

OVERDOSAGE

Reports of acute toxicity and/or death following overdosage of glucocorticoids are rare. In the event of overdosage, no specific antidote is available; treatment is supportive and symptomatic.
The intraperitoneal LD_{50} of dexamethasone acetate in female mice was 424 mg/kg.

DOSAGE AND ADMINISTRATION

For intramuscular, intralesional, intra-articular, and soft tissue injection.
Dosage Requirements Are Variable and Must Be Individualized on the Basis of the Disease and the Response of the Patient.
Dosage in children under 12 has not been established.
Intramuscular Injection
Dosage ranges from 1 to 2 mL, equivalent to 8 to 16 mg of dexamethasone. If further treatment is needed, dosage may be repeated at intervals of 1 to 3 weeks.
Intralesional Injection
The usual dose is 0.1 to 0.2 mL, equivalent to 0.8 to 1.6 mg of dexamethasone, per injection site.
Intra-articular and Soft Tissue Injection
The dose varies, depending on the location and the severity of inflammation. The usual dose is 0.5 to 2 mL, equivalent to 4 to 16 mg of dexamethasone. If further treatment is needed, dosage may be repeated at intervals of 1 to 3 weeks. Frequent intra-articular injection may result in damage to joint tissues.

HOW SUPPLIED

No. 7644—Sterile Suspension DECADRON-LA, 8 mg dexamethasone equivalent per mL, is a sterile white suspension, and is supplied as follows:
NDC 0006-7644-01 in 1 mL vials
NDC 0006-7644-03 in 5 mL vials.

Storage
Sensitive to heat. Do not autoclave.
Protect from freezing.
A.H.F.S. Category: 68:04
DC 7350017 Issued March 1988

DECASPRAY® Topical Aerosol   ℞
(Dexamethasone, MSD), U.S.P.

DESCRIPTION

Topical Aerosol DECASPRAY® (Dexamethasone, MSD) is a topical steroid preparation, each 25 g of which contains 10 mg of dexamethasone. The topical corticosteroids constitute a class of primarily synthetic steroids used as anti-inflammatory and anti-pruritic agents.
Dexamethasone is 9-fluoro-11β, 17, 21-trihydroxy-16α-methylpregna-1, 4-diene-3, 20 dione. Its empirical formula is $C_{22}H_{29}FO_5$ and its structural formula is:

Dexamethasone has a molecular weight of 392.47.
The inactive ingredients are isopropyl myristate, and isobutane. Each second of spray dispenses approximately 0.075 mg of dexamethasone.

CLINICAL PHARMACOLOGY

Topical corticosteroids share anti-inflammatory, anti-pruritic, and vasoconstrictive actions.
The mechanism of anti-inflammatory activity of the topical corticosteroids is unclear. Various laboratory methods, including vasoconstrictor assays, are used to compare and predict potencies and/or clinical efficacies of the topical corticosteroids. There is some evidence to suggest that a recognizable correlation exists between vasoconstrictor potency and therapeutic efficacy in man.
Pharmacokinetics
The extent of percutaneous absorption of topical corticosteroids is determined by many factors including the vehicle, the integrity of the epidermal barrier, and the use of occlusive dressings.
Topical corticosteroids can be absorbed from normal intact skin. Inflammation and/or other disease processes in the skin increase percutaneous absorption. Occlusive dressings substantially increase the percutaneous absorption of topical corticosteroids. Thus, occlusive dressings may be a valuable therapeutic adjunct for treatment of resistant dermatoses. (See DOSAGE AND ADMINISTRATION.)
Once absorbed through the skin, topical corticosteroids are handled through pharmacokinetic pathways similar to systemically administered corticosteroids. Corticosteroids are bound to plasma proteins in varying degrees. Corticosteroids are metabolized primarily in the liver and are then excreted by the kidneys. Some of the topical corticosteroids and their metabolites are also excreted into the bile.

INDICATIONS AND USAGE

DECASPRAY Topical Aerosol is indicated for relief of the inflammatory and pruritic manifestations of corticosteroid-responsive dermatoses.

CONTRAINDICATIONS

Topical corticosteroids are contraindicated in those patients with a history of hypersensitivity to any of the components of the preparation.

WARNINGS

Avoid spraying in eyes or nose. Contents under pressure. Do not puncture or burn. Keep out of reach of children. Use only as directed. Intentional misuse by deliberately concentrating and inhaling the contents can be harmful or fatal.

PRECAUTIONS

General
Systemic absorption of topical corticosteroids has produced reversible hypothalamic-pituitary-adrenal (HPA) axis suppression, manifestations of Cushing's syndrome, hyperglycemia, and glycosuria in some patients.
Conditions which augment systemic absorption include the application of the more potent corticosteroids, use over large surface areas, prolonged use, and the addition of occlusive dressings.
Therefore, patients receiving a large dose of a potent topical corticosteroid applied to a large surface area or under an

occlusive dressing should be evaluated periodically for evidence of HPA axis suppression by using urinary free cortisol and ACTH stimulation tests. If HPA axis suppression is noted, an attempt should be made to withdraw the drug, to reduce the frequency of application, or to substitute a less potent corticosteroid.
Recovery of HPA axis function is generally prompt and complete upon discontinuation of the drug. Infrequently, signs and symptoms of corticosteroid withdrawal may occur, requiring supplemental systemic corticosteroids.
Children may absorb proportionally larger amounts of topical corticosteroids and thus be more susceptible to systemic toxicity (See PRECAUTIONS, *Pediatric Use*).
If irritation develops, topical corticosteroids should be discontinued and appropriate therapy instituted.
In the presence of dermatological infections, the use of an appropriate antifungal or antibacterial agent should be instituted. If a favorable response does not occur promptly, the corticosteroid should be discontinued until the infection has been adequately controlled.
The product is not for ophthalmic use. However, if applied to the eyelids or skin near the eyes, the drug may enter the eyes. In patients with a history of herpes simplex keratitis ocular exposure to corticosteroids may lead to a recurrence. Prolonged ocular exposure may cause steroid glaucoma.
A few individuals may be sensitive to one or more of the components of this product. If any reaction indicating sensitivity is observed, discontinue use.
Generally, occlusive dressings should not be used on weeping or exudative lesions.
If occlusive dressing therapy is used, inspect lesions between dressings for development of infection. If infection develops, the technique should be discontinued and appropriate antimicrobial therapy instituted.
When large areas of the body are covered with an occlusive dressing, thermal homeostasis may be impaired. If elevation of body temperature occurs, use of the occlusive dressing should be discontinued.
CAUTION: Flammable. Do not use around open flame or while smoking.
Information for the Patient
Patients using topical corticosteroids should receive the following information and instructions:
1. This medication is to be used as directed by the physician. It is for external use only. Avoid contact with the eyes.
2. Patients should be advised not to use this medication for any disorder other than that for which it was prescribed.
3. The treated skin area should not be bandaged or otherwise covered or wrapped so as to be occlusive unless directed by the physician.
4. Patients should report any signs of local adverse reactions, especially under occlusive dressing.
5. Parents of pediatric patients should be advised not to use tight-fitting diapers or plastic pants on a child being treated in the diaper area, as these garments may constitute occlusive dressings.
Laboratory Tests
The following tests may be helpful in evaluating the HPA axis suppression:
● Urinary free cortisol test
● ACTH stimulation test
Carcinogenesis, Mutagenesis, and
Impairment of Fertility
Long-term animal studies have not been performed to evaluate the carcinogenic potential or the effect on fertility of topical corticosteroids.
Studies to determine mutagenicity with prednisolone and hydrocortisone have revealed negative results.
Pregnancy
Pregnancy Category C: Corticosteroids are generally teratogenic in laboratory animals when administered systemically at relatively low dosage levels. The more potent corticosteroids have been shown to be teratogenic after dermal application in laboratory animals. There are no adequate and well-controlled studies in pregnant women on teratogenic effects from topically applied corticosteroids. Therefore, topical corticosteroids should be used during pregnancy only if the potential benefit justifies the potential risk to the fetus. Drugs of this class should not be used extensively on pregnant patients, in large amounts, or for prolonged periods of time.
Nursing Mothers
It is not known whether topical administration of corticosteroids could result in sufficient systemic absorption to produce detectable quantities in breast milk. Systemically administered corticosteroids are secreted into breast milk in quantities *not* likely to have a deleterious effect on the in-

Continued on next page

Merck Sharp & Dohme—Cont.

fant. Nevertheless, caution should be exercised when topical corticosteroids are administered to a nursing woman.

Pediatric Use

Pediatric patients may demonstrate greater susceptibility to topical corticosteroid-induced HPA axis suppression and Cushing's syndrome than mature patients because of a larger skin surface area to body weight ratio.

Hypothalamic-pituitary-adrenal (HPA) axis suppression, Cushing's syndrome, and intracranial hypertension have been reported in children receiving topical corticosteroids. Manifestations of adrenal suppression in children include linear growth retardation, delayed weight gain, low plasma cortisol levels, and absence of response to ACTH stimulation. Manifestations of intracranial hypertension include bulging fontanelles, headaches, and bilateral papilledema.

Administration of topical corticosteroids to children should be limited to the least amount compatible with an effective therapeutic regimen. Chronic corticosteroid therapy may interfere with the growth and development of children.

ADVERSE REACTIONS

The following adverse reactions are reported infrequently with topical corticosteroids, but may occur more frequently with the use of occlusive dressings. These reactions are listed in an approximate decreasing order of occurrence:

Burning
Itching
Irritation
Dryness
Folliculitis
Hypertrichosis
Acneiform eruptions
Hypopigmentation
Perioral dermatitis
Allergic contact dermatitis
Maceration of the skin
Secondary infection
Skin atrophy
Striae
Miliaria

OVERDOSAGE

Topically applied corticosteroids can be absorbed in sufficient amounts to produce systemic effects (See PRECAUTIONS).

DOSAGE AND ADMINISTRATION

Patients should be instructed in the correct way to use DECASPRAY. The preparation is readily applied, even on hairy areas. It does not have to be rubbed into the skin.

Optimal effects will be obtained with DECASPRAY when these directions are followed:

1. Keep the affected area clean to reduce the possibility of infection.
2. Shake the container *gently* once or twice each time before using. Hold it about six inches from the area to be treated. Effective medication may be obtained with the container held either upright or inverted, since it is fitted with a special valve that dispenses approximately the same dosage in either position.
3. Spray each four inch square of affected area for one or two seconds three or four times a day, depending on the nature of the condition and the response to therapy.
4. When a favorable response is obtained, reduce dosage gradually and eventually discontinue.
5. Occlusive dressings may be used for the management of psoriasis or recalcitrant conditions.

HOW SUPPLIED

No. 7623X—DECASPRAY is supplied as follows:
NDC 0006-7623-25 in a 25 g pressurized container.
A.H.F.S. Category: 84:06
DC 6005318   Issued April 1983
COPYRIGHT © MERCK & CO., INC., 1983
All rights reserved

DEMSER® Capsules   ℞
(Metyrosine, MSD), U.S.P.

DESCRIPTION

DEMSER® (Metyrosine, MSD) is (−)-α-methyl-*L*-tyrosine or (α-MPT). It has the following structural formula:
[See Chemical Formula at top of next column].

Metyrosine is a white, crystalline compound of molecular weight 195. It is very slightly soluble in water, acetone, and methanol, and insoluble in chloroform and benzene. It is

---

$$HO \text{---} \underset{\bullet}{\bigcirc} \text{---} CH_2 \text{---} \underset{NH_2}{\overset{CH_3}{\underset{|}{\overset{|}{C}}}} \text{---} COOH$$

soluble in acidic aqueous solutions. It is also soluble in alkaline aqueous solutions, but is subject to oxidative degradation under these conditions.

DEMSER is supplied as capsules, for oral administration. Each capsule contains 250 mg metyrosine. Inactive ingredients are colloidal silicon dioxide, gelatin, hydroxypropyl cellulose, magnesium stearate, and titanium dioxide. The capsules may also contain any combination of D&C Red 33, D&C Yellow 10, FD&C Blue 1, and FD&C Blue 2.

CLINICAL PHARMACOLOGY

DEMSER inhibits tyrosine hydroxylase, which catalyzes the first transformation in catecholamine biosynthesis, i.e., the conversion of tyrosine to dihydroxyphenylalanine (DOPA). Because the first step is also the rate-limiting step, blockade of tyrosine hydroxylase activity results in decreased endogenous levels of catecholamines, usually measured as decreased urinary excretion of catecholamines and their metabolites.

In patients with pheochromocytoma, who produce excessive amounts of norepinephrine and epinephrine, administration of one to four grams of DEMSER per day has reduced catecholamine biosynthesis from about 35 to 80 percent as measured by the total excretion of catecholamines and their metabolites (metanephrine and vanillylmandelic acid). The maximum biochemical effect usually occurs within two to three days, and the urinary concentration of catecholamines and their metabolites usually returns to pretreatment levels within three to four days after DEMSER is discontinued. In some patients the total excretion of catecholamines and catecholamine metabolites may be lowered to normal or near normal levels (less than 10 mg/24 hours). In most patients the duration of treatment has been two to eight weeks, but several patients have received DEMSER for periods of one to 10 years.

Most patients with pheochromocytoma treated with DEMSER experience decreased frequency and severity of hypertensive attacks with their associated headache, nausea, sweating, and tachycardia. In patients who respond, blood pressure decreases progressively during the first two days of therapy with DEMSER; after withdrawal, blood pressure usually increases gradually to pretreatment values within two to three days.

Metyrosine is well absorbed from the gastrointestinal tract. From 53 to 88 percent (mean 69 percent) was recovered in the urine as unchanged drug following maintenance oral doses of 600 to 4000 mg/24 hours in patients with pheochromocytoma or essential hypertension. Less than 1% of the dose was recovered as catechol metabolites. These metabolites are probably not present in sufficient amounts to contribute to the biochemical effects of metyrosine. The quantities excreted, however, are sufficient to interfere with accurate determination of urinary catecholamines determined by routine techniques.

Plasma half-life of metyrosine determined over an 8-hour period after single oral doses was 3.4–3.7 hours in three patients.

For further information, refer to: Sjoerdsma, A.; Engelman, K.; Waldman, T. A.; Cooperman, L. H.; Hammond, W. G.: Pheochromocytoma: Current concepts of diagnosis and treatment, Ann. Intern. Med. 65: 1302–1326, Dec. 1966.

INDICATIONS AND USAGE

DEMSER is indicated in the treatment of patients with pheochromocytoma for:
1. Preoperative preparation of patients for surgery
2. Management of patients when surgery is contraindicated
3. Chronic treatment of patients with malignant pheochromocytoma.

DEMSER is not recommended for the control of essential hypertension.

CONTRAINDICATIONS

DEMSER is contraindicated in persons known to be hypersensitive to this compound.

WARNINGS

Maintain Fluid Volume During and After Surgery

When DEMSER is used preoperatively, alone or especially in combination with alpha-adrenergic blocking drugs, adequate intravascular volume must be maintained intraoperatively (especially after tumor removal) and postoperatively to avoid hypotension and decreased perfusion of vital organs resulting from vasodilatation and expanded volume capacity. Following tumor removal, large volumes of plasma may be

---

needed to maintain blood pressure and central venous pressure within the normal range.

In addition, life-threatening arrhythmias may occur during anesthesia and surgery, and may require treatment with a beta blocker or lidocaine. During surgery, patients should have continuous monitoring of blood pressure and electrocardiogram.

Intraoperative Effects

While the preoperative use of DEMSER in patients with pheochromocytoma is thought to decrease intraoperative problems with blood pressure control, DEMSER does not eliminate the danger of hypertensive crises or arrhythmias during manipulation of the tumor, and the alpha-adrenergic blocking drug, phentolamine, may be needed.

Interaction with Alcohol

DEMSER may add to the sedative effects of alcohol and other CNS depressants, e.g., hypnotics, sedatives, and tranquilizers. (See PRECAUTIONS, *Information for Patients and Drug Interactions.*)

PRECAUTIONS

General

Metyrosine Crystalluria: Crystalluria and urolithiasis have been found in dogs treated with DEMSER (Metyrosine, MSD) at doses similar to those used in humans, and crystalluria has also been observed in a few patients. To minimize the risk of crystalluria, patients should be urged to maintain water intake sufficient to achieve a daily urine volume of 2000 mL or more, particularly when doses greater than 2 g per day are given. Routine examination of the urine should be carried out. Metyrosine will crystallize as needles or rods. If metyrosine crystalluria occurs, fluid intake should be increased further. If crystalluria persists, the dosage should be reduced or the drug discontinued.

Relatively Little Data Regarding Long-term Use: The total human experience with the drug is quite limited and few patients have been studied long-term. Chronic animal studies have not been carried out. Therefore, suitable laboratory tests should be carried out periodically in patients requiring prolonged use of DEMSER and caution should be observed in patients with impaired hepatic or renal function.

Information for Patients

When receiving DEMSER, patients should be warned about engaging in activities requiring mental alertness and motor coordination, such as driving a motor vehicle or operating machinery. DEMSER may have additive sedative effects with alcohol and other CNS depressants, e.g., hypnotics, sedatives, and tranquilizers.

Patients should be advised to maintain a liberal fluid intake. (See PRECAUTIONS, *General.*)

Drug Interactions

Caution should be observed in administering DEMSER to patients receiving phenothiazines or haloperidol because the extrapyramidal effects of these drugs can be expected to be potentiated by inhibition of catecholamine synthesis.

Concurrent use of DEMSER with alcohol or other CNS depressants can increase their sedative effects. (See WARNINGS and PRECAUTIONS, *Information for Patients.*)

Laboratory Test Interference

Spurious increases in urinary catecholamines may be observed in patients receiving DEMSER due to the presence of metabolites of the drug.

Carcinogenesis, Mutagenesis, Impairment of Fertility

Long-term carcinogenic studies in animals and studies on mutagenesis and impairment of fertility have not been performed with metyrosine.

Pregnancy

Pregnancy Category C. Animal reproduction studies have not been conducted with DEMSER. It is also not known whether DEMSER can cause fetal harm when administered to a pregnant woman or can affect reproduction capacity. DEMSER should be given to a pregnant woman only if clearly needed.

Nursing Mothers

It is not known whether DEMSER is excreted in human milk. Because many drugs are excreted in human milk, caution should be exercised when DEMSER is administered to a nursing woman.

Pediatric Use

Safety and effectiveness in children under 12 years of age have not been established.

ADVERSE REACTIONS

Central Nervous System

Sedation: The most common adverse reaction to DEMSER is moderate to severe sedation, which has been observed in almost all patients. It occurs at both low and high dosages. Sedative effects begin within the first 24 hours of therapy, are maximal after two to three days, and tend to wane during the next few days. Sedation usually is not obvious after one week unless the dosage is increased, but at dosages greater than 2000 mg/day some degree of sedation or fatigue may persist.

In most patients who experience sedation, temporary changes in sleep pattern occur following withdrawal of the drug. Changes consist of insomnia that may last for two or three days and feelings of increased alertness and ambition. Even patients who do not experience sedation while on DEMSER may report symptoms of psychic stimulation when the drug is discontinued.

Extrapyramidal Signs: Extrapyramidal signs such as drooling, speech difficulty, and tremor have been reported in approximately 10 percent of patients. These occasionally have been accompanied by trismus and frank parkinsonism.

Anxiety and Psychic Disturbances: Anxiety and psychic disturbances such as depression, hallucinations, disorientation, and confusion may occur. These effects seem to be dose-dependent and may disappear with reduction of dosage.

Diarrhea

Diarrhea occurs in about 10 percent of patients and may be severe. Anti-diarrheal agents may be required if continuation of DEMSER is necessary.

Miscellaneous

Infrequently, slight swelling of the breast, galactorrhea, nasal stuffiness, decreased salivation, dry mouth, headache, nausea, vomiting, abdominal pain, and impotence or failure of ejaculation may occur. Crystalluria (see PRECAUTIONS) and transient dysuria and hematuria have been observed in a few patients. Hematologic disorders (including eosinophilia, anemia, thrombocytopenia, and thrombocytosis), increased SGOT levels, peripheral edema, and hypersensitivity reactions such as urticaria and pharyngeal edema have been reported rarely.

OVERDOSAGE

Signs of metyrosine overdosage include those central nervous system effects observed in some patients even at low dosages.

At doses exceeding 2000 mg/day, some degree of sedation or feeling of fatigue may persist. Doses of 2000–4000 mg/day can result in anxiety or agitated depression, neuromuscular effects (including fine tremor of the hands, gross tremor of the trunk, tightening of the jaw with trismus), diarrhea, and decreased salivation with dry mouth.

Reduction of drug dose or cessation of treatment results in the disappearance of these symptoms.

The acute toxicity of metyrosine was 442 mg/kg and 752 mg/kg in the female mouse and rat respectively.

DOSAGE AND ADMINISTRATION

The recommended initial dosage of DEMSER for adults and children 12 years of age and older is 250 mg orally four times daily. This may be increased by 250 mg to 500 mg every day to a maximum of 4.0 g/day in divided doses. When used for preoperative preparation, the optimally effective dosage of DEMSER should be given for at least five to seven days. Optimally effective dosages of DEMSER usually are between 2.0 and 3.0 g/day, and the dose should be titrated by monitoring clinical symptoms and catecholamine excretion. In patients who are hypertensive, dosage should be titrated to achieve normalization of blood pressure and control of clinical symptoms. In patients who are usually normotensive, dosage should be titrated to the amount that will reduce urinary metanephrines and/or vanillylmandelic acid by 50 percent or more.

If patients are not adequately controlled by the use of DEMSER, an alpha-adrenergic blocking agent (phenoxybenzamine) should be added.

Use of DEMSER in children under 12 years of age has been limited and a dosage schedule for this age group cannot be given.

HOW SUPPLIED

No. 3355—Capsules DEMSER, 250 mg, are opaque, two-toned blue capsules coded MSD 690 on one side and DEMSER on the other. They are supplied as follows:
NDC 0006-0690-68 bottles of 100.

Shown in *Product Identification Section, page 418*
A.H.F.S. Category: 92:00
DC 7111505   Issued September 1985
COPYRIGHT© MERCK & CO., INC., 1985
All rights reserved

DIUPRES® Tablets   ℞
(Reserpine-Chlorothiazide, MSD), U.S.P.

WARNING

This fixed combination drug is not indicated for initial therapy of hypertension. Hypertension requires therapy titrated to the individual patient. If the fixed combination represents the dosage so determined, its use may be more convenient in patient management. The treatment of hypertension is not static, but must be re-evaluated as conditions in each patient warrant.

DESCRIPTION

DIUPRES® (Reserpine-Chlorothiazide, MSD) combines two antihypertensives: DIURIL® (Chlorothiazide, MSD) and reserpine.

Chlorothiazide

Chlorothiazide is a diuretic and antihypertensive. Its chemical name is 6-chloro-2*H*-1,2,4-benzothiadiazine-7-sulfonamide 1,1-dioxide. Its empirical formula is $C_7H_6ClN_3O_4S_2$ and its structural formula is:

Chlorothiazide is a white, or practically white, crystalline powder with a molecular weight of 295.72, which is very slightly soluble in water, but readily soluble in dilute aqueous sodium hydroxide. It is soluble in urine to the extent of about 150 mg per 100 mL at pH 7.

Reserpine

The chemical name of reserpine is 11,17α-dimethoxy-18β-[(3, 4, 5-trimethoxybenzoyl)oxy]-3β,   20α-yohimban- 16 β-carboxylic acid methylester. It is a crystalline alkaloid derived from Rauwolfia serpentina. Its empirical formula is $C_{33}H_{40}N_2O_9$ and its structural formula is:

Reserpine is a white or pale buff to slightly yellowish, odorless, crystalline powder with a molecular weight of 608.69, is insoluble in water and freely soluble in glacial acetic acid. DIUPRES is supplied as tablets in two strengths for oral use: DIUPRES-250, contains 250 mg of chlorothiazide and 0.125 mg of reserpine.

DIUPRES-500, contains 500 mg of chlorothiazide and 0.125 mg of reserpine.

Each tablet contains the following inactive ingredients: FD&C Red 3, gelatin, lactose, magnesium stearate, starch and talc.

CLINICAL PHARMACOLOGY

Chlorothiazide

The mechanism of the antihypertensive effect of thiazides is unknown. Chlorothiazide does not usually affect normal blood pressure.

Chlorothiazide affects the distal renal tubular mechanism of electrolyte reabsorption. At maximal therapeutic dosage all thiazides are approximately equal in their diuretic efficacy. Chlorothiazide increases excretion of sodium and chloride in approximately equivalent amounts. Natriuresis may be accompanied by some loss of potassium and bicarbonate.

After oral use diuresis begins within 2 hours, peaks in about 4 hours and lasts about 6 to 12 hours.

Reserpine

Reserpine has antihypertensive, bradycardic, and tranquilizing properties. It lowers arterial blood pressure by depletion of catecholamines. Reserpine is beneficial in relieving anxiety, tension, and headache in the hypertensive patient. It acts at the hypothalamic level of the central nervous system to promote relaxation without hypnosis or analgesia. The sleep pattern shown by the electroencephalogram following barbiturates does not occur with this drug. In laboratory animals spontaneous activity and response to external stimuli are decreased, but confusion or difficulty of movement is not evident.

The bradycardic action of reserpine promotes relaxation and may eliminate sinus tachycardia. It is most pronounced in subjects with sinus tachycardia and usually is not prominent in persons with a normal pulse rate.

Miosis, relaxation of the nictitating membrane, ptosis, hypothermia, and increased gastrointestinal activity are noted in animals given reserpine, sometimes in subclinical doses. None of these effects, except increased gastrointestinal activity, has been found to be clinically significant in man with therapeutic doses.

Pharmocokinetics and Metabolism

Chlorothiazide

Chlorothiazide is not metabolized but is eliminated rapidly by the kidney. The plasma half-life of chlorothiazide is 45–120 minutes. After oral doses, 20–24 percent is excreted unchanged in the urine. Chlorothiazide crosses the placental but not the blood-brain barrier and is excreted in breast milk.

Reserpine

Oral reserpine is rapidly absorbed from the gastrointestinal tract. Methylreserpate and trimethoxybenzoic acid are the primary metabolites which result from the hydrolytic cleavage of reserpine. Maximal blood levels are achieved approximately 2 hours after the oral dosage of ³H-reserpine to six normal volunteers; within 96 hours approximately 8 percent was excreted in urine and 62 percent in feces. Reserpine appears in human breast milk. Reserpine crosses the placental barrier in guinea pigs.

INDICATION AND USAGE

Hypertension (see box warning).

Use in Pregnancy. Routine use of diuretics during normal pregnancy is inappropriate and exposes mother and fetus to unnecessary hazard. Diuretics do not prevent development of toxemia of pregnancy and there is no satisfactory evidence that they are useful in the treatment of toxemia.

Edema during pregnancy may arise from pathologic causes or from the physiologic and mechanical consequences of pregnancy. Thiazides are indicated in pregnancy when edema is due to pathologic causes, just as they are in the absence of pregnancy (see PRECAUTIONS, *Pregnancy*). Dependent edema in pregnancy, resulting from restriction of venous return by the gravid uterus, is properly treated through elevation of the lower extremities and use of support stockings. Use of diuretics to lower intravascular volume in this instance is illogical and unnecessary. During normal pregnancy there is hypervolemia which is not harmful to the fetus or the mother in the absence of cardiovascular disease. However, it may be associated with edema, rarely generalized edema. If such edema causes discomfort, increased recumbency will often provide relief. Rarely this edema may cause extreme discomfort which is not relieved by rest. In these instances, a short course of diuretic therapy may provide relief and be appropriate.

CONTRAINDICATIONS

Chlorothiazide is contraindicated in anuria.

DIUPRES is contraindicated in hypersensitivity to chlorothiazide or other sulfonamide-derived drugs or to reserpine. Electroshock therapy should not be given to patients while on reserpine, as severe and even fatal reactions have been reported with minimal convulsive electroshock dosage. After discontinuing reserpine, allow at least seven days before starting electroshock therapy.

Active peptic ulcer, ulcerative colitis, and active mental depression, especially suicidal tendencies, are contraindications to reserpine therapy.

WARNINGS

Chlorothiazide

Use with caution in severe renal disease. In patients with renal disease, thiazides may precipitate azotemia. Cumulative effects of the drug may develop in patients with impaired renal function.

Thiazides should be used with caution in patients with impaired hepatic function or progressive liver disease, since minor alterations of fluid and electrolyte balance may precipitate hepatic coma.

Thiazides may add to or potentiate the action of other antihypertensive drugs.

Sensitivity reactions may occur in patients with or without a history of allergy or bronchial asthma.

The possibility of exacerbation or activation of systemic lupus erythematosus has been reported.

Lithium generally should not be given with diuretics (see PRECAUTIONS, *Drug Interactions*).

Reserpine

The occurrence of mental depression due to reserpine in doses of 0.25 mg daily or less is unusual. In any event, DIUPRES should be discontinued at the first sign of depression.

Continued on next page

Merck Sharp & Dohme—Cont.

PRECAUTIONS

General
Chlorothiazide

All patients receiving diuretic therapy should be observed for evidence of fluid or electrolyte imbalance: namely, hyponatremia, hypochloremic alkalosis, and hypokalemia. Serum and urine electrolyte determinations are particularly important when the patient is vomiting excessively or receiving parenteral fluids. Warning signs or symptoms of fluid and electrolyte imbalance, irrespective of cause, include dryness of mouth, thirst, weakness, lethargy, drowsiness, restlessness, muscle pains or cramps, muscular fatigue, hypotension, oliguria, tachycardia, and gastrointestinal disturbances such as nausea and vomiting.

Hypokalemia may develop, especially with brisk diuresis, when severe cirrhosis is present or after prolonged therapy. Interference with adequate oral electrolyte intake will contribute to hypokalemia. Hypokalemia may cause cardiac arrhythmia and may also sensitize or exaggerate the response of the heart to the toxic effects of digitalis (e.g., increased ventricular irritability). Hypokalemia may be avoided or treated by use of potassium sparing diuretics or potassium supplements such as foods with a high potassium content.

Although any chloride deficit is generally mild and usually does not require specific treatment except under extraordinary circumstances (as in liver disease or renal disease), chloride replacement may be required in the treatment of metabolic alkalosis.

Dilutional hyponatremia may occur in edematous patients in hot weather. Appropriate therapy is water restriction, rather than administration of salt, except in rare instances when the hyponatremia is life threatening. In actual salt depletion, appropriate replacement is the therapy of choice.

Hyperuricemia may occur or acute gout may be precipitated in certain patients receiving thiazides.

In diabetic patients dosage adjustments of insulin or oral hypoglycemic agents may be required. Hyperglycemia may occur with thiazide diuretics. Thus latent diabetes mellitus may become manifest during thiazide therapy.

The antihypertensive effect of the drug may be enhanced in the postsympathectomy patient.

If progressive renal impairment becomes evident, consider withholding or discontinuing diuretic therapy.

Thiazides have been shown to increase the urinary excretion of magnesium; this may result in hypomagnesemia.

Thiazides may decrease urinary calcium excretion. Thiazides may cause intermittent and slight elevation of serum calcium in the absence of known disorders of calcium metabolism. Marked hypercalcemia may be evidence of hidden hyperparathyroidism. Thiazides should be discontinued before carrying out tests for parathyroid function.

Increases in cholesterol and triglyceride levels may be associated with thiazide diuretic therapy.

Reserpine

Since reserpine may increase gastric secretion and motility, it should be used cautiously in patients with a history of peptic ulcer, ulcerative colitis, or other gastrointestinal disorder. This compound may precipitate biliary colic in patients with gallstones, or bronchial asthma in susceptible persons. Reserpine may cause hypotension including orthostatic hypotension.

Anxiety or depression, as well as psychosis, may develop during reserpine therapy. If depression is present when therapy is begun, it may be aggravated. Mental depression is unusual with reserpine doses of 0.25 mg daily or less. In any case, DIUPRES should be discontinued at the first sign of depression. Extreme caution should be used in treating patients with a history of mental depression, and the possibility of suicide should be kept in mind.

As with most antihypertensive therapy, caution should be exercised when treating hypertensive patients with renal insufficiency, since they adjust poorly to lowered blood pressure.

When two or more antihypertensives are given, the individual dosages may have to be reduced to prevent excessive drop in blood pressure. In hypertensive patients with coronary artery disease, it is important to avoid a precipitous drop in blood pressure.

Laboratory Tests

Periodic determination of serum electrolytes to detect possible electrolyte imbalance should be done at appropriate intervals.

Drug Interactions
Chlorothiazide

When given concurrently the following drugs may interact with thiazide diuretics.

Alcohol, barbiturates, or narcotics—potentiation of orthostatic hypotension may occur.

Antidiabetic drugs (oral agents and insulin)—dosage adjustment of the antidiabetic drug may be required.

Other antihypertensive drugs—additive effect or potentiation.

Corticosteroids, ACTH—intensified electrolyte depletion, particularly hypokalemia.

Pressor amines (e.g., norepinephrine)—possible decreased response to pressor amines but not sufficient to preclude their use.

Skeletal muscle relaxants, nondepolarizing (e.g., tubocurarine)—possible increased responsiveness to the muscle relaxant.

Lithium—generally should not be given with diuretics. Diuretic agents reduce the renal clearance of lithium and add a high risk of lithium toxicity. Refer to the package insert for lithium preparations before use of such preparations with DIUPRES.

Non-steroidal Anti-inflammatory Drugs—In some patients, the administration of a non-steroidal anti-inflammatory agent can reduce the diuretic, natriuretic, and antihypertensive effects of loop, potassium-sparing and thiazide diuretics. Therefore, when DIUPRES and non-steroidal anti-inflammatory agents are used concomitantly, the patient should be observed closely to determine if the desired effect of the diuretic is obtained.

Reserpine

In hypertensive patients on reserpine therapy significant hypotension and bradycardia may develop during surgical anesthesia. The anesthesiologist should be aware that reserpine has been taken, since it may be necessary to give vagal blocking agents parenterally to prevent or reverse hypotension and/or bradycardia.

Use reserpine cautiously with digitalis and quinidine; cardiac arrhythmias have occurred with reserpine preparations.

Barbiturates enhance the central nervous system depressant effects of reserpine.

Drug/Laboratory Test Interactions

Thiazides should be discontinued before carrying out tests for parathyroid function (see PRECAUTIONS, *General*).

Carcinogenesis, Mutagenesis,
Impairment of Fertility

Long-term carcinogenic or mutagenic studies have not been done with DIUPRES.

In a two-litter study in the rat at an oral dose of 50.0/0.25 mg/kg, the combination of chlorothiazide/reserpine did not impair fertility or produce abnormalities in the fetus.

Chlorothiazide

Carcinogenic studies have not been done with chlorothiazide.

Chlorothiazide was not mutagenic *in vitro*, in the Ames microbial mutagen test at a maximum concentration of 5 mg/plate using Strains TA98 and TA100. Chlorothiazide did not produce any significant mutagenicity in the dominant lethal assay in the mouse after 8 oral doses of 50 mg/kg or single intraperitoneal doses of 525 or 644 mg/kg, although early fetal deaths and preimplantation losses were increased beyond control values. In the test using *Aspergillus nidulans*, chlorothiazide was negative and did not induce disjunction. Chlorothiazide had no effect on fertility in a two-litter study in rats at doses up to 60 mg/kg/day (2 times the maximum recommended human dose).

Reserpine

Reserpine at a concentration of 1 to 5000 mcg/plate had no mutagenic activity against four strains of S. typhimurium *in vitro* in the Ames microbial mutagen test with or without metabolic activation. Reserpine did not induce malignant transformation of mouse fibroblasts *in vitro* at concentrations of 0.3 to 10 mcg/mL.

A few chromosomal aberrations were induced by reserpine *in vitro* in cultured mouse mammary carcinoma cells but were considered negative in this study. The drug did not produce chromosomal aberrations in human peripheral leucocyte cultures although an increase in mitotic figures occurred. One study reported chromosomal aberrations and dominant lethal mutations in mice at doses up to 10 mg/kg of reserpine in the form of a pharmaceutical preparation. Another study did not show dominant lethal mutations in mice at IP doses of 0.92 and 4.6 mg/kg of reserpine.

Reserpine did not impair fertility in a two-litter study in the rat at an oral dose of 0.25 mg/kg (35 times the maximum recommended human dose).

Rodent studies have shown that reserpine is an animal tumorigen, causing an increased incidence of mammary fibroadenomas in female mice, malignant tumors of the seminal vesicle in male mice, and malignant adrenal medullary tumors in male rats. These findings arose in two year studies in which the drug was administered in the feed at concentrations of 5 and 10 ppm—about 100 to 300 times the usual human dose. The breast neoplasms are thought to be related to reserpine's prolactin-elevating effect. Several other prolactin-elevating drugs have also been associated with an increased incidence of mammary neoplasia in rodents.

The extent to which these findings indicate a risk to humans is uncertain. Tissue culture experiments show that about one-third of human breast tumors are prolactin-dependent *in vitro*, a factor of considerable importance if the use of the drug is contemplated in a patient with previously detected breast cancer. The possibility of an increased risk of breast cancer in reserpine users has been studied extensively; however, no firm conclusion has emerged. Although a few epidemiologic studies have suggested a slightly increased risk (less than twofold in all studies except one) in women who have used reserpine, other studies of generally similar design have not confirmed this. Epidemiologic studies conducted using other drugs (neuroleptic agents) that, like reserpine, increase prolactin levels and therefore would be considered rodent mammary carcinogens, have not shown an association between chronic administration of the drug and human mammary tumorigenesis. While long-term clinical observation has not suggested such an association, the available evidence is considered too limited to be conclusive at this time. An association of reserpine intake with pheochromocytoma or tumors of the seminal vesicles has not been explored.

Pregnancy
Teratogenic Effects—Pregnancy Category C: There are no adequate and well-controlled studies in pregnant women. DIUPRES may cause fetal harm when given to a pregnant woman. DIUPRES should be used during pregnancy only if the potential benefit justifies the potential risk to the fetus. (See INDICATIONS AND USAGE.)

Reserpine: Reproduction studies in rats have shown that reserpine is teratogenic at doses of 1–2 mg/kg (125–250 times the maximum recommended human dose) IM or IP given early in pregnancy. A variety of abnormalities was produced including anophthalmia, absence of the axial skeleton, hydronephrosis, etc. Pregnancy in rabbits was interrupted when doses as low as 0.04 mg/kg (10 times the maximum recommended human dose) were given early or late in pregnancy.

Chlorothiazide: Thiazides cross the placental barrier and appear in cord blood.

Reproduction studies in the rabbit, the mouse and the rat at doses up to 500 mg/kg/day (25 times the maximum recommended human dose) showed no evidence of external abnormalities of the fetus due to chlorothiazide. Chlorothiazide given in a two-litter study in rats at doses up to 60 mg/kg/day (2 times the maximum recommended human dose) did not impair fertility or produce birth abnormalities in the offspring.

Nonteratogenic Effects

Reserpine: Reserpine has been demonstrated to cross the placental barrier in guinea pigs with depression of adrenal catecholamine stores in the newborn. There is some evidence that side effects such as nasal congestion, lethargy, depressed Moro reflex, and bradycardia may appear in infants born of reserpine-treated mothers.

Chlorothiazide: These may include fetal or neonatal jaundice, thrombocytopenia, and possibly other adverse reactions which have occurred in the adult.

Nursing Mothers

Thiazides and reserpine appear in breast milk. Because of the potential for serious adverse reactions in nursing infants from DIUPRES, a decision should be made whether to discontinue nursing or to discontinue the drug, taking into account the importance of the drug to the mother.

Pediatric Use

Safety and effectiveness of DIUPRES in children has not been established.

ADVERSE REACTIONS

The following adverse reactions have been reported and, within each category, are listed in order of decreasing severity.

Chlorothiazide

Body as a Whole: Weakness.

Cardiovascular: Hypotension including orthostatic hypotension (may be aggravated by alcohol, barbiturates, narcotics or antihypertensive drugs).

Digestive: Pancreatitis, jaundice (intrahepatic cholestatic jaundice), diarrhea, vomiting, sialadenitis, cramping, constipation, gastric irritation, nausea, anorexia.

Hematologic: Aplastic anemia, agranulocytosis, leukopenia, hemolytic anemia, thrombocytopenia.

Hypersensitivity: Anaphylactic reactions, necrotizing angiitis (vasculitis and cutaneous vasculitis), respiratory distress including pneumonitis and pulmonary edema, photosensitivity, fever, urticaria, rash, purpura.

Metabolic: Electrolyte imbalance (see PRECAUTIONS), hyperglycemia, glycosuria, hyperuricemia.

Musculoskeletal: Muscle spasm.

Nervous System/Psychiatric: Vertigo, paresthesias, dizziness, headache, restlessness.

Renal: Renal failure, renal dysfunction, interstitial nephritis. (See WARNINGS.)

Special Senses: Transient blurred vision, xanthopsia.

Whenever adverse reactions are moderate or severe, thiazide dosage should be reduced or therapy withdrawn.

Reserpine

Cardiovascular: Angina pectoris, arrhythmia, premature ventricular contractions, other direct cardiac effects (e.g., fluid retention, congestive heart failure), bradycardia.

Digestive: Vomiting, diarrhea, nausea, hypersecretion and increased motility, anorexia, dryness of mouth, increased salivation.
Hematologic: Thrombocytopenic purpura, excessive bleeding following prostatic surgery.
Hypersensitivity: Pruritis, rash, flushing of skin.
Metabolic: Weight gain.
Musculoskeletal: Muscular aches.
Nervous System/Psychiatric: Mental depression, dull sensorium, syncope, paradoxical anxiety, excessive sedation, nightmares, headache, dizziness, nervousness, parkinsonism (usually reversible with decreased dosage or discontinuance of therapy).
Respiratory: Dyspnea, epistaxis, nasal congestion, enhanced susceptibility to colds.
Special Senses: Optic atrophy, uveitis, deafness, glaucoma, conjunctival injection, blurred vision.
Urogenital: Dysuria, impotence, decreased libido, non-puerperal lactation.

OVERDOSAGE

Overdosage may lead to excessive sedation, mental depression, severe hypotension, extrapyramidal reactions.
There is no specific antidote. In the event of overdosage, symptomatic and supportive measures should be employed. Emesis should be induced or gastric lavage performed. Correct dehydration, electrolyte imbalance, hepatic coma and hypotension by established procedures. If required, give oxygen or artificial respiration for respiratory impairment. In the event of severe hypotension from the reserpine component, intravenous use of a vasopressor is indicated [e.g., ARAMINE® (Metaraminol Bitartrate, MSD), levarterenol, phenylephrine]. Anticholinergics may be needed to relieve gastrointestinal distress from reserpine. Because the effects of the rauwolfia alkaloids are prolonged, the patient should be closely observed for at least 72 hours.
The oral LD_{50} of chlorothiazide is 8.5 g/kg, greater than 10 g/kg, and greater than 1 g/kg, in the mouse, rat and dog, respectively. The oral LD_{50} of reserpine in the mouse is 390 mg/kg.

DOSAGE AND ADMINISTRATION

The initial dosage of DIUPRES should conform to the dosages of the individual components established during titration (see box warning).
The usual adult dosage of DIUPRES-250® is 1 or 2 tablets once or twice a day; that of DIUPRES-500® is 1 tablet once or twice a day. Dosage may require adjustment according to the blood pressure response of the patient.

HOW SUPPLIED

No. 3261—Tablets DIUPRES-250 are pink, round, scored, compressed tablets, coded MSD 230. Each tablet contains 250 mg of chlorothiazide and 0.125 mg of reserpine. They are supplied as follows:
NDC 0006-0230-68 in bottles of 100
NDC 0006-0230-82 in bottles of 1000
    Shown in Product Identification Section, page 418
No. 3262—Tablets DIUPRES-500 are pink, round, scored, compressed tablets, coded MSD 405. Each tablet contains 500 mg of chlorothiazide and 0.125 mg of reserpine. They are supplied as follows:
NDC 0006-0405-68 in bottles of 100
NDC 0006-0405-82 in bottles of 1000
    Shown in Product Identification Section, page 418
Storage
Keep container tightly closed. Protect from light.
    A.H.F.S. Category: 24:08
    DC 7398838 Issued October 1987
COPYRIGHT © MERCK & CO., INC., 1986
All rights reserved

DIURIL® Sodium Intravenous   ℞
(Chlorothiazide Sodium, MSD), U.S.P.

DESCRIPTION

Intravenous Sodium DIURIL® (Chlorothiazide Sodium, MSD) is a diuretic and antihypertensive. It is 6-chloro-2*H*-1,2,4-benzothiadiazine-7-sulfonamide 1,1-dioxide monosodium salt and its molecular weight is 317.70. Its empirical formula is $C_7H_5ClN_3NaO_4S_2$ and its structural formula is:

Intravenous Sodium DIURIL is a sterile lyophilized white powder and is supplied in a vial containing:

Chlorothiazide sodium equivalent
  to chlorothiazide ....0.5 g
Inactive ingredients:
  Mannitol ....0.25 g
Sodium hydroxide to adjust pH, with 0.4 mg thimerosal (mercury derivative) added as preservative.
DIURIL (Chlorothiazide, MSD) is a diuretic and antihypertensive. It is 6-chloro-2*H*-1,2,4-benzothiadiazine-7-sulfonamide 1,1-dioxide. Its empirical formula is $C_7H_6ClN_3N_3O_4S_2$ and its structural formula is:

It is a white, or practically white, crystalline powder with a molecular weight of 295.72, which is very slightly soluble in water, but readily soluble in dilute aqueous sodium hydroxide. It is soluble in urine to the extent of about 150 mg per 100 mL at pH 7.

CLINICAL PHARMACOLOGY

The mechanism of the antihypertensive effect of thiazides is unknown. DIURIL does not usually affect normal blood pressure.
DIURIL affects the distal renal tubular mechanism of electrolyte reabsorption. At maximal therapeutic dosage all thiazides are approximately equal in their diuretic efficacy. DIURIL increases excretion of sodium and chloride in approximately equivalent amounts. Natriuresis may be accompanied by some loss of potassium and bicarbonate.
After oral use diuresis begins within 2 hours, peaks in about 4 hours and lasts about 6 to 12 hours. Following intravenous use of Sodium DIURIL, onset of the diuretic action occurs in 15 minutes and the maximal action in 30 minutes.
Pharmacokinetics and Metabolism
DIURIL is not metabolized but is eliminated rapidly by the kidney; 96 percent of an intravenous dose is excreted unchanged in the urine within 23 hours. The plasma half-life of chlorothiazide is 45–120 minutes. Chlorothiazide crosses the placental but not the blood-brain barrier and is excreted in breast milk.

INDICATIONS AND USAGE

Intravenous Sodium DIURIL is indicated as adjunctive therapy in edema associated with congestive heart failure, hepatic cirrhosis, and corticosteroid and estrogen therapy.
Intravenous Sodium DIURIL has also been found useful in edema due to various forms of renal dysfunction such as nephrotic syndrome, acute glomerulonephritis, and chronic renal failure.
Use in Pregnancy. Routine use of diuretics during normal pregnancy is inappropriate and exposes mother and fetus to unnecessary hazard. Diuretics do not prevent development of toxemia of pregnancy and there is no satisfactory evidence that they are useful in the treatment of toxemia.
Edema during pregnancy may arise from pathologic causes or from the physiologic and mechanical consequences of pregnancy. Thiazides are indicated in pregnancy when edema is due to pathologic causes, just as they are in the absence of pregnancy (see PRECAUTIONS, *Pregnancy*). Dependent edema in pregnancy, resulting from restriction of venous return by the gravid uterus, is properly treated through elevation of the lower extremities and use of support stockings. Use of diuretics to lower intravascular volume in this instance is illogical and unnecessary. During normal pregnancy there is hypervolemia which is not harmful to the fetus or the mother in the absence of cardiovascular disease. However, it may be associated with edema, rarely generalized edema. If such edema causes discomfort, increased recumbency will often provide relief. Rarely this edema may cause extreme discomfort which is not relieved by rest. In these instances, a short course of diuretic therapy may provide relief and be appropriate.

CONTRAINDICATIONS

Anuria.
Hypersensitivity to any component of this product or to other sulfonamide-derived drugs.

WARNINGS

Intravenous use in infants and children has been limited and is not generally recommended.
Use with caution in severe renal disease. In patients with renal disease, thiazides may precipitate azotemia. Cumulative effects of the drug may develop in patients with impaired renal function.
Thiazides should be used with caution in patients with impaired hepatic function or progressive liver disease, since minor alterations of fluid and electrolyte balance may precipitate hepatic coma.
Thiazides may add to or potentiate the action of other antihypertensive drugs.
Sensitivity reactions may occur in patients with or without a history of allergy or bronchial asthma.
The possibility of exacerbation or activation of systemic lupus erythematosus has been reported.
Lithium generally should not be given with diuretics (see PRECAUTIONS, *Drug Interactions*).

PRECAUTIONS

General
All patients receiving diuretic therapy should be observed for evidence of fluid or electrolyte imbalance: namely, hyponatremia, hypochloremic alkalosis, and hypokalemia. Serum and urine electrolyte determinations are particularly important when the patient is vomiting excessively or receiving parenteral fluids. Warning signs or symptoms of fluid and electrolyte imbalance, irrespective of cause, include dryness of mouth, thirst, weakness, lethargy, drowsiness, restlessness, muscle pains or cramps, muscular fatigue, hypotension, oliguria, tachycardia, and gastrointestinal disturbances such as nausea and vomiting.
Hypokalemia may develop especially with brisk diuresis, when severe cirrhosis is present or after prolonged therapy. Interference with adequate oral electrolyte intake will also contribute to hypokalemia. Hypokalemia may cause cardiac arrhythmias and may also sensitize or exaggerate the response of the heart to the toxic effects of digitalis (e.g., increased ventricular irritability). Hypokalemia may be avoided or treated by use of potassium sparing diuretics or potassium supplements such as foods with a high potassium content.
Although any chloride deficit is generally mild and usually does not require specific treatment except under extraordinary circumstances (as in liver disease or renal disease), chloride replacement may be required in the treatment of metabolic alkalosis.
Dilutional hyponatremia may occur in edematous patients in hot weather; appropriate therapy is water restriction, rather than administration of salt, except in rare instances when the hyponatremia is life threatening. In actual salt depletion, appropriate replacement is the therapy of choice.
Hyperuricemia may occur or acute gout may be precipitated in certain patients receiving thiazides.
In diabetic patients dosage adjustments of insulin or oral hypoglycemic agents may be required. Hyperglycemia may occur with thiazide diuretics. Thus latent diabetes mellitus may become manifest during thiazide therapy.
The antihypertensive effects of the drug may be enhanced in the postsympathectomy patient.
If progressive renal impairment becomes evident, consider withholding or discontinuing diuretic therapy.
Thiazides have been shown to increase the urinary excretion of magnesium; this may result in hypomagnesemia.
Thiazides may decrease urinary calcium excretion. Thiazides may cause intermittent and slight elevation of serum calcium in the absence of known disorders of calcium metabolism. Marked hypercalcemia may be evidence of hidden hyperparathyroidism. Thiazides should be discontinued before carrying out tests for parathyroid function.
Increases in cholesterol and triglyceride levels may be associated with thiazide diuretic therapy.
Laboratory Tests
Periodic determination of serum electrolytes to detect possible electrolyte imbalance should be done at appropriate intervals.
Drug Interactions
When given concurrently the following drugs may interact with thiazide diuretics.
Alcohol, barbiturates, or narcotics —potentiation of orthostatic hypotension may occur.
Antidiabetic drugs —(oral agents and insulin)—dosage adjustment of the antidiabetic drug may be required.
Other antihypertensive drugs —additive effect or potentiation.
Corticosteroids, ACTH —intensified electrolyte depletion, particularly hypokalemia.
Pressor amines (e.g., norepinephrine) —possible decreased response to pressor amines but not sufficient to preclude their use.
Skeletal muscle relaxants, nondepolarizing (e.g., tubocurarine) —possible increased responsiveness to the muscle relaxant.
Lithium —generally should not be given with diuretics. Diuretic agents reduce the renal clearance of lithium and add a

Continued on next page

Merck Sharp & Dohme—Cont.

high risk of lithium toxicity. Refer to the package insert for lithium preparations before use of such preparations with Sodium DIURIL.

Non-steroidal Anti-inflammatory Drugs —In some patients, the administration of a non-steroidal anti-inflammatory agent can reduce the diuretic, natriuretic, and antihypertensive effects of loop, potassium-sparing and thiazide diuretics. Therefore, when Sodium DIURIL and non-steroidal anti-inflammatory agents are used concomitantly, the patient should be observed closely to determine if the desired effect of the diuretic is obtained.

Drug/Laboratory Test Interactions

Thiazides should be discontinued before carrying out tests for parathyroid function (see PRECAUTIONS, *General*).

Carcinogenesis, Mutagenesis, Impairment of Fertility

Carcinogenic studies have not been done with chlorothiazide.

Chlorothiazide was not mutagenic *in vitro*, in the Ames microbial mutagen test at a maximum concentration of 5 mg/plate using Strains TA98 and TA100. Chlorothiazide did not produce any significant mutagenicity in the dominant lethal assay in the mouse after 8 oral doses of 50 mg/kg or single intraperitoneal doses of 525 or 644 mg/kg, although early fetal deaths and preimplantation losses were increased beyond control values. In a test using *Aspergillus nidulans*, chlorothiazide was negative and did not induce disjunction. Chlorothiazide had no effect on fertility in a two-litter study in rats at doses up to 60 mg/kg/day (2 times the maximum recommended human dose).

Pregnancy

Teratogenic Effects —Pregnancy Category B: Reproduction studies in the rabbit, the mouse and the rat at doses up to 500 mg/kg/day (25 times the maximum recommended human dose) showed no evidence of external abnormalities of the fetus due to chlorothiazide.

Chlorothiazide given in a two-litter study in rats at doses up to 60 mg/kg/day (2 times the usual daily maximum recommended human dose) did not impair fertility or produce birth abnormalities in the offspring.

There are no adequate and well-controlled studies with Intravenous Sodium DIURIL in pregnant women; however, thiazides cross the placental barrier and appear in cord blood. Since animal reproduction studies are not always predictive of human response, Intravenous Sodium DIURIL should be used during pregnancy only if clearly needed. (See INDICATIONS AND USAGE.)

Nonteratogenic Effects: These may include fetal or neonatal jaundice, thrombocytopenia, and possibly other adverse reactions which have occurred in the adult.

Nursing Mothers

Because of the potential for serious adverse reactions in nursing infants from Intravenous Sodium DIURIL, a decision should be made whether to discontinue nursing or to discontinue the drug, taking into account the importance of the drug to the mother.

Pediatric Use

Safety and effectiveness of Intravenous Sodium DIURIL in children has not been established.

ADVERSE REACTIONS

The following adverse reactions have been reported and, within each category, are listed in order of decreasing severity.

Body as a Whole: Weakness.

Cardiovascular: Hypotension including orthostatic hypotension (may be aggravated by alcohol, barbiturates, narcotics or antihypertensive drugs).

Digestive: Pancreatitis, jaundice (intrahepatic cholestatic jaundice), diarrhea, vomiting, sialadenitis, cramping, constipation, gastric irritation, nausea, anorexia.

Hematologic: Aplastic anemia, agranulocytosis, leukopenia, hemolytic anemia, thrombocytopenia.

Hypersensitivity: Anaphylactic reactions, necrotizing angiitis (vasculitis and cutaneous vasculitis), respiratory distress including pneumonitis and pulmonary edema, photosensitivity, fever, urticaria, rash, purpura.

Metabolic: Electrolyte imbalance (see PRECAUTIONS), hyperglycemia, glycosuria, hyperuricemia.

Musculoskeletal: Muscle spasm.

Nervous System/Psychiatric: Vertigo, paresthesias, dizziness, headache, restlessness.

Special Senses: Transient blurred vision, xanthopsia.

Renal: Renal failure, renal dysfunction, interstitial nephritis (see WARNINGS); hematuria (following intravenous use). Whenever adverse reactions are moderate or severe, thiazide dosage should be reduced or therapy withdrawn.

OVERDOSAGE

The most common signs and symptoms observed are those caused by electrolyte depletion (hypokalemia, hypochlore-

mia, hyponatremia) and dehydration resulting from excessive diuresis. If digitalis has also been administered, hypokalemia may accentuate cardiac arrhythmias.

In the event of overdosage, symptomatic and supportive measures should be employed. Correct dehydration, electrolyte imbalance, hepatic coma and hypotension by established procedures. If required, give oxygen or artificial respiration for respiratory impairment.

The intravenous LD_{50} of chlorothiazide in the mouse is 1.1 g/kg.

DOSAGE AND ADMINISTRATION

Intravenous Sodium DIURIL should be reserved for patients unable to take oral medication or for emergency situations. Therapy should be individualized according to patient response. Use the smallest dosage necessary to achieve the required response.

Intravenous use in infants and children has been limited and is not generally recommended.

When medication can be taken orally, therapy with DIURIL tablets or oral suspension may be substituted for intravenous therapy, using the same dosage schedule as for the parenteral route.

Add 18 mL of Sterile Water for Injection to the vial to form an isotonic solution for intravenous injection. Never add less than 18 mL. Unused solution may be stored at room temperature for 24 hours, after which it must be discarded. Parenteral drug products should be inspected visually for particulate matter and discoloration prior to use whenever solution and container permit. The solution is compatible with dextrose or sodium chloride solutions for intravenous infusion. Avoid simultaneous administration of solutions of chlorothiazide with whole blood or its derivatives.

Extravasation must be rigidly avoided. Do not give subcutaneously or intramuscularly.

The usual adult dosage is 0.5 to 1.0 g once or twice a day. Many patients with edema respond to intermittent therapy, i.e., administration on alternate days or on three to five days each week. With an intermittent schedule, excessive response and the resulting undesirable electrolyte imbalance are less likely to occur.

HOW SUPPLIED

No. 3250—Intravenous Sodium DIURIL is a dry, sterile lyophilized white powder usually in plug form, supplied in vials containing chlorothiazide sodium equivalent to 0.5 g of chlorothiazide.

NDC 0006-3250-32.

Storage

Store reconstituted solution at room temperature and discard unused portion after 24 hours.

A.H.F.S. Category: 40:28

DC 7413527   Issued February 1988

DIURIL® Tablets   ℞
(Chlorothiazide, MSD), U.S.P.
DIURIL® Oral Suspension   ℞
(Chlorothiazide, MSD), U.S.P.

DESCRIPTION

DIURIL® (Chlorothiazide, MSD) is a diuretic and antihypertensive. It is 6-chloro-2*H* -1,2,4 -benzothiadiazine-7-sulfonamide 1,1-dioxide. Its empirical formula is $C_7H_6ClN_3O_4S_2$ and its structural formula is:

It is a white, or practically white, crystalline powder with a molecular weight of 295.72, which is very slightly soluble in water, but readily soluble in dilute aqueous sodium hydroxide. It is soluble in urine to the extent of about 150 mg per 100 mL at pH 7.

DIURIL is supplied as 250 mg and 500 mg tablets, for oral use. Each tablet contains the following inactive ingredients: gelatin, magnesium stearate, starch and talc. The 250 mg tablet also contains lactose.

Oral Suspension DIURIL contains 250 mg of chlorothiazide per 5 mL, alcohol 0.5 percent, with methylparaben 0.12 percent, propylparaben 0.02 percent, and benzoic acid 0.1 percent added as preservatives. The inactive ingredients are D&C Yellow 10, flavors, glycerin, purified water, sodium saccharin, sucrose and tragacanth.

CLINICAL PHARMACOLOGY

The mechanism of the antihypertensive effect of thiazides is unknown. DIURIL does not usually affect normal blood pressure.

DIURIL affects the distal renal tubular mechanism of electrolyte reabsorption. At maximal therapeutic dosage all thiazides are approximately equal in their diuretic efficacy. DIURIL increases excretion of sodium and chloride in approximately equivalent amounts. Natriuresis may be accompanied by some loss of potassium and bicarbonate.

After oral use diuresis begins within 2 hours, peaks in about 4 hours and lasts about 6 to 12 hours.

Pharmacokinetics and Metabolism

DIURIL is not metabolized but is eliminated rapidly by the kidney. The plasma half-life of chlorothiazide is 45–120 minutes. After oral doses, 20–24 percent of the dose is excreted unchanged in the urine. Chlorothiazide crosses the placental but not the blood-brain barrier and is excreted in breast milk.

INDICATIONS AND USAGE

DIURIL is indicated as adjunctive therapy in edema associated with congestive heart failure, hepatic cirrhosis, and corticosteroid and estrogen therapy.

DIURIL has also been found useful in edema due to various forms of renal dysfunction such as nephrotic syndrome, acute glomerulonephritis, and chronic renal failure.

DIURIL is indicated in the management of hypertension either as the sole therapeutic agent or to enhance the effectiveness of other antihypertensive drugs in the more severe forms of hypertension.

Use in Pregnancy. Routine use of diuretics during normal pregnancy is inappropriate and exposes mother and fetus to unnecessary hazard. Diuretics do not prevent development of toxemia of pregnancy and there is no satisfactory evidence that they are useful in the treatment of toxemia.

Edema during pregnancy may arise from pathologic causes or from the physiologic and mechanical consequences of pregnancy. Thiazides are indicated in pregnancy when edema is due to pathologic causes, just as they are in the absence of pregnancy (see PRECAUTIONS, *Pregnancy*). Dependent edema in pregnancy, resulting from restriction of venous return by the gravid uterus, is properly treated through elevation of the lower extremities and use of support stockings. Use of diuretics to lower intravascular volume in this instance is illogical and unnecessary. During normal pregnancy there is hypervolemia which is not harmful to the fetus or the mother in the absence of cardiovascular disease. However, it may be associated with edema, rarely generalized edema. If such edema causes discomfort, increased recumbency will often provide relief. Rarely this edema may cause extreme discomfort which is not relieved by rest. In these instances, a short course of diuretic therapy may provide relief and be appropriate.

CONTRAINDICATIONS

Anuria.

Hypersensitivity to this product or to other sulfonamide-derived drugs.

WARNINGS

Use with caution in severe renal disease. In patients with renal disease, thiazides may precipitate azotemia. Cumulative effects of the drug may develop in patients with impaired renal function.

Thiazides should be used with caution in patients with impaired hepatic function or progressive liver disease, since minor alterations of fluid and electrolyte balance may precipitate hepatic coma.

Thiazides may add to or potentiate the action of other antihypertensive drugs.

Sensitivity reactions may occur in patients with or without a history of allergy or bronchial asthma.

The possibility of exacerbation or activation of systemic lupus erythematosus has been reported.

Lithium generally should not be given with diuretics (see PRECAUTIONS, *Drug Interactions*).

PRECAUTIONS

General

All patients receiving diuretic therapy should be observed for evidence of fluid or electrolyte imbalance: namely, hyponatremia, hypochloremic alkalosis, and hypokalemia. Serum and urine electrolyte determinations are particularly important when the patient is vomiting excessively or receiving parenteral fluids. Warning signs or symptoms of fluid and electrolyte imbalance, irrespective of cause, include dryness of mouth, thirst, weakness, lethargy, drowsiness, restlessness, muscle pains or cramps, muscular fatigue, hypotension, oliguria, tachycardia, and gastrointestinal disturbances such as nausea and vomiting.

Hypokalemia may develop, especially with brisk diuresis, when severe cirrhosis is present or after prolonged therapy. Interference with adequate oral electrolyte intake will also contribute to hypokalemia. Hypokalemia may cause cardiac arrhythmias and may also sensitize or exaggerate the response of the heart to the toxic effects of digitalis (e.g., increased ventricular irritability). Hypokalemia may be avoided or treated by use of potassium sparing diuretics or potassium supplements such as foods with a high potassium content.

Although any chloride deficit is generally mild and usually does not require specific treatment except under extraordinary circumstances (as in liver disease or renal disease), chloride replacement may be required in the treatment of metabolic alkalosis.

Dilutional hyponatremia may occur in edematous patients in hot weather; appropriate therapy is water restriction, rather than administration of salt, except in rare instances when the hyponatremia is life threatening. In actual salt depletion, appropriate replacement is the therapy of choice.

Hyperuricemia may occur or acute gout may be precipitated in certain patients receiving thiazides.

In diabetic patients dosage adjustments of insulin or oral hypoglycemic agents may be required. Hyperglycemia may occur with thiazide diuretics. Thus latent diabetes mellitus may become manifest during thiazide therapy.

The antihypertensive effects of the drug may be enhanced in the post-sympathectomy patient.

If progressive renal impairment becomes evident, consider withholding or discontinuing diuretic therapy.

Thiazides have been shown to increase the urinary excretion of magnesium; this may result in hypomagnesemia.

Thiazides may decrease urinary calcium excretion. Thiazides may cause intermittent and slight elevation of serum calcium in the absence of known disorders of calcium metabolism. Marked hypercalcemia may be evidence of hidden hyperparathyroidism. Thiazides should be discontinued before carrying out tests for parathyroid function.

Increases in cholesterol and triglyceride levels may be associated with thiazide diuretic therapy.

Laboratory Tests
Periodic determination of serum electrolytes to detect possible electrolyte imbalance should be done at appropriate intervals.

Drug Interactions
When given concurrently the following drugs may interact with thiazide diuretics.

Alcohol, barbiturates, or narcotics—potentiation of orthostatic hypotension may occur.

Antidiabetic drugs (oral agents and insulin)—dosage adjustment of the antidiabetic drug may be required.

Other antihypertensive drugs—additive effect or potentiation.

Corticosteroids, ACTH—intensified electrolyte depletion, particularly hypokalemia.

Pressor amines (e.g., norepinephrine)—possible decreased response to pressor amines but not sufficient to preclude their use.

Skeletal muscle relaxants, nondepolarizing (e.g., tubocurarine)—possible increased responsiveness to the muscle relaxant.

Lithium—generally should not be given with diuretics. Diuretic agents reduce the renal clearance of lithium and add a high risk of lithium toxicity. Refer to the package insert for lithium preparations before use of such preparations with DIURIL.

Non-steroidal Anti-inflammatory Drugs—In some patients, the administration of a non-steroidal anti-inflammatory agent can reduce the diuretic, natriuretic, and antihypertensive effects of loop, potassium-sparing and thiazide diuretics. Therefore, when DIURIL and non-steroidal anti-inflammatory agents are used concomitantly, the patient should be observed closely to determine if the desired effect of the diuretic is obtained.

Drug/Laboratory Test Interactions
Thiazides should be discontinued before carrying out tests for parathyroid function (see PRECAUTIONS, *General*).

Carcinogenesis, Mutagenesis, Impairment of Fertility
Carcinogenic studies have not been done with chlorothiazide.

Chlorothiazide was not mutagenic *in vitro* in the Ames microbial mutagen test at a maximum concentration of 5 mg/plate using Strains TA98 and TA100. Chlorothiazide did not produce any significant mutagenicity in the dominant lethal assay in the mouse after 8 oral doses of 50 mg/kg or single intraperitoneal doses of 525 or 644 mg/kg, although early fetal deaths and preimplantation losses were increased beyond control values. In a test using *Aspergillus nidulans*, chlorothiazide was negative and did not induce disjunction. Chlorothiazide had no effect on fertility in a two-litter study in rat at doses up to 60 mg/kg/ day (2 times the maximum recommended human dose).

Pregnancy
Teratogenic Effects—Pregnancy Category B: Reproduction studies in the rabbit, the mouse and the rat at doses up to 500 mg/kg/day (25 times the maximum recommended human dose) showed no evidence of external abnormalities of the fetus due to chlorothiazide.

Chlorothiazide given in a two-litter study in rats at doses up to 60 mg/kg/day (2 times the maximum recommended human dose) did not impair fertility.

There are no adequate and well-controlled studies with DIURIL in pregnant women; however, thiazides cross the placental barrier and appear in cord blood. Since animal reproduction studies are not always predictive of human response, DIURIL should be used during pregnancy only if clearly needed. (See INDICATIONS AND USAGE.)

Nonteratogenic Effects: These may include fetal or neonatal jaundice, thrombocytopenia, and possibly other adverse reactions which have occurred in the adult.

Nursing Mothers
Because of the potential for serious adverse reactions in nursing infants from DIURIL, a decision should be made whether to discontinue nursing or to discontinue the drug, taking into account the importance of the drug to the mother.

ADVERSE REACTIONS

The following adverse reactions have been reported and, within each category, are listed in order of decreasing severity.

Body as a Whole: Weakness.
Cardiovascular: Hypotension including orthostatic hypotension (may be aggravated by alcohol, barbiturates, narcotics or antihypertensive drugs).
Digestive: Pancreatitis, jaundice (intrahepatic cholestatic jaundice), diarrhea, vomiting, sialadenitis, cramping, constipation, gastric irritation, nausea, anorexia.
Hematologic: Aplastic anemia, agranulocytosis, leukopenia, hemolytic anemia, thrombocytopenia.
Hypersensitivity: Anaphylactic reactions, necrotizing angiitis (vasculitis and cutaneous vasculitis), respiratory distress including pneumonitis and pulmonary edema, photosensitivity, fever, urticaria, rash, purpura.
Metabolic: Electrolyte imbalance (see PRECAUTIONS), hyperglycemia, glycosuria, hyperuricemia.
Musculoskeletal: Muscle spasm.
Nervous System/Psychiatric: Vertigo, paresthesias, dizziness, headache, restlessness.
Renal: Renal failure, renal dysfunction, interstitial nephritis. (See WARNINGS.)
Special Senses: Transient blurred vision, xanthopsia.
Whenever adverse reactions are moderate or severe, thiazide dosage should be reduced or therapy withdrawn.

OVERDOSAGE

The most common signs and symptoms observed are those caused by electrolyte depletion (hypokalemia, hypochloremia, hyponatremia) and dehydration resulting from excessive diuresis. If digitalis has also been administered, hypokalemia may accentuate cardiac arrhythmias.

In the event of overdosage, symptomatic and supportive measures should be employed. Emesis should be induced or gastric lavage performed. Correct dehydration, electrolyte imbalance, hepatic coma and hypotension by established procedures. If required, give oxygen or artificial respiration for respiratory impairment.

The oral LD_{50} of chlorothiazide is 8.5 g/kg, greater than 10 g/kg, and greater than 1 g/kg, in the mouse, rat and dog respectively.

DOSAGE AND ADMINISTRATION

Therapy should be individualized according to patient response. Use the smallest dosage necessary to achieve the required response.

Adults
For Diuresis
The usual adult dosage is 0.5 to 1.0 g once or twice a day. Many patients with edema respond to intermittent therapy, i.e., administration on alternate days or on three to five days each week. With an intermittent schedule, excessive response and the resulting undesirable electrolyte imbalance are less likely to occur.
For Control of Hypertension
The usual adult starting dosage is 0.5 or 1.0 g a day as a single or divided dose. Dosage is increased or decreased according to blood pressure response. Rarely some patients may require up to 2.0 g a day in divided doses.

Infants and Children
The usual oral pediatric dosage is based on 10 mg of DIURIL per pound of body weight per day in two doses. Infants under 6 months of age may require up to 15 mg per pound per day in two doses.

On this basis, infants up to 2 years of age may be given 125 to 375 mg daily in two doses (2.5 to 7.5 mL, or $\frac{1}{2}$ to $1\frac{1}{2}$ teaspoonfuls of the oral suspension daily). Children from 2 to 12 years of age may be given 375 mg to 1.0 g daily in two doses (7.5 to 20 mL, or $1\frac{1}{2}$ to 4 teaspoonfuls of oral suspension daily). Dosage in both age groups should be based on body weight.

HOW SUPPLIED

No. 3244—Tablets DIURIL, 250 mg, are white, round, scored, compressed tablets, coded MSD 214. They are supplied as follows:
NDC 0006-0214-68 bottles of 100.
NDC 0006-0214-82 bottles of 1000.
Shown in Product Identification Section, page 418
No. 3245—Tablets DIURIL, 500 mg, are white, round, scored, compressed tablets, coded MSD 432. They are supplied as follows:
NDC 0006-0432-68 bottles of 100.
NDC 0006-0432-28 unit dose packages of 100.
NDC 0006-0432-82 bottles of 1000.
NDC 0006-0432-86 bottles of 5000.
Shown in Product Identification Section, page 418
No. 3239—Oral Suspension DIURIL, 250 mg of chlorothiazide per 5 mL, is a yellow, creamy suspension, and is supplied as follows:
NDC 0006-3239-66 bottles of 237 mL.
Storage
Oral Suspension DIURIL must be protected from freezing.
     A.H.F.S. Category: 40:28
     DC 7398750   Issued October 1987

DOLOBID® Tablets   ℞
(Diflunisal, MSD), U.S.P.

DESCRIPTION

Diflunisal is 2', 4'-difluoro-4-hydroxy-3-biphenylcarboxylic acid. Its empirical formula is $C_{13}H_8F_2O_3$ and its structural formula is:

Diflunisal has a molecular weight of 250.20. It is a stable, white, crystalline compound with a melting point of 211–213°C. It is practically insoluble in water at neutral or acidic pH. Because it is an organic acid, it dissolves readily in dilute alkali to give a moderately stable solution at room temperature. It is soluble in most organic solvents including ethanol, methanol, and acetone.

DOLOBID® (Diflunisal, MSD) is available in 250 and 500 mg tablets for oral administration. Tablets DOLOBID contain the following inactive ingredients: cellulose, FD&C Yellow 6 hydroxypropyl cellulose, hydroxypropyl methylcellulose, magnesium stearate, starch, talc, and titanium dioxide.

CLINICAL PHARMACOLOGY

Action
DOLOBID is a non-steroidal drug with analgesic, anti-inflammatory and antipyretic properties. It is a peripherally-acting non-narcotic analgesic drug. Habituation, tolerance and addiction have not been reported.

Diflunisal is a difluorophenyl derivative of salicylic acid. Chemically, diflunisal differs from aspirin (acetylsalicylic acid) in two respects. The first of these two is the presence of a difluorophenyl substituent at carbon 1. The second difference is the removal of the 0-acetyl group from the carbon 4 position. Diflunisal is not metabolized to salicylic acid, and the fluorine atoms are not displaced from the difluorophenyl ring structure.

The precise mechanism of the analgesic and anti-inflammatory actions of diflunisal is not known. Diflunisal is a prostaglandin synthetase inhibitor. In animals, prostaglandins sensitize afferent nerves and potentiate the action of bradykinin in inducing pain. Since prostaglandins are known to be among the mediators of pain and inflammation, the mode of action of diflunisal may be due to a decrease of prostaglandins in peripheral tissues.

Pharmacokinetics and Metabolism
DOLOBID is rapidly and completely absorbed following oral administration with peak plasma concentrations occurring between 2 to 3 hours. The drug is excreted in the urine as two soluble glucuronide conjugates accounting for about 90% of

Continued on next page

Information on the Merck Sharp & Dohme products listed on these pages is the full prescribing information from product circulars in use August 31, 1989.

Merck Sharp & Dohme—Cont.

the administered dose. Little or no diflunisal is excreted in the feces. Diflunisal appears in human milk in concentrations of 2–7% of those in plasma. More than 99% of diflunisal in plasma is bound to proteins.

As is the case with salicylic acid, concentration-dependent pharmacokinetics prevail when DOLOBID is administered; a doubling of dosage produces a greater than doubling of drug accumulation. The effect becomes more apparent with repetitive doses. Following single doses, peak plasma concentrations of 41 ± 11 μg/mL (mean $\pm$ S.D.) were observed following 250 mg doses, 87 ± 17 μg/mL were observed following 500 mg and 124 ± 11 μg/mL following single 1000 mg doses. However, following administration of 250 mg b.i.d., a mean peak level of 56 ± 14 μg/mL was observed on day 8, while the mean peak level after 500 mg b.i.d. for 11 days was 190 ± 33 μg/mL. In contrast to salicylic acid which has a plasma half-life of $2\frac{1}{2}$ hours, the plasma half-life of diflunisal is 3 to 4 times longer (8 to 12 hours), because of a difluorophenyl substituent at carbon 1. Because of its long half-life and nonlinear pharmacokinetics, several days are required for diflunisal plasma levels to reach steady state following multiple doses. For this reason, an initial loading dose is necessary to shorten the time to reach steady state levels, and 2 to 3 days of observation are necessary for evaluating changes in treatment regimens if a loading dose is not used.

Studies in baboons to determine passage across the blood-brain barrier have shown that only small quantities of diflunisal, under normal or acidotic conditions are transported into the cerebrospinal fluid (CSF). The ratio of blood/CSF concentrations after intravenous doses of 50 mg/kg or oral doses of 100 mg/kg of diflunisal was 100:1. In contrast, oral doses of 500 mg/kg of aspirin resulted in a blood/CSF ratio of 5:1.

Mild to Moderate Pain
DOLOBID is a peripherally-acting analgesic agent with a long duration of action. DOLOBID produces significant analgesia within 1 hour and maximum analgesia within 2 to 3 hours.

Consistent with its long half-life, clinical effects of DOLOBID mirror its pharmacokinetic behavior, which is the basis for recommending a loading dose when instituting therapy. Patients treated with DOLOBID, on the first dose, tend to have a slower onset of pain relief when compared with drugs achieving comparable peak effects. However, DOLOBID produces longer-lasting responses than the comparative agents.

Comparative single dose clinical studies have established the analgesic efficacy of DOLOBID at various dose levels relative to other analgesics. Analgesic effect measurements were derived from hourly evaluations by patients during eight and twelve-hour postdosing observation periods. The following information may serve as a guide for prescribing DOLOBID.

DOLOBID 500 mg was comparable in analgesic efficacy to aspirin 650 mg, acetaminophen 600 mg or 650 mg, and acetaminophen 650 mg with propoxyphene napsylate 100 mg. Patients treated with DOLOBID had longer lasting responses than the patients treated with the comparative analgesics.

DOLOBID 1000 mg was comparable in analgesic efficacy to acetaminophen 600 mg with codeine 60 mg. Patients treated with DOLOBID had longer lasting responses than the patients who received acetaminophen with codeine.

A loading dose of 1000 mg provides faster onset of pain relief, shorter time to peak analgesic effect, and greater peak analgesic effect than an initial 500 mg dose.

In contrast to the comparative analgesics, a significantly greater proportion of patients treated with DOLOBID did not remedicate and continued to have a good analgesic effect eight to twelve hours after dosing. Seventy-five percent (75%) of patients treated with DOLOBID continued to have a good analgesic response at four hours. When patients having a good analgesic response at four hours were followed, 78% of these patients continued to have a good analgesic response at eight hours and 64% at twelve hours.

Chronic Anti-inflammatory Therapy in Osteoarthritis and Rheumatoid Arthritis
In the controlled, double-blind clinical trials in which DOLOBID (500 mg to 1000 mg a day) was compared with anti-inflammatory doses of aspirin (2–4 grams a day), patients treated with DOLOBID had a significantly lower incidence of tinnitus and of adverse effects involving the gastrointestinal system than patients treated with aspirin. (See also *Effect on Fecal Blood Loss*).

Osteoarthritis
The effectiveness of DOLOBID for the treatment of osteoarthritis was studied in patients with osteoarthritis of the hip and/or knee. The activity of DOLOBID was demonstrated by clinical improvement in the signs and symptoms of disease activity.

In a double-blind multicenter study of 12 weeks' duration in which dosages were adjusted according to patient response, DOLOBID, 500 or 750 mg daily, was shown to be comparable in effectiveness to aspirin, 2000 or 3000 mg daily. In open-label extensions of this study to 24 or 48 weeks, DOLOBID continued to show similar effectiveness and generally was well tolerated.

Rheumatoid Arthritis
In controlled clinical trials, the effectiveness of DOLOBID was established for both acute exacerbations and long-term management of rheumatoid arthritis. The activity of DOLOBID was demonstrated by clinical improvement in the signs and symptoms of disease activity.

In a double-blind multicenter study of 12 weeks' duration in which dosages were adjusted according to patient response, DOLOBID 500 or 750 mg daily was comparable in effectiveness to aspirin 2,600 or 3,900 mg daily. In open-label extensions of this study to 52 weeks, DOLOBID continued to be effective and was generally well tolerated.

DOLOBID 500, 750, or 1000 mg daily was compared with aspirin 2000, 3000, or 4000 mg daily in a multicenter study of 8 weeks' duration in which dosages were adjusted according to patient response. In this study, DOLOBID was comparable in efficacy to aspirin.

In a double-blind multicenter study of 12 weeks' duration in which dosages were adjusted according to patient needs, DOLOBID 500 or 750 mg daily and ibuprofen 1600 or 2400 mg daily were comparable in effectiveness and tolerability.

In a double-blind multicenter study of 12 weeks' duration, DOLOBID 750 mg daily was comparable in efficacy to naproxen 750 mg daily. The incidence of gastrointestinal adverse effects and tinnitus was comparable for both drugs. This study was extended to 48 weeks on an open-label basis. DOLOBID continued to be effective and generally well tolerated.

In patients with rheumatoid arthritis, DOLOBID and gold salts may be used in combination at their usual dosage levels. In clinical studies, DOLOBID added to the regimen of gold salts usually resulted in additional symptomatic relief but did not alter the course of the underlying disease.

Antipyretic Activity
DOLOBID is not recommended for use as an antipyretic agent. In single 250 mg, 500 mg, or 750 mg doses, DOLOBID produced measurable but not clinically useful decreases in temperature in patients with fever; however, the possibility that it may mask fever in some patients, particularly with chronic or high doses, should be considered.

Uricosuric Effect
In normal volunteers, an increase in the renal clearance of uric acid and a decrease in serum uric acid was observed when DOLOBID was administered at 500 mg or 750 mg daily in divided doses. Patients on long-term therapy taking DOLOBID at 500 mg to 1000 mg daily in divided doses showed a prompt and consistent reduction across studies in mean serum uric acid levels, which were lowered as much as 1.4 mg%. It is not known whether DOLOBID interferes with the activity of other uricosuric agents.

Effect on Platelet Function
As an inhibitor of prostaglandin synthetase, DOLOBID has a dose-related effect on platelet function and bleeding time. In normal volunteers, 250 mg b.i.d. for 8 days had no effect on platelet function, and 500 mg b.i.d., the usual recommended dose, had a slight effect. At 1000 mg b.i.d., which exceeds the maximum recommended dosage, however, DOLOBID inhibited platelet function. In contrast to aspirin, these effects of DOLOBID were reversible, because of the absence of the chemically labile and biologically reactive 0-acetyl group at the carbon 4 position. Bleeding time was not altered by a dose of 250 mg b.i.d., and was only slightly increased at 500 mg b.i.d. At 1000 mg b.i.d., a greater increase occurred, but was not statistically significantly different from the change in the placebo group.

Effect on Fecal Blood Loss
When DOLOBID was given to normal volunteers at the usual recommended dose of 500 mg twice daily, fecal blood loss was not significantly different from placebo. Aspirin at 1000 mg four times daily produced the expected increase in fecal blood loss. DOLOBID at 1000 mg twice daily (NOTE: exceeds the recommended dosage) caused a statistically significant increase in fecal blood loss, but this increase was only one-half as large as that associated with aspirin 1300 mg twice daily.

Effect on Blood Glucose
DOLOBID did not affect fasting blood sugar in diabetic patients who were receiving tolbutamide or placebo.

INDICATIONS AND USAGE

DOLOBID is indicated for acute or long-term use for symptomatic treatment of the following:

1. Mild to moderate pain
2. Osteoarthritis
3. Rheumatoid arthritis

CONTRAINDICATIONS

Patients who are hypersensitive to this product.
Patients in whom acute asthmatic attacks, urticaria, or rhinitis are precipitated by aspirin or other non-steroidal anti-inflammatory drugs.

WARNINGS

Peptic ulceration and gastrointestinal bleeding have been reported in patients receiving DOLOBID. Fatalities have occurred rarely. Gastrointestinal bleeding is associated with higher morbidity and mortality in patients acutely ill with other conditions, the elderly and patients with hemorrhagic disorders. In patients with active gastrointestinal bleeding or an active peptic ulcer, the physician must weigh the benefits of therapy with DOLOBID against possible hazards, institute an appropriate ulcer regimen, and carefully monitor the patient's progress. When DOLOBID is given to patients with a history of either upper or lower gastrointestinal tract disease, it should be given only after consulting the ADVERSE REACTIONS section and under close supervision.

Risk of GI Ulcerations, Bleeding and Perforation with NSAID Therapy
Serious gastrointestinal toxicity such as bleeding, ulceration, and perforation, can occur at any time, with or without warning symptoms, in patients treated chronically with NSAID therapy. Although minor upper gastrointestinal problems, such as dyspepsia, are common, usually developing early in therapy, physicians should remain alert for ulceration and bleeding in patients treated chronically with NSAIDs even in the absence of previous GI tract symptoms. In patients observed in clinical trials of several months to two years duration, symptomatic upper GI ulcers, gross bleeding or perforation appear to occur in approximately 1% of patients treated for 3–6 months, and in about 2–4% of patients treated for one year. Physicians should inform patients about the signs and/or symptoms of serious GI toxicity and what steps to take if they occur.

Studies to date have not identified any subset of patients not at risk of developing peptic ulceration and bleeding. Except for a prior history of serious GI events and other risk factors known to be associated with peptic ulcer disease, such as alcoholism, smoking, etc., no risk factors (e.g., age, sex) have been associated with increased risk. Elderly or debilitated patients seem to tolerate ulceration or bleeding less well than other individuals and most spontaneous reports of fatal GI events are in this population. Studies to date are inconclusive concerning the relative risk of various NSAIDs in causing such reactions. High doses of any NSAID probably carry a greater risk of these reactions, although controlled clinical trials showing this do not exist in most cases. In considering the use of relatively large doses (within the recommended dosage range), sufficient benefit should be anticipated to offset the potential increased risk of GI toxicity.

PRECAUTIONS

General
Because serious GI tract ulceration and bleeding can occur without warning symptoms, physicians should follow chronically treated patients for the signs and symptoms of ulceration and bleeding and should inform them of the importance of this follow-up (see WARNINGS, *Risk of GI Ulcerations, Bleeding and Perforation with NSAID Therapy*).

Although DOLOBID has less effect on platelet function and bleeding time than aspirin, at higher doses it is an inhibitor of platelet function; therefore, patients who may be adversely affected should be carefully observed when DOLOBID is administered (see CLINICAL PHARMACOLOGY).

Because of reports of adverse eye findings with agents of this class, it is recommended that patients who develop eye complaints during treatment with DOLOBID have ophthalmologic studies.

Peripheral edema has been observed in some patients taking DOLOBID. Therefore, as with other drugs in this class, DOLOBID should be used with caution in patients with compromised cardiac function, hypertension, or other conditions predisposing to fluid retention.

Acetylsalicylic acid has been associated with Reye syndrome. Because diflunisal is a derivative of salicylic acid, the possibility of its association with Reye syndrome cannot be excluded.

Hypersensitivity Syndrome
A potentially life-threatening, apparent hypersensitivity syndrome has been reported. This multisystem syndrome includes constitutional symptoms (fever, chills), and cutaneous findings (see ADVERSE REACTIONS, *Dermatologic*). It may also include involvement of major organs (changes in liver function, jaundice, leukopenia, thrombocytopenia,

eosinophilia, disseminated intravascular coagulation, renal impairment, including renal failure), and less specific findings (adenitis, arthralgia, myalgia, arthritis, malaise, anorexia, disorientation). If evidence of hypersensitivity occurs, therapy with DOLOBID should be discontinued.

Renal Effects
As with other non-steroidal anti-inflammatory drugs, long term administration of diflunisal to animals has resulted in renal papillary necrosis and other abnormal renal pathology. In humans, there have been reports of acute interstitial nephritis with hematuria and proteinuria and occasionally nephrotic syndrome.

A second form of renal toxicity has been seen in patients with prerenal and renal conditions leading to a reduction in renal blood flow or blood volume, where the renal prostaglandins have a supportive role in the maintenance of renal perfusion. In these patients administration of an NSAID may cause a dose dependent reduction in prostaglandin formation and may precipitate overt renal decompensation. Patients at greatest risk of this reaction are those with conditions such as renal or hepatic dysfunction, diabetes mellitus, advanced age, extracellular volume depletion from any cause, congestive heart failure, septicemia, pyelonephritis, or concomitant use of any nephrotoxic drug. DOLOBID or other NSAIDs should be given with caution and renal function should be monitored in any patient who may have reduced renal reserve. Discontinuation of NSAID therapy is typically followed by recovery to the pretreatment state.
Since DOLOBID is eliminated primarily by the kidneys, patients with significantly impaired renal function should be closely monitored; a lower daily dosage should be anticipated to avoid excessive drug accumulation.

Information for Patients
DOLOBID, like other drugs of its class, is not free of side effects. The side effects of these drugs can cause discomfort and, rarely, there are more serious side effects such as gastrointestinal bleeding, which may result in hospitalization and even fatal outcomes.
NSAIDs (Non-Steroidal Anti-Inflammatory Drugs) are often essential agents in the management of arthritis and have a major role in the treatment of pain, but they also may be commonly employed for conditions which are less serious. Physicians may wish to discuss with their patients the potential risks (see WARNINGS, PRECAUTIONS and ADVERSE REACTIONS) and likely benefits of NSAID treatment, particularly when the drugs are used for less serious conditions where treatment without NSAIDs may represent an acceptable alternative to both the patient and physician.

Laboratory Tests
Liver Function Tests: As with other non-steroidal anti-inflammatory drugs, borderline elevations of one or more liver tests may occur in up to 15% of patients. These abnormalities may progress, may remain essentially unchanged, or may be transient with continued therapy. The SGPT (ALT) test is probably the most sensitive indicator of liver dysfunction. Meaningful (3 times the upper limit of normal) elevations of SGPT or SGOT (AST) occurred in controlled clinical trials in less than 1% of patients. A patient with symptoms and/or signs suggesting liver dysfunction, or in whom an abnormal liver test has occurred, should be evaluated for evidence of the development of more severe hepatic reactions while on therapy with DOLOBID. Severe hepatic reactions, including jaundice, have been reported with DOLOBID as well as with other non-steroidal anti-inflammatory drugs. Although such reactions are rare, if abnormal liver tests persist or worsen, if clinical signs and symptoms consistent with liver disease develop, or if systemic manifestations occur (e.g., eosinophilia, rash, etc.), DOLOBID should be discontinued, since liver reactions can be fatal.

Drug Interactions
DOLOBID prolongs the prothrombin time in patients who are on oral anticoagulants. DOLOBID has not been shown to interact with tolbutamide. DOLOBID interacts with hydrochlorothiazide, furosemide, acetaminophen, aspirin, indomethacin, sulindac and naproxen (see below).
Oral Anticoagulants: In some normal volunteers, the concomitant administration of DOLOBID and warfarin, acenocoumarol, or phenprocoumon resulted in prolongation of prothrombin time. This may occur because diflunisal competitively displaces coumarins from protein binding sites. Accordingly, when DOLOBID is administered with oral anticoagulants, the prothrombin time should be closely monitored during and for several days after concomitant drug administration. Adjustment of dosage of oral anticoagulants may be required.
Tolbutamide: In diabetic patients receiving DOLOBID and tolbutamide, no significant effects were seen on tolbutamide plasma levels or fasting blood glucose.
Hydrochlorothiazide: In normal volunteers, concomitant administration of DOLOBID and hydrochlorothiazide resulted in significantly increased plasma levels of hydrochlorothiazide. DOLOBID decreased the hyperuricemic effect of hydrochlorothiazide.
Furosemide: In normal volunteers, the concomitant administration of DOLOBID and furosemide had no effect on the diuretic activity of furosemide. DOLOBID decreased the hyperuricemic effect of furosemide.
Antacids: Concomitant administration of antacids may reduce plasma levels of DOLOBID. This effect is small with occasional doses of antacids, but may be clinically significant when antacids are used on a continuous schedule.
Acetaminophen: In normal volunteers, concomitant administration of DOLOBID and acetaminophen resulted in an approximate 50% increase in plasma levels of acetaminophen. Acetaminophen had no effect on plasma levels of DOLOBID. Since acetaminophen in high doses has been associated with hepatotoxicity, concomitant administration of DOLOBID and acetaminophen should be used cautiously, with careful monitoring of patients.
Concomitant administration of DOLOBID and acetaminophen in dogs, but not in rats, at approximately 2 times the recommended maximum human therapeutic dose of each (40-52 mg/kg/day of DOLOBID/acetaminophen), resulted in greater gastrointestinal toxicity than when either drug was administered alone. The clinical significance of these findings has not been established.
Drug Interactions: Non-steroidal Anti-inflammatory Drugs
The administration of diflunisal to normal volunteers receiving indomethacin decreased the renal clearance and significantly increased the plasma levels of indomethacin. In some patients the combined use of indomethacin and DOLOBID has been associated with fatal gastrointestinal hemorrhage. Therefore, indomethacin and DOLOBID should not be used concomitantly.
Since no further clinical data are available about the safety and effectiveness of DOLOBID when used in combination with other non-steroidal anti-inflammatory drugs, no recommendation for their concomitant use can be made. The following information was obtained from studies in normal volunteers.
Aspirin: In normal volunteers, a small decrease in diflunisal levels was observed when multiple doses of DOLOBID and aspirin were administered concomitantly.
Sulindac: The concomitant administration of DOLOBID and sulindac in normal volunteers resulted in lowering of the plasma levels of the active sulindac sulfide metabolite by approximately one-third.
Naproxen: The concomitant administration of DOLOBID and naproxen in normal volunteers had no effect on the plasma levels of naproxen, but significantly decreased the urinary excretion of naproxen and its glucuronide metabolite. Naproxen had no effect on plasma levels of DOLOBID.
Carcinogenesis, Mutagenesis,
Impairment of Fertility
Diflunisal did not affect the type or incidence of neoplasia in a 105-week study in the rat given doses up to 40 mg/kg/day (equivalent to approximately 1.3 times the maximum recommended human dose), or in long-term carcinogenic studies in mice given diflunisal at doses up to 80 mg/kg/day (equivalent to approximately 2.7 times the maximum recommended human dose). It was concluded that there was no carcinogenic potential for DOLOBID.
Diflunisal passes the placental barrier to a minor degree in the rat. Diflunisal had no mutagenic activity after oral administration in the dominant lethal assay, in the Ames microbial mutagen test or in the V-79 Chinese hamster lung cell assay.
No evidence of impaired fertility was found in reproduction studies in rats at doses up to 50 mg/kg/day.
Pregnancy
Pregnancy Category C. A dose of 60 mg/kg/day of diflunisal (equivalent to two times the maximum human dose) was maternotoxic, embryotoxic, and teratogenic in rabbits. In three of six studies in rabbits, evidence of teratogenicity was observed at doses ranging from 40 to 50 mg/kg/day. Teratology studies in mice, at doses up to 45 mg/kg/day, and in rats at doses up to 100 mg/kg/day, revealed no harm to the fetus due to diflunisal. Aspirin and other salicylates have been shown to be teratogenic in a wide variety of species, including the rat and rabbit, at doses ranging from 50 to 400 mg/kg/day (approximately one to eight times the human dose). There are no adequate and well controlled studies with diflunisal in pregnant women. DOLOBID should be used during the first two trimesters of pregnancy only if the potential benefit justifies the potential risk to the fetus. Because of the known effect of drugs of this class on the human fetal cardiovascular system (closure of ductus arteriosus), use during the third trimester of pregnancy is not recommended.
In rats at a dose of one and one-half times the maximum human dose, there was an increase in the average length of gestation. Similar increases in the length of gestation have been observed with aspirin, indomethacin, and phenylbutazone, and may be related to inhibition of prostaglandin synthetase. Drugs of this class may cause dystocia and delayed parturition in pregnant animals.
Nursing Mothers
Diflunisal is excreted in human milk in concentrations of 2–7% of those in plasma. Because of the potential for serious adverse reactions in nursing infants from DOLOBID, a decision should be made whether to discontinue nursing or to discontinue the drug, taking into account the importance of the drug to the mother.
Pediatric Use
The adverse effects observed following diflunisal administration to neonatal animals appear to be species, age, and dose-dependent. At dose levels approximately 3 times the usual human therapeutic dose, both aspirin (200 to 400 mg/kg/day) and diflunisal (80 mg/kg/day) resulted in death, leukocytosis, weight loss, and bilateral cataracts in neonatal (4 to 5-day-old) beagle puppies after 2 to 10 doses. Administration of an 80 mg/kg/day dose of diflunisal to 25-day-old puppies resulted in lower mortality, and did not produce cataracts. In newborn rats, a 400 mg/kg/day dose of aspirin resulted in increased mortality and some cataracts, whereas the effects of diflunisal administration at doses up to 140 mg/kg/day were limited to a decrease in average body weight gain.
Safety and effectiveness in infants and children have not been established, and use of the drug in children below the age of 12 years is not recommended.

ADVERSE REACTIONS

The adverse reactions observed in controlled clinical trials encompass observations in 2,427 patients.
Listed below are the adverse reactions reported in the 1,314 of these patients who received treatment in studies of two weeks or longer. Five hundred thirteen patients were treated for at least 24 weeks, 255 patients were treated for at least 48 weeks, and 46 patients were treated for 96 weeks. In general, the adverse reactions listed below were 2 to 14 times less frequent in the 1,113 patients who received short-term treatment for mild to moderate pain.

Incidence Greater Than 1%

Gastrointestinal
The most frequent types of adverse reactions occurring with DOLOBID are gastrointestinal: these include nausea*, vomiting, dyspepsia*, gastrointestinal pain*, diarrhea*, constipation, and flatulence.
Psychiatric
Somnolence, insomnia.
Central Nervous System
Dizziness.
Special Senses
Tinnitus.
Dermatologic
Rash*.
Miscellaneous
Headache*, fatigue/tiredness.

Incidence Less Than 1 in 100

The following adverse reactions, occurring less frequently than 1 in 100, were reported in clinical trials or since the drug was marketed. The probability exists of a causal relationship between DOLOBID and these adverse reactions.
Dermatologic
Erythema multiforme, exfoliative dermatitis, Stevens-Johnson syndrome, toxic epidermal necrolysis, urticaria, pruritus, sweating, dry mucous membranes, stomatitis, photosensitivity.
Gastrointestinal
Peptic ulcer, gastrointestinal bleeding, anorexia, eructation, gastrointestinal perforation, gastritis.
Liver function abnormalities; jaundice, sometimes with fever; cholestasis; hepatitis.
Hematologic
Thrombocytopenia; agranulocytosis; hemolytic anemia.
Genitourinary
Dysuria; renal impairment, including renal failure; interstitial nephritis; hematuria; proteinuria.
Psychiatric
Nervousness, depression, hallucinations, confusion, disorientation.
Central Nervous System
Vertigo; light-headedness; paresthesias.
Special Senses
Transient visual disturbances including blurred vision.
Hypersensitivity Reactions
Acute anaphylactic reaction with bronchospasm; angioedema.
Hypersensitivity vasculitis.
Hypersensitivity syndrome (see PRECAUTIONS).
Miscellaneous
Asthenia, edema.

---

*Incidence between 3% and 9%. Those reactions occurring in 1% to 3% are not marked with an asterisk.

Continued on next page

Merck Sharp & Dohme—Cont.

Causal Relationship Unknown

Other reactions have been reported in clinical trials or since the drug was marketed, but occurred under circumstances where a causal relationship could not be established. However, in these rarely reported events, that possibility cannot be excluded. Therefore, these observations are listed to serve as alerting information to physicians.

Respiratory
Dyspnea.
Cardiovascular
Palpitation, syncope.
Musculoskeletal
Muscle cramps.
Genitourinary
Nephrotic syndrome.
Miscellaneous
Chest pain.

Potential Adverse Effects

In addition, a variety of adverse effects not observed with DOLOBID in clinical trials or in marketing experience, but reported with other non-steroidal analgesic/anti-inflammatory agents, should be considered potential adverse effects of DOLOBID.

OVERDOSAGE

Cases of overdosage have occurred and deaths have been reported. Most patients recovered without evidence of permanent sequelae. The most common signs and symptoms observed with overdosage were drowsiness, vomiting, nausea, diarrhea, hyperventilation, tachycardia, sweating, tinnitus, disorientation, stupor and coma. Diminished urine output and cardiorespiratory arrest have also been reported. The lowest dosage of DOLOBID at which a death has been reported was 15 grams without the presence of other drugs. In a mixed drug overdose, ingestion of 7.5 grams of DOLOBID resulted in death.

In the event of overdosage, the stomach should be emptied by inducing vomiting or by gastric lavage, and the patient carefully observed and given symptomatic and supportive treatment. Because of the high degree of protein binding, hemodialysis may not be effective.

DOSAGE AND ADMINISTRATION

Concentration-dependent pharmacokinetics prevail when DOLOBID is administered; a doubling of dosage produces a greater than doubling of drug accumulation. The effect becomes more apparent with repetitive doses.

For mild to moderate pain, an initial dose of 1000 mg followed by 500 mg every 12 hours is recommended for most patients. Following the initial dose, some patients may require 500 mg every 8 hours.

A lower dosage may be appropriate depending on such factors as pain severity, patient response, weight, or advanced age; for example, 500 mg initially, followed by 250 mg every 8–12 hours.

For osteoarthritis and rheumatoid arthritis, the suggested dosage range is 500 mg to 1000 mg daily in two divided doses. The dosage of DOLOBID may be increased or decreased according to patient response.

Maintenance doses higher than 1500 mg a day are not recommended.

DOLOBID may be administered with water, milk or meals. Tablets should be swallowed whole, not crushed or chewed.

HOW SUPPLIED

Tablets DOLOBID are capsule-shaped, film-coated tablets supplied as follows:

No. 3390—250 mg peach colored, coded MSD 675
NDC 0006-0675-28 unit dose package of 100
NDC 0006-0675-61 unit of use bottles of 60
(6505-01-164-0581, 250 mg 60's)

Shown in Product Identification Section, page 418

No. 3392—500 mg orange colored, coded MSD 697
NDC 0006-0697-28 unit dose package of 100
NDC 0006-0697-61 unit of use bottles of 60
(6505-01-144-9724, 500 mg 60's).

Shown in Product Identification Section, page 418

A.H.F.S. Category: 28:08
DC 7327724   Issued October 1988

EDECRIN® Tablets   ℞
(Ethacrynic Acid, MSD), U.S.P.
Intravenous
SODIUM EDECRIN®   ℞
(Ethacrynate Sodium, MSD), U.S.P.

EDECRIN® (Ethacrynic Acid, MSD) is a potent diuretic which, if given in excessive amounts, may lead to profound diuresis with water and electrolyte depletion. Therefore, careful medical supervision is required, and dose and dose schedule must be adjusted to the individual patient's needs (see DOSAGE AND ADMINISTRATION).

DESCRIPTION

Ethacrynic acid is an unsaturated ketone derivative of an aryloxyacetic acid. It is designated chemically as [2,3-dichloro-4-(2-methylene-1-oxobutyl)phenoxy] acetic acid, and has a molecular weight of 303.14. Ethacrynic acid is a white, or practically white, crystalline powder, very slightly soluble in water, but soluble in most organic solvents such as alcohols, chloroform, and benzene. Its empirical formula is $C_{13}H_{12}Cl_2O_4$ and its structural formula is:

Ethacrynate sodium, the sodium salt of ethacrynic acid, is soluble in water at 25°C to the extent of about 7 percent. Solutions of the sodium salt are relatively stable at about pH 7 at room temperature for short periods, but as the pH or temperature increases the solutions are less stable. The molecular weight of ethacrynate sodium is 325.12. Its empirical formula is $C_{13}H_{11}Cl_2NaO_4$ and its structural formula is:

EDECRIN is supplied as 25 mg and 50 mg tablets for oral use. Each tablet contains the following inactive ingredients: colloidal silicon dioxide, lactose, magnesium stearate, starch and talc. The 50 mg tablet also contains D&C Yellow 10, FD&C Blue 1 and FD&C Yellow 6. Intravenous SODIUM EDECRIN® (Ethacrynate Sodium, MSD) is a sterile freeze-dried powder and is supplied in a vial containing:

Ethacrynate sodium equivalent to ethacrynic
acid .... 50.0 mg
Inactive ingredients:
Mannitol .... 62.5 mg
with 0.1 mg thimerosal (mercury derivative) added as preservative.

CLINICAL PHARMACOLOGY

Pharmacokinetics and Metabolism

EDECRIN acts on the ascending limb of the loop of Henle and on the proximal and distal tubules. Urinary output is usually dose dependent and related to the magnitude of fluid accumulation. Water and electrolyte excretion may be increased several times over that observed with thiazide diuretics, since EDECRIN inhibits reabsorption of a much greater proportion of filtered sodium than most other diuretic agents. Therefore, EDECRIN is effective in many patients who have significant degrees of renal insufficiency (see WARNINGS concerning deafness). EDECRIN has little or no effect on glomerular filtration or on renal blood flow, except following pronounced reductions in plasma volume when associated with rapid diuresis.

The electrolyte excretion pattern of ethacrynic acid varies from that of the thiazides and mercurial diuretics. Initial sodium and chloride excretion is usually substantial and chloride loss exceeds that of sodium. With prolonged administration, chloride excretion declines, and potassium and hydrogen ion excretion may increase. EDECRIN is effective whether or not there is clinical acidosis or alkalosis.

Although EDECRIN, in carefully controlled studies in animals and experimental subjects, produces a more favorable sodium/potassium excretion ratio than the thiazides, in patients with increased diuresis excessive amounts of potassium may be excreted.

Onset of action is rapid, usually within 30 minutes after an oral dose of EDECRIN or within 5 minutes after an intravenous injection of SODIUM EDECRIN. After oral use, diuresis peaks in about 2 hours and lasts about 6 to 8 hours.

The sulfhydryl binding propensity of ethacrynic acid differs somewhat from that of the organomercurials. Its mode of action is not by carbonic anhydrase inhibition.

Ethacrynic acid does not cross the blood-brain barrier.

INDICATIONS AND USAGE

EDECRIN is indicated for treatment of edema when an agent with greater diuretic potential than those commonly employed is required.

1. Treatment of the edema associated with congestive heart failure, cirrhosis of the liver, and renal disease, including the nephrotic syndrome.
2. Short-term management of ascites due to malignancy, idiopathic edema, and lymphedema.
3. Short-term management of hospitalized pediatric patients, other than infants, with congenital heart disease or the nephrotic syndrome.
4. Intravenous SODIUM EDECRIN is indicated when a rapid onset of diuresis is desired, e.g., in acute pulmonary edema, or when gastrointestinal absorption is impaired or oral medication is not practicable.

CONTRAINDICATIONS

All diuretics, including ethacrynic acid, are contraindicated in anuria. If increasing electrolyte imbalance, azotemia, and/or oliguria occur during treatment of severe, progressive renal disease, the diuretic should be discontinued.

In a few patients this diuretic has produced severe, watery diarrhea. If this occurs, it should be discontinued and not used again.

Until further experience in infants is accumulated, therapy with oral and parenteral EDECRIN is contraindicated.

Hypersensitivity to any component of this product.

WARNINGS

The effects of EDECRIN on electrolytes are related to its renal pharmacologic activity and are dose dependent. The possibility of profound electrolyte and water loss may be avoided by weighing the patient throughout the treatment period, by careful adjustment of dosage, by initiating treatment with small doses, and by using the drug on an intermittent schedule when possible. When excessive diuresis occurs, the drug should be withdrawn until homeostasis is restored. When excessive electrolyte loss occurs, the dosage should be reduced or the drug temporarily withdrawn.

Initiation of diuretic therapy with EDECRIN in the cirrhotic patient with ascites is best carried out in the hospital. When maintenance therapy has been established, the individual can be satisfactorily followed as an outpatient.

EDECRIN should be given with caution to patients with advanced cirrhosis of the liver, particularly those with a history of previous episodes of electrolyte imbalance or hepatic encephalopathy. Like other diuretics it may precipitate hepatic coma and death.

Too vigorous a diuresis, as evidenced by rapid and excessive weight loss, may induce an acute hypotensive episode. In elderly cardiac patients, rapid contraction of plasma volume and the resultant hemoconcentration should be avoided to prevent the development of thromboembolic episodes, such as cerebral vascular thromboses and pulmonary emboli which may be fatal. Excessive loss of potassium in patients receiving digitalis glycosides may precipitate digitalis toxicity. Care should also be exercised in patients receiving potassium-depleting steroids.

A number of possibly drug-related deaths have occurred in critically ill patients refractory to other diuretics. These generally have fallen into two categories: (1) patients with severe myocardial disease who have been receiving digitalis and presumably developed acute hypokalemia with fatal arrhythmia; (2) patients with severely decompensated hepatic cirrhosis with ascites, with or without accompanying encephalopathy, who were in electrolyte imbalance and died because of intensification of the electrolyte defect.

Deafness, tinnitus, and vertigo with a sense of fullness in the ears have occurred, most frequently in patients with severe impairment of renal function. These symptoms have been associated most often with intravenous administration and with doses in excess of those recommended. The deafness has usually been reversible and of short duration (one to 24 hours). However, in some patients the hearing loss has been permanent. A number of these patients were also receiving drugs known to be ototoxic. EDECRIN may increase the ototoxic potential of other drugs (see PRECAUTIONS, subsection *Drug Interactions*).

Lithium generally should not be given with diuretics (see PRECAUTIONS, subsection *Drug Interactions*).

PRECAUTIONS

General

Weakness, muscle cramps, paresthesias, thirst, anorexia, and signs of hyponatremia, hypokalemia, and/or hypochloremic alkalosis may occur following vigorous or excessive diuresis and these may be accentuated by rigid salt restriction. Rarely tetany has been reported following vigorous diuresis. *During therapy with ethacrynic acid, liberalization of salt intake and supplementary potassium chloride are often necessary.*

When a metabolic alkalosis may be anticipated, e.g., in cirrhosis with ascites, the use of potassium chloride or a potassium-sparing agent before and during therapy with EDECRIN may mitigate or prevent the hypokalemia.

Loop diuretics have been shown to increase the urinary excretion of magnesium; this may result in hypomagnesemia. The safety and efficacy of ethacrynic acid in hypertension have not been established. However, the dosage of coadministered antihypertensive agents may require adjustment. Orthostatic hypotension may occur in patients receiving other antihypertensive agents when given ethacrynic acid. EDECRIN has little or no effect on glomerular filtration or on renal blood flow, except following pronounced reductions in plasma volume when associated with rapid diuresis. A transient increase in serum urea nitrogen may occur. Usually, this is readily reversible when the drug is discontinued. As with other diuretics used in the treatment of renal edema, hypoproteinemia may reduce responsiveness to ethacrynic acid and the use of salt-poor albumin should be considered. A number of drugs, including ethacrynic acid, have been shown to displace warfarin from plasma protein; a reduction in the usual anticoagulant dosage may be required in patients receiving both drugs.

EDECRIN may increase the risk of gastric hemorrhage associated with corticosteroid treatment.

Laboratory Tests

Frequent serum electrolyte, CO_2 and BUN determinations should be performed early in therapy and periodically thereafter during active diuresis. Any electrolyte abnormalities should be corrected or the drug temporarily withdrawn.

Increases in blood glucose and alterations in glucose tolerance tests have been observed in patients receiving EDECRIN.

Drug Interactions

Lithium generally should not be given with diuretics because they reduce its renal clearance and add a high risk of lithium toxicity. Read circulars for lithium preparations before use of such concomitant therapy.

EDECRIN may increase the ototoxic potential of other drugs such as aminoglycoside and some cephalosporin antibiotics. Their concurrent use should be avoided.

A number of drugs, including ethacrynic acid, have been shown to displace warfarin from plasma protein; a reduction in the usual anticoagulant dosage may be required in patients receiving both drugs.

In some patients, the administration of a non-steroidal anti-inflammatory agent can reduce the diuretic, natriuretic, and antihypertensive effects of loop, potassium-sparing and thiazide diuretics. Therefore, when EDECRIN and non-steroidal anti-inflammatory agents are used concomitantly, the patient should be observed closely to determine if the desired effect of the diuretic is obtained.

Carcinogenesis, Mutagenesis, Impairment of Fertility

There was no evidence of a tumorigenic effect in a 79-week oral chronic toxicity study in rats at doses up to 45 times the human dose.

Ethacrynic acid had no effect on fertility in a two-litter study in rats or a two-generation study in mice at 10 times the human dose.

Pregnancy

Pregnancy Category B: Reproduction studies in the mouse and rabbit at doses up to 50 times the human dose showed no evidence of external abnormalities of the fetus due to EDECRIN.

In a two-litter study in the dog and rat, oral doses of 5 or 20 mg/kg/day (2½ or 10 times the human dose), respectively, did not interfere with pregnancy or with growth and development of the pups. Although there was reduction in the mean body weights of the fetuses in a teratogenic study in the rat at a dose level of 100 mg/kg (50 times the human dose), there was no effect on mortality or postnatal development. Functional and morphologic abnormalities were not observed. There are, however, no adequate and well-controlled studies in pregnant women. Since animal reproduction studies are not always predictive of human response, EDECRIN should be used during pregnancy only if clearly needed.

Nursing Mothers

It is not known whether this drug is excreted in human milk. Because many drugs are excreted in human milk and because of the potential for serious adverse reactions in nursing infants from EDECRIN, a decision should be made whether to discontinue nursing or to discontinue the drug, taking into account the importance of the drug to the mother.

Pediatric Use

For information on oral use in pediatrics, other than infants, see INDICATIONS AND USAGE and DOSAGE AND ADMINISTRATION.

Safety and effectiveness in infants have not been established (see CONTRAINDICATIONS).

Safety and effectiveness of intravenous use in children have not been established (see DOSAGE AND ADMINISTRATION, *Intravenous Use*).

ADVERSE REACTIONS

Gastrointestinal

Anorexia, malaise, abdominal discomfort or pain, dysphagia, nausea, vomiting, and diarrhea have occurred. These are more frequent with large doses or after one to three months of continuous therapy. A few patients have had sudden onset of profuse, watery diarrhea. Discontinue EDECRIN if diarrhea is severe and do not give it again. Gastrointestinal bleeding has occurred in some patients. Rarely, acute pancreatitis has been reported.

Metabolic

Reversible hyperuricemia and acute gout have been reported. Acute symptomatic hypoglycemia with convulsions occurred in two uremic patients who received doses above those recommended. Hyperglycemia has been reported. Rarely, jaundice and abnormal liver function tests have been reported in seriously ill patients receiving multiple drug therapy, including EDECRIN.

Hematologic

Agranulocytosis or severe neutropenia has been reported in a few critically ill patients also receiving agents known to produce this effect. Thrombocytopenia has been reported rarely. Henoch-Schönlein purpura has been reported rarely in patients with rheumatic heart disease receiving multiple drug therapy, including EDECRIN.

Special Senses (See WARNINGS)

Deafness, tinnitus and vertigo with a sense of fullness in the ears, and blurred vision have occurred.

Central Nervous System

Headache, fatigue, apprehension, confusion.

Miscellaneous

Skin rash, fever, chills, hematuria.

SODIUM EDECRIN occasionally has caused local irritation and pain after intravenous use.

OVERDOSAGE

Overdosage may lead to excessive diuresis with electrolyte depletion and dehydration.

In the event of overdosage, symptomatic and supportive measures should be employed. Emesis should be induced or gastric lavage performed. Correct dehydration, electrolyte imbalance, hepatic coma, and hypotension by established procedures. If required, give oxygen or artificial respiration for respiratory impairment.

In the mouse, the oral LD_{50} of ethacrynic acid is 627 mg/kg and the intravenous LD_{50} of ethacrynate sodium is 175 mg/kg.

DOSAGE AND ADMINISTRATION

Dosage must be regulated carefully to prevent a more rapid or substantial loss of fluid or electrolyte than is indicated or necessary. The magnitude of diuresis and natriuresis is largely dependent on the degree of fluid accumulation present in the patient. Similarly, the extent of potassium excretion is determined in large measure by the presence and magnitude of aldosteronism.

Oral Use

EDECRIN is available for oral use as 25 mg and 50 mg tablets.

Dosage: To Initiate Diuresis

In Adults: The smallest dose required to produce gradual weight loss (about 1 to 2 pounds per day) is recommended. Onset of diuresis usually occurs at 50 to 100 mg for adults. After diuresis has been achieved, the minimally effective dose (usually from 50 to 200 mg daily) may be given on a continuous or intermittent dosage schedule. Dosage adjustments are usually in 25 to 50 mg increments to avoid derangement of water and electrolyte excretion.

The patient should be weighed under standard conditions before and during the institution of diuretic therapy with this compound. Small alterations in dose should effectively prevent a massive diuretic response. The following schedule may be helpful in determining the smallest effective dose.

    Day 1—50 mg (single dose) after a meal
    Day 2—50 mg twice daily after meals, if necessary
    Day 3—100 mg in the morning and 50 to 100 mg following the afternoon or evening meal, depending upon response to the morning dose

A few patients may require initial and maintenance doses as high as 200 mg twice daily. These higher doses, which should be achieved gradually, are most often required in patients with severe, refractory edema.

In children (excluding infants, see CONTRAINDICATIONS): The initial dose should be 25 mg. Careful stepwise increments in dosage of 25 mg should be made to achieve effective maintenance.

Maintenance Therapy

It is usually possible to reduce the dosage and frequency of administration once dry weight has been achieved.

EDECRIN (Ethacrynic Acid, MSD) may be given intermittently after an effective diuresis is obtained with the regimen outlined above. Dosage may be on an alternate daily schedule or more prolonged periods of diuretic therapy may be interspersed with rest periods. Such an intermittent dosage schedule allows time for correction of any electrolyte imbalance and may provide a more efficient diuretic response. The chloruretic effect of this agent may give rise to retention of bicarbonate and a metabolic alkalosis. This may be corrected by giving chloride (ammonium chloride or arginine chloride). Ammonium chloride should not be given to cirrhotic patients.

EDECRIN has additive effects when used with other diuretics. For example, a patient who is on maintenance dosage of an oral diuretic may require additional intermittent diuretic therapy, such as an organomercurial, for the maintenance of basal weight. The intermittent use of EDECRIN orally may eliminate the need for injections of organocurials. Small doses of EDECRIN may be added to existing diuretic regimens to maintain basal weight. This drug may potentiate the action of carbonic anhydrase inhibitors, with augmentation of natriuresis and kaliuresis. Therefore, when adding EDECRIN the initial dose and changes of dose should be in 25 mg increments, to avoid electrolyte depletion. Rarely, patients who failed to respond to ethacrynic acid have responded to older established agents.

While many patients do not require supplemental potassium, the use of potassium chloride or potassium-sparing agents, or both, during treatment with EDECRIN is advisable, especially in cirrhotic or nephrotic patients and in patients receiving digitalis.

Salt liberalization usually prevents the development of hyponatremia and hypochloremia. During treatment with EDECRIN, salt may be liberalized to a greater extent than with other diuretics. Cirrhotic patients, however, usually require at least moderate salt restriction concomitant with diuretic therapy.

Intravenous Use

Intravenous SODIUM EDECRIN is for intravenous use when oral intake is impractical or in urgent conditions, such as acute pulmonary edema.

The usual intravenous dose for the average sized adult is 50 mg, or 0.5 to 1.0 mg per kg of body weight. Usually only one dose has been necessary; occasionally a second dose at a new injection site, to avoid possible thrombophlebitis, may be required. A single intravenous dose not exceeding 100 mg has been used in critical situations.

Insufficient pediatric experience precludes recommendation for this age group.

To reconstitute the dry material, add 50 mL of 5 percent Dextrose Injection, or Sodium Chloride Injection to the vial. Occasionally, some 5 percent Dextrose Injection solutions may have a low pH (below 5). The resulting solution with such a diluent may be hazy or opalescent. Intravenous use of such a solution is not recommended. Inspect the vial containing Intravenous SODIUM EDECRIN for particulate matter and discoloration before use.

The solution may be given slowly through the tubing of a running infusion or by direct intravenous injection over a period of several minutes. Do not mix this solution with whole blood or its derivatives. Discard unused reconstituted solution after 24 hours.

SODIUM EDECRIN should not be given subcutaneously or intramuscularly because of local pain and irritation.

HOW SUPPLIED

No. 3321—Tablets EDECRIN, 25 mg, are white, capsule shaped, scored tablets, coded MSD 65. They are supplied as follows:

NDC 0006-0065-68 in bottles of 100.

    Shown in Product Identification Section, page 418

No. 3322—Tablets EDECRIN, 50 mg, are green, capsule shaped, scored tablets, coded MSD 90. They are supplied as follows:

NDC 0006-0090-68 in bottles of 100.

    Shown in Product Identification Section, page 418

No. 3330—Intravenous SODIUM EDECRIN is a dry white material either in a plug form or as a powder. It is supplied in vials containing ethacrynate sodium equivalent to 50 mg of ethacrynic acid, **NDC 0006-3330-50.**

Continued on next page

Information on the Merck Sharp & Dohme products listed on these pages is the full prescribing information from product circulars in use August 31, 1989.

Merck Sharp & Dohme—Cont.

A.H.F.S. Category: 40:28
DC 7413624   Issued October 1985
COPYRIGHT © MERCK & CO., INC., 1984
All rights reserved

ELAVIL® Tablets   ℞
(Amitriptyline HCl, MSD), U.S.P.
ELAVIL® Injection   ℞
(Amitriptyline HCl, MSD), U.S.P.

DESCRIPTION

Amitriptyline HCl is 3-(10,11-dihydro-5H-dibenzo [a,d] cycloheptene-5-ylidene)-N,N-dimethyl-1-propanamine hydrochloride. Its empirical formula is $C_{20}H_{23}N \cdot HCl$ and its structural formula is:

· HCl

$CHCH_2CH_2N(CH_3)_2$

Amitriptyline HCl, a dibenzocycloheptadiene derivative, has a molecular weight of 313.87. It is a white, odorless, crystalline compound which is freely soluble in water.
ELAVIL® (Amitriptyline HCl, MSD) is supplied as 10 mg, 25 mg, 50 mg, 75 mg, 100 mg, and 150 mg tablets and as a sterile solution for intramuscular use. Inactive ingredients of the tablets are calcium phosphate, cellulose, colloidal silicon dioxide, hydroxypropyl cellulose, hydroxypropyl methylcellulose, lactose, magnesium stearate, starch, stearic acid, talc, and titanium dioxide. Tablets ELAVIL 10 mg also contain FD&C Blue 1. Tablets ELAVIL 25 mg also contain D&C Yellow 10, FD&C Blue 1, and FD&C Yellow 6. Tablets ELAVIL 50 mg also contain D&C Yellow 10, FD&C Yellow 6 and iron oxide. Tablets ELAVIL 75 mg also contain FD&C Yellow 6. Tablets ELAVIL 100 mg also contain FD&C Blue 2 and FD&C Red 40. Tablets ELAVIL 150 mg also contain FD&C Blue 2 and FD&C Yellow 6. Each milliliter of the sterile solution contains:
Amitriptyline hydrochloride..10 mg
Dextrose..44 mg
Water for Injection, q.s...1 mL
Added as preservatives:
Methylparaben ....1.5 mg
Propylparaben ....0.2 mg

ACTIONS

ELAVIL is an antidepressant with sedative effects. Its mechanism of action in man is not known. It is not a monoamine oxidase inhibitor and it does not act primarily by stimulation of the central nervous system.
Amitriptyline inhibits the membrane pump mechanism responsible for uptake of norepinephrine and serotonin in adrenergic and serotonergic neurons. Pharmacologically this action may potentiate or prolong neuronal activity since reuptake of these biogenic amines is important physiologically in terminating transmitting activity. This interference with the reuptake of norepinephrine and/or serotonin is believed by some to underlie the antidepressant activity of amitriptyline.

INDICATIONS

For the relief of symptoms of depression. Endogenous depression is more likely to be alleviated than are other depressive states.

CONTRAINDICATIONS

ELAVIL is contraindicated in patients who have shown prior hypersensitivity to it.
It should not be given concomitantly with monoamine oxidase inhibitors. Hyperpyretic crises, severe convulsions, and deaths have occurred in patients receiving tricyclic antidepressant and monoamine oxidase inhibiting drugs simultaneously. When it is desired to replace a monoamine oxidase inhibitor with ELAVIL, a minimum of 14 days should be allowed to elapse after the former is discontinued. ELAVIL should then be initiated cautiously with gradual increase in dosage until optimum response is achieved.
This drug is not recommended for use during the acute recovery phase following myocardial infarction.

WARNINGS

ELAVIL may block the antihypertensive action of guanethidine or similarly acting compounds.

It should be used with caution in patients with a history of seizures and, because of its atropine-like action, in patients with a history of urinary retention, angle-closure glaucoma or increased intraocular pressure. In patients with angle-closure glaucoma, even average doses may precipitate an attack.
Patients with cardiovascular disorders should be watched closely. Tricyclic antidepressant drugs, including ELAVIL, particularly when given in high doses, have been reported to produce arrhythmias, sinus tachycardia, and prolongation of the conduction time. Myocardial infarction and stroke have been reported with drugs of this class.
Close supervision is required when ELAVIL is given to hyperthyroid patients or those receiving thyroid medication. ELAVIL may enhance the response to alcohol and the effects of barbiturates and other CNS depressants. In patients who may use alcohol excessively, it should be borne in mind that the potentiation may increase the danger inherent in any suicide attempt or overdosage. Delirium has been reported with concurrent administration of amitriptyline and disulfiram.
Usage in Pregnancy—Safe use of ELAVIL during pregnancy and lactation has not been established; therefore, in administering the drug to pregnant patients, nursing mothers, or women who may become pregnant, the possible benefits must be weighed against the possible hazards to mother and child.
Animal reproduction studies have been inconclusive and clinical experience has been limited.
Usage in Children—In view of the lack of experience with the use of this drug in children, it is not recommended at the present time for patients under 12 years of age.

PRECAUTIONS

Schizophrenic patients may develop increased symptoms of psychosis; patients with paranoid symptomatology may have an exaggeration of such symptoms. Depressed patients, particularly those with known manic-depressive illness, may experience a shift to mania or hypomania. In these circumstances the dose of amitriptyline may be reduced or a major tranquilizer such as perphenazine may be administered concurrently.
When ELAVIL is given with anticholinergic agents or sympathomimetic drugs, including epinephrine combined with local anesthetics, close supervision and careful adjustment of dosages are required.
Hyperpyrexia has been reported when ELAVIL is administered with anticholingeric agents or with neuroleptic drugs, particularly during hot weather.
Paralytic ileus may occur in patients taking tricyclic antidepressants in combination with anticholinergic-type drugs.
Cimetidine is reported to reduce hepatic metabolism of certain tricyclic antidepressants, thereby delaying elimination and increasing steady-state concentrations of these drugs. Clinically significant effects have been reported with the tricyclic antidepressants when used concomitantly with cimetidine. Increases in plasma levels of tricyclic antidepressants, and in the frequency and severity of side effects, particularly anticholinergic, have been reported when cimetidine was added to the drug regimen. Discontinuation of cimetidine in well-controlled patients receiving tricyclic antidepressants and cimetidine may decrease the plasma levels and efficacy of the antidepressants.
Caution is advised if patients receive large doses of ethchlorvynol concurrently. Transient delirium has been reported in patients who were treated with one gram of ethchlorvynol and 75-150 mg of ELAVIL.
The possibility of suicide in depressed patients remains until significant remission occurs. Potentially suicidal patients should not have access to large quantities of this drug. Prescriptions should be written for the smallest amount feasible.
Concurrent administration of ELAVIL and electroshock therapy may increase the hazards associated with such therapy. Such treatment should be limited to patients for whom it is essential.
When possible, the drug should be discontinued several days before elective surgery.
Both elevation and lowering of blood sugar levels have been reported.
ELAVIL should be used with caution in patients with impaired liver function.
Information for Patients
While on therapy with ELAVIL, patients should be advised as to the possible impairment of mental and/or physical abilities required for performance of hazardous tasks, such as operating machinery or driving a motor vehicle.

ADVERSE REACTIONS

Within each category the following adverse reactions are listed in order of decreasing severity. Included in the listing are a few adverse reactions which have not been reported with this specific drug. However, pharmacological similari-

ties among the tricyclic antidepressant drugs require that each of the reactions be considered when amitriptyline is administered.
Cardiovascular: Myocardial infarction; stroke; heart block; arrhythmias; hypotension, particularly orthostatic hypotension; hypertension; tachycardia; palpitation.
CNS and Neuromuscular: Coma; seizures; hallucinations; delusions; confusional states; disorientation; incoordination; ataxia; tremors; peripheral neuropathy; numbness, tingling, and paresthesias of the extremities; extrapyramidal symptoms; dysarthria; disturbed concentration; excitement; anxiety; insomnia; restlessness; nightmares; drowsiness; dizziness; weakness; fatigue; headache; syndrome of inappropriate ADH (antidiuretic hormone) secretion; tinnitus; alteration in EEG patterns.
Anticholinergic: Paralytic ileus; hyperpyrexia; urinary retention, dilatation of the urinary tract; constipation; blurred vision, disturbance of accommodation, increased intraocular pressure, mydriasis; dry mouth.
Allergic: Skin rash; urticaria; photosensitization; edema of face and tongue.
Hematologic: Bone marrow depression including agranulocytosis, leukopenia, thrombocytopenia; purpura; eosinophilia.
Gastrointestinal: Rarely hepatitis (including altered liver function and jaundice); nausea; epigastric distress; vomiting; anorexia; stomatitis; peculiar taste; diarrhea; parotid swelling; black tongue.
Endocrine: Testicular swelling and gynecomastia in the male; breast enlargement and galactorrhea in the female; increased or decreased libido; elevation and lowering of blood sugar levels.
Other: Alopecia; edema; weight gain or loss; urinary frequency; increased perspiration.
Withdrawal Symptoms: After prolonged administration, abrupt cessation of treatment may produce nausea, headache, and malaise. Gradual dosage reduction has been reported to produce, within two weeks, transient symptoms including irritability, restlessness, and dream and sleep disturbance. These symptoms are not indicative of addiction. Rare instances have been reported of mania or hypomania occurring within 2–7 days following cessation of chronic therapy with tricyclic antidepressants.

DOSAGE AND ADMINISTRATION

Oral Dosage
Dosage should be initiated at a low level and increased gradually, noting carefully the clinical response and any evidence of intolerance.
Initial Dosage for Adults—For outpatients 75 mg of amitriptyline HCl a day in divided doses usually is satisfactory. If necessary, this may be increased to a total of 150 mg per day. Increases are made preferably in the late afternoon and/or bedtime doses. A sedative effect may be apparent before the antidepressant effect is noted, but an adequate therapeutic effect may take as long as 30 days to develop.
An alternate method of initiating therapy in outpatients is to begin with 50 to 100 mg amitriptyline HCl at bedtime. This may be increased by 25 or 50 mg as necessary in the bedtime dose to a total of 150 mg per day.
Hospitalized patients may require 100 mg a day initially. This can be increased gradually to 200 mg a day if necessary. A small number of hospitalized patients may need as much as 300 mg a day.
Adolescent and Elderly Patients—In general, lower dosages are recommended for these patients. Ten mg 3 times a day with 20 mg at bedtime may be satisfactory in adolescent and elderly patients who do not tolerate higher dosages.
Maintenance—The usual maintenance dosage of amitriptyline HCl is 50 to 100 mg per day. In some patients 40 mg per day is sufficient. For maintenance therapy the total daily dosage may be given in a single dose preferably at bedtime. When satisfactory improvement has been reached, dosage should be reduced to the lowest amount that will maintain relief of symptoms. It is appropriate to continue maintenance therapy 3 months or longer to lessen the possibility of relapse.
Intramuscular Dosage
Initially, 20 to 30 mg (2 to 3 mL) four times a day.
When ELAVIL injection is administered intramuscularly, the effects may appear more rapidly than with oral administration.
When ELAVIL injection is used for initial therapy in patients unable or unwilling to take ELAVIL tablets, the tablets should replace the injection as soon as possible.
Usage in Children
In view of the lack of experience with the use of this drug in children, it is not recommended at the present time for patients under 12 years of age.
Plasma Levels
Because of the wide variation in the absorption and distribution of tricyclic antidepressants in body fluids, it is difficult to directly correlate plasma levels and therapeutic effect. However, determination of plasma levels may be useful in

identifying patients who appear to have toxic effects and may have excessively high levels, or those in whom lack of absorption or noncompliance is suspected. Adjustments in dosage should be made according to the patient's clinical response and not on the basis of plasma levels.*

OVERDOSAGE

Manifestations—High doses may cause temporary confusion, disturbed concentration, or transient visual hallucinations. Overdosage may cause drowsiness; hypothermia; tachycardia and other arrhythmic abnormalities, such as bundle branch block; ECG evidence of impaired conduction; congestive heart failure; dilated pupils; disorders of ocular motility; convulsions; severe hypotension; stupor; and coma. Other symptoms may be agitation, hyperactive reflexes, muscle rigidity, vomiting, hyperpyrexia, or any of those listed under ADVERSE REACTIONS.

All patients suspected of having taken an overdosage should be admitted to a hospital as soon as possible. *Treatment* is symptomatic and supportive. Empty the stomach as quickly as possible by emesis followed by gastric lavage upon arrival at the hospital. Following gastric lavage, activated charcoal may be administered. Twenty to 30 g of activated charcoal may be given every four to six hours during the first 24 to 48 hours after ingestion. An ECG should be taken and close monitoring of cardiac function instituted if there is any sign of abnormality. Maintain an open airway and adequate fluid intake; regulate body temperature.

The intravenous administration of 1–3 mg of physostigmine salicylate is reported to reverse the symptoms of tricyclic antidepressant poisoning. Because physostigmine is rapidly metabolized, the dosage of physostigmine should be repeated as required particularly if life threatening signs such as arrhythmias, convulsions, and deep coma recur or persist after the initial dosage of physostigmine. Because physostigmine itself may be toxic, it is not recommended for routine use. Standard measures should be used to manage circulatory shock and metabolic acidosis. Cardiac arrhythmias may be treated with neostigmine, pyridostigmine, or propranolol. Should cardiac failure occur, the use of digitalis should be considered. Close monitoring of cardiac function for not less than five days is advisable.

Anticonvulsants may be given to control convulsions. Amitriptyline increases the CNS depressant action but not the anticonvulsant action of barbiturates; therefore, an inhalation anesthetic, diazepam, or paraldehyde is recommended for control of convulsions.

Dialysis is of no value because of low plasma concentrations of the drug.

Since overdosage is often deliberate, patients may attempt suicide by other means during the recovery phase.

Deaths by deliberate or accidental overdosage have occurred with this class of drugs.

HOW SUPPLIED

No. 3287—Tablets ELAVIL, 10 mg, are blue, round, film coated tablets, coded MSD 23. They are supplied as follows:
NDC 0006-0023-68 bottles of 100
(6505-00-079-7453, 10 mg 100's)
NDC 0006-0023-28 unit dose packages of 100
NDC 0006-0023-82 bottles of 1000.
Shown in Product Identification Section, page 418
No. 3288—Tablets ELAVIL, 25 mg, are yellow, round, film coated tablets, coded MSD 45. They are supplied as follows:
NDC 0006-0045-68 bottles of 100
(6505-00-082-2659, 25 mg 100's)
NDC 0006-0045-28 unit dose packages of 100
(6505-00-118-2509, 25 mg individually sealed 100's)
NDC 0006-0045-82 bottles of 1000
(6505-00-724-6358, 25 mg 1000's)
NDC 0006-0045-86 bottles of 5000.
Shown in Product Identification Section, page 418
No. 3320—Tablets ELAVIL, 50 mg, are beige, round, film coated tablets, coded MSD 102. They are supplied as follows:
NDC 0006-0102-68 bottles of 100
NDC 0006-0102-28 unit dose packages of 100
NDC 0006-0102-82 bottles of 1000.
Shown in Product Identification Section, page 418
No. 3348—Tablets ELAVIL, 75 mg, are orange, round, film coated tablets, coded MSD 430. They are supplied as follows:
NDC 0006-0430-68 bottles of 100
NDC 0006-0430-28 unit dose packages of 100.
Shown in Product Identification Section, page 418
No. 3349—Tablets ELAVIL, 100 mg, are mauve, round, film

*Hollister, L. E., J. Amer. Med. Ass. *241*: 2530–2533, June 8, 1979.

coated tablets, coded MSD 435. They are supplied as follows:
NDC 0006-0435-68 bottles of 100
NDC 0006-0435-28 unit dose packages of 100.
Shown in Product Identification Section, page 418
No. 3351—Tablets ELAVIL, 150 mg, are blue, capsule shaped, film coated tablets, coded MSD 673. They are supplied as follows:
NDC 0006-0673-30 bottles of 30
NDC 0006-0673-68 bottles of 100
NDC 0006-0673-28 unit dose packages of 100.
Shown in Product Identification Section, page 418
No. 3286—Injection ELAVIL, 10 mg/mL, is a clear, colorless solution, and is supplied as follows:
NDC 0006-3286-10 in 10 mL vials.
Storage
Store Tablets ELAVIL in a well-closed container. Avoid storage at temperatures above 30°C (104°F). In addition, tablets ELAVIL 10 mg must be protected from light and stored in a well-closed, light-resistant container.
Protect Injection ELAVIL from freezing and avoid storage above 40°C (104°F).

METABOLISM

Studies in man following oral administration of ^{14}C-labeled drug indicated that amitriptyline is rapidly absorbed and metabolized. Radioactivity of the plasma was practically negligible, although significant amounts of radioactivity appeared in the urine by 4 to 6 hours and one-half to one-third of the drug was excreted within 24 hours.

Amitriptyline is metabolized by N-demethylation and bridge hydroxylation in man, rabbit, and rat. Virtually the entire dose is excreted as glucuronide or sulfate conjugate of metabolites, with little unchanged drug appearing in the urine. Other metabolic pathways may be involved.

A.H.F.S. Category: 28:16:04
DC 7398128   Issued July 1986

ELSPAR®   ℞
(Asparaginase, MSD)

WARNING

IT IS RECOMMENDED THAT ASPARAGINASE BE ADMINISTERED TO PATIENTS ONLY IN A HOSPITAL SETTING UNDER THE SUPERVISION OF A PHYSICIAN WHO IS QUALIFIED BY TRAINING AND EXPERIENCE TO ADMINISTER CANCER CHEMOTHERAPEUTIC AGENTS, BECAUSE OF THE POSSIBILITY OF SEVERE REACTIONS, INCLUDING ANAPHYLAXIS AND SUDDEN DEATH. THE PHYSICIAN MUST BE PREPARED TO TREAT ANAPHYLAXIS AT EACH ADMINISTRATION OF THE DRUG.
IN THE TREATMENT OF EACH PATIENT THE PHYSICIAN MUST WEIGH CAREFULLY THE POSSIBILITY OF ACHIEVING THERAPEUTIC BENEFIT VERSUS THE RISK OF TOXICITY. THE FOLLOWING DATA SHOULD BE THOROUGHLY REVIEWED BEFORE ADMINISTERING THE COMPOUND.

DESCRIPTION

ELSPAR® (Asparaginase, MSD) contains the enzyme L-asparagine amidohydrolase, type EC-2, derived from *Escherichia coli*. It is a white crystalline powder that is freely soluble in water and practically insoluble in methanol, acetone and chloroform. Its activity is expressed in terms of International Units (I.U.) according to the recommendation of the International Union of Biochemistry. The specific activity of ELSPAR is at least 225 I.U. per milligram of protein and each vial contains 10,000 I.U. of asparaginase and 80 mg of mannitol, an inactive ingredient, as a sterile, white lyophilized plug or powder for intravenous or intramuscular injection after reconstitution.

CLINICAL PHARMACOLOGY

Action
In a significant number of patients with acute leukemia, particularly lymphocytic, the malignant cells are dependent on an exogenous source of asparagine for survival. Normal cells, however, are able to synthesize asparagine and thus are affected less by the rapid depletion produced by treatment with the enzyme asparaginase. This is a unique approach to therapy based on a metabolic defect in asparagine synthesis of some malignant cells. ELSPAR, derived from *Escherichia coli*, is effective in inducing remissions in some patients with acute lymphocytic leukemia.

Asparagine Dependence Test
An asparagine dependence test has been utilized during the investigational studies. In this test leukemic cells obtained from some marrow cultures could be shown to require asparagine in *vitro*, suggesting sensitivity to asparaginase therapy in *vivo*. However, present data indicate that the correlation between asparagine dependence in such tests and the final

response to therapy is sufficiently poor that the test is not recommended as a basis for selection of patients for treatment.

Pharmacokinetics and Metabolism
In a study in patients with metastatic cancer and leukemia, initial plasma levels of L-asparaginase following intravenous administration were correlated to dose. Daily administration resulted in a cumulative increase in plasma levels. Plasma half-life varied from 8 to 30 hours; it did not appear to be influenced by dosage, either single or repetitive, and could not be correlated with age, sex, surface area, renal or hepatic function, diagnosis or extent of disease. Apparent volume of distribution was approximately 70–80% of estimated plasma volume. There was some slow movement of asparaginase from vascular to extravascular, extracellular space. L-asparaginase was detected in the lymph. Cerebrospinal fluid levels were less than 1% of concurrent plasma levels. Only trace amounts appeared in the urine.

In a study in which patients with leukemia and metastatic cancer received intramuscular L-asparaginase, peak plasma levels of asparaginase were reached 14 to 24 hours after dosing. Plasma half-life was 39 to 49 hours. No asparaginase was detected in the urine.

INDICATIONS AND USAGE

ELSPAR is indicated in the therapy of patients with acute lymphocytic leukemia. This agent is useful primarily in combination with other chemotherapeutic agents in the induction of remissions of the disease in children. ELSPAR should not be used as the sole induction agent unless combination therapy is deemed inappropriate. ELSPAR is not recommended for maintenance therapy.

CONTRAINDICATIONS

ELSPAR is contraindicated in patients with pancreatitis or a history of pancreatitis. Acute hemorrhagic pancreatitis, in some instances fatal, has been reported following asparaginase administration. Asparaginase is also contraindicated in patients who have had previous anaphylactic reactions to it.

WARNINGS

Allergic reactions to asparaginase are frequent and may occur during the primary course of therapy. They are not completely predictable on the basis of the intradermal skin test. Anaphylaxis and death have occurred even in a hospital setting with experienced observers.

Once a patient has received ELSPAR as part of a treatment regimen, retreatment with this agent at a later time is associated with increased risk of hypersensitivity reactions. In patients found by skin testing to be hypersensitive to asparaginase, and in any patient who has received a previous course of therapy with asparaginase, therapy with this agent should be instituted or reinstituted only after successful desensitization, and then only if in the judgement of the physician the possible benefit is greater than the increased risk. Desensitization itself may be hazardous. (See DOSAGE AND ADMINISTRATION, *Intradermal Skin Test.*)

In view of the unpredictability of the adverse reactions to asparaginase, it is recommended that this product be used in a hospital setting. Asparaginase has an adverse effect on liver function in the majority of patients. Therapy with asparaginase may increase pre-existing liver impairment caused by prior therapy or the underlying disease. Because of this there is a possibility that asparaginase may increase the toxicity of other medications.

The administration of ELSPAR *intravenously concurrently with or immediately before* a course of vincristine and prednisone may be associated with increased toxicity. (See DOSAGE AND ADMINISTRATION, *Recommended Induction Regimens.*)

PRECAUTIONS

General
This drug may be a contact irritant and both powder and solution must be handled and administered with care. Inhalation of dust or vapors and contact with skin or mucous membranes, especially those of the eyes, must be avoided. In case of contact, wash with copious amounts of water for at least 15 minutes.

Asparaginase has been reported to have immunosuppressive activity in animal experiments. Accordingly, the possibility that use of the drug in man may predispose to infection should be considered.

Continued on next page

Merck Sharp & Dohme—Cont.

Asparaginase toxicity is reported to be greater in adults than in children.

Laboratory Tests

The fall in circulating lymphoblasts often is quite marked; normal or below normal leukocyte counts are noted frequently within the first several days after initiating therapy. This may be accompanied by a marked rise in serum uric acid. The possible development of uric acid nephropathy should be borne in mind. Appropriate preventive measures should be taken, e.g., allopurinol, increased fluid intake, alkalization of urine. As a guide to the effects of therapy, the patient's peripheral blood count and bone marrow should be monitored frequently.

Frequent serum amylase determinations should be obtained to detect early evidence of pancreatitis. If pancreatitis occurs, therapy should be stopped and not reinstituted.

Blood sugar should be monitored during therapy with ELSPAR because hyperglycemia may occur.

Drug Interactions

Tissue culture and animal studies indicate that ELSPAR can diminish or abolish the effect of methotrexate on malignant cells. This effect on methotrexate activity persists as long as plasma asparagine levels are suppressed. These results would seem to dictate against the clinical use of methotrexate with ELSPAR, or during the period following ELSPAR therapy when plasma asparagine levels are below normal.

Drug/Laboratory Test Interactions

L-asparaginase has been reported to interfere with the interpretation of thyroid function tests by producing a rapid and marked reduction in serum concentrations of thyroxine-binding globulin within two days after the first dose. Serum concentrations of thyroxine-binding globulin returned to pretreatment values within four weeks of the last dose of L-asparaginase.

Animal Toxicology

A one-month intravenous toxicity study of ELSPAR in dogs at doses of 250, 1000, and 2000 I.U./kg/day revealed reduced serum total protein and albumin with loss of body weight at the highest dose level and anorexia, emesis, and diarrhea at all dosage levels. A similar study in monkeys at doses of 100, 300, and 1000 I.U./kg/day also revealed reduction of serum total protein and albumin and body weight loss at all dosage levels. Bromsulfalein retention and fatty changes in the liver were noted in monkeys that were given 300 and 1000 I.U./kg/day. The rabbit was unusually sensitive to ELSPAR since a single intravenous dose of 1000 I.U./kg caused hypocalcemia associated with necrosis of the parathyroid cells, convulsions, and death in about one third of the animals. Some rabbits that died showed small thymic and lymph node hemorrhages and necrosis of the germinal centers in the lymph nodes and spleen. The intravenous administration of calcium gluconate alleviated or prevented the adverse effects.

Changes in the pancreatic islets (not pancreatitis) ranging from edema to necrosis were observed in the rabbits in the acute intravenous toxicity studies (doses of 12,500 to 50,000 I.U./kg) but not in rabbits that received 1000 I.U./kg. The anatomical changes and the hypocalcemia found in the rabbits were not observed in the subacute intravenous studies in the dogs and monkeys.

Carcinogenesis, Mutagenesis, Impairment of Fertility

The intraperitoneal injection of 2500 I.U./kg/ day for 4 days in newborn Swiss mice resulted in a small increase in pulmonary adenomas; lymphatic leukemia was not increased. L-asparaginase at concentrations of 152-909 I.U./plate was not mutagenic in the Ames microbial mutagen test with or without metabolic activation.

There are no adequate studies on the effects of asparaginase on fertility.

Pregnancy

Pregnancy Category C. In mice and rats ELSPAR has been shown to retard the weight gain of mothers and fetuses when given in doses of more than 1000 I.U./kg (the recommended human dose). Resorptions, gross abnormalities and skeletal abnormalities were observed. A similar study in rats of the intravenous administration of 50 or 100 I.U./kg (one-twentieth or one-tenth of the human dose) to pregnant rabbits on Day 8 and 9 of gestation resulted in dose dependent embryotoxicity and gross abnormalities. There are no adequate and well-controlled studies in pregnant women. ELSPAR should be used during pregnancy only if the potential benefit justifies the potential risk to the fetus.

Nursing Mothers

It is not known whether this drug is secreted in human milk. Because many drugs are secreted in human milk and because of the potential for serious adverse reactions in nursing infants from ELSPAR, a decision should be made whether to discontinue nursing or to discontinue the drug, taking into account the importance of the drug to the mother.

ADVERSE REACTIONS

Allergic reactions, including skin rashes, urticaria, arthralgia, respiratory distress, and acute anaphylaxis have been reported. (See WARNINGS.) Acute reactions have occurred in the absence of a positive skin test and during continued maintenance of therapeutic serum levels of ELSPAR.

In children with advanced leukemia, a lower incidence of anaphylaxis has been reported with intramuscular administration, although there was a higher incidence of milder hypersensitivity reactions than with intravenous administration.

Fatal hyperthermia has been reported.

Pancreatitis, sometimes fulminant and fatal, has occurred during or following therapy with ELSPAR.

Hyperglycemia with glucosuria and polyuria has been reported in low incidence. Serum and urine acetone usually have been absent or negligible in these patients; this syndrome thus resembles hyperosmolar, nonketotic, hyperglycemia induced by a variety of other agents. This complication usually responds to discontinuance of ELSPAR, judicious use of intravenous fluid, and insulin, but may be fatal on occasion.

In addition to hypofibrinogenemia, depression of various other clotting factors has been reported. Most marked has been a decrease in plasma levels of factors V and VIII with a variable decrease in factors VII and IX. A decrease in circulating platelets has occurred in low incidence which, together with the increased levels of fibrin degradation products in the serum, may indicate development of a consumption coagulopathy. Bleeding has been a problem in only a minority of patients with demonstrable coagulopathy. However, intracranial hemorrhage and fatal bleeding associated with low fibrinogen levels have been reported. Increased fibrinolytic activity, apparently compensatory in nature, also has occurred.

Some patients have shown central nervous system effects consisting of depression, somnolence, fatigue, coma, confusion, agitation, and hallucinations varying from mild to severe. Rarely, a Parkinson-like syndrome has occurred, with tremor and a progressive increase in muscular tone. These side effects usually have reversed spontaneously after treatment was stopped. Therapy with ELSPAR is associated with an increase in blood ammonia during the conversion of asparagine to asparatic acid by the enzyme. No clear correlation exists between the degree of elevation of blood ammonia levels and the appearance of CNS changes. Chills, fever, nausea, vomiting, anorexia, abdominal cramps, weight loss, headache, and irritability may occur and usually are mild. Azotemia, usually pre-renal, occurs frequently. Acute renal shut down and fatal renal insufficiency have been reported during treatment. Proteinuria has occurred infrequently.

A variety of liver function abnormalities have been reported, including elevations of SGOT, SGPT, alkaline phosphatase, bilirubin (direct and indirect), and depression of serum albumin, cholesterol (total and esters), and plasma fibrinogen. Increases and decreases of total lipids have occurred. Marked hypoalbuminemia associated with peripheral edema has been reported. However, these abnormalities usually are reversible on discontinuance of therapy and some reversal may occur during the course of therapy. Fatty changes in the liver have been documented by biopsy. Malabsorption syndrome has been reported.

Rarely, transient bone marrow depression has been observed, as evidenced by a delay in return of hemoglobin or hematocrit levels to normal in patients undergoing hematologic remission of leukemia. Marked leukopenia has been reported.

OVERDOSAGE

The acute intravenous LD_{50} of ELSPAR for mice was about 500,000 I.U./kg and for rabbits about 22,000 I.U./kg.

DOSAGE AND ADMINISTRATION

As a component of selected multiple agent induction regimens, ELSPAR may be administered by either the intravenous or the intramuscular route. When administered intravenously this enzyme should be given over a period of not less than thirty minutes through the side arm of an already running infusion of Sodium Chloride Injection or Dextrose Injection 5% (D_5W). ELSPAR has little tendency to cause phlebitis when given intravenously. Anaphylactic reactions require the immediate use of epinephrine, oxygen, and intravenous steroids.

When administering ELSPAR intramuscularly, the volume at a single injection site should be limited to 2 ml. If a volume greater than 2 ml is to be administered, two injection sites should be used.

Unfavorable interactions of ELSPAR with some antitumor agents have been demonstrated. It is recommended therefore, that ELSPAR be used in combination regimens only by physicians familiar with the benefits and risks of a given regimen. During the period of its inhibition of protein synthesis and cell replication ELSPAR may interfere with the action of drugs such as methotrexate which require cell replication for their lethal effect. ELSPAR may interfere with the enzymatic detoxification of other drugs, particularly in the liver.

Recommended Induction Regimens:

When using chemotherapeutic agents in combination for the induction of remissions in patients with acute lymphocytic leukemia, regimens are sought which provide maximum chance of success while avoiding excessive cumulative toxicity or negative drug interactions.

One of the following combination regimens incorporating ELSPAR is recommended for acute lymphocytic leukemia in children:

In the regimens below, Day 1 is considered to be the first day of therapy.

Regimen I

Prednisone 40 mg/square meter of body surface area per day orally in three divided doses for 15 days, followed by tapering of the dosage as follows:

20 mg/square meter for 2 days, 10 mg/square meter for 2 days, 5 mg/square meter for 2 days, 2.5 mg/square meter for 2 days and then discontinue.

Vincristine sulfate 2 mg/square meter of body surface area intravenously once weekly on Days 1, 8, and 15 of the treatment period. The maximum single dose should not exceed 2.0 mg.

Asparaginase 1,000 I.U./kg/day intravenously for ten successive days beginning on Day 22 of the treatment period.

Regimen II

Prednisone 40 mg/square meter of body surface area per day orally in three divided doses for 28 days (the total daily dose should be to the nearest 2.5 mg), following which the dosage of prednisone should be discontinued gradually over a 14 day period.

Vincristine sulfate 1.5 mg/square meter of body surface area intravenously weekly for four doses, on Days 1, 8, 15, and 22 of the treatment period. The maximum single dose should not exceed 2.0 mg.

Asparaginase 6,000 I.U./square meter of body surface area intramuscularly on Days 4, 7, 10, 13, 16, 19, 22, 25, and 28 of the treatment period. When a remission is obtained with either of the above regimens, appropriate maintenance therapy must be instituted. ELSPAR should not be used as part of a maintenance regimen. The above regimens do not preclude a need for special therapy directed toward the prevention of central nervous system leukemia.

It should be noted that ELSPAR has been used in combination regimens other than those recommended above. It is important to keep in mind that ELSPAR administered intravenously concurrently with or immediately before a course of vincristine and prednisone may be associated with increased toxicity. Physicians using a given regimen should be thoroughly familiar with its benefits and risks. Clinical data are insufficient for a recommendation concerning the use of combination regimens in adults. Asparaginase toxicity is reported to be greater in adults than in children.

Use of ELSPAR as the sole induction agent should be undertaken only in an unusual situation when a combined regimen is inappropriate because of toxicity or other specific patient-related factors, or in cases refractory to other therapy. When ELSPAR is to be used as the sole induction agent for children or adults the recommended dosage regimen is 200 I.U./kg/ day intravenously for 28 days. When complete remissions were obtained with this regimen, they were of short duration, 1 to 3 months. ELSPAR has been used as the sole induction agent in other regimens. Physicians using a given regimen should be thoroughly familiar with its benefits and risks.

Patients undergoing induction therapy must be carefully monitored and the therapeutic regimen adjusted according to response and toxicity.

Such adjustments should always involve decreasing dosages of one or more agents or discontinuation depending on the degree of toxicity. Patients who have received a course of ELSPAR, if retreated, have an increased risk of hypersensitivity reactions. Therefore, retreatment should be undertaken only when the benefit of such therapy is weighed against the increased risk.

Intradermal Skin Test:

Because of the occurrence of allergic reactions, an intradermal skin test should be performed prior to the initial administration of ELSPAR and when ELSPAR is given after an interval of a week or more has elapsed between doses. The skin test solution may be prepared as follows: Reconstitute the contents of a 10,000 I.U. vial with 5.0 ml of diluent. From this solution (2,000 I.U./ml) withdraw 0.1 ml and inject it into another vial containing 9.9 ml of diluent, yielding a skin test solution of approximately 20.0 I.U./ml. Use 0.1 ml of this solution (about 2.0 I.U.) for the intradermal skin test. The skin test site should be observed for at least one hour for the appearance of a wheal or erythema either of which indicates a positive reaction. An allergic reaction even to the skin test dose in certain sensitized individuals may rarely occur. A negative skin test reaction does not preclude the possibility of the development of an allergic reaction.

Desensitization:

Desensitization should be performed before administering the first dose of ELSPAR on initiation of therapy in positive reactors, and on retreatment of any patient in whom such therapy is deemed necessary after carefully weighing the increased risk of hypersensitivity reactions. Rapid desensitization of the patient may be attempted with progressively increasing amounts of intravenously administered ELSPAR provided adequate precautions are taken to treat an acute allergic reaction should it occur. One reported schedule begins with a total of 1 I.U. given intravenously and doubles the dose every 10 minutes, provided no reaction has occurred, until the accumulated total amount given equals the planned doses for that day.

For convenience the following table is included to calculate the number of doses necessary to reach the patient's total dose for that day:

Injection Number	ELSPAR Dose in I.U.	Accumulated Total Dose
1	1	1
2	2	3
3	4	7
4	8	15
5	16	31
6	32	63
7	64	127
8	128	255
9	256	511
10	512	1023
11	1024	2047
12	2048	4095
13	4096	8191
14	8192	16383
15	16384	32767
16	32768	65535
17	65536	131071
18	131072	262143

For example: A patient weighing 20 kg who is to receive 200 I.U./kg (total dose 4000 I.U.) would receive injections 1 through 12 during desensitization.

DIRECTIONS FOR RECONSTITUTION

Parenteral drug products should be inspected visually for particulate matter and discoloration prior to administration whenever solution and container permit. When reconstituted, ELSPAR should be a clear, colorless solution. If the solution becomes cloudy, discard.

For Intravenous Use

Reconstitute with Sterile Water for Injection or with Sodium Chloride Injection. The volume recommended for reconstitution is 5 ml for the 10,000 unit vials. Ordinary shaking during reconstitution does not inactivate the enzyme. This solution may be used for direct intravenous administration within an eight hour period following restoration. For administration by infusion, solutions should be diluted with the isotonic solutions, Sodium Chloride Injection or Dextrose Injection 5%. These solutions should be infused within eight hours and only if clear.

Occasionally, a very small number of gelatinous fiber-like particles may develop on standing. Filtration through a 5.0 micron filter during administration will remove the particles with no resultant loss in potency. Some loss of potency has been observed with the use of a 0.2 micron filter.

For Intramuscular Use

When ELSPAR is administered intramuscularly according to the schedule cited in the induction regimen, reconstitution is carried out by adding 2 ml Sodium Chloride Injection to the 10,000 unit vial. The resulting solution should be used within eight hours and only if clear.

HOW SUPPLIED

No. 4612 — ELSPAR is a white lyophilized plug or powder supplied as follows:

NDC 0006-4612-00 in a sterile 10 ml vial containing 10,000 I.U. of asparaginase and 80 mg mannitol, an inactive ingredient.

Personnel preparing ELSPAR should avoid drug contact with skin, mucous membranes, or eyes and avoid inhaling the dust or vapor.

Store at 2–8°C (36–46°F). ELSPAR does not contain a preservative. Unused, reconstituted solution should be stored at 2 to 8°C (36 to 46°F) and discarded after eight hours, or sooner if it becomes cloudy.

A.H.F.S. Category: 44:00

DC 7407109   Issued September 1983

FLEXERIL® Tablets   ℞

(Cyclobenzaprine HCl, MSD), U.S.P.

DESCRIPTION

Cyclobenzaprine hydrochloride is a white, crystalline tricyclic amine salt with the empirical formula $C_{20}H_{21}N \cdot HCl$ and a molecular weight of 311.9. It has a melting point of 217°C, and a pK_a of 8.47 at 25°C. It is freely soluble in water and alcohol, sparingly soluble in isopropanol, and insoluble in hydrocarbon solvents. If aqueous solutions are made alkaline, the free base separates. Cyclobenzaprine HCl is designated chemically as 3-(5H-dibenzo[a,d]cyclohepten-5-ylidene)-N, N-dimethyl-1-propanamine hydrochloride, and has the following structural formula:

$$HCCH_2CH_2N(CH_3)_2 \cdot HCl$$

FLEXERIL® (Cyclobenzaprine HCl, MSD) is supplied as 10 mg tablets for oral administration.

Tablets FLEXERIL contain the following inactive ingredients: hydroxypropyl cellulose, hydroxypropyl methylcellulose, iron oxide, lactose, magnesium stearate, starch, and titanium dioxide.

CLINICAL PHARMACOLOGY

Cyclobenzaprine HCl relieves skeletal muscle spasm of local origin without interfering with muscle function. It is ineffective in muscle spasm due to central nervous system disease. Cyclobenzaprine reduced or abolished skeletal muscle hyperactivity in several animal models. Animal studies indicate that cyclobenzaprine does not act at the neuromuscular junction or directly on skeletal muscle. Such studies show that cyclobenzaprine acts primarily within the central nervous system at brain stem as opposed to spinal cord levels, although its action on the latter may contribute to its overall skeletal muscle relaxant activity. Evidence suggests that the net effect of cyclobenzaprine is a reduction of tonic somatic motor activity, influencing both gamma (γ) and alpha (α) motor systems.

Pharmacological studies in animals showed a similarity between the effects of cyclobenzaprine and the structurally related tricyclic antidepressants, including reserpine antagonism, norepinephrine potentiation, potent peripheral and central anticholinergic effects, and sedation. Cyclobenzaprine caused slight to moderate increase in heart rate in animals.

Cyclobenzaprine is well absorbed after oral administration, but there is a large intersubject variation in plasma levels. Cyclobenzaprine is eliminated quite slowly with a half-life as long as one to three days. It is highly bound to plasma proteins, is extensively metabolized primarily to glucuronide-like conjugates, and is excreted primarily via the kidneys. No significant effect on plasma levels or bioavailability of FLEXERIL or aspirin was noted when single or multiple doses of the two drugs were administered concomitantly. Concomitant administration of FLEXERIL and aspirin is usually well tolerated and no unexpected or serious clinical or laboratory adverse effects have been observed. No studies have been performed to indicate whether FLEXERIL enhances the clinical effect of aspirin or other analgesics, or whether analgesics enhance the clinical effect of FLEXERIL in acute musculoskeletal conditions.

Clinical Studies

Controlled clinical studies show that FLEXERIL significantly improves the signs and symptoms of skeletal muscle spasm as compared with placebo. The clinical responses include improvement in muscle spasm as determined by palpation, reduction in local pain and tenderness, increased range of motion, and less restriction in activities of daily living. When daily observations were made, clinical improvement was observed as early as the first day of therapy.

Eight double-blind controlled clinical studies were performed in 642 patients comparing FLEXERIL, diazepam*, and placebo. Muscle spasm, local pain and tenderness, limitation of motion, and restriction in activities of daily living were evaluated. In three of these studies there was a significantly greater improvement with FLEXERIL than with diazepam, while in the other studies the improvement following both treatments was comparable.

Although the frequency and severity of adverse reactions observed in patients treated with FLEXERIL were comparable to those observed in patients treated with diazepam, dry mouth was observed more frequently in patients treated with FLEXERIL and dizziness more frequently in those treated with diazepam. The incidence of drowsiness, the most frequent adverse reaction, was similar with both drugs. Analysis of the data from controlled studies shows that FLEXERIL produces clinical improvement whether or not sedation occurs.

---

*VALIUM® (diazepam, Roche)

Surveillance Program

A post-marketing surveillance program was carried out in 7607 patients with acute musculoskeletal disorders, and included 297 patients treated for 30 days or longer. The overall effectiveness of FLEXERIL was similar to that observed in the double-blind controlled studies; the overall incidence of adverse effects was less (see ADVERSE REACTIONS).

INDICATIONS AND USAGE

FLEXERIL is indicated as an adjunct to rest and physical therapy for relief of muscle spasm associated with acute, painful musculoskeletal conditions.

Improvement is manifested by relief of muscle spasm and its associated signs and symptoms, namely, pain, tenderness, limitation of motion, and restriction in activities of daily living.

FLEXERIL (Cyclobenzaprine HCl, MSD) should be used only for short periods (up to two or three weeks) because adequate evidence of effectiveness for more prolonged use is not available and because muscle spasm associated with acute, painful musculoskeletal conditions is generally of short duration and specific therapy for longer periods is seldom warranted.

FLEXERIL has not been found effective in the treatment of spasticity associated with cerebral or spinal cord disease, or in children with cerebral palsy.

CONTRAINDICATIONS

Hypersensitivity to the drug.

Concomitant use of monoamine oxidase inhibitors or within 14 days after their discontinuation.

Acute recovery phase of myocardial infarction, and patients with arrhythmias, heart block or conduction disturbances, or congestive heart failure.

Hyperthyroidism.

WARNINGS

Cyclobenzaprine is closely related to the tricyclic antidepressants, e.g., amitriptyline and imipramine. In short term studies for indications other than muscle spasm associated with acute musculoskeletal conditions, and usually at doses somewhat greater than those recommended for skeletal muscle spasm, some of the more serious central nervous system reactions noted with the tricyclic antidepressants have occurred (see WARNINGS, below, and ADVERSE REACTIONS).

FLEXERIL may interact with monoamine oxidase (MAO) inhibitors. Hyperpyretic crisis, severe convulsions, and deaths have occurred in patients receiving tricyclic antidepressants and MAO inhibitor drugs.

Tricyclic antidepressants have been reported to produce arrhythmias, sinus tachycardia, prolongation of the conduction time leading to myocardial infarction and stroke.

FLEXERIL may enhance the effects of alcohol, barbiturates, and other CNS depressants.

PRECAUTIONS

General

Because of its atropine-like action, FLEXERIL should be used with caution in patients with a history of urinary retention, angle-closure glaucoma, increased intraocular pressure, and in patients taking anticholinergic medication.

Information for Patients

FLEXERIL may impair mental and/or physical abilities required for performance of hazardous tasks, such as operating machinery or driving a motor vehicle.

Drug Interactions

FLEXERIL may enhance the effects of alcohol, barbiturates, and other CNS depressants.

Tricyclic antidepressants may block the antihypertensive action of guanethidine and similarly acting compounds.

Carcinogenesis, Mutagenesis, Impairment of Fertility

In rats treated with FLEXERIL for up to 67 weeks at doses of approximately 5 to 40 times the maximum recommended human dose, pale, sometimes enlarged, livers were noted and there was a dose-related hepatocyte vacuolation with lipidosis. In the higher dose groups this microscopic change was seen after 26 weeks and even earlier in rats which died prior to 26 weeks; at lower doses, the change was not seen until after 26 weeks.

Continued on next page

Information on the Merck Sharp & Dohme products listed on these pages is the full prescribing information from product circulars in use August 31, 1989.

Merck Sharp & Dohme—Cont.

Cyclobenzaprine did not affect the onset, incidence or distribution of neoplasia in an 81-week study in the mouse or in a 105-week study in the rat.

At oral doses of up to 10 times the human dose, cyclobenzaprine did not adversely affect the reproductive performance or fertility of male or female rats. Cyclobenzaprine did not demonstrate mutagenic activity in the male mouse at dose levels of up to 20 times the human dose.

Pregnancy

Pregnancy Category B: Reproduction studies have been performed in rats, mice and rabbits at doses up to 20 times the human dose, and have revealed no evidence of impaired fertility or harm to the fetus due to FLEXERIL. There are, however, no adequate and well-controlled studies in pregnant women. Because animal reproduction studies are not always predictive of human response, this drug should be used during pregnancy only if clearly needed.

Nursing Mothers

It is not known whether this drug is excreted in human milk. Because cyclobenzaprine is closely related to the tricyclic antidepressants, some of which are known to be excreted in human milk, caution should be exercised when FLEXERIL is administered to a nursing woman.

Pediatric Use

Safety and effectiveness of FLEXERIL in children below the age of 15 have not been established.

ADVERSE REACTIONS

The following list of adverse reactions is based on the experience in 473 patients treated with FLEXERIL in controlled clinical studies, 7607 patients in the post-marketing surveillance program, and reports received since the drug was marketed. The overall incidence of adverse reactions among patients in the surveillance program was less than the incidence in the controlled clinical studies.

The adverse reactions reported most frequently with FLEXERIL were drowsiness, dry mouth and dizziness. The incidence of these common adverse reactions was lower in the surveillance program than in the controlled clinical studies:

	Clinical Studies	Surveillance Program
drowsiness	39%	16%
dry mouth	27%	7%
dizziness	11%	3%

Among the less frequent adverse reactions, there was no appreciable difference in incidence in controlled clinical studies or in the surveillance program. Adverse reactions which were reported in 1% to 3% of the patients were: fatigue/tiredness, asthenia, nausea, constipation, dyspepsia, unpleasant taste, blurred vision, headache, nervousness, and confusion.

Incidence Less Than 1 in 100

The following adverse reactions have been reported at an incidence of less than 1 in 100:

Body as a Whole: Syncope; facial edema; malaise.

Cardiovascular: Tachycardia; arrhythmia; vasodilatation; palpitation; hypotension.

Digestive: Vomiting; anorexia; diarrhea; gastrointestinal pain; gastritis; thirst; flatulence; edema of the tongue; abnormal liver function and rare reports of hepatitis, jaundice and cholestasis.

Musculoskeletal: Local weakness.

Nervous System and Psychiatric: Ataxia; vertigo; dysarthria; tremors; hypertonia; convulsions; muscle twitching; disorientation; insomnia; depressed mood; abnormal sensations; anxiety; agitation; abnormal thinking and dreaming; hallucinations; excitement; paresthesia.

Skin: Sweating; skin rash; urticaria.

Special Senses: Ageusia; tinnitus.

Urogenital: Urinary frequency and/or retention.

Causal Relationship Unknown

Other reactions, reported rarely for FLEXERIL under circumstances where a causal relationship could not be established or reported for other tricyclic drugs, are listed to serve as alerting information to physicians:

Body as a Whole: Chest pain; edema.

Cardiovascular: Hypertension; myocardial infarction; heart block; stroke.

Digestive: Paralytic ileus; tongue discoloration; stomatitis; parotid swelling.

Endocrine: Inappropriate ADH syndrome.

Hematic and Lymphatic: Purpura; bone marrow depression; leukopenia; eosinophilia; thrombocytopenia.

Metabolic, Nutritional and Immune: Elevation and lowering of blood sugar levels; weight gain or loss.

Musculoskeletal: Myalgia.

Nervous System and Psychiatric: Decreased or increased libido; abnormal gait; delusions; peripheral neuropathy; Bell's palsy; alteration in EEG patterns; extrapyramidal symptoms.

Respiratory: Dyspnea.

Skin: Pruritus; photosensitization; alopecia.

Urogenital: Impaired urination; dilatation of urinary tract; impotence; testicular swelling; gynecomastia; breast enlargement; galactorrhea.

DRUG ABUSE AND DEPENDENCE

Pharmacologic similarities among the tricyclic drugs require that certain withdrawal symptoms be considered when FLEXERIL is administered, even though they have not been reported to occur with this drug. Abrupt cessation of treatment after prolonged administration may produce nausea, headache, and malaise. These are not indicative of addiction.

OVERDOSAGE

Manifestations: High doses may cause temporary confusion, disturbed concentration, transient visual hallucinations, agitation, hyperactive reflexes, muscle rigidity, vomiting, or hyperpyrexia, in addition to anything listed under ADVERSE REACTIONS. Based on the known pharmacologic actions of the drug, overdosage may cause drowsiness, hypothermia, tachycardia and other cardiac rhythm abnormalities such as bundle branch block, ECG evidence of impaired conduction, and congestive heart failure. Other manifestations may be dilated pupils, convulsions, severe hypotension, stupor, and coma.

The acute oral LD_{50} of FLEXERIL is approximately 338 and 425 mg/kg in mice and rats, respectively.

Treatment: Treatment is symptomatic and supportive. Empty the stomach as quickly as possible by emesis, followed by gastric lavage. After gastric lavage, activated charcoal may be administered. Twenty to 30 g of activated charcoal may be given every four to six hours during the first 24 to 48 hours after ingestion. An ECG should be taken and close monitoring of cardiac function must be instituted if there is any evidence of dysrhythmia. Maintenance of an open airway, adequate fluid intake, and regulation of body temperature are necessary.

The intravenous administration of 1-3 mg of physostigmine salicylate is reported to reverse symptoms of poisoning by atropine and other drugs with anticholinergic activity. Physostigmine may be helpful in the treatment of cyclobenzaprine overdose. Because physostigmine is rapidly metabolized, the dosage of physostigmine should be repeated as required, particularly if life-threatening signs such as arrhythmias, convulsions, and deep coma recur or persist after the initial dosage of physostigmine. Because physostigmine itself may be toxic, it is not recommended for routine use. Standard medical measures should be used to manage circulatory shock and metabolic acidosis. Cardiac arrhythmias may be treated with neostigmine, pyridostigmine, or propranolol. When signs of cardiac failure occur, the use of a short-acting digitalis preparation should be considered. Close monitoring of cardiac function for not less than five days is advisable.

Anticonvulsants may be given to control seizures.

Dialysis is probably of no value because of low plasma concentrations of the drug.

Since overdosage is often deliberate, patients may attempt suicide by other means during the recovery phase. Deaths by deliberate or accidental overdosage have occurred with this class of drugs.

DOSAGE AND ADMINISTRATION

The usual dosage of FLEXERIL is 10 mg three times a day, with a range of 20 to 40 mg a day in divided doses. Dosage should not exceed 60 mg a day. Use of FLEXERIL for periods longer than two or three weeks is not recommended. (See INDICATIONS AND USAGE.)

HOW SUPPLIED

No. 3358—Tablets FLEXERIL, 10 mg, are butterscotch yellow, D-shaped, film coated tablets, coded MSD 931. They are supplied as follows:

NDC 0006-0931-68 in bottles of 100

NDC 0006-0931-28 unit dose packages of 100

NDC 0006-0931-30 BACK-PACK® unit-of-use package of 30.

Shown in Product Identification Section, page 418

A.H.F.S. Category: 12:20

DC 7399210   Issued March 1986

FLOROPRYL® Sterile Ophthalmic Ointment   ℞

(Isoflurophate, MSD), U.S.P.

For Topical Application into the

   Conjunctival Sac Only

DESCRIPTION

FLOROPRYL® (Isoflurophate, MSD) is available as 0.025% sterile ophthalmic ointment in polyethylene mineral oil gel. Isoflurophate has a molecular weight of 184.15 and is known chemically as bis (1-methylethyl) phosphorofluoridate. Its empirical formula is $C_6H_{14}FO_3P$ and its structural formula is:

$$(CH_3)_2CH-O-\underset{\underset{O}{\|}}{\overset{\overset{F}{|}}{P}}-O-CH(CH_3)_2$$

CLINICAL PHARMACOLOGY

FLOROPRYL is a cholinesterase inhibitor with sustained activity. Application to the eye produces intense miosis and ciliary muscle contraction due to inhibition of cholinesterase, allowing acetylcholine to accumulate at sites of cholinergic transmission.

FLOROPRYL *irreversibly* inactivates cholinesterase. Thus, following use of FLOROPRYL in the eye, cholinesterase must be either regenerated or supplied from depots elsewhere in the body before ophthalmic action dependent on cholinesterase returns.

If given systemically in sufficient amounts, FLOROPRYL reduces plasma cholinesterase to zero. However, when applied locally to the eye, plasma cholinesterase is usually reduced only slightly.

INDICATIONS AND USAGE

Open-angle glaucoma (FLOROPRYL should be used in glaucoma only when shorter-acting miotics have proven inadequate.)

Conditions obstructing aqueous outflow, such as synechial formation, that are amenable to miotic therapy

Following iridectomy

Accommodative esotropia (accommodative convergent strabismus)

CONTRAINDICATIONS

Hypersensitivity to any component of this product.

Because of the toxicity of cholinesterase inhibitors in general, FLOROPRYL is contraindicated in women who are or who may become pregnant. If this drug is used during pregnancy, or if the patient becomes pregnant while taking this drug, the patient should be apprised of the potential hazard to the fetus.

Because miotics may aggravate inflammation, FLOROPRYL should not be used in active uveal inflammation and/or glaucoma associated with iridocyclitis.

WARNINGS

In patients receiving cholinesterase inhibitors such as FLOROPRYL, succinylcholine should be administered with extreme caution before and during general anesthesia because of possible respiratory and cardiovascular collapse.

Because of possible adverse additive effects, FLOROPRYL should be administered only with extreme caution to patients with myasthenia gravis who are receiving systemic anticholinesterase therapy; conversely, extreme caution should be exercised in the use of an anticholinesterase drug for the treatment of myasthenia gravis patients who are already undergoing topical therapy with cholinesterase inhibitors.

PRECAUTIONS

General

FLOROPRYL should be used with caution in patients with chronic angle-closure (narrow-angle) glaucoma or in patients with narrow angles, because of the possibility of producing pupillary block and increasing angle blockage.

Gonioscopy is recommended prior to medication with FLOROPRYL.

When an intraocular inflammatory process is present, the intensity and persistence of miosis and ciliary muscle contraction that result from anticholinesterase therapy require abstention from, or cautious use of, FLOROPRYL.

Systemic effects are infrequent when FLOROPRYL is applied carefully. The hands should be washed immediately following application.

Discontinue FLOROPRYL if salivation, urinary incontinence, diarrhea, profuse sweating, muscle weakness, respiratory difficulties, shock, or cardiac irregularities occur.

Persons receiving cholinesterase inhibitors who are exposed to organophosphate-type insecticides and pesticides (gardeners, organophosphate plant or warehouse workers, farmers, residents of communities which are undergoing insecticide spraying or dusting, etc.) should be warned of the added systemic effects possible from absorption through the respiratory tract or skin. Wearing of respiratory masks, frequent washing, and clothing changes may be advisable.

Anticholinesterase drugs should be used with extreme caution, if at all, in patients with marked vagotonia, bronchial asthma, spastic gastrointestinal disturbances, peptic ulcer, pronounced bradycardia and hypotension, recent myocardial infarction, epilepsy, parkinsonism, and other disorders that may respond adversely to vagotonic effects.

After long-term use of FLOROPRYL, dilation of blood vessels and resulting greater permeability increase the possibility of hyphema during ophthalmic surgery. Therefore, this drug should be discontinued before surgery.

Despite observance of all precautions and the use of only the recommended dose, there is some evidence that repeated administration may cause depression of the concentration of cholinesterase in the serum and erythrocytes, with resultant systemic effects.

Drug Interactions
See WARNINGS regarding possible drug interactions of FLOROPRYL with succinylcholine or with other anticholinesterase agents.

Carcinogenesis, Mutagenesis, Impairment of Fertility
Long-term studies in animals have not been performed to evaluate the effects of FLOROPRYL on fertility or carcinogenic potential.

Pregnancy
Pregnancy Category X: See CONTRAINDICATIONS.

Nursing Mothers
It is not known whether this drug is excreted in human milk. Because of the potential for serious adverse reactions in nursing infants from FLOROPRYL, a decision should be made whether to discontinue nursing or to discontinue the drug, taking into account the importance of the drug to the mother.

Pediatric Use
The occurrence of iris cysts is more frequent in children. (See ADVERSE REACTIONS and DOSAGE AND ADMINISTRATION.)

Extreme caution should be exercised in children receiving FLOROPRYL who may require general anesthesia (see WARNINGS).

Since FLOROPRYL is a potent cholinesterase inhibitor it should be kept out of the reach of children.

ADVERSE REACTIONS

Stinging, burning, lacrimation, lid muscle twitching, conjunctival and ciliary redness, brow ache, headache, and induced myopia with visual blurring may occur.

As with all miotic therapy, retinal detachment has been reported occasionally.

Activation of latent iritis or uveitis may occur.

Iris cysts may form, enlarge, and obscure vision. Occurrence is more frequent in children. The iris cyst usually shrinks upon discontinuance of the miotic. Rarely, the cyst may rupture or break free into the aqueous. Frequent examination for this occurrence is advised.

Prolonged use may cause conjunctival thickening and obstruction of nasolacrimal canals.

Systemic effects, which occur rarely, are suggestive of increased cholinergic activity. Such effects may include nausea, vomiting, abdominal cramps, diarrhea, urinary incontinence, salivation, sweating, difficulty in breathing, bradycardia, or cardiac irregularities. Medical management of systemic effects may be indicated (see TREATMENT OF ADVERSE EFFECTS).

Lens opacities have been reported in patients on miotic therapy. Routine slit-lamp examinations, including the lens, should accompany prolonged use.

Paradoxical increase in intraocular pressure may follow anticholinesterase application. This may be alleviated by pupil-dilating medication.

TREATMENT OF ADVERSE EFFECTS

If FLOROPRYL is taken systemically by accident, or if systemic effects occur after topical application in the eye or from accidental skin contact, atropine sulfate in a dose (for adults) of 0.4 to 0.6 mg or more should be given parenterally (intravenously if necessary). The recommended dosage of atropine in infants and children up to 12 years of age is 0.01 mg/kg repeated every two hours as needed until the desired effect is obtained, or adverse effects of atropine preclude further usage. The maximum single dose should not exceed 0.4 mg.

The use of much larger doses of atropine in treating anticholinesterase intoxication in adults has been reported in the literature. Initially 2 to 6 mg may be given followed by 2 mg every hour or more often, as long as muscarinic effects con-

tinue. The greater possibility of atropinization with large doses, particularly in sensitive individuals, should be borne in mind.

Pralidoxime* chloride has been reported to be useful in treatment of systemic effects due to cholinesterase inhibitors. However, its use is recommended in addition to and not as a substitute for atropine.

A short-acting barbiturate is indicated if convulsions occur that are not entirely relieved by atropine. Barbiturate dosage should be carefully adjusted to avoid central respiratory depression. Marked weakness or paralysis of muscles of respiration should be treated promptly by artificial respiration and maintenance of a clear airway.

The oral LD_{50} of FLOROPRYL is 37 mg/kg in the mouse, 5–10 mg/kg in the rat, and 4–10 mg/kg in the rabbit.

DOSAGE AND ADMINISTRATION

FLOROPRYL *is intended solely for topical use in the conjunctival sac.*

Isoflurophate hydrolyzes in the presence of water to form hydrofluoric acid. To prevent absorption of moisture and loss of potency, the ointment tube should be kept tightly closed; the tip of the tube should not be washed or allowed to touch the eyelid or other moist surface.

Whenever possible, FLOROPRYL should be applied at night before retiring to lessen blurring of vision. As it is an extremely potent drug, it should be used with great care and only by those familiar with its use and thoroughly indoctrinated in the technic of application.

The required dose is applied in the conjunctival sac, with the patient supine, care being taken not to touch the cornea with the tip of the tube. *Wash the hands immediately after administration.*

FLOROPRYL *should not be used more often than directed. Caution is necessary to avoid overdosage.*

Keep frequency of use to a minimum in all patients, but especially in children, to reduce the chance of iris cyst development (see ADVERSE REACTIONS). If tolerance develops, another miotic should be used. FLOROPRYL may be resumed later.

Glaucoma
For initial therapy $\frac{1}{4}$ inch strip of ophthalmic ointment FLOROPRYL 0.025 per cent is placed in the glaucomatous eye every 8 to 72 hours. A decrease in intraocular pressure should occur within a few hours. During this period, keep the patient under supervision and make tonometric examinations at least hourly for 3 or 4 hours to be sure that no immediate rise in pressure occurs (see ADVERSE REACTIONS).

Strabismus
Essentially equal visual acuity of both eyes is a prerequisite to successful treatment. For initial evaluation FLOROPRYL may be used as a diagnostic aid to determine if an accomodative factor exists. This is especially useful preoperatively in young children and in patients with normal hypermetropic refractive errors. Not more than $\frac{1}{4}$ inch strip of ointment is administered every night for 2 weeks. If the eyes become straighter, an accommodative factor is demonstrated. This technic may supplement or complement standard testing with atropine and trial with glasses for the accommodative factor.

In esotropia uncomplicated by amblyopia or anisometropia, ophthalmic ointment FLOROPRYL may be used in both eyes, not more than $\frac{1}{4}$ inch strip at a time every night for 2 weeks, as too severe a degree of miosis may interfere with vision. The dosage is then reduced to from $\frac{1}{4}$ inch strip every other day to $\frac{1}{4}$ inch strip once a week for 2 months, after which the patient's status should be re-evaluated.

If benefit can not be maintained with a dosage interval of at least 48 hours, therapy with FLOROPRYL should be stopped. Frequency of administration and duration of maintenance therapy depend on how long the eyes remain straight without medication. Intervals between administration should be gradually increased to the greatest length compatible with good results. Therapy may need to be continued for many years in some patients; in others, it has been possible to discontinue therapy after several months.

HOW SUPPLIED

No. 7742—Sterile Ophthalmic Ointment FLOROPRYL 0.025 per cent is an opaque white, smooth, unctuous ointment and is supplied as follows:
NDC 0006-7742-04 in a 3.5 g tube.

Storage
Protect from moisture, freezing and excessive heat.

A.H.F.S. Category: 52:20

DC 7413720   Issued October 1987

* PROTOPAM® Chloride (Pralidoxime Chloride). Ayerst Laboratories.

HEP–B–GAMMAGEE®   ℞
(Hepatitis B Immune Globulin [Human], MSD), U.S.P.

DESCRIPTION

HEP-B-GAMMAGEE® [Hepatitis B Immune Globulin (Human), MSD] is a sterile solution of human immunoglobulin (10–18% protein) intended for intramuscular injection. The high levels of antibody to hepatitis B surface antigen (anti-HBs) found in the product are derived from a small group of well-monitored individuals who were hyperimmunized with hepatitis B vaccine. The potency is adjusted by the addition of IgG obtained from large pools of normal plasma. Each unit of plasma was found to be nonreactive when tested for hepatitis B surface antigen (HBsAg) by an FDA approved test. The pooled plasma is processed by MSD and/or Armour Pharmaceutical Company using Cohn cold ethanol fractionation procedures. The product is dissolved in 0.3 molar glycine and contains thimerosal (mercury derivative) 1:10,000 added as a preservative. The solution has a pH of 6.8 ± 0.4 adjusted with hydrochloric acid or sodium hydroxide. Each vial of HEP-B-GAMMAGEE contains anti-HBs equivalent to or exceeding the potency of anti-HBs in a U.S. reference Hepatitis B Immune Globulin (Office of Biologics Research and Review FDA).

There is no evidence to suggest that the causative virus of AIDS (HIV) has been transmitted by HEP-B-GAMMAGEE prepared by the Cohn cold ethanol process.

CLINICAL PHARMACOLOGY

Hepatitis B Immune Globulin (Human) provides passive immunization for individuals exposed to the hepatitis B virus (HBV) as evidenced by a reduction in the attack rate of hepatitis B following its use. The administration of the usual recommended dose of HEP-B-GAMMAGEE generally results in a detectable level of circulating antibody to hepatitis B surface antigen (anti-HBs) which persists for approximately 2 months or longer. Peak serum levels of anti-HBs are seen at 3–7 days after intramuscular administration of hepatitis B immunoglobulin. The half-life of this antibody ranges from 17.5–25 days. The possibility of hepatitis B transmission is remote, as it is with other immune globulins prepared by the cold ethanol process.

INDICATIONS AND USAGE

HEP-B-GAMMAGEE is indicated for post-exposure prophylaxis following either parenteral exposure, direct mucous membrane contact, sexual exposure or oral ingestion involving HBsAg-positive materials such as blood, plasma or serum. Such exposures might occur by accidental "needlestick", accidental splash, or a pipetting accident. HEP-B-GAMMAGEE is also indicated for post-exposure prophylaxis in infants born to hepatitis B-positive (HBsAg-positive) mothers.

CONTRAINDICATIONS

Hypersensitivity to any component of the product.

WARNINGS

Persons with isolated immunoglobulin A deficiency have the potential for developing antibodies to immunoglobulin A and could have anaphylactic reactions to subsequent administration of blood products that contain immunoglobulin A. Therefore, as with any immunoglobulin preparation, Hepatitis B Immune Globulin (Human) should be given to such persons only if the expected benefits outweigh the potential risks.

In patients who have severe thrombocytopenia or any coagulation disorder that would contraindicate intramuscular injections, Hepatitis B Immune Globulin (Human) should be given only if the expected benefits outweigh the potential risks.

PRECAUTIONS

General
HEP-B-GAMMAGEE should be given with caution to patients with a history of prior systemic allergic reactions following the administration of human immune globulin preparations. Hypersensitivity reactions to injections of immunoglobulin occur rarely. The incidence of these reactions may be increased in patients receiving large intramuscular doses

Continued on next page

Merck Sharp & Dohme—Cont.

or in patients receiving repeated injections of immunoglobulin.

HEP-B-GAMMAGEE *must not be administered intravenously* because of the potential for serious reactions. Injections should be made intramuscularly. Care should be taken to draw back on the plunger of the syringe before injection in order to be certain that the needle is not in a blood vessel. Epinephrine should be available for treatment of acute allergic symptoms.

Drug Interactions

Antibodies present in immunoglobulin preparations may interfere with the immune response to live virus vaccines such as measles, mumps, and rubella. Therefore, vaccination with live virus vaccines should be deferred until approximately three months after administration of Hepatitis B Immune Globulin (Human). It may be necessary to revaccinate persons who received Hepatitis B Immune Globulin (Human) shortly after live virus vaccination.

Pregnancy

Pregnancy Category C. Animal reproduction studies have not been conducted with HEP-B-GAMMAGEE. It is also not known whether HEP-B-GAMMAGEE can cause fetal harm when administered to a pregnant woman or can affect reproduction capacity. HEP-B-GAMMAGEE should be given to a pregnant woman only if clearly needed.

Nursing Mothers

It is not known whether this drug is excreted in human milk. Because many drugs are excreted in human milk, caution should be exercised when HEP-B-GAMMAGEE is administered to a nursing woman.

ADVERSE REACTIONS

Local pain and tenderness at the injection site, urticaria and angioedema may occur. Anaphylactic reactions, although rare, have been reported following the injection of human immunoglobulin preparations. Anaphylaxis is more likely to occur if Hepatitis B Immune Globulin (Human) is given intravenously; therefore, Hepatitis B Immune Globulin (Human) must be administered *only* intramuscularly. In highly allergic individuals, repeated injections may lead to anaphylactic shock.

OVERDOSAGE

Although no data are available, clinical experience with other immunoglobulin preparations suggests that the only manifestations would be pain and tenderness at the injection site.

DOSAGE AND ADMINISTRATION

Parenteral drug products should be inspected visually for particulate matter and discoloration prior to administration, whenever solution and container permit. HEP-B-GAMMAGEE is a clear, very slightly amber, moderately viscous liquid.

HEP-B-GAMMAGEE is administered *intramuscularly. It must not be injected intravenously.*

It is important to use a separate sterile syringe and needle for each individual patient to prevent transmission of hepatitis B and other infectious agents from one person to another.

Known or Presumed Exposure to HBsAg

There are no prospective studies directly testing the efficacy of a combination of Hepatitis B Immune Globulin (Human) and hepatitis B vaccine (HEPTAVAX-B® (Hepatitis B Vaccine, MSD) or RECOMBIVAX HB® [Hepatitis B Vaccine (Recombinant), MSD]) in preventing clinical hepatitis B following percutaneous, ocular or mucous membrane exposure to hepatitis B virus. However, since most persons with such exposures (e.g., health-care workers) are candidates for the hepatitis B vaccine and since combined Hepatitis B Immune Globulin (Human) plus vaccine is more efficacious than Hepatitis B Immune Globulin (Human) alone in perinatal exposures, the following guidelines are recommended for persons who have been exposed to hepatitis B virus such as through (1) percutaneous (needlestick), ocular, mucous membrane exposure to blood known or presumed to contain HBsAg, (2) human bites by known or presumed HBsAg carriers, that penetrate the skin, or (3) following intimate sexual contact with known or presumed HBsAg carriers:

Recommendations for adults who have not been previously vaccinated against hepatitis B:

Hepatitis B Immune Globulin (Human) (0.06 mL/kg) should be given intramuscularly as soon as possible after exposure and within 24 hours if possible. Hepatitis B vaccine (see HEPTAVAX-B (Hepatitis B Vaccine, MSD) or RECOMBIVAX HB [Hepatitis B Vaccine (Recombinant), MSD] circular for appropriate dosage recommendations) should be given intramuscularly within 7 days of exposure and second

and third doses given one and six months, respectively, after the first dose.

Recommendations for adults who have been previously vaccinated against hepatitis B:

Prior recipients of a recommended course of hepatitis B vaccine should have their anti-HBs titer checked promptly. For those with known adequate antibody (10 MIU/mL anti-HBs, approximately equal to 10 SRU) nothing is required. Those with inadequate or unknown titers should receive a dose of Hepatitis B Immune Globulin (Human) and a dose of hepatitis B vaccine simultaneously at two different sites as soon as possible.

Dosage for Infants Born of HBsAg Positive Mothers:

Infants born to HBsAg positive mothers are at high risk of becoming chronic carriers of hepatitis B virus and of developing the chronic sequelae of hepatitis B virus infection. Well-controlled studies have shown that administration of three 0.5 mL doses of Hepatitis B Immune Globulin (Human) starting at birth is 75% effective in preventing establishment of the chronic carrier state in these infants during the first year of life. Protection can be transient, whereupon the effectiveness of the Hepatitis B Immune Globulin (Human) would decline thereafter. Results from clinical studies indicate that administration of one 0.5 mL dose of Hepatitis B Immune Globulin (Human) at birth and the recommended three doses of HEPTAVAX-B (Hepatitis B Vaccine, MSD) or RECOMBIVAX HB [Hepatitis B Vaccine (Recombinant), MSD] (see Table below), were effective in preventing establishment of the chronic carrier state in infants born to HBsAg and HBeAg positive mothers.

Testing for HBsAg and anti-HBs is recommended at 12–15 months of age. If HBsAg is not detectable, and anti-HBs is present, the child has been protected.

The recommended dosage for infants born to HBsAg positive mothers is as follows:

Treatment	Birth	Within 7 days	1 month	6 months
Hepatitis B vaccine** (pediatric formulation)		0.5 mL*	0.5 mL	0.5 mL
Hepatitis B Immune Globulin (Human)	0.5 mL	—	—	—

* The first dose of hepatitis B vaccine may be given at birth at the same time as Hepatitis B Immune Globulin (Human); but should be administered in the opposite anterolateral thigh.

** See DOSAGE AND ADMINISTRATION section of HEPTAVAX-B (Hepatitis B Vaccine, MSD) or RECOMBIVAX HB [Hepatitis B Vaccine (Recombinant), MSD] circular.

HOW SUPPLIED

No. 4692—HEP-B-GAMMAGEE is supplied as follows:
NDC 0006-4692-00 in 5 mL vials.
Store at 2–8°C (35.6–46.4°F). Do not freeze. Do not use after expiration date.

A.H.F.S. Category: 80:04
DC 7413907   Issued January 1988
COPYRIGHT © MERCK & CO., INC., 1988
All rights reserved

HEPTAVAX–B®   ℞
(Hepatitis B Vaccine, MSD), U.S.P.

DESCRIPTION

HEPTAVAX-B® (Hepatitis B Vaccine, MSD) is a non-infectious formalin-inactivated subunit viral vaccine derived from surface antigen (HBsAg or Australia antigen) of hepatitis B virus. The antigen is harvested and purified from the plasma of human carriers of hepatitis B virus according to methods developed by Merck Sharp and Dohme Research Laboratories.

The starting plasma from which the antigen is extracted is obtained from a small, closely monitored population of asymptomatic HBsAg-positive donors. Periodically each donor is required to undergo a health examination, and appropriate laboratory tests are performed prior to each plasmapheresis.

The vaccine production process uses purification and inactivation steps which are known to remove or inactivate not only infectious hepatitis B virus particles, but also representatives of all known groups of animal viruses. Such groups include rhabdo-, pox-, toga-, reo-, herpes-, corona-, myxo-, picorna-, parvo-, and retrovirus; delta agent, and slow viruses.

Initial purification is accomplished by double ultracentrifugation. This is followed by an inactivation process consisting of three sequential treatments using pepsin, 8 Molar urea, and formalin. Each of these treatments alone has been shown to inactivate 10^5 or more infectious doses of hepatitis B virus/mL, and one or more of the treatments also has been shown to inactivate members of many other virus groups, including those listed above. In addition, studies in chimpanzees and humans show that hepatitis B vaccine produced according to this process does not transmit the agent(s) of non-A/non-B hepatitis. Follow-up data from clinical trials of HEPTAVAX-B provide no evidence to suggest transmission of Acquired Immune Deficiency Syndrome (AIDS) by this vaccine, even when the vaccine has been used routinely in infants in Alaska. Each of the three sequential treatments, pepsin, urea, and formalin, have been shown to inactivate retroviruses, including HTLV-I, HTLV-II, HTLV-III and LAV, which have been associated with AIDS. Other studies have shown that individuals who have received this vaccine showed no rise in antibodies to HTLV-I, HTLV-II, HTLV-III or LAV. Other studies have shown no detectable HTLV DNA in this vaccine.

Each lot of hepatitis B vaccine is tested for sterility and is inoculated into cell cultures and several species of animals including chimpanzees, to rule out the presence of adventitious viruses.

HEPTAVAX-B is a sterile suspension for intramuscular injection; however, it may be administered subcutaneously to persons at risk of hemorrhage following intramuscular injections (see DOSAGE AND ADMINISTRATION). Each 1.0 mL dose of the adult formulation vaccine contains 20 mcg of hepatitis B surface antigen formulated in an alum adjuvant, and thimerosal (mercury derivative) 1:20,000 added as a preservative. Each 0.5 mL dose of the pediatric formulation vaccine contains 10 mcg of hepatitis B surface antigen formulated in an alum adjuvant, and thimerosal (mercury derivative) 1:20,000 added as a preservative. The vaccine is prepared without regard to subtype. HEPTAVAX-B is indicated for immunization of persons at risk of infection from hepatitis B virus including all known subtypes.

CLINICAL PHARMACOLOGY

Hepatitis B virus is one of at least three hepatitis viruses that cause a systemic infection, with a major pathology in the liver. The others are hepatitis A virus, and non-A, non-B hepatitis viruses.

Hepatitis B virus is an important cause of viral hepatitis. There is no specific treatment for this disease. The incubation period for type B hepatitis is relatively long; six weeks to six months may elapse between exposure and the onset of clinical symptoms. The prognosis following infection with hepatitis B virus is variable and dependent on at least three factors: (1) Age—Infants and younger children usually experience milder initial disease than older persons; (2) Dose of Virus—The higher the dose, the more likely acute icteric hepatitis B will result; and, (3) Severity of Associated Underlying Disease—Underlying malignancy or pre-existing hepatic disease predisposes to increased mortality and morbidity.

Persistence of viral infection (the chronic hepatitis B virus carrier state) occurs in 5–10% of persons following acute hepatitis B, and occurs more frequently after initial anicteric hepatitis B than after initial icteric disease. Consequently, carriers of hepatitis B surface antigen (HBsAg) frequently give no history of recognized acute hepatitis. It has been estimated that more than 170 million people in the world today are persistently infected with hepatitis B virus. The Centers for Disease Control (CDC) estimates that there are approximately 0.7 to 1.0 million chronic carriers of hepatitis B virus in the USA and that this pool of carriers grows by 2%–3% (8,000 to 16,000 individuals) annually. Chronic carriers represent the largest human reservoir of hepatitis B virus.

The serious complications and sequelae of hepatitis B virus infection include massive hepatic necrosis, cirrhosis of the liver, chronic active hepatitis, and hepatocellular carcinoma. Chronic carriers of HBsAg appear to be at increased risk of developing hepatocellular carcinoma, which accounts for 80 to 90 percent of primary liver carcinomas. Although a number of etiologic factors are associated with development of hepatocellular carcinoma, the single most important etiologic factor appears to be active infection with the hepatitis B virus.

There is also evidence that several diseases other than hepatitis have been associated with hepatitis B virus infection through an immunologic mechanism involving antigen antibody complexes. Such diseases include a syndrome with rash, urticaria, and arthralgia resembling serum sickness; polyarteritis nodosa; membranous glomerulonephritis; and infantile papular acrodermatitis.

Although the vehicles for transmission of the virus are predominantly blood and blood products, viral antigen has also been found in tears, saliva, breast milk, urine, semen and vaginal secretions. Hepatitis B virus is quite stable and capable of surviving for days on environmental surfaces. Infection may occur when hepatitis B virus, transmitted by infected body fluids, is implanted via mucous surfaces or percutaneously introduced through accidental or deliberate breaks in the skin.

Transmission of hepatitis B virus infection is often associated with close interpersonal contact with an infected individual and with crowded living conditions. In such circumstances, transmission by inoculation via routes other than overt parenteral ones may be quite common. Infection in infancy by the hepatitis B virus usually leads to the chronic carrier state. Perinatal transmission of hepatitis B infection from infected mother to child, at or shortly after birth, can occur if the mother is a hepatitis B surface antigen (HBsAg) carrier or if the mother has an acute hepatitis B infection in the third trimester. Among infants born to women in whom sera are positive for both the hepatitis B surface antigen and the e antigen, 85–90% are infected and become chronic carriers.

Hepatitis B is endemic throughout the world and is a serious medical problem in population groups at increased risk. (Refer to INDICATIONS AND USAGE)

Numerous epidemiological studies have shown that persons who develop anti-HBs following active infection with the hepatitis B virus are protected against the disease on re-exposure to the virus.

Clinical studies established that HEPTAVAX-B when injected into the deltoid muscle induced protective levels of antibody in greater than 90% of healthy individuals who received the recommended 3 dose regimen. A lower response rate (81%) to vaccine may be obtained if the vaccine is administered as a buttock injection. A protective antibody (anti-HBs) level has been defined by the Immunization Practices Advisory Committee as 1) 10 or more sample ratio units (SRU) as determined by radioimmunoassay or 2) a positive result as determined by enzyme immunoassay. Note: 10 SRU is comparable to 10 mIU/mL of antibody.

Responsiveness to the vaccine is age dependent. The seroconversion rate for children 1–10 years of age was 100%. In contrast, seroconversion rates for adults ranged from 92 to 96% for those 20 to 49 years of age and 77% for those 50 years of age or older. Immunocompromised and immunosuppressed persons respond less well than do healthy individuals. Studies among hemodialysis patients show that approximately 60 percent of those who receive three 40 μg doses of the vaccine develop anti-HBs.

These studies show that vaccine-induced levels of anti-HBs also are lower and tend to remain at protective levels for shorter periods in hemodialysis patients than do levels in healthy adults. Protective efficacy of the vaccine was not demonstrated in hemodialysis patients in a large double-blind clinical study in which the overall attack rate for hepatitis B was low. Nevertheless, the Immunization Practices Advisory Committee (ACIP) in reviewing these data recommended that the vaccine continue to be used in hemodialysis patients as an adjunctive measure to reduce the rate of transmission of hepatitis B.

The protective efficacy of HEPTAVAX-B has been demonstrated in adults at high risk of contracting hepatitis B infection.

In two clinical trials efficacy was 98% for individuals whose anti-HBs titers were equal to or greater than 10 SRU after the recommended 3 doses of vaccine. These individuals were protected against acute hepatitis B, chronic antigenemia and asymptomatic infections (excluding seroconversion for anti-HBc). Efficacy among all vaccine recipients without regard to the level of antibody response was 82–87%.

In one of the above studies involving individuals at high risk of contracting hepatitis B infection, there was evidence of protective immunity in approximately 78% of vaccinated subjects following 2 doses of the 3 dose regimen. However, the third dose was required to raise the proportion of seroconverters to 92%, induce higher titers, and provide an extended period of protection.

In a third study, conducted in medical staff at hemodialysis units, protective antibody developed in 96% of vaccine recipients after administration of three doses of vaccine. Additionally, this study demonstrated the subtype cross-protection of HEPTAVAX-B. A lot of the vaccine selected to contain only the *ad* antigenic subtype induced protection against infection from the *ay* subtype hepatitis B virus. These results confirm that monovalent HBsAg/*ad* vaccine can provide protection in populations at high risk of infection with the *ay* subtype virus (e.g., patients and staff in hemodialysis units and users of illicit injectable drugs).

A protective level of anti-HBs (≥ 10 SRU) is produced in greater than 90% of healthy individuals when the 3 dose regimen of HEPTAVAX-B is administered in the deltoid muscle. In regard to serologic confirmation of post-vaccination immunity and revaccination of nonresponders, the Immunization Practices Advisory Committee has issued the following recommendations:

Testing for immunity following vaccination is not recommended routinely but is advised for persons whose subsequent management depends on knowing their immune status, such as dialysis patients and staff, and for persons in whom a suboptimal response may be anticipated, such as those who have received vaccine in the buttock.

Revaccination of persons who do not respond to the primary series (nonresponders) produces adequate antibody in only one-third when the primary vaccination has been given in the deltoid. Therefore, revaccination of non-responders to deltoid injection is not recommended routinely. For persons who did not respond to a primary vaccine series given in the buttock, preliminary data from two small studies suggest that revaccination in the arm induces adequate antibody in over 75%. Revaccination should be strongly considered for such persons.

Adverse reactions in individuals who have received a fourth or fifth injection have been similar in type and severity to those of the initial three dose series (see ADVERSE REACTIONS).

The duration of protection and need for booster doses are not yet defined. Studies have shown that anti-HBs levels may fall below 10 SRU in some vaccinees over a period of 3–4 years. In one study, 71% of adults who initially responded to the vaccine with protective levels of anti-HBs retained levels of ≥ 10 SRU over 4½ years. Among those in this population who lost antibody, protection against chronic antigenemia and hepatitis appeared to persist. Individuals who remain at high risk of exposure to hepatitis B virus may wish to periodically determine their anti-HBs level. If antibody levels fall below 10 SRU, administration of an additional dose of HEPTAVAX-B should be considered.

Recent studies have established the relative efficacies of immune globulin and/or hepatitis B vaccine in infants born to HBsAg-positive, HBeAg-positive mothers; following accidental percutaneous or permucosal exposure to HBsAg positive blood, or sexual exposure to HBsAg-positive persons (See DOSAGE AND ADMINISTRATION).

It has been demonstrated that Hepatitis B Immune Globulin, when administered simultaneously with HEPTAVAX-B at separate body sites, did not interfere with the induction of protective antibodies against hepatitis B virus elicited by the vaccine.

Reports in the literature describe a more virulent form of hepatitis B (case fatality rates of up to 12%) associated with superinfections or coinfections by delta virus, an incomplete RNA virus. Delta virus can only infect and cause illness in persons infected with hepatitis B virus since the delta agent requires a coat of HBsAg in order to become infectious. Therefore, persons immune to hepatitis B virus infection should also be immune to delta virus infection.

Interchangeability of Plasma-Derived and Recombinant Hepatitis B Vaccines

Unlike plasma-derived vaccine, recombinant-derived vaccine is produced in yeast by the hepatitis B virus gene which codes for the hepatitis B surface antigen (HBsAg). Like plasma-derived vaccine, recombinant-derived vaccine is a protein aggregate or particle visible by electron microscopy containing important vaccine antigen epitopes as determined by monoclonal antibody analyses.

Recombinant-derived vaccine has been shown by *in vitro* analyses to induce antibodies (anti-HBs) which are biochemically and immunologically comparable by extent of binding, and both avidity and affinity of binding to virus-derived antigen, to antibodies induced by plasma-derived vaccine. In cross absorption studies, the spectra of antibodies induced in man to plasma-derived or to recombinant hepatitis B vaccines were indistinguishable.

The recommended doses of HEPTAVAX-B and RECOMBIVAX HB® [Hepatitis B Vaccine (Recombinant), MSD] have resulted in similar seroconversion rates in healthy persons; the geometric mean titers (GMTs) following RECOMBIVAX HB [Hepatitis B Vaccine (Recombinant), MSD] have been lower in some studies and equivalent in others but were many times greater than the minimum level associated with protection (≥ 10 mIU/mL). A single injection of the recommended dose of RECOMBIVAX HB [Hepatitis B Vaccine (Recombinant), MSD] induced significant anamnestic antibody responses in 97% of 31 healthy adults vaccinated 5 to 7 years previously with HEPTAVAX-B.

There have been no clinical studies in which a three-dose vaccine series was initiated with HEPTAVAX-B and completed with RECOMBIVAX HB [Hepatitis B Vaccine (Recombinant), MSD], or vice versa. However, based on the comparability of the plasma-derived and recombinant-derived vaccines in extensive *in vitro* and *in vivo* studies as described above, it is possible to interchange the use of these two vaccines (but see CONTRAINDICATIONS).

INDICATIONS AND USAGE

HEPTAVAX-B is indicated for immunization against infection caused by all known subtypes of hepatitis B virus. HEPTAVAX-B will not prevent hepatitis caused by other agents, such as hepatitis A virus, non-A, non-B hepatitis viruses, or other viruses known to infect the liver.

Vaccination is recommended in persons of all ages, especially those who are or will be at increased risk of infection with hepatitis B virus, for example:

- **Health Care Personnel**
  Dentists and oral surgeons.
  Physicians and surgeons.
  Nurses.
  Paramedical personnel and custodial staff who may be exposed to the virus via blood or other patient specimens.
  Dental hygienists and dental nurses.
  Laboratory personnel handling blood, blood products and other patient specimens.
  Dental, medical and nursing students.
- *Selected Patients and Patient Contacts*
  Patients and staff in hemodialysis units and hematology/oncology units.
  Patients requiring frequent and/or large volume blood transfusions or clotting factor concentrates (e.g., persons with hemophilia, thalassemia).
  Clients (residents) and staff of institutions for the mentally handicapped.
  Classroom contacts of deinstitutionalized mentally handicapped persons who have persistent hepatitis B antigenemia and who show aggressive behavior.
  Household and other intimate contacts of persons with persistent hepatitis B antigenemia.
- *Infants Born to HBsAg Positive Mothers* (See DOSAGE AND ADMINISTRATION)
- *Populations with high incidence of the disease,* such as:
  Alaskan Eskimos.
  Indochinese refugees.
  Haitian refugees.
- *Military Personnel identified as being at increased risk*
- *Morticians and Embalmers*
- *Blood bank and plasma fractionation workers*
- *Persons at Increased Risk of the Disease Due to Their Sexual Practices,* such as:
  Persons who repeatedly contract sexually transmitted diseases.
  Homosexually active males.
  Female prostitutes.
- *Prisoners*
- *Users of illicit injectable drugs*

Revaccination
See CLINICAL PHARMACOLOGY

CONTRAINDICATIONS

Hypersensitivity to any component of the vaccine.

WARNINGS

Persons with immuno-deficiency or those receiving immunosuppressive therapy require larger vaccine doses and respond less well than do healthy individuals. Refer to DOSAGE AND ADMINISTRATION for use in such individuals. Because of the long incubation period for hepatitis B, it is possible for unrecognized infection to be present at the time HEPTAVAX-B is given. HEPTAVAX-B may not prevent hepatitis B in such patients.

Patients who develop symptoms suggestive of hypersensitivity after an injection should not receive further injections of HEPTAVAX-B (see CONTRAINDICATIONS and ADVERSE REACTIONS).

PRECAUTIONS

General
As with any parenteral vaccine, epinephrine should be available for immediate use should an anaphylactoid reaction occur.

Any serious active infection is reason for delaying use of HEPTAVAX-B, except when, in the opinion of the physician, withholding the vaccine entails a greater risk.

Caution and appropriate care should be exercised in administering HEPTAVAX-B to individuals with severely compromised cardiopulmonary status or to others in whom a febrile or systemic reaction could pose a significant risk.

Pregnancy
Pregnancy Category C. Animal reproduction studies have not been conducted with HEPTAVAX-B. It is also not known whether HEPTAVAX-B can cause fetal harm when administered to a pregnant woman or can affect reproductive capacity. HEPTAVAX-B should be given to a pregnant woman only if clearly needed.

Nursing Mothers
Studies in 12 lactating women have failed to reveal evidence of this vaccine being secreted in breast milk.

Pediatric Use
HEPTAVAX-B has been shown to be well-tolerated and highly immunogenic in infants and children of all ages. New-

Continued on next page

Information on the Merck Sharp & Dohme products listed on these pages is the full prescribing information from product circulars in use August 31, 1989.

Merck Sharp & Dohme—Cont.

borns also respond well; maternally transferred antibodies do not interfere with the active immune response to the vaccine. See DOSAGE AND ADMINISTRATION for recommended pediatric dosage and for recommended dosage for infants born to HBsAg positive mothers.

ADVERSE REACTIONS

HEPTAVAX-B is generally well tolerated. No serious adverse reactions attributable to vaccination were reported during the course of clinical trials involving administration of HEPTAVAX-B to over 19,000 individuals. There was no tendency towards increasing frequency or severity of complaints with successive doses of the vaccine. As with any vaccine, there is the possibility that broad use of the vaccine could reveal rare adverse reactions not observed in clinical trials.

In three double-blind placebo-controlled studies among 3,350 persons, the overall rates of adverse reactions reported by vaccine recipients (24.3%, 21.5% and 22.8%) did not differ significantly from those of placebo recipients (21.4%, 18.7% and 21.9%). Approximately half of all reported reactions were injection site soreness, which occurred somewhat more frequently among vaccine recipients.

In another group of studies, 3,516 doses of vaccine were administered to 1,255 healthy adults. Vaccinees were monitored for 5 days after each dose, and the following adverse reactions were reported:

	% of doses
BODY AS A WHOLE	
Injection site reactions, consisting principally of soreness, and including erythema, swelling, warmth and induration	12.3
Fatigue/asthenia	1.9
Malaise	0.8
Fever (≥ 100°F)	1.8
Chills	0.4
Sensation of warmth	0.4
Irritability	0.1
Diaphoresis	0.1
DIGESTIVE SYSTEM	
Gastrointestinal illness including anorexia, nausea, vomiting, abdominal pain and diarrhea	2.0
Abdominal cramps	0.3
HEMATOLOGIC AND LYMPHATIC SYSTEM	
Adenitis	0.1
MUSCULOSKELETAL SYSTEM	
Myalgia	1.2
Arthralgia	0.7
NERVOUS SYSTEM	
Headache	3.1
Dizziness	0.5
Disturbed sleep	0.2
Paresthesia	0.2
RESPIRATORY SYSTEM	
Upper respiratory illness	2.5
INTEGUMENTARY SYSTEM	
Rash (non-specific)	0.3

In a double-blind, placebo-controlled, clinical trial of 1,330 health-care workers, the frequency of elevations in SGPT (ALT) in vaccine recipients was not significantly different from that in placebo recipients. In marketed use of the vaccine, non-specific abnormalities in SGPT (ALT) and other liver function tests have been reported, but no causal relationship has been established.

Body as a Whole
Soreness, swelling and pain in the injected arm.

The following additional adverse reactions have been reported with use of the marketed vaccine:

Hypersensitivity Reactions
Anaphylaxis; and symptoms of immediate hypersensitivity including urticaria, edema, angioedema, and pruritus have been reported rarely within the first few hours after vaccination. An apparent hypersensitivity syndrome of delayed onset has been reported rarely, days to weeks after vaccination. This has included the following findings: arthritis (usually transient), fever, and dermatologic reactions such as urticaria, erythema multiforme, or ecchymoses (see WARNINGS).

Nervous System
Neurological disorders such as: optic neuritis; myelitis, including transverse myelitis; acute radiculoneuropathy, including Guillain-Barré syndrome; peripheral neuropathy, including Bell's Palsy and herpes zoster; and vertigo.

Hematologic
Thrombocytopenia with or without purpura.

Special Senses
Tinnitus, visual disturbances.

Integumentary System
Flushing.

DOSAGE AND ADMINISTRATION

Do not inject intravenously or intradermally.
HEPTAVAX-B is for intramuscular injection. The deltoid muscle is the preferred site for intramuscular injection in adults. Data suggest that injections given in the buttocks frequently are given into fatty tissue instead of into muscle. Such injections may result in a lower seroconversion rate than is expected. The anterolateral thigh is the recommended site for intramuscular injection in infants and children.

HEPTAVAX-B may be administered subcutaneously to persons at risk of hemorrhage following intramuscular injections. The immune responses and clinical reactions following intramuscular and subcutaneous administration of HEPTAVAX-B have been shown to be comparable. However, when other aluminum-adsorbed vaccines have been administered subcutaneously, an increased incidence of local reactions including subcutaneous nodules has been observed. Therefore, subcutaneous administration should be used only in persons (e.g., hemophiliacs) at risk of hemorrhage following intramuscular injections.

Shake well before withdrawal and use. Thorough agitation at the time of administration is necessary to maintain suspension of the vaccine.

Parenteral drug products should be inspected visually for particulate matter and discoloration prior to administration. After thorough agitation, HEPTAVAX-B is a slightly opaque, white suspension.

The immunization regimen consists of 3 doses of vaccine given according to the following schedule:

  1st dose: at elected date
  2nd dose: 1 month later
  3rd dose: 6 months after the first dose

The volume of vaccine to be given on each occasion is as follows:
[See table below].
Revaccination—(see CLINICAL PHARMACOLOGY).

Dosage For Infants Born of HBsAg Positive Mothers
Infants born to HBsAg positive mothers are at high risk of becoming chronic carriers of hepatitis B virus and of developing the chronic sequelae of hepatitis B virus infection. Well-controlled studies have shown that administration of three 0.5 mL doses of Hepatitis B Immune Globulin starting at birth is 75% effective in preventing establishment of the chronic carrier state in these infants during the first year of life. Protection can be transient, whereupon the effectiveness of the Hepatitis B Immune Globulin would decline thereafter. Results from clinical studies indicate that administration of one 0.5 mL dose of Hepatitis B Immune Globulin at birth and three 20 mcg (1.0 mL) doses of HEPTAVAX-B, the first dose given within one week after birth, was 85–93% effective in preventing establishment of the chronic carrier state in infants born to HBsAg and HBeAg positive mothers. Preliminary data from studies using one 0.5 mL dose of Hepatitis B Immune Globulin and three 10 mcg (0.5 mL) doses of HEPTAVAX-B in the same type of population indicate that this lower dose of vaccine is equally effective.

Testing for HBsAg and anti-HBs is recommended at 12–15 months. If HBsAg is not detectable, and anti-HBs is present, the child has been protected.

The recommended dosage for infants born to HBsAg positive mothers is as follows:

Treatment	Birth	Within 7 days	1 month	6 months
HEPTAVAX-B pediatric formulation 10 mcg/0.5 mL		0.5 mL*	0.5 mL	0.5 mL
HEPATITIS B IMMUNE GLOBULIN	0.5 mL	—	—	—

*The first dose of HEPTAVAX-B may be given at birth at the same time as Hepatitis B Immune Globulin, but should be administered in the opposite anterolateral thigh. This procedure may be preferable to ensure absorption of the vaccine.

Known or Presumed Exposure to HBsAg
There are no prospective studies directly testing the efficacy of a combination of Hepatitis B Immune Globulin and HEPTAVAX-B in preventing clinical hepatitis B following percutaneous, ocular or mucous membrane exposure to hepatitis B virus. However, since most persons with such exposures (e.g., health care workers) are candidates for the hepatitis B vaccine and since combined hepatitis B Immune Globulin plus vaccine is more efficacious than Hepatitis B Immune Globulin alone in perinatal exposures, the following guidelines are recommended for persons who have been exposed to hepatitis B virus such as through (1) percutaneous (needlestick), ocular, mucous membrane exposure to blood known or presumed to contain HBsAg, (2) human bites by known or presumed HBsAg carriers, that penetrate the skin, or (3) following intimate sexual contact with known or presumed HBsAg carriers:

Hepatitis B Immune Globulin (0.06 mL/kg) should be given as soon as possible after exposure and within 24 hours if possible. Hepatitis B vaccine 1.0 mL (20 mcg/1.0 mL) should be given intramuscularly within 7 days of exposure and second and third doses given one and six months, respectively, after the first dose.

The vaccine is used as supplied; no dilution or reconstitution is necessary. It is important to use a separate sterile syringe and needle for each individual patient to prevent transmission of hepatitis and other infectious agents from one person to another.

3.0 mL Vial
For Syringe Use Only: Withdraw the recommended dose from the vial using a sterile needle and syringe free of preservatives, antiseptics, and detergents.

HOW SUPPLIED

No. 4720—HEPTAVAX-B, Adult Formulation, is supplied as a multi-dose vial of vaccine, 20 mcg/1.0 mL, NDC 0006-4720-00 in 3 mL vials (6505-01-139-5000, 3 mL).
No. 4736—HEPTAVAX-B, Pediatric Formulation, is supplied as a one dose vial of vaccine, 10 mcg/0.5 mL, NDC 0006-4736-00 in 0.5 mL vials.

Storage
Store unopened and opened vials at 2–8°C (35.6–46.4°F). Storage above or below the recommended temperature may reduce potency.
Do not freeze since freezing destroys potency.
          A.H.F.S. Category: 80:12
    DC 7409209   Issued April 1988
COPYRIGHT © MERCK & CO., INC., 1985
All rights reserved

HUMORSOL® Sterile Ophthalmic Solution   ℞
(Demecarium Bromide, MSD), U.S.P.
For Topical Application into the
Conjunctival Sac Only

DESCRIPTION

Ophthalmic Solution HUMORSOL® (Demecarium Bromide, MSD) is a sterile solution supplied in two dosage strengths: 0.125 percent and 0.25 percent. The inactive ingredients are sodium chloride and water for injection; benzalkonium chloride 1:5000 is added as preservative. Demecarium bromide is a quaternary ammonium compound with a molecular weight of 716.60. Its chemical name is 3,3'-[1,10-decanediylbis [(methylimino)carbonyloxy]] bis [*N,N,N*-trimethylbenzenaminium] dibromide. Its empirical formula is $C_{32}H_{52}Br_2N_4O_4$ and its structural formula is:
[See Chemical Formula at top of next column].

CLINICAL PHARMACOLOGY

HUMORSOL is a cholinesterase inhibitor with sustained activity. It acts mainly on true (erythrocyte) cholinesterase.

HEPTAVAX-B

Group	Formulation	Initial	1 month	6 months
Younger Children (Birth to 10 years of age)	Pediatric 10 mcg/0.5 mL	0.5 mL	0.5 mL	0.5 mL
Adults and Older Children	Adult 20 mcg/1.0 mL	1.0 mL	1.0 mL	1.0 mL
Dialysis Patients and Immunocompromised Patients	Adult 20 mcg/1.0 mL	2.0 mL*	2.0 mL*	2.0 mL*

*Two 1.0 mL doses given at different sites.

Application of HUMORSOL to the eye produces intense miosis and ciliary muscle contraction due to inhibition of cholinesterase, allowing acetylcholine to accumulate at sites of cholinergic transmission. These effects are accompanied by increased capillary permeability of the ciliary body and iris, increased permeability of the blood-aqueous barrier, and vasodilation. Myopia may be induced or, if present, may be augmented by the increased refractive power of the lens that results from the accommodative effect of the drug. HUMORSOL indirectly produces some of the muscarinic and nicotinic effects of acetylcholine as quantities of the latter accumulate.

INDICATIONS AND USAGE

Open-angle glaucoma (HUMORSOL should be used in glaucoma only when shorter-acting miotics have proved inadequate.)
Conditions obstructing aqueous outflow, such as synechial formation, that are amenable to miotic therapy
Following iridectomy
Accommodative esotropia (accommodative convergent strabismus)

CONTRAINDICATIONS

Hypersensitivity to any component of this product.
Because of the toxicity of cholinesterase inhibitors in general, HUMORSOL is contraindicated in women who are or who may become pregnant. If this drug is used during pregnancy, or if the patient becomes pregnant while taking this drug, the patient should be apprised of the potential hazard to the fetus.
Because miotics may aggravate inflammation, HUMORSOL should not be used in active uveal inflammation and/or glaucoma associated with iridocyclitis.

WARNINGS

In patients receiving cholinesterase inhibitors such as HUMORSOL, succinylcholine should be administered with extreme caution before and during general anesthesia.
Because of possible adverse additive effects, HUMORSOL should be administered only with extreme caution to patients with myasthenia gravis who are receiving systemic anticholinesterase therapy; conversely, extreme caution should be exercised in the use of an anticholinesterase drug for the treatment of myasthenia gravis patients who are already undergoing topical therapy with cholinesterase inhibitors.

PRECAUTIONS

General
Gonioscopy is recommended prior to medication with HUMORSOL.
HUMORSOL should be used with caution in patients with chronic angle-closure (narrow-angle) glaucoma or in patients with narrow angles, because of the possibility of producing pupillary block and increasing angle blockage.
When an intraocular inflammatory process is present, the intensity and persistence of miosis and ciliary muscle contraction that result from anticholinesterase therapy require abstention from, or cautious use of, HUMORSOL.
Systemic effects are infrequent when HUMORSOL is instilled carefully. Compression of the lacrimal duct for several seconds immediately following instillation minimizes drainage into the nasal chamber with its extensive absorption surface. Wash the hands immediately after instillation.
Discontinue HUMORSOL if salivation, urinary incontinence, diarrhea, profuse sweating, muscle weakness, respiratory difficulties, shock, or cardiac irregularities occur.
Persons receiving cholinesterase inhibitors who are exposed to organophosphate-type insecticides and pesticides (gardeners, organophosphate plant or warehouse workers, farmers, residents of communities which are undergoing insecticide spraying or dusting, etc.) should be warned of the added systemic effects possible from absorption through the respiratory tract or skin. Wearing of respiratory masks, frequent washing, and clothing changes may be advisable.
Anticholinesterase drugs should be used with extreme caution, if at all, in patients with marked vagotonia, bronchial asthma, spastic gastrointesinal disturbances, peptic ulcer, pronounced bradycardia and hypotension, recent myocardial infarction, epilepsy, parkinsonism, and other disorders that may respond adversely to vagotonic effects.

After long-term use of HUMORSOL, dilation of blood vessels and resulting greater permeability increase the possibility of hyphema during ophthalmic surgery. Therefore, this drug should be discontinued before surgery.
Despite observance of all precautions and the use of only the recommended dose, there is some evidence that repeated administration may cause depression of the concentration of cholinesterase in the serum and erythrocytes, with resultant systemic effects.
Drug Interactions
See WARNINGS regarding possible drug interactions of HUMORSOL with succinylcholine or with other anticholinesterase agents.
Carcinogenesis, Mutagenesis, Impairment of Fertility
Long-term studies in animals have not been performed to evaluate the effects of HUMORSOL on fertility or carcinogenic potential.
Pregnancy
Pregnancy Category X: See CONTRAINDICATIONS.
Nursing Mothers
It is not known whether this drug is excreted in human milk. Because of the potential for serious adverse reactions in nursing infants from HUMORSOL, a decision should be made whether to discontinue nursing or to discontinue the drug, taking into account the importance of the drug to the mother.
Pediatric Use
The occurrence of iris cysts is more frequent in children. (See ADVERSE REACTIONS and DOSAGE AND ADMINISTRATION.)
Extreme caution should be exercised in children receiving HUMORSOL who may require general anesthesia (see WARNINGS).
Since HUMORSOL is a potent cholinesterase inhibitor it should be kept out of the reach of children.

ADVERSE REACTIONS

Stinging, burning, lacrimation, lid muscle twitching, conjunctival and ciliary redness, brow ache, headache, and induced myopia with visual blurring may occur.
Activation of latent iritis or uveitis may occur.
As with all miotic therapy, retinal detachment has been reported occasionally.
Iris cysts may form, enlarge, and obscure vision. Occurrence is more frequent in children. The iris cyst usually shrinks upon discontinuance of the miotic. Rarely, the cyst may rupture or break free into the aqueous. Frequent examination for this occurrence is advised.
Lens opacities have been reported in patients on miotic therapy. Routine slit-lamp examinations, including the lens, should accompany prolonged use.
Paradoxical increase in intraocular pressure may follow anticholinesterase instillation. This may be alleviated by pupil-dilating medication.
Prolonged use may cause conjunctival thickening and obstruction of nasolacrimal canals.
Systemic effects, which occur rarely, are suggestive of increased cholinergic activity. Such effects may include nausea, vomiting, abdominal cramps, diarrhea, urinary incontinence, salivation, sweating, difficulty in breathing, bradycardia, or cardiac irregularities. Medical management of systemic effects may be indicated (see TREATMENT OF ADVERSE EFFECTS).

TREATMENT OF ADVERSE EFFECTS

If HUMORSOL is taken systemically by accident, or if systemic effects occur after topical application in the eye or from accidental skin contact, administer atropine sulfate parenterally (intravenously if necessary) in a dose (for adults) of 0.4 to 0.6 mg or more. The recommended dosage of atropine in infants and children up to 12 years of age is 0.01 mg/kg repeated every two hours as needed until the desired effect is obtained, or adverse effects of atropine preclude further usage. The maximum single dose should not exceed 0.4 mg.
The use of much larger doses of atropine in treating anticholinesterase intoxication in adults has been reported in the literature. Initially 2 to 6 mg may be given followed by 2 mg every hour or more often, as long as muscarinic effects continue. The greater possibility of atropinization with large doses, particularly in sensitive individuals, should be borne in mind.
Pralidoxime* chloride has been reported to be useful in treating systemic effects due to cholinesterase inhibitors. However, its use is recommended in addition to and not as substitute for atropine.
A short-acting barbiturate is indicated if convulsions occur that are not entirely relieved by atropine. Barbiturate dosage should be carefully adjusted to avoid central respiratory depression. Marked weakness or paralysis of muscles of res-

---

*PROTOPAM® Chloride (Pralidoxime Chloride). Ayerst Laboratories

piration should be treated promptly by artificial respiration and maintenance of a clear airway.
The oral LD_{50} of HUMORSOL is 2.96 mg/kg in the mouse.

DOSAGE AND ADMINISTRATION

HUMORSOL *is intended solely for topical use in the conjunctival sac.*
As HUMORSOL is an extremely potent drug, the physician should thoroughly familiarize himself with its use and the technic of instillation.
The required dose is applied in the conjunctival sac, with the patient supine, care being taken not to touch the cornea with the tip of the OCUMETER** ophthalmic dispenser. *The patient or person administering the medication should apply continuous gentle pressure on the lacrimal duct with the index finger for several seconds immediately following instillation of the drops. This is to prevent drainage overflow of solution into the nasal and pharyngeal spaces, which might cause systemic absorption. Wash the hands immediately after administration.*
HUMORSOL *should not be used more often than directed. Caution is necessary to avoid overdosage.*
Initial titration and dosage adjustments with HUMORSOL must be individualized to obtain maximal therapeutic effect. The patient must be closely observed during the initial period. If the response is not adequate within the first 24 hours, other measures should be considered.
Keep frequency of use to a minimum in all patients, but especially in children, to reduce the chance of iris cyst development (see ADVERSE REACTIONS).
Glaucoma
For initial therapy with HUMORSOL (0.125 percent or 0.25 percent) place 1 drop (children) or 1 or 2 drops (adults) in the glaucomatous eye. A decrease in intraocular pressure should occur within a few hours. During this period, keep the patient under supervision and make tonometric examinations at least hourly for 3 or 4 hours to be sure that no immediate rise in pressure occurs (see ADVERSE REACTIONS).

Duration of effect varies with the individual. The usual dosage can vary from as much as 1 or 2 drops twice a day to as little as 1 or 2 drops twice a week. The 0.125 percent strength used twice a day usually results in smooth control of the physiologic diurnal variation in intraocular pressure. This is probably the preferred dosage for most wide (open) angle glaucoma patients.

Strabismus
Essentially equal visual acuity of both eyes is a prerequisite to the successful treatment of esotropia with HUMORSOL. For initial evaluation it may be used as a diagnostic aid to determine if an accommodative factor exists. This is especially useful preoperatively in young children and in patients with normal hypermetropic refractive errors. One drop is given daily for 2 weeks, then 1 drop every 2 days for 2 to 3 weeks. If the eyes become straighter, an accommodative factor is demonstrated. This technic may supplement or complement standard testing with atropine and trial with glasses for the accommodative factor.

In esotropia uncomplicated by amblyopia or anisometropia, HUMORSOL may be instilled in both eyes, *not more than 1 drop at a time every day for 2 to 3 weeks*, as too severe a degree of miosis may interfere with vision. Then reduce the dosage to 1 drop every other day for 3 to 4 weeks and reevaluate the patient's status.
HUMORSOL may be continued in a dosage of 1 drop every 2 days to 1 drop twice a week. (The latter dosage may be maintained for several months.) Evaluate the patient's condition every 4 to 12 weeks. If improvement continues, change the schedule to 1 drop once a week and eventually to a trial without medication. However, if after 4 months, control of the condition still requires 1 drop every 2 days, therapy with HUMORSOL should be stopped.

HOW SUPPLIED

Sterile Ophthalmic Solution HUMORSOL is a clear, colorless, aqueous solution and is supplied in a 5 mL white, opaque, plastic OCUMETER ophthalmic dispenser with a controlled-drop tip:
No. 3255—0.125 percent solution.
  NDC 0006-3255-03.
No. 3267—0.25 percent solution.
  NDC 0006-3267-03.

**Registered trademark of MERCK & CO., Inc.

Continued on next page

Merck Sharp & Dohme—Cont.

Storage
Protect from freezing and excessive heat.

A.H.F.S. Category: 52:20
DC 7414311 Issued October 1987
COPYRIGHT © MERCK & CO., INC., 1987
All rights reserved

HYDELTRASOL® Injection, Sterile ℞
(Prednisolone Sodium Phosphate, MSD), U.S.P.

DESCRIPTION

Prednisolone sodium phosphate, a synthetic adrenocortical steroid, is a white or slightly yellow powder that is slightly hygroscopic and is freely soluble in water. The molecular weight is 484.39. It is designated chemically as 11β, 17-dihydroxy-21-(phosphonooxy) pregna-1,4-diene-3,20-dione disodium salt. The empirical formula is $C_{21}H_{27}Na_2O_8P$ and the structural formula is:

HYDELTRASOL® (Prednisolone Sodium Phosphate, MSD) injection is a sterile solution (pH 7.0 to 8.0) for intravenous, intramuscular, intra-articular, intralesional, and soft tissue administration.
Each milliliter contains prednisolone sodium phosphate equivalent to 20 mg prednisolone phosphate. Inactive ingredients per mL: niacinamide, 25 mg; sodium hydroxide to adjust pH; disodium edetate, 0.5 mg; Water for Injection, q.s. 1 mL. Sodium bisulfite, 1 mg, and phenol, 5 mg, added as preservatives.

ACTIONS

HYDELTRASOL injection has a rapid onset but short duration of action when compared with less soluble preparations. Because of this, it is suitable for the treatment of acute disorders responsive to adrenocortical steroid therapy.
Naturally occurring glucocorticoids (hydrocortisone and cortisone), which also have salt-retaining properties, are used as replacement therapy in adrenocortical deficiency states. Their synthetic analogs, including prednisolone, are primarily used for their potent anti-inflammatory effects in disorders of many organ systems.
Glucocorticoids cause profound and varied metabolic effects. In addition, they modify the body's immune responses to diverse stimuli.
At equipotent anti-inflammatory doses, prednisolone has less tendency to cause salt and water retention than either hydrocortisone or cortisone.

INDICATIONS

A. By intravenous or intramuscular injection when oral therapy is not feasible:
1. *Endocrine disorders*
   Primary or secondary adrenocortical insufficiency (hydrocortisone or cortisone is the drug of choice; synthetic analogs may be used in conjunction with mineralocorticoids where applicable; in infancy, mineralocorticoid supplementation is of particular importance)
   Acute adrenocortical insufficiency (hydrocortisone or cortisone is the drug of choice; mineralocorticoid supplementation may be necessary, particularly when synthetic analogs are used)
   Preoperatively, and in the event of serious trauma or illness, in patients with known adrenal insufficiency or when adrenocortical reserve is doubtful
   Congenital adrenal hyperplasia
   Nonsuppurative thyroiditis
   Hypercalcemia associated with cancer
2. *Rheumatic disorders*
   As adjunctive therapy for short-term administration (to tide the patient over an acute episode or exacerbation) in:
   Post-traumatic osteoarthritis
   Synovitis of osteoarthritis
   Rheumatoid arthritis, including juvenile rheumatoid arthritis (selected cases may require low-dose maintenance therapy)
   Acute and subacute bursitis
   Epicondylitis
   Acute nonspecific tenosynovitis
   Acute gouty arthritis

   Psoriatic arthritis
   Ankylosing spondylitis
3. *Collagen diseases*
   During an exacerbation or as maintenance therapy in selected cases of:
   Systemic lupus erythematosus
   Acute rheumatic carditis
   Systemic dermatomyositis (polymyositis)
4. *Dermatologic diseases*
   Pemphigus
   Severe erythema multiforme (Stevens-Johnson syndrome)
   Exfoliative dermatitis
   Bullous dermatitis herpetiformis
   Severe seborrheic dermatitis
   Severe psoriasis
   Mycosis fungoides
5. *Allergic states*
   Control of severe or incapacitating allergic conditions intractable to adequate trials of conventional treatment in:
   Bronchial asthma
   Contact dermatitis
   Atopic dermatitis
   Serum sickness
   Seasonal or perennial allergic rhinitis
   Drug hypersensitivity reactions
   Urticarial transfusion reactions
   Acute noninfectious laryngeal edema (epinephrine is the drug of first choice)
6. *Ophthalmic diseases*
   Severe acute and chronic allergic and inflammatory processes involving the eye, such as:
   Herpes zoster ophthalmicus
   Iritis, iridocyclitis
   Chorioretinitis
   Diffuse posterior uveitis and choroiditis
   Optic neuritis
   Sympathetic ophthalmia
   Anterior segment inflammation
   Allergic conjunctivitis
   Keratitis
   Allergic corneal marginal ulcers
7. *Gastrointestinal diseases*
   To tide the patient over a critical period of the disease in:
   Ulcerative colitis (Systemic therapy)
   Regional enteritis (Systemic therapy)
8. *Respiratory diseases*
   Symptomatic sarcoidosis
   Berylliosis
   Fulminating or disseminated pulmonary tuberculosis when used concurrently with appropriate antituberculous chemotherapy
   Loeffler's syndrome not manageable by other means
   Aspiration pneumonitis
9. *Hematologic disorders*
   Acquired (autoimmune) hemolytic anemia
   Idiopathic thrombocytopenic purpura in adults (I.V. only; I.M. administration is contraindicated)
   Secondary thrombocytopenia in adults
   Erythroblastopenia (RBC anemia)
   Congenital (erythroid) hypoplastic anemia
10. *Neoplastic diseases*
    For palliative management of:
    Leukemias and lymphomas in adults
    Acute leukemia of childhood
11. *Edematous states*
    To induce diuresis or remission of proteinuria in the nephrotic syndrome, without uremia, of the idiopathic type, or that due to lupus erythematosus
12. *Miscellaneous*
    Tuberculous meningitis with subarachnoid block or impending block when used concurrently with appropriate antituberculous chemotherapy
    Trichinosis with neurologic or myocardial involvement.

B. By intra-articular or soft tissue injection:
   As adjunctive therapy for short-term administration (to tide the patient over an acute episode or exacerbation) in:
   Synovitis of osteoarthritis
   Rheumatoid arthritis
   Acute and subacute bursitis
   Acute gouty arthritis
   Epicondylitis
   Acute nonspecific tenosynovitis
   Post-traumatic osteoarthritis.

C. By intralesional injection:
   Keloids
   Localized hypertrophic, infiltrated, inflammatory lesions of: lichen planus, psoriatic plaques, granuloma annulare, and lichen simplex chronicus (neurodermatitis)
   Discoid lupus erythematosus
   Necrobiosis lipoidica diabeticorum
   Alopecia areata
   May also be useful in cystic tumors of an aponeurosis or tendon (ganglia).

CONTRAINDICATIONS

Systemic fungal infections (see WARNINGS regarding amphotericin B)
Hypersensitivity to any component of this product, including sulfites (see WARNINGS).

WARNINGS

Because rare instances of anaphylactoid reactions have occurred in patients receiving parenteral corticosteroid therapy, appropriate precautionary measures should be taken prior to administration, especially when the patient has a history of allergy to any drug. Anaphylactoid and hypersensitivity reactions have been reported for Injection HYDELTRASOL (see ADVERSE REACTIONS).
Injection HYDELTRASOL contains sodium bisulfite, a sulfite that may cause allergic-type reactions including anaphylactic symptoms and life-threatening or less severe asthmatic episodes in certain susceptible people. The overall prevalence of sulfite sensitivity in the general population is unknown and probably low. Sulfite sensitivity is seen more frequently in asthmatic than in nonasthmatic people.
Corticosteroids may exacerbate systemic fungal infections and therefore should not be used in the presence of such infections unless they are needed to control drug reactions due to amphotericin B. Moreover, there have been cases reported in which concomitant use of amphotericin B and hydrocortisone was followed by cardiac enlargement and congestive failure.
In patients on corticosteroid therapy subjected to any unusual stress, increased dosage of rapidly acting corticosteroids before, during, and after the stressful situation is indicated.
Drug-induced secondary adrenocortical insufficiency may result from too rapid withdrawal of corticosteroids and may be minimized by gradual reduction of dosage. This type of relative insufficiency may persist for months after discontinuation of therapy; therefore, in any situation of stress occurring during that period, hormone therapy should be reinstituted. If the patient is receiving steroids already, dosage may have to be increased. Since mineralocorticoid secretion may be impaired, salt and/or a mineralocorticoid should be administered concurrently.
Corticosteroids may mask some signs of infection, and new infections may appear during their use. There may be decreased resistance and inability to localize infection when corticosteroids are used. Moreover, corticosteroids may affect the nitroblue-tetrazolium test for bacterial infection and produce false negative results.
In cerebral malaria, a double-blind trial has shown that the use of corticosteroids is associated with prolongation of coma and a higher incidence of pneumonia and gastrointestinal bleeding.
Corticosteroids may activate latent amebiasis. Therefore, it is recommended that latent or active amebiasis be ruled out before initiating corticosteroid therapy in any patient who has spent time in the tropics or any patient with unexplained diarrhea.
Prolonged use of corticosteroids may produce posterior subcapsular cataracts, glaucoma with possible damage to the optic nerves, and may enhance the establishment of secondary ocular infections due to fungi or viruses.
Usage in pregnancy. Since adequate human reproduction studies have not been done with corticosteroids, use of these drugs in pregnancy or in women of childbearing potential requires that the anticipated benefits be weighed against the possible hazards to the mother and embryo or fetus. Infants born of mothers who have received substantial doses of corticosteroids during pregnancy should be carefully observed for signs of hypoadrenalism.
Corticosteroids appear in breast milk and could suppress growth, interfere with endogenous corticosteroid production, or cause other unwanted effects. Mothers taking pharmacologic doses of corticosteroids should be advised not to nurse.
Average and large doses of cortisone or hydrocortisone can cause elevation of blood pressure, salt and water retention, and increased excretion of potassium. These effects are less likely to occur with the synthetic derivatives except when used in large doses. Dietary salt restriction and potassium supplementation may be necessary. All corticosteroids increase calcium excretion.
Administration of live virus vaccines, including smallpox, is contraindicated in individuals receiving immunosuppressive doses of corticosteroids. If inactivated viral or bacterial vaccines are administered to individuals receiving immunosuppressive doses of corticosteroids, the expected serum antibody response may not be obtained. However, immunization procedures may be undertaken in patients who are receiving corticosteroids as replacement therapy, e.g., for Addison's disease.
The use of HYDELTRASOL injection in active tuberculosis should be restricted to those cases of fulminating or disseminated tuberculosis in which the corticosteroid is used for the management of the disease in conjunction with appropriate antituberculous regimen.

If corticosteroids are indicated in patients with latent tuberculosis or tuberculin reactivity, close observation is necessary as reactivation of the disease may occur. During prolonged corticosteroid therapy, these patients should receive chemoprophylaxis.

Literature reports suggest an apparent association between use of corticosteroids and left ventricular free wall rupture after a recent myocardial infarction; therefore, therapy with corticosteroids should be used with great caution in these patients.

PRECAUTIONS

This product, like many other steroid formulations, is sensitive to heat. Therefore, it should not be autoclaved when it is desirable to sterilize the exterior of the vial.

Following prolonged therapy, withdrawal of corticosteroids may result in symptoms of the corticosteroid withdrawal syndrome including fever, myalgia, arthralgia, and malaise. This may occur in patients even without evidence of adrenal insufficiency.

There is an enhanced effect of corticosteroids in patients with hypothyroidism and in those with cirrhosis.

Corticosteroids should be used cautiously in patients with ocular herpes simplex for fear of corneal perforation.

The lowest possible dose of corticosteroid should be used to control the condition under treatment, and when reduction in dosage is possible, the reduction must be gradual.

Psychic derangements may appear when corticosteroids are used, ranging from euphoria, insomnia, mood swings, personality changes, and severe depression to frank psychotic manifestations. Also, existing emotional instability or psychotic tendencies may be aggravated by corticosteroids.

Aspirin should be used cautiously in conjunction with corticosteroids in hypoprothrombinemia.

Steroids should be used with caution in nonspecific ulcerative colitis, if there is a probability of impending perforation, abscess, or other pyogenic infection, also in diverticulitis, fresh intestinal anastomoses, active or latent peptic ulcer, renal insufficiency, hypertension, osteoporosis, and myasthenia gravis. Signs of peritoneal irritation following gastrointestinal perforation in patients receiving large doses of corticosteroids may be minimal or absent. Fat embolism has been reported as a possible complication of hypercortisonism.

When large doses are given, some authorities advise that antacids be administered between meals to help to prevent peptic ulcer.

Growth and development of infants and children on prolonged corticosteroid therapy should be carefully followed.

Steroids may increase or decrease motility and number of spermatozoa in some patients.

Phenytoin, phenobarbital, ephedrine, and rifampin may enhance the metabolic clearance of corticosteroids, resulting in decreased blood levels and lessened physiologic activity, thus requiring adjustment in corticosteroid dosage.

The prothrombin time should be checked frequently in patients who are receiving corticosteroids and coumarin anticoagulants at the same time because of reports that corticosteroids have altered the response to these anticoagulants. Studies have shown that the usual effect produced by adding corticosteroids is inhibition of response to coumarins, although there have been some conflicting reports of potentiation not substantiated by studies.

When corticosteroids are administered concomitantly with potassium-depleting diuretics, patients should be observed closely for development of hypokalemia.

Intra-articular injection of a corticosteroid may produce systemic as well as local effects.

Appropriate examination of any joint fluid present is necessary to exclude a septic process.

A marked increase in pain accompanied by local swelling, further restriction of joint motion, fever, and malaise is suggestive of septic arthritis. If this complication occurs and the diagnosis of sepsis is confirmed, appropriate antimicrobial therapy should be instituted.

Injection of a steroid into an infected site is to be avoided. Corticosteroids should not be injected into unstable joints.

Patients should be impressed strongly with the importance of not overusing joints in which symptomatic benefit has been obtained as long as the inflammatory process remains active.

Frequent intra-articular injection may result in damage to joint tissues.

The slower rate of absorption by intramuscular administration should be recognized.

ADVERSE REACTIONS

Fluid and electrolyte disturbances
Sodium retention
Fluid retention
Congestive heart failure in susceptible patients
Potassium loss
Hypokalemic alkalosis

Hypertension
Musculoskeletal
Muscle weakness
Steroid myopathy
Loss of muscle mass
Osteoporosis
Vertebral compression fractures
Aseptic necrosis of femoral and humeral heads
Pathologic fracture of long bones
Tendon rupture
Gastrointestinal
Peptic ulcer with possible subsequent perforation and hemorrhage
Perforation of the small and large bowel, particularly in patients with inflammatory bowel disease
Pancreatitis
Abdominal distention
Ulcerative esophagitis
Dermatologic
Impaired wound healing
Thin fragile skin
Petechiae and ecchymoses
Erythema
Increased sweating
May suppress reactions to skin tests
Burning or tingling, especially in the perineal area (after I.V. injection)
Other cutaneous reactions, such as allergic dermatitis, urticaria, angioneurotic edema
Neurologic
Convulsions
Increased intracranial pressure with papilledema (pseudotumor cerebri) usually after treatment
Vertigo
Headache
Psychic disturbances
Endocrine
Menstrual irregularities
Development of cushingoid state
Suppression of growth in children
Secondary adrenocortical and pituitary unresponsiveness, particularly in times of stress, as in trauma, surgery, or illness
Decreased carbohydrate tolerance
Manifestations of latent diabetes mellitus
Increased requirements for insulin or oral hypoglycemic agents in diabetics
Hirsutism
Ophthalmic
Posterior subcapsular cataracts
Increased intraocular pressure
Glaucoma
Exophthalmos
Metabolic
Negative nitrogen balance due to protein catabolism
Cardiovascular
Myocardial rupture following recent myocardial infarction (see WARNINGS).
Other
Anaphylactoid or hypersensitivity reactions
Thromboembolism
Weight gain
Increased appetite
Nausea
Malaise
The following *additional* adverse reactions are related to parenteral corticosteroid therapy:
Rare instances of blindness associated with intralesional therapy around the face and head
Hyperpigmentation or hypopigmentation
Subcutaneous and cutaneous atrophy
Sterile abscess
Postinjection flare (following intra-articular use)
Charcot-like arthropathy.

OVERDOSAGE

Reports of acute toxicity and/or death following overdosage of glucocorticoids are rare. In the event of overdosage, no specific antidote is available; treatment is supportive and symptomatic.

The intraperitoneal LD_{50} of prednisolone phosphate disodium in female mice was 1190 mg/kg.

DOSAGE AND ADMINISTRATION

For intravenous, intramuscular, intra-articular, intralesional, and soft tissue injection.
DOSAGE REQUIREMENTS ARE VARIABLE AND MUST BE INDIVIDUALIZED ON THE BASIS OF THE DISEASE AND THE RESPONSE OF THE PATIENT.
Intravenous and Intramuscular Injection
HYDELTRASOL injection can be given directly from the vial, or it can be added to Sodium Chloride Injection or Dextrose Injection and given by intravenous drip.

Benzyl alcohol as a preservative has been associated with toxicity in premature infants. Solutions used for intravenous administration or further dilution of this product should be preservative-free when used in the neonate, especially the premature infant.

When it is mixed with an infusion solution, sterile precautions should be observed. Since infusion solutions generally do not contain preservatives, mixtures should be used within 24 hours.

The initial dosage varies from 4 to 60 mg a day depending on the disease being treated. In less severe diseases doses lower than 4 mg may suffice, while in severe diseases doses higher than 60 mg may be required. Usually the daily parenteral dose of HYDELTRASOL injection is the same as the daily oral dose of prednisolone and the dosage interval is every 4 to 8 hours.

The initial dosage should be maintained or adjusted until the patient's response is satisfactory. If a satisfactory clinical response does not occur after a reasonable period of time, discontinue HYDELTRASOL injection and transfer the patient to other therapy.

After a favorable initial response, the proper maintenance dosage should be determined by decreasing the initial dosage in small amounts to the lowest dosage that maintains an adequate clinical response.

Patients should be observed closely for signs that might require dosage adjustment, including changes in clinical status resulting from remissions or exacerbations of the disease, individual drug responsiveness, and the effect of stress (e.g., surgery, infection, trauma). During stress it may be necessary to increase dosage temporarily.

If the drug is to be stopped after more than a few days of treatment, it usually should be withdrawn gradually.

Intra-articular, Intralesional, and Soft Tissue Injection
Intra-articular, intralesional, and soft tissue injections are generally employed when the affected joints or areas are limited to one or two sites. Dosage and frequency of injection vary depending on the condition being treated and the site of injection. The usual dose is from 2 to 30 mg. The frequency usually ranges from once every three to five days to once every two to three weeks. Frequent intra-articular injection may result in damage to joint tissues.

Some of the usual single doses are:
[See table on next page.]

HYDELTRASOL injection is particularly recommended for use in conjunction with one of the less soluble, longer-acting steroids, such as HYDELTRA-T.B.A.® (Prednisolone Tebutate, MSD) suspension or HYDROCORTONE® Acetate (Hydrocortisone Acetate, MSD) sterile suspension, available for intra-articular and soft tissue injection.

HOW SUPPLIED

No. 7577X—Injection HYDELTRASOL, 20 mg prednisolone phosphate equivalent per mL, is a clear, colorless to slightly yellow solution, and is supplied as follows:
NDC 0006-7577-02 in 2 mL vials
NDC 0006-7577-03 in 5 mL vials
(6505-00-890-1496 20 mg/mL 5 mL vial).
Storage
Sensitive to heat. Do not autoclave.
Protect from light. Store container in carton until contents have been used.

    A.H.F.S. Category: 68:04
    DC 7407225   Issued March 1988

HYDELTRA–T.B.A.® Sterile Suspension   ℞
(Prednisolone Tebutate, MSD), U.S.P.

For intra-articular, intralesional, and soft tissue injection only.

NOT FOR INTRAVENOUS USE
DESCRIPTION

Prednisolone tebutate, a synthetic adrenocortical steroid, is a white to slightly yellow powder sparingly soluble in alcohol, freely soluble in chloroform, and very slightly soluble in water. The molecular weight is 476.61 (monohydrate). It is designated chemically as 11β,17- dihydroxy - 21 - [(3,3-dimethyl-1-oxobutyl)oxy] pregna-1,4-diene-3,20-dione. The empirical formula is $C_{27}H_{38}O_6$ and the structural formula is:
[See Chemical Formula at top of next column].
HYDELTRA-T.B.A.® (Prednisolone Tebutate, MSD) sterile suspension is a white to slightly yellow suspension (pH 6.0 to

Continued on next page

Information on the Merck Sharp & Dohme products listed on these pages is the full prescribing information from product circulars in use August 31, 1989.

Merck Sharp & Dohme—Cont.

8.0) that settles upon standing. Each mL contains prednisolone tebutate, 20 mg. Inactive ingredients per mL: sodium citrate, 1 mg; polysorbate 80, 1 mg; sorbitol solution, 0.5 mL (equal to 450 mg d-sorbitol); Water for Injection, q.s., 1 mL. Benzyl alcohol, 9 mg, added as preservative.

ACTIONS

HYDELTRA-T.B.A. has a slow onset but long duration of action when compared with more soluble preparations. Because of its slight solubility, it is suitable for intra-articular, intralesional, and soft tissue injection where its anti-inflammatory effects are confined mainly to the area in which it has been injected, although it is capable of producing systemic hormonal effects.

Naturally occurring glucocorticoids (hydrocortisone and cortisone), which also have salt-retaining properties, are used as replacement therapy in adrenocortical deficiency states. Their synthetic analogs, including prednisolone, are primarily used for their potent anti-inflammatory effects in disorders of many organ systems.

Glucocorticoids cause profound and varied metabolic effects. In addition, they modify the body's immune responses to diverse stimuli.

INDICATIONS

A. By intra-articular or soft tissue injection:
As adjunctive therapy for short-term administration (to tide the patient over an acute episode or exacerbation) in:
     Synovitis of osteoarthritis
     Rheumatoid arthritis
     Acute and subacute bursitis
     Acute gouty arthritis
     Epicondylitis
     Acute nonspecific tenosynovitis
     Post-traumatic osteoarthritis
B. By intralesional injection:
May be useful in cystic tumors of an aponeurosis or tendon (ganglia).

CONTRAINDICATIONS

Systemic fungal infections
Hypersensitivity to any component of this product

WARNINGS

Because rare instances of anaphylactoid reactions have occurred in patients receiving parenteral corticosteroid therapy, appropriate precautionary measures should be taken prior to administration, especially when the patient has a history of allergy to any drug. Anaphylactoid and hypersensitivity reactions have been reported for Sterile Suspension HYDELTRA-T.B.A. (see ADVERSE REACTIONS).

In patients on corticosteroid therapy subjected to any unusual stress, increased dosage of rapidly acting corticosteroids before, during, and after the stressful situation is indicated.

Drug-induced secondary adrenocortical insufficiency may result from too rapid withdrawal of corticosteroids and may be minimized by gradual reduction of dosage. This type of relative insufficiency may persist for months after discontinuation of therapy; therefore, in any situation of stress occurring during that period, hormone therapy should be reinstituted. If the patient is receiving steroids already, dosage may have to be increased. Since mineralocorticoid secretion may be impaired, salt and/or a mineralocorticoid should be administered concurrently.

Corticosteroids may mask some signs of infection, and new infections may appear during their use. There may be decreased resistance and inability to localize infection when corticosteroids are used. Moreover, corticosteroids may affect the nitroblue-tetrazolium test for bacterial infection and produce false negative results.

In cerebral malaria, a double-blind trial has shown that the use of corticosteroids is associated with prolongation of coma and a higher incidence of pneumonia and gastrointestinal bleeding.

Corticosteroids may activate latent amebiasis. Therefore, it is recommended that latent or active amebiasis be ruled out before initiating corticosteroid therapy in any patient who has spent time in the tropics or any patient with unexplained diarrhea.

Prolonged use of corticosteroids may produce posterior subcapsular cataracts, glaucoma with possible damage to the optic nerves, and may enhance the establishment of secondary ocular infections due to fungi or viruses.

Usage in pregnancy. Since adequate human reproduction studies have not been done with corticosteroids, use of these drugs in pregnancy or in women of childbearing potential requires that the anticipated benefits be weighed against the possible hazards to the mother and embryo or fetus. Infants born of mothers who have received substantial doses of corticosteroids during pregnancy should be carefully observed for signs of hypoadrenalism.

Corticosteroids appear in breast milk and could suppress growth, interfere with endogenous corticosteroid production, or cause other unwanted effects. Mothers taking pharmacologic doses of corticosteroids should be advised not to nurse.

Average and large doses of cortisone or hydrocortisone can cause elevation of blood pressure, salt and water retention, and increased excretion of potassium. These effects are less likely to occur with the synthetic derivatives except when used in large doses. Dietary salt restriction and potassium supplementation may be necessary. All corticosteroids increase calcium excretion.

Administration of live virus vaccines, including smallpox, is contraindicated in individuals receiving immunosuppressive doses of corticosteroids. If inactivated viral or bacterial vaccines are administered to individuals receiving immunosuppressive doses of corticosteroids, the expected serum antibody response may not be obtained.

If corticosteroids are indicated in patients with latent tuberculosis or tuberculin reactivity, close observation is necessary as reactivation of the disease may occur. During prolonged corticosteroid therapy, these patients should receive chemoprophylaxis.

Literature reports suggest an apparent association between use of corticosteroids and left ventricular free wall rupture after a recent myocardial infarction; therefore, therapy with corticosteroids should be used with great caution in these patients.

PRECAUTIONS

This product, like many other steroid formulations, is sensitive to heat. Therefore, it should not be autoclaved when it is desirable to sterilize the exterior of the vial.

Following prolonged therapy, withdrawal of corticosteroids may result in symptoms of the corticosteroid withdrawal syndrome including fever, myalgia, arthralgia, and malaise.

This may occur in patients even without evidence of adrenal insufficiency.

There is an enhanced effect of corticosteroids in patients with hypothyroidism and in those with cirrhosis.

Corticosteroids should be used cautiously in patients with ocular herpes simplex for fear of corneal perforation.

Psychic derangements may appear when corticosteroids are used, ranging from euphoria, insomnia, mood swings, personality changes, and severe depression to frank psychotic manifestations. Also, existing emotional instability or psychotic tendencies may be aggravated by corticosteroids.

Aspirin should be used cautiously in conjunction with corticosteroids in hypoprothrombinemia.

Steroids should be used with caution in nonspecific ulcerative colitis, if there is a probability of impending perforation, abscess, or other pyogenic infection, also in diverticulitis, fresh intestinal anastomoses, active or latent peptic ulcer, renal insufficiency, hypertension, osteoporosis, and myasthenia gravis. Signs of peritoneal irritation following gastrointestinal perforation in patients receiving large doses of corticosteroids may be minimal or absent. Fat embolism has been reported as a possible complication of hypercortisonism.

When large doses are given, some authorities advise that antacids be administered between meals to help to prevent peptic ulcer.

Growth and development of infants and children on prolonged corticosteroid therapy should be carefully followed.

Steroids may increase or decrease motility and number of spermatozoa in some patients.

Phenytoin, phenobarbital, ephedrine, and rifampin may enhance the metabolic clearance of corticosteroids, resulting in decreased blood levels and lessened physiologic activity, thus requiring adjustment in corticosteroid dosage.

The prothrombin time should be checked frequently in patients who are receiving corticosteroids and coumarin anticoagulants at the same time because of reports that corticosteroids have altered the response to these anticoagulants. Studies have shown that the usual effect produced by adding corticosteroids is inhibition of response to coumarins, although there have been some conflicting reports of potentiation not substantiated by studies.

When corticosteroids are administered concomitantly with potassium-depleting diuretics, patients should be observed closely for development of hypokalemia.

Intra-articular injection of a corticosteroid may produce systemic as well as local effects.

Appropriate examination of any joint fluid present is necessary to exclude a septic process.

A marked increase in pain accompanied by local swelling, further restriction of joint motion, fever, and malaise is suggestive of septic arthritis. If this complication occurs and the diagnosis of sepsis is confirmed, appropriate antimicrobial therapy should be instituted.

Injection of a steroid into an infected site is to be avoided.
Corticosteroids should not be injected into unstable joints.

Patients should be impressed strongly with the importance of not overusing joints in which symptomatic benefit has been obtained as long as the inflammatory process remains active.

Frequent intra-articular injection may result in damage to joint tissues.

ADVERSE REACTIONS

Fluid and electrolyte disturbances
     Sodium retention
     Fluid retention
     Congestive heart failure in susceptible patients
     Potassium loss
     Hypokalemic alkalosis
     Hypertension
Musculoskeletal
     Muscle weakness
     Steroid myopathy
     Loss of muscle mass
     Osteoporosis
     Vertebral compression fractures
     Aseptic necrosis of femoral and humeral heads
     Pathologic fracture of long bones
     Tendon rupture
Gastrointestinal
     Peptic ulcer with possible subsequent perforation and hemorrhage
     Perforation of the small and large bowel, particularly in patients with inflammatory bowel disease
     Pancreatitis
     Abdominal distention
     Ulcerative esophagitis
Dermatologic
     Impaired wound healing
     Thin fragile skin
     Petechiae and ecchymoses
     Erythema

	Doses	
Site of Injection	Amount of Injection (mL)	Amount of Prednisolone Phosphate (mg)
Large Joints (e.g., Knee)	0.5 to 1	10 to 20
Small Joints (e.g., Interphalangeal, Temporomandibular)	0.2 to 0.25	4 to 5
Bursae	0.5 to 0.75	10 to 15
Tendon Sheaths	0.1 to 0.25	2 to 5
Soft Tissue Infiltration	0.5 to 1.5	10 to 30
Ganglia	0.25 to 0.5	5 to 10

Increased sweating

May suppress reactions to skin tests

Other cutaneous reactions, such as allergic dermatitis, urticaria, angioneurotic edema

Neurologic

Convulsions

Increased intracranial pressure with papilledema (pseudotumor cerebri) usually after treatment

Vertigo

Headache

Psychic disturbances

Endocrine

Menstrual irregularities

Development of cushingoid state

Suppression of growth in children

Secondary adrenocortical and pituitary unresponsiveness, particularly in times of stress, as in trauma, surgery, or illness

Decreased carbohydrate tolerance

Manifestations of latent diabetes mellitus

Increased requirements for insulin or oral hypoglycemic agents in diabetics

Hirsutism

Ophthalmic

Posterior subcapsular cataracts

Increased intraocular pressure

Glaucoma

Exophthalmos

Metabolic

Negative nitrogen balance due to protein catabolism

Cardiovascular

Myocardial rupture following recent myocardial infarction (see WARNINGS).

Other

Anaphylactoid or hypersensitivity reactions

Thromboembolism

Weight gain

Increased appetite

Nausea

Malaise

Foreign body granulomatous reactions involving the synovium have been reported with repeated injections of HYDELTRA-T.B.A.

Localized pain and swelling, sometimes distal to the site of injection and persisting for several days, have been reported. The following *additional* adverse reactions are related to injection of corticosteroids:

Rare instances of blindness associated with intralesional therapy around the face and head

Hyperpigmentation or hypopigmentation

Subcutaneous and cutaneous atrophy

Sterile abscess

Postinjection flare (following intra-articular use)

Charcot-like arthropathy

DOSAGE AND ADMINISTRATION

> *For intra-articular, intralesional, and soft tissue injection only.*

NOT FOR INTRAVENOUS USE

DOSAGE AND FREQUENCY OF INJECTION ARE VARIABLE AND MUST BE INDIVIDUALIZED ON THE BASIS OF THE DISEASE AND THE RESPONSE OF THE PATIENT.

The initial dose varies from 4 to 40 mg depending on the disease being treated and the size of the area to be injected. Frequency of injection depends on symptomatic response, and usually is once every two or three weeks. Severe conditions may require injection once a week. Frequent intra-articular injection may result in damage to joint tissues. If satisfactory clinical response does not occur after a reasonable period of time, discontinue HYDELTRA-T.B.A. sterile suspension and transfer the patient to other therapy.

Patients should be observed closely for signs that might require dosage adjustment, including changes in clinical status resulting from remissions or exacerbations of the disease, and individual drug responsiveness.

For rapid onset of action, a soluble adrenocortical hormone preparation, such as DECADRON® Phosphate (Dexamethasone Sodium Phosphate, MSD) injection or HYDELTRASOL® (Prednisolone Sodium Phosphate, MSD) injection, may be given with HYDELTRA-T.B.A.

If desired, a local anesthetic may be used, and may be injected before HYDELTRA-T.B.A., or mixed in a syringe with HYDELTRA-T.B.A. and given simultaneously.

If used prior to intra-articular injection of the steroid, inject most of the anesthetic into the soft tissues of the surrounding area and instill a small amount into the joint.

If given together, mixing should be done in the injection syringe by drawing the steroid in *first*, then the anesthetic. In this way, the anesthetic will not be introduced inadvertently

into the vial of steroid. *The mixture must be used immediately and any unused portion discarded.*

Some of the usual single doses are:

Large Joints (e.g., Knee)	20 mg (1 mL), occasionally 30 mg (1.5 mL). Doses over 40 mg (2 mL) not recommended.
Small Joints (e.g., Interphalangeal, Temporomandibular)	8 to 10 mg (0.4 to 0.5 mL).
Bursae	20 to 30 mg (1 to 1.5 mL).
Tendon Sheaths	4 to 10 mg (0.2 to 0.5 mL).
Ganglia	10 to 20 mg (0.5 to 1 mL).

HOW SUPPLIED

No. 7572—Sterile Suspension HYDELTRA-T.B.A., 20 mg per mL, is a white, milky suspension, and is supplied as follows:

NDC 0006-7572-01 in 1 mL vials (6505-00-225-7499 1 mL vial)

NDC 0006-7572-03 in 5 mL vials (6505-00-890-1353 5 mL vial).

Storage

Sensitive to heat. Do not autoclave.

Protect from freezing.

Protect from light. Store container in carton until contents have been used.

A.H.F.S. Category: 68:04

DC 7349124   Issued March 1988

HYDROCORTONE®   ℞

Acetate Sterile Suspension

(Hydrocortisone Acetate, MSD), U.S.P.

For intra-articular, intralesional, and soft tissue injection only.

NOT FOR INTRAVENOUS USE

DESCRIPTION

Hydrocortisone acetate, a synthetic adrenocortical steroid, is a white to practically white, odorless, crystalline powder. It is insoluble in water and slightly soluble in alcohol and chloroform. The molecular weight is 404.50. It is designated chemically as 21-(acetyloxy)-11β,17-dihydroxypregn-4-ene-3,20-dione. The empirical formula is $C_{23}H_{32}O_6$ and the structural formula is:

HYDROCORTONE® Acetate (Hydrocortisone Acetate, MSD) sterile suspension is a sterile suspension of hydrocortisone acetate (pH 5.0 to 7.0) in a suitable aqueous medium. It is supplied in two strengths, one containing 25 mg hydrocortisone acetate per milliliter, the other containing 50 mg per milliliter. Inactive ingredients per mL: sodium chloride, 9 mg; polysorbate 80, 4 mg; sodium carboxymethylcellulose, 5 mg; and Water for Injection, q.s., 1 mL. Benzyl alcohol, 9 mg, added as preservative.

ACTIONS

HYDROCORTONE Acetate sterile suspension has a slow onset but long duration of action when compared with more soluble preparations. Because of its insolubility, it is suitable for intra-articular, intralesional, and soft tissue injection where its anti-inflammatory effects are confined mainly to the area in which it has been injected, although it is capable of producing systemic hormonal effects.

Naturally occurring glucocorticoids (hydrocortisone and cortisone), which also have salt-retaining properties, are used as replacement therapy in adrenocortical deficiency

states. They are also used for their potent anti-inflammatory effect in disorders of many organ systems.

Glucocorticoids cause profound and varied metabolic effects. In addition, they modify the body's immune responses to diverse stimuli.

INDICATIONS

A. By intra-articular or soft tissue injection:

As adjunctive therapy for short-term administration (to tide the patient over an acute episode or exacerbation) in:

Synovitis of osteoarthritis

Rheumatoid arthritis

Acute and subacute bursitis

Acute gouty arthritis

Epicondylitis

Acute nonspecific tenosynovitis

Post-traumatic osteoarthritis

B. By intralesional injection:

Keloids

Localized hypertrophic, infiltrated, inflammatory lesions of: lichen planus, psoriatic plaques, granuloma annulare, and lichen simplex chronicus (neurodermatitis)

Discoid lupus erythematosus

Necrobiosis lipoidica diabeticorum

Alopecia areata

May also be useful in cystic tumors of an aponeurosis or tendon (ganglia).

CONTRAINDICATIONS

Systemic fungal infections

Hypersensitivity to any component of this product

WARNINGS

Because rare instances of anaphylactoid reactions have occurred in patients receiving parenteral corticosteroid therapy, appropriate precautionary measures should be taken prior to administration, especially when the patient has a history of allergy to any drug.

In patients on corticosteroid therapy subjected to any unusual stress, increased dosage of rapidly acting corticosteroids before, during, and after the stressful situation is indicated.

Drug-induced secondary adrenocortical insufficiency may result from too rapid withdrawal of corticosteroids and may be minimized by gradual reduction of dosage. This type of relative insufficiency may persist for months after discontinuation of therapy; therefore, in any situation of stress occurring during that period, hormone therapy should be reinstituted. If the patient is receiving steroids already, dosage may have to be increased. Since mineralocorticoid secretion may be impaired, salt and/or a mineralocorticoid should be administered concurrently.

Corticosteroids may mask some signs of infection, and new infections may appear during their use. There may be decreased resistance and inability to localize infection when corticosteroids are used. Moreover, corticosteroids may affect the nitroblue-tetrazolium test for bacterial infection and produce false negative results.

In cerebral malaria, a double-blind trial has shown that the use of corticosteroids is associated with prolongation of coma and a higher incidence of pneumonia and gastrointestinal bleeding.

Corticosteroids may activate latent amebiasis. Therefore, it is recommended that latent or active amebiasis be ruled out before initiating corticosteroid therapy in any patient who has spent time in the tropics or any patient with unexplained diarrhea.

Prolonged use of corticosteroids may produce posterior subcapsular cataracts, glaucoma with possible damage to the optic nerves, and may enhance the establishment of secondary ocular infections due to fungi or viruses.

Usage in pregnancy: Since adequate human reproduction studies have not been done with corticosteroids, use of these drugs in pregnancy or in women of childbearing potential requires that the anticipated benefits be weighed against the possible hazards to the mother and embryo or fetus. Infants born of mothers who have received substantial doses of corticosteroids during pregnancy should be carefully observed for signs of hypoadrenalism.

Corticosteroids appear in breast milk and could suppress growth, interfere with endogenous corticosteroid production, or cause other unwanted effects. Mothers taking pharmacologic doses of corticosteroids should be advised not to nurse. Average and large doses of cortisone or hydrocortisone can cause elevation of blood pressure, salt and water retention,

Continued on next page

Information on the Merck Sharp & Dohme products listed on these pages is the full prescribing information from product circulars in use August 31, 1989.

Merck Sharp & Dohme—Cont.

and increased excretion of potassium. These effects are less likely to occur with the synthetic derivatives except when used in large doses. Dietary salt restriction and potassium supplementation may be necessary. All corticosteroids increase calcium excretion.

Administration of live virus vaccines, including smallpox, is contraindicated in individuals receiving immunosuppressive doses of corticosteroids. If inactivated viral or bacterial vaccines are administered to individuals receiving immunosuppressive doses of corticosteroids, the expected serum antibody response may not be obtained.

If corticosteroids are indicated in patients with latent tuberculosis or tuberculin reactivity, close observation is necessary as reactivation of the disease may occur. During prolonged corticosteroid therapy, these patients should receive chemoprophylaxis.

Literature reports suggest an apparent association between use of corticosteroids and left ventricular free wall rupture after a recent myocardial infarction; therefore, therapy with corticosteroids should be used with great caution in these patients.

PRECAUTIONS

This product, like many other steroid formulations, is sensitive to heat. Therefore, it should not be autoclaved when it is desirable to sterilize the exterior of the vial.

Following prolonged therapy, withdrawal of corticosteroids may result in symptoms of the corticosteroid withdrawal syndrome including fever, myalgia, arthralgia, and malaise. This may occur in patients even without evidence of adrenal insufficiency.

There is an enhanced effect of corticosteroids in patients with hypothyroidism and in those with cirrhosis.

Corticosteroids should be used cautiously in patients with ocular herpes simplex for fear of corneal perforation.

Psychic derangements may appear when corticosteroids are used, ranging from euphoria, insomnia, mood swings, personality changes, and severe depression to frank psychotic manifestations. Also, existing emotional instability or psychotic tendencies may be aggravated by corticosteroids.

Aspirin should be used cautiously in conjunction with corticosteroids in hypoprothrombinemia.

Steroids should be used with caution in nonspecific ulcerative colitis, if there is a probability of impending perforation, abscess, or other pyogenic infection, also in diverticulitis, fresh intestinal anastomoses, active or latent peptic ulcer, renal insufficiency, hypertension, osteoporosis, and myasthenia gravis. Signs of peritoneal irritation following gastrointestinal perforation in patients receiving large doses of corticosteroids may be minimal or absent. Fat embolism has been reported as a possible complication of hypercortisonism.

When large doses are given, some authorities advise that antacids be administered between meals to help to prevent peptic ulcer.

Growth and development of infants and children on prolonged corticosteroid therapy should be carefully followed.

Steroids may increase or decrease motility and number of spermatozoa in some patients.

Phenytoin, phenobarbital, ephedrine, and rifampin may enhance the metabolic clearance of corticosteroids resulting in decreased blood levels and lessened physiologic activity, thus requiring adjustment in corticosteroid dosage.

The prothrombin time should be checked frequently in patients who are receiving corticosteroids and coumarin anticoagulants at the same time because of reports that corticosteroids have altered the response to these anticoagulants. Studies have shown that the usual effect produced by adding corticosteroids is inhibition of response to coumarins, although there have been some conflicting reports of potentiation not substantiated by studies.

When corticosteroids are administered concomitantly with potassium-depleting diuretics, patients should be observed closely for development of hypokalemia.

Intra-articular injection of a corticosteroid may produce systemic as well as local effects.

Appropriate examination of any joint fluid present is necessary to exclude a septic process.

A marked increase in pain accompanied by local swelling, further restriction of joint motion, fever, and malaise is suggestive of septic arthritis. If this complication occurs and the diagnosis of sepsis is confirmed, appropriate antimicrobial therapy should be instituted.

Injection of a steroid into an infected site is to be avoided.

Corticosteroids should not be injected into unstable joints. Patients should be impressed strongly with the importance of not overusing joints in which symptomatic benefit has been obtained as long as the inflammatory process remains active.

Frequent intra-articular injection may result in damage to joint tissues.

ADVERSE REACTIONS

Fluid and electrolyte disturbances
  Sodium retention
  Fluid retention
  Congestive heart failure in susceptible patients
  Potassium loss
  Hypokalemic alkalosis
  Hypertension
Musculoskeletal
  Muscle weakness
  Steroid myopathy
  Loss of muscle mass
  Osteoporosis
  Vertebral compression fractures
  Aseptic necrosis of femoral and humeral heads
  Pathologic fracture of long bones
  Tendon rupture
Gastrointestinal
  Peptic ulcer with possible subsequent perforation and hemorrhage
  Perforation of the small and large bowel, particularly in patients with inflammatory bowel disease
  Pancreatitis
  Abdominal distention
  Ulcerative esophagitis
Dermatologic
  Impaired wound healing
  Thin fragile skin
  Petechiae and ecchymoses
  Erythema
  Increased sweating
  May suppress reactions to skin tests
  Other cutaneous reactions, such as allergic dermatitis, urticaria, angioneurotic edema
Neurologic
  Convulsions
  Increased intracranial pressure with papilledema (pseudotumor cerebri) usually after treatment
  Vertigo
  Headache
  Psychic disturbances
Endocrine
  Menstrual irregularities
  Development of cushingoid state
  Suppression of growth in children
  Secondary adrenocortical and pituitary unresponsiveness, particularly in times of stress, as in trauma, surgery, or illness
  Decreased carbohydrate tolerance
  Manifestations of latent diabetes mellitus
  Increased requirements for insulin or oral hypoglycemic agents in diabetics
  Hirsutism
Ophthalmic
  Posterior subcapsular cataracts
  Increased intraocular pressure
  Glaucoma
  Exophthalmos
Metabolic
  Negative nitrogen balance due to protein catabolism
Cardiovascular
  Myocardial rupture following recent myocardial infarction (see WARNINGS).
Other
  Anaphylactoid or hypersensitivity reactions
  Thromboembolism
  Weight gain
  Increased appetite
  Nausea
  Malaise
The following *additional* adverse reactions are related to injection of corticosteroids:
  Rare instances of blindness associated with intralesional therapy around the face and head
  Hyperpigmentation or hypopigmentation
  Subcutaneous and cutaneous atrophy
  Sterile abscess
  Postinjection flare (following intra-articular use)
  Charcot-like arthropathy.

OVERDOSAGE

Reports of acute toxicity and/or death following overdosage of glucocorticoids are rare. In the event of overdosage, no specific antidote is available; treatment is supportive and symptomatic.

DOSAGE AND ADMINISTRATION

For intra-articular, intralesional, and soft tissue injection only

NOT FOR INTRAVENOUS USE

DOSAGE AND FREQUENCY OF INJECTION ARE VARIABLE AND MUST BE INDIVIDUALIZED ON THE BASIS OF THE DISEASE AND THE RESPONSE OF THE PATIENT.

The initial dose varies from 5 to 75 mg depending on the disease being treated and the size of the area to be injected. Frequency of injection depends on symptomatic response, and usually is once every two or three weeks. Severe conditions may require injection once a week. Frequent intra-articular injection may result in damage to joint tissues. If satisfactory clinical response does not occur after a reasonable period of time, discontinue HYDROCORTONE Acetate sterile suspension and transfer the patient to other therapy.

Patients should be observed closely for signs that might require dosage adjustment, including changes in clinical status resulting from remissions or exacerbations of the disease, and individual drug responsiveness.

Some of the usual single doses are:

Large Joints (e.g., Knee)	25 mg, occasionally 37.5 mg. Doses over 50 mg not recommended
Small Joints (e.g, Interphalangeal, Temporomandibular)	10 to 25 mg
Bursae	25 to 37.5 mg
Tendon Sheaths	5 to 12.5 mg
Soft Tissue Infiltration	25 to 50 mg, occasionally 75 mg
Ganglia	12.5 to 25 mg

For rapid onset of action, a soluble adrenocortical hormone preparation, such as DECADRON® Phosphate (Dexamethasone Sodium Phosphate, MSD) injection or HYDELTRASOL® (Prednisolone Sodium Phosphate, MSD) injection, may be given with HYDROCORTONE Acetate sterile suspension.

If desired, a local anesthetic may be used, and may be injected before HYDROCORTONE Acetate sterile suspension or mixed in a syringe with HYDROCORTONE Acetate sterile suspension and given simultaneously.

If used prior to intra-articular injection of the steroid, inject most of the anesthetic into the soft tissues of the surrounding area and instill a small amount into the joint.

If given together, mixing should be done in the injection syringe by drawing the steroid in *first*, then the anesthetic. In this way, the anesthetic will not be introduced inadvertently into the vial of steroid. *The mixture must be used immediately and any unused portion discarded.*

HOW SUPPLIED

No. 7501—Sterile suspension HYDROCORTONE Acetate is a white, mobile suspension, containing 25 mg hydrocortisone acetate in each mL, and is supplied as follows:
NDC 0006-7501-03 in 5 mL vials.
No. 7519—Sterile suspension HYDROCORTONE Acetate is a white, mobile suspension, containing 50 mg hydrocortisone acetate in each mL, and is supplied as follows:
NDC 0006-7519-03 in 5 mL vials.
Storage
Sensitive to heat. Do not autoclave.
Protect from freezing.
    A.H.F.S. Category: 68:04
    DC 7348726   Issued March 1988

HYDROCORTONE® Phosphate Injection, Sterile   ℞
(Hydrocortisone Sodium Phosphate, MSD), U.S.P.

DESCRIPTION

Hydrocortisone sodium phosphate, a synthetic adrenocortical steroid, is a white to light yellow, odorless or practically odorless powder. It is freely soluble in water and is exceedingly hygroscopic. The molecular weight is 486.41. It is designated chemically as 11β, 17-dihydroxy-21-(phosphonooxy) pregn-4-ene-3,20-dione disodium salt. The empirical formula is $C_{21}H_{29}Na_2O_8P$ and the structural formula is:
[See Chemical Formula at top of next column]
HYDROCORTONE® Phosphate (Hydrocortisone Sodium Phosphate, MSD) injection is a sterile solution (pH 7.5 to 8.5) for intravenous, intramuscular, and subcutaneous administration.
Each milliliter contains hydrocortisone sodium phosphate

equivalent to 50 mg hydrocortisone. Inactive ingredients per mL: 8 mg creatinine, 10 mg sodium citrate, sodium hydroxide to adjust pH, and Water for Injection, q.s. 1 mL, with 3.2 mg sodium bisulfite, 1.5 mg methylparaben, and 0.2 mg propylparaben added as preservatives.

ACTIONS

HYDROCORTONE Phosphate injection has a rapid onset but short duration of action when compared with less soluble preparations. Because of this, it is suitable for the treatment of acute disorders responsive to adrenocortical steroid therapy.

Naturally occurring glucocorticoids (hydrocortisone and cortisone), which also have salt-retaining properties, are used as replacement therapy in adrenocortical deficiency states. They are also used for their potent anti-inflammatory effects in disorders of many organ systems.

Glucocorticoids cause profound and varied metabolic effects. In addition, they modify the body's immune responses to diverse stimuli.

INDICATIONS

When oral therapy is not feasible:

1. *Endocrine disorders*

Primary or secondary adrenocortical insufficiency (hydrocortisone or cortisone is the drug of choice; synthetic analogs may be used in conjunction with mineralocorticoids where applicable; in infancy, mineralocorticoid supplementation is of particular importance)

Acute adrenocortical insufficiency (hydrocortisone or cortisone is the drug of choice; mineralocorticoid supplementation may be necessary, particularly when synthetic analogs are used)

Preoperatively, and in the event of serious trauma or illness, in patients with known adrenal insufficiency or when adrenocortical reserve is doubtful

Shock unresponsive to conventional therapy if adrenocortical insufficiency exists or is suspected
Congenital adrenal hyperplasia
Nonsuppurative thyroiditis
Hypercalcemia associated with cancer

2. *Rheumatic disorders*

As adjunctive therapy for short-term administration (to tide the patient over an acute episode or exacerbation) in:
Post-traumatic osteoarthritis
Synovitis of osteoarthritis
Rheumatoid arthritis, including juvenile rheumatoid arthritis (selected cases may require low-dose maintenance therapy)
Acute and subacute bursitis
Epicondylitis
Acute nonspecific tenosynovitis
Acute gouty arthritis
Psoriatic arthritis
Ankylosing spondylitis

3. *Collagen diseases*

During an exacerbation or as maintenance therapy in selected cases of:
Systemic lupus erythematosus
Acute rheumatic carditis
Systemic dermatomyositis (polymyositis)

4. *Dermatologic diseases*
Pemphigus
Severe erythema multiforme (Stevens-Johnson syndrome)
Exfoliative dermatitis
Bullous dermatitis herpetiformis
Severe seborrheic dermatitis
Severe psoriasis
Mycosis fungoides

5. *Allergic states*

Control of severe or incapacitating allergic conditions intractable to adequate trials of conventional treatment in:
Bronchial asthma
Contact dermatitis
Atopic dermatitis
Serum sickness
Seasonal or perennial allergic rhinitis
Drug hypersensitivity reactions
Urticarial transfusion reactions
Acute noninfectious laryngeal edema (epinephrine is the drug of first choice)

6. *Ophthalmic diseases*

Severe acute and chronic allergic and inflammatory processes involving the eye, such as:
Herpes zoster ophthalmicus
Iritis, iridocyclitis
Chorioretinitis
Diffuse posterior uveitis and choroiditis
Optic neuritis
Sympathetic ophthalmia
Anterior segment inflammation
Allergic conjunctivitis
Keratitis
Allergic corneal marginal ulcers

7. *Gastrointestinal diseases*

To tide the patient over a critical period of the disease in:
Ulcerative colitis (Systemic therapy)
Regional enteritis (Systemic therapy)

8. *Respiratory diseases*
Symptomatic sarcoidosis
Berylliosis
Fulminating or disseminated pulmonary tuberculosis when used concurrently with appropriate antituberculous chemotherapy
Loeffler's syndrome not manageable by other means
Aspiration pneumonitis

9. *Hematologic disorders*
Acquired (autoimmune) hemolytic anemia
Idiopathic thrombocytopenic purpura in adults (I.V. only; I.M. administration is contraindicated)
Secondary thrombocytopenia in adults
Erythroblastopenia (RBC anemia)
Congenital (erythroid) hypoplastic anemia

10. *Neoplastic diseases*

For palliative management of:
Leukemias and lymphomas in adults
Acute leukemia of childhood

11. *Edematous states*

To induce diuresis or remission of proteinuria in the nephrotic syndrome, without uremia, of the idiopathic type, or that due to lupus erythematosus

12. *Miscellaneous*

Tuberculous meningitis with subarachnoid block or impending block when used concurrently with appropriate antituberculous chemotherapy
Trichinosis with neurologic or myocardial involvement

CONTRAINDICATIONS

Systemic fungal infections (see WARNINGS regarding amphotericin B)
Hypersensitivity to any component of this product, including sulfites (see WARNINGS).

WARNINGS

Because rare instances of anaphylactoid reactions have occurred in patients receiving parenteral corticosteroid therapy, appropriate precautionary measures should be taken prior to administration, especially when the patient has a history of allergy to any drug. Anaphylactoid and hypersensitivity reactions have been reported for Injection HYDROCORTONE Phosphate (see ADVERSE REACTIONS).

Injection HYDROCORTONE Phosphate contains sodium bisulfite, a sulfite that may cause allergic-type reactions including anaphylactic symptoms and life-threatening or less severe asthmatic episodes in certain susceptible people. The overall prevalence of sulfite sensitivity in the general population is unknown and probably low. Sulfite sensitivity is seen more frequently in asthmatic than in nonasthmatic people.

Corticosteroids may exacerbate systemic fungal infections and therefore should not be used in the presence of such infections unless they are needed to control drug reactions due to amphotericin B. Moreover, there have been cases reported in which concomitant use of amphotericin B and hydrocortisone was followed by cardiac enlargement and congestive failure.

In patients on corticosteroid therapy subjected to any unusual stress, increased dosage of rapidly acting corticosteroids before, during, and after the stressful situation is indicated.

Drug-induced secondary adrenocortical insufficiency may result from too rapid withdrawal of corticosteroids and may be minimized by gradual reduction of dosage. This type of relative insufficiency may persist for months after discontinuation of therapy; therefore, in any situation of stress occurring during that period, hormone therapy should be reinstituted. If the patient is receiving steroids already, dosage may have to be increased. Since mineralocorticoid secretion may be impaired, salt and/or a mineralocorticoid should be administered concurrently.

Corticosteroids may mask some signs of infection, and new infections may appear during their use. There may be decreased resistance and inability to localize infection when corticosteroids are used. Moreover, corticosteroids may af-

fect the nitroblue-tetrazolium test for bacterial infection and produce false negative results.

In cerebral malaria, a double-blind trial has shown that the use of corticosteroids is associated with prolongation of coma and a higher incidence of pneumonia and gastrointestinal bleeding.

Corticosteroids may activate latent amebiasis. Therefore, it is recommended that latent or active amebiasis be ruled out before initiating corticosteroid therapy in any patient who has spent time in the tropics or any patient with unexplained diarrhea.

Prolonged use of corticosteroids may produce posterior subcapsular cataracts, glaucoma with possible damage to the optic nerves, and may enhance the establishment of secondary ocular infections due to fungi or viruses.

Usage in pregnancy. Since adequate human reproduction studies have not been done with corticosteroids, use of these drugs in pregnancy or in women of childbearing potential requires that the anticipated benefits be weighed against the possible hazards to the mother and embryo or fetus. Infants born of mothers who have received substantial doses of corticosteroids during pregnancy should be carefully observed for signs of hypoadrenalism.

Corticosteroids appear in breast milk and could suppress growth, interfere with endogenous corticosteroid production, or cause other unwanted effects. Mothers taking pharmacologic doses of corticosteroids should be advised not to nurse. Average and large doses of cortisone or hydrocortisone can cause elevation of blood pressure, salt and water retention, and increased excretion of potassium. These effects are less likely to occur with the synthetic derivatives except when used in large doses. Dietary salt restriction and potassium supplementation may be necessary. All corticosteroids increase calcium excretion.

Administration of live virus vaccines, including smallpox, is contraindicated in individuals receiving immunosuppressive doses of corticosteroids. If inactivated viral or bacterial vaccines are administered to individuals receiving immunosuppressive doses of corticosteroids, the expected serum antibody response may not be obtained. However, immunization procedures may be undertaken in patients who are receiving corticosteroids as replacement therapy, e.g., for Addison's disease.

The use of HYDROCORTONE Phosphate injection in active tuberculosis should be restricted to those cases of fulminating or disseminated tuberculosis in which the corticosteroid is used for the management of the disease in conjunction with an appropriate antituberculous regimen.

If corticosteroids are indicated in patients with latent tuberculosis or tuberculin reactivity, close observation is necessary as reactivation of the disease may occur. During prolonged corticosteroid therapy, these patients should receive chemoprophylaxis.

Literature reports suggest an apparent association between use of corticosteroids and left ventricular free wall rupture after a recent myocardial infarction; therefore, therapy with corticosteroids should be used with great caution in these patients.

PRECAUTIONS

This product, like many other steroid formulations, is sensitive to heat. Therefore, it should not be autoclaved when it is desirable to sterilize the exterior of the vial.

Following prolonged therapy, withdrawal of corticosteroids may result in symptoms of the corticosteroid withdrawal syndrome including fever, myalgia, arthralgia, and malaise. This may occur in patients even without evidence of adrenal insufficiency.

There is an enhanced effect of corticosteroids in patients with hypothyroidism and in those with cirrhosis.

Corticosteroids should be used cautiously in patients with ocular herpes simplex for fear of corneal perforation.

The lowest possible dose of corticosteroid should be used to control the condition under treatment, and when reduction in dosage is possible, the reduction must be gradual.

Psychic derangements may appear when corticosteroids are used, ranging from euphoria, insomnia, mood swings, personality changes, and severe depression to frank psychotic manifestations. Also, existing emotional instability or psychotic tendencies may be aggravated by corticosteroids.

Aspirin should be used cautiously in conjunction with corticosteroids in hypoprothrombinemia.

Steroids should be used with caution in nonspecific ulcerative colitis, if there is a probability of impending perforation, abscess, or other pyogenic infection, also in diverticulitis, fresh intestinal anastomoses, active or latent peptic ulcer, renal insufficiency, hypertension, osteoporosis, and my-

Continued on next page

Information on the Merck Sharp & Dohme products listed on these pages is the full prescribing information from product circulars in use August 31, 1989.

Merck Sharp & Dohme—Cont.

asthenia gravis. Signs of peritoneal irritation following gastrointestinal perforation in patients receiving large doses of corticosteroids may be minimal or absent. Fat embolism has been reported as a possible complication of hypercortisonism.

When large doses are given, some authorities advise that antacids be administered between meals to help to prevent peptic ulcer.

Growth and development of infants and children on prolonged corticosteroid therapy should be carefully followed. Steroids may increase or decrease motility and number of spermatozoa in some patients.

Phenytoin, phenobarbital, ephedrine, and rifampin may enhance the metabolic clearance of corticosteroids, resulting in decreased blood levels and lessened physiologic activity, thus requiring adjustment in corticosteroid dosage.

The prothrombin time should be checked frequently in patients who are receiving corticosteroids and coumarin anticoagulants at the same time because of reports that corticosteroids have altered the response to these anticoagulants. Studies have shown that the usual effect produced by adding corticosteroids is inhibition of response to coumarins, although there have been some conflicting reports of potentiation not substantiated by studies.

When corticosteroids are administered concomitantly with potassium-depleting diuretics, patients should be observed closely for development of hypokalemia.

Injection of a steroid into an infected site is to be avoided. The slower rate of absorption by intramuscular administration should be recognized.

ADVERSE REACTIONS

Fluid and electrolyte disturbances
  Sodium retention
  Fluid retention
  Congestive heart failure in susceptible patients
  Potassium loss
  Hypokalemic alkalosis
  Hypertension
Musculoskeletal
  Muscle weakness
  Steroid myopathy
  Loss of muscle mass
  Osteoporosis
  Vertebral compression fractures
  Aseptic necrosis of femoral and humeral heads
  Pathologic fracture of long bones
  Tendon rupture
Gastrointestinal
  Peptic ulcer with possible subsequent perforation and hemorrhage
  Perforation of the small and large bowel, particularly in patients with inflammatory bowel disease
  Pancreatitis
  Abdominal distention
  Ulcerative esophagitis
Dermatologic
  Impaired wound healing
  Thin fragile skin
  Petechiae and ecchymoses
  Erythema
  Increased sweating
  May suppress reactions to skin tests
  Burning or tingling, especially in the perineal area (after I.V. injection)
  Other cutaneous reactions, such as allergic dermatitis, urticaria, angioneurotic edema
Neurologic
  Convulsions
  Increased intracranial pressure with papilledema (pseudotumor cerebri) usually after treatment
  Vertigo
  Headache
  Psychic disturbances
Endocrine
  Menstrual irregularities
  Development of cushingoid state
  Suppression of growth in children
  Secondary adrenocortical and pituitary unresponsiveness, particularly in times of stress, as in trauma, surgery, or illness
  Decreased carbohydrate tolerance
  Manifestations of latent diabetes mellitus
  Increased requirements for insulin or oral hypoglycemic agents in diabetics
  Hirsutism
Ophthalmic
  Posterior subcapsular cataracts
  Increased intraocular pressure
  Glaucoma
  Exophthalmos

Metabolic
  Negative nitrogen balance due to protein catabolism
Cardiovascular
  Myocardial rupture following recent myocardial infarction (see WARNINGS).
Other
  Anaphylactoid or hypersensitivity reactions
  Thromboembolism
  Weight gain
  Increased appetite
  Nausea
  Malaise

The following *additional* adverse reactions are related to parenteral corticosteroid therapy:
  Rare instances of blindness associated with intralesional therapy around the face and head
  Hyperpigmentation or hypopigmentation
  Subcutaneous and cutaneous atrophy
  Sterile abscess

OVERDOSAGE

Reports of acute toxicity and/or death following overdosage of glucocorticoids are rare. In the event of overdosage, no specific antidote is available; treatment is supportive and symptomatic.

The intraperitoneal LD_{50} of hydrocortisone in female mice was 1740 mg/kg.

DOSAGE AND ADMINISTRATION

For intravenous, intramuscular, and subcutaneous injection.
HYDROCORTONE Phosphate injection can be given directly from the vial, or it can be added to Sodium Chloride Injection or Dextrose Injection and administered by intravenous drip.

Benzyl alcohol as a preservative has been associated with toxicity in premature infants. Solutions used for intravenous administration or further dilution of this product should be preservative-free when used in the neonate, especially the premature infant.

When it is mixed with an infusion solution, sterile precautions should be observed. Since infusion solutions generally do not contain preservatives, mixtures should be used within 24 hours.

DOSAGE REQUIREMENTS ARE VARIABLE AND MUST BE INDIVIDUALIZED ON THE BASIS OF THE DISEASE AND THE RESPONSE OF THE PATIENT.

The initial dosage varies from 15 to 240 mg a day depending on the disease being treated. In less severe diseases doses lower than 15 mg may suffice, while in severe diseases doses higher than 240 mg may be required. Usually the parenteral dosage ranges are one-third to one-half the oral dose given every 12 hours. However, in certain overwhelming, acute, life-threatening situations, administration in dosages exceeding the usual dosages may be justified and may be in multiples of the oral dosages.

The initial dosage should be maintained or adjusted until the patient's response is satisfactory. If a satisfactory clinical response does not occur after a reasonable period of time, discontinue HYDROCORTONE Phosphate injection and transfer the patient to other therapy.

After a favorable initial response, the proper maintenance dosage should be determined by decreasing the initial dosage in small amounts to the lowest dosage that maintains an adequate clinical response.

Patients should be observed closely for signs that might require dosage adjustment, including changes in clinical status resulting from remissions or exacerbations of the disease, individual drug responsiveness, and the effect of stress (e.g., surgery, infection, trauma). During stress it may be necessary to increase dosage temporarily.

If the drug is to be stopped after more than a few days of treatment, it usually should be withdrawn gradually.

HOW SUPPLIED

No. 7633—Injection HYDROCORTONE Phosphate, 50 mg hydrocortisone equivalent per mL, is a clear, light yellow solution, and is supplied as follows:
NDC 0006-7633-04 in 2 mL multiple dose vials.
NDC 0006-7633-10 in 10 mL multiple dose vials.
Storage
Sensitive to heat. Do not autoclave.
A.H.F.S. Category: 68:04
DC 7349523   Issued March 1988

HYDROCORTONE® Tablets   ℞
(Hydrocortisone, MSD), U.S.P.

DESCRIPTION

Glucocorticoids are adrenocortical steroids, both naturally occurring and synthetic, which are readily absorbed from the gastrointestinal tract.

Hydrocortisone is a white to practically white, odorless, crystalline powder, very slightly soluble in water. The molecular weight is 362.47. It is designated chemically as 11β,17,21-trihydroxypregn-4-ene-3,20-dione. The empirical formula is $C_{21}H_{30}O_5$ and the structural formula is:

Hydrocortisone is believed to be the principal hormone secreted by the adrenal cortex.
HYDROCORTONE® (Hydrocortisone, MSD) tablets are supplied in two potencies, 10 mg and 20 mg.
Inactive ingredients are lactose, magnesium stearate, and starch.

ACTIONS

Naturally occurring glucocorticoids (hydrocortisone and cortisone), which also have salt-retaining properties, are used as replacement therapy in adrenocortical deficiency states. They are also used for their potent anti-inflammatory effects in disorders of many organ systems.

Glucocorticoids cause profound and varied metabolic effects. In addition, they modify the body's immune responses to diverse stimuli.

INDICATIONS

1. *Endocrine Disorders*
  Primary or secondary adrenocortical insufficiency (hydrocortisone or cortisone is the first choice; synthetic analogs may be used in conjunction with mineralocorticoids where applicable; in infancy mineralocorticoid supplementation is of particular importance)
  Congenital adrenal hyperplasia
  Nonsuppurative thyroiditis
  Hypercalcemia associated with cancer
2. *Rheumatic Disorders*
  As adjunctive therapy for short-term administration (to tide the patient over an acute episode or exacerbation) in:
  Psoriatic arthritis
  Rheumatoid arthritis, including juvenile rheumatoid arthritis (selected cases may require low-dose maintenance therapy)
  Ankylosing spondylitis
  Acute and subacute bursitis
  Acute nonspecific tenosynovitis
  Acute gouty arthritis
  Post-traumatic osteoarthritis
  Synovitis of osteoarthritis
  Epicondylitis
3. *Collagen Diseases*
  During an exacerbation or as maintenance therapy in selected cases of—
  Systemic lupus erythematosus
  Acute rheumatic carditis
  Systemic dermatomyositis (polymyositis)
4. *Dermatologic Diseases*
  Pemphigus
  Bullous dermatitis herpetiformis
  Severe erythema multiforme (Stevens-Johnson syndrome)
  Exfoliative dermatitis
  Mycosis fungoides
  Severe psoriasis
  Severe seborrheic dermatitis
5. *Allergic States*
  Control of severe or incapacitating allergic conditions intractable to adequate trials of conventional treatment:
  Seasonal or perennial allergic rhinitis
  Bronchial asthma
  Contact dermatitis
  Atopic dermatitis
  Serum sickness
  Drug hypersensitivity reactions
6. *Ophthalmic Diseases*
  Severe acute and chronic allergic and inflammatory processes involving the eye and its adnexa, such as—
  Allergic conjunctivitis
  Keratitis
  Allergic corneal marginal ulcers
  Herpes zoster ophthalmicus
  Iritis and iridocyclitis
  Chorioretinitis
  Anterior segment inflammation

Diffuse posterior uveitis and choroiditis
Optic neuritis
Sympathetic ophthalmia

7. *Respiratory Diseases*
Symptomatic sarcoidosis
Loeffler's syndrome not manageable by other means
Berylliosis
Fulminating or disseminated pulmonary tuberculosis when used concurrently with appropriate antituberculous chemotherapy
Aspiration pneumonitis

8. *Hematologic Disorders*
Idiopathic thrombocytopenic purpura in adults
Secondary thrombocytopenia in adults
Acquired (autoimmune) hemolytic anemia
Erythroblastopenia (RBC anemia)
Congenital (erythroid) hypoplastic anemia

9. *Neoplastic Diseases*
For palliative management of:
Leukemias and lymphomas in adults
Acute leukemia of childhood

10. *Edematous States*
To induce a diuresis or remission of proteinuria in the nephrotic syndrome, without uremia, of the idiopathic type or that due to lupus erythematosus

11. *Gastrointestinal Diseases*
To tide the patient over a critical period of the disease in:
Ulcerative colitis
Regional enteritis

12. *Miscellaneous*
Tuberculous meningitis with subarachnoid block or impending block when used concurrently with appropriate antituberculous chemotherapy
Trichinosis with neurologic or myocardial involvement

CONTRAINDICATIONS

Systemic fungal infections
Hypersensitivity to this product

WARNINGS

In patients on corticosteroid therapy subjected to unusual stress, increased dosage of rapidly acting corticosteroids before, during, and after the stressful situation is indicated.
Drug-induced secondary adrenocortical insufficiency may result from too rapid wthdrawal of corticosteroids and may be minimized by gradual reduction of dosage. This type of relative insufficiency may persist for months after discontinuation of therapy; therefore, in any situation of stress occurring during that period, hormone therapy should be reinstituted. If the patient is receiving steroids already, dosage may have to be increased. Since mineralocorticoid secretion may be impaired, salt and/or a mineralocorticoid should be administered concurrently.
Corticosteroids may mask some signs of infection, and new infections may appear during their use. There may be decreased resistance and inability to localize infection when corticosteroids are used. Moreover, corticosteroids may affect the nitroblue-tetrazolium test for bacterial infection and produce false negative results.
In cerebral malaria, a double-blind trial has shown that the use of corticosteroids is associated with prolongation of coma and a higher incidence of pneumonia and gastrointestinal bleeding.
Corticosteroids may activate latent amebiasis. Therefore, it is recommended that latent or active amebiasis be ruled out before initiating corticosteroid therapy in any patient who has spent time in the tropics or any patient with unexplained diarrhea.
Prolonged use of corticosteroids may produce posterior subcapsular cataracts, glaucoma with possible damage to the optic nerves, and may enhance the establishment of secondary ocular infections due to fungi or viruses.
Usage in pregnancy: Since adequate human reproduction studies have not been done with corticosteroids, use of these drugs in pregnancy or in women of childbearing potential requires that the anticipated benefits be weighed against the possible hazards to the mother and embryo or fetus. Infants born of mothers who have received substantial doses of corticosteroids during pregnancy should be carefully observed for signs of hypoadrenalism.
Corticosteroids appear in breast milk and could suppress growth, interfere with endogenous corticosteroid production, or cause other unwanted effects. Mothers taking pharmacologic doses of corticosteroids should be advised not to nurse.
Average and large doses of hydrocortisone or cortisone can cause elevation of blood pressure, salt and water retention, and increased excretion of potassium. These effects are less likely to occur with the synthetic derivatives except when used in large doses. Dietary salt restriction and potassium supplementation may be necessary. All corticosteroids increase calcium excretion.
Administration of live virus vaccines, including smallpox, is contraindicated in individuals receiving immunosuppressive doses of corticosteroids. If inactivated viral or bacterial vaccines are administered to individuals receiving immunosuppressive doses of corticosteroids, the expected serum antibody response may not be obtained. However, immunization procedures may be undertaken in patients who are receiving corticosteroids as replacement therapy, e.g., for Addison's disease.
The use of HYDROCORTONE tablets in active tuberculosis should be restricted to those cases of fulminating or disseminated tuberculosis in which the corticosteroid is used for the management of the disease in conjunction with an appropriate antituberculous regimen.
If corticosteroids are indicated in patients with latent tuberculosis or tuberculin reactivity, close observation is necessary as reactivation of the disease may occur. During prolonged corticosteroid therapy, these patients should receive chemoprophylaxis.
Literature reports suggest an apparent association between use of corticosteroids and left ventricular free wall rupture after a recent myocardial infarction; therefore, therapy with corticosteroids should be used with great caution in these patients.

PRECAUTIONS

Following prolonged therapy, withdrawal of corticosteroids may result in symptoms of the corticosteroid withdrawal syndrome including fever, myalgia, arthralgia, and malaise. This may occur in patients even without evidence of adrenal insufficiency.
There is an enhanced effect of corticosteroids in patients with hypothyroidism and in those with cirrhosis.
Corticosteroids should be used cautiously in patients with ocular herpes simplex because of possible corneal perforation.
The lowest possible dose of corticosteroid should be used to control the condition under treatment, and when reduction in dosage is possible, the reduction should be gradual.
Psychic derangements may appear when corticosteroids are used, ranging from euphoria, insomnia, mood swings, personality changes, and severe depression, to frank psychotic manifestations. Also, existing emotional instability or psychotic tendencies may be aggravated by corticosteroids.
Aspirin should be used cautiously in conjunction with corticosteroids in hypoprothrombinemia.
Steroids should be used with caution in nonspecific ulcerative colitis, if there is a probability of impending perforation, abscess, or other pyogenic infection, diverticulitis, fresh intestinal anastomoses, active or latent peptic ulcer, renal insufficiency, hypertension, osteoporosis, and myasthenia gravis. Signs of peritoneal irritation following gastrointestinal perforation in patients receiving large doses of corticosteroids may be minimal or absent. Fat embolism has been reported as a possible complication of hypercortisonism.
When large doses are given, some authorities advise that corticosteroids be taken with meals and antacids taken between meals to help to prevent peptic ulcer.
Growth and development of infants and children on prolonged corticosteroid therapy should be carefully observed.
Steroids may increase or decrease motility and number of spermatozoa in some patients.
Phenytoin, phenobarbital, ephedrine, and rifampin may enhance the metabolic clearance of corticosteroids, resulting in decreased blood levels and lessened physiologic activity, thus requiring adjustment in corticosteroid dosage.
The prothrombin time should be checked frequently in patients who are receiving corticosteroids and coumarin anticoagulants at the same time because of reports that corticosteroids have altered the response to these anticoagulants. Studies have shown that the usual effect produced by adding corticosteroids is inhibition of response to coumarins, although there have been some conflicting reports of potentiation not substantiated by studies.
When corticosteroids are administered concomitantly with potassium-depleting diuretics, patients should be observed closely for development of hypokalemia.

ADVERSE REACTIONS

Fluid and Electrolyte Disturbances
Sodium retention
Fluid retention
Congestive heart failure in susceptible patients
Potassium loss
Hypokalemic alkalosis
Hypertension
Musculoskeletal
Muscle weakness
Steroid myopathy
Loss of muscle mass
Osteoporosis
Vertebral compression fractures
Aseptic necrosis of femoral and humeral heads
Pathologic fracture of long bones
Tendon rupture

Gastrointestinal
Peptic ulcer with possible perforation and hemorrhage
Perforation of the small and large bowel, particularly in patients with inflammatory bowel disease
Pancreatitis
Abdominal distention
Ulcerative esophagitis
Dermatologic
Impaired wound healing
Thin fragile skin
Petechiae and ecchymoses
Erythema
Increased sweating
May suppress reactions to skin tests
Other cutaneous reactions, such as allergic dermatitis, urticaria, angioneurotic edema
Neurologic
Convulsions
Increased intracranial pressure with papilledema (pseudotumor cerebri) usually after treatment
Vertigo
Headache
Psychic disturbances
Endocrine
Menstrual irregularities
Development of cushingoid state
Suppression of growth in children
Secondary adrenocortical and pituitary unresponsiveness, particularly in times of stress, as in trauma, surgery, or illness
Decreased carbohydrate tolerance
Manifestations of latent diabetes mellitus
Increased requirements for insulin or oral hypoglycemic agents in diabetics
Hirsutism
Ophthalmic
Posterior subcapsular cataracts
Increased intraocular pressure
Glaucoma
Exophthalmos
Metabolic
Negative nitrogen balance due to protein catabolism
Cardiovascular
Myocardial rupture following recent myocardial infarction (see WARNINGS).
Other
Hypersensitivity
Thromboembolism
Weight gain
Increased appetite
Nausea
Malaise

OVERDOSAGE

Reports of acute toxicity and/or death following overdosage of glucocorticoids are rare. In the event of overdosage, no specific antidote is available; treatment is supportive and symptomatic.
The intraperitoneal LD_{50} of hydrocortisone in female mice was 1740 mg/kg.

DOSAGE AND ADMINISTRATION

For oral administration
DOSAGE REQUIREMENTS ARE VARIABLE AND MUST BE INDIVIDUALIZED ON THE BASIS OF THE DISEASE AND THE RESPONSE OF THE PATIENT.
The initial dosage varies from 20 to 240 mg a day depending on the disease being treated. In less severe diseases doses lower than 20 mg may suffice, while in severe diseases doses higher than 240 mg may be required. The initial dosage should be maintained or adjusted until the patient's response is satisfactory. If satisfactory clinical response does not occur after a reasonable period of time, discontinue HYDROCORTONE tablets and transfer the patient to other therapy.
After a favorable initial response, the proper maintenance dosage should be determined by decreasing the initial dosage in small amounts to the lowest dosage that maintains an adequate clinical response.
Patients should be observed closely for signs that might require dosage adjustment, including changes in clinical status resulting from remissions or exacerbations of the disease, individual drug responsiveness, and the effect of stress (e.g, surgery, infection, trauma). During stress it may be necessary to increase dosage temporarily.

Continued on next page

Merck Sharp & Dohme—Cont.

If the drug is to be stopped after more than a few days of treatment, it usually should be withdrawn gradually.

HOW SUPPLIED

No. 7604—Tablets HYDROCORTONE, 10 mg each, are white, oval shaped compressed tablets, scored on one side, coded MSD 619, and are supplied as follows:
NDC 0006-0619-68 in bottles of 100.
  Shown in Product Identification Section, page 418
No. 7602—Tablets HYDROCORTONE, 20 mg each, are white, oval shaped compressed tablets, scored on one side, coded MSD 625, and are supplied as follows:
NDC 0006-0625-68 in bottles of 100.
  Shown in Product Identification Section, page 418
  A.H.F.S. Category: 68:04
  DC 7414424   Issued March 1988

HydroDIURIL® Tablets   ℞
(Hydrochlorothiazide, MSD), U.S.P.

DESCRIPTION

HydroDIURIL® (Hydrochlorothiazide, MSD) is a diuretic and antihypertensive. It is the 3,4-dihydro derivative of chlorothiazide. Its chemical name is 6-chloro-3,4-dihydro- '2H -1, 2, 4-benzothiadiazine-7-sulfonamide 1,1-dioxide. Its empirical formula is $C_7H_8ClN_3O_4S_2$ and its structural formula is:

It is a white, or practically white, crystalline powder with a molecular weight of 297.72, which is slightly soluble in water, but freely soluble in sodium hydroxide solution.
HydroDIURIL is supplied as 25 mg, 50 mg and 100 mg tablets for oral use. Each tablet contains the following inactive ingredients: calcium phosphate, FD&C Yellow 6, gelatin, lactose, magnesium stearate, starch and talc.

CLINICAL PHARMACOLOGY

The mechanism of the antihypertensive effect of thiazides is unknown. HydroDIURIL does not usually affect normal blood pressure.
HydroDIURIL affects the distal renal tubular mechanism of electrolyte reabsorption. At maximal therapeutic dosage all thiazides are approximately equal in their diuretic efficacy. HydroDIURIL increases excretion of sodium and chloride in approximately equivalent amounts. Natriuresis may be accompanied by some loss of potassium and bicarbonate.
After oral use diuresis begins within 2 hours, peaks in about 4 hours and lasts about 6 to 12 hours.
Pharmacokinetics and Metabolism
HydroDIURIL is not metabolized but is eliminated rapidly by the kidney. When plasma levels have been followed for at least 24 hours, the plasma half-life has been observed to vary between 5.6 and 14.8 hours. At least 61 percent of the oral dose is eliminated unchanged within 24 hours. Hydrochlorothiazide crosses the placental but not the blood-brain barrier and is excreted in breast milk.

INDICATIONS AND USAGE

HydroDIURIL is indicated as adjunctive therapy in edema associated with congestive heart failure, hepatic cirrhosis, and corticosteroid and estrogen therapy.
HydroDIURIL has also been found useful in edema due to various forms of renal dysfunction such as nephrotic syndrome, acute glomerulonephritis, and chronic renal failure.
HydroDIURIL is indicated in the management of hypertension either as the sole therapeutic agent or to enhance the effectiveness of other antihypertensive drugs in the more severe forms of hypertension.
Use in Pregnancy. Routine use of diuretics during normal pregnancy is inappropriate and exposes mother and fetus to unnecessary hazard. Diuretics do not prevent development of toxemia of pregnancy and there is no satisfactory evidence that they are useful in the treatment of toxemia.
Edema during pregnancy may arise from pathologic causes or from the physiologic and mechanical consequences of pregnancy. Thiazides are indicated in pregnancy when edema is due to pathologic causes, just as they are in the absence of pregnancy (see PRECAUTIONS, *Pregnancy*). Dependent edema in pregnancy, resulting from restriction of venous return by the gravid uterus, is properly treated through elevation of the lower extremities and use of support stockings. Use of diuretics to lower intravascular volume in

this instance is illogical and unnecessary. During normal pregnancy there is hypervolemia which is not harmful to the fetus or the mother in the absence of cardiovascular disease. However, it may be associated with edema, rarely generalized edema. If such edema causes discomfort, increased recumbency will often provide relief. Rarely this edema may cause extreme discomfort which is not relieved by rest. In these instances, a short course of diuretic therapy may provide relief and be appropriate.

CONTRAINDICATIONS

Anuria.
Hypersensitivity to this product or to other sulfonamide-derived drugs.

WARNINGS

Use with caution in severe renal disease. In patients with renal disease, thiazides may precipitate azotemia. Cumulative effects of the drug may develop in patients with impaired renal function.
Thiazides should be used with caution in patients with impaired hepatic function or progressive liver disease, since minor alterations of fluid and electrolyte balance may precipitate hepatic coma.
Thiazides may add to or potentiate the action of other antihypertensive drugs.
Sensitivity reactions may occur in patients with or without a history of allergy or bronchial asthma.
The possibility of exacerbation or activation of systemic lupus erythematosus has been reported.
Lithium generally should not be given with diuretics (see PRECAUTIONS, *Drug Interactions*).

PRECAUTIONS

General
All patients receiving diuretic therapy should be observed for evidence of fluid or electrolyte imbalance: namely, hyponatremia, hypochloremic alkalosis, and hypokalemia. Serum and urine electrolyte determinations are particularly important when the patient is vomiting excessively or receiving parenteral fluids. Warning signs or symptoms of fluid and electrolyte imbalance, irrespective of cause, include dryness of mouth, thirst, weakness, lethargy, drowsiness, restlessness, muscle pains or cramps, muscular fatigue, hypotension, oliguria, tachycardia, and gastrointestinal disturbances such as nausea and vomiting.
Hypokalemia may develop, especially with brisk diuresis, when severe cirrhosis is present or after prolonged therapy. Interference with adequate oral electrolyte intake will also contribute to hypokalemia. Hypokalemia may cause cardiac arrhythmia and may also sensitize or exaggerate the response of the heart to the toxic effects of digitalis (e.g., increased ventricular irritability). Hypokalemia may be avoided or treated by use of potassium sparing diuretics or potassium supplements such as foods with a high potassium content.
Although any chloride deficit is generally mild and usually does not require specific treatment except under extraordinary circumstances (as in liver disease or renal disease), chloride replacement may be required in the treatment of metabolic alkalosis.
Dilutional hyponatremia may occur in edematous patients in hot weather; appropriate therapy is water restriction, rather than administration of salt, except in rare instances when the hyponatremia is life threatening. In actual salt depletion, appropriate replacement is the therapy of choice.
Hyperuricemia may occur or acute gout may be precipitated in certain patients receiving thiazides.
In diabetic patients dosage adjustments of insulin or oral hypoglycemic agents may be required. Hyperglycemia may occur with thiazide diuretics. Thus latent diabetes mellitus may become manifest during thiazide therapy.
The antihypertensive effects of the drug may be enhanced in the post-sympathectomy patient.
If progressive renal impairment becomes evident, consider withholding or discontinuing diuretic therapy.
Thiazides have been shown to increase the urinary excretion of magnesium; this may result in hypomagnesemia.
Thiazides may decrease urinary calcium excretion. Thiazides may cause intermittent and slight elevation of serum calcium in the absence of known disorders of calcium metabolism. Marked hypercalcemia may be evidence of hidden hyperparathyroidism. Thiazides should be discontinued before carrying out tests for parathyroid function.
Increases in cholesterol and triglyceride levels may be associated with thiazide diuretic therapy.
Laboratory Tests
Periodic determination of serum electrolytes to detect possible electrolyte imbalance should be done at appropriate intervals.

Drug Interactions
When given concurrently the following drugs may interact with thiazide diuretics.
Alcohol, barbiturates, or narcotics —potentiation of orthostatic hypotension may occur.
Antidiabetic drugs —(oral agents and insulin)—dosage adjustment of the antidiabetic drug may be required.
Other antihypertensive drugs —additive effect or potentiation.
Corticosteroids, ACTH —intensified electrolyte depletion, particularly hypokalemia.
Pressor amines (e.g., norepinephrine) —possible decreased response to pressor amines but not sufficient to preclude their use.
Skeletal muscle relaxants, nondepolarizing (e.g., tubocurarine) —possible increased responsiveness to the muscle relaxant.
Lithium —generally should not be given with diuretics. Diuretic agents reduce the renal clearance of lithium and add a high risk of lithium toxicity. Refer to the package insert for lithium preparations before use of such preparations with HydroDIURIL.
Non-steroidal Anti-inflammatory Drugs —In some patients, the administration of a non-steroidal anti-inflammatory agent can reduce the diuretic, natriuretic, and antihypertensive effects of loop, potassium-sparing and thiazide diuretics. Therefore, when HydroDIURIL and non-steroidal anti-inflammatory agents are used concomitantly, the patient should be observed closely to determine if the desired effect of the diuretic is obtained.
Drug/Laboratory Test Interactions
Thiazides should be discontinued before carrying out tests for parathyroid function (see PRECAUTIONS, *General*).
Carcinogenesis, Mutagenesis, Impairment of Fertility
Hydrochlorothiazide is currently under study in the U.S. Carcinogenesis Testing Program.
Hydrochlorothiazide was not mutagenic *in vitro*, in the Ames microbial mutagen test at a maximum concentration of 5 mg/plate using Strains TA98 and TA100. Urine samples of patients treated with hydrochlorothiazide did not have mutagenic activity in the Ames test.
The ability of a number of drugs to induce nondisjunction and crossing-over was measured using *Aspergillus nidulans*. A large number of drugs, including hydrochlorothiazide, induced nondisjunction.
Hydrochlorothiazide had no effect on fertility in a two-litter study in rats at doses of 4-5.6 mg/kg/day (up to 2 times the maximum recommended human dose).
Pregnancy
Teratogenic Effects—Pregnancy Category B: Reproduction studies in the rabbit, the mouse and the rat at doses up to 100 mg/kg/day (50 times the maximum human dose) showed no evidence of external abnormalities of the fetus due to hydrochlorothiazide. Hydrochlorothiazide given in a two-litter study in rats at doses of 4–5.6 mg/kg/day (approximately 1–2 times the maximum recommended human dose) did not impair fertility or produce birth abnormalities in the offspring. There are no adequate and well-controlled studies with HydroDIURIL in pregnant women; however, thiazides cross the placental barrier and appear in cord blood. Since animal reproduction studies are not always predictive of human response, HydroDIURIL should be used during pregnancy only if clearly needed. (See INDICATIONS AND USAGE.)
Nonteratogenic effects: These may include fetal or neonatal jaundice, thrombocytopenia, and possibly other adverse reactions which have occurred in the adult.
Nursing Mothers
Because of the potential for serious adverse reactions in nursing infants from HydroDIURIL, a decision should be made whether to discontinue nursing or to discontinue the drug, taking into account the importance of the drug to the mother.

ADVERSE REACTIONS

The following adverse reactions have been reported and, within each category, are listed in order of decreasing severity.
Body as a Whole: Weakness.
Cardiovascular: Hypotension including orthostatic hypotension (may be aggravated by alcohol, barbiturates, narcotics or antihypertensive drugs).
Digestive: Pancreatitis, jaundice (intrahepatic cholestatic jaundice), diarrhea, vomiting, sialadenitis, cramping, constipation, gastric irritation, nausea, anorexia.
Hematologic: Aplastic anemia, agranulocytosis, leukopenia, hemolytic anemia, thrombocytopenia.
Hypersensitivity: Anaphylactic reactions, necrotizing angiitis (vasculitis and cutaneous vasculitis), respiratory distress including pneumonitis and pulmonary edema, photosensitivity, fever, urticaria, rash, purpura.
Metabolic: Electrolyte imbalance (see PRECAUTIONS), hyperglycemia, glycosuria, hyperuricemia.

Musculoskeletal: Muscle spasm.

Nervous System/Psychiatric: Vertigo, paresthesias, dizziness, headache, restlessness.

Renal: Renal failure, renal dysfunction, interstitial nephritis. (See WARNINGS.)

Special Senses: Transient blurred vision, xanthopsia.

Whenever adverse reactions are moderate or severe, thiazide dosage should be reduced or therapy withdrawn.

OVERDOSAGE

The oral LD_{50} of hydrochlorothiazide is greater than 10 g/kg in the mouse and rat.

The most common signs and symptoms observed are those caused by electrolyte depletion (hypokalemia, hypochloremia, hyponatremia) and dehydration resulting from excessive diuresis. If digitalis has also been administered, hypokalemia may accentuate cardiac arrhythmias.

In the event of overdosage, symptomatic and supportive measures should be employed. Emesis should be induced or gastric lavage performed. Correct dehydration, electrolyte imbalance, hepatic coma and hypotension by established procedures. If required, give oxygen or artificial respiration for respiratory impairment.

DOSAGE AND ADMINISTRATION

Therapy should be individualized according to patient response. Use the smallest dosage necessary to achieve the required response.

Adults

For Diuresis

The usual adult dosage is 50 to 100 mg once or twice a day. Many patients with edema respond to intermittent therapy, i.e., administration on alternate days or on three to five days each week. With an intermittent schedule, excessive response and the resulting undesirable electrolyte imbalance are less likely to occur.

For Control of Hypertension

The usual adult starting dosage is 50 or 100 mg a day as a single or divided dose. Dosage is increased or decreased according to blood pressure response. Rarely some patients may require up to 200 mg a day in divided doses.

Patients usually do not require doses in excess of 50 mg of hydrochlorothiazide daily when used concomitantly with other antihypertensive agents.

Infants and Children

The usual pediatric dosage is based on 1.0 mg of HydroDIU-RIL per pound of body weight per day in two doses. Infants under 6 months of age may require up to 1.5 mg per pound per day in two doses.

On this basis, infants up to 2 years of age may be given 12.5 to 37.5 mg daily in two doses. Children from 2 to 12 years of age may be given 37.5 to 100 mg daily in two doses. Dosage in both age groups should be based on body weight.

HOW SUPPLIED

No. 3263—Tablets HydroDIURIL, 25 mg, are peach-colored, round, scored, compressed tablets, coded MSD 42. They are supplied as follows:

NDC 0006-0042-68 bottles of 100

NDC 0006-0042-28 unit dose packages of 100

NDC 0006-0042-82 bottles of 1000.

Shown in Product Identification Section, page 418

No. 3264—Tablets HydroDIURIL, 50 mg, are peach-colored, round, scored, compressed tablets, coded MSD 105. They are supplied as follows:

NDC 0006-0105-68 bottles of 100

NDC 0006-0105-28 unit dose packages of 100

NDC 0006-0105-82 bottles of 1000

NDC 0006-0105-86 bottles of 5000.

Shown in Product Identification Section, page 418

No. 3340—Tablets HydroDIURIL, 100 mg, are peach-colored, round, scored, compressed tablets, coded MSD 410. They are supplied as follows:

NDC 0006-0410-68 bottles of 100.

Shown in Product Identification Section, page 418

A.H.F.S. Category: 40:28

DC 7398042   Issued October 1987

COPYRIGHT © MERCK & CO., INC., 1986

All rights reserved

HYDROPRES® Tablets   ℞

(Reserpine-Hydrochlorothiazide, MSD), U.S.P.

---

apy titrated to the individual patient. If the fixed combination represents the dosage so determined, its use may be more convenient in patient management. The treatment of hypertension is not static, but must be re-evaluated as conditions in each patient warrant.

DESCRIPTION

HYDROPRES® (Reserpine-Hydrochlorothiazide, MSD) combines two antihypertensives: HydroDIURIL® (Hydrochlorothiazide, MSD) and reserpine.

Hydrochlorothiazide

Hydrochlorothiazide is a diuretic and antihypertensive. It is the 3,4-dihydro derivative of chlorothiazide. Its chemical name is 6-chloro-3,4-dihydro-2H-1,2,4-benzothiadiazine-7-sulfonamide 1,1-dioxide. Its empirical formula is $C_7H_8ClN_3O_4S_2$ and its structural formula is:

Hydrochlorothiazide is a white, or practically white, crystalline powder with a molecular weight of 297.72, which is slightly soluble in water, but freely soluble in sodium hydroxide solution.

Reserpine

The chemical name for reserpine is (11, 17α-dimethoxy -18β-[(3,4,5-trimethoxybenzoyl) oxy]-3β, 20α-yohimban-16β-carboxylic acid methyl ester). It is a crystalline alkaloid derived from Rauwolfia serpentina. Its empirical formula is $C_{33}H_{40}N_2O_9$ and its structural formula is:

Reserpine is a white or pale buff to slightly yellowish, odorless, crystalline powder with a molecular weight of 608.69, is insoluble in water, and freely soluble in glacial acetic acid.

HYDROPRES is supplied as tablets in two strengths for oral use:

HYDROPRES 25, contains 25 mg of hydrochlorothiazide and 0.125 mg of reserpine.

HYDROPRES 50, contains 50 mg of hydrochlorothiazide and 0.125 mg of reserpine.

Each tablet contains the following inactive ingredients: calcium phosphate, D&C Yellow 10, FD&C Blue 1, FD&C Yellow 6, lactose, magnesium stearate, starch and talc.

CLINICAL PHARMACOLOGY

Hydrochlorothiazide

The mechanism of the antihypertensive effect of thiazides is unknown. Hydrochlorothiazide does not usually affect normal blood pressure.

Hydrochlorothiazide affects the distal renal tubular mechanism of electrolyte reabsorption. At maximal therapeutic dosage all thiazides are approximately equal in their diuretic efficacy.

Hydrochlorothiazide increases excretion of sodium and chloride in approximately equivalent amounts. Natriuresis may be accompanied by some loss of potassium and bicarbonate. After oral use, diuresis begins within 2 hours, peaks in about 4 hours and lasts about 6 to 12 hours.

Reserpine

Reserpine has antihypertensive, bradycardic, and tranquilizing properties. It lowers arterial blood pressure by depletion of catecholamines. Reserpine is beneficial in relieving anxiety, tension, and headache in the hypertensive patient. It acts at the hypothalamic level of the central nervous system to promote relaxation without hypnosis or analgesia. The sleep pattern shown by the electroencephalogram following barbiturates does not occur with this drug. In laboratory animals spontaneous activity and response to external stimuli are decreased, but confusion or difficulty of movement is not evident.

The bradycardic action of reserpine promotes relaxation and may eliminate sinus tachycardia. It is most pronounced in subjects with sinus tachycardia and usually is not prominent in persons with a normal pulse rate.

Miosis, relaxation of the nictitating membrane, ptosis, hypothermia, and increased gastrointestinal activity are noted in animals given reserpine, sometimes in subclinical doses.

None of these effects, except increased gastrointestinal activity, has been found to be clinically significant in man with therapeutic doses.

Pharmacokinetics and Metabolism

Hydrochlorothiazide

Hydrochlorothiazide is not metabolized but is eliminated rapidly by the kidney. When plasma levels have been followed for at least 24 hours, the plasma half-life has been observed to vary between 5.6 and 14.8 hours. At least 61 percent of the oral dose is eliminated unchanged within 24 hours. Hydrochlorothiazide crosses the placental but not the blood-brain barrier and is excreted in breast milk.

Reserpine

Oral reserpine is rapidly absorbed from the gastrointestinal tract. Methylreserpate and trimethoxybenzoic acid are the primary metabolites which result from the hydrolytic cleavage of reserpine. Maximal blood levels were achieved approximately 2 hours after the oral dosage of ³H-reserpine to six normal volunteers; within 96 hours approximately 8 percent was excreted in urine and 62 percent in feces. Reserpine appears in human breast milk. Reserpine crosses the placental barrier in guinea pigs.

INDICATION AND USAGE

Hypertension (see box warning).

Use in Pregnancy. Routine use of diuretics during normal pregnancy is inappropriate and exposes mother and fetus to unnecessary hazard. Diuretics do not prevent development of toxemia of pregnancy and there is no satisfactory evidence that they are useful in the treatment of toxemia.

Edema during pregnancy may arise from pathologic causes or from the physiologic and mechanical consequences of pregnancy. Thiazides are indicated in pregnancy when edema is due to pathologic causes, just as they are in the absence of pregnancy (see PRECAUTIONS, *Pregnancy*). Dependent edema in pregnancy, resulting from restriction of venous return by the gravid uterus, is properly treated through elevation of the lower extremities and use of support stockings. Use of diuretics to lower intravascular volume in this instance is illogical and unnecessary. During normal pregnancy there is hypervolemia which is not harmful to the fetus or the mother in the absence of cardiovascular disease. However, it may be associated with edema, rarely generalized edema. If such edema causes discomfort, increased recumbency will often provide relief. Rarely this edema may cause extreme discomfort which is not relieved by rest. In these instances, a short course of diuretic therapy may provide relief and be appropriate.

CONTRAINDICATIONS

Hydrochlorothiazide is contraindicated in anuria.

HYDROPRES is contraindicated in hypersensitivity to hydrochlorothiazide or other sulfonamide-derived drugs or to reserpine.

Electroshock therapy should not be given to patients while on reserpine, as severe and even fatal reactions have been reported with minimal convulsive electroshock dosage. After discontinuing reserpine, allow at least seven days before starting electroshock therapy.

Active peptic ulcer, ulcerative colitis, and active mental depression, especially suicidal tendencies, are contraindications to reserpine therapy.

WARNINGS

Hydrochlorothiazide

Use with caution in severe renal disease. In patients with renal disease, thiazides may precipitate azotemia. Cumulative effects of the drug may develop in patients with impaired renal function.

Thiazides should be used with caution in patients with impaired hepatic function or progressive liver disease, since minor alterations of fluid and electrolyte balance may precipitate hepatic coma.

Thiazides may add to or potentiate the action of other antihypertensive drugs.

Sensitivity reactions may occur in patients with or without a history of allergy or bronchial asthma.

The possibility of exacerbation or activation of systemic lupus erythematosus has been reported.

Lithium generally should not be given with diuretics (see PRECAUTIONS, *Drug Interactions*).

Reserpine

The occurrence of mental depression due to reserpine in doses of 0.25 mg daily or less is unusual. In any event, HY-

Continued on next page

Information on the Merck Sharp & Dohme products listed on these pages is the full prescribing information from product circulars in use August 31, 1989.

Merck Sharp & Dohme—Cont.

DROPRES should be discontinued at the first sign of depression.

PRECAUTIONS

General

Hydrochlorothiazide

All patients receiving diuretic therapy should be observed for evidence of fluid or electrolyte imbalance: namely, hyponatremia, hypochloremic alkalosis, and hypokalemia. Serum and urine electrolyte determinations are particularly important when the patient is vomiting excessively or receiving parenteral fluids. Warning signs or symptoms of fluid and electrolyte imbalance irrespective of cause, include dryness of mouth, thirst, weakness, lethargy, drowsiness, restlessness, muscle pains or cramps, muscular fatigue, hypotension, oliguria, tachycardia, and gastrointestinal disturbances such as nausea and vomiting.

Hypokalemia may develop, especially with brisk diuresis, when severe cirrhosis is present or after prolonged therapy. Interference with adequate oral electrolyte intake will contribute to hypokalemia. Hypokalemia may cause cardiac arrhythmia and may also sensitize or exaggerate the response of the heart to the toxic effects of digitalis (e.g., increased ventricular irritability). Hypokalemia may be avoided or treated by use of potassium sparing diuretic or potassium supplements such as foods with a high potassium content.

Although any chloride deficit is generally mild and usually does not require specific treatment except under extraordinary circumstances (as in liver disease or renal disease), chloride replacement may be required in the treatment of metabolic alkalosis.

Dilutional hyponatremia may occur in edematous patients in hot weather. Appropriate therapy is water restriction, rather than administration of salt, except in rare instances when the hyponatremia is life threatening. In actual salt depletion, appropriate replacement is the therapy of choice.

Hyperuricemia may occur or acute gout may be precipitated in certain patients receiving thiazides.

In diabetic patients dosage adjustment of insulin or oral hypoglycemic agents may be required. Hyperglycemia may occur with thiazide diuretics. Thus latent diabetes mellitus may become manifest during thiazide therapy.

The antihypertensive effect of the drug may be enhanced in the postsympathectomy patient.

If progressive renal impairment becomes evident, consider withholding or discontinuing diuretic therapy.

Thiazides have been shown to increase the urinary excretion of magnesium; this may result in hypomagnesemia.

Thiazides may decrease urinary calcium excretion. Thiazides may cause intermittent and slight elevation of serum calcium in the absence of known disorders of calcium metabolism. Marked hypercalcemia may be evidence of hidden hyperparathyroidism. Thiazides should be discontinued before carrying out tests for parathyroid function.

Increases in cholesterol and triglyceride levels may be associated with thiazide diuretic therapy.

Reserpine

Since reserpine may increase gastric secretion and motility, it should be used cautiously in patients with a history of peptic ulcer, ulcerative colitis, or other gastrointestinal disorder. This compound may precipitate biliary colic in patients with gallstones, or bronchial asthma in susceptible persons. Reserpine may cause hypotension including orthostatic hypotension.

Anxiety or depression, as well as psychosis, may develop during reserpine therapy. If depression is present when therapy is begun, it may be aggravated. Mental depression is unusual with reserpine doses of 0.25 mg daily or less. In any case, HYDROPRES should be discontinued at the first sign of depression. Extreme caution should be used in treating patients with a history of mental depression, and the possibility of suicide should be kept in mind.

As with most antihypertensive therapy, caution should be exercised when treating hypertensive patients with renal insufficiency, since they adjust poorly to lowered blood pressure.

When two or more antihypertensives are given, the individual dosages may have to be reduced to prevent excessive drop in blood pressure. In hypertensive patients with coronary artery disease, it is important to avoid a precipitous drop in blood pressure.

Laboratory Tests

Periodic determination of serum electrolytes to detect possible electrolyte imbalance should be done at appropriate intervals.

Drug Interactions

Hydrochlorothiazide

When given concurrently the following drugs may interact with thiazide diuretics.

Alcohol, barbiturates, or narcotics —potentiation of orthostatic hypotension may occur.

Antidiabetic drugs (oral agents and insulin) —dosage adjustment of the antidiabetic drug may be required.

Other antihypertensive drugs —additive effect or potentiation.

Corticosteroids, ACTH —intensified electrolyte depletion, particularly hypokalemia.

Pressor amines (e.g., norepinephrine) —possible decreased response to pressor amines but not sufficient to preclude their use.

Skeletal muscle relaxants, nondepolarizing (e.g., tubocurarine) —possible increased responsiveness to the muscle relaxant.

Lithium —generally should not be given with diuretics. Diuretic agents reduce the renal clearance of lithium and add a high risk of lithium toxicity. Refer to the package insert for lithium preparations before use of such preparations with HYDROPRES.

Non-steroidal Anti-inflammatory Drugs —In some patients, the administration of a non-steroidal anti-inflammatory agent can reduce the diuretic, natriuretic, and antihypertensive effects of loop, potassium-sparing and thiazide diuretics. Therefore, when HYDROPRES and non-steroidal anti-inflammatory agents are used concomitantly, the patient should be observed closely to determine if the desired effect of the diuretic is obtained.

Reserpine

In hypertensive patients on reserpine therapy significant hypotension and bradycardia may develop during surgical anesthesia. The anesthesiologist should be aware that reserpine has been taken, since it may be necessary to give vagal blocking agents parenterally to prevent or reverse hypotension and/or bradycardia.

Use reserpine cautiously with digitalis and quinidine; cardiac arrhythmias have occurred with reserpine preparations.

Barbiturates enhance the central nervous system depressant effects of reserpine.

Drug/Laboratory Test Interactions

Thiazides should be discontinued before carrying out tests for parathyroid function (see PRECAUTIONS, *General*).

Carcinogenesis, Mutagenesis, Impairment of Fertility

Long-term carcinogenic or mutagenic studies have not been done with HYDROPRES.

In a two-litter study in the rat at an oral dose of 5.0/0.25 mg/kg, the combination of hydrochlorothiazide/reserpine did not impair fertility or produce abnormalities in the fetus.

Hydrochlorothiazide

Hydrochlorothiazide is currently under study in the U.S. Carcinogenesis Testing Program.

Hydrochlorothiazide was not mutagenic *in vitro*, in the Ames microbial mutagen test at a maximum concentration of 5 mg/plate using Strains TA98 and TA100. Urine samples from patients treated with hydrochlorothiazide did not have mutagenic activity in the Ames test.

The ability of a number of drugs to induce nondisjunction and crossing-over was measured with *Aspergillus nidulans*. A large number of drugs, including hydrochlorothiazide, induced nondisjunction.

Hydrochlorothiazide had no effect on fertility in a two-litter study in rats at doses of 4–5.6 mg/kg/day (up to 2 times the maximum recommended human dose).

Reserpine

Reserpine at a concentration of 1 to 5000 mcg/plate had no mutagenic activity against four strains of S. typhimurium *in vitro* in the Ames microbial mutagen test with or without metabolic activation. Reserpine did not induce malignant transformation of mouse fibroblasts *in vitro* at concentrations of 0.3 to 10 mcg/mL.

A few chromosomal aberrations were induced by reserpine *in vitro* in cultured mouse mammary carcinoma cells but were considered negative in this study. The drug did not produce chromosomal aberrations in human peripheral leucocyte cultures although an increase in mitotic figures occurred. One study reported chromosomal aberrations and dominant lethal mutations in mice at doses up to 10 mg/kg of reserpine in the form of a pharmaceutical preparation. Another study did not show dominant lethal mutations in mice at IP doses of 0.92 and 4.6 mg/kg of reserpine.

Reserpine did not impair fertility in a two-litter study in the rat at an oral dose of 0.25 mg/kg (35 times the maximum recommended human dose).

Rodent studies have shown that reserpine is an animal tumorigen, causing an increased incidence of mammary fibroadenomas in female mice, malignant tumors of the seminal vesicles in male mice, and malignant adrenal medullary tumors in male rats. These findings arose in 2 year studies in which the drug was administered in the feed at concentrations of 5 and 10 ppm—about 100 to 300 times the usual human dose. The breast neoplasms are thought to be related to reserpine's prolactin-elevating effect. Several other prolactin-elevating drugs have also been associated with an increased incidence of mammary neoplasia in rodents. The extent to which these findings indicate a risk to humans is uncertain. Tissue culture experiments show that about one-third of human breast tumors are prolactin-dependent *in vitro*, a factor of considerable importance if the use of the drug is contemplated in a patient with previously detected breast cancer. The possibility of an increased risk of breast cancer in reserpine users has been studied extensively; however, no firm conclusion has emerged. Although a few epidemiologic studies have suggested a slightly increased risk (less than twofold in all studies except one) in women who have used reserpine, other studies of generally similar design have not confirmed this. Epidemiologic studies conducted using other drugs (neuroleptic agents) that, like reserpine, increase prolactin levels and therefore would be considered rodent mammary carcinogens, have not shown an association between chronic administration of the drug and human mammary tumorigenesis. While long-term clinical observation has not suggested such an association, the available evidence is considered too limited to be conclusive at this time. An association of reserpine intake with pheochromocytoma or tumors of the seminal vesicles has not been explored.

Pregnancy

Teratogenic Effects —Pregnancy Category C: HYDROPRES may cause fetal harm when given to a pregnant woman. There are no adequate and well-controlled studies in pregnant women. HYDROPRES should be used during pregnancy only if the potential benefit justifies the potential risk to the fetus. (See INDICATIONS AND USAGE.)

Reserpine: Reproduction studies in rats have shown that reserpine is teratogenic at doses of 1-2 mg/kg (125 to 250 times the maximum recommended human dose) IM or IP given early in pregnancy. A variety of abnormalities was produced including anophthalmia, absence of the axial skeleton, hydronephrosis, etc. Pregnancy in rabbits was interrupted when doses as low as 0.04 mg/kg (10 times the maximum recommended human dose) were given early or late in pregnancy.

Hydrochlorothiazide: Thiazides cross the placental barrier and appear in cord blood.

Reproduction studies in the rabbit, the mouse and the rat at doses up to 100 mg/kg/day (50 times the maximum recommended human dose) showed no evidence of external abnormalities of the fetus due to hydrochlorothiazide. Hydrochlorothiazide given in a two-litter study in rats at doses of 4-5.6 mg/kg/day (approximately 1-2 times the maximum recommended human dose) did not impair fertility or produce abnormalities in the offspring.

Nonteratogenic Effects

Reserpine: Reserpine has been demonstrated to cross the placental barrier in guinea pigs with depression of adrenal catecholamine stores in the newborn. There is some evidence that side effects such as nasal congestion, lethargy, depressed Moro reflex, and bradycardia may appear in infants born of reserpine-treated mothers.

Hydrochlorothiazide: These may include fetal or neonatal jaundice, thrombocytopenia, and possibly other adverse reactions which have occurred in the adult.

Nursing Mothers

Thiazides and reserpine appear in breast milk. Because of the potential for serious adverse reactions in nursing infants from HYDROPRES, a decision should be made whether to discontinue nursing or to discontinue the drug, taking into account the importance of the drug to the mother.

Pediatric Use

Safety and effectiveness of HYDROPRES in children has not been established.

ADVERSE REACTIONS

The following adverse reactions have been reported and, within each category, are listed in order of decreasing severity.

Hydrochlorothiazide

Body as a Whole: Weakness.

Cardiovascular: Hypotension including orthostatic hypotension (may be aggravated by alcohol, barbiturates, narcotics or antihypertensive drugs).

Digestive: Pancreatitis, jaundice (intrahepatic cholestatic jaundice), diarrhea, vomiting, sialadenitis, cramping, constipation, gastric irritation, nausea, anorexia.

Hematologic: Aplastic anemia, agranulocytosis, leukopenia, hemolytic anemia, thrombocytopenia.

Hypersensitivity: Anaphylactic reactions, necrotizing angiitis (vasculitis and cutaneous vasculitis), respiratory distress including pneumonitis and pulmonary edema, photosensitivity, fever, urticaria, rash, purpura.

Metabolic: Electrolyte imbalance (see PRECAUTIONS), hyperglycemia, glycosuria, hyperuricemia.

Musculoskeletal: Muscle spasm.

Nervous System/Psychiatric: Vertigo, paresthesias, dizziness, headache, restlessness.

Renal: Renal failure, renal dysfunction, interstitial nephritis. (See WARNINGS.)

Special Senses: Transient blurred vision, xanthopsia.

Whenever adverse reactions are moderate or severe, thiazide dosage should be reduced or therapy withdrawn.

Reserpine
Cardiovascular: Angina pectoris, arrhythmia, premature ventricular contractions, other direct cardiac effects (e.g., fluid retention, congestive heart failure); bradycardia.
Digestive: Vomiting, diarrhea, nausea, hypersecretion and increased motility, anorexia, dryness of mouth, increased salivation.
Hematologic: Thrombocytopenic purpura, excessive bleeding following prostatic surgery.
Hypersensitivity: Pruritus, rash, flushing of skin.
Metabolic: Weight gain.
Musculoskeletal: Muscular aches.
Nervous System/Psychiatric: Mental depression, dull sensorium, syncope, paradoxical anxiety, excessive sedation, nightmares, headache, dizziness, nervousness, parkinsonism (usually reversible with decreased dosage or discontinuance of therapy).
Respiratory: Dyspnea, epistaxis, nasal congestion, enhanced susceptibility to colds.
Special Senses: Optic atrophy, uveitis, deafness, glaucoma, conjunctival injection, blurred vision.
Urogenital: Dysuria, impotence, decreased libido, non-puerperal lactation.

OVERDOSAGE

Overdosage may lead to excessive sedation, mental depression, severe hypotension, extrapyramidal reactions.
There is no specific antidote. In the event of overdosage, symptomatic and supportive measures should be employed. Emesis should be induced or gastric lavage performed. Correct dehydration, electrolyte imbalance, hepatic coma and hypotension by established procedures. If required, give oxygen or artificial respiration for respiratory impairment. In the event of severe hypotension from the reserpine component, intravenous use of a vasopressor is indicated [e.g., AR-AMINE® (Metaraminol Bitartrate, MSD), levarterenol, phenylephrine]. Anticholinergics may be needed to relieve gastrointestinal distress from reserpine. Because the effects of the rauwolfia alkaloids are prolonged, the patient should be closely observed for at least 72 hours.
The oral LD$_{50}$ of hydrochlorothiazide is greater than 10 g/kg in the mouse and rat. The oral LD$_{50}$ of reserpine in the mouse is 390 mg/kg.

DOSAGE AND ADMINISTRATION

The initial dosage of HYDROPRES should conform to the dosages of the individual components established during titration (see box warning).
The usual adult dosage of HYDROPRES 25 is 1 or 2 tablets once a day; that of HYDROPRES 50 is 1 tablet once a day. Patients usually do not require doses in excess of 50 mg of hydrochlorothiazide daily when combined with other antihypertensive agents. Dosage may require adjustment according to the blood pressure response of the patient.

HOW SUPPLIED

No. 3265—Tablets HYDROPRES 25 are green, round, scored, compressed tablets, coded MSD 53. Each tablet contains 25 mg of hydrochlorothiazide and 0.125 mg of reserpine. They are supplied as follows:
NDC 0006-0053-68 in bottles of 100
NDC 0006-0053-82 in bottles of 1000.
Shown in Product Identification Section, page 418
No. 3266—Tablets HYDROPRES 50 are green, round, scored, compressed tablets, coded MSD 127. Each tablet contains 50 mg of hydrochlorothiazide and 0.125 mg of reserpine. They are supplied as follows:
NDC 0006-0127-68 in bottles of 100
NDC 0006-0127-82 in bottles of 1000.
Shown in Product Identification Section, page 418
Storage
Keep container tightly closed. Protect from light.
A.H.F.S. Category: 24:08
DC 7414638 Issued October 1987
COPYRIGHT © MERCK & CO., INC., 1986
All rights reserved

INDOCIN® Capsules, Oral Suspension and ℞
Suppositories
(Indomethacin, MSD), U.S.P.
INDOCIN® SR Capsules ℞
(Indomethacin, MSD), U.S.P.

DESCRIPTION

INDOCIN® (Indomethacin, MSD) cannot be considered a simple analgesic and should not be used in conditions other than those recommended under INDICATIONS.
INDOCIN is supplied in four dosage forms. Capsules INDOCIN for oral administration contain either 25 mg or 50 mg of indomethacin and the following inactive ingredients: colloi-

dal silicon dioxide, FD & C Blue 1, FD & C Red 3, gelatin, lactose, lecithin, magnesium stearate, and titanium dioxide. Capsules INDOCIN SR for sustained release oral administration contain 75 mg of indomethacin and the following inactive ingredients: cellulose, confectioner's sugar, FD & C Blue 1, FD & C Blue 2, FD & C Red 3, gelatin, hydroxypropyl methylcellulose, magnesium stearate, polyvinyl acetate-crotonic acid copolymer, starch, and titanium dioxide. Suspension INDOCIN for oral use contains 25 mg of indomethacin per 5 mL, alcohol 1%, and sorbic acid 0.1% added as a preservative and the following inactive ingredients: antifoam AF emulsion, flavors, purified water, sodium hydroxide or hydrochloric acid to adjust pH, sorbitol solution, tragacanth. Suppositories INDOCIN for rectal use contain 50 mg of indomethacin and the following inactive ingredients: butylated hydroxyanisole, butylated hydroxytoluene, edetic acid, glycerin, polyethylene glycol 3350, polyethylene glycol 8000 and sodium chloride. Indomethacin is a non-steroidal anti-inflammatory indole derivative designated chemically as 1-(4-chlorobenzoyl)-5-methoxy-2-methyl-1*H*-indole-3-acetic acid. Indomethacin is practically insoluble in water and sparingly soluble in alcohol. It has a pKa of 4.5 and is stable in neutral or slightly acidic media and decomposes in strong alkali. The suspension has a pH of 4.0–5.0. The structural formula is:

CLINICAL PHARMACOLOGY

INDOCIN is a non-steroidal drug with anti-inflammatory, antipyretic and analgesic properties. Its mode of action, like that of other anti-inflammatory drugs, is not known. However, its therapeutic action is not due to pituitary-adrenal stimulation.
INDOCIN is a potent inhibitor of prostaglandin synthesis *in vitro*. Concentrations are reached during therapy which have been demonstrated to have an effect *in vivo* as well. Prostaglandins sensitize afferent nerves and potentiate the action of bradykinin in inducing pain in animal models. Moreover, prostaglandins are known to be among the mediators of inflammation. Since indomethacin is an inhibitor of prostaglandin synthesis, its mode of action may be due to a decrease of prostaglandins in peripheral tissues.
INDOCIN has been shown to be an effective anti-inflammatory agent, appropriate for long-term use in rheumatoid arthritis, ankylosing spondylitis, and osteoarthritis.
INDOCIN affords relief of symptoms; it does not alter the progressive course of the underlying disease.
INDOCIN suppresses inflammation in rheumatoid arthritis as demonstrated by relief of pain, and reduction of fever, swelling and tenderness. Improvement in patients treated with INDOCIN for rheumatoid arthritis has been demonstrated by a reduction in joint swelling, average number of joints involved, and morning stiffness; by increased mobility as demonstrated by a decrease in walking time; and by improved functional capability as demonstrated by an increase in grip strength.
Indomethacin has been reported to diminish basal and CO$_2$ stimulated cerebral blood flow in healthy volunteers following acute oral and intravenous administration. In one study after one week of treatment with orally administered indomethacin, this effect on basal cerebral blood flow had disappeared. The clinical significance of this effect has not been established.
Capsules INDOCIN have been found effective in relieving the pain, reducing the fever, swelling, redness, and tenderness of acute gouty arthritis. Capsules INDOCIN rather than Capsules INDOCIN SR are recommended for treatment of acute gouty arthritis—see INDICATIONS.
Following single oral doses of Capsules INDOCIN 25 mg or 50 mg, indomethacin is readily absorbed, attaining peak plasma concentrations of about 1 and 2 mcg/mL, respectively, at about 2 hours. Orally administered Capsules INDOCIN are virtually 100% bioavailable, with 90% of the dose absorbed within 4 hours. A single 50 mg dose of Oral Suspension INDOCIN was found to be bioequivalent to a 50 mg INDOCIN capsule when each was administered with food.
Capsules INDOCIN SR 75 mg are designed to release 25 mg of the drug initially and the remaining 50 mg over approximately 12 hours (90% of dose absorbed by 12 hours). When measured over a 24-hour period, the cumulative amount and time-course of indomethacin absorption from a single Capsule INDOCIN SR are comparable to those of 3 doses of 25 mg Capsules INDOCIN given at 4–6 hour intervals.
Plasma concentrations of indomethacin fluctuate less and are more sustained following administration of Capsules INDOCIN SR than following administration of 25 mg Capsules INDOCIN given at 4–6 hour intervals. In multiple-dose comparisons, the mean daily steady-state plasma level of indomethacin attained with daily administration of Cap-

sules INDOCIN SR 75 mg was indistinguishable from that following Capsules INDOCIN 25 mg given at 0, 6 and 12 hours daily. However, there was a significant difference in indomethacin plasma levels between the two dosage regimens especially after 12 hours.
Controlled clinical studies of safety and efficacy in patients with osteoarthritis have shown that one Capsule INDOCIN SR was clinically comparable to one 25 mg Capsule INDOCIN t.i.d.; and in controlled clinical studies in patients with rheumatoid arthritis, one Capsule INDOCIN SR taken in the morning and one in the evening were clinically indistinguishable from one 50 mg Capsule INDOCIN t.i.d.
Indomethacin is eliminated via renal excretion, metabolism, and biliary excretion. Indomethacin undergoes appreciable enterohepatic circulation. The mean half-life of indomethacin is estimated to be about 4.5 hours. With a typical therapeutic regimen of 25 or 50 mg t.i.d., the steady-state plasma concentrations of indomethacin are an average 1.4 times those following the first dose.
The rate of absorption is more rapid from the rectal suppository than from Capsules INDOCIN. Ordinarily, therefore, the total amount absorbed from the suppository would be expected to be at least equivalent to the capsule. In controlled clinical trials, however, the amount of indomethacin absorbed was found to be somewhat less (80–90%) than that absorbed from Capsules INDOCIN. This is probably because some subjects did not retain the material from the suppository for the one hour necessary to assure complete absorption. Since the suppository dissolves rather quickly rather than melting slowly, it is seldom recovered in recognizable form if the patient retains the suppository for more than a few minutes.
Indomethacin exists in the plasma as the parent drug and its desmethyl, desbenzoyl, and desmethyl-desbenzoyl metabolites, all in the unconjugated form. About 60 percent of an oral dosage is recovered in urine as drug and metabolites (26 percent as indomethacin and its glucuronide), and 33 percent is recovered in feces (1.5 percent as indomethacin).
About 99% of indomethacin is bound to protein in plasma over the expected range of therapeutic plasma concentrations.
In a gastroscopic study in 45 healthy subjects, the number of gastric mucosal abnormalities was significantly higher in the group receiving Capsules INDOCIN than in the group taking Suppositories INDOCIN or placebo.
In a double-blind comparative clinical study involving 175 patients with rheumatoid arthritis, however, the incidence of upper gastrointestinal adverse effects with Suppositories or Capsules INDOCIN was comparable. The incidence of lower gastrointestinal adverse effects was greater in the suppository group.

INDICATIONS

Indomethacin has been found effective in active stages of the following:
1. Moderate to severe rheumatoid arthritis including acute flares of chronic disease.
2. Moderate to severe ankylosing spondylitis.
3. Moderate to severe osteoarthritis.
4. Acute painful shoulder (bursitis and/or tendinitis).
5. Acute gouty arthritis.
Capsules INDOCIN SR are recommended for all of the indications for Capsules INDOCIN except acute gouty arthritis. INDOCIN may enable the reduction of steroid dosage in patients receiving steroids for the more severe forms of rheumatoid arthritis. In such instances the steroid dosage should be reduced slowly and the patients followed very closely for any possible adverse effects.
The use of INDOCIN in conjunction with aspirin or other salicylates is not recommended. Controlled clinical studies have shown that the combined use of INDOCIN and aspirin does not produce any greater therapeutic effect than the use of INDOCIN alone. Furthermore, in one of these clinical studies, the incidence of gastrointestinal side effects was significantly increased with combined therapy (see DRUG INTERACTIONS).

CONTRAINDICATIONS

INDOCIN should not be used in:
Patients who are hypersensitive to this product.
Patients in whom acute asthmatic attacks, urticaria, or rhinitis are precipitated by aspirin or other non-steroidal anti-inflammatory agents.
Suppositories INDOCIN are contraindicated in patients with a history of proctitis or recent rectal bleeding.

Continued on next page

Information on the Merck Sharp & Dohme products listed on these pages is the full prescribing information from product circulars in use August 31, 1989.

Merck Sharp & Dohme—Cont.

WARNINGS

General:

Because of the variability of the potential of INDOCIN to cause adverse reactions in the individual patient, the following are strongly recommended:

1. The lowest possible effective dose for the individual patient should be prescribed. Increased dosage tends to increase adverse effects, particularly in doses over 150–200 mg/day, without corresponding increase in clinical benefits.
2. Careful GI instructions to, and observations of, the individual patient are essential to the prevention of serious adverse reactions. As advancing years appear to increase the possibility of adverse reactions, INDOCIN should be used with greater care in the aged.
3. Effectiveness of INDOCIN in children has not been established. INDOCIN should not be prescribed for children 14 years of age and younger unless toxicity or lack of efficacy associated with other drugs warrants the risk.
   In experience with more than 900 children reported in the literature or to Merck Sharp and Dohme who were treated with Capsules INDOCIN, side effects in children were comparable to those reported in adults. Experience in children has been confined to the use of Capsules INDOCIN. If a decision is made to use indomethacin for children two years of age or older, such patients should be monitored closely and periodic assessment of liver function is recommended. There have been cases of hepatotoxicity reported in children with juvenile rheumatoid arthritis, including fatalities.
   If indomethacin treatment is instituted, a suggested starting dose is 2 mg/kg/day given in divided doses. Maximum daily dosage should not exceed 4 mg/kg/day or 150–200 mg/day, whichever is less. As symptoms subside, the total daily dosage should be reduced to the lowest level required to control symptoms, or the drug should be discontinued.
4. If Capsules INDOCIN SR are used for initial therapy or during dosage adjustment, observe the patient closely (see DOSAGE AND ADMINISTRATION).

Gastrointestinal Effects:

Single or multiple ulcerations, including perforation and hemorrhage of the esophagus, stomach, duodenum or small and large intestine, have been reported to occur with INDOCIN. Fatalities have been reported in some instances. Rarely, intestinal ulceration has been associated with stenosis and obstruction.

Gastrointestinal bleeding without obvious ulcer formation and perforation of pre-existing sigmoid lesions (diverticulum, carcinoma, etc.) have occurred. Increased abdominal pain in ulcerative colitis patients or the development of ulcerative colitis and regional ileitis have been reported to occur rarely.

Because of the occurrence, and at times severity, of gastrointestinal reactions to INDOCIN, the prescribing physician must be continuously alert for any sign or symptom signaling a possible gastrointestinal reaction. The risks of continuing therapy with INDOCIN in the face of such symptoms must be weighed against the possible benefits to the individual patient.

INDOCIN should not be given to patients with active gastrointestinal lesions or with a history of recurrent gastrointestinal lesions except under circumstances which warrant the very high risk and where patients can be monitored very closely.

The gastrointestinal effects may be reduced by giving Capsules INDOCIN or Capsules INDOCIN SR immediately after meals, with food, or with antacids.

Risk of GI Ulcerations, Bleeding and Perforation with NSAID Therapy

Serious gastrointestinal toxicity such as bleeding, ulceration, and perforation, can occur at any time, with or without warning symptoms, in patients treated chronically with NSAID therapy. Although minor upper gastrointestinal problems, such as dyspepsia, are common, usually developing early in therapy, physicians should remain alert for ulceration and bleeding in patients treated chronically with NSAIDs even in the absence of previous GI tract symptoms. In patients observed in clinical trials of several months to two years duration, symptomatic upper GI ulcers, gross bleeding or perforation appear to occur in approximately 1% of patients treated for 3–6 months, and in about 2–4% of patients treated for one year. Physicians should inform patients about the signs and/or symptoms of serious GI toxicity and what steps to take if they occur.

Studies to date have not identified any subset of patients not at risk of developing peptic ulceration and bleeding. Except for a prior history of serious GI events and other risk factors known to be associated with peptic ulcer disease, such as alcoholism, smoking, etc., no risk factors (e.g., age, sex) have been associated with increased risk. Elderly or debilitated patients seem to tolerate ulceration or bleeding less well

than other individuals and most spontaneous reports of fatal GI events are in this population. Studies to date are inconclusive concerning the relative risk of various NSAIDs in causing such reactions. High doses of any NSAID probably carry a greater risk of these reactions, although controlled clinical trials showing this do not exist in most cases. In considering the use of relatively large doses (within the recommended dosage range), sufficient benefit should be anticipated to offset the potential increased risk of GI toxicity.

Renal Effects:

As with other non-steroidal anti-inflammatory drugs, long term administration of indomethacin to animals has resulted in renal papillary necrosis and other abnormal renal pathology. In humans, there have been reports of acute interstitial nephritis with hematuria, proteinuria, and occasionally nephrotic syndrome.

A second form of renal toxicity has been seen in patients with prerenal and renal conditions leading to a reduction in renal blood flow or blood volume, where the renal prostaglandins have a supportive role in the maintenance of renal perfusion. In these patients administration of an NSAID may cause a dose dependent reduction in prostaglandin formation and may precipitate overt renal decompensation. Patients at greatest risk of this reaction are those with conditions such as renal or hepatic dysfunction, diabetes mellitus, advanced age, extracellular volume depletion from any cause, congestive heart failure, septicemia, pyelonephritis, or concomitant use of any nephrotoxic drug. INDOCIN or other NSAIDs should be given with caution and renal function should be monitored in any patient who may have reduced renal reserve. Discontinuation of NSAID therapy is typically followed by recovery to the pretreatment state.

Increases in serum potassium concentration, including hyperkalemia, have been reported, even in some patients without renal impairment. In patients with normal renal function, these effects have been attributed to a hyporeninemic-hypoaldosteronism state (see PRECAUTIONS, *Drug Interactions*).

Since INDOCIN is eliminated primarily by the kidneys, patients with significantly impaired renal function should be closely monitored; a lower daily dosage should be anticipated to avoid excessive drug accumulation.

Ocular Effects:

Corneal deposits and retinal disturbances, including those of the macula, have been observed in some patients who had received prolonged therapy with INDOCIN. The prescribing physician should be alert to the possible association between the changes noted and INDOCIN. It is advisable to discontinue therapy if such changes are observed. Blurred vision may be a significant symptom and warrants a thorough ophthalmological examination. Since these changes may be asymptomatic, ophthalmologic examination at periodic intervals is desirable in patients where therapy is prolonged.

Central Nervous System Effects:

INDOCIN may aggravate depression or other psychiatric disturbances, epilepsy, and parkinsonism, and should be used with considerable caution in patients with these conditions. If severe CNS adverse reactions develop, INDOCIN should be discontinued.

INDOCIN may cause drowsiness; therefore, patients should be cautioned about engaging in activities requiring mental alertness and motor coordination, such as driving a car. INDOCIN may also cause headache. Headache which persists despite dosage reduction requires cessation of therapy with INDOCIN.

Use in Pregnancy and the Neonatal Period

INDOCIN is not recommended for use in pregnant women, since safety for use has not been established, and because of the known effect of drugs of this class on the human fetal cardiovascular system (closure of the ductus arteriosus) during the third trimester of pregnancy.

Teratogenic studies were conducted in mice and rats at dosages of 0.5, 1.0, 2.0, and 4.0 mg/kg/day. Except for retarded fetal ossification at 4 mg/kg/day considered secondary to the decreased average fetal weights, no increase in fetal malformations was observed as compared with control groups. Other studies in mice reported in the literature using higher doses (5 to 15 mg/kg/day) have described maternal toxicity and death, increased fetal resorptions, and fetal malformations. Comparable studies in rodents using high doses of aspirin have shown similar maternal and fetal effects.

As with other non-steroidal anti-inflammatory agents which inhibit prostaglandin synthesis, indomethacin has been found to delay parturition in rats.

In rats and mice, 4.0 mg/kg/day given during the last three days of gestation caused a decrease in maternal weight gain and some maternal and fetal deaths. An increased incidence of neuronal necrosis in the diencephalon in the live-born fetuses was observed. At 2.0 mg/kg/day, no increase in neuronal necrosis was observed as compared to the control groups. Administration of 0.5 or 4.0 mg/kg/day during the first three days of life did not cause an increase in neuronal necrosis at either dose level.

Use in Nursing Mothers

INDOCIN is excreted in the milk of lactating mothers. INDOCIN is not recommended for use in nursing mothers.

PRECAUTIONS

INDOCIN may mask the usual signs and symptoms of infection. Therefore, the physician must be continually on the alert for this and should use the drug with extra care in the presence of existing controlled infection.

Fluid retention and peripheral edema have been observed in some patients taking INDOCIN. Therefore, as with other non-steroidal anti-inflammatory drugs, INDOCIN should be used with caution in patients with cardiac dysfunction, hypertension, or other conditions predisposing to fluid retention.

In a study of patients with severe heart failure and hyponatremia, INDOCIN was associated with significant deterioration of circulatory hemodynamics, presumably due to inhibition of prostaglandin dependent compensatory mechanisms. INDOCIN, like other non-steroidal anti-inflammatory agents, can inhibit platelet aggregation. This effect is of shorter duration than that seen with aspirin and usually disappears within 24 hours after discontinuation of INDOCIN. INDOCIN has been shown to prolong bleeding time (but within the normal range) in normal subjects. Because this effect may be exaggerated in patients with underlying hemostatic defects, INDOCIN should be used with caution in persons with coagulation defects.

As with other non-steroidal anti-inflammatory drugs, borderline elevations of one or more liver tests may occur in up to 15% of patients. These abnormalities may progress, may remain essentially unchanged, or may be transient with continued therapy. The SGPT (ALT) test is probably the most sensitive indicator of liver dysfunction. Meaningful (3 times the upper limit of normal) elevations of SGPT or SGOT (AST) occurred in controlled clinical trials in less than 1% of patients. A patient with symptoms and/or signs suggesting liver dysfunction, or in whom an abnormal liver test has occurred, should be evaluated for evidence of the development of more severe hepatic reaction while on therapy with INDOCIN. Severe hepatic reactions, including jaundice and cases of fatal hepatitis, have been reported with INDOCIN as with other non-steroidal anti-inflammatory drugs. Although such reactions are rare, if abnormal liver tests persist or worsen, if clinical signs and symptoms consistent with liver disease develop, or if systemic manifestations occur (e.g., eosinophilia, rash, etc.), INDOCIN should be discontinued.

Information for Patients

INDOCIN, like other drugs of its class, is not free of side effects. The side effects of these drugs can cause discomfort and, rarely, there are more serious side effects such as gastrointestinal bleeding, which may result in hospitalization and even fatal outcomes.

NSAIDs (Non-steroidal Anti-inflammatory Drugs) are often essential agents in the management of arthritis; but they also may be commonly employed for conditions which are less serious.

Physicians may wish to discuss with their patients the potential risks (see WARNINGS, PRECAUTIONS and ADVERSE REACTIONS) and likely benefits of NSAID treatment, particularly when the drugs are used for less serious conditions where treatment without NSAIDs may represent an acceptable alternative to both the patient and physician.

Laboratory Tests

Because serious GI tract ulceration and bleeding can occur without warning symptoms, physicians should follow chronically treated patients for the signs and symptoms of ulceration and bleeding and should inform them of the importance of this follow-up (see WARNINGS, *Risk of GI Ulcerations, Bleeding and Perforation with NSAID Therapy*).

Carcinogenesis, Mutagenesis, Impairment of Fertility

In an 81-week chronic oral toxicity study in the rat at doses up to 1 mg/kg/day, indomethacin had no tumorigenic effect. Indomethacin produced no neoplastic or hyperplastic changes related to treatment in carcinogenic studies in the rat (dosing period 73–110 weeks) and the mouse (dosing period 62–88 weeks) at doses up to 1.5 mg/kg/day.

Indomethacin did not have any mutagenic effect in *in vitro* bacterial tests (Ames test and *E. coli* with or without metabolic activation) and a series of *in vivo* tests including the host-mediated assay, sex-linked recessive lethals in *Drosophila*, and the micronucleus test in mice.

Indomethacin at dosage levels up to 0.5 mg/kg/day had no effect on fertility in mice in a two generation reproduction study or a two litter reproduction study in rats.

Drug Interactions

In normal volunteers receiving indomethacin, the administration of diflunisal decreased the renal clearance and significantly increased the plasma levels of indomethacin. In some patients, combined use of INDOCIN and diflunisal has been associated with fatal gastrointestinal hemorrhage. Therefore, diflunisal and INDOCIN should not be used concomitantly.

In a study in normal volunteers, it was found that chronic concurrent administration of 3.6 g of aspirin per day decreases indomethacin blood levels approximately 20%.

Clinical studies have shown that INDOCIN does not influence the hypoprothrombinemia produced by anticoagulants. However, when any additional drug, including INDOCIN, is added to the treatment of patients on anticoagulant therapy, the patients should be observed for alterations of the prothrombin time.

When INDOCIN is given to patients receiving probenecid, the plasma levels of indomethacin are likely to be increased. Therefore, a lower total daily dosage of INDOCIN may produce a satisfactory therapeutic effect. When increases in the dose of INDOCIN are made, they should be made carefully and in small increments.

Caution should be used if INDOCIN is administered simultaneously with methotrexate. INDOCIN has been reported to decrease the tubular secretion of methotrexate and to potentiate its toxicity.

Capsules INDOCIN 50 mg t.i.d. produced a clinically relevant elevation of plasma lithium and reduction in renal lithium clearance in psychiatric patients and normal subjects with steady state plasma lithium concentrations. This effect has been attributed to inhibition of prostaglandin synthesis. As a consequence, when INDOCIN and lithium are given concomitantly, the patient should be carefully observed for signs of lithium toxicity. (Read circulars for lithium preparations before use of such concomitant therapy.) In addition, the frequency of monitoring serum lithium concentration should be increased at the outset of such combination drug treatment.

In some patients, the administration of INDOCIN can reduce the diuretic, natriuretic, and, antihypertensive effects of loop, potassium-sparing, and thiazide diuretics. Therefore, when INDOCIN and diuretics are used concomitantly, the patient should be observed closely to determine if the desired effect of the diuretic is obtained.

INDOCIN reduces basal plasma renin activity (PRA), as well as those elevations of PRA induced by furosemide administration, or salt or volume depletion. These facts should be considered when evaluating plasma renin activity in hypertensive patients.

It has been reported that the addition of triamterene to a maintenance schedule of INDOCIN resulted in reversible acute renal failure in two of four healthy volunteers. INDOCIN and triamterene should not be administered together. INDOCIN and potassium-sparing diuretics each may be associated with increased serum potassium levels. The potential effects of INDOCIN and potassium-sparing diuretics on potassium kinetics and renal function should be considered when these agents are administered concurrently.

Most of the above effects concerning diuretics have been attributed, at least in part, to mechanisms involving inhibition of prostaglandin synthesis by INDOCIN.

Blunting of the antihypertensive effect of beta-adrenoceptor blocking agents by non-steroidal anti-inflammatory drugs including INDOCIN has been reported. Therefore, when using these blocking agents to treat hypertension, patients should be observed carefully in order to confirm that the desired therapeutic effect has been obtained. There are reports that INDOCIN can reduce the antihypertensive effect of captopril in some patients.

False-negative results in the dexamethasone suppression test (DST) in patients being treated with INDOCIN have been reported. Thus, results of the DST should be interpreted with caution in these patients.

Pediatric Use
Effectiveness in children 14 years of age and younger has not been established (see WARNINGS).

ADVERSE REACTIONS

The adverse reactions for Capsules INDOCIN listed in the following table have been arranged into two groups: (1) incidence greater than 1%; and (2) incidence less than 1%. The incidence for group (1) was obtained from 33 double-blind controlled clinical trials reported in the literature (1,092 patients). The incidence for group (2) was based on reports in clinical trials, in the literature, and on voluntary reports since marketing. The probability of a causal relationship exists between INDOCIN and these adverse reactions, some of which have been reported only rarely.

In controlled clinical trials, the incidence of adverse reactions to Capsules INDOCIN SR and equal 24-hour doses of Capsules INDOCIN were similar.

The adverse reactions reported with Capsules INDOCIN may occur with use of the suppositories. In addition, rectal irritation and tenesmus have been reported in patients who have received the suppositories.

The adverse reactions reported with Capsules INDOCIN may also occur with use of the suspension.

[See table above].

Causal relationship unknown: Other reactions have been reported but occurred under circumstances where a causal relationship could not be established. However, in these rarely reported events, the possibility cannot be excluded.

Incidence greater than 1%	Incidence less than 1%	
GASTROINTESTINAL		
nausea* with or without vomiting	anorexia	gastrointestinal bleeding without obvious ulcer formation and perforation of pre-existing sigmoid lesions (diverticulum, carcinoma, etc.)
dyspepsia* (including indigestion, heartburn and epigastric pain)	bloating (includes distention)	
	flatulence	
	peptic ulcer	
	gastroenteritis	
	rectal bleeding	
diarrhea	proctitis	development of ulcerative colitis and regional ileitis
abdominal distress or pain	single or multiple ulcerations, including perforation and hemorrhage of the esophagus, stomach, duodenum or small and large intestines	ulcerative stomatitis
constipation		toxic hepatitis and jaundice (some fatal cases have been reported)
	intestinal ulceration associated with stenosis and obstruction	
CENTRAL NERVOUS SYSTEM		
headache (11.7%)	anxiety (includes nervousness)	light-headedness
dizziness*	muscle weakness	syncope
vertigo	involuntary muscle movements	paresthesia
somnolence	insomnia	aggravation of epilepsy and parkinsonism
depression and fatigue (including malaise and listlessness)	muzziness	depersonalization
	psychic disturbances including psychotic episodes	coma
	mental confusion	peripheral neuropathy
	drowsiness	convulsions
		dysarthria
SPECIAL SENSES		
tinnitus	ocular—corneal deposits and retinal disturbances, including those of the macula, have been reported in some patients on prolonged therapy with INDOCIN	blurred vision
		diplopia
		hearing disturbances, deafness

[Continued following page]

Therefore, these observations are being listed to serve as alerting information to physicians:
Cardiovascular: Thrombophlebitis
Hematologic: Although there have been several reports of leukemia, the supporting information is weak.
Genitourinary: Urinary frequency.

OVERDOSAGE

The following symptoms may be observed following overdosage: nausea, vomiting, intense headache, dizziness, mental confusion, disorientation, or lethargy. There have been reports of paresthesias, numbness, and convulsions.
Treatment is symptomatic and supportive. The stomach should be emptied as quickly as possible if the ingestion is recent. If vomiting has not occurred spontaneously, the patient should be induced to vomit with syrup of ipecac. If the patient is unable to vomit, gastric lavage should be performed. Once the stomach has been emptied, 25 or 50 g of activated charcoal may be given. Depending on the condition of the patient, close medical observation and nursing care may be required. The patient should be followed for several days because gastrointestinal ulceration and hemorrhage have been reported as adverse reactions of indomethacin. Use of antacids may be helpful.
The oral LD_{50} of indomethacin in mice and rats (based on 14 day mortality response) was 50 and 12 mg/kg, respectively.

DOSAGE AND ADMINISTRATION

INDOCIN is available as 25 and 50 mg Capsules INDOCIN, 75 mg Capsules INDOCIN SR for oral use, Oral Suspension INDOCIN, containing 25 mg of indomethacin per 5 mL, and 50 mg Suppositories INDOCIN for rectal use. Capsules INDOCIN SR 75 mg once a day can be substituted for Capsules INDOCIN 25 mg t.i.d. However, there will be significant differences between the two dosage regimens in indomethacin blood levels, especially after 12 hours (see CLINICAL PHARMACOLOGY). In addition, Capsules INDOCIN SR 75 mg b.i.d. can be substituted for Capsules INDOCIN 50 mg t.i.d. Capsules INDOCIN SR may be substituted for all the indications for Capsules INDOCIN except acute gouty arthritis. Adverse reactions appear to correlate with the size of the dose of INDOCIN in most patients but not all. Therefore,

every effort should be made to determine the smallest effective dosage for the individual patient.
Always give Capsules INDOCIN, Capsules INDOCIN SR, or Oral Suspension INDOCIN with food, immediately after meals, or with antacids to reduce gastric irritation.
Pediatric Use
INDOCIN ordinarily should not be prescribed for children 14 years of age and under (see WARNINGS).
Adult Use
Dosage Recommendations for Active Stages of the Following:
1. Moderate to severe rheumatoid arthritis including acute flares of chronic disease; moderate to severe ankylosing spondylitis; and moderate to severe osteoarthritis.
   Suggested Dosage:
   Capsules INDOCIN 25 mg b.i.d. or t.i.d. If this is well tolerated, increase the daily dosage by 25 or by 50 mg, if required by continuing symptoms, at weekly intervals until a satisfactory response is obtained or until a total daily dose of 150–200 mg is reached. DOSES ABOVE THIS AMOUNT GENERALLY DO NOT INCREASE THE EFFECTIVENESS OF THE DRUG.

In patients who have persistent night pain and/or morning stiffness, the giving of a large portion, up to a maximum of 100 mg, of the total daily dose at bedtime, either orally or by rectal suppositories, may be helpful in affording relief. The total daily dose should not exceed 200 mg. In acute flares of chronic rheumatoid arthritis, it may be necessary to increase the dosage by 25 mg or, if required, by 50 mg daily.
If Capsules INDOCIN SR 75 mg are used for initiating indomethacin treatment, one capsule daily should be the usual starting dose in order to observe patient tolerance since 75 mg per day is the maximum recommended starting dose for indomethacin (see above). If Capsules INDOCIN SR are used to increase the daily dose, patients should be observed for possible signs and symptoms of intolerance since the daily increment will exceed the daily increment recommended for

Continued on next page

Information on the Merck Sharp & Dohme products listed on these pages is the full prescribing information from product circulars in use August 31, 1989.

Merck Sharp & Dohme—Cont.

the other dosage forms. For patients who require 150 mg of INDOCIN per day and have demonstrated acceptable tolerance, INDOCIN SR may be prescribed as one capsule twice daily.

If minor adverse effects develop as the dosage is increased, reduce the dosage rapidly to a tolerated dose and OBSERVE THE PATIENT CLOSELY.

If severe adverse reactions occur, STOP THE DRUG. After the acute phase of the disease is under control, an attempt to reduce the daily dose should be made repeatedly until the patient is receiving the smallest effective dose or the drug is discontinued.

Careful instructions to, and observations of, the individual patient are essential to the prevention of serious, irreversible, including fatal, adverse reactions.

As advancing years appear to increase the possibility of adverse reactions, INDOCIN should be used with greater care in the aged.

2. Acute painful shoulder (bursitis and/or tendinitis).
   Initial Dose:
   75–150 mg daily in 3 or 4 divided doses.
   The drug should be discontinued after the signs and symptoms of inflammation have been controlled for several days. The usual course of therapy is 7–14 days.

3. Acute gouty arthritis.
   Suggested Dosage:
   Capsules INDOCIN 50 mg t.i.d. until pain is tolerable. The dose should then be rapidly reduced to complete cessation of the drug. Definite relief of pain has been reported within 2 to 4 hours. Tenderness and heat usually subside in 24 to 36 hours, and swelling gradually disappears in 3 to 5 days.

HOW SUPPLIED

No. 3316—Capsules INDOCIN, 25 mg are opaque blue and white capsules, coded MSD 25. They are supplied as follows:

NDC 0006-0025-68 bottles of 100
(6505-00-926-2154, 25 mg 100's)
NDC 0006-0025-78 unit of use bottles of 100
NDC 0006-0025-28 unit dose packages of 100
(6505-00-118-2776, 25 mg individually sealed 100's)
NDC 0006-0025-82 bottles of 1000
(6505-00-931-0680, 25 mg 1000's).

Shown in Product Identification Section, page 418

No. 3317—Capsules INDOCIN, 50 mg are opaque blue and white capsules, coded MSD 50. They are supplied as follows:

NDC 0006-0050-68 bottles of 100
NDC 0006-0050-28 unit dose packages of 100.

Shown in Product Identification Section, page 418

No. 3376—Oral Suspension INDOCIN, 25 mg per 5 mL, is an off-white suspension with a pineapple coconut mint flavor. It is supplied as follows:

NDC 0006-3376-66 in bottles of 237 mL.

No. 3370—Capsules INDOCIN SR, 75 mg each, are capsules with an opaque blue cap and clear body containing a mixture of blue and white pellets, coded MSD 693. They are supplied as follows:

NDC 0006-0693-31 unit of use bottles of 30
(6505-01-135-7391, 75 mg 30's)
NDC 0006-0693-61 unit of use bottles of 60
(6505-01-137-4629, 75 mg 60's).

Shown in Product Identification Section, page 418

No. 3354—Suppositories INDOCIN, 50 mg each, are white, opaque, rectal suppositories and are supplied as follows:

NDC 0006-0150-30, boxes of 30.

Shown in Product Identification Section, page 418

Storage

Store Oral Suspension INDOCIN below 30°C (86°F). Avoid temperatures above 50°C (122°F). Protect from freezing.
Store Suppositories INDOCIN below 30°C (86°F). Avoid transient temperatures above 40°C (104°F).

Suppositories INDOCIN are distributed by:
MERCK SHARP & DOHME, Division of Merck & Co., INC.
West Point, Pa. 19486
Manufactured by:
MERCK SHARP & DOHME

CARDIOVASCULAR		
none	hypertension	congestive heart failure
	hypotension	arrhythmia;
	tachycardia	palpitations
	chest pain	
METABOLIC		
none	edema	hyperglycemia
	weight gain	glycosuria
	fluid retention	hyperkalemia
	flushing or sweating	
INTEGUMENTARY		
none	pruritus	exfoliative dermatitis
	rash; urticaria	erythema nodosum
	petechiae or	loss of hair
	ecchymosis	Stevens-Johnson
		syndrome
		erythema multiforme
		toxic epidermal
		necrolysis
HEMATOLOGIC		
none	leukopenia	aplastic anemia
	bone marrow	hemolytic anemia
	depression	agranulocytosis
	anemia secondary	thrombocytopenic
	to obvious or	purpura
	occult	disseminated intravascular
	gastrointestinal	coagulation
	bleeding	
HYPERSENSITIVITY		
none	acute anaphylaxis	dyspnea
	acute respiratory	asthma
	distress	purpura
	rapid fall in blood	angiitis
	pressure	pulmonary edema
	resembling a	
	shock-like state	
	angioedema	
GENITOURINARY		
none	hematuria	BUN elevation
	vaginal bleeding	renal insufficiency,
	proteinuria	including renal
	nephrotic syndrome	failure
	interstitial nephritis	
MISCELLANEOUS		
none	epistaxis	
	breast changes,	
	including	
	enlargement and	
	tenderness, or	
	gynecomastia	

*Reactions occurring in 3% to 9% of patients treated with INDOCIN. (Those reactions occurring in less than 3% of the patients are unmarked.)

(Italia) S.p.A.
27100—Pavia, Italy
Capsules and Oral Suspension INDOCIN® and Capsules INDOCIN® SR are distributed and manufactured by:
MERCK SHARP & DOHME, Division of Merck & Co., INC.
West Point, Pa. 19486
    A.H.F.S. Category: 28:08
    DC 7342917   Issued March 1989
COPYRIGHT © MERCK & CO., INC., 1988
All rights reserved

INDOCIN® I.V.   ℞
(Indomethacin Sodium Trihydrate, MSD)

DESCRIPTION

Sterile INDOCIN® I.V. (Indomethacin Sodium Trihydrate, MSD) for intravenous administration is lyophilized indomethacin sodium trihydrate. Each vial contains indomethacin sodium trihydrate equivalent to 1 mg indomethacin as a white to yellow lyophilized powder or plug. Variations in the size of the lyophilized plug and the intensity of color have no relationship to the quality or amount of indomethacin present in the vial.

Indomethacin sodium trihydrate is designated chemically as 1-(4-chlorobenzoyl)-5- methoxy-2-methyl-1H -indole-3-acetic acid, sodium salt, trihydrate. Its molecular weight is 433.82. Its empirical formula is $C_{19}H_{15}ClNNaO_4 \cdot 3H_2O$ and its structural formula is:

CLINICAL PHARMACOLOGY

Although the exact mechanism of action through which indomethacin causes closure of a patent ductus arteriosus is not known, it is believed to be through inhibition of prostaglandin synthesis. Indomethacin has been shown to be a potent inhibitor of prostaglandin synthesis, both *in vitro* and *in vivo*. In human newborns with certain congenital heart malformations, PGE 1 dilates the ductus arteriosus. In fetal and newborn lambs, E type prostaglandins have also been shown to maintain the patency of the ductus, and as in human newborns, indomethacin causes its constriction.

Studies in healthy young animals and in premature infants with patent ductus arteriosus indicated that, after the first dose of intravenous indomethacin, there was a transient reduction in cerebral blood flow velocity and cerebral blood flow. The clinical significance of this effect has not been established.

In double-blind placebo-controlled studies of INDOCIN I.V. in 460 small pre-term infants, weighing 1750 g or less, the infants treated with placebo had a ductus closure rate after 48 hours of 25 to 30 percent, whereas those treated with IN-DOCIN I.V. had a 75 to 80 percent closure rate. In one of these studies, a multicenter study, involving 405 pre-term infants, later re-opening of the ductus arteriosus occurred in 26 percent of infants treated with INDOCIN I.V., however, 70 percent of these closed subsequently without the need for surgery or additional indomethacin.

Pharmacokinetics and Metabolism

The disposition of indomethacin following intravenous administration (0.2 mg/kg) in pre-term neonates with patent ductus arteriosus has not been extensively evaluated. Even though the plasma half-life of indomethacin was variable among premature infants, it was shown to vary inversely with postnatal age and weight. In one study, of 28 infants who could be evaluated, the plasma half-life in those infants less than 7 days old averaged 20 hours (range: 3–60 hours, n = 18). In infants older than 7 days, the mean plasma half-life of indomethacin was 12 hours (range: 4–38 hours, n = 10). Grouping the infants by weight, mean plasma half-life in those weighing less than 1000 g was 21 hours (range: 9–60 hours, n = 10); in those weighing more than 1000 g, the mean plasma half-life was 15 hours (range: 3–52 hours, n = 18).

Following intravenous administration in adults, indomethacin is eliminated via renal excretion, metabolism, and biliary excretion. Indomethacin undergoes appreciable enterohepatic circulation. The mean plasma half-life of indomethacin is 4.5 hours. In the absence of enterohepatic circulation, it is 90 minutes.

In adults, about 99 percent of indomethacin is bound to protein in plasma over the expected range of therapeutic plasma concentrations. The percent bound in neonates has not been studied. In controlled trials in premature infants, however, no evidence of bilirubin displacement has been observed as evidenced by increased incidence of bilirubin encephalopathy (kernicterus).

INDICATIONS AND USAGE

INDOCIN I.V. is indicated to close a hemodynamically significant patent ductus arteriosus in premature infants weighing between 500 and 1750 g when after 48 hours usual medical management (e.g., fluid restriction, diuretics, digitalis, respiratory support, etc.) is ineffective. Clear-cut clinical evidence of a hemodynamically significant patent ductus arteriosus should be present, such as respiratory distress, a continuous murmur, a hyperactive precordium, cardiomegaly and pulmonary plethora on chest x-ray.

CONTRAINDICATIONS

INDOCIN I.V. is contraindicated in: infants with proven or suspected infection that is untreated; infants who are bleeding, especially those with active intracranial hemorrhage or gastrointestinal bleeding; infants with thrombocytopenia; infants with coagulation defects; infants with or who are suspected of having necrotizing enterocolitis; infants with significant impairment of renal function; infants with congenital heart disease in whom patency of the ductus arteriosus is necessary for satisfactory pulmonary or systemic blood flow (e.g., pulmonary atresia, severe tetralogy of Fallot, severe coarctation of the aorta).

WARNINGS

Gastrointestinal Effects:
In the collaborative study, major gastrointestinal bleeding was no more common in those infants receiving indomethacin than in those infants on placebo. However, minor gastrointestinal bleeding (i.e., chemical detection of blood in the stool) was more commonly noted in those infants treated with indomethacin. Severe gastrointestinal effects have been reported in adults with various arthritic disorders treated chronically with oral indomethacin. [For further information, see package circular for Capsules INDOCIN® (Indomethacin, MSD)].

Central Nervous System Effects:
Prematurity per se, is associated with an increased incidence of spontaneous intraventricular hemorrhage. Because indomethacin may inhibit platelet aggregation, the potential for intraventricular bleeding may be increased. However, in the large multi-center study of INDOCIN I.V. (see CLINICAL PHARMACOLOGY), the incidence of intraventricular hemorrhage in babies treated with INDOCIN I.V. was not significantly higher than in the control infants.

Renal Effects:
INDOCIN I.V. may cause significant reduction in urine output (50 percent or more) with concomitant elevations of blood urea nitrogen and creatinine, and reductions in glomerular filtration rate and creatinine clearance. These effects in most infants are transient, disappearing with cessation of therapy with INDOCIN I.V. However, because adequate renal function can depend upon renal prostaglandin synthesis, INDOCIN I.V. may precipitate renal insufficiency, including acute renal failure, especially in infants with other conditions that may adversely affect renal function (e.g., extracellular volume depletion from any cause, congestive heart failure, sepsis, concomitant use of any nephrotoxic drug, hepatic dysfunction). When significant suppression of urine volume occurs after a dose of INDOCIN I.V., no additional dose should be given until the urine output returns to normal levels.

INDOCIN I.V. in pre-term infants may suppress water excretion to a greater extent than sodium excretion. When this occurs, a significant reduction in serum sodium values (i.e., hyponatremia) may result. Infants should have serum electrolyte determinations done during therapy with INDOCIN I.V. Renal function and serum electrolytes should be monitored (see PRECAUTIONS, *Drug Interactions* and DOSAGE AND ADMINISTRATION).

PRECAUTIONS

General
INDOCIN (Indomethacin, MSD) may mask the usual signs and symptoms of infection. Therefore, the physician must be continually on the alert for this and should use the drug with extra care in the presence of existing controlled infection. Severe hepatic reactions have been reported in adults treated chronically with oral indomethacin for arthritic disorders. [For further information, see package circular for Capsules INDOCIN (Indomethacin, MSD)]. If clinical signs and symptoms consistent with liver disease develop in the neonate, or if systemic manifestations occur, INDOCIN I.V. should be discontinued.

INDOCIN I.V. may inhibit platelet aggregation. In one small study, platelet aggregation was grossly abnormal after indomethacin therapy (given orally to premature infants to close the ductus arteriosus). Platelet aggregation returned to normal by the tenth day. Premature infants should be observed for signs of bleeding.

The drug should be administered carefully to avoid extravascular injection or leakage as the solution may be irritating to tissue.

Drug Interactions
Since renal function may be reduced by INDOCIN I.V., consideration should be given to reduction in dosage of those medications that rely on adequate renal function for their elimination. Because the half-life of digitalis (given frequently to pre-term infants with patent ductus arteriosus and associated cardiac failure) may be prolonged when given concomitantly with indomethacin, the infant should be observed closely; frequent ECGs and serum digitalis levels may be required to prevent or detect digitalis toxicity early. Furthermore, in one study of premature infants treated with INDOCIN I.V. and also receiving either gentamicin or amikacin, both peak and trough levels of these aminoglycosides were significantly elevated.

Therapy with indomethacin may blunt the natriuretic effect of furosemide. This response has been attributed to inhibition of prostaglandin synthesis by non-steroidal anti-inflammatory drugs. In a study of 19 premature infants with patent ductus arteriosus treated with either INDOCIN I.V. alone or a combination of INDOCIN I.V. and furosemide, results showed that infants receiving both INDOCIN I.V. and furosemide had significantly higher urinary output, higher levels of sodium and chloride excretion, and higher glomerular filtration rates than did those infants receiving INDOCIN I.V. alone. In this study, the data suggested that therapy with furosemide helped to maintain renal function in the premature infant when INDOCIN I.V. was added to the treatment of patent ductus arteriosus.

Neonatal Effects
In rats and mice, oral indomethacin 4.0 mg/kg/day given during the last three days of gestation caused a decrease in maternal weight gain and some maternal and fetal deaths. An increased incidence of neuronal necrosis in the diencephalon in the live-born fetuses was observed. At 2.0 mg/kg/day, no increase in neuronal necrosis was observed as compared to the control groups. Administration of 0.5 or 4.0 mg/kg/day during the first three days of life did not cause an increase in neuronal necrosis at either dose level. Pregnant rats, given 2.0 mg/kg/day and 4.0 mg/kg/day during the last trimester of gestation, delivered offspring whose pulmonary blood vessels were both reduced in number and excessively muscularized. These findings are similar to those observed in the syndrome of persistent pulmonary hypertension of the newborn.

ADVERSE REACTIONS

In a double-blind placebo-controlled trial of 405 premature infants weighing less than or equal to 1750 g with evidence of large ductal shunting, in those infants treated with indomethacin (n = 206), there was a statistically significantly greater incidence of bleeding problems, including gross or microscopic bleeding into the gastrointestinal tract, oozing from the skin after needle stick, pulmonary hemorrhage, and disseminated intravascular coagulopathy. There was no statistically significant difference between treatment groups with reference to intracranial hemorrhage.

The infants treated with indomethacin sodium trihydrate also had a significantly higher incidence of transient oliguria and elevations of serum creatinine (greater than or equal to 1.8 mg/dL) than did the infants treated with placebo.

The incidences of retrolental fibroplasia (grades III and IV) and pneumothorax in infants treated with INDOCIN I.V. were no greater than in placebo controls and were statistically significantly lower than in surgically-treated infants. The following additional adverse reactions in infants have been reported from the collaborative study, anecdotal case reports, and from other studies using rectal, oral, or intravenous indomethacin for treatment of patent ductus arteriosus. The rates are based on the experience of 849 indomethacin-treated infants reported in the medical literature, regardless of the route of administration. One year follow-up is available on 175 infants and shows no long-term sequelae which could be attributed to indomethacin. In controlled clinical studies, only electrolyte imbalance and renal dysfunction (of the reactions listed below) occurred statistically significantly more frequently after INDOCIN I.V. than after placebo.

Renal: renal dysfunction in 41 percent of infants, including one or more of the following: reduced urinary output; reduced urine sodium, chloride, or potassium, urine osmolality, free water clearance, or glomerular filtration rate; elevated serum creatinine or BUN; uremia.

Gastrointestinal: gastrointestinal bleeding*, vomiting, abdominal distention, transient ileus, localized perforation(s) of the small and/or large intestine.

Metabolic: hyponatremia*, elevated serum potassium*, reduction in blood sugar, including hypoglycemia, increased weight gain (fluid retention).

Coagulation: decreased platelet aggregation (see PRECAUTIONS).

---

*Incidence 3–9 percent. Those reactions which are unmarked occurred in 1–3 percent of patients.

The following adverse reactions have also been reported in infants treated with indomethacin, however, a causal relationship to therapy with INDOCIN I.V. has not been established:

Cardiovascular: intracranial bleeding**, bradycardia, pulmonary hypertension.
Respiratory: apnea, exacerbation of pre-existing pulmonary infection.
Metabolic: acidosis/alkalosis.
Hematologic: disseminated intravascular coagulation.
Gastrointestinal: necrotizing enterocolitis.
Ophthalmic: retrolental fibroplasia.**

A variety of additional adverse experiences have been reported in adults treated with oral indomethacin for moderate to severe rheumatoid arthritis, osteoarthritis, ankylosing spondylitis, acute painful shoulder and acute gouty arthritis (see section ADDITIONAL ADVERSE REACTIONS—ADULTS). Their relevance to the pre-term neonate receiving indomethacin for patent ductus arteriosus is unknown, however, the possibility exists that these experiences may be associated with the use of INDOCIN I.V. in pre-term neonates.

DOSAGE AND ADMINISTRATION

FOR INTRAVENOUS ADMINISTRATION ONLY.
Dosage recommendations for closure of the ductus arteriosus depends on the age of the infant at the time of therapy. A course of therapy is defined as three intravenous doses of INDOCIN I.V. given at 12–24 hour intervals, with careful attention to urinary output. If anuria or marked oliguria (urinary output < 0.6 mL/kg/hr) is evident at the scheduled time of the second or third dose of INDOCIN I.V., no additional doses should be given until laboratory studies indicate that renal function has returned to normal (see WARNINGS, *Renal Effects*).
Dosage according to age is as follows:

AGE at 1st dose	DOSAGE (mg/kg)		
	1st	2nd	3rd
Less than 48 hours	0.2	0.1	0.1
2–7 days	0.2	0.2	0.2
over 7 days	0.2	0.25	0.25

If the ductus arteriosus closes or is significantly reduced in size after an interval of 48 hours or more from completion of the first course of INDOCIN I.V., no further doses are necessary. If the ductus arteriosus re-opens, a second course of 1–3 doses may be given, each dose separated by a 12–24 hour interval as described above.

If the infant remains unresponsive to therapy with INDOCIN I.V. after 2 courses, surgery may be necessary for closure of the ductus arteriosus. If severe adverse reactions occur, STOP THE DRUG.

Directions for Use
Parenteral drug products should be inspected visually for particulate matter and discoloration prior to administration whenever solution and container permit.

The solution should be prepared only with 1 to 2 mL of preservative-free sterile Sodium Chloride Injection, 0.9 percent or preservative-free Sterile Water for Injection. Benzyl alcohol as a preservative has been associated with toxicity in newborns. Therefore, all diluents should be preservative-free. If 1 mL of diluent is used, the concentration of indomethacin in the solution will equal approximately 0.1 mg/0.1 mL; if 2 mL of diluent are used, the concentration of the solution will equal approximately 0.05 mg/0.1 mL. Any unused portion of the solution should be discarded because there is no preservative contained in the vial. A fresh solution should be prepared just prior to each administration. Once reconstituted, the indomethacin solution may be injected intravenously over 5–10 seconds.

Further dilution with intravenous infusion solutions is not recommended. INDOCIN I.V. is not buffered, and reconstitution with solutions at pH values below 6.0 may result in precipitation of the insoluble indomethacin free acid moiety.

HOW SUPPLIED

No. 3406—Sterile INDOCIN I.V. is a lyophilized white to yellow powder or plug supplied as single dose vials contain-

---

**Incidence in both indomethacin and placebo-treated infants 3–9 percent. Those reactions which are unmarked occurred in less than 3 percent.

Continued on next page

Information on the Merck Sharp & Dohme products listed on these pages is the full prescribing information from product circulars in use August 31, 1989.

Merck Sharp & Dohme—Cont.

ing indomethacin sodium trihydrate, equivalent to 1 mg indomethacin.
NDC 0006-3406-17.
Storage
Store below 30°C (86°F). *Protect from light.* Store container in carton until contents have been used.

ADDITIONAL ADVERSE REACTIONS—ADULTS

The following adverse reactions have been reported in adults treated with oral indomethacin for moderate to severe rheumatoid arthritis, osteoarthritis, ankylosing spondylitis, acute painful shoulder and acute gouty arthritis. Complaints not of relevance in the treatment of the premature infant, such as anorexia, psychic disturbances, and blurred vision, are not listed.

Incidence 1% to 3%	Incidence less than 1%	
GASTROINTESTINAL		
diarrhea	bloating (includes	gastrointestinal
constipation	distention)	bleeding without
	flatulence	obvious ulcer
	peptic ulcer	formation and
	gastroenteritis	perforation of
	rectal bleeding	pre-existing sigmoid
	proctitis	lesions
	single or multiple	development of
	ulcerations, includ-	ulcerative stomatitis
	ing perforation and	toxic hepatitis and
	hemorrhage of the	jaundice (some fatal
	esophagus, stomach,	cases have been
	duodenum or small	reported)
	and large intestines	
	intestinal ulceration	
	associated with	
	stenosis and	
	obstruction	
CENTRAL NERVOUS SYSTEM		
none	involuntary muscle	aggravation of epilepsy
	movements	coma
		peripheral neuropathy
		convulsions
SPECIAL SENSES		
none	hearing disturbances,	
	deafness	
CARDIOVASCULAR		
none	hypertension	arrhythmia
	hypotension	congestive heart fail-
	tachycardia	ure
		thrombophlebitis
METABOLIC		
none	edema	hyperglycemia
	weight gain	glycosuria
	flushing	hyperkalemia
INTEGUMENTARY		
none	rash; urticaria	exfoliative dermatitis
	petechiae or	erythema nodosum
	ecchymosis	loss of hair
		Stevens-Johnson
		syndrome
		erythema multiforme
		toxic epidermal
		necrolysis
HEMATOLOGIC		
none	leukopenia	aplastic anemia
	bone marrow	hemolytic anemia
	depression	agranulocytosis
	anemia secondary to	thrombocytopenic
	obvious or occult	purpura
	gastrointestinal	
	bleeding	
HYPERSENSITIVITY		
none	acute anaphylaxis	dyspnea
	acute respiratory	asthma
	distress	purpura
	rapid fall in blood	angiitis
	pressure resembling	pulmonary edema
	a shock-like state	
GENITOURINARY		
none	hematuria	renal insufficiency,
	vaginal bleeding	including renal
		failure
MISCELLANEOUS		
none	epistaxis	
	breast changes,	
	including en-	
	largement and	
	tenderness, or	
	gynecomastia	

See package circular for Capsules INDOCIN (Indomethacin, MSD) for additional information concerning adverse reactions and other cautionary statements.
    A.H.F.S. Category: 28:08
    DC 7414810   Issued June 1988
COPYRIGHT © MERCK & CO., INC., 1985

INVERSINE® Tablets   ℞
(Mecamylamine HCl, MSD), U.S.P.

DESCRIPTION

INVERSINE® (Mecamylamine HCl, MSD) is a potent, oral antihypertensive agent and ganglion blocker, and is a secondary amine. It is $N,2,3,3$-tetramethylbicyclo[2.2.1] heptan-2-amine hydrochloride. Its empirical formula is $C_{11}H_{21}N$ · HCl and its structural formula is:

$$NHCH_3 \cdot HCl$$
$$CH_2 \begin{cases} -CH_3 \\ -CH_3 \\ CH_3 \end{cases}$$

It is a white, odorless, or practically odorless, crystalline powder, is highly stable, soluble in water and has a molecular weight of 203.75.
INVERSINE is supplied as tablets for oral use, each containing 2.5 mg mecamylamine HCl. Inactive ingredients are acacia, calcium phosphate, D&C Yellow 10, FD&C Yellow 6, lactose, magnesium stearate, starch, and talc.

CLINICAL PHARMACOLOGY

Mecamylamine reduces blood pressure in both normotensive and hypertensive individuals. It has a gradual onset of action ($\frac{1}{2}$ to 2 hours) and a long-lasting effect (usually 6 to 12 hours or more). A small oral dosage often produces a smooth and predictable reduction of blood pressure. Although this antihypertensive effect is predominantly orthostatic, the supine blood pressure is also significantly reduced.
Pharmacokinetics and Metabolism
Mecamylamine is almost completely absorbed from the gastrointestinal tract, resulting in consistent lowering of blood pressure in most patients with hypertensive cardiovascular disease. Mecamylamine is excreted slowly in the urine in the unchanged form. The rate of its renal elimination is influenced markedly by urinary pH. Alkalinization of the urine reduces, and acidification promotes, renal excretion of mecamylamine.
Mecamylamine crosses the blood-brain and placental barriers.

INDICATIONS AND USAGE

For the management of moderately severe to severe essential hypertension and in uncomplicated cases of malignant hypertension.

CONTRAINDICATIONS

INVERSINE should not be used in mild, moderate, labile hypertension and may prove unsuitable in uncooperative patients. It is contraindicated in coronary insufficiency or recent myocardial infarction.
INVERSINE should be given with great discretion, if at all, when renal insufficiency is manifested by a rising or elevated BUN. The drug is contraindicated in uremia. Patients receiving antibiotics and sulfonamides should generally not be treated with ganglion blockers. Other contraindications are glaucoma, organic pyloric stenosis or hypersensitivity to the product.

WARNINGS

Mecamylamine, a secondary amine, readily penetrates into the brain and thus may produce central nervous sytem effects. Tremor, choreiform movements, mental aberrations, and convulsions may occur rarely. These have occurred most often when large doses of INVERSINE were used, especially in patients with cerebral or renal insufficiency.
When ganglion blockers or other potent antihypertensive drugs are discontinued suddenly, hypertensive levels return. In patients with malignant hypertension and others, this may occur abruptly and may cause fatal cerebral vascular accidents or acute congestive heart failure. When INVERSINE is withdrawn, this should be done gradually and other antihypertensive therapy usually must be substituted. On the other hand, the effects of INVERSINE sometimes may last from hours to days after therapy is discontinued.

PRECAUTIONS

General
The patient's condition should be evaluated carefully, particularly as to renal and cardiovascular function. When renal, cerebral, or coronary blood flow is deficient, any additional impairment, which might result from added hypotension, must be avoided. The use of INVERSINE in patients with marked cerebral and coronary arteriosclerosis or after a recent cerebral accident requires caution.
The action of INVERSINE may be potentiated by excessive heat, fever, infection, hemorrhage, pregnancy, anesthesia, surgery, vigorous exercise, other antihypertensive drugs, alcohol, and salt depletion as a result of diminished intake or increased excretion due to diarrhea, vomiting, excessive sweating, or diuretics.
During therapy with INVERSINE, sodium intake should not be restricted but, if necessary, the dosage of the ganglion blocker must be adjusted.
Since urinary retention may occur in patients on ganglion blockers, caution is required in patients with prostatic hypertrophy, bladder neck obstruction, and urethral stricture. Frequent loose bowel movements with abdominal distention and decreased borborygmi may be the first signs of paralytic ileus. If these are present, INVERSINE should be discontinued immediately and remedial steps taken.
Information for Patients
INVERSINE may cause dizziness, lightheadedness, or fainting, especially when rising from a lying or sitting position. This effect may be increased by alcoholic beverages, exercise, or during hot weather. Getting up slowly may help alleviate such a reaction.
Drug Interactions
Patients receiving antibiotics and sulfonamides generally should not be treated with ganglion blockers.
The action of INVERSINE may be potentiated by anesthesia, other antihypertensive drugs and alcohol.
Carcinogenesis, Mutagenesis, Impairment of Fertility
Long-term studies in animals have not been performed to evaluate the effects upon fertility, mutagenic or carcinogenic potential of INVERSINE.
Pregnancy
Pregnancy Category C. Animal reproduction studies have not been conducted with INVERSINE. It is not known whether INVERSINE can cause fetal harm when given to a pregnant woman or can affect reproductive capacity. INVERSINE should be given to a pregnant woman only if clearly needed.
Nursing Mothers
Because of the potential for serious adverse reactions in nursing infants from INVERSINE, a decision should be made whether to discontinue nursing or to discontinue the drug, taking into account the importance of the drug to the mother.

ADVERSE REACTIONS

The following adverse reactions have been reported and within each category are listed in order of decreasing severity.
Gastrointestinal: Ileus, constipation (sometimes preceded by small, frequent liquid stools), vomiting, nausea, anorexia, glossitis and dryness of mouth.
Cardiovascular: Orthostatic dizziness and syncope, postural hypotension.
Nervous System/Psychiatric: Convulsions, choreiform movements, mental aberrations, tremor, and paresthesias (see WARNINGS).
Respiratory: Interstitial pulmonary edema and fibrosis.
Urogenital: Urinary retention, impotence, decreased libido.
Special Senses: Blurred vision, dilated pupils.
Miscellaneous: Weakness, fatigue, sedation.

OVERDOSAGE

Signs of overdosage include: hypotension (which may progress to peripheral vascular collapse), postural hypotension, nausea, vomiting, diarrhea, constipation, paralytic ileus, urinary retention, dizziness, anxiety, dry mouth, mydriasis, blurred vision, or palpitations. A rise in intraocular pressure may occur.
Pressor amines may be used to counteract excessive hypotension. Since patients being treated with ganglion blockers are more than normally reactive to pressor amines, small doses of the latter are recommended to avoid excessive response. The oral LD_{50} of mecamylamine in the mouse is 92 mg/kg.

DOSAGE AND ADMINISTRATION

Therapy is usually started with one 2.5 mg tablet of INVERSINE twice a day. This initial dosage should be modified by increments of one 2.5 mg tablet at intervals of not less than 2 days until the desired blood pressure response occurs (the criterion being a dosage just under that which causes signs of mild postural hypotension).

The average total daily dosage of INVERSINE is 25 mg, usually in three divided doses. However, as little as 2.5 mg daily may be sufficient to control hypertension in some patients. A range of two to four or even more doses may be required in severe cases when smooth control is difficult to obtain. In severe or urgent cases, larger increments at smaller intervals may be needed. Partial tolerance may develop in certain patients, requiring an increase in the daily dosage of INVERSINE.

Administration of INVERSINE after meals may cause a more gradual absorption and smoother control of excessively high blood pressure. The timing of doses in relation to meals should be consistent. Since the blood pressure response to antihypertensive drugs is increased in the early morning, the larger dose should be given at noontime and perhaps in the evening. The morning dose, as a rule, should be relatively small and in some instances may even be omitted.

The *initial regulation of dosage* should be determined by blood pressure readings in the erect position at the time of maximal effect of the drug, as well as by other signs and symptoms of orthostatic hypertension.

The *effective maintenance dosage* should be regulated by blood pressure readings in the erect position and by limitation of dosage to that which causes slight faintness or dizziness in this position. If the patient or a relative can use a sphygmomanometer, instructions may be given to reduce or omit a dose if readings fall below a designated level or if faintness or lightheadedness occurs. *However, no change should be instituted without the knowledge of the physician.* Close supervision and education of the patient, as well as critical adjustment of dosage, are essential to successful therapy.

Other Antihypertensive Agents

When INVERSINE is given with other antihypertensive drugs, the dosage of these other agents, as well as that of INVERSINE, should be reduced to avoid excessive hypotension. However, thiazides should be continued in their usual dosage, while that of INVERSINE is decreased by at least 50 percent.

HOW SUPPLIED

No. 3219—Tablets INVERSINE, 2.5 mg, are yellow, round, scored, compressed tablets, coded MSD 52. They are supplied as follows:

NDC 0006-0052-68 in bottles of 100.

Shown in Product Identification Section, page 418
A.H.F.S. Category: 24:08
DC 6041721 Issued September 1985
COPYRIGHT © MERCK & CO., INC., 1985
All rights reserved

LACRISERT® Sterile Ophthalmic Insert   ℞
(Hydroxypropyl Cellulose Ophthalmic Insert, MSD)

DESCRIPTION

LACRISERT® (Hydroxypropyl Cellulose Ophthalmic Insert, MSD) is a rod-shaped, water soluble, ophthalmic preparation made of hydroxypropyl cellulose, 5 mg. LACRISERT contains no preservatives or other ingredients. It is about 1.27 mm in diameter by about 3.5 mm long.

LACRISERT is supplied in packages of 60 units, together with illustrated instructions and a special applicator for removing LACRISERT from the unit dose blister and inserting it into the eye. A spare applicator is included in each package.

ACTIONS

LACRISERT acts to stabilize and thicken the precorneal tear film and prolong the tear film breakup time which is usually accelerated in patients with dry eye states. LACRISERT also acts to lubricate and protect the eye. LACRISERT usually reduces the signs and symptoms resulting from moderate to severe dry eye syndromes.

INDICATIONS

LACRISERT is indicated in patients with moderate to severe dry eye syndromes, including keratoconjunctivitis sicca. LACRISERT is indicated especially in patients who remain symptomatic after an adequate trial of therapy with artificial tear solutions.

LACRISERT is also indicated for patients with:
    Exposure keratitis
    Decreased corneal sensitivity
    Recurrent corneal erosions

LACRISERT usually reduces the signs and symptoms resulting from moderate to severe dry eye syndromes, such as conjunctival hyperemia, corneal and conjunctival staining with rose bengal, exudation, itching, burning, foreign body sensation, smarting, photophobia, dryness and blurred or cloudy

vision. Progressive visual deterioration which occurs in some patients may be retarded, halted, or sometimes reversed.

In a multicenter crossover study the 5 mg LACRISERT administered once a day during the waking hours was compared to artificial tears used four or more times daily. There was a significant prolongation of tear film breakup time and a significant decrease in foreign body sensation associated with dry eye syndrome in patients during treatment with inserts as compared to artificial tears. Improvement, as measured by amelioration of symptoms, by slit lamp examination and by rose bengal staining of the cornea and conjunctiva, was greater in most patients with moderate to severe symptoms during treatment with LACRISERT. Patient comfort was usually better with LACRISERT than with artificial tears solution, and most patients preferred LACRISERT.

In most patients treated with LACRISERT for over one year, improvement was observed as evidenced by amelioration of symptoms generally associated with keratoconjunctivitis sicca such as burning, tearing, foreign body sensation, itching, photophobia and blurred or cloudy vision.

During studies in healthy volunteers, a thickened precorneal tear film was usually observed through the slit lamp while LACRISERT was present in the conjunctival sac.

CONTRAINDICATIONS

LACRISERT is contraindicated in patients who are hypersensitive to hydroxypropyl cellulose.

WARNINGS

Instructions for inserting and removing LACRISERT should be carefully followed.

PRECAUTIONS

Because this product may produce transient blurring of vision, patients should be instructed to exercise caution when operating hazardous machinery or driving a motor vehicle. If improperly placed in the inferior cul-de-sac, LACRISERT may result in corneal abrasion (see DOSAGE AND ADMINISTRATION).

ADVERSE REACTIONS

The following adverse reactions have been reported in patients treated with LACRISERT, but were in most instances mild and transient:
    Transient blurring of vision (See PRECAUTIONS)
    Ocular discomfort or irritation
    Matting or stickiness of eyelashes
    Photophobia
    Hypersensitivity
    Edema of the eyelids
    Hyperemia

DOSAGE AND ADMINISTRATION

One LACRISERT ophthalmic insert in each eye once daily is usually sufficient to relieve the symptoms associated with moderate to severe dry eye syndromes. Individual patients may require more flexibility in the use of LACRISERT; some patients may require twice daily use for optimal results. Clinical experience with LACRISERT indicates that in some patients several weeks may be required before satisfactory improvement of symptoms is achieved.

LACRISERT is inserted into the inferior cul-de-sac of the eye beneath the base of the tarsus, not in apposition to the cornea. Illustrated instructions are included in each package. While in the licensed practitioner's office, the patient should read the instructions, then practice insertion and removal of LACRISERT until proficiency is achieved.

NOTE: Occasionally LACRISERT is inadvertently expelled from the eye, especially in patients with shallow conjunctival fornices. The patient should be cautioned against rubbing the eye(s) containing LACRISERT, especially upon awakening, so as not to dislodge or expel the insert. If required, another LACRISERT ophthalmic insert may be inserted. If experience indicates that transient blurred vision develops in an individual patient, the patient may want to remove LACRISERT a few hours after insertion to avoid this. Another LACRISERT ophthalmic insert may be inserted if needed.

If LACRISERT causes worsening of symptoms, the patient should be instructed to inspect the conjunctival sac to make certain LACRISERT is in the proper location, deep in the inferior cul-de-sac of the eye beneath the base of the tarsus. If these symptoms persist, LACRISERT should be removed and the patient should contact the practitioner.

HOW SUPPLIED

No. 3380—LACRISERT, a rod-shaped, water-soluble, ophthalmic preparation made of hydroxypropyl cellulose, 5 mg, is supplied as follows:

NDC 0006-3380-60 in packages containing 60 unit doses, two reusable applicators and a storage container.
Store below 30°C (86°F).
DC 7189405 Issued November 1984
Copyright © MERCK & CO., INC., 1985
All rights reserved

M-M-R®II   ℞
(Measles, Mumps, and Rubella Virus Vaccine Live, MSD), U.S.P.

DESCRIPTION

M-M-R® II (Measles, Mumps, and Rubella Virus Vaccine Live, MSD) is a live virus vaccine for immunization against measles (rubeola), mumps and rubella (German measles). M-M-R II is a sterile lyophilized preparation of (1) ATTENUVAX® (Measles Virus Vaccine Live, MSD), a more attenuated line of measles virus, derived from Enders' attenuated Edmonston strain and grown in cell cultures of chick embryo; (2) MUMPSVAX® (Mumps Virus Vaccine Live, MSD), the Jeryl Lynn (B level) strain of mumps virus grown in cell cultures of chick embryo; and (3) MERUVAX® II (Rubella Virus Vaccine Live, MSD), the Wistar RA 27/3 strain of live attenuated rubella virus grown in human diploid cell (WI-38) culture. The vaccine viruses are the same as those used in the manufacture of ATTENUVAX (Measles Virus Vaccine Live, MSD), MUMPSVAX (Mumps Virus Vaccine Live, MSD) and MERUVAX II (Rubella Virus Vaccine Live, MSD). The three viruses are mixed before being lyophilized. The product contains no preservative.

The reconstituted vaccine is for subcutaneous administration. When reconstituted as directed, the dose for injection is 0.5 mL and contains not less than the equivalent of 1,000 $TCID_{50}$ (tissue culture infectious doses) of the U.S. Reference Measles Virus; 5,000 $TCID_{50}$ of the U.S. Reference Mumps Virus; and 1,000 $TCID_{50}$ of the U.S. Reference Rubella Virus. Each dose contains approximately 25 mcg of neomycin. The product contains no preservative. Sorbitol and hydrolized gelatin are added as stabilizers.

CLINICAL PHARMACOLOGY

Clinical studies of 279 triple seronegative children, 11 months to 7 years of age, demonstrated that M-M-R II is highly immunogenic and generally well tolerated. In these studies, a single injection of the vaccine induced measles hemagglutination-inhibition (HI) antibodies in 95 percent, mumps neutralizing antibodies in 96 percent, and rubella HI antibodies in 99 percent of susceptible persons.

The RA 27/3 rubella strain in M-M-R II elicits higher immediate post-vaccination HI, complement-fixing and neutralizing antibody levels than other strains of rubella vaccine and has been shown to induce a broader profile of circulating antibodies including anti-theta and anti-iota precipitating antibodies. The RA 27/3 rubella strain immunologically simulates natural infection more closely than other rubella vaccine viruses. The increased levels and broader profile of antibodies produced by RA 27/3 strain rubella virus vaccine appear to correlate with greater resistance to subclinical reinfection with the wild virus, and provide greater confidence for lasting immunity.

Vaccine induced antibody levels following administration of M-M-R II have been shown to persist for at least two years without substantial decline. Antibody levels after immunization with M-M-R (Measles, Mumps, and Rubella Virus Vaccine Live, MSD), containing the HPV-77 strain of rubella, have persisted for 10.5 years without substantial decline. If the present pattern continues, it will provide a basis for the expectation that immunity following vaccination will be permanent. However, continued surveillance will be required to demonstrate this point.

INDICATIONS AND USAGE

M-M-R II is indicated for simultaneous immunization against measles, mumps, and rubella in persons 15 months of age or older. A booster is not needed.

Infants who are less than 15 months of age may fail to respond to the measles component of the vaccine due to presence in the circulation of residual measles antibody of maternal origin; the younger the infant, the lower the likelihood of seroconversion. In geographically isolated or other relatively inaccessible populations for whom immunization programs are logistically difficult, and in population groups in which natural measles infection may occur in a significant proportion of infants before 15 months of age, it may be desirable to

Continued on next page

Merck Sharp & Dohme—Cont.

give the vaccine to infants at an earlier age. Infants vaccinated under these conditions at less than 12 months of age should be revaccinated after reaching 15 months of age. There is some evidence to suggest that infants immunized at less than one year of age may not develop sustained antibody levels when later reimmunized. The advantage of early protection must be weighed against the chance for failure to respond adequately on reimmunization.

Previously unimmunized children of susceptible pregnant women should receive live attenuated rubella vaccine, because an immunized child will be less likely to acquire natural rubella and introduce the virus into the household.

Non-Pregnant Adolescent and Adult Females

Immunization of susceptible non-pregnant adolescent and adult females of childbearing age with live attenuated rubella virus vaccine is indicated if certain precautions are observed (see below and PRECAUTIONS). Vaccinating susceptible postpubertal females confers individual protection against subsequently acquiring rubella infection during pregnancy, which in turn prevents infection of the fetus and consequent congenital rubella injury.

Women of childbearing age should be advised not to become pregnant for three months after vaccination and should be informed of the reasons for this precaution.*

It is recommended that rubella susceptibility be determined by serologic testing prior to immunization.** If immune, as evidenced by a specific rubella antibody titer of 1:8 or greater (hemagglutination-inhibition test), vaccination is unnecessary. Congenital malformations do occur in up to seven percent of all live births. Their chance appearance after vaccination could lead to misinterpretation of the cause, particularly if the prior rubella-immune status of vaccinees is unknown.

Postpubertal females should be informed of the frequent occurrence of generally self-limited arthralgia and/or arthritis beginning 2 to 4 weeks after vaccination (see ADVERSE REACTIONS).

Postpartum Women

It has been found convenient in many instances to vaccinate rubella-susceptible women in the immediate postpartum period. (See *Nursing Mothers*).

Revaccination: Children vaccinated when younger than 12 months of age should be revaccinated. Based on available evidence, there is no reason to routinely revaccinate persons who were vaccinated originally when 12 months of age or older. However, persons should be revaccinated if there is evidence to suggest that initial immunization was ineffective.

Use with other Vaccines

Routine administration of DTP (diphtheria, tetanus, pertussis) and/or OPV (oral poliovirus vaccine) concomitantly with measles, mumps and rubella vaccines is not recommended because there are insufficient data relating to the simultaneous administration of these antigens. However, the American Academy of Pediatrics has noted that in some circumstances, particularly when the patient may not return, some practitioners prefer to administer all these antigens on a single day. If done, separate sites and syringes should be used for DTP and M-M-R II.

M-M-R II should not be given less than one month before or after administration of other virus vaccines.

CONTRAINDICATIONS

Do not give M-M-R II to pregnant females; the possible effects of the vaccine on fetal development are unknown at this time. If vaccination of postpubertal females is undertaken, pregnancy should be avoided for three months following vaccination. (See PRECAUTIONS, *Pregnancy*).

Anaphylactoid reaction to neomycin (each dose of reconstituted vaccine contains approximately 25 mcg of neomycin).

*NOTE: The Immunization Practices Advisory Committee (ACIP) has recommended "In view of the importance of protecting this age group against rubella, reasonable precautions in a rubella immunization program include asking females if they are pregnant, excluding those who say they are, and explaining the theoretical risks to the others."

**NOTE: The Immunization Practices Advisory Committee (ACIP) has stated "When practical, and when reliable laboratory services are available, potential vaccinees of childbearing age can have serologic tests to determine susceptibility to rubella. . . . However, routinely performing serologic tests for all females of childbearing age to determine susceptibility so that vaccine is given only to proven susceptibles is expensive and has been ineffective in some areas. Accordingly, the ACIP believes that rubella vaccination of a woman who is not known to be pregnant and has no history of vaccination is justifiable without serologic testing."

History of anaphylactoid reaction to eggs (see HYPERSENSITIVITY TO EGGS below).

Any febrile respiratory illness or other active febrile infection.

Active untreated tuberculosis.

Patients receiving immunosuppressive therapy. This contraindication does not apply to patients who are receiving corticosteroids as replacement therapy, e.g., for Addison's disease.

Individuals with blood dyscrasias, leukemia, lymphomas of any type, or other malignant neoplasms affecting the bone marrow or lymphatic systems.

Primary immunodeficiency states, including cellular immune deficiencies, hypogammaglobulinemic and dysgammaglobulinemic states.

Individuals with a family history of congenital or hereditary immunodeficiency, until the immune competence of the potential vaccine recipient is demonstrated.

HYPERSENSITIVITY TO EGGS

Live measles vaccine and live mumps vaccine are produced in chick embryo cell culture. Persons with a history of anaphylactic or other immediate reactions (e.g., hives, swelling of the mouth and throat, difficulty breathing, hypotension, or shock) subsequent to egg ingestion should not be vaccinated. Evidence indicates that persons are not at increased risk if they have egg allergies that are not anaphylactic in nature. Such persons may be vaccinated in the usual manner. There is no evidence to indicate that persons with allergies to chickens or feathers are at increased risk of reaction to the vaccine.

PRECAUTIONS

General

Adequate treatment provisions including epinephrine, should be available for immediate use should an anaphylactoid reaction occur.

Due caution should be employed in administration of M-M-R II to persons with a history of febrile convulsions, cerebral injury or any other condition in which stress due to fever should be avoided. The physician should be alert to the temperature elevation which may occur following vaccination. (See ADVERSE REACTIONS).

Vaccination should be deferred for at least 3 months following blood or plasma transfusions, or administration of human immune serum globulin.

Excretion of small amounts of the live attenuated rubella virus from the nose or throat has occurred in the majority of susceptible individuals 7–28 days after vaccination. There is no confirmed evidence to indicate that such virus is transmitted to susceptible persons who are in contact with the vaccinated individuals. Consequently, transmission through close personal contact, while accepted as a theoretical possibility, is not regarded as a significant risk. However, transmission of the rubella vaccine virus to infants via breast milk has been documented (see *Nursing Mothers*).

There are no reports of transmission of live attenuated measles or mumps viruses from vaccinees to susceptible contacts. It has been reported that live attenuated measles, mumps and rubella virus vaccines given individually may result in a temporary depression of tuberculin skin sensitivity. Therefore, if a tuberculin test is to be done, it should be administered either before or simultaneously with M-M-R II.

As for any vaccine, vaccination with M-M-R II may not result in seroconversion in 100% of susceptible persons given the vaccine.

Pregnancy

Pregnancy Category C

Animal reproduction studies have not been conducted with M-M-R II. It is also not known whether M-M-R II can cause fetal harm when administered to a pregnant woman or can affect reproduction capacity. Therefore, the vaccine should not be administered to pregnant females; furthermore, pregnancy should be avoided for three months following vaccination (see CONTRAINDICATIONS).

In counseling women who are inadvertently vaccinated when pregnant or who become pregnant within 3 months of vaccination, the physician should be aware of the following: (1) In a 10 year survey involving over 700 pregnant women who received rubella vaccine within 3 months before or after conception (of whom 189 received the Wistar RA 27/3 strain), none of the newborns had abnormalities compatible with congenital rubella syndrome; (2) Although mumps virus is capable of infecting the placenta and fetus, there is no good evidence that it causes congenital malformations in humans. Mumps vaccine virus also has been shown to infect the placenta, but the virus has not been isolated from the fetal tissues from susceptible women who were vaccinated and underwent elective abortions; and (3) Reports have indicated that contracting of natural measles during pregnancy enhances fetal risk. Increased rates of spontaneous abortion, stillbirth, congenital defects and prematurity have been observed subsequent to natural measles during pregnancy.

There are no adequate studies of the attenuated (vaccine) strain of measles virus in pregnancy. However, it would be prudent to assume that the vaccine strain of virus is also capable of inducing adverse fetal effects.

Nursing Mothers

It is not known whether measles or mumps vaccine virus is secreted in human milk. Recent studies have shown that lactating postpartum women immunized with live attenuated rubella vaccine may secrete the virus in breast milk and transmit it to breast-fed infants. In the infants with serological evidence of rubella infection, none exhibited severe disease; however, one exhibited mild clinical illness typical of acquired rubella. Caution should be exercised when M-M-R II is administered to a nursing woman.

ADVERSE REACTIONS

Because of the slightly acidic pH (6.2–6.6) of the vaccine, patients may complain of burning and/or stinging of short duration at the injection site.

The adverse clinical reactions associated with the use of M-M-R II are those expected to follow administration of the monovalent vaccines given separately. These may include malaise, sore throat, headache, fever, rash, nausea, and vomiting; mild local reactions such as erythema, induration, tenderness and regional lymphadenopathy; parotitis, orchitis, nerve deafness, thrombocytopenia and purpura; allergic reactions such as wheal and flare at the injection site or urticaria; polyneuritis; and arthralgia and/or arthritis (usually transient and rarely chronic).

Moderate fever [101–102.9°F (38.3–39.4°C)] occurs occasionally, and high fever [above 103°F (39.4°C)] occurs less commonly. On rare occasions, children developing fever may exhibit febrile convulsions. Rash occurs infrequently and is usually minimal, but rarely may be generalized.

Forms of optic neuritis, including retrobulbar neuritis, papillitis, and retinitis may infrequently follow viral infections, and have been reported to occur 1 to 3 weeks following inoculation with some live virus vaccines.

Clinical experience with live attenuated measles, mumps and rubella virus vaccines given individually indicates that encephalitis and other nervous system reactions have occurred very rarely. These might occur also with M-M-R II. Experience from more than 80 million doses of all live measles vaccines given in the U.S. through 1975 indicates that significant central nervous system reactions such as encephalitis and encephalopathy, occurring within 30 days after vaccination, have been temporally associated with measles vaccine approximately once for every million doses. In no case has it been shown that reactions were actually caused by vaccine. The Center for Disease Control has pointed out that "a certain number of cases of encephalitis may be expected to occur in a large childhood population in a defined period of time even when no vaccines are administered". However, the data suggest the possibility that some of these cases may have been caused by measles vaccines. The risk of such serious neurological disorders following live measles virus vaccine administration remains far less than that for encephalitis and encephalopathy with natural measles (one per two thousand reported cases).

There have been isolated reports of ocular palsies and Guillain-Barre syndrome occurring after immunization with vaccines containing live attenuated measles virus. The ocular palsies have occurred approximately 3–24 days following vaccination. No definite causal relationship has been established between either of these events and vaccination. Isolated reports of polyneuropathy including Guillain-Barré syndrome have also been reported after immunization with rubella containing vaccines.

There have been reports of subacute sclerosing panencephalitis (SSPE) in children who did not have a history of natural measles but did receive measles vaccine. Some of these cases may have resulted from unrecognized measles in the first year of life or possibly from the measles vaccination. Based on estimated nationwide measles vaccine distribution, the association of SSPE cases to measles vaccination is about one case per million vaccine doses distributed. This is far less than the association with natural measles, 6–22 cases of SSPE per million cases of measles. The results of a retrospective case-controlled study conducted by the Center for Disease Control suggest that the overall effect of measles vaccine has been to protect against SSPE by preventing measles with its inherent higher risk of SSPE.

Local reactions characterized by marked swelling, redness and vesiculation at the injection site of attenuated live measles virus vaccines, and systemic reactions including atypical measles, have occurred in persons who received killed measles vaccine previously. M-M-R II was not given under this condition in clinical trials. Rarely, more severe reactions that require hospitalization, including prolonged high fevers and extensive local reactions, have been reported. Panniculitis has been reported rarely following administration of measles vaccine.

Arthralgia and/or arthritis (usually transient and rarely chronic), and polyneuritis are features of natural rubella and vary in frequency and severity with age and sex, being greatest in adult females and least in prepubertal children. This type of involvement as well as myalgia and paresthesia, have also been reported following administration of MERUVAX II (Rubella Virus Vaccine Live, MSD).

Chronic arthritis has been associated with natural rubella infection and has been related to persistent virus and/or viral antigen isolated from body tissues. Only rarely have vaccine recipients developed chronic joint symptoms.

Following vaccination in children, reactions in joints are uncommon and generally of brief duration. In women, incidence rates for arthritis and arthralgia are generally higher than those seen in children (children: 0–3%; women: 12–20%), and the reactions tend to be more marked and of longer duration. Symptoms may persist for a matter of months or on rare occasions for years. In adolescent girls, the reactions appear to be intermediate in incidence between those seen in children and in adult women. Even in older women (35–45 years), these reactions are generally well tolerated and rarely interfere with normal activities.

DOSAGE AND ADMINISTRATION

FOR SUBCUTANEOUS ADMINISTRATION
Do not inject intravenously.

The dosage of vaccine is the same for all persons. Inject the total volume of the single dose vial (about 0.5 mL) or 0.5 mL of the 10 dose vial of reconstituted vaccine subcutaneously, preferably into the outer aspect of upper arm. *Do not give immune globulin (IG) concurrently with* M-M-R II.

During shipment, to insure that there is no loss of potency, the vaccine must be maintained at a temperature of 10°C (50°F) or less.

Before reconstitution, store M-M-R II at 2–8°C (35.6–46.4°F). *Protect from light.*

CAUTION: A sterile syringe free of preservatives, antiseptics, and detergents should be used for each injection and/or reconstitution of the vaccine because these substances may inactivate the live virus vaccine. A 25 gauge, ⅝″ needle is recommended.

To reconstitute, use only the diluent supplied, since it is free of preservatives or other antiviral substances which might inactivate the vaccine.

Single Dose Vial—First withdraw the entire volume of diluent into the syringe to be used for reconstitution. Inject all the diluent in the syringe into the vial of lyophilized vaccine, and agitate to mix thoroughly. Withdraw the entire contents into a syringe and inject the total volume of restored vaccine subcutaneously.

It is important to use a separate sterile syringe and needle for each individual patient to prevent transmission of hepatitis B and other infectious agents from one person to another.

10 Dose Vial (available only to government agencies/institutions)

Withdraw the entire contents (7 mL) of the diluent vial into the sterile syringe to be used for reconstitution, and introduce into the 10 dose vial of lyophilized vaccine. Agitate to ensure thorough mixing. The outer labeling suggests "For Jet Injector or Syringe Use". Use with separate sterile syringes is permitted for containers of 10 doses or less. The vaccine and diluent do not contain preservatives; therefore, the user must recognize the potential contamination hazards and exercise special precautions to protect the sterility and potency of the product. The use of aseptic techniques and proper storage prior to and after restoration of the vaccine and subsequent withdrawal of the individual doses is essential. Use 0.5 mL of the reconstituted vaccine for subcutaneous injection.

It is important to use a separate sterile syringe and needle for each individual patient to prevent transmission of hepatitis B and other infectious agents from one person to another.

Each dose contains not less than the equivalent of 1,000 TCID$_{50}$ of the U.S. Reference Measles Virus, 5,000 TCID$_{50}$ of the U.S. Reference Mumps Virus and 1,000 TCID$_{50}$ of the U.S. Reference Rubella Virus.

Parenteral drug products should be inspected visually for particulate matter and discoloration prior to administration. M-M-R II, when reconstituted, is clear yellow.

HOW SUPPLIED

No. 4749—M-M-R II is supplied as a single-dose vial of lyophilized vaccine, **NDC** 0006-4749-00, and a vial of diluent.

No. 4681/4309—M-M-R II is supplied as follows: (1) a box of 10 single-dose vials of lyophilized vaccine (package A), **NDC** 0006-4681-00; and (2) a box of 10 vials of diluent (package B). To conserve refrigerator space, the diluent may be stored separately at room temperature (6505-00-165-6519, Ten Pack).

Available only to government agencies/institutions

No. 4682X—M-M-R II is supplied as one 10 dose vial of lyophilized vaccine, **NDC** 0006-4682-00, and one 7 mL vial of diluent.

Storage

It is recommended that the vaccine be used as soon as possible after reconstitution. Protect vaccine from light at all times, since such exposure may inactivate the virus. Store reconstituted vaccine in the vaccine vial in a dark place at 2–8°C (35.6–46.4°F) and discard if not used within 8 hours.

A.H.F.S. Category: 80:12
DC 7416510 Issued October 1986
Copyright © MERCK & CO., INC., 1985
All rights reserved

M-R-VAX®II ℞
(Measles and Rubella Virus Vaccine Live, MSD), U.S.P.

DESCRIPTION

M-R-VAX® II (Measles and Rubella Virus Vaccine Live, MSD) is a live virus vaccine for immunization against measles (rubeola) and rubella (German measles).

M-R-VAX II is a sterile lyophilized preparation of (1) ATTENUVAX® (Measles Virus Vaccine Live, MSD), a more attenuated line of measles virus, derived from Enders' attenuated Edmonston strain and grown in cell cultures of chick embryo; and (2) MERUVAX® II (Rubella Virus Vaccine Live, MSD), the Wistar RA 27/3 strain of live attenuated rubella virus grown in human diploid cell (WI-38) culture. The vaccine viruses are the same as those used in the manufacture of ATTENUVAX (Measles Virus Vaccine Live, MSD) and MERUVAX II (Rubella Virus Vaccine Live, MSD). The two viruses are mixed before being lyophilized. The product contains no preservative.

The reconstituted vaccine is for subcutaneous administration. When reconstituted as directed, the dose for injection is 0.5 mL and contains not less than the equivalent of 1,000 TCID$_{50}$ (tissue culture infectious doses) of the U.S. Reference Measles Virus; and 1,000 TCID$_{50}$ of the U.S. Reference Rubella Virus. Each dose contains approximately 25 mcg of neomycin. The product contains no preservative. Sorbitol and hydrolized gelatin are added as stabilizers.

CLINICAL PHARMACOLOGY

Clinical studies of 237 double seronegative children, 10 months to 10 years of age, demonstrated that M-R-VAX II is highly immunogenic and generally well tolerated. In these studies, a single injection of the vaccine induced measles hemagglutination-inhibition (HI) antibodies in 95 percent and rubella HI antibodies in 99 percent of susceptible persons.

The RA 27/3 rubella strain in M-R-VAX II elicits higher immediate post-vaccination HI, complement-fixing and neutralizing antibody levels than other strains of rubella vaccine and has been shown to induce a broader profile of circulating antibodies including anti-theta and anti-iota precipitating antibodies. The RA 27/3 rubella strain immunologically simulates natural infection more closely than other rubella vaccine viruses. The increased levels and broader profile of antibodies produced by RA 27/3 strain rubella virus vaccine appear to correlate with greater resistance to subclinical reinfection with the wild virus, and provide greater confidence for lasting immunity.

Vaccine induced antibody levels following administration of M-R-VAX II have been shown to persist for at least two years without substantial decline. Antibody levels after immunization with M-R-VAX (Measles and Rubella Virus Vaccine Live, MSD), containing the HPV-77 strain of rubella, have persisted for 9 years without substantial decline. If the present pattern continues, it will provide a basis for the expectation that immunity following vaccination will be permanent. However, continued surveillance will be required to demonstrate this point.

INDICATIONS AND USAGE

M-R-VAX II is indicated for simultaneous immunization against measles and rubella in persons 15 months of age or older. A booster is not needed.

Infants who are less than 15 months of age may fail to respond to the measles component of the vaccine due to presence in the circulation of residual measles antibody of maternal origin; the younger the infant, the lower the likelihood of seroconversion. In geographically isolated or other relatively inaccessible populations for whom immunization programs are logistically difficult, and in population groups in which natural measles infection may occur in a significant proportion of infants before 15 months of age, it may be desirable to give the vaccine to infants at an earlier age. Infants vaccinated under these conditions at less than 12 months of age should be revaccinated after reaching 15 months of age. There is some evidence to suggest that infants immunized at less than one year of age may not develop sustained antibody levels when later reimmunized. The advantage of early protection must be weighed against the chance for failure to respond adequately on reimmunization.

Previously unimmunized children of susceptible pregnant women should receive live attenuated rubella vaccine, because an immunized child will be less likely to acquire natural rubella and introduce the virus into the household.

Non-Pregnant Adolescent and Adult Females

Immunization of susceptible non-pregnant adolescent and adult females of childbearing age with live attenuated rubella virus vaccine is indicated if certain precautions are observed (see below and PRECAUTIONS). Vaccinating susceptible postpubertal females confers individual protection against subsequently acquiring rubella infection during pregnancy, which in turn prevents infection of the fetus and consequent congenital rubella injury.

Women of childbearing age should be advised not to become pregnant for three months after vaccination and should be informed of the reason for this precaution.*

It is recommended that rubella susceptibility be determined by serologic testing prior to immunization.** If immune, as evidenced by a specific rubella antibody titer of 1:8 or greater (hemagglutination-inhibition test), vaccination is unnecessary. Congenital malformations do occur in up to seven percent of all live births. Their chance appearance after vaccination could lead to misinterpretation of the cause, particularly if the prior rubella-immune status of vaccinees is unknown.

Postpubertal females should be informed of the frequent occurrence of generally self-limited arthralgia and/or arthritis beginning 2 to 4 weeks after vaccination (see ADVERSE REACTIONS).

Postpartum Women

It has been found convenient in many instances to vaccinate rubella-susceptible women in the immediate postpartum period. (See *Nursing Mothers*).

Revaccination: Children vaccinated when younger than 12 months of age should be revaccinated. Based on available evidence, there is no reason to routinely revaccinate persons who were vaccinated originally when 12 months of age or older. However, persons should be revaccinated if there is evidence to suggest that initial immunization was ineffective.

Use with other Vaccines

Routine administration of DTP (diphtheria, tetanus, pertussis) and/or OPV (oral poliovirus vaccine) concomitantly with measles, mumps and rubella vaccines is not recommended because there are insufficient data relating to the simultaneous administration of these antigens. However, the American Academy of Pediatrics has noted that in some circumstances, particularly when the patient may not return, some practitioners prefer to administer all these antigens on a single day. If done, separate sites and syringes should be used for DTP and M-R-VAX II.

M-R-VAX II should not be given less than one month before or after administration of other virus vaccines.

CONTRAINDICATIONS

Do not give M-R-VAX II to pregnant females; the possible effects of the vaccine on fetal development are unknown at this time. If vaccination of postpubertal females is undertaken, pregnancy should be avoided for three months following vaccination. (See PRECAUTIONS, *Pregnancy*).

Anaphylactoid reaction to neomycin (each dose of reconstituted vaccine contains approximately 25 mcg of neomycin). History of anaphylactoid reaction to eggs (see HYPERSENSITIVITY TO EGGS below).

Any febrile respiratory illness or other active febrile infection.

---

*NOTE: The Immunization Practices Advisory Committee (ACIP) has recommended "In view of the importance of protecting this age group against rubella, reasonable precautions in a rubella immunization program include asking females if they are pregnant, excluding those who say they are, and explaining the theoretical risks to the others."

**NOTE: The Immunization Practices Advisory Committee (ACIP) has stated "When practical, and when reliable laboratory services are available, potential vaccinees of childbearing age can have serologic tests to determine susceptibility to rubella. . . . However, routinely performing serologic tests for all females of childbearing age to determine susceptibility so that vaccine is given only to proven susceptibles is expensive and has been ineffective in some areas. Accordingly, the ACIP believes that rubella vaccination of a woman who is not known to be pregnant and has no history of vaccination is justifiable without serologic testing."

Continued on next page

Merck Sharp & Dohme—Cont.

Active untreated tuberculosis.

Patients receiving immunosuppressive therapy. This contraindication does not apply to patients who are receiving corticosteroids as replacement therapy, e.g., for Addison's disease.

Individuals with blood dyscrasias, leukemia, lymphomas of any type, or other malignant neoplasms affecting the bone marrow or lymphatic systems.

Primary immunodeficiency states, including cellular immune deficiencies, hypogammaglobulinemic and dysgammaglobulinemic states.

Individuals with a family history of congenital or hereditary immunodeficiency, until the immune competence of the potential vaccine recipient is demonstrated.

HYPERSENSITIVITY TO EGGS

Live measles vaccine is produced in chick embryo cell culture. Persons with a history of anaphylactic or other immediate reactions (e.g., hives, swelling of the mouth and throat, difficulty breathing, hypotension, or shock) subsequent to egg ingestion should not be vaccinated. Evidence indicates that persons not at increased risk if they have egg allergies that are not anaphylactic in nature. Such persons may be vaccinated in the usual manner. There is no evidence to indicate that persons with allergies to chickens or feathers are at increased risk of reaction to the vaccine.

PRECAUTIONS

General

Adequate treatment provisions including epinephrine, should be available for immediate use should an anaphylactoid reaction occur.

Due caution should be employed in administration of M-R-VAX II to persons with a history of febrile convulsions, cerebral injury or any other condition in which stress due to fever should be avoided. The physician should be alert to the temperature elevation which may occur following vaccination. (See ADVERSE REACTIONS).

Vaccination should be deferred for at least 3 months following blood or plasma transfusions, or administration of human immune serum globulin.

Excretion of small amounts of the live attenuated rubella virus from the nose or throat has occurred in the majority of susceptible individuals 7–28 days after vaccination. There is no confirmed evidence to indicate that such virus is transmitted to susceptible persons who are in contact with the vaccinated individuals. Consequently, transmission through close personal contact, while accepted as a theoretical possibility, is not regarded as a significant risk. However, transmission of the rubella vaccine virus to infants via breast milk has been documented (see *Nursing Mothers*).

There are no reports of transmission of live attenuated measles virus from vaccinees to susceptible contacts.

It has been reported that live attenuated measles and rubella virus vaccines given individually may result in a temporary depression of tuberculin skin sensitivity. Therefore, if a tuberculin test is to be done, it should be administered either before or simultaneously with M-R-VAX II.

As for any vaccine, vaccination with M-R-VAX II may not result in seroconversion in 100% of susceptible persons given the vaccine.

Pregnancy

Pregnancy Category C

Animal reproduction studies have not been conducted with M-R-VAX II. It is also not known whether M-R-VAX II can cause fetal harm when administered to a pregnant woman or can affect reproduction capacity. Therefore, the vaccine should not be administered to pregnant females; futhermore, pregnancy should be avoided for three months following vaccination (see CONTRAINDICATIONS).

In counseling women who are inadvertently vaccinated when pregnant or who become pregnant within 3 months of vaccination, the physician should be aware of the following: (1) In a 10 year survey involving over 700 pregnant women who received rubella vaccine within 3 months before or after conception, (of whom 189 received the Wistar RA 27/3 strain), none of the newborns had abnormalities compatible with congenital rubella syndrome; (2) Reports have indicated that contracting of natural measles during pregnancy enhances fetal risk. Increased rates of spontaneous abortion, stillbirth, congenital defects and prematurity have been observed subsequent to natural measles during pregnancy. There are no adequate studies of the attenuated (vaccine) strain of measles virus in pregnancy. However, it would be prudent to assume that the vaccine strain of virus is also capable of inducing adverse fetal effects.

Nursing Mothers

It is not known whether measles vaccine virus is secreted in human milk. Recent studies have shown that lactating postpartum women immunized with live attenuated rubella vaccine may secrete the virus in breast milk and transmit it to breast-fed infants. In the infants with serological evidence of rubella infection, none exhibited severe disease; however, one exhibited mild clinical illness typical of acquired rubella. Caution should be exercised when M-R-VAX II is administered to a nursing woman.

ADVERSE REACTIONS

Because of the slightly acidic pH (6.2–6.6) of the vaccine, patients may complain of burning and/or stinging of short duration at the injection site.

The adverse clinical reactions associated with the use of M-R-VAX II are those expected to follow administration of the monovalent vaccines given separately. These may include malaise, sore throat, headache, fever, rash, nausea, and vomiting; mild local reactions such as erythema, induration, tenderness and regional lymphadenopathy; thrombocytopenia and purpura; allergic reactions such as wheal and flare at the injection site or urticaria; polyneuritis, and arthralgia and/or arthritis (usually transient and rarely chronic).

Moderate fever [101–102.9°F (38.3–39.4°C)] occurs occasionally, and high fever [above 103°F (39.4°C)] occurs less commonly. On rare occasions, children developing fever may exhibit febrile convulsions. Rash occurs infrequently and is usually minimal, but rarely may be generalized.

Forms of optic neuritis, including retrobulbar neuritis, papillitis, and retinitis may infrequently follow viral infections, and have been reported to occur 1 to 3 weeks following inoculation with some live virus vaccines.

Clinical experience with live attenuated measles and rubella virus vaccines given individually indicates that encephalitis and other nervous system reactions have occurred very rarely. These might occur also with M-R-VAX II.

Experience from more than 80 million doses of all live measles vaccines given in the U.S. through 1975 indicates that significant central nervous system reactions such as encephalitis and encephalopathy, occurring within 30 days after vaccination, have been temporally associated with measles vaccine approximately once for every million doses. In no case has it been shown that reactions were actually caused by vaccine. The Center for Disease Control has pointed out that "a certain number of cases of encephalitis may be expected to occur in a large childhood population in a defined period of time even when no vaccines are administered". However, the data suggest the possibility that some of these cases may have been caused by measles vaccines. The risk of such serious neurological disorders following live measles virus vaccine administration remains far less than that for encephalitis and encephalopathy with natural measles (one per two thousand reported cases).

There have been isolated reports of ocular palsies and Guillain-Barré syndrome occurring after immunization with vaccines containing live attenuated measles virus. The ocular palsies have occurred approximately 3–24 days following vaccination. No definite causal relationship has been established between either of these events and vaccination. Isolated reports of polyneuropathy including Guillain-Barré syndrome have also been reported after immunization with rubella containing vaccines.

There have been reports of subacute sclerosing panencephalitis (SSPE) in children who did not have a history of natural measles but did receive measles vaccine. Some of these cases may have resulted from unrecognized measles in the first year of life or possibly from the measles vaccination. Based on estimated nationwide measles vaccine distribution, the association of SSPE cases to measles vaccination is about one case per million vaccine doses distributed. This is far less than the association with natural measles, 6–22 cases of SSPE per million cases of measles. The results of a retrospective case-controlled study conducted by the Center for Disease Control suggest that the overall effect of measles vaccine has been to protect against SSPE by preventing measles with its inherent higher risk of SSPE.

Local reactions characterized by marked swelling, redness and vesiculation at the injection site of attenuated live measles virus vaccines, and systemic reactions including atypical measles, have occurred in persons who received killed measles vaccine previously. M-R-VAX II was not given under this condition in clinical trials. Rarely, more severe reactions that require hospitalization, including prolonged high fevers and extensive local reactions, have been reported. Panniculitis has been reported rarely following administration of measles vaccine.

Arthralgia and/or arthritis (usually transient and rarely chronic), and polyneuritis are features of natural rubella and vary in frequency and severity with age and sex, being greatest in adult females and least in prepubertal children. This type of involvement as well as myalgia and paresthesia have also been reported following administration of MERUVAX II (Rubella Virus Vaccine Live, MSD).

Chronic arthritis has been associated with natural rubella infection and has been related to persistent virus and/or viral antigen isolated from body tissues. Only rarely have vaccine recipients developed chronic joint symptoms.

Following vaccination in children, reactions in joints are uncommon and generally of brief duration. In women, incidence rates for arthritis and arthralgia are generally higher than those seen in children (children: 0–3%; women: 12–20%), and the reactions tend to be more marked and of longer duration. Symptoms may persist for a matter of months or on rare occasions for years. In adolescent girls, the reactions appear to be intermediate in incidence between those seen in children and in adult women. Even in older women (35–45 years), these reactions are generally well tolerated and rarely interfere with normal activities.

DOSAGE AND ADMINISTRATION

FOR SUBCUTANEOUS ADMINISTRATION

Do not inject intravenously

The dosage of vaccine is the same for all persons. Inject the total volume of the single dose vial (about 0.5 mL) or 0.5 mL of the multiple dose vial of reconstituted vaccine subcutaneously, preferably into the outer aspect of upper arm. *Do not give immune globulin (IG) concurrently with M-R-VAX II.*

During shipment, to insure that there is no loss of potency, the vaccine must be maintained at a temperature of 10°C (50°F) or less.

Before reconstitution, store M-R-VAX II at 2–8°C (35.6–46.4°F). *Protect from light.*

CAUTION: A sterile syringe free of preservatives, antiseptics, and detergents should be used for each injection and/or reconstitution of the vaccine because these substances may inactivate the live virus vaccine. A 25 gauge, ⅝″ needle is recommended.

To reconstitute, use only the diluent supplied, since it is free of preservatives or other antiviral substances which might inactivate the vaccine.

Single Dose Vial —First withdraw the entire volume of diluent into the syringe to be used for reconstitution. Inject all the diluent in the syringe into the vial of lyophilized vaccine, and agitate to mix thoroughly. Withdraw the entire contents into a syringe and inject the total volume of restored vaccine subcutaneously.

It is important to use a separate sterile syringe and needle for each individual patient to prevent transmission of hepatitis B and other infectious agents from one person to another.

10 Dose Vial (available only to government agencies/institutions) —Withdraw the entire contents (7 mL) of the diluent vial into the sterile syringe to be used for reconstitution, and introduce into the 10 dose vial of lyophilized vaccine. Agitate to ensure thorough mixing. The outer labeling suggests "For Jet Injector or Syringe Use". Use with separate sterile syringes is permitted for containers of 10 doses or less. The vaccine and diluent do not contain preservatives; therefore, the user must recognize the potential contamination hazards and exercise special precautions to protect the sterility and potency of the product. The use of aseptic techniques and proper storage prior to and after restoration of the vaccine and subsequent withdrawal of the individual doses is essential. Use 0.5 mL of the reconstituted vaccine for subcutaneous injection.

It is important to use a separate sterile syringe and needle for each individual patient to prevent transmission of hepatitis B and other infectious agents from one person to another.

50 Dose Vial (available only to government agencies/institutions) —Withdraw the entire contents (30 mL) of diluent vial into the sterile syringe to be used for reconstitution and introduce into the 50 dose vial of lyophilized vaccine. Agitate to ensure thorough mixing. With full aseptic precautions, attach the vial to the sterilized multidose jet injector apparatus. Use 0.5 mL of the reconstituted vaccine for subcutaneous injection.

Each dose contains not less than the equivalent of 1,000 $TCID_{50}$ of the U.S. Reference Measles Virus and 1,000 $TCID_{50}$ of the U.S. Reference Rubella Virus.

Parenteral drug products should be inspected visually for particulate matter and discoloration prior to administration. M-R-VAX II, when reconstituted, is clear yellow.

HOW SUPPLIED

No. 4751—M-R-VAX II is supplied as a single-dose vial of lyophilized vaccine, **NDC** 0006-4751-00, and a vial of diluent. No. 4677/4309—M-R-VAX II is supplied as follows: (1) a box of 10 single-dose vials of lyophilized vaccine (package A), **NDC** 0006-4677-00; and (2) a box of 10 vials of diluent (package B). To conserve refrigerator space, the diluent may be stored separately at room temperature.

Available only to government agencies/institutions:

No. 4678—M-R-VAX II is supplied as one 10 dose vial of lyophilized vaccine, **NDC** 0006-4678-00, and one 7 mL vial of diluent.

No. 4679—M-R-VAX II is supplied as one 50 dose vial of ly-ophilized vaccine, **NDC** 0006-4679-00, and one 30 mL vial of diluent.

Storage

It is recommended that the vaccine be used as soon as possible after reconstitution. Protect vaccine from light at all times, since such exposure may inactivate the virus. Store reconstituted vaccine in the vaccine vial in a dark place at 2–8°C (35.6–46.4°F) and discard if not used within 8 hours.

A.H.F.S. Category: 80:12

DC 7417112   Issued October 1986

COPYRIGHT © MERCK & CO., INC., 1985

All rights reserved

MEFOXIN®   ℞
(Cefoxitin Sodium, MSD), U.S.P.

DESCRIPTION

MEFOXIN® (Sterile Cefoxitin Sodium, MSD) is a semi-synthetic, broad-spectrum cepha antibiotic for parenteral administration. It is derived from cephamycin C, which is produced by *Streptomyces lactamdurans*. It is the sodium salt of 3-(hydroxymethyl)-7α- methoxy-8-oxo -7- [2- (2-thienyl) acetamido]-5-thia-1-azabicyclo [4.2.0] oct-2- ene-2-carboxylate carbamate (ester). The empirical formula is $C_{16}H_{16}N_3NaO_7S_2$, and the structural formula is:

MEFOXIN contains approximately 53.8 mg (2.3 milliequivalents) of sodium per gram of cefoxitin activity. Solutions of MEFOXIN range from colorless to light amber in color. The pH of freshly constituted solutions usually ranges from 4.2 to 7.0.

CLINICAL PHARMACOLOGY

Clinical Pharmacology

After intramuscular administration of a 1 gram dose of MEFOXIN to normal volunteers, the mean peak serum concentration was 24 mcg/mL. The peak occurred at 20 to 30 minutes. Following an intravenous dose of 1 gram, serum concentrations were 110 mcg/mL at 5 minutes, declining to less than 1 mcg/mL at 4 hours. The half-life after an intravenous dose is 41 to 59 minutes; after intramuscular administration, the half-life is 64.8 minutes. Approximately 85 percent of cefoxitin is excreted unchanged by the kidneys over a 6-hour period, resulting in high urinary concentrations. Following an intramuscular dose of 1 gram, urinary concentrations greater than 3000 mcg/mL were observed. Probenecid slows tubular excretion and produces higher serum levels and increases the duration of measurable serum concentrations.

Cefoxitin passes into pleural and joint fluids and is detectable in antibacterial concentrations in bile.

Clinical experience has demonstrated that MEFOXIN can be administered to patients who are also receiving carbenicillin, kanamycin, gentamicin, tobramycin, or amikacin (see PRECAUTIONS and ADMINISTRATION).

Microbiology

The bactericidal action of cefoxitin results from inhibition of cell wall synthesis. Cefoxitin has *in vitro* activity against a wide range of gram-positive and gram-negative organisms. The methoxy group in the 7α position provides MEFOXIN with a high degree of stability in the presence of beta-lactamases, both penicillinases and cephalosporinases, of gram-negative bacteria. Cefoxitin is usually active against the following organisms *in vitro* and in clinical infections:

Gram-positive
  Staphylococcus aureus, including penicillinase and non-penicillinase producing strains.
  Staphylococcus epidermidis
  Beta-hemolytic and other streptococci (most strains of enterococci, e.g., *Streptococcus faecalis,* are resistant)
  Streptococcus pneumoniae
Gram-negative
  Escherichia coli
  Klebsiella species (including *K. pneumoniae*)
  Hemophilus influenzae
  Neisseria gonorrhoeae, including penicillinase and non-penicillinase producing strains
  Proteus mirabilis
  Morganella morganii
  Proteus vulgaris
  Providencia species, including *Providencia rettgeri*
Anaerobic organisms
  Peptococcus species

Peptostreptococcus species
Clostridium species
  Bacteroides species, including the *B. fragilis* group (includes *B. fragilis, B. distasonis, B. ovatus, B. thetaiotaomicron, B. vulgatus*)

MEFOXIN is inactive *in vitro* against most strains of *Pseudomonas aeruginosa* and enterococci and many strains of *Enterobacter cloacae.*

Methicillin-resistant staphylococci are almost uniformly resistant to MEFOXIN.

Susceptibility Tests

For fast-growing aerobic organisms, quantitative methods that require measurements of zone diameters give the most precise estimates of antibiotic susceptibility. One such procedure* has been recommended for use with discs to test susceptibility to cefoxitin. Interpretation involves correlation of the diameters obtained in the disc test with minimal inhibitory concentration (MIC) values for cefoxitin.

Reports from the laboratory giving results of the standardized single disc susceptibility test* using a 30 mcg cefoxitin disc should be interpreted according to the following criteria: Organisms producing zones of 18 mm or greater are considered susceptible, indicating that the tested organism is likely to respond to therapy.

Organisms of intermediate susceptibility produce zones of 15 to 17 mm, indicating that the tested organism would be susceptible if high dosage is used or if the infection is confined to tissues and fluids (e.g., urine) in which high antibiotic levels are attained.

Resistant organisms produce zones of 14 mm or less, indicating that other therapy should be selected.

The cefoxitin disc should be used for testing cefoxitin susceptibility.

Cefoxitin has been shown by *in vitro* tests to have activity against certain strains of *Enterobacteriaceae* found resistant when tested with the cephalosporin class disc. For this reason, the cefoxitin disc should not be used for testing susceptibility to cephalosporins, and cephalosporin discs should not be used for testing susceptibility to cefoxitin.

Dilution methods, preferably the agar plate dilution procedure, are most accurate for susceptibility testing of obligate anaerobes.

A bacterial isolate may be considered susceptible if the MIC value for cefoxitin† is not more than 16 mcg/mL. Organisms are considered resistant if the MIC is greater than 32 mcg/mL.

INDICATIONS AND USAGE

Treatment

MEFOXIN is indicated for the treatment of serious infections caused by susceptible strains of the designated microorganisms in the diseases listed below.

(1) Lower respiratory tract infections, including pneumonia and lung abscess, caused by *Streptococcus pneumoniae,* other streptococci (excluding enterococci, e.g., *Streptococcus faecalis*), *Staphylococcus aureus* (penicillinase and non-penicillinase producing), *Escherichia coli, Klebsiella* species, *Hemophilus influenzae,* and *Bacteroides* species.

(2) Genitourinary infections. Urinary tract infections caused by *Escherichia coli, Klebsiella* species, *Proteus mirabilis,* indole-positive Proteus (which include the organisms now called *Morganella morganii* and *Proteus vulgaris),* and *Providencia* species (including *Providencia rettgeri).* Uncomplicated gonorrhea due to *Neisseria gonorrhoeae* (penicillinase and non-penicillinase producing).

(3) Intra-abdominal infections, including peritonitis and intra-abdominal abscess, caused by *Escherichia coli, Klebsiella* species, *Bacteroides* species including the *Bacteroides fragilis* group**, and *Clostridium* species.

(4) Gynecological infections, including endometritis, pelvic cellulitis, and pelvic inflammatory disease caused by *Escherichia coli, Neisseria gonorrhoeae* (penicillinase and non-penicillinase producing), *Bacteroides* species including the *Bacteroides fragilis* group**, *Clostridium* species, *Peptococcus* species, *Peptostreptococcus* species, and Group B streptococci.

(5) Septicemia caused by *Streptococcus pneumoniae, Staphylococcus aureus* (penicillinase and non-penicillinase produc-

---

* Bauer, A. W.; Kirby, W. M. M.; Sherris, J. C.; Turck, M.: Antibiotic susceptibility testing by a standardized single disc method, Amer. J. Clin. Path. 45 : 493–496, Apr. 1966. Standardized disc susceptibility test, Federal Register 37 : 20527–20529, 1972. National Committee for Clinical Laboratory Standards: Approved Standard: ASM-2, Performance Standards for Antimicrobial Disc Susceptibility Tests, July 1975.

† Determined by the ICS agar dilution method (Ericsson and Sherris, Acta Path. Microbiol. Scand. (B) Suppl. No. 217, 1971) or any other method that has been shown to give equivalent results.

---

ing), *Escherichia coli, Klebsiella* species, and *Bacteroides* species including the *Bacteroides fragilis* group.**

(6) Bone and joint infections caused by *Staphylococcus aureus* (penicillinase and non-penicillinase producing).

(7) Skin and skin structure infections caused by *Staphylococcus aureus* (penicillinase and non-penicillinase producing), *Staphylococcus epidermidis,* streptococci (excluding enterococci, e.g., *Streptococcus faecalis*), *Escherichia coli, Proteus mirabilis, Klebsiella* species, *Bacteroides* species including the *Bacteroides fragilis* group**, *Clostridium* species, *Peptococcus* species, and *Peptostreptococcus* species.

Appropriate culture and susceptibility studies should be performed to determine the susceptibility of the causative organisms to MEFOXIN. Therapy may be started while awaiting the results of these studies.

In randomized comparative studies, MEFOXIN and cephalothin were comparably safe and effective in the management of infections caused by gram-positive cocci and gram-negative rods susceptible to the cephalosporins. MEFOXIN has a high degree of stability in the presence of bacterial beta-lactamases, both penicillinases and cephalosporinases.

Many infections caused by aerobic and anaerobic gram-negative bacteria resistant to some cephalosporins respond to MEFOXIN. Similarly, many infections caused by aerobic and anaerobic bacteria resistant to some penicillin antibiotics (ampicillin, carbenicillin, penicillin G) respond to treatment with MEFOXIN. Many infections caused by mixtures of susceptible aerobic and anaerobic bacteria respond to treatment with MEFOXIN.

Prevention

When compared to placebo in randomized controlled studies in patients undergoing gastrointestinal surgery, vaginal hysterectomy, abdominal hysterectomy and cesarean section, the prophylactic use of MEFOXIN resulted in a significant reduction in the number of postoperative infections. The prophylactic administration of MEFOXIN may reduce the incidence of certain postoperative infections in patients undergoing surgical procedures (e.g., hysterectomy, gastrointestinal surgery and transurethral prostatectomy) that are classified as contaminated or potentially contaminated.

The perioperative use of MEFOXIN may be effective in surgical patients in whom subsequent infection at the operative site would present a serious risk, e.g., prosthetic arthroplasty.

Effective prophylactic use depends on the time of administration. MEFOXIN usually should be given one-half to one hour before the operation, which is sufficient time to achieve effective levels in the wound during the procedure. Prophylactic administration should usually be stopped within 24 hours since continuing administration of any antibiotic increases the possibility of adverse reactions but, in the majority of surgical procedures, does not reduce the incidence of subsequent infection. However, in patients undergoing prosthetic arthroplasty, it is recommended that MEFOXIN be continued for 72 hours after the surgical procedure.

If there are signs of infection, specimens for culture should be obtained for identification of the causative organism so that appropriate treatment may be instituted.

CONTRAINDICATIONS

MEFOXIN is contraindicated in patients who have shown hypersensitivity to cefoxitin and the cephalosporin group of antibiotics.

WARNINGS

BEFORE THERAPY WITH 'MEFOXIN' IS INSTITUTED, CAREFUL INQUIRY SHOULD BE MADE TO DETERMINE WHETHER THE PATIENT HAS HAD PREVIOUS HYPERSENSITIVITY REACTIONS TO CEFOXITIN, CEPHALOSPORINS, PENICILLINS, OR OTHER DRUGS. THIS PRODUCT SHOULD BE GIVEN WITH CAUTION TO PENICILLIN-SENSITIVE PATIENTS. ANTIBIOTICS SHOULD BE ADMINISTERED WITH CAUTION TO ANY PATIENT WHO HAS DEMONSTRATED SOME FORM OF ALLERGY, PARTICULARLY TO DRUGS. IF AN ALLERGIC REACTION TO 'MEFOXIN' OCCURS, DISCONTINUE THE DRUG. SERIOUS HYPERSENSITIVITY REACTIONS MAY REQUIRE EPINEPHRINE AND OTHER EMERGENCY MEASURES.

Pseudomembranous colitis has been reported with virtually all antibiotics (including cephalosporins); therefore, it is important to consider its diagnosis in patients who develop diarrhea in association with antibiotic use. This colitis may range from mild to life threatening in severity.

** *B. fragilis, B. distasonis, B. ovatus, B. thetaiotaomicron, B. vulgatus.*

Continued on next page

Merck Sharp & Dohme—Cont.

Treatment with broad-spectrum antibiotics alters normal flora of the colon and may permit overgrowth of clostridia. Studies indicate a toxin produced by *Clostridium difficile* is one primary cause of antibiotic-associated colitis. Mild cases of pseudomembranous colitis may respond to drug discontinuance alone. In more severe cases, management may include sigmoidoscopy, appropriate bacteriological studies, fluid, electrolyte and protein supplementation, and the use of a drug such as oral vancomycin as indicated. Isolation of the patient may be advisable. Other causes of colitis should also be considered.

PRECAUTIONS

General
The total daily dose should be reduced when MEFOXIN is administered to patients with transient or persistent reduction of urinary output due to renal insufficiency (see DOSAGE), because high and prolonged serum antibiotic concentrations can occur in such individuals from usual doses. Antibiotics (including cephalosporins) should be prescribed with caution in individuals with a history of gastrointestinal disease, particularly colitis.
As with other antibiotics, prolonged use of MEFOXIN may result in overgrowth of nonsusceptible organisms. Repeated evaluation of the patient's condition is essential. If superinfection occurs during therapy, appropriate measures should be taken.
Drug Interactions
Increased nephrotoxicity has been reported following concomitant administration of cephalosporins and aminoglycoside antibiotics.
Drug/Laboratory Test Interactions
As with cephalothin, high concentrations of cefoxitin (> 100 micrograms/mL) may interfere with measurement of serum and urine creatinine levels by the Jaffé reaction, and produce false increases of modest degree in the levels of creatinine reported. Serum samples from patients treated with cefoxitin should not be analyzed for creatinine if withdrawn within 2 hours of drug administration.
High concentrations of cefoxitin in the urine may interfere with measurement of urinary 17-hydroxy-corticosteroids by the Porter-Silber reaction, and produce false increases of modest degree in the levels reported.
A false-positive reaction for glucose in the urine may occur. This has been observed with CLINITEST* reagent tablets.
Carcinogenesis, Mutagenesis, Impairment of Fertility
Long-term studies in animals have not been performed with cefoxitin to evaluate carcinogenic or mutagenic potential. Studies in rats treated intravenously with 400 mg/kg of cefoxitin (approximately three times the maximum recommended human dose) revealed no effects on fertility or mating ability.
Pregnancy
Pregnancy Category B. Reproduction studies performed in rats and mice at parenteral doses of approximately one to seven and one-half times the maximum recommended human dose did not reveal teratogenic or fetal toxic effects, although a slight decrease in fetal weight was observed. There are, however, no adequate and well-controlled studies in pregnant women. Because animal reproduction studies are not always predictive of human response, this drug should be used during pregnancy only if clearly needed.
In the rabbit, cefoxitin was associated with a high incidence of abortion and maternal death. This was not considered to be a teratogenic effect but an expected consequence of the rabbit's unusual sensitivity to antibiotic-induced changes in the population of the microflora of the intestine.

* Registered trademark of Ames Company, Division of Miles Laboratories, Inc.

Nursing Mothers
MEFOXIN is excreted in human milk in low concentrations. Caution should be exercised when MEFOXIN is administered to a nursing woman.
Pediatric Use
Safety and efficacy in infants from birth to three months of age have not yet been established. In children three months of age and older, higher doses of MEFOXIN have been associated with an increased incidence of eosinophilia and elevated SGOT.

ADVERSE REACTIONS

MEFOXIN is generally well tolerated. The most common adverse reactions have been local reactions following intravenous or intramuscular injection. Other adverse reactions have been encountered infrequently.
Local Reactions
Thrombophlebitis has occurred with intravenous administration. Pain, induration, and tenderness after intramuscular injections have been reported.
Allergic Reactions
Rash (including exfoliative dermatitis), pruritus, eosinophilia, fever, and other allergic reactions including anaphylaxis have been noted.
Cardiovascular
Hypotension
Gastrointestinal
Diarrhea, including documented pseudomembranous colitis which can appear during or after antibiotic treatment. Nausea and vomiting have been reported rarely.
Blood
Eosinophilia, leukopenia, including granulocytopenia, neutropenia, anemia, including hemolytic anemia, thrombocytopenia, and bone marrow depression. A positive direct Coombs test may develop in some individuals, especially those with azotemia.
Liver Function
Transient elevations in SGOT, SGPT, serum LDH, serum alkaline phosphatase; and jaundice have been reported.
Renal Function
Elevations in serum creatinine and/or blood urea nitrogen levels have been observed. As with the cephalosporins, acute renal failure has been reported rarely. The role of MEFOXIN in changes in renal function tests is difficult to assess, since factors predisposing to prerenal azotemia or to impaired renal function usually have been present.

OVERDOSAGE

The acute intravenous LD_{50} in the adult female mouse and rabbit was about 8.0 g/kg and greater than 1.0 g/kg respectively. The acute intraperitoneal LD_{50} in the adult rat was greater than 10.0 g/kg.

DOSAGE

TREATMENT
Adults
The usual adult dosage range is 1 gram to 2 grams every six to eight hours. Dosage and route of administration should be determined by susceptibility of the causative organisms,

Table 2—Maintenance Dosage of MEFOXIN in Adults with Reduced Renal Function

Renal Function	Creatinine Clearance (mL/min)	Dose (grams)	Frequency
Mild impairment	50–30	1–2	every 8–12 hours
Moderate impairment	29–10	1–2	every 12–24 hours
Severe impairment	9–5	0.5–1	every 12–24 hours
Essentially no function	< 5	0.5–1	every 24–48 hours

severity of infection, and the condition of the patient (see Table 1 for dosage guidelines).
[See table below].
MEFOXIN may be used in patients with reduced renal function with the following dosage adjustments:
In adults with renal insufficiency, an initial loading dose of 1 gram to 2 grams may be given. After a loading dose, the recommendations for *maintenance dosage* (Table 2) may be used as a guide.
[See table above].
When only the serum creatinine level is available, the following formula (based on sex, weight, and age of the patient) may be used to convert this value into creatinine clearance. The serum creatinine should represent a steady state of renal function.

Males:
$$\frac{\text{Weight (kg)} \times (140 - \text{age})}{72 \times \text{serum creatinine (mg/100 mL)}}$$

Females: $0.85 \times$ above value

In patients undergoing hemodialysis, the loading dose of 1 to 2 grams should be given after each hemodialysis, and the maintenance dose should be given as indicated in Table 2. Antibiotic therapy for group A beta-hemolytic streptococcal infections should be maintained for at least 10 days to guard against the risk of rheumatic fever or glomerulonephritis. In staphylococcal and other infections involving a collection of pus, surgical drainage should be carried out where indicated.
The recommended dosage of MEFOXIN **for uncomplicated gonorrhea** is 2 grams intramuscularly, with 1 gram of BENEMID® (Probenecid, MSD) given by mouth at the same time or up to ½ hour before MEFOXIN.
Infants and Children
The recommended dosage in children three months of age and older is 80 to 160 mg/kg of body weight per day divided into four to six equal doses. The higher dosages should be used for more severe or serious infections. The total daily dosage should not exceed 12 grams.
At this time no recommendation is made for children from birth to three months of age (See PRECAUTIONS).
In children with renal insufficiency the dosage and frequency of dosage should be modified consistent with the recommendations for adults (see Table 2).
PREVENTION
General
For prophylactic use in surgery, the following doses are recommended:
Adults:
1) 2 grams administered intravenously or intramuscularly just prior to surgery (approximately one-half to one hour before the initial incision).
2) 2 grams every 6 hours after the first dose for no more than 24 hours (continued for 72 hours after prosthetic arthroplasty).
Children (3 months and older):
30 to 40 mg/kg doses may be given at the times designated above.
Obstetric-Gynecologic
For prophylactic use in vaginal hysterectomy, a single 2.0 gram dose administered intramuscularly one-half to one hour prior to surgery is recommended.
For patients undergoing cesarean section, a single 2.0 gram dose should be administered intravenously as soon as the umbilical cord is clamped. A 3-dose regimen may be more effective than a single dose regimen in preventing postoperative infection (esp. endometritis) following cesarean section. Such a regimen would consist of 2.0 grams given intravenously as soon as the umbilical cord is clamped, followed by 2.0 grams 4 and 8 hours after the initial dose.
Transurethral prostatectomy patients:
One gram administered just prior to surgery; 1 gram every 8 hours for up to five days.

PREPARATION OF SOLUTION

Table 3 is provided for convenience in constituting MEFOXIN for both intravenous and intramuscular administration.
[See table on next page].
For intravenous use, 1 gram should be constituted with at least 10 mL of Sterile Water for Injection, and 2 grams, with 10 or 20 mL. The 10 gram bulk package should be constituted with 43 or 93 mL of Sterile Water for Injection or any of the solutions listed under the *Intravenous* portion of the COM-

Table 1—Guidelines for Dosage of MEFOXIN

Type of Infection	Daily Dosage	Frequency and Route
Uncomplicated forms* of infections such as pneumonia, urinary tract infection, cutaneous infection	3–4 grams	1 gram every 6–8 hours IV or IM
Moderately severe or severe infections	6–8 grams	1 gram every 4 hours *or* 2 grams every 6–8 hours IV
Infections commonly needing antibiotics in higher dosage (e.g., gas gangrene)	12 grams	2 grams every 4 hours *or* 3 grams every 6 hours IV

*Including patients in whom bacteremia is absent or unlikely

PATIBILITY AND STABILITY section. CAUTION: THE 10 GRAM BULK STOCK SOLUTION IS NOT FOR DIRECT INFUSION. One or 2 grams of MEFOXIN for infusion may be constituted with 50 or 100 mL of 0.9 percent Sodium Chloride Injection, 5 percent or 10 percent Dextrose Injection, or any of the solutions listed under the *Intravenous* portion of the COMPATIBILITY AND STABILITY section.

Benzyl alcohol as a preservative has been associated with toxicity in neonates. While toxicity has not been demonstrated in infants greater than three months of age, in whom use of MEFOXIN may be indicated, small infants in this age range may also be at risk for benzyl alcohol toxicity. Therefore, diluent containing benzyl alcohol should not be used when MEFOXIN is constituted for administration to infants. *For ADD-Vantage®† vials,* see separate INSTRUCTIONS FOR USE OF MEFOXIN IN ADD-Vantage® VIALS. MEFOXIN in ADD-Vantage® vials should be constituted with ADD-Vantage® diluent containers containing 50 mL or 100 mL of either 0.9 percent Sodium Chloride Injection or 5 percent Dextrose Injection. MEFOXIN in ADD-Vantage® vials is for IV use only.

For intramuscular use, each gram of MEFOXIN may be constituted with 2 mL of Sterile Water for Injection, or — **For intramuscular use ONLY:** each gram of MEFOXIN may be constituted with 2 mL of 0.5 percent lidocaine hydrochloride solution** (without epinephrine) to minimize the discomfort of intramuscular injection.

ADMINISTRATION

MEFOXIN may be administered intravenously or intramuscularly after constitution.

Parenteral drug products should be inspected visually for particulate matter and discoloration prior to administration whenever solution and container permit.

Intravenous Administration

The intravenous route is preferable for patients with bacteremia, bacterial septicemia, or other severe or life-threatening infections, or for patients who may be poor risks because of lowered resistance resulting from such debilitating conditions as malnutrition, trauma, surgery, diabetes, heart failure, or malignancy, particularly if shock is present or impending.

For intermittent intravenous administration, a solution containing 1 gram or 2 grams in 10 mL of Sterile Water for Injection can be injected over a period of three to five minutes. Using an infusion system, it may also be given over a longer period of time through the tubing system by which the patient may be receiving other intravenous solutions. However, during infusion of the solution containing MEFOXIN, it is advisable to temporarily discontinue administration of any other solutions at the same site.

For the administration of higher doses by continuous intravenous infusion, a solution of MEFOXIN may be added to an intravenous bottle containing 5 percent Dextrose Injection, 0.9 percent Sodium Chloride Injection, 5 percent Dextrose and 0.9 percent Sodium Chloride Injection, or 5 percent Dextrose Injection with 0.02 percent sodium bicarbonate solution. BUTTERFLY† or scalp vein-type needles are preferred for this type of infusion.

Solutions of MEFOXIN, like those of most beta-lactam antibiotics, should not be added to aminoglycoside solutions (e.g., gentamicin sulfate, tobramycin sulfate, amikacin sulfate) because of potential interaction. However, MEFOXIN and aminoglycosides may be administered separately to the same patient.

COMPATIBILITY AND STABILITY

Intravenous

MEFOXIN, as supplied in vials or the bulk package and constituted to 1 gram/10 mL with Sterile Water for Injection, Bacteriostatic Water for Injection (see PREPARATION OF SOLUTION), 0.9 percent Sodium Chloride Injection, or 5 percent Dextrose Injection, maintains satisfactory potency for 24 hours at room temperature, for one week under refrigeration (below 5°C), and for at least 30 weeks in the frozen state.

These primary solutions may be further diluted in 50 to 1000 mL of the following solutions and maintain potency for 24 hours at room temperature and at least 48 hours under refrigeration:

**See package circular of manufacturer for detailed information concerning contraindications, warnings, precautions, and adverse reactions.

† Registered trademark of Abbott Laboratories, Inc.

Intramuscular Administration

As with all intramuscular preparations, MEFOXIN should be injected well within the body of a relatively large muscle such as the upper outer quadrant of the buttock (i.e., gluteus maximus); aspiration is necessary to avoid inadvertent injection into a blood vessel.

MEFOXIN — Table 3—Preparation of Solution

Strength	Amount of Diluent to be Added (mL)*	Approximate Withdrawable Volume (mL)	Approximate Average Concentration (mg/mL)
1 gram Vial	2 (Intramuscular)	2.5	400
2 gram Vial	4 (Intramuscular)	5	400
1 gram Vial	10 (IV)	10.5	95
2 gram Vial	10 or 20 (IV)	11.1 or 21.0	180 or 95
1 gram Infusion Bottle	50 or 100 (IV)	50 or 100	20 or 10
2 gram Infusion Bottle	50 or 100 (IV)	50 or 100	40 or 20
10 gram Bulk	43 or 93 (IV)	49 or 98.5	200 or 100

*Shake to dissolve and let stand until clear.

Sterile Water for Injection‡
0.9 percent Sodium Chloride Injection
5 percent or 10 percent Dextrose Injection‡
5 percent Dextrose and 0.9 percent Sodium Chloride Injection
5 percent Dextrose Injection with 0.02 percent sodium bicarbonate solution
5 percent Dextrose Injection with 0.2 percent or 0.45 percent saline solution
Ringer's Injection‡
Lactated Ringer's Injection‡
5 percent dextrose in Lactated Ringer's Injection‡
5 percent or 10 percent invert sugar in water
10 percent invert sugar in saline solution
5 percent Sodium Bicarbonate Injection
Neut (sodium bicarbonate)*‡
M/6 sodium lactate solution
NORMOSOL-M in D5-W*‡
IONOSOL B w/Dextrose 5 percent*‡
POLYONIC M 56 in 5 percent Dextrose**
Mannitol 5% and 2.5%
Mannitol 10%‡
ISOLYTE*** E
ISOLYTE*** E with 5% dextrose

MEFOXIN, as supplied in infusion bottles and constituted with 50 to 100 mL of 0.9 percent Sodium Chloride Injection, or 5 percent or 10 percent Dextrose Injection, maintains satisfactory potency for 24 hours at room temperature or for 1 week under refrigeration (below 5°C).

MEFOXIN is supplied in single dose ADD-Vantage® vials and should be prepared as directed in the accompanying INSTRUCTIONS FOR USE OF MEFOXIN IN ADD-Vantage® VIALS using ADD-Vantage® diluent containers containing 50 mL or 100 mL of either 0.9 percent Sodium Chloride Injection or 5 percent Dextrose Injection. When prepared with either of these diluents, MEFOXIN maintains satisfactory potency for 24 hours at room temperature. Limited studies with solutions of MEFOXIN in 0.9 percent Sodium Chloride Injection, Lactated Ringer's Injection, and 5 percent Dextrose Injection in VIAFLEX† intravenous bags show stability for 24 hours at room temperature, 48 hours under refrigeration or 26 weeks in the frozen state and 24 hours at room temperature thereafter. Also, solutions of MEFOXIN in 0.9 percent Sodium Chloride Injection show similar stability in plastic tubing, drip chambers, and volume control devices of common intravenous infusion sets. After constitution with Sterile Water for Injection and subsequent storage in disposable plastic syringes, MEFOXIN is stable for 24 hours at room temperature and 48 hours under refrigeration.

After the periods mentioned above, any unused solutions or frozen material should be discarded. Do not refreeze.

Intramuscular

MEFOXIN, as constituted with Sterile Water for Injection, Bacteriostatic Water for Injection, or 0.5 percent or 1 percent lidocaine hydrochloride solution (without epinephrine), maintains satisfactory potency for 24 hours at room temperature, for one week under refrigeration (below 5°C), and for at least 30 weeks in the frozen state.

After the periods mentioned above, any unused solutions or frozen material should be discarded. Do not refreeze.

MEFOXIN has also been found compatible when admixed in intravenous infusions with the following:
Heparin 0.1 units/mL at room temperature—8 hours
Heparin 100 units/mL at room temperature—24 hours
M.V.I.†† concentrate at room temperature 24 hours; under refrigeration 48 hours
BEROCCA††† C-500 at room temperature 24 hours; under refrigeration 48 hours

* Registered trademark of Abbott Laboratories.
** Registered trademark of Cutter Laboratories, Inc.
*** Registered trademark of American Hospital Supply Corporation.
‡ In these solutions, MEFOXIN has been found to be stable for a period of one week under refrigeration.
† Registered trademark of Travenol Laboratories, Inc.
†† Registered trademark of USV Pharmaceutical Corp.
††† Registered trademark of Roche Laboratories.

Insulin in Normal Saline at room temperature 24 hours; under refrigeration 48 hours
Insulin in 10% invert sugar at room temperature 24 hours; under refrigeration 48 hours

HOW SUPPLIED

Sterile MEFOXIN is a dry white to off-white powder supplied in vials and infusion bottles containing cefoxitin sodium as follows:
No. 3356—1 gram cefoxitin equivalent
NDC 0006-3356-71 in trays of 10 vials (6505-01-189-3960, 1 g 10's).
NDC 0006-3356-45 in trays of 25 vials.
No. 3368—1 gram cefoxitin equivalent
NDC 0006-3368-71 in trays of 10 infusion bottles (6505-01-195-0649, 1 g 10's).
No. 3357—2 gram cefoxitin equivalent
NDC 0006-3357-73 in trays of 10 vials (6505-01-189-3961, 2 g 10's).
NDC 0006-3357-53 in trays of 25 vials (6505-01-104-6393, 2 g 25's).
No. 3369—2 gram cefoxitin equivalent
NDC 0006-3369-73 in trays of 10 infusion bottles (6505-01-185-2624, 2 g 10's).
No. 3388—10 gram cefoxitin equivalent
NDC 0006-3388-67 in trays of 6 bulk bottles (6505-01-263-0730, 10 g 6's).
No. 3548—1 gram cefoxitin equivalent
NDC 0006-3548-45 in trays of 25 ADD-Vantage® vials.
No. 3549—2 gram cefoxitin equivalent
NDC 0006-3549-53 in trays of 25 ADD-Vantage® vials.
Special storage instructions
MEFOXIN in the dry state should be stored below 30°C. Avoid exposure to temperatures above 50°C. The dry material as well as solutions tend to darken, depending on storage conditions; product potency, however, is not adversely affected.

A.H.F.S. Category: 8:12.28
DC 7057126   Issued July 1988
COPYRIGHT © MERCK & CO., INC., 1984
All rights reserved

MEFOXIN® Premixed Intravenous Solution   ℞
(Cefoxitin Sodium Injection, MSD)

DESCRIPTION

Cefoxitin sodium is a semi-synthetic, broad-spectrum cepha antibiotic for parenteral administration. It is derived from cephamycin C, which is produced by *Streptomyces lactamdurans*. It is the sodium salt of 3-(hydroxymethyl)-7α-methoxy-8-oxo-7-[2-(2-thienyl)acetamido]-5-thia-1-azabicyclo [4.2.0] oct-2-ene-2-carboxylate carbamate (ester). The empirical formula is $C_{16}H_{16}N_3NaO_7S_2$, and the structural formula is:

Cefoxitin sodium contains approximately 53.8 mg (2.3 milliequivalents) of sodium per gram of cefoxitin activity.
Premixed Intravenous Solution MEFOXIN® (Cefoxitin Sodium Injection, MSD) is supplied as a sterile, nonpyrogenic, frozen solution of cefoxitin sodium in an iso-osmotic

Continued on next page

Merck Sharp & Dohme—Cont.

diluent in plastic containers. Each 50 mL contains cefoxitin sodium equivalent to either 1 gram or 2 grams of cefoxitin in 5% Dextrose (2.5 g dextrose hydrous USP, Water for Injection q.s. to 50 mL). The pH is adjusted with sodium bicarbonate and may be adjusted with hydrochloric acid. The pH is approximately 6.5. After thawing, the solution is intended for intravenous use only. Solutions of MEFOXIN range from colorless to light amber.

The plastic container is fabricated from specially formulated polyvinyl chloride. Solutions in contact with the plastic container can leach out certain of the container's chemical components, e.g., di-2-ethylhexyl phthalate (DEHP), in very small amounts (up to 5 parts per million) within the expiration period. The safety of the plastic has been demonstrated by animal tests according to the USP biological tests for plastic containers, as well as by tissue culture toxicity studies.

MEFOXIN is also available in dry powder form in vials and infusion bottles containing sterile cefoxitin sodium equivalent to either 1 gram or 2 grams of cefoxitin, and in vials for pharmacy bulk use containing sterile cefoxitin sodium equivalent to 10 grams of cefoxitin, for constitution and either intravenous or intramuscular administration (see appropriate product circular).

CLINICAL PHARMACOLOGY

Clinical Pharmacology
Following an intravenous dose of 1 gram of cefoxitin, serum concentrations were 110 mcg/mL at 5 minutes, declining to less than 1 mcg/mL at 4 hours. The half-life after an intravenous dose is 41 to 59 minutes. Approximately 85 percent of cefoxitin is excreted unchanged by the kidneys over a 6-hour period, resulting in high urinary concentrations. Probenecid slows tubular excretion and produces higher serum levels and increases the duration of measurable serum concentrations.

Cefoxitin passes into pleural and joint fluids and is detectable in antibacterial concentrations in bile.

Clinical experience has demonstrated that cefoxitin can be administered to patients who are also receiving carbenicillin, kanamycin, gentamicin, tobramycin, or amikacin (see PRECAUTIONS and ADMINISTRATION).

Microbiology
The bactericidal action of cefoxitin results from inhibition of cell wall synthesis. Cefoxitin has *in vitro* activity against a wide range of gram-positive and gram-negative organisms. The methoxy group in the 7α position provides MEFOXIN with a high degree of stability in the presence of beta-lactamases, both penicillinases and cephalosporinases, of gram-negative bacteria. Cefoxitin is usually active against the following organisms *in vitro* and in clinical infections:

Gram-positive
Staphylococcus aureus, including penicillinase and non-penicillinase producing strains
Staphylococcus epidermidis
Beta-hemolytic and other streptococci (most strains of enterococci, e.g., *Streptococcus faecalis*, are resistant)
Streptococcus pneumoniae

Gram-negative
Escherichia coli
Klebsiella species (including *K. pneumoniae*)
Hemophilus influenzae
Neisseria gonorrhoeae, including penicillinase and non-penicillinase producing strains
Proteus mirabilis
Morganella morganii
Proteus vulgaris
Providencia species, including *Providencia rettgeri*

Anaerobic organisms
Peptococcus species
Peptostreptococcus species
Clostridium species
Bacteroides species, including the *B. fragilis* group (includes *B. fragilis, B. distasonis, B. ovatus, B. thetaiotaomicron, B. vulgatus*)

MEFOXIN is inactive *in vitro* against most strains of *Pseudomonas aeruginosa* and enterococci and many strains of *Enterobacter cloacae*.

Methicillin-resistant staphylococci are almost uniformly resistant to MEFOXIN.

Susceptibility Tests
For fast-growing aerobic organisms, quantitative methods that require measurements of zone diameters give the most precise estimates of antibiotic susceptibility. One such procedure* has been recommended for use with discs to test susceptibility to cefoxitin. Interpretation involves correlation of the diameters obtained in the disc test with minimal inhibitory concentration (MIC) values for cefoxitin.

Reports from the laboratory giving results of the standardized single disc susceptibility test* using a 30 mcg cefoxitin disc should be interpreted according to the following criteria:
Organisms producing zones of 18 mm or greater are considered susceptible, indicating that the tested organism is likely to respond to therapy.

Organisms of intermediate susceptibility produce zones of 15 to 17 mm, indicating that the tested organism would be susceptible if high dosage is used or if the infection is confined to tissues and fluids (e.g., urine) in which high antibiotic levels are attained.

Resistant organisms produce zones of 14 mm or less, indicating that other therapy should be selected.

The cefoxitin disc should be used for testing cefoxitin susceptibility.

Cefoxitin has been shown by *in vitro* tests to have activity against certain strains of *Enterobacteriaceae* found resistant when tested with the cephalosporin class disc. For this reason, the cefoxitin disc should not be used for testing susceptibility to cephalosporins, and cephalosporin discs should not be used for testing susceptibility to cefoxitin.

Dilution methods, preferably the agar plate dilution procedure, are most accurate for susceptibility testing of obligate anaerobes.

A bacterial isolate may be considered susceptible if the MIC value for cefoxitin** is not more than 16 mcg/mL. Organisms are considered resistant if the MIC is greater than 32 mcg/mL.

INDICATIONS AND USAGE

MEFOXIN, supplied as a premixed solution in plastic containers, is intended for intravenous use only. For indications specifically concerning the intramuscular use of cefoxitin (e.g., gonococcal urethritis) or for adverse reactions associated only with intramuscular administration, please refer to the product circular for MEFOXIN (Sterile Cefoxitin Sodium, MSD) supplied as dry powder.

Treatment
MEFOXIN is indicated for the treatment of serious infections caused by susceptible strains of the designated microorganisms in the diseases listed below.

(1) **Lower respiratory tract infections,** including pneumonia and lung abscess, caused by *Streptococcus pneumoniae,* other streptococci (excluding enterococci, e.g., *Streptococcus faecalis*), *Staphylococcus aureus* (penicillinase and non-penicillinase producing), *Escherichia coli, Klebsiella* species, *Hemophilus influenzae,* and *Bacteroides* species.

(2) **Genitourinary infections.** Urinary tract infections caused by *Escherichia coli, Klebsiella* species, *Proteus mirabilis,* indole-positive Proteus , (which include *Morganella morganii* and *Proteus vulgaris*), and *Providencia* species (including *Providencia rettgeri*). Uncomplicated gonorrhea due to *Neisseria gonorrhoeae* (penicillinase and non-penicillinase producing).

(3) **Intra-abdominal infections,** including peritonitis and intra-abdominal abscess, caused by *Escherichia coli, Klebsiella* species, *Bacteroides* species including the *Bacteroides fragilis* group***, and *Clostridium* species.

(4) **Gynecological infections,** including endometritis, pelvic cellulitis, and pelvic inflammatory disease caused by *Escherichia coli, Neisseria gonorrhoeae* (penicillinase and non-penicillinase producing), *Bacteroides* species including the *Bacteroides fragilis* group***, *Clostridium* species, *Peptococcus* species, *Peptostreptococcus* species, and Group B streptococci.

(5) **Septicemia** caused by *Streptococcus pneumoniae, Staphylococcus aureus* (penicillinase and non-penicillinase producing), *Escherichia coli, Klebsiella* species, and *Bacteroides* species including the *Bacteroides fragilis* group.***

(6) **Bone and joint infections** caused by *Staphylococcus aureus* (penicillinase and non-penicillinase producing).

(7) **Skin and skin structure infections** caused by *Staphylococcus aureus* (penicillinase and non-penicillinase producing), *Staphylococcus epidermidis,* streptococci (excluding enterococci, e.g., *Streptococcus faecalis*), *Escherichia coli, Proteus mirabilis, Klebsiella* species, *Bacteroides* species including the *Bacteroides fragilis* group***, *Clostridium* species, *Peptococcus* species, and *Peptostreptococcus* species.

Appropriate culture and susceptibility studies should be performed to determine the susceptibility of the causative organisms to MEFOXIN. Therapy may be started while awaiting the results of these studies.

In randomized comparative studies, cefoxitin and cephalothin were comparably safe and effective in the management

---

* Bauer, A. W.; Kirby, W. M. M.; Sherris, J. C.; Turck, M.: Antibiotic susceptibility testing by a standardized single disc method, Amer. J. Clin. Path. *45* : 493–496, Apr. 1966. Standardized disc susceptibility test, Federal Register *37* : 20527–20529, 1972. National Committee for Clinical Laboratory Standards: Approved Standard: M2-A3, Performance Standards for Antimicrobial Disk Susceptibility Tests, 1984.

** Determined by the ICS agar dilution method (Ericsson and Sherris, Acta Path. Microbiol. Scand. [B] Suppl. No. 217, 1971) or any other method that has been shown to give equivalent results.

*** *B. fragilis, B. distasonis, B. ovatus, B. thetaiotaomicron, B. vulgatus.*

---

of infections caused by gram-positive cocci and gram-negative rods susceptible to the cephalosporins. MEFOXIN has a high degree of stability in the presence of bacterial beta-lactamases, both penicillinases and cephalosporinases.

Many infections caused by aerobic and anaerobic gram-negative bacteria resistant to some cephalosporins respond to MEFOXIN. Similarly, many infections caused by aerobic and anaerobic bacteria resistant to some penicillin antibiotics (ampicillin, carbenicillin, penicillin G) respond to treatment with MEFOXIN. Many infections caused by mixtures of susceptible aerobic and anaerobic bacteria respond to treatment with MEFOXIN.

Prevention
When compared to placebo in randomized controlled studies in patients undergoing gastrointestinal surgery, vaginal hysterectomy, abdominal hysterectomy and cesarean section, the prophylactic use of cefoxitin resulted in a significant reduction in the number of postoperative infections.

The prophylactic administration of MEFOXIN may reduce the incidence of certain postoperative infections in patients undergoing surgical procedures (e.g., hysterectomy, gastrointestinal surgery and transurethral prostatectomy) that are classified as contaminated or potentially contaminated.

The perioperative use of MEFOXIN may be effective in surgical patients in whom infection at the operative site would present a serious risk, e.g., prosthetic arthroplasty.

Effective prophylactic use depends on the time of administration. MEFOXIN usually should be given one-half to one hour before the operation, which is sufficient time to achieve effective levels in the wound during the procedure. Prophylactic administration should usually be stopped within 24 hours since continuing administration of any antibiotic increases the possibility of adverse reactions but, in the majority of surgical procedures, does not reduce the incidence of subsequent infection. However, in patients undergoing prosthetic arthroplasty, it is recommended that MEFOXIN be continued for 72 hours after the surgical procedure.

If there are signs of infection, specimens for culture should be obtained for identification of the causative organism so that appropriate treatment may be instituted.

CONTRAINDICATIONS

MEFOXIN is contraindicated in patients who have shown hypersensitivity to cefoxitin and the cephalosporin group of antibiotics.

WARNINGS

BEFORE THERAPY WITH 'MEFOXIN' IS INSTITUTED, CAREFUL INQUIRY SHOULD BE MADE TO DETERMINE WHETHER THE PATIENT HAS HAD PREVIOUS HYPERSENSITIVITY REACTIONS TO CEFOXITIN, CEPHALOSPORINS, PENICILLINS, OR OTHER DRUGS. THIS PRODUCT SHOULD BE GIVEN WITH CAUTION TO PENICILLIN-SENSITIVE PATIENTS. ANTIBIOTICS SHOULD BE ADMINISTERED WITH CAUTION TO ANY PATIENT WHO HAS DEMONSTRATED SOME FORM OF ALLERGY, PARTICULARLY TO DRUGS. IF AN ALLERGIC REACTION TO 'MEFOXIN' OCCURS, DISCONTINUE THE DRUG. SERIOUS HYPERSENSITIVITY REACTIONS MAY REQUIRE EPINEPHRINE AND OTHER EMERGENCY MEASURES.

Pseudomembranous colitis has been reported with virtually all antibiotics (including cephalosporins); therefore, it is important to consider its diagnosis in patients who develop diarrhea in association with antibiotic use. This colitis may range from mild to life threatening in severity.

Treatment with broad-spectrum antibiotics alters normal flora of the colon and may permit overgrowth of clostridia. Studies indicate a toxin produced by *Clostridium difficile* is one primary cause of antibiotic-associated colitis.

Mild cases of pseudomembranous colitis may respond to drug discontinuance alone. In more severe cases, management may include sigmoidoscopy, appropriate bacteriological studies, fluid, electrolyte and protein supplementation, and the use of a drug such as oral vancomycin as indicated. Isolation of the patient may be advisable. Other causes of colitis should also be considered.

PRECAUTIONS

General
The total daily dose should be reduced when MEFOXIN is administered to patients with transient or persistent reduction of urinary output due to renal insufficiency (see DOSAGE), because high and prolonged serum antibiotic concentrations can occur in such individuals from usual doses.

Antibiotics (including cephalosporins) should be prescribed with caution in individuals with a history of gastrointestinal disease, particularly colitis.

As with other antibiotics, prolonged use of MEFOXIN may result in overgrowth of nonsusceptible organisms. Repeated evaluation of the patient's condition is essential. If superinfection occurs during therapy, appropriate measures should be taken.

Do not use unless solution is clear and seal is intact.

Drug Interactions
Increased nephrotoxicity has been reported following concomitant administration of cephalosporins and aminoglycoside antibiotics.

Drug/Laboratory Test Interactions
As with cephalothin, high concentrations of cefoxitin (> 100 micrograms/mL) may interfere with measurement of serum and urine creatinine levels by the Jaffé reaction, and produce false increases of modest degree in the levels of creatinine reported. Serum samples from patients treated with cefoxitin should not be analyzed for creatinine if withdrawn within 2 hours of drug administration.

High concentrations of cefoxitin in the urine may interfere with measurement of urinary 17-hydroxy-corticosteroids by the Porter-Silber reaction, and produce false increases of modest degree in the levels reported.

A false-positive reaction for glucose in the urine may occur. This has been observed with CLINITEST* reagent tablets.

Carcinogenesis, Mutagenesis, Impairment of Fertility
Long term studies in animals have not been performed with cefoxitin to evaluate carcinogenic or mutagenic potential. Studies in rats treated intravenously with 400 mg/kg of cefoxitin (approximately three times the maximum recommended human dose) revealed no effects on fertility or mating ability.

Pregnancy
Pregnancy Category B. Reproduction studies performed in rats and mice at parenteral doses of approximately one to seven and one-half times the maximum recommended human dose did not reveal teratogenic or fetal toxic effects, although a slight decrease in fetal weight was observed. There are, however, no adequate and well-controlled studies in pregnant women. Because animal reproduction studies are not always predictive of human response, this drug should be used during pregnancy only if clearly needed.

In the rabbit, cefoxitin was associated with a high incidence of abortion and maternal death. This was not considered to be a teratogenic effect but an expected consequence of the rabbit's unusual sensitivity to antibiotic-induced changes in the population of the microflora of the intestine.

Nursing Mothers
Cefoxitin is excreted in human milk in low concentrations. Caution should be exercised when MEFOXIN is administered to a nursing woman.

Pediatric Use
Safety and efficacy in infants from birth to three months of age have not yet been established. In children three months of age and older, higher doses of cefoxitin have been associated with an increased incidence of eosinophilia and elevated SGOT.

ADVERSE REACTIONS

Cefoxitin is generally well tolerated. The most common adverse reactions have been local reactions following intravenous injection. Other adverse reactions have been encountered infrequently.

Local Reactions
Thrombophlebitis has occurred with intravenous administration.

Allergic Reactions
Rash (including exfoliative dermatitis), pruritus, eosinophilia, fever, and other allergic reactions including anaphylaxis have been noted.

Cardiovascular
Hypotension

Gastrointestinal
Diarrhea, including documented pseudomembranous colitis which can appear during or after antibiotic treatment. Nausea and vomiting have been reported rarely.

Blood
Eosinophilia, leukopenia including granulocytopenia, neutropenia, anemia, including hemolytic anemia, thrombocytopenia, and bone marrow depression. A positive direct Coombs test may develop in some individuals, especially those with azotemia.

Liver Function
Transient elevations in SGOT, SGPT, serum LDH, and serum alkaline phosphatase; and jaundice have been reported.

Renal Function
Elevations in serum creatinine and/or blood urea nitrogen levels have been observed. As with the cephalosporins, acute renal failure has been reported rarely. The role of MEFOXIN in changes in renal function tests is difficult to assess, since factors predisposing to prerenal azotemia or to impaired renal function usually have been present.

----

* Registered trademark of Ames Company, Division of Miles Laboratories, Inc.

Table 1—Guidelines for Dosage of MEFOXIN

Type of Infection	Daily Dosage	Frequency and Route
Uncomplicated forms* of infections such as pneumonia, urinary tract infection, cutaneous infection	3–4 grams	1 gram every 6–8 hours IV
Moderately severe or severe infections	6–8 grams	1 gram every 4 hours *or* 2 grams every 6–8 hours IV
Infections commonly needing antibiotics in higher dosage (e.g., gas gangrene)	12 grams	2 grams every 4 hours *or* 3 grams every 6 hours IV

* Including patients in whom bacteremia is absent or unlikely.

Table 2—Maintenance Dosage of MEFOXIN in Adults with Reduced Renal Function

Renal Function	Creatinine Clearance (mL/min)	Dose (grams)	Frequency
Mild impairment	50–30	1–2	every 8–12 hours
Moderate impairment	29–10	1–2	every 12–24 hours
Severe impairment	9–5	0.5–1	every 12–24 hours
Essentially no function	<5	0.5–1	every 24–48 hours

OVERDOSAGE

The acute intravenous LD_{50} in the adult female mouse and rabbit was about 8.0 g/kg and greater than 1.0 g/kg respectively. The acute intraperitoneal LD_{50} in the adult rat was greater than 10.0 g/kg.

DOSAGE

TREATMENT
Adults
The usual adult dosage range is 1 gram to 2 grams every six to eight hours. Dosage and route of administration should be determined by susceptibility of the causative organisms, severity of infection, and the condition of the patient (see Table 1 for dosage guidelines).

MEFOXIN may be used in patients with reduced renal function with the following dosage adjustments:

In adults with renal insufficiency, an initial loading dose of 1 gram to 2 grams may be given. After a loading dose, the recommendations for *maintenance dosage* (Table 2) may be used as a guide.

When only the serum creatinine level is available, the following formula (based on sex, weight, and age of the patient) may be used to convert this value into creatinine clearance. The serum creatinine should represent a steady state of renal function.

Males:
$$\frac{\text{Weight (kg)} \times (140 - \text{age})}{72 \times \text{serum creatinine (mg/100 mL)}}$$

Females: $0.85 \times$ above value

In patients undergoing hemodialysis, the loading dose of 1 to 2 grams should be given after each hemodialysis, and the maintenance dose should be given as indicated in Table 2. Antibiotic therapy for group A beta-hemolytic streptococcal infections should be maintained for at least 10 days to guard against the risk of rheumatic fever or glomerulonephritis. In staphylococcal and other infections involving a collection of pus, surgical drainage should be carried out where indicated.

Infants and Children
The recommended dosage in children three months of age and older is 80 to 160 mg/kg of body weight per day divided into four to six equal doses. The higher dosages should be used for more severe or serious infections. The total daily dosage should not exceed 12 grams.

At this time no recommendation is made for children from birth to three months of age (see PRECAUTIONS).

In children with renal insufficiency the dosage and frequency of dosage should be modified consistent with the recommendations for adults (see Table 2).

PREVENTION
General
For prophylactic use in surgery, the following doses are recommended:

Adults:
(1) 2 grams administered intravenously just prior to surgery (approximately one-half to one hour before the initial incision).
(2) 2 grams every 6 hours after the first dose for no more than 24 hours (continued for 72 hours after prosthetic arthroplasty).

Children (3 months and older):
30 to 40 mg/kg doses may be given at the times designated above.

Cesarean section patients:
A single 2 gram dose should be administered intravenously as soon as the umbilical cord is clamped. A 3-dose regimen may be more effective than a single dose regimen in preventing postoperative infection (esp. endometritis) following cesarean section. Such a regimen would consist of 2 grams given intravenously as soon as the umbilical cord is clamped, followed by 2 grams 4 and 8 hours after the initial dose.

Transurethral prostatectomy patients:
One gram administered just prior to surgery; 1 gram every 8 hours for up to five days.
[See table above].

ADMINISTRATION

This premixed solution is for intravenous use only. Thaw the container at room temperature. After thawing, check for minute leaks by squeezing the bag firmly. If leaks are found or if the seal is not intact, discard the solution since sterility may be compromised. Additives should not be introduced into this solution.

Parenteral drug products should be inspected visually for particulate matter and discoloration prior to administration, whenever solution and container permit. Do not use if the solution is cloudy or a precipitate has formed. Solutions of MEFOXIN tend to darken, depending on storage conditions; product potency, however, is not adversely affected.

The intravenous route is preferred for patients with bacteremia, bacterial septicemia, or other severe or life-threatening infections, or for patients who may be poor risks because of lowered resistance resulting from such debilitating conditions as malnutrition, trauma, surgery, diabetes, heart failure, or malignancy, particularly if shock is present or impending.

Premixed Intravenous Solution MEFOXIN supplied as a sterile, nonpyrogenic, frozen solution in plastic containers is to be administered as a continuous or intermittent intravenous infusion. Scalp vein type needles are preferred for this type of infusion.

Use sterile equipment. It is recommended that the intravenous administration apparatus be replaced at least once every 48 hours.

CAUTION: Do not use plastic containers in series connections. Such use would result in air embolism due to residual air being drawn from the primary container before administration of the fluid from the secondary container is complete.

Preparation for administration:
1. Suspend container from eyelet support.
2. Remove plastic protector from outlet port at bottom of container.
3. Attach administration set. Refer to complete directions accompanying set.

MEFOXIN may be administered through the tubing system by which the patient may be receiving other intravenous solutions. However, during infusion of the solution containing MEFOXIN, it is advisable to temporarily discontinue administration of any other solutions at the same site.

Solutions of MEFOXIN, like those of most beta-lactam antibiotics, should not be added to aminoglycoside solutions (e.g.,

Continued on next page

Information on the Merck Sharp & Dohme products listed on these pages is the full prescribing information from product circulars in use August 31, 1989.

Merck Sharp & Dohme—Cont.

gentamicin sulfate, tobramycin sulfate, amikacin sulfate) because of potential interaction. However, MEFOXIN and aminoglycosides may be administered separately to the same patient.

STABILITY

MEFOXIN, as supplied premixed in 5% Dextrose in plastic containers, maintains satisfactory potency after thawing for 24 hours at room temperature and 5 days if stored under refrigeration [2 to 8°C (35.6 to 46.4°F)]. After these periods, any unused thawed solutions should be discarded.
DO NOT REFREEZE.

HOW SUPPLIED

Premixed Intravenous Solution MEFOXIN is supplied in single dose plastic containers containing cefoxitin sodium as follows:
No. 2B3506—1 gram cefoxitin equivalent in 50 mL 5% Dextrose
NDC 0006-3506-24 in boxes of 24.
No. 2B3507—2 gram cefoxitin equivalent in 50 mL 5% Dextrose
NDC 0006-3507-25 in boxes of 24.
Special storage instructions
Do not store above −20°C (−4°F). After thawing, do not refreeze.
Manufactured for:
MERCK SHARP & DOHME
DIV OF MERCK & CO., INC., WEST POINT, PA 19486, USA
By:
TRAVENOL LABORATORIES, INC.
Deerfield, Illinois 60015
     A.H.F.S. Category 8:12.28
     DC7407409   Issued January 1989
COPYRIGHT © MERCK & CO., INC., 1985
All rights reserved

MEPHYTON® Tablets   ℞
(Phytonadione, MSD), U.S.P.
Vitamin K₁

DESCRIPTION

Phytonadione is a vitamin which is a clear, yellow to amber, viscous, and nearly odorless liquid. It is insoluble in water, soluble in chloroform and slightly soluble in ethanol. It has a molecular weight of 450.70.
Phytonadione is 2-methyl-3-phytyl-1, 4-naphthoquinone. Its empirical formula is $C_{31}H_{46}O_2$ and its structural formula is:

MEPHYTON® (Phytonadione, MSD) tablets containing 5 mg of phytonadione are yellow, compressed tablets, scored on one side. Inactive ingredients are acacia, calcium phosphate, colloidal silicon dioxide, lactose, magnesium stearate, starch, and talc.

CLINICAL PHARMACOLOGY

MEPHYTON tablets possess the same type and degree of activity as does naturally-occurring vitamin K, which is necessary for the production via the liver of active prothrombin (factor II), proconvertin (factor VII), plasma thromboplastin component (factor IX), and Stuart factor (factor X). The prothrombin test is sensitive to the levels of three of these four factors—II, VII, and X. The mechanism by which vitamin K promotes formation of these clotting factors in the liver is not known.
Oral phytonadione is adequately absorbed from the gastrointestinal tract only if bile salts are present. After absorption, phytonadione is initially concentrated in the liver, but the concentration declines rapidly. Very little vitamin K accumulates in tissues. Little is known about the metabolic fate of vitamin K. Almost no free unmetabolized vitamin K appears in bile or urine.
In normal animals and humans, phytonadione is virtually devoid of pharmacodynamic activity. However, in animals and humans deficient in vitamin K, the pharmacological action of vitamin K is related to its normal physiological function; that is, to promote the hepatic biosynthesis of vitamin K-dependent clotting factors.
MEPHYTON tablets generally exert their effect within 6 to 10 hours.

INDICATIONS AND USAGE

MEPHYTON is indicated in the following coagulation disorders which are due to faulty formation of factors II, VII, IX and X when caused by vitamin K deficiency or interference with vitamin K activity.
MEPHYTON tablets are indicated in:
—anticoagulant-induced prothrombin deficiency caused by coumarin or indanedione derivatives;
—hypoprothrombinemia secondary to antibacterial therapy;
—hypoprothrombinemia secondary to administration of salicylates;
—hypoprothrombinemia secondary to obstructive jaundice or biliary fistulas but only if bile salts are administered concurrently, since otherwise the oral vitamin K will not be absorbed.

CONTRAINDICATION

Hypersensitivity to any component of this medication.

WARNINGS

An immediate coagulant effect should not be expected after administration of phytonadione.
Phytonadione will not counteract the anticoagulant action of heparin.
When vitamin K₁ is used to correct excessive anticoagulant-induced hypoprothrombinemia, anticoagulant therapy still being indicated, the patient is again faced with the clotting hazards existing prior to starting the anticoagulant therapy. Phytonadione is not a clotting agent, but overzealous therapy with vitamin K₁ may restore conditions which originally permitted thromboembolic phenomena. Dosage should be kept as low as possible, and prothrombin time should be checked regularly as clinical conditions indicate.
Repeated large doses of vitamin K are not warranted in liver disease if the response to initial use of the vitamin is unsatisfactory. Failure to respond to vitamin K may indicate a congenital coagulation defect or that the condition being treated is unresponsive to vitamin K.

PRECAUTIONS

General
Temporary resistance to prothrombin-depressing anticoagulants may result, especially when larger doses of phytonadione are used. If relatively large doses have been employed, it may be necessary when reinstituting anticoagulant therapy to use somewhat larger doses of the prothrombin-depressing anticoagulant, or to use one which acts on a different principle, such as heparin sodium.
Laboratory Tests
Prothrombin time should be checked regularly as clinical conditions indicate.
Carcinogenesis, Mutagenesis, Impairment of Fertility
Studies of carcinogenicity or impairment of fertility have not been performed with MEPHYTON. MEPHYTON at concentrations up to 2000 mcg/plate with or without metabolic activation, was negative in the Ames microbial mutagen test.
Pregnancy
Pregnancy Category C: Animal reproduction studies have not been conducted with MEPHYTON. It is also not known whether MEPHYTON can cause fetal harm when administered to a pregnant woman or can affect reproduction capacity. MEPHYTON should be given to a pregnant woman only if clearly needed.
Pediatric Use
Safety and effectiveness in children have not been established with MEPHYTON. Hemolysis, jaundice, and hyperbilirubinemia in newborns, particularly in premature infants, have been reported with vitamin K.
Nursing Mothers
It is not known whether this drug is excreted in human milk. Because many drugs are excreted in human milk, caution should be exercised when MEPHYTON is administered to a nursing woman.

ADVERSE REACTIONS

Transient "flushing sensations" and "peculiar" sensations of taste have been observed with parenteral phytonadione, as well as rare instances of dizziness, rapid and weak pulse, profuse sweating, brief hypotension, dyspnea, and cyanosis.
Hyperbilirubinemia has been observed in the newborn following administration of parenteral phytonadione. This has occurred rarely and primarily with doses above those recommended.

OVERDOSAGE

The intravenous and oral LD_{50}s in the mouse are approximately 1.17 g/kg and greater than 24.18 g/kg, respectively.

DOSAGE AND ADMINISTRATION

MEPHYTON
Summary of Dosage Guidelines
(See circular text for details)

Adults	Initial Dosage
Anticoagulant-Induced Prothrombin Deficiency (caused by coumarin or indanedione derivatives)	2.5 mg–10 mg or up to 25 mg (rarely 50 mg)
Hypoprothrombinemia due to other causes (Antibiotics; Salicylates or other drugs; Factors limiting absorption or synthesis)	2.5 mg–25 mg or more (rarely up to 50 mg)

Anticoagulant-Induced Prothrombin Deficiency in Adults
To correct excessively prolonged prothrombin times caused by oral anticoagulant therapy—2.5 to 10 mg or up to 25 mg initially is recommended. In rare instances 50 mg may be required. Frequency and amount of subsequent doses should be determined by prothrombin time response or clinical condition. (See WARNINGS.) If, in 12 to 48 hours after oral administration, the prothrombin time has not been shortened satisfactorily, the dose should be repeated.
Hypoprothrombinemia Due to Other Causes in Adults
If possible, discontinuation or reduction of the dosage of drugs interfering with coagulation mechanisms (such as salicylates, antibiotics) is suggested as an alternative to administering concurrent MEPHYTON. The severity of the coagulation disorder should determine whether the immediate administration of MEPHYTON is required in addition to discontinuation or reduction of interfering drugs.
A dosage of 2.5 to 25 mg or more (rarely up to 50 mg) is recommended, the amount and route of administration depending upon the severity of the condition and response obtained. The oral route should be avoided when the clinical disorder would prevent proper absorption. Bile salts must be given with the tablets when the endogenous supply of bile to the gastrointestinal tract is deficient.

HOW SUPPLIED

No. 7776—Tablets MEPHYTON, 5 mg vitamin K₁, are yellow, round, scored, compressed tablets, coded MSD 43. They are supplied as follows:
NDC 0006-0043-68 bottles of 100.
     Shown in Product Identification Section, page 418
Storage:
Protect from light.
         A.H.F.S. Category: 88:24
     DC 7469512   Issued August 1986
COPYRIGHT © MERCK & CO., Inc., 1986
All rights reserved

MERUVAX®II   ℞
(Rubella Virus Vaccine Live, MSD), U.S.P.
(Wistar RA 27/3 Strain)

DESCRIPTION

MERUVAX® II (Rubella Virus Vaccine Live, MSD) is a live virus vaccine for immunization against rubella (German measles).
MERUVAX II is a sterile lyophilized preparation of the Wistar Institute RA 27/3 strain of live attenuated rubella virus. The virus was adapted to and propagated in human diploid cell (WI-38) culture.
The reconstituted vaccine is for subcutaneous administration. When reconstituted as directed, the dose for injection is 0.5 mL and contains not less than the equivalent of 1,000 $TCID_{50}$ (tissue culture infectious doses) of the U.S. Reference Rubella Virus. Each dose also contains approximately 25 mcg of neomycin. The product contains no preservative. Sorbitol and hydrolized gelatin are added as stabilizers.

CLINICAL PHARMACOLOGY

MERUVAX II produces a modified, non-communicable rubella infection in susceptible persons.
Extensive clinical trials of rubella virus vaccines, prepared using RA 27/3 strain rubella virus, have been carried out in more than 28,000 human subjects (approximately 11,000 with MERUVAX II) in the U.S.A. and more than 20 additional countries. A single injection of the vaccine has been shown to induce rubella hemagglutination-inhibiting (HI) antibodies in 97% or more of susceptible persons. The RA 27/3 rubella strain elicits higher immediate post-vaccination HI, complement-fixing and neutralizing antibody levels than other strains of rubella vaccine and has been shown to induce a broader profile of circulating antibodies including

anti-theta and anti-iota precipitating antibodies. The RA 27/3 rubella strain immunologically simulates natural infection more closely than other rubella vaccine viruses. The increased levels and broader profile of antibodies produced by RA 27/3 strain rubella virus vaccine appear to correlate with greater resistance to subclinical reinfection with the wild virus, and provide greater confidence for lasting immunity.

Vaccine-induced antibody levels have been shown to persist for at least 10 years without substantial decline. If the present pattern continues, it will provide a basis for the expectation that immunity following vaccination will be permanent. However, continued surveillance will be required to demonstrate this point.

INDICATIONS AND USAGE†

1. *Children Between 12 Months of Age and Puberty*
MERUVAX II is indicated for immunization against rubella (German measles) in persons from 12 months of age to puberty. A booster is not needed. It is not recommended for infants younger than 12 months because they may retain maternal rubella neutralizing antibodies that may interfere with the immune response. Children in kindergarten and the first grades of elementary school deserve priority for vaccination because often they are epidemiologically the major source of virus dissemination in the community. A history of rubella illness is usually not reliable enough to exclude children from immunization.

Previously unimmunized children of susceptible pregnant women should receive live attenuated rubella vaccine, because an immunized child will be less likely to acquire natural rubella and introduce the virus into the household.

2. *Adolescent and Adult Males*
Vaccination of adolescent or adult males may be a useful procedure in preventing or controlling outbreaks of rubella in circumscribed population groups (e.g., military bases and schools).

3. *Non-Pregnant Adolescent and Adult Females*
Immunization of susceptible non-pregnant adolescent and adult females of childbearing age with live attenuated rubella virus vaccine is indicated if certain precautions are observed (see below and PRECAUTIONS). Vaccinating susceptible postpubertal females confers individual protection against subsequently acquiring rubella infection during pregnancy, which in turn prevents infection of the fetus and consequent congenital rubella injury.

Women of childbearing age should be advised not to become pregnant for three months after vaccination and should be informed of the reason for this precaution.*

It is recommended that rubella susceptibility be determined by serologic testing prior to immunization.** If immune, as evidenced by a specific rubella antibody titer of 1:8 or greater (hemagglutination-inhibition test), vaccination is unnecessary. Congenital malformations do occur in up to seven percent of all live births. Their chance appearance after vaccination could lead to misinterpretation of the cause, particularly if the prior rubella-immune status of vaccinees is unknown.

Postpubertal females should be informed of the frequent occurrence of generally self-limited arthralgia and/or arthritis beginning 2 to 4 weeks after vaccination (see ADVERSE REACTIONS).

4. *Postpartum Women*
It has been found convenient in many instances to vaccinate rubella-susceptible women in the immediate postpartum period (see *Nursing Mothers*).

---

† Based in part on the recommendation for rubella vaccine use of the Immunization Practices Advisory Committee (ACIP), Morbidity and Mortality Weekly Report: *33* (22): 301-310, 315-318, June 8, 1984.

*NOTE: The Immunization Practices Advisory Committee (ACIP) has recommended "In view of the importance of protecting this age group against rubella, reasonable precautions in a rubella immunization program include asking females if they are pregnant, excluding those who say they are, and explaining the theoretical risks to the others."

**NOTE: The Immunization Practices Advisory Committee (ACIP) has stated "When practical, and when reliable laboratory services are available, potential vaccinees of childbearing age can have serologic tests to determine susceptibility to rubella.... However, routinely performing serologic tests for all females of childbearing age to determine susceptibility so that vaccine is given only to proven susceptibles is expensive and has been ineffective in some areas. Accordingly, the ACIP believes that rubella vaccination of a woman who is not known to be pregnant and has no history of vaccination is justifiable without serologic testing."

Revaccination:
Children vaccinated when younger than 12 months of age should be revaccinated. Based on available evidence, there is no reason to routinely revaccinate persons who were vaccinated originally when 12 months of age or older. However, persons should be revaccinated if there is evidence to suggest that initial immunization was ineffective.

Use with Other Vaccines
Routine administration of DTP (diphtheria, tetanus, pertussis) and/or OPV (oral poliovirus vaccine) concomitantly with measles, mumps and rubella vaccines is not recommended because there are insufficient data relating to the simultaneous administration of these antigens. However, the American Academy of Pediatrics has noted that in some circumstances, particularly when the patient may not return, some practitioners prefer to administer all these antigens on a single day. If done, separate sites and syringes should be used for DTP and MERUVAX II.

MERUVAX II should not be given less than one month before or after administration of other virus vaccines.

CONTRAINDICATIONS

Do not give MERUVAX II to pregnant females; the possible effects of the vaccine on fetal development are unknown at this time. If vaccination of postpubertal females is undertaken, pregnancy should be avoided for three months following vaccination. (See PRECAUTIONS, *Pregnancy*).

Anaphylactoid reaction to neomycin (each dose of reconstituted vaccine contains approximately 25 mcg of neomycin).

Any febrile respiratory illness or other active febrile infection.

Active untreated tuberculosis.

Patients receiving immunosuppressive therapy. This contraindication does not apply to patients who are receiving corticosteroids as replacement therapy, e.g., for Addison's disease.

Individuals with blood dyscrasias, leukemia, lymphomas of any type, or other malignant neoplasms affecting the bone marrow or lymphatic systems.

Primary immunodeficiency states, including cellular immune deficiencies, hypogammaglobulinemic and dysgammaglobulinemic states.

Individuals with a family history of congenital or hereditary immunodeficiency, until the immune competence of the potential vaccine recipient is demonstrated.

PRECAUTIONS

General
Adequate treatment provisions including epinephrine, should be available for immediate use should an anaphylactoid reaction occur.

Excretion of small amounts of the live attenuated rubella virus from the nose or throat has occurred in the majority of susceptible individuals 7-28 days after vaccination. There is no confirmed evidence to indicate that such virus is transmitted to susceptible persons who are in contact with the vaccinated individuals. Consequently, transmission through close personal contact, while accepted as a theoretical possibility, is not regarded as a significant risk. However, transmission of the vaccine virus to infants via breast milk has been documented (see *Nursing Mothers*).

There is no evidence that live rubella virus vaccine given after exposure to natural rubella virus will prevent illness.

There is, however, no contraindication to vaccinating children already exposed to natural rubella.

Vaccination should be deferred for at least three months following blood or plasma transfusions, or administration of human immune serum globulin. However, susceptible postpartum patients who received blood products may receive MERUVAX II prior to discharge provided that a repeat HI titer is drawn 6-8 weeks after vaccination to insure seroconversion. Similarly, although studies with other live rubella virus vaccines suggest that MERUVAX II may be given in the immediate postpartum period to those non-immune women who have received anti-Rho (D) globulin (human) without interfering with vaccine effectiveness, a follow-up post-vaccination HI titer should also be determined.

It has been reported that attenuated rubella virus vaccine, live, may result in a temporary depression of tuberculin skin sensitivity. Therefore, if a tuberculin test is to be done, it should be administered either before or simultaneously with MERUVAX II.

As for any vaccine, vaccination with MERUVAX II may not result in seroconversion in 100% of susceptible persons given the vaccine.

Pregnancy
Pregnancy Category C
Animal reproduction studies have not been conducted with MERUVAX II. It is also not known whether MERUVAX II can cause fetal harm when administered to a pregnant woman or can affect reproduction capacity. There is evidence suggesting transmission of rubella vaccine viruses to products of conception. Therefore, rubella vaccine should not be administered to pregnant females (see CONTRAINDICATIONS).

In counseling women who are inadvertently vaccinated when pregnant or who become pregnant within 3 months of vaccination, the physician should be aware of the following: In a 10 year survey involving over 700 pregnant women who received rubella vaccine within 3 months before or after conception, (of whom 189 received the Wistar RA 27/3 strain) none of the newborns had abnormalities compatible with congenital rubella syndrome.

Nursing Mothers
Recent studies have shown that lactating postpartum women immunized with live attenuated rubella vaccine may secrete the virus in breast milk and transmit it to breast-fed infants. In the infants with serological evidence of rubella infection, none exhibited severe disease; however, one exhibited mild clinical illness typical of acquired rubella. Caution should be exercised when MERUVAX II is administered to a nursing woman.

ADVERSE REACTIONS

Because of the slightly acidic pH (6.2-6.6) of the vaccine, patients may complain of burning and/or stinging of short duration at the injection site.

Symptoms of the same kind as those seen following natural rubella may occur after vaccination. These include regional lymphadenopathy, urticaria, rash, malaise, sore throat, fever, headache, nausea, vomiting, polyneuritis, and arthralgia and/or arthritis (usually transient and rarely chronic). Local pain, wheal and flare, induration, and erythema may occur at the site of injection. Reactions are usually mild and transient.

Moderate fever [101-102.9°F (38.3-39.4°C)] occurs occasionally, and high fever [over 103°F (39.4°C)] occurs less commonly.

Chronic arthritis has been associated with natural rubella infection and has been related to persistent virus and/or viral antigen isolated from body tissues. Only rarely have vaccine recipients developed chronic joint symptoms.

Following vaccination in children, reactions in joints are uncommon and generally of brief duration. In women, incidence rates for arthritis and arthralgia are generally higher than those seen in children (children: 0-3%; women: 12-20%) and the reactions tend to be more marked and of longer duration. Symptoms may persist for a matter of months or on rare occasions for years. In adolescent girls, the reactions appear to be intermediate in incidence between those seen in children and in adult women. Even in older women (35-45 years), these reactions are generally well tolerated and rarely interfere with normal activities. Myalgia and paresthesia have been reported rarely after administration of MERUVAX II.

Forms of optic neuritis, including retrobulbar neuritis and papillitis may infrequently follow viral infections, and have been reported to occur 1 to 3 weeks following inoculation with some live virus vaccines.

Isolated reports of polyneuropathy including Guillain-Barré syndrome have been reported after immunization with rubella containing vaccines.

Clinical experience with live rubella vaccines thus far indicates that encephalitis and other nervous system reactions have occurred very rarely in subjects who were given the vaccines, but a cause and effect relationship has not been established.

In view of the decreases in platelet counts that have been reported, thrombocytopenic purpura is a theoretical hazard.

DOSAGE AND ADMINISTRATION

FOR SUBCUTANEOUS ADMINISTRATION
Do not inject intravenously
The dosage of vaccine is the same for all persons. Inject the total volume of the single dose vial (about 0.5 mL) or 0.5 mL of the multiple dose vial of reconstituted vaccine subcutaneously, preferably into the outer aspect of upper arm. *Do not give immune globulin (IG) concurrently with* MERUVAX II.
To insure that there is no loss of potency during shipment, the vaccine must be maintained at a temperature of 10°C (50°F) or less.
Before reconstitution, store MERUVAX II at 2-8°C (35.6-46.4°F). *Protect from light.*
CAUTION: A sterile syringe free of preservatives, antiseptics, and detergents should be used for each injection and/or reconstitution of the vaccine because these substances may inactivate the live virus vaccine. A 25 gauge, 5/8" needle is recommended.
To reconstitute, use only the diluent supplied, since it is free of preservatives or other antiviral substances which might inactivate the vaccine.

Continued on next page

Merck Sharp & Dohme—Cont.

Single Dose Vial—First withdraw the entire volume of diluent into the syringe to be used for reconstitution. Inject all the diluent in the syringe into the vial of lyophilized vaccine, and agitate to mix thoroughly. Withdraw the entire contents into a syringe and inject the total volume of restored vaccine subcutaneously.

It is important to use a separate sterile syringe and needle for each individual patient to prevent transmission of hepatitis B and other infectious agents from one person to another.

10 Dose Vial (available only to government agencies/institutions)—Withdraw the entire contents (7 mL) of the diluent vial into the sterile syringe to be used for reconstitution, and introduce into the 10 dose vial of lyophilized vaccine. Agitate to ensure thorough mixing. The outer labeling suggests "For Jet Injector or Syringe Use". Use with separate sterile syringes is permitted for containers of 10 doses or less. The vaccine and diluent do not contain preservatives; therefore, the user must recognize the potential contamination hazards and exercise special precautions to protect the sterility and potency of the product. The use of aseptic techniques and proper storage prior to and after restoration of the vaccine and subsequent withdrawal of the individual doses is essential. Use 0.5 mL of the reconstituted vaccine for subcutaneous injection.

It is important to use a separate sterile syringe and needle for each individual patient to prevent transmission of hepatitis B and other infectious agents from one person to another.

50 Dose Vial (available only to government agencies/institutions)—Withdraw the entire contents (30 mL) of diluent vial into the sterile syringe to be used for reconstitution and introduce into the 50 dose vial of lyophilized vaccine. Agitate to ensure thorough mixing. With full aseptic precautions, attach the vial to the sterilized multidose jet injector apparatus. Use 0.5 mL of the reconstituted vaccine for subcutaneous injection.

Each dose contains not less than the equivalent of 1,000 $TCID_{50}$ of the U.S. Reference Rubella Virus.

Parenteral drug products should be inspected visually for particulate matter and discoloration prior to administration. MERUVAX II, when reconstituted, is clear yellow.

HOW SUPPLIED

No. 4747—MERUVAX II is supplied as a single-dose vial of lyophilized vaccine,
NDC 0006-4747-00, and a vial of diluent.
No. 4673/4309—MERUVAX II is supplied as follows: (1) a box of 10 single-dose vials of lyophilized vaccine (package A), NDC 0006-4673-00; and (2) a box of 10 vials of diluent (package B). To conserve refrigerator space, the diluent may be stored separately at room temperature.
(6505-00-145-0180, Ten Pack).
Available only to government agencies/institutions:
No. 4674—MERUVAX II is supplied as one 10 dose vial of lyophilized vaccine,
NDC 0006-4674-00, and one 7 mL vial of diluent.
No. 4675—MERUVAX II is supplied as one 50 dose vial of lyophilized vaccine,
NDC 0006-4675-00, and one 30 mL vial of diluent.
(6505-01-222-6468, 50 Dose).
Storage
It is recommended that the vaccine be used as soon as possible after reconstitution. Protect vaccine from light at all times, since such exposure may inactivate the virus. Store reconstituted vaccine in the vaccine vial in a dark place at 2–8°C (35.6–46.4°F) and discard if not used within 8 hours.

A.H.F.S. Category: 80:12
DC 7415512 Issued October 1986
COPYRIGHT © MERCK & CO., INC., 1985
All rights reserved

MEVACOR® Tablets   ℞
(Lovastatin, MSD)

DESCRIPTION

MEVACOR® (Lovastatin, MSD), is a cholesterol lowering agent isolated from a strain of *Aspergillus terreus*. After oral ingestion, lovastatin, which is an inactive lactone, is hydrolyzed to the corresponding β-hydroxyacid form. This is a principal metabolite and an inhibitor of 3-hydroxy-3-methylglutaryl-coenzyme A (HMG-CoA) reductase. This enzyme catalyzes the conversion of HMG-CoA to mevalonate, which is an early and rate limiting step in the biosynthesis of cholesterol.

Lovastatin is [1S-[1α(R*),3α,7β,8β(2S*,4S*),8aβ]]-1,2,3,7,8,8a -hexahydro-3,7-dimethyl-8-[2-(tetrahydro-4-hydroxy-6-oxo-2H -pyran-2-yl)ethyl]-1-napthalenyl 2-methylbutanoate.

The empirical formula of lovastatin is $C_{24}H_{36}O_5$ and its molecular weight is 404.55. Its structural formula is:

Lovastatin is a white, nonhygroscopic crystalline powder that is insoluble in water and sparingly soluble in ethanol, methanol, and acetonitrile.

Tablets MEVACOR are supplied as 20 mg and 40 mg tablets for oral administration. In addition to the active ingredient lovastatin, each tablet contains the following inactive ingredients: cellulose, lactose, magnesium stearate, and starch. Butylated hydroxyanisole (BHA) is added as a preservative. Tablets MEVACOR 20 mg also contain FD&C Blue 2. Tablets MEVACOR 40 mg also contain D&C Yellow 10 and FD&C Blue 2.

CLINICAL PHARMACOLOGY

The involvement of low-density lipoprotein (LDL) cholesterol in atherogenesis has been well-documented in clinical and pathological studies, as well as in many animal experiments. Epidemiological studies have established that high LDL (low-density lipoprotein) cholesterol and low HDL (high-density lipoprotein) cholesterol are both risk factors for coronary heart disease. The Lipid Research Clinics Coronary Primary Prevention Trial (LRC-CPPT), coordinated by the National Institutes of Health (NIH) studied men aged 35–59 with cholesterol levels 265 mg/dL or greater, and triglyceride levels not more than 300 mg/dL. This seven-year, double-blind, placebo-controlled study demonstrated that lowering LDL cholesterol with diet and cholestyramine decreased the combined rate of coronary heart disease death plus non-fatal myocardial infarction.

MEVACOR has been shown to reduce both normal and elevated LDL cholesterol concentrations. The effect of lovastatin-induced changes in lipoprotein levels, including reduction of serum cholesterol, on cardiovascular morbidity or mortality has not been established.

LDL is formed from VLDL and is catabolized predominantly by the high affinity LDL receptor. The mechanism of the LDL-lowering effect of MEVACOR may involve both reduction of VLDL cholesterol concentration, and induction of the LDL receptor, leading to reduced production and/or increased catabolism of LDL cholesterol. Apolipoprotein B also falls substantially during treatment with MEVACOR. Since each LDL particle contains one molecule of apolipoprotein B, and since little apolipoprotein B is found in other lipoproteins, this strongly suggests that MEVACOR does not merely cause cholesterol to be lost from LDL, but also reduces the concentration of circulating LDL particles. In addition, MEVACOR increases HDL cholesterol and reduces VLDL cholesterol and plasma triglycerides (see Tables I–IV under *Clinical Studies*).

MEVACOR is a specific inhibitor of HMG-CoA reductase, the enzyme which catalyzes the conversion of HMG-CoA to mevalonate. However, at therapeutic doses, the enzyme is not completely blocked, thereby allowing biologically necessary amounts of mevalonate to be available. The conversion of HMG-CoA to mevalonate is an early step in the biosynthetic pathway for cholesterol.

Although cholesterol is the precursor of all steroid hormones, lovastatin has been shown to have no effect on steroidogenesis.

Pharmacokinetics
Lovastatin is a lactone which is readily hydrolyzed *in vivo* to the corresponding β-hydroxyacid, a potent inhibitor of HMG-CoA reductase. Inhibition of HMG-CoA reductase is the basis for an assay in pharmacokinetic studies of the β-hydroxyacid metabolites (active inhibitors) and, following base hydrolysis, active plus latent inhibitors (total inhibitors) in plasma following administration of lovastatin.

Following an oral dose of ^{14}C-labeled lovastatin in man, 10% of the dose was excreted in urine and 83% in feces. The latter represents absorbed drug equivalents excreted in bile, as well as any unabsorbed drug. Absorption of lovastatin, estimated relative to an intravenous reference dose, in each of four animal species tested, averaged about 30% of an oral dose. Studies in the dog have indicated that the availability of the absorbed drug to the general circulation is limited by extensive first-pass extraction in the liver, its primary site of action, with subsequent excretion of drug equivalents in the bile. As a consequence of extensive hepatic extraction of lovastatin, the availability of drug to the general circulation

is low and variable. In a single dose study in four hypercholesterolemic patients, it was estimated that less than 5% of an oral dose of lovastatin reaches the general circulation as active inhibitors. Following administration of lovastatin tablets the coefficient of variation, based on between-subject variability, was approximately 40% for the area under the curve of total inhibitory activity in the general circulation. Both lovastatin and its β-hydroxyacid metabolite are highly bound (>95%) to human plasma proteins. Animal studies demonstrated that lovastatin crosses the blood-brain and placental barriers.

The major active metabolites present in human plasma are the β-hydroxyacid of lovastatin, its 6'-hydroxy derivative, and two unidentified metabolites. Peak plasma concentrations of both active and total inhibitors were attained within 2 to 4 hours of dose administration. While the recommended therapeutic dose range is 20 to 80 mg/day, linearity of inhibitory activity in the general circulation was established by a single dose study employing lovastatin tablet dosages from 60 to as high as 120 mg. With a once-a-day dosing regimen, plasma concentrations of total inhibitors over a dosing interval achieved a steady state between the second and third days of therapy and were about 1.5 times those following a single dose. When lovastatin was given under fasting conditions, plasma concentrations of total inhibitors were on average about two-thirds those found when lovastatin was administered immediately after a standard test meal.

Clinical Studies
MEVACOR has been shown to be highly effective in reducing total and LDL cholesterol in heterozygous familial and non-familial forms of hypercholesterolemia. A marked response was seen within 2 weeks, and the maximum therapeutic response occurred within 4–6 weeks. The response was maintained indefinitely during continuation of therapy. Single daily doses given in the evening were more effective than the same dose given in the morning, perhaps because cholesterol is synthesized mainly at night.

In multicenter, double-blind studies in patients with familial or non-familial hypercholesterolemia, MEVACOR, administered in doses ranging from 20 mg q.p.m. to 40 mg b.i.d., was compared to placebo. MEVACOR consistently and significantly decreased total plasma cholesterol (TOTAL-C), LDL cholesterol (LDL-C), total cholesterol/HDL cholesterol (TOTAL-C/HDL-C) ratio and LDL cholesterol/HDL cholesterol (LDL-C/HDL-C) ratio (p < 0.01). In addition, MEVACOR increased total HDL cholesterol (HDL-C) and decreased VLDL cholesterol (VLDL-C) and plasma triglycerides (TRIG.) (see Tables I and II for dose response results).
[See table on top right next page].

MEVACOR was compared to cholestyramine in a randomized open parallel study and to probucol in a double-blind, parallel study. Both studies were performed with patients with hypercholesterolemia who were at high risk of myocardial infarction. At all dosage levels tested, MEVACOR produced a significantly greater reduction of total plasma cholesterol, and total cholesterol/HDL cholesterol ratio when compared to cholestyramine or probucol (p < 0.01). The increase in HDL cholesterol was also significantly greater with MEVACOR than with probucol (p < 0.01), but not cholestyramine (see Tables III & IV).
[See table on bottom left next page].

INDICATIONS AND USAGE

MEVACOR is indicated as an adjunct to diet for the reduction of elevated total and LDL cholesterol levels in patients with primary hypercholesterolemia (Types IIa and IIb[1]), when the response to diet and other nonpharmacological measures alone has been inadequate.

---

[1] Fredrickson, D.S.: Fat transport in lipoproteins—an integrated approach to mechanism and disorders, N.Eng.J.Med. 276:34, 1967.
Fredrickson classification: Type IIa—elevation of LDL; Type IIb—elevation of LDL and VLDL.

After establishing that the elevation in plasma lipids represents a primary disorder not due to secondary conditions such as poorly-controlled diabetes mellitus, hypothyroidism, the nephrotic syndrome, liver disease, or dysproteinemias, it should ideally be determined that patients for whom treatment with lovastatin is being considered have an elevated LDL-C level as the cause for an elevated total serum cholesterol. This may be particularly relevant for patients with total triglycerides over 400 mg/dL or with markedly elevated HDL-C values, where non-LDL lipoprotein fractions may contribute significantly to total cholesterol levels without apparent increase in cardiovascular risk. In most patients LDL-C may be estimated according to the following equation:

LDL-C = Total cholesterol − [0.16 × (triglycerides) + HDL-C]

When total triglycerides are greater than 400 mg/dL this equation is less accurate. In such patients, LDL cholesterol may be obtained by ultracentrifugation.

Lovastatin has not been studied in patients with Type III hyperlipoproteinemia[2] or with total cholesterol elevations due to elevated intermediate density lipoproteins.

---

[2] Fredrickson, D.S.: Fat transport in lipoproteins—an integrated approach to mechanism and disorders, N.Eng.J.Med. 276 :34, 1967.
Fredrickson classification: Type III—elevation of IDL (intermediate density lipoprotein).

The effect of lovastatin-induced changes in lipoprotein levels, including reduction of serum cholesterol, on cardiovascular morbidity or mortality has not been established. MEVACOR may be useful to reduce elevated LDL cholesterol levels in patients with combined hypercholesterolemia and hypertriglyceridemia.

CONTRAINDICATIONS

Hypersensitivity to any component of this medication. Active liver disease or unexplained persistent elevations of serum transaminases.
Pregnancy and lactation.
Atherosclerosis is a chronic process and the discontinuation of lipid-lowering drugs during pregnancy should have little impact on the outcome of long-term therapy of primary hypercholesterolemia. Moreover, cholesterol and other products of the cholesterol biosynthesis pathway are essential components for fetal development, including synthesis of steroids and cell membranes. Because of the ability of inhibitors of HMG-CoA reductase such as MEVACOR to decrease the synthesis of cholesterol and possibly other products of the cholesterol biosynthesis pathway, MEVACOR may cause fetal harm when administered to a pregnant woman. Therefore, lovastatin is contraindicated during pregnancy. Lovastatin should be administered to women of childbearing age only when such patients are highly unlikely to conceive. If the patient becomes pregnant while taking this drug, lovastatin should be discontinued and the patient should be apprised of the potential hazard to the fetus.

WARNINGS

Liver Dysfunction

Marked persistent increases (to more than 3 times the upper limit of normal) in serum transaminases occurred in 1.9% of adult patients who received lovastatin for at least one year in clinical trials (see ADVERSE REACTIONS). When the drug was interrupted or discontinued in these patients, the transaminase levels usually fell slowly to pretreatment levels. The increases usually appeared 3 to 12 months after the start of therapy with lovastatin, and were not associated with jaundice or other clinical signs or symptoms. There was no evidence of hypersensitivity. A liver biopsy was done in one of these patients and showed areas of focal hepatitis. In this patient, transaminase levels returned to normal following discontinuation of therapy. Some of these patients had abnormal liver function tests prior to lovastatin therapy and/or consumed substantial quantities of alcohol.

It is recommended that liver function tests be performed before treatment begins, every 4–6 weeks during the first 15 months of therapy with lovastatin and periodically thereafter in all patients. Special attention should be paid to patients who develop elevated serum transaminase levels, and in these patients, measurements should be repeated promptly and then performed more frequently. If the transaminase levels show evidence of progression, particularly if they rise to three times the upper limit of normal and are persistent, the drug should be discontinued. Liver biopsy should be considered if elevations are persistent beyond the discontinuation of the drug.

TABLE I
FAMILIAL HYPERCHOLESTEROLEMIA STUDY
DOSE RESPONSE OF MEVACOR
(Percent Change from Baseline After 6 Weeks)

DOSAGE	N	TOTAL-C (mean)	LDL-C (mean)	HDL-C (mean)	LDL-C/ HDL-C (mean)	TOTAL-C/ HDL-C (mean)	TRIG. (median)
Placebo	21	−1	−2	+1	−1	0	+3
MEVACOR							
20 mg q.p.m.	20	−18	−19	+10	−26	−24	−7
40 mg q.p.m.	21	−24	−27	+10	−32	−29	−22
10 mg b.i.d.	19	−22	−25	+6	−28	−25	−11
20 mg b.i.d.	20	−27	−31	+12	−38	−34	−18
40 mg b.i.d.	20	−34	−39	+8	−43	−38	−12

TABLE II
NON-FAMILIAL HYPERCHOLESTEROLEMIA STUDY
DOSE RESPONSE OF MEVACOR
(Percent Change from Baseline After 6 Weeks)

DOSAGE	N	TOTAL-C (mean)	LDL-C (mean)	HDL-C (mean)	LDL-C/ HDL-C (mean)	TOTAL-C/ HDL-C (mean)	VLDL-C (median)	TRIG. (median)
Placebo	20	+5	+9	+4	+7	+3	−14	−3
MEVACOR								
20 mg q.p.m.	20	−18	−22	+11	−29	−24	−30	−17
40 mg q.p.m.	20	−19	−21	+4	−20	−19	−31	−20
10 mg b.i.d.	19	−18	−24	+3	−25	−20	−2	−15
20 mg b.i.d.	18	−29	−34	+6	−36	−31	−31	−23
40 mg b.i.d.	21	−32	−39	+13	−46	−39	−31	−27

The drug should be used with caution in patients who consume substantial quantities of alcohol and/or have a past history of liver disease. Active liver disease or unexplained transaminase elevations are contraindications to the use of lovastatin.

As with other lipid-lowering agents, moderate (less than three times the upper limit of normal) elevations of serum transaminases have been reported following therapy with MEVACOR (see ADVERSE REACTIONS). These changes appeared soon after initiation of therapy with MEVACOR, were often transient, were not accompanied by any symptoms and interruption of treatment was not required.

Skeletal Muscle

Several cases of rhabdomyolysis have been associated with lovastatin therapy alone, when combined with immunosuppressive therapy including cyclosporine in cardiac transplant patients, and when combined in non-transplant patients with either gemfibrozil or lipid-lowering doses (≥ 1 g/day) of nicotinic acid. Acute renal failure from rhabdomyolysis has been seen more commonly with the lovastatin-gemfibrozil combination, and has also been reported in transplant patients receiving lovastatin plus cyclosporine.

Rhabdomyolysis with or without renal impairment has been reported in seriously ill patients receiving erythromycin concomitantly with lovastatin. Therefore, patients receiving concomitant lovastatin and erythromycin should be carefully monitored.

Fulminant rhabdomyolysis has been seen as early as three weeks after initiation of combined therapy with gemfibrozil and lovastatin, but may be seen after several months. For these reasons, it is felt that, in most subjects who have had an unsatisfactory lipid response to either drug alone, the possible benefits of combined therapy with lovastatin and gemfibrozil do not outweigh the risks of severe myopathy, rhabdomyolysis, and acute renal failure. While it is not known whether this interaction occurs with fibrates other than gemfibrozil, myopathy and rhabdomyolysis have occasionally been associated with the use of other fibrates alone, including clofibrate. Therefore, the combined use of lovastatin with other fibrates should generally be avoided.

Physicians contemplating combined therapy with lovastatin and lipid-lowering doses of nicotinic acid or with immunosuppressive drugs should carefully weigh the potential benefits and risks and should carefully monitor patients for any signs and symptoms of muscle pain, tenderness, or weakness, particularly during the initial months of therapy and during any periods of upward dosage titration of either drug. Periodic CPK determinations may be considered in such situations, but there is no assurance that such monitoring will prevent the occurrence of severe myopathy. The monitoring of lovastatin drug and metabolite levels may be considered in transplant patients who are treated with immunosuppressives and lovastatin.

Lovastatin therapy should be temporarily withheld or discontinued in any patient with an acute, serious condition suggestive of a myopathy or having a risk factor predisposing to the development of renal failure secondary to rhabdomyolysis, including: severe acute infection, hypotension, major surgery, trauma, severe metabolic, endocrine and electrolyte disorders, and uncontrolled seizures.

Myalgia has been associated with lovastatin therapy. Transient, mildly elevated creatine phosphokinase levels are commonly seen in lovastatin-treated patients. However, in clinical trials, approximately 0.5% of patients developed a myopathy, i.e., myalgia or muscle weakness associated with markedly elevated CPK levels. Myopathy should be considered in any patient with diffuse myalgias, muscle tenderness or weakness, and/or marked elevation of CPK. Patients should be advised to report promptly unexplained muscle pain, tenderness or weakness, particularly if accompanied by malaise or fever. Lovastatin therapy should be discontinued if markedly elevated CPK levels occur or myopathy is diagnosed or suspected.

Most of the patients who have developed myopathy (including rhabdomyolysis) while taking lovastatin were receiving concomitant therapy with immunosuppressive drugs, gemfibrozil or lipid-lowering doses of nicotinic acid. In clinical trials, about 30 percent of patients on concomitant immunosuppressive therapy including cyclosporine developed myopathy; the corresponding percentages for gemfibrozil and niacin were approximately 5 percent and 2 percent respectively.

In six patients with cardiac transplants taking immunosuppressive therapy including cyclosporine concomitantly with lovastatin 20 mg/day, the average plasma level of active metabolites derived from lovastatin was elevated to approximately four times the expected levels. Because of an apparent relationship between increased plasma levels of active metabolites derived from lovastatin and myopathy, the daily dosage in patients taking immunosuppressants should not exceed 20 mg/day (see DOSAGE AND ADMINISTRATION). Even at this dosage, the benefits and risks of using lovastatin in patients taking immunosuppressants should be carefully considered.

PRECAUTIONS

General

Before instituting therapy with MEVACOR, an attempt

TABLE III
MEVACOR vs. Cholestyramine
(Percent Change from Baseline After 12 Weeks)

TREATMENT	N	TOTAL-C (mean)	LDL-C (mean)	HDL-C (mean)	LDL-C/ HDL-C (mean)	TOTAL-C/ HDL-C (mean)	VLDL-C (median)	TRIG. (median)
MEVACOR								
20 mg. b.i.d.	85	−27	−32	+9	−36	−31	−34	−21
40 mg b.i.d.	88	−34	−42	+8	−44	−37	−31	−27
Cholestyramine								
12 g b.i.d.	88	−17	−23	+8	−27	−21	+2	+11

TABLE IV
MEVACOR vs. Probucol
(Percent Change from Baseline After 14 Weeks)

TREATMENT	N	TOTAL-C (mean)	LDL-C (mean)	HDL-C (mean)	LDL-C/ HDL-C (mean)	TOTAL-C/ HDL-C (mean)	VLDL-C (median)	TRIG. (median)
MEVACOR								
40 mg q.p.m.	47	−25	−32	+9	−38	−31	−37	−18
80 mg q.p.m.	49	−30	−37	+11	−42	−36	−27	−17
40 mg b.i.d.	47	−33	−40	+12	−45	−39	−40	−25
Probucol								
500 mg b.i.d.	97	−10	−8	−23	+26	+23	−13	+1

Continued on next page

Information on the Merck Sharp & Dohme products listed on these pages is the full prescribing information from product circulars in use August 31, 1989.

Merck Sharp & Dohme—Cont.

should be made to control hypercholesterolemia with appropriate diet, exercise, weight reduction in obese patients, and to treat other underlying medical problems (see INDICATIONS AND USAGE).

Eye

There was a high prevalence of baseline lenticular opacities in the patient population included in the clinical trials with lovastatin. During these trials the appearance of new opacities was noted. The causal relationship of lovastatin to these findings has not been established.

Of 431 patients examined with slit lamp at baseline and during therapy with lovastatin, 34 had opacities reported at the final examination (5–15 months after starting lovastatin) that were not noted at baseline. On the other hand, in 45 patients, opacities observed at baseline were not noted at the final examination, so that the prevalence did not increase.

Patients with Lens Opacities

N	Baseline(%)	New	Lost	Final Exam(%)
431	147 (34.1%)	34	45	136 (31.6%)

There was no clinically significant change in visual acuity in the patients who had new opacities reported, nor was any patient, including those with opacities noted at baseline, discontinued from therapy because of a decrease in visual acuity. Nevertheless, until further experience is obtained, it is recommended that patients placed on lovastatin therapy be examined with a slit lamp before or shortly after initiation of treatment, and annually thereafter.

Homozygous Familial Hypercholesterolemia

MEVACOR is less effective in patients with the rare homozygous familial hypercholesterolemia, possibly because these patients have no functional LDL receptors. MEVACOR appears to be more likely to raise serum transaminases (see ADVERSE REACTIONS) in these homozygous patients.

Drug Interactions

Immunosuppressive Drugs, Gemfibrozil, Niacin (Nicotinic Acid), Erythromycin: See WARNINGS, *Skeletal Muscle*.

Coumarin Anticoagulants: In a clinical trial in warfarin-treated patients designed specifically to observe a potential effect of lovastatin on the prothrombin time, lovastatin in dosages up to 40 mg b.i.d. did not produce any consistent alteration of the anticoagulant action of warfarin. However, since the drug was marketed, clinically evident bleeding and/or increased prothrombin time have been reported in a few patients taking coumarin anticoagulants concomitantly with lovastatin. The causal relationship to lovastatin is unclear. Nevertheless, it is recommended that in patients taking anticoagulants, prothrombin time be determined before starting lovastatin and frequently enough during early therapy to insure that no significant alteration of prothrombin time occurs. Once a stable prothrombin time has been documented, prothrombin times can be monitored at the intervals usually recommended for patients on coumarin anticoagulants. If the dose of lovastatin is changed, the same procedure should be repeated. Lovastatin therapy has not been associated with bleeding or with changes in prothrombin time in patients not taking anticoagulants.

Antipyrine: Antipyrine is a model for drugs metabolized by the microsomal hepatic enzyme system (cytochrome P450 system). Because lovastatin had no effect on the pharmacokinetics of antipyrine, interactions with other drugs metabolized via this mechanism are not expected.

Propranolol: In normal volunteers, there was no clinically significant pharmacokinetic or pharmacodynamic interaction with concomitant administration of single doses of lovastatin and propranolol.

Digoxin: In patients with hypercholesterolemia, concomitant administration of lovastatin and digoxin resulted in no effect on digoxin plasma concentrations.

Other Concomitant Therapy: Although specific interaction studies were not performed, in clinical studies, lovastatin was used concomitantly with beta blockers, calcium channel blockers, diuretics and nonsteroidal anti-inflammatory drugs (NSAIDs) without evidence of clinically significant adverse interactions.

Drug/Laboratory Test Interactions

Lovastatin may elevate creatine phosphokinase and transaminase levels (see ADVERSE REACTIONS). This should be considered in the differential diagnosis of chest pain in a patient on therapy with lovastatin.

Carcinogenesis, Mutagenesis, Impairment of Fertility

In a 21-month carcinogenic study in mice, a statistically significant (p < 0.05) increase in the incidence of hepatocellular carcinomas and adenomas was observed at doses of 500 mg/kg/day (312 times the maximum recommended human dose) of lovastatin. These changes were not seen in mice given doses of 20 and 100 mg/kg/day (12.5 and 62.5 times the maximum recommended human dose).

A statistically significant increase (p ≤ 0.05) in the incidence of pulmonary adenomas was seen in female mice receiving 500 mg/kg/day (312 times the maximum recommended human dose); no similar changes were seen in males at any dose or in females receiving 20 or 100 mg/kg/day (12.5 or 62.5 times the maximum recommended human dose). Because the incidence of pulmonary tumors was within the range of untreated animals in studies of similar duration, the relationship of this latter change to treatment is not known.

In addition, an increase in the incidence of papilloma in the non-glandular mucosa of the stomach was observed in mice receiving 100 and 500 mg/kg/day (62.5 and 312 times the maximum recommended human dose); no increase was seen at a dosage of 20 mg/kg/day (12.5 times the maximum recommended human dose). The glandular mucosa was not affected. The human stomach contains only glandular mucosa. Importantly, there is a strong association between this change and hyperplasia of the squamous epithelium (acanthosis) in this region; acanthosis is a characteristic change observed in the non-glandular mucosa of rodents treated with HMG-CoA reductase inhibitors and is most probably a result of inhibition of the reductase in this tissue.

Similar squamous epithelium is found in the esophagus and ano-rectal junction of the mouse and rat; however, no evidence of a similar drug-induced hyperplastic response was observed in these tissues in studies of up to 21 months in the mouse given up to 500 mg/kg/day (312 times the maximum recommended human dose), or in a study of 24 months in the rat given 180 mg/kg/day (112 times the maximum recommended human dose).

In a 24 month carcinogenicity study in rats, there was a positive dose response relationship for hepatocellular carcinogenicity in males (unadjusted p=0.025). However, because the incidence of hepatocellular carcinogenicity observed in male rats in this study is similar to that observed spontaneously in this strain of rat, the implications of this finding are unclear. No evidence of mutagenicity was observed in a microbial mutagen test using mutant strains of *Salmonella typhimurium* with or without rat or mouse liver metabolic activation. In addition, no evidence of damage to genetic material was noted in an *in vitro* alkaline elution assay using rat or mouse hepatocytes, a V-79 mammalian cell forward mutation study, an *in vitro* chromosome aberration study in CHO cells, or an *in vivo* chromosomal aberration assay in mouse bone marrow.

No drug related effects on fertility were found in studies with rats.

Pregnancy

Pregnancy Category X

See CONTRAINDICATIONS.

Lovastatin has been shown to produce skeletal malformations in the rat fetus at doses of 800 mg/kg/day (500 times the maximum recommended human dose). At similar doses in mice, an increase in skeletal malformations was observed. These individual changes are within the range of those observed spontaneously in this strain of mouse. No drug-induced changes were seen in either species at doses of up to 80 mg/kg/day (50 times the maximum recommended human dose). No evidence of malformations was noted in rabbits at up to 15 mg/kg/day (highest tolerated dose—about 9 times the maximum recommended human dose). There are no data in pregnant women.

Nursing Mothers

Studies in rats have shown that lovastatin is excreted in the milk. It is not known whether this drug is excreted in human milk. Because many drugs are excreted in human milk and because of the potential for serious adverse reactions in nursing infants from MEVACOR, women taking lovastatin should not nurse their infants (see CONTRAINDICATIONS).

Pediatric Use

Safety and effectiveness in children have not been established. Because children are not likely to benefit from cholesterol lowering for at least a decade and because experience with this drug is limited (no studies in subjects below the age of 20 years), treatment of children with lovastatin is not recommended at this time.

ADVERSE REACTIONS

MEVACOR is generally well tolerated; adverse reactions usually have been mild and transient. Less than 1% of patients were discontinued from controlled clinical studies due to adverse experiences attributable to MEVACOR. About 2% of patients were discontinued from all studies (controlled and uncontrolled) due to adverse experiences attributable to MEVACOR; about one-third of these patients were discontinued due to increases in serum transaminases.

Clinical Adverse Experiences

Adverse experiences reported in patients treated with MEVACOR in controlled clinical studies are shown in the table below:

Laboratory Tests

Marked persistent increases of serum transaminases have been noted (see WARNINGS).

About 11% of patients had elevations of creatine phosphokinase (CPK) levels of at least twice the normal value on one or more occasions. The corresponding values for the control agents were cholestyramine, 9 percent and probucol, 2 percent. This was attributable to the noncardiac fraction of CPK. Large increases in CPK have sometimes been reported (see WARNINGS, *Skeletal Muscle*).

Concomitant Therapy

In controlled clinical studies in which lovastatin was administered concomitantly with cholestyramine, no adverse reactions peculiar to this concomitant treatment were observed. The adverse reactions that occurred were limited to those reported previously with lovastatin or cholestyramine. Other lipid-lowering agents were not administered concomitantly with lovastatin during controlled clinical studies. In uncontrolled clinical studies, most of the patients who have developed myopathy were receiving concomitant therapy with immunosuppressive drugs, gemfibrozil or niacin (nicotinic acid) (see WARNINGS, *Skeletal Muscle*).

Uncontrolled Clinical Studies

The adverse experiences observed in uncontrolled studies were similar to those seen in controlled clinical studies. Abnormal liver function tests were observed at a higher incidence than in the controlled studies (see WARNINGS, *Liver Dysfunction*). Myopathy (myalgia with marked CPK elevations) was reported in approximately 0.5 percent of patients (see WARNINGS, *Skeletal Muscle*).

Causal Relationship Unclear

Nervous System

Peripheral neuropathy has been reported; the relationship to lovastatin is uncertain. Visual evoked response, nerve conduction measurements and electromyography in over 30 patients showed no evidence of neurotoxic effects of lovastatin.

Special Senses

Of 431 patients examined with slit lamp at baseline and during therapy with lovastatin, 34 had opacities reported at the final examination (5–15 months after starting lovastatin) that were not noted at baseline. On the other hand, in 45 patients, opacities observed at baseline were not noted at the final examination, so that the prevalence did not increase (see PRECAUTIONS).

Post-Marketing Experience

Additional adverse experiences occurring since the drug was marketed are listed below.

	MEVACOR (N = 613) %	Placebo (N = 82) %	Cholestyramine (N = 88) %	Probucol (N = 97) %
Gastrointestinal				
Constipation	4.9	—	34.1	2.1
Diarrhea	5.5	4.9	8.0	10.3
Dyspepsia	3.9	—	13.6	3.1
Flatus	6.4	2.4	21.6	2.1
Abdominal pain/cramps	5.7	2.4	5.7	5.2
Heartburn	1.6	—	8.0	—
Nausea	4.7	3.7	9.1	6.2
Musculoskeletal				
Muscle cramps	1.1	—	1.1	—
Myalgia	2.4	1.2	—	—
Nervous System/Psychiatric				
Dizziness	2.0	1.2	—	1.0
Headache	9.3	4.9	4.5	8.2
Skin				
Rash/pruritus	5.2	—	4.5	—
Special Senses				
Blurred vision	1.5	—	1.1	3.1
Dysgeusia	0.8	—	1.1	—

Clinical Adverse Experiences
Gastrointestinal: Hepatitis, cholestatic jaundice, anorexia, vomiting.
Hypersensitivity Reactions: An apparent hypersensitivity syndrome has been reported rarely which has included one or more of the following features: anaphylaxis, angioedema, lupus-like syndrome, polymyalgia rheumatica, thrombocytopenia, leukopenia, hemolytic anemia, positive ANA, ESR increase, arthritis, arthralgia, urticaria, asthenia, and photosensitivity.
Nervous System/Psychiatric: Paresthesia.
Causal Relationship Unknown
Gastrointestinal: Pancreatitis, stomatitis.
Skin: Alopecia.
Nervous System/Psychiatric: Depression, insomnia.
Metabolic: Edema.
Clinical Laboratory Test Findings
Liver Function Tests: Liver function test abnormalities, including elevated alkaline phosphatase and bilirubin.

OVERDOSAGE

The oral LD_{50} of MEVACOR in mice is 20 g/kg.
Five healthy human volunteers have received up to 200 mg of lovastatin as a single dose without clinically significant adverse experiences. A few cases of accidental overdosage have been reported; no patients had any specific symptoms, and all patients recovered without sequelae. The maximum dose taken was fifty-two 20 mg tablets (1.04 g).
Until further experience is obtained, no specific treatment of overdosage with MEVACOR can be recommended.
The dialyzability of lovastatin and its metabolites in man is not known at present.

DOSAGE AND ADMINISTRATION

The patient should be placed on a standard cholesterol-lowing diet before receiving MEVACOR and should continue on this diet during treatment with MEVACOR. MEVACOR should be given with meals.
The recommended starting dose is 20 mg once a day given with the evening meal. The recommended dosing range is 20–80 mg/day in single or divided doses; the maximum recommended dose is 80 mg/day. Adjustments of dosage should be made at intervals of 4 weeks or more. Doses should be individualized according to the patient's response (see Tables I to IV under CLINICAL PHARMACOLOGY, *Clinical Studies* for dose response results).
For those patients with severely elevated serum cholesterol levels (i.e., > 300 mg/dL [7.8 mmol/L] on diet), MEVACOR may be initiated at 40 mg/day.
In patients taking immunosuppressive drugs concomitantly with lovastatin (see WARNINGS, *Skeletal Muscle*), the maximum recommended dosage is 20 mg/day.
Cholesterol levels should be monitored periodically and consideration should be given to reducing the dosage of MEVACOR if cholesterol levels fall below the targeted range.
Concomitant Therapy
Preliminary evidence suggests that the cholesterol-lowering effects of lovastatin and the bile acid sequestrant, cholestyramine, are additive.
Dosage in Patients with Renal Insufficiency
Because MEVACOR does not undergo significant renal excretion, modification of dosage should not be necessary in patients with renal insufficiency.

HOW SUPPLIED

No. 3561—Tablets MEVACOR 20 mg are light blue, octagonal tablets, coded MSD 731. They are supplied as follows:
NDC 0006-0731-61 unit of use bottles of 60
(6505-01-267-2497, 20 mg 60's)
NDC 0006-0731-28 unit dose packages of 100.
   Shown in Product Identification Section, page 418
No. 3562—Tablets MEVACOR 40 mg are green, octagonal tablets, coded MSD 732. They are supplied as follows:
NDC 0006-0732-61 unit of use bottles of 60.
   Shown in Product Identification Section, page 418
Storage
Store between 5–30°C (41–86°F). Tablets MEVACOR 20 mg must be protected from light and stored in a well-closed, light-resistant container.
Distributed by:
MERCK SHARP & DOHME
DIV OF MERCK & CO., INC.,
WEST POINT, PA 19486, USA
Manufactured by:
MERCK SHARP & DOHME, CAGUAS,
Division of Merck Sharp & Dohme
Quimica de Puerto Rico, Inc.
Caguas, Puerto Rico, 00626
Certain manufacturing operations
have been performed by other firms.

A.H.F.S. Category: 24:06
DC 7526507 Issued March 1989
COPYRIGHT © MERCK & CO., INC., 1987, 1989
All rights reserved

MIDAMOR® Tablets   ℞
(Amiloride HCl, MSD), U.S.P.

DESCRIPTION

Amiloride HCl, an antikaliuretic-diuretic agent, is a pyrazine-carbonyl-guanidine that is unrelated chemically to other known antikaliuretic or diuretic agents. It is the salt of a moderately strong base (pKa 8.7). It is designated chemically as 3,5-diamino-6-chloro-N-(diaminomethylene) pyrazinecarboxamide monohydrochloride, dihydrate and has a molecular weight of 302.14. Its empirical formula is $C_6H_8ClN_7O \cdot HCl \cdot 2H_2O$ and its structural formula is:

MIDAMOR® (Amiloride HCl, MSD) is available for oral use as tablets containing 5 mg of anhydrous amiloride HCl. Each tablet contains the following inactive ingredients: calcium phosphate, D&C Yellow 10, iron oxide, lactose, magnesium stearate and starch.

CLINICAL PHARMACOLOGY

MIDAMOR is a potassium-conserving (antikaliuretic) drug that possesses weak (compared with thiazide diuretics) natriuretic, diuretic, and antihypertensive activity. These effects have been partially additive to the effects of thiazide diuretics in some clinical studies. When administered with a thiazide or loop diuretic, MIDAMOR has been shown to decrease the enhanced urinary excretion of magnesium which occurs when a thiazide or loop diuretic is used alone. MIDAMOR has potassium-conserving activity in patients receiving kaliuretic-diuretic agents.
MIDAMOR is not an aldosterone antagonist and its effects are seen even in the absence of aldosterone.
MIDAMOR exerts its potassium sparing effect through the inhibition of sodium reabsorption at the distal convoluted tubule, cortical collecting tubule and collecting duct; this decreases the net negative potential of the tubular lumen and reduces both potassium and hydrogen secretion and their subsequent excretion. This mechanism accounts in large part for the potassium sparing action of amiloride.
MIDAMOR usually begins to act within 2 hours after an oral dose. Its effect on electrolyte excretion reaches a peak between 6 and 10 hours and lasts about 24 hours. Peak plasma levels are obtained in 3 to 4 hours and the plasma half-life varies from 6 to 9 hours. Effects on electrolytes increase with single doses of amiloride HCl up to approximately 15 mg. Amiloride HCl is not metabolized by the liver but is excreted unchanged by the kidneys. About 50 percent of a 20 mg dose of MIDAMOR is excreted in the urine and 40 percent in the stool within 72 hours. MIDAMOR has little effect on glomerular filtration rate or renal blood flow. Because amiloride HCl is not metabolized by the liver, drug accumulation is not anticipated in patients with hepatic dysfunction, but accumulation can occur if the hepatorenal syndrome develops.

INDICATIONS AND USAGE

MIDAMOR is indicated as adjunctive treatment with thiazide diuretics or other kaliuretic-diuretic agents in congestive heart failure or hypertension to:
  a. help restore normal serum potassium levels in patients who develop hypokalemia on the kaliuretic diuretic
  b. prevent development of hypokalemia in patients who would be exposed to particular risk if hypokalemia were to develop, e.g., digitalized patients or patients with significant cardiac arrhythmias.
The use of potassium-conserving agents is often unnecessary in patients receiving diuretics for uncomplicated essential hypertension when such patients have a normal diet.
MIDAMOR has little additive diuretic or antihypertensive effect when added to a thiazide diuretic.
MIDAMOR should rarely be used alone. It has weak (compared with thiazides) diuretic and antihypertensive effects. Used as single agents, potassium sparing diuretics, including MIDAMOR, result in an increased risk of hyperkalemia (approximately 10% with amiloride). MIDAMOR should be used alone only when persistent hypokalemia has been documented and only with careful titration of the dose and close monitoring of serum electrolytes.

CONTRAINDICATIONS

Hyperkalemia
MIDAMOR should not be used in the presence of elevated serum potassium levels (greater than 5.5 mEq per liter).

Antikaliuretic Therapy or Potassium Supplementation
MIDAMOR should not be given to patients receiving other potassium-conserving agents, such as spironolactone or triamterene. Potassium supplementation in the form of medication, potassium-containing salt substitutes or a potassium-rich diet should not be used with MIDAMOR except in severe and/or refractory cases of hypokalemia. Such concomitant therapy can be associated with rapid increases in serum potassium levels. If potassium supplementation is used, careful monitoring of the serum potassium level is necessary.
Impaired Renal Function
Anuria, acute or chronic renal insufficiency, and evidence of diabetic nephropathy are contraindications to the use of MIDAMOR. Patients with evidence of renal functional impairment (blood urea nitrogen [BUN] levels over 30 mg per 100 mL or serum creatinine levels over 1.5 mg per 100 mL) or diabetes mellitus should not receive the drug without careful, frequent and continuing monitoring of serum electrolytes, creatinine, and BUN levels. Potassium retention associated with the use of an antikaliuretic agent is accentuated in the presence of renal impairment and may result in the rapid development of hyperkalemia.
Hypersensitivity
MIDAMOR is contraindicated in patients who are hypersensitive to this product.

WARNINGS

Hyperkalemia

> Like other potassium-conserving agents, amiloride may cause hyperkalemia (serum potassium levels greater than 5.5 mEq per liter) which, if uncorrected, is potentially fatal. Hyperkalemia occurs commonly (about 10%) when amiloride is used without a kaliuretic diuretic. This incidence is greater in patients with renal impairment, diabetes mellitus (with or without recognized renal insufficiency), and in the elderly. When MIDAMOR is used concomitantly with a thiazide diuretic in patients without these complications, the risk of hyperkalemia is reduced to about 1–2 percent. It is thus essential to monitor serum potassium levels carefully in any patient receiving amiloride, particularly when it is first introduced, at the time of diuretic dosage adjustments, and during any illness that could affect renal function.

The risk of hyperkalemia may be increased when potassium-conserving agents, including MIDAMOR, are administered concomitantly with an angiotensin-converting enzyme inhibitor. (See PRECAUTIONS, *Drug Interactions.*) Warning signs or symptoms of hyperkalemia include paresthesias, muscular weakness, fatigue, flaccid paralysis of the extremities, bradycardia, shock, and ECG abnormalities. Monitoring of the serum potassium level is essential because mild hyperkalemia is not usually associated with an abnormal ECG. When abnormal, the ECG in hyperkalemia is characterized primarily by tall, peaked T waves or elevations from previous tracings. There may also be lowering of the R wave and increased depth of the S wave, widening and even disappearance of the P wave, progressive widening of the QRS complex, prolongation of the PR interval, and ST depression.
Treatment of hyperkalemia: If hyperkalemia occurs in patients taking MIDAMOR, the drug should be discontinued immediately. If the serum potassium level exceeds 6.5 mEq per liter, active measures should be taken to reduce it. Such measures include the intravenous administration of sodium bicarbonate solution or oral or parenteral glucose with a rapid-acting insulin preparation. If needed, a cation exchange resin such as sodium polystyrene sulfonate may be given orally or by enema. Patients with persistent hyperkalemia may require dialysis.
Diabetes Mellitus
In diabetic patients, hyperkalemia has been reported with the use of all potassium-conserving diuretics, including MIDAMOR, even in patients without evidence of diabetic nephropathy. Therefore, MIDAMOR should be avoided, if possible, in diabetic patients and, if it is used, serum electrolytes and renal function must be monitored frequently. MIDAMOR should be discontinued at least three days before glucose tolerance testing.
Metabolic or Respiratory Acidosis
Antikaliuretic therapy should be instituted only with caution in severely ill patients in whom respiratory or metabolic acidosis may occur, such as patients with cardiopulmonary disease or poorly controlled diabetes. If MIDAMOR is given to these patients, frequent monitoring of acid-base balance is

Continued on next page

Information on the Merck Sharp & Dohme products listed on these pages is the full prescribing information from product circulars in use August 31, 1989.

Merck Sharp & Dohme—Cont.

necessary. Shifts in acid-base balance alter the ratio of extracellular/intracellular potassium, and the development of acidosis may be associated with rapid increases in serum potassium levels.

PRECAUTIONS

General
Electrolyte Imbalance and BUN Increases
Hyponatremia and hypochloremia may occur when MIDAMOR is used with other diuretics and increases in BUN levels have been reported. These increases usually have accompanied vigorous fluid elimination, especially when diuretic therapy was used in seriously ill patients, such as those who had hepatic cirrhosis with ascites and metabolic alkalosis, or those with resistant edema. Therefore, when MIDAMOR is given with other diuretics to such patients, careful monitoring of serum electrolytes and BUN levels is important. In patients with pre-existing severe liver disease, hepatic encephalopathy, manifested by tremors, confusion, and coma, and increased jaundice, have been reported in association with diuretics, including amiloride HCl.

Drug Interactions
When amiloride HCl is administered concomitantly with an angiotensin-converting enzyme inhibitor, the risk of hyperkalemia may be increased. Therefore, if concomitant use of these agents is indicated because of demonstrated hypokalemia, they should be used with caution and with frequent monitoring of serum potassium. (See WARNINGS.)
Lithium generally should not be given with diuretics because they reduce its renal clearance and add a high risk of lithium toxicity. Read circulars for lithium preparations before use of such concomitant therapy.
In some patients, the administration of a non-steroidal anti-inflammatory agent can reduce the diuretic, natriuretic, and antihypertensive effects of loop, potassium-sparing and thiazide diuretics. Therefore, when MIDAMOR and non-steroidal anti-inflammatory agents are used concomitantly, the patient should be observed closely to determine if the desired effect of the diuretic is obtained. Since indomethacin and potassium-sparing diuretics, including MIDAMOR, each may be associated with increased serum potassium levels, the potential effects on potassium kinetics and renal function should be considered when these agents are administered concurrently.

Carcinogenicity, Mutagenicity, Impairment of Fertility
There was no evidence of a tumorigenic effect when amiloride HCl was administered for 92 weeks to mice at doses up to 10 mg/kg/day (25 times the maximum daily human dose). Amiloride HCl has also been administered for 104 weeks to male and female rats at doses up to 6 and 8 mg/kg/day (15 and 20 times the maximum daily dose for humans, respectively) and showed no evidence of carcinogenicity.
Amiloride HCl was devoid of mutagenic activity in various strains of *Salmonella typhimurium* with or without a mammalian liver microsomal activation system (Ames test).

Pregnancy
Pregnancy Category B. Teratogenicity studies with amiloride HCl in rabbits and mice given 20 and 25 times the maximum human dose, respectively, revealed no evidence of harm to the fetus, although studies showed that the drug crossed the placenta in modest amounts. Reproduction studies in rats at 20 times the expected maximum daily dose for humans showed no evidence of impaired fertility. At approximately 5 or more times the expected maximum daily dose for humans, some toxicity was seen in adult rats and rabbits and a decrease in rat pup growth and survival occurred. There are, however, no adequate and well-controlled studies in pregnant women. Because animal reproduction studies are not always predictive of human response, this drug should be used during pregnancy only if clearly needed.

Nursing Mothers
Studies in rats have shown that amiloride is excreted in milk in concentrations higher than that found in blood, but it is not known whether MIDAMOR is excreted in human milk. Because many drugs are excreted in human milk and because of the potential for serious adverse reactions in nursing infants from MIDAMOR, a decision should be made whether to discontinue nursing or to discontinue the drug, taking into account the importance of the drug to the mother.

Pediatric Use
Safety and effectiveness in children have not been established.

ADVERSE REACTIONS

MIDAMOR is usually well tolerated and, except for hyperkalemia (serum potassium levels greater than 5.5 mEq per liter—see WARNINGS), significant adverse effects have been reported infrequently. Minor adverse reactions were reported relatively frequently (about 20%) but the relationship of many of the reports to amiloride HCl is uncertain and the

overall frequency was similar in hydrochlorothiazide treated groups. Nausea/anorexia, abdominal pain, flatulence, and mild skin rash have been reported and probably are related to amiloride. Other adverse experiences that have been reported with amiloride are generally those known to be associated with diuresis, or with the underlying disease being treated.
The adverse reactions for MIDAMOR listed in the following table have been arranged into two groups: (1) incidence greater than one percent; and (2) incidence one percent or less. The incidence for group (1) was determined from clinical studies conducted in the United States (837 patients treated with MIDAMOR). The adverse effects listed in group (2) include reports from the same clinical studies and voluntary reports since marketing. The probability of a causal relationship exists between MIDAMOR and these adverse reactions, some of which have been reported only rarely.

Incidence > 1%	Incidence ≤ 1%
Body as a Whole	
Headache*	Back pain
Weakness	Chest pain
Fatigability	Neck/shoulder ache
	Pain, extremities
Cardiovascular	
None	Angina pectoris
	Orthostatic hypotension
	Arrhythmia
	Palpitation
Digestive	
Nausea/anorexia*	Jaundice
Diarrhea*	GI bleeding
Vomiting*	Abdominal fullness
Abdominal pain	GI disturbance
Gas pain	Thirst
Appetite changes	Heartburn
Constipation	Flatulence
	Dyspepsia
Metabolic	
Elevated serum potassium levels (> 5.5 mEq per liter)†	None
Integumentary	
None	Skin rash
	Itching
	Dryness of mouth
	Pruritus
	Alopecia
Musculoskeletal	
Muscle cramps	Joint pain
	Leg ache
Nervous	
Dizziness	Paresthesia
Encephalopathy	Tremors
	Vertigo
Psychiatric	
None	Nervousness
	Mental confusion
	Insomnia
	Decreased libido
	Depression
	Somnolence
Respiratory	
Cough	Shortness of breath
Dyspnea	
Special Senses	
None	Visual disturbances
	Nasal congestion
	Tinnitus
	Increased intraocular pressure
Urogenital	
Impotence	Polyuria
	Dysuria
	Urinary frequency
	Bladder spasms

Causal Relationship Unknown
Other reactions have been reported but occurred under circumstances where a causal relationship could not be established. However, in these rarely reported events, that possibility cannot be excluded. Therefore, these observations are listed to serve as alerting information to physicians.

*   Reactions occurring in 3% to 8% of patients treated with MIDAMOR. (Those reactions occurring in less than 3% of the patients are unmarked.)
†   See WARNINGS.

Activation of probable pre-existing peptic ulcer
Aplastic anemia
Neutropenia
Abnormal liver function

OVERDOSAGE

No data are available in regard to overdosage in humans. The oral LD_{50} of amiloride hydrochloride (calculated as the base) is 56 mg/kg in mice and 36 to 85 mg/kg in rats, depending on the strain.
It is not known whether the drug is dialyzable.
The most likely signs and symptoms to be expected with overdosage are dehydration and electrolyte imbalance. These can be treated by established procedures. Therapy with MIDAMOR should be discontinued and the patient observed closely. There is no specific antidote. Emesis should be induced or gastric lavage performed. Treatment is symptomatic and supportive. If hyperkalemia occurs, active measures should be taken to reduce the serum potassium levels.

DOSAGE AND ADMINISTRATION

MIDAMOR should be administered with food.
MIDAMOR, one 5 mg tablet daily, should be added to the usual antihypertensive or diuretic dosage of a kaliuretic diuretic. The dosage may be increased to 10 mg per day, if necessary. More than two 5 mg tablets of MIDAMOR daily usually are not needed, and there is little controlled experience with such doses. If persistent hypokalemia is documented with 10 mg, the dose can be increased to 15 mg, then 20 mg, with careful monitoring of electrolytes.
In treating patients with congestive heart failure after an initial diuresis has been achieved, potassium loss may also decrease and the need for MIDAMOR should be reevaluated. Dosage adjustment may be necessary. Maintenance therapy may be on an intermittent basis.
If it is necessary to use MIDAMOR alone (see INDICATIONS), the starting dosage should be one 5 mg tablet daily. This dosage may be increased to 10 mg per day, if necessary. More than two 5 mg tablets usually are not needed, and there is little controlled experience with such doses. If persistent hypokalemia is documented with 10 mg, the dose can be increased to 15 mg, then 20 mg, with careful monitoring of electrolytes.

HOW SUPPLIED

No. 3381—Tablets MIDAMOR, 5 mg, are yellow, diamond-shaped, compressed tablets, coded MSD 92. They are supplied as follows:
NDC 0006-0092-68 bottles of 100.
    Shown in Product Identification Section, page 418
Storage
Protect from moisture, freezing and excessive heat.
      A.H.F.S. Category: 40:28
      DC 7212513   Issued May 1988
COPYRIGHT © MERCK & CO., INC., 1985
All rights reserved

MINTEZOL® Chewable Tablets   ℞
(Thiabendazole, MSD), U.S.P.

MINTEZOL® Suspension   ℞
(Thiabendazole, MSD), U.S.P.

DESCRIPTION

MINTEZOL® (Thiabendazole, MSD) is an anthelmintic provided as 500 mg chewable tablets, and as a suspension, containing 500 mg thiabendazole per 5 mL. The suspension also contains sorbic acid 0.1% added as a preservative. Inactive ingredients in the tablets are acacia, calcium phosphate, flavors, lactose, magnesium stearate, mannitol, methylcellulose, and sodium saccharin. Inactive ingredients in the suspension are an antifoam agent, flavors, polysorbate, purified water, sorbitol solution, and tragacanth.
Thiabendazole is a white to off-white odorless powder with a molecular weight of 201.26, which is practically insoluble in water but readily soluble in dilute acid and alkali. Its chemical name is 2-(4-thiazolyl)-1*H*-benzimidazole. The empirical formula is $C_{10}H_7N_3S$ and the structural formula is:

CLINICAL PHARMACOLOGY

In man, thiabendazole is rapidly absorbed and peak plasma concentration is reached within 1 to 2 hours after the oral administration of a suspension. It is metabolized almost completely to the 5-hydroxy form which appears in the urine as glucuronide or sulfate conjugates. In 48 hours, about 5% of the administered dose is recovered from the feces and about 90% from the urine. Most is excreted in the first 24 hours.

Mechanism of Action

The precise mode of action of thiabendazole on the parasite is unknown, but it may inhibit the helminth-specific enzyme fumarate reductase.

Thiabendazole is vermicidal and/or vermifugal against *Ascaris lumbricoides* ("common roundworm"), *Strongyloides stercoralis* (threadworm), *Necator americanus*, and *Ancylostoma duodenale* (hookworm), *Trichuris trichiura* (whipworm), *Ancylostoma braziliense* (dog and cat hookworm), *Toxocara canis* and *Toxocara cati* (ascarids), and *Enterobius vermicularis* (pinworm).

Its effect on larvae of *Trichinella spiralis* that have migrated to muscle is questionable.

Thiabendazole also suppresses egg and/or larval production and may inhibit the subsequent development of those eggs or larvae which are passed in the feces.

INDICATIONS AND USAGE

MINTEZOL is indicated for the treatment of:
    Strongyloidiasis (threadworm)
    Cutaneous larva migrans (creeping eruption)
    Visceral larva migrans
    Trichinosis: Relief of symptoms and fever and a reduction of eosinophilia have followed the use of MINTEZOL during the invasion stage of the disease.

Although not indicated as primary therapy, when enterobiasis (pinworm) occurs with any of the conditions listed above, additional therapy is not required for most patients. MINTEZOL should be used only in the following infestations when more specific therapy is not available or cannot be used or when further therapy with a second agent is desirable: Uncinariasis (hookworm: *Necator americanus* and *Ancylostoma duodenale*); Trichuriasis (whipworm); Ascariasis (large roundworm).

CONTRAINDICATION

Hypersensitivity to this product.

WARNINGS

If hypersensitivity reactions occur, the drug should be discontinued immediately and not be resumed. Erythema multiforme has been associated with thiabendazole therapy; in severe cases (Stevens-Johnson syndrome), fatalities have occurred.

Because CNS side effects may occur quite frequently, activities requiring mental alertness should be avoided.

PRECAUTIONS

General

MINTEZOL is not suitable for the treatment of mixed infections with ascaris because it may cause these worms to migrate.

Ideally, supportive therapy is indicated for anemic, dehydrated or malnourished patients prior to initiation of the anthelmintic therapy.

In the presence of hepatic or renal dysfunction, patients should be carefully monitored.

MINTEZOL should be used only in patients in whom susceptible worm infestation has been diagnosed and should not be used prophylactically.

Information for Patients

Because CNS side effects may occur quite frequently, activities requiring mental alertness should be avoided.

Laboratory Tests

Rarely, a transient rise in cephalin flocculation and SGOT has occurred in patients receiving MINTEZOL.

Drug Interactions

Thiabendazole may compete with other drugs, such as theophylline, for sites of metabolism in the liver, thus elevating the serum levels of such compounds to potentially toxic levels. Therefore, when concomitant use of thiabendazole and xanthine derivatives is anticipated, it may be necessary to monitor blood levels and/or reduce the dosage of such compounds. Such concomitant use should be administered under careful medical supervision.

Carcinogenesis, Mutagenesis, Impairment of Fertility

Thiabendazole has been used in numerous short- and long-term studies in animals at doses up to 15 times the usual human dose and was without carcinogenic effects. It did not adversely affect fertility in the mouse at $2\frac{1}{2}$ times the usual human dose or in the rat at a dose equivalent to the usual human dose. Thiabendazole had no mutagenic activity in *in vitro* microbial mutagen test, the micronucleus test and the host mediated assay *in vivo*.

Pregnancy

Pregnancy Category C: Reproduction and teratogenic studies done in the rabbit at a dose up to 15 times the usual human dose, in the rat at a dose equivalent to the human dose, and in the mouse at a dose up to $2\frac{1}{2}$ times the usual human dose, revealed no evidence of harm to the fetus. In an addi-

Therapeutic Regimens

Indication	Regimen	Comments
*STRONGYLOIDIASIS	2 doses per day for 2 successive days.	A single dose of 20 mg/lb or 50 mg/kg may be employed as an alternative schedule, but a higher incidence of side effects should be expected.
CUTANEOUS LARVA MIGRANS (Creeping Eruption)	2 doses per day for 2 successive days.	If active lesions are still present 2 days after completion of therapy, a second course is recommended.
VISCERAL LARVA MIGRANS	2 doses per day for 7 successive days.	Safety and efficacy data on the seven-day treatment course are limited.
*TRICHINOSIS	2 doses per day for 2–4 successive days according to the response of the patient.	The optimal dosage for the treatment of trichinosis has not been established.
Other Indications * Intestinal roundworms (including Ascariasis, Uncinariasis and Trichuriasis)	2 doses per day for 2 successive days.	A single dose of 20 mg/lb or 50 mg/kg may be employed as an alternative schedule, but a higher incidence of side effects should be expected.

* Clinical experience with thiabendazole for treatment of each of these conditions in children weighing less than 30 lbs has been limited.

tional study in the mouse, no defects were observed when thiabendazole was given in an aqueous suspension, at a dose 10 times the usual human dose; however, cleft palate and axial skeletal defects were observed when thiabendazole was suspended in olive oil and given at the same dose. There are no adequate and well controlled studies in pregnant women. MINTEZOL should be used during pregnancy only if the potential benefit justifies the potential risk to the fetus.

Nursing Mothers

It is not known whether this drug is excreted in human milk. Because of the potential for serious adverse reactions in nursing infants from MINTEZOL, a decision should be made whether to discontinue nursing or to discontinue the drug, taking into account the importance of the drug to the mother.

Pediatric Use

The safety and effectiveness of thiabendazole for the treatment of Strongyloidiasis, Ascariasis, Uncinariasis, Trichuriasis and Trichinosis in children weighing less than 30 lbs has been limited.

ADVERSE REACTIONS

Gastrointestinal: anorexia, nausea, vomiting, diarrhea, epigastric distress, jaundice, cholestasis and parenchymal liver damage.

Central Nervous System: dizziness, weariness, drowsiness, giddiness, headache, numbness, hyperirritability, convulsions, collapse, psychic disturbances.

Special Senses: tinnitus, abnormal sensation in eyes, xanthopsia, blurring of vision, drying of mucous membranes (mouth, eyes, etc.).

Cardiovascular: hypotension.

Metabolic: hyperglycemia.

Hematologic: transient leukopenia.

Genitourinary: hematuria, enuresis, malodor of the urine, crystalluria.

Hypersensitivity: pruritus, fever, facial flush, chills, conjunctival injection, angioedema, anaphylaxis, skin rashes (including perianal), erythema multiforme (including Stevens-Johnson syndrome), and lymphadenopathy.

Miscellaneous: appearance of live Ascaris in the mouth and nose.

OVERDOSAGE

Overdosage may be associated with transient disturbances of vision and psychic alterations.

There is no specific antidote in the event of overdosage. Therefore, symptomatic and supportive measures should be employed. Emesis should be induced or gastric lavage performed carefully.

The oral LD_{50} of MINTEZOL is 3.6 g/kg, 3.1 g/kg and 3.8 g/kg in the mouse, rat, and rabbit respectively.

DOSAGE AND ADMINISTRATION

The recommended maximum daily dose of MINTEZOL is 3 grams.

MINTEZOL should be given after meals if possible. Tablets MINTEZOL should be chewed before swallowing. Dietary

restriction, complementary medications and cleansing enemas are not needed.

The usual dosage schedule for all conditions is two doses per day. The dosage is determined by the patient's weight. A weight-dose chart follows:

Weight	Each Dose	
	g	mL
30 lb	0.25	2.5
	($\frac{1}{2}$ tablet)	($\frac{1}{2}$ teaspoon)
50 lb	0.5	5.0
	(1 tablet)	(1 teaspoon)
75 lb	0.75	7.5
	($1\frac{1}{2}$ tablets)	($1\frac{1}{2}$ teaspoons)
100 lb	1.0	10.0
	(2 tablets)	(2 teaspoons)
125 lb	1.25	12.5
	($2\frac{1}{2}$ tablets)	($2\frac{1}{2}$ teaspoons)
150 lb & over	1.5	15.0
	(3 tablets)	(3 teaspoons)

The regimen for each indication follows:
[See table above].

HOW SUPPLIED

No. 3331 — MINTEZOL Suspension, 500 mg per 5 mL, is white to off-white and is supplied as follows:
NDC 0006-3331-60 in bottles of 120 mL
(6505-00-935-5835, 0.5 g/5 mL, 120 mL).
No. 3332 — MINTEZOL Chewable Tablets, 500 mg, are white to off-white, orange-flavored, round, scored, compressed tablets, coded MSD 907. They are supplied as follows:
NDC 0006-0907-36 in boxes of 36 strip packaged, individually foil-wrapped tablets
(6505-01-226-9909, 500 mg chewable, 36's).
Shown in Product Identification Section, page 418
A.H.F.S. Category: 8:08
DC 7528210 Issued June 1985
COPYRIGHT © MERCK & CO., INC., 1983
All rights reserved

MODURETIC® Tablets
(Amiloride HCl-Hydrochlorothiazide, MSD), U.S.P. ℞

DESCRIPTION

MODURETIC® (Amiloride HCl-Hydrochlorothiazide, MSD) combines the potassium-conserving action of amiloride HCl with the natriuretic action of hydrochlorothiazide.

Amiloride HCl is designated chemically as 3,5-diamino-6- chloro -*N*- (diaminomethylene) pyrazinecarboxamide monohydrochloride, dihydrate and has a molecular

Continued on next page

Information on the Merck Sharp & Dohme products listed on these pages is the full prescribing information from product circulars in use August 31, 1989.

Merck Sharp & Dohme—Cont.

weight of 302.14. Its empirical formula is $C_6H_8ClN_7O \cdot HCl \cdot 2H_2O$ and its structural formula is:

Hydrochlorothiazide is designated chemically as 6-chloro-3,4-dihydro-2H-1,2,4-benzothiadiazine-7-sulfonamide 1,1-dioxide. Its empirical formula is $C_7H_8ClN_3O_4S_2$ and its structural formula is:

It is a white, or practically white, crystalline powder with a molecular weight of 297.72, which is slightly soluble in water, but freely soluble in sodium hydroxide solution. MODURETIC is available for oral use as tablets containing 5 mg of anhydrous amiloride HCl and 50 mg of hydrochlorothiazide. Each tablet contains the following inactive ingredients: calcium phosphate, FD&C Yellow 6, guar gum, lactose, magnesium stearate and starch.

CLINICAL PHARMACOLOGY

MODURETIC provides diuretic and antihypertensive activity (principally due to the hydrochlorothiazide component), while acting through the amiloride component to prevent the excessive potassium loss that may occur in patients receiving a thiazide diuretic. Due to its amiloride component, the urinary excretion of magnesium is less with MODURETIC than with a thiazide or loop diuretic used alone (see PRECAUTIONS). The onset of the diuretic action of MODURETIC is within 1 to 2 hours and this action appears to be sustained for approximately 24 hours.

Amiloride HCl
Amiloride HCl is a potassium-conserving (antikaliuretic) drug that possesses weak (compared with thiazide diuretics) natriuretic, diuretic, and antihypertensive activity. These effects have been partially additive to the effects of thiazide diuretics in some clinical studies. Amiloride HCl has potassium-conserving activity in patients receiving kaliuretic-diuretic agents.
Amiloride HCl is not an aldosterone antagonist and its effects are seen even in the absence of aldosterone.
Amiloride HCl exerts its postassium sparing effect through the inhibition of sodium reabsorption at the distal convoluted tubule, cortical collecting tubule and collecting duct; this decreases the net negative potential of the tubular lumen and reduces both potassium and hydrogen secretion and their subsequent excretion. This mechanism accounts in large part for the potassium sparing action of amiloride. Amiloride HCl usually begins to act within 2 hours after an oral dose. Its effect on electrolyte excretion reaches a peak between 6 and 10 hours and lasts about 24 hours. Peak plasma levels are obtained in 3 to 4 hours and the plasma half-life varies from 6 to 9 hours. Effects on electrolytes increase with single doses of amiloride HCl up to approximately 15 mg.
Amiloride HCl is not metabolized by the liver but is excreted unchanged by the kidneys. About 50 percent of a 20 mg dose of amiloride HCl is excreted in the urine and 40 percent in the stool within 72 hours. Amiloride HCl has little effect on glomerular filtration rate or renal blood flow. Because amiloride HCl is not metabolized by the liver, drug accumulation is not anticipated in patients with hepatic dysfunction, but accumulation can occur if the hepatorenal syndrome develops.

Hydrochlorothiazide
The mechanism of the antihypertensive effect of thiazides is unknown. Thiazides do not usually affect normal blood pressure.
Hydrochlorothiazide is a diuretic and antihypertensive. It affects the distal renal tubular mechanism of electrolyte reabsorption. Hydrochlorothiazide increases excretion of sodium and chloride in approximately equivalent amounts. Natriuresis may be accompanied by some loss of potassium and bicarbonate.
After oral use diuresis begins within two hours, peaks in about four hours and lasts about 6 to 12 hours.
Hydrochlorothiazide is not metabolized but is eliminated rapidly by the kidney. When plasma levels have been followed for at least 24 hours, the plasma half-life has been observed to vary between 5.6 and 14.8 hours. At least 61 percent of the oral dose is eliminated unchanged within 24 hours. Hydrochlorothiazide crosses the placental but not the blood-brain barrier and is excreted in breast milk.

INDICATIONS AND USAGE

MODURETIC is indicated in those patients with hypertension or with congestive heart failure who develop hypokalemia when thiazides or other kaliuretic diuretics are used alone, or in whom maintenance of normal serum potassium levels is considered to be clinically important, e.g., digitalized patients, or patients with significant cardiac arrhythmias.
The use of potassium-conserving agents is often unnecessary in patients receiving diuretics for uncomplicated essential hypertension when such patients have a normal diet.
MODURETIC may be used alone or as an adjunct to other antihypertensive drugs, such as methyldopa or beta blockers. Since MODURETIC enhances the action of these agents, dosage adjustments may be necessary to avoid an excessive fall in blood pressure and other unwanted side effects.
This fixed combination drug is not indicated for the initial therapy of edema or hypertension except in individuals in whom the development of hypokalemia cannot be risked.

CONTRAINDICATIONS

Hyperkalemia
MODURETIC should not be used in the presence of elevated serum potassium levels (greater than 5.5 mEq per liter).
Antikaliuretic Therapy or Potassium Supplementation
MODURETIC should not be given to patients receiving other potassium-conserving agents, such as spironolactone or triamterene. Potassium supplementation in the form of medication, potassium-containing salt substitutes or a potassium-rich diet should not be used with MODURETIC except in severe and/or refractory cases of hypokalemia. Such concomitant therapy can be associated with rapid increases in serum potassium levels. If potassium supplementation is used, careful monitoring of the serum potassium level is necessary.
Impaired Renal Function
Anuria, acute or chronic renal insufficiency, and evidence of diabetic nephropathy are contraindications to the use of MODURETIC. Patients with evidence of renal functional impairment (blood urea nitrogen [BUN] levels over 30 mg per 100 mL or serum creatinine levels over 1.5 mg per 100 mL) or diabetes mellitus should not receive the drug without careful, frequent and continuing monitoring of serum electrolytes, creatinine, and BUN levels. Potassium retention associated with the use of an antikaliuretic agent is accentuated in the presence of renal impairment and may result in the rapid development of hyperkalemia.
Hypersensitivity
MODURETIC is contraindicated in patients who are hypersensitive to this product, or to other sulfonamide-derived drugs.

WARNINGS

Hyperkalemia

> Like other potassium-conserving diuretic combinations, MODURETIC may cause hyperkalemia (serum potassium levels greater than 5.5 mEq per liter). In patients without renal impairment or diabetes mellitus, the risk of hyperkalemia with MODURETIC is about 1-2 percent. This risk is higher in patients with renal impairment or diabetes mellitus (even without recognized diabetic nephropathy). Since hyperkalemia, if uncorrected, is potentially fatal, it is essential to monitor serum potassium levels carefully in any patient receiving MODURETIC, particularly when it is first introduced, at the time of dosage adjustments, and during any illness that could affect renal function.

The risk of hyperkalemia may be increased when potassium-conserving agents, including MODURETIC, are administered concomitantly with an angiotensin-converting enzyme inhibitor. (See PRECAUTIONS, *Drug Interactions*.) Warning signs or symptoms of hyperkalemia include paresthesias, muscular weakness, fatigue, flaccid paralysis of the extremities, bradycardia, shock, and ECG abnormalities. Monitoring of the serum potassium level is essential because mild hyperkalemia is not usually associated with an abnormal ECG. When abnormal, the ECG in hyperkalemia is characterized primarily by tall, peaked T waves or elevations from previous tracings. There may also be lowering of the R wave and increased depth of the S wave, widening and even disappearance of the P wave, progressive widening of the QRS complex, prolongation of the PR interval, and ST depression.
Treatment of hyperkalemia: If hyperkalemia occurs in patients taking MODURETIC, the drug should be discontinued immediately. If the serum potassium level exceeds 6.5 mEq per liter, active measures should be taken to reduce it. Such measures include the intravenous administration of sodium bicarbonate solution or oral or parenteral glucose with a rapid-acting insulin preparation. If needed, a cation exchange resin such as sodium polystyrene sulfonate may be

given orally or by enema. Patients with persistent hyperkalemia may require dialysis.
Diabetes Mellitus
In diabetic patients, hyperkalemia has been reported with the use of all potassium-conserving diuretics, including amiloride HCl, even in patients without evidence of diabetic nephropathy. Therefore, MODURETIC should be avoided, if possible, in diabetic patients and, if it is used, serum electrolytes and renal function must be monitored frequently. MODURETIC should be discontinued at least three days before glucose tolerance testing.
Metabolic or Respiratory Acidosis
Antikaliuretic therapy should be instituted only with caution in severely ill patients in whom respiratory or metabolic acidosis may occur, such as patients with cardiopulmonary disease or poorly controlled diabetes. If MODURETIC is given to these patients, frequent monitoring of acid-base balance is necessary. Shifts in acid-base balance alter the ratio of extracellular/intracellular potassium, and the development of acidosis may be associated with rapid increases in serum potassium levels.

PRECAUTIONS

General
Electrolyte Imbalance and BUN Increases
Determination of serum electrolytes to detect possible electrolyte imbalance should be performed at appropriate intervals.
Patients should be observed for clinical signs of fluid or electrolyte imbalance: i.e., hyponatremia, hypochloremic alkalosis, and hypokalemia. Serum and urine electrolyte determinations are particularly important when the patient is vomiting excessively or receiving parenteral fluids. Warning signs or symptoms of fluid and electrolyte imbalance, irrespective of cause, include dryness of mouth, thirst, weakness, lethargy, drowsiness, restlessness, seizures, muscle pains or cramps, muscular fatigue, hypotension, oliguria, tachycardia, and gastrointestinal disturbances such as nausea and vomiting.
Hyponatremia and hypochloremia may occur during the use of thiazides and other diuretics. Any chloride deficit during thiazide therapy is generally mild and may be lessened by the amiloride HCl component of MODURETIC. Hypochloremia usually does not require specific treatment except under extraordinary circumstances (as in liver disease or renal disease). Dilutional hyponatremia may occur in edematous patients in hot weather; appropriate therapy is water restriction, rather than administration of salt, except in rare instances when the hyponatremia is life threatening. In actual salt depletion, appropriate replacement is the therapy of choice.
Hypokalemia may develop during thiazide therapy, especially with brisk diuresis, when severe cirrhosis is present, during concomitant use of corticosteroids or ACTH, or after prolonged therapy. However, this usually is prevented by the amiloride HCl component of MODURETIC.
Interference with adequate oral electrolyte intake will also contribute to hypokalemia. Hypokalemia may cause cardiac arrhythmia and may also sensitize or exaggerate the response of the heart to the toxic effects of digitalis (e.g., increased ventricular irritability).
Thiazides have been shown to increase the urinary excretion of magnesium; this may result in hypomagnesemia. Amiloride HCl, a component of MODURETIC, has been shown to decrease the enhanced urinary excretion of magnesium which occurs when a thiazide or loop diuretic is used alone.
Increases in BUN levels have been reported with amiloride HCl and with hydrochlorothiazide. These increases usually have accompanied vigorous fluid elimination, especially when diuretic therapy was used in seriously ill patients, such as those who had hepatic cirrhosis with ascites and metabolic alkalosis, or those with resistant edema. Therefore, when MODURETIC is given to such patients, careful monitoring of serum electrolyte and BUN levels is important. In patients with pre-existing severe liver disease, hepatic encephalopathy, manifested by tremors, confusion, and coma, and increased jaundice, have been reported in association with diuretic therapy including amiloride HCl and hydrochlorothiazide.
In patients with renal disease, diuretics may precipitate azotemia. Cumulative effects of the components of MODURETIC may develop in patients with impaired renal function. If renal impairment becomes evident, MODURETIC should be discontinued (see CONTRAINDICATIONS and WARNINGS).
Drug Interactions
In some patients, the administration of a non-steroidal anti-inflammatory agent can reduce the diuretic, natriuretic, and antihypertensive effects of loop, potassium-sparing and thiazide diuretics. Therefore, when MODURETIC and non-steroidal anti-inflammatory agents are used concomitantly, the patient should be observed closely to determine if the desired effect of the diuretic is obtained. Since indomethacin and potassium-sparing diuretics, including MODURETIC, each may be associated with increased serum potassium levels,

the potential effects on potassium kinetics and renal function should be considered when these agents are administered concurrently.

Amiloride HCl
When amiloride HCl is administered concomitantly with an angiotensin-converting enzyme inhibitor, the risk of hyperkalemia may be increased. Therefore, if concomitant use of these agents is in indicated because of demonstrated hypokalemia, they should be used with caution and with frequent monitoring of serum potassium. (See WARNINGS.)

Hydrochlorothiazide
When given concurrently the following drugs may interact with thiazide diuretics.

Alcohol, barbiturates, or narcotics —potentiation of orthostatic hypotension may occur.

Antidiabetic drugs (oral agents and insulin)—dosage adjustment of the antidiabetic drug may be required.

Other antihypertensive drugs —additive effect or potentiation.

Corticosteroids, ACTH —intensified electrolyte depletion, particularly hypokalemia.

Pressor amines (e.g., norepinephrine) —possible decreased response to pressor amines but not sufficient to preclude their use.

Skeletal muscle relaxants, nondepolarizing (e.g., tubocurarine) —possible increased responsiveness to the muscle relaxant.

Lithium —generally should not be given with diuretics. Diuretic agents reduce the renal clearance of lithium and add a high risk of lithium toxicity. Refer to the package insert for lithium preparations before use of such preparations with MODURETIC.

Metabolic and Endocrine Effects
In diabetic patients, insulin requirements may be increased, decreased, or unchanged due to the hydrochlorothiazide component. Diabetes mellitus that has been latent may become manifest during administration of thiazide diuretics. Because calcium excretion is decreased by thiazides, MODURETIC should be discontinued before carrying out tests for parathyroid function. Pathologic changes in the parathyroid glands, with hypercalcemia and hypophosphatemia have been observed in a few patients on prolonged thiazide therapy; however, the common complications of hyperparathyroidism such as renal lithiasis, bone resorption, and peptic ulceration have not been seen.

Hyperuricemia may occur or acute gout may be precipitated in certain patients receiving thiazide therapy.

Other Precautions
In patients receiving thiazides, sensitivity reactions may occur with or without a history of allergy or bronchial asthma. The possibility of exacerbation or activation of systemic lupus erythematosus has been reported with the use of thiazides.
Increases in cholesterol and triglyceride levels may be associated with thiazide diuretic therapy.

Carcinogenicity, Mutagenicity, Impairment of Fertility
Long-term studies in animals have not been performed to evaluate the effects upon fertility, mutagenicity or carcinogenic potential of MODURETIC.

Amiloride HCl
There was no evidence of a tumorigenic effect when amiloride HCl was administered for 92 weeks to mice at doses up to 10 mg/kg/day (25 times the maximum daily human dose). Amiloride HCl has also been administered for 104 weeks to male and female rats at doses up to 6 and 8 mg/kg/day (15 and 20 times the maximum daily dose for humans, respectively) and showed no evidence of carcinogenicity. Amiloride HCl was devoid of mutagenic activity in various strains of *Salmonella typhimurium* with or without a mammalian liver microsomal activation system (Ames test).

Hydrochlorothiazide
Hydrochlorothiazide is currently under study in the U.S. Carcinogenesis Testing Program.
Hydrochlorothiazide was not mutagenic *in vitro*, in the Ames microbial mutagen test at a maximum concentration of 5 mg/plate using Strains TA98 and TA100. Urine samples of patients treated with hydrochlorothiazide did not have mutagenic activity in the Ames test.
The ability of a number of drugs to induce nondisjunction and crossing-over was measured using *Aspergillus nidulans*. A large number of drugs, including hydrochlorothiazide, induced nondisjunction.
Hydrochlorothiazide had no effect on fertility in a two-litter study in rats at doses of 4–5.6 mg/kg/day (up to 2 times the maximum recommended human dose).

Pregnancy
Pregnancy Category B. Teratogenicity studies have been performed with combinations of amiloride HCl and hydrochlorothiazide in rabbits and mice at doses up to 25 times the expected maximum daily dose for humans and have revealed no evidence of harm to the fetus. No evidence of impaired fertility in rats was apparent at dosage levels up to 25 times the expected maximum human daily dose. A perinatal and postnatal study in rats showed a reduction in maternal body weight gain during and after gestation at a daily dose of 25 times the expected maximum daily dose for humans. The

body weights of alive pups at birth and at weaning were also reduced at this dose level. There are no adequate and well controlled studies in pregnant women. Because animal reproduction studies are not always predictive of human responses, and because of the data listed below with the individual components, this drug should be used during pregnancy only if clearly needed.

Amiloride HCl
Teratogenicity studies with amiloride HCl in rabbits and mice given 20 and 25 times the maximum human dose, respectively, revealed no evidence of harm to the fetus, although studies showed that the drug crossed the placenta in modest amounts. Reproduction studies in rats at 20 times the expected maximum daily dose for humans showed no evidence of impaired fertility. At approximately 5 or more times the expected maximum daily dose for humans, some toxicity was seen in adult rats and rabbits and a decrease in rat pup growth and survival occurred.

Hydrochlorothiazide
Teratogenic Effects: Reproduction studies in the rabbit, the mouse and the rat at doses up to 100 mg/kg/day (50 times the maximum human dose) showed no evidence of external abnormalities of the fetus due to hydrochlorothiazide. Hydrochlorothiazide given in a two-litter study in rats at doses of 4–5.6 mg/kg/day (approximately 1–2 times the maximum recommended human dose) did not impair fertility or produce birth abnormalities in the offspring.
Thiazides cross the placental barrier and appear in the cord blood.
Nonteratogenic Effects: These may include fetal or neonatal jaundice, thrombocytopenia, and possibly other adverse reactions which have occurred in the adult.

Nursing Mothers
Studies in rats have shown that amiloride is excreted in milk in concentrations higher than that found in blood, but it is not known whether amiloride HCl is excreted in human milk. However, thiazides appear in breast milk. Because of the potential for serious adverse reactions in nursing infants, a decision should be made whether to discontinue nursing or to discontinue the drug, taking into account the importance of the drug to the mother.

Pediatric Use
Safety and effectiveness in children have not been established.

ADVERSE REACTIONS

MODURETIC is usually well tolerated and significant clinical adverse effects have been reported infrequently. The risk of hyperkalemia (serum potassium levels greater than 5.5 mEq per liter) with MODURETIC is about 1–2 percent in patients without renal impairment or diabetes mellitus (see WARNINGS). Minor adverse reactions to amiloride HCl have been reported relatively frequently (about 20%) but the relationship of many of the reports to amiloride HCl is uncertain and the overall frequency was similar in hydrochlorothiazide treated groups. Nausea/anorexia, abdominal pain, flatulence, and mild skin rash have been reported and probably are related to amiloride. Other adverse experiences that have been reported with MODURETIC are generally those known to be associated with diuresis, thiazide therapy, or with the underlying disease being treated. Clinical trials have not demonstrated that combining amiloride and hydrochlorothiazide increases the risk of adverse reactions over those seen with the individual components.
The adverse reactions for MODURETIC listed in the following table have been arranged into two groups: (1) incidence greater than one percent; and (2) incidence one percent or less. The incidence for group (1) was determined from clinical studies conducted in the United States (607 patients treated with MODURETIC). The adverse effects listed in group (2) include reports from the same clinical studies and voluntary reports since marketing. The probability of a causal relationship exists between MODURETIC and these adverse reactions, some of which have been reported only rarely.

Incidence >1%	Incidence ≤1%
Body as a Whole	
Headache*	Malaise
Weakness*	Chest pain
Fatigue/tiredness	Back pain
	Syncope
Cardiovascular	
Arrhythmia	Tachycardia
	Digitalis toxicity
	Orthostatic hypotension
	Angina pectoris
Digestive	
Nausea/anorexia*	Constipation
Diarrhea	GI bleeding
Gastrointestinal pain	GI disturbance
Abdominal pain	Appetite changes
	Abdominal fullness
	Hiccups
	Thirst
	Vomiting
	Anorexia
	Flatulence
Metabolic	
Elevated serum potassium levels (>5.5 mEq per liter)†	Gout
	Dehydration
	Symptomatic hyponatremia**
Integumentary	
Rash*	Flushing
Pruritus	Diaphoresis
Musculoskeletal	
Leg ache	Muscle cramps/spasm
	Joint pain
Nervous	
Dizziness*	Paresthesia/numbness
	Stupor
	Vertigo
Psychiatric	
None	Insomnia
	Nervousness
	Depression
	Sleepiness
	Mental confusion
Respiratory	
Dyspnea	None
Special Senses	
None	Bad taste
	Visual disturbance
	Nasal congestion
Urogenital	
None	Impotence
	Nocturia
	Dysuria
	Incontinence
	Renal dysfunction including renal failure

Other adverse reactions that have been reported with the individual components and within each category are listed in order of decreasing severity:

Amiloride —*Body as a Whole:* Painful extremities, neck/shoulder ache, fatigability; *Cardiovascular:* Palpitation; *Digestive:* Activation of probable pre-existing peptic ulcer, abnormal liver function, jaundice, dyspepsia, heartburn; *Hematologic:* Aplastic anemia, neutropenia; *Integumentary:* Alopecia, itching, dry mouth; *Nervous System/Psychiatric:* Encephalopathy, tremors, decreased libido; *Respiratory:* Shortness of breath, cough; *Special Senses:* Increased intraocular pressure, tinnitus; *Urogenital:* Bladder spasms, polyuria, urinary frequency.

Hydrochlorothiazide —*Digestive:* Pancreatitis, jaundice (intrahepatic cholestatic jaundice), sialadenitis, cramping, gastric irritation; *Hematologic:* Aplastic anemia, agranulocytosis, leukopenia, hemolytic anemia, thrombocytopenia;

Hypersensitivity: Anaphylactic reactions, necrotizing angiitis (vasculitis, cutaneous vasculitis), respiratory distress including pneumonitis and pulmonary edema, photosensitivity, fever, urticaria, purpura; *Metabolic:* Electrolyte imbalance (see PRECAUTIONS), hyperglycemia, glycosuria, hyperuricemia; *Nervous System/Psychiatric:* Restlessness; *Special Senses:* Transient blurred vision, xanthopsia; *Urogenital:* Interstitial nephritis (see WARNINGS).

OVERDOSAGE

No data are available in regard to overdosage in humans. The oral LD₅₀ of the combination drug is 189 and 422 mg/kg for female mice and female rats, respectively.
It is not known whether the drug is dialyzable.
No specific information is available on the treatment of overdosage with MODURETIC, and no specific antidote is available. Treatment is symptomatic and supportive. Therapy with MODURETIC should be discontinued and the patient observed closely. Suggested measures include induction of emesis and/or gastric lavage.
Amiloride HCl: No data are available in regard to overdosage in humans.
The oral LD₅₀ of amiloride HCl (calculated as the base) is 56 mg/kg in mice and 36 to 85 mg/kg in rats, depending on the strain.

---

* Reactions occurring in 3% to 8% of patients treated with MODURETIC. (Those reactions occurring in less than 3% of the patients are unmarked.)
† See WARNINGS.
**See PRECAUTIONS.

Continued on next page

Information on the Merck Sharp & Dohme products listed on these pages is the full prescribing information from product circulars in use August 31, 1989.

Merck Sharp & Dohme—Cont.

The most common signs and symptoms to be expected with overdosage are dehydration and electrolyte imbalance. If hyperkalemia occurs, active measures should be taken to reduce the serum potassium levels.

Hydrochlorothiazide: The oral LD$_{50}$ of hydrochlorothiazide is greater than 10.0 g/kg in both mice and rats.

The most common signs and symptoms observed are those caused by electrolyte depletion (hypokalemia, hypochloremia, hyponatremia) and dehydration resulting from excessive diuresis. If digitalis has also been administered, hypokalemia may accentuate cardiac arrhythmias.

DOSAGE AND ADMINISTRATION

MODURETIC should be administered with food.

The usual starting dosage is 1 tablet a day. The dosage may be increased to 2 tablets a day, if necessary. More than 2 tablets of MODURETIC daily usually are not needed and there is no controlled experience with such doses. The daily dose is usually given as a single dose but may be given in divided doses. Once an initial diuresis has been achieved, dosage adjustment may be necessary. Maintenance therapy may be on an intermittent basis.

HOW SUPPLIED

No. 3385—Tablets MODURETIC are peach-colored, diamond-shaped, scored, compressed tablets, coded MSD 917. Each tablet contains 5 mg of anhydrous amiloride HCl and 50 mg of hydrochlorothiazide. They are supplied as follows:
NDC 0006-0917-68 in bottles of 100
(6505-01-139-1498 100's)
NDC 0006-0917-28 unit dose packages of 100.

Shown in Product Identification Section, page 418

Storage
Protect from moisture, freezing and excessive heat.

A.H.F.S. Category: 40:28
DC 7168018   Issued May 1988
COPYRIGHT © MERCK & CO., INC., 1988
All rights reserved

MUMPSVAX®   ℞
(Mumps Virus Vaccine Live, MSD), U.S.P.
Jeryl Lynn Strain

DESCRIPTION

MUMPSVAX® (Mumps Virus Vaccine Live, MSD) is a live virus vaccine for immunization against mumps.

MUMPSVAX is a sterile lyophilized preparation of the Jeryl Lynn (B level) strain of mumps virus. The virus was adapted to and propagated in cell cultures of chick embryo free of avian leukosis virus and other adventitious agents.

The reconstituted vaccine is for subcutaneous administration. When reconstituted as directed, the dose for injection is 0.5 mL and contains not less than the equivalent of 5,000 TCID$_{50}$ (tissue culture infectious doses) of the U.S. Reference Mumps Virus. Each dose contains approximately 25 mcg of neomycin. The product contains no preservative. Sorbitol and hydrolized gelatin are added as stabilizers.

CLINICAL PHARMACOLOGY

MUMPSVAX produces a modified, non-communicable mumps infection in susceptible persons. Extensive clinical trials have demonstrated that MUMPSVAX is highly immunogenic and well tolerated. A single injection of the vaccine has been shown to induce mumps neutralizing antibodies in approximately 97 percent of susceptible children and approximately 93 percent of susceptible adults. The pattern of antibody response closely resembles that observed for natural mumps. Although the antibody level is significantly lower than that following natural infection, it is protective and long lasting. Vaccine-induced antibody levels have been shown to persist for at least 15 years with a rate of decline comparable to that seen in natural infection. If the present pattern continues, it will provide a basis for the expectation that immunity following vaccination will be permanent. However, continued surveillance will be required to demonstrate this point.

INDICATIONS AND USAGE

MUMPSVAX is indicated for immunization against mumps in persons 12 months of age or older. Most adults are likely to have been infected naturally and generally may be considered immune, even if they did not have clinically recognizable disease. A booster is not needed. It is not recommended for infants younger than 12 months because they may retain maternal mumps neutralizing antibodies which may interfere with the immune response.

Evidence indicates that the vaccine will not offer protection when given after exposure to natural mumps. Passively ac-

quired antibody can interfere with the response to live, attenuated-virus vaccines. Therefore, administration of mumps virus vaccine should be deferred until approximately three months after passive immunization.

Revaccination: Children vaccinated when younger than 12 months of age should be revaccinated. Based on available evidence, there is no reason to routinely revaccinate persons who were vaccinated originally when 12 months of age or older. However, persons should be revaccinated if there is evidence to suggest that initial immunization was ineffective.

Use with other Vaccines
Routine administration of DTP (diphtheria, tetanus, pertussis) and/or OPV (oral poliovirus vaccine) concomitantly with measles, mumps and rubella vaccine is not recommended because there are insufficient data relating to the simultaneous administration of these antigens. However, the American Academy of Pediatrics has noted that in some circumstances, particularly when the patient may not return, some practitioners prefer to administer all these antigens on a single day. If done, separate sites and syringes should be used for DTP and MUMPSVAX.

MUMPSVAX should not be given less than one month before or after administration of other virus vaccines.

CONTRAINDICATIONS

Do not give MUMPSVAX to pregnant females; the possible effects of the vaccine on fetal development are unknown at this time. If vaccination of postpubertal females is undertaken, pregnancy should be avoided for three months following vaccination (see PRECAUTIONS, *Pregnancy*).

Anaphylactoid reaction to neomycin (each dose of reconstituted vaccine contains approximately 25 mcg of neomycin).

History of anaphylactoid reaction to eggs (see HYPERSENSITIVITY TO EGGS below).

Any febrile respiratory illness or other active febrile infection.

Active untreated tuberculosis.

Patients receiving immunosuppressive therapy. This contraindication does not apply to patients who are receiving corticosteroids as replacement therapy, e.g., for Addison's disease.

Individuals with blood dyscrasias, leukemia, lymphomas of any type, or other malignant neoplasms affecting the bone marrow or lymphatic systems.

Primary immunodeficiency states, including cellular immune deficiencies, hypogammaglobulinemic and dysgammaglobulinemic states.

Individuals with a family history of congenital or hereditary immunodeficiency, until the immune competence of the potential vaccine recipient is demonstrated.

HYPERSENSITIVITY TO EGGS

Live mumps vaccine is produced in chick embryo cell culture. Persons with a history of anaphylactic or other immediate reactions (e.g., hives, swelling of the mouth and throat, difficulty breathing, hypotension, or shock) subsequent to egg ingestion should be vaccinated only with extreme caution. Evidence indicates that persons are not at increased risk if they have egg allergies that are not anaphylactic in nature. Such persons may be vaccinated in the usual manner. There is no evidence to indicate that persons with allergies to chickens or feathers are at increased risk of reaction to the vaccine.

PRECAUTIONS

General
Adequate treatment provisions including epinephrine, should be available for immediate use should an anaphylactoid reaction occur.

Vaccination should be deferred for at least 3 months following blood or plasma transfusions, or administration of human immune serum globulin.

There are no reports of transmission of live mumps virus from vaccinees to susceptible contacts.

It has been reported that mumps virus vaccine, live, may result in a temporary depression of tuberculin skin sensitivity. Therefore, if a tuberculin test is to be done, it should be administered either before or simultaneously with MUMPSVAX.

As for any vaccine, vaccination with MUMPSVAX may not result in seroconversion in 100% of susceptible persons given the vaccine.

Pregnancy
Pregnancy Category C
Animal reproduction studies have not been conducted with MUMPSVAX. It is also not known whether MUMPSVAX can cause fetal harm when administered to a pregnant woman or can affect reproduction capacity. Therefore, mumps virus vaccine should not be given to persons known to be pregnant; furthermore, pregnancy should be avoided for three months following vaccination. Although mumps

virus is capable of infecting the placenta and fetus, there is no good evidence that it causes congenital malformations in humans. Mumps vaccine virus also has been shown to infect the placenta, but the virus has not been isolated from the fetal tissues from susceptible women who were vaccinated and underwent elective abortions.

Nursing Mothers
It is not known whether mumps vaccine virus is secreted in human milk. Therefore, because many drugs are excreted in human milk, caution should be exercised when MUMPSVAX is administered to a nursing woman.

ADVERSE REACTIONS

Because of the slightly acidic pH (6.2–6.6) of the vaccine, patients may complain of burning and/or stinging of short duration at the injection site.

Mild fever occurs occasionally. Fever above 103°F (39.4°C) is uncommon.

Parotitis has been reported to occur in very low incidence, and orchitis rarely, in persons who were vaccinated. In most instances investigated, prior exposure to natural mumps was established. In other instances, whether or not this was due to vaccine or to prior natural mumps exposure or to other causes has not been established.

Reports of purpura and allergic reactions such as wheal and flare at the injection site or urticaria have been extremely rare.

Forms of optic neuritis, including retrobulbar neuritis and papillitis may infrequently follow viral infections, and have been reported to occur 1 to 3 weeks following inoculation with some live virus vaccines.

Very rarely encephalitis, febrile seizures, nerve deafness and other nervous system reactions have occurred in vaccinees. A cause-effect relationship has not been established.

DOSAGE AND ADMINISTRATION

FOR SUBCUTANEOUS ADMINISTRATION
Do not inject intravenously
The dosage of vaccine is the same for all persons. Inject the total volume (about 0.5 mL) of reconstituted vaccine subcutaneously, preferably into the outer aspect of upper arm. *Do not give immune serum globulin (ISG) concurrently with* MUMPSVAX.

During shipment, to insure that there is no loss of potency, the vaccine must be maintained at a temperature of 10°C (50°F) or less.

Before reconstitution, store MUMPSVAX at 2–8°C (35.6–46.4°F). *Protect from light.*

CAUTION: A sterile syringe free of preservatives, antiseptics, and detergents should be used for each injection and/or reconstitution of the vaccine because these substances may inactivate the live virus vaccine. A 25 gauge, ⅝″ needle is recommended.

To reconstitute, use only the diluent supplied, since it is free of preservatives or other antiviral substances which might inactivate the vaccine.

Single Dose Vial—First withdraw the entire volume of diluent into the syringe to be used for reconstitution. Inject all the diluent in the syringe into the vial of lyophilized vaccine, and agitate to mix thoroughly. Withdraw the entire contents into a syringe and inject the total volume of restored vaccine subcutaneously.

It is important to use a separate sterile syringe and needle for each individual patient to prevent transmission of hepatitis B and other infectious agents from one person to another.

10 Dose Vial (available only to government agencies/institutions)—Withdraw the entire contents (7 mL) of the diluent vial into the sterile syringe to be used for reconstitution, and introduce into the 10 dose vial of lyophilized vaccine. Agitate to ensure thorough mixing. The outer labeling suggests "For Jet Injector or Syringe Use". Use with separate sterile syringes is permitted for containers of 10 doses or less. The vaccine and diluent do not contain preservatives; therefore, the user must recognize the potential contamination hazards and exercise special precautions to protect the sterility and potency of the product. The use of aseptic techniques and proper storage prior to and after restoration of the vaccine and subsequent withdrawal of the individual doses is essential. Use 0.5 mL of the reconstituted vaccine for subcutaneous injection.

It is important to use a separate sterile syringe and needle for each individual patient to prevent transmission of hepatitis B and other infectious agents from one person to another.

50 Dose Vial (available only to government agencies/institutions)—Withdraw the entire contents (30 mL) of the diluent vial into the sterile syringe to be used for reconstitution and introduce into the 50 dose vial of lyophilized vaccine. Agitate to ensure thorough mixing. With full aseptic precautions, attach the vial to the sterilized multidose jet injector apparatus. Use 0.5 mL of the reconstituted vaccine for subcutaneous injection.

Each dose of MUMPSVAX contains not less than the equivalent of 5,000 TCID$_{50}$ of the U.S. Reference Mumps Virus. Parenteral drug products should be inspected visually for particulate matter and discoloration prior to administration. MUMPSVAX, when reconstituted, is clear yellow.

HOW SUPPLIED

No. 4753—MUMPSVAX is supplied as a single-dose vial of lyophilized vaccine, **NDC** 0006-4753-00, and a vial of diluent. No. 4584X/4309—MUMPSVAX is supplied as follows: (1) a box of 10 single-dose vials of lyophilized vaccine (package A), **NDC** 0006-4584-00; and (2) a box of 10 vials of diluent (package B). To conserve refrigerator space, the diluent may be stored separately at room temperature.

Available only to government agencies/institutions:

No. 4664X—MUMPSVAX is supplied as one 10 dose vial of lyophilized vaccine, **NDC** 0006-4664-00, and one 7 mL vial of diluent.

No. 4593X—MUMPSVAX is supplied as one 50 dose vial of lyophilized vaccine, **NDC** 0006-4593-00, and one 30 mL vial of diluent.

Storage

It is recommended that the vaccine be used as soon as possible after reconstitution. Protect vaccine from light at all times, since such exposure may inactivate the virus. Store reconstituted vaccine in the vaccine vial in a dark place at 2–8°C (35.6–46.4°F) and discard if not used within 8 hours.

A.H.F.S. Category: 80:12
DC 7075407 Issued October 1984
COPYRIGHT © MERCK & CO., INC., 1985
All rights reserved

MUSTARGEN®, Trituration of ℞
(Mechlorethamine HCl for Injection, MSD), U.S.P.

DESCRIPTION

MUSTARGEN® (Mechlorethamine HCl, MSD), an antineoplastic nitrogen mustard also known as HN2 hydrochloride, is a nitrogen analog of sulfur mustard. It is a white, crystalline, hygroscopic powder that is very soluble in water and also soluble in alcohol.

Mechlorethamine hydrochloride is designated chemically as 2-chloro-N-(2-chloroethyl)-N-methylethanamine hydrochloride. The molecular weight is 192.52 and the melting point is 108–111°C. The empirical formula is $C_5H_{11}Cl_2N \cdot HCl$, and the structural formula is: $CH_3N(CH_2CH_2Cl)_2 \cdot HCl$.

Trituration of MUSTARGEN is a sterile, white crystalline powder for injection by the intravenous or intracavitary routes after dissolution. Each vial of MUSTARGEN contains 10 mg of mechlorethamine hydrochloride triturated with sodium chloride q.s. 100 mg. When dissolved with 10 mL Sterile Water for Injection or 0.9% Sodium Chloride Injection, the resulting solution has a pH of 3–5 at a concentration of 1 mg mechlorethamine HCl per mL.

CLINICAL PHARMACOLOGY

Mechlorethamine, a biologic alkylating agent, has a cytotoxic action which inhibits rapidly proliferating cells.

Pharmacokinetics and Metabolism

In water or body fluids, mechlorethamine undergoes rapid chemical transformation and combines with water or reactive compounds of cells, so that the drug is no longer present in active form a few minutes after administration.

INDICATIONS AND USAGE

Before using MUSTARGEN *see CONTRAINDICATIONS, WARNINGS, PRECAUTIONS, ADVERSE REACTIONS, DOSAGE AND ADMINISTRATION, and HOW SUPPLIED, Special Handling.*

MUSTARGEN, administered intravenously, is indicated for the palliative treatment of Hodgkin's disease (Stages III and IV), lymphosarcoma, chronic myelocytic or chronic lymphocytic leukemia, polycythemia vera, mycosis fungoides, and bronchogenic carcinoma.

MUSTARGEN, administered intrapleurally, intraperitoneally, or intrapericardially, is indicated for the palliative treatment of metastatic carcinoma resulting in effusion.

CONTRAINDICATIONS

The use of MUSTARGEN is contraindicated in the presence of known infectious diseases and in patients who have had previous anaphylactic reactions to MUSTARGEN.

WARNINGS

Extravasation of the drug into subcutaneous tissues results in a painful inflammation. The area usually becomes indurated and sloughing may occur. If leakage of drug is obvious, prompt infiltration of the area with sterile isotonic sodium thiosulfate ($\frac{1}{6}$ molar) and application of an ice compress for 6 to 12 hours may minimize the local reaction. For a $\frac{1}{6}$ molar solution of sodium thiosulfate, use 4.14 g of sodium thiosulfate per 100 mL of Sterile Water for Injection or 2.64 g of anhydrous sodium thiosulfate per 100 mL or dilute 4 mL of Sodium Thiosulfate Injection (10%) with 6 mL of Sterile Water for Injection.

Before using MUSTARGEN, *an accurate histologic diagnosis of the disease, a knowledge of its natural course, and an adequate clinical history are important. The hematologic status of the patient must first be determined. It is essential to understand the hazards and therapeutic effects to be expected. Careful clinical judgment must be exercised in selecting patients. If the indication for its use is not clear, the drug should not be used.*

As nitrogen mustard therapy may contribute to extensive and rapid development of amyloidosis, it should be used only if foci of acute and chronic suppurative inflammation are absent.

Usage in Pregnancy

Mechlorethamine hydrochloride can cause fetal harm when administered to a pregnant woman. MUSTARGEN has been shown to produce fetal malformations in the rat and ferret when given as single subcutaneous injections of 1 mg/kg (2–3 times the maximum recommended human dose). There are no adequate and well controlled studies in pregnant women. If this drug is used during pregnancy, or if the patient becomes pregnant while taking this drug, the patient should be apprised of the potential hazard to the fetus. Women of childbearing potential should be advised to avoid becoming pregnant.

PRECAUTIONS

General

This drug is highly toxic and both powder and solution must be handled and administered with care. Since MUSTARGEN is a powerful vesicant, it is intended primarily for intravenous use, and in most instances is given by this route. Inhalation of dust or vapors and contact with skin or mucous membranes, especially those of the eyes, must be avoided. Rubber gloves should be worn when handling MUSTARGEN. (See DOSAGE AND ADMINISTRATION and HOW SUPPLIED, *Special Handling*.)

Because of the toxicity of MUSTARGEN, and the unpleasant side effects following its use, the potential risk and discomfort from the use of this drug in patients with inoperable neoplasms or in the terminal stage of the disease must be balanced against the limited gain obtainable. These gains will vary with the nature and the status of the disease under treatment. The routine use of MUSTARGEN in all cases of widely disseminated neoplasms is to be discouraged.

The use of MUSTARGEN in patients with leukopenia, thrombocytopenia, and anemia, due to invasion of the bone marrow by tumor carries a greater risk. In such patients a good response to treatment with disappearance of the tumor from the bone marrow may be associated with improvement of bone marrow function. However, in the absence of a good response or in patients who have been previously treated with chemotherapeutic agents, hematopoiesis may be further compromised, and leukopenia, thrombocytopenia and anemia may become more severe and lead to the demise of the patient.

Tumors of bone and nervous tissue have responded poorly to therapy. Results are unpredictable in disseminated and malignant tumors of different types.

Precautions must be observed with the use of MUSTARGEN and x-ray therapy or other chemotherapy in alternating courses. Hematopoietic function is characteristically depressed by either form of therapy, and neither MUSTARGEN following x-ray therapy nor x-ray therapy subsequent to the drug should be given until bone marrow function has recovered. In particular, irradiation of such areas as sternum, ribs, and vertebrae shortly after a course of nitrogen mustard may lead to hematologic complications.

MUSTARGEN has been reported to have immunosuppressive activity. Therefore, it should be borne in mind that use of the drug may predispose the patient to bacterial, viral or fungal infection.

Hyperuricemia may develop during therapy with MUSTARGEN. The problem of urate precipitation should be anticipated, particularly in the treatment of the lymphomas, and adequate methods for control of hyperuricemia should be instituted and careful attention directed toward adequate fluid intake before treatment.

Since drug toxicity, especially sensitivity to bone marrow failure, seems to be more common in chronic lymphatic leukemia than in other conditions, the drug should be given in this condition with great caution, if at all.

Extreme caution must be used in exceeding the average recommended dose. (See OVERDOSAGE.)

Laboratory Tests

Many abnormalities of renal, hepatic, and bone marrow function have been reported in patients with neoplastic disease and receiving mechlorethamine. It is advisable to check renal, hepatic, and bone marrow functions frequently.

Carcinogenesis, Mutagenesis, Impairment of Fertility

Therapy with alkylating agents such as MUSTARGEN may be associated with an increased incidence of a second malignant tumor, especially when such therapy is combined with other antineoplastic agents or radiation therapy.

Young-adult female RF mice were injected intravenously with four doses of 2.4 mg/kg of mechlorethamine (0.1% solution) at 2-week intervals with observations for up to 2 years. An increased incidence of thymic lymphomas and pulmonary adenomas was observed. Painting mechlorethamine on the skin of mice for periods up to 33 weeks resulted in squamous cell tumors in 9 of 33 mice.

Mechlorethamine induced mutations in the Ames test, in *E. coli*, and *Neurospora crassa*. Mechlorethamine caused chromosome aberrations in a variety of plant and mammalian cells. Dominant lethal mutations were produced in ICR/Ha Swiss mice.

Mechlorethamine impaired fertility in the rat at a daily dose of 500 mg/kg intravenously for two weeks.

Pregnancy

Pregnancy Category D. See WARNINGS.

Nursing Mothers

It is not known whether this drug is excreted in human milk. Because many drugs are excreted in human milk and because of the potential for serious adverse reactions in nursing infants from MUSTARGEN, a decision should be made whether to discontinue nursing or to discontinue the drug, taking into account the importance of the drug to the mother.

Pediatric Use

Safety and effectiveness in children have not been established by well-controlled studies. Use of MUSTARGEN in children has been quite limited. MUSTARGEN has been used in Hodgkin's disease, stages III and IV, in combination with other oncolytic agents (MOPP schedule). The MOPP chemotherapy combination includes mechlorethamine, vincristine, procarbazine, and prednisone or prednisolone.

ADVERSE REACTIONS

Clinical use of MUSTARGEN *usually is accompanied by toxic manifestations.*

Local Toxicity

Thrombosis and thrombophlebitis may result from direct contact of the drug with the intima of the injected vein. Avoid high concentration and prolonged contact with the drug, especially in cases of elevated pressure in the antebrachial vein (e.g., in mediastinal tumor compression from severe vena cava syndrome).

Systemic Toxicity

General: Hypersensitivity reactions, including anaphylaxis, have been reported. Nausea, vomiting and depression of formed elements in the circulating blood are dose-limiting side effects and usually occur with the use of full doses of MUSTARGEN. Jaundice, alopecia, vertigo, tinnitus and diminished hearing may occur infrequently. Rarely, hemolytic anemia associated with such diseases as the lymphomas and chronic lymphocytic leukemia may be precipitated by treatment with alkylating agents including MUSTARGEN. Also, various chromosomal abnormalities have been reported in association with nitrogen mustard therapy.

MUSTARGEN is given preferably at night in case sedation for side effects is required. Nausea and vomiting usually occur 1 to 3 hours after use of the drug. Emesis may disappear in the first 8 hours, but nausea may persist for 24 hours. Nausea and vomiting may be so severe as to precipitate vascular accidents in patients with a hemorrhagic tendency. Premedication with antiemetics, in addition to sedatives, may help control severe nausea and vomiting. Anorexia, weakness and diarrhea may also occur.

Hematologic: The usual course of MUSTARGEN (total dose of 0.4 mg/kg either given as a single intravenous dose or divided into two or four daily doses of 0.2 or 0.1 mg/kg respectively) generally produces a lymphocytopenia within 24 hours after the first injection; significant granulocytopenia occurs within 6 to 8 days and lasts for 10 days to 3 weeks. Agranulocytosis appears to be relatively infrequent and recovery from leukopenia in most cases is complete within two weeks of the maximum reduction. Thrombocytopenia is variable but the time course of the appearance and recovery from reduced platelet counts generally parallels the sequence of granulocyte levels. In some cases severe thrombocytopenia may lead to bleeding from the gums and gastroin-

Continued on next page

Merck Sharp & Dohme—Cont.

testinal tract, petechiae, and small subcutaneous hemorrhages; these symptoms appear to be transient and in most cases disappear with return to a normal platelet count. However, a severe and even uncontrollable depression of the hematopoietic system occasionally may follow the usual dose of MUSTARGEN, particularly in patients with widespread disease and debility and in patients previously treated with other antineoplastic agents or x-ray. Persistent pancytopenia has been reported. In rare instances, hemorrhagic complications may be due to hyperheparinemia. Erythrocyte and hemoglobin levels may decline during the first 2 weeks after therapy but rarely significantly. Depression of the hematopoietic system may be found up to 50 days or more after starting therapy.

Integumentary: Occasionally, a maculopapular skin eruption occurs, but this may be idiosyncratic and does not necessarily recur with subsequent courses of the drug. Erythema multiforme has been observed. Herpes zoster, a common complicating infection in patients with lymphomas, may first appear after therapy is instituted and on occasion may be precipitated by treatment. Further treatment should be discontinued during the acute phase of this illness to avoid progression to generalized herpes zoster.

Reproductive: Since the gonads are susceptible to MUSTARGEN, treatment may be followed by delayed catamenia, oligomenorrhea, or temporary or permanent amenorrhea. Impaired spermatogenesis, azoospermia, and total germinal aplasia have been reported in male patients treated with alkylating agents, especially in combination with other drugs. In some instances spermatogenesis may return in patients in remission, but this may occur only several years after intensive chemotherapy has been discontinued. Patients should be warned of the potential risk to their reproductive capacity.

OVERDOSAGE

With total doses exceeding 0.4 mg/kg of body weight for a single course, severe leukopenia, anemia, thrombocytopenia and a hemorrhagic diathesis with subsequent delayed bleeding may develop. Death may follow. The only treatment in instances of excessive dosage appears to be repeated blood product transfusions, antibiotic treatment of complicating infections and general supportive measures.

The intravenous LD_{50} of MUSTARGEN is 2 mg/kg and 1.6 mg/kg in the mouse and rat, respectively.

DOSAGE AND ADMINISTRATION

Intravenous Administration

The dosage of MUSTARGEN varies with the clinical situation, the therapeutic response and the magnitude of hematologic depression. A total dose of 0.4 mg/kg of body weight for each course usually is given either as a single dose or in divided doses of 0.1 to 0.2 mg/kg per day. Dosage should be based on ideal dry body weight. The presence of edema or ascites must be considered so that dosage will be based on actual weight unaugmented by these conditions.

The margin of safety in therapy with MUSTARGEN is narrow and considerable care must be exercised in the matter of dosage. Repeated examinations of blood are *mandatory* as a guide to subsequent therapy. (See OVERDOSAGE.)

Within a few minutes after intravenous injection, MUSTARGEN undergoes chemical transformation, combines with reactive compounds, and is no longer present in its active form in the blood stream. Subsequent courses should not be given until the patient has recovered hematologically from the previous course; this is best determined by repeated studies of the peripheral blood elements awaiting their return to normal levels. It is often possible to give repeated courses of MUSTARGEN as early as three weeks after treatment.

Preparation of Solution for Intravenous Administration

This drug is highly toxic and both powder and solution must be handled and administered with care. Since MUSTARGEN is a powerful vesicant, it is intended primarily for intravenous use, and in most instances is given by this route. Inhalation of dust or vapors and contact with skin or mucous membranes, especially those of the eyes, must be avoided. Rubber gloves should be worn when handling MUSTARGEN. Should accidental eye contact occur, copious irrigation with water, normal saline or a balanced salt ophthalmic irrigating solution should be instituted immediately, followed by prompt ophthalmologic consultation. Should accidental skin contact occur, the affected part must be irrigated immediately with copious amounts of water, for at least 15 minutes, followed by 2 percent sodium thiosulfate solution. (See also box warning and *Special Handling.*)

Each vial of MUSTARGEN contains 10 mg of mechlorethamine hydrochloride triturated with sodium chloride q.s. 100 mg. In neutral or alkaline aqueous solution it undergoes rapid chemical transformation and is highly unstable. Although solutions prepared according to instructions are

acidic and do not decompose as rapidly, they should be prepared immediately before each injection since they will decompose on standing. When reconstituted, MUSTARGEN is a clear colorless solution. *Do not use if the solution is discolored or if droplets of water are visible within the vial prior to reconstitution.*

Using a sterile 10 mL syringe, inject 10 mL of Sterile Water for Injection or 10 mL Sodium Chloride Injection into a vial of MUSTARGEN. With the needle (syringe attached) still in the rubber stopper, shake the vial several times to dissolve the drug completely. The resultant solution contains 1 mg of mechlorethamine hydrochloride per mL.

Parenteral drug products should be inspected visually for particulate matter and discoloration prior to administration whenever solution and container permit.

Special Handling

Due to the drug's toxic and mutagenic properties, appropriate precautions including the use of appropriate safety equipment are recommended for the preparation of MUSTARGEN for parenteral administration. The National Institutes of Health presently recommends that the preparation of injectable anti-neoplastic drugs should be performed in a Class II laminar flow biological safety cabinet and that personnel preparing drugs of this class should wear surgical gloves and a closed front surgical-type gown with knit cuffs. Several other guidelines for proper handling and disposal of anti-cancer drugs have been published and should be considered. There is no general agreement that all of the procedures recommended in the guidelines are necessary or appropriate.

Accidental contact: Should accidental eye contact occur, copious irrigation with water, normal saline or a balanced salt ophthalmic irrigating solution should be instituted immediately, followed by prompt ophthalmologic consultation. Should accidental skin contact occur, the affected part must be irrigated immediately with copious amounts of water, for at least 15 minutes, followed by 2 percent sodium thiosulfate solution. (See also box warning.)

Technique for Intravenous Administration

Withdraw into the syringe the calculated volume of solution required for a single injection. *Dispose of any remaining solution after neutralization (see below).* Although the drug may be injected directly into any suitable vein, it is injected preferably into the rubber or plastic tubing of a flowing intravenous infusion set. This reduces the possibility of severe local reactions due to extravasation or high concentration of the drug. Injecting the drug into the tubing rather than adding it to the entire volume of the infusion fluid minimizes a chemical reaction between the drug and the solution. The rate of injection apparently is not critical provided it is completed within a few minutes.

Intracavitary Administration

Nitrogen mustard has been used by intracavitary administration with varying success in certain malignant conditions for the control of pleural, peritoneal, and pericardial effusions caused by malignant cells.

The technic and the dose used by any of these routes varies. Therefore, if MUSTARGEN is given by the intracavitary route, the published articles concerning such use should be consulted. *Because of the inherent risks involved, the physician should be experienced in the appropriate injection technics, and be thoroughly aware of the indications, dosages, hazards, and precautions as set forth in the published literature. When using MUSTARGEN by the intracavitary route, the general precautions concerning this agent should be borne in mind.*

As a general guide, reference is made especially to the technics of Weisberger et al. Intracavitary use is indicated in the presence of pleural, peritoneal, or pericardial effusion due to metastatic tumors. Local therapy with nitrogen mustard is used only when malignant cells are demonstrated in the effusion. Intracavitary injection is not recommended when the accumulated fluid is chylous in nature, since results are likely to be poor.

Paracentesis is first performed with most of the fluid being removed from the pleural or peritoneal cavity. The intracavitary use of MUSTARGEN may exert at least some of its effect through production of a chemical poudrage. Therefore, the removal of excess fluid allows the drug to more easily contact the peritoneal and pleural linings. For intrapleural or intrapericardial injection nitrogen mustard is introduced directly through the thoracentesis needle. For intraperitoneal injection it is given through a rubber catheter inserted into the trocar used for paracentesis or through a No. 18 gauge needle inserted at another site. This drug should be injected slowly, with frequent aspiration to ensure that a free flow of fluid is present. If fluid cannot be aspirated, pain and necrosis due to injection of solution outside the cavity may occur. Free flow of fluid also is necessary to prevent injection into a loculated pocket and to ensure adequate dissemination of nitrogen mustard.

The usual dose of nitrogen mustard for intracavitary injection is 0.4 mg/kg of body weight, though 0.2 mg/kg (or 10 to 20 mg) has been used by the intrapericardial route. The solution is prepared, as previously described for intravenous injection, by adding 10 mL of Sterile Water for Injection or

10 mL of Sodium Chloride Injection to the vial containing 10 mg of mechlorethamine hydrochloride. (Amounts of diluent of 50 to 100 mL of normal saline have also been used.) The position of the patient should be changed every 5 to 10 minutes for an hour after injection to obtain more uniform distribution of the drug throughout the serous cavity. The remaining fluid may be removed from the pleural or peritoneal cavity by paracentesis 24 to 36 hours later. The patient should be followed carefully by clinical and x-ray examination to detect reaccumulation of fluid.

Pain occurs rarely with intrapleural use; it is common with intraperitoneal injection and is often associated with nausea, vomiting, and diarrhea of 2 to 3 days duration. Transient cardiac irregularities may occur with intrapericardial injection. Death, possibly accelerated by nitrogen mustard, has been reported following the use of this agent by the intracavitary route. Although absorption of MUSTARGEN when given by the intracavitary route is probably not complete because of its rapid deactivation by body fluids, the systemic effect is unpredictable. The acute side effects such as nausea and vomiting are usually mild. Bone marrow depression is generally milder than when the drug is given intravenously. Care should be taken to avoid use by the intracavitary route when other agents which may suppress bone marrow function are being used systemically.

Neutralization of Equipment and Unused Solution

To clean rubber gloves, tubing, glassware, etc., after giving MUSTARGEN, soak them in an aqueous solution containing equal volumes of sodium thiosulfate (5%) and sodium bicarbonate (5%) for 45 minutes. Excess reagents and reaction products are washed away easily with water. Any unused injection solution should be neutralized by mixing with an equal volume of sodium thiosulfate/sodium bicarbonate solution. Allow the mixture to stand for 45 minutes. Vials that have contained MUSTARGEN should be treated in the same way with thiosulfate/bicarbonate solution before disposal.

HOW SUPPLIED

No. 7753—Trituration of MUSTARGEN is a white crystalline powder, each vial containing 10 mg mechlorethamine hydrochloride with sodium chloride q.s. 100 mg, and is supplied as follows:

NDC 0006-7753-31 in treatment sets of 4 vials.

Storage

Store at room temperature. Solutions of mechlorethamine HCl decompose on standing; therefore, solutions of the drug should be prepared immediately before use.

A.H.F.S. Category: 10:00

DC 7417928   Issued July 1987

MYOCHRYSINE® Injection   ℞
(Gold Sodium Thiomalate, MSD), U.S.P.

Physicians planning to use MYOCHRYSINE® (Gold Sodium Thiomalate, MSD) should thoroughly familiarize themselves with its toxicity and its benefits. The possibility of toxic reactions should always be explained to the patient before starting therapy. Patients should be warned to report promptly any symptoms suggesting toxicity. Before each injection of MYOCHRYSINE, the physician should review the results of laboratory work, and see the patient to determine the presence or absence of adverse reactions since some of these can be severe or even fatal.

DESCRIPTION

MYOCHRYSINE is a sterile aqueous solution of gold sodium thiomalate. It contains 0.5 percent benzyl alcohol added as a preservative. The pH of the product is 5.8–6.5.

Gold sodium thiomalate is a mixture of the mono- and disodium salts of gold thiomalic acid. The structural formula is:

$$\begin{array}{l} CH_2COO^- \\ | \\ Au\!-\!S\!-\!CHCOO^- \end{array} \cdot \; xNa^+ \; \cdot \; (2\!-\!x)H^+$$

mercaptobutanedioic acid, monogold (1+) sodium salt

The molecular weight for $C_4H_3AuNa_2O_4S$ (the disodium salt) is 390.07 and for $C_4H_4AuNaO_4S$ (the monosodium salt) is 368.09.

MYOCHRYSINE is supplied as a solution for intramuscular injection containing 25 mg or 50 mg of gold sodium thiomalate per mL.

CLINICAL PHARMACOLOGY

The mode of action of gold sodium thiomalate is unknown. The predominant action appears to be a suppressive effect on the synovitis of active rheumatoid disease.

INDICATIONS AND USAGE

MYOCHRYSINE is indicated in the treatment of selected cases of active rheumatoid arthritis— both adult and juvenile type. The greatest benefit occurs in the early active stage. In late stages of the illness when cartilage and bone damage have occurred, gold can only check the progression of rheumatoid arthritis and prevent further structural damage to joints. It cannot repair damage caused by previously active disease.

MYOCHRYSINE should be used only as *one part* of a complete program of therapy; alone it is not a complete treatment.

CONTRAINDICATIONS

Severe toxicity resulting from previous exposure to gold or other heavy metals.
Severe debilitation.
Systemic lupus erythematosus.

WARNINGS

Before treatment is started, the patient's hemoglobin, erythrocyte, white blood cell, differential and platelet counts should be determined, and urinalysis should be done to serve as basic reference. Urine should be analyzed for protein and sediment changes prior to each injection. Complete blood counts including platelet estimation should be made before every second injection throughout treatment. The occurrence of purpura or ecchymoses at any time always requires a platelet count.

Danger signals of possible gold toxicity include: rapid reduction of hemoglobin, leukopenia below 4000 WBC/cu mL, eosinophilia above 5 percent, platelet decrease below 100,000/cu mL, albuminuria, hematuria, pruritus, skin eruption, stomatitis, or persistent diarrhea. No additional injections of MYOCHRYSINE should be given unless further studies show these abnormalities to be caused by conditions other than gold toxicity.

PRECAUTIONS

General
Gold salts should not be used concomitantly with penicillamine.

The safety of coadministration with cytotoxic drugs has not been established.

Caution is indicated in the use of MYOCHRYSINE in patients with the following:

1. a history of blood dyscrasias such as granulocytopenia or anemia caused by drug sensitivity,
2. allergy or hypersensitivity to medications,
3. skin rash,
4. previous kidney or liver disease,
5. marked hypertension,
6. compromised cerebral or cardiovascular circulation.

Diabetes mellitus or congestive heart failure should be under control before gold therapy is instituted.

Carcinogenicity
Renal adenomas have been reported in long-term toxicity studies of rats receiving MYOCHRYSINE at high dose levels (2 mg/kg weekly for 45 weeks, followed by 6 mg/kg daily for 47 weeks), approximately 2 to 42 times the usual human dose. These adenomas are histologically similar to those produced in rats by chronic administration of experimental gold compounds and other heavy metals, such as lead. No reports have been received of renal adenomas in man in association with the use of MYOCHRYSINE.

Pregnancy
Pregnancy Category C.
MYOCHRYSINE has been shown to be teratogenic during the organogenetic period in rats and rabbits when given in doses, respectively, of 140 and 175 times the usual human dose. Hydrocephaly and microphthalmia were the malformations observed in rats when MYOCHRYSINE was administered subcutaneously at a dose of 25 mg/kg/day from day 6 through day 15 of gestation. In rabbits, limb malformations and gastroschisis were the malformations observed when MYOCHRYSINE was administered subcutaneously at doses of 20–45 mg/kg/day from day 6 through day 18 of gestation. There are no adequate and well-controlled studies in pregnant women. MYOCHRYSINE should be used during pregnancy only if the potential benefit to the mother justifies the potential risk to the fetus.

Nursing Mothers
The presence of gold has been demonstrated in the milk of lactating mothers. In addition, gold has been found in the serum and red blood cells of a nursing infant. In view of the above findings and because of the potential for serious adverse reactions in nursing infants from MYOCHRYSINE, a decision should be made whether to discontinue nursing or to discontinue the drug, taking into account the importance of the drug to the mother. The slow excretion and persistence of gold in the mother, even after therapy is discontinued, must also be kept in mind.

ADVERSE REACTIONS

A variety of adverse reactions may develop during the initial phase (weekly injections) of therapy or during maintenance treatment. Adverse reactions are observed most frequently when the cumulative dose of MYOCHRYSINE administered is between 400 and 800 mg. Very uncommonly, complications occur days to months after cessation of treatment.

Cutaneous reactions: Dermatitis is the most common reaction. *Any eruption, especially if pruritic, that develops during treatment with MYOCHRYSINE should be considered a reaction to gold until proven otherwise.* Pruritus often exists before dermatitis becomes apparent, and therefore should be considered a warning signal of impending cutaneous reaction. The most serious form of cutaneous reaction is generalized exfoliative dermatitis which may lead to alopecia and shedding of nails. Gold dermatitis may be aggravated by exposure to sunlight or an actinic rash may develop.

Mucous membrane reactions: Stomatitis is the second most common adverse reaction. Shallow ulcers on the buccal membranes, on the borders of the tongue, and on the palate or in the pharynx may occur as the only adverse reaction, or along with dermatitis. Sometimes diffuse glossitis or gingivitis develops. A metallic taste may precede these oral mucous membrane reactions and should be considered a warning signal.

Conjunctivitis is a rare reaction.

Renal reactions: Gold may be toxic to the kidney and produce a nephrotic syndrome or glomerulitis with hematuria. These renal reactions are usually relatively mild and subside completely if recognized early and treatment is discontinued. They may become severe and chronic if treatment is continued after onset of the reaction. Therefore, it is important to perform a *urinalysis before every injection*, and to discontinue treatment promptly if proteinuria or hematuria develops.

Hematologic reactions: Blood dyscrasia due to gold toxicity is rare, but because of the potential serious consequences it must be constantly watched for and recognized early by frequent blood examinations done throughout treatment. Granulocytopenia; thrombocytopenia, with or without purpura; hypoplastic and aplastic anemia; and eosinophilia have all been reported. These hematologic disorders may occur separately or in combinations.

Nitritoid and allergic reactions: Reactions of the "nitritoid type" which may resemble anaphylactoid effects have been reported. Flushing, fainting, dizziness and sweating are most frequently reported. Other symptoms that may occur include: nausea, vomiting, malaise and weakness.

More severe, but less common effects include: anaphylactic shock, syncope, bradycardia, thickening of the tongue, difficulty in swallowing and breathing, and angioneurotic edema. These effects may occur almost immediately after injection or as late as 10 minutes following injection. They may occur at any time during the course of therapy and if observed, treatment with MYOCHRYSINE should be discontinued.

Miscellaneous reactions: Gastrointestinal reactions have been reported, including nausea, vomiting, anorexia, abdominal cramps and diarrhea. Ulcerative enterocolitis, which can be severe or even fatal, has been reported rarely.

There have been rare reports of reactions involving the eye such as iritis, corneal ulcers, and gold deposits in ocular tissues. Peripheral and central nervous system complications have been reported rarely. Peripheral neuropathy, with or without fasciculations, sensorimotor effects (including Guillain-Barré syndrome) and elevated spinal fluid protein have been reported. Central nervous system complications have included confusion, hallucinations and seizures. Usually these signs and symptoms cleared upon discontinuation of gold therapy.

Hepatitis, jaundice, with or without cholestasis, gold bronchitis, pulmonary injury manifested by interstitial pneumonitis and fibrosis, partial or complete hair loss and fever have also been reported.

Sometimes arthralgia occurs for a day or two after an injection of MYOCHRYSINE; this reaction usually subsides after the first few injections.

MANAGEMENT OF ADVERSE REACTIONS

Treatment with MYOCHRYSINE should be discontinued immediately when toxic reactions occur. Minor complications such as localized dermatitis, mild stomatitis, or slight proteinuria generally require no other therapy and resolve spontaneously with suspension of MYOCHRYSINE. Moderately severe skin and mucous membrane reactions often benefit from topical corticosteroids, oral antihistaminics, and soothing or anesthetic lotions.

If stomatitis or dermatitis becomes severe or more generalized, systemic corticosteroids (generally, prednisone 10 to 40 mg daily in divided doses) may provide symptomatic relief. For serious renal, hematologic, pulmonary, and enterocolitic complications, high doses of systemic corticosteroids (prednisone 40 to 100 mg daily in divided doses) are recommended. The optimum duration of corticosteroid treatment varies with the response of the individual patient. Therapy may be required for many months when adverse effects are unusually severe or progressive.

In patients whose complications do not improve with high-dose corticosteroid treatment, or who develop significant steroid-related adverse reactions, a chelating agent may be given to enhance gold excretion. Dimercaprol (BAL) has been used successfully, but patients must be monitored carefully as numerous untoward reactions may attend its use. Corticosteroids and a chelating agent may be used concomitantly.

MYOCHRYSINE *should not be reinstituted after severe or idiosyncratic reactions.*

MYOCHRYSINE may be readministered following resolution of mild reactions, using a reduced dosage schedule. If an initial test dose of 5 mg MYOCHRYSINE is well-tolerated, progressively larger doses (5 to 10 mg increments) may be given at weekly to monthly intervals until a dose of 25 to 50 mg is reached.

DOSAGE AND ADMINISTRATION

MYOCHRYSINE should be administered only by intramuscular injection, preferably intragluteally. It should be given with the patient lying down. He should remain recumbent for approximately 10 minutes after the injection.

Therapeutic effects from MYOCHRYSINE occur slowly. Early improvement, often limited to a reduction in morning stiffness, may begin after six to eight weeks of treatment, but beneficial effects may not be observed until after months of therapy.

Parenteral drug products should be inspected visually for particulate matter and discoloration prior to administration. Do not use if material has darkened. Color should not exceed pale yellow.

For the adult of average size the following dosage schedule is suggested:

Weekly Injections	
1st injection	10 mg
2nd injection	25 mg
3rd and subsequent injections, 25 to 50 mg	

until there is toxicity or major clinical improvement, or, in the absence of either of these, the cumulative dose of MYOCHRYSINE reaches one gram.

MYOCHRYSINE is continued until the cumulative dose reaches one gram unless toxicity or major clinical improvement occurs. If significant clinical improvement occurs before a cumulative dose of one gram has been administered, the dose may be decreased or the interval between injections increased as with maintenance therapy. Maintenance doses of 25 to 50 mg every other week for two to 20 weeks are recommended. If the clinical course remains stable, injections of 25 to 50 mg may be given every third and subsequently every fourth week indefinitely. Some patients may require maintenance treatment at intervals of one to three weeks. Should the arthritis exacerbate during maintenance therapy, weekly injections may be resumed temporarily until disease activity is suppressed.

Should a patient fail to improve during initial therapy (cumulative dose of one gram), several options are available:

1— the patient may be considered to be unresponsive and MYOCHRYSINE is discontinued
2— the same dose (25 to 50 mg) of MYOCHRYSINE may be continued for approximately ten additional weeks
3— the dose of MYOCHRYSINE may be increased by increments of 10 mg every one to four weeks, not to exceed 100 mg in a single injection.

If significant clinical improvement occurs using option 2 or 3, the maintenance schedule described above should be initiated. If there is no significant improvement or if toxicity occurs, therapy with MYOCHRYSINE should be stopped. The higher the individual dose of MYOCHRYSINE, the greater the risk of gold toxicity. Selection of one of these options for chrysotherapy should be based upon a number of factors, including the physician's experience with gold salt therapy, the course of the patient's condition, the choice of alternative treatments, and the availability of the patient for the close supervision required.

Continued on next page

Merck Sharp & Dohme—Cont.

Juvenile Rheumatoid Arthritis

The pediatric dose of MYOCHRYSINE is proportional to the adult dose on a weight basis. After the initial test dose of 10 mg, the recommended dose for children is one mg per kilogram body weight, not to exceed 50 mg for a single injection. Otherwise, the guidelines given above for administration to adults also apply to children.

Concomitant Drug Therapy—Gold salts should not be used concomitantly with penicillamine.

The safety of coadministration with cytotoxic drugs has not been established. Other measures, such as salicylates, other non-steroidal anti-inflammatory drugs, or systemic corticosteroids, may be continued when MYOCHRYSINE is initiated. After improvement commences, analgesic and anti-inflammatory drugs may be discontinued slowly as symptoms permit.

HOW SUPPLIED

Injection MYOCHRYSINE is a clear colorless to light yellow solution, depending on potency, which must be protected from light. It is supplied as follows:

No. 7764—25 mg of gold sodium thiomalate per mL as NDC 0006-7764-64 in boxes of 6 x 1 mL ampuls.

No. 7762—50 mg of gold sodium thiomalate per mL as NDC 0006-7762-64 in boxes of 6 x 1 mL ampuls

NDC 0006-7762-10 in 10 mL vials

(6505-00-973-8579, 10 mL vial).

Storage

Protect from light.

Store container in carton until contents have been used.

A.H.F.S. Category: 60:00

DC 6015526   Revised June 1987

COPYRIGHT © MERCK & CO., INC. 1985

All rights reserved

NEODECADRON® Sterile Ophthalmic Ointment ℞
(Neomycin Sulfate-Dexamethasone Sodium Phosphate, MSD), U.S.P.

DESCRIPTION

Sterile ophthalmic ointment NEODECADRON® (Neomycin Sulfate-Dexamethasone Sodium Phosphate, MSD) is a topical corticosteroid-antibiotic ointment for use in certain disorders of the anterior segment of the eye.

Ophthalmic ointment NEODECADRON contains in each gram: dexamethasone sodium phosphate equivalent to 0.5 mg (0.05%) dexamethasone phosphate and neomycin sulfate equivalent to 3.5 mg neomycin base. Inactive ingredients: white petrolatum and mineral oil.

Dexamethasone sodium phosphate is an inorganic ester of dexamethasone. Its empirical formula is $C_{22}H_{28}FNa_2O_8P$. Neomycin sulfate is the sulfate salt of neomycin, an antibacterial substance produced by the growth of *Streptomyces fradiae* Waksman (Fam. Streptomycetaceae).

CLINICAL PHARMACOLOGY

Dexamethasone sodium phosphate, a corticosteroid, suppresses the inflammatory response to a variety of agents, and it probably delays or slows healing. Since corticosteroids may inhibit the body's defense mechanism against infection, a concomitant antimicrobial drug may be used when this inhibition is considered to be clinically significant in a particular case.

Neomycin sulfate, the anti-infective component in the combination, is included to provide action against specific organisms susceptible to it. Neomycin sulfate is considered active mainly against gram-negative organisms, except *Bacteroides* spp. and *Pseudomonas aeruginosa*, which are resistant. Gram-positive organisms except for *Staphylococcus aureus* are usually resistant.

When a decision to administer both a corticosteroid and an antimicrobial is made, the administration of such drugs in combination has the advantage of greater patient compliance and convenience, with the added assurance that the appropriate dosage of both drugs is administered, plus assured compatibility of ingredient when both types of drug are in the same formulation and, particularly, that the correct volume of drug is delivered and retained.

The relative potency of corticosteroids depends on the molecular structure, concentration, and release from the vehicle.

INDICATIONS AND USAGE

For steroid-responsive inflammatory ocular conditions for which a corticosteroid is indicated and where bacterial infection or a risk of bacterial ocular infection exists.

Ocular steroids are indicated in inflammatory conditions of the palpebral and bulbar conjunctiva, cornea, and anterior segment of the globe where the inherent risk of steroid use in certain infective conjunctivitides is accepted to obtain a diminution in edema and inflammation. They are also indicated in chronic anterior uveitis and corneal injury from chemical, radiation, or thermal burns, or penetration of foreign bodies.

The use of a combination drug with an anti-infective component is indicated where the risk of infection is high or where there is an expectation that potentially dangerous numbers of bacteria will be present in the eye.

The particular anti-infective drug in this product is active against the following common bacterial eye pathogens:

    Staphylococcus aureus
    Escherichia coli
    Haemophilus influenzae
    Klebsiella/Enterobacter species
    Neisseria species

The product does not provide adequate coverage against:

    Pseudomonas aeruginosa
    Serratia marcescens
    Streptococci, including *Streptococcus pneumoniae*

CONTRAINDICATIONS

Epithelial herpes simplex keratitis (dendritic keratitis), acute infectious stages of vaccinia, varicella, and many other viral diseases of the cornea and conjunctiva. Mycobacterial infection of the eye. Fungal diseases of ocular structures. Hypersensitivity to a component of the medication (hypersensitivity to the antibiotic component occurs at a higher rate than for other components).

The use of these combinations is always contraindicated after uncomplicated removal of a corneal foreign body.

WARNINGS

Prolonged use may result in glaucoma, with damage to the optic nerve, defects in visual acuity and fields of vision, and posterior subcapsular cataract formation. Prolonged use may suppress the host response and thus increase the hazard of secondary ocular infections. In those diseases causing thinning of the cornea or sclera, perforations have been known to occur with the use of topical corticosteroids. In acute purulent conditions of the eye, corticosteroids may mask infection or enhance existing infection. If these products are used for 10 days or longer, intraocular pressure should be routinely monitored even though it may be difficult in children and uncooperative patients.

Employment of corticosteroid medication in the treatment of herpes simplex requires great caution: periodic slit-lamp microscopy is recommended.

Any substance (e.g. neomycin sulfate) may occasionally cause cutaneous sensitization. If any reaction indicating such sensitivity is observed, discontinue use.

PRECAUTIONS

The initial prescriptions and renewal of the medication order beyond 8 grams should be made by a physician only after examination of the patient with the aid of magnification, such as slit-lamp biomicroscopy and, where appropriate, fluorescein staining.

The possibility of persistent fungal infections of the cornea should be considered after prolonged corticosteroid dosing.

Usage in Pregnancy

Safety of intensive or protracted use of topical corticosteroids during pregnancy has not been substantiated.

ADVERSE REACTIONS

Adverse reactions have occurred with corticosteroid/anti-infective combination drugs which can be attributed to the corticosteroid component, the anti-infective component, or the combination. Exact incidence figures are not available since no denominator of treated patients is available.

Reactions occurring most often from the presence of the anti-infective ingredient are allergic sensitizations. The reactions due to the corticosteroid component in decreasing order of frequency are: elevation of intraocular pressure (IOP) with possible development of glaucoma, and infrequent optic nerve damage; posterior subcapsular cataract formation; and delayed wound healing.

Secondary Infection: The development of secondary infection has occurred after use of combinations containing corticosteroids and antimicrobials. Fungal infections of the cornea are particularly prone to develop coincidentally with long-term applications of corticosteroid. The possibility of fungal invasion must be considered in any persistent corneal ulceration where corticosteroid treatment has been used. Secondary bacterial ocular infection following suppression of host responses also occurs.

DOSAGE AND ADMINISTRATION

The duration of treatment will vary with the type of lesion and may extend from a few days to several weeks, according to therapeutic response. Relapses, more common in chronic active lesions than in self-limited conditions, usually respond to retreatment.

Apply a thin coating of ophthalmic ointment NEODECADRON three or four times a day. When a favorable response is observed, reduce the number of daily applications to two, and later to one a day as maintenance dose if this is sufficient to control symptoms.

Not more than 8 grams should be prescribed initially and the prescription should not be refilled without further evaluation as outlined in PRECAUTIONS above.

Ophthalmic ointment NEODECADRON is particularly convenient when an eye pad is used. It may also be the preparation of choice for patients in whom therapeutic benefit depends on prolonged contact of the active ingredients with ocular tissues.

HOW SUPPLIED

No. 7617—Sterile Ophthalmic Ointment NEODECADRON is a clear, unctuous ointment, and is supplied as follows:

NDC 0006-7617-04 in 3.5 g tubes

(6505-00-823-7956 0.05% 3.5 g)

A.H.F.S. Category: 52:08

DC 6167722   Issued June 1982

NEODECADRON® Sterile Ophthalmic Solution ℞
(Neomycin Sulfate-Dexamethasone Sodium Phosphate, MSD), U.S.P.

DESCRIPTION

Ophthalmic solution NEODECADRON® (Neomycin Sulfate-Dexamethasone Sodium Phosphate, MSD) is a topical corticosteroid-antibiotic solution for use in certain disorders of the anterior segment of the eye.

Each milliliter of buffered ophthalmic solution NEODECADRON in the OCUMETER® ophthalmic dispenser contains: dexamethasone sodium phosphate equivalent to 1 mg (0.1%) dexamethasone phosphate, and neomycin sulfate equivalent to 3.5 mg neomycin base. Inactive ingredients: creatinine, sodium citrate, sodium borate, polysorbate 80, disodium edetate, hydrochloric acid to adjust pH to 6.6–7.2, and water for injection. Benzalkonium chloride 0.02% and sodium bisulfite 0.1% added as preservatives.

Dexamethasone sodium phosphate is a water soluble, inorganic ester of dexamethasone. Its empirical formula is $C_{22}H_{28}FNa_2O_8P$. It is approximately three thousand times more soluble in water at 25°C than hydrocortisone.

Neomycin sulfate is the sulfate salt of neomycin, an antibacterial substance produced by the growth of *Streptomyces fradiae* Waksman (Fam. Streptomycetaceae).

CLINICAL PHARMACOLOGY

Dexamethasone sodium phosphate, a corticosteroid, suppresses the inflammatory response to a variety of agents, and it probably delays or slows healing. Since corticosteroids may inhibit the body's defense mechanism against infection, a concomitant antimicrobial drug may be used when this inhibition is considered to be clinically significant in a particular case. Neomycin sulfate, the anti-infective component in the combination, is included to provide action against specific organisms susceptible to it. Neomycin sulfate is considered active mainly against gram-negative organisms, except *Bacteroides* spp. and *Pseudomonas aeruginosa*, which are resistant. Gram-positive organisms except for *Staphylococcus aureus* are usually resistant.

When a decision to administer both a corticosteroid and an antimicrobial is made, the administration of such drugs in combination has the advantage of greater patient compliance and convenience, with the added assurance that the appropriate dosage of both drugs is administered, plus assured compatibility of ingredients when both types of drug are in the same formulation and, particularly, that the correct volume of drug is delivered and retained.

The relative potency of corticosteroids depends on the molecular structure, concentration, and release from the vehicle.

INDICATIONS AND USAGE

For steroid-responsive inflammatory ocular conditions for which a corticosteroid is indicated and where bacterial infection or a risk of bacterial ocular infection exists.

Ocular steroids are indicated in inflammatory conditions of the palpebral and bulbar conjunctiva, cornea, and anterior segment of the globe where the inherent risk of steroid use in certain infective conjunctivitides is accepted to obtain a diminution in edema and inflammation. They are also indicated in chronic anterior uveitis and corneal injury from chemical, radiation, or thermal burns, or penetration of foreign bodies. The use of a combination drug with an anti-infective component is indicated where the risk of infection is high or where there is an expectation that potentially dangerous numbers of bacteria will be present in the eye.

The particular anti-infective drug in this product is active against the following common bacterial eye pathogens:

Staphylococcus aureus
Escherichia coli
Haemophilus influenzae
Klebsiella/Enterobacter species
Neisseria species

The product does not provide adequate coverage against:

Pseudomonas aeruginosa
Serratia marcescens
Streptococci, including *Streptococcus pneumoniae*

CONTRAINDICATIONS

Epithelial herpes simplex keratitis (dendritic keratitis), acute infectious stages of vaccinia, varicella, and many other viral diseases of the cornea and conjunctiva. Mycobacterial infection of the eye. Fungal diseases of ocular structures. Hypersensitivity to any component of this product, including sulfites (see WARNINGS). (Hypersensitivity to the antibiotic component occurs at a higher rate than for other components.)

The use of these combinations is always contraindicated after uncomplicated removal of a corneal foreign body.

WARNINGS

Prolonged use may result in glaucoma, with damage to the optic nerve, defects in visual acuity and fields of vision, and posterior subcapsular cataract formation. Prolonged use may suppress the host response and thus increase the hazard of secondary ocular infections. In those diseases causing thinning of the cornea or sclera, perforations have been known to occur with the use of topical corticosteroids. In acute purulent conditions of the eye, corticosteroids may mask infection or enhance existing infection. If these products are used for 10 days or longer, intraocular pressure should be routinely monitored even though it may be difficult in children and uncooperative patients.

Employment of corticosteroid medication in the treatment of herpes simplex requires great caution: periodic slit-lamp microscopy is recommended.

Any substance (e.g., neomycin sulfate) may occasionally cause cutaneous sensitization. If any reaction indicating such sensitivity is observed, discontinue use.

Ophthalmic Solution NEODECADRON contains sodium bisulfite, a sulfite that may cause allergic-type reactions including anaphylactic symptoms and life-threatening or less severe asthmatic episodes in certain susceptible people. The overall prevalence of sulfite sensitivity in the general population is unknown and probably low. Sulfite sensitivity is seen more frequently in asthmatic than in nonasthmatic people.

PRECAUTIONS

The initial prescription and renewal of the medication order beyond 20 milliliters should be made by a physician only after examination of the patient with the aid of magnification, such as slit-lamp biomicroscopy and, where appropriate, fluorescein staining.

The possibility of persistent fungal infections of the cornea should be considered after prolonged corticosteroid dosing.

Usage in Pregnancy

Safety of intensive or protracted use of topical corticosteroids during pregnancy has not been substantiated.

ADVERSE REACTIONS

Adverse reactions have occurred with corticosteroid/anti-infective combination drugs which can be attributed to the corticosteroid component, the anti-infective component, the combination, or any other component of the product. Exact incidence figures are not available since no denominator of treated patients is available.

Reactions occurring most often from the presence of the anti-infective ingredient are allergic sensitizations. The reactions due to the corticosteroid component in decreasing order of frequency are: elevation of intraocular pressure (IOP) with possible development of glaucoma, and infrequent optic nerve damage; posterior subcapsular cataract formation; and delayed wound healing.

Secondary Infection: The development of secondary infection has occurred in use of combinations containing corticosteroids and antimicrobials. Fungal infections of the cornea are particularly prone to develop coincidentally with long-term applications of corticosteroid. The possibility of fungal invasion must be considered in any persistent corneal ulceration where corticosteroid treatment has been used. Secondary bacterial ocular infection following suppression of host responses also occurs.

DOSAGE AND ADMINISTRATION

The duration of treatment will vary with the type of lesion and may extend from a few days to several weeks, according to therapeutic response. Relapses, more common in chronic active lesions than in self-limited conditions, usually respond to retreatment.

Instill one or two drops of ophthalmic solution NEODECADRON into the conjunctival sac every hour during the day and every two hours during the night as initial therapy. When a favorable response is observed, reduce dosage to one drop every four hours. Later, further reduction in dosage to one drop three or four times daily may suffice to control symptoms.

Not more than 20 milliliters should be prescribed initially and the prescription should not be refilled without further evaluation as outlined in PRECAUTIONS above.

HOW SUPPLIED

Sterile ophthalmic solution NEODECADRON is a clear, colorless to pale yellow solution.

No. 7639—Ophthalmic solution NEODECADRON is supplied as follows:

NDC 0006-7639-03 in 5 mL white opaque, plastic OCUMETER ophthalmic dispenser with a controlled drop tip. (6505-01-039-4352 0.1% 5 mL).

A.H.F.S. Category: 52:08

DC 7261319   Issued February 1987

NEODECADRON® Topical Cream   ℞
(Neomycin Sulfate-Dexamethasone Sodium Phosphate, MSD), U.S.P.

DESCRIPTION

NEODECADRON® (Neomycin Sulfate-Dexamethasone Sodium Phosphate, MSD) Topical Cream is a topical steroid-antibiotic preparation.

NEODECADRON Topical Cream contains in each gram: dexamethasone sodium phosphate equivalent to 1 mg (0.1%) dexamethasone phosphate, and neomycin sulfate equivalent to 3.5 mg neomycin base, in a greaseless bland base. Inactive ingredients: stearyl alcohol, cetyl alcohol, mineral oil, polyoxyl 40 stearate, sorbitol solution, methyl polysilicone emulsion, creatinine, disodium edetate, sodium citrate, sodium hydroxide to adjust pH, and purified water. Methylparaben 0.15%, sodium bisulfite 0.25%, and sorbic acid 0.1% added as preservatives.

Dexamethasone sodium phosphate is 9-fluoro-11β,17-dihydroxy-16α-methyl-21-(phosphonooxy)pregna-1,4-diene-3,20-dione disodium salt. Its empirical formula is $C_{22}H_{28}FNa_2O_8P$ and its structural formula is:

Dexamethasone sodium phosphate has a molecular weight of 516.41.

Glucocorticoids are adrenocortical steroids, both naturally occurring and synthetic. Dexamethasone is a synthetic analog of naturally occurring glucocorticoids (hydrocortisone and cortisone).

Neomycin sulfate is the sulfate salt of neomycin, an antibacterial substance produced by the growth of *Streptomyces fradiae* Waksman (Fam. Streptomycetaceae).

CLINICAL PHARMACOLOGY

Topical corticosteroids share anti-inflammatory, anti-pruritic, and vasoconstrictive actions.

The mechanism of anti-inflammatory activity of the topical corticosteroids is unclear. Various laboratory methods, including vasoconstrictor assays, are used to compare and predict potencies and/or clinical efficacies of the topical corticosteroids. There is some evidence to suggest that a recognizable correlation exists between vasoconstrictor potency and therapeutic efficacy in man.

Pharmacokinetics

The extent of percutaneous absorption of topical corticosteroids is determined by many factors including the vehicle, the integrity of the epidermal barrier, and the use of occlusive dressings.

Topical corticosteroids can be absorbed from normal intact skin. Inflammation and/or other disease processes in the skin increase percutaneous absorption. Occlusive dressings substantially increase the percutaneous absorption of topical corticosteroids. Thus, occlusive dressings may be a valuable therapeutic adjunct for treatment of resistant dermatoses. (See DOSAGE AND ADMINISTRATION.)

Once absorbed through the skin, topical corticosteroids are handled through pharmacokinetic pathways similar to systemically administered corticosteroids. Corticosteroids are bound to plasma proteins in varying degrees. Corticosteroids are metabolized primarily in the liver and are then excreted by the kidneys. Some of the topical corticosteroids and their metabolites are also excreted into the bile.

The antibiotic component, neomycin, is bactericidal to many gram-positive and gram-negative bacteria.

INDICATIONS AND USAGE

For the treatment of corticosteroid-responsive dermatoses with secondary infection. It has not been demonstrated that this steroid-antibiotic combination provides greater benefit than the steroid component alone after 7 days of treatment (see WARNINGS).

CONTRAINDICATIONS

Hypersensitivity to any component of this product, including sulfites (see WARNINGS).

WARNINGS

Topical Cream NEODECADRON contains sodium bisulfite, a sulfite that may cause allergic-type reactions including anaphylactic symptoms and life-threatening or less severe asthmatic episodes in certain susceptible people. The overall prevalence of sulfite sensitivity in the general population is unknown and probably low. Sulfite sensitivity is seen more frequently in asthmatic than in nonasthmatic people.

Because of the concern of nephrotoxicity and ototoxicity associated with neomycin, this combination product should not be used over a wide area or for extended periods of time.

PRECAUTIONS

General

Systemic absorption of topical corticosteroids has produced reversible hypothalamic-pituitary-adrenal (HPA) axis suppression, manifestations of Cushing's syndrome, hyperglycemia, and glycosuria in some patients.

Conditions which augment systemic absorption include the application of the more potent corticosteroids, use over large surface areas, prolonged use, and the addition of occlusive dressings.

Therefore, patients receiving a large dose of a potent topical corticosteroid applied to a large surface area or under an occlusive dressing should be evaluated periodically for evidence of HPA axis suppression by using urinary free cortisol and ACTH stimulation tests. If HPA axis suppression is noted, an attempt should be made to withdraw the drug, to reduce the frequency of application, or to substitute a less potent corticosteroid.

Recovery of HPA axis function is generally prompt and complete upon discontinuation of the drug. Infrequently, signs and symptoms of corticosteroid withdrawal may occur, requiring supplemental systemic corticosteroids.

Children may absorb proportionally larger amounts of topical corticosteroids and thus be more susceptible to systemic toxicity (see PRECAUTIONS, *Pediatric Use*).

Corticosteroids may mask some signs of infection, and new infections may appear during their use. There may be decreased resistance and inability to localize infection when corticosteroids are used. Therefore, patients with bacterial infections should also be given appropriate antibiotic therapy if Topical Cream NEODECADRON. Moreover, corticosteroids may affect the nitroblue-tetrazolium test for bacterial infection and produce false-negative results.

Corticosteroid therapy exerts its major immunosuppressive effects by impairing the normal function of the T-lymphocyte population and macrophages. When T-cell and/or macrophage function is impaired, latent disease may be activated or there may be an exacerbation of intercurrent infections due to pathogens, including those caused by Candida, Mycobacterium, Ameba, Toxoplasma, Strongyloides, Pneumocystis, Cryptococcus, Nocardia, etc. Products containing steroids should be used with caution in patients with impaired T-cell function or in patients receiving other immunosuppressive therapy.

In the presence of dermatological infections, the use of an appropriate antifungal or antibacterial agent should be instituted. If a favorable response does not occur promptly, the

Continued on next page

Merck Sharp & Dohme—Cont.

corticosteroid should be discontinued until the infection has been adequately controlled.

If irritation develops, topical corticosteroids should be discontinued and appropriate therapy instituted.

This product is not for ophthalmic use. However, if applied to the eyelids or skin near the eyes, the drug may enter the eyes. In patients with a history of herpes simplex keratitis, ocular exposure to corticosteroids may lead to a recurrence. Prolonged ocular exposure may cause steroid glaucoma.

A few individuals may be sensitive to one or more of the components of this product. Sensitivity to neomycin may occasionally develop, especially when it is applied to abraded skin. If any reaction indicating sensitivity is observed, discontinue use. There are reports in the current medical literature that indicate an increase in the prevalence of persons sensitive to neomycin.

Generally, occlusive dressings should not be used on weeping or exudative lesions.

If the occlusive dressing technique is employed, caution should be exercised with regard to the use of plastic films which are often inflammable and may pose a suffocation hazard for children.

When large areas of the body are covered with an occlusive dressing, thermal homeostasis may be impaired. If elevation of body temperature occurs, use of the occlusive dressing should be discontinued.

Information for the Patient
Patients using topical corticosteroids should receive the following information and instructions:
1. This medication is to be used as directed by the physician. It is for external use only. Avoid contact with the eyes.
2. Patients should be advised not to use this medication for any disorder other than that for which it was prescribed.
3. The treated skin area should not be bandaged or otherwise covered or wrapped so as to be occlusive unless directed by the physician.
4. Patients should report any signs of local adverse reactions, especially under occlusive dressings.
5. Parents of pediatric patients should be advised not to use tight-fitting diapers or plastic pants on a child being treated in the diaper area, as these garments may constitute occlusive dressings.

Laboratory Tests
The following tests may be helpful in evaluating the HPA axis suppression:
- Urinary free cortisol test
- ACTH stimulation test

Carcinogenesis, Mutagenesis and Impairment of Fertility
Long-term animal studies have not been performed to evaluate the carcinogenic potential or the effect on fertility of Topical Cream NEODECADRON.

Studies to determine mutagenicity with prednisolone and hydrocortisone have revealed negative results.

Pregnancy
Pregnancy Category C: Corticosteroids are generally teratogenic in laboratory animals when administered systemically at relatively low dosage levels. The more potent corticosteroids have been shown to be teratogenic after dermal application in laboratory animals. There are no adequate and well controlled studies in pregnant women on teratogenic effects from topically applied corticosteroids. Therefore, topical corticosteroids should be used during pregnancy only if the potential benefit justifies the potential risk to the fetus. Drugs of this class should not be used extensively on pregnant patients, in large amounts, or for prolonged periods of time.

Nursing Mothers
It is not known whether topical administration of corticosteroids could result in sufficient systemic absorption to produce detectable quantities in breast milk. Systemically administered corticosteroids are secreted into breast milk in quantities *not* likely to have a deleterious effect on the infant. Nevertheless, caution should be exercised when topical corticosteroids are administered to a nursing woman.

Pediatric Use
Pediatric patients may demonstrate greater susceptibility to topical corticosteroid-induced HPA axis suppression and Cushing's syndrome than mature patients because of a larger skin surface area to body weight ratio.

Hypothalamic-pituitary-adrenal (HPA) axis suppression, Cushing's syndrome, and intracranial hypertension have been reported in children receiving topical corticosteroids. Manifestations of adrenal suppression in children include linear growth retardation, delayed weight gain, low plasma cortisol levels, and absence of response to ACTH stimulation. Manifestations of intracranial hypertension include bulging fontanelles, headaches, and bilateral papilledema.

Administration of topical corticosteroids to children should be limited to the least amount compatible with an effective therapeutic regimen. Chronic corticosteroid therapy may interfere with the growth and development of children.

ADVERSE REACTIONS

The following adverse reactions are reported infrequently with topical corticosteroids, but may occur more frequently with the use of occlusive dressings. These reactions are listed in an approximate decreasing order of occurrence:
Burning
Itching
Irritation
Dryness
Folliculitis
Hypertrichosis
Acneiform eruptions
Hypopigmentation
Perioral dermatitis
Allergic contact dermatitis
Maceration of the skin
Secondary infection
Skin atrophy
Striae
Miliaria
Prevalence of neomycin hypersensitivity is increasing. Ototoxicity and nephrotoxicity have been reported with prolonged use or use of large amounts of topical neomycin preparations.

OVERDOSAGE

Topically applied corticosteroids can be absorbed in sufficient amounts to produce systemic effects (see PRECAUTIONS).

DOSAGE AND ADMINISTRATION

Apply to the affected area as a thin film three or four times daily.

Before using NEODECADRON Topical Cream in the *ear*, clean the aural canal thoroughly and sponge dry. Confirm that the eardrum is intact. With a cotton-tipped applicator, apply a thin coating of the cream to the affected canal area two or three times a day. When a favorable response is obtained, reduce the number of daily applications to one or two, and eventually discontinue.

HOW SUPPLIED

No. 7607—Topical Cream NEODECADRON is a white cream, and is supplied as follows:
NDC 0006-7607-12 in 15 g tubes
NDC 0006-7607-24 in 30 g tubes
A.H.F.S. Category: 84:06
DC 7612426   Issued September 1988
COPYRIGHT © MERCK & CO. INC., 1985
All rights reserved

NOROXIN® Tablets   ℞
(Norfloxacin, MSD)

DESCRIPTION

NOROXIN® (Norfloxacin, MSD) is a synthetic, broad-spectrum antibacterial agent for oral administration. Norfloxacin, a fluoroquinolone, is 1-ethyl-6-fluoro-1, 4-dihydro-4-oxo-7-(1-piperazinyl)-3-quinolinecarboxylic acid. Its empirical formula is $C_{16}H_{18}FN_3O_3$ and the structural formula is:

Norfloxacin is a white to pale yellow crystalline powder with a molecular weight of 319.34 and a melting point of about 221°C. It is freely soluble in glacial acetic acid, and very slightly soluble in ethanol, methanol and water.

NOROXIN is available in 400 mg tablets. Each tablet contains the following inactive ingredients: cellulose, croscarmellose sodium, iron oxide, hydroxypropyl cellulose, hydroxypropyl methylcellulose, magnesium stearate, and titanium dioxide.

Norfloxacin, a fluoroquinolone, differs from quinolones by having a fluorine atom at the 6 position and a piperazine moiety at the 7 position. Examples of antibacterial drugs which are quinolones include nalidixic acid and cinoxacin.

CLINICAL PHARMACOLOGY

In fasting healthy volunteers, at least 30–40% of an oral dose of NOROXIN is absorbed. Absorption is rapid following single doses of 200 mg and 400 mg. At the respective doses, mean peak serum and plasma concentrations of 0.8 and 1.5 mcg/mL are attained approximately one hour after dosing.

The presence of food may decrease absorption. The effective half-life of norfloxacin in serum and plasma is 3–4 hours. Steady-state concentrations of norfloxacin will be attained within two days of dosing.

In healthy elderly volunteers (65–75 years of age with normal renal function for their age), norfloxacin is eliminated more slowly because of their slightly decreased renal function. Drug absorption appears unaffected. However, the effective half-life of norfloxacin in these elderly subjects is 4 hours.

The disposition of norfloxacin in patients with creatinine clearance rates greater than $30\ mL/min/1.73m^2$ is similar to that in healthy volunteers. In patients with creatinine clearance rates equal to or less than $30\ mL/min/1.73m^2$, the renal elimination of norfloxacin decreases so that the effective serum half-life is 6.5 hours. In these patients, alteration of dosage is necessary (see DOSAGE AND ADMINISTRATION). Drug absorption appears unaffected by decreasing renal function.

Norfloxacin is eliminated through metabolism, biliary excretion, and renal excretion. After a single 400 mg dose of NOROXIN, mean antimicrobial activities equivalent to 278, 773, and 82 mcg of norfloxacin/g of feces were obtained at 12, 24, and 48 hours, respectively. Renal excretion occurs by both glomerular filtration and tubular secretion as evidenced by the high rate of renal clearance (approximately 275 mL/min). Within 24 hours of drug administration, 26 to 32% of the administered dose is recovered in the urine as norfloxacin with an additional 5–8% being recovered in the urine as six active metabolites of lesser antimicrobial potency. Only a small percentage (less than 1%) of the dose is recovered thereafter. Fecal recovery accounts for another 30% of the administered dose.

Two to three hours after a single 400 mg dose, urinary concentrations of 200 mcg/mL or more are attained in the urine. In healthy volunteers, mean urinary concentrations of norfloxacin remain above 30 mcg/mL for at least 12 hours following a 400 mg dose. The urinary pH may affect the solubility of norfloxacin. Norfloxacin is least soluble at urinary pH of 7.5 with greater solubility occurring at pHs above and below this value. The serum protein binding of norfloxacin is between 10 and 15%.

The following are mean concentrations of norfloxacin in various fluids and tissues measured 1 to 4 hours post-dose after two 400 mg doses, unless otherwise indicated:

Renal Parenchyma	7.3 µg/g
Prostate	2.5 µg/g
Seminal Fluid	2.7 µg/mL
Testicle	1.6 µg/g
Uterus/Cervix	3.0 µg/g
Vagina	4.3 µg/g
Fallopian Tube	1.9 µg/g
Bile	6.9 µg/mL (after two 200 mg doses)

Microbiology
Norfloxacin has *in vitro* activity against a broad spectrum of gram-positive and gram-negative aerobic bacteria. The fluorine atom at the 6 position provides increased potency against gram-negative organisms and the piperazine moiety at the 7 position is responsible for antipseudomonal activity. Norfloxacin inhibits bacterial deoxyribonucleic acid synthesis and is bactericidal. At the molecular level three specific events are attributed to NOROXIN in *E. coli* cells:
1) inhibition of the ATP-dependent DNA supercoiling reaction catalyzed by DNA gyrase,
2) inhibition of the relaxation of supercoiled DNA,
3) promotion of double-stranded DNA breakage.

Resistance to norfloxacin due to spontaneous mutation *in vitro* is a rare occurrence (range: 10^{-9} to 10^{-12} cells). Resistance of the organism has developed during therapy with norfloxacin in less than 1% of patients treated. Organisms in which development of resistance is greatest are the following:
Pseudomonas aeruginosa
Klebsiella pneumoniae
Acinetobacter species
Enterococci
For this reason, when there is a lack of satisfactory clinical response, culture and susceptibility testing should be done. Nalidixic acid resistant organisms are generally susceptible to norfloxacin *in vitro*; however, these organisms may have higher MICs to norfloxacin than nalidixic acid susceptible strains. There is generally no cross-resistance between norfloxacin and other classes of antibacterial agents. Therefore, norfloxacin demonstrates activity against indicated organisms resistant to the aminoglycosides (including gentamicin), penicillins, cephalosporins, tetracyclines, macrolides, and sulfonamides, including combinations of sulfamethoxazole and trimethoprim. Antagonism has been demonstrated *in vitro* between norfloxacin and nitrofurantoin.

While *in vitro* studies have demonstrated the susceptibility of most strains of the following organisms, clinical efficacy for infections other than those included in the INDICATIONS AND USAGE section has not been documented.

Aerobic Bacteria
Gram-positive bacteria including:
Streptococcus faecalis (enterococcus)
Staphylococcus aureus (including both penicillinase-producing and methicillin-resistant strains)
Staphylococcus epidermidis
Staphylococcus saprophyticus
Bacillus cereus
Gram-negative bacteria including:
Acinetobacter calcoaceticus
Aeromonas species
Alcaligenes species
Campylobacter species
Citrobacter diversus
Citrobacter freundii
Edwardsiella tarda
Enterobacter aerogenes
Enterobacter cloacae
Escherichia coli
Flavobacterium species
Hafnia alvei
Klebsiella oxytoca
Klebsiella pneumoniae
Klebsiella rhinoscleromatis
Morganella morganii
Neisseria gonorrhoeae
Proteus mirabilis
Proteus vulgaris
Providencia alcalifaciens
Providencia rettgeri
Providencia stuartii
Pseudomonas aeruginosa
Salmonella typhi
Salmonella species
Serratia marcescens
Shigella species
Vibrio cholerae
Vibrio parahemolyticus
Yersinia enterocolitica
Other
Unreaplasma urealyticum
NOROXIN is not generally active against obligate anaerobes.
Susceptibility Tests
Quantitative methods that require measurement of zone diameters give precise estimates of bacterial susceptibility. One such procedure has been recommended for use with discs to test susceptibility to norfloxacin.
Reports from the laboratory giving results of the standard single disc susceptibility test with a 10 mcg norfloxacin disc should be interpreted according to the following criteria.
Susceptible organisms produce zones of 13 mm or greater, indicating that the test organism is likely to respond to therapy.
Resistant organisms produce zones of 12 mm or less, indicating that other therapy should be selected.
A bacterial isolate may be considered susceptible if the MIC value for norfloxacin is equal to or less than 16 mcg/mL. Organisms are considered resistant if the MIC is equal to or greater than 32 mcg/mL.
The standardized quality control procedure requires use of control organisms. The 10 mcg norfloxacin disc should give the zone diameters listed below for the quality control strains.

Organism	ATCC®	Zone Size Range
E. coli	25922	28–35 mm
P. aeruginosa	27853	22–29 mm
S. aureus	25923	17–28 mm

Dilution susceptibility tests should give MICs between the ranges listed below for the quality control strains.

Organism	ATCC®	MIC (mcg/mL)
E. coli	25922	0.03–0.125
S. aureus	29213	0.5 –2.0
S. faecalis	29212	2.0 –8.0
P. aeruginosa	27853	1.0 –4.0

Based on urinary concentrations of norfloxacin achieved in man, breakpoint criteria have been established as listed below.

Category	Zone Diameter (mm)	Recommended MIC Breakpoint (mcg/mL)
Susceptible	≥ 13	≤ 16
Resistant	≤ 12	≥ 32

Norfloxacin susceptibility test results should not be used to predict susceptibility to other less potent quinolone antibacterial agents such as nalidixic acid.

INDICATIONS AND USAGE

Treatment
NOROXIN is indicated for the treatment of adults with complicated and uncomplicated urinary tract infections that are caused by susceptible strains of the designated microorganisms listed below:
Escherichia coli; Klebsiella pneumoniae; Enterobacter cloacae*; Proteus mirabilis; indole positive *Proteus* species* (which may include the organisms now called *Proteus vulgaris*, Providencia rettgeri *,* and *Morganella morganii*) *; *Pseudomonas aeruginosa; Citrobacter freundii*; Staphylococcus aureus*, Staphylococcus epidermidis*;* and group D streptococci.
NOTE: Specimens for culture and susceptibility testing should be obtained prior to and during treatment if clinical response warrants. However, NOROXIN may be used to initiate therapy in urinary tract infections prior to the availability of laboratory results.

CONTRAINDICATIONS

NOROXIN is contraindicated in patients with a history of hypersensitivity to norfloxacin or the quinolone group of antibacterial agents (e.g., nalidixic acid and cinoxacin).

WARNINGS

Norfloxacin should not be used in children or pregnant women.
The oral administration of single doses of norfloxacin, 6 times the recommended human clinical dose, caused lameness in immature dogs. Histologic examination of the weight-bearing joints of these dogs revealed permanent lesions of the cartilage. Related drugs (e.g., nalidixic acid and cinoxacin) also produced erosions of the cartilage in weight-bearing joints and other signs of arthropathy in immature animals of various species.

PRECAUTIONS

Needle shaped crystals were found in the urine of some volunteers who received either placebo, 800 mg norfloxacin, or 1600 mg norfloxacin (at or twice the recommended daily dose, respectively) while participating in a double-blind, crossover study comparing single doses of norfloxacin with placebo. While crystalluria is not expected to occur under usual conditions with a dosage regimen of 400 mg b.i.d., as a precaution, the daily recommended dosage should not be exceeded and the patient should drink sufficient fluids to ensure a proper state of hydration and adequate urinary output.
Alteration in dosage regimen is necessary for patients with impaired renal function (see DOSAGE AND ADMINISTRATION).
Convulsions have been reported rarely with norfloxacin although no causal relationship has been established. Convulsions, increased intracranial pressure, and toxic psychoses have been reported with other drugs in this class. If these reactions occur in patients receiving norfloxacin, the drug should be discontinued and appropriate measures instituted. The effects of norfloxacin on brain function or on the electrical activity of the brain have not been tested. Until more information becomes available, quinolones should be used with caution in patients with known factors which predispose to seizures.
Drug Interactions
Diminished urinary excretion of norfloxacin has been reported during the concomitant administration of probenecid and norfloxacin.
The concomitant use of nitrofurantoin is not recommended since nitrofurantoin may antagonize the antibacterial effect of NOROXIN in the urinary tract.
The concomitant administration of norfloxacin with antacids is not recommended.
Information for Patients
Patients should be advised to take NOROXIN one hour before or two hours after a meal. Patients should also be advised to drink fluids liberally and not to take antacids concomitantly or within 2 hours after dosing.
NOROXIN may cause dizziness or lightheadedness; therefore, patients should know how they react to norfloxacin before they operate an automobile or machinery or engage in activities requiring mental alertness and coordination.
Carcinogenesis, Mutagenesis, Impairment of Fertility
No increase in neoplastic changes was observed with norfloxacin as compared to controls in a study in rats, lasting up to 96 weeks at doses 8–9 times the usual human dose.
Norfloxacin was tested for mutagenic activity in a number of *in vivo* and *in vitro* tests. Norfloxacin had no mutagenic effect in the dominant lethal test in mice and did not cause chromosomal aberrations in hamsters or rats at doses 30–60 times the usual dose. Norfloxacin had no mutagenic activity *in vitro* in the Ames microbial mutagen test, Chinese hamster fibroblasts and V-79 mammalian cell assay. Although norfloxacin was weakly positive in the Rec-assay for DNA

*Efficacy for this organism in this organ system was studied in fewer than 10 infections.

repair, all other mutagenic assays were negative including a more sensitive test (V-79).
Norfloxacin did not adversely affect the fertility of male and female mice at oral doses up to 33 times the usual human dose.
Pregnancy
Pregnancy Category C: Norfloxacin has been shown to produce embryonic loss in monkeys when given in doses 10 times the maximum human dose (400 mg b.i.d.), with peak plasma levels that are 2 to 3 times those obtained in humans. There has been no evidence of a teratogenic effect in any of the animal species tested (rat, rabbit, mouse, monkey) at 6–50 times the human dose. There were no adequate and well controlled studies in pregnant women. Since norfloxacin, like other drugs in this class, causes arthropathy in immature animals, it should not be used in pregnant women (see WARNINGS).
Nursing Mothers
It is not known whether norfloxacin is excreted in human milk.
When a 200 mg dose of NOROXIN was administered to nursing mothers, norfloxacin was not detected in human milk. However, because the dose studied was low, because other drugs in this class are secreted in human milk, and because of the potential for serious adverse reactions from norfloxacin in nursing infants, a decision should be made to discontinue nursing or to discontinue the drug, taking into account the importance of the drug to the mother.
Pediatric Use
Norfloxacin should not be used in children because it causes arthropathy in juvenile animals (see WARNINGS).

ADVERSE REACTIONS

In clinical trials, NOROXIN was generally well tolerated. The incidence of subjects reporting drug related adverse experiences in clinical trials involving 1127 subjects was 3.4%. However, the incidence figures below were calculated without reference to drug relationship.
The most common adverse experiences (1%–3%) were either gastrointestinal or neurological: nausea 2.8%, headache 2.7%, and dizziness 1.8%.
Additional reactions (0.3%–1%) were: fatigue, rash, abdominal pain, dyspepsia, somnolence, depression, insomnia, constipation, flatulence, and heartburn.
Less frequent reactions included: dry mouth, diarrhea, fever, vomiting, and erythema.
CNS effects characterized as generalized seizures and myoclonus have been reported rarely with NOROXIN. A causal relationship to NOROXIN has not been established (see PRECAUTIONS). Visual disturbances have been reported with drugs in this class.
Abnormal laboratory values observed in these 1127 subjects in clinical trials were eosinophilia 1.8%, elevation of ALT (SGPT) and AST (SGOT) 1.8%, increased alkaline phosphatase 1.4%, and decreased WBC or neutrophil count 1.2%. Those occurring less frequently included increased BUN, serum creatinine, and LDH, and decreased hematocrit.
The following additional adverse reactions have been reported since the drug was marketed:
Hypersensitivity Reactions
Hypersensitivity reactions have been reported including anaphylactoid reactions, angioedema, urticaria, Stevens-Johnson syndrome and arthralgia.
Skin
Photosensitivity
Gastrointestinal
Pseudomembranous colitis

OVERDOSAGE

The acute oral LD$_{50}$ values in male and female mice and male and female rats were greater than 4 g/kg.
In the event of acute overdosage, the stomach should be emptied by inducing vomiting or by gastric lavage, and the patient carefully observed and given symptomatic and supportive treatment. Adequate hydration must be maintained.

DOSAGE AND ADMINISTRATION

Tablets NOROXIN should be taken one hour before or two hours after a meal with a glass of water. Patients receiving NOROXIN should be well hydrated (see PRECAUTIONS).
Normal Renal Function
The recommended dosage of NOROXIN is:
Uncomplicated urinary tract infections: 400 mg twice daily for 7 to 10 days.

Continued on next page

Merck Sharp & Dohme—Cont.

Complicated urinary tract infections: 400 mg twice daily for 10 to 21 days.

Maximum total daily dosage should not exceed 800 mg per day.

Renal Impairment

NOROXIN may be used for the treatment of urinary tract infections in patients with renal insufficiency. In patients with a creatinine clearance rate of 30 mL/min/1.73m² or less, the recommended dosage is one 400 mg tablet once daily for the duration given above. At this dosage, the urinary concentration exceeds the MICs for most urinary pathogens susceptible to norfloxacin, even when the creatinine clearance is less than 10 mL/min/1.73m².

When only the serum creatinine level is available, the following formula (based on sex, weight, and age of the patient) may be used to convert this value into creatinine clearance. The serum creatinine should represent a steady state of renal function.

Males: $= \dfrac{(\text{weight in kg}) \times (140 - \text{age})}{(72) \times \text{serum creatinine (mg/100 mL)}}$

Females: $= (0.85) \times (\text{above value})$

Elderly

Elderly patients with a creatinine clearance of greater than 30 mL/min/1.73m² should receive the dosages recommended under *Normal Renal Function.*

Elderly patients with a creatinine clearance of 30 mL/min/1.73m² or less should receive 400 mg once daily as recommended under *Renal Impairment.*

HOW SUPPLIED

No. 3522—Tablets NOROXIN 400 mg are dark pink, oval shaped, film-coated tablets, coded MSD 705 on one side and NOROXIN on the other. They are supplied as follows:

NDC 0006-0705-68 bottles of 100
NDC 0006-0705-20 unit of use bottles of 20
NDC 0006-0705-28 unit dose packages of 100.

Shown in Product Identification Section, page 418

Storage

Tablets NOROXIN should be stored in a tightly-closed container. Avoid storage at temperatures above 40℃ (104°F).

ANIMAL PHARMACOLOGY

Norfloxacin and related drugs have been shown to cause arthropathy in immature animals of most species tested (see WARNINGS).

Crystalluria has occurred in laboratory animals tested with norfloxacin. In dogs, needle shaped drug crystals were seen in the urine at doses of 50 mg/kg/day. In rats, crystals were reported following doses of 200 mg/kg/day.

Embryo lethality and slight maternotoxicity (vomiting and anorexia) were observed in cynomolgus monkeys at doses of 150 mg/kg/day or higher.

Ocular toxicity, seen with some related drugs, was not observed in any norfloxacin treated animals.

A.H.F.S. Category: 8:36
DC 7455407   Issued January 1988
COPYRIGHT © MERCK & CO., INC., 1986
All rights reserved

PEPCID® Tablets   ℞
(Famotidine, MSD)
PEPCID® Oral Suspension   ℞
(Famotidine for Oral Suspension, MSD)
PEPCID® I.V.   ℞
(Famotidine, MSD)

DESCRIPTION

The active ingredient in PEPCID® (Famotidine, MSD), is a histamine H_2-receptor antagonist. Famotidine is 3-[[[2-[(aminoiminomethyl) amino] -4- thiazolyl] methyl]-thio]-*N*-(aminosulfonyl) propanimidamide. The empirical formula of famotidine is $C_8H_{15}N_7O_2S_3$ and its molecular weight is 337.43. Its structural formula is:

[See Chemical Formula at top of next column].

Famotidine is a white to pale yellow crystalline compound that is freely soluble in glacial acetic acid, slightly soluble in methanol, very slightly soluble in water, and practically insoluble in ethanol.

Famotidine is supplied in three dosage forms: PEPCID Tablets, PEPCID Oral Suspension, and PEPCID I.V.

Each tablet for oral administration contains either 20 mg or 40 mg of famotidine and the following inactive ingredients: hydroxypropyl cellulose, hydroxypropyl methylcellulose, iron oxides, magnesium stearate, microcrystalline cellulose, starch, talc, titanium dioxide.

Each 5 mL of the oral suspension when prepared as directed contains 40 mg of famotidine and the following inactive ingredients: citric acid, flavors, microcrystalline cellulose and carboxymethylcellulose sodium, sucrose and xanthan gum. Added as preservatives are sodium benzoate 0.1%, sodium methylparaben 0.1%, and sodium propylparaben 0.02%.

Each mL of the solution for intravenous injection contains 10 mg of famotidine and the following inactive ingredients: L-aspartic acid 4 mg, mannitol 20 mg, and Water for Injection q.s. 1 mL. The multidose injection also contains benzyl alcohol 0.9% added as preservative.

CLINICAL PHARMACOLOGY

GI Effects

PEPCID is a competitive inhibitor of histamine H_2-receptors. The primary clinically important pharmacologic activity of PEPCID is inhibition of gastric secretion. Both the acid concentration and volume of gastric secretion are suppressed by PEPCID, while changes in pepsin secretion are proportional to volume output.

In normal volunteers and hypersecretors, PEPCID inhibited basal and nocturnal gastric secretion, as well as secretion stimulated by food and pentagastrin. After oral administration, the onset of the antisecretory effect occurred within one hour; the maximum effect was dose-dependent, occurring within one to three hours. Duration of inhibition of secretion by doses of 20 and 40 mg was 10 to 12 hours.

After intravenous administration, the maximum effect was achieved within 30 minutes. Single intravenous doses of 10 and 20 mg inhibited nocturnal secretion for a period of 10 to 12 hours. The 20 mg dose was associated with the longest duration of action in most subjects.

Single evening oral doses of 20 and 40 mg inhibited basal and nocturnal acid secretion in all subjects; mean nocturnal gastric acid secretion was inhibited by 86% and 94%, respectively, for a period of at least 10 hours. The same doses given in the morning suppressed food-stimulated acid secretion in all subjects. The mean suppression was 76% and 84% respectively 3 to 5 hours after administration, and 25% and 30% respectively 8 to 10 hours after administration. In some subjects who received the 20 mg dose, however, the antisecretory effect was dissipated within 6–8 hours. There was no cumulative effect with repeated doses. The nocturnal intragastric pH was raised by evening doses of 20 and 40 mg of PEPCID to mean values of 5.0 and 6.4, respectively. When PEPCID was given after breakfast, the basal daytime interdigestive pH at 3 and 8 hours after 20 or 40 mg of PEPCID was raised to about 5.

PEPCID had little or no effect on fasting or postprandial serum gastrin levels. Gastric emptying and exocrine pancreatic function were not affected by PEPCID.

Other Effects

Systemic effects of PEPCID in the CNS, cardiovascular, respiratory or endocrine systems have not been found to date. Serum prolactin levels did not rise after intravenous 20 mg bolus doses of PEPCID. No antiandrogenic effects have been detected.

Pharmacokinetics

PEPCID is incompletely absorbed. The bioavailability of oral doses is 40–45%. PEPCID Tablets and PEPCID Oral Suspension are bioequivalent. Bioavailability may be slightly increased by food, or slightly decreased by antacids; however, these effects are of no clinical consequence. PEPCID undergoes minimal first-pass metabolism. After oral doses,

peak plasma levels occur in 1–3 hours. Plasma levels after multiple doses are similar to those after single doses. Fifteen to 20% of PEPCID in plasma is protein bound. PEPCID has an elimination half-life of 2.5–3.5 hours. PEPCID is eliminated by renal (65–70%) and metabolic (30–35%) routes. Renal clearance is 250–450 mL/min, indicating some tubular excretion. Twenty-five to 30% of an oral dose and 65–70% of an intravenous dose are recovered in the urine as unchanged compound. The only metabolite identified in man is the S-oxide.

There is a close relationship between creatinine clearance values and the elimination half-life of PEPCID. In patients with severe renal insufficiency, i.e., creatinine clearance less than 10 mL/min, PEPCID elimination half-life may exceed 20 hours and adjustment of dose or dosing intervals may be necessary (see PRECAUTIONS, DOSAGE AND ADMINISTRATION).

In elderly patients, there are no clinically significant age-related changes in the pharmacokinetics of PEPCID.

Clinical Studies

Duodenal Ulcer

In a U.S. multicenter, double-blind study in outpatients with endoscopically confirmed duodenal ulcer, orally administered PEPCID was compared to placebo. As shown in the table below, 70% of patients treated with PEPCID 40 mg h.s. were healed by week 4.

Outpatients with endoscopically confirmed healed ulcers

	PEPCID 40 mg h.s. (N = 89)	PEPCID 20 mg b.i.d. (N = 84)	Placebo h.s. (N = 97)
Week 2	*32%	*38%	17%
Week 4	*70%	*67%	31%

*Statistically significantly different than placebo (p < 0.001)

Patients not healed by week 4 were continued in the study. By week 8, 83% of patients treated with PEPCID had healed versus 45% of patients treated with placebo. The incidence of ulcer healing with PEPCID was significantly higher than with placebo at each time point based on proportion of endoscopically confirmed healed ulcers.

In this study, time to relief of daytime and nocturnal pain was significantly shorter for patients receiving PEPCID than for patients receiving placebo; patients receiving PEPCID also took less antacid than the patients receiving placebo.

Long-Term Maintenance

Treatment of Duodenal Ulcers

PEPCID, 20 mg p.o. h.s. was compared to placebo h.s. as maintenance therapy in two double-blind, multicenter studies of patients with endoscopically confirmed healed duodenal ulcers. In the U.S. study the observed ulcer incidence within 12 months in patients treated with placebo was 2.4 times greater than in the patients treated with PEPCID. The 89 patients treated with PEPCID had a cumulative observed ulcer incidence of 23.4% compared to an observed ulcer incidence of 56.6% in the 89 patients receiving placebo (p < 0.01). These results were confirmed in an international study where the cumulative observed ulcer incidence within 12 months in the 307 patients treated with PEPCID was 35.7%, compared to an incidence of 75.5% in the 325 patients treated with placebo (p < 0.01).

Gastric Ulcer

In both a U.S. and an international multicenter, double-blind study in patients with endoscopically confirmed active benign gastric ulcer, orally administered PEPCID, 40 mg h.s., was compared to placebo h.s. Antacids were permitted during the studies, but consumption was not significantly different between the PEPCID and placebo groups. As shown in the table below, the incidence of ulcer healing (dropouts counted as unhealed) with PEPCID was statistically significantly better than placebo at weeks 6 and 8 in the U.S. study, and at weeks 4, 6 and 8 in the international study, based on the number of ulcers that healed, confirmed by endoscopy. [See table below.]

Time to complete relief of daytime and nighttime pain was statistically significantly shorter for patients receiving PEPCID than for patients receiving placebo; however, in neither study was there a statistically significant difference in the proportion of patients whose pain was relieved by the end of the study (week 8).

Pathological Hypersecretory Conditions (e.g., Zollinger-Ellison Syndrome, Multiple Endocrine Adenomas)

In studies of patients with pathological hypersecretory conditions such as Zollinger-Ellison Syndrome with or without multiple endocrine adenomas, PEPCID significantly inhibited gastric acid secretion and controlled associated symptoms. Doses from 20 to 160 mg q 6 h maintained basal acid secretion below 10 mEq/hr; initial doses were titrated to the individual patient need and subsequent adjustments were necessary with time in some patients. PEPCID was well tolerated at these high dose levels for prolonged periods (greater than 12 months) in eight patients, and there were no cases reported of gynecomastia, increased prolactin levels, or impotence which were considered to be due to the drug.

Patients with endoscopically
confirmed healed ulcers

	U.S. Study		International Study	
	PEPCID 40 mg h.s. (N=74)	Placebo h.s. (N=75)	PEPCID 40 mg h.s. (N=149)	Placebo h.s. (N=145)
Week 4	45%	39%	**47%	31%
Week 6	**66%	44%	**65%	46%
Week 8	*78%	64%	**80%	54%

*,** Statistically significantly better than placebo (p ≤ 0.05, p ≤ 0.01 respectively)

INDICATIONS AND USAGE

PEPCID is indicated in:

1. *Short term treatment of active duodenal ulcer.* Most patients heal within 4 weeks; there is rarely reason to use PEPCID at full dosage for longer than 6 to 8 weeks. Studies have not assessed the safety of famotidine in uncomplicated active duodenal ulcer for periods of more than eight weeks.
2. *Maintenance therapy for duodenal ulcer patients at reduced dosage after healing of an active ulcer.* Controlled studies have not extended beyond one year.
3. *Short term treatment of active benign gastric ulcer.* Most patients heal within 6 weeks. Studies have not assessed the safety or efficacy of famotidine in uncomplicated active benign gastric ulcer for periods of more than 8 weeks.
4. *Treatment of pathological hypersecretory conditions (e.g., Zollinger-Ellison Syndrome, multiple endocrine adenomas).* PEPCID I.V. is indicated in some hospitalized patients with pathological hypersecretory conditions or intractable ulcers, or as an alternative to the oral dosage forms for short-term use in patients who are unable to take oral medication.

CONTRAINDICATIONS

Hypersensitivity to any component of these products.

PRECAUTIONS

General

Symptomatic response to therapy with PEPCID does not preclude the presence of gastric malignancy.

Patients with Severe Renal Insufficiency

Longer intervals between doses or lower doses may need to be used in patients with severe renal insufficiency (creatinine clearance < 10 mL/min) to adjust for the longer elimination half-life of famotidine. (See CLINICAL PHARMACOLOGY and DOSAGE AND ADMINISTRATION.) However, currently, no drug-related toxicity has been found with high plasma concentrations of famotidine.

Information for Patients

The patient should be instructed to shake the oral suspension vigorously for 5–10 seconds prior to each use. Unused constituted oral suspension should be discarded after 30 days.

Drug Interactions

No drug interactions have been identified. Studies with famotidine in man, in animal models, and *in vitro* have shown no significant interference with the disposition of compounds metabolized by the hepatic microsomal enzymes, e.g., cytochrome P450 system. Compounds tested in man include warfarin, theophylline, phenytoin, diazepam, aminopyrine and antipyrine. Indocyanine green as an index of hepatic drug extraction has been tested and no significant effects have been found.

Carcinogenesis, Mutagenesis, Impairment of Fertility

In a 106 week study in rats and a 92 week study in mice given oral doses of up to 2000 mg/kg/day (approximately 2500 times the recommended human dose for active duodenal ulcer), there was no evidence of carcinogenic potential for PEPCID.

Famotidine was negative in the microbial mutagen test (Ames test) using *Salmonella typhimurium* and *Escherichia coli* with or without rat liver enzyme activation at concentrations up to 10,000 mcg/plate. In *in vivo* studies in mice, with a micronucleus test and a chromosomal aberration test, no evidence of a mutagenic effect was observed.

In studies with rats given oral doses of up to 2000 mg/kg/day or intravenous doses of up to 200 mg/kg/day fertility and reproductive performance were not affected.

Pregnancy

Pregnancy Category B

Reproductive studies have been performed in rats and rabbits at oral doses of up to 2000 and 500 mg/kg/day respectively and in both species at I.V. doses of up to 200 mg/kg/day, and have revealed no significant evidence of impaired fertility or harm to the fetus due to PEPCID. While no direct fetotoxic effects have been observed, sporadic abortions occurring only in mothers displaying marked decreased food intake were seen in some rabbits at oral doses of 200 mg/kg/day (250 times the usual human dose) or higher. There are, however, no adequate or well-controlled studies in pregnant women. Because animal reproductive studies are not always predictive of human response, this drug should be used during pregnancy only if clearly needed.

Nursing Mothers

Studies performed in lactating rats have shown that famotidine is secreted into breast milk. Transient growth depression was observed in young rats suckling from mothers treated with maternotoxic doses of at least 600 times the usual human dose. It is not known whether this drug is secreted into human milk. Because many drugs are secreted into human milk and because of the potential for serious adverse reactions in nursing infants from PEPCID, a decision should be made whether to discontinue nursing or dis-

continue the drug, taking into account the importance of the drug to the mother.

Pediatric Use

Safety and effectiveness in children have not been established.

Use in Elderly Patients

No dosage adjustment is required based on age (see CLINICAL PHARMACOLOGY, *Pharmacokinetics*). Dosage adjustment in the case of severe renal impairment may be necessary.

ADVERSE REACTIONS

The adverse reactions listed below have been reported during domestic and international clinical trials in approximately 2500 patients. In those controlled clinical trials in which PEPCID Tablets were compared to placebo, the incidence of adverse experiences in the group which received PEPCID Tablets, 40 mg at bedtime, was similar to that in the placebo group.

The following adverse reactions have been reported to occur in more than 1% of patients on therapy with PEPCID in controlled clinical trials, and may be causally related to the drug: headache (4.7%), dizziness (1.3%), constipation (1.2%) and diarrhea (1.7%).

The following other adverse reactions have been reported infrequently in clinical trials or since the drug was marketed. The relationship to therapy with PEPCID has been unclear in many cases. Within each category the adverse reactions are listed in order of decreasing severity:

Body as a Whole: fever, asthenia, fatigue

Cardiovascular: palpitation

Gastrointestinal: cholestatic jaundice, liver enzyme abnormalities, vomiting, nausea, abdominal discomfort, anorexia, dry mouth

Hematologic: thrombocytopenia

Hypersensitivity: anaphylaxis, angioedema, orbital or facial edema, urticaria, rash, conjunctival injection

Musculoskeletal: musculoskeletal pain, arthralgia

Nervous System/Psychiatric: grand mal seizure; psychic disturbances including depression, anxiety, decreased libido, hallucinations; paresthesia; insomnia; somnolence

Respiratory: bronchospasm

Skin: alopecia, acne, pruritus, dry skin, flushing

Special Senses: tinnitus, taste disorder

The adverse reactions reported for PEPCID Tablets may also occur with PEPCID Oral Suspension or PEPCID I.V. In addition, transient irritation at the injection site has been observed with PEPCID I.V.

AV block has been reported with other H$_2$-receptor antagonists, but not with famotidine.

OVERDOSAGE

There is no experience to date with deliberate overdosage. Doses of up to 640 mg/day have been given to patients with pathological hypersecretory conditions with no serious adverse effects. In the event of overdosage, treatment should be symptomatic and supportive. Unabsorbed material should be removed from the gastrointestinal tract, the patient should be monitored, and supportive therapy should be employed.

The oral LD$_{50}$ of famotidine in male and female rats and mice was greater than 3000 mg/kg and the minimum lethal acute oral dose in dogs exceeded 2000 mg/kg. Famotidine did not produce overt effects at high oral doses in mice, rats, cats and dogs, but induced significant anorexia and growth depression in rabbits starting with 200 mg/kg/day orally. The intravenous LD$_{50}$ of famotidine for mice and rats ranged from 254–563 mg/kg and the minimum lethal single I.V. dose in dogs was approximately 300 mg/kg. Signs of acute intoxication in I.V. treated dogs were emesis, restlessness, pallor of mucous membranes or redness of mouth and ears, hypotension, tachycardia and collapse.

DOSAGE AND ADMINISTRATION

Duodenal Ulcer

Acute Therapy: The recommended adult oral dosage for active duodenal ulcer is 40 mg once a day at bedtime. Most patients heal within 4 weeks; there is rarely reason to use PEPCID at full dosage for longer than 6 to 8 weeks. A regimen of 20 mg b.i.d. is also effective.

Maintenance Therapy: The recommended oral dose is 20 mg once a day at bedtime.

Benign Gastric Ulcer

Acute Therapy: The recommended adult oral dosage for active benign gastric ulcer is 40 mg once a day at bedtime.

Pathological Hypersecretory Conditions (e.g., Zollinger-Ellison Syndrome, Multiple Endocrine Adenomas)

The dosage of PEPCID in patients with pathological hypersecretory conditions varies with the individual patient. The recommended adult oral starting dose for pathological hypersecretory conditions is 20 mg q 6 h. In some patients, a higher starting dose may be required. Doses should be ad-

justed to individual patient needs and should continue as long as clinically indicated. Doses up to 160 mg q 6 h have been administered to some patients with severe Zollinger-Ellison Syndrome.

Oral Suspension

PEPCID Oral Suspension may be substituted for PEPCID Tablets in any of the above indications. Each five mL contains 40 mg of famotidine after constitution of the powder with 46 mL of Purified Water as directed.

Directions for Preparing PEPCID Oral Suspension

Prepare suspension at time of dispensing. Slowly add 46 mL of Purified Water. Shake vigorously for 5–10 seconds immediately after adding the water and immediately before use.

Stability of PEPCID Oral Suspension

Unused constituted oral suspension should be discarded after 30 days.

Intravenous Administration

In some hospitalized patients with pathological hypersecretory conditions or intractable ulcers, or in patients who are unable to take oral medication, PEPCID I.V. may be administered. The recommended dosage is 20 mg q 12 h.

Preparation of PEPCID Intravenous Solutions

Dilute 2 mL of PEPCID I.V. (solution containing 10 mg/mL) with 0.9% Sodium Chloride Injection or other compatible intravenous solution to a total volume of either 5 mL or 10 mL and inject over a period of not less than 2 minutes.

Preparation of PEPCID Intravenous Infusion Solutions

PEPCID I.V. may also be administered as an infusion, 2 mL diluted with 100 mL of 5% dextrose or other compatible solution, and infused over a 15–30 minute period.

Stability of PEPCID I.V.

PEPCID I.V. is stable for 48 hours at room temperature when added to or diluted with most commonly used intravenous solutions, e.g., Water for Injection, 0.9% Sodium Chloride Injection, 5% and 10% Dextrose Injection, Lactated Ringer's Injection, or Sodium Bicarbonate Injection, 5%. Parenteral drug products should be inspected visually for particulate matter and discoloration prior to administration whenever solution and container permit.

Concomitant Use of Antacids

Antacids may be given concomitantly if needed.

Dosage Adjustment for Patients with Severe Renal Insufficiency

In patients with severe renal insufficiency, i.e., with a creatinine clearance less than 10 mL/min, the elimination half-life of PEPCID may exceed 20 hours, reaching approximately 24 hours in anuric patients. Although no relationship of adverse effects to high plasma levels has been established, to avoid excess accumulation of the drug, the dose of PEPCID may be reduced to 20 mg h.s. or the dosing interval may be prolonged to 36–48 hours as indicated by the patient's clinical response.

HOW SUPPLIED

No. 3535—Tablets PEPCID, 20 mg, are beige colored, U-shaped, film-coated tablets coded MSD 963. They are supplied as follows:

NDC 0006-0963-31 unit of use bottles of 30

NDC 0006-0963-28 unit dose package of 100.

Shown in Product Identification Section, page 418

No. 3536—Tablets PEPCID, 40 mg, are light brownish-orange, U-shaped, film-coated tablets coded MSD 964. They are supplied as follows:

NDC 0006-0964-31 unit of use bottles of 30 (6505-01-257-3164, 40 mg 30's)

NDC 0006-0964-28 unit dose package of 100.

Shown in Product Identification Section, page 418

No. 3538—Oral Suspension PEPCID is a white to off-white powder containing 400 mg of famotidine for constitution. When constituted as directed, PEPCID Oral Suspension is a smooth, mobile, off-white, homogeneous suspension with a cherry-banana-mint flavor, containing 40 mg of famotidine per 5 mL.

NDC 0006-3538-92, bottles containing 400 mg famotidine. FOR INTRAVENOUS USE ONLY

No. 3539—Injection PEPCID I.V. 10 mg per 1 mL, is a non-preserved, clear, colorless solution and is supplied as follows:

NDC 0006-3539-04, 10 × 2 mL single dose vials.

No. 3541—Injection PEPCID I.V. 10 mg per 1 mL, is a clear, colorless solution and is supplied as follows:

NDC 0006-3541-14, 4 mL vials.

Storage

Avoid storage of PEPCID Tablets at temperatures above 40°C (104°F).

Avoid storage of the powder for oral suspension at temperatures above 40°C (104°F). After constitution store the suspen-

Continued on next page

Information on the Merck Sharp & Dohme products listed on these pages is the full prescribing information from product circulars in use August 31, 1989.

Merck Sharp & Dohme—Cont.

sion below 30°C (86°F). Do not freeze. Discard unused suspension after 30 days.

Store PEPCID I.V. at 2–8°C (35.6–46.4°F). If solution freezes, bring to room temperature; allow sufficient time to solubilize all the components.

When diluted as recommended (see DOSAGE AND ADMINISTRATION) PEPCID I.V. is stable for 48 hours at room temperature.

A.H.F.S. Category: 56:40
DC 7545308 Issued November 1988
COPYRIGHT © MERCK & CO., INC., 1986, 1988
All rights reserved

PERIACTIN® Tablets   ℞
(Cyproheptadine HCl, MSD), U.S.P.
PERIACTIN® Syrup   ℞
(Cyproheptadine HCl, MSD), U.S.P.

DESCRIPTION

PERIACTIN® (Cyproheptadine HCl, MSD) is an antihistaminic and antiserotonergic agent.

Cyproheptadine hydrochloride is a white to slightly yellowish, crystalline solid, with a molecular weight of 350.89, which is soluble in water, freely soluble in methanol, sparingly soluble in ethanol, soluble in chloroform, and practically insoluble in ether. It is the sesquihydrate of 4-(5H-dibenzo [a,d] cyclohepten-5-ylidene)-1-methylpiperidine hydrochloride. The empirical formula of the anhydrous salt is $C_{21}H_{21}N \cdot HCl$ and the structural formula of the anhydrous salt is:

PERIACTIN is available in tablets, containing 4 mg of cyproheptadine hydrochloride, and as a syrup in which 5 mL contains 2 mg of cyproheptadine hydrochloride, with a pH range of 3.5 to 4.5.

The tablets also contain the following inactive ingredients: calcium phosphate, lactose, magnesium stearate, and starch. The syrup contains the following inactive ingredients: D & C Yellow 10, artificial flavors, glycerin, purified water, sodium saccharin, and sucrose.

CLINICAL PHARMACOLOGY

PERIACTIN is a serotonin and histamine antagonist with anticholinergic and sedative effects. Antiserotonin and antihistamine drugs appear to compete with serotonin and histamine, respectively, for receptor sites.

Pharmacokinetics and Metabolism
After a single 4 mg oral dose of ^{14}C-labelled cyproheptadine HCl in normal subjects, given as tablets or syrup, 2-20% of the radioactivity was excreted in the stools. Only about 34% of the stool radioactivity was unchanged drug, corresponding to less than 5.7% of the dose. At least 40% of the administered radioactivity was excreted in the urine. No significant difference in the mean urinary excretion exists between the tablet and syrup formulations. No detectable amounts of unchanged drug were present in the urine of patients on chronic 12-20 mg daily doses of PERIACTIN Syrup. The principle metabolite found in human urine has been identified as a quaternary ammonium glucuronide conjugate of cyproheptadine. Elimination is diminished in renal insufficiency.

INDICATIONS AND USAGE

Perennial and seasonal allergic rhinitis
Vasomotor rhinitis
Allergic conjunctivitis due to inhalant allergens and foods
Mild, uncomplicated allergic skin manifestations of urticaria and angioedema
Amelioration of allergic reactions to blood or plasma
Cold urticaria
Dermatographism
As therapy for anaphylactic reactions *adjunctive* to epinephrine and other standard measures after the acute manifestations have been controlled.

CONTRAINDICATIONS

Newborn or Premature Infants
This drug should *not* be used in newborn or premature infants.

Nursing Mothers
Because of the higher risk of antihistamines for infants generally and for newborns and prematures in particular, antihistamine therapy is contraindicated in nursing mothers.

Other Conditions
Hypersensitivity to cyproheptadine and other drugs of similar chemical structure:
  Monoamine oxidase inhibitor therapy
  (see DRUG INTERACTIONS)
  Angle-closure glaucoma
  Stenosing peptic ulcer
  Symptomatic prostatic hypertrophy
  Bladder neck obstruction
  Pyloroduodenal obstruction
  Elderly, debilitated patients

WARNINGS

Children
Overdosage of antihistamines, particularly in infants and children, may produce hallucinations, central nervous system depression, convulsions, and death.

Antihistamines may diminish mental alertness; conversely, particularly in the young child, they may occasionally produce excitation.

CNS Depressants
Antihistamines may have additive effects with alcohol and other CNS depressants, e.g., hypnotics, sedatives, tranquilizers, antianxiety agents.

Activities Requiring Mental Alertness
Patients should be warned about engaging in activities requiring mental alertness and motor coordination, such as driving a car or operating machinery.

Antihistamines are more likely to cause dizziness, sedation, and hypotension in elderly patients.

PRECAUTIONS

General
Cyproheptadine has an atropine-like action and, therefore, should be used with caution in patients with:
  History of bronchial asthma
  Increased intraocular pressure
  Hyperthyroidism
  Cardiovascular disease
  Hypertension

Information for Patients
Antihistamines may diminish mental alertness; conversely, particularly in the young child, they may occasionally produce excitation.

Patients should be warned about engaging in activities requiring mental alertness and motor coordination, such as driving a car or operating machinery.

Drug Interactions
MAO inhibitors prolong and intensify the anticholinergic effects of antihistamines.

Antihistamines may have additive effects with alcohol and other CNS depressants, e.g., hypnotics, sedatives, tranquilizers, antianxiety agents.

Carcinogenesis, Mutagenesis, Impairment of Fertility
Long-term carcinogenic studies have not been done with cyproheptadine.

Cyproheptadine had no effect on fertility in a two-litter study in rats or a two generation study in mice at about 10 times the human dose.

Cyproheptadine did not produce chromosome damage in human lymphocytes or fibroblasts *in vitro;* high doses (10^{-4} M) were cytotoxic. Cyproheptadine did not have any mutagenic effect in the Ames microbial mutagen test; concentrations of above 500 mcg/plate inhibited bacterial growth.

Pregnancy
Pregnancy Category B: Reproduction studies have been performed in rabbits, mice, and rats at oral or subcutaneous doses up to 32 times the maximum recommended human oral dose and have revealed no evidence of impaired fertility or harm to the fetus due to cyproheptadine. Cyproheptadine has been shown to be fetotoxic in rats when given by intraperitoneal injection in doses four times the maximum recommended human oral dose. Two studies in pregnant women, however, have not shown that cyproheptadine increases the risk of abnormalities when administered during the first, second and third trimesters of pregnancy. No teratogenic effects were observed in any of the newborns. Nevertheless, because the studies in humans cannot rule out the possibility of harm, cyproheptadine should be used during pregnancy only if clearly needed.

Nursing Mothers
It is not known whether this drug is excreted in human milk. Because many drugs are excreted in human milk, and because of the potential for serious adverse reactions in nursing infants from PERIACTIN, a decision should be made whether to discontinue nursing or to discontinue the drug, taking into account the importance of the drug to the mother (see CONTRAINDICATIONS).

Pediatric Use
Safety and effectiveness in children below the age of two have not been established. See CONTRAINDICATIONS, *Newborn Premature Infants,* and WARNINGS, *Children.*

ADVERSE REACTIONS

Adverse reactions which have been reported with the use of antihistamines are as follows:

Central Nervous System: Sedation and sleepiness (often transient), dizziness, disturbed coordination, confusion, restlessness, excitation, nervousness, tremor, irritability, insomnia, paresthesias, neuritis, convulsions, euphoria, hallucinations, hysteria, faintness.

Integumentary: Allergic manifestation of rash and edema, excessive perspiration, urticaria, photosensitivity.

Special Senses: Acute labyrinthitis, blurred vision, diplopia, vertigo, tinnitus.

Cardiovascular: Hypotension, palpitation, tachycardia, extrasystoles, anaphylactic shock.

Hematologic: Hemolytic anemia, leukopenia, agranulocytosis, thrombocytopenia.

Digestive System: Dryness of mouth, epigastric distress, anorexia, nausea, vomiting, diarrhea, constipation, jaundice.

Genitourinary: Urinary frequency, difficult urination, urinary retention, early menses.

Respiratory: Dryness of nose and throat, thickening of bronchial secretions, tightness of chest and wheezing, nasal stuffiness.

Miscellaneous: Fatigue, chills, headache.

OVERDOSAGE

Antihistamine overdosage reactions may vary from central nervous system depression to stimulation especially in children. Also, atropine-like signs and symptoms (dry mouth; fixed, dilated pupils; flushing, etc.) as well as gastrointestinal symptoms may occur.

If vomiting has not occurred spontaneously the patient should be induced to vomit with syrup of ipecac.

If the patient is unable to vomit, perform gastric lavage followed by activated charcoal. Isotonic or ½ isotonic saline is the lavage of choice. Precautions against aspiration must be taken especially in infants and children.

When life threatening CNS signs and symptoms are present, intravenous physostigmine salicylate may be considered. Dosage and frequency of administration are dependent on age, clinical response, and recurrence after response. (See package circulars for physostigmine products.)

Saline cathartics, as milk of magnesia, by osmosis draw water into the bowel and, therefore, are valuable for their action in rapid dilution of bowel content.

Stimulants should *not* be used.

Vasopressors may be used to treat hypotension.

The oral LD_{50} of cyproheptadine is 123 mg/kg, and 295 mg/kg in the mouse and rat, respectively.

DOSAGE AND ADMINISTRATION

DOSAGE SHOULD BE INDIVIDUALIZED ACCORDING TO THE NEEDS AND THE RESPONSE OF THE PATIENT. Each PERIACTIN tablet contains 4 mg of cyproheptadine hydrochloride. Each 5 mL of PERIACTIN syrup contains 2 mg of cyproheptadine hydrochloride.

Although intended primarily for administration to children, the syrup is also useful for administration to adults who cannot swallow tablets.

Children
The total daily dosage for children may be calculated on the basis of body weight or body area using approximately 0.25 mg/kg/day (0.11 mg/lb/day) or 8 mg per square meter of body surface (8 mg/M²). In small children for whom the calculation of dosage based upon body size is most important, it may be necessary to use PERIACTIN syrup to permit accurate dosage.

Age 2 to 6 years
The usual dose is 2 mg (½ tablet or 1 teaspoon) two or three times a day, adjusted as necessary to the size and response of the patient. The dose is not to exceed 12 mg a day.

Age 7 to 14 years
The usual dose is 4 mg (1 tablet or 2 teaspoons) two or three times a day, adjusted as necessary to the size and response of the patient. The dose is not to exceed 16 mg a day.

Adults
The total daily dose for adults should not exceed 0.5 mg/kg/day (0.23 mg/lb/day).

The therapeutic range is 4 to 20 mg a day, with the majority of patients requiring 12 to 16 mg a day. An occasional patient may require as much as 32 mg a day for adequate relief. It is suggested that dosage be initiated with 4 mg (1 tablet or 2 teaspoons) three times a day and adjusted according to the size and response of the patient.

HOW SUPPLIED

No. 3276—Tablets PERIACTIN, containing 4 mg of cyproheptadine hydrochloride each, are white, round, scored, compressed tablets, coded MSD 62. They are supplied as follows: NDC 0006-0062-68 bottles of 100 (6505-00-890-1884 4 mg 100's).

Shown in Product Identification Section, page 419
No. 3289X—Syrup PERIACTIN, 2 mg per 5 mL is a clear, yellow, syrupy liquid. Contains alcohol 5%, with sorbic acid 0.1% added as preservative and is supplied as follows: NDC 0006-3289-74 bottles of 473 mL.

Storage
Store Tablets PERIACTIN in a well-closed container. Avoid storage at temperatures above 40℃ (104°F).
Store Syrup PERIACTIN in a container which is kept tightly closed. Avoid storage at temperatures below −20℃ (−4°F) and above 40℃ (104°F).

A.H.F.S. Category: 4:00
DC 7398317 Issued May 1986
COPYRIGHT © MERCK & CO., INC., 1985
All rights reserved

PNEUMOVAX® 23 ℞
(Pneumococcal Vaccine Polyvalent, MSD)

DESCRIPTION

PNEUMOVAX® 23 (Pneumococcal Vaccine Polyvalent, MSD), is a sterile, liquid vaccine for intramuscular or subcutaneous injection. It consists of a mixture of highly purified capsular polysaccharides from the 23 most prevalent or invasive pneumococcal types accounting for at least 90% of pneumococcal blood isolates and at least 85% of all pneumococcal isolates from sites which are generally sterile as determined by ongoing surveillance of U.S. data.

PNEUMOVAX 23 is manufactured according to methods developed by the MERCK SHARP & DOHME Research Laboratories. Each 0.5 mL dose of vaccine contains 25 μg of each polysaccharide type dissolved in isotonic saline solution containing 0.25% phenol as preservative.

Type 6B pneumococcal polysaccharide exhibits somewhat greater stability in purified form than does Type 6A. A high degree of cross-reactivity between the two types has been demonstrated in adult volunteers. Therefore, Type 6B has replaced Type 6A, which had been used in the 14-valent vaccine. Although contained in the 14-valent vaccine, Type 25 is not included in PNEUMOVAX 23 because it has recently become a rare isolate in many parts of the world including the United States, Canada and Europe.
[See table above].

CLINICAL PHARMACOLOGY

Pneumococcal infection is a leading cause of death throughout the world and a major cause of pneumonia, meningitis, and otitis media. The emergence of strains of pneumococci with increased resistance to one or more of the common antibiotics and recent isolations of pneumococci with multiple antibiotic resistance emphasize the importance of vaccine prophylaxis against pneumococcal disease. Based on projection from limited observations in the United States, it has been estimated that 400,000 to 500,000 cases of pneumococcal pneumonia may occur annually. The overall case fatality rate ranges from 5–10%. Populations at high risk are the elderly; individuals with immune deficiencies; patients with asplenia or splenic deficiencies, including sickle cell anemia and other severe hemoglobinopathies; alcoholics; and patients with the following diseases: Hodgkin's disease, multiple myeloma and nephrotic syndrome. About 25% of all persons with pneumococcal pneumonia develop bacteremia. Death occurs in about 28% of these bacteremic patients over 50 years of age. Of all patients with pneumococcal bacteremia who died despite treatment with penicillin or tetracycline, as many as 60% died within five days of onset of the illness.

The annual incidence of pneumococcal meningitis is approximately 1.5 to 2.5 per 100,000 population. One-half of the cases occur in children, in whom the fatality rate is about 40%. Children with sickle cell disease have been estimated to have a risk of pneumococcal meningitis nearly 600 times greater than normal children. Other illnesses caused by

23 Pneumococcal Capsular Types Included in PNEUMOVAX 23

Nomenclature																									Pneumococcal Types
Danish	1	2	3	4	5	6B	7F	8	9N	9V	10A	11A	12F	14	15B	17F	18C	19F	19A	20	22F	23F	33F		
U.S.	1	2	3	4	5	26	51	8	9	68	34	43	12	14	54	17	56	19	57	20	22	23	70		

pneumococci include acute exacerbations of chronic bronchitis, sinusitis, arthritis and conjunctivitis.

Invasive pneumococcal disease causes high morbidity and mortality in spite of effective antimicrobial control by antibiotics. These effects of pneumococcal disease appear due to irreversible physiologic damage caused by the bacteria during the first 5 days following onset of illness, and occur irrespective of antimicrobial therapy. Vaccination offers an effective means of further reducing the mortality and morbidity of this disease.

At present, there are 83 known pneumococcal capsular types. However, the preponderance of pneumococcal diseases is caused by only some capsular types. For example, a 10-year (1952–1962) surveillance at a New York medical center, showed that 56% of all deaths due to pneumococcal pneumonia were caused by 6 capsular types and that approximately 78% of all pneumococcal pneumonias were caused by 12 capsular types. Such unequal distribution of pneumococcal capsular types causing disease has been shown throughout the world. It is on the basis of this information that the pneumococcal vaccine is composed of 23 capsular types, designed to provide coverage of approximately 90% of the most frequently reported types.

It has been established that the purified pneumococcal capsular polysaccharides induce antibody production and that such antibody is effective in preventing pneumococcal disease. Studies in humans have demonstrated the immunogenicity (antibody-stimulating capability) of each of the 23 capsular types when tested in polyvalent vaccines. Adults of all ages responded immunologically to the vaccines. Earlier studies with 12- and 14-valent pneumococcal vaccines in children two years of age and older and in adults showed immunogenic responses. Protective capsular type-specific antibody levels develop by the third week following vaccination.

The protective efficacy of pneumococcal vaccines containing 6 and 12 capsular polysaccharides was investigated in controlled studies of gold miners in South Africa, in whom there is a high attack rate for pneumococcal pneumonia. Capsular type-specific attack rates for pneumococcal pneumonia were observed for the period from 2 weeks through about 1 year after vaccination. The rates for pneumonia caused by the same capsular types represented in the vaccines are given in the table. Protective efficacy was 76% and 92%, respectively, in the two studies for the capsular types represented.
[See table below].

In similar studies carried out by Dr. R. Austrian and associates using similar pneumococcal vaccines prepared for the National Institute of Allergy and Infectious Diseases, the reduction in pneumonias caused by the capsular types contained in the vaccines was 79%. Reduction in type-specific pneumococcal bacteremia was 82%. A preliminary report suggests that in patients with sickle cell anemia and/or anatomical or functional asplenia, the vaccine was highly effective in persons over two years of age in preventing severe pneumococcal disease and bacteremia.

The duration of protective effect of PNEUMOVAX 23 is presently unknown, but it has been shown in previous studies with other pneumococcal vaccines that antibody induced by the vaccine may persist for as long as 5 years. Type-specific antibody levels induced by PNEUMOVAX (Pneumococcal Vaccine, Polyvalent, MSD) (14-valent) have been observed to decline over a 42-month period of observation, but remain significantly above prevaccination levels in almost all recipients who manifest an initial response.

INDICATIONS AND USAGE

PNEUMOVAX 23 is indicated for immunization against pneumococcal disease caused by those pneumococcal types included in the vaccine. Effectiveness of the vaccine in the prevention of pneumococcal pneumonia and pneumococcal bacteremia has been demonstrated in controlled trials. PNEUMOVAX 23 *will not immunize against capsular types of pneumococcus other than those contained in the vaccine.*

Use in selected individuals over 2 years of age as follows: (1) patients who have anatomical asplenia or who have splenic dysfunction due to sickle cell disease or other causes; (2) persons with chronic illnesses in which there is an increased risk of pneumococcal disease, such as functional impairment of cardiorespiratory, hepatic and renal systems; (3) persons 50 years of age or older; (4) patients with other chronic illnesses who may be at greater risk of developing pneumococcal infection or experiencing more severe pneumococcal illness as a result of alcohol abuse or coexisting diseases including diabetes mellitus, chronic cerebrospinal fluid leakage, or conditions associated with immunosuppression; (5) patients with Hodgkin's disease if immunization can be given at least 10 days prior to treatment. For maximal antibody response immunization should be given at least 14 days prior to the start of treatment with radiation or chemotherapy. Immunization of patients less than 10 days prior to or during treatment is not recommended. (see CONTRAINDICATIONS.)

Use in communities. Persons over 2 years of age as follows: (1) closed groups such as those in residential schools, nursing homes and other institutions. (To decrease the likelihood of acute outbreaks of pneumococcal disease in closed institutional populations where there is increased risk that the disease may be severe, vaccination of the entire closed population should be considered where there are no other contraindications.); (2) groups epidemiologically at risk in the community when there is a generalized outbreak in the population due to a single pneumococcal type included in the vaccine; (3) patients at high risk of influenza complications, particularly pneumonia.

PNEUMOVAX 23 may not be effective in preventing infection resulting from basilar skull fracture or from external communication with cerebrospinal fluid.

Simultaneous administration of pneumococcal polysaccharide vaccine and whole-virus influenza vaccine gives satisfactory antibody response without increasing the occurrence of adverse reactions. Simultaneous administration of the pneumococcal vaccine and split-virus influenza vaccine may also be expected to yield satisfactory results.

Revaccination
Revaccination of adults is not recommended. Adults previously immunized with any polyvalent pneumococcal vaccine should not receive PNEUMOVAX 23 or PNEUMOVAX (Pneumococcal Vaccine, Polyvalent, MSD) (14-valent) since an increased incidence and severity of adverse reactions among healthy adults receiving such reinjections have been noted, most likely due to sustained high antibody levels.

Certain groups of children at very high risk for pneumococcal disease (e.g., children with sickle cell disease or nephrotic syndrome) may have lower peak levels of antibody response and/or more rapid rates of decline in antibody levels than do healthy adults. However, insufficient data are available at this time to permit formulation of guidelines for reimmunization of high-risk children.

CONTRAINDICATIONS

Hypersensitivity to any component of the vaccine. Epinephrine injection (1:1000) must be immediately available should an acute anaphylactoid reaction occur due to any component of the vaccine.

Revaccination of adults is contraindicated. Adults previously immunized with any polyvalent pneumococcal vaccine should not receive PNEUMOVAX 23 or PNEUMOVAX (Pneumococcal Vaccine, Polyvalent, MSD) (14-valent) since an increased incidence and severity of adverse reactions among healthy adults receiving such reinjections have been noted, most likely due to sustained high antibody levels.

Patients with Hodgkin's disease immunized less than 7 to 10 days prior to immunosuppressive therapy have in some instances been found to have post-immunization antibody levels below their pre-immunization levels. Because of these results, immunization less than 10 days prior to or during treatment is contraindicated.

Patients with Hodgkin's disease who have received extensive chemotherapy and/or nodal irradiation have been shown to have an impaired antibody response to a 12-valent pneumococcal vaccine. Because, in some intensively treated patients, administration of that vaccine depressed pre-existing levels of antibody to some pneumococcal types, PNEUMOVAX 23

Continued on next page

Information on the Merck Sharp & Dohme products listed on these pages is the full prescribing information from product circulars in use August 31, 1989.

PNEUMOVAX 23

Number of Capsular Types in Pneumococcal Vaccine	Rate/1000 for Pneumonia Caused by Homologous Capsular Types		Protective Efficacy
	Vaccinated Group	Control Group	
6	9.2	38.3	76%
12	1.8	22.0	92%

Merck Sharp & Dohme—Cont.

is not recommended at this time for patients who have received these forms of therapy for Hodgkin's disease.

WARNINGS

If the vaccine is used in persons receiving immunosuppressive therapy, the expected serum antibody response may not be obtained.

Intradermal administration may cause severe local reactions.

PRECAUTIONS

General

Caution and appropriate care should be exercised in administering PNEUMOVAX 23 to individuals with severely compromised cardiac and/or pulmonary function in whom a systemic reaction would pose a significant risk.

Any febrile respiratory illness or other active infection is reason for delaying use of PNEUMOVAX 23, except when, in the opinion of the physician, withholding the agent entails even greater risk.

In patients who require penicillin (or other antibiotic) prophylaxis against pneumococcal infection, such prophylaxis should not be discontinued after vaccination with PNEUMOVAX 23.

Pregnancy

Pregnancy Category C: Animal reproduction studies have not been conducted with PNEUMOVAX 23. It is also not known whether PNEUMOVAX 23 can cause fetal harm when administered to a pregnant woman or can affect reproduction capacity. PNEUMOVAX 23 should be given to a pregnant woman only if clearly needed.

Nursing Mothers

It is not known whether this drug is excreted in human milk. Because many drugs are excreted in human milk, caution should be exercised when PNEUMOVAX 23 is administered to a nursing woman.

Pediatric Use

Children less than 2 years of age do not respond satisfactorily to the capsular types of PNEUMOVAX 23 that are most often the cause of pneumococcal disease in this age group. Safety and effectiveness in children below the age of 2 years have not been established. Accordingly, PNEUMOVAX 23 is not recommended in this age group.

ADVERSE REACTIONS

Local erythema and soreness at the injection site, usually of less than 48 hours duration, occurs commonly; local induration occurs less commonly. In a study of PNEUMOVAX 22 (containing 22 capsular types) in 29 adults, 21 (71%) showed local reaction characterized principally by local soreness and/or induration at the injection site within 2 days after vaccination.

Rash, urticaria, arthralgia, serum sickness, and adenitis have been reported rarely.

Low grade fever (less than 100.9°F) occurs occasionally and is usually confined to the 24-hour period following vaccination. Although rare, fever over 102°F has been reported. Malaise, myalgia, and asthenia also have been reported.

Patients with otherwise stabilized idiopathic thrombocytopenic purpura have, on rare occasions, experienced a relapse in their thrombocytopenia, occurring 2 to 14 days after vaccination, and lasting up to 2 weeks.

Reactions of greater severity, duration, or extent are unusual. Neurological disorders such as paresthesias and acute radiculoneuropathy including Guillain-Barré syndrome have been rarely reported in temporal association with administration of pneumococcal vaccine. No cause and effect relationship has been established. Rarely, anaphylactoid reactions have been reported.

DOSAGE AND ADMINISTRATION

Do not inject intravenously. Intradermal administration should be avoided.

Parenteral drug products should be inspected visually for particulate matter and discoloration prior to administration, whenever solution and container permit. PNEUMOVAX 23 is a clear, colorless solution.

Administer a single 0.5 mL dose of PNEUMOVAX 23 subcutaneously or intramuscularly (preferably in the deltoid muscle or lateral mid-thigh), with appropriate precautions to avoid intravascular administration.

Single-Dose and 5-Dose Vials

For Syringe Use Only: Withdraw 0.5 mL from the vial using a sterile needle and syringe free of preservatives, antiseptics and detergents.

It is important to use a separate sterile syringe and needle for each individual patient to prevent transmission of hepatitis B and other infectious agents from one person to another. Store unopened and opened vials at 2–8°C (35.6–46.4°F). The vaccine is used directly as supplied. No dilution or reconstitution is necessary. Phenol 0.25% added as preservative. All vaccine must be discarded after the expiration date.

HOW SUPPLIED

No. 4739—PNEUMOVAX 23 contains one 5-dose vial of liquid vaccine, **NDC** 0006-4739-00. For use with syringe only (6505-01-092-0391).

No. 4741—PNEUMOVAX 23 is supplied as follows: **NDC** 0006-4741-00. A box of 5 individual cartons, each containing a single-dose vial of vaccine.

A.H.F.S. Category: 80:12

DC 7497404   Issued September 1988

PRIMAXIN®   ℞
(Imipenem-Cilastatin Sodium, MSD)

DESCRIPTION

PRIMAXIN® (Imipenem-Cilastatin Sodium, MSD) is a formulation of imipenem, a thienamycin antibiotic, and cilastatin sodium, the inhibitor of the renal dipeptidase, dehydropeptidase I, with sodium bicarbonate added as a buffer. PRIMAXIN is a potent broad spectrum antibacterial agent for intravenous administration.

Imipenem (N-formimidoylthienamycin monohydrate) is a crystalline derivative of thienamycin, which is produced by *Streptomyces cattleya.* Its chemical name is [5R -[5α, 6α (R *)]]-6-(1-hydroxyethyl)-3-[[2-[(iminomethyl)amino] ethyl] thio]-7-oxo-1-azabicyclo [3.2.0] hept-2-ene-2-carboxylic acid monohydrate. It is an off-white, nonhygroscopic crystalline compound with a molecular weight of 317.37. It is sparingly soluble in water, and slightly soluble in methanol. Its empirical formula is $C_{12}H_{17}N_3O_4S \cdot H_2O$, and its structural formula is:

Cilastatin sodium is the sodium salt of a derivatized heptenoic acid. Its chemical name is [R- [R*,S*- (Z)]]-7-[(2-amino-2-carboxyethyl)thio]-2-[[(2, 2-dimethylcyclopropyl) carbonyl]amino]-2-heptenoic acid, monosodium salt. It is an off-white to yellowish-white, hygroscopic, amorphous compound with a molecular weight of 380.43. It is very soluble in water and in methanol. Its empirical formula is

$C_{16}H_{25}N_2O_5S$ Na, and its structural formula is:

PRIMAXIN is buffered to provide solutions in the pH range of 6.5 to 7.5. There is no significant change in pH when solutions are prepared and used as directed. (See COMPATIBILITY AND STABILITY.) PRIMAXIN 250 contains 18.8 mg of sodium (0.8 mEq) and PRIMAXIN 500 contains 37.5 mg of sodium (1.6 mEq). Solutions of PRIMAXIN range from colorless to yellow. Variations of color within this range do not affect the potency of the product.

CLINICAL PHARMACOLOGY

Intravenous Administration

Intravenous infusion of PRIMAXIN over 20 minutes results in peak plasma levels of imipenem antimicrobial activity that range from 14 to 24 mcg/mL for the 250 mg dose, from 21 to 58 mcg/mL for the 500 mg dose and from 41 to 83 mcg/mL for the 1000 mg dose. At these doses, plasma levels of imipenem antimicrobial activity decline to below 1 mcg/mL or less in 4 to 6 hours. Peak plasma levels of cilastatin following a 20-minute intravenous infusion of PRIMAXIN, range from 15 to 25 mcg/mL for the 250 mg dose, from 31 to 49 mcg/mL for the 500 mg dose and from 56 to 88 mcg/mL for the 1000 mg dose.

General

The plasma half-life of each component is approximately 1 hour. The binding of imipenem to human serum proteins is approximately 20% and that of cilastatin is approximately 40%. Approximately 70% of the administered imipenem is recovered in the urine within 10 hours after which no further urinary excretion is detectable. Urine concentrations of imipenem in excess of 10 mcg/mL can be maintained for up to 8 hours with PRIMAXIN at the 500 mg dose. Approximately 70% of the cilastatin sodium dose is recovered in the urine within 10 hours of administration of PRIMAXIN.

No accumulation of PRIMAXIN in plasma or urine is observed with regimens administered as frequently as every 6 hours in patients with normal renal function.

Imipenem, administered alone, is metabolized in the kidneys by dehydropeptidase I resulting in relatively low levels in urine. Cilastatin sodium, an inhibitor of this enzyme, effectively prevents renal metabolism of imipenem so that when imipenem and cilastatin sodium are given concomitantly fully adequate antibacterial levels of imipenem are achieved in the urine.

After a 1 gram dose of PRIMAXIN, the following average levels of imipenem were measured (usually at 1 hour postdose except where indicated) in the tissues and fluids listed: [See table below].

Microbiology

The bactericidal activity of imipenem results from the inhibition of cell wall synthesis. Its greatest affinity is for penicillin binding proteins (PBP) 1A, 1B, 2, 4, 5, and 6 of *Escherichia coli,* and 1A, 1B, 2, 4 and 5 of *Pseudomonas aeruginosa.* The lethal effect is related to binding to PBP 2 and PBP 1B. Imipenem has *in vitro* activity against a wide range of gram-positive and gram-negative organisms.

Imipenem has a high degree of stability in the presence of beta-lactamases, both penicillinases and cephalosporinases produced by gram-negative and gram-positive bacteria. It is a potent inhibitor of beta-lactamases from certain gram-negative bacteria which are inherently resistant to most beta-lactam antibiotics, e.g., *Pseudomonas aeruginosa, Serratia* spp., and *Enterobacter* spp.

In vitro, imipenem is active against most strains of clinical isolates of the following microorganisms:

Gram-positive:

Group D streptococci (including enterococci e.g., *Streptococcus faecalis*)

    NOTE: Imipenem is inactive against *Streptococcus faecium.*

Streptococcus pyogenes (Group A streptococci)

Streptococcus agalactiae (Group B streptococci)

Group C streptococci

Group G streptococci

Viridans streptococci

Streptococcus pneumoniae (formerly *Diplococcus pneumoniae*)

Staphylococcus aureus including penicillinase producing strains

Staphylococcus epidermidis including penicillinase producing strains

    NOTE: Many strains of methicillin-resistant staphylococci are resistant to imipenem.

Gram-negative:

Escherichia coli

Proteus mirabilis

Proteus vulgaris

Tissue or Fluid	N	Imipenem Level mcg/mL or mcg/g	Range
Vitreous Humor	3	3.4 (3.5 hours post dose)	2.88–3.6
Aqueous Humor	5	2.99 (2 hours post dose)	2.4–3.9
Lung Tissue	8	5.6 (median)	3.5–15.5
Sputum	1	2.1	—
Pleural	1	22.0	—
Peritoneal	12	23.9 S.D. ±5.3 (2 hours post dose)	—
Bile	2	5.3 (2.25 hours post dose)	4.6 to 6.0
CSF (uninflamed)	5	1.0 (4 hours post dose)	0.26–2.0
CSF (inflamed)	7	2.6 (2 hours post dose)	0.5–5.5
Fallopian Tubes	1	13.6	—
Endometrium	1	11.1	—
Myometrium	1	5.0	—
Bone	10	2.6	0.4–5.4
Interstitial Fluid	12	16.4	10.0–22.6
Skin	12	4.4	NA
Fascia	12	4.4	NA

Morganella morganii
Providencia rettgeri
Providencia stuartii
Citrobacter spp.
Klebsiella spp. including *K. pneumoniae* and *K. oxytoca*
Enterobacter spp.
Hafnia spp. including *H. alvei*
Serratia marcescens
Serratia spp. including *S. liquefaciens*
Haemophilus parainfluenzae
H. influenzae
Gardnerella vaginalis
Acinetobacter spp.
Pseudomonas aeruginosa

   NOTE: Imipenem is inactive against *P. maltophilia* and some strains of *P. cepacia.*

Anaerobes:
Bacteroides spp. including *Bacteroides bivius, Bacteroides fragilis, Bacteroides melaninogenicus*
Clostridium spp. including *C. perfringens*
Eubacterium spp.
Fusobacterium spp.
Peptococcus spp.
Peptostreptococcus spp.
Propionibacterium spp. including *P. acnes*
Actinomyces spp.
Veillonella spp.

Imipenem has been shown to be active *in vitro* against the following microorganisms; however, clinical efficacy has not yet been established.

Gram-positive:
Listeria monocytogenes
Nocardia spp.

Gram-negative:
Salmonella spp.
Shigella spp.
Yersinia spp. including *Yersinia enterocolitica, Yersinia pseudotuberculosis*
Bordetella bronchiseptica
Campylobacter spp.
Achromobacter spp.
Alcaligenes spp.
Moraxella spp.
Pasteurella multocida
Aeromonas hydrophila
Plesiomonas shigelloides
Neisseria gonorrhoeae (including penicillinase-producing strains)

Anaerobes:
Bacteroides asaccharolyticus
Bacteroides disiens
Bacteroides distasonis
Bacteroides ovatus
Bacteroides thetaiotaomicron
Bacteroides vulgatus

In vitro tests show imipenem to act synergistically with aminoglycoside antibiotics against some isolates of *Pseudomonas aeruginosa.*

Susceptibility Testing
Quantitative methods that require measurement of zone diameters give the most precise estimate of antibiotic susceptibility. One such procedure has been recommended for use with discs to test susceptibility to imipenem.

Reports from the laboratory giving results of the standard single-disc susceptibility test with a 10 mcg imipenem disc should be interpreted according to the following criteria.

Fully susceptible organisms produce zones of 16 mm or greater, indicating that the test organism is likely to respond to doses of 2 g per day or less (see **DOSAGE AND ADMINISTRATION.**)

Moderately susceptible organisms produce zones of 14 to 15 mm and are expected to be susceptible if the maximum recommended dosage is used or if infection is confined to tissues and fluids in which high antibiotic levels are attained.

Resistant organisms produce zones of 13 mm or less, indicating that other therapy should be selected.

A bacterial isolate may be considered fully susceptible if the MIC value for imipenem is equal to or less than 4 mcg/mL. Organisms are considered moderately susceptible if the MIC value is 8 mcg/mL. Organisms are considered resistant if the MIC is equal to or greater than 16 mcg/mL.

The standardized quality control procedure requires use of control organisms. The 10 mcg imipenem disc should give the zone diameters listed below for the quality control strains.

Organism	ATCC	Zone Size Range
E. coli	25922	26–32 mm
Ps. aeruginosa	27853	20–28 mm

Dilution susceptibility tests should give MICs between the ranges listed below for the quality control strains.

Organism	ATCC	MIC (mcg/mL)
E. coli	25922	0.06–0.25
S. aureus	29213	0.015–0.06
S. faecalis	29212	0.5–2.0
Ps. aeruginosa	27853	1.0–4.0

Based on blood levels of imipenem achieved in man, breakpoint criteria have been adopted for imipenem.

Category	Zone Diameter (mm)	Recommended MIC Breakpoint (mcg/mL)
Fully Susceptible	≥ 16	≤ 4
Moderately Susceptible	14–15	8
Resistant	≤ 13	≥ 16

INDICATIONS AND USAGE

PRIMAXIN is indicated for the treatment of serious infections caused by susceptible strains of the designated microorganisms in the diseases listed below:

(1) **Lower respiratory tract infections.** *Staphylococcus aureus* (penicillinase producing strains), *Escherichia coli, Klebsiella* species, *Enterobacter* species, *Haemophilus influenzae, Haemophilus parainfluenzae*, Acinetobacter* species, *Serratia marcescens.*

(2) **Urinary tract infections** (Complicated and uncomplicated). *Staphylococcus aureus* (penicillinase producing strains)*, Group D streptococci (enterococci), *Escherichia coli, Klebsiella* species, *Enterobacter* species, *Proteus vulgaris*, Providencia rettgeri*, Morganella morganii*, Pseudomonas aeruginosa.*

(3) **Intra-abdominal infections.** *Staphylococcus aureus* (penicillinase producing strains)*, *Staphylococcus epidermidis,* Group D streptococci (enterococci), *Escherichia coli, Klebsiella* species, *Enterobacter* species, *Proteus* species (indole positive and indole negative), *Morganella morganii*, Pseudomonas aeruginosa, Citrobacter* species, *Clostridium* species, Gram-positive anaerobes, including *Peptococcus* species, *Peptostreptococcus* species, *Eubacterium* species, *Propionibacterium* species*, *Bifidobacterium* species, *Bacteroides* species, including *B. fragilis, Fusobacterium* species.

(4) **Gynecologic infections.** *Staphylococcus aureus* (penicillinase producing strains)*, *Staphylococcus epidermidis,* Group B streptococci, Group D streptococci (enterococci), *Escherichia coli, Klebsiella* species*, *Proteus* species (indole positive and indole negative), *Enterobacter* species*, Gram-positive anaerobes, including *Peptococcus* species*, *Peptostreptococcus* species, *Propionibacterium* species*, *Bifidobacterium* species*, *Bacteroides* species, *B. fragilis*, Gardnerella vaginalis.*

(5) **Bacterial septicemia.** *Staphylococcus aureus* (penicillinase producing strains), Group D streptococci (enterococci), *Escherichia coli, Klebsiella* species, *Pseudomonas aeruginosa, Serratia* species*, *Enterobacter* species, *Bacteroides* species, *B. fragilis*.*

(6) **Bone and joint infections.** *Staphylococcus aureus* (penicillinase producing strains), *Staphylococcus epidermidis,* Group D streptococci (enterococci), *Enterobacter* species, *Pseudomonas aeruginosa.*

(7) **Skin and skin structure infections.** *Staphylococcus aureus* (penicillinase producing strains), *Staphylococcus epidermidis,* Group D streptococci (enterococci), *Escherichia coli, Klebsiella* species, *Enterobacter* species, *Proteus vulgaris, Providencia rettgeri*, Morganella morganii, Pseudomonas aeruginosa, Serratia* species, *Citrobacter* species, *Acinetobacter* species, Gram-positive anaerobes, including *Peptococcus* species and *Peptostreptococcus* species, *Bacteroides* species, including *B. fragilis, Fusobacterium* species*.

(8) **Endocarditis.** *Staphylococcus aureus* (penicillinase producing strains).

(9) **Polymicrobic infections.** PRIMAXIN is indicated for polymicrobic infections including those in which *S. pneumoniae* (pneumonia, septicemia), Group A beta-hemolytic streptococcus (skin and skin structure), or non-penicillinase-producing *S. aureus* is one of the causative organisms. However, monobacterial infections due to these organisms are usually treated with narrower spectrum antibiotics, such as penicillin G.

Because of its broad spectrum of bactericidal activity against gram-positive and gram-negative aerobic and anaerobic bacteria, PRIMAXIN is useful for the treatment of mixed infections and as presumptive therapy prior to the identification of the causative organisms.

Although clinical improvement has been observed in patients with cystic fibrosis, chronic pulmonary disease, and lower respiratory tract infections caused by *Pseudomonas*

* Efficacy for this organism in this organ system was studied in fewer than 10 infections.

aeruginosa, bacterial eradication may not necessarily be achieved.

As with other beta-lactam antibiotics, some strains of *Pseudomonas aeruginosa* may develop resistance fairly rapidly on treatment with PRIMAXIN. When clinically appropriate during therapy of *Pseudomonas aeruginosa* infections, periodic susceptibility testing should be done.

Infections resistant to other antibiotics, for example, cephalosporins, penicillin, and aminoglycosides, have been shown to respond to treatment with PRIMAXIN.

CONTRAINDICATIONS

PRIMAXIN is contraindicated in patients who have shown hypersensitivity to any component of this product.

WARNINGS

SERIOUS AND OCCASIONALLY FATAL HYPERSENSITIVITY (anaphylactic) REACTIONS HAVE BEEN REPORTED IN PATIENTS RECEIVING THERAPY WITH BETA-LACTAMS. THESE REACTIONS ARE MORE APT TO OCCUR IN PERSONS WITH A HISTORY OF SENSITIVITY TO MULTIPLE ALLERGENS.

THERE HAVE BEEN REPORTS OF PATIENTS WITH A HISTORY OF PENICILLIN HYPERSENSITIVITY WHO HAVE EXPERIENCED SEVERE HYPERSENSITIVITY REACTIONS WHEN TREATED WITH ANOTHER BETA-LACTAM. BEFORE INITIATING THERAPY WITH 'PRIMAXIN,' CAREFUL INQUIRY SHOULD BE MADE CONCERNING PREVIOUS HYPERSENSITIVITY REACTIONS TO PENICILLINS, CEPHALOSPORINS, OTHER BETA-LACTAMS, AND OTHER ALLERGENS. IF AN ALLERGIC REACTION TO 'PRIMAXIN' OCCURS, DISCONTINUE THE DRUG. SERIOUS HYPERSENSITIVITY REACTIONS MAY REQUIRE EPINEPHRINE AND OTHER EMERGENCY MEASURES.

Pseudomembranous colitis has been reported with virtually all antibiotics, including PRIMAXIN; therefore it is important to consider its diagnosis in patients who develop diarrhea in association with antibiotic use. This colitis may range in severity from mild to life threatening.

Mild cases of pseudomembranous colitis may respond to drug discontinuance alone. In more severe cases, management may include sigmoidoscopy, appropriate bacteriological studies, fluid, electrolyte and protein supplementation, and the use of a drug such as oral vancomycin, as indicated. Isolation of the patient may be advisable. Other causes of colitis should also be considered.

PRECAUTIONS

General
CNS adverse experiences such as confusional states, myoclonic activity, and seizures have been reported during treatment with PRIMAXIN, especially when recommended dosages were exceeded. These experiences have occurred most commonly in patients with CNS disorders (e.g., brain lesions or history of seizures) and/or compromised renal function. However, there have been reports of CNS adverse experiences in patients who had no recognized or documented underlying CNS disorder or compromised renal function.

Patients with severe or marked impairment of renal function, whether or not undergoing hemodialysis, had a higher risk of seizure activity when receiving maximum recommended doses than those with no impairment of renal function; therefore, maximum recommended doses should be used only where clearly indicated (see **DOSAGE AND ADMINISTRATION**).

Patients with creatinine clearances of ≤ 5 mL/min/1.73 m² should not receive PRIMAXIN unless hemodialysis is instituted within 48 hours.

For patients on hemodialysis, PRIMAXIN is recommended only when the benefit outweighs the potential risk of seizures.

Close adherence to recommended dosage and dosage schedules is urged, especially in patients with known factors that predispose to convulsive activity. Anticonvulsant therapy should be continued in patients with known seizure disorder. If focal tremors, myoclonus, or seizures occur, patients should be evaluated neurologically, placed on anticonvulsant therapy if not already instituted, and the dosage of PRIMAXIN re-examined to determine whether it should be decreased or the antibiotic discontinued.

As with other antibiotics, prolonged use of PRIMAXIN may result in overgrowth of nonsusceptible organisms. Repeated evaluation of the patient's condition is essential. If superinfection occurs during therapy, appropriate measures should be taken.

Continued on next page

Merck Sharp & Dohme—Cont.

While PRIMAXIN possesses the characteristic low toxicity of the beta-lactam group of antibiotics, periodic assessment of organ system function during prolonged therapy is advisable.

Drug Interactions

Since concomitant administration of PRIMAXIN and probenecid results in only minimal increases in plasma levels of imipenem and plasma half-life, it is not recommended that probenecid be given with PRIMAXIN.

PRIMAXIN should not be mixed with or physically added to other antibiotics. However, PRIMAXIN may be administered concomitantly with other antibiotics, such as aminoglycosides.

Carcinogenesis, Mutagenesis, Impairment of Fertility

Gene toxicity studies were performed in a variety of bacterial and mammalian tests *in vivo* and *in vitro*. The tests were: V79 mammalian cell mutation assay (PRIMAXIN alone and imipenem alone), Ames test (cilastatin sodium alone), unscheduled DNA synthesis assay (PRIMAXIN) and *in vivo* mouse cytogenicity test (PRIMAXIN). None of these tests showed any evidence of genetic damage.

Reproduction tests in male and female rats were performed with PRIMAXIN at dosage levels up to 8 times the usual human dose. Slight decreases in live fetal body weight were restricted to the highest dosage level. No other adverse effects were observed on fertility, reproductive performance, fetal viability, growth or postnatal development of pups. Similarly, no adverse effects on the fetus or on lactation were observed when PRIMAXIN was administered to rats late in gestation.

Pregnancy

Pregnancy Category C. Teratogenicity studies with cilastatin sodium in rabbits and rats at 10 and 33 times the usual human dose, respectively, showed no evidence of adverse effect on the fetus. No evidence of teratogenicity or adverse effect on postnatal growth or behavior was observed in rats given imipenem at dosage levels up to 30 times the usual human dose. Similarly, no evidence of adverse effect on the fetus was observed in teratology studies in rabbits with imipenem at dosage levels at the usual human dose.

Teratology studies with PRIMAXIN at doses up to 11 times the usual human dose in pregnant mice and rats during the period of major organogenesis revealed no evidence of teratogenicity.

Data from preliminary studies suggests an apparent intolerance to PRIMAXIN (including emesis, inappetence, body weight loss, diarrhea and death) at doses equivalent to the average human dose in pregnant rabbits and cynomolgus monkeys that is not seen in non-pregnant animals in these or other species. In other studies, PRIMAXIN was well tolerated in equivalent or higher doses (up to 11 times the average human dose) in pregnant rats and mice. Further studies are underway to evaluate these findings.

There are, however, no adequate and well-controlled studies in pregnant women. PRIMAXIN should be used during pregnancy only if the potential benefit justifies the potential risk to the fetus.

Nursing Mothers

It is not known whether this drug is excreted in human milk. Because many drugs are excreted in human milk, caution should be exercised when PRIMAXIN is administered to a nursing woman.

Pediatric Use

Safety and effectiveness in infants and children below 12 years of age have not yet been established.

ADVERSE REACTIONS

PRIMAXIN is generally well tolerated. Many of the 1,723 patients treated in clinical trials were severely ill and had multiple background diseases and physiological impairments, making it difficult to determine causal relationship of adverse experiences to therapy with PRIMAXIN.

Local Adverse Reactions

Adverse local clinical reactions that were reported as possibly, probably or definitely related to therapy with PRIMAXIN were:

    Phlebitis/thrombophlebitis—3.1%
    Pain at the injection site—0.7%
    Erythema at the injection site—0.4%
    Vein induration—0.2%
    Infused vein infection—0.1%

Systemic Adverse Reactions

The most frequently reported systemic adverse clinical reactions that were reported as possibly, probably, or definitely related to PRIMAXIN were nausea (2.0%), diarrhea (1.8%), vomiting (1.5%), rash (0.9%), fever (0.5%), hypotension (0.4%), seizures (0.4%) (see *PRECAUTIONS*), dizziness (0.3%), pruritus (0.3%), urticaria (0.2%), somnolence (0.2%). Additional adverse systemic clinical reactions reported as possibly, probably or definitely drug related occurring in less than 0.2% of the patients or reported since the drug was

marketed are listed within each body system in order of decreasing severity: *Gastrointestinal*—pseudomembranous colitis (see WARNINGS), hemorrhagic colitis, hepatitis (rarely), gastroenteritis, abdominal pain, glossitis, tongue papillar hypertrophy, heartburn, pharyngeal pain, increased salivation; *CNS*—encephalopathy, tremor, confusion, myoclonus, paresthesia, vertigo, headache, psychic disturbances; *Special Senses*—transient hearing loss in patients with impaired hearing, tinnitus, taste perversion; *Respiratory*—chest discomfort, dyspnea, hyperventilation, thoracic spine pain; *Cardiovascular*—palpitations, tachycardia; *Skin*—toxic epidermal necrolysis (rarely), erythema multiforme, facial edema, flushing, cyanosis, hyperhidrosis, skin texture changes, candidiasis, pruritus vulvae; *Body as a whole*—polyarthralgia, asthenia/weakness; *Renal*—acute renal failure (rarely), oliguria/anuria, polyuria. The role of PRIMAXIN in changes in renal function is difficult to assess, since factors predisposing to pre-renal azotemia or to impaired renal function usually have been present.

Adverse Laboratory Changes

Adverse laboratory changes without regard to drug relationship that were reported during clinical trials or reported since the drug was marketed were:

Hepatic: Increased SGPT, SGOT, alkaline phosphatase, bilirubin and LDH.

Hemic: Increased eosinophils, positive Coombs test, decreased WBC and neutrophils including agranulocytosis, increased WBC, increased platelets, decreased platelets, decreased hemoglobin and hematocrit, increased monocytes, abnormal prothrombin time, increased lymphocytes, increased basophils.

Electrolytes: Decreased serum sodium, increased potassium, increased chloride.

Renal: Increased BUN, creatinine.

Urinalysis: Presence of urine protein, urine red blood cells, urine white blood cells, urine casts, urine bilirubin, and urine urobilinogen.

OVERDOSAGE

The intravenous LD_{50} of imipenem is greater than 2000 mg/kg in the rat and approximately 1500 mg/kg in the mouse.

The intravenous LD_{50} of cilastatin sodium is approximately 5000 mg/kg in the rat and approximately 8700 mg/kg in the mouse.

The intravenous LD_{50} of PRIMAXIN is approximately 1000 mg/kg in the rat and approximately 1100 mg/kg in the mouse.

Information on overdosage in humans is not available.

DOSAGE AND ADMINISTRATION

The dosage recommendations for PRIMAXIN represent the quantity of imipenem to be administered. An equivalent amount of cilastatin is also present in the solution. Each 250 mg or 500 mg dose should be given by intravenous administration over 20 to 30 minutes. Each 1000 mg dose should be infused over 40 to 60 minutes. In patients who develop nausea during the infusion, the rate of infusion may be slowed. The total daily dosage for PRIMAXIN should be based on the type or severity of infection and given in equally divided doses based on consideration of degree of susceptibility of the pathogen(s), renal function and body weight. Patients with impaired renal function, as judged by creatinine clearance ≤ 70 mL/min/1.73 m^2, require adjustment of dosage as described in the succeeding section of these guidelines.

Dosage regimens in column A in the Table for Adults with Normal Renal Functions are recommended for infections caused by fully susceptible organisms which represent the majority of pathogenic species. Dosage regimens in column B of this Table are recommended for infections caused by organisms with moderate susceptibility to imipenem, primarily some strains of *Ps. aeruginosa*.

Doses cited in the Table below are based on a body weight of 70 kg. A further proportionate reduction in dose administered must be made for patients with a body weight less than 70 kg by multiplying the selected dose by the patient's weight in kg divided by 70.

INTRAVENOUS DOSAGE SCHEDULE FOR ADULTS WITH NORMAL RENAL FUNCTION

Type or Severity of Infection	A Fully Susceptible Organisms including gram-positive and gram-negative aerobes and anaerobes	B Moderately susceptible organisms, primarily some strains of *Ps. aeruginosa*
Mild	250 mg q6h	500 mg q6h
Moderate	500 mg q8h	500 mg q6h
	500 mg q6h	1 g q8h

Severe, life threatening	500 mg q6h	1 g q8h 1 g q6h
Uncomplicated urinary tract infection	250 mg q6h	250 mg q6h
Complicated urinary tract infection	500 mg q6h	500 mg q6h

Due to the high antimicrobial activity of PRIMAXIN, it is recommended that the maximum total daily dosage not exceed 50 mg/kg/day or 4.0 g/day, whichever is lower. There is no evidence that higher doses provide greater efficacy. However, patients over twelve years of age with cystic fibrosis and normal renal function have been treated with PRIMAXIN at doses up to 90 mg/kg/day in divided doses, not exceeding 4.0 g/day.

INTRAVENOUS DOSAGE SCHEDULE FOR ADULTS WITH IMPAIRED RENAL FUNCTION

Patients with creatinine clearance of ≤ 70 mL/min/1.73 m^2 require adjustment of the dosage of PRIMAXIN as indicated in the Table below. Creatinine clearance may be calculated from serum creatinine concentration by the following equation:

$$T_{cc}\text{ (Males)} = \frac{\text{(wt. in kg) (140 } - \text{ age)}}{(72)\text{ (creatinine in mg/dL)}}$$

$$T_{cc}\text{ (Females)} = 0.85 \times \text{above value}$$

Column A of the following Table shows maximum dosages recommended in each category of impaired renal function for infections caused by fully susceptible organisms which represent the majority of pathogenic species. The maximum dosages in column B are recommended only for infections caused by organisms with moderate susceptibility to imipenem, primarily some strains of *Ps. aeruginosa*. Doses cited are based on a body weight of 70 kg. A further proportionate reduction in dose administered must be made for patients with a body weight less than 70 kg by multiplying the selected dose by the patient's weight in kg divided by 70.

Patients with creatinine clearance ≤ 5 mL/min/1.73 m^2 should not receive PRIMAXIN unless hemodialysis is instituted within 48 hours. There is inadequate information to recommend usage of PRIMAXIN for patients undergoing peritoneal dialysis.

[See table on next page].

Patients with creatinine clearances of 6 to 20 mL/min/1.73 m^2 should be treated with 250 mg (or 3.5 mg/kg whichever is lower) every 12 hours for most pathogens. When the 500 mg dose is used in these patients, there may be an increased risk of seizures.

Similar dosage and safety considerations apply in the treatment of patients with creatinine clearances of ≤ 5 mL/min/1.73 m^2 who are undergoing hemodialysis. Both imipenem and cilastatin are cleared from the circulation during hemodialysis. The patient should receive PRIMAXIN after hemodialysis and at 12 hour intervals timed from the end of that hemodialysis session. Dialysis patients, especially those with background CNS disease, should be carefully monitored; for patients on hemodialysis, PRIMAXIN is recommended only when the benefit outweighs the potential risk of seizures (see PRECAUTIONS).

PREPARATION OF SOLUTION

Infusion Bottles

Contents of the infusion bottles of PRIMAXIN Powder should be restored with 100 mL of diluent (see list of diluents under COMPATIBILITY AND STABILITY) and shaken until a clear solution is obtained.

Vials

Contents of the vials must be suspended and transferred to 100 mL of an appropriate infusion solution.

A suggested procedure is to add approximately 10 mL from the appropriate infusion solution (see list of diluents under COMPATIBILITY AND STABILITY) to the vial. Shake well and transfer the resulting suspension to the infusion solution container.

CAUTION: THE SUSPENSION IS NOT FOR DIRECT INFUSION.

Repeat with an additional 10 mL of infusion solution to ensure complete transfer of vial contents to the infusion solution. **The resulting mixture should be agitated until clear.**

ADD-Vantage ®† Vials

See separate INSTRUCTIONS FOR USE OF 'PRIMAXIN' IN ADD-Vantage® VIALS.

PRIMAXIN in ADD-Vantage® vials should be reconstituted with ADD-Vantage® diluent containers containing 100 mL of either 0.9 percent Sodium Chloride Injection or 100 mL 5 percent Dextrose Injection.

Maximum Recommended Intravenous Dosage of PRIMAXIN in Adults With Impaired Renal Function

Creatinine Clearance (mL/min/ 1.73 m^2)	Renal Function	A Fully Susceptible Organisms including gram-positive and gram-negative aerobes and anaerobes	B Moderately Susceptible organisms, primarily some strains of *Ps. aeruginosa*
31–70	Mild Impairment	500 mg q8h	500 mg q6h
21–30	Moderate Impairment	500 mg q12h	500 mg q8h
6–20	Severe to Marked Impairment	250 mg q12h See Text Below	500 mg q12h See Text Below
0–5	None, but on Hemodialysis		

COMPATIBILITY AND STABILITY

Before reconstitution:
The dry powder should be stored at a temperature below 30°C.
Reconstituted solutions:
Solutions of PRIMAXIN range from colorless to yellow. Variations of color within this range do not affect the potency of the product.
PRIMAXIN, as supplied in infusion bottles and vials and reconstituted as above with the following diluents, maintains satisfactory potency for four hours at room temperature or for 24 hours under refrigeration (5°C) (note exception below). Solutions of PRIMAXIN should not be frozen.

  0.9% Sodium Chloride Injection*
  5% or 10% Dextrose Injection
  5% Dextrose Injection with 0.02% sodium bicarbonate solution
  5% Dextrose and 0.9% Sodium Chloride Injection
  5% Dextrose Injection with 0.225% or 0.45% saline solution
  NORMOSOL†–M in D5-W
  5% Dextrose Injection with 0.15% potassium chloride solution
  Mannitol 2.5%, 5% and 10%

PRIMAXIN is supplied in single dose ADD-Vantage® vials and should be prepared as directed in the accompanying INSTRUCTIONS FOR USE OF 'PRIMAXIN' IN ADD-Vantage® VIALS using ADD-Vantage® diluent containers containing 100 mL of either 0.9 percent Sodium Chloride Injection or 5 percent Dextrose Injection. When prepared with either of these diluents, PRIMAXIN maintains satisfactory potency for 8 hours at room temperature.
PRIMAXIN should not be mixed with or physically added to other antibiotics. However, PRIMAXIN may be administered concomitantly with other antibiotics, such as aminoglycosides.

HOW SUPPLIED

PRIMAXIN is supplied as a sterile powder mixture in vials and infusion bottles containing imipenem (anhydrous equivalent) and cilastatin sodium as follows:

No. 3514—250 mg imipenem equivalent and 250 mg cilastatin equivalent and 10 mg sodium bicarbonate as a buffer
NDC 0006-3514-74 in trays of 10 vials.
(6505-01-232-3116 vial, 10's).
No. 3516—500 mg imipenem equivalent and 500 mg cilastatin equivalent and 20 mg sodium bicarbonate as a buffer
NDC 0006-3516-75 in trays of 10 vials
(6505-01-232-3115 vial, 10's).
No. 3515—250 mg imipenem equivalent and 250 mg cilastatin equivalent and 10 mg sodium bicarbonate as a buffer
NDC 0006-3515-74 in trays of 10 infusion bottles.
(6505-01-246-4126 infusion bottle, 10's).
No. 3517—500 mg imipenem equivalent and 500 mg cilastatin equivalent and 20 mg sodium bicarbonate as a buffer
NDC 0006-3517-75 in trays of 10 infusion bottles.
(6505-01-234-0240 infusion bottle, 10's).
No. 3551—250 mg imipenem equivalent and 250 mg cilastatin equivalent and 10 mg sodium bicarbonate as a buffer
NDC 0006-3551-74 in trays of 10 ADD-Vantage® vials.
NDC 0006-3551-58 in trays of 25 ADD-Vantage® vials.
No. 3552—500 mg imipenem equivalent and 500 mg cilastatin equivalent and 20 mg sodium bicarbonate as a buffer

NDC 0006-3552-75 in trays of 10 ADD-Vantage® vials.
(6505-01-276-4591 500 mg ADD-Vantage®, 10's).
NDC 0006-3552-59 in trays of 25 ADD-Vantage® vials.
(6505-01-279-9627 500 mg ADD-Vantage®, 25's).

A.H.F.S. Category: 8:12.28
DC 7362409   Issued January 1989
COPYRIGHT© MERCK & CO., INC., 1987
All rights reserved

PRINIVIL® Tablets   ℞
(Lisinopril, MSD)

DESCRIPTION

PRINIVIL® (Lisinopril, MSD), a synthetic peptide derivative, is an oral long-acting angiotensin converting enzyme inhibitor. Lisinopril is chemically described as (S)-1-[N^2-(1-carboxy-3-phenylpropyl)-L-lysyl]-L-proline dihydrate. Its empirical formula is $C_{21}H_{31}N_3O_5 \cdot 2H_2O$ and its structural formula is:

Lisinopril is a white to off-white, crystalline powder, with a molecular weight of 441.52. It is soluble in water and sparingly soluble in methanol and practically insoluble in ethanol.
PRINIVIL is supplied as 5 mg, 10 mg, 20 mg and 40 mg tablets for oral administration. In addition to the active ingredient lisinopril, each tablet contains the following inactive ingredients: calcium phosphate, mannitol, magnesium stearate, and starch. The 10 mg, 20 mg and 40 mg tablets also contain iron oxide.

CLINICAL PHARMACOLOGY

Mechanism of Action
Lisinopril inhibits angiotensin-converting enzyme (ACE) in human subjects and animals. ACE is a peptidyl dipeptidase that catalyzes the conversion of angiotensin I to the vasoconstrictor substance, angiotensin II. Angiotensin II also stimulates aldosterone secretion by the adrenal cortex. Inhibition of ACE results in decreased plasma angiotensin II which leads to decreased vasopressor activity and to decreased aldosterone secretion. The latter decrease may result in a small increase of serum potassium. In hypertensive patients with normal renal function treated with PRINIVIL alone for up to 24 weeks, the mean increase in serum potassium was approximately 0.1 mEq/L; however, approximately 15 percent of patients had increases greater than 0.5 mEq/L and approximately six percent had a decrease greater than 0.5 mEq/L. In the same study, patients treated with PRINIVIL and hydrochlorothiazide for up to 24 weeks had a mean decrease in serum potassium of 0.1 mEq/L; approximately 4 percent of patients had increases greater than 0.5 mEq/L and approximately 12 percent had a decrease greater than 0.5 mEq/L. (See PRECAUTIONS.) Removal of angiotensin II negative feedback on renin secretion leads to increased plasma renin activity.
ACE is identical to kininase, an enzyme that degrades bradykinin. Whether increased levels of bradykinin, a potent vasodepressor peptide, play a role in the therapeutic effects of PRINIVIL remains to be elucidated.
While the mechanism through which PRINIVIL lowers blood pressure is believed to be primarily suppression of the renin-angiotensin-aldosterone system, PRINIVIL is antihypertensive even in patients with low-renin hypertension. Although PRINIVIL was antihypertensive in all races studied, black hypertensive patients (usually a low-renin hypertensive population) had a smaller average response to monotherapy than non-black patients.
Concomitant administration of PRINIVIL and hydrochlorothiazide further reduced blood pressure in black and non-black patients and any racial difference in blood pressure response was no longer evident.
Pharmacokinetics and Metabolism
Following oral administration of PRINIVIL, peak serum concentrations of lisinopril occur within about 7 hours. Declining serum concentrations exhibit a prolonged terminal phase which does not contribute to drug accumulation. This terminal phase probably represents saturable binding to ACE and is not proportional to dose. Lisinopril does not appear to be bound to other serum proteins.
Lisinopril does not undergo metabolism and is excreted unchanged entirely in the urine. Based on urinary recovery, the mean extent of absorption of lisinopril is approximately 25 percent, with large intersubject variability (6–60 percent) at all doses tested (5–80 mg). Lisinopril absorption is not influenced by the presence of food in the gastrointestinal tract.
Upon multiple dosing, lisinopril exhibits an effective half-life of accumulation of 12 hours.
Impaired renal function decreases elimination of lisinopril, which is excreted principally through the kidneys, but this decrease becomes clinically important only when the glomerular filtration rate is below 30 mL/min. Above this glomerular filtration rate, the elimination half-life is little changed. With greater impairment, however, peak and trough lisinopril levels increase, time to peak concentration increases and time to attain steady state is prolonged. Older patients, on average, have (approximately doubled) higher blood levels and area under the plasma concentration time curve (AUC) than younger patients. (See DOSAGE AND ADMINISTRATION.) Lisinopril can be removed by hemodialysis.
Studies in rats indicate that lisinopril crosses the blood-brain barrier poorly. Multiple doses of lisinopril in rats do not result in accumulation in any tissues. Milk of lactating rats contains radioactivity following administration of ^{14}C lisinopril. By whole body autoradiography, radioactivity was found in the placenta following administration of labeled drug to pregnant rats, but none was found in the fetuses.
Pharmacodynamics
Administration of PRINIVIL to patients with hypertension results in a reduction of supine and standing blood pressure to about the same extent with no compensatory tachycardia. Symptomatic postural hypotension is usually not observed although it can occur and should be anticipated in volume and/or salt-depleted patients. (See WARNINGS.) When given together with thiazide-type diuretics, the blood pressure lowering effects of the two drugs are approximately additive.
In most patients studied, onset of antihypertensive activity was seen at one hour after oral administration of an individual dose of PRINIVIL, with peak reduction of blood pressure achieved by six hours. Although an antihypertensive effect was observed 24 hours after dosing with recommended single daily doses, the effect was more consistent and the mean effect was considerably larger in some studies with doses of 20 mg or more than with lower doses. However, at all doses studied, the mean antihypertensive effect was substantially smaller 24 hours after dosing than it was six hours after dosing.
In some patients achievement of optimal blood pressure reduction may require two to four weeks of therapy.
The antihypertensive effects of PRINIVIL are maintained during long-term therapy. Abrupt withdrawal of PRINIVIL has not been associated with a rapid increase in blood pressure or a significant increase in blood pressure compared to pretreatment levels.
Two dose-response studies utilizing a once daily regimen were conducted in 438 mild to moderate hypertensive patients not on a diuretic. Blood pressure was measured 24 hours after dosing. An antihypertensive effect of PRINIVIL was seen with 5 mg in some patients. However, in both studies blood pressure reduction occurred sooner and was greater in patients treated with 10, 20, or 80 mg of PRINIVIL. In controlled clinical studies, PRINIVIL 20–80 mg has been compared in patients with mild to moderate hypertension to hydrochlorothiazide 12.5–50 mg and with atenolol 50–200 mg; and in patients with moderate to severe hypertension to metoprolol 100–200 mg. It was superior to hydrochlorothiazide in effects on systolic and diastolic blood pressure in a population that was 3/4 Caucasian. PRINIVIL was approximately equivalent to atenolol and metoprolol in effects on

Continued on next page

Information on the Merck Sharp & Dohme products listed on these pages is the full prescribing information from product circulars in use August 31, 1989.

---

*PRIMAXIN has been found to be stable in 0.9% Sodium Chloride Injection for 10 hours at room temperature or 48 hours under refrigeration.
†Registered trademark of Abbott Laboratories, Inc.

Merck Sharp & Dohme—Cont.

diastolic blood pressure and had somewhat greater effects on systolic blood pressure.

PRINIVIL had similar effectiveness and adverse effects in younger and older (> 65 years) patients. It was less effective in blacks than in Caucasians.

In hemodynamic studies in patients with essential hypertension, blood pressure reduction was accompanied by a reduction in peripheral arterial resistance with little or no change in cardiac output and in heart rate. In a study in nine hypertensive patients, following administration of PRINIVIL, there was an increase in mean renal blood flow that was not significant. Data from several small studies are inconsistent with respect to the effect of PRINIVIL on glomerular filtration rate in hypertensive patients with normal renal function, but suggest that changes, if any, are not large.

In patients with renovascular hypertension PRINIVIL has been shown to be well tolerated and effective in controlling blood pressure (see PRECAUTIONS).

INDICATIONS AND USAGE

PRINIVIL is indicated for the treatment of hypertension. It may be used alone as initial therapy or concomitantly with other classes of antihypertensive agents.

In using PRINIVIL, consideration should be given to the fact that another angiotensin converting enzyme inhibitor, captopril, has caused agranulocytosis, particularly in patients with renal impairment or collagen vascular disease, and that available data are insufficient to show that PRINIVIL does not have a similar risk. (See WARNINGS.)

CONTRAINDICATIONS

PRINIVIL is contraindicated in patients who are hypersensitive to this product and in patients with a history of angioedema related to previous treatment with an angiotensin converting enzyme inhibitor.

WARNINGS

Angioedema

Angioedema of the face, extremities, lips, tongue, glottis and/or larynx has been reported in patients treated with angiotensin converting enzyme inhibitors, including PRINIVIL. In such cases PRINIVIL should be promptly discontinued and the patient carefully observed until the swelling disappears. In instances where swelling has been confined to the face and lips the condition has generally resolved without treatment, although antihistamines have been useful in relieving symptoms. Angioedema associated with laryngeal edema may be fatal. **Where there is involvement of the tongue, glottis or larynx, likely to cause airway obstruction, appropriate therapy, e.g., subcutaneous epinephrine solution 1:1000 (0.3 mL to 0.5 mL) should be promptly administered.** (See ADVERSE REACTIONS.)

Hypotension

Excessive hypotension was rarely seen in uncomplicated hypertensive patients but is a possible consequence of the use of PRINIVIL in salt/volume-depleted persons, such as those treated vigorously with diuretics or patients on dialysis. (See PRECAUTIONS, Drug Interactions and ADVERSE REACTIONS.) In patients with severe congestive heart failure, with or without associated renal insufficiency, excessive hypotension has been observed and may be associated with oliguria and/or progressive azotemia, and rarely with acute renal failure and/or death. Because of the potential fall in blood pressure in these patients, therapy should be started under very close medical supervision. Such patients should be followed closely for the first two weeks of treatment and whenever the dose of PRINIVIL and/or diuretic is increased. Similar considerations apply to patients with ischemic heart or cerebrovascular disease in whom an excessive fall in blood pressure could result in a myocardial infarction or cerebrovascular accident.

If hypotension occurs, the patient should be placed in supine position and, if necessary, receive an intravenous infusion of normal saline. A transient hypotensive response is not a contraindication to further doses which usually can be given without difficulty once the blood pressure has increased after volume expansion.

Neutropenia/Agranulocytosis

Another angiotensin converting enzyme inhibitor, captopril, has been shown to cause agranulocytosis and bone marrow depression, rarely in uncomplicated patients but more frequently in patients with renal impairment especially if they also have a collagen vascular disease. Available data from clinical trials of PRINIVIL are insufficient to show that PRINIVIL does not cause agranulocytosis at similar rates. Periodic monitoring of white blood cell counts in patients with collagen vascular disease and renal disease should be considered.

PRECAUTIONS

General

Impaired Renal Function: As a consequence of inhibiting the renin-angiotensin-aldosterone system, changes in renal function may be anticipated in susceptible individuals. In patients with severe congestive heart failure whose renal function may depend on the activity of the renin-angiotensin-aldosterone system, treatment with angiotensin converting enzyme inhibitors, including PRINIVIL, may be associated with oliguria and/or progressive azotemia and rarely with acute renal failure and/or death.

In hypertensive patients with unilateral or bilateral renal artery stenosis, increases in blood urea nitrogen and serum creatinine may occur. Experience with another angiotensin converting enzyme inhibitor suggests that these increases are usually reversible upon discontinuation of PRINIVIL and/or diuretic therapy. In such patients renal function should be monitored during the first few weeks of therapy. Some hypertensive patients with no apparent pre-existing renal vascular disease have developed increases in blood urea nitrogen and serum creatinine, usually minor and transient, especially when PRINIVIL has been given concomitantly with a diuretic. This is more likely to occur in patients with pre-existing renal impairment. Dosage reduction of PRINIVIL and/or discontinuation of the diuretic may be required.

Evaluation of the hypertensive patient should always include assessment of renal function. (See DOSAGE AND ADMINISTRATION.)

Hyperkalemia: In clinical trials hyperkalemia (serum potassium greater than 5.7 mEq/L) occurred in approximately 2.2 percent of hypertensive patients and 4.0 percent of patients with congestive heart failure. In most cases these were isolated values which resolved despite continued therapy. Hyperkalemia was a cause of discontinuation of therapy in approximately 0.1 percent of hypertensive patients. Risk factors for the development of hyperkalemia include renal insufficiency, diabetes mellitus, and the concomitant use of potassium-sparing diuretics, potassium supplements and/or potassium-containing salt substitutes, which should be used cautiously, if at all, with PRINIVIL. (See *Drug Interactions.*)

Surgery/Anesthesia: In patients undergoing major surgery or during anesthesia with agents that produce hypotension, PRINIVIL may block angiotensin II formation secondary to compensatory renin release. If hypotension occurs and is considered to be due to this mechanism, it can be corrected by volume expansion.

Information for Patients

Angioedema: Angioedema, including laryngeal edema, may occur especially following the first dose of PRINIVIL. Patients should be so advised and told to report immediately any signs or symptoms suggesting angioedema (swelling of face, extremities, eyes, lips, tongue, difficulty in swallowing or breathing) and to take no more drug until they have consulted with the prescribing physician.

Symptomatic Hypotension: Patients should be cautioned to report lightheadedness especially during the first few days of therapy. If actual syncope occurs, the patients should be told to discontinue the drug until they have consulted with the prescribing physician.

All patients should be cautioned that excessive perspiration and dehydration may lead to an excessive fall in blood pressure because of reduction in fluid volume. Other causes of volume depletion such as vomiting or diarrhea may also lead to a fall in blood pressure; patients should be advised to consult with their physician.

Hyperkalemia: Patients should be told not to use salt substitutes containing potassium without consulting their physician.

Neutropenia: Patients should be told to report promptly any indication of infection (e.g., sore throat, fever) which may be a sign of neutropenia.

NOTE: As with many other drugs, certain advice to patients being treated with PRINIVIL is warranted. This information is intended to aid in the safe and effective use of this medication. It is not a disclosure of all possible adverse or intended effects.

Drug Interactions

Hypotension—Patients on Diuretic Therapy: Patients on diuretics and especially those in whom diuretic therapy was recently instituted, may occasionally experience an excessive reduction of blood pressure after initiation of therapy with PRINIVIL. The possibility of hypotensive effects with PRINIVIL can be minimized by either discontinuing the diuretic or increasing the salt intake prior to initiation of treatment with PRINIVIL. If it is necessary to continue the diuretic, initiate therapy with PRINIVIL at a dose of 5 mg daily, and provide close medical supervision after the initial dose for at least two hours and until blood pressure has stabilized for at least an additional hour. (See WARNINGS, and DOSAGE AND ADMINISTRATION.) When a diuretic is added to the therapy of a patient receiving PRINIVIL, an additional antihypertensive effect is usually observed. Studies with ACE inhibitors in combination with diuretics indicate that the dose of the ACE inhibitor can be reduced when it is given with a diuretic. (See DOSAGE AND ADMINISTRATION.)

Indomethacin: In a study in 36 patients with mild to moderate hypertension where the antihypertensive effects of PRINIVIL alone were compared to PRINIVIL given concomitantly with indomethacin, the use of indomethacin was associated with a reduced effect, although the difference between the two regimens was not significant.

Other Agents: PRINIVIL has been used concomitantly with nitrates and/or digoxin without evidence of clinically significant adverse interactions. No clinically important pharmacokinetic interactions occurred when PRINIVIL was used concomitantly with propranolol or hydrochlorothiazide. The presence of food in the stomach does not alter the bioavailability of PRINIVIL.

Agents Increasing Serum Potassium: PRINIVIL attenuates potassium loss caused by thiazide-type diuretics. Use of PRINIVIL with potassium-sparing diuretics (e.g., spironolactone, triamterene, or amiloride), potassium supplements, or potassium-containing salt substitutes may lead to significant increases in serum potassium. Therefore, if concomitant use of these agents is indicated because of demonstrated hypokalemia, they should be used with caution and with frequent monitoring of serum potassium.

Carcinogenesis, Mutagenesis, Impairment of Fertility

There was no evidence of a tumorigenic effect when lisinopril was administered for 105 weeks to male and female rats at doses up to 90 mg/kg/day (about 56 times* the maximum recommended daily human dose) or when lisinopril was administered for 92 weeks to (male and female) mice at doses up to 135 mg/kg/day (about 84 times* the maximum recommended daily human dose).

Lisinopril was not mutagenic in the Ames microbial mutagen test with or without metabolic activation. It was also negative in a forward mutation assay using Chinese hamster lung cells. Lisinopril did not produce single strand DNA breaks in an *in vitro* alkaline elution rat hepatocyte assay. In addition, lisinopril did not produce increases in chromosomal aberrations in an *in vitro* test in Chinese hamster ovary cells or in an *in vivo* study in mouse bone marrow. There were no adverse effects on reproductive performance in male and female rats treated with up to 300 mg/kg/day of lisinopril.

Pregnancy

Pregnancy Category C. Lisinopril was not teratogenic in mice treated on days 6–15 of gestation with up to 1,000 mg/kg/day (625 times the maximum recommended human dose). There was an increase in fetal resorptions at doses down to 100 mg/kg; at doses of 1000 mg/kg this was prevented by saline supplementation. There was no fetotoxicity or teratogenicity in rats treated with up to 300 mg/kg/day (188 times the maximum recommended dose) of lisinopril at days 6–17 of gestation. In rats receiving lisinopril from day 15 of gestation through day 21 postpartum, there was an increased incidence in pup deaths on days 2–7 postpartum and a lower average body weight of pups on day 21 postpartum. The increase in pup deaths and decrease in pup weight did not occur with maternal saline supplementation.

Lisinopril, at doses up to 1 mg/kg/day, was not teratogenic when given throughout the organogenic period in saline supplemented rabbits. Saline supplementation (physiologic saline in place of tap water) was used to eliminate maternotoxic effects and enable evaluation of the teratogenic potential at the highest possible dosage level. The rabbit has been shown to be extremely sensitive to angiotensin converting enzyme inhibitors (captopril and enalapril) with maternal and fetotoxic effects apparent at or below the recommended therapeutic dosage levels in man.

Fetotoxicity was demonstrated in rabbits by an increased incidence of fetal resorptions at an oral dose of lisinopril at 1 mg/kg/day and by an increased incidence of incomplete ossification at the lowest dose tested (0.1 mg/kg/day). A single intravenous dose of 15 mg/kg of lisinopril administered to pregnant rabbits on gestation days 16, 21 or 26 resulted in 88 percent to 100 percent fetal death.

By whole body autoradiography, radioactivity was found in the placenta following administration of labeled lisinopril to pregnant rats, but none was found in the fetuses.

Human Experience: There are no adequate and well-controlled studies of lisinopril in pregnant women. However, data are available that show drugs of this class cross the human placenta. Because the risk of fetal toxicity with the use of ACE inhibitors has not been clearly defined (see below), PRINIVIL should be used during pregnancy only if the potential benefit justifies the potential risk to the fetus.

Post-marketing experience with all ACE inhibitors thus far suggests the following with regard to pregnancy outcome. Inadvertent exposure limited to the first trimester of pregnancy has not been reported to affect fetal outcome adversely. Fetal exposure during the second and third trimesters of pregnancy has been associated with fetal and neonatal morbidity and mortality.

When ACE inhibitors are used during the later stages of pregnancy, there have been reports of hypotension and decreased renal perfusion in the newborn. Oligohydramnios in the mother has also been reported, presumably representing decreased renal function in the fetus. Infants exposed *in utero* to ACE inhibitors should be closely observed for hypotension, oliguria and hyperkalemia. If oliguria occurs, attention should be directed toward support of blood pressure and renal perfusion with the administration of fluids and pressors as appropriate. Problems associated with prematurity such as patent ductus arteriosus have occurred in association with maternal use of ACE inhibitors but it is not clear whether they are related to ACE inhibition, maternal hypertension or the underlying prematurity.

Another ACE inhibitor, enalapril, has been removed from the neonatal circulation by peritoneal dialysis and theoretically may be removed by exchange transfusion, although there is no experience with the latter procedure. There is no experience with either of these procedures for removing lisinopril or other ACE inhibitors from the neonatal circulation.

Nursing Mothers
Milk of lactating rats contains radioactivity following administration of ^{14}C lisinopril. It is not known whether this drug is secreted in human milk. Because many drugs are secreted in human milk, caution should be exercised when PRINIVIL is given to a nursing mother.

Pediatric Use
Safety and effectiveness in children have not been established.

---

*Based on patient weight of 50 kg

ADVERSE REACTIONS

PRINIVIL has been found to be generally well tolerated in controlled clinical trials involving 2003 patients and subjects.

The most frequent clinical adverse experiences in controlled trials with PRINIVIL were: dizziness (6.3 percent), headache (5.3 percent), fatigue (3.3 percent), diarrhea (3.2 percent), upper respiratory symptoms (3.0 percent) and cough (2.9 percent), all of which were more frequent than in placebo-treated patients. For the most part, adverse experiences were mild and transient in nature. Discontinuation of therapy was required in 6.0 percent of patients. In clinical trials, the overall frequency of adverse experiences could not be related to total daily dosage within the recommended therapeutic dosage range.

For adverse experiences which occurred in more than one percent of patients and subjects treated with PRINIVIL or PRINIVIL plus hydrochlorothiazide in controlled clinical trials, comparative incidence data are listed in the table below.
[See table above].

Clinical adverse experiences occurring in 0.3 to 1.0 percent of patients treated with PRINIVIL monotherapy in the controlled trials and rarer, serious, possibly drug-related events reported in uncontrolled studies or marketing experience included:
Body as a Whole: Chest discomfort, fever, flushing.
Cardiovascular: Angina pectoris, orthostatic hypotension, rhythm disturbances, tachycardia, peripheral edema, palpitation.
Digestive: Abdominal pain, anorexia, constipation, flatulence.
Metabolism: Gout.
Musculoskeletal: Joint pain, shoulder pain.
Nervous System/Psychiatric: Depression, somnolence, insomnia, stroke.
Respiratory System: Bronchitis, sinusitis, pharyngeal pain.
Urogenital: Oliguria, progressive azotemia, acute renal failure.
Other: Blurred vision, pruritus, urinary tract infection, vasculitis of the legs.
Angioedema: Angioedema has been reported in patients receiving PRINIVIL (0.1 percent). Angioedema associated with laryngeal edema may be fatal. If angioedema of the face, extremities, lips, tongue, glottis and/or larynx occurs, treatment with PRINIVIL should be discontinued and appropriate therapy instituted immediately. (See WARNINGS.)
Hypotension: In hypertensive patients, hypotension occurred in 1.2 percent and syncope occurred in 0.1 percent of patients. Hypotension or syncope was a cause for discontinuation of therapy in 0.5 percent of hypertensive patients. (See WARNINGS.)
In patients with congestive heart failure, hypotension occurred in 5.0 percent and syncope occurred in 1.0 percent of patients. These adverse experiences were causes for discontinuation of therapy in 1.3 percent of these patients.
Clinical Laboratory Test Findings
Serum Electrolytes: Hyperkalemia (see PRECAUTIONS).
Creatinine, Blood Urea Nitrogen: Minor increases in blood urea nitrogen and serum creatinine, reversible upon discontinuation of therapy, were observed in about 2.0 percent of patients with essential hypertension treated with PRINIVIL alone. Increases were more common in patients receiving

	PRINIVIL (n=2003*) Incidence (discontinuation)	PRINIVIL/ Hydrochlorothiazide (n=644) Incidence (discontinuation)	Placebo (n=207) Incidence
		Percent of Patients in Controlled Studies	
Dizziness	6.3 (0.6)	9.0 (0.9)	1.9
Headache	5.3 (0.2)	4.3 (0.5)	1.9
Fatigue	3.3 (0.2)	3.9 (0.5)	1.0
Diarrhea	3.2 (0.3)	2.6 (0.3)	2.4
Upper Respiratory Symptoms	3.0 (0.0)	4.5 (0.0)	0.0
Cough	2.9 (0.4)	4.5 (0.8)	1.0
Nausea	2.3 (0.3)	2.5 (0.2)	2.4
Hypotension	1.8 (0.8)	1.6 (0.5)	0.5
Rash	1.5 (0.4)	1.6 (0.2)	0.5
Orthostatic Effects	1.4 (0.0)	3.4 (0.2)	1.0
Asthenia	1.3 (0.4)	2.0 (0.2)	1.0
Chest Pain	1.3 (0.1)	1.2 (0.2)	1.4
Vomiting	1.3 (0.2)	1.4 (0.0)	0.5
Dyspnea	1.1 (0.0)	0.5 (0.2)	1.4
Dyspepsia	1.0 (0.0)	1.9 (0.0)	0.0
Paresthesia	0.8 (0.0)	2.0 (0.2)	0.0
Impotence	0.7 (0.2)	1.6 (0.3)	0.0
Muscle Cramps	0.6 (0.0)	2.8 (0.6)	0.5
Back Pain	0.5 (0.0)	1.1 (0.0)	1.4
Nasal Congestion	0.3 (0.0)	1.2 (0.0)	0.0
Decreased Libido	0.2 (0.1)	1.2 (0.0)	0.0
Vertigo	0.1 (0.0)	1.1 (0.2)	0.0

*Includes 420 patients treated for congestive heart failure who were receiving concomitant digitalis and/or diuretic therapy.

concomitant diuretics and in patients with renal artery stenosis. (See PRECAUTIONS.) Reversible minor increases in blood urea nitrogen and serum creatinine were observed in approximately 9.1 percent of patients with congestive heart failure on concomitant diuretic therapy. Frequently, these abnormalities resolved when the dosage of the diuretic was decreased.

Hemoglobin and Hematocrit: Small decreases in hemoglobin and hematocrit (mean decreases of approximately 0.4 g percent and 1.3 vol percent, respectively) occurred frequently in patients treated with PRINIVIL but were rarely of clinical importance in patients without some other cause of anemia. In clinical trials, less than 0.1 percent of patients discontinued therapy due to anemia.
Other (Causal Relationship Unknown): Rarely, elevations of liver enzymes and/or serum bilirubin have occurred.
Overall, 2.0 percent of patients discontinued therapy due to laboratory adverse experiences, principally elevations in blood urea nitrogen (0.6 percent), serum creatinine (0.5 percent) and serum potassium (0.4 percent).

OVERDOSAGE

The oral LD_{50} of lisinopril is greater than 20 g/kg in mice and rats. The most likely manifestation of overdosage would be hypotension, for which the usual treatment would be intravenous infusion of normal saline solution. Lisinopril can be removed by hemodialysis.

DOSAGE AND ADMINISTRATION

Initial Therapy: In patients with uncomplicated essential hypertension not on diuretic therapy, the recommended initial dose is 10 mg once a day. Dosage should be adjusted according to blood pressure response. The usual dosage range is 20 to 40 mg per day administered in a single daily dose. The antihypertensive effect may diminish toward the end of the dosing interval regardless of the administered dose, but most commonly with a dose of 10 mg daily. This can be evaluated by measuring blood pressure just prior to dosing to determine whether satisfactory control is being maintained for 24 hours. If it is not, an increase in dose should be considered. Doses up to 80 mg have been used but do not appear to give a greater effect. If blood pressure is not controlled with PRINIVIL alone, a low dose of a diuretic may be added. Hydrochlorothiazide 12.5 mg has been shown to provide an additive effect. After the addition of a diuretic, it may be possible to reduce the dose of PRINIVIL.
Diuretic Treated Patients: In hypertensive patients who are currently being treated with a diuretic, symptomatic hypotension may occur occasionally following the initial dose of PRINIVIL. The diuretic should be discontinued, if possible, for two to three days before beginning therapy with PRINIVIL to reduce the likelihood of hypotension. (See WARNINGS.) The dosage of PRINIVIL should be adjusted according to blood pressure response. If the patient's blood pressure is not controlled with PRINIVIL alone, diuretic therapy may be resumed as described above.
If the diuretic cannot be discontinued, an initial dose of 5 mg should be used under medical supervision for at least two hours and until blood pressure has stabilized for at least an

additional hour. (See WARNINGS and PRECAUTIONS, *Drug Interactions*.)
Concomitant administration of PRINIVIL with potassium supplements, potassium salt substitutes, or potassium-sparing diuretics may lead to increases of serum potassium (see PRECAUTIONS).
Use in Elderly: In general, blood pressure response and adverse experiences were similar in younger and older patients given similar doses of PRINIVIL. Pharmacokinetic studies, however, indicate that maximum blood levels and area under the plasma concentration time curve (AUC) are doubled in older patients so that dosage adjustments should be made with particular caution.
Dosage Adjustment in Renal Impairment: The usual dose of PRINIVIL (10 mg) is recommended for patients with a creatinine clearance > 30 mL/min (serum creatinine of up to approximately 3 mg/dL). For patients with creatinine clearance ≥ 10 mL/min ≤ 30 mL/min (serum creatinine ≥ 3 mg/dL), the first dose is 5 mg once daily. For patients with creatinine clearance < 10 mL/min (usually on hemodialysis) the recommended initial dose is 2.5 mg. The dosage may be titrated upward until blood pressure is controlled or to a maximum of 40 mg daily.

Renal Status	Creatinine-Clearance mL/min	Initial Dose mg/day
Normal Renal Function to Mild Impairment	> 30 mL/min	10 mg
Moderate to Severe Impairment	≥ 10 ≤ 30 mL/min	5 mg
Dialysis Patients	< 10 mL/min	2.5 mg*

*Dosage or dosing interval should be adjusted depending on the blood pressure response.

HOW SUPPLIED

No. 3577—Tablets PRINIVIL, 5 mg, are white, shield shaped, scored, compressed tablets, with code MSD 19 on one side and PRINIVIL on the other. They are supplied as follows:
NDC 0006-0019-28 unit dose packages of 100
NDC 0006-0019-58 unit of use bottles of 100.
Shown in Product Identification Section, page 419
No. 3578—Tablets PRINIVIL, 10 mg, are light yellow, shield shaped, compressed tablets, with code MSD 106 on one side and PRINIVIL on the other. They are supplied as follows:
NDC 0006-0106-28 unit dose packages of 100

Continued on next page

Merck Sharp & Dohme—Cont.

NDC 0006-0106-31 unit of use bottles of 30
NDC 0006-0106-58 unit of use bottles of 100.
   Shown in Product Identification Section, page 419
No. 3579—Tablets PRINIVIL, 20 mg, are peach, shield shaped, compressed tablets, with code MSD 207 on one side and PRINIVIL on the other. They are supplied as follows:
NDC 0006-0207-28 unit dose packages of 100
NDC 0006-0207-31 unit of use bottles of 30
NDC 0006-0207-58 unit of use bottles of 100.
   Shown in Product Identification Section, page 419
No. 3580—Tablets PRINIVIL, 40 mg, are rose red, shield shaped, compressed tablets, with code MSD 237 on one side and PRINIVIL on the other. They are supplied as follows:
NDC 0006-0237-58 unit of use bottles of 100.
   Shown in Product Identification Section, page 419
Storage
Protect from moisture, freezing and excessive heat.
Dispense in a tight container, if product package is subdivided.

A.H.F.S. Category: 24:08
DC 7507509 Issued February 1989
COPYRIGHT © MERCK & CO., INC., 1988
All rights reserved

PRINZIDE® Tablets ℞
(Lisinopril-Hydrochlorothiazide, MSD)

DESCRIPTION

PRINZIDE® (Lisinopril-Hydrochlorothiazide, MSD) combines an angiotensin converting enzyme inhibitor, lisinopril, and a diuretic, hydrochlorothiazide.
Lisinopril, a synthetic peptide derivative, is an oral long-acting angiotensin converting enzyme inhibitor. It is chemically described as (S)-1-$[N^2$-(1-carboxy-3-phenylpropyl)-L-lysyl]-L-proline dihydrate. Its empirical formula is $C_{21}H_{31}N_3O_5 \cdot 2H_2O$ and its structural formula is:

Lisinopril is a white to off-white, crystalline powder, with a molecular weight of 441.52. It is soluble in water, sparingly soluble in methanol, and practically insoluble in ethanol.
Hydrochlorothiazide is 6-chloro-3,4-dihydro-$2H$-1,2,4-benzothiadiazine-7-sulfonamide 1,1-dioxide. Its empirical formula is $C_7H_8ClN_3O_4S_2$ and its structural formula is:

Hydrochlorothiazide is a white, or practically white, crystalline powder with a molecular weight of 297.72, which is slightly soluble in water, but freely soluble in sodium hydroxide solution.
PRINZIDE is available for oral use in two tablet combinations of lisinopril with hydrochlorothiazide: PRINZIDE 12.5, containing 20 mg lisinopril and 12.5 mg hydrochlorothiazide and; PRINZIDE 25, containing 20 mg lisinopril and 25 mg hydrochlorothiazide.
Inactive ingredients are calcium phosphate, iron oxide, magnesium stearate, mannitol, and starch.

CLINICAL PHARMACOLOGY

Lisinopril-Hydrochlorothiazide
As a result of its diuretic effects, hydrochlorothiazide increases plasma renin activity, increases aldosterone secretion, and decreases serum potassium. Administration of lisinopril blocks the renin-angiotensin aldosterone axis and tends to reverse the potassium loss associated with the diuretic.
In clinical studies, the extent of blood pressure reduction seen with the combination of lisinopril and hydrochlorothiazide was approximately additive. The combination appeared somewhat less effective in black patients, but relatively few black patients were studied. In most patients, the antihypertensive effect of PRINZIDE was sustained for at least 24 hours.
In a randomized, controlled comparison, the mean antihypertensive effects of PRINZIDE 12.5 and PRINZIDE 25 were similar, suggesting that many patients who respond adequately to the latter combination may be controlled with PRINZIDE 12.5. (See DOSAGE AND ADMINISTRATION.)

Concomitant administration of lisinopril and hydrochlorothiazide has little or no effect on the bioavailability of either drug. The combination tablet is bioequivalent to concomitant administration of the separate entities.
Lisinopril
Mechanism of Action
Lisinopril inhibits angiotensin-converting enzyme (ACE) in human subjects and animals. ACE is a peptidyl dipeptidase that catalyzes the conversion of angiotensin I to the vasoconstrictor substance, angiotensin II. Angiotensin II also stimulates aldosterone secretion by the adrenal cortex. Inhibition of ACE results in decreased plasma angiotensin II which leads to decreased vasopressor activity and to decreased aldosterone secretion. The latter decrease may result in a small increase of serum potassium. Removal of angiotensin II negative feedback on renin secretion leads to increased plasma renin activity. In hypertensive patients with normal renal function treated with lisinopril alone for up to 24 weeks, the mean increase in serum potassium was less than 0.1 mEq/L; however, approximately 15 percent of patients had increases greater than 0.5 mEq/L and approximately six percent had a decrease greater than 0.5 mEq/L. In the same study, patients treated with lisinopril plus a thiazide diuretic showed essentially no change in serum potassium. (See PRECAUTIONS.)
ACE is identical to kininase, an enzyme that degrades bradykinin. Whether increased levels of bradykinin, a potent vasodepressor peptide, play a role in the therapeutic effects of lisinopril remains to be elucidated.
While the mechanism through which lisinopril lowers blood pressure is believed to be primarily suppression of the renin-angiotensin-aldosterone system, lisinopril is antihypertensive even in patients with low-renin hypertension. Although lisinopril was antihypertensive in all races studied, black hypertensive patients (usually a low-renin hypertensive population) had a smaller average response to lisinopril monotherapy than non-black patients.
Pharmacokinetics and Metabolism
Following oral administration of lisinopril, peak serum concentrations occur within about 7 hours. Declining serum concentrations exhibit a prolonged terminal phase which does not contribute to drug accumulation. This terminal phase probably represents saturable binding to ACE and is not proportional to dose. Lisinopril does not appear to be bound to other serum proteins.
Lisinopril does not undergo metabolism and is excreted unchanged entirely in the urine. Based on urinary recovery, the mean extent of absorption of lisinopril is approximately 25 percent, with large intersubject variability (6–60 percent) at all doses tested (5–80 mg). Lisinopril absorption is not influenced by the presence of food in the gastrointestinal tract. Upon multiple dosing, lisinopril exhibits an effective half-life of accumulation of 12 hours.
Impaired renal function decreases elimination of lisinopril, which is excreted principally through the kidneys, but this decrease becomes clinically important only when the glomerular filtration rate is below 30 mL/min. Above this glomerular filtration rate, the elimination half-life is little changed. With greater impairment, however, peak and trough lisinopril levels increase, time to peak concentration increases and time to attain steady state is prolonged. Older patients, on average, have (approximately doubled) higher blood levels and area under the plasma concentration time curve (AUC) than younger patients. (See DOSAGE AND ADMINISTRATION.) Lisinopril can be removed by hemodialysis.
Studies in rats indicate that lisinopril crosses the blood-brain barrier poorly. Multiple doses of lisinopril in rats do not result in accumulation in any tissues. However, milk of lactating rats contains radioactivity following administration of ^{14}C lisinopril. By whole body autoradiography, radioactivity was found in the placenta following administration of labeled drug to pregnant rats, but none was found in the fetuses.
Pharmacodynamics
Administration of lisinopril to patients with hypertension results in a reduction of supine and standing blood pressure to about the same extent with no compensatory tachycardia. Symptomatic postural hypotension is usually not observed although it can occur and should be anticipated in volume and/or salt-depleted patients. (See WARNINGS.)
In most patients studied, onset of antihypertensive activity was seen at one hour after oral administration of an individual dose of lisinopril, with peak reduction of blood pressure achieved by six hours.
In some patients achievement of optimal blood pressure reduction may require two to four weeks of therapy.
At recommended single daily doses, antihypertensive effects have been maintained for at least 24 hours, after dosing, although the effect at 24 hours was substantially smaller than the effect six hours after dosing.
The antihypertensive effects of lisinopril have continued during long-term therapy. Abrupt withdrawal of lisinopril has not been associated with a rapid increase in blood pressure; nor with a significant overshoot of pretreatment blood pressure.

In hemodynamic studies in patients with essential hypertension, blood pressure reduction was accompanied by a reduction in peripheral arterial resistance with little or no change in cardiac output and in heart rate. In a study in nine hypertensive patients, following administration of lisinopril, there was an increase in mean renal blood flow that was not significant. Data from several small studies are inconsistent with respect to the effect of lisinopril on glomerular filtration rate in hypertensive patients with normal renal function, but suggest that changes, if any, are not large.
In patients with renovascular hypertension lisinopril has been shown to be well tolerated and effective in controlling blood pressure (see PRECAUTIONS).
Hydrochlorothiazide
The mechanism of the antihypertensive effect of thiazides is unknown. Thiazides do not usually affect normal blood pressure.
Hydrochlorothiazide is a diuretic and antihypertensive. It affects the distal renal tubular mechanism of electrolyte reabsorption. Hydrochlorothiazide increases excretion of sodium and chloride in approximately equivalent amounts. Natriuresis may be accompanied by some loss of potassium and bicarbonate.
After oral use diuresis begins within two hours, peaks in about four hours and lasts about 6 to 12 hours.
Hydrochlorothiazide is not metabolized but is eliminated rapidly by the kidney. When plasma levels have been followed for at least 24 hours, the plasma half-life has been observed to vary between 5.6 and 14.8 hours. At least 61 percent of the oral dose is eliminated unchanged within 24 hours. Hydrochlorothiazide crosses the placental but not the blood-brain barrier.

INDICATIONS AND USAGE

PRINZIDE is indicated for the treatment of hypertension in patients for whom combination therapy is appropriate.
This fixed dose combination is not indicated for initial therapy. Patients already receiving a diuretic when lisinopril is initiated, or given a diuretic and lisinopril simultaneously, can develop symptomatic hypotension. In the initial titration of the individual entities, it is important, if possible, to stop the diuretic for several days before starting lisinopril or, if this is not possible, begin lisinopril at a low initial dose. (See DOSAGE AND ADMINISTRATION.)
In using PRINZIDE, consideration should be given to the fact that an angiotensin converting enzyme inhibitor, captopril, has caused agranulocytosis, particularly in patients with renal impairment or collagen vascular disease, and that available data are insufficient to show that lisinopril does not have a similar risk. (See WARNINGS.)

CONTRAINDICATIONS

PRINZIDE is contraindicated in patients who are hypersensitive to any component of this product and in patients with a history of angioedema related to previous treatment with an angiotensin converting enzyme inhibitor. Because of the hydrochlorothiazide component, this product is contraindicated in patients with anuria or hypersensitivity to other sulfonamide-derived drugs.

WARNINGS

Angioedema
Angioedema of the face, extremities, lips, tongue, glottis and/or larynx has been reported rarely in patients treated with angiotensin converting enzyme inhibitors, including lisinopril. In such cases PRINZIDE should be promptly discontinued and the patient carefully observed until the swelling disappears. In instances where swelling has been confined to the face and lips the condition has generally resolved without treatment, although antihistamines have been useful in relieving symptoms. Angioedema associated with laryngeal edema may be fatal. **Where there is involvement of the tongue, glottis or larynx, likely to cause airway obstruction, subcutaneous epinephrine solution 1:1000 (0.3 mL to 0.5 mL) should be promptly administered and/or other appropriate therapy should be instituted.** (See ADVERSE REACTIONS.)
Hypotension and Related Effects
Excessive hypotension was rarely seen in uncomplicated hypertensive patients but is a possible consequence of lisinopril use in salt/volume-depleted persons, such as those treated vigorously with diuretics or patients on dialysis. (See PRECAUTIONS, *Drug Interactions* and ADVERSE REACTIONS.)
Syncope has been reported in 0.8 percent of patients receiving PRINZIDE. In patients with hypertension receiving lisinopril alone, the incidence of syncope was 0.1 percent. The overall incidence of syncope may be reduced by proper titration of the individual components. (See PRECAUTIONS, *Drug Interactions*, ADVERSE REACTIONS and DOSAGE AND ADMINISTRATION.)

In patients with severe congestive heart failure, with or without associated renal insufficiency, excessive hypotension has been observed and may be associated with oliguria and/or progressive azotemia, and rarely with acute renal failure and/or death. Because of the potential fall in blood pressure in these patients, therapy should be started under very close medical supervision. Such patients should be followed closely for the first two weeks of treatment and whenever the dose of lisinopril and/or diuretic is increased. Similar considerations apply to patients with ischemic heart or cerebrovascular disease in whom an excessive fall in blood pressure could result in a myocardial infarction or cerebrovascular accident.

If hypotension occurs, the patient should be placed in supine position and, if necessary, receive an intravenous infusion of normal saline. A transient hypotensive response is not a contraindication to further doses which usually can be given without difficulty once the blood pressure has increased after volume expansion.

Neutropenia/Agranulocytosis
Another angiotensin converting enzyme inhibitor, captopril, has been shown to cause agranulocytosis and bone marrow depression, rarely in uncomplicated patients but more frequently in patients with renal impairment, especially if they also have a collagen vascular disease. Available data from clinical trials of lisinopril are insufficient to show that lisinopril does not cause agranulocytosis at similar rates. Periodic monitoring of white blood cell counts in patients with collagen vascular disease and renal disease should be considered.

Hydrochlorothiazide
Thiazides should be used with caution in severe renal disease. In patients with renal disease, thiazides may precipitate azotemia. Cumulative effects of the drug may develop in patients with impaired renal function.

Thiazides should be used with caution in patients with impaired hepatic function or progressive liver disease, since minor alterations of fluid and electrolyte balance may precipitate hepatic coma.

Sensitivity reactions may occur in patients with or without a history of allergy or bronchial asthma.

The possibility of exacerbation or activation of systemic lupus erythematosus has been reported.

Lithium generally should not be given with thiazides (see PRECAUTIONS, *Drug Interactions, Hydrochlorothiazide*).

PRECAUTIONS

General
Lisinopril
Impaired Renal Function: As a consequence of inhibiting the renin-angiotensin-aldosterone system, changes in renal function may be anticipated in susceptible individuals. In patients with severe congestive heart failure whose renal function may depend on the activity of the renin-angiotensin-aldosterone system, treatment with angiotensin converting enzyme inhibitors, including lisinopril, may be associated with oliguria and/or progressive azotemia and rarely with acute renal failure and/or death.

In hypertensive patients with unilateral or bilateral renal artery stenosis, increases in blood urea nitrogen and serum creatinine may occur. Experience with another angiotensin converting enzyme inhibitor suggests that these increases are usually reversible upon discontinuation of lisinopril and /or diuretic therapy. In such patients renal function should be monitored during the first few weeks of therapy.

Some hypertensive patients with no apparent pre-existing renal vascular disease have developed increases in blood urea and serum creatinine, usually minor and transient, especially when lisinopril has been given concomitantly with a diuretic. This is more likely to occur in patients with pre-existing renal impairment. Dosage reduction of lisinopril and/or discontinuation of the diuretic may be required.

Evaluation of the hypertensive patient should always include assessment of renal function. (See DOSAGE AND ADMINISTRATION.)

Hyperkalemia: In clinical trials hyperkalemia (serum potassium greater than 5.7 mEq/L) occurred in approximately 1.4 percent of hypertensive patients treated with lisinopril plus hydrochlorothiazide. In most cases these were isolated values which resolved despite continued therapy. Hyperkalemia was not a cause of discontinuation of therapy. Risk factors for the development of hyperkalemia include renal insufficiency, diabetes mellitus, and the concomitant use of potassium-sparing diuretics, potassium supplements and/or potassium-containing salt substitutes, which should be used cautiously if at all with PRINZIDE. (See *Drug Interactions*.)

Surgery/Anesthesia: In patients undergoing major surgery or during anesthesia with agents that produce hypotension, lisinopril may block angiotensin II formation secondary to compensatory renin release. If hypotension occurs and is considered to be due to this mechanism, it can be corrected by volume expansion.

Hydrochlorothiazide
Periodic determination of serum electrolytes to detect possible electrolyte imbalance should be performed at appropriate intervals.

All patients receiving thiazide therapy should be observed for clinical signs of fluid or electrolyte imbalance: namely, hyponatremia, hypochloremic alkalosis, and hypokalemia. Serum and urine electrolyte determinations are particularly important when the patient is vomiting excessively or receiving parenteral fluids. Warning signs or symptoms of fluid and electrolyte imbalance, irrespective of cause, include dryness of mouth, thirst, weakness, lethargy, drowsiness, restlessness, muscle pains or cramps, muscular fatigue, hypotension, oliguria, tachycardia, and gastrointestinal disturbances such as nausea and vomiting.

Hypokalemia may develop, especially with brisk diuresis, when severe cirrhosis is present, or after prolonged therapy. Interference with adequate oral electrolyte intake will also contribute to hypokalemia. Hypokalemia may cause cardiac arrhythmia and may also sensitize or exaggerate the response of the heart to the toxic effects of digitalis (e.g., increased ventricular irritability). Because lisinopril reduces the production of aldosterone, concomitant therapy with lisinopril attenuates the diuretic-induced potassium loss (see *Drug Interactions, Agents Increasing Serum Potassium*). Although any chloride deficit is generally mild and usually does not require specific treatment, except under extraordinary circumstances (as in liver disease or renal disease), chloride replacement may be required in the treatment of metabolic alkalosis.

Dilutional hyponatremia may occur in edematous patients in hot weather; appropriate therapy is water restriction, rather than administration of salt except in rare instances when the hyponatremia is life-threatening. In actual salt depletion, appropriate replacement is the therapy of choice.

Hyperuricemia may occur or frank gout may be precipitated in certain patients receiving thiazide therapy.

In diabetic patients dosage adjustments of insulin or oral hypoglycemic agents may be required. Hyperglycemia may occur with thiazide diuretics. Thus latent diabetes mellitus may become manifest during thiazide therapy.

The antihypertensive effects of the drug may be enhanced in the postsympathectomy patient.

If progressive renal impairment becomes evident consider withholding or discontinuing diuretic therapy.

Thiazides have been shown to increase the urinary excretion of magnesium; this may result in hypomagnesemia.

Thiazides may decrease urinary calcium excretion. Thiazides may cause intermittent and slight elevation of serum calcium in the absence of known disorders of calcium metabolism. Marked hypercalcemia may be evidence of hidden hyperparathyroidism. Thiazides should be discontinued before carrying out tests for parathyroid function.

Increases in cholesterol and triglyceride levels may be associated with thiazide diuretic therapy.

Information for Patients
Angioedema: Angioedema, including laryngeal edema, may occur especially following the first dose of lisinopril. Patients should be so advised and told to report immediately any signs or symptoms suggesting angioedema (swelling of face, extremities, eyes, lips, tongue, difficulty in swallowing or breathing) and to take no more drug until they have consulted with the prescribing physician.

Symptomatic Hypotension: Patients should be cautioned to report lightheadedness especially during the first few days of therapy. If actual syncope occurs, the patients should be told to discontinue the drug until they have consulted with the prescribing physician.

All patients should be cautioned that excessive perspiration and dehydration may lead to an excessive fall in blood pressure because of reduction in fluid volume. Other causes of volume depletion such as vomiting or diarrhea may also lead to a fall in blood pressure; patients should be advised to consult with their physician.

Hyperkalemia: Patients should be told not to use salt substitutes containing potassium without consulting their physician.

Neutropenia: Patients should be told to report promptly any indication of infection (e.g., sore throat, fever) which may be a sign of neutropenia.

NOTE: As with many other drugs, certain advice to patients being treated with PRINZIDE is warranted. This information is intended to aid in the safe and effective use of this medication. It is not a disclosure of all possible adverse or intended effects.

Drug Interactions
Lisinopril
Hypotension—Patients on Diuretic Therapy: Patients on diuretics and especially those in whom diuretic therapy was recently instituted, may occasionally experience an excessive reduction of blood pressure after initiation of therapy with lisinopril. The possibility of hypotensive effects with lisinopril can be minimized by either discontinuing the diuretic or increasing the salt intake prior to initiation of treatment with lisinopril. If it is necessary to continue the diuretic, initiate therapy with lisinopril at a dose of 5 mg

daily, and provide close medical supervision after the initial dose for at least two hours and until blood pressure has stabilized for at least an additional hour. (See WARNINGS, and DOSAGE AND ADMINISTRATION.)

When a diuretic is added to the therapy of a patient receiving lisinopril, an additional antihypertensive effect is usually observed. (See DOSAGE AND ADMINISTRATION.)

Indomethacin: In a study in 36 patients with mild to moderate hypertension where the antihypertensive effects of lisinopril alone were compared to lisinopril given concomitantly with indomethacin, the use of indomethacin was associated with a reduced effect, although the difference between the two regimens was not significant.

Other Agents: Lisinopril has been used concomitantly with nitrates and/or digoxin without evidence of clinically significant adverse interactions. No meaningful clinically important pharmacokinetic interactions occurred when lisinopril was used concomitantly with propranolol, digoxin, or hydrochlorothiazide. The presence of food in the stomach does not alter the bioavailability of lisinopril.

Agents Increasing Serum Potassium: Lisinopril attenuates potassium loss caused by thiazide-type diuretics. Use of lisinopril with potassium-sparing diuretics (e.g., spironolactone, triamterene, or amiloride), potassium supplements, or potassium-containing salt substitutes may lead to significant increases in serum potassium. Therefore, if concomitant use of these agents is indicated, because of demonstrated hypokalemia, they should be used with caution and with frequent monitoring of serum potassium.

Hydrochlorothiazide
When administered concurrently the following drugs may interact with thiazide diuretics.

Alcohol, barbiturates, or narcotics —potentiation of orthostatic hypotension may occur.

Antidiabetic drugs (oral agents and insulin)—dosage adjustment of the antidiabetic drug may be required.

Other antihypertensive drugs —additive effect or potentiation.

Corticosteroids, ACTH —intensified electrolyte depletion, particularly hypokalemia.

Pressor amines (e.g., norepinephrine) —possible decreased response to pressor amines but not sufficient to preclude their use.

Skeletal muscle relaxants, nondepolarizing (e.g., tubocurarine) —possible increased responsiveness to the muscle relaxant.

Lithium —should not generally be given with diuretics. Diuretic agents reduce the renal clearance of lithium and add a high risk of lithium toxicity. Refer to the package insert for lithium preparations before use of such preparations with PRINZIDE.

Non-steroidal Anti-inflammatory Drugs —In some patients, the administration of a non-steroidal anti-inflammatory agent can reduce the diuretic, natriuretic, and antihypertensive effects of loop, potassium-sparing and thiazide diuretics. Therefore, when PRINZIDE and non-steroidal anti-inflammatory agents are used concomitantly, the patient should be observed closely to determine if the desired effect of PRINZIDE is obtained.

Carcinogenesis, Mutagenesis, Impairment of Fertility
Lisinopril-Hydrochlorothiazide
Lisinopril in combination with hydrochlorothiazide was not mutagenic in a microbial mutagen test using *Salmonella typhimurium* (Ames test) or *Escherichia coli* with or without metabolic activation or in a forward mutation assay using Chinese hamster lung cells. Lisinopril-hydrochlorothiazide did not produce DNA single strand breaks in an *in vitro* alkaline elution rat hepatocyte assay. In addition, it did not produce increases in chromosomal aberrations in an *in vitro* test in Chinese hamster ovary cells or in an *in vivo* study in mouse bone marrow.

Lisinopril
There was no evidence of a tumorigenic effect when lisinopril was administered for 105 weeks to male and female rats at doses up to 90 mg/kg/day (about 56 times* the maximum recommended daily human dose). Lisinopril has also been administered for 92 weeks to (male and female) mice at doses up to 135 mg/kg/day (about 84 times* the maximum recommended daily human dose) and showed no evidence of carcinogenicity.

Lisinopril was not mutagenic in the Ames microbial mutagen test with or without metabolic activation. It was also negative in a forward mutation assay using Chinese hamster lung cells. Lisinopril did not produce single strand DNA breaks in an *in vitro* alkaline elution rat hepatocyte assay. In addition, lisinopril did not produce increases in chromosomal aberrations in an *in vitro* test in Chinese hamster ovary cells or in an *in vivo* study in mouse bone marrow.

Continued on next page

Information on the Merck Sharp & Dohme products listed on these pages is the full prescribing information from product circulars in use August 31, 1989.

Merck Sharp & Dohme—Cont.

There were no adverse effects on reproductive performance in male and female rats treated with up to 300 mg/kg/day of lisinopril.

_____

*Based on patient weight of 50 kg

Hydrochlorothiazide

Hydrochlorothiazide is currently under study in the U.S. Carcinogenesis Testing Program.

Hydrochlorothiazide was not mutagenic in the *in vitro* Ames mutagenicity assay of *Salmonella typhimurium* strains TA98, TA100, TA1535, TA1537 and TA1538 or in *in vivo* mutagenicity assays of mouse germinal cell chromosomes and Chinese hamster bone marrow cell chromosomes. It was, however, mutagenic in inducing non-disjunction (96% frequency) in diploid strains of *Aspergillus nidulans*.

Hydrochlorothiazide had no adverse effect on fertility of male or female mice or rats in studies in which these species were exposed to doses of up to 4 and 100 mg/kg/day, respectively.

Pregnancy

Lisinopril-Hydrochlorothiazide

Pregnancy Category C. Teratogenicity studies were conducted in mice and rats with up to 90 mg/kg/day of lisinopril (56 times the maximum recommended human dose) in combination with 10 mg/kg/day of hydrochlorothiazide (2.5 times the maximum recommended human dose). Maternal or fetotoxic effects were not seen in mice with the combination. In rats decreased maternal weight gain and decreased fetal weight occurred down to 3/10 mg/kg/day (the lowest dose tested). Associated with the decreased fetal weight was a delay in fetal ossification. The decreased fetal weight and delay in fetal ossification were not seen in saline-supplemented animals given 90/10 mg/kg/day.

There are no adequate and well-controlled studies of PRINZIDE in pregnant women. PRINZIDE should be used during pregnancy only if the potential benefit justifies the potential risk to the fetus.

Lisinopril

Lisinopril was not teratogenic in mice treated on days 6-15 of gestation with up to 1,000 mg/kg/day (625 times the maximum recommended human dose). There was an increase in fetal resorptions at doses down to 100 mg/kg; at doses of 1000 mg/kg this was prevented by saline supplementation. By whole body autoradiography, radioactivity was found in the placenta following administration of labeled drug to pregnant rats, but none was found in the fetuses. There was no fetotoxicity or teratogenicity in rats treated with up to 300 mg/kg/day (188 times the maximum recommended dose) of lisinopril on days 6-17 of gestation. However, in rats receiving lisinopril from day 15 of gestation through day 21 postpartum, there was an increased incidence of pup deaths on days 2-7 postpartum and a lower average body weight of pups on day 21 postpartum. The increase in pup deaths and decrease in pup weight did not occur with maternal saline supplementation.

Lisinopril, at doses up to 1 mg/kg/day, was not teratogenic when given throughout the organogenic period in saline-supplemented rabbits. Saline supplementation (physiologic saline in place of tap water) was used to eliminate maternotoxic effects and enable evaluation of the teratogenic potential at the highest possible dosage level. The rabbit has been shown to be extremely sensitive to angiotensin converting enzyme inhibitors (captopril and enalapril) with maternal and fetotoxic effects apparent at or below the recommended therapeutic dosage levels in man.

Fetotoxicity was demonstrated in rabbits by an increased incidence of fetal resorptions at a dose of lisinopril of 1 mg/kg/day and by an increased incidence of incomplete ossi-

fication at 0.1 mg/kg/day (the lowest dose tested). A single intravenous dose of 15 mg/kg of lisinopril administered to pregnant rabbits on gestation days 16, 21 or 26 resulted in 88 percent to 100 percent fetal death.

By whole body autoradiography, radioactivity was found in the placenta following administration of labeled lisinopril to pregnant rats, but none was found in the fetuses.

Human Experience: There are no adequate and well-controlled studies of lisinopril in pregnant women. However, data are available that show drugs of this class cross the human placenta. Because the risk of fetal toxicity with the use of ACE inhibitors has not been clearly defined (see below), lisinopril should be used during pregnancy only if the potential benefit justifies the potential risk to the fetus.

Post-marketing experience with all ACE inhibitors thus far suggests the following with regard to pregnancy outcome. Inadvertent exposure limited to the first trimester of pregnancy has not been reported to affect fetal outcome adversely. Fetal exposure during the second and third trimesters of pregnancy has been associated with fetal and neonatal morbidity and mortality.

When ACE inhibitors are used during the later stages of pregnancy, there have been reports of hypotension and decreased renal perfusion in the newborn. Oligohydramnios in the mother has also been reported, presumably representing decreased renal function in the fetus. Infants exposed *in utero* to ACE inhibitors should be closely observed for hypotension, oliguria and hyperkalemia. If oliguria occurs, attention should be directed toward support of blood pressure and renal perfusion with the administration of fluids and pressors as appropriate. Problems associated with prematurity such as patent ductus arteriosus have occurred in association with maternal use of ACE inhibitors but it is not clear whether they are related to ACE inhibition, maternal hypertension or the underlying prematurity.

Another ACE inhibitor, enalapril, has been removed from the neonatal circulation by peritoneal dialysis and theoretically may be removed by exchange transfusion, although there is no experience with the latter procedure. There is no experience with either of these procedures for removing lisinopril or other ACE inhibitors from the neonatal circulation.

Hydrochlorothiazide

There was no evidence of harm to the fetus when hydrochlorothiazide was administered to pregnant mice and rats during organogenesis at doses up to 3000 and 1350 mg/kg/day, respectively.

Thiazides cross the placental barrier and appear in cord blood. They may cause fetal or neonatal jaundice, thrombocytopenia, and possibly other adverse reactions which have occurred in the adult.

Nursing Mothers

It is not known whether lisinopril is secreted in human milk. However, milk of lactating rats contains radioactivity following administration of ^{14}C lisinopril. In another study, lisinopril was present in rat milk at levels similar to plasma levels in the dams. Thiazides do appear in human milk. Because of the potential for serious reactions in nursing infants from hydrochlorothiazide and the unknown effects of lisinopril in infants, a decision should be made whether to discontinue nursing or to discontinue PRINZIDE, taking into account the importance of the drug to the mother.

Pediatric Use

Safety and effectiveness in children have not been established.

ADVERSE REACTIONS

PRINZIDE has been evaluated for safety in 930 patients, including 100 patients treated for 50 weeks or more.

	Percent of Patients in Controlled Studies	
	Lisinopril-Hydrochlorothiazide (n=930) Incidence (discontinuation)	Placebo (n=207) Incidence
Dizziness	7.5 (0.8)	1.9
Headache	5.2 (0.3)	1.9
Cough	3.9 (0.6)	1.0
Fatigue	3.7 (0.4)	1.0
Orthostatic Effects	3.2 (0.1)	1.0
Diarrhea	2.5 (0.2)	2.4
Nausea	2.2 (0.1)	2.4
Upper Respiratory Infection	2.2 (0.0)	0.0
Muscle Cramps	2.0 (0.4)	0.5
Asthenia	1.8 (0.2)	1.0
Paresthesia	1.5 (0.1)	0.0
Hypotension	1.4 (0.3)	0.5
Vomiting	1.4 (0.1)	0.5
Dyspepsia	1.3 (0.0)	0.0
Rash	1.2 (0.1)	0.5
Impotence	1.2 (0.3)	0.0

In clinical trials with PRINZIDE no adverse experiences peculiar to this combination drug have been observed. Adverse experiences that have occurred have been limited to those that have been previously reported with lisinopril or hydrochlorothiazide.

The most frequent clinical adverse experiences in controlled trials (including open label extensions) with any combination of lisinopril and hydrochlorothiazide were: dizziness (7.5 percent), headache (5.2 percent), cough (3.9 percent), fatigue (3.7 percent) and orthostatic effects (3.2 percent), all of which were more common than in placebo-treated patients. Generally, adverse experiences were mild and transient in nature; but see WARNINGS regarding angioedema and excessive hypotension or syncope. Discontinuation of therapy due to adverse effects was required in 4.4 percent of patients, principally because of dizziness, cough, fatigue and muscle cramps.

Adverse experiences occurring in greater than one percent of patients treated with lisinopril plus hydrochlorothiazide in controlled clinical trials are shown below.

[See table below.]

Clinical adverse experiences occurring in 0.3 to 1.0 percent of patients in controlled trials included:

Body as a Whole: Chest pain, abdominal pain, syncope, chest discomfort, fever, trauma, virus infection.

Cardiovascular: Palpitation, orthostatic hypotension.

Digestive: Gastrointestinal cramps, dry mouth, constipation, heartburn.

Musculoskeletal: Back pain, shoulder pain, knee pain, back strain, myalgia, foot pain.

Nervous/Psychiatric: Decreased libido, vertigo, depression, somnolence.

Respiratory: Common cold, nasal congestion, influenza, bronchitis, pharyngeal pain, dyspnea, pulmonary congestion, chronic sinusitis, allergic rhinitis, pharyngeal discomfort.

Skin: Flushing, pruritus, skin inflammation, hyperhidrosis.

Special Senses: Blurred vision, tinnitus, otalgia.

Urogenital: Urinary tract infection.

Angioedema: Angioedema of the face, extremities, lips, tongue, glottis and/or larynx has been reported rarely. (See WARNINGS.)

Hypotension: In clinical trials, adverse effects relating to hypotension occurred as follows: hypotension (1.4), orthostatic hypotension (0.5), other orthostatic effects (3.2). In addition syncope occurred in 0.8 percent of patients. (See WARNINGS.)

Clinical Laboratory Test Findings

Serum Electrolytes: (See PRECAUTIONS.)

Creatinine, Blood Urea Nitrogen: Minor reversible increases in blood urea nitrogen and serum creatinine were observed in patients with essential hypertension treated with PRINZIDE. More marked increases have also been reported and were more likely to occur in patients with renal artery stenosis. (See PRECAUTIONS.)

Serum Uric Acid, Glucose, Magnesium, Cholesterol, Triglycerides and Calcium: (See PRECAUTIONS.)

Hemoglobin and Hematocrit: Small decreases in hemoglobin and hematocrit (mean decreases of approximately 0.5 g percent and 1.5 vol percent, respectively) occurred frequently in hypertensive patients treated with PRINZIDE but were rarely of clinical importance unless another cause of anemia coexisted. In clinical trials, 0.4 percent of patients discontinued therapy due to anemia.

Other (Causal Relationship Unknown): Rarely, elevations of liver enzymes and/or serum bilirubin have occurred.

Other adverse reactions that have been reported with the individual components are listed below:

Lisinopril —Lisinopril has been evaluated for safety in 2003 patients. In clinical trials adverse reactions which occurred with lisinopril were also seen with PRINZIDE. In addition, the following were reported: *Cardiovascular:* Angina pectoris, rhythm disturbances, tachycardia, peripheral edema. *Digestive:* Anorexia, flatulence. *Metabolism:* Gout. *Musculoskeletal:* Joint pain. *Nervous System/Psychiatric:* Insomnia, stroke. *Urogenital:* Oliguria, progressive azotemia, acute renal failure. *Other:* Vasculitis.

Hydrochlorothiazide —*Body as a Whole:* Weakness; *Digestive:* Anorexia, gastric irritation, cramping, jaundice (intrahepatic cholestatic jaundice), pancreatitis, sialadenitis, constipation; *Hematologic:* Leukopenia, agranulocytosis, thrombocytopenia, aplastic anemia, hemolytic anemia; *Musculoskeletal:* Muscle spasm; *Nervous System/Psychiatric:* Restlessness; *Renal:* Renal failure, renal dysfunction, interstitial nephritis (see WARNINGS); *Special Senses:* Xanthopsia; *Hypersensitivity:* Purpura, photosensitivity, urticaria, necrotizing angiitis (vasculitis and cutaneous vasculitis), respiratory distress including pneumonitis and pulmonary edema, anaphylactic reactions.

OVERDOSAGE

No specific information is available on the treatment of overdosage with PRINZIDE. Treatment is symptomatic and supportive. Therapy with PRINZIDE should be discontinued and the patient observed closely. Suggested measures include induction of emesis and/or gastric lavage, and correction of dehydration, electrolyte imbalance and hypotension by established procedures.

Lisinopril

The oral LD_{50} of lisinopril is greater than 20 g/kg in mice and rats. The most likely manifestation of overdosage would be hypotension, for which the usual treatment would be intravenous infusion of normal saline solution.

Lisinopril can be removed by hemodialysis.

Hydrochlorothiazide

The oral LD_{50} of hydrochlorothiazide is greater than 10.0 g/kg in both mice and rats. The most common signs and symptoms observed are those caused by electrolyte depletion (hypokalemia, hypochloremia, hyponatremia) and dehydration resulting from excessive diuresis. If digitalis has also been administered, hypokalemia may accentuate cardiac arrhythmias.

DOSAGE AND ADMINISTRATION

DOSAGE MUST BE INDIVIDUALIZED. THE FIXED COMBINATION IS NOT FOR INITIAL THERAPY. IT MAY BE SUBSTITUTED FOR THE TITRATED INDIVIDUAL COMPONENTS. ALTERNATIVELY, PATIENTS WHO HAVE RECEIVED LISINOPRIL MONOTHERAPY 20 OR 40 MG MAY BE GIVEN 'PRINZIDE' 12.5, THEN 'PRINZIDE' 25, THUS TITRATING THE HYDROCHLOROTHIAZIDE COMPONENT USING THE COMBINATION.

The usual dose is one or two tablets of PRINZIDE 12.5 or PRINZIDE 25 once daily. (See INDICATIONS AND USAGE and WARNINGS.) However, because data from a clinical trial suggest that the mean group antihypertensive response is similar when lisinopril 20 mg is combined with hydrochlorothiazide 12.5 mg or 25 mg, patients whose blood pressure is controlled with lisinopril 20 mg plus hydrochlorothiazide 25 mg ordinarily should be given a trial of PRINZIDE 12.5 before PRINZIDE 25 is used. (See CLINICAL PHARMACOLOGY, *Lisinopril-Hydrochlorothiazide*.)

Patients usually do not require doses in excess of 50 mg of hydrochlorothiazide daily, particularly when it is combined with other antihypertensive agents.

For lisinopril monotherapy the recommended initial dose in patients not on diuretics is 10 mg of lisinopril once a day. Dosage should be adjusted according to blood pressure response. The usual dosage range of lisinopril is 20 to 40 mg administered in a single daily dose; the maximum recommended dose is 80 mg in a single daily dose. Blood pressure should be measured at the interdosing interval to ensure that there is an adequate antihypertensive response at that time. If blood pressure is not controlled with lisinopril alone, a diuretic may be added. Hydrochlorothiazide 12.5 mg has been shown to provide an additive effect. After addition of the diuretic it may be possible to reduce the dose of lisinopril. In patients who are currently being treated with a diuretic, symptomatic hypotension occasionally may occur following the initial dose of lisinopril. The diuretic should, if possible, be discontinued for two to three days before beginning therapy with lisinopril to reduce the likelihood of hypotension. (See WARNINGS.) If the patient's blood pressure is not controlled with lisinopril alone, diuretic therapy may be resumed.

If the diuretic cannot be discontinued an initial dose of 5 mg of lisinopril should be used under medical supervision for at least two hours and until blood pressure has stabilized for at least an additional hour. (See WARNINGS and PRECAUTIONS, *Drug Interactions*.)

Concomitant administration of PRINZIDE with potassium supplements, potassium salt substitutes, or potassium sparing diuretics may lead to increases of serum potassium (see PRECAUTIONS).

Dosage Adjustment in Renal Impairment

The usual dose of PRINZIDE is recommended for patients with a creatinine clearance > 30 mL/min (serum creatinine of up to approximately 3 mg/dL).

When concomitant diuretic therapy is required in patients with severe renal impairment, a loop diuretic, rather than a thiazide diuretic is preferred for use with lisinopril; therefore, for patients with severe renal dysfunction the lisinopril-hydrochlorothiazide combination tablet is not recommended.

HOW SUPPLIED

No. 3594—Tablets PRINZIDE 12.5, are yellow, round, fluted-edge tablets, coded MSD 140 on one side and PRINZIDE on the other. Each tablet contains 20 mg of lisinopril and 12.5 mg of hydrochlorothiazide. They are supplied as follows:
NDC 0006-0140-31 unit of use bottles of 30
NDC 0006-0140-58 unit of use bottles of 100.
Shown in Product Identification Section, page 419
No. 3595—Tablets PRINZIDE 25, are orange, round, fluted-edge tablets, coded MSD 142 on one side and PRINZIDE on the other. Each tablet contains 20 mg of lisinopril and 25 mg of hydrochlorothiazide. They are supplied as follows:
NDC 0006-0142-31 unit of use bottles of 30
NDC 0006-0142-58 unit of use bottles of 100.
Shown in Product Identification Section, page 419
Storage
Avoid storage at temperatures above 40°C (104°F).
Dispense in a well-closed container, if product package is subdivided.

A.H.F.S. Category: 24:08
DC 7615001 Issued January 1989
COPYRIGHT © MERCK & CO., INC., 1989
All rights reserved

RECOMBIVAX HB® ℞
[Hepatitis B Vaccine (Recombinant), MSD]

DESCRIPTION

RECOMBIVAX HB® [Hepatitis B Vaccine (Recombinant), MSD] is a non-infectious subunit viral vaccine derived from Hepatitis B surface antigen (HBsAg) produced in yeast cells. A portion of the hepatitis B virus gene, coding for HBsAg, is cloned into yeast, and the vaccine for hepatitis B is produced from cultures of this recombinant yeast strain according to methods developed in the Merck Sharp & Dohme Research Laboratories.

The antigen is harvested and purified from fermentation cultures of a recombinant strain of the yeast *Saccharomyces cerevisiae* containing the gene for the *adw* subtype of HBsAg. The HBsAg protein is released from the yeast cells by cell disruption and purified by a series of physical and chemical methods. The vaccine contains no detectable yeast DNA but may contain up to 4% yeast protein. The vaccine produced by the Merck method has been shown to be comparable to the plasma-derived vaccine in terms of animal potency (mouse, monkey, and chimpanzee) and protective efficacy (chimpanzee and human).

The vaccine against hepatitis B, prepared from recombinant yeast cultures, is free of association with human blood or blood products.

Each lot of hepatitis B vaccine is tested for safety, in mice and guinea pigs, and for sterility.

RECOMBIVAX HB is a sterile suspension for intramuscular injection; however, it may be administered subcutaneously to persons at risk of hemorrhage following intramuscular injections (see DOSAGE AND ADMINISTRATION). Each 1.0 mL dose of the adult formulation vaccine contains 10 mcg of hepatitis B surface antigen adsorbed onto approximately 0.5 mg of aluminum hydroxide; each 0.5 mL dose of the pediatric formulation vaccine contains 5 mcg of hepatitis B surface antigen adsorbed onto approximately 0.25 mg of aluminum hydroxide. Both formulations contain thimerosal (mercury derivative) 1:20,000 added as a preservative. Both preparations have been treated with formaldehyde prior to adsorption onto alum. The vaccine is of the *adw* subtype. RECOMBIVAX HB is indicated for immunization of persons at risk of infection from hepatitis B virus including all known subtypes.

CLINICAL PHARMACOLOGY

Hepatitis B virus is one of at least three hepatitis viruses that cause a systemic infection, with a major pathology in the liver. The others are hepatitis A virus, and non-A, non-B hepatitis viruses.

Hepatitis B virus is an important cause of viral hepatitis. There is no specific treatment for this disease. The incubation period for hepatitis B is relatively long; six weeks to six months may elapse between exposure and the onset of clinical symptoms. The prognosis following infection with hepatitis B virus is variable and dependent on at least three factors: (1) Age—Infants and younger children usually experience milder initial disease than older persons; (2) Dose of virus—The higher the dose, the more likely acute icteric hepatitis B will result; and, (3) Severity of associated underlying disease—underlying malignancy or pre-existing hepatic disease predisposes to increased mortality and morbidity.

Persistence of viral infection (the chronic hepatitis B virus carrier state) occurs in 5–10% of persons following acute hepatitis B, and occurs more frequently after initial anicteric hepatitis B than after initial icteric disease. Consequently, carriers of hepatitis B surface antigen (HBsAg) frequently give no history of having had recognized acute hepatitis. It has been estimated that more than 170 million people in the world today are persistently infected with hepatitis B virus. The Centers for Disease Control (CDC) estimates that there are approximately 0.5 to 1.0 million chronic carriers of hepatitis B virus in the USA and that this pool of carriers grows by 2%–3% (8,000 to 16,000 individuals) annually. Chronic carriers represent the largest human reservoir of hepatitis B virus.

The serious complications and sequelae of hepatitis B virus infection include massive hepatic necrosis, cirrhosis of the liver, chronic active hepatitis, and hepatocellular carci-

noma. Chronic carriers of HBsAg appear to be at increased risk of developing hepatocellular carcinoma. Although a number of etiologic factors are associated with development of hepatocellular carcinoma, the single most important etiologic factor appears to be active infection with the hepatitis B virus.

There is also evidence that several diseases other than hepatitis have been associated with hepatitis B virus infection through an immunologic mechanism involving antigen-antibody complexes. Such diseases include a syndrome with rash, urticaria, and arthralgia resembling serum sickness; periarteritis nodosa; membranous glomerulonephritis; and infantile papular acrodermatitis.

Although the vehicles for transmission of the virus are often blood and blood products, viral antigen has also been found in tears, saliva, breast milk, urine, semen and vaginal secretions. Hepatitis B virus is capable of surviving for days on environmental surfaces exposed to body fluids containing hepatitis B virus. Infection may occur when hepatitis B virus, transmitted by infected body fluids, is implanted via mucous surfaces or percutaneously introduced through accidental or deliberate breaks in the skin.

Transmission of hepatitis B virus infection is often associated with close interpersonal contact with an infected individual and with crowded living conditions. In such circumstances, transmission by inoculation via routes other than overt percutaneous ones may be quite common. Perinatal transmission of hepatitis B infection from infected mother to child, at or shortly after birth, can occur if the mother is a hepatitis B surface antigen (HBsAg) carrier or if the mother has an acute hepatitis B infection in the third trimester. Infection in infancy by the hepatitis B virus usually leads to the chronic carrier state. Among infants born to women whose sera are positive for both the hepatitis B surface antigen and the e antigen, 85–90% are infected and become chronic carriers. Well-controlled studies have shown that administration of three 0.5 mL doses of Hepatitis B Immune Globulin (Human) starting at birth is 75% effective in preventing establishment of the chronic carrier state in these infants during the first year of life. However, the protective effect of Hepatitis B Immune Globulin (Human) is transient. Hepatitis B is endemic throughout the world and is a serious medical problem in population groups at increased risk. (Refer to INDICATIONS AND USAGE.)

Numerous epidemiological studies have shown that persons who develop anti-HBs following active infection with the hepatitis B virus are protected against the disease on reexposure to the virus.

Clinical studies have established that RECOMBIVAX HB when injected into the deltoid muscle induced protective levels of antibody in greater than 90% of 564 healthy adults and teenagers who received the recommended 3 dose regimen. Studies with hepatitis B vaccine derived from plasma have shown that a lower response rate (81%) to vaccine may be obtained if the vaccine is administered as a buttock injection. Seroconversion rates and geometric mean antibody titers were measured 1 to 2 months after the 3rd dose. A protective antibody (anti-HBs) level has been defined as 1) 10 or more sample ratio units (SRU) as determined by radioimmunoassay or 2) a positive result as determined by enzyme immunoassay. Note: 10 SRU is comparable to 10 mIU/mL of antibody.

Responsiveness to the vaccine was age dependent. The seroconversion rate for 73 children 1–10 years of age was 100%. In contrast, seroconversion rates for 453 adults 20 to 39 years of age ranged from 95 to 99% and for 56 adults 40 years of age or older were 91%.

The protective efficacy of RECOMBIVAX HB has been demonstrated in neonates born of mothers positive for both HBsAg and HBeAg (a core-associated antigenic complex which correlates with high infectivity). In a clinical study of infants who received one dose of Hepatitis B Immune Globulin at birth followed by the recommended three dose regimen of RECOMBIVAX HB, efficacy in prevention of chronic hepatitis B infection was 94% in 93 infants at six months and 93% in 57 infants at nine months as compared to the infection rate in untreated historical controls. Significantly fewer neonates became chronically infected when given one dose of Hepatitis B Immune Globulin at birth followed by the recommended three dose regimen of RECOMBIVAX HB when compared to historical controls who received only a single dose of Hepatitis B Immune Globulin. Testing for HBsAg and anti-HBs is recommended at 12–15 months of age. If HBsAg is not detectable, and anti-HBs is present, the child has been protected.

As demonstrated in the above study, Hepatitis B Immune Globulin, when administered simultaneously with RECOMBIVAX HB at separate body sites, did not interfere with the

Continued on next page

Information on the Merck Sharp & Dohme products listed on these pages is the full prescribing information from product circulars in use August 31, 1989.

Merck Sharp & Dohme—Cont.

induction of protective antibodies against hepatitis B virus elicited by the vaccine.

The duration of protective effect of RECOMBIVAX HB is unknown at present, and the need for booster doses is not yet defined.

Reports in the literature describe a more virulent form of hepatitis B associated with superinfections or coinfections by delta virus, an imcomplete RNA virus. Delta virus can only infect and cause illness in persons infected with hepatitis B virus since the delta agent requires a coat of HBsAg in order to become infectious. Therefore, persons immune to hepatitis B virus infection should also be immune to delta virus infection.

Interchangeability of Plasma-Derived and Recombinant Hepatitis B Vaccines

Recombinant-derived vaccine is produced in yeast by the hepatitis B virus gene which codes for the hepatitis B surface antigen (HBsAg). Like plasma-derived vaccine, recombinant-derived vaccine is a protein aggregate or particle visible by electron microscopy containing important vaccine antigen epitopes as determined by monoclonal antibody analyses.

Recombinant-derived vaccine has been shown by *in vitro* analyses to induce antibodies (anti-HBs) which are biochemically and immunologically comparable by extent of binding, and both avidity and affinity of binding to virus-derived antigen, to antibodies induced by plasma-derived vaccine. In cross absorption studies, the spectra of antibodies induced in man to plasma-derived or to recombinant hepatitis B vaccines were indistinguishable.

The recommended doses of HEPTAVAX-B® (Hepatitis B Vaccine, MSD) and RECOMBIVAX HB have resulted in similar seroconversion rates in healthy persons; the geometric mean titers (GMTs) following RECOMBIVAX HB have been lower in some studies and equivalent in others but were many times greater than the minimum level associated with protection (≥ 10 mIU/mL). A single injection of the recommended dose of RECOMBIVAX HB induced significant anamnestic antibody responses in 97% of 31 healthy adults vaccinated 5 to 7 years previously with HEPTAVAX-B (Hepatitis B Vaccine, MSD).

There have been no clinical studies in which a three-dose vaccine series was initiated with HEPTAVAX-B (Hepatitis B Vaccine, MSD) and completed with RECOMBIVAX HB, or vice versa. However, based on the comparability of the plasma-derived and recombinant-derived vaccines in extensive *in vitro* and *in vivo* studies as described above, it is possible to interchange the use of these two vaccines (but see CONTRA-INDICATIONS).

INDICATIONS AND USAGE

RECOMBIVAX HB is indicated for immunization against infection caused by all known subtypes of hepatitis B virus. RECOMBIVAX HB will not prevent hepatitis caused by other agents, such as hepatitis A virus, non-A, non-B hepatitis viruses, or other viruses known to infect the liver.

Vaccination is recommended in persons of all ages, who are or will be at increased risk of infection with hepatitis B virus. In areas with high prevalence of infection, most of the population are at risk of acquiring hepatitis B infection at a young age. Therefore, vaccination should be targeted to prevent such transmission. In areas of low prevalence, vaccination should be limited to those who are in groups identified as being at increased risk of infection, for example:
- *Health Care Personnel*
  Dentists and oral surgeons.
  Physicians and surgeons.
  Nurses.
  Paramedical personnel and custodial staff who may be exposed to the virus via blood or other patient specimens.
  Dental hygienists and dental nurses.
  Laboratory personnel handling blood, blood products, and other patient specimens.
  Dental, medical and nursing students.
- *Selected Patients and Patient Contacts*
  Staff in hemodialysis units and hematology/oncology units.
  Patients requiring frequent and/or large volume blood tranfusions or clotting factor concentrates (e.g., persons with hemophilia, thalassemia).
  Clients (residents) and staff of institutions for the mentally handicapped.
  Classroom contacts of deinstitutionalized mentally handicapped persons who have persistent hepatitis B surface antigenemia and who show aggressive behavior.
  Household and other intimate contacts of persons with persistent hepatitis B surface antigenemia.
- *Infants Born to HBsAg Positive Mothers whether HBeAg positive or negative (See DOSAGE AND ADMINISTRATION)*

- Sub-populations with a known high incidence of the disease, such as:
  Alaskan Eskimos.
  Indochinese refugees.
  Haitian refugees.
- *Military Personnel identified as being at increased risk*
- *Morticians and Embalmers*
- *Blood bank and plasma fractionation workers*
- *Persons at Increased Risk of the Disease Due to Their Sexual Practices*, such as:
  Persons who repeatedly contract sexually transmitted diseases.
  Homosexually active males.
  Female prostitutes.
- *Prisoners*
- *Users of illicit injectable drugs*

Revaccination
See CLINICAL PHARMACOLOGY

CONTRAINDICATIONS

Hypersensitivity to yeast or any component of the vaccine.

WARNINGS

Patients who develop symptoms suggestive of hypersensitivity after an injection should not receive further injections of RECOMBIVAX HB (see CONTRAINDICATIONS).

Because of the long incubation period for hepatitis B, it is possible for unrecognized infection to be present at the time RECOMBIVAX HB is given. RECOMBIVAX HB may not prevent hepatitis B in such patients.

PRECAUTIONS

General
As with any percutaneous vaccine, epinephrine should be available for immediate use should an anaphylactoid reaction occur.

Any serious active infection is reason for delaying use of RECOMBIVAX HB except when in the opinion of the physician, withholding the vaccine entails a greater risk.

Caution and appropriate care should be exercised in administering RECOMBIVAX HB to individuals with severely compromised cardiopulmonary status or to others in whom a febrile or systemic reaction could pose a significant risk.

Pregnancy
Pregnancy Category C: Animal reproduction studies have not been conducted with RECOMBIVAX HB. It is also not known whether RECOMBIVAX HB can cause fetal harm when administered to a pregnant woman or can affect reproduction capacity. RECOMBIVAX HB should be given to a pregnant woman only if clearly needed.

Nursing Mothers
It is not known whether RECOMBIVAX HB is excreted in human milk. Because many drugs are excreted in human milk, cautions should be exercised when RECOMBIVAX HB is administered to a nursing woman.

Pediatric Use
RECOMBIVAX HB has been shown to be usually well-tolerated and highly immunogenic in infants and children of all ages. Newborns also respond well; maternally transferred antibodies do not interfere with the active immune response to the vaccine. See DOSAGE AND ADMINISTRATION for recommended pediatric dosage and for recommended dosage for infants born to HBsAg positive mothers.

ADVERSE REACTIONS

RECOMBIVAX HB is generally well-tolerated. No serious adverse reactions attributable to the vaccine have been reported during the course of clinical trials. No adverse experiences were reported during clinical trials which could be related to changes in the titers of antibodies to yeast. As with any vaccine, there is the possibility that broad use of the vaccine could reveal adverse reactions not observed in clinical trials.

In a group of studies, 3258 doses of vaccine were administered to 1252 healthy adults who were monitored for 5 days after each dose. Injection site and systemic complaints were reported following 17% and 15% of the injections, respectively. The following adverse reactions were reported:

Incidence Equal to or
Greater Than 1% of Injections
LOCAL REACTION (INJECTION SITE)
Injection site reactions consisting principally of soreness, and including pain, tenderness, pruritus, erythema, ecchymosis, swelling, warmth, and nodule formation.
BODY AS A WHOLE
The most frequent systemic complaints include fatigue/weakness; headache; fever ($\geq 100°$F); and malaise.
DIGESTIVE SYSTEM
Nausea; and diarrhea
RESPIRATORY SYSTEM
Pharyngitis; and upper respiratory infection

Incidence Less than 1% of Injections
BODY AS A WHOLE
Sweating; achiness; sensation of warmth; lightheadedness; chills; and flushing
DIGESTIVE SYSTEM
Vomiting; abdominal pains/cramps; dyspepsia; and diminished appetite
RESPIRATORY SYSTEM
Rhinitis; influenza; and cough
NERVOUS SYSTEM
Vertigo/dizziness; and paresthesia
INTEGUMENTARY SYSTEM
Pruritus; rash (non-specified); angioedema; and urticaria
MUSCULOSKELETAL SYSTEM
Arthralgia including monoarticular; myalgia; back pain; neck pain; shoulder pain; and neck stiffness
HEMIC/LYMPHATIC SYSTEM
Lymphadenopathy
PSYCHIATRIC/BEHAVIORAL
Insomnia/Disturbed sleep
SPECIAL SENSES
Earache
UROGENITAL SYSTEM
Dysuria
CARDIOVASCULAR SYSTEM
Hypotension
The following additional adverse reactions have been reported with use of the marketed vaccine:
Hypersensitivity
Anaphylaxis and symptoms of immediate hypersensitivity reactions including rash, pruritus, urticaria, edema, angioedema, dyspnea, chest discomfort, bronchial spasm, palpitation, or symptoms consistent with a hypotensive episode have been reported within the first few hours after vaccination. An apparent hypersensitivity syndrome (serum-sickness-like) of delayed onset has been reported days to weeks after vaccination, including: arthralgia/arthritis (usually transient), fever, and dermatologic reactions such as urticaria, erythema multiforme, ecchymoses and erythema nodosum (See WARNINGS and PRECAUTIONS).
Special Senses
Optic Neuritis.
Potential ADVERSE EFFECTS:
In addition, a variety of adverse effects, not observed in clinical trials with RECOMBIVAX HB, have been reported with HEPTAVAX-B (plasma-derived hepatitis B vaccine). Those listed below are to serve as alerting information to physicians:
  Nervous System: Neurological disorders such as myelitis including transverse myelitis; acute radiculoneuropathy including Guillain-Barré syndrome; peripheral neuropathy, including Bell's Palsy and herpes zoster.
  Hematologic
  Thrombocytopenia
  Special Senses
  Tinnitus, visual disturbances

DOSAGE AND ADMINISTRATION

Do not inject intravenously or intradermally.
RECOMBIVAX HB is for intramuscular injection. The *deltoid muscle* is the preferred site for intramuscular injection in adults. Data suggests that injections given in the buttocks frequently are given into fatty tissue instead of into muscle. Such injections have resulted in a lower seroconversion rate than was expected. The *anterolateral thigh* is the recommended site for intramuscular injection in infants and young children.

RECOMBIVAX HB may be administered subcutaneously to persons at risk of hemorrhage following intramuscular injections. However, when other aluminum-adsorbed vaccines have been administered subcutaneously, an increased incidence of local reactions including subcutaneous nodules has been observed. Therefore, subcutaneous administration should be used only in persons (e.g., hemophiliacs) at risk of hemorrhage following intramuscular injections.

Shake well before withdrawal and use. Thorough agitation at the time of administration is necessary to maintain suspension of the vaccine.

Parenteral drug products should be inspected visually for particulate matter and discoloration prior to administration. After thorough agitation, RECOMBIVAX HB is a slightly opaque, white suspension. The immunization regimen consists of 3 doses of vaccine given according to the following schedule:
  1st dose: at elected date
  2nd dose: 1 month later
  3rd dose: 6 months after the first dose
The volume of vaccine to be given on each occasion is as follows:
[See table on next page].
Revaccination
Whenever revaccination or administration of a booster dose is appropriate, RECOMBIVAX HB may be used (see CLINICAL PHARMACOLOGY).

Group	Formulation	Initial	1 month	6 months
Younger Children (Birth to 10 years of age)	Pediatric 5 mcg/0.5 mL	0.5 mL	0.5 mL	0.5 mL
Adults and Older Children	Adult 10 mcg/1.0 mL	1.0 mL	1.0 mL	1.0 mL

Dosage For Infants Born of HBsAg Positive Mothers

The recommended treatment regimen for infants born of HBsAg positive mothers is as follows:

Treatment	Birth	Within 7 days	1 month	6 months
RECOMBIVAX HB (Pediatric dose 5 mcg/0.5 mL)	0.5 mL*		0.5 mL	0.5 mL
HEPATITIS B IMMUNE GLOBULIN	0.5 mL	—	—	

* The first 0.5 mL dose of RECOMBIVAX HB may be given at birth at the same time as Hepatitis B Immune Globulin, but should be administered in the opposite anterolateral thigh. This procedure may be preferable to ensure absorption of the vaccine.

Known or Presumed Exposure to HBsAg

There are no prospective studies directly testing the efficacy of a combination of Hepatitis B Immune Globulin (Human) and RECOMBIVAX HB in preventing clinical hepatitis B following percutaneous, ocular or mucous membrane exposure to hepatitis B virus. However, since most persons with such exposures (e.g., health-care workers) are candidates for RECOMBIVAX HB and since combined Hepatitis B Immune Globulin (Human) plus vaccine is more efficacious than Hepatitis B Immune Globulin (Human) alone in perinatal exposures, the following guidelines are recommended for persons who have been exposed to hepatitis B virus such as through (1) percutaneous (needlestick), ocular, mucous membrane exposure to blood known or presumed to contain HBsAg, (2) human bites by known or presumed HBsAg carriers, that penetrate the skin, or (3) following intimate sexual contact with known or presumed HBsAg carriers:

Hepatitis B Immune Globulin (Human) (0.06 mL/kg) should be given intramuscularly as soon as possible after exposure and within 24 hours if possible. RECOMBIVAX HB (see dosage recommendation) should be given intramuscularly at a separate site within 7 days of exposure and second and third doses given one and six months, respectively, after the first dose.

The vaccine should be used as supplied; no dilution or reconstitution is necessary. The full recommended dose of the vaccine should be used.

It is important to use a separate sterile syringe and needle for each individual patient to prevent transmission of hepatitis and other infectious agents from one person to another.

For Syringe Use Only: Withdraw the recommended dose from the vial using a sterile needle and syringe free of preservatives, antiseptics, and detergents.

HOW SUPPLIED

No. 4773—RECOMBIVAX HB, Adult Formulation, is supplied as a multi-dose vial of vaccine, 10 mcg/1 mL, **NDC** 0006-4773-00 in 3 mL vials.
(6505-01-266-3780 10 mcg/mL, 3 mL).
No. 4775—RECOMBIVAX HB, Adult Formulation, is supplied as a single-dose vial of vaccine, 10 mcg/1 mL, **NDC** 0006-4775-00 in a 1 mL vial.
No. 4769—RECOMBIVAX HB, Pediatric Formulation, is supplied as a single dose vial of vaccine, 5 mcg/0.5 mL, **NDC** 0006-4769-00 in 0.5 mL vials.
Storage
Store vials at 2–8°C (35.6°–46.4°F). Storage above or below the recommended temperature may reduce potency.
Do not freeze since freezing destroys potency.
A.H.F.S. Category: 80:12
DC 7462203 Issued December 1988
COPYRIGHT © MERCK & CO., INC., 1986
All rights reserved

SINEMET® Tablets   ℞
(Carbidopa-Levodopa, MSD), U.S.P.

DESCRIPTION

When SINEMET® (Carbidopa-Levodopa, MSD) is to be given to patients who are being treated with levodopa, levodopa must be discontinued at least eight hours before therapy with SINEMET is started. In order to re-duce adverse reactions, it is necessary to individualize therapy. See the WARNINGS and DOSAGE AND ADMINISTRATION sections before initiating therapy.

Carbidopa, an inhibitor of aromatic amino acid decarboxylation, is a white, crystalline compound, slightly soluble in water, with a molecular weight of 244.3. It is designated chemically as (—)-L-α-hydrazino -α- methyl -β- (3, 4- dihydroxybenzene) propanoic acid monohydrate, and has the following structural formula:

Tablet content is expressed in terms of anhydrous carbidopa which has a molecular weight of 226.3.

Levodopa, an aromatic amino acid, is a white, crystalline compound, slightly soluble in water, with a molecular weight of 197.2. It is designated chemically as (—)-L-α-amino-β-(3,4-dihydroxybenzene) propanoic acid, and has the following structural formula:

SINEMET is supplied as tablets in three strengths:
SINEMET 25-100, containing 25 mg of carbidopa and 100 mg of levodopa
SINEMET 10-100, containing 10 mg of carbidopa and 100 mg of levodopa
SINEMET 25-250, containing 25 mg of carbidopa and 250 mg of levodopa.
Inactive ingredients are cellulose, magnesium stearate, and starch. Tablets SINEMET 10-100 and 25-250 also contain FD&C Blue 2. Tablets SINEMET 25-100 also contain D&C Yellow 10 and FD&C Yellow 6.

ACTIONS

Current evidence indicates that symptoms of Parkinson's disease are related to depletion of dopamine in the corpus striatum. Administration of dopamine is ineffective in the treatment of Parkinson's disease apparently because it does not cross the blood-brain barrier. However, levodopa, the metabolic precursor of dopamine, does cross the blood-brain barrier, and presumably is converted to dopamine in the basal ganglia. This is thought to be the mechanism whereby levodopa relieves symptoms of Parkinson's disease.

When levodopa is administered orally it is rapidly converted to dopamine in extracerebral tissues so that only a small portion of a given dose is transported unchanged to the central nervous system. For this reason, large doses of levodopa are required for adequate therapeutic effect and these may often be attended by nausea and other adverse reactions, some of which are attributable to dopamine formed in extracerebral tissues.

Since levodopa competes with certain amino acids, the absorption of levodopa may be impaired in some patients on a high protein diet.

Carbidopa inhibits decarboxylation of peripheral levodopa. It does not cross the blood-brain barrier and does not affect the metabolism of levodopa within the central nervous system.

Since its decarboxylase inhibiting activity is limited to extracerebral tissues, administration of carbidopa with levodopa makes more levodopa available for transport to the brain. In dogs, reduced formation of dopamine in extracerebral tissues, such as the heart, provides protection against the development of dopamine-induced cardiac arrhythmias. Clinical studies tend to support the hypothesis of a similar protective effect in humans although controlled data are too limited at the present time to draw firm conclusions.

Carbidopa reduces the amount of levodopa required by about 75 percent and, when administered with levodopa, increases both plasma levels and the plasma half-life of levodopa, and decreases plasma and urinary dopamine and homovanillic acid.

In clinical pharmacologic studies, simultaneous administration of carbidopa and levodopa produced greater urinary excretion of levodopa in proportion to the excretion of dopamine than administration of the two drugs at separate times.

Pyridoxine hydrochloride (vitamin B_6), in oral doses of 10 mg to 25 mg, may reverse the effects of levodopa by increasing the rate of aromatic amino acid decarboxylation. Carbidopa inhibits this action of pyridoxine.

INDICATIONS

SINEMET is indicated in the treatment of the symptoms of idiopathic Parkinson's disease (paralysis agitans), postencephalitic parkinsonism, and symptomatic parkinsonism which may follow injury to the nervous system by carbon monoxide intoxication and manganese intoxication. SINEMET is indicated in these conditions to permit the administration of lower doses of levodopa with reduced nausea and vomiting, with more rapid dosage titration, with a somewhat smoother response, and with supplemental pyridoxine (vitamin B_6).

The incidence of levodopa-induced nausea and vomiting is less with SINEMET than with levodopa. In many patients this reduction in nausea and vomiting will permit more rapid dosage titration.

In some patients a somewhat smoother antiparkinsonian effect results from therapy with SINEMET than with levodopa. However, patients with markedly irregular ("on-off") responses to levodopa have not been shown to benefit from SINEMET.

Since carbidopa prevents the reversal of levodopa effects caused by pyridoxine, SINEMET can be given to patients receiving supplemental pyridoxine (vitamin B_6).

Although the administration of carbidopa permits control of parkinsonism and Parkinson's disease with much lower doses of levodopa, there is no conclusive evidence at present that this is beneficial other than in reducing nausea and vomiting, permitting more rapid titration, and providing a somewhat smoother response to levodopa. *Carbidopa does not decrease adverse reactions due to central effects of levodopa. By permitting more levodopa to reach the brain, particularly when nausea and vomiting is not a dose-limiting factor, certain adverse CNS effects, e.g., dyskinesias, may occur at lower dosages and sooner during therapy with SINEMET than with levodopa.*

Certain patients who responded poorly to levodopa have improved when SINEMET was substituted. This is most likely due to decreased peripheral decarboxylation of levodopa which results from administration of carbidopa rather than to a primary effect of carbidopa on the nervous system. Carbidopa has not been shown to enhance the intrinsic efficacy of levodopa in parkinsonian syndromes.

In considering whether to give SINEMET to patients already on levodopa who have nausea and /or vomiting, the practitioner should be aware that, while many patients may be expected to improve, some do not. Since one cannot predict which patients are likely to improve, this can only be determined by a trial of therapy. It should be further noted that in controlled trials comparing SINEMET with levodopa, about half of the patients with nausea and/or vomiting on levodopa improved spontaneously despite being retained on the same dose of levodopa during the controlled portion of the trial.

CONTRAINDICATIONS

Monoamine oxidase inhibitors and SINEMET should not be given concomitantly. These inhibitors must be discontinued at least two weeks prior to initiating therapy with SINEMET.

SINEMET is contraindicated in patients with known hypersensitivity to this drug, and in narrow angle glaucoma.

Because levodopa may activate a malignant melanoma, it should not be used in patients with suspicious, undiagnosed skin lesions or a history of melanoma.

WARNINGS

When patients are receiving levodopa, it must be discontinued at least eight hours before SINEMET is started. SINEMET should be substituted at a dosage that will provide approximately 25 percent of the previous levodopa dosage (see DOSAGE AND ADMINISTRATION). Patients who are taking SINEMET should be instructed not to take additional levodopa unless it is prescribed by the physician.

As with levodopa, SINEMET may cause involuntary movements and mental disturbances. These reactions are thought to be due to increased brain dopamine following administration of levodopa. All patients should be observed carefully for the development of depression with concomitant suicidal tendencies. Patients with past or current psychoses should

Continued on next page

Merck Sharp & Dohme—Cont.

be treated with caution. *Because carbidopa permits more levodopa to reach the brain and, thus, more dopamine to be formed, dyskinesias may occur at lower dosages and sooner with* SINEMET *than with levodopa.* The occurrence of dyskinesias may require dosage reduction.

SINEMET should be administered cautiously to patients with severe cardiovascular or pulmonary disease, bronchial asthma, renal, hepatic or endocrine disease.

Care should be exercised in administering SINEMET, as with levodopa, to patients with a history of myocardial infarction who have residual atrial, nodal, or ventricular arrhythmias. In such patients, cardiac function should be monitored with particular care during the period of initial dosage adjustment, in a facility with provisions for intensive cardiac care.

As with levodopa there is a possibility of upper gastrointestinal hemorrhage in patients with a history of peptic ulcer.

A symptom complex resembling the neuroleptic malignant syndrome including muscular rigidity, elevated body temperature, mental changes, and increased serum creatine phosphokinase has been reported when antiparkinsonian agents were withdrawn abruptly. Therefore, patients should be observed carefully when the dosage of SINEMET is reduced abruptly or discontinued, especially if the patient is receiving neuroleptics.

Usage in Pregnancy and Lactation: Although the effects of SINEMET on human pregnancy and lactation are unknown, both levodopa and combinations of carbidopa and levodopa have caused visceral and skeletal malformations in rabbits. Use of SINEMET in women of childbearing potential requires that the anticipated benefits of the drug be weighed against possible hazards to mother and child. SINEMET should not be given to nursing mothers.

Usage in Children: The safety of SINEMET in patients under 18 years of age has not been established.

PRECAUTIONS

As with levodopa, periodic evaluations of hepatic, hematopoietic, cardiovascular, and renal function are recommended during extended therapy.

Patients with chronic wide angle glaucoma may be treated cautiously with SINEMET provided the intraocular pressure is well controlled and the patient is monitored carefully for changes in intraocular pressure during therapy.

Laboratory Tests

Abnormalities in laboratory tests may include elevations of liver function tests such as alkaline phosphatase, SGOT (AST), SGPT (ALT), lactic dehydrogenase, and bilirubin. Abnormalities in protein-bound iodine, blood urea nitrogen and positive Coombs test have also been reported. Commonly, levels of blood urea nitrogen, creatinine, and uric acid are lower during administration of SINEMET than with levodopa.

SINEMET may cause a false-positive reaction for urinary ketone bodies when a test tape is used for determination of ketonuria. This reaction will not be altered by boiling the urine specimen. False-negative tests may result with the use of glucose-oxidase methods of testing for glucosuria.

Drug Interactions

Caution should be exercised when the following drugs are administered concomitantly with SINEMET:

Symptomatic postural hypotension can occur when SINEMET is added to the treatment of a patient receiving antihypertensive drugs. Therefore, when therapy with SINEMET is started, dosage adjustment of the antihypertensive drug may be required. For patients receiving monoamine oxidase inhibitors, see CONTRAINDICATIONS.

There have been rare reports of adverse reactions, including hypertension and dyskinesia, resulting from the concomitant use of tricyclic antidepressants and SINEMET.

Phenothiazines and butyrophenones may reduce the therapeutic effects of levodopa. In addition, the beneficial effects of levodopa in Parkinson's disease have been reported to be reversed by phenytoin and papaverine. Patients taking these drugs with SINEMET should be carefully observed for loss of therapeutic response.

ADVERSE REACTIONS

The most common serious adverse reactions occurring with SINEMET are choreiform, dystonic, and other involuntary movements. Other serious adverse reactions are mental changes including paranoid ideation and psychotic episodes, depression with or without development of suicidal tendencies, and dementia. Convulsions also have occurred; however, a causal relationship with SINEMET has not been established.

A common but less serious effect is nausea.

Less frequent adverse reactions are cardiac irregularities and/or palpitation, orthostatic hypotensive episodes, brady-

kinetic episodes (the "on-off" phenomenon), anorexia, vomiting, and dizziness.

Rarely, gastrointestinal bleeding, development of duodenal ulcer, hypertension, phlebitis, hemolytic and non-hemolytic anemia, thrombocytopenia, leukopenia, and agranulocytosis have occurred.

Laboratory tests which have been reported to be abnormal are alkaline phosphatase, SGOT (AST), SGPT (ALT), lactic dehydrogenase, bilirubin, blood urea nitrogen, protein-bound iodine, and Coombs test.

Other adverse reactions that have been reported with levodopa are:

Nervous System: ataxia, numbness, increased hand tremor, muscle twitching, muscle cramps, blepharospasm (which may be taken as an early sign of excess dosage, consideration of dosage reduction may be made at this time), trismus, activation of latent Horner's syndrome.

Psychiatric: confusion, sleepiness, insomnia, nightmares, hallucinations, delusions, agitation, anxiety, euphoria.

Gastrointestinal: dry mouth, bitter taste, sialorrhea, dysphagia, bruxism, hiccups, abdominal pain and distress, constipation, diarrhea, flatulence, burning sensation of tongue.

Metabolic: weight gain or loss, edema.

Integumentary: malignant melanoma (see also CONTRAINDICATIONS), flushing, increased sweating, dark sweat, skin rash, loss of hair.

Genitourinary: urinary retention, urinary incontinence, dark urine, priapism.

Special Senses: diplopia, blurred vision, dilated pupils, oculogyric crises.

Miscellaneous: weakness, faintness, fatigue, headache, hoarseness, malaise, hot flashes, sense of stimulation, bizarre breathing patterns, neuroleptic malignant syndrome.

DOSAGE AND ADMINISTRATION

The optimum daily dosage of SINEMET must be determined by careful titration in each patient. SINEMET tablets are available in a 1:4 ratio of carbidopa to levodopa (SINEMET 25-100) as well as a 1:10 ratio (SINEMET 25-250 and SINEMET 10-100). Tablets of the two ratios may be given separately or combined as needed to provide the optimum dosage. Studies show that peripheral dopa decarboxylase is saturated by carbidopa at approximately 70 to 100 mg a day. Patients receiving less than this amount of carbidopa are more likely to experience nausea and vomiting.

Usual Initial Dosage

Dosage is best initiated with one tablet of SINEMET 25-100 three times a day. This dosage schedule provides 75 mg of carbidopa per day. Dosage may be increased by one tablet every day or every other day, as necessary, until a dosage of eight tablets of SINEMET 25-100 a day is reached.

If SINEMET 10-100 is used, dosage may be initiated with one tablet three or four times a day. However, this will not provide an adequate amount of carbidopa for many patients. Dosage may be increased by one tablet every day or every other day until a total of eight tablets (2 tablets q.i.d.) is reached.

How to Transfer Patients from Levodopa

Levodopa must be discontinued at least eight hours before starting SINEMET (Carbidopa-Levodopa, MSD). A daily dosage of SINEMET should be chosen that will provide approximately 25 percent of the previous levodopa dosage. Patients who are taking less than 1500 mg of levodopa a day should be started on one tablet of SINEMET 25-100 three or four times a day. The suggested starting dosage for most patients taking more than 1500 mg of levodopa is one tablet of SINEMET 25-250 three or four times a day.

Maintenance

Therapy should be individualized and adjusted according to the desired therapeutic response. At least 70 to 100 mg of carbidopa per day should be provided. When a greater proportion of carbidopa is required, one tablet of SINEMET 25-100 may be substituted for each tablet of SINEMET 10-100. When more levodopa is required, SINEMET 25-250 should be substituted for SINEMET 25-100 or SINEMET 10-100. If necessary, the dosage of SINEMET 25-250 may be increased by one-half or one tablet every day or every other day to a maximum of eight tablets a day. Experience with total daily dosages of carbidopa greater than 200 mg is limited.

Because both therapeutic and adverse responses occur more rapidly with SINEMET than with levodopa alone, patients should be monitored closely during the dose adjustment period. Specifically, involuntary movements will occur more rapidly with SINEMET than with levodopa. The occurrence of involuntary movements may require dosage reduction. Blepharospasm may be a useful early sign of excess dosage in some patients.

Current evidence indicates that other standard drugs for Parkinson's disease (except levodopa) may be continued while SINEMET is being administered, although their dosage may have to be adjusted.

If general anesthesia is required, SINEMET may be continued as long as the patient is permitted to take fluids and medication by mouth. If therapy is interrupted temporarily,

the usual daily dosage may be administered as soon as the patient is able to take oral medication.

OVERDOSAGE

Management of acute overdosage with SINEMET is basically the same as management of acute overdosage with levodopa; however, pyridoxine is not effective in reversing the actions of SINEMET.

General supportive measures should be employed, along with immediate gastric lavage. Intravenous fluids should be administered judiciously and an adequate airway maintained. Electrocardiographic monitoring should be instituted and the patient carefully observed for the development of arrhythmias; if required, appropriate antiarrhythmic therapy should be given. The possibility that the patient may have taken other drugs as well as SINEMET should be taken into consideration. To date, no experience has been reported with dialysis; hence, its value in overdosage is not known.

HOW SUPPLIED

No. 3365—Tablets SINEMET 25-100 are yellow, oval, scored tablets, coded MSD 650. They are supplied as follows:

NDC 0006-0650-68 bottles of 100
(6505-01-097-1233 100's)
NDC 0006-0650-28 unit dose packages of 100.
Shown in Product Identification Section, page 419

No. 3346—Tablets SINEMET 10-100 are dark dapple-blue, oval, scored, uncoated tablets, coded MSD 647. They are supplied as follows:

NDC 0006-0647-68 bottles of 100
(6505-01-020-8280 100's)
NDC 0006-0647-28 unit dose packages of 100.
Shown in Product Identification Section, page 419

No. 3347—Tablets SINEMET 25-250 are light dapple-blue, oval, scored, uncoated tablets, coded MSD 654. They are supplied as follows:

NDC 0006-0654-68 bottles of 100
(6505-01-020-8279 100's)
NDC 0006-0654-28 unit dose packages of 100.
Shown in Product Identification Section, page 419

Storage

Tablets SINEMET 10-100 and Tablets SINEMET 25-250 must be protected from light.

A.H.F.S. Category: 92:00
DC 7399117   Issued April 1988
COPYRIGHT © MERCK & CO., INC., 1985

TIMOLIDE® Tablets   ℞
(Timolol Maleate-Hydrochlorothiazide, MSD), U.S.P.

DESCRIPTION

TIMOLIDE® (Timolol Maleate-Hydrochlorothiazide, MSD) is for the treatment of hypertension. It combines the antihypertensive activity of two agents: a non-selective beta-adrenergic receptor blocking agent (timolol maleate) and a diuretic (hydrochlorothiazide).

Timolol maleate is (S)-1-[(1, 1-dimethylethyl) amino]-3-[[4- (4-morpholinyl)-1, 2, 5-thiadiazol -3- yl] oxy]-2-propanol, (Z)-butenedioate (1:1) salt. Its empirical formula is $C_{13}H_{24}N_4O_3S \cdot C_4H_4O_4$ and its structural formula is:

Timolol maleate has a molecular weight of 432.49. It is a white, odorless, crystalline powder which is soluble in water, methanol, and alcohol.

Hydrochlorothiazide is 6-chloro-3,4-dihydro-2H-1,2,4-benzothiadiazine-7-sulfonamide 1, 1- dioxide. Its empirical formula is $C_7H_8ClN_3O_4S_2$ and its structural formula is:

Hydrochlorothiazide has a molecular weight of 297.72. It is a white, or practically white, crystalline powder which is slightly soluble in water, but freely soluble in sodium hydroxide solution.

TIMOLIDE is supplied as tablets containing 10 mg of timolol maleate and 25 mg of hydrochlorothiazide for oral administration. Inactive ingredients are cellulose, FD&C Blue 2, magnesium stearate, and starch.

CLINICAL PHARMACOLOGY

TIMOLIDE

Timolol maleate and hydrochlorothiazide have been used singly and concomitantly for the treatment of hypertension. The antihypertensive effects of these agents are additive. The two components of TIMOLIDE have similar dosage schedules, and studies have shown that there is no interference with bioavailability when these agents are given together in the single combination tablet. Therefore, this combination provides a convenient formulation for the concomitant administration of these two entities.

In controlled clinical trials with TIMOLIDE in selected patients with mild to moderate essential hypertension, about 90 percent had a good to excellent response. In patients with more severe hypertension, TIMOLIDE may be administered with other antihypertensives such as ALDOMET® (Methyldopa, MSD) or a vasodilator.

Although the mechanisms of action of timolol maleate and hydrochlorothiazide in the treatment of hypertension have not been established, they are thought to be different; for example, hydrochlorothiazide increases plasma renin activity while timolol maleate reduces plasma renin activity.

Timolol Maleate

Timolol maleate is a beta$_1$ and beta$_2$ (non-selective) adrenergic receptor blocking agent that does not have significant intrinsic sympathomimetic, direct myocardial depressant, or local anesthetic activity.

Pharmacodynamics

Clinical pharmacology studies have confirmed the beta-adrenergic blocking activity as shown by (1) changes in resting heart rate and response of heart rate to changes in posture; (2) inhibition of isoproterenol-induced tachycardia; (3) alteration of the response to the Valsalva maneuver and amyl nitrite administration; and (4) reduction of heart rate and blood pressure changes on exercise.

Timolol maleate decreases the positive chronotropic, positive inotropic, bronchodilator, and vasodilator responses caused by beta-adrenergic receptor agonists. The magnitude of this decreased response is proportional to the existing sympathetic tone and the concentration of timolol maleate at receptor sites.

In normal volunteers, the reduction in heart rate response to a standard exercise was dose dependent over the test range of 0.5 to 20 mg, with a peak reduction at 2 hours of approximately 30% at higher doses.

Beta-adrenergic receptor blockade reduces cardiac output in both healthy subjects and patients with heart disease. In patients with severe impairment of myocardial function beta-adrenergic receptor blockade may inhibit the stimulatory effect of the sympathetic nervous system necessary to maintain adequate cardiac function.

Beta-adrenergic receptor blockade in the bronchi and bronchioles results in increased airway resistance from unopposed parasympathetic activity. Such an effect in patients with asthma or other bronchospastic conditions is potentially dangerous.

Clinical studies indicate that timolol maleate at a dosage of 20–60 mg/day reduces blood pressure without causing postural hypotension in most patients with essential hypertension. Administration of timolol maleate to patients with hypertension results initially in a decrease in cardiac output, little immediate change in blood pressure, and an increase in calculated peripheral resistance. With continued administration of timolol maleate blood pressure decreases within a few days, cardiac output usually remains reduced, and peripheral resistance falls toward pretreatment levels. Plasma volume may decrease or remain unchanged during therapy with timolol maleate. In the majority of patients with hypertension timolol maleate also decreases plasma renin activity. Dosage adjustment to achieve optimal antihypertensive effect may require a few weeks. When therapy with timolol maleate is discontinued, the blood pressure tends to return to pretreatment levels gradually. In most patients the antihypertensive activity of timolol maleate is maintained with long-term therapy and is well tolerated.

The mechanism of the antihypertensive effects of beta-adrenergic receptor blocking agents is not established at this time. Possible mechanisms of action include reduction in cardiac output, reduction in plasma renin activity, and a central nervous system sympatholytic action.

Pharmacokinetics and Metabolism

Timolol maleate is rapidly and nearly completely absorbed (about 90%) following oral ingestion. Detectable plasma levels of timolol occur within one-half hour and peak plasma levels occur in about one to two hours. The drug half-life in plasma is approximately 4 hours and this is essentially unchanged in patients with moderate renal insufficiency. Timolol is partially metabolized by the liver and timolol and its metabolites are excreted by the kidney. Timolol is not extensively bound to plasma proteins; i.e., <10% by equilibrium dialysis and approximately 60% by ultrafiltration. An *in vitro* hemodialysis study, using ^{14}C timolol added to human plasma or whole blood, showed that timolol was readily dialyzed from these fluids; however, a study of patients with renal failure showed that timolol did not dialyze readily. Plasma levels following oral administration are about half those following intravenous administration indicating approximately 50% first pass metabolism. The level of beta sympathetic activity varies widely among individuals, and no simple correlation exists between the dose or plasma level of timolol maleate and its therapeutic activity. Therefore, objective clinical measurements such as reduction of heart rate and/or blood pressure should be used as guides in determining the optimal dosage for each patient.

Hydrochlorothiazide

Hydrochlorothiazide is a diuretic and antihypertensive agent. It affects the renal tubular mechanism of electrolyte reabsorption. Hydrochlorothiazide increases excretion of sodium and chloride in approximately equivalent amounts. Natriuresis may be accompanied by some loss of potassium and bicarbonate. The mechanism of the antihypertensive effect of thiazides may be related to the excretion and redistribution of body sodium. Hydrochlorothiazide usually does not cause clinically important changes in normal blood pressure.

INDICATIONS AND USAGE

TIMOLIDE is indicated for the treatment of hypertension. **This fixed combination drug is not indicated for initial therapy of hypertension. If the fixed combination represents the dose titrated to an individual patient's needs, it may be more convenient than the separate components.**

CONTRAINDICATIONS

TIMOLIDE is contraindicated in patients with bronchial asthma or with a history of bronchial asthma, or severe chronic obstructive pulmonary disease (see WARNINGS); sinus bradycardia; second and third degree atrioventricular block; overt cardiac failure (see WARNINGS); cardiogenic shock; anuria; hypersensitivity to this product or to sulfonamide-derived drugs.

WARNINGS

Cardiac Failure

Sympathetic stimulation may be essential for support of the circulation in individuals with diminished myocardial contractility, and its inhibition by beta-adrenergic receptor blockade may precipitate more severe failure. Although beta blockers should be avoided in overt congestive heart failure, they can be used, if necessary, with caution in patients with a history of failure who are well-compensated, usually with digitalis and diuretics. Both digitalis and timolol maleate slow AV conduction. If cardiac failure persists, therapy with TIMOLIDE should be withdrawn.

In Patients Without a History of Cardiac Failure continued depression of the myocardium with beta-blocking agents over a period of time can, in some cases, lead to cardiac failure. At the first sign or symptom of cardiac failure, patients receiving TIMOLIDE should be digitalized and/or be given additional diuretic therapy. Observe the patient closely. If cardiac failure continues, despite adequate digitalization and diuretic therapy, TIMOLIDE should be withdrawn.

Renal and Hepatic Disease and Electrolyte Disturbances

Since timolol maleate is partially metabolized in the liver and excreted mainly by the kidneys, dosage reductions may be necessary when hepatic and/or renal insufficiency is present.

Although the pharmacokinetics of timolol maleate are not greatly altered by renal impairment, marked hypotensive responses have been seen in patients with marked renal impairment undergoing dialysis after 20 mg doses. Dosing in such patients should therefore be especially cautious.

In patients with renal disease, thiazides may precipitate azotemia, and cumulative effects may develop in the presence of impaired renal function. If progressive renal impairment becomes evident, TIMOLIDE should be discontinued.

In patients with impaired hepatic function or progressive liver disease, even minor alterations in fluid and electrolyte balance may precipitate hepatic coma. Hepatic encephalopathy, manifested by tremors, confusion, and coma, has been reported in association with diuretic therapy including hydrochlorothiazide.

Exacerbation of Ischemic Heart Disease Following Abrupt Withdrawal —Hypersensitivity to catecholamines has been observed in patients withdrawn from beta blocker therapy; exacerbation of angina and, in some cases, myocardial infarction have occurred after *abrupt* discontinuation of such therapy. When discontinuing chronically administered timolol maleate, particularly in patients with ischemic heart disease, the dosage should be gradually reduced over a period of one to two weeks and the patient should be carefully monitored. If angina markedly worsens or acute coronary insufficiency develops, timolol maleate administration should be reinstituted promptly, at least temporarily, and other measures appropriate for the management of unstable angina should be taken. Patients should be warned against interruption or discontinuation of therapy without the physician's advice. Because coronary artery disease is common and may be unrecognized, it may be prudent not to discontinue timolol maleate therapy abruptly even in patients treated only for hypertension.

Obstructive Pulmonary Disease

PATIENTS WITH CHRONIC OBSTRUCTIVE PULMONARY DISEASE (e.g., CHRONIC BRONCHITIS, EMPHYSEMA) OF MILD OR MODERATE SEVERITY, BRONCHOSPASTIC DISEASE OR A HISTORY OF BRONCHOSPASTIC DISEASE (OTHER THAN BRONCHIAL ASTHMA OR A HISTORY OF BRONCHIAL ASTHMA, IN WHICH 'TIMOLIDE' IS CONTRAINDICATED, see CONTRAINDICATIONS), SHOULD IN GENERAL NOT RECEIVE BETA BLOCKERS, INCLUDING 'TIMOLIDE'. However, if TIMOLIDE is necessary in such patients, then the drug should be administered with caution since it may block bronchodilation produced by endogenous and exogenous catecholamine stimulation of beta$_2$ receptors.

Major Surgery

The necessity or desirability of withdrawal of beta-blocking therapy prior to major surgery is controversial. Beta-adrenergic receptor blockade impairs the ability of the heart to respond to beta-adrenergically mediated reflex stimuli. This may augment the risk of general anesthesia in surgical procedures. Some patients receiving beta-adrenergic receptor blocking agents have been subject to protracted severe hypotension during anesthesia. Difficulty in restarting and maintaining the heartbeat has also been reported. For these reasons, in patients undergoing elective surgery, some authorities recommend gradual withdrawal of beta-adrenergic receptor blocking agents.

If necessary during surgery, the effects of beta-adrenergic blocking agents may be reversed by sufficient doses of such agonists as isoproterenol, dopamine, dobutamine or levarterenol (see OVERDOSAGE).

Metabolic and Endocrine Effects

Beta-adrenergic blockade may mask certain clinical signs (e.g., tachycardia) of hyperthyroidism. Patients suspected of developing thyrotoxicosis should be managed carefully to avoid abrupt withdrawal of beta blockade which might precipitate a thyroid storm. Thiazides may decrease serum PBI levels without signs of thyroid disturbance.

Beta-adrenergic receptor blocking agents may mask the signs and symptoms of acute hypoglycemia. Therefore, TIMOLIDE should be administered with caution to patients subject to spontaneous hypoglycemia, or to diabetic patients (especially those with labile diabetes) who are receiving insulin or oral hypoglycemic agents. Insulin requirements in diabetic patients may be increased, decreased, or unchanged by thiazides. Diabetes mellitus which has been latent may become manifest during administration of thiazide diuretics. Because calcium excretion is decreased by thiazides, TIMOLIDE should be discontinued before carrying out tests for parathyroid function. Pathologic changes in the parathyroid glands, with hypercalcemia and hypophosphatemia, have been observed in a few patients on prolonged thiazide therapy; however, the common complications of hyperparathyroidism such as renal lithiasis, bone resorption, and peptic ulceration have not been seen.

Hyperuricemia may occur or acute gout may be precipitated in certain patients receiving thiazide therapy.

PRECAUTIONS

General

Electrolyte and Fluid Balance Status: Periodic determination of serum electrolytes to detect possible electrolyte imbalance should be performed at appropriate intervals.

Patients should be observed for clinical signs of fluid or electrolyte imbalance, i.e., hyponatremia, hypochloremic alkalosis, and hypokalemia. Serum and urine electrolyte determinations are particularly important when the patient is vomiting excessively or receiving parenteral fluids. Warning signs or symptoms of fluid and electrolyte imbalance include dryness of the mouth, thirst, weakness, lethargy, drowsiness, restlessness, muscle pains or cramps, muscular fatigue, hypotension, oliguria, tachycardia, and gastrointestinal disturbances such as nausea and vomiting.

Hypokalemia may develop, especially with brisk diuresis, when severe cirrhosis is present, or during concomitant use of corticosteroids or ACTH.

Interference with adequate oral electrolyte intake will also contribute to hypokalemia. Hypokalemia can sensitize or exaggerate the response of the heart to the toxic effects of digitalis (e.g., increased ventricular irritability). Hypokale-

Continued on next page

Merck Sharp & Dohme—Cont.

mia may be avoided or treated by use of potassium supplements or foods with a high potassium content.

Any chloride deficit during thiazide therapy is generally mild and usually does not require specific treatment except under extraordinary circumstances (as in liver disease or renal disease). Dilutional hyponatremia may occur in edematous patients in hot weather; appropriate therapy is water restriction rather than administration of salt except in rare instances when the hyponatremia is life threatening. In actual salt depletion, appropriate replacement is the therapy of choice.

Thiazides have been shown to increase urinary excretion of magnesium, which may result in hypomagnesemia.

Muscle Weakness: Beta-adrenergic blockade has been reported to potentiate muscle weakness consistent with certain myasthenic symptoms (e.g., diplopia, ptosis, and generalized weakness). Timolol has been reported rarely to increase muscle weakness in some patients with myasthenia gravis or myasthenic symptoms.

Cerebrovascular Insufficiency: Because of potential effects of beta-adrenergic blocking agents relative to blood pressure and pulse, these agents should be used with caution in patients with cerebrovascular insufficiency. If signs or symptoms suggesting reduced cerebral blood flow are observed, consideration should be given to discontinuing these agents.

Drug Interactions

TIMOLIDE may potentiate the action of other antihypertensive agents used concomitantly. Close observation of the patient is recommended when TIMOLIDE is administered to patients receiving catecholamine-depleting drugs such as reserpine, because of possible additive effects and the production of hypotension and/or marked bradycardia, which may produce vertigo, syncope, or postural hypotension.

Blunting of the antihypertensive effect of beta-adrenoceptor blocking agents by non-steroidal anti-inflammatory drugs has been reported. In some patients, the administration of a non-steroidal anti-inflammatory agent can reduce the diuretic, natriuretic, and antihypertensive effects of loop, potassium-sparing and thiazide diuretics. Therefore, when TIMOLIDE and non-steroidal anti-inflammatory agents are used concomitantly, the patient should be observed closely to determine if the desired therapeutic effect has been obtained.

Literature reports suggest that oral calcium antagonists may be used in combination with beta-adrenergic blocking agents when heart function is normal, but should be avoided in patients with impaired cardiac function. Hypotension, AV conduction disturbances, and left ventricular failure have been reported in some patients receiving beta-adrenergic blocking agents when an oral calcium antagonist was added to the treatment regimen. Hypotension was more likely to occur if the calcium antagonist were a dihydropyridine derivative, e.g., nifedipine, while left ventricular failure and AV conduction disturbances were more likely to occur with either verapamil or diltiazem.

Intravenous calcium antagonists should be used with caution in patients receiving beta-adrenergic blocking agents. The concomitant use of beta-adrenergic blocking agents with digitalis and either diltiazem or verapamil may have additive effects in prolonging AV conduction time.

Thiazides may decrease arterial responsiveness to norepinephrine. This diminution is not sufficient to preclude the therapeutic effectiveness of norepinephrine. Thiazides may increase the responsiveness to tubocurarine.

Lithium generally should not be given with diuretics because they reduce its renal clearance and add a high risk of lithium toxicity. Read circulars for lithium preparations before use of such preparations with TIMOLIDE.

Other Precautions

In patients receiving thiazides, sensitivity reactions may occur with or without a history of allergy or bronchial asthma. The possible exacerbation or activation of systemic lupus erythematosus has been reported. The antihypertensive effects of thiazides may be enhanced in the post-sympathectomy patient.

Increases in cholesterol and triglyceride levels may be associated with thiazide diuretic therapy.

Carcinogenesis, Mutagenesis, Impairment of Fertility

In a two-year study of timolol maleate in rats, there was a statistically significant ($P \leq 0.05$) increase in the incidence of adrenal pheochromocytomas in male rats administered 300 times the maximum recommended human dose (1 mg/kg/day). Similar differences were not observed in rats administered doses equivalent to 25 or 100 times the maximum recommended human dose. In a lifetime study in mice, there were statistically significant ($P \leq 0.05$) increases in the incidence of benign and malignant pulmonary tumors and benign uterine polyps in female mice at 500 mg/kg/day, but not at 5 or 50 mg/kg/day. There was also a significant increase in mammary adenocarcinomas at the 500 mg/kg/day dose. This was associated with elevations in serum prolactin which occurred in female mice administered timolol at 500 mg/kg, but not at doses of 5 or 50 mg/kg/day. An increased

incidence of mammary adenocarcinomas in rodents has been associated with administration of several other therapeutic agents which elevate serum prolactin, but no correlation between serum prolactin levels and mammary tumors has been established in man. Furthermore, in adult human female subjects who received oral dosages of up to 60 mg of timolol maleate, the maximum recommended human oral dosage, there were no clinically meaningful changes in serum prolactin.

There was a statistically significant increase ($P \leq 0.05$) in the overall incidence of neoplasms in female mice at the 500 mg/kg/day dosage level.

Timolol maleate was devoid of mutagenic potential when evaluated *in vivo* (mouse) in the micronucleus test and cytogenetic assay (doses up to 800 mg/kg) and *in vitro* in a neoplastic cell transformation assay (up to 100 μg /mL). In Ames tests the highest concentrations of timolol employed, 5000 or 10,000 μg/plate, were associated with statistically significant elevations ($P \leq 0.05$) of revertants observed with tester strain TA100 (in seven replicate assays), but not in the remaining three strains. In the assays with tester strain TA100, no consistent dose response relationship was observed, nor did the ratio of test to control revertants reach 2. A ratio of 2 is usually considered the criterion for a positive Ames test.

Reproduction and fertility studies in rats showed no adverse effect on male or female fertility at doses up to 150 times the maximum recommended human dose.

Pregnancy

Pregnancy Category C. Combinations of timolol maleate and hydrochlorothiazide were studied for teratogenic potential in the mouse and rabbit. The timolol maleate/hydrochlorothiazide combinations were administered orally to pregnant mice and pregnant rabbits at dosage levels of 1/2.5, 4/10, or 8/10 mg/kg/day. No teratogenic, embryotoxic, fetotoxic, or maternotoxic effects attributable to treatment were observed in either species. There are no adequate and well-controlled studies in pregnant women with TIMOLIDE. Because of the data listed below with the individual components, TIMOLIDE should be used during pregnancy only if the potential benefit justifies the potential risk to the fetus.

Timolol Maleate: Teratogenicity studies with timolol maleate in mice and rabbits at doses up to 50 mg/kg/day (50 times the maximum recommended human dose) showed no evidence of fetal malformations. Although delayed fetal ossification was observed at this dose in rats, there were no adverse effects on postnatal development of offspring. Doses of 1000 mg/kg/day (1,000 times the maximum recommended human dose) were maternotoxic in mice and resulted in an increased number of fetal resorptions. Increased fetal resorptions were also seen in rabbits at doses of 100 times the maximum recommended human dose, in this case without apparent maternotoxicity.

Hydrochlorothiazide: TIMOLIDE contains hydrochlorothiazide. Thiazides cross the placental barrier and appear in cord blood. The possible hazards to the fetus include fetal or neonatal jaundice, thrombocytopenia, and possibly other adverse reactions which have occurred in the adult.

Nursing Mothers

Because of the potential for serious adverse reactions from timolol and hydrochlorothiazide in nursing infants, a decision should be made whether to discontinue nursing or to discontinue the drug, taking into account the importance of the drug to the mother.

Pediatric Use

Safety and effectiveness in children have not been established.

ADVERSE REACTIONS

TIMOLIDE is usually well tolerated in properly selected patients. Most adverse effects have been mild and transient. The adverse reactions listed in the following table were spontaneously reported and have been arranged into two groups: (1) incidence greater than 1%; and (2) incidence less than 1%. The incidence was obtained from clinical studies conducted in the United States (257 patients treated with TIMOLIDE).

Incidence Greater Than 1%	Incidence Less Than 1%
BODY AS A WHOLE	
fatigue/tiredness (1.9%)	chest pain
	headache
asthenia (1.9%)	
CARDIOVASCULAR	
hypotension (1.6%)	arrhythmia
bradycardia (1.2%)	syncope
	cardiac failure
DIGESTIVE SYSTEM	
none	diarrhea
	dyspepsia
	nausea
	gastrointestinal pain
	constipation
INTEGUMENTARY	
none	rash
	increased pigmentation
	dry mucous membranes
MUSCULOSKELETAL	
none	myalgia
NERVOUS SYSTEM	
dizziness (1.2%)	none
PSYCHIATRIC	
none	insomnia
	decreased libido
	nervousness
	confusion
	trouble concentrating
	somnolence
RESPIRATORY	
bronchial spasm (1.6%)	rales
dyspnea (1.2%)	
UROGENITAL	
none	renal colic

The following additional adverse effects have been reported in clinical experience with the drug: cerebral ischemia, cerebral vascular accident, gout, muscle cramps, oculogyric crisis, worsening of chronic obstructive pulmonary disease, earache, and impotence.

Other adverse reactions that have been reported with the individual components are listed below:

Timolol Maleate—Body as a Whole: extremity pain, decreased exercise tolerance, weight loss, fever; *Cardiovascular:* cardiac arrest, cerebral vascular accident, worsening of angina pectoris, sinoatrial block, AV block, worsening of arterial insufficiency, Raynaud's phenomenon, claudication, palpitations, vasodilatation, cold hands and feet, edema; *Digestive:* hepatomegaly, elevated liver function tests, vomiting; *Hematologic:* nonthrombocytopenic purpura; *Endocrine:* hyperglycemia, hypoglycemia; *Skin:* skin irritation, pruritus, sweating, alopecia; *Musculoskeletal:* arthralgia; *Nervous System:* local weakness, vertigo, paresthesia, increase in signs and symptoms of myasthenia gravis; *Psychiatric:* depression, nightmares, hallucinations; *Respiratory:* cough; *Special Senses:* visual disturbances, diplopia, ptosis, eye irritation, dry eyes, tinnitus; *Urogenital:* urination difficulties. There have been reports of retroperitoneal fibrosis in patients receiving timolol maleate and in patients receiving other beta-adrenergic blocking agents. A causal relationship between this condition and therapy with beta-adrenergic blocking agents has not been established.

Hydrochlorothiazide—Body as a Whole: weakness; *Digestive:* anorexia, gastric irritation, vomiting, cramping, jaundice (intrahepatic cholestatic jaundice), pancreatitis, sialadenitis; *Nervous System/Psychiatric:* vertigo, paresthesias, restlessness; *Hematologic:* Leukopenia, agranulocytosis, thrombocytopenia, aplastic anemia, hemolytic anemia; *Cardiovascular:* orthostatic hypotension (may be aggravated by alcohol, barbiturates, or narcotics); *Hypersensitivity:* purpura, photosensitivity, urticaria, necrotizing angiitis (vasculitis, cutaneous vasculitis), fever, respiratory distress including pneumonitis and pulmonary edema, anaphylactic reactions; *Metabolic:* hyperglycemia, glycosuria, hyperuricemia, electrolyte imbalance (see PRECAUTIONS); *Musculoskeletal:* muscle spasm; *Special Senses:* transient blurred vision, xanthopsia.

Potential Adverse Effects: In addition, a variety of adverse effects not observed in clinical trials with timolol maleate, but reported with other beta-adrenergic blocking agents, should be considered potential adverse effects of timolol maleate: *Nervous System:* Reversible mental depression progressing to catatonia; an acute reversible syndrome characterized by disorientation for time and place, short-term memory loss, emotional lability, slightly clouded sensorium, and decreased performance on neuropsychometrics; *Cardiovascular:* Intensification of AV block (see CONTRAINDICATIONS); *Digestive:* Mesenteric arterial thrombosis, ischemic colitis; *Hematologic:* Agranulocytosis, thrombocytopenic purpura; *Allergic:* Erythematous rash, fever combined with aching and sore throat, laryngospasm with respiratory distress; *Miscellaneous:* Peyronie's disease.

There have been reports of a syndrome comprising psoriasiform skin rash, conjunctivitis sicca, otitis, and sclerosing serositis attributed to the beta-adrenergic receptor blocking agent, practolol. This syndrome has not been reported with TIMOLIDE or BLOCADREN® (Timolol Maleate, MSD).

Clinical Laboratory Test Findings: Clinically important changes in standard laboratory parameters were rarely associated with the administration of TIMOLIDE. The changes in laboratory parameters were not progressive and usually were not associated with clinical manifestations. The most common changes were increases in serum triglycerides and uric acid and decreases in serum potassium and chloride. Decreases in HDL cholesterol have been reported.

OVERDOSAGE

No data are available in regard to overdosage in humans. Pretreatment of mice with hydrochlorothiazide (5 mg/kg) did not alter the LD_{50} of timolol (1320 mg/kg compared to 1300 mg/kg without pretreatment).

No specific information is available on the treatment of overdosage with TIMOLIDE, and no specific antidote is available. Treatment is symptomatic and supportive. Therapy with TIMOLIDE should be discontinued and the patient observed closely. Suggested measures include induction of emesis and/or gastric lavage, and correction of dehydration, electrolyte imbalance, and hypotension by established procedures.

Timolol Maleate

No data are available in regard to overdosage in humans. The oral LD_{50} of the drug is 1190 and 900 mg/kg in female mice and female rats, respectively.

An *in vitro* hemodialysis study, using ^{14}C timolol added to human plasma or whole blood, showed that timolol was readily dialyzed from these fluids; however, a study of patients with renal failure showed that timolol did not dialyze readily.

The most common signs and symptoms to be expected with overdosage with a beta-adrenergic receptor blocking agent are symptomatic bradycardia, hypotension, bronchospasm, and acute cardiac failure. If overdosage occurs the following therapeutic measures should be considered:

(1) *Gastric lavage.*

(2) *Symptomatic bradycardia:* Use atropine sulfate intravenously in a dosage of 0.25 mg to 2 mg to induce vagal blockade. If bradycardia persists, intravenous isoproterenol hydrochloride should be administered cautiously. In refractory cases the use of a transvenous cardiac pacemaker may be considered.

(3) *Hypotension:* Use sympathomimetic pressor drug therapy, such as dopamine, dobutamine or levarterenol. In refractory cases the use of glucagon hydrochloride has been reported to be useful.

(4) *Bronchospasm:* Use isoproterenol hydrochloride. Additional therapy with aminophylline may be considered.

(5) *Acute cardiac failure:* Conventional therapy with digitalis, diuretics, and oxygen should be instituted immediately. In refractory cases the use of intravenous aminophylline is suggested. This may be followed, if necessary, by glucagon hydrochloride which has been reported to be useful.

(6) *Heart block (second or third degree):* Use isoproterenol hydrochloride or a transvenous cardiac pacemaker.

Hydrochlorothiazide

The most common signs and symptoms observed with hydrochlorothiazide overdosage are those caused by electrolyte depletion (hypokalemia, hypochloremia, hyponatremia) and dehydration resulting from excessive diuresis. If digitalis has also been administered, hypokalemia may accentuate cardiac arrhythmias.

DOSAGE AND ADMINISTRATION

The recommended starting and maintenance dosage is 1 tablet twice a day or 2 tablets once a day. If the antihypertensive response is not satisfactory, another antihypertensive agent may be added.

HOW SUPPLIED

No. 3373—Tablets TIMOLIDE 10-25 are light blue, flat, hexagonal-shaped, compressed tablets, with MSD 67 code on one side and TIMOLIDE on the other. Each tablet contains 10 mg of timolol maleate and 25 mg of hydrochlorothiazide. They are supplied as follows:

NDC 0006-0067-68 bottles of 100.

Shown in Product Identification Section, page 419

Storage

Store in a well-closed container, protected from light.

A.H.F.S. Category: 24:08
DC 7244226   Issued August 1987
COPYRIGHT © MERCK & CO., INC., 1985
All rights reserved

TIMOPTIC® Sterile Ophthalmic Solution   ℞
(Timolol Maleate, MSD), U.S.P.

DESCRIPTION

TIMOPTIC® (Timolol Maleate, MSD) Ophthalmic Solution is a non-selective beta-adrenergic receptor blocking agent. Its chemical name is (S)- 1- [(1, 1-dimethylethyl)amino] -3- [[4- (4- morpholinyl) -1, 2, 5-thiadiazol-3-yl]oxy] -2- propanol, (Z)- butenedioate (1:1) salt. Timolol maleate possesses an asymmetric carbon atom in its structure and is provided as

the levo isomer. The nominal optical rotation of timolol maleate is:
$[\alpha]^{25}_{405 \text{ nm}}$ in 0.1N HCl (C = 5%) = −12.2°.

Its empirical formula is $C_{13}H_{24}N_4O_3S \cdot C_4H_4O_4$ and its structural formula is:

Timolol maleate has a molecular weight of 432.49. It is a white, odorless, crystalline powder which is soluble in water, methanol, and alcohol. TIMOPTIC is stable at room temperature.

TIMOPTIC Ophthalmic Solution is supplied as a sterile, isotonic, buffered, aqueous solution of timolol maleate in two dosage strengths: Each mL of TIMOPTIC 0.25% contains 2.5 mg of timolol (3.4 mg of timolol maleate). Each mL of TIMOPTIC 0.5% contains 5.0 mg of timolol (6.8 mg of timolol maleate). Inactive ingredients: monobasic and dibasic sodium phosphate, sodium hydroxide to adjust pH, and water for injection. Benzalkonium chloride 0.01% is added as preservative.

CLINICAL PHARMACOLOGY

Timolol maleate is a $beta_1$ and $beta_2$ (non-selective) adrenergic receptor blocking agent that does not have significant intrinsic sympathomimetic, direct myocardial depressant, or local anesthetic (membrane-stabilizing) activity.

Beta-adrenergic receptor blockade reduces cardiac output in both healthy subjects and patients with heart disease. In patients with severe impairment of myocardial function beta-adrenergic receptor blockade may inhibit the stimulatory effect of the sympathetic nervous system necessary to maintain adequate cardiac function.

Beta-adrenergic receptor blockade in the bronchi and bronchioles results in increased airway resistance from unopposed para-sympathetic activity. Such an effect in patients with asthma or other bronchospastic conditions is potentially dangerous.

TIMOPTIC Ophthalmic Solution, when applied topically in the eye, has the action of reducing elevated as well as normal intraocular pressure, whether or not accompanied by glaucoma. Elevated intraocular pressure is a major risk factor in the pathogenesis of glaucomatous visual field loss. The higher the level of intraocular pressure, the greater the likelihood of glaucomatous visual field loss and optic nerve damage.

The onset of reduction in intraocular pressure following administration of TIMOPTIC can usually be detected within one-half hour after a single dose. The maximum effect usually occurs in one to two hours and significant lowering of intraocular pressure can be maintained for periods as long as 24 hours with a single dose. Repeated observations over a period of one year indicate that the intraocular pressure-lowering effect of TIMOPTIC is well maintained.

The precise mechanism of the ocular hypotensive action of TIMOPTIC is not clearly established at this time. Tonography and fluorophotometry studies in man suggest that its predominant action may be related to reduced aqueous formation. However, in some studies a slight increase in outflow facility was also observed. Unlike miotics, TIMOPTIC reduces intraocular pressure with little or no effect on accommodation or pupil size. Thus, changes in visual acuity due to increased accommodation are uncommon, and dim or blurred vision and night blindness produced by miotics are not evident. In addition, in patients with cataracts the inability to see around lenticular opacities when the pupil is constricted is avoided.

In the clinical studies which are reported below, ocular pressure reductions to less than 22 mmHg were used as a reasonable reference point to allow comparisons between treatments. Reduction of ocular pressure to just below 22 mmHg may not be optimal for all patients; therapy should be individualized.

In controlled multiclinic studies in patients with untreated intraocular pressures of 22 mmHg or greater, TIMOPTIC 0.25 percent or 0.5 percent administered twice a day produced a greater reduction in intraocular pressure than 1, 2, 3, or 4 percent pilocarpine solution administered four times a day or 0.5, 1, or 2 percent epinephrine hydrochloride solution administered twice a day.

In the multiclinic studies comparing TIMOPTIC with pilocarpine, 61 percent of patients treated with TIMOPTIC had intraocular pressure reduced to less than 22 mmHg compared to 32 percent of patients treated with pilocarpine. For patients completing these studies, the mean reduction in pressure at the end of the study from pretreatment was 30.7 percent for patients treated with TIMOPTIC and 21.7 percent for patients treated with pilocarpine.

In the multiclinic studies comparing TIMOPTIC with epinephrine, 69 percent of patients treated with TIMOPTIC had intraocular pressure reduced to less than 22 mmHg com-

pared to 42 percent of patients treated with epinephrine. For patients completing these studies, the mean reduction in pressure at the end of the study from pretreatment was 33.2 percent for patients treated with TIMOPTIC and 28.1 percent for patients treated with epinephrine.

In these studies, TIMOPTIC was generally well tolerated and produced fewer and less severe side effects than either pilocarpine or epinephrine. A slight reduction of resting heart rate in some patients receiving TIMOPTIC (mean reduction 2.9 beats/minute standard deviation 10.2) was observed.

TIMOPTIC has also been used in patients with glaucoma wearing conventional (PMMA) hard contact lenses, and has generally been well tolerated. TIMOPTIC has not been studied in patients wearing lenses made with materials other than PMMA.

INDICATIONS AND USAGE

TIMOPTIC Ophthalmic Solution has been shown to be effective in lowering intraocular pressure and may be used in:
Patients with chronic open-angle glaucoma
Patients with aphakic glaucoma
Some patients with secondary glaucoma
Other patients with elevated intraocular pressure who are at sufficient risk to require lowering of the ocular pressure.
Clinical trials have also shown that in patients who respond inadequately to multiple antiglaucoma drug therapy the addition of TIMOPTIC may produce a further reduction in intraocular pressure.

CONTRAINDICATIONS

TIMOPTIC is contraindicated in patients with bronchial asthma or with a history of bronchial asthma, or severe chronic obstructive pulmonary disease (see WARNINGS); sinus bradycardia; second and third degree atrioventricular block; overt cardiac failure (see WARNINGS); cardiogenic shock; hypersensitivity to any component of this product.

WARNINGS

As with other topically applied ophthalmic drugs, this drug may be absorbed systemically.

The same adverse reactions found with systemic administration of beta-adrenergic blocking agents may occur with topical administration. For example, severe respiratory reactions and cardiac reactions, including death due to bronchospasm in patients with asthma, and rarely death in association with cardiac failure, have been reported following administration of TIMOPTIC (Timolol Maleate, MSD) (see CONTRAINDICATIONS).

Cardiac Failure

Sympathetic stimulation may be essential for support of the circulation in individuals with diminished myocardial contractility, and its inhibition by beta-adrenergic receptor blockade may precipitate more severe failure.

In Patients Without a History of Cardiac Failure continued depression of the myocardium with beta-blocking agents over a period of time can, in some cases, lead to cardiac failure. At the first sign or symptom of cardiac failure TIMOPTIC should be discontinued.

Obstructive Pulmonary Disease

PATIENTS WITH CHRONIC OBSTRUCTIVE PULMONARY DISEASE (e.g., CHRONIC BRONCHITIS, EMPHYSEMA) OF MILD OR MODERATE SEVERITY, BRONCHOSPASTIC DISEASE OR A HISTORY OF BRONCHOSPASTIC DISEASE (OTHER THAN BRONCHIAL ASTHMA OR A HISTORY OF BRONCHIAL ASTHMA, IN WHICH 'TIMOPTIC' IS CONTRAINDICATED, see CONTRAINDICATIONS), SHOULD IN GENERAL NOT RECEIVE BETA BLOCKERS, INCLUDING 'TIMOPTIC'. However, if TIMOPTIC is necessary in such patients, then the drug should be administered with caution since it may block bronchodilation produced by endogenous and exogenous catecholamine stimulation of $beta_2$ receptors.

Major Surgery

The necessity or desirability of withdrawal of beta-adrenergic blocking agents prior to major surgery is controversial. Beta-adrenergic receptor blockade impairs the ability of the heart to respond to beta-adrenergically mediated reflex stimuli. This may augment the risk of general anesthesia in surgical procedures. Some patients receiving beta-adrenergic receptor blocking agents have been subject to protracted severe hypotension during anesthesia. Difficulty in restarting and maintaining the heartbeat has also been reported. For these reasons, in patients undergoing elective surgery,

Continued on next page

Merck Sharp & Dohme—Cont.

some authorities recommend gradual withdrawal of beta-adrenergic receptor blocking agents.

If necessary during surgery, the effects of beta-adrenergic blocking agents may be reversed by sufficient doses of such agonists as isoproterenol, dopamine, dobutamine or levarterenol (see OVERDOSAGE).

Diabetes Mellitus

Beta-adrenergic blocking agents should be administered with caution in patients subject to spontaneous hypoglycemia or to diabetic patients (especially those with labile diabetes) who are receiving insulin or oral hypoglycemic agents. Beta-adrenergic receptor blocking agents may mask the signs and symptoms of acute hypoglycemia.

Thyrotoxicosis

Beta-adrenergic blocking agents may mask certain clinical signs (e.g., tachycardia) of hyperthyroidism. Patients suspected of developing thyrotoxicosis should be managed carefully to avoid abrupt withdrawal of beta-adrenergic blocking agents which might precipitate a thyroid storm.

PRECAUTIONS

General

Patients who are receiving a beta-adrenergic blocking agent orally and TIMOPTIC should be observed for a potential additive effect either on the intraocular pressure or on the known systemic effects of beta blockade.

Patients should not receive two topical ophthalmic beta-adrenergic blocking agents concurrently (see DOSAGE AND ADMINISTRATION).

Because of potential effects of beta-adrenergic blocking agents relative to blood pressure and pulse, these agents should be used with caution in patients with cerebrovascular insufficiency. If signs or symptoms suggesting reduced cerebral blood flow develop following initiation of therapy with TIMOPTIC, alternative therapy should be considered.

Muscle Weakness: Beta-adrenergic blockade has been reported to potentiate muscle weakness consistent with certain myasthenic symptoms (e.g., diplopia, ptosis, and generalized weakness). Timolol has been reported rarely to increase muscle weakness in some patients with myasthenia gravis or myasthenic symptoms.

In patients with angle-closure glaucoma, the immediate objective of treatment is to reopen the angle. This requires constricting the pupil with a miotic. TIMOPTIC has little or no effect on the pupil. When TIMOPTIC is used to reduce elevated intraocular pressure in angle-closure glaucoma, it should be used with a miotic and not alone.

As with the use of other antiglaucoma drugs, diminished responsiveness to TIMOPTIC after prolonged therapy has been reported in some patients. However, in one long-term study in which 96 patients have been followed for at least 3 years, no significant difference in mean intraocular pressure has been observed after initial stabilization.

Drug Interactions

Although TIMOPTIC used alone has little or no effect on pupil size, mydriasis resulting from concomitant therapy with TIMOPTIC and epinephrine has been reported occasionally.

Close observation of the patient is recommended when a beta blocker is administered to patients receiving catecholamine-depleting drugs such as reserpine, because of possible additive effects and the production of hypotension and/or marked bradycardia, which may produce vertigo, syncope, or postural hypotension.

Caution should be used in the coadministration of beta-adrenergic blocking agents, such as TIMOPTIC, and oral or intravenous calcium antagonists, because of possible atrioventricular conduction disturbances, left ventricular failure, and hypotension. In patients with impaired cardiac function, coadministration should be avoided.

The concomitant use of beta-adrenergic blocking agents with digitalis and calcium antagonists may have additive effects in prolonging atrioventricular conduction time.

Animal Studies

No adverse ocular effects were observed in rabbits and dogs administered TIMOPTIC topically in studies lasting one and two years respectively.

Carcinogenesis, Mutagenesis, Impairment of Fertility

In a two-year oral study of timolol maleate in rats, there was a statistically significant (P ≤ 0.05) increase in the incidence of adrenal pheochromocytomas in male rats administered 300 times the maximum recommended human oral dose* (1 mg/kg/day). Similar differences were not observed in rats administered oral doses equivalent to 25 or 100 times the maximum recommended human oral dose. In a lifetime oral study in mice, there were statistically significant (P ≤ 0.05) increases in the incidence of benign and malignant pulmonary tumors and benign uterine polyps in female mice at 500 mg/kg/day, but not at 5 or 50 mg/kg/day. There was also a significant increase in mammary adenocarcinomas at the 500 mg/kg/day dose. This was associated with elevations in

serum prolactin which occurred in female mice administered timolol at 500 mg/kg, but not at doses of 5 or 50 mg/kg/day. An increased incidence of mammary adenocarcinomas in rodents has been associated with administration of several other therapeutic agents which elevate serum prolactin, but no correlation between serum prolactin levels and mammary tumors has been established in man. Furthermore, in adult human female subjects who received oral dosages of up to 60 mg of timolol maleate, the maximum recommended human oral dosage, there were no clinically meaningful changes in serum prolactin.

Timolol maleate was devoid of mutagenic potential when evaluated *in vivo* (mouse) in the micronucleus test and cytogenetic assay (doses up to 800 mg/kg) and *in vitro* in a neoplastic cell transformation assay (up to 100 μg/mL). In Ames tests the highest concentrations of timolol employed, 5000 or 10,000 μg/plate, were associated with statistically significant elevations (P ≤ 0.05) of revertants observed with tester strain TA100 (in seven replicate assays), but not in the remaining three strains. In the assays with tester strain TA100, no consistent dose response relationship was observed, nor did the ratio of test to control revertants reach 2. A ratio of 2 is usually considered the criterion for a positive Ames test.

Reproduction and fertility studies in rats showed no adverse effect on male or female fertility at doses up to 150 times the maximum recommended human oral dose.

Pregnancy

Pregnancy Category C. Teratogenicity studies with timolol in mice and rabbits at doses up to 50 mg/kg/day (50 times the maximum recommended human oral dose) showed no evidence of fetal malformations. Although delayed fetal ossification was observed at this dose in rats, there were no adverse effects on postnatal development of offspring. Doses of 1000 mg/kg/day (1,000 times the maximum recommended human oral dose) were maternotoxic in mice and resulted in an increased number of fetal resorptions. Increased fetal resorptions were also seen in rabbits at doses of 100 times the maximum recommended human oral dose, in this case without apparent maternotoxicity. There are no adequate and well-controlled studies in pregnant women. TIMOPTIC should be used during pregnancy only if the potential benefit justifies the potential risk to the fetus.

Nursing Mothers

Because of the potential for serious adverse reactions from timolol in nursing infants, a decision should be made whether to discontinue nursing or to discontinue the drug, taking into account the importance of the drug to the mother.

Pediatric Use

Safety and effectiveness in children have not been established by adequate and well-controlled studies.

ADVERSE REACTIONS

TIMOPTIC Ophthalmic Solution is usually well tolerated. The following adverse reactions have been reported either in clinical trials of up to 3 years duration prior to release in 1978 or since the drug has been marketed.

BODY AS A WHOLE

Headache, asthenia, chest pain.

CARDIOVASCULAR

Bradycardia, arrhythmia, hypotension, syncope, heart block, cerebral vascular accident, cerebral ischemia, cardiac failure, palpitation, cardiac arrest.

DIGESTIVE

Nausea, diarrhea.

NERVOUS SYSTEM/PSYCHIATRIC

Dizziness, depression, increase in signs and symptoms of myasthenia gravis, paresthesia.

SKIN

Hypersensitivity, including localized and generalized rash; urticaria.

RESPIRATORY

Bronchospasm (predominantly in patients with pre-existing bronchospastic disease), respiratory failure, dyspnea, nasal congestion.

ENDOCRINE

Masked symptoms of hypoglycemia in insulin-dependent diabetics (See WARNINGS).

SPECIAL SENSES

Signs and symptoms of ocular irritation, including conjunctivitis, blepharitis, keratitis, blepharoptosis, decreased corneal sensitivity, visual disturbances including refractive changes (due to withdrawal of miotic therapy in some cases), diplopia, ptosis.

Causal Relationship Unknown: The following adverse effects have been reported, and a causal relationship to ther-

apy with TIMOPTIC has not been established: *Body as a Whole:* Fatigue; *Cardiovascular:* Hypertension, pulmonary edema, worsening of angina pectoris; *Digestive:* Dyspepsia, anorexia, dry mouth; *Nervous System/Psychiatric:* Behavioral changes including confusion, hallucinations, anxiety, disorientation, nervousness, somnolence, and other psychic disturbances; *Skin:* Alopecia; *Special Senses:* Aphakic cystoid macular edema; *Urogenital:* Retroperitoneal fibrosis, impotence.

The following additional adverse effects have been reported in clinical experience with oral timolol maleate, and may be considered potential effects of ophthalmic timolol maleate: *Body as a Whole:* Extremity pain, decreased exercise tolerance, weight loss; *Cardiovascular:* Edema, worsening of arterial insufficiency, Raynaud's phenomenon, vasodilatation; *Digestive:* Gastrointestinal pain, hepatomegaly, vomiting; *Hematologic:* Nonthrombocytopenic purpura; *Endocrine:* Hyperglycemia, hypoglycemia; *Skin:* Pruritus, skin irritation, increased pigmentation, sweating, cold hands and feet; *Musculoskeletal:* Arthralgia, claudication; *Nervous System/Psychiatric:* Vertigo, local weakness, decreased libido, nightmares, insomnia, diminished concentration; *Respiratory:* Rales, cough, bronchial obstruction; *Special Senses:* Tinnitus, dry eyes; *Urogenital:* Urination difficulties.

Potential Adverse Effects: In addition, a variety of adverse effects have been reported with other beta-adrenergic blocking agents and may be considered potential effects of ophthalmic timolol maleate: *Digestive:* Mesenteric arterial thrombosis, ischemic colitis; *Hematologic:* Agranulocytosis, thrombocytopenic purpura; *Nervous System:* Reversible mental depression progressing to catatonia; an acute reversible syndrome characterized by disorientation for time and place, short-term memory loss, emotional lability, slightly clouded sensorium, and decreased performance on neuropsychometrics; *Allergic:* Erythematous rash, fever combined with aching and sore throat, laryngospasm with respiratory distress; *Urogenital:* Peyronie's disease.

There have been reports of a syndrome comprising psoriasiform skin rash, conjunctivitis sicca, otitis and sclerosing serositis attributed to the beta-adrenergic receptor blocking agent, practolol. This syndrome has not been reported with timolol maleate.

OVERDOSAGE

No data are available in regard to overdosage in humans. The oral LD_{50} of the drug is 1190 and 900 mg/kg in female mice and female rats, respectively.

An *in vitro* hemodialysis study, using ^{14}C timolol added to human plasma or whole blood, showed that timolol was readily dialyzed from these fluids; however, a study of patients with renal failure showed that timolol did not dialyze readily.

The most common signs and symptoms to be expected with overdosage with administration of a systemic beta-adrenergic receptor blocking agent are symptomatic bradycardia, hypotension, bronchospasm, and acute cardiac failure. The following therapeutic measures should be considered:

(1) *Gastric lavage:* If ingested.

(2) *Symptomatic bradycardia:* Use atropine sulfate intravenously in a dosage of 0.25 mg to 2 mg to induce vagal blockade. If bradycardia persists, intravenous isoproterenol hydrochloride should be administered cautiously. In refractory cases the use of a transvenous cardiac pacemaker may be considered.

(3) *Hypotension:* Use sympathomimetic pressor drug therapy, such as dopamine, dobutamine or levarterenol. In refractory cases the use of glucagon hydrochloride has been reported to be useful.

(4) *Bronchospasm:* Use isoproterenol hydrochloride. Additional therapy with aminophylline may be considered.

(5) *Acute cardiac failure:* Conventional therapy with digitalis, diuretics, and oxygen should be instituted immediately. In refractory cases the use of intravenous aminophylline is suggested. This may be followed if necessary by glucagon hydrochloride which has been reported to be useful.

(6) *Heart block (second or third degree):* Use isoproterenol hydrochloride or a transvenous cardiac pacemaker.

DOSAGE AND ADMINISTRATION

TIMOPTIC Ophthalmic Solution is available in concentrations of 0.25 and 0.5 percent. The usual starting dose is one drop of 0.25 percent TIMOPTIC in the affected eye(s) twice a day. If the clinical response is not adequate, the dosage may be changed to one drop of 0.5 percent solution in the affected eye(s) twice a day.

Since in some patients the pressure-lowering response to TIMOPTIC may require a few weeks to stabilize, evaluation should include a determination of intraocular pressure after approximately 4 weeks of treatment with TIMOPTIC.

If the intraocular pressure is maintained at satisfactory levels, the dosage schedule may be changed to one drop once a day in the affected eye(s). Because of diurnal variations in

---

*The maximum recommended single oral dose is 30 mg of timolol. One drop of TIMOPTIC 0.5% contains about 1/150 of this dose which is about 0.2 mg.

There was a statistically significant increase (P ≤ 0.05) in the overall incidence of neoplasms in female mice at the 500 mg/kg/day dosage level.

intraocular pressure, satisfactory response to the once-a-day dose is best determined by measuring the intraocular pressure at different times during the day.

Dosages above one drop of 0.5 percent TIMOPTIC twice a day generally have not been shown to produce further reduction in intraocular pressure. If the patient's intraocular pressure is still not at a satisfactory level on this regimen, concomitant therapy with pilocarpine and other miotics, and/or epinephrine, and/or systemically administered carbonic anhydrase inhibitors, such as acetazolamide, can be instituted.

When a patient is transferred from another topical ophthalmic beta-adrenergic blocking agent, that agent should be discontinued after proper dosing on one day and treatment with TIMOPTIC started on the following day with 1 drop of 0.25 percent TIMOPTIC in the affected eye(s) twice a day. The dose may be increased to one drop of 0.5 percent TIMOPTIC twice a day if the clinical response is not adequate.

When a patient is transferred from a single antiglaucoma agent, other than a topical ophthalmic beta-adrenergic blocking agent, continue the agent already being used and add one drop of 0.25 percent TIMOPTIC in the affected eye(s) twice a day. On the following day, discontinue the previously used antiglaucoma agent completely and continue with TIMOPTIC. If a higher dosage of TIMOPTIC is required, substitute one drop of 0.5 percent solution in the affected eye(s) twice a day.

When a patient is transferred from several concomitantly administered antiglaucoma agents, individualization is required. If any of the agents is an ophthalmic beta-adrenergic blocker, it should be discontinued before starting TIMOPTIC. Additional adjustments should involve one agent at a time and usually should be made at intervals of not less than one week. A recommended approach is to continue the agents being used and to add one drop of 0.25 percent TIMOPTIC in the affected eye(s) twice a day. On the following day, discontinue one of the other antiglaucoma agents. The remaining antiglaucoma agents may be decreased or discontinued according to the patient's response to treatment. If a higher dosage of TIMOPTIC is required, substitute one drop of 0.5 percent solution in the affected eye(s) twice a day. The physician may be able to discontinue some or all of the other antiglaucoma agents.

HOW SUPPLIED

Sterile Ophthalmic Solution TIMOPTIC is a clear, colorless to light yellow solution.

No. 3366—TIMOPTIC Ophthalmic Solution, 0.25% timolol equivalent, is supplied in a white, opaque, plastic OCUMETER® ophthalmic dispenser with a controlled drop tip as follows:

NDC 0006-3366-32, 2.5 mL
NDC 0006-3366-03, 5 mL
(6505-01-069-6518, 0.25% 5 mL)
NDC 0006-3366-10, 10 mL
NDC 0006-3366-12, 15 mL.

No. 3367—TIMOPTIC Ophthalmic Solution, 0.5% timolol equivalent, is supplied in a white, opaque, plastic OCUMETER ophthalmic dispenser with a controlled drop tip as follows:

NDC 0006-3367-32, 2.5 mL
NDC 0006-3367-03, 5 mL
(6505-01-069-6519, 0.5% 5 mL)
NDC 0006-3367-10, 10 mL
NDC 0006-3367-12, 15 mL.
Storage
Protect from light. Store at room temperature.
      A.H.F.S. Category: 52:36
      DC 7115426   Issued October 1986
COPYRIGHT © MERCK & CO., INC., 1985
All rights reserved

TIMOPTIC®   ℞
(Timolol Maleate, MSD)
in OCUDOSE® (Dispenser)
Preservative-Free Sterile Ophthalmic Solution
in a Sterile Ophthalmic Unit Dose Dispenser

DESCRIPTION

Timolol maleate is a non-selective beta-adrenergic receptor blocking agent. Its chemical name is (S)-1-[(1,1-dimethylethyl)amino]-3-[[4-(4-morpholinyl)-1,2,5-thiadiazol-3-yl]oxy]-2-propanol, (Z)-butenedioate (1:1) salt. Timolol maleate possesses an asymmetric carbon atom in its structure and is provided as the levo isomer. The nominal optical rotation of timolol maleate is
$[\alpha]^{25}_{405\ nm}$ in 0.1N HCl (C = 5%) = −12.2°.

Its empirical formula is $C_{13}H_{24}N_4O_3S \cdot C_4H_4O_4$ and its structural formula is:
[See Chemical Formula at top of next column].

Timolol maleate has a molecular weight of 432.49. It is a white, odorless, crystalline powder which is soluble in water, methanol, and alcohol. Timolol maleate is stable at room temperature.

Timolol maleate ophthalmic solution is supplied in two formulations: Ophthalmic Solution TIMOPTIC® (Timolol Maleate, MSD), which contains the preservative, benzalkonium chloride; and Ophthalmic Solution TIMOPTIC® (Timolol Maleate, MSD), the preservative-free formulation.

Preservative-free Ophthalmic Solution TIMOPTIC is supplied in OCUDOSE®, a unit dose container as a sterile, isotonic, buffered, aqueous solution of timolol maleate in two dosage strengths: Each mL of Preservative-free TIMOPTIC in OCUDOSE 0.25% contains 2.5 mg of timolol (3.4 mg of timolol maleate). Each mL of Preservative-free TIMOPTIC in OCUDOSE 0.5% contains 5.0 mg of timolol (6.8 mg of timolol maleate). Inactive ingredients: monobasic and dibasic sodium phosphate, sodium hydroxide to adjust pH, and water for injection.

CLINICAL PHARMACOLOGY

Timolol maleate is a $beta_1$ and $beta_2$ (non-selective) adrenergic receptor blocking agent that does not have significant intrinsic sympathomimetic, direct myocardial depressant, or local anesthetic (membrane-stabilizing) activity.

Beta-adrenergic receptor blockade reduces cardiac output in both healthy subjects and patients with heart disease. In patients with severe impairment of myocardial function beta-adrenergic receptor blockade may inhibit the stimulatory effect of the sympathetic nervous system necessary to maintain adequate cardiac function.

Beta-adrenergic receptor blockade in the bronchi and bronchioles results in increased airway resistance from unopposed parasympathetic activity. Such an effect in patients with asthma or other bronchospastic conditions is potentially dangerous.

TIMOPTIC (Timolol Maleate, MSD), when applied topically in the eye, has the action of reducing elevated as well as normal intraocular pressure, whether or not accompanied by glaucoma. Elevated intraocular pressure is a major risk factor in the pathogenesis of glaucomatous visual field loss. The higher the level of intraocular pressure, the greater the likelihood of glaucomatous visual field loss and optic nerve damage.

The onset of reduction in intraocular pressure following administration of TIMOPTIC (Timolol Maleate, MSD) can usually be detected within one-half hour after a single dose. The maximum effect usually occurs in one to two hours and significant lowering of intraocular pressure can be maintained for periods as long as 24 hours with a single dose. Repeated observations over a period of one year indicate that the intraocular pressure-lowering effect of TIMOPTIC (Timolol Maleate, MSD) is well maintained.

The precise mechanism of the ocular hypotensive action of TIMOPTIC (Timolol Maleate, MSD) is not clearly established at this time. Tonography and fluorophotometry studies in man suggest that its predominant action may be related to reduced aqueous formation. However, in some studies a slight increase in outflow facility was also observed. Unlike miotics, TIMOPTIC (Timolol Maleate, MSD) reduces intraocular pressure with little or no effect on accommodation or pupil size. Thus, changes in visual acuity due to increased accommodation are uncommon, and dim or blurred vision and night blindness produced by miotics are not evident. In addition, in patients with cataracts the inability to see around lenticular opacities when the pupil is constricted is avoided.

Clinical studies have shown that the mean percent reductions in intraocular pressure with Preservative-free TIMOPTIC and TIMOPTIC (Timolol Maleate, MSD) were similar. Preservative-free TIMOPTIC was generally well tolerated. In the clinical studies which are reported below, ocular pressure reductions to less than 22 mmHg were used as a reasonable reference point to allow comparisons between treatments. Reduction of ocular pressure to just below 22 mmHg may not be optimal for all patients; therapy should be individualized.

In controlled multiclinic studies in patients with untreated intraocular pressures of 22 mmHg or greater, TIMOPTIC (Timolol Maleate, MSD) 0.25 percent or 0.5 percent administered twice a day produced a greater reduction in intraocular pressure than 1, 2, 3, or 4 percent pilocarpine solution administered four times a day or 0.5, 1, or 2 percent epinephrine hydrochloride solution administered twice a day.

In the multiclinic studies comparing TIMOPTIC (Timolol Maleate, MSD) with pilocarpine, 61 percent of patients treated with TIMOPTIC (Timolol Maleate, MSD) had intra-

ocular pressure reduced to less than 22 mmHg compared to 32 percent of patients treated with pilocarpine. For patients completing these studies, the mean reduction in pressure at the end of the study from pretreatment was 30.7 percent for patients treated with TIMOPTIC (Timolol Maleate, MSD) and 21.7 percent for patients treated with pilocarpine.

In the multiclinic studies comparing TIMOPTIC (Timolol Maleate, MSD) with epinephrine, 69 percent of patients treated with TIMOPTIC (Timolol Maleate, MSD) had intraocular pressure reduced to less than 22 mmHg compared to 42 percent of patients treated with epinephrine. For patients completing these studies, the mean reduction in pressure at the end of the study from pretreatment was 33.2 percent for patients treated with TIMOPTIC (Timolol Maleate, MSD) and 28.1 percent for patients treated with epinephrine.

In these studies, TIMOPTIC (Timolol Maleate, MSD) was generally well tolerated and produced fewer and less severe side effects than either pilocarpine or epinephrine. A slight reduction of resting heart rate in some patients receiving TIMOPTIC (Timolol Maleate, MSD) (mean reduction 2.9 beats/minute standard deviation 10.2) was observed.

TIMOPTIC (Timolol Maleate, MSD) has also been used in patients with glaucoma wearing conventional (PMMA) hard contact lenses, and has generally been well tolerated. TIMOPTIC (Timolol Maleate, MSD) has not been studied in patients wearing lenses made with materials other than PMMA.

INDICATIONS AND USAGE

TIMOPTIC (Timolol Maleate, MSD) has been shown to be effective in lowering intraocular pressure. Clinical studies have shown that the mean percent reductions in intraocular pressure with Preservative-free TIMOPTIC and TIMOPTIC (Timolol Maleate, MSD) are similar. When a patient is sensitive to the preservative, benzalkonium chloride, or when use of a preservative-free topical medication is advisable, Preservative-free TIMOPTIC may be used in:

     Patients with chronic open-angle glaucoma
     Patients with aphakic glaucoma
     Some patients with secondary glaucoma
     Other patients with elevated intraocular pressure who are at sufficient risk to require lowering of the ocular pressure. Clinical trials have also shown that in patients who respond inadequately to multiple antiglaucoma drug therapy the addition of TIMOPTIC (Timolol Maleate, MSD) may produce a further reduction of intraocular pressure.

CONTRAINDICATIONS

Preservative-free TIMOPTIC in OCUDOSE is contraindicated in patients with bronchial asthma or with a history of bronchial asthma, or severe chronic obstructive pulmonary disease (see WARNINGS); sinus bradycardia; second and third degree atrioventricular block; overt cardiac failure (see WARNINGS); cardiogenic shock; hypersensitivity to any component of this product.

WARNINGS

As with other topically applied ophthalmic drugs, this drug may be absorbed systemically.

The same adverse reactions found with systemic administration of beta-adrenergic blocking agents may occur with topical administration. For example, severe respiratory reactions and cardiac reactions, including death due to bronchospasm in patients with asthma, and rarely death in association with cardiac failure, have been reported following administration of TIMOPTIC (Timolol Maleate, MSD) (see CONTRAINDICATIONS).

Cardiac Failure
Sympathetic stimulation may be essential for support of the circulation in individuals with diminished myocardial contractility, and its inhibition by beta-adrenergic receptor blockade may precipitate more severe failure.

In Patients Without a History of Cardiac Failure continued depression of the myocardium with beta-blocking agents over a period of time can, in some cases, lead to cardiac failure. At the first sign or symptom of cardiac failure Preservative-free TIMOPTIC in OCUDOSE should be discontinued.

Obstructive Pulmonary Disease
PATIENTS WITH CHRONIC OBSTRUCTIVE PULMONARY DISEASE (e.g., CHRONIC BRONCHITIS, EMPHYSEMA) OF MILD OR MODERATE SEVERITY, BRONCHOSPASTIC DISEASE OR A HISTORY OF BRONCHOSPASTIC DISEASE (OTHER THAN BRONCHIAL ASTHMA OR A HISTORY OF BRONCHIAL ASTHMA, IN WHICH 'Preservative-free TIMOPTIC in OCUDOSE' IS CONTRAINDI-

Continued on next page

Information on the Merck Sharp & Dohme products listed on these pages is the full prescribing information from product circulars in use August 31, 1989.

Merck Sharp & Dohme—Cont.

CATED, see CONTRAINDICATIONS), SHOULD IN GENERAL NOT RECEIVE BETA BLOCKERS, INCLUDING 'Preservative-free TIMOPTIC in OCUDOSE'. However, if Preservative-free TIMOPTIC in OCUDOSE is necessary in such patients, then the drug should be administered with caution since it may block bronchodilation produced by endogenous and exogenous catecholamine stimulation of beta₂ receptors.

Major Surgery
The necessity or desirability of withdrawal of beta-adrenergic blocking agents prior to major surgery is controversial. Beta-adrenergic receptor blockade impairs the ability of the heart to respond to beta-adrenergically mediated reflex stimuli. This may augment the risk of general anesthesia in surgical procedures. Some patients receiving beta-adrenergic receptor blocking agents have been subject to protracted severe hypotension during anesthesia. Difficulty in restarting and maintaining the heartbeat has also been reported. For these reasons, in patients undergoing elective surgery, some authorities recommend gradual withdrawal of beta-adrenergic receptor blocking agents.

If necessary during surgery, the effects of beta-adrenergic blocking agents may be reversed by sufficient doses of such agonists as isoproterenol, dopamine, dobutamine or levarterenol (see OVERDOSAGE).

Diabetes Mellitus
Beta-adrenergic blocking agents should be administered with caution in patients subject to spontaneous hypoglycemia or to diabetic patients (especially those with labile diabetes) who are receiving insulin or oral hypoglycemic agents. Beta-adrenergic receptor blocking agents may mask the signs and symptoms of acute hypoglycemia.

Thyrotoxicosis
Beta-adrenergic blocking agents may mask certain clinical signs (e.g., tachycardia) of hyperthyroidism. Patients suspected of developing thyrotoxicosis should be managed carefully to avoid abrupt withdrawal of beta-adrenergic blocking agents which might precipitate a thyroid storm.

PRECAUTIONS

General
Patients who are receiving a beta-adrenergic blocking agent orally and Preservative-free TIMOPTIC in OCUDOSE should be observed for a potential additive effect either on the intraocular pressure or on the known systemic effects of beta blockade.
Patients should not receive two topical ophthalmic beta-adrenergic blocking agents concurrently (see DOSAGE AND ADMINISTRATION).
Because of potential effects of beta-adrenergic blocking agents relative to blood pressure and pulse, these agents should be used with caution in patients with cerebrovascular insufficiency. If signs or symptoms suggesting reduced cerebral blood flow develop following initiation of therapy with Preservative-free TIMOPTIC in OCUDOSE, alternative therapy should be considered.
Muscle Weakness: Beta-adrenergic blockade has been reported to potentiate muscle weakness consistent with certain myasthenic symptoms (e.g., diplopia, ptosis, and generalized weakness). Timolol has been reported rarely to increase muscle weakness in some patients with myasthenia gravis or myasthenic symptoms.
In patients with angle-closure glaucoma, the immediate objective of treatment is to reopen the angle. This requires constricting the pupil with a miotic. TIMOPTIC (Timolol Maleate, MSD) has little or no effect on the pupil. When Preservative-free TIMOPTIC in OCUDOSE is used to reduce elevated intraocular pressure in angle-closure glaucoma, it should be used with a miotic and not alone.
As with the use of other antiglaucoma drugs, diminished responsiveness to TIMOPTIC (Timolol Maleate, MSD) after prolonged therapy has been reported in some patients. However, in one long-term study in which 96 patients have been followed for at least 3 years, no significant difference in mean intraocular pressure has been observed after initial stabilization.
Information for Patients
Patients should be instructed about the use of Preservative-free TIMOPTIC in OCUDOSE.
Since sterility cannot be maintained after the individual unit is opened, patients should be instructed to use the product immediately after opening, and to discard the individual unit and any remaining contents immediately after use.
Drug Interactions
Although TIMOPTIC (Timolol Maleate, MSD) used alone has little or no effect on pupil size, mydriasis resulting from concomitant therapy with TIMOPTIC (Timolol Maleate, MSD) and epinephrine has been reported occasionally.
Close observation of the patient is recommended when a beta blocker is administered to patients receiving catecholamine-depleting drugs such as reserpine, because of possible addi-

tive effects and the production of hypotension and/or marked bradycardia, which may produce vertigo, syncope, or postural hypotension.
Caution should be used in the coadministration of beta-adrenergic blocking agents, such as Preservative-free TIMOPTIC in OCUDOSE, and oral or intravenous calcium antagonists, because of possible atrioventricular conduction disturbances, left ventricular failure, and hypotension. In patients with impaired cardiac function, coadministration should be avoided.
The concomitant use of beta-adrenergic blocking agents with digitalis and calcium antagonists may have additive effects in prolonging atrioventricular conduction time.
Animal Studies
No adverse ocular effects were observed in rabbits and dogs administered TIMOPTIC (Timolol Maleate, MSD) topically in studies lasting one and two years respectively.
Carcinogenesis, Mutagenesis, Impairment of Fertility
In a two-year oral study of timolol maleate in rats, there was a statistically significant (P ≤ 0.05) increase in the incidence of adrenal pheochromocytomas in male rats administered 300 times the maximum recommended human oral dose* (1 mg/kg/day). Similar differences were not observed in rats administered oral doses equivalent to 25 or 100 times the maximum recommended human oral dose. In a lifetime oral study in mice, there were statistically significant (P ≤ 0.05) increases in the incidence of benign and malignant pulmonary tumors and benign uterine polyps in female mice at 500 mg/kg/day, but not at 5 or 50 mg/kg/day. There was also a significant increase in mammary adenocarcinomas at the 500 mg/kg/day dose. This was associated with elevations in serum prolactin which occurred in female mice administered timolol at 500 mg/kg, but not at doses of 5 or 50 mg/kg/day. An increased incidence of mammary adenocarcinomas in rodents has been associated with administration of several other therapeutic agents which elevate serum prolactin, but no correlation between serum prolactin levels and mammary tumors has been established in man. Furthermore, in adult human female subjects who received oral dosages of up to 60 mg of timolol maleate, the maximum recommended human oral dosage, there were no clinically meaningful changes in serum prolactin.

There was a statistically significant increase (P ≤ 0.05) in the overall incidence of neoplasms in female mice at the 500 mg/kg/day dosage level.
Timolol maleate was devoid of mutagenic potential when evaluated *in vivo* (mouse) in the micronucleus test and cytogenetic assay (doses up to 800 mg/kg) and *in vitro* in a neoplastic cell transformation assay (up to 100 µg/mL). In Ames tests the highest concentrations of timolol employed, 5000 or 10,000 µg/plate, were associated with statistically significant elevations (P ≤ 0.05) of revertants observed with tester strain TA 100 (in seven replicate assays), but not in the remaining three strains. In the assays with tester strain TA 100, no consistent dose response relationship was observed, nor did the ratio of test to control revertants reach 2. A ratio of 2 is usually considered the criterion for a positive Ames test.
Reproduction and fertility studies in rats showed no adverse effect on male or female fertility at doses up to 150 times the maximum recommended human oral dose.

Pregnancy
Pregnancy Category C. Teratogenicity studies with timolol in mice and rabbits at doses up to 50 mg/kg/day (50 times the maximum recommended human oral dose) showed no evidence of fetal malformations. Although delayed fetal ossification was observed at this dose in rats, there were no adverse effects on postnatal development of offspring. Doses of 1000 mg/kg/day (1,000 times the maximum recommended human oral dose) were maternotoxic in mice and resulted in an increased number of fetal resorptions. Increased fetal resorptions were also seen in rabbits at doses of 100 times the maximum recommended human oral dose, in this case without apparent maternotoxicity. There are no adequate and well-controlled studies in pregnant women. Preservative-free TIMOPTIC in OCUDOSE should be used during pregnancy only if the potential benefit justifies the potential risk to the fetus.
Nursing Mothers
Because of the potential for serious adverse reactions from timolol in nursing infants, a decision should be made whether to discontinue nursing or to discontinue the drug, taking into account the importance of the drug to the mother.
Pediatric Use
Safety and effectiveness in children have not been established by adequate and well-controlled studies.

*The maximum recommended single oral dose is 30 mg of timolol. One drop of Preservative-free TIMOPTIC in OCUDOSE 0.5% contains about 1/150 of this dose which is about 0.2 mg.

ADVERSE REACTIONS
Preservative-free TIMOPTIC in OCUDOSE Ophthalmic Solution is usually well tolerated. The following adverse reactions have been reported with TIMOPTIC (Timolol Maleate, MSD), either in clinical trials of up to 3 years duration prior to release in 1978 or since the drug has been marketed, and may be expected to occur with Preservative-free TIMOPTIC.
BODY AS A WHOLE
Headache, asthenia, chest pain.
CARDIOVASCULAR
Bradycardia, arrhythmia, hypotension, syncope, heart block, cerebral vascular accident, cerebral ischemia, cardiac failure, palpitation, cardiac arrest.
DIGESTIVE
Nausea, diarrhea.
NERVOUS SYSTEM/PSYCHIATRIC
Dizziness, depression, increase in signs and symptoms of myasthenia gravis, paresthesia.
SKIN
Hypersensitivity, including localized and generalized rash; urticaria.
RESPIRATORY
Bronchospasm (predominantly in patients with pre-existing bronchospastic disease), respiratory failure, dyspnea, nasal congestion.
ENDOCRINE
Masked symptoms of hypoglycemia in insulin-dependent diabetics (See WARNINGS).
SPECIAL SENSES
Signs and symptoms of ocular irritation, including conjunctivitis, blepharitis, keratitis, blepharoptosis, decreased corneal sensitivity, visual disturbances including refractive changes (due to withdrawal of miotic therapy in some cases), diplopia, ptosis.
Causal Relationship Unknown: The following adverse effects have been reported, and a causal relationship to therapy with ophthalmic timolol maleate has not been established: *Body as a Whole:* Fatigue; *Cardiovascular:* Hypertension, pulmonary edema, worsening of angina pectoris; *Digestive:* Dyspepsia, anorexia, dry mouth; *Nervous System/Psychiatric:* Behavioral changes including confusion, hallucinations, anxiety, disorientation, nervousness, somnolence, and other psychic disturbances; *Skin:* Alopecia; *Special Senses:* Aphakic cystoid macular edema; *Urogenital:* Retroperitoneal fibrosis, impotence.
The following additional adverse effects have been reported in clinical experience with oral timolol maleate, and may be considered potential adverse effects of ophthalmic timolol maleate: *Body as a Whole:* Extremity pain, decreased exercise tolerance, weight loss; *Cardiovascular:* Edema, worsening of arterial insufficiency, Raynaud's phenomenon, vasodilatation; *Digestive:* Gastrointestinal pain, hepatomegaly, vomiting; *Hematologic:* Nonthrombocytopenic purpura; *Endocrine:* Hyperglycemia, hypoglycemia; *Skin:* Pruritus, skin irritation, increased pigmentation, sweating, cold hands and feet; *Musculoskeletal:* Arthralgia, claudication; *Nervous System/Psychiatric:* Vertigo, local weakness, decreased libido, nightmares, insomnia, diminished concentration; *Respiratory:* Rales, cough, bronchial obstruction; *Special Senses:* Tinnitus, dry eyes; *Urogenital:* Urination difficulties.
Potential Adverse Effects: In addition, a variety of adverse effects have been reported with other beta-adrenergic blocking agents and may be considered potential effects of ophthalmic timolol maleate: *Digestive:* Mesenteric arterial thrombosis, ischemic colitis; *Hematologic:* Agranulocytosis, thrombocytopenic purpura; *Nervous System:* Reversible mental depression progressing to catatonia; an acute reversible syndrome characterized by disorientation for time and place, short-term memory loss, emotional lability, slightly clouded sensorium, and decreased performance on neuropsychometrics; *Allergic:* Erythematous rash, fever combined with aching and sore throat, laryngospasm with respiratory distress; *Urogenital:* Peyronie's disease.
There have been reports of a syndrome comprising psoriasiform skin rash, conjunctivitis sicca, otitis and sclerosing serositis attributed to the beta-adrenergic receptor blocking agent, practolol. This syndrome has not been reported with timolol maleate.

OVERDOSAGE

No data are available in regard to overdosage in humans. The oral LD₅₀ of timolol maleate is 1190 and 900 mg/kg in female mice and female rats, respectively.
An *in vitro* hemodialysis study, using ¹⁴C timolol added to human plasma or whole blood, showed that timolol was readily dialyzed from these fluids; however, a study of patients with renal failure showed that timolol did not dialyze readily.
The most common signs and symptoms to be expected with overdosage with administration of a systemic beta-adrenergic receptor blocking agent are symptomatic bradycardia, hypotension, bronchospasm, and acute cardiac failure. The

following additional therapeutic measures should be considered:

(1) *Gastric lavage:* If ingested.

(2) *Symptomatic bradycardia:* Use atropine sulfate intravenously in a dosage of 0.25 mg to 2 mg to induce vagal blockade. If bradycardia persists, intravenous isoproterenol hydrochloride should be administered cautiously. In refractory cases the use of a transvenous cardiac pacemaker may be considered.

(3) *Hypotension:* Use sympathomimetic pressor drug therapy, such as dopamine, dobutamine or levarterenol. In refractory cases the use of glucagon hydrochloride has been reported to be useful.

(4) *Bronchospasm:* Use isoproterenol hydrochloride. Additional therapy with aminophylline may be considered.

(5) *Acute cardiac failure:* Conventional therapy with digitalis, diuretics, and oxygen should be instituted immediately. In refractory cases the use of intravenous aminophylline is suggested. This may be followed if necessary by glucagon hydrochloride which has been reported to be useful.

(6) *Heart block (second or third degree):* Use isoproterenol hydrochloride or a transvenous cardiac pacemaker.

DOSAGE AND ADMINISTRATION

Preservative-free TIMOPTIC in OCUDOSE is a sterile solution that does not contain a preservative. The solution from one individual unit is to be used immediately after opening for administration to one or both eyes. Since sterility cannot be guaranteed after the individual unit is opened, the remaining contents should be discarded immediately after administration.

Preservative-free TIMOPTIC in OCUDOSE is available in concentrations of 0.25 and 0.5 percent. The usual starting dose is one drop of 0.25 percent Preservative-free TIMOPTIC in OCUDOSE in the affected eye(s) administered twice a day. Apply enough gentle pressure on the individual container to obtain a single drop of solution. If the clinical response is not adequate, the dosage may be changed to one drop of 0.5 percent solution in the affected eye(s) administered twice a day. Since in some patients the pressure-lowering response to Preservative-free TIMOPTIC in OCUDOSE may require a few weeks to stabilize, evaluation should include a determination of intraocular pressure after approximately 4 weeks of treatment with Preservative-free TIMOPTIC in OCUDOSE.

If the intraocular pressure is maintained at satisfactory levels, the dosage schedule may be changed to one drop once a day in the affected eye(s). Because of diurnal variations in intraocular pressure, satisfactory response to the once-a-day dose is best determined by measuring the intraocular pressure at different times during the day.

Dosages above one drop of 0.5 percent TIMOPTIC (Timolol Maleate, MSD) twice a day generally have not been shown to produce further reduction in intraocular pressure. If the patient's intraocular pressure is not at a satisfactory level during treatment with Preservative-free TIMOPTIC in OCUDOSE 0.5 percent, concomitant therapy with pilocarpine and other miotics, and/or epinephrine, and/or systemically administered carbonic anhydrase inhibitors, such as acetazolamide, can be instituted taking into consideration that the preparation(s) used concomitantly may contain one or more preservatives.

When a patient is transferred from another topical ophthalmic beta-adrenergic blocking agent, that agent should be discontinued after proper dosing on one day and treatment with Preservative-free TIMOPTIC in OCUDOSE started on the following day with one drop of 0.25 percent Preservative-free TIMOPTIC in OCUDOSE in the affected eye(s) twice a day. The dose may be increased to one drop of 0.5 percent Preservative-free TIMOPTIC in OCUDOSE twice a day if the clinical response is not adequate.

When a patient is transferred from a single antiglaucoma agent, other than a topical ophthalmic beta-adrenergic blocking agent, continue the agent already being used and add one drop of 0.25 percent Preservative-free TIMOPTIC in OCUDOSE in the affected eye(s) twice a day. On the following day, discontinue the previously used antiglaucoma agent completely and continue with Preservative-free TIMOPTIC in OCUDOSE. If a higher dosage of Preservative-free TIMOPTIC in OCUDOSE is required, substitute one drop of 0.5 percent solution in the affected eye(s) twice a day.

When a patient is transferred from several concomitantly administered antiglaucoma agents, individualization is required. If any of the agents is an ophthalmic beta-adrenergic blocker, it should be discontinued before starting Preservative-free TIMOPTIC in OCUDOSE. Additional adjustments should involve one agent at a time and usually should be made at intervals of not less than one week. A recommended approach is to continue the agents being used and to add one drop of 0.25 percent Preservative-free TIMOPTIC in OCUDOSE in the affected eye(s) twice a day. On the following day, discontinue one of the other antiglaucoma agents. The remaining antiglaucoma agents may be decreased or discontinued according to the patient's response to treatment. If a

higher dosage of Preservative-free TIMOPTIC in OCUDOSE is required, substitute one drop of 0.5 percent solution in the affected eye(s) twice a day. The physician may be able to discontinue some or all of the other antiglaucoma agents.

HOW SUPPLIED

Preservative-free Sterile Ophthalmic Solution TIMOPTIC in OCUDOSE is a clear, colorless to light yellow solution.

No. 3542—Preservative-free TIMOPTIC, 0.25% timolol equivalent, is supplied in OCUDOSE, a clear polyethylene unit dose container. Each individual unit contains 0.45 mL of solution, and is available in a foil laminate overwrapped pouch as follows:

NDC 0006-3542-60; 60 Individual Unit Doses.

No. 3543—Preservative-free TIMOPTIC, 0.5% timolol equivalent, is supplied in OCUDOSE, a clear polyethylene unit dose container. Each individual unit contains 0.45 mL of solution, and is available in a foil laminate overwrapped pouch as follows:

NDC 0006-3543-60; 60 Individual Unit Doses.

Storage

Store Preservative-free TIMOPTIC in OCUDOSE at room temperature.

Because evaporation can occur through the unprotected polyethylene unit dose container and prolonged exposure to direct light can modify the product, the unit dose container should be kept in the protective foil overwrap and used within one month after the foil package has been opened.

Manufactured by:

MERCK SHARP & DOHME, Division of Merck & Co., INC.

West Point, Pa. 19486

Filled by:

PACO

Lakewood, NJ 08701

A.H.F.S. Category: 52:36

DC 7475303   Issued November 1986

COPYRIGHT © MERCK & CO., INC., 1986

All rights reserved

TONOCARD® Tablets   ℞
(Tocainide HCl, MSD)

WARNINGS

Blood Dyscrasias: Agranulocytosis, bone marrow depression, leukopenia, neutropenia, aplastic/hypoplastic anemia, thrombocytopenia and sequelae such as septicemia and septic shock have been reported in patients receiving TONOCARD. Most of these patients received TONOCARD within the recommended dosage range. Fatalities have occurred (with approximately 25 percent mortality in reported agranulocytosis cases). Since most of these events have been noted during the first 12 weeks of therapy, it is recommended that complete blood counts, including white cell, differential and platelet counts be performed, optimally, at weekly intervals for the first three months of therapy; and frequently thereafter. Complete blood counts should be performed promptly if the patient develops any signs of infection (such as fever, chills, sore throat, or stomatitis), bruising, or bleeding. If any of these hematologic disorders is identified, TONOCARD should be discontinued and appropriate treatment should be instituted if necessary. Blood counts usually return to normal within one month of discontinuation. Caution should be used in patients with pre-existing marrow failure or cytopenia of any type. (See ADVERSE REACTIONS.)

Pulmonary Fibrosis: Pulmonary fibrosis, interstitial pneumonitis, fibrosing alveolitis, pulmonary edema, and pneumonia have been reported in patients receiving TONOCARD. Many of these events occurred in patients who were seriously ill. Fatalities have been reported. The experiences are usually characterized by bilateral infiltrates on x-ray and are frequently associated with dyspnea and cough. Fever may or may not be present. Patients should be instructed to promptly report the development of any pulmonary symptoms such as exertional dyspnea, cough or wheezing. Chest x-rays are advisable at that time. If these pulmonary disorders develop, TONOCARD should be discontinued. (See ADVERSE REACTIONS.)

DESCRIPTION

TONOCARD* (Tocainide HCl, MSD) is a primary amine analog of lidocaine with antiarrhythmic properties useful in the treatment of ventricular arrhythmias. The chemical name for tocainide hydrochloride is 2-amino-*N*-(2,6-dimethylphenyl) propanamide hydrochloride. Its empir-

---

* Registered trademark of Astra Pharmaceutical Products, Inc.

ical formula is $C_{11}H_{16}N_2O \cdot HCl$, with a molecular weight of 228.72. The structural formula is:

Tocainide hydrochloride is a white crystalline powder with a bitter taste and is freely soluble in water. It is supplied as 400 mg and 600 mg tablets for oral administration. Each tablet contains the following inactive ingredients: hydroxypropyl methylcellulose, iron oxide, magnesium stearate, methylcellulose, polyethylene glycol, and titanium dioxide.

CLINICAL PHARMACOLOGY

Action

Tocainide, like lidocaine, produces dose dependent decreases in sodium and potassium conductance, thereby decreasing the excitability of myocardial cells. In experimental animal models, the dose-related depression of sodium current is more pronounced in ischemic tissue than in normal tissue.

Electrophysiology

Tocainide is a Class I antiarrhythmic compound with electrophysiologic properties in man similar to those of lidocaine, but dissimilar from quinidine, procainamide, and disopyramide.

In studies of isolated dog Purkinje fibers, tocainide in concentrations of 1–50 mcg/mL had no significant effect on resting membrane potential, but reduced the amplitude and rate of depolarization (dv/dt) of the action potential. Tocainide decreased the effective refractory period (ERP) to a lesser extent than the action potential duration (APD) resulting in an increase in the ERP/APD ratio.

In patients with cardiac disease, TONOCARD produced no clinically significant changes in sinus nodal function, effective refractory periods, or intracardiac conduction times when studied under electrophysiologic testing procedures. Tocainide, like lidocaine, characteristically does not prolong ventricular depolarization (QRS duration) or repolarization (QT intervals) as measured by electrocardiography. Theoretically, therefore, TONOCARD may be useful in the treatment of ventricular arrhythmias associated with a prolonged QT interval.

Patients who respond to lidocaine also respond to TONOCARD in a majority of cases. Failure to respond to lidocaine usually predicts failure to respond to TONOCARD, but there are exceptions to this.

In a controlled comparison with quinidine, 600 mg b.i.d. of TONOCARD produced a mean reduction of 42 percent in PVC count, compared to a 54 percent reduction by quinidine 300 mg every 6 hours. Among all patients entered into the study, about one-fifth of tocainide recipients and one-third of quinidine recipients had 75 percent or greater reductions in PVC count or had elimination of ventricular tachycardia.

Pharmacokinetics

Following oral administration of tocainide, peak plasma concentrations occur within 0.5 to 2 hours. The average plasma half-life in patients is approximately 15 hours. Although the effective plasma concentration may vary from patient to patient, the usual therapeutic plasma range (as defined by 50–80 percent PVC suppression) is 4–10 mcg/mL (18–45 micromole/L), expressed as tocainide hydrochloride. Tocainide is approximately 10 percent bound to plasma protein.

In contrast to lidocaine, tocainide undergoes negligible first pass hepatic degradation. Following oral administration, the bioavailability of TONOCARD approaches 100 percent. The extent of its bioavailability is unaffected by food. Tocainide has no cardioactive metabolites. Approximately 40 percent of the administered dose of tocainide is excreted unchanged in the urine. Acidification of the urine has not been shown to significantly alter tocainide excretion in the urine, but alkalinization of the urine results in a significant decrease in the percent of tocainide excreted unchanged in the urine. Animal data indicate that tocainide crosses the blood-brain barrier; however, it has less lipid solubility than lidocaine.

Hemodynamics

Cardiac catheterization studies in man utilizing intravenous tocainide infusions (0.5–0.75 mg/kg/min over 15 min) have shown that tocainide usually produces a small degree of depression of parameters of left ventricular function, such as left ventricular dP/dt, and left ventricular end diastolic pressure. There were usually no changes in cardiac output or clinical evidence of increasing congestive heart failure in the

Continued on next page

Information on the Merck Sharp & Dohme products listed on these pages is the full prescribing information from product circulars in use August 31, 1989.

Merck Sharp & Dohme—Cont.

well-compensated patients studied. Small but statistically significant increases in aortic and pulmonary arterial pressures have been consistently observed and are probably related to small increases in vascular resistance. When used concomitantly with a beta-blocking drug, tocainide further reduced cardiac index and left ventricular dP/dt and further increased pulmonary wedge pressure.

No clinically significant changes in heart rate, blood pressure, or signs of myocardial depression were observed in a study of 72 post-myocardial infarction patients receiving long-term therapy with oral TONOCARD at usual doses (400 mg q8h). When tocainide was administered orally at a dose of 120 mg/kg to anesthetized dogs (14 times the initial maximum dose recommended for humans), a negative inotropic effect was observed: the rate of change of left ventricular pressure decreased by up to 29 percent of control at 3 hours after administration. This effect was not observed at lower doses (60 mg/kg). Tocainide has been used safely in patients with acute myocardial infarction and various degrees of congestive heart failure. It has, however, a small negative inotropic effect and can increase peripheral resistance slightly. It therefore should be used cautiously in patients with known heart failure, particularly if a beta blocker is given as well. (See PRECAUTIONS).

INDICATIONS AND USAGE

TONOCARD is indicated for the treatment of life-threatening ventricular arrhythmias. However, because TONOCARD has the potential to produce serious and sometimes fatal hematologic disorders (0.18 percent in clinical trials) particularly leukopenia, agranulocytosis or aplastic/hypoplastic anemia as well as pulmonary fibrosis (sometimes fatal), the risk/benefit decision is most difficult (see Box WARNINGS). The use of TONOCARD should be reserved for patients in whom, in the opinion of the physician, the benefits of treatment outweigh the risks, keeping in mind the possible alternative therapies for the patient.

Like all other antiarrhythmics, tocainide has not been shown to prevent sudden death in patients with serious ventricular ectopic activity, and also, like all other antiarrhythmics, it has potentially serious adverse effects, including the ability to worsen arrhythmias. It is therefore essential that each patient given tocainide be evaluated electrocardiographically and clinically prior to, and during, tocainide therapy to determine whether the response to tocainide supports continued treatment.

CONTRAINDICATIONS

Patients who are hypersensitive to this product or to local anesthetics of the amide type.
Patients with second or third degree atrioventricular block in the absence of an artificial ventricular pacemaker.

WARNINGS

Acceleration of Ventricular Rate: Acceleration of ventricular rate occurs infrequently when antiarrhythmics are administered to patients with atrial flutter or fibrillation (see ADVERSE REACTIONS).

PRECAUTIONS

General
In patients with known heart failure or minimal cardiac reserve, TONOCARD should be used with caution because of the potential for aggravating the degree of heart failure.
Caution should be used in the institution or continuation of antiarrhythmic therapy in the presence of signs of increasing depression of cardiac conductivity.
In patients with severe liver or kidney disease, the rate of drug elimination may be significantly decreased (see DOSAGE AND ADMINISTRATION).
Since antiarrhythmic drugs may be ineffective in patients with hypokalemia, the possibility of a potassium deficit should be explored and, if present, the deficit should be corrected.
Like all other oral antiarrhythmics, TONOCARD has been reported to increase arrhythmias in some patients (see ADVERSE REACTIONS).
Information for Patients
Patients should be instructed to promptly report the development of bruising or bleeding; any signs of infections such as fever, chills, sore throat, or soreness and ulcers in the mouth; or any pulmonary symptoms, such as exertional dyspnea, cough, or wheezing; rash.
Laboratory Tests
As with other antiarrhythmics, abnormal liver function tests, particularly in the early stages of therapy, have been reported. Periodic monitoring of liver function should be

considered. Hepatitis and jaundice have been reported in some patients.
Drug Interactions
Tocainide and lidocaine are pharmacodynamically similar. The concomitant use of these two agents may cause an increased incidence of adverse reactions, including central nervous system adverse reactions such as seizure.
Specific interaction studies with cimetidine, digoxin, metoprolol and warfarin have been conducted, no clinically significant interaction was seen with cimetidine, digoxin or warfarin; but tocainide and metoprolol had additive effects on wedge pressure and cardiac index. TONOCARD has also been used in open studies with digitalis, beta-blocking agents, other antiarrhythmic agents, anticoagulants, and diuretics, without evidence of clinically significant interactions. Nevertheless, caution should be exercised in the use of multiple drug therapy.
TONOCARD is equally effective in digitalized and non-digitalized patients. In 17 patients with refractory ventricular arrhythmias on concomitant therapy, serum digoxin levels (1.1 ± 0.4 ng/mL) remained in the expected normal range (0.5–2.5 ng/mL) during tocainide administration.
Carcinogenesis, Mutagenesis, Impairment of Fertility
The carcinogenic potential of tocainide was studied in mice using oral doses up to 300 mg/kg/day (about 6 times the maximum recommended human dose) for up to 94 weeks in males and 102 weeks in females and in rats at doses up to 200 mg/kg/day for 24 months. Tocainide did not affect the type or incidence of neoplasia in the two studies.
Tocainide did not show any mutagenic potential when evaluated *in vivo* in the micronucleus test using mice at oral doses up to 187.5 mg/kg/day (about 7 times the usual human dose). Also, no mutagenic activity was seen *in vitro* in the Ames microbial mutagen test or in the mouse lymphoma forward mutation assay.
Reproduction and fertility studies in rats showed no adverse effects on male or female fertility at oral doses up to 200 mg/kg/day (about 8 times the usual human dose).
Pregnancy
Pregnancy Category C. In a teratogenicity study in rabbits, tocainide was administered orally at doses of 25, 50, and 100 mg/kg/day (about 1 to 4 times the usual human dose). No evidence of a drug-related teratogenic effect was noted; however, these doses were maternotoxic and produced a dose-related increase in abortions and stillbirths. In a teratogenicity study in rats, an oral dose of 300 mg/kg/day (about 12 times the usual human dose) showed no evidence of treatment-related fetal malformations, but maternotoxicity and an increase in fetal resorptions were noted. An oral dose of 30 mg/kg/day (about twice the usual human dose) did not produce any adverse effects.
In reproduction studies in rats at maternotoxic oral doses of 200 and 300 mg/kg/day (about 8 and 12 times the usual human dose, respectively), dystocia, and delayed parturition occurred which was accompanied by an increase in stillbirths and decreased survival in offspring during the first week postpartum. Growth and viability of surviving offspring were not affected for the remainder of the lactation period.
There are no adequate and well-controlled studies in pregnant women. TONOCARD should be used during pregnancy only if the potential benefit justifies the potential risk to the fetus.
Nursing Mothers
It is not known whether tocainide is secreted in human milk. Because many drugs are secreted in human milk and because of the potential for serious adverse reactions in nursing infants from TONOCARD, a decision should be made whether to discontinue nursing or to discontinue the drug, taking into account the importance of the drug to the mother.
Pediatric Use
Safety and effectiveness in children have not been established.

ADVERSE REACTIONS

TONOCARD commonly produces minor, transient, nervous system and gastrointestinal adverse reactions, but is otherwise generally well tolerated. TONOCARD has been evaluated in both short-term (n = 1,358) and long-term (n = 262) controlled studies as well as a compassionate use program. Dosages were lower in most of the controlled studies (1200 mg/day) and higher in the compassionate use program (1800 mg and more). In long-term (2–6 months) controlled studies, the most frequent adverse reactions were dizziness/vertigo (15.3 percent), nausea (14.5 percent), paresthesia (9.2 percent), and tremor (8.4 percent). These reactions were generally mild, transient, dose-related and reversible with a reduction in dosage, by taking the drug with food, or by therapy discontinuation. Tremor, when present, may be useful as a clinical indicator that the maximum dose is being approached. Adverse reactions leading to therapy discontinuation occurred in 21 percent of patients in long-term con-

trolled trials and were usually related to the nervous system or digestive system.
Adverse reactions occurring in greater than one percent of patients from the short-term and long-term controlled studies appear in the following table:

	Percent of Patients Controlled Studies	
	Short-term (n = 1,358)	Long-term (n = 262)
BODY AS A WHOLE		
Tiredness/drowsiness/fatigue/ lethargy/lassitude/ sleepiness	1.6	0.8
Hot/cold feelings	0.5	1.5
CARDIOVASCULAR		
Hypotension	3.4	2.7
Bradycardia	1.8	0.4
Palpitations	1.8	0.4
Chest pain	1.6	0.4
Conduction disorders	1.5	0.0
Left ventricular failure	1.4	0.0
DIGESTIVE		
Nausea	15.2	14.5
Vomiting	8.3	4.6
Anorexia	1.2	1.9
Diarrhea/loose stools	0.0	3.8
NERVOUS SYSTEM/PSYCHIATRIC		
Dizziness/vertigo	8.0	15.3
Paresthesia	3.5	9.2
Tremor	2.9	8.4
Confusion/disorientation/ hallucinations	2.1	2.7
Headache	2.1	4.6
Nervousness	1.5	0.4
Altered mood/awareness	1.5	3.4
Incoordination/unsteadiness/ walking disturbances	1.2	0.0
Anxiety	1.1	1.5
Ataxia	0.2	3.0
SKIN		
Diaphoresis	5.1	2.3
Rash/skin lesion	0.4	8.4
SPECIAL SENSES		
Blurred vision/visual disturbances	1.3	1.5
Tinnitus/hearing loss	0.4	1.5
Nystagmus	0.0	1.1

An additional group of about 2,000 patients has been treated in a program allowing for the use of TONOCARD under compassionate use circumstances. These patients were seriously ill with the large majority on multiple drug therapy, and comparatively high doses of TONOCARD were used. Fifty-four percent of the patients continued in the program for one year or longer, and 12 percent were treated for longer than three years, with the longest duration of therapy being nine years. Adverse reactions leading to therapy discontinuation occurred in 12 percent of patients (usually central nervous system effects or rash). A tabulation of adverse reactions occurring in one percent or more of patients follows:

	Percent of Patients Compassionate Use (n = 1,927)
CARDIOVASCULAR	
Increased ventricular arrhythmias/PVCs	10.9
CHF/progression of CHF	4.0
Tachycardia	3.2
Hypotension	1.8
Conduction disorders	1.3
Bradycardia	1.0
DIGESTIVE	
Nausea	24.6
Anorexia	11.3
Vomiting	9.0
Diarrhea/loose stools	6.8
MUSCULOSKELETAL	
Arthritis/arthralgia	4.7
Myalgia	1.7
NERVOUS SYSTEM/PSYCHIATRIC	
Dizziness/vertigo	25.3
Tremor	21.6
Nervousness	11.5
Confusion/disorientation/ hallucinations	11.2
Altered mood/awareness	11.0
Ataxia	10.8
Paresthesia	9.2

SKIN

Rash/skin lesion	12.2
Diaphoresis	8.3
Lupus	1.6

SPECIAL SENSES

Blurred vision/vision disturbances	10.0
Nystagmus	1.1

Adverse reactions occurring in less than one percent of patients in either the controlled studies or the compassionate use program or since the drug was marketed are as follows:

Body as a Whole: Septicemia; septic shock; syncope; vasovagal episodes; edema; fever; chills; cinchonism; asthenia; malaise.

Cardiovascular: Ventricular fibrillation; extension of acute myocardial infarction; cardiogenic shock; pulmonary embolism; angina; AV block; hypertension; claudication; increased QRS duration; pleurisy/pericarditis; prolonged QT interval; right bundle branch block; cardiomegaly; sinus arrest; vasculitis; orthostatic hypotension; cold extremities.

Digestive: Hepatitis, jaundice (see PRECAUTIONS), abnormal liver function tests; pancreatitis; abdominal pain/discomfort; constipation; dysphagia; gastrointestinal symptoms (including dyspepsia); stomatitis; dry mouth; thirst.

Hematologic: Agranulocytosis; bone marrow depression; aplastic/hypoplastic anemia; hemolytic anemia; anemia; leukopenia; neutropenia; thrombocytopenia; eosinophilia.

Metabolic and Immune: Hypersensitivity Reaction (including some of the following symptoms or signs: rash, fever, joint pains, abnormal liver function tests, eosinophilia); increased ANA.

Musculoskeletal: Muscle cramps; muscle twitching/spasm; neck pain; pain radiating from neck; pressure on shoulder.

Nervous System/Psychiatric: Coma; convulsions/seizures; myasthenia gravis; depression; psychosis; psychic disturbances; agitation; decreased mental acuity; dysarthria; impaired memory; increased stuttering/slurred speech; insomnia/sleeping disturbances; local anesthesia; dream abnormalities.

Respiratory: Respiratory arrest; pulmonary edema; pulmonary fibrosis; fibrosing alveolitis; pneumonia; interstitial pneumonitis; dyspnea; hiccough; yawning.

Skin: Stevens-Johnson syndrome; exfoliative dermatitis; erythema multiforme; urticaria; alopecia; pruritus; pallor/flushed face.

Special Senses: Diplopia; earache; taste perversion/smell perversion.

Urogenital: Urinary retention; polyuria/increased diuresis.

Agranulocytosis, bone marrow depression, leukopenia, neutropenia, aplastic/hypoplastic anemia, and thrombocytopenia have been reported (0.18 percent) in patients receiving TONOCARD in controlled trials and the compassionate use program. Most of these events have been noted during the first 12 weeks of therapy. (See Box WARNINGS).

Pulmonary fibrosis, interstitial pneumonitis, fibrosing alveolitis, pulmonary edema, and pneumonia, possibly drug related, have been reported in patients receiving TONOCARD. The incidence of pulmonary fibrosis (including interstitial pneumonitis and fibrosing alveolitis) was 0.11 percent in controlled trials and the compassionate use program. These events usually occurred in seriously ill patients. Symptoms of these pulmonary disorders and/or x-ray changes usually occurred following 3–18 weeks of therapy. Fatalities have been reported. (See Box WARNINGS.)

A number of disorders, in which a causal relationship with TONOCARD has not been established, have been reported in seriously ill patients. These include: renal failure, renal dysfunction, myocardial infarction, cerebrovascular accidents and transient ischemic attacks. These disorders may be related to the patients underlying condition.

DRUG ABUSE AND DEPENDENCE

Drug withdrawal after chronic treatment has not shown any indication of psychological or physical dependence.

OVERDOSAGE

The initial and most important signs and symptoms of overdosage would be expected to be related to the central nervous system. Other adverse reactions, such as gastrointestinal disturbances, may follow. (See ADVERSE REACTIONS). Should convulsions or cardiopulmonary depression or arrest develop, the patency of the airway and adequacy of ventilation must be assured immediately. Should convulsions persist despite ventilatory therapy with oxygen, small increments of anticonvulsive agents may be given intravenously. Examples of such agents include a benzodiazepine (e.g., diazepam), an ultra-short-acting barbiturate (e.g., thiopental or thiamylal), or a short-acting barbiturate (e.g., pentobarbital or secobarbital).

The oral LD_{50} of tocainide was calculated to be about 800 mg/kg in mice, 1000 mg/kg in rats, and 230 mg/kg in guinea pigs; deaths were usually preceded by convulsions.

Studies in normal individuals to date indicate that tocainide has a hemodialysis clearance approximately equivalent to its renal clearance.

DOSAGE AND ADMINISTRATION

The dosage of TONOCARD must be individualized on the basis of antiarrhythmic response and tolerance, both of which are dose related. Clinical and electrocardiographic evaluation (including Holter monitoring if necessary for evaluation) are needed to determine whether the desired antiarrhythmic response has been obtained and to guide titration and dose adjustment. Adverse effects appearing shortly after dosing, for example, suggest a need for dividing the dose further with a shorter dose-interval. Loss of arrhythmia control prior to the next dose suggests use of a shorter dose interval and/or a dose increase. Absence of a clear response suggests reconsideration of therapy.

The recommended initial dosage is 400 mg every 8 hours. The usual adult dosage is between 1200 and 1800 mg/day in a three dose daily divided regimen. Doses beyond 2400 mg per day have been administered infrequently. Patients who tolerate the t.i.d. regimen may be tried on a twice daily regimen with careful monitoring.

Some patients, particularly those with renal or hepatic impairment, may be adequately treated with less than 1200 mg/day.

HOW SUPPLIED

No. 3409—Tablets TONOCARD, 400 mg, are oval, yellow, scored, film-coated tablets, coded MSD 707. They are supplied as follows:

NDC 0006-0707-68 bottles of 100
(6505-01-203-6240 100's)
NDC 0006-0707-28 unit dose packages of 100.
Shown in Product Identification Section, page 419

No. 3410—Tablets TONOCARD, 600 mg, are oblong, yellow, scored, film-coated tablets, coded MSD 709. They are supplied as follows:

NDC 0006-0709-68 bottles of 100
(6505-01-206-0273 100's)
NDC 0006-0709-28 unit dose packages of 100.
Shown in Product Identification Section, page 419

A.H.F.S. Category: 24:04
DC 7369908 Issued June 1989
COPYRIGHT © MERCK & CO., INC., 1987, 1989
All rights reserved

TRIAVIL® Tablets
(Perphenazine-Amitriptyline HCl, MSD), U.S.P.

℞

DESCRIPTION

TRIAVIL® (Perphenazine-Amitriptyline HCl, MSD), a broad-spectrum psychotherapeutic agent for the management of outpatients and hospitalized patients with psychoses or neuroses characterized by mixtures of anxiety or agitation with symptoms of depression, is a combination of perphenazine and ELAVIL® (Amitriptyline HCl, MSD). Since such mixed syndromes can occur in patients with various degrees of intensity of mental illness, TRIAVIL tablets are provided in multiple combinations to afford dosage flexibility for optimum management.

TRIAVIL is a combination of perphenazine, a piperazine phenothiazine, and ELAVIL (Amitriptyline HCl, MSD), a dibenzocycloheptadiene.

Perphenazine

Perphenazine is 4-[3-(2-chloro-10*H*-phenothiazin-10-yl)-propyl]-1-piperazineethanol. Its empirical formula is $C_{21}H_{26}ClN_3OS$ and its structural formula is:

Perphenazine has a molecular weight of 403.97. It is a white, odorless, bitter-tasting powder that is insoluble in water.

ELAVIL (Amitriptyline HCl, MSD)

Amitriptyline hydrochloride is 3-(10,11-dihydro-5*H*-dibenzo[a,d]cyclohepten-5-ylidene)-*N,N*-dimethyl-1-propanamine hydrochloride. Its empirical formula is $C_{20}H_{23}N \cdot HCl$ and its structural formula is:

Amitriptyline HCl, a dibenzocycloheptadiene derivative, has a molecular weight of 313.87. It is a white, odorless, crystalline compound which is freely soluble in water.

Tablets TRIAVIL are supplied in 5 potencies:
TRIAVIL 2-10, containing 2 mg of perphenazine and 10 mg of amitriptyline HCl.
TRIAVIL 2-25, containing 2 mg of perphenazine and 25 mg of amitriptyline HCl.
TRIAVIL 4-10, containing 4 mg of perphenazine and 10 mg of amitriptyline HCl.
TRIAVIL 4-25, containing 4 mg of perphenazine and 25 mg of amitriptyline HCl.
TRIAVIL 4-50, containing 4 mg of perphenazine and 50 mg of amitriptyline HCl.

Inactive ingredients are calcium phosphate, cellulose, hydroxypropyl cellulose, hydroxypropyl methylcellulose, lactose, magnesium stearate, starch, talc, and titanium dioxide. TRIAVIL 2-10 also contains FD&C Blue 1. TRIAVIL 2-25 and 4-50 also contain FD&C Yellow 6. TRIAVIL 4-10 also contains iron oxide. TRIAVIL 4-25 also contains D&C Yellow 10 and FD&C Yellow 6.

ACTIONS

Perphenazine—In common with all members of the piperazine group of phenothiazine derivatives, perphenazine has greater behavioral potency than phenothiazine derivatives of other groups without a corresponding increase in autonomic, hematologic, or hepatic side effects.

Extrapyramidal effects, however, may occur more frequently. These effects are interpreted as neuropharmacologic. They usually regress after discontinuation of the drug. Perphenazine is a potent tranquilizer and also a potent antiemetic. Orally, its milligram potency is about five or six times that of chlorpromazine with respect to behavioral effects. It is capable of alleviating symptoms of anxiety, tension, psychomotor excitement, and other manifestations of emotional stress without apparent dulling of mental acuity.

ELAVIL (Amitriptyline HCl, MSD) is an antidepressant with sedative effects. Its mechanism of action in man is not known. It is not a monoamine oxidase inhibitor and it does not act primarily by stimulation of the central nervous system.

INDICATIONS

TRIAVIL is recommended for treatment of (1) patients with *moderate to severe anxiety and/or agitation and depressed mood*, (2) patients with *depression in whom anxiety and/or agitation are severe*, and (3) patients with *depression and anxiety in association with chronic physical disease*. In many of these patients anxiety masks the depressive state so that, although therapy with a tranquilizer appears to be indicated, the administration of a tranquilizer alone will not be adequate.

Schizophrenic patients who have associated depressive symptoms should be considered for therapy with TRIAVIL.

Many patients presenting symptoms such as agitation, anxiety, insomnia, psychomotor retardation, functional somatic complaints, a feeling of tiredness, loss of interest, and anorexia have responded well to therapy with TRIAVIL.

CONTRAINDICATIONS

TRIAVIL is contraindicated in depression of the central nervous system from drugs (barbiturates, alcohol, narcotics, analgesics, antihistamines); in the presence of evidence of bone marrow depression; and in patients known to be hypersensitive to phenothiazines or amitriptyline.

It should not be given concomitantly with monoamine oxidase inhibitors. Hyperpyretic crises, severe convulsions, and deaths have occurred in patients receiving tricyclic antidepressants and monoamine oxidase inhibitors simultaneously. When it is desired to replace a monoamine oxidase inhibitor with TRIAVIL, a minimum of 14 days should be allowed to elapse after the former is discontinued. TRIAVIL should then be initiated cautiously with gradual increase in dosage until optimum response is achieved.

Amitriptyline HCl is not recommended for use during the acute recovery phase following myocardial infarction.

WARNINGS

Tardive dyskinesia

Tardive dyskinesia, a syndrome consisting of potentially irreversible, involuntary dyskinetic movements may develop in patients treated with neuroleptic (antipsychotic) drugs. Although the prevalence of the syndrome appears to be high-

Continued on next page

Merck Sharp & Dohme—Cont.

est among the elderly, especially elderly women, it is impossible to rely upon prevalence estimates to predict, at the inception of neuroleptic treatment, which patients are likely to develop the syndrome. Whether neuroleptic drug products differ in their potential to cause tardive dyskinesia is unknown.

Both the risk of developing the syndrome and the likelihood that it will become irreversible are believed to increase as the duration of treatment and the total cumulative dose of neuroleptic drugs administered to the patient increase. However, the syndrome can develop, although much less commonly, after relatively brief treatment periods at low doses. There is no known treatment for established cases of tardive dyskinesia, although the syndome may remit, partially or completely, if neuroleptic treatment is withdrawn. Neuroleptic treatment, itself, however, may suppress (or partially suppress) the signs and symptoms of the syndrome and thereby may possibly mask the underlying disease process. The effect that symptomatic suppression has upon the long-term course of the syndrome is unknown.

Given these considerations, neuroleptics should be prescribed in a manner that is most likely to minimize the occurrence of tardive dyskinesia. Chronic neuroleptic treatment should generally be reserved for patients who suffer from a chronic mental illness that, 1) is known to respond to neuroleptic drugs, and, 2) for whom alternative, equally effective, but potentially less harmful treatments are *not* available or appropriate. In patients who do require chronic treatment, the smallest dose and the shortest duration of treatment producing a satisfactory clinical response should be sought. The need for continued treatment should be reassessed periodically.

If signs and symptoms of tardive dyskinesia appear in a patient on neuroleptics, drug discontinuation should be considered. However, some patients may require treatment despite the presence of the syndrome.

(For further information about the description of tardive dyskinesia and its clinical detection, please refer to the section on ADVERSE REACTIONS).

Neuroleptic Malignant Syndrome (NMS)

A potentially fatal symptom complex sometimes referred to as Neuroleptic Malignant Syndrome (NMS) has been reported in association with antipsychotic drugs. Clinical manifestations of NMS are hyperpyrexia, muscle rigidity, altered mental status and evidence of autonomic instability (irregular pulse or blood pressure, tachycardia, diaphoresis, and cardiac dysrhythmias).

The diagnostic evaluation of patients with this syndrome is complicated. In arriving at a diagnosis, it is important to identify cases where the clinical presentation includes both serious medical illness (e.g., pneumonia, systemic infection, etc.) and untreated or inadequately treated extrapyramidal signs and symptoms (EPS). Other important considerations in the differential diagnosis include central anticholinergic toxicity, heat stroke, drug fever and primary central nervous system (CNS) pathology.

The management of NMS should include 1) immediate discontinuation of antipsychotic drugs and other drugs not essential to concurrent therapy, 2) intensive symptomatic treatment and medical monitoring, and 3) treatment of any concomitant serious medical problems for which specific treatments are available. There is no general agreement about specific pharmacological treatment regimens for uncomplicated NMS.

If a patient requires antipsychotic drug treatment after recovery from NMS, the potential reintroduction of drug therapy should be carefully considered. The patient should be carefully monitored, since recurrences of NMS have been reported.

General

TRIAVIL should not be given concomitantly with guanethidine or similarly acting compounds, since amitriptyline, like other tricyclic antidepressants, may block the antihypertensive effect of these compounds.

Because of the atropine-like activity of amitriptyline, TRIAVIL should be used with caution in patients with a history of urinary retention, or with angle-closure glaucoma or increased intraocular pressure. In patients with angle-closure glaucoma, even average doses may precipitate an attack.

It should be used with caution also in patients with convulsive disorders. Dosage of anticonvulsive agents may have to be increased.

Patients with cardiovascular disorders should be watched closely. Tricyclic antidepressants, including amitriptyline HCl, particularly when given in high doses, have been reported to produce arrhythmias, sinus tachycardia, and prolongation of the conduction time. Myocardial infarction and stroke have been reported with drugs of this class.

Close supervision is required when amitriptyline HCl is given to hyperthyroid patients or those receiving thyroid medication.

TRIAVIL may enhance the response to alcohol and the effects of barbiturates and other CNS depressants. In patients who may use alcohol excessively, it should be borne in mind that the potentiation may increase the danger inherent in any suicide attempt or overdosage. Delirium has been reported with concurrent administration of amitriptyline and disulfiram.

Usage in Pregnancy—TRIAVIL is not recommended for use in pregnant patients or in nursing mothers at this time. Reproduction studies in rats have shown no fetal abnormalities; however, clinical experience and follow-up in pregnancy have been limited, and the possibility of adverse effects on fetal development must be considered.

Usage in Children—Since dosage for children has not been established, TRIAVIL is not recommended for use in children.

PRECAUTIONS

General

The possibility of suicide in depressed patients remains during treatment and until significant remission occurs. Such patients should not have access to large quantities of this drug.

Perphenazine

As with all phenothiazine compounds, perphenazine should not be used indiscriminately. Caution should be observed in giving it to patients who have previously exhibited severe adverse reactions to other phenothiazines.

Some of the untoward actions of perphenazine tend to appear more frequently when high doses are used. However, as with other phenothiazine compounds, patients receiving perphenazine in any dosage should be kept under close supervision.

The antiemetic effect of perphenazine may obscure signs of toxicity due to overdosage of other drugs, or render more difficult the diagnosis of disorders such as brain tumors or intestinal obstruction.

A significant, not otherwise explained, rise in body temperature may suggest individual intolerance to perphenazine, in which case TRIAVIL should be discontinued.

Neuroleptic drugs elevate prolactin levels; the elevation persists during chronic administration. Tissue culture experiments indicate that approximately one third of human breast cancers are prolactin dependent *in vitro*, a factor of potential importance if the prescription of these drugs is contemplated in a patient with a previously detected breast cancer. Although disturbances such as galactorrhea, amenorrhea, gynecomastia, and impotence have been reported, the clinical significance of elevated serum prolactin levels is unknown for most patients. An increase in mammary neoplasms has been found in rodents after chronic administration of neuroleptic drugs. Neither clinical studies nor epidemiologic studies conducted to date, however, have shown an association between chronic administration of these drugs and mammary tumorigenesis; the available evidence is considered too limited to be conclusive at this time.

ELAVIL (Amitriptyline HCl, MSD)

Depressed patients, particularly those with known manic depressive illness, may experience a shift to mania or hypomania. Patients with paranoid symptomatology may have an exaggeration of such symptoms. The tranquilizing effect of TRIAVIL seems to reduce the likelihood of these effects.

Concurrent administration of amitriptyline HCl and electroshock therapy may increase the hazards associated with such therapy. Such treatment should be limited to patients for whom it is essential.

Discontinue the drug several days before elective surgery if possible.

Both elevation and lowering of blood sugar levels have been reported.

ELAVIL (Amitriptyline HCl, MSD) should be used with caution in patients with impaired liver function.

Information for Patients

While on therapy with TRIAVIL, patients should be advised as to the possible impairment of mental and/or physical abilities required for performance of hazardous tasks, such as operating machinery or driving a motor vehicle.

Drug Interactions

Perphenazine

If hypotension develops, epinephrine should not be employed, as its action is blocked and partially reversed by perphenazine.

Phenothiazines may potentiate the action of central nervous system depressants (opiates, analgesics, antihistamines, barbiturates, alcohol) and atropine. In concurrent therapy with any of these, TRIAVIL should be given in reduced dosage. Phenothiazines also may potentiate the action of heat and phosphorous insecticides.

ELAVIL (Amitriptyline HCl, MSD)

When ELAVIL (Amitriptyline HCl, MSD) is given with anticholinergic agents or sympathomimetic drugs, including epinephrine combined with local anesthetics, close supervision and careful adjustment of dosages are required.

Hyperpyrexia has been reported when ELAVIL (Amitriptyline HCl, MSD) is administered with anticholinergic agents or with neuroleptic drugs, particularly during hot weather. Paralytic ileus may occur in patients taking tricyclic antidepressants in combination with anticholinergic-type drugs. Cimetidine is reported to reduce hepatic metabolism of certain tricyclic antidepressants, thereby delaying elimination and increasing steady-state concentrations of these drugs. Clinically significant effects have been reported with the tricyclic antidepressants when used concomitantly with cimetidine. Increases in plasma levels of tricyclic antidepressants, and in the frequency and severity of side effects, particularly anticholinergic, have been reported when cimetidine was added to the drug regimen. Discontinuation of cimetidine in well-controlled patients receiving tricyclic antidepressants and cimetidine may decrease the plasma levels and efficacy of the antidepressants.

Caution is advised if patients receive large doses of etchlorvynol concurrently. Transient delirium has been reported in patients who were treated with 1 g of ethchlorvynol and 75-150 mg of ELAVIL (Amitriptyline HCl, MSD).

ADVERSE REACTIONS

To date, clinical evaluation of TRIAVIL has not revealed any adverse reactions peculiar to the combination. The adverse reactions that occurred were limited to those that have been reported previously for perphenazine and amitriptyline.

Treatment with TRIAVIL is commonly associated with sedation, hypotension, neurological impairments, and dry mouth.

Perphenazine

The common acute neurological effects of neuroleptic drugs, including perphenazine, consist of dystonia, akathisia or motor restlessness, and pseudoparkinsonism.

More chronic use of neuroleptics may be associated with the development of tardive dyskinesia. The salient features of this syndrome are described in the WARNINGS section and below.

The following adverse reactions have been reported and, within each category, are listed in order of decreasing severity.

Neurological:

Tardive dyskinesia:

The syndrome is characterized by involuntary choreoathetoid movements which variously involve the tongue, face, mouth, lips, or jaw (e.g., protrusion of the tongue, puffing of cheeks, puckering of the mouth, chewing movements), trunk and extremities. The severity of the syndrome and the degree of impairment produced vary widely.

The syndrome may become clinically recognizable either during treatment, upon dosage reduction, or upon withdrawal of treatment. Movements may decrease in intensity and may disappear altogether if further treatment with neuroleptics is withheld. It is generally believed that reversibility is more likely after short rather than long term neuroleptic exposure. Consequently, early detection of tardive dyskinesia is important. To increase the likelihood of detecting the syndrome at the earliest possible time, the dosage of neuroleptic drug should be reduced periodically (if clinically possible) and the patient observed for signs of the disorder. It has been suggested that fine vermicular movements of the tongue may be an early sign of the syndrome, and that the full-blown syndrome may not develop if medication is stopped when lingual vermiculation appears.

1. Dystonia

This may present as acute, reversible torticollis, opisthotonos, carpopedal spasm, trismus, dysphagia, respiratory difficulty, oculogyric crisis, and protrusion of the tongue. Treatment consists of the parenteral administration of either an anticholinergic antiparkinsonian agent or diphenhydramine.

2. Akathisia

Akathisia presents as constant motor restlessness. The patient with akathisia often complains, *when asked*, about his/her inability to stop moving. Akathisia should *not* be treated with an increased dose of neuroleptic; rather, the dose of antipsychotic may be lowered until the motor restlessness has subsided. The efficacy of anticholinergic treatment of this side effect is unestablished.

3. Pseudoparkinsonism

Pseudoparkinsonism refers to a drug-induced state similar to the classic syndrome. Generally, anticholinergic antiparkinsonian agents (i.e., benztropine, biperiden, procyclidine, or trihexphenidyl) and amantadine are helpful in alleviating symptoms that cannot be managed by neuroleptic dose reduction. The value of prophylactic antiparkinsonian drug therapy has not been established. The need for continued use of antiparkinsonian medication should be re-evaluated periodically.

Cardiovascular: Hypotension, hypertension, tachycardia, peripheral edema, occasional change in pulse rate, ECG abnormalities (quinidine-like effect), reversed epinephrine effect.

CNS and Neuromuscular: Neuroleptic malignant syndrome (see WARNINGS); extrapyramidal symptoms, including acute dyskinesia (see *Neurological*); reactivation of psychoses and production of catatonic-like states; paradoxical excitement; ataxia; muscle weakness; hypnotic effects; mild insomnia; lassitude; headache; hyperflexia; altered cerebrospinal fluid proteins.

Autonomic: Urinary frequency or incontinence, dry mouth or salivation, nasal congestion.

Allergic: Anaphylactoid reactions, laryngeal edema, asthma, angioneurotic edema.

Hematologic: Blood dyscrasias including pancytopenia, agranulocytosis, leukopenia, thrombocytopenic purpura, eosinophilia.

Gastrointestinal: Liver damage (jaundice, biliary stasis), obstipation, vomiting, nausea, constipation, anorexia.

Dermatologic: Eczema up to exfoliative dermatitis, urticaria, erythema, itching, photosensitivity.

Ophthalmic: Pigmentation of the cornea and lens, blurred vision.

Endocrine: Lactation, galactorrhea, hyperglycemia, gynecomastia, disturbances in menstrual cycle.

Other: False-positive pregnancy tests, including immunologic.

Other adverse reactions that should be considered because they have been reported with various phenothiazine compounds, but not with perphenazine, include:

CNS and Neuromuscular: Grand mal convulsions, cerebral edema.

Gastrointestinal: Polyphagia.

Dermatologic: Photophobia, pigmentation.

Ophthalmic: Pigmentary retinopathy.

Endocrine: Failure of ejaculation.

ELAVIL (Amitriptyline HCl, MSD)

Within each category the following adverse reactions are listed in order of decreasing severity. Included in the listing are a few adverse reactions which have not been reported with this specific drug. However, pharmacological similarities among the tricyclic antidepressant drugs require that each of the reactions be considered when amitriptyline is administered.

Cardiovascular: Myocardial infarction; stroke; heart block; arrhythmias; hypotension, particularly orthostatic hypotension; hypertension; tachycardia; palpitation.

CNS and Neuromuscular: Coma; seizures; hallucinations; delusions; confusional states; disorientation; incoordination; ataxia; tremors; peripheral neuropathy; numbness, tingling, and paresthesias of the extremities; extrapyramidal symptoms; dysarthria; disturbed concentration; excitement; anxiety; insomnia; restlessness; nightmares; drowsiness; dizziness; weakness; fatigue; headache; syndrome of inappropriate ADH (antidiuretic hormone) secretion; tinnitus; alteration in EEG patterns.

Anticholinergic: Paralytic ileus; hyperpyrexia; urinary retention, dilatation of the urinary tract; constipation; blurred vision, disturbance of accommodation, increased intraocular pressure, mydriasis; dry mouth.

Allergic: Skin rash; urticaria; photosensitization; edema of face and tongue.

Hematologic: Bone marrow depression including agranulocytosis, leukopenia, thrombocytopenia; purpura; eosinophilia.

Gastrointestinal: Rarely hepatitis (including altered liver function and jaundice); nausea; epigastric distress; vomiting; anorexia; stomatitis; peculiar taste; diarrhea; parotid swelling; black tongue.

Endocrine: Testicular swelling and gynecomastia in the male; breast enlargement and galactorrhea in the female; increased or decreased libido; elevation and lowering of blood sugar levels.

Other: Alopecia; edema; weight gain or loss; urinary frequency; increased perspiration.

Withdrawal Symptoms: After prolonged administration, abrupt cessation of treatment may produce nausea, headache, and malaise. Gradual dosage reduction has been reported to produce within two weeks, transient symptoms including irritability, restlessness, and dream and sleep disturbance. These symptoms are not indicative of addiction. Rare instances have been reported of mania or hypomania occurring within 2-7 days following cessation of chronic therapy wih tricyclic antidepressants.

DOSAGE AND ADMINISTRATION

Since dosage for children has not been established, TRIAVIL is not recommended for use in children.

The total daily dose of TRIAVIL should not exceed four tablets of the 4-50 or eight tablets of any other dosage strength.

Initial Dosage

In psychoneurotic patients when anxiety and depression are of such a degree as to warrant combined therapy, one tablet of TRIAVIL 2-25 or TRIAVIL 4-25 three or four times a day or one tablet of TRIAVIL 4-50 twice a day is recommended. *In more severely ill patients with schizophrenia,* TRIAVIL 4-25 is recommended in an initial dose of two tablets three

times a day. If necessary, a fourth dose may be given at bedtime.

In elderly patients and adolescents, and some other patients in whom anxiety tends to predominate, TRIAVIL 4-10 may be administered three or four times a day initially, then adjusted as required for subsequent adequate therapy.

Maintenance Dosage

Depending on the condition being treated, therapeutic response may take from a few days to a few weeks or even longer. After a satisfactory response is noted, dosage should be reduced to the smallest amount necessary to obtain relief from the symptoms for which TRIAVIL is being administered. A useful maintenance dosage is one tablet of TRIAVIL 2-25 or 4-25 two to four times a day or one tablet of TRIAVIL 4-50 twice a day. TRIAVIL 2-10 and 4-10 can be used to increase flexibility in adjusting maintenance dosage to the lowest amount consistent with relief of symptoms. In some patients, maintenance dosage is required for many months.

OVERDOSAGE

Manifestations—High doses may cause temporary confusion, disturbed concentration, or transient visual hallucinations. Overdosage may cause drowsiness; hypothermia; tachycardia and other arrhythmic abnormalities, such as bundle branch block; ECG evidence of impaired conduction; congestive heart failure; dilated pupils; disorders of ocular motility; convulsions; severe hypotension; stupor; and coma. Other symptoms may be agitation, hyperactive reflexes, muscle rigidity, vomiting, hyperpyrexia, or any of the adverse reactions listed for perphenazine or amitriptyline.

Levarterenol (norepinephrine) may be used to treat hypotension, but not epinephrine.

All patients suspected of having taken an overdosage should be admitted to a hospital as soon as possible. *Treatment* is symptomatic and supportive. Empty the stomach as quickly as possible by emesis followed by gastric lavage upon arrival at the hospital. Saline emetics should not be used as the antiemetic effect of perphenazine may cause retention of the saline load and subsequent hypernatremia. Following gastric lavage, activated charcoal may be administered. Twenty to 30 g of activated charcoal may be given every four to six hours during the first 24 to 48 hours after ingestion. An ECG should be taken and close monitoring of cardiac function instituted if there is any sign of abnormality. Maintain an open airway and adequate fluid intake; regulate body temperature.

The intravenous administration of 1–3 mg of physostigmine salicylate is reported to reverse the symptoms of tricyclic antidepressant poisoning. Because physostigmine is rapidly metabolized, the dosage of physostigmine should be repeated as required particularly if life threatening signs such as arrhythmias, convulsions, and deep coma recur or persist after the initial dosage of physostigmine. On this basis, in severe overdosage with perphenazine-amitriptyline combinations, symptomatic treatment of central anticholinergic effects with physostigmine salicylate should be considered. Because physostigmine itself may be toxic, it is not recommended for routine use.

Standard measures should be used to manage circulatory shock and metabolic acidosis. Cardiac arrhythmias may be treated with neostigmine, pyridostigmine, or propranolol. Should cardiac failure occur, the use of digitalis should be considered. Close monitoring of cardiac function for not less than five days is advisable.

Anticonvulsants may be given to control convulsions. Amitriptyline and perphenazine increase the CNS depressant action but not the anticonvulsant action of barbiturates; therefore, an inhalation anesthetic, diazepam, or paraldehyde is recommended for control of convulsions. The management of acute symptoms of parkinsonism resulting from perphenazine intoxication may be treated with appropriate doses of COGENTIN® (Benztropine Mesylate, MSD) or diphenhydramine hydrochloride.*

Dialysis is of no value because of low plasma concentrations of the drug.

Since overdosage is often deliberate, patients may attempt suicide by other means during the recovery phase.

Deaths by deliberate or accidental overdosage have occurred with this class of drugs.

HOW SUPPLIED

No. 3328—Tablets TRIAVIL 2-10 are blue, triangular, film

----

*BENADRYL® (Diphenhydramine Hydrochloride), Parke, Davis & Co.

coated tablets, coded MSD 914. They are supplied as follows:

NDC 0006-0914-68 bottles of 100
NDC 0006-0914-28 unit dose package of 100
NDC 0006-0914-74 bottles of 500.
  Shown in Product Identification Section, page 419
No. 3311—Tablets TRIAVIL 2-25 are orange, triangular, film coated tablets, coded MSD 921. They are supplied as follows:
NDC 0006-0921-68 bottles of 100
NDC 0006-0921-28 unit dose package of 100
NDC 0006-0921-74 bottles of 500.
(6505-01-210-4467 500's)
  Shown in Product Identification Section, page 419
No. 3310—Tablets TRIAVIL 4-10 are salmon, triangular, film coated tablets, coded MSD 934. They are supplied as follows:
NDC 0006-0934-68 bottles of 100
NDC 0006-0934-28 unit dose package of 100
NDC 0006-0934-74 bottles of 500.
  Shown in Product Identification Section, page 419
No. 3312—Tablets TRIAVIL 4-25 are yellow, triangular, film coated tablets, coded MSD 946. They are supplied as follows:
NDC 0006-0946-68 bottles of 100
(6505-01-210-4468 100's)
NDC 0006-0946-28 unit dose package of 100
NDC 0006-0946-74 bottles of 500.
  Shown in Product Identification Section, page 419
No. 3364—Tablets TRIAVIL 4-50 are orange, diamond shaped, film coated tablets, coded MSD 517. They are supplied as follows:
NDC 0006-0517-60 bottles of 60
NDC 0006-0517-68 bottles of 100
NDC 0006-0517-28 unit dose package of 100.
  Shown in Product Identification Section, page 419
Storage
Store Tablets TRIAVIL in a well-closed container. Avoid storage at temperatures above 40°C (104°F). In addition, Tablets TRIAVIL 2–10 must be protected from light and stored in a well-closed, light-resistant container.
  A.H.F.S. Categories: 28:16:04, 28:16:08
  DC 7398429   Issued July 1987
COPYRIGHT © MERCK & CO., INC. 1985
All rights reserved

TURBINAIRE®—see under
DECADRON® Phosphate, TURBINAIRE®
(Dexamethasone Sodium Phosphate, MSD)

URECHOLINE® Tablets   ℞
(Bethanechol Chloride, MSD), U.S.P.
URECHOLINE® Injection   ℞
(Bethanechol Chloride, MSD), U.S.P.

DESCRIPTION

URECHOLINE® (Bethanechol Chloride, MSD), a cholinergic agent, is a synthetic ester which is structurally and pharmacologically related to acetylcholine.

It is designated chemically as 2-[(aminocarbonyl)oxy]-*N, N, N*-trimethyl-1-propanaminium chloride. Its empirical formula is $C_7H_{17}ClN_2O_2$ and its structural formula is:

$$\left[\begin{array}{c} CH_3CH-CH_2N^+(CH_3)_3 \\ | \\ OCONH_2 \end{array} \right] Cl^-$$

It is a white, hygroscopic crystalline compound having a slight amine-like odor, freely soluble in water, and has a molecular weight of 196.68.

URECHOLINE is supplied as 5 mg, 10 mg, 25 mg, and 50 mg tablets for oral use. Inactive ingredients in the tablets are calcium phosphate, lactose, magnesium stearate, and starch. Tablets URECHOLINE 10 mg also contain FD&C Red 3 and FD&C Red 40. Tablets URECHOLINE 25 mg and 50 mg also contain D&C Yellow 10 and FD&C Yellow 6.

URECHOLINE is also supplied as a sterile solution **for subcutaneous use only.** The sterile solution is essentially neutral. Each milliliter contains bethanechol chloride, 5 mg, and Water for Injection, q.s., 1 mL. It may be autoclaved at 120° C for 20 minutes without discoloration or loss of potency.

CLINICAL PHARMACOLOGY

Bethanechol chloride acts principally by producing the effects of stimulation of the parasympathetic nervous system. It increases the tone of the detrusor urinae muscle, usually producing a contraction sufficiently strong to initiate micturition and empty the bladder. It stimulates gastric motility,

Continued on next page

Information on the Merck Sharp & Dohme products listed on these pages is the full prescribing information from product circulars in use August 31, 1989.

Merck Sharp & Dohme—Cont.

increases gastric tone, and often restores impaired rhythmic peristalsis.

Stimulation of the parasympathetic nervous system releases acetylcholine at the nerve endings. When spontaneous stimulation is reduced and therapeutic intervention is required, acetylcholine can be given, but it is rapidly hydrolyzed by cholinesterase, and its effects are transient. Bethanechol chloride is not destroyed by cholinesterase and its effects are more prolonged than those of acetylcholine.

Effects on the GI and urinary tracts sometimes appear within 30 minutes after oral administration of bethanechol chloride, but more often 60–90 minutes are required to reach maximum effectiveness. Following oral administration, the usual duration of action of bethanechol is one hour, although large doses (300–400 mg) have been reported to produce effects for up to six hours. Subcutaneous injection produces a more intense action on bladder muscle than does oral administration of the drug.

Because of the selective action of bethanechol, nicotinic symptoms of cholinergic stimulation are usually absent or minimal when orally or subcutaneously administered in therapeutic doses, while muscarinic effects are prominent. Muscarinic effects usually occur within 5–15 minutes after subcutaneous injection, reach a maximum in 15–30 minutes, and disappear within two hours. Doses that stimulate micturition and defecation and increase peristalsis do not ordinarily stimulate ganglia or voluntary muscles. Therapeutic test doses in normal human subjects have little effect on heart rate, blood pressure, or peripheral circulation.

Bethanechol chloride does not cross the blood-brain barrier because of its charged quaternary amine moiety. The metabolic fate and mode of excretion of the drug have not been elucidated.

A clinical study* was conducted on the relative effectiveness of oral and subcutaneous doses of bethanechol chloride on the stretch response of bladder muscle in patients with urinary retention. Results showed that 5 mg of the drug given subcutaneously stimulated a response that was more rapid in onset and of larger magnitude than an oral dose of 50 mg, 100 mg, or 200 mg. All the oral doses, however, had a longer duration of effect than the subcutaneous dose. Although the 50 mg oral dose caused little change in intravesical pressure in this study, this dose has been found in other studies to be clinically effective in the rehabilitation of patients with decompensated bladders.

INDICATIONS AND USAGE

For the treatment of acute postoperative and postpartum nonobstructive (functional) urinary retention and for neurogenic atony of the urinary bladder with retention.

CONTRAINDICATIONS

Hypersensitivity to URECHOLINE tablets or to any component of URECHOLINE injection, hyperthyroidism, peptic ulcer, latent or active bronchial asthma, pronounced bradycardia or hypotension, vasomotor instability, coronary artery disease, epilepsy, and parkinsonism.

URECHOLINE should not be employed when the strength or integrity of the gastrointestinal or bladder wall is in question, or in the presence of mechanical obstruction; when increased muscular activity of the gastrointestinal tract or urinary bladder might prove harmful, as following recent urinary bladder surgery, gastrointestinal resection and anastomosis, or when there is possible gastrointestinal obstruction; in bladder neck obstruction, spastic gastrointestinal disturbances, acute inflammatory lesions of the gastrointestinal tract, or peritonitis; or in marked vagotonia.

WARNING

The sterile solution is for subcutaneous use only. It should never be given intramuscularly or intravenously. Violent symptoms of cholinergic over-stimulation, such as circulatory collapse, fall in blood pressure, abdominal cramps, bloody diarrhea, shock, or sudden cardiac arrest are likely to occur if the drug is given by either of these routes. Although rare, these same symptoms have occurred after subcutaneous injection, and may occur in cases of hypersensitivity or overdosage.

PRECAUTIONS

General

In urinary retention, if the sphincter fails to relax as URECHOLINE contracts the bladder, urine may be forced up the ureter into the kidney pelvis. If there is bacteriuria, this may cause reflux infection.

*Diokno, A. C.; Lapides, J., Urol. *10:* 23–24, July 1977.

Information for Patients

URECHOLINE tablets should preferably be taken one hour before or two hours after meals to avoid nausea or vomiting. Dizziness, lightheadedness or fainting may occur, especially when getting up from a lying or sitting position.

Drug Interactions

Special care is required if this drug is given to patients receiving ganglion blocking compounds because a critical fall in blood pressure may occur. Usually, severe abdominal symptoms appear before there is such a fall in the blood pressure.

Carcinogenesis, Mutagenesis, Impairment of Fertility

Long-term studies in animals have not been performed to evaluate the effects upon fertility, mutagenic or carcinogenic potential of URECHOLINE.

Pregnancy

Pregnancy Category C. Animal reproduction studies have not been conducted with URECHOLINE. It is also not known whether URECHOLINE can cause fetal harm when administered to a pregnant woman or can affect reproduction capacity. URECHOLINE should be given to a pregnant woman only if clearly needed.

Nursing Mothers

It is not known whether this drug is secreted in human milk. Because many drugs are secreted in human milk and because of the potential for serious adverse reactions from URECHOLINE in nursing infants, a decision should be made whether to discontinue nursing or to discontinue the drug, taking into account the importance of the drug to the mother.

Pediatric Use

Safety and effectiveness in children have not been established.

ADVERSE REACTIONS

Adverse reactions are rare following oral administration of bethanechol, but are more common following subcutaneous injection. Adverse reactions are more likely to occur when dosage is increased.

The following adverse reactions have been observed: *Body as a Whole:* malaise; *Digestive:* abdominal cramps or discomfort, colicky pain, nausea and belching, diarrhea, borborygmi, salivation; *Renal:* urinary urgency; *Nervous System:* headache; *Cardiovascular:* a fall in blood pressure with reflex tachycardia, vasomotor response; *Skin:* flushing producing a feeling of warmth, sensation of heat about the face, sweating; *Respiratory:* bronchial constriction, asthmatic attacks; *Special Senses:* lacrimation, miosis.

OVERDOSAGE

Early signs of overdosage are abdominal discomfort, salivation, flushing of the skin ("hot feeling"), sweating, nausea and vomiting.

Atropine is a specific antidote. The recommended dose for adults is 0.6 mg (1/100 grain). Repeat doses can be given every two hours, according to clinical response. The recommended dosage in infants and children up to 12 years of age is 0.01 mg/kg (to a maximum single dose of 0.4 mg) repeated every two hours as needed until the desired effect is obtained, or adverse effects of atropine preclude further usage. Subcutaneous injection of atropine is preferred except in emergencies when the intravenous route may be employed. When URECHOLINE is administered subcutaneously, a syringe containing a dose of atropine sulfate should always be available to treat symptoms of toxicity.

The oral LD_{50} of bethanechol chloride is 1510 mg/kg in the mouse.

DOSAGE AND ADMINISTRATION

Dosage and route of administration must be individualized, depending on the type and severity of the condition to be treated.

Preferably give the drug when the stomach is empty. If taken soon after eating, nausea and vomiting may occur.

Oral—The usual adult dosage is 10 to 50 mg three or four times a day. The minimum effective dose is determined by giving 5 or 10 mg initially and repeating the same amount at hourly intervals until satisfactory response occurs or until a maximum of 50 mg has been given. The effects of the drug sometimes appear within 30 minutes and usually within 60 to 90 minutes. They persist for about an hour.

Subcutaneous—The usual dose is 1 mL (5 mg), although some patients respond satisfactorily to as little as 0.5 mL (2.5 mg). The minimum effective dose is determined by injecting 0.5 mL (2.5 mg) initially and repeating the same amount at 15 to 30 minute intervals to a maximum of four doses until satisfactory response is obtained, unless disturbing reactions appear. The minimum effective dose may be repeated thereafter three or four times a day as required.

Rarely, single doses up to 2 mL (10 mg) may be required. Such large doses may cause severe reactions and should be used only after adequate trial of single doses of 0.5 to 1 mL

(2.5 to 5 mg) has established that smaller doses are not sufficient.

URECHOLINE is usually effective in 5 to 15 minutes after subcutaneous injection.

If necessary, the effects of the drug can be abolished promptly by atropine (see OVERDOSAGE).

Parenteral drug products should be inspected visually for particulate matter and discoloration prior to administration, whenever solution and container permit.

HOW SUPPLIED

Tablets URECHOLINE are round, compressed tablets, scored on one side. They are supplied as follows:

No. 7785—5 mg, white in color, coded MSD 403.
NDC 0006-0403-68 in bottles of 100
NDC 0006-0403-28 unit dose packages of 100.
   Shown in Product Identification Section, page 419
No. 7787—10 mg, pink in color, coded MSD 412.
NDC 0006-0412-68 in bottles of 100
(6505-00-616-7856 10 mg 100's)
NDC 0006-0412-28 unit dose packages of 100.
(6505-01-153-3547, 10 mg individually sealed 100's).
   Shown in Product Identification Section, page 419
No. 7788—25 mg, yellow in color, coded MSD 457.
NDC 0006-0457-68 in bottles of 100
NDC 0006-0457-28 unit dose packages of 100.
   Shown in Product Identification Section, page 419
No. 7790 — 50 mg, yellow in color, coded MSD 460.
NDC 0006-0460-68 in bottles of 100
NDC 0006-0460-28 in unit dose packages of 100.
   Shown in Product Identification Section, page 419
No. 7786—Injection URECHOLINE, 5 mg per mL, is a clear, colorless solution, and is supplied as follows:
NDC 0006-7786-29 in box of 6 × 1 mL vials
(6505-00-616-8947 in box of 6 × 1 mL vials).

Storage

Store Tablets URECHOLINE in a tightly-closed container. Avoid storage at temperatures above 40°C (104°F). Avoid storage of Injection URECHOLINE at temperatures below −20°C (−4°F) and above 40°C (104°F).

A.H.F.S. Category: 12:04
DC 6208430 Issued May 1986
COPYRIGHT © MERCK & CO., INC., 1984
All rights reserved

VASERETIC® Tablets   ℞
(Enalapril Maleate–Hydrochlorothiazide, MSD)

DESCRIPTION

VASERETIC® (Enalapril Maleate-Hydrochlorothiazide, MSD) combines an angiotensin converting enzyme inhibitor, enalapril maleate, and a diuretic, hydrochlorothiazide. Enalapril maleate is the maleate salt of enalapril, the ethyl ester of a long-acting angiotensin converting enzyme inhibitor, enalaprilat. Enalapril maleate is chemically described as (*S*)-1-[*N*-[1-(ethoxycarbonyl)-3-phenylpropyl]-L-alanyl]-L-proline, (*Z*)-2-butenedioate salt (1:1). Its empirical formula is $C_{20}H_{28}N_2O_5 \cdot C_4H_4O_4$, and its structural formula is:

Enalapril maleate is a white to off-white crystalline powder with a molecular weight of 492.53. It is sparingly soluble in water, soluble in ethanol, and freely soluble in methanol. Enalapril is a pro-drug; following oral administration, it is bioactivated by hydrolysis of the ethyl ester to enalaprilat, which is the active angiotensin converting enzyme inhibitor. Hydrochlorothiazide is 6-chloro-3,4-dihydro-2*H*-1, 2, 4-benzothiadiazine-7-sulfonamide 1,1-dioxide. Its empirical formula is $C_7H_8ClN_3O_4S_2$ and its structural formula is:

It is a white, or practically white, crystalline powder with a molecular weight of 297.72, which is slightly soluble in water, but freely soluble in sodium hydroxide solution.

VASERETIC is available for oral use as tablets containing 10 mg of enalapril maleate, 25 mg of hydrochlorothiazide and the following inactive ingredients: iron oxides, lactose, magnesium stearate, starch and other ingredients.

CLINICAL PHARMACOLOGY

As a result of its diuretic effects, hydrochlorothiazide increases plasma renin activity, increases aldosterone secretion, and decreases serum potassium. Administration of enalapril maleate blocks the renin-angiotensin-aldosterone axis and tends to reverse the potassium loss associated with the diuretic.

In clinical studies, the extent of blood pressure reduction seen with the combination of enalapril maleate and hydrochlorothiazide was approximately additive. The antihypertensive effect of VASERETIC was usually sustained for at least 24 hours.

Concomitant administration of enalapril maleate and hydrochlorothiazide has little, or no effect on the bioavailability of either drug. The combination tablet is bioequivalent to concomitant administration of the separate entities.

Enalapril Maleate

Mechanism of Action: Enalapril, after hydrolysis to enalaprilat, inhibits angiotensin-converting enzyme (ACE) in human subjects and animals. ACE is a peptidyl dipeptidase that catalyzes the conversion of angiotensin I to the vasoconstrictor substance, angiotensin II. Angiotensin II also stimulates aldosterone secretion by the adrenal cortex. Inhibition of ACE results in decreased plasma angiotensin II, which leads to decreased vasopressor activity and to decreased aldosterone secretion. Although the latter decrease is small, it results in small increases of serum potassium. In hypertensive patients treated with enalapril maleate alone for up to 48 weeks, mean increases in serum potassium of approximately 0.2 mEq/L were observed. In patients treated with enalapril maleate plus a thiazide diuretic, there was essentially no change in serum potassium. (See PRECAUTIONS.) Removal of angiotensin II negative feedback on renin secretion leads to increased plasma renin activity.

ACE is identical to kininase, an enzyme that degrades bradykinin. Whether increased levels of bradykinin, a potent vasodepressor peptide, play a role in the therapeutic effects of enalapril remains to be elucidated.

While the mechanism through which enalapril lowers blood pressure is believed to be primarily suppression of the renin-angiotensin-aldosterone system, enalapril is antihypertensive even in patients with low-renin hypertension. Although enalapril was antihypertensive in all races studied, black hypertensive patients (usually a low-renin hypertensive population) had a smaller average response to enalapril maleate monotherapy than non-black patients. In contrast, hydrochlorothiazide was more effective in black patients than enalapril. Concomitant administration of enalapril maleate and hydrochlorothiazide was equally effective in black and non-black patients.

Pharmacokinetics and Metabolism: Following oral administration of enalapril maleate, peak serum concentrations of enalapril occur within about one hour. Based on urinary recovery, the extent of absorption of enalapril is approximately 60 percent. Enalapril absorption is not influenced by the presence of food in the gastrointestinal tract. Following absorption, enalapril is hydrolyzed to enalaprilat, which is a more potent angiotensin converting enzyme inhibitor than enalapril; enalaprilat is poorly absorbed when administered orally. Peak serum concentrations of enalaprilat occur three to four hours after an oral dose of enalapril maleate. Excretion of enalapril and enalaprilat is primarily renal. Approximately 94 percent of the dose is recovered in the urine and feces as enalaprilat or enalapril. The principal components in urine are enalaprilat, accounting for about 40 percent of the dose, and intact enalapril. There is no evidence of metabolites of enalapril, other than enalaprilat. The serum concentration profile of enalaprilat exhibits a prolonged terminal phase, apparently representing a small fraction of the administered dose that has been bound to ACE. The amount bound does not increase with dose, indicating a saturable site of binding. The effective half-life for accumulation of enalaprilat following multiple doses of enalapril maleate is 11 hours.

The disposition of enalapril and enalaprilat in patients with renal insufficiency is similar to that in patients with normal renal function until the glomerular filtration rate is 30 mL/min or less. With renal function ≤ 30 mL/min, peak and trough enalaprilat levels increase, time to peak concentration increases and time to steady state may be delayed. The effective half-life of enalaprilat following multiple doses of enalapril maleate is prolonged at this level of renal insufficiency. Enalaprilat is dialyzable at the rate of 62 mL/min. Studies in dogs indicate that enalapril crosses the blood-brain barrier poorly, if at all; enalaprilat does not enter the brain. Multiple doses of enalapril maleate in rats do not result in accumulation in any tissues. Milk of lactating rats contains radioactivity following administration of ^{14}C enalapril maleate. Radioactivity was found to cross the placenta following administration of labeled drug to pregnant hamsters.

Pharmacodynamics: Administration of enalapril maleate to patients with hypertension of severity ranging from mild to severe results in a reduction of both supine and standing blood pressure usually with no orthostatic component. Symptomatic postural hypotension is infrequent with enalapril alone but it can be anticipated in volume-depleted patients, such as patients treated with diuretics. In clinical trials with enalapril and hydrochlorothiazide administered

concurrently, syncope occurred in 1.3 percent of patients. (See WARNINGS and DOSAGE AND ADMINISTRATION.) In most patients studied, after oral administration of a single dose of enalapril maleate, onset of antihypertensive activity was seen at one hour with peak reduction of blood pressure achieved by four to six hours.

At recommended doses, antihypertensive effects of enalapril maleate monotherapy have been maintained for at least 24 hours. In some patients the effects may diminish toward the end of the dosing interval; this was less frequently observed with concomitant administration of enalapril maleate and hydrochlorothiazide.

Achievement of optimal blood pressure reduction may require several weeks of enalapril therapy in some patients. The antihypertensive effects of enalapril have continued during long term therapy. Abrupt withdrawal of enalapril has not been associated with a rapid increase in blood pressure.

In hemodynamic studies in patients with essential hypertension, blood pressure reduction produced by enalapril was accompanied by a reduction in peripheral arterial resistance with an increase in cardiac output and little or no change in heart rate. Following administration of enalapril maleate, there is an increase in renal blood flow; glomerular filtration rate is usually unchanged. The effects appear to be similar in patients with renovascular hypertension.

In a clinical pharmacology study, indomethacin or sulindac was administered to hypertensive patients receiving enalapril maleate. In this study there was no evidence of a blunting of the antihypertensive action of enalapril maleate.

Hydrochlorothiazide

The mechanism of the antihypertensive effect of thiazides is unknown. Thiazides do not usually affect normal blood pressure. Hydrochlorothiazide is a diuretic and antihypertensive. It affects the distal renal tubular mechanism of electrolyte reabsorption. Hydrochlorothiazide increases excretion of sodium and chloride in approximately equivalent amounts. Natriuresis may be accompanied by some loss of potassium and bicarbonate. After oral use diuresis begins within two hours, peaks in about four hours and lasts about 6 to 12 hours. Hydrochlorothiazide is not metabolized but is eliminated rapidly by the kidney. When plasma levels have been followed for at least 24 hours, the plasma half-life has been observed to vary between 5.6 and 14.8 hours. At least 61 percent of the oral dose is eliminated unchanged within 24 hours. Hydrochlorothiazide crosses the placental but not the blood-brain barrier.

INDICATIONS AND USAGE

VASERETIC is indicated for the treatment of hypertension in patients for whom combination therapy is appropriate. **This fixed dose combination is not indicated for initial therapy. Patients already receiving a diuretic when enalapril is initiated, or given a diuretic and enalapril simultaneously, can develop symptomatic hypotension. In the initial titration of the individual entities, it is important, if possible, to stop the diuretic for several days before starting enalapril or, if this is not possible, begin enalapril at a low initial dose (see DOSAGE AND ADMINISTRATION). This fixed dose combination is not suitable for titration but may be substituted for the individual components if the titrated doses are the same as those in the combination.**

In using VASERETIC, consideration should be given to the fact that another angiotensin converting enzyme inhibitor, captopril, has caused agranulocytosis, particularly in patients with renal impairment or collagen vascular disease, and that available data are insufficient to show that enalapril does not have a similar risk. (See WARNINGS.)

CONTRAINDICATIONS

VASERETIC is contraindicated in patients who are hypersensitive to any component of this product and in patients with a history of angioedema related to previous treatment with an angiotensin converting enzyme inhibitor. Because of the hydrochlorothiazide component, this product is contraindicated in patients with anuria or hypersensitivity to other sulfonamide-derived drugs.

WARNINGS

Hypotension: Excessive hypotension was rarely seen in uncomplicated hypertensive patients but is a possible consequence of enalapril use in severely salt/volume depleted persons such as those treated vigorously with diuretics or patients on dialysis.

Syncope has been reported in 1.3 percent of patients receiving VASERETIC. In patients receiving enalapril alone, the incidence of syncope is 0.5 percent. The overall incidence of syncope may be reduced by proper titration of the individual components. (See PRECAUTIONS, *Drug Interactions,* ADVERSE REACTIONS and DOSAGE AND ADMINISTRATION.)

In patients with severe congestive heart failure, with or without associated renal insufficiency, excessive hypotension has been observed and may be associated with oliguria and/or progressive azotemia, and rarely with acute renal failure and/or death. Because of the potential fall in blood pressure in these patients, therapy should be started under very close medical supervision. Such patients should be followed closely for the first two weeks of treatment and whenever the dose of enalapril and/or diuretic is increased. Similar considerations may apply to patients with ischemic heart or cerebrovascular disease, in whom an excessive fall in blood pressure could result in a myocardial infarction or cerebrovascular accident.

If hypotension occurs, the patient should be placed in supine position and, if necessary, receive an intravenous infusion of normal saline. A transient hypotensive response is not a contraindication to further doses which usually can be given without difficulty once the blood pressure has increased after volume expansion.

Angioedema: Angioedema of the face, extremities, lips, tongue, glottis and/or larynx has been reported in patients treated with angiotensin converting enzyme inhibitors, including enalapril. In such cases VASERETIC should be promptly discontinued and the patient carefully observed until the swelling disappears. In instances where swelling has been confined to the face and lips the condition has generally resolved without treatment, although antihistamines have been useful in relieving symptoms. Angioedema associated with laryngeal edema may be fatal. **Where there is involvement of the tongue, glottis or larynx, likely to cause airway obstruction, appropriate therapy, e.g., subcutaneous epinephrine solution 1:1000 (0.3 mL to 0.5 mL) should be promptly administered.** (See ADVERSE REACTIONS.)

Neutropenia/Agranulocytosis: Another angiotensin converting enzyme inhibitor, captopril, has been shown to cause agranulocytosis and bone marrow depression, rarely in uncomplicated patients but more frequently in patients with renal impairment especially if they also have a collagen vascular disease. Available data from clinical trials of enalapril are insufficient to show that enalapril does not cause agranulocytosis at similar rates. Foreign marketing experience has revealed several cases of neutropenia or agranulocytosis in which a causal relationship to enalapril cannot be excluded. Periodic monitoring of white blood cell counts in patients with collagen vascular disease and renal disease should be considered.

Hydrochlorothiazide

Thiazides should be used with caution in severe renal disease. In patients with renal disease, thiazides may precipitate azotemia. Cumulative effects of the drug may develop in patients with impaired renal function.

Thiazides should be used with caution in patients with impaired hepatic function or progressive liver disease, since minor alterations of fluid and electrolyte balance may precipitate hepatic coma.

Sensitivity reactions may occur in patients with or without a history of allergy or bronchial asthma.

The possibility of exacerbation or activation of systemic lupus erythematosus has been reported.

Lithium generally should not be given with thiazides (see PRECAUTIONS, *Drug Interactions, Hydrochlorothiazide*).

PRECAUTIONS

General

Enalapril Maleate

Impaired Renal Function: As a consequence of inhibiting the renin-angiotensin-aldosterone system, changes in renal function may be anticipated in susceptible individuals. In patients with severe congestive heart failure whose renal function may depend on the activity of the renin-angiotensin-aldosterone system, treatment with angiotensin converting enzyme inhibitors, including enalapril, may be associated with oliguria and/or progressive azotemia and rarely with acute renal failure and/or death.

In clinical studies in hypertensive patients with unilateral or bilateral renal artery stenosis, increases in blood urea nitrogen and serum creatinine were observed in 20 percent of patients. These increases were almost always reversible upon discontinuation of enalapril and/or diuretic therapy. In such patients renal function should be monitored during the first few weeks of therapy.

Some patients with hypertension or heart failure with no apparent pre-existing renal vascular disease have developed increases in blood urea and serum creatinine, usually minor and transient, especially when enalapril has been given concomitantly with a diuretic. This is more likely to occur in patients with pre-existing renal impairment. Dosage reduction of enalapril and/or discontinuation of the diuretic may be required.

Continued on next page

Information on the Merck Sharp & Dohme products listed on these pages is the full prescribing information from product circulars in use August 31, 1989.

Merck Sharp & Dohme—Cont.

Evaluation of the hypertensive patient should always include assessment of renal function.

Hyperkalemia: Elevated serum potassium (greater than 5.7 mEq/L) was observed in approximately one percent of hypertensive patients in clinical trials treated with enalapril alone. In most cases these were isolated values which resolved despite continued therapy, although hyperkalemia was a cause of discontinuation of therapy in 0.28 percent of hypertensive patients. Hyperkalemia was less frequent (approximately 0.1 percent) in patients treated with enalapril plus hydrochlorothiazide. Risk factors for the development of hyperkalemia include renal insufficiency, diabetes mellitus, and the concomitant use of potassium-sparing diuretics, potassium supplements and/or potassium-containing salt substitutes, which should be used cautiously, if at all, with enalapril. (See *Drug Interactions.*)

Surgery/Anesthesia: In patients undergoing major surgery or during anesthesia with agents that produce hypotension, enalapril may block angiotensin II formation secondary to compensatory renin release. If hypotension occurs and is considered to be due to this mechanism, it can be corrected by volume expansion.

Hydrochlorothiazide

Periodic determination of serum electrolytes to detect possible electrolyte imbalance should be performed at appropriate intervals. All patients receiving thiazide therapy should be observed for clinical signs of fluid or electrolyte imbalance: namely hyponatremia, hypochloremic alkalosis, and hypokalemia. Serum and urine electrolyte determinations are particularly important when the patient is vomiting excessively or receiving parenteral fluids. Warning signs or symptoms of fluid and electrolyte imbalance, irrespective of cause, include dryness of mouth, thirst, weakness, lethargy, drowsiness, restlessness, muscle pains or cramps, muscular fatigue, hypotension, oliguria, tachycardia, and gastrointestinal disturbances such as nausea and vomiting.

Hypokalemia may develop, especially with brisk diuresis, when severe cirrhosis is present, or after prolonged therapy. Interference with adequate oral electrolyte intake will also contribute to hypokalemia. Hypokalemia may cause cardiac arrhythmia and may also sensitize or exaggerate the response of the heart to the toxic effects of digitalis (e.g., increased ventricular irritability). Because enalapril reduces the production of aldosterone, concomitant therapy with enalapril attenuates the diuretic-induced potassium loss (see *Drug Interactions, Agents Increasing Serum Potassium*).

Although any chloride deficit is generally mild and usually does not require specific treatment except under extraordinary circumstances (as in liver disease or renal disease), chloride replacement may be required in the treatment of metabolic alkalosis.

Dilutional hyponatremia may occur in edematous patients in hot weather; appropriate therapy is water restriction, rather than administration of salt except in rare instances when the hyponatremia is life-threatening. In actual salt depletion, appropriate replacement is the therapy of choice.

Hyperuricemia may occur or frank gout may be precipitated in certain patients receiving thiazide therapy.

In diabetic patients dosage adjustments of insulin or oral hypoglycemic agents may be required. Hyperglycemia may occur with thiazide diuretics. Thus latent diabetes mellitus may become manifest during thiazide therapy.

The antihypertensive effects of the drug may be enhanced in the postsympathectomy patient.

If progressive renal impairment becomes evident consider withholding or discontinuing diuretic therapy.

Thiazides have been shown to increase the urinary excretion of magnesium; this may result in hypomagnesemia.

Thiazides may decrease urinary calcium excretion. Thiazides may cause intermittent and slight elevation of serum calcium in the absence of known disorders of calcium metabolism. Marked hypercalcemia may be evidence of hidden hyperparathyroidism. Thiazides should be discontinued before carrying out tests for parathyroid function.

Increases in cholesterol and triglyceride levels may be associated with thiazide diuretic therapy.

Information for Patients

Angioedema: Angioedema, including laryngeal edema, may occur especially following the first dose of enalapril. Patients should be so advised and told to report immediately any signs or symptoms suggesting angioedema (swelling of face, extremities, eyes, lips, tongue, difficulty in swallowing or breathing) and to take no more drug until they have consulted with the prescribing physician.

Hypotension: Patients should be cautioned to report lightheadedness especially during the first few days of therapy. If actual syncope occurs, the patients should be told to discontinue the drug until they have consulted with the prescribing physician.

All patients should be cautioned that excessive perspiration and dehydration may lead to an excessive fall in blood pressure because of reduction in fluid volume. Other causes of volume depletion such as vomiting or diarrhea may also lead to a fall in blood pressure; patients should be advised to consult with the physician.

Hyperkalemia: Patients should be told not to use salt substitutes containing potassium without consulting their physician.

Neutropenia: Patients should be told to report promptly any indication of infection (e.g., sore throat, fever) which may be a sign of neutropenia.

NOTE: As with many other drugs, certain advice to patients being treated with VASERETIC is warranted. This information is intended to aid in the safe and effective use of this medication. It is not a disclosure of all possible adverse or intended effects.

Drug Interactions

Enalapril Maleate

Hypotension —Patients on Diuretic Therapy: Patients on diuretics and especially those in whom diuretic therapy was recently instituted, may occasionally experience an excessive reduction of blood pressure after initiation of therapy with enalapril. The possibility of hypotensive effects with enalapril can be minimized by either discontinuing the diuretic or increasing the salt intake prior to initiation of treatment with enalapril. If it is necessary to continue the diuretic, provide medical supervision for at least two hours and until blood pressure has stabilized for at least an additional hour. (See WARNINGS, and DOSAGE AND ADMINISTRATION.)

Agents Causing Renin Release: The antihypertensive effect of enalapril is augmented by antihypertensive agents that cause renin release (e.g., diuretics).

Other Cardiovascular Agents: Enalapril has been used concomitantly with beta adrenergic-blocking agents, methyldopa, nitrates, calcium-blocking agents, hydralazine and prazosin without evidence of clinically significant adverse interactions.

Agents Increasing Serum Potassium: Enalapril attenuates diuretic-induced potassium loss. Potassium-sparing diuretics (e.g., spironolactone, triamterene, or amiloride), potassium supplements, or potassium-containing salt substitutes may lead to significant increases in serum potassium. Therefore, if concomitant use of these agents is indicated because of demonstrated hypokalemia they should be used with caution and with frequent monitoring of serum potassium.

Lithium: See WARNINGS, *Hydrochlorothiazide*; PRECAUTIONS, *Drug Interactions, Hydrochlorothiazide.*

Hydrochlorothiazide

When administered concurrently the following drugs may interact with thiazide diuretics:

Alcohol, barbiturates, or narcotics —potentiation of orthostatic hypotension may occur.

Antidiabetic drugs (oral agents and insulin)—dosage adjustment of the antidiabetic drug may be required.

Other antihypertensive drugs —additive effect or potentiation.

Corticosteroids, ACTH —intensified electrolyte depletion, particularly hypokalemia.

Pressor amines (e.g., norepinephrine) —possible decreased response to pressor amines but not sufficient to preclude their use.

Skeletal muscle relaxants, nondepolarizing (e.g., tubocurarine) —possible increased responsiveness to the muscle relaxant.

Lithium —should not generally be given with diuretics. Diuretic agents reduce the renal clearance of lithium and add a high risk of lithium toxicity. Refer to the package insert for lithium preparations before use of such preparations with VASERETIC.

Non-steroidal Anti-inflammatory Drugs —In some patients, the administration of a non-steroidal anti-inflammatory agent can reduce the diuretic, natriuretic, and antihypertensive effects of loop, potassium-sparing and thiazide diuretics. Therefore, when VASERETIC and non-steroidal anti-inflammatory agents are used concomitantly, the patient should be observed closely to determine if the desired effect of the diuretic is obtained.

Carcinogenesis, Mutagenesis,
Impairment of Fertility

Enalapril in combination with hydrochlorothiazide was not mutagenic in the Ames microbial mutagen test with or without metabolic activation. Enalapril-hydrochlorothiazide did not produce DNA single strand breaks in an *in vitro* alkaline elution assay in rat hepatocytes or chromosomal aberrations in an *in vivo* mouse bone marrow assay.

Enalapril Maleate

There was no evidence of a tumorigenic effect when enalapril was administered for 106 weeks to rats at doses up to 90 mg/kg/day (150 times* the maximum daily human dose). Enalapril has also been administered for 94 weeks to male and female mice at doses up to 90 and 180 mg/kg/day, respectively, (150 and 300 times* the maximum daily dose for humans) and showed no evidence of carcinogenicity.

---

* Based on patient weight of 50 kg

Neither enalapril maleate nor the active diacid was mutagenic in the Ames microbial mutagen test with or without metabolic activation. Enalapril was also negative in the following genotoxicity studies: rec-assay, reverse mutation assay with *E. coli*, sister chromatid exchange with cultured mammalian cells, and the micronucleus test with mice, as well as in an *in vivo* cytogenic study using mouse bone marrow.

There were no adverse effects on reproductive performance in male and female rats treated with 10 to 90 mg/kg/day of enalapril.

Hydrochlorothiazide

Hydrochlorothiazide is currently under study in the U.S. Carcinogenesis Testing Program.

Hydrochlorothiazide was not mutagenic *in vitro*, in the Ames microbial mutagen test at a maximum concentration of 5 mg/plate using Strains TA98 and TA100. Urine samples from patients treated with hydrochlorothiazide did not have mutagenic activity in the Ames test. The ability of a number of drugs to induce nondisjunction and crossing-over was measured using *Aspergillus nidulans.* A large number of drugs, including hydrochlorothiazide, induced nondisjunction. Hydrochlorothiazide had no effect on fertility in a two-litter study in rats at doses of 4–5.6 mg/kg/day (up to 2 times the usual daily human dose).

Pregnancy

Pregnancy Category C. There was no teratogenicity in rats given up to 90 mg/kg/day of enalapril (150 times the maximum human dose) in combination with 10 mg/kg/day of hydrochlorothiazide (2½ times the maximum human dose) or in mice given up to 30 mg/kg/day of enalapril (50 times the maximum human dose) in combination with 10 mg/kg/day of hydrochlorothiazide (2½ times the maximum human dose). At these doses, fetotoxicity expressed as a decrease in average fetal weight occurred in both species. No fetotoxicity occurred at lower doses; 30/10 mg/kg/day of enalapril-hydrochlorothiazide in rats and 10/10 mg/kg/day of enalapril-hydrochlorothiazide in mice.

There are no adequate and well-controlled studies of VASERETIC in pregnant women. VASERETIC should be used during pregnancy only if the potential benefit justifies the potential risk to the fetus.

Enalapril Maleate

There was no fetotoxicity or teratogenicity in rats treated with up to 200 mg/kg/day of enalapril (333 times the maximum human dose). Fetotoxicity, expressed as a decrease in average fetal weight, occurred in rats given 1200/mg/kg/day of enalapril, but did not occur when these animals were supplemented with saline. Enalapril was not teratogenic in rabbits. However, maternal and fetal toxicity occurred in some rabbits at doses of 1 mg/kg/day or more. Saline supplementation prevented the maternal and fetal toxicity seen at doses of 3 and 10 mg/kg/day, but not at 30 mg/kg/day (50 times the maximum human dose). Radioactivity was found to cross the placenta following administration of labeled drug to pregnant hamsters.

Human Experience: There are no adequate and well-controlled studies of enalapril in pregnant women. However, data are available that show enalapril crosses the human placenta. Because the risk of fetal toxicity with the use of ACE inhibitors has not been clearly defined (see below), enalapril should be used during pregnancy only if the potential benefit justifies the potential risk to the fetus.

Post-marketing experience with all ACE inhibitors thus far suggests the following with regard to pregnancy outcome. Inadvertent exposure limited to the first trimester of pregnancy has not been reported to affect fetal outcome adversely. Fetal exposure during the second and third trimesters of pregnancy has been associated with fetal and neonatal morbidity and mortality.

When ACE inhibitors are used during the later stages of pregnancy, there have been reports of hypotension and decreased renal perfusion in the newborn. Oligohydramnios in the mother has also been reported, presumably representing decreased renal function in the fetus. Infants exposed *in utero* to ACE inhibitors should be closely observed for hypotension, oliguria and hyperkalemia. If oliguria occurs, attention should be directed toward support of blood pressure and renal perfusion with the administration of fluids and pressors as appropriate. Problems associated with prematurity such as patent ductus arteriosus have occurred in association with maternal use of ACE inhibitors, but it is not clear whether they are related to ACE inhibition, maternal hypertension or the underlying prematurity.

Enalapril has been removed from the neonatal circulation by peritoneal dialysis and may theoretically be removed by exchange transfusion, although there is no experience with the latter procedure.

Hydrochlorothiazide

Teratogenic Effects: Reproduction studies in the rabbit, the mouse and the rat at doses up to 100 mg/kg/day (50 times the human dose) showed no evidence of external abnormalities of the fetus due to hydrochlorothiazide. Hydrochlorothiazide given in a two-litter study in rats at doses of 4–5.6

mg/kg/day (approximately 1–2 times the usual daily human dose) did not impair fertility or produce birth abnormalities in the offspring.

Thiazides cross the placental barrier and appear in cord blood.

Nonteratogenic Effects: These may include fetal or neonatal jaundice, thrombocytopenia, and possibly other adverse reactions which have occurred in the adult.

Nursing Mothers

It is not known whether enalapril is secreted in human milk, however, thiazides do appear in human milk. Milk of lactating rats contains radioactivity following administration of ^{14}C enalapril maleate. Because of the potential for serious reactions in nursing infants from hydrochlorothiazide, a decision should be made whether to discontinue nursing or to discontinue VASERETIC, taking into account the importance of the drug to the mother.

Pediatric Use

Safety and effectiveness in children have not been established.

ADVERSE REACTIONS

VASERETIC has been evaluated for safety in more than 1500 patients, including over 300 patients treated for one year or more. In clinical trials with VASERETIC no adverse experiences peculiar to this combination drug have been observed. Adverse experiences that have occurred, have been limited to those that have been previously reported with enalapril or hydrochlorothiazide.

The most frequent clinical adverse experiences in controlled trials were: dizziness (8.6 percent), headache (5.5 percent), fatigue (3.9 percent) and cough (3.5 percent). Generally, adverse experiences were mild and transient in nature. Adverse experiences occurring in greater than two percent of patients treated with VASERETIC in controlled clinical trials are shown below.

	Percent of Patients in Controlled Studies	
	VASERETIC (n=1580) Incidence (discontinuation)	Placebo (n=230) Incidence
Dizziness	8.6 (0.7)	4.3
Headache	5.5 (0.4)	9.1
Fatigue	3.9 (0.8)	2.6
Cough	3.5 (0.4)	0.9
Muscle Cramps	2.7 (0.2)	0.9
Nausea	2.5 (0.4)	1.7
Asthenia	2.4 (0.3)	0.9
Orthostatic Effects	2.3 (<0.1)	0.0
Impotence	2.2 (0.5)	0.5
Diarrhea	2.1 (<0.1)	1.7

Clinical adverse experiences occurring in 0.5 to 2.0 percent of patients in controlled trials included: *Body As A Whole:* Syncope, chest pain, abdominal pain; *Cardiovascular:* Orthostatic hypotension, palpitation, tachycardia; *Digestive:* Vomiting, dyspepsia, constipation, flatulence, dry mouth; *Nervous/Psychiatric:* Insomnia, nervousness, paresthesia, somnolence, vertigo; *Skin:* Pruritus, rash; *Other:* Dyspnea, gout, back pain, arthralgia, hyperhidrosis, decreased libido, tinnitus, urinary tract infection.

Angioedema: Angioedema has been reported in patients receiving VASERETIC (0.6 percent). Angioedema associated with laryngeal edema may be fatal. If angioedema of the face, extremities, lips, tongue, glottis and/or larynx occurs, treatment with VASERETIC should be discontinued and appropriate therapy instituted immediately. (See WARNINGS.)

Hypotension: In clinical trials, adverse effects relating to hypotension occurred as follows: hypotension (0.9 percent), orthostatic hypotension (1.5 percent), other orthostatic effects (2.3 percent). In addition syncope occurred in 1.3 percent of patients. (See WARNINGS.)

Clinical Laboratory Test Findings

Serum Electrolytes: (See PRECAUTIONS.)

Creatinine, Blood Urea Nitrogen: In controlled clinical trials minor increases in blood urea nitrogen and serum creatinine, reversible upon discontinuation of therapy, were observed in about 0.6 percent of patients with essential hypertension treated with VASERETIC. More marked increases have been reported in other enalapril experience. Increases are more likely to occur in patients with renal artery stenosis. (See PRECAUTIONS.)

Serum Uric Acid, Glucose, Magnesium, and Calcium: (See PRECAUTIONS.)

Hemoglobin and Hematocrit: Small decreases in hemoglobin and hematocrit (mean decreases of approximately 0.3 g percent and 1.0 vol percent, respectively) occur frequently in hypertensive patients treated with VASERETIC but are rarely of clinical importance unless another cause of anemia coexists. In clinical trials, less than 0.1 percent of patients discontinued therapy due to anemia.

Other (Causal Relationship Unknown): Rarely, elevations of liver enzymes and/or serum bilirubin have occurred.

Other adverse reactions that have been reported with the individual components are listed below and, within each category, are in order of decreasing severity.

*Enalapril Maleate —*Enalapril has been evaluated for safety in more than 10,000 patients. In clinical trials adverse reactions which occurred with enalapril were also seen with VASERETIC. However, since enalapril has been marketed, the following adverse reactions have been reported:

Cardiovascular: Cardiac arrest; myocardial infarction or cerebrovascular accident, possibly secondary to excessive hypotension in high risk patients (see WARNINGS, *Hypotension*): pulmonary embolism and infarction; rhythm disturbances, atrial fibrillation; hypotension; angina pectoris; *Digestive:* Ileus, pancreatitis, hepatitis or cholestatic jaundice, melena, anorexia, glossitis; *Hematologic:* Rare cases of neutropenia, thrombocytopenia and bone marrow depression have been reported in which a causal relationship to enalapril cannot be excluded; *Nervous System/Psychiatric:* Depression, confusion, ataxia; *Renal:* Renal failure, oliguria, renal dysfunction, (see PRECAUTIONS and DOSAGE AND ADMINISTRATION); *Respiratory:* Bronchospasm, pneumonia, bronchitis, rhinorrhea, asthma, upper respiratory infection; *Skin:* Herpes zoster, alopecia, flushing, photosensitivity; *Other:* Vasculitis, blurred vision, taste alteration. A symptom complex has been reported which may include fever, myalgia and arthralgia; an elevated erythrocyte sedimentation rate may be present. Rash or other dermatologic manifestations may occur. These symptoms have disappeared after discontinuation of therapy.

Hydrochlorothiazide —Body as a Whole: Weakness; *Digestive:* Pancreatitis, jaundice (intrahepatic cholestatic jaundice), sialadenitis, cramping, gastric irritation, anorexia; *Hematologic:* Aplastic anemia, agranulocytosis, leukopenia, hemolytic anemia, thrombocytopenia; *Hypersensitivity:* Purpura, photosensitivity, urticaria, necrotizing angiitis (vasculitis and cutaneous vasculitis), fever, respiratory distress including pneumonitis and pulmonary edema, anaphylactic reactions; *Musculoskeletal:* Muscle spasm; *Nervous system/Psychiatric:* Restlessness; *Renal:* Renal failure, renal dysfunction, interstitial nephritis (see WARNINGS); *Special Senses:* Transient blurred vision, xanthopsia.

OVERDOSAGE

No specific information is available on the treatment of overdosage with VASERETIC. Treatment is symptomatic and supportive. Therapy with VASERETIC should be discontinued and the patient observed closely. Suggested measures include induction of emesis and/or gastric lavage, and correction of dehydration, electrolyte imbalance and hypotension by established procedures.

*Enalapril Maleate —*The oral LD_{50} of enalapril is 2000 mg/kg in mice and rats. The most likely manifestation of overdosage would be hypotension, for which the usual treatment would be intravenous infusion of normal saline solution. Enalaprilat may be removed from general circulation by hemodialysis.

*Hydrochlorothiazide —*The oral LD_{50} of hydrochlorothiazide is greater than 10.0 g/kg in both mice and rats. The most common signs and symptoms observed are those caused by electrolyte depletion (hypokalemia, hypochloremia, hyponatremia) and dehydration resulting from excessive diuresis. If digitalis has also been administered, hypokalemia may accentuate cardiac arrhythmias.

DOSAGE AND ADMINISTRATION

DOSAGE MUST BE INDIVIDUALIZED. THE FIXED COMBINATION IS NOT FOR INITIAL THERAPY. THE DOSE OF 'VASERETIC' SHOULD BE DETERMINED BY THE TITRATION OF THE INDIVIDUAL COMPONENTS.

Once the patient has been successfully titrated with the individual components as described below, VASERETIC (one or two 10-25 tablets once daily) may be substituted if the titrated doses are the same as those in the fixed combination. (See INDICATIONS AND USAGE and WARNINGS.)

Patients usually do not require doses in excess of 50 mg of hydrochlorothiazide daily when combined with other antihypertensive agents. Therefore, since each tablet of VASERETIC includes 25 mg of hydrochlorothiazide, the daily dose of VASERETIC should not exceed two tablets. If further blood pressure control is indicated, additional doses of enalapril or other nondiuretic antihypertensive agents should be considered.

For enalapril monotherapy the recommended initial dose in patients not on diuretics is 5 mg of enalapril once a day. Dosage should be adjusted according to blood pressure response. The usual dosage range of enalapril is 10 to 40 mg per day administered in a single dose or two divided doses. In some patients treated once daily, the antihypertensive effects may diminish toward the end of the dosing interval. In such patients, an increase in dosage or twice daily administration

should be considered. If blood pressure is not controlled with enalapril alone, a diuretic may be added.

In patients who are currently being treated with a diuretic, symptomatic hypotension occasionally may occur following the initial dose of enalapril. The diuretic should, if possible, be discontinued for two to three days before beginning therapy with enalapril to reduce the likelihood of hypotension. (See WARNINGS.) If the patient's blood pressure is not controlled with enalapril alone, diuretic therapy may be resumed.

If the diuretic cannot be discontinued an initial dose of 2.5 mg of enalapril should be used under medical supervision for at least two hours and until blood pressure has stabilized for at least an additional hour. (See WARNINGS and PRECAUTIONS, *Drug Interactions*.)

Concomitant administration of VASERETIC with potassium supplements, potassium salt substitutes, or potassium sparing agents may lead to increases of serum potassium. (See PRECAUTIONS.)

Dosage Adjustment in Renal Impairment: The usual dose of VASERETIC is recommended for patients with a creatinine clearance > 30 mL/min (serum creatinine of up to approximately 3 mg/dL).

When concomitant diuretic therapy is required in patients with severe renal impairment, a loop diuretic, rather than a thiazide diuretic is preferred for use with enalapril; therefore, for patients with severe renal dysfunction the enalapril maleate-hydrochlorothiazide combination tablet is not recommended.

HOW SUPPLIED

No. 3418—Tablets VASERETIC 10-25, are rust, squared capsule-shaped, compressed tablets, coded MSD 720 on one side and VASERETIC on the other. Each tablet contains 10 mg of enalapril maleate and 25 mg of hydrochlorothiazide. They are supplied as follows:

NDC 0006-0720-68 bottles of 100 (with desiccant).

Shown in Product Identification Section, page 419

Storage

Store below 30°C (86°F) and avoid transient temperatures above 50°C (122°F). Keep container tightly closed. Protect from moisture.

Dispense in a tight container, if product package is subdivided.

A.H.F.S. Category: 24:08

DC 7432305   Issued February 1989

COPYRIGHT © MERCK & CO., INC., 1989

All rights reserved

VASOTEC® I.V. Injection   ℞
(Enalaprilat, MSD)

DESCRIPTION

VASOTEC® I.V. (Enalaprilat, MSD) is a sterile aqueous solution for intravenous administration. Enalaprilat is an angiotensin converting enzyme inhibitor. It is chemically described as (S)-1-[N-(1-carboxy-3-phenylpropyl)-L-alanyl]-L-proline dihydrate. Its empirical formula is $C_{18}H_{24}N_2O_5 \cdot 2H_2O$ and its structural formula is:

Enalaprilat is a white to off-white, crystalline powder with a molecular weight of 384.43. It is sparingly soluble in methanol and slightly soluble in water.

Each milliliter of VASOTEC I.V. contains 1.25 mg enalaprilat (anhydrous equivalent); sodium chloride to adjust tonicity; sodium hydroxide to adjust pH; water for injection, q.s.; with benzyl alcohol, 9 mg, added as a preservative.

CLINICAL PHARMACOLOGY

Enalaprilat, an angiotensin-converting enzyme (ACE) inhibitor when administered intravenously, is the active metabolite of the orally administered pro-drug, enalapril maleate. Enalaprilat is poorly absorbed orally.

Mechanism of Action

Intravenous enalaprilat, or oral enalapril, after hydrolysis to enalaprilat, inhibits ACE in human subjects and animals. ACE is a peptidyl dipeptidase that catalyzes the conversion of angiotensin I to the vasoconstrictor substance, angioten-

Continued on next page

Information on the Merck Sharp & Dohme products listed on these pages is the full prescribing information from product circulars in use August 31, 1989.

Merck Sharp & Dohme—Cont.

sin II. Angiotensin II also stimulates aldosterone secretion by the adrenal cortex. Inhibition of ACE results in decreased plasma angiotensin II, which leads to decreased vasopressor activity and to decreased aldosterone secretion. Although the latter decrease is small, it results in small increases of serum potassium. In hypertensive patients treated with enalapril alone for up to 48 weeks, mean increases in serum potassium of approximately 0.2 mEq/L were observed. In patients treated with enalapril plus a thiazide diuretic, there was essentially no change in serum potassium. (See PRECAUTIONS.) Removal of angiotensin II negative feedback on renin secretion leads to increased plasma renin activity. ACE is identical to kininase, an enzyme that degrades bradykinin. Whether increased levels of bradykinin, a potent vasodepressor peptide, play a role in the therapeutic effects of enalaprilat remains to be elucidated.

While the mechanism through which enalaprilat lowers blood pressure is believed to be primarily suppression of the renin-angiotensin-aldosterone system, enalaprilat has antihypertensive activity even in patients with low-renin hypertension. In clinical studies, black hypertensive patients (usually a low-renin hypertensive population) had a smaller average response to enalaprilat monotherapy than non-black patients.

Pharmacokinetics and Metabolism

Following intravenous administration of a single dose, the serum concentration profile of enalaprilat is polyexponential with a prolonged terminal phase, apparently representing a small fraction of the administered dose that has been bound to ACE. The amount bound does not increase with dose, indicating a saturable site of binding. The effective half-life for accumulation of enalaprilat, as determined from oral administration of multiple doses of enalapril maleate, is approximately 11 hours. Excretion of enalaprilat is primarily renal with more than 90 percent of an administered dose recovered in the urine as unchanged drug within 24 hours. Enalaprilat is poorly absorbed following oral administration. The disposition of enalaprilat in patients with renal insufficiency is similar to that in patients with normal renal function until the glomerular filtration rate is 30 mL/min or less. With renal function ≤30 mL/min, peak and trough enalaprilat levels increase, time to peak concentration increases and time to steady state may be delayed. The effective half-life of enalaprilat is prolonged at this level of renal insufficiency. (See DOSAGE AND ADMINISTRATION.) Enalaprilat is dialyzable at the rate of 62 mL/min.

Studies in dogs indicate that enalaprilat does not enter the brain, and that enalapril crosses the blood-brain barrier poorly, if at all. Multiple doses of enalapril maleate in rats do not result in accumulation in any tissues. Milk in lactating rats contains radioactivity following administration of ^{14}C enalapril maleate. Radioactivity was found to cross the placenta following administration of labeled drug to pregnant hamsters.

Pharmacodynamics

VASOTEC I.V. results in the reduction of both supine and standing systolic and diastolic blood pressure, usually with no orthostatic component. Symptomatic postural hypotension is therefore infrequent, although it might be anticipated in volume-depleted patients (see WARNINGS). The onset of action usually occurs within fifteen minutes of administration with the maximum effect occurring within one to four hours. The abrupt withdrawal of enalaprilat has not been associated with a rapid increase in blood pressure.

The duration of hemodynamic effects appears to be dose-related. However, for the recommended dose, the duration of action in most patients is approximately six hours.

Following administration of enalapril, there is an increase in renal blood flow; glomerular filtration rate is usually unchanged. The effects appear to be similar in patients with renovascular hypertension.

INDICATIONS AND USAGE

VASOTEC I.V. is indicated for the treatment of hypertension when oral therapy is not practical.

VASOTEC I.V. has been studied with only one other antihypertensive agent, furosemide, which showed approximately additive effects on blood pressure. Enalapril, the pro-drug of enalaprilat, has been used extensively with a variety of other antihypertensive agents, without apparent difficulty except for occasional hypotension.

In using VASOTEC I.V., consideration should be given to the fact that another angiotensin converting enzyme inhibitor, captopril, has caused agranulocytosis, particularly in patients with renal impairment or collagen vascular disease, and that available data are insufficient to show that VASOTEC I.V. does not have a similar risk. (See WARNINGS.)

CONTRAINDICATIONS

VASOTEC I.V. is contraindicated in patients who are hyper-

sensitive to any component of this product and in patients with a history of angioedema related to previous treatment with an angiotensin converting enzyme inhibitor.

WARNINGS

Hypotension

Excessive hypotension was rarely seen in uncomplicated hypertensive patients but is a possible consequence of enalaprilat use in severely salt/volume depleted persons such as those treated vigorously with diuretics or patients on dialysis. (See PRECAUTIONS, *Drug Interactions* and ADVERSE REACTIONS.) In patients with severe congestive heart failure, with or without associated renal insufficiency, excessive hypotension has been observed and may be associated with oliguria and/or progressive azotemia, and rarely with acute renal failure and/or death. Because of the potential fall in blood pressure in these patients, therapy should be started under very close medical supervision. Such patients should be followed closely whenever the dose of enalaprilat is adjusted and/or diuretic is increased. Similar considerations may apply to patients with ischemic heart or cerebrovascular disease, in whom an excessive fall in blood pressure could result in a myocardial infarction or cerebrovascular accident.

If hypotension occurs, the patient should be placed in supine position and, if necessary, receive an intravenous infusion of normal saline. A transient hypotensive response is not a contraindication to further doses which usually can be given without difficulty once the blood pressure has increased after volume expansion.

Angioedema

Angioedema of the face, extremities, lips, tongue, glottis and/or larynx has been reported in patients treated with angiotensin converting enzyme inhibitors, including enalapril. In such cases VASOTEC I.V. should be promptly discontinued and the patient carefully observed until the swelling disappears. In instances where swelling has been confined to the face and lips the condition has generally resolved without treatment, although antihistamines have been useful in relieving symptoms. Angioedema associated with laryngeal edema may be fatal. **Where there is involvement of the tongue, glottis or larynx, likely to cause airway obstruction, appropriate therapy, e.g., subcutaneous epinephrine solution 1:1000 (0.3 mL to 0.5 mL) should be promptly administered.** (See ADVERSE REACTIONS.)

Neutropenia/Agranulocytosis

Another angiotensin converting enzyme inhibitor, captopril, has been shown to cause agranulocytosis and bone marrow depression, rarely in uncomplicated patients but more frequently in patients with renal impairment especially if they also have a collagen vascular disease. Available data from clinical trials of enalapril are insufficient to show that enalapril does not cause agranulocytosis in similar rates. Foreign marketing experience has revealed several cases of neutropenia, or agranulocytosis in which a causal relationship to enalapril cannot be excluded. Periodic monitoring of white blood cell counts in patients with collagen vascular disease and renal disease should be considered.

PRECAUTIONS

General

Impaired Renal Function: As a consequence of inhibiting the renin-angiotensin-aldosterone system, changes in renal function may be anticipated in susceptible individuals. In patients with severe congestive heart failure whose renal function may depend on the activity of the renin-angiotensin-aldosterone system, treatment with angiotensin converting enzyme inhibitors, including enalapril or enalaprilat, may be associated with oliguria and/or progressive azotemia and rarely with acute renal failure and/or death.

In clinical studies in hypertensive patients with unilateral or bilateral renal artery stenosis, increases in blood urea nitrogen and serum creatinine were observed in 20 percent of patients receiving enalapril. These increases were almost always reversible upon discontinuation of enalapril or enalaprilat and/or diuretic therapy. In such patients renal function should be monitored during the first few weeks of therapy.

Some hypertensive patients with no apparent pre-existing renal vascular disease have developed increases in blood urea and serum creatinine, usually minor and transient, especially when enalapril has been given concomitantly with a diuretic. This is more likely to occur in patients with pre-existing renal impairment. Dosage reduction of enalaprilat and/or discontinuation of the diuretic may be required.

Evaluation of the hypertensive patient should always include assessment of renal function. (See DOSAGE AND ADMINISTRATION.)

Hyperkalemia: Elevated serum potassium (greater than 5.7 mEq/L) was observed in approximately one percent of hypertensive patients in clinical trials receiving enalapril. In most

cases these were isolated values which resolved despite continued therapy. Hyperkalemia was a cause of discontinuation of therapy in 0.28 percent of hypertensive patients. Risk factors for the development of hyperkalemia include renal insufficiency, diabetes mellitus, and the concomitant use of potassium-sparing agents or potassium supplements, which should be used cautiously, if at all, with VASOTEC I.V. (See *Drug Interactions.*)

Surgery/Anesthesia: In patients undergoing major surgery or during anesthesia with agents that produce hypotension, enalapril may block angiotensin II formation secondary to compensatory renin release. If hypotension occurs and is considered to be due to this mechanism, it can be corrected by volume expansion.

Drug Interactions

Hypotension—Patients on Diuretic Therapy: Patients on diuretics and especially those in whom diuretic therapy was recently instituted, may occasionally experience an excessive reduction of blood pressure after initiation of therapy with enalaprilat. The possibility of hypotensive effects with enalaprilat can be minimized by administration of an intravenous infusion of normal saline, discontinuing the diuretic or increasing the salt intake prior to initiation of treatment with enalaprilat. If it is necessary to continue the diuretic, provide close medical supervision for at least one hour after the initial dose of enalaprilat. (See WARNINGS.)

Agents Causing Renin Release: The antihypertensive effect of VASOTEC I.V. appears to be augmented by antihypertensive agents that cause renin release (e.g., diuretics).

Other Cardiovascular Agents: VASOTEC I.V. has been used concomitantly with digitalis, beta adrenergic-blocking agents, methyldopa, nitrates, calcium-blocking agents, hydralazine and prazosin without evidence of clinically significant adverse interactions.

Agents Increasing Serum Potassium: VASOTEC I.V. attenuates potassium loss caused by thiazide-type diuretics. Potassium-sparing diuretics (e.g., spironolactone, triamterene, or amiloride), potassium supplements, or potassium-containing salt substitutes may lead to significant increases in serum potassium. Therefore, if concomitant use of these agents is indicated because of demonstrated hypokalemia, they should be used with caution and with frequent monitoring of serum potassium.

Lithium: A few cases of lithium toxicity have been reported in patients receiving concomitant enalapril and lithium and were reversible upon discontinuation of both drugs. Although a causal relationship has not been established, it is recommended that caution be exercised when lithium is used concomitantly with enalapril and serum lithium levels should be monitored frequently.

Carcinogenesis, Mutagenesis, Impairment of Fertility

Carcinogenicity studies have not been done with VASOTEC I.V.

VASOTEC I.V. is the bioactive form of its ethyl ester, enalapril maleate. There was no evidence of a tumorigenic effect when enalapril was administered orally for 106 weeks to rats at doses up to 90 mg/kg/day (150 times* the maximum daily human dose). Enalapril has also been administered for 94 weeks to male and female mice at oral doses up to 90 and 180 mg/kg/day, respectively (150 and 300 times* the maximum oral daily dose for humans), and showed no evidence of carcinogenicity.

VASOTEC I.V. was not mutagenic in the Ames microbial mutagen test with or without metabolic activation. Enalapril showed no drug-related changes in the following genotoxicity studies: rec-assay, reverse mutation assay with *E. coli*, sister chromatid exchange with cultured mammalian cells, the micronucleus test with mice, and in an *in vivo* cytogenic study using mouse bone marrow. There were no adverse effects on reproductive performance in male and female rats treated with 10 to 90 mg enalapril/kg/day.

Pregnancy

Pregnancy Category C. No reproductive or teratogenicity studies have been performed with VASOTEC I.V. Radioactivity was found to cross the placenta following oral administration of labeled enalapril to pregnant hamsters.

Studies with oral enalapril showed no fetotoxicity or teratogenicity in rats treated with up to 200 mg/kg/day. Fetotoxicity, expressed as a decrease in average fetal weight, occurred in rats given 1200 mg/kg/day of enalapril, but did not occur when these animals were supplemented with saline. Enalapril was not teratogenic in rabbits. However, maternal and fetal toxicity occurred in some rabbits at doses of 1 mg/kg/day or more. Saline supplementation prevented the maternal and fetal toxicity seen at doses of 3 and 10 mg/kg/day, but not at 30 mg/kg/day.

Human Experience: There are no adequate and well-controlled studies in pregnant women. However, data are available that show enalapril crosses the human placenta. Because the risk of fetal toxicity with the use of ACE inhibitors has not been clearly defined (see below), VASOTEC I.V. should be used during pregnancy only if the potential benefit justifies the potential risk to the fetus.

*Based on patient weight of 50 kg

Post-marketing experience with all ACE inhibitors thus far suggests the following with regard to pregnancy outcome. Inadvertent exposure limited to the first trimester of pregnancy has not been reported to affect fetal outcome adversely. Fetal exposure during the second and third trimesters of pregnancy has been associated with fetal and neonatal morbidity and mortality.

When ACE inhibitors are used during the later stages of pregnancy, there have been reports of hypotension and decreased renal perfusion in the newborn. Oligohydramnios in the mother has also been reported, presumably representing decreasing renal function in the fetus. Infants exposed *in utero* to ACE inhibitors should be closely observed for hypotension, oliguria and hyperkalemia. If oliguria occurs, attention should be directed toward support of blood pressure and renal perfusion with the administration of fluids and pressors as appropriate. Problems associated with prematurity such as patent ductus arteriosus have occurred in association with maternal use of ACE inhibitors but it is not clear whether they are related to ACE inhibition, maternal hypertension or the underlying prematurity.

Enalapril has been removed from the neonatal circulation by peritoneal dialysis and theoretically may be removed by exchange transfusion, although there is no experience with the latter procedure.

Nursing Mothers
Milk in lactating rats contains radioactivity following administration of ^{14}C enalapril maleate. It is not known whether this drug is secreted in human milk. Because many drugs are secreted in human milk, caution should be exercised when VASOTEC I.V. is given to a nursing mother.

Pediatric Use
Safety and effectiveness in children have not been established.

ADVERSE REACTIONS

VASOTEC I.V. has been found to be generally well tolerated in controlled clinical trials involving 349 patients (168 with hypertension, 153 with congestive heart failure and 28 with coronary artery disease). The most frequent clinically significant adverse experience was hypotension (3.4 percent), occurring in eight patients (5.2 percent) with congestive heart failure, three (1.8 percent) with hypertension and one with coronary artery disease. Other adverse experiences occurring in greater than one percent of patients were: headache (2.9 percent) and nausea (1.1 percent).

Adverse experiences occurring in 0.5 to 1.0 percent of patients in controlled clinical trials included: myocardial infarction, fatigue, dizziness, fever, rash and constipation.

Enalapril Maleate
Since enalapril is converted to enalaprilat, those adverse experiences associated with enalapril might also be expected to occur with VASOTEC I.V.

The following adverse experiences have been reported with enalapril and, within each category, are listed in order of decreasing severity.

Body As A Whole: Syncope, orthostatic effects, chest pain, abdominal pain, asthenia.

Cardiovascular: Cardiac arrest; myocardial infarction or cerebrovascular accident, possibly secondary to excessive hypotension in high risk patients (see WARNINGS, *Hypotension*); pulmonary embolism and infarction; rhythm disturbances; atrial fibrillation; orthostatic hypotension; angina pectoris; palpitation.

Digestive: Ileus, pancreatitis, hepatitis or cholestatic jaundice, melena, diarrhea, vomiting, dyspepsia, anorexia, glossitis.

Nervous/Psychiatric: Depression, vertigo, confusion, ataxia, somnolence, insomnia, nervousness, paresthesia.

Respiratory: Bronchospasm, dyspnea, pneumonia, bronchitis, cough, rhinorrhea, asthma, upper respiratory infection.

Skin: Herpes zoster, pruritus, alopecia, flushing, photosensitivity.

Urogenital: Renal failure, oliguria, renal dysfunction (see PRECAUTIONS and DOSAGE AND ADMINISTRATION), urinary tract infection, impotence.

Other: Vasculitis, muscle cramps, hyperhidrosis, blurred vision, taste alteration, tinnitus.

A symptom complex has been reported which may include fever, myalgia and arthralgia; an elevated erythrocyte sedimentation rate may be present. Rash or other dermatologic manifestations may occur. These symptoms have disappeared after discontinuation of therapy.

Angioedema: Angioedema has been reported in patients receiving enalapril (0.2 percent). Angioedema associated with laryngeal edema may be fatal. If angioedema of the face, extremities, lips, tongue, glottis and/or larynx occurs, treatment with enalapril should be discontinued and appropriate therapy instituted immediately. (See WARNINGS.)

Hypotension: Combining the results of clinical trials in patients with hypertension or congestive heart failure, hypotension (including postural hypotension, and other orthostatic effects) was reported in 2.3 percent of patients following the initial dose of enalapril or during extended therapy.

In the hypertensive patients, hypotension occurred in 0.9 percent and syncope occurred in 0.5 percent of patients. Hypotension or syncope was a cause for discontinuation of therapy in 0.1 percent of hypertensive patients. (See WARNINGS.)

Clinical Laboratory Test Findings
Serum Electrolytes: Hyperkalemia (see PRECAUTIONS), hyponatremia.

Creatinine, Blood Urea Nitrogen: In controlled clinical trials minor increases in blood urea nitrogen and serum creatinine, reversible upon discontinuation of therapy, were observed in about 0.2 percent of patients with essential hypertension treated with enalapril alone. Increases are more likely to occur in patients receiving concomitant diuretics or in patients with renal artery stenosis. (See PRECAUTIONS.)

Hemoglobin and Hematocrit: Small decreases in hemoglobin and hematocrit (mean decreases of approximately 0.3 g percent and 1.0 vol percent, respectively) occur frequently in hypertensive patients treated with enalapril but are rarely of clinical importance unless another cause of anemia coexists. In clinical trials, less than 0.1 percent of patients discontinued therapy due to anemia.

Other (Causal Relationship Unknown): In marketing experience, rare cases of neutropenia, thrombocytopenia and bone marrow depression have been reported.

Liver Function Tests: Elevations of liver enzymes and/or serum bilirubin have occurred.

OVERDOSAGE

In clinical studies, some hypertensive patients received a maximum dose of 80 mg of enalaprilat intravenously over a fifteen minute period. At this high dose, no adverse effects beyond those as associated with the recommended dosages were observed.

The intravenous LD_{50} of enalaprilat is 3740–5890 mg/kg in female mice.

The most likely manifestation of overdosage would be hypotension, for which the usual treatment would be intravenous infusion of normal saline solution.

Enalaprilat may be removed from general circulation by hemodialysis.

DOSAGE AND ADMINISTRATION

FOR INTRAVENOUS ADMINISTRATION ONLY

The dose in hypertension is 1.25 mg every six hours administered intravenously over a five minute period. A clinical response is usually seen within 15 minutes. Peak effects after the first dose may not occur for up to four hours after dosing. The peak effects of the second and subsequent doses may exceed those of the first.

No dosage regimen for VASOTEC I.V. has been clearly demonstrated to be more effective in treating hypertension than 1.25 mg every six hours. However, in controlled clinical studies in hypertension, doses as high as 5 mg every six hours were well tolerated for up to 36 hours. There has been inadequate experience with doses greater than 20 mg per day.

In studies of patients with hypertension, VASOTEC I.V. has not been administered for periods longer than 48 hours. In other studies, patients have received VASOTEC I.V. for as long as seven days.

The dose for patients being converted to VASOTEC I.V. from oral therapy for hypertension with enalapril maleate is 1.25 mg every six hours. For conversion from intravenous to oral therapy, the recommended initial dose of Tablets VASOTEC® (Enalapril Maleate, MSD) is 5 mg once a day with subsequent dosage adjustments as necessary.

Patients on Diuretic Therapy
For patients on diuretic therapy the recommended starting dose for hypertension is 0.625 mg administered intravenously over a five minute period. A clinical response is usually seen within 15 minutes. Peak effects after the first dose may not occur for up to four hours after dosing, although most of the effect is usually apparent within the first hour. If after one hour there is an inadequate clinical response, the 0.625 mg dose may be repeated. Additional doses of 1.25 mg may be administered at six hour intervals.

For conversion from intravenous to oral therapy, the recommended initial dose of Tablets VASOTEC (Enalapril Maleate, MSD) for patients who have responded to 0.625 mg of enalaprilat every six hours is 2.5 mg once a day with subsequent dosage adjustment as necessary.

Dosage Adjustment in Renal Impairment
The usual dose of 1.25 mg of enalaprilat every six hours is recommended for patients with a creatinine clearance > 30 mL/min (serum creatinine of up to approximately 3 mg/dL). For patients with creatinine clearance ≤ 30 mL/min (serum creatinine ≥ 3 mg/dL), the initial dose is 0.625 mg. (See WARNINGS.)

If after one hour there is an inadequate clinical response, the 0.625 mg dose may be repeated. Additional doses of 1.25 mg may be administered at six hour intervals.

For dialysis patients, the initial dose should be 0.625 mg q.6.h.

For conversion from intravenous to oral therapy, the recommended initial dose of Tablets VASOTEC (Enalapril Maleate, MSD) is 5 mg once a day for patients with creatinine clearance > 30 mL/min and 2.5 mg once daily for patients with creatinine clearance ≤ 30 mL/min. Dosage should then be adjusted according to blood pressure response.

Administration
VASOTEC I.V. should be administered as a slow intravenous infusion, as indicated above, over at least five minutes. It may be administered as provided or diluted with up to 50 mL of a compatible diluent.

Parenteral drug products should be inspected visually for particulate matter and discoloration prior to use whenever solution and container permit.

Compatibility and Stability
VASOTEC I.V. as supplied and mixed with the following intravenous diluents has been found to maintain full activity for 24 hours at room temperature:
5 percent Dextrose Injection
0.9 percent Sodium Chloride Injection
0.9 percent Sodium Chloride Injection in 5 percent Dextrose
5 percent Dextrose in Lactated Ringer's Injection
McGaw ISOLYTE* E.

HOW SUPPLIED

No. 3508—VASOTEC I.V., 1.25 mg per mL, is a clear, colorless solution and is supplied in vials containing 2 mL.
NDC 0006-3508-04, 2 mL vials.
Storage
Store below 30°C (86°F).

A.H.F.S. Category: 24:08
DC 7494605 Issued February 1989
COPYRIGHT © MERCK & CO., INC., 1989
All rights reserved

VASOTEC® Tablets ℞
(Enalapril Maleate, MSD)

DESCRIPTION

VASOTEC® (Enalapril Maleate, MSD) is the maleate salt of enalapril, the ethyl ester of a long-acting angiotensin converting enzyme inhibitor, enalaprilat. Enalapril maleate is chemically described as (S)-1-[N-[1-(ethoxycarbonyl)-3-phenylpropyl]-L-alanyl]-L-proline, (Z)-2-butenedioate salt (1:1). Its empirical formula is $C_{20}H_{28}N_2O_5 \bullet C_4H_4O_4$, and its structural formula is:

Enalapril maleate is a white to off-white, crystalline powder with a molecular weight of 492.53. It is sparingly soluble in water, soluble in ethanol, and freely soluble in methanol. Enalapril is a pro-drug; following oral administration, it is bioactivated by hydrolysis of the ethyl ester to enalaprilat, which is the active angiotensin converting enzyme inhibitor. Enalapril maleate is supplied as 2.5 mg, 5 mg, 10 mg, and 20 mg tablets for oral administration. In addition to the active ingredient enalapril maleate, each tablet contains the following inactive ingredients: lactose, magnesium stearate, starch, and other ingredients. The 2.5 mg, 10 mg and 20 mg tablets also contain iron oxides.

CLINICAL PHARMACOLOGY

Mechanism of Action
Enalapril, after hydrolysis to enalaprilat, inhibits angiotensin-converting enzyme (ACE) in human subjects and animals. ACE is a peptidyl dipeptidase that catalyzes the conversion of angiotensin I to the vasoconstrictor substance, angiotensin II. Angiotensin II also stimulates aldosterone secretion by the adrenal cortex. The beneficial effects of enalapril in hypertension and heart failure appear to result primarily from suppression of the renin-angiotensin-aldosterone system. Inhibition of ACE results in decreased plasma angiotensin II, which leads to decreased vasopressor activity and to decreased aldosterone secretion. Although the latter decrease is small, it results in small increases of serum potassium. In hypertensive patients treated with VASOTEC alone for up to 48 weeks, mean increases in serum potassium of

* Registered trademark of American Hospital Supply Corporation.

Continued on next page

Merck Sharp & Dohme—Cont.

approximately 0.2 mEq/L were observed. In patients treated with VASOTEC plus a thiazide diuretic, there were essentially no change in serum potassium. (See PRECAUTIONS.) Removal of angiotensin II negative feedback on renin secretion leads to increased plasma renin activity.

ACE is identical to kininase, an enzyme that degrades bradykinin. Whether increased levels of bradykinin, a potent vasodepressor peptide, play a role in the therapeutic effects of VASOTEC remains to be elucidated.

While the mechanism through which VASOTEC lowers blood pressure is believed to be primarily suppression of the renin-angiotensin-aldosterone system, VASOTEC is antihypertensive even in patients with low-renin hypertension. Although VASOTEC was antihypertensive in all races studied, black hypertensive patients (usually a low-renin hypertensive population) had a smaller average response to enalapril monotherapy than non-black patients.

Pharmacokinetics and Metabolism

Following oral administration of VASOTEC, peak serum concentrations of enalapril occur within about one hour. Based on urinary recovery, the extent of absorption of enalapril is approximately 60 percent. Enalapril absorption is not influenced by the presence of food in the gastrointestinal tract. Following absorption, enalapril is hydrolyzed to enalaprilat, which is a more potent angiotensin converting enzyme inhibitor than enalapril; enalaprilat is poorly absorbed when administered orally. Peak serum concentrations of enalaprilat occur three to four hours after an oral dose of enalapril maleate. Excretion of VASOTEC is primarily renal. Approximately 94 percent of the dose is recovered in the urine and feces as enalaprilat or enalapril. The principal components in urine are enalaprilat, accounting for about 40 percent of the dose, and intact enalapril. There is no evidence of metabolites of enalapril, other than enalaprilat.

The serum concentration profile of enalaprilat exhibits a prolonged terminal phase, apparently representing a small fraction of the administered dose that has been bound to ACE. The amount bound does not increase with dose, indicating a saturable site of binding. The effective half-life for accumulation of enalaprilat following multiple doses of enalapril maleate is 11 hours.

The disposition of enalapril and enalaprilat in patients with renal insufficiency is similar to that in patients with normal renal function until the glomerular filtration rate is 30 mL/min or less. With renal function ≤ 30 mL/min, peak and trough enalaprilat levels increase, time to peak concentration increases and time to steady state may be delayed. The effective half-life of enalaprilat following multiple doses of enalapril maleate is prolonged at this level of renal insufficiency. (See DOSAGE AND ADMINISTRATION.) Enalaprilat is dialyzable at the rate of 62 mL/min.

Studies in dogs indicate that enalapril crosses the blood-brain barrier poorly, if at all; enalaprilat does not enter the brain. Multiple doses of enalapril maleate in rats do not result in accumulation in any tissues. Milk of lactating rats contains radioactivity following administration of ^{14}C enalapril maleate. Radioactivity was found to cross the placenta following administration of labeled drug to pregnant hamsters.

Pharmacodynamics and Clinical Effects

Hypertension: Administration of VASOTEC to patients with hypertension of severity ranging from mild to severe results in a reduction of both supine and standing blood pressure usually with no orthostatic component. Symptomatic postural hypotension is therefore infrequent, although it might be anticipated in volume-depleted patients. (See WARNINGS.)

In most patients studied, after oral administration of a single dose of enalapril, onset of antihypertensive activity was seen at one hour with peak reduction of blood pressure achieved by four to six hours.

At recommended doses, antihypertensive effects have been maintained for at least 24 hours. In some patients the effects may diminish toward the end of the dosing interval (see DOSAGE AND ADMINISTRATION).

In some patients achievement of optimal blood pressure reduction may require several weeks of therapy.

The antihypertensive effects of VASOTEC have continued during long term therapy. Abrupt withdrawal of VASOTEC has not been associated with a rapid increase in blood pressure.

In hemodynamic studies in patients with essential hypertension, blood pressure reduction was accompanied by a reduction in peripheral arterial resistance with an increase in cardiac output and little or no change in heart rate. Following administration of VASOTEC, there is an increase in renal blood flow; glomerular filtration rate is usually unchanged. The effects appear to be similar in patients with renovascular hypertension.

When given together with thiazide-type diuretics, the blood pressure lowering effects of VASOTEC are approximately additive.

In a clinical pharmacology study, indomethacin or sulindac was administered to hypertensive patients receiving VASOTEC. In this study there was no evidence of a blunting of the antihypertensive action of VASOTEC.

Heart Failure: In trials in patients treated with digitalis and diuretics, treatment with enalapril resulted in decreased systemic vascular resistance, blood pressure, pulmonary capillary wedge pressure, and heart size, and increased cardiac output and exercise tolerance. Heart rate was unchanged or slightly reduced, and mean ejection fraction was unchanged or increased. There was a beneficial effect on severity of heart failure as measured by the New York Heart Association (NYHA) classification and on symptoms of dyspnea and fatigue. Hemodynamic effects were observed after the first dose, and appeared to be maintained in uncontrolled studies lasting as long as four months. Effects on exercise tolerance, heart size, and severity and symptoms of heart failure were observed in placebo-controlled studies lasting from eight weeks to over one year.

A Scandinavian multicenter trial compared the effects of enalapril and placebo on mortality in 253 patients with severe heart failure (NYHA Class IV) and radiographic evidence of cardiomegaly who were maintained on therapy with diuretics and digitalis. Other vasodilators were used as needed. In the enalapril group, the reduction in all-cause mortality was 40 percent after six months and 31 percent after one year. There was an improvement in NYHA classification, a reduction in heart size, and a lessened need for concomitant vasodilator therapy in the enalapril group.

INDICATIONS AND USAGE

Hypertension

VASOTEC is indicated for the treatment of hypertension. VASOTEC is effective alone or in combination with other antihypertensive agents, especially thiazide-type diuretics. The blood pressure lowering effects of VASOTEC and thiazides are approximately additive.

Heart Failure

VASOTEC is indicated as adjunctive therapy in the management of heart failure, in patients who are not responding adequately to diuretics and digitalis.

In a multicenter placebo-controlled trial in patients with severe heart failure (New York Heart Association Class IV) and radiographic evidence of cardiomegaly who were maintained on therapy with diuretics and digitalis, patients who received VASOTEC had a 40 percent reduction in mortality after six months and a 31 percent reduction after one year. (See CLINICAL PHARMACOLOGY.)

VASOTEC is to be used with diuretics and digitalis.

In using VASOTEC consideration should be given to the fact that another angiotensin converting enzyme inhibitor, captopril, has caused agranulocytosis, particularly in patients with renal impairment or collagen vascular disease, and that available data are insufficient to show that VASOTEC does not have a similar risk. (See WARNINGS.)

CONTRAINDICATIONS

VASOTEC is contraindicated in patients who are hypersensitive to this product and in patients with a history of angioedema related to previous treatment with an angiotensin converting enzyme inhibitor.

WARNINGS

Angioedema

Angioedema of the face, extremities, lips, tongue, glottis and/or larynx has been reported in patients treated with angiotensin converting enzyme inhibitors, including VASOTEC. In such cases VASOTEC should be promptly discontinued and the patient carefully observed until the swelling disappears. In instances where swelling has been confined to the face and lips the condition has generally resolved without treatment, although antihistamines have been useful in relieving symptoms. Angioedema associated with laryngeal edema may be fatal. **Where there is involvement of the tongue, glottis or larynx, likely to cause airway obstruction, appropriate therapy, e.g., subcutaneous epinephrine solution 1:1000 (0.3 mL to 0.5 mL) should be promptly administered.** (See ADVERSE REACTIONS.)

Hypotension

Excessive hypotension is rare in uncomplicated hypertensive patients treated with VASOTEC alone. Heart failure patients given VASOTEC commonly have some reduction in blood pressure, especially with the first dose, but discontinuation of therapy for continuing symptomatic hypotension usually is not necessary when dosing instructions are followed; caution should be observed when initiating therapy. (See DOSAGE AND ADMINISTRATION.) Patients at risk for excessive hypotension, sometimes associated with oliguria and/or progressive azotemia, and rarely with acute renal failure and/or death, include those with the following conditions or characteristics: heart failure, hyponatremia, high dose diuretic therapy, recent intensive diuresis or increase in diuretic dose, renal dialysis, or severe volume and/or salt depletion of any etiology. It may be advisable to eliminate the diuretic (except in heart failure patients), reduce the diuretic dose or increase salt intake cautiously before initiating therapy with VASOTEC in patients at risk for excessive hypotension who are able to tolerate such adjustments. (See PRECAUTIONS, Drug Interactions and ADVERSE REACTIONS.) In patients at risk for excessive hypotension, therapy should be started under very close medical supervision and such patients should be followed closely for the first two weeks of treatment and whenever the dose of enalapril and/or diuretic is increased. Similar considerations may apply to patients with ischemic heart or cerebrovascular disease, in whom an excessive fall in blood pressure could result in a myocardial infarction or cerebrovascular accident.

If excessive hypotension occurs, the patient should be placed in supine position and, if necessary, receive an intravenous infusion of normal saline. A transient hypotensive response is not a contraindication to further doses of VASOTEC which usually can be given without difficulty once the blood pressure has stabilized. If symptomatic hypotension develops, a dose reduction or discontinuation of VASOTEC or concomitant diuretic may be necessary.

Neutropenia/Agranulocytosis

Another angiotensin converting enzyme inhibitor, captopril, has been shown to cause agranulocytosis and bone marrow depression, rarely in uncomplicated patients but more frequently in patients with renal impairment especially if they also have a collagen vascular disease. Available data from clinical trials of enalapril are insufficient to show that enalapril does not cause agranulocytosis at similar rates. Foreign marketing experience has revealed several cases of neutropenia or agranulocytosis in which a causal relationship to enalapril cannot be excluded. Periodic monitoring of white blood cell counts in patients with collagen vascular disease and renal disease should be considered.

PRECAUTIONS

General

Impaired Renal Function: As a consequence of inhibiting the renin-angiotensin-aldosterone system, changes in renal function may be anticipated in susceptible individuals. In patients with severe heart failure whose renal function may depend on the activity of the renin-angiotensin-aldosterone system, treatment with angiotensin converting enzyme inhibitors, including VASOTEC, may be associated with oliguria and/or progressive azotemia and rarely with acute renal failure and/or death.

In clinical studies in hypertensive patients with unilateral or bilateral renal artery stenosis, increases in blood urea nitrogen and serum creatinine were observed in 20 percent of patients. These increases were almost always reversible upon discontinuation of enalapril and/or diuretic therapy. In such patients renal function should be monitored during the first few weeks of therapy.

Some patients with hypertension or heart failure with no apparent pre-existing renal vascular disease have developed increases in blood urea and serum creatinine, usually minor and transient, especially when VASOTEC has been given concomitantly with a diuretic. This is more likely to occur in patients with pre-existing renal impairment. Dosage reduction and/or discontinuation of the diuretic and/or VASOTEC may be required.

Evaluation of patients with hypertension or heart failure should always include assessment of renal function. (See DOSAGE AND ADMINISTRATION.)

Hyperkalemia: Elevated serum potassium (greater than 5.7 mEq/L) was observed in approximately one percent of hypertensive patients in clinical trials. In most cases these were isolated values which resolved despite continued therapy. Hyperkalemia was a cause of discontinuation of therapy in 0.28 percent of hypertensive patients. In clinical trials in heart failure, hyperkalemia was observed in 3.8 percent of patients but was not a cause for discontinuation. Risk factors for the development of hyperkalemia include renal insufficiency, diabetes mellitus, and the concomitant use of potassium-sparing diuretics, potassium supplements and/or potassium-containing salt substitutes, which should be used cautiously, if at all, with VASOTEC. (See Drug Interactions.)

Surgery/Anesthesia: In patients undergoing major surgery or during anesthesia with agents that produce hypotension, enalapril may block angiotensin II formation secondary to compensatory renin release. If hypotension occurs and is considered to be due to this mechanism, it can be corrected by volume expansion.

Information for Patients

Angioedema: Angioedema, including laryngeal edema, may occur especially following the first dose of enalapril. Patients should be so advised and told to report immediately any signs or symptoms suggesting angioedema (swelling of face, extremities, eyes, lips, tongue, difficulty in swallowing or breathing) and to take no more drug until they have consulted with the prescribing physician.

Hypotension: Patients should be cautioned to report lightheadedness especially during the first few days of therapy. If actual syncope occurs, the patients should be told to discontinue the drug until they have consulted with the prescribing physician.

All patients should be cautioned that excessive perspiration and dehydration may lead to an excessive fall in blood pressure because of reduction in fluid volume. Other causes of volume depletion such as vomiting or diarrhea may also lead to a fall in blood pressure; patients should be advised to consult with the physician.

Hyperkalemia: Patients should be told not to use salt substitutes containing potassium without consulting their physician.

Neutropenia: Patients should be told to report promptly any indication of infection (e.g., sore throat, fever) which may be a sign of neutropenia.

NOTE: As with many other drugs, certain advice to patients being treated with enalapril is warranted. This information is intended to aid in the safe and effective use of this medication. It is not a disclosure of all possible adverse or intended effects.

Drug Interactions

Hypotension—Patients on Diuretic Therapy: Patients on diuretics and especially those in whom diuretic therapy was recently instituted, may occasionally experience an excessive reduction of blood pressure after initiation of therapy with enalapril. The possibility of hypotensive effects with enalapril can be minimized by either discontinuing the diuretic or increasing the salt intake prior to initiation of treatment with enalapril. If it is necessary to continue the diuretic, provide close medical supervision after the initial dose for at least two hours and until blood pressure has stabilized for at least an additional hour. (See WARNINGS and DOSAGE AND ADMINISTRATION.)

Agents Causing Renin Release: The antihypertensive effect of VASOTEC is augmented by antihypertensive agents that cause renin release (e.g., diuretics).

Other Cardiovascular Agents: VASOTEC has been used concomitantly with beta adrenergic-blocking agents, methyldopa, nitrates, calcium-blocking agents, hydralazine, prazosin and digoxin without evidence of clinically significant adverse interactions.

Agents Increasing Serum Potassium: VASOTEC attenuates potassium loss caused by thiazide-type diuretics. Potassium-sparing diuretics (e.g., spironolactone, triamterene, or amiloride), potassium supplements, or potassium-containing salt substitutes may lead to significant increases in serum potassium. Therefore, if concomitant use of these agents is indicated because of demonstrated hypokalemia, they should be used with caution and with frequent monitoring of serum potassium. Potassium sparing agents should generally not be used in patients with heart failure receiving VASOTEC.

Lithium: A few cases of lithium toxicity have been reported in patients receiving concomitant VASOTEC and lithium and were reversible upon discontinuation of both drugs. Although a causal relationship has not been established, it is recommended that caution be exercised when lithium is used concomitantly with VASOTEC and serum lithium levels should be monitored frequently.

Carcinogenesis, Mutagenesis, Impairment of Fertility

There was no evidence of a tumorigenic effect when enalapril was administered for 106 weeks to rats at doses up to 90 mg/kg/day (150 times* the maximum daily human dose). Enalapril has also been administered for 94 weeks to male and female mice at doses up to 90 and 180 mg/kg/day, respectively, (150 and 300 times* the maximum daily dose for humans) and showed no evidence of carcinogenicity.

Neither enalapril maleate nor the active diacid was mutagenic in the Ames microbial mutagen test with or without metabolic activation. Enalapril was also negative in the following genotoxicity studies: rec-assay, reverse mutation assay with *E. coli*, sister chromatid exchange with cultured mammalian cells, and the micronucleus test with mice, as well as in an *in vivo* cytogenetic study using mouse bone marrow.

There were no adverse effects on reproductive performance in male and female rats treated with 10 to 90 mg/kg/day of enalapril.

Pregnancy

Pregnancy Category C. There was no fetotoxicity or teratogenicity in rats treated with up to 200 mg/kg/day of enalapril (333 times the maximum human dose). Fetotoxicity, expressed as a decrease in average fetal weight, occurred in rats given 1200 mg/kg/day of enalapril, but did not occur when these animals were supplemented with saline. Enalapril was not teratogenic in rabbits. However, maternal and fetal toxicity occurred in some rabbits at doses of 1 mg/kg/day or more. Saline supplementation prevented the maternal and fetal toxicity seen at doses of 3 and 10 mg/kg/day, but not at 30 mg/kg/day (50 times the maximum human dose).

_____
* Based on patient weight of 50 kg

Radioactivity was found to cross the placenta following administration of labeled enalapril to pregnant hamsters.

Human Experience: There are no adequate and well-controlled studies of enalapril in pregnant women. However, data are available that show enalapril crosses the human placenta. Because the risk of fetal toxicity with the use of ACE inhibitors has not been clearly defined (see below), VASOTEC should be used during pregnancy only if the potential benefit justifies the potential risk to the fetus.

Post-marketing experience with all ACE inhibitors thus far suggests the following with regard to pregnancy outcome. Inadvertent exposure limited to the first trimester of pregnancy has not been reported to affect fetal outcome adversely. Fetal exposure during the second and third trimesters of pregnancy has been associated with fetal and neonatal morbidity and mortality.

When ACE inhibitors are used during the later stages of pregnancy, there have been reports of hypotension and decreased renal perfusion in the newborn. Oligohydramnios in the mother has also been reported, presumably representing decreased renal function in the fetus. Infants exposed *in utero* to ACE inhibitors should be closely observed for hypotension, oliguria and hyperkalemia. If oliguria occurs, attention should be directed toward support of blood pressure and renal perfusion with the administration of fluids and pressors as appropriate. Problems associated with prematurity such as patent ductus arteriosus have occurred in association with maternal use of ACE inhibitors but it is not clear whether they are related to ACE inhibition, maternal hypertension or the underlying prematurity.

Enalapril has been removed from the neonatal circulation by peritoneal dialysis and theoretically may be removed by exchange transfusion, although there is no experience with the latter procedure.

Nursing Mothers

Milk in lactating rats contains radioactivity following administration of ^{14}C enalapril maleate.

It is not known whether this drug is secreted in human milk. Because many drugs are secreted in human milk, caution should be exercised when VASOTEC is given to a nursing mother.

Pediatric Use

Safety and effectiveness in children have not been established.

ADVERSE REACTIONS

VASOTEC has been evaluated for safety in more than 10,000 patients, including over 1000 patients treated for one year or more. VASOTEC has been found to be generally well tolerated in controlled clinical trials involving 2987 patients. For the most part, adverse experiences were mild and transient in nature. In clinical trials, discontinuation of therapy due to clinical adverse experiences was required in 3.3 percent of patients with hypertension and in 5.7 percent of patients with heart failure. The frequency of adverse experiences was not related to total daily dosage within the usual dosage ranges. In patients with hypertension the overall percentage of patients treated with VASOTEC reporting adverse experiences was comparable to placebo.

HYPERTENSION

Adverse experiences occurring in greater than one percent of patients with hypertension treated with VASOTEC in controlled clinical trials are shown below. In patients treated with VASOTEC, the maximum duration of therapy was three years; in placebo treated patients the maximum duration of therapy was 12 weeks.

	VASOTEC (n = 2314) Incidence (discontinuation)	Placebo (n = 230) Incidence
Body As A Whole		
Fatigue	3.0 (<0.1)	2.6
Orthostatic Effects	1.2 (<0.1)	0.0
Asthenia	1.1 (0.1)	0.9
Digestive		
Diarrhea	1.4 (<0.1)	1.7
Nausea	1.4 (0.2)	1.7
Nervous/Psychiatric		
Headache	5.2 (0.3)	9.1
Dizziness	4.3 (0.4)	4.3
Respiratory		
Cough	1.3 (0.1)	0.9
Skin		
Rash	1.4 (0.4)	0.4

HEART FAILURE

Adverse experiences occurring in greater than one percent of patients with heart failure treated with VASOTEC are shown below. The incidences represent the experiences from both controlled and uncontrolled clinical trials (maximum duration of therapy was approximately one year). In the placebo treated patients, the incidences reported are from the controlled trials (maximum duration of therapy is 12 weeks). The percentage of patients with severe heart failure

---

(NYHA Class IV) was 29 percent and 43 percent for patients treated with VASOTEC and placebo, respectively.

	VASOTEC (n = 673) Incidence (discontinuation)	Placebo (n = 339) Incidence
Body As A Whole		
Orthostatic Effects	2.2 (0.1)	0.3
Syncope	2.2 (0.1)	0.9
Chest Pain	2.1 (0.0)	2.1
Fatigue	1.8 (0.0)	1.8
Abdominal Pain	1.6 (0.4)	2.1
Asthenia	1.6 (0.1)	0.3
Cardiovascular		
Hypotension	6.7 (1.9)	0.6
Orthostatic Hypotension	1.6 (0.1)	0.3
Angina Pectoris	1.5 (0.1)	1.8
Myocardial Infarction	1.2 (0.3)	1.8
Digestive		
Diarrhea	2.1 (0.1)	1.2
Nausea	1.3 (0.1)	0.6
Vomiting	1.3 (0.0)	0.9
Nervous/Psychiatric		
Dizziness	7.9 (0.6)	0.6
Headache	1.8 (0.1)	0.9
Vertigo	1.6 (0.1)	1.2
Respiratory		
Cough	2.2 (0.0)	0.6
Bronchitis	1.3 (0.0)	0.9
Dyspnea	1.3 (0.0)	0.4
Pneumonia	1.0 (0.0)	2.4
Skin		
Rash	1.3 (0.0)	2.4
Urogenital		
Urinary Tract Infection	1.3 (0.0)	2.4

Other serious clinical adverse experiences occurring since the drug was marketed or adverse experiences occurring in 0.5 to 1.0 percent of patients with hypertension or heart failure in clinical trials are listed below and, within each category, are in order of decreasing severity.

Cardiovascular: Cardiac arrest; myocardial infarction or cerebrovascular accident, possibly secondary to excessive hypotension in high risk patients (see WARNINGS, *Hypotension*); pulmonary embolism and infarction; rhythm disturbances; atrial fibrillation; palpitation.

Digestive: Ileus, pancreatitis, hepatitis or cholestatic jaundice, melena, anorexia, dyspepsia, constipation, glossitis.

Nervous/Psychiatric: Depression, confusion, ataxia, somnolence, insomnia, nervousness, paresthesia.

Urogenital: Renal failure, oliguria, renal dysfunction (see PRECAUTIONS and DOSAGE AND ADMINISTRATION), impotence.

Respiratory: Bronchospasm, rhinorrhea, asthma, upper respiratory infection.

Skin: Herpes zoster, pruritus, alopecia, flushing, photosensitivity.

Other: Vasculitis, muscle cramps, hyperhidrosis, blurred vision, taste alteration, tinnitus.

A symptom complex has been reported which may include fever, myalgia and arthralgia; an elevated erythrocyte sedimentation rate may be present. Rash or other dermatologic manifestations may occur. These symptoms have disappeared after discontinuation of therapy.

Angioedema: Angioedema has been reported in patients receiving VASOTEC (0.2 percent). Angioedema associated with laryngeal edema may be fatal. If angioedema of the face, extremities, lips, tongue, glottis and/or larynx occurs, treatment with VASOTEC should be discontinued and appropriate therapy instituted immediately. (See WARNINGS.)

Hypotension: In the hypertensive patients, hypotension occurred in 0.9 percent and syncope occurred in 0.5 percent of patients following the initial dose or during extended therapy. Hypotension or syncope was a cause for discontinuation of therapy in 0.1 percent of hypertensive patients. In heart failure patients, hypotension occurred in 6.7 percent and syncope occurred in 2.2 percent of patients. Hypotension or syncope was a cause for discontinuation of therapy in 1.9 percent of patients with heart failure. (See WARNINGS.)

Clinical Laboratory Test Findings

Serum Electrolytes: Hyperkalemia (see PRECAUTIONS), hyponatremia.

Creatinine, Blood Urea Nitrogen: In controlled clinical trials minor increases in blood urea nitrogen and serum creatinine, reversible upon discontinuation of therapy, were observed in about 0.2 percent of patients with essential hypertension treated with VASOTEC alone. Increases are more

Continued on next page

Merck Sharp & Dohme—Cont.

likely to occur in patients receiving concomitant diuretics or in patients with renal artery stenosis. (See PRECAUTIONS.) In patients with heart failure who were also receiving diuretics with or without digitalis increases in blood urea nitrogen or serum creatinine, usually reversible upon discontinuation of VASOTEC and/or other concomitant diuretic therapy, were observed in about 11 percent of patients. Increases in blood urea nitrogen or creatinine were a cause for discontinuation in 1.2 percent of patients.

Hemoglobin and Hematocrit: Small decreases in hemoglobin and hematocrit (mean decreases of approximately 0.3 g percent and 1.0 vol percent, respectively) occur frequently in either hypertension or congestive heart failure patients treated with VASOTEC but are rarely of clinical importance unless another cause of anemia coexists. In clinical trials, less than 0.1 percent of patients discontinued therapy due to anemia.

Other (Causal Relationship Unknown): In marketing experience, rare cases of neutropenia, thrombocytopenia, and bone marrow depression have been reported.

Liver Function Tests: Elevations of liver enzymes and/or serum bilirubin have occurred.

OVERDOSAGE

Limited data are available in regard to overdosage in humans.

The oral LD_{50} of enalapril is 2000 mg/kg in mice and rats. The most likely manifestation of overdosage would be hypotension, for which the usual treatment would be intravenous infusion of normal saline solution.

Enalaprilat may be removed from general circulation by hemodialysis.

DOSAGE AND ADMINISTRATION

Hypertension
In patients who are currently being treated with a diuretic, symptomatic hypotension occasionally may occur following the initial dose of VASOTEC. The diuretic should, if possible, be discontinued for two to three days before beginning therapy with VASOTEC to reduce the likelihood of hypotension. (See WARNINGS.) If the patient's blood pressure is not controlled with VASOTEC alone, diuretic therapy may be resumed.

If the diuretic cannot be discontinued an initial dose of 2.5 mg should be used under medical supervision for at least two hours and until blood pressure has stabilized for at least an additional hour. (See WARNINGS and PRECAUTIONS, *Drug Interactions.*)

The recommended initial dose in patients not on diuretics is 5 mg once a day. Dosage should be adjusted according to blood pressure response. The usual dosage range is 10 to 40 mg per day administered in a single dose or two divided doses. In some patients treated once daily, the antihypertensive effect may diminish toward the end of the dosing interval. In such patients, an increase in dosage or twice daily administration should be considered. If blood pressure is not controlled with VASOTEC alone, a diuretic may be added. Concomitant administration of VASOTEC with potassium supplements, potassium salt substitutes, or potassium-sparing diuretics may lead to increases of serum potassium (see PRECAUTIONS).

Dosage Adjustment in Hypertensive Patients with Renal Impairment
The usual dose of enalapril is recommended for patients with a creatinine clearance > 30 mL/min (serum creatinine of up to approximately 3 mg/dL). For patients with creatinine clearance ≤ 30 mL/min (serum creatinine ≥ 3 mg/dL), the first dose is 2.5 mg once daily. The dosage may be titrated upward until blood pressure is controlled or to a maximum of 40 mg daily.

Renal Status	Creatinine-Clearance mL/min	Initial Dose mg/day
Normal Renal Function	> 80 mL/min	5 mg
Mild Impairment	≤ 80 > 30 mL/min	5 mg
Moderate to Severe Impairment	≤ 30 mL/min	2.5 mg
Dialysis Patients	—	2.5 mg on dialysis days*

* Dosage on nondialysis days should be adjusted depending on the blood pressure response.

Heart Failure
VASOTEC is indicated as adjunctive therapy with diuretics and digitalis. The recommended starting dose is 2.5 mg once or twice daily. After the initial dose of VASOTEC, the pa-

tient should be observed under medical supervision for at least two hours and until blood pressure has stabilized for at least an additional hour. (See WARNINGS and PRECAUTIONS, *Drug Interactions.*) If possible, the dose of the diuretic should be reduced which may diminish the likelihood of hypotension. The appearance of hypotension after the initial dose of VASOTEC does not preclude subsequent careful dose titration with the drug, following effective management of the hypotension. The usual therapeutic dosing range for the treatment of heart failure is 5 to 20 mg daily given in two divided doses. The maximum daily dose is 40 mg. Once daily dosing has been effective in a controlled study, but nearly all patients in this study were given 40 mg, the maximum recommended daily dose, and there has been much more experience with twice daily dosing. In addition, patients in the mortality trial received therapy twice daily (see below). Dosage may be adjusted depending upon clinical or hemodynamic response. (See WARNINGS.)

In a placebo-controlled study which demonstrated reduced mortality in patients with severe heart failure (NYHA Class IV), patients were treated with 2.5–40 mg per day of VASOTEC, almost always administered in two divided doses. (See CLINICAL PHARMACOLOGY, *Pharmacodynamics and Clinical Effects.*)

Dosage Adjustment in Heart Failure Patients with Renal Impairment or Hyponatremia
In heart failure patients with hyponatremia (serum sodium less than 130 mEq/L) or with serum creatinine greater than 1.6 mg/dL, therapy should be initiated at 2.5 mg daily under close medical supervision. (See DOSAGE AND ADMINISTRATION, *Heart Failure,* WARNINGS and PRECAUTIONS, *Drug Interactions.*) The dose may be increased to 2.5 mg b.i.d., then 5 mg b.i.d. and higher as needed, usually at intervals of four days or more if at the time of dosage adjustment there is not excessive hypotension or significant deterioration of renal function. The maximum daily dose is 40 mg.

HOW SUPPLIED

No. 3411—Tablets VASOTEC, 2.5 mg, are yellow, biconvex barrel shaped, scored, compressed tablets with code MSD 014 on one side and VASOTEC on the other. They are supplied as follows:
NDC 0006-0014-68 bottles of 100 (with desiccant)
NDC 0006-0014-28 unit dose packages of 100.
    Shown in Product Identification Section, page 419
No. 3412—Tablets VASOTEC, 5 mg, are white, barrel shaped, scored, compressed tablets, with code MSD 712 on one side and VASOTEC on the other. They are supplied as follows:
NDC 0006-0712-68 bottles of 100 (with desiccant)
(6505-01-236-8880, 5 mg 100's)
NDC 0006-0712-28 unit dose packages of 100.
    Shown in Product Identification Section, page 419
No. 3413—Tablets VASOTEC, 10 mg, are salmon, barrel shaped, compressed tablets, with code MSD 713 on one side and VASOTEC on the other. They are supplied as follows:
NDC 0006-0713-68 bottles of 100 (with desiccant)
(6505-01-236-8881, 10 mg 100's)
NDC 0006-0713-28 unit dose packages of 100.
    Shown in Product Identification Section, page 419
No. 3414—Tablets VASOTEC, 20 mg, are peach, barrel shaped, compressed tablets, with code MSD 714 on one side and VASOTEC on the other. They are supplied as follows:
NDC 0006-0714-68 bottles of 100 (with desiccant)
(6505-01-237-0545, 20 mg 100's)
NDC 0006-0714-28 unit dose packages of 100.
    Shown in Product Identification Section, page 419
Storage
Store below 30°C (86°F) and avoid transient temperatures above 50°C (122°F). Keep container tightly closed. Protect from moisture.
Dispense in a tight container, if product package is subdivided.

    A.H.F.S. Categories: 24:04, 24:08
    DC 7575817 Issued February 1989
COPYRIGHT © MERCK & CO., INC. 1987, 1989
All rights reserved

VIVACTIL® Tablets   ℞
(Protriptyline HCl, MSD), U.S.P.

DESCRIPTION

Protriptyline HCl is *N*-methyl-5*H*-dibenzo[*a,d*]-cycloheptene-5-propanamine hydrochloride. Its empirical formula is $C_{19}H_{21}N \bullet HCl$ and its structural formula is:

H CH₂CH₂CH₂NHCH₃ • HCl

Protriptyline HCl, a dibenzocycloheptene derivative, has a molecular weight of 299.84. It is a white to yellowish powder that is freely soluble in water and soluble in dilute HCl.
VIVACTIL® (Protriptyline HCl, MSD) is supplied as 5 mg and 10 mg film coated tablets. Inactive ingredients are calcium phosphate, cellulose, guar gum, hydroxypropyl cellulose, hydroxypropyl methylcellulose, lactose, magnesium stearate, starch, talc, and titanium dioxide. Tablets VIVACTIL 5 mg and 10 mg also contain FD&C Yellow 6. Tablets VIVACTIL 10 mg also contain D&C Yellow 10.

ACTIONS

VIVACTIL is an antidepressant agent. The mechanism of its antidepressant action in man is not known. It is not a monoamine oxidase inhibitor, and it does not act primarily by stimulation of the central nervous system.
VIVACTIL has been found in some studies to have a more rapid onset of action than imipramine or amitriptyline. The initial clinical effect may occur within one week. Sedative and tranquilizing properties are lacking. The rate of excretion is slow.

INDICATIONS

VIVACTIL is indicated for the treatment of symptoms of mental depression in patients who are under close medical supervision. Its activating properties make it particularly suitable for withdrawn and anergic patients.

CONTRAINDICATIONS

VIVACTIL is contraindicated in patients who have shown prior hypersensitivity to it.
It should not be given concomitantly with a monoamine oxidase inhibiting compound. Hyperpyretic crises, severe convulsions, and deaths have occurred in patients receiving tricyclic antidepressant and monoamine oxidase inhibiting drugs simultaneously. When it is desired to substitute VIVACTIL for a monoamine oxidase inhibitor, a minimum of 14 days should be allowed to elapse after the latter is discontinued. VIVACTIL should then be initiated cautiously with gradual increase in dosage until optimum response is achieved.
This drug should not be used during the acute recovery phase following myocardial infarction.

WARNINGS

VIVACTIL may block the antihypertensive effect of guanethidine or similarly acting compounds.
VIVACTIL should be used with caution in patients with a history of seizures, and, because of its autonomic activity, in patients with a tendency to urinary retention, or increased intraocular tension.
Tachycardia and postural hypotension may occur more frequently with VIVACTIL than with other antidepressant drugs. VIVACTIL should be used with caution in elderly patients and patients with cardiovascular disorders; such patients should be observed closely because of the tendency of the drug to produce tachycardia, hypotension, arrhythmias, and prolongation of the conduction time. Myocardial infarction and stroke have occurred with drugs of this class.
On rare occasions, hyperthyroid patients or those receiving thyroid medication may develop arrhythmias when this drug is given.
In patients who may use alcohol excessively, it should be borne in mind that the potentiation may increase the danger inherent in any suicide attempt or overdosage.

Usage in Children
This drug is not recommended for use in children because safety and effectiveness in the pediatric age group have not been established.

Usage in Pregnancy
Safe use in pregnancy and lactation has not been established; therefore, use in pregnant women, nursing mothers or women who may become pregnant requires that possible benefits be weighed against possible hazards to mother and child.
In mice, rats, and rabbits, doses about ten times greater than the recommended human doses had no apparent adverse effects on reproduction.

PRECAUTIONS

When protriptyline HCl is used to treat the depressive component of schizophrenia, psychotic symptoms may be aggravated. Likewise, in manic-depressive psychosis, depressed patients may experience a shift toward the manic phase if they are treated with an antidepressant drug. Paranoid delusions, with or without associated hostility, may be exaggerated. In any of these circumstances, it may be advisable to reduce the dose of VIVACTIL or to use a major tranquilizing drug concurrently.

Symptoms, such as anxiety or agitation, may be aggravated in overactive or agitated patients.

When VIVACTIL is given with anticholinergic agents or sympathomimetic drugs, including epinephrine combined with local anesthetics, close supervision and careful adjustment of dosages are required.

Hyperpyrexia has been reported when tricyclic antidepressants are administered with anticholinergic agents or with neuroleptic drugs, particularly during hot weather.

Cimetidine is reported to reduce hepatic metabolism of certain tricyclic antidepressants, thereby delaying elimination and increasing steady-state concentrations of these drugs. Clinically significant effects have been reported with the tricyclic antidepressants when used concomitantly with cimetidine. Increases in plasma levels of tricyclic antidepressants, and in the frequency and severity of side effects, particularly anticholinergic, have been reported when cimetidine was added to the drug regimen. Discontinuation of cimetidine in well-controlled patients receiving tricyclic antidepressants and cimetidine may decrease the plasma levels and efficacy of the antidepressants.

It may enhance the response to alcohol and the effects of barbiturates and other CNS depressants.

The possibility of suicide in depressed patients remains during treatment and until significant remission occurs. This type of patient should not have access to large quantities of the drug.

Concurrent administration of VIVACTIL and electroshock therapy may increase the hazards of therapy. Such treatment should be limited to patients for whom it is essential. Discontinue the drug several days before elective surgery, if possible.

Both elevation and lowering of blood sugar levels have been reported.

Information for Patients

While on therapy with VIVACTIL, patients should be advised as to the possible impairment of mental and/or physical abilities required for performance of hazardous tasks, such as operating machinery or driving a motor vehicle.

ADVERSE REACTIONS

Within each category the following adverse reactions are listed in order of decreasing severity. Included in the listing are a few adverse reactions which have not been reported with this specific drug. However, the pharmacological similarities among the tricyclic antidepressant drugs require that each of the reactions be considered when protriptyline is administered. VIVACTIL is more likely to aggravate agitation and anxiety and produce cardiovascular reactions such as tachycardia and hypotension.

Cardiovascular: Myocardial infarction; stroke; heart block; arrhythmias; hypotension, particularly orthostatic hypotension; hypertension; tachycardia; palpitation.

Psychiatric: Confusional states (especially in the elderly) with hallucinations, disorientation, delusions, anxiety, restlessness, agitation; hypomania; exacerbation of psychosis; insomnia, panic, and nightmares.

Neurological: Seizures; incoordination; ataxia; tremors; peripheral neuropathy; numbness, tingling, and paresthesias of extremities; extrapyramidal symptoms; drowsiness; dizziness; weakness and fatigue; headache; syndrome of inappropriate ADH (antidiuretic hormone) secretion; tinnitus; alteration in EEG patterns.

Anticholinergic: Paralytic ileus; hyperpyrexia; urinary retention, delayed micturition, dilatation of the urinary tract; constipation; blurred vision, disturbance of accommodation, increased intraocular pressure, mydriasis; dry mouth and rarely associated sublingual adenitis.

Allergic: Drug fever; petechiae, skin rash, urticaria, itching, photosensitization (avoid excessive exposure to sunlight); edema (general, or of face and tongue).

Hematologic: Agranulocytosis; bone marrow depression; leukopenia; thrombocytopenia; purpura; eosinophilia.

Gastrointestinal: Nausea and vomiting; anorexia; epigastric distress; diarrhea; peculiar taste; stomatitis; abdominal cramps; black tongue.

Endocrine: Impotence, increased or decreased libido; gynecomastia in the male; breast enlargement and galactorrhea in the female; testicular swelling; elevation or depression of blood sugar levels.

Other: Jaundice (simulating obstructive); altered liver function; parotid swelling; alopecia; flushing; weight gain or loss, urinary frequency, nocturia; perspiration.

Withdrawal Symptoms: Though not indicative of addiction, abrupt cessation of treatment after prolonged therapy may produce nausea, headache, and malaise.

DOSAGE AND ADMINISTRATION

Dosage should be initiated at a low level and increased gradually, noting carefully the clinical response and any evidence of intolerance.

Usual Adult Dosage—Fifteen to 40 mg a day divided in 3 or 4 doses. If necessary, dosage may be increased to 60 mg a

day. Dosages above this amount are not recommended. Increases should be made in the morning dose.

Adolescent and Elderly Patients—In general, lower dosages are recommended for these patients. Five mg 3 times a day may be given initially, and increased gradually if necessary. In elderly patients, the cardiovascular system must be monitored closely if the daily dose exceeds 20 mg.

When satisfactory improvement has been reached, dosage should be reduced to the smallest amount that will maintain relief of symptoms.

Minor adverse reactions require reduction in dosage. Major adverse reactions or evidence of hypersensitivity require prompt discontinuation of the drug.

Usage in Children—This drug is not recommended for use in children because safety and effectiveness in the pediatric age group have not been established.

OVERDOSAGE

Manifestations—High doses may cause temporary confusion, disturbed concentration, or transient visual hallucinations. Overdosage may cause drowsiness; hypothermia; tachycardia and other arrhythmic abnormalities, for example, bundle branch block; ECG evidence of impaired conduction; congestive heart failure; dilated pupils; convulsions; severe hypotension; stupor; and coma. Other symptoms may be agitation, hyperactive reflexes, muscle rigidity, vomiting, hyperpyrexia, or any of those listed under ADVERSE REACTIONS.

Experience in the management of overdosage with protriptyline is limited. The following recommendations are based on the management of overdosage with other tricyclic antidepressants.

All patients suspected of having taken an overdosage should be admitted to a hospital as soon as possible. *Treatment* is symptomatic and supportive. Empty the stomach as quickly as possible by emesis followed by gastric lavage upon arrival at the hospital. Following gastric lavage, activated charcoal may be administered. Twenty to 30 g of activated charcoal may be given every four to six hours during the first 24 to 48 hours after ingestion. An ECG should be taken and close monitoring of cardiac function instituted if there is any sign of abnormality. Maintain an open airway and adequate fluid intake; regulate body temperature.

The intravenous administration of 1-3 mg of physostigmine salicylate is reported to reverse the symptoms of other tricyclic antidepressant poisoning in humans. Because physostigmine is rapidly metabolized, the dosage of physostigmine should be repeated as required particularly if life threatening signs such as arrhythmias, convulsions, and deep coma recur or persist after the initial dosage of physostigmine. Because physostigmine itself may be toxic, it is not recommended for routine use.

Standard measures should be used to manage circulatory shock and metabolic acidosis. Cardiac arrhythmias may be treated with neostigmine, pyridostigmine, or propranolol. Should cardiac failure occur, the use of digitalis should be considered. Close monitoring of cardiac function for not less than five days is advisable.

Anticonvulsants may be given to control convulsions.

Dialysis is of no value because of low plasma concentrations of the drug.

Since overdosage is often deliberate, patients may attempt suicide by other means during the recovery phase.

Deaths by deliberate or accidental overdosage have occurred with this class of drugs.

HOW SUPPLIED

No. 3313—Tablets VIVACTIL, 5 mg, are orange, oval, film coated tablets, coded MSD 26. They are supplied as follows: NDC 0006-0026-68 bottles of 100.

   Shown in Product Identification Section, page 419

No. 3314—Tablets VIVACTIL, 10 mg, are yellow, oval, film coated tablets, coded MSD 47. They are supplied as follows: NDC 0006-0047-68 bottles of 100

(6505-00-462-7353, 10 mg 100's)

NDC 0006-0047-28 unit dose packages of 100.

   Shown in Product Identification Section, page 419

Storage

Store Tablets VIVACTIL in a tightly closed container. Avoid storage at temperatures above 40°C (104°F).

METABOLISM

Metabolic studies indicate that protriptyline is well absorbed from the gastrointestinal tract and is rapidly sequestered in tissues. Relatively low plasma levels are found after administration, and only a small amount of unchanged drug is excreted in the urine of dogs and rabbits. Preliminary studies indicate that demethylation of the secondary amine moiety occurs to a significant extent, and that metabolic transformation probably takes place in the liver. It penetrates the brain rapidly in mice and rats, and moreover that which is present in the brain is almost all unchanged drug.

Studies on the disposition of radioactive protriptyline in human test subjects showed significant plasma levels within 2 hours, peaking at 8 to 12 hours, then declining gradually. Urinary excretion studies in the same subjects showed significant amounts of radioactivity in 2 hours. The rate of excretion was slow. Cumulative urinary excretion during 16 days accounted for approximately 50% of the drug. The fecal route of excretion did not seem to be important.

   A.H.F.S. Category: 28:16:04

   DC 7398519 Issued July 1986

Information on the Merck Sharp & Dohme products listed on these pages is the full prescribing information from product circulars in use August 31, 1989.

Mericon Industries, Inc.
8819 N. PIONEER ROAD
PEORIA, IL 61615

ORAZINC CAPSULES   OTC
(zinc sulfate USP)

(See PDR For Nonprescription Drugs)

ORAZINC LOZENGES   OTC
(zinc gluconate)

(See PDR For Nonprescription Drugs)

Merieux Institute, Inc.
P. O. BOX 523980
MIAMI, FL 33152-3980

IMOGAM® RABIES   ℞
[ĭm′o-găm]
(Rabies Immune Globulin-Human)

NDC 50361-180-20 2ml (300IU) pediatric vial
NDC 50361-180-10 10ml (1500IU) adult vial
Supplied in tamper proof plastic box.

IMOVAX® RABIES   ℞
[ĭm′o-vak]
(Rabies Vaccine Human Diploid Cell)

NDC 50361-250-10 1ml IM pre-exposure/post-exposure single dose vial
Supplied in tamper proof unit dose plastic box containing disposable syringe with 1 ml of Sterile Water for Injection U.S.P. for reconstitution and sterile disposable needles for reconstitution and administration, and 1 ml vial of lyophilized vaccine.

IMOVAX® RABIES I.D.
[ĭm′o-vak I.D.]
(Rabies Vaccine Human Diploid Cell)

NDC 50361-251-20 0.1ml I.D. pre-exposure immunization only intradermal syringe.
Supplied in a box containing tamperproof vacuum sealed glass tube holding syringe that contains 0.1ml of lyophilized Rabies Vaccine; a vial of Sterile Water for Injection U.S.P. for reconstitution of the vaccine.
The potency of IMOVAX® RABIES I.D. is equal to or greater than 2.5 I.U./ml of rabies antigen. A 0.1ml intradermal dose contains at least 0.25 I.U. Three 0.1ml I.D. are required for pre-exposure immunization.

MONO-VACC® TEST (O.T.)   ℞
[mon′ō-vak]
TUBERCULIN, MONO-VACC® TEST (O.T.)
(old tuberculin)
Multiple Puncture Device

NDC 50361-770-40   25 tests per box.
Supplied in plastic tamper proof box of 25 tests/box. Also available test reading cards in English, Spanish, Vietnamese and Chinese.

Continued on next page

Merieux—Cont.

MULTITEST CMI®   ℞
[mul'ti-test]
(Skin Test Antigens for Cellular Hypersensitivity)

NDC 50361-780-80

DESCRIPTION
Skin Test Antigens for Cellular Hypersensitivity, MULTI-TEST CMI® is a disposable, plastic applicator consisting of eight sterile test heads preloaded with the following seven delayed hypersensitivity skin test antigens and glycerin negative control for precutaneous administration: Tetanus Toxoid Antigen, Diphtheria Toxoid Antigen, Streptococcus Antigen, Old Tuberculin, Candida Antigen, Trichophyton Antigen, and Proteus Antigen.
MULTITEST CMI® provides a quick, convenient and uniform procedure for delayed cutaneous hypersensitivity testing.
Supplied in box of 10 individual cartons containing one preloaded MULTITEST CMI® per carton.

EDUCATIONAL MATERIAL

Booklets
"Rabies Concepts for Medical Professionals", Daniel Fishbein, Leigh Sawyer, William G. Winkler, Editors. Chapters dealing with rabies in humans, animals, diagnosis, pre and post-exposure prophylaxis, etiology, glossary and bibliography. 1 each free to: Physicians, Pharmacists, Public Health Officials and Veterinarians. For additional quantities and prices, please write or call.
Newsletter
"IMMUNEWS", Merieux Institute, Inc., Editor. Quarterly newsletter on recently published articles on rabies, coverage of rabies conferences and rabies enzootic and epizootic updates. Free by subscription only (no charge). 1 copy each to: Physicians, Pharmacists, Public Health Officials and Veterinarians.
Video Cassettes
"Play it Safe", Merieux Institute, Inc., Editor. A 30 second Public Service Announcement available for Professional Organization, ie, State or County Medical Societies for commercial. T.V. broadcast warning about rabies danger and prophylaxis available in ½" or ¾" V.H.S. Suitable for duplication for T.V. broadcast and with space available to identify Medical or Pharmaceutical Society, Public Health Agency or Veterinary Society. Available on a No Charge loan basis for duplication. Call or write for additional information.
"Rabies 100 Years After Pasteur", Institut Merieux, Editor. A 20 minute ½" or ¾" V.H.S. cassette color film on progress made in rabies prevention and treatment since Pasteur's first vaccination in 1885. This, and "Rabies/LaRage" are available free of charge for showing at group functions, society meetings, etc. Allow 7 weeks (minimum) prior to desired date. Call or write for additional information.
"The Problem Of Rabies In Wildlife", Dr. Harvey R. Fischman, Editor-in-Chief, The Johns Hopkins University School of Hygiene and Public Health. A 70 minute ½" or ¾" V.H.S. cassette color film. Available free of charge; allow 7 weeks (minimum) prior to desired date. Call or write for additional information.
Charts
"Rabies-What to do in an Emergency", Merieux Institute, Inc., Editor. Wall chart and pocket chart with ACIP/CDC recommendations on what to do in rabies exposure. Free to: Physicians, Pharmacists, Public Health Officials and Veterinarians.

IDENTIFICATION PROBLEM?
Consult PDR's
Product Identification Section
where you'll find over 1700
products pictured actual size
and in full color.

Merrell Dow U.S.A.
Division of Merrell Dow Pharmaceuticals Inc.
CINCINNATI, OH 45242-9553

AVC™   ℞
(sulfanilamide)
Cream/Suppositories

CAUTION: Federal law prohibits dispensing without prescription.

DESCRIPTION
AVC™ is a preparation for vaginal administration for the treatment of *Candida albicans* infections and available in the following forms:
AVC Cream
Each tube contains:
Sulfanilamide 15.0%
in a water-miscible, non-staining base made from lactose, propylene glycol, stearic acid, diglycol stearate, methylparaben, propylparaben, trolamine, and water; buffered with lactic acid to an acid pH of approximately 4.3.
AVC Suppositories
Each suppository contains:
Sulfanilamide .... 1.05 g
with lactose, in a base made from polyethylene glycol 400, polysorbate 80, polyethylene glycol 3350, and glycerin; buffered with lactic acid to an acid pH of approximately 4.5. AVC Suppositories have an inert, white, non-staining covering, which dissolves promptly in the vagina. The covering is composed of gelatin, glycerin, water, methylparaben, propylparaben, and coloring.
Sulfanilamide is an anti-infective agent. It is *p*-aminobenzenesulfonamide with the chemical structure:

$$H_2N\!-\!\!\langle\ \rangle\!-\!SO_2NH_2$$

Sulfanilamide occurs as a white odorless crystalline powder with a slightly bitter taste and sweet aftertaste. It is slightly soluble in water, alcohol, acetone, glycerin, propylene glycol, hydrochloric acid, and solutions of potassium and sodium hydroxide. It is practically insoluble in chloroform, ether, benzene, and petroleum ether.

CLINICAL PHARMACOLOGY
Sulfanilamide has been a useful ingredient of vaginal formulations for about four decades. It blocks certain metabolic processes essential for the growth of susceptible bacteria. In AVC, the sulfanilamide is in a specially compounded base buffered to the pH (about 4.3) of the normal vagina to encourage the presence of the normally occurring Döederlein's bacilli of the vagina.
The use of AVC for the treatment of vulvovaginitis caused by *Candida albicans* is supported by three clinical investigations. The three studies show AVC with sulfanilamide to be significantly more effective (p ≤ 0.01) than placebo as follows:
> In Study I, the ratio of effectiveness was 71% for the AVC with sulfanilamide versus 49% for placebo with 30 days of treatment;
> In Study II, the percentages were 48% and 24%, respectively, with 15 days of treatment;
> In Study III, the percentages were 66% versus 33%, respectively, with 30 days of treatment.

INDICATIONS AND USAGE
For the treatment of vulvovaginitis caused by *Candida albicans*. (See CLINICAL PHARMACOLOGY.)

CONTRAINDICATIONS
AVC should not be used in patients known to be sensitive to this product or to the sulfonamides.

PRECAUTIONS
General
Because sulfonamides are absorbed from the vaginal mucosa, the usual precautions for oral sulfonamides apply. Patients should be observed for skin rash or evidence of systemic toxicity, and if these develop, the medications should be discontinued.
Deaths associated with administration of oral sulfonamides have reportedly occurred from hypersensitivity reactions, agranulocytosis, aplastic anemia, and other blood dyscrasias. Goiter production, diuresis, and hypoglycemia have reportedly occurred rarely in patients receiving oral sulfonamides. Cross-sensitivity may exist with these agents. Rats appear to be especially susceptible to the goitrogenic effects of sulfonamides, and long-term administration has reportedly produced thyroid malignancies in this species.
Vaginal applicators or inserters should be used with caution after the seventh month of pregnancy.
Information For Patients
The doctor should advise the patient that in the event unusual local itching and burning occur, or other unusual symptoms develop, medication should be discontinued and not re-started without further consultation.

Drug Interactions
Drug interactions have not been documented with AVC.
Carcinogenesis, Mutagenesis, Impairment of Fertility
No data are available on long-term potential of AVC for carcinogenicity, mutagenicity, or impairment of fertility in animals or humans.
Pregnancy
Teratogenic Effects
Pregnancy Category C
Animal reproductive studies have been conducted with sulfonamides, including sulfanilamide (see below). It is not known whether AVC can cause fetal harm when administered to a pregnant woman or can affect reproductive capacity. AVC should be given to a pregnant woman only if clearly needed.
Sulfonamides, including sulfanilamide, readily pass through the placenta and reach fetal circulation. The concentration in the fetus is from 50–90% of that in the maternal blood and if high enough, can cause toxic effects. The safe use of sulfonamides, including sulfanilamide, in pregnancy has not been established. The teratogenic potential of most sulfonamides has not been thoroughly investigated in either animals or humans. However, a significant increase in the incidence of cleft palate and other bony abnormalities of offspring has been observed when certain sulfonamides of the short, intermediate, and long-acting types (including sulfanilamide) were given to pregnant rats and mice at high oral doses (seven to 25 times the human therapeutic oral dose).
Nursing Mothers
Sulfanilamide should be avoided in nursing mothers because absorbed sulfonamides will appear in maternal milk, and have caused kernicterus in the newborn. Because of the potential for serious adverse reactions in nursing infants from sulfonamides, a decision should be made whether to discontinue nursing or to discontinue the drug.
Pediatric Use
Safety and effectiveness of AVC in children have not been established.

ADVERSE REACTIONS
Local sensitivity reactions such as increased discomfort or a burning sensation have occasionally been reported following the use of topical sulfonamides. With the use of AVC Cream, sensitivity reactions (only local) were reported for 0.2% of the investigational patients.
Treatment should be discontinued if either local or systemic manifestations of sulfonamide toxicity or sensitivity occur.

DRUG ABUSE AND DEPENDENCE
Tolerance, abuse, or dependence with AVC have not been reported.

OVERDOSAGE
There have been no reports of accidental overdosage with AVC.
The acute oral LD$_{50}$ of sulfanilamide is 3700–4200 mg/kg in mice.
The minimum human lethal dose of AVC has not been established.
It is not known if AVC is dialyzable.

DOSAGE AND ADMINISTRATION
One applicatorful (about 6 g) or one suppository intravaginally once or twice daily. Improvements in symptoms should occur within a few days, but treatment should be continued for a period of 30 days.
Douching with a suitable solution before insertion may be recommended for hygienic purposes.

HOW SUPPLIED
AVC *Cream*
NDC 0068-0099-04   4 oz tube with applicator
Store at room temperature, below 86°F. Protect from cold. Product darkens with age. Potency is maintained throughout labeled shelf life when stored as directed.
AVC *Suppositories*
NDC 0068-0098-16   Box of 16 white gelatin suppositories with inserter
Store at room temperature, below 86°F. Protect from excessive cold and moisture.
> *Product Information as of September, 1986*
Suppositories are Manufactured by
R. P. Scherer, North America
Clearwater, Florida 33518 for
MERRELL DOW U.S.A.
Division of Merrell Dow Pharmaceuticals Inc.
Cincinnati, Ohio 45242-9553

CANTIL®   ℞
[kăn'til]
(mepenzolate bromide USP)
Tablets

CAUTION: Federal law prohibits dispensing without prescription.

DESCRIPTION

Cantil (mepenzolate bromide USP) chemically is 3-[(hydroxydiphenylacetyl) oxy]-1,1- dimethylpiperidinium bromide and has the following structure:

Mepenzolate bromide occurs as a white or light cream-colored powder, which is freely soluble in methanol, slightly soluble in water and chloroform, and practically insoluble in ether.

Each yellow tablet contains 25 mg mepenzolate bromide USP. This tablet also contains inactive ingredients: corn starch, FD&C Yellow No. 5 (tartrazine, See PRECAUTIONS), glucose, lactose, magnesium stearate, microcrystalline cellulose, and sucrose.

CLINICAL PHARMACOLOGY

Cantil diminishes gastric acid and pepsin secretion. Cantil also suppresses spontaneous contractions of the colon. Pharmacologically, it is a post-ganglionic parasympathetic inhibitor.

Radiotracer studies in which Cantil-^{14}C was used in animals and humans indicate that absorption following oral administration, as with other quaternary ammonium compounds, is low. Between 3 and 22% of an orally administered dose is excreted in the urine over a 5-day period, with the majority of the radioactivity appearing on Day 1. The remainder appears in the next 5 days in the feces and presumably has not been absorbed.

INDICATION

Cantil is indicated for use as adjunctive therapy in the treatment of peptic ulcer. Cantil has not been shown to be effective in contributing to the healing of peptic ulcer, decreasing the rate of recurrence or preventing complications.

CONTRAINDICATIONS

Glaucoma, obstructive uropathy (for example, bladder neck obstruction due to prostatic hypertrophy), obstructive disease of the gastrointestinal tract (for example, pyloroduodenal stenosis, achalasia), paralytic ileus, intestinal atony of the elderly or debilitated patient, unstable cardiovascular status in acute hemorrhage, severe ulcerative colitis, toxic megacolon complicating ulcerative colitis, myasthenia gravis, allergic or idiosyncratic reactions to Cantil or related compounds.

WARNINGS

In the presence of high environmental temperature, heat prostration (fever and heat stroke due to decreased sweating) can occur with use of Cantil.

Cantil may produce drowsiness or blurred vision. The patient should be cautioned regarding activities requiring mental alertness such as operating a motor vehicle or other machinery or performing hazardous work while taking this drug.

With overdosage, a curare-like action may occur, i.e., neuromuscular blockade leading to muscular weakness and possible paralysis.

It should be noted that the use of anticholinergic drugs in the treatment of gastric ulcer may produce a delay in gastric emptying time and may complicate such therapy (antral stasis).

Pregnancy

Reproduction studies in rats and rabbits have shown no evidence of impaired fertility or harm to the animal fetus. Information on possible adverse effects in the pregnant female is limited to uncontrolled data derived from marketing experience. Such experience has revealed no reports of the effect of Cantil on human pregnancies. No controlled studies to establish the safety of the drug in pregnancy have been performed.

Pediatric Use

Since there is no adequate experience in children who have received this drug, safety and efficacy in children have not been established. Newborn animal studies have been undertaken that show that younger animals are more sensitive to the toxic effects of mepenzolate bromide than are older animals.

PRECAUTIONS

Use Cantil with caution in the elderly and in all patients with:

    Autonomic neuropathy
    Hepatic or renal disease
    Ulcerative colitis. Large doses may suppress intestinal motility to the point of producing a paralytic ileus and for this reason precipitate or aggravate "toxic megacolon," a serious complication of the disease.

Hyperthyroidism, coronary heart disease, congestive heart failure, "cardiac tachyarrhythmias," tachycardia, hypertension, and prostatic hypertrophy.

Hiatal hernia associated with reflux esophagitis, since anticholinergic drugs may aggravate this condition.

This product contains FD&C Yellow No. 5 (tartrazine), which may cause allergic-type reactions (including bronchial asthma) in certain susceptible individuals. Although the overall incidence of FD&C Yellow No. 5 (tartrazine) sensitivity in the general population is low, it is frequently seen in patients who also have aspirin hypersensitivity.

Nursing Mothers

It is not known whether this drug is secreted in human milk. As a general rule, nursing should not be undertaken while a patient is on a drug since many drugs are excreted in human milk.

ADVERSE REACTIONS

Xerostomia, decreased sweating, urinary hesitancy and retention, blurred vision, tachycardia, palpitations, dilatation of the pupil, cycloplegia, increased ocular tension, loss of taste, headaches, nervousness, mental confusion, drowsiness, weakness, dizziness, insomnia, nausea, vomiting, constipation, bloated feeling, impotence, suppression of lactation, severe allergic reaction or drug idiosyncrasies including anaphylaxis, urticaria and other dermal manifestations.

OVERDOSAGE

The symptoms of overdosage with Cantil progress from an intensification of the usual adverse effects to CNS disturbances (from restlessness and excitement to psychotic behavior), circulatory changes (flushing, fall in blood pressure, circulatory failure), respiratory failure, paralysis, and coma. Measures to be taken are (1) immediate lavage of the stomach and (2) injection of physostigmine 0.5 to 2 mg intravenously, repeated as necessary up to a total of 5 mg. Fever may be treated symptomatically (alcohol sponging, ice packs). Excitement of a degree that demands attention may be managed with sodium thiopental 2% solution given slowly intravenously or chloral hydrate (100–200 ml of a 2% solution) by rectal infusion. In the event of progression of the curare-like effect to paralysis of the respiratory muscles, artificial respiration should be instituted and maintained until effective respiratory action returns.

DOSAGE AND ADMINISTRATION

Usual Adult Dose: 1 or 2 tablets three times a day preferably with meals and 1 or 2 tablets at bedtime. Begin with the lower dosage when possible and adjust subsequently according to the patient's response.

Since there is no adequate experience in children who have received this drug, safety and efficacy in children have not been established.

DRUG INTERACTIONS

Concomitant administration of anticholinergic drugs and any other drugs which would increase the anticholinergic effects of Cantil is to be avoided.

HOW SUPPLIED

Tablets (25 mg) debossed MERRELL 37: bottles of 100.

Product Information as of April, 1985
Shown in Product Identification Section, page 419

CEPHULAC® (lactulose) Syrup   ℞
[sĕf′ū-lăk]
FOR ORAL OR RECTAL ADMINISTRATION

CAUTION: Federal law prohibits dispensing without prescription.

DESCRIPTION

Cephulac (lactulose) is a synthetic disaccharide in syrup form for oral or rectal administration. Each 15 mL of Cephulac contains: 10 g lactulose (and less than 2.2 g galactose, less than 1.2 g lactose, and 1.2 g or less of other sugars). Also contains FD&C Blue No. 1, FD&C Yellow No. 6, water and flavoring. A minimal quantity of sodium hydroxide is used to adjust pH when necessary. The pH range is 3.0 to 7.0.

Cephulac is a colonic acidifier for treatment and prevention of portal-systemic encephalopathy.

The chemical name for lactulose is 4-0-β-D-galactopyranosyl-D-fructofuranose. It has the following structural formula:

[See Chemical Formula at top of next column].

CLINICAL PHARMACOLOGY

Lactulose causes a decrease in blood ammonia concentration and reduces the degree of portal-systemic encephalopathy.

These actions are considered to be results of the following:

    Bacterial degradation of lactulose in the colon acidifies the colonic contents.

    This acidification of colonic contents results in the retention of ammonia in the colon as the ammonium ion. Since the colonic contents are then more acid than the blood, ammonia can be expected to migrate from the blood into the colon to form the ammonium ion.

The molecular weight is 342.30. It is freely soluble in water.

The acid colonic contents convert NH_3 to the ammonium ion $[NH_4]^+$, trapping it and preventing its absorption.

The laxative action of the metabolites of lactulose then expels the trapped ammonium ion from the colon.

Experimental data indicate that lactulose is poorly absorbed. Lactulose given orally to man and experimental animals resulted in only small amounts reaching the blood. Urinary excretion has been determined to be 3% or less and is essentially complete within 24 hours.

When incubated with extracts of human small intestinal mucosa, lactulose was not hydrolyzed during a 24-hour period and did not inhibit the activity of these extracts on lactose. Lactulose reaches the colon essentially unchanged. There it is metabolized by bacteria with the formation of low molecular weight acids that acidify the colon contents.

INDICATIONS AND USAGE

For the prevention and treatment of portal-systemic encephalopathy, including the stages of hepatic pre-coma and coma. Controlled studies have shown that lactulose syrup therapy reduces the blood ammonia levels by 25–50%; this is generally paralleled by an improvement in the patients' mental state and by an improvement in EEG patterns. The clinical response has been observed in about 75% of patients, which is at least as satisfactory as that resulting from neomycin therapy. An increase in patients' protein tolerance is also frequently observed with lactulose therapy. In the treatment of chronic portal-systemic encephalopathy, Cephulac has been given for over 2 years in controlled studies.

CONTRAINDICATIONS

Since Cephulac contains galactose (less than 2.2 g/15 mL), it is contraindicated in patients who require a low galactose diet.

WARNINGS

A theoretical hazard may exist for patients being treated with lactulose syrup who may be required to undergo electrocautery procedures during proctoscopy or colonoscopy. Accumulation of H_2 gas in significant concentration in the presence of an electrical spark may result in an explosive reaction. Although this complication has not been reported with lactulose, patients on lactulose therapy undergoing such procedures should have a thorough bowel cleansing with a non-fermentable solution. Insufflation of CO_2 as an additional safeguard may be pursued but is considered to be a redundant measure.

PRECAUTIONS

General

Since Cephulac contains galactose (less than 2.2 g/15 mL) and lactose (less than 1.2 g/15 mL), it should be used with caution in diabetics.

In the overall management of portal-systemic encephalopathy it should be recognized that there is serious underlying liver disease with complications such as electrolyte disturbance (e.g., hypokalemia) for which other specific therapy may be required.

Infants receiving lactulose may develop hyponatremia and dehydration.

Drug Interactions

There have been conflicting reports about the concomitant use of neomycin and lactulose syrup. Theoretically, the elimination of certain colonic bacteria by neomycin and possibly other anti-infective agents may interfere with the desired degradation of lactulose and thus prevent the acidification of colonic contents. Thus the status of the lactulose-treated patient should be closely monitored in the event of concomitant oral anti-infective therapy.

Results of preliminary studies in humans and rats suggest that nonabsorbable antacids given concurrently with lac-

Continued on next page

Merrell Dow—Cont.

tulose may inhibit the desired lactulose-induced drop in colonic pH. Therefore, a possible lack of desired effect of treatment should be taken into consideration before such drugs are given concomitantly with Cephulac.

Other laxatives should not be used, especially during the initial phase of therapy for portal-systemic encephalopathy, because the loose stools resulting from their use may falsely suggest that adequate Cephulac dosage has been achieved.

Carcinogenesis, Mutagenesis, Impairment of Fertility
There are no known human data on long-term potential for carcinogenicity, mutagenicity, or impairment of fertility. There are no known animal data on long-term potential for mutagenicity.

Administration of lactulose syrup in the diet of mice for 18 months in concentrations of 3 and 10 percent (V/W) did not produce any evidence of carcinogenicity.

In studies in mice, rats, and rabbits, doses of lactulose syrup up to 6 or 12 mL/kg/day produced no deleterious effects on breeding, conception, or parturition.

Pregnancy
Teratogenic Effects
Pregnancy Category B
Reproduction studies have been performed in mice, rats, and rabbits at doses up to 2 or 4 times the usual human oral dose and have revealed no evidence of impaired fertility or harm to the fetus due to Cephulac. There are, however, no adequate and well-controlled studies in pregnant women. Because animal reproduction studies are not always predictive of human response, this drug should be used during pregnancy only if clearly needed.

Nursing Mothers
It is not known whether this drug is excreted in human milk. Because many drugs are excreted in human milk, caution should be exercised when Cephulac is administered to a nursing woman.

Pediatric Use
Very little information on the use of lactulose in young children and adolescents has been recorded. (See DOSAGE AND ADMINISTRATION.)

ADVERSE REACTIONS
Precise frequency data are not available.
Cephulac may produce gaseous distention with flatulence or belching and abdominal discomfort such as cramping in about 20% of patients. Excessive dosage can lead to diarrhea with potential complications such as loss of fluids, hypokalemia, and hypernatremia. Nausea and vomiting have been reported.

OVERDOSAGE
Signs and Symptoms
There have been no reports of accidental overdosage. In the event of overdosage it is expected that diarrhea and abdominal cramps would be the major symptoms. Medication should be terminated.

Oral LD$_{50}$
The acute oral LD$_{50}$ of the drug is 48.8 mL/kg in mice and greater than 30 mL/kg in rats.

Dialysis
Dialysis data are not available for lactulose. Its molecular similarity to sucrose, however, would suggest it should be dialyzable.

DOSAGE AND ADMINISTRATION
Oral
Adult: The usual adult, oral dosage is 2 to 3 tablespoonfuls (30 to 45 mL, containing 20 g to 30 g of lactulose) three or four times daily. The dosage may be adjusted every day or two to produce 2 or 3 soft stools daily.

Hourly doses of 30 to 45 mL of Cephulac may be used to induce the rapid laxation indicated in the initial phase of the therapy of portal-systemic encephalopathy. When the laxative effect has been achieved, the dose of Cephulac may then be reduced to the recommended daily dose. Improvement in the patient's condition may occur within 24 hours but may not begin before 48 hours or even later.

Continuous long-term therapy is indicated to lessen the severity and prevent the recurrence of portal-systemic encephalopathy. The dose of Cephulac for this purpose is the same as the recommended daily dose.

Pediatric: Very little information on the use of lactulose in young children and adolescents has been recorded. As with adults, the subjective goal in proper treatment is to produce 2 or 3 soft stools daily. On the basis of information available, the recommended initial daily oral dose in infants is 2.5 to 10 mL in divided doses. For older children and adolescents the total daily dose is 40 to 90 mL. If the initial dose causes diarrhea, the dose should be reduced immediately. If diarrhea persists, lactulose should be discontinued.

Rectal
When the adult patient is in the impending coma or coma stage of portal-systemic encephalopathy and the danger of aspiration exists, or when the necessary endoscopic or intubation procedures physically interfere with the administra-

tion of the recommended oral doses, Cephulac may be given as a retention enema via a rectal balloon catheter. Cleansing enemas containing soap suds or other alkaline agents should not be used.

Three hundred mL of Cephulac should be mixed with 700 mL of water or physiologic saline and retained for 30 to 60 minutes. Cephulac enema may be repeated every 4 to 6 hours. If the enema is inadvertently evacuated too promptly, it may be repeated immediately.

The goal of treatment is reversal of the coma stage in order that the patient may be able to take oral medication. Reversal of coma may take place within 2 hours of the first enema in some patients. Cephulac, given orally in the recommended doses, should be started before Cephulac by enema is stopped entirely.

HOW SUPPLIED
NDC 0068-0413-16
  1 pint bottles
NDC 0068-0413-64
  2 quart bottles
NDC 0068-0413-39
  30 mL unit dose cups in trays of 10 cups
Cephulac contains lactulose 667 mg/mL (10 g/15 mL).
Store at room temperature, 59°-86°F (15°-30°C).
Under recommended storage conditions, a normal darkening of color may occur. Such darkening is characteristic of sugar solutions and does not affect therapeutic action. Prolonged exposure to temperatures above 86°F (30°C) or to direct light may cause extreme darkening and turbidity which may be pharmaceutically objectionable. If this condition develops, do not use.
Prolonged exposure to freezing temperatures may cause change to a semisolid, too viscous to pour. Viscosity will return to normal upon warming to room temperature.

Product Information as of January, 1988
Shown in Product Identification Section, page 419

CHRONULAC® ℞
[*krŏn 'ū-lăk*]
(lactulose)
Syrup

CAUTION: Federal law prohibits dispensing without prescription.

DESCRIPTION
Chronulac (lactulose) is a synthetic disaccharide in syrup form for oral administration. Each 15 mL of Chronulac contains: 10 g lactulose (and less than 2.2 g galactose, less than 1.2 g lactose, and 1.2 g or less of other sugars). Also contains FD&C Blue No. 1, FD&C Yellow No. 6, water and flavoring. A minimal quantity of sodium hydroxide is used to adjust pH when necessary. The pH range is 3.0 to 7.0.
Chronulac is a colonic acidifier which promotes laxation.
The chemical name for lactulose is 4-0-β-D-galactopyranosyl-D-fructofuranose. It has the following structural formula:

The molecular weight is 342.30. It is freely soluble in water.

CLINICAL PHARMACOLOGY
Chronulac is poorly absorbed from the gastrointestinal tract and no enzyme capable of hydrolysis of this disaccharide is present in human gastrointestinal tissue. As a result, oral doses of Chronulac reach the colon virtually unchanged. In the colon, Chronulac is broken down primarily to lactic acid, and also to small amounts of formic and acetic acids, by the action of colonic bacteria, which results in an increase in osmotic pressure and slight acidification of the colonic contents. This in turn causes an increase in stool water content and softens the stool.

Since Chronulac does not exert its effect until it reaches the colon, and since transit time through the colon may be slow, 24 to 48 hours may be required to produce the desired bowel movement.

Chronulac given orally to man and experimental animals resulted in only small amounts reaching the blood. Urinary excretion has been determined to be 3% or less and is essentially complete within 24 hours.

INDICATIONS AND USAGE
For the treatment of constipation. In patients with a history of chronic constipation, lactulose syrup (Chronulac) therapy increases the number of bowel movements per day and the number of days on which bowel movements occur.

CONTRAINDICATIONS
Since Chronulac contains galactose (less than 2.2 g/15 mL), it is contraindicated in patients who require a low galactose diet.

WARNINGS
A theoretical hazard may exist for patients being treated with lactulose syrup who may be required to undergo electrocautery procedures during proctoscopy or colonoscopy. Accumulation of H_2 gas in significant concentration in the presence of an electrical spark may result in an explosive reaction. Although this complication has not been reported with lactulose, patients on lactulose therapy undergoing such procedures should have a thorough bowel cleansing with a non-fermentable solution. Insufflation of CO_2 as an additional safeguard may be pursued but is considered to be a redundant measure.

PRECAUTIONS
General
Since Chronulac contains galactose (less than 2.2 g/15 mL) and lactose (less than 1.2 g/15 mL), it should be used with caution in diabetics.

Information for Patients
In the event that an unusual diarrheal condition occurs, contact your physician.

Laboratory Tests
Elderly, debilitated patients who receive Chronulac for more than six months should have serum electrolytes (potassium, chloride, carbon dioxide) measured periodically.

Drug Interactions
Results of preliminary studies in humans and rats suggest that nonabsorbable antacids given concurrently with lactulose may inhibit the desired lactulose-induced drop in colonic pH. Therefore, a possible lack of desired effect of treatment should be taken into consideration before such drugs are given concomitantly with Chronulac.

Carcinogenesis, Mutagenesis, Impairment of Fertility
There are no known human data on long-term potential for carcinogenicity, mutagenicity, or impairment of fertility. There are no known animal data on long-term potential for mutagenicity.

Administration of lactulose syrup in the diet of mice for 18 months in concentrations of 3 and 10 percent (V/W) did not produce any evidence of carcinogenicity.

In studies in mice, rats, and rabbits doses of lactulose syrup up to 6 or 12 mL/kg/day produced no deleterious effects in breeding, conception, or parturition.

Pregnancy
Teratogenic Effects
Pregnancy Category B
Reproduction studies have been performed in mice, rats, and rabbits at doses up to 3 or 6 times the usual human oral dose and have revealed no evidence of impaired fertility or harm to the fetus due to Chronulac. There are, however, no adequate and well-controlled studies in pregnant women. Because animal reproduction studies are not always predictive of human response, this drug should be used during pregnancy only if clearly needed.

Nursing Mothers
It is not known whether this drug is excreted in human milk. Because many drugs are excreted in human milk, caution should be exercised when Chronulac is administered to a nursing mother.

Pediatric Use
Safety and effectiveness in children have not been established.

ADVERSE REACTIONS
Precise frequency data are not available.
Initial dosing may produce flatulence and intestinal cramps, which are usually transient. Excessive dosage can lead to diarrhea with potential complications such as loss of fluids, hypokalemia, and hypernatremia.
Nausea and vomiting have been reported.

OVERDOSAGE
Signs and Symptoms
There have been no reports of accidental overdosage. In the event of overdosage, it is expected that diarrhea and abdominal cramps would be the major symptoms. Medication should be terminated.

Oral LD$_{50}$
The acute oral LD$_{50}$ of the drug is 48.8 mL/kg in mice and greater than 30 mL/kg in rats.

Dialysis
Dialysis data are not available for lactulose. Its molecular similarity to sucrose, however, would suggest that it should be dialyzable.

DOSAGE AND ADMINISTRATION
The usual dose is 1 to 2 tablespoonfuls (15 to 30 mL, containing 10 g to 20 g of lactulose) daily. The dose may be increased to 60 mL daily if necessary. Twenty-four to 48 hours may be required to produce a normal bowel movement.
Note: Some patients have found that Chronulac may be more acceptable when mixed with fruit juice, water, or milk.

HOW SUPPLIED

NDC 0068-0409-08
  8 fl oz bottles
NDC 0068-0409-30
  30 mL unit dose cups in trays of 10 cups
NDC 0068-0409-32
  1 quart bottles
Chronulac contains lactulose 667 mg/mL (10 g/15 mL).
Store at room temperature, 59°–86°F (15°–30°C).
Under recommended storage conditions, a normal darkening of color may occur. Such darkening is characteristic of sugar solutions and does not affect therapeutic action. Prolonged exposure to temperatures above 86°F (30°C) or to direct light may cause extreme darkening and turbidity which may be pharmaceutically objectionable. If this condition develops, do not use.
Prolonged exposure to freezing temperatures may cause change to a semisolid, too viscous to pour. Viscosity will return to normal upon warming to room temperature.
Product Information as of January, 1988
Shown in Product Identification Section, page 419

CLOMID®   ℞
[*klǎhm′ĭd*]
(clomiphene citrate tablets USP)

For prescribing information, write to:
Professional Information Department
MERRELL DOW U.S.A.
Division of Merrell Dow Pharmaceuticals Inc.
Cincinnati, Ohio 45242-9553, U.S.A.
   Shown in Product Identification Section, page 419

HIPREX®   ℞
[*hĭp′rĕx*]
(methenamine hippurate)

CAUTION: Federal law prohibits dispensing without prescription.

DESCRIPTION

Each yellow capsule-shaped tablet contains 1 g methenamine hippurate which is the hippuric acid salt of methenamine (hexamethylenetetramine). The tablet also contains inactive ingredients: FD&C Yellow No. 5 (tartrazine, See PRECAUTIONS), magnesium stearate, povidone, and saccharin sodium.

ACTIONS

Microbiology: Hiprex (methenamine hippurate) has antibacterial activity because the methenamine component is hydrolyzed to formaldehyde in acid urine. Hippuric acid, the other component, has some antibacterial activity and also acts to keep the urine acid. The drug is generally active against *E. coli*, enterococci and staphylococci. *Enterobacter aerogenes* is generally resistant. The urine must be kept sufficiently acid for urea-splitting organisms such as *Proteus* and *Pseudomonas* to be inhibited.
Human Pharmacology: Within ½ hour after ingestion of a single 1-gram dose of Hiprex, antibacterial activity is demonstrable in the urine. Urine has continuous antibacterial activity when Hiprex is administered at the recommended dosage schedule of 1 gram twice daily. Over 90% of methenamine moiety is excreted in the urine within 24 hours after administration of a single 1-gram dose. Similarly, the hippurate moiety is rapidly absorbed and excreted, and it reaches the urine by both tubular secretion and glomerular filtration. This action may be important in older patients or in those with some degree of renal impairment.

INDICATIONS

Hiprex is indicated for prophylactic or suppressive treatment of frequently recurring urinary tract infections when long-term therapy is considered necessary. This drug should only be used after eradication of the infection by other appropriate antimicrobial agents.

CONTRAINDICATIONS

Hiprex (methenamine hippurate) is contraindicated in patients with renal insufficiency, severe hepatic insufficiency, or severe dehydration. Methenamine preparations should not be given to patients taking sulfonamides because some sulfonamides may form an insoluble precipitate with formaldehyde in the urine.

WARNINGS

Large doses of methenamine (8 grams daily for 3 to 4 weeks) have caused bladder irritation, painful and frequent micturition, albuminuria, and gross hematuria.

PRECAUTIONS

1. Care should be taken to maintain an acid pH of the urine, especially when treating infections due to urea-splitting organisms such as *Proteus* and strains of *Pseudomonas*.

2. In a few instances in one study, the serum transaminase levels were slightly elevated during treatment but returned to normal while the patients were still taking Hiprex. Because of this report, it is recommended that liver function studies be performed periodically on patients taking the drug, especially those with liver dysfunction.
3. *Use in Pregnancy:* In early pregnancy the safe use of Hiprex is not established. In the last trimester, safety is suggested, but not definitely proved. No adverse effects on the fetus were seen in studies in pregnant rats and rabbits. Hiprex taken during pregnancy can interfere with laboratory tests of urine estriol (resulting in unmeasurably low values) when acid hydrolysis is used in the laboratory procedure. This interference is due to the presence in the urine of methenamine and/or formaldehyde. Enzymatic hydrolysis, in place of acid hydrolysis, will circumvent this problem.
4. This product contains FD&C Yellow No. 5 (tartrazine), which may cause allergic-type reactions (including bronchial asthma) in certain susceptible individuals. Although the overall incidence of FD&C Yellow No. 5 (tartrazine) sensitivity in the general population is low, it is frequently seen in patients who also have aspirin hypersensitivity.

ADVERSE REACTIONS

Minor adverse reactions have been reported in less than 3.5% of patients treated. These reactions have included nausea, upset stomach, dysuria, and rash.

DOSAGE AND ADMINISTRATION

1 tablet (1.0 g) twice daily (morning and night) for adults and children over 12 years of age.
½ to 1 tablet (0.5 to 1.0 g) twice daily (morning and night) for children 6 to 12 years of age.
Since the antibacterial activity of Hiprex is greater in acid urine, restriction of alkalinizing foods and medications is desirable. If necessary, as indicated by urinary pH and clinical response, supplemental acidification of the urine should be instituted. The efficacy of therapy should be monitored by repeated urine cultures.

HOW SUPPLIED

1-gram scored, capsule-shaped yellow tablets debossed MERRELL 277 in bottles of 100
   Product Information as of April, 1985
   Shown in Product Identification Section, page 419

LORELCO® Tablets   ℞
[*lō-rĕl-cō*]
(probucol)

CAUTION: Federal law prohibits dispensing without prescription.

DESCRIPTION

Lorelco (probucol) film-coated tablets for oral administration contain 250 mg or 500 mg of probucol per tablet. Each tablet also contains as inactive ingredients: corn starch, ethylcellulose, glycerin, hydroxypropyl cellulose, hydroxypropyl methylcellulose 2910, iron oxide, lactose, magnesium stearate, microcrystalline cellulose, polysorbate 80, talc, and titanium dioxide. Lorelco is an agent for the reduction of elevated serum cholesterol. The chemical name is 4,4′-[(1-methylethylidene)bis(thio)]bis[2,6-bis(1,1-dimethylethyl)phenol]. Its chemical structure does not resemble that of any other available cholesterol-lowering agent. It is lipophilic.

CLINICAL PHARMACOLOGY

Lorelco lowers total serum cholesterol and has relatively little effect on serum triglycerides. Patients responding to probucol exhibit a decrease in low-density lipoprotein (LDL) cholesterol. Cholesterol is reduced not only in the LDL fraction, but also in the high-density lipoprotein (HDL) fraction with proportionately greater effect on the high-density portion. Epidemiologic studies have shown that both low HDL-cholesterol and high LDL-cholesterol are independent risk factors for coronary heart disease. The risk of lowering HDL-cholesterol while lowering LDL-cholesterol remains unknown. There is little or no effect reported on very low-density lipoprotein (VLDL).
Studies on the mode of action of Lorelco indicate that it increases the fractional rate of LDL catabolism. This effect may be linked to the observed increased excretion of fecal bile acids, a final metabolic pathway for the elimination of cholesterol from the body. Lorelco also exhibits inhibition of early stages of cholesterol biosynthesis and slight inhibition of absorption of dietary cholesterol. There is no increase in the cyclic precursors of cholesterol, namely desmosterol and 7-dehydrocholesterol. On this basis, it is concluded that

Lorelco does not affect the later stages of cholesterol biosynthesis.
Absorption of Lorelco from the gastrointestinal tract is limited and variable. When it is administered with food, peak blood levels are higher and less variable. With continuous administration in a dosage of 500 mg b.i.d., the blood levels of an individual gradually increase over the first three to four months and thereafter remain fairly constant. In 116 patients treated with Lorelco for periods of three months to one year, the mean blood level was 23.6 ± 17.2 mcg/mL ($\pm$ S.D.) ranging to 78.3 mcg/mL. Levels observed after seven years of treatment in 40 patients yielded an average value of 21.5 ± 16.5 mcg/mL ($\pm$ S.D.) ranging to 62.0 mcg/mL. In a separate study in eight patients, blood levels averaged 19.0 mcg/mL at the end of 12 months of treatment. Six weeks after cessation of therapy, the average had fallen by 60%. After six months, the average had fallen by 80%.
In December 1984, a National Institutes of Health Consensus Development Conference Panel[1] concluded that lowering definitely elevated blood cholesterol levels (specifically blood levels of LDL-cholesterol) will reduce the risk of heart attacks due to coronary heart disease. The effect of probucol-induced reduction of serum cholesterol or triglyceride levels, or reduction of HDL-cholesterol levels on morbidity or mortality due to coronary heart disease has not been established.

INDICATIONS AND USAGE

Serious animal toxicity has been encountered with probucol. See WARNINGS and ANIMAL PHARMACOLOGY AND TOXICOLOGY sections. Probucol is not an innocuous drug and strict attention should be paid to the INDICATIONS, CONTRAINDICATIONS, and WARNINGS.
Drug therapy should not be used for the routine treatment of elevated blood lipids for the prevention of coronary heart disease. Dietary therapy specific for the type of hyperlipidemia is the initial treatment of choice. Excess body weight may be an important factor and should be addressed prior to any drug therapy. Physical exercise can be an important ancillary measure. Contributory disease such as hypothyroidism or diabetes mellitus should be looked for and adequately treated. The use of drugs should be considered only when reasonable attempts have been made to obtain satisfactory results with nondrug methods. If the decision ultimately is to use drugs, the patient should be instructed that this does not reduce the importance of adhering to diet.
The selection of patients for cholesterol-lowering drug therapy should take into account other important coronary risk factors such as smoking, hypertension, and diabetes mellitus. Consideration should be given to the efficacy, safety, and compliance factors for each of the cholesterol-lowering drugs prior to selecting the one most appropriate for an individual patient.
Lorelco may be indicated for the reduction of elevated serum cholesterol in patients with primary hypercholesterolemia (Types IIa and IIb hyperlipoproteinemia),[2] whose elevated LDL-cholesterol has not responded adequately to diet, weight reduction and control of diabetes mellitus. Lorelco may be useful to lower elevated LDL-cholesterol that occurs in those patients with combined hypercholesterolemia and hypertriglyceridemia (Type IIb) due to elevation of both LDL and VLDL, but it is not indicated where hypertriglyceridemia is the abnormality of most concern. After establishing that the elevation in serum total cholesterol represents a primary lipid disorder, it should be determined that patients being considered for treatment with Lorelco have an elevated LDL-cholesterol as the cause for an elevated total serum cholesterol. This may be particularly relevant for patients with elevated triglycerides or with markedly elevated HDL-cholesterol values, where non-LDL fractions may contribute significantly to total cholesterol levels without apparent increase in cardiovascular risk. In most patients, LDL-cholesterol may be estimated according to the following equation:
LDL-cholesterol = Total cholesterol − [(0.16 × triglycerides) + HDL-cholesterol]
When total triglycerides are greater than 400 mg/dL, this equation is less accurate. In such patients, LDL-cholesterol may be obtained by ultracentrifugation.
It is not always possible to predict from the lipoprotein type or other factors which patients will exhibit favorable results. Lipid levels, including HDL-cholesterol, should be periodically assessed.
The effect of probucol-induced reduction of serum cholesterol or triglyceride levels, or reduction of HDL-cholesterol levels on morbidity or mortality due to coronary heart disease has not been established.

CONTRAINDICATIONS

(See also WARNINGS and PRECAUTIONS.) Lorelco is contraindicated in patients who are known to have a hypersensi-

Continued on next page

Information on Merrell Dow products is based on labeling in effect in June, 1989.

Merrell Dow—Cont.

tivity to it. Lorelco is contraindicated in patients with evidence of recent or progressive myocardial damage or findings suggestive of serious ventricular arrhythmias or with unexplained syncope or syncope of cardiovascular origin. Lorelco is contraindicated in patients with an abnormally long QT interval.

WARNINGS

SERIOUS ANIMAL TOXICITY HAS BEEN ENCOUNTERED WITH PROBUCOL IN RHESUS MONKEYS FED AN ATHEROGENIC DIET AND IN BEAGLE DOGS. (SEE ANIMAL PHARMACOLOGY AND TOXICOLOGY SECTION.)

Prolongation of the QT interval can occur in patients on Lorelco. Serious arrhythmias have been seen in association with an abnormally long QT interval in patients on Lorelco alone and in patients on Lorelco and a concomitant antiarrhythmic drug. The following precautions are deemed prudent:

1. Patients should be advised to adhere to a low cholesterol, low fat diet at the start of treatment with Lorelco and throughout the treatment period.
2. An ECG should be done prior to starting treatment and repeated at appropriate intervals during treatment. If an abnormally long QT interval is observed, the possible benefits and risks should be carefully considered before making a decision to continue Lorelco.

Lorelco therapy should be discontinued or not started if the QT interval at an observed heart rate on a resting ECG is persistently more than one of the values listed below:

Observed Heart Rate	QT Interval in sec (15% above the upper limit of normal)*	
(beats/min)	Males	Females
40	0.56	0.58
50	0.52	0.53
60	0.49	0.50
70	0.45	0.47
80	0.43	0.44
86	0.42	0.43
92	0.40	0.41
100	0.39	0.40
109	0.37	0.38
120	0.36	0.36
133	0.34	0.35

*Values calculated from Burch GE, Winsor T. A primer of electrocardiography. Philadelphia, PA: Lea and Febiger; 1958; p. 272 (Table 6).

3. Patients developing unexplained syncope or syncope of cardiovascular origin should have Lorelco therapy discontinued and should have ECG surveillance.
4. Drugs that prolong the QT interval are more likely to be associated with ventricular tachycardia after:
   a. An increase in the dose of the drug.
   b. Addition of a second drug that prolongs the QT interval (including tricyclic antidepressants, class I and III antiarrhythmics, and phenothiazines).
   c. Hypokalemia or hypomagnesemia.
   d. Severe bradycardia due to intrinsic heart disease or drug effects on the atrial rate (beta-blockers) or AV block (digoxin).
   e. Development of recent or acute myocardial infarction, ischemia, or inflammation.

The use of Lorelco in patients receiving any of these drugs should be based on the conclusion that alternate methods of hypocholesterolemic therapy are either ineffective or not tolerated, and the potential benefits of cholesterol lowering outweigh the risk of serious arrhythmia.

The following conditions should be resolved or corrected prior to initiation of therapy with Lorelco:
   a. Hypokalemia
   b. Hypomagnesemia
   c. Severe bradycardia due to intrinsic heart disease or drug effects on the atrial rate (beta-blockers) or AV block (digoxin).
   d. Recent or acute myocardial infarction, ischemia, or inflammation.

PRECAUTIONS

General: Before instituting therapy with Lorelco, adequate baseline studies should be performed to determine that the patient has persistently elevated total and LDL-cholesterol levels representing a primary lipid disorder, and that the increased cholesterol is not due to secondary conditions such as hypothyroidism, poorly controlled diabetes mellitus, obstructive liver disease, nephrotic syndrome, or dysproteinemias. Serum lipid levels, including HDL-cholesterol, should be determined after an overnight fast before treatment, during an adequate trial of diet and weight reduction therapy prior to addition of drug therapy, and periodically during combined diet and drug therapy, including assessment during the first several months of drug treatment. A

favorable trend in lipid levels should be evident during the first three to four months of administration of Lorelco, and if satisfactory lipid alteration is not achieved, the drug should be discontinued. Lorelco lowers serum total and LDL-cholesterol, and also lowers HDL-cholesterol in most patients with elevated LDL-cholesterol. Epidemiologic studies within hypercholesterolemic populations have shown that serum HDL-cholesterol is an independent, inversely correlated, risk factor for coronary heart disease (see CLINICAL PHARMACOLOGY). Human studies which will attempt to confirm or deny the hypothesis that drug-induced alteration in HDL-cholesterol affects cardiovascular risk are currently under evaluation. It is not known whether probucol-induced reduction of serum HDL-cholesterol will affect cardiovascular risk since no long-term, controlled clinical trials of Lorelco for the prevention of coronary heart disease, similar to the LRC-CPPT (See CLINICAL STUDIES), have been performed. The probable benefits obtained from LDL-cholesterol reduction must be weighed against the possible risk of a reduction in HDL-cholesterol when assessing the response of each patient receiving Lorelco treatment. If satisfactory lipid alteration is not achieved, the drug should be discontinued.

Information for Patients: The patient should be instructed to adhere to a prudent diet. Females should be cautioned against becoming pregnant for at least six months after discontinuing Lorelco and should not breast-feed their infants during therapy with Lorelco.

Laboratory Tests: The physician should schedule periodic blood lipid determinations and periodic ECGs. (See WARNINGS.)

Elevations of the serum transaminases (SGOT, SGPT), bilirubin, alkaline phosphatase, creatine phosphokinase, uric acid, blood urea nitrogen and blood glucose above the normal range were observed on one or more occasions in various patients treated with Lorelco. Most often these were transient and/or could have been related to the patient's clinical state or other modes of therapy. Although the basis for the relationship between Lorelco and these abnormalities is not firm, the possibility that some of these are drug related cannot be excluded. In the controlled trials, the incidence of abnormal laboratory values was no higher in the patients treated with Lorelco than in the patients who received placebo. If abnormal laboratory tests persist or worsen, if clinical signs consistent with the abnormal laboratory tests develop, or if systemic manifestations occur, Lorelco should be discontinued.

Drug Interactions: The addition of clofibrate to Lorelco is not recommended, since the lowering effect on mean serum levels of either LDL or total cholesterol is generally not significantly additive and, in some patients, there may be a pronounced lowering of HDL-cholesterol.

Neither oral hypoglycemic agents nor oral anticoagulants alter the effect of Lorelco on serum cholesterol. The dosage of these agents is not usually modified when given with Lorelco.

Monkeys fed a high fat, high cholesterol diet admixed with probucol exhibited serious toxicity. (See WARNINGS and ANIMAL PHARMACOLOGY AND TOXICOLOGY sections.) Prolongation of the QT interval can occur in patients on Lorelco and serious arrhythmias have been seen in association with an abnormally long QT interval in patients on Lorelco. The addition of a second drug that prolongs the QT interval (including tricyclic antidepressants, class I and III antiarrhythmics, and phenothiazines) may increase the risk of serious arrhythmia. (See CONTRAINDICATIONS AND WARNINGS.)

Carcinogenesis, Mutagenesis, Impairment of Fertility
In chronic studies of two years' duration in rats, no toxicity or carcinogenicity was observed. These results are consistent with the lack of any adverse effect on fertility and the negative findings in tests for mutagenic activity in rats.

Pregnancy:
Teratogenic Effects
Pregnancy—Category B: Reproduction studies have been performed in rats and rabbits at doses up to 50 times the human dose, and have revealed no evidence of impaired fertility or harm to the fetus due to probucol. There are, however, no adequate and well-controlled studies in pregnant women. Because animal reproduction studies are not always predictive of human response, this drug should be used during pregnancy only if clearly needed. Furthermore, if a patient wishes to become pregnant, it is recommended that the drug be withdrawn and birth control procedures be used for at least six months because of persistence of the drug in the body for prolonged periods. (See CLINICAL PHARMACOLOGY.)

Labor and Delivery: The effect of Lorelco on human labor and delivery is unknown.

Nursing Mothers: It is not known whether this drug is excreted in human milk, but it is likely, since such excretion has been shown in animals. It is recommended that nursing not be undertaken while a patient is on Lorelco.

Pediatric Use: Safety and effectiveness in children have not been established.

ADVERSE REACTIONS

Gastrointestinal
diarrhea or loose stools, flatulence, abdominal pain, nausea, vomiting, indigestion, gastrointestinal bleeding

Cardiovascular
prolongation of the QT interval on ECG, syncope, ventricular arrhythmias (ventricular tachycardia, torsades de pointes, ventricular fibrillation), sudden death.

Neurologic
headache, dizziness, paresthesia, insomnia, tinnitus, peripheral neuritis

Hematologic
eosinophilia, low hemoglobin and/or hematocrit, thrombocytopenia

Dermatologic
rash, pruritus, ecchymosis, petechiae, hyperhidrosis, fetid sweat

Genitourinary
impotency, nocturia

Ophthalmic
conjunctivitis, tearing, blurred vision

Endocrine
enlargement of multinodular goiter

Idiosyncrasies
observed with initiation of therapy and characterized by dizziness, palpitations, syncope, nausea, vomiting and chest pain

Other
diminished sense of taste and smell, anorexia, angioneurotic edema

DRUG ABUSE AND DEPENDENCE

No evidence of abuse potential has been associated with Lorelco, nor is there evidence of psychological or physical dependence in humans.

OVERDOSAGE

There is a single report of a 15-kg, three-year-old, male child who ingested 5 g of probucol. Emesis was induced by ipecac. The child remained well, apart from a brief episode of loose stools and flatulence. No specific information is available on the treatment of overdosage with Lorelco and no specific antidote is available. Probucol is not dialyzable. Treatment is symptomatic and supportive. Probucol has shown no identifiable acute toxicity in mice and rats. In these animals, the LD$_{50}$ (oral) is in excess of 5 g/kg of body weight.

DOSAGE AND ADMINISTRATION

For adult use only. The recommended and maximal dose is 1000 mg daily given in two divided doses of 500 mg each (two 250 mg tablets or one 500 mg tablet) with the morning and evening meals.

HOW SUPPLIED

250 mg round, white, film-coated tablets imprinted with either the DOW diamond trademark over the code number 51 or LORELCO 250. Bottles of 120 (NDC 0068-0051-52)
500 mg capsule-shaped, white, film-coated tablets, marked LORELCO 500. Bottles of 100 (NDC 0068-0053-61)
Keep well closed. Store in a dry place. Avoid excessive heat. Dispense in well-closed light-resistant containers with child-resistant closures.

ANIMAL PHARMACOLOGY AND TOXICOLOGY

In rhesus monkeys, administration of probucol in diets containing unusually high amounts of cholesterol and saturated fat resulted in the death of four of eight animals after several weeks. Premonitory syncope was frequently observed and was associated with a pronounced prolongation of the QT intervals (30 to 50% longer than that observed in untreated monkeys). Serum levels of probucol greater than 20 mcg/mL were generally associated with some prolongation in the QT interval in the cholesterol-fed monkey. A 75 msec or greater increase in QT interval from control values was usually seen at 40 mcg/mL and above. Blood levels in humans receiving Lorelco average approximately 20 mcg/mL and not uncommonly reach levels of 40 mcg/mL and higher. Rhesus monkeys fed normal (low fat) chow and receiving probucol three to thirty times the human dose equivalent achieved blood levels only one-third those of many human subjects. No adverse effects were detected in these monkeys over an eighth-year period of continuous drug administration. In another study in rhesus monkeys, an atherogenic diet was fed for two years and daily treatment with probucol, separated in time from the atherogenic meal, was carried out during the second year. Serum probucol levels ranged 20 to 50 mcg/mL in five of ten monkeys, and less in the remaining animals. Marked prolongation of the QT$_c$ interval in the ECG or syncopal behavior was never observed over the entire one-year treatment period. Regression of gross aortic lesions comparable to that observed in a parallel group of monkeys receiving cholestyramine was seen in animals receiving probucol. It should be emphasized that both HDL-cholesterol and LDL-cholesterol were markedly reduced in this regression study. During the performance of a two-year chronic study involving 32 probucol-treated dogs (beagles), there were 12 fatalities.

Subsequent experiments have indicated that probucol sensitizes the canine myocardium to epinephrine, resulting in ventricular fibrillation in many dogs. Among the animal species in which probucol has been studied, the dog is peculiar with respect to the phenomenon of sudden death due to the sensitization of the myocardium to epinephrine. In contrast to findings in the dog, injections of epinephrine to probucol-treated monkeys did not induce ventricular fibrillation.

In other studies, monkeys were given probucol either before and after, or only after myocardial infarction induced by coronary artery ligation. In these studies, there was no difference between probucol- and placebo-treated groups with respect to either survival or detailed blind quantitation of myocardial changes (gross and histopathologic).

Probucol has shown no identifiable toxicity in mice and rats. In these animals, the LD_{50} (oral) is in excess of 5 g/kg of body weight. In chronic studies of two years' duration in rats, no toxicity or carcinogenicity was observed.

From studies in rats, dogs, and monkeys, it is known that probucol accumulates slowly in adipose tissue. Approximately 90% of probucol administered orally is unabsorbed. For that which is absorbed, the biliary tract is the major pathway for clearance from the body and very little is excreted by way of the kidneys.

Myocardial injury was produced in various groups of rats by one of the following procedures: aortic coarctation, coronary ligation, or cobalt or isoproterenol injection. After probucol administration, no deleterious effects related to treatment occurred as measured by survival and microscopic examination of myocardial damage.

Probucol was administered to minipigs beginning ten days before ligation of coronary artery and continued for 60 days after surgery. Challenge with epinephrine at the end of 60 days failed to induce ventricular fibrillation in any of the coronary-ligated, probucol-treated minipigs.

CLINICAL STUDIES

In a multicenter, randomized, double-blind study, the LRC-CPPT[3], hypercholesterolemic patients treated with an oral bile acid sequestrant (cholestyramine) and a cholesterol-lowering diet experienced average total and LDL-cholesterol reductions greater than those obtained in the placebo group treated with diet alone. The cumulative seven-year incidence of the primary end point—combined incidence of definite CHD death and/or definite nonfatal myocardial infarction—was 7% in the cholestyramine group and 8.6% in the placebo group. This was a 19% reduction in risk (P less than 0.05, single-tail test) of the primary end point reflecting a 24% reduction in definite CHD death and a 19% reduction in nonfatal myocardial infarction.

The subjects included in the study were middle-aged men (35–59 years old) with serum cholesterol levels at least 265 mg/dL and no previous history of heart disease. It is not clear to what extent these findings can be extrapolated to other segments of the hypercholesterolemic population not studied.

The bile acid sequestrant, cholestyramine, was used in the above trial. Caution should be exercised in extrapolating these results to Lorelco since it differs from cholestyramine with regard to its mode of action, spectrum of cholesterol-lowering potency, effect on HDL-cholesterol, and possible toxicity. The effect of probucol-induced reduction of serum cholesterol levels on morbidity or mortality due to coronary heart disease has not been established.

REFERENCES

1. Consensus Development Panel. Lowering blood cholesterol to prevent heart disease. *JAMA.* 1985; 253:2080–2086.
2. Fredrickson DS, Levy RI. Lees RS. Fat transport in lipoproteins—an integrated approach to mechanisms and disorders. *N. Engl J Med.* 1967; 276:34–44.
3. The Lipid Research Clinics Program. The Lipid Research Clinics coronary primary prevention trial results: I. Reduction in incidence of coronary heart disease. *JAMA.* 1984; 251:351–364.

Product Information as of June, 1988

Shown in Product Identification Section, page 419

NORPRAMIN®   ℞

[nŏr´prăm-ĭn]

(desipramine hydrochloride tablets USP)

CAUTION: Federal law prohibits dispensing without prescription.

DESCRIPTION

Norpramin (desipramine hydrochloride USP) is an antidepressant drug of the tricyclic type, and is chemically:

5H-Dibenz[b,f]azepine-5-propanamine, 10, 11-dihydro-N-methyl-, monohydrochloride

[See Chemical Formula at top of next column].

INACTIVE INGREDIENTS

The following inactive ingredients are contained in all dosage strengths: acacia, calcium carbonate, corn starch, D&C

Red No. 30 and D&C Yellow No. 10 (except 10 mg and 150 mg), FD&C Blue No. 1, FD&C Red No. 3, FD&C Yellow No. 6, hydrogenated soy oil, iron oxide, light mineral oil, magnesium stearate, mannitol, polyethylene glycol 8000, pregelatinized corn starch, sodium benzoate (except 150 mg), sucrose, talc, titanium dioxide, and other ingredients.

CLINICAL PHARMACOLOGY

Mechanism of Action

Available evidence suggests that many depressions have a biochemical basis in the form of a relative deficiency of neurotransmitters such as norepinephrine and serotonin. Norepinephrine deficiency may be associated with relatively low urinary 3-methoxy-4-hydroxyphenyl glycol (MHPG) levels, while serotonin deficiencies may be associated with low spinal fluid levels of 5-hydroxyindoleacetic acid.

While the precise mechanism of action of the tricyclic antidepressants is unknown, a leading theory suggests that they restore normal levels of neurotransmitters by blocking the re-uptake of these substances from the synapse in the central nervous system. Evidence indicates that the secondary amine tricyclic antidepressants, including Norpramin, may have greater activity in blocking the re-uptake of norepinephrine. Tertiary amine tricyclic antidepressants, such as amitriptyline, may have greater effect on serotonin re-uptake.

Norpramin (desipramine hydrochloride) is not a monoamine oxidase (MAO) inhibitor and does not act primarily as a central nervous system stimulant. It has been found in some studies to have a more rapid onset of action than imipramine. Earliest therapeutic effects may occasionally be seen in 2 to 5 days, but full treatment benefit usually requires 2 to 3 weeks to obtain.

Metabolism

Tricyclic antidepressants, such as desipramine hydrochloride, are rapidly absorbed from the gastrointestinal tract. Tricyclic antidepressants or their metabolites are to some extent excreted through the gastric mucosa and reabsorbed from the gastrointestinal tract. Desipramine is metabolized in the liver and approximately 70% is excreted in the urine. The rate of metabolism of tricyclic antidepressants varies widely from individual to individual, chiefly on a genetically determined basis. Up to a thirty-sixfold difference in plasma level may be noted among individuals taking the same oral dose of desipramine. In general, the elderly metabolize tricyclic antidepressants more slowly than do younger adults.

Certain drugs, particularly the psychostimulants and the phenothiazines, increase plasma levels of concomitantly administered tricyclic antidepressants through competition for the same metabolic enzyme systems. Concurrent administration of cimetidine and tricyclic antidepressants can produce clinically significant increases in the plasma concentrations of the tricyclic antidepressants. Conversely, decreases in plasma levels of the tricyclic antidepressants have been reported upon discontinuation of cimetidine which may result in the loss of the therapeutic efficacy of the tricyclic antidepressant. Other substances, particularly barbiturates and alcohol, induce liver enzyme activity and thereby reduce tricyclic antidepressant plasma levels. Similar effects have been reported with tobacco smoke.

Research on the relationship of plasma level to therapeutic response with the tricyclic antidepressants has produced conflicting results. While some studies report no correlation, many studies cite therapeutic levels for most tricyclics in the range of 50 to 300 nanograms per milliliter. The therapeutic range is different for each tricyclic antidepressant. For desipramine, an optimal range of therapeutic plasma levels has not been established.

INDICATIONS

Norpramin (desipramine hydrochloride) is indicated for relief of symptoms in various depressive syndromes, especially endogenous depression.

CONTRAINDICATIONS

Desipramine hydrochloride should not be given in conjunction with, or within 2 weeks of, treatment with an MAO inhibitor drug; hyperpyretic crises, severe convulsions, and death have occurred in patients taking MAO inhibitors and tricyclic antidepressants. When Norpramin (desipramine hydrochloride) is substituted for an MAO inhibitor, at least 2 weeks should elapse between treatments. Norpramin should then be started cautiously and should be increased gradually.

The drug is contraindicated in the acute recovery period following myocardial infarction. It should not be used in those who have shown prior hypersensitivity to the drug. Cross sensitivity between this and other dibenzazepines is a possibility.

WARNINGS

1. Extreme caution should be used when this drug is given in the following situations:

   a. In patients with cardiovascular disease, because of the possibility of conduction defects, arrhythmias, tachycardias, strokes, and acute myocardial infarction.

   b. In patients with a history of urinary retention or glaucoma, because of the anticholinergic properties of the drug.

   c. In patients with thyroid disease or those taking thyroid medication, because of the possibility of cardiovascular toxicity, including arrhythmias.

   d. In patients with a history of seizure disorder, because this drug has been shown to lower the seizure threshold.

2. This drug is capable of blocking the antihypertensive effect of guanethidine and similarly acting compounds.

3. USE IN PREGNANCY

   Safe use of desipramine hydrochloride during pregnancy and lactation has not been established; therefore, if it is to be given to pregnant patients, nursing mothers, or women of childbearing potential, the possible benefits must be weighed against the possible hazards to mother and child. Animal reproductive studies have been inconclusive.

4. USE IN CHILDREN

   Norpramin (desipramine hydrochloride) is not recommended for use in children since safety and effectiveness in the pediatric age group have not been established. (See ADVERSE REACTIONS, Cardiovascular.)

5. The patient should be cautioned that this drug may impair the mental and/or physical abilities required for the performance of potentially hazardous tasks such as driving a car or operating machinery.

6. In patients who may use alcohol excessively, it should be borne in mind that the potentiation may increase the danger inherent in any suicide attempt or overdosage.

PRECAUTIONS

1. It is important that this drug be dispensed in the least possible quantities to depressed outpatients, since suicide has been accomplished with this class of drug. Ordinary prudence requires that children not have access to this drug or to potent drugs of any kind; if possible, this drug should be dispensed in containers with child-resistant safety closures. Storage of this drug in the home must be supervised responsibly.

2. If serious adverse effects occur, dosage should be reduced or treatment should be altered.

3. Norpramin (desipramine hydrochloride) therapy in patients with manic-depressive illness may induce a hypomanic state after the depressive phase terminates.

4. The drug may cause exacerbation of psychosis in schizophrenic patients.

5. Close supervision and careful adjustment of dosage are required when this drug is given concomitantly with anticholinergic or sympathomimetic drugs.

6. Patients should be warned that while taking this drug their response to alcoholic beverages may be exaggerated.

7. Clinical experience in the concurrent administration of ECT and antidepressant drugs is limited. Thus, if such treatment is essential, the possibility of increased risk relative to benefits should be considered.

8. If Norpramin (desipramine hydrochloride) is to be combined with other psychotropic agents such as tranquilizers or sedative/hypnotics, careful consideration should be given to the pharmacology of the agents employed since the sedative effects of Norpramin and benzodiazepines (e.g., chlordiazepoxide or diazepam) are additive. Both the sedative and anticholinergic effects of the major tranquilizers are also additive to those of Norpramin.

9. Concurrent administration of cimetidine and tricyclic antidepressants can produce clinically significant increases in the plasma levels of the tricyclic antidepressants (see CLINICAL PHARMACOLOGY, *Metabolism*). Conversely, decreases in plasma levels of the tricyclic antidepressants have been reported upon discontinuation of cimetidine which may result in the loss of the therapeutic efficacy of the tricyclic antidepressant.

10. This drug should be discontinued as soon as possible prior to elective surgery because of the possible cardiovascular effects. Hypertensive episodes have been observed during surgery in patients taking desipramine hydrochloride.

11. Both elevation and lowering of blood sugar levels have been reported.

12. Leukocyte and differential counts should be performed in any patient who develops fever and sore throat during therapy; the drug should be discontinued if there is evidence of pathologic neutrophil depression.

Continued on next page

Information on Merrell Dow products is based on labeling in effect in June, 1989.

Merrell Dow—Cont.

ADVERSE REACTIONS

Note: Included in the following listing are a few adverse reactions that have not been reported with this specific drug. However, the pharmacologic similarities among the tricyclic antidepressant drugs require that each of the reactions be considered when Norpramin (desipramine hydrochloride) is given.

Cardiovascular: hypotension, hypertension, tachycardia, palpitation, arrhythmias, heart block, myocardial infarction, stroke. There has been a report of an "acute collapse" and "sudden death" in an eight-year old (18 kg) male, treated for two years for hyperactivity. (See WARNINGS, Use in Children.)

Psychiatric: confusional states (especially in the elderly) with hallucinations, disorientation, delusions; anxiety, restlessness, agitation; insomnia and nightmares; hypomania; exacerbation of psychosis.

Neurologic: numbness, tingling, paresthesias of extremities; incoordination, ataxia, tremors; peripheral neuropathy; extrapyramidal symptoms; seizures; alteration in EEG patterns; tinnitus.

Anticholinergic: dry mouth, and rarely associated sublingual adenitis; blurred vision, disturbance of accommodation, mydriasis, increased intraocular pressure; constipation, paralytic ileus; urinary retention, delayed micturition, dilatation of urinary tract.

Allergic: skin rash, petechiae, urticaria, itching, photosensitization (avoid excessive exposure to sunlight), edema (of face and tongue or general), drug fever, cross sensitivity with other tricyclic drugs.

Hematologic: bone marrow depressions including agranulocytosis, eosinophilia, purpura, thrombocytopenia.

Gastrointestinal: anorexia, nausea and vomiting, epigastric distress, peculiar taste, abdominal cramps, diarrhea, stomatitis, black tongue.

Endocrine: gynecomastia in the male, breast enlargement and galactorrhea in the female; increased or decreased libido, impotence, painful ejaculation, testicular swelling; elevation or depression of blood sugar levels; syndrome of inappropriate antidiuretic hormone secretion (SIADH).

Other: jaundice (simulating obstructive), altered liver function; weight gain or loss; perspiration, flushing, urinary frequency, nocturia; parotid swelling; drowsiness, dizziness, weakness and fatigue, headache; alopecia.

Withdrawal Symptoms: Though not indicative of addiction, abrupt cessation of treatment after prolonged therapy may produce nausea, headache, and malaise.

DOSAGE AND ADMINISTRATION

Not recommended for use in children.

Lower dosages are recommended for elderly patients and adolescents. Lower dosages are also recommended for outpatients compared to hospitalized patients, who are closely supervised. Dosage should be initiated at a low level and increased according to clinical response and any evidence of intolerance. Following remission, maintenance medication may be required for a period of time and should be at the lowest dose that will maintain remission.

Usual Adult Dose

The usual adult dose is 100 to 200 mg per day. In more severely ill patients, dosage may be further increased gradually to 300 mg/day if necessary. Dosages above 300 mg/day are not recommended.

Dosage should be initiated at a lower level and increased according to tolerance and clinical response.

Treatment of patients requiring as much as 300 mg should generally be initiated in hospitals, where regular visits by the physician, skilled nursing care, and frequent electrocardiograms (ECG's) are available.

The best available evidence of impending toxicity from very high doses of Norpramin is prolongation of the QRS or QT intervals on the ECG. Prolongation of the PR interval is also significant, but less closely correlated with plasma levels. Clinical symptoms of intolerance, especially drowsiness, dizziness, and postural hypotension, should also alert the physician to the need for reduction in dosage. Plasma desipramine measurement would constitute the optimal guide to dosage monitoring.

Initial therapy may be administered in divided doses or a single daily dose.

Maintenance therapy may be given on a once-daily schedule for patient convenience and compliance.

Adolescent and Geriatric Dose

The usual adolescent and geriatric dose is 25 to 100 mg daily. Dosage should be initiated at a lower level and increased according to tolerance and clinical response to a usual maximum of 100 mg daily. In more severely ill patients, dosage may be further increased to 150 mg/day. Doses above 150 mg/day are not recommended in these age groups.

Initial therapy may be administered in divided doses or a single daily dose.

Maintenance therapy may be given on a once-daily schedule for patient convenience and compliance.

OVERDOSAGE

There is no specific antidote for desipramine, nor are there specific phenomena of diagnostic value characterizing poisoning by the drug.

Within an hour of ingestion the patient may become agitated or stuporous and then comatose. Hypotension, shock, and renal shutdown may ensue. Grand mal seizures, both early and late after ingestion, have been reported. Hyperactive reflexes, hyperpyrexia, muscle rigidity, vomiting, and ECG evidence of impaired conduction may occur. Serious disturbances of cardiac rate, rhythm, and output can occur. The precepts of early evacuation of the ingested material and subsequent support of respiration (airway and movement), circulation, and renal output apply.

The principles of management of coma and shock by means of the mechanical respirator, cardiac pacemaker, monitoring of central venous pressure, and regulation of fluid and acid-base balance are well known in most medical centers and are not further discussed here.

Because CNS involvement, respiratory depression, and cardiac arrhythmia can occur suddenly, hospitalization and close observation are generally advisable, even when the amount ingested is thought to be small or the initial degree of intoxication appears slight or moderate. Most patients with ECG abnormalities should have continuous cardiac monitoring for at least 72 hours and be closely observed until well after cardiac status has returned to normal; relapses may occur after apparent recovery.

The slow intravenous administration of physostigmine salicylate has been reported to reverse most of the anticholinergic cardiovascular and CNS effects of overdose with tricyclic antidepressants. In adults, 1 to 3 mg has been reported to be effective. In children, the dose should be started with 0.5 mg and repeated at 5-minute intervals to determine the minimum effective dose; no more than 2 mg should be given. Because of the short duration of action of physostigmine, the effective dose should be repeated at 30-minute to 60-minute intervals, as necessary. Rapid injection should be avoided to reduce the possibility of physostigmine-induced convulsions.

Other possible therapeutic considerations include:

(a) Dialysis: Desipramine is found in low concentration in the serum, even after a massive oral dose. *In vitro* experiments in which blood bank blood was used indicate that it is very poorly dialyzed. Because of indications that the drug is secreted in gastric juice, constant gastric lavage has been suggested.

(b) Pharmacologic treatment of shock: Since desipramine potentiates the action of such vasopressor agents as levarterenol and metaraminol, they should be used only with caution.

(c) Pharmacologic control of seizures: Intravenous barbiturates are the treatment of choice for the control of grand mal seizures. One may, alternatively, consider the parenteral use of diphenylhydantoin, which has less central depressant effect but also has an effect on heart rhythm that has not yet been fully defined.

(d) Pharmacologic control of cardiac function: Severe disturbances of cardiac rate, rhythm, and output are probably the initiating events in shock. Intravascular volume must be maintained by i.v. fluids. Digitalization should be carried out early in view of the fact that a positive inotropic effect can be achieved without increase in cardiac work. Many of the cardiodynamic effects of digitalis are the exact opposite of those of massive doses of desipramine (animal studies).

HOW SUPPLIED

10 mg blue coated tablets imprinted 68-7
  NDC 0068-0007-01: bottles of 100
25 mg yellow coated tablets imprinted MERRELL 11 or NORPRAMIN 25
  NDC 0068-0011-01: bottles of 100
  NDC 0068-0011-61: unit dose dispenser of 100
  NDC 0068-0011-10: bottles of 1000
50 mg green coated tablets imprinted MERRELL 15 or NORPRAMIN 50
  NDC 0068-0015-01: bottles of 100
  NDC 0068-0015-61: unit dose dispenser of 100
  NDC 0068-0015-10: bottles of 1000
75 mg orange coated tablets imprinted MERRELL 19 or NORPRAMIN 75
  NDC 0068-0019-01: bottles of 100
100 mg peach coated tablets imprinted MERRELL 20 or NORPRAMIN 100
  NDC 0068-0020-01: bottles of 100
150 mg white coated tablets imprinted MERRELL 21 or NORPRAMIN 150
  NDC 0068-0021-50: bottles of 50

Norpramin tablets should be stored at room temperature, preferably below 86°F (30°C). Protect from excessive heat.

Product Information as of January, 1989

Shown in Product Identification Section, page 419

QUINAMM™ 260 mg   ℞
[*kwĭn 'ăm*]
(quinine sulfate tablets)

CAUTION: Federal law prohibits dispensing without prescription.

DESCRIPTION

Quinamm is available as tablets for oral administration. Each tablet contains 260 mg quinine sulfate. Also contains, as inactive ingredients: corn starch, pregelatinized starch, sodium starch glycolate, sucrose, and zinc stearate.

Neuromuscular Agent

Quinine sulfate has the following structural formula:

Quinine sulfate occurs as a white, crystalline powder, which darkens on exposure to light. It is odorless and has a persistent, very bitter taste. It is slightly soluble in water, alcohol, chloroform, and ether.

CLINICAL PHARMACOLOGY

Quinine, a cinchona alkaloid, acts on skeletal muscle by three mechanisms: it increases the refractory period by direct action on the muscle fiber, it decreases the excitability of the motor end-plate, an action similar to that of curare, and it affects the distribution of calcium within the muscle fiber. Quinine is readily absorbed when given orally. Absorption occurs mainly from the upper part of the small intestine, and is almost complete even in patients with marked diarrhea. The cinchona alkaloids in large measure are metabolically degraded in the body, especially in the liver; less than 5% of an administered dose is excreted unaltered in the urine. It is reported that there is no accumulation of the drugs in the body upon continued administration. The metabolic degradation products are excreted in the urine, where many of them have been identified as hydroxy derivatives, but small amounts also appear in the feces, gastric juice, bile, and saliva. Renal excretion of quinine is twice as rapid when the urine is acidic as when it is alkaline, due to the greater tubular reabsorption of the alkaloidal base that occurs in an alkaline media. Excretion is also limited by the binding of a large fraction of cinchona alkaloids to plasma proteins.

Peak plasma concentrations of cinchona alkaloids occur within 1 to 3 hours after a single oral dose. The half-life is 4 to 5 hours. After chronic administration of total daily doses of 1 g of drug, the average plasma quinine concentration is approximately 7 μg/ml. After termination of quinine therapy, the plasma level falls rapidly and only a negligible concentration is detectable after 24 hours.

A large fraction (approximately 70%) of the plasma quinine is bound to proteins. This explains in part why the concentration of alkaloid in cerebrospinal fluid is only 2 to 5% of that in the plasma. However, it can traverse the placental membrane and readily reach fetal tissues.

Tinnitus and impairment of hearing rarely should occur at plasma quinine concentrations of less than 10 μg/ml. While this level would not be anticipated from use of 1 or 2 tablets of Quinamm daily, an occasional patient may have some evidence of cinchonism on this dosage, such as tinnitus. (See WARNINGS section.)

INDICATIONS AND USAGE

For the prevention and treatment of nocturnal recumbency leg muscle cramps.

CONTRAINDICATIONS

Quinamm may cause fetal harm when administered to a pregnant woman. Congenital malformations in the human have been reported with the use of quinine, primarily with large doses (up to 30 g) for attempted abortion. In about half of these reports, the malformation was deafness related to auditory nerve hypoplasia. Among the other abnormalities reported were limb anomalies, visceral defects, and visual changes. In animal tests, teratogenic effects were found in rabbits and guinea pigs and were absent in mice, rats, dogs, and monkeys. Quinamm is contraindicated in women who are or may become pregnant. If this drug is used during pregnancy, or if the patient becomes pregnant while taking this drug, the patient should be apprised of the potential hazard to the fetus.

Because of the quinine content, Quinamm is contraindicated in patients with known quinine hypersensitivity and in patients with glucose-6-phosphate dehydrogenase (G-6-PD) deficiency.

Since thrombocytopenic purpura may follow the administration of quinine in highly sensitive patients, a history of this occurrence associated with previous quinine ingestion contraindicates its further use. Recovery usually occurs following withdrawal of the medication and appropriate therapy. This drug should not be used in patients with tinnitus or optic neuritis or in patients with a history of blackwater fever.

WARNINGS

Repeated doses or overdosage of quinine in some individuals may precipitate a cluster of symptoms referred to as cinchonism. Such symptoms, in the mildest form, include ringing in the ears, headache, nausea, and slightly disturbed vision; however, when medication is continued or after large single doses, symptoms also involve the gastrointestinal tract, the nervous and cardiovascular systems, and the skin.

Hemolysis (with the potential for hemolytic anemia) has been associated with a G-6-PD deficiency in patients taking quinine. Quinamm should be stopped immediately if evidence of hemolysis appears.

If symptoms occur, drug should be discontinued and supportive measures instituted. In case of overdosage, see OVERDOSAGE section of prescribing information.

PRECAUTIONS

General

Quinamm should be discontinued if there is any evidence of hypersensitivity. (See CONTRAINDICATIONS.) Cutaneous flushing, pruritus, skin rashes, fever, gastric distress, dyspnea, ringing in the ears, and visual impairment are the usual expressions of hypersensitivity, particularly if only small doses of quinine have been taken. Extreme flushing of the skin accompanied by intense, generalized pruritus is the most common form. Hemoglobinuria and asthma from quinine are rare types of idiosyncrasy.

In patients with atrial fibrillation, the administration of quinine requires the same precautions as those for quinidine. (See *Drug Interactions.*)

Drug Interactions

Increased plasma levels of digoxin have been demonstrated in individuals after concomitant quinine administration. Increased plasma levels of digitoxin have been demonstrated in individuals after concomitant quinidine administration. It is therefore recommended that plasma levels of digoxin or digitoxin be determined periodically for those individuals taking either of these glycosides and Quinamm concomitantly.

Concurrent use of aluminum-containing antacids may delay or decrease absorption of quinine.

Cinchona alkaloids, including quinine, have the potential to depress the hepatic enzyme system that synthesizes the vitamin K-dependent factors. The resulting hypoprothrombinemic effect may enhance the action of warfarin and other oral anticoagulants.

The effects of neuromuscular blocking agents (particularly pancuronium, succinylcholine, and tubocurarine) may be potentiated with quinine, and result in respiratory difficulties.

Urinary alkalizers (such as acetazolamide and sodium bicarbonate) may increase quinine blood levels with potential for toxicity.

Drug/Laboratory Interactions

Quinine may produce an elevated value for urinary 17-ketogenic steroids when the Zimmerman method is used.

Carcinogenesis, Mutagenesis, Impairment of Fertility

A study of quinine sulfate administered in drinking water (0.1%) to rats for periods up to 20 months showed no evidence of neoplastic changes.

Mutation studies of quinine (dihydrochloride) in male and female mice gave negative results by the micronucleus test. Intraperitoneal injections (0.5 mM/kg) were given twice, 24 hours apart. Direct *Salmonella typhimurium* tests were negative; when mammalian liver homogenate was added, positive results were found.

Mutation studies of quinine hydrochloride, 100 mg/kg, p.o. in Chinese hamsters showed no genotoxic activity in the sister chromatid exchange (SCE) test, micronucleus test, or chromosome aberration test. In mice given quinine hydrochloride, 100 mg/kg, p.o., the micronucleus test and chromosome aberration test were negative; the SCE test exhibited an increase of SCEs/cell. Tests were repeated in two inbred strains of mice using 55, 75, and 110 mg/kg p.o. The effect was more pronounced in these mice and the increase in SCEs/cell demonstrated a linear dose relationship. One of the inbred strains had positive micronucleus test findings. The chromosome aberration test also revealed an increase of chromatid breaks. The Ames test system results were negative for point mutation.

No information relating to the effect of quinine upon fertility in animal or in man has been found.

Pregnancy

Category X. See CONTRAINDICATIONS.

Nonteratogenic Effects

Because quinine crosses the placenta in humans, the potential for fetal effects is present. Stillbirths in mothers taking quinine have been reported in which no obvious cause for the fetal deaths was shown. Quinine in toxic amounts has been associated with abortion. Whether this action is always due to direct effect on the uterus is questionable.

Nursing Mothers

Caution should be exercised when Quinamm is given to nursing women because quinine is excreted in breast milk (in small amounts).

ADVERSE REACTIONS

The following adverse reactions have been reported with Quinamm in therapeutic or excessive dosage. (Individual or multiple symptoms may represent cinchonism or hypersensitivity.)

Hematologic: acute hemolysis, thrombocytopenic purpura, agranulocytosis, hypoprothrombinemia

CNS: visual disturbances, including blurred vision with scotomata, photophobia, diplopia, diminished visual fields, and disturbed color vision; tinnitus, deafness, and vertigo; headache, nausea, vomiting, fever, apprehension, restlessness, confusion, and syncope

Dermatologic/allergic: cutaneous rashes (urticarial, the most frequent type of allergic reaction, papular, or scarlatinal), pruritus, flushing of the skin, sweating, occasional edema of the face

Respiratory: asthmatic symptoms

Cardiovascular: anginal symptoms

Gastrointestinal: nausea and vomiting (may be CNS-related), epigastric pain, hepatitis

DRUG ABUSE AND DEPENDENCE

Tolerance, abuse, or dependence with Quinamm has not been reported.

OVERDOSAGE

The more common signs and symptoms of overdosage are tinnitus, dizziness, skin rash, and gastrointestinal disturbance (intestinal cramping). With higher doses, cardiovascular and CNS effects may occur, including headache, fever, vomiting, apprehension, confusion, and convulsions. Other effects are listed in the ADVERSE REACTIONS section. Fatalities with quinine have been reported from single oral doses of 2 to 8 grams; a single fatality reported with a dose of 1.5 grams may reflect an idiosyncratic effect. Several cases of blindness following large overdoses of quinine, with partial recovery of vision in each instance, have been reported. Tinnitus and impaired hearing may occur at plasma quinine concentrations over 10 μg/ml. This level would not be normally attained with the use of 1 or 2 Quinamm tablets daily, but in a hypersensitive patient, as little as 0.3 g of quinine may produce tinnitus.

Treatment

Treatment for overdosage should include initially efforts to remove any residual Quinamm from the stomach by gastric lavage or by emesis induced with syrup of ipecac. The blood pressure should be supported and measures used to maintain renal function. Artificial respiration may be needed. Sedatives, oxygen, and other supportive measures should be used as necessary.

Fluid and electrolyte balance with intravenous fluids should be maintained. Acidification of the urine will promote renal excretion of quinine. In the presence of hemoglobinuria, however, acidification of the urine may augment renal blockade. Quinine should be readily dialyzable by hemodialysis and/or hemoperfusion procedures.

Evidence of angioedema or asthma may require the use of epinephrine, corticosteroids, and antihistamines. In the acute phase of toxic amaurosis caused by quinine, vasodilators administered intravenously may have a salutary effect. Stellate block has also been used effectively for quinine-associated blindness. Residual visual impairment occasionally yields to vasodilators.

DOSAGE AND ADMINISTRATION

1 tablet upon retiring. If needed, 2 tablets may be taken nightly—1 following the evening meal and 1 upon retiring. After several consecutive nights in which recumbency leg cramps do not occur, Quinamm may be discontinued in order to determine whether continued therapy is needed.

HOW SUPPLIED

NDC 0068-0547-15

260 mg tablets in bottles of 100. Tablets are round, white, debossed W one side, Merrell 547 other side.

Store at room temperature, below 86°F (30°C).

Product Information as of December, 1984
Shown in Product Identification Section, page 419

RIFADIN®   ℞

[rĭf'ă-dĭn]

(rifampin capsules)

and

RIFADIN® I.V.

(rifampin for injection)

CAUTION: Federal law prohibits dispensing without prescription.

DESCRIPTION

Rifadin (rifampin) capsules for oral administration contain 150 mg or 300 mg rifampin per capsule. The 150 mg capsules also contain, as inactive ingredients: corn starch, edible white ink, FD&C Blue No. 1, FD&C Red No. 3, FD&C Red No. 40, gelatin, magnesium stearate, and titanium dioxide. The 300 mg capsules also contain, as inactive ingredients: corn starch, D&C Red No. 28, FD&C Blue No. 1, FD&C Red No. 40, gelatin, magnesium stearate, and titanium dioxide.

Rifadin I.V. (rifampin for injection) contains rifampin 600 mg, sodium formaldehyde sulfoxylate 10 mg, and sodium hydroxide to adjust pH.

Rifampin is a semisynthetic antibiotic derivative of rifamycin B. The chemical name for rifampin is 3-(4-methyl-1-piperazinyl-iminomethyl)-rifamycin SV. Its chemical structure is:

Rifampin USP is a red-brown crystalline powder soluble in water, freely soluble in chloroform, and soluble in ethyl acetate and in methanol. Its molecular weight is 822.95.

CLINICAL PHARMACOLOGY

Human Pharmacology—Oral

Rifampin is readily absorbed from the gastrointestinal tract. Peak blood levels in normal adults vary widely from individual to individual. The peak level averages 7 μg/mL but may vary from 4 to 32 μg/mL. Absorption of rifampin is reduced when the drug is ingested with food.

In normal subjects, the biological half-life of rifampin in serum averages about 3 hours after a 600 mg oral dose, with increases up to 5.1 hours reported after a 900 mg dose. With repeated administration, the half-life decreases and reaches average values of approximately 2–3 hours. It does not differ in patients with renal failure at doses not exceeding 600 mg daily and, consequently, no dosage adjustment is required. Refer to WARNINGS for information regarding patients with hepatic insufficiency.

After absorption, rifampin is rapidly eliminated in the bile, and an enterohepatic circulation ensues. During this process, rifampin undergoes progressive deacetylation so that nearly all the drug in the bile is in this form in about 6 hours. This metabolite is microbiologically active. Intestinal reabsorption is reduced by deacetylation, and elimination is facilitated. Up to 30% of a dose is excreted in the urine, with about half of this being unchanged drug.

Rifampin is widely distributed throughout the body. It is present in effective concentrations in many organs and body fluids, including cerebrospinal fluid. Rifampin is about 80% protein bound. Most of the unbound fraction is not ionized and therefore diffuses freely into tissues.

Serum Levels in Children

In one recent study, children 6–58 months old were given rifampin suspended in simple syrup or as dry powder mixed with applesauce at a dose of 10 mg/kg body weight. Peak serum levels of 10.7 and 11.5 μg/mL were obtained 1 hour after preprandial ingestion of the drug suspension and the applesauce mixture, respectively. The calculated $t_{1/2}$ for both preparations was 2.9 hrs. It should be noted that in other studies in children, at doses of 10 mg/kg body weight, mean peak serum levels of 3.5 μg/mL to 15 μg/mL have been reported.

Human Pharmacology—I.V.

After intravenous administration of a 300 or 600 mg dose of rifampin infused over 30 minutes to healthy male volunteers (n = 12), mean peak plasma concentrations were 9.0 and 17.5 μg/mL, respectively. The average plasma concentrations in these volunteers remained detectable for 8 and 12 hours, respectively (see table).

Rifampin Dosage I.V.	Plasma Concentrations (μg/mL)					
	30 min.	1 h	2 h	4 h	8 h	12 h
300 mg	8.9	4.9	4.0	2.5	< 2	< 2
600 mg	17.4	11.7	9.4	6.4	3.5	< 2

Continued on next page

Information on Merrell Dow products is based on labeling in effect in June, 1989.

Merrell Dow—Cont.

Plasma concentrations after the 600 mg dose, which were disproportionately higher (up to 30% greater than expected) than those found after the 300 mg dose, indicated that the elimination of larger doses was not as rapid.

After repeated once-a-day infusions (3 h duration) of 600 mg in patients (n = 5) for 7 days, concentrations of I.V. rifampin decrease from 5.8 μg/mL 8 hours after the infusion on day 1 to 2.6 μg/mL 8 hours after the infusion on day 7.

The rifampin dose is widely distributed throughout the body. It is present in effective concentrations in many organs and body fluids, including cerebrospinal fluid. Rifampin is about 80% protein bound. Most of the unbound fraction is not ionized and therefore diffuses freely into tissues.

Rifampin is rapidly eliminated in the bile and undergoes progressive enterohepatic circulation and deacetylation to the primary metabolite, 25-desacetyl-rifampin. This metabolite is microbiologically active. Less than 30% of the dose is excreted as rifampin or metabolites. Serum concentrations do not differ in patients with renal failure and, consequently, no dosage adjustment is required.

Serum Concentrations of Rifampin in Children
In patients 0.25–12.8 years old (n = 12), the mean peak serum concentration of rifampin at the end of a 30 minute infusion of approximately 300 mg/m^2 was 26 μg/mL. In these patients, peak concentrations 1–4 days after initiation of therapy ranged from 11.7 to 41.5 μg/mL; peak concentrations 5–14 days after initiation of therapy were 13.6 to 37.4 μg/mL. The serum half-life of rifampin decreased significantly from (1.34–3.24) hours early in therapy to (1.17–3.19) hours 5–14 days after therapy was initiated.

Microbiology
Rifampin inhibits DNA-dependent RNA polymerase activity in susceptible cells. Specifically, it interacts with bacterial RNA polymerase but does not inhibit the mammalian enzyme. Rifampin is particularly active against rapidly growing extracellular organisms but has been demonstrated to have intracellular bactericidal activity against susceptible organisms as well.

Cross-resistance to rifampin has been shown only with other rifamycins.

Rifampin has bactericidal activity against slow and intermittently growing *M. tuberculosis*. It also has significant activity against *Neisseria meningitidis* (see INDICATIONS AND USAGE).

In the treatment of both tuberculosis and the meningococcal carrier state (see INDICATIONS AND USAGE), the small number of resistant cells present within large populations of susceptible cells can rapidly become predominant. In addition, resistance to rifampin has been determined to occur as single-step mutations of the DNA-dependent RNA polymerase. Since resistance can emerge rapidly, appropriate susceptibility tests should be performed in the event of persistent positive cultures.

Rifampin has been shown to have initial *in vitro* activity against the following organisms; however, clinical efficacy has not been established (see INDICATIONS AND USAGE): *Mycobacterium leprae, Haemophilus influenzae, Staphylococcus aureus,* and *Staphylococcus epidermidis.* Both penicillinase-producing and non-penicillinase-producing strains, and β-lactam resistant staphylococci (Methicillin Resistant *S. aureus*/MRSA) are initially susceptible to rifampin *in vitro.*

Susceptibility Testing
Use only diagnostic products and methods approved by the Food and Drug Administration for rifampin susceptibility testing of *Mycobacterium tuberculosis* and *Neisseria meningitidis.* Consult the Food and Drug Administration-approved labeling of the diagnostic products for interpretation criteria and quality control parameters.

For the other organisms listed in the microbiology subsection of the labeling, *in vitro* susceptibility testing should be assessed by standardized methods[1,2] currently being developed by the National Committee for Clinical Laboratory Standards.

INDICATIONS AND USAGE
Tuberculosis: Rifampin is indicated in the treatment of all forms of tuberculosis. Rifadin® (rifampin) must always be used in conjunction with at least one other antituberculosis drug. Frequently used regimens are rifampin and isoniazid; rifampin, isoniazid, and pyrazinamide; rifampin, isoniazid, and ethambutol; and rifampin and ethambutol.
Rifadin I.V. is indicated for the initial treatment and retreatment of tuberculosis when the drug cannot be taken by mouth.

Meningococcal Carriers: Rifampin is indicated for the treatment of asymptomatic carriers of *N. meningitidis* to eliminate meningococci from the nasopharynx. Rifampin is not indicated for the treatment of meningococcal infection because of the possibility of the rapid emergence of resistant organisms. (See WARNINGS.)

Rifampin should not be used indiscriminately, and therefore diagnostic laboratory procedures, including serotyping and susceptibility testing, should be performed for establishment of the carrier state and the correct treatment. So that the usefulness of rifampin in the treatment of asymptomatic meningococcal carriers is preserved, the drug should be used only when the risk of meningococcal disease is high.

In the treatment of both tuberculosis and the meningococcal carrier state, the small number of resistant cells present within large populations of susceptible cells can rapidly become predominant. Since resistance can emerge rapidly, susceptibility tests should be performed in the event of persistent positive cultures.

CONTRAINDICATIONS
Rifampin is contraindicated in patients with a history of hypersensitivity to any of the rifamycins. (See WARNINGS.)

WARNINGS
Rifampin has been shown to produce liver dysfunction. Fatalities associated with jaundice have occured in patients with liver disease and in patients taking rifampin with other hepatotoxic agents. Patients with impaired liver function should only be given rifampin in cases of necessity and then with caution and under strict medical supervision.

In these patients, careful monitoring of liver function, especially serum glutamic pyruvic transaminase (SGPT) and serum glutamic oxaloacetic transaminase (SGOT) should be carried out prior to therapy and then every two to four weeks during therapy. If signs of hepatocellular damage occur, rifampin should be withdrawn.

In some cases, hyperbilirubinemia resulting from competition between rifampin and bilirubin for excretory pathways of the liver at the cell level can occur in the early days of treatment. An isolated report showing a moderate rise in bilirubin and/or transaminase level is not in itself an indication for interrupting treatment; rather, the decision should be made after repeating the tests, noting trends in the levels, and considering them in conjunction with the patient's clinical condition.

Rifampin has enzyme-inducing properties, including induction of delta amino levulinic acid synthetase. Isolated reports have associated porphyria exacerbation with rifampin administration.

The possibility of rapid emergence of resistant meningococci restricts the use of Rifadin to short-term treatment of the asymptomatic carrier state. Rifadin is not to be used for the treatment of meningococcal disease.

PRECAUTIONS
General
For the treatment of tuberculosis, rifampin is usually administered on a daily basis. High doses of rifampin (greater than 600 mg) given once or twice weekly have resulted in a high incidence of adverse reactions, including the "flu syndrome" (fever, chills and malaise), hematopoietic reactions (leukopenia, thrombocytopenia, or acute hemolytic anemia), cutaneous, gastrointestinal, and hepatic reactions, shortness of breath, shock and renal failure. Recent studies indicate that regimens using twice-weekly doses of rifampin 600 mg plus isoniazid 15 mg/kg are much better tolerated.

Intermittent therapy may be used if the patient cannot or will not self-administer drugs on a daily basis. Patients on intermittent therapy should be closely monitored for compliance and cautioned against intentional or accidental interruption of prescribed therapy because of the increased risk of serious adverse reactions.

Rifadin I.V.
For intravenous infusion only. Must not be administered by intramuscular or subcutaneous route. Avoid extravasation during injection; local irritation and inflammation due to extravascular infiltration of the infusion have been observed. If these occur, the infusion should be discontinued and restarted at another site.

Information for Patients
The patient should be told that this medication may cause the urine, feces, saliva, sputum, sweat and tears to turn red-orange. Permanent discoloration of soft contact lenses may occur.

The patient should be advised that the reliability of oral contraceptives may be affected; consideration should be given to using alternative contraceptive measures.

Laboratory Tests
A complete blood count (CBC) should be obtained prior to instituting therapy and periodically throughout the course of therapy. Because of a possible transient rise in transaminase and bilirubin values, blood for baseline clinical chemistries should be obtained before rifampin dosing.

Drug Interactions
Rifampin has liver enzyme-inducing properties and may reduce the activity of a number of drugs, including anticoagulants, corticosteroids, cyclosporine, cardiac glycoside preparations, quinidine, oral contraceptives, oral hypoglycemic agents (sulfonylureas), dapsone, narcotics and analgesics. Rifampin also has been reported to diminish the effects of concurrently administered methadone, barbiturates, diazepam, verapamil, beta-adrenergic blockers, clofibrate, proges-

tins, disopyramide, mexiletine, theophylline, chloramphenicol and anticonvulsants. It may be necessary to adjust the dosages of these drugs if they are given concurrently with rifampin.

Patients using oral contraceptives should be advised to change to non-hormonal methods of birth control during rifampin therapy. Also, diabetes may become more difficult to control.

When rifampin is taken with para-aminosalicylic acid (PAS), rifampin levels in the serum may decrease. Therefore, the drugs should be taken at least 8 hours apart.

Probenecid has been reported to increase rifampin blood levels. Halothane, when given concomitantly with rifampin, has been reported to increase the hepatotoxicity of both drugs. Ketoconazole, when given concomitantly with rifampin, has been reported to diminish the serum concentrations of both drugs. Dosage should be adjusted if indicated by the patient's clinical condition. An interaction has also been reported with rifampin-isoniazid and Vitamin D.

Drug/Laboratory Interactions
Therapeutic levels of rifampin have been shown to inhibit standard microbiological assays for serum folate and Vitamin B$_{12}$. Thus, alternate assay methods should be considered. Transient abnormalities in liver function tests (e.g., elevation in serum bilirubin, abnormal bromsulphalein (BSP) excretion, alkaline phosphatase and serum transaminases), and reduced biliary excretion of contrast media used for visualization of the gallbladder have also been observed. Therefore, these tests should be performed before the morning dose of rifampin.

Carcinogenesis, Mutagenesis, Impairment of Fertility
There are no known human data on long-term potential for carcinogenicity, mutagenicity, or impairment of fertility. A few cases of accelerated growth of lung carcinoma have been reported in man, but a causal relationship with the drug has not been established. An increase in the incidence of hepatomas in female mice (of a strain known to be particularly susceptible to the spontaneous development of hepatomas) was observed when rifampin was administered in doses 2 to 10 times the average daily human dose for 60 weeks followed by an observation period of 46 weeks. No evidence of carcinogenicity was found in male mice of the same strain, mice of a different strain, or rats, under similar experimental conditions.

Rifampin has been reported to possess immunosuppressive potential in rabbits, mice, rats, guinea pigs, human lymphocytes *in vitro*, and humans. Antitumor activity *in vitro* has also been shown with rifampin.

There was no evidence of mutagenicity in bacteria, *Drosophila melanogaster*, or mice, nor did rifampin induce chromosome aberrations in human lymphocytes treated *in vitro*. However, an increase in chromatid breaks was noted when whole-blood cell cultures were treated with rifampin.

Pregnancy—Teratogenic Effects
Pregnancy—Category C: Rifampin has been shown to be teratogenic in rodents give oral doses of rifampin 15 to 25 times the human dose. Although rifampin has been reported to cross the placental barrier and appear in cord blood, the effect of Rifadin, alone or in combination with other antituberculosis drugs, on the human fetus is not known. Neonates of rifampin-treated mothers should be carefully observed for any evidence of adverse effects. Isolated cases of fetal malformations have been reported; however, there are no adequate and well-controlled studies in pregnant women. Rifampin should be used during pregnancy only if the potential benefit justifies the potential risk to the fetus.

Rifampin in oral doses of 150 to 250 mg/kg produced teratogenic effects in mice and rats. Malformations were primarily cleft palate in the mouse and spina bifida in the rat. The incidence of these anomalies was dose-dependent. When rifampin was given to pregnant rabbits in doses up to 20 times the usual daily human dose, imperfect osteogenesis and embryotoxicity were reported.

When administered during the last few weeks of pregnancy, rifampin can cause post-natal hemorrhages in the mother and infant for which treatment with Vitamin K may be indicated.

Nursing Mothers
Because of the potential for tumorigenicity shown for rifampin in animal studies a decision should be made whether to discontinue nursing or to discontinue the drug, taking into account the importance of the drug to the mother.

Pediatric Use—See CLINICAL PHARMACOLOGY—Serum *Levels in Children;* see also DOSAGE AND ADMINISTRATION

ADVERSE REACTIONS
Gastrointestinal
Heartburn, epigastric distress, anorexia, nausea, vomiting, jaundice, flatulence, cramps and diarrhea have been noted in some patients. Although *C. difficile* has been shown *in vitro* to be sensitive to rifampin, pseudomembranous colitis has been reported with the use of rifampin (and other broad spectrum antibiotics). Therefore, it is important to consider this diagnosis in patients who develop diarrhea in association with antibiotic use. Rarely, hepatitis or a shock-like

syndrome with hepatic involvement and abnormal liver function tests has been reported.

Hematologic

Thrombocytopenia has occurred primarily with high dose intermittent therapy, but has also been noted after resumption of interrupted treatment. It rarely occurs during well supervised daily therapy. This effect is reversible if the drug is discontinued as soon as purpura occurs. Cerebral hemorrhage and fatalities have been reported when rifampin administration has been continued or resumed after the appearance of purpura.

Transient leukopenia, hemolytic anemia and decreased hemoglobin have been observed.

Central Nervous System

Headache, fever, drowsiness, fatigue, ataxia, dizziness, inability to concentrate, mental confusion, behavioral changes, muscular weakness, pains in extremities and generalized numbness have been observed.

Rare reports of myopathy have also been observed.

Ocular

Visual disturbances have been observed.

Endocrine

Menstrual disturbances have been observed.

Renal

Elevations in BUN and serum uric acid have been reported. Rarely, hemolysis hemoglobinuria, hematuria, renal insufficiency and acute renal failure have been noted. These are generally considered to be hypersensitivity reactions. They usually occur during intermittent therapy or when treatment is resumed following intentional or accidental interruption of a daily dosage regimen, and are reversible when rifampin is discontinued and appropriate therapy instituted.

Dermatologic

Cutaneous reactions are mild and self-limiting and do not appear to be hypersensitivity reactions. Typically, they consist of flushing and itching with or without a rash. More serious cutaneous reactions which may be due to hypersensitivity occur but are uncommon.

Hypersensitivity Reactions

Occasionally, pruritus, urticaria, rash, pemphigoid reaction, eosinophilia, sore mouth, sore tongue and conjunctivitis have been observed.

Miscellaneous

Edema of the face and extremities has been reported. Other reactions reported to have occurred with intermittent dosage regimens include "flu" syndrome (such as episodes of fever, chills, headache, dizziness and bone pain), shortness of breath, wheezing, decrease in blood pressure and shock. The "flu" syndrome may also appear if rifampin is taken irregularly by the patient or if daily administration is resumed after a drug free interval.

OVERDOSAGE

Signs and Symptoms:

Nausea, vomiting and increasing lethargy will probably occur within a short time after ingestion; unconsciousness may occur when there is severe hepatic disease. Brownish-red or orange discoloration of the skin, urine, sweat, saliva, tears and feces will occur, and its intensity is proportional to the amount ingested.

Liver enlargement, possibly with tenderness, may develop within a few hours after severe overdosage; jaundice may develop rapidly. Hepatic involvement may be more marked in patients with prior impairment of hepatic function. Other physical findings remain essentially normal.

Bilirubin levels may increase rapidly with severe overdosage; hepatic enzyme levels may be affected, especially with prior impairment of hepatic function. A direct effect upon the hematopoietic system, electrolyte levels, or acid-base balance is unlikely.

Acute Toxicity

In animal studies, the LD_{50} of rifampin is approximately 885 mg/kg in the mouse, 1720 mg/kg in the rat, and 2120 mg/kg in the rabbit.

Non-fatal overdoses with as high as 12 g of rifampin have been reported. In one patient who swallowed 12 g of rifampin, vomiting occurred four times within 1 hour of ingestion of rifampin. Gastric lavage with 20 liters of water was initiated 5 hours after ingestion. Twelve hours after ingestion of rifampin, a plasma concentration of 400 μg of rifampin/mL was measured by microbiological assay. The plasma concentration fell to 64 μg/mL on the following day, and to 0.1 μg/mL on the third day. Urinary rifampin concentration was 313 μg/mL approximately 30 hours after ingestion of the drug, 625 μg/mL after 36 hours, and 78 μg/mL after 40 hours. By the fourth day following the dose, only 0.1 μg/mL rifampin was present in the urine. There was biochemical evidence of mild impairment of liver function. Liver function tests had returned to normal within 5 days, and the patient's recovery was described as uneventful.

One case of fatal overdose is known: a 26-year-old man died after self-administering 60 g of rifampin.

Treatment

Since nausea and vomiting are likely to be present, gastric lavage is probably preferable to induction of emesis. Following evacuation of the gastric contents, the instillation of activated charcoal slurry into the stomach may help absorb any remaining drug from the gastrointestinal tract. Antiemetic medication may be required to control severe nausea/vomiting.

Active diuresis (with measured intake and output) will help promote excretion of the drug. Hemodialysis may be of value in some patients. In patients with previously adequate hepatic function, reversal of liver enlargement and of impaired hepatic excretory function probably will be noted within 72 hours, with a rapid return toward normal thereafter.

DOSAGE AND ADMINISTRATION

Rifampin can be administered by the oral route or by I.V. infusion (see INDICATIONS AND USAGE).

Tuberculosis

Adults: 600 mg in a single daily administration, oral or I.V.

Children: 10–20 mg/kg not to exceed 600 mg/day, oral or I.V.

It is recommended that oral rifampin be administered once daily, either one hour before, or two hours after a meal.

In the treatment of tuberculosis, rifampin should always be administered with at least one other antituberculosis drug. In general, therapy for tuberculosis should be continued for 6 to 9 months or until at least 6 months have elapsed from conversion of sputum to culture negativity. In patients who cannot be relied on for compliance, intermittent therapy with 600 mg/day two or three times/week under close supervision may be prescribed and substituted for the daily regimen after 1–2 months of an initial daily phase of therapy.

The *9-Month Regimen* ordinarily consists of rifampin and isoniazid, usually supplemented during the initial phase by pyrazinamide, streptomycin or ethambutol.

The *6-Month Regimen* ordinarily consists of an initial *2-month* phase of rifampin, isoniazid and pyrazinamide, and, if clinically indicated, streptomycin or ethambutol; followed by *4 months* of rifampin and isoniazid.

Either of the above regimens is recommended as standard therapy.

The above recommendations apply to patients with drug-susceptible organisms. Patients with drug-resistant organisms may require longer treatment with other drug regimens.

Meningococcal Carriers

Adults For adults, it is recommended that 600 mg rifampin be administered twice daily for 2 days.

Infants and Children Children 1 month of age or older: 10 mg/kg every 12 hours for 2 days.

Children under 1 month of age: 5 mg/kg every 12 hours for 2 days.

Preparation of Solution for I.V. Infusion

Reconstitute the lyophilized powder by transferring 10 mL of sterile water for injection to a vial containing 600 mg of rifampin for injection. Swirl vial gently to completely dissolve the antibiotic. The resultant solution contains 60 mg rifampin activity per mL and is stable at room temperature for 24 hours. Withdraw a volume equivalent to the amount of rifampin calculated to be administered and add to 500 mL of infusion medium. Mix well and infuse at a rate allowing for complete infusion in 3 hours. In some cases, the amount of rifampin calculated to be administered may be added to 100 mL of infusion medium and infused in 30 minutes. The 500 mL and 100 mL dilutions are also stable at room temperature for 24 hours.

CAUTION: Dextrose 5% for injection is the recommended infusion medium. Sterile Saline may be used when dextrose is contraindicated, but the stability of rifampin is slightly reduced. Other solutions are not recommended.

Preparation of Extemporaneous Oral Suspension

For pediatric and adult patients in whom capsule swallowing is difficult or where lower doses are needed, a liquid suspension may be prepared as follows:

Rifadin 1% w/v suspension (10 mg/mL) can be compounded using one of five syrups—Simple Syrup (Syrup NF), Simple Syrup (Humco Laboratories), Simple Syrup (Whiteworth Inc.), Wild Cherry Syrup (Eli Lilly and Company), and Syrpalta® Syrup (Emerson Laboratories).

1. Empty contents of four Rifadin 300 mg capsules or eight Rifadin 150 mg capsules onto a piece of weighing paper.
2. If necessary, gently crush the capsule contents with a spatula to produce a fine powder.
3. Transfer rifampin powder blend to a 4-ounce amber glass prescription bottle.
4. Rinse the paper and spatula with 20 mL of one of the above-mentioned syrups and add the rinse to the bottle. Shake vigorously.
5. Add 100 mL of syrup to the bottle and shake vigorously.

This compounding procedure results in a 1% w/v suspension containing 10 mg rifampin/mL. Stability studies indicate that the suspension is stable when stored at room temperature (25 ± 3°C) or in a refrigerator (2–8°C) for four weeks. This extemporaneously prepared suspension must be shaken well prior to administration.

HOW SUPPLIED

150 mg maroon and scarlet capsules imprinted "RIFADIN 150".

Bottles of 30 (NDC 0068-0510-30)

300 mg maroon and scarlet capsules imprinted "RIFADIN 300".

Bottles of 30 (NDC 0068-0508-30)

Bottles of 60 (NDC 0068-0508-60)

Bottles of 100 (NDC 0068-0508-61)

Storage: Keep tightly closed. Store in a dry place. Avoid excessive heat.

Rifadin I.V. (rifampin for injection) is available in glass vials containing 600 mg rifampin (NDC 0068-0597-01).

Storage: Avoid excessive heat (temperatures above 40°C or 104°F). Protect from light.

1. National Committee for Clinical Laboratory Standards, Approved Standard: Performance Standards for Antimicrobial Disk Susceptibility Tests (M2-T4), December 1988.
2. National Committee for Clinical Laboratory Standards, Approved Standard: Methods for Dilution Antimicrobial Susceptibility Tests for Bacteria that Grow Aerobically (M7-T2), December 1988.

Product Information as of May, 1989

Rifadin 150 mg capsules are manufactured by:

MERRELL DOW PHARMACEUTICALS (CANADA) INC.

Richmond Hill, Ontario, L4C 5H2 CANADA for

MERRELL DOW U.S.A.

Division of Merrell Dow Pharmaceuticals Inc.

Cincinnati, Ohio 45215

Rifadin I.V. (rifampin for injection) is manufactured by:

GRUPPO LEPETIT S.p.A.

Milan, Italy for

MERRELL DOW U.S.A.

Division of Merrell Dow Pharmaceuticals Inc.

Cincinnati, Ohio 45215

Shown in Product Identification Section, page 419

RIFAMATE® ℞

[rĭf'ăh-māt]

rifampin and isoniazid

Capsules

CAUTION: Federal law prohibits dispensing without prescription.

> ### WARNING
> Severe and sometimes fatal hepatitis associated with isoniazid therapy may occur and may develop even after many months of treatment. The risk of developing hepatitis is age related. Approximate case rates by age are: 0 per 1,000 for persons under 20 years of age, 3 per 1,000 for persons in the 20–34 year age group, 12 per 1,000 for persons in the 35–49 year age group, 23 per 1,000 for persons in the 50–64 year age group, and 8 per 1,000 for persons over 65 years of age. The risk of hepatitis is increased with daily consumption of alcohol. Precise data to provide a fatality rate for isoniazid-related hepatitis are not available; however, in a U.S. Public Health Service Surveillance Study of 13,838 persons taking isoniazid, there were 8 deaths among 174 cases of hepatitis. Therefore, patients given isoniazid should be carefully monitored and interviewed at monthly intervals. Serum transaminase concentration becomes elevated in about 10–20 percent of patients, usually during the first few months of therapy, but it can occur at any time. Usually enzyme levels return to normal despite continuance of drug, but in some cases progressive liver dysfunction occurs. Patients should be instructed to report immediately any of the prodromal symptoms of hepatitis, such as fatigue, weakness, malaise, anorexia, nausea, or vomiting. If these symptoms appear or if signs suggestive of hepatic damage are detected, isoniazid should be discontinued promptly, since continued use of the drug in these cases has been reported to cause a more severe form of liver damage.
> Patients with tuberculosis should be given appropriate treatment with alternative drugs. If isoniazid must be reinstituted, it should be reinstituted only after symptoms and laboratory abnormalities have cleared. The drug should be restarted in very small and gradually increasing doses and should be withdrawn immediately if there is any indication of recurrent liver involvement. Treatment should be deferred in persons with acute hepatic diseases.

DESCRIPTION

Rifamate is a combination capsule containing 300 mg rifampin and 150 mg isoniazid. The capsules also contain as inactive ingredients: colloidal silicon dioxide, FD&C Blue No. 1, FD&C Red No. 40, gelatin, magnesium stearate, sodium starch glycolate, and titanium dioxide.

Continued on next page

Information on Merrell Dow products is based on labeling in effect in June, 1989.

Merrell Dow—Cont.

Rifampin is a semisynthetic antibiotic derivative of rifamycin B. Specifically, rifampin is the hydrazone, 3-(4-methylpiperazinylimino-methyl) rifamycin SV.

Isoniazid is the hydrazide of isonicotinic acid. It exists as colorless or white crystals or as a white, crystalline powder that is water soluble, odorless, and slowly affected by exposure to air and light.

ACTIONS

Rifampin

Rifampin inhibits DNA-dependent RNA polymerase activity in susceptible cells. Specifically, it interacts with bacterial RNA polymerase but does not inhibit the mammalian enzyme. This is the mechanism of action by which rifampin exerts its therapeutic effect. Rifampin cross resistance has only been shown with other rifamycins.

In a study of 14 normal human adult males, peak blood levels of rifampin occured $1 \frac{1}{2}$ to 3 hours following oral administration of two Rifamate capsules. The peaks ranged from 6.9 to 14 mcg/ml with an average of 10 mcg/ml.

In normal subjects the $T\frac{1}{2}$ (biological half-life) of rifampin in blood is approximately 3 hours. Elimination occurs mainly through the bile and, to a much lesser extent the urine.

Isoniazid

Isoniazid acts against actively growing tubercle bacilli.

After oral administration isoniazid produces peak blood levels within 1 to 2 hours which decline to 50% or less within 6 hours. It diffuses readily into all body fluids (cerebrospinal, pleural, and ascitic fluids), tissues, organs and excreta (saliva, sputum, and feces). The drug also passes through the placental barrier and into milk in concentrations comparable to those in the plasma. From 50 to 70% of a dose of isoniazid is excreted in the urine in 24 hours.

Isoniazid is metabolized primarily by acetylation and dehydrazination. The rate of acetylation is genetically determined. Approximately 50% of Blacks and Caucasians are "slow inactivators"; the majority of Eskimos and Orientals are "rapid inactivators."

The rate of acetylation does not significantly alter the effectiveness of isoniazid. However, slow acetylation may lead to higher blood levels of the drug, and thus an increase in toxic reactions.

Pyridoxine deficiency (B_6) is sometimes observed in adults with high doses of isoniazid and is considered probably due to its competition with pyridoxal phosphate for the enzyme apotryptophanase.

INDICATIONS

For pulmonary tuberculosis in which organisms are susceptible, and when the patient has been titrated on the individual components and it has therefore been established that this fixed dosage is therapeutically effective.

This fixed-dosage combination drug is not recommended for initial therapy of tuberculosis or for preventive therapy.

In the treatment of tuberculosis, small numbers of resistant cells, present within large populations of susceptible cells, can rapidly become the predominating type. Since rapid emergence of resistance can occur, culture and susceptibility tests should be performed in the event of persistent positive cultures.

This drug is *not* indicated for the treatment of meningococcal infections or asymptomatic carriers of *N. meningitidis* to eliminate meningococci from the nasopharynx.

CONTRAINDICATIONS

Previous isoniazid-associated hepatic injury; severe adverse reactions to isoniazid, such as drug fever, chills, and arthritis; acute liver disease of any etiology.

A history of previous hypersensitivity reaction to any of the rifamycins or to isoniazid, including drug-induced hepatitis.

WARNINGS

Rifamate (rifampin-isoniazid) is a combination of two drugs, each of which has been associated with liver dysfunction. Liver function tests should be performed prior to therapy with Rifamate and periodically during treatment.

Rifampin

Rifampin has been shown to produce liver dysfunction. There have been fatalities associated with jaundice in patients with liver disease or receiving rifampin concomitantly with other hepatoxic agents. Since an increased risk may exist for individuals with liver disease, benefits must be weighed carefully against the risk of further liver damage. Several studies of tumorigenicity potential have been done in rodents. In one strain of mice known to be particularly susceptible to the spontaneous development of hepatomas, rifampin given at a level 2–10 times the maximum dosage used clinically, resulted in a significant increase in the occurrence of hepatomas in female mice of this strain after one year of administration. There was no evidence of tumorigenicity in the males of this strain, in males or females of another mouse strain, or in rats.

Isoniazid

See the boxed warning.

PRECAUTIONS

Rifampin

Rifampin is not recommended for intermittent therapy; the patient should be cautioned against intentional or accidental interruption of the daily dosage regimen since rare renal hypersensitivity reactions have been reported when therapy was resumed in such cases.

Rifampin has been observed to increase the requirements for anticoagulant drugs of the coumarin type. The cause of the phenomenon is unknown. In patients receiving anticoagulants and rifampin concurrently, it is recommended that the prothrombin time be performed daily or as frequently as necessary to establish and maintain the required dose of anticoagulant.

Urine, feces, saliva, sputum, sweat and tears may be colored red-orange by rifampin and its metabolites. Soft contact lenses may be permanently stained. Individuals to be treated should be made aware of these possibilities.

It has been reported that the reliability of oral contraceptives may be affected in some patients being treated for tuberculosis with rifampin in combination with at least one other antituberculosis drug. In such cases, alternative contraceptive measures may need to be considered.

It has also been reported that rifampin given in combination with other antituberculosis drugs may decrease the pharmacologic activity of methadone, oral hypoglycemics, digitoxin, quinidine, disopyramide, dapsone and corticosteroids. In these cases, dosage adjustment of the interacting drugs is recommended.

Therapeutic levels of rifampin have been shown to inhibit standard assays for serum folate and vitamin B_{12}. Alternative methods must be considered when determining folate and vitamin B_{12} concentrations in the presence of rifampin.

Since rifampin has been reported to cross the placental barrier and appear in cord blood and in maternal milk, neonates and newborns of rifampin-treated mothers should be carefully observed for any evidence of untoward effects.

Isoniazid

All drugs should be stopped and an evaluation of the patient should be made at the first sign of a hypersensitivity reaction.

Use of isoniazid should be carefully monitored in the following:

1. Patients who are receiving phenytoin (diphenylhydantoin) concurrently. Isoniazid may decrease the excretion of phenytoin or may enhance its effects. To avoid phenytoin intoxication, appropriate adjustment of the anticonvulsant dose should be made.

2. Daily users of alcohol. Daily ingestion of alcohol may be associated with a higher incidence of isoniazid hepatitis.

3. Patients with current chronic liver disease or severe renal dysfunction.

Periodic ophthalmoscopic examination during isoniazid therapy is recommended when visual symptoms occur.

Usage in Pregnancy and Lactation

Rifampin

Although rifampin has been reported to cross the placental barrier and appear in cord blood, the effect of rifampin, alone or in combination with other antituberculosis drugs, on the human fetus is not known. An increase in congenital malformations, primarily spina bifida and cleft palate, has been reported in the offspring of rodents given oral doses of 150–250 mg/kg/day of rifampin during pregnancy.

The possible teratogenic potential in women capable of bearing children should be carefully weighed against the benefits of therapy.

Isoniazid

It has been reported that in both rats and rabbits, isoniazid may exert an embryocidal effect when administered orally during pregnancy, although no isoniazid-related congenital anomalies have been found in reproduction studies in mammalian species (mice, rats, and rabbits). Isoniazid should be prescribed during pregnancy only when therapeutically necessary. The benefit of preventive therapy should be weighed against a possible risk to the fetus. Preventive treatment generally should be started after delivery because of the increased risk of tuberculosis for new mothers.

Since isoniazid is known to cross the placental barrier and to pass into maternal breast milk, neonates and breast-fed infants of isoniazid treated mothers should be carefully observed for any evidence of adverse effects.

Carcinogenesis:

Isoniazid has been reported to induce pulmonary tumors in a number of strains of mice.

ADVERSE REACTIONS

Rifampin

Nervous system reactions: headache, drowsiness, fatigue, ataxia, dizziness, inability to concentrate, mental confusion, visual disturbances, muscular weakness, pain in extremities and generalized numbness.

Gastrointestinal disturbances: in some patients heartburn, epigastric distress, anorexia, nausea, vomiting, gas, cramps, and diarrhea.

Hepatic reactions: transient abnormalities in liver function tests (e.g. elevations in serum bilirubin, BSP, alkaline phosphatase, serum transaminases) have been observed. Rarely, hepatitis or a shocklike syndrome with hepatic involvement and abnormal liver function tests.

Hematologic reactions: thrombocytopenia, transient leukopenia, hemolytic anemia, eosinophilia and decreased hemoglobin have been observed. Thrombocytopenia has occurred when rifampin and ethambutol were administered concomitantly according to an intermittent dose schedule twice weekly and in high doses.

Allergic and immunological reactions: occasionally pruritus, urticaria, rash, pemphigoid reaction, eosinophilia, sore mouth, sore tongue and exudative conjunctivitis. Rarely, hemolysis, hemoglobinuria, hematuria, renal insufficiency or acute renal failure have been reported which are generally considered to be hypersensitivity reactions. These have usually occurred during intermittent therapy or when treatment was resumed following intentional or accidental interruption of a daily dosage regimen and were reversible when rifampin was discontinued and appropriate therapy instituted.

Although rifampin has been reported to have an immunosuppressive effect in some animal experiments, available human data indicate that this has no clinical significance.

Metabolic reactions: elevations in BUN and serum uric acid have occurred.

Miscellaneous reactions: fever and menstrual disturbances have been noted.

Isoniazid

The most frequent reactions are those affecting the nervous system and the liver.

Nervous system reactions: Peripheral neuropathy is the most common toxic effect. It is dose-related, occurs most often in the malnourished and in those predisposed to neuritis (e.g., alcoholics and diabetics), and is usually preceded by paresthesias of the feet and hands. The incidence is higher in "slow inactivators".

Other neurotoxic effects, which are uncommon with conventional doses, are convulsions, toxic encephalopathy, optic neuritis and atrophy, memory impairment, and toxic psychosis.

Gastrointestinal reactions: Nausea, vomiting, and epigastric distress.

Hepatic reactions: Elevated serum transaminases (SGOT; SGPT), bilirubinemia, bilirubinuria, jaundice, and occasionally severe and sometimes fatal hepatitis. The common prodromal symptoms are anorexia, nausea, vomiting, fatigue, malaise, and weakness. Mild and transient elevation of serum transaminase levels occurs in 10 to 20 percent of persons taking isoniazid. The abnormality usually occurs in the first 4 to 6 months of treatment but can occur at any time during therapy. In most instances, enzyme levels return to normal with no necessity to discontinue medication. In occasional instances, progressive liver damage occurs, with accompanying symptoms. In these cases, the drug should be discontinued immediately. The frequency of progressive liver damage increases with age. It is rare in persons under 20, but occurs in up to 2.3 percent of those over 50 years of age.

Hematologic reactions: agranulocytosis, hemolytic sideroblastic or aplastic anemia, thrombocytopenia and eosinophilia.

Hypersensitivity reactions: fever, skin eruptions (morbilliform, maculopapular, purpuric, or exfoliative), lymphadenopathy and vasculitis.

Metabolic and endocrine reactions: pyridoxine deficiency, pellagra, hyperglycemia, metabolic acidosis, and gynecomastia.

Miscellaneous reactions: rheumatic syndrome and systemic lupus erythematosus-like syndrome.

OVERDOSAGE

Rifampin

Signs and Symptoms

Nausea, vomiting, and increasing lethargy will probably occur within a short time after ingestion; actual unconsciousness may occur with severe hepatic involvement. Brownish-red or orange discoloration of the skin, urine, sweat, saliva, tears, and feces is proportional to amount ingested.

Liver enlargement, possibly with tenderness, can develop within a few hours after severe overdosage and jaundice may develop rapidly. Hepatic involvement may be more marked in patients with prior impairment of hepatic function. Other physical findings remain essentially normal.

Direct and total bilirubin levels may increase rapidly with severe overdosage; hepatic enzyme levels may be affected, especially with prior impairment of hepatic function. A direct effect upon hemopoietic system, electrolyte levels or acid-base balance is unlikely.

Isoniazid

Signs and Symptoms

Isoniazid overdosage produces signs and symptoms within 30 minutes to 3 hours. Nausea, vomiting, dizziness, slurring of speech, blurring of vision, visual hallucinations (including bright colors and strange designs), are among the early manifestations. With marked overdosage, respiratory distress and CNS depression, progressing rapidly from stupor to profound coma, are to be expected, along with severe, intractable seizures. Severe metabolic acidosis, acetonuria, and hyperglycemia are typical laboratory findings.

Rifamate (rifampin and isoniazid capsules)

Treatment

The airway should be secured and adequate respiratory exchange established. Only then should gastric emptying (lavage-aspiration) be attempted; this may be difficult because of seizures. Since nausea and vomiting are likely to be present, gastric lavage is probably preferable to induction of emesis. Activated charcoal slurry instilled into the stomach following evacuation of gastric contents can help absorb any remaining drug in the GI tract. Antiemetic medication may be required to control severe nausea and vomiting.

Blood samples should be obtained for immediate determination of gases, electrolytes, BUN, glucose, etc. Blood should be typed and crossmatched in preparation for possible hemodialysis.

Rapid control of metabolic acidosis is fundamental to management. Intravenous sodium bicarbonate should be given at once and repeated as needed, adjusting subsequent dosage on the basis of laboratory findings (i.e. serum sodium, pH, etc.). At the same time, anticonvulsants should be given intravenously (i.e. barbiturates, diphenylhydantoin, diazepam) as required, and large doses of intravenous pyridoxine.

Forced osmotic diuresis must be started early and should be continued for some hours after clinical improvement to hasten renal clearance of drug and help prevent relapse. Fluid intake and output should be monitored.

Bile drainage may be indicated in presence of serious impairment of hepatic function lasting more than 24–48 hours. Under these circumstances, and for severe cases extra-corporeal hemodialysis may be required; if this is not available, peritoneal dialysis can be used along with forced diuresis.

Along with measures based on initial and repeated determination of blood gases and other laboratory tests as needed, meticulous respiratory and other intensive care should be utilized to protect against hypoxia, hypotension, aspiration, pneumonitis, etc.

In patients with previously adequate hepatic function, reversal of liver enlargement and impaired hepatic excretory function probably will be needed within 72 hours, with rapid return toward normal thereafter.

Untreated or inadequately treated cases of gross isoniazid overdosage can terminate fatally, but good response has been reported in most patients brought under adequate treatment within the first few hours after drug ingestion.

DOSAGE AND ADMINISTRATION

In general, therapy should be continued until bacterial conversion and maximal improvement have occured.

Adults: Two Rifamate (rifampin-isoniazid) capsules (600 mg rifampin, 300 mg isoniazid) once daily, administered one hour before or two hours after a meal.

Concomitant administration of pyridoxine (B_6) is recommended in the malnourished, in those predisposed to neuropathy (e.g. diabetics) and in adolescents.

Susceptibility Testing

Rifampin

Rifampin susceptibility powders are available for both direct and indirect methods of determining the susceptibility of strains of mycobacteria. The MIC's of susceptible clinical isolates when determined in 7H10 or other non-egg-containing media have ranged from 0.1 to 2 mcg/ml.

Quantitative methods that require measurement of zone diameters give the most precise estimates of antibiotic susceptibility. One such procedure has been recommended for use with discs for testing susceptibility to rifampin. Interpretations correlate zone diameters from the disc test with MIC (minimal inhibitory concentration) values for rifampin.

HOW SUPPLIED

Capsules (opaque red), containing 300 mg rifampin and 150 mg isoniazid; bottles of 60 (NDC 0068-0509-60).

Product Information as of April, 1985
Shown in Product Identification Section, page 419

SELDANE® ℞

[sĕl′dān]
(terfenadine)
60 mg Tablets

CAUTION: Federal law prohibits dispensing without prescription.

DESCRIPTION

Seldane (terfenadine) is available as tablets for oral administration. Each tablet contains 60 mg terfenadine. Tablets also contain, as inactive ingredients: corn starch, gelatin, lactose, magnesium stearate, and sodium bicarbonate.

Terfenadine is a histamine H_1-receptor antagonist with the chemical name α-[4-(1,1-Dimethylethyl) phenyl]-4-(hydroxydiphenylmethyl)-1-piperidinebutanol. The molecular weight is 471.68. The molecular formula is $C_{32}H_{41}NO_2$.

It has the following chemical structure:

Terfenadine occurs as a white to off-white crystalline powder. It is freely soluble in chloroform, soluble in ethanol, and very slightly soluble in water.

CLINICAL PHARMACOLOGY

Terfenadine is chemically and pharmacologically distinct from other antihistamines.

Histamine skin wheal studies have shown that Seldane in single and repeated doses of 60 mg in 64 subjects has an antihistaminic effect beginning at 1–2 hours, reaching its maximum at 3–4 hours, and lasting in excess of 12 hours.

Clinical trials of Seldane involved about 2,600 patients, most receiving either Seldane, another antihistamine and/or placebo in double-blind, randomized controlled comparisons. The four best controlled and largest trials each lasted 7 days and involved about 1,000 total patients in comparisons of Seldane (60 mg b.i.d.) with an active drug (chlorpheniramine, 4 mg t.i.d.; dexchlorpheniramine, 2 mg t.i.d.; or clemastine 1 mg b.i.d.). In the four trials, about 50–70% of Seldane or other antihistamine recipients had moderate to complete relief of symptoms, compared with 30–50% of placebo recipients, with a significant difference favoring the active drugs in each study. In these studies, Seldane was associated with less frequent drowsiness than the other antihistamines; the frequency of drowsiness with Seldane was similar to the frequency with placebo. None of these studies showed a difference between Seldane and other antihistamines in the frequency of anticholinergic effects. In studies which included 52 subjects in whom EEG assessments were made, no depressant effects have been observed.

Animal studies have demonstrated that terfenadine is a peripheral specific histamine H_1-receptor antagonist. In these animal studies, no sedative or anticholinergic effects were observed at effective antihistaminic doses. Radioactive disposition and autoradiographic studies in rats and radioligand binding studies with guinea pig brain H_1-receptors indicate that, at effective antihistamine doses, neither terfenadine nor its metabolites penetrate the blood brain barrier well.

Pharmacokinetic studies in 27 male subjects, using ^{14}C-labeled terfenadine, demonstrated that an oral dose of terfenadine is well absorbed from the gastrointestinal tract and rapidly and extensively biotransformed. Following administration of a single 60 mg Seldane tablet, detectable plasma levels were observed within one-half hour. Plasma levels peaked at about 2 hours after administration; a distribution half-life of 3.4 hours was followed by an elimination half-life of 20.25 hours. Terfenadine is extensively (97%) bound to human serum protein. Elimination studies in 6 male volunteers showed that fecal excretion accounted for 60% of the dose while 40% of the dose was eliminated via the urine. Almost all of the dose was eliminated in the form of metabolic products.

Following administration of single doses of 60 or 180 mg of Seldane, a linear response was observed in maximum plasma concentration. Area under the curve (AUC) calculations, however, indicate a nearly four-fold increase in response for a three-fold increase in dose.

INDICATIONS AND USAGE

Seldane is indicated for the relief of symptoms associated with seasonal allergic rhinitis such as sneezing, rhinorrhea, pruritus, and lacrimation.

CONTRAINDICATIONS

Seldane is contraindicated in patients with a known hypersensitivity to terfenadine or any of its ingredients.

PRECAUTIONS

Information for patients

Patients taking Seldane should receive the following information and instructions. Antihistamines are prescribed to reduce allergic symptoms. Patients should be questioned about pregnancy or lactation before starting Seldane therapy, since the drug should be used in pregnancy or lactation only if the potential benefit justifies the potential risk to fetus or baby. Patients should be instructed to take Seldane only as needed and not to exceed the prescribed dose. Patients should also be instructed to store this medication in a tightly closed container in a cool, dry place, away from heat or direct sunlight, and away from children.

Carcinogenesis, mutagenesis, impairment of fertility

Oral doses of terfenadine, corresponding to 63 times the recommended human daily dose, in mice for 18 months or in rats for 24 months, revealed no evidence of tumorigenicity. Microbial and micronucleus test assays with terfenadine have revealed no evidence of mutagenesis.

Reproduction and fertility studies in rats showed no effects on male or female fertility at oral doses of up to 21 times the human daily dose. At 63 times the human daily dose there was a small but significant reduction in implants and at 125 times the human daily dose reduced implants and increased post-implantation losses were observed, which were judged to be secondary to maternal toxicity.

Pregnancy Category C

There was no evidence of animal teratogenicity. Reproduction studies have been performed in rats at doses 63 times and 125 times the human daily dose and have revealed decreased pup weight gain and survival when terfenadine was administered throughout pregnancy and lactation. There are no adequate and well-controlled studies in pregnant women. Seldane should be used during pregnancy only if the potential benefit justifies the potential risk to the fetus.

Nonteratogenic effects

Seldane is not recommended for nursing women. The drug has caused decreased pup weight gain and survival in rats given doses 63 times and 125 times the human daily dose throughout pregnancy and lactation. Effects on pups exposed to Seldane only during lactation are not known, and there are no adequate and well-controlled studies in women during lactation.

Pediatric use

Safety and effectiveness of Seldane in children below the age of 12 years have not been established.

General

Consideration should be given to potential anticholinergic (drying) effects in patients with lower airway disease, including asthma.

ADVERSE REACTIONS

Experience from clinical studies, including both controlled and uncontrolled studies involving more than 2,400 patients who received Seldane, provides information on adverse experience incidence for periods of a few days up to six months. The usual dose in these studies was 60 mg twice daily, but in a small number of patients, the dose was as low as 20 mg twice a day, or as high as 600 mg daily.

In controlled clinical studies using the recommended dose of 60 mg b.i.d., the incidence of reported adverse effects in patients receiving Seldane was similar to that reported in patients receiving placebo.

[See table on top next page].

In addition to the more frequent side effects reported in clinical trials (See Table), adverse effects have been reported at a lower incidence in clinical trials and/or spontaneously during marketing of Seldane that warrant listing as possibly associated with drug administration. These include: alopecia (hair loss or thinning), anaphylaxis, angioedema, arrhythmia (including ventricular tachyarrhythmia), bronchospasm, confusion, depression, galactorrhea, hypotension, insomnia, menstrual disorders (including dysmenorrhea), musculoskeletal symptoms, nightmares, palpitation, paresthesia, photosensitivity, prolonged QT interval, seizures, sweating, syncope, tachycardia, tremor, urinary frequency, and visual disturbances. In clinical trials, several instances of mild, or in one case, moderate transaminase elevations were seen in patients receiving Seldane. Mild elevations were also seen in placebo treated patients. Marketing experiences include isolated reports of jaundice, cholestatic hepatitis, and hepatitis; in most cases available information is incomplete. In neither the clinical trials nor marketing experience is a causal relationship of liver abnormalities to Seldane use clear.

OVERDOSAGE

Several cases of overdosage have been reported. Generally, signs and symptoms were absent or mild (e.g., headache, nausea, confusion). However, a severe ventricular arrhythmia (torsade de pointes) developed 15 hours after ingestion of 56 tablets (3360 mg) of Seldane, 14 capsules (7000 mg) of cephalexin, and 2 tablets (1200 mg) of ibuprofen. This progressed to ventricular fibrillation which responded well to defibrillation and lidocaine.

Therefore, in cases of overdosage, cardiac monitoring for at least 24 hours is recommended, along with standard measures to remove any unabsorbed drug. It is not known if Seldane is dialyzable.

Treatment of the signs and symptoms of overdosage should be symptomatic and supportive after the acute stage.

Oral LD_{50} values for terfenadine were greater than 5000 mg/kg in mature mice and rats. The oral LD_{50} was 438

Continued on next page

Information on Merrell Dow products is based on labeling in effect in June, 1989.

Merrell Dow—Cont.

ADVERSE EVENTS REPORTED IN CLINICAL TRIALS

Percent of Patients Reporting

Adverse Event	Controlled Studies*			All Clinical Studies**	
	Seldane N = 781	Placebo N = 665	Control N = 626***	Seldane N = 2462	Placebo N = 1478
Central Nervous System					
Drowsiness	9.0	8.1	18.1	8.5	8.2
Headache	6.3	7.4	3.8	15.8	11.2
Fatigue	2.9	0.9	5.8	4.5	3.0
Dizziness	1.4	1.1	1.0	1.5	1.2
Nervousness	0.9	0.2	0.6	1.7	1.0
Weakness	0.9	0.6	0.2	0.6	0.5
Appetite Increase	0.6	0.0	0.0	0.5	0.0
Gastrointestinal System					
Gastrointestinal Distress (Abdominal distress, Nausea, Vomiting, Change in Bowel habits)	4.6	3.0	2.7	7.6	5.4
Eye, Ear, Nose, and Throat					
Dry Mouth/Nose/Throat	2.3	1.8	3.5	4.8	3.1
Cough	0.9	0.2	0.5	2.5	1.7
Sore Throat	0.5	0.3	0.5	3.2	1.6
Epistaxis	0.0	0.8	0.2	0.7	0.4
Skin					
Eruption (including rash and urticaria) or itching	1.0	1.7	1.4	1.6	2.0

* Duration of treatment in "CONTROLLED STUDIES" was usually 7–14 DAYS.
** Duration of treatment in "ALL CLINICAL STUDIES" was up to 6 months.
*** CONTROL DRUGS: Chlorpheniramine (291 patients), d-Chlorpheniramine (189 patients), Clemastine (146 patients)

mg/kg in newborn rats. Single doses as high as ten times (600 mg) the recommended therapeutic dose in adults have been well tolerated.

DOSAGE AND ADMINISTRATION

The usual dosage for adults and children 12 years and older is 60 mg (1 tablet) twice daily.

HOW SUPPLIED

NDC 0068-0723-61

60 mg tablets in bottles of 100. Tablets are round, white, and debossed "SELDANE". Store tablets at controlled room temperature (59°–86°F) (15°–30°C). Protect from exposure to temperatures above 104°F (40°C) and moisture.

Product Information as of June, 1988
Shown in Product Identification Section, page 419

TACE®   ℞
[tās]
(CHLOROTRIANISENE USP)
12 mg and 25 mg
Capsules

CAUTION: Federal law prohibits dispensing without prescription.

WARNINGS

1. ESTROGENS HAVE BEEN REPORTED TO INCREASE THE RISK RATIO FOR ENDOMETRIAL CARCINOMA.

Three independent case control studies have reported an increased risk ratio of endometrial cancer in postmenopausal women exposed to exogenous estrogens for prolonged periods.[1-3] This reported risk was independent of the other risk factors studied. Additionally, the incidence rates of endometrial cancer have increased since 1969 in 8 different areas of the United States with population-based cancer reporting systems, an increase that may (or may not) be related to the expanded use of estrogens during the last decade.[4]

The 3 case control studies reported that the estimated risk ratio for endometrial cancer in estrogen users was about 4.5 to 13.9 times greater than in nonusers. The risk appeared to depend on both duration of treatment[1] and on estrogen dose.[3] In view of these reports, when estrogens are used for the treatment of menopausal symptoms, the lowest dose that will control symptoms should be utilized and medication should be discontinued as soon as possible. When prolonged treatment is medically indicated, the patient should be reassessed on at least a semiannual basis to determine the need for continued therapy. Although the evidence must be considered preliminary, one study suggests that cyclic administration of low doses of estrogen may carry less risk than continuous administration;[3] it therefore appears prudent to utilize such a regimen.

Close clinical surveillance of all women taking estrogens is important. In all cases of undiagnosed persistent or recurring abnormal vaginal bleeding, adequate diagnostic measures should be undertaken to rule out malignancy.

There is no evidence at present that "natural" estrogens are more or less hazardous than "synthetic" estrogens at equiestrogenic doses.

2. ESTROGENS SHOULD NOT BE USED DURING PREGNANCY. The use of exogenous estrogens and progestagens during early pregnancy has been reported to damage the offspring. An association has been reported between *in utero* exposure of the female fetus to diethylstilbestrol, a nonsteroidal estrogen, and an increased risk of the postpubertal development of an ordinarily rare form of vaginal or cervical cancer.[5,6] This risk for diethylstilbestrol was recently estimated to be in the range of 0.14 to 1.4 per 1000 exposures,[7] consistent with a previous risk estimate of not greater than 4 per 1000 exposures.[8] Furthermore, a high percentage of such females exposed *in utero* (30 to over 90%) has been reported to have vaginal adenosis, epithelial changes of the vagina and cervix.[9-12] Although these changes are histologically benign, it is not known whether they are precursors of adenocarcinoma. Although similar data are not available with the use of other estrogens, it cannot be presumed they would not induce similar changes. Several reports suggest a possible association between fetal exposure to exogenous estrogens and progestagens and congenital anomalies, including congenital heart defects and limb reduction defects.[13-16] One case control study[16] estimated a 4.7 fold increased risk of limb reduction defects in infants exposed *in utero* to exogenous steroids (oral contraceptives, hormone withdrawal tests for pregnancy, or attempted treatment for threatened abortion). Some of these exposures were very short and involved only a few days of treatment. The data suggest that the risk of limb reduction defects in exposed fetuses is somewhat less than 1 per 1000.

This product is not for use in therapy of threatened or habitual abortion.

If TACE (CHLOROTRIANISENE USP) is used during pregnancy, or if the patient becomes pregnant while taking this drug, she should be apprised of the potential risks to the fetus, and the advisability of pregnancy continuation.

DESCRIPTION

TACE (CHLOROTRIANISENE USP) is a long-acting, synthetic estrogen in capsule form suitable for oral administration.

Each green, soft gelatin capsule contains 12 mg of chlorotrianisene. This capsule also contains inactive ingredients: corn oil (solvent), FD&C Blue No. 1, FD&C Yellow No. 5 (tartrazine, See PRECAUTIONS), gelatin, glycerin, methylparaben, propylparaben, titanium dioxide, and water. Each two-tone green, hard gelatin capsule contains 25 mg of chlorotrianisene. This capsule also contains inactive ingredients: FD&C Blue No. 1 or FD&C Green No. 3, FD&C Blue No. 2, FD&C Red No. 40, FD&C Yellow No. 5 (tartrazine, See PRECAUTIONS), FD&C Yellow No. 6, gelatin, iron oxide, magnesium stearate, titanium dioxide, and tristearin (solvent).

Chemistry

Generic name: Chlorotrianisene USP

Chemical name:

Benzene, 1, 1′, 1″-(1-chloro-1-ethenyl-2-ylidene) tris [4-methoxyl]-, Chlorotris (p-methoxyphenyl) ethylene.

Structural Formula:

Chlorotrianisene occurs as small, white crystals or as a crystalline powder. It is odorless. It is slightly soluble in alcohol and very slightly soluble in water.

INDICATIONS AND USAGE

1. Postpartum breast engorgement—Although estrogens have been widely used for the prevention of postpartum breast engorgement, controlled studies have demonstrated that the incidence of significant painful engorgement in patients not receiving such hormonal therapy is low and usually responsive to appropriate analgesic or other supportive therapy. Consequently, the benefit to be derived from estrogen therapy for this indication must be carefully weighed against the potential risk of puerperal thromboembolism associated with the use of estrogens.[17]
2. Prostatic carcinoma—palliative therapy of advanced disease.
3. Moderate to severe *vasomotor* symptoms associated with the menopause. (There is no well-documented evidence that estrogens are effective for nervous symptoms or depression which might occur during menopause and they should not be used to treat these conditions.)
4. Atrophic vaginitis.
5. Kraurosis vulvae.
6. Female hypogonadism.

TACE (CHLOROTRIANISENE USP) HAS NOT BEEN SHOWN TO BE EFFECTIVE FOR ANY PURPOSE DURING PREGNANCY, AND ITS USE MAY HAVE POTENTIAL RISKS TO THE FETUS. (SEE BOXED WARNING.)

The lowest effective dose appropriate for the specific indication should be utilized. Studies of the addition of a progestin for seven or more days of a cycle of estrogen administration have reported a lowered incidence of endometrial hyperplasia. Morphological and biochemical studies of endometrium suggest that 10 to 13 days of progestin are needed to provide maximal maturation of the endometrium and to eliminate any hyperplastic changes. Whether this will provide protection from endometrial carcinoma has not been clearly established. There are possible additional risks which may be associated with the inclusion of progestin in estrogen replacement regimens. The potential risks include adverse effects on carbohydrate and lipid metabolism. The choice of progestin and dosage may be important in minimizing these adverse effects. (See WARNINGS and PRECAUTIONS.)

CONTRAINDICATIONS

TACE (CHLOROTRIANISENE USP) should not be used in women or men with any of the following conditions:

1. Known or suspected cancer of the breast except in appropriately selected patients being treated for metastatic disease.
2. Known or suspected estrogen-dependent neoplasia.
3. Known or suspected pregnancy (See Boxed Warning.)
4. Undiagnosed abnormal genital bleeding.
5. Active thrombophlebitis or thromboembolic disorders.
6. A past history of thrombophlebitis, thrombosis, or thromboembolic disorders (except when used in treatment of prostatic malignancy).

WARNINGS

1. *Induction of malignant neoplasms.* Long-term continuous administration of natural and synthetic estrogens in certain animal species increases the frequency of carcinomas of the breast, cervix, vagina, and liver. There are now reports that estrogens increase the risk of carcinoma of the endometrium in humans. (See Boxed Warning.)

At the present time there is no satisfactory evidence that estrogens given to post-menopausal women increase the risk of cancer of the breast,[18] although a recent long-term follow-up of a single physician's practice has raised this possibility.[19] Because of the animal data, there is a need for caution in prescribing estrogens for women with a strong family history of breast cancer or who have breast nodules, fibrocystic disease, or abnormal mammograms.

2. *Gallbladder disease.* A recent study has reported a two to threefold increase in the risk of surgically confirmed gall-

bladder disease in women receiving post-menopausal estrogens,[18] similar to the twofold increase previously noted in users of oral contraceptives.[20] In the case of oral contraceptives the increased risk appeared after a period of use.[20]

3. *Effects similar to those caused by estrogen-progestagen oral contraceptives.* There are several adverse effects reported in association with oral contraceptives, most of which have not been documented as consequences of post-menopausal estrogen therapy, although it has been reported that there is an increased risk of thrombosis in men receiving high doses of estrogens for prostatic cancer and in women receiving estrogens for postpartum breast engorgement.[17,21–23] The possibility that the adverse effects reported in association with oral contraceptives may be associated with larger doses of estrogen cannot be excluded.

　a. *Thromboembolic disease.* Studies have now shown that users of oral contraceptives have an increased risk of various thromboembolic, thrombotic, and vascular diseases, such as thrombophlebitis, pulmonary embolism, stroke, and myocardial infarction.[24–31] Cases of retinal thrombosis, mesenteric thrombosis, and optic neuritis have been reported in oral contraceptive users. There is evidence that the risk of several of these adverse reactions is related to the dose of the drug.[32,33] An increased risk of post-surgery thromboembolic complications has also been reported in users of oral contraceptives.[34,35] If feasible, estrogen should be discontinued at least 4 weeks before surgery of the type associated with an increased risk of thromboembolism, or during periods of prolonged immobilization. While an increased rate of thromboembolic and thrombotic disease in postmenopausal users of estrogens has not been found,[18,36] this does not rule out the possibility that such an increase may be present, or that subgroups of women who have underlying risk factors, or who are receiving relatively large doses of estrogens may have an increased risk. Therefore, estrogens should not be used in persons with active thrombophlebitis or thromboembolic disorders, and they should not be used (except in treatment of malignancy) in persons with a history of such disorders. They should be used with caution in patients with cerebral vascular or coronary artery disease and only for those in whom estrogens are needed.
Doses of estrogen (5 mg conjugated estrogens per day), comparable to those used to treat cancer of the prostate and breast, have been reported in a large prospective clinical trial in men[37] to increase the risk of nonfatal myocardial infarction, pulmonary embolism, and thrombophlebitis. When estrogen doses of this size are used, any of the thromboembolic and thrombotic adverse effects associated with oral contraceptive use should be considered as a risk.

　b. *Hepatic adenoma.* Benign hepatic adenomas have been reported to be associated with the use of oral contraceptives.[38–40] Although benign and rare, these may rupture and may cause death through intra-abdominal hemorrhage. Such lesions have not yet been reported in association with other estrogen or progestagen preparations but should be considered in estrogen users having abdominal pain and tenderness, abdominal mass, or hypovolemic shock. Hepatocellular carcinoma has also been reported in women taking estrogen-containing oral contraceptives.[39] The relationship of this malignancy to these drugs is not known at this time.

　c. *Elevated blood pressure.* Increased blood pressure is not uncommon in women using oral contraceptives and there is now a report that this may occur with use of estrogens in the menopause[41] and blood pressure should be monitored with estrogen use, especially if high doses are used.

　d. *Glucose tolerance.* A worsening of glucose tolerance has been observed in a significant percentage of patients on estrogen-containing oral contraceptives. For this reason diabetic patients should be carefully observed while receiving estrogen.

4. *Hypercalcemia.* Administration of estrogens may lead to hypercalcemia in patients with breast cancer and bone metastases. If this occurs, the drug should be stopped and appropriate measures taken to reduce the serum calcium level.

PRECAUTIONS (See also INDICATIONS.)
A.　General Precautions
1. A complete medical and family history should be taken prior to the initiation of any estrogen therapy. The pretreatment and periodic physical examinations should include special reference to blood pressure, breasts, abdomen, and pelvic organs, and should include a Papanicolaou smear. As a general rule, estrogen should not be prescribed for longer than 1 year without another physical examination being performed.
2. Fluid retention—Because estrogens may cause some degree of fluid retention, conditions that might be influenced by this factor such as epilepsy, migraine, and cardiac or renal dysfunction require careful observation.

3. Certain patients may develop undesirable manifestations of excessive estrogenic stimulation, such as abnormal or excessive uterine bleeding, mastodynia, etc.
4. Oral contraceptives have been reported to be associated with an increased incidence of mental depression. Although it is not clear whether this is possibly due to the estrogenic or progestagenic component of the contraceptive, patients with a history of depression should be carefully observed.
5. Patients having pre-existing uterine leiomyomata should be observed for increased growth of myomata during estrogen therapy.
6. The pathologist should be advised of estrogen therapy when relevent specimens are submitted.
7. Patients with a past history of jaundice during pregnancy have an increased risk of recurrence of jaundice while receiving estrogen-containing oral contraceptive therapy. If jaundice develops in any patient receiving estrogen, the medication should be discontinued while the cause is investigated.
8. Estrogens may be poorly metabolized in patients with impaired liver function and they should be administered with caution in such patients.
9. Because estrogens influence the metabolism of calcium and phosphorus, they should be used with caution in patients with metabolic bone diseases that are associated with hypercalcemia or in patients with renal insufficiency.
10. Because of the effects of estrogens on epiphyseal closure, they should be used judiciously in young patients in whom bone growth is not complete.
11. Judicious assessment of the following changes in certain endocrine and liver function tests is necessary for patients receiving large doses of estrogen.
　a. Increased sulfobromophthalein retention.
　b. Increased prothrombin and factors VII, VIII, IX, and X; decreased antithrombin 3; increased norepinephrine-induced platelet aggregability.
　c. Increased thyroid binding globulin (TBG) leading to increased circulating total thyroid hormone, as measured by PBI, T4 by column, or T4 by radioimmunoassay. Free T3 resin uptake is decreased, reflecting the elevated TBG; free T4 concentration is unaltered.
　d. Impaired glucose tolerance.
　e. Decreased pregnanediol excretion.
　f. Reduced response to metyrapone test.
　g. Reduced serum folate concentration.
　h. Increased serum triglyceride, phospholipid, or cholesterol.
12. This product contains FD&C Yellow No. 5 (tartrazine), which may cause allergic-type reactions (including bronchial asthma) in certain susceptible individuals. Although the overall incidence of FD&C Yellow No. 5 (tartrazine) sensitivity in the general population is low, it is frequently seen in patients who also have aspirin hypersensitivity.

B.　Information For The Patient
A patient package insert accompanies this drug product. This insert is available from pharmacists who carry this product and from the company upon request.

C.　Pregnancy Category X
See Contraindications and Boxed Warning.

D.　Nursing Mothers
As a general principle, the administration of any drug to nursing mothers should be done only when clearly necessary since many drugs are excreted in human milk.

ADVERSE REACTIONS

(See Warnings regarding reports of induction of neoplasia, adverse effects on the fetus, increased incidence of gallbladder disease, and adverse effects similar to those of oral contraceptives, including thromboembolism.) The following additional adverse reactions have been reported with estrogenic therapy including oral contraceptives:
1. *Genitourinary system*
Breakthrough bleeding, spotting, change in menstrual flow and cycle.
Dysmenorrhea.
Premenstrual-like syndrome.
Amenorrhea during and after treatment.
Increase in size of uterine fibromyomata.
Vaginal candidiasis.
Change in cervical eversion and in degree of cervical secretion.
Cystitis-like syndrome.
2. *Breasts*
Tenderness, enlargement, secretion.
3. *Gastrointestinal*
Nausea, vomiting.
Abdominal cramps, bloating.
Cholestatic jaundice.

4. *Skin*
Chloasma or melasma, which may persist when drug is discontinued.
Erythema multiforme.
Erythema nodosum.
Hemorrhagic eruption.
Loss of scalp hair.
Hirsutism.
Urticaria.
5. *Eyes*
Steepening of corneal curvature.
Intolerance to contact lenses.
6. *CNS*
Headache, migraine, dizziness.
Mental depression.
Chorea.
7. *Miscellaneous*
Increase or decrease in weight.
Reduced carbohydrate tolerance.
Aggravation of porphyria.
Edema.
Changes in libido and/or potency.

ACUTE OVERDOSAGE
Numerous reports of ingestion of large doses of estrogen-containing oral contraceptives by young children indicate that serious ill effects usually do not occur. Overdosage of estrogen may cause nausea, and withdrawal bleeding may occur in females.

DOSAGE AND ADMINISTRATION
Given for a few days
Prevention of postpartum breast engorgement.
　The usual dosage is one 12 mg capsule four times daily for 7 days, or two 25 mg capsules every six hours for 6 doses. For immediate postpartum use, the first dose should be given within 8 hours after delivery.
Given chronically
Inoperable progressing prostatic cancer.
　The usual dosage is 12 to 25 mg daily (one or two 12 mg capsules or one 25 mg capsule).
Given cyclically for short-term use only
　For treatment of moderate to severe *vasomotor* symptoms, atrophic vaginitis, or kraurosis vulvae associated with the menopause.
The lowest dose that will control symptoms should be chosen and medication should be discontinued as promptly as possible.
Administration should be cyclic (*e.g.*, 3 weeks on and 1 week off).
Attempts to discontinue or taper medication should be made at 3-month to 6-month intervals.
　The usual dosage range for vasomotor symptoms associated with the menopause is 12 to 25 mg daily (one or two 12 mg capsules or one 25 mg capsule) for 30 days; one or more courses may be prescribed.
The usual dosage range for atrophic vaginitis or kraurosis vulvae is 12 to 25 mg daily (one or two 12 mg capsules or one 25 mg capsule) for 30 to 60 days.
Given cyclically
For female hypogonadism.
The usual dosage is 12 to 25 mg daily (one or two 12 mg capsules or one 25 mg capsule) for 21 days. This course may, if desired, be followed immediately by the intramuscular injection of 100 mg of progesterone; alternatively, an oral progestogen such as medroxyprogesterone may be given during the last 5 days of TACE (CHLOROTRIANISENE USP) therapy. The next course may begin on the 5th day of the induced uterine bleeding.
Treated patients with an intact uterus should be monitored closely for signs of endometrial cancer, and appropriate diagnostic measures should be taken to rule out malignancy in the event of persistent or recurrent abnormal vaginal bleeding.

HOW SUPPLIED
TACE 12 mg (CHLOROTRIANISENE CAPSULES USP) green capsules imprinted MERRELL 690
　NDC 0068-0690-61; bottles of 100
TACE 25 mg (CHLOROTRIANISENE CAPSULES USP) two-tone green capsules imprinted MERRELL 691
　NDC 0068-0691-60; bottles of 60
References and *Information for Patients* appear following the Prescribing Information for TACE 72 mg Capsules.
　　　Product Information as of June, 1986.
　Shown in Product Identification Section, page 419

Continued on next page

Information on Merrell Dow products is based on labeling in effect in June, 1989.

Merrell Dow—Cont.

TACE®

[tās]
(CHLOROTRIANISENE USP)
72 mg Capsules

℞

CAUTION: Federal law prohibits dispensing without prescription.

WARNINGS

> **1. ESTROGENS HAVE BEEN REPORTED TO INCREASE THE RISK RATIO FOR ENDOMETRIAL CARCINOMA.**
>
> Three independent case control studies have reported an increased risk ratio of endometrial cancer in postmenopausal women exposed to exogenous estrogens for prolonged periods.[1-3] This reported risk was independent of the other risk factors studied. Additionally, the incidence rates of endometrial cancer have increased since 1969 in 8 different areas of the United States with population-based cancer reporting systems, an increase that may [or may not] be related to the expanded use of estrogens during the last decade.[4]
>
> The 3 case control studies reported that the estimated risk ratio for endometrial cancer in estrogen users was about 4.5 to 13.9 times greater than in nonusers. The risk appeared to depend on both duration of treatment[1] and on estrogen dose.[3] In view of these reports, when estrogens are used for the treatment of menopausal symptoms, the lowest dose that will control symptoms should be utilized and medication should be discontinued as soon as possible. When prolonged treatment is medically indicated, the patient should be reassessed on at least a semi-annual basis to determine the need for continued therapy. Although the evidence must be considered preliminary, one study suggests that cyclic administration of low doses of estrogen may carry less risk than continuous administration;[3] it therefore appears prudent to utilize such a regimen.
>
> Close clinical surveillance of all women taking estrogens is important. In all cases of undiagnosed persistent or recurring abnormal vaginal bleeding, adequate diagnostic measures should be undertaken to rule out malignancy.
>
> There is no evidence at present that "natural" estrogens are more or less hazardous than "synthetic" estrogens at equiestrogenic doses.
>
> **2. ESTROGENS SHOULD NOT BE USED DURING PREGNANCY.**
>
> The use of exogenous estrogens and progestagens during early pregnancy has been reported to damage the offspring. An association has been reported between *in utero* exposure of the female fetus to diethylstilbestrol, a non-steroidal estrogen, and an increased risk of the post-pubertal development of an ordinarily rare form of vaginal or cervical cancer.[5,6] This risk for diethylstilbestrol was recently estimated to be in the range of 0.14 to 1.4 per 1000 exposures,[7] consistent with a previous risk estimate of not greater than 4 per 1000 exposures.[8] Furthermore, a high percentage of such females exposed *in utero* (30 to over 90%) has been reported to have vaginal adenosis, epithelial changes of the vagina and cervix.[9-12] Although these changes are histologically benign, it is not known whether they are precursors of adenocarcinoma. Although similar data are not available with the use of other estrogens, it cannot be presumed they would not induce similar changes.
>
> Several reports suggest a possible association between fetal exposure to exogenous estrogens and progestagens and congenital anomalies, including congenital heart defects and limb reduction defects.[13-16] One case control study[16] estimated a 4.7 fold increased risk of limb reduction defects in infants exposed *in utero* to exogenous steroids (oral contraceptives, hormone withdrawal tests for pregnancy, or attempted treatment for threatened abortion). Some of these exposures were very short and involved only a few days of treatment. The data suggest that the risk of limb reduction defects in exposed fetuses is somewhat less than 1 per 1000.
>
> This product is not for use in therapy of threatened or habitual abortion.
>
> If TACE (CHLOROTRIANISENE USP) is used during pregnancy, or if the patient becomes pregnant while taking this drug, she should be apprised of the potential risks to the fetus, and the advisability of pregnancy continuation.

DESCRIPTION

TACE (CHLOROTRIANISENE USP) is a long-acting, synthetic estrogen in capsule form suitable for oral administration.

Each two-tone green and yellow soft gelatin capsule contains 72 mg of TACE (CHLOROTRIANISENE) in Dispex®, an emulsifiable vehicle containing corn oil, sorbitan trioleate, polysorbate 80, and benzyl benzoate. This capsule also contains other inactive ingredients: FD&C Blue No. 1, FD&C Yellow No. 5 (tartrazine, See PRECAUTIONS), gelatin, glycerin, iron oxide, methylparaben, propylparaben, sorbitol, titanium dioxide, and water.

Chemistry
Generic name: Chlorotrianisene USP
Chemical name: Benzene, 1, 1', 1''-(1-chloro-1-ethenyl-2-ylidene) tris [4-methoxy]-. Chlorotris (*p*-methoxyphenyl) ethylene.
Structural Formula:

CH₃O— ⬡ —OCH₃
          C=C
CH₃O— ⬡   Cl

Chlorotrianisene occurs as small, white crystals or as a crystalline powder. It is odorless. It is slightly soluble in alcohol and very slightly soluble in water.

INDICATIONS AND USAGE

Postpartum breast engorgement—Although estrogens have been widely used for the prevention of postpartum breast engorgement, controlled studies have demonstrated that the incidence of significant painful engorgement in patients not receiving such hormonal therapy is low and usually responsive to appropriate analgesic or other supportive therapy. Consequently, the benefit to be derived from estrogen therapy for this indication must be carefully weighed against the potential risk of puerperal thromboembolism associated with the use of estrogens.[17]

TACE (CHLOROTRIANSENE USP) HAS NOT BEEN SHOWN TO BE EFFECTIVE FOR ANY PURPOSE DURING PREGNANCY, AND ITS USE MAY HAVE POTENTIAL RISKS TO THE FETUS. (SEE BOXED WARNING.)
The lowest effective dose appropriate for the specific indication should be utilized. Studies of the addition of a progestin for seven or more days of a cycle of estrogen administration have reported a lowered incidence of endometrial hyperplasia. Morphological and biochemical studies of endometrium suggest that 10 to 13 days of progestin are needed to provide maximal maturation of the endometrium and to eliminate any hyperplastic changes. Whether this will provide protection from endometrial carcinoma has not been clearly established. There are possible additional risks which may be associated with the inclusion of progestin in estrogen replacement regimens. The potential risks include adverse effects on carbohydrate and lipid metabolism. The choice of progestin and dosage may be important in minimizing these adverse effects. (See WARNINGS and PRECAUTIONS.)

CONTRAINDICATIONS

TACE (CHLOROTRIANSENE USP) should not be used in women or men with any of the following conditions:
1. Known or suspected cancer of the breast except in appropriately selected patients being treated for metastatic disease.
2. Known or suspected estrogen-dependent neoplasia.
3. Known or suspected pregnancy. (See Boxed Warning.)
4. Undiagnosed abnormal genital bleeding.
5. Active thrombophlebitis or thromboembolic disorders.
6. A past history of thrombophlebitis, thrombosis, or thromboembolic disorders (except when used in treatment of prostatic malignancy).

WARNINGS

1. *Induction of malignant neoplasms.* Long-term continuous administration of natural and synthetic estrogens in certain animal species increases the frequency of carcinomas of the breast, cervix, vagina, and liver. There are now reports that estrogens increase the risk of carcinoma of the endometrium in humans. (See Boxed Warning.)
At the present time there is no satisfactory evidence that estrogens given to postmenopausal women increase the risk of cancer of the breast,[18] although a recent long-term follow-up of a single physician's practice has raised this possibility.[19] Because of the animal data, there is a need for caution in prescribing estrogens for women with a strong family history of breast cancer or who have breast nodules, fibrocystic disease, or abnormal mammograms.
2. *Gallbladder disease.* A recent study has reported a two to threefold increase in the risk of surgically confirmed gallbladder disease in women receiving postmenopausal estrogens,[18] similar to the twofold increase previously noted in users of oral contraceptives.[20] In the case of oral contraceptives the increased risk appeared after a period of use.[20]

3. *Effects similar to those caused by estrogen-progestagen oral contraceptives.* There are several adverse effects reported in association with oral contraceptives, most of which have not been documented as consequences of postmenopausal estrogen therapy, although it has been reported that there is an increased risk of thrombosis in men receiving high doses of estrogens for prostatic cancer and in women receiving estrogens for postpartum breast engorgement.[17,21-23] The possibility that the adverse effects reported in association with oral contraceptives may be associated with larger doses of estrogen cannot be excluded.
a. *Thromboembolic disease.* Studies have now shown that users of oral contraceptives have an increased risk of various thromboembolic, thrombotic, and vascular diseases, such as thrombophlebitis, pulmonary embolism, stroke, and myocardial infarction.[24-31] Cases of retinal thrombosis, mesenteric thrombosis, and optic neuritis have been reported in oral contraceptive users. There is evidence that the risk of several of these adverse reactions is related to the dose of the drug.[32,33] An increased risk of post-surgery thromboembolic complications has also been reported in users of oral contraceptives.[34,35] If feasible, estrogen should be discontinued at least 4 weeks before surgery of the type associated with an increased risk of thromboembolism, or during periods of prolonged immobilization. While an increased rate of thromboembolic and thrombotic disease in postmenopausal users of estrogens has not been found,[18,36] this does not rule out the possibility that such an increase may be present, or that subgroups of women who have underlying risk factors, or who are receiving relatively large doses of estrogens may have an increased risk. Therefore, estrogens should not be used in persons with active thrombophlebitis or thromboembolic disorders, and they should not be used (except in treatment of malignancy) in persons with a history of such disorders. They should be used with caution in patients with cerebral vascular or coronary artery disease and only for those in whom estrogens are needed.
Doses of estrogen (5 mg conjugated estrogens per day), comparable to those used to treat cancer of the prostate and breast, have been reported in a large prospective clinical trial in men[37] to increase the risk of nonfatal myocardial infarction, pulmonary embolism, and thrombophlebitis. When estrogen doses of this size are used, any of the thromboembolic and thrombotic adverse effects associated with oral contraceptive use should be considered as a risk.
b. *Hepatic adenoma.* Benign hepatic adenomas have been reported to be associated with the use of oral contraceptives.[38-40] Although benign and rare, these may rupture and may cause death through intra-abdominal hemorrhage. Such lesions have not yet been reported in association with other estrogen or progestagen preparations but should be considered in estrogen users having abdominal pain and tenderness, abdominal mass, or hypovolemic shock. Hepatocellular carcinoma has also been reported in women taking estrogen-containing oral contraceptives.[39] The relationship of this malignancy to these drugs is not known at this time.
c. *Elevated blood pressure.* Increased blood pressure is not uncommon in women using oral contraceptives and there is now a report that this may occur with use of estrogens in the menopause[41] and blood pressure should be monitored with estrogen use, especially if high doses are used.
d. *Glucose tolerance.* A worsening of glucose tolerance has been observed in a significant percentage of patients on estrogen-containing oral contraceptives. For this reason diabetic patients should be carefully observed while receiving estrogen.
4. *Hypercalcemia.* Administration of estrogens may lead to hypercalcemia in patients with breast cancer and bone metastases. If this occurs, the drug should be stopped and appropriate measures taken to reduce the serum calcium level.

PRECAUTIONS (See also INDICATIONS.)

A. General Precautions
1. A complete medical and family history should be taken prior to the initiation of any estrogen therapy. The pretreatment and periodic physical examinations should include special reference to blood pressure, breasts, abdomen, and pelvic organs, and should include a Papanicolaou smear. As a general rule, estrogen should not be prescribed for longer than 1 year without another physical examination being performed.
2. Fluid retention—Because estrogens may cause some degree of fluid retention, conditions that might be influenced by this factor such as epilepsy, migraine, and cardiac or renal dysfunction require careful observation.
3. Certain patients may develop undesirable manifestations of excessive estrogenic stimulation, such as abnormal or excessive uterine bleeding, mastodynia, etc.
4. Oral contraceptives have been reported to be associated with an increased incidence of mental depression. Although it is not clear whether this is possibly due to the estrogenic or progestagenic component of the contracep-

tive, patients with a history of depression should be carefully observed.

5. Patients having pre-existing uterine leiomyomata should be observed for increased growth of myomata during estrogen therapy.

6. The pathologist should be advised of estrogen therapy when relevant specimens are submitted.

7. Patients with a past history of jaundice during pregnancy have an increased risk of recurrence of jaundice while receiving estrogen-containing oral contraceptive therapy. If jaundice develops in any patient receiving estrogen, the medication should be discontinued while the cause is investigated.

8. Estrogens may be poorly metabolized in patients with impaired liver function and they should be administered with caution in such patients.

9. Because estrogens influence the metabolism of calcium and phosphorus, they should be used with caution in patients with metabolic bone diseases that are associated with hypercalcemia or in patients with renal insufficiency.

10. Because of the effects of estrogens on epiphyseal closure, they should be used judiciously in young patients in whom bone growth is not complete.

11. Judicious assessment of the following changes in certain endocrine and liver function tests is necessary for patients receiving large doses of estrogen.
    a. Increased sulfobromophthalein retention.
    b. Increased prothrombin and factors VII, VIII, IX and X; decreased antithrombin 3; increased norepinephrine-induced platelet aggregability.
    c. Increased thyroid binding globulin (TBG) leading to increased circulating total thyroid hormone, as measured by PBI, T4 by column, or T4 by radioimmunoassay. Free T3 resin uptake is decreased, reflecting the elevated TBG; free T4 concentration is unaltered.
    d. Impaired glucose tolerance.
    e. Decreased pregnanediol excretion.
    f. Reduced response to metyrapone test.
    g. Reduced serum folate concentration.
    h. Increased serum triglyceride, phospholipid, or cholesterol.

12. This product contains FD&C Yellow No. 5 (tartrazine), which may cause allergic-type reactions (including bronchial asthma) in certain susceptible individuals. Although the overall incidence of FD&C Yellow No. 5 (tartrazine) sensitivity in the general population is low, it is frequently seen in patients who also have aspirin hypersensitivity.

B. Information For The Patient
A patient package insert accompanies this drug product. This insert is available from pharmacists who carry this product and from the company upon request.

C. Pregnancy Category X
See Contraindications and Boxed Warning.

D. Nursing Mothers
As a general principle, the administration of any drug to nursing mothers should be done only when clearly necessary since many drugs are excreted in human milk.

ADVERSE REACTIONS

(See Warnings regarding reports of induction of neoplasia, adverse effects on the fetus, increased incidence of gallbladder disease, and adverse effects similar to those of oral contraceptives, including thromboembolism.) The following additional adverse reactions have been reported with estrogenic therapy including oral contraceptives.

1. *Genitourinary system*
Breakthrough bleeding, spotting, change in menstrual flow and cycle.
Dysmenorrhea.
Premenstrual-like syndrome.
Amenorrhea during and after treatment.
Increase in size of uterine fibromyomata.
Vaginal candidiasis.
Change in cervical eversion and in degree of cervical secretion.
Cystitis-like syndrome.

2. *Breasts*
Tenderness, enlargement, secretion.

3. *Gastrointestinal*
Nausea, vomiting.
Abdominal cramps, bloating.
Cholestatic jaundice.

4. *Skin*
Chloasma or melasma, which may persist when drug is discontinued.
Erythema multiforme.
Erythema nodosum.
Hemorrhagic eruption.
Loss of scalp hair.
Hirsutism.
Urticaria.

5. *Eyes*
Steepening of corneal curvature.
Intolerance to contact lenses.

6. *CNS*
Headache, migraine, dizziness.
Mental depression.
Chorea.

7. *Miscellaneous*
Increase or decrease in weight.
Reduced carbohydrate tolerance.
Aggravation of porphyria.
Edema.
Changes in libido and/or potency.

ACUTE OVERDOSAGE

Numerous reports of ingestion of large doses of estrogen-containing oral contraceptives by younger children indicate that serious ill effects usually do not occur. Overdosage of estrogen may cause nausea, and withdrawal bleeding may occur in females.

DOSAGE AND ADMINISTRATION

Given for a few days
Prevention of postpartum breast engorgement.
The usual dosage is 1 TACE 72 mg capsule twice daily for 2 days. The first dose should be given as soon as possible after delivery but within 8 hours.

HOW SUPPLIED

TACE 72 mg (CHLOROTRIANSENE CAPSULES USP) green and yellow capsules imprinted MERRELL 692
NDC 0068-0692-48: packages of 48 capsules.

REFERENCES

1. Ziel, H.K. and Finkel, W.D.: Increased risk of endometrial carcinoma among users of conjugated estrogens. New Eng. J. Med. 293:1167–1170, 1975.
2. Smith, D.C., Prentice, R., Thompson, D.J., and Hermann, W.L.: Association of exogenous estrogen and endometrial carcinoma. New Eng. J. Med. 293:1164–1167, 1975.
3. Mack, T.M., Pike, M.C., Henderson, B.E., Pfeffer, R.I., Gerkins, V.R., Arthur, M., and Brown, S.E.: Estrogens and endometrial cancer in a retirement community. New Eng. J. Med. 294:1262–1267, 1976.
4. Weiss, N.S., Szekely, D.R., and Austin, D.F.: Increasing incidence of endometrial cancer in the United States. New Eng. J. Med. 294:1259–1262, 1976.
5. Herbst, A.L., Ulfelder, H., and Poskanzer, D.C.: Adenocarcinoma of the vagina. New Eng. J. Med. 284:878–881, 1971.
6. Greenwald, P., Barlow, J.J., Nasca, P.C., and Burnett, W.S.: Vaginal cancer after maternal treatment with synthetic estrogens. New Eng. J. Med. 285:390–392, 1971.
7. Herbst, A.L., Cole, P., Colton, T., Robboy, S.J., and Scully, R.E.: Age-incidence and risk of diethylstilbestrol-related clear cell adenocarcinoma of the vagina and cervix. Amer. J. Obstet. Gynec. 128:43–50, 1977.
8. Lanier, A.P., Noller, K.L., Decker, D.G., Elveback, L.R., and Kurland, L.T.: Cancer and stilbestrol. A follow-up of 1719 persons exposed to estrogens in utero and born 1943–1959. Mayo Clin. Proc. 48:793–799, 1973.
9. Herbst, A.L., Kurman, R.J., and Scully, R.E.: Vaginal and cervical abnormalities after exposure to stilbestrol in utero. Obstet. Gynec. 40:287–298, 1972.
10. Herbst, A.L., Poskanzer, D.C., Robboy, S.J., Friedlander, L., and Scully, R.E.: Prenatal exposure to stilbestrol. A prospective comparison of exposed female offspring with unexposed controls. New Eng. J. Med. 292:334–339, 1975.
11. Stafl, A., Mattingly, R.F., Foley, D.V., and Fetherston, W.C.: Clinical diagnosis of vaginal adenosis. Obstet. Gynec. 43:118–128, 1974.
12. Sherman, A.I., Goldrath, M., Berlin, A., Vakhariya, V., Banooni, F., Michaels, W., Goodman, P., and Brown, S: Cervical-vaginal adenosis after in utero exposure to synthetic estrogens. Obstet. Gynec. 44:531–545, 1974.
13. Gal, I., Kirman, B., and Stern, J.: Hormone pregnancy tests and congenital malformation. Nature 216:83, 1967.
14. Levy, E.P., Cohen, A., and Fraser, F.C.: Hormone treatment during pregnancy and congenital heart defects. Lancet 1:611, 1973.
15. Nora, J.J. and Nora, A.H.: Birth defects and oral contraceptives. Lancet 1:941–942, 1973.
16. Janerich, D.T., Piper, J.M., and Glebatis, D.M.: Oral contraceptives and congenital limb-reduction defects. New Eng J. Med. 291:697–700, 1974.
17. Daniel, D.G., Campbell, H., and Turnbull, A.C.: Puerperal thromboembolism and suppression of lactation. Lancet 2:287–289, 1967.
18. Boston Collaborative Drug Surveillance Program: Surgically confirmed gall bladder disease, venous thromboembolism, and breast tumors in relation to post menopausal estrogen therapy. New Eng. J. Med. 290:15–19, 1974.
19. Hoover, R., Gray, L.A., Sr., Cole, P., and MacMahon, B.: Menopausal estrogens and breast cancer. New Eng. J. Med. 295:401–405, 1976.
20. Boston Collaborative Drug Surveillance Program: Oral contraceptives and venous thromboembolic disease, surgically confirmed gallbladder disease, and breast tumors. Lancet 1:1399–1404, 1973.
21. Bailar, J.C., III: Thromboembolism and oestrogen therapy. Lancet 2:560, 1967.
22. The Veterans Administration Cooperative Urological Research Group: Carcinoma of the prostate: Treatment comparisons. J. Urol. 98:516–522, 1967.
23. Blackard, C.E., Doe, R.P., Mellinger, G.T., and Byar, D.P.: Incidence of cardiovascular disease and death in patients receiving diethylstilbestrol for carcinoma of the prostate. Cancer 26:249–256, 1970.
24. Royal College of General Practitioners: Oral contraception and thromboembolic disease. J. Roy. Coll. Gen. Pract. 13:267–269, 1967.
25. Inman, W.H.W. and Vessey, M.P.: Investigation of deaths from pulmonary, coronary, and cerebral thrombosis and embolism in women of childbearing age. Brit. Med. J. 2:193–199, 1968.
26. Vessey, M.P. and Doll, R.: Investigation of relation between use of oral contraceptives and thromboembolic disease. A further report, Brit. Med. J. 2:651–657, 1969.
27. Sartwell, P.E., Masi, A.T., Arthes, F.G., Greene, G.R., and Smith, H.E.: Thromboembolism and oral contraceptives: An epidemiological case-control study. Amer. J. Epidem. 90:365–380, 1969.
28. Collaborative Group for the Study of Stroke in Young Women: Oral contraception and increased risk of cerebral ischemia or thrombosis. New Eng. J. Med. 288:871–878, 1973.
29. Collaborative Group for the Study of Stroke in Young Women: Oral contraceptives and stroke in young women: Associated risk factors. J.A.M.A. 231:718–722, 1975.
30. Mann, J.I. and Inman, W.H.W.: Oral contraceptives and death from myocardial infarction. Brit. Med. J. 2:245–248, 1975.
31. Mann, J.I., Vessey, M.P., Thorogood, M., and Doll, R.: Myocardial infarction in young women with special reference in oral contraceptive practice. Brit. Med. J. 2:241–245, 1975.
32. Inman, W.H.W., Vessey, M.P., Westerholm, B., and Engelund, A.: Thromboembolic disease and the steroidal content of oral contraceptives. A report to the Committee on Safety of Drugs. Brit. Med. J. 2:203–209, 1970.
33. Stolley, P.D., Tonascia, J.A., Tockman, M.S., Sartwell, P.E., Rutledge, A.H., and Jacobs, M.P.: Thrombosis with low-estrogen oral contraceptives. Amer. J. Epidem. 102:197–208, 1975.
34. Vessey, M.P., Doll, R., Fairbairn, A.S., and Glober, G.: Post-operative thromboembolism and the use of the oral contraceptives. Brit. Med. J. 3:123–126, 1970.
35. Greene, G.R. and Sartwell, P.E.: Oral contraceptive use in patients with thromboembolism following surgery, trauma, or infection. Amer. J. Public Health 62:680–685, 1972.
36. Rosenberg, L., Armstrong, B., Phil, D., and Jick, H.: Myocardial infarction and estrogen therapy in post-menopausal women. New Eng. J. Med. 294:1256–1259, 1976.
37. Coronary Drug Project Research Group: The coronary drug project: Initial findings leading to modifications of its research protocol. J.A.M.A. 214:1303–1313, 1970.
38. Baum, J., Holtz, F., Bookstein, J.J., and Klein, E.W.: Possible association between benign hepatomas and oral contraceptives. Lancet 2:926–928, 1973.
39. Mays, E.T., Christopherson, W.M., Mahr, M.M., and Williams, H.C.: Hepatic changes in young women ingesting contraceptive steroids. Hepatic hemorrhage and primary hepatic tumors. J.A.M.A. 235:730–732, 1976.
40. Edmondson, H., Henderson, A.B., and Benton, B.: Liver-cell adenomas associated with the use of oral contraceptives. New Eng. J. Med. 294:470–472, 1976.
41. Pfeffer, R.I. and Van Den Noort, S.: Estrogen use and stroke risk in postmenopausal women. Amer. J. Epidem. 103:445–456, 1976.

Product Information as of June, 1986

Manufactured by
R.P. Scherer, North America
Clearwater, Florida 33518 for
MERRELL DOW PHARMACEUTICALS INC.
Subsidiary of The Dow Chemical Company
Cincinnati, Ohio 45215, U.S.A.

Continued on next page

Merrell Dow—Cont.

TACE®   ℞
(CHLOROTRIANISENE)
12 mg, 25 mg and 72 mg Capsules

INFORMATION FOR PATIENTS

> TACE (CHLOROTRIANISENE) is a synthetic estrogen
> supplied in 12 mg, 25 mg, and 72 mg capsules.

What You Should Know About Estrogens: Estrogens are female hormones produced by the ovaries. The ovaries make several different kinds of estrogens. In addition, scientists have been able to make a variety of synthetic estrogens. As far as we know, all these estrogens have many similar properties and therefore much the same usefulness, side effects, and risks. This leaflet is intended to help you understand what estrogens are sometimes used for, the risks involved in their use, and how to use them as safely as possible.
This leaflet includes important information about estrogens, but not all the information. If you want to know more, you can ask your doctor or pharmacist to let you read the package insert for this product prepared for the doctor.

USES OF ESTROGEN
Estrogens are prescribed by doctors for a number of purposes, including:
1.   To provide estrogen during a period of adjustment when a woman's ovaries produce it in decreased amounts in order to prevent certain uncomfortable symptoms of estrogen deficiency. (All women normally produce less estrogen, generally between the ages of 45 and 55; this is called the menopause.)
2.   To prevent symptoms of estrogen deficiency when a woman's ovaries have been removed surgically before the natural menopause.
3.   To prevent pregnancy. (Estrogens are given along with a progestagen, another female hormone; these combinations are called oral contraceptives or birth control pills. Patient labeling is available to women taking oral contraceptives and they will not be discussed in this leaflet.) *This product is not intended to prevent pregnancy.*
4.   To treat certain cancers in women and men. *This product is not intended to treat cancers in women.*
5.   To prevent painful swelling of the breasts after pregnancy in women who choose not to nurse their babies.
THERE IS NO PROPER USE OF TACE IN A PREGNANT WOMAN.

ESTROGENS IN THE MENOPAUSE
In the natural course of their lives, all women eventually experience a decrease in estrogen production. This usually occurs between ages 45 and 55 but may occur earlier or later. Sometimes the ovaries may need to be removed before or during natural menopause by an operation, producing a "surgical menopause."
When the amount of estrogen in the blood begins to decrease, many women may develop typical symptoms: feelings of warmth in the face, neck, and chest or sudden intense episodes of heat and sweating throughout the body (called "hot flashes" or "hot flushes"). These symptoms are sometimes very uncomfortable. A few women eventually develop changes in the vagina (called "atrophic vaginitis") which cause discomfort, especially during and after intercourse. Estrogens can be prescribed to treat these symptoms of the menopause. It is estimated that considerably more than half of all women undergoing the menopause have only mild symptoms or no symptoms at all and therefore do not need estrogens. Other women may need estrogens for a few months, while their bodies adjust to lower estrogen levels. Sometimes the need will be for periods longer than six months. In an attempt to avoid overstimulation of the uterus (womb), estrogens are usually given cyclically during each month of use, that is, three weeks of pills followed by one week without pills.
Sometimes women experience nervous symptoms or depression during menopause. There is no well-documented evidence that estrogens are effective for such symptoms and they should not be used to treat them, although other treatment may be needed.
You may have heard that taking estrogens for long periods (years) after the menopause will keep your skin soft and supple and keep you feeling young. There is no evidence that this is so, however, and such long-term treatment carries important risks.

ESTROGENS TO PREVENT SWELLING OF THE BREASTS AFTER PREGNANCY
If you do not breast feed your baby after delivery, your breasts may fill up with milk and become engorged and painful. This usually begins about 3 to 4 days after delivery and may last for a few days to up to a week or more. Sometimes the discomfort is severe, but usually it is not and can be controlled by pain relieving drugs such as aspirin and by binding the breasts up tightly. Estrogens can be used to try to prevent the breasts from filling up.
While this treatment is usually successful in reducing amount of filling, in many cases the breasts fill up to some degree in spite of treatment. The daily dose of estrogens needed to prevent pain and swelling of the breasts is larger than the dose needed to treat symptoms of the menopause and this may increase your chances of developing blood clots in the legs or lungs. (See below.) Therefore, it is important that you discuss the benefits and the risks of estrogen use with your doctor if you have decided not to breast feed your baby.

THE DANGERS OF ESTROGENS
1.   *Cancer of the uterus.* Several independent studies have reported an increased risk ratio of endometrial cancer (cancer of the lining of the uterus) if estrogens are used in the post-menopausal period for more than a year. Women taking estrogens are reported to have roughly 5 to 10 times as great a chance of getting this cancer as women who take no estrogens. To put this another way, while a postmenopausal woman not taking estrogens has 1 chance in 1,000 each year of getting cancer of the uterus, a woman taking estrogens has 5 to 10 chances in 1,000 each year. For this reason *it is important to take estrogens only when you really need them.* The risk of this cancer is reported to be greater the longer estrogens are used and also seems to be greater when larger doses are taken. For this reason, *it is important to take the lowest dose of estrogen that will control symptoms and to take it only as long as it is needed.* If estrogens are needed for longer periods of time, your doctor will want to reevaluate your need for estrogens at least every six months.
Women using estrogens should report any irregular vaginal bleeding to their doctors; such bleeding may be of no importance, but it can be an early warning of cancer of the uterus. If you have undiagnosed vaginal bleeding, you should not use estrogens until a diagnosis is made that there is no cancer of the uterus.
If you have had your uterus completely removed (total hysterectomy), there is no danger of developing cancer of the uterus.
2.   *Other possible cancers.* Long-term continuous administration of estrogens in certain animal species increases the frequency of cancers of the breast, cervix, vagina, and liver. At present there is no satisfactory evidence that women using estrogen in the menopause have an increased risk of such tumors, but there is no way yet to be sure they do not; and one study raises the possibility that use of estrogens in the menopause may increase the risk of breast cancer many years later. This is a further reason to use estrogens only when clearly needed. While you are taking estrogens, it is important that you go to your doctor at least every six months for an examination. Also, if members of your family have had breast cancer or if you have breast nodules or abnormal mammograms (breast x-rays), your doctor may wish to carry out more frequent examinations of your breasts.
3.   *Gall bladder disease.* Women who use estrogens after menopause are reported to be more likely to develop gall bladder disease needing surgery than women who do not use estrogens. Birth control pills have a similar effect.
4.   *Abnormal blood clotting.* Oral contraceptives increase the risk of blood clotting in various parts of the body. This can result in a stroke (if the clot is in the brain), a heart attack (clot in a blood vessel of the heart), or a pulmonary embolus (a clot which forms in the legs or pelvis, then breaks off and travels to the lungs). Any of these can be fatal.
At this time use of estrogens in the menopause is not known to cause such blood clotting, but the possibility that such clotting in association with oral contraceptives may be associated with larger doses of estrogen cannot be excluded. It is recommended that if you have had clotting in the legs or lungs or a heart attack or stroke while you were using estrogens or birth control pills, you should not use estrogens (unless they are being used to treat cancer of the breast or prostate). If you have had a stroke or heart attack or if you have angina pectoris, estrogens should be used with caution and only if clearly needed (for example, if you have severe symptoms of the menopause).
The larger doses of estrogen used to prevent swelling of the breasts after pregnancy have been reported to increase the risk of clotting in the legs and lungs.
Special Warning About Pregnancy: You should not receive estrogen if you are pregnant. It has been reported that there is a greater than usual chance that the developing child will be born with a birth defect, although the possibility remains fairly small. It is also reported that a female child may have an increased risk of developing cancer of the vagina or cervix later in life (in the teens or twenties). Every possible effort should be made to avoid exposure to TACE during pregnancy. If exposure occurs, see your doctor.
Other Effects of Estrogens: In addition to the serious reported risks of estrogens described above, estrogens have the following side effects and potential risks:
1.   *Nausea and vomiting.* The most common side effect of estrogen therapy is nausea. Vomiting is less common.
2.   *Effects on breasts.* Estrogens may cause breast tenderness or enlargement and may cause the breasts to secrete a liquid. These effects are not dangerous.
3.   *Effects on the uterus.* Estrogens may cause benign fibroid tumors of the uterus to get larger.
Some women will have menstrual bleeding when estrogens are stopped. But if the bleeding occurs on days you are still taking estrogens you should report this to your doctor.
4.   *Effects on liver.* Women taking oral contraceptives develop on rare occasions a tumor of the liver which can rupture and bleed into the abdomen. So far, these tumors have not been reported in women using estrogens in the menopause, but you should report any swelling or unusual pain or tenderness in the abdomen to your doctor immediately. Women with a past history of jaundice (yellowing of the skin and white parts of the eyes) may get jaundice again during estrogen use. If this occurs, stop taking estrogens and see your doctor.
5.   *Other effects.* Estrogens may cause excess fluid to be retained in the body. This may make some conditions worse, such as epilepsy, migraine, heart disease, or kidney disease.

SUMMARY
Estrogens have important uses, but they have reported risks of potentially serious conditions developing as well. You must decide, with your doctor, whether the risks are acceptable to you in view of the benefits of treatment. Except where your doctor has prescribed TACE for use in special cases of cancer of the prostate, you should not use TACE if you have cancer of the breast or uterus, are pregnant, have undiagnosed abnormal vaginal bleeding, clotting in the legs or lungs, have had a stroke, heart attack or angina, or clotting in the legs or lungs in the past while you were taking estrogens.
You can use TACE as safely as possible by understanding that your doctor will require regular physical examinations while you are taking it and will try to discontinue the drug as soon as possible and use the smallest dose possible. Be alert for signs of trouble including:
1.   Abnormal bleeding from the vagina.
2.   Pains in the calves or chest or sudden shortness of breath, or coughing blood (indicating possible clots in the legs, heart, or lungs).
3.   Severe headache, dizziness, fainting, or changes in vision (indicating possible developing clots in the brain or eye).
4.   Breast lumps. (You should ask your doctor how to examine your own breasts.)
5.   Jaundice (yellowing of the skin).
6.   Mental depression.
Based on his or her assessment of your medical needs, your doctor has prescribed this drug for you. Do not give this drug to anyone else.

HOW SUPPLIED
TACE (CHLOROTRIANISENE) is a long-acting synthetic estrogen in capsule form. The capsule is suitable for taking by mouth.
Each two-tone green and yellow, soft gelatin capsule imprinted MERRELL 692 contains 72 mg of chlorotrianisene in Dispex®, an emulsifiable vehicle containing corn oil, sorbitan trioleate, polysorbate 80, and benzyl benzoate. This capsule also contains other inactive ingredients: FD&C Blue No. 1, FD&C Yellow No. 5 (tartrazine) as a color additive, gelatin, glycerin, iron oxide, methylparaben, propylparaben, sorbitol, titanium dioxide, and water.

Patient Information as of April, 1985
Shown in Product Identification Section, page 419

> **Information on Merrell Dow products is based on labeling in effect in June, 1989.**

Miles Inc.
Consumer Healthcare Division
P.O. BOX 340
ELKHART, IN 46515

ALKA–MINTS® Chewable Antacid
Rich in Calcium

(See PDR For Nonprescription Drugs)

ALKA–SELTZER® Effervescent
Antacid & Pain Reliever With
Specially Buffered Aspirin
[*al-kuh-selt-sir*]

ACTIVE INGREDIENTS
Each tablet contains: aspirin 325 mg., heat treated sodium bicarbonate 1916 mg., citric acid 1000 mg. ALKA-SELTZER® in water contains principally the antacid sodium citrate and the analgesic sodium acetylsalicylate. Buffered pH is between 6 and 7.

INACTIVE INGREDIENTS
None.

INDICATIONS
ALKA-SELTZER® Effervescent Antacid & Pain Reliever is an analgesic and an antacid and is indicated for relief of sour stomach, acid indigestion or heartburn with headache or body aches and pains. Also for fast relief of upset stomach with headache from overindulgence in food and drink—especially recommended for taking before bed and again on arising. Effective for pain relief alone: headache or body and muscular aches and pains.

ACTIONS
When the ALKA-SELTZER® Effervescent Antacid & Pain Reliever tablet is dissolved in water, the acetylsalicylate ion differs from acetylsalicylic acid chemically, physically and pharmacologically. Being fat insoluble, it is not absorbed by the gastric mucosal cells. Studies and observations in animals and man including radiochrome determinations of fecal blood loss, measurement of ion fluxes and direct visualization with gastrocamera, have shown that, as contrasted with acetylsalicylic acid, the acetylsalicylate ion delivered in the solution does not alter gastric mucosal permeability to permit back-diffusion of hydrogen ion, and gastric damage and acute gastric mucosal lesions are therefore not seen after administration of the product.

ALKA-SELTZER® Effervescent Antacid & Pain Reliever has the capacity to neutralize gastric hydrochloric acid quickly and effectively. In-vitro, 154 ml. of 0.1 N hydrochloric acid are required to decrease the pH of one tablet of ALKA-SELTZER® Effervescent Antacid & Pain Reliever in solution to 4.0. Measured against the in vitro standard established by the Food and Drug Administration one tablet neutralizes 17.2 mEq of acid. In vivo, the antacid activity of two ALKA-SELTZER® Antacid & Pain Reliever tablets is comparable to that of 10 ml. of milk of magnesia. ALKA-SELTZER® Effervescent Antacid & Pain Reliever is able to resist pH changes caused by the continuing secretion of acid in the normal individual and to maintain an elevated pH until emptying occurs.

ALKA-SELTZER® Effervescent Antacid & Pain Reliever provides highly water soluble acetylsalicylate ions which are fat insoluble. Acetylsalicylate ions are not absorbed from the stomach. They empty from the stomach and thereby become available for absorption from the duodenum. Thus, fast drug absorption and high plasma acetylsalicylate levels are achieved. Plasma levels of salicylate following the administration of ALKA-SELTZER® Effervescent Antacid & Pain Reliever solution (acetylsalicylate ion equivalent to 648 mg. acetylsalicylic acid) can reach 29 mg./liter in 10 minutes and rise to peak levels as high as 55 mg./liter within 30 minutes.

WARNINGS
Children and teenagers should not use this medicine for chicken pox or flu symptoms before a doctor is consulted about Reye Syndrome, a rare but serious illness reported to be associated with aspirin. As with any drug, if you are pregnant or nursing a baby, seek the advice of a health professional before using this product. Except under the advice and supervision of a physician, do not take more than, Adults: 8 tablets in a 24 hour period. (60 years of age or older: 4 tablets in a 24 hour period), or use the maximum dosage for more than 10 days. Do not use if you are allergic to aspirin or have asthma, if you have a coagulation (bleeding) disease, or if you are on a sodium restricted diet. Each tablet contains 567 mg. of sodium.

Keep this and all drugs out of the reach of children.

DOSAGE AND ADMINISTRATION
ALKA-SELTZER® Effervescent Antacid & Pain Reliever is taken in solution, approximately three ounces of water per tablet is sufficient.

Adults: 2 tablets every 4 hours. CAUTION: If symptoms persist or recur frequently, or if you are under treatment for ulcer, consult your physician.

PROFESSIONAL LABELING
ASPIRIN FOR MYOCARDIAL INFARCTION
INDICATION
The Aspirin contained in ALKA-SELTZER is indicated to reduce the risk of death and/or non-fatal myocardial infarction in patients with a previous infarction or unstable angina pectoris.

CLINICAL TRIALS
The indication is supported by the results of six, large, randomized multicenter, placebo-controlled studies[1-7] involving 10,816 predominantly male, post-myocardial infarction (MI) patients and one randomized placebo-controlled study of 1,266 men with unstable angina. Therapy with aspirin was begun at intervals after the onset of acute MI varying from less than 3 days to more than 5 years and continued for periods of from less than one year to four years. In the unstable angina study, treatment was started within 1 month after the onset of unstable angina and continued for 12 weeks and complicating conditions such as congestive heart failure were not included in the study.

Aspirin therapy in MI patients was associated with about a 20 percent reduction in the risk of subsequent death and/or non-fatal reinfarction, a median absolute decrease of 3 percent from the 12 to 22 percent event rates in the placebo groups. In aspirin-treated unstable angina patients the reduction in risk was about 50 percent, a reduction in event rate of 5 percent from the 10 percent rate in the placebo group over the 12 weeks of the study.

Daily dosage of aspirin in the post-myocardial infarction studies was 300 mg in one study and 900 to 1500 mg in five studies. A dose of 325 mg was used in the study of unstable angina.

ADVERSE REACTIONS
Gastrointestinal Reactions: Symptoms and signs of gastrointestinal irritation were not significantly increased in subjects treated for unstable angina with buffered aspirin in solution. (ALKA-SELZER®.) Doses of 1000 mg per day of aspirin tablets caused gastrointestinal symptoms and bleeding that in some cases were clinically significant. In the largest post-infarction study (the Aspirin Myocardial Infarction Study (AMIS) with 4,500 people), the percentage incidences of gastrointestinal symptoms for the aspirin (1000 mg of a standard, solid-tablet formulation) and placebo-treated subjects, respectively, were: stomach pain (14.5%; 4.4%); heartburn (11.9%; 4.8%); nausea and/or vomiting (7.6%; 2.1%); hospitalization for gastrointestinal disorder (4.9%; 3.5%). In the AMIS and other trials, aspirin treated patients had increased rates of gross gastrointestinal bleeding. As with all aspirin products ALKA-SELTZER® is contraindicated in patients with aspirin sensitivity, with asthma, or with coagulation disease.

CARDIOVASCULAR AND BIOCHEMICAL
In the AMIS trial, the dosage of 1000 mg per day of aspirin was associated with small increases in systolic blood pressure (BP) (average 1.5 to 2.1 mm) and diastolic BP (0.5 to 0.6 mm), depending upon whether maximal or last available readings were used. Blood urea nitrogen and uric acid levels were also increased, but by less than 1.0 mg%. Subjects with marked hypertension or renal insufficiency had been excluded from the trial so that the clinical importance of these observations for such subjects or for any subjects treated over more prolonged periods is not known. It is recommended that patients placed on long-term aspirin treatment, even at doses of 300 mg per day, be seen at regular intervals to assess changes in these measurements.

SODIUM IN BUFFERED ASPIRIN FOR SOLUTION FORMULATIONS
One tablet daily of buffered aspirin in solution adds 567 mg of sodium to that in the diet and may not be tolerated by patients with active sodium-retaining states such as congestive heart or renal failure. This amount of sodium adds about 30 percent to the 70 to 90 meq intake suggested as appropriate for dietary treatment of essential hypertension in the 1984 Report of the Joint National Committee on Detection, Evaluation, and Treatment of High Blood Pressure[8].

DOSAGE AND ADMINISTRATION
Although most of the studies used dosages exceeding 300 mg, daily, two trials used only 300 mg and pharmacologic data indicate that this dose inhibits platelet function fully. Therefore, 300 mg or a conventional 325 mg aspirin dose daily is a reasonable, routine dose that would minimize gastrointestinal adverse reactions. This use of aspirin applies to both solid, oral dosage forms (buffered and plain aspirin) and buffered aspirin in solution.

REFERENCES
(1) Elwood, P. C., et al., "A Randomized Controlled Trial of Acetysalicylic Acid in the Secondary Prevention of Mortality from Myocardial Infarction," *British Medical Journal* 1:436–440, 1974.
(2) The Coronary Drug Project Research Group, "Aspirin in Coronary Heart Disease," *Journal of Chronic Diseases*, 29:625–642, 1976.
(3) Breddin, K., et al., "Secondary Prevention of Myocardial Infarction: A Comparison of Acetylsalicylic Acid, Phenprocoumon or Placebo," *International Congress Series* 470:263–268, 1979.
(4) Aspirin Myocardial Infarction Study Research Group, "A Randomized, Controlled Trial of Aspirin in Persons Recovered from Myocardial Infarction," *Journal American Medical Association* 245:661–669, 1980.
(5) Elwood, P. C., and P. M. Sweetnam, "Aspirin and Secondary Mortality after Myocardial Infarction." *Lancet* pp. 1313–1315, December 22–29, 1979.
(6) The Persantine-Aspirin Reinfarction Study Research Group, "Persantine and Aspirin in Coronary Heart Disease," *Circulation*, 62: 449–460, 1980.
(7) Lewis, H. D., et al., "Protective Effects of Aspirin Against Acute Myocardial Infarction and Death in Men with Unstable Angina, Results of a Veterans Administration Cooperative Study," *New England Journal of Medicine* 309:396–403, 1983.
(8) "1984 Report of the Joint National Committee on Detection, Evaluation, Treatment of High Blood Pressure," U.S. Department of Health and Human Services and United States Public Health Service, National Institutes of Health.

HOW SUPPLIED
Tablets: foil sealed; box of 12, 24, 36 and 72 in twin packs; card of 96 in twin packs; carton of 100 in twin packs.

Flavored ALKA-SELTZER®
Effervescent Antacid & Pain Reliever
[al-kuh-selt-sir]

ACTIVE INGREDIENTS
Each tablet contains: Aspirin 325 mg, heat treated sodium bicarbonate 1710 mg, citric acid 1220 mg. Alka-Seltzer in water contains principally the antacid sodium citrate and the analgesic sodium acetylsalicylate.

INACTIVE INGREDIENTS
Flavors, Saccharin Sodium.

INDICATIONS
SPARKLING FRESH TASTE!
Flavored Alka-Seltzer®
For speedy relief of ACID INDIGESTION, SOUR STOMACH or HEARTBURN with HEADACHE, or BODY ACHES AND PAINS. Also for fast relief of UPSET STOMACH with HEADACHE from overindulgence in food and drink—especially recommended for taking before bed and again on arising. EFFECTIVE FOR PAIN RELIEF ALONE: HEADACHE or BODY and MUSCULAR ACHES and PAINS.

WARNINGS
Children and teenagers should not use this medicine for chicken pox and flu symptoms before a doctor is consulted about Reye Syndrome, a rare but serious illness reported to be associated with aspirin.

As with any drug, if you are pregnant or nursing a baby, seek the advice of a health professional before using this product. Except under the advice and supervision of a physician: Do not take more than, ADULTS: 6 tablets in a 24-hour period, (60 years of age or older: 4 tablets in a 24-hour period), or use the daily maximum dosage for more than 10 days. Do not use if you are allergic to aspirin or have asthma, if you have a coagulation (bleeding) disease, or if you are on a sodium restricted diet. Each tablet contains 506 mg of sodium.
KEEP this and all drugs out of the reach of children.

DIRECTIONS
Alka-Seltzer must be dissolved in water before taking. ADULTS: 2 tablets every 4 hours. CAUTION: If symptoms persist or recur frequently or if you are under treatment for ulcer, consult your physician.

PROFESSIONAL LABELING
ASPIRIN FOR MYOCARDIAL INFARCTION
INDICATION
The Aspirin contained in Alka-Seltzer is indicated to reduce the risk of death and/or non-fatal myocardial infarction in patients with a previous infarction or unstable angina pectoris.

CLINICAL TRIALS
The indication is supported by the results of six, large, randomized multicenter, placebo-controlled studies[1-7] involving 10,816, predominantly male, post-myocardial infarction (MI) patients and one randomized placebo-controlled study of 1,266 men with unstable angina. Therapy with aspirin was begun at intervals after the onset of acute MI varying from less than 3 days to more than 5 years and continued for periods of from less than one year to four years. In the unstable angina study, treatment was started within 1 month after the onset of unstable angina and continued for 12 weeks and complicating conditions such as congestive heart failure were not included in the study.

Aspirin therapy in MI patients was associated with about a 20 percent reduction in the risk of subsequent death and/or non-fatal reinfarction, a median absolute decrease of 3 percent from the 12 to 22 percent event rates in the placebo groups. In aspirin-treated unstable angina patients the reduction in risk was about 50 percent, a reduction in event rate of 5 percent from the 10 percent rate in the placebo group over the 12 week of the study.

Daily dosage of aspirin in the post-myocardial infarction studies was 300 mg in one study and 900 to 1500 mg in five studies. A dose of 325 mg was used in the study of unstable angina.

ADVERSE REACTIONS
Gastrointestinal Reactions: Symptoms and signs of gastrointestinal irritation were not significantly increased in subjects treated for unstable angina with buffered aspirin in solution (ALKA-SELTZER®). Doses of 1000 mg per day of aspirin tablets caused gastrointestinal symptoms and bleed-

Continued on next page

Miles Consumer Healthcare—Cont.

ing that in some cases were clinically significant. In the largest post-infarction study (the Aspirin Myocardial Infarction Study (AMIS) with 4,500 people), the percentage incidences of gastrointestinal symptoms for the aspirin (1000 mg of a standard, solid-tablet formulation) and placebo-treated subjects, respectively, were: stomach pain (14.5%; 4.4%); heartburn (11.9%; 4.8%); nausea and/or vomiting (7.6%; 2.1%); hospitalization for gastrointestinal disorder (4.9%; 3.5%). In the AMIS and other trials, aspirin treated patients had increased rates of gross gastrointestinal bleeding. As with all aspirin products Alka-Seltzer is contraindicated in patients with aspirin sensitivity, with asthma, or with coagulation disease.

Cardiovascular and Biochemical: In the AMIS trial, the dosage of 1000 mg per day of aspirin was associated with small increases in systolic blood pressure (BP) (average 1.5 to 2.1 mm) and diastolic BP (0.5 to 0.6 mm), depending upon whether maximal or last available readings were used. Blood urea nitrogen and uric acid levels were also increased, but by less than 1.0 mg%. Subjects with marked hypertension or renal insufficiency had been excluded from the trial so that the clinical importance of these observations for such subjects or for any subjects treated over more prolonged periods is not known. It is recommended that patients placed on long-term aspirin treatment, even at doses of 300 mg per day, be seen at regular intervals to assess changes in these measurements.

Sodium in Buffered Aspirin for Solution Formulations: One tablet daily of flavored buffered aspirin in solution adds 506 mg of sodium to that in the diet and may not be tolerated by patients with active sodium-retaining states such as congestive heart or renal failure. This amount of sodium adds about 30 percent to the 70 to 90 meq intake suggested as appropriate for dietary treatment of essential hypertension in the 1984 Report of the Joint National Committee on Detection, Evaluation, and Treatment of High Blood Pressure[8].

DOSAGE AND ADMINISTRATION

Although most of the studies used dosages exceeding 300 mg, daily, two trials used only 300 mg and pharmacologic data indicate that this dose inhibits platelet function fully. Therefore, 300 mg or a conventional 325 mg aspirin dose daily is a reasonable, routine dose that would minimize gastrointestinal adverse reactions. This use of aspirin applies to both solid, oral dosage forms (buffered and plain aspirin) and buffered aspirin in solution.

REFERENCES

(1) Elwood, P. C., et al., A Randomized Controlled Trial of Acetysalicylic Acid in the Secondary Prevention of Mortality from Myocardial Infarction," *British Medical Journal* 1:436–440, 1974.
(2) The Coronary Drug Project Research Group, "Aspirin in Coronary Heart Disease," *Journal of Chronic Diseases,* 29:625–642, 1976.
(3) Breddin K., et al., "Secondary Prevention of Myocardial Infarction: A Comparison of Acetysalicylic Acid, Phenprocoumon or Placebo," *Int. Congr. Series* 470:263–268, 1979.
(4) Aspirin Myocardial Infarction Study Research Group, "A Randomized, Controlled Trial of Aspirin in Persons Recovered from Myocardial Infarction," *Journal American Medical Association* 245:661–669, 1980.
(5) Elwood, P. C., and P. M. Sweetnam, "Aspirin and Secondary Mortality after Myocardial Infarction," *Lancet* pp. 1313–1315, December 22–29, 1979.
(6) The Persantine-Aspirin Reinfarction Study Research Group, "Persantine and Aspirin in Coronary Heart Disease," *Circulation,* 62: 449–460, 1980.
(7) Lewis, H. D., et al., "Protective Effects of Aspirin Against Acute Myocardial Infarction and Death in Men with Unstable Angina, Results of a Veterans Administration Cooperative Study," *New England Journal of Medicine* 309:396–403, 1983.
(8) "1984 Report of the Joint National Committee on Detection, Evaluation, Treatment of High Blood Pressure," U.S. Department of Health and Human Services and United States Public Health Service, National Institutes of Health.

HOW SUPPLIED

Tablets: foil sealed; box of 12, 24, and 36 in twin packs.

ALKA-SELTZER® Effervescent Antacid
[al-kuh-selt-sir]

ACTIVE INGREDIENTS

Each tablet contains heat treated sodium bicarbonate 958 mg., citric acid 832 mg., potassium bicarbonate 312 mg. ALKA-SELTZER® Effervescent Antacid in water contains principally the antacids sodium citrate and potassium citrate.

INACTIVE INGREDIENTS
A tableting aid.

INDICATIONS
ALKA-SELTZER® Effervescent Antacid is indicated for relief of acid indigestion, sour stomach or heartburn.

ACTIONS
The ALKA-SELTZER® Effervescent Antacid solution provides quick and effective neutralization of gastric acid. Measured by the in vitro standard established by the Food and Drug Administration one tablet will neutralize 10.6 mEq of acid.

WARNINGS
Except under the advice and supervision of a physician, do not take more than: Adults: 8 tablets in a 24 hour period (60 years of age or older: 7 tablets in a 24 hour period), Children 4 tablets in a 24 hour period; or use the maximum dosage of this product for more than 2 weeks.
Do not use this product if you are on a sodium restricted diet. Each tablet contains 311 mg. of sodium.
Keep this and all drugs out of the reach of children. As with any drug, if you are pregnant or nursing a baby, seek the advice of a health professional before using this product.

DOSAGE AND ADMINISTRATION
ALKA-SELTZER® Effervescent Antacid is taken in solution; approximately 3 oz. of water per tablet is sufficient. Adults: one or two tablets every 4 hours as needed. Children: ½ the adult dosage.

HOW SUPPLIED
Tablets: foil sealed; box of 20 and 36 in twin packs.

ALKA-SELTZER® Extra Strength
Antacid & Pain Reliever

ACTIVE INGREDIENTS
Each tablet contains: Aspirin 500mg, heat treated sodium bicarbonate 1985mg, citric acid 1000mg. Alka-Seltzer in water contains principally the antacid sodium citrate and the analgesic sodium acetylsalicylate.

INACTIVE INGREDIENTS
Flavors

INDICATIONS
For speedy relief of acid indigestion, sour stomach or heartburn with headache or body aches and pains. Also, for fast relief of upset stomach with headache from overindulgence in food and drink—especially recommended for taking before bed and again on arising. Effective for pain relief alone: Headache or body and muscular aches and pains.

WARNINGS
Children and teenagers should not use this medicine for chicken pox or flu symptoms before a doctor is consulted about Reye Syndrome, a rare but serious illness reported to be associated with aspirin. As with any drug, if you are pregnant or nursing a baby, seek the advice of a health professional before using this product. Except under the advice and supervision of a physician: Do not take more than, Adults: 7 tablets in a 24-hour period (60 years of age or older, 4 tablets in a 24-hour period), or use the daily maximum dosage for more than 10 days. Do not use if you are allergic to aspirin or have asthma, if you have a coagulation (bleeding) disease, or if you are on a sodium restricted diet. Each tablet contains 588mg of sodium. Keep this and all drugs out of the reach of children.

DOSAGE AND ADMINISTRATION
Extra Strength Alka-Seltzer must be dissolved in water before taking. Adults: 2 tablets every 4 hours. Caution: If symptoms persist, or recur frequently, or if you are under treatment for ulcer, consult your physician.

HOW SUPPLIED
Tablets: foil sealed; Boxes of 12 and 24 in twin packs.

ALKA-SELTZER® ADVANCED FORMULA EFFERVESCENT ANTACID & NON-ASPIRIN PAIN RELIEVER

(See PDR For Nonprescription Drugs)

ALKA-SELTZER PLUS® Cold Medicine

(See PDR For Nonprescription Drugs)

ALKA-SELTZER PLUS®
Night-Time Cold Medicine

(See PDR For Nonprescription Drugs)

BACTINE® Antiseptic · Anesthetic First Aid Spray
[bak-tēn]

(See PDR For Nonprescription Drugs)

BACTINE® First Aid Antibiotic Ointment

(See PDR For Nonprescription Drugs)

BACTINE® Hydrocortisone (0.5%) Skin Care Cream
[bak-tēn]

(See PDR For Nonprescription Drugs)

BIOCAL™ 500 mg Tablets
Calcium Supplement

(See PDR For Nonprescription Drugs)

BUGS BUNNY® Children's Chewable Vitamins (Sugar Free)

(See PDR For Nonprescription Drugs)

BUGS BUNNY® Children's Chewable Vitamins + Minerals with Iron and Calcium (Sugar Free)

(See PDR For Nonprescription Drugs)

BUGS BUNNY® Plus Iron Children's Chewable Vitamins (Sugar Free)

(See PDR For Nonprescription Drugs)

BUGS BUNNY® With Extra C Children's Chewable Vitamins (Sugar Free)
Multivitamin Supplement

(See PDR For Nonprescription Drugs)

FLINTSTONES® Children's Chewable Vitamins

(See PDR For Nonprescription Drugs)

FLINTSTONES® Plus Iron Children's Chewable Vitamins

(See PDR For Nonprescription Drugs)

FLINTSTONES® COMPLETE
With Iron, Calcium & Minerals
Children's Chewable Vitamins

(See PDR For Nonprescription Drugs)

FLINTSTONES® With Extra C Children's Chewable Vitamins (Sugar Free)
Multivitamin Supplement

(See PDR For Nonprescription Drugs)

MILES® NERVINE
NIGHTTIME SLEEP-AID

(See PDR For Nonprescription Drugs)

ONE–A–DAY® Essential Vitamins
with Beta Carotene

(See PDR For Nonprescription Drugs)

ONE–A–DAY® Maximum Formula
Vitamins and Minerals with Beta Carotene

(See PDR For Nonprescription Drugs)

ONE–A–DAY® Plus Extra C
Vitamins with Beta Carotene

(See PDR For Nonprescription Drugs)

ONE–A–DAY STRESSGARD® Stress Formula Vitamins with Beta Carotene

(See PDR For Nonprescription Drugs)

ONE–A–DAY WITHIN® Multivitamin for Women with Calcium, Extra Iron, Zinc and Beta Carotene

(See PDR For Nonprescription Drugs)

Miles Inc.
Cutter Biological
**400 MORGAN LANE
WEST HAVEN, CT 06516**

GAMASTAN®   ℞
[găm′as-tan″]
Immune Globulin (Human) U.S.P.

2 ml., 10 ml. vials.

IMMUNE GLOBULIN INTRAVENOUS (HUMAN)   ℞
GAMIMUNE® N

DESCRIPTION
Immune Globulin Intravenous (Human)—Gamimune® N is a sterile 4.5–5.5% solution of human protein in 9–11% maltose; it contains no preservative. Each milliliter (mL) contains approximately 50 mg of protein, not less than 98% of which has the electrophoretic mobility of gamma globulin. Not less than 90% of the gamma globulin is monomer. Also present are traces of IgA and IgM. The distribution of IgG subclasses is similar to that found in normal serum. Gamimune N has a buffer capacity of 16.5 mEq/L of solution ($\sim$ 0.3 mEq/g of protein). The calculated osmolality is 309 milliosmoles per kilogram of solvent (water) and the calculated osmolarity is 278 milliosmoles per liter of solution.
The product is made by cold ethanol fractionation of large pools of human plasma; each individual unit of plasma used in the pool has been tested and found non-reactive for hepatitis B surface antigen (HBsAg) by an FDA approved method. Part of the fractionation may be performed by another licensed manufacturer. The immunoglobulin is isolated from Cohn Effluent III by diafiltration and ultrafiltration. The protein has not been chemically modified other than in the adjustment of the pH of the solution to 4.0–4.5.[1] Isotonicity is achieved by the addition of maltose. The product is intended for intravenous administration.

CLINICAL PHARMACOLOGY
Gamimune N supplies a broad spectrum of opsonic and neutralizing IgG antibodies for the prevention or attenuation of a wide variety of infectious diseases. As Gamimune N is administered intravenously, essentially 100% of the infused IgG antibodies are immediately available in the recipient's circulation.[2] A relatively rapid fall in serum IgG level in the first week post-infusion is to be expected; this decrease averages 40% of the peak level achieved immediately post-infusion and is mainly due to the equilibration of IgG between the plasma and the extravascular space.[2,10,11,14] The *in vivo* half-life of Gamimune N equals or exceeds the three week half-life reported for IgG in the literature, but individual patient variation in half-life has been observed.[2] Thus, this variable as well as the amount of immune globulin administered per dose is important in determining the frequency of administration of the drug for each individual patient.
While Gamimune N has been shown to be effective in some cases of idiopathic thrombocytopenic purpura (ITP) (see INDICATIONS AND USAGE) the mechanism of action has not been fully elucidated.
The intravenous administration of solutions of maltose has been studied by several investigators.[4–8] Healthy subjects tolerated the infusions well, and no adverse effects were observed at a rate of 0.25 g maltose/kg body weight per hour.[5] In safety studies conducted by Cutter Biological, infusions of 10% maltose administered at 0.27–0.62 g maltose/kg per hour[8] to normal subjects produced either mild side effects (e.g., headache) or no adverse reaction.[2] Following intravenous administrations of maltose, maltose was detected in the peripheral blood; there was a dose-dependent excretion of maltose and glucose in the urine and a mild diuretic effect.[2] These alterations were well tolerated without significant adverse effects.[2] The highest recommended infusion rate, 0.08 mL/kg body weight per minute (see DOSAGE AND ADMINISTRATION), is equivalent to 0.48 g maltose/kg body weight per hour.

The buffer capacity of Immune Globulin Intravenous (Human)—Gamimune® N is 16.5 mEq/L ($\sim$ 0.3 mEq/g protein); a dose of 150–400 mg/kg (3–8 mL/kg) body weight therefore represents an acid load of 0.0495–0.1320 mEq/kg body weight. The total buffering capacity of whole blood in a normal individual is 45–50 mEq/L of blood, or 3.6 mEq/kg body weight.[9] Thus, the acid load delivered in the largest dose of Gamimune N would be neutralized by the buffering capacity of whole blood alone, even if the dose were infused instantaneously. (An infusion usually lasts several hours.)
In Phase I human studies, no change in arterial blood pH measurements was detected following the intravenous administration of Gamimune N at a dose of 150 mg/kg body weight;[2] following a dose of 400 mg/kg body weight in 37 patients, there were no clinically important differences in mean venous pH or bicarbonate measurements in patients who received Gamimune N compared with those who received a chemically modified intravenous immunoglobulin preparation with a pH of 6.8.[2]
In patients with limited or compromised acid-base compensatory mechanisms, consideration should be given to the effect of the additional acid load Gamimune N might present.

INDICATIONS AND USAGE
Primary Humoral Immunodeficiency
Gamimune N is efficacious in the treatment of primary immunodeficiency states in which severe impairment of antibody forming capacity has been shown, such as: congenital agammaglobulinemias, common variable immunodeficiency, Wiskott-Aldrich syndrome, x-linked immunodeficiency with hyper IgM, and severe combined immunodeficiencies.[3,12–15] Gamimune N is especially useful when high levels or rapid elevation of circulating antibodies are desired or when intramuscular injections are contraindicated.
Idiopathic Thrombocytopenic Purpura (ITP)
In clinical situations in which a rapid rise in platelet count is needed to control bleeding or to allow a patient with ITP to undergo surgery, administration of Immune Globulin Intravenous (Human)—Gamimune® N should be considered; in patients in whom a response is achieved, the rise of platelets is generally rapid (within 1–5 days), transient (most often lasting from several days to several weeks) and should not be considered curative. It is presently not possible to predict which patients with ITP will respond to therapy, although the increase in platelet counts in children seems to be better than that of adults.
Two different dosing regimens of Immune Globulin Intravenous (Human)—Gamimune N, have been studied in clinical investigations: a regimen consisting of 400 mg/kg body weight daily for five consecutive days, and a high dose treatment regimen consisting of 1,000 mg/kg body weight administered on either one day or two consecutive days.
In clinical studies of Gamimune N, 5 of 6 (83.3%) children and 12 of 16 (75%) adults with acute or chronic ITP treated with 400 mg/kg body weight for five consecutive days demonstrated clinically significant platelet increments of $\geq 30,000/\text{mm}^3$ over baseline. The mean platelet count in children with ITP rose from $27,800/\text{mm}^3$ at baseline to $297,000/\text{mm}^3$ (range $50,000$–$455,000/\text{mm}^3$) and the mean platelet count in adults with ITP rose from $27,900/\text{mm}^3$ at baseline to $124,900/\text{mm}^3$ (range $11,000$–$341,000/\text{mm}^3$). Two of three children with acute ITP rapidly went into complete remission. However, childhood ITP may respond spontaneously without treatment.
Thirteen of 14 children (92.9%) and 26 of 29 adults (89.7%) with acute or chronic ITP treated with Gamimune N 1,000 mg/kg body weight administered on either one day or two consecutive days responded to treatment with clinically significant platelet increments of $\geq 30,000/\text{mm}^3$ over baseline. This included 3 of 3 patients with ITP that were human immunodeficiency virus (HIV) antibody positive and 2 of 2 patients with ITP were pregnant. The mean platelet count in children with ITP treated with Gamimune N 1,000 mg/kg body weight on 1 day or 2 consecutive days rose from $44,400/\text{mm}^3$ at baseline to $285,600/\text{mm}^3$ (range $89,000$–$473,000/\text{mm}^3$) and the mean platelet count in adults with ITP treated with the regimen rose from $23,400/\text{mm}^3$ at baseline to $173,100/\text{mm}^3$ (range $28,000$–$709,000/\text{mm}^3$). Two patients, one each with acute adult and chronic childhood ITP, entered complete remission with treatment.
Six of the 29 adult patients with ITP received IGIV, pH 4.25 1,000 mg/kg on 1 day or 2 consecutive days to increase the platelet count prior to splenectomy. Mean platelet counts rose from $14,500/\text{mm}^3$ at baseline to $129,300/\text{mm}^3$ (range $51,000$–$242,000/\text{mm}^3$) prior to surgery.
The duration of the platelet rise following treatment of ITP with either treatment regimen of Immune Globulin Intravenous (Human)—Gamimune® N was variable, ranging from several days to 12 months or more. Some ITP patients have demonstrated continuing responsiveness over many months to intermittent infusions of Gamimune N 400–1,000 mg/kg body weight, administered as a single maintenance dose, at intervals as indicated by the platelet count.

CONTRAINDICATIONS
Gamimune N is contraindicated in individuals who are known to have had an anaphylactic or severe systemic response to Immune Globulin (Human). Individuals with selective IgA deficiencies who have known antibody against IgA (anti-IgA antibody) should not receive Gamimune N since these patients may experience severe reactions to the IgA which may be present.[13]

WARNINGS
Gamimune N should be administered only intravenously as the intramuscular and subcutaneous routes have not been evaluated.
Gamimune N may, on rare occasions, cause a precipitous fall in blood pressure and a clinical picture of anaphylaxis, even when the patient is not known to be sensitive to immune globulin preparations. These reactions may be related to the rate of infusion. Accordingly, the infusion rate given under DOSAGE AND ADMINISTRATION should be closely followed, at least until the physician has had sufficient experience with a given patient. The patient's vital signs should be monitored continuously and careful observation made for any symptoms throughout the entire infusion. Epinephrine should be available for the treatment of an acute anaphylactic reaction.

PRECAUTIONS
General
Any vial that has been entered should be used promptly. Partially used vials should be discarded. Do not use if turbid. Solution which has been frozen should not be used.
Drug Interactions
If dilution is required, Gamimune N may be diluted with 5% dextrose in water (D5/W). No other drug interactions or compatibilities have been evaluated. It is recommended that infusion of Gamimune N be given by a separate line, by itself, without mixing with other intravenous fluids or medications the patient might be receiving.
Pregnancy Category C
Animal reproduction studies have not been conducted with Gamimune N. It is not known whether Gamimune N can cause fetal harm when administered to a pregnant woman or can affect reproduction capacity. Gamimune N should be given to a pregnant woman only if clearly needed.

ADVERSE REACTIONS
In a study of 37 patients with immunodeficiency syndromes receiving Gamimune N at a monthly dose of 400 mg/kg body weight, reactions were seen in 5.2% of the infusions of Immune Globulin Intravenous (Human)—Gamimune® N. Symptoms reported with Gamimune N included malaise, a feeling of faintness, fever, chills, headache, nausea, vomiting, chest tightness, dyspnea and chest, back or hip pain. In addition, mild erythema following infiltration of Immune Globulin Intravenous (Human)—Gamimune N at the infusion site was reported in some cases.
In studies of Gamimune N administered at a dose of 400 mg/kg body weight in the treatment of adult and pediatric patients with ITP, systemic reactions were noted in only 4 of 154 (2.6%) infusions, and all but one occurred at rates of infusion greater than 0.04 mL/kg body weight per minute. The symptoms reported included chest tightness, a sense of tachycardia (pulse was 84 beats per minute), and a burning sensation in the head; these symptoms were all mild and transient.
In studies of Gamimune H administered at a dose of 1,000 mg/kg body weight either as a single dose or as two doses on consecutive days in the treatment of adult and pediatric patients with ITP, adverse reactions were noted in only 25 of 251 (10%) infusions. Symptoms reported included headache, nausea, fever, chills, back pain, chest tightness, shortness of breath. In children, the high dose regimen has been well-tolerated at the highest rates of infusion. In adults, however, the frequency of adverse reactions tended to increase with infusion rates in excess of 0.06 mL/kg/min. In general, reactions reported with infusion of Gamimune N in these studies were reported as mild or moderate, and responded to slowing of the infusion rate.
In the studies undertaken to date, other types of reactions have not been reported with Gamimune N. It may be, however, that adverse effects will be similar to those previously reported with intravenous and intramuscular immunoglobulin administration. Potential reactions therefore, may also include anxiety, flushing, wheezing, abdominal cramps, myalgias, arthralgia, and dizziness; rash has been reported only rarely. Reactions to intravenous immunoglobulin tend to be related to the rate of infusion.
True anaphylactic reactions to Gamimune N may occur in recipients with documented prior histories of severe allergic reactions to intramuscular immunoglobulin, but some patients may tolerate cautiously administered intravenous immunoglobulin without adverse effects.[2,16] Very rarely an anaphylactoid reaction may occur in patients with no prior

Continued on next page

Miles-Cutter—Cont.

history of severe allergic reactions to either intramuscular or intravenous immunoglobulin.[2]

DOSAGE AND ADMINISTRATION

Primary Humoral Immunodeficiency

The usual dosage of Immune Globulin Intravenous (Human)—Gamimune N® for prophylaxis in primary immunodeficiency syndromes is 100–200 mg/kg (2–4 mL/kg) of body weight administered approximately once a month by intravenous infusion. The dosage may be given more frequently or increased as high as 400 mg/kg (8 mL/kg) body weight, if the clinical response is inadequate, or the level of IgG achieved in the circulation is felt to be insufficient. The minimum level of IgG required for protection has not been determined.

Idiopathic Thrombocytopenic Purpura

Induction: An increase in platelet count has been observed in children and some adults with acute or chronic ITP receiving Gamimune N 400 mg/kg body weight daily for five days, or alternatively, 1,000 mg/kg body weight daily for 1 day or 2 consecutive days. In the latter treatment regimen, if an adequate increase in the platelet count is observed at 24 hours, the second dose of 1,000 mg/kg body weight may be withheld. The high dose regimen (1,000 mg/kg × 1–2 days) is not recommended for individuals with expanded fluid volumes or where fluid volume may be a concern. With both treatment regimens, a response usually occurs within several days and is maintained for a variable period of time. In general, a response is seen less often in adults than in children.

Maintenance: In adults and children with ITP, if after induction therapy the platelet count falls to less than 30,000/mm³ and/or the patient manifests clinically significant bleeding, Gamimune N 400 mg/kg body weight may be given as a single infusion. If an adequate response does not result, the dose can be increased to 800–1,000 mg/kg of body weight given as a single infusion. Maintenance infusions may be administered intermittently as clinically indicated to maintain a platelet count greater than 30,000/mm³.

Investigations indicate that Gamimune N is well-tolerated and less likely to produce side effects when infused at the indicated rate. It is recommended that Gamimune N be infused by itself at a rate of 0.01 to 0.02 mL/kg body weight per minute for 30 minutes; if well-tolerated, the rate may be **gradually** increased to a maximum of 0.08 mL/kg body weight per minute. If side effects occur, the rate may be reduced, or the infusion interrupted until symptoms subside. The infusion may then be resumed at the rate which is comfortable for the patient.

Parenteral drug products should be inspected visually for particulate matter and discoloration prior to administration, whenever solution and container permit.

HOW SUPPLIED

Immune Globulin Intravenous (Human)—Gamimune® N is supplied in the following sizes:

Size	Grams Protein
10 mL	0.5
50 mL	2.5
100 mL	5.0
250 mL	12.5

STORAGE

Store at 2–8°C (35–46°F). Do not freeze. Do not use after expiration date.

CAUTION

U.S. Federal law prohibits dispensing without a prescription.

LIMITED WARRANTY

A number of factors beyond our control could reduce the efficacy of this product or even result in an ill effect following its use. These include improper storage and handling of the product after it leaves our hands, diagnosis, dosage, method of administration, and biological differences in individual patients. Because of these factors, it is important that this product be stored properly and that the directions be followed carefully during use.

The foregoing statement is made in lieu of any other warranty, express or implied, including any warranty of merchantability or fitness. Representatives of the Company are not authorized to vary the terms of this warranty or the contents of any printed labeling for this product except by printed notice from the Company's headquarters. The prescriber and user of this product must accept the terms hereof.

REFERENCES

1. Tenold RA, inventor; Cutter Laboratories, assignee. Intravenously injectable immune serum globulin. U.S. Patent 4,396,608 August 2, 1983.
2. Data on file at Miles Inc., Cutter Biological.
3. Ochs HD, Buckley RH, Pirofsky B, et al: Safety and patient acceptability of intravenous immune globulin in 10% maltose. Lancet 2(8205):1158–9, 1980.
4. Berg G, Matzkies F: Wirkung von Maltose nach intravenoser Dauerinfusion auf den Stoffwechsel. Z Ernahrungswiss 15:255–62, 1976.
5. Forster H, Hoos I, Boecker S: Versuche mit Probanden zur parenteralen Verwertung von Maltose. Z Ernahrungswiss 15(3):284–93, 1976.
6. Finke C, Reinauer H: Utilization of maltose and oligosaccharides after intravenous infusion in man. Nutr Metab 21(Suppl 1):115–7, 1977.
7. Young EA, Drummond A, Cioletti L, et al: Metabolism of continuously infused intravenous maltose. Clin Res 25(3):543A, 1977.
8. Soroff HS, Hansen LM, Sasvary D, et al: Clinical pharmacology and metabolism of maltose in normal human volunteers. Clin Res 26(3):286A, 1978.
9. Guyton AC: Textbook of Medical Physiology. 5th ed. Philadelphia, W.B. Saunders Company, 1976, pp 499–500.
10. Pirofsky B, Campbell SM, Montanaro A: Individual patients variation in the kinetics of intravenous immunoglobulin administration. J Clin Immunol 2 (2):7S–14S, 1982.
11. Pirofsky B: Intravenous immune globulin therapy in hypogammaglobulinemia. Amer J Med 76(3A): 53–60, 1984.
12. Nolte MT, Pirofsky B, Gerritz GA, et al: Intravenous immunoglobulin therapy for antibody deficiency. Clin Exp Immunol 36:237–43, 1979.
13. Buckley RH: Immunoglobulin replacement therapy: indications and contraindications for use and variable IgG levels achieved. In: Alving BM (ed.): Immunoglobulins: characteristics and uses of intravenous preparations. Washington, D.C., U.S. Government Printing Office (1980), pp 3–8.
14. Pirofsky B, Anderson CJ, Bardana EJ Jr.: Therapeutic and detrimental effects of intravenous immunoglobulin therapy. In: Alving BM (ed.): Immunoglobulins: characteristics and uses of intravenous preparations. Washington, D.C., U.S. Government Printing Office (1980), pp 15–22.
15. Ochs HD: Intravenous immunoglobulin therapy of patients with primary immunodeficiency syndromes: efficacy and safety of a new modified immune globulin preparation. In: Alvin BM (ed.): Immunoglobulins: characteristics and uses of intravenous preparations. Washington, D.C., U.S. Government Printing Office (1980), pp 9–14.
16. Peerless AG, Stiehm ER: Intravenous gammaglobulin for reaction to intramuscular preparation. Lancet 2(8347):461, 1983.

U.S. License No. 8
Miles Inc.
Cutter Biological
Elkhart, IN 46515 USA

HYPERAB®   ℞
[hī′per-ab″]
(Rabies Immune Globulin—Human)
2 ml. (300 IU) pediatric vial
10 ml. (1500 IU) adult vial

HYPERHEP®   ℞
[hī′per-hep″]
(Hepatitis B Immune Globulin—Human)
1 ml., 5 ml. vials

HYPER–TET®   ℞
[hī′per-tet″]
(Tetanus Immune Globulin—Human U.S.P.)
250 units vial or prefilled disposable syringe

HypRho®–D Mini–Dose   ℞
[hī″prō-d′]
Rh₀(D) Immune Globulin (Human)

DESCRIPTION

Rh₀(D) Immune Globulin (Human)—HypRho®-D Mini-Dose—is a sterile solution of immune globulin containing antibodies to Rh₀(D) which is for intramuscular injection only. It is prepared from human venous plasma collected from carefully screened donors. It contains 15–18% protein stabilized with 0.21–0.32 M glycine and preserved with 80–120 μg/mL thimerosal (a mercury derivative), as measured by mercury assay. The pH is adjusted with sodium carbonate.

One dose of HypRho-D Mini-Dose contains not less than one-sixth the quantity of Rh₀(D) antibody contained in one standard dose of Rh₀(D) Immune Globulin (Human), USP and it will suppress the immunizing potential of 2.5 mL of Rh₀(D) positive packed red blood cells or the equivalent of whole blood (5 mL). The quantity of Rh₀(D) antibody in HypRho-D Mini-Dose is not less than one-sixth of that contained in 1 mL of the U.S. Food and Drug Administration Reference Rh₀(D) Immune Globulin (Human).

Each individual unit of plasma used in the manufacturing of this product has been tested and found nonreactive for hepatitis B surface antigen (HBsAg) and negative for antibody to human immunodeficiency virus (HIV) by FDA approved tests.

CLINICAL PHARMACOLOGY

Rh sensitization may occur in nonsensitized Rh₀(D) negative women following transplacental hemorrhage resulting from spontaneous or induced abortions.[1–2] The risk of sensitization is higher in women undergoing induced abortions than in those aborting spontaneously.[1–3]

HypRho-D Mini-Dose is used to prevent the formation of anti-Rh₀(D) antibody in Rh₀(D) negative women who are exposed to the Rh₀(D) antigen at the time of spontaneous or induced abortion (up to 12 weeks gestation).[3–5] HypRho-D Mini-Dose suppresses the stimulation of active immunity by Rh₀(D) positive fetal erythrocytes that may enter the maternal circulation at the time of termination of the pregnancy. The amount of anti-Rh₀(D) in HypRho-D Mini-Dose has been shown to effectively prevent maternal isosensitization to the Rh₀(D) antigens following spontaneous or induced abortion occurring up to the 12th week of gestation.[6–8] After the 12th week of gestation, a standard dose of Rh₀(D) Immune Globulin (Human), USP—HypRho®-D is indicated.

INDICATIONS AND USAGE

Rh₀(D) Immune Globulin (Human)—HypRho®-D Mini-Dose is recommended to prevent the isoimmunization of Rh₀(D) negative women at the time of spontaneous or induced abortion of up to 12 weeks gestation provided the following criteria are met:

1. The mother must be Rh₀(D) negative and must not already be sensitized to the Rh₀(D) antigen.
2. The father is not known to be Rh₀(D) negative.
3. Gestation is not more than 12 weeks at termination.

Note: Rh₀(D) Immune Globulin (Human) prophylaxis is not indicated if the fetus or father can be determined to be Rh negative. If the Rh status of the fetus is unknown, the fetus must be assumed to be Rh₀(D) positive, and HypRho-D Mini-Dose should be administered to the mother.

FOR ABORTIONS OR MISCARRIAGES OCCURRING AFTER 12 WEEKS GESTATION, A STANDARD DOSE OF Rh₀(D) IMMUNE GLOBULIN (HUMAN), USP IS INDICATED.

HypRho-D Mini-Dose should be administered within three hours or as soon as possible after spontaneous passage or surgical removal of the products of conception. However, if HypRho-D Mini-Dose is not given within this time period, consideration should still be given to its administration since clinical studies in male volunteers have demonstrated the effectiveness of Rh₀(D) Immune Globulin (Human), USP in preventing isoimmunization as long as 72 hours after infusion of Rh₀(D) positive red cells.[9]

CONTRAINDICATIONS

None known.

WARNINGS

NEVER ADMINISTER HYPRHO-D MINI-DOSE INTRAVENOUSLY. INJECT ONLY INTRAMUSCULARLY. ADMINISTER ONLY TO WOMEN POST-ABORTION OR POST-MISCARRIAGE OF UP TO 12 WEEKS GESTATION.

HypRho-D Mini-Dose should be given with caution to patients with a history of prior systemic allergic reactions following the administration of human immune globulin preparations or in patients who are known to have had an allergic response to thimerosal.

The attending physician who wishes to administer HypRho-D Mini-Dose to persons with isolated immunoglobulin A (IgA) deficiency must weigh the benefits of immunization against the potential risks of hypersensitivity reactions. Such persons have increased potential for developing antibodies to IgA and could have anaphylactic reactions to subsequent administration of blood products that contain IgA.

As with all preparations administered by the intramuscular route, bleeding complications may be encountered in patients with thrombocytopenia or other bleeding disorders.

PRECAUTIONS

General

Although systemic reactions to immunoglobulin preparations are rare, epinephrine should be available for treatment of acute anaphylactic symptoms.

Drug Interactions

Other antibodies in the Rh₀(D) Immune Globulin (Human)—HypRho®-D Mini-Dose preparation may interfere with the response to live vaccines such as measles, mumps, polio or rubella. Therefore, immunization with live vaccines should not be given within three months after HypRho-D Mini-Dose administration.

Pregnancy Category C

Animal reproduction studies have not been conducted with HypRho-D Mini-Dose. It is also not known whether HypRho-D Mini-Dose can cause fetal harm when administered to a pregnant woman or can affect reproduction capacity.

It should be again noted, however, that HypRho-D Mini-Dose is **not** indicated for use during pregnancy and it should be administered only post-abortion or post-miscarriage.

ADVERSE REACTIONS

Reactions to HypRho-D Mini-Dose are infrequent in $Rh_o(D)$ negative individuals and consist primarily of slight soreness at the site of injection and slight temperature elevation. While sensitization to repeated injections of human globulin is extremely rare, it has occurred.

DOSAGE AND ADMINISTRATION

One syringe of HypRho-D Mini-Dose provides sufficient antibody to prevent Rh sensitization to 2.5 mL $Rh_o(D)$ positive packed red cells or the equivalent (5 mL) of whole blood. This dose is sufficient to provide protection against maternal Rh sensitization for women undergoing spontaneous or induced abortion of up to 12 weeks gestation.

HypRho-D Mini-Dose should be administered within three hours or as soon as possible following spontaneous or induced abortion. If prompt administration is not possible, HypRho-D Mini-Dose should be given within 72 hours following termination of the pregnancy.

Parenteral drug products should be inspected visually for particulate matter and discoloration prior to administration, whenever solution and container permit.

HOW SUPPLIED

Each HypRho-D Mini-Dose package contains:

Ten single dose prefilled syringes of HypRho-D Mini-Dose, a package insert giving directions for use, and patient identification cards.

STORAGE

Store at 2°–8°C (35°–46°F). Do not freeze.

CAUTION

U.S. Federal law prohibits dispensing without prescription.

LIMITED WARRANTY

A number of factors beyond our control could reduce the efficacy of this product or even result in an ill effect following its use. These include improper storage and handling of the product after it leaves our hands, diagnosis, dosage, method of administration, and biological differences in individual patients. Because of these factors, it is important that this product be stored properly and that the directions be followed carefully during use.

The foregoing statement is made in lieu of any other warranty, express or implied, including any warranty of merchantability or fitness. Representatives of the Company are not authorized to vary the terms of this warranty or the contents of any printed labeling for this product except by printed notice from the Company's headquarters. The prescriber and user of this product must accept the terms hereof.

REFERENCES

1. Queenan JT, Shah S, Kubarych SF, *et al:* Role of induced abortion in rhesus immunisation. *Lancet* 1(7704): 815–7, 1971.
2. Goldman JA, Eckerling B: Prevention of Rh immunization after abortion with anti-Rh_o(D)-immunoglobulin. *Obstet Gynecol* 40(3):366–70, 1972.
3. The selective use of Rh_o(D) immune globulin (RhIG). *ACOG Tech Bull* 61, 1981.
4. Prevention of Rh sensitization. *WHO Tech Rep Ser* 468, 1971.
5. Recommendation of the Public Health Service Advisory Committee on Immunization Practices: Rh immune globulin. *Morbid Mortal Wkly Rep* 21(15):126–7, 1972.
6. Stewart FH, Burnhill MS, Bozorgi N: Reduced dose of Rh immunoglobulin following first trimester pregnancy termination. *Obstet Gynecol* 51(3):318–22, 1978.
7. McMaster conference on prevention of Rh immunization, 28-30 September, 1977. *Vox Sang* 36(1):50–64, 1979.
8. Simonovits I: Efficiency of anti-D IgG prevention after induced abortion. *Vox Sang* 26(4):361–7, 1974.
9. Freda VJ, Gorman JG, Pollack W: Prevention of Rh-hemolytic disease with Rh-immune globulin. *Am J Obstet Gynecol* 128(4):456–60, 1977.

14-7621-053
(Rev Sept 1988)

HypRho®-D   ℞

[hī"prō-d']
$Rh_o(D)$ Immune
Globulin (Human), USP

DESCRIPTION

$Rh_o(D)$ Immune Globulin (Human), USP—HypRho®-D is a sterile solution of immune globulin containing antibodies to $Rh_o(D)$ which is intended for intramuscular injection. It contains 15–18% protein stabilized with 0.21–0.32 M glycine and is preserved with 80–120 μg/mL thimerosal (a mercury derivative), as measured by mercury assay. The pH is adjusted with sodium carbonate. The potency is equal to or greater than that of the U.S. Food and Drug Administration Reference $Rh_o(D)$ Immune Globulin (Human), USP. Each single dose vial or syringe contains sufficient anti-$RH_o(D)$ (approximately 300 μg^*) to effectively suppress the immunizing potential of 15 mL of $Rh_o(D)$ positive red blood cells.[2–4]

This product has been prepared from large pools of human venous plasma. Each individual unit of plasma has been tested and found nonreactive for hepatitis B surface antigen (HBsAg) and negative for antibody to human immunodeficiency virus (HIV) by FDA approved tests.

*A full dose of $Rh_o(D)$ Immune Globulin (Human), USP has traditionally been referred to as a "300 μg" dose and this usage is employed here for convenience in terminology. **It should not be construed as the actual anti-D content.** Each full dose of $RH_o(D)$ Immune Globulin (Human), USP must contain at least as much anti-D as 1mL of the U.S. Reference $Rh_o(D)$ Immune Globulin (Human), USP. Studies performed at the FDA have shown that the U.S. Reference contains 820 international units (IU) of anti-D per mL. When the conversion factor determined for the International (WHO) Reference Preparation[1] is used, 820 IU per mL is equivalent to 164 μg per mL of anti-D.

CLINICAL PHARMACOLOGY

HypRho-D is used to prevent isoimmunization in the $Rh_o(D)$ negative individual exposed to $Rh_o(D)$ positive blood as the result of a fetomaternal hemorrhage occurring during a delivery of an $Rh_o(D)$ positive infant, abortion (either spontaneous or induced), or following amniocentesis or abdominal trauma. Similarly, immunization resulting in the production of anti-$Rh_o(D)$ following transfusion of Rh positive red cells to an $Rh_o(D)$ negative recipient may be prevented by administering $Rh_o(D)$ Immune Globulin (Human), USP.[5,6]

Rh hemolytic disease of the newborn is the result of the active immunization of an $Rh_o(D)$ negative mother by $Rh_o(D)$ positive red cells entering the maternal circulation during a previous delivery, abortion, amniocentesis, abdominal trauma, or as a result of red cell transfusion.[7,8] HypRho-D acts by suppressing the immune response of $Rh_o(D)$ negative individuals to $Rh_o(D)$ positive red blood cells. The mechanism of action of HypRho-D is not fully understood.

The administration of $Rh_o(D)$ Immune Globulin (Human), USP within 72 hours of a full-term delivery of an $Rh_o(D)$ positive infant by an $Rh_o(D)$ negative mother reduces the incidence of Rh isoimmunization from 12–13% to 1–2%. The 1–2% treatment failures are probably due to isoimmunization occurring during the latter part of pregnancy or following delivery.[10] Bowman, *et al,*[11] have reported that the incidence of isoimmunization can be further reduced from approximately 1.6% to less than 0.1% by administering $Rh_o(D)$ Immune Globulin in two doses, one antenatal at 28 weeks gestation and another following delivery.

INDICATIONS AND USAGE

Pregnancy and Other Obstetric Conditions

$Rh_o(D)$ Immune Globulin (Human), USP—HypRho-D is recommended for the prevention of Rh hemolytic disease of the newborn by its administration to the $Rh_o(D)$ negative mother within 72 hours after birth of an $Rh_o(D)$ positive infant,[12] providing the following criteria are met:

1. The mother must be $Rh_o(D)$ negative, and must not already be sensitized to the $Rh_o(D)$ factor.

2. Her child must be $Rh_o(D)$ positive, and should have a negative direct antiglobulin test (see PRECAUTIONS).

If HypRho-D is administered antepartum, it is essential that the mother receive another dose of HypRho-D after delivery of an $Rh_o(D)$ positive infant.

If the father can be determined to be $Rh_o(D)$ negative, HypRho-D need not be given.

HypRho-D should be administered within 72 hours to all nonimmunized $Rh_o(D)$ negative women who have underdone spontaneous or induced abortion, following ruptured tubal pregnancy, amniocentesis or abdominal trauma unless the blood group of the fetus or the father is known to be $Rh_o(D)$ negative.[7,8] If the fetal blood group cannot be determined, one must assume that it is $Rh_o(D)$ positive,[2] and HypRho-D should be administered to the mother.

Transfusion

HypRho-D may be used to prevent isoimmunization in $Rh_o(D)$ negative individuals who have been transfused with $Rh_o(D)$ positive red blood cells or blood components containing red blood cells.[5,13]

CONTRAINDICATIONS

None known.

WARNINGS

NEVER ADMINISTER HypRho-D INTRAVENOUSLY. INJECT ONLY INTRAMUSCULARLY. NEVER ADMINISTER TO THE NEONATE.

$Rh_o(D)$ Immune Globulin (Human), USP should be given with caution to patients with a history of prior systemic allergic reactions following the administration of human immunoglobulin preparations or to patients who are known to have had an allergic respose to thimerosal.

The attending physician who wishes to administer $Rh_o(D)$ Immune Globulin (Human), USP to persons with isolated immunoglobulin A (IgA) deficiency must weigh the benefits of immunization against the potential risks of hypersensitivity reactions. Such persons have increased potential for developing antibodies to IgA and could have anaphylactic reactions to subsequent administration of blood products that contain IgA.

As with all preparations administered by the intramuscular route, bleeding complications may be encountered in patients with thrombocytopenia or other bleeding disorders.

PRECAUTIONS

General

A large fetomaternal hemorrhage late in pregnancy or following delivery may cause a weak mixed field positive D^u test result. If there is any doubt about the mother's Rh type, she should be given $RH_o(D)$ Immune Globulin (Human), USP. A screening test to detect fetal red blood cells may be helpful in such cases.

If more than 15 mL of D positive fetal red blood cells are present in the mother's circulation, more than a single dose of $Rh_o(D)$ Immune Globulin (Human), USP—HypRho®-D is required. Failure to recognize this may result in the administration of an inadequate dose.

Although systemic reactions to human immunoglobulin preparations are rare, epinephrine should be available for treatment of acute anaphylactic reactions.

Drug Interactions

Other antibodies in the $Rh_o(D)$ Immune Globulin (Human), USP preparation may interfere with the response to live vaccines such as measles, mumps, polio or rubella. Therefore, immunization with live vaccines should not be given within three months after $Rh_o(D)$ Immune Globulin (Human), USP administration.

Drug/Laboratory Interactions

Babies born of women given $Rh_o(D)$ Immune Globulin (Human), USP antepartum may have a weakly positive direct antiglobulin test at birth.

Passively acquired anti-$Rh_o(D)$ may be detected in maternal serum if antibody screening tests are performed subsequent to antepartum or post partum administration of $Rh_o(D)$ Immune Globulin (Human), USP.

Pregnancy Category C

Animal reproduction studies have not been conducted with HypRho-D. It is also not known whether HypRho-D can cause fetal harm when administered to a pregnant woman or can affect reproduction capacity. HypRho-D should be given to a pregnant woman only if clearly needed.

ADVERSE REACTIONS

Reactions to $Rh_o(D)$ Immune Globulin (Human), USP are infrequent in $Rh_o(D)$ negative individuals and consist primarily of slight soreness at the site of injection and slight temperature elevation. While sensitization to repeated injections of human immune globulin is extremely rare, it has occurred. Elevated bilirubin levels have been reported in some individuals receiving multiple doses of $Rh_o(D)$ Immune Globulin (Human), USP following mismatched tranfusions. This is believed to be due to a relatively rapid rate of foreign red cell destruction.

DOSAGE AND ADMINISTRATION

Pregnancy and Other Obstetric Conditions

1. For postpartum prophylaxis, administer one vial or syringe of HypRho-D (300 μg^*), preferably within 72 hours of delivery. Although a lesser degree of protection is afforded if Rh antibody is administered beyond the 72-hour period, HypRho-D may still be given.[7,14] Full-term deliveries can vary in their dosage requirements depending on the magnitude of the fetomaternal hemorrhage. One 300 μg^* vial or syringe of HypRho-D provides sufficient antibody to prevent Rh sensitization if the volume of red blood cells that has entered the circulation is 15 mL or less.[2–4] In instances where a large (greater than 30 mL of whole blood or 15 mL red blood cells) fetomaternal hemorrhage is suspected, a fetal red cell count by an approved laboratory technique (e.g., modified Kleihauer-Betke acid elution stain technique) should be performed to determine the dosage of immune globulin required.[8,15] The red blood cell volume of the calculated fetomaternal hemorrhage is divided by 15 mL to obtain the number of vials or syringes of $Rh_o(D)$ Immune Globulin (Human), USP—HypRho®-D for administration.[3,8,13] If more than 15 mL of red cells is suspected or if the dose calculation results in a fraction, administer the next higher whole number of vials or syringes (e.g., if 1.4, give 2 vials or syringes).

2. For antenatal prophylaxis, one 300 μg^* vial or syringe of HypRho(D) is administered at approximately 28 weeks gestation. This must be followed by another 300 μg^* dose, preferably within 72 hours following delivery, if the infant is Rh positive.

Continued on next page

Miles-Cutter—Cont.

3. Following threatened abortion at any stage of gestation with continuation of pregnancy, it is recommended that 300 μg* of HypRho-D be given. If more than 15 mL of red cells is suspected due to fetomaternal hemorrhage, the same dose modification in #1 above applies.

4. Following miscarriage, abortion, or termination of ectopic pregnancy at or beyond 13 weeks gestation, it is recommended that 300 μg* of HypRho-D be given. If more than 15 mL of red blood cells is suspected due to fetomaternal hemorrhage, the same dose modification in #1 above applies. If pregnancy is terminated prior to 13 weeks gestation, a single dose of Mini-Dose Rh₀(D) (approximately 50 μg*) may be used instead of HypRho-D.

5. Following amniocentesis at either 15 to 18 weeks gestation or during the third trimester, or following abdominal trauma in the second or third trimester, it is recommended that 300 μg* of HypRho-D be administered. If there is a fetomaternal hemorrhage in excess of 15 mL of red cells, the same dose modification in #1 applies.

If abdominal trauma, amniocentesis, or other adverse event requires the administration of HypRho-D at 13 to 18 weeks gestation, another 300 μg* dose should be given at 26 to 28 weeks. To maintain protection throughout pregnancy, the level of passively acquired anti-Rh₀(D) should not be allowed to fall below the level required to prevent an immune response to Rh positive red cells. The half life of IgG is 23 to 26 days. In any case, a dose of HypRho-D should be given within 72 hours after delivery if the baby is Rh positive. If delivery occurs within three weeks after the last dose, the postpartum dose may be withheld unless there is a femomaternal hemorrhage in excess of 15 mL of red blood cells.[16]

*See footnote under DESCRIPTION.

Transfusion

In the case of a transfusion of Rh₀(D) positive red cells to an Rh₀(D) negative recipient, the volume of Rh positive whole blood administered is multiplied by the hematocrit of the donor uniting the volume of red blood cells transfused. The volume of red blood cells is divided by 15 mL which provides the number of vials or syringes of HypRho-D to be administered.

If the dose calculated results in a fraction, the next higher whole number of vials or syringes should be administered (e.g., if 1.4, give 2 vials or 2 syringes). HypRho-D should be administered within 72 hours after an incompatible transfusion, but preferably as soon as possible.

Injection Procedure

DO NOT INJECT INTRAVENOUSLY. DO NOT INJECT NEONATE.

A. Single Vial or Syringe Dose

INJECT ENTIRE CONTENTS OF THE VIAL OR SYRINGE INTO THE INDIVIDUAL INTRAMUSCULARLY.

B. Multiple Vial or Syringe Dose

1. Calculate the number of vials or syringes of Rh₀(D) Immune Globulin (Human), USP—HypRho®-D to be given (See Dosage section above).

2. The total volume of HypRho-D can be given in divided doses at different sites at one time or the total dose may be divided and injected at intervals, provided the total dosage is given within 72 hours of the fetomaternal hemorrhage or transfusion. USING STERILE TECHNIQUE, INJECT THE ENTIRE CONTENTS OF THE CALCULATED NUMBER OF VIALS OR SYRINGES INTRAMUSCULARLY INTO THE PATIENT.

Parenteral drug products should be inspected visually for particulate matter and discoloration prior to administration, whenever solution and container permit.

HOW SUPPLIED

HypRho-D is available in vials and in syringes as follows:

Product Code	Contents
621-10	Ten single dose vials of HypRho-D. Package insert giving directions for use and patient identification cards.
621-15	One single dose vial of HypRho-D. Package insert giving directions for use, an injection form and a patient identification card.
621-22	Ten single dose syringes of HypRho-D. Package insert giving directions for use, patient identification cards, and patient information booklets.
621-25	Five single dose syringes of HypRho-D. Package insert giving directions for use, patient identification cards, and patient information booklets.

STORAGE

Store at 2–8°C (35–46°F). Do not freeze.

CAUTION

U.S. Federal law prohibits dispensing without a prescription.

LIMITED WARRANTY

A number of factors beynd our control could reduce the efficacy of this product or even result in an ill effect following its use. These include improper storage and handling of the product after it leaves our hands, diagnosis, dosage, method of administration, and biological differences in individual patients. Because of these factors, it is important that this product be stored properly and that the directions be followed carefully during use.

The foregoing statement is made in lieu of any other warranty, express or implied, including any warranty of merchantability or fitness.

Representatives of the Company are not authorized to vary the terms of this warranty or the contents of any printed labeling for this product except by printed notice from the Company's headquarters. The prescriber and user of this product must accept the terms hereof.

REFERENCES

1. Gunson HH, Bowell PJ, Kirkwood TBL: Collaborative study to recalibrate the International Reference Preparation of Anti-D Immunoglobulin. *J Clin Pathol* 33:249–53, 1980.
2. Rh₀(D) immune globulin (human). *Med Lett Drugs Ther* 16(1):3–4, 1974.
3. Pollack W, Ascari WQ, Kochesky RJ, *et al:* Studies on Rh prophylaxis I. Relationship between doses of anti-Rh and size of antigenic stimulus. *Transfusion* 11(6):333–9, 1971.
4. Unpublished data in files of Cutter Biological.
5. Pollack W, Asceri WQ, Crispen JF, *et al:* Studies on Rh prophylaxis. II. Rh immune prophylaxis after transfusion with Rh-positive blood. *Transfusion* 11 (6):340–4, 1971.
6. Keith LG, Houser GH: Anti-Rh immune globulin after a massive transfusion accident. *Transfusion* 11(3):176, 1971.
7. The selective use of Rh₀(D) Immune Globulin (RHIG). *ACOG Tech Bull* 61, 1981.
8. Current uses of Rh₀ immune globulin and detection of antibodies. *ACOG Tech Bull* 35, 1976.
9. Pollack W: Rh hemolytic disease of the newborn; its cause and prevention. *Prog Clin Biol Res* 70:185–203, 1981.
10. Bowman JM, Chown B, Lewis M, *et al:* Rh isoimmunization during pregnancy: antenatal prophylaxis. *Can Med Assoc J* 118(6):623–7, 1978.
11. Bowman JM, Pollock JM: Antenatal prophylaxis of Rh isommunization: 28-weeks-gestation service program. *Can Med Assoc J* 118(6):627–30, 1978.
12. Ascari WQ, Allen AE, Baker WJ, et al: Rh-o(D) immune globulin (human): evaluation in women at risk of Rh immunization. *JAMA* 205(1): 1–4, 1968.
13. Prevention of Rh sensitization, *WHO Tech Rep Ser* 468:25, 1971.
14. Samson D. Mollison PL: Effect on primary Rh immunization of delayed administration of anti-Rh. *Immunology* 28:349–57, 175.
15. Finn R, Harper DT, Stallings, SA, et al: Transplacental hemorrhage. *Transfusion* 3(2):114–24, 1963.
16. Garraty G (ed): Hemolytic disease of the newborn. Arlington, VA, American Association of Blood Banks, 78, 1984.

14-7621-002
(Rev Feb 1988)

KOATE®-HS   ℞

[kō'ate]

Antihemophilic Factor (Human)

(Factor VIII, AHF, AHG)

A heat-treated in solution, stable, purified dried concentrate of human Antihemophilic Factor.

250 AHF units, approx., with 10 ml Sterile Water for Injection, U.S.P., sterile filter needle, and transfer needle.

500 AHF units, approx., with 20 ml Sterile Water for Injection, U.S.P., sterile filter needle, and transfer needle.

1000 AHF units, approx., with 30 ml or 40 ml Sterile Water for Injection, U.S.P., sterile filter needle, and transfer needle.

KOATE®-HP   ℞

[kō'ate]

Antihemophilic Factor (Human)

(Factor VIII, AHF, AHG)

A stable, dried concentrate of human Antihemophlic Factor (AHF, Factor VIII, AHG) which has been chromatographically purified.

250 AHF units, approx., with 5 ml Sterile Water for Injection, U.S.P., sterile filter needle, transfer needle, and administration set

500 AHF units, approx., with 5 ml Sterile Water for Injection, U.S.P., sterile filter needle, transfer needle, and administration set.

1000 AHF units, approx., with 10 ml Sterile Water for Injection, U.S.P., sterile filter needle, transfer needle, and administration set.

1500 AHF units, approx., with 10 ml Sterile Water for Injection, U.S.P., sterile filter needle, transfer needle, and administration set.

KONYNE®-HT   ℞

[kō'nine-HT]

(Factor IX Complex-Heat Treated)

500 unit vial, approx., with 20 ml sterile water for Injection, U.S.P., sterile filter needle, and transfer needle.

1000 unit vial, approx., with 40 ml sterile water for Injection, U.S.P., sterile filter needle, and transfer needle.

PLAGUE VACCINE, U.S.P.   ℞

20 ml. vials

ALPHA₁-PROTEINASE INHIBITOR   ℞
(HUMAN)
PROLASTIN®

[pro-las'tin]

DESCRIPTION

Alpha₁-Proteinase Inhibitor (Human), PROLASTIN®, is a sterile, stable, lyophilized preparation of purified human Alpha₁-Proteinase Inhibitor (alpha₁-PI) also known as alpha₁-antitrypsin, Alpha₁-Proteinase Inhibitor (Human) is intended for use in therapy of congenital alpha₁-antitrypsin deficiency.

Alpha₁-Proteinase Inhibitor (Human) is prepared from pooled human plasma of normal donors by modification and refinements of the cold ethanol method of Cohn.[1] Each unit of plasma has been tested and found nonreactive for hepatitis B surface antigen (HBsAg) and negative for antibody to human immunodeficiency virus (HIV) by FDA approved tests. In addition, in order to reduce the potential risk of transmission of infectious agents, Alpha₁-Proteinase Inhibitor (Human) has been heat-treated in solution at 60±0.5°C for not less than 10 hours. However, no procedure has been found to be totally effective in removing viral infectivity from plasma fractionation products.

The specific activity of Alpha₁-Proteinase Inhibitor (Human) is ≥0.35 mg functional alpha₁-PI/mg protein and when reconstituted, the concentration of alpha₁-PI is ≥20 mg/mL. When reconstituted, Alpha₁-Proteinase Inhibitor (Human) has a pH of 6.6–7.4, a sodium content of 100–210 mEq/L, a chloride content of 60–180 mEq/L, a sodium phosphate content of 0.015–0.025 M, a polyethylene glycol content of NMT 5 ppm, and NMT 0.1% sucrose, Alpha₁-Proteinase Inhibitor (Human) contains small amounts of other plasma proteins including alpha₂-plasmin inhibitor, alpha₁-antichymotrypsin, C₁-esterase inhibitor, haptoglobin, antithrombin III, alpha₁-lipoprotein, albumin, and IgA.[1]

Each vial of Alpha₁-Proteinase Inhibitor (Human) contains the labeled amount of functionally active alpha₁-PI in milligrams per vial (mg/vial), as determined by capacity to neutralize porcine pancreatic elastase.[1] Alpha₁-Proteinase Inhibitor (Human) contains no preservative and must be administered by the intravenous route.

CLINICAL PHARMACOLOGY

Alpha₁-antitrypsin deficiency is a chronic hereditary, usually fatal, autosomal recessive disorder in which a low concentration of alpha₁-PI (alpha₁-antitrypsin) is associated with slowly progressive, severe, panacinar emphysema that most often manifests itself in the third to fourth decades of life.[2-9] [Although the terms "Alpha₁-Proteinase Inhibitor" and "alpha₁-antitrypsin" are used interchangeably in the scientific literature, the hereditary disorder associated with a reduction in the serum level of alpha₁-PI is conventionally referred to as "alpha₁-antitrypsin deficiency" while the deficient protein is referred to as "Alpha₁-Proteinase Inhibitor"[10]. The emphysema is typically worse in the lower lung zones.[4,8,9] The pathogenesis of development of emphysema in alpha₁-antitrypsin deficiency is not well understood at this time. It is believed, however, to be due to a chronic biochemical imbalance between elastase (an enzyme capable of degrading elastin tissues, released by inflammatory cells, primarily neutrophils, in the lower respiratory tract) and alpha₁-PI (the principal inhibitor of neutrophil elastase) which is deficient in alpha₁-antitrypsin disease.[11-15] As a result, it is believed that alveolar structures are unprotected from chronic exposure to elastase released from a chronic, low level burden of neutrophils in the lower respiratory tract, resulting in progressive degradation of elastin tissues.[11-15] The eventual outcome is the development of emphysema. Neonatal hepatitis with cholestatic jaundice appears in approxiately 10% of newborns with alpha₁-antitrypsin deficiency.[15] In some adults, alpha₁-antitrypsin deficiency is complicated by cirrhosis.[15]

A large number of phenotypic variants of alpha$_1$-antitrypsin deficiency exists.[15] The most severely affected individuals are those with the PiZZ variant, typically characterized by alpha$_1$-PI serum levels <35% normal.[15] Epidemiologic studies of individuals with various phenotypes of alpha$_1$-antitrypsin deficiency have demonstrated that individuals with endogenous serum levels of alpha$_1$-PI ≤ 50 mg/dL (based on commercial standards) have a risk of >80% of developing emphysema over a lifetime.[3–6,8,9,16] However, individuals with endogenous alpha$_1$-PI levels > 80 mg/dL in general, do not manifest an increased risk for development of emphysema above the general population background risk.[5,15] From these observations, it is believed that the "threshold" level of alpha$_1$-PI in the serum required to provide adequate anti-elastase activity in the lung of individuals with alpha$_1$-antitrypsin deficiency is about 80 mg/dL (based on commercial standards for immunologic assay of alpha$_1$-PI).[12,15,17]

In clinical studies of Alpha$_1$-Proteinase Inhibitor (Human), PROLASTIN®, 23 subjects with the PiZZ variant of congenital deficiency of alpha$_1$-antitrypsin deficiency and documented destructive lung disease participated in a study of acute and/or chronic replacement therapy with Alpha$_1$-Proteinase Inhibitor (Human).[18] The mean *in vivo* recovery of alpha$_1$-PI was 4.2 mg (immunologic) dL per mg (functional)/kg body weight administered.[18,19] The half-life of alpha$_1$-PI *in vivo* was approximately 4.5 days.[18,19] Based on these observations, a program of chronic replacement therapy was developed. Nineteen of the subjects in these studies received Alpha$_1$-Proteinase Inhibitor (Human) replacement therapy, 60 mg/kg body weight, once weekly for up to 26 weeks (average 24 weeks of therapy). With this schedule of replacement therapy, blood levels of alpha$_1$-PI were maintained above 80 mg/dL (based on the commercial standards for alpha$_1$-PI immunologic assay).[18–20] Within a few weeks of commencing this program, bronchoalveolar lavage studies demonstrated significantly increased levels of alpha$_1$-PI and functional antineutrophil elastase capacity in the epithelial lining fluid of the lower respiratory tract of the lung, as compared to levels prior to commencing the program of chronic replacement therapy with Alpha$_1$-Proteinase Inhibitor (Human).[18–20]

All 23 individuals who participated in the investigations were immunized with Hepatitis B Vaccine and received a single dose of Hepatitis B Immune Globulin (Human) on entry into the investigation. Although no other steps were taken to prevent hepatitis, neither hepatitis B nor non-A, non-B hepatitis occurred in any of the subjects.[18–19] All subjects remained seronegative for HIV antibody. None of the subjects developed any detectable antibody to alpha$_1$-PI or other serum protein.

Long term controlled clinical trials to evaluate the effect of chronic replacement therapy with Alpha$_1$-Proteinase Inhibitor (Human), PROLASTIN® on the development of or progression of emphysema in patients with congenital alpha$_1$-antitrypsin deficiency, have not been performed. Estimates of the sample size required of this rare disorder and the slow progressive nature of the clinical course have been considered impediments in the ability to conduct such a trial.[21] Studies to monitor the long term effects will continue as part of the post approval process.

INDICATIONS AND USAGE
Congenital Alpha$_1$-Antitrypsin Deficiency
Alpha$_1$-Proteinase Inhibitor (Human) is indicated for chronic replacement therapy of individuals having congenital deficiency of alpha$_1$-PI (alpha$_1$-antitrypsin deficiency) with clinically demonstrable panacinar emphysema. Clinical and biochemical studies have demonstrated that with such therapy, it is possible to increase plasma levels of alpha$_1$-PI, and that levels of functionally active alpha$_1$-PI in the lung epithelial lining fluid are increased proportionately.[18–20] As some individuals with alpha$_1$-antitrypsin deficiency will not go on to develop panacinar emphysema, only those with early evidence of such disease should be considered for chronic replacement therapy with Alpha$_1$-Proteinase Inhibitor (Human).[22] Subjects with the PiMZ or PiMS phenotypes of alpha$_1$-antitrypsin deficiency should not be considered for such treatment as they appear to be at small risk for panacinar emphysema.[23] Clinical data are not available as to the long-term effects derived from chronic replacement therapy of individuals with alpha$_1$-antitrypsin deficiency with Alpha$_1$-Proteinase Inhibitor (Human). Only adult subjects have received Alpha$_1$-Proteinase Inhibitor (Human) to date.

Alpha$_1$-Proteinase Inhibitor (Human) is not indicated for use in patients other than those with PiZZ, PiZ(null), or Pi(null) (null) phenotypes.

CONTRAINDICATIONS
Individuals with selective IgA deficiencies who have known antibody against IgA (anti-IgA antibody) should not receive Alpha$_1$-Proteinase Inhibitor (Human), PROLASTIN®, since these patients may experience severe reactions, including anaphylaxis, to IgA which may be present.

WARNINGS
Alpha$_1$-Proteinase Inhibitor (Human) is purified from large pools of fresh human plasma obtained from many paid donors. Although each unit of plasma has been found nonreactive for hepatitis B surface antigen (HBsAg) using an FDA approved test, the presence of viruses in such pools must be assumed.

Alpha$_1$-Proteinase Inhibitor (Human) has been heat-treated in solution at 60°C for 10 hours in order to reduce the potential for transmission of infectious agents.[1] No procedure has been found to be totally effective in removing viral infectivity from plasma products. No cases of hepatitis, either hepatitis B or non-A, non-B hepatitis have been recorded to date in individuals receiving Alpha$_1$-Proteinase Inhibitor (Human).[18] However, as all individuals received prophylaxis against hepatitis B, no conclusion can be drawn at this time regarding potential transmission of hepatitis B virus.

PRECAUTIONS
General
1. Administer within 3 hours after reconstitution. Do not refrigerate after reconstitution.
2. Administer only by the intravenous route.
3. As with any colloid solution there will be an increase in plasma volume following intravenous administration of Alpha$_1$-Proteinase Inhibitor (Human), PROLASTIN® [23] Caution should therefore be used in patients at risk for circulatory overload.
4. It is recommended that in preparation for receiving Alpha$_1$-Proteinase Inhibitor (Human) recipients be immunized against hepatitis B using a licensed Hepatitis B Vaccine according to the manufacturer's recommendations. Should it become necessary to treat an individual with Alpha$_1$-Proteinase Inhibitor (Human), and time is insufficient for adequate antibody response to vaccination, individuals should receive a single dose of Hepatitis B Immune Globulin (Human), 0.06 mL/kg body weight, intramuscularly, at the time of administration of the initial dose of Hepatitis B Vaccine.
5. Alpha$_1$-Proteinase Inhibitor (Human) should be given alone, without mixing with other agents or diluting solutions.
6. Administration equipment and any reconstituted Alpha$_1$-Proteinase Inhibitor (Human) not used should be appropriately discarded.

Carcinogenesis, Mutagenesis, Impairment of Fertility
Long term studies in animals to evaluate carcinogenesis, mutagenesis or impairment of fertility have not been conducted.

Pregnancy Category C
Animal reproduction studies have not been conducted with Alpha$_1$-Proteinase Inhibitor (Human), PROLASTIN®. It is also not known whether PROLASTIN can cause fetal harm when administered to a pregnant woman or can affect reproduction capacity. PROLASTIN should be given to a pregnant woman only if clearly needed.

Pediatric Use
Safety and effectiveness in children have not been established.

ADVERSE REACTIONS
Therapeutic administration of Alpha$_1$-Proteinase Inhibitor (Human), 60 mg/kg weekly, has been demonstrated to be well tolerated. In clinical studies, 6 reactions were observed with 517 infusions of Alpha$_1$-Proteinase Inhibitor (Human), or 1.16%. None of the reactions was severe.[18] The adverse reactions reported included delayed fever (maximum temperature rise was 38.9°C, resolving spontaneously over 24 hours) occurring up to 12 hours following treatment (0.77%), lightheadedness (0.19%), and dizziness (0.19%).[18] Mild transient leukocytosis and dilutional anemia several hours after infusion has also been noted.[18]

DOSAGE AND ADMINISTRATION
Each bottle of Alpha$_1$-Proteinase Inhibitor (Human) has the functional activity, as determined by inhibition of porcine pancreatic elastase,[1] stated on the label of the bottle.

The "threshold" level of alpha$_1$-PI in the serum believed to provide adequate anti-elastase activity in the lung of individuals with alpha$_1$-antitrypsin deficiency is 80 mg/dL (based on commercial standards for alpha$_1$-PI immunologic assay).[12,15,17] However, assays of alpha$_1$-PI based on commercial standards measure antigenic activity of alpha$_1$-PI whereas the labeled potency value of alpha$_1$-PI is expressed as actual functional activity, *i.e.*, actual capacity to neutralize porcine pancreatic elastase. As functional activity may be less than antigenic activity serum levels of alpha$_1$-PI determined using commercial immunologic assays may not accurately reflect actual functional alpha$_1$-PI levels. Therefore, although it may be helpful to monitor serum levels of alpha$_1$-PI in individuals receiving Alpha$_1$-Proteinase Inhibitor (Human), PROLASTIN®, using currently available commercial assays of antigenic activity, results of these assays should not be used to determine the required therapeutic dosage.

The recommended dosage of Alpha$_1$-Proteinase Inhibitor (Human) is 60 mg/kg body weight administered once weekly.

This dose is intended to increase and maintain a level of functional alpha$_1$-PI in the epithelial lining of the lower respiratory tract providing adequate anti-elastase activity in the lung of individuals with alpha$_1$-antitrypsin deficiency. Alpha$_1$-Proteinase Inhibitor (Human) may be given at a rate of 0.08 mL/kg/min or greater and must be administered intravenously. The recommended dosage of 60 mg/kg takes approximately 30 minutes to infuse.

Parenteral drug products should be inspected visually for particulate matter and discoloration prior to administration, whenever solution and container permit.

Reconstitution
1. Warm the unopened diluent and concentrate to room temperature (NMT 37°C, 99°F).
2. After removing the plastic flip-top caps (Fig. A), aseptically cleanse rubber stoppers of both bottles.
3. Remove the protective cover from the plastic transfer needle cartridge with tamper-proof seal and penetrate the stopper of the diluent bottle (Fig. B).
4. Remove the remaining portion of the plastic cartridge. Invert the diluent bottle and penetrate the rubber seal on the concentrate bottle (Fig. C) with the needle at an angle.
5. The vacuum will draw the diluent into the concentrate bottle. For best results, and to avoid foaming, hold the diluent bottle at an angle to the concentrate bottle in order to direct the jet of diluent against the wall of the concentrate bottle (Fig. C).
6. After removing the diluent bottle and transfer needle (Fig. D), gently swirl the concentrate bottle until the powder is completely dissolved (Fig. E).
7. Swab top of reconstituted bottle of Alpha$_1$-Proteinase Inhibitor (Human), PROLASTIN® again.
8. Attach the sterile filter needle provided to syringe. With filter needle in place, insert syringe into reconstituted bottle of PROLASTIN® and withdraw PROLASTIN® solution into syringe (Fig. F).
9. To administer PROLASTIN®, replace filter needle with appropriate injection needle and follow procedure for I.V. administration.
10. The contents of more than one bottle of PROLASTIN® may be drawn into the same syringe before administration. If more than one bottle of PROLASTIN® is used, withdraw contents from bottles using aseptic technique. Place contents into an administration container (plastic minibag or glass bottle) using a syringe.* Avoid pushing an I.V. administration set spike into the product container stopper as this has been known to force the stopper into the vial, with a resulting loss of sterility.

*For a patient of average weight (about 70 kg), the volume needed will exceed the limit of one syringe.

Fig. A   Fig. B   Fig. C

Fig. D   Fig. E   Fig. F

HOW SUPPLIED
Alpha$_1$-Proteinase Inhibitor (Human), PROLASTIN®, is supplied in the following single dose vials with the total alpha$_1$-PI functional activity, in milligrams, stated on the label of each vial. A suitable volume of Sterile Water for Injection, USP is provided.

Product Code	Approximate Alpha$_1$-PI Functional Activity	Diluent
601-30	500 mg	20 mL
601-35	1000 mg	40 mL

STORAGE
Alpha$_1$-Proteinase Inhibitor (Human) should be stored under refrigeration (2–8°C; 35–46°F). Freezing should be avoided as breakage of the diluent bottle might occur.

Continued on next page

Miles-Cutter—Cont.

CAUTION
U.S. Federal law prohibits dispensing without a prescription.

LIMITED WARRANTY
A number of factors beyond our control could reduce the efficacy of this product or even result in an ill effect following its use. These include improper storage and handling of the product after it leaves our hands, diagnosis, dosage, method of administration, and biological differences in individual patients. Because of these factors, it is important that this product be stored properly, that the direcitons be followed carefully during use, and that the risk of transmitting viruses be carefully weighed before the product is prescribed. No warranty, express or implied, including any warranty of merchantability or fitness is made. Representatives of the Company are not authorized to vary the terms of the contents of the printed labeling, including the package insert, for this product except by printed notice from the Company's headquarters. Prescriber and user of this product must accept the terms hereof.

REFERENCES
1. Coan MH, Brockway WJ, Eguizabal H, et al: Preparation and properties of alpha$_1$-proteinase inhibitor concentrate from human plasma. *Vox Sang* 48(6):333–42, 1985.
2. Laurell CB, Eriksson S: The electrophoretic alpha$_1$-globulin pattern of serum in alpha$_1$-antitrypsin deficiency. *Scand J Clin Lab Invest* 15:132–40, 1963.
3. Eriksson S: Pulmonary emphysema and alpha$_1$-antitrypsin deficiency. *Acta Med Scand* 175(2):197–205, 1964.
4. Eriksson S: Studies in alpha$_1$-antitrypsin deficiency. *Acta Med Scand Suppl* 432:1–85, 1965.
5. Kueppers F, Black LF: Alpha$_1$-antitrypsin and its deficiency. *Am Rev Respir Dis* 110(2):176–94, 1974.
6. Morse JO: Alpha$_1$-antitrypsin deficiency. *N Engl J Med* 299:1045–8; 1099–105, 1978.
7. Black LF, Kueppers F: Alpha$_1$-antitrypsin deficiency in nonsmokers. *Am Rev Respir Dis* 117(3):421–8, 1978.
8. Tobin JM, Cook PJ, Hutchinson DC: Alpha$_1$-antitrypsin deficiency: the clinical and physiological features of pulmonary emphysema in subjects homozygous for Pi type Z. A survey by the British Thoracic Association. *Br J Dis Chest* 77(1):14–27, 1983.
9. Larsson C: Natural history and life expectancy in severe alpha$_1$-antitrypsin deficiency, Pi Z. *Acta Med Scand* 204(5):345–51, 1978.
10. Pannell R, Johnson D, Travis J: Isolation and properties of human plasma alpha$_1$-proteinase inhibitor. *Biochemistry* 13(26):5439–45, 1974.
11. Lieberman J: Elastase, collagenase, emphysema, and alpha$_1$-antitrypsin deficiency. *Chest* 70(1):62–7, 1976.
12. Gadek JE, Fells GA, Zimmerman RL, et al: Antielastases of the human alveolar structures: Implications for the protease-antiprotease theory of emphysema. *J Clin Invest* 68(4):889–98, 1981.
13. Beatty K, Bieth J, Travis J: Kinetics of association of serine proteinases with native and oxidized alpha-1-proteinase inhibitor and alpha-1-antichymotrypsin. *J Biol Chem* 255(9):3931–4, 1980.
14. Janoff A, White R, Carp H, et al: : Lung injury induced by leukocytic proteases. *Am J Pathol* 97(1):111–36, 1979.
15. Gadek JE, Crystal RG: Alpha$_1$-antitrypsin deficiency. In: Stanbury JB, Wyngaarden JB, Frederickson DS, et al, eds.: *The Metabolic Basis of Inherited Disease* 5th ed. New York, McGraw-Hill, 1983, p. 1450–67.
16. Larsson C, Dirksen H, Sundstrom G, et al: Lung function studies in asymptomatic individuals with moderately (Pi SZ) and severely (Pi Z) reduced levels of alpha$_1$-antitrypsin. *Scand J Respir Dis* 57(6):267–80, 1976.
17. Gadek JE, Klein HG, Holland PV, et al: Replacement therapy of alpha$_1$-antitrypsin deficiency: reversal of protease-antiprotease imbalance within the alveolar structures of PiZ subjects. *J Clin Invest* 68(5):1158–65, 1981.
18. Data on file, Cutter Biological.
19. Wewars M, Casolaro A, Sellers S, et al: Pulmonary Branch, NHLBI, alpha$_1$-antitrypsin (AAT) deficiency replacement study: Chronic augmentation of the antineutrophil elastase capacity of the lower respiratory tract of AAT deficient individuals with a weekly infusion of AAT. (abstract) *Am Rev Respir Dis* 133(4:2):A103, 1986.
20. Wewars MD, Casolaro MA, Crystal RG: Comparison of alpha-1-antitrypsin levels and antineutrophil elastase capacity of blood and lung in a patient with the alpha-1-antitrypsin phenotype null-null before and during alpha-1-antitrypsin augmentation therapy. *Am Rev Respir* 135(3):539-43, 1987.
21. Burrows B: A clinical trial of efficacy of antiproteolytic therapy: can it be done? *Am Rev Respir Dis* 127(2:2):S42–3, 1983.
22. Cohen AB: Unravelling the mysteries of alpha$_1$-antitrypsin deficiency. *N Engl J Med* 314(12):778–9, 1986.
23. Finlayson JS: Albumin products. *Semin Thromb Hemost* 6(2);85-120, 1980.

U.S. License No. 8
Canadian License No. 24   14-7601-001
Issued Nov. 1988

Miles Inc.
Pharmaceutical Division
400 MORGAN LANE
WEST HAVEN, CT 06516

PRODUCT IDENTIFICATION CODES
To provide an accurate identification of Miles Inc. Pharmaceutical Division products, each solid dosage form is coded with the name Miles and a 3 digit product identification number.

PRODUCT	PRODUCT IDENTIFICATION CODE NUMBER
ORAL DOSAGE FORMS	
Adalat Capsules 10 mg (nifedipine/Miles)	811
Adalat Capsules 20 mg (nifedipine/Miles)	821
Biltricide Tablets 600 mg (praziquantel)	521
Cipro Tablets 250 mg (ciprofloxacin HCl/Miles)	512
Cipro Tablets 500 mg (ciprofloxacin HCl/Miles)	513
Cipro Tablets 750 mg (ciprofloxacin HCl/Miles)	514
Decholin® Tablets 250 mg (dehydrocholic acid)	121
Lithane® Tablets 300 mg (lithium carbonate)	951
Mycelex® Troche 10 mg (clotrimazole)	095
Niclocide® Chewable Tablets 500 mg (niclosamide)	721
Stilphostrol® Tablets 50 mg (diethylstilbestrol diphosphate)	132
NON-ORAL DOSAGE FORMS	
Domeboro® Tablets (aluminum sulfate, calcium acetate)	411
Mycelex®-G Vaginal Tablets 100 mg (clotrimazole)	093
Mycelex®-G 500 mg Vaginal Tablets (clotrimazole)	097
Nimotop® Capsules 30 mg (nimodipine/Miles)	855

ADALAT®   ℞
Capsules
(nifedipine/Miles)
For Oral Use

PRODUCT OVERVIEW

KEY FACTS
Adalat (nifedipine) is a vasospecific antianginal drug of the calcium channel blocker class. The hemodynamic and electrophysiological actions of Adalat make it especially appropriate in patients with angina and coexisting cardiovascular conditions. (see Mechanism of Action section below.)

MAJOR USES
Adalat can be used in patients with vasospastic angina and in angina suggestive of a vasospastic component, as well as in patients with chronic stable angina without vasospasm who are unresponsive or intolerant to beta blockers and/or organic nitrates.

SAFETY INFORMATION
Careful monitoring of blood pressure is suggested during initial administration and titration, since Adalat decreases peripheral vascular resistance. Patients only rarely discontinue Adalat therapy because of its adverse effects, and unwanted effects on the cardiovascular system are usually not serious.

PRESCRIBING INFORMATION
ADALAT®   ℞
Capsules
(nifedipine/Miles)
For Oral Use

DESCRIPTION
ADALAT (nifedipine) is an antianginal drug belonging to a new class of pharmacological agents, the calcium channel blockers. Nifedipine is 3, 5-pyridinedicarboxylic acid, 1,4-dihydro-2, 6-dimethyl-4-(2-nitrophenyl)-, dimethyl ester, $C_{17}H_{18}N_2O_6$, and has the structural formula:

Nifedipine is a yellow crystalline substance, practically insoluble in water but soluble in ethanol. It has a molecular weight of 346.3. ADALAT CAPSULES are formulated as soft gelatin capsules for oral administration each containing 10 mg or 20 mg of nifedipine. Inert ingredients in the formulations are: glycerin; peppermint oil; polyethylene glycol 400; soft gelatin capsules (which may contain FDC Yellow No. 6 and Red Ferric Oxide, and other inert ingredients), and water. The 10 mg capsules also contain saccharin sodium.

CLINICAL PHARMACOLOGY
ADALAT is a calcium ion influx inhibitor (slow channel blocker or calcium ion antagonist) and inhibits the transmembrane influx of calcium ions into cardiac muscle and smooth muscle. The contractile processes of cardiac muscle and vascular smooth muscle are dependent upon the movement of extracellular calcium ions into these cells through specific ion channels. ADALAT selectively inhibits calcium ion influx across the cell membrane of cardiac muscle and vascular smooth muscle without changing serum calcium concentrations.

Mechanism of Action
The precise means by which this inhibition relieves angina has not been fully determined, but includes at least the following two mechanisms:

1) Relaxation and prevention of coronary artery spasm
ADALAT dilates the main coronary arteries and coronary arterioles, both in normal and ischemic regions, and is a potent inhibitor of coronary artery spasm, whether spontaneous or ergonovine-induced. This property increases myocardial oxygen delivery in patients with coronary artery spasm, and is responsible for the effectiveness of ADALAT in vasospastic (Prinzmetal's or variant) angina. Whether this effect plays any role in classical angina is not clear, but studies of exercise tolerance have not shown an increase in the maximum exercise rate-pressure product, a widely accepted measure of oxygen utilization. This suggests that, in general, relief of spasm or dilation of coronary arteries is not an important factor in classical angina.

2) Reduction of oxygen utilization
ADALAT regularly reduces arterial pressure at rest and at a given level of exercise by dilating peripheral arterioles and reducing the total peripheral resistance (afterload) against which the heart works. This unloading of the heart reduces myocardial energy consumption and oxygen requirements and probably accounts for the effectiveness of ADALAT in chronic stable angina.

Pharmacokinetics and Metabolism
ADALAT is rapidly and fully absorbed after oral administration. The drug is detectable in serum 10 minutes after oral administration, and peak blood levels occur in approximately 30 minutes. It is highly bound by serum proteins. ADALAT® is extensively converted to inactive metabolites and approximately 80 percent of ADALAT and metabolites are eliminated via the kidneys. The half-life of nifedipine in plasma is approximately two hours. There is no information on the effects of renal or hepatic impairment on excretion or metabolism of ADALAT.

Hemodynamics
Like other slow channel blockers, ADALAT exerts a negative inotropic effect on isolated myocardial tissue. This rarely, if ever, seen in intact animals or man, probably because of reflex responses to its vasodilating effects. In man, ADALAT causes decreased peripheral vascular resistance and a fall in systolic and diastolic pressure, usually modest (5–10mm Hg systolic), but sometimes larger. There is usually a small increase in heart rate, a reflex response to vasodilation. Measurements of cardiac function in patients with normal ventricular function have generally found a small increase in cardiac index without major effects on ejection fraction, left ventricular and diastolic pressure (LVEDP) or volume (LVEDV). In patients with impaired ventricular function, most acute studies have shown some increase in ejection fraction and reduction in left ventricular filing pressure.

Electrophysiologic Effects
Although like other members of its class, ADALAT decreases sinoatrial node function and atrioventricular conduction in isolated myocardial preparations, such effects have not been seen in studies in intact animals or in man. In formal electrophysiologic studies, predominantly in patients

with normal conduction systems, ADALAT has had no tendency to prolong atrioventricular conduction, prolong sinus node recovery time, or slow sinus rate.

INDICATIONS AND USAGE

I. Vasospastic Angina

ADALAT (nifedipine) is indicated for the management of vasospastic angina confirmed by any of the following criteria: 1) classical pattern of angina at rest accompanied by ST segment elevation, 2) angina or coronary artery spasm provoked by ergonovine, or 3) angiographically demonstrated coronary artery spasm. In those patients who have had angiography, the presence of significant fixed obstructive disease is not incompatible with the diagnosis of vasospastic angina, provided that the above criteria are satisfied. ADALAT may also be used where the clinical presentation suggests a possible vasospastic component but where vasospasm has not been confirmed, e.g., where pain has a variable threshold on exertion or in unstable angina where electrocardiographic findings are compatible with intermittent vasospasm, or when angina is refractory to nitrates and/or adequate doses of beta blockers.

II. Chronic Stable Angina

(Classical Effort-Associated Angina)

ADALAT is indicated for the management of chronic stable angina (effort-associated angina) without evidence of vasospasm in patients who remain symptomatic despite adequate doses of beta blockers and/or organic nitrates or who cannot tolerate those agents.

In chronic stable angina (effort-associated angina) ADALAT has been effective in controlled trials of up to eight weeks duration in reducing angina frequency and increasing exercise tolerance, but confirmation of sustained effectiveness and evaluation of long term safety in these patients are incomplete.

Controlled studies in small numbers of patients suggest concomitant use of ADALAT® and beta blocking agents may be beneficial in patients with chronic stable angina, but available information is not sufficient to predict with confidence the effects of concurrent treatment, especially in patients with compromised left ventricular function or cardiac conduction abnormalities. When introducing such concomitant therapy, care must be taken to monitor blood pressure closely since severe hypotension can occur from the combined effects of the drugs. (See WARNINGS).

CONTRAINDICATIONS

Known hypersensitivity reaction to ADALAT.

WARNINGS

Excessive Hypotension

Although in most patients, the hypotensive effect of ADALAT is modest and well tolerated, occasional patients have had exessive and poorly tolerated hypotension. These responses have usually occurred during initial titration or at the time of subsequent upward dosage adjustment, and may be more likely in patients on concomitant beta blockers. Severe hypotension and/or increased fluid volume requirements have been reported in patients receiving ADALAT together with a beta blocking agent who underwent coronary artery bypass surgery using high dose fentanyl anesthesia. The interaction with high dose fentanyl appears to be due to the combination of ADALAT and a beta blocker, but the possibility that it may occur with ADALAT alone, with low doses of fentanyl, in other surgical procedures, or with other narcotic analgesics can not be ruled out. In ADALAT treated patients where surgery using high dose fentanyl anesthesia is contemplated, the physician should be aware of these potential problems and, if the patient's condition permits, sufficient time (at least 36 hours) should be allowed for ADALAT to be washed out of the body prior to surgery.

Increased Angina

Occasional patients have developed well documented increased frequency, duration or severity of angina on starting ADALAT or at the time of dosage increases. The mechanism of this response is not established but could result from decreased coronary perfusion associated with decreased diastolic pressure with increased heart rate, or from increased demand resulting from increased heart rate alone.

Beta Blocker Withdrawal

Patients recently withdrawn from beta blockers may develop a withdrawal syndrome with increased angina, probably related to increased sensitivity to catecholamines. Initiation of ADALAT treatment will not prevent this occurrence and might be expected to exacerbate it by provoking reflex catecholamine release. There have been occasional reports of increased angina in a setting of beta blocker withdrawal and ADALAT initiation. It is important to taper beta blockers if possible rather than stopping them abruptly before beginning ADALAT.

Congestive Heart Failure

Rarely, patients, usually receiving a beta blocker, have developed heart failure after beginning ADALAT. Patients with tight aortic stenosis may be at greater risk for such an event, as the unloading effect of ADALAT® would be expected to be of less benefit to these patients, owing to their fixed impedance to flow across the aortic valve.

PRECAUTIONS

General: Hypotension: Because ADALAT decreases peripheral vascular resistance, careful monitoring of blood pressure during the initial administration and titration of ADALAT is suggested. Close observation is especially recommended for patients already taking medications that are known to lower blood pressure. (See WARNINGS).

Peripheral edema: Mild to moderate peripheral edema, typically associated with arterial vasodilation and not due to left ventricular dysfunction, occurs in about one in ten patients treated with ADALAT (nifedipine). This edema occurs primarily in the lower extremities and usually responds to diuretic therapy. With patients whose angina is complicated by congestive heart failure, care should be taken to differentiate this peripheral edema from the effects of increasing left ventricular dysfunction.

Laboratory tests: Rare, usually transient, but occasionally significant elevations of enzymes such as alkaline phosphatase, CPK, LDH, SGOT and SGPT have been noted. The relationship to ADALAT therapy is uncertain in most cases, but probable in some. These laboratory abnormalities have rarely been associated with clinical symptoms, however, cholestasis with or without jaundice has been reported. Rare instances of allergic hepatitis have been reported.

ADALAT, like other calcium channel blockers, decreases platelet aggregation *in vitro*. Limited clinical studies have demonstrated a moderate but statistically significant decrease in platelet aggregation and increase in bleeding time in some ADALAT patients. This is thought to be a function of inhibition of calcium transport across the platelet membrane. No clinical significance for these findings has been demonstrated.

Although ADALAT has been used safely in patients with renal dysfunction and has been reported to exert a beneficial effect in certain cases, rare, reversible elevations in BUN and serum creatinine have been reported in patients with pre-existing chronic renal insufficiency. The relationship to ADALAT therapy is uncertain in most cases, but probable in some.

Drug Interactions: Beta-adrenergic blocking agents: (See INDICATIONS and WARNINGS). Experience in over 1400 patients in a non-comparative clinical trial has shown that concomitant administration of ADALAT and beta-blocking agents is usually well tolerated, but there have been occasional literature reports suggesting that the combination may increase the likelihood of congestive heart failure, severe hypotension or exacerbation of angina.

Long acting nitrates: ADALAT may be safely co-administered with nitrates, but there have been no controlled studies to evaluate the antianginal effectiveness of this combination.

Digitalis: Administration of ADALAT with digoxin increased digoxin levels in nine of twelve normal volunteers. The average increase was 45%. Another investigator found no increase in digoxin levels in thirteen patients with coronary artery disease. In an uncontrolled study of over two hundred patients with congestive heart failure during which digoxin blood levels were not measured, digitalis toxicity was not observed. Since there have been isolated reports of patients with elevated digoxin levels, it is recommended that digoxin levels be monitored when initiating, adjusting, and discontinuing ADALAT to avoid possible over- or underdigitalization.

Coumarin anticoagulants: There have been rare reports of increased prothrombin time in patients taking coumarin anticoagulants to whom ADALAT® was administered. However, the relationship to ADALAT therapy is uncertain.

Cimetidine: A study in six healthy volunteers has shown a significant increase in peak nifedipine plasma levels (80%) and area-under-the-curve (74%) after a one week course of cimetidine at 1000 mg per day and nifedipine at 40 mg per day. Ranitidine produced smaller, non-significant increases. The effect may be mediated by the known inhibition of cimetidine on hepatic cytochrome P-450, the enzyme system probably responsible for the first-pass metabolism of nifedipine. If nifedipine therapy is initiated in a patient currently receiving cimetidine, cautious titration is advised.

Carcinogenesis, mutagenesis, impairment of fertility: Nifedipine was administered orally to rats for two years and was not shown to be carcinogenic. When given to rats prior to mating, nifedipine caused reduced fertility at a dose approximately 30 times the maximum recommended human dose. *In vitro* mutagenicity studies were negative.

Pregnancy: Pregnancy category C. Nifedipine has been shown to be teratogenic in rats when given in doses 30 times the maximum recommended human dose. Nifedipine was embryotoxic (increased fetal resorptions, decreased fetal weight, increased stunted forms, increased fetal deaths, decreased neonatal survival) in rats, mice and rabbits at doses of from 3 to 10 times the maximum recommended human dose. In pregnant monkeys, doses ⅔ and twice the maximum recommended human dose resulted in small placentas and underdeveloped chorionic villi. In rats doses three times maximum human dose and higher caused prolongation of pregnancy. There are no adequate and well controlled studies in pregnant women. ADALAT should be used during pregnancy only if the potential benefit justifies the potential risk to the fetus.

ADVERSE REACTIONS

In multiple-dose U.S. and foreign controlled studies in which adverse reactions were reported spontaneously, adverse effects were frequent but generally not serious and rarely required discontinuation of therapy or dosage adjustment. Most were expected consequences of the vasodilator effects of ADALAT.

Adverse Reactions	ADALAT (%) (N = 226)	Placebo (%) (N = 235)
Dizziness, lightheadedness, giddiness	27	15
Flushing, heat sensation	25	8
Headache	23	20
Weakness	12	10
Nausea, heartburn	11	8
Muscle cramps, tremor	8	3
Peripheral edema	7	1
Nervousness, mood changes	7	4
Palpitation	7	5
Dyspnea, cough, wheezing	6	3
Nasal congestion, sore throat	6	8

There is also a large uncontrolled experience in over 2100 patients in the United States. Most of the patients had vasospastic or resistant angina pectoris, and about half had concomitant treatment with beta-adrenergic blocking agents. The most common adverse events were:

Incidence Approximately 10%
Cardiovascular: peripheral edema
Central Nervous System: dizziness or lightheadedness
Gastrointestinal: nausea
Systemic: headache and flushing, weakness

Incidence Approximately 5%
Cardiovascular: transient hypotension

Incidence 2% or Less
Cardiovascular: palpitation
Respiratory: nasal and chest congestion, shortness of breath
Gastrointestinal: diarrhea, constipation, cramps, flatulence
Musculoskeletal: inflammation, joint stiffness, muscle cramps
Central Nervous System: shakiness, nervousness, jitteriness, sleep disturbances, blurred vision, difficulties in balance
Other: dermatitis, pruritus, urticaria, fever, sweating, chills, sexual difficulties

Incidence Approximately 0.5%
Cardiovascular: syncope. Syncopal episodes did not recur with reduction in the dose of ADALAT® or concomitant antianginal medication.

Incidence Less Than 0.5%
Hematologic: thrombocytopenia, anemia, leukopenia, purpura
Gastrointestinal: allergic hepatitis
Oral: gingival hyperplasia
Other: erythromelalgia

Several of these side effects appear to be dose related. Peripheral edema occurred in about one in 25 patients at doses less than 60 mg per day and in about one patient in eight at 120 mg per day or more. Transient hypotension, generally of mild to moderate severity and seldom requiring discontinuation of therapy, occurred in one of 50 patients at less than 60 mg per day and in one of 20 patients at 120 mg per day or more. Very rarely, introduction of ADALAT therapy was associated with an increase in anginal pain, possibly due to associated hypotension.

In addition, more serious adverse events were observed, not readily distinguishable from the natural history of the disease in these patients. It remains possible, however, that some or many of these events were drug related. Myocardial infarction occurred in about 4% of patients and congestive heart failure or pulmonary edema in about 2%. Ventricular arrhythmias or conduction disturbances each occurred in fewer than 0.5% of patients.

In a subgroup of over 1000 patients receiving ADALAT with concomitant beta blocker therapy, the pattern and incidence of adverse experiences was not different from that of the entire group of ADALAT treated patients (See PRECAUTIONS).

In a subgroup of approximately 250 patients with a diagnosis of congestive heart failure as well as angina, dizziness or lightheadedness, peripheral edema, headache or flushing each occurred in one in eight patients. Hypotension occurred in about one in 20 patients. Syncope occurred in approximately one patient in 250. Myocardial infarction or symptoms of congestive heart failure each occurred in about one

Continued on next page

Miles Pharm. Div.—Cont.

patient in 15. Atrial or ventricular dysrhythmias each occurred in about one patient in 150.

OVERDOSAGE

Although there is no well documented experience with ADALAT® overdosage, available data suggest that gross overdosage could result in excessive peripheral vasodilation with subsequent marked and probably prolonged systemic hypotension. Clinically significant hypotension due to ADALAT overdosage calls for active cardiovascular support including monitoring of cardiac and respiratory function, elevation of extremities, and attention to circulating fluid volume and urine output. A vasoconstrictor (such as norepinephrine) may be helpful in restoring vascular tone and blood pressure, provided that there is no contraindication to its use. Clearance of ADALAT would be expected to be prolonged in patients with impaired liver function. Since ADALAT is highly protein-bound, dialysis is not likely to be of benefit.

DOSAGE AND ADMINISTRATION

The dosage of ADALAT needed to suppress angina and that can be tolerated by the patient must be established by titration. Excessive doses can result in hypotension. The starting dose is one 10 mg capsule, swallowed whole, 3 times/day. The usual effective dose range is 10–20 mg three times daily. Some patients, especially those with evidence of coronary artery spasm, respond only to higher doses, more frequent administration, or both. In such patients, doses of 20–30 mg three or four times daily may be effective. Doses above 120 mg daily are rarely necessary. More than 180 mg per day is not recommended.

In most cases, ADALAT titration should proceed over a 7–14 day period so that the physician can assess the response to each dose level and monitor the blood pressure before proceeding to higher doses.

If symptoms so warrant, titration may proceed more rapidly provided that the patient is assessed frequently. Based on the patient's physical activity level, attack frequency, and sublingual nitroglycerin consumption, the dose of ADALAT may be increased from 10 mg t.i.d. to 20 mg t.i.d. and then to 30 mg t.i.d. over a three-day period.

In hospitalized patients under close observation, the dose may be increased in 10 mg increments over four to six-hour periods as required to control pain and arrhythmias due to ischemia. A single dose should rarely exceed 30 mg.

No "rebound effect" has been observed upon discontinuation of ADALAT. However, if discontinuation of ADALAT is necessary, sound clinical practice suggests that the dosage should be decreased gradually with close physician supervision.

Co-Administration with Other Antianginal Drugs

Sublingual nitroglycerin may be taken as required for the control of acute manifestations of angina, particularly during ADALAT titration. See **Precautions, Drug Interactions,** for information on co-administration of ADALAT with beta blockers or long acting nitrates.

HOW SUPPLIED

ADALAT soft gelatin capsules are supplied in:

Bottles of 100:   10 mg (NDC 0026-8811-51) orange
     20 mg (NDC 0026-8821-51)
     orange and light brown

Bottles of 300:   10 mg (NDC 0026-8811-18) orange
     20 mg (NDC 0026-8821-18)
     orange and light brown

Unit dose packages   10 mg (NDC 0026-8811-48) orange
of 100:   20 mg (NDC 0026-8821-48) orange and
     light brown

The capsules are identified as follows: 10 mg (Miles 811), 20 mg (Miles 821).

The capsules should be protected from light and moisture and stored at controlled room temperature 59° to 77°F (15° to 25°C). Dispense in tight, light resistant containers (USP).

Encapsulated by
R.P. Scherer N.A.
Clearwater, FL 33518
Manufactured by
Miles Inc.
Pharmaceutical Division
400 Morgan Lane
West Haven, CT 06516
PD 100678   BAY a 1040   0650   Rev. 10/88
Shown in Product Identification Section, page 419

ANA–KIT®
ANAPHYLAXIS EMERGENCY TREATMENT KIT   ℞

DESCRIPTION

Epinephrine Injection, USP, (1:1000), contained in a sterile, 1 mL syringe, designed to deliver 2 doses of 0.3 mL each. Product is intended for subcutaneous or intramuscular use. Each mL of Epinephrine Injection, USP, (1:1000) contains 1 mg *l*-epinephrine as the hydrochloride, 8.5 mg sodium chlo-

ride, not more than 5 mg chlorobutanol (chloral derivative) and 1.5 mg sodium bisulfite.

Epinephrine is a sympathomimetic catecholamine. Its naturally occurring levo isomer, which is twenty times as active as the *d* isomer, is now obtained in pure form by separation from the synthetically produced racemate.

Chemically, epinephrine is β-(3,4-dihydroxyphenyl)-α-methylaminoethanol with the following structure:

Chlo-Amine® Chlorpheniramine Maleate Tablets: 4 chewable tablets, each containing 2 mg chlorpheniramine maleate, USP, for oral administration. Contains FD&C Yellow No. 6 (Sunset Yellow) as a color additive. Chlorpheniramine maleate is an antihistamine having the chemical name γ-(4-chlorophenyl)-N,N-dimethyl-2-pyridinepropanamine, (Z)-2-butenedioate(1:1) with the following structure:

DEVICES: 2 sterile pads containing isopropyl alcohol 70% by volume. One tourniquet.

CLINICAL PHARMACOLOGY

EPINEPHRINE: The most valuable drug for the emergency treatment of severe allergic reactions is epinephrine. The vasoconstrictor effect of epinephrine on the capillary directly antagonizes the generalized vasodilation produced by histamine. Epinephrine reverses the increased permeability of dilated capillaries to plasma. The shock of severe allergic reactions is due to the loss of circulating blood volume by pooling in the dilated capillary beds and loss of plasma into the tissues. Epinephrine quickly restores circulating blood volume and blood pressure by constricting the capillary bed. The itching during episodes of hives or angioedema is promptly relieved by epinephrine. Epinephrine is a powerful relaxer of the smooth muscle of the bronchioles, stomach, intestine, pregnant uterus and urinary bladder wall. The bronchospasm, wheezing and dyspnea of the acute allergic reactions are relieved. Where abdominal cramping, defecation or involuntary urination have occurred during severe allergic attacks, epinephrine rapidly produces relief. Subcutaneously or intramuscularly administered epinephrine has a rapid onset and short duration of action. Subcutaneous administration during asthmatic attacks may produce bronchodilation within 5 to 10 minutes, and maximal effects may occur within 20 minutes.

CHLO-AMINE: Chlo-Amine is an effective agent in nullifying the characteristic effects of histamine and is especially valuable in the prophylaxis and relief of many allergic symptoms. It is readily absorbed from the intestinal tract and released into the tissues from the bloodstream. This action is both prompt and sustained. Elimination of the drug is such that there is a low incidence of side effects.

INDICATIONS AND USAGE

HOLLISTER-STIER Anaphylaxis Emergency Treatment Kit (Ana-Kit®) is indicated for use by adult and pediatric patients under the following situations:

1. Allergic reactions including anaphylactic shock due to stinging insects (primarily of the Hymenoptera order, which includes bees, wasps, hornets, yellow jackets, bumble bees, and fire ants.

2. Severe allergic or anaphylactoid reactions due to allergy injections, exposures to pollens, dusts, molds, foods, drugs, and exercise or unknown substances (so-called idiopathic anaphylaxis).

3. Severe, life-threatening asthma attacks characterized by wheezing, dyspnea and inability to breathe.

In the sensitive patient, severe allergic reactions and anaphylactic shock may occur within minutes of the insect sting or exposure to an allergenic substance.

Symptoms may include bronchoconstriction, wheezing, sneezing, hoarseness, urticaria, angioedema, erythema, pruritis, tachycardia, thready pulse, falling blood pressure, sense of oppression or impending doom, disorientation, cramping abdominal pain, incontinance, faintness, loss of consciousness.

The Ana-Kit is compactly designed to be carried and used by patients when severe symptoms arise, and the patient is out of reach of immediate attention by a doctor or hospital.

CONTRAINDICATIONS

EPINEPHRINE: Epinephrine must not be given intra-arterially as marked vasoconstriction may result in gangrene. **This unit is not intended for intravenous use.** Further dilution would be necessary and is not practical with this emergency syringe.

Epinephrine Injection, USP, (1:1000) must not be used if there is hypersensitivity to any of the components.

Epinephrine is contraindicated in narrow-angle glaucoma; cardiogenic, traumatic, or hemorrhagic shock; cardiac dilation; cerebral arteriosclerosis; and organic brain damage. Epinephrine should not be used to counteract circulatory collapse or hypotension due to phenothiazines, since such agents may reverse the pressor effect of epinephrine, leading to a further lowering of blood pressure.

Epinephrine should not be administered concomitantly with other sympathomimetic agents, since the effects are additive and may be detrimental to the patient.

CHLO-AMINE: No known contraindications.

WARNINGS

EPINEPHRINE: Overdosage or accidental intravenous administration of conventional subcutaneous doses may induce severe or fatal hypertension, or cerebrovascular hemorrhage. Fatalities may also occur from pulmonary edema resulting from peripheral constriction and cardiac stimulation. The marked pressor effects may be counteracted by use of rapidly acting vasodilators, such as the nitrites and alpha-adrenergic blockers.

Deaths have been reported in asthmatics treated with epinephrine following the use of isoproterenol or orciprenaline. Epinephrine is the preferred treatment for serious allergic or other emergency situations even though this product contains sodium bisulfite, a sulfite that may in other products cause allergic-type reactions including anaphylactic symptoms or life-threatening or less severe asthmatic episodes in certain susceptible persons. The alternatives to using epinephrine in a life-threatening situation may not be satisfactory. The presence of a sulfite(s) in this product should not deter administration of the drug for treatment of serious allergic or other emergency situations.

Epinephrine must be administered with great caution, if at all, in patients with cardiac arrhythmias, coronary artery or organic heart disease, and hypertension. In patients with coronary insufficiency or ischemic heart disease, epinephrine may precipitate or aggravate angina pectoris as well as produce potentially fatal ventricular arrhythmias. Epinephrine should be administered only with great caution to elderly patients, those with diabetes mellitus, hyperthyroidism or psychoneurotic disorders; also to those with longstanding bronchial asthma or emphysema if such individuals may also have degenerative heart disease, and to pregnant women (see "Pregnancy").

CHLO-AMINE®: Chlorpheniramine maleate should be used with extreme caution in patients with stenosing peptic ulcer, pyloroduodenal obstruction, prostatic hypertrophy, or bladder neck obstruction. These compounds have an atropine-like action and therefore should be used with caution in patients with a history of increased intraocular pressure, cardiovascular disease, or hypertension. The asthmatic patient should take the chlorpheniramine maleate tablets with caution.

PRECAUTIONS

GENERAL: Hollister-Stier Ana-Kit® is not intended to be a substitute for medical attention or hospital care. The kit is designed to be compact and easy to carry, and to provide emergency treatment when medical care is not immediately available. Highly sensitive individuals should have the kit readily available at all times. Because of its small size it can be carried by outdoor sportsmen, golfers, gardeners, or any sensitive individual who may be exposed to stinging insects (wasps, hornets, yellow jackets, fire ants or bees) or other potentially life-threatening allergens. The drugs in the Ana-Kit®, when used as directed immediately following exposure to an allergen, may prove life-saving. Certain changes in the emergency instructions and in the kit itself may be made by the doctor according to the needs of the patient. IN ALL CASES THE PHYSICIAN SHOULD INSTRUCT THE PATIENT, AND/OR ANY OTHER PERSON WHO MIGHT BE IN A POSITION TO ADMINISTER THE EPINEPHRINE, IN THE PROPER USE OF THE SYRINGE AND THE OTHER COMPONENTS OF THIS KIT.

The effects of epinephrine may be potentiated by **tricyclic antidepressants,** sodium levothyroxine, and certain antihistamines, notably chlorpheniramine, tripeiennamine, and diphenhydramine.

Carcinogenesis, Mutagenesis, Impairment of Fertility: There are no data from either animal or human studies regarding the carcinogenicity or mutagenicity of epinephrine or Chlo-Amine, and no studies have been conducted to determine their potential for the impairment of fertility.

Pregnancy: Teratogenic Effects. Pregnancy Category C—Epinephrine has been shown to be teratogenic in rats and hamsters at dose levels hundreds of times as high as the maximal human dose. Although there are no adequate or well-controlled studies in pregnant women, epinephrine crosses the placenta and its use during pregnancy may cause anoxia in the fetus. Epinephrine should be used in pregnancy only if the potential benefit justifies the potential risk to the fetus. **Pediatric Use:** Administer Epinephrine or Chlo-Amine with caution to infants and children (see "Dosage and Administration"). Syncope has occurred following the administration of epinephrine to asthmatic children.

INFORMATION FOR PATIENTS: Complete patient information, including dosage, directions for proper administration, and precautions, can be found at the end of this package insert, as well as inside each Ana-Kit® kit.

ADVERSE REACTIONS

EPINEPHRINE: Adverse reactions include transient, moderate anxiety, apprehensiveness, restlessness, tremor, weakness, dizziness, sweating, palpitations, pallor, nausea and vomiting, headache, and respiratory difficulties. These symptoms occur in some persons receiving therapeutic doses of epinephrine, but are more likely to occur, or to occur in exaggerated form, in those with hypertension or hyperthyroidism. Excessive doses cause acute hypertension and cardiac arrhythmias.

CHLO-AMINE: Drowsiness, dizziness, blurred vision, dry mouth and gastrointestinal upsets may occur. Patients should not drive or operate machinery after taking the drug. Large doses produce central nervous system depression and occasionally tremors or convulsions. Reports of hematological disorders are rare.

OVERDOSAGE

EPINEPHRINE: Epinephrine is rapidly inactivated in the body, and treatment is primarily supportive. If necessary, pressor effects may be counteracted by rapidly acting vasodilators or alpha-adrenergic blocking drugs. If prolonged hypotension follows such measures, it may be necessary to administer another pressor drug, such as levarterenol.

If an epinephrine overdose induces pulmonary edema that interferes with respiration, treatment consists of a rapidly acting alpha-adrenergic blocking drug such as phentolamine and/or intermittent positive-pressure respiration.

Epinephrine overdosage can also cause transient bradycardia followed by tachycardia, and these may be accompanied by potentially fatal cardiac arrhythmias. Ventricular premature contractions may appear within one minute after injection and may be followed by multifocal ventricular tachycardia (prefibrillation rhythm). Subsidence of the ventricular effects may be followed by atrial tachycardia and occasionally by atrioventricular block. Treatment of arrhythmias consists of administration of beta-adrenergic blocking drug such as propranolol.

Overdosage sometimes also results in extreme pallor and coldness of the skin, metabolic acidosis, and kidney failure. Suitable corrective measures must be taken.

CHLO-AMINE: Overdose symptoms may be sedation, apnea, cardiovascular collapse to stimulation, insomnia, hallucinations, tremors or convulsions. Also there may be dizziness, tinnitus, ataxia, blurred vision, hypotension, dry mouth, flushing, and abdominal symptoms.

Treatment—The patient should be induced to vomit, preferably with ipecac syrup—and large amounts of water. Prevent aspiration of vomitus. Gastric lavage may be necessary using activated charcoal and saline. Hyperosmotic cathartics such as Milk of Magnesia may hasten elimination of residual cling. Vasopressors can be used to correct hypotension. Diazepan may be used to control seizures. Hyperpyrexia can be treated with cool sponges or a hypothermic blanket.

DOSAGE AND ADMINISTRATION

The physician who prescribes the Ana-Kit® should review the package insert in detail with the patient. This review should include the proper use of the 2-dose epinephrine syringe to insure that subcutaneous or intramuscular injections are given into the deltoid region of the arm or the anterolateral aspect of the thigh. See also the PATIENT DIRECTIONS FOR USE.

EPINEPHRINE: For subcutaneous or intramuscular injection only.

Adults and children over 12 years: 0.3 mL; 6–12 years: 0.2 mL; 2–6 years: 0.15 mL; Infants to 2 years: 0.05 to 0.1 mL. When syringe is properly set up, as directed in the Patient Instruction Sheet, a 0.3 mL dose is administered when plunger is pushed until it stops. Syringe barrel has 0.1 mL graduations so that smaller doses can be measured. (Operation of syringe is explained in the Patient Directions For Use section at the end of this package insert.)

If after 10 minutes from the first injection symptoms are not noticeably improved, administer a second dose of epinephrine from the syringe.

CHLO-AMINE: Tablets are chewable antihistamines. Adults and children over 12 years: 4 tablets; children 6–12 years: 2 tablets; children under 6 years: 1 tablet.

HOW SUPPLIED

HOLLISTER-STIER ANAPHYLAXIS EMERGENCY TREATMENT KIT (ANA-KIT®) CONTAINS:

SYRINGE: One sterile syringe containing 1 mL Epinephrine Injection, USP, (1:1000). Syringe delivers two 0.3 mL doses.

TABLETS: Four 2 mg chewable Chlo-Amine® tablets, Chlorpheniramine Maleate Tablets.

DEVICES: Two sterile pads containing 70% isopropyl alcohol (by volume) and 1 tourniquet.

PROTECT FROM LIGHT. KEEP AT ROOM TEMPERATURE, APPROX. 25°C (77°F), PROTECT FROM FREEZING.

CAUTION: U.S. Federal Law Prohibits Dispensing Without Prescription.

Epinephrine Mfg. by: Wyeth Laboratories, Inc.,
Philadelphia, PA 19101
Pkgd. and Dist. by:
Hollister-Stier
Miles Inc.
Pharmaceutical Division
Spokane, WA 99207 USA

PATIENT DIRECTIONS FOR USE
ANA-KIT® Anaphylaxis Emergency Treatment Kit
(Please read entire direction sheet before an emergency arises.)

The Ana-Kit® **IS TO BE USED ONLY WHEN PRESCRIBED BY A PHYSICIAN,** for patients who are highly allergic to pollens, foods, dusts, insect stings, and drugs which may produce a life-threatening anaphylactic reaction, or have severe asthma attacks.

IN THE EVENT OF A LIFE-THREATENING SITUATION, FOLLOW THESE STEPS IMMEDIATELY TO ADMINISTER THE EPINEPHRINE.

1. Remove red rubber needle cover. Hold syringe upright and push plunger to expel air and excess epinephrine (plunger will stop).
2. Rotate rectangular plunger ¼ turn to the right. Plunger will align with slot in barrel of syringe. Wipe injection site with alcohol swab.
3. Insert needle straight into arm or thigh as illustrated.
4. Push plunger until it stops. Syringe will inject a 0.3 mL dose for adults and children over 12 years.
   Children: Syringe barrel has 0.1 mL graduations so that smaller doses can be measured. Administer to infants to 2 years: 0.05 to 0.1 mL; 2–6 years: 0.15 mL; and 6–12 years: 0.2 mL.

ONCE THE INITIAL EPINEPHRINE INJECTION HAS BEEN ADMINISTERED, FOLLOW THESE ADDITIONAL STEPS.

1. CONTACT PHYSICIAN, IF POSSIBLE.
2. REMOVE STINGER if stung by insect. (Use fingernails. DO NOT push, pinch or squeeze, or further imbed the stinger into the skin as this may cause further venom to be injected.)
3. APPLY TOURNIQUET. If exposure to life-threatening agent was by injection (allergic extract, drug) or insect sting on an arm or leg, place tourniquet between injection or sting site and body. (If exposure is elsewhere—neck, face, or body—proceed immediately to Step 5.)
4. TIGHTEN TOURNIQUET. To tighten, pull on the end of ONE STRING. Then, at least every ten minutes, loosen the tourniquet by pulling on the small metal ring.
5. CHEW AND SWALLOW CHLO-AMINE TABLETS. For adults and children over 12 years, take 4 tablets; children 6–12 years take 2 tablets; children under 6 years take 1 tablet. These tablets are chewable antihistamine which is generally tolerated.
6. PREPARE SYRINGE FOR A POSSIBLE SECOND INJECTION. Turn the rectangular plunger ¼ turn to the right to line up with rectangular slot in the syringe. (A slight wiggling may aid the turning and alignment of the plunger.)
7. THE SECOND INJECTION. If after 10 minutes from the first injection symptoms are not noticeably improved, a second injection is required.

Cleanse skin area with alcohol swab and make second injection as in STEPS 3 and 4 for the first epinephrine injection. (A small amount of epinephrine will remain in syringe after the second dose and cannot be expelled.) **Note:** Dispose of syringe and remaining contents if second injection is not required.

8. APPLY ICE PACKS IF AVAILABLE, AT THE SITE OF THE DRUG OR ALLERGY INJECTION, OR INSECT STING (if applicable).
9. KEEP PATIENT WARM AND AVOID EXERTION.

PRECAUTIONS

EPINEPHRINE: For subcutaneous or intramuscular injection only. **Not intended for intravenious use.**

Epinephrine Injection, USP, contains sodium bisulfite. Patients with a suspected sulfite sensitivity should consult their physician well in advance before the need to use this product becomes critical.

Epinephrine is light sensitive and should be stored in box provided. KEEP AT ROOM TEMPERATURE, approximately 25°C (77°F). Protect from freezing. Do not try to force air out of the syringe until you are ready to use the epinephrine. This may rupture the seal and allow the epinephrine solution to contact the metal promoting deterioration. Never remove rubber protector over needle until ready to use syringe as this may cause needle and contents to become contaminated. Any epinephrine solution in contact with the needle may cause rusting of the metal.

Periodically check contents of the syringe. If discoloration or precipitate is present, DO NOT USE. Obtain replacement syringe from physician. Periodically check expiration date on syringe. If expiration date is near, re-order new syringe and discard outdated syringe after new syringe has been received.

CHLO-AMINE: As with any drug, if you are pregnant or nursing a baby, seek the advice of a health professional before using this product.

Patients should not drive or operate machinery after taking Chlo-Amine. Drowsiness, dizziness, blurred vision, dry mouth and gastrointestinal upsets may occur. Keep out of reach of children.

The asthmatic patient should take the chlorpheniramine maleate tablets with caution.

LIMITED WARRANTY: A number of factors beyond our control could reduce the efficacy of this product or even result in an ill effect following its use. These include storage and handling of the product after it leaves our hands, diagnosis, dosage, method of administration and biological differences in individual patients. Because of these factors, it is important that this product be stored properly and that the directions be followed carefully during use.

The foregoing statement is made in lieu of any other warranty, express or implied, including any warranty of merchantability or fitness. Representatives of the Company are not authorized to vary the terms of this warranty or the contents of any printed labeling for this product except by printed notice from the Company's Spokane, WA office. The prescriber and user of this product must accept the terms hereof.

Epinephrine Mfg. by: Wyeth Laboratories, Inc.,
Philadelphia, PA 19101
Pkgd. and Dist. by:
Hollister-Stier
Miles Inc.
Pharmaceutical Division
Spokane, WA 99207 USA

Phys: 471103 M02 10/89   © 1988 Miles Inc.
Cr. Ref. 471104

AZLIN®   ℞
Sterile azlocillin sodium
for intravenous use.

PRODUCT OVERVIEW

KEY FACTS

AZLIN® is a semisynthetic broad spectrum penicillin antibiotic for parenteral administration. A bactericidal antibiotic, AZLIN® acts by interfering with cell wall synthesis. It is active against *Pseudomonas aeruginosa* and other *Pseudomonas* species, many of which are resistant to other broad spectrum antibiotics. AZLIN® is also active *in vitro* against many strains of the organisms (see Clinical Pharmacology).

MAJOR USES

AZLIN® is primarily indicated for treatment of serious infections caused by susceptible strains of *P. aeruginosa*. It has been proven effective in treatment of infections of the

Continued on next page

Miles Pharm. Div.—Cont.

lower respiratory tract, urinary tract, skin and skin structure, bones and joints, including osteomyelitis, and bacterial septicemia. In certain severe infections when the causative organisms are unknown and *Pseudomonas aeruginosa* is suspected, AZLIN® may be administered with an aminoglycoside or cephalosporin antibiotic as initial therapy. As soon as results of culture and susceptibility tests become available, antimicrobial therapy should be adjusted as indicated.

SAFETY INFORMATION

AZLIN® is contraindicated in patients with a history of hypersensitivity reactions to any of the penicillins. Although AZLIN® shares with other penicillins the low potential for toxicity, as with any potent drug, periodic assessment of organ system functions, including renal, hepatic and hematopoietic, is advisable during prolonged therapy.

PRESCRIBING INFORMATION

AZLIN®   ℞
Sterile azlocillin sodium
for intravenous use.

DESCRIPTION

AZLIN® (sterile azlocillin sodium) is a semisynthetic broad spectrum penicillin antibiotic for parenteral administration. It is the monosodium salt of 6-D-2 (2-OXO-imidazolidine-1-carboxamido)-2-phenyl-acetamido-penicillanic acid.
Structural Formula:

Empirical Formula: $C_{20}H_{22}N_5O_6S$ Na

AZLIN® has a molecular weight of 483.5 and contains 49.8 mg (2.17 mEq) of sodium per one gram of azlocillin activity. The dosage form is supplied as a sterile white to pale yellow powder, which is freely soluble in water. When reconstituted, aqueous solutions of AZLIN® are clear and range from colorless to pale yellow with a pH of 6.0 to 8.0.

CLINICAL PHARMACOLOGY

Intravenous Administration. In healthy adult volunteers, mean serum levels of azlocillin 30 minutes after a 5–10 minute intravenous injection of 1g, 2g, or 5g are 35, 106 and 256 mcg/ml, respectively. Serum levels, as noted below, lack dose proportionality:
[See table below].
After an intravenous infusion (30 min) of 2g or 3g azlocillin, mean serum levels 5 minutes after dosing are 130 mcg/ml (73–189) and 180 mcg/ml (133–235), respectively.
[See table below].
Following intravenous infusion (30 min) of a 3g dose of azlocillin every 6 hours for 5 days, mean peak serum concentrations were higher than 150 mcg/ml; trough levels were between 4–12 mcg/ml. From the first to the last day of dosing, the serum half-life increased from 61 minutes to approximately 77 minutes.
General. As with other penicillins, azlocillin is excreted primarily by the kidney through glomerular filtration and tubular secretion. The rate of elimination is dose dependent and also related to the status of renal function. In patients with normal renal function, 50 to 70% of the administered dose is recovered from the urine within 24 hours after dosing. Two hours after an intravenous injection of 2g, concentrations of active drug in urine generally exceed 4000 mcg/ml. By 4–8 hours after injection, concentrations are still above 500 mcg/ml. The serum elimination half-life of azlocillin is dose dependent and ranges from approximately

55 minutes after an intravenous dose of 2g to about 70 minutes after intravenous dose of 5g. Probenecid interferes with the renal tubular secretion of azlocillin, thereby increasing serum concentrations and prolonging serum half-life of the antibiotic.
In patients with reduced renal function, the serum half-life of azlocillin is prolonged, depending on degree of renal impairment. Dosage adjustments are usually not necessary except in patients with moderate to severe renal impairment. (See Dosage and Administration). As with other penicillins, azlocillin is metabolized only slightly; less than 10% of the administered dose is found in the urine in the form of the penicilloate or penilloate. The drug is readily removed from the serum by hemodialysis.
Following an intravenous dose of 2g azlocillin, peak concentrations of active drug in bile generally exceed 1000 mcg/ml. The bile levels are approximately 15 times higher than the corresponding serum levels. Biliary excretion is reduced in patients with common bile duct obstruction.
Following parenteral administration, the apparent volume of distribution is approximately 20% of body weight. The drug is present in active form in the serum, urine, bile, bronchial and wound secretions, bone and other tissues. As with other penicillins, penetration into the cerebrospinal fluid (CSF) is generally poor, however, higher CSF concentrations are obtained in the presence of meningeal inflammation.
The serum level of uric acid has been noted to be depressed in some patients receiving azlocillin; this effect appears to be transient.
Protein binding studies indicate that the degree of azlocillin binding is low (25–45%) and depends upon testing methods and concentrations of drug studied.

Microbiology

Azlocillin is a bactericidal antibiotic which acts by interfering with synthesis of cell wall components. It is active against *Pseudomonas aeruginosa* and other species of Pseudomonas, many of which are resistant to other broad spectrum antibiotics. Azlocillin is also active *in vitro* against many strains of the following organisms, however, clinical efficacy for infections other than those included in the indication section has not been documented:

Gram-negative bacteria
Escherichia coli
Proteus mirabilis
Proteus vulgaris
Morganella morganii (formerly *P. morganii*)
Providencia rettgeri (formerly *P. rettgeri*)
Providencia stuartii
Enterobacter species
Shigella species
Haemophilus influenzae
Haemophilus parainfluenzae
Neisseria species
Citrobacter species
Some strains of *Klebsiella, Serratia, Salmonella,* and *Acinetobacter* are also susceptible.

Gram-positive bacteria
Staphylococcus aureus (non-penicillinase producing strains)
Beta-hemolytic streptococci (Groups A and B)
Streptococcus pneumoniae (formerly *Diplococcus pneumoniae*)
Streptococcus faecalis (enterococcus)
Listeria monocytogenes

Anaerobic Organisms
Peptococcus species
Peptostreptococcus species
Clostridium species
Bacteroides species (including *B. fragilis* group)
Fusobacterium species
Veillonella species
Eubacterium species

Azlocillin is inactive against penicillinase-producing strains of *Staphylococcus aureus* and is susceptible to inactivation by beta-lactamases produced by the Enterobacteriaceae.
In vitro studies have shown that azlocillin combined with an aminoglycoside (e.g., gentamicin, tobramycin, amikacin, sisomicin) acts synergistically against many strains of *Pseudomonas aeruginosa.*
Azlocillin is slightly more active when tested at alkaline pH and, as with other penicillins, has reduced activity when tested *in vitro* with increasing inoculum. The minimal bactericidal concentration (MBC) may exceed the minimal inhibitory concentration (MIC) by four-fold or more depending on medium used. Resistance to azlocillin *in vitro* develops slowly (multiple step mutation). Some strains of *Pseudomonas aeruginosa* have developed resistance fairly rapidly.

Susceptibility Tests

Quantitative methods that require measurement of zone diameters give good estimates of bacterial susceptibility. One such procedure* has been recommended for use with discs to test susceptibility to antimicrobials. When the causative organism is tested by the Kirby-Bauer disc diffusion method, a 75 mcg azlocillin disc should give a zone of 18 mm or greater to indicate susceptibility. Zone sizes of 14 mm or less indicate resistance. Zone sizes of 15 to 17 mm indicate intermediate susceptibility. With this procedure, a report from the laboratory of "Susceptible" indicates that the infecting organism is likely to respond to therapy. A report of "Resistant" indicates that the infecting organism is not likely to respond to therapy; other therapy should be selected. A report of "Intermediate Susceptibility" suggests that the organism may be susceptible if the infection is confined to tissues and fluids (e.g., urine), in which high antibiotic levels are attained. The azlocillin disc should be used for testing susceptibility to azlocillin. Standardized procedure requires use of control organisms. The 75 mcg azlocillin disc should give zone diameters between 24 and 30 mm for *P. aeruginosa* ATCC 27853. For *E. coli* ATCC 25922 the zone diameters should be between 21 and 24 mm.

* Bauer, A.W., Kirby, W.M., Sherris, J.C., and Turck, M.: Antibiotic Testing by a Standardized Single Disc Method, Am. J. Clin. Pathol., 45:493, 1966; Standardized Disc Susceptibility Test, FEDERAL REGISTER, 39: 19182–19184, 1974.

In certain conditions, it may be desirable to do additional susceptibility testing by broth or agar dilution techniques. Dilution methods, preferably the agar plate dilution procedure, are most accurate for susceptibility testing of obligate anaerobes. *Pseudomonas* species and the *Enterobacteriaceae* are considered susceptible if the MIC of azlocillin is no greater than 64 mcg/ml and are considered resistant if the MIC is greater than 128 mcg/ml. The MIC values of azlocillin for the control strains are the following:
   P. aeruginosa ATCC 27853, 4–8 mcg/ml and
   E. coli ATCC 25922, 8–16 mcg/ml.
Azlocillin standard is available for broth or agar dilution studies.

INDICATIONS AND USAGE

AZLIN® is indicated primarily for the treatment of serious infections caused by susceptible strains of *Pseudomonas aeruginosa* in the conditions listed below:
LOWER RESPIRATORY TRACT INFECTIONS including pneumonia and lung abscess.
URINARY TRACT INFECTIONS both complicated and uncomplicated of the lower and upper urinary tract.
SKIN AND SKIN STRUCTURE INFECTIONS including ulcers, abscesses, burns and severe external otitis.
BONE AND JOINT INFECTIONS including osteomyelitis.
BACTERIAL SEPTICEMIA
Azlocillin has also been shown to be effective for the treatment of Lower Respiratory Tract Infections caused by *Escherichia coli* and *Haemophilus influenzae;* Urinary Tract In-

AZLIN®

AZLOCILLIN SERUM LEVELS IN ADULTS (mcg/ml) 5–10 MIN IV INJECTION

DOSE	5 min	15 min	30 min	1 hr	2 hr	3 hr	4 hr	6 hr	8 hr
1g			35 (29–41)	22 (18–26)	9.4 (7.2–14)	4.3 (2.6–6.8)	2.2 (1.2–4.0)		
2g	239 (142–363)	139 (85–188)	106 (83–134)	47 (30–60)	19 (16–26)	12 (8.7–13)	7.4 (5.7–11)	2.1 (1.8–2.9)	0.5 (0–0.7)
5g	527 (470–604)	353 (258–440)	256 (184–287)	174 (116–231)	85 (43–121)	55 (26–91)	33 (15–58)	7.7 (1.6–19)	4.1 (1.4–7.8)

AZLIN®

AZLOCILLIN SERUM LEVELS IN ADULTS (mcg/ml) 30 MIN IV INFUSION

DOSE	0	5 min	15 min	30 min	45 min	1 hr	1.5 hr	2 hr	3 hr	4 hr	6 hr	8 hr
2g	165 (55–278)	130 (73–189)	104 (62–175)	85 (42–121)	62 (23–85)	49 (27–82)	36 (19–57)	26 (13–48)	13 (5–25)	6 (2–11)	2 (1–4)	1 (1–4)
3g	214 (155–273)	180 (133–235)	139 (119–186)	104 (61–159)	82 (58–121)	68 (38–94)	58 (35–74)	39 (17–53)	24 (9–36)	10 (3–14)	3 (1–5)	1 (1–4)

fections and Skin Structure Infections caused by *Escherichia coli*, *Proteus mirabilis* or *Streptococcus faecalis;* and Septicemia caused by *Escherichia coli.*

Appropriate culture and susceptibility tests should be performed before treatment in order to isolate and identify organisms causing infections and to determine their susceptibility to azlocillin. Therapy with AZLIN® may be initiated before results of these tests are known; once results become available, appropriate therapy should be continued.

In certain severe infections, when the causative organisms are unknown and *Pseudomonas aeruginosa* is suspected, AZLIN® may be administered in conjunction with an aminoglycoside or a cephalosporin antibiotic as initial therapy. As soon as results of culture and susceptibility tests become available, antimicrobial therapy should be adjusted as indicated. Culture and susceptibility testing, performed periodically during therapy, will provide information on the therapeutic effect of the antimicrobial and will monitor for the possible emergence of bacterial resistance.

AZLIN® has been used effectively in combination with an aminoglycoside antibiotic for the treatment of life-threatening infections caused by *Pseudomonas aeruginosa* including acute pulmonary exacerbation in patients with cystic fibrosis. For the treatment of febrile episodes in immunosuppressed patients with granulocytopenia, AZLIN® should be combined with an aminoglycoside or a cephalosporin antibiotic.

CONTRAINDICATIONS

AZLIN® is contraindicated in patients with a history of hypersensitivity reactions to any of the penicillins.

WARNINGS

Serious and occasionally fatal hypersensitivity (anaphylactic) reactions have occurred in patients receiving a penicillin. These reactions are more apt to occur in individuals with a history of sensitivity to multiple allergens. There have been reports of individuals with a history of penicillin hypersensitivity reactions who have experienced severe hypersensitivity reactions when treated with a cephalosporin. Before therapy with azlocillin is instituted, careful inquiry should be made to determine whether the patient has had previous hypersensitivity reactions to penicillins, cephalosporins or other drugs. Antibiotics should be used with caution in any patient who has demonstrated some form of allergy, particularly to drugs.

If an allergic reaction occurs during therapy with azlocillin, the drug should be discontinued. SERIOUS ANAPHYLACTOID REACTIONS REQUIRE IMMEDIATE EMERGENCY TREATMENT WITH EPINEPHRINE. OXYGEN, INTRAVENOUS STEROIDS, AND AIRWAY MANAGEMENT, INCLUDING INTUBATION, SHOULD ALSO BE PROVIDED AS INDICATED.

PRECAUTIONS

Although AZLIN® shares with other penicillins the low potential for toxicity, as with any potent drug, periodic assessment of organ system functions, including renal, hepatic and hematopoietic, is advisable during prolonged therapy. Bleeding manifestations have occurred in some patients receiving beta-lactam antibiotics. These reactions have been associated with abnormalities of coagulation tests, such as clotting time, platelet aggregation and prothrombin time

and are more likely to occur in patients with renal impairment. Although AZLIN® has rarely been associated with any bleeding abnormalities, the possibility of this occurring should be kept in mind, particularly in patients with severe renal impairment receiving maximum doses of the drug. AZLIN® has only rarely been reported to cause hypokalemia; however, the possibility of this occurring should also be kept in mind, particularly when treating patients with fluid and electrolyte imbalance. Periodic monitoring of serum potassium may be advisable in patients receiving prolonged therapy.

AZLIN® is a monosodium salt containing only 49.8 mg (2.17 mEq) of sodium per gram of azlocillin. This should be considered when treating patients requiring restricted salt intake. As with any penicillin, an allergic reaction, including anaphylaxis, may occur during AZLIN® administration, particularly in a hypersensitive individual.

The rapid intravenous administration of AZLIN® has been associated with transient chest discomfort. Therefore, the drug should not be infused over a period of less than five minutes.

As with other antibiotics, prolonged use of AZLIN® may result in overgrowth of non-susceptible organisms. If this occurs, appropriate measures should be taken.

AZLIN®, along with other ureidopenicillins, has been reported in one study to prolong neuromuscular blockage of vecuronium. Caution is indicated when azlocillin is used perioperatively.

Interactions with Drugs and Laboratory Tests

As with other penicillins, the mixing of azlocillin with an aminoglycoside in solutions for parenteral administration can result in substantial inactivation of the aminoglycoside. Probenecid interferes with the renal tubular secretion of azlocillin, thereby increasing serum concentrations and prolonging serum half-life of the antibiotic.

The serum level of uric acid has been noted to be depressed in some patients receiving azlocillin; this effect appears to be transient.

High urine concentrations of azlocillin may produce false positive protein reactions (pseudoproteinuria) with the following methods: sulfosalicylic acid and boiling test, acetic acid test, biuret reaction, and nitric acid test. The bromphenol blue (Multi-stix®) reagent strip test has been reported to be reliable.

Pregnancy Category B

Reproduction studies have been performed in rats and mice at doses up to 2 times the human dose, and have revealed no evidence of impaired fertility or harm to the fetus, due to AZLIN®. There are however no adequate and well controlled studies in pregnant women. Because animal reproductive studies are not always predictive of human response, this drug should be used during pregnancy only if clearly needed. Azlocillin crosses the placenta and is found in cord blood and amniotic fluid.

Nursing Mothers

Azlocillin is detected in low concentrations in the milk of nursing mothers, therefore caution should be exercised when AZLIN® is administered to a nursing woman.

Drug Abuse and Dependence

Neither AZLIN® abuse nor AZLIN® dependence has been reported.

ADVERSE REACTIONS

As with other penicillins, the following adverse reactions may occur:

Hypersensitivity reactions: skin rash, pruritus, urticaria, arthralgia, myalgia, drug fever, chills, chest discomfort, and anaphylactic reactions.

Central nervous system: headache, giddiness, neuromuscular hyperirritability or convulsive seizures.

Gastro-intestinal disturbances: disturbances of taste and smell, stomatitis, flatulence, nausea, vomiting and diarrhea, epigastric pain.

Hemic and Lymphatic Systems: thrombocytopenia, leukopenia, neutropenia, eosinophilia and reduction of hemoglobin or hematocrit. Prolongation of prothrombin time and bleeding time.

Abnormalities of hepatic and renal function tests: elevation of serum aspartate aminotransferase (SGOT), serum alanine aminotransferase (SGPT), serum alkaline phosphatase, serum LDH, serum bilirubin. Elevation of serum creatinine and/or BUN, hypernatremia. Reduction in serum potassium and uric acid.

Local reactions: pain and thrombophlebitis with intravenous administration.

OVERDOSAGE

As with other penicillins, AZLIN® in overdosage has the potential to cause neuromuscular hyperirritability or convulsive seizures. Hemodialysis, if necessary, will aid in removal of the drug from the blood.

DOSAGE AND ADMINISTRATION

AZLIN® (sterile azlocillin sodium) may be administered by slow intravenous injection (5 min or longer) or by intravenous infusion (30 min).

The recommended adult dosage for serious infections is 200–300 mg/kg per day given in 4 to 6 divided doses. The usual dose is 3g given every 4 hours (18g/day). For life-threatening infections, up to 350 mg/kg per day may be administered, but the total daily dosage should ordinarily not exceed 24g.

[See table below].

For patients with life-threatening infections, 4g may be administered every 4 hours (24g/day).

Dosage for any individual patient must take into consideration the site and severity of infection, the susceptibility of the organisms causing infection, and the status of the patient's host defense mechanisms.

The duration of therapy depends upon the severity of infection. Generally, AZLIN® should be continued for at least 2 days after the signs and symptoms of infection have disappeared. The usual duration is 10 to 14 days; however, in difficult and complicated infections, more prolonged therapy may be required (e.g., osteomyelitis).

In certain deep-seated infections, involving abscess formation, appropriate surgical drainage should be performed in conjunction with antimicrobial therapy.

Patients with Impaired Renal Function

The rate of elimination of azlocillin is dose dependent and related to the degree of renal function impairment. After an intravenous dose of 5g, the serum half-life is approximately 1 hour in patients with creatinine clearances above 80 ml/min, 2.0 hr in those with clearances of 30–79 ml/min, 4.0 hr in those with clearances of 10–29 ml/min and approximately 5.9 hr in patients with clearances of less than 10 ml/min. Dosage adjustments of AZLIN® are not required in patients with mild impairment of renal function. For patients with a creatinine clearance of ≤ 30 ml/min (serum creatinine of approximately 3.0 mg% or greater), the following dosage guide may be used.

[See table bottom left].

For patients undergoing hemodialysis for renal failure, 3g may be administered after each dialysis and then every 12 hours.

For patients with renal failure, particularly those with concomitant hepatic insufficiency, measurement of serum levels of azlocillin will provide additional guidance for adjusting dosage.

Intravenous Administration

AZLIN® may be administered intravenously by intermittent infusion or by direct slow intravenous injection.

Infusion. Each gram of azlocillin should be reconstituted by vigorous shaking with at least 10 ml of Sterile Water for Injection, 5% Dextrose Injection or 0.9% Sodium Chloride Injection. The dissolved drug should be further diluted to desired volume (50-100 ml) with an appropriate intravenous solution. (See Compatibility and Stability section). The solution of reconstituted drug may then be administered over a period of 30 minutes by direct infusion or through a Y-type intravenous infusion set which may already be in place. If this method or the "piggyback" method of administration is used, it is advisable to discontinue temporarily the administration of any other solutions during the infusion of AZLIN®.

AZLIN® DOSAGE GUIDE (ADULTS)

Condition	Daily Dosage Range	Usual Daily Dosage	Frequency and Route of Administration
Urinary tract infection (uncomplicated)	100–125 mg/kg	8g	2g every 6 hours IV
Urinary tract infection (complicated)	150–200 mg/kg	12g	3g every 6 hours IV
Lower respiratory tract infection	225–300 mg/kg	16–18g	3g every 4 hours or 4g every 6 hours IV
Skin & skin structure infection	225–300 mg/kg	16–18g	3g every 4 hours or 4g every 6 hours IV
Bone & joint infection	225–300 mg/kg	16–18g	3g every 4 hours or 4g every 6 hours IV
Septicemia	225–300 mg/kg	16–18g	3g every 4 hours or 4g every 6 hours IV

AZLIN® DOSAGE GUIDE FOR PATIENTS WITH IMPAIRED RENAL FUNCTION

Creatinine Clearance ml/min	Urinary Tract Infection (Uncomplicated)	Urinary Tract Infection (Complicated)	Serious Systemic Infection
> 30	Usual Recommended Dosage		
10–30	1.5 g every 12 hours	1.5g every 8 hours	2g every 8 hours
< 10	1.5 g every 12 hours	2g every 12 hours	3g every 12 hours

Continued on next page

Miles Pharm. Div.—Cont.

Intravenous Solution   Stability

	10 mg/ml		50 mg/ml	
	Controlled Room Temperature	Refrigeration	Controlled Room Temperature	Refrigeration
Sterile Water for Injection, USP	96 hours	168 hours	24 hours	48 hours
0.9% Sodium Chloride Injection, USP	96 hours	168 hours	24 hours	96 hours
5% Dextrose Injection, USP	96 hours	168 hours	24 hours	72 hours
5% Dextrose in 0.225% Sodium Chloride Injection, USP	96 hours	168 hours	24 hours	72 hours
Lactated Ringer's Injection, USP	24 hours	96 hours	24 hours	48 hours
5% Dextrose in 0.45% Sodium Chloride Injection, USP	96 hours	168 hours	24 hours	72 hours

Unused portion must be discarded after the time period stated.

Injection. The reconstituted solution of AZLIN® may also be injected directly into a vein or into intravenous tubing; when administered in this way, the injection should be given slowly over a period of 5 minutes or longer. To minimize venous irritation, the concentration of drug should not exceed 10%.

When AZLIN® is given in combination with another antimicrobial, such as an aminoglycoside, each drug should be given separately in accordance with the recommended dosage and routes of administration for each drug.

After reconstitution and prior to administration, AZLIN® as with other parenteral drugs, should be inspected visually for particulate matter and discoloration.

Pediatric Use

Only limited data are available on the safety and effectiveness of AZLIN® in the treatment of infants with documented serious infection. Until further experience is gained, the drug should not be used in the newborn period.

In children with acute pulmonary exacerbation of cystic fibrosis, azlocillin may be administered at a dose of 75 mg/kg every 4 hours (450 mg/kg/day). The total daily dosage should not exceed 24g. The drug may be infused intravenously over a period of about 30 minutes.

COMPATIBILITY AND STABILITY

AZLIN® at concentrations of up to 10 mg/ml and up to 50 mg/ml is stable (loss of potency less than 10%) when stored in the following intravenous solutions for the time periods stated. When stored under refrigeration (2-8°C). AZLIN® at concentrations up to 100 mg/ml is stable for 24 hours. [See table above].

HOW SUPPLIED

AZLIN® (sterile azlocillin sodium) is a white to pale yellow powder supplied in vials and infusion bottles. Each vial contains azlocillin sodium equivalent to 2g, 3g or 4g azlocillin. Each infusion bottle contains azlocillin sodium equivalent to 2g, 3g or 4g azlocillin.

AZLIN® vials and infusion bottles should be stored at or below 30°C (86°F). The powder as well as the reconstituted solution of drug may darken slightly, depending upon storage conditions, but potency is not affected.

	NDC Number
2g Vial	0026-8311-30
3g Vial	0026-8312-35
3g Piggyback	0026-8312-36
4g Vial	0026-8314-35
4g Piggyback	0026-8314-36

Miles Inc.
Pharmaceutical Division
400 Morgan Lane
West Haven, CT 06516 USA
©1988 Miles Inc.
PD100692   BAY e 6905   Rev. 10/88

BILTRICIDE®   ℞
(praziquantel)

DESCRIPTION

BILTRICIDE® (praziquantel) is a trematodicide provided in tablet form for the oral treatment of schistosome infections and infections due to liver fluke.

BILTRICIDE® (praziquantel) is 2-(cyclohexylcarbonyl)-1,2,3,6,7, 11b-hexahydro4H-pyrazino [2, 1-a] isoquinolin-4-one with the molecular formula; $C_{19}H_{24}N_2O_2$. The structural formula is as follows:
[See Chemical Formula at top of next column].

Praziquantel is a colorless crystalline powder of bitter taste. The compound is stable under normal conditions and melts at 136-140°C with decomposition. The active substance is hygroscopic. Praziquantel is easily soluble in chloroform and dimethylsulfoxide, soluble in ethanol and very slightly soluble in water.

BILTRICIDE® lacquered tablets contain 600 mg of praziquantel. Inactive ingredients: corn starch, magnesium stearate, microcrystalline cellulose, povidone and sodium lauryl sulfate.

CLINICAL PHARMACOLOGY

BILTRICIDE® induces a rapid contraction of schistosomes by a specific effect on the permeability of the cell membrane. The drug further causes vacuolization and disintegration of the schistosome tegument.

After oral administration BILTRICIDE® is rapidly absorbed (80%), subjected to a first pass effect, metabolized and eliminated by the kidneys. Maximal serum concentration is achieved 1-3 hours after dosing. The half-life of praziquantel in serum is 0.8-1.5 hours.

INDICATIONS AND USAGE

BILTRICIDE® is indicated for the treatment of infections due to: all species of schistosoma (eg. *Schistosoma mekongi, Schistosoma japonicum, Schistosoma mansoni* and *Schistosoma hematobium)*, and infections due to the liver flukes, *Clonorchis sinensis/Opisthorchis viverrini* (approval of this indication was based on studies in which the two species were not differentiated).

CONTRAINDICATIONS

BILTRICIDE® should not be given to patients who previously have shown hypersensitivity to the drug. Since parasite destruction within the eye may cause irreparable lesions, ocular cysticercosis should not be treated with this compound.

PRECAUTIONS

Information for the patient: Patients should be warned not to drive a car and not to operate machinery on the day of BILTRICIDE® treatment and the following day.

Minimal increases in liver enzymes have been reported in some patients.

When schistosomiasis or fluke infection is found to be associated with cerebral cysticercosis it is advised to hospitalize the patient for the duration of treatment.

Drug Interactions: No data are available regarding interaction of BILTRICIDE® with other drugs.

Mutagenesis, Carcinogenesis: Mutagenic effects in Salmonella tests found by one laboratory have not been confirmed in the same tested strain by other laboratories. Long term carcinogenicity studies in rats and golden hamsters did not reveal any carcinogenic effect.

Pregnancy Category B: Reproduction studies have been performed in rats and rabbits at doses up to 40 times the human dose and have revealed no evidence of impaired fertility or harm to the fetus due to BILTRICIDE®. There are, however, no adequate and well-controlled studies in pregnant women. An increase of the abortion rate was found in rats at three times the single human therapeutic dose. While animal reproduction studies are not always predictive of human response, this drug should be used during pregnancy only if clearly needed.

Nursing mothers: BILTRICIDE® appeared in the milk of nursing women at a concentration of about ¼ that of maternal serum. Women should not nurse on the day of BILTRICIDE® treatment and during the subsequent 72 hours.

Pediatric use: Safety in children under 4 years of age has not been established.

ADVERSE EFFECTS

In general BILTRICIDE® is very well tolerated. Side effects are usually mild and transient and do not require treatment. The following side effects were observed generally in order of severity: malaise, headache, dizziness, abdominal discomfort with or without nausea, rise in temperature and, rarely, urticaria. Such symptoms can, however, also result from the infection itself. Such side effects may be more frequent and/ or serious in patients with a heavy worm burden. In patients with liver impairment caused by the infection, no adverse effects of BILTRICIDE® have occurred which would necessitate restriction in use.

OVERDOSAGE

In rats and mice the acute LD_{50} was about 2,500 mg/kg. No data are available in humans. In the event of overdose a fast-acting laxative should be given.

DOSAGE AND ADMINISTRATION

The dosage recommended for the treatment of schistosomiasis is: 3×20 mg/kg bodyweight as a one day treatment. The recommended dose for clonorchiasis and opisthorchiasis is: 3×25 mg/kg as a one day treatment. The tablets should be washed down unchewed with some liquid during meals. Keeping the tablets or segments thereof in the mouth can reveal a bitter taste which can promote gagging or vomiting. The interval between the individual doses should not be less than 4 and not more than 6 hours.

HOW SUPPLIED

BILTRICIDE® is supplied as a 600 mg white, film-coated, oblong tablet with three scores. When broken each of the four segments contains 150 mg of active ingredient so that the dosage can be easily adjusted to the patient's body-weight.

Segments are broken off by pressing the score (notch) with thumbnails. If ¼ of a tablet is required, this is best achieved by breaking the segment from the outer end.
BILTRICIDE® is available in bottles of 6.

	NDC
6	0026-2521-06

STORAGE CONDITIONS

Store below 86°F (30°C).

Miles Inc.
Pharmaceutical Division
400 Morgan Lane
West Haven, CT 06516 USA
Made in Germany
© 1989 Miles Inc.
PD100709   0765   EMBAY 8440   3/89
Shown in Product Identification Section, page 419

CIPRO®   ℞
(ciprofloxacin HCl/Miles)
TABLETS

DESCRIPTION

CIPRO® (ciprofloxacin HCl/Miles) is a synthetic broad spectrum antibacterial agent for oral administration. Ciprofloxacin, a fluoroquinolone, is available as the monohydrochloride monohydrate salt of 1-cyclopropyl-6-fluoro-1,4-dihydro-4-oxo-7-(1-piperazinyl)-3-quinolinecarboxylic acid. It is a faintly yellowish to light yellow crystalline powder with a molecular weight of 385.8. Its empirical formula is $C_{17}H_{18}FN_3O_3 \cdot HCl \cdot H_2O$ and its chemical structure is as follows:

CIPRO® is available in 250-mg, 500-mg and 750-mg (ciprofloxacin equivalent) film-coated tablets. The inactive ingredients are starch, microcrystalline cellulose, silicon dioxide, crospovidone, magnesium stearate, hydroxypropyl methylcellulose, titanium dioxide, polyethylene glycol and water. Ciprofloxacin differs from other quinolones in that it has a fluorine atom at the 6-position, a piperazine moiety at the 7-position, and a three-carbon ring at the 1-position. Examples of other antibacterial drugs in the quinolone class are nalidixic acid, cinoxacin, and norfloxacin.

CLINICAL PHARMACOLOGY

CIPRO® tablets are rapidly and well absorbed from the gastrointestinal tract after oral administration. The absolute bioavailability is approximately 70% with no substantial loss by first pass metabolism. Serum concentrations increase proportionately with the dose as shown:

Dose (mg)	Maximum Serum Concentration (mcg/mL)	Area Under Curve (AUC) (mcg·hr/mL)
250	1.2	4.8
500	2.4	11.6
750	4.3	20.2
1000	5.4	30.8

Maximum serum concentrations are attained 1 to 2 hours after oral dosing. Mean concentrations 12 hours after dosing with 250, 500, or 750 mg are 0.1, 0.2, and 0.4 mcg/mL, respectively. The serum elimination half-life in subjects with normal renal function is approximately 4 hours.

Approximately 40 to 50% of an orally administered dose is excreted in the urine as unchanged drug. After a 250-mg oral dose, urine concentrations of ciprofloxacin usually exceed 200 mcg/mL during the first two hours and are approximately 30 mcg/mL at 8 to 12 hours after dosing. The urinary excretion of ciprofloxacin is virtually complete within 24 hours after dosing. The renal clearance of ciprofloxacin, which is approximately 300 mL/minute, exceeds the normal glomerular filtration rate of 120 mL/minute. Thus, active tubular secretion would seem to play a significant role in its elimination. Co-administration of probenecid with ciprofloxacin results in a 50% reduction in the ciprofloxacin renal clearance and a 50% increase in its concentration in the systemic circulation. Although bile concentrations of ciprofloxacin are several fold higher than serum concentrations after oral dosing, only a small amount of the dose administered is recovered from the bile. Approximately 20 to 35% of an oral dose is recovered from the feces within 5 days after dosing. Ciprofloxacin is also metabolized. Four metabolites have been identified in human urine which together account for approximately 15% of an oral dose. The metabolites have antimicrobial activity, but are less active than unchanged ciprofloxacin.

When CIPRO® is given concomitantly with food, there is a delay in the absorption of the drug, resulting in peak concentrations that are closer to 2 hours after dosing rather than 1 hour. The overall absorption, however, is not substantially affected. Concurrent administration of antacids containing magnesium hydroxide or aluminum hydroxide does, however, substantially interfere with the bioavailability of ciprofloxacin (SEE PRECAUTIONS).

Concomitant administration of ciprofloxacin with theophylline may prolong the serum elimination half-life of theophylline, elevate serum theophylline levels, and may increase the risk of a patient developing CNS adverse reactions (SEE PRECAUTIONS).

In patients with reduced renal function, the half-life of ciprofloxacin is slightly prolonged. Dosage adjustments may be required. (SEE DOSAGE AND ADMINISTRATION).

The binding of ciprofloxacin to serum proteins is 20 to 40% which is not likely to be high enough to cause significant protein binding interactions with other drugs.

After oral administration ciprofloxacin is widely distributed throughout the body. Tissue concentrations often exceed serum concentrations in both men and women, particularly in genital tissue. Ciprofloxacin is present in active form in the saliva, nasal secretions, sputum, skin blister fluid, lymph, peritoneal fluid, bile and prostatic secretions. The drug diffuses into the cerebrospinal fluid (CSF), however CSF concentrations are generally only about 10% of peak serum concentrations. Ciprofloxacin has been detected in skin, fat, muscle, cartilage, and bone.

Microbiology: Ciprofloxacin has *in vitro* activity against a wide range of gram-negative and gram-positive organisms. The bactericidal action of ciprofloxacin results from interference with the enzyme DNA gyrase needed for the synthesis of bacterial DNA.

While *in vitro* studies have demonstrated the susceptibility of most strains of the following micro-organisms, clinical efficacy for infections other than those included in the INDICATIONS AND USAGE section has not been documented:

Gram-Negative: *Escherichia coli; Klebsiella* species (including *Klebsiella pneumoniae* and *Klebsiella oxytoca); Enterobacter* species; *Citrobacter* species; *Edwardsiella tarda; Salmonella* species; *Shigella* species; *Proteus mirabilis; Proteus vulgaris; Providencia stuartii; Providencia rettgeri; Morganella morganii; Serratia* species (including *Serratia marcescens); Yersinia enterocolitica; Pseudomonas aeruginosa; Acinetobacter* species; *Haemophilus influenzae; Haemophilus parainfluenzae; Haemophilus ducreyi; Neisseria gonorrhoeae, Neisseria meningitidis; Moraxella (Branhamella) catarrhalis; Campylobacter* species; *Aeromonas* species; *Vibrio* species (including *V. cholerae); Brucella melitensis; Pasteurella multocida;* and *Legionella* species.

Gram-Positive: *Staphylococcus aureus* (including methicillin-susceptible and methicillin-resistant strains); coagulase-negative *Staphylococcus* species (including *Staphylococcus epidermidis); Streptococcus pyogenes;* and *Streptococcus pneumoniae.*

Most strains of streptococci including *Streptococcus faecalis* are only moderately susceptible to ciprofloxacin as are *Mycobacterium tuberculosis* and *Chlamydia trachomatis.*

Most strains of *Pseudomonas cepacia* and some strains of *Pseudomonas maltophilia* are resistant to ciprofloxacin as are most anaerobic bacteria, including *Bacteroides fragilis* and *Clostridium difficile.*

Ciprofloxacin is slightly less active when tested at acidic pH. The inoculum size has little effect when tested *in vitro*. The minimal bactericidal concentration (MBC) generally does not exceed the minimal inhibitory concentration (MIC) by more than a factor of 2. Resistance to ciprofloxacin *in vitro* develops slowly (multiple-step mutation). Rapid one-step development of resistance has not been observed.

Ciprofloxacin does not cross-react with other antimicrobial agents such as beta-lactams or aminoglycosides.

In vitro studies have shown that additive activity often results when ciprofloxacin is combined with other antimicrobial agents such as beta-lactams, aminoglycosides, clindamycin, or metronidazole.

Susceptibility Tests

Diffusion Techniques: Quantitative methods that require measurement of zone diameters give the most precise estimates of antibiotic susceptibility. One such procedure recommended for use with the 5-mcg ciprofloxacin disk is the National Committee for Clinical Laboratory Standards (NCCLS) approved procedure. Only a 5-mcg ciprofloxacin disk should be used, and it should not be used for testing susceptibility to less active quinolones; there are no suitable surrogate disks.

Results of laboratory tests using 5-mcg ciprofloxacin disks should be interpreted using the following criteria:

Zone Diameter (mm)	Interpretation
≥ 21	(S) Susceptible
16–20	(I) Intermediate (Moderately Susceptible)
≤ 15	(R) Resistant

Dilution Techniques: Broth and agar dilution methods, such as those recommended by the NCCLS, may be used to determine the minimum inhibitory concentration (MIC) of ciprofloxacin. MIC test results should be interpreted according to the following criteria:

MIC (mcg/mL)	Interpretation
≤ 1	(S) Susceptible
> 1-≤ 2	(I) Intermediate (Moderately Susceptible)
> 2	(R) Resistant

For any susceptibility test, a report of "susceptible" indicates that the pathogen is likely to respond to ciprofloxacin therapy. A report of "resistant" indicates that the pathogen is not likely to respond. A report of "intermediate" (moderately susceptible) indicates that the pathogen is expected to be susceptible to ciprofloxacin if high doses are used, or if the infection is confined to tissues and fluids in which high ciprofloxacin levels are obtained. The Quality Control strains should have the following assigned daily ranges for ciprofloxacin.

QC STRAINS	DISK ZONE DIAMETER (mm)	MIC (mcg/mL)
S. aureus (ATCC 25923)	22–30	
S. aureus (ATCC 29213)		0.25–1.0
E. coli (ATCC 25922)	30–40	0.008–0.03
P. aeruginosa (ATCC 27853)	25–33	0.25–1.0

INDICATIONS AND USAGE

CIPRO® is indicated for the treatment of infections caused by susceptible strains of the designated microorganisms in the conditions listed below:

Lower Respiratory Infections caused by *Escherichia coli, Klebsiella pneumoniae, Enterobacter cloacae, Proteus mirabilis, Pseudomonas aeruginosa, Haemophilus influenzae, Haemophilus parainfluenzae,* and *Streptococcus pneumoniae.*

Skin and Skin Structure Infections caused by *Escherichia coli, Klebsiella pneumoniae, Enterobacter cloacae, Proteus mirabilis, Proteus vulgaris, Providencia stuartii, Morganella morganii, Citrobacter freundii, Pseudomonas aeruginosa, Staphylococcus aureus,* (penicillinase and nonpenicillinase-producing strains), *Staphylococcus epidermidis,* and *Streptococcus pyogenes.*

Bone and Joint Infections caused by *Enterobacter cloacae, Serratia marcescens,* and *Pseudomonas aeruginosa.*

Urinary Tract Infections caused by *Escherichia coli, Klebsiella pneumoniae, Enterobacter cloacae, Serratia marcescens, Proteus mirabilis, Providencia rettgeri, Morganella morganii, Citrobacter diversus, Citrobacter freundii, Pseudomonas aeruginosa, Staphylococcus epidermidis,* and *Streptococcus faecalis.*

Infectious diarrhea caused by *Escherichia coli* (enterotoxigenic strains), *Campylobacter jejuni, Shigella flexneri** and *Shigella sonnei** when antibacterial therapy is indicated.

* Efficacy for this organism in this organ system was studied in fewer than 10 infections.

Appropriate culture and susceptibility tests should be performed before treatment in order to isolate and identify organisms causing infection and to determine their susceptibility to ciprofloxacin. Therapy with CIPRO® may be initiated before results of these tests are known; once results become available appropriate therapy should be continued. As with

other drugs, some strains of *Pseudomonas aeruginosa* may develop resistance fairly rapidly during treatment with ciprofloxacin. Culture and susceptibility testing performed periodically during therapy will provide information not only on the therapeutic effect of the antimicrobial agent but also on the possible emergence of bacterial resistance.

CONTRAINDICATIONS

A history of hypersensitivity to ciprofloxacin is a contraindication to its use. A history of hypersensitivity to other quinolones may also contraindicate the use of ciprofloxacin.

WARNINGS

CIPROFLOXACIN SHOULD NOT BE USED IN CHILDREN OR PREGNANT WOMEN. The oral administration of ciprofloxacin caused lameness in immature dogs. Histopathological examination of the weight-bearing joints of these dogs revealed permanent lesions of the cartilage. Related drugs such as nalidixic acid, cinoxacin and norfloxacin also produced erosions of cartilage of weight-bearing joints and other signs of arthropathy in immature animals of various species (SEE ANIMAL PHARMACOLOGY).

PRECAUTIONS

General: As with other quinolones, ciprofloxacin may cause central nervous system (CNS) stimulation which may lead to tremor, restlessness, lightheadedness, confusion, and very rarely to hallucinations or convulsive seizures. Therefore, ciprofloxacin should be used with caution in patients with known or suspected CNS disorders, such as severe cerebral arteriosclerosis or epilepsy, or other factors which predispose to seizures. (SEE ADVERSE REACTIONS).

Anaphylactic reactions following the first dose, have been reported in patients receiving therapy with quinolones. Some reactions were accompanied by cardiovascular collapse, loss of consciousness, tingling, pharyngeal or facial edema, dyspnea, urticaria, and itching. Only a few patients had a history of hypersensitivity reaction. Anaphylactic reactions may require epinephrine and other emergency measures. Ciprofloxacin should be discontinued at the first sign of hypersensitivity or allergy.

Severe hypersensitivity reactions characterized by rash, fever, eosinophilia, jaundice, and hepatic necrosis with fatal outcome have been reported rarely (less than one per million prescriptions) in patients receiving ciprofloxacin along with other drugs. The possibility that these reactions were related to ciprofloxacin cannot be excluded. Ciprofloxacin should be discontinued at the first appearance of a skin rash or any sign of other hypersensitivity reaction.

Crystals of ciprofloxacin have been observed rarely in the urine of human subjects but more frequently in the urine of laboratory animals (SEE ANIMAL PHARMACOLOGY). Crystalluria related to ciprofloxacin has been reported only rarely in man because human urine is usually acidic. Patients receiving ciprofloxacin should be well hydrated and alkalinity of the urine should be avoided. The recommended daily dose should not be exceeded.

Alteration of the dosage regimen is necessary for patients with impairment of renal function. (SEE DOSAGE AND ADMINISTRATION).

Drug Interactions: Concurrent administration of ciprofloxacin with theophylline may lead to elevated plasma concentrations of theophylline and prolongation of its elimination half-life. This may result in increased risk of theophylline-related adverse reactions. If concomitant use cannot be avoided, plasma levels of theophylline should be monitored and dosage adjustments made as appropriate.

Antacids containing magnesium hydroxide or aluminum hydroxide may interfere with the absorption of ciprofloxacin resulting in serum and urine levels lower than desired; concurrent administration of these agents with ciprofloxacin should be avoided.

Probenecid interferes with renal tubular secretion of ciprofloxacin and produces an increase in the level of ciprofloxacin in the serum. This should be considered if patients are receiving both drugs concomitantly.

As with other broad spectrum antibiotics prolonged use of ciprofloxacin may result in overgrowth of nonsusceptible organisms. Repeated evaluation of the patient's condition and microbial susceptibility testing is essential. If superinfection occurs during therapy, appropriate measures should be taken.

Information for Patients: Patients should be advised that ciprofloxacin may be taken with or without meals. The preferred time of dosing is two hours after a meal. Patients should also be advised to drink fluids liberally and not take antacids containing magnesium or aluminum concomitantly or within two hours after dosing.

Ciprofloxacin may cause dizziness and lightheadedness; therefore patients should know how they react to this drug before they operate an automobile or machinery or engage in activities requiring mental alertness or coordination.

Continued on next page

Miles Pharm. Div.—Cont.

Carcinogenesis, Mutagenesis, Impairment of Fertility: Eight *in vitro* mutagenicity tests have been conducted with ciprofloxacin and the test results are listed below:

Salmonella/Microsome Test (Negative)

E. coli DNA Repair Assay (Negative)

Mouse Lymphoma Cell Forward Mutation Assay (Positive)

Chinese Hamster V$_{79}$ Cell HGPRT Test (Negative)

Syrian Hamster Embryo Cell Transformation Assay (Negative)

Saccharomyces cerevisiae Point Mutation Assay (Negative)

Saccharomyces cerevisiae Mitotic Crossover and Gene Conversion Assay (Negative)

Rat Hepatocyte DNA Repair Assay (Positive)

Thus 2 of the 8 tests were positive but results of the following 3 *in vitro* test systems gave negative results:

Rat Hepatocyte DNA Repair Assay

Micronucleus Test (Mice)

Dominant Lethal Test (Mice)

Long term carcinogenicity studies in animals have not yet been completed.

Pregnancy—Pregnancy Category C: Reproduction studies have been performed in rats and mice at doses up to 6 times the usual daily human dose and have revealed no evidence of impaired fertility or harm to the fetus due to ciprofloxacin. In rabbits, as with most antimicrobial agents, ciprofloxacin (30 and 100 mg/kg orally) produced gastro-intestinal disturbances resulting in maternal weight loss and an increased incidence of abortion. No teratogenicity was observed at either dose. After intravenous administration, at doses up to 20 mg/kg, no maternal toxicity was produced and no embryotoxicity or teratogenicity was observed. There are, however, no adequate and well-controlled studies in pregnant women. SINCE CIPROFLOXACIN, LIKE OTHER DRUGS IN ITS CLASS, CAUSES ARTHROPATHY IN IMMATURE ANIMALS, IT SHOULD NOT BE USED IN PREGNANT WOMEN (SEE WARNINGS).

Nursing Mothers: It is not known whether ciprofloxacin is excreted in human milk, however it is known that ciprofloxacin is excreted in the milk of lactating rats and that other drugs of this class are excreted in human milk. Because of this and because of the potential for serious adverse reactions from ciprofloxacin in nursing infants, a decision should be made to discontinue nursing or to discontinue the drug, taking into account the importance of the drug to the mother.

Pediatric Use: Ciprofloxacin should not be used in children because it causes arthropathy in immature animals (SEE WARNINGS).

ADVERSE REACTIONS

Ciprofloxacin is generally well-tolerated. During clinical investigation, 2,799 patients received 2,868 courses of the drug. Adverse events that were considered likely to be drug related occurred in 7.3% of courses, possibly related in 9.2%, and remotely related in 3.0%. Ciprofloxacin was discontinued because of an adverse event in 3.5% of courses, primarily involving the gastrointestinal system (1.5%), skin (0.6%), and central nervous system (0.4%).

The most frequently reported events, drug related or not, were nausea (5.2%), diarrhea (2.3%), vomiting (2.0%), abdominal pain/discomfort (1.7%), headache (1.2%), restlessness (1.1%), and rash (1.1%).

Additional events that occurred in less than 1% of ciprofloxacin courses are listed below. Those typical of quinolones are italicized.

GASTROINTESTINAL: *(See above),* painful oral mucosa, oral candidiasis, dysphagia, intestinal perforation, gastrointestinal bleeding.

CENTRAL NERVOUS SYSTEM: *(See above),* dizziness, lightheadedness, insomnia, nightmares, hallucinations, manic reaction, irritability, tremor, ataxia, convulsive seizures, lethargy, drowsiness, weakness, malaise, anorexia, phobia, depersonalization, depression, paresthesia.

SKIN/HYPERSENSITIVITY: *(See above),* pruritus, urticaria, photosensitivity, flushing, fever, chills, angioedema, edema of the face, neck, lips, conjunctivae or hands; cutaneous candidiasis, hyperpigmentation, erythema nodosum.

SPECIAL SENSES: *blurred vision, disturbed vision (change in color perception, overbrightness of lights), decreased visual acuity, diplopia, eye pain, tinnitus, bad taste.*

MUSCULOSKELETAL: *joint or back pain, joint stiffness,* achiness, neck or chest pain, flare up of gout.

RENAL/UROGENITAL: *interstitial nephritis, nephritis, renal failure,* polyuria, urinary retention, urethral bleeding, vaginitis, acidosis.

CARDIOVASCULAR: palpitations, atrial flutter, ventricular ectopy, syncope, hypertension, angina pectoris, myocardial infarction, cardiopulmonary arrest, cerebral thrombosis.

RESPIRATORY: epistaxis, laryngeal or pulmonary edema, hiccough, hemoptysis, dyspnea, bronchospasm, pulmonary embolism.

Most of these events were described as only mild or moderate in severity, abated soon after the drug was discontinued, and required no treatment.

In several instances nausea, vomiting, tremor, restlessness, agitation or palpitations were judged by investigators to be related to elevated plasma levels of theophylline possibly as a result of drug interaction with ciprofloxacin.

Other adverse events reported in the postmarketing phase include anaphylactoid reactions, Stevens-Johnson syndrome, exfoliative dermatitis, toxic epidermal necrolysis, hepatic necrosis, postural hypotension, possible exacerbation of myasthenia gravis, confusion, dysphasia, nystagmus, pseudomembranous colitis, dyspepsia, flatulence, and constipation. Also reported were agranulocytosis; elevation of serum triglycerides, serum cholesterol, blood glucose, serum potassium; prolongation of prothrombin time; albuminuria; candiduria, vaginal candidiasis; and renal calculi (See Precautions).

Adverse Laboratory Changes: Changes in laboratory parameters listed as adverse events without regard to drug relationship:

Hepatic—Elevations of: ALT (SGPT) (1.9%), AST (SGOT) (1.7%), Alkaline Phosphatase (0.8%), LDH (0.4%), serum bilirubin (0.3%).

Hematologic—eosinophilia (0.6%), leukopenia (0.4%), decreased blood platelets (0.1%), elevated blood platelets (0.1%), pancytopenia (0.1%).

Renal—Elevations of: Serum creatinine (1.1%), BUN (0.9%). CRYSTALLURIA, CYLINDRURIA AND HEMATURIA HAVE BEEN REPORTED.

Other changes occurring in less than 0.1% of courses were: Elevation of serum gammaglutamyl transferase, elevation of serum amylase, reduction in blood glucose, elevated uric acid, decrease in hemoglobin, anemia, bleeding diathesis, increase in blood monocytes, leukocytosis.

OVERDOSAGE

Information on overdosage in humans is not available. In the event of acute overdosage the stomach should be emptied by inducing vomiting or by gastric lavage, and the patient carefully observed and given supportive treatment. Adequate hydration must be maintained. In the event of serious toxic reactions from overdosage, hemodialysis or peritoneal dialysis may aid in the removal of ciprofloxacin from the body, particularly if renal function is compromised.

DOSAGE AND ADMINISTRATION

The usual adult dosage for patients with urinary tract infections is 250 mg every 12 hours. For patients with complicated infections caused by organisms not highly susceptible, 500 mg may be administered every 12 hours.

Respiratory tract infections, skin and skin structure infections, and bone and joint infections may be treated with 500 mg every 12 hours. For more severe or complicated infections, a dosage of 750 mg may be given every 12 hours.

	Strength	NDC Code	Tablet Identification
Bottles of 50:	250 mg	NDC 0026-8512-50	Miles 512
	500 mg	NDC 0026-8513-50	Miles 513
	750 mg	NDC 0026-8514-50	Miles 514
Unit Dose	250 mg	NDC 0026-8512-48	Miles 512
Packages of 100	500 mg	NDC 0026-8513-48	Miles 513
	750 mg	NDC 0026-8514-48	Miles 514

The recommended dosage for Infectious Diarrhea is 500 mg every 12 hours.

[See table below].

The determination of dosage for any particular patient must take into consideration the severity and nature of the infection, the susceptibility of the causative organism, the integrity of the patient's host-defense mechanisms, and the status of renal function.

The duration of treatment depends upon the severity of infection. Generally ciprofloxacin should be continued for at least 2 days after the signs and symptoms of infection have disappeared. The usual duration of 7 to 14 days, however for severe or complicated infections more prolonged therapy may be required. Bone and joint infections may require treatment for 4 to 6 weeks or longer. Infectious Diarrhea may be treated for 5–7 days.

Impaired Renal Function: Ciprofloxacin is eliminated primarily by renal excretion, however the drug is also metabolized and partially excreted through the biliary system of the liver. These alternate pathways of drug elimination appear to compensate for the reduced renal excretion in patients with renal impairment. Nonetheless, some modification of dosage is recommended, particularly for patients with severe renal dysfunction. The following table provides dosage guidelines for use in patients with renal impairment, however, monitoring of serum drug levels provide the most reliable basis for dosage adjustment.

RECOMMENDED STARTING AND MAINTENANCE DOSES FOR PATIENTS WITH IMPAIRED RENAL FUNCTION

Creatinine Clearance (mL/min)	Dose
>50	See Usual Dosage
30–50	250–500 mg q 12 h
5–29	250–500 mg q 18 h
Patients on hemodialysis or Peritoneal dialysis	250–500 mg q 24 h (after dialysis)

When only the serum creatinine concentration is known, the following formula may be used to estimate creatinine clearance.

Men: Creatinine clearance

$$\text{(mL/min)} = \frac{\text{Weight (kg)} \times (140 - \text{age})}{72 \times \text{serum creatinine (mg/mL)}}$$

Women: $0.85 \times$ the value calculated for men.

The serum creatinine should represent a steady state of renal function.

In patients with severe infections and severe renal impairment, a unit dose of 750 mg may be administered at the intervals noted above; however patients should be carefully monitored and the serum ciprofloxacin concentration should be measured periodically. Peak concentrations (1–2 hours after dosing) above 5 mcg/mL should be avoided.

For patients with changing renal function or for patients with renal impairment and hepatic insufficiency, measurement of serum concentrations of ciprofloxacin will provide additional guidance for adjusting dosage.

HOW SUPPLIED

CIPRO® (ciprofloxacin HCl/Miles) is available as round, slightly yellowish film-coated tablets containing 250 mg ciprofloxacin. The 250-mg tablet is coded with the word "Miles" on one side and "512" on the reverse side. CIPRO® is also available as capsule shaped, slightly yellowish film-coated tablets containing 500 mg or 750 mg ciprofloxacin. The 500-mg tablet is coded with the word "Miles" on one side and "513" on the reverse side; the 750-mg tablet is coded with the word "Miles" on one side and "514" on the reverse side. Each tablet strength is available in bottles of 50's and in Unit Dose packages of 100.

[See table above].

Store below 86°F (30°C).

ANIMAL PHARMACOLOGY

Ciprofloxacin and related drugs have been shown to cause arthropathy in immature animals of most species tested (SEE WARNINGS). Damage of weight bearing joints was observed in juvenile dogs and rats. In young beagles 100 mg/kg ciprofloxacin given daily for 4 weeks caused degenerative articular changes of the knee joint. At 30 mg/kg the effect on the joint was minimal. In a subsequent study in beagles, removal of weight bearing from the joint reduced the lesions but did not totally prevent them.

Crystalluria, sometimes associated with secondary nephropathy, occurs in laboratory animals dosed with ciprofloxacin. This is primarily related to the reduced solubility of ciprofloxacin under alkaline conditions, which predominate in the urine of test animals; in man, crystalluria is rare since

DOSAGE GUIDELINES

Location of Infection	Type or Severity	Unit Dose	Frequency	Daily Dose
Urinary Tract	Mild/Moderate	250 mg	q 12 h	500 mg
	Severe/Complicated	500 mg	q 12 h	1000 mg
Respiratory Tract Bone and Joint Skin & Skin Structure	Mild/Moderate	500 mg	q 12 h	1000 mg
	Severe/Complicated	750 mg	q 12 h	1500 mg
Infectious Diarrhea	Mild/Moderate/Severe	500 mg	q 12 h	1000 mg

human urine is typically acidic. In rhesus monkeys, crystalluria without nephropathy has been noted after single oral doses as low as 30 mg/kg. After 6 months of dosing at 30 mg/kg/day, no nephropathological changes were noted; however, nephropathy was observed after dosing at 90 mg/kg/day for the same duration.

Ocular toxicity seen with some related drugs has not been observed in ciprofloxacin-treated animals.

Miles Inc.
Pharmaceutical Division
400 Morgan Lane
West Haven, CT 06516 USA
© 1989 Miles Inc.

PZ100706   1/89   Bay o 9867   5202-2-A-U.S.-2   0723
Shown in Product Identification Section, page 419

DECHOLIN® Tablets
(dehydrocholic acid)

DESCRIPTION
Each tablet contains 250 mg dehydrocholic acid.
Inactive Ingredients: Corn starch, gelatin, lactose, magnesium stearate, potato starch and talc.

INDICATIONS
For relief of occasional constipation (irregularity). This product generally produces bowel movement in 6–12 hours.

WARNINGS
Do not use laxative products when abdominal pain, nausea, or vomiting are present unless directed by a doctor.
If you have noticed a sudden change in bowel habits that persists over a period of 2 weeks, consult a doctor before using a laxative.
Laxative products should not be used for a period longer than 1 week unless directed by a doctor.
Rectal bleeding or failure to have a bowel movement after use of a laxative may indicate a serious condition. Discontinue use and consult your doctor.
KEEP THIS AND ALL MEDICATIONS OUT OF THE REACH OF CHILDREN.

WARNING
As with any drug, if you are pregnant or nursing a baby, seek the advice of a health professional before using this product.

DOSAGE AND ADMINISTRATION
Adults and children 12 years of age and over: oral dosage is 250 to 500 milligrams three times a day, not to exceed 1500 milligrams in 24 hours. Children under 12 years of age: consult a doctor.

HOW SUPPLIED
White tablets coded with number 121-Miles in bottles of 100.
Store at controlled room temperature (59°–86°F.).
PL 102049   0788   4/89
Shown in Product Identification Section, page 419

DOMEBORO® Powder Packets,
Effervescent Tablets (acid pH)
Astringent Wet Dressing

One packet or tablet dissolved in a pint of water makes a modified Burow's Solution approximately equivalent to a 1:40 dilution, two packets or tablets a 1:20 dilution, and four packets or tablets a 1:10 dilution.
Buffered to an acid pH.

CONTAINS
Aluminum sulfate and calcium acetate.

INDICATIONS
A soothing wet dressing for relief of inflammatory conditions of the skin such as insect bites, poison ivy, swellings and bruises, athlete's foot and diaper rash.

DIRECTIONS
Dissolve one or two packets or tablets in a pint (large glass) of water and stir. When the powder disperses, shake resulting mixture. Do not strain or filter. Bandage the site of application loosely. Pour mixture on bandage every few minutes to keep dressing moist. Apply the dressing for four treatment periods of 30 minutes each day or as directed by physician. Do not use plastic or other impervious material to prevent evaporation without consulting your physician.

CAUTION
Keep away from eyes. For external use only. Store below 86°F. (30°C.).

HOW SUPPLIED
Powder Packets: Boxes of 12 and 100. Each packet contains 2.2 gm. Individually foil-wrapped *Tablets:* Boxes of 12, 100 and 1000.
White tablets coded with number 411-Miles.
Shown in Product Identification Section, page 419

DTIC–Dome® ℞
(dacarbazine)
Sterile

> ### WARNING
> It is recommended that DTIC-Dome (dacarbazine) be administered under the supervision of a qualified physician experienced in the use of cancer chemotherapeutic agents.
> 1. Hemopoietic depression is the most common toxicity with DTIC-Dome (See Warnings).
> 2. Hepatic necrosis has been reported (See Warnings).
> 3. Studies have demonstrated this agent to have a carcinogenic and teratogenic effect when used in animals.
> 4. In treatment of each patient, the physician must weigh carefully the possibility of achieving therapeutic benefit against the risk of toxicity.

DESCRIPTION
DTIC-Dome Sterile (dacarbazine) is a colorless to an ivory colored solid which is light sensitive. Each vial contains 100mg of dacarbazine, or 200mg of dacarbazine (the active ingredient), anhydrous citric acid and mannitol. DTIC-Dome is reconstituted and administered intravenously (pH 3-4). DTIC-Dome is an anticancer agent. Chemically, DTIC-Dome is 5-(3, 3-dimethyl-l-triazeno)-imidazole-4-carboxamide (DTIC).

$C_6H_{10}N_6O$

CLINICAL PHARMACOLOGY
After intravenous administration of DTIC-Dome, the volume of distribution exceeds total body water content suggesting localization in some body tissue, probably the liver. Its disappearance from the plasma is biphasic with initial half-life of 19 minutes and a terminal half-life of 5 hours. In a patient with renal and hepatic dysfunctions, the half-lives were lengthened to 55 minutes and 7.2 hours. The average cumulative excretion of unchanged DTIC in the urine is 40% of the injected dose in 6 hours. DTIC is subject to renal tubular secretion rather than glomerular filtration. At therapeutic concentrations DTIC is not appreciably bound to human plasma protein.

In man, DTIC is extensively degraded. Besides unchanged DTIC, 5-aminoimidazole -4 carboxamide (AIC) is a major metabolite of DTIC excreted in the urine. AIC is not derived endogenously but from the injected DTIC, because the administration of radioactive DTIC labeled with ^{14}C in the imidazole portion of the molecule (DTIC-2-^{14}C) gives rise to AIC-2-^{14}C.[1]

Although the exact mechanism of action of DTIC-Dome is not known, three hypotheses have been offered:
1. inhibition of DNA synthesis by acting as a purine analog
2. action as an alkylating agent
3. interaction with SH groups

INDICATIONS AND USAGE
DTIC-Dome is indicated in the treatment of metastatic malignant melanoma. In addition, DTIC-Dome is also indicated for Hodgkin's disease as a secondary-line therapy when used in combination with other effective agents.

CONTRAINDICATIONS
DTIC-Dome is contraindicated in patients who have demonstrated a hypersensitivity to it in the past.

WARNINGS
Hemopoietic depression is the most common toxicity with DTIC-Dome and involves primarily the leukocytes and platelets, although, anemia may sometimes occur. Leukopenia and thrombocypenia may be severe enough to cause death. The possible bone marrow depression requires careful monitoring of white blood cells, red blood cells, and platelet levels. Hemopoietic toxicity may warrant temporary suspension or cessation of therapy with DTIC-Dome.

Hepatic toxicity accompanied by hepatic vein thrombosis and hepatocellular necrosis resulting in death, has been reported. The incidence of such reactions has been low; approximately 0.01% of patients treated. This toxicity has been observed mostly when DTIC-Dome has been administered concomitantly with other anti-neoplastic drugs; however, it has also been reported in some patients treated with DTIC-Dome alone.

Anaphylaxis can occur following the administration of DTIC-Dome.

PRECAUTIONS
Hospitalization is not always necessary but adequate laboratory study capability must be available. Extravasation of the drug subcutaneously during intravenous administration may result in tissue damage and severe pain. Local pain, burning sensation, and irritation at the site of injection may be relieved by locally applied hot packs.

Carcinogenicity of DTIC was studied in rats and mice. Proliferative endocardial lesions, including fibrosarcomas and sarcomas were induced by DTIC in rats. In mice, administration of DTIC resulted in the induction of angiosarcomas of the spleen.

Pregnancy Category C—DTIC-Dome has been shown to be teratogenic in rats when given in doses 20 times the human daily dose on day 12 of gestation. DTIC when administered in 10 times the human daily dose to male rats (twice weekly for 9 weeks) did not affect the male libido, although female rats mated to male rats had higher incidence of resorptions than controls. In rabbits, DTIC daily dose 7 times the human daily dose given on Days 6–15 of gestation resulted in fetal skeletal anomalies. There are no adequate and well controlled studies in pregnant women. DTIC-Dome should be used during pregnancy only if the potential benefit justifies the potential risk to the fetus.

It is not known whether this drug is excreted in human milk. Because many drugs are excreted in human milk and because of the potential for tumorigenicity shown for DTIC-Dome in animal studies, a decision should be made whether to discontinue nursing or to discontinue the drug, taking into account the importance of the drug to the mother.

ADVERSE REACTIONS
Symptoms of anorexia, nausea, and vomiting are the most frequently noted of all toxic reactions. Over 90% of patients are affected with the initial few doses. The vomiting lasts 1–12 hours and is incompletely and unpredictably palliated with phenobarbital and/or prochlorperazine. Rarely, intractable nausea and vomiting have necessitated discontinuance of therapy with DTIC-Dome. Rarely, DTIC-Dome has caused diarrhea. Some helpful suggestions include restricting the patient's oral intake of food for 4–6 hours prior to treatment. The rapid toleration of these symptoms suggests that a central nervous system mechanism may be involved, and usually these symptoms subside after the first 1 or 2 days.

There are a number of minor toxicities that are infrequently noted. Patients have experienced an influenza-like syndrome of fever to 39°C, myalgias and malaise. These symptoms occur usually after large single doses, may last for several days, and they may occur with successive treatments. Alopecia has been noted as has facial flushing and facial paresthesia. There have been few reports of significant liver or renal function test abnormalities in man. However, these abnormalities have been observed more frequently in animal studies.

Erythematous and urticarial rashes have been observed infrequently after administration of DTIC-Dome. Rarely, photosensitivity reactions may occur.

OVERDOSAGE
Give supportive treatment and monitor blood cell counts.

DOSAGE AND ADMINISTRATION
MALIGNANT MELANOMA—The recommended dosage is 2 to 4.5mg/kg/day for 10 days. Treatment may be repeated at 4 week intervals.[2]

An alternate recommended dosage is 250mg/square meter body surface/day I.V. for 5 days. Treatment may be repeated every 3 weeks.[3,4]

HODGKIN'S DISEASE: The recommended dosage of DTIC-Dome in the treatment of Hodgkin's Disease is 150mg/square meter body surface/day for 5 days, in combination with other effective drugs. Treatment may be repeated every 4 weeks.[5] An alternative recommended dosage is 375mg/square meter body surface on day 1, in combination with other effective drugs, to be repeated every 15 days.[6]

DTIC-Dome (dacarbazine) 100mg/vial and 200mg/vial are reconstituted with 9.9 ml and 19.7 ml, respectively, of Sterile Water for Injection, U.S.P. The resulting solution contains 10mg/ml of dacarbazine having a pH of 3.0 to 4.0. The calculated dose of the resulting solution is drawn into a syringe and administered *only* intravenously.

The reconstituted solution may be further diluted with 5% dextrose injection, U.S.P. or sodium chloride injection, U.S.P. and administered as an intravenous infusion.

After reconstitution and prior to use, the solution in the vial may be stored at 4°C for up to 72 hours or at normal room conditions (temperature and light) for up to 8 hours. If the reconstituted solution is further diluted in 5% dextrose, injection, U.S.P. or sodium chloride injection, U.S.P., the resulting solution may be stored at 4°C for up to 24 hours or at normal room conditions for up to 8 hours.

Procedures for proper handling and disposal of anticancer drugs should be considered. Several guidelines on this subject have been published.[7-12] There is no general agreement

Continued on next page

Miles Pharm. Div.—Cont.

that all of the procedures recommended in the guidelines are necessary or appropriate.

HOW SUPPLIED

10 ml vials containing 100mg or 20 ml vials containing 200 mg of DTIC-Dome as sterile dacarbazine in boxes of 12. Store in refrigerator 2°C to 8°C (36°F to 46°F).

REFERENCES

1. Loo, T.J., et al.: Mechanism of action and pharmacology studies with DTIC (NSC-45388). Cancer Treatment Reports 60: 149–152, 1976.
2. Nathanson, L., et al.: Characteristics of prognosis and response to an imidazole carboxamide in malignant melanoma. Clinical Pharmacology and Therapeutics 12: 955–962, 1971.
3. Costanza, M.E., et al.: Therapy of malignant melanoma with an imidazole carboxamide and bischloroethyl nitrosourea. Cancer 30: 1457–1461, 1972.
4. Luce, J.K., et al.: Clinical trials with the antitumor agent 5-(3, 3-dimethyl-l-triazeno) imidazole-4-carboxamide (NSC-45388). Cancer Chemotherapy Reports 54: 119–124, 1970.
5. Bonadonna, G., et al.: Combined Chemotherapy (MOPP or ABVD)—radiotherapy approach in advanced Hodgkin's disease. Cancer Treatment Reports 61: 769–777, 1977.
6. Santoro, A., and Bonadonna, G.: Prolonged disease-free survival in MOPP-resistant Hodgkin's disease after treatment with adriamycin, bleomycin, vinblastine and decarbazine (ABVD). Cancer Chemotherapy Pharmacol. 2: 101–105, 1979.
7. Recommendations for the Safe Handling of Parenteral Antineoplastic Drugs. NIH Publication No. 83-2621. For sale by the Superintendent of Documents, U.S. Government Printing Office, Washington, D.C. 20402.
8. AMA Council Report. Guidelines for Handling Parenteral Antineoplastics. JAMA, March 15, 1985.
9. National Study Commission on Cytotoxic Exposure—Recommendations for Handling Cytotoxic Agents. Available from Louis P. Jeffrey, Sc. D., Director of Pharmacy Services, Rhode Island Hospital, 593 Eddy Street, Providence, Rhode Island 02902.
10. Clinical Oncological Society of Australia: Guidelines and recommendations for safe handling of antineoplastic agents. Med. J. Australia 1: 426–428, 1983.
11. Jones, R.B., et al.: Safe handling of chemotherapeutic agents: A report from the Mount Sinai Medical Center. Ca-A Cancer Journal for Clinicians Sept./Oct. 258–263, 1983.
12. American Society of Hospital Pharmacists technical assistance bulletin on handling cytotoxic drugs in hospitals. Am. J. Hosp. Pharm. 42: 131–137, 1985.

Manufactured by:
Ben Venue Laboratories
Bedford, Ohio 44146
Distributed by:
Miles Inc.
Pharmaceutical Division
400 Morgan Lane
West Haven, CT 06516

PD100688   0561   6/88

LITHANE®   ℞
(lithium carbonate)
TABLETS

For Control of Manic Episodes
in Manic-Depressive Psychosis

Warning

> Lithium toxicity is closely related to serum lithium levels, and can occur at doses close to therapeutic levels. Facilities for prompt and accurate serum lithium determinations should be available before initiating therapy.

DESCRIPTION

Lithium carbonate is a white, light, alkaline powder with molecular formula Li_2CO_3 and molecular weight 73.89. Lithium is an element of the alkali-metal group with atomic number 3, atomic weight 6.94, and an emission line at 671 nm on the flame photometer. Lithane® tablets contain the following inactive ingredients: Corn Starch, Dibasic Calcium Phosphate, FD & C Yellow No. 5 Dye, Lake, FD & C Blue No. 1 Dye, Lake, Magnesium Stearate, Polyethylene Glycol, Sodium Lauryl Sulfate.

ACTIONS

Preclinical studies have shown that lithium alters sodium transport in nerve and muscle cells and effects a shift toward intraneuronal metabolism of catecholamines, but the spe-

cific biochemical mechanism of lithium action in mania is unknown.

INDICATIONS

Lithium carbonate is indicated in the treatment of manic episodes of manic-depressive illness. Maintenance therapy prevents or diminishes the intensity of subsequent episodes in those manic-depressive patients with a history of mania.
Typical symptoms of mania include pressure of speech, motor hyperactivity, reduced need for sleep, flight of ideas, grandiosity, elation, poor judgment, aggressiveness, and possibly hostility. When given to a patient experiencing a manic episode, lithium may produce a normalization of symptomatology within 1 to 3 weeks.

WARNINGS

Lithium should generally not be given to patients with significant renal or cardiovascular disease, severe debilitation or dehydration, or sodium depletion, and to patients receiving diuretics, since the risk of lithium toxicity is very high in such patients. If the psychiatric indication is life-threatening, and if such a patient fails to respond to other measures, lithium treatment may be undertaken with extreme caution, including daily serum lithium determinations and adjustment to the usually low doses ordinarily tolerated by these individuals. In such instances, hospitalization is a necessity. Chronic lithium therapy may be associated with diminution of renal concentrating ability, occasionally presenting as nephrogenic diabetes insipidus, with polyuria and polydipsia. Such patients should be carefully managed to avoid dehydration with resulting lithium retention and toxicity. This condition is usually reversible when lithium is discontinued. Morphologic changes with glomerular and interstitial fibrosis and nephron atrophy have been reported in patients on chronic lithium therapy. Morphologic changes have also been seen in manic-depressive patients never exposed to lithium. The relationship between renal functional and morphologic changes and their association with lithium therapy have not been established.
When kidney function is assessed, for baseline data prior to starting lithium therapy or thereafter, routine urinalysis and other tests may be used to evaluate tubular function (e.g. urine specific gravity or osmolality following a period of water deprivation, or 24 hour urine volume) and glomerular function (e.g. serum creatinine or creatinine clearance). During lithium therapy, progressive or sudden changes in renal function, even within the normal range, indicate the need for reevaluation of treatment.
Lithium therapy has been reported in some cases to be associated with morphologic changes in the kidneys. The relationship between such changes and renal function has not been established.
An encephalopathic syndrome (characterized by weakness, lethargy, fever, tremulousness and confusion, extrapyramidal symptoms, leukocytosis, elevated serum enzymes, BUN and FBS) followed by irreversible brain damage has occurred in a few patients treated with lithium plus haloperidol. A causal relationship between these events and the concomitant administration of lithium and haloperidol has not been established; however, patients receiving such combined therapy should be monitored closely for early evidence of neurologic toxicity and treatment discontinued promptly if such signs appear. The possibility of similar adverse interactions with other antipsychotic medication exists.
Lithium toxicity is closely related to serum lithium levels, and can occur at doses close to therapeutic levels (see DOSAGE AND ADMINISTRATION).
Outpatients and their families should be warned that the patient must discontinue lithium carbonate therapy and contact his physician if such clinical signs of lithium toxicity as diarrhea, vomiting, tremor, mild ataxia, drowsiness, or muscular weakness occur.
Lithium carbonate may impair mental and/or physical abilities. Caution patients about activities requiring alertness (e.g., operating vehicles or machinery).
Lithium may prolong the effects of neuromuscular blocking agents. Therefore, neuromuscular blocking agents should be given with caution to patients receiving lithium.
Usage in Pregnancy: Adverse effects on nidation in rats, embryo viability in mice, and metabolism in vitro of rat testis and human spermatozoa have been attributed to lithium, as have teratogenicity in submammalian species and cleft palates in mice. Studies in rats, rabbits, and monkeys have shown no evidence of lithium-induced teratology.
In humans, lithium carbonate may cause fetal harm when administered to a pregnant woman. Data from lithium birth registries suggest an increase in cardiac and other anomalies, especially Ebstein' anomaly. If this drug is used during pregnancy, or if a patient becomes pregnant while taking this drug, the patient should be apprised of the potential hazard to the fetus.
There are lithium birth registries in the United States and elsewhere; however there is at the present time insufficient data to determine the effects of lithium carbonate on human fetuses. Therefore, at this point, lithium should not be used in pregnancy, especially the first trimester, unless in the

opinion of the physician, the potential benefits outweigh the possible hazards.
Usage in Nursing Mothers: Lithium is excreted in human milk. Nursing should not be undertaken during lithium therapy except in rare and unusual circumstances where, in the view of the physician, the potential benefits to the mother outweigh possible hazards to the child.
Usage in Children: Since information regarding the safety and effectiveness of lithium carbonate in children under 12 years of age is not available, its use in such patients is not recommended at this time.

PRECAUTIONS

The ability to tolerate lithium is greater during the acute manic phase and decreases when manic symptoms subside (see DOSAGE AND ADMINISTRATION).
Caution should be used when lithium and diuretics are used concomitantly because diuretic-induced sodium loss may reduce the renal clearance of lithium and increase serum lithium levels with risk of lithium toxicity. Patients receiving such combined therapy should have serum lithium levels monitored closely and the lithium dosage adjusted if necessary.
The distribution space of lithium approximates that of total body water. Lithium is primarily excreted in urine with insignificant excretion in feces. Renal excretion of lithium is proportional to its plasma concentration. The half-life of elimination of lithium is approximately 24 hours. Lithium decreases sodium reabsorption by the renal tubules which could lead to sodium depletion. Therefore, it is essential for the patient to maintain a normal diet, including salt, and an adequate fluid intake (2500–3000 ml) at least during the initial stabilization period. Decreased tolerance to lithium has been reported to ensue from protracted sweating or diarrhea and, if such occur, supplemental fluid and salt should be administered.
In addition to sweating and diarrhea, concomitant infection with elevated temperatures may also necessitate a temporary reduction or cessation of medication.
Previously existing underlying thyroid disorders do not necessarily constitute a contraindication to lithium treatment; where hypothyroidism exists, careful monitoring of thyroid function during lithium stabilization and maintenance allows for correction of changing thyroid parameters, if any; where hypothroidism occurs during lithium stabilization and maintenance, supplemental thyroid treatment may be used.
This product contains FD&C Yellow No. 5 (tartrazine) which may cause allergic-type reactions (including bronchial asthma) in certain susceptible individuals. Although the over-all incidence of FD&C Yellow No. 5 (tartrazine) sensitivity in the general population is low, it is frequently seen in patients who also have aspirin hypersensitivity.
Indomethacin has been reported to increase steady state plasma lithium levels from 30 to 59 percent. There is also some evidence that other nonsteroidal anti-inflammatory agents may have a similar effect. When such combinations are used, increased plasma lithium level monitoring is recommended.

ADVERSE REACTIONS

Adverse reactions are seldom encountered at serum lithium levels below 1.5 mEq./l., except in the occasional patient sensitive to lithium. Mild to moderate toxic reactions may occur at levels from 1.5–2.5 mEq./l., and moderate to severe reactions may be seen at levels from 2.0–2.5 mEq./l., depending upon individual response to the drug.
Fine hand tremor, polyuria, and mild thirst may occur during initial therapy for the acute manic phase, and may persist throughout treatment. Transient and mild nausea and general discomfort may also appear during the first few days of lithium administration.
These side effects are an inconvenience rather than a disabling condition, and usually subside with continued treatment or a temporary reduction or cessation of dosage. If persistent, a cessation of dosage is indicated.
Diarrhea, vomiting, drowsiness, muscular weakness, and lack of coordination may be early signs of lithium intoxication, and can occur at lithium levels below 2.0 mEq./l. At higher levels, giddiness, ataxia, blurred vision, tinnitus, and a large output of dilute urine may be seen. Serum lithium levels above 3.0 mEq./l. may produce a complex clinical picture involving multiple organs and organ systems. Serum lithium levels should not be permitted to exceed 2.0 mEq./l, during the acute treatment phase.
The following reactions have been reported and appear to be related to serum lithium levels, including levels within the therapeutic range:
Neurological: Cases of pseudotumor cerebri (increased intracranial pressure and papilledema) have been reported with lithium use. If undetected, this condition may result in enlargement of the blind spot, constriction of visual fields and eventual blindness due to optic atrophy. Lithium should be discontinued, if clinically possible, if this syndrome occurs.

MEZLOCILLIN SERUM LEVELS IN ADULTS (mcg/mL) 5 MIN. IV INJECTION

DOSE	0	5 min.	10 min.	20 min.	30 min.	1 hr.	2 hr.	3 hr.	4 hr.	6 hr.	8 hr.
1g	149 (132–185)	100 (64–143)	66 (47–87)	50 (31–87)	40 (22–83)	18 (8–31)	5.3 (3.3–7.7)	2.5 (1.7–3.7)	1.7 (0.7–2.8)	0.5 (0–1.2)	0.1 (0–0.2)
2g	314 (207–362)	253 (161–364)	161 (113–214)	117 (76–174)	82 (55–112)	56 (23–88)	20 (7.5–32)	11 (3.8–16)	4.4 (1.6–8.7)	1.5 (0.5–2.6)	0.6 (0.1–1.4)
5g	547 (268–854)	411 (199–597)	357 (246–456)	250 (203–353)	226 (190–333)	131 (104–193)	76 (59–104)	31 (20–40)	13 (6.4–17)	4.6 (2.1–9.4)	1.9 (1.1–3.6)

MEZLIN®   MEZLOCILLIN SERUM LEVELS IN ADULTS (mcg/mL) 30 MIN. IV INFUSION

DOSE	0	5 min.	15 min.	30 min.	45 min.	1 hr.	2 hr.	3 hr.	4 hr.	6 hr.	8 hr.
3g	263 (87–489)	170 (63–371)	141 (75–301)	109 (56–288)	79 (41–135)	57 (28–100)	26 (14–55)	12 (5.8–26)	4.4 (2.2–6.5)	1.6 (1.0–3.4)	<1

Neuromuscular: tremor, muscle hyperirritability (fasciculations, twitching, clonic movements of whole limbs), ataxia, choreo-athetotic movements, hyperactive deep tendon reflexes.

Central Nervous System: blackout spells, epileptiform seizures, slurred speech, dizziness, vertigo, incontinence of urine or feces, somnolence, psychomotor retardation, restlessness, confusion stupor, coma.

Cardiovascular: cardiac arrhythmia, hypotension, peripheral circulatory collapse.

Gastrointestinal: anorexia, nausea, vomiting, diarrhea.

Genitourinary: albuminuria, oliguria, polyuria, glycosuria.

Dermatologic: drying and thinning of hair, anesthesia of skin, chronic folliculitis, xerosis cutis, alopecia, and exacerbation of psoriasis.

Autonomic Nervous System: blurred vision, dry mouth.

Thyroid Abnormalities: Euthyroid goiter and/or hypothyroidism (including myxedema) accompanied by lower T_3 and T_4. I^{131} iodine uptake may be elevated. (See **Precautions**.) Paradoxically, rare cases of hyperthroidism have been reported.

EEG. Changes: diffuse slowing, widening of frequency spectrum, potentiation and disorganization of background rhythm.

EKG. Changes: reversible flattening, isoelectricity or inversion of T-waves.

Miscellaneous: fatigue, lethargy, tendency to sleep, dehydration, weight loss, transient scotomata.

Miscellaneous reactions unrelated to dosage are: transient electroencephalographic and electrocardiographic changes, leucocytosis, headache, diffuse non-toxic goiter with or without hypothyroidism, transient hyperglycemia, generalized pruritus with or without rash, cutaneous ulcers, albuminuria, worsening of organic brain syndromes, excessive weight gain, edematous swelling of ankles or wrists, and thirst or polyuria, sometimes resembling diabetes insipidus, and metallic taste. A single report has been received of the development of painful discoloration of fingers and toes and coldness of the extremities within one day of the starting of treatment of lithium. The mechanism through which these symptoms (resembling Raynaud's Syndrome) developed is not known. Recovery followed discontinuance.

DOSAGE AND ADMINISTRATION

Acute Mania: Optimal patient response to lithium carbonate usually can be established and maintained with 600 mg t.i.d. Such doses will normally produce an effective serum lithium level ranging between 1.0 and 1.5 mEq./l. Dosage must be individualized according to serum levels and clinical response. Regular monitoring of the patient's clinical state and of serum lithium levels is necessary. Serum levels should be determined twice per week during the acute phase, and until the serum level and clinical condition of the patient have been stabilized.

Long term Control: The desirable lithium levels are 0.6 to 1.2 mEq./l. Dosage will vary from one individual to another, but usually 300 mg t.i.d. or q.i.d. will maintain this level. Serum lithium levels in uncomplicated cases receiving maintenance therapy during remission should be monitored at least every two months.

Patients abnormally sensitive to lithium may exhibit toxic signs at serum levels of 1.0 to 1.5 mEq./l. Elderly patients often respond to reduced dosage, and may exhibit signs of toxicity at serum levels ordinarily tolerated by other patients.

N.B.: Blood samples for serum lithium determinations should be drawn immediately prior to the next dose when lithium concentrations are relatively stable (i.e., 8–12 hours after the previous dose). Total reliance must not be placed on serum levels alone. Accurate patient evaluation requires both clinical and laboratory analysis.

OVERDOSAGE

The toxic levels for lithium are close to the therapeutic levels. It is therefore important that patients and their families be cautioned to watch for early toxic symptoms and to discontinue the drug and inform the physician should they occur. Toxic symptoms are listed in detail under ADVERSE REACTIONS.

Treatment: No specific antidote for lithium poisoning is known. Early symptoms of lithium toxicity can usually be treated by reduction or cessation of dosage of the drug and resumption of the treatment at a lower dose after 24 to 48 hours. In severe cases of lithium poisoning, the first and foremost goal of treatment consists of elimination of this ion from the organism.

Treatment is essentially the same as that used in barbiturate poisoning: 1) lavage, 2) correction of fluid and electrolyte imbalance, and 3) regulation of kidney functioning. Urea, mannitol, and aminophylline all produce significant increases in lithium excretion. Hemodialysis is an effective and rapid means of removing the ion from the severely toxic patient. Infection prophylaxis, regular chest X-rays, and preservation of adequate respiration are essential.

HOW SUPPLIED

Lithane® (lithium carbonate) is available as round green scored tablets containing 300 mg of lithium carbonate embossed with the word "MILES" and the three digit code 951, in bottles of 100.

PD100591   Revised July 1983
Manufactured for
Miles Inc.
Pharmaceutical Division
400 Morgan Lane
West Haven, CT 06516
by Pfizer, Inc., New York, N.Y. 10017
©1980, Miles Inc.
Shown in Product Identification Section, page 419

MEZLIN®   ℞
Sterile mezlocillin sodium
for intravenous or intramuscular use.
BAYPEN®

DESCRIPTION

MEZLIN® (sterile mezlocillin sodium) is a semisynthetic broad spectrum penicillin antibiotic for parenteral administration. It is the monohydrate sodium salt of 6-{D-2 [3-(methyl-sulfonyl)-2-OXO- imidazolidine-1-carboxamido]-2-phenyl acetamido} penicillanic acid.

Structural Formula:

Empirical Formula: $C_{21}H_{24}N_5O_8S_2Na \cdot H_2O$
MEZLIN® has a molecular weight of 579.6 and contains 42.6 mg (1.85 mEq) of sodium per one gram of mezlocillin activity. The dosage form is supplied as a sterile white to pale yellow crystalline powder, which is freely soluble in water. When reconstituted, solutions of MEZLIN® are clear and range from colorless to pale yellow with a pH of 4.5 to 8.0.

CLINICAL PHARMACOLOGY

Intravenous Administration. In healthy adult volunteers, mean serum levels of mezlocillin 5 minutes after a 5-minute intravenous injection of 1g, 2g, or 5g are 100, 253, or 411 mcg/mL, respectively. Serum levels, as noted below, lack dose proportionality.
[See table above].
Fifteen minutes after a 4g intravenous injection (2–5 min.), the concentration in serum is 254 mcg/mL; 1 hour and 4 hours later levels are 93 mcg/mL and 9.1 mcg/mL, respectively:
[See table below].
After an intravenous infusion (15 min.) of 3g, mean levels 15 minutes after dosing are 269 mcg/mL (170–280).
A 30-minute intravenous infusion of 3g produces mean peak concentrations of 263 mcg/mL; 1 hour and 4 hours later the concentrations are 57 mcg/mL and 4.4 mcg/mL, respectively:
[See table above].
Following intravenous infusion (2 hr.) of a 3g dose of mezlocillin every 4 hours for 7 days, mean peak serum concentrations are higher than 100 mcg/mL, and levels above 50 mcg/mL are maintained throughout dosing.

Intramuscular Administration. MEZLIN® is rapidly absorbed after intramuscular injection. In healthy volunteers, the mean peak serum concentration occurs approximately 45 minutes after a single dose of 1g and is about 15 mcg/mL. The oral administration of 1g probenecid before injection produces an increase in mezlocillin serum levels of about 50%. After repetitive intramuscular doses of 1g mezlocillin every 6 hours, peak levels in the serum generally range between 35 and 45 mcg/mL. The relationship between the pharmacokinetics of intramuscular and intravenous dosing has not yet been clearly established.

General. As with other penicillins, mezlocillin is excreted primarily by glomerular filtration and tubular secretion. The rate of elimination is dose dependent and related to the degree of renal functional impairment. In patients with normal renal function, approximately 55% of the administered dose is recovered from the urine within the first 6 hours after dosing. Two hours after an intravenous injection of 2g, concentrations of active drug in urine generally exceed 4000 mcg/mL. By 4–6 hours after injection, concentrations usually decline to a range of about 50 to 200 mcg/mL. The serum elimination half-life of mezlocillin after intravenous dosing is approximately 55 minutes.

In patients with reduced renal function, the half-life is only slightly prolonged. Dosage adjustments are usually not necessary except in patients with severe renal impairment. (See Dosage and Administration). As with other penicillins, mezlocillin is metabolized only slightly; less than 10% of the drug excreted in the urine is in the form of the penicilloate or penilloate. The drug is readily removed from the serum by hemodialysis and, to a lesser extent, by peritoneal dialysis. Up to 26% of a dose of mezlocillin is recovered from the bile of patients with normal liver function. Following intravenous doses of 2 to 5g, concentrations of active drug in bile generally range from 500 to 2500 mcg/mL. The biliary excretion of mezlocillin is reduced in patients with common bile duct obstruction.

Mezlocillin is not appreciably absorbed when given orally. Following parenteral administration, the apparent volume of distribution is approximately equal to the extracellular fluid volume. The drug is present in active form in the serum, urine, bile, peritoneal fluid, pleural fluid, bronchial and wound secretions, bone and other tissues. As with other penicillins, penetration into the cerebrospinal fluid (CSF) is generally poor, however higher CSF concentrations are obtained in the presence of meningeal inflammation.

Protein binding studies indicate that the degree of mezlocillin binding is low (16–42%) and depends upon testing methods and concentrations of drug studied.

Microbiology
Mezlocillin is a bactericidal antibiotic which acts by interfering with synthesis of cell wall components. It is active

Continued on next page

MEZLIN®

MEZLOCILLIN SERUM LEVELS IN ADULTS (mcg/mL) 2–5 MIN. IV INJECTION

DOSE	0	15 min.	30 min.	45 min.	1 hr.	2 hr.	3 hr.	4 hr.	6 hr.
4g	—	254 (155–400)	163 (99–260)	122 (78–215)	93 (67–133)	47 (22–96)	20 (8–45)	9.1 (6–13)	8.4 (5–17)

Miles Pharm. Div.—Cont.

against a variety of gram-negative and gram-positive bacteria, including aerobic and anaerobic strains. Mezlocillin is usually active *in vitro* against most strains of the following organisms:

Gram-negative bacteria

Escherichia coli	*Klebsiella* species (including K. pneumoniae)
Proteus mirabilis	*Enterobacter* species
Proteus vulgaris	*Shigella* species*
Morganella morganii (formerly *P. morganii*)	*Pseudomonas aeruginosa* (and other species)
Providencia rettgeri (formerly *Proteus rettgeri*)	*Haemophilus influenzae*
Providencia stuartii	*Haemophilus parainfluenzae*
Citrobacter species*	*Neisseria* species

Many strains of *Serratia, Salmonella**, and *Acinetobacter** are also susceptible.

Gram-positive bacteria

Staphylococcus aureus (non-penicillinase producing strains)
Beta-hemolytic *streptococci* (Groups A and B)
Streptococcus pneumoniae (formerly *Diplococcus Pneumoniae*)
Streptococcus faecalis (enterococcus)

Anaerobic Organisms

Peptococcus species	*Fusobacterium* species*
Peptostreptococcus species	*Veillonella* species*
Clostridium species*	*Eubacterium* species*

Bacteroides species (including *B. fragilis* group)

* Mezlocillin has been shown to be active *in vitro* against these organisms, however clinical efficacy has not yet been established.

Noteworthy is mezlocillin's broadened spectrum of *in vitro* activity against important pathogenic aerobic gram-negative bacteria, including strains of *Pseudomonas, Klebsiella, Enterobacter, Serratia, Proteus, Escherichia* and *Haemophilus*, as well as *Bacteroides* and other anaerobes; and its excellent inhibitory effect against gram-positive organisms including *Streptococcus faecalis* (enterococcus). It is inactive against penicillinase-producing strains of *Staphylococcus aureus*.

In vitro studies have shown that mezlocillin combined with an aminoglycoside (e.g., gentamicin, tobramycin, amikacin, sisomicin) acts synergistically against strains of *Streptococcus faecalis* and *Pseudomonas aeruginosa*. In some instances, this combination also acts synergistically *in vitro* against other gram-negative bacteria such as *Serratia, Klebsiella* and *Acinetobacter* species.

Mezlocillin is slightly more active when tested at alkaline pH and, as with other penicillins, has reduced activity when tested *in vitro* with increasing inoculum. The minimum bactericidal concentration (MBC) generally exceeds the minimum inhibitory concentration (MIC) by a factor of 2 or 3. Resistance to mezlocillin *in vitro* develops slowly (multiple step mutation). Some strains of *Pseudomonas aeruginosa* have developed resistance fairly rapidly. Mezlocillin is not stable in the presence of penicillinase and strains of *Staphylococcus aureus* resistant to penicillin are also resistant to mezlocillin.

Susceptibility Tests

Quantitative methods that require measurement of zone diameters give good estimates of bacterial susceptibility. One such procedure* has been recommended for use with discs to test susceptibility to antimicrobials, When the causative organism is tested by the Kirby-Bauer method of disc susceptibility, a 75 mcg mezlocillin disc should give a zone of 18 mm or greater to indicate susceptibility. Zone sizes of 14 mm or less indicate resistance. Zone sizes of 15 to 17 mm indicate intermediate susceptibility. Susceptible strains of *Haemophilus* and *Neisseria* species give zones of ≥ 29 mm, resistant strains ≤ 28 mm. With this procedure, a report from the laboratory of "Susceptible" indicates that the infecting organism is likely to respond to therapy. A report of "Resistant" indicates that the infecting organism is not likely to respond to therapy; other therapy should be selected. A report of "Intermediate Susceptibility" suggests that the organism may be susceptible if the infection is confined to tissues and fluids (e.g., urine), in which high antibiotic levels are attained. The mezlocillin disc should be used for testing susceptibility to mezlocillin. In certain conditions, it may be desirable to do additional susceptibility testing by broth or agar dilution techniques. Dilution methods, preferably the agar plate dilution procedure, are most accurate for susceptibility testing of obligate anaerobes. *Enterobacteriaceae, Pseudomonas* species and *Acinetobacter* species are considered susceptible if the MIC of mezlocillin is no greater than 64 mcg/mL and are considered resistant if the MIC is greater than 128 mcg/mL. *Haemophilus* and *Neisseria* species are considered susceptible if the MIC of mezlocillin is less than or equal to 1 mcg/mL. Mezlocillin standard is available for broth or agar dilution studies.

* Bauer, A.W., Kirby, W.M., Sherris, J.C. and Turck, M.: Antibiotic Testing by a Standardized Single Disc Method, Am. J. Clin. Pathol., 45:493, 1966. Standardized Disc Susceptibility Test, FEDERAL REGISTER 39: 19182–19184, 1974.

INDICATIONS AND USAGE

MEZLIN® is indicated for the treatment of serious infections caused by susceptible strains of the designated microorganisms in the conditions listed below:

LOWER RESPIRATORY TRACT INFECTIONS including pneumonia and lung abscess caused by *Haemophilus influenzae, Klebsiella* species including *K. pneumoniae, Proteus mirabilis, Pseudomonas* species including *P. aeruginosa, E. coli,* and *Bacteroides* species including *B. fragilis.*

INTRA-ABDOMINAL INFECTIONS including acute cholecystitis, cholangitis, peritonitis, hepatic abscess and intra-abdominal abscess caused by susceptible *E. coli, Proteus mirabilis, Klebsiella* species, *Pseudomonas* species, *S. faecalis* (enterococcus), *Bacteroides* species, *Peptococcus* species, and *Peptostreptococcus* species.

URINARY TRACT INFECTIONS caused by susceptible *E. coli, Proteus mirabilis,* the indole positive *Proteus* species, *Morganella morganii; Klebsiella* species, *Enterobacter* species, *Serratia* species, *Pseudomonas* species, *S. faecalis* (enterococcus).
Uncomplicated gonorrhea due to susceptible *Neisseria gonorrhoeae.*

GYNECOLOGICAL INFECTIONS including endometritis, pelvic cellulitis, and pelvic inflammatory disease associated with susceptible *Neisseria gonorrhoeae, Peptococcus* species, *Peptostreptococcus* species, *Bacteroides* species, *E. coli, Proteus mirabilis, Klebsiella* species, and *Enterobacter* species.

SKIN AND SKIN STRUCTURE INFECTIONS caused by susceptible *S. faecalis* (enterococcus), *E. coli, Proteus mirabilis,* the indole positive *Proteus* species, *Proteus vulgaris,* and *Providencia rettgeri; Klebsiella* species, *Enterobacter* species, *Pseudomonas* species, *Peptococcus* species, and *Bacteroides* species.

SEPTICEMIA including bacteremia caused by susceptible *E. coli, Klebsiella* species, *Enterobacter* species, *Pseudomonas* species, *Bacteroides* species, and *Peptococcus* species.

Mezlocillin has also been shown to be effective for the treatment of infections caused by *Streptococcus* species including Group A Beta-hemolytic *Streptococcus* and *Streptococcus pneumoniae* (formerly *Diplococcus pneumoniae*) however, infections caused by these organisms are ordinarily treated with more narrow spectrum penicillins.

Appropriate culture and susceptibility tests should be performed before treatment in order to isolate and identify organisms causing infection and to determine their susceptibility to mezlocillin. Therapy with MEZLIN® may be initiated before results of these tests are known; once results become available, appropriate therapy should be continued.

Mezlocillin's broad spectrum of activity makes it particularly useful for treating mixed infections caused by susceptible strains of both gram-negative and gram-positive aerobic or anaerobic bacteria. It is not effective, however, against infections caused by penicillinase-producing *Staphylococcus aureus.*

In certain severe infections, when the causative organisms are unknown, MEZLIN® may be administered in conjunction with an aminoglycoside or a cephalosporin antibiotic as initial therapy. As soon as results of culture and susceptibility tests become available, antimicrobial therapy should be adjusted if indicated. Culture and sensitivity testing, performed periodically during therapy, will provide information on the therapeutic effect of the antimicrobal and will monitor for the possible emergence of bacterial resistance.

MEZLIN® has been used effectively in combination with an aminoglycoside antibiotic for the treatment of life-threatening infections caused by *Pseudomonas aeruginosa*. For the treatment of febrile episodes in immunosuppressed patients with granulocytopenia, MEZLIN® should be combined with an aminoglycoside or a cephalosporin antibiotic.

Prevention: The administration of MEZLIN® perioperatively (preoperatively, intraoperatively, and postoperatively) may reduce the incidence of infections in patients undergoing surgical procedures (e.g. vaginal hysterectomy and colorectal surgery) that may be classified as contaminated or potentially contaminated. Effective perioperative use for surgery depends on the time of administration. To achieve effective tissue levels, MEZLIN® should be given 1/2 hour to 1 1/2 hours before surgery.

In patients undergoing Caesarean section, intraoperative (after clamping the umbilical cord) and postoperative use of MEZLIN® may reduce the incidence of certain postoperative infections. (See DOSAGE AND ADMINISTRATION section.)

For patients undergoing colorectal surgery, preoperative bowel preparation by mechanical cleansing as well as with a non-absorbable antibiotic (e.g. neomycin) is recommended.

If there are signs of infection, specimens for culture should be obtained for identification of the causative organism so that appropriate therapy may be instituted.

CONTRAINDICATIONS

MEZLIN® is contraindicated in patients with a history of hypersensitivity reactions to any of the penicillins.

WARNINGS

Serious and occasionally fatal hypersensitivity (anaphylactic) reactions have occurred in patients receiving a penicillin. These reactions are more apt to occur in individuals with a history of sensitivity to multiple allergens. There have been reports of individuals with a history of penicillin hypersensitivity reactions who have experienced severe hypersensitivity reactions when treated with a cephalosporin. Before therapy with mezlocillin is instituted, careful inquiry should be made to determine whether the patient has had previous hypersensitivity reactions to penicillins, cephalosporins or other drugs. Antibiotics should be used with caution in any patient who has demonstrated some form of allergy, particularly to drugs.

If an allergic reaction occurs during therapy with mezlocillin, the drug should be discontinued. SERIOUS ANAPHYLACTOID REACTIONS REQUIRE IMMEDIATE EMERGENCY TREATMENT WITH EPINEPHRINE. OXYGEN, INTRAVENOUS STERIODS, AND AIRWAY MANAGEMENT, INCLUDING INTUBATION, SHOULD ALSO BE PROVIDED AS INDICATED.

PRECAUTIONS

General

Although MEZLIN® shares with other pencillins the low potential for toxicity, as with any potent drug, periodic assessment of organ system functions, including renal, hepatic and hematopoietic, is advisable during prolonged therapy. MEZLIN® has been reported rarely to cause acute interstitial nephritis.

Bleeding manifestations have occurred in some patients receiving beta-lactam antibiotics. These reactions have been associated with abnormalities of coagulation tests such as clotting time, platelet aggregation and prothrombin time and are more likely to occur in patients with renal impairment. Although MEZLIN® has rarely been associated with any clinical bleeding, the possibility of this occurring should be kept in mind, particularly in patients with severe renal impairment receiving maximum doses of the drug.

MEZLIN® has only rarely been reported to cause hypokalemia; however, the possibility of this occurring should also be kept in mind, particularly when treating patients with fluid and electrolyte imbalance. Periodic monitoring of serum potassium may be advisable in patients receiving prolonged therapy.

MEZLIN® is a monosodium salt containing only 42.6 mg (1.85 mEq) of sodium per gram of mezlocillin. This should be considered when treating patients requiring restricted salt intake.

As with any penicillin, an allergic reaction, including anaphylaxis, may occur during MEZLIN® administration, particularly in a hypersensitive individual.

As with other antibiotics, prolonged use of MEZLIN® may result in overgrowth of non-susceptible organisms. If this occurs, appropriate measures should be taken.

MEZLIN®, along with other ureidopenicillins, has been reported in one study to prolong neuromuscular blockage of vecuronium. Caution is indicated when mezlocillin is used perioperatively.

Antimicrobials used in high doses for short periods to treat gonorrhea may mask or delay the symptoms of incubating syphilis. Therefore, prior to treatment, patients with gonorrhea should also be evaluated for syphilis. Specimens for dark field examination should be obtained from any suspected primary lesion and serologic tests should be performed. Patients treated with MEZLIN® should undergo follow-up serologic tests three months after therapy.

Interactions with Drugs and Laboratory Tests

As with other penicillins, the mixing of mezlocillin with a aminoglycoside in solutions for parenteral administration can result in substantial inactivation of the aminoglycoside. Probenecid interferes with the renal tubular secretion of mezlocillin, thereby increasing serum concentrations and prolonging serum half-life of the antibiotic.

High urine concentrations of mezlocillin may produce false positive protein reactions (pseudoproteinuria) with the following methods: sulfosalicyclic acid and boiling test, acetic acid test, biuret reaction, and nitric acid test. The bromphenol blue (Multi-stix®) reagent strip test has been reported to be reliable.

Pregnancy Category B

Reproduction studies have been performed in rats and mice at doses up to 2 times the human dose, and have revealed no evidence of impaired fertility or harm to the fetus, due to MEZLIN®. There are however no adequate and well controlled studies in pregnant women. Because animal reproductive studies are not always predictive of human response, this drug should be used during pregnancy only if clearly needed. Mezlocillin crosses the placenta and is found in low concentrations in cord blood and amniotic fluid.

Nursing Mothers

Mezlocillin is detected in low concentrations in the milk of

MEZLIN® DOSAGE GUIDE (ADULTS)

Condition	Daily Dosage Range	Usual Daily Dosage	Frequency and Route of Administration
Urinary tract infection (uncomplicated)	100–125 mg/kg	6–8g	1.5–2g every 6 hours IV or IM
Urinary tract infection (complicated) Lower respiratory tract infection	150–200 mg/kg	12g	3g every 6 hours IV
Intra-abdominal infection Gynecological infection Skin & skin structure infection Septicemia	225–300 mg/kg	16–18g	4g every 6 hours or 3g every 4 hours IV

MEZLIN® DOSAGE GUIDE FOR PATIENTS WITH IMPAIRED RENAL FUNCTION

Creatinine Clearance mL/min.	Urinary Tract Infection (Uncomplicated)	Urinary Tract Infection (Complicated)	Serious Systemic Infection
>30	Usual Recommended Dosage		
10–30	1.5g every 8 hours	1.5g every 6 hours	3g every 8 hours
<10	1.5g every 8 hours	1.5g every 8 hours	2g every 8 hours

nursing mothers, therefore caution should be exercised when MEZLIN® is administered to a nursing woman.

ADVERSE REACTIONS

As with other penicillins, the following adverse reactions may occur:

Hypersensitivity reactions: skin rash, pruritus, urticaria, drug fever, acute interstitial nephritis and anaphylactic reactions.

Gastrointestinal distrubances: abnormal taste sensation, nausea, vomiting and diarrhea. If diarrhea persists, pseudomembranous colitis should be considered.

Hemic and Lymphatic Systems: thrombocytopenia, leukopenia, neutropenia, eosinophilia, reduction of hemoglobin or hematocrit, and positive Coombs' test.

Abnormalities of hepatic and renal function tests: elevation of serum aspartate aminotransferase (SGOT), serum alanine aminotransferase (SGPT), serum alkaline phosphatase, serum bilirubin. Elevation of serum creatinine and/or BUN. Reduction in serum potassium.

Central nervous system: convulsive seizures or neuromuscular hyperirritability.

Local reactions: thrombophlebitis with intravenous administration, pain with intramuscular injection.

OVERDOSAGE

As with other penicillins, MEZLIN® in overdosage has the potential to cause neuromusuclar hyperirritability or convulsive seizures. Hemodialysis, if necessary, will aid in removal of the drug from the blood.

DOSAGE AND ADMINISTRATION

MEZLIN® (sterile mezlocillin sodium) may be administered intravenously or intramuscularly. For serious infections, the intravenous route of administration should be used. Intramuscular doses should not exceed 2g per injection.

The recommended adult dosage for serious infections is 200–300 mg/kg per day given in 4 to 6 divided doses. The usual dose is 3g given every 4 hours (18g/day) or 4g given every 6 hours (16g/day). For life-threatening infections, up to 350 mg/kg per day may be administered, but the total daily dosage should ordinarily not exceed 24g.

[See table above].

For patients with life-threatening infections, 4g may be administered every 4 hours (24g/day).

Dosage for any individual patient must take into consideration the site and severity of infection, the susceptibility of the organisms causing infection, and the status of the patient's host defense mechanism.

The duration of therapy depends upon the severity of infection. Generally, MEZLIN® should be continued for at least 2 days after the signs and symptoms of infection have disappeared. The usual duration is 7 to 10 days; however, in difficult and complicated infections, more prolonged therapy may be required. Antibiotic therapy for Group A beta-hemolytic streptococcal infections should be maintained for at least 10 days to reduce the risk of rheumatic fever or glomerulonephritis.

In certain deep-seated infections, involving abscess formation, appropriate surgical drainage should be performed in conjunction with antimicrobial therapy.

For acute, uncomplicated gonococcal urethritis, the usual dose is 1–2g given once intravenously or by intramuscular injection. Probenecid 1g may be given orally at the time of dosing or up to ½-hour before. (For full prescribing information, refer to probenecid package insert).

Prevention

To prevent postoperative infection in contaminated or potentially contaminated surgery, the following doses are recommended:

4g IV given ½ hour to 1½ hours prior to the start of surgery
4g IV given 6 hours and 12 hours later.

Caesarean Section Patients.

The first dose of 4g is given intravenously as soon as the umbilical cord is clamped. The second and third doses of 4g should be given intravenously 4 and 8 hours, respectively, after the first dose.

Patients with Impaired Renal Function

The rate of elimination of mezlocillin is dose dependent and related to the degree of renal function impairment. After an intravenous dose of 3g the serum half-life is approximately 1 hour in patients with creatinine clearances above 60 mL/min, 1.3 hr. in those with clearances of 30–59 mL/min., 1.6 hr. in those with clearances of 10–29 mL/min. and approximately 3.6 hr. in patients with clearances of less than 10 mL/min. Dosage adjustments of MEZLIN® are not required in patients with mild impairment of renal function. For patients with a creatinine clearance of ≤30 mL/min. (serum creatinine of approximately 3.0 mg% or greater), the following dosage guide may be used.

[See table above].

For life-threatening infections, 3g may be given every 6 hours to patients with creatinine clearances between 10–30 mL/min. and 2g every 6 hours to those with clearances less than 10 mL/min.

For patients with serious systemic infection undergoing hemodialysis for renal failure, 3–4g may be administered after each dialysis and then every 12 hours. Patients undergoing peritoneal dialysis may receive 3g every 12 hours.

For patients with renal failure and hepatic insufficiency, measurement of serum levels of mezlocillin will provide additional guidance for adjusting dosage.

Intravenous Administration

MEZLIN® may be administered intravenously by intermittent infusion or by direct intravenous injection.

Infusion. Each gram of mezlocillin should be reconstituted by vigorous shaking with at least 10 mL of Sterile Water for Injection, 5% Dextrose Injection or 0.9% Sodium Chloride Injection. The dissolved drug should be further diluted to desired volume (50–100 mL) with an appropriate intravenous solution. (See Compatibility and Stability section.) The solution of reconstituted drug may then be administered over a period of 30 minutes by direct infusion, or through a Y-type intravenous infusion set which may already be in place. If this method or the "piggyback" method of administration is used, it is advisable to discontinue temporarily the administration of any other solutions during the infusion of MEZLIN®.

Injection. The reconstituted solution of MEZLIN® may also be injected directly into a vein or into intravenous tubing; when administered this way, the injection should be given slowly over a period of 3–5 minutes. To minimize venous irritation, the concentration of drug should not exceed 10%.

When MEZLIN® is given in combination with another antimicrobial, such as an aminoglycoside, each drug should be given separately in accordance with the recommended dosage and routes of administration for each drug.

Intramuscular Administration

Each gram of mezlocillin may be reconstituted by vigorous shaking with 3–4 mL of sterile water for injection or with 3–4 mL of 0.5 or 1.0% lidocaine hydrochloride solution (without epinephrine). (For full prescribing information, refer to lidocaine package insert). Intramuscular doses of MEZLIN® should not exceed 2g per injection.

As with all intramuscular preparations, MEZLIN® should be injected well within the body of a relatively large muscle, such as the upper outer quadrant of the buttock (i.e., gluteus maximus); aspiration will help avoid unintentional injection into a blood vessel. Slow injection (12–15 sec.) will minimize the discomfort associated with intramuscular administration.

Infants and Children

Only limited data are available on the safety and effectiveness of MEZLIN® in the treatment of infants and children with documented serious infection. In the event a child has an infection for which MEZLIN® may be judged particularly appropriate, the following dosage guide may be used:

[See table below].

For infants beyond one month of age and children up to the age of 12 years, 50 mg/kg may be administered every 4 hours (300 mg/kg/day).

The drug may be infused intravenously over 30-minutes or be given by intramuscular injection.

COMPATIBILITY AND STABILITY

MEZLIN® at concentrations of 10 mg/mL and 100 mg/mL is stable (loss of potency less than 10%) in the following intravenous solutions for the time periods stated.

[See table top left next page]

If precipitation should occur under refrigeration, the product should be warmed to 37°C for 20 minutes in a water bath and shaken well.

*This solution is stable from 10 mg/mL to 50 mg/mL under refrigeration.

MEZLIN® at concentrations up to 250 mg/mL is stable for 24 hours at room temperature in the following diluents:
  Sterile Water for Injection, USP
  0.9% Sodium Chloride Injection, USP
  0.5% and 1.0% Lidocaine Hydrochloride solution (without epinephrine)

MEZLIN® is stable for up to 28 days when frozen at −12°C at concentrations up to 100 mg/mL in the following diluents:
  Sterile Water for Injection, USP
  0.9% Sodium Chloride Injection, USP or 5% Dextrose Injection, USP

HOW SUPPLIED

MEZLIN® (sterile mezlocillin sodium) is a white to pale yellow crystalline powder supplied as listed below:

MEZLIN® is available in vials, infusion bottles, pharmacy bulk packages and ADD-Vantage® vials containing mezlocillin sodium equivalent to mezlocillin, as specified:

	NC Number
1g Vial	0026-8211-10
2g Vial	0026-8212-30
2g Infusion Bottle	0026-8212-36
3g Vial	0026-8213-35
3g Infusion Bottle	0026-8213-36
3g ADD-Vantage® Vial	0026-8213-19
4g Vial	0026-8214-35
4g Infusion Bottle	0026-8214-36
4g ADD-Vantage® Vial	0026-8214-19
20g Pharmacy Bulk Package	0026-8220-31

Unreconstituted MEZLIN® should be stored at temperatures not exceeding 86°F (30°C). The powder as well as the reconstituted solution of drug may darken slightly, depend-

MEZLIN DOSAGE GUIDE (NEWBORNS)

BODY WEIGHT	AGE	
(gm)	≤7 DAYS	>7 DAYS
≤2000	75 mg/kg every 12 hours (150 mg/kg/day)	75 mg/kg every 8 hours (225 mg/kg/day)
>2000	75 mg/kg every 12 hours (150 mg/kg/day)	75 mg/kg every 6 hours (300 mg/kg/day)

Continued on next page

Miles Pharm. Div.—Cont.

INTRAVENOUS SOLUTION

STABILITY

INTRAVENOUS SOLUTION	Controlled Room Temperature	Refrigeration
Sterile Water for Injection, USP	48 hours	7 days
0.9% Sodium Chloride Injection, USP	48 hours	7 days
5% Dextrose Injection, USP	48 hours	7 days
5% Dextrose in 0.225% Sodium Chloride Injection, USP	72 hours	7 days
Lactated Ringer's Injection, USP	24 hours	7 days
5% Dextrose in Electrolyte #75 Injection	72 hours	7 days
5% Dextrose in 0.45% Sodium Chloride Injection, USP*	48 hours	48 hours
Ringer's Injection	24 hours	24 hours
10% Dextrose Injection	24 hours	24 hours
5% Fructose Injection	24 hours	24 hours

ing upon storage conditions, but potency is not affected, Miles Inc.

Miles Inc.
Pharmaceutical Division
400 Morgan Lane
West Haven, CT 06516 USA
Made in Germany
PD100669 1/89 BAY f 1353 5202/4/A/US/MILES 0714
© 1989 Miles Inc.

MEZLIN® ℞
(sterile mezlocillin sodium)
PHARMACY BULK PACKAGE—NOT FOR DIRECT INFUSION
BAYPEN®

DESCRIPTION

A pharmacy bulk package is a container of a sterile preparation for parenteral use that contains many single doses. The contents are intended for use in a pharmacy admixture program and are restricted to the preparation of admixtures for intravenous infusion, or the filling of empty sterile syringes for intravenous injection for patients with individualized dosing requirements (see Dosage and Administration section)

MEZLIN® (sterile mezlocillin sodium) is a semisynthetic broad spectrum penicillin antibiotic for parenteral administration. It is the monohydrate sodium salt of 6-{D-2 [3-(methyl-sulfonyl) -2-OXO-imidazolidine-1-carboxamido]-2- phenyl acetamido} penicillanic acid.

Structural Formula:

Empirical Formula: $C_{21}H_{24}N_5O_8S_2Na \cdot H_2O$
MEZLIN® has a molecular weight of 579.6 and contains 42.6 mg (1.85 mEq) of sodium per one gram of mezlocillin activity. The dosage form is supplied as a sterile white to pale yellow crystalline powder, which is freely soluble in water. When reconstituted, solutions of MEZLIN® are clear and range from colorless to pale yellow with a pH of 4.5 to 8.0.

CLINICAL PHARMACOLOGY

Intravenous Administration. In healthy adult volunteers, mean serum levels of mezlocillin 5 minutes after a 5-minute intravenous injection of 1g, 2g, or 5g are 100, 253, or 411 mcg/ml, respectively. Serum levels, as noted below, lack dose proportionality at:
[See table below].
Fifteen minutes after a 4g intravenous injection (2.5 min), the concentration in serum is 254 mcg/ml; 1 hour and 4 hours later levels are 93 mcg/ml and 9.1 mcg/ml, respectively:
[See table top next page].
After an intravenous infusion (15 min) of 3g, mean levels 15 minutes after dosing are 269 mcg/ml (170–280).
A 30-minute intravenous infusion of 3g produces mean peak concentrations of 263 mcg/ml; 1 hour and 4 hours later the concentrations are 57 mcg/ml and 4.4 mcg/ml, respectively:
[See table bottom next page].
Following intravenous infusion (2 hr) of a 3g dose of mezlocillin every 4 hours for 7 days, mean peak serum concentrations are higher than 100 mcg/ml, and levels above 50 mcg/ml are maintained throughout dosing.
Intramuscular Administration. MEZLIN® is rapidly absorbed after intramuscular injection. In healthy volunteers,

the mean peak serum concentration occurs approximately 45 minutes after a single dose of 1g and is about 15 mcg/ml. The oral administration of 1g probenecid before injection produces an increase in mezlocillin serum levels of about 50%. After repetitive intramuscular doses of 1g mezlocillin every 6 hours, peak levels in the serum generally range between 35 and 45 mcg/ml. The relationship between the pharmacokinetics of intramuscular and intravenous dosing has not yet been clearly established.

General. As with other penicillins, mezlocillin is excreted primarily by glomerular filtration and tubular secretion. The rate of elimination is dose dependent and related to the degree of renal functional impairment. In patients with normal renal function, approximately 55% of the administered dose is recovered from the urine within the first 6 hours after dosing. Two hours after an intravenous injection of 2g, concentrations of active drug in urine generally exceed 4000 mcg/ml. By 4–6 hours after injection, concentrations usually decline to a range of about 50 to 200 mcg/ml. The serum elimination half-life of mezlocillin after intravenous dosing is approximately 55 minutes.

In patients with reduced renal function, the half-life is only slightly prolonged. Dosage adjustments are usually not necessary except in patients with severe renal impairment. (See Dosage and Administration). As with other penicillins, mezlocillin is metabolized only slightly; less than 10% of the drug excreted in the urine is in the form of the penicilloate or penilloate. The drug is readily removed from the serum by hemodialysis and, to a lesser extent, by peritoneal dialysis. Up to 26% of a dose of mezlocillin is recovered from the bile of patients with normal liver function. Following intravenous doses of 2 to 5g, concentrations of active drug in bile generally range from 500 to 2500 mcg/ml. The biliary excretion of mezlocillin is reduced in patients with common bile duct obstruction.

Mezlocillin is not appreciably absorbed when given orally. Following parenteral administration, the apparent volume of distribution is approximately equal to the extracellular fluid volume. The drug is present in active form in the serum, urine, bile, peritoneal fluid, pleural fluid, bronchial and wound secretions, bone and other tissues. As with other penicillins, penetration into the cerebrospinal fluid (CSF) is generally poor, however higher CSF concentrations are obtained in the presence of meningeal inflammation.

Protein binding studies indicate that the degree of mezlocillin binding is low (16–42%) and depends upon testing methods and concentrations of drug studied.

Microbiology
Mezlocillin is a bactericidal antibiotic which acts by interfering with synthesis of cell wall components. It is active against a variety of gram-negative and gram-positive bacteria, including aerobic and anaerobic strains. Mezlocillin is usually active in vitro against most strains of the following organisms:

Gram-negative bacteria
Escherichia coli
Proteus mirabilis
Proteus vulgaris
Morganella morganii (formerly *P. morganii*)
Providencia rettgeri (formerly *Proteus rettgeri*)
Providencia stuartii
Citrobacter species*
Klebsiella species (including *K. pneumoniae*)
Enterobacter species
Shigella species*
Pseudomonas aeruginosa (and other species)
Haemophilus influenzae
Haemophilus parainfluenzae
Neisseria species

Many strains of *Serratia*, *Salmonella**, and *Acinetobacter** are also susceptible.
Gram-positive bacteria
Staphylococcus aureus (non-penicillinase producing strains)
Beta-hemolytic *streptococci* (Groups A and B)
Streptococcus pneumoniae (formerly *Diplococcus pneumoniae*)
Streptococcus faecalis (enterococcus)
Anaerobic Organisms
Peptococcus species
Peptostreptococcus species
Clostridium species*
Bacteroides species (including *B. fragilis* group)
Fusobacterium species*
Veillonella species*
Eubacterium species*
*Mezlocillin has been shown to be active in vitro against these organisms, however clinical efficacy has not yet been established.
Noteworthy is mezlocillin's broadened spectrum of in vitro activity against important pathogenic aerobic gram-negative bacteria, including strains of *Pseudomonas*, *Klebsiella*, *Enterobacter*, *Serratia*, *Proteus*, *Escherichia* and *Haemophilus*, as well as *Bacteroides* and other anaerobes; and its excellent inhibitory effect against gram-positive organisms including *Streptococcus faecalis* (enterococcus). It is inactive against penicillinase-producing strains of *Staphylococcus aureus*.

In vitro studies have shown that mezlocillin combined with an aminoglycoside (e.g., gentamicin, tobramycin, amikacin, sisomicin) acts synergistically against strains of *Streptococcus faecalis* and *Pseudomonas aeruginosa*. In some instances, this combination also acts synergistically in vitro against other gram-negative bacteria such as *Serratia*, *Klebsiella* and *Acinetobacter* species.

Mezlocillin is slightly more active when tested at alkaline pH and, as with other penicillins, has reduced activity when tested in vitro with increasing inoculum. The minimum bactericidal concentration (MBC) generally exceeds the minimum inhibitory concentration (MIC) by a factor of 2 or 3. Resistance to mezlocillin in vitro develops slowly (multiple step mutation). Some strains of *Pseudomonas aeruginosa* have developed resistance fairly rapidly. Mezlocillin is not stable in the presence of penicillinase and strains of *Staphylococcus aureus* resistant to penicillin are also resistant to mezlocillin.

Susceptibility Tests
Quantitative methods that require measurement of zone diameters give good estimates of bacterial susceptibility. One such procedure* has been recommended for use with discs to test susceptibility to antimicrobials. When the causative organism is tested by the Kirby-Bauer method of disc susceptibility, a 75 mcg mezlocillin disc should give a zone of 18 mm or greater to indicate susceptibility. Zone sizes of 14 mm or less indicate resistance. Zone sizes of 15 to 17 mm indicate intermediate susceptibility. Susceptible strains of *Haemophilus* and *Neisseria* species give zones of ≥ 29 mm, resistant strains ≤ 28 mm. With this procedure, a report from the laboratory of "Susceptible" indicates that the infecting organism is likely to respond to therapy. A report of "Resistant" indicates that the infecting organism is not likely to respond to therapy; other therapy should be selected. A report of "Intermediate Susceptibility" suggests that the organism may be susceptible if the infection is confined to tissues and fluids (e.g., urine), in which high antibiotic levels are attained. The mezlocillin disc should be used for testing susceptibility to mezlocillin. In certain conditions, it may be desirable to do additional susceptibility testing by broth or agar dilution techniques. Dilution methods, preferably the agar plate dilution procedure, are most accurate for susceptibility testing of obligate anaerobes. Enterobacteriaceae, *Pseudomonas* and *Acinetobacter* species are considered susceptible if the MIC of mezlocillin is no greater than 64 mcg/ml and are considered resistant if the MIC is greater than 128 mcg/ml. *Haemophilus* species and *Neisseria* species are considered susceptible if the MIC of mezlocillin is less than or equal to 1 mcg/ml. Mezlocillin standard is available for broth or agar dilution studies.
*Bauer, A.W., Kirby, W.M., Sherris, J.C. and Turck, M.: Antibiotic Testing by a Standardized Single Disc Method, Am. J. Clin. Pathol., 45:493, 1966; Standardized Disc Susceptibility Test, FEDERAL REGISTER, 39: 19182–19184, 1974.

MEZLOCILLIN SERUM LEVELS IN ADULTS (mcg/ml) 5 MIN IV INJECTION

DOSE	0	5 min	10 min	20 min	30 min	1 hr	2 hr	3 hr	4 hr	6 hr	8 hr
1g	149 (132–185)	100 (64–143)	66 (47–87)	50 (31–87)	40 (22–83)	18 (8–31)	5.3 (3.3–7.7)	2.5 (1.7–3.7)	1.7 (0.7–2.8)	0.5 (0–1.2)	0.1 (0–0.2)
2g	314 (207–362)	253 (161–364)	161 (113–214)	117 (76–174)	82 (55–112)	56 (23–88)	20 (7.5–32)	11 (3.8–16)	4.4 (1.6–8.7)	1.5 (0.5–2.6)	0.6 (0.1–1.4)
5g	547 (268–854)	411 (199–597)	357 (246–456)	250 (203–353)	226 (190–333)	131 (104–193)	76 (59–104)	31 (20–40)	13 (6.4–17)	4.6 (2.1–9.4)	1.9 (1.1–3.6)

MEZLOCILLIN SERUM LEVELS IN ADULTS (mcg/ml) 2–5 MIN IV INJECTION

DOSE	0	15 min	30 min	45 min	1 hr	2 hr	3 hr	4 hr	6 hr
4g	—	254 (155–400)	163 (99–260)	122 (78–215)	93 (67–133)	47 (22–96)	20 (8–45)	9.1 (6–13)	8.4 (5–17)

INDICATIONS AND USAGE

MEZLIN® is indicated for the treatment of serious infections caused by susceptible strains of the designated microorganisms in the conditions listed below:

LOWER RESPIRATORY TRACT INFECTIONS including pneumonia and lung abscess caused by *Haemophilus influenzae, Klebsiella* species including *K. pneumoniae, Proteus mirabilis, Pseudomonas* species including *P. aeruginosa, E. coli,* and *Bacteroides* species including *B. fragilis.*

INTRA-ABDOMINAL INFECTIONS including acute cholecystitis, cholangitis, peritonitis, hepatic abscess and intraabdominal abscess caused by susceptible *E. coli, Proteus mirabilis, Klebsiella* species, *Pseudomonas* species, *S. faecalis* (enterococcus), *Bacteroides* species, *Peptococcus* species, and *Peptostreptococcus* species.

URINARY TRACT INFECTIONS caused by susceptible *E. coli, Proteus mirabilis,* the indole positive *Proteus* species, *Morganella morganii; Klebsiella* species, *Enterobacter* species, *Serratia* species, *Pseudomonas* species, *S. faecalis* (enterococcus).

Uncomplicated gonorrhea due to susceptible *Neisseria gonorrhoeae.*

GYNECOLOGICAL INFECTIONS including endometritis, pelvic cellulitis, and pelvic inflammatory disease associated with susceptible *Neisseria gonorrhoeae, Peptococcus* species, *Peptostreptococcus* species, *Bacteroides* species, *E. coli, Proteus mirabilis, Klebsiella* species, and *Enterobacter* species.

SKIN AND SKIN STRUCTURE INFECTIONS caused by susceptible *S. faecalis* (enterococcus), *E. coli, Proteus mirabilis,* the indole positive *Proteus* species, *Proteus vulgaris,* and *Providencia rettgeri; Klebsiella* species, *Enterobacter* species, *Pseudomonas* species, *Peptococcus* species, and *Bacteroides* species.

SEPTICEMIA including bacteremia caused by susceptible *E. coli, Klebsiella* species, *Enterobacter* species, *Pseudomonas* species, *Bacteroides* species, and *Peptococcus* species.

Mezlocillin has also been shown to be effective for the treatment of infections caused by *Streptococcus* species including Group A Beta-hemolytic *Streptococcus* and *Streptococcus pneumoniae* (formerly *Diplococcus pneumoniae*) however, infections caused by these organisms are ordinarily treated with more narrow spectrum penicillins.

Appropriate culture and susceptibility tests should be performed before treatment in order to isolate and identify organisms causing infection and to determine their susceptibility to mezlocillin. Therapy with MEZLIN® may be initiated before results of these tests are known; once results become available, appropriate therapy should be continued.

Mezlocillin's broad spectrum of activity makes it particularly useful for treating mixed infections caused by susceptible strains of both gram-negative and gram-positive aerobic or anaerobic bacteria. It is not effective, however, against infections caused by penicillinase-producing *Staphylococcus aureus.*

In certain severe infections, when the causative organisms are unknown, MEZLIN® may be administered in conjunction with an aminoglycoside or a cephalosporin antibiotic as initial therapy. As soon as results of culture and susceptibility tests become available, antimicrobial therapy should be adjusted if indicated. Culture and sensitivity testing, performed periodically during therapy, will provide information on the therapeutic effect of the antimicrobial and will monitor for the possible emergence of bacterial resistance.

MEZLIN® has been used effectively in combination with an aminoglycoside antibiotic for the treatment of life-threatening infections caused by *Pseudomonas aeruginosa.* For the treatment of febrile episodes in immunosuppressed patients with granulocytopenia, MEZLIN® should be combined with an aminoglycoside or a cephalosporin antibiotic.

Prevention: The administration of MEZLIN® perioperatively (preoperatively, intraoperatively, and postoperatively) may reduce the incidence of infections in patients undergoing surgical procedures (e.g. vaginal hysterectomy and colorectal surgery) that may be classified as contaminated or potentially contaminated. Effective perioperative use for surgery depends on the time of administration. To achieve effective tissue levels, MEZLIN® should be given ½ hour to 1½ hours before surgery.

In patients undergoing Caesarean section, intraoperative (after clamping the umbilical cord) and postoperative use of MEZLIN® may reduce the incidence of certain postoperative infections. See DOSAGE AND ADMINISTRATION section.

For patients undergoing colorectal surgery, preoperative bowel preparation by mechanical cleansing as well as with a non-absorbable antibiotic (e.g. neomycin) is recommended. If there are signs of infection, specimens for culture should be obtained for identification of the causative organism so that appropriate therapy may be instituted.

CONTRAINDICATIONS

MEZLIN® is contraindicated in patients with a history of hypersensitivity reactions to any of the penicillins.

WARNINGS

Serious and occasionally fatal hypersensitivity (anaphylactic) reactions have occurred in patients receiving a penicillin. These reactions are more apt to occur in individuals with a history of sensitivity to multiple allergens. There have been reports of individuals with a history of penicillin hypersensitivity reactions who have experienced severe hypersensitivity reactions when treated with a cephalosporin. Before therapy with mezlocillin is instituted, careful inquiry should be made to determine whether the patient has had previous hypersensitivity reactions to penicillins, cephalosporins or other drugs. Antibiotics should be used with caution in any patient who has demonstrated some form of allergy, particularly to drugs.

If an allergic reaction occurs during therapy with mezlocillin, the drug should be discontinued. SERIOUS ANAPHYLACTOID REACTIONS REQUIRE IMMEDIATE EMERGENCY TREATMENT WITH EPINEPHRINE. OXYGEN, INTRAVENOUS STERIODS, AND AIRWAY MANAGEMENT, INCLUDING INTUBATION, SHOULD BE PROVIDED AS INDICATED.

PRECAUTIONS

General

Although MEZLIN® shares with other pencillins the low potential for toxicity, as with any potent drug, periodic assessment of organ system functions, including renal, hepatic and hematopoietic, is advisable during prolonged therapy. MEZLIN® has been reported rarely to cause acute interstitial nephritis.

Bleeding manifestations have occurred in some patients receiving beta-lactam antibiotics. These reactions have been associated with abnormalities of coagulation tests, such as clotting time, platelet aggregation and prothrombin time and are more likely to occur in patients with renal impairment. Although MEZLIN has rarely been associated with clinical bleeding, the possibility of this occurring should be kept in mind, particularly in patients with severe renal impairment receiving maximum doses of the drug.

MEZLIN® has only rarely been reported to cause hypokalemia, however, the possibility of this occurring should also be kept in mind, particularly when treating patients with fluid and electrolyte imbalance. Periodic monitoring of serum potassium may be advisable in patients receiving prolonged therapy.

MEZLIN® is a monosodium salt containing only 42.6 mg (1.85 mEq) of sodium per gram of mezlocillin. This should be considered when treating patients requiring restricted salt intake.

As with any penicillin, an allergic reaction, including anaphylaxis, may occur during MEZLIN® administration, particularly in a hypersensitive individual.

As with other antibiotics, prolonged use of MEZLIN® may result in overgrowth of non-susceptible organisms. If this occurs, appropriate measures should be taken.

MEZLIN®, along with other ureidopenicillins, has been reported in one study to prolong neuromuscular blockage of vecuronium. Caution is indicated when mezlocillin is used perioperatively.

Antimicrobials used in high doses for short periods to treat gonorrhea may mask or delay the symptoms of incubating syphilis. Therefore, prior to treatment, patients with gonorrhea should also be evaluated for syphilis. Specimens for dark field examination should be obtained from any suspected primary lesion and serologic tests should be performed. Patients treated with MEZLIN® should undergo follow-up serologic tests three months after therapy.

Interactions with Drugs and Laboratory Tests

As with other penicillins, the mixing of mezlocillin with an aminoglycoside in solutions for parenteral administration can result in substantial inactivation of the aminoglycoside. Probenecid interferes with the renal tubular secretion of mezlocillin, thereby increasing serum concentrations and prolonging serum half-life of the antibiotic.

High urine concentrations of mezlocillin may produce false positive protein reactions (pseudoproteinuria) with the following methods: sulfosalicyclic acid and boiling test, acetic acid test, biuret reaction, and nitric acid test. The bromphenol blue (Multi-stix®) reagent strip test has been reported to be reliable.

Pregnancy Category B

Reproduction studies have been performed in rats and mice at doses up to 2 times the human dose, and have revealed no evidence of impaired fertility or harm to the fetus, due to MEZLIN®. There are however no adequate and well controlled studies in pregnant women. Because animal reproductive studies are not always predictive of human response, this drug should be used during pregnancy only if clearly needed. Mezlocillin crosses the placenta and is found in low concentrations in cord blood and amniotic fluid.

Nursing Mothers

Mezlocillin is detected in low concentrations in the milk of nursing mothers. Therefore caution should be exercised when MEZLIN® is administered to a nursing woman.

ADVERSE REACTIONS

As with other penicillins, the following adverse reactions may occur:

Hypersensitivity reactions: skin rash, pruritus, urticaria, drug fever, acute interstitial nephritis and anaphylactic reactions.

Gastrointestinal disturbances: abnormal taste sensation, nausea, vomiting and diarrhea. If diarrhea persists, pseudomembranous colitis should be considered.

Hematologic and Lymphatic Systems: thrombocytopenia, leukopenia, neutropenia, eosinophilia, reduction of hemoglobin or hematocrit, and positive Coombs' test.

Abnormalities of hepatic and renal function tests: elevation of serum aspartate aminotransferase (SGOT), serum alanine aminotransferase (SGPT), serum alkaline phosphatase, serum bilirubin. Elevation of serum creatinine and/or BUN. Reduction in serum potassium.

Central nervous system: convulsive seizures or neuromuscular hyperirritability.

Local reactions: thrombophlebitis with intravenous administration, pain with intramsucular injection.

OVERDOSAGE

As with other penicillins, MEZLIN® in overdosage has the potential to cause neuromusuclar hyperirritability or convulsive seizures. Hemodialysis, if necessary, will aid in removal of the drug from the blood.

DOSAGE AND ADMINISTRATION

MEZLIN® (sterile mezlocillin sodium) may be administered intravenously or intramuscularly. For serious infections, the intravenous route of administration should be used. Intramuscular doses should not exceed 2g per injection.

The 20g pharmacy bulk package is intended for the preparation of solutions for intravenous use. When intramuscular administration is required, the MEZLIN® vial should be used.

The recommended adult dosage for serious infections is 200–300 mg/kg per day given in 4 to 6 divided doses. The usual dose is 3g given every 4 hours (18g/day) or 4g given every 6 hours (16g/day). For life-threatening infections, up to 350 mg/kg per day may be administered, but the total daily dosage should ordinarily not exceed 24g.

[See table top next page].

For patients with life-threatening infections, 4g may be administered every 4 hours (24g/day).

Dosage for any individual patient must take into consideration the site and severity of infection, the susceptibility of the organisms causing infection, and the status of the patient's host defense mechanism.

The duration of therapy depends upon the severity of infection. Generally, MEZLIN® should be continued for at least 2 days after the signs and symptoms of infection have disappeared. The usual duration is 7 to 10 days; however, in difficult and complicated infections, more prolonged therapy may be required. Antibiotic therapy for Group A Beta-hemolytic streptococcal infections should be maintained for at least 10 days to reduce the risk of rheumatic fever or glomerulonephritis.

In certain deep-seated infections, involving abscess formation, appropriate surgical drainage should be performed in conjunction with antimicrobial therapy.

MEZLOCILLIN SERUM LEVELS IN ADULTS (mcg/ml) 30 MIN IV INFUSION

DOSE	0	5 min	15 min	30 min	45 min	1 hr	2 hr	3 hr	4 hr	6 hr	8 hr
3g	263 (87–489)	170 (63–371)	141 (75–301)	109 (56–288)	79 (41–135)	57 (28–100)	26 (14–55)	12 (5.8–26)	4.4 (2.2–6.5)	1.6 (1.0–3.4)	<1

Continued on next page

Miles Pharm. Div.—Cont.

MEZLIN® DOSAGE GUIDE (ADULTS)

Condition	Daily Dosage Range	Usual Daily Dosage	Frequency and Route of Administration
Urinary tract infection (uncomplicated)	100–125 mg/kg	6-8g	1.5–2g every 6 hours IV or IM
Urinary tract infection (complicated)	150–200 mg/kg	12g	3g every 6 hours IV
Lower respiratory tract infection			
Intra-abdominal infection			4g every 6 hours or 3g every 4 hours IV
Gynecological infection	225–300 mg/kg	16–18g	
Skin & skin structure infection			
Septicemia			

MEZLIN® DOSAGE GUIDE FOR PATIENTS WITH IMPAIRED RENAL FUNCTION

Creatinine Clearance ml/min	Urinary Tract Infection (Uncomplicated)	Urinary Tract Infection (Complicated)	Serious Systemic Infection
> 30	Usual Recommended Dosage		
10–30	1.5g every 8 hours	1.5g every 6 hours	3g every 8 hours
< 10	1.5g every 8 hours	1.5g every 8 hours	2g every 8 hours

For acute, uncomplicated gonococcal urethritis, the usual dose is 1–2g given once intravenously or by intramuscular injection. Probenecid 1g may be given orally at the time of dosing or up to ½-hour before. (For full prescribing information, refer to probenecid package insert).

Prevention

To prevent postoperative infection in contaminated or potentially contaminated surgery, the following doses are recommended:

4g IV given ½ hour to 1½ hours prior to the start of surgery.

4g IV given 6 hours and 12 hours later.

Caesarean Section Patients

The first dose of 4g is given intravenously as soon as the umbilical cord is clamped. The second and third doses of 4g should be given intravenously 4 and 8 hours, respectively, after the first dose.

Patients with Impaired Renal Function

The rate of elimination of mezlocillin is dose dependent and related to the degree of renal function impairment. After an intravenous dose of 3g, the serum half-life is approximately 1 hour in patients with creatinine clearances above 60 ml/min, 1.3 hr in those with clearances of 30–59 ml/min, 1.6 hr in those with clearances of 10–29 ml/min and approximately 3.6 hr in patients with clearances of less than 10 ml/min. Dosage adjustments of MEZLIN® are not required in patients with mild impairment of renal function. For patients with a creatinine clearance of ≤ 30 ml/min (serum creatinine of approximately 3.0 mg% or greater), the following dosage guide may be used.

[See table above].

For life-threatening infections, 3g may be given every 6 hours to patients with creatinine clearances between 10–30 ml/min and 2g every 6 hours to those with clearances less than 10 ml/min.

For patients with serious systemic infection undergoing hemodialysis for renal failure, 3–4g may be administered after each dialysis and then every 12 hours. Patients undergoing peritoneal dialysis may receive 3g every 12 hours.

For patients with renal failure and hepatic insufficiency, measurement of serum levels of mezlocillin will provide additional guidance for adjusting dosage.

Directions for Proper Use of 20 gram Pharmacy Bulk Package

A pharmacy bulk package is a container of a sterile preparation for parenteral use that contains many single doses. The contents are intended for use in a pharmacy admixture program and are restricted to the preparation of admixtures for intravenous infusion, or the filling of empty sterile syringes for intravenous injection for patients with individualized dosing requirements.

THE CLOSURE SHALL BE PENETRATED ONLY ONE TIME AFTER RECONSTITUTION with a suitable sterile transfer set or dispensing device which allows measured dispensing of the contents. The pharmacy bulk package is to be used only in a suitable work area such as a laminar flow hood or an equivalent clean air compounding area.

Reconstitute by vigorous shaking with 186 ml of Sterile Water for Injection, 5% Dextrose Injection or 0.9% Sodium Chloride Injection resulting in a solution containing approximately 100 mg/ml which may be stored at controlled room temperature or under refrigeration. Within 8 hours of reconstitution, the desired dosages should be withdrawn and may be further diluted with an appropriate intravenous solution (see Compatability & Stability section).

Intravenous Administration

MEZLIN® may be administered intravenously by intermittent infusion or by direct intravenous injection.

Infusion: The dissolved drug may be further diluted to desired volume (50–100 ml) with an appropriate intravenous solution (See Compatibility and Stability section). The solution of reconstituted drug may then be administered over a period of 30 minutes by direct infusion, or through a Y-type intravenous infusion set which may already be in place. If this method or the "piggyback" method of administration is used, it is advisable to discontinue temporarily the administration of any other solutions during the infusion of MEZLIN®.

Injection. The reconstituted solution of MEZLIN® may also be injected directly into a vein or into intravenous tubing; when administered this way, the injection should be given slowly over a period of 3–5 minutes. To minimize venous irritation, the concentration of drug should not exceed 10%. When MEZLIN® is given in combination with another antimicrobial, such as an aminoglycoside, each drug should be given separately in accordance with the recommended dosage and routes of administration for each drug.

Intramuscular Administration

For intramuscular administration, please refer to the Dosage and Administration section of the MEZLIN® vial package insert.

Infants and Children

Only limited data are available on the safety and effectiveness of MEZLIN® in the treatment of infants and children with documented serious infection. In the event a child has an infection for which MEZLIN® may be judged particularly appropriate, the following dosage guide may be used:

MEZLIN DOSAGE GUIDE (NEWBORNS)

BODY WEIGHT (gm)	AGE ≤7 DAYS	>7 DAYS
≤2000	75 mg/kg every 12 hours (150 mg/kg/day)	75 mg/kg every 8 hours (225 mg/kg/day)
>2000	75 mg/kg every 12 hours (150 mg/kg/day)	75 mg/kg every 6 hours (300 mg/kg/day)

For infants beyond one month of age and children up to the age of 12 years, 60 mg/kg may be administered every 4 hours (300 mg/kg/day).

The drug may be infused intravenously over 30-minutes or be given by intramuscular injection.

COMPATIBILITY AND STABILITY

MEZLIN® at concentrations of 10 mg/ml and 100 mg/ml is stable (loss of potency less than 10%) in the following intravenous solutions for the time periods stated (includes time retained in pharmacy bulk package after reconstitution): [See table below].

If precipitation should occur under refrigeration, the product should be warmed to 37°C for 20 minutes in a water bath and shaken well.

*This solution is stable from 10 mg/ml to 50 mg/ml under refrigeration.

MEZLIN® is stable for up to 28 days when frozen at −12°C at concentrations up to 100 mg/ml in the following diluents:

Sterile Water for Injection, USP

0.9% Sodium Chloride Injection, USP or 5% Dextrose Injection, USP

HOW SUPPLIED

MEZLIN® (sterile mezlocillin sodium) is a white to pale yellow crystalline powder supplied as listed below:

MEZLIN® is available in vials, infusion bottles, pharmacy bulk packages and ADD-Vantage® vials containing mezlocillin sodium equivalent to mezlocillin, as specified.

	NDC Number
1g Vial	0026-8211-10
2g Vial	0026-8212-30
2g Infusion Bottle	0026-8212-36
3g Vial	0026-8213-35
3g Infusion Bottle	0026-8213-36
3g ADD-Vantage Vial	0026-8213-19
4g Vial	0026-8214-35
4g Infusion Bottle	0026-8214-36
4g ADD-Vantage Vial	0026-8214-19
20g Pharmacy Bulk Package	0026-8220-31

Unreconstituted MEZLIN® should be stored at temperatures not exceeding 30°C (86°F). The powder as well as the reconstituted solution of drug may darken slightly, depending upon storage conditions, but potency is not affected.

Miles Inc.
Pharmaceutical Division
400 Morgan Lane
West Haven, CT 06516 USA
Made in Germany
Issued: November 1987
PD100668 BAY f 1353   5202/4/A/US/2 0223

MITHRACIN®   ℞
(plicamycin)

FOR INTRAVENOUS USE

WARNING

IT IS RECOMMENDED THAT MITHRACIN (plicamycin) BE ADMINISTERED ONLY TO HOSPITALIZED PATIENTS BY OR UNDER THE SUPERVISION OF A QUALIFIED PHYSICIAN WHO IS EXPERIENCED IN THE USE OF CANCER CHEMOTHERAPEUTIC AGENTS, BECAUSE OF THE POSSIBILITY OF SEVERE REACTIONS. FACILITIES FOR THE DETERMINATION OF NECESSARY LABORATORY STUDIES MUST BE AVAILABLE.

SEVERE THROMBOCYTOPENIA, A HEMORRHAGIC TENDENCY AND EVEN DEATH MAY RESULT FROM THE USE OF MITHRACIN. ALTHOUGH SEVERE TOXICITY IS MORE APT TO OCCUR IN PATIENTS WHO HAVE FAR-ADVANCED DISEASE OR ARE OTHERWISE CONSIDERED POOR RISKS FOR THERAPY, SERIOUS TOXICITY MAY ALSO OCCASIONALLY OCCUR EVEN IN PATIENTS WHO ARE IN RELATIVELY GOOD CONDITION.

IN THE TREATMENT OF EACH PATIENT, THE PHYSICIAN MUST WEIGH CAREFULLY THE POSSIBILITY OF ACHIEVING THERAPEUTIC BENEFIT VERSUS THE RISK OF TOXICITY WHICH MAY OCCUR WITH MITHRACIN THERAPY. THE FOLLOWING DATA CONCERNING THE USE OF MITHRACIN IN THE TREATMENT OF TESTICULAR TUMORS, HYPERCALCEMIC AND/OR HYPERCALCIURIC CONDITIONS ASSOCIATED WITH VARIOUS ADVANCED MALIGNANCIES, SHOULD BE THOROUGHLY REVIEWED BEFORE ADMINISTERING THIS COMPOUND.

INTRAVENOUS SOLUTION	Controlled Room Temperature	Refrigeration
Sterile Water for Injection, USP	48 hours	7 days
0.9% Sodium Chloride Injection, USP	48 hours	7 days
5% Dextrose Injection, USP	48 hours	7 days
5% Dextrose in 0.225% Sodium Chloride Injection, USP	72 hours	7 days
Lactated Ringer's Injection, USP	72 hours	7 days
5% Dextrose in Electrolyte #75 Injection	72 hours	7 days
5% Dextrose in 0.45% Sodium Chloride Injection, USP*	48 hours	48 hours
Ringer's Injection	24 hours	24 hours
10% Dextrose Injection	24 hours	24 hours
5% Fructose Injection	24 hours	24 hours

DESCRIPTION

Mithracin is a yellow crystalline compound which is produced by a microorganism, *Streptomyces plicatus*. Mithracin is available in vials as a freeze-dried, sterile preparation for intravenous administration. Each vial contains 2500 mcg (2.5 mg) of Mithracin with 100 mg of mannitol and sufficient disodium phosphate to adjust to pH 7. After reconstitution with sterile water for injection, the solution has a pH of 7. The drug is unstable in acid solutions with a pH below 4. Mithracin is an antineoplastic agent. It has an empirical formula of $C_{52}H_{76}O_{24}$. The following structural formula has been proposed for this compound.
[See Chemical Formula below].

CLINICAL PHARMACOLOGY

Although the exact mechanism by which Mithracin causes tumor inhibition is not yet known, studies have indicated that this compound forms a complex with deoxyribonucleic acid (DNA) and inhibits cellular ribonucleic acid (RNA) and enzymic RNA synthesis. The binding of Mithracin to DNA in the presence of $Mg++$ (or other divalent cations) is responsible for the inhibition of DNA-dependent or DNA-directed RNA synthesis. This action presumably accounts for the biological properties of Mithracin.

Mithracin shows potent cytotoxicity against malignant cells of human origin (Hela cells) growing in tissue culture. Mithracin is lethal to Hela cells in 48 hours at concentrations as low as 0.5 micrograms per milliliter of tissue culture medium. Mithracin has shown significant anti-tumor activity against experimental leukemia in mice when administered intraperitoneally.

Plicamycin may lower serum calcium levels; the exact mechanism (or mechanisms) by which the drug exerts this effect is unknown. It appears that plicamycin may block the hypercalcemic action of pharmacologic doses of vitamin D. It has also been suggested that plicamycin may lower calcium serum levels by inhibiting the effect of parathyroid hormone upon osteoclasts. Plicamycin's inhibition of DNA-dependent RNA synthesis appears to render osteoclasts unable to fully respond to parathyroid hormone with the biosynthesis necessary for osteolysis. Decreases in serum phosphate levels and urinary calcium excretion accompany the lowering of serum calcium concentrations.

Radioautography studies[1] with ^{3}H-labeled plicamycin in C3H mice show that the greatest concentrations of the isotope are in the Kupffer cells of the liver and cells of the renal tubules. Plicamycin is rapidly cleared from the blood within the first 2 hours and excretion is also rapid. Sixty-seven percent of measured excretion occurs within 4 hours, 75% within 8 hours, and 90% is recovered in the first 24 hours after injection. There is no evidence of protein binding, nor is there any evidence of metabolism of the carbohydrate moiety of the drug to carbon dioxide and water with loss through respiration. Plicamycin crosses the blood-brain barrier; the concentration found in brain tissue is low but it persists longer than in other tissues. The experimental results in animals correlate closely with results achieved in man.[2]

INDICATIONS

Mithracin is a potent antineoplastic agent which has been shown to be useful in the treatment of carefully selected hospitalized patients with malignant tumors of the testis in whom successful treatment by surgery and/or radiation is impossible. Also, on the basis of limited clinical experience to date, it may be considered in the treatment of certain symptomatic patients with hypercalcemia and hypercalciuria associated with a variety of advanced neoplasms.

The use of Mithracin in other types of neoplastic disease is not recommended at the present time.

CONTRAINDICATIONS

Mithracin (plicamycin) is contraindicated in patients with thrombocytopenia, thrombocytopathy, coagulation disorder or an increased susceptibility to bleeding due to other causes. Mithracin should not be administered to any patient with impairment of bone marrow function.

Mithracin may cause fetal harm when administered to a pregnant woman. Mithracin is contraindicated in women who are or may become pregnant. If this drug is used during pregnancy or if the patient becomes pregnant while taking this drug, the patient should be apprised of the potential hazard to the fetus.

PRECAUTIONS

General: Mithracin should be administered only to patients who ar hospitalized and who can be observed carefully and frequently during and after therapy.

Severe thrombocytopenia, a hemorrhagic tendency and even death may result from the use of Mithracin. Although severe toxicity is more apt to occur in patients who have far-advanced disease or are otherwise considered poor risks for therapy, serious toxicity may also occasionally occur even in patients who are in relatively good condition.

Electrolyte imbalance, especially hypocalcemia, hypokalemia, and hypophosphatemia, should be corrected with appropriate electrolyte therapy prior to treatment with Mithracin.

Mithracin should be used with extreme caution in patients with significant impairment of renal or hepatic function.

Mithracin should not normally be administered to patients who are pregnant or to mothers who are breast feeding.

In the treatment of each patient, the physician must weigh carefully the possibility of achieving therapeutic benefit versus the risk of toxicity which may occur with Mithracin therapy.

Laboratory Tests: The following laboratory studies should be obtained frequently during therapy and for several days following the last dose: platelet count, prothrombin time, bleeding time. The occurrence of thrombocytopenia or a significant prolongation of prothrombin time or bleeding time is an indication for the termination of therapy.

Carcinogenesis, mutagenesis, impairment of fertility: No long-term studies in animals have been performed to evaluate the carcinogenic potential of Mithracin. Histologic evidence of inhibition of spermatogenesis was observed in a substantial number of male rats receiving doses of 0.6 mg/kg/day and above.

Pregnancy Category X: See "Contraindications" section.

Nursing Mothers: It is not known whether this drug is excreted in human milk. Because many drugs are excreted in human milk and because of the potential for serious adverse reactions in nursing infants from Mithracin, a decision should be made whether to discontinue nursing or to discontinue the drug, taking into account the importance of the drug to the mother.

ADVERSE REACTIONS

THE MOST IMPORTANT FORM OF TOXICITY ASSOCIATED WITH THE USE OF MITHRACIN CONSISTS OF A BLEEDING SYNDROME WHICH USUALLY BEGINS WITH AN EPISODE OF EPISTAXIS. This bleeding tendency may only consist of a single or several episodes of epistaxis and progress no further. However, in some cases, this hemorrhagic syndrome can start with an episode of hematemesis which may progress to more wide-spread hemorrhage in the gastrointestinal tract or to a more generalized bleeding tendency. This hemorrhagic diathesis is most likely due to abnormalities in multiple clotting factors.

A detailed analysis of the clinical data in 1,160 patients treated with Mithracin indicates that the hemorrhagic syndrome is dose related. With doses of 30 mcg/kg/day or less for 10 or fewer doses, the incidence of bleeding episodes has been 5.4% with an associated drug-related mortality rate of 1.6%. With doses greater than 30 mcg/kg/day and/or for more than 10 doses, a significantly larger number of bleeding episodes occurred (11.9%) and the associated drug-related mortality rate was also significantly higher (5.7%).

The most common side effects reported with the use of Mithracin consist of gastrointestinal symptoms: anorexia, nausea, vomiting, diarrhea, and stomatitis. Other less frequently reported side effects include fever, drowsiness, weakness, lethargy, malaise, headache, depression, phlebitis, facial flushing, and skin rash.

The following laboratory abnormalities have been reported during therapy with Mithracin (plicamycin) and in most instances were reversible following cessation of treatment:

Hematologic Abnormalities: Depression of platelet count, white count, hemoglobin and prothrombin content; elevation of clotting time and bleeding time; abnormal clot retraction. Thrombocytopenia may be rapid in onset and may occur at any time during therapy or within several days following the last dose. With the occurrence of severe thrombocytopenia, the infusion of platelet concentrates or platelet-rich plasma may be helpful in elevating the platelet count.

The occurrence of leukopenia with the use of Mithracin is relatively uncommon, occurring only in approximately 6% of patients.

It has been uncommon for abnormalities in clotting time or clot retraction to be demonstrated prior to the onset of an overt bleeding episode noted in some patients treated with Mithracin. Nevertheless, the performance of these tests periodically is recommended because in a few instances, an abnormality in one of these studies may have served as a warning to terminate therapy because of impeding serious toxicity.

Abnormal Liver Function Tests: Increased levels of serum glutamic oxalacetic transaminase, serum glutamic pyruvic transaminase, lactic dehydrogenase, alkaline phosphatase, serum bilirubin, ornithine carbamyl transferase, isocitric dehydrogenase, and increased retention of bromsulphalein.

Abnormal Renal Function Tests: Increased blood urea nitrogen and serum creatinine; proteinuria.

Abnormalities in Electrolyte Concentrations: Depression of serum calcium, phosphorus, and potassium.

OVERDOSAGE

Generally, adverse effects following the use of Mithracin, especially the hemorrhagic syndrome, are dose related. Therefore, following administration of an overdose, patients can be expected to experience an exaggeration of the usual adverse effects. Close monitoring of the hematologic picture, including factors involved in the clotting mechanism, hepatic and renal functions, and serum electrolytes, is necessary. No specific antidote for Mithracin is known. Management of overdosage would include general supportive measures to sustain the patient through the period of toxicity.

DOSAGE

The daily dose of Mithracin is based on the patient's body weight. If a patient has abnormal fluid retention such as edema, hydrothorax or ascites, the patient's ideal weight rather than actual body weight should be used to calculate the dose.

Treatment of Testicular Tumors: In the treatment of patients with testicular tumors the recommended daily dose of Mithracin (plicamycin) is 25 to 30 mcg (0.025–0.030 mg) per kilogram of body weight. Therapy should be continued for a period of 8 to 10 days unless significant side effects or toxicity occur during therapy. A course of therapy consisting of more than 10 daily doses is not recommended. Individual daily doses should not exceed 30 mcg (0.030 mg) per kilogram of body weight.

In those patients with responsive tumors, some degree of tumor regression is usually evident within 3 or 4 weeks following the initial course of therapy. If tumor masses remain unchanged following an initial course of therapy, additional courses of therapy at monthly intervals are warranted.

When a significant tumor regression is obtained, it is suggested that additional courses of therapy be given at monthly intervals until a complete regression of tumor masses is achieved or until definite tumor progression or new tumor masses occur in spite of continued courses of therapy.

Treatment of Hypercalcemia and Hypercalciuria: Reversal of hypercalcemia and hypercalciuria can usually be achieved with Mithracin at doses considerably lower than those recommended for use in the treatment of testicular tumors. In hypercalcemia and hypercalciuria associated with advanced malignancy the recommended course of treatment with Mithracin is 25 mcg (0.025 mg) per kilogram of body weight per day for 3 or 4 days.

If the desired degree of reversal of hypercalcemia or hypercalciuria is not achieved with the initial course of therapy, additional courses of therapy may then be administered at intervals of one week or more to achieve the desired result or to maintain serum calcium and urinary calcium excretion at normal levels. It may be possible to maintain normal calcium balance with single, weekly doses or with a schedule of 2 or 3 doses per week.

NOTE: BECAUSE OF THE DRUG'S TOXICITY AND THE LIMITED CLINICAL EXPERIENCE TO DATE IN THESE INDICATIONS, THE FOLLOWING RECOMMENDATIONS SHOULD BE KEPT IN MIND BY THE PHYSICIAN.
1. CONSIDER CASES OF HYPERCALCEMIA AND HYPERCALCIURIA NOT RESPONSIVE TO CONVENTIONAL TREATMENT.
2. APPLY SAME CONTRAINDICATIONS AND PRECAUTIONARY MEASURES AS IN ANTI-TUMOR TREATMENT.
3. RENAL FUNCTION SHOULD BE CAREFULLY MONITORED BEFORE, DURING, AND AFTER TREATMENT.
4. BENEFITS OF USE DURING PREGNANCY OR IN WOMEN OF CHILD-BEARING AGE SHOULD BE WEIGHED AGAINST POTENTIAL TOXICITY TO EMBRYO OR FETUS.

ADMINISTRATION

By IV administration only. The appropriate daily dose of Mithracin should be diluted in one liter of 5% Dextrose Injection, USP or Sodium Chloride Injection, USP and administered by slow intravenous infusion over a period of 4 to 6 hours. Rapid direct intravenous injection of Mithracin should be avoided as it may be associated with a higher incidence and greater severity of gastrointestinal side effects. Extravasation of solutions of Mithracin may cause local irritation and cellulitis at injection sites. Should thrombophlebitis or perivascular cellulitis occur, the infusion should be terminated and reinstituted at another site. The application of moderate heat to the site of extravasation may help to disperse the compound and minimize discomfort and local

Continued on next page

Miles Pharm. Div.—Cont.

tissue irritation. The use of antiemetic compounds prior to and during treatment with Mithracin may be helpful in relieving nausea and vomiting.

Procedures for proper handling and disposal of anti-cancer drugs should be considered. Several guidelines on this subject have been published.[3-8] There is no general agreement that all of the procedures recommended in the guidelines are necessary or appropriate.

HOW SUPPLIED

Mithracin is available in vials as a freeze-dried preparation for intravenous administration. Each vial contains 2500 mcg (2.5 mg) of Mithracin with 100 mg of mannitol and sufficient disodium phosphate to adjust to pH 7. These vials should be stored at refrigerator temperatures between 2°C. to 8°C. (36°F. to 46°F.).

To reconstitute, add aseptically 4.9 ml of Sterile Water for Injection to the contents of the vial and shake to dissolve. Each ml of the resulting solution will then contain 500 mcg (0.5 mg) of Mithracin. NOTE: 1 mg (milligram)=1000 mcg (micrograms). AFTER REMOVAL OF THE APPROPRIATE DOSE, THE REMAINING UNUSED SOLUTION MUST BE DISCARDED, FRESH SOLUTIONS MUST BE PREPARED IN THE ABOVE MANNER EACH DAY OF THERAPY.

ANIMAL PHARMACOLOGY AND TOXICOLOGY

In mice the average intravenous LD_{50} of Mithracin is 2,000 mcg/kg of body weight. When administered orally, it is not toxic to mice even at doses 100 times greater than the intravenous LD_{50}. In rats the average intravenous LD_{50} of Mithracin is 1,700 mcg/kg of body weight. It is not toxic to rats when administered orally at doses 17 times greater than the intravenous LD_{50}. In dogs and monkeys Mithracin is essentially non-toxic when administered intravenously for 24 days at daily doses as high as 50 and 24 mcg/kg of body weight, respectively. However, at higher doses of 100 mcg/kg/day intravenously it is lethal to dogs and monkeys. Signs of toxicity in dogs and monkeys included anorexia, vomiting, listlessness, nelena, anemia, lymphopenia, elevated alkaline phosphatase, serum glutamic oxalacetic transaminase, serum glutamic pyruvic transaminase values, hypochloremia, and azotemia. Dogs also showed marked thrombocytopenia, hyponatremia, hypokalemia, hypocalcemia, and decreased prothrombin consumption. Necropsy findings consisted of necrosis of lymphoid tissue and multiple generalized hemorrhages. Mithracin (plicamycin) was only mildly irritating when injected intramuscularly in rabbits and subcutaneously in guinea pigs. Histologic evidence of inhibition of spermatogenesis was observed in a substantial number of male rats receiving doses of 0.6 mg/kg/day and above. This preclinical finding of selective drug effect constituted the scientific rationale for clinical trials in testicular tumors.

Clinical Reports:

Treatment of Patients with Inoperable Testicular Tumors:

In a combined series of 305 patients with inoperable testicular tumors treated with Mithracin, 33 patients (10.8%) showed a complete disappearance of tumor masses and an additional 80 patients (26.2%) responded with significant partial regression of tumor masses. The longest duration of a continuing complete response is now over 8½ years. The therapeutic responses in this series of patients have been summarized by type of testicular tumor in the accompanying table.

[See table below].

Mithracin may be useful in the treatment of patients with testicular tumors which are resistant to other chemotherapeutic agents. Prior radiation therapy or prior chemotherapy did not alter the response rate with Mithracin. This suggests that there is no significant cross resistance between Mithracin (plicamycin) and other chemotherapeutic agents.

Treatment of Patients with Hypercalcemia and Hypercalciuria: A limited number of patients with hypercalcemia

(range: 12.0–25.8 mg%) and patients with hypercalciuria (range 215–492 mg/day) associated with malignant disease were treated with Mithracin. Hypercalcemia and hypercalciuria were promptly reversed in all patients. In some patients, the primary malignancy was of non-testicular origin.

REFERENCES

1. Kennedy, B.D., et al: Cancer Res.27:1534, 1967.
2. Ransohoff, J., et al: Cancer Chemother. Rep. 49:51, 1965.
3. Recommendations for the Safe Handling of Parenteral Antieoplastic Drugs. NIH Publication No. 83-2621. For sale by the Superintendent of Documents, U.S. Government Printing Office, Washington, D.C. 20402.
4. AMA Council Report. Guidelines for Handling Parenteral Antineoplastics. JAMA, March 15, 1985.
5. National Study Commission on Cytotoxic Exposure—Recommendations for Handling Cytotoxic Agents. Available from Louis P. Jeffrey, Sc.D., Director of Pharmacy Services, Rhode Island Hospital, 593 Eddy Street, Providence, Rhode Island 02902.
6. Clinical Oncological Society of Australia: Guidelines and recommendations for safe handling of antineoplastic agents. Med J Australia 1:426–428, 1983.
7. Jones, R.B., et al: Safe handling of chemotherapeutic agents: A report from the Mount Sinai Medical Center. Ca—A Cancer Journal for Clinicians, Sept/Oct. 258–263, 1983.
8. American Society of Hospital Pharmacists technical assistance bulletin on handling cytotoxic drugs in hospitals. Am J Hosp Pharm 42:131–137, 1985.

Manufactured for
Miles Inc.
Pharmaceutical Division
400 Morgan Lane
West Haven, CT 06516
by Pfizer Laboratories, New York, N.Y. 10017
PD100654   Revised October 1986

MYCELEX® 1%   ℞
(clotrimazole) Cream
For dermatologic use only

PRODUCT OVERVIEW

KEY FACTS

Mycelex®-1% (dermatologic Cream) contains 10 mg clotrimazole in a vanishing cream base. Clotrimazole is a broad spectrum antifungal which exhibits fungicidal activity in vitro against *Candida albicans* and other species of the genus *Candida*. No single-step or multiple-step resistance to clotrimazole has developed during successive passages of *Candida albicans*.

MAJOR USES

Mycelex®-1% (Dermatologic Cream) is a clinically proven effective antifungal indicated for the topical treatment of the following dermal infections; tinea pedis, tinea cruris, and tinea corporis, due to *Trichophyton rubrum*, *Trichophyton mentagrophytes; Epidermophyton floccosum* and *Microsporum canis;* candidiasis due to *Candida albicans;* and tinea versicolor due to *Malassezia furfur.*

SAFETY INFORMATION

Mycelex® Cream is contraindicated in individuals who have shown hypersensitivity to any of its components. Mycelex Cream is not for ophthalmic use.

PRESCRIBING INFORMATION

MYCELEX® 1%   ℞
(clotrimazole) Cream
For dermatologic use only

DESCRIPTION

Mycelex Cream 1% contains clotrimazole, a synthetic antifungal agent having the chemical name [1-(o-Chloro-a,a-diphenylbenzyl)imidazole]: the empirical formula

$C_{22}H_{17}CIN_2$; a molecular weight of 344.84; and the chemical structure:

[See Chemical Formula below].

Clotrimazole is an odorless, white crystalline substance. It is practically insoluble in water, sparingly soluble in ether and very soluble in polyethylene glycol 400, ethanol and chloroform.

Each gram of Mycelex Cream contains 10 mg clotrimazole, dispersed in an emulsion vehicle composed of sorbitan monostearate, polysorbate 60, cetyl esters wax, cetostearyl alcohol, 2-octyldodecanol, purified water; benzyl alcohol (1%) as preservative.

CLINICAL PHARMACOLOGY

Clotrimazole is a broad-spectrum antifungal agent that is used for the treatment of dermal infections caused by various species of pathogenic dermatophytes, yeasts, and *Malassezia furfur*. The primary action of clotrimazole is against dividing and growing organisms.

In vitro, clotrimazole exhibits fungistatic and fungicidal activity against isolates of *Trichophyton rubrum, Trichophyton mentagrophytes, Epidermophyton floccosum, Microsporum canis,* and *Candida* species, including *Candida albicans.* In general, the *in vitro* activity of clotrimazole corresponds to that of tolnaftate and griseofulvin against the mycelia of dermatophytes (*Trichophyton, Microsporum,* and *Epidermophyton),* and to that of the polyenes (amphotericin B and nystatin) against budding fungi (*Candida*). Using an *in vivo* (mouse) and an *in vitro* (mouse kidney homogenate) testing system, clotrimazole and miconazole were equally effective in preventing the growth of the pseudomycelia and mycelia of *Candida albicans.*

Strains of fungi having a natural resistance to clotrimazole are rare. Only a single isolate of *Candida guilliermondi* has been reported to have primary resistance to clotrimazole. No single-step or multiple-step resistance to clotrimazole has developed during successive passages of *Candida albicans* and *Trichophyton mentagrophytes.* No appreciable change in sensitivity was detected after successive passage of isolates of *C. albicans, C. krusei,* or *C. pseudotropicalis* in liquid or solid media containing clotrimazole. Also, resistance could not be developed in chemically induced mutant strains of polyene-resistant isolates of *C. albicans.* Slight, reversible resistance was noted in three isolates of *C. albicans* tested by one investigator. There is a single report that records the clinical emergence of a *C. albicans* strain with considerable resistance to flucytosine and miconazole, and with cross-resistance to clotrimazole, the strain remained sensitive to nystatin and amphotericin B.

In studies of the mechanism of action, the minimum fungicidal concentration of clotrimazole caused leakage of intracellular phosphorus compounds into the ambient medium with concomitant breakdown of cellular nucleic acids and accelerated potassium efflux. Both these events began rapidly and extensively after addition of the drug.

Clotrimazole appears to be well absorbed in humans following oral administration and is eliminated mainly as inactive metabolites. Following topical and vaginal administration, however, clotrimazole appears to be minimally absorbed. Six hours after the application of radioactive clotrimazole 1% cream and 1% solution onto intact and acutely inflamed skin, the concentration of clotrimazole varied from 100 mcg/cm in the stratum corneum to 0.5 to 1 mcg/cm in the stratum reticulare, and 0.1 mcg/cm in the subcutis. No measurable amount of radioactivity (≤ 0.001 mcg/ml) was found in the serum within 48 hours after application under occlusive dressing of 0.5 ml of the solution or 0.8 g of the cream. Only 0.5% or less of the applied radioactivity was excreted in the urine.

Following intravaginal administration of 100mg ^{14}C-clotrimazole vaginal tablets to nine adult females, an average peak serum level, corresponding to only 0.03 μg equivalents/ml of clotrimazole, was reached one to two days after application. After intravaginal administration of 5 g of 1% ^{14}C-clotrimazole vaginal cream, containing 50 mg active drug, to five subjects (one with candida colpitis), serum levels corresponding to approximately 0.01 μg equivalents/ml were reached between 8 and 24 hours after application.

MITHRACIN
RESULTS IN 305 TESTICULAR TUMOR CASES BY TUMOR TYPE

TYPE OF TESTICULAR TUMOR	TOTAL	COMPLETE RESPONSE	PARTIAL RESPONSE	NO RESPONSE
EMBRYONAL CELL	173	26	42	105
TERATOMA	5	0	1	4
TERATOCARCINOMA	23	0	5	18
SEMINOMA	18	0	7	11
CHORIOCARCINOMA	13	1	6	6
MIXED TUMOR	73	6	19	48
TOTALS	305	33	80	192

INDICATIONS AND USAGE

Mycelex® Cream is indicated for the topical treatment of the following dermal infections: tinea pedis, tinea cruris, and tinea corporis due to *Trichophyton rubrum, Trichophyton mentagrophytes, Epidermophyton floccosum,* and *Microsporum canis;* candidiasis due to *Candida albicans,* and tinea versicolor due to *Malassezia furfur.*

CONTRAINDICATIONS

Mycelex® Cream is contraindicated in individuals sensitive to its components.

WARNINGS

Mycelex Cream is not for ophthalmic use.

PRECAUTIONS

General: If irritation or sensitivity develops with the use of Mycelex Cream, treatment should be discontinued and appropriate therapy instituted.

Information For Patients:
The patient should be advised to:
1. Use the medication for the full treatment time even though the symptoms may have improved. Notify the physician if there is no improvement after four weeks of treatment.
2. Inform the physician if the area of application shows signs of increased irritation (redness, itching, burning, blistering, swelling, oozing) indicative of possible sensitization.
3. Avoid the use of occlusive wrappings or dressings.
4. Avoid sources of infection or reinfection.

Laboratory Tests: If there is lack of response to Mycelex® Cream, appropriate microbiological studies should be repeated to confirm the diagnosis and rule out other pathogens before instituting another course of antimycotic therapy.

Drug Interactions: Synergism or antagonism between clotrimazole and nystatin, or amphotericin B, or flucytosine against strains of *C. albicans* has not been reported.

Carcinogenesis, mutagenesis, impairment of fertility: An 18-month oral dosing study with clotrimazole in rats has not revealed any carcinogenic effect.

In tests for mutagenesis, chromosomes of the spermatophores of Chinese hamsters which had been exposed to clotrimazole were examined for structural changes during the metaphase. Prior to testing, the hamsters had received five oral clotrimazole doses of 100 mg/kg body weight. The results of this study showed that clotrimazole had no mutagenic effect.

Usage in Pregnancy: Pregnancy Category B: The disposition of ^{14}C-clotrimazole has been studied in humans and animals. Clotrimazole is very poorly absorbed following dermal application or intravaginal administration to humans. (See Clinical Pharmacology.)

In clinical trials, use of vaginally applied clotrimazole in pregnant women in their second and third trimesters has not been associated with ill effects. There are, however, no adequate and well-controlled studies in pregnant women during the first trimester of pregnancy.

Studies in pregnant rats with intravaginal doses up to 100 mg/kg have revealed no evidence of harm to the fetus due to clotrimazole.

High oral doses of clotrimazole in rats and mice ranging from 50 to 120 mg/kg resulted in embryotoxicity (possibly secondary to maternal toxicity), impairment of mating, decreased litter size and number of viable young and decreased pup survival to weaning. However, clotrimazole was not teratogenic in mice, rabbits and rats at oral doses up to 200, 180 and 100 mg/kg, respectively. Oral absorption in the rat amounts to approximately 90% of the administered dose. Because animal reproduction studies are not always predictive of human response, this drug should be used only if clearly indicated during the first trimester of pregnancy.

Nursing Mothers: It is not known whether this drug is excreted in human milk. Because many drugs are excreted in human milk, caution should be exercised when clotrimazole is used by a nursing woman.

Pediatric Use: Safety and effectiveness in children have been established for clotrimazole when used as indicated and in the recommended dosage.

ADVERSE REACTIONS

The following adverse reactions have been reported in connection with the use of the cream and solution forms of this product: erythema, stinging, blistering, peeling, edema, pruritus, urticaria, burning, and general irritation of the skin.

OVERDOSAGE

Acute overdosage with topical application of clotrimazole is unlikely and would not be expected to lead to a life-threatening situation.

DOSAGE AND ADMINISTRATION

Gently massage sufficient Mycelex® Cream into the affected and surrounding skin areas twice a day, in the morning and evening.

Clinical improvement, with relief of pruritus, usually occurs within the first week of treatment with Mycelex. If the patient shows no clinical improvement after four weeks of treatment with Mycelex, the diagnosis should be reviewed.

HOW SUPPLIED

Mycelex Cream 1% is supplied in 15, 30, and (2 × 45) gram tubes.
Store below 86°F (30°C). Avoid Freezing.

	NDC Numbers
15g	0026-3091-61
30g	0026-3091-59
2 × 45g	0026-3091-67

Miles Inc.
Pharmaceutical Division
400 Morgan Lane
West Haven, CT 06516 USA
Caution: Federal (USA) law prohibits dispensing without a prescription.
PD100670   Bay 5097   0228
U.S. Patents No. 3,660,577 and 3,705,172.
© 1988 Miles Inc.

MYCELEX®   ℞
(clotrimazole)
Troche

PRODUCT OVERVIEW

KEY FACTS

MYCELEX® Troche is a slow-dissolving tablet (lozenge) containing 10 mg of clotrimazole, a synthetic antifungal agent for topical use in the mouth. Clotrimazole is a broad-spectrum antifungal which exhibits fungicidal activity *in vitro* against *Candida albicans* and other species of the genus *Candida*. No single-step or multiple-step resistance to clotrimazole has developed during successive passages of *Candida albicans* in the laboratory.

MAJOR USES

MYCELEX® Troche has been proven effective in the treatment of oropharyngeal candidiasis (oral thrush) in patients over 3 years of age.

SAFETY INFORMATION

MYCELEX® Troches are contra-indicated in patients who are hypersensitive to any of its components. MYCELEX Troches are not indicated for the treatment of systemic mycoses. Since elevated SGOT levels have been reported, periodic assessment of hepatic function is advisable, particularly, in patients with pre-existing hepatic impairment.

PRESCRIBING INFORMATION

MYCELEX®   ℞
(clotrimazole)
Troche

DESCRIPTION

Each Mycelex® Troche contains 10 mg clotrimazole [1(o-chloro-α, α-diphenylbenzyl) imidazole], a synthetic antifungal agent, for topical use in the mouth.
Structural Formula:

Chemical Formula:
$C_{22}H_{17}ClN_2$
The troche dosage form is a large, slowly dissolving tablet (lozenge) containing 10 mg of clotrimazole dispersed in dextrose, microcrystalline cellulose, povidone, and magnesium stearate.

CLINICAL PHARMACOLOGY

Clotrimazole is a broad-spectrum antifungal agent that inhibits the growth of pathogenic yeasts by altering the permeability of cell membranes. It exhibits fungicidal activity *in vitro* against *Candida albicans* and other species of the genus *Candida*. No single-step or multiple-step resistance to clotrimazole has developed during successive passages of *Candida albicans* in the laboratory.

After oral administration of a 10 mg clotrimazole troche to healthy volunteers concentrations sufficient to inhibit most species of *Candida* persist in saliva for up to three hours following the approximately 30 minutes needed for a troche to dissolve. The long term effective concentration of drug in saliva appears to be related to the slow release of clotrimazole from the oral mucosa to which the drug is apparently bound. Repetitive dosing at three hour intervals maintains effective salivary levels above the minimum inhibitory concentration of most strains of *Candida*. In another study the mean serum concentrations were 4.98 ± 3.7 and 3.23 ± 1.4 nanograms/ml at 30 and 60 minutes respectively.

INDICATIONS AND USAGE

Mycelex Troches are indicated for the local treatment of oropharyngeal candidiasis. The diagnosis should be confirmed by a KOH smear and/or culture prior to treatment.

CONTRAINDICATIONS

Mycelex Troches are contraindicated in patients who are hypersensitive to any of its components.

WARNING

Mycelex Troches are not indicated for the treatment of systemic mycoses.

PRECAUTIONS

Abnormal liver function tests have been reported in patients treated with clotrimazole troches; elevated SGOT levels were reported in about 15% of patients in the clinical trials. In most cases the elevations were minimal and it was often impossible to distinguish effects of clotrimazole from those of other therapy and the underlying disease (malignancy in most cases). Periodic assessment of hepatic function is advisable particularly in patients with pre-existing hepatic impairment.

Since patients must be instructed to allow each troche to dissolve slowly in the mouth in order to achieve maximum effect of the medication, they must be of such an age and physical and/or mental condition to comprehend such instructions.

Carcinogenesis: An 18 month dosing study with clotrimazole in rats has not revealed any carcinogenic effect.

Usage in Pregnancy: Pregnancy Category C: Clotrimazole has been shown to be embryotoxic in rats and mice when given in doses 100 times the adult human dose (in mg/kg), possibly secondary to maternal toxicity. The drug was not teratogenic in mice, rabbits, and rats when given in doses up to 200, 180, and 100 times the human dose.

Clotrimazole given orally to mice from nine weeks before mating through weaning at a dose 120 times the human dose was associated with impairment of mating, decreased number of viable young, and decreased survival to weaning. No effects were observed at 60 times the human dose. When the drug was given to rats during a similar time period at 50 times the human dose, there was a slight decrease in the number of pups per litter and decreased pup viability.

There are no adequate and well controlled studies in pregnant women. Clotrimazole troches should be used during pregnancy only if the potential benefit justifies the potential risk to the fetus.

Pediatric Use: Safety and effectiveness of clotrimazole in children below the age of 3 years have not been established; therefore, its use in such patients is not recommended.

ADVERSE REACTIONS

Abnormal liver function tests have been reported in patients treated with clotrimazole troches; elevated SGOT levels were reported in about 15% of patients in the clinical trials (see **Precautions** section).

Nausea and vomiting was reported in about one in twenty patients.

OVERDOSE

No data available.

DRUG ABUSE AND DEPENDENCE

No data available.

DOSAGE AND ADMINISTRATION

Mycelex® Troches are administered only as a lozenge that must be dissolved slowly in the mouth. The recommended dose is one troche five times a day for fourteen consecutive days. Only limited data are available on the safety and effectiveness of the clotrimazole troche after prolonged administration; therefore, therapy should be limited to short term use, if possible.

HOW SUPPLIED

Mycelex® Troches, white discoid, uncoated tablets are supplied in bottles of 70 and 140. Each tablet will be identified with the following: Miles 095.
Store below 86°F (30°C), avoid freezing.

Miles Inc.
Pharmaceutical Division
400 Morgan Lane
West Haven, CT 06516
PD100685   BAY 5097   0477
Shown in Product Identification Section, page 419

Continued on next page

Miles Pharm. Div.—Cont.

MYCELEX®-G 1%   ℞
(clotrimazole) Vaginal Cream

PRODUCT OVERVIEW

KEY FACTS
Mycelex®-G-1% Vaginal Cream is an effective vaginal antifungal cream. Each applicatorful of Mycelex-G-1% Vaginal Cream contains approximately 50 mg of clotrimazole. Clotrimazole is a broad spectrum antifungal which exhibits fungicidal activity *in vitro* against *Candida albicans* and other species of the genus *Candida*. No single-step or multiple-step resistance to clotrimazole has developed during successive passages of *Candida albicans*.

MAJOR USES
Mycelex®-G-1% Vaginal Cream has been proven clinically effective for the local treatment of patients with vulvovaginal candidiasis.

SAFETY INFORMATION
Mycelex®-G-1% Vaginal Cream is contraindicated in women who have shown hypersensitivity to any of the components. If there is a lack of response to treatment with Mycelex®-G-1% Vaginal Cream, appropriate microbiological studies should be repeated to confirm the diagnosis and rule out other pathogens before instituting another course of antimycotic therapy. No adequate and well-controlled studies in pregnany women during the first trimester of pregnancy.

PRESCRIBING INFORMATION

MYCELEX®-G 1%   ℞
(clotrimazole) Vaginal Cream

DESCRIPTION
Mycelex-G is clotrimazole [1-(o-Chloro-α,α-diphenylbenzyl) imidazole], a synthetic antifungal agent having the chemical formula, $C_{22}H_{17}ClN_2$, and following chemical structure:

Each applicatorful of Mycelex-G Vaginal Cream contains approximately 50 mg. clotrimazole dispersed in sorbitan monostearate, polysorbate 60, cetyl esters wax, cetostearyl alcohol, 2-octyldodecanol, purified water, and as a preservative, benzyl alcohol (1%).

ACTIONS
Clotrimazole is a broad spectrum antifungal agent that inhibits the growth of pathogenic yeasts. Clotrimazole exhibits fungicidal activity *in vitro* against *Candida albicans* and other species of the genus *Candida*.
No single-step or multiple-step resistance to clotrimazole has developed during successive passages of *Candida albicans*.

INDICATIONS
Mycelex-G Vaginal Cream is indicated for the local treatment of patients with vulvovaginal candidiasis (moniliasis). As Mycelex-G Vaginal Cream has been shown to be effective only for candidal vulvovaginitis, the diagnosis should be confirmed by KOH smears and/or cultures. Other pathogens commonly associated with vulvovaginitis (*Trichomonas* and *Hemophilus vaginalis*) should be ruled out by appropriate laboratory methods.
Studies have shown that women taking oral contraceptives had a cure rate similar to those not taking oral contraceptives.

CONTRAINDICATIONS
Mycelex-G Vaginal Cream is contraindicated in women who have shown hypersensitivity to any of the components of the preparation.

PRECAUTIONS
Laboratory Tests: If there is a lack of response to Mycelex-G Vaginal Cream, appropriate microbiological studies should be repeated to confirm the diagnosis and rule out other pathogens before instituting another course of antimycotic therapy.
Usage in Pregnancy: While Mycelex-G Vaginal Cream has not been studied in the first trimester of pregnancy, use in the second and third trimesters has not been associated with ill effects.
Application of ^{14}C labeled clotrimazole has shown negligible absorption (peak serum level of 0.01 mcg/ml 24 hours after insertion of vaginal cream containing 50 mg. of active drug) from both normal and inflamed human vaginal mucosa.

ADVERSE REACTIONS
Three (0.5%) of the 653 patients treated with Mycelex-G Vaginal Cream reported complaints during therapy that were possibly drug related. Vaginal burning occurred in one patient; erythema, irritation and burning in another; intercurrent cystitis was reported in the third.

DOSAGE AND ADMINISTRATION
Mycelex-G Vaginal Cream has been found to be effective when used from seven to fourteen days; studies have shown that patients treated for fourteen days had a significantly higher cure rate. The recommended dose is one applicatorful a day for seven to fourteen consecutive days; using the applicator supplied, insert one applicatorful of cream (approximately 5 grams) intravaginally preferably at bedtime.
Store below 86°F (30°C).

HOW SUPPLIED
Mycelex-G Vaginal Cream 1% is supplied in 45 and 90 gram tubes with a measured-dose applicator, for seven-day and for fourteen-day treatments.

	NDC
45g	0026-3094-45
90g	0026-3094-46

Caution: Federal (USA) law prohibits dispensing without prescription.
Miles Inc.
Pharmaceutical Division
400 Morgan Lane
West Haven, CT 06516 USA
PD100679   2/88   BAY 5097
© 1988 Miles Inc.

MYCELEX®-G 100 mg   ℞
(clotrimazole) Vaginal Tablets

PRODUCT OVERVIEW

KEY FACTS
Mycelex®-G 100 mg is an effective vaginal antifungal tablet containing 100 mg of clotrimazole (the active ingredient). Clotrimazole is a broad spectrum antifungal which exhibits fungicidal activity *in vitro* against *Candida albicans* and other species of the genus *Candida*. No single-step or multiple-step resistance to clotrimazole has developed during successive passages of *Candida albicans*.

MAJOR USES
Mycelex®-G 100 Vaginal Tablet has been proven clinically effective for the local treatment of vulvovaginal candidiasis.

SAFETY INFORMATION
Mycelex®-G 100 mg Vaginal Tablet is contraindicated in women who have shown hypersensitivity to any of the components. If there is a lack of response to treatment with Mycelex-G 100mg Vaginal Tablets, appropriate microbiological studies should be repeated to confirm the diagnosis and rule out other pathogens before instituting another course of antimycotic therapy. No adequate and well-controlled studies in pregnant women during the first trimester of pregnancy.

PRESCRIBING INFORMATION

MYCELEX®-G 100 mg   ℞
(clotrimazole) Vaginal Tablets

DESCRIPTION
Mycelex-G is clotrimazole [1-(o-Chloro-α, α-diphenylbenzyl) imidazole], a synthetic antifungal agent having the chemical formula, $C_{22}H_{17}ClN_2$.
Each Mycelex-G Vaginal Tablet contains 100 mg clotrimazole dispersed in lactose, povidone, corn starch and magnesium stearate.

ACTIONS
Clotrimazole is a broad-spectrum antifungal agent that inhibits the growth of pathogenic yeasts. Clotrimazole exhibits fungicidal activity *in vitro* against *Candida albicans* and other species of the genus *Candida*.
No single-step or multiple-step resistance to clotrimazole has developed during successive passages of *Candida albicans*.

INDICATIONS
Mycelex-G Vaginal Tablets are indicated for the local treatment of vulvovaginal candidiasis. The diagnosis should be confirmed by KOH smears and/or cultures. Other pathogens commonly associated with vulvovaginitis (*Trichomonas* and *Hemophilus vaginalis)* should be ruled out by appropriate laboratory methods.

CONTRAINDICATIONS
Mycelex-G Vaginal Tablets are contraindicated in women who have shown hypersensitivity to any components of the preparation.

PRECAUTIONS
Laboratory Tests: If there is a lack of response to Mycelex-G Vaginal Tablets, appropriate microbiological studies should be repeated to confirm the diagnosis and rule out other pathogens before instituting another course of antimycotic therapy.
Application of ^{14}C-labeled clotrimazole has shown negligible absorption (peak of 0.03 mcg/ml of serum 24 hours after insertion of a 100 mg tablet) from both normal and inflamed human vaginal mucosa.
Usage in Pregnancy: While Mycelex-G Vaginal Tablets have not been studied in the first trimester of pregnancy, use in the second and third trimesters has not been associated with ill effects. Follow-up reports now available on 71 neonates of 117 pregnant patients reveal no adverse effects or complications attributable to Mycelex-G therapy.

ADVERSE REACTIONS
Eighteen (1.6%) of the 1116 patients treated with Mycelex-G in double-blind studies reported complaints during therapy that were possibly drug-related. Mild burning occured in six patients while other complaints, such as skin rash, itching, vulval irritation, lower abdominal cramps and bloating, slight cramping, slight urinary frequency, and burning or irritation in the sexual partner, occurred rarely.

DOSAGE AND ADMINISTRATION
The recommended dose is one tablet a day for seven consecutive days. Recent studies indicate that an alternative regimen of two tablets a day for three consecutive days is similarly effective in non-pregnant patients; however, in pregnant patients the three-day treatment course did not prove to be effective and is therefore not recommended. They should receive the seven-day treatment. Using the applicator supplied, insert one or two tablets intravaginally preferably at bedtime.
In the event of treatment failure, other pathogens commonly responsible for vaginitis should be ruled out before instituting another course of antimycotic therapy. There are no studies to show whether a second course of clotrimazole would be effective in patients who fail to respond to the initial course.

HOW SUPPLIED
Mycelex-G Vaginal Tablets are 100 mg, white, bullet-shaped, uncoated tablets, debossed with the word Miles and the number 093 supplied in a strip of seven tablets with a plastic applicator and patient instructions.
Do not store above 35°C (95°F).
U.S. Patent No. 3,660,577 and 3,705,172.
Miles Inc.
Pharmaceutical Division
400 Morgan Lane
West Haven, CT 06516 USA
PD100699   BAY 5097   11/88
© 1988 Miles Inc.

0661

Shown in Product Identification Section, page 419

MYCELEX®-G 500 mg   ℞
brand of clotrimazole
Vaginal Tablet

PRODUCT OVERVIEW

KEY FACTS
Mycelex®-G 500 mg is an effective antifungal containing 500 mg of clotrimazole (the active ingredient). Clotrimazole is a broad spectrum antifungal which exhibits fungicidal activity *in vitro* against *Candida albicans* and other species of the genus *Candida*. No single-step or multiple-step resistance to clotrimazole has developed during successive passages of *Candida albicans*.

MAJOR USES
Mycelex®-G 500 mg has proved to be clinically effective for local treatment of vulvovaginal candidiasis when one day therapy is felt warranted. In the case of severe vulvovaginal candidiasis longer antimycotic therapy such as Mycelex®-G 100 mg tablets or Mycelex®-G Cream is recommended.

SAFETY INFORMATION
Mycelex®-G 500 Vaginal Tablets are contraindicated in women who have shown hypersensitivity to any components of the compound. If there is a lack of response to treatment with Mycelex®-G 500 mg, appropriate microbiological studies should be repeated to confirm the diagnosis and rule out other pathogens before instituting another course of antimycotic therapy. No adequate and well-controlled studies in pregnant women during the first trimester of pregnancy.

PRESCRIBING INFORMATION

MYCELEX®-G 500mg   ℞
brand of clotrimazole
Vaginal Tablet

DESCRIPTION
Each Mycelex®-G 500 mg Vaginal Tablet contains 500 mg clotrimazole (the active ingredient) dispersed in lactose, microcrystalline cellulose, lactic acid, corn starch, crospovidone, calcium lactate, magnesium stearate, silicon dioxide and hydroxypropyl methylcellulose. Chemically, clotrimazole is [1-(o-Chloro-α, α-diphenylbenzyl) imidazole], a synthetic antifungal agent having the chemical formul $C_{22}H_{17}ClN_2$; a molecular weight of 344.84; and the following

chemical structure:

Clotrimazole is an odorless, white crystalline substance, practically insoluble in water, sparingly soluble in ether, soluble in carbon tetrachloride, and very soluble in ethanol and chloroform.

CLINICAL PHARMACOLOGY

Serum levels and levels in vaginal secretions of clotrimazole were measured in six healthy volunteers who had one 500 mg vaginal tablet inserted. Although serum levels of clotrimazole were higher than those in other volunteers given 100 mg and 200 mg vaginal tablets these levels did not exceed 10 nanograms/ml. It has been estimated that three to ten percent of a vaginal dose of clotrimazole may be absorbed, but the drug rapidly and efficiently degrades to microbiologically inactive metabolites. The clotrimazole concentrations remaining in vaginal secretions were still in the mg/ml range for 48 hours and in two of the six subjects at 72 hours.

The findings of high clotrimazole concentrations in vaginal secretions for up to 72 hours and low concentrations in the serum suggest that nearly all the clotrimazole given in the 500 mg vaginal tablet remains in the vagina for 48 hours, and in some cases 72 hours, in fungicidal concentrations.

Clotrimazole is a broad-spectrum antifungal agent. It has been postulated that the compound affects the permeability characteristics of the membrane allowing the leakage of essential intracellular components with a consequent inhibition of the synthesis of such macromolecules as protein, lipid, DNA, and polysaccharides.

At concentrations as low as 2–5 µg/ml, clotrimazole exhibits fungicidal activity *in vitro* against *Candida albicans* and other species of the genus *Candida.*

No single-step or multiple-step resistance to clotrimazole has developed during successive passages of *Candida albicans.*

INDICATIONS

Mycelex®-G 500 mg Vaginal Tablets are indicated for the local treatment of vulvovaginal candidiasis when one day therapy is felt warranted. In the case of severe vulvovaginitis due to candidiasis, longer antimycotic therapy is recommended. The diagnosis should be confirmed by KOH smears and/or cultures. Other pathogens commonly associated with vulvovaginitis, *Trichomonas* and *Gardnerella (Haemophilus) vaginalis* should be ruled out by appropriate laboratory methods.

CONTRAINDICATIONS

Mycelex®-G 500 mg Vaginal Tablets are contraindicated in women who have shown hypersensitivity to any components of the preparation.

WARNINGS

None.

PRECAUTIONS

If there is a lack of response to Mycelex®-G 500 mg Vaginal Tablets, appropriate microbiological studies should be repeated to confirm the diagnosis and rule out other pathogens before instituting another course of antimycotic therapy.

CARCINOGENESIS

No long term studies in animals have been performed to evaluate the carcinogenic potential of Mycelex®-G 500 mg Vaginal Tablets intravaginally. A long term study in rats (Wistar strains) where clotrimazole was administered orally provided no indication of carcinogenicity.

USAGE IN PREGNANCY

Pregnancy Category B: The disposition of ^{14}C-clotrimazole has been studied in humans and animals. Clotrimazole is poorly absorbed following intravaginal administration to humans, whereas it is rather well absorbed after oral administration.

In clinical trials, use of vaginally applied clotrimazole in pregnant women in their second and third trimesters has not been associated with ill effects. There are, however, no adequate and well-controlled studies in pregnant women during the first trimester of pregnancy.

Studies in pregnant rats given repeated intravaginal doses up to 100 mg/kg/day have revealed no evidence of harm to the fetus due to clotrimazole.

Repeated high oral doses of clotrimazole in rats and mice ranging from 50 to 120 mg/kg resulted in embryotoxicity (possibly secondary to maternal toxicity), impairment of mating, decreased litter size and number of viable young and decreased pup survival to weaning. However, clotrimazole was not teratogenic in mice, rabbits and rats at oral doses up to 200, 180 and 100 mg/kg, respectively. Oral absorption in the rat amounts to approximately 90% of the administered dose.

Because animal reproduction studies are not always predictive of human response, this drug should be used only if clearly indicated during the first trimester of pregnancy.

ADVERSE REACTIONS

Of 297 patients in double-blind studies with the 500 mg vaginal tablet, 3 of 149 patients treated with active drug and 3 of 148 patients treated with placebo reported complaints during therapy that were possibly drug related. In the active drug group, vomiting occurred in one patient, vaginal soreness with coitus in another, and complaints of vaginal irritation, itching, burning and dyspareunia in the third patient. In the placebo group, clitoral irritation occurred in one patient and dysuria, described as remotely related to drug, in the other. A third patient in the placebo group developed bacterial vaginitis which the investigator classed as possibly related to drug.

Eighteen (1.6%) of the 1116 patients treated with Mycelex®-G in other formulations in double-blind studies reported complaints during therapy that were possibly drug-related. Mild burning occurred in six patients while other complaints such as skin rash, itching, vulval irritation, lower abdominal cramps and bloating, slight cramping, slight urinary frequency, and burning or irritation in the sexual partner, occurred rarely.

OVERDOSAGE

No data available.

DRUG ABUSE AND DEPENDENCE

Drug abuse and dependence with Mycelex®-G 500 mg Vaginal Tablets has not been reported.

DOSAGE AND ADMINISTRATION

The recommended dose is one tablet inserted intravaginally one time only, preferably at bedtime. In the event of treatment failure, that is, persistence of signs and symptoms of vaginitis after five days, other pathogens commonly responsible for vaginitis should be ruled out before instituting another course of antimycotic therapy.

HOW SUPPLIED

Mycelex-G 500 mg Vaginal Tablets are white, bullet shaped, uncoated tablets, coded with Miles on one side and 097 on the other, supplied as a single 500 mg tablet with plastic applicator and patient instructions, or in twin pack with Mycelex 1% cream 7 g tube.

Store Below 30°C (86°F).

U.S. Patent Numbers 3,660,577; 3,705,172; 3,839,573; 4,457,938.

Manufactured by

Miles Inc.

Pharmaceutical Division

400 Morgan Lane

West Haven, CT 06516

PD100689   6/88   BAY 5097   0563

© 1988 Miles Inc.

NICLOCIDE®   ℞
(niclosamide)
Chewable Tablets

DESCRIPTION

NICLOCIDE (niclosamide) is an anthelmintic provided in chewable tablet form at a strength of 500 mg per tablet. Niclosamide is 2′, 5-Dichloro-4′-nitrosalicylanilide. Inactive ingredients: corn starch, magnesium stearate, povidone, sodium lauryl sulfate, sodium saccharin, talc and vanillin. The empirical formula is $C_{13}H_8Cl_2N_2O_4$ with the following structural formula:

CLINICAL PHARMACOLOGY

NICLOCIDE inhibits oxidative phosphorylation in the mitochondria of cestodes. Both *in vitro* and *in vivo*, the scolex and proximal segments are killed on contact with the drug. The scolex of the tapeworm, loosened from the gut wall, may be digested in the intestine, and thus may not be identified in the feces even after extensive purging.

The use of NICLOCIDE has not been associated with the development of anemia, leukopenia or thrombocytopenia nor have there been any effects on normal renal and hepatic functions.

INDICATIONS AND USAGE

NICLOCIDE (niclosamide) is indicated for the treatment of tapeworm infections by *Taenia saginata* (beef tapeworm), *Diphyllobothrium latum* (fish tapeworm) and *Hymenolepis nana* (dwarf tapeworm).

CONTRAINDICATIONS

NICLOCIDE™ Tablets are contraindicated in individuals who have shown hypersensitivity to any of its components.

PRECAUTIONS

NICLOCIDE affects the cestodes of the intestine only. It is without effect in cysticercosis.

Drug Interactions: No data are available regarding interaction of niclosamide with other drugs.

Carcinogenesis, mutagenesis, impairment of fertility:

Carcinogenicity Potential: Although carcinogenicity studies on niclosamide *per se* have not been done, long-term feeding studies on its ethanolamine salt in rats and mice did not show carcinogenicity. Mutagenicity tests have not been performed.

Pregnancy: Pregnancy Category B: Reproduction studies in rabbits and rats at doses of 25 times the human therapeutic dose and in mice at 12 times the human therapeutic dose, have revealed no evidence of impaired fertility or harm to the fetus due to niclosamide. There are, however, no adequate and well-controlled studies in pregnant women. Because animal studies are not always predictive of human response, the drug should be used during pregnancy only if clearly needed.

Nursing Mothers: No studies are available.

Pediatric Use: In children under 2 years of age, the safety of the drug has not been established.

ADVERSE REACTIONS

The incidence of side effects has been reported as follows: nausea/vomiting 4.1%, abdominal discomfort including loss of appetite 3.4%, diarrhea 1.6%, drowsiness, dizziness, and or headache 1.4%, and skin rash including pruritus ani 0.3%. Other side effects listed in decreasing order of frequency were: oral irritation, fever, rectal bleeding, weakness, bad taste in mouth, sweating, palpitations, constipation, alopecia, edema of an arm, backache and irritability. There was also one instance of a transient rise in SGOT in an i.v. narcotic addict. Two cases of urticaria reported may be related to the breakdown products of the tapeworm. All side effects were mild or moderate and transitory and did not necessitate discontinuation of the treatment.

OVERDOSAGE

Insufficient data are available. In the event of overdose a fast-acting laxative and enema should be given. Vomiting should not be induced.

DOSAGE AND ADMINISTRATION

1. *Taenia saginata* and *Diphyllobothrium latum*
   a. Adults: 4 tablets (2.0 g) chewed thoroughly in a single dose.
   b. Children weighing more than 34 kg (75 lbs): 3 tablets (1.5 g) chewed thoroughly in a single dose.
   c. Children weighing between 11 and 34 kg (25 to 75 lbs): 2 tablets (1.0 g) chewed thoroughly in a single dose.
2. *Hymenolepis nana*
   a. Adults: 4 tablets (2.0 g) chewed thoroughly as a single daily dose for 7 days.
   b. Children weighing more than 34 kg (75 lbs): 3 tablets (1.5g) chewed thoroughly on the first day, then 2 tablets (1.0 g) daily for next 6 days.
   c. Children weighing between 11 and 34 kg (25 to 75 lbs): 2 tablets (1.0 g) to be chewed thoroughly on the first day, then one tablet (0.5 g) daily for next 6 days.

   T. saginata and *D. latum* infections are usually due to a single adult worm and require an intermediate host in their life cycle. With *Hymenolepis nana* multiple infections are the rule. No intermediate host is required; both larval and adult stages of the worm may be found in the human intestine where the complete life cycle occurs. Since the drug is more effective against the mature than the larval stage, therapy must be extended over several days to cover all stages of maturation.

   Patients with *H. nana* must be instructed to observe strict personal and environmental hygiene to avoid autoinfection with this parasite.
3. NICLOCIDE™ must be thoroughly chewed and then swallowed with a little water. No special dietary restrictions are necessary before or after treatment. The best time to take the drug is after a light meal (e.g., breakfast). A mild laxative may be desirable in constipated patients to achieve a normal bowel movement. Young children should have the tablets crushed to a fine powder and mixed with a small amount of water to form a paste.

   NICLOCIDE has a vanilla taste which is not unpleasant to most persons.

   NICLOCIDE is suitable for administration on an ambulatory or outpatient basis.
4. Follow-up:

   As the vermicidal action of NICLOCIDE renders the tapeworm, especially the scolex and proximal segments, vulnerable to destruction during their passage through the gut, it is not always possible to identify the

Continued on next page

Miles Pharm. Div.—Cont.

scolex in stools. The sooner the tapeworm is passed and examined after treatment, the better the chance of identification of the scolex. Segments and/or ova of beef or fish tapeworm may be present in the stool for up to 3 days after therapy. Persistent *T. saginata* or *D. latum* segments and/ or ova on the seventh day post therapy indicate failure. A second identical course of treatment may be given at that time.

No patient should be considered cured unless the stool has been negative for a minimum of three months.

HOW SUPPLIED

NICLOCIDE is available as round, light yellow chewable tablets, scored on one side, coded with the word Miles and number 721, each containing 500 mg of niclosamide, and is supplied in boxes of 4 tablets.

Storage Conditions: Store below 86°F (30°C), avoid freezing.

Miles Inc.
Pharmaceutical Division
400 Morgan Lane
West Haven, CT 06516

PD100697   BAY 2353 0617   June 1985
Shown in Product Identification Section, page 419

NIMOTOP®   ℞
(nimodipine/Miles)
CAPSULES
For Oral Use

DESCRIPTION

Nimotop® (nimodipine) belongs to the class of pharmacological agents known as calcium channel blockers. Nimodipine is isopropyl (2 - methoxyethyl) 1, 4 - dihydro - 2, 6 - dimethyl - 4 - (3 - nitrophenyl) - 3, 5 - pyridine - dicarboxylate. It has a molecular weight of 418.5 and a molecular formula of $C_{21}H_{26}N_2O_7$. The structural formula is:

Nimodipine is a yellow crystalline substance, practically insoluble in water.
NIMOTOP® capsules are formulated as soft gelatin capsules for oral administration. Each liquid filled capsule contains 30 mg of nimodipine in a vehicle of glycerin, peppermint oil, purified water and polyethylene glycol 400. The soft gelatin capsule shell contains gelatin, glycerin, purified water and titanium dioxide.

CLINICAL PHARMACOLOGY

Mechanism of Action: Nimodipine is a calcium channel blocker. The contractile processes of smooth muscle cells are dependent upon calcium ions, which enter these cells during depolarization as slow ionic transmembrane currents. Nimodipine inhibits calcium ion transfer into these cells and thus inhibits contractions of vascular smooth muscle. In animal experiments, nimodipine had a greater effect on cerebral arteries than on arteries elsewhere in the body perhaps because it is highly lipophilic, allowing it to cross the blood-brain barrier: concentrations of nimodipine as high as 12.5 ng/mL have been detected in the cerebrospinal fluid of nimodipine treated subarachnoid hemorrhage (SAH) patients.
Based on animal experiments, it was hoped that nimodipine would prevent cerebral arterial spasm in SAH patients. While the clinical studies described below demonstrate a favorable effect by nimodipine on the severity of neurological deficits caused by cerebral vasospasm following SAH, there is no arteriographic evidence that the drug either prevents or relieves the spasm of these arteries. The actual mechanism of action in humans is, therefore, unknown.
Pharmacokinetics and Metabolism: In man, nimodipine is rapidly absorbed after oral administration, and peak concentrations are generally attained within one hour. The terminal elimination half-life is approximately 8 to 9 but earlier elimination rates are much more rapid, equivalent to a half life of 1–2 hours; a consequence is the need for frequent (every 4 hours) dosing. There were no signs of accumulation when nimodipine was given three times a day for seven days. Nimodipine is over 95% bound to plasma proteins. The binding as concentration independent over the range of 10 ng/mL to 10 μg/mL. Nimodipine is eliminated almost exclusively in the form of metabolites and less than 1% is recovered in the urine as unchanged drug. Numerous metabolites, all of which are either inactive or considerably less active than the parent compound, have been identified. Because of a high first-pass metabolism, the bioavailability of nimodipine averages 13% after oral administration. The bioavailability is significantly increased in patients with hepatic disease, with C_{max} approximately double that in normals which necessitates lowering the dose in this group of patients (see Dosage and Administration). The influence of food on the pharmacokinetics of nimodipine capsules has not been studied.

Clinical Trials: Nimodipine has been shown, in 4 randomized, placebo-controlled trials, to reduce the severity of neurologic deficits resulting from vasospasm in patients who have had a recent subarachnoid hemorrhage (SAH). The trials used doses ranging from 20–30 mg to 90 mg every 4 hours, with drug given to 21 days in 3 studies, and for at least 18 days in the other. Three of the 4 trials followed patients for 3–6 months. Three of the trials studied relatively well patients, with all or most patients in Hunt and Hess Grades I–II (essentially free of focal deficits after the initial bleed); the fourth studied much sicker patients, Hunt and Hess Grades III–V. Two studies, one domestic, one French, were similar in design, with relatively unimpaired SAH patients randomized to nimodipine or placebo. In each, a judgment was made as to whether any late-developing deficit was due to spasm or other causes, and the deficits were graded. Both studies showed significantly fewer severe deficits due to spasm in the nimodipine group; the second (French) study showed fewer spasm-related deficits of all severities. No effect was seen on deficits not related to spasm.
[See table below].
A Canadian study entered much sicker patients, who had a high rate of death and disability, and used a dose of 90 mg every 4 hours, but was otherwise similar to the first two studies. Analysis of delayed ischemic deficits, many of which result from spasm, showed a significant reduction in spasm-related deficits. Among analyzed patients (72 nimodipine, 82 placebo), there were the following outcomes.
[See table above].
A fourth, large, study was performed in the United Kingdom in SAH patients with all grades of severity (but about 90% were in Grades I–III). Outcomes were not defined as spasm related or not but there was a significant reduction in the overall rate of infarction and severely disabling neurological outcome at 3 months:

	Nimodipine	Placebo
Total patients	278	276
Good recovery	199*	169
Moderate disability	24	16
Severe disability	12**	31
Death	43***	60

  * p = 0.0444—good and moderate vs severe and dead
 ** p = 0.001—severe disability
*** p = 0.056—death

A dose-ranging study comparing 30, 60 and 90 mg doses found a generally low rate of spasm-related neurological deficits but no significant relation of response to dose.
The effect of nimodipine on mortality is not yet clear. The large United Kingdom study showed near-significantly improved survival. The two smaller studies (domestic, French) had too few deaths to contribute to this question. The Canadian study, despite showing markedly decreased spasm-related deficits, showed overall (all patients randomized) greater 90 day mortality, 49/91 (54%) on nimodipine vs 39/97 (39%) on placebo, a significant difference. Most of the deaths appeared, in this very severely ill group (Hunt and Hess Grades III–V), to be consequences of SAH, but a drug effect cannot be ruled out. In this study 90 mg every 4 hours was the dose used, perhaps too high for the very ill population studied. The 90 mg dose is not recommended nor is treatment of Hunt and Hess Grades IV–V patients.

INDICATIONS AND USAGE

Nimotop® (nimodipine) is indicated for the improvement of neurological deficits due to spasm following subarachnoid hemorrhage from ruptured congenital intracranial aneurysms in patients who are in good neurological condition post-ictus (e.g. Hunt and Hess Grades I–III). Oral Nimotop® therapy should begin within 96 hours of the subarachnoid hemorrhage and continue for 21 days.

CONTRAINDICATIONS

None known.

PRECAUTIONS

General: Blood Pressure: Nimodipine has the hemodynamic effects expected of a calcium channel blocker, although they are generally not marked. In patients with subarachnoid hemorrhage given Nimotop® in clinical studies about 5% were reported to have had lowering of the blood pressure and about 1% left the study because of this (not all could be attributed to nimodipine). Nevertheless, blood pressure should be carefully monitored during treatment with Nimotop® based on its known pharmacology and the known effects of calcium channel blockers.
Hepatic Disease: The metabolism of Nimotop® is decreased in patients with impaired hepatic function. Such patients should have their blood pressure and pulse rate monitored closely and should be given a lower dose (see Dosage and Administration).
Laboratory Test Interactions: None known.
Drug Interaction: It is possible that the cardiovascular action of other calcium channel blockers could be enhanced by the addition of Nimotop®.
In Europe, Nimotop® was observed to occasionally intensify the effect of antihypertensive compounds taken concomitantly by patients suffering from hypertension: this phenomenon was not observed in North American clinical trials.
Carcinogenesis, Mutagenesis, Impairment of Fertility: In a two-year study, higher incidences of adenocarcinoma of the uterus and Leydig-cell adenoma of the testes were observed in rats given a diet containing 1800 ppm nimodipine (equivalent to 91 to 121 mg/kg/day nimodipine) than in placebo controls. The differences were not statistically significant; however, the higher rates were well within historical control range for these tumors in the Wistar strain. Nimodipine was found not to be carcinogenic in a 91-week mouse study but the high dose of 1800 ppm nimodipine-in-feed (546 to 774 mg/kg/day) shortened the life expectancy of the animals. Mutagenic studies, including the Ames, micronucleus and dominant lethal tests were negative.
Nimodipine did not impair the fertility and general reproductive performance of male and female Wistar rats following oral doses of up to 30 mg/kg/day when administered daily for more than 10 weeks in the males and 3 weeks in the females prior to mating and continued to day 7 of pregnancy. This dose in a rat is about 4 times the equivalent clinical dose of 60 mg q4h in a 50 kg patient.
Pregnancy: Category C. Nimodipine has been shown to have a teratogenic effect in Himalayan rabbits. Incidences of malformations and stunted fetuses were increased at oral (by gavage) doses of 1 and 10 mg/kg/day administered from day 6 through day 18 of pregnancy but not at 3.0 mg/kg/day in one of two identical rabbit studies. In the second increased incidence of stunted fetuses was seen at 1.0 mg/kg/day but not at higher doses. Nimodipine was embryotoxic, causing resorption and stunted growth of fetuses, in Long Evans rats at 100 mg/kg/day administered by gavage from day 6 through day 15 of pregnancy. In two other rat studies, doses of 30 mg/kg/day nimodipine administered by gavage from day 16 of gestation and continued until sacrifice (day 20 of pregnancy or day 21 post partum) were associated with higher incidences of skeletal variation, stunted

	Delayed Ischemic Deficits (DID)		Permanent Deficits	
	Nimodipine n (%)	Placebo n (%)	Nimodipine n (%)	Placebo n (%)
DID Spasm alone	8 (11)*	25 (31)	5 (7)*	22 (27)
DID Spasm Contributing	18 (25)	21 (26)	16 (22)	17 (21)
DID Without Spasm	7 (10)	8 (10)	6 (8)	7 (9)
No DID	39 (54)	28 (34)	45 (63)	36 (44)

*P = 0.001, nimodipine vs placebo

Study	Dose	Grade*	Number Analyzed	Any Deficit Due to Spasm	Numbers With Severe Deficit
1.	20–30 mg	I–II	Nimodipine 56	13	1
			Placebo 60	16	8**
2.	60 mg	I–III	Nimodipine 31	4	2
			Placebo 39	11	10**

Patients

*Hunt and Hess Grade
**p = 0.03

fetuses and stillbirths but no malformations. There are no adequate and well controlled studies in pregnant women to directly assess the effect on human fetuses. Nimodipine should be used during pregnancy only if the potential benefit justifies the potential risk to the fetus.

Nursing Mothers: Nimodipine and/or its metabolites have been shown to appear in rat milk at concentrations much higher than in maternal plasma. It is not known whether the drug is excreted in human milk. Because many drugs are excreted in human milk, nursing mothers are advised not to breast feed their babies when taking the drug.

Pediatric Use: Safety and effectiveness in children have not been established.

ADVERSE REACTIONS

Adverse experiences were reported by 92 of 823 patients with subarachnoid hemorrhage (11.2%) who were given nimodipine. The most frequently reported adverse experience was decreased blood pressure in 4.4% of these patients. Twenty-nine of 479 (6.1%) placebo treated patients also reported adverse experiences. The events reported with a frequency greater than 1% are displayed below by dose.

[See table right].

There were no other adverse experiences reported by the patients who were given 0.35 mg/kg q4h, 30 mg q4h or 120 mg q4h. Adverse experiences with an incidence rate of less than 1% in the 60 mg q4h dose group were: hepatitis; itching; gastrointestinal hemorrhage; thrombocytopenia; anemia; palpitations; vomiting; flushing; diaphoresis; wheezing; phenytoin toxicity; lightheadedness; dizziness; rebound vasospasm; jaundice; hypertension; hematoma.

Adverse experiences with an incidence rate less than 1% in the 90 mg q4h dose group were: itching; gastrointestinal hemorrhage; thrombocytopenia; neurological deterioration; vomiting; diaphoresis; congestive heart failure; hyponatremia; decreasing platelet count; disseminated intravascular coagulation; deep vein thrombosis.

As can be seen from the table, side effects that appear related to nimodipine use based on increased incidence with higher dose or a higher rate compared to placebo control, included decreased blood pressure, edema and headaches which are known pharmacologic actions of calcium channel blockers. It must be noted, however, that SAH is frequently accompanied by alterations in consciousness which lead to an under reporting of adverse experiences. Patients who received nimodipine in clinical trials for other indications reported flushing (2.1%), headache (4.1%) and fluid retention (0.3%), typical responses to calcium channel blockers. As a calcium channel blocker, nimodipine may have the potential to exacerbate heart failure in susceptible patients or to interfere with A-V conduction, but these events were not observed. No clinically significant effects on hematologic factors, renal or hepatic function or carbohydrate metabolism have been causally associated with oral nimodipine. Isolated cases of non-fasting elevated serum glucose levels (0.8%), elevated LDH levels (0.4%), decreased platelet counts (0.3%), elevated alkaline phosphatase levels (0.2%) and elevated SGPT levels (0.2%) have been reported rarely.

DRUG ABUSE AND DEPENDENCE

There have been no reported instances of drug abuse or dependence with Nimotop®.

OVERDOSAGE

There have been no reports of overdosage from the oral administration of Nimotop®. Symptoms of overdosage would be expected to be related to cardiovascular effects such as excessive peripheral vasodilation with marked systemic hypotension. Clinically significant hypotension due to Nimotop® overdosage may require active cardiovascular support. Norepinephrine or dopamine may be helpful in restoring blood pressure. Since Nimotop® is highly protein-bound, dialysis is not likely to be of benefit.

DOSAGE AND ADMINISTRATION

Nimotop® is given orally in the form of ivory colored, soft gelatin 30 mg capsules for subarachnoid hemorrhage.

The oral dose is 60 mg (two 30 mg capsules) every 4 hours for 21 consecutive days. Oral Nimotop® therapy should commence within 96 hours of the subarachnoid hemorrhage.

If the capsule cannot be swallowed, e.g., at the time of surgery, or if the patient is unconscious, a hole should be made in both ends of the capsule with an 18 gauge needle, and the contents of the capsule extracted into a syringe. The contents should then be emptied into the patient's *in situ* naso-gastric tube and washed down the tube with 30 mL of normal saline (0.9%).

Patients with hepatic failure have substantially reduced clearance and approximately doubled C_{max}. Dosage should be reduced to 30 mg every 4 hours, with close monitoring of blood pressure and heart rate.

HOW SUPPLIED

Each ivory colored, soft gelatin NIMOTOP® capsule is imprinted with the word Miles and Miles 855 and contains 30 mg of nimodipine. The 30 mg capsules are packaged in unit dose foil pouches and supplied in cartons containing 100 capsules. The capsules should be stored in the manufac-

Sign/Symptom	Nimodipine 0.35 mg/kg (n = 82)	30 mg (n = 71)	60 mg (n = 494)	90 mg (n = 172)	120 mg (n = 4)	Placebo (n = 479)
Decreased Blood Pressure	1 (1.2)	0	19 (3.8)	14 (8.1)	2 (50.0)	6 (1.2)
Abnormal Liver Function Test	1 (1.2)	0	2 (0.4)	1 (0.6)	0	7 (1.5)
Edema	0	0	2 (0.4)	2 (1.2)	0	3 (0.6)
Diarrhea	0	3 (4.2)	0	3 (1.7)	0	3 (0.6)
Rash	2 (2.4)	0	3 (0.6)	2 (1.2)	0	3 (0.6)
Headache	0	1 (1.4)	6 (1.2)	0	0	1 (0.2)
Gastrointestinal Symptoms	2 (2.4)	0	0	2 (1.2)	0	0
Nausea	1 (1.2)	1 (1.4)	6 (1.2)	1 (0.6)	0	0
Dyspnea	1 (1.2)	0	0	0	0	0
EKG Abnormalities	0	1 (1.4)	0	1 (0.6)	0	0
Tachycardia	0	1 (1.4)	0	0	0	0
Bradycardia	0	0	5 (1.0)	1 (0.6)	0	0
Muscle Pain/Cramp	0	1 (1.4)	1 (0.2)	1 (0.6)	0	0
Acne	0	1 (1.4)	0	0	0	0
Depression	0	1 (1.4)	0	0	0	0

DOSE q4h — Number of Patients (%)

turer's original foil package at a controlled room temperature of 59°F to 86°F (15°C to 30°C).

Capsules should be protected from light and freezing.

	Strength	NDC Code	Capsule Identification
Unit Dose Package of 100:	30 mg	0026-2855-48	Miles 855

Manufactured by: Miles Inc.
Pharmaceutical Division
400 Morgan Lane
West Haven, CT 06516
Encapsulated by: R.P. Scherer North America
Division of R.P. Scherer Corp.
Clearwater, FL 33518
PD100667   1/89   BAY e 9736   5202-7-A-U.S.-1   0703
© 1989 Miles Inc.

Shown in Product Identification Section, page 419

Otic DOMEBORO® Solution (acid pH)   ℞
(acetic acid 2%)

INGREDIENTS
Aluminum Sulfate, Boric Acid, Calcium Carbonate, Glacial Acetic Acid, Purified Water, and Sodium Hydroxide.

INDICATIONS
For the treatment of superficial infections of the external auditory canal caused by organisms susceptible to the action of the antimicrobial.

PRECAUTIONS
If undue irritation or sensitivity develops, discontinue treatment.

CAUTION
Federal (U.S.A.) law prohibits dispensing without prescription.

For external use only. Not for ophthalmic use. Store below 86°F (30°C), avoid freezing.

USUAL DOSAGE
Instill 4–6 drops in the ear every 2 to 3 hours.

HOW SUPPLIED
2 fl. oz. (60 cc.) plastic squeeze bottle with otic tip.

STILPHOSTROL®   ℞
(diethylstilbestrol diphosphate)

DESCRIPTION
STILPHOSTROL (diethylstilbestrol diphosphate) is available as tablets containing 50 mg diethylstilbestrol diphosphate, colored white to off-white with grey to tan mottling. STILPHOSTROL is also available for intravenous administration as a sterile solution in 5 ml ampules containing 0.25 gram diethylstilbestrol diphosphate as its sodium salt. The solution is clear, colorless to light straw-colored, with a pH of 9.0 to 10.5, and may darken with age and exposure to heat and light.

STILPHOSTROL is a phosphoryiated, nonsteroidal estrogen with the chemical name: Diethylstilbestrol 4,4-Diphosphoric ester, an empirical formula of $C_{18}H_{22}O_8P_2$, and the following structural formula:

CLINICAL PHARMACOLOGY
Putative receptor proteins for estrogens have been detected in estrogen-responsive tissues. Estrogens are first bound to a cytoplasmic receptor protein. Following modification, the estrogen-protein complex is translocated to the nucleus where ultimate binding of the estrogen containing complex occurs. As a result of such binding characteristic metabolic alterations ensue.

In the male patient with androgenic hormone dependent conditions such as metastatic carcinoma of the prostate gland, estrogens counter the androgenic influence by competing for the receptor sites. As a result of treatment with estrogens, metastatic lesions in the bone may also show improvement.

It has been demonstrated in animal studies that diethylstilbestrol diphosphate is rapidly hydrolysed to diethylstilbestrol through phosphatase activity in the blood and tissues. When diethylstilbestrol diphosphate (92 mg/kg body wt.) was injected intravenously into rabbits over a period of 2 to 3 minutes, free diethylstilbestrol appeared in the blood stream as early as 5 minutes after termination of injection, and within 15 minutes had reached a concentration of 16.3 ug/ml of plasma. This was followed by a rapid decline in concentration, only 1.2 ug/ml remaining after 2 hours.[1] It is, therefore, expected that the high concentration of serum acid phosphate in patients with prostatic carcinoma will hydrolyse diethylstilbestrol diphosphate to free, active diethylstilbestrol.

Diethylstilbestrol is metabolized by the body in much the same manner as the endogenous hormones. Inactivation of estrogen is carried out mainly in the liver. A certain proportion of the estrogen reaching that organ is excreted into the bile, only to be reabsorbed from the intestine. During this enterohepatic circulation, degradation of estrogen occurs through conversion to less active products, through oxidation to nonestrogenic substances, and through conjugation with sulfuric and glucuronic acids. These water-soluble conjugates are strong acids and are thus fully ionized in the body fluids; penetration into cells is therefore limited, and excretion by the kidney is favored because little tubular reabsorption is possible.

INDICATION AND USAGE
STILPHOSTROL (diethylstilbestrol diphosphate) is indicated for the treatment of prostatic carcinoma—palliative therapy of advanced disease.

CONTRAINDICATIONS
Estrogens should not be used in men with any of the following conditions:
1. Known or suspected cancer of the breast except in appropriately selected patients being treated for metastatic disease.
2. Known or suspected estrogen-dependent neoplasia.
3. Active thrombophlebitis or thromboembolic disorders.
STILPHOSTROL IS NOT INDICATED IN THE TREATMENT OF ANY DISORDER IN WOMEN.

WARNINGS
1. Induction of malignant neoplasms: Long-term continuous administration of natural and synthetic estrogens in certain animal species increases the frequency of carcinomas of the breast, cervix, vagina, and liver.
2. Gallbladder disease: A study has reported a 2- to 3-fold increase in the risk of surgically confirmed gallbladder disease in women receiving postmenopausal estrogens,[2] similar to a 2-fold increase previously noted in users of oral contraceptives.[3,9]

Continued on next page

Miles Pharm. Div.—Cont.

3. Effects similar to those caused by estrogen-progestogen oral contraceptives: There are several serious adverse effects of oral contraceptives. It has been shown that there is an increased risk of thrombosis in men receiving estrogens for prostatic cancer and women for postpartum breast engorgement.[4–7].

a. Thromboembolic disease: It is now well established that users of oral contraceptives have an increased risk of various thromboembolic and thrombotic vascular diseases, such as thrombophlebitis, pulmonary embolism, stroke, and myocardial infarction.[8–16] Cases of retinal thrombosis, mesenteric thrombosis, and optic neuritis have been reported in oral contraceptive users. There is evidence that the risk of several of these adverse reactions is related to the dose of the drug.[17,18] An increased risk of postsurgery thromboembolic complications has also been reported in users of oral contraceptives.[19,20] If feasible, estrogen should be discontinued at least 4 weeks before surgery of the type associated with an increased risk of thromboembolism or during periods of prolonged immobilization.

Estrogens should not be used in persons with active thrombophlebitis or thromboembolic disorders. They should be used with caution in patients with cerebral vascular or coronary artery disease and only for those in whom estrogens are clearly indicated.

Large doses of estrogen (5 mg conjugated estrogens per day), comparable to those used to treat cancer of the prostate, have been shown in a large prospective clinical trial in men[21] to increase the risk of nonfatal myocardial infarction, pulmonary embolism and thrombophlebitis. When estrogen doses of this size are used, any of the thromboembolic and thrombotic adverse effects associated with oral contraceptive use should be considered a clear risk.

b. Hepatic adenoma: Benign hepatic adenomas appear to be associated with the use of oral contraceptives.[22–24] Although benign, and rare, these may rupture and may cause death through intra-abdominal hemorrhage. Such lesions have not yet been reported in association with other estrogen or progestogen preparations but should be considered in estrogen users having abdominal pain and tenderness, abdominal mass, or hypovolemic shock. Hepatocellular carcinoma has also been reported in women taking estrogen-containing oral contraceptives.[23] The relationship of this malignancy to these drugs is not known at this time.

c. Elevated blood pressure: Women using oral contraceptives sometimes experience increased blood pressure which, in most cases, returns to normal on discontinuing the drug. There is now a report that this may occur with use of estrogens in the menopause[25] and blood pressure should be monitored with estrogen use, especially if high doses are used.

d. Glucose tolerance: A worsening of glucose tolerance has been observed in a significant percentage of patients on estrogen-containing oral contraceptives. For this reason, diabetic patients should be carefully observed while receiving estrogen.

4. Hypercalcemia: Administration of estrogens may lead to severe hypercalcemia in patients with breast cancer and bone metastases. If this occurs, the drug should be stopped and appropriate measures taken to reduce the serum calcium level.

PRECAUTIONS

General:

1. A complete medical and family history should be taken prior to the initiation of any estrogen therapy. The pretreatment and periodic physical examinations should include special reference to blood pressure, breasts, abdomen and pelvic organs. As a general rule, estrogen should not be prescribed for longer than one year without another physical examination being performed.

2. Fluid retention—Because estrogens may cause some degree of fluid retention, conditions which might be influenced by this factor such as asthma, epilepsy, migraine, and cardiac or renal dysfunction, require careful observation.

3. Certain patients may develop undesirable manifestations of excessive estrogenic stimulation, such as gynecomastia.

4. Oral contraceptives appear to be associated with an increased incidence of mental depression. Although it is not clear whether this is due to the estrogenic or progestogenic component of the contraceptive, patients with a history of depression should be carefully observed.

5. If jaundice develops in any patient receiving estrogen, the medication should be discontinued while the cause is investigated.

6. Estrogens may be poorly metabolized in patients with impaired liver function and they should be administered with caution in such patients.

7. Because estrogens influence the metabolism of calcium and phosphorus, they should be used with caution in patients with metabolic bone diseases that are associated with hypercalcemia or in patients with renal insufficiency.

Information for Patients:

1. Stilphostrol should not be used by women.

2. The following side effects have been reported in patients being treated with Stilphostrol. If they occur they should be reported promptly to your physician:
- Mood changes, depression
- Nervousness, dizziness
- Loss of appetite, nausea, vomiting, abdominal cramps, bloating
- Skin rash
- Chest pain and shortness of breath
- Numbness or tingling about the nose or mouth
- Fluid accumulation
- Swelling or tenderness of breasts
- Disturbances of vision
- Frequent or uncomfortable urination
- Painful swelling of extremities

3. The patient should consult a physician regularly for evaluation of blood pressure and heart rate.

4. Diabetic patients should monitor urines very carefully. Test of blood sugar may be necessary as well.

5. The following clinical problems are associated with the use of Stilphostrol:
- Hepatic cutaneous prophyria
- Erythema nodosum
- Erythema multiforme

A significant association has been shown between the use of estrogen containing drugs and the following serious reactions:
1. Thrombophlebitis
2. Pulmonary embolism
3. Cerebral thrombosis
4. There is suggestive evidence that there may be a relationship with coronary thrombosis.

The following adverse reactions are known to have occurred in patients receiving estrogens:
- Change in body weight
- Headache
- Loss of sex drive
- Post injection flare
- Aggravation of migraine headaches
- Loss of scalp hair
- Hemorrhagic eruption
- Fatigue
- Backache

Drug/Laboratory Test Interactions:

1. The pathologist should be advised of estrogen therapy when relevant specimens are submitted.

2. Certain endocrine and liver function tests may be affected by estrogen-containing oral contraceptives.

The following similar changes may be expected with larger doses of estrogen.

a. Increased sulfobromophthalein retention.

b. Increased prothrombin and factors VII, VIII, IX, and X; decreased antithrombin 3; incresed norepinephrine-induced platelet aggregability.

c. Increased thyroid binding globulin (TBG) leading to increased circulating total thyroid hormone, as measured by PBI, T4 by column, or T4 by radioimmunoassay. Free T3 resin uptake is decreased, reflecting the elevated TBG; free T4 concentration is unaltered.

d. Impaired glucose tolerance.

e. Reduced response to metyrapone test.

f. Reduced serum folate concentration.

g. Increased serum triglyceride and phospholipid concentration.

Carcinogenesis, mutagenesis, impairment of fertility: (See Warnings regarding induction of neoplasia.)

Pregnancy: Pregnancy Category X. STILPHOSTROL IS NOT INDICATED IN THE TREATMENT OF ANY DISORDER IN WOMEN.

Pediatric Use: Because of the effects of estrogen on epiphyseal closure, they should be used judiciously in young patients in whom bone growth is not complete.

ADVERSE REACTIONS

(See Warnings regarding induction of neoplasia, increased incidence of gallbladder disease, and adverse effects similar to those of oral contraceptives, including thromboembolism.)

The following additional adverse reactions have been reported with estrogenic therapy, including oral contraceptives:

1. Breasts: Tenderness, enlargement, secretion.

2. Gastrointestinal: Nausea, vomiting; abdominal cramps, bloating; cholestatic jaundice.

3. Skin: Chloasma or melasma which may persist when drug is discontinued; erythema multiforme, erythema nodosum; hemorrhagic eruption; loss of scalp hair; hirsutism.

4. Eyes: Steepening of corneal curvature; intolerance to contact lenses.

5. CNS: Headache, migraine, dizziness, mental depression; chorea.

6. Miscellaneous: Increase or decrease in weight; reduced carbohydrate tolerance; aggravation of porphyria; edema; changes in libido; transient itching and burning sensation in the perineal region.

OVERDOSAGE

Numerous reports of ingestion of large doses of estrogen-containing oral contraceptives by young children indicate that acute serious ill effects do not occur. Overdosage of estrogen may cause nausea.

DOSAGE AND ADMINISTRATION

Inoperable, progressing prostatic cancer.

STILPHOSTROL Tablets 50 mg: Start with one tablet three times a day and increase this dose level to four or more tablets three times a day, depending on the tolerance of the patient. Maximum daily dose not to exceed one gram. Alternatively, if relief is not obtained with high oral dosages, STILPHOSTROL may be administered intravenously. STILPHOSTROL solution must be diluted before intravenous infusion.

STILPHOSTROL Ampules 0.25 gram: It is recommended that 0.5 gram (2 amupules) dissolved in approximately 250 ml of normal saline for injection USP, or 5% dextrose for injection USP, be given intravenously the first day, and that each day thereafter one gram (4 ampules) be similarly administered in approximately 250 to 500 ml of normal saline for injection USP, or 5% dextrose for injection USP.

The infusion should be administered slowly (20–30 drops per minute) during the first 10–15 minutes and then the rate of flow adjusted so that the entire amount is given in a period of about one hour. This procedure should be followed for five days or more depending on the response of the patient. Following the first intensive course of therapy, 0.25–0.5 gram (1 or 2 ampules) may be administered in a similar manner once or twice weekly or maintenance obtained with STILPHOSTROL Tablets.

Stability of Solution: After reconstitution, if storage is desired, the solution should be kept at room temperature and away from direct light. Under these conditions the solution is stable for about 5 days, so long as cloudiness or evidence of a precipitate has not occurred.

HOW SUPPLIED

STILPHOSTROL Tablets–Bottles of 50 tablets.

Each scored tablet, white to off-white with grey to tan mottling, contains diethylstilbestrol diphosphate 50 mg. Each tablet is identified with: Miles 132.

STORAGE: Store at controlled room temperature (59°–86°F), protect from light.

STILPHOSTROL Ampules—Boxes of 20 ampules.

Each 5 ml ampule contains diethylstilbestrol diphosphate 0.25 gram as a solution of its sodium salt.

STORAGE: Store at controlled room temperature (50°–86°F), protect from light.

REFERENCES

1. Johnson, W., et al: Proc. Soc. Exp. Biol. Med. 106:327–330, 1961.
2. Boston Collaborative Drug Surveillance Program: N. Eng. J. Med. 290:15–19, 1974.
3. Boston Collaborative Drug Surveillance Program: Lancet 1:1399–1404, 1973.
4. Daniel, D.G., et al: Lancet 2:287–289, 1967.
5. The Veterans Administration Cooperative Urological Research Group: J. Urol. 98:516–522, 1967.
6. Bailar, J.C.: Lancet 2-560, 1967.
7. Blackard, C., et al: Cancer 26:249–256, 1970.
8. Royal College of General Practitioners: R. Coll. Gen. Pract. 13:267–279, 1967.
9. Royal College of General Practitioners: Oral Contraceptives and Health, New York, Pitman Corp., 1974.
10. Inman, W.H.W., et al: Br. Med. J. 2:193–199, 1968.
11. Vessey, M.P., et al: Br. Med. J. 2:651–657, 1969.
12. Sartwell, P.E., et al: Am.J. Epidemiol. 90:365–380, 1969.
13. Collaborative Group for the Study of Stroke in Young Women: N. Eng. J. Med. 288:871–878, 1973.
14. Collaborative Group for the Study of Stroke in Young Women: J.A.M.A. 231:718–722, 1975.
15. Mann, J.I., et al: Br. Med. J. 2:245–248, 1975.
16. Mann, J.I., et al: Br. Med. J. 2:241–245, 1975.
17. Inman, W.H.W., et al: Br. Med. J. 2:203–209, 1970.
18. Stolley, P.D., et al: Am. J. Epidemiol. 102:197–208, 1975.
19. Vessey, M.P., et al: Br. Med. J. 3:123–126, 1970.
20. Greene, G.R., et al: Am. J. Public Health 62:680–685, 1972.
21. Coronary Drug Project Research Group: J.A.M.A. 214:1303–1313, 1970.
22. Baum, J., et al: Lancet 2:926–928, 1973.
23. Mays, E.T., et al: J.A.M.A. 235:730–732, 1976.
24. Edmonson, H.A., et al: N. Eng. J. Med. 294:470–472, 1976.
25. Pfeffer, R.I., et al: M. J. Epidemiol. 103:445–456, 1976.

Ampules manufactured by:
Ben Venue Laboratories, Inc.
Bedford, OH 44146
Distributed by
Miles Inc.
Pharmaceutical Division
400 Morgan Lane
West Haven, CT 06516
PD 100708   0760   Rev 3/89
Shown in Product Identification Section, page 419

TRIDESILON® 0.05%   ℞
(desonide)
creme

DESCRIPTION

Tridesilon® Creme contains microdispersed desonide (the active ingredient) in a compatible vehicle buffered to the pH range of normal skin. Each gram of Tridesilon® Creme contains 0.5 milligrams of desonide. Tridesilon® Creme is applied topically.

Tridesilon® (desonide) is a non-fluorinated corticosteroid. Chemically, desonide is Pregna-1,4-diene-3,20-dione,11,21-dihydroxy-16,17-[(1-methylethylidene)bis(oxy)]-,(11β,16α)- with the following structural formula:

The vehicle for Tridesilon® Creme 0.05% contains glycerin, sodium lauryl sulfate, aluminum sulfate, calcium acetate, dextrin, purified water, cetyl stearyl alcohol, synthetic beeswax, (B-wax), white petrolatum, and light mineral oil. Preserved with methylparaben.

EMPIRICAL FORMULA	MOLECULAR WEIGHT	CAS REGISTRY NUMBER
$C_{24}H_{32}O_6$	416.51	638-94-8

CLINICAL PHARMACOLOGY

Topical corticosteroids share anti-inflammatory, anti-pruritic and vasoconstrictive actions.

The mechanism of anti-inflammatory activity of the topical corticosteroids is unclear. Various laboratory methods, including vasoconstrictor assays, are used to compare and predict potencies and/or clinical efficacies of the topical corticosteroids. There is some evidence to suggest that a recognizable correlation exists between vasoconstrictor potency and therapeutic efficacy in man.

Pharmacokinetics

The extent of percutaneous absorption of topical corticosteroids is determined by many factors including the vehicle, the integrity of the epidermal barrier, and the use of occlusive dressings.

Topical corticosteroids can be absorbed from normal intact skin. Inflammation and/or other disease processes in the skin increase percutaneous absorption. Occlusive dressings substantially increase the percutaneous absorption of topical corticosteroids. Thus, occlusive dressings may be a valuable therapeutic adjunct for treatment of resistant dermatoses. (See DOSAGE AND ADMINISTRATION).

Once absorbed through the skin, topical corticosteroids are handled through pharmacokinetic pathways similar to systemically administered corticosteroids. Corticosteroids are bound to plasma proteins in varying degrees. Corticosteroids are metabolized primarily in the liver and are then excreted by the kidneys. Some of the topical corticosteroids and their metabolites are also excreted into the bile.

INDICATIONS AND USAGE

Topical corticosteroids are indicated for the relief of the inflammatory and pruritic manifestations of corticosteroid-responsive dermatoses.

CONTRAINDICATIONS

Topical corticosteroids are contraindicated in those patients with a history of hypersensitivity to any of the components of the preparation.

PRECAUTIONS

General

Systemic absorption of topical corticosteroids has produced reversible hypothalmic-pituitary-adrenal (HPA) axis suppression, manifestations of Cushing's syndrome, hyperglycemia, and glycosuria in some patients.

Conditions which augment systemic absorption include the application of the more potent steroids, use over large surface areas, prolonged use, and the addition of occlusive dressings.

Therefore, patients receiving a large dose of a potent topical steroid applied to a large surface area or under an occlusive dressing should be evaluated periodically for evidence of HPA axis suppression by using the urinary free cortisol and ACTH stimulation tests. If HPA axis suppression is noted, an attempt should be made to withdraw the drug, to reduce the frequency of application, or to substitute a less potent steroid.

Recovery of HPA axis function is generally prompt and complete upon discontinuation of the drug. Infrequently, signs and symptoms of steroid withdrawal may occur, requiring supplemental systemic corticosteroids.

Children may absorb proportionally larger amounts of topical corticosteroids and thus be more susceptible to systemic toxicity. (See PRECAUTIONS—Pediatric Use).

If irritation develops, topical corticosteroids should be discontinued and appropriate therapy instituted.

In the presence of dermatological infections, the use of an appropriate antifungal or antibacterial agent should be instituted. If a favorable response does not occur promptly, the corticosteroid should be discontinued until the infection has been adequately controlled.

Information for the Patient

Patients using topical corticosteroids should receive the following information and instructions:

1. This medication is to be used as directed by the physician. It is for external use only. Avoid contact with eyes.

2. Patients should be advised not to use this medication for any disorder other than for which it was prescribed.

3. The treated skin area should not be bandaged or otherwise covered or wrapped as to be occlusive unless directed by the physician.

4. Patients should report any signs of local adverse reactions especially under occlusive dressing.

5. Parents of pediatric patients should be advised not to use tightfitting diapers or plastic pants on a child being treated in the diaper area, as these garments may constitute occlusive dressings.

Laboratory Tests

The following tests may be helpful in evaluating the HPA axis suppression:

Urinary free cortisol test
ACTH stimulation test

Carcinogenesis, Mutagenesis, and Impairment of Fertility

Long-term animal studies have not been performed to evaluate the carcinogenic potential or the effect on fertility of topical corticosteroids.

Studies to determine mutagenicity with prednisolone and hydrocortisone have revealed negative results.

Pregnancy Category C

Corticosteroids are generally teratogenic in laboratory animals when administered systemically at relatively low dosage levels. The more potent corticosteroids have been shown to be teratogenic after dermal application in laboratory animals. There are no adequate and well-controlled studies in pregnant women on teratogenic effects from topically applied corticosteroids. Therefore, topical corticosteroids should be used during pregnancy only if the potential benefit justifies the potential risk to the fetus. Drugs of this class should not be used extensively on pregnant patients, in large amounts, or for prolonged periods of time.

Nursing Mothers

It is not known whether topical administration of corticosteroids could result in sufficient systemic absorption to produce detectable quantities in breast milk. Systemically administered corticosteroids are secreted into breast milk in quantities *not* likely to have a deleterious effect on the infant. Nevertheless, caution should be exercised when topical corticosteroids are administered to a nursing woman.

Pediatric Use

Pediatric patients may demonstrate greater susceptibility to topical corticosteroid-induced HPA axis suppression and Cushing's syndrome than mature patients because of a larger skin surface area to body weight ratio.

Hypothalamic-pituitary-adrenal (HPA) axis suppression. Cushing's syndrome, and intracranial hypertension have been reported in children receiving topical corticosteroids. Manifestations of adrenal supression in children include linear growth retardation, delayed weight gain, low plasma cortisol levels, and absence of response to ACTH stimulation. Manifestations of intracranial hypertension include bulging fontanelles, headaches, and bilateral papilledema.

Administration of topical corticosteroids to children should be limited to the least amount compatible with an effective therapeutic regimen. Chronic corticosteroid therapy may interfere with the growth and development of children.

ADVERSE REACTIONS

The following local adverse reactions are reported infrequently with topical corticosteroids, but may occur more frequently with the use of occlusive dressings. These reactions are listed in an approximate decreasing order of occurrence:

Burning
Itching
Irritation
Dryness
Folliculitis
Hypertrichosis
Acneiform eruptions
Hypopigmentation
Perioral dermatitis
Allergic contact dermatitis
Maceration of the skin
Secondary infection
Skin atrophy
Striae
Miliaria

OVERDOSAGE

Topically applied corticosteroids can be absorbed in sufficient amounts to produce systemic effects. (See PRECAUTIONS).

DOSAGE AND ADMINISTRATION

Topical corticosteroids are generally applied to the affected area as a thin film from two to four times daily depending on the severity of the condition.

Occlusive dressings may be used for management of psoriasis or recalcitrant conditions.

If an infection develops, the use of occlusive dressings should be discontinued and appropriate antimicrobial therapy instituted.

HOW SUPPLIED

Tridesilon® (desonide) Cream 0.05% is supplied in 15 and 60 gram tubes and in 5 pound jars. It is a white semi-solid. **Store below 86°F (30°C), avoid freezing.**

	NDC Number
15g	0026-5561-61
60g	0026-5561-62
5lb	0026-5561-92

Miles Inc.
Pharmaceutical Division
400 Morgan Lane
West Haven, CT 06516 USA

CAUTION

Federal (USA) law prohibits dispensing without a prescription.

© 1988 Miles Inc.   PD100672   0229

TRIDESILON® 0.05%   ℞
(desonide)
ointment

DESCRIPTION

Tridesilon® Ointment contains microdispersed desonide (the active ingredient) in white petrolatum. Each gram of Tridesilon® Ointment contains 0.5 miligrams of desonide. Tridesilon® Ointment is applied topically.

Tridesilon® (desonide) is a non-fluorinated corticosteroid. Chemically, desonide is Pregna-1,4-diene-3,20-dione,11,21-dihydroxy-16,17-[(1-methylethylidene)bis(oxy)]-,11β,16α)- with the following structural formula:

EMPIRICAL FORMULA	MOLECULAR WEIGHT	CAS REGISTRY NUMBER
$C_{24}H_{32}O_6$	416.51	638-94-8

CLINICAL PHARMACOLOGY

Topical corticosteroids share anti-inflammatory, anti-puritic and vasoconstrictive actions.

The mechanism of anti-inflammatory activity of the topical corticosteroids is unclear. Various laboratory methods, including vasoconstrictor assays, are used to compare and predict potencies and/or clinical efficacies of the topical corticosteroids. There is some evidence to suggest that a recognizable correlation exists between vasoconstrictor potency and therapeutic efficacy in man.

Pharmacokinetics

The extent of percutaneous absorption of topical corticosteroids is determined by many factors including the vehicle, the integrity of the epidermal barrier, and the use of occlusive dressings.

Topical corticosteroids can be absorbed from normal intact skin. Inflammation and/or other disease processes in the skin increase percutaneous absorption. Occlusive dressings substantially increase the percutaneous absorption of topical corticosteroids. Thus, occlusive dressings may be a valuable therapeutic adjunct for treatment of resistant dermatoses. (See DOSAGE AND ADMINISTRATION).

Once absorbed through the skin, topical corticosteroids are handled through pharmacokinetic pathways similar to systemically administered corticosteroids. Corticosteroids are bound to plasma proteins in varying degrees. Corticosteroids are metabolized primarily in the liver and are then excreted by the kidneys. Some of the topical corticosteroids and their metabolites are also excreted into the bile.

Continued on next page

Miles Pharm. Div.—Cont.

INDICATIONS AND USAGE

Topical corticosteroids are indicated for the relief of the inflammatory and pruritic manifestations of corticosteroid-responsive dermatoses.

CONTRAINDICATIONS

Topical corticosteroids are contraindicated in those patients with a history of hypersensitivity to any of the components of the preparation.

PRECAUTIONS

General

Systemic absorption of topical corticosteroids has produced reversible hypothalamic-pituitary-adrenal (HPA) axis suppression, manifestations of Cushing's syndrome, hyperglycemia, and glycosuria in some patients.

Conditions which augment systemic absorption include the application of the more potent steroids, use over large surface areas, prolonged use, and the addition of occlusive dressings.

Therefore, patients receiving a large dose of a potent topical steroid applied to a large surface area or under an occlusive dressing should be evaluated periodically for evidence of HPA axis suppression by using the urinary free cortisol and ACTH stimulation tests. If HPA axis suppression is noted, an attempt should be made to withdraw the drug, to reduce the frequency of application, or to substitute a less potent steroid.

Recovery of HPA axis functions is generally prompt and complete upon discontinuation of the drug. Infrequently, signs and symptoms of steroid withdrawal may occur, requiring supplemental systemic corticosteroids.

Children may absorb proportionally larger amounts of topical corticosteroids and thus be more susceptible to systemic toxicity. (See PRECAUTIONS—Pediatric Use).

If irritation develops, topical corticosteroids should be discontinued and appropriate therapy instituted.

In the presence of dermatological infections, the use of an appropriate antifungal or antibacterial agent should be instituted. If a favorable response does not occur promptly, the corticosteroid should be discontinued until the infection has been adequately controlled.

Information for the Patient

Patients using topical corticosteroids should receive the following information and instructions:

1. This medication is to be used as directed by the physician. It is for external use only. Avoid contact with the eyes.
2. Patients should be advised not to use this medication for any disorder other than for which it was prescribed.
3. The treated skin area should not be bandaged or otherwise covered or wrapped so as to be occlusive unless directed by the physician.
4. Patients should report any signs of local adverse reactions especially under occlusive dressing.
5. Parents of pediatric patients should be advised not to use tight-fitting diapers or plastic pants on a child being treated in the diaper area, as these garments may constitute occlusive dressings.

Laboratory Tests

The following tests may be helpful in evaluating the HPA axis suppression.
Urinary free cortisol test
ACTH stimulation test

Carcinogenesis, Mutagenesis, and Impairment of Fertility

Long-term animal studies have not been performed to evaluate the carcinogenic potential or the effect on fertility of topical corticosteroids.

Studies to determine mutagenicity with prednisolone and hydrocortisone have revealed negative results.

Pregnancy Category C

Corticosteroids are generally teratogenic in laboratory animals when administered systemically at relatively low dosage levels. The more potent corticosteroids have been shown to be teratogenic after dermal application in laboratory animals. There are no adequate and well-controlled studies in pregnant women on teratogenic effects from topically applied corticosteroids. Therefore, topical corticosteroids should be used during pregnancy only if the potential benefit justifies the potential risk to the fetus. Drugs of this class should not be used extensively on pregnant patients, in large amounts, or for prolonged periods of time.

Nursing Mothers

It is not known whether topical administration of corticosteroids could result in sufficient systemic absorption to produce detectable quantities in breast milk. Systemically administered corticosteroids are secreted into breast milk in quantities *not* likely to have a deleterious effect on the infant. Nevertheless, caution should be exercised when topical corticosteroids are administered to a nursing woman.

Pediatric Use

Pediatric patients may demonstrate greater susceptibility to topical corticosteroid-induced HPA axis and Cushing's syndrome than mature patients because of a larger skin surface area to body weight ratio.

Hypothalmic-pituitary-adrenal (HPA) axis suppression, Cushing's syndrome, and intracranial hypertension have been reported in children receiving topical corticosteroids. Manifestations of adrenal suppression in children include linear growth retardation, delayed weight gain, low plasma cortisol levels, and absence of response to ACTH stimulation. Manifestations of intracranial hypertension include bulging fontanelles, headaches, and bilateral papilledema.

Administration of topical costicosteroids to children should be limited to the least amount compatible with an effective therapeutic regimen. Chronic corticosteroid therapy may interfere with the growth and development of children.

ADVERSE REACTIONS

The following local adverse reactions are reported infrequently with topical corticosteroids, but may occur more frequently with the use of occlusive dressings. These reactions are listed in an approximate decreasing order of occurrence:

Burning
Itching
Irritation
Dryness
Folliculitis
Hypertrichosis
Acneiform eruptions
Hypopigmentation
Perioral dermatitis
Allergic contact dermatitis
Maceration of the skin
Secondary infection
Skin atrophy
Striae
Miliaria

OVERDOSAGE

Topically applied corticosteroids can be absorbed in sufficient amounts to produce systemic effects. (See PRECAUTIONS).

DOSAGE AND ADMINISTRATION

Topical corticosteroids are generally applied to the affected area as a thin film from two to four times daily depending on the severity of the condition.

Occlusive dressings may be used for the management of psoriasis or recalcitrant conditions.

If an infection develops, the use of occlusive dressings should be discontinued and appropriate antimicrobial therapy instituted.

HOW SUPPLIED

Tridesilon® (desonide) Ointment 0.05% is supplied in 15 and 60 gram tubes. It is white or faintly yellowish, transparent semisolid.

Store below 86°F (30°C). Avoid freezing.

	NDC Number
15g	0026-5591-61
60g	0026-5591-62

Miles Inc.
Pharmaceutical Division
400 Morgan Lane
West Haven, CT 06516 USA
CAUTION: Federal (USA) law prohibits dispensing without a prescription.
PD100671   0227
© 1988 Miles Inc.

TRIDESILON® 0.05%   ℞
Otic
(desonide 0.05%–acetic acid 2%)
solution

DESCRIPTION

Otic Tridesilon® Solution contains desonide 0.05% and acetic acid 2% (the active ingredients) in a compatible vehicle buffered to the pH range of the normal ear. Otic Tridesilon® Solution is instilled into the external auditory canal. Tridesilon® (desonide) is a non-fluorinated corticosteroid. Chemically, desonide is Pregna-1,4-diene-3,20-dione,11,21-dihydroxy-16,17-[(1-methylethylidene)bis(oxy)]-,(11β,16α)- with the following structural formula:

EMPIRICAL FORMULA	MOLECULAR WEIGHT	CAS REGISTRY NUMBER
$C_{24}H_{32}O_6$	416.51	638-94-8

Acetic acid is an astringent and antimicrobial agent. Chemically, it is $C_2H_4O_2$ with the following structural formula:

The base is composed of purified water, propylene glycol, sodium acetate, and citric acid.

CLINICAL PHARMACOLOGY

Topical corticosteroids share anti-inflammatory, anti-pruritic and vasoconstrictive actions.

The mechanism of anti-inflammatory activity of the topical corticosteroids is unclear. Various laboratory methods, including vasoconstrictor assays, are used to compare and predict potencies and/or clinical efficacies of the topical corticosteroids. There is some evidence to suggest that a recognizable correlation exists between vasoconstrictor potency and therapeutic efficacy in man.

Pharmacokinetics

The extent of percutaneous absorption of topical corticosteroids is determined by many factors including the vehicle, the integrity of the epidermal barrier, and the use of occlusive dressings.

Topical corticosteroids can be absorbed from normal intact skin. Inflammation and/or other disease processes in the skin increase percutaneous absorption. Occlusive dressings substantially increase the percutaneous absorption of topical corticosteroids.

Once absorbed through the skin, topical corticosteroids are handled through pharmacokinetic pathways similar to systemically administered corticosteroids. Corticosteroids are bound to plasma proteins in varying degrees. Corticosteroids are metabolized primarily in the liver and are then excreted by the kidneys. Some of the topical corticosteroids and their metabolites are also excreted into the bile.

INDICATIONS AND USAGE

Otic Tridesilon Solution is indicated for the treatment of superficial infections of the external auditory canal caused by organisms susceptible to the action of the antimicrobial and accompanied by inflammation.

CONTRAINDICATIONS

Otic Tridesilon Solution (desonide 0.05%-acetic acid 2%) is contraindicated in those patients who have shown hypersensitivity to any of the components of the preparation. Perforated tympanic membranes are frequently considered a contraindication to the use of external ear canal medication.

PRECAUTIONS

General

Systemic absorption of topical corticosteroids has produced reversible hypothalamic-pituitary-adrenal (HPA) axis suppression, manifestations of Cushing's syndrome, hyperglycemia, and glycosuria in some patients.

Conditions which augment systemic absorption include the application of the more potent steroids, use over large surface areas, prolonged use, and the addition of occlusive dressings.

Children may absorb proportionally larger amounts of topical corticosteroids and thus be more susceptible to systemic toxicity. (See PRECAUTIONS—Pediatric Use).

If irritation develops, the product should be discontinued and appropriate therapy instituted.

If infection persists or new infection appears, appropriate therapy should be instituted. If a favorable response does not occur promptly, the corticosteroid should be discontinued until the infection has been adequately controlled.

Information for the Patient

Patients using topical corticosteroids should receive the following information and instructions:

1. This medication is to be used as directed by the physician. It is for external use only. Avoid contact with the eyes.
2. Patients should be advised not to use this medication for any disorder other than for which it was prescribed.

Laboratory Tests

The following tests may be helpful in evaluating the HPA axis suppression:
Urinary free cortisol test
ACTH stimulation test

Carcinogenesis, Mutagenesis, and Impairment of Fertility

Long-term animal studies have not been preformed to evaluate the carcinogenic potential or the effect on fertility of topical corticosteroids.

Studies to determine mutagenicity with prednisolone and hydrocortisone have revealed negative results.

Pregnancy Category C

Corticosteroids are generally teratogenic in laboratory animals when administered systemically at relatively low dosage levels. The more potent corticosteroids have been shown to be teratogenic after dermal application in laboratory animals. There are no adequate and well-controlled studies in pregnant women on teratogenic effects from topically applied corticosteroids. Therefore, topical corticosteroids should be used during pregnancy only if the potential benefit justifies the potential risk to the fetus. Drugs of this class should not be used extensively on pregnant patients, in large amounts, or for prolonged periods of time.

Nursing Mothers
It is not known whether topical administration of corticosteroids could result in sufficient systemic absorption to produce detectable quantities in breast milk. Systemically administered corticosteroids are secreted into breast milk in quantities *not* likely to have a deleterious effect on the infant. Nevertheless, caution should be exercised when topical corticosteroids are administered to a nursing woman.

Pediatric Use
Pediatric patients may demonstrate greater susceptibility to topical corticosteroid-induced HPA axis suppression and Cushing's syndrome than mature patients because of a larger skin surface area to body weight ratio.

Hypothalamic-pituitary-adrenal (HPA) axis suppression. Cushing's syndrome, and intracranial hypertension have been reported in children receiving topical corticosteroids. Manifestations of adrenal suppression in children include linear growth retardation, delayed weight gain, low plasma cortisol levels, and absence of response to ACTH stimulation. Manifestations of intracranial hypertension include bulging fontanelles, headaches, and bilateral papilledema.

Administration of topical corticosteroids to children should be limited to the least amount compatible with an effective therapeutic regimen.

Chronic corticosteroid therapy may interfere with the growth and development of children.

ADVERSE REACTIONS
The following local adverse reactions may occur infrequently with otic use of topical corticosteroids. These reactions are listed in an approximate decreasing order of occurrence.

Burning	Hypopigmentation
Itching	Allergic contact dermatitis
Irritation	Maceration of the skin
Dryness	Secondary infection
Folliculitis	Skin atrophy
Hypertrichosis	

OVERDOSAGE
Topically applied corticosteroids can be absorbed in sufficient amounts to produce systemic effects. (See PRECAUTIONS).

DOSAGE AND ADMINISTRATION
All ceruminous material and debris should be carefully removed to permit Otic Tridesilon® Solution (desonide 0.05%–acetic acid 2%) to contact the infected surfaces. Instill 3 to 4 drops into the ear 3 to 4 times daily. If preferred, a gauze or cotton wick saturated with the solution may be inserted in the ear canal and allowed to remain in situ. It should be kept moist by further addition of the solution, as required.

HOW SUPPLIED
Otic Tridesilon® Solution (desonide 0.05%—acetic acid 2%) is supplied in 10cc bottles with dropper.
Otic Tridesilon® is a clear colorless solution.

	NDC Number
10 mL	0026-7210-10

Store below 86°F (30°C), avoid freezing.
Miles Inc.
Pharmaceutical Division
400 Morgan Lane
West Haven, CT 06516 USA
CAUTION: Federal (USA) law prohibits dispensing without a prescription. For external use only.
PD100698   10/88   0627
© 1988 Miles Inc.

IDENTIFICATION PROBLEM?
Consult PDR's
Product Identification Section
where you'll find over 1700
products pictured actual size
and in full color.

Milex Products, Inc.
**5915 NORTHWEST HIGHWAY
CHICAGO, IL 60631**

AMINO-CERV™ ℞
[ah-me'no-serv]
pH 5.5 Cervical Creme

ACTIVE INGREDIENTS
Urea 8.34%, Sodium Propionate 0.50%, Methionine 0.83%, Cystine 0.35%, Inositol 0.83%, Benzalkonium Chloride 0.000004%. Buffered to pH of 5.5 in a water-miscible creme base.

DESCRIPTION
An AMINO-ACID and UREA creme specifically formulated for cervical treatment: Cervicitis (mild), postpartum cervicitis, postpartum cervical tears, post cauterization, post cryosurgery and post conization.

ADVANTAGES
METHIONINE and CYSTINE are amino-acids necessary for wound healing and forming of epithelial tissue. INOSITOL acts as an essential growth factor and promotes epithelialization.

UREA aids in debridement, dissolves the coagulum and promotes epithelialization. Its solvent action on fibroblasts prevents the formation of excessive tissue—thus preventing stenosis when used as directed.

BENZALKONIUM CHLORIDE serves to lower surface tension and thus aids in spreading the medication. Along with SODIUM PROPIONATE it also exerts a bacteriostatic effect.

AMINO-CERV is geared to the higher pH of the healthy cervix in contrast with pH 4 vaginal preparations. With its pH factor of 5.5 Amino-Cerv promotes faster healing of the cervix, yet will not adversely affect a healthy vagina.

DIRECTIONS
When immediate postpartum bleeding has subsided (usually from 24 to 48 hours after delivery), one Milex-Jector full of AMINO-CERV creme should be applied nightly for four weeks. In mild CERVICITIS (not requiring cautery or cryosurgery) one applicatorful of AMINO-CERV should be injected in the vagina nightly upon retiring for 2 weeks.

A small amount of AMINO-CERV should be applied immediately after HOT CAUTERIZATION, HOT CONIZATION and CRYOSURGERY. One applicatorful should be injected nightly upon retiring for 2 to 4 weeks (the duration of treatment depends on extent of cauterization or hot conization or cryosurgery). During the weekly office visit for (2 to 4 visits) the physician should again apply a small amount of AMINO-CERV with a probe or applicator. The canal is to be completely probed on the last visit.

After COLD CONING, one applicatorful should be injected upon retiring about 24 hours after surgery and nightly thereafter for four weeks. During the four weekly office visits following cold coning, a small amount of AMINO-CERV should be applied with a probe or applicator into the canal by the physician. The canal is to be completely probed on the last visit.

Reasons For Variation of Directions:
(1) After hot conization, cauterization and cryosurgery immediate use of AMINO-CERV is indicated to aid in dissolving dead or burned tissue.
(2) After cold coning, there is no dead tissue to slough off. Therefore, a wait of 24 hours or longer is desirable for normal healing to take place and for some fibroblasts to be laid down before applying the AMINO-CERV (which has a solvent action on both the fibroblasts and the absorbable sutures). When NONABSORBABLE sutures are used, AMINO-CERV can be used immediately.

CONTRAINDICATIONS
Deleterious side effects have not been a problem at the doses recommended. The usual precautions against allergic reactions should be observed.

STORAGE
Store at room temperature.

PACKAGING
2¾ oz. tube with Milex-Jector (2 weeks supply, 14 applications).
Available only on hospital direct orders: 5½ oz. tube with MILEX-JECTOR (4 weeks supply, 28 applications).

PRO-CEPTION
[pro-sep'shun]

DESCRIPTION
PRO-CEPTION is a precoital douche to help promote conception. It provides in a convenient form supplementary nutrient immediately available to the sperm for metabolism and movement. Also effective for removal of a thick tenacious mucous plug of the cervix.

DIRECTIONS
The screw cap is used as a measuring device and filled level with the powder which is then dissolved in eight ounces of lukewarm water. The woman is told to douche while in a recumbent position and to retain the solution (10 to 15 minutes). Following coitus the patient should remain recumbent for two hours or more. May be used as a companion with Milex Oligospermia Cups.

CONTRAINDICATIONS
None.

PACKAGING
Available in 12 douche container.

Minnetonka Medical
Minnetonka, Inc.
**P.O. BOX 1A
MINNETONKA, MN 55343**

TRANS-PLANTAR™ ℞
Salicylic Acid USP, 21%

DESCRIPTION
TRANS-PLANTAR™ Dermal Patch Delivery System contains Salicylic Acid USP, 21%, evenly dispersed in an adhesive patch composed of natural non-sensitizing Karaya, Polyethylene Glycol-300 USP, Propylene Glycol USP and Quaternium-15. *See also under TRANS-VER-SAL® Delivery System For Verruca Treatment.*

CLINICAL PHARMACOLOGY
The pharmacologic activity of the TRANS-PLANTAR™ delivery system is attributed to Salicylic Acid USP (21%). *See also under TRANS-VER-SAL® Delivery System For Verruca Treatment.*

INDICATIONS AND USAGE
The TRANS-PLANTAR™ delivery system is for the treatment of verruca plantaris.
This product is not for use on moles, birthmarks, uro-genital warts and warts with hair.

CONTRAINDICATIONS, PRECAUTIONS, ADVERSE REACTIONS
See under TRANS-VER-SAL® Delivery System For Verruca Treatment.

PATIENT INSTRUCTIONS
These are provided on the back panel of dispensing package.

DOSAGE AND ADMINISTRATION
TRANS-PLANTAR™ patches are applied once each day before retiring. *See also under TRANS-VER-SAL® Delivery System For Verruca Treatment.*

HOW SUPPLIED
The TRANS-PLANTAR™ system is supplied in a carton of 25 patches, 20mm in diameter (NDC #53309-203-04). Each carton also contains 25 securing tapes and one cleaning file.
STORE BETWEEN 40–100°F (4–37.8°C). DO NOT FREEZE.
U.S. Patent 4,778,786 ● Minnetonka, Inc.
Licensed Under Patent 4,675,009 ● LecTec Corporation
Shown in Product Identification Section, page 419

TRANS–VER–SAL® ℞
**Salicylic Acid, USP 15%
in Karaya Gum Base
Delivery Patch System for Verruca Treatment**

DESCRIPTION
TRANS-VER-SAL®, Dermal Patch Delivery System,* contains Salicylic Acid USP, 15%, evenly dispersed in an adhesive patch composed of natural non-sensitizing Karaya, Polyethylene Glycol-300 USP, Propylene Glycol USP and Quaternium-15. The system is designed to be applied topically to verrucous tissue and provide constant and controlled release of the active drug over an eight-hour treatment period. Each patch is covered with a polyethylene moisture barrier which creates a beneficial occlusive effect.
TRANS-VER-SAL® patches are sealed in moisture resistant, polyester-foil-polyethylene laminate. Upon application, the patches are held in place with skin compatible adhesive tapes provided in kit. A cleaning file is also supplied to aid in the removal of the sloughed verrucous tissue.

CLINICAL PHARMACOLOGY
The pharmacologic activity of the TRANS-VER-SAL® delivery system is attributed to Salicylic Acid USP (15%). The structural formula of Salicylic Acid is:
[See Chemical Formula at top of next page].
While the exact mode of action of Salicylic Acid in verruca treatment is unknown, its activity appears to be due to a

Continued on next page

Minnetonka Medical—Cont.

keratolytic action which results in mechanical removal of stratum corneum cells infected with the papilloma virus. The application of Salicylic Acid by a transdermal delivery system provides for a more steady release of the drug into the stratum corneum than traditional collodion formulas which tend to unload their concentration of Salicylic Acid after the solvents evaporate.

A moisture barrier which covers each patch maintains a hydrated environment to allow for a better penetration of the active drug and increased sloughing of keratolized verrucous tissue.

INDICATIONS AND USAGE

The TRANS-VER-SAL® delivery system is clinically proven effective for the treatment of common verruca infections. See DOSAGE AND ADMINISTRATION for information on frequency and duration of use.

This product is not for use on moles, birthmarks, uro-genital warts and warts with hair.

CONTRAINDICATIONS

TRANS-VER-SAL® patches should not be used by patients with diabetes or impaired blood circulation unless directed by physician.

PRECAUTIONS

TRANS-VER-SAL® patches are for external, dermal use only. Patches should not be applied in contact with eyes or mucous membranes. The patches should be trimmed carefully so as not to come in contact with normal skin surrounding verrucae. Treatment should be discontinued if excessive irritation of surrounding skin occurs.

Patient Instructions: *See back panel of dispensing package.*

ADVERSE REACTIONS

Localized irritation will occur if TRANS-VER-SAL® patches are applied in contact with normal skin surrounding verrucous tissue. In the event of such a reaction, the irritation should be allowed to subside by temporarily discontinuing treatment. Upon resuming treatment, TRANS-VER-SAL® patches should be carefully trimmed so as to contact only verrucous tissue.

DOSAGE AND ADMINISTRATION

TRANS-VER-SAL® patches are applied once each day before retiring. The verrucous tissue should first be cleaned of debris with the emery file provided and then moistened with warm water using a cotton tipped applicator. The patch is then removed from the clear strip, trimmed to size (if necessary), and applied to the wart with the occlusive top film facing up. The patch is then secured with the adhesive tape provided.

The TRANS-VER-SAL® patch should be left in place overnight and discarded in the morning. This procedure is to be repeated each day until verruca resolution is complete. Generally, visible clinical improvement will occur during the first two to four weeks of treatment. Complete resolution may be expected after six to twelve weeks of therapy. As the verruca is diminishing, it is important that the patch be trimmed accordingly to avoid contact with normal skin.

HOW SUPPLIED

The TRANS-VER-SAL® system is supplied in cartons of 40 patches of either 6mm diameter (NDC #53309-202-04) or 12mm in diameter (NDC #53309-202-06). Each carton also contains 42 securing tapes and one emery file.

Store BELOW 100°F (37.8°C).

PATIENT INSTRUCTIONS

These are provided with each package.

CAUTION

Federal law prohibits dispensing without prescription.

PRODUCT AVAILABILITY

Two sizes of transdermal patches facilitate the treatment of various sizes of infections.

TRANS-VER-SAL® 6mm: 6mm patches, 40 ea. Complete with 42 tapes and one file.

TRANS-VER-SAL® 12mm: 12mm patches, 40 ea. Complete with 42 tapes and one file.

DETAILED PATIENT LABELING

Directions for use—Use at night before retiring.

1. PREPARE MEDICATED PATCH. Lift a patch from the clear strip, leaving the top plastic film in place. If the patch is bigger than the wart, trim it to a size which will cover only the wart surface.

2. PREPARE TREATMENT SITE. Clean skin, then smooth wart surface with emery file supplied.

3. MOISTEN THE WART. Apply a drop of warm water to the wart, keeping the surrounding skin dry.

4. APPLY MEDICATED PATCH. Keep plastic film on the top of patch facing up. Apply sticky bottom side to the wart.

5. SECURE THE PATCH. Use a strip of the tape provided to hold the patch in place.

Remove the patch in the morning (after about 8 hours) and discard.

Continue using TRANS-VER-SAL® patches nightly as directed or until your physician has determined the wart is gone.

For further information, please contact:
MINNETONKA MEDICAL
MINNETONKA, INC., Distributor
P.O. BOX 1A, Minnetonka, Minnesota 55343
(612)448-4181 ● (800)345-8084

*U.S. Patent 4,778,786 Minnetonka, Inc. Licensed Under Patent 4,675,009 LecTec Corp.
©1988 MINNETONKA, INC.

Shown in Product Identification Section, page 419

EDUCATIONAL MATERIAL

Video
TRANS-VER-SAL® Patient Education Videotape, FREE to physicians
Samples available upon request, (800) 345-8084 or (612) 448-4181 in Minnesota, FREE to physicians
TRANS-PLANTAR™ Samples available upon request, (800) 345-8084 or (612) 448-4181 in Minnesota. FREE to physicians.

Mission Pharmacal Company
1325 E. DURANGO ST.
SAN ANTONIO, TX 78210

CALCET®
[kăl 'cet]
Calcium Supplement
NDC-0178-0251-01

COMPOSITION

Each tablet contains:

	% US RDA*	
Calcium Lactate		240 mg.
Calcium Gluconate		240 mg.
Calcium Carbonate		240 mg.
(Calcium	15	152.8 mg.)
Vitamin D	25	100. Units

* Percent of U.S. Recommended Daily Allowance for adults and children 4 or more years of age.

INDICATIONS

CALCET® tablets are indicated as a daily supplement to provide a dietary source of calcium. CALCET® tablets are of particular value in people who have milk allergies, in people who have low calcium leg cramps or calcium deficiencies due to low dietary calcium.

DOSAGE

TWO CALCET® TABLETS AT BEDTIME as a general or prenatal supplement. In calcium deficiency states or in nocturnal leg cramping, dosage should be increased to TWO CALCET® TABLETS AT BEDTIME plus one tablet mid-morning and one tablet mid-afternoon.

HOW SUPPLIED

CALCET® tablets are supplied as yellow, oval shaped, coated tablets in bottles of 100 tablets.

LITERATURE AVAILABLE

Yes.

CALCET PLUS™
[kăl 'cet]
Calcium-Iron-Zinc-Multivitamin
NDC 0178-0252-60

COMPOSITION

Each tablet contains:

			%USRDA*
Vitamin C (Calcium Ascorbate, Ascorbic Acid)	500	mg.	800
Vitamin B₁ (Thiamine Mononitrate)	2.25	mg.	150
Vitamin B₂ (Riboflavin)	2.55	mg.	150
Vitamin B₃ (Niacinamide)	30.0	mg.	150
Vitamin B₅ (d-Calcium Pantothenate)	15.0	mg.	150
Vitamin B₆ (Pyridoxine Hydrochloride)	3.0	mg.	150
Vitamin B₁₂ (Crystalline on Resin)	9	mcg.	150
Folic Acid	0.8	mg.	200
Vitamin A (Vitamin A Acetate)	5000	USPU	100
Vitamin D	400	USPU	100
Vitamin E (d-Alpha Tocopheryl Acetate or Acid Succinate)	30	USPU	100
Calcium (Calcium Ascorbate, Calcium Carbonate)	152.8	mg.	15
Iron (Ferrous Fumarate)	18.0	mg.	100
Zinc (Zinc Sulfate, dried)	15.0	mg.	100

* USRDA: U.S. recommended daily allowance for adults and children 4 or more years of age.

INDICATIONS

CALCET PLUS tablets are indicated as adjunctive therapy in osteoporosis, pre- and post-operative patients, low calcium leg cramping, for patients with milk allergies and nursing mothers.

DOSAGE

Two CALCET PLUS tablets at bedtime.

HOW SUPPLIED

CALCET PLUS tablets are supplied as white, oval shaped, coated tablets in bottles of 60's.

LITERATURE AVAILABLE

Yes.

CITRACAL®
[sit 'ra-cal]
Calcium Citrate

DESCRIPTION

CITRACAL® is a clinically proven more bioavailable source of calcium, ideal as a calcium supplement and as an aluminum-free phosphate binder for:
1) end stage renal disease
2) mild to moderate renal insufficiency
3) renal osteodystrophy
Each tablet contains:
950 mg. Calcium Citrate, Ultra Dense
200 mg. Calcium ....20% USRDA
USRDA: U.S. recommended daily allowance for adults and children 4 or more years of age.
Ingredients: Major: Calcium citrate.
Citracal™ tablets contain no lactose, salt, starch, nitrates, preservatives, artifical flavors or colors.

DIRECTIONS FOR USE

Take 2 to 4 tablets a day or as recommended by your physician.
STORE AT ROOM TEMPERATURE.
KEEP OUT OF THE REACH OF CHILDREN.

HOW SUPPLIED

CITRACAL® NDC 0178-0800-01 is supplied as white, bolus shaped, sugar coated tablets in bottles of 100 tablets each.
For Product Information call: 1-800-531-3333
In Texas: 1-800-292-7364

CITRACAL® LIQUITAB
[sit 'ra-cal lĭc 'wĭ-tab]
Presolubilized Calcium Citrate
Effervescent Citrus Flavored Tablets

DESCRIPTION

CITRACAL® LIQUITAB is a presolubilized form of calcium citrate which provides superior bioavailabilty and exceptional aluminum free phosphate binding. CITRACAL® LIQUITAB is the best choice in calcium supplementation and in end stage renal patients.
Each tablet contains:
2376 mg. Calcium Citrate,
500 mg. Calcium ....50% USRDA*
*USRDA: U.S. recommended daily allowance for adults and children 4 or more years of age.

DIRECTIONS FOR USE

Dissolve 1 tablet or amount recommended by your physician, in a glass of water.
STORE AT ROOM TEMPERATURE. KEEP OUT OF THE REACH OF CHILDREN.
For product information call: 1-800-531-3333
In Texas: 1-800-292-7364

COMPETE®
[kŏm 'pēt]
Multivitamins with Iron and Zinc
NDC-0178-0221-01

DESCRIPTION
COMPETE® is a multivitamin with iron and zinc formulated to provide an especially well tolerated group of nutritional components for the active, stressful lifestyle of the 1980's. COMPETE® provides 150% of the U.S.R.D.A. of all components except vitamins A and D, which have been maintained at a 100% level, and vitamin B_6 which is provided in a level of 1028% U.S.R.D.A. for the particular needs of today's active woman using birth control tablets.

Composition: Each tablet contains:

	Quantity/ Tablet	%USRDA
Vitamin A	5000 I.U.	100%
Vitamin D	400 I.U.	100%
Vitamin E	45 I.U.	150%
Vitamin C	90 mg	150%
Folic Acid	0.4 mg	150%
Thiamine Mononitrate	2.25 mg	150%
Riboflavin	2.6 mg	150%
Niacinamide	30 mg	150%
Pyridoxine HCl	25.0 mg	1028%
Vitamin B_{12}	9 mcg	150%
Iron (As Ferrous Gluconate 233 mg)	27 mg	150%
Zinc (As Zinc Sulfate)	22.5 mg	150%

DOSAGE
One tablet at bedtime as directed by your physician.

WARNING
KEEP THIS AND ALL MEDICATIONS OUT OF THE REACH OF CHILDREN.
In case of accidental overdose, seek professional assistance or contact a poison control center immediately.

PRECAUTION
Folic Acid, especially in doses above 0.1 mg. daily, may obscure pernicious anemia in that hematologic remission may occur while neurological manifestations remain progressive.

HOW SUPPLIED
COMPETE® is supplied as orange, football-shaped, sugar coated tablets in bottles of 100.

FERRALET®
[fer "a-lét]
Ferrous Gluconate
NDC-0178-0082-01

COMPOSITION
Each tablet contains:

		% US RDA*
Ferrous Gluconate	320 mg	
(Iron	37.0 mg.)	206.0

*Percent of U.S. recommended daily allowance for adults and children 4 or more years of age.

DESCRIPTION
The FERRALET® tablet contains only one active ingredient, iron, as ferrous gluconate. FERRALET® is particularly well tolerated in most patients because ferrous gluconate is non-astringent, non-irritating, and will not precipitate protein from aqueous media. FERRALET® provides a more efficient source of ferrous ion because of the low ionization constant of ferrous gluconate, coupled with high solubility and stability over the entire pH range of the gastrointestinal tract. FERRALET® provides utilizable iron throughout the entire length of the intestinal absorption bed. With FERRALET®, heavy iron loading is not necessary due to the superior efficiency of the iron component. The result of moderate ferrous ion dosage is usually improved patient acceptance and excellent dosage continuity. FERRALET® is manufactured in a unique, easy to swallow shape, to further enhance patient acceptance of the product. FERRALET® has a tailored disintegration rate to minimize gastric intolerance with a rapid dissolution rate to assure rapid availability for absorption.

INDICATIONS
Anemias amenable to iron therapy.

DOSAGE
One to three tablets a day depending upon the severity of the anemia and the particular toleration of the patient.

HOW SUPPLIED
FERRALET® is packaged in bottles of 100 tablets.

LITERATURE AVAILABLE
Yes.

FOSFREE®
[fos 'frē]
Calcium—Vitamins—Iron
NDC-0178-0031-01

COMPOSITION
Each tablet contains:

		One Tablet	% US RDA
Calcium Lactate		250.0 mg.	
Calcium Gluconate		250.0 mg.	
Calcium Carbonate		300.0 mg.	
(Calcium		175.7 mg.)	17
Ferrous Gluconate		125.0 mg.	
(Iron		14.5 mg.)	80
Vitamin D_2		150.0 USP U. optional	
Vitamin A Acetate	1500.0 USP U.		30
Ascorbic Acid (C)		50.0 mg.	83
Pyridoxine HCl (B_6)		3.0 mg.	123
Thiamine Mononitrate (B_1)		5.0 mg.	306
Riboflavin (B_2)		2.0 mg.	117
Niacinamide (B_3)		10.0 mg.	50
d-Calcium Pantothenate (B_5)		1.0 mg.	9
Vitamin B_{12} (Crystalline on resin)		2.0 mcg.	33

ACTION AND USES
FOSFREE® tablets are primarily indicated as a prenatal, postpartum or geriatric supplement particularly when soluble calcium salt supplementation is desired. FOSFREE® is a specific for hypocalcemic tetany (nocturnal leg cramping).

ADMINISTRATION AND DOSAGE
One or two FOSFREE® tablets at bedtime as a general or prenatal supplement. In calcium deficiency states or in nocturnal leg cramping, dosage should be increased to two FOSFREE® tablets at bedtime plus one tablet mid-morning and one tablet mid-afternoon.

HOW SUPPLIED
FOSFREE® is supplied as yellow capsule shaped coated tablets in bottles of 100 tablets.

LITERATURE AVAILABLE
Yes.

IROMIN-G®
[i 'rō-min]
Hematinic Supplement
NDC-0178-0081-01

COMPOSITION
Each tablet contains:

	% US RDA	
Ferrous Gluconate		260 mg.
(Iron	214	30 mg.)
Ascorbic Acid (C)	166	100.0 mg.
Thiamine Mononitrate (B_1)	333	5.0 mg.
Pyridoxine HCl (B_6)	1028	25.0 mg.
Riboflavin (B_2)	117	2.0 mg.
Niacinamide	50	10.0 mg.
Folic Acid	200	0.8 mg.
d-Calcium Pantothenate	9	1.0 mg.
Vitamin B_{12} (Crystalline on resin)	33	2.0 mcg.
Vitamin A Acetate	80	4000.0 USP U.
Vitamin D_2	Optional	400.0 USP U.
Calcium Carbonate		70.0 mg.
Calcium Gluconate		100.0 mg.
Calcium Lactate		100.0 mg.
(Calcium	5	50.0 mg.)

ACTION AND USES
Secondary anemias, and as a supplement for the prenatal, teenage and geriatric diet.

ADMINISTRATION AND DOSAGE
One to three tablets daily after meals or as directed by a physician.

PRECAUTION
Folic Acid, especially in doses above 0.1 mg. daily, may obscure pernicious anemia in that hematologic remission may occur while neurological manifestations remain progressive.

SIDE EFFECTS
IROMIN-G® is virtually free of side effects when given in the recommended dosage. The rare constipation, diarrhea, or gastric upset can usually be controlled by dosage adjustment.

HOW SUPPLIED
IROMIN-G® is supplied as red football shaped coated tablets in bottles of 100 tablets.

LITERATURE AVAILABLE
Yes.

MEDILAX™
[mĕd 'i-laks]
Phenolphthalein tablets, U.S.P.
NDC 0178-0095-24

COMPOSITION
Each tablet contains:
Phenolphthalein U.S.P. .... 120 mg

ACTION AND USES
MEDILAX™ extra strength laxative tablets are recommended for relief of occasional constipation with a mild overnight action. MEDILAX™ is a chewable tablet in citrus flavor. MEDILAX™ contains NeutraSweet®.

DOSAGE AND ADMINISTRATION
Adults oral dosage is 1 to 2 tablets daily in a single or divided dose with a full glass of water.

PRECAUTION
Do not use laxative products when abdominal pain, nausea, or vomiting are present unless directed by your doctor. MEDILAX™ may cause pink to red urine coloration in patients with alkaline urine. Keep this and all medications out of the reach of children. Phenylketonurics: Contains Phenylalanine 1.5 mg per tablet.

HOW SUPPLIED
MEDILAX™ is supplied in yellow scored tablets in film strip package of 24 tablets.
LITERATURE AVAILABLE.
Yes.

MISSION PHARMACAL UROLOGICALS

CALCIBIND®   ℞
[kal 'sē-bīnd]
Cellulose Sodium Phosphate
Oral Powder

DESCRIPTION
Cellulose Sodium Phosphate (CSP), the active ingredient in CALCIBIND®, is a synthetic compound made by phosphorylation of cellulose and has the following structural formula:

Where n indicates the degree of polymerization and has an average value of approximately 3000. The molecular weight of CSP monomer is 286.1 and the average molecular weight of the polymer is 858,000.
It has an inorganic bound phosphate of 31–36%, free phosphate of 3.5%, sodium content of approximately 11% and a calcium binding capacity of 1.8 mmol of Ca per gram of the oral powder. It has excellent ion exchange properties, the sodium ion exchanging for calcium. When taken orally, CSP binds calcium, the complex of calcium and cellulose phosphate being excreted in feces. The dosage of CALCIBIND® is powder for oral administration.

HOW SUPPLIED
CALCIBIND® NDC 0178-0255-30 is available for oral administration in bottles of 300 grams of CSP bulk powder.

LITHOSTAT®   ℞
[lith 'o-stat]
Acetohydroxamic Acid (AHA)

DESCRIPTION
Acetohydroxamic acid (AHA) is a stable, synthetic compound derived from hydroxylamine and ethyl acetate. Its molecular structure is similar to urea:
[See Chemical Formula at top of next page].

Continued on next page

Mission—Cont.

ACETOHYDROXAMIC ACID (AHA)

AHA is weakly acidic, highly soluble in water, and chelates metals - notably iron. The molecular weight is 75.068. AHA has a PKA of 9.32 and a melting point of 89–91°C. Available as 250 mg tablets.

HOW SUPPLIED

LITHOSTAT®, NDC 0178-0500-01, is available for oral administration as 250 mg scored tablets, in unit of use packages of 100 tablets.

THIOLA™   ℞

[thi-ól-a]
Tiopronin Tablets

DESCRIPTION

THIOLA™ (Tiopronin) is a reducing and complexing thiol compound. Tiopronin is N-(2-Mercaptopropionyl) glycine and has the following structure:

Tiopronin has the empirical formula $C_5H_9NO_3S$ and a molecular weight of 163.20. It has one asymmetric center and therefore exists as dl (racemic) mixture.
Tiopronin is a white crystalline powder which is freely soluble in water.
THIOLA™ tablets are white sugar coated tablets, each containing 100 mg. of Tiopronin and are taken orally.

HOW SUPPLIED

THIOLA™ (NDC 0178-0900-01), is available for oral administration as 100 mg. round, white, sugar coated tablets in bottles of 100 tablets each.
For product information call: 1-800-531-3333
In Texas call: 1-800-292-7364

UROCIT®-K   ℞

[yu'ro-cĭt kay]
Potassium Citrate
WAX MATRIX TABLETS

DESCRIPTION

Urocit®-K is a citrate salt of potassium. Its empirical formula is $K_3C_6H_5O_7 \cdot H_2O$, and its structural formula is:

Potassium citrate is a white granular powder that is soluble in water at 154g/100 ml, almost insoluble in alcohol, and insoluble in organic solvents.
Urocit®-K is supplied as wax matrix tablets, containing 5 meq (540 mg) potassium citrate each, for oral administration.

HOW SUPPLIED

Urocit®-K (NDC 0178-0600-01) is available for oral administration in tablet form (5 meq potassium citrate/tablet), in bottles each containing 100 tablets.

MISSION PRENATAL SERIES

MISSION PRENATAL®
Vitamins—Iron—Calcium—.4 mg. Folic Acid
NDC 0178-132-01

MISSION PRENATAL® F.A.
Vitamins—Iron—Calcium—.8 mg. Folic Acid and Zinc
NDC 0178-0153-01

MISSION PRENATAL® H.P.
Vitamins—Iron—Calcium—0.8 mg. Folic Acid
NDC 0178-0161-01

COMPOSITION

Each tablet contains:

	%U.S.R.D.A.	
Ferrous Gluconate		260 mg.
(Iron	214	30 mg.)
Ascorbic Acid (C)	167	100.0 mg.
Thiamine Mononitrate (B₁)	270	5.0 mg.

*† Pyridoxine HCl (B₆)	99		3.0 mg.
Riboflavin (B₂)	100		2.0 mg.
Niacinamide	50		10.0 mg.
d-Calcium Pantothenate	9		1.0 mg.
Vitamin B₁₂ (Crystalline on Resin)	25		2.0 mcg.
*† Folic Acid	50		0.4 mg.
Vitamin A Acetate	50		4000.0 USPU
Vitamin D₂	100		400.0 USPU
Calcium Carbonate			70.0 mg.
Calcium Gluconate			100.0 mg.
Calcium Lactate			100.0 mg.
(Calcium	4		50.0 mg.)
Zinc (as Zinc Sulfate)	100		15.0 mg.

*Pyridoxine HCL—Mission® Prenatal F.A. =10mg., 329%U.S.R.D.A.
*Folic Acid—Mission® Prenatal F.A. =.8mg., 100%U.S.R.D.A.
†Pyridoxine HCL—Mission®Prenatal H.P. =25 mg., 1250%U.S.R.D.A.
†Folic Acid—Mission® Prenatal H.P. =1.0 mg., 125%U.S.R.D.A.
Zinc—only in Mission® Prenatal F.A.

INDICATIONS

ALL MISSION® PRENATALS are prenatal and postpartum supplements.

DOSAGE

Take one tablet at bedtime or as directed by your physician. Keep this and all medications out of the reach of children.

PRECAUTION

Folic acid, especially in doses above 0.1 mg. daily, may obscure pernicious anemia in that hematologic remission may occur while neurological manifestations remain progressive.

HOW SUPPLIED

MISSION® PRENATAL is supplied as pink, football-shaped, sugar coated tablets in bottles of 100.
MISSION® PRENATAL F.A. is supplied as blue, football-shaped, sugar coated tablets in bottles of 100.
MISSION® PRENATAL H.P. is supplied as green, football-shaped, sugar-coated tablets in bottles of 100.

MISSION PRENATAL™ Rx   ℞

Prenatal Supplement with
Vitamins and Minerals
NDC 0178-0007-01

COMPOSITION

Each Tablet Contains:

		%USRDA*
Vitamin A (as Vitamin A Acetate)	8000 I.U.	100
Vitamin D	400 I.U.	100
Vitamin C (as Ascorbic Acid, Calcium Ascorbate)	240 mg.	400
Vitamin B₁ (as Thiamine Mononitrate)	4 mg.	216
Vitamin B₂ (as Riboflavin)	2 mg.	100
Vitamin B₃ (as Niacinamide)	20 mg.	100
Vitamin B₅ (as Calcium Pantothenate)	10 mg.	100
Vitamin B₆ (as Pyridoxine Hydrochloride)	20 mg.	658
Vitamin B₁₂ (as Cyanocobalamine on resin)	8 mcg.	100
Folic Acid	1 mg.	125
Iron (as Ferrous Fumarate)	60 mg.	333
Calcium (as Calcium Carbonate and Calcium Ascorbate)	175 mg.	13.5
Iodine (as Potassium Iodide)	0.3 mg.	200
Zinc (as Zinc Sulfate, dried)	15 mg.	100
Copper (as Cupric Oxide)	2 mg.	100

* USRDA: U.S. recommended daily allowance for pregnant or lactating women.

INDICATIONS

MISSION PRENATAL Rx is a prenatal and postpartum supplement.

DOSAGE

Take one tablet at bedtime or as directed by your physician.

CAUTION

Federal law prohibits dispensing without a prescription.

HOW SUPPLIED

MISSION PRENATAL Rx is supplied as pink, football shape, film-coated tablets in bottles of 100.

LITERATURE AVAILABLE

Yes.

MISSION® SURGICAL SUPPLEMENT

A dietary supplement for pre-surgical and post-surgical patients. NDC 0178-0168-01

COMPOSITION

Each tablet contains:

		%USRDA*	
Ascorbic Acid (C)	500.0 mg	833	
Thiamine Mononitrate (B₁)	2.5 mg	150	
Riboflavin (B₂)	2.6 mg	150	
Niacinamide (B₃)	30.0 mg	150	
Calcium Pantothenate (B₅)	16.3 mg	150	
Pyridoxine Hydrochloride (B₆)	3.6 mg	150	
Vitamin B₁₂	9.0 mcg	150	
Vitamin A Acetate	5000 USPU	100	
Vitamin D₂	400 USPU	100	
Vitamin E Acetate or Acid Succinate	45 IU	150	
Iron (as Ferrous Gluconate)	27.0 mg	150	
Zinc (as Zinc Sulfate)	22.5 mg	150	

*USRDA: U.S. Recommended Daily Allowance for adults and children 4 or more years of age.

ACTION AND USES

A dietary supplement specifically designed to provide the vitamin and mineral nutritional assistance needed by the pre- and post-surgical patient for optimal recovery from the stress of surgery.

ADMINISTRATION AND DOSAGE

One tablet at bedtime or as directed by physician.

WARNING

<u>KEEP THIS AND ALL MEDICATIONS OUT OF THE REACH OF CHILDREN.</u> In case of accidental overdose, seek professional assistance or contact a poison control center immediately.

HOW SUPPLIED

MISSION® PRE-SURGICAL is supplied as a light green, bolus-shaped, sugar coated tablet in bottles of 100.

LITERATURE AVAILABLE

Yes.

PRULET®

[prŭ-let']
Phenolphthalein Tablets U.S.P.
NDC 0178-0090-01

COMPOSITION

Each tablet contains:
Phenolphthalein U.S.P. .... 60 mg.

ACTION AND USES

PRULET® is a mild and gentle, effective laxative for patients with atonic or hypotonic bowel syndrome.
PRULET® is a chewable tablet in lemon—lime flavor.

ADMINISTRATION AND DOSAGE

Take one to three tablets administered at bedtime; then adjust to need.

CONTRAINDICATIONS

Not to be taken in the presence of nausea, vomiting, abdominal pains, or other symptoms of appendicitis.

PRECAUTIONS

Phenolphthalein is known to produce skin eruptions in sensitized individuals. If a skin rash or eruption appears, do not take this or any other preparation containing phenolphthalein. PRULET® may cause pink to red urine coloration in patients with an alkaline urine.

HOW SUPPLIED

PRULET® is supplied in green scored tablets in film strip packages of 12 and 40 tablets.

LITERATURE AVAILABLE

Yes.

SUPAC®
[sŭ'pac]
Analgesic Compound
NDC-0178-0100-01

COMPOSITION
Each tablet contains:

Acetaminophen	160 mg.
Aspirin	230 mg.
Caffeine	33 mg.
Calcium Gluconate	60 mg.

ACTION AND USES
For temporary relief of pain accompanying simple head colds, temporary relief of pain accompanying menstruation, sinus and tension headache, minor traumatic pain, tooth extractions, arthritic and rheumatic pain syndromes.

ADMINISTRATION AND DOSAGE
Adults—One or two tablets. This dose may be repeated in 4 hours. Do not exceed 4 tablets at a single dose or 16 tablets in a 24 hour period. Children—6 to 12 years of age, ½ of the maximum adult dose or dosage; 3 to 6 years of age, ⅓ of the maximum adult dose or dosage.

PRECAUTIONS
If pain persists for more than 10 days, or redness is present, or in conditions affecting children under 12 years of age, physicians should be alert to other possible complications.

HOW SUPPLIED
SUPAC® is supplied as white scored tablets in bottles of 100 and 1000 tablets.

LITERATURE AVAILABLE
Yes.

THERABID®
[thĕr'a-bid]
Therapeutic Multivitamin
NDC 0178-0171-01

COMPOSITION
Each Tablet Contains:

		% US RDA
Ascorbic Acid (Vitamin C)	500 mg.	833
Thiamine Mononitrate (Vitamin B₁)	15 mg.	1000
Riboflavin (Vitamin B₂)	10 mg.	588
Niacinamide (Vitamin B₃)	100 mg.	500
Calcium Pantothenate (Vitamin B₅)	20 mg.	200
Pyridoxine Hydrochloride (Vitamin B₆)	10 mg.	500
Vitamin B₁₂	5 mcg.	83
Vitamin A Acetate	5,000 U.	100
Vitamin D	200 U.	50
Vitamin E (as Vitamin E Acetate or Acid Succinate)	30 IU	100

ACTION AND USES
THERABID® is a therapeutic multivitamin preparation.

ADMINISTRATION AND DOSAGE
One to two tablets per day or at the discretion of the physician.

PRECAUTIONS
Do not exceed a dosage of four tablets per day.

HOW SUPPLIED
THERABID® is supplied as green capsule shaped sugar coated tablets in bottles of 100 tablets.

LITERATURE AVAILABLE
Yes.

THERA–GESIC®
[ther'a-jē-zik]
Analgesic Creme Balm
Methyl Salicylate and Menthol

DESCRIPTION
THERA-GESIC® contains Methyl Salicylate and Menthol in a rapidly absorbed greaseless base.

ACTIONS
Topical analgesic, counterirritant.

INDICATIONS
For the temporary relief of pain associated with musculo-skeletal soreness and discomfort; additionally, as a topical adjunct in arthritis, rheumatism, and bursitis.

CONTRAINDICATIONS
Do not use in patients with Aspirin or Salicylate idiosyncrasy.

WARNINGS
Use only as directed. Keep away from children to avoid accidental poisoning. Keep away from eyes, mucous membranes, broken or irritated skin. If skin irritation develops, or if pain lasts 10 days or more, or if redness is present, discontinue use and consult a physician. <u>DO NOT SWALLOW.</u> If swallowed, induce vomiting, call a physician.

PRECAUTIONS
Do not use excessive amounts of THERA-GESIC® or occlude a fresh application of THERA-GESIC®. Do not heat pack THERA-GESIC® covered skin. For use by adults only.

ADVERSE REACTIONS
Adverse reactions related to the Salicylate and Menthol components are possible. These include excessive irritation, tinnitus, nausea or vomiting if excessive or extreme dosage is employed.

DOSAGE AND ADMINISTRATION
Gently massage THERA-GESIC® in thin applications into the sore or painful area as well as into the area immediately surrounding the painful area. The number of thin applications applied controls the intensity of the action of THERA-GESIC®. One application provides a mild effect, two provide a strong effect and three applications provide a very strong effect. Once THERA-GESIC® has penetrated the skin, the area may be washed, leaving the area dry, clean and free from the typical wintergreen odor without decreasing the effectiveness of the product. If you intend to bandage or wrap the area, the area should be washed first to avoid excessive irritation.

HOW SUPPLIED

NDC-0178-0320-03	Tubes–3 oz.
NDC-0178-0320-05	Tubes–5 oz.

Muro Pharmaceutical, Inc.
890 EAST STREET
TEWKSBURY, MA 01876-9987

BROMFED® CAPSULES ℞
[brŏm'fĕd]

A light green and clear capsule containing white beads. Timed-Release.
Each capsule contains:

Brompheniramine maleate	12 mg
Pseudoephedrine hydrochloride	120 mg

in a specially prepared base to provide prolonged action.

BROMFED-PD® CAPSULES ℞

A dark green and clear capsule containing white beads. Timed-Release.
Each capsule contains:

Brompheniramine maleate	6 mg
Pseudoephedrine hydrochloride	60 mg

in a specially prepared base to provide prolonged action.

BROMFED® and **BROMFED-PD® CAPSULES** also contain inactive ingredients: benzyl alcohol, butyl paraben, carboxymethylcellulose sodium, D & C yellow #10, edetate calcium disodium, FD&C blue #1, FD&C yellow #6, gelatin, methyl paraben, pharmaceutical glaze, propyl paraben, sodium lauryl sulfate, sodium propionate, starch, sucrose and other ingredients.

BROMFED® TABLETS ℞

A white scored tablet.
Each tablet contains:

Brompheniramine maleate	4 mg
Pseudoephedrine hydrochloride	60 mg

Also contains as inactive ingredients colloidal silicon dioxide, lactose, magnesium stearate, microcrystalline cellulose and sodium starch glycolate.

BROMFED contains ingredients of the following therapeutic classes: antihistamine and decongestant.

CLINICAL PHARMACOLOGY
Brompheniramine maleate is an alkylamine type antihistamine. This group of antihistamines are among the most active histamine antagonists and are generally effective in relatively low doses. The drugs are not so prone to produce drowsiness and are among the most suitable agents for day time use; but again, a significant proportion of patients do experience this effect. Pseudoephedrine hydrochloride is a sympathomimetic which acts predominently on alpha receptors and has little action on beta receptors. It therefore functions as an oral nasal decongestant with minimal CNS stimulation.

INDICATIONS
For the temporary relief of symptoms of seasonal and perennial allergic rhinitis, and vasomotor rhinitis, including nasal obstruction (congestion).

CONTRAINDICATIONS
Hypersensitivity to any of the ingredients. Also contraindicated in patients with severe hypertension, severe coronary artery disease, patients on MAO inhibitor therapy, patients with narrow-angle glaucoma, urinary retention, peptic ulcer and during an asthmatic attack.

WARNINGS
Considerable caution should be exercised in patients with hypertension, diabetes mellitus, ischemic heart disease, hyperthyroidism, increased intraocular pressure and prostatic hypertrophy. The elderly (60 years or older) are more likely to exhibit adverse reactions.
Antihistamines may cause excitability, especially in children. At dosages higher than the recommended dose, nervousness, dizziness or sleeplessness may occur.

PRECAUTIONS
General: Caution should be exercised in patients with high blood pressure, heart disease, diabetes or thyroid disease. The antihistamine in this product may exhibit additive effects with other CNS depressants, including alcohol.
Information for Patients: Antihistamine may cause drowsiness and ambulatory patients who operate machinery or motor vehicles should be cautioned accordingly.
Drug Interactions: MAO inhibitors and beta adrenergic blockers increase the effects of sympathomimetics. Sympathomimetics may reduce the antihypertensive effects of methyldopa, mecamylamine, reserpine and veratrum alkaloids. Concomitant use of antihistamines with alcohol and other CNS depressants may have an additive effect.
Pregnancy: The safety of use of this product in pregnancy has not been established.

ADVERSE REACTIONS
Adverse reactions include drowsiness, lassitude, nausea, giddiness, dryness of mouth, blurred vision, cardiac palpitations, flushing, increased irritability or excitement (especially in children).

DOSAGE AND ADMINISTRATION
BROMFED® CAPSULES Adults and children over 12 years of age—1 capsule every 12 hours.
BROMFED-PD® CAPSULES Children 6 to 12 years of age—1 capsule every 12 hours.
BROMFED® TABLETS Adults and children 12 and over: One tablet every 4 hours not to exceed 6 doses in 24 hours. Children 6 to 12 years: One-half tablet every 4 hours not to exceed 6 doses in 24 hours. Do not give to children under 6 years except under the advice and supervision of a physician.

HOW SUPPLIED
BROMFED® CAPSULES. Bottle of 100 (NDC 0451-4000-50) and 500 (NDC 0451-4000-60). Each capsule is coded "BROMFED" "MURO 12-120".
BROMFED-PD® CAPSULES. Bottle of 100 (NDC 0451-4001-50) and 500 (NDC 0451-4001-60). Each capsule is coded "BROMFED-PD" "MURO 6-60".
BROMFED® TABLETS. Bottle of 100 (NDC 0451-4060-50). Each tablet is coded "MURO 4060" on one side and scored on the reverse side.
Dispense in tight containers as defined in USP. Store between 15°–30°C (59°–86°F).
CAUTION: FEDERAL (U.S.A.) LAW PROHIBITS DISPENSING WITHOUT A PRESCRIPTION.

BROMFED® SYRUP
[brŏm'fĕd]

(See PDR For Nonprescription Drugs)

BROMFED®–DM COUGH SYRUP ℞
[brŏm'fĕd]

Each teaspoonful contains:

Brompheniramine maleate	2 mg
Pseudoephedrine hydrochloride	30 mg
Dextromethorphan hydrobromide	10 mg

HOW SUPPLIED
0451-4101-16—16 fl. oz. (480 mL)

GUAIFED® CAPSULES ℞
[gwī'ah-fed]

A white opaque and clear capsule containing white beads.
Each capsule contains:

Pseudoephedrine hydrochloride	120 mg

in a specially prepared base to provide prolonged action.

Guaifenesin	250 mg

designed for immediate release to provide rapid action.

Continued on next page

Muro—Cont.

GUAIFED–PD® CAPSULE   ℞

A blue and clear capsule containing white beads.
Each capsule contains:
Pseudoephedrine hydrochloride .... 60 mg
in a specially prepared base to provide prolonged action.
Guaifenesin .... 300 mg
designed for immediate release to provide rapid action.

GUAIFED® and GUAIFED–PD® CAPSULES also contain
as inactive ingredients: Benzyl Alcohol, Butyl Paraben, Edetate Calcium Disodium, Gelatin, Methyl Paraben, Pharmaceutical Glaze, Propyl Paraben, Sodium Lauryl Sulfate, Sodium Propionate, Starch, Sucrose, Titanium Dioxide, FD&C Blue #1 (GUAIFED-PD only) and other ingredients.

GUAIFED® and GUAIFED–PD® contains ingredients of the following therapeutic classes: nasal decongestant and expectorant.

CLINICAL PHARMACOLOGY

Pseudoephedrine hydrochloride is a sympathomimetic which acts predominantly on alpha adrenergic receptors in the mucosa of the respiratory tract, producing vasoconstriction and has little action on beta receptors. It therefore functions as an oral nasal decongestant with minimal CNS stimulation. Pseudoephedrine hydrochloride also increases sinus drainage and secretions. Guaifenesin is an expectorant which increases the output of phlegm (sputum) and bronchial secretions by reducing adhesiveness and surface tension. The increased flow of less viscid secretions promotes ciliary action and changes a dry, unproductive cough to one that is more productive and less frequent.

INDICATIONS

For temporary relief of nasal congestion and dry non-productive cough associated with the common cold and other respiratory allergies. Helps drainage of the bronchial tubes by thinning the mucus.

CONTRAINDICATIONS

This product is contraindicated in patients with a known hypersensitivity to any of its ingredients. Also contraindicated in patients with severe hypertension, severe coronary artery disease and patients on MAO inhibitor therapy. Should not be used during pregnancy or in nursing mothers. Considerable caution should be exercised in patients with hypertension, diabetes mellitus, ischemic heart disease, hyperthyroidism, increased intraocular pressure and prostatic hypertrophy. The elderly (60 years or older) are more likely to exhibit adverse reactions. At dosages higher than the recommended dose, nervousness, dizziness or sleeplessness may occur.

PRECAUTIONS

General: Caution should be exercised in patients with high blood pressure, heart disease, diabetes or thyroid disease and in patients who exhibit difficulty in urination due to enlargement of the prostate gland. Check with a physician if symptoms do not improve within 7 days or if accompanied by high fever, rash or persistent headache.
Drug Interactions: Do not take this product if you are presently taking a prescription drug for high blood pressure or depression, without first consulting a physician. MAO inhibitors and beta adrenergic blockers may increase the effect of sympathomimetics. Sympathomimetics may reduce the antihypertensive effects of methyldopa, mecamylamine, reserpine and veratrum alkaloids. Pseudoephedrine hydrochloride may increase the possibility of cardiac arrhythmias in patients presently taking digitalis glycosides.
Pregnancy: Pregnancy Catagory B. It has been shown that pseudoephedrine hydrochloride can cause reduced average weight, length, and rate of skeletal ossification in the animal fetus.
Nursing Mothers: Pseudoephedrine is excreted in breast milk; use by nursing mother is not recommended because of the higher than usual risk of side effects from sympathomimetic amines for infants, especially newborn and premature infants.
Geriatrics: Pseudoephedrine should be used with caution in the elderly because they may be more sensitive to the effects of the sympathomimetics.

WARNINGS

Do not take this product for persistent or chronic cough such as occurs with smoking, asthma, or emphysema, or where cough is accompanied by excessive secretions except under the advice and supervision of a physician. This medication should be taken a few hours prior to bedtime to minimize the possibility of sleeplessness. Take this medication with a glass of water after each dose, to help loosen mucus in the lungs.

ADVERSE REACTIONS

Adverse reactions include nausea, cardiac palpitations, increased irritability or excitement, headache, dizziness, tachycardia, diarrhea, drowsiness, stomach pain, seizures, slowed heart rate, shortness of breath and/or troubled breathing.

OVERDOSAGE

KEEP THIS AND ALL DRUGS OUT OF THE REACH OF CHILDREN. IN CASE OF SUSPECTED OVERDOSE, IMMEDIATELY CALL YOUR REGIONAL POISON CONTROL CENTER and/or SEEK PROFESSIONAL ASSISTANCE.
Symptoms of overdosage may be caused by pseudoephedrine. Symptoms of overdosage with pseudoephedrine include anxiety, tenseness, respiratory difficulty, headache and awareness of the slow forceful heartbeat.

TREATMENT OF OVERDOSE

The stomach should be emptied promptly by emetics and/or gastric lavage. The installation of activated charcoal also should be considered. Cardiac function and serum electrolytes should be monitored and treatment instigated if indicated. If convulsions or marked CNS excitement occurs, diazepam may be used.

DOSAGE AND ADMINISTRATION

GUAIFED® CAPSULES Adults and children over 12 years of age: 1 capsule every 12 hours.
GUAIFED–PD® CAPSULES Adults and children over 12 years of age: 1 or 2 capsules every 12 hours. Children 6 to 12 years of age—1 capsule every 12 hours.

HOW SUPPLIED

GUAIFED® CAPSULES Bottle of 100 (NDC 0451-4002-50) and 500 (NDC 0451-4002-60). Each capsule is coded "GUAIFED" "MURO 120-250".
GUAIFED–PD® CAPSULES Bottle of 100 (NDC 0451-4003-50) and 500 (NDC 0451-4003-60). Each capsule is coded "GUAIFED-PD" "MURO 60-300".
Dispense in tight containers as defined in USP. Store at controlled room temperature, between 15°–30°C (59°–86°F).
Dispense in child resistant container.
Keep this and all drugs out of reach of children.
CAUTION: FEDERAL (U.S.A.) LAW PROHIBITS DISPENSING WITHOUT A PRESCRIPTION.

IOTUSS® LIQUID   Ⓒ ℞
[ī'ō-tŭs]

Each teaspoonful contains:
Iodinated glycerol, 30 mg (15 mg organically bound iodine), codeine phosphate, (Warning: may be habit forming), 10 mg.

HOW SUPPLIED
NDC 0451-6500-16—16 fl. oz. (473mL)

IOTUSS–DM® LIQUID   ℞
[ī'ō-tŭs]

Each teaspoonful contains:
Iodinated glycerol, 30 mg (15 mg organically bound iodine), dextromethorphan hydrobromide, 10 mg.

HOW SUPPLIED
NDC 0451-8200-16—16 fl. oz. (473 mL)

LIQUID PRED® SYRUP   ℞

Each teaspoonful contains:
Prednisone 5mg/5mL

HOW SUPPLIED
NDC-0451-1201-04–4 fl. oz. (120 mL)
NDC-0451-1201-08–8 fl. oz. (240 mL)

PRELONE® SYRUP   ℞
(Prednisolone 5 mg and 15 mg per 5 mL)

Each 5 mL of *PRELONE* Syrup contains **5 mg** or **15 mg** of prednisolone for oral administration. Benzoic acid 0.1% is added as a preservative. It also contains: citric acid, edetate disodium, glycerin, propylene glycol, purified water, sodium saccharin, (sorbitol in 5mg dosage) sucrose in 15 mg dosage) artificial flavor. The **15 mg** dosage of PRELONE SYRUP also contains FD&C blue #1 and red #40, and alcohol 5%.

HOW SUPPLIED
PRELONE Syrup containing **5 mg** of Prednisolone in each 5 mL (teaspoonful) is dye-free, grape flavored clear liquid and is supplied in 120 mL and 240 mL bottles. NDC #0451-2205-04 and 0451-2205-08 respectively.
PRELONE Syrup containing **15 mg** of Prednisolone in each 5 mL (teaspoonful) is red, cherry flavored clear liquid and is supplied in 240 mL bottles. NDC #0451-1500-08.

SALINEX NASAL MIST AND DROPS
[sal'i-nĕx]
(Buffered isotonic sodium chloride solution)

(See PDR For Nonprescription Drugs)

Mylan Pharmaceuticals Inc.
781 CHESTNUT RIDGE ROAD
P.O. BOX 4310
MORGANTOWN, WV 26505-4310

The following list of Mylan products is provided to facilitate identification. It includes the color(s) and identification codes for all tablets and capsules.

PRODUCT GENERIC NAME Description Color(s)	IDENTIFICATION CODE (Front/Back*)
ALLOPURINOL Tablets, USP, 100 mg. ℞ White	M31/Blank
ALLOPURINOL Tablets, USP, 300 mg. ℞ White	M71/Blank
AMITRIPTYLINE HYDROCHLORIDE Tablets, USP, 10 mg. ℞ Pink	M77/Blank
AMITRIPTYLINE HYDROCHLORIDE Tablets, USP, 25 mg. ℞ Lt. Green	M51/Blank
AMITRIPTYLINE HYDROCHLORIDE Tablets, USP, 50 mg. ℞ Brown	M36/Blank
AMITRIPTYLINE HYDROCHLORIDE Tablets, USP, 75 mg. ℞ Purple	M37/Blank
AMITRIPTYLINE HYDROCHLORIDE Tablets, USP, 100 mg. ℞ Orange	M38/Blank
AMITRIPTYLINE HYDROCHLORIDE Tablets, USP, 150 mg. ℞ Flesh	M39/Blank
AMOXICILLIN TRIHYDRATE Capsules, USP, 250 mg. ℞ Caramel & Buff	MYLAN 204
AMOXICILLIN TRIHYDRATE Capsules, USP, 500 mg. ℞ Buff & Buff	MYLAN 205
AMOXICILLIN TRIHYDRATE for Oral Suspension, USP, 125 mg./5 ml. ℞	—
AMOXICILLIN TRIHYDRATE for Oral Suspension, USP, 250 mg./5 ml. ℞	—
AMPICILLIN TRIHYDRATE Capsules, USP, 250 mg. ℞ Scarlet & Lt. Gray	MYLAN 115
AMPICILLIN TRIHYDRATE Capsules, USP, 500 mg. ℞ Scarlet & Lt. Gray	MYLAN 116
AMPICILLIN TRIHYDRATE for Oral Suspension, USP, 125 mg./5 ml. ℞	—
AMPICILLIN TRIHYDRATE for Oral Suspension, USP, 250 mg./5 ml. ℞	—
CHLORDIAZEPOXIDE and AMITRIPTYLINE HYDROCHLORIDE Tablets, USP, 5 mg./12.5 mg. Ⓒ/℞ Green	MYLAN/211
CHLORDIAZEPOXIDE and AMITRIPTYLINE HYDROCHLORIDE Tablets, USP, 10 mg./25 mg. Ⓒ/℞ White	MYLAN/277
CHLOROTHIAZIDE Tablets, USP, 250 mg. ℞ White	MYLAN 150/250
CHLOROTHIAZIDE Tablets, USP, 500 mg. ℞ White	MYLAN 162/Blank
CHLORPROPAMIDE Tablets, USP, 100 mg. ℞ Green	MYLAN 197/100
CHLORPROPAMIDE Tablets, USP, 250 mg. ℞ Green	MYLAN 210/250
CHLORTHALIDONE Tablets, USP, 25 mg. ℞ Lt. Yellow	MYLAN 222/25
CHLORTHALIDONE Tablets, USP, 50 mg. ℞ Lt. Green	MYLAN 213/50
CLONIDINE HYDROCHLORIDE Tablets, USP, 0.1 mg. ℞ White	MYLAN 152/Blank

CLONIDINE HYDROCHLORIDE	MYLAN 186/Blank
Tablets, USP, 0.2 mg. ℞	
White	
CLONIDINE HYDROCHLORIDE	MYLAN 199/Blank
Tablets, USP, 0.3 mg. ℞	
White	
CLONIDINE HYDROCHLORIDE and	M1/Blank
CHLORTHALIDONE	
Tablets, USP, 0.1 mg./15 mg. ℞	
Yellow	
CLONIDINE HYDROCHLORIDE and	M27/Blank
CHLORTHALIDONE	
Tablets, USP, 0.2 mg./15 mg. ℞	
Yellow	
CLONIDINE HYDROCHLORIDE and	M72/Blank
CHLORTHALIDONE	
Tablets, USP, 0.3 mg./15 mg. ℞	
Yellow	
CLORAZEPATE DIPOTASSIUM	M30/Blank
Tablets, 3.75 mg. ℂ/℞	
Blue	
CLORAZEPATE DIPOTASSIUM	M40/Blank
Tablets, 7.5 mg. ℂ/℞	
Peach	
CLORAZEPATE DIPOTASSIUM	M70/Blank
Tablets, 15 mg. ℂ/℞	
Pink	
CYPROHEPTADINE HYDROCHLORIDE	MYLAN 100/4
Tablets, USP, 4 mg. ℞	
White	
DIAZEPAM	MYLAN 271/Scored
Tablets, USP, 2 mg. ℂ/℞	
White	
DIAZEPAM	MYLAN 345/Scored
Tablets, USP, 5 mg. ℂ/℞	
Orange	
DIAZEPAM	MYLAN 477/Scored
Tablets, USP, 10 mg. ℂ/℞	
Green	
DIPHENOXYLATE HYDRO-	MYLAN 415/Blank
CHLORIDE and ATROPINE SULFATE	
Tablets, USP, 2.5 mg./0.025 mg. ℂ/℞	
White	
DOXEPIN HYDROCHLORIDE	MYLAN 1049
Capsules, USP, 10 mg. ℞	
Buff & Buff	
DOXEPIN HYDROCHLORIDE	MYLAN 3125
Capsules, USP, 25 mg. ℞	
Ivory & White	
DOXEPIN HYDROCHLORIDE	MYLAN 4250
Capsules, USP, 50 mg. ℞	
Ivory & Ivory	
DOXEPIN HYDROCHLORIDE	MYLAN 5375
Capsules, USP, 75 mg. ℞	
Brt. Lt. Green & Brt. Lt. Green	
DOXEPIN HYDROCHLORIDE	MYLAN 6410
Capsules, USP, 100 mg. ℞	
Brt. Lt. Green & White	
DOXYCYCLINE HYCLATE	MYLAN 145
Capsules, USP, 50 mg. ℞	
Aqua Blue & White	
DOXYCYCLINE HYCLATE	MYLAN 148
Capsules, USP, 100 mg. ℞	
Aqua Blue & Aqua Blue	
DOXYCYCLINE HYCLATE	MYLAN 167/100
Tablets, USP, 100 mg. ℞	
Beige	
ERYTHROMYCIN ETHYLSUCCINATE	M400/Blank
Tablets, USP, 400 mg. ℞	
Beige	
ERYTHROMYCIN STEARATE	MYLAN 106/250
Tablets, USP, 250 mg. ℞	
Pink	
ERYTHROMYCIN STEARATE	MYLAN 107/500
Tablets, USP, 500 mg. ℞	
Pink	
FENOPROFEN CALCIUM	M471/Blank
Tablets, USP, 600 mg. ℞	
Orange	
FLUPHENAZINE HYDROCHLORIDE	M/4
Tablets, USP, 1 mg. ℞	
Pink	
FLUPHENAZINE HYDROCHLORIDE	M/9
Tablets, USP, 2.5 mg. ℞	
Yellow	
FLUPHENAZINE HYDROCHLORIDE	M/74
Tablets, USP, 5 mg. ℞	
Green	
FLUPHENAZINE HYDROCHLORIDE	M/97
Tablets, USP, 10 mg. ℞	
Pink	
FLURAZEPAM HYDROCHLORIDE	MYLAN 4415
Capsules, USP, 15 mg. ℂ/℞	
White & Powder Blue	

FLURAZEPAM HYDROCHLORIDE	MYLAN 4430
Capsules, USP, 30 mg. ℂ/℞	
Powder Blue & Powder Blue	
FUROSEMIDE	MYLAN 208/20
Tablets, USP, 20 mg. ℞	
White	
FUROSEMIDE	MYLAN 216/40
Tablets, USP, 40 mg. ℞	
White	
FUROSEMIDE	MYLAN 232/80
Tablets, USP, 80 mg. ℞	
White	
HALOPERIDOL	MYLAN 351/Scored
Tablets, USP, 0.5 mg. ℞	
Orange	
HALOPERIDOL	MYLAN 257/Scored
Tablets, USP, 1.0 mg. ℞	
Orange	
HALOPERIDOL	MYLAN 214/Scored
Tablets, USP, 2 mg. ℞	
Orange	
HALOPERIDOL	MYLAN 327/Scored
Tablets, USP, 5 mg. ℞	
Orange	
IBUPROFEN	MYLAN/401
Tablets, USP, 400 mg. ℞	
White	
IBUPROFEN	MYLAN/601
Tablets, USP, 600 mg. ℞	
White	
IBUPROFEN	MYLAN/801
Tablets, USP, 800 mg. ℞	
White	
INDOMETHACIN	MYLAN 143
Capsules, USP, 25 mg. ℞	
Lt. Green & Lt. Green	
INDOMETHACIN	MYLAN 147
Capsules, USP, 50 mg. ℞	
Lt. Green & Lt. Green	
LORAZEPAM	M/321
Tablets, USP, 0.5 mg. ℂ/℞	
White	
LORAZEPAM	MYLAN 457/Blank
Tablets, USP, 1.0 mg. ℂ/℞	
White	
LORAZEPAM	MYLAN 777/Blank
Tablets, USP, 2.0 mg ℂ/℞	
White	
MAPROTILINE HYDROCHLORIDE	M/60
Tablets, USP, 25 mg. ℞	
White	
MAPROTILINE HYDROCHLORIDE	M/87
Tablets, USP, 50 mg. ℞	
Blue	
MAPROTILINE HYDROCHLORIDE	M/92
Tablets, USP, 75 mg. ℞	
White	
MECLOFENAMATE SODIUM	MYLAN 2150
Capsules, USP, 50 mg. ℞	
Coral & Coral	
MECLOFENAMATE SODIUM	MYLAN 3000
Capsules, USP, 100 mg. ℞	
Coral & White	
METHYCLOTHIAZIDE	M29/Blank
Tablets, USP, 5 mg. ℞	
Blue	
METHYLDOPA	MYLAN/611
Tablets, USP, 250 mg. ℞	
Beige	
METHYLDOPA	MYLAN/421
Tablets, USP, 500 mg. ℞	
Beige	
METHYLDOPA	MYLAN/507
and HYDROCHLOROTHIAZIDE	
Tablets, USP, 250 mg./15 mg. ℞	
Green	
METHYLDOPA	MYLAN/711
and HYDROCHLOROTHIAZIDE	
Tablets, USP, 250 mg./25 mg. ℞	
White	
PENICILLIN V POTASSIUM	MYLAN 111/250
Tablets (Oval), USP, 250 mg. ℞	
White	
PENICILLIN V POTASSIUM	MYLAN 195/250
Tablets (Round), USP, 250 mg. ℞	
White	
PENICILLIN V POTASSIUM	MYLAN 198/500
Tablets (Oval), USP, 500 mg. ℞	
White	
PENICILLIN V POTASSIUM	MYLAN 112/500
Tablets (Round), USP, 500 mg. ℞	
White	
PENICILLIN V POTASSIUM	—
For Oral Solution, USP, 125 mg./5 ml. ℞	
PENICILLIN V POTASSIUM	—
For Oral Solution, USP, 250 mg./5 ml. ℞	

PERPHENAZINE & AMITRIPTYLINE	MYLAN/330
HYDROCHLORIDE	
Tablets, USP, 2 mg./10 mg. ℞	
White	
PERPHENAZINE & AMITRIPTYLINE	MYLAN/442
HYDROCHLORIDE	
Tablets, USP, 2 mg./25 mg. ℞	
Purple	
PERPHENAZINE & AMITRIPTYLINE	MYLAN/727
HYDROCHLORIDE	
Tablets, USP, 4 mg./10 mg. ℞	
Blue	
PERPHENAZINE & AMITRIPTYLINE	MYLAN/574
HYDROCHLORIDE	
Tablets, USP, 4 mg./25 mg. ℞	
Orange	
PERPHENAZINE & AMITRIPTYLINE	MYLAN/73
HYDROCHLORIDE	
Tablets, USP, 4 mg./50 mg. ℞	
Purple	
PRAZOSIN HYDROCHLORIDE	MYLAN 1101
Capsules, USP, 1 mg. ℞	
Dk. Green/Brown	
PRAZOSIN HYDROCHLORIDE	MYLAN 2302
Capsules, USP, 2 mg. ℞	
Brown/Brown	
PRAZOSIN HYDROCHLORIDE	MYLAN 3205
Capsules, USP, 5 mg. ℞	
Lt. Blue/Brown	
PROBENECID	MYLAN 156/500
Tablets, USP. 500 mg. ℞	
Yellow	
PROPOXYPHENE HYDROCHLORIDE	MYLAN/130
and ACETAMINOPHEN	
Tablets, USP, 65 mg./ 650 mg. ℂ/℞	
Reddish Orange	
PROPOXYPHENE NAPSYLATE	MYLAN/155
and ACETAMINOPHEN	
Tablets, USP, 100 mg./650 mg. ℂ/℞	
Pink	
PROPOXYPHENE NAPSYLATE	MYLAN/521
and ACETAMINOPHEN	
Tablets, USP, 100 mg./650 mg. ℂ/℞	
White	
PROPRANOLOL HYDROCHLORIDE	MYLAN 182/10
Tablets, USP, 10 mg. ℞	
Orange	
PROPRANOLOL HYDROCHLORIDE	MYLAN 183/20
Tablets, USP, 20 mg. ℞	
Blue	
PROPRANOLOL HYDROCHLORIDE	MYLAN 184/40
Tablets, USP, 40 mg. ℞	
Green	
PROPRANOLOL HYDROCHLORIDE	MYLAN 187/60
Tablets, USP, 60 mg. ℞	
Pink	
PROPRANOLOL HYDROCHLORIDE	MYLAN 185/80
Tablets, USP, 80 mg. ℞	
Yellow	
PROPRANOLOL HYDROCHLO-	MYLAN 731/Scored
RIDE and HYDROCHLOROTHIAZIDE	
Tablets, 40 mg./25 mg. ℞	
White	
PROPRANOLOL HYDROCHLO-	MYLAN 347/Scored
RIDE and HYDROCHLOROTHIAZIDE	
Tablets, 80 mg./25 mg. ℞	
White	
RESERPINE	MYLAN 175/Blank
and CHLOROTHIAZIDE	
Tablets, USP, 0.125 mg./250 mg. ℞	
Lt. Orange	
RESERPINE	MYLAN 176/Blank
and CHLOROTHIAZIDE	
Tablets, USP, 0.125 mg./500 mg. ℞	
Lt. Orange	
SPIRONOLACTONE	MYLAN 146/25
Tablets, USP, 25 mg. ℞	
White	
SPIRONOLACTONE and	MYLAN 141/Blank
HYDROCHLOROTHIAZIDE	
Tablets, 25 mg./25 mg. ℞	
Ivory	
TEMAZEPAM	MYLAN 4010
Capsules, 15 mg. ℂ/℞	
Peach & Peach	
TEMAZEPAM	MYLAN 5050
Capsules, 30 mg. ℂ/℞	
Yellow & Yellow	
TETRACYCLINE HYDROCHLORIDE	MYLAN 101
Capsules, USP, 250 mg. ℞	
Medium Orange & Yellow	
TETRACYCLINE HYDROCHLORIDE	MYLAN 102
Capsules, USP, 500 mg. ℞	
Black & Yellow	

Continued on next page

Mylan—Cont.

THIORIDAZINE HYDROCHLORIDE Tablets, USP, 10 mg. ℞ *Orange*	M54/10
THIORIDAZINE HYDROCHLORIDE Tablets, USP, 25 mg. ℞ *Orange*	M58/25
THIORIDAZINE HYDROCHLORIDE Tablets, USP, 50 mg. ℞ *Orange*	M59/50
THIORIDAZINE HYDROCHLORIDE Tablets, USP, 100 mg. ℞ *Orange*	M61/100
THIOTHIXENE Capsules, USP, 1 mg. ℞ *Caramel & Powder Blue*	MYLAN 1001
THIOTHIXENE Capsules, USP, 2 mg. ℞ *Caramel & Yellow*	MYLAN 2002
THIOTHIXENE Capsules, USP, 5 mg. ℞ *Caramel & White*	MYLAN 3005
THIOTHIXENE Capsules, USP, 10 mg. ℞ *Caramel & Peach*	MYLAN 5010
TOLAZAMIDE Tablets, USP, 250 mg. ℞ *White*	MYLAN 217/250
TOLAZAMIDE Tablets, USP, 500 mg. ℞ *White*	MYLAN 551/Blank
TOLBUTAMIDE Tablets, USP, 500 mg. ℞ *White*	MYLAN 215/500
VERAPAMIL Tablets, USP, 80 mg. ℞ *White*	MYLAN 512/Blank
VERAPAMIL Tablets, USP, 120 mg. ℞ *White*	MYLAN 772/Blank

*Front/Back Side for Tablets
or Left and Right Side
for Capsules.

Natren, Inc.
10935 CAMARILLO STREET
NORTH HOLLYWOOD, CA 91602

BIFIDO FACTOR™
(bifidobacterium bifidum)

(See PDR For Nonprescription Drugs)

BULGARICUM I.B.™
(lactobacillus bulgaricus)

(See PDR For Nonprescription Drugs)

LIFE START®
(bifidobacterium infantis)

(See PDR For Nonprescription Drugs)

M.F.A.™ Milk Free Acidophilus
(lactobacillus acidophilus)

(See PDR For Nonprescription Drugs)

SUPERDOPHILUS®
(lactobacillus acidophilus)

(See PDR For Nonprescription Drugs)

Products are cross-indexed by
generic and chemical names
in the
YELLOW SECTION

Nature's Bounty, Inc.
90 ORVILLE DRIVE
BOHEMIA, NY 11716

ENER-B®
Intra-nasal Vitamin B-12 Gel
Dietary Supplement

DESCRIPTION
ENER-B® is the first intra-nasal application for Vitamin B-12. Each delivery supplies 400 mcg. of Vitamin B-12. This method of delivery provides the highest Vitamin B-12 blood levels that can be obtained without a prescription. Clinical tests show that ENER-B produced 8.4 to 10 times more Vitamin B-12 in the blood than tablets.

Measured Vitamin B-12 Increase in Blood Levels

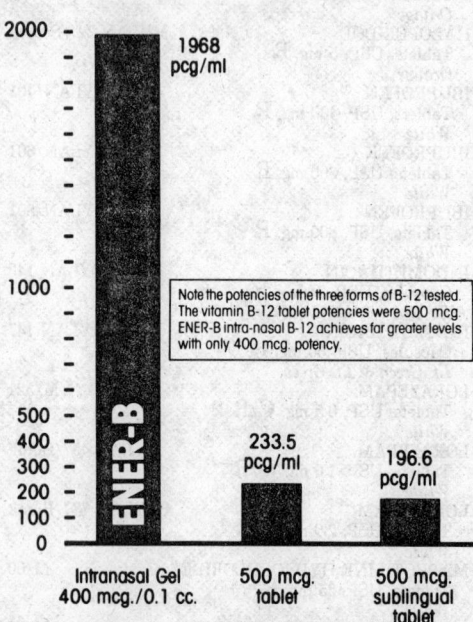

Note the potencies of the three forms of B-12 tested. The vitamin B-12 tablet potencies were 500 mcg. ENER-B intra-nasal B-12 achieves far greater levels with only 400 mcg. potency.

Intranasal Gel 400 mcg./0.1 cc.	500 mcg. tablet	500 mcg. sublingual tablet
1968 pcg/ml	233.5 pcg/ml	196.6 pcg/ml
Maximum blood levels achieved in 1.6 hours	Maximum B-12 blood levels in 25.6 hours	Maximum B-12 blood levels in 5.7 hours

Clinical Test results are available by writing Nature's Bounty.

POTENCY AND ADMINISTRATION
Each nasal applicator delivers $\frac{1}{10}$ cc of gel into the nose which adheres to the mucous membranes providing 400 mcg. of Vitamin B-12. Odorless and non-irritating to the nose.

DIRECTIONS
As a dietary supplement, one unit every two to three days.

HOW SUPPLIED
Packages of 12 unit doses. Supplies 400 mcg. of B-12 each.

Nordisk-USA
3202 TOWER OAKS BLVD.
SUITE 100
ROCKVILLE, MD 20852

HUMAN AND PURIFIED PORK INSULIN PRODUCTS

INSULATARD® NPH
[in 'sŭl-ă''tard nph]
U-100 Purified Pork, Purified Pork insulin isophane
suspension.

DESCRIPTION
Insulatard NPH insulin is produced from the pork insulin molecule and has low immunogenic potential. Insulatard NPH contains no excess protamine and can be mixed reliably with Nordisk Velosulin without altering the time course of either component insulin. The resultant mixtures (NPH & Regular) impose no usage restrictions on the mixer or user regarding the timing of the injection of the combination of insulins.

Insulatard® NPH is a suspension of protamine insulin crystals. It has a slower onset of action than Velosulin® (Regular) Insulin. The effect on the blood sugar begins approximately 1½ hours after the injection and lasts up to approximately 24 hours, having its maximum effect between the 4th and 12th hour.

The time course of action of any insulin may vary considerably in different individuals, or at different times in the same individual. Because of this variation, the time periods listed here should be considered as general guidelines only.

Insulin is an anabolic hormone. Its action is primarily concerned with the metabolism of carbohydrates, but also affects protein and fat metabolism. Insulin facilitates the cellular uptake of glucose and its metabolism in insulin-responsive tissue (e.g. liver, muscle, adipose, and nervous tissue). Insulin also inhibits the breakdown of fat, the production of ketones and increases the uptake of amino acids. The administration of the proper doses of insulin to patients with abnormal or absent beta cell function (reduced capacity, abnormal responsiveness or inability to produce endogenous insulin) restores the patient's ability to metabolize glucose and establish near normal carbohydrate, fat, and protein metabolism.

MAJOR USES
Insulatard NPH is indicated in the treatment of insulin-requiring diabetes mellitus. The route of administration of Insulatard NPH is via subcutaneous injection.

SAFETY INFORMATION
Insulatard NPH is a safe and an appropriate insulin to use or dispense for the diabetic patient when NPH insulin is indicated. As with any insulin product in achieving glycemic control, careful monitoring and changes in daily dosage or timing of injections may be necessary.

WARNING
ANY CHANGE OF INSULIN SHOULD BE MADE CAUTIOUSLY ONLY UNDER MEDICAL SUPERVISION. WHEN CHANGING TO PURIFIED PORK INSULIN FROM ANY OTHER INSULIN A DOSAGE ADJUSTMENT, IF ANY, IS LIKELY TO BE A REDUCTION TO AVOID HYPOGLYCEMIA. CHANGES IN PURITY, STRENGTH (U-40, U-80, U-100), BRAND (MANUFACTURER), TYPE (LENTE, NPH, REGULAR, ETC.) AND/ OR SPECIES SOURCE (BEEF, PORK, BEEF/ PORK) MAY RESULT IN THE NEED FOR A CHANGE IN DOSAGE. IT IS NOT POSSIBLE TO IDENTIFY WHICH PATIENTS WILL REQUIRE A REDUCTION IN DOSAGE TO AVOID HYPOGLYCEMIA WHEN USING THIS INSULIN. ADJUSTMENT MAY BE NEEDED WITH THE FIRST DOSE OR OVER A PERIOD OF SEVERAL WEEKS. (SEE DOSAGE ADJUSTMENT SECTION). BE AWARE OF THE POSSIBILITY OF SYMPTOMS OF EITHER HYPOGLYCEMIA OR HYPERGLYCEMIA. SEE SECTIONS ENTITLED INSULIN REACTION AND HYPERGLYCEMIA.

INSULIN USE IN DIABETES
Your physician has explained that you have diabetes and that your treatment involves injections of insulin. Insulin is normally produced by the pancreas, a gland that lies behind the stomach. Without insulin, glucose (a simple sugar made from digested food) is trapped in the bloodstream and cannot enter the cells of the body. Some patients who don't make enough of their own insulin, or who cannot use the insulin they do make properly, must take insulin by injection in order to control their blood glucose levels.

Each case of diabetes is different and requires direct and continued medical supervision. Your physician has told you the type, strength and amount of insulin you should use and the time(s) at which you should inject it, and has also discussed with you a diet and exercise schedule. You should contact your physician if you experience any difficulties or if you have questions.

TYPES OF INSULINS
Standard and purified animal insulins as well as human insulins are available. Standard and purified insulins differ in their degree of purification and content of noninsulin material. Standard and purified insulins also vary in species source: they may be of beef, pork, or mixed beef and pork origin. Human insulin is identical in structure to the insulin produced by the human pancreas, and thus differs from animal insulins. Insulins vary in time of action and in strength; see PRODUCT DESCRIPTION and SYRINGES for additional information.

Your physician has prescribed the insulin that is right for you; be sure you have purchased the correct insulin and check it carefully before you use it.

MIXING TWO TYPES OF INSULIN
Different insulins should be mixed only under instruction from a physician. Hypodermic syringes may vary in the amount of space between the bottom line and the needle ("dead space"), so if you are mixing two types of insulin be sure to discuss any change in the model and brand of syringe you are using with your physician or pharmacist. When you are mixing two types of insulin, always draw the Regular (clear) insulin into the syringe first.

SYRINGES

Use the correct syringe

The volume of the dose depends on the number of units of insulin per ml. Insulatard® NPH Human is only available in the U-100 strength (100 units per ml). Make sure that you understand the markings on your syringe and use only a syringe marked for U-100.

Disposable Syringes

Disposable syringes and needles require no sterilization provided the package is intact. They should be used only once and discarded.

Reusable Syringes

Reusable syringes and needles must be sterile when used. The best method of sterilization is to boil the syringe, plunger and needle in water for 5 minutes. If this is not possible, as when travelling, the parts may be sterilized by immersion for at least 5 minutes in a sterilizing liquid like ethyl alcohol, 70%. Do not use bathing, rubbing or medicated alcohol for sterilization. Remove all liquid from the syringe by pushing the plunger in and out several times and leave it to dry if alcohol has been used for sterilization.

IMPORTANT

Failure to comply with the above and the following antiseptic measures may lead to infections at the injection site.

PREPARING THE INJECTION

Rotate the vial carefully to obtain a uniformly cloudy suspension of the crystals. Avoid heavy foaming. Do not use a vial if the insulin remains clear after it has been shaken. Also do not use it if you see lumps that float or stick to the sides.

1. Clean your hands and the injection site with soap and water or with alcohol. Wipe the rubber stopper with an alcohol swab. (Note: remove the tamper-resistant cap at first use. If the cap has already been removed, do not use this product, return it to your pharmacy.)
2. For insulin suspensions, roll the vial of insulin gently in your hands to mix it. Vigorous shaking immediately before the dose is drawn into the syringe may result in the formation of bubbles or foam which could cause dosage errors.
3. Pull back the plunger until the black tip reaches the marking for the number of units you will inject.
4. Push the needle through the rubber stopper into the vial.
5. Push the plunger all the way in. This inserts air into the bottle.
6. Turn the vial and syringe upside down and slowly pull the plunger back to a few units beyond the correct dose.
7. If there are air bubbles, flick the syringe firmly with your finger to raise the air bubbles to the needle, then slowly push the plunger to the correct unit marking.
8. Lift the vial off the syringe.

GIVING THE INJECTION

1. The following areas are suitable for subcutaneous insulin injection: thighs, upper arms, buttocks, abdomen. Do not change areas without consulting your physician. The actual point of injection should be changed each time; injection sites should be about an inch apart.
2. The injection site should be clean and dry. Pinch up skin area to be injected and hold it firmly.
3. Hold the syringe like a pencil and push the needle quickly and firmly into the pinched-up area. If you go straight in it will probably sting less. Pull back the plunger slightly. If blood comes into the syringe, the needle has entered a blood vessel. Remove the needle and make the injection in another spot.
4. If blood does not appear in the syringe, release skin and push plunger all the way in to inject insulin beneath the skin. Do not inject into a muscle unless your physician has advised it. You should never inject insulin into a vein.
5. Remove needle. If slight bleeding occurs, press lightly with a dry cotton swab for a few seconds—do not rub.

USAGE IN PREGNANCY

It is particularly important to maintain good control of your diabetes during pregnancy and special attention must be paid to your diet, exercise and insulin regimens. If you are pregnant or nursing a baby, consult your physician or nurse educator.

INSULIN REACTION

Insulin reaction (too little sugar in the blood, also called hypoglycemia) can occur if you take too much insulin, miss a meal or exercise or work harder than normal. The symptoms, which usually come on suddenly, are hunger, dizziness, and sweating. Personality change or confusion may also occur. Eating sugar or a sugar-sweetened product will normally correct the condition.

If symptoms persist, call a physician; an insulin reaction can lead to unconsciousness. If a reaction results in loss of consciousness, emergency medical care should be obtained immediately. If you have had repeated reactions or if an insulin reaction has led to a loss of consciousness, contact your physician.

DIABETIC KETOACIDOSIS AND COMA

Diabetic ketoacidosis may develop if your body has too little insulin. The most common causes are acute illness or infection or failure to take enough insulin by injection. If you are ill, you should check your urine for ketones. The symptoms of diabetic ketoacidosis usually come on gradually, over a period of hours or days, and include a drowsy feeling, flushed face, thirst and loss of appetite. Notify a physician immediately if the urine test is positive for ketones (acetone) or if you have any of these symptoms. More severe symptoms are fast, heavy breathing and rapid pulse; if these symptoms occur, you should have medical attention right away.

ADVERSE REACTIONS

Insulin allergy occurs very rarely, but when it does, it may cause a serious reaction including a general skin rash over the body, shortness of breath, fast pulse, sweating, and a drop in blood pressure. If any of these symptoms develop you should seek emergency medical care.

In a very few diabetics, the skin where insulin has been injected may become red, swollen and itchy. This is called a local reaction. It may occur if the injection is not properly made, if the skin is sensitive to the cleansing solution or if the patient is allergic to insulin. If you have a local reaction, notify your physician.

Patients with severe systemic allergic reactions to insulin (i.e. generalized urticaria, angioedema, anaphylaxis) should be skin tested with each new preparation to be used prior to initiation of therapy with that preparation.

IMPORTANT NOTES

1. A change in the type, strength, species or purity of insulin could require a dosage adjustment. Any change in insulin should be made under medical supervision.
2. You may have learned how to test your urine or your blood for glucose. It is important to do these tests regularly and to record the results for review with your physician or nurse educator.
3. If you have an acute illness, especially with vomiting or fever, continue taking your insulin. If possible, stay on your regular diet. If you have trouble eating, drink fruit juices, regular soft drinks, or clear soups; if you can, eat small amounts of bland foods. Test your urine for glucose and ketones and, if possible, test your blood glucose. Note the results and contact your physician for possible insulin dose adjustment. If you have severe and prolonged vomiting, seek emergency medical care.
4. You should always carry identification which states that you have diabetes.

Always consult your physician if you have any questions about your condition or the use of insulin.

Helpful information for people with diabetes is published by American Diabetes Association, 1660 Duke St., Alexandria, VA 22314.

HOW SUPPLIED

10 ml vials
100 units per ml.
NDC # 50445-200-01
Brochures, Time Action Profile Charts, Samples—Free to Physicians.

INSULATARD® NPH HUMAN

[in 'sŭl-ă "tard nph hyōō 'men]
U-100 Human, Human insulin isophane suspension (semi-synthetic)

DESCRIPTION

Insulatard NPH Human insulin is produced semi-synthetically by enzymatic conversion of the pork insulin molecule and has low immunogenic potential. Insulatard NPH Human contains no excess protamine and can be mixed reliably with Velosulin Human without altering the time course of either component insulin. The resultant mixtures (NPH & Regular) impose no usage restrictions on the mixer or user regarding the timing of the injection of the combination of insulins. Insulatard NPH Human and Velosulin Human may be mixed in the same syringe without loss of effectiveness, whether used immediately or used over extended periods of time (five minutes, two days, two weeks).

Insulatard® NPH Human is a suspension of protamine insulin crystals. It has a slower onset of action than Velosulin® Human (Regular) Insulin. The effect on the blood sugar begins approximately $1\frac{1}{2}$ hours after the injection and lasts up to approximately 24 hours, having its maximum effect between the 4th and 12th hour.

The time course of action of any insulin may vary considerably in different individuals, or at different times in the same individual. Because of this variation, the time periods listed here should be considered as general guidelines only.

Insulin is an anabolic hormone. Its action is primarily concerned with the metabolism of carbohydrates, but also affects protein and fat metabolism. Insulin facilitates the cellular uptake of glucose and its metabolism in insulin-responsive tissue (e.g. liver, muscle, adipose, and nervous tissue).

Insulin also inhibits the breakdown of fat, the production of ketones and increases the uptake of amino acids. The administration of the proper doses of insulin to patients with abnormal or absent beta cell function (reduced capacity, abnormal responsiveness or inability to produce endogenous insulin) restores the patient's ability to metabolize glucose and establish near normal carbohydrate, fat, and protein metabolism.

WARNING

Any change of insulin should be made cautiously and only under medical supervision. Changes in purity, strength (U-40, U-80, U-100), brand (manufacturer), type (lente, NPH, regular, etc.) and/or species source (beef, pork, beef/pork, human) may result in the need for a change in dosage. Adjustment may be needed with the first dose or over a period of several weeks.

Be aware that symptoms of hypoglycemia (low blood glucose) or hyperglycemia (high blood glucose) may indicate the need for dosage adjustment. Please read sections entitled "Insulin Reaction" and "Diabetic Ketoacidosis and Coma".

INSULIN USE IN DIABETES

Your physician has explained that you have diabetes and that your treatment involves injections of insulin. Insulin is normally produced by the pancreas, a gland that lies behind the stomach. Without insulin, glucose (a simple sugar made from digested food) is trapped in the bloodstream and cannot enter the cells of the body. Some patients who don't make enough of their own insulin, or who cannot use the insulin they do make properly, must take insulin by injection in order to control their blood glucose levels.

Each case of diabetes is different and requires direct and continued medical supervision. Your physician has told you the type, strength and amount of insulin you should use and the time(s) at which you should inject it, and has also discussed with you a diet and exercise schedule. You should contact your physician if you experience any difficulties or if you have questions.

TYPES OF INSULINS

Standard and purified animal insulins as well as human insulins are available. Standard and purified insulins differ in their degree of purification and content of noninsulin material. Standard and purified insulins also vary in species source: they may be of beef, pork, or mixed beef and pork origin. Human insulin is identical in structure to the insulin produced by the human pancreas, and thus differs from animals insulins. Insulins vary in time of action and in strength; see PRODUCT DESCRIPTION and SYRINGES for additional information.

Your physician has prescribed the insulin that is right for you; be sure you have purchased the correct insulin and check it carefully before you use it.

MIXING TWO TYPES OF INSULIN

Different insulins should be mixed only under instruction from a physician. Hypodermic syringes may vary in the amount of space between the bottom line and the needle ("dead space"), so if you are mixing two types of insulin be sure to discuss any change in the model and brand of syringe you are using with your physician or pharmacist. When you are mixing two types of insulin, always draw the Regular (clear) insulin into the syringe first.

SYRINGES

Use the correct syringe

The volume of the dose depends on the number of units of insulin per ml. Insulatard® NPH Human is only available in the U-100 strength (100 units per ml). Make sure that you understand the markings on your syringe and use only a syringe marked for U-100.

Disposable Syringes

Disposable syringes and needles require no sterilization provided the package is intact. They should be used only once and discarded.

Reusable Syringes

Reusable syringes and needles must be sterile when used. The best method of sterilization is to boil the syringe, plunger and needle in water for 5 minutes. If this is not possible, as when travelling, the parts may be sterilized by immersion for at least 5 minutes in a sterilizing liquid like ethyl alcohol, 70%. Do not use bathing, rubbing or medicated alcohol for sterilization. Remove all liquid from the syringe by pushing the plunger in and out several times and leave it to dry if alcohol has been used for sterilization.

IMPORTANT

Failure to comply with the above and the following antiseptic measures may lead to infections at the injection site.

PREPARING THE INJECTION

Rotate the vial carefully to obtain a uniformly cloudy suspension of the crystals. Avoid heavy foaming. Do not use a vial if the insulin remains clear after it has been shaken. Also do not use it if you see lumps that float or stick to the sides.

Continued on next page

Nordisk-USA—Cont.

1. Clean your hands and the injection site with soap and water or with alcohol. Wipe the rubber stopper with an alcohol swab. (Note: remove the tamper-resistant cap at first use. If the cap has already been removed, do not use this product, return it to your pharmacy.)
2. For insulin suspensions, roll the vial of insulin gently in your hands to mix it. Vigorous shaking immediately before the dose is drawn into the syringe may result in the formation of bubbles or foam which could cause dosage errors.
3. Pull back the plunger until the black tip reaches the marking for the number of units you will inject.
4. Push the needle through the rubber stopper into the vial.
5. Push the plunger all the way in. This inserts air into the bottle.
6. Turn the vial and syringe upside down and slowly pull the plunger back to a few units beyond the correct dose.
7. If there are air bubbles, flick the syringe firmly with your finger to raise the air bubbles to the needle, then slowly push the plunger to the correct unit marking.
8. Lift the vial off the syringe.

GIVING THE INJECTION

1. The following areas are suitable for subcutaneous insulin injection: thighs, upper arms, buttocks, abdomen. Do not change areas without consulting your physician. The actual point of injection should be changed each time; injection sites should be about an inch apart.
2. The injection site should be clean and dry. Pinch up skin area to be injected and hold it firmly.
3. Hold the syringe like a pencil and push the needle quickly and firmly into the pinched-up area. If you go straight in it will probably sting less. Pull back the plunger slightly. If blood comes into the syringe, the needle has entered a blood vessel. Remove the needle and make the injection in another spot.
4. If blood does not appear in the syringe, release skin and push plunger all the way in to inject insulin beneath the skin. Do not inject into a muscle unless your physician has advised it. You should never inject insulin into a vein.
5. Remove needle. If slight bleeding occurs, press lightly with a dry cotton swab for a few seconds—do not rub.

USAGE IN PREGNANCY

It is particularly important to maintain good control of your diabetes during pregnancy and special attention must be paid to your diet, exercise and insulin regimens. If you are pregnant or nursing a baby, consult your physician or nurse educator.

INSULIN REACTION

Insulin Reaction (too little sugar in the blood, also called hypoglycemia) can occur if you take too much insulin, miss a meal or exercise or work harder than normal. The symptoms, which usually come on suddenly, are hunger, dizziness, and sweating. Personality change or confusion may also occur. Eating sugar or a sugar-sweetened product will normally correct the condition.

If symptoms persist, call a physician; an insulin reaction can lead to unconsciousness. If a reaction results in loss of consciousness, emergency medical care should be obtained immediately. If you have had repeated reactions or if an insulin reaction has led to a loss of consciousness, contact your physician.

DIABETIC KETOACIDOSIS AND COMA

Diabetic ketoacidosis may develop if your body has too little insulin. The most common causes are acute illness or infection or failure to take enough insulin by injection. If you are ill, you should check your urine for ketones. The symptoms of diabetic ketoacidosis usually come on gradually, over a period of hours or days, and include a drowsy feeling, flushed face, thirst and loss of appetite. Notify a physician immediately if the urine test is positive for ketones (acetone) or if you have any of these symptoms. More severe symptoms are fast, heavy breathing and rapid pulse; if these symptoms occur, you should have medical attention right away.

ADVERSE REACTIONS

Insulin allergy occurs very rarely, but when it does, it may cause a serious reaction including a general skin rash over the body, shortness of breath, fast pulse, sweating, and a drop in blood pressure. If any of these symptoms develop you should seek emergency medical care.

In a very few diabetics, the skin where insulin has been injected may become red, swollen and itchy. This is called a local reaction. It may occur if the injection is not properly made, if the skin is sensitive to the cleansing solution or if the patient is allergic to insulin. If you have a local reaction, notify your physician.

Patients with severe systemic allergic reactions to insulin (i.e. generalized urticaria, angioedema, anaphylaxis) should be skin tested with each new preparation to be used prior to initiation of therapy with that preparation.

IMPORTANT NOTES

1. A change in the type, strength, species or purity of insulin could require a dosage adjustment. Any change in insulin should be made under medical supervision.
2. You may have learned how to test your urine or your blood for glucose. It is important to do these tests regularly and to record the results for review with your physician or nurse educator.
3. If you have an acute illness, especially with vomiting or fever, continue taking your insulin. If possible, stay on your regular diet. If you have trouble eating, drink fruit juices, regular soft drinks, or clear soups; if you can, eat small amounts of bland foods. Test your urine for glucose and ketones and, if possible, test your blood glucose. Note the results and contact your physician for possible insulin dose adjustment. If you have severe and prolonged vomiting, seek emergency medical care.
4. You should always carry identification which states that you have diabetes.

Always consult your physician if you have any questions about your condition or the use of insulin.

Helpful information for people with diabetes is published by American Diabetes Association, 1660 Duke St., Alexandria, VA 22314.

HOW SUPPLIED

10 ml vials
100 units per ml
NDC #50445-222-01
Brochures, Time Action Profile Charts, Samples-Free to Physicians.

MIXTARD®

[mix ' tard]
U-100, 70% Isophane purified pork insulin suspension and 30% purified pork insulin injection

DESCRIPTION

MIXTARD is a standard mixture of 30% VELOSULIN (corresponding to Regular insulin) and 70% INSULATARD NPH. The content of VELOSULIN gives the preparation a rapid onset of effect on the blood sugar, approximately ½ hour after the injection.

Mixtard is produced from the pork insulin molecule and has low immunogenic potential. Mixtard is a unique and stable premixture of 30% regular acting (Velosulin) and 70% intermediate acting (Insulatard NPH) purified pork insulins for more convenient and accurate insulin administration. Mixtard provides the rapid onset (½ hour) of Regular insulin and sustained duration (up to 24 hours) of NPH insulin.

Insulin is an anabolic hormone. Its action is primarily concerned with the metabolism of carbohydrates, but also affects protein and fat metabolism. Insulin facilitates the cellular uptake of glucose and its metabolism in insulin-responsive tissue (e.g. liver, muscle, adipose, and nervous tissue). Insulin also inhibits the breakdown of fat, the production of ketones and increases the uptake of amino acids. The administration of the proper doses of insulin to patients with abnormal or absent beta cell function (reduced capacity, abnormal responsiveness or inability to produce endogenous insulin) restores the patient's ability to metabolize glucose and establish near normal carbohydrate, fat, and protein metabolism.

MAJOR USES

Mixtard is indicated in the treatment of insulin-requiring diabetes mellitus. The route of administration for Mixtard is via subcutaneous injection. Mixtard is ideal for diabetic patients who have difficulty in mixing insulins. These patients include: elderly diabetics, diabetics with impaired vision or neurologic handicaps, or those diabetic patients simply unable to follow mixing instructions.

WARNING

ANY CHANGE OF INSULIN SHOULD BE MADE CAUTIOUSLY ONLY UNDER MEDICAL SUPERVISION. WHEN CHANGING TO PURIFIED PORK INSULIN FROM ANY OTHER INSULIN A DOSAGE ADJUSTMENT, IF ANY, IS LIKELY TO BE A REDUCTION TO AVOID HYPOGLYCEMIA. CHANGES IN PURITY, STRENGTH (U-40, U-80, U-100), BRAND (MANUFACTURER), TYPE (LENTE, NPH, REGULAR, ETC.) AND/ OR SPECIES SOURCE (BEEF, PORK, BEEF/ PORK) MAY RESULT IN THE NEED FOR A CHANGE IN DOSAGE. IT IS NOT POSSIBLE TO IDENTIFY WHICH PATIENTS WILL REQUIRE A REDUCTION IN DOSAGE TO AVOID HYPOGLYCEMIA WHEN USING THIS INSULIN. ADJUSTMENT MAY BE NEEDED WITH THE FIRST DOSE OR OVER A PERIOD OF SEVERAL WEEKS. (SEE DOSAGE ADJUSTMENT SECTION). BE AWARE OF THE POSSIBILITY OF SYMPTOMS OF EITHER HYPOGLYCEMIA OR HYPERGLYCEMIA. SEE SECTIONS ENTITLED INSULIN REACTION AND HYPERGLYCEMIA.

INSULIN USE IN DIABETES

Your physician has explained that you have diabetes and that your treatment involves injections of insulin. Insulin is

normally produced by the pancreas, a gland that lies behind the stomach. Without insulin, glucose (a simple sugar made from digested food) is trapped in the bloodstream and cannot enter the cells of the body. Some patients who don't make enough of their own insulin, or who cannot use the insulin they do make properly, must take insulin by injection in order to control their blood glucose levels.

Each case of diabetes is different and requires direct and continued medical supervision. Your physician has told you the type, strength and amount of insulin you should use and the time(s) at which you should inject it, and has also discussed with you a diet and exercise schedule. You should contact your physician if you experience any difficulties or if you have questions.

TYPES OF INSULINS

Standard and purified animal insulins as well as human insulins are available. Standard and purified insulins differ in their degree of purification and content of noninsulin material. Standard and purified insulins also vary in species source: they may be of beef, pork, or mixed beef and pork origin. Human insulin is identical in structure to the insulin produced by the human pancreas, and thus differs from animals insulins. Insulins vary in time of action and in strength; see PRODUCT DESCRIPTION and SYRINGES for additional information.

Your physician has prescribed the insulin that is right for you; be sure you have purchased the correct insulin and check it carefully before you use it.

MIXING TWO TYPES OF INSULIN

Different insulins should be mixed only under instruction from a physician. Hypodermic syringes may vary in the amount of space between the bottom line and the needle ("dead space"), so if you are mixing two types of insulin be sure to discuss any change in the model and brand of syringe you are using with your physician or pharmacist. When you are mixing two types of insulin, always draw the Regular (clear) insulin into the syringe first.

SYRINGES

Use the correct syringe

The volume of the dose depends on the number of units of insulin per ml. Insulatard® NPH Human is only available in the U-100 strength (100 units per ml). Make sure that you understand the markings on your syringe and use only a syringe marked for U-100.

Disposable Syringes

Disposable syringes and needles require no sterilization provided the package is intact. They should be used only once and discarded.

Reusable Syringes

Reusable syringes and needles must be sterile when used. The best method of sterilization is to boil the syringe, plunger and needle in water for 5 minutes. If this is not possible, as when travelling, the parts may be sterilized by immersion for at least 5 minutes in a sterilizing liquid like ethyl alcohol, 70%. Do not use bathing, rubbing or medicated alcohol for sterilization. Remove all liquid from the syringe by pushing the plunger in and out several times and leave it to dry if alcohol has been used for sterilization.

IMPORTANT

Failure to comply with the above and the following antiseptic measures may lead to infections at the injection site.

PREPARING THE INJECTION

Rotate the vial carefully to obtain a uniform cloudy suspension of the crystals. Avoid heavy foaming. Do not use a vial if the insulin remains clear after it has been shaken. Also do not use it if you see lumps that float or stick to the sides.

1. Clean your hands and the injection site with soap and water or with alcohol. Wipe the rubber stopper with an alcohol swab. (Note: remove the tamper-resistant cap at first use. If the cap has already been removed, do not use this product, return it to your pharmacy.)
2. For insulin suspensions, roll the vial of insulin gently in your hands to mix it. Vigorous shaking immediately before the dose is drawn into the syringe may result in the formation of bubbles or foam which could cause dosage errors.
3. Pull back the plunger until the black tip reaches the marking for the number of units you will inject.
4. Push the needle through the rubber stopper into the vial.
5. Push the plunger all the way in. This inserts air into the bottle.
6. Turn the vial and syringe upside down and slowly pull the plunger back to a few units beyond the correct dose.
7. If there are air bubbles, flick the syringe firmly with your finger to raise the air bubbles to the needle, then slowly push the plunger to the correct unit marking.
8. Lift the vial off the syringe.

GIVING THE INJECTION

1. The following areas are suitable for subcutaneous insulin injection: thighs, upper arms, buttocks, abdomen. Do not change areas without consulting your physician. The ac-

tual point of injection should be changed each time; injection sites should be about an inch apart.

2. The injection site should be clean and dry. Pinch up skin area to be injected and hold it firmly.

3. Hold the syringe like a pencil and push the needle quickly and firmly into the pinched-up area. If you go straight in it will probably sting less. Pull back the plunger slightly. If blood comes into the syringe, the needle has entered a blood vessel. Remove the needle and make the injection in another spot.

4. If blood does not appear in the syringe, release skin and push plunger all the way in to inject insulin beneath the skin. Do not inject into a muscle unless your physician has advised it. You should never inject insulin into a vein.

5. Remove needle. If slight bleeding occurs, press lightly with a dry cotton swab for a few seconds—**do not rub.**

USAGE IN PREGNANCY

It is particularly important to maintain good control of your diabetes during pregnancy and special attention must be paid to your diet, exercise and insulin regimens. If you are pregnant or nursing a baby, consult your physician or nurse educator.

INSULIN REACTION

Insulin reaction (too little sugar in the blood, also called hypoglycemia) can occur if you take too much insulin, miss a meal or exercise or work harder than normal. The symptoms, which usually come on suddenly, are hunger, dizziness, and sweating. Personality change or confusion may also occur. Eating sugar or a sugar-sweetened product will normally correct the condition.

If symptoms persist, call a physician; an insulin reaction can lead to unconsciousness. If a reaction results in loss of consciousness, emergency medical care should be obtained immediately. If you have had repeated reactions or if an insulin reaction has led to a loss of consciousness, contact your physician.

DIABETIC KETOACIDOSIS AND COMA

Diabetic ketoacidosis may develop if your body has too little insulin. The most common causes are acute illness or infection or failure to take enough insulin by injection. If you are ill, you should check your urine for ketones. The symptoms of diabetic ketoacidosis usually come on gradually, over a period of hours or days, and include a drowsy feeling, flushed face, thirst and loss of appetite. Notify a physician immediately if the urine test is positive for ketones (acetone) or if you have any of these symptoms. More severe symptoms are fast, heavy breathing and rapid pulse; if these symptoms occur, you should have medical attention right away.

ADVERSE REACTIONS

Insulin allergy occurs very rarely, but when it does, it may cause a serious reaction including a general skin rash over the body, shortness of breath, fast pulse, sweating, and a drop in blood pressure. If any of these symptoms develop you should seek emergency medical care.

In a very few diabetics, the skin where insulin has been injected may become red, swollen and itchy. This is called a local reaction. It may occur if the injection is not properly made, if the skin is sensitive to the cleansing solution or if the patient is allergic to insulin. If you have a local reaction, notify your physician.

Patients with severe systemic allergic reactions to insulin (i.e. generalized urticaria, angioedema, anaphylaxis) should be skin tested with **each** new preparation to be used prior to initiation of therapy with that preparation.

IMPORTANT NOTES

1. A change in the type, strength, species or purity of insulin could require a dosage adjustment. Any change in insulin should be made under medical supervision.

2. You may have learned how to test your urine or your blood for glucose. It is important to do these tests regularly and to record the results for review with your physician or nurse educator.

3. If you have an acute illness, especially with vomiting or fever, continue taking your insulin. If possible, stay on your regular diet. If you have trouble eating, drink fruit juices, regular soft drinks, or clear soups; if you can, eat small amounts of bland foods. Test your urine for glucose and ketones and, if possible, test your blood glucose. Note the results and contact your physician for possible insulin dose adjustment. If you have severe and prolonged vomiting, seek emergency medical care.

4. You should always carry identification which states that you have diabetes.

Always consult your physician if you have any questions about your condition or the use of insulin.

Helpful information for people with diabetes is published by American Diabetes Association, 1660 Duke St., Alexandria, VA 22314.

HOW SUPPLIED

10 ml vials
100 units per ml.
NDC #50445-300-01
Brochures, Time Action Profile Charts, Samples - Free to physicians.

MIXTARD® HUMAN 70/30

[mix'tard hyōō'men 70/30]
U-100, 70% Human insulin isophane suspension and 30% Human insulin injection
(semi-synthetic)

DESCRIPTION

Mixtard Human 70/30 is a standard mixture of 30% Velosulin Human (corresponding to Regular insulin) and 70% Insulatard NPH Human. The content of Velosulin Human gives the preparation a rapid onset of effect on the blood sugar, approx. $\frac{1}{2}$ hour after the injection. The content of Insulatard NPH Human gives it a duration of up to 24 hours, depending on the size of the dose. The maximal effect lies between the 4th and the 8th hour after injection.

Insulin is an anabolic hormone. Its action is primarily concerned with the metabolism of carbohydrates, but also affects protein and fat metabolism. Insulin facilitates the cellular uptake of glucose and its metabolism in insulin-responsive tissue (e.g. liver, muscle, adipose, and nervous tissue). Insulin also inhibits the breakdown of fat, the production of ketones and increases the uptake of amino acids. The administration of the proper doses of insulin to patients with abnormal or absent beta cell function (reduced capacity, abnormal responsiveness or inability to produce endogenous insulin) restores the patient's ability to metabolize glucose and establish near normal carbohydrate, fat, and protein metabolism.

Mixtard Human 70/30 is indicated in the treatment of insulin-requiring diabetes mellitus. The route of administration for Mixtard Human 70/30 is via subcutaneous injection. Mixtard Human 70/30 is ideal for diabetic patients who have difficulty in mixing insulins. These patients include: elderly diabetics, diabetics with impaired vision or neurologic handicaps, or those diabetic patients simply unable to follow mixing instructions.

WARNING

ANY CHANGE OF INSULIN SHOULD BE MADE CAUTIOUSLY ONLY UNDER MEDICAL SUPERVISION. WHEN CHANGING TO PURIFIED PORK INSULIN FROM ANY OTHER INSULIN A DOSAGE ADJUSTMENT, IF ANY, IS LIKELY TO BE A REDUCTION TO AVOID HYPOGLYCEMIA. CHANGES IN PURITY, STRENGTH (U-40, U-80, U-100), BRAND (MANUFACTURER), TYPE (LENTE, NPH, REGULAR, ETC.) AND/ OR SPECIES SOURCE (BEEF, PORK, BEEF/ PORK) MAY RESULT IN THE NEED FOR A CHANGE IN DOSAGE. IT IS NOT POSSIBLE TO IDENTIFY WHICH PATIENTS WILL REQUIRE A REDUCTION IN DOSAGE TO AVOID HYPOGLYCEMIA WHEN USING THIS INSULIN. ADJUSTMENT MAY BE NEEDED WITH THE FIRST DOSE OR OVER A PERIOD OF SEVERAL WEEKS. (SEE DOSAGE ADJUSTMENT SECTION). BE AWARE OF THE POSSIBILITY OF SYMPTOMS OF EITHER HYPOGLYCEMIA OR HYPERGLYCEMIA. SEE SECTIONS ENTITLED INSULIN REACTION AND HYPERGLYCEMIA.

INSULIN USE IN DIABETES

Your physician has explained that you have diabetes and that your treatment involves injections of insulin. Insulin is normally produced by the pancreas, a gland that lies behind the stomach. Without insulin, glucose (a simple sugar made from digested food) is trapped in the bloodstream and cannot enter the cells of the body. Some patients who don't make enough of their own insulin, or who cannot use the insulin they do make properly, must take insulin by injection in order to control their blood glucose levels.

Each case of diabetes is different and requires direct and continued medical supervision. Your physician has told you the type, strength and amount of insulin you should use and the time(s) at which you should inject it, and has also discussed with you a diet and exercise schedule. You should contact your physician if you experience any difficulties or if you have questions.

TYPES OF INSULINS

Standard and purified animal insulins as well as human insulins are available. Standard and purified insulins differ in their degree of purification and content of noninsulin material. Standard and purified insulins also vary in species source: they may be of beef, pork, or mixed beef and pork origin. Human insulin is identical in structure to the insulin produced by the human pancreas, and thus differs from animal insulins. Insulins vary in time of action and in strength; see PRODUCT DESCRIPTION and SYRINGES for additional information.

Your physician has prescribed the insulin that is right for you; be sure you have purchased the correct insulin and check it carefully before you use it.

MIXING TWO TYPES OF INSULIN

Different insulins should be mixed only under instruction from a physician. Hypodermic syringes may vary in the amount of space between the bottom line and the needle ("dead space"), so if you are mixing two types of insulin be sure to discuss any change in the model and brand of syringe you are using with your physician or pharmacist. When you are mixing two types of insulin, always draw the Regular (clear) insulin into the syringe first.

SYRINGES

Use the correct syringe

The volume of the dose depends on the number of units of insulin per ml. Insulatard® NPH Human is only available in the U-100 strength (100 units per ml). Make sure that you understand the markings on your syringe and use only a syringe marked for U-100.

Disposable Syringes

Disposable syringes and needles require no sterilization provided the package is intact. They should be used only once and discarded.

Reusable Syringes

Reusable syringes and needles must be sterile when used. The best method of sterilization is to boil the syringe, plunger and needle in water for 5 minutes. If this is not possible, as when travelling, the parts may be sterilized by immersion for at least 5 minutes in a sterilizing liquid like ethyl alcohol, 70%. Do not use bathing, rubbing or medicated alcohol for sterilization. Remove all liquid from the syringe by pushing the plunger in and out several times and leave it to dry if alcohol has been used for sterilization.

IMPORTANT

Failure to comply with the above and the following antiseptic measures may lead to infections at the injection site.

PREPARING THE INJECTION

Rotate the vial carefully to obtain a uniformly cloudy suspension of the crystals. Avoid heavy foaming. Do not use a vial if the insulin remains clear after it has been shaken. Also do not use it if you see lumps that float or stick to the sides.

1. Clean your hands and the injection site with soap and water or with alcohol. Wipe the rubber stopper with an alcohol swab. (Note: remove the tamper-resistant cap at first use. If the cap has already been removed, do not use this product; return it to your pharmacy.)

2. For insulin suspensions, roll the vial of insulin gently in your hands to mix it. Vigorous shaking immediately before the dose is drawn into the syringe may result in the formation of bubbles or foam which could cause dosage errors.

3. Pull back the plunger until the black tip reaches the marking for the number of units you will inject.

4. Push the needle through the rubber stopper into the vial.

5. Push the plunger all the way in. This inserts air into the bottle.

6. Turn the vial and syringe upside down and slowly pull the plunger back to a few units beyond the correct dose.

7. If there are air bubbles, flick the syringe firmly with your finger to raise the air bubbles to the needle, then slowly push the plunger to the correct unit marking.

8. Lift the vial off the syringe.

GIVING THE INJECTION

1. The following areas are suitable for subcutaneous insulin injection: thighs, upper arms, buttocks, abdomen. Do not change areas without consulting your physician. The actual point of injection should be changed each time; injection sites should be about an inch apart.

2. The injection site should be clean and dry. Pinch up skin area to be injected and hold it firmly.

3. Hold the syringe like a pencil and push the needle quickly and firmly into the pinched-up area. If you go straight in it will probably sting less. Pull back the plunger slightly. If blood comes into the syringe, the needle has entered a blood vessel. Remove the needle and make the injection in another spot.

4. If blood does not appear in the syringe, release skin and push plunger all the way in to inject insulin beneath the skin. Do not inject into a muscle unless your physician has advised it. You should never inject insulin into a vein.

5. Remove needle. If slight bleeding occurs, press lightly with a dry cotton swab for a few seconds—**do not rub.**

USAGE IN PREGNANCY

It is particularly important to maintain good control of your diabetes during pregnancy and special attention must be paid to your diet, exercise and insulin regimens. If you are pregnant or nursing a baby, consult your physician or nurse educator.

Continued on next page

Nordisk-USA—Cont.

INSULIN REACTION

Insulin reaction (too little sugar in the blood, also called hypoglycemia) can occur if you take too much insulin, miss a meal or exercise or work harder than normal. The symptoms, which usually come on suddenly, are hunger, dizziness, and sweating. Personality change or confusion may also occur. Eating sugar or a sugar-sweetened product will normally correct the condition.

If symptoms persist, call a physician; an insulin reaction can lead to unconsciousness. If a reaction results in loss of consciousness, emergency medical care should be obtained immediately. If you have had repeated reactions or if an insulin reaction has led to a loss of consciousness, contact your physician.

DIABETIC KETOACIDOSIS AND COMA

Diabetic ketoacidosis may develop if your body has too little insulin. The most common causes are acute illness or infection or failure to take enough insulin by injection. If you are ill, you should check your urine for ketones. The symptoms of diabetic ketoacidosis usually come on gradually, over a period of hours or days, and include a drowsy feeling, flushed face, thirst and loss of appetite. Notify a physician immediately if the urine test is positive for ketones (acetone) or if you have any of these symptoms. More severe symptoms are fast, heavy breathing and rapid pulse; if these symptoms occur, you should have medical attention right away.

ADVERSE REACTIONS

Insulin allergy occurs very rarely, but when it does, it may cause a serious reaction including a general skin rash over the body, shortness of breath, fast pulse, sweating, and a drop in blood pressure. If any of these symptoms develop you should seek emergency medical care.

In a very few diabetics, the skin where insulin has been injected may become red, swollen and itchy. This is called a local reaction. It may occur if the injection is not properly made, if the skin is sensitive to the cleansing solution or if the patient is allergic to insulin. If you have a local reaction, notify your physician.

Patients with severe systemic allergic reactions to insulin (i.e. generalized urticaria, angioedema, anaphylaxis) should be skin tested with **each** new preparation to be used prior to initiation of therapy with that preparation.

IMPORTANT NOTES

1. A change in the type, strength, species or purity of insulin could require a dosage adjustment. Any change in insulin should be made under medical supervision.
2. You may have learned how to test your urine or your blood for glucose. It is important to do these tests regularly and to record the results for review with your physician or nurse educator.
3. If you have an acute illness, especially with vomiting or fever, continue taking your insulin. If possible, stay on your regular diet. If you have trouble eating, drink fruit juices, regular soft drinks, or clear soups; if you can, eat small amounts of bland foods. Test your urine for glucose and ketones and, if possible, test your blood glucose. Note the results and contact your physician for possible insulin dose adjustment. If you have severe and prolonged vomiting, seek emergency medical care.
4. You should always carry identification which states that you have diabetes.

Always consult your physician if you have any questions about your condition or the use of insulin.

Helpful information for people with diabetes is published by American Diabetes Association, 1660 Duke St., Alexandria, VA 22314.

HOW SUPPLIED

10 ml vials
100 units per ml.
NDC #50445-333-01
Brochures, Time Action Profile Charts, Samples-Free to Physicians.

VELOSULIN®

[*vĕl "ō´sul "in*]
**U-100 Purified Pork, Purified Pork Injection
(regular)**

DESCRIPTION

Velosulin is produced from the pork insulin molecule and has low immunogenic potential. Velosulin is the only buffered regular acting animal species insulin, making the product beneficial for insulin infusion pump therapy. Velosulin can be mixed with Nordisk Insulatard NPH reliably without usage restrictions and without loss of effectiveness over extended periods of time.

Insulin is an anabolic hormone. Its action is primarily concerned with the metabolism of carbohydrates, but also affects protein and fat metabolism. Insulin facilitates the cellular uptake of glucose and its metabolism in insulin-responsive tissue (e.g. liver, muscle, adipose, and nervous tissue). Insulin also inhibits the breakdown of fat, the production of ketones and increases the uptake of amino acids. The administration of the proper doses of insulin to patients with abnormal or absent beta cell function (reduced capacity, abnormal responsiveness or inability to produce endogenous insulin) restores the patient's ability to metabolize glucose and establish near normal carbohydrate, fat, and protein metabolism.

VELOSULIN has a rapid onset of effect on the blood sugar, approximately $\frac{1}{2}$ hour after the injection. The effect lasts up to approximately 8 hours with a maximal effect between the 1st and 3rd hour.

WARNING

ANY CHANGE OF INSULIN SHOULD BE MADE CAUTIOUSLY ONLY UNDER MEDICAL SUPERVISION. WHEN CHANGING TO PURIFIED PORK INSULIN FROM ANY OTHER INSULIN A DOSAGE ADJUSTMENT, IF ANY, IS LIKELY TO BE A REDUCTION TO AVOID HYPOGLYCEMIA. CHANGES IN PURITY, STRENGTH (U-40, U-80, U-100), BRAND (MANUFACTURER), TYPE (LENTE, NPH, REGULAR, ETC.) AND/ OR SPECIES SOURCE (BEEF, PORK, BEEF/ PORK) MAY RESULT IN THE NEED FOR A CHANGE IN DOSAGE. IT IS NOT POSSIBLE TO IDENTIFY WHICH PATIENTS WILL REQUIRE A REDUCTION IN DOSAGE TO AVOID HYPOGLYCEMIA WHEN USING THIS INSULIN. ADJUSTMENT MAY BE NEEDED WITH THE FIRST DOSE OR OVER A PERIOD OF SEVERAL WEEKS. (SEE DOSAGE ADJUSTMENT SECTION). BE AWARE OF THE POSSIBILITY OF SYMPTOMS OF EITHER HYPOGLYCEMIA OR HYPERGLYCEMIA. SEE SECTIONS ENTITLED INSULIN REACTION AND HYPERGLYCEMIA.

INSULIN USE IN DIABETES

Your physician has explained that you have diabetes and that your treatment involves injections of insulin. Insulin is normally produced by the pancreas, a gland that lies behind the stomach. Without insulin, glucose (a simple sugar made from digested food) is trapped in the bloodstream and cannot enter the cells of the body. Some patients who don't make enough of their own insulin, or who cannot use the insulin they do make properly, must take insulin by injection in order to control their blood glucose levels. The usual route of administration for Velosulin is via subcutaneous injection. Velosulin may occasionally be given intravenously by medical personnel. Patients trained in the use of insulin infusion pump devices may also use Velosulin in their device.

Each case of diabetes is different and requires direct and continued medical supervision. Your physician has told you the type, strength and amount of insulin you should use and the time(s) at which you should inject it, and has also discussed with you a diet and exercise schedule. You should contact your physician if you experience any difficulties or if you have questions.

TYPES OF INSULINS

Standard and purified animal insulins as well as human insulins are available. Standard and purified insulins differ in their degree of purification and content of noninsulin material. Standard and purified insulins also vary in species source: they may be of beef, pork, or mixed beef and pork origin. Human insulin is identical in structure to the insulin produced by the human pancreas, and thus differs from animals insulins. Insulins vary in time of action and in strength; see PRODUCT DESCRIPTION and SYRINGES for additional information.

Your physician has prescribed the insulin that is right for you; be sure you have purchased the correct insulin and check it carefully before you use it.

MIXING TWO TYPES OF INSULIN

Different insulins should be mixed only under instruction from a physician. Hypodermic syringes may vary in the amount of space between the bottom line and the needle ("dead space"), so if you are mixing two types of insulin be sure to discuss any change in the model and brand of syringe you are using with your physician or pharmacist. When you are mixing two types of insulin, always draw the Regular (clear) insulin into the syringe first.

SYRINGES

Use the correct syringe
The volume of the dose depends on the number of units of insulin per ml. Insulatard® NPH Human is only available in the U-100 strength (100 units per ml). Make sure that you understand the markings on your syringe and use only a syringe marked for U-100.

Disposable Syringes
Disposable syringes and needles require no sterilization provided the package is intact. They should be used only once and discarded.

Reusable Syringes
Reusable syringes and needles must be sterile when used. The best method of sterilization is to boil the syringe, plunger and needle in water for 5 minutes. If this is not possible, as when travelling, the parts may be sterilized by immersion for at least 5 minutes in a sterilizing liquid like ethyl alcohol, 70%. Do not use bathing, rubbing or medicated alcohol for sterilization. Remove all liquid from the syringe by pushing the plunger in and out several times and leave it to dry if alcohol has been used for sterilization.

IMPORTANT

Failure to comply with the above and the following antiseptic measures may lead to infections at the injection site.

PREPARING THE INJECTION

Do not use the preparation if the color has become other than water clear or if the liquid has become viscous.

1. Clean your hands and the injection site with soap and water or with alcohol. Wipe the rubber stopper with an alcohol swab. (Note: remove the tamper-resistant cap at first use. If the cap has already been removed, do not use this product, return it to your pharmacy.)
2. For insulin suspensions, roll the vial of insulin gently in your hands to mix it. Vigorous shaking immediately before the dose is drawn into the syringe may result in the formation of bubbles or foam which could cause dosage errors.
3. Pull back the plunger until the black tip reaches the marking for the number of units you will inject.
4. Push the needle through the rubber stopper into the vial.
5. Push the plunger all the way in. This inserts air into the bottle.
6. Turn the vial and syringe upside down and slowly pull the plunger back to a few units beyond the correct dose.
7. If there are air bubbles, flick the syringe firmly with your finger to raise the air bubbles to the needle, then slowly push the plunger to the correct unit marking.
8. Lift the vial off the syringe.

GIVING THE INJECTION

1. The following areas are suitable for subcutaneous insulin injection: thighs, upper arms, buttocks, abdomen. Do not change areas without consulting your physician. The actual point of injection should be changed each time; injection sites should be about an inch apart.
2. The injection site should be clean and dry. Pinch up skin area to be injected and hold it firmly.
3. Hold the syringe like a pencil and push the needle quickly and firmly into the pinched-up area. If you go straight in it will probably sting less. Pull back the plunger slightly. If blood comes into the syringe, the needle has entered a blood vessel. Remove the needle and make the injection in another spot.
4. If blood does not appear in the syringe, release skin and push plunger all the way in to inject insulin beneath the skin. Do not inject into a muscle unless your physician has advised it. You should never inject insulin into a vein.
5. Remove needle. If slight bleeding occurs, press lightly with a dry cotton swab for a few seconds—**do not rub.**

USAGE IN PREGNANCY

It is particularly important to maintain good control of your diabetes during pregnancy and special attention must be paid to your diet, exercise and insulin regimens. If you are pregnant or nursing a baby, consult your physician or nurse educator.

INSULIN REACTION

Insulin reaction (too little sugar in the blood, also called hypoglycemia) can occur if you take too much insulin, miss a meal or exercise or work harder than normal. The symptoms, which usually come on suddenly, are hunger, dizziness, and sweating. Personality change or confusion may also occur. Eating sugar or a sugar-sweetened product will normally correct the condition.

If symptoms persist, call a physician; an insulin reaction can lead to unconsciousness. If a reaction results in loss of consciousness, emergency medical care should be obtained immediately. If you have had repeated reactions or if an insulin reaction has led to a loss of consciousness, contact your physician.

DIABETIC KETOACIDOSIS AND COMA

Diabetic ketoacidosis may develop if your body has too little insulin. The most common causes are acute illness or infection or failure to take enough insulin by injection. If you are ill, you should check your urine for ketones. The symptoms of diabetic ketoacidosis usually come on gradually, over a period of hours or days, and include a drowsy feeling, flushed face, thirst and loss of appetite. Notify a physician immediately if the urine test is positive for ketones (acetone) or if you have any of these symptoms. More severe symptoms are fast, heavy breathing and rapid pulse; if these symptoms occur, you should have medical attention right away.

ADVERSE REACTIONS

Insulin allergy occurs very rarely, but when it does, it may cause a serious reaction including a general skin rash over the body, shortness of breath, fast pulse, sweating, and a drop in blood pressure. If any of these symptoms develop you should seek emergency medical care.

In a very few diabetics, the skin where insulin has been injected may become red, swollen and itchy. This is called a local reaction. It may occur if the injection is not properly made, if the skin is sensitive to the cleansing solution or if the patient is allergic to insulin. If you have a local reaction, notify your physician.

Patients with severe systemic allergic reactions to insulin (i.e. generalized urticaria, angioedema, anaphylaxis) should be skin tested with **each** new preparation to be used prior to initiation of therapy with that preparation.

IMPORTANT NOTES

1. A change in the type, strength, species or purity of insulin could require a dosage adjustment. Any change in insulin should be made under medical supervision.
2. You may have learned how to test your urine or your blood for glucose. It is important to do these tests regularly and to record the results for review with your physician or nurse educator.
3. If you have an acute illness, especially with vomiting or fever, continue taking your insulin. If possible, stay on your regular diet. If you have trouble eating, drink fruit juices, regular soft drinks, or clear soups; if you can, eat small amounts of bland foods. Test your urine for glucose and ketones and, if possible, test your blood glucose. Note the results and contact your physician for possible insulin dose adjustment. If you have severe and prolonged vomiting, seek emergency medical care.
4. You should always carry identification which states that you have diabetes.

Always consult your physician if you have any questions about your condition or the use of insulin.

Helpful information for people with diabetes is published by American Diabetes Association, 1660 Duke St., Alexandria, VA 22314.

HOW SUPPLIED

10 ml vials
100 units per ml.
NDC # 50445-100-01
Brochures, Time Action Profile Charts, Samples—Free to Physicians.

VELOSULIN® HUMAN

[věl "ŏ 'sul "in hyōō 'men]
U-100 Human, Human insulin injection
(semi-synthetic)

DESCRIPTION

Velosulin Human insulin is produced semi-synthetically by enzymatic conversion of the pork insulin molecule and has low immunogenic potential. Velosulin Human is the only buffered regular acting human insulin, making the product beneficial for insulin infusion pump therapy. Velosulin Human can be mixed with Nordisk Insulatard NPH Human reliably without usage restrictions, and without loss of effectiveness over extended periods of time.

Velosulin® Human is a clear solution of insulin. It has a rapid onset of action, approximately ½ hour after the injection. The effect lasts up to approximately 8 hours with a maximal effect between the 1st and 3rd hour.

The time course of action of any insulin may vary considerably in different individuals, or at different times in the same individual. Because of this variation, the time periods listed here should be considered as general guidelines only.

Insulin is an anabolic hormone. Its action is primarily concerned with the metabolism of carbohydrates, but also affects protein and fat metabolism. Insulin facilitates the cellular uptake of glucose and its metabolism in insulin-responsive tissue (e.g. liver, muscle, adipose, and nervous tissue). Insulin also inhibits the breakdown of fat, the production of ketones and increases the uptake of amino acids. The administration of the proper doses of insulin to patients with abnormal or absent beta cell function (reduced capacity, abnormal responsiveness or inability to produce endogenous insulin) restores the patient's ability to metabolize glucose and establish near normal carbohydrate, fat, and protein metabolism.

WARNING

Any change of insulin should be made cautiously and only under medical supervision. Changes in purity, strength (U-40, U-80, U-100), brand (manufacturer), type (lente, NPH, regular, etc.) and/or species source (beef, pork, beef/pork, human) may result in the need for a change in dosage. Adjustment may be needed with the first dose or over a period of several weeks.

Be aware that symptoms of hypoglycemia (low blood sugar) or hyperglycemia (high blood glucose) may indicate the need for dosage adjustment. Please read sections entitled "Insulin Reaction" and "Diabetic Ketoacidosis and Coma."

INSULIN USE IN DIABETES

Your physician has explained that you have diabetes and that your treatment involves injections of insulin. Insulin is normally produced by the pancreas, a gland that lies behind the stomach. Without insulin, glucose (a simple sugar made from digested food) is trapped in the bloodstream and cannot

enter the cells of the body. Some patients who don't make enough of their own insulin, or who cannot use the insulin they do make properly, must take insulin by injection in order to control their blood glucose levels. The usual route of administration for Velosulin Human is via subcutaneous injection. Velosulin Human may occasionally be given intravenously by medical personnel. Patients trained in the use of insulin infusion pump devices may also use Velosulin Human in their device.

Each case of diabetes is different and requires direct and continued medical supervision. Your physician has told you the type, strength and amount of insulin you should use and the time(s) at which you should inject it, and has also discussed with you a diet and exercise schedule. You should contact your physician if you experience any difficulties or if you have questions.

TYPES OF INSULINS

Standard and purified animal insulins as well as human insulins are available. Standard and purified insulins differ in their degree of purification and content of noninsulin material. Standard and purified insulins also vary in species source: they may be of beef, pork, or mixed beef and pork origin. Human insulin is identical in structure to the insulin produced by the human pancreas, and thus differs from animals insulins. Insulins vary in time of action and in strength; see PRODUCT DESCRIPTION and SYRINGES for additional information.

Your physician has prescribed the insulin that is right for you; be sure you have purchased the correct insulin and check it carefully before you use it.

MIXING TWO TYPES OF INSULIN

Different insulins should be mixed only under instruction from a physician. Hypodermic syringes may vary in the amount of space between the bottom line and the needle ("dead space"), so if you are mixing two types of insulin be sure to discuss any change in the model and brand of syringe you are using with your physician or pharmacist. When you are mixing two types of insulin, always draw the Regular (clear) insulin into the syringe first.

SYRINGES

Use the correct syringe
The volume of the dose depends on the number of units of insulin per ml. Insulatard® NPH Human is only available in the U-100 strength (100 units per ml). Make sure that you understand the markings on your syringe and use only a syringe marked for U-100.

Disposable Syringes
Disposable syringes and needles require no sterilization provided the package is intact. They should be used only once and discarded.

Reusable Syringes
Reusable syringes and needles must be sterile when used. The best method of sterilization is to boil the syringe, plunger and needle in water for 5 minutes. If this is not possible, as when travelling, the parts may be sterilized by immersion for at least 5 minutes in a sterilizing liquid like ethyl alcohol, 70%. Do not use bathing, rubbing or medicated alcohol for sterilization. Remove all liquid from the syringe by pushing the plunger in and out several times and leave it to dry if alcohol has been used for sterilization.

IMPORTANT

Failure to comply with the above and the following antiseptic measures may lead to infections at the injection site.

PREPARING THE INJECTION

Do not use the preparation if the color has become other than water clear or if the liquid has become viscous.

1. Clean your hands and the injection site with soap and water or with alcohol. Wipe the rubber stopper with an alcohol swab. (Note: remove the tamper-resistant cap at first use. If the cap has already been removed, do not use this product, return it to your pharmacy.)
2. For insulin suspensions, roll the vial of insulin gently in your hands to mix it. Vigorous shaking immediately before the dose is drawn into the syringe may result in the formation of bubbles or foam which could cause dosage errors.
3. Pull back the plunger until the black tip reaches the marking for the number of units you will inject.
4. Push the needle through the rubber stopper into the vial.
5. Push the plunger all the way in. This inserts air into the bottle.
6. Turn the vial and syringe upside down and slowly pull the plunger back to a few units beyond the correct dose.
7. If there are air bubbles, flick the syringe firmly with your finger to raise the air bubbles to the needle, then slowly push the plunger to the correct unit marking.
8. Lift the vial off the syringe.

GIVING THE INJECTION

1. The following areas are suitable for subcutaneous insulin injection: thighs, upper arms, buttocks, abdomen. Do not change areas without consulting your physician. The ac-

tual point of injection should be changed each time; injection sites should be about an inch apart.
2. The injection site should be clean and dry. Pinch up skin area to be injected and hold it firmly.
3. Hold the syringe like a pencil and push the needle quickly and firmly into the pinched-up area. If you go straight in it will probably sting less. Pull back the plunger slightly. If blood comes into the syringe, the needle has entered a blood vessel. Remove the needle and make the injection in another spot.
4. If blood does not appear in the syringe, release skin and push plunger all the way in to inject insulin beneath the skin. Do not inject into a muscle unless your physician has advised it. You should never inject insulin into a vein.
5. Remove needle. If slight bleeding occurs, press lightly with a dry cotton swab for a few seconds—do not rub.

USAGE IN PREGNANCY

It is particularly important to maintain good control of your diabetes during pregnancy and special attention must be paid to your diet, exercise and insulin regimens. If you are pregnant or nursing a baby, consult your physician or nurse educator.

INSULIN REACTION

Insulin reaction (too little sugar in the blood, also called hypoglycemia) can occur if you take too much insulin, miss a meal or exercise or work harder than normal. The symptoms, which usually come on suddenly, are hunger, dizziness, and sweating. Personality change or confusion may also occur. Eating sugar or a sugar-sweetened product will normally correct the condition.

If symptoms persist, call a physician; an insulin reaction can lead to unconsciousness. If a reaction results in loss of consciousness, emergency medical care should be obtained immediately. If you have had repeated reactions or if an insulin reaction has led to a loss of consciousness, contact your physician.

DIABETIC KETOACIDOSIS AND COMA

Diabetic ketoacidosis may develop if your body has too little insulin. The most common causes are acute illness or infection or failure to take enough insulin by injection. If you are ill, you should check your urine for ketones.The symptoms of diabetic ketoacidosis usually come on gradually, over a period of hours or days, and include a drowsy feeling, flushed face, thirst and loss of appetite. Notify a physician immediately if the urine test is positive for ketones (acetone) or if you have any of these symptoms. More severe symptoms are fast, heavy breathing and rapid pulse; if these symptoms occur, you should have medical attention right away.

ADVERSE REACTIONS

Insulin allergy occurs very rarely, but when it does, it may cause a serious reaction including a general skin rash over the body, shortness of breath, fast pulse, sweating, and a drop in blood pressure. If any of these symptoms develop you should seek emergency medical care.

In a very few diabetics, the skin where insulin has been injected may become red, swollen and itchy. This is called a local reaction. It may occur if the injection is not properly made, if the skin is sensitive to the cleansing solution or if the patient is allergic to insulin. If you have a local reaction, notify your physician.

Patients with severe systemic allergic reactions to insulin (i.e. generalized urticaria, angioedema, anaphylaxis) should be skin tested with **each** new preparation to be used prior to initiation of therapy with that preparation.

IMPORTANT NOTES

1. A change in the type, strength, species or purity of insulin could require a dosage adjustment. Any change in insulin should be made under medical supervision.
2. You may have learned how to test your urine or your blood for glucose. It is important to do these tests regularly and to record the results for review with your physician or nurse educator.
3. If you have an acute illness, especially with vomiting or fever, continue taking your insulin. If possible, stay on your regular diet. If you have trouble eating, drink fruit juices, regular soft drinks, or clear soups; if you can, eat small amounts of bland foods. Test your urine for glucose and ketones and, if possible, test your blood glucose. Note the results and contact your physician for possible insulin dose adjustment. If you have severe and prolonged vomiting, seek emergency medical care.
4. You should always carry identification which states that you have diabetes.

Always consult your physician if you have any questions about your condition or the use of insulin.

Helpful information for people with diabetes is published by American Diabetes Association, 1660 Duke St., Alexandria, VA 22314.

Continued on next page

Nordisk-USA—Cont.

HOW SUPPLIED

10 ml vials
100 units per ml.
NDC #50445-111-01
Brochures, Time Action Profile Charts, Samples-Free to
Physicians

Norwich Eaton
Pharmaceuticals, Inc.

A Procter & Gamble Company
NORWICH, NY 13815-0231

Literature on Norwich Eaton products sent to physicians on
request.
Information on these Norwich Eaton products is based on
labeling in effect June 1, 1989. Further information on these
and other Norwich Eaton products may be obtained by direct
inquiry to Medical Department,
Norwich Eaton Pharmaceuticals, Inc.
P.O. Box 191, Norwich, NY 13815-0191.

BUPRENEX®   Ⓒ ℞

[būp'rĕn-ex]
(buprenorphine hydrochloride)
INJECTABLE

DESCRIPTION

Buprenex (buprenorphine hydrochloride) is a narcotic under
the Controlled Substances Act due to its chemical derivation
from thebaine. Chemically, it is 17-(cyclopropylmethyl)-α-
(1,1-dimethylethyl)-4, 5-epoxy-18, 19-dihydro-3-hydroxy-
6-methoxy-α-methyl-6, 14-ethenomorphinan-7-methanol,
hydrochloride [5α, 7α(S)]. Buprenorphine hydrochloride is a
white powder, weakly acidic and with limited solubility in
water. Buprenex is a clear, sterile, injectable agonist-antagonist analgesic intended for intravenous or intramuscular
administration. Each ml of Buprenex contains 0.324 mg buprenorphine hydrochloride (equivalent to 0.3 mg buprenorphine), 50 mg anhydrous dextrose, water for injection and
HCl to adjust pH. Buprenorphine hydrochloride has the
molecular formula, $C_{29}H_{41}NO_4 \cdot HCl$, and the following structure:

Molecular weight: 504.09

CLINICAL PHARMACOLOGY

Buprenex is a parenteral opioid analgesic with 0.3 mg Buprenex being approximately equivalent to 10 mg morphine
sulfate in analgesic and respiratory depressant effects. Pharmacological effects occur as soon as 15 minutes after intramuscular injection and persist for 6 hours or longer. Peak
pharmacologic effects usually are observed at 1 hour. When
used intravenously, the times to onset and peak effect are
shortened.
The limits of sensitivity of available analytical methodology
precluded demonstration of bioequivalence between intramuscular and intravenous routes of administration. In postoperative patients, pharmacokinetic studies have shown
elimination half-lives ranging from 1.2–7.2 hours (mean 2.2
hours) after intravenous administration of 0.3 mg of buprenorphine.
Buprenorphine, in common with morphine and other phenolic opioid analgesics, is metabolized by the liver and its
clearance is related to hepatic blood flow. Studies in patients
anesthetized with 0.5% halothane have shown that this anesthetic decreases hepatic blood flow by about 30%.
Mechanism of Analgesic Action: Buprenex exerts its analgesic effect via high affinity binding to μ subclass opiate receptors in the central nervous system. Although Buprenex
may be classified as a partial agonist, under the conditions of
recommended use it behaves very much like classical μ agonists such as morphine. One unusual property of Buprenex
observed in *in vitro* studies is its very slow rate of dissociation
from its receptor. This could account for its longer duration

of action than morphine, the unpredictability of its reversal
by opioid antagonists, and its low level of manifest physical
dependence.
Narcotic Antagonist Activity: Buprenorphine demonstrates narcotic antagonist activity and has been shown to be
equipotent with naloxone as an antagonist of morphine in
the mouse tail flick test.
Cardiovascular Effects: Buprenex may cause a decrease or,
rarely, an increase in pulse rate and blood pressure in some
patients.
Effects on Respiration: Under usual conditions of use, both
Buprenex and morphine show similar dose-related respiratory depressant effects. A therapeutic dose of Buprenex (0.3
mg buprenorphine) can decrease respiratory rate in an
equivalent manner to an equianalgesic dose of morphine
(10mg). (See WARNINGS.)

INDICATIONS AND USAGE

Buprenex is indicated for the relief of moderate to severe
pain.

CONTRAINDICATIONS

Buprenex should not be administered to patients who have
been shown to be hypersensitive to the drug.

WARNINGS

Impaired Respiration: As with other potent opioids, clinically significant respiratory depression may occur within the
recommended dose range in patients receiving therapeutic
doses of buprenorphine. Buprenex should be used with caution in patients with compromised respiratory function (e.g.,
chronic obstructive pulmonary disease, cor pulmonale, decreased respiratory reserve, hypoxia, hypercapnia, or preexisting respiratory depression). Particular caution is advised
if Buprenex is administered to patients taking or recently
receiving drugs with CNS/respiratory depressant effects. In
patients with the physical and/or pharmacological risk factors above, the dose should be reduced by approximately one-
half.
**NALOXONE MAY NOT BE EFFECTIVE IN REVERS-
ING THE RESPIRATORY DEPRESSION PRODUCED
BY BUPRENEX. THEREFORE, AS WITH OTHER PO-
TENT OPIOIDS, THE PRIMARY MANAGEMENT OF
OVERDOSE SHOULD BE THE REESTABLISHMENT
OF ADEQUATE VENTILATION WITH MECHANICAL
ASSISTANCE OF RESPIRATION, IF REQUIRED.**
**Interaction with Other Central Nervous System Depress-
ants:** Patients receiving Buprenex in the presence of other
narcotic analgesics, general anesthetics, antihistamines,
benzodiazepines, phenothiazines, other tranquilizers, seda-
tive/hypnotics or other CNS depressants (including alcohol)
may exhibit increased CNS depression. When such combined
therapy is contemplated, it is particularly important that
the dose of one or both agents be reduced.
Head Injury and Increased Intracranial Pressure: Buprenex, like other potent analgesics, may itself elevate cerebrospinal fluid pressure and should be used with caution in
head injury, intracranial lesions and other circumstances
where cerebrospinal pressure may be increased. Buprenex
can produce miosis and changes in the level of consciousness
which may interfere with patient evaluation.
Use in Ambulatory Patients: Buprenex may impair the
mental or physical abilities required for the performance of
potentially dangerous tasks such as driving a car or operating machinery. Therefore, Buprenex should be administered
with caution to ambulatory patients who should be warned
to avoid such hazards.
Use in Narcotic-Dependent Patients: Because of the narcotic antagonist activity of Buprenex, use in the physically
dependent individual may result in withdrawal effects.

PRECAUTIONS

General: Buprenex should be administered with caution in
the elderly or debilitated and those with severe impairment
of hepatic, pulmonary, or renal function; myxedema or hypothyroidism; adrenal cortical insufficiency (e.g., Addison's
disease); CNS depression or coma; toxic psychoses; prostatic
hypertrophy or urethral stricture; acute alcoholism, delirium tremens; or kyphoscoliosis.
Because Buprenex is metabolized by the liver, the activity of
Buprenex may be increased and/or extended in those individuals with impaired hepatic function or those receiving
other agents known to decrease hepatic clearance.
Buprenex has been shown to increase intracholedochal pressure to a similar degree as other opioid analgesics, and thus
should be administered with caution to patients with dysfunction of the biliary tract.
Information for Patients: The effects of Buprenex, particularly drowsiness, may be potentiated by other centrally acting agents such as alcohol or benzodiazepines. It is particularly important that in these circumstances patients must
not drive or operate machinery. Buprenex has some pharmacologic effects similar to morphine which in susceptible patients may lead to self-administration of the drug when pain
no longer exists. Patients must not exceed the dosage of Buprenex prescribed by their physician. Patients should be
urged to consult their physician if other prescription medica-

tions are currently being used or are prescribed for future
use.
Drug Interactions: Drug interactions common to other potent opioid analgesics also may occur with Buprenex. Particular care should be taken when Buprenex is used in combination with central nervous system depressant drugs (see
WARNINGS). Although specific information is not presently
available, caution should be exercised when Buprenex is
used in combination with MAO inhibitors. There have been
reports of respiratory and cardiovascular collapse in patients
who received therapeutic doses of diazepam and Buprenex. A
suspected interaction between Buprenex and phenprocoumon resulting in purpura has been reported.
Carcinogenesis, Mutagenesis, Impairment of Fertility: The
effects of Buprenex on fertility and gestation indices were
investigated in rats by the subcutaneous and intramuscular
routes at doses 10 to 1,000 times the proposed human doses.
Dystocia was noted in dams treated with 1,000 times the
human dose. No effects on fertility or gestation were noted in
these Segment 1 studies.
Pregnancy: Pregnancy Category C. Reproduction studies
have been performed in the rat at doses which ranged from
10 to 1,000 times the proposed human dose by the subcutaneous and intramuscular routes and 160 times the proposed
human dose by the intravenous routes. By the intramuscular
route, Buprenex produced mild but statistically significant
($p < 0.05$) post-implantation losses and early fetal deaths at
10 and 100 but not 1,000 times the proposed human dose. No
fetal malformations were noted in rats at any dose when
Buprenex was administered by subcutaneous, intramuscular, or intravenous routes. In rabbits, intramuscularly administered Buprenex produced a dose-related trend for extra
rib formation which attained statistical significance ($p <
0.01$) at 1,000 times the proposed human dose. By the intrave-
nous route, doses in rats of 40 and 160 times the proposed
human dose of Buprenex caused a slight increase in post-
implantation losses that may have been treatment-related.
No major fetal malformations were noted in drug treated
groups when administered by intramuscular or intravenous
routes.
There are no adequate and well-controlled studies in pregnant women. Buprenex should be used during pregnancy
only if the potential benefit justifies the potential risk to the
fetus.
Labor and Delivery: The safety of Buprenex given during
labor and delivery has not been established.
Nursing Mothers: An apparent lack of milk production
during general reproduction studies with Buprenex in rats
caused decreased viability and lactation indices. It is unknown at this time whether or not Buprenex is excreted in
human milk. Despite the lack of specific knowledge on this
issue, it is reasonable to assume that Buprenex will enter
human milk and caution should be exercised in the use of
Buprenex when it is administered to nursing mothers.
Pediatric Use: Safety and effectiveness in children have not
been established.

ADVERSE REACTIONS

The most frequent side effect in clinical studies involving
1,133 patients was sedation which occurred in approximately two-thirds of the patients. Although sedated, these
patients could easily be aroused to an alert state.
**Other less frequent adverse reactions occurring in 5–10% of
the patients were:**

Nausea	Dizziness/Vertigo

Occurring in 1–5% of the patients:

Sweating	Headache
Hypotension	Nausea/Vomiting
Vomiting	Hypoventilation
Miosis	

**The following adverse reactions were reported to have oc-
curred in less than 1% of the patients:**
CNS Effect: confusion, blurred vision, euphoria, weakness/
fatigue, dry mouth, nervousness, depression, slurred speech,
paresthesia.
Cardiovascular: hypertension, tachycardia, bradycardia.
Gastrointestinal: constipation.
Respiratory: dyspnea, cyanosis.
Dermatological: pruritus.
Ophthalmological: diplopia, visual abnormalities.
Miscellaneous: injection site reaction, urinary retention,
dreaming, flushing/warmth, chills/cold, tinnitus, conjunctivitis, Wenckebach block, and psychosis.
Other effects observed infrequently include malaise, hallucinations, depersonalization, coma, dyspepsia, flatulence, apnea, rash, amblyopia, tremor, and pallor.
The following reactions have been reported to occur rarely:
loss of appetite, dysphoria/agitation, diarrhea, urticaria,
and convulsions/ lack of muscle coordination.
In the United Kingdom, buprenorphine kydrochloride was
made available under monitored release regulation during
the first year of sale, and yielded data from 1,736 physicians
on 9,123 patients (17,120 administrations). No important
new adverse effects attributable to buprenorphine hydrochloride were observed.

DRUG ABUSE AND DEPENDENCE

Buprenorphine hydrochloride is a partial agonist of the morphine type: *i.e.*, it has certain opioid properties which may lead to psychic dependence of the morphine type due to an opiate-like euphoric component of the drug. Direct dependence studies have shown little physical dependence upon withdrawal of the drug. However, caution should be used in prescribing to individuals who are known to be drug abusers or ex-narcotic addicts. The drug may not substitute in acutely dependent narcotic addicts due to its antagonist component and may induce withdrawal symptoms.

OVERDOSAGE

Manifestations: Clinical experience with Buprenex overdosage has been insufficient to define the signs of this condition at this time. Although the antagonist activity of buprenorphine may become manifest at doses somewhat above the recommended therapeutic range, doses in the recommended therapeutic range may produce clinically significant respiratory depression in certain circumstances. (See WARNINGS.)
Treatment: The respiratory and cardiac status of the patients should be monitored carefully. Primary attention should be given to the reestablishment of adequate respiratory exchange through provision of a patent airway and institution of assisted or controlled ventilation. Oxygen, intravenous fluids, vasopressors, and other supportive measures should be employed as indicated. Doxapram, a respiratory stimulant, may be used. NALOXONE MAY NOT BE EFFECTIVE IN REVERSING THE RESPIRATORY DEPRESSION PRODUCED BY BUPRENEX. THEREFORE, AS WITH OTHER POTENT OPIOIDS, THE PRIMARY MANAGEMENT OF OVERDOSE SHOULD BE THE REESTABLISHMENT OF ADEQUATE VENTILATION WITH MECHANICAL ASSISTANCE OF RESPIRATION, IF REQUIRED.

DOSAGE AND ADMINISTRATION

The usual dosage for persons 13 years of age and over is 1 ml Buprenex (0.3 mg buprenorphine) given by deep intramuscular or slow (over at least 2 minutes) intravenous injection at up to 6-hour intervals, as needed. Repeat once (up to 0.3 mg) if required, 30 to 60 minutes after initial dosage, giving consideration to previous dose pharmacokinetics, and thereafter only as needed. In high-risk patients (e.g., elderly, debilitated, presence of respiratory disease, etc.) and or in patients where other CNS depressants are present, such as in the immediate postoperative period, the dose should be reduced by approximately one-half. Extra caution should be exercised with the intravenous route of administration, particularly with the initial dose.
Occasionally, it may be necessary to administer single doses of up to 0.6 mg depending on the severity of the pain and the response of the patient. This dose should only be given I.M. and only to patients who are not in a high risk category (see WARNINGS and PRECAUTIONS). At this time, there are insufficient data to recommend single doses greater than 0.6 mg for long-term use.
Parenteral drug products should be inspected visually for particulate matter and discoloration prior to administration, whenever solution and container permit.

HOW SUPPLIED

Buprenex (buprenorphine hydrochloride) is supplied in clear glass snap-ampuls of 1 ml (0.3 mg buprenorphine). NDC 0149-0757-01
Avoid excessive heat (over 104°F or 40°C). Protect from prolonged exposure to light.

CAUTION

Federal law prohibits dispensing without prescription.
Manufactured by:
Reckitt & Colman Pharmaceutical Division
Kingston-upon-Hull HU8 7DS
England
Distributed by:
Norwich Eaton Pharmaceuticals, Inc.
under license from Reckitt & Colman Products, Limited
Buprenex® is a trademark of Reckitt & Colman (Overseas) Limited.
REVISED NOVEMBER 1987

                          BUP-P7

COMHIST® LA   ℞
[kŏm´hist]

DESCRIPTION

Each COMHIST LA yellow and clear capsule for oral administration contains:
chlorpheniramine maleate	4 mg
phenyltoloxamine citrate	50 mg
phenylephrine hydrochloride	20 mg

in a special base to provide a prolonged therapeutic effect.
This product contains ingredients of the following therapeutic classes: antihistamine and decongestant.
Chlorpheniramine maleate is an antihistamine having the chemical name γ-(4-chlorophenyl)-N,N-dimethyl-2-pyridinepropanamine,(Z)-2-butenedioate(1:1) with the following structure:

Phenyltoloxamine citrate is an antihistamine having the chemical name N,N-dimethyl-2-(α-phenyl-o-tolyloxy) ethylamine dihydrogen citrate with the following structure:

Phenylephrine hydrochloride is a decongestant having the chemical name 3-hydroxy-α[(methylamino)methyl]benzenemethanol hydrochloride with the following structure:

INACTIVE INGREDIENTS

Each capsule contains FD&C Blue #2, edible black ink, gelatin, sugar spheres, D&C Yellow #10, FD&C Yellow #6, and other ingredients.

CLINICAL PHARMACOLOGY

Chlorpheniramine maleate is an alkylamine-type antihistamine while phenyltoloxamine citrate belongs to the ethanolamine chemical class. The antihistamines in COMHIST LA act by competing with histamine for H_1 histamine receptor sites, thereby preventing the action of histamine on the cell. Clinically, chlorpheniramine and phenyltoloxamine suppress the histamine-mediated symptoms of allergic rhinitis, relieving sneezing, rhinorrhea, and itching of the eyes, nose, and throat.
Phenylephrine hydrochloride is an α-adrenergic receptor agonist (sympathomimetic) which produces vasoconstriction by stimulating α-receptors within the mucosa of the respiratory tract. Clinically, phenylephrine shrinks swollen mucous membranes, reduces tissue hyperemia, edema, and nasal congestion, and increases nasal airway patency.

INDICATIONS AND USAGE

COMHIST LA is indicated for the relief of rhinorrhea and congestion associated with seasonal and/or perennial allergic rhinitis and vasomotor rhinitis.

CONTRAINDICATIONS

COMHIST LA is contraindicated in persons hypersensitive to any of its components. It should not be administered to children under 12 years of age, patients with severe hypertension, narrow angle glaucoma, or asthmatic symptoms, or patients taking monoamine oxidase inhibitors.

WARNINGS

Chlorpheniramine maleate and phenyltoloxamine citrate should be used with extreme caution in patients with stenosing peptic ulcer, pyloroduodenal obstruction, prostatic hypertrophy, or bladder neck obstruction. These compounds have an atropine-like action and therefore should be used with caution in patients with a history of bronchial asthma, increased intraocular pressure, cardiovascular disease, or hypertension. Sympathomimetic amines should be used with caution in patients with hypertension, diabetes mellitus, heart disease, increased intraocular pressure, hyperthyroidism, or prostatic hypertrophy.

PRECAUTIONS

Information for Patients: This product may cause sedation. Patients should be cautioned against engaging in activities requiring mental alertness, such as driving a car or operating machinery.
Drug Interactions: The sedative effects of chlorpheniramine maleate and phenyltoloxamine citrate are additive to the CNS depressant effects of alcohol, hypnotics, sedatives, and tranquilizers. COMHIST LA should not be used in patients taking monoamine oxidase inhibitors.
Pregnancy: Pregnancy Category C. Animal reproduction studies have not been conducted with COMHIST LA. It is also not known whether COMHIST LA can cause fetal harm when administered to a pregnant woman or can affect reproduction capacity. COMHIST LA should be given to pregnant woman only if clearly needed.
Nursing Mothers: It is not known whether the drugs in COMHIST LA are excreted in human milk. Because many drugs are excreted in human milk and because of the potential for serious adverse reactions in nursing infants, a decision should be made whether to discontinue nursing or to discontinue the product, taking into account the importance of the drug to the mother.
Pediatric Use: Safety and effectiveness of COMHIST LA in children below the age of 12 have not been established.

ADVERSE REACTIONS

General: Urticaria, drug rash, dryness of mouth, nose, and throat.
Cardiovascular System: Hypotension, headache, palpitations.
Hematologic System: Thrombocytopenia, agranulocytosis, leukopenia.
Nervous System: Sedation, dizziness, excitation (especially in children), nervousness, insomnia, blurred vision, convulsions.
Gastrointestinal System: Epigastric distress, anorexia, nausea, vomiting, diarrhea, constipation.
Genitourinary System: Urinary frequency, urinary retention.
Respiratory System: Thickening of bronchial secretions, tightness of chest and wheezing, nasal stuffiness.

OVERDOSAGE

The treatment of overdosage should provide symptomatic and supportive care. If the amount ingested is considered dangerous or excessive, induce vomiting with ipecac syrup unless the patient is convulsing, comatose, or has lost the gag reflex, in which case perform gastric lavage using a large-bore tube. If indicated, follow with activated charcoal and a saline cathartic. Since the effects of COMHIST LA may last up to 12 hours, treatment should be continued for at least that length of time.

DOSAGE AND ADMINISTRATION

Adults and children 12 years of age and older—1 capsule every 8 to 12 hours; not recommended for children under 12 years of age.

HOW SUPPLIED

COMHIST LA is available as a yellow and clear capsule imprinted "COMHIST LA" and "01490446".
NDC 0149-0446-01 Bottle of 100

CAUTION

Federal law prohibits dispensing without prescription.
Manufactured for
Norwich Eaton Pharmaceuticals, Inc.
by KV Pharmaceutical Company
St. Louis, Missouri 63144
REVISED SEPTEMBER 1985   COMLA-X7

DANTRIUM®   ℞
[dan´trē-um]
(dantrolene sodium)
CAPSULES

Dantrium (dantrolene sodium) has a potential for hepatotoxicity, and should not be used in conditions other than those recommended. Symptomatic hepatitis (fatal and non-fatal) has been reported at various dose levels of the drug. The incidence reported in patients taking up to 400 mg/day is much lower than in those taking doses of 800 mg or more per day. Even sporadic short courses of these higher dose levels within a treatment regimen markedly increased the risk of serious hepatic injury. Liver dysfunction as evidenced by blood chemical abnormalities alone (liver enzyme elevations) has been observed in patients exposed to Dantrium for varying periods of time. Overt hepatitis has occurred at varying intervals after initiation of therapy, but has been most frequently observed between the third and twelfth month of therapy. The risk of hepatic injury appears to be greater in females, in patients over 35 years of age, and in patients taking other medication(s) in addition to Dantrium (dantrolene sodium). Dantrium should be used only in conjunction with appropriate monitoring of hepatic function including frequent determination of SGOT or SGPT. If no observable benefit is derived from the administration of Dantrium after a total of 45 days, therapy should be discontinued. The lowest possible effective dose for the individual patient should be prescribed.

DESCRIPTION

The chemical formula of Dantrium (dantrolene sodium) is hydrated 1-[[[5-(4-nitrophenyl)-2-furanyl]methylene]amino]-2, 4-imidazolidinedione sodium salt. It is an orange powder, slightly soluble in water, but due to its slightly acidic nature the solubility increases somewhat in alkaline solution. The anhydrous salt has a molecular weight of 336. The hydrated salt contains approximately 15% water ($3\frac{1}{2}$ moles) and has a molecular weight of 399. The structural formula for the hydrated salt is: [See formula next page]

Continued on next page

Norwich Eaton—Cont.

Dantrium is supplied in capsules of 25 mg, 50 mg, and 100 mg.

Inactive Ingredients: Each capsule contains edible black ink, gelatin, lactose, magnesium stearate, FD&C Red #3, starch, talc, titanium dioxide, and may contain one or more of the following: FD&C Blue #2, D&C Red #33, iron oxide red, D&C Yellow #10, FD&C Yellow #6, iron oxide yellow.

CLINICAL PHARMACOLOGY

In isolated nerve-muscle preparation, Dantrium has been shown to produce relaxation by affecting the contractile response of the skeletal muscle at a site beyond the myoneural junction, directly on the muscle itself. In skeletal muscle, Dantrium dissociates the excitation-contraction coupling, probably by interfering with the release of Ca^{++} from the sarcoplasmic reticulum. This effect appears to be more pronounced in fast muscle fibers as compared to slow ones, but generally affects both. A central nervous system effect occurs, with drowsiness, dizziness and generalized weakness occasionally present. Although Dantrium does not appear to directly affect the CNS, the extent of its indirect effect is unknown. The absorption of Dantrium after oral administration in humans is incomplete and slow but consistent, and dose-related blood levels are obtained. The duration and intensity of skeletal muscle relaxation is related to the dosage and blood levels. The mean biologic half-life of Dantrium in adults is 8.7 hours after a 100-mg dose. Specific metabolic pathways in the degradation and elimination of Dantrium in human subjects have been established. Metabolic patterns are similar in adults and children. In addition to the parent compound, dantrolene, which is found in measurable amounts in blood and urine, the major metabolites noted in body fluids are the 5-hydroxy analog and the acetamido analog. Since Dantrium is probably metabolized by hepatic microsomal enzymes, enhancement of its metabolism by other drugs is possible. However, neither phenobarbital nor diazepam appears to affect Dantrium metabolism.

Clinical experience in the management of fulminant human malignant hyperthermia, as well as experiments conducted in malignant hyperthermia susceptible swine, have revealed that the administration of intravenous dantrolene, combined with indicated supportive measures, is effective in reversing the hypermetabolic process of malignant hyperthermia. Known differences between human and swine malignant hyperthermia are minor. The prophylactic administration of oral or intravenous dantrolene to malignant hyperthermia susceptible swine will attenuate or prevent the development of signs of malignant hyperthermia in a manner dependent upon the dosage of dantrolene administered and the intensity of the malignant hyperthermia triggering stimulus. Limited clinical experience with the administration of oral dantrolene to patients judged malignant hyperthermia susceptible, when combined with clinical experience in the use of intravenous dantrolene for the treatment of malignant hyperthermia and data derived from the above cited animal model experiments, suggests that oral dantrolene will also attenuate or prevent the development of signs of human malignant hyperthermia, provided that currently accepted practices in the management of such patients are adhered to (see INDICATIONS AND USAGE); intravenous dantrolene should also be available for use should the signs of malignant hyperthermia appear.

INDICATIONS AND USAGE

In Chronic Spasticity:
Dantrium is indicated in controlling the manifestations of clinical spasticity resulting from upper motor neuron disorders (e.g., spinal cord injury, stroke, cerebral palsy, or multiple sclerosis). It is of particular benefit to the patient whose functional rehabilitation has been retarded by the sequelae of spasticity. Such patients must have presumably reversible spasticity where relief of spasticity will aid in restoring residual function. Dantrium is not indicated in the treatment of skeletal muscle spasm resulting from rheumatic disorders. If improvement occurs, it will ordinarily occur within the dosage titration (see DOSAGE AND ADMINISTRATION), and will be manifested by a decrease in the severity of spasticity and the ability to resume a daily function not quite attainable without Dantrium.

Occasionally, subtle but meaningful improvement in spasticity may occur with Dantrium therapy. In such instances, information regarding improvement should be solicited from the patient and those who are in constant daily contact and attendance with him. Brief withdrawal of Dantrium for a period of 2 to 4 days will frequently demonstrate exacerbation of the manifestations of spasticity and may serve to confirm a clinical impression.

A decision to continue the administration of Dantrium on a long-term basis is justified if introduction of the drug into the patient's regimen:

     produces a significant reduction in painful and/or disabling spasticity such as clonus, or

     permits a significant reduction in the intensity and/or degree of nursing care required, or

     rids the patient of any annoying manifestation of spasticity considered important by the patient himself.

In Malignant Hyperthermia:
Oral Dantrium is also indicated preoperatively to prevent or attenuate the development of signs of malignant hyperthermia in known, or strongly suspect, malignant hyperthermia susceptible patients who require anesthesia and/or surgery. Currently accepted clinical practices in the management of such patients must still be adhered to (careful monitoring for early signs of malignant hyperthermia, minimizing exposure to triggering mechanisms and prompt use of intravenous dantrolene sodium and indicated supportive measures should signs of malignant hyperthermia appear); see also the package insert for Dantrium (dantrolene sodium) Intravenous.

Oral Dantrium should be administered following a malignant hyperthermic crisis to prevent recurrence of the signs of malignant hyperthermia.

CONTRAINDICATIONS

Active hepatic disease, such as hepatitis and cirrhosis, is a contraindication for use of Dantrium. Dantrium is contraindicated where spasticity is utilized to sustain upright posture and balance in locomotion or whenever spasticity is utilized to obtain or maintain increased function.

WARNINGS

It is important to recognize that fatal and non-fatal liver disorders of an idiosyncratic or hypersensitivity type may occur with Dantrium therapy.

At the start of Dantrium therapy, it is desirable to do liver function studies (SGOT, SGPT, alkaline phosphatase, total bilirubin) for a baseline or to establish whether there is pre-existing liver disease. If baseline liver abnormalities exist and are confirmed, there is a clear possibility that the potential for Dantrium hepatotoxicity could be enhanced, although such a possibility has not yet been established.

Liver function studies (e.g., SGOT or SGPT) should be performed at appropriate intervals during Dantrium therapy. If such studies reveal abnormal values, therapy should generally be discontinued. Only where benefits of the drug have been of major importance to the patient, should reinitiation or continuation of therapy be considered. Some patients have revealed a return to normal laboratory values in the face of continued therapy while others have not.

If symptoms compatible with hepatitis, accompanied by abnormalities in liver function tests or jaundice appear, Dantrium should be discontinued. If caused by Dantrium and detected early, the abnormalities in liver function characteristically have reverted to normal when the drug was discontinued.

Dantrium therapy has been reinstituted in a few patients who have developed clinical and/or laboratory evidence of hepatocellular injury. If such reinstitution of therapy is done, it should be attempted only in patients who clearly need Dantrium and only after previous symptoms and laboratory abnormalities have cleared. The patient should be hospitalized and the drug should be restarted in very small and gradually increasing doses. Laboratory monitoring should be frequent and the drug should be withdrawn immediately if there is any indication of recurrent liver involvement. Some patients have reacted with unmistakable signs of liver abnormality upon administration of a challenge dose, while others have not.

Dantrium should be used with particular caution in females and in patients over 35 years of age in view of apparent greater likelihood of drug-induced, potentially fatal, hepatocellular disease in these groups.

Long-term safety of Dantrium in humans has not been established. Chronic studies in rats, dogs and monkeys at dosages greater than 30 mg/kg/day showed growth or weight depression and signs of hepatopathy and possible occlusion nephropathy, all of which were reversible upon cessation of treatment. Sprague-Dawley female rats fed dantrolene sodium for 18 months at dosage levels of 15, 30, and 60 mg/kg/day showed an increased incidence of benign and malignant mammary tumors compared with concurrent controls and, at the highest dosage, an increase in the incidence of hepatic lymphangiomas and hepatic angiosarcomas. These effects were not seen in 2½-year studies in Sprague-Dawley or Fischer 344 rats or in 2-year studies in mice of the HaM/ICR strain. Carcinogenicity in humans cannot be fully excluded, so that this possible risk of chronic administration must be weighed against the benefits of the drug (i.e., after a brief trial) for the individual patient.

USAGE IN PREGNANCY

The safety of Dantrium for use in women who are or who may become pregnant has not been established. Dantrium should not be used in nursing mothers.

Usage in Children: The long-term safety of Dantrium in children under the age of 5 years has not been established. Because of the possibility that adverse effects of the drug could become apparent only after many years, a benefit-risk consideration of the long-term use of Dantrium is particularly important in pediatric patients.

Drug Interactions: While a definite drug interaction with estrogen therapy has not yet been established, caution should be observed if the two drugs are to be given concomitantly. Hepatotoxicity has occurred more often in women over 35 years of age receiving concomitant estrogen therapy. There are very rare reports of cardiovascular collapse in patients treated simultaneously with verapamil and dantrolene sodium. The combination of therapeutic doses of intravenous dantrolene sodium and verapamil in halothane/α-chloralose anesthetized swine has resulted in ventricular fibrillation and cardiovascular collapse in association with marked hyperkalemia. Until the relevance of these findings to humans is established, the combination of dantrolene sodium and verapamil is not recommended during the management of malignant hyperthermia.

PRECAUTIONS

Dantrium should be used with caution in patients with impaired pulmonary function, particularly those with obstructive pulmonary disease, and in patients with severely impaired cardiac function due to myocardial disease. It should be used with caution in patients with a history of previous liver disease or dysfunction (see WARNINGS).

Patients should be cautioned against driving a motor vehicle or participating in hazardous occupations while taking Dantrium. Caution should be exercised in the concomitant administration of tranquilizing agents.

Dantrium might possibly evoke a photosensitivity reaction; patients should be cautioned about exposure to sunlight while taking it.

ADVERSE REACTIONS

The most frequently occurring side effects of Dantrium have been drowsiness, dizziness, weakness, general malaise, fatigue, and diarrhea. These are generally transient, occurring early in treatment, and can often be obviated by beginning with a low dose and increasing dosage gradually until an optimal regimen is established. Diarrhea may be severe and may necessitate temporary withdrawal of Dantrium therapy. If diarrhea recurs upon readministration of Dantrium, therapy should probably be withdrawn permanently.

Other less frequent side effects, listed according to system are:

Gastrointestinal: Constipation, GI bleeding, anorexia, swallowing difficulty, gastric irritation, abdominal cramps.
Hepatobiliary: Hepatitis (see WARNINGS).
Neurologic: Speech disturbance, seizure, headache, light-headedness, visual disturbance, diplopia, alteration of taste, insomnia.
Cardiovascular: Tachycardia, erratic blood pressure, phlebitis.
Psychiatric: Mental depression, mental confusion, increased nervousness.
Urogenital: Increased urinary frequency, crystalluria, hematuria, difficult erection, urinary incontinence and/or nocturia, difficult urination and/or urinary retention.
Integumentary: Abnormal hair growth, acne-like rash, pruritus, urticaria, eczematoid eruption, sweating.
Musculoskeletal: Myalgia, backache.
Respiratory: Feeling of suffocation.
Special Senses: Excessive tearing.
Hypersensitivity: Pleural effusion with pericarditis.
Other: Chills and fever.

DOSAGE AND ADMINISTRATION

For Use in Chronic Spasticity:
Prior to the administration of Dantrium, consideration should be given to the potential response to treatment. A decrease in spasticity sufficient to allow a daily function not otherwise attainable should be the therapeutic goal of treatment with Dantrium. Refer to INDICATIONS AND USAGE section for description of response to be anticipated.

It is important to establish a therapeutic goal (regain and maintain a specific function such as therapeutic exercise program, utilization of braces, transfer maneuvers, etc.) before beginning Dantrium therapy. Dosage should be increased until the maximum performance compatible with the dysfunction due to underlying disease is achieved. No further increase in dosage is then indicated.

Usual Dosage: It is important that the dosage be titrated and individualized for maximum effect. The lowest dose compatible with optimal response is recommended.

In view of the potential for liver damage in long-term Dantrium use, therapy should be stopped if benefits are not evident within 45 days.

Adults: Begin therapy with 25 mg once daily; increase to 25 mg two, three, or four times daily and then by increments of 25 mg up to as high as 100 mg two, three, or four times daily if necessary. As most patients will respond to a dose of 400 mg/day or less, rarely should doses higher than 400 mg/day be used (see Box Warning.)

Each dosage level should be maintained for four to seven days to determine the patient's response. The dose should not be increased beyond, and may even have to be reduced to, the amount at which the patient received maximal benefit without adverse effects.

Children: A similar approach should be utilized starting with 0.5 mg/kg of body weight twice daily; this is increased to 0.5 mg/kg three or four times daily and then by increments of 0.5 mg/kg up to as high as 3.0 mg/kg two, three, or four times daily, if necessary. Doses higher than 100 mg four times daily should not be used in children.

For Malignant Hyperthermia:

Preoperatively: Administer 4 to 8 mg/kg/day of oral Dantrium in 3 or 4 divided doses for one or two days prior to surgery, with the last dose being given approximately 3 to 4 hours before scheduled surgery with a minimum of water. This dosage will usually be associated with skeletal muscle weakness and sedation (sleepiness or drowsiness); adjustment can usually be made within the recommended dosage range to avoid incapacitation or excessive gastrointestinal irritation (including nausea and/or vomiting).

Post Crisis Follow-up:

Oral Dantrium should also be administered following a malignant hyperthermia crisis, in doses of 4 to 8 mg/kg per day in four divided doses, for a one to three day period to prevent recurrence of the manifestations of malignant hyperthermia.

OVERDOSAGE

For acute overdosage, general supportive measures should be employed along with immediate gastric lavage.

Intravenous fluids should be administered in fairly large quantities to avert the possibility of crystalluria. An adequate airway should be maintained and artificial resuscitation equipment should be at hand. Electrocardiographic monitoring should be instituted, and the patient carefully observed. To date, no experience has been reported with dialysis and its value in Dantrium overdosage is not known.

HOW SUPPLIED

Dantrium (dantrolene sodium) is available in:

25-mg opaque, orange and light brown capsules:
NDC 0149-0030-05 bottle of 100
NDC 0149-0030-66 bottle of 500
NDC 0149-0030-77 hospital unit-dose strips in boxes of 100
50-mg opaque, orange and dark brown capsules:
NDC 0149-0031-05 bottle of 100
100-mg opaque, orange and light brown capsules:
NDC 0149-0033-05 bottle of 100
NDC 0149-0033-77 hospital unit-dose strips in boxes of 100
Address medical inquiries to Norwich Eaton Pharmaceuticals, Inc., Medical Department, Norwich, NY 13815.

CAUTION

Federal law prohibits dispensing without prescription.
Manufactured by
Eaton Laboratories, Inc.
Manati, Puerto Rico 00701
Distributed by
Norwich Eaton Pharmaceuticals, Inc.
REVISED AUGUST 1988   DANCP-P9

DANTRIUM®   ℞
[dan'trē-um]
INTRAVENOUS
(dantrolene sodium
for injection)

DESCRIPTION

Dantrium Intravenous is a sterile, nonpyrogenic, lyophilized formulation of dantrolene sodium for injection. Dantrium Intravenous is supplied in 70 ml vials containing 20 mg dantrolene sodium, 3000 mg mannitol, and sufficient sodium hydroxide to yield a pH of approximately 9.5 when reconstituted with 60 ml sterile water for injection USP (without a bacteriostatic agent).

Dantrolene is classified as a direct-acting skeletal muscle relaxant. Chemically, Dantrium is hydrated 1-[[[5-(4-nitrophenyl)-2-furanyl]methylene]amino]-2,4-imidazolidinedione sodium salt. The structural formula for the hydrated salt is:

The hydrated salt contains approximately 15% water (3½ moles) and has a molecular weight of 399. The anhydrous salt (dantrolene) has a molecular weight of 336.

CLINICAL PHARMACOLOGY

In isolated nerve-muscle preparations, Dantrium produces skeletal muscle relaxation by directly affecting the contractile response of the muscle at a site beyond the myoneural junction. In skeletal muscle, Dantrium dissociates excitation-contraction coupling, probably by interfering with the release of CA^{++} from the sarcoplasmic reticulum. The administration of intravenous Dantrium to human volunteers is associated with loss of grip strength and weakness in the legs, as well as subjective CNS complaints (see also PRECAUTIONS, Information for Patients). Information concerning the passage of Dantrium across the blood-brain barrier is not available.

In the anesthetic-induced malignant hyperthermia (MH) syndrome, evidence points to an intrinsic abnormality of skeletal muscle tissue. In affected humans, it has been postulated that "triggering agents" (e.g., general anesthetics and depolarizing neuromuscular blocking agents) produce a change within the cell which results in an elevated myoplasmic calcium. This elevated myoplasmic calcium activates acute cellular catabolic processes that cascade to the MH crisis.

It is hypothesized that addition of Dantrium to the "triggered" malignant hyperthermic muscle cell reestablishes a normal level of ionized calcium in the myoplasm. Inhibition of calcium release from the sarcoplasmic reticulum by Dantrium reestablishes the myoplasmic calcium equilibrium, increasing the percentage of bound calcium. In this way, physiologic, metabolic, and biochemical changes associated with the MH crisis may be reversed or attenuated.

Experimental results in malignant hyperthermia susceptible (MHS) swine show that prophylactic administration of intravenous or oral dantrolene prevents or attenuates the development of vital sign and blood gas changes characteristic of malignant hyperthermia (MH) in a dose related manner. The efficacy of intravenous dantrolene in the treatment of human and porcine MH crisis, when considered along with prophylactic experiments in MHS swine, lends support to prophylactic use of oral or intravenous dantrolene in MHS humans. When prophylactic intravenous dantrolene is administered as directed, whole bloood concentrations remain at a near steady state level for 3 or more hours after the infusion is completed. Clinical experience has shown that early vital sign and/or blood gas changes characteristic of MH may appear during or after anesthesia and surgery despite the prophylactic use of dantrolene and adherence to currently accepted patient management practices. These signs are compatible with attenuated MH and respond to the administration of additional i.v. dantrolene (see DOSAGE AND ADMINISTRATION). The administration of the recommended prophylactic dose of intravenous dantrolene to healthy volunteers was not associated with clinically significant cardiorespiratory changes.

Specific metabolic pathways for the degradation and elimination of Dantrium in humans have been established. Dantrolene is found in measurable amounts in blood and urine. Its major metabolites in body fluids are 5-hydroxy dantrolene and an acetylamino metabolite of dantrolene. Another metabolite with an unknown structure appears related to the latter. Dantrium may also undergo hydrolysis and subsequent oxidation forming nitrophenylfuroic acid.

The mean biologic half-life of Dantrium after intravenous administration is variable, between 4 to 8 hours under most experimental conditions. Based on assays of whole blood and plasma, slightly greater amounts of dantrolene are associated with red blood cells than with the plasma fraction of blood. Significant amounts of dantrolene are bound to plasma proteins, mostly albumin, and this binding is readily reversible.

Cardiopulmonary depression has not been observed in MHS swine following the administration of up to 7.5 mg/kg i.v. dantrolene. This is twice the amount needed to maximally diminish twitch response to single supramaximal peripheral nerve stimulation (95% inhibition). A transient, inconsistent, depressant effect on gastrointestinal smooth muscles has been observed at high doses.

INDICATIONS AND USAGE

Dantrium Intravenous is indicated, along with appropriate supportive measures, for the management of the fulminant hypermetabolism of skeletal muscle characteristic of MH crisis in patients of all ages. Dantrium Intravenous should be administered by continuous rapid intravenous push as soon as the MH reaction is recognized (i.e., tachycardia, tachypnea, central venous desaturation, hypercarbia, metabolic acidosis, skeletal muscle rigidity, increased utilization of anesthesia circuit carbon dioxide absorber, cyanosis and mottling of the skin, and, in many cases, fever).

Dantrium Intravenous is also indicated preoperatively, and sometimes postoperatively, to prevent or attenuate the development of clinical and laboratory signs of malignant hyperthermia in individuals judged to be malignant hyperthermia susceptible.

CONTRAINDICATIONS

None.

WARNINGS

The use of Dantrium Intravenous in the management of MH crisis is not a substitute for previously known supportive measures. These measures must be individualized, but it will usually be necessary to discontinue the suspect triggering agents, attend to increased oxygen requirements, manage the metabolic acidosis, institute cooling when necessary, monitor urinary output, and monitor for electrolyte imbalance.

Since the effect of disease state and other drugs on the consequences of Dantrium-related skeletal muscle weakness, including possible respiratory depression, cannot be predicted, patients who receive i.v. Dantrium preoperatively should have vital signs monitored.

If patients judged malignant hyperthermia susceptible are administered intravenous or oral Dantrium preoperatively, anesthetic preparation must still follow a standard MHS regimen, including the avoidance of known triggering agents. Monitoring for early clinical and metabolic signs of MH is indicated because attenuation of MH, rather than prevention, is possible. These signs usually call for the administration of additional i.v. dantrolene.

PRECAUTIONS

General: Care must be taken to prevent extravasation of Dantrium solution into the surrounding tissues due to the high pH of the intravenous formulation.

When mannitol is used for prevention or treatment of late renal complications of MH, the 3 g of mannitol needed to dissolve each 20 mg vial of i.v. Dantrium should be taken into consideration.

Information for Patients: Based upon data in human volunteers, it will sometimes be appropriate to tell patients who receive Dantrium Intravenous that decrease in grip strength and weakness of leg muscles, especially walking down stairs, can be expected postoperatively. In addition, symptoms such as "lightheadedness" may be noted. Since some of these symptoms may persist for up to 48 hours, patients must not operate an automobile or engage in other hazardous activity during this time. Caution is also indicated at meals on the day of administration because difficulty swallowing and choking has been reported.

Drug Interactions: Dantrium is metabolized by the liver, and it is theoretically possible that its metabolism may be enhanced by drugs known to induce hepatic microsomal enzymes. However, neither phenobarbital nor diazepam appears to affect Dantrium metabolism. Binding to plasma protein is not significantly altered by diazepam, diphenylhydantoin, or phenylbutazone. Binding to plasma proteins is reduced by warfarin and clofibrate and increased by tolbutamide.

The combination of therapeutic doses of intravenous dantrolene sodium and verapamil in halothane/α-chloralose anesthetized swine has resulted in ventricular fibrillation and cardiovascular collapse in association with marked hyperkalemia. It is recommended that the combination of intravenous dantrolene sodium and calcium channel blockers, such as verapamil, not be used together during the management of malignant hyperthermia crisis until the relevance of these findings to humans is established.

Carcinogenesis, Mutagenesis, and Impairment of Fertility: Studies of Dantrium in animals to evaluate mutagenic potential and the effect on fertility have not been conducted. Sprague-Dawley female rats fed Dantrium for 18 months at dosage levels of 15, 30, and 60 mg/kg/day showed an increased incidence of benign and malignant mammary tumors compared with concurrent controls. At the highest dosage, there was an increase in the incidence of hepatic lymphangiomas and hepatic angiosarcomas. These effects were not seen in 30-month studies in Sprague-Dawley or Fischer-344 rats or in 24-month studies in mice of the HaM/ICR strain., Although the possibility that the drug may be carcinogenic in humans cannot be fully excluded, the risks associated with administration of Dantrium Intravenous in a life-threatening crisis would appear to be minimal.

Usage In Pregnancy: Pregnancy Category C: Dantrium has been shown to be embryocidal in the rabbit and has been shown to decrease pup survival in the rat when given at doses seven times the human oral dose. There are no adequate and well-controlled studies in pregnant women. Dantrium Intravenous should be used during pregnancy only if the potential benefit justifies the potential risk to the fetus.

Labor and Delivery: In one controlled study, 100 mg per day of prophylactic oral Dantrium was administered to term pregnant patients awaiting labor and delivery. Dantrolene readily crossed the placenta, with maternal and fetal whole blood levels approximately equal at delivery; neonatal levels then fell approximately 50% per day for 2 days before declining sharply. No neonatal respiratory and neuromuscular side effects were detected at low dose. More data, at higher

Continued on next page

Norwich Eaton—Cont.

doses, are needed before more definitive conclusions can be made.

ADVERSE REACTIONS

There have been occasional reports of death following MH crisis even when treated with intravenous dantrolene; incidence figures are not available (the predantrolene mortality of MH crisis was approximately 50%). Most of these deaths can be accounted for by late recognition, delayed treatment, inadequate dosage, lack of supportive therapy, intercurrent disease and/or the development of delayed complications such as renal failure or disseminated intravascular coagulopathy. In some cases there are insufficient data to completely rule out therapeutic failure of dantrolene.

There are rare reports of fatality in MH crisis, despite initial satisfactory response to i.v. dantrolene, which involve patients who could not be weaned from dantrolene after initial treatment.

The following adverse reactions are in approximate order of severity:

There are rare reports of pulmonary edema developing during the treatment of MH crisis in which the diluent volume and mannitol needed to deliver i.v. dantrolene possibly contributed.

There have been reports of thrombophlebitis following administration of intravenous dantrolene; actual incidence figures are not available.

There have been rare reports of urticaria and erythema possibly associated with the administration of i.v. Dantrium.

None of the serious reactions occasionally reported with long-term oral Dantrium use, such as hepatitis, seizures, and pleural effusion with pericarditis, have been reasonably associated with short-term Dantrium Intravenous therapy.

OVERDOSAGE

Because Dantrium Intravenous must be administered at a low concentration in a large volume of fluid, acute toxicity of Dantrium could not be assessed in animals. In 14-day (subacute) studies, the intravenous formulation of Dantrium was relatively non-toxic to rats at doses of 10 mg/kg/day and 20 mg/kg/day. While 10 mg/kg/day in dogs for 14 days evoked little toxicity, 20 mg/kg/day for 14 days caused hepatic changes of questionable biologic significance.

No data are available to define the symptomatology of an overdose of Dantrium Intravenous. If an overdose is suspected, treatment is symptomatic and supportive. There is no known antidote.

DOSAGE AND ADMINISTRATION

As soon as the MH reaction is recognized, all anesthetic agents should be discontinued; the administration of 100% oxygen is recommended. Dantrium Intravenous should be administered by continuous rapid intravenous push beginning at a minimum dose of 1 mg/kg, and continuing until symptoms subside or the maximum cumulative dose of 10 mg/kg has been reached. If the physiologic and metabolic abnormalities reappear, the regimen may be repeated. It is important to note that administration of Dantrium Intravenous should be continuous until symptoms subside. The effective dose to reverse the crisis is directly dependent upon the individual's degree of susceptibility to MH, the amount and time of exposure to the triggering agent, and the time elapsed between onset of the crisis and initiation of treatment.

Children's Dose: Experience to date indicates that the dose of Dantrium Intravenous for children is the same as for adults.

Preoperatively: Dantrium Intravenous and/or Dantrium Capsules may be administered preoperatively to patients judged MH susceptible as part of the overall patient management to prevent or attenuate the development of clincal and laboratory signs of MH.

Dantrium Intravenous: The recommended prophylactic dose of Dantrium Intravenous is 2.5 mg/kg, starting approximately 1¼ hours before anticipated anesthesia and infused over approximately 1 hour. This dose should prevent or attenuate the development of clinical and laboratory signs of MH provided that the usual precautions, such as avoidance of established MH triggering agents, are followed.

Additional Dantrium Intravenous may be indicated during anesthesia and surgery because of the appearance of early clinical and/or blood gas signs of MH or because of prolonged surgery (see also CLINICAL PHARMACOLOGY, WARNINGS, and PRECAUTIONS). Additional doses must be individualized.

Oral Administration of Dantrium Capsules: Administer 4 to 8 mg/kg/day of oral Dantrium in 3 or 4 divided doses for one or two days prior to surgery, with the last dose being given with a minimum of water approximately 3 to 4 hours before scheduled surgery. Adjustment can usually be made within the recommended dosage range to avoid incapacitation (weakness, drowsiness, etc.) or excessive

gastrointestinal irritation (nausea and/or vomiting). See also the package insert for Dantrium (dantrolene sodium) Capsules.

Post Crisis Follow-up: Dantrium Capsules, 4 to 8 mg/kg/day, in four divided doses should be administered for one to three days following a malignant hyperthermia crisis to prevent recurrence of the manifestations of malignant hyperthermia.

Intravenous Dantrium may be used postoperatively to prevent or attenuate the recurrence of signs of MH when oral Dantrium administration is not practical. The i.v. dose of Dantrium in the postoperative period must be individualized, starting with 1 mg/kg or more as the clinical situation dictates.

PREPARATION

Each vial of Dantrium Intravenous should be reconstituted by adding 60 ml of *sterile water for injection USP (without a bacteriostatic agent), and the vial shaken until the solution is clear.* 5% Dextrose Injection U.S.P, 0.9% Sodium Chloride Injection U.S.P, and other acidic solutions are not compatible with Dantrium Intravenous and should not be used. The contents of the vial must be *protected from direct light and used within 6 hours* after reconstitution. Store reconstituted solutions at controlled room temperature (59°F to 86°F or 15°C to 30°C).

Reconstituted Dantrium Intravenous should *not* be transferred to large glass bottles for prophylactic infusion due to precipitate formation observed with the use of some glass bottles as reservoirs.

For prophylactic infusion, the required number of individual vials of Dantrium Intravenous should be reconstituted as outlined above. The contents of individual vials are then transferred to a larger volume sterile intravenous plastic bag. Stability data on file at Norwich Eaton Pharmaceuticals, Inc. indicate commercially available sterile plastic bags are acceptable drug delivery devices. However, it is recommended that the prepared infusion be inspected carefully for cloudiness and/or precipitation prior to dispensing and administration. Such solutions should not be used. While stable for 6 hours, it is recommended that the infusion be prepared immediately prior to the anticipated dosage administration time.

Parenteral drug products should be inspected visually for particulate matter and discoloration prior to administration.

HOW SUPPLIED

Dantrium Intravenous (NDC 0149-0734-02) is available in vials containing a sterile lyophilized mixture of 20 mg dantrolene sodium, 3000 mg mannitol, and sufficient sodium hydroxide to yield a pH of approximately 9.5 when reconstituted with 60 ml sterile water for injection USP (without a bacteriostatic agent).

Store unreconstituted product at controlled room temperature (59°F to 86°F or 15°C to 30°C) and avoid prolonged exposure to light.

Address medical inquiries to Norwich Eaton Pharmaceuticals Inc., Medical Department, P.O. Box 191, Norwich, NY 13815-0191.

CAUTION

Federal law prohibits dispensing with prescription.
Manufactured by
Eaton Laboratories, Inc.
Manati, Puerto Rico 00701
Distributed by
Norwich Eaton Pharmaceuticals, Inc.
REVISED FEBRUARY 1989   DANTIV-P5

DIDRONEL®   ℞
[dī'drō-nel]
(etidronate disodium)

DESCRIPTION

Didronel tablets contain either 200 mg or 400 mg of etidronate disodium, the disodium salt of (1-hydroxyethylidene) diphosphonic acid, for oral administration. This compound, also known as EHDP, regulates bone metabolism. It is a white powder, highly soluble in water, with a molecular weight of 250 and the following structural formula:

$$HO - \overset{\displaystyle \overset{ONa}{|}}{\underset{\displaystyle \underset{O}{|}}{P}} - \overset{\displaystyle \overset{OH}{|}}{\underset{\displaystyle \underset{CH_3}{|}}{C}} - \overset{\displaystyle \overset{ONa}{|}}{\underset{\displaystyle \underset{O}{|}}{P}} - OH$$

Inactive Ingredients: Each tablet contains magnesium stearate, microcrystalline cellulose, and starch.

CLINICAL PHARMACOLOGY

Didronel acts primarily on bone. It can inhibit the formation, growth and dissolution of hydroxyapatite crystals and their amorphous precursors by chemisorption to calcium phosphate surfaces. Inhibition of crystal resorption occurs at lower doses than are required to inhibit crystal growth. Both effects increase as the dose increases.

Didronel is not metabolized. Absorption averages about 1% of an oral dose of 5 mg/kg body weight/day. This increases to about 2.5% at 10 mg/kg/day and 6% at 20 mg/kg/day. Most of the absorbed drug is cleared from the blood within 6 hours. Within 24 hours about half of the absorbed dose is excreted in the urine. The remainder is chemically adsorbed to bone, especially to areas of elevated osteogenesis, and is slowly eliminated. Unabsorbed drug is excreted intact in the feces. Didronel therapy does not adversely affect serum levels of parathyroid hormone or calcium. Hyperphosphatemia has been observed in Didronel patients, usually in association with doses of 10–20 mg/kg/day. No adverse effects have been traced to this, and it is not a contraindication for therapy. It is apparently due to drug-related increased tubular reabsorption of phosphate by the kidney. Serum phosphate levels generally return to normal 2–4 weeks posttherapy.

PAGET'S DISEASE: Paget's disease of bone (osteitis deformans) is an idiopathic, progressive disease characterized by abnormal and accelerated bone metabolism in one or more bones. Signs and symptoms may include bone pain and/or deformity, neurologic disorders, elevated cardiac output and other vascular disorders, and increased serum alkaline phosphatase and/or urinary hydroxyproline levels. Bone fractures are common in patients with Paget's disease.

Didronel slows accelerated bone turnover (resorption and accretion) in pagetic lesions and, to a lesser extent, in normal bone. This has been demonstrated histologically, scintigraphically, biochemically, and through calcium kinetic and balance studies. Reduced bone turnover is often accompanied by symptomatic improvement, including reduced bone pain. Also, the incidence of pagetic fractures may be reduced, and elevated cardiac output and other vascular disorders may be improved by Didronel therapy.

HETEROTOPIC OSSIFICATION: Heterotopic ossification, also referred to as myositis ossificans (circumscripta, progressiva or traumatica), ectopic calcification, periarticular ossification, or paraosteoarthropathy, is characterized by metaplastic osteogenesis. It usually presents with signs of localized inflammation or pain, elevated skin temperature, and redness. When tissues near joints are involved, functional loss may also be present.

Heterotopic ossification may occur for no known reason as in myositis ossificans progressiva or may follow a wide variety of surgical, occupational, and sports trauma (e.g., hip arthroplasty, spinal cord injury, head injury, burns and severe thigh bruises). Heterotopic ossification has also been observed in non-traumatic conditions (e.g., infections of the central nervous system, peripheral neuropathy, tetanus, biliary cirrhosis, Peyronie's disease, as well as in association with a variety of benign and malignant neoplasms).

Clinical trials have demonstrated the efficacy of Didronel in heterotopic ossification following total hip replacement, or due to spinal cord injury.

—*Heterotopic ossification complicating total hip replacement* typically develops radiographically 3–8 weeks postoperatively in the pericapsular area of the affected hip joint. The overall incidence is about 50%; about one-third of these cases are clinically significant.

—*Heterotopic ossification due to spinal cord injury* typically develops radiographically 1–4 months after injury. It occurs below the level of injury, usually at major joints. The overall incidence is about 40%; about one-half of these cases are clinically significant.

Didronel chemisorbs to calcium hydroxyapatite crystals and their amorphous precursors, blocking the aggregation, growth and mineralization of these crystals. This is thought to be the mechanism by which Didronel prevents or retards heterotopic ossification. There is no evidence Didronel affects mature heterotopic bone.

INDICATIONS AND USAGE

PAGET'S DISEASE: Didronel is indicated for the treatment of symptomatic Paget's disease of bone. Didronel therapy usually arrests or significantly impedes the disease process as evidenced by:

—Symptomatic relief, including decreased pain and/or increased mobility (experienced by 3 out of 5 patients).

—Reductions in serum alkaline phosphatase and urinary hydroxyproline levels (30% or more in 4 out of 5 patients).

—Histomorphometry showing reduced numbers of osteoclasts and osteoblasts, and more lamellar bone formation.

—Bone scans showing reduced radionuclide uptake at pagetic lesions.

In addition, reductions in pagetically elevated cardiac output and skin temperature have been observed in some patients. Also, the incidence of pagetic fractures may be reduced when Didronel is administered intermittently over a period of years.

In many patients, the disease process will be suppressed for a period of at least one year following cessation of therapy. The upper limit of this period has not been determined.

Didronel's effects have not been studied in patients with asymptomatic Paget's disease. However, Didronel treatment of such patients may be warranted if extensive involvement threatens irreversible neurologic damage, major joints, or major weight-bearing bones.

HETEROTOPIC OSSIFICATION: Didronel is indicated in the prevention and treatment of heterotopic ossification following total hip replacement or due to spinal cord injury. Didronel reduces the incidence of clinically important heterotopic bone by about two-thirds. Among those patients who form heterotopic bone, Didronel retards the progression of immature lesions and reduces the severity by at least half. Follow-up data (at least nine months posttherapy) suggest these benefits persist.

In total hip replacement patients, Didronel does not promote loosening of the prosthesis or impede trochanteric reattachment.

In spinal cord injury patients, Didronel does not inhibit fracture healing or stabilization of the spine.

CONTRAINDICATIONS

None known.

WARNINGS

In Paget's patients the response to therapy may be of slow onset and continue for months after Didronel therapy is discontinued. Dosage should not be increased prematurely. A 90-day drug-free interval should be provided between courses of therapy.

Heterotopic ossification: No specific warnings.

PRECAUTIONS

General: Patients should maintain an adequate nutritional status, particularly an adequate intake of calcium and vitamin D.

Therapy has been withheld from some patients with enterocolitis since diarrhea may be experienced, particularly at higher doses.

Didronel is not metabolized and is excreted intact via the kidney. There is no experience to specifically guide treatment in patients with impaired renal function. Didronel dosage should be reduced when reductions in glomerular filtration rates are present. Patients with renal impairment should be closely monitored.

Didronel suppresses bone turnover, and may retard mineralization of osteoid laid down during the bone accretion process. These effects are dose and time dependent. Osteoid, which may accumulate noticeably at doses of 10–20 mg/kg/day, mineralizes normally posttherapy. In patients with fractures, especially of long bones, it may be advisable to delay or interrupt treatment until callus is evident.

In Paget's patients, treatment regimens exceeding the recommended (see DOSAGE AND ADMINISTRATION) daily maximum dose of 20 mg/kg or continuous administration of medication for periods greater than 6 months may be associated with an increased risk of fracture.

Long bones predominantly affected by lytic lesions, particularly in those patients unresponsive to Didronel therapy, may be especially prone to fracture. Patients with predominantly lytic lesions should be monitored radiographically and biochemically to permit termination of Didronel in those patients unresponsive to treatment.

Carcinogenesis: Long-term studies in rats have indicated that Didronel is not carcinogenic.

Pregnancy: Teratogenic Effects: Pregnancy Category B. Reproduction/teratology studies performed in rats and rabbits at doses up to five times the maximum human dose by the intended route of administration have revealed no evidence of impaired fertility or harm to the fetus due to Didronel. At doses of twenty-two times the maximum human dose, a decrease in live fetuses was observed in rats. The only incidence of malformations occurred in rats at exaggerated doses following parenteral administration and were skeletal in nature. These malformations were deemed to be the result of pharmacological action of the drug. There are no adequate, well-controlled studies in pregnant women. Because animal reproduction studies are not always predictive of human response, this drug should be used during pregnancy only if clearly needed.

Nursing Mothers: It is not known whether this drug is excreted in human milk. Because many drugs are excreted in human milk, caution should be exercised when Didronel is administered to a nursing woman.

Pediatric Use: Safety and effectiveness in children have not been established. Children have been treated with Didronel, at doses recommended for adults, to prevent heterotopic ossifications or soft tissue calcifications. A rachitic syndrome has been reported infrequently at doses of 10 mg/kg/day and more for prolonged periods approaching or exceeding a year. The epiphyseal radiologic changes associated with retarded mineralization of new osteoid and cartilage, and occasional symptoms reported, have been reversible when medication is discontinued.

ADVERSE REACTIONS

The incidence of gastrointestinal complaints (diarrhea, nausea) is the same for Didronel at 5 mg/kg/day as for placebo, about 1 patient in 15. At 10–20 mg/kg/day the incidence may increase to 2 or 3 in 10. These complaints are often alleviated by dividing the total daily dose.

Hypersensitivity reactions, including angioedema/urticaria, rash and/or pruritis have been reported rarely.

In Paget's patients, increased or recurrent bone pain at pagetic sites, and/or the onset of pain at previously asymptomatic sites has been reported. At 5 mg/kg/day about 1 patient in 10 (verus 1 in 15 in the placebo group) report these phenomena. At higher doses the incidence rises to about 2 in 10. When therapy continues, pain resolves in some patients but persists in others.

Heterotopic ossification: No specific adverse reactions.

OVERDOSAGE

Clinical experience with Didronel overdosage is extremely limited. Decreases in serum calcium following substantial overdosage may be expected in some patients. Signs and symptoms of hypocalcemia also may occur in some of these patients. In one event, an 18–year–old female who ingested an estimated single dose of 4,000–6,000 mg (67–100 mg/kg) of Didronel was reported to be mildly hypocalcemic (7.52 mg/dl) and experienced paresthesia of the fingers. Some patients may develop vomiting and expel the drug.

Gastric lavage may remove unabsorbed drug. Standard procedures for treating hypocalcemia, including the administration of Ca++ intravenously, would be expected to restore physiologic amounts of ionized calcium and relieve signs and symptoms of hypocalcemia. Such treatment has been effective.

DOSAGE AND ADMINISTRATION

Didronel should be taken as a single, oral dose. However, should gastrointestinal discomfort occur, the dose may be divided. To maximize absorption, patients should avoid taking the following items within two hours of dosing:

—Food, especially those high in calcium, such as milk or milk products.

—Vitamins with mineral supplements or antacids which are high in metals such as calcium, iron, magnesium or aluminum.

PAGET'S DISEASE

Initial Treatment Regimens: 5–10 mg/kg/day, not to exceed 6 months, or 11–20 mg/kg/day, not to exceed 3 months.

The recommended initial dose is 5 mg/kg/day for a period not to exceed six months. Doses above 10 mg/kg/day should be reserved for when 1) lower doses are ineffective or 2) there is an overriding need to suppress rapid bone turnover (especially when irreversible neurologic damage is possible) or reduce elevated cardiac output. Doses in excess of 20 mg/kg/day are not recommended.

Retreatment Guidelines: Retreatment should be initiated only after: 1) a Didronel-free period of at least 90 days and 2) there is biochemical, symptomatic or other evidence of active disease process. It is advisable to monitor patients every 3–6 months although some patients may go drug free for extended periods. Retreatment regimens are the same as for initial treatment. For most patients the original dose will be adequate for retreatment. If not, consideration should be given to increasing the dose within the recommended guidelines.

HETEROTOPIC OSSIFICATION: The following treatment regimens have been shown to be effective:

—Total Hip Replacement Patients: 20 mg/kg/day for 1 month before and 3 months after surgery (4 months total).

—Spinal Cord Injured Patients: 20 mg/kg/day for 2 weeks followed by 10 mg/kg/day for 10 weeks (12 weeks total). Didronel therapy should begin as soon as medically feasible following the injury, preferably prior to evidence of heterotopic ossification.

Retreatment has not been studied.

HOW SUPPLIED

Didronel is available as 200-mg, white, rectangular tablets with "P&G" on one face and "402" on the other.

  NDC 0149-0405-60 bottle of 60

400-mg, white, scored, capsule-shaped tablets with "N E" on one face and "406" on the other.

  NDC 0149-0406-60 bottle of 60

CAUTION

Federal law prohibits dispensing without prescription.
REVISED JUNE 1988

DID-P8

Shown in Product Identification Section, page 420

DIDRONEL® I.V. INFUSION   ℞

[dī'-drō-nel]
(etidronate disodium)

DILUTE BEFORE USE

DESCRIPTION

Didronel I.V. Infusion is a clear, colorless, sterile solution of etidronate disodium, the disodium salt of (1-hydroxyethylidene) diphosphonic acid. Each 6-ml ampule contains a 5% solution of 300 mg etidronate disodium in water for injection for slow intravenous infusion.

Etidronate disodium is a white powder, highly soluble in water, with a molecular weight of 250 and the following structural formula:

[See Chemical Formula at top of next column].

$$HO\!-\!\overset{\overset{\displaystyle ONa}{|}}{\underset{\underset{\displaystyle O}{|}}{P}}\!-\!\overset{\overset{\displaystyle OH}{|}}{\underset{\underset{\displaystyle CH_3}{|}}{C}}\!-\!\overset{\overset{\displaystyle ONa}{|}}{\underset{\underset{\displaystyle O}{|}}{P}}\!-\!OH$$

CLINICAL PHARMACOLOGY

Didronel acts primarily on bone. Its major pharmacologic action is the reduction of normal and abnormal bone resorption. Secondarily, it reduces bone formation since formation is coupled to resorption. This reduces bone turnover, but the reduction of bone turnover, *per se,* is not the important action in the reduction of hypercalcemia.

Didronel's reduction of abnormal bone resorption is responsible for its therapeutic benefit in hypercalcemia. The antiresorptive action of Didronel has been demonstrated under a variety of conditions, although the exact mechanism(s) is not fully understood. It may be related to the drug's inhibition of hydroxyapatite crystal dissolution and/or its action on bone resorbing cells. The number of osteoclasts in active bone turnover sites is substantially reduced after Didronel therapy is administered. Didronel also can inhibit the formation and growth of hydroxyapatite crystals and their amorphous precursors at concentrations in excess of those required to inhibit crystal dissolution.

Etidronate disodium is not metabolized. A large fraction of the infused dose is excreted rapidly and unchanged in the urine. The mean residence time in the exchangeable pool is approximately 8.7 ± 1.0 hours. The mean volume of distribution at steady-state in normal humans is 1370 ± 203 ml/kg while the plasma half-life $(t\frac{1}{2})$ is 6.0 ± 0.7 hours. In these same subjects, nonrenal clearance from the exchangeable pool amounts to 30–50% of the infused dose. This nonrenal clearance is considered to be due to uptake of the drug by bone; subsequently the drug is slowly eliminated through bone turnover. The half-life of the dose on bone is in excess of 90 days.

Hyperphosphatemia, which is often observed in association with oral Didronel medication at doses of 10–20 mg/kg/day, occurs less frequently, in association with intravenous medication of patients with hypercalcemia of malignancy.

Hyperphosphatemia is apparently due to increased tubular reabsorption of phosphate by the kidney. No adverse effects have been associated with Didronel-related hyperphosphatemia and its occurrence is not a contraindication to therapy. Serum phosphate elevations usually return to normal 2–4 weeks after medication is discontinued.

The responsiveness of animal tumors susceptible to four commonly employed classes or subclasses of chemotherapeutic agents, antitumor antibiotics (doxorubicin), a classic alkylating agent (cyclophosphamide), a nitrosourea (carmustine), and a pyrimidine antagonist (5-fluorouracil), were not adversely altered by the concurrent administration of intravenous Didronel.

Hypercalcemia of Malignancy: Hypercalcemia of malignancy is usually related to increased bone resorption associated with the presence of neoplastic tissue. It occurs in 8 to 20% of patients with malignant disease. Whereas hypercalcemia is more often seen in patients with demonstrable osteolytic, osteoblastic, or mixed metastatic tumors in bone, discrete skeletal lesions cannot be demonstrated in at least 30% of patients.

Patients with certain types of neoplasms, such as carcinoma of the breast, bronchogenic carcinoma, renal cell carcinoma, cancers of the head and neck, lymphomas, and multiple myeloma, are especially prone to developing hypercalcemia.

As hypercalcemia of malignancy evolves, the renal tubules develop a diminished capacity to concentrate urine. The resultant polyuria and nocturia decrease the extracellular fluid volume. This decrease may be aggravated by vomiting and reduced fluid intake. Thus, the ability of the kidney to eliminate excess calcium is compromised. Renal impairment can eventually cause nitrogen retention, acidosis, renal failure, and further decrease in excretion of calcium. Didronel I.V. Infusion, by inhibiting excessive bone resorption, interrupts this process. Salt loading and use of "high ceiling" or "loop" diuretics may be used to promote calcium excretion, because the rate of renal calcium excretion is directly related to the rate of sodium excretion.

The physiologic derangements induced by excessive serum calcium are due to increased levels of ionized calcium. The pathophysiologic effects of excessive serum calcium are heightened by reductions in serum albumin which normally binds a fraction (about 40%) of the total serum calcium. In patients with hypercalcemia of malignancy, serum albumin is often reduced and this tends to mask the magnitude of the increase in the level of ionized calcium. By reducing the flow of calcium from resorbing bone, Didronel I.V. Infusion effectively reduces total and ionized serum calcium.

In the principal clinical study of Didronel for hypercalcemia of malignancy, patients with elevated calcium levels (10.1–17.4 mg/dl) were treated simultaneously with daily administrations of intravenous Didronel over a 3-day period

Continued on next page

Norwich Eaton—Cont.

and up to 3000 ml of saline and 80 mg of loop diuretic. The response to treatment for these patients was compared with that from patients treated with saline and loop diuretics alone. In terms of total serum calcium changes, 88% of patients treated with Didronel I.V. Infusion as described, had reductions of serum calcium of 1 mg/dl or more. Total serum calcium returned to normal in 63% of patients within 7 days compared to 33% of patients treated with hydration alone. Reductions in urinary calcium excretion, which accompany reductions in excessive bone resorption, became apparent after 24 hours. This was accompanied or followed by maximum decreases in serum calcium which were observed, most frequently, 72 hours after the first infusion.

The physiologically important component of serum calcium is the ionized portion. In most institutions, this cannot be measured directly. It is important to recognize that factors influencing the ratio of free and bound calcium such as serum proteins, particularly albumin, may complicate the interpretation of total serum calcium measurements. If indicated, a corrected serum calcium value should be calculated using an established algorithm.

When the total serum calcium values are adjusted for serum albumin levels, there was a return to normocalcemia in 24% of Didronel-treated patients and in 7% of patients treated with saline infusion. Eighty-seven percent of patients receiving Didronel and 67% of patients on saline had albumin-adjusted serum calcium levels returned to normal or reduced by at least 1 mg/dl.

In the above mentioned study, a second course of Didronel I.V. Infusion was tried in a small number of patients who had a recurrence of hypercalcemia following an initial response to a 3-day infusion of the drug. All patients who received a second 3-day course of Didronel I.V. Infusion showed a decrease of total serum calcium of at least 1 mg/dl. Normalization of total serum calcium occurred in 11 out of 14 patients.

Didronel I.V. Infusion does not appear to alter renal tubular reabsorption of calcium, and does not affect hypercalcemia in patients with hyperparathyroidism where increased calcium reabsorption may be a factor in the hypercalcemia. Limited clinical study results suggest that continuation of Didronel therapy with oral tablets may maintain clinically acceptable serum calcium levels and prolong normocalcemia.

INDICATIONS AND USAGE

Didronel I.V. Infusion, together with achievement and maintenance of adequate hydration, is indicated for the treatment of hypercalcemia of malignancy inadequately managed by dietary modification and/or oral hydration.

In the treatment of hypercalcemia of malignancy, it is important to initiate rehydration with saline together with "high ceiling" or "loop" diuretics if indicated to restore urine output. This also is intended to increase the renal excretion of calcium and initiate a reduction in serum calcium. Since increased bone resorption is usually the underlying cause of an increased flux of calcium into the vascular compartment, concurrent therapy with Didronel I.V. Infusion is recommended as soon as there is a restoration of urine output. Since Didronel is excreted by the kidney, it is important to know that renal function is adequate to handle not only the increased fluid load but also the excretion of the drug itself. (See WARNINGS.)

Didronel I.V. Infusion is also indicated for the treatment of hypercalcemia of malignancy which persists after adequate hydration has been restored. Patients with and without metastases and with a variety of tumors have been responsive to treatment with Didronel I.V. Infusion. Adequate hydration of patients should be maintained, but in aged patients and in those with cardiac failure, care must be taken to avoid overhydration.

CONTRAINDICATIONS

In patients with Class Dc and higher renal functional impairment (serum creatinine greater than 5.0 mg/dl) Didronel I.V. Infusion should be withheld.

WARNINGS

Occasional mild to moderate abnormalities in renal function (elevated BUN and/or serum creatinine) have been observed when Didronel I.V. Infusion was given as directed to patients with hypercalcemia of malignancy. These changes were reversible or remained stable, without worsening, after completion of the course of Didronel I.V. Infusion. In some patients with pre-existing renal impairment or in those who had received potentially nephrotoxic drugs, further depression of renal function was sometimes seen. This suggests that Didronel I.V. Infusion may produce or aggravate the depression of renal function in approximately 8 of 203 treatment courses when used to treat hypercalcemia of malignancy. Therefore, it is recommended that appropriate monitoring of renal function with serum creatinine and/or BUN be carried out with Didronel I.V. Infusion treatment.

The effects of Didronel I.V. Infusion administration on renal function in patients with serum creatinine greater than 2.5 mg/dl (Class Cc and higher, Classification of Renal Functional Impairment, Council on the Kidney in Cardiovascular Disease, American Heart Association, Ann. Int. Med. 75:251–52, 1971) has not been systematically examined in controlled trials.

Since Didronel is excreted by the kidney, it is important to know that renal function is adequate to handle not only the increased fluid load but also the excretion of the drug itself. Since these capacities are impaired in patients with underlying renal disease and since experience with Didronel I.V. Infusion in patients with serum creatinine > 2.5 mg/dl is limited, the use of Didronel I.V. Infusion in such patients should occur only after a careful assessment of renal status or potential risks and potential benefits. (See WARNINGS.) Reduction of the dose of Didronel I.V. Infusion, if used at all, may be advisable in Class Cc renal functional impairment (serum creatinine 2.5 to 4.9 mg/dl); and, Didronel I.V. Infusion be used only if the potential benefit of hypercalcemia correction will substantially exceed the potential for worsening of renal function. In patients with Class Dc and higher renal functional impairment (serum creatinine greater than 5.0 mg/dl) Didronel I.V. Infusion should be withheld.

PRECAUTIONS

General: Hypercalcemia may cause or exacerbate impaired renal function. In clinical trials, while elevations of serum creatinine or blood urea nitrogen were seen in patients with hypercalcemia of malignancy prior to treatment with Didronel I.V. Infusion, these measurements improved in some patients or remained unchanged in most patients. Nevertheless, elevations in serum creatinine during treatment with Didronel I.V. Infusion have been observed in approximately 10% of patients.

In animal preclinical studies, administration of Didronel I.V. Infusion in amounts or at rates in excess of those recommended produced transient hypocalcemia or induced proximal renal tubular damage.

In the principal clinical trial of Didronel I.V. Infusion 33 of 185 patients (18%) treated one or more times with Didronel I.V. Infusion had serum calcium values below the lower limits of normal. When adjusted for levels of reduced serum albumin, less than 1% of the 185 patients are estimated to have hypocalcemic ionized serum calcium levels. No adverse effects have been traced to hypocalcemia.

The hypercalcemia of hyperparathyroidism is refractory to Didronel I.V. Infusion. It is possible for this disease to coexist in patients with malignancy.

Carcinogenesis, Mutagenesis, Impairment of Fertility: Long-term studies in rats indicate that Didronel is not carcinogenic.

Pregnancy: Teratogenic Effects: Pregnancy Category C. Animal reproduction studies have not been conducted with Didronel I.V. Infusion. It is also not known whether Didronel I.V. Infusion can cause fetal harm when administered to a pregnant woman or can affect reproduction capacity. Didronel I.V. Infusion should be given to a pregnant woman only if clearly needed.

Nursing Mothers: It is not known whether this drug is excreted in human milk. Because many drugs are excreted in human milk, caution should be exercised when Didronel I.V. Infusion is administered to a nursing woman.

Pediatric Use: Safety and effectiveness in children have not been established.

ADVERSE REACTIONS

Hypercalcemia of malignancy is frequently associated with abnormal elevations of serum creatinine and BUN. One-third of the patients participating in multiclinic trials had such elevations before receiving Didronel I.V. Infusion. In these trials, the elevations of BUN or serum creatinine improved in some patients, or remained unchanged in most patients; however, in approximately 10% of patients, occasional mild to moderate abnormalities in renal function (increases of > 0.5 mg/dl serum creatinine) were observed during or immediately after treatment. The possibility that Didronel I.V. Infusion contributed to these changes cannot be excluded (see WARNINGS).

Of patients who participated in the controlled hypercalcemia trials, 10 of 221 (5%) treatment courses reported a metallic or altered taste, or loss of taste, which usually disappeared within hours, during and/or shortly after Didronel I.V. Infusion. A few patients with Paget's Disease of bone have reported allergic skin rashes in association with oral Didronel medication.

OVERDOSAGE

Rapid intravenous administration of Didronel at doses above 27 mg/kg has produced ECG changes and bleeding problems in animals. These abnormalities are probably related to marked and/or rapid decreases in ionized calcium levels in blood and tissue fluids. They are thought to be due to chelation of calcium by massive amounts of the diphosphonate. These abnormalities have been shown to be reversible in animal studies by the administration of ionizable calcium salts.

Similar problems are not expected to occur in humans treated with Didronel I.V. Infusion used as recommended (see DOSAGE AND ADMINISTRATION). Moreover, signs and symptoms of hypocalemia such as paresthesias and carpopedal spasms have not been reported. The chelation effects of the diphosphonate, should they occur in man, should be reversible with the intravenous administration of calcium gluconate.

Administration of intravenous etidronate disodium at doses and possibly at rates in excess of those recommended has been reported to be associated with renal insufficiency.

DOSAGE AND ADMINISTRATION

Didronel I.V. Infusion: The recommended dose of Didronel I.V. Infusion is 7.5 mg/kg body weight/day for three successive days. **This daily dose must be diluted in at least 250 ml of sterile normal saline.** Stability studies show that diluted solution stored at controlled room temperature (59°F to 86°F or 15°C to 30°C) shows no loss of drug for a 48-hour period. THE DILUTED DOSE OF DIDRONEL I.V. INFUSION SHOULD BE ADMINISTERED INTRAVENOUSLY OVER A PERIOD OF AT LEAST 2 HOURS. Didronel I.V. Infusion may be added to volumes of fluid greater than 250 ml when this is convenient.

REGARDLESS OF THE VOLUME OF SOLUTION IN WHICH DIDRONEL I.V. INFUSION IS DILUTED, SLOW INFUSION IS IMPORTANT TO SAFETY. The minimum infusion time of two hours at the recommended dose, or smaller doses, should be observed. The usual course of treatment is one infusion of 7.5 mg/kg body weight/day on each of 3 consecutive days but some patients have been treated for up to 7 days. When patients are treated for more than 3 days, there may be an increased possibility of producing hypocalcemia.

Retreatment with Didronel I.V. Infusion may be appropriate if hypercalcemia recurs. There should be at least a seven-day interval between courses of treatment with Didronel I.V. Infusion. The dose and manner of retreatment is the same as that for initial treatment. Retreatment for more than three days has not been adequately studied. The safety and efficacy of more than two courses of therapy with Didronel I.V. Infusion have not been studied. In the presence of renal impairment, reduction of the dose may be advisable.

Parenteral drug products should be inspected visually for particulate matter and discoloration prior to administration whenever solution and container permit.

Didronel Oral Tablets: Didronel (etidronate disodium) tablets may be started on the day following the last dose of Didronel I.V. Infusion. The recommended oral dose of Didronel for patients who have had hypercalcemia is 20 mg/kg body weight/day for 30 days. If serum calcium levels remain normal or at clinically acceptable levels, treatment may be extended. Treatment for more than 90 days has not been adequately studied and is not recommended. Please consult the package insert pertaining to oral Didronel tablets for additional prescribing information.

HOW SUPPLIED

Didronel I.V. Infusion is supplied in 6 ml ampules as a 5% solution containing 300 mg etidronate disodium.

NDC 0149-0457-01 carton of 6 ampules.

Avoid excessive heat (over 104°F or 40°C) for undiluted product.

Address medical inquiries to Norwich Eaton Pharmaceuticals, Inc., Medical Department, P.O. Box 191, Norwich, NY 13815-0191.

CAUTION

Federal law prohibits dispensing without prescription.
Manufactured by
Taylor Pharmacal Company
Decatur, Illinois 62525
for **Norwich Eaton Pharmaceuticals, Inc.**
FEBRUARY 1987   DIDIV-P3

ENTEX®   ℞

[n'tex]
(phenylephrine hydrochloride/phenylpropanolamine hydrochloride/guaifenesin)

DESCRIPTION

Each ENTEX orange and white capsule for oral administration contains:

phenylephrine hydrochloride	5 mg
phenylpropanolamine hydrochloride	45 mg
guaifenesin	200 mg

This product contains ingredients of the following therapeutic classes: decongestant and expectorant.

Phenylephrine hydrochloride is a decongestant having the chemical name, 3-hydroxy-α-[(methylamino)methyl]benzenemethanol hydrochloride, with the following structure:

[See Chemical Formula at top of next page].

Phenylpropanolamine hydrochloride is a decongestant having the chemical name, benzenemethanol, α-(1-aminoethyl)-, hydrochloride (R*, S*), (±), with the following structure:

Guaifenesin is an expectorant having the chemical name, 1,2-propanediol,3-(2-methoxyphenoxy)-, with the following structure:

INACTIVE INGREDIENTS

Each capsule contains edible black ink, gelatin, FD&C Red #3, silica gel, starch, titanium dioxide, FD&C Yellow #6, and may contain zinc stearate.

CLINICAL PHARMACOLOGY

Phenylephrine hydrochloride and phenylpropanolamine hydrochloride are α-adrenergic receptor agonists (sympathomimetics) which produce vasoconstriction by stimulating α-receptors within the mucosa of the respiratory tract. Clinically, phenylephrine and phenylpropanolamine shrink swollen mucous membranes, reduce tissue hyperemia, edema, and nasal congestion, and increase nasal airway patency. Guaifenesin promotes lower respiratory tract drainage by thinning bronchial secretions, lubricates irritated respiratory tract membranes through increased mucous flow, and facilitates removal of viscous, inspissated mucus. As a result, sinus and bronchial drainage is improved, and dry, nonproductive coughs become more productive and less frequent.

INDICATIONS AND USAGE

ENTEX is indicated for the symptomatic relief of sinusitis, bronchitis, pharyngitis, and coryza when these conditions are associated with nasal congestion and viscous mucus in the lower respiratory tract.

CONTRAINDICATIONS

ENTEX is contraindicated in individuals with known hypersensitivity to sympathomimetics, severe hypertension, or in patients receiving monoamine oxidase inhibitors.

WARNINGS

Sympathomimetic amines should be used with caution in patients with hypertension, diabetes mellitus, heart disease, peripheral vascular disease, increased intraocular pressure, hyperthyroidism, or prostatic hypertrophy.

PRECAUTIONS

Drug Interactions: ENTEX should not be used in patients taking monoamine oxidase inhibitors or other sympathomimetics.
Drug/Laboratory Test Interactions: Guaifenesin has been reported to interfere with clinical laboratory determinations of urinary 5-hydroxyindoleacetic acid (5-HIAA) and urinary vanillylmandelic acid (VMA).
Pregnancy: Pregnancy Category C. Animal reproduction studies have not been conducted with ENTEX. It is also not known whether ENTEX can cause fetal harm when administered to a pregnant woman or can affect reproduction capacity. ENTEX should be given to a pregnant woman only if clearly needed.
Nursing Mothers: It is not known whether the drugs in ENTEX are excreted in human milk. Because many drugs are excreted in human milk and because of the potential for serious adverse reactions in nursing infants, a decision should be made whether to discontinue nursing or to discontinue the product, taking into account the importance of the drug to the mother.
Pediatric Use: Safety and effectiveness of ENTEX capsules in children below the age of 12 have not been established.

ADVERSE REACTIONS

Possible adverse reactions include nervousness, insomnia, restlessness, headache, nausea, or gastric irritation. These reactions seldom, if ever, require discontinuation of therapy. Urinary retention may occur in patients with prostatic hypertrophy.

OVERDOSAGE

The treatment of overdosage should provide symptomatic and supportive care. If the amount ingested is considered dangerous or excessive, induce vomiting with ipecac syrup unless the patient is convulsing, comatose, or has lost the gag reflex, in which case perform gastric lavage using a large-bore tube. If indicated, follow with activated charcoal and a saline cathartic.

DOSAGE AND ADMINISTRATION

Adults and children 12 years of age and older—one capsule four times daily (every 6 hours) with food or fluid. ENTEX is not recommended for children under 12 years of age.

HOW SUPPLIED

ENTEX orange and white capsules are imprinted with "ENTEX" and "0149 0412".
NDC 0149-0412-01 Bottle of 100
NDC 0149-0412-05 Bottle of 500

CAUTION

Federal law prohibits dispensing without prescription.
REVISED SEPTEMBER 1985   ENXCP-P6

ENTEX® LIQUID   ℞
[n 'tex]
(phenylephrine hydrochloride/phenylpropanolamine hydrochloride/guaifenesin)

DESCRIPTION

Each 5 ml (one teaspoonful) for oral administration contains
phenylephrine hydrochloride ....5 mg
phenylpropanolamine hydrochloride ....20 mg
guaifenesin ....100 mg
alcohol 5%
This product contains ingredients of the following therapeutic classes: decongestant and expectorant.
Phenylephrine hydrochloride is a decongestant having the chemical name, 3-hydroxy-α-[(methylamino)methyl]benzenemethanol hydrochloride, with the following structure:

Phenylpropanolamine hydrochloride is a decongestant having the chemical name, benzenemethanol, α-(1-aminoethyl)-, hydrochloride (R*, S*), ($\pm$), with the following structure:

Guaifenesin is an expectorant having the chemical name, 1,2-propanediol, 3-(2-methoxyphenoxy)-, with the following structure:

Inactive Ingredients: ENTEX LIQUID contains citric acid, flavoring, glycerin, purified water, saccharin sodium, sodium benzoate, sodium chloride, sorbitol solution, sucrose, and FD&C Yellow #6.

CLINICAL PHARMACOLOGY

Phenylephrine hydrochloride and phenylpropanolamine hydrochloride are α-adrenergic receptor agonists (sympathomimetics) which produce vasoconstriction by stimulating α-receptors within the mucosa of the respiratory tract. Clinically, phenylephrine and phenylpropanolamine shrink swollen mucous membranes, reduce tissue hyperemia, edema, and nasal congestion, and increase nasal airway patency. Guaifenesin promotes lower respiratory tract drainage by thinning bronchial secretions, lubricates irritated respiratory tract membranes through increased mucous flow, and facilitates removal of viscous, inspissated mucus. As a result, sinus and bronchial drainage is improved, and dry, nonproductive coughs become more productive and less frequent.

INDICATIONS AND USAGE

ENTEX LIQUID is indicated for the symptomatic relief of sinusitis, bronchitis, pharyngitis, and coryza when these conditions are associated with nasal congestion and inspissated mucus in the lower respiratory tract.

CONTRAINDICATIONS

ENTEX LIQUID is contraindicated in individuals with hypersensitivity to sympathomimetics, severe hypertension, or in patients receiving monoamine oxidase inhibitors.

WARNINGS

Sympathomimetic amines should be used with caution in patients with hypertension, diabetes mellitus, heart disease, peripheral vascular disease, increased intraocular pressure, hyperthyroidism, or prostatic hypertrophy.

PRECAUTIONS

Drug Interactions: ENTEX LIQUID should not be used in patients taking monoamine oxidase inhibitors or other sympathomimetics.
Drug/Laboratory Test Interactions: Guaifenesin has been reported to interfere with clinical laboratory determinations of urinary 5-hydroxyindoleacetic acid (5-HIAA) and urinary vanillylmandelic acid (VMA).
Pregnancy: Pregnancy Category C. Animal reproduction studies have not been conducted with ENTEX LIQUID. It is also not known whether ENTEX LIQUID can cause fetal harm when administered to a pregnant woman or can affect reproduction capacity. ENTEX LIQUID should be given to a pregnant woman only if clearly needed.
Nursing Mothers: It is not known whether the drugs in EXTEX LIQUID are excreted in human milk. Because many drugs are excreted in human milk and because of the potential for serious adverse reactions in nursing infants, a decision should be made whether to discontinue nursing or to discontinue the product, taking into account the importance of the drug to the mother.
Pediatric Use: Safety and effectiveness of ENTEX LIQUID in children below the age of 2 have not been established.

ADVERSE REACTIONS

Possible adverse reactions include nervousness, insomnia, restlessness, headache, nausea, or gastric irritation. These reactions seldom, if ever, require discontinuation of therapy. Urinary retention may occur in patients with prostatic hypertrophy.

OVERDOSAGE

The treatment of overdosage should provide symptomatic and supportive care. If the amount ingested is considered dangerous or excessive, induce vomiting with ipecac syrup unless the patient is convulsing, comatose, or has lost the gag reflex, in which case perform gastric lavage using a large-bore tube. If indicated, follow with activated charcoal and a saline cathartic.

DOSAGE AND ADMINISTRATION

All dosage should be administered four times daily (every 6 hours).
Children:
2 to under 4 years ....½ teaspoonful (2.5 ml)
4 to under 6 years ....1 teaspoonful (5.0 ml)
6 to under 12 years ....1½ teaspoonfuls (7.5 ml)
Adults and children 12 years of age and older: 2 teaspoonfuls (10.0 ml)

HOW SUPPLIED

ENTEX LIQUID is available as an orange-colored, pleasant-tasting liquid.
NDC 0149-0414-16 16 FL. OZ. (1 Pint) bottle

CAUTION

Federal law prohibits dispensing without prescription.
REVISED SEPTEMBER 1985   ENXLQ-P5

ENTEX® LA   ℞
[n 'tex]
(phenylpropanolamine hydrochloride/guaifenesin)

DESCRIPTION

Each Entex LA orange scored, long-acting tablet for oral administration contains
phenylpropanolamine hydrochloride ....75 mg
guaifenesin ....400 mg
in a special base to provide a prolonged therapeutic effect. This product contains ingredients of the following therapeutic classes: decongestant and expectorant.
Phenylpropanolamine hydrochloride is a decongestant having the chemical name, benzenemethanol, α-(1-aminoethyl)-, hydrochloride (R*, S*), ($\pm$), with the following structure:

Guaifenesin is an expectorant having the chemical name, 1,2-propanediol, 3-(2-methoxyphenoxy)-, with the following structure:

Inactive Ingredients: Each tablet contains carbomer 934P, compressible sugar, docusate sodium, FD&C Yellow No. 6 Aluminum Lake, hydroxypropyl cellulose, hydroxypropyl

Continued on next page

Norwich Eaton—Cont.

methylcellulose, polyethylene glycol, silicon dioxide, stearic acid, titanium dioxide, and zinc stearate.

CLINICAL PHARMACOLOGY

Phenylpropanolamine hydrochloride is an α-adrenergic receptor agonist (sympathomimetic) which produces vasoconstriction by stimulating α-receptors within the mucosa of the respiratory tract. Clinically, phenylpropanolamine shrinks swollen mucous membranes, reduces tissue hyperemia, edema, and nasal congestion, and increases nasal airway patency. Guaifenesin promotes lower respiratory tract drainage by thinning bronchial secretions, lubricates irritated respiratory tract membranes through increased mucous flow, and facilitates removal of viscous, inspissated mucus. As a result, sinus and bronchial drainage is improved, and dry, nonproductive coughs become more productive and less frequent.

INDICATIONS AND USAGE

Entex LA is indicated for the symptomatic relief of sinusitis, bronchitis, pharyngitis, and coryza when these conditions are associated with nasal congestion and viscous mucus in the lower respiratory tract.

CONTRAINDICATIONS

Entex LA is contraindicated in individuals with known hypersensitivity to sympathomimetics, severe hypertension, or in patients receiving monoamine oxidase inhibitors.

WARNINGS

Sympathomimetic amines should be used with caution in patients with hypertension, diabetes mellitus, heart disease, peripheral vascular disease, increased intraocular pressure, hyperthyroidism, or prostatic hypertrophy.

PRECAUTIONS

Information for Patients: Do not crush or chew Entex LA tablets prior to swallowing.
Drug Interactions: Entex LA should not be used in patients taking monoamine oxidase inhibitors or other sympathomimetics.
Drug/Laboratory Test Interactions: Guaifenesin has been reported to interfere with clinical laboratory determinations of urinary 5-hydroxyindoleacetic acid (5-HIAA) and urinary vanillylmandelic acid (VMA).
Pregnancy: Pregnancy Category C. Animal reproduction studies have not been conducted with Entex LA. It is also not known whether Entex LA can cause fetal harm when administered to a pregnant woman or can affect reproduction capacity. Entex LA should be given to a pregnant woman only if clearly needed.
Nursing Mothers: It is not known whether the drugs in Entex LA are excreted in human milk. Because many drugs are excreted in human milk and because of the potential for serious adverse reactions in nursing infants, a decision should be made whether to discontinue nursing or to discontinue the product, taking into account the importance of the drug to the mother.
Pediatric Use: Safety and effectiveness of Entex LA tablets in children below the age of 6 have not been established.

ADVERSE REACTIONS

Possible adverse reactions include nervousness, insomnia, restlessness, headache, nausea, or gastric irritation. These reactions seldom, if ever, require discontinuation of therapy. Urinary retention may occur in patients with prostatic hypertrophy.

OVERDOSAGE

The treatment of overdosage should provide symptomatic and supportive care. If the amount ingested is considered dangerous or excessive, induce vomiting with ipecac syrup unless the patient is convulsing, comatose, or has lost the gag reflex, in which case perform gastric lavage using a large-bore tube. If indicated, follow with activated charcoal and a saline cathartic. Since the effects of Entex LA may last up to 12 hours, treatment should be continued for at least that length of time.

DOSAGE AND ADMINISTRATION

Adults and children 12 years of age and older—one tablet twice daily (every 12 hours); children 6 to under 12 years—one-half (½) tablet twice daily (every 12 hours). Entex LA is not recommended for children under 6 years of age. Tablets may be broken in half for ease of administration without affecting release of medication but should not be crushed or chewed prior to swallowing.

HOW SUPPLIED

Entex LA is available as an orange, scored tablet coded with "ENTEX LA" on one side and "0149 0436" on the scored side.
NDC 0149-0436-01 bottle of 100
NDC 0149-0436-05 bottle of 500

CAUTION
Federal law prohibits dispensing without prescription.

ENXLA-Y1

Manufactured by
Eaton Laboratories, Inc.
Manati, Puerto Rico 00701
Distributed by
Norwich Eaton Pharmaceuticals, Inc.
REVISED JULY 1988
Shown in Product Identification Section, page 420

FURACIN® SOLUBLE DRESSING   ℞
[*fewr 'a sin*]
(nitrofurazone)

DESCRIPTION

Chemically, Furacin is nitrofurazone, 2-[(5-nitro-2-furanyl)methylene]hydrazinecarboxamide, with the following structure:

$$O_2N \quad CH = NNHCONH_2$$

Furacin Soluble Dressing is a preparation containing 0.2% nitrofurazone in Solubase® (a water-soluble base of polyethylene glycols 3350, 900, and 300).
Furacin Soluble Dressing is an antibacterial agent for topical use.

CLINICAL PHARMACOLOGY

Furacin Soluble Dressing (nitrofurazone) is a nitrofuran that is bactericidal for most pathogens commonly causing surface infections, including *Staphylococcus aureus, Streptococcus, Escherichia coli, Clostridium perfringens, Aerobacter aerogenes,* and *Proteus.*
Furacin Soluble Dressing inhibits a number of bacterial enzymes, especially those involved in the aerobic and anaerobic degradation of glucose and pyruvate. The activity appears to involve the pyruvate dehydrogenase system as well as citrate synthetase, malate dehydrogenase, glutathione reductase, and pyruvate decarboxylase. Glutathione reductase inhibition may be caused by control of pentose phosphate metabolism. Although Furacin Soluble Dressing inhibits a variety of enzymes, it is not considered to be a general enzyme inactivator since many enzymes are not inhibited by this compound.

INDICATIONS AND USAGE

Furacin Soluble Dressing is a topical antibacterial agent indicated for adjunctive therapy of patients with second- and third-degree burns when bacterial resistance to other agents is a real or potential problem.
It is also indicated in skin grafting where bacterial contamination may cause graft rejection and/or donor site infection particularly in hospitals with historical resistant-bacteria epidemics.
There is no known evidence of effectiveness of this product in the treatment of minor burns or surface bacterial infections involving wounds, cutaneous ulcers, or the various pyodermas.

CONTRAINDICATIONS

Known sensitization to any of the components of this preparation is a contraindication for use.

WARNINGS

Nitrofurazone has been shown to produce mammary tumors when fed at high doses to female Sprague-Dawley rats. The relevance of this to topical use in humans is unknown.
Furacin Soluble Dressing should be used with caution in patients with known or suspected renal impairment. The polyethylene glycols in the base can be absorbed through denuded skin and may not be excreted normally by the compromised kidney. This may lead to symptoms of progressive renal impairment such as increased BUN, anion gap, and metabolic acidosis. (NOTE: Furacin (nitrofurazone) Topical Cream does not contain polyethylene glycols.)

PRECAUTIONS

General: Use of topical antimicrobials occasionally allows overgrowth of nonsusceptible organisms including fungi. If this occurs, or if irritation, sensitization or superinfection develops, treatment with Furacin Soluble Dressing should be discontinued and appropriate therapy instituted.
Carcinogenesis, mutagenesis, and impairment of fertility: Nitrofurazone has been shown to produce mammary tumors when fed at high doses to female Sprague-Dawley rats. The relevance of this to topical use in humans is unknown. Dietary dosage levels of 60 and 30 mg/kg/day shortened the onset time of the typical mammary gland tumors associated with older female rats. These tumors exhibited the same histological characteristics seen in the spontaneously occurring tumors, and were seen only in the female animals. No mammary tumors were seen in rats treated with nitrofurazone orally in the diet for 1 year at levels of approximately 11 mg/kg/day. Spermatogenic arrest was noted in the male rats

---

in dietary dosage levels of 30 mg/kg/day and above, after one year on test.
Pregnancy: Pregnancy Category C: Nitrofurazone has been shown to have an embryocidal effect in rabbits when given in oral doses thirty times the human dose. There are no adequate and well controlled studies in pregnant women. Furacin Soluble Dressing should be used during pregnancy only if the potential benefit justifies the potential risk to the fetus.
Nursing mothers: It is not known whether this drug is excreted in human milk. Because many drugs are excreted in human milk and because of the potential for tumorigenicity shown for nitrofurazone in animal studies, a decision should be made whether to discontinue nursing or to discontinue the drug, taking into account the importance of the drug to the mother.
Pediatric use: Safety and effectiveness in children have not been established.

ADVERSE REACTIONS

Instances of clinical skin reactions have been reported for patients treated with Furacin formulations. Symptoms appear as varying degrees of contact dermatitides such as rash, pruritus, and local edema. Although the exact incidence of such reactions is difficult to determine, historically, a survey of world literature and clinical data generated by Norwich Eaton indicates an overall incidence of approximately 1%. Allergic reactions to Furacin Soluble Dressing should be treated symptomatically.

DOSAGE AND ADMINISTRATION

Burns: Apply directly to the lesion with a spatula, or first place on gauze. Impregnated gauze may be used. Reapply depending on the preferred dressing technique. Flushing the dressing with sterile saline facilitates its removal.

PREPARATION OF IMPREGNATED GAUZE

Sterile gauze strips are placed in a tray and covered with Furacin Soluble Dressing. Repeat the procedure, adding several layers of gauze for each layer of Furacin Soluble Dressing. Sprinkling a little sterile water on each layer of dressing will minimize any color change from autoclaving. Cover the tray very loosely and autoclave at 121°C for 30 minutes at 15 to 20 pounds pressure.
To impregnate bandage rolls, place some Furacin Soluble Dressing in the bottom of a glass jar. Stand rolls on end. Place more Furacin Soluble Dressing on top. Cover top of jar with aluminum foil. Autoclave at 121°C for 45 minutes at 15 to 20 pounds pressure. Do not store impregnated bandage rolls for more than 24 hours.
Autoclaving more than once is not recommended.

HOW SUPPLIED

Furacin Soluble Dressing is available in:
NDC 0149-0704-12 tube of 28 grams
NDC 0149-0704-11 tube of 56 grams
NDC 0149-0704-61 jar of 454 grams

ANIMAL TOXICOLOGY

The oral administration of nitrofurazone for 7 days to rats at extremely high dosage levels of 240 mg/kg/day produced severe hepatorenal lesions whereas only renal changes were seen when the dosage level was reduced to 60 mg/kg/day for 60 days.
Dogs treated orally with nitrofurazone for 400 days at levels of 11 mg/kg/day showed no toxic effects related to drug treatment. The single intravenous administration in dogs of 20, 35, or 75 mg/kg nitrofurazone produced clinical signs of lacrimation, salivation, emesis, diarrhea, excitation, weakness, ataxia, and weight loss, whereas 100 mg/kg produced convulsions and death.
There was no evidence of toxicosis in rhesus monkeys treated with doses of nitrofurazone as high as 58 mg/kg/day for 10 weeks and 23 mg/kg/day for 63 weeks.
The peroral LD_{50} of nitrofurazone in mice and rats is 747 and 590 mg/kg respectively.
For bacterial sensitivity tests: Furacin Sensi-Discs are available from BBL, Division of BioQuest.
REVISED SEPTEMBER 1986   FSD-P1

FURACIN® TOPICAL CREAM   ℞
[*fewr 'a-sin*]
(nitrofurazone)

DESCRIPTION

Chemically, Furacin is nitrofurazone, 2-[(5-nitro-2-furanyl)methylene]hydrazinecarboxamide, with the following structure:

$$O_2N \quad CH = NNHCONH_2$$

Furacin Topical Cream is a preparation containing 0.2% Furacin in a water-miscible base consisting of glycerin, cetyl alcohol, mineral oil, an ethoxylated fatty alcohol, methylparaben, propylparaben, and purified water.

Furacin Topical Cream is an antibacterial agent for topical use.

CLINICAL PHARMACOLOGY

Furacin Topical Cream is a nitrofuran that is bactericidal for most pathogens commonly causing surface infections, including *Staphylococcus aureus, Streptococcus, Escherichia coli, Clostridium perfringens, Aerobacter aerogenes,* and *Proteus.*

Furacin Topical Cream inhibits a number of bacterial enzymes, especially those involved in the aerobic and anaerobic degradation of glucose and pyruvate. The activity appears to involve the pyruvate dehydrogenase system as well as citrate synthetase, malate dehydrogenase, glutathione reductase, and pyruvate decarboxylase. Glutathion reductase inhibition may be caused by control of pentose phosphate metabolism. Although Furacin Topical Cream inhibits a variety of enzymes, it is not considered to be a general enzyme inactivator since many enzymes are not inhibited by this compound.

INDICATIONS AND USAGE

Furacin Topical Cream is a topical antibacterial agent indicated for adjunctive therapy of patients with second- and third-degree burns when bacterial resistance to other agents is a real or potential problem.

It is also indicated in skin grafting where bacterial contamination may cause graft rejection and/or donor site infection particularly in hospitals with historical resistant-bacteria epidemics.

There is no known evidence of effectiveness of this product in the treatment of minor burns or surface bacterial infections involving wounds, cutaneous ulcers or the various pyodermas.

CONTRAINDICATIONS

Known sensitization to any of the components of this preparation is a contraindication for use.

WARNINGS

None

PRECAUTIONS

General: Use of Furacin Topical Cream occasionally allows overgrowth of nonsusceptible organisms including fungi and *Pseudomonas.* If this occurs, or if irritation, sensitization or superinfection develops, treatment with Furacin Topical Cream should be discontinued and appropriate therapy instituted.

Information for Patients: Patients should be told to use Furacin Topical Cream only as directed by a physician. Patients should be advised to discontinue the drug and contact a physician should rash or irritation occur.

Carcinogenesis, Mutagenesis, and Impairment of Fertility: Nitrofurazone has been shown to produce mammary tumors when fed at high doses to female Sprague-Dawley rats. The relevance of this to topical use in humans is unknown. Dietary dosage levels of 60 and 30 mg/kg/day shortened the onset time of the typical mammary gland tumors associated with older female rats. These tumors exhibited the same histological characteristics seen in the spontaneously occurring tumors, and were seen only in the female animals. No mammary tumors were seen in rats treated with nitrofurazone orally in the diet for 1 year at levels approximately 11 mg/kg/day. Spermatogenic arrest was noted in the male rats in dietary dosage levels of 30 mg/kg/day and above, after one year on test.

Pregnancy: Pregnancy Category C: Nitrofurazone, when administered orally to pregnant rabbits, caused a slight increase in the frequency of still-births when given in doses thirty times the human dose. There are no adequate and well controlled studies in pregnant women. Furacin Topical Cream should be used during pregnancy only if the potential benefit justifies the potential risk to the fetus.

Nursing Mothers: It is not known whether this drug is excreted in human milk. Because many drugs are excreted in human milk and because of the potential for tumorigenicity shown for nitrofurazone in animal studies, a decision should be made whether to discontinue nursing or to discontinue the drug, taking into account the importance of the drug to the mother.

ADVERSE REACTIONS

Instances of clinical skin reactions have been reported for patients treated with Furacin formulations. Symptoms appear as varying degrees of contact dermatitides such as rash, pruritus, and local edema. Although the exact incidence of such reactions is difficult to determine, historically, a survey of world literature and clinical data generated by Norwich Eaton indicates an overall incidence of approximately 1%. Allergic reactions to Furacin Topical Cream should be treated symptomatically.

DOSAGE AND ADMINISTRATION

Apply Furacin Topical Cream directly to the lesion, or first place on gauze. Reapply once daily or every few days, depending on the usual dressing technique.

HOW SUPPLIED

Furacin Topical Cream is available in:
NDC 0149-0777-15 tube of 14 grams
NDC 0149-0777-12 tube of 28 grams
NDC 0149-0777-61 jar of 368 grams
Storage: Avoid exposure to direct sunlight, strong fluorescent lighting, alkaline materials, and excessive heat (over 104°F or 40°C).

ANIMAL TOXICOLOGY

The oral administration of nitrofurazone for 7 days to rats at extremely high dosage levels of 240 mg/kg/day produced severe hepatorenal lesions whereas only renal changes were seen when the dosage level was reduced to 60 mg/kg/day for 60 days.

Dogs treated orally with nitrofurazone for 400 days at levels of 11 mg/kg/day showed no toxic effects related to drug treatment.

There was no evidence of toxicosis in rhesus monkeys treated with doses of nitrofurazone as high as 58 mg/kg/day for 10 weeks and 23 mg/kg/day for 63 weeks.

The peroral LD_{50} of nitrofurazone in mice and rats is 747 and 590 mg/kg respectively.

For bacterial sensitivity tests: Furacin Sensi-Discs are available from BBL, Division of BioQuest.

CAUTION

Federal law prohibits dispensing without prescription.
REVISED SEPTEMBER 1986   FTC-P5

FUROXONE®   ℞
[fewr-ox 'ōne]
(furazolidone)

DESCRIPTION

Furoxone (furazolidone) is one of the synthetic antimicrobial nitrofurans. It is a stable, yellow, crystalline compound with the following structure:

$$O_2N - \text{(ring)} - CH=N - N - \overset{C=O}{\underset{H_2C - CH_2}{\quad}}$$

3-(5-nitrofurfurylideneamino)-2-oxazolidinone

Inactive Ingredients: Furoxone tablets contain calcium pyrophosphate, FD&C Blue #2, FD&C Red #3, magnesium stearate, starch, and sucrose. Furoxone liquid contains carboxymethylcellulose sodium, flavors, glycerin, magnesium aluminum silicate, methylparaben, propylparaben, purified water, and saccharin sodium.

ACTION

Furoxone has a broad antibacterial spectrum covering the majority of gastrointestinal tract pathogens including *E. coli,* staphylococci, *Salmonella, Shigella, Proteus, Aerobacter aerogenes, Vibrio cholerae* [9,10,11] and *Giardia lamblia.* [5,6] Its bactericidal activity is based upon its interference with several bacterial enzyme systems; this antimicrobial action minimizes the development of resistant organisms. It neither significantly alters the normal bowel flora nor results in fungal overgrowth. The brown color found in the urine with adequate dosage is of no clinical significance.

INDICATIONS

Indicated in the specific and symptomatic treatment of bacterial or protozoal diarrhea and enteritis caused by susceptible organisms. Furoxone products are well tolerated, have a very low incidence of adverse reactions.

CONTRAINDICATINS

1. To obviate an Antabuse® (disulfiram)-like reaction which may occur in some patients, the ingestion of alcohol should be avoided during or within four days after Furoxone therapy (see ADVERSE REACTIONS).
2. IN GENERAL, MAOI DRUGS, TYRAMINE-CONTAINING FOODS AND INDIRECTLY-ACTING SYMPATHOMIMETIC AMINES ARE CONTRAINDICATED OR SHOULD BE USED WITH CAUTION IN PATIENTS RECEIVING FUROXONE (SEE PRECAUTIONS).
3. INFANTS UNDER 1 MONTH SHOULD NOT RECEIVE FUROXONE (SEE ADVERSE REACTIONS AND DOSAGE FOR CHILDREN).[4] THE FUROXONE CONCENTRATION IN THE BREAST MILK OF LACTATING WOMEN HAS NOT BEEN DETERMINED, THEREFORE THE SAFETY IN THIS CIRCUMSTANCE HAS NOT BEEN ESTABLISHED.
4. Prior sensitivity to Furoxone is a contraindication.

WARNINGS

(See CONTRAINDICATIONS listed above.)

Use In Pregnancy: The safety of Furoxone during the childbearing age has not been established; as with any potent antibacterial, Furoxone must be administered with caution during the childbearing age. However, animal breeding studies have revealed no evidence of teratogenicity following the administration of Furoxone for long periods of time and at doses far in excess of those recommended for the human. There have been no clinical reports regarding this possible adverse effect on the fetus or the newborn infant.

PRECAUTIONS

Monoamine Oxidase Inhibition:[7] Effective inhibition of monoamine oxidase by furazolidone has been demonstrated experimentally in man by the enhancement of tyramine and amphetamine sensitivity and by the directly measured monoamine oxidase inhibition.

A period of five days of furazolidone administration in the recommended doses in these patients was required to give an enhancement of the tyramine and amphetamine sensitivities by two to threefold. Administration of furazolidone in the recommended dose of 400 mg/day for a period of five days should not subject the adult patient to an undue hazard of hypertensive crisis due to monoamine oxidase inhibition. Hypertensive crises have never been reported even after the peroral administration of larger doses and/or for longer periods of time. Controlled studies reveal no signs or symptoms of hypertensive crisis even after the peroral administration of Furoxone in doses of 400 mg/day in excessive of 48 consecutive months.[8]

If administered in doses larger than recommended or in excess of five days, the indications must be weighed against the possible hazards of hypertensive crisis related to the accumulation of monoamine oxidase inhibition. If indications are sufficient, the patients should be informed of drugs and foods which predispose to hypertensive crises:
(A) Other known MAOI drugs; however, when indicated they should be prescribed with caution and at a reduced dosage.
(B) Tyramine-containing foods such as broad beans, yeast extracts, strong unpasteurized cheeses, beer, wine, pickled herring, chicken livers, and fermented products are contraindicated.
(C) Indirectly-acting sympathomimetic amines such as those found in nasal decongestants (phenylephrine, ephedrine) and anorectics (amphetamines) are contraindicated.
(D) Likewise, sedatives, antihistamines, tranquilizers, and narcotics should be used in reduced dosages and with caution.

Orthostatic hypotension and hypoglycemia may occur.

Carcinogenesis, Mutagenesis, Impairment of Fertility: Furazolidone has shown evidence of tumorigenic activity in several studies involving chronic, high-dose oral administration to rodents. Promotion of the development of mammary neoplasia has been demonstrated in rats of two strains. Prominent among the findings in mice was that furazolidone caused significant increases in malignant lung tumors. The relevance of these animal findings, particularly in relationship to short-term therapy in humans, is not established.

ADVERSE REACTIONS

A few hypersensitivity reactions to Furoxone have been reported including a fall in blood pressure, urticaria, fever, arthralgia, and a vesicular morbilliform rash. These reactions subsided following withdrawal of the drug.

Nausea, emesis, headache, or malaise occur occasionally and may be minimized or eliminated by reduction in dosage or withdrawal of the drug.

Rarely, individuals receiving Furoxone have exhibited an Antabuse® (disulfiram)-like reaction to alcohol characterized by flushing, slight temperature elevation, dyspnea, and in some instances, a sense of constriction within the chest. All symptomatology disappeared within 24 hours with no lasting ill effects. During nine years of clinical use and approximately 3.5 million courses of therapy (in the U.S.A. alone) in the published literature and documented case reports 43 cases have been reported—of which 14 were produced under experimental conditions with planned doses of the compound in excess of those recommended.

Three of these experienced a fall in blood pressure necessitating active therapy. Indications are that levarterenol (Levophed®) may be used to combat such hypotensive episodes since human studies show that this drug is not potentiated in patients treated with Furoxone. (Indirectly acting pressor agents should be avoided.) The ingestion of alcohol in any form should be avoided during Furoxone therapy and for four days thereafter to prevent this reaction.

Furoxone may cause mild reversible intravascular hemolysis in certain ethnic groups of Mediterranean and Near-Eastern origin, and Negroes.[1,3] This is due to an intrinsic defect of red blood cell metabolism in a small percentage of these ethnic groups, making them unusually susceptible to hemolysis by numerous compounds.[2] It is necessary to observe such patients closely while receiving Furoxone and to discontinue its use if there is any indication of hemolysis.

Should not be administered to infants under 1 month of age because of the possibility of producing a hemolytic anemia due to immature enzyme systems (glutathione instability) in the early neonatal period.[4]

Continued on next page

Norwich Eaton—Cont.

Colitis, proctitis, anal pruritus, staphylococcic enteritis, renal or hepatic toxicity have not been a significant problem with Furoxone.

DOSAGE AND ADMINISTRATION

FUROXONE TABLETS, 100 mg each, are brown and scored to facilitate adjustment of dosage.

Average Adult Dosage: One 100-mg tablet four times daily.
Average Dosage for Children: Those 5 years of age or older should receive 25 to 50 mg ($\frac{1}{4}$ to $\frac{1}{2}$ tablet) four times daily. The tablet dosage may be crushed and given in a spoonful of corn syrup.

FUROXONE LIQUID composition: each 15 ml tablespoonful contains Furoxone 50 mg per 15 ml (3.33 mg per ml) in a light-yellow aqueous vehicle. Suitable flavoring, suspending and preservative agents complete the formulation. (See Inactive Ingredients.) It is stable in storage. Prior to administering Furoxone Liquid shake the bottle vigorously. It should be dispensed in amber bottles.

Average Adult Dosage: Two tablespoonfuls four times daily.
Average Dosage for Children:
5 years or older—$\frac{1}{2}$ to 1 tablespoonful four times daily (7.5–15.0 ml)
1 to 4 years old—1 to $1\frac{1}{2}$ teaspoonfuls four times daily (5.0–7.5 ml)
1 month to 1 year—$\frac{1}{2}$ to 1 teaspoonful four times daily (2.5–5.0 ml)

This dosage is based on an average dose of 5 mg of Furoxone per Kg (2.3 mg per lb) of body weight given in four equally divided doses during 24 hours. The maximal dose of 8.8 mg of Furoxone per Kg (4 mg per lb) of body weight per 24 hours should probably not be exceeded because of the possibility of producing nausea or emesis. If these are severe, the dosage should be reduced.

The average case of diarrhea treated with Furoxone will respond within 2 to 5 days of therapy. Occasional patients may require a longer term of therapy. If satisfactory clinical response is not obtained within 7 days it indicates that the pathogen is refractory to Furoxone and the drug should be discontinued. Adjunctive therapy with other antibacterial agents or bismuth salts is not contraindicated. (N.B. Refer to WARNINGS.)

In order to administer furazolidone in doses larger than recommended or in excess of five days the indications must be weighed against the possible hazards of hypertensive crisis related to the accumulation of monoamine oxidase inhibition. If indications are sufficient, the patient should be informed of drugs and foods which predispose to hypertensive crises. (See PRECAUTIONS.)

HOW SUPPLIED

Furoxone Tablets, 100 mg each, coded "Eaton 072", are supplied in amber bottles containing 20 and 100 tablets. (Should be dispensed in amber bottles.)
Furoxone Liquid is supplied in amber bottles containing 60 ml and 473 ml. (Should be dispensed in amber bottles.)

REFERENCES

(1) Kellermeyer, R.S., Tarlov, A.R., Schrier, S.L., and Alving, A.S.J. Lab. Clin. Med. 52:827–828 (Nov) 1958.
(2) Tarlov et al. Arch. Int. Med. 109:209–234, 1962.
(3) Kellermeyer et al. J.A.M.A. 180: No. 5, 388–394, 1962.
(4) Zinkham, Pediatrics 23:18–32, 1959; Gross & Hurwitz, Pediatrics 22:453, 1958.
(5) Fallas Vargas, M. un Nuevo Tratamiento para la Giardiasis (A New Treatment for Giardiasis). Rev. Med. Costa Rica 19:269–284 (July) 1962.
(6) Webster, B. H. Furazolidone in the Treatment of Giardiasis. Amer. J. Dig. Diseases 5:618–622 (July) 1960.
(7) Oates, J.A., Pettinger, W.A. Inhibition of Monoamine Oxidase by Furazolidone in Man. Data on file: Office of the Medical Director, Norwich Eaton Pharmaceuticals, Inc. Available upon request.
(8) Kirsner, Joseph B., M.D., Ph.D. Data on file: Office of the Medical Director, Norwich Eaton Pharmaceuticals, Inc. Available upon request.
(9) Neogy, K.N., et al. Furazolidone in Cholera, Journ. Indian Med. Assoc. 48:137, 1967.
(10) Chaudhuri, R.N. et al. Furazolidone in Cholera, Lancet 2:909 (Oct 30) 1965.
(11) Curlin, G. Comparison of Antibiotic Regimens in Cholera. Abstracts of papers, Epidemiological Intelligence Service Conference, Atlanta, Ga., April 11–14, 1967, p. 11.

FUROXONE (FURAZOLIDONE) SENSI-DISCS for laboratory determination of bacterial sensitivity are available from BBL, division of BioQuest.

CAUTION

Federal law prohibits dispensing without prescription. Literature available to physicians on request.
REVISED APRIL 1985   FUROX-P4

MACRODANTIN® CAPSULES   ℞
[mak″rō-dan′tin]
(nitrofurantoin macrocrystals)

PRODUCT OVERVIEW

KEY FACTS

MACPAC™ is a unique 28-capsule Macrodantin compliance package, available in both 50 mg and 100 mg strengths. MACPAC is specially designed to aid patient compliance with Macrodantin therapy. MACPAC contains seven portable blister cards, each containing four capsules labelled breakfast, lunch, dinner and bedtime. MACPAC also contains a concise UTI information booklet that discusses the symptoms, causes and prevention of urinary tract infections and a reminder card which encourages patients to complete the full course of therapy to help prevent a relapse.

MAJOR USES

Macrodantin is specifically indicated for the treatment of urinary tract infections when due to susceptible strains of *E. coli*, enterococci, *S. aureus* (it is not indicated for the treatment of associated renal cortical or perinephric abscesses), and certain susceptible strains of *Klebsiella*, *Enterobacter* and *Proteus* species.

SAFETY INFORMATION

Anuria, oliguria, or significant impairment of renal function (creatinine clearance under 40 ml per minute) are contraindications. Macrodantin is contraindicated in pregnant patients at term (during labor and delivery) as well as in infants under one month of age. The drug is also contraindicated in those patients with known hypersenitivity to nitrofurantoin. Although serious adverse reactions have been reported, the most common adverse reactions are gastrointestinal effects (ie, nausea, emesis, and anorexia) which can be minimized by reduction of dosage. **Before prescribing, please consult full prescribing information.**

PRESCRIBING INFORMATION

MACRODANTIN® CAPSULES   ℞
[mak″rō-dan′tin]
(nitrofurantoin macrocrystals)

DESCRIPTION

Macrodantin (nitrofurantoin macrocrystals) is a synthetic chemical of controlled crystal size. It is a stable, yellow crystalline compound. Macrodantin is an antibacterial agent for specific urinary tract infections. It is available in 25-mg, 50-mg, and 100-mg capsules for oral administration.

1-[[(5-NITRO-2-FURANYL)METHYLENE]AMINO]-2,4-IMIDAZOLIDINEDIONE

INACTIVE INGREDIENTS: Each capsule contains edible black ink, gelatin, lactose, starch, talc, titanium dioxide, and may contain FD&C Yellow #6 and and D&C Yellow #10.

CLINICAL PHARMACOLOGY

Macrodantin is a larger crystal form of Furadantin® (nitrofurantoin). The absorption of Macrodantin is slower and its excretion somewhat less when compared to Furandantin. Blood concentrations at therapeutic dosage are usually low. Many patients who cannot tolerate microcrystalline nitrofurantion are able to take Macrodantin without nausea. It is highly soluble in urine, to which it may impart a brown color.

Following a dose regimen of 100 mg q.i.d. for 7 days, average urinary drug recoveries (0-24 hours) on day 1 and day 7 were 37.9% and 35.0%.

Unlike many drugs, the presence of food or agents delaying gastric emptying can increase the bioavailability of Macrodantin, presumably by allowing better dissolution in gastric juices.

Microbiology: Macrodantin, *in vitro*, is bacteriostatic in low concentrations (5-10 mcg/ml) and is considered bactericidal in higher concentrations. Its mode of action is presumed to be interference with several bacterial enzyme systems. Bacteria develop only a limited resistance to furan derivatives.

While *in vitro* studies have demonstrated the susceptibility of most strains of the following organisms, clinical efficacy for infections other than those included in the INDICATIONS AND USAGE section has not been documented: *Escherichia coli*, enterococci (e.g., *Streptococcus faecalis*), *Staphylococcus aureus*, *Staphylococcus epidermidis*.

Note: Some strains of *Enterobacter* species and *Klebsiella* species are resistant to Macrodantin. It is not active against most strains of *Proteus* and *Serratia* species. It has no activity against *Pseudomonas* species.

Antagonism has been demonstrated between nitrofurantoin and both nalidixic acid and oxolinic acid *in vitro*.

Susceptibility Tests—Quantitative methods that require measurement of zone diameters give the most precise estimates of antimicrobial susceptibility. One recommended procedure, (NCCLS, ASM-2)*, uses a disc containing 300 micrograms for testing susceptibility; interpretations correlate zone diameters of this disc test with MIC values for nitrofurantoin. Reports from the laboratory should be interpreted according to the following criteria:

Susceptible organisms produce zones of 17 mm or greater, indicating that the tested organism is likely to respond to therapy.

Organisms of intermediate susceptibility produce zones of 15 to 16 mm, indicating that the tested organism would be susceptible if high dosage is used.

Resistant organisms produce zones of 14 mm or less, indicating that other therapy should be selected.

A bacterial isolate may be considered susceptible if the MIC value for nitrofurantoin is 25 micrograms per ml or less. Organisms are considered resistant if the MIC is not less than 100 micrograms per ml or more.

*National Committee for Clinical Laboratory Standards. Approved Standard: ASM-2, Performance Standards for Antimicrobial Disc Susceptibility Tests, July, 1975.

NOTE

Specimens for culture and susceptibility testing should be obtained prior to and during the drug administration.

INDICATIONS AND USAGE

Macrodantin is specifically indicated for the treatment of urinary tract infections when due to susceptible strains of *E. coli*, enterococci, *S. aureus* (it is not indicated for the treatment of associated renal cortical or perinephric abscesses), and certain susceptible strains of *Klebsiella*, *Enterobacter* and *Proteus* species.

CONTRAINDICATIONS

Anuria, oliguria, or significant impairment of renal function (creatinine clearance under 40 ml per minute) are contraindications. Treatment of this type of patient carries an increased risk of toxicity and is much less effective because of impaired excretion of the drug.

The drug is contraindicated in pregnant patients at term (during labor and delivery) as well as in infants under one month of age because of the possibility of hemolytic anemia in the fetus or in the newborn infant due to immature erythrocyte enzyme systems (glutathione instability).

Macrodantin is also contraindicated in those patients with known hypersensitivity to nitrofurantoin.

WARNINGS: ACUTE, SUBACUTE, OR CHRONIC PULMONARY REACTIONS HAVE BEEN OBSERVED IN PATIENTS TREATED WITH NITROFURANTOIN. IF THESE REACTIONS OCCUR, MACRODANTIN SHOULD BE DISCONTINUED AND APPROPRIATE MEASURES TAKEN. REPORTS HAVE CITED PULMONARY REACTIONS AS A CONTRIBUTING CAUSE OF DEATH.

CHRONIC PULMONARY REACTIONS (DIFFUSE INTERSTITIAL PNEUMONITIS OR PULMONARY FIBROSIS, OR BOTH) CAN DEVELOP INSIDIOUSLY. THESE REACTIONS OCCUR RARELY AND GENERALLY IN PATIENTS RECEIVING THERAPY FOR SIX MONTHS OR LONGER. CLOSE MONITORING OF THE PULMONARY CONDITION OF PATIENTS RECEIVING LONG-TERM THERAPY IS WARRANTED AND REQUIRES THAT THE BENEFITS OF THERAPY BE WEIGHED AGAINST POTENTIAL RISKS. (SEE RESPIRATORY REACTIONS.)

Hepatitis, including chronic active hepatitis, occurs rarely. Fatalities have been reported. The onset of chronic active hepatitis may be insidious, and patients receiving long-term therapy should be monitored periodically for changes in liver function. If hepatitis occurs, the drug should be withdrawn immediately and appropriate measures taken.

Peripheral neuropathy, which may become severe or irreversible, has occurred. Fatalities have been reported. Conditions such as renal impairment (creatinine clearance under 40 ml per minute), anemia, diabetes mellitus, electrolyte imbalance, vitamin B deficiency, and dibilitating disease may enhance the occurence of peripheral neuropathy.

Cases of hemolytic anemia of the primaquine sensitivity type have been induced by nitrofurantoin. Hemolysis appears to be linked to a glucose-6-phosphate dehydrogenase deficiency in the red blood cells of the affected patients. This deficiency is found in 10 percent of Negroes and a small percentage of ethnic groups of Mediterranean and Near Eastern origin. Hemolysis is an indication for discontinuing Macrodantin; hemolysis ceases when the drug is withdrawn.

PRECAUTIONS

Drug Interactions: Magnesium trisilicate, when administered concomitantly with Macrodantin, reduces both the rate and extent of absorption. The mechanism for this interaction probably is adsorption of drug onto the surface of magnesium trisilicate.

Uricosuric drugs such as probenecid and sulfinpyrazone may inhibit renal tubular secretion of Macrodantin. The resulting increase in serum levels may increase toxicity and the decreased urinary levels could lessen its efficacy as a urinary tract antibacterial.

Carcinogensis, Mutagenesis: Nitrofurantoin, when fed to female Holzman rats at levels of 0.3% in a commercial diet for up to 44.5 weeks, was not carcinogenic. Nitrofurantoin was not carcinogenic when female Sprague-Dawley rats were fed a commercial diet with nitrofurantoin levels at 0.1% to 0.187% (total cumulative, 9.25 g) for 75 weeks. Further studies of the effects chronic administration to rodents are in progress.

Results of microbial *in vitro* tests using *Escherichia coli, Salmonella typhimurium,* and *Aspergillus nidulans* suggest that nitrofurantoin is a weak mutagen. Results of a dominant lethal assay in the mouse were negative.

Impairment of Fertility: The administration of high doses of nitrofurantoin to rats causes temporary spermatogenic arrest; this is reversible on discontinuing the drug. Doses of 10 mg/kg or greater in healthy human males may, in certain unpredictable instances, produce slight to moderate spermatogenic arrest with a decrease in sperm count.

Pregnancy: The safety of Macrodantin during pregnancy and lactation has not been established. Use of this drug in women of childbearing potential requires that the anticipated benefit be weighed against the possible risks.

Labor and Delivery: See CONTRAINDICATIONS.

Nursing Mothers: Nitrofurantoin has been detected in breast milk, in trace amounts. Caution should be exercised when Macrodantin is administered to a nursing woman, especially if the infant is known or suspected to have a glucose-6-phosphate dehydrogenase deficiency.

Pediatric Use: Contraindicated in infants under one month of age. (See CONTRAINDICATIONS.)

ADVERSE REACTIONS

Respiratory: CHRONIC, SUBACUTE, OR ACUTE PULMONARY HYPERSENSITIVITY REACTIONS MAY OCCUR.
CHRONIC PULMONARY REACTIONS OCCUR GENERALLY IN PATIENTS WHO HAVE RECEIVED CONTINUOUS TREATMENT FOR SIX MONTHS OR LONGER. MALAISE, DYSPNEA ON EXERTION, COUGH, AND ALTERED PULMONARY FUNCTION ARE COMMON MANIFESTATIONS WHICH CAN OCCUR INSIDIOUSLY. RADIOLOGIC AND HISTOLOGIC FINDINGS OF DIFFUSE INTERSTITIAL PNEUMONITIS OR FIBROSIS, OR BOTH, ARE ALSO COMMON MANIFESTATIONS OF THE CHRONIC PULMONARY REACTION. FEVER IS RARELY PROMINENT.
THE SEVERITY OF CHRONIC PULMONARY REACTIONS AND THEIR DEGREE OF RESOLUTION APPEAR TO BE RELATED TO THE DURATION OF THERAPY AFTER THE FIRST CLINICAL SIGNS APPEAR. PULMONARY FUNCTION MAY BE IMPAIRED PERMANENTLY, EVEN AFTER CESSATION OF THERAPY. THE RISK IS GREATER WHEN CHRONIC PULMONARY REACTIONS ARE NOT RECOGNIZED EARLY.
In subacute pulmonary reactions, fever and eosinophilia occur less often than in the acute form. Upon cessation of therapy, recovery may require several months. If the symptoms are not recognized as being drug-related and nitrofurantoin therapy is not stopped, the symptoms may become more severe.
Acute pulmonary reactions are commonly manifested by fever, chills, cough, chest pain, dyspnea, pulmonary infiltration with consolidation or pleural effusion on x-ray, and eosinophilia. Acute reactions usually occur within the first week of treatment and are reversible with cessation of therapy. Resolution often is dramatic. (See WARNINGS.)

Gastrointestinal: Hepatitis, including chronic active hepatitis, and cholestatic jaundice occur rarely.
Nausea, emesis, and anorexia occur most often. Abdominal pain and diarrhea are less common gastrointestinal reactions. These dose-related reactions can be minimized by reduction of dosage.

Neurologic: Peripheral neuropathy, which may become severe or irreversible, has occurred. Fatalities have been reported. Conditions such as renal impairment (creatinine clearance under 40 ml per minute), anemia, diabetes mellitus, electrolyte imbalance, vitamin B deficiency, and debilitating diseases may increase the possibility of peripheral neuropathy.
Less frequent reactions, of unknown causal relationship, are nystagmus, vertigo, dizziness, asthenia, headache, and drowsiness.

Dermatologic: Exfoliative dermititis and erythema multiforme (including Stevens-Johnson Syndrome) have been reported rarely. Transient alopecia also has been reported.

Allergic Reactions: Lupus-like syndrome associated with pulmonary reaction to nitrofurantoin has been reported. Also, angioedema, maculopapular, erythematous or eczematous eruptions, urticaria, rash, and pruritus have occurred. Anaphylaxis, sialadentitis, pancreatitis, arthralgia, myalgia, drug fever, and chills or chills and fever have been reported.

Hematologic: Agranulocytosis, leukopenia, granulocytopenia, hemolytic anemia, thrombocytopenia, glucose-6-phosphate dehydrogenase deficiency anemia, megaloblastic anemia, and eosinophilia have occurred. Cessation of therapy has returned the blood picture to normal. Aplastic anemia has been reported rarely.

Miscellaneous reactions: As with other antimicrobial agents, superinfections by resistant organisms, e.g., *Pseudomonas,* may occur. However, these are limited to the genitourinary tract because suppression of normal bacterial flora does not occur elsewhere in the body.

OVERDOSAGE

Occasional incidents of acute overdosage of Macrodantin have not resulted in any specific symptoms other than vomiting. In case vomiting does not occur soon after an excessive dose, induction of emesis is recommended. There is no specific antidote, but a high fluid intake should be maintained to promote urinary excretion of the drug.

DOSAGE AND ADMINISTRATION

Macrodantin should be given with food to improve drug absorption and, in some patients, tolerance.

Adults: 50–100 mg four times a day—the lower dosage level is recommended for uncomplicated urinary tract infections.

Children: 5–7 mg/kg of body weight per 24 hours, given in four divided doses (contraindicated under one month of age). Therapy should be continued for one week or for at least 3 days after sterility of the urine is obtained. Continued infection indicates the need for reevaluation.
For long-term suppressive therapy in adults, a reduction of dosage to 50–100 mg at bedtime may be adequate. For long-term suppressive therapy in children, doses as low as 1 mg/kg per 24 hours, given in a single or in two divided doses, may be adequate. **SEE WARNINGS SECTION REGARDING RISKS ASSOCIATED WITH LONG-TERM THERAPY.**

HOW SUPPLIED

Macrodantin is available as follows:
25-mg opaque, white capsule imprinted with one black line encircling the capsule and coded "Macrodantin 25 mg" and "0149-0007".

NDC 0149-0007-05   bottle of 100
50-mg opaque, yellow and white capsule imprinted with two black lines encircling the capsule and coded "Macrodantin 50 mg" and "0149-0008".*

NDC 0149-0008-05   bottle of 100
NDC 0149-0008-25 MACPAC™, box of 7 DAYCARD™ blisters, 4 capsules each.
NDC 0149-0008-66   bottle of 500
NDC 0149-0008-67   bottle of 1000
NDC 0149-0008-77   hospital unit-dose strips in box of 100
100-mg opaque, yellow capsule imprinted with three black lines encircling the capsule and coded "Macrodantin 100 mg" and "0149 0009".*

NDC 0149-0009-05   bottle of 100
NDC 0149-0009-23 MACPAC™, box of 7 DAYCARD™ blisters, 4 capsules each.
NDC 0149-0009-66   bottle of 500
NDC 0149-0009-67   bottle of 1000
NDC 0149-0009-77   hospital unit-dose strips in box of 100

*capsule design, registered trademark of Eaton Laboratories, Inc.

Furadantin/Macrodantin Sensi-Discs for the laboratory determination of bacterial sensitivity are available from BBL, Division of BioQuest. For information on nitrofurantoin assays in blood, serum, and urine, write or call the Medical Department. Literature sent to physicians on request. Address medical inquires to Norwich Eaton Pharmaceuticals, Inc. Medical Department, P.O. Box 191, Norwich, NY 13815-0191.

CAUTION

Federal law prohibits dispensing without prescription.
Manufactured by
Eaton Laboratories, Inc.
Manati, Puerto Rico 00701
Distributed by
Norwich Eaton Pharmaceuticals, Inc.
REVISED MAY 1988   MACRO-U1
Shown in Product Identification Section, page 420

TOLEREX™
[tol ′ur-ex]

Nutritional Information And Use Instructions
Tolerex™ is a patented, nutritionally complete elemental diet formulated for the nutritional management of patients with impaired digestion and/or malabsorption.

COMPOSITION
Tolerex is a chemically defined diet composed of all essential nutrients in simple, readily absorbable form: free amino acids, predigested carbohydrates, safflower oil, vitamins, minerals, electrolytes and trace elements. One 80-gram packet provides 300 Calories and 0.98 grams of available nitrogen with a caloric density of 1 Calorie per ml when diluted with 255 ml water to a total standard dilution volume of 300 ml:

	Amount per 80 g	Amount per 1000 ml (Standard dilution)	Energy Distribution
Total energy (Calories)	300	1000	
Amino acids (free base equivalent)	6.18 g	20.6 g	8.2%
Carbohydrate (dry basis)	67.9 g	226.3 g	90.5%
Fat	0.435 g	1.45 g	1.3%
Linoleic acid	0.348 g	1.16 g	1.0%

Six 80-g packets of Tolerex supply 5.88 grams of available nitrogen, 2.61 grams fat, 407 grams carbohydrate, and the following vitamins, minerals, electrolytes and amino acid profile:

Vitamins, Minerals and Trace Elements	Per 1000 ml (Standard dilution)	Per 6 Packets (480 Grams)	% U.S. RDA Per 6 Packets
Vitamin A	2778 IU	5000 IU	100
Vitamin D₃	222 IU	400 IU	100
Vitamin E	16.7 IU	30 IU	100
Vitamin C	33.3 mg	60 mg	100
Folic Acid	0.22 mg	0.4 mg	100
Thiamine	0.83 mg	1.5 mg	100
Riboflavin	0.94 mg	1.7 mg	100
Niacin	11.1 mg	20 mg	100
Vitamin B₆	1.11 mg	2 mg	100
Vitamin B₁₂	3.33 mcg	6 mcg	100
Biotin	0.17 mcg	0.3 mcg	100
Pantothenic Acid	5.55 mg	10 mg	100
Vitamin K₁	37.2 mcg	67 mcg	*
Choline	40.9 mcg	73.7 mg	*
Calcium	0.55 g	1 g	100
Phosphorus	0.55 g	1 g	100
Iodine	83.3 mcg	150 mcg	100
Iron	10 mg	18 mg	100
Magnesium	222 mg	400 mg	100
Copper	1.11 mg	2 mg	100
Zinc	8.33 mg	15 mg	100
Manganese	1.56 mg	2.81 mg	*
Selenium†	83.3 mcg	150 mcg	*
Molybdenum†	83.3 mcg	150 mcg	*
Chromium†	27.8 mcg	50 mcg	*

* No U.S. RDA established
† Represents amounts of these elements added.

Electrolytes	mEq per 1000 ml (Standard dilution)	Wt per 1000 ml (Standard dilution)
CATIONS		
Sodium	20.4	468 mg
Potassium	30.0	1172 mg
Calcium	27.7	556 mg
Magnesium	18.3	222 mg
Manganese	0.057	1.56 mg
Iron	0.358	10 mg
Copper	0.035	1.11 mg
Zinc	0.255	8.33 mg
Selenium†	0.002*	83.3 mcg
Molybdenum†	0.002**	83.3 mcg
Chromium†	0.002	27.8 mcg
ANIONS		
Chloride	26.8	950 mg
Phosphorus	54.0‡	556 mg
Acetate	18.7	1106 mg
Iodide	0.0007	83.3 mcg

† Represents amounts of these elements added.
* Calculated as Selenite SeO₃⁻²
** Calculated as Molybdate MoO₄⁻²
‡ Calculated as Phosphate PO₄⁻³

Amino Acid Profile	% Total Amino Acids
ESSENTIAL	
L-Isoleucine	4.55
L-Leucine	7.20
L-Valine	5.02
L-Lysine	5.41
L-Methionine	4.66
L-Phenylalanine	5.18
L-Threonine	4.55
L-Tryptophan	1.41
Total essential amino acids	37.98
NON-ESSENTIAL	
L-Alanine	4.85
L-Arginine	8.87
L-Aspartic Acid	10.35

Continued on next page

Norwich Eaton—Cont.

L-Glutamine	17.07
Glycine	7.91
L-Histidine	2.21
L-Proline	6.48
L-Serine	3.34
L-Tyrosine	0.94
Total non-essential amino acids	62.02

In the standard solution of 1 Calorie/ml, Tolerex has a pH of approximately 5.5 and an average osmolality of 550 mOsm/kg.

ACTIONS AND USES

Tolerex is a nutritionally complete, elemental diet that is rapidly utilized, since absorption can take place without the aid of peptidases. Tolerex is absorbed within the first 100 cm of functional small intestine. It is essentially a no-residue diet. There is minimal stimulation of biliary, pancreatic, and intestinal secretions, because of its free L-amino acid nitrogen (protein) source, glucose oligosaccharide primary energy source, and low fat content. The low fat content also permits rapid gastric emptying and minimizes gastric residuals, thus reducing the possibility of aspiration.

The balanced amino acid profile of Tolerex allows optimum utilization and retention of its readily absorbed, elemental nitrogen source.

Tolerex is useful as a maintenance diet in the dietary management of patients suffering from intractable diarrhea, impaired digestion and absorption which are secondary to a variety of diseases and disorders such as gastrointestinal disease, e.g. inflammatory bowel disease, cancer, intestinal atresia; and conditions leading to partial function of the gastrointestinal tract, e.g. malnutrition, pancreatitis, fistula, partial obstruction, short-gut syndrome. Tolerex is also useful as an aid in preparing the bowel for diagnostic and surgical procedures, and as a transition diet between parenteral and normal oral feeding. It is well tolerated by patients with known food sensitivities because it contains crystalline pure amino acids rather than whole protein or protein derivatives. Tolerex has been proven useful as an elimination diet for patients undergoing diagnosis of specific food allergens.

One packet diluted with 255 ml (8½ oz.) of water makes a single serving. Six packets of Tolerex mixed thoroughly with 1530 ml of water provide a full day's supply for the average adult with 1800 Calories, 5.88 grams available nitrogen, 2.61 grams fat, and 408 grams carbohydrate. Tolerex is a perishable liquid food when in solution. A full day's supply may be prepared at one time and stored in the refrigerator for up to 24 hours; shake the liquid briefly before serving. Do not leave at room temperature for more than 8 hours.

Tolerex may be administered via a nasogastric, esophagostomy, gastrostomy, or jejunostomy feeding tube. Because of the diet's homogeneity and low viscosity, small bore feeding tubes (16 gauge catheter or #5 French feeding tube) may be used to optimize patient tolerance. It is suggested that the diet be given at room temperature by continous drip technique using a suitable infusion pump. At the 1 Calorie per ml dilution, Tolerex supplies most of the daily fluid requirements. Additional fluids should be given when necessary to maintain adequate urine output.

During the first two days of use, Tolerex may need to be overdiluted for the osmotically sensitive patient, gradually concentrating up to full strength. The following administration schedule will facilitate GI adaptation, in most patients, within three days:

[See table below.]

If diarrhea is encountered, provide an antidiarrheal agent, which will often allow uninterrupted titration of the diet. Regress the rate and/or strength of the diet if needed. Then continue with progressive schedule until desired caloric/nitrogen intake is achieved.

Tolerex may also be given orally, but should be flavored and served chilled over ice. Vivonex® Flavor Packets are specifically developed for this purpose, although other flavoring agents may be used if their contribution to the elemental and nutritional qualities of the diet are kept in mind. Tolerex should be sipped slowly, preferably with a straw, when served as a beverage. Initiate oral feeding with a dilute solution, e.g. one packet diluted with 555 ml (18½ oz.) water, and gradually increase volume and concentration.

Oral feedings of elemental diets are sometimes met by poor patient acceptance due to the lack of the usual appetite cues of normal meals. Varying the available flavors, serving chilled over ice with a straw, and educating and motivating the patient as to the therapeutic importance of this form of

	Amount per 80.4 g		Amount per 1000 ml (standard dilution)		Energy Distribution
Total energy (Calories)	300		1000		
Amino acids (free base equivalent)	11.46	g	38.20	g	15.3%
Carbohydrate (dry basis)	61.67	g	205.57	g	82.2%
Fat	0.83	g	2.77	g	2.5%
Linoleic acid	0.65	g	2.17	g	2.0%

diet, are reportedly effective in improving patient acceptability.

PRECAUTIONS

DO NOT ADMINISTER TOLEREX™ PARENTERALLY. For use only under medical supervision.

Nausea, vomiting, abdominal cramps and distension, and diarrhea have been reported. Nausea is usually due to a high feeding rate, while diarrhea may be caused by a high diet concentration, low serum albumin, and concomitant medication. If intolerance is encountered, consider: 1) reverting one step in the above administration schedule, and then continuing slowly with a progressive schedule until desired caloric and nitrogen intake is achieved, 2) giving Tolerex at room temperature, 3) repleting the patient's serum albumin level within normal range, 4) using a continuous drip technique, and 5) monitoring the patient's medication for potential GI side effects. Local water conditions have also been implicated in instances of diarrhea. Using sterile water in diet preparation has been reported to be effective in this circumstance. Aspiration is an uncommon complication with Tolerex because of its low fat content. However, the likelihood of aspiration may be reduced by radiologically confirming the anatomic position of the feeding tube, elevating the head of the bed 30° while the patient is receiving diet intragastrically, and limiting the administration rate to 150 ml/hour or less, depending upon patient tolerance. Jejunal administration should also be considered.

Diabetics receiving this diet should be closely monitored. Use in children may require adjusting the daily consumption to meet the Recommended Daily Allowance for the age group involved.

Additional professional and technical information is available through your local Norwich Eaton representative.

SUPPLY INFORMATION

Tolerex (**NDC** 0149-0458-01) is available in cartons of six 80-g sealed packets for individual servings. Each packet provides 300 Calories in a total volume of 300 ml when mixed with 255 ml water.

Vivonex Flavor Packets are available in Vanilla (**NDC** 0149-0054-02), Strawberry (**NDC** 0149-0056-02), Orange-Pineapple (**NDC** 0149-0058-02), and Lemon-Lime (**NDC** 0149-0057-02) flavors.

Revised May 1989   TOLX-P3

Patent No. 3,697,287

VIVONEX®

[vī´vō-nex″]
FLAVOR PACKETS—Lemon-Lime, Orange-Pineapple, Strawberry or Vanilla
NONNUTRITIVE

Exclusively for use with Vivonex T.E.N., and Tolerex

VIVONEX® T.E.N.

[vī´vō-nex]
Elemental Diet For TOTAL ENTERAL NUTRITION
an effective substitute for intravenous feeding (TPN)

Vivonex® T.E.N. is a high nitrogen, elemental diet for total enteral nutrition. Vivonex T.E.N. is an effective substitute for intravenous feeding (TPN), except in patients where enteral feeding may be contraindicated (i.e., less than 60 cm of functioning small intestine). Its high essential to nonessential amino acid ratio (52:48), enhanced branched-chain amino acid content (33% of total amino acids), and optimal quantity of protein-sparing carbohydrate in a 175:1 Calorie to nitrogen ratio, make it especially useful in stressed, catabolic patients. Vivonex T.E.N. will further benefit those patients requiring a low residue feeding that permits maximal absorption with minimal digestion.

INDICATIONS

Vivonex T.E.N. is recommended in the dietary management of the following conditions:
- Stress
  - multiple trauma
  - burns
  - immediate postoperative malnutrition
  - sepsis
- Impaired digestion and absorption
  - inflammatory bowel disease
  - cancer
  - intestinal atresia
  - pancreatitis
  - fistula
  - partial obstruction
  - short-gut syndrome
- Malnutrition and cachexia
- Bowel preparation prior to diagnostic and surgical procedures
- Transition diet between parenteral and normal oral feeding
- Food sensitivities

COMPOSITION

Vivonex T.E.N. is a chemically defined diet composed of all essential nutrients in simple, readily absorbable form: free amino acids, predigested carbohydrates, safflower oil, vitamins, minerals, electrolytes, and trace elements. One 80.4-gram packet provides 300 Calories and 1.71 grams of available nitrogen with a caloric density of 1 Calorie per ml when diluted with 250 ml water to a total standard dilution volume of 300 ml:

[See table above.]

Ten 80.4-gram packets of Vivonex T.E.N. meet or exceed the quantity of nutrients and energy required by the average catabolic adult: 17.1 grams of available nitrogen, 115 grams amino acids, 8.33 grams fat, 617 grams carbohydrate, and the following vitamins, minerals, electrolytes, and amino acid profile:

[See table on next page.]

Electrolytes	mEq per 1000 ml (standard dilution)	Wt. Per 1000 ml (standard dilution)
Cations		
Sodium	20	460 mg
Potassium	20	782 mg
Calcium	25	500 mg
Magnesium	16.5	200 mg
Manganese	0.034	937 mcg
Iron	0.322	9 mg
Copper	0.032	1 mg
Zinc	0.306	10 mg
Selenium†	0.001*	50 mcg
Molybdenum†	0.001**	50 mcg
Chromium†	0.001	17 mcg
Anions		
Chloride	23.1	819 mg
Phosphorus	48.5‡	500 mg
Acetate	31.0	1830 mg
Iodide	0.0006	75 mcg

† Represents amounts of these elements added
* Calculated as Selenite, SeO_3^{-2}
** Calculated as Molybdate, MoO_4^{-2}
‡ Calculated as Phosphate, PO_4^{-3}

Amino Acid Profile	% Total Amino Acids
Essential	
L-Isoleucine	8.27
L-Leucine	16.56
L-Valine	8.27
L-Lysine	5.10
L-Methionine	3.66
L-Phenylalanine	5.16
L-Threonine	4.00
L-Tryptophan	1.28
Total essential amino acids	52.30
Non-essential	
L-Alanine	5.18
L-Arginine	7.64
L-Aspartic Acid	7.01

Day	Strength	Approx. Rate (ml/hour)	Tolerex (No. of Packets)	†	Total Water (ml)	=	Volume (ml)	Calories (Cal.)	Nitrogen (g)
1	½	75	3		1,665		1,800	900	3
2	⅔	75	4		1,620		1,800	1,200	4
3	Full	75	6		1,530		1,800	1,800	6

L-Glutamine	12.85
Glycine	4.01
L-Histidine	2.36
L-Proline	4.88
L-Serine	2.93
L-Tryosine	0.84
Total nonessential amino acids	47.70
Branched-chain amino acids	
(Isoleucine, Leucine, Valine)	33.10
Aromatic amino acids	6.00
(Phenylalanine, Tyrosine)	
Branched-chain: Aromatic amino acid molar ratio	7.4 : 1

In the standard dilution of 1 Calorie/ml, Vivonex T.E.N. has a pH of approximately 5.0 and an average osmolality of 630 mOsm/kg.

MIXING AND STORAGE

To prepare 300 ml of full strength diet (1 packet):
1. Add 1 packet of diet to 250 ml of warm water in a 1 pint container.
2. Cover and shake for 20 seconds.

Any remaining undissolved particles will dissolve spontaneously after standing 5–10 minutes.

NOTE: For larger quantities the container should be no more than ¾ full after diet is added to water, and more time may be required to shake product into solution. Vivonex T.E.N. can also be blenderized if desired.

Vivonex T.E.N. is a perishable liquid food when in solution. A full day's supply may be prepared at one time and stored in the refrigerator for up to 48 hours; shake the liquid briefly before serving. Do not leave at room temperature for more than 8 hours.

Feeding Tube Administration: VIVONEX T.E.N. may be administered via a nasogastric, nasointestinal, esophagostomy, gastrostomy, or jejunostomy feeding tube. Because of its homogeneity and low viscosity, small bore feeding tubes (16 gauge catheter or #5 French tube) may be used to optimize patient tolerance. The diet should be given at room temperature by continuous drip technique, using the Vivonex® Acutrol® Enteral Feeding System, the Vivonex® Delivery System, or a suitable infusion pump. At the 1 Calorie per ml dilution, Vivonex T.E.N. supplies most of the daily fluid requirements. Additional fluids should be given when necessary to maintain hydration and adequate urine output.

Generally, patient tolerance is optimized with any enteral diet by beginning with a dilute solution, titrating up to the desired calorie and nitrogen input. Although a more aggressive administration schedule may be considered, especially for gastric feeding or patients with a serum albumin level greater than 3.5 g/dl, the following schedule has been found to facilitate adaptation in most patients:
[See table below].

Once full strength T.E.N. is being administered, nutrient intake can be increased by raising the continuous flow rate in 25 ml increments and/or raising the concentration, e.g., one packet + 150 ml water = 200 ml of 1.5 Cal/ml diet. Diarrhea is the most common side effect with any liquid diet. Concomitant use of an antidiarrheal will often allow uninterrupted titration of the diet. However, in some instances, it may be necessary to revert one step to a more dilute solution, maintaining the patient at the last tolerated rate until free of symptoms for eight hours. Then, continue with progressive schedule until desired calorie and nitrogen intake is achieved.

ORAL ADMINISTRATION

For oral use, Vivonex T.E.N. should be flavored and served chilled over ice. Vivonex Flavor Packets were specifically developed for this purpose, although other flavoring agents may be used if their contribution to the elemental and nutritional qualities of the diet are kept in mind. Vivonex T.E.N. should be sipped slowly, preferably through a straw, when served as a beverage. Initiate oral feeding with dilute solution, e.g., one packet diluted with 550 ml (18⅓ oz.), and gradually increase volume and concentration.

Oral feedings of elemental diets are sometimes met with poor patient acceptance because of taste and the lack of the usual appetite cues of normal meals. Varying the available flavors, serving chilled over ice and sipping through a straw, and educating and motivating the patient as to the therapeutic importance of this form of diet, are reportedly effective in improving patient acceptability.

PRECAUTIONS

DO NOT ADMINISTER VIVONEX T.E.N. PARENTERALLY. For use only under medical supervision. Nausea, vomiting, abdominal cramps, distention, and diarrhea are

Vitamins, Minerals and Trace Elements	Per 1000 ml (standard dilution)		Per 10 Packets (804 Grams)		% U.S. RDA Per 10 Packets
Vitamin A	2500	IU	7500	IU	150
Vitamin D₃	200	IU	600	IU	150
Vitamin E	15	IU	45	IU	150
Vitamin C	60	mg	180	mg	300
Folic Acid	0.4	mg	1.2	mg	300
Thiamine	1.5	mg	4.5	mg	300
Riboflavin	1.7	mg	5.1	mg	300
Niacin	20	mg	60	mg	300
Vitamin B₆	2	mg	6	mg	300
Vitamin B₁₂	6	mcg	18	mcg	300
Biotin	0.3	mg	0.9	mg	300
Pantothenic Acid	10	mg	30	mg	300
Vitamin K₁	22.3	mcg	67	mcg	*
Choline	73.7	mg	221	mg	
Calcium	0.5	g	1.5	g	150
Phosphorus	0.5	g	1.5	g	150
Iodine	75	mcg	225	mcg	150
Iron	9	mg	27	mg	150
Magnesium	200	mg	600	mg	150
Copper	1	mg	3	mg	150
Zinc	10	mg	30	mg	200
Manganese	0.94	mg	2.81	mg	*
Selenium†	50	mcg	150	mcg	*
Molybdenum†	50	mcg	150	mcg	*
Chromium†	16.67	mcg	50	mcg	*

* No U.S. RDA established.
† Represents amounts of these elements added.

possible. Nausea and diarrhea are usually due to feeding rate or diet concentration. Local water conditions may be implicated in instances of diarrhea. Preparing diet with deionized or distilled water may be effective in this circumstance.

Aspiration is an uncommon complication with Vivonex T.E.N. because of its low fat content. However, radiologically confirm the anatomic position of the feeding tube, elevate the head of the bed 30° while the patient is receiving diet intragastrically, and control the administration to 150 ml/hour or less, depending upon patient tolerance. Jejunal administration should also be considered.

Diabetics and patients with renal insufficiency receiving this diet should be closely monitored. Use in children may require adjusting the daily consumption to meet the Recommended Daily Allowance for the age group involved.

SUPPLY INFORMATION

Vivonex T.E.N. (NDC 0149-0067-01) is available in cartons of ten 80.4-gram sealed packets, each providing 300 Calories.

Vivonex Flavor Packets are available in Vanilla (NDC 0149-0054-02), Strawberry (NDC 0149-0056-02), Orange-Pineapple (NDC 0149-0058-02), and Lemon-Lime (NDC 0149-0057-02) flavors.

The Vivonex Acutrol Enteral Feeding System (NDC 0149-0065-06) is a one-liter, universal, gravity feeding system offering a unique rapid-fill funnel cap, easy-to-read fluid level graduations, macro-drip sight chamber, precise control roller clamp, universal luer adapter, and a built-in burette.

The Vivonex Delivery System (NDC 0149-0050-10) is a disposable, gravity-drip tube feeding system with one liter capacity, complete with micro-drop cannula and connecting tubing.

Additional professional and technical information on all Vivonex products is available through local Norwich Eaton Pharmaceuticals representatives.

REVISED MAY 1986   VIVTEN-P4

EDUCATIONAL MATERIAL

Norwich Eaton offers a wide range of educational services to the medical profession free of charge. Please write to the Director of Medical Relations, Norwich Eaton Pharmaceuticals, Inc., Norwich, NY 13815-0231, for further information.

- **The Norwich Eaton Audio-Visual Library**—more than 350 film, slide and videotape programs are available on free-loan (Directory available upon request)
- **Professional Speaker Bureaus** (Urinary Tract Infection, Nutrition, Clinical Management of Pain, and Nutritional Support of Aids Patients)
- **Patient Education Brochures and Films**
- **ACOG Physician Placement Service**
- **AUA Physician Placement Service**

Nutripharm Laboratories, Inc.
185 INDUSTRIAL PARKWAY
SUITE G
SOMERVILLE, NJ 08876

ISOCOM®   ℞

CAUTION

Federal law prohibits dispensing without prescription.

DESCRIPTION

Each capsule contains Isometheptene Mucate 65 mg., Dichloralphenazone 100 mg., and Acetaminophen 325 mg. Isometheptene Mucate is a white crystalline powder having a characteristic aromatic odor and bitter taste. It is an unsaturated aliphatic amine with sympathomimetic properties. Dichloralphenazone is a white microcrystalline powder, with slight odor and tastes saline at first, becoming acrid. It is a mild sedative.
Acetaminophen, a non-salycylate, occurs as a white, odorless, crystalline powder possessing a slightly bitter taste.

ACTIONS

Isometheptene Mucate, a sympathomimetic amine, acts by constricting dilated cranial and cerebral arterioles, thus reducing the stimuli that lead to vascular headaches. Dichloralphenazone, a mild sedative, reduces the patient's emotional reaction to the pain of both vascular and tension headaches. Acetaminophen raises the threshold to painful stimuli, thus exerting an analgesic effect against all types of headaches.

INDICATIONS

For relief of vascular and tension headaches.

Based on a review for this drug (isometheptene mucate), The National Academy of Sciences—National Research Council and/or other information, FDA has classified the other indication as "possibly" effective in the treatment of migraine headache.
Final classification of the less-than-effective indication requires further investigation.

CONTRAINDICATIONS

Isocom is contraindicated in Glaucoma and/or severe cases of renal disease, hypertension, organic heart disease, hepatic disease and in those patients who are on monoamineoxidase (MAO) inhibitor therapy.

PRECAUTIONS

Caution should be observed in hypertension, peripheral vascular disease and after recent cardiovascular attacks.

Continued on next page

Day	Strength	Approx. Rate (ml/hour)	Vivonex T.E.N. (no. of packets)	+	Water (ml)	=	Total Volume (ml)	Calories (Cal.)	Nitrogen (g)
1	½	50	2	+	1100	=	1200	600	3.42
2	½	100	4	+	2200	=	2400	1200	6.84
3	¾	100	6	+	2100	=	2400	1800	10.26
4	Full	100	8	+	2000	=	2400	2400	13.68

Nutripharm—Cont.

ADVERSE REACTIONS
Transient dizziness and skin rash may appear in hypersensitive patients. This can usually be eliminated by reducing the dose.

DOSAGE AND ADMINISTRATION
FOR RELIEF OF MIGRAINE HEADACHE: The usual adult dose is two capsules at once, followed by one capsule every hour until relieved, up to 5 capsules within a twelve hour period.

FOR RELIEF OF TENSION HEADACHE: The usual adult dose is one or two capsules every four hours up to 8 capsules a day.

HOW SUPPLIED
Bottles of 50 capsules, NDC 51081-424-05, bottles of 100 capsules, NDC 51081-424-10, bottles of 250 capsules, NDC 51081-424-25.

NUTRIPHARM LABORATORIES, INC.
Somerville, N.J. 08876

Organon Inc.
375 MT. PLEASANT AVE.
WEST ORANGE, NJ 07052

Below are listed the currently available products. For a complete catalog and price list, direct inquiries to Customer Service. For specific product information, direct inquiries to the Professional Services Department.

BCG Vaccine, USP   ℞
Tice Strain

Distributed by Organon Inc.
(See Organon Teknika Section for complete product information.)

CALDEROL®   ℞
[kal-dah'rol]
(calcifediol capsules, USP)

DESCRIPTION
Calderol® Capsules contain calcifediol, USP, which is the colorless, crystalline monohydrate of 25-hydroxycholecalciferol prepared by chemical synthesis and is identical to the natural vitamin metabolite. Calcifediol has a calculated molecular weight of 418.67 and is soluble in organic solvents but relatively insoluble in water. Chemically, calcifediol is (5Z,7E)-9,10-secocholesta-5,7,10(19)-triene-3β,25-diol monohydrate. The structural formula is represented below:

The other names frequently used for 25-hydroxycholecalciferol are 25-hydroxyvitamin D_3, 25-HCC, 25-OHCC, and 25-OHD$_3$.

Calderol® for oral administration is available in two strengths: a white capsule containing 20 μg calcifediol and an orange capsule containing 50 μg calcifediol.

Each 20 μg. and 50 μg. capsule contains: gelatin, glycerin, corn oil, methyleneipropyl paraben, purified water, and titanium dioxide as inactive ingredients.

Each 50 μg. capsule also contains: FD&C yellow #6 (sunset yellow) as a color additive.

CLINICAL PHARMACOLOGY
The natural supply of vitamin D in man mainly depends on the ultraviolet rays of the sun for conversion of 7-dehydrocholesterol to vitamin D_3 (cholecalciferol). It is now known that vitamin D_3 must first be converted to 25-OHD$_3$ (25-hydroxycholecalciferol) by a vitamin D_3-25-hydroxylase enzyme (25-OHase) present in the liver. 25-Hydroxycholecalciferol is the major transport form of vitamin D_3 and can be readily monitored in the serum. It is further converted to 1,25-dihydroxycholecalciferol (1,25-(OH)$_2D_3$) and 24,25-dihydroxycholecalciferol (24,25-(OH)$_2D_3$) in the kidney. 1,25-(OH)$_2D_3$ stimulates resorption of calcium from bone and increases intestinal calcium absorption. The physiologic role of 24,25-(OH)$_2D_3$ has not been clearly established. The metabolic activity of calcifediol in clinical use appears to be related not only to its conversion to other metabolites but also due to its intrinsic activity.

When administered orally, calcifediol is rapidly absorbed from the intestine, with peak 25-OHD$_3$ concentrations in the serum reported after about 4 hours. 25-Hydroxycholecalciferol is known to be transported in blood, bound to a specific plasma protein. The terminal half-life of orally administered calcifediol in the serum is about 16 days.

INDICATIONS AND USAGE
Calderol® (calcifediol) is indicated in the treatment and management of metabolic bone disease or hypocalcemia associated with chronic renal failure in patients undergoing renal dialysis.

In studies to date it has been shown to increase serum calcium levels, to decrease alkaline phosphatase and parathyroid hormone levels in some patients, to decrease subperiosteal bone resorption in some patients, and to decrease histological signs of hyperparathyroid bone disease and mineralization defects in some patients.

CONTRAINDICATIONS
Calderol® (calcifediol) should not be given to patients with hypercalcemia or evidence of vitamin D toxicity.

WARNINGS
Since calcifediol is a metabolite of vitamin D, vitamin D and its derivatives should be withheld during treatment.

Aluminum carbonate or hydroxide gels should be used to control serum phosphorus levels in patients undergoing dialysis.

Overdosage of any form of vitamin D is dangerous (see also **Overdosage**). Progressive hypercalcemia may be so severe as to require emergency attention. Chronic hypercalcemia can lead to generalized vascular calcification, nephrocalcinosis, and other soft-tissue calcification. The serum calcium times phosphorus (Ca $\times$ P) product should not be allowed to exceed 70. Radiographic and/or slit lamp evaluation of suspect anatomical regions may be useful in the early detection of this condition.

PRECAUTIONS
i) *General:* Excessive dosage of Calderol® (calcifediol) induces hypercalcemia and in some instances hypercalciuria; therefore, early in treatment during dosage adjustment, serum calcium should be determined frequently (at least weekly). Should hypercalcemia develop, the drug should be discontinued immediately. After achieving normocalcemia, the drug may be readministered at a lower dosage. Calderol® should be given cautiously to patients receiving digitalis, because hypercalcemia in such patients may precipitate cardiac arrhythmias.

ii) *Information for the Patient:* The patient and his or her parents or spouse should be informed about compliance with dosage instructions, adherence to instructions about diet, calcium supplementation, phosphate binder usage, and avoidance of non approved prescription drugs. Patients should also be informed about the symptoms of hypercalcemia (see **Adverse Reactions**).

iii) *Essential Laboratory Tests:* Serum calcium, phosphorus and alkaline phosphatase and 24-hour urinary calcium and phosphorus should be determined periodically. During the initial phase of the medication, serum calcium should be determined more frequently (at least weekly).

iv) *Drug Interactions:* Cholestyramine has been reported to reduce absorption of fat-soluble vitamins; as such, it may impair intestinal absorption of calcifediol. The administration of anticonvulsants has been shown to affect the calcifediol requirements in some patients.

v) *Carcinogenesis, Mutagenesis, Impairment of Fertility:* - Long-term studies in animals have not been completed to evaluate the carcinogenic potential of Calderol®. No significant effects of calcifediol on fertility and/or general reproductive performances were reported.

vi) *Use in Pregnancy:* Teratogenic effects:

Pregnancy Category C: Calcifediol has been shown to be teratogenic in rabbits when given in doses of 6 to 12 times the human dose. There are no adequate and well-controlled studies in pregnant women. Calderol® should be used during pregnancy only if the potential benefit justifies potential risk to the fetus.

When calcifediol was given orally to bred rabbits on the 6th through the 18th day of gestation, gross visceral and skeletal examination of pups indicated that the compound was teratogenic at doses of 25 and 50 μg/kg/day. A dose of 5 μg/kg/day was not teratogenic. In a similar study in rats, calcifediol was not teratogenic at doses up to and including 60 μg/kg/day.

vii) *Labor and Delivery:* The effect of this drug on the mother and the fetus during labor and delivery is not known.

viii) *Nursing Mothers:* It is not known whether this drug is excreted in human milk. Because many drugs are excreted in human milk, caution should be exercised when Calderol® is administered to a nursing woman.

ix) *Pediatric Use:* The safety and effectiveness of Calderol® in children have not been established.

ADVERSE REACTIONS
Since calcifediol is an active metabolite of vitamin D, adverse effects are, in general, similar to those encountered with excessive vitamin D intake. The early and late signs and symptoms of vitamin D intoxication associated with hypercalcemia include:

a. *Early:* Weakness, headache, somnolence, nausea, vomiting, dry mouth, constipation, muscle pain, bone pain, and metallic taste.

b. *Late:* Polyuria, polydipsia, anorexia, irritability, weight loss, nocturia, conjunctivitis (calcific), pancreatitis, photophobia, rhinorrhea, pruritus, hyperthermia, decreased libido, elevated BUN, albuminuria, hypercholesterolemia, elevated SGOT and SGPT, ectopic calcification, hypertension, cardiac arrhythmias, and, rarely, overt psychosis.

OVERDOSAGE
Administration of Calderol® (calcifediol) to patients in excess of their daily requirements can cause hypercalcemia, hypercalciuria, and hyperphosphatemia. High intake of calcium and phosphate concomitant with Calderol® may lead to similar abnormalities.

Treatment of Hypercalcemia and Overdosages: General treatment of hypercalcemia (greater than 1 μg/dl above the upper limit of the normal range) consists of discontinuation of therapy with Calderol®. Serum calcium measurements should be performed regularly until normocalcemia ensues. Hypercalcemia usually resolves in two to four weeks. When serum calcium levels have returned to within normal limits, therapy with Calderol® may be reinstituted at a dosage lower than prior therapy. Serum calcium levels should be obtained at least weekly after all dosage changes and subsequent dosage titration. Persistent or markedly elevated calcium levels in dialysis patients may be corrected by dialysis against a calcium-free dialysate.

Treatment of Accidental Overdosage: The treatment of acute accidental overdosage of Calderol® should consist of general supportive measures. If drug ingestion is discovered within a relatively short time, induction of emesis or gastric lavage may be of benefit in preventing further absorption. If the drug has passed through the stomach, the administration of mineral oil may promote fecal elimination. Serial serum calcium determination, rate of urinary calcium excretion, and an assessment of electrocardiographic abnormalities due to hypercalcemia should be obtained. Such monitoring is critical in patients receiving digitalis. Discontinuation of supplemental calcium and a low calcium diet are also indicated in accidental overdosage. Because the conversion of calcifediol to 1.25-(OH)$_2D_3$ is tightly regulated by the body's needs, further measures are probably unnecessary. Should persistent and marked hypercalcemia occur, however, there are a variety of therapeutic measures that may be considered, depending on the patient's underlying condition. These include the use of drugs such as phosphates and corticosteroids as well as measures to induce an appropriate forced diuresis. The use of peritoneal dialysis against a calcium-free dialysate may also be considered.

The Oral LD$_{50}$ in the rat is > 320 μg/kg.

DOSAGE AND ADMINISTRATION
The optimal daily dose of Calderol® (calcifediol) must be carefully determined for each patient. The recommended initial dosage of Calderol® is based on the assumption that each patient is receiving an adequate daily intake of calcium from dietary sources or from the addition of calcium supplements. The RDA for calcium in adults is 1000 mg. To ensure that each patient receives an adequate daily intake of calcium, the physician should either prescribe a calcium supplement or instruct the patients in proper dietary measures.

Chronic Renal Failure—Dialysis Patients: The recommended initial dose of Calderol® is 300 to 350 μg of calcifediol weekly, administered on a daily or alternate-day schedule. If a satisfactory response in the biochemical parameters and clinical manifestations of the disease state is not observed, dosage may be increased at four-week intervals. During this titration period, serum calcium levels should be obtained at least weekly, and if hypercalcemia is noted, the drug should be discontinued until normocalcemia ensues.

Some patients with normal serum calcium levels may respond to doses of 20 μg of calcifediol every other day. Most patients respond to doses between 50 and 100 μg daily or between 100 and 200 μg on alternate days.

HOW SUPPLIED
Calderol® (calcifediol capsules, USP) are available in the following strengths and package sizes:

Strength	Packaged	NDC Number
20 μg	Bottle of 60	0052-0472-60
	(white, soft elastic capsules)	
50 μg	Bottle of 60	0052-0474-60
	(orange, soft elastic capsules)	
	Caution: Federal law prohibits	
	dispensing without prescription.	

Organon Inc., W. Orange, NJ 07052

Revised 2/88

Shown in Product Identification Section, page 420

CORTROPHIN®—Zinc ℞
ACTH
(sterile corticotropin zinc hydroxide suspension, USP)

HOW SUPPLIED
Vials, 5 mL (40 USP Units/mL).

CORTROSYN® ℞

Cosyntropin is α 1–24 corticotropin, a synthetic subunit of ACTH.

HOW SUPPLIED
Box containing: 10 Vials of Cortrosyn® (Cosyntropin) for injection 0.25 mg
10 ampuls of solvent (sodium chloride for injection, USP)

COTAZYM® ℞
[kōt′a zīm]
(pancrelipase capsules, USP)

DESCRIPTION
Cotazym (Pancrelipase, USP) is a powder containing enzymes obtained from the pancreas of the hog. These include amylase and protease but principally lipase. Each capsule contains:
Lipase—8,000 USP Units
Protease—30,000 USP Units
Amylase—30,000 USP Units
Precipitated calcium carbonate 25 mg.
Each capsule also contains the inactive ingredients: cornstarch, gelatin, magnesium stearate, talc, FD&C green #3, FD&C yellow #10 as coloring and titanium dixoide.

INDICATIONS AND USAGE
It is indicated in conditions where pancreatic enzymes are either absent or deficient with resultant inadequate fat digestion. Such conditions include but are not limited to chronic pancreatitis, pancreatectomy, cystic fibrosis and steatorrhea of diverse etiologies.

CONTRAINDICATIONS
Known hypersensitivity to pork protein.

PRECAUTIONS
In the event that capsules are opened for any reason care should be taken so that powder is not inhaled or spilled on hands since it may prove irritating to the skin or mucous membranes.

ADVERSE REACTIONS
No adverse reactions have been reported. It should be noted, however, that extremely high doses of exogenous pancreatic enzymes have been associated with hyperuricosuria and hyperuricemia.

DOSAGE AND ADMINISTRATION
One to three capsules just prior to each meal or snack. Individual cases may require higher dosage and dietery adjustment.

STORAGE
Not to exceed 25℃ (77°F). Dry place when opened.

DISPENSE
In tight container as defined in the USP.

SUPPLIED
Cotazym capsules (regular) bottles of 100 and 500. NDC # 0052-0381-91, NDC # 0052-0381-95.
Shown in Product Identification Section, page 420

COTAZYM®-S ℞
[kōt′a zīm-s]
(pancrelipase, USP)
Enteric coated spheres

HOW SUPPLIED
Bottles of 100 capsules
Bottles of 500 capsules
Shown in Product Identification Section, page 420

DECA–DURABOLIN® ℞
(nandrolone decanoate injection, USP)

HOW SUPPLIED
50 mg/mL—2 mL vials, 1 mL prefilled syringe.
100 mg/mL—2 mL vials, 1 mL prefilled syringe.
200 mg/mL—1 mL vials, 1 mL prefilled syringe.

DURABOLIN® ℞
(nandrolone phenpropionate injection, USP)

HOW SUPPLIED
25 mg/mL—5 mL vials.
50 mg/mL—2 mL vials.

HEPARIN SODIUM ℞
Injection, USP
(From Beef Lung)

HOW SUPPLIED
1,000 USP Units/mL (aqueous) Vials, 10 mL and 30 mL
5,000 USP Units/mL (aqueous) Vials, 1 mL single use only and 10 mL
10,000 USP Units/mL (aqueous) Vials, 1 mL single use only and 4 mL

HEXADROL® Elixir ℞
(dexamethasone elixir, USP)

Each 5 mL contains: 0.5 mg dexamethasone with 5% alcohol.

HOW SUPPLIED
Elixir (0.5 mg/5 mL)—Bottle of 120 mL

HEXADROL® ℞
(dexamethasone tablets, USP)

HOW SUPPLIED
Tablets (0.5 mg yellow, scored)—bottle of 100
Tablets (0.75 mg white, scored)—bottle of 100
Tablets (1.5 mg peach, scored)—bottle of 100
Tablets (4 mg green, scored)—bottle of 100
Tablets (4 mg green, scored)—Box of 100
(10 strips-10 per strip)
Shown in Product Identification Section, page 420

HEXADROL® ℞
Therapeutic Pack
(dexamethasone tablets, USP)

HOW SUPPLIED
Each pack contains: 6 × 1.5 mg tablets, (peach scored); 8 × 0.75 mg tablets, (white, scored).
Shown in Product Identification Section, page 420

HEXADROL® ℞
Phosphate Injection
(dexamethasone sodium phosphate injection, USP)

HOW SUPPLIED
Available in three potencies:
4 mg/mL—1 mL vials single use only, 5 mL vials, 1 mL prefilled syringe.
10 mg/mL—10 mL vials, 1 mL prefilled syringe.
20 mg/mL—5 mL vial, 5 mL prefilled syringe.

HYDROCORTISONE, USP ℞
Micronized Powder
Non-Sterile: For Prescription Compounding Only

HOW SUPPLIED
Available in 10, 25 and 100 gram containers.

LIQUAEMIN® Sodium ℞
(heparin sodium injection, USP)
from porcine intestinal mucosa

HOW SUPPLIED
1,000 USP Units/mL Vials, 10 mL & 30 mL
5,000 USP Units mL Vials, 1 mL single use only & 10 mL
10,000 USP Units/mL Vials, 1 mL single use only & 4 mL
20,000 USP Units/mL Vials, 1 mL, single use only, 2 mL & 5 mL
40,000 USP Units/mL Vials, 1 mL single use only

NORCURON® ℞
(vecuronium bromide) for injection

> THIS DRUG SHOULD BE ADMINISTERED BY ADEQUATELY TRAINED INDIVIDUALS FAMILIAR WITH ITS ACTIONS, CHARACTERISTICS, AND HAZARDS.

DESCRIPTION
NORCURON® (vecuronium bromide) for injection is a nondepolarizing neuromuscular blocking agent of intermediate duration, chemically designated as piperidinium, 1-[(2β, 3α, 5α, 16β, 17β)-3, 17-bis(acetyloxy)-2-(1- piperidinyl) androstan-16-yl]-1-methyl-, bromide. The structural formula is:

Its chemical formula is $C_{34}H_{57}BrN_2O_4$ with molecular weight 637.74.
Norcuron® is supplied as a sterile nonpyrogenic freeze-dried buffered cake of very fine microscopic crystalline particles for intravenous injection only. Each 10 mL vial contains 10 mg vecuronium bromide. Each vial also contains 20.75 mg citric acid anhydrous, 16.25 mg sodium phosphate dibasic anhydrous, 97 mg mannitol (to adjust tonicity), sodium hydroxide and/or phosphoric acid to buffer and adjust to a pH of 4. Bacteriostatic water for injection, USP, when supplied, contains 0.9% w/v BENZYL ALCOHOL, WHICH IS NOT FOR USE IN NEWBORNS.

CLINICAL PHARMACOLOGY
Norcuron® (vecuronium bromide) for injection is a nondepolarizing neuromuscular blocking agent possessing all of the characteristic pharmacological actions of this class of drugs (curariform). It acts by competing for cholinergic receptors at the motor end-plate. The antagonism to acetylcholine is inhibited and neuro-muscular block is reversed by acetylcholinesterase inhibitors such as neostigmine, edrophonium, and pyridostigmine. Norcuron® is about ⅓ more potent than pancuronium; the duration of neuromuscular blockade produced by Norcuron® is shorter than that of pancuronium at initially equipotent doses. The time to onset of paralysis decreases and the duration of maximum effect increases with increasing Norcuron® doses. The use of a peripheral nerve stimulator is of benefit in assessing the degree of muscular relaxation.
The ED_{90} (dose required to produce 90% suppression of the muscle twitch response with balanced anesthesia) has averaged 0.057 mg/kg (0.049 to 0.062 mg/kg in various studies). An initial Norcuron® dose of 0.08 to 0.10 mg/kg generally produces first depression of twitch in approximately 1 minute, good or excellent intubation conditions within 2.5 to 3 minutes, and maximum neuromuscular blockade within 3 to 5 minutes of injection in most patients. Under balanced anesthesia, the time to recovery to 25% of control (clinical duration) is approximately 25 to 40 minutes after injection and recovery is usually 95% complete approximately 45–65 minutes after injection of intubating dose. The neuromuscular blocking action of Norcuron® is slightly enhanced in the presence of potent inhalation anesthetics. If Norcuron® is first administered more than 5 minutes after the start of the inhalation of enflurane, isoflurane, or halothane, or when steady state has been achieved, the intubating dose of Norcuron® may be decreased by approximately 15% (see **DOSAGE AND ADMINISTRATION** section). Prior administration of succinylcholine may enhance the neuromuscular blocking effect of Norcuron® and its duration of action. With succinylcholine as the intubating agent, initial doses of 0.04–0.06 mg/kg of Norcuron® will produce complete neuromuscular block with clinical duration of action of 25–30 minutes. If succinylcholine is used prior to Norcuron®, the administration of Norcuron® should be delayed until the patient starts recovering from succinylcholine- induced neuromuscular blockade. The effect of prior use of other nondepolarizing neuromuscular blocking agents on the activity of Norcuron® has not been studied (see **Drug Interactions**). Repeated administration of maintenance doses of Norcuron® may be administered at approximately 12 to 15 minute intervals. Halothane anesthesia increases the clinical duration of the maintenance dose only slightly. Under enflurane a maintenance dose of 0.010 mg/kg is approximately equal to 0.015 mg/kg dose under balanced anesthesia.
The recovery index (time from 25% to 75% recovery) is approximately 15–25 minutes under balanced or halothane

Continued on next page

Organon—Cont.

anesthesia. When recovery from Norcuron® neuromuscular blocking effect begins, it proceeds more rapidly than recovery from pancuronium. Once spontaneous recovery has started, the neuromuscular block produced by Norcuron® is readily reversed with various anticholinesterase agents, e.g. pyridostigmine, neostigmine, or edrophonium in conjunction with an anticholinergic agent such as atropine or glycopyrrolate. Rapid recovery is a finding consistent with Norcuron®'s short elimination half-life.

Pharmacokinetics: At clinical doses of 0.04–0.10 mg/kg, 60–80% of Norcuron® is usually bound to plasma protein. The distribution half-life following a single intravenous dose (range 0.025–0.280 mg/kg) is approximately 4 minutes. Elimination half-life over this same dosage range is approximately 65–75 minutes in healthy surgical patients and in renal failure patients undergoing transplant surgery. In late pregnancy, elimination half-life may be shortened to approximately 35–40 minutes. The volume of distribution at steady state is approximately 300–400 mL/kg; systemic rate of clearance is approximately 3–4.5 mL/minute/kg. In man, urine recovery of Norcuron® varies from 3–35% within 24 hours. Data derived from patients requiring insertion of a T-tube in the common bile duct suggests that 25–50% of a total intravenous dose of vecuronium may be excreted in bile within 42 hours. Only unchanged Norcuron® (vecuronium bromide) for injection has been detected in human plasma following clinical use. One metabolite, 3-deacetyl vecuronium, has been recovered in the urine of some patients in quantities that account for up to 10% of injected dose; 3-deacetyl vecuronium has also been recovered by T-tube in some patients accounting for up to 25% of the injected dose.

This metabolite has been judged by animal screening (dogs and cats) to have 50% or more of the potency of Norcuron®; equipotent doses are of approximately the same duration as Norcuron® in dogs and cats. Biliary excretion accounts for about half the dose of Norcuron® within 7 hours in the anesthetized rat. Circulatory bypass of the liver (cat preparation) prolongs recovery from Norcuron®. Limited data derived from patients with cirrhosis or cholestasis suggests that some measurements of recovery may be doubled in such patients. In patients with renal failure, measurements of recovery do not differ significantly from similar measurements in healthy patients.

Studies involving routine hemodynamic monitoring in good risk surgical patients reveal that the administration of Norcuron® in doses up to three times that needed to produce clinical relaxation (0.15 mg/kg) did not produce clinically significant changes in systolic, diastolic or mean arterial pressure. The heart rate, under similar monitoring, remained unchanged in some studies and was lowered by a mean of up to 8% in other studies. A large dose of 0.28 mg/kg administered during a period of no stimulation, while patients were being prepared for coronary artery bypass grafting, was not associated with alterations in rate-pressure-product or pulmonary capillary wedge pressure. Systemic vascular resistance was lowered slightly and cardiac output was increased insignificantly. (The drug has not been studied in patients with hemodynamic dysfunction secondary to cardiac valvular disease). Limited clinical experience with use of Norcuron® during surgery for pheochromocytoma has shown that administration of this drug is not associated with changes in blood pressure or heart rate.

Unlike other nondepolarizing skeletal muscle relaxants, Norcuron® has no clinically significant effects on hemodynamic parameters. Norcuron® will not counteract those hemodynamic changes or known side effects produced by or associated with anesthetic agents, other drugs or various other factors known to alter hemodynamics.

INDICATIONS AND USAGE

Norcuron® is indicated as an adjunct to general anesthesia, to facilitate endotracheal intubation and to provide skeletal muscle relaxation during surgery or mechanical ventilation.

CONTRAINDICATIONS

Norcuron® is contraindicated in patients known to have a hypersensitivity to it.

WARNINGS

NORCURON® SHOULD BE ADMINISTERED IN CAREFULLY ADJUSTED DOSAGE BY OR UNDER THE SUPERVISION OF EXPERIENCED CLINICIANS WHO ARE FAMILIAR WITH ITS ACTIONS AND THE POSSIBLE COMPLICATIONS THAT MIGHT OCCUR FOLLOWING ITS USE. THE DRUG SHOULD NOT BE ADMINISTERED UNLESS FACILITIES FOR INTUBATION, ARTIFICIAL RESPIRATION, OXYGEN THERAPY, AND REVERSAL AGENTS ARE IMMEDIATELY AVAILABLE, THE CLINICIAN MUST BE PREPARED TO ASSIST OR CONTROL RESPIRATION. In patients who are known to have myasthemia gravis or the myasthenic (Eaton-Lambert) syndrome, small doses of Norcuron® may have profound effects. In such patients, a peripheral nerve stimulator and use of a small test dose may be of value in monitoring the response to administration of muscle relaxants.

PRECAUTIONS

General: Limited data on histamine assay and available clinical experience indicate that hypersensitivity reactions such as bronchospasm, flushing, redness, hypotension, tachycardia, and other reactions commonly associated with histamine release are unlikely to occur.

Renal Failure: Norcuron® is well tolerated without clinically significant prolongation of neuromuscular blocking effect in patients with renal failure who have been optimally prepared for surgery by dialysis. Under emergency conditions in anephric patients some prolongation of neuromuscular blockade may occur; herefore, if anephric patients cannot be prepared for non-elective surgery, a lower initial dose of Norcuron® should be considered.

Altered Circulation Time: Conditions associated with slower circulation time in cardiovascular disease, old age, edematous states resulting in increased volume of distribution may contribute to a delay in onset time, therefore dosage should not be increased.

Hepatic Disease: Limited experience in patients with cirrhosis or cholestasis has revealed prolonged recovery time in keeping with the role the liver plays in Norcuron® metabolism and excretion (see **Pharmacokinetics**). Data currently available do not permit dosage recommendations in patients with impaired liver function.

Long-term Use in I.C.U.: In the intensive care unit, in rare cases, long-term use of neuromuscular blocking drugs to facilitate mechanical ventilation may be associated with prolonged paralysis and/or skeletal muscle weakness, that may be first noted during attempts to wean such patients from the ventilator. Typically, such patients receive other drugs such as broad spectrum antibiotics, narcotics and/or steroids and may have electrolyte imbalance and diseases which lead to electrolyte imbalance, hypoxic episodes of varying duration, acid-base imbalance and extreme debilitation, any of which may enhance the actions of a neuromuscular blocking agent. Additionally, patients immobilized for extended periods frequently develop symptoms consistent with disuse muscle atrophy. Therefore, when there is a need for long-term mechanical ventilation, the benefits-to-risk ratio of neuromuscular blockade must be considered.

Continuous infusion or intermittent bolus dosing to support mechanical ventilation, has not been studied sufficiently to support dosage recommendations.

UNDER THE ABOVE CONDITIONS, APPROPRIATE MONITORING, SUCH AS USE OF A PERIPHERAL NERVE STIMULATOR, TO ASSESS THE DEGREE OF NEUROMUSCULAR BLOCKADE, MAY PRECLUDE INADVERTENT EXCESS DOSING.

Severe Obesity or Neuromuscular Disease: Patients with severe obesity or neuromuscular disease may pose airway and/or ventilatory problems requiring special care before, during and after the use of neuromuscular blocking agents such as Norcuron®.

Malignant Hyperthermia: Many drugs used in anesthetic practice are suspected of being capable of triggering a potentially fatal hypermetabolism of skeletal muscle known as malignant hyperthermia. There are insufficient data derived from screening in susceptible animals (swine) to establish whether or not Norcuron® is capable of triggering malignant hyperthermia.

C.N.S.: Norcuron® has no known effect on consciousness, the pain threshold or cerebration. Administration must be accompanied by adequate anesthesia or sedation.

Drug Interactions: Prior administration of succinylcholine may enhance the neuromuscular blocking effect of Norcuron® (vecuronium bromide) for injection and its duration of action. If succinylcholine is used before Norcuron®, the administration of Norcuron® should be delayed until the succinylcholine effect shows signs of wearing off. With succinylcholine as the intubating agent, initial doses of 0.04–0.06 mg/kg of Norcuron® may be administered to produce complete neuromuscular block with clinical duration of action of 25–30 minutes (see **CLINICAL PHARMACOLOGY**). The use of Norcuron® before succinylcholine, in order to attenuate some of the side effects of succinylcholine, has not been sufficiently studied.

Other nondepolarizing neuromusclar blocking agents (pancuronium, d-tubocurarine, metocurine, and gallamine) act in the same fashion as does Norcuron®, therefore these drugs and Norcuron® may manifest an additive effect when used together. There are insufficient data to support concomitant use of Norcuron® and other competitive muscle relaxants in the same patient.

Inhalational Anesthetics: Use of volatile inhalational anesthetics such as enflurane, isoflurane, and halothane with Norcuron® will enhance neuromuscular blockade. Potentiation is most prominent with use of enflurane and isoflurane. With the above agents the initial dose of Norcuron® may be the same as with balanced anesthesia unless the inhalational anesthetic has been administered for a sufficient time at a sufficient dose to have reached clinical equilibrium (see **CLINICAL PHARMACOLOGY**).

Antibiotics: Parenteral/intraperitoneal administration of high doses of certain antibiotics may intensify or produce neuromuscular block on their own. The following antibiotics have been associated with various degrees of paralysis: aminoglycosides (such as neomycin, streptomycin, kanamycin, gentamicin, and dihydrostreptomycin); tetracyclines; bacitracin; polymyxin B; colistin; and sodium colistimethate. If these or other newly introduced antibiotics are used in conjunction with Norcuron®, unexpected prolongation of neuromuscular block should be considered a possibility.

Other: Experience concerning injection of quinidine during recovery from use of other muscle relaxants suggests that recurrent paralysis may occur. This possibility must also be considered for Norcuron®. Norcuron® induced neuromuscular blockade has been counteracted by alkalosis and enhanced by acidosis in experimental animals (cat). Electrolyte imbalance and diseases which lead to electrolyte imbalance, such as adrenal cortical insufficiency, have been shown to alter neuromuscular blockade. Depending on the nature of the imbalance, either enhancement or inhibition may be expected. Magnesium salts, administered for the management of toxemia of pregnancy, may enhance the neuromuscular blockade.

Drug/laboratory test interactions: None known

Carcinogenesis, Mutagensis, Impairment of Fertility: Long-term studies in animals have not been performed to evaluate carcinogenic or mutagenic potential or impairment of fertility.

Pregnancy: Pregnancy Category C: Animal reproduction studies have not been conducted with Norcuron®. It is also not known whether Norcuron® can cause fetal harm when administered to a pregnant woman or can affect reproduction capacity. Norcuron® should be given to a pregnant woman only if clearly needed.

Pediatric Use: Infants under 1 year of age but older than 7 weeks, also tested under halothane anesthesia, are moderately more sensitive to Norcuron® on a mg/kg basis than adults and take about 1½ times as long to recover. Information presently available does not permit recommendations for usage in neonates.

ADVERSE REACTIONS

Norcuron® was well tolerated and produced no adverse reactions during extensive clinical trials. The most frequent adverse reaction to nondepolarizing blocking agents as a class consists of an extension of the drug's pharmacological action beyond the time period needed. This may vary from skeletal muscle weakness to profound and prolonged skeletal muscle paralysis resulting in respiration insufficiency or apnea.

Inadequate reversal of the neuromuscular blockade is possible with Norcuron® as with all curariform drugs. These adverse reactions are managed by manual or mechanical ventilation until recovery is judged adequate. Little or no increase in intensity of blockade or duration of action of Norcuron® is noted from the use of thiobarbiturates, narcotic analgesics, nitrous oxide, or droperidol. See **OVERDOSAGE** for discussion of other drugs used in anesthetic practice which also cause respiratory depression.

Prolonged paralysis and/or skeletal muscle weakness have been reported after long-term use to support mechanical ventilation in the intensive care unit. (see **PRECAUTIONS**).

Bronchospasm, flushing, redness, hypotension and tachycardia have been reported in very rare instances.

OVERDOSAGE

The possibility of iatrogenic overdosage can be minimized by carefully monitoring muscle twitch response to peripheral nerve stimulation.

Excessive doses of Norcuron® produced enhanced pharmacological effects. Residual neuromuscular blockade beyond the time period needed may occur with Norcuron® as with other neuromuscular blockers. This may be manifested by skeletal muscle weakness, decreased respiratory reserve, low tidal volume, or apnea. A peripheral nerve stimulator may be used to assess the degree of residual neuromuscular blockade from other causes of decreased respiratory reserve. Respiratory depression may be due either wholly or in part to other drugs used during the conduct of general anesthesia such as narcotics, thiobarbiturates and other central nervous system depressants. Under such circumstances the primary treatment is maintenance of a patent airway and manual or mechanical ventilation until complete recovery of normal respiration is assured. Regonol® (pyridostigmine bromide) injection, neostigmine, or edrophonium, in conjunction with atropine or glycopyrrolate will usually antagonize the skeletal muscle relaxant action of Norcuron®. Satisfactory reversal can be judged by adequacy of skeletal muscle tone and by adequacy of respiration. A peripheral nerve stimulator may also be used to monitor restoration of twitch height. Failure of prompt reversal (within 30 minutes) may occur in the presence of extreme debilitation, carcinomatosis, and with concomitant use of certain broad spectrum antibiotics, or anesthetic agents and other drugs which enhance neuromuscular blockade or cause respiratory depression of their own. Under such circumstances the management is the same as that of prolonged neuromuscular blockade. Ventilation must be supported by artificial means until the patient has resumed control of his respiration. Prior to the use of reversal agents, reference should be made to the specific package insert of the reversal agent.

DOSAGE AND ADMINISTRATION

Norcuron® (vecuronium bromide) for injection is for intravenous use only. This drug should be administered by or under the supervision of experienced clinicians familar with the use of neuromuscular blocking agents. Dosage must be individualized in each case. The dosage information which follows is derived from studies based upon units of drug per unit of body weight and is intended to serve as a guide only, especially regarding enhancement of neuromuscular blockade of Norcuron® by volatile anesthetics and by prior use of succinylcholine (see **PRECAUTIONS/Drug Interactions**). Parenteral drug products should be inspected visually for particulate matter and discoloration prior to administration whenever solution and container permit.

To obtain maximum clinical benefits of Norcuron® and to minimize the possibility of overdosage, the monitoring of muscle twitch response to peripheral nerve stimulation is advised.

The recommended initial dose of Norcuron® is 0.08 to 0.10 mg/kg (1.4 to 1.75 times the ED_{90}) given as an intravenous bolus injection. This dose can be expected to produce good or excellent non-emergency intubation conditions in 2.5 to 3 minutes after injection. Under balanced anesthesia, clinically required neuromuscular blockade lasts approximately 25–30 minutes with recovery to 25% of control achieved approximately 25 to 40 minutes after injection and recovery to 95% of control achieved approximately 45–65 minutes after injection. In the presence of potent inhalation anesthetics, the neuromuscular blocking effect of Norcuron® is enhanced. If Norcuron® is first administered more than 5 minutes after the start of inhalation agent or when steady state has been achieved, the initial Norcuron® dose may be reduced by approximately 15%, i.e., 0.060 to 0.085 mg/kg.

Prior administration of succinylcholine may enhance the neuromuscular blocking effect and duration of action of Norcuron®. If intubation is performed using succinylcholine, a reduction of initial dose of Norcuron® to 0.04–0.06 mg/kg with inhalation anesthesia and 0.05–0.06 mg/kg with balanced anesthesia may be required.

During prolonged surgical procedures, maintenance doses of 0.010 to 0.015 mg/kg of Norcuron® are recommended; after the initial Norcuron® injection, the first maintenance dose will generally be required within 25 to 40 minutes. However, clinical criteria should be used to determine the need for maintenance doses. Since Norcuron® lacks clinically important cumulative effects, subsequent maintenance doses, if required, may be administered at relatively regular intervals for each patient, ranging approximately from 12 to 15 minutes under balanced anesthesia, slightly longer under inhalation agents. (If less frequent administration is desired, higher maintenance doses may be administered.)

Should there be reason for the selection of larger doses in individual patients, initial doses ranging from 0.15 mg/kg up to 0.28 mg/kg have been administered during surgery under halothane anesthesia without ill effects to the cardiovascular system being noted as long as ventilation is properly maintained (see **CLINICAL PHARMACOLOGY**).

Use by Continuous Infusion: After an intubating dose of 80–100 µg/kg, a continuous infusion of 1 µg/kg/min can be initiated approximately 20–40 min later. Infusion of Norcuron® should be initiated only after early evidence of spontaneous recovery from the bolus dose. Long-term intravenous infusion to support mechanical ventilation in the intensive care unit has not been studied sufficiently to support dosage recommendations. (see **PRECAUTIONS**)

The infusion of Norcuron® should be individualized for each patient. The rate of administration should be adjusted according to the patient's twitch response as determined by peripheral nerve stimulation. An initial rate of 1 µg/kg/min is recommended, with the rate of the infusion adjusted thereafter to maintain a 90% suppression of twitch response. Average infusion rates may range from 0.8 to 1.2 µg/kg/min. Inhalation anesthetics, particularly enflurane and isoflurane may enhance the neuromuscular blocking action of nondepolarizing muscle relaxants. In the presence of steady-state concentrations of enflurane or isoflurane, it may be necessary to reduce the rate of infusion 25–60 percent, 45–60 min after the intubating dose. Under halothane anesthesia it may not be necessary to reduce the rate of infusion.

Spontaneous recovery and reversal of neuromuscular blockade following discontinuation of Norcuron® infusion may be expected to proceed at rates comparable to that following a single bolus dose (see **CLINICAL PHARMACOLOGY**). Infusion solutions of Norcuron® can be prepared by mixing Norcuron® with an appropriate infusion solution such as 5% glucose in water, 0.9% NaCl, 5% glucose in saline, or Lactated Ringers. Unused portions of infusion solutions should be discarded.

Infusion rates of Norcuron® can be individualized for each patient using the following table:

Drug Delivery Rate	Infusion Delivery Rate	
(µg/kg/min)	(mL/kg/min)	
	0.1 mg/mL*	0.2 mg/mL†
0.7	0.007	0.0035
0.8	0.008	0.0040
0.9	0.009	0.0045
1.0	0.010	0.0050
1.1	0.011	0.0055
1.2	0.012	0.0060
1.3	0.013	0.0065

* 10 mg of Norcuron® in 100 mL solution
† 20 mg of Norcuron® in 100 mL solution

The following table is a guideline for mL/min delivery for a solution of 0.1 mg/mL (10 mg in 100 mL) with an infusion pump.

NORCURON® INFUSION RATE —mL/MIN

Amount of Drug µg/kg/min	Patient Weight—kg						
	40	50	60	70	80	90	100
0.7	0.28	0.35	0.42	0.49	0.56	0.63	0.70
0.8	0.32	0.40	0.48	0.56	0.64	0.72	0.80
0.9	0.36	0.45	0.54	0.63	0.72	0.81	0.90
1.0	0.40	0.50	0.60	0.70	0.80	0.90	1.00
1.1	0.44	0.55	0.66	0.77	0.88	0.99	1.10
1.2	0.48	0.60	0.72	0.84	0.96	1.08	1.20
1.3	0.52	0.65	0.78	0.91	1.04	1.17	1.30

NOTE: If a concentration of 0.2 mg/mL is used (20 mg in 100 mL), the rate should be decreased by one-half.

Dosage in Children: Older children (10 to 17 years of age) have approximately the same dosage requirements (mg/kg) as adults and may be managed the same way. Younger children (1 to 10 years of age) may require a slightly higher initial dose and may also require supplementation slightly more often than adults. Infants under one year of age but older than 7 weeks are moderately more sensitive to Norcuron® on a mg/kg basis than adults and take about 1½ times as long to recover. See also subsection of **PRECAUTIONS** titled **Pediatric Use.** Information presently available does not permit recommendation on usage in neonates (see **PRECAUTIONS**). There are insufficient data concerning continuous infusion of vecuronium in children, therefore, no dosing recommendation can be made.

COMPATIBILITY

Norcuron® is compatible in solution with:
0.9% NaCl solution
5% glucose in water
Sterile water for injection
5% glucose in saline
Lactated Ringers
Use within 24 hours of mixing with the above solutions. Parenteral drug products should be inspected visually for particulate matter and discoloration prior to administration whenever solution and container permit.

HOW SUPPLIED

10 mL vials (10 mg of vecuronium bromide) and 10 mL prefilled syringes of diluent (bacteriostatic water for injection, USP). 22g 1¼" needle.

Boxes of 10	NDC No. 0052-0441-60

10 mL vials (10 mg vecuronium bromide) and 10 mL vials of diluent (bacteriostatic water for injection, USP).

Boxes of 10	NDC No. 0052-0441-17

10 mL vials (10 mg vecuronium bromide) only; DILUENT NOT SUPPLIED.

Boxes of 10	NDC No. 0052-0441-15

STORAGE

15–30°C (59–86°F). Protect from light.

AFTER RECONSTITUTION

- When reconstituted with supplied bacteriostatic water for injection: CONTAINS BENZYL ALCOHOL, WHICH IS NOT INTENDED FOR USE IN NEWBORNS. Use within 5 days. May be stored at room temperature or refrigerated.
- When reconstituted with sterile water for injection or other compatible I.V. solutions: Refrigerate vial. Use within 24 hours. Single use only. Discard unused portion.

Manufactured for ORGANON INC.
By BEN VENUE LABORATORIES, INC.
BEDFORD OHIO 44146
or by
ORGANON INC.
WEST ORANGE, NEW JERSEY 07052
PTD. IN USA-440,441   5310117 REVISED 3/89

PAVULON®   ℞
[pāv-u-lon]
(pancuronium bromide) injection

HOW SUPPLIED

2 mL ampuls—2 mg/mL—boxes of 25
5 mL ampuls—2 mg/mL—boxes of 25
10 mL vials—1 mg/mL—boxes of 25

PREGNYL®   ℞
(chorionic gonadotropin for injection, U.S.P.)

DESCRIPTION

Human chorionic gonadotropin (HCG), a polypeptide hormone produced by the human placenta, is composed of an alpha and a beta sub-unit. The alpha sub-unit is essentially identical to the alpha sub-units of the human pituitary gonadotropins, luteinizing hormone (LH) and follicle-stimulating hormone (FSH), as well as to the alpha sub-unit of human thyroid-stimulating hormone (TSH). The beta sub-units of these hormones differ in amino acid sequence.

PREGNYL® (chorionic gonadotropin for injection, USP) is a highly purified pyrogen free preparation obtained from the urine of pregnant females. It is standardized by a biological assay procedure. It is available for intramuscular injection in multiple dose vials containing 10,000 USP units of sterile dried powder with 5 mg. monobasic sodium phosphate and 4.4 mg. dibasic sodium phosphate. If required, pH is adjusted with sodium hydroxide and/or phosphoric acid. Each package also contains a 10 mL vial of solvent (water for injection with 0.56% sodium chloride and 0.9% benzyl alcohol). If required, pH is adjusted with sodium hydroxide and/or hydrochloric acid.

CLINICAL PHARMACOLOGY

The action of HCG is virtually identical to that of pituitary LH although HCG appears to have a small degree of FSH activity as well. It stimulates production of gonadal steroid hormones by stimulating the interstitial cells, (Leydig cells) of the testis to produce androgens and the corpus luteum of the ovary to produce progesterone.

Androgen stimulation in the male leads to the development of secondary sex characteristics and may stimulate testicular descent when no anatomical impediment to descent is present. This descent is usually reversible when HCG is discontinued. During the normal menstrual cycle, LH participates with FSH in the development and maturation of the normal ovarian follicle and the mid-cycle LH surge triggers ovulation. HCG can substitute for LH in this function.

During a normal pregnancy, HCG secreted by the placenta maintains the corpus luteum after LH secretion decreases, supporting continued secretion of estrogen and progesterone and preventing menstruation. HCG HAS NO KNOWN EFFECT ON FAT MOBILIZATION, APPETITE OR SENSE OF HUNGER, OR BODY FAT DISTRIBUTION.

INDICATIONS

HCG HAS NOT BEEN DEMONSTRATED TO BE EFFECTIVE ADJUNCTIVE THERAPY IN THE TREATMENT OF OBESITY. THERE IS NO SUBSTANTIAL EVIDENCE THAT IT INCREASES WEIGHT LOSS BEYOND THAT RESULTING FROM CALORIC RESTRICTION, THAT IT CAUSES A MORE ATTRACTIVE OR "NORMAL" DISTRIBUTION OF FAT, OR THAT IT DECREASES THE HUNGER AND DISCOMFORT ASSOCIATED WITH CALORIE-RESTRICTED DIETS.

1. Prepubertal cryptorchidism not due to anatomical obstruction. In general, HCG is thought to induce testicular descent in situations when descent would have occurred at puberty. HCG thus may help predict whether or not orchiopexy will be needed in the future. Although, in some cases, descent following HCG administration is permanent, in most cases, the response is temporary. Therapy is usually instituted between the ages 4 and 9.
2. Selected cases of hypogonadotropic hypogonadism (hypogonadism secondary to a pituitary deficiency) in males.
3. Induction of ovulation and pregnancy in the anovulatory, infertile woman in whom the cause of anovulation is secondary and not due to primary ovarian failure and who has been appropriately pretreated with human menotropins.

CONTRAINDICATIONS

Precocious puberty, prostatic carcinoma or other androgen-dependent neoplasm, prior allergic reaction to HCG.

Continued on next page

Organon—Cont.

WARNINGS

HCG should be used in conjunction with human menopausal gonadotropins only by physicians experienced with infertility problems who are familiar with the criteria for patient selection, contraindications, warnings, precautions and adverse reactions described in the package insert for menotropins.

The principal serious adverse reactions during this use are: (1) Ovarian hyperstimulation, a syndrome of sudden ovarian enlargement, ascites with or without pain, and/or pleural effusion, (2) Rupture of ovarian cysts with resultant hemoperitoneum, (3) Multiple births, and (4) Arterial thromboembolism.

PRECAUTIONS

1. Induction of androgen secretion by HCG may induce precocious puberty in patients treated for cryptorchidism. Therapy should be discontinued if signs of precocious puberty occur.
2. Since androgens may cause fluid retention, HCG should be used with caution in patients with cardiac or renal disease, epilepsy, migraine, or asthma.

ADVERSE REACTIONS

Headache, irritability, restlessness, depression, fatigue, edema, precocious puberty, gynecomastia, pain at the site of injection.

DOSAGE AND ADMINISTRATION

(Intramuscular Use Only): The dosage regimen employed in any particular case will depend upon the indication for use, the age and weight of the patient, and the physician's preference. The following regimens have been advocated by various authorities:

Prepubertal cryptorchidism not due to anatomical obstruction.
1. 4,000 U.S.P. Units three times weekly for three weeks.
2. 5,000 U.S.P. Units every second day for four injections.
3. 15 injections of 500 to 1,000 U.S.P. Units over a period of six weeks.
4. 500 U.S.P. Units three times weekly for four to six weeks. If this course of treatment is not successful, another series is begun one month later, giving 1,000 U.S.P. Units per injection.

Selected cases of hypogonadotropic hypogonadism in males.
1. 500 to 1,000 U.S.P. Units three times a week for three weeks, followed by the same dose twice a week for three weeks.
2. 4,000 U.S.P. Units three times weekly for six to nine months, following which the dosage may be reduced to 2,000 U.S.P. Units three times weekly for an additional three months.

Induction of ovulation and pregnancy in the anovulatory, infertile woman in whom the cause of anovulation is secondary and not due to primary ovarian failure and who has been appropriately pre-treated with human menotropins. (See prescribing information for menotropins for dosage and administration for that drug product). 5,000 to 10,000 U.S.P. Units one day following the last dose of menotropins. (A dosage of 10,000 U.S.P. Units is recommended in the labeling for menotropins).

IMPORTANT: USE COMPLETELY AFTER RECONSTITUTION. RECONSTITUTED SOLUTION IS STABLE FOR 90 DAYS WHEN REFRIGERATED.

HOW SUPPLIED

Two-vial package containing:

1–10 mL lyophilized multiple dose vial containing:
10,000 USP Units chorionic gonadotropin per vial (NDC 0052-0315-10)

1–10 mL vial of solvent containing:
water for injection with 0.56% sodium chloride and 0.9% benzyl alcohol (NDC 0052-0325-10.)

When reconstituted, each 10 mL vial contains:

Chorionic gonadotropin	10,000 USP Units
Monobasic sodium phosphate	5 mg.
Dibasic sodium phosphate	4.4 mg.
Sodium chloride	0.56%
Benzyl alcohol	0.9%

If required pH adjusted with sodium hydroxide and/or phosphoric acid.

CAUTION

Federal law prohibits dispensing without prescription.

STORAGE

Store at 15°–30°C (59°–86°F) Reconstituted material will remain stable for 90 days when refrigerated.

DIRECTIONS FOR RECONSTITUTION

Two vial package: Withdraw sterile air from lyophilized vial and inject into diluent vial. Remove 1–10 mL from diluent and add to lyophilized vial; agitate gently until powder is completely dissolved in solution.

Parenteral drug products should be inspected visually for particulate matter and discoloration prior to administration, whenever solution and container permit.

Revised 4/88

REGONOL®   ℞
[re-gō-nol]
(pyridostigmine bromide) injection, USP

HOW SUPPLIED

5 mg/mL: 2 mL ampuls—boxes of 25—NDC-0052-0460-02
5 mL vials—boxes of 25—NDC-0052-0460-05

REVERSOL®   ℞
(edrophonium chloride injection, USP)

HOW SUPPLIED

10 mL multidose vials-boxes of 25, NDC 0052-0466-34.

SUCCINYLCHOLINE CHLORIDE INJECTION   ℞
USP

HOW SUPPLIED

20 mg/mL–10 mL vials, boxes of 25.

WIGRAINE®   ℞

DESCRIPTION

Wigraine® Tablet: Each tablet contains the following:

Ergotamine Tartrate, USP	1 mg
Caffeine, USP	100 mg

Each tablet also contains: Lactose, Magnesium Stearate, Microcrystalline Cellulose, Purified Water and Starch as inactive ingredients.

Wigraine® tablets are uncoated and prepared to insure rapid disintegration (by an exclusive manufacturing process) and facilitate quick absorption. Rapid onset of effect is important for the satisfactory treatment of acute attacks of vascular headaches.

Wigraine® Suppository: Each suppository contains the following:

Ergotamine tartrate, USP	2 mg
Caffeine, USP	100 mg
Tartaric Acid	21.5 mg

Wigraine® suppositories contain the active ingredients in a synthetic cocoa butter base which melts rapidly at room temperature.

CLINICAL PHARMACOLOGY

Ergotamine is an alpha adrenergic blocking agent with a direct stimulating effect on the smooth muscle of peripheral and cranial blood vessels and produces depression of central vasomotor centers. The compound also has the properties of serotonin antagonism. In comparison to hydrogenated ergotamine, the adrenergic blocking actions are less pronounced and vasoconstrictive actions are greater. Caffeine, also a cranial vasoconstrictor is added to further enhance the vasoconstrictive effect without the necessity of increasing ergotamine dosage.

INDICATIONS AND USAGE

Wigraine® is indicated as therapy to abort or prevent vascular headaches such as migraine, migraine variants, or so-called histamine cephalalgia.

CONTRAINDICATIONS

Wigraine® can cause fetal harm when administered to a pregnant women. It can produce prolonged uterine contractions which can result in abortion. Wigraine® is contraindicated in women who are or may become pregnant. If this is used during pregnancy, or if the patient becomes pregnant while taking this drug, the patient should be advised of the potential hazard to the fetus.

Peripheral vascular disease, coronary heart disease, hypertension, impaired hepatic or renal function, sepsis, and hypersensitivity to any of the components.

PRECAUTIONS

Although signs and symptoms of ergotism rarely develop even after long term intermittent use of the orally or rectally administered drugs, care should be exercised to remain within the limits of recommended dosage.

Pregnancy Category X. See Contraindications section.

Nursing Mothers. It is not known whether the ergotamine tartrate in Wigraine® is excreted in human milk. Because some ergot alkoids have been found in the milk of nursing mothers resulting in symptoms of ergotism in their children, a decision should be made whether to discontinue nursing or to discontinue the drug, taking into account the importance of the drug to the mother.

Pediatric Usage. Safety and effectiveness in children have not been established.

ADVERSE REACTIONS

In order of decreasing severity: precordial distress and pain, muscle pains in the extremities, numbness and tingling in fingers and toes, transient tachycardia or bradycardia, vomiting, nausea, weakness in the legs, diarrhea, localized edema and itching.

DOSAGE AND ADMINISTRATION

Best results are obtained if the tablets or suppositories are administered at the first sign of an attack. Wigraine® tablet: the average adult dose is 2 tablets at the start of a vascular headache (migraine) attack; followed by 1 additional tablet every ½ hour if needed, up to 6 tablets per attack. Total weekly dosage should not exceed 10 tablets. Wigraine® suppository: the maximum adult dose is 2 suppositories for an individual attack. In carefully selected patients, with due consideration of maximum dosage recommendations, administration of the drug at bedtime may be an appropriate short-term preventive measure.

OVERDOSAGE

The toxic effects of an acute overdosage of Wigraine® are due primarily to the ergotamine component. The amount of caffeine is such that its toxic effects will be overshadowed by those of ergotamine. Symptoms include vomiting, numbness, tingling, pain and cyanosis of the extremities associated with diminished or absent peripheral pulses, hypertension or hypotension, drowsiness, stupor, coma, convulsions and shock. Treatment consists of removal of the offending drug by induction of emesis, gastric lavage and catharsis. Maintenance of adequate pulmonary ventilation, correction of hypotension, and control of convulsions are important considerations. Treatment of peripheral vasospasm should consist of warmth, but not heat, and protection of the ischemic limbs. Vasodilators may be used with benefit but caution must be exercised to avoid aggravating an already existing hypotension. The LD50 limits of the various components as outlined in NIOSH 1978 Registry of Toxic Effects of Chemical Substances, published by U.S. Department of Health, Education and Welfare are as follows: Ergotamine Tartrate IV LD50 in rats = 80mg/Kg, Caffeine IV LD50 in rats = 105mg/Kg.

HOW SUPPLIED

Wigraine® tablets are white tablets embossed with "ORGANON 542" on one side. They are individually foil stripped and packaged in boxes of 20's NDC #0052-0542-20 and 100's NDC #0052-0542-91. Wigraine® suppositories are individualIy foil wrapped and packaged in boxes of 12. NDC #0052-0548-12.

STORAGE

Wigraine® tablets should be stored at a maximum of 30°C (86°F) and the suppositories should be refrigerated at 2°-8°C (36°-46°F).

CAUTION

Federal law prohibits dispensing without prescription.
Shown in Product Identification Section, page 420
ISSUED 4/87

ZYMASE™   ℞
(pancrelipase, USP)
enteric coated spheres

DESCRIPTION

Zymase capsules contain enteric coated spheres of pancrelipase, a substance containing enzymes, principally lipase, with amylase and protease obtained from the pancreas of the hog. Each capsule contains not less than:

Lipase—12,000 USP Units
Protease—24,000 USP Units
Amylase—24,000 USP Units

Each capsule also contains: Gelatin, purified water, starch, talc, titanium dioxide, FD&C Green #3, FD&C Yellow #10, and other inactive ingredients.

CLINICAL PHARMACOLOGY

Zymase is protected against inactivation by gastric acidity, and active enzymes are released in the duodenum. The enzymes promote hydrolysis of fats into glycerol and fatty acids, protein into proteases and derived substances, and starch into dextrans and sugars.

INDICATIONS AND USAGE

Zymase is indicated in conditions where pancreatic enzymes are either absent or deficient with resultant inadequate fat digestion. Such conditions include but are not limited to chronic pancreatitis, pancreatectomy, cystic fibrosis and steatorrhea of diverse etiologies.

CONTRAINDICATIONS

Known hypersensitivity to pork protein.

PRECAUTIONS

To maintain enteric coating integrity, do not chew or crush spheres.

ADVERSE REACTIONS

No adverse reactions have been reported. It should be noted, however, that extremely high does of exogenous pancreatic enzymes have been associated with hyperuricosuria and hyperuricemia.

DOSAGE AND ADMINISTRATION

One to two capsules with each meal or snack. Individual cases may require higher dosage and dietary adjustment. Where swallowing of capsules is difficult, capsules may be opened and the spheres taken with liquids or soft foods which do not require chewing.

STORAGE

Not to exceed 25°C (77°F). Dry place when opened.

DISPENSE

In tight container as defined in the USP.

Shown in Product Identification Section, page 420

Organon Teknika Corporation
100 AKZO AVENUE
DURHAM, NC 27704

BCG VACCINE, USP   ℞
FOR PERCUTANEOUS USE
TICE™ BCG VACCINE

DESCRIPTION

BCG vaccine is a live culture preparation of the Bacillus Calmette-Guerin (BCG) strain of *Mycobacterium bovis* and is a substrain of the Pasteur Institute strain designed for use as an active immunizing agent against tuberculosis. The vaccine is a preservative-free, freeze-dried ampule for percutaneous application.

CLINICAL PHARMACOLOGY

BCG vaccine stimulates the reticuloendothelial system (RES) to produce activated cells, especially macrophages, that prevent the multiplication of virulent mycobacteria (1). Although antibodies against mycobacteria are also produced they are not active in establishing anti-tuberculosis immunity. Many clinical trials on the protective effect of BCG vaccine against tuberculosis have been published. Summaries of the most recent works are available (2,3).

INDICATIONS AND USAGE

BCG vaccine is indicated for tuberculin negative persons who are exposed to risks of tuberculosis infection. Clinical evidence (4) has demonstrated a large reduction in the incidence of tuberculosis in vaccinated persons as compared to unvaccinated controls. The American Academy of Pediatrics, Committee on the Control of Infectious Diseases (5) advises BCG vaccine for children who live in, or plan to travel in, areas where tuberculosis is prevalent or are in situations where there is likelihood of exposure to adults with active or recently arrested pulmonary or renal tuberculosis (i.e., arrested less than five years). It is also recommended in population groups in which there is a high incidence of tuberculosis infection, and for children of tuberculous mothers (6,7,8). Health workers exposed to repeated or increased risks and others working in institutions serving populations having relatively high endemic prevalence of tuberculosis should be considered for vaccination. BCG vaccine should not be used as a substitute for established programs of control, case-finding measures, and proper treatment, but should be used to complement these measures.

CONTRAINDICATIONS

BCG vaccine for the prevention of tuberculosis should not ordinarily be given to persons with impaired immune responses, whether they be congenital, disease produced, drug or therapy induced (i.e. cytotoxic drugs and radiation used in cancer therapy). The concurrent use of steroid drugs requires caution because of the possibility of the vaccine establishing a systemic infection. If necessary the infection can be halted by use of anti-tuberculosis drugs (9).

WARNINGS

BCG Vaccine should not be used in infants, children or adults with severe immune deficiency syndromes. Children with family history of immune deficiency disease should not be vaccinated; if they are, then full anti-tuberculosis chemotherapy should be given. A recent case was treated with transfer factor (4, 10).

PRECAUTIONS

General Information:
DO NOT INJECT INTRAVENOUSLY OR SUBCUTANEOUSLY OR INTRADERMALLY.
1) Normal Reaction: The intensity and duration of the local reaction depends on the depth of penetration of the multiple-puncture disc and individual variations in patients' tissue reactions. The initial skin lesions usually appear within 10–14 days and consist of small red papules at the site. The

papules reach maximum diameter (about 3mm) after 4 to 6 weeks, after which they may scale and then slowly subside. Six months afterwards there is usually no visible sign of the vaccination, but on occasion a faintly discernible pattern of the disc points may be visible. On people whose skin tends to keloid formation, there may be slightly more visible evidence of the vaccination.

Vaccination is recommended only for those tuberculin negative to a recent skin test to 5TU. Otherwise, vaccination of persons highly sensitive to mycobacterial antigens can result in hypersensitivity reactions including fever, anorexia, myalgia, and neuralgia, which lasts a few days.

After BCG vaccination, it is usually not possible to clearly distinguish between a tuberculin reaction caused by persistent postvaccination sensitivity and one caused by virulent suprainfection. Caution is advised in attributing a positive skin test to BCG vaccination. A sharp rise in the tuberculin reaction since the latest test should be further investigated (except in the immediate postvaccination period).

2) Information for Patients: Keep vaccinated person away from people with active tuberculosis for six to twelve weeks after vaccination to allow the protection to develop fully. Keep the vaccination site clean until the local reaction has disappeared.

3) Drug Interaction: Immune suppressive drugs may interfere with the development of the immune response and should be used only with medical supervision.

4) Pregnancy: Although no harmful effects of BCG on the fetus have been observed (11), it is prudent to avoid vaccination during pregnancy unless there is an immediate excessive risk of unavoidable exposure to infective tuberculosis.

5) Adverse Reactions: Vaccination with the percutaneous concentration of BCG vaccine has eliminated the major portion of the few untoward side effects seen after intradermal methods of vaccination. Occasionally, lymphadenopathy of the regional lymph node, that spontaneously resolves itself, is seen in young children. Only rarely does the node create a fistula followed by a short period of drainage. The usual treatment is to maintain cleanliness of the site of drainage and allow the lesion to heal spontaneously without medical intervention.

Other rare events are osteomyelitis, lupoid reactions, disseminated BCG infection, and death. Osteomyelitis has been reported to occur in 1 per 1,000,000 vaccinees. Disseminated BCG infection and death are very rare (1 per 10,000,000 vaccinees) (12) and occur almost exclusively in children with impaired immune responses.

6) Overdosage: Accidental overdosages if treated immediately with anti-tuberculosis drugs show no complications (13). If the vaccination is allowed to progress it can still be treated successfully with anti-tuberculosis drugs but complications can include regional adenitis, lupus vulgaris, subcutaneous cold abscesses, ocular lesions, and others (14).

DOSAGE AND ADMINISTRATION

Preparing For Use: Using sterile methods, one cc of sterile water for injection (without preservative) is added to each ampule of vaccine. Draw mixture into syringe and expel into ampule 3 times to insure thorough mixing.

Parenteral drug products should be inspected visually for particulate matter and discoloration prior to administration, whenever solution and container permit. The vaccine is to be administered by a licensed medical practitioner after fully explaining the risks and benefits to the vaccinee, parent or guardian. After vaccine is prepared, the immunizing dose of 0.2–0.3 cc is dropped on the cleansed surface of the skin, and a percutaneous procedure using multiple-puncture disc applied through vaccine (5). After vaccination the vaccine should flow into the wounds and dry. No dressing is required, however, it is recommended that the site be kept dry for 24 hours.

Reconstituted vaccine should be kept refrigerated, protected from exposure to light and used within 8 hours. Vaccination should be repeated in those who remain tuberculin negative to 5 TU of tuberculin after 2–3 months. In infants less than one month old the dosage of vaccine should be reduced to one half, preferably by using 2 cc sterile water when reconstituting. If indications for vaccination persist, these children should receive a full dose after one year of age if they remain tuberculin negative to 5 TU on skin testing.

HOW SUPPLIED

BCG vaccine is supplied in 2 ml ampule. When reconstituted with one ml of diluent it will yield one ml of BCG vaccine at the original concentration. Vaccine is to be stored at 2°C to 8°C (36 to 46°F) and protected from light.

REFERENCES

1) Youmans, G.P.; *Tuberculosis,* W. B. Saunders Co., Philadelphia, Pa. 1979.
2) Rosenthal, Sol Roy; *BCG Vaccine: Tuberculosis-Cancer,* P.S.G. Publishing Co., Littleton, Mass. 1980.
3) Rosenthal, S.R. and R.G. Crispen, *BCG Vaccine,* University of Illinois, 1971.
4) Fourth Report, Medical Research Council: BCG Vaccine and Vole Bacillus Vaccines in the Prevention of Tuberculosis in Adolescence and Early Adult Life, *Bull WHO* 46:371, 1972.
5) Committee on the Control of Infectious Diseases, American Acadamy of Pediatrics, 17 edition, 1974.
6) Gellis, S. Sidney and B.M. Kagen; *Current Pediatric Therapy-5:* W.B. Saunders Co., Philadelphia, Pa., 1971.
7) Kempe, C.H., H.K. Silver and D. O'Brien: *Current Pediatric Diagnosis and Treatment,* 2nd edition.
8) Kendig, E.L.; The Place of BCG Vaccine in the Management of Infants Born of Tuberculous Mothers, *New England Journal of Medicine,* 281:520, 1969.
9) Crispen, R.G. and Y.S. Lee; Qualitative Measurement of Drug Effects on Mycobacteria, 16th Interscience Conference on Antimicrobial Agents and Chemotherapy, 1976.
10) Sharma, M.R., N. Foroozanfar and F.A. Ala; Progressive BCG Infection in an Immunodeficient Child Treated with Transfer Factor; *Clinical Immunology and Immunopathology,* 10:369, 1978.
11) Fourestier; M., G. Baissette, L. Bergerson, and E. Saint-Germain; BCG et grossesse, *Rev. Tuberc.* (Paris) 15, 278, 1951.
12) Mande, R.; *BCG Vaccination,* Dawsons, London, 1968.
13) Griffith, A.H.; Ten Cases of BCG Overdose Treated with Isoniazid; *Tubercle* 44:247, 1963.
14) Watkins, S.M.; Unusual Complication of BCG Vaccination, *British Medical Journal.* 1:442, 1971.

Manufactured by:
Organon Teknika Corporation
100 Akzo Avenue
Durham, NC 27704
U.S. License No. 956
Manufactured at Chicago, IL 60607
Distributed by: Organon, Inc.
West Orange, NJ 07052

Ortho Pharmaceutical Corporation
RARITAN, NJ 08869-0602

ACI–JEL® Therapeutic Vaginal Jelly   ℞

DESCRIPTION

ACI-JEL Vaginal Jelly is a bland, non-irritating, water-dispersible, buffered acid jelly for intravaginal use. ACI-JEL is classified as a Vaginal Therapeutic Jelly. ACI-JEL contains 0.921% glacial acetic acid ($C_2H_4O_2$), 0.025% oxyquinoline sulfate ($C_{18}H_{16}N_2O_6S$), 0.7% ricinoleic acid ($C_{18}H_{34}O_3$), and 5% glycerin ($C_3H_8O_3$) compounded with tragacanth, acacia, propylparaben, potassium hydroxide, stannous chloride, egg albumen, potassium bitartrate, perfume and purified water. ACI-JEL is formulated to pH 3.9–4.1.

CLINICAL PHARMACOLOGY

ACI-JEL acts to restore and maintain normal vaginal acidity through its buffer action.

INDICATIONS AND USAGE

ACI-JEL is indicated as adjunctive therapy in those cases where restoration and maintenance of vaginal acidity are desirable.

CONTRAINDICATIONS

None known.

WARNINGS

No serious adverse reactions or potential safety hazards have been reported with the use of ACI-JEL.

PRECAUTIONS

General: No special care is required for the safe and effective use of ACI-JEL. *Drug Interactions:* No incidence of drug interactions have been reported with concomitant use of ACI-JEL and any other medications. *Laboratory Tests:* The monitoring of vaginal acidity (pH) may be helpful in following the patient's response. (The normal vaginal pH has been shown to be in the range of 4.0 to 5.0.) *Carcinogenesis:* No long-term studies in animals have been performed to evaluate carcinogenic potential. *Pregnancy:* Pregnancy Category C. Animal reproduction studies have not been conducted with ACI-JEL. It is also not known whether ACI-JEL can cause fetal harm when administered to a pregnant woman or can affect reproduction capacity. ACI-JEL should be given to a pregnant woman only if clearly needed. *Nursing Mothers:* It is not known whether this drug is excreted in human milk. Because many drugs are excreted in human milk, caution should be exercised when ACI-JEL is administered to a nursing woman.

ADVERSE REACTIONS

Occasional cases of local stinging and burning have been reported.

Continued on next page

Ortho Pharm.—Cont.

DOSAGE AND ADMINISTRATION
The usual dose is one applicatorful, administered intravaginally, morning and evening. Duration of treatment may be determined by the patient's response to therapy.

HOW SUPPLIED
85g Tube with ORTHO® Measured-Dose Applicator.
NDC 0062-5421-01

CONCEPTROL™ Single Use Contraceptives

(See PDR For Nonprescription Drugs)

DELFEN® Contraceptive Foam

(See PDR For Nonprescription Drugs)

DIENESTROL Cream   ℞

(See ORTHO® Dienestrol Cream)

GYNOL II® Contraceptive Jelly

(See PDR For Nonprescription Drugs)

LIPPES LOOP™   ℞
Intrauterine Device

DESCRIPTION
The LIPPES LOOP is made of polyethylene in the shape of a double S. Four different sizes are manufactured to allow for the variability in the size of the uterus. (See below.) A fine, double thread or "tail" made of polyethylene suture (monofilament) is attached to the lower end to facilitate removal. In addition, palpation of the tail through the cervix by the patient, or visualization by the physician, can assist in determining whether or not an undetected expulsion has occurred. A LIPPES LOOP comes prepackaged and sterilized with an introducer, together with an insertion tube in a polyethylene pouch. The insertion tube is equipped with a flange to aid in gauging the depth to which the insertion tube should be inserted through the cervical canal and into the uterine cavity. The four available sizes are as follows:
Loop A—22.2 mm. Blue thread. For those women who cannot tolerate a larger size device.
Loop B—27.5 mm. WITH REDUCED RADII. Black thread. Suggested for women who have had premature pregnancy losses and multiparous females whose uteri sound out less than 6 cm.
Loop C—30 mm. WITH REDUCED RADII. Yellow thread. Suggested for use when Loop D is removed for bleeding or pain. The physician is advised to wait two to four weeks between removing a loop for bleeding and reinserting a second loop.
Loop D—30 mm. White thread. Suggested for use in women with one or more children.
Mode of Action or Principles of IUD Design:
The exact mechanism of action of the LIPPES LOOP is not known. However, it is believed to interfere in some manner with nidation in the endometrium, probably through foreign body reaction in the uterus.

INDICATIONS AND USAGE
LIPPES LOOP is indicated for contraception.

CONTRAINDICATIONS
IUD's should not be inserted when the following conditions exist:
1. Pregnancy or suspicion of pregnancy.
2. Abnormalities of the uterus resulting in distortion of the uterine cavity.
3. Pelvic inflammatory disease or a history of repeated pelvic inflammatory disease.
4. Postpartum endometritis or infected abortion in the past three months.
5. Known or suspected uterine or cervical malignancy including unresolved, abnormal "Pap" smear.
6. Genital bleeding of unknown etiology.
7. Cervicitis until infection is controlled.

WARNINGS
1. Pregnancy. a. Long-term effects. Long-term effects on the offspring when pregnancy occurs with LIPPES LOOP in place are unknown.
b. Septic abortion. Reports have indicated an increased incidence of septic abortion associated in some instances with septicemia, septic shock, and death in patients becoming pregnant with an IUD in place. Most of these reports have been associated with the mid-trimester of pregnancy. In some cases, the initial symptoms have been insidious and not easily recognized. If pregnancy should occur with an IUD in place, the IUD should be removed if the string is visible or, if removal proves to be or would be difficult, termination of the pregnancy should be considered and offered the patient as an option, bearing in mind that the risks associated with an elective abortion increase with gestational age.
c. Continuation of pregnancy. If the patient chooses to continue the pregnancy, she must be warned of the increased risk of spontaneous abortion and of the increased risk of sepsis, including death, if the pregnancy continues with the IUD in place. The patient must be closely observed and she must be advised to report all abnormal symptoms, such as flu-like syndrome, fever, abdominal cramping and pain, bleeding, or vaginal discharge, immediately because generalized symptoms of septicemia may be insidious.
2. Ectopic pregnancy. a. A pregnancy that occurs with an IUD in place is more likely to be ectopic than a pregnancy occurring without an IUD in place. Accordingly, patients who become pregnant while using the IUD should be carefully evaluated for the possibility of an ectopic pregnancy.
b. Special attention should be directed to patients with delayed menses, slight metrorrhagia and/or unilateral pelvic pain, and to those patients who wish to terminate a pregnancy because of IUD failure, to determine whether ectopic pregnancy has occurred.
3. Pelvic infection. An increased risk of pelvic infection has been reported with the IUD in place. Although the etiology of this risk is not understood, it has been suggested that the tail may act as a mechanism for the passage of vaginal bacteria into the uterus. This, at times, may result in the development of bilateral or unilateral tubo-ovarian abscesses or general peritonitis. Pelvic infection may lead to hospitalization or surgery and infertility. Appropriate aerobic and anaerobic bacteriological studies should be done and antibiotic therapy initiated. The IUD should be removed and the continuing treatment reassessed based upon the results of culture and sensitivity tests.
Because of the increased risk of pelvic infection, the physician may wish each woman who has an IUD in place to have a periodic cervical vaginal "Pap" smear and pelvic exam. All "Pap" smears should include specific evaluation for actinomycosis.
4. Effect on future fertility. An increased risk of tubal infertility, with or without prior symptoms of pelvic infection, has been associated with the use of IUD's, particularly inert IUD's, including the LIPPES LOOP. This risk appears to be greatest for nulliparous women and those exposed to multiple sexual partners. The decision to use an IUD must be made by the physician and patient with appropriate regard for the possibility of future infertility. This consideration is especially important for women, particularly nulliparous women, who may wish to have children at a later date.
5. Embedment. Partial penetration or lodging of the IUD in the endometrium can result in difficult removals.
6. Perforation. Partial or total perforation of the uterine wall or cervix may occur with the use of IUDs. The possibility of perforation must be kept in mind during insertion and at the time of any subsequent examination. If perforation occurs, the IUD should be removed. Adhesions, foreign body reactions, and intestinal obstruction may result if an IUD is left in the peritoneal cavity. There are a few reports that there has been migration after insertion apparently in the absence of perforation at insertion. In any event, it is possible for the IUD to perforate outside the uterus.

PRECAUTIONS
1. Patient counseling. Prior to insertion, the physician, nurse or other trained health professional must provide the patient with the Patient Brochure. The patient should be given the opportunity to read the brochure and discuss fully any questions she may have concerning the IUD as well as other methods of contraception.
2. Patient evaluation and clinical considerations. a. A complete medical history should be obtained to determine conditions that might influence the selection of an IUD. Physical examination should include a pelvic examination, "Pap" smear, gonorrhea culture and, if indicated, appropriate tests for other forms of venereal disease. Papanicolaou smears should include specific evaluation for actinomycosis.
b. The uterus should be carefully sounded prior to insertion to determine the degree of patency of the endocervical canal and the internal os, and the direction and depth of the uterine cavity. In occasional cases, severe cervical stenosis may be encountered. Do not use excessive force to overcome this resistance.
c. The uterus should sound to a depth of 6 to 8 centimeters (cm). Insertion of an IUD into a uterine cavity measuring less than 6.5 cm by sounding may increase the incidence of expulsion, bleeding, pain and perforation.
d. The possibility of insertion in the presence of an existing undetermined pregnancy is reduced if insertion is performed during or shortly following a menstrual period. The IUD should not be inserted postpartum or postabortion until involution of the uterus is completed. The incidence of perforation and expulsion is greater if involution is not completed.
e. IUD's should be used with caution in those patients who have anemia or a history of menorrhagia or hypermenorrhea. Patients experiencing menorrhagia and/or metrorrhagia following IUD insertion may be at risk for the development of hypochromic microcytic anemia. Also, IUD's should be used with caution in patients receiving anticoagulants or having a coagulopathy.
f. Syncope, bradycardia, or other neurovascular episodes may occur during insertion or removal of IUD's especially in patients with a previous disposition to these conditions.
g. Patients with valvular or congenital heart disease are more prone to develop subacute bacterial endocarditis than patients who do not have valvular or congenital heart disease. Use of an IUD in these patients may represent a potential source of septic emboli.
h. Use of an IUD in those patients with cervicitis should be postponed until treatment has cured the infection (see CONTRAINDICATIONS Section).
i. Since an IUD may be expelled or displaced, patients should be reexamined and evaluated shortly after the first postinsertion menses, but definitely within three months after insertion. Thereafter, annual examination with appropriate medical and laboratory examination should be carried out.
j. The patient should be told that some bleeding and cramps may occur during the first few weeks after insertion, but if these symptoms continue or are severe, she should report them to her physician. The patient should be instructed on how to check to make certain that the thread still protrudes from the cervix, and she should be cautioned that there is no contraceptive protection if the IUD is expelled. She should be instructed to check the tail as often as possible, but at least after each menstrual period. The patient should be cautioned not to pull on the thread and displace the IUD. If partial expulsion occurs, removal is indicated and a new IUD may be inserted.
k. The use of medical diathermy (shortwave and microwave) in patients with metal-containing IUD's may cause heat injury to the surrounding tissue. Therefore, medical diathermy to the abdominal and sacral areas should not be used.
[LIPPES LOOP contains no metals. This section does not apply to LIPPES LOOP].

ADVERSE REACTIONS
These adverse reactions are not listed in any order of frequency or severity.
Reported adverse reactions include: endometritis, spontaneous abortion, septic abortion, septicemia, perforation of the uterus and cervix, embedment, migration resulting in partial or complete perforation, fragmentation of the IUD, pelvic infection (pelvic inflammatory disease), future infertility, vaginitis, leukorrhea, cervical erosion, pregnancy, ectopic pregnancy, difficult removal, complete or partial expulsion of the IUD, intermenstrual spotting, prolongation of menstrual flow, anemia, pain and cramping, dysmenorrhea, backaches, dyspareunia, neurovascular episodes, including bradycardia and syncope secondary to insertion. Perforation into the abdomen has been followed by abdominal adhesions, intestinal penetration, intestinal obstruction, and cystic masses in the pelvis.

DIRECTIONS FOR USE
Preinsertion
1. It is imperative that sterile technique be maintained throughout the insertion procedure.
2. Perform a thorough pelvic examination to determine freedom from overt disease and to determine position and shape of the uterus. RULE OUT PREGNANCY AND OTHER CONTRAINDICATIONS.
3. With a speculum in place, gently insert a sterile sound to determine the depth and direction of the uterine canal. Be sure to determine the position of the uterus before insertion. Occasionally a tenaculum is required if the uterine canal needs to be straightened. If a stenotic cervix must be dilated, use a sterile Hank's dilator rather than a Hegar's; dilation to a Hank's 16 to 18 should be sufficient.
Insertion
Caution: It is generally felt that perforations are caused at the time of insertion, although the perforation may not be detected until some time later. The position of the uterus should be determined during the preinsertion examination. Great care must be exercised during the preinsertion sounding and subsequent insertion. No attempt should be made to force the insertion. There are a few reports, however, that there has been migration after insertion apparently in the absence of perforation at insertion. In any event, it is possible for the IUD to perforate outside the uterus.
1. How to prepare the LIPPES LOOP Intrauterine Double-S inserter.
Using sterile gloves, hold tube in one hand and with the other draw LOOP into inserter by pulling the push rod. As the LOOP is drawn into the inserter you will encounter some resistance. It is important to use a slow steady pulling action until all but the bulbous tip of the LOOP is entirely within the inserter. At this point, insure that both the flat surface of the bulbous tip and the inserter flange are in a horizontal plane.

Do this not more than one minute before insertion.

2. How to insert LIPPES LOOP Intrauterine Double-S. Insert the loaded inserter gently through the endocervical canal, with the flange in a horizontal plane. DO NOT FORCE THE INSERTION. If resistance is encountered, do not proceed; perforation of the uterus may occur. If the flange makes contact with the cervix WITHOUT the inserter touching the fundal wall, withdraw ¼ inch before pressing the push rod to release the device in utero. Should the inserter touch the fundal wall BEFORE the flange makes contact, withdraw ½ inch prior to pressing the push rod to release the device in utero. With the inserter now in place, proceed, and WITHOUT UNDUE PRESSURE, push the rod slowly as far as it will go. LIPPES LOOP Intrauterine Double-S should now be in place. Withdraw the inserter tube and push rod from the cervical os until the tail is visible. Cut the tail leaving it as long as possible.

Time of Insertion

LIPPES LOOP Intrauterine Double-S should be inserted preferably the last one or two days of a normal menstrual period or the two days following the last day.

The expulsion and perforation rate may be increased when insertions are made before normal uterine involution occurs (usually four to six weeks postpartum or postabortion).

To Remove

To remove LIPPES LOOP Intrauterine Double-S, pull gently on the exposed tail. On those rare occasions that the tail is not available, the device should be carefully removed.

CLINICAL STUDIES

Different event rates have been recorded with the use of different IUD's. Inasmuch as these rates are usually derived from separate studies conducted by different investigators in several population groups, they cannot be compared with precision. Furthermore, event rates tend to be lower as clinical experience is expanded, possibly due to retention in the clinical study of those patients who accept the treatment regimen and do not discontinue due to adverse reactions or pregnancy. In clinical trials conducted by the Population Council with the LIPPES LOOP, use effectiveness was determined as follows for women, as tabulated by the life table method. (Rates are expressed as events per 100 women through 12 and 24 months of use). This experience is based on 198,257 woman/months of use, including 121,489 woman/months of use in first year after insertion, and 76,768 woman/months of use in second year after insertion. LIPPES LOOP Intrauterine Double-S devices are manufactured in four different sizes, and the figures given above represent the totals for the four sizes. The following table presents these figures individually for each size LOOP:
[See table above].

TABLE II
LOOP A
(Annual Rates Per 100 Users)

	12 Months	24 Months (cumulative)
Pregnancy	5.3	9.7
Expulsion	23.9	27.7
Medical Removal	12.2	20.0
Continuation Rate	75.2	63.6

TABLE III
LOOP B
(Annual Rates Per 100 Users)

	12 Months	24 Months (cumulative)
Pregnancy	3.4	6.3
Expulsion	18.9	24.9
Medical Removal	15.1	23.8
Continuation Rate	74.6	59.2

TABLE IV
LOOP C
(Annual Rates Per 100 Users)

	12 Months	24 Months (cumulative)
Pregnancy	3.0	4.8
Expulsion	19.1	24.6
Medical Removal	14.3	22.1
Continuation Rate	76.5	62.8

TABLE V
LOOP D
(Annual Rates Per 100 Users)

	12 Months	24 Months (cumulative)
Pregnancy	2.7	4.2
Expulsion	12.7	16.0
Medical Removal	15.2	23.3
Continuation Rate	77.4	65.6

MASSE'® Breast Cream

(See PDR For Nonprescription Drugs)

TABLE I

LIPPES LOOP Size	Number Woman/Months	Woman/Months of Use 1st Year After Insertion	Woman/Months of Use 2nd Year After Insertion
A	13,453	8,751	4,702
B	12,463	9,660	2,803
C	50,775	31,032	19,743
D	121,566	72,046	49,520

Tables II–V below give the pregnancy, expulsion, medical removal and continuation rates for each individual size LOOP:

MONISTAT® 7 Vaginal Cream ℞
(miconazole nitrate 2%)

DESCRIPTION

MONISTAT 7 Vaginal Cream (miconazole nitrate 2%) is a water-miscible, white cream containing as the active ingredient, 2% miconazole nitrate, 1-[2,4-dichloro-β-(2,4-dichlorobenzyloxy) phenethyl] imidazole nitrate.

ACTIONS

MONISTAT 7 Vaginal Cream exhibits fungicidal activity in vitro against species of the genus Candida. The pharmacologic mode of action is unknown.

INDICATIONS

MONISTAT 7 Vaginal Cream is indicated for the local treatment of vulvovaginal candidiasis (moniliasis). As MONISTAT 7 Vaginal Cream is effective only for candidal vulvovaginitis, the diagnosis should be confirmed by KOH smears and/or cultures. Other pathogens commonly associated with vulvovaginitis (Trichomonas and Haemophilus vaginalis [Gardnerella]) should be ruled out by appropriate laboratory methods.

MONISTAT 7 is effective in both pregnant and non-pregnant women, as well as in women taking oral contraceptives. (See PRECAUTIONS.)

CONTRAINDICATIONS

Patients known to be hypersensitive to this drug.

PRECAUTIONS

General: Discontinue drug if sensitization or irritation is reported during use. Laboratory Tests: If there is a lack of response to MONISTAT 7, appropriate microbiological studies should be repeated to confirm the diagnosis and rule out other pathogens.

Pregnancy: Since MONISTAT is absorbed in small amounts from the human vagina, it should be used in the first trimester of pregnancy only when the physician considers it essential to the welfare of the patient.

Clinical studies, during which MONISTAT was used for 14 days, included 209 pregnant patients. Follow-up reports now available in 117 of these patients reveal no adverse effects or complications attributable to MONISTAT therapy in infants born to these women.

ADVERSE REACTIONS

During clinical studies with MONISTAT for a 14-day regimen, 39 of the 528 patients (7.4%) treated with MONISTAT reported complaints during therapy that were possibly drug-related. Most complaints were reported during the first week of therapy. Vulvovaginal burning, itching or irritation occurred in 6.6%, while other complaints such as vaginal burning, pelvic cramps, hives, skin rash and headache occurred rarely (each less than 0.2% patient incidence). The therapy-related dropout rate was 0.9%.

CLINICAL

Statistical analysis of randomized clinical trials, conducted to determine the shortest effective course of therapy with MONISTAT, demonstrates that a regimen of seven or more days has a cure rate equivalent to the 14-day regimen.

The graphic representation of this conclusion plots Days of Therapy versus Cure Rates. The solid line represents the

DOSE RESPONSE CURVE

mean therapeutic cure rate and the shaded area represents the 95% confidence interval.

DOSAGE AND ADMINISTRATION

One applicatorful is administered intravaginally once daily at bedtime for seven days. Course of therapy may be repeated after other pathogens have been ruled out by appropriate smears and cultures.

HOW SUPPLIED

MONISTAT 7 Vaginal Cream is available in 1.59 oz. (45 g) tubes (NDC 0062-5431-07) with ORTHO® Measured-Dose Applicator.

Shown in Product Identification Section, page 420

MONISTAT® 3 ℞
(miconazole nitrate, 200 mg)
Vaginal Suppositories

DESCRIPTION

MONISTAT 3 Vaginal Suppositories are white to off-white suppositories, each containing the antifungal agent, miconazole nitrate, 1-[2,4-Dichloro-β-[(2,4-dichlorobenzyl)oxy]phenethyl]-imidazole mononitrate, 200 mg, in a hydrogenated vegetable oil base. Miconazole nitrate for vaginal use is also available as MONISTAT 7 Vaginal Cream and MONISTAT 7 Vaginal Suppositories.

MICONAZOLE NITRATE

CLINICAL PHARMACOLOGY

Miconazole nitrate exhibits fungicidal activity in vitro against species of the genus Candida. The pharmacologic mode of action is unknown. Following intravaginal administration of miconazole nitrate, small amounts are absorbed. Administration of a single dose of miconazole nitrate suppositories (100mg) to healthy subjects resulted in a total recovery from the urine and feces of 0.85% (±0.43%) of the administered dose.

Animal studies indicate that the drug crossed the placenta and doses above those used in humans result in embryo and feto-toxicity (80 mg/kg, orally), although this has not been reported in human subjects (See PRECAUTIONS).

In multi-center clinical trials in 440 women with vulvovaginal candidiasis, the efficacy of treatment with the MONISTAT 3 Vaginal Suppository for 3 days was compared with treatment for 7 days with MONISTAT 7 Vaginal Cream. The clinical cure rates (free of microbiological evidence and clinical signs and symptoms of candidiasis at 8–10 days and 30–35 days post-therapy) were numerically lower, although not statistically different, with the 3-Day Suppository when compared with the 7-Day Cream.

INDICATIONS AND USAGE

MONISTAT 3 Vaginal Suppositories are indicated for the local treatment of vulvovaginal candidiasis (moniliasis). Effectiveness in pregnancy and in diabetic patients has not been established. As MONISTAT is effective only for candidal vulvovaginitis, the diagnosis should be confirmed by KOH smear and/or cultures. Other pathogens commonly associated with vulvovaginitis (Trichomonas and Haemophilus vaginalis [Gardnerella]) should be ruled out by appropriate laboratory methods.

CONTRAINDICATIONS

Patients known to be hypersensitive to this drug.

PRECAUTIONS

General: Discontinue drug if sensitization or irritation is reported during use. The base contained in the suppository formulation may interact with certain latex products, such as that used in vaginal contraceptive diaphragms. Concurrent use is not recommended. MONISTAT 7 Vaginal Cream may be considered for use under these conditions.

Continued on next page

Ortho Pharm.—Cont.

Laboratory Tests: If there is a lack of response to MONISTAT 3 Vaginal Suppositories, appropriate microbiological studies (standard KOH smear and/or cultures) should be repeated to confirm the diagnosis and rule out other pathogens.

Carcinogenesis, Mutagenesis, Impairment of Fertility: Long-term animal studies to determine carcinogenic potential have not been performed.

Fertility (Reproduction): Oral administration of miconazole nitrate in rats has been reported to produce prolonged gestation. However, this effect was not observed in oral rabbit studies. In addition, signs of fetal and embryo toxicity were reported in rat and rabbit studies, and dystocia was reported in rat studies after oral doses at and above 80 mg per kg. Intravaginal administration did not produce these effects in rats.

Pregnancy: Since imidazoles are absorbed in small amounts from the human vagina, they should not be used in the first trimester of pregnancy unless the physician considers it essential to the welfare of the patient.

Clinical studies, during which miconazole nitrate vaginal cream and suppositories were used for up to 14 days, were reported to include 514 pregnant patients. Follow-up reports available in 471 of these patients reveal no adverse effects or complications attributable to miconazole nitrate therapy in infants born to these women.

Nursing Mothers: It is not known whether miconazole nitrate is excreted in human milk. Because many drugs are excreted in human milk, caution should be exercised when miconazole nitrate is administered to a nursing woman.

ADVERSE REACTIONS

During clinical studies with the MONISTAT 3 Vaginal Suppository (miconazole nitrate, 200 mg) 301 patients were treated. The incidence of vulvovaginal burning, itching or irritation was 2%. Complaints of cramping (2%) and headaches (1.3%) were also reported. Other complaints (hives, skin rash) occurred with less than a 0.5% incidence. The therapy-related dropout rate was 0.3%.

OVERDOSE

Overdose of miconazole nitrate in humans has not been reported to date. In mice, rats, guinea pigs and dogs, the oral LD 50 values were found to be 578.1, > 640, 275.9 and > 160 mg/kg, respectively.

DOSAGE AND ADMINISTRATION

MONISTAT 3 Vaginal Suppositories: One suppository (miconazole nitrate, 200 mg) is inserted intravaginally once daily at bedtime for three consecutive days. Before prescribing another course of therapy, the diagnosis should be reconfirmed by smears and/or cultures to rule out other pathogens.

HOW SUPPLIED

MONISTAT 3 Suppositories (miconazole nitrate, 200 mg) are available as 2.5 gm, elliptically shaped white to off-white suppositories in packages of three (NDC 0062-5437-01) with a vaginal applicator. Store at 59°–86° F (15–30° C).

Shown in Product Identification Section, page 420

MONISTAT® 7 Vaginal Suppositories   ℞
(100 mg miconazole nitrate)

DESCRIPTION

MONISTAT 7 Vaginal Suppositories are white to off-white suppositories, each containing the antifungal agent, miconazole nitrate, 1-[2,4-Dichloro-β-(2,4-dichlorobenzyl) oxy]phenethyl]-imidazole mononitrate, 100 mg, in a hydrogenated vegetable oil base. Miconazole nitrate for vaginal use is also available as MONISTAT 7 Vaginal Cream.

MICONAZOLE NITRATE

CLINICAL PHARMACOLOGY

Miconazole nitrate exhibits fungicidal activity *in vitro* against species of the genus *Candida*. The pharmacologic mode of action is unknown. Following intravaginal administration of MONISTAT 7 Vaginal Suppositories or MONISTAT 7 Vaginal Cream, small amounts are absorbed. Administration of a single dose of MONISTAT 7 Vaginal Suppositories to healthy subjects resulted in a total recovery from the urine and feces of 0.85% (±0.43%) of the adminis-

tered dose. For MONISTAT 7 Vaginal Cream the corresponding figure was 1.03% (±0.51%) of the administered dose.

Animal studies indicate that the drug crossed the placenta and doses above those used in humans result in embryo and feto-toxicity (80 mg/kg-orally) although this has not been reported in human subjects (see Precautions).

INDICATIONS AND USAGE

MONISTAT 7 Vaginal Suppositories are indicated for the local treatment of vulvovaginal candidiasis (moniliasis). Effectiveness in pregnancy has not been established. As MONISTAT 7 is effective only for candidal vulvovaginitis, the diagnosis should be confirmed by KOH smear and/or cultures. Other pathogens commonly associated with vulvovaginitis *(Trichomonas* and *Haemophilus vaginalis [Gardnerella*]) should be ruled out by appropriate laboratory methods.

Clinical: Statistical analyses of randomized clinical trials, conducted to determine the shortest effective course of therapy with miconazole nitrate vaginal cream and suppositories, demonstrate that a regimen of seven or more days had a cure rate equivalent to a 14-day regimen.

The graphic representation of this conclusion plots Days of Therapy versus Cure Rate for miconazole nitrate vaginal cream. (Results were similar with suppositories.) The solid line represents the mean therapeutic cure rate and the shaded area represents the 95% confidence interval.

DOSE RESPONSE CURVE

CONTRAINDICATIONS

Patients known to be hypersensitive to this drug.

PRECAUTIONS

General: Discontinue drug if sensitization or irritation is reported during use. The base contained in the suppository formulation may interact with certain latex products, such as that used in vaginal contraceptive diaphragms. Concurrent use is not recommended. MONISTAT 7 Vaginal Cream may be considered for use under these conditions.

Laboratory Tests: If there is a lack of response to MONISTAT 7, appropriate microbiological studies (standard KOH smear and/or cultures) should be repeated to confirm the diagnosis and rule out other pathogens.

Carcinogenesis, Mutagenesis, Impairment of Fertility: Long-term animal studies to determine carcinogenic potential have not been performed.

Fertility (reproduction): Oral administration of miconazole nitrate in rats has been reported to produce prolonged gestation. However, this effect was not observed in oral rabbit studies. In addition, signs of fetal and embryotoxicity were reported in rat and rabbit studies and dystocia in rat studies after oral doses at and above 80 mg per kg. Intravaginal administration did not produce these effects in rats.

Pregnancy: Since imidazoles are absorbed in small amounts from the human vagina, they should not be used in the first trimester of pregnancy unless the physician considers it essential to the welfare of the patient.

Clinical studies, during which miconazole nitrate vaginal cream and suppositories were used for up to 14 days, were reported to include 487 pregnant patients. Follow-up reports available on 446 of these patients reveal no adverse effects or complications attributable to miconazole nitrate therapy in infants born to these women.

Nursing Mothers: It is not known whether miconazole nitrate is excreted in human milk. Because many drugs are excreted in human milk, caution should be exercised when miconazole nitrate is administered to a nursing woman.

ADVERSE REACTIONS

During clinical studies with miconazole nitrate cream for a 14-day regimen, 39 of the 528 patients (7.4%) treated with miconazole nitrate cream reported complaints during therapy that were possibly drug-related. Most complaints were reported during the first week of therapy. Vulvovaginal burning, itching or irritation occurred in 6.6%, while other complaints such as vaginal burning, pelvic cramps, hives,

skin rash and headache occurred rarely (each less than 0.2% patient incidence). The therapy-related dropout rate was 0.9%.

During clinical studies with regimens which varied from 1 to 14 days, 1,057 patients were treated with miconazole nitrate suppositories. The incidence of vulvovaginal burning, itching or irritation was 0.5%, while complaints of skin rash occurred at only a 0.2% incidence.

OVERDOSE

Overdosage of miconazole nitrate in humans has not been reported to date. In mice, rats, guinea pigs and dogs, the oral LD_{50} values were found to be 578.1, > 640, 275.9 and > 160 mg/kg, respectively.

DOSAGE AND ADMINISTRATION

MONISTAT 7 Vaginal Suppositories: One suppository (100 mg miconazole nitrate) is inserted intravaginally once daily at bedtime for seven days. Before prescribing another course of therapy, the diagnosis should be reconfirmed by smears and/or cultures to rule out other pathogens.

HOW SUPPLIED

MONISTAT 7 Vaginal Suppositories are available as 2.5gm (100 mg miconazole nitrate) elliptically shaped white to off-white suppositories in packages of seven (NDC 0062-5432-01) with a vaginal applicator. Store at 59°–86°F (13°–30°C).

Shown in Product Identification Section, page 420

MONISTAT®   ℞
(miconazole nitrate)
DUAL-PAK®

3 DAY SUPPOSITORY THERAPY
MONISTAT® 3
(miconazole nitrate, 200 mg)
Vaginal Suppositories

DESCRIPTION

MONISTAT 3 Vaginal Suppositories are white to off-white suppositories, each containing the antifungal agent, miconazole nitrate, 1-[2,4-Dichloro-β-[(2,4-dichlorobenzyl)oxy]phenethyl]-imidazole mononitrate, 200 mg., in a hydrogenated vegetable oil base. Miconazole nitrate for vaginal use is also available as MONISTAT 7 Vaginal Cream and MONISTAT 7 Vaginal Suppositories.

MICONAZOLE NITRATE

CLINICAL PHARMACOLOGY

Miconazole nitrate exhibits fungicidal activity *in vitro* against species of the genus *Candida*. The pharmacologic mode of action is unknown. Following intravaginal administration of miconazole nitrate, small amounts are absorbed. Administration of a single dose of miconazole nitrate suppositories (100 mg) to healthy subjects resulted in a total recovery from the urine and feces of 0.85% (±0.43%) of the administered dose.

Animal studies indicate that the drug crossed the placenta and doses above those used in humans result in embryo and feto-toxicity (80 mg/kg, orally), although this has not been reported in human subjects (See PRECAUTIONS).

In multi-center clinical trials in 440 women with vulvovaginal candidiasis, the efficacy of treatment with the MONISTAT 3 Vaginal Suppository for 3 days was compared with treatment for 7 days with MONISTAT 7 Vaginal Cream. The clinical cure rates (free of microbiological evidence and clinical signs and symptoms of candidiasis at 8–10 days and 30–35 days post-therapy) were numerically lower, although not statistically different, with the 3-Day Suppository when compared with the 7-Day Cream.

INDICATIONS AND USAGE

MONISTAT 3 Vaginal Suppositories are indicated for the local treatment of vulvovaginal candidiasis (moniliasis). Effectiveness in pregnancy and in diabetic patients has not been established. As MONISTAT is effective only for candidal vulvovaginitis, the diagnosis should be confirmed by KOH smear and/or cultures. Other pathogens commonly associated with vulvovaginitis (*Trichomonas* and *Haemophilus vaginalis* [*Gardnerella*]) should be ruled out by appropriate laboratory methods.

CONTRAINDICATIONS

Patients known to be hypersensitive to this drug.

PRECAUTIONS

General: Discontinue drug if sensitization or irritation is reported during use. The base contained in the suppository formulation may interact with certain latex products, such as that used in vaginal contraceptive diaphragms. Concurrent use is not recommended. MONISTAT 7 Vaginal Cream may be considered for use under these conditions. Laboratory Tests: If there is a lack of response to MONISTAT 3 Vaginal Suppositories, appropriate microbiological studies (standard KOH smear and/or cultures) should be repeated to confirm the diagnosis and rule out other pathogens.

Carcinogenesis, Mutagenesis, Impairment of Fertility: Long-term animal studies to determine carcinogenic potential have not been performed.

Fertility (Reproduction): Oral administration of miconazole nitrate in rats has been reported to produce prolonged gestation. However, this effect was not observed in oral rabbit studies. In addition, signs of fetal and embryo toxicity were reported in rat and rabbit studies, and dystocia was reported in rat studies after oral doses at and above 80 mg per kg. Intravaginal administration did not produce these effects in rats.

Pregnancy: Since imidazoles are absorbed in small amounts from the human vagina, they should not be used in the first trimester of pregnancy unless the physician considers it essential to the welfare of the patient.

Clinical studies, during which miconazole nitrate vaginal cream and suppositories were used for up to 14 days, were reported to include 514 pregnant patients. Follow-up reports available in 471 of these patients reveal no adverse effects or complications attributable to miconazole nitrate therapy in infants born to these women.

Nursing Mothers: It is not known whether miconazole nitrate is excreted in human milk. Because many drugs are excreted in human milk, caution should be exercised when miconazole nitrate is administered to a nursing woman.

ADVERSE REACTIONS

During clinical studies with the MONISTAT 3 Vaginal Suppository (miconazole nitrate, 200 mg) 301 patients were treated. The incidence of vulvovaginal burning, itching or irritation was 2%. Complaints of cramping (2%) and headaches (1.3%) were also reported. Other complaints (hives, skin rash) occurred with less than a 0.5% incidence. The therapy-related dropout rate was 0.3%.

OVERDOSE

Overdose of miconazole nitrate in humans has not been reported to date. In mice, rats, guinea pigs and dogs, the oral LD 50 values were found to be 578.1, > 640, 275.9 and > 160 mg/kg, respectively.

DOSAGE AND ADMINISTRATION

MONISTAT 3 Vaginal Suppositories: One suppository (miconazole nitrate, 200 mg) is inserted intravaginally once daily at bedtime for three consecutive days. Before prescribing another course of therapy, the diagnosis should be reconfirmed by smears and/or cultures to rule out other pathogens.

HOW SUPPLIED

MONISTAT 3 Suppositories (miconazole nitrate, 200 mg) are available as 2.5 gm, elliptically shaped white to off-white suppositories in packages of three (NDC 0062-5437-01) with a vaginal applicator. Store at 59–86°F (15–30°C).

7 DAY CREAM THERAPY
MONISTAT-DERM®
(miconazole nitrate 2%)
Cream and Lotion
For Topical Use Only

DESCRIPTION

MONISTAT-DERM (miconazole nitrate 2%) Cream and Lotion each contain miconazole nitrate* 2%, formulated into a water-miscible base consisting of pegoxol 7 stearate, peglicol 5 oleate, mineral oil, benzoic acid, butylated hydroxynisole and purified water.

ACTIONS

Miconazole nitrate is a synthetic antifungal agent which inhibits the growth of the common dermatophytes, *Trichophyton rubrum, Trichophyton mentagrophytes,* and *Epidermophyton floccosum,* the yeast-like fungus, *Candida albicans,* and the organism responsible for tinea versicolor *(Malessezia furfur).*

INDICATIONS

For topical application in the treatment of tinea pedis (athlete's foot), tinea cruris, and tinea corporis caused by *Trichophyton rubrum, Tichophyton mentagrophytes,* and *Epidermophyton floccosum,* in the treatment of cutaneous candidiasis (moniliasis), and in the treatment of tinea versicolor.

CONTRAINDICATIONS

MONISTAT-DERM (miconazole nitrate 2%) Cream and Lotion have no known contraindications.

PRECAUTIONS

If a reaction suggesting sensitivity or chemical irritation should occur, use of the medication should be discontinued.

For external use only. Avoid introduction of MONISTAT-DERM Cream and Lotion into the eyes.

ADVERSE REACTIONS

There have been isolated reports of irritation, burning, maceration, and allergic contact dermatitis associated with the application of MONISTAT-DERM.

DOSAGE AND ADMINISTRATION

Sufficient MONISTAT-DERM Cream should be applied to cover affected areas twice daily (morning and evening) in patients with tinea pedis, tinea cruris, tinea corporis, and cutaneous candidiasis, and once daily in patients with tinea versicolor. It is preferable to use MONISTAT-DERM Lotion in intertriginous areas; if the cream is used, it should be applied sparingly and smoothed in well to avoid maceration effects.

Early relief of symptoms (2 to 3 days) is experienced by the majority of patients and clinical improvement may be seen fairly soon after treatment is begun; however, *Candida* infections and tinea cruris and corporis should be treated for two weeks and tinea pedis for one month in order to reduce the possibility of recurrence. If a patient shows no clinical improvement after a month of treatment, the diagnosis should be redetermined. Patients with tinea versicolor usually exhibit clinical and mycological clearing after two weeks of treatment.

HOW SUPPLIED

MONISTAT-DERM (miconazole nitrate 2%) Cream containing miconazole nitrate at 2% strength is supplied in 15 g., (NDC 0062-5434-02), 1 oz. (NDC 0062-5434-01) and 3 oz. (NDC 0062-5434-03) tubes. MONISTAT-DERM (miconazole nitrate 2%) Lotion containing miconazole nitrate at 2% w/w strength is supplied in polyethylene squeeze bottles in quantities of 30 ml. (NDC 0062-5435-02) and 60 ml. (NDC-0062-5435-05).

*Chemical name: 1-[2,4-dichloro-β-{(2,4- dichlorobenzyl) oxy}phenethyl] imidazole mononitrate.

Shown in Product Identification Section, page 420

ORTHOCLONE OKT®3 Sterile Solution ℞
(muromonab-CD3)
For Intravenous Use Only

WARNING

Only physicians experienced in immunosuppressive therapy and management of renal transplant patients should use ORTHOCLONE OKT3 (muromonab-CD3). Patients receiving ORTHOCLONE OKT3 should be managed in facilities equipped and staffed for cardiopulmonary resuscitation.

Severe pulmonary edema has occurred in patients with fluid overload prior to treatment with ORTHOCLONE OKT3.

DESCRIPTION

ORTHOCLONE OKT3 (muromonab-CD3) Sterile Solution is a murine monoclonal antibody to the T3 (CD3) antigen of human T cells which functions as an immunosuppressant. It is for intravenous use only. The antibody is a biochemically purified IgG$_{2a}$ immunoglobulin with a heavy chain of approximately 50,000 daltons and a light chain of approximately 25,000 daltons. It is directed to a glycoprotein with a molecular weight of 20,000 in the human T cell surface which is essential for T cell functions. Because it is a monoclonal antibody preparation, ORTHOCLONE OKT3 Sterile Solution is a homogeneous, reproducible antibody product with consistent, measurable reactivity to human T cells.

Each 5 ml ampule of ORTHOCLONE OKT3 Sterile Solution contains 5 mg (1 mg/ml) of muromonab-CD3 in a clear colorless solution which may contain a few fine translucent protein particles. Each ampule contains a buffered solution (pH 7.0 ±0.5) of monobasic sodium phosphate (2.25 mg), dibasic sodium phosphate (9.0 mg), sodium chloride (43 mg) and polysorbate 80 (1.0 mg) in water for injection.

The proper name, muromonab-CD3, is derived from the descriptive term murine monoclonal antibody. The CD3 designation identifies the specificity of the antibody as the Cell Differentiation (CD) cluster 3 defined by the First International Workshop on Human Leukocyte Differentiation Antigens.

CLINICAL PHARMACOLOGY

ORTHOCLONE OKT3 reverses graft rejection, most probably by blocking the function of all T cells which play a major role in acute renal rejection.

ORTHOCLONE OKT3 reacts with and blocks the function of a 20,000 dalton molecule (CD3) in the membrane of human T cells that has been associated *in vitro* with the antigen recognition structure of T cells and is essential for signal transduction. In *in vitro* cytolytic assays, ORTHOCLONE OKT3 blocks both the generation and function of effector cells. It is a potent mitogen *in vitro* in calf serum, but this mitogenicity

is markedly reduced in human serum. ORTHOCLONE OKT3 thus blocks all known T cell functions.

In vivo, ORTHOCLONE OKT3 reacts with most peripheral blood T cells and T cells in body tissues, but has not been found to react with other hematopoietic elements or other tissues of the body.

In all patients studied, a rapid and concomitant decrease in the number of circulating CD3 positive, CD4 positive and CD8 positive T cells was observed within minutes after the administration of ORTHOCLONE OKT3 (muromonab-CD3). Between days two and seven increasing numbers of circulating CD4 positive and CD8 positive cells have been observed in patients although CD3 positive cells are not detectable. The presence of these CD4 and CD8 positive cells has not been found to affect the clinical course of the patient. CD3 positive cells reappear rapidly and reach pre-treatment levels within a week after termination of ORTHOCLONE OKT3 therapy. Increasing numbers of CD3 positive cells have been observed in some patients during the second week of ORTHOCLONE OKT3 therapy, possibly as a result of the development of neutralizing antibodies to ORTHOCLONE OKT3.

Antibodies to ORTHOCLONE OKT3 have been observed, occurring with an incidence of 21% (n=43) for IgM, 86% (n=43) for IgG and 29% (n=35) for IgE. The mean time of appearance of IgG antibodies was 20±2 (mean ±SD) days. Early IgG antibodies appeared towards the end of the second week of treatment in 3% (n=86) of the patients. Serum levels of ORTHOCLONE OKT3 are measurable using an enzyme-linked immunosorbent assay (ELISA). During treatment with 5 mg per day for 14 days, mean serum trough levels of the drug rose over the first three days and then averaged 0.9 µg/ml on days 3 to 14. The levels obtained during therapy have been shown to block T cell effector functions *in vitro.*

Following administration of ORTHOCLONE OKT3 *in vivo,* leukocytes have been observed in cerebrospinal and peritoneal fluids. The mechanism for this effect is not understood.

INDICATIONS AND USAGE

ORTHOCLONE OKT3 is indicated for the treatment of acute allograft rejection in renal transplant patients.

In a controlled randomized clinical trial, ORTHOCLONE OKT3 was significantly more effective than conventional high dose steroid therapy in reversing acute renal allograft rejection. In this trial, 122 evaluable patients undergoing acute rejection of cadaveric renal transplants were treated either with ORTHOCLONE OKT3 daily for a mean of 14 days, with concomitant lowering of the dosage of azathioprine and maintenance steroids (62 patients), or with conventional high dose steroids (60 patients). ORTHOCLONE OKT3 reversed 94% of the rejections compared to a 75% reversal rate obtained with conventional high dose steroid treatment (p=0.006). The one year Kaplan-Meier (actuarial) estimates of graft survival rates for these patients who had acute rejection were 62% and 45% for ORTHOCLONE OKT3 and steroid treated patients, respectively (p=0.04). At two years the rates were 56% and 42%, respectively (p=0.06).

One- and two-year patient survivals were not significantly different between the two groups, being 85% and 75% for ORTHOCLONE OKT3 treated patients and 90% and 85% for steroid treated patients.

In additional open clinical trials, the observed rate of reversal of acute renal allograft rejection was 92% (n=126) for ORTHOCLONE OKT3 therapy. ORTHOCLONE OKT3 also was effective in reversing acute renal allograft rejections in 65% (n=225) of cases where steroids and lymphocyte immune globulin preparations were contraindicated or were not successful (rescue).

The dosage of other immunosuppressive agents used in conjunction with ORTHOCLONE OKT3 should be lowered to minimal levels (See DOSAGE AND ADMINISTRATION Section).

CONTRAINDICATIONS

ORTHOCLONE OKT3 (muromonab-CD3) should not be used in patients who are hypersensitive to this or any other product of murine origin nor in patients who are in fluid overload, as evidenced by chest x-ray or a greater than 3 percent weight gain within the week prior to planned ORTHOCLONE OKT3 administration.

WARNINGS

SEE BOXED WARNING

Immunosuppressive therapy can lead to increased susceptibility to infection. Further, lymphomas have been reported following immunosuppressive therapy, and data suggest that their occurrence is related to the intensity and duration of immunosuppression rather than the use of specific agents. Significant fever, chills, dyspnea and malaise may occur $\frac{1}{2}$ to 6 hours after the first dose of ORTHOCLONE OKT3. Therefore, the injection of the first dose should be performed in a facility where the patient can be closely monitored and which is equipped and staffed for cardio-pulmonary resusci-

Continued on next page

Ortho Pharm.—Cont.

tation. The most serious first-dose reaction—potentially fatal severe pulmonary edema—has occurred infrequently (4.7% of the initial 107 patients and 0.0% in the subsequent 311 patients treated with first-dose restrictions). In each case of severe pulmonary edema, fluid overload was present before treatment. Therefore, patients should be evaluated for fluid overload by chest x-ray or weight gain of greater than 3%. Weight should be brought to a value less than or equal to 3% above the minimum weight in the prior week before ORTHOCLONE OKT3 treatment is initiated. Reactions to the first dose may be minimized by using the recommended steroid regimen (See DOSAGE AND ADMINISTRATION Section).

This formulation of ORTHOCLONE OKT3 contains polysorbate 80 and must not be used for the *in vitro* treatment of bone marrow.

PRECAUTIONS

General

If the patient temperature exceeds 37.8°C (100°F), it should be lowered by antipyretics before ORTHOCLONE OKT3 administration.

Use a low protein-binding 0.2 or 0.22 micrometer (μm) filter to prepare the injections (See ADMINISTRATION INSTRUCTIONS).

ORTHOCLONE OKT3 is a heterologous protein and induces detectable antibodies in most patients. Only limited data are available regarding retreatment with ORTHOCLONE OKT3. The presence of antibodies to ORTHOCLONE OKT3 could limit its efficacy following readministration and possibly cause serious adverse reactions. Caution should be used if retreatment is considered.

Physicians should be aware that an aseptic meningitis syndrome was identified during a post-marketing survey of 143 patients. The most commonly reported symptoms in this survey are: fever (87%), headache (42%), neck stiffness (13%) and photophobia (10%), which have occurred most often during the first three days of ORTHOCLONE OKT3 therapy. Seizures are reported in two patients. In this survey, of the twelve patients who had undergone lumbar puncture, ten were evaluable. The cerebrospinal fluid in these patients showed leukocytosis (8/9)—mainly polymorphonuclear in 4, elevated protein (6/7), and decreased glucose (2/8). One patient had a culture positive for enterovirus. All other viral, bacterial and fungal cultures performed were negative. One of the ten patients had a concomitant urinary tract infection. Although all patients in this survey with this syndrome had a benign course and have recovered, infection must be considered in the differential diagnosis of an immunosuppressed transplant patient with any signs or symptoms of meningitis.

Information for patients: Patients should be informed of the expected first dose ORTHOCLONE OKT3 (muromonab-CD3) effects, which are markedly reduced on successive days of ORTHOCLONE OKT3 treatment.

Laboratory tests: Chest x-ray taken within 24 hours before initiating ORTHOCLONE OKT3 treatment must be clear of fluid. WBCs and differentials should be monitored at intervals during treatment with ORTHOCLONE OKT3. The effect of ORTHOCLONE OKT3 on circulating T cells expressing the CD3 antigen should be monitored by an *in vitro* assay.

Carcinogenesis: Long term studies have not been performed in laboratory animals to evaluate the carcinogenic potential of ORTHOCLONE OKT3.

Pregnancy category C: Animal reproductive studies have not been conducted with ORTHOCLONE OKT3. It is also not known whether ORTHOCLONE OKT3 can cause fetal harm when administered to a pregnant woman or can affect reproduction capacity. ORTHOCLONE OKT3 should be given to a pregnant woman only if clearly needed.

Pediatric use: Safety and effectiveness in children have not been established. Although no adequate controlled studies have been conducted in children, patients as young as two years of age have received ORTHOCLONE OKT3 with no unexpected adverse effects.

ADVERSE REACTIONS

Determinations of adverse experiences with ORTHOCLONE OKT3 have been primarily documented in clinical trials of renal rejection following cadaveric transplantation. These patients were simultaneously receiving low-dose immunosuppressive therapy, primarily azathioprine and corticosteroids.

Compared to conventional treatment, patients treated with ORTHOCLONE OKT3 experienced increased adverse reactions during the first two days of treatment. During this period the majority of patients experienced pyrexia (73%) of which 2% were 40.0°C (104°F) or above, and chills (57%). In addition, other adverse experiences occurring in more than 8% of the patients during the first two days of ORTHOCLONE OKT3 therapy included dyspnea (21%), chest pain (14%), vomiting (13%), wheezing (11%), nausea (11%), diarrhea (10%), and tremor (10%). Similar adverse effects were observed in the additional open clinical studies.

Potentially fatal severe pulmonary edema was reported following the first dose in less than 2% of the cases and was always associated with fluid overload. It is therefore essential that patients receiving ORTHOCLONE OKT3 not be in fluid overload and remain under close medical supervision for 48 hours after the first dose administration. The first dose should be administered as detailed in the DOSAGE AND ADMINISTRATION Section.

In the ORTHOCLONE OKT3 treated patients in the randomized controlled trial, the most common infections observed in the first 45 days following start of ORTHOCLONE OKT3 therapy were due to cytomegalovirus (19%) and Herpes simplex (27%). Other severe and life-threatening infections seen in these patients during this period were *Staphylococcus epidermidis* (4.8%), *Pneumocystis carinii* (3.1%), Legionella (1.6%), Cryptococcus (1.6%), Serratia (1.6%) and gram-negative bacteria (1.6%). The incidence of infections was not statistically different with ORTHOCLONE OKT3 than with high dose steroids.

Additional clinically significant adverse reactions were observed whose causal relationship to ORTHOCLONE OKT3 therapy is unclear. They were anaphylaxis (1 patient), serum sickness (2 patients) and lymphoma (2 patients).

A monoclonal B-lymphoproliferative disorder, similar to Epstein-Barr virus (EBV) associated B-lymphoproliferation, occurred in one of 22 bone marrow transplantation patients treated for graft-versus-host disease with ORTHOCLONE OKT3. This patient also received treatment with corticosteroids, cyclosporine, methotrexate and anti-thymocyte globulin. One patient with acute renal rejection was diagnosed as having generalized lymphoma three weeks after receiving three days of ORTHOCLONE OKT3. This patient also received treatment with high dose steroids, cyclosporine, antithymocyte globulin and azathioprine. Long term risk for increased incidence of lymphoma or other malignancies has not been determined.

In a post-marketing survey of 143 patients, an aseptic meningitis syndrome has been identified. The symptoms reported in the survey are fever (87%), headache (42%), neck stiffness (13%) and photophobia (10%). A combination of the above four symptoms occurred in 6% of the patients. This syndrome has been reported to occur usually within three days of initiation of ORTHOCLONE OKT3 therapy. All patients in the survey with this syndrome had a benign course and have recovered.

In the 9 months post-licensure, 11 patients (0.4%) of an estimated 2500 patients treated with ORTHOCLONE OKT3 were reported to have seizures; ten occurred during the first 3 days of ORTHOCLONE OKT3 therapy. Eight of the 10 patients had either known seizure disorder, hypoglycemia or were concurrently on dialysis. Cerebrospinal fluid in at least two of 11 patients, who had lumbar puncture, showed leukocytosis and elevated protein. One of the 11 patients was subsequently retreated with ORTHOCLONE OKT3 on two occasions without additional seizures. One patient with a past history of seizure disorder developed refractory generalized seizures two days after transplantation and initiation of prophylactic ORTHOCLONE OKT3 therapy and died one day later. The causal relationship between ORTHOCLONE OKT3 and seizure is unknown.

OVERDOSAGE

The maximum amount of ORTHOCLONE OKT3 that can safely be administered in single or multiple doses has not been determined.

DOSAGE AND ADMINISTRATION

The recommended dose of ORTHOCLONE OKT3 for the treatment of acute renal allograft rejection is 5 mg per day for 10 to 14 days. Treatment should begin once acute renal rejection is diagnosed.

Patients should be monitored closely for 48 hours after the first dose is administered. Intravenous methylprednisolone sodium succinate 1.0 mg/kg given prior to ORTHOCLONE OKT3 administration and intravenous hydrocortisone sodium succinate 100 mg given 30 minutes after ORTHOCLONE OKT3 administration is strongly recommended to decrease the incidence of reactions to the first dose. Acetaminophen and antihistamines can be given concomitantly with ORTHOCLONE OKT3 to reduce early reactions. Patient temperature should not exceed 37.8°C (100°F) at the time of first ORTHOCLONE OKT3 administration (See TABLE I).

Conventional concomitant immunosuppressive therapy should be lowered during ORTHOCLONE OKT3 administration to a daily dose of prednisone 0.5 mg/kg and azathioprine 25 mg. Retrospective analysis of open label studies suggest that cyclosporine should be discontinued at the start of ORTHOCLONE OKT3 (muromonab-CD3) therapy. Maintenance immunosuppression, including cyclosporine if indicated, should be resumed approximately three days prior to cessation of ORTHOCLONE OKT3 therapy.

TABLE I
Suggested Prevention And Treatment Of ORTHOCLONE OKT3 First Dose Effects

Adverse Reaction	Effective Prevention or Palliation	Supportive Treatment
1. Severe pulmonary edema	• Clear chest x-ray within 24 hrs. preinjection	• Prompt intubation and oxygenation
	• Weight restriction to ≤3% gain over 7 days preinjection	• 24 hr. close observation
2. Fever, chills	• 1.0 mg/kg methylprednisolone sodium succinate preinjection	• Cooling blanket
	• Fever reduction below 37.8°C (100°F) preinjection	• Acetaminophen p.r.n.
3. Respiratory Effects	• 100 mg hydrocortisone sodium succinate 30 min. postinjection	• Additional 100 mg hydrocortisone sodium succinate p.r.n.

ADMINISTRATION INSTRUCTIONS

1. Parenteral drug products should be inspected visually for particulate matter and discoloration prior to administration. Because ORTHOCLONE OKT3 is a protein solution, it may develop a few fine translucent particles which have been shown not to affect its potency.
2. Prepare ORTHOCLONE OKT3 for injection by drawing solution into a syringe through a low protein-binding 0.2 or 0.22 micrometer (μm) filter. Discard filter and attach needle for IV bolus injection.
3. Administer ORTHOCLONE OKT3 as an IV bolus in less than one minute. Do not administer by intravenous infusion or in conjunction with other drug solutions.

HOW SUPPLIED

ORTHOCLONE OKT3 is supplied as a sterile solution in packages of 5 ampules (NDC 0062-7102-01). Each 5 ml ampule contains 5 mg of muromonab-CD3.

Storage: Store in a refrigerator at 2 to 8°C (36 to 46°F). **DO NOT FREEZE OR SHAKE.**

REFERENCES

1. Kung, P.C., Goldstein, G., Reinherz, E.L. and Schlossman, S.F. (1979), "Monoclonal Antibodies Defining Distinctive Human T Cell Surface Antigens". Science *206*: 347–349.
2. ORTHO Multicenter Transplant Study Group (1985), "A Randomized Clinical Trial of OKT3 Monoclonal Antibody for Acute Rejection of Cadaveric Renal Transplants". New England Journal of Medicine. *313*: 337–342.
3. Nomenclature Subcommittee, (1984), "Differentiation Human Leukocyte Antigens: A Proposed Nomenclature". Immunology Today *5*, No. 6.: 158–159.

ORTHO PHARMACEUTICAL CORPORATION
BIOTECH DIVISION
Raritan, New Jersey 08869, USA

©OPC 1986.   Revised April 1987
Shown in Product Identification Section, page 420

ORTHO-CREME® Contraceptive Cream

(See PDR For Nonprescription Drugs)

ORTHO™ DIAPHRAGM KITS

DESCRIPTION

ORTHO Diaphragm Kits include three different types in a variety of sizes.

1. The ALL-FLEX* Arcing Spring Diaphragm is a molded, buff-colored, latex vaginal diaphragm containing a distortion-free, dual spring-within-a-spring which provides unique arcing action no matter where the rim is compressed. It is ideal not only where ordinary diaphragms are indicated, but also in patients with mild cystocele, rectocele or retroversion.
2. The ORTHO* Coil Spring Diaphragm is a molded latex vaginal diaphragm. The rim encases a tension-adjusted, cadmium-plated coil spring.
3. The ORTHO-WHITE* Flat Spring Diaphragm is a molded, pure white, latex vaginal diaphragm containing a flat, watch-type spring which allows compressibility in one plane only, thus facilitating insertion.

ORTHO Diaphragms are used in conjunction with spermicides, e.g., GYNOL II* Contraceptive Jelly, ORTHO-GYNOL* Contraceptive Jelly or ORTHO-CREME* Contraceptive Cream in conception control.

ACTION

These diaphragms when properly fitted serve two purposes:
a. To stop the sperm from entering the cervical canal;
b. To hold the spermicide.

INDICATIONS

ORTHO Diaphragms, in conjunction with an appropriate spermicide, are indicated for the prevention of pregnancy in women who elect to use diaphragms as a method of contraception.

PRECAUTIONS

Although an association has not been established between diaphragm use and toxic shock syndrome (TSS), symptoms of this condition have been reported in a few women using diaphragms. In most of these cases, the women wore a diaphragm continuously for more than 24 hours. Therefore, continuous wearing of the diaphragm for more than 24 hours is not recommended.

Primary symptoms of TSS are sudden high fever (usually 102°F or more) and vomiting, diarrhea, fainting or near fainting when standing up, dizziness or a rash that looks like a sunburn. There may also be other signs of TSS, such as aching of muscles and joints, redness of the eyes, sore throat and weakness. The patient should be instructed that if she has sudden high fever and one or more of the other symptoms, she should remove her diaphragm and consult her physician immediately.

INSTRUCTIONS

1. Proper placement of the diaphragm is vital for effectiveness.
2. To be fully effective the diaphragm should never be used without contraceptive cream or jelly. This contraceptive cream or jelly must be spread around the inner surface of the diaphragm as well as around the rim.
3. The diaphragm may be inserted up to six hours before intercourse. If more than six hours has elapsed between insertion of the diaphragm and intercourse, additional contraceptive jelly or cream must be applied. The diaphragm should not be removed to apply this additional cream or jelly.
4. The diaphragm should not be removed nor should the patient douche for six hours after intercourse. The diaphragm should not remain in position for more than 24 hours.

HOW SUPPLIED

All ORTHO Diaphragm Kits are available individually and contain a sample tube of GYNOL II Contraceptive Jelly. Each diaphragm is contained in an attractive plastic compact.
1. The ALL-FLEX Arcing Spring Diaphragm is available in sizes 55mm through 95mm in 5mm increments.
2. The ORTHO Coil Spring Diaphragm is available in sizes 50mm through 105mm in 5mm increments.
3. The ORTHO-WHITE Flat Spring Diaphragm is available in sizes 55mm through 95mm in 5mm increments.
*Trademark

ORTHO® Dienestrol Cream   ℞

1. ESTROGENS HAVE BEEN REPORTED TO INCREASE THE RISK OF ENDOMETRIAL CARCINOMA.

Three independent case control studies have shown an increased risk of endometrial cancer in postmenopausal women exposed to exogenous estrogens for prolonged periods.[1-3] This risk was independent of the other known risk factors for endometrial cancer. These studies are further supported by the finding that incidence rates of endometrial cancer have increased sharply since 1969 in eight different areas of the United States with population-based cancer reporting systems, an increase which may be related to the rapidly expanding use of estrogens during the last decade.[4]

The three case control studies reported that the risk of endometrial cancer in estrogen users was about 4.5 to 13.9 times greater than in nonusers. The risk appears to depend on both duration of treatment[1] and on estrogen dose.[3] In view of these findings, when estrogens are used for the treatment of menopausal symptoms, the lowest dose that will control symptoms should be utilized and medication should be discontinued as soon as possible. When prolonged treatment is medically indicated, the patient should be reassessed on at least a semiannual basis to determine the need for continued therapy. Although the evidence must be considered preliminary, one study suggests that cyclic administration of low doses of estrogen may carry less risk than continuous administration;[3] it therefore appears prudent to utilize such a regimen.

Close clinical surveillance of all women taking estrogens is important. In all cases of undiagnosed persistent or recurring abnormal vaginal bleeding, adequate diagnostic measures should be undertaken to rule out malignancy.

There is no evidence at present that "natural" estrogens are more or less hazardous than "synthetic" estrogens at equiestrogenic doses.

2. ESTROGENS SHOULD NOT BE USED DURING PREGNANCY

The use of female sex hormones, both estrogens and progestogens, during early pregnancy may seriously damage the offspring. It has been shown that females exposed *in utero* to diethylstilbestrol, a non-steroidal estrogen, have an increased risk of developing in later life a form of vaginal or cervical cancer that ordinarily is extremely rare.[5,6] This risk has been estimated as not greater than 4 per 1000 exposures.[7] Furthermore, a high percentage of such exposed women (from 30 to 90 percent) have been found to have vaginal adenosis,[8-12] epithelial changes of the vagina and cervix. Although these changes are histologically benign, it is not known whether they are precursors of malignancy. Although similar data are not available with the use of other estrogens, it cannot be presumed they would not induce similar changes.

Several reports suggest an association between intrauterine exposure to female sex hormones and congenital anomalies, including congenital heart defects and limb reduction defects.[13-16] One case control study[16] estimated a 4.7 fold increased risk of limb reduction defects in infants exposed in utero to sex hormones (oral contraceptives, hormone withdrawal tests for pregnancy, or attempted treatment for threatened abortion). Some of these exposures were very short and involved only a few days of treatment. The data suggest that the risk of limb reduction defects in exposed fetuses is somewhat less than 1 per 1000.

In the past, female sex hormones have been used during pregnancy in an attempt to treat threatened or habitual abortion. There is considerable evidence that estrogens are ineffective for these indications, and there is no evidence from well controlled studies that progestogens are effective for these uses.

If ORTHO Dienestrol Cream is used during pregnancy, or if the patient becomes pregnant while using this drug, she should be apprised of the potential risks to the fetus, and the advisability of pregnancy continuation.

DESCRIPTION

ORTHO Dienestrol Cream
Cream for Intravaginal use only
Active ingredient: Dienestrol 0.01%.
Dienestrol is a synthetic, non-steroidal estrogen. It is compounded in a cream base suitable for intravaginal use only. The cream base is composed of glyceryl monostearate, peanut oil, glycerin, benzoic acid, glutamic acid, butylated hydroxyanisole, citric acid, sodium hydroxide and water. The pH is approximately 4.3.

CLINICAL PHARMACOLOGY

Systemic absorption and mode of action are undetermined.

INDICATIONS AND USAGE

ORTHO Dienestrol Cream is indicated in the treatment of atrophic vaginitis and kraurosis vulvae.

ORTHO DIENESTROL CREAM HAS NOT BEEN SHOWN TO BE EFFECTIVE FOR ANY PURPOSE DURING PREGNANCY AND ITS USE MAY CAUSE SEVERE HARM TO THE FETUS (*SEE* BOXED WARNING).

CONTRAINDICATIONS

Estrogens may cause fetal harm when administered to a pregnant woman (see Boxed Warning). Estrogens are contraindicated in women who are or may become pregnant. If this drug is used during pregnancy, or if the patient becomes pregnant while using this drug, the patient should be apprised of the potential hazard to the fetus.

Estrogens should also not be used in women with any of the following conditions:
1. Known or suspected cancer of the breast.
2. Known or suspected estrogen-dependent neoplasia.
3. Undiagnosed abnormal genital bleeding.
4. Active thrombophlebitis or thromboembolic disorders.
5. A past history of thrombophlebitis, thrombosis, or thromboembolic disorders associated with previous estrogen use.

WARNINGS

1. *Induction of malignant neoplasms.* Long-term continuous administration of natural and synthetic estrogens in certain animal species increases the frequency of carcinomas of the breast, cervix, vagina, and liver. There is now evidence that estrogens increase the risk of carcinoma of the endometrium in humans. (*See* Boxed Warning.)

At the present time there is no satisfactory evidence that estrogens given to postmenopausal women increase the risk of cancer of the breast,[18] although a recent long-term followup of a single physician's practice has raised this possibility.[18a] Because of the animal data, there is a need for caution in prescribing estrogens for women with a strong family history of breast cancer or who have breast nodules, fibrocystic disease, or abnormal mammograms.

2. *Gall bladder disease.* A recent study has reported a 2 to 3-fold increase in the risk of surgically confirmed gall bladder disease in women receiving postmenopausal estrogens,[18] similar to the 2-fold increase previously noted in users of oral contraceptives.[19,24] In the case of oral contraceptives the increased risk appeared after two years of use.[24]

3. *Effects similar to those caused by estrogen-progestogen oral contraceptives.* There are several serious adverse effects of oral contraceptives, most of which have not, up to now, been documented as consequences of postmenopausal estrogen therapy. This may reflect the comparatively low doses of estrogen used in postmenopausal women. It would be expected that the larger doses of estrogen used to treat prostatic or breast cancer or postpartum breast engorgement are more likely to result in these adverse effects, and, in fact, it has been shown that there is an increased risk of thrombosis in men receiving estrogens for prostatic cancer and women for postpartum breast engorgement.[20-23]

a. *Thromboembolic disease.* It is now well established that users of oral contraceptives have an increased risk of various thromboembolic and thrombotic vascular diseases, such as thrombophlebitis, pulmonary embolism, stroke, and myocardial infarction.[24-31] Cases of retinal thrombosis, mesenteric thrombosis, and optic neuritis have been reported in oral contraceptive users. There is evidence that the risk of several of these adverse reactions is related to the dose of the drug.[32,33] An increased risk of postsurgery thromboembolic complications has also been reported in users of oral contraceptives.[34,35] If feasible, estrogen should be discontinued at least 4 weeks before surgery of the type associated with an increased risk of thromboembolism, or during periods of prolonged immobilization.

While an increased rate of thromboembolic and thrombotic disease in postmenopausal users of estrogens has not been found,[18,36] this does not rule out the possibility that such an increase may be present or that subgroups of women who have underlying risk factors or who are receiving relatively large doses of estrogens may have increased risk. Therefore estrogens should not be used in persons with active thrombophlebitis or thromboembolic disorders, and they should not be used (except in treatment of malignancy) in persons with a history of such disorders in association with estrogen use. They should be used with caution in patients with cerebral vascular or coronary artery disease and only for those in whom estrogens are clearly needed.

Large doses of estrogen (5 mg conjugated estrogens per day), comparable to those used to treat cancer of the prostate and breast, have been shown in a large prospective clinical trial in men to increase the risk of nonfatal myocardial infarction, pulmonary embolism and thrombophlebitis. When estrogen doses of this size are used, any of the thromboembolic and thrombotic adverse effects associated with oral contraceptive use should be considered a clear risk.

b. *Hepatic adenoma.* Benign hepatic adenomas appear to be associated with the use of oral contraceptives.[38-40] Although benign, and rare, these may rupture and may cause death through intra-abdominal hemorrhage. Such lesions have not yet been reported in association with other estrogen or progestogen preparations but should be considered in estrogen users having abdominal pain and tenderness, abdominal mass, or hypovolemic shock. Hepatocellular carcinoma has also been reported in women taking estrogen-containing oral contraceptives.[39] The relationship of this malignancy to these drugs is not known at this time.

c. *Elevated blood pressure.* Increased blood pressure is not uncommon in women using oral contraceptives. There is now a report that this may occur with use of estrogens during menopause.[41] Blood pressure should be monitored with estrogen use, especially if high doses are used.

d. *Glucose tolerance.* A worsening of glucose tolerance has been observed in a significant percentage of patients on estrogen-containing oral contraceptives. For this reason, diabetic patients should be carefully observed while receiving estrogen.

4. *Hypercalcemia.* Administration of estrogens may lead to severe hypercalcemia in patients with breast cancer and bone metastases. If this occurs, the drug should be stopped and appropriate measures taken to reduce the serum calcium level.

PRECAUTIONS

A. General

1. A complete medical and family history should be taken prior to the initiation of any estrogen therapy. The pretreatment and periodic physical examinations should include special reference to blood pressure, breasts, abdomen, and pelvic organs, and should include a Papanicolaou smear. As a general rule, estrogen should not be prescribed for longer than one year without another physical examination being performed.

Continued on next page

Ortho Pharm.—Cont.

2. Fluid retention—Because estrogens may cause some degree of fluid retention, conditions which might be influenced by this factor such as epilepsy, migraine, and cardiac or renal dysfunction, require careful observation.

3. Certain patients may develop undesirable manifestations of excessive estrogenic stimulation, such as abnormal or excessive uterine bleeding, mastodynia, etc.

4. Oral contraceptives appear to be associated with an increased incidence of mental depression.[24] Although it is not clear whether this is due to the estrogenic or progestogenic component of the contraceptive, patients with a history of depression should be carefully observed.

5. Preexisting uterine leiomyomata may increase in size during estrogen use.

6. The pathologist should be advised of estrogen therapy when relevant specimens are submitted.

7. Patients with a past history of jaundice during pregnancy have an increased risk of recurrence of jaundice while receiving estrogen-containing oral contraceptive therapy. If jaundice develops in any patient receiving estrogen, the medication should be discontinued while the cause is investigated.

8. Estrogens may be poorly metabolized in patients with impaired liver function and they should be administered with caution in such patients.

9. Because estrogens influence the metabolism of calcium and phosphorus, they should be used with caution in patients with metabolic bone diseases that are associated with hypercalcemia or in patients with renal insufficiency.

10. Because of the effects of estrogens on epiphyseal closure, they should be used judiciously in young patients in whom bone growth is not complete.

11. The lowest effective dose appropriate for the specific indication should be utilized. Studies of the addition of a progestin for seven or more days of a cycle of estrogen administration have reported a lowered incidence of endometrial hyperplasia. Morphological and biochemical studies of endometrium suggest that 10 to 13 days of progestin are needed to provide maximal maturation of the endometrium and to eliminate any hyperplastic changes. Whether this will provide protection from endometrial carcinoma has not been clearly established. There are possible additional risks which may be associated with the inclusion of progestin in estrogen replacement regimens. The potential risks include adverse effects on carbohydrate and lipid metabolism. The choice of progestin and dosage may be important in minimizing these adverse effects.

B. Information for Patients: See text of Patient Package Information which is reproduced below.

C. Drug/Laboratory Test Interactions

Certain endocrine and liver function tests may be affected by estrogen-containing oral contraceptives. The following similar changes may be expected with larger doses of estrogen:

1. Increased sulfobromophthalein retention.
2. Increased prothrombin and factors VII, VIII, IX and X; decreased antithrombin 3; increased norepinephrine-induced platelet aggregability.
3. Increased thyroid-binding globulin (TBG) leading to increased circulating total thyroid hormone, as measured by PBI, T4 by column, or T4 by radioimmunoassay. Free T3 resin uptake is decreased, reflecting the elevated TBG; free T4 concentration is unaltered.
4. Impaired glucose tolerance.
5. Decreased pregnanediol excretion.
6. Reduced response to metyrapone test.
7. Reduced serum folate concentration.
8. Increased serum triglyceride and phospholipid concentration.

D. Carcinogenesis, Mutagenesis, Impairment of Fertility: See "Warnings" section for information on carcinogenesis, mutagenesis and impairment of fertility.

E. Pregnancy:
Teratogenic Effects.
Pregnancy Category X.
See "Contraindications" section.

F. Nursing Mothers: It is not known whether this drug is excreted in human milk. Because many drugs are excreted in human milk, caution should be exercised when estrogens are administered to a nursing woman.

ADVERSE REACTIONS

(See Warnings regarding induction of neoplasia, adverse effects on the fetus, increased incidence of gall bladder disease, and adverse effects similar to those of oral contraceptives, including thromboembolism.) The following additional adverse reactions have been reported with estrogenic therapy, including oral contraceptives:

1. *Genitourinary system.*
Increase in size of uterine fibromyomata.
Vaginal candidiasis.
Breakthrough bleeding, spotting, change in menstrual flow.
Dysmenorrhea.

Premenstrual-like syndrome.
Amenorrhea during and after treatment.
Change in cervical eversion and in degree of cervical secretion.
Cystitis-like syndrome.

2. *Breasts.*
Tenderness, enlargement, secretion.

3. *Gastrointestinal.*
Cholestatic jaundice.
Nausea, vomiting.
Abdominal cramps, bloating.

4. *Skin.*
Erythema multiforme.
Erythema nodosum.
Hemorrhagic eruption.
Loss of scalp hair.
Hirsutism.
Chloasma or melasma which may persist when drug is discontinued.

5. *Eyes.*
Steepening of corneal curvature.
Intolerance to contact lenses.

6. *CNS.*
Mental depression.
Headache, migraine, dizziness.
Chorea.

7. *Miscellaneous.*
Reduced carbohydrate tolerance.
Aggravation of porphyria.
Edema.
Changes in libido.
Increase or decrease in weight.

OVERDOSAGE

Numerous reports of ingestion of large doses of estrogen-containing oral contraceptives by young children indicate that serious ill effects do not occur. Overdosage of estrogen may cause nausea, and withdrawal bleeding may occur in females.

DOSAGE AND ADMINISTRATION

Given cyclically for short term use only:
For treatment of atrophic vaginitis, or kraurosis vulvae associated with the menopause.

The lowest dose that will control symptoms should be chosen and medication should be discontinued as promptly as possible.

Attempts to discontinue or taper medication should be made at 3 to 6 month intervals.

The usual dosage range is one or two applicatorsful per day for one or two weeks, then gradually reduced to one half initial dosage for a similar period. A maintenance dosage of one applicatorful, one to three times a week, may be used after restoration of the vaginal mucosa has been achieved.

Treated patients with an intact uterus should be monitored closely for signs of endometrial cancer and appropriate diagnostic measures should be taken to rule out malignancy in the event of persistent or recurring abnormal vaginal bleeding.

SUPPLIED

Available in 2.75 oz. (78g) tubes with or without ORTHO® Measured-Dose Applicator.
With applicator: NDC 0062-5450-77
Without applicator: NDC 0062-5450-00
Store at controlled room temperature.

1. Ziel, H.K. and W.D. Finkle, "Increased Risk of Endometrial Carcinoma Among Users of Conjugated Estrogens," *New England Journal of Medicine,* 293:1167–1170, 1975.
2. Smith, D.C., R. Prentic, D.J. Thompson, and W.L. Hermann, "Association of Exogenous Estrogen and Endometrial Carcinoma," *New England Journal of Medicine,* 293:1164–1167, 1975.
3. Mack, T.M., M.C. Pike, B.E. Henderson, R.I. Pfeffer, V.R. Gerkins, M. Arthur, and S.E. Brown, "Estrogens and Endometrial Cancer in a Retirement Community," *New England Journal of Medicine,* 294:1267–1287, 1976.
4. Weiss, N.S., D.R. Szekely and D.F. Austin, "Increasing Incidence of Endometrial Cancer in the United States," *New England Journal of Medicine,* 294:1259–1262, 1976.
5. Herbst, A.L., H. Ulfelder and D.C. Poskanzer, "Adenocarcinoma of Vagina," *New England Journal of Medicine,* 284:878–881, 1971.
6. Greenwald, P., J. Barlow, P. Nasca, and W. Burnett, "Vaginal Cancer after Maternal Treatment with Synthetic Estrogens," *New England Journal of Medicine,* 285:390–392, 1971.
7. Lanier, A., K. Noller, D. Decker, L. Elveback, and L. Kurland, "Cancer and Stilbestrol. A Follow-up of 1719 Persons Exposed to Estrogens in Utero and Born 1943–1959," *Mayo Clinic Proceedings,* 48:793–799, 1973.
8. Herbst, A., R. Kurman, and R. Scully, "Vaginal and Cervical Abnormalities After Exposure to Stilbestrol In Utero," *Obstetrics and Gynecology,* 40:287–298, 1972.
9. Herbst, A., S. Robboy, G. Macdonald, and R. Scully, "The Effects of Local Progesterone on Stilbestrol-Associated Vaginal Adenosis," *American Journal of Obstetrics and Gynecology* 118:607–615, 1974.
10. Herbst, A., D. Poskanzer, S. Robboy, L. Friedlander, and R. Scully, "Prenatal Exposure to Stilbestrol, A Prospective Comparison of Exposed Female Offspring with Unexposed Controls," *New England Journal of Medicine,* 292:334–339, 1975.
11. Staffi, A., R. Mattingly, D. Foley, and W. Fetherston, "Clinical Diagnosis of Vaginal Adenosis," *Obstetrics and Gynecology,* 43:118–128, 1974.
12. Sherman, A.I., M. Goldrath, A. Berlin, V. Vakhariya, F. Banooni, W. Michaels, P. Goodman, S. Brown, "Cervical-Vaginal Adenosis After *In Utero* Exposure to Synthetic Estrogens," *Obstetrics and Gynecology,* 44:531–545, 1974.
13. Gal, I., B. Kirman, and J. Stern, "Hormone Pregnancy Tests and Congenital Malformation," *Nature,* 216:83, 1967.
14. Levy, E.P., A. Cohen, and F.C. Fraser, "Hormone Treatment During Pregnancy and Congenital Heart Defects," *Lancet,* 1:611, 1973.
15. Nora, J. and A. Nora, "Birth Defects and Oral Contraceptives," *Lancet,* 1:941–942, 1973.
16. Janerich, D.T., J.M. Piper, and D.M. Glebatis, "Oral Contraceptives and Congenital Limb-Reduction Defects," *New England Journal of Medicine,* 291:697–700, 1974.
17. "Estrogens for Oral or Parenteral Use," *Federal Register,* 40:8212, 1975.
18. Boston Collaborative Drug Surveillance Program, "Surgically Confirmed Gall Bladder Disease, Venous Thromboembolism and Breast Tumors in Relation to Post-Menopausal Estrogen Therapy," *New England Journal of Medicine,* 290:15–19, 1974.
18a. Hoover, R., L.A. Gray, Sr., P. Cole, and B. MacMahon, "Menopausal Estrogens and Breast Cancer," *New England Journal of Medicine,* 295:401–405, 1976.
19. Boston Collaborative Drug Surveillance Program, "Oral Contraceptives and Venous Thromboembolic Disease, Surgically Confirmed Gall Bladder Disease, and Breast Tumors," *Lancet* 1:1399–1404, 1973.
20. Daniel, D.G., H. Campbell, and A.C. Turnbull, "Puerperal Thromboembolism and Suppression of Lactation," *Lancet,* 2:287–289, 1967.
21. The Veterans Administration Cooperative Urological Research Group, "Carcinoma of the Prostate: Treatment Comparisons," *Journal of Urology,* 98:516–522, 1967.
22. Bailer, J.C., "Thromboembolism and Oestrogen Therapy," *Lancet,* 2:560, 1967.
23. Blackard, C., R. Doe, G. Mellinger, and D. Byar, "Incidence of Cardiovascular Disease and Death In Patients Receiving Diethylstilbestrol for Carcinoma of the Prostate," *Cancer,* 26:249–256, 1970.
24. Royal College of General Practitioners, "Oral Contraception and Thromboembolic Disease," *Journal of the Royal College of General Practitioners,* 13:267–279, 1967.
25. Inman, W.H.W. and M.P. Vessey, "Investigation of Deaths from Pulmonary, Coronary, and Cerebral Thrombosis and Embolism in Women of Child-Bearing Age," *British Medical Journal,* 2:193–199, 1968.
26. Vessey, M.P. and R. Doll, "Investigation of Relation Between Use of Oral Contraceptives and Thromboembolic Disease, A Further Report," *British Medical Journal,* 2:651–657, 1969.
27. Sartwell, P.E., A.T. Masi, F.G. Arthes, G.R. Greene, and H.E. Smith, "Thromboembolism and Oral Contraceptives: An Epidemiological Case Control Study," *American Journal of Epidemiology,* 90:365–380, 1969.
28. Collaborative Group for the Study of Stroke In Young Women, "Oral Contraception and Increased Risk of Cerebral Ischemia or Thrombosis," *New England Journal of Medicine,* 288:871–878, 1973.
29. Collaborative Group for the Study of Stroke in Young Women, "Oral Contraceptives and Stroke in Young Women: Associated Risk Factors," *Journal of the American Medical Association,* 231:718–722, 1975.
30. Mann, J.I. and W.H.W. Inman, "Oral Contraceptives and Death from Myocardial Infarction," *British Medical Journal,* 2:245–248, 1975.
31. Mann, J.I., M.P. Vessey, M. Thorogood, and R. Doll., "Myocardial Infarction in Young Women with Special Reference to Oral Contraceptive Practice," *British Medical Journal,* 2:241–245, 1975.
32. Inman, W.H.W., V.P. Vessey, B. Westerholm, and A. Engelund, "Thromboembolic Disease and the Steroidal Content of Oral Contraceptives," *British Medical Journal,* 2:203–209, 1970.
33. Stolley, P.D., J.A. Tonascia, M.S. Tockman, P.E. Sartwell, A.H. Rutledge, and M.P. Jacobs, "Thrombosis with Low-Estrogen Oral Contraceptives," *American Journal of Epidemiology,* 102:197–208, 1975.
34. Vessey, M.P., R. Doll, A.S. Fairbairn, and G. Glober, "Post-Operative Thromboembolism and the Use of the Oral Contraceptives," *British Medical Journal,* 3:123–126, 1970.
35. Greene, G.R. and P.E. Sartwell, "Oral Contraceptive Use in Patients with Thromboembolism Following Surgery, Trauma or Infection," *American Journal of Public Health,* 62:680–685, 1972.
36. Rosenberg, L., M.B. Armstrong and H. Jick, "Myocardial Infarction and Estrogen Therapy in Postmenopausal

Women," *New England Journal of Medicine*, 294:1256–1259, 1976.

37. Coronary Drug Project Research Group, "The Coronary Drug Project: Initial Findings Leading to Modifications of Its Research Protocol," *Journal of the American Medical Association*, 214:1303–1313, 1970.

38. Baum, J., F. Holtz, J.J. Bookstein, and E.W. Klein, "Possible Association between Benign Hepatomas and Oral Contraceptives," *Lancet*, 2:926–928, 1973.

39. Mays, E.T., W.M. Christopherson, M.M. Mahr, and H.C. Williams, "Hepatic Changes in Young Women Ingesting Contraceptive Steroids, Hepatic Hemorrhage and Primary Hepatic Tumors." *Journal of the American Medical Association*, 235:730–782, 1976.

40. Edmondson, H.A., B. Henderson, and B. Benton, "Liver Cell Adenomas Associated with the Use of Oral Contraceptives," *New England Journal of Medicine*, 294:470–472, 1976.

41. Pfeffer, R.I. and S. Van Den Noore, "Estrogen Use and Stroke Risk in Postmenopausal Women," *American Journal of Epidemiology*, 103:445–456, 1976.

PATIENT INFORMATION ABOUT ESTROGENS

Estrogens are female hormones produced by the ovaries. The ovaries make several different kinds of estrogens. In addition, scientists have been able to make a variety of synthetic estrogens. As far as we know, all these synthetic estrogens have similar properties and therefore much the same usefulness, side effects, and risks. This leaflet is intended to help you understand what estrogens are used for, some of the risks involved in their use, and to help minimize these risks. This leaflet includes important information about estrogens, but not all the information. If you want to know more, you can ask your doctor or pharmacist to let you read the package insert prepared for the doctor.

USES OF ESTROGEN

THERE IS NO PROPER USE OF ESTROGENS IN A PREGNANT WOMAN

Estrogens are prescribed by doctors for a number of purposes, including:

1. To provide estrogen during a period of adjustment when a woman's ovaries no longer produce it, in order to prevent certain uncomfortable symptoms of estrogen deficiency. (All women normally decrease the production of estrogens, generally between the ages of 45 and 55; this is called the menopause.)

2. To prevent symptoms of estrogen deficiency when a woman's ovaries have been removed surgically before the natural menopause.

3. To prevent pregnancy. (Estrogens are given along with a progestogen, another female hormone; these combinations are called oral contraceptives or birth control pills. Patient labeling is available to women taking oral contraceptives and they will not be discussed in this leaflet.)

4. To treat certain cancers in women and men.

5. To prevent painful swelling of the breasts after pregnancy in women who choose not to nurse their babies.

ESTROGENS IN THE MENOPAUSE

In the natural course of their lives, all women eventually experience a decrease in estrogen production. This usually occurs between ages 45 and 55 but may occur earlier or later. Sometimes the ovaries may need to be removed by an operation before natural menopause, producing a "surgical menopause."

When the amount of estrogen in the blood begins to decrease, many women may develop typical symptoms: Feelings of warmth in the face, neck, and chest or sudden intense episodes of heat and sweating throughout the body (called "hot flashes" or "hot flushes"). These symptoms are sometimes very uncomfortable. A few women eventually develop changes in the vagina (called "atrophic vaginitis") which cause discomfort, especially during and after intercourse. Estrogens can be prescribed to treat these symptoms of the menopause. It is estimated that considerably more than half of all women undergoing the menopause have only mild symptoms or no symptoms at all and therefore do not need estrogens. Other women may need estrogens for a few months, while their bodies adjust to lower estrogen levels. Sometimes the need will be for periods longer than six months. In an attempt to avoid over-stimulation of the uterus (womb), estrogens are usually given cyclically during each month of use, that is three weeks of pills followed by one week without pills.

Sometimes women experience nervous symptoms or depression during menopause. There is no evidence that estrogens are effective for such symptoms and they should not be used to treat them, although other treatment may be needed.

You may have heard that taking estrogens for long periods (years) after the menopause will keep your skin soft and supple and keep you feeling young. There is no evidence that this is so, however, and such long-term treatment carries important risks.

Estrogens to Prevent Swelling of the Breasts After Pregnancy: If you do not breast-feed your baby after delivery, your breasts may fill up with milk and become painful and engorged. This usually begins about three to four days after delivery and may last for a few days to up to a week or more. Sometimes the discomfort is severe, but usually it is not and can be controlled by pain-relieving drugs such as aspirin and by binding the breasts up tightly. Estrogens can be used to try to prevent the breasts from filling up. While this treatment is sometimes successful, in many cases the breasts fill up to some degree in spite of treatment. The dose of estrogens needed to prevent pain and swelling of the breasts is much larger than the dose needed to treat symptoms of the menopause and this may increase your chances of developing blood clots in the legs or lungs (see below). Therefore, it is important that you discuss the benefits and the risks of estrogen use with your doctor if you have decided not to breast-feed your baby.

Some of the Dangers of Estrogen:

1. *Cancer of the uterus.* If estrogens are used in the postmenopausal period for more than a year, there is an increased risk of *endometrial cancer* (cancer of the uterus). Women taking estrogens have roughly five to ten times as great a chance of getting this cancer as women who take no estrogens. To put this another way, while a postmenopausal woman not taking estrogens has one chance in 1,000 each year of getting cancer of the uterus, a woman taking estrogens has five to ten chances in 1,000 each year. For this reason *it is important to take estrogens only when you really need them.*

The risk of this cancer is greater the longer estrogens are used and also seems to be greater when larger doses are taken. For this reason *it is important to take the lowest dose of estrogen that will control symptoms and to take it only as long as it is needed.* If estrogens are needed for longer periods of time, your doctor will want to reevaluate your need for estrogens at least every six months.

Women using estrogens should report any irregular vaginal bleeding to their doctors; such bleeding may be of no importance, but it can be an early warning of cancer of the uterus. If you have undiagnosed vaginal bleeding, you should not use estrogens until a diagnosis is made and you are certain there is no cancer of the uterus.

If you have had your uterus completely removed (total hysterectomy), there is no danger of developing cancer of the uterus.

2. *Other possible cancers.* Estrogens can cause development of other tumors in animals, such as tumors of the breast, cervix, vagina, or liver, when given for a long time. At present there is no good evidence that women using estrogen in the menopause have an increased risk of such tumors, but there is no way yet to be sure they do not; and one study raises the possibility that use of estrogens in the menopause may increase the risk of breast cancer many years later. This is a further reason to use estrogens only when clearly needed. While you are taking estrogens, it is important that you go to your doctor at least once a year for a physical examination. Also, if members of your family have had breast cancer or if you have breast nodules or abnormal mammograms (breast x-rays), your doctor may wish to carry out more frequent examinations of your breasts.

3. *Gall bladder disease.* Women who use estrogens after menopause are more likely to develop gall bladder disease needing surgery than women who do not use estrogens. Birth control pills have a similar effect.

4. *Abnormal blood clotting.* Oral contraceptives, some of which contain estrogens, increase the risk of blood clotting in various parts of the body. This can result in a stroke (if the clot is in the brain), a heart attack (clot in a blood vessel of the heart), or a pulmonary embolus (a clot which forms in the legs or pelvis, then breaks off and travels to the lungs). Any of these can be fatal. Blood clots may result in the loss of a limb, paralysis or loss of sight, depending on where the blood clot is formed or lodges if it breaks loose.

The larger doses of estrogen used to prevent swelling of the breasts after pregnancy have been reported to cause clotting in the legs and lungs.

It is recommended that if you have had any blood clotting disorders including clotting in the legs or lungs, or a heart attack or stroke, you should not use estrogens.

Special Warning About Pregnancy: You should not receive estrogen if you are pregnant. If this should occur, there is a greater than usual chance that the developing child will be born with a birth defect, although the possibility remains fairly small. A female child then may have an increased risk of developing cancer of the vagina or cervix later in life (in the teens or twenties). Every possible effort should be made to avoid exposure to estrogens during pregnancy. If exposure occurs, see your doctor.

Some Other Effects of Estrogens: In addition to the serious known risks of estrogens described above, estrogens have the following side effects and potential risks:

1. *Nausea and vomiting.* The most common side effect of estrogen therapy is nausea. Vomiting is less common.

2. *Effects on breasts.* Estrogens may cause breast tenderness or enlargement and may cause the breasts to secrete a liquid.

3. *Effects on the uterus.* Estrogens may cause benign fibroid tumors of the uterus to get larger.

Some women will have menstrual bleeding when estrogens are stopped. But if the bleeding occurs on days you are still taking estrogens you should report this to your doctor.

4. *Effects on liver.* Women taking estrogens develop on rare occasions a tumor of the liver which can rupture and bleed into the abdomen. You should report any swelling or unusual pain or tenderness in the abdomen to your doctor immediately.

Women with a past history of jaundice (yellowing of the skin and white parts of the eyes) may get jaundice again during estrogen use.

5. *Other effects.* Estrogens may cause excess fluid to be retained in the body. This may make some conditions worse, such as epilepsy, migraine, heart disease, or kidney disease. If any of the above occur, stop taking estrogens and call your doctor.

SUMMARY

Estrogens have important uses, but they have serious risks as well. You must decide, with your doctor, whether the risks are acceptable to you in view of the benefits of treatment. Except where your doctor has prescribed estrogens for use in special cases of cancer of the breast or prostate, you should not use estrogens if you have cancer of the breast or uterus, are pregnant, have undiagnosed abnormal vaginal bleeding, blood clotting disorders including clotting in the legs or lungs, or have had a stroke, heart attack or angina.

You must understand that your doctor will require regular physical examinations while you are taking them and will try to discontinue the drug as soon as possible and use the smallest dose possible. You can help minimize the risk by being alert for signs of trouble including:

1. Abnormal bleeding from the vagina.
2. Pains in the calves or chest or sudden shortness of breath, or coughing blood (indicating possible clots in the legs, heart or lungs).
3. Severe headache, dizziness, faintness, or changes in vision (indicating possible developing clots in the brain or eye).
4. Breast lumps (you should ask your doctor how to examine your own breasts).
5. Jaundice (yellowing of the skin).
6. Mental depression.
7. *Any* other unusual condition or problem.

Based on his or her assessment of your medical needs, your doctor has prescribed this drug for you. Do not give the drug to anyone else.

HOW SUPPLIED

Available in 2.75 oz. (78g) tubes with or without ORTHO® Measured-Dose Applicator.
With applicator: NDC 0062-5450-77
Without applicator: NDC 0062-5450-00
Store at controlled room temperature.

ORTHO® Personal Lubricant

(See PDR For Nonprescription Drugs)

ORTHO-GYNOL® Contraceptive Jelly

(See PDR For Nonprescription Drugs)

ORTHO–NOVUM® Tablets   ℞
(norethindrone/mestranol) or
(norethindrone/ethinyl estradiol)
and

MODICON® Tablets   ℞
(norethindrone/ethinyl estradiol)
and

MICRONOR® Tablets   ℞
(norethindrone)

DESCRIPTION

COMBINATION ORAL CONTRACEPTIVES

Each of the following products is a combination oral contraceptive containing the progestational compound norethindrone and the estrogenic compound ethinyl estradiol: ORTHO-NOVUM 7/7/7 □ 21 Tablets and ORTHO-NOVUM 7/7/7□ 28 Tablets: Each white tablet contains 0.5 mg of norethindrone and 0.035 mg of ethinyl estradiol. Inactive ingredients include lactose, magnesium stearate, and pregelatinized starch. Each light peach tablet contains 0.75 mg of norethindrone and 0.035 mg of ethinyl estradiol. Inactive ingredients include FD&C Yellow No. 6, lactose, magnesium stearate, and pregelatinized starch. Each peach tablet contains 1 mg of norethindrone and 0.035 mg of ethinyl estradiol. Inactive ingredients include FD&C Yellow No. 6, lactose, magnesium stearate, and pregelatinized starch. Each green tablet in the ORTHO-NOVUM 7/7/7 □ 28 package contains only inert ingredients, as follows: D&C Yellow No. 10 Aluminum Lake, FD&C Blue No. 2 Aluminum Lake,

Continued on next page

Ortho Pharm.—Cont.

lactose, magnesium stearate, microcrystalline cellulose and pregelatinized starch.

ORTHO-NOVUM 10/11 □ 21 Tablets and ORTHO-NOVUM 10/11 □ 28 Tablets: Each white tablet contains 0.5 mg of norethindrone and 0.035 mg of ethinyl estradiol. Inactive ingredients include lactose, magnesium stearate, and pregelatinized starch. Each peach tablet contains 1 mg norethindrone and 0.035 mg of ethinyl estradiol. Inactive ingredients include FD&C Yellow No. 6, lactose, magnesium stearate, and pregelatinized starch. Each green tablet in the ORTHO-NOVUM 10/11 □ 28 package contains only inert ingredients, as listed under green tablets in ORTHO-NOVUM 7/7/7 □ 28.

ORTHO-NOVUM 1/35 □ 21 Tablets and ORTHO-NOVUM 1/35 □ 28 Tablets: Each peach tablet contains 1 mg of norethindrone and 0.035 mg of ethinyl estradiol. Inactive ingredients include FD&C Yellow No. 6, lactose, magnesium stearate and pregelatinized starch. Each green tablet in the ORTHO-NOVUM 1/35 □ 28 package contains only inert ingredients, as listed under green tablets in ORTHO-NOVUM 7/7/7 □ 28.

MODICON 21 Tablets and MODICON 28 Tablets: Each white tablet contains 0.5 mg of norethindrone and 0.035 mg of ethinyl estradiol. Inactive ingredients include lactose, magnesium stearate, and pregelatinized starch. Each green tablet in the MODICON 28 package contains only inert ingredients, as listed under green tablets in ORTHO-NOVUM 7/7/7 □ 28.

Each of the following products is a combination oral contraceptive containing the progestational compound norethindrone and the estrogenic compound mestranol:

ORTHO-NOVUM 1/50 □ 21 Tablets and ORTHO-NOVUM 1/50 □ 28 Tablets: Each yellow tablet contains 1 mg of norethindrone and 0.05 mg of mestranol. Inactive ingredients include D&C Yellow No. 10, lactose, magnesium stearate, and pregelatinized starch. Each green tablet in the ORTHO-NOVUM 1/50 □ 28 package contains only inert ingredients, as listed under green tablets in ORTHO-NOVUM 7/7/7 □ 28.

ORTHO-NOVUM 1/80 □ 21 Tablets and ORTHO-NOVUM 1/80 □ 28 tablets: Each white tablet contains 1 mg of norethindrone and 0.08 mg of mestranol. Inactive ingredients include lactose, magnesium stearate and pregelatinized starch. Each green tablet in the ORTHO-NOVUM 1/80 □ 28 package contains only inert ingredients, as listed under green tablets in ORTHO-NOVUM 7/7/7 □ 28.

ORTHO-NOVUM 2 mg □ 21 Tablets each contain 2 mg of norethindrone and 0.10 mg of mestranol. Inactive ingredients include lactose, magnesium stearate, and pregelatinized starch.

PROGESTOGEN-ONLY ORAL CONTRACEPTIVE

The following product is a progestogen-only oral contraceptive containing the progestational compound norethindrone: MICRONOR Tablets: Each tablet contains 0.35 mg of norethindrone. Inactive ingredients include D&C Green No. 5, D&C Yellow No. 10, lactose, magnesium stearate, povidone and starch.

The chemical name for norethindrone is 17-hydroxy-19-nor-17α-pregn-4-en-20-yn-3-one, for ethinyl estradiol is 19-nor-17α-pregna-1,3,5(10)-trien-20-yne-3,17-diol, and for mestranol is 3-methoxy-19-nor-17α-pregna, 1,3,5(10)-trien-20-yn-17-ol.

CLINICAL PHARMACOLOGY
COMBINATION ORAL CONTRACEPTIVES

Combination oral contraceptives act by suppression of gonadotropins. Although the primary mechanism of this action is inhibition of ovulation, other alterations include changes in the cervical mucus (which increase the difficulty of sperm entry into the uterus) and the endometrium (which reduce the likelihood of implantation).

CLINICAL PHARMACOLOGY
PROGESTOGEN-ONLY ORAL CONTRACEPTIVES

The primary mechanism through which MICRONOR prevents conception is not known, but progestogen-only contraceptives are known to alter the cervical mucus, exert a progestational effect on the endometrium, interfering with implantation, and, in some patients, suppress ovulation.

INDICATIONS AND USAGE

ORTHO-NOVUM 7/7/7 □ 21, ORTHO-NOVUM 7/7/7 □ 28, ORTHO-NOVUM 10/11 □ 21, ORTHO-NOVUM 10/11 □ 28, ORTHO-NOVUM 1/35 □ 21, ORTHO-NOVUM 1/35 □ 28, MODICON 21, MODICON 28, ORTHO-NOVUM 1/50 □ 21, ORTHO-NOVUM 1/50 □ 28, ORTHO-NOVUM 1/80 □ 21, ORTHO-NOVUM 1/80 □ 28, and MICRONOR are indicated for the prevention of pregnancy in women who elect to use this product as a method of contraception.

Oral contraceptives are highly effective. Table I lists the typical accidental pregnancy rates for users of combination oral contraceptives and other methods of contraception. The efficacy of these contraceptive methods, except sterilization, depends upon the reliability with which they are used. Correct and consistent use of methods can result in lower failure rates.

ORTHO-NOVUM 2 mg □ 21 is indicated for the treatment of hypermenorrhea. It is indicated for contraception only when lower dose formulations prove unacceptable.

TABLE I: LOWEST EXPECTED AND TYPICAL FAILURE RATES DURING THE FIRST YEAR OF CONTINUOUS USE OF A METHOD

% of Women Experiencing an Accidental Pregnancy in the First Year of Continuous Use

Method	Lowest Expected*	Typical**
(No contraception)	(89)	(89)
Oral contraceptives		3
combined	0.1	N/A***
progestin only	0.5	N/A***
Diaphragm with spermicidal cream or jelly	3	18
Spermicides alone (foam, creams, jellies and vaginal suppositories)	3	21
Vaginal sponge		
nulliparous	5	18
multiparous	>8	>28
IUD (medicated)	1	6#
Condom without spermicides	2	12
Periodic abstinence (all methods)	2–10	20
Female sterilization	0.2	0.4
Male sterilization	0.1	0.15

Adapted from J. Trussell and K. Kost, Table II, ref. #1.
* The authors' best guess of the percentage of women expected to experience an accidental pregnancy among couples who initiate a method (not necessarily for the first time) and who use it consistently and correctly during the first year if they do not stop for any other reason.
** This term represents "typical" couples who initiate use of a method (not necessarily for the first time), who experience an accidental pregnancy during the first year if they do not stop for any other reason.
*** N/A—Data not available
# Combined typical rate for both medicated and non-medicated IUD. The rate for medicated IUD alone is not available.

CONTRAINDICATIONS

Oral contraceptives should not be used in women who currently have the following conditions:
- Thrombophlebitis or thromboembolic disorders
- A past history of deep vein thrombophlebitis or thromboembolic disorders
- Cerebral vascular or coronary artery disease
- Known or suspected carcinoma of the breast
- Carcinoma of the endometrium or other known or suspected estrogen-dependent neoplasia
- Undiagnosed abnormal genital bleeding
- Cholestatic jaundice of pregnancy or jaundice with prior pill use
- Hepatic adenomas or carcinomas
- Known or suspected pregnancy

WARNINGS

> Cigarette smoking increases the risk of serious cardiovascular side effects from oral contraceptive use This risk increases with age and with heavy smoking (15 or more cigarettes per day) and is quite marked in women over 35 years of age Women who use oral contraceptives should be strongly advised not to smoke.

The use of oral contraceptives is associated with increased risks of several serious conditions including myocardial infarction, thromboembolism, stroke, hepatic neoplasia, and gallbladder disease, although the risk of serious morbidity or mortality is very small in healthy women without underlying factors. The risk of morbidity and mortality increases significantly in the presence of other underlying risk factors such as hypertension, hyperlipidemias, obesity and diabetes. Practitioners prescribing oral contraceptives should be familiar with the following information relating to these risks. The information contained in this package insert is principally based on studies carried out in patients who used oral contraceptives with higher formulations of estrogens and progestogens than those in common use today. The effect of long term use of the oral contraceptives with lower formulations of both estrogens and progestogens remains to be determined.

Throughout this labeling, epidemiological studies reported are of two types: retrospective or case control studies and prospective or cohort studies. Case control studies provide a measure of the relative risk of a disease, namely, a *ratio* of the incidence of a disease among oral contraceptive users to that among nonusers. The relative risk does not provide information on the actual clinical occurrence of a disease. Cohort studies provide a measure of attributable risk, which is the *difference* in the incidence of disease between oral contraceptive users and nonusers. The attributable risk does provide information about the actual occurrence of a disease in the population (Adapted from refs. 2 and 3 with the author's permission). For further information, the reader is referred to a text on epidemiological methods.

1. THROMBOEMBOLIC DISORDERS AND OTHER VASCULAR PROBLEMS
a. Myocardial Infarction

An increased risk of myocardial infarction has been associated with oral contraceptive use. This risk is primarily in smokers or women with other underlying risk factors for coronary artery disease such as hypertension, hypercholesterolemia, morbid obesity, and diabetes. The relative risk of heart attack for current oral contraceptive users has been estimated to be two to six (4–10). The risk is very low under the age of 30.

Smoking in combination with oral contraceptive use has been shown to contribute substantially to the incidence of myocardial infarctions in women in their mid-thirties or older with smoking accounting for the majority of excess cases (11). Mortality rates associated with circulatory disease have been shown to increase substantially in smokers, especially in those 35 years of age and older among women who use oral contraceptives.

CIRCULATORY DISEASE MORTALITY RATES PER 100,000 WOMEN YEARS BY AGE, SMOKING STATUS AND ORAL CONTRACEPTIVE USE

TABLE II. (Adapted from P.M. Layde and V. Beral, ref. #12.)

Oral contraceptives may compound the effects of well-known risk factors, such as hypertension, diabetes, hyperlipidemias, age and obesity (13). In particular, some progestogens are known to decrease HDL cholesterol and cause glucose intolerance, while estrogens may create a state of hyperinsulinism (14–18). Oral contraceptives have been shown to increase blood pressure among users (see section 9 in Warnings). Similar effects on risk factors have been associated with an increased risk of heart disease. Oral contraceptives must be used with caution in women with cardiovascular disease risk factors.

b. Thromboembolism

An increased risk of thromboembolic and thrombotic disease associated with the use of oral contraceptives is well established. Case control studies have found the relative risk of users compared to non-users to be 3 for the first episode of superficial venous thrombosis, 4 to 11 for deep vein thrombosis or pulmonary embolism, and 1.5 to 6 for women with predisposing conditions for venous thromboembolic disease (2,3,19–24). Cohort studies have shown the relative risk to be somewhat lower, about 3 for new cases and about 4.5 for new cases requiring hospitalization (25). The risk of thromboembolic disease associated with oral contraceptives is not related to length of use and disappears after pill use is stopped (2).

A two- to four-fold increase in relative risk of post-operative thromboembolic complications has been reported with the use of oral contraceptives (9). The relative risk of venous thrombosis in women who have predisposing conditions is twice that of women without such medical conditions (26). If feasible, oral contraceptives should be discontinued at least four weeks prior to and for two weeks after elective surgery of a type associated with an increase in risk of thromboembolism and during and following prolonged immobilization. Since the immediate postpartum period is also associated with an increased risk of thromboembolism, oral contraceptives should be started no earlier than four weeks after delivery in women who elect not to breast feed.

c. Cerebrovascular diseases

Oral contraceptives have been shown to increase both the relative and attributable risks of cerebrovascular events (thrombotic and hemorrhagic strokes), although, in general, the risk is greatest among older (> 35 years), hypertensive women who also smoke. Hypertension was found to be a risk factor for both users and non-users, for both types of strokes, and smoking interacted to increase the risk of stroke (27–29). In a large study, the relative risk of thrombotic strokes has been shown to range from 3 for normotensive users to 14 for users with severe hypertension (30). The relative risk of hemorrhagic stroke is reported to be 1.2 for non-smokers who used oral contraceptives, 2.6 for smokers who did not use oral contraceptives, 7.6 for smokers who used oral contraceptives, 1.8 for normotensive users and 25.7 for users with severe hypertension (30). The attributable risk is also greater in older women (3).

d. Dose-related risk of vascular disease from oral contraceptives

A positive association has been observed between the amount of estrogen and progestogen in oral contraceptives and the risk of vascular disease (31–33). A decline in serum high density lipoproteins (HDL) has been reported with many progestational agents (14–16). A decline in serum high density lipoproteins has been associated with an increased incidence of ischemic heart disease. Because estrogens increase HDL cholesterol, the net effect of an oral contraceptive depends on a balance achieved between doses of estrogen and progestogen and the activity of the progestogen used in the contraceptive. The activity and amount of both hormones should be considered in the choice of an oral contraceptive.

Minimizing exposure to estrogen and progestogen is in keeping with good principles of therapeutics. For any particular estrogen/progestogen combination, the dosage regimen prescribed should be one which contains the least amount of estrogen and progestogen that is compatible with a low failure rate and the needs of the individual patient. New acceptors of oral contraceptives agents should be started on preparations containing 0.035 mg or less of estrogen.

e. Persistence of risk of vascular disease

There are two studies which have shown persistence of risk of vascular disease for ever-users of oral contraceptives.

In a study in the United States, the risk of developing myocardial infarction after discontinuing oral contraceptives persists for at least 9 years for women 40–49 years who had used oral contraceptives for five or more years, but this increased risk was not demonstrated in other age groups (8). In another study in Great Britain, the risk of developing cerebrovascular disease persisted for at least 6 years after discontinuation of oral contraceptives, although excess risk was very small (34). However, both studies were performed with oral contraceptive formulations containing 50 micrograms or higher of estrogens.

2. ESTIMATES OF MORTALITY FROM CONTRACEPTIVE USE

One study gathered data from a variety of sources which have estimated the mortality rate associated with different methods of contraception at different ages (Table III). These estimates include the combined risk of death associated with contraceptive methods plus the risk attributable to pregnancy in the event of method failure. Each method of contraception has its specific benefits and risks. The study concluded that with the exception of oral contraceptive users 35 and older who smoke and 40 and older who do not smoke, mortality associated with all methods of birth control is low and below that associated with childbirth. However, smokers 35 and older and non-smokers 40 and older who use oral contraceptives have a significant increase in mortality higher than those using other methods of birth control. These facts must be weighed in conjunction with failure rates for other methods and the risk associated with subsequent pregnancy. (See Table I.)

[See table above].

3. CARCINOMA OF THE REPRODUCTIVE ORGANS

Numerous epidemiological studies have been performed on the incidence of breast, endometrial, ovarian and cervical cancer in women using oral contraceptives. While there are conflicting reports the overall evidence in the literature suggests that use of oral contraceptives is not associated with an increase in the risk of developing breast cancer (36,38). The Cancer and Steroid Hormone (CASH) study (36,79) also showed no latent effect on the risk of breast cancer for at least a decade following long term use. Some studies have shown a slightly increased relative risk of developing breast cancer (37,39–43).

Some studies suggest that oral contraceptive use has been associated with an increase in the risk of cervical intraepithelial neoplasia in some populations of women (45–48). However, there continues to be controversy about the extent to which such findings may be due to differences in sexual behavior and other factors.

In spite of many studies of the relationship between oral contraceptive use and breast and cervical cancers, a cause and effect relationship has not been established.

4. HEPATIC NEOPLASIA

Benign hepatic adenomas are associated with oral contraceptive use, although the incidence of benign tumors is rare in the United States. Indirect calculations have estimated the

TABLE III—ANNUAL NUMBER OF BIRTH-RELATED OR METHOD-RELATED DEATHS ASSOCIATED WITH CONTROL OF FERTILITY PER 100,000 NON-STERILE WOMEN, BY FERTILITY CONTROL METHOD ACCORDING TO AGE

Method of control and outcome	15–19	20–24	25–29	30–34	35–39	40–44
No fertility control methods*	7.0	7.4	9.1	14.8	25.7	28.2
Oral contraceptives non-smoker**	0.3	0.5	0.9	1.9	13.8	31.6
Oral contraceptives smoker**	2.2	3.4	6.6	13.5	51.1	117.2
IUD**	0.8	0.8	1.0	1.0	1.4	1.4
Condom*	1.1	1.6	0.7	0.2	0.3	0.4
Diaphragm/spermicide*	1.9	1.2	1.2	1.3	2.2	2.8
Periodic abstinence*	2.5	1.6	1.6	1.7	2.9	3.6

* Deaths are birth related
** Deaths are method related

Adapted from H.W. Ory, ref. #35.

attributable risk to be in the range of 3.3 cases/100,000 for users, a risk that increases after four or more years of use especially with oral contraceptives of higher dose (49). Rupture of benign, hepatic adenomas may cause death through intra-abdominal hemorrhage (50,51).

Studies from Britain have shown an increased risk of developing hepatocellular carcinoma (52–54) in long-term (> 8 years) oral contraceptive users. However, these cancers are rare in the U.S. and the attributable risk (the excess incidence) of liver cancers in oral contraceptive users approaches less than one per million users.

5. OCULAR LESIONS

There have been clincial case reports of retinal thrombosis associated with the use of oral contraceptives. Oral contraceptives should be discontinued if there is unexplained partial or complete loss of vision; onset of proptosis or diplopia; papilledema; or retinal vascular lesions. Appropriate diagnostic and therapeutic measures should be undertaken immediately.

6. ORAL CONTRACEPTIVE USE BEFORE OR DURING EARLY PREGNANCY: RISK OF BIRTH DEFECTS

Extensive epidemiological studies have revealed no increased risk of birth defects in women who have used oral contraceptives prior to pregnancy (56,57). The majority of recent studies also do not indicate a teratogenic effect, particularly in so far as cardiac anomalies and limb reduction defects are concerned (55,56,58,59), when taken inadvertently during early pregnancy.

The administration of oral contraceptives to induce withdrawal bleeding should not be used as a test for pregnancy. Oral contraceptives should not be used during pregnancy to treat threatened or habitual abortion.

It is recommended that for any patient who has missed two consecutive periods (or after 45 days from the last menstrual period if the progestogen-only oral contraceptives are used), pregnancy should be ruled out before continuing oral contraceptive use. If the patient has not adhered to the prescribed schedule, the possibility of pregnancy should be considered at the time of the first missed period or upon missing one MICRONOR Tablet. Oral contraceptive use should be discontinued until pregnancy is ruled out.

7. GALLBLADDER DISEASE

Earlier studies have reported an increased lifetime relative risk of gallbladder surgery in users of oral contraceptives and estrogens (60,61). More recent studies, however, have shown that the relative risk of developing gallbladder disease among oral contraceptive users may be minimal (62–64). The recent findings of minimal risk may be related to the use of oral contraceptive formulations containing lower hormonal doses of estrogens and progestogens.

8. CARBOHYDRATE AND LIPID METABOLIC EFFECTS

Oral contraceptives have been shown to cause a decrease in glucose tolerance in a significant percentage of users (17). This effect has been shown to be directly related to estrogen dose (65). Progestogens increase insulin secretion and create insulin resistance, this effect varying with different progestational agents (17,66). However, in the non-diabetic woman, oral contraceptives appear to have no effect on fasting blood glucose (67). Because of these demonstrated effects, prediabetic and diabetic women in particular should be carefully monitored while taking oral contraceptives.

A small proportion of women will have persistent hypertriglyceridemia while on the pill. As discussed earlier (see Warnings 1a. and 1d.), changes in serum triglycerides and lipoprotein levels have been reported in oral contraceptive users.

9. ELEVATED BLOOD PRESSURE

An increase in blood pressure has been reported in women taking oral contraceptives (68) and this increase is more likely in older oral contraceptive users (69) and with extended duration of use (61). Data from the Royal College of General Practitioners (12) and subsequent randomized trials have shown that the incidence of hypertension increases with increasing progestational activity.

Women with a history of hypertension or hypertension-related diseases, or renal disease (70) should be encouraged to use another method of contraception. If women elect to use oral contraceptives, they should be monitored closely and if significant elevation of blood pressure occurs, oral contraceptives should be discontinued. For most women, elevated blood pressure will return to normal after stopping oral contraceptives, and there is no difference in the occurrence of hypertension between former and never users (68–71).

10. HEADACHE

The onset or exacerbation of migraine or development of headache with a new pattern which is recurrent, persistent or severe requires discontinuation of oral contraceptives and evaluation of the cause.

11. BLEEDING IRREGULARITIES

Breakthrough bleeding and spotting are sometimes encountered in patients on oral contraceptives, especially during the first three months of use. Non-hormonal causes should be considered and adequate diagnostic measures taken to rule out malignancy or pregnancy in the event of breakthrough bleeding, as in the case of any abnormal vaginal bleeding. If pathology has been excluded, time or a change to another formulation may solve the problem. In the event of amenorrhea, pregnancy should be ruled out.

An alteration in menstrual patterns is likely to occur in women using progestogen-only contraceptives. The amount and duration of flow, cycle length, breakthrough bleeding, spotting and amenorrhea will probably be quite variable. Bleeding irregularities occur more frequently with the use of progestogen-only oral contraceptives than with the combinations and the dropout rate due to such conditions is higher. Some women may encounter post-pill amenorrhea or oligomenorrhea, especially when such a condition was preexistent.

12. ECTOPIC PREGNANCY

Ectopic as well as intrauterine pregnancy may occur in contraceptive failures. However, in progestogen-only oral contraceptive failures, the ratio of ectopic to intrauterine pregnancies is higher than in women who are not receiving oral contraceptives, since the drugs are more effective in preventing intrauterine than ectopic pregnancies.

PRECAUTIONS

1. PHYSICAL EXAMINATION AND FOLLOW UP

A complete medical history and physical examination should be taken prior to the initiation or reinstitution of oral contraceptives and at least annually during use of oral contraceptives. These physical examinations should include special reference to blood pressure, breasts, abdomen and pelvic organs, including cervical cytology, and relevant laboratory tests. In case of undiagnosed, persistent or recurrent abnormal vaginal bleeding, appropriate diagnostic measures should be conducted to rule out malignancy. Women with a strong family history of breast cancer or who have breast nodules should be monitored with particular care.

2. LIPID DISORDERS

Women who are being treated for hyperlipidemias should be followed closely if they elect to use oral contraceptives. Some progestogens may elevate LDL levels and may render the control of hyperlipidemias more difficult.

3. LIVER FUNCTION

If jaundice develops in any woman receiving such drugs, the medication should be discontinued. Steroid hormones may be poorly metabolized in patients with impaired liver function.

4. FLUID RETENTION

Oral contraceptives may cause some degree of fluid retention. They should be prescribed with caution, and only with careful monitoring, in patients with conditions which might be aggravated by fluid retention.

Continued on next page

Ortho Pharm.—Cont.

5. EMOTIONAL DISORDERS
Women with a history of depression should be carefully observed and the drug discontinued if depression recurs to a serious degree.

6. CONTACT LENSES
Contact lens wearers who develop visual changes or changes in lens tolerance should be assessed by an ophthalmologist.

7. DRUG INTERACTIONS
Reduced efficacy and increased incidence of breakthrough bleeding and menstrual irregularies have been associated with concomitant use of rifampin. A similar assocation, though less marked, has been suggested with barbiturates, phenylbutazone, phenytoin sodium, and possibly with griseofulvin, ampicillin and tetracyclines (72).

8. INTERACTIONS WITH LABORATORY TESTS
Certain endocrine and liver function tests and blood components may be affected by oral contraceptives:
a. Increased prothrombin and factors VII, VIII, IX, and X; decreased antithrombin 3; increased norepinephrine-induced platelet aggregability.
b. Increased thyroid binding globulin (TBG) leading to increased circulating total thyroid hormone, as measured by protein-bound iodine (PBI), T4 by column or by radio-immunoassay. Free T3 resin uptake is decreased, reflecting the elevated TBG, free T4 concentration is unaltered.
c. Other binding proteins may be elevated in serum.
d. Sex-binding globulins are increased and result in elevated levels of total circulating sex steroids and corticoids; however, free or biologically active levels remain unchanged.
e. Triglycerides may be increased.
f. Glucose tolerance may be decreased.
g. Serum folate levels may be depressed by oral contraceptive therapy. This may be of clinical significance if a woman becomes pregnant shortly after discontinuing oral contraceptives

9. CARCINOGENESIS
See WARNINGS section.

10. PREGNANCY
Pregnancy Category X. See CONTRAINDICATIONS and WARNINGS sections.

11. NURSING MOTHERS
Small amounts of oral contraceptive steroids have been identified in the milk of nursing mothers and a few adverse effects on the child have been reported, including jaundice and breast enlargement. In addition, oral contraceptives given in the postpartum period may interfere with lactation by decreasing the quantity and quality of breast milk. If possible, the nursing mother should be advised not to use oral contraceptives but to use other forms of contraception until she has completely weaned her child.

INFORMATION FOR THE PATIENT
See Patient Labeling Printed Below

ADVERSE REACTIONS
An increased risk of the following serious adverse reactions has been associated with the use of oral contraceptives (see Warnings section).
• Thrombophlebitis and venous thrombosis with or without embolism
• Arterial thromboembolism
• Pulmonary embolism
• Myocardial infarction
• Cerebral hemorrhage
• Cerebral thrombosis
• Hypertension
• Gallbladder disease
• Hepatic adenomas or benign liver tumors
The following adverse reactions have been reported in patients receiving oral contraceptives and are believed to be drug-related:
• Nausea
• Vomiting
• Gastrointestinal symptoms (such as abdominal cramps and bloating)
• Breakthrough bleeding
• Spotting
• Change in menstrual flow
• Amenorrhea
• Temporary infertility after discontinuance of treatment
• Edema
• Melasma which may persist
• Breast changes: tenderness, enlargement, and secretion
• Change in weight (increase or decrease)
• Change in cervical erosion and secretion
• Diminution in lactation when given immediately postpartum
• Cholestatic jaundice
• Migraine
• Rash (allergic)
• Mental depression
• Reduced tolerance to carbohydrates
• Vaginal candidiasis

• Change in corneal curvature (steepening)
• Intolerance to contact lenses
The following adverse reactions have been reported in users of oral contraceptives and the association has been neither confirmed nor refuted:
• Pre-menstrual-like syndrome
• Cataracts
• Changes in appetite
• Cystitis-like syndrome
• Headache
• Nervousness
• Dizziness
• Hirsutism
• Loss of scalp hair
• Erythema multiforme
• Erythema nodosum
• Hemorrhagic eruption
• Vaginitis
• Porphyria
• Impaired renal function
• Hemolytic uremic syndrome
• Acne
• Changes in libido
• Colitis

OVERDOSAGE
Serious ill effects have not been reported following acute ingestion of large doses of oral contraceptives by young children. Overdosage may cause nausea, and withdrawal bleeding may occur in females.

NON-CONTRACEPTIVE HEALTH BENEFITS
The following non-contraceptive health benefits related to the use of combination oral contraceptives are supported by epidemiological studies which largely utilized oral contraceptive formulations containing estrogen doses exceeding 0.035 mg of estrogen (73–78).
Effects on menses:
• increased menstrual cycle regularity
• decreased blood loss and decreased incidence of iron deficiency anemia
• decreased incidence of dysmenorrhea
Effects related to inhibition of ovulation:
• decreased incidence of functional ovarian cysts
• decreased incidence of ectopic pregnancies
Other effects:
• decreased incidence of fibroadenomas and fibrocystic disease of the breast
• decreased incidence of acute pelvic inflammatory disease
• decreased incidence of endometrial cancer
• decreased incidence of ovarian cancer

DOSAGE AND ADMINISTRATION
To achieve maximum contraceptive effectiveness, ORTHO-NOVUM Tablets, MODICON Tablets and MICRONOR must be taken exactly as directed and at intervals not exceeding 24 hours.

21-Day Regimen (Sunday Start)
When taking ORTHO-NOVUM 7/7/7 □ 21, the first white tablet should be taken on the first Sunday after menstruation begins. If period begins on Sunday, the first white tablet is taken on that day. If switching directly from another oral contraceptive, the first white tablet should be taken on the first Sunday after the last ACTIVE tablet of the previous product. Tablets are taken as follows: One white tablet daily for 7 days, then one light peach tablet daily for 7 days, then one peach tablet daily for 7 days. For subsequent cycles, no tablets are taken for seven days, then a white tablet is taken the next day (Sunday), etc.
When taking ORTHO-NOVUM 10/11 □ 21, the first white tablet should be taken on the first Sunday after menstruation begins. If period begins on Sunday, the first white tablet is taken on that day. If switching directly from another oral contraceptive, the first white tablet shold be taken on the first Sunday after the last ACTIVE tablet of the previous product. Tablets are taken as follows: One white tablet daily for 10 days, then one peach tablet daily for 11 days. For subsequent cycles, no tablets are taken for 7 days, then a white tablet is taken the next day (Sunday), etc. If first starting oral contraceptives more than 5 days from the onset of menses, contraceptive reliance should not be placed on these products until after the first 7 consecutive days of administration. The use of ORTHO-NOVUM 7/7/7 □ 21 and ORTHO-NOVUM 10/11 □ 21 for contraception may be initiated postpartum. When the tablets are administered during the postpartum period, the increased risk of thromboembolic disease associated with the postpartum period must be considered. (See CONTRAINDICATIONS AND WARNINGS concerning thromboembolic disease.) The possibility of ovulation and conception prior to initiation of medication should be considered. If the patient misses more than one tablet, the patient should begin taking tablets again as soon as remembered and another method of contraception used for the balance of that tablet cycle.

21-Day Regimen (21 days on, 7 days off)
The dosage of ORTHO-NOVUM 1/35 □ 21, MODICON 21, ORTHO-NOVUM 1/50 □ 21, ORTHO-NOVUM 1/80 □ 21

and ORTHO-NOVUM 2 mg □ 21 for the initial cycle of therapy is one tablet administered daily from the 5th day through the 25th day of the menstrual cycle, counting the first day of menstrual flow as "Day 1." The use of these products for contraception may be initiated postpartum. When the tablets are administered during the postpartum period, the increased risk of thromboembolic disease associated with the postpartum period must be considered. (See CONTRAINDICATIONS and WARNINGS concerning thromboembolic disease.) If ORTHO-NOVUM 1/35 □ 21, MODICON 21, ORTHO-NOVUM 1/50 □ 21, ORTHO-NOVUM 1/80 □ 21, and ORTHO-NOVUM 2 mg □ 21 are first taken later than the fifth day of the first menstrual cycle of medication or postpartum, contraceptive reliance should not be placed on these products until after the first seven consecutive days of administration. For subsequent cycles, no tablets are taken for 7 days, then a new course is started of one tablet a day for 21 days. The dosage regimen then continues with 7 days of no medication, followed by 21 days of medication, instituting a three-weeks-on, one-week-off dosage regimen. The possibility of ovulation and conception prior to initiation of medication should be considered. If the patient misses more than one tablet, the patient should begin taking tablets again as soon as remembered and another method of contraception used for the balance of that tablet cycle.
ORTHO-NOVUM 2 mg □ 21: Following three months of treatment of hypermenorrhea, medication may be discontinued to determine the need for further therapy.
(See discussion of Dose-Related Risk of Vascular Disease from Oral Contraceptives.)

28-Day Regimen (Sunday Start)
When taking ORTHO-NOVUM 7/7/7 □ 28, the first white tablet should be taken on the first Sunday after menstruation begins. If period begins on Sunday, the first white tablet is taken on that day. If switching directly from another oral contraceptive, the first white tablet should be taken on the first Sunday after the last ACTIVE tablet of the previous product. Tablets are taken without interruption as follows: One white tablet daily for 7 days, one light peach tablet daily for 7 days, one peach tablet daily for 7 days, then one green tablet daily for 7 days. After 28 tablets have been taken, a white tablet is then taken the next day (Sunday), etc.
When taking ORTHO-NOVUM 10/11 □ 28, the first white tablet should be taken on the first Sunday after menstruation begins. If period begins on Sunday, the first white tablet is taken on that day. If switching directly from another oral contraceptive, the first white tablet should be taken on the first Sunday after the last ACTIVE tablet of the previous product. Tablets are taken without interruption as follows: one white tablet daily for 10 days, one peach tablet daily for 11 days, then one green tablet daily for 7 days. After 28 tablets have been taken, a white tablet is then taken the next day (Sunday), etc.
When taking ORTHO-NOVUM 1/35 □ 28, the first peach tablet should be taken on the first Sunday after mestruation begins. When taking MODICON 28 or ORTHO-NOVUM 1/80 □ 28, the first white tablet should be taken on the first Sunday after menstruation begins. When taking ORTHO-NOVUM 1/50 □ 28, the first yellow tablet should be taken on the first Sunday after menstruation begins. If period begins on Sunday, the first peach tablet, white tablet or yellow tablet is taken on that day. If switching directly from another oral contraceptive, the first peach, white or yellow tablet should be taken on the first Sunday after the last ACTIVE tablet of the previous product. Tablets are taken without interruption as follows: One peach, white or yellow tablet daily for 21 days, then one green tablet daily for 7 days. After 28 tablets have been taken, a peach, white or yellow tablet is then taken the next day (Sunday), etc. If first starting oral contraceptives more than 5 days from the onset of menses, contraceptive reliance should not be placed on these products until after the first 7 consecutive days of administration.
The use of ORTHO-NOVUM 7/7/7 □ 28, ORTHO-NOVUM 10/11 □ 28, ORTHO-NOVUM 1/35 □ 28, MODICON 28, ORTHO-NOVUM 1/50 □ 28, and ORTHO-NOVUM 1/80 □ 28 for contraception may be initiated postpartum. When the tablets are administered during the postpartum period, the increased risk of thromboembolic disease associated with the postpartum period must be considered. (See CONTRAINDICATIONS and WARNINGS concerning thromboembolic disease.) The possibility of ovulation and conception prior to initiation of medication should be considered. If the patient misses more than one tablet, the patient should begin taking tablets again as soon as remembered and another method of contraception used for the balance of that tablet cycle.

MICRONOR (Continuous Regimen)
MICRONOR (norethindrone) is administered on a continuous daily dosage regimen starting on the first day of menstruation, i.e., one tablet each day, every day of the year. Tablets should be taken at the same time each day and continued daily. The patient should be advised that if prolonged bleeding occurs, she should consult her physician.
The use of MICRONOR for contraception may be initiated postpartum (see WARNINGS section). When MICRONOR is administered during the postpartum period, the increased

risk of thromboembolic disease associated with the post-partum period must be considered. (See CONTRAINDI-CATIONS and WARNINGS concerning thromboembolic disease.)

If the patient misses one tablet, MICRONOR should be discontinued immediately and a method of nonhormonal contraception should be used until menses has appeared or pregnancy has been excluded.

Alternatively, if the patient has taken the tablets correctly, and if menses does not appear when expected, a nonhormonal method of contraception should be substituted until an appropriate diagnostic procedure is performed to rule out pregnancy.

All Oral Contraceptives

Breakthrough bleeding, spotting, and amenorrhea are frequent reasons for patients discontinuing oral contraceptives. In breakthrough bleeding, as in all cases of irregular bleeding from the vagina, nonfunctional causes should be borne in mind. In undiagnosed persistent or recurrent abnormal bleeding from the vagina, adequate diagnostic measures are indicated to rule out pregnancy or malignancy. If pathology has been excluded, time or a change to another formulation may solve the problem. Changing to an oral contraceptive with a higher estrogen content, while potentially useful in minimizing menstrual irregularity, should be done only if necessary since this may increase the risk of thromboembolic disease.

Use of oral contraceptives in the event of a missed menstrual period:

1. If the patient has not adhered to the prescribed schedule, the possibility of pregnancy should be considered at the time of the first missed period (or upon missing one MICRONOR Tablet) and oral contraceptive use should be discontinued until pregnancy is ruled out.

2. If the patient has adhered to the prescribed regimen and misses two consecutive periods (or after 45 days from the last menstrual period if the progestogen-only oral contraceptives are used), pregnancy should be ruled out before continuing oral contraceptive use.

HOW SUPPLIED

ORTHO-NOVUM 7/7/7 □ 21 Tablets are available in a DIALPAK™ Tablet Dispenser (NDC 0062-1780-15) containing 21 tablets, as follows: 7 white tablets (0.5 mg norethindrone and 0.035 mg ethinyl estradiol), 7 light peach tablets (0.75 norethindrone and 0.035 mg ethinyl estradiol) and 7 peach tablets (1 mg norethindrone and 0.035 mg ethinyl estradiol). The white tablets are unscored with "Ortho" and "535" debossed on each side; the light peach tablets are unscored with "Ortho" and "75" debossed on each side; the peach tablets are unscored with "Ortho" and "135" debossed on each side.

ORTHO-NOVUM 7/7/7 □ 21 is available for clinic usage in a VERIDATE™ Tablet Dispenser (unfilled) and VERIDATE Refills (NDC 0062-1780-20).

ORTHO-NOVUM 7/7/7 □ 28 Tablets are available in a DIALPAK Tablet Dispenser (NDC 0062-1781-15) containing 28 tablets as follows: 7 white, 7 light peach and 7 peach tablets as described under ORTHO-NOVUM 7/7/7 □ 21, and 7 green tablets containing inert ingredients.

ORTHO-NOVUM 7/7/7 □ 28 is available for clinic usage in a VERIDATE Tablet Dispenser (unfilled) and VERIDATE Refills (NDC 0062-1781-20).

ORTHO-NOVUM 10/11 □ 21 Tablets are available in a DIALPAK Tablet Dispenser (NDC 0062-1770-15) containing 21 tablets, as follows: 10 white tablets (0.5 mg norethindrone and 0.035 mg ethinyl estradiol) and 11 peach tablets (1 mg norethindrone and 0.035 mg ethinyl estradiol). The white tablets are unscored with "Ortho" and "535" debossed on each side; the peach tablets are unscored with "Ortho" and "135" debossed on each side.

ORTHO-NOVUM 10/11 □ 21 is available for clinic usage in a VERIDATE Tablet Dispenser (unfilled) and VERIDATE Refills (NDC 0062-1770-20).

ORTHO-NOVUM 10/11 □ 28 Tablets are available in a DIALPAK Tablet dispenser (NDC 0062-1771-15) containing 28 tablets, as follows: 10 white and 11 peach tablets as described under ORTHO-NOVUM 10/11 □ 21, and 7 green tablets containing inert ingredients.

ORTHO-NOVUM 10/11 □ 28 is available for clinic usage in a VERIDATE Tablet Dispenser (unfilled) and VERIDATE Refills (NDC 0062-1771-20).

ORTHO-NOVUM 1/35 □ 21 Tablets are available in a DIALPAK Tablet Dispenser (NDC 0062-1760-15) containing 21 peach tablets (1 mg norethindrone and 0.035 mg ethinyl estradiol) which are unscored with "Ortho" and "135" debossed on each side.

ORTHO-NOVUM 1/35 □ 21 is available for clinic usage in a VERIDATE Tablet Dispenser (unfilled) and VERIDATE Refills (NDC 0062-1760-20).

ORTHO-NOVUM 1/35 □ 28 Tablets are available in a DIALPAK Tablet Dispenser (NDC 0062-1761-15) containing 28 tablets, as follows: 21 peach tablets as described under ORTHO-NOVUM 1/35 □ 21, and 7 green tablets containing inert ingredients.

ORTHO-NOVUM 1/35 □ 28 is available for clinic usage in a VERIDATE Tablet Dispenser (unfilled) and VERIDATE Refills (NDC 0062-1761-20).

MODICON 21 Tablets are available in a DIALPAK Tablet Dispenser (NDC 0062-1712-15) containing 21 white tablets (0.5 mg norethindrone and 0.035 mg ethinyl estradiol) which are unscored with "Ortho" and "535" debossed on each side.

MODICON 28 Tablets are available in a DIALPAK Tablet Dispenser (NDC 0062-1714-15) containing 28 tablets, as follows: 21 white tablets as described under MODICON 21, and 7 green tablets containing inert ingredients.

MODICON 28 is available for clinic usage in a VERIDATE Tablet Dispenser (unfilled) and VERIDATE Refills (NDC 0062-1714-20).

ORTHO-NOVUM 1/50 □ 21 Tablets are available in a DIALPAK Tablet Dispenser (NDC 0062-1331-15) containing 21 yellow tablets (1 mg norethindrone and 0.05 mg mestranol) which are unscored with "Ortho" and "150" debossed on each side.

ORTHO-NOVUM 1/50 □ 21 is available for clinic usage in a VERIDATE Tablet Dispenser (unfilled) and VERIDATE Refills (NDC 0062-1331-20).

ORTHO-NOVUM 1/50 □ 28 Tablets are available in a DIALPAK Tablet Dispenser (NDC 0062-1332-15) containing 28 tablets, as follows: 21 yellow tablets as described under ORTHO-NOVUM 1/50 □ 21, and 7 green tablets containing inert ingredients.

ORTHO-NOVUM 1/50 □ 28 is available for clinic usage in a VERIDATE Tablet Dispenser (unfilled) and VERIDATE Refills (NDC 0062-1332-20).

MICRONOR Tablets are available in a DIALPAK Tablet Dispenser (NDC 0062-1411-01) containing 28 lime tablets (0.35 mg norethindrone) which are unscored with "Ortho" and "0.35" debossed on each side.

MICRONOR is available for clinic usage in a VERIDATE Tablet Dispenser (unfilled) and VERIDATE Refills (NDC 0062-1411-23).

Manufacture and shipment of the following products by Ortho Pharmaceutical Corporation was discontinued as of October 1988:

ORTHO-NOVUM 1/80 □ 21 Tablets are available in a DIALPAK Tablet Dispenser (NDC 0062-1390-15) containing 21 white tablets (1 mg norethindrone and 0.08 mg mestranol) which are unscored with "Ortho" and "1" debossed on each side.

ORTHO-NOVUM 1/80 □ 28 Tablets are available in a DIALPAK Tablet Dispenser (NDC 0062-1391-15) containing 28 tablets, as follows: 21 white tablets as described under ORTHO-NOVUM 1/80 □ 21, and 7 green tablets containing inert ingredients.

ORTHO-NOVUM 1/80 □ 28 is available for clinic usage in a VERIDATE Tablet Dispenser (unfilled) and VERIDATE Refills (NDC 0062-1391-20).

ORTHO-NOVUM 2 mg □ 21 Tablets are available in a DIALPAK Tablet Dispenser (NDC 0062-1351-08) containing 21 white tablets (2 mg norethindrone and 0.10 mg mestranol) which are unscored with "Ortho" and "2" debossed on each side.

REFERENCES

1. Reproduced with permission of the Population Council from J. Trussell and K. Kost: Contraceptive failure in the United States: A critical review of the literature. Studies in Family Planning, 18 (5), September–October 1987. **2.** Stadel BV. Oral contraceptives and cardiovascular disease. (Pt. 1). N Engl J Med 1981; 305:612–618. **3.** Stadel BV. Oral contraceptives and cardiovascular disease. (Pt. 2). N Engl J Med 1981; 305:672–677. **4.** Adam SA, Thorogood M. Oral contraception and myocardial infarction revisted: the effects of new preparations and prescribing patterns. Br J Obstet Gynecol 1981; 88:838–845. **5.** Mann JI, Inman WH. Oral contraceptives and death from myocardial infarction. Br Med J 1975; 2(5965):245–248. **6.** Mann JI, Vessel MP, Thorogood M, Doll R. Myocardial infarction in young women with special reference to oral contraceptive practice. Br Med J 1975; 2(5956):241–245. **7.** Royal College of General Practitioners' Oral Contraception Study: Further analyses of mortality in oral contraceptive users. Lancet 1981; 1:541–546. **8.** Slone D, Shapiro S, Kaufman DW, Rosenberg L, Miettinen OS, Stolley PD. Risk of myocardial infarction in relation to current and discontinued use of oral contraceptives. N Engl J Med 1981; 305:420–424. **9.** Vessey MP. Femal hormones and vascular disease-an epidemiological overview. Br J Fam Plann 1980; 6:1–12. **10.** Russell-Briefel RG, Ezzati TM, Fulwood R. Perlman JA, Murphy RS. Cardiovascular risk status and oral contraceptive use, United States, 1976–80. Prevent Med 1986; 15:352–362. **11.** Goldbaum GM, Kendrick JS, Hogelin GC, Gentry EM. The relative impact of smoking and oral contraceptive use on women in the United States. JAMA 1987; 258:1339–1342. **12.** Layde PM, Beral V. Further analyses of mortality in oral contraceptive users: Royal College of General Practitioners' Oral Contraception Study. (Table 5) Lancet 1981; 1:541–546. **13.** Knopp RH. Arteriosclerosis risk: the roles of oral contraceptives and postmenopausal estrogens. J Reprod Med 1986; 31(9) (Supplement):913–921. **14.** Krauss RM, Roy S. Mishell DR, Casagrande J, Pike MC.

Effects of two low-dose oral contraceptives on serum lipids and lipoproteins: Differential changes in high-density lipoproteins subclasses. Am J Obstet 1983; 145:446–452. **15.** Wahl P, Walden C, Knopp R. Hoover J, Wallace R, Heiss G, Rifkind B. Effect of estrogen/progestin potency on lipid/lipoprotein cholesterol. N. Engl J Med 1983; 308:862–867. **16.** Wynn V. Niththyananthan R. The effect of progestin in combined oral contraceptives on serum lipids with special reference to high density lipoproteins. Am J Obstet Gynecol 1982; 142:766–771. **17.** Wynn V, Godsland I. Effects of oral contraceptives on carbohydrate metabolism. J Reprod Med 1986; 31(9)(Supplement):892–897. **18.** La Rosa JC. Atherosclerotic risk factors in cardiovascular disease. J. Reprod Med 1986; 31(9)(Supplement):906–912. **19.** Inman WH, Vessey MP. Investigation of death from pulmonary, coronary, and cerebral thrombosis and embolism in women of childbearing age. Br Med J. 1968; 2(5599):193–199. **20.** Maquire MG, Tonascia J, Sartwell PE, Stolley PD, Tockman MS. Increased risk of thrombosis due to oral contraceptives: a further report. Am J Epidemiol 1979; 110(2):188–195. **21.** Pettiti DB, Wingerd J, Pellegrin F, Ramacharan S. Risk of vascular disease in women: smoking, oral contraceptives, non-contraceptive estrogens, and other factors. JAMA 1979; 242:1150–1154. **22.** Vessey MP, Doll R. Investigation of relation between use of oral contraceptives and thromboembolic disease. Br Med J 1968; 2(5599):199–205. **23.** Vessey MP, Doll R. Investigation of relation between use of oral contraceptives and thromboembolic disease. A further report. Br Med J 1969; 2(5658):651–657. **24.** Porter JB, Hunter JR, Danielson DA, Jick H. Stergachis A. Oral contraceptives and non-fatal vascular disease-recent experience. Obstet Gynecol 1982; 59(3):299–302. **25.** Vessey M, Doll R, Petro R, Johnson B, Wiggins P. A long-term follow-up study of women using different methods of contraception: an interim report. J Biosocial Sci 1976; 8:375–427. **26.** Royal College of General Practitioners: Oral Contraceptives, venous thrombosis, and varicose veins. J Royal Coll Gen Pract 1978; 28:393–399. **27.** Collaborative Group for the Study of Stroke in Young Women; Oral contraception and increased risk of cerebral ischemia or thrombosis. N Engl J Med 1973; 288:871–878. **28.** Petitti DB, Wingerd J. Use of oral contraceptives, cigarette smoking, and risk of subarachnoid hemorrhage. Lancet 1978; 2:234–236. **29.** Inman WH. Oral contraceptives and fatal subarachnoid hemorrhage. Br Med J 1979; 2(6203):1468–70. **30.** Collaborative Group for the Study of Stroke in Young Women: Oral Contraceptives and stroke in young women: associated risk factors. JAMA 1975; 231:718–722. **31.** Inman WH, Vessey MP, Westerholm B, Engelund A. Thromboembolic disease and the steroidal content of oral contraceptives. A report to the Committee on Safety of Drugs. Br Med J. 1970; 2:203–209. **32.** Meade TW, Greenberg G. Thompson SG. Progestogens and cardiovascular reactions associated with oral contraceptives and a comparison of the safety of 50- and 35-mcg oestrogen preparations. Br Med J 1980; 280(6224):1157–1161. **33.** Kay CR. Progestogens and arterial disease-evidence from the Royal College of General Practitioners' Study. Am J Obstet Gynecol 1982; 142:762–765. **34.** Royal College of General Practitioners: Incidence of arterial disease among oral contraceptive users. J Royal Coll Gen Pract 1983; 33:75–82. **35.** Ory HW. Mortality associated with fertility and fertility control: 1983. Family Planning Perspectives 1983; 15:50–56. **36.** The Cancer and Steroid Hormone Study of the Centers for Disease Control and the National Institute of Child Health and Human Development: Oral-contraceptive use and the risk of breast cancer. N Engl J Med 1986; 315:405–411. **37.** Pike MC, Henderson BE, Krailo MD, Duke A, Roy S. Breast cancer in young women and use of oral contraceptives: possible modifying effect of formulation and age at use. Lancest 1983; 2:926–929. **38.** Paul C, Skegg DG, Spears GFS, Kaldor JM. Oral contraceptives and breast cancer: A national study. Br Med J 1986; 293:723–725. **39.** Miller DR, Rosenberg L, Kaufman DW, Schottenfeld D, Stolley PD, Shapiro S. Breast cancer risk in relation to early oral contraceptive use. Obstet Gynecol 1986; 68:863–868. **40.** Olson H, Olson KL, Moller TR, Ranstam J, Holm P. Oral contraceptive use and breast cancer in young women in Sweden (letter). Lancet 1985; 2:748–749. **41.** McPherson K, Vessey M, Neil A, Doll R, Jones L, Roberts M. Early contraceptive use and breast cancer: Results of another case-control study. Br J Cancer 1987; 56:653–660. **42.** Huggins GR, Zucker PF. Oral contraceptives and neoplasia: 1987 update. Fertil Steril 1987; 47:733–761. **43.** McPherson K, Drife JO. The pill and breast cancer: why the uncertainty? Br Med J 1986; 293:709–710. **44.** Shapiro S. Oral contraceptives-time to take stock. N Engl J Med 1987; 315:450–451. **45.** Ory H, Naib Z, Conger SB, Hatcher RA, Tyler CW. Contraceptive choice and prevalence of cervical dysplasia and carcinoma in situ. Am J Obstet Gynecol 1976; 124:573–577. **46.** Vessey MP, Lawless M, McPherson K, Yeates D. Neoplasia of the cervix uteri and contraception: a possible adverse effect of the pill. Lancet 1983; 2930. **47.** Brinton LA, Huggins GR, Lehman HF, Malli K, Savitz DA, Trapido E, Rosenthal J,

Continued on next page

Ortho Pharm.—Cont.

Hoover R. Long term use of oral contraceptives and risk of invasive cervical cancer. Int J Cancer 1986; 38 :339–344. **48.** WHO Collaborative Study of Neoplasia and Steroid Contraceptives: Invasive cervical cancer and combined oral contraceptives. Br Med J 1985; 290 :961–965. **49.** Rooks JB, Ory HW, Ishak KG, Strauss LT, Greenspan JR, Hill AP, Tyler CW. Epidemiology of hepatocellular adenoma: the role of oral contraceptive use. JAMA 1979; 242 :644–648. **50.** Bein NN, Goldsmith HS. Recurrent massive hemorrhage from benign hepatic tumors secondary to oral contraceptives. Br J Surg 1977; 64 :433–435. **51.** Klatskin G, Hepatic tumors: possible relationship to use of oral contraceptives. Gastroenterology 1977; 73 :366–394. **52.** Henderson BE, Preston-Martin S, Edmondson HA, Peters RL, Pike MC. Hepatocellular carcinoma and oral contraceptives. Br J Cancer 1983; 48 :437–440. **53.** Neuberger J, Forman D, Doll R, Williams R. Oral contraceptives and hepatocellular carcinoma. Br Med J 1986; 292 :1355–1357. **54.** Forman D, Vincent TJ, Doll R. Cancer of the liver and oral contraceptives. Br Med J 1986; 292 :1357–1361. **55.** Harlap S, Eldor J. Births following oral contraceptive failures. Obstet Gyncecol 1980; 55 : 447–452. **56.** Savolainen E, Saksela E, Saxen L. Teratogenic hazards of oral contraceptives analyzed in a national malformation register. Am J Obstet Gynecol 1981; 140 :521–524. **57.** Janerich DT, Piper JM, Glebatis DM. Oral contraceptives and birth defects. Am J Epidemiol 1980; 112 :73–79. **58.** Ferencz C, Matanoski GM, Wilson PD, Rubin JD, Neill CA, Gutberlet R. Maternal hormone therapy and congenital heart disease. Teratology 1980; 21 :225–239. **59.** Rothman KJ, Fyler DC, Goldbatt A, Kreidberg MB. Exogenous hormones and other drug exposures of children with congenital heart disease. Am J Epidemiol 1979; 109 :433–439. **60.** Boston Collaborative Drug Surveillance Program: Oral contraceptives and venous thromboembolic disease, surgically confirmed gallbladder disease, and breast tumors. Lancet 1973; 1 :1399–1404. **61.** Royal College of General Practitioners: Oral contraceptives and health. New York, Pittman 1974. **62.** Layde PM, Vessey MP, Yeates D. Risk of gall bladder disease: a cohort study of young women attending family planning clinics. J Epidemiol Community Health 1982; 36 :274–278. **63.** Rome Group for Epidemiology and Prevention of Cholelithiasis (GREPCO): Prevalence of gallstone disease in an Italian adult female population. Am J Epidemiol 1984; 119 :796–805. **64.** Storm BL, Tamragouri RT, Morse ML, Lazar EL, West SL, Stolley PD, Jones JK. Oral contraceptives and other risk factors for gall bladder disease. Clin Pharmacol Ther 1986; 39 :335–341. **65.** Wynn V. Adams PW, Godsland IF, Melrose J, Niththyananthan R, Oakley NW, Seedj A. Comparison of effects of different combined oral-contraceptive formulations on carbohydrate and lipid metabolism. Lancet 1979; 1 :1045–1049. **66.** Wynn V. Effect of progesterone and progestins on carbohydrate metabolism. In: Progesterone and Progestin. Bardin CW, Milgrom E, Mauvis-Jarvis P. eds. New York, Raven Press 1983; pp. 395–410. **67.** Perlman JA, Roussell-Briefel RG, Ezzati TM, Lieberknecht G. Oral glucose tolerance and the potency of oral contraceptive progestogens. J Chronic Dis 1985:38 :857–864. **68.** Royal College of General Practitioners' Oral contraception Study: Effect on hypertension and benign breast disease of progestogen component in combined oral contraceptives. Lancet 1977; 1 :624. **69.** Fisch IR, Frank J. Oral contraceptives and blood pressure. JAMA 1977; 237 :2499–2503. **70.** Laragh AJ. Oral contraceptive induced hypertension-nine years later. Am J Obstet Gynecol 1976; 126 :141–147. **71.** Ramcharan S. Peritz E, Pellegrin FA, Williams WT. Incidence of hypertension in the Walnut Creek Contraceptive Drug Study cohort: In: Pharmacology of steroid contraceptive drugs. Garattini S, Berendes HW. Eds. New York, Raven Press, 1977; pp. 277–288, (Monographs of the Mario Negri Institute for Pharmacological Research Milan). **72.** Stockley I. Interactions with oral contraceptives. J Pharm 1976; 216 :140–143. **73.** The Cancer and Steroid Hormone Study of the Centers for Disease Control and the National Institute of Child Health and Human Development: Oral contraceptive use and the risk of ovarian cancer. JAMA 1983; 249 :1596–1599. **74.** The Cancer and Steroid Hormone Study of the Centers for Disease Control and the National Institute of Child Health and Human Development: Combination oral contraceptive use and the risk of endometrial cancer. JAMA 1987; 257 :796–800. **75.** Ory HW. Functional ovarian cysts and oral contraceptives: negative association confirmed surgically. JAMA 1974; 228 :68–69. **76.** Ory WH, Cole P, MacMahon B, Hoover R. Oral contraceptives and reduced risk of benign breast disease. N Engl J Med 1976; 294 :419–422. **77.** Ory HW. The noncontraceptive health benefits from oral contraceptive use. Fam Plann Perspect 1982; 14 :182–184. **78.** Ory HW, Forrest JD, Lincoln R. Making choices: Evaluating the health risks and benefits of birth control methods. New York, The Alan Guttmacher Institute, 1983; p. 1. **79.** Schlesselman J, Stadel BV, Murray P, Lai S. Breast cancer in relation to early use of oral contraceptives JAMA 1988; 259 :1828–1833.

Brief Summary Patient Package Insert

Oral contraceptives, also known as "birth control pills" or "the pill", are taken to prevent pregnancy and when taken correctly, have a failure rate of less than 1% per year when used without missing any pills. The typical failure rate of large numbers of pill users is less than 3% per year when women who miss pills are included. For most women oral contraceptives are also free of serious or unpleasant side effects. However, forgetting to take pills considerably increases the chances of pregnancy.

For the majority of women, oral contraceptives can be taken safely. But there are some women who are at high risk of developing certain serious diseases that can be fatal or may cause temporary or permanent disability. The risks associated with taking oral contraceptives increase significantly if you:

● smoke
● are over the age of 40
● have high blood pressure, diabetes, high cholesterol
● have or have had clotting disorders, heart attack, stroke, angina pectoris, cancer of the breast or sex organs, jaundice or malignant or benign liver tumors.

You should not take the pill if you suspect you are pregnant or have unexplained vaginal bleeding.

> **Cigarette smoking increases the risk of serious cardiovascular side effects from oral contraceptive use. This risk increases with age and with heavy smoking (15 or more cigarettes per day) and is quite marked in women over 35 years of age. Women who use oral contraceptives are strongly advised not to smoke.**

Most side effects of the pill are not serious. The most common such effects are nausea, vomiting, bleeding between menstrual periods, weight gain, breast tenderness, and difficulty wearing contact lenses. These side effects, especially nausea and vomiting, may subside within the first three months of use.

The serious side effects of the pill occur very infrequently, especially if you are in good health and are young. However, you should know that the following medical conditions have been associated with or made worse by the pill:

1. Blood clots in the legs (thrombophlebitis), lungs (pulmonary embolism), stoppage or rupture of a blood vessel in the brain (stroke), blockage of blood vessels in the heart (heart attack or angina pectoris) or other organs of the body. As mentioned above, smoking increases the risk of heart attacks and strokes and subsequent serious medical consequences.
2. Liver tumors, which may rupture and cause severe bleeding. A possible but not definite association has been found with the pill and liver cancer. However, liver cancers are extremely rare. The chance of developing liver cancer from using the pill is thus even rarer.
3. High blood pressure, although blood pressure usually returns to normal when the pill is stopped.

The symptoms associated with these serious side effects are discussed in the detailed leaflet given to you with your supply of pills. Notify your doctor or health care provider if you notice any unusual physical disturbances while taking the pill. In addition, drugs such as rifampin, as well as some anticonvulsants and some antibiotics may decrease oral contraceptive effectiveness.

Studies to date of women taking the pill have not shown an increase in the incidence of cancer of the breast or cervix. There is, however, insufficient evidence to rule out the possibility that pills may cause such cancers.

Taking the combination pill provides some important noncontraceptive benefits. These include less painful menstruation, less menstrual blood loss and anemia, fewer pelvic infections, and fewer cancers of the ovary and the lining of the uterus.

Be sure to discuss any medical condition you may have with your health care provider. Your health care provider will take a medical and family history before prescribing oral contraceptives and will examine you. You should be reexamined at least once a year while taking oral contraceptives. Your pharmacist should have given you the detailed patient information labeling which gives you further information which you should read and discuss with your health care provider.

Detailed Patient Labeling

PLEASE NOTE: This labeling is revised from time to time as important new medical information becomes available. Therefore, please review this labeling carefully.

The following oral contraceptive products contain a combination of an estrogen and progestogen, the two kinds of female hormones:

ORTHO-NOVUM 7/7/7 □ 21 Day Regimen and
ORTHO-NOVUM 7/7/7 □ 28 Day Regimen
Each white tablet contains 0.5 mg norethindrone and 0.035 mg ethinyl estradiol. Each light peach tablet contains 0.75 mg norethindrone and 0.035 mg ethinyl estradiol. Each peach tablet contains 1 mg norethindrone and 0.035 mg ethinyl estradiol. Each green tablet in ORTHO-NOVUM 7/7/7 □ 28 Day Regimen contains inert ingredients.

ORTHO-NOVUM 10/11 □ 21 Day Regimen and
ORTHO-NOVUM 10/11 □ 28 Day Regimen
Each white tablet contains 0.5 mg norethindrone and 0.035 mg ethinyl estradiol. Each peach tablet contains 1 mg norethindrone and 0.035 mg ethinyl estradiol. Each green tablet in ORTHO-NOVUM 10/11 □ 28 Day Regimen contains inert ingredients.

ORTHO-NOVUM 1/35 □ 21 Day Regimen and
ORTHO-NOVUM 1/35 □ 28 Day Regimen
Each peach tablet contains 1 mg norethindrone and 0.035 mg ethinyl estradiol. Each green tablet in ORTHO-NOVUM 1/35 □ 28 Day Regimen contains inert ingredients.

MODICON 21 Day Regimen and MODICON 28 Day Regimen
Each white tablet contains 0.5 mg norethindrone and 0.035 mg ethinyl estradiol. Each green tablet in MODICON 28 Day Regimen contains inert ingredients.

ORTHO-NOVUM 1/50 □ 21 Day Regimen and
ORTHO-NOVUM 1/50 □ 28 Day Regimen
Each yellow tablet contains 1 mg norethindrone and 0.05 mg mestranol. Each green tablet in ORTHO-NOVUM 1/50 □ 28 Day Regimen contains inert ingredients.

ORTHO-NOVUM 1/80 □ 21 Day Regimen and
ORTHO-NOVUM 1/80 □ 28 Day Regimen.
Each white tablet contains 1 mg norethindrone and 0.08 mg mestranol. Each green tablet in ORTHO-NOVUM 1/80 □ 28 Day Regimen contains inert ingredients.

ORTHO-NOVUM 2 mg □ 21 Day Regimen
Each tablet contains 2 mg norethindrone and 0.10 mg mestranol.

PROGESTOGEN-ONLY ORAL CONTRACEPTIVE

The following oral contraceptive product contains only a progestogen and is often called the "mini-pill":
MICRONOR 28 Day Regimen
Each tablet contains 0.35 mg norethindrone.

INTRODUCTION

Any woman who considers using oral contraceptives (the birth control pill or the pill) should understand the benefits and risks of using this form of birth control. This patient labeling will give you much of the information you will need to make this decision and will also help you determine if you are at risk of developing any of the serious side effects of the pill. It will tell you how to use the pill properly so that it will be as effective as possible. However, this labeling is not a replacement for a careful discussion between you and your health care provider. You should discuss the information provided in this labeling with him or her, both when you first start taking the pill and during your revisits. You should follow your health care provider's advice with regard to regular check-ups while you are on the pill.

EFFECTIVENESS OF ORAL CONTRACEPTIVES

Oral contraceptives or "birth control pills" or "the pill" are used to prevent pregnancy and are more effective than other non-surgical methods of birth control. When they are taken correctly, the chance of becoming pregnant is less than 1% (1 pregnancy per 100 women per year of use) when used perfectly, without missing any pills. Typical failure rates are actually 3% per year. The chance of becoming pregnant increases with each missed pill during a menstrual cycle.

In comparison, typical failure rates for other methods of birth control during the first year of use are as follows:

IUD: 6%
Diaphragm with spermicides: 18%
Spermicides alone: 21%
Vaginal sponge: 18% to 30%
Condom alone: 12%
Periodic abstinence: 20%
No methods: 89%

WHO SHOULD NOT TAKE ORAL CONTRACEPTIVES

> **Cigarette smoking increases the risk of serious cardiovascular side effects from oral contraceptive use. This risk increases with age and with heavy smoking (15 or more cigarettes per day) and is quite marked in women over 35 years of age. Women who use oral contraceptives are strongly advised not to smoke.**

Some women should not use the pill. For example, you should not take the pill if you are pregnant or think you may be pregnant. You should also not use the pill if you have any of the following conditions:

● A history of heart attack or stroke
● Blood clots in the legs (thrombophlebitis), lungs (pulmonary embolism), or eyes
● A history of blood clots in the deep veins of your legs
● Chest pain (angina pectoris)
● Known or suspected breast cancer or cancer of the lining of the uterus, cervix or vagina
● Unexplained vaginal bleeding (until a diagnosis is reached by your doctor)
● Yellowing of the whites of the eyes or of the skin (jaundice) during pregnancy or during previous use of the pill

- Liver tumor (benign or cancerous)
- Known or suspected pregnancy

Tell your health care provider if you have ever had any of these conditions. Your health care provider can recommend a safer method of birth control.

OTHER CONSIDERATIONS BEFORE TAKING ORAL CONTRACEPTIVES

Tell your health care provider if you have or have had:
- Breast nodules, fibrocystic disease of the breast, an abnormal breast x-ray or mammogram
- Diabetes
- Elevated cholesterol or triglycerides
- High blood pressure
- Migraine or other headaches or epilepsy
- Mental depression
- Gallbladder, heart or kidney disease
- History of scanty or irregular menstrual periods

Women with any of these conditions should be checked often by their health care provider if they choose to use oral contraceptives.

Also, be sure to inform your doctor or health care provider if you smoke or are on any medications.

RISKS OF TAKING ORAL CONTRACEPTIVES

1. Risk of developing blood clots

Blood clots and blockage of blood vessels are the most serious side effects of taking oral contraceptives. In particular, a clot in the legs can cause thrombophlebitis and a clot that travels to the lungs can cause a sudden blocking of the vessel carrying blood to the lungs. Rarely, clots occur in the blood vessels of the eye and may cause blindness, double vision, or impaired vision.

If you take oral contraceptives and need elective surgery, need to stay in bed for a prolonged illness or have recently delivered a baby, you may be at risk of developing blood clots. You should consult your doctor about stopping oral contraceptives three to four weeks before surgery and not taking oral contraceptives for two weeks after surgery or during bed rest. You should also not take oral contraceptives soon after delivery of a baby. It is advisable to wait for at least four weeks after delivery if you are not breast feeding. If you are breast feeding, you should wait until you have weaned your child before using the pill. (See also the section on Breast Feeding in General Precautions.)

The risk of circulatory disease in oral contraceptive users may be higher in users of high dose pills and may be greater with longer duration of oral contraceptive use. In addition, some of these increased risks may continue for a number of years after stopping oral contraceptives. The risk of abnormal blood clotting increases with age in both users and nonusers of oral contraceptives, but the increased risk from the oral contraceptive appears to be present at all ages. For women aged 20 to 44 it is estimated that about 1 in 2,000 using oral contraceptives will be hospitalized each year because of abnormal clotting. Among nonusers in the same age group, about 1 in 20,000 would be hospitalized each year. For oral contraceptive users in general, it has been estimated that in women between the ages of 15 and 34 the risk of death due to a circulatory disorder is about 1 in 12,000 per year, whereas for nonusers the rate is about 1 in 50,000 per year. In the age group 35 to 44, the risk is estimated to be about 1 in 2,500 per year for oral contraceptive users and about 1 in 10,000 per year for nonusers.

2. Heart attacks and strokes

Oral contraceptives may increase the tendency to develop strokes (stoppage or rupture of blood vessels in the brain) and angina pectoris and heart attacks (blockage of blood vessels in the heart). Any of these conditions can cause death or disability.

Smoking greatly increases the possibility of suffering heart attacks and strokes. Furthermore, smoking and the use of oral contraceptives greatly increase the chances of developing and dying of heart disease.

3. Gallbladder disease

Oral contraceptive users probably have a greater risk than nonusers of having gallbladder disease, although this risk may be related to pills containing high doses of estrogens.

4. Liver tumors

In rare cases, oral contraceptives can cause benign but dangerous liver tumors. These benign liver tumors can rupture and cause fatal internal bleeding. In addition, a possible but not definite association has been found with the pill and liver cancers in two studies, in which a few women who developed these very rare cancers were found to have used oral contraceptives for long periods. However, liver cancers are rare.

5. Cancer of the reproductive organs

There is, at present, no confirmed evidence that oral contraceptives increase the risk of cancer of the reproductive organs in human studies. While there is some conflict among studies regarding breast cancer and oral contraceptive use, the majority of studies have found no overall increase in the risk of developing breast cancer. However, women who use oral contraceptives and have a strong family history of breast cancer or who have breast nodules or abnormal mammograms should be closely followed by their doctors.

ANNUAL NUMBER OF BIRTH-RELATED OR METHOD-RELATED DEATHS ASSOCIATED WITH CONTROL OF FERTILITY PER 100,000 NONSTERILE WOMEN, BY FERTILITY CONTROL METHOD ACCORDING TO AGE

Method of control and outcome	15–19	20–24	25–29	30–34	35–39	40–44
No fertility control methods*	7.0	7.4	9.1	14.8	25.7	28.2
Oral contraceptives non-smoker**	0.3	0.5	0.9	1.9	13.8	31.6
Oral contraceptives smoker**	2.2	3.4	6.6	13.5	51.1	117.2
IUD**	0.8	0.8	1.0	1.0	1.4	1.4
Condom*	1.1	1.6	0.7	0.2	0.3	0.4
Diaphragm/spermicide*	1.9	1.2	1.2	1.3	2.2	2.8
Periodic abstinence*	2.5	1.6	1.6	1.7	2.9	3.6

* Deaths are birth-related
** Deaths are method-related

Some studies have found an increase in the incidence of cancer of the cervix in women who use oral contraceptives. However, this finding may be related to factors other than the use of oral contraceptives.

ESTIMATED RISK OF DEATH FROM A BIRTH CONTROL METHOD OR PREGNANCY

All methods of birth control and pregnancy are associated with a risk of developing certain diseases which may lead to disability or death. An estimate of the number of deaths associated with different methods of birth control and pregnancy has been calculated and is shown in the following table. [See table above].

In the above table, the risk of death from any birth control method is less than the risk of childbirth, except for oral contraceptive users over the age of 35 who smoke and pill users over the age of 40 even if they do not smoke. It can be seen in the table that for women aged 15 to 39, the risk of death was highest with pregnancy (7–26 deaths per 100,000 women, depending on age). Among pill users who do not smoke, the risk of death was always lower than that associated with pregnancy for any age group, although over the age of 40, the risk increases to 32 deaths per 100,000 women, compared to 28 associated with pregnancy at that age. However, for pill users who smoke and are over the age of 35, the estimated number of deaths exceeds those for other methods of birth control. If a woman is over the age of 40 and smokes, her estimated risk of death is four times higher (117/100,000 women) than the estimated risk associated with pregnancy (28/100,000 women) in that age group.

Moreover, if you do not smoke and are under the age of 35, the possible risk of death from oral contraceptive use is extremely low when you consider the failure rate associated with other methods of contraception such as the condom or diaphragm and the resulting pregnancy-associated risk.

WARNING SIGNALS

If any of these adverse effects occur while you are taking oral contraceptives, call your doctor immediately:
- Sharp chest pain, coughing of blood, or sudden shortness of breath (indicating a possible clot in the lung)
- Pain in the calf (indicating a possible clot in the leg)
- Crushing chest pain or heaviness in the chest (indicating a possible heart attack)
- Sudden severe headache or vomiting, dizziness or fainting, disturbances of vision or speech, weakness, or numbness in an arm or leg (indicating a possible stroke)
- Sudden partial or complete loss of vision (indicating a possible clot in the eye)
- Breast lumps (indicating possible breast cancer or fibrocystic disease of the breast; ask your doctor or health care provider to show you how to examine your breasts)
- Severe pain or tenderness in the stomach area (indicating a possibly ruptured liver tumor)
- Difficulty in sleeping, weakness, lack of energy, fatigue, or change in mood (possibly indicating severe depression)
- Jaundice or a yellowing of the skin or eyeballs, accompanied frequently by fever, fatigue, loss of appetite, dark colored urine, or light colored bowel movements (indicating possible liver problems)

SIDE EFFECTS OF ORAL CONTRACEPTIVES

1. Vaginal bleeding

Irregular vaginal bleeding or spotting may occur while you are taking the pills. Irregular bleeding may vary from slight staining between menstrual periods to breakthrough bleeding which is a flow much like a regular period. Irregular bleeding occurs most often during the first few months of oral contraceptive use, but may also occur after you have been taking the pill for some time. Such bleeding may be temporary and usually does not indicate any serious problems. It is important to continue taking your pills on schedule. If the bleeding occurs in more than one cycle or lasts for more than a few days, talk to your doctor or health care provider.

2. Contact lenses

If you wear contact lenses and notice a change in vision or an inability to wear your lenses, contact your doctor or health care provider.

3. Fluid retention

Oral contraceptives may cause edema (fluid retention) with swelling of the fingers or ankles and may raise your blood pressure. If you experience fluid retention, contact your doctor or health care provider.

4. Melasma

A spotty darkening of the skin is possible, particularly of the face, which may persist.

5. Other side effects

Other side effects may include nausea and vomiting, change in appetite, headache, nervousness, depression, dizziness, loss of scalp hair, rash, and vaginal infections.

If any of these side effects bother you, call your doctor or health care provider.

GENERAL PRECAUTIONS

1. Missed periods and use of oral contraceptives before or during early pregnancy

There may be times when you may not menstruate regularly after you have completed taking a cycle of pills. If you have taken your pills regularly and miss one menstrual period, continue taking your pills for the next cycle but be sure to inform your health care provider before doing so. If you have not taken the pills daily as instructed and missed a menstrual period, or if you are taking MICRONOR and missed one tablet, you may be pregnant. If you missed two consecutive menstrual periods, or if you are taking MICRONOR and it is 45 days or more from the start of your last menstrual period, you may be pregnant. Check with your health care provider immediately to determine whether you are pregnant. Do not continue to take oral contraceptives until you are sure you are not pregnant, but continue to use another method of contraception.

There is no conclusive evidence that oral contraceptive use is associated with an increase in birth defects, when taken inadvertently during early pregnancy. Previously, a few studies had reported that oral contraceptives might be associated with birth defects, but these findings have not been seen in more recent studies. Nevertheless, oral contraceptives or any other drugs should not be used during pregnancy unless clearly necessary and prescribed by your doctor. You should check with your doctor about risks to your unborn child of any medication taken during pregnancy.

2. While breast feeding

If you are breast feeding, consult your doctor before starting oral contraceptives. Some of the drug will be passed on to the child in the milk. A few adverse effects on the child have been reported, including yellowing of the skin (jaundice) and breast enlargement. In addition, oral contraceptives may decrease the amount and quality of your milk. If possible, do not use oral contraceptives while breast feeding. You should use another method of contraception since breast feeding provides only partial protection from becoming pregnant and this partial protection decreases significantly as you breast feed for longer periods of time. You should consider starting oral contraceptives only after you have weaned your child completely.

3. Laboratory tests

If you are scheduled for any laboratory tests, tell your doctor you are taking birth control pills. Certain blood tests may be affected by birth control pills.

4. Drug interactions

Certain drugs may interact with birth control pills to make them less effective in preventing pregnancy or cause an increase in breakthrough bleeding. Such drugs include rifampin, drugs used for epilepsy such as barbiturates (for example, phenobarbital) and phenytoin (Dilantin is one brand of this drug), phenylbutazone (Butazolidin is one brand) and possibly certain antibiotics. You may need to use additional contraception when you take drugs which can make oral contraceptives less effective.

HOW TO TAKE ORAL CONTRACEPTIVES

1. General Instructions

You must take your pill every day according to the instructions. Oral contraceptives are most effective if taken no more

Continued on next page

Ortho Pharm.—Cont.

than 24 hours apart. Take your pill at the same time every day so that you are less likely to forget to take it. You will then maintain an effective dose of the oral contraceptive in your body.

ORTHO-NOVUM 7/7/7—Sunday-Start Package:

21-Day Regimen: The first white tablet should be taken on the first Sunday after the menstrual period begins. If period begins on Sunday, begin taking tablets that day. If switching directly from another oral contraceptive, take the first white tablet on the first Sunday after your last ACTIVE tablet of the previous product. Take one white tablet at the same time each day for 7 consecutive days, take one light peach tablet daily for 7 days, then take one peach tablet daily for 7 days. When newly starting oral contraceptives, if the Sunday you begin ORTHO-NOVUM 7/7/7 is more than 5 days from the start of your menstrual period, it is important that you use another method of birth control until you have taken a white tablet daily for seven consecutive days. After taking your last peach tablet, wait for seven days during which time a menstrual period usually occurs. After the seven-day waiting period, on Sunday, start taking a white tablet each day for the next 7 days; a light peach tablet for the next 7 days; then a peach tablet for the next 7 days, thus using a three-weeks-on, one-week-off regimen.

28-Day Regimen: The first white tablet should be taken on the first Sunday after the menstrual period begins. If period begins on Sunday, begin taking tablets that day. If switching directly from another oral contraceptive, take the first white tablet on the first Sunday after your last ACTIVE tablet of the previous product. Take one white tablet at the same time each day for 7 consecutive days, take one light peach tablet daily for 7 days, take one peach tablet daily for 7 days, then take one green tablet daily for 7 days, during which time your period usually occurs. When newly starting oral contraceptives, if the Sunday you begin ORTHO-NOVUM 7/7/7 is more than 5 days from the start of your menstrual period, it is important that you use another method of birth control until you have taken a white tablet daily for seven consecutive days. After 28 tablets have been taken, (last green tablet will always be taken on Saturday) take the first tablet (white) from your next package the following day (Sunday) whether or not you are still menstruating. With the 28-day regimen, tablets are taken every day of the year.

ORTHO-NOVUM 10/11—Sunday-Start Package:

21-Day Regimen: The first white tablet should be taken on the first Sunday after the menstrual period begins. If period begins on Sunday, begin taking tablets that day. If switching directly from another oral contraceptive, take the first white tablet on the first Sunday after your last ACTIVE tablet of the previous product. Take one white tablet at the same time each day for 10 consecutive days, then take one peach tablet daily for 11 days. When newly starting oral contraceptives, if the Sunday you begin ORTHO-NOVUM 10/11 is more than 5 days from the start of your menstrual period, it is important that you use another method of birth control until you have taken a white tablet daily for seven consecutive days. After taking your last peach tablet, wait for seven days during which time a menstrual period usually occurs. After the seven-day waiting period, on Sunday, start taking a white tablet each day for the next 10 days, then a peach tablet for the next 11 days, thus using a three-weeks-on, one-week-off regimen.

28-Day Regimen: The first white tablet should be taken on the first Sunday after the menstrual period begins. If period begins on Sunday, begin taking tablets that day. If switching directly from another oral contraceptive, take the first white tablet on the first Sunday after your last ACTIVE tablet of the previous product. Take one white tablet at the same time each day for 10 days, take one peach tablet daily for 11 days, then take one green tablet daily for 7 days, during which time your period usually occurs. When newly starting oral contraceptives, if the Sunday you begin ORTHO-NOVUM 10/11 is more than 5 days from the start of your menstrual period, it is important that you use another method of birth control until you have taken a white tablet daily for seven consecutive days. After 28 tablets have been taken, (last green tablet will always be taken on a Saturday) take the first tablet (white) from your next package the following day (Sunday) whether or not you are still menstruating. With the 28-day regimen, pills are taken every day of the year.

ORTHO-NOVUM 1/35, MODICON, ORTHO-NOVUM 1/50, ORTHO-NOVUM 1/80 and ORTHO-NOVUM 2 mg

21-day Regimen: Counting the first day of menstrual flow as "Day 1," take one tablet daily from the 5th through the 25th day of the menstrual cycle. If the first tablet is taken later than the 5th day of the menstrual cycle or postpartum, contraceptive reliance should not be placed on ORTHO-NOVUM or MODICON until after the first seven consecutive days of administration. Take a tablet the same time each day, preferably at bedtime, for 21 days, then wait for 7 days during which time a menstrual period usually

occurs. Following the 7-day waiting period, start taking a tablet each day for the next 21 days, thus using a three-weeks-on, one-week-off dosage regimen.

When ORTHO-NOVUM 2 mg □ 21 Tablets are used for the treatment of hypermenorrhea, your physician will discuss the regimen with you.

ORTHO-NOVUM 1/35, MODICON, ORTHO-NOVUM 1/50 and ORTHO-NOVUM 1/80.

28-Day Regimen: The first white, yellow or peach tablet should be taken on the first Sunday after the menstrual period begins. If period begins on Sunday, begin taking tablets that day. If switching directly from another oral contraceptive, take the first white, yellow or peach tablet on the first Sunday after your last ACTIVE tablet of the previous product. Take one white, yellow or peach tablet at the same time each day for 21 consecutive days, then take one green tablet daily for 7 days during which time your menstrual period usually occurs. When newly starting oral contraceptives, if the Sunday you begin ORTHO-NOVUM 1/35, MODICON, ORTHO-NOVUM 1/50 or ORTHO-NOVUM 1/80 is more than 5 days from the start of your menstrual period, it is important that you use another method of birth control until you have taken a white, yellow or peach tablet daily for seven consecutive days. After 28 tablets have been taken, (last green tablet will always be taken on a Saturday) take the first tablet (white, yellow or peach) from your next package the following day (Sunday) whether or not you are still menstruating. With the 28-day regimen, pills are taken every day of the year.

MICRONOR—Continuous Regimen

The first MICRONOR Tablet should be taken on the first day of the menstrual period. Take one tablet at the same time each day without interruption for as long as contraceptive protection is desired.

The effectiveness of progestogen-only oral contraceptives, such as MICRONOR, is lower than that of the combination oral contraceptives containing both estrogen and progestogen. If 100 women utilized an estrogen-containing oral contraceptive for a period of one year, generally less than one pregnancy would be expected to occur; however, if MICRONOR had been utilized, approximately three pregnancies might occur.

Women who participated in the clinical studies with MICRONOR and who had not taken other oral contraceptives before starting MICRONOR had a higher pregnancy rate (four women out of 100), particularly during the first six months of therapy, and to a large extent because they did not take their tablets correctly.

Of course, if you don't take your tablets as directed, or forget to take them every day, the chance you may become pregnant is naturally greater.

MICRONOR (norethindrone) will probably cause some changes in your menstrual pattern. Your cycle, that is the time between menstrual periods, will vary. For example, you might have a 28-day cycle, followed by a 17-day cycle, followed by a 35-day cycle, etc. This is common with MICRONOR.

While using MICRONOR, your period may be longer or shorter than before. If bleeding lasts more than eight days, be sure to let your doctor know.

If your doctor has scheduled you for surgery, or you need prolonged bed rest, he or she may suggest that you stop taking the pill four weeks before surgery to avoid an increased risk of blood clots. It is also advisable not to start oral contraceptives sooner than four weeks after delivery of a baby.

2. If you forget to take your pill

Combination Oral Contraceptives

If you miss only one combination pill in a cycle, the chance of becoming pregnant is small. Take the missed pill as soon as you realize that you have forgotten it and continue to take your tablets for the rest of that cycle as directed. Since the risk of pregnancy increases with each additional pill you skip, it is very important that you take one pill a day. If you should miss more than one tablet, do not take those tablets missed, but begin taking tablets again as soon as remembered and use another method of contraception for the balance of that tablet cycle.

MICRONOR Tablets

If you miss one MICRONOR Tablet in a cycle, you may become pregnant. Check with your doctor immediately. Oral contraceptives should not be taken by pregnant women.

3. Pregnancy due to pill failure

The incidence of pill failure resulting in pregnancy is approximately one percent (i.e., one pregnancy per 100 women per year) if taken every day as directed, but more typical failure rates are about 3%. If failure does occur, the risk to the fetus is minimal.

4. Pregnancy after stopping the pill

There may be some delay in becoming pregnant after you stop using oral contraceptives, especially if you had irregular menstrual cycles before you used oral contraceptives. It may be advisable to postpone conception until you begin menstruating regularly once you have stopped taking the pill and desire pregnancy.

There does not appear to be any increase in birth defects in newborn babies when pregnancy occurs soon after stopping the pill.

5. Overdosage

Serious ill effects have not been reported following ingestion of large doses of oral contraceptives by young children. Overdosage may cause nausea and withdrawal bleeding in females. In case of overdosage, contact your health care provider or pharmacist.

6. Other information

Your health care provider will take a medical and family history before prescribing oral contraceptives and will examine you. You should be reexamined at least once a year. Be sure to inform your health care provider if there is a family history of any of the conditions listed previously in this leaflet. Be sure to keep all appointments with your health care provider, because this is a time to determine if there are early signs of side effects of oral contraceptive use.

Do not use the drug for any condition other than the one for which it was prescribed. This drug has been prescribed specifically for you; do not give it to others who may want birth control pills.

HEALTH BENEFITS FROM ORAL CONTRACEPTIVES

In addition to preventing pregnancy, use of combination oral contraceptives may provide certain benefits. They are:

- menstrual cycles may become more regular
- blood flow during menstruation may be lighter and less iron may be lost. Therefore, anemia due to iron deficiency is less likely to occur.
- pain or other symptoms during menstruation may be encountered less frequently
- ectopic (tubal) pregnancy may occur less frequently
- noncancerous cysts or lumps in the breast may occur less frequently
- acute pelvic inflammatory disease may occur less frequently
- oral contraceptive use may provide some protection against developing two forms of cancer: cancer of the ovaries and cancer of the lining of the uterus.

If you want more information about birth control pills, ask your doctor or pharmacist. They have a more technical leaflet called the Professional Labeling, which you may wish to read. The professional labeling is also published in a book entitled *Physicians' Desk Reference,* available in many book stores and public libraries.

Shown in Product Identification Section, page 420

PROTOSTAT®   ℞
(metronidazole) Tablets

WARNING

Metronidazole has been shown to be carcinogenic in mice and rats. *(See Warnings.)* Unnecessary use of this drug should be avoided. Its use should be reserved for the conditions described in the *Indications And Usage* section below.

DESCRIPTION

PROTOSTAT (metronidazole) is a 1-(β-hydroxyethyl)-2-methyl-5-nitroimidazole. Both the 250 mg and 500 mg tablets include the following inactive ingredients: Lactose, magnesium stearate, microcrystalline cellulose, povidone, sodium starch glycolate, and stearic acid. Metronidazole is classified therapeutically as an antiprotozoal *(Trichomonas),* and antibacterial (antianaerobic) agent. It occurs as pale yellow crystals that are slightly soluble in water and alcohol. Metronidazole has the following structural formula:

CLINICAL PHARMACOLOGY

Metronidazole is usually well absorbed after oral administration, with peak plasma concentrations occurring between one and two hours. An average elimination half-life is 8 hours in healthy humans. Plasma concentrations of metronidazole are proportional to the administered dose. Oral administration of 250 mg., 500 mg., or 2,000 mg. produced peak plasma concentrations of 6 mcg/ml, 12 mcg/ml, and 40 mcg/ml, respectively. Studies reveal no significant bioavailability differences between males and females; however, because of weight differences, the resulting plasma levels in males are generally lower.

Metronidazole is the major component appearing in the plasma, with lesser quantities of the 2-hydroxymethyl metabolite also being present. Less than 20% of the circulating metronidazole is bound to plasma proteins. Both the parent compound and the metabolite possess *in vitro* trichomonacidal activity and *in vitro* bactericidal activity against most strains of anaerobic bacteria.

The major route of elimination of metronidazole and its metabolites is via the urine (60-80% of the dose), with fecal excretion accounting for 6-15% of the dose. The metabolites that appear in the urine result primarily from side-chain oxidation [1-(β-hydroxyethyl)-2-hydroxymethyl-5-nitroimidazole and 2-methyl-5-nitroimidazole-1-yl-acetic acid] and glucuronide conjugation, with unchanged metronidazole accounting for approximately 20% of the total. Renal clearance of metronidazole is approximately 10 ml/min/1.73m².

Decreased renal function does not alter the single-dose pharmacokinetics of metronidazole. However, plasma clearance of metronidazole is decreased in patients with decreased liver function.

Metronidazole appears in cerebrospinal fluid, saliva, and breast milk in concentrations similar to those found in plasma. Bactericidal concentrations of metronidazole have also been detected in pus from hepatic abscesses.

Microbiology: Metronidazole possesses direct trichomonacidal and amoebicidal activity against *Trichomonas Vaginalis* and *Entamoeba histolytica.* The *in vitro* minimal inhibitory concentration (MIC) for most strains of these organisms is 1 mcg/ml or less. Metronidazole's mechanism of antiprotozoal action is unknown.

Anaerobic Bacteria: Metronidazole is active *in vitro* against obligate anaerobes, but does not appear to possess any clinically relevant activity against facultative anaerobes or obligate aerobes. Against susceptible organisms, metronidazole is generally bactericidal at concentrations equal to or slightly higher than the minimal inhibitory concentrations (MIC). Metronidazole has been shown to have *in vitro* and clinical activity against the following organisms:

Anaerobic gram-negative bacilli, including:
Bacteroides species, including the *Bacteroides fragilis* group (*B. fragilis, B. distasonis, B. ovatus, B. thetaiotaomicron, B. vulgatus*)
Fusobacterium species
Anaerobic gram-positive bacilli, including:
Clostridium species and susceptible strains of *Eubacterium*
Anaerobic gram-positive cocci, including:
Peptococcus species
Peptostreptococcus species

Susceptibility tests: Bacteriologic studies should be performed to determine the causative organisms and their susceptibility to metronidazole; however, the rapid, routine susceptibility testing of individual isolates of anaerobic bacteria is not always practical, and therapy may be started while awaiting these results.

Quantitative methods give the most precise estimates of susceptibility to antibacterial drugs. A standardized agar dilution method and a broth microdilution method are recommended.[1]

Control strains are recommended for standardized susceptibility testing. Each time the test is performed, one or more of the following strains should be included: *Clostridium perfringens* ATCC 13124, *Bacteroides fragilis* ATCC 25285, and *Bacteroides thetaiotaomicron* ATCC 29741. The mode metronidazole MIC's for those three strains are reported to be 0.25, 0.25, and 0.5 mcg/ml, respectively.

A clinical laboratory is considered under acceptable control if the results of the control strains are within one doubling dilution of the mode MIC's reported for metronidazole.

A bacterial isolate may be considered susceptible if the MIC value for metronidazole is not more than 16 mcg/ml. An organism is considered resistant if the MIC is greater than 16 mcg/ml. A report of "resistant" from the laboratory indicates that the infecting organism is not likely to respond to therapy.

INDICATIONS AND USAGE

Symptomatic Trichomoniasis: PROTOSTAT is indicated for the treatment of symptomatic trichomoniasis in females and males when the presence of trichomonad has been confirmed by appropriate laboratory procedures (wet smears and/or cultures).

Asymptomatic Trichomoniasis: PROTOSTAT is indicated in the treatment of asymptomatic females when the organism is associated with endocervicitis, cervicitis, or cervical erosion. Since there is evidence that presence of the trichomonad can interfere with accurate assessment of abnormal cytological smears, additional smears should be performed after eradication of the parasite.

Treatment of Asymptomatic Consorts: *T. vaginalis* infection is a venereal disease. Therefore, asymptomatic sexual partners of treated patients should be treated simultaneously if the organism has been found to be present in order to prevent reinfection of the partner. The decision as to whether to treat an asymptomatic male partner with a negative culture or one in whom no culture has been attempted is an individual one. In making this decision, it should be noted that there is evidence that women may become reinfected if the consort is not treated. Also, since there can be considerable difficulty in isolating the organism from the asymptomatic male car-

rier, negative smears and cultures cannot be relied upon in this regard. In any event, the consort should be treated with PROTOSTAT in cases of reinfection.

Amebiasis: PROTOSTAT is indicated in the treatment of acute intestinal amoebiasis (amoebic dysentery) and amoebic liver abscess.

In amoebic liver abscess, PROTOSTAT therapy does not obviate the need for aspiration or drainage of pus.

Anaerobic Bacterial Infections: PROTOSTAT is indicated in the treatment of serious infections caused by susceptible anaerobic bacteria. Indicated surgical procedures should be performed in conjunction with PROTOSTAT therapy. In a mixed aerobic and anaerobic infection, antibiotics appropriate for the treatment of aerobic infection should be used in addition to PROTOSTAT. In the treatment of most serious anaerobic infections the intravenous form of metronidazole is usually administered initially. This may be followed by oral therapy with PROTOSTAT at the discretion of the physician.

INTRA-ABDOMINAL INFECTION, including peritonitis, intra-abdominal abscess, and liver abscess, caused by *Bacteroides* species including the *B. fragilis* group (*B. fragilis, B. distasonis, B. ovatus, B. thetaiotaomicron, B. vulgatus), Clostridium* species, *Eubacterium* species, *Peptococcus* species, and *Peptostreptococcus* species.

SKIN AND SKIN STRUCTURE INFECTIONS caused by *Bacteroides* species including the *B. fragilis* group, *Clostridium* species, *Peptococcus* species, *Peptostreptococcus* species, and *Fusobacterium* species.

GYNECOLOGIC INFECTIONS, including endometritis, endomyometritis, tubo-ovarian abscess, and post-surgical vaginal cuff infection, caused by *Bacteroides* species including the *B. fragilis* group, *Clostridium* species, *Peptococcus* species, and *Peptostreptococcus* species.

BACTERIAL SEPTICEMIA caused by *Bacteroides* species including the *B. fragilis* group, and *Clostridium* species.

BONE AND JOINT INFECTIONS, as adjunctive therapy, caused by *Bacteroides* species including the *B. fragilis* group.

CENTRAL NERVOUS SYSTEM (CNS) INFECTIONS, including meningitis and brain abscess, caused by *Bacteroides* species including the *B. fragilis* group.

LOWER RESPIRATORY TRACT INFECTIONS, including pneumonia, empyema, and lung abscess, caused by *Bacteroides* species including the *B. fragilis* group.

ENDOCARDITIS caused by *Bacteroides* species including the *B. fragilis* group.

CONTRAINDICATIONS

PROTOSTAT is contraindicated in patients with a prior history of hypersensitivity to metronidazole or other nitroimidazole derivatives. PROTOSTAT is contraindicated during the first trimester of pregnancy. (*See Warnings.*)

WARNINGS

Convulsive Seizures and Peripheral Neuropathy: Convulsive seizures and peripheral neuropathy, the latter characterized mainly by numbness or paresthesia of an extremity, have been reported in patients treated with metronidazole. The appearance of abnormal neurologic signs demands the prompt discontinuation of PROTOSTAT therapy. PROTOSTAT should be administered with caution to patients with central nervous system diseases.

Tumorigenicity Studies in Rodents: Metronidazole has shown evidence of carcinogenic activity in a number of studies involving chronic, oral administration in mice and rats. Prominent among the effects in the mouse was the promotion of pulmonary tumorigenesis. This has been observed in all six reported studies in that species, including one study in which the animals were dosed on an intermittent schedule (administration during every fourth week only). At very high dose levels (approx. 500mg/kg/day) there was a statistically significant increase in the incidence of malignant liver tumors in males. Also, the published results of one of the mouse studies indicated an increase in the incidence of malignant lymphomas as well as pulmonary neoplasms associated with lifetime feeding of the drug. All these effects are statistically significant.

Several long-term oral dosing studies in the rats have been completed. There was a statistically significant increase in the incidence of various neoplasms, particularly in mammary and hepatic tumors, among female rats administered metronidazole over those noted in the concurrent female control groups.

Two lifetime tumorigenicity studies in hamsters have been performed and reported to be negative.

Mutagenicity Studies: Although metronidazole has shown mutagenic activity in a number of *in vitro* assay systems, studies in mammals (*in vivo*) have failed to demonstrate a potential for genetic damage.

PRECAUTIONS

General: Patients with severe hepatic disease metabolize metronidazole slowly, with resultant accumulation of metronidazole and its metabolites in the plasma. Accordingly, for such patients, doses below those usually recommended should be administered cautiously.

Known or previously unrecognized candidiasis may present more prominent symptoms during therapy with PROTOSTAT and requires treatment with a candicidal agent.

Information for Patients: Alcoholic beverages should be avoided while taking metronidazole and at least one day afterward. (*See Drug Interactions.*)

Laboratory Tests: PROTOSTAT (metronidazole) is a nitroimidazole and should be used with care in patients with evidence of, or history of, blood dyscrasia. A mild leukopenia has been observed during its administration; however, no persistent hematologic abnormalities attributable to metronidazole have been observed in clinical studies. Total and differential leukocyte counts are recommended before and after therapy for trichomoniasis and amoebiasis, especially if a second course of therapy is necessary, and before and after therapy for anaerobic infection.

Drug Interactions: Metronidazole has been reported to potentiate the anticoagulant effect of coumarin and warfarin resulting in a prolongation of prothrombin time. This possible drug interaction should be considered when PROTOSTAT is prescribed for patients on this type of anticoagulant therapy.

The simultaneous administration of drugs that decrease microsomal liver enzyme activity, such as cimetidine, may prolong the half-life and decrease plasma clearance of metronidazole.

Alcoholic beverages should not be consumed during metronidazole therapy and for at least one day afterward because abdominal cramps, nausea, vomiting, headache, and flushing may occur.

Drug/Laboratory Test Interactions: Metronidazole may interfere with certain types of determinations of serum chemistry values, such as aspartate aminotransferase (AST, SGOT), alanine aminotransferase (ALT, SGPT), lactate dehydrogenase (LDH), triglycerides, and hexokinase glucose. Values of zero may be observed. All of the assays in which interference has been reported involve enzymatic coupling of the assay to oxidation-reduction of nicotine adenine dinucleotide (NAD NADH). Interference is due to the similarity in absorbance peaks of NADH (340 nm) and metronidazole (322 nm) at pH 7.

Carcinogenesis: (See Warnings.)

Pregnancy: Teratogenic Effects—Pregnancy Category B: Metronidazole crosses the placental barrier and enters the fetal circulation rapidly. Reproduction studies have been performed in rats at doses up to five times the human dose and have revealed no evidence of impaired fertility or harm to the fetus due to metronidazole. Metronidazole administered intraperitoneally to pregnant mice at approximately the human dose caused fetotoxicity; administered orally to pregnant mice, no fetotoxicity was observed. There are, however, no adequate and well-controlled studies in pregnant women. Because animal reproduction studies are not always predictive of human response, and because metronidazole is a carcinogen in rodents, this drug should be used during pregnancy only if clearly needed (see Contraindications). Use of PROTOSTAT for trichomoniasis in the second and third trimesters should be restricted to those in whom local palliative treatment has been inadequate to control symptoms.

Nursing Mothers: Because of the potential for tumorigenicity shown for metronidazole in mouse and rat studies, a decision should be made whether to discontinue nursing or to discontinue the drug, taking into account the importance of the drug to the mother. Metronidazole is secreted in breast milk in concentrations similar to those found in plasma.

Pediatric Use: Safety and effectiveness in children have not been established, except for the treatment of amebiasis.

ADVERSE REACTIONS

The two most serious adverse reactions reported in patients treated with PROTOSTAT (metronidazole) have been convulsive seizures and peripheral neuropathy, the latter characterized mainly by numbness or paresthesia of an extremity. Since persistent peripheral neuropathy has been reported in some patients receiving prolonged administration of PROTOSTAT, patients should be specifically warned about these reactions and should be told to stop the drug and report immediately to their physicians if any neurologic symptoms occur.

The most common adverse reactions reported have been referable to the gastrointestinal tract, particularly nausea reported by about 12% of patients, sometimes accompanied by headache, anorexia, and occasionally vomiting; diarrhea, epigastric distress; and abdominal cramping. Constipation has also been reported.

The following reactions have also been reported during treatment with PROTOSTAT (metronidazole):

Mouth: A sharp, unpleasant metallic taste is not unusual. Furry tongue, glossitis, and stomatitis have occurred; these may be associated with a sudden overgrowth of *Candida* which may occur during effective therapy.

Continued on next page

Ortho Pharm.—Cont.

Hematopoietic: Reversible neutropenia (leukopenia); rarely, reversible thrombocytopenia.

Cardiovascular: Flattening of the T-wave may be seen in electrocardiographic tracings.

Central Nervous System: Convulsive seizures, peripheral neuropathy, dizziness, vertigo, incoordination, ataxia, confusion, irritability, depression, weakness, and insomnia.

Hypersensitivity: Urticaria, erythematous rash, flushing, nasal congestion, dryness of mouth (or vagina or vulva), and fever.

Renal: Dysuria, cystitis, polyuria, incontinence, and a sense of pelvic pressure. Instances of darkened urine have been reported by approximately one patient in 100,000. Although the pigment which is probably responsible for this phenomenon has not been positively identified, it is almost certainly a metabolite of metronidazole and seems to have no clinical significance.

Other: Proliferation of *Candida* in the vagina, dyspareunia, decrease of libido, proctitis, and fleeting joint pains sometimes resembling "serum sickness." If patients receiving PROTOSTAT drink alcoholic beverages, they may experience abdominal distress, nausea, vomiting, flushing, or headache. A modification of the taste of alcoholic beverages has also been reported.

Crohn's disease patients are known to have an increased incidence of gastrointestinal and certain extraintestinal cancers. There have been some reports in the medical literature of breast and colon cancer in Crohn's disease patients who have been treated with metronidazole at high doses for extended periods of time. A cause and effect relationship has not been established. Crohn's disease is not an approved indication for metronidazole.

OVERDOSAGE

Single oral doses of metronidazole, up to 15 g, have been reported in suicide attempts and accidental overdoses. Symptoms reported include nausea, vomiting, and ataxia. Oral metronidazole has been used as a radiation sensitizer in the treating of malignant tumors. Neurotoxic effects, including seizures and peripheral neuropathy, have been reported after 5 to 7 days of doses of 6 to 10.4 g every other day.

Treatment: There is no specific antidote for PROTOSTAT overdose; therefore, management of the patient should consist of symptomatic and supportive therapy.

DOSAGE AND ADMINISTRATION

Trichomoniasis:

In The Female: One-day treatment—two grams of PROTOSTAT given either as a single dose or in two divided doses of one gram each given in the same day.

Seven-day course of treatment—250 mg three times daily for seven consecutive days. There is some indication from controlled comparative studies that cure rates as determined by vaginal smears, signs and symptoms, may be higher after a seven-day course of treatment than after a one-day treatment regimen.

The dosage regimen should be individualized. Single-dose treatment can assure compliance, especially if administered under supervision, in those patients who cannot be relied on to continue the seven-day regimen.

A seven-day course of treatment may minimize reinfection of the female long enough to treat sexual contacts. Further, some patients may tolerate one course of therapy better than the other.

Pregnant patients should not be treated during the first trimester with either regimen. If treated during the second or third trimester, the one-day course of therapy should not be used, as it results in higher serum levels which reach the fetal circulation. *(See Contraindications and Precautions.)*

When repeated courses of the drug are required, it is recommended that an interval of four to six weeks elapse between courses and that the presence of the trichomonad be reconfirmed by appropriate laboratory measures. Total and differential leukocyte counts should be made before and after treatment.

In The Male: Treatment should be individualized as for the female.

Amebiasis: Adults: For Acute Intestinal Amebiasis (Acute Amebic Dysentery):

750 mg. orally 3 times daily for 5 to 10 days.

For Amebic Liver Abscess: 500 mg or 750 mg orally 3 times daily for 5 to 10 days.

Children: 35 to 50 mg/kg of body weight/24 hours divided into 3 doses, orally for 10 days.

Anaerobic Bacterial Infections: In the treatment of most serious anaerobic infections the intravenous form of metronidazole is usually administered initially.

Following intravenous therapy, oral metronidazole may be used when conditions warrant based upon the severity of the disease and the response of the patient to intravenous treatment.

The usual adult *oral* dosage is 7.5 mg/kg every six hours (approximately 500 mg for a 70 kg adult). A maximum of 4.0 g should not be exceeded during a 24-hour period.

The usual duration of therapy is 7 to 10 days; however, infections of the bone and joint, lower respiratory tract, and endocardium may require longer treatment.

Patients with severe hepatic disease metabolize metronidazole slowly, with resultant accumulation of metronidazole and its metabolites in the plasma. Accordingly, for such patients, doses below those usually recommended should be administered cautiously. Close monitoring of plasma metronidazole levels[2] and toxicity is recommended.

The dose of PROTOSTAT should not be specifically reduced in anuric patients since accumulated metabolites may be rapidly removed by dialysis.

HOW SUPPLIED

Available in tablets containing 250 mg and 500 mg of metronidazole, USP. PROTOSTAT 250 mg is a white to off-white capsule-shaped, convex tablet. Each 250 mg PROTOSTAT Tablet is scored on one side and imprinted with ORTHO 1570 on the other side, packaged in a bottle of 100 tablets (NDC 0062-1570-01). PROTOSTAT 500 mg is a white to off-white capsule-shaped, convex tablet. Each 500 mg PROTOSTAT tablet is scored on one side and imprinted with ORTHO 1571 on the other side, packaged in a bottle of 50 tablets (NDC 0062-1571-01).

Dispense in well-closed, light-resistant containers as defined in the USP.

Store below 86°F (30°C).

1. Proposed standard: PSM-11—Proposed Reference Dilution Procedure for Antimicrobic Susceptibility Testing of Anaerobic Bacteria, National Committee for Clinical Laboratory Standards, and Sutter, et al: Collaborative Evaluation of a Proposed Reference Dilution Method of Susceptibility Testing of Anaerobic Bacteria, Antimicrob. Agents Chemother. *16*:495-502 (Oct.) 1979; and Talley, et al: *In Vitro* Activity of Thienamycin Antimicrob. Agents Chemother. *14*:436-438 (Sept.) 1978.

2. Ralph, E.D., and Kirby, W.M.M.: Bioassay of Metronidazole With Either Anaerobic or Aerobic Incubation, J. Infect. Dis. *132*:587-591 (Nov.) 1975; or Gulaid, et al: Determination of Metronidazole and Its Major Metabolites in Biological Fluids by High Pressure Liquid Chromatography, Br. J. Clin. Pharmacol. *6*:430-432, 1978.

Shown in Product Identification Section, page 420

SULTRIN™ Triple Sulfa Cream ℞
(sulfathiazole/sulfacetamide/
sulfabenzamide/urea)

SULTRIN™ Triple Sulfa ℞
Vaginal Tablets
(sulfathiazole/sulfacetamide/
sulfabenzamide)

DESCRIPTION

SULTRIN Cream contains sulfathiazole (Benzenesulfonamide,4-amino-N-2-thiazolyl-N[1]-2-thiazolylsulfanilamide) 3.42%, sulfacetamide (Acetamide,N-[(4-aminophenyl) sulfonyl]-N-Sulfanilylacetamide) 2.86%, sulfabenzamide (Benzamide,N-[(4-aminophenyl) sulfonyl]-N-Sulfanilylbenzamide) 3.7% and urea (carbamide) 0.64%, compounded with glyceryl monostearate, cetyl alcohol 2%, stearic acid, cholesterol, lanolin, lecithin, peanut oil, propylparaben, propylene glycol, diethylaminoethyl stearamide, phosphoric acid, methylparaben and purified water.

Each SULTRIN Tablet contains sulfathiazole (Benzenesulfonamide,4-amino-N -2- thiazolyl-N[1]-2-thiazolylsulfanilamide) 172.5 mg, sulfacetamide (Acetamide,N-[(4-aminophenyl)sulfonyl] -N- Sulfanilylacetamide) 143.75 mg and sulfabenzamide (Benzamide,N-[(4-aminophenyl)sulfonyl]-N-Sulfanilylbenzamide) 184.0 mg, compounded with urea, lactose, guar gum, starch and magnesium stearate.

SULTRIN Cream and SULTRIN Tablets are topical antibacterial preparations available for intravaginal administration.

CLINICAL PHARMACOLOGY

The mode of action of SULTRIN is not completely known. SULTRIN Cream and SULTRIN Tablets are topical antibacterial preparations used intravaginally against *Haemophilus (Gardnerella) vaginalis* bacteria. Indirect effects, such as lowering the vaginal pH, may be equally important mechanisms.

INDICATIONS AND USAGE

SULTRIN Cream and SULTRIN Tablets are indicated for the treatment of vaginitis caused by *Haemophilus (Gardnerella) vaginalis* bacteria.

The diagnosis of a *Haemophilus (Gardnerella) vaginalis* vaginitis should be firmly established before initiation of treatment with SULTRIN.

CONTRAINDICATIONS

SULTRIN is contraindicated in the following circumstances: kidney disease; hypersensitivity to sulfonamides; in pregnancy at term and during the nursing period because sulfonamides cross the placenta, are excreted in breast milk and may cause Kernicterus.

WARNINGS

Deaths associated with the administration of sulfonamides have been reported from hypersensitivity reactions, agranulocytosis, aplastic anemia and other blood dyscrasias.

The presence of clinical signs such as sore throat, fever, pallor, purpura or jaundice may be early indications of serious blood disorders.

PRECAUTIONS

Because sulfonamides may be absorbed from the vaginal mucosa, the usual precautions for oral sulfonamides apply. Patients should be observed for skin rash or evidence of systemic toxicity, and if these develop, the medications should be discontinued.

Laboratory tests: Standard office diagnostic procedures for vaginitis are usually sufficient to establish the diagnosis of *Haemophilus (Gardnerella) vaginalis* and to rule out a trichomonal or monilial infection. These include noting a fish-like odor upon addition of 10% KOH to vaginal discharge and microscopic identification of "clue cells" in a wet mount preparation. If cultures are obtained, care must be taken to use appropriate media and methods for *Haemophilus (Gardnerella) vaginalis.*

Carcinogenesis, mutagenesis, impairment of fertility: The sulfonamides bear certain chemical similarities to some goitrogens. Rats appear to be especially susceptible to the goitrogenic effects of sulfonamides, and long-term administration has produced thyroid malignancies in this species.

Pregnancy:

Teratogenic Effects: Pregnancy Category C: The safe use of sulfonamides in pregnancy has not been established. The teratogenicity potential of most sulfonamides has not been thoroughly investigated in either animals or humans. However, a significant increase in the incidence of cleft palate and other bony abnormalities of offspring has been observed when certain sulfonamides of the short, intermediate and long-acting types were given to pregnant rats and mice at high oral doses (7 to 25 times the human therapeutic dose).

Nursing Mothers: Because of the potential for serious adverse reactions in nursing infants from SULTRIN, a decision should be made whether to discontinue nursing or to discontinue the drug, taking into account the importance of the drug to the mother. See CONTRAINDICATIONS.

Pediatric use: Safety and effectiveness in children have not been established.

ADVERSE REACTIONS

There has been one reported case of Agranulocystosis in a patient receiving SULTRIN Cream. The most frequent adverse reactions to SULTRIN are localized irritation and/or allergy including rare reports of Stevens Johnson syndrome which may be fatal.

DOSAGE AND ADMINISTRATION

SULTRIN Cream. One full applicator intravaginally twice daily for four to six days. This course of therapy may be repeated if necessary; the dosage may be reduced one-half to one-quarter.

SULTRIN Vaginal Tablets. One tablet intravaginally before retiring and again in the morning for ten days. This course may be repeated, if necessary.

HOW SUPPLIED

Cream—78 g tubes with the ORTHO* Measured-Dose Applicator.

Vaginal Tablets (as white, capsule-shaped tablets with the Ortho Shield and the word "Ortho" debossed on one side)—Package of twenty foil-wrapped tablets with vaginal applicator.

NDC 0062-5440-77; SULTRIN Cream
NDC 0062-5441-64; SULTRIN Tablets
REVISED JANUARY 1988   643-10-380-4

TERAZOL® 3 ℞
Vaginal Suppositories 80 mg
(terconazole)

DESCRIPTION

TERAZOL 3 Vaginal Suppositories are white to off-white suppositories for intravaginal administration containing 80 mg of the antifungal agent terconazole, *cis* -1-[4-[[2-(2,4-dichlorophenyl)-2-(1H-1,2, 4-triazol-1-ylmethyl)-1,3-dioxolan-4-yl]methoxy]phenyl]-4-(1-methylethyl) piperazine, in triglycerides derived from coconut and/or palm kernel oil (a base of hydrogenated vegetable oils) and butylated hydroxyanisole.

TERCONAZOLE

$C_{26}H_{31}Cl_2N_5O_3$

Terconazole, a triazole derivative, is a white to almost white powder with a molecular weight of 532.47. It is insoluble in water; sparingly soluble in ethanol; and soluble in butanol.

CLINICAL PHARMACOLOGY

Microbiology: Terconazole exhibits fungicidal activity *in vitro* against *Candida albicans*. The MIC values for terconazole against most species of lactic acid bacteria typically found in the human vagina were ≥ 128 mcg/ml, therefore, these beneficial bacteria are not affected by drug treatment. The exact pharmacologic mode of action of terconazole is uncertain; however, it may exert its antifungal activity by the disruption of normal fungal cell membrane permeability. No resistance to terconazole has developed during successive passages of *C. albicans*.

Human Pharmacology: Following intravaginal administration of terconazole in humans, absorption ranged from 5–8% in three hysterectomized subjects and 12–16% in two non-hysterectomized subjects with tubal ligations. Following oral (30 mg) administration of ^{14}C-labelled terconazole, the half-life of elimination from the blood for the parent terconazole was 6.9 hours (range 4.0–11.3). Terconazole is extensively metabolized; the plasma AUC for terconazole compared to the AUC for total radioactivity was 0.6%. Total radioactivity was eliminated from the blood with a half-life of 52.2 hours (range 44–60). Excretion of radioactivity was both by renal (32–56%) and fecal (47–52%) routes.

Photosensitivity reactions were observed in some normal volunteers following repeated dermal application of terconazole 2.0% and 0.8% creams under conditions of filtered artificial ultraviolet light.

Photosensitivity reactions have not been observed in U.S. and foreign clinical trials in patients who were treated vaginally with terconazole suppositories or cream.

INDICATIONS AND USAGE

TERAZOL 3 Vaginal Suppositories are indicated for the local treatment of vulvovaginal candidiasis (moniliasis). As TERAZOL 3 Vaginal Suppositories are effective only for vulvovaginitis caused by the genus *Candida*, the diagnosis should be confirmed by KOH smears and/or cultures.

CONTRAINDICATIONS

Patients known to be hypersensitive to terconazole or to any components of the suppository.

WARNINGS

None.

PRECAUTIONS

General: Discontinue use and do not retreat with terconazole if sensitization, irritation, fever, chills or flu-like symptoms are reported during use. The base contained in the suppository formulation may interact with certain rubber latex products, such as those used in vaginal contraceptive diaphragms, therefore concurrent use is not recommended. If there is lack of response to TERAZOL 3 Vaginal Suppositories, appropriate microbiological studies (standard KOH smear and/or cultures) should be repeated to confirm the diagnosis and rule out other pathogens.

Drug Interactions: The therapeutic effect of TERAZOL 3 Vaginal Suppositories is not affected by oral contraceptive usage.

Carcinogenesis, Mutagenesis, Impairment of Fertility

Carcinogenesis: Studies to determine the carcinogenic potential of terconazole have not been performed.

Mutagenicity: Terconazole was not mutagenic when tested *in vitro* for induction of microbial point mutations (Ames test), or for inducing cellular transformation, or *in vivo* for chromosome breaks (micronucleus test) or dominant lethal mutations in mouse germ cells.

Impairment of Fertility: No impairment of fertility occurred when female rats were administered terconazole orally up to 40 mg/kg/day.

Pregnancy: Pregnancy Category C

There was no evidence of teratogenicity when terconazole was administered orally up to 40 mg/kg/day (25 × the recommended intravaginal human dose) in rats, or 20 mg/kg/day in rabbits, or subcutaneously in rats up to 20 mg/kg/day. Dosages at or below 10 mg/kg/day produced no embryotoxicity; however, there was a delay in fetal ossification at 10 mg/kg/day in rats. There was some evidence of embryotoxicity in rabbits and rats at 20–40 mg/kg. In rats this was reflected as a decrease in litter size and number of viable young and reduced fetal weight. There was also delay in ossification and an increased incidence of skeletal variants.

The no-effect oral dose of 10 mg/kg/day resulted in a mean peak plasma level of terconazole in pregnant rats of 0.176 mcg/ml which exceeds by 44 times the mean peak plasma level (0.004 mcg/ml) seen in normal subjects after intravaginal administration of terconazole. This assessment does not account for possible exposure of the fetus through direct transfer of terconazole from the irritated vagina to the fetus by diffusion across amniotic membranes.

Since terconazole is absorbed from the human vagina, it should not be used in the first trimester of pregnancy unless the physician considers it essential to the welfare of the patient.

Nursing Mothers: It is not known whether terconazole is excreted in human milk. Animal studies hve shown that rat off-spring exposed via the milk of treated (40 mg/kg/orally) dams showed decreased survival during the first few postpartum days. Because many drugs are excreted in human milk, and because of the potential for adverse reaction in nursing infants from terconazole, a decision should be made whether to discontinue nursing or to discontinue the drug, taking into account the importance of the drug to the mother.

Pediatric Use: Safety and efficacy in children have not been established.

ADVERSE REACTIONS

During controlled clinical studies conducted in the United States, 284 patients with vulvovaginal candidiasis were treated with terconazole 80 mg vaginal suppositories. Based on comparative analyses with placebo (295 patients) the adverse experiences considered adverse reactions most likely related to terconazole 80 mg vaginal suppositories were headache (30.3% vs 20.7% with placebo) and pain of the female genitalia (4.2% vs 0.7% with placebo). Adverse reactions that were reported but were not statistically significantly different from placebo were burning (15.2% vs 11.2% with placebo) and body pain (3.9% vs 1.7% with placebo). Fever (2.8% vs 1.4% with placebo) and chills (1.8% vs 0.7% with placebo) have also been reported. The therapy-related dropout rate was 3.5% and the placebo therapy-related dropout rate was 2.7%. The adverse drug experience on terconazole most frequently causing discontinuation was burning (2.5% vs 1.4% with placebo) and pruritus (1.8% vs 1.4% with placebo).

DOSAGE AND ADMINISTRATION

One TERAZOL 3 Vaginal Suppository (80 mg terconazole) is administered intravaginally once daily at bedtime for three consecutive days. Before prescribing another course of therapy, the diagnosis should be reconfirmed by smears and/or cultures and other pathogens commonly associated with vulvovaginitis ruled out. The therapeutic effect of TERAZOL 3 Vaginal Suppositories is not affected by menstruation.

HOW SUPPLIED

TERAZOL 3 (terconazole) Vaginal Suppositories 80 mg are available as 2.5 g, elliptically shaped white to off-white suppositories in packages of three (NDC 0062-5351-01) with a vaginal applicator. Store at Controlled Room Temperature (59°F–86°F or 15°C–30°C).

643-10-302-5   REVISED JANUARY 1989

Shown in Product Identification Section, page 420

TERAZOL® 7   ℞
Vaginal Cream 0.4%
(terconazole)

DESCRIPTION

TERAZOL 7 Vaginal Cream is a white to off-white, water washable cream for intravaginal administration containing 0.4% of the antifungal agent terconazole, *cis*-1-[4-[[2-(2,4-dichlorophenyl)-2-(1H-1, 2, 4-triazol-1-ylmethyl)-1,3-dioxolan-4-yl]methoxy]phenyl]-4-(1-methylethyl) piperazine, compounded in a cream base consisting of butylated hydroxyanisole, cetyl alcohol, isopropyl myristate, polysorbate 60, polysorbate 80, propylene glycol, stearyl alcohol, and purified water.

TERCONAZOLE

$C_{26}H_{31}Cl_2N_5O_3$

Terconazole, a triazole derivative, is a white to almost white powder with a molecular weight of 532.47. It is insoluble in water; sparingly soluble in ethanol; and soluble in butanol.

CLINICAL PHARMACOLOGY

Microbiology: Terconazole exhibits fungicidal activity *in vitro* against *Candida albicans*. Antifungal activity also has been demonstrated against other fungi. The MIC values for

terconazole against most species of lactic acid bacteria typically found in the human vagina were ≥ 128 mcg/ml, therefore these beneficial bacteria are not affected by drug treatment.

The exact pharmacologic mode of action of terconazole is uncertain; however, it may exert its antifungal activity by the disruption of normal fungal cell membrane permeability. No resistance to terconazole has developed during successive passages of *C. albicans*.

Human Pharmacology: Following intravaginal administration of terconazole in humans, absorption ranged from 5–8% in three hysterectomized subjects and 12–16% in two non-hysterectomized subjects with tubal ligations.

Following oral (30 mg) administration of ^{14}C-labelled terconazole, the half-life of elimination from the blood for the parent terconazole was 6.9 hours (range 4.0–11.3). Terconazole is extensively metabolized; the plasma AUC for terconazole compared to the AUC for total radioactivity was 0.6%. Total radioactivity was eliminated from the blood with a half-life of 52.2 hours (range 44–60). Excretion of radioactivity was both by renal (32–56%) and fecal (47–52%) routes.

Photosensitivity reactions were observed in some normal volunteers following repeated dermal application of terconazole, 2.0% and 0.8% creams under conditions of filtered artificial ultraviolet light. Photosensitivity reactions have not been observed in U.S. and foreign clinical trials in patients who were treated with terconazole 0.4% vaginal cream.

INDICATIONS AND USAGE

TERAZOL 7 Vaginal Cream is indicated for the local treatment of vulvovaginal candidiasis (moniliasis). As TERAZOL 7 Vaginal Cream is effective only for vulvovaginitis caused by the genus *Candida*, the diagnosis should be confirmed by KOH smears and/or cultures.

CONTRAINDICATIONS

Patients known to be hypersensitive to terconazole or to any of the components of the cream.

WARNINGS

None.

PRECAUTIONS

General: Discontinue use and do not retreat with terconazole if sensitization, irritation, fever, chills or flu-like symptoms are reported during use. If there is lack of response to TERAZOL 7 Vaginal Cream, appropriate microbiological studies (standard KOH smear and/or cultures) should be repeated to confirm the diagnosis and rule out other pathogens.

Drug Interactions: The therapeutic effect of TERAZOL 7 Vaginal Cream is not affected by oral contraceptive usage.

Carcinogenesis, Mutagenesis, Impairment of Fertility:

Carcinogenesis: Studies to determine the carcinogenic potential of terconazole have not been performed.

Mutagenicity: Terconazole was not mutagenic when tested *in vitro* for induction of microbial point mutations (Ames test) or for inducing cellular transformation, or *in vivo* for chromosome breaks (micronucleus test) or dominant lethal mutations in mouse germ cells.

Impairment of Fertility: No impairment of fertility occurred when female rats were administered terconazole orally up to 40 mg/kg/day.

Pregnancy: Pregnancy Category C.

There was no evidence of teratogenicity when terconazole was administered orally up to 40 mg/kg/day (100 × the recommended intravaginal human dose) in rats, or 20 mg/kg/day in rabbits, or subcutaneously in rats up to 20 mg/kg/day.

Dosages at or below 10 mg/kg/day produced no embryotoxicity; however, there was a delay in fetal ossification at 10 mg/kg/day in rats. There was some evidence of embryotoxicity in rabbits and rats at 20–40 mg/kg. In rats this was reflected as a decrease in litter size and number of viable young and reduced fetal weight. There was also delay in ossification and increased incidence of skeletal variants.

The no-effect oral dose of 10 mg/kg/day resulted in a mean peak plasma level of terconazole in pregnant rats of 0.176 mcg/ml which exceeds by 44 times the mean peak plasma levels (0.004 mcg/ml) seen in normal subjects after intravaginal administration of terconazole. This safety assessment does not account for possible exposure of the fetus through direct transfer of terconazole from the irritated vagina to the fetus by diffusion across amniotic membranes.

Since terconazole is absorbed from the human vagina, it should not be used in the first trimester of pregnancy unless the physician considers it essential to the welfare of the patient.

Nursing Mothers: It is not known whether this drug is excreted in human milk. Animal studies have shown that rat off-spring exposed via the milk of treated (40 mg/kg/orally) dams showed decreased survival during the first few postpartum days, but overall pup weight and weight gain were

Continued on next page

Ortho Pharm.—Cont.

comparable to or greater than controls throughout lactation. Because many drugs are excreted in human milk, and because of the potential for adverse reaction in nursing infants from terconazole, a decision should be made whether to discontinue nursing or to discontinue the drug, taking into account the importance of the drug to the mother.

Pediatric Use: Safety and efficacy in children have not been established.

ADVERSE REACTIONS
During controlled clinical studies conducted in the United States, 521 patients with vulvovaginal candidiasis were treated with terconazole 0.4% vaginal cream. Based on comparative analyses with placebo, the adverse experiences considered most likely related to terconazole 0.4% vaginal cream were headaches (26% vs 17% with placebo) and body pain (2.1% vs 0% with placebo). Vulvovaginal burning (5.2%), itching (2.3%) or irritation (3.1%) occurred less frequently with terconazole 0.4% vaginal cream than with the vehicle placebo. Fever (1.7% vs 0.5% with placebo) and chills (0.4% vs 0.0% with placebo) have also been reported. The therapy-related dropout rate was 1.9%. The adverse drug experience on terconazole most frequently causing discontinuation was vulvovaginal itching (0.6%), which was lower than the incidence for placebo (0.9%).

OVERDOSAGE
Overdose of terconazole in humans has not been reported to date. In the rat, the oral LD 50 values were found to be 1741 and 849 mg/kg for the male and female, respectively. The oral LD 50 values for the male and female dog were ≃1280 and ≥640 mg/kg, respectively.

DOSAGE AND ADMINISTRATION
One full applicator (5 g) of TERAZOL 7 Vaginal Cream (20 mg terconazole) is administered intravaginally once daily at bedtime for seven consecutive days. Before prescribing another course of therapy, the diagnosis should be reconfirmed by smears and/or cultures and other pathogens commonly associated with vulvovaginitis ruled out. The therapeutic effect of TERAZOL 7 Vaginal Cream is not affected by menstruation.

HOW SUPPLIED
TERAZOL® 7 (terconazole) Vaginal Cream 0.4% is available in 45 g (NDC 0062-5350-01) tubes with an ORTHO™ Measured-Dose Applicator. Store at Controlled Room Temperature (59°F–86°F).

643-10-300-5   Revised January 1989
Shown in Product Identification Section, page 420

EDUCATIONAL MATERIAL

THE ORTHO FILM LIBRARY
Ortho Pharmaceutical Corporation can provide a number of educational films on a free-loan basis to hospitals, medical schools and health care professionals for use in training and educational programs.
These films, which are available directly from the distributor, KAROL MEDIA, 22 Riverview Drive, Wayne, New Jersey 07470, or by calling (201) 628-9111 are:
Modern Obstetrics: Cesarean Section
Modern Obstetrics: Diabetes in Pregnancy
Modern Obstetrics: Fetal Evaluation
Modern Obstetrics: Normal Labor and Delivery—no printed narration available
Modern Obstetrics: Postpartum Hemorrhage
Modern Obstetrics: Pre-Eclampsia—Eclampsia
Chorionic Villi Sampling—no printed narration available
Printed narrations of these Modern Obstetrics films are available upon written request from: Professional Affairs Department, Ortho Pharmaceutical Corporation, Route 202, P.O. Box 300, Raritan, New Jersey 08869-0602.

Products are
listed alphabetically
in the
PINK SECTION.

Ortho Pharmaceutical Corporation
DERMATOLOGICAL DIVISION
P.O. BOX 300
ROUTE 202
RARITAN, NJ 08869-0602

ERYCETTE™   ℞
(erythromycin 2%)
TOPICAL SOLUTION

DESCRIPTION
Erythromycin is an antibiotic produced from a strain of *Streptomyces erythraeus*. It is basic and readily forms salts with acids. Each ml of ERYCETTE (erythromycin 2%) Topical Solution contains 20 mg of erythromycin base in a vehicle consisting of alcohol (66%) and propylene glycol. It may contain citric acid to adjust pH. Each pledget is filled to contain 0.8 ml. ERYCETTE is not USP with regard to minimum volume.

ACTIONS
Although the mechanism by which ERYCETTE Solution acts in reducing inflammatory lesions of acne vulgaris is unknown, it is presumably due to its antibiotic action.

INDICATIONS
ERYCETTE Solution is indicated for the topical control of acne vulgaris.

CONTRAINDICATIONS
ERYCETTE Solution is contraindicated in persons who have shown hypersensitivity to any of its ingredients.

PRECAUTIONS
General: The use of antibiotic agents may be associated with the overgrowth of antibiotic-resistant organisms. If this occurs, administration of this drug should be discontinued and appropriate measures taken.
Information for Patients: ERYCETTE Solution is for external use only and should be kept away from the eyes, nose, mouth, and other mucous membranes. Concomitant topical acne therapy should be used with caution because a cumulative irritant effect may occur, especially with the use of peeling, desquamating, or abrasive agents. Each pledget should be used once and discarded.
Carcinogenesis, Mutagenesis, Impairment of Fertility: Long-term animal studies to evaluate carcinogenic potential, mutagenicity, or the effect on fertility of erythromycin have not been performed.
Pregnancy: Pregnancy Category C. Animal reproduction studies have not been conducted with erythromycin. It is also not known whether erythromycin can cause fetal harm when administered to a pregnant woman or can affect reproduction capacity. Erythromycin should be given to a pregnant woman only if clearly needed.
Nursing Mothers: It is not known whether erythromycin is excreted in human milk after topical application. However, this is reported to occur with oral and parenteral administration. Therefore, caution should be exercised when erhthromycin is administered to a nursing woman.

ADVERSE REACTIONS
Adverse conditions reported include dryness, tenderness, pruritis, desquamation, erythema, oiliness, and burning sensation. Irritation of the eyes has also been reported. A case of generalized urticarial reaction, possibly related to the drug, which required the use of systemic steroid therapy has been reported.

DOSAGE AND ADMINISTRATION
The ERYCETTE pledget should be rubbed over the affected area twice a day after the skin is thoroughly washed with warm water and soap and patted dry. Acne lesions on the face, neck, shoulders, chest and back may be treated in this manner. Additional pledgets may be used, if needed. Each pledget should be used once and discarded.

HOW SUPPLIED
ERYCETTE (erythromycin 2%) Topical Solution is supplied as foil-covered saturated pledgets (swabs) in boxes of 60 (NDC 0062-1185-01).
Store at controlled room temperature (59°–86°F).

GRIFULVIN V®   ℞
(griseofulvin microsize)
Tablets/Suspension

DESCRIPTION
Griseofulvin is an antibiotic derived from a species of *Penicillium*. Each GRIFULVIN V Tablet contains either 250 mg or 500 mg of griseofulvin microsize, and also contains calcium stearate, colloidal silicon dioxide, starch, and wheat gluten. Additionally, the 250 mg tablet also contains dibasic calcium phosphate. Each 5 ml of GRIFULVIN V Suspension contains

---

125 mg of griseofluvin microsize and also contains alcohol 0.008%, docusate sodium, FD&C Red No. 40, FD&C Yellow No. 6, flavors, magnesium aluminium silicate, menthol, methylparaben, propylene glycol, propylparaben, saccharin sodium, simethicone emulsion, sodium alginate, sucrose, and purified water.

CLINICAL PHARMACOLOGY
GRIFULVIN V (griseofulvin microsize) acts systemically to inhibit the growth of *Trichophyton*, *Microsporum* and *Epidermophyton* genera of fungi. Fungistatic amounts are deposited in the keratin, which is gradually exfoliated and replaced by noninfected tissue.
Griseofulvin absorption from the gastrointestinal tract varies considerably among individuals, mainly because of insolubility of the drug in aqueous media of the upper G.I. tract. The peak serum level found in fasting adults given 0.5 gm. occurs at about four hours and ranges between 0.5 and 2.0 mcg./ml.
It should be noted that some individuals are consistently "poor absorbers" and tend to attain lower blood levels at all times. This may explain unsatisfactory therapeutic results in some patients. Better blood levels can probably be attained in most patients if the tablets are administered after a meal with a high fat content.

INDICATIONS AND USAGE
Major indications for GRIFULVIN V griseofulvin microsize are:
   Tinea capitis (ringworm of the scalp)
   Tinea corporis (ringworm of the body)
   Tinea pedis (athlete's foot)
   Tinea unguium (onychomycosis; ringworm of the nails)
   Tinea cruris (ringworm of the thigh)
   Tinea barbae (barber's itch)
GRIFULVIN V (griseofulvin microsize) inhibits the growth of those genera of fungi that commonly cause ringworm infections of the hair, skin, and nails, such as:
   Trichophyton rubrum
   Trichophyton tonsurans
   Trichophyton mentagrophytes
   Trichophyton interdigitalis
   Trichophyton verrucosum
   Trichophyton sulphureum
   Trichophyton schoenleini
   Microsporum audouini
   Microsporum canis
   Microsporum gypseum
   Epidermophyton floccosum
   Trichophyton megnini
   Trichophyton gallinae
   Trichophyton crateriform
Note: Prior to therapy, the type of fungi responsible for the infection should be indentified. The use of the drug is not justified in minor or trivial infections which will respond to topical antifungal agents alone.
It is *not* effective in:
   Bacterial infections
   Candidiasis (Moniliasis)
   Histoplasmosis
   Actinomycosis
   Sporotrichosis
   Chromoblastomycosis
   Coccidioidomycosis
   North American Blastomycosis
   Cryptococcosis (Torulosis)
   Tinea versicolor
   Nocardiosis

CONTRAINDICATIONS
This drug is contraindicated in patients with porphyria, hepatocellular failure, and in individuals with a history of hypersensitivity to griseofulvin.
Two cases of conjoined twins have been reported in patients taking griseofulvin during the first trimester of pregnancy. Griseofulvin should not be prescribed to pregnant patients.

WARNINGS
Prophylactic Usage: Safety and efficacy of prophylactic use of this drug has not been established.
Chronic feeding of griseofulvin, at levels ranging from 0.5-2.5% of the diet, resulted in the development of liver tumors in several strains of mice, particularly in males. Smaller particle sizes result in an enhanced effect. Lower oral dosage levels have not been tested. Subcutaneous administration of relatively small doses of griseofulvin once a week during the first three weeks of life has also been reported to induce hepatomata in mice. Although studies in other animal species have not yielded evidence of tumorigenicity, these studies were not of adequate design to form a basis for conclusions in this regard.
In subacute toxicity studies, orally administered griseofulvin produced hepatocellar necrosis in mice, but this has not been seen in other species. Disturbances in porphyrin metabolism have been reported in griseofulvin-treated laboratory animals. Griseofulvin has been reported to have a colchicine-like effect on mitosis and cocarcinogenicity with methyl-

cholanthrene in cutaneous tumor induction in laboratory animals.

Reports of animal studies in the Soviet literature state that a griseofulvin preparation was found to be embryotoxic and teratogenic on oral administration to pregnant Wistar rats. Rat reproduction studies done thus far in the United States and Great Britain have been inconclusive in this regard, and additional animal reproduction studies are underway. Pups with abnormalities have been reported in the litters of a few bitches treated with griseofulvin.

Suppression of spermatogenesis has been reported to occur in rats but investigation in man failed to confirm this.

PRECAUTIONS

Patients on prolonged therapy with any potent medication should be under close observation. Periodic monitoring of organ system function, including renal, hepatic and hemopoietic, should be done.

Since griseofulvin is derived from species of penicillin, the possibility of cross sensitivity with penicillin exists; however, known penicillin-sensitive patients have been treated without difficulty.

Since a photosensitivity reaction is occasionally associated with griseofulvin therapy, patients should be warned to avoid exposure to intense natural or artificial sunlight. Should a photosensitivity reaction occur, lupus erythematosus may be aggravated.

Drug Interactions: Patients on warfarin-type anticoagulant therapy may require dosage adjustment of the anticoagulant during and after griseofulvin therapy. Concomitant use of barbiturates usually depresses griseofulvin activity and may necessitate raising the dosage.

The concomitant administration of griseofulvin has been reported to reduce the efficacy of oral contraceptives and to increase the incidence of breakthrough bleeding.

ADVERSE REACTIONS

When adverse reactions occur, they are most commonly of the hypersensitivity type such as skin rashes, urticaria and rarely, angioneurotic edema, and may necessitate withdrawal of therapy and appropriate countermeasures. Paresthesias of the hands and feet have been reported rarely after extended therapy. Other side effects reported occasionally are oral thrush, nausea, vomiting, epigastric distress, diarrhea; headache, fatigue, dizziness, insomnia, mental confusion and impairment of performance of routine activities. Proteinuria and leukopenia have been reported rarely. Administration of the drug should be discontinued if granulocytopenia occurs.

When rare, serious reactions occur with griseofulvin, they are usually associated with high dosages, long periods of therapy, or both.

DOSAGE AND ADMINISTRATION

Accurate diagnosis of the infecting organism is essential. Identification should be made either by direct microscopic examination of a mounting of infected tissue in a solution of potassium hydroxide or by culture on an appropriate medium.

Medication must be continued until the infecting organism is completely eradicated as indicated by appropriate clinical or laboratory examination. Representative treatment periods are tinea capitis, 4 to 6 weeks; tinea corporis, 2 to 4 weeks; tinea pedis, 4 to 8 weeks; tinea unguium—depending on rate of growth—fingernails, at least 4 months; toenails, at least 6 months.

General measures in regard to hygiene should be observed to control sources of infection or reinfection. Concomitant use of appropriate topical agents is usually required, particularly in treatment of tinea pedis since in some forms of athlete's foot, yeasts and bacteria may be involved. Griseofulvin will not eradicate the bacterial or monilial infection.

Adults: A daily dose of 500 mg. will give a satisfactory response in most patients with tinea corporis, tinea cruris, and tinea capitis.

For those fungus infections more difficult to eradicate such as tinea pedis and tinea unguium, a daily dose of 1.0 gram is recommended.

Children: Approximately 5 mg. per pound of body weight per day is an effective dose for most children. On this basis the following dosage schedule for children is suggested:

Children weighing 30 to 50 pounds—125 mg. to 250 mg. daily.

Children weighing over 50 pounds—250 mg. to 500 mg. daily.

HOW SUPPLIED

GRIFULVIN V (griseofulvin microsize) 250 mg. Tablets in bottles of 100 (NDC 0062-0211-60) (white, scored, imprinted "ORTHO 211").

GRIFULVIN V (griseofulvin microsize) 500 mg. Tablets in bottles of 100 (NDC 0062-0214-60) and 500 (NDC 0062-0214-70) (white, scored, imprinted "ORTHO 214").

Dispense GRIFULVIN V tablets in well-closed container as defined in the official compendia.

GRIFULVIN V (griseofulvin microsize) Suspension 125 mg. per 5 cc. in bottles of 4 fl. oz. (NDC 0062-0206-04).

Dispense GRIFULVIN V suspension in tight, light-resistant container as defined in the official compendia.

STORE AT ROOM TEMPERATURE

MECLAN®   ℞
(meclocycline sulfosalicylate)
Cream 1%
For Topical Use Only

DESCRIPTION

MECLAN (meclocycline sulfosalicylate) Cream 1% is a homogeneous smooth yellow cream, each gram of which contains meclocycline sulfosalicylate equivalent to 10 mg. of meclocycline activity in an aqueous cream vehicle consisting of glyceryl stearate, propylene glycol stearate, caprylic/capric triglyceride, paraffin, trihydroxystearin, polysorbate 40, sorbitol solution, propyl gallate, sorbic acid, sodium formaldehyde sulfoxylate, perfume, and water. The vehicle is pharmaceutically compatible with both oil- and water-based systems.

Chemically meclocycline sulfosalicylate is [4S-(4α, 4aα, 5α, 5aα, 12aα)]-7-chloro-4-(dimethyl-amino) - 1, 4,4a,5,5a,6,11,- 12a -octahydro- 3,5,10,12,12a-pentahydroxy-6-methylene-1, 11-dioxo-2-naphthacenecarboxamide 5-sulfosalicylate.

ACTIONS (CLINICAL PHARMACOLOGY)

The mode of action of MECLAN Cream in the treatment of acne is not fully understood. However, it appears that meclocycline possesses a localized effect, since it is not absorbed through the skin in sufficient quantities to be detected systemically. In subtotal body inunction studies, up to 40 times the average treatment dose was applied to 20 human subjects daily for 28 days. No measurable amounts of meclocycline appeared in the blood (0.1 microgram/ml. level of detectability) or urine (0.02 microgram/ml. level of detectability).

INDICATION

MECLAN Cream (meclocycline sulfosalicylate) is indicated for topical application in the treatment of acne vulgaris.

CONTRAINDICATIONS

MECLAN is contraindicated in persons who have shown hypersensitivity to any of its ingredients or to any of the other tetracyclines.

WARNINGS

Although no absorption has been demonstrated by 28-day inunction studies in humans, the possibility exists that significant percutaneous absorption may result from prolonged use. Therefore, caution is advised in administering MECLAN (meclocycline sulfosalicylate) to persons with hepatic or renal dysfunction.

Contains sodium formaldehyde sulfoxylate, a sulfite-producing agent that may cause allergic-type reactions including anaphylactic symptoms and life-threatening or less severe asthmatic episodes in certain susceptible people. The overall prevalence of sulfite sensitivity in the general population is unknown and probably low. Sulfite sensitivity is seen more frequently in asthmatic than in nonasthmatic people.

PRECAUTIONS

This drug is for external use only and should be kept out of the eyes, nose, and mouth. It should be used with caution by patients who are sensitive to formaldehyde.

Pregnancy: Pregnancy Category B. Reproduction studies have been performed in rats and rabbits at oral doses up to 1000 times the human dose (assuming the human dose to be one gram of cream per day) and have revealed no evidence of impaired fertility or harm to the fetus due to meclocycline sulfosalicylate. There was, however, a slight delay in ossification in rabbits when meclocycline was applied topically. There are no adequate and well-controlled studies in pregnant women. Because animal reproduction studies are not always predictive of human response, this drug should be used during pregnancy only if clearly needed.

Nursing Mothers: It is not known whether this drug is excreted in human milk. Because many drugs are excreted in human milk, caution should be exercised when meclocycline sulfosalicylate is administered to a nursing woman.

ADVERSE REACTIONS

MECLAN is well tolerated by the skin. In the clinical trials there was one report of acute contact dermatitis. There were isolated reports of skin irritation. Temporary follicular staining may occur with excessive application. Patch testing has demonstrated no photosensitivity or contact allergy potential.

DOSAGE AND ADMINISTRATION

It is recommended that MECLAN be applied to the affected area twice daily, morning and evening. Less frequent application may be used depending on patient response. Excessive use of MECLAN Cream may cause staining of some fabrics.

HOW SUPPLIED

MECLAN (meclocycline sulfosalicylate) Cream 1% is supplied in 20 gram (NDC 0062-0675-80) and 45 gram (NDC 0062-0675-01) sealed tubes.

MONISTAT-DERM™   ℞
(miconazole nitrate 2%)
Cream and Lotion
For Topical Use Only

DESCRIPTION

MONISTAT-DERM (miconazole nitrate 2%) Cream and Lotion each contain miconazole nitrate* 2%, formulated into a water-miscible base consisting of pegoxol 7 stearate, peglicol 5 oleate, mineral oil, benzoic acid, and butylated hydroxyanisole and purified water.

*Chemical name: 1-[2,4-dichloro-β-{(2,4-dichlorobenzyl)oxy} phenethyl] imidazole mononitrate.

ACTIONS

Miconazole nitrate is a synthetic antifungal agent which inhibits the growth of the common dermatophytes, *Trichophyton rubrum, Trichophyton mentagrophytes,* and *Epidermophyton floccosum,* the yeast-like fungus. *Candida albicans,* and the organism responsible for tinea versicolor *(Malassezia furfur).*

INDICATIONS

For topical application in the treatment of tinea pedis (athlete's foot), tinea cruris, and tinea corporis caused by *Trichophyton rubrum, Trichophyton mentagrophytes,* and *Epidermophyton floccosum,* in the treatment of cutaneous candidiasis (moniliasis), and in the treatment of tinea versicolor.

CONTRAINDICATIONS

MONISTAT-DERM (miconazole nitrate 2%) Cream and Lotion have no known contraindications.

PRECAUTIONS

If a reaction suggesting sensitivity or chemical irritation should occur, use of the medication should be discontinued. For external use only. Avoid introduction of MONISTAT-DERM Cream and Lotion into the eyes.

ADVERSE REACTIONS

There have been isolated reports of irritation, burning, maceration, and allergic contact dermatitis associated with application of MONISTAT-DERM.

DOSAGE AND ADMINISTRATION

Sufficient MONISTAT-DERM Cream should be applied to cover affected areas twice daily (morning and evening) in patients with tinea pedis, tinea cruris, tinea corporis, and cutaneous candidiasis, and once daily in patients with tinea versicolor. It is preferable to use MONISTAT-DERM Lotion in intertriginous areas; if the cream is used, it should be applied sparingly and smoothed in well to avoid maceration effects.

Early relief of symptoms (2 to 3 days) is experienced by the majority of patients and clinical improvement may be seen fairly soon after treatment is begun; however, *Candida* infections and tinea cruris and corporis should be treated for two weeks and tinea pedis for one month in order to reduce the possibility of recurrence. If a patient shows no clinical improvement after a month of treatment, the diagnosis should be redetermined. Patients with tinea versicolor usually exhibit clinical and mycological clearing after two weeks of treatment.

HOW SUPPLIED

MONISTAT-DERM (miconazole nitrate 2%) Cream containing miconazole nitrate at 2% strength is supplied in 15 g. (NDC 0062-5434-02), 1 oz. (NDC 0062-5434-01) and 3 oz. (NDC 0062-5434-03) tubes. MONISTAT-DERM (miconazole nitrate 2%) Lotion containing miconazole nitrate at 2% w/w strength is supplied in polyethylene squeeze bottles in quantities of 30 ml. (NDC 0062-5435-02) and 60 ml. (NDC 0062-5435-05).

PERSA-GEL® 5% & 10%   ℞
(benzoyl peroxide)
acetone-base gel
PERSA-GEL W 5% & 10%
(benzoyl peroxide)
water-base gel

DESCRIPTION

PERSA-GEL and PERSA-GEL W 5% and 10% (benzoyl peroxide 5% and 10%) are topical gel preparations for use in the treatment of acne vulgaris. Benzoyl peroxide is an oxidizing agent which possesses antibacterial properties and is classified as a keratolytic.

PERSA-GEL contains benzoyl peroxide 5% or 10% as the active ingredient in a gel base containing acetone, carbomer

Continued on next page

Ortho Derm.—Cont.

940, trolamine, sodium lauryl sulfate, propylene glycol and purified water.

PERSA-GEL W contains benzoyl peroxide 5% or 10% as the active ingredient in a gel base containing purified water, carbomer, 934P sodium hydroxide, hydroxypropyl methylcellulose 2906, and laureth 4.

CLINICAL PHARMACOLOGY

The mechanism of action of benzoyl peroxide has not been determined but may be related to its antibacterial activity against **Propionibacterium acnes** and its ability to cause drying and peeling. Benzoyl peroxide reduces the concentration of free fatty acids in the sebum. Little is known about the percutaneous penetration, metabolism, and excretion of benzoyl peroxide, although it is likely that benzoic acid is a major metabolite. There is no evidence of systemic toxicity caused by benzoyl peroxide in humans.

INDICATIONS AND USAGE

These products are indicated for the topical treatment of acne vulgaris.

CONTRAINDICATIONS

These products are contraindicated in patients with a history of hypersensitivity to any of the components of the preparations.

PRECAUTIONS

General: For external use only. If severe irritation develops, discontinue use and institute appropriate therapy. After the reaction clears, treatment may often be resumed with less frequent application. This preparation should not be used in or near the eyes or on mucous membranes.

Information for Patients: Avoid contact with eyes, eyelids, lips and mucous membranes. If accidental contact occurs, rinse with water. May bleach hair and colored fabrics. If excessive irritation develops, discontinue use and consult your physician.

Carcinogenesis, Mutagenesis, Impairment of Fertility: Data from several studies using mice known to be highly susceptible to cancer suggest that benzoyl peroxide acts as a tumor promotor. The clinical significance of these findings to humans is unknown.

Pregnancy: Pregnancy Category C: Animal reproduction studies have not been conducted with benzoyl peroxide. It is also not known whether benzoyl peroxide can cause fetal harm when administered to a pregnant woman or can affect reproduction capacity. Benzoyl peroxide should be used by a pregnant woman only if clearly needed. There are no data available on the effect of benzoyl peroxide on the growth, development and functional maturation of the unborn child.

Nursing Mothers: It is not known whether this drug is excreted in human milk. Because many drugs are excreted in human milk, caution should be exercised when benzoyl peroxide is administered to a nursing woman.

Pediatric Use: Safety and effectiveness in children have not been established.

ADVERSE REACTIONS

Allergic contact dermatitis has been reported with topical benzoyl peroxide therapy.

DOSAGE AND ADMINISTRATION

PERSA-GEL or PERSA-GEL W 5% or 10% should be applied once or twice daily to affected areas after washing with a mild cleanser and water. The degree of drying and peeling can be adjusted by modification of the dosage schedule.

HOW SUPPLIED

PERSA-GEL 5%, 1.5 oz. tubes
(NDC 0062-8610-31)
PERSA-GEL 5%, 3 oz. tubes
(NDC 0062-8610-03)
PERSA-GEL 10%, 1.5 oz. tubes
(NDC 0062-8600-31)
PERSA-GEL 10%, 3 oz. tubes
(NDC 0062-8600-03)
PERSA-GEL W 5% 1.5 oz. tubes
(NDC 0062-8630-31)
PERSA-GEL W 5% 3.0 oz. tubes
(NDC 0062-8630-03)
PERSA-GEL W 10% 1.5 oz. tubes
(NDC 0062-8620-31)
PERSA-GEL W 10% 3.0 oz. tubes
(NDC 0062-8620-03)
Store at controlled room temperature (59°– 86°F).

RETIN-A™   ℞
(tretinoin)
Cream●Gel●Liquid
For Topical Use Only

DESCRIPTION

RETIN-A Gel. Cream and Liquid, containing tretinoin are used for the topical treatment of acne vulgaris. RETIN-A Gel contains tretinoin (tretinoic acid, vitamin A acid) in either of two strengths. 0.025% or 0.01% by weight, in a gel vehicle of butylated hydroxytoluene, hydroxypropyl cellulose and alcohol 90% w/w. RETIN-A (tretinoin) Cream contains tretinoin in either of three strengths. 0.1%, 0.05%, or 0.025% by weight, in a hydrophilic cream vehicle of stearic acid, isopropyl myristate, polyoxyl 40 stearate, stearyl alcohol, xanthan gum, sorbic acid, butylated hydroxytoluene, and purified water. RETIN-A Liquid contains tretinoin 0.05% by weight polyethylene glycol 400, butylated hydroxytoluene and alcohol 55%. Chemically, tretinoin is all-trans-retinoic acid.

CLINICAL PHARMACOLOGY

Although the exact mode of action of tretinoin is unknown, current evidence suggests that topical tretinoin decreases cohesiveness of follicular epithelial cells with decreased microcomedo formation. Additionally, tretinoin stimulates mitotic activity and increased turnover of follicular epithelial cells causing extrusion of the comedones.

INDICATIONS AND USAGE

RETIN-A is indicated for topical application in the treatment of acne vulgaris.

CONTRAINDICATIONS

Use of the product should be discontinued if hypersensitivity to any of the ingredients is noted.

PRECAUTIONS

General: If a reaction sugesting sensitivity or chemical irritation occurs, use of the medication should be discontinued. Exposure to sunlight, including sunlamps, should be minimized during the use of RETIN-A, and patients with sunburn should be advised not to use the product until fully recovered because of heightened susceptibility to sunlight as a result of the use of tretinoin. Patients who may be required to have considerable sun exposure due to occupation and those with inherent sensitivity to the sun should exercise particular caution. Use of sunscreen products and protective clothing over treated areas may be prudent when exposure cannot be avoided. Weather extremes, such as wind or cold, also may be irritating to patients under treatment with tretinoin.

RETIN-A (tretinoin) acne treatment should be kept away from the eyes, the mouth, angles of the nose, and mucous membranes. Topical use may induce severe local erythema and peeling at the site of application. If the degree of local irritation warrants, patients should be directed to use the medication less frequently, discontinue use temporarily, or discontinue use altogether. Tretinoin has been reported to cause severe irritation on eczematous skin and should be used with utmost caution in patients with this condition.

Drug Interactions: Concomitant topical medication, medicated or abrasive soaps and cleansers, soaps and cosmetics that have a strong drying effect, and products with high concentrations of alcohol, astringents, spices or lime should be used with caution because of possible interaction with tretinoin. Particular caution should be exercised in using preparations containing sulfur, resorcinol, or salicylic acid with RETIN-A. It also is advisable to "rest" a patient's skin until the effects of such preparations subside before use of RETIN-A is begun.

Carcinogenesis: Long-term animal studies to determine the carcinogenic potential of tretinoin have not been performed. Studies in hairless albino mice suggest that tretinoin may accelerate the tumorigenic potential of ultraviolet radiation. Although the significance to man is not clear, patients should avoid or minimize exposure to sun.

Pregnancy: Pregnancy Category B. Reproduction studies performed in rats and rabbits at dermal doses up to 50 times the human dose (assuming the human dose to be 500 mg of gel per day) have revealed no evidence of impaired fertility or harm to the fetus due to tretinoin (retinoic acid). There was, however, a slightly higher incidence of irregularly contoured or partially ossified skull bones in some rat and rabbit fetuses. There are no adequate and well-controlled studies in pregnant women. Because animal reproduction studies are not always predictive of human response, this drug should be used during pregnancy only if clearly needed.

Nursing Mothers: It is not known whether this drug is excreted in human milk. Nevertheless, a decision should be made whether to discontinue nursing or to discontinue the drug taking into account the importance of the drug to the mother.

ADVERSE REACTIONS

The skin of certain sensitve individuals may become excessively red, edematous, blistered, or crusted. If these effects occur, the medication should either be discontinued until the integrity of the skin is restored, or the medication should be adjusted to a level the patient can tolerate. True contact allergy to topical tretinoin is rarely encountered. Temporary hyper- or hypopigmentation has been reported with repeated application of RETIN-A. Some individuals have been reported to have heightened susceptibility to sunlight while under treatment with RETIN-A. To date, all adverse effects of RETIN-A have been reversible upon discontinuance of therapy (see Dosage and Administration Section).

OVERDOSAGE

If medication is applied excessively, no more rapid or better results will be obtained and marked redness, peeling, or discomfort may occur. Oral ingestion of the drug may lead to the same side effects as those associated with excessive oral intake of Vitamin A.

DOSAGE AND ADMINISTRATION

RETIN-A Gel, Cream or Liquid should be applied once a day, before retiring, to the skin where acne lesions appear, using enough to cover the entire affected area lightly. Liquid: The liquid may be applied using a fingertip gauze pad or cotton swab. If gauze or cotton is employed care should be taken not to oversaturate it to the extent that the liquid would run into areas where treatment is not intended. Gel: Excessive application results in "pilling" of the gel which minimizes the likelihood of overapplication by the patient.

Application may cause a transitory feeling of warmth or slight stinging. In cases where it has been necessary to temporarily discontinue therapy or to reduce the frequency of application, therapy may be resumed or frequency of application increased when the patients become able to tolerate the treatment.

Alterations of vehicle, drug concentration, or dose frequency should be closely monitored by careful observation of the clinical therapeutic response and skin tolerance.

During the early weeks of therapy, an *apparent* exacerbation of inflammatory lesions may occur. This is due to the action of the medication on deep, previously unseen lesions and should not be considered a reason to discontinue therapy. Therapeutic results should be noticed after two to three weeks but more than six weeks of therapy may be required before definite beneficial effects are seen.

Once the acne lesions have responded satisfactorily, it may be possible to maintain the improvement with less frequent applications, or other dosage forms.

Patients treated with RETIN-A (tretinoin) acne treatment may use cosmetics, but the areas to be treated should be cleansed thoroughly before the medication is applied.
(See Precautions)

HOW SUPPLIED

RETIN-A (tretinoin) is supplied as:
1. A 0.025% Gel in tubes of 15 grams (NDC 0062-0475-42) and 45 grams (NDC 0062-0475-45), and a 0.01% Gel in tubes of 15 grams (NDC 0062-0575-44) and 45 grams (NDC 0062-0575-46).
2. A 0.1% Cream in tubes of 20 grams (NDC 0062-0275-23) and 45 grams (NDC 0062-0275-01), a 0.05% Cream in tubes of 20 grams (NDC 0062-0175-12) and 45 grams (NDC 0062-0175-13), and a 0.025% Cream in tubes of 20 grams (NDC 0062-0165-01) and 45 grams (NDC 0062-0165-02).
3. A 0.05% Liquid in amber bottles containing 28 ml (NDC 0062-0075-07).

STORAGE CONDITIONS

RETIN-A Liquid, 0.05%, and RETIN-A Gel 0.025% and 0.01%: store below 86°F. RETIN-A-Cream. 0.1%, 0.05%, and 0.025% store below 80°F.

SPECTAZOLE™   ℞
(econazole nitrate 1%)
Cream
For Topical Use Only

DESCRIPTION

SPECTAZOLE Cream contains the antifungal agent, econazole nitrate 1%, in a water-miscible base consisting of pegoxol 7 stearate, peglicol 5 oleate, mineral oil, benzoic acid, butylated hydroxyanisole, and purified water. The white to off-white soft cream is for topical use only.

Chemically, econazole nitrate is 1-[2-{(4-chlorophenyl)methoxy}-2-(2,4-dichlorophenyl)ethyl]-1H-imidazole mononitrate. Its structure is as follows:

CLINICAL PHARMACOLOGY

After topical application to the skin of normal subjects, systemic absorption of econazole nitrate is extremely low. Although most of the applied drug remains on the skin surface, drug concentrations were found in the stratum corneum which, by far, exceeded the minimum inhibitory concentration for dermatophytes. Inhibitory concentrations were achieved in the epidermis and as deep as the middle region of the dermis. Less than 1% of the applied dose was recovered in the urine and feces.

Microbiology: In *in-vitro* studies, econazole nitrate exhibits broad-spectrum antifungal activity against the dermatophytes, *Trichophyton rubrum, Trichophyton mentagrophytes, Trichophyton tonsurans, Microsporum canis, Microsporum audouini, Microsporum gypseum,* and *Epidermophyton floccosum,* the yeasts, *Candida albicans* and *Pityrosporum orbiculare* (the organism responsible for tinea versicolor), and certain gram positive bacteria.

INDICATIONS AND USAGE
SPECTAZOLE Cream is indicated for topical application in the treatment of tinea pedis, tinea cruris, and tinea corporis caused by *Trichophyton rubrum, Trichophyton mentagrophytes, Trichophyton tonsurans, Microsporum canis, Microsporum audouini, Microsporum gypseum,* and *Epidermophyton floccosum,* in the treatment of cutaneous candidiasis, and in the treatment of tinea versicolor.

CONTRAINDICATIONS
SPECTAZOLE Cream is contraindicated in individuals who have shown hypersensitivity to any of its ingredients.

WARNINGS
SPECTAZOLE is not for ophthalmic use.

PRECAUTIONS
General: If a reaction suggesting sensitivity or chemical irritation should occur, use of the medication should be discontinued.
For external use only. Avoid introduction of SPECTAZOLE Cream into the eyes.
Carcinogenicity Studies: Long-term animal studies to determine carcinogenic potential have not been performed.
Fertility (Reproduction): Oral administration of econazole nitrate in rats has been reported to produce prolonged gestation. Intravaginal administration in humans has not shown prolonged gestation or other adverse reproductive effects attributable to econazole nitrate therapy.
Pregnancy: Pregnancy Category C. Econazole nitrate has not been shown to be teratogenic when administered orally to mice, rabbits or rats. Fetotoxic or embryotoxic effects were observed in Segment I oral studies with rats receiving 10 to 40 times the human dermal dose. Similar effects were observed in Segment II or Segment III studies with mice, rabbits and/or rats receiving oral doses 80 or 40 times the human dermal dose.
Econazole should be used in the first trimester of pregnancy only when the physician considers it essential to the welfare of the patient. The drug should be used during the second and third trimesters of pregnancy only if clearly needed.
Nursing Mothers: It is not known whether econazole nitrate is excreted in human milk. Following oral administration of econazole nitrate to lactating rats, econazole and/or metabolites were excreted in milk and were found in nursing pups. Also, in lactating rats receiving large oral doses (40 or 80 times the human dermal dose), there was a reduction in post partum viability of pups and survival to weaning; however, at these high doses, maternal toxicity was present and may have been a contributing factor. Caution should be exercised when econazole nitrate is administered to a nursing woman.

ADVERSE REACTIONS
During clinical trials, 12 (3.3%) of 366 patients treated with econazole nitrate 1% cream reported side effects, consisting mainly of burning, itching, stinging and erythema.

OVERDOSE
Overdosage of econazole nitrate in humans has not been reported to date. In mice, rats, guinea pigs and dogs, the oral LD 50 values were found to be 462, 668, 272, and > 160 mg/kg, respectively.

DOSAGE AND ADMINISTRATION
Sufficient SPECTAZOLE Cream should be applied to cover affected areas twice daily (morning and evening) in patients with tinea pedis, tinea cruris, tinea corporis, and cutaneous candidiasis, and once daily in patients with tinea versicolor. Early relief of symptoms is experienced by the majority of patients and clinical improvement may be seen fairly soon after treatment is begun; however, candidal infections and tinea cruris and corporis should be treated for two weeks and tinea pedis for one month in order to reduce the possibility of recurrence. If a patient shows no clinical improvement after the treatment period, the diagnosis should be redetermined. Patients with tinea versicolor usually exhibit clinical and mycological clearing after two weeks of treatment.

HOW SUPPLIED
SPECTAZOLE (econazole nitrate 1%) Cream is supplied in tubes of 15 grams (NDC 0062-5460-02), 30 grams (NDC 0062-5460-01), and 85 grams (NDC 0062-5460-03).
Store SPECTAZOLE Cream below 86°F.

Products are cross-indexed by
generic and chemical names in the
YELLOW SECTION

Owen Laboratories
Division of Dermatological Products of Texas, Inc.
SAN ANTONIO, TX 78296
An Affiliate of Alcon Laboratories, Inc.
FORT WORTH, TX 76134

BENZAC® 5 & 10 Gel   ℞
BENZAC W® 2½, 5 & 10 Water Base Gel   ℞
BENZAC W® WASH 5 & 10   ℞
(benzoyl peroxide)

DESCRIPTION
BENZAC® (benzoyl peroxide) 5 and 10 are topical alcohol-base preparations and BENZAC W® 2½, 5 and 10 and BENZAC W® Wash 5 and 10 are topical water-base preparations for use in the treatment of acne vulgaris. Benzoyl peroxide is an oxidizing agent which possesses antibacterial properties and is classified as keratolytic.
BENZAC® 5 and BENZAC® 10 contain, respectively, benzoyl peroxide 5% and 10% as the active ingredient in a gel base containing alcohol 12% (w/w), polyoxyethylene lauryl ether 6%, dimethicone, carbomer 940, fragrance and purified water. May contain sodium hydroxide and/or citric acid (for pH adjustment).
BENZAC W® 2½, BENZAC W® 5 and BENZAC W® 10 contain, respectively, benzoyl peroxide 2½%, 5% and 10% as the active ingredient in a gel base containing dioctyl sodium sulfosuccinate, edetate disodium, poloxamer 182, carbomer 940, propylene glycol, silicon dioxide and purified water. May also contain citric acid and/or sodium hydroxide to adjust pH.
BENZAC W® Wash 5 and BENZAC W® Wash 10 contain, respectively, benzoyl peroxide 5% and 10% as the active ingredient in a vehicle consisting of sodium C14-16 olefin sulfonate, carbomer 940 and purified water.

CLINICAL PHARMACOLOGY
The mechanism of action of benzoyl peroxide has not been determined but may be related to its antibacterial activity against *Propionibacterium acnes* and its ability to cause drying and peeling. Benzoyl peroxide reduces the concentration of free fatty acids in the sebum. Little is known about the percutaneous penetration, metabolism, and excretion of benzoyl peroxide, although it is likely that benzoic acid is a major metabolite. There is no evidence of systemic toxicity caused by benzoyl peroxide in humans.

INDICATIONS AND USAGE
BENZAC® 5 and 10 and BENZAC W® 2½, 5 and 10 are indicated for the topical treatment of acne vulgaris.
BENZAC W® Wash 5 and 10 are indicated for the topical treatment of mild to moderate acne vulgaris. In severe, complicated acne, BENZAC W® Wash 5 and 10 may be used as an adjunct to other therapeutic regimens.

CONTRAINDICATIONS
These preparations are contraindicated in patients with a history of hypersensitivity to any of their components.

PRECAUTIONS
General: For external use only. If severe irritation develops, discontinue use and institute appropriate therapy. After the reaction clears, treatment may often be resumed with less frequent application. These preparations should not be used in or near the eyes or on mucous membranes.
Information for patients: Avoid contact with eyes, eyelids, lips and mucous membranes. If accidental contact occurs, rinse with water. Contact with any colored material (including hair and fabric) may result in bleaching or discoloration. Concurrent use with PABA-containing sunscreens may result in transient discoloration of the skin. If excessive irritation develops, discontinue use and consult your physician.
Carcinogensis, Mutagenesis, Impairment of Fertility: There is no evidence in the published literature that benzoyl peroxide is carcinogenic, mutagenic or that it impairs fertility.
Pregnancy: Teratogenic Effects: Pregnancy Category C: Animal reproduction studies have not been conducted with benzoyl peroxide. It is not known whether benzoyl peroxide can cause fetal harm when administered to a pregnant woman or can affect reproduction capacity. Benzoyl peroxide should be used by a pregnant woman only if clearly needed. There are no available data on the effect of benzoyl peroxide on the later growth, development and functional maturation of the unborn child.
Nursing Mothers: It is not known whether this drug is excreted in human milk. Because many drugs are excreted in human milk, caution should be exercised when benzoyl peroxide is administered to a nursing woman.
Pediatric Use: Safety and effectiveness in children have not been established.

ADVERSE REACTIONS
Allergic contact dermatitis and dryness have been reported with topical benzoyl peroxide therapy.

OVERDOSAGE
If excessive scaling, erythema or edema occur, the use of this preparation should be discontinued. To hasten resolution of the adverse effects, cool compresses may be used. After symptoms and signs subside, a reduced dosage schedule may be cautiously tried if the reaction is judged to be due to excessive use and not allergenicity.

DOSAGE AND ADMINISTRATION
BENZAC® 5 or 10 or BENZAC W® 2½, 5 or 10 should be applied once or twice daily to cover affected areas after washing with a mild cleanser and water. Wash with BENZAC W® Wash 5 or 10 once or twice daily, avoiding contact with eyes and mucous membranes. Wet the area of application. Apply BENZAC W® Wash 5 or 10 to the hands and wash the affected areas. Rinse with water and dry. The degree of drying and peeling can be adjusted by modification of the dosage schedule.

HOW SUPPLIED
BENZAC® 5 Gel
60 gm tubes—**NDC** 0299-3655-01
BENZAC® 10 Gel
60 gm tubes—**NDC** 0299-3665-01
BENZAC W® 2½ Water Base Gel
60 gm tubes—**NDC** 0299-3590-60
90 gm tubes—**NDC** 0299-3590-90
BENZAC W® 5 Water Base Gel
60 gm tubes—**NDC** 0299-3600-01
90 gm tubes—**NDC** 0299-3600-09
BENZAC W® 10 Water Base Gel
60 gm tubes—**NDC** 0299-3610-01
90 gm tubes—**NDC** 0299-3610-09
BENZAC W® Wash 5
4 oz. plastic bottles—**NDC** 0299-3670-04
8 oz. plastic bottles—**NDC** 0299-3670-08
BENZAC W® Wash 10
8 oz. plastic bottles—**NDC** 0299-3672-08
Store BENZAC W® and BENZAC W® Wash at controlled room temperature (59°–86°F). Store BENZAC® below 75°F.

CETAPHIL®
Gentle Skin Cleanser—Soap Substitute

COMPOSITION
Contains water, cetyl alcohol, propylene glycol, sodium lauryl sulfate, stearyl alcohol, methylparaben, propylparaben and butylparaben.

ACTION AND USES
CETAPHIL® Cleanser is a gentle, non-irritating cleanser for sensitive skin. CETAPHIL is non-alkaline and provides gentle, thorough cleansing without the irritancy of harsh soaps. The unique oil-free formula is particularly well-suited for atopic dermatitis, diaper dermatitis and other eczematous skin conditions. Its emollient quality helps soften as it cleanses, providing comfort for sensitive, irritated skin.

ADMINISTRATION AND DOSAGE
CETAPHIL can be used with or without water.
Without water: Apply a liberal amount to the skin and rub gently to produce a slight lather. Remove excess with a soft cloth, leaving a thin film of CETAPHIL on the skin. The emollient quality will leave the skin soft and moist.
With water: Apply to the skin and rub gently. Rinse.

HOW SUPPLIED
CETAPHIL® Cleanser 8 oz. (PIC 0299-3921-08);
CETAPHIL® Cleanser 16 oz. (PIC 0299-3921-16).

DESOWEN®   ℞
(desonide)
Cream 0.05%/Ointment 0.05%

DESCRIPTION
DesOwen® Cream and Ointment contain the topical corticosteroid, desonide, a nonfluorinated corticosteroid. It has the chemical name: Pregna-1,4-diene-3,20-dione,11, 21-dihydroxy-16,17-[(1-methylethylidene)bis(oxy)]-,(11β, 16α)-; the molecular formula: $C_{24}H_{32}O_6$; molecular weight: 416.51; CAS-638-94-8. The structural formula is:

Each gram of DesOwen Cream contains 0.5 mg of desonide microdispersed in a compatible vehicle buffered to the pH range of normal skin. It contains propylene glycol, polysorbate 60, emulsifying wax, isopropyl palmitate, stearic acid, synthetic beeswax, citric acid, sodium hydroxide, and puri-

Continued on next page

Owen—Cont.

fied water. It is preserved with sorbic acid and potassium sorbate.

Each gram of DesOwen Ointment contains 0.5 mg of desonide in a base consisting of mineral oil and polyethylene.

CLINICAL PHARMACOLOGY

Topical corticosteroids share anti-inflammatory, anti-pruritic, and vasoconstrictive actions.

The mechanism of anti-inflammatory activity of the topical corticosteroids is unclear. Various laboratory methods, including vasoconstrictor assays, are used to compare and predict potencies and/or clinical efficacies of the topical corticosteroids. There is some evidence to suggest that a recognizable correlation exists between vasoconstrictor potency and therapeutic efficacy in man.

Pharmacokinetics: The extent of percutaneous absorption of topical corticosteroids is determined by many factors including the vehicle, the integrity of the epidermal barrier, and the use of occlusive dressings.

Topical corticosteroids can be absorbed from normal intact skin. Inflammation and/or other disease processes in the skin increase percutaneous absorption. Occlusive dressings substantially increase the percutaneous absorption of topical corticosteroids.

Thus, occlusive dressings may be a valuable therapeutic adjunct for treatment of resistant dermatoses. (See DOSAGE AND ADMINISTRATION.)

Once absorbed through the skin, topical corticosteroids are handled through pharmacokinetic pathways similar to systemically administered corticosteroids. Corticosteroids are bound to plasma proteins in varying degrees. Corticosteroids are metabolized primarily in the liver and are then excreted by the kidneys. Some of the topical corticosteroids and their metabolites are also excreted into the bile.

INDICATIONS AND USAGE

DesOwen Cream 0.05% and Ointment 0.05% (desonide) are indicated for the relief of the inflammatory and pruritic manifestations of corticosteroid-responsive dermatoses.

CONTRAINDICATIONS

Topical corticosteroids are contraindicated in those patients with a history of hypersensitivity to any of the components of the preparation.

PRECAUTIONS

General: Systemic absorption of topical corticosteroids has produced reversible hypothalamic-pituitary-adrenal (HPA) axis suppression, manifestations of Cushing's syndrome, hyperglycemia, and glucosuria in some patients.

Conditions which augment systemic absorption include the application of the more potent steroids, use over large surface areas, prolonged use, and the addition of occlusive dressings.

Therefore, patients receiving a large dose of a potent topical steroid applied to a large surface area or under an occlusive dressing should be evaluated periodically for evidence of HPA axis suppression by using the urinary free cortisol and ACTH stimulation tests. If HPA axis suppression is noted, an attempt should be made to withdraw the drug, to reduce the frequency of application, or to substitute a less potent steroid.

Recovery of HPA axis function is generally prompt and complete upon discontinuation of the drug. Infrequently, signs and symptoms of steroid withdrawal may occur, requiring supplemental systemic corticosteroids.

Children may absorb proportionally larger amounts of topical corticosteroids and thus be more susceptible to systemic toxicity (See PRECAUTIONS—PEDIATRIC USE).

If irritation develops, topical corticosteroids should be discontinued and appropriate therapy instituted.

In the presence of dermatological infections, the use of an appropriate antifungal or antibacterial agent should be instituted. If a favorable response does not occur promptly, the corticosteroids should be discontinued until the infection has been adequately controlled.

Information for the Patient: Patients using topical corticosteroids should receive the following information and instructions:

1. This medication is to be used as directed by the physician. It is for external use only. Avoid contact with the eyes.
2. Patients should be advised not to use this medication for any disorder other than for which it was prescribed.
3. The treated skin area should not be bandaged or otherwise covered or wrapped as to be occlusive unless directed by the physician.
4. Patients should report any signs of local adverse reactions especially under occlusive dressing.
5. Parents of pediatric patients should be advised not to use tight-fitting diapers or plastic pants on a child being treated in the diaper area, as these garments may constitute occlusive dressings.

Laboratory Tests: The following tests may be helpful in evaluating the HPA axis suppression:

    Urinary free cortisol test
    ACTH stimulation test

Carcinogenesis, Mutagenesis, and Impairment of Fertility: Long-term animal studies have not been performed to evaluate the carcinogenic potential or the effect on fertility of topical corticosteroids.

Studies to determine mutagenicity with prednisolone and hydrocortisone have revealed negative results.

Pregnancy Category C: Corticosteroids are generally teratogenic in laboratory animals when administered systemically at relatively low dosage levels. The more potent corticosteroids have been shown to be teratogenic after dermal application in laboratory animals. There are no adequate and well controlled studies in pregnant women on teratogenic effects from topically applied corticosteroids. Therefore, topical corticosteroids should be used during pregnancy only if the potential benefit justifies the potential risk to the fetus. Drugs of this class should not be used extensively on pregnant patients, in large amounts, or for prolonged periods of time.

Nursing Mothers: It is not known whether topical administration of corticosteroids could result in sufficient systemic absorption to produce detectable quantities in breast milk. Systemically administered corticosteroids are secreted into breast milk, in quantities *not* likely to have a deleterious effect on the infant. Nevertheless, caution should be exercised when topical corticosteroids are administered to a nursing woman.

Pediatric Use: *Pediatric patients may demonstrate greater susceptibility to topical corticosteroid-induced HPA axis suppression and Cushing's syndrome than mature patients because of a larger skin surface area to body weight ratio.*

Hypothalamic-pituitary-adrenal (HPA) axis suppression, Cushing's syndrome, and intracranial hypertension have been reported in children receiving topical corticosteroids. Manifestations of adrenal suppression in children include linear growth retardation, delayed weight gain, low plasma cortisol levels, and absence of response to ACTH stimulation. Manifestations of intracranial hypertension include bulging fontanelles, headaches, and bilateral papilledema.

Administration of topical corticosteroids to children should be limited to the least amount compatible with an effective therapeutic regimen. Chronic corticosteroid therapy may interfere with the growth and development of children.

ADVERSE REACTIONS

The following local adverse reactions are reported infrequently with topical corticosteroids, but may occur more frequently with the use of occlusive dressings. These reactions are listed in an approximate decreasing order of occurrence: burning, itching, irritation, dryness, folliculitis, hypertrichosis, acneiform eruptions, hypopigmentation, perioral dermatitis, allergic contact dermatitis, maceration of the skin, secondary infection, skin atrophy, striae and miliaria.

OVERDOSAGE

Topically applied corticosteroids can be absorbed in sufficient amounts to produce systemic effects (See PRECAUTIONS).

DOSAGE AND ADMINISTRATION

DesOwen Cream 0.05% or Ointment 0.05% (desonide) should be applied to the affected area as a thin film two or three times daily depending on the severity of the condition.

Occlusive dressings may be used for the management of psoriasis or recalcitrant conditions.

If an infection develops, the use of occlusive dressings should be discontinued and appropriate antimicrobial therapy instituted.

HOW SUPPLIED

DesOwen Cream 0.05% (desonide) is supplied in tubes containing:

15 g NDC 0299-5770-15
60 g NDC 0299-5770-60

DesOwen Ointment 0.05% (desonide) is supplied in tubes containing:

15 g NDC 0299-5775-15
60 g NDC 0299-5775-60

CAUTION: Federal law prohibits dispensing without prescription.

Storage Conditions: Store below 86° F. Do not freeze.

IONIL® Shampoo
Therapeutic Salicylic Acid Shampoo

COMPOSITION

Salicylic acid, water, laureth-23, SD alcohol 40 12%; laureth-4, benzalkonium chloride, tetrasodium EDTA.

ACTION AND USES

IONIL® Shampoo relieves the itching, irritation, and flaking associated with dandruff, seborrheic dermatitis, and psoriasis of the scalp. IONIL contains no anionic detergents or soaps making it gentle enough for daily use.

ADMINISTRATION AND DOSAGE

Wet hair, apply IONIL, and massage into scalp. Don't expect as much initial sudsing as with anionic non-medicated shampoos. Rinse, then apply IONIL again and massage into a lather. Allow to remain in hair for about five minutes before rinsing.

CAUTION

For external use only. Avoid contact with eyes. Upon accidental contact with eyes, flush with clear water. Keep this and all drugs out of the reach of children. If accidentally swallowed, seek professional assistance.

HOW SUPPLIED

4 oz. (PIC 0299-3730-02), 8 oz. (PIC 0299-3730-04), 16 oz. (PIC 0299-3730-05), and 32 oz. (PIC 0299-3730-06) bottles.

IONIL® PLUS Shampoo
Therapeutic Shampoo

COMPOSITION

ACTIVE: Salicylic Acid 2%. INACTIVE: Water, Sodium Laureth Sulfate, Lauramide DEA, Quaternium-22, Talloweth-60 Myristyl Glycol, Laureth-23, TEA Lauryl Sulfate, Glycol Distearate, Laureth-4, TEA-Abietoyl Hydrolyzed Collagen, DMDM Hydantoin, Tetrasodium EDTA, Sodium Hydroxide, Fragrance, FD&C Blue No. 1.

ACTION AND USES

IONIL PLUS Shampoo relieves the itching, irritation and flaking associated with dandruff, seborrheic dermatitis, and psoriasis of the scalp. IONIL PLUS shampoo is gentle enough for daily use and leaves hair manageable.

ADMINISTRATION AND DOSAGE

Wet hair, apply IONIL PLUS and massage into scalp. Let lather stand one minute, then rinse. Repeat application, if needed. May be used daily.

CAUTION

For external use only. Rinse eyes with water if contact is made. Keep this and all drugs out of the reach of children.

HOW SUPPLIED

4 oz. (PIC 0299-3731-04) and 8 oz. (PIC 0299-3731-08) bottles.

IONIL® T Shampoo
Therapeutic Coal Tar and Salicylic Acid Shampoo

COMPOSITION

OWENTAR® (coal tar solution), salicylic acid, water, laureth-23, laureth-4, SD alcohol 40 12%, isopropyl alcohol 4%, benzalkonium chloride, tetrasodium EDTA.

ACTION AND USES

IONIL® T therapeutically relieves the itching and flaking associated with dandruff, seborrheic dermatitis, and psoriasis of the scalp. IONIL T contains no anionic detergents or soaps making it gentle enough for daily use.

ADMINISTRATION AND DOSAGE

Wet hair, apply IONIL T, and massage into scalp. Don't expect as much initial sudsing as the anionic non-medicated shampoos. Rinse, then apply IONIL T again and massage into a lather. Allow to remain in hair for about five minutes before rinsing.

CAUTION

For external use only. Avoid contact with eyes. Upon accidental contact with eyes flush with clear water. Keep this and all drugs out of the reach of children.

HOW SUPPLIED

4 oz. (PIC 0299-3750-02), 8 oz. (PIC 0299-3750-04), 16 oz. (PIC 0299-3750-05), and 32 oz. (PIC 0299-3750-06) bottles.

IONIL T® PLUS Shampoo
Therapeutic Tar Shampoo

COMPOSITION

ACTIVE: OWENTAR® II (equivalent to 2% crude coal tar). INACTIVE: Water, Sodium Laureth Sulfate, Lauramide DEA, Quaternium-22, Laureth-23, Talloweth-60 Myristyl Glycol, TEA Lauryl Sulfate, Glycol Distearate, Laureth-4, TEA-Abietoyl Hydrolyzed Collagen, DMDM Hydantoin, Disodium EDTA, Fragrance, FD&C Blue No. 1, Ext. D&C Yellow No. 7.

ACTION AND USES

IONIL T PLUS Shampoo therapeutically relieves the itching and flaking associated with dandruff, seborrheic dermatitis, and psoriasis of the scalp. Will not discolor white or light colored hair. IONIL T PLUS is gentle enough for daily use and leaves hair manageable.

ADMINISTRATION AND DOSAGE

Wet hair, apply IONIL T PLUS, and massage into scalp. Let lather stand one minute and then rinse. Repeat application, if needed. May be used daily.

CAUTION

For external use only. Rinse eyes with water if contact is made. Keep this and all drugs out of the reach of children.

HOW SUPPLIED

4 oz. (PIC 0299-3752-04) and 8 oz. (PIC 0299-3752-08) bottles.

LOCOID®   ℞
(hydrocortisone butyrate)
Cream 0.1%
Ointment 0.1%

CAUTION: Federal law prohibits dispensing without prescription.

DESCRIPTION

LOCOID cream and ointment contain the topical corticosteroid, hydrocortisone butyrate, a non-fluorinated ester of hydrocortisone. It has the chemical name: pregn-4-ene-3,20-dione, 11,21-dihydroxy-17-[(1-oxobutyl)oxy]-, (11_β)-; the empirical formula: $C_{25}H_{36}O_6$; the molecular weight: 432.54 and the CAS registry number: 13609-67-1.

LOCOID® Cream 0.1%
Each gram of LOCOID cream contains 1 mg of hydrocortisone butyrate in a hydrophilic base consisting of cetostearyl alcohol, ceteth-20, mineral oil, white petrolatum, citric acid, sodium citrate, methylparaben (preservative) and purified water.

LOCOID® Ointment 0.1%
Each gram of LOCOID ointment contains 1 mg of hydrocortisone butyrate in a base consisting of mineral oil and polyethylene.

CLINICAL PHARMACOLOGY

Topical corticosteroids share anti-inflammatory, anti-pruritic and vasoconstrictive actions.

The mechanism of anti-inflammatory activity of the topical corticosteroids is unclear. Various laboratory methods, including vasoconstrictor assays, are used to compare and predict potencies and/or clinical efficacies of the topical corticosteroids. There is some evidence to suggest that a recognizable correlation exists between vasoconstrictor potency and therapeutic efficacy in man.

Pharmacokinetics
The extent of percutaneous absorption of topical corticosteroids is determined by many factors including the vehicle, the integrity of the epidermal barrier, and the use of occlusive dressings.

Topical corticosteroids can be absorbed from normal intact skin. Inflammation and/or other disease processes in the skin increase percutaneous absorption. Occlusive dressings substantially increase the percutaneous absorption of topical corticosteroids.

Thus, occlusive dressings may be a valuable therapeutic adjunct for treatment of resistant dermatoses. (See DOSAGE AND ADMINISTRATION.)

Once absorbed through the skin, topical corticosteroids are handled through pharmacokinetic pathways similar to systemically administered corticosteroids. Corticosteroids are bound to plasma proteins in varying degrees. Corticosteroids are metabolized primarily in the liver and are then excreted by the kidneys. Some of the topical corticosteroids and their metabolites are also excreted into the bile.

INDICATIONS AND USAGE

LOCOID cream 0.1% and ointment 0.1% (hydrocortisone butyrate) are indicated for the relief of the inflammatory and pruritic manifestations of corticosteroid-responsive dermatoses.

CONTRAINDICATIONS

Topical corticosteroids are contraindicated in those patients with a history of hypersensitivity to any of the components of the preparation.

PRECAUTIONS

General: Systemic absorption of topical corticosteroids has produced reversible hypothalamic-pituitary-adrenal (HPA) axis suppression, manifestations of Cushing's syndrome, hyperglycemia, and glucosuria in some patients.

Conditions which augment systemic absorption include the application of the more potent steroids, use over large surface areas, prolonged use, and the addition of occlusive dressings.

Therefore, patients receiving a large dose of a potent topical steroid applied to a large surface area or under an occlusive dressing should be evaluated periodically for evidence of HPA axis suppression by using the urinary free cortisol and ACTH stimulation tests. If HPA axis suppression is noted, an attempt should be made to withdraw the drug, to reduce the frequency of application, or to substitute a less potent steroid.

Recovery of HPA axis function is generally prompt and complete upon discontinuation of the drug. Infrequently, signs and symptoms of steroid withdrawal may occur, requiring supplemental systemic corticosteroids.

Children may absorb proportionally larger amounts of topical corticosteroids and thus be more susceptible to systemic toxicity (See PRECAUTIONS—PEDIATRIC USE).

If irritation develops, topical corticosteroids should be discontinued and appropriate therapy instituted.

In the presence of dermatological infections, the use of an appropriate antifungal or antibacterial agent should be instituted. If a favorable response does not occur promptly, the corticosteroid should be discontinued until the infection has been adequately controlled.

Information for the patient
Patients using topical corticosteroids should receive the following information and instructions:

1. This medication is to be used as directed by the physician. It is for external use only. Avoid contact with the eyes.
2. Patients should be advised not to use this medication for any disorder other than for which it was prescribed.
3. The treated skin area should not be bandaged or otherwise covered or wrapped as to be occlusive unless directed by the physician.
4. Patients should report any signs of local adverse reactions especially under occlusive dressing.
5. Parents of pediatric patients should be advised not to use tight-fitting diapers or plastic pants on a child being treated in the diaper area, as these garments may constitute occlusive dressings.

Laboratory tests
The following tests may be helpful in evaluating the HPA axis suppression:
Urinary free cortisol test
ACTH stimulation test

Carcinogenesis, mutagenesis, and impairment of fertility
Long-term animal studies have not been performed to evaluate the carcinogenic potential or the effect on fertility of topical corticosteroids.

Studies to determine mutagenicity with prednisolone and hydrocortisone have revealed negative results.

Pregnancy category C
Corticosteroids are generally teratogenic in laboratory animals when administered systemically at relatively low dosage levels. The more potent corticosteroids have been shown to be teratogenic after dermal application in laboratory animals. There are no adequate and well-controlled studies in pregnant women on teratogenic effects from topically applied corticosteroids. Therefore, topical corticosteroids should be used during pregnancy only if the potential benefit justifies the potential risk to the fetus. Drugs of this class should not be used extensively on pregnant patients, in large amounts, or for prolonged periods of time.

Nursing mothers
It is not known whether topical administration of corticosteroids could result in sufficient systemic absorption to produce detectable quantities in breast milk. Systemically administered corticosteroids are secreted into breast milk, in quantities not likely to have a deleterious effect on the infant. Nevertheless, caution should be exercised when topical corticosteroids are administered to a nursing woman.

Pediatric use
Pediatric patients may demonstrate greater susceptibility to topical corticosteroid-induced HPA axis suppression and Cushing's syndrome than mature patients because of a larger skin surface area to body weight ratio.

Hypothalamic-pituitary-adrenal (HPA) axis suppression, Cushing's syndrome, and intracranial hypertension have been reported in children receiving topical corticosteroids. Manifestations of adrenal suppression in children include linear growth retardation, delayed weight gain, low plasma cortisol levels, and absence of response to ACTH stimulation. Manifestations of intracranial hypertension include bulging fontanelles, headaches, and bilateral papilledema.

Administration of topical corticosteroids to children should be limited to the least amount compatible with an effective therapeutic regimen. Chronic corticosteroid therapy may interfere with the growth and development of children.

ADVERSE REACTIONS

The following local adverse reactions are reported infrequently with topical corticosteroids, but may occur more frequently with the use of occlusive dressings. These reactions are listed in an approximate decreasing order of occurrence: burning, itching, irritation, dryness, folliculitis, hypertrichosis, acneiform eruptions, hypopigmentation, perioral dermatitis, allergic contact dermatitis, maceration of the skin, secondary infection, skin atrophy, striae, miliaria.

OVERDOSAGE

Topically applied corticosteroids can be absorbed in sufficient amounts to produce systemic effects (See PRECAUTIONS).

DOSAGE AND ADMINISTRATION

LOCOID cream 0.1% or LOCOID ointment 0.1% (hydrocortisone butyrate) should be applied to the affected area as a thin film two to three times daily depending on the severity of the condition.

Occlusive dressings may be used for the management of psoriasis or recalcitrant conditions.

If an infection develops, the use of occlusive dressings should be discontinued and appropriate antimicrobial therapy instituted.

HOW SUPPLIED

LOCOID cream 0.1% (hydrocortisone butyrate) is supplied in tubes containing:
15 g NDC 0299-2000-15
45 g NDC 0299-2000-45
60 g NDC 0299-2000-60
LOCOID ointment 0.1% (hydrocortisone butyrate) is supplied in tubes containing:
15 g NDC 0299-2010-15
45 g NDC 0299-2010-45

STORAGE CONDITIONS

LOCOID cream 0.1%: Store between 46° and 77°F (8° and 25°C).
LOCOID ointment 0.1%: Store below 86°F (30°C).
Avoid freezing.
Manufactured under
license from Gist-Brocades, N.V.
Delft-Netherlands

NUTRACORT®   ℞
(hydrocortisone)
Cream 1%
Lotion 1% & 2.5%

DESCRIPTION

NUTRACORT® cream and lotion are topical hydrocortisone preparations. Hydrocortisone is therapeutically classed as an anti-inflammatory and anti-pruritic agent. Hydrocortisone is a white crystalline powder that is very slightly soluble in water and ether and sparingly soluble in acetone and alcohol.

Chemical Name: Pregn-4-ene-3,20-dione, 11, 17, 21-trihydroxy-,(11_β)-.
Empirical Formula: $C_{21}H_{30}O_5$
Molecular Weight: 362.47
NUTRACORT® Cream 1% contains: Hydrocortisone 1.0% (10 mg/g) in a cream base containing propylene glycol, polysorbate 60, emulsifying wax, synthetic beeswax, stearic acid, isopropyl palmitate, sorbic acid, potassium sorbate, propyl gallate, citric acid and/or sodium hydroxide (to adjust pH), purified water and certified color.
NUTRACORT® Lotion 1% contains: Hydrocortisone 1.0% (10 mg/mL) in a lotion base containing sodium lauryl sulfate, light mineral oil, cetyl alcohol, stearyl alcohol, methylparaben, propylparaben, sorbitan monostearate, glyceryl stearate SE, edetate sodium, purified water and certified color. May contain citric acid and/or sodium hydroxide for pH adjustment.
NUTRACORT® Lotion 2.5% contains: Hydrocortisone 2.5% (25 mg/mL) in a lotion base containing sodium lauryl sulfate, light mineral oil, cetyl alcohol, stearyl alcohol, methylparaben, propylparaben, sorbitan monostearate, glyceryl stearate SE, edetate disodium, purified water and certified colors. May contain citric acid and/or sodium hydroxide for pH adjustment.

CLINICAL PHARMACOLOGY

Topical corticosteroids share anti-inflammatory, anti-pruritic and vasoconstrictive actions.

The mechanism of anti-inflammatory activity of the topical corticosteroids is unclear. Various laboratory methods, including vasoconstrictor assays, are used to compare and predict potencies and/or clinical efficacies of the topical corticosteroids. There is some evidence to suggest that a recognizable correlation exists between vasoconstrictor potency and therapeutic efficacy in man.

Pharmacokinetics: The extent of percutaneous absorption of topical corticosteroids is determined by many factors including the vehicle, the integrity of the epidermal barrier, and the use of occlusive dressings.

Topical corticosteroids can be absorbed from normal intact skin. Inflammation and/or other disease processes in the skin increase percutaneous absorption. Occlusive dressings substantially increase the percutaneous absorption of topical corticosteroids. Thus, occlusive dressings may be a valuable therapeutic adjunct for treatment of resistant dermatoses. (See DOSAGE AND ADMINISTRATION.)

Once absorbed through the skin, topical corticosteroids are handled through pharmacokinetic pathways similar to systemically administered corticosteroids. Corticosteroids are bound to plasma proteins in varying degrees. Corticosteroids are metabolized primarily in the liver and are then excreted by the kidneys. Some of the topical corticosteroids and their metabolites are also excreted into the bile.

Continued on next page

Owen—Cont.

INDICATIONS AND USAGE
Topical corticosteroids are indicated for the relief of the inflammatory and pruritic manifestations of corticosteroid-responsive dermatoses.

CONTRAINDICATIONS
Topical corticosteroids are contraindicated in those patients with a history of hypersensitivity to any of the components of the preparation.

PRECAUTIONS
General: Systemic absorption of topical corticosteroids has produced reversible hypothalamic-pituitary-adrenal (HPA) axis suppression, manifestations of Cushing's syndrome, hyperglycemia, and glucosuria in some patients.
Conditions which augment systemic absorption include the application of the more potent steroids, use over large surface areas, prolonged use, and the addition of occlusive dressings.
Therefore, patients receiving a large dose of a potent topical steroid applied to a large surface area or under an occlusive dressing should be evaluated periodically for evidence of HPA axis suppression by using the urinary free cortisol and ACTH stimulation tests. If HPA axis suppression is noted, an attempt should be made to withdraw the drug, to reduce the frequency of application, or to substitute a less potent steroid. Recovery of HPA axis function is generally prompt and complete upon discontinuation of the drug. Infrequently, signs and symptoms of steroid withdrawal may occur, requiring supplemental systemic corticosteroids.
Children may absorb proportionally larger amounts of topical corticosteroids and thus be more susceptible to systemic toxicity. (See PRECAUTIONS—Pediatric Use.)
If irritation develops, topical corticosteroids should be discontinued and appropriate therapy instituted.
In the presence of dermatological infections, the use of an appropriate antifungal or antibacterial agent should be instituted. If a favorable response does not occur promptly, the corticosteroid should be discontinued until the infection has been adequately controlled.
Information for the Patient: Patients using topical corticosteroids should receive the following information and instructions:
1. This medication is to be used as directed by the physician. It is for external use only. Avoid contact with the eyes.
2. Patients should be advised not to use this medication for any disorder other than for which it was prescribed.
3. The treated skin area should not be bandaged or otherwise covered or wrapped as to be occlusive unless directed by the physician.
4. Patients should report any signs of local adverse reactions especially under occlusive dressing.
5. Parents of pediatric patients should be advised not to use tight-fitting diapers or plastic pants on a child being treated in the diaper area, as these garments may constitute occlusive dressings.
Laboratory Tests: The following tests may be helpful in evaluating the HPA axis suppression:
Urinary free cortisol test
ACTH stimulation test
Carcinogenesis, Mutagenesis, and Impairment of Fertility: Long-term animal studies have not been performed to evaluate the carcinogenic potential or the effect on fertility of topical corticosteroids.
Studies to determine mutagencity with prednisolone and hydrocortisone have revealed negative results.
Pregnancy Category C: Corticosteroids are generally teratogenic in laboratory animals when administered systemically at relatively low dosage levels. The more potent corticosteroids have been shown to be teratogenic after dermal application in laboratory animals. There are no adequate and well-controlled studies in pregnant women on teratogenic effects from topically applied corticosteroids. Therefore, topical corticosteroids should be used during pregnancy only if the potential benefit justifies the potential risk to the fetus. Drugs of this class should not be used extensively on pregnant patients, in large amounts, or for prolonged periods of time.
Nursing Mothers: It is not known whether topical administration of corticosteroids could result in sufficient systemic absorption to produce detectable quantities in breast milk. Systemically administered corticosteroids are secreted into breast milk in quantities *not* likely to have a deleterious effect on the infant. Nevertheless, caution should be exercised when topical corticosteroids are administered to a nursing woman.
Pediatric Use: *Pediatric patients may demonstrate greater susceptibility to topical corticosteroid-induced HPA axis suppression and Cushing's syndrome than mature patients because of a larger skin surface area to body weight ratio.*
Hypothalamic-pituitary-adrenal (HPA) axis suppression, Cushing's syndrome, and intracranial hypertension have been reported in children receiving topical corticosteroids.

Manifestations of adrenal suppression in children include linear growth retardation, delayed weight gain, low plasma cortisol levels, and absence of response to ACTH stimulation. Manifestations of intracranial hypertension include bulging fontanelles, headaches, and bilateral papilledema.
Administration of topical corticosteroids to children should be limited to the least amount compatible with an effective therapeutic regimen. Chronic corticosteroid therapy may interfere with the growth and development of children.

ADVERSE REACTIONS
The following local adverse reactions are reported infrequently with topical corticosteroids, but may occur more frequently with the use of occlusive dressings. These reactions are listed in an approximate decreasing order of occurrence:
Burning, Itching, Irritation, Dryness, Folliculitis, Hypertrichosis, Acneiform eruptions, Hypopigmentation, Perioral dermatitis, Allergic contact dermatitis, Maceration of the skin, Secondary infection, Skin Atrophy, Striae, Miliaria.

OVERDOSAGE
Topically applied corticosteroids can be absorbed in sufficient amounts to produce systemic effects (See PRECAUTIONS).

DOSAGE AND ADMINISTRATION
Topical corticosteroids are generally applied to the affected area as a thin film from three to four times daily depending on the severity of the condition.
Occlusive dressings may be used for the management of psoriasis or recalcitrant conditions.
If an infection develops, the use of occlusive dressings should be discontinued and appropriate antimicrobial therapy instituted.

HOW SUPPLIED
NUTRACORT® Cream 1% is supplied in high density polyethylene (HDPE) tubes:
30g **NDC** 0299-5821-30
60g **NDC** 0299-5821-60
and in polypropylene jars:
4 oz. **NDC** 0299-5821-04
NUTRACORT® Lotion 1% is supplied in HDPE bottles:
2 fl. oz. **NDC** 0299-5830-01
4 fl. oz. **NDC** 0299-5830-02
NUTRACORT® Lotion 2.5% is supplied in HDPE bottles:
2 fl. oz. **NDC** 0299-5825-01
4 fl. oz. **NDC** 0299-5825-02
Store at room temperature.

NUTRADERM® Lotion
Skin-Lubricant—Moisturizer

NUTRADERM® Cream
Moisturizer—Emollient

COMPOSITION
Lotion contains mineral oil in water, sorbitan stearate, stearyl alcohol, sodium lauryl sulfate, cetyl alcohol, carbomer 940, methylparaben triethanolamine, propylparaben and fragrance.
Cream contains mineral oil in water, sorbitan stearate, stearyl alcohol, cetyl alcohol, sorbitol, isopropyl palmitate, cetyl esters wax, sodium lauryl sulfate, dimethicone, methylparabens, propylparaben, citric acid and fragrance.

ACTIONS AND USES
NUTRADERM® Lotion lubricates and moisturizes the skin through hydration. It helps retain the normal moisture balance of the skin and helps the protective action of skin lipids. Indicated for generalized dryness and itching associated with chapped or chafed skin, sunburn, winter-itch, aging, heat rash, diaper rash and detergent hands.

ADMINISTRATION AND DOSAGE
Apply freely to dry skin areas as necessary.

HOW SUPPLIED
NUTRADERM Lotion 8 oz. (PIC 0299-5880-04), NUTRADERM Lotion 16 oz. (PIC 0299-5880-05) plastic bottles; also available as NUTRADERM Cream 3 oz. (PIC 0299-5850-30) plastic tubes; NUTRADERM Cream 1 lb. (PIC 0299-5850-05) plastic jar.

Products are cross-indexed
by product classifications
in the
BLUE SECTION

Paddock Laboratories, Inc.
3101 LOUISIANA AVENUE NORTH
MINNEAPOLIS, MN 55427

ACTIDOSE with SORBITOL™   OTC
[*act 'ĭ-dose*]
(Activated Charcoal Suspension)

Actidose (Activated charcoal) is supplied in bottles containing 25 grams and 50 grams activated charcoal suspension. Each milliliter contains 208 mg (0.208 grams) activated charcoal and 400 mg (0.4 grams) sorbitol.

ACTIDOSE–AQUA   OTC
[*act 'ĭ'dose a–qua*]
(Activated Charcoal Suspension)

Actidose-Aqua (Activated Charcoal) is supplied in bottles containing 25 grams and 50 grams activated charcoal suspension. Each milliliter contains 208 mg (0.208 grams) activated charcoal in aqueous suspension.

ETS–2%™   ℞
(Erythromycin Topical Solution)

DESCRIPTION
Erythromycin is an antibiotic produced from a strain of Streptomyces erythraeus. It is basic and readily forms salts with acids. Erythromycin 2 percent Topical Solution containing 20 mg/ml erythromycin base in a clear solution vehicle of 66 percent alcohol, propylene glycol and citric acid.

CLINICAL PHARMACOLOGY
Although the mechanism by which Erythromycin Solution acts in reducing inflammatory lesions of acne vulgaris is unknown, it is presumably due to its antibiotic action.

INDICATIONS AND USAGE
Erythromycin Solution is indicated for the topical control of acne vulgaris.

CONTRAINDICATIONS
Erythromycin Solution is contraindicated in persons who have shown hypersensitivity to erythromycin or any of the other listed ingredients.

WARNING
The safe use of Erythromycin Solution during pregnancy or lactation has not been established.

PRECAUTIONS
Erythromycin Solution is recommended for external use only and should be kept away from the eyes, nose, mouth and other mucous membranes. Concomitant topical acne therapy should be used with caution because a cumulative irritancy effect may occur, especially with the use of peeling, desquamating or abrasive agents.
The use of antibiotic agents may be associated with the overgrowth of antibiotic-resistant organisms. If this occurs, administration of this drug should be discontinued and appropriate measures taken.

ADVERSE REACTIONS
Adverse conditions reported include dryness, tenderness, pruritus, desquamation, erythema, oiliness, and burning sensation. Irritation of the eyes has also been reported. A case of generalized urticarial reaction, possibly related to the drug, which required the use of systemic steroid therapy has been reported.

DOSAGE AND ADMINISTRATION
Erythromycin Solution should be applied to the affected area each morning and evening after the skin is thoroughly washed with warm water and soap and patted dry. Apply contents by tilting bottle and rubbing applicator over affected area until skin is thoroughly wet. Close tightly after each use.

HOW SUPPLIED
Bottles of 2 fl. oz. (59 ml). Store at controlled room temperature (59°F–86°F). NDC 0574-0014-02

CAUTION
Federal law prohibits dispensing without prescription.

EMULSOIL®
(Self-Emulsifying Castor Oil)

(See PDR For Nonprescription Drugs)

GLUTOSE®
(Dextrose Gel)
For Insulin Reactions

(See PDR For Nonprescription Drugs)

IPECAC SYRUP

(See PDR For Nonprescription Drugs)

NYSTATIN, USP   ℞
**For Extemporaneous Preparation
of Oral Suspension**

DESCRIPTION
Nystatin, USP is an antifungal antibiotic which is both fungistatic and fungicidal *in vitro* against a wide variety of yeasts and yeast-like fungi. It is a polyene antibiotic of undetermined structural formula that is obtained from *Streptomyces noursei*. Nystatin, USP, which contains no excipients or preservatives, is a ready-to-use non-sterile powder for oral administration available in bottles of 50-million, 150-million, 500-million and 5-billion units.

CLINICAL PHARMACOLOGY
Nystatin probably acts by binding to sterols in the cell membrane of the fungus with a resultant change in membrane permeability allowing leakage of intracellular components. It is absorbed very sparingly following oral administration, with no detectable blood levels when given in the recommended doses. Most of the orally administered nystatin is passed unchanged in the stool.

INDICATIONS AND USAGE
For the treatment of infections of the oral cavity caused by *Candida albicans* (monilia).

CONTRAINDICATIONS
Hypersensitivity to the drug.

ADVERSE REACTIONS
Large oral doses of nystatin have occasionally produced diarrhea, gastrointestinal distress, nausea and vomiting.

DOSAGE AND ADMINISTRATION
Adults and older children: Add ⅛ tsp. (500,000 units) of nystatin, USP to approximately ½ to 1 cup (120 to 240 ml, or 4 to 8 oz.) of water and stir well. The entire dose should then be used to thoroughly rinse the mouth and the dose should be retained in the mouth as long as possible before swallowing. This dose should be given orally four times daily, and should be continued for at least 48 hours after perioral symptoms have disappeared and cultures have returned to normal. One-eighth tsp. of nystatin, USP is equivalent to the recommended dose for adults and children of Nystatin Oral Suspension (4 to 6 ml, or 400,000 to 600,000 units). This product contains no preservative and therefore should be used immediately after mixing and should not be stored.

HOW SUPPLIED
Bottles containing 50-million units, 150-million units, 500-million units and 5-billion units—(1 billion units is approximately 170 to 200 g depending on potency of the powder).
    NDC 0574-0403-05—50-Million Units
    NDC 0574-0403-15—150-Million Units
    NDC 0574-0403-50—500-Million Units
    NDC 0574-0403-01—5-Billion Units
Store under refrigeration 2–8°C (36–46°F) in tight light-resistant containers.
Note: The potency of this product cannot be assured for longer than 90 days after the container is first opened.
                                  6/85

Palisades Pharmaceuticals, Inc.
**219 COUNTY ROAD
TENAFLY, NEW JERSEY 07670**

PALS™
**Internal Deodorant
Chlorophyllin Copper Complex**
['pals]

DESCRIPTION
PALS™ is a safe and effective internal deodorant. Each coated tablet contains 100 mg. of Chlorophyllin Copper Complex, achieving the desired effect with just one or two tablets daily.

INDICATIONS
PALS™ is indicated for the control of odors from colostomies and ileostomies, and as an aid to reduce fecal and urinary odor due to incontinence.

ACTION AND ADMINISTRATION
INCONTINENT PATIENTS
The odor problem due to incontinence, generally associated with hospitals and nursing homes, can be easily reduced or eliminated completely by the use of PALS™.
When taking PALS™ for odor due to incontinence, it is recommended that patients take one or two tablets at meal-

time to get the effective dosage. It may take up to two weeks before the desired effect is first noticeable.
OSTOMY PATIENTS
Because the odor problems of ileostomy patients are different than the problems faced by colostomy patients, due to the nature and frequency of the discharge, the best dosage schedule may also be different.
Ileostomy: In ileostomy patients, one-half of a PALS™ tablet or more after every meal is usually the most effective dosage schedule since discharge may occur more than once a day.
Colostomy: In colostomy patients, one or two PALS™ once daily is usually more effective than several smaller doses because contents are more exposed to breakdown in the colon and elimination is generally once a day.
In both colostomy and ileostomy patients, it may take up to a week to get the desired odor control because the effect of PALS™ is cumulative. Once reached, the level of odor control can easily be maintained at the recommended dose.

DIRECTIONS
Adults and children over the age of 12: Up to two tablets, by mouth, taken daily. Children under 12: Consult a physician. Ostomy patients may take PALS™ orally or place the tablet directly in their ostomy appliance.

ADVERSE REACTIONS
No adverse reactions have been reported from the use of Chlorophyllin Copper Complex at the recommended dosage over an extended period of time. However, the patient may experience a mild laxative effect and the fecal discharge is usually a dark green.

WARNINGS
KEEP THIS AND ALL MEDICATION OUT OF THE REACH OF CHILDREN

HOW SUPPLIED
Oral tablets of PALS™ 100 mg. in bottles of 30's NDC# 53159-016-30, 100's NDC#53159-016-01, 1000's NDC#53159-016-10, and travel paks of 30's NDC#53159-016-40.
No Doctor's prescription is necessary.
PALISADES PHARMACEUTICALS, INC.
219 County Road, Tenafly, N.J. 07670
Shown in Product Identification Section, page 420

SCLEROMATE™   ℞
[skle ″ro-māt]
MORRHUATE SODIUM INJECTION U.S.P.

DESCRIPTION
Morrhuate Sodium Injection, U.S.P. is a mixture of the sodium salts of the saturated and unsaturated fatty acids of Cod Liver Oil. SCLEROMATE Morrhuate Sodium Injection, U.S.P. is prepared by the saponification of selected Cod Liver Oils, it is overlaid with filtered Nitrogen to prevent discoloration that occurs on exposure to oxygen. Morrhuate Sodium occurs as a pale-yellowish, granular powder with a slight fishy odor and is soluable in water and in alcohol.
NOTE: Solid matter may develop a hazy appearance on standing and the injection should not be used if the solid matter does not dissolve completely on warming. The pH of the injection is adjusted to approximately 9.5.

CLINICAL PHARMACOLOGY
Morrhuate Sodium, when injected into the vein, causes inflammation of the intima and formation of a thrombus. This blood clot occludes the injected vein and fibrous tissue develops, resulting in the obliteration of the vein.

INDICATIONS AND USAGE
Morrhuate Sodium Injection is used for the obliteration of primary varicosed veins that consist of simple dilation with competent valves.
Sclerotherapy should not be used in patients with significant valvular or deep vein incompetence. (See Precautions.)
Although a Morrhuate Sodium has been used as a sclerosing agent for the treatment of internal hemorrhoids, there is no substantial evidence that the drug is useful for this purpose. Most patients with symptomatic primary varicosed veins should be treated initially with compression stockings. If this treatment is inadequate, surgery may be required. Sclerosing agents may be useful as a supplement to venous ligation to obliterate residual varicosed veins or in patients who have conditions which increase the risk of surgery. However, many clinicians consider sclerotherapy if not effective may decrease the potential success of later surgery, should this be required.

CONTRAINDICATIONS
Morrhuate Sodium is contraindicated in patients who have shown a previous hypersensitivity reaction to the drug or to the fatty acids of cod liver oil. Continued administration of the drug is contraindicated when an unusual local reaction at the injection site or a systemic reaction occurs.
Thrombosis induced by Morrhuate Sodium may extend into the deep venous system in patients with significant valvular

incompetence, therefore, valvular competency, deep vein patency, and deep vein competency should be determined by angiography and/or by tests such as the Trendelenberg and Perthes before injection of sclerosing agents. The drug is contraindicated for obliterations of superficial veins in patients with persistent occlusion of the deep veins. Morrhuate Sodium is also contraindicated in patients with acute superficial thrombophlebitis; underlying arterial disease; varicosities caused by abdominal and pelvic tumors, uncontrolled diabetes melitus, thyrotoxicosis, tuberculosis, neoplasms, asthma, sepsis, blood dyscrasias, acute respiratory or skin disease; and in bedridden patients. Treatment with Morrhuate Sodium should be delayed in patients with acute local or systemic infections (including infected ulcers). Extensive therapy with the drug is inadvisable in patients who are severely debilitated or senile.

PRECAUTIONS
Burning or cramping sensations indicate local reactions. Urticaria may result. Sloughing and necrosis of tissue may occur with extravasation of the drug. Technique development is essential for optimal success in sclerotherapy, therefore the drug should be administered only by a physician familiar with proper injection technique. Drowsiness and headache may occur rarely. Pulmonary embolism has been reported.
Rarely, patients may have, or may develop hypersensitivity to Morrhuate Sodium, characterized by dizziness, weakness, vascular collapse, asthma, respiratory depression, gastrointestinal disturbances (i.e., Nausea, vomiting), and urticaria. Anaphylactic reactions may occur within a few minutes after injection of the drug and are most likely to occur when therapy is reinstituted after an interval of several weeks. Morrhuate Sodium should only be administered when adequate facilities, drugs (i.e., epinephrine, antihistamines, corticosteroids), and personnel are available for the treatment of anaphylactic reactions.

PREGNANCY
Safety in use of Morrhuate Sodium during pregnancy has not been established.

DOSAGE
Morrhuate Sodium is administered only by INTRAVENOUS Injection. Care must be taken to avoid extravasation. (see Precautions.) Specialized references should be consulted for specific procedures and techniques of administration. When small veins are injected, or the injection solution is cold, or if solid matter has separated in the solution, the ampul or vial should be warmed by immersing in hot water. The solution should become clear on warming; only a clear solution should be used. Because the solution froths easily, a large bore needle should be used to fill the syringe, however, a small bore needle should be used for the injection.
To determine possible sensitivity to the drug, some clinicians recommend injection of 0.25–1 ml of 5% Morrhuate Sodium injection into a varicosity 24 hours before administration of a large dose.
Dosage of Morrhuate Sodium depends on the size and degree of varicosity. The usual adult dose for obliteration of small or medium veins is 50–100mg (1–2ml of the 5% injection). For large veins, 150–250 (3–5ml of the injection) is used. The drug may be given as multiple injections at one time or in single doses. Therapy may be repeated at 5–7 day intervals, according to the patient's response. Following injection of Morrhuate Sodium, the vein promptly becomes hard and swollen for 2–4 inches, depending on the size and response of the vein. After 24 hours, the vein is hard and slightly tender to the touch (with little or no periphlebitis). The skin around the injection becomes light-bronze; this color usually disappears shortly. An aching sensation and feeling of stiffness usually occur and last approximately 48 hours.

HOW SUPPLIED
MORRHUATE SODIUM INJECTION 5%
NDC-53159-003-25   5ml Ampuls in boxes of 25's
NDC-53159-003-01   30ml Multiple use Vials
NDC-53159-003-10   10ml fill in 20ml Multiple use Vials

STORAGE
Store below 40 degrees C. (104 degrees F.) preferably in a refrigerator, or between 15–30 degrees C. (59–86 degrees F.)
Rev. July 1985
Shown in Product Identification Section, page 420

YOCON®   ℞
[yō′kon]
(brand of yohimbine hydrochloride)

DESCRIPTION
Yohimbine is a 3α-15α-20β-17α-hydroxy Yohimbine-16α-carboxylic acid methyl ester. The alkaloid is found in Rubaceae and related trees. Also in Rauwolfia Serpentina (L) Benth.

Continued on next page

Palisades—Cont.

Yohimbine is an indolalkylamine alkaloid with chemical similarity to reserpine. It is a crystalline powder, odorless. Each compressed tablet contains (1/12 gr.) 5.4 mg of Yohimbine Hydrochloride.

ACTION

Yohimbine blocks presynaptic alpha-2 adrenergic receptors. Its action on peripheral blood vessels resembles that of reserpine, though it is weaker and of short duration. Yohimbine's peripheral autonomic nervous system effect is to increase parasympathetic (cholinergic) and decrease sympathetic (adrenergic) activity. It is to be noted that in male sexual performance, erection is linked to cholinergic activity and to alpha-2 adrenergic blockade which may theoretically result in increased penile inflow, decreased penile outflow or both. Yohimbine exerts a stimulating action on the mood and may increase anxiety. Such actions have not been adequately studied or related to dosage although they appear to require high doses of the drug. Yohimbine has a mild anti-diuretic action, probably via stimulation of hypothalmic centers and release of posterior pituitary hormone.

Reportedly, Yohimbine exerts no significant influence on cardiac stimulation and other effects mediated by β-adrenergic receptors, its effect on blood pressure, if any, would be to lower it; however, no adequate studies are at hand to quantitate this effect in terms of Yohimbine dosage.

INDICATIONS

YOCON is indicated as a sympathicolytic and mydriatic. It may have activity as an aphrodisiac.

CONTRAINDICATIONS

Renal diseases, and patient's sensitive to the drug. In view of the limited and inadequate information at hand, no precise tabulation can be offered of additional contra-indications.

WARNING

Generally, this drug is not proposed for use in females and certainly must not be used during pregnancy. Neither is this drug proposed for use in pediatric, geriatric or cardio-renal patients with gastric or duodenal ulcer history. Nor should it be used in conjunction with mood-modifying drugs such as antidepressants, or in psychiatric patients in general.

ADVERSE REACTIONS

Yohimbine readily penetrates the (CNS) and produces a complex pattern of responses in lower doses than required to produce peripheral α-adrenergic blockade. These include, anti-diuresis, a general picture of central excitation including elevation of blood pressure and heart rate increased motor activity, irritability and tremor. Sweating, nausea and vomiting are common after parenteral administration of the drug.[1,2] Also dizziness, headache, skin flushing reported when used orally.[1,3]

DOSAGE AND ADMINISTRATION

Experimental dosage reported in treatment of erectile impotence:[1,3,4] 1 tablet (5.4 mg) 3 times a day, to adult males taken orally. Occasional side effects reported with this dosage are nausea, dizziness or nervousness. In the event of side effects dosage is to be reduced to ½ tablet 3 times a day, followed by gradual increases to 1 tablet 3 times a day. Reported therapy not more than 10 weeks[3].

HOW SUPPLIED

Oral tablets of Yocon® 1/12 gr 5.4 mg in bottles of 100's **NDC** 53159-001-01 and 1000's **NDC** 53159-001-10.

REFERENCES

1. A. Morales et al., New England Journal of Medicine: 1221. November 12, 1981.
2. Goodman, Gilman —The Pharmacological basis of Therapeutics 6th ed., p. 176-188, McMillan
3. Weekly Urological Clinical letter, 27:2, July 4, 1983.
4. A. Morales et al., The Journal of Urology 128 : 45-47, 1982.
Rev. January 1985

Shown in Product Identification Section, page 420

Par Pharmaceutical, Inc.
ONE RAM RIDGE ROAD
SPRING VALLEY, NY 10977

COMPLETE LISTING OF PAR PRODUCTS

Par Pharmaceutical, Inc. manufactures tablets and capsules with an identification system that consists of the letters PAR and the NDC product numbers or product strength imprinted or embossed on the surface. To expedite product identification, an alphabetical listing of Par's products is provided below. Each product comes in a variety of packaging specifications, with the most common being 100's, 500's and 1000's.

Imprint numbers same as NDC numbers except where indicated otherwise.

NDC # 49884-	Product
104	Allopurinol Tablets 100 mg.
105	Allopurinol Tablets 300 mg.
117	Amiloride HCl Tablets 5 mg.
128	Amiloride with Hydrochlorothiazide 5mg/50mg.
164	Benztropine Mesylate Tablets 0.5 mg.
165	Benztropine Mesylate Tablets 1.0 mg.
166	Benztropine Mesylate Tablets 2.0 mg.
246	Carisoprodol & Aspirin Compound Tablets
265	Chlordiazepoxide and Amitriptyline Tablets 5 mg/12.5 mg.
266	Chlordiazepoxide and Amitriptyline Tablets 10 mg/25 mg.
077	Chlorpropamide Tablets 100 mg.
078	Chlorpropamide Tablets 250 mg.
016	Chlorzoxazone Tablets 250 mg.
082	Chlorzoxazone Caplets 500 mg.
110	Clonidine HCl Tablets 0.1 mg.
111	Clonidine HCl Tablets 0.2 mg.
112	Clonidine HCl Tablets 0.3 mg.
113	Clonidine HCl and Chlorthalidone Tablets 0.1 mg/15 mg.
115	Clonidine HCl and Chlorthalidone Tablets 0.2 mg/15 mg.
116	Clonidine HCl and Chlorthalidone Tablets 0.3 mg/15 mg.
043	Cyproheptadine HCl Tablets 4 mg.
083	Dexamethasone Tablets 0.25 mg.
084	Dexamethasone Tablets 0.5 mg.
085	Dexamethasone Tablets 0.75 mg.
086	Dexamethasone Tablets 1.5 mg.
087	Dexamethasone Tablets 4 mg.
129	Dexamethasone Tablets 6 mg.
045	Dexchlorpheniramine Maleate Tablets 4 mg. (I.D. Code #4)
046	Dexchlorpheniramine Maleate Tablets 6 mg. (I.D. Code #6)
190	Diazepam Tablets 2 mg.
191	Diazepam Tablets 5 mg.
192	Diazepam Tablets 10 mg.
042	Dipyridamole Tablets 25 mg. (I.D. Code #25)
031	Dipyridamole Tablets 50 mg. (I.D. Code #50)
065	Dipyridamole Tablets 75 mg. (I.D. Code #75)
217	Doxepin HCl Capsules 10 mg.
218	Doxepin HCl Capsules 25 mg.
219	Doxepin HCl Capsules 50 mg.
220	Doxepin HCl Capsules 75 mg.
221	Doxepin HCl Capsules 100 mg.
222	Doxepin HCl Capsules 150 mg.
066	Doxylamine Succinate Tablets 25 mg.
287	Fenoprofen Calcium Capsules 200 mg.
288	Fenoprofen Calcium Capsules 300 mg.
286	Fenoprofen Calcium Tablets 600 mg.
193	Flurazepam HCl Capsules 15 mg.
194	Flurazepam HCl Capsules 30 mg.
223	Haloperidol Tablets 0.5 mg.
224	Haloperidol Tablets 1 mg.
225	Haloperidol Tablets 2 mg.
226	Haloperidol Tablets 5 mg.
227	Haloperidol Tablets 10 mg.
228	Haloperidol Tablets 20 mg.
029	Hydralazine HCl Tablets 10 mg.
027	Hydralazine HCl Tablets 25 mg.
028	Hydralazine HCl Tablets 50 mg.
121	Hydralazine HCl Tablets 100 mg.
143	Hydra-Zide (Hydralazine HCl & Hydrochlorothiazide) Capsules 25mg/25 mg.
144	Hydra-Zide (Hydralazine HCl & Hydrochlorothiazide) Capsules 50 mg/50 mg.
145	Hydra-Zide (Hydralazine HCl & Hydrochlorothiazide) Capsules 100 mg/50 mg.
147	Hydroflumethiazide Tablets 50 mg.
148	Hydroflumethiazide with Reserpine Tablets 50 mg/0.125 mg.
012	Hydroxyzine HCl Tablets 10 mg.
013	Hydroxyzine HCl Tablets 25 mg.
014	Hydroxyzine HCl Tablets 50 mg.
069	Hydroxyzine Pamoate Capsules 25 mg.
070	Hydroxyzine Pamoate Capsules 50 mg.
071	Hydroxyzine Pamoate Capsules 100 mg.
161	Ibuprofen Tablets 300 mg.
162	Ibuprofen Tablets 400 mg.
163	Ibuprofen Tablets 600 mg.
216	Ibuprofen Tablets 800 mg.
054	Imipramine HCl Tablets 10 mg.
055	Imipramine HCl Tablets 25 mg.
056	Imipramine HCl Tablets 50 mg.
067	Indomethacin Capsules 25 mg.
068	Indomethacin Capsules 50 mg.
020	Isosorbide Dinitrate Tablets 5 mg.
021	Isosorbide Dinitrate Tablets 10 mg.
022	Isosorbide Dinitrate Tablets 20 mg.
009	Isosorbide Dinitrate Tablets 30 mg.
025	Isosorbide Dinitrate Tablets 40 mg. S.A.
237	Leucovorin Calcium Tablets 5 mg.
238	Leucovorin Calcium Tablets 25 mg.
206	Lorazepam Tablets 0.5 mg.
207	Lorazepam Tablets 1 mg.
208	Lorazepam Tablets 2 mg.
034	Meclizine HCl Tablets 12.5 mg.
035	Meclizine HCl Tablets 25 mg.
015	Meclizine HCl Tablets 50 mg.
263	Meclofenamate Sodium Capsules 50 mg.
264	Meclofenamate Sodium Capsules 100 mg.
289	Megestrol Acetate Tablets 20 mg.
290	Megestrol Acetate Tablets 40 mg.
176	Meprobamate and Aspirin Tablets 200 mg/325 mg.
258	Metaproterenol Sulfate Tablets 10 mg.
259	Metaproterenol Sulfate Tablets 20 mg.
249	Methocarbamol 400 mg. and Aspirin 325 mg. Tablets
177	Methyclothiazide Tablets 2.5 mg.
178	Methyclothiazide Tablets 5 mg.
150	Methyldopa Tablets 125 mg.
151	Methyldopa Tablets 250 mg.
152	Methyldopa Tablets 500 mg.
202	Methyldopa and Chlorothiazide Tablets 250 mg/150 mg.
203	Methyldopa and Chlorothiazide Tablets 250 mg/250 mg.
186	Methyldopa with Hydrochlorothiazide Tablets 250 mg/15 mg.
187	Methyldopa with Hydrochlorothiazide Tablets 250 mg/25 mg.
188	Methyldopa with Hydrochlorothiazide Tablets 500 mg/30 mg.
189	Methyldopa with Hydrochlorothiazide Tablets 500 mg/50 mg.
158	Methylprednisolone Tablets 16 mg.
159	Methylprednisolone Tablets 24 mg.
160	Methylprednisolone Tablets 32 mg.
132	Metoclopramide HCl Tablets 10 mg.
095	Metronidazole Compressed Tablets 250 mg.
114	Metronidazole Compressed Tablets 500 mg.
229	Metronidazole Film Coated Tablets 250 mg. (I.D. Code #130)
230	Metronidazole Film Coated Tablets 500 mg. (I.D. Code #131)
256	Minoxidil Tablets 2.5 mg.
257	Minoxidil Tablets 10 mg.
119	Nystatin Tablets 500,000 Units
213	Orphengesic® Tablets (Orphenadrine Citrate with Caffeine and Aspirin) 25 mg/30 mg/385 mg.
214	Orphengesic® Forte Tablets (Orphenadrine Citrate with Caffeine & Aspirin) 50 mg/60 mg/770 mg.
030	Par Decon Tablets (Phenylpropanolamine HCl 40 mg. with Phenylephrine HCl 10 mg., Phenyltoxamine Citrate 15 mg. and Chlorpheniramine Maleate 5 mg.) (S.A.)
181	Perphenazine and Amitriptyline Tablets 2 mg/10 mg.
182	Perphenazine and Amitriptyline Tablets 2 mg/25 mg.
183	Perphenazine and Amitriptyline Tablets 4 mg/10 mg.
184	Perphenazine and Amitriptyline Tablets 4 mg/25 mg.
185	Perphenazine and Amitriptyline Tablets 4 mg/50 mg.
118	Propantheline Bromide Tablets 15 mg.
106	Propranolol HCl Tablets 10 mg.
107	Propranolol HCl Tablets 20 mg.
108	Propranolol HCl Tablets 40 mg.
109	Propranolol HCl Tablets 80 mg.
247	Salsalate Tablets 500 mg.

248	Salsalate Tablets 750 mg.
170	Sulfinpyrazone Tablets 100 mg.
171	Sulfinpyrazone Capsules 200 mg.
240	Temazepam Capsules 15 mg.
241	Temazepam Capsules 30 mg.
096	Thioridazine HCl Tablets 10 mg.
097	Thioridazine HCl Tablets 15 mg.
098	Thioridazine HCl Tablets 25 mg.
099	Thioridazine HCl Tablets 50 mg.
101	Thioridazine HCl Tablets 100 mg.
102	Thioridazine HCl Tablets 150 mg.
103	Thioridazine HCl Tablets 200 mg.
122	Tolazamide Tablets 100 mg.
123	Tolazamide Tablets 250 mg.
124	Tolazamide Tablets 500 mg.
279	Triamterene and Hydrochlorothiazide Tablets 75 mg/50 mg.
038	Trichlormethiazide Tablets 2 mg.
039	Trichlormethiazide Tablets 4 mg.
125	Valproic Acid Capsules 250 mg.

Parke-Davis
Division of Warner-Lambert Company
201 TABOR ROAD
MORRIS PLAINS, NEW JERSEY
07950

PARCODE®
(Parke-Davis Accurate Recognition Code)

Code Number   **Product Name**

1   **Nitrogard Buccal Tablets, 1 mg**
Each tablet contains 1 mg nitroglycerin.

2   **Nitrogard Buccal Tablets, 2 mg**
Each tablet contains 2 mg nitroglycerin.

3   **Nitrogard Buccal Tablets, 3 mg**
Each tablet contains 3 mg nitroglycerin.

001   **Peritrate® Tablets**
Each tablet contains 20 mg pentaerythritol tetranitrate.

002-003   *Unassigned*

004   **Peritrate® SA Sustained Action Tablets**
Each tablet contains 80 mg pentaerythritol tetranitrate (20 mg in the immediate release layer and 60 mg in the sustained release base).

005-006   *Unassigned*

007   **Dilantin® Infatabs®**
Each tablet contains 50 mg phenytoin sodium, USP.

008   **Peritrate® Tablets**
Each tablet contains 40 mg pentaerythritol tetranitrate.

009-012   *Unassigned*

013   **Peritrate® Tablets**
Each tablet contains 10 mg pentaerythritol tetranitrate.

014-069   *Unassigned*

070   ***Propranolol Hydrochloride Tablets, USP**
Each tablet contains 10 mg propranolol hydrochloride, USP.

071   ***Propranolol Hydrochloride Tablets, USP**
Each tablet contains 20 mg propranolol hydrochloride, USP.

072   ***Propranolol Hydrochloride Tablets, USP**
Each tablet contains 40 mg propranolol hydrochloride, USP.

073   ***Propranolol Hydrochloride Tablets, USP**
Each tablet contains 60 mg propranolol hydrochloride, USP

074   ***Propranolol Hydrochloride Tablets, USP**
Each tablet contains 80 mg propranolol hydrochloride, USP.

075-110   *Unassigned*

111-   **Ergostat® Sublingual Tablets**
Each tablet contains 2 mg ergotamine tartrate.

112-120   *Unassigned*

121   ***Chlorthalidone Tablets, USP**
Each tablet contains 50 mg chlorthalidone, USP.

122   *Unassigned*

123   ***Chlorthalidone Tablets, USP**
Each tablet contains 25 mg chlorthalidone, USP.

124-140   *Unassigned*

141   ***Diazepam Tablets, USP**
Each tablet contains 2 mg diazepam, USP.

142   ***Diazepam Tablets, USP**
Each tablet contains 5 mg diazepam, USP.

143   ***Diazepam Tablets, USP**
Each tablet contains 10 mg diazepam, USP.

144-165   *Unassigned*

166   **Mandelamine® Tablets**
Each tablet contains 0.5 gram methenamine mandelate, USP.

167   **Mandelamine® Tablets**
Each tablet contains 1.0 gram methenamine mandelate, USP.

168-176   *Unassigned*

177   **Sinubid ® Tablets**
Each tablet contains 600 mg acetaminophen, 100 mg phenylpropanolamine hydrochloride, and 66 mg phenyltoloxamine citrate.

178-179   *Unassigned*

180   **Pyridium® Tablets**
Each tablet contains 100 mg phenazopyridine hydrochloride, USP.

181   **Pyridium® Tablets**
Each tablet contains 200 mg phenazopyridine hydrochloride, USP.

182   **Pyridium® Plus Tablets**
Each tablet contains 150 mg phenazopyridine hydrochloride (Pyridium®), 0.3 mg hyoscyamine hydrobromide, and 15 mg butabarbital.

183-199   *Unassigned*

200   **Brondecon® Tablets**
Each tablet contains 200 mg oxtriphylline and 100 mg guaifenesin.

201   *Unassigned*

202   **Procan® SR Tablets, 250 mg**
Each sustained-release tablet contains 250 mg procainamide hydrochloride.

203   *Unassigned*

204   **Procan® SR Tablets, 500 mg**
Each sustained-release tablet contains 500 mg procainamide hydrochloride.

205   **Procan® SR Tablets, 750 mg**
Each sustained-release tablet contains 750 mg procainamide hydrochloride.

206   *Unassigned*

207   **Procan® SR Tablets, 1000 mg**
Each sustained-release tablet contains 1000 mg procainamide hydrochloride.

208-209   *Unassigned*

210   **Choledyl® Tablets**
Each tablet contains 100 mg oxtriphylline, USP.

211   **Choledyl® Tablets**
Each tablet contains 200 mg oxtriphylline, USP.

212-213   *Unassigned*

214   **Choledyl® SA Tablets**
Each sustained-action tablet contains 400 mg oxtriphylline, USP.

215-220   *Unassigned*

221   **Choledyl® SA Tablets**
Each sustained-action tablet contains 600 mg oxtriphylline, USP.

222-230   *Unassigned*

231   **Tedral® SA Tablets**
Each sustained-action tablet contains 180 mg anhydrous theophylline (90 mg in the immediate release layer and 90 mg in the sustained-release layer); 48 mg ephedrine hydrochloride (16 mg in the immediate release layer and 32 mg in the sustained-release layer); 25 mg phenobarbital in the immediate release layer.

232-236   *Unassigned*

237   **Zarontin® Capsules**
Each capsule contains 250 mg ethosuximide, USP.

238-250   *Unassigned*

251   **Proloid® Tablets**
Each tablet contains ½ grain thyroglobulin, USP.

252   **Proloid® Tablets**
Each tablet contains 1 grain thyroglobulin, USP.

253   **Proloid® Tablets**
Each tablet contains 1½ grains thyroglobulin, USP.

254   **Proloid® Tablets**
Each tablet contains 3 grains thyroglobulin, USP.

255-256   *Unassigned*

257   **Proloid® Tablets**
Each tablet contains 2 grains thyroglobulin, USP.

258-259   *Unassigned*

260   **Euthroid®-½ Tablets**
Each tablet contains 30 mcg levothyroxine sodium (T_4), 7.5 mcg liothyronine sodium (T_3).

261   **Euthroid®-1 Tablets**
Each tablet contains 60 mcg levothyroxine sodium (T_4), 15 mcg liothyronine sodium (T_3).

262   **Euthroid®-2 Tablets**
Each tablet contains 120 mcg levothyroxine sodium (T_4), 30 mcg liothyronine sodium (T_3).

263   **Euthroid®-3 Tablets**
Each tablet contains 180 mcg levothyroxine sodium (T_4), 45 mcg liothyronine sodium (T_3).

264-269   *Unassigned*

270   **Nardil® Tablets**
Each tablet contains 15 mg phenelzine sulfate, USP.

271   ***Amitriptyline Hydrochloride Tablets**
Each tablet contains 100 mg amitriptyline hydrochloride, USP.

272   ***Amitriptyline Hydrochloride Tablets**
Each tablet contains 10 mg amitriptyline hydrochloride, USP.

273   ***Amitriptyline Hydrochloride Tablets**
Each tablet contains 25 mg amitriptyline hydrochloride, USP.

274   ***Amitriptyline Hydrochloride Tablets**
Each tablet contains 50 mg amitriptyline hydrochloride, USP.

275   ***Amitriptyline Hydrochloride Tablets**
Each tablet contains 75 mg amitriptyline hydrochloride, USP.

276   **℞ Centrax® Tablets**
Each tablet contains 10 mg prazepam.

277   *Unassigned*

278   ***Amitriptyline Hydrochloride Tablets**
Each tablet contains 150 mg amitriptyline hydrochloride, USP.

279-281   *Unassigned*

282   **Natafort® Filmseal®**
Each tablet represents vitamin A (acetate), 6,000 IU; vitamin D 400 IU; folic acid, 1 mg; vitamin B_1 (thiamine mononitrate), 3 mg; vitamin B_2 (riboflavin), 2 mg; vitamin B_6 (pyridoxine hydrochloride), 15 mg; vitamin B_{12} (cyanocobalamin), crystalline, 6 mcg; vitamin C (ascorbic acid), 120 mg; nicotinamide (niacinamide), 20 mg; vitamin E (*dl*-alpha tocopheryl acetate), 30 IU; calcium (as calcium carbonate), 350 mg; magnesium (as magnesium oxide), 100 mg; iodine (as potassium iodide), 0.15 mg; iron (as ferrous fumarate), 65 mg; zinc (as zinc oxide), 25 mg.

283-319   *Unassigned*

320   **Parsidol® Tablets**
Each tablet contains 10 mg ethopropazine hydrochloride, USP.

321   **Parsidol® Tablets**
Each tablet contains 50 mg ethopropazine hydrochloride, USP.

322-336   *Unassigned*

337   **Eldec® Kapseals®**
Each capsule represents vitamin A (acetate), (0.5 mg) 1,667 IU; vitamin C (ascorbic acid), 66.7 mg; vitamin B_1 (thiamine mononitrate), 10 mg; vitamin B_2 (riboflavin), 0.87 mg; vitamin B_6 (pyridoxine hydrochloride), 0.67 mg; nicotinamide (niacinamide), 16.7 mg; *dl*-panthenol, 10 mg; ferrous sulfate, dried, 16.7 mg; iodine (as potassium iodide), 0.05 mg; calcium carbonate, 66.7 mg; vitamin E (*dl*-alpha tocopheryl acetate), (10 mg) 10 IU; vitamin B_{12} (cyanocobalamin), 2 mcg; folic acid, 0.33 mg. The Kapseal is a Dark Blue No. 1 capsule with Light Blue opaque band.

338-361   *Unassigned*

362   **Dilantin® Kapseals®**
Each Kapseal contains 100 mg extended phenytoin sodium, USP. The Kapseal is a No. 3 capsule with Orange band. (The Orange band on White cap-

Continued on next page

This product information was prepared in August, 1989. On these and other Parke-Davis Products, information may be obtained by addressing PARKE-DAVIS, Division of Warner-Lambert Company, Morris Plains, New Jersey 07950.

Parke-Davis—Cont.

sule is a trademark registered in the US Patent Office.)

363-
364 *Unassigned*
365 Dilantin® Kapseals®
Each Kapseal contains 30 mg extended phenytoin sodium, USP. The Kapseal is a No. 4 capsule with Pink opaque band.

366-
372 *Unassigned*
373 Benadryl® Kapseals®
Each Kapseal contains 50 mg diphenhydramine hydrochloride. The Kapseal is a Pink No. 4 capsule with White opaque band. (The White band on Pink capsule is a trademark registered in the US Patent Office.)

374 *Unassigned*
375 Dilantin® with Phenobarbital (¼ grain) Kapseals®
Each Kapseal contains Dilantin (phenytoin sodium), 100 mg; phenobarbital, 16 mg (¼ grain). The Kapseal is a No. 3 capsule with Garnet band.

376-
378 *Unassigned*
379 Chloromycetin® Kapseals®
Each Kapseal contains 250 mg chloramphenicol. The Kapseal is a White opaque No. 2 capsule with Gray opaque band. (The Gray band on White capsule is a trademark registered in the US Patent Office.)

380-
392 *Unassigned*
393 Milontin® Kapseals®
Each Kapseal contains 500 mg phensuximide, USP. The Kapseal is a Light Orange No. 0 capsule with Orange band.

394-
401 *Unassigned*
402 *Ampicillin Capsules, USP, 250 mg
Each capsule contains ampicillin trihydrate equivalent to 250 mg ampicillin.
403 *Unassigned*
404 *Ampicillin Capsules, USP, 500 mg
Each capsule contains ampicillin trihydrate equivalent to 500 mg ampicillin.
405-
406 *Unassigned*
407 *Tetracycline Hydrochloride Capsules, USP, 250 mg
Each capsule contains 250 mg tetracycline hydrochloride, USP.

408-
436 *Unassigned*
437 Estrovis® Tablets
Each tablet contains 100 mcg quinestrol.

438-
439 *Unassigned*
440 *Furosemide Tablets, USP, 20 mg
Each tablet contains 20 mg furosemide, USP.
441 *Furosemide Tablets, USP, 40 mg
Each tablet contains 40 mg furosemide, USP.
442 *Furosemide Tablets, USP, 80 mg
Each tablet contains 80 mg furosemide, USP.
443 *Clonidine Hydrochloride Tablets, USP, 0.1 mg
Each tablet contains 0.1 mg clonidine hydrochloride, USP.
444 *Clonidine Hydrochloride Tablets, USP, 0.2 mg
Each tablet contains 0.2 mg clonidine hydrochloride, USP.
445 *Clonidine Hydrochloride Tablets, USP, 0.3 mg
Each tablet contains 0.3 mg clonidine hydrochloride, USP.

446-
470 *Unassigned*
471 Benadryl® Capsules
Each capsule contains 25 mg diphenhydramine hydrochloride.

472-
489 *Unassigned*
490 Easprin® Enteric Coated Tablets
Each tablet contains 15 grains (975 mg) aspirin, USP.

491-
524 *Unassigned*
525 Celontin® Kapseals®
Each Kapseal contains 300 mg methsuximide, USP. The Kapseal is a Yellow Tint No. 2 capsule with Orange band.

526-
528 *Unassigned*
529 Humatin® Capsules
Each capsule contains paromomycin sulfate, USP, equivalent to 250 mg paromomycin.
530 *Unassigned*
531 Dilantin® with Phenobarbital (½ grain) Kapseals®
Each Kapseal contains Dilantin (phenytoin sodium), 100 mg; phenobarbital, 32 mg (½ grain). The Kapseal is a No. 3 capsule with Black band.

532-
533 *Unassigned*
534 Natabec® with Fluoride Kapseals®
Each Kapseal represents vitamin A (acetate) (1.2 mg), 4,000 IU*; vitamin D (ergocalciferol) (10 mcg), 400 IU; vitamin C (ascorbic acid), 50 mg; thiamine mononitrate (vitamin B₁), 3 mg; riboflavin (vitamin B₂), 2.0 mg; nicotinamide (niacinamide), 20 mg; vitamin B₆ (pyridoxine hydrochloride), 3 mg; vitamin B₁₂, crystalline (cyanocobalamin), 5 mcg; ferrous sulfate, 150 mg; calcium carbonate, 600 mg; sodium fluoride, 2.2 mg.

*International Units
The Kapseal is a Pastel Pink No. 0 capsule with Ruby Red opaque band.

535-
536 *Unassigned*
537 Celontin® (Half Strength) Kapseals®
Each Kapseal contains 150 mg methsuximide, USP. The Kapseal is a Yellow Tint No. 4 capsule with Brown opaque band.

538-
539 *Unassigned*
540 Ponstel® Kapseals®
Each Kapseal contains 250 mg mefenamic acid. The Kapseal is an Ivory opaque No. 1 capsule with Light Blue opaque band. The blue band on ivory capsule combination is a Parke-Davis trademark.

541-
546 *Unassigned*
547 Natabec ℞® Kapseals®
Each Kapseal represents vitamin A (acetate) (1.2 mg), 4,000 IU; Vitamin D (10 mcg) 400 IU; ascorbic acid, 50 mg; thiamine mononitrate, 3 mg; riboflavin, 2 mg; pyridoxine hydrochloride, 3 mg; cyanocobalamin, 5 mcg; niacinamide, 10 mg; folic acid, 1 mg; calcium carbonate, precipitated, 600 mg; iron* 30 mg.

*Supplied as dried ferrous sulfate.
The Kapseal is a Blue opaque No. 0 capsule with Pink opaque band. The banded capsule is a Warner-Lambert trademark registered in the US Patent Office.

548-
551 *Unassigned*
552 ℂCentrax® Capsules
Each capsule contains 5 mg prazepam.
553 ℂCentrax® Capsules
Each capsule contains 10 mg prazepam.
554 ℂCentrax® Capsules
Each capsule contains 20 mg prazepam.

555-
556 *Unassigned*
557 *Verapamil Hydrochloride Tablets
Each tablet contains 80 mg verapamil hydrochloride.

558-
572 *Unassigned*
573 *Verapamil Hydrochloride Tablets
Each tablet contains 120 mg verapamil hydrochloride.

574-
606 *Unassigned*
607 *ℂPhenobarbital Tablets, USP
Each tablet contains 60 mg (1 grain) phenobarbital.

608-
617 *Unassigned*
618 Placebo tablet in Norlestrin 28 1/50.
619-
621 *Unassigned*
622 Ferrous Fumarate Tablets
Each tablet contains 75 mg ferrous fumarate, USP.

623-
633 *Unassigned*
634 *ℂAcetaminophen with Codeine Phosphate Tablets, No. 2
Each tablet contains 300 mg acetaminophen and 15 mg (¼ grain) codeine phosphate.
635 *ℂAcetaminophen with Codeine Phosphate Tablets, No. 3

Each tablet contains 300 mg acetaminophen and 30 mg (½ grain) codeine phosphate.
636 *Unassigned*
637 *ℂAcetaminophen with Codeine Phosphate Tablets, No. 4
Each tablet contains 300 mg acetaminophen and 60 mg (1 grain) codeine phosphate.
638 Tabron® Filmseal®
Each tablet represents ferrous fumarate, 304.2 mg (represents 100 mg of elemental iron); vitamin C (ascorbic acid), 500 mg; vitamin B₁ (thiamine mononitrate), 6 mg; vitamin B₂ (riboflavin), 6 mg; vitamin B₆ (pyridoxine hydrochloride), 5 mg; vitamin B₁₂ (cyanocobalamin), crystalline, 25 mcg; folic acid, 1 mg; nicotinamide (niacinamide), 30 mg; calcium pantothenate, 10 mg; vitamin E (dl-alpha tocopheryl acetate), (30 mg), 30 IU; docusate sodium, 50 mg.

639-
647 *Unassigned*
648 *Penicillin V Potassium Tablets, USP, 250 mg
Each tablet contains penicillin V potassium equivalent to 250 mg (400,000 units) penicillin V.

649-
668 *Unassigned*
669 Lopid® Capsules
Each capsule contains 300 mg gemfibrozil.

670-
671 *Unassigned*
672 *Erythromycin Stearate Filmseals
Each Filmseal® contains 250 mg erythromycin as erythromycin stearate.
673 *Penicillin V Potassium Tablets, USP, 500 mg
Each tablet contains penicillin V potassium equivalent to 500 mg (800,000 units) penicillin V.

674-
691 *Unassigned*
692 *ℂPropoxyphene Hydrochloride Capsules, USP
Each capsule contains 65 mg propoxyphene hydrochloride.

693-
695 *Unassigned*
696 ERYC® Capsules
Each capsule contains 250 mg erythromycin, USP.
697 *Tetracycline Hydrochloride Capsules, USP, 500 mg
Each capsule contains 500 mg tetracycline hydrochloride, USP.
698 *ℂPhenobarbital Tablets, USP
Each tablet contains 100 mg (1½ grains) phenobarbital.
699 *ℂPhenobarbital Tablets, USP
Each tablet contains 15 mg (¼ grain) phenobarbital.
700 *ℂPhenobarbital Tablets, USP
Each tablet contains 30 mg (½ grain) phenobarbital.

701 *Unassigned*
702 *Hydrochlorothiazide Tablets, USP
Each tablet contains 25 mg hydrochlorothiazide.

703-
709 *Unassigned*
710 *Hydrochlorothiazide Tablets, USP
Each tablet contains 50 mg hydrochlorothiazide.

711 *Unassigned*
712 *Spironolactone with Hydrochlorothiazide Tablets
Each tablet contains 25 mg spironolactone and 25 mg hydrochlorothiazide.
713 *Spironolactone Tablets, USP
Each tablet contains 25 mg spironolactone, USP.

714-
724 *Unassigned*
725 *ℂAspirin with Codeine Phosphate Tablets, No. 2
Each tablet contains codeine phosphate, ¼ grain; aspirin, 325 mg.
726 *ℂAspirin with Codeine Phosphate Tablets, No. 3
Each tablet contains codeine phosphate, ½ grain; aspirin, 325 mg.
727 *ℂAspirin with Codeine Phosphate Tablets, No. 4
Each tablet contains codeine phosphate, 1 grain; aspirin, 325 mg.

728-
729 *Unassigned*
730 *Amoxicillin Capsules 250 mg
Each capsule contains 250 mg amoxicillin.
731 *Amoxicillin Capsules 500 mg
Each capsule contains 500 mg amoxicillin.

732-
736 *Unassigned*

737 **Lopid® Tablets**
    Each tablet contains 600 mg gemfibrozil.

738-
812 *Unassigned*
813 ***Doxycycline Hyclate Tablets, USP**
    Each tablet contains 100 mg doxycycline hyclate, USP.

814-
828 *Unassigned*
829 ***Doxycycline Hyclate Capsules, USP**
    Each capsule contains 50 mg doxycycline hyclate, USP.

830 ***Doxycycline Hyclate Capsules, USP**
    Each capsule contains 100 mg doxycycline hyclate, USP.

831-
848 *Unassigned*
849 ***Quinidine Sulfate Tablets, USP**
    Each tablet contains 3 grains (200 mg) quinidine sulfate.

850 ***Quinidine Gluconate Tablets/Duraquin®**
    Each scored, white, sustained-release tablet contains 330 mg quinidine gluconate.

851-
864 *Unassigned*
865 ***Methyldopa Tablets, USP**
    Each tablet contains 250 mg methyldopa, USP.
866 ***Methyldopa Tablets, USP**
    Each tablet contains 500 mg methyldopa, USP.

867-
881 *Unassigned*
882 **Norlutin® Tablets**
    Each tablet contains 5 mg norethindrone, USP.

883-
886 *Unassigned*
887 ***Indomethacin Capsules, USP**
    Each capsule contains 25 mg indomethacin, USP.
888 ***Indomethacin Capsules, USP**
    Each capsule contains 50 mg indomethacin, USP.

889-
900 *Unassigned*
901 **Norlestrin® 2.5/50 Tablets**
    Each tablet contains norethindrone acetate, 2.5 mg; ethinyl estradiol, 50 mcg.

902-
903 *Unassigned*
904 **Norlestrin® 1/50 Tablets**
    Each tablet contains norethindrone acetate, 1 mg; ethinyl estradiol, 50 mcg.

905-
914 *Unassigned*
915 **Loestrin® 1/20 Tablets**
    Each tablet contains norethindrone acetate, 1 mg; ethinyl estradiol, 20 mcg.
916 **Loestrin® 1.5/30 Tablets**
    Each tablet contains norethindrone acetate, 1.5 mg; ethinyl estradiol, 30 mcg.

917 *Unassigned*
918 **Norlutate® Tablets**
    Each tablet contains 5 mg norethindrone acetate.
919 ***Erythromycin Stearate Filmseals**
    Each Filmseal® contains 500 mg erythromycin as erythromycin stearate.

920-
999 *Unassigned*

* Effective July 1, 1987, all Parke-Davis Generics were transferred to Warner Chilcott Laboratories, a new division of Warner-Lambert Company. Please refer to the Manufacturer' Index for a complete listing of Warner Chilcott products.

* Effective July 1, 1987, all Parke-Davis Generics were transferred to Warner Chilcott Laboratories, a new division of Warner-Lambert Company. Please refer to the Manufacturer' Index for a complete listing of Warner Chilcott products.

* Effective July 1, 1987, all Parke-Davis Generics were transferred to Warner Chilcott Laboratories, a new division of Warner-Lambert Company. Please refer to the Manufacturers' Index for a complete listing of Warner Chilcott products.

ADRENALIN® CHLORIDE SOLUTION ℞
[ă-drĕn′ă-lĭn″ chlō′rĭde]
(Epinephrine Injection, USP), 1:1000

DESCRIPTION
A sterile solution intended for subcutaneous or intramuscular injection. When diluted, it may also be administered intracardially or intravenously. Each milliliter contains 1 mg Adrenalin (epinephrine) as the hydrochloride dissolved in Water for Injection, USP, with sodium chloride added for isotonicity. The ampoules contain not more than 0.1% so-

dium bisulfite as an antioxidant, and the air in the ampoule has been displaced by nitrogen. The Steri-Vials® contain 0.5% Chloretone® (chlorobutanol) (chloroform derivative) as a preservative and not more than 0.15% sodium bisulfite as an antioxidant. Epinephrine is the active principle of the adrenal medulla, chemically described as (−)-3,4-Dihydroxy-α-[(methylamino) methyl] benzyl alcohol.

CLINICAL PHARMACOLOGY
Adrenalin (epinephrine) is a sympathomimetic drug. It activates an adrenergic receptive mechanism on effector cells and imitates all actions of the sympathetic nervous system except those on the arteries of the face and sweat glands. Epinephrine acts on both alpha and beta receptors and is the most potent alpha receptor activator.

INDICATIONS AND USAGE
In general, the most common uses of epinephrine are to relieve respiratory distress due to bronchospasm, to provide rapid relief of hypersensitivity reactions to drugs and other allergens, and to prolong the action of infiltration anesthetics. Its cardiac effects may be of use in restoring cardiac rhythm in cardiac arrest due to various causes, but it is not used in cardiac failure or in hemorrhagic, traumatic, or cardiogenic shock.

Epinephrine is used as a hemostatic agent. It is also used in treating mucosal congestion of hay fever, rhinitis, and acute sinusitis; to relieve bronchial asthmatic paroxysms; in syncope due to complete heart block or carotid sinus hypersensitivity; for symptomatic relief of serum sickness, urticaria, angioneurotic edema; for resuscitation in cardiac arrest following anesthetic accidents; in simple (open angle) glaucoma; for relaxation of uterine musculature and to inhibit uterine contractions. Epinephrine Injection can be utilized to prolong the action of intraspinal and local anesthetics (see Contraindications).

CONTRAINDICATIONS
Epinephrine is contraindicated in narrow angle (congestive) glaucoma, shock, during general anesthesia with halogenated hydrocarbons or cyclopropane and in individuals with organic brain damage. Epinephrine is also contraindicated with local anesthesia of certain areas, eg, fingers, toes, because of the danger of vasoconstriction producing sloughing of tissue; in labor because it may delay the second stage; in cardiac dilatation and coronary insufficiency.

WARNINGS
Administer with caution to elderly people; to those with cardiovascular disease, hypertension, diabetes or hyperthyroidism; in psychoneurotic individuals, and in pregnancy.
Patients with long-standing bronchial asthma and emphysema who have developed degenerative heart disease should be administered the drug with extreme caution.
Overdosage or inadvertent intravenous injection of epinephrine may cause cerebrovascular hemorrhage resulting from the sharp rise in blood pressure.
Fatalities may also result from pulmonary edema because of the peripheral constriction and cardiac stimulation produced. Rapidly acting vasodilators such as nitrites, or alpha blocking agents may counteract the marked pressor effects of epinephrine.
Epinephrine is the preferred treatment for serious allergic or other emergency situations even though this product contains sodium bisulfite, a sulfite that may in other products cause allergic-type reactions including anaphylactic symptoms or life-threatening or less severe asthmatic episodes in certain susceptible persons. The alternatives to using epinephrine in a life-threatening situation may not be satisfactory. The presence of a sulfite in this product should not deter administration of the drug for treatment of serious allergic or other emergency situations.

PRECAUTIONS
General: Adrenalin (epinephrine injection) should be protected from exposure to light. Do not remove ampoules or syringes from carton until ready to use. The solution should not be used if it is brown in color or contains a precipitate. Epinephrine is readily destroyed by alkalies and oxidizing agents. In the latter category are oxygen, chlorine, bromine, iodine, permanganates, chromates, nitrites and salts of easily reducible metals, especially iron.
Drug Interactions: Use of epinephrine with excessive doses of digitalis, mercurial diuretics, or other drugs that sensitize the heart to arrhythmias is not recommended. Anginal pain may be induced when coronary insufficiency is present.
The effects of epinephrine may be potentiated by tricyclic antidepressants; certain antihistamines, eg, diphenhydramine, tripelennamine, d-chlorpheniramine; and sodium l-thyroxine.
Usage in Pregnancy: Pregnancy Category C. Adrenalin (epinephrine) has been shown to be teratogenic in rats when given in doses about 25 times the human dose. There are no adequate and well controlled studies in pregnant women. Adrenalin should be used during pregnancy only if the potential benefit justifies the potential risk to the fetus.

ADVERSE REACTIONS
Transient and minor side effects of anxiety, headache, fear and palpitations often occur with therapeutic doses, especially in hyperthyroid individuals. Repeated local injections can result in necrosis at sites of injection from vascular constriction. "Epinephrine-fastness" can occur with prolonged use.

DOSAGE AND ADMINISTRATION
Subcutaneously or intramuscularly—0.2 to 1 ml (mg). Start with a small dose and increase if required.
Note: The subcutaneous is the preferred route of administration. If given intramuscularly, injection into the buttocks should be avoided.
For bronchial asthma and certain allergic manifestations, eg, angioedema, urticaria, serum sickness, anaphylactic shock, use epinephrine subcutaneously. For bronchial asthma in pediatric patients, administer 0.01 mg/kg or 0.3 mg/m^2 to a maximum of 0.5 mg subcutaneously, repeated every four hours if required.
For cardiac resuscitation—A dose of 0.5 ml (0.5 mg) diluted to 10 ml with sodium chloride injection can be administered intravenously or intracardially to restore myocardial contractility. External cardiac massage should follow intracardial administration to permit the drug to enter coronary circulation. The drug should be used secondarily to unsuccessful attempts with physical or electromechanical methods.
Ophthalmologic use (for producing conjunctival decongestion, to control hemorrhage, produce mydriasis and reduce intraocular pressure)—use a concentration of 1:10,000 (0.1 mg/ml) to 1:1,000 (1 mg/ml).
Intraspinal use (Amp 88)—Usual dose is 0.2 to 0.4 ml (0.2 to 0.4 mg) added to anesthetic spinal fluid mixture (may prolong anesthetic action by limiting absorption). For use with local anesthetic—Epinephrine 1:100,000 (0.01 mg /ml) to 1:20,000 (0.05 mg/ml) is the usual concentration employed with local anesthetics.

HOW SUPPLIED
N 0071-4188-03 (Amp 88) Sterile solution containing 1 mg Adrenalin (epinephrine) as the hydrochloride in each 1-ml ampoule (1:1000). For intramuscular or subcutaneous use. When diluted, it may also be administered intracardially, intravenously, or intraspinally. Supplied in packages of ten.
N 0071-4011-13 (S.V. 11) Sterile solution containing 1 mg Adrenalin (epinephrine) as the hydrochloride (1:1000). For intramuscular or subcutaneous use. When diluted, it may also be administered intracardially or intravenously. Supplied in a 30 ml Steri-Vial® (rubber-diaphragm-capped vial.)
4188G041

ANUSOL-HC® ℞
[ăn′ū-sŏl″]
(Hydrocortisone Acetate Cream, USP) 1%

Caution—Federal law prohibits dispensing without prescription.

DESCRIPTION
The topical corticosteroids constitute a class of primarily synthetic steroids used as anti-inflammatory and anti-pruritic agents. Anusol-HC® (Hydrocortisone Acetate Cream, USP) 1% is a topical corticosteroid with micronized hydrocortisone acetate 1% (active ingredient) in a buffered, water-washable cream containing the following inactive ingredients: citric acid, USP; glyceryl stearate; imidurea, NF; methylparaben, NF; mineral oil, USP; PEG-100 stearate; polysorbate 60, NF; propylene glycol, USP; propylparaben, NF; purified water, USP; sodium citrate, USP hydrous, sorbitan monostearate, NF; and white petrolatum, USP. Hydrocortisone acetate has the chemical name Pregn-4-ene-3,20-dione, 21-(acetyloxy)-11, 17-dihydroxy-, (11β).

CLINICAL PHARMACOLOGY
Topical corticosteroids share anti-inflammatory, anti-pruritic and vasoconstrictive actions.
The mechanism of anti-inflammatory activity of the topical corticosteroids is unclear. Various laboratory methods, including vasoconstrictor assays, are used to compare and predict potencies and/or clinical efficacies of the topical corticosteroids. There is some evidence to suggest that a recognizable correlation exists between vasoconstrictor potency and therapeutic efficacy in man.
Pharmacokinetics: The extent of percutaneous absorption of topical corticosteroids is determined by many factors in-

Continued on next page

This product information was prepared in August, 1989. On these and other Parke-Davis Products, information may be obtained by addressing PARKE-DAVIS, Division of Warner-Lambert Company, Morris Plains, New Jersey 07950.

Parke-Davis—Cont.

cluding the vehicle, the integrity of the epidermal barrier, and the use of occlusive dressings.

Topical corticosteroids can be absorbed from normal intact skin. Inflammation and/or other disease processes in the skin increase percutaneous absorption. Occlusive dressings substantially increase the percutaneous absorption of topical corticosteroids. Thus, occlusive dressings may be a valuable therapeutic adjunct for treatment of resistant dermatoses (see DOSAGE AND ADMINISTRATION).

Once absorbed through the skin, topical corticosteroids are handled through pharmacokinetic pathways similar to systemically administered corticosteroids. Corticosteroids are bound to plasma proteins in varying degrees. Corticosteroids are metabolized primarily in the liver and are then excreted by the kidneys. Some of the topical corticosteroids and their metabolites are also excreted into the bile.

INDICATIONS AND USAGE

Topical corticosteroids are indicated for the relief of the inflammatory and pruritic manifestations of corticosteroid-responsive dermatoses.

CONTRAINDICATIONS

Topical corticosteroids are contraindicated in those patients with a history of hypersensitivity to any of the components of the preparation.

PRECAUTIONS

General: Systemic absorption of topical corticosteroids has produced reversible hypothalamic-pituitary-adrenal (HPA) axis suppression, manifestations of Cushing's syndrome, hyperglycemia, and glucosuria in some patients.

Conditions which augment systemic absorption include the application of the more potent steroids, use over large surface areas, prolonged use, and the addition of occlusive dressings.

Therefore, patients receiving a large dose of a potent topical steroid applied to a large surface area or under an occlusive dressing should be evaluated periodically for evidence of HPA axis suppression by using the urinary free cortisol and ACTH stimulation tests. If HPA axis suppression is noted, an attempt should be made to withdraw the drug, to reduce the frequency of application, or to substitute a less potent steroid.

Recovery of HPA axis function is generally prompt and complete upon discontinuation of the drug. Infrequently, signs and symptoms of steroid withdrawal may occur, requiring supplemental systemic corticosteroids.

Children may absorb proportionally larger amounts of topical corticosteroids and thus be more susceptible to systemic toxicity (see PRECAUTIONS—Pediatric Use).

If irritation develops, topical corticosteroids should be discontinued and appropriate therapy instituted. In the presence of dermatological infections, the use of an appropriate antifungal or antibacterial agent should be instituted. If a favorable response does not occur promptly, the corticosteroid should be discontinued until the infection has been adequately controlled.

Information for the Patient: Patients using topical corticosteroids should receive the following information and instructions:

1. This medication is to be used as directed by the physician. It is for external use only. Avoid contact with the eyes.
2. Patients should be advised not to use this medication for any disorder other than for which it has been prescribed.
3. The treated skin area should not be bandaged or otherwise covered or wrapped as to be occlusive unless directed by the physician.
4. Patients should report any signs of local adverse reactions especially under occlusive dressing.
5. Parents of pediatric patients should be advised not to use tight-fitting diapers or plastic pants on a child being treated in the diaper area, as these garments may constitute occlusive dressings.

Laboratory Tests: The following tests may be helpful in evaluating the HPA axis suppression:

    Urinary free cortisol test
    ACTH stimulation test

Carcinogenesis, Mutagenesis, and Impairment of Fertility: Long-term animal studies have not been performed to evaluate the carcinogenic potential or the effect on fertility of topical corticosteroids. Studies to determine mutagenicity with prednisolone and hydrocortisone have revealed negative results.

Pregnancy Category C: Corticosteroids are generally teratogenic in laboratory animals when administered systemically at relatively low dosage levels. The more potent corticosteroids have been shown to be teratogenic after dermal application in laboratory animals. There are no adequate and well-controlled studies in pregnant women on teratogenic effects from topically applied corticosteroids.

Therefore, topical corticosteroids should be used during pregnancy only if the potential benefit justifies the potential risk to the fetus. Drugs of this class should not be used exten-

sively on pregnant patients, in large amounts, or for prolonged periods of time.

Nursing Mothers: It is not known whether topical administration of corticosteroids could result in sufficient systemic absorption to produce detectable quantities in breast milk. Systemically administered corticosteroids are secreted into breast milk in quantities not likely to have a deleterious effect on the infant. Nevertheless, caution should be exercised when topical corticosteroids are administered to a nursing woman.

Pediatric Use: PEDIATRIC PATIENTS MAY DEMONSTRATE GREATER SUSCEPTIBILITY TO TOPICAL CORTICOSTEROID-INDUCED HPA AXIS SUPPRESSION AND CUSHING'S SYNDROME THAN MATURE PATIENTS BECAUSE OF A LARGER SKIN SURFACE AREA IN BODY WEIGHT RATIO.

Hypothalamic-pituitary-adrenal (HPA) axis suppression, Cushing's syndrome, and intracranial hypertension have been reported in children receiving topical corticosteroids. Manifestations of adrenal suppression in children include linear growth retardation, delayed weight gain, low plasma cortisol levels, and absence of response to ACTH stimulation. Manifestations of intracranial hypertension include bulging fontanelles, headaches, and bilateral papilledema.

Administration of topical corticosteroids to children should be limited to the least amount compatible with an effective therapeutic regimen. Chronic corticosteroid therapy may interfere with the growth and development of children.

ADVERSE REACTIONS

The following local adverse reactions are reported infrequently with topical corticosteroids, but may occur more frequently with the use of occlusive dressings. These reactions are listed in an approximate decreasing order of occurrence:

Burning
Itching
Irritation
Dryness
Folliculitis
Hypertrichosis
Acneiform eruptions
Hypopigmentation
Perioral dermatitis
Allergic contact dermatitis
Maceration of the skin
Secondary infection
Skin atrophy
Striae
Miliaria

OVERDOSAGE

Topically applied corticosteroids can be absorbed in sufficient amounts to produce systemic effects. (See PRECAUTIONS).

DOSAGE AND ADMINISTRATION

Topical corticosteroids are generally applied to the affected area as a thin film from two to four times daily depending on the severity of the condition.

Occlusive dressings may be used for the management of psoriasis or recalcitrant conditions. If an infection develops, the use of occlusive dressings should be discontinued and appropriate antimicrobial therapy instituted.

HOW SUPPLIED

Anusol-HC® (Hydrocortisone Acetate Cream, USP) 1% is supplied in one-ounce tubes (N-0071-3124-13).

Store at controlled room temperature 15°–30°C (59°–86°F).

3124G010

Shown in Product Identification Section, page 421

ANUSOL-HC® 25-mg SUPPOSITORIES   ℞
[ăn ′ū-sŏl ″]
(Hydrocortisone Acetate)

DESCRIPTION

Each Anusol-HC 25-mg Suppository contains 25 mg hydrocortisone acetate in a hydrogenated cocoglyceride base. Hydrocortisone acetate is a corticosteroid. Chemically, hydrocortisone acetate is pregn-4-ene-3, 20-dione, 21-(acetyloxy)-11, 17-dihydroxy-, (11β)-.

CLINICAL PHARMACOLOGY

In normal subjects, about 26 percent of hydrocortisone acetate is absorbed when the hydrocortisone acetate suppository is applied to the rectum. Absorption of hydrocortisone acetate may vary across abraded or inflamed surfaces.

Topical steroids are primarily effective because of their anti-inflammatory, antipruritic and vasoconstrictive action.

INDICATIONS AND USAGE

For use in inflamed hemorrhoids, post irradiation (factitial) proctitis, as an adjunct in the treatment of chronic ulcerative colitis, cryptitis, other inflammatory conditions of the anorectum, and pruritus ani.

CONTRAINDICATION

Anusol-HC suppositories are contraindicated in those patients with a history of hypersensitivity to any of the components.

PRECAUTIONS

Do not use unless adequate proctologic examination is made. If irritation develops, the product should be discontinued and appropriate therapy instituted.

In the presence of an infection, the use of an appropriate antifungal or antibacterial agent should be instituted. If a favorable response does not occur promptly, the corticosteroid should be discontinued until the infection has been adequately controlled.

No long-term studies in animals have been performed to evaluate the carcinogenic potential of corticosteroid suppositories.

Pregnancy Category C

In laboratory animals, topical steroids have been associated with an increase in the incidence of fetal abnormalities when gestating females have been exposed to rather low dosage levels. There are no adequate and well-controlled studies in pregnant women. Anusol-HC suppositories should only be used during pregnancy if the potential benefit justifies the risk to the fetus. Drugs of this class should not be used extensively on pregnant patients, in large amounts, or for prolonged periods of time.

It is not known whether this drug is excreted in human milk, and because many drugs are excreted in human milk and because of the potential for serious adverse reactions in nursing infants from Anusol-HC suppositories, a decision should be made whether to discontinue nursing or to discontinue the drug, taking into account the importance of the drug to the mother.

ADVERSE REACTIONS

The following local adverse reactions have been reported with corticosteroid suppositories:

1. Burning
2. Itching
3. Irritation
4. Dryness
5. Folliculitis
6. Hypopigmentation
7. Allergic Contact Dermatitis
8. Secondary infection

DRUG ABUSE AND DEPENDENCE

Drug abuse and dependence have not been reported in patients treated with Anusol-HC suppositories.

OVERDOSAGE

If signs and symptoms of systemic overdosage occur discontinue use.

DOSAGE AND ADMINISTRATION

Usual dosage: One suppository in the rectum morning and night for two weeks, in nonspecific proctitis. In more severe cases, one suppository three times daily; or two suppositories twice daily. In factitial proctitis, recommended therapy is six to eight weeks or less, according to response.

HOW SUPPLIED

Anusol-HC 25-mg Suppositories are off-white, smooth surfaced, rod shaped with one rounded end. Package of 12 suppositories (N-0071-1726-07) and package of 24 suppositories (N-0071-1726-13).

Store below 30° C (86° F). Protect from freezing.

Caution—Federal law prohibits dispensing without prescription.

1726G010

Shown in Product Identification Section, page 421

APLISOL®   ℞
[ă ′plĭ-sŏl ″]
(tuberculin purified protein
derivative, diluted
[Stabilized Solution])

For complete product information, consult Diagnostic Products Information Section.

APLITEST®   ℞
[ă ′plĭ-tĕst ″]
(tuberculin purified protein
derivative)
Multiple-Puncture Device

For complete product information, consult Diagnostic Products Information Section.

BENADRYL® ℞
[bĕ'nă-dril]
(Diphenhydramine Hydrochloride Capsules, USP)

DESCRIPTION

Benadryl (diphenhydramine hydrochloride) is an antihistamine drug having the chemical name 2-(Diphenylmethoxy)-N, N-dimethylethylamine hydrochloride and has the empirical formula $C_{17}H_{21}NO \cdot HCl$ (molecular weight 291.82). It occurs as a white, crystalline powder and is freely soluble in water and alcohol.

Each Benadryl capsule contains 25 mg or 50 mg diphenhydramine hydrochloride for oral administration.

The 25-mg capsule also contains lactose, NF and magnesium stearate, NF. The capsule shell and/or band contains D&C red No. 28; FD&C blue No. 1; FD&C red No. 3; FD&C red No. 40; gelatin, NF; colloidal silicon dioxide, NF; and sodium lauryl sulfate, NF.

The 50-mg capsule also contains confectioner's sugar, NF and talc, USP. The capsule shell and/or band contains FD&C blue No. 1; FD&C red No. 3; gelatin, NF; glyceryl monooleate; colloidal silicon dioxide, NF; sodium bisulfite, NF; sodium lauryl sulfate, NF; and titanium dioxide, USP.

CLINICAL PHARMACOLOGY

Diphenhydramine hydrochloride is an antihistamine with anticholinergic (drying) and sedative effects. Antihistamines appear to compete with histamine for cell receptor sites on effector cells.

A single oral dose of diphenhydramine hydrochloride is quickly absorbed with maximum activity occurring in approximately one hour. The duration of activity following an average dose of Benadryl is from four to six hours. Diphenhydramine is widely distributed throughout the body, including the CNS. Little, if any, is excreted unchanged in the urine; most appears as the degradation products of metabolic transformation in the liver, which are almost completely excreted within 24 hours.

INDICATIONS AND USAGE

Benadryl in the oral form is effective for the following indications:

Antihistaminic: For allergic conjunctivitis due to foods; mild, uncomplicated allergic skin manifestations of urticaria and angioedema; amelioration of allergic reactions to blood or plasma; dermatographism; as therapy for anaphylactic reactions *adjunctive* to epinephrine and other standard measures after the acute manifestations have been controlled.

Motion sickness: For active and prophylactic treatment of motion sickness.

Antiparkinsonism: For parkinsonism (including drug-induced) in the elderly unable to tolerate more potent agents; mild cases of parkinsonism (including drug-induced) in other age groups; in other cases of parkinsonism (including drug-induced) in combination with centrally acting anticholinergic agents.

CONTRAINDICATIONS

Use in Newborn or Premature Infants
This drug should *not* be used in newborn or premature infants.

Use in Nursing Mothers
Because of the higher risk of antihistamines for infants generally, and for newborns and prematures in particular, antihistamine therapy is contraindicated in nursing mothers. Antihistamines are also contraindicated in the following conditions:

Hypersensitivity to diphenhydramine hydrochloride and other antihistamines of similar chemical structure.

WARNINGS

Antihistamines should be used with considerable caution in patients with narrow-angle glaucoma, stenosing peptic ulcer, pyloroduodenal obstruction, symptomatic prostatic hypertrophy, or bladder-neck obstruction.

Use in Children
In infants and children, especially, antihistamines in *overdosage* may cause hallucinations, convulsions, or death.

As in adults, antihistamines may diminish mental alertness in children. In the young child, particularly, they may produce excitation.

Use in the Elderly (approximately 60 years or older).
Antihistamines are more likely to cause dizziness, sedation, and hypotension in elderly patients.

PRECAUTIONS

General: Diphenhydramine hydrochloride has an atropine-like action and therefore should be used with caution in patients with a history of bronchial asthma, increased intraocular pressure, hyperthyroidism, cardiovascular disease or hypertension.

Information for Patients: Patients taking diphenhydramine hydrochloride should be advised that this drug may cause drowsiness and has an additive effect with alcohol.

Patients should be warned about engaging in activities requiring mental alertness such as driving a car or operating appliances, machinery, etc.

Drug Interactions: Diphenhydramine hydrochloride has additive effects with alcohol and other CNS depressants (hypnotics, sedatives, tranquilizers, etc).

CAUTION—Patients taking monoamine oxidase inhibitors should not receive antihistamine therapy concurrently. MAO inhibitors prolong and intensify the anticholinergic (drying) effects of antihistamines.

Carcinogenesis, Mutagenesis, Impairment of Fertility: Long-term studies in animals to determine mutagenic and carcinogenic potential have not been performed.

Pregnancy: Pregnancy Category B. Reproduction studies have been performed in rats and rabbits at doses up to 5 times the human dose and have revealed no evidence of impaired fertility or harm to the fetus due to diphenhydramine hydrochloride. There are, however, no adequate and well-controlled studies in pregnant women. Because animal reproduction studies are not always predictive of human response, this drug should be used during pregnancy only if clearly needed.

ADVERSE REACTIONS

The most frequent adverse reactions are underscored.
1. *General:* Urticaria, drug rash, anaphylactic shock, photosensitivity, excessive perspiration, chills, dryness of mouth, nose, and throat.
2. *Cardiovascular System:* Hypotension, headache, palpitations, tachycardia, extrasystoles.
3. *Hematologic System:* Hemolytic anemia, thrombocytopenia, agranulocytosis.
4. *Nervous System:* <u>Sedation, sleepiness, dizziness, disturbed coordination</u>, fatigue, confusion, restlessness, excitation, nervousness, tremor, irritability, insomnia, euphoria, paresthesia, blurred vision, diplopia, vertigo, tinnitus, acute labyrinthitis, neuritis, convulsions.
5. *GI System:* <u>Epigastric distress</u>, anorexia, nausea, vomiting, diarrhea, constipation.
6. *GU System:* Urinary frequency, difficult urination, urinary retention, early menses.
7. *Respiratory System:* <u>Thickening of bronchial secretions</u>, tightness of chest and wheezing, nasal stuffiness.

OVERDOSAGE

Antihistamine overdosage reactions may vary from central nervous system depression to stimulation. Stimulation is particularly likely in children. Atropine-like signs and symptoms, dry mouth; fixed, dilated pupils; flushing, and gastrointestinal symptoms may also occur.

If vomiting has not occurred spontaneously the patient should be induced to vomit. This is best done by having him drink a glass of water or milk after which he should be made to gag. Precautions against aspiration must be taken, especially in infants and children.

If vomiting is unsuccessful gastric lavage is indicated within 3 hours after ingestion and even later if large amounts of milk or cream were given beforehand. Isotonic or ½ isotonic saline is the lavage solution of choice.

Saline cathartics, as milk of magnesia, by osmosis draw water into the bowel and therefore are valuable for their action in rapid dilution of food content.

Stimulants should not be used.

Vasopressors may be used to treat hypotension.

DOSAGE AND ADMINISTRATION

DOSAGE SHOULD BE INDIVIDUALIZED ACCORDING TO THE NEEDS AND THE RESPONSE OF THE PATIENT.

A single oral dose of diphenhydramine hydrochloride is quickly absorbed with maximum activity occurring in approximately one hour. The duration of activity following an average dose of Benadryl is from four to six hours.

ADULTS: 25 to 50 mg three or four times daily. The nighttime sleep-aid dosage is 50 mg at bedtime.

CHILDREN: (over 20 lb): 12.5 to 25 mg three to four times daily. Maximum daily dosage not to exceed 300 mg. For physicians who wish to calculate the dose on the basis of body weight or surface area, the recommended dosage is 5 mg/kg/24 hours or 150 mg/m²/24 hours.

Data are not available on the use of diphenhydramine hydrochloride as a nighttime sleep-aid in children under 12 years. The basis for determining the most effective dosage regimen will be the response of the patient to medication and the condition under treatment.

In motion sickness, full dosage is recommended for prophylactic use, the first dose to be given 30 minutes before exposure to motion and similar doses before meals and upon retiring for the duration of exposure.

HOW SUPPLIED

Benadryl 50 mg (P-D 373)—each banded capsule (Kapseals®) contains 50 mg diphenhydramine hydrochloride. Available as a pink capsule with white band in bottles of 100 (N 0071-0373-24), 1000 (N 0071-0373-32), and unit dose 100 (N 0071-0373-40).

Benadryl 25 mg (P-D 471)—each capsule contains 25 mg diphenhydramine hydrochloride. Available as a pink/white capsule in bottles of 100 (N 0071-0471-24), 1000 (N 0071-0471-32), and unit dose 100 (N 0071-0471-40).

Storage Conditions:
Store at controlled room temperature 15°–30°C (59°–86°F). Protect from moisture.

Caution—Federal law prohibits dispensing without prescription.

Shown in Product Identification Section, page 421
0373G214

BENADRYL® ℞
[bĕ'nă-dril]
(Diphenhydramine Hydrochloride Injection, USP)

DESCRIPTION

Benadryl (diphenhydramine hydrochloride) is an antihistamine drug having the chemical name 2-(Diphenylmethoxy)-N, N-dimethylethylamine hydrochloride. It occurs as a white crystalline powder, is freely soluble in water and alcohol and has a molecular weight of 291.82. The molecular formula is $C_{17}H_{21}NO \cdot HCl$.

Benadryl in the parenteral form is a sterile, pyrogen-free solution available in two concentrations: 10 mg and 50 mg of diphenhydramine hydrochloride per mL. The solutions for parenteral use have been adjusted to a pH between 5.0 and 6.0 with either sodium hydroxide or hydrochloric acid. The multidose Steri-Vials® contain 0.1 mg/mL benzethonium chloride as a germicidal agent.

CLINICAL PHARMACOLOGY

Diphenhydramine hydrochloride is an antihistamine with anticholinergic (drying) and sedative side effects. Antihistamines appear to compete with histamine for cell receptor sites on effector cells.

Benadryl in the injectable form has a rapid onset of action. Diphenhydramine hydrochloride is widely distributed throughout the body, including the CNS. A portion of the drug is excreted unchanged in the urine, while the rest is metabolized via the liver. Detailed information on the pharmacokinetics of Diphenhydramine Hydrochloride Injection is not available.

INDICATIONS AND USAGE

Benadryl in the injectable form is effective for the following conditions when Benadryl in the oral form is impractical.

Antihistaminic: For amelioration of allergic reactions to blood or plasma, in anaphylaxis as an adjunct to epinephrine and other standard measures after the acute symptoms have been controlled, and for other uncomplicated allergic conditions of the immediate type when oral therapy is impossible or contraindicated.

Motion Sickness: For active treatment of motion sickness.

Antiparkinsonism: For use in parkinsonism, when oral therapy is impossible or contraindicated, as follows: parkinsonism in the elderly who are unable to tolerate more potent agents, mild cases of parkinsonism in other age groups, and in other cases of parkinsonism in combination with centrally acting anticholinergic agents.

CONTRAINDICATIONS

Use in Newborn or Premature Infants
This drug should *not* be used in newborn or premature infants.

Use in Nursing Mothers
Because of the higher risk of antihistamines for infants generally, and for newborns and prematures in particular, antihistamine therapy is contraindicated in nursing mothers.

Antihistamines are also contraindicated in the following conditions:
Hypersensitivity to diphenhydramine hydrochloride and other antihistamines of similar chemical structure.

WARNINGS

Antihistamines should be used with considerable caution in patients with narrow-angle glaucoma, stenosing peptic ulcer, pyloroduodenal obstruction, symptomatic prostatic hypertrophy, or bladder-neck obstruction.

Use in Children
In infants and children, especially, antihistamines in *overdosage* may cause hallucinations, convulsions, or death.

As in adults, antihistamines may diminish mental alertness in children. In the young child, particularly, they may produce excitation.

Use in the Elderly (approximately 60 years or older)
Antihistamines are more likely to cause dizziness, sedation, and hypotension in elderly patients.

Continued on next page

This product information was prepared in August, 1989. On these and other Parke-Davis Products, information may be obtained by addressing PARKE-DAVIS, Division of Warner-Lambert Company, Morris Plains, New Jersey 07950.

Parke-Davis—Cont.

PRECAUTIONS

General: Diphenhydramine hydrochloride has an atropine-like action and therefore should be used with caution in patients with a history of bronchial asthma, increased intraocular pressure, hyperthyroidism, cardiovascular disease or hypertension. Use with caution in patients with lower respiratory disease, including asthma.

Information for Patients: Patients taking diphenhydramine hydrochloride should be advised that this drug may cause drowsiness and has an additive effect with alcohol. Patients should be warned about engaging in activities requiring mental alertness such as driving a car or operating appliances, machinery, etc.

Drug Interactions: Diphenhydramine hydrochloride has additive effects with alcohol and other CNS depressants (hypnotics, sedatives, tranquilizers, etc).

MAO inhibitors prolong and intensify the anticholinergic (drying) effects of antihistamines.

Carcinogenesis, Mutagenesis, Impairment of Fertility: Long-term studies in animals to determine mutagenic and carcinogenic potential have not been performed.

Pregnancy: Pregnancy Category B. Reproduction studies have been performed in rats and rabbits at doses up to 5 times the human dose and have revealed no evidence of impaired fertility or harm to the fetus due to diphenhydramine hydrochloride. There are, however, no adequate and well-controlled studies in pregnant women. Because animal reproduction studies are not always predictive of human response, this drug should be used during pregnancy only if clearly needed.

ADVERSE REACTIONS

The most frequent adverse reactions are underscored.

1. *General:* Urticaria, drug rash, anaphylactic shock, photosensitivity, excessive perspiration, chills, dryness of mouth, nose, and throat
2. *Cardiovascular System:* Hypotension, headache, palpitations, tachycardia, extrasystoles
3. *Hematologic System:* Hemolytic anemia, thrombocytopenia, agranulocytosis
4. *Nervous System:* Sedation, sleepiness, dizziness, disturbed coordination, fatigue, confusion, restlessness, excitation, nervousness, tremor, irritability, insomnia, euphoria, paresthesia, blurred vision, diplopia, vertigo, tinnitus, acute labyrinthitis, neuritis, convulsions
5. *GI System:* Epigastric distress, anorexia, nausea, vomiting, diarrhea, constipation
6. *GU System:* Urinary frequency, difficult urination, urinary retention, early menses
7. *Respiratory System:* Thickening of bronchial secretions, tightness of chest and wheezing, nasal stuffiness

OVERDOSAGE

Antihistamine overdosage reactions may vary from central nervous system depression to stimulation. Stimulation is particularly likely in children. Atropine-like signs and symptoms, dry mouth; fixed, dilated pupils; flushing, and gastrointestinal symptoms may also occur.

Stimulants should not be used.

Vasopressors may be used to treat hypotension.

DOSAGE AND ADMINISTRATION

Benadryl in the injectable form is indicated when the oral form is impractical.

Parenteral drug products should be inspected visually for particulate matter and discoloration prior to administration, whenever solution and container permit.

DOSAGE SHOULD BE INDIVIDUALIZED ACCORDING TO THE NEEDS AND THE RESPONSE OF THE PATIENT.

Children: 5 mg/kg/24 hr or 150 mg/m²/24 hr. Maximum daily dosage is 300 mg. Divide into four doses, administered intravenously or deeply intramuscularly.

Adults: 10 to 50 mg intravenously or deeply intramuscularly; 100 mg if required; maximum daily dosage is 400 mg.

HOW SUPPLIED

Benadryl in parenteral form is supplied as:

Benadryl Steri-Vials®—sterile, pyrogen-free solution containing 10 mg diphenhydramine hydrochloride in each milliliter of solution with 0.1 mg/mL benzethonium chloride as a germicidal agent. Available in 10-mL (N 0071-4015-10) and 30-mL (N 0071-4015-13) Steri-Vials (rubber-diaphragm-capped vials).

Sterile, pyrogen-free solution containing 50 mg diphenhydramine hydrochloride in each milliliter of solution with 0.1 mg/mL benzethonium chloride as a germicidal agent. Available in 10-mL (N-0071-4402-10) Steri-Vials.

Benadryl Steri-Dose®—sterile, pyrogen-free solution containing 50 mg diphenhydramine hydrochloride in a 1-mL disposable syringe (Steri-Dose). Available in packages of ten individually cartoned syringes (N 0071-4259-40) and in packages of two trays of 5 syringes (N 0071-4259-41).

Benadryl Ampoule—sterile, pyrogen-free solution containing 50 mg diphenhydramine hydrochloride in a 1-mL ampoule. Available in packages of ten (N 0071-4259-03).

STORAGE CONDITIONS

Store at controlled room temperature 15°–30°C (59°–86°F). Protect from freezing and light.

Caution—Federal law prohibits dispensing without prescription.

4259G013

CELONTIN® KAPSEALS®   ℞

[cĕ″lŏn'tĭn]

(methsuximide capsules, USP)

DESCRIPTION

Celontin (methsuximide) is an anticonvulsant succinimide, chemically designated as N,2-Dimethyl-2-phenylsuccinimide.

Each Celontin capsule contains 150 mg or 300 mg methsuximide, USP. Also contains starch, NF. The capsule and band contain citric acid, USP; colloidal silicon dioxide, NF; D&C yellow No. 10; FD&C red No. 3; FD&C yellow No. 6 (Sunset Yellow); gelatin, NF; glyceryl monooleate; sodium benzoate, NF; sodium lauryl sulfate NF. The 150-mg capsule and band also contain FD&C blue No. 1; titanium dioxide, USP. The 300-mg capsule and band also contain polyethylene glycol 200.

ACTION

Methsuximide suppresses the paroxysmal three-cycle-per-second spike and wave activity associated with lapses of consciousness which is common in absence (petit mal) seizures. The frequency of epileptiform attacks is reduced, apparently by depression of the motor cortex and elevation of the threshold of the central nervous system to convulsive stimuli.

INDICATION

Celontin is indicated for the control of absence (petit mal) seizures that are refractory to other drugs.

CONTRAINDICATION

Methsuximide should not be used in patients with a history of hypersensitivity to succinimides.

WARNINGS

Blood dyscrasias, including some with fatal outcome, have been reported to be associated with the use of succinimides; therefore, periodic blood counts should be performed.

It has been reported that succinimides have produced morphological and functional changes in animal liver. For this reason, methsuximide should be administered with extreme caution to patients with known liver or renal disease. Periodic urinalysis and liver function studies are advised for all patients receiving the drug.

Cases of systemic lupus erythematosus have been reported with the use of succinimides. The physician should be alert to this possibility.

USAGE IN PREGNANCY

The effects of Celontin in human pregnancy and nursing infants are unknown.

Recent reports suggest an association between the use of anticonvulsant drugs by women with epilepsy and an elevated incidence of birth defects in children born to these women. Data are more extensive with respect to phenytoin and phenobarbital, but these are also the most commonly prescribed anticonvulsants; less systematic or anecdotal reports suggest a possible similar association with the use of all known anticonvulsant drugs.

The reports suggesting an elevated incidence of birth defects in children of drug-treated epileptic women cannot be regarded as adequate to prove a definite cause-and-effect relationship. There are intrinsic methodologic problems in obtaining adequate data on drug teratogenicity in humans; the possibility also exists that other factors, eg, genetic factors or the epileptic condition itself, may be more important than drug therapy in leading to birth defects. The great majority of mothers on anticonvulsant medication deliver normal infants. It is important to note that anticonvulsant drugs should not be discontinued in patients in whom the drug is administered to prevent major seizures because of the strong possibility of precipitating status epilepticus with attendant hypoxia and threat to life. In individual cases where the severity and frequency of the seizure disorder are such that the removal of medication does not pose a serious threat to the patient, discontinuation of the drug may be considered prior to and during pregnancy, although it cannot be said with any confidence that even minor seizures do not pose some hazard to the developing embryo or fetus.

The prescribing physician will wish to weigh these considerations in treating or counseling epileptic women of childbearing potential.

Hazardous Activities: Methsuximide may impair the mental and/or physical abilities required for the performance of potentially hazardous tasks, such as driving a motor vehicle

---

or other such activity requiring alertness; therefore, the patient should be cautioned accordingly.

PRECAUTIONS

It is recommended that the physician withdraw the drug slowly on the appearance of unusual depression, aggressiveness, or other behavioral alterations.

As with other anticonvulsants, it is important to proceed slowly when increasing or decreasing dosage, as well as when adding or eliminating other medication. Abrupt withdrawal of anticonvulsant medication may precipitate absence (petit mal) status.

Methsuximide, when used alone in mixed types of epilepsy, may increase the frequency of grand mal seizures in some patients.

ADVICE TO THE PHARMACIST AND PATIENT: Since methsuximide has a relatively low melting temperature (124°F), storage conditions which may promote high temperatures (closed cars, delivery vans, or storage near steam pipes) should be avoided. Do not dispense or use capsules that are not full or in which contents have melted. Effectiveness may be reduced. Protect from excessive heat (104°F).

ADVERSE REACTIONS

Gastrointestinal System: Gastrointestinal symptoms occur frequently and have included nausea or vomiting, anorexia, diarrhea, weight loss, epigastric and abdominal pain, and constipation.

Hemopoietic System: Hemopoietic complications associated with the administration of methsuximide have included eosinophilia, leukopenia, monocytosis, and pancytopenia.

Nervous System: Neurologic and sensory reactions reported during therapy with methsuximide have included drowsiness, ataxia or dizziness, irritability and nervousness, headache, blurred vision, photophobia, hiccups, and insomnia. Drowsiness, ataxia, and dizziness have been the most frequent side effects noted. Psychologic abnormalities have included confusion, instability, mental slowness, depression, hypochondriacal behavior, and aggressiveness. There have been rare reports of psychosis, suicidal behavior, and auditory hallucinations.

Integumentary System: Dermatologic manifestations which have occurred with the administration of methsuximide have included urticaria, Stevens-Johnson syndrome, and pruritic erythematous rashes.

Other: Miscellaneous reactions reported include periorbital edema and hyperemia.

DOSAGE AND ADMINISTRATION

Optimum dosage of Celontin must be determined by trial. A suggested dosage schedule is 300 mg per day for the first week. If required, dosage may be increased thereafter at weekly intervals by 300 mg per day for the three weeks following to a daily dosage of 1.2 g. Because therapeutic effect and tolerance vary among patients, therapy with Celontin must be individualized according to the response of each patient. Optimal dosage is that amount of Celontin which is barely sufficient to control seizures so that side effects may be kept to a minimum. The smaller capsule (150 mg) facilitates administration to small children.

Celontin may be administered in combination with other anticonvulsants when other forms of epilepsy coexist with absence (petit mal).

HOW SUPPLIED

N 0071-0525-24 (P-D 525)—Celontin Kapseals, #1 capsule each containing 300 mg methsuximide; bottles of 100.

N 0071-0537-24 (P-D 537)—Celontin Kapseals, Half Strength, #4 capsule each containing 150 mg methsuximide, bottles of 100.

Store at controlled room temperature 15°–30°C (59°–86°F). Protect from light and moisture.

0537G013

Shown in Product Identification Section, page 421

CENTRAX®   ℂⱽ ℞

[cĕn'trăx]

(prazepam capsules and tablets, USP)

DESCRIPTION

Centrax (prazepam) is a benzodiazepine derivative. Chemically, prazepam is 7-chloro-1-(cyclopropylmethyl)-1, 3-dihydro-5-phenyl-2H-1, 4-benzodiazepin-2-one, and has a molecular weight of 324.8.

Each Centrax capsule contains 5 mg, 10 mg, or 20 mg prazepam, USP. Also contains lactose, NF; magnesium stearate, NF; sodium lauryl sulfate, NF. The capsule contains colloidal silicon dioxide, NF; gelatin, NF; sodium lauryl sulfate, NF; titanium dioxide, USP. The Centrax 5-mg capsule also contains D&C yellow No. 10; FD&C blue No.1; FD&C yellow No. 6 (sunset yellow). The Centrax 10-mg capsule also contains FD&C blue No. 1; FD&C green No. 3. The Centrax 20-mg capsule also contains D&C yellow No. 10; FD&C yellow No. 6 (sunset yellow).

Each Centrax tablet contains 10 mg prazepam, USP. Also contains corn starch, NF, FD&C blue No. 2, aluminum lake;

lactose, NF; magnesium stearate, NF; microcrystalline cellulose, NF.

CLINICAL PHARMACOLOGY

Studies in normal subjects have shown that Centrax (prazepam) has depressant effects on the central nervous system. Oral administration of single doses as high as 60 mg and of divided doses up to 100 mg three times a day (300 mg total daily dosage) were without toxic effects.

Single, oral doses of Centrax (prazepam) in normal subjects produced average peak blood levels of the major metabolite norprazepam at 6 hours postadministration, with significant amounts still present after 48 hours. Prazepam was slowly absorbed over a prolonged period; rather constant blood levels were maintained on multiple-dose schedules; and excretion was prolonged. The mean half-life of norprazepam measured in subjects given 10 mg prazepam three times a day for one week was 63 ($\pm$ 15 SD) hours before and 70 ($\pm$ 10 SD) hours after multiple dosing—a nonsignificant difference. Human metabolism studies showed that prior to elimination from the body, prazepam is metabolized in large part to 3-hydroxyprazepam and oxazepam.

INDICATIONS

Centrax is indicated for the management of anxiety disorders or for the short-term relief of the symptoms of anxiety. Anxiety or tension associated with the stress of everyday life usually does not require treatment with an anxiolytic.

The effectiveness of Centrax in long-term use, that is, more than 4 months, has not been assessed by systematic clinical studies. The physician should periodically reassess the usefulness of the drug for the individual patient.

CONTRAINDICATIONS

Centrax (prazepam) is contraindicated in patients with a known hypersensitivity to the drug and in those with acute narrow-angle glaucoma.

WARNINGS

Centrax (prazepam) is not recommended in psychotic states and in those psychiatric disorders in which anxiety is not a prominent feature.

Patients taking Centrax should be cautioned against engaging in hazardous occupations requiring mental alertness, such as operating dangerous machinery including motor vehicles.

Since Centrax has a central nervous system depressant effect, patients should be advised against the simultaneous ingestion of alcohol and other CNS-depressant drugs during Centrax therapy.

Physical and Psychological Dependence: Withdrawal symptoms, similar in character to those noted with barbiturates and alcohol (convulsions, tremor, abdominal and muscle cramps, vomiting and sweating), have occurred following abrupt discontinuance of benzodiazepines. The more severe withdrawal symptoms have usually been limited to those patients who received excessive doses over an extended period of time. Generally milder withdrawal symptoms (e.g., dysphoria and insomnia) have been reported following abrupt discontinuance of benzodiazepines taken continuously at therapeutic levels for several months. Consequently, after extended therapy, abrupt discontinuation should generally be avoided and a gradual dosage tapering schedule followed. Addiction-prone individuals (such as drug addicts or alcoholics) should be under careful surveillance when receiving prazepam or other psychotropic agents because of the predisposition of such patients to habituation and dependence.

PRECAUTIONS

Information for Patients:

To assure the safe and effective use of benzodiazepines, patients should be informed that since benzodiazepines may produce psychological and physical dependence, it is advisable that they consult with their physician before either increasing the dose or abruptly discontinuing this drug. Patients should also be advised to inform their physician if they are nursing, pregnant, planning to become pregnant or become pregnant while on this medication and about any alcohol consumption or medication they are taking. In addition, as with all CNS-acting agents, patients should be cautioned against driving or engaging in hazardous activities requiring mental alertness until they experience how this medication affects them.

Usage in Pregnancy and Lactation: An increased risk of congenital malformations associated with the use of minor tranquilizers (chlordiazepoxide, diazepam, and meprobamate) during the first trimester of pregnancy has been suggested in several studies. Prazepam, a benzodiazepine derivative, has not been studied adequately to determine whether it, too, may be associated with an increased risk of fetal abnormality. Because use of these drugs is rarely a matter of urgency, their use during this period should almost always be avoided. The possibility that a woman of childbearing potential may be pregnant at the time of institution of therapy should be considered. Patients should be advised that if they become pregnant during therapy or intend to become pregnant, they should communicate with their physicians

about the desirability of discontinuing the drug. In view of their molecular size, prazepam and its metabolites are probably excreted in human milk. Therefore, this drug should not be given to nursing mothers.

In those patients in whom a degree of depression accompanies the anxiety, suicidal tendencies may be present and protective measures may be required. The least amount of drug that is feasible should be available to the patient at any one time.

Patients taking Centrax (prazepam) for prolonged periods should have blood counts and liver function tests periodically. The usual precautions in treating patients with impaired renal or hepatic functions should also be observed. Hepatomegaly and cholestasis were observed in chronic toxicity studies in rats and dogs.

In elderly or debilitated patients, the initial dose should be small, and increments should be made gradually, in accordance with the response of the patient, to preclude ataxia or excessive sedation.

If Centrax is to be combined with other psychotropic agents or anticonvulsant drugs, careful consideration should be given to the pharmacology of the agents to be employed—particularly with known compounds which may potentiate the action of Centrax, such as phenothiazines, narcotics, barbiturates, MAO inhibitors and other antidepressants. *Pediatric Use:* Safety and effectiveness in patients below the age of 18 have not been established.

ADVERSE REACTIONS

The side effects most frequently reported during double-blind, placebo-controlled trials employing a typical 30-mg divided total daily dosage and the percent incidence in the prazepam group were fatigue (11.6%), dizziness (8.7%), weakness (7.7%), drowsiness (6.8%), lightheadedness (6.8%), and ataxia (5.0%). Less frequently reported were headache, confusion, tremor, vivid dreams, slurred speech, palpitation, stimulation, dry mouth, diaphoresis, and various gastrointestinal complaints. Other side effects included pruritus, transient skin rashes, swelling of feet, joint pains, various genitourinary complaints, blurred vision, and syncope. Single, nightly dose, controlled trials of variable dosages showed a dose-related incidence of these same side effects. Transient and reversible aberrations of liver function tests have been reported, as have been slight decreases in blood pressure and increases in body weight.

These findings are characteristic of benzodiazepine drugs.

OVERDOSAGE

As in the management of overdosage with any drug, it should be borne in mind that multiple agents may have been taken. Vomiting should be induced if it has not occurred spontaneously. Immediate gastric lavage is also recommended. General supportive care, including frequent monitoring of vital signs and close observation of the patient, is indicated. Hypotension, though unlikely, may be controlled with Levophed® (levarterenol bitartrate), or Aramine® (metaraminol bitartrate).

DOSAGE AND ADMINISTRATION

Centrax (prazepam) is administered orally in divided doses. The usual daily dose is 30 mg. The dose should be adjusted gradually within the range of 20 mg to 60 mg daily in accordance with the response of the patient. In elderly or debilitated patients it is advisable to initiate treatment at a divided daily dose of 10 mg to 15 mg (see Precautions). Centrax may also be administered as a single, daily dose at bedtime. The recommended starting nightly dose is 20 mg. The response of the patient to several days' treatment will permit the physician to adjust the dose upwards or, occasionally, downwards to maximize antianxiety effect with a minimum of daytime drowsiness. The optimum dosage will usually range from 20 mg to 40 mg.

DRUG INTERACTIONS

If Centrax (prazepam) is to be combined with other drugs acting on the central nervous system, careful consideration should be given to the pharmacology of the agents to be employed. The actions of the benzodiazepines may be potentiated by barbiturates, narcotics, phenothiazines, monoamine oxidase inhibitors, or other antidepressants.

If Centrax (prazepam) is used to treat anxiety associated with somatic disease states, careful attention must be paid to possible drug interaction with concomitant medication.

HOW SUPPLIED

Centrax 5 mg—Each capsule contains 5 mg prazepam. Available in bottles of 100 (N 0710-0552-24), and 500 (N 0710-0552-30). Centrax 10 mg—Each capsule contains 10 mg prazepam. Available in bottles of 100 (N 0710-0553-24), and 500 (N 0710-0553-30). Centrax 20 mg—Each capsule contains 20 mg prazepam. Available in bottles of 100 (N 0710-0554-24). Also supplied as Centrax Tablets (prazepam tablets, USP) 10 mg light blue, scored tablets in bottles of 100 (N 0710-0276-24) and unit dose (N 0710-0276-40).

Direct Medical Inquiries to:
Parke-Davis, Div Warner-Lambert Inc
c/o Warner-Lambert Co
201 Tabor Road, Morris Plains, NJ 07950.
Attn: Medical Affairs Dept

0552G126

Shown in Product Identification Section, page 421

CHLOROMYCETIN® CREAM, 1%   ℞

[chlō "rō-my-cē 'tĭn]
(chloramphenicol cream, USP) 1%

DESCRIPTION

Each gram of Chloromycetin Cream, 1%, contains 10 mg chloramphenicol with 0.1% propylparaben in a water-miscible ointment base of liquid petrolatum, cetyl alcohol, sodium lauryl sulfate, sodium phosphate buffer, and water.

CLINICAL PHARMACOLOGY

Chloramphenicol is a broad-spectrum antibiotic originally isolated from *Streptomyces venezuelae.* It is primarily bacteriostatic and acts by inhibition of protein synthesis by interfering with the transfer of activated amino acids from soluble RNA to ribosomes. Development of resistance to chloramphenicol can be regarded as minimal for staphylococci and many other species of bacteria.

INDICATIONS AND USAGE

Chloromycetin (chloramphenicol) Cream, 1%, is indicated for the treatment of surface skin infections caused by bacteria susceptible to chloramphenicol. Deeper cutaneous infections should be treated with appropriate systemic antibiotics.

CONTRAINDICATION

This product is contraindicated in persons sensitive to any of its components.

WARNINGS

Bone marrow hypoplasia, including aplastic anemia and death, has been reported following the local application of chloramphenicol.

PRECAUTIONS

The prolonged use of antibiotics may occasionally result in overgrowth of nonsusceptible organisms, including fungi. If new infections appear during medication, the drug should be discontinued and appropriate measures should be taken. In all except very superficial infections, the topical use of chloramphenicol should be supplemented by appropriate systemic medication.

ADVERSE REACTIONS

Signs of local irritation with subjective symptoms of itching or burning, angioneurotic edema, urticaria, vesicular and maculopapular dermatitis have been reported in patients sensitive to chloramphenicol and are causes for discontinuing the medication. Similar sensitivity reactions to other materials in topical preparations may also occur. Blood dyscrasias have been reported in association with the use of chloramphenicol (See WARNINGS).

DOSAGE AND ADMINISTRATION

Apply to the infected area three or four times daily after cleansing.

HOW SUPPLIED

N 0071-3166-13
Chloromycetin Cream, 1% is supplied in 1 ounce tubes.
Store between 15°-30°C (59°-86°F).
Chloromycetin, brand of chloramphenicol. Reg US Pat Off
Caution—Federal law prohibits dispensing without prescription.
September 1987
Manufactured by
Parke-Davis
Scarborough, Ontario, Canada
Distributed by
PARKE-DAVIS
Div of Warner-Lambert Co
Morris Plains, NJ 07950 USA   3166G013

CHLOROMYCETIN®   ℞

[chlō "rō-my-cē 'tĭn]
HYDROCORTISONE OPHTHALMIC
(Chloramphenicol and Hydrocortisone Acetate for Suspension, USP)

> **WARNING**
> Bone marrow hypoplasia including aplastic anemia and
> death has been reported following local application of

Continued on next page

This product information was prepared in August, 1989. On these and other Parke-Davis Products, information may be obtained by addressing PARKE-DAVIS, Division of Warner-Lambert Company, Morris Plains, New Jersey 07950.

Parke-Davis—Cont.

chloramphenicol. Chloramphenicol should not be used when less potentially dangerous agents would be expected to provide effective treatment.

DESCRIPTION

Chloromycetin® Hydrocortisone Ophthalmic (Chloramphenicol and Hydrocortisone Acetate for Suspension, USP) is a sterile, buffered antibiotic/antiinflammatory dry mixture for suspension for ophthalmic administration. Each vial of Chloromycetin Hydrocortisone Ophthalmic contains 12.5 mg chloramphenicol and 25 mg hydrocortisone acetate with boric acid-sodium borate buffer, cholesterol, methylcellulose, sodium chloride, and Phemerol® (benzethonium chloride), 0.1 mg per ml, in the suspension when prepared as directed. A 5 ml vial of Sterile Distilled Water is included in each package for use as a diluent in the preparation of a suspension of Chloromycetin Hydrocortisone suitable for ophthalmic use.

The chemical names for chloramphenicol are:

(1) Acetamide,2,2-dichloro-N-[2-hydroxy-1-(hydroxymethyl)-2-(4-nitrophenyl) ethyl]-, and

(2) D-*threo* -(–)-2,2-Dichloro-N-[β-hydroxy-α-(hydroxymethyl)-*p* -nitrophenethyl] acetamide

The chemical names for hydrocortisone acetate are:

(1) Pregn-4-ene-3,20-dione,21-(acetyloxy)-11,17-dihydroxy-,(11β)-, and

(2) 17-Hydroxycorticosterone 21-acetate

CLINICAL PHARMACOLOGY

Corticoids suppress the inflammatory response to a variety of agents and they probably delay or slow healing. Since corticoids may inhibit the body's defense mechanism against infection, a concomitant antimicrobial drug may be used when this inhibition is considered to be clinically significant in a particular case.

The antiinfective component in this combination is included to provide action against specific organisms susceptible to it. Chloramphenicol is considered active against a wide spectrum of gram-negative and gram-positive organisms such as *Escherichia coli, Hemophilus influenzae, Staphylococcus aureus, Streptococcus hemolyticus,* and *Moraxella lacunata* (Morax-Axenfeld bacillus). Development of resistance to chloramphenicol can be regarded as minimal for staphylococci and many other species of bacteria. Chloramphenicol is primarily bacteriostatic and acts by inhibition of protein synthesis by interfering with the transfer of activated amino acids from soluble RNA to ribosomes. It has been noted that chloramphenicol is found in measurable amounts in the aqueous humor following local application to the eye.

When a decision to administer both a corticoid and an antimicrobial is made, the administration of such drugs in combination has the advantage of greater patient compliance and convenience, with the added assurance that the appropriate dosage of both drugs is administered, plus assured compatibility of ingredients when both types of drug are in the same formulation and, particularly, that the correct volume of drug is delivered and retained.

The relative potency of corticosteroids depends on the molecular structure, concentration, and release from the vehicle.

INDICATIONS AND USAGE

Chloramphenicol should be used only in those serious infections for which less potentially dangerous drugs are ineffective or contraindicated. Bacteriological studies should be performed to determine the causative organisms and their sensitivity to chloramphenicol (See Box Warning).

For steroid-responsive inflammatory ocular conditions for which a corticosteroid is indicated and where bacterial infection or a risk of bacterial ocular infection exists.

Ocular steroids are indicated in inflammatory conditions of the palpebral and bulbar conjunctiva, cornea, and anterior segment of the globe where the inherent risk of steroid use in certain infective conjunctivitides is accepted to obtain a diminution in edema and inflammation. They are also indicated in chronic anterior uveitis and corneal injury from chemical, radiation, thermal burns, or penetration of foreign bodies. The use of a combination drug with an antiinfective component is indicated where the risk of infection is high or where there is an expectation that potentially dangerous numbers of bacteria will be present in the eye.

The particular antiinfective drug in this product is active against the following common bacterial eye pathogens:

Staphylococcus aureus

Streptococci, including *Streptococcus pneumoniae*

Escherichia coli

Hemophilus influenzae

Klebsiella/Enterobacter species

Moraxella lacunata (Morax-Axenfeld bacillus)

Neisseria species

The product does not provide adequate coverage against:

Pseudomonas aeruginosa

Serratia marcescens

CONTRAINDICATIONS

Epithelial herpes simplex keratitis (dendritic keratitis), vaccinia, varicella, and many other viral diseases of the cornea and conjunctiva. Mycobacterial infection of the eye. Fungal diseases of ocular structures. Hypersensitivity to a component of the medication. (Hypersensitivity to the antibiotic component occurs at a higher rate than for other components).

The use of these combinations is always contraindicated after uncomplicated removal of a corneal foreign body.

WARNINGS

SEE BOX WARNING

Prolonged use of steroids may result in glaucoma, with damage to the optic nerve, defects in visual acuity and fields of vision, and posterior subcapsular cataract formation. Prolonged use may suppress the host response and thus increase the hazard of secondary ocular infections. In those diseases causing thinning of the cornea or sclera, perforations have been known to occur with the use of topical steroids. In acute purulent conditions of the eye, steroids may mask infection or enhance existing infection. If these products are used for 10 days or longer, intraocular pressure should be routinely monitored even though it may be difficult in children and uncooperative patients.

Employment of steroid medication in the treatment of herpes simplex requires great caution.

PRECAUTIONS

The initial prescription and renewal of the medication order beyond 20 milliliters should be made by a physician only after examination of the patient with the aid of magnification, such as slit lamp biomicroscopy and, where appropriate, fluorescein staining.

The possibility of persistent fungal infections of the cornea should be considered after prolonged steroid dosing.

The prolonged use of antibiotics may occasionally result in overgrowth of nonsusceptible organisms, including fungi. If new infections appear during medication, the drug should be discontinued and appropriate measures should be taken.

In all serious infections the topical use of chloramphenicol should be supplemented by appropriate systemic medication.

ADVERSE REACTIONS

Blood dyscrasias have been reported in association with the use of chloramphenicol. (See **Warnings**).

Adverse reactions have occurred with steroid /antiinfective combination drugs which can be attributed to the steroid component, the antiinfective component, or the combination. Exact incidence figures are not available since no denominator of treated patients is available.

Reactions occurring most often from the presence of the antiinfective ingredient are allergic sensitizations. The reactions due to the steroid component in decreasing order of frequency are: elevation of intraocular pressure (IOP) with possible development of glaucoma, and infrequent optic nerve damage; posterior subcapsular cataract formation; and delayed wound healing.

Secondary Infection: The development of secondary infection has occurred after use of combinations containing steroids and antimicrobials. Fungal infections of the cornea are particularly prone to develop coincidentally with long-term applications of steroid. The possibility of fungal invasion must be considered in any persistent corneal ulceration where steroid treatment has been used.

Secondary bacterial ocular infection following suppression of host responses also occurs.

DOSAGE AND ADMINISTRATION

Two drops applied to the affected eye every three hours, or more frequently if deemed advisable by the prescribing physician. Administration should be continued day and night for the first 48 hours, after which the interval between applications may be increased. Treatment should be continued for at least 48 hours after the eye appears normal.

Directions for dispensing—Add 5 ml sterile distilled water to contents of vial under aseptic conditions. Shake to make uniform suspension. Place sterile dropper in vial. Each ml of suspension prepared as directed contains 2.5 mg Chloromycetin (chloramphenicol) and 5 mg Hydrocortisone Acetate. Not more than 20 milliliters should be prescribed initially and the prescription should not be refilled without further evaluation as outlined in Precautions above.

HOW SUPPLIED

N 0071-3228-36 Chloromycetin Hydrocortisone Ophthalmic (Chloramphenicol and Hydrocortisone Acetate for Suspension, USP) is supplied in a package containing dry ingredients in a 5 ml vial and a vial containing 5 ml of Sterile Distilled Water for use as a diluent in preparation of the ophthalmic suspension. After dispensing, the product may be stored at room temperature for a period of not more than 10 days. A sterilized dropper-cap assembly for use with the vial is included in the package.

Chloromycetin, brand of chloramphenicol, Reg US Pat Off.

3228G014

WARNING

Serious and fatal blood dyscrasias (aplastic anemia, hypoplastic anemia, thrombocytopenia, and granulocytopenia) are known to occur after the administration of chloramphenicol. In addition, there have been reports of aplastic anemia attributed to chloramphenicol which later terminated in leukemia. Blood dyscrasias have occurred after both short-term and prolonged therapy with this drug. Chloramphenicol must not be used when less potentially dangerous agents will be effective, as described in the Indications section. *It must not be used in the treatment of trivial infections or where it is not indicated, as in colds, influenza, infections of the throat; or as a prophylactic agent to prevent bacterial infections.*

Precautions: It is essential that adequate blood studies be made during treatment with the drug. While blood studies may detect early peripheral blood changes, such as leukopenia, reticulocytopenia, or granulocytopenia, before they become irreversible, such studies cannot be relied on to detect bone marrow depression prior to development of aplastic anemia. To facilitate appropriate studies and observation during therapy, it is desirable that patients be hospitalized.

DESCRIPTION

Chloramphenicol is an antibiotic that is clinically useful for, *and should be reserved for,* serious infections caused by organisms susceptible to its antimicrobial effects when less potentially hazardous therapeutic agents are ineffective or contraindicated. Sensitivity testing is essential to determine its indicated use, but may be performed concurrently with therapy initiated on clinical impression that one of the indicated conditions exists (see Indications and Usage section). Each capsule contains 250 mg chloramphenicol. Also contains lactose, NF. The capsule shell and/or band contains gelatin, NF; colloidal silicon dioxide, NF; glyceryl monooleate; gray Opatint OD-7502; sodium lauryl sulfate, NF; titanium dioxide USP.

CLINICAL PHARMACOLOGY

In vitro chloramphenicol exerts mainly a bacteriostatic effect on a wide range of gram-negative and gram-positive bacteria and is active *in vitro* against rickettsiae, the lymphogranuloma psittacosis group, and *Vibrio cholerae.* It is particularly active against *Salmonella typhi* and *Hemophilus influenzae.* The mode of action is through interference or inhibition of protein synthesis in intact cells and in cell-free systems.

Chloramphenicol administered orally is absorbed rapidly from the intestinal tract. In controlled studies in adult volunteers using the recommended dosage of 50 mg/kg/day, a dosage of 1 g every 6 hours for 8 doses was given. Using the microbiological assay method, the average peak serum level was 11.2 mcg/ml one hour after the first dose. A cumulative effect gave a peak rise to 18.4 mcg/ml after the fifth dose of 1 g. Mean serum levels ranged from 8 to 14 mcg/ml over the 48-hour period. Total urinary excretion of chloramphenicol in these studies ranged from a low of 68% to a high of 99% over a three-day period. From 8 to 12% of the antibiotic excreted is in the form of free chloramphenicol; the remainder consists of microbiologically inactive metabolites, principally the conjugate with glucuronic acid. Since the glucuronide is excreted rapidly, most chloramphenicol detected in the blood is in the microbiologically active free form. Despite the small proportion of unchanged drug excreted in the urine, the concentration of free chloramphenicol is relatively high, amounting to several hundred mcg/ml in patients receiving divided doses of 50 mg/kg/day. Small amounts of active drug are found in bile and feces. Chloramphenicol diffuses rapidly, but its distribution is not uniform. Highest concentrations are found in liver and kidney, and lowest concentrations are found in brain and cerebrospinal fluid. Chloramphenicol enters cerebrospinal fluid even in the absence of meningeal inflammation, appearing in concentrations about half of those found in the blood. Measurable levels are also detected in pleural and in ascitic fluids, saliva, milk, and in the aqueous and vitreous humors. Transport across the placental barrier occurs with somewhat lower concentration in cord blood of newborn infants than in maternal blood.

INDICATIONS AND USAGE

In accord with the concepts in the warning box and this indications section, chloramphenicol must be used only in those serious infections for which less potentially dangerous

drugs are ineffective or contraindicated. However, chloramphenicol may be chosen to initiate antibiotic therapy on the clinical impression that one of the conditions below is believed to be present; *in vitro* sensitivity tests should be performed concurrently so that the drug may be discontinued as soon as possible if less potentially dangerous agents are indicated by such tests. The decision to continue use of chloramphenicol rather than another antibiotic when both are suggested by *in vitro* studies to be effective against a specific pathogen should be based upon severity of the infection, susceptibility of the pathogen to the various antimicrobial drugs, efficacy of the various drugs in the infection, and the important additional concepts contained in the Warning Box above:

1. Acute infections caused by *Salmonella typhi*
Chloramphenicol is a drug of choice.* It is not recommended for the routine treatment of the typhoid carrier state.

2. Serious infections caused by susceptible strains in accordance with the concepts expressed above:
a. *Salmonella* species
b. *H influenzae*, specifically meningeal infections
c. Rickettsia
d. Lymphogranuloma-psittacosis group
e. Various gram-negative bacteria causing bacteremia, meningitis, or other serious gram-negative infections
f. Other susceptible organisms which have been demonstrated to be resistant to all other appropriate antimicrobial agents.

3. Cystic fibrosis regimens

CONTRAINDICATIONS

Chloramphenicol is contraindicated in individuals with a history of previous hypersensitivity and/or toxic reaction to it. *It must not be used in the treatment of trivial infections or where it is not indicated, as in colds, influenza, infections of the throat; or as a prophylactic agent to prevent bacterial infections.*

---

* In the treatment of typhoid fever, some authorities recommend that chloramphenicol be administered at therapeutic levels for 8 to 10 days after the patient has become afebrile to lessen the possibility of relapse.

PRECAUTIONS

1. Baseline blood studies should be followed by periodic blood studies approximately every two days during therapy. The drug should be discontinued upon appearance of reticulocytopenia, leukopenia, thrombocytopenia, anemia, or any other blood study findings attributable to chloramphenicol. However, it should be noted that such studies do not exclude the possible later appearance of the irreversible type of bone marrow depression.

2. Repeated courses of the drug should be avoided if at all possible. Treatment should not be continued longer than required to produce a cure with little or no risk of relapse of the disease.

3. Concurrent therapy with other drugs that may cause bone marrow depression should be avoided.

4. Excessive blood levels may result from administration of the recommended dose to patients with impaired liver or kidney function, including that due to immature metabolic processes in the infant. The dosage should be adjusted accordingly or, preferably, the blood concentration should be determined at appropriate intervals.

5. There are no studies to establish the safety of this drug in pregnancy.

6. Since chloramphenicol readily crosses the placental barrier, caution in use of the drug is particularly important during pregnancy at term or during labor because of potential toxic effects on the fetus ("gray syndrome").

7. Precaution should be used in therapy of premature and full-term infants to avoid "gray syndrome" toxicity. (See Adverse Reactions.) Serum drug levels should be carefully followed during therapy of the newborn infant.

8. Precaution should be used in therapy during lactation because of the possibility of toxic effects on the nursing infant.

9. The use of this antibiotic, as with other antibiotics, may result in an overgrowth of nonsusceptible organisms, including fungi. If infections caused by nonsusceptible organisms appear during therapy, appropriate measures should be taken.

ADVERSE REACTIONS

1. Blood Dyscrasias

The most serious adverse effect of chloramphenicol is bone marrow depression. Serious and fatal blood dyscrasias (aplastic anemia, hypoplastic anemia, thrombocytopenia, and granulocytopenia) are known to occur after the administration of chloramphenicol. An irreversible type of marrow depression leading to aplastic anemia with a high rate of mortality is characterized by the appearance weeks or months after therapy of bone marrow aplasia or hypoplasia. Peripherally, pancytopenia is most often observed, but in a small number of cases only one or two of the three major cell types (erythrocytes, leukocytes, platelets) may be depressed.

A reversible type of bone marrow depression, which is dose-related, may occur. This type of marrow depression is characterized by vacuolization of the erythroid cells, reduction of reticulocytes, and leukopenia, and responds promptly to the withdrawal of chloramphenicol.

An exact determination of the risk of serious and fatal blood dyscrasias is not possible because of lack of accurate information regarding (1) the size of the population at risk, (2) the total number of drug-associated dyscrasias, and (3) the total number of nondrug-associated dyscrasias.

In a report to the California State Assembly by the California Medical Association and the State Department of Public Health in January 1967, the risk of fatal aplastic anemia was estimated at 1:24,200 to 1:40,500 based on two dosage levels. There have been reports of aplastic anemia attributed to chloramphenicol which later terminated in leukemia. Paroxysmal nocturnal hemoglobinuria has also been reported.

2. Gastrointestinal Reactions

Nausea, vomiting, glossitis and stomatitis, diarrhea, and enterocolitis may occur in low incidence.

3. Neurotoxic Reactions

Headache, mild depression, mental confusion, and delirium have been described in patients receiving chloramphenicol. Optic and peripheral neuritis have been reported, usually following long-term therapy. If this occurs, the drug should be promptly withdrawn.

4. Hypersensitivity Reactions

Fever, macular and vesicular rashes, angioedema, urticaria, and anaphylaxis may occur. Herxheimer reactions have occurred during therapy for typhoid fever.

5. "Gray Syndrome"

Toxic reactions including fatalities have occurred in the premature and newborn; the signs and symptoms associated with these reactions have been referred to as the "gray syndrome". One case of "gray syndrome" has been reported in an infant born to a mother having received chloramphenicol during labor. One case has been reported in a 3-month-old infant. The following summarizes the clinical and laboratory studies that have been made on these patients:

(a) In most cases, therapy with chloramphenicol had been instituted within the first 48 hours of life.
(b) Symptoms first appeared after 3 to 4 days of continued treatment with high doses of chloramphenicol.
(c) The symptoms appeared in the following order:
   (1) abdominal distention with or without emesis;
   (2) progressive pallid cyanosis;
   (3) vasomotor collapse, frequently accompanied by irregular respiration;
   (4) death within a few hours of onset of these symptoms.
(d) The progression of symptoms from onset to exitus was accelerated with higher dose schedules.
(e) Preliminary blood serum level studies revealed unusually high concentrations of chloramphenicol (over 90 mcg/ml after repeated doses).
(f) Termination of therapy upon early evidence of the associated symptomatology frequently reversed the process with complete recovery.

DOSAGE AND ADMINISTRATION

Dosage Recommendations For Oral Chloramphenicol Preparations

The majority of microorganisms susceptible to chloramphenicol will respond to a concentration between 5 and 20 mcg/ml. The desired concentration of active drug in blood should fall within this range over most of the treatment period. Dosage of 50 mg/kg/day divided into 4 doses at intervals of 6 hours will usually achieve and sustain levels of this magnitude.

Except in certain circumstances (eg, premature and newborn infants and individuals with impairment of hepatic or renal function), lower doses may not achieve these concentrations. Chloramphenicol, like other potent drugs, should be prescribed at recommended doses known to have therapeutic activity. Close observation of the patient should be maintained and in the event of any adverse reactions, dosage should be reduced or the drug discontinued, if other factors in the clinical situation permit.

Adults

Adults should receive 50 mg/kg/day (approximately one 250-mg capsule per each 10 lbs body weight) in divided doses at 6-hour intervals. In exceptional cases, patients with infections due to moderately resistant organisms may require increased dosage up to 100 mg/kg/day to achieve blood levels inhibiting the pathogen, but these high doses should be decreased as soon as possible. Adults with impairment of hepatic or renal function or both may have reduced ability to metabolize and excrete the drug. In instances of impaired metabolic processes, dosages should be adjusted accordingly. (See discussion under Newborn Infants.) Precise control of concentration of the drug in the blood should be carefully followed in patients with impaired metabolic processes by the available microtechniques (information available on request).

Children

Dosage of 50 mg/kg/day divided into 4 doses at 6-hour intervals yields blood levels in the range effective against most susceptible organisms. Severe infections (eg, bacteremia or meningitis), especially when adequate cerebrospinal fluid concentrations are desired, may require dosage up to 100 mg/kg/day; however, it is recommended that dosage be reduced to 50 mg/kg/day as soon as possible. Children with impaired liver or kidney function may retain excessive amounts of the drug.

Newborn Infants

(See section titled "Gray Syndrome" under Adverse Reactions.)

A total of 25 mg/kg/day in 4 equal doses at 6-hour intervals usually produces and maintains concentrations in blood and tissues adequate to control most infections for which the drug is indicated. Increased dosage in these individuals, demanded by severe infections, should be given only to maintain the blood concentration within a therapeutically effective range. After the first two weeks of life, full-term infants ordinarily may receive up to a total of 50 mg/kg/day equally divided into 4 doses at 6-hour intervals. **These dosage recommendations are extremely important because blood concentration in all premature infants and full-term infants under two weeks of age differs from that of other infants.** This difference is due to variations in the maturity of the metabolic functions of the liver and the kidneys.

When these functions are immature (or seriously impaired in adults), high concentrations of the drug are found which tend to increase with succeeding doses.

Infants and Children with Immature Metabolic Processes

In young infants and other children in whom immature metabolic functions are suspected, a dose of 25 mg/kg/day will usually produce therapeutic concentrations of the drug in the blood. In this group particularly, the concentration of the drug in the blood should be carefully following by microtechniques. (Information available on request.)

HOW SUPPLIED

Kapseals No. 379, Chloromycetin (Chloramphenicol Capsules), each contain 250 mg chloramphenicol.
N 0071-0379-09 Bottles of 16.
N 0071-0379-24 Bottles of 100.
N 0071-0379-40 Unit dose packages of 100 (10/10's).
AHFS 8:12.08   **0379G101**

Chloromycetin, brand of chloramphenicol.
Reg. US Pat Off

STORAGE

Store at a room temperature below 86°F(30°C). Protect from moisture and excessive heat.
Caution—Federal law prohibits dispensing without prescription.
Shown in Product Identification Section, page 421

CHLOROMYCETIN® OPHTHALMIC   ℞

[chlō"rō-my-cē'tin]
(Chloramphenical for Ophthalmic Solution, USP)

> **WARNING**
> Bone marrow hypoplasia including aplastic anemia and death have been reported following local application of chloramphenicol. Chloramphenicol should not be used when less potentially dangerous agents would be expected to provide effective treatment.

DESCRIPTION

Each vial of Chloromycetin Ophthalmic contains 25 mg of Chloromycetin (chloramphenicol) with boric acid-sodium borate buffer. Sodium hydroxide may have been added for adjustment of pH. A 15 ml bottle of Sterile Distilled Water is included in each package for use as a diluent in the preparation of a solution of Chloromycetin suitable for ophthalmic use. By varying the quantity of diluent used solutions ranging in strength from 0.16% to 0.5% may be prepared. Both the powder for solution and the diluent contain no preservatives. Sterile powder.
The chemical names for chloramphenicol are:
(1) Acetamide,2,2-dichloro-*N*-[2-hydroxy-1-(hydroxymethyl)-2-(4-nitrophenyl) ethyl]-, and
(2) D-*three*-(–)-2,2-Dichloro-*N*-[β-hydroxy-α-(hydroxymethyl)-*p*-nitrophenethyl] acetamide

Continued on next page

This product information was prepared in August, 1989. On these and other Parke-Davis Products, information may be obtained by addressing PARKE-DAVIS, Division of Warner-Lambert Company, Morris Plains, New Jersey 07950.

Parke-Davis—Cont.

CLINICAL PHARMACOLOGY

Chloramphenicol is a broad-spectrum antibiotic originally isolated from *Streptomyces venezuelae*. It is primarily bacteriostatic and acts by inhibition of protein synthesis by interfering with the transfer of activated amino acids from soluble RNA to ribosomes. It has been noted that chloramphenicol is found in measurable amounts in the aqueous humor following local application to the eye. Development of resistance to chloramphenicol can be regarded as minimal for staphylococci and many other species of bacteria.

INDICATIONS AND USAGE

Chloramphenicol should be used only in those serious infections for which less potentially dangerous drugs are ineffective or contraindicated. Bacteriological studies should be performed to determine the causative organisms and their sensitivity to chloramphenicol (See Box Warning).

Chloromycetin (chloramphenicol) Ophthalmic is indicated for the treatment of surface ocular infections involving the conjunctiva and/or cornea caused by chloramphenicol-susceptible organisms.

The particular antiinfective drug in this product is active against the following common bacterial eye pathogens:

Staphylococcus aureus
Streptococci, including *Streptococcus pneumoniae*
Escherichia coli
Haemophilus influenzae
Klebsiella/Enterobacter species
Moraxella lacunata (Morax-Axenfeld bacillus)
Neisseria species
The product does not provide adequate coverage against:
Pseudomonas aeruginosa
Serratia marcescens

CONTRAINDICATIONS

This product is contraindicated in persons sensitive to any of its components.

WARNINGS

SEE BOX WARNING

PRECAUTIONS

The prolonged use of antibiotics may occasionally result in overgrowth of nonsusceptible organisms, including fungi. If new infections appear during medication, the drug should be discontinued and appropriate measures should be taken. In all serious infections the topical use of chloramphenicol should be supplemented by appropriate systemic medication.

ADVERSE REACTIONS

Blood dyscrasias have been reported in association with the use of chloramphenicol (See WARNINGS). Transient burning or stinging sensations may occur with use of Chloromycetin Ophthalmic Solution.

DOSAGE AND ADMINISTRATION

Two drops applied to the affected eye every three hours, or more frequently if deemed advisable by the prescribing physician. Administration should be continued day and night for the first 48 hours, after which the interval between applications may be increased. Treatment should be continued for at least 48 hours after the eye appears normal.

Directions for dispensing—Prepare solution by adding sterile distilled water to the vial as follows:

Strength of solution desired	Add sterile distilled water
0.5%	5 ml
0.25%	10 ml
0.16%	15 ml

Solutions remain stable at room temperature for ten days.

HOW SUPPLIED

N 0071-3213-35 Chloromycetin (chloramphenicol) Ophthalmic is supplied in a package containing dry ingredients in a 15 ml vial and also a vial containing 15 ml of Sterile Distilled Water for use as a diluent in preparing the solution for ophthalmic use. A sterilized dropper-cap assembly for use on the vial of solution is included in the package.
Store below 30°C (86°F).
Chloromycetin, brand of chloramphenicol. Reg US Pat Off
3213G012

CHLOROMYCETIN® ℞
[chlō ″rō-my-cē ′tĭn]
OPHTHALMIC OINTMENT, 1%
(chloramphenicol ophthalmic ointment, USP)

> **WARNING**
> Bone marrow hypoplasia including aplastic anemia and death has been reported following local application of chloramphenicol. Chloramphenicol should not be used when less potentially dangerous agents would be expected to provide effective treatment.

DESCRIPTION

Each gram of Chloromycetin Ophthalmic Ointment, 1% contains 10 mg chloramphenicol in a special base of liquid petrolatum and polyethylene. It contains no preservatives. Sterile ointment.
The chemical names for chloramphenicol are:
(1) Acetamide,2,2-dichloro-*N*-[2-hydroxy-1-(hydroxymethyl)-2-(4-nitrophenyl) ethyl]-, and
(2) D-*threo*-(-)-2,2-Dichloro-*N*-[β-hydroxy-α-(hydroxymethyl)-*p*-nitrophenethyl] acetamide

CLINICAL PHARMACOLOGY

Chloramphenicol is a broad-spectrum antibiotic originally isolated from *Streptomyces venezuelae*. It is primarily bacteriostatic and acts by inhibition of protein synthesis by interfering with the transfer of activated amino acids from soluble RNA to ribosomes. It has been noted that chloramphenicol is found in measurable amounts in the aqueous humor following local application to the eye. Development of resistance to chloramphenicol can be regarded as minimal for staphylococci and many other species of bacteria.

INDICATIONS AND USAGE

Chloramphenicol should be used only in those serious infections for which less potentially dangerous drugs are ineffective or contraindicated. Bacteriological studies should be performed to determine the causative organisms and their sensitivity to chloramphenicol (See Box Warning).

Chloromycetin (chloramphenicol) Ophthalmic Ointment, 1% is indicated for the treatment of surface ocular infections involving the conjunctiva and/or cornea caused by chloramphenicol-susceptible organisms.

The particular antiinfective drug in this product is active against the following common bacterial eye pathogens:

Staphylococcus aureus
Streptococci, including *Streptococcus pneumoniae*
Escherichia coli
Haemophilus influenzae
Klebsiella/Enterobacter species
Moraxella lacunata (Morax-Axenfeld bacillus)
Neisseria species
The product does not provide adequate coverage against:
Pseudomonas aeruginosa
Serratia marcescens

CONTRAINDICATIONS

This product is contraindicated in persons sensitive to any of its components.

WARNINGS

SEE BOX WARNING
Ophthalmic ointments may retard corneal wound healing.

PRECAUTIONS

The prolonged use of antibiotics may occasionally result in overgrowth of nonsusceptible organisms, including fungi. If new infections appear during medication, the drug should be discontinued and appropriate measures should be taken. In all serious infections the topical use of chloramphenicol should be supplemented by appropriate systemic medication.

ADVERSE REACTIONS

Blood dyscrasias have been reported in association with the use of chloramphenicol (See WARNINGS).

Allergic or inflammatory reactions due to individual hypersensitivity and occasional burning or stinging may occur with the use of Chloromycetin Ophthalmic Ointment. Blood dyscrasias have been reported in association with the use of chloramphenicol (See WARNINGS).

DOSAGE AND ADMINISTRATION

A small amount of ointment placed in the lower conjunctival sac every three hours, or more frequently if deemed advisable by the prescribing physician. Administration should be continued day and night for the first 48 hours, after which the interval between applications may be increased. Treatment should be continued for at least 48 hours after the eye appears normal.

HOW SUPPLIED

N 0071-3070-07
Chloromycetin Ophthalmic Ointment, 1% (Chloramphenicol Ophthalmic Ointment, USP) is supplied, sterile, in ophthalmic ointment tubes of 3.5 grams.
Chloromycetin, brand of chloramphenicol. Reg US Pat Off
AHFS Category 52:04.04   **3070G022**

CHLOROMYCETIN® OTIC ℞
[chlō ″rō-my-cē ′tĭn ō ′-tĭc]
(chloramphenicol otic)

> **WARNING**
> Bone marrow hypoplasia including aplastic anemia and death has been reported following local application of chloramphenicol. Chloramphenicol should not be used when less potentially dangerous agents would be expected to provide effective treatment.

DESCRIPTION

Each milliliter of Chloromycetin Otic contains 5 mg (0.5%) chloramphenicol in propylene glycol. Sterile.
The chemical names for chloramphenicol are:
(1) Acetamide,2,2-dichloro -*N* - [2-hydroxy-1-(hydroxymethyl) -2- (4-nitro-phenyl) ethyl]-, and
(2) D- *threo* -(—) -2,2 -Dichloro -*N* - [β-hydroxy-α(hydroxymethyl)-*p* -nitrophenethyl]acetamide

CLINICAL PHARMACOLOGY

Chloramphenicol is a broad-spectrum antibiotic originally isolated from *Streptomyces venezuelae*. It is primarily bacteriostatic and acts by inhibition of protein synthesis by interfering with the transfer of activated amino acids from soluble RNA to ribosomes. Development of resistance to chloramphenicol can be regarded as minimal for staphylococci and many other species of bacteria.

INDICATIONS AND USAGE

Chloromycetin (chloramphenicol) Otic is indicated for the treatment of surface infections of the external auditory canal caused by susceptible strains of various gram-positive and gram-negative organisms including:
Staphylococcus aureus, *Escherichia coli*, *Hemophilus influenzae*, *Pseudomonas aeruginosa*, *Aerobacter aerogenes*, *Klebsiella pneumoniae* and *Proteus* species.
Deeper infections should be treated with appropriate systemic antibiotics.

CONTRAINDICATIONS

This product is contraindicated in persons sensitive to any of its components.
Perforated tympanic membrane is considered a contraindication to the use of any medication in the external ear canal.

WARNINGS

SEE BOX WARNING.
Discontinue promptly if sensitization or irritation occurs.

PRECAUTIONS

The prolonged use of antibiotics may occasionally result in overgrowth of nonsusceptible organisms, including fungi. If new infections appear during medication, the drug should be discontinued and appropriate measures should be taken.
In all serious infections, the topical use of chloramphenicol should be supplemented by appropriate systemic medication.
The possibility of the occurrence of ototoxicity must be considered if this product is allowed to enter the middle ear.

ADVERSE REACTION

Signs of local irritation with subjective symptoms of itching or burning, angioneurotic edema, urticaria, vesicular and maculopapular dermatitis have been reported in patients sensitive to chloramphenicol and are causes for discontinuing the medication. Similar sensitivity reactions to other materials in topical preparations may also occur. Blood dyscrasias have been reported in association with the use of chloramphenicol (See WARNINGS).

DOSAGE AND ADMINISTRATION

Instill 2 or 3 drops into the affected ear three times daily.

HOW SUPPLIED

N0071-3313-35 Chloromycetin (chloramphenicol) Otic is supplied in 15 mL vials with droppers.
Store below 30°C (86°F).
Chloromycetin, brand of chloramphenicol, Reg US Pat Off.
Caution—Federal law prohibits dispensing without prescription.
3313G023

ORAL SUSPENSION
CHLOROMYCETIN® PALMITATE ℞
[chlō″rō-my-ce´tĭn păl´mĭ-tāte″]
(chloramphenicol palmitate oral
suspension, USP)

WARNING

Serious and fatal blood dyscrasias (aplastic anemia, hypoplastic anemia, thrombocytopenia, and granulocytopenia) are known to occur after the administration of chloramphenicol. In addition, there have been reports of aplastic anemia attributed to chloramphenicol which later terminated in leukemia. Blood dyscrasias have occurred after both short-term and prolonged therapy with this drug. Chloramphenicol must not be used when less potentially dangerous agents will be effective, as described in the Indications section. *It must not be used in the treatment of trivial infections or where it is not indicated, as in colds, influenza, infections of the throat; or as a prophylactic agent to prevent bacterial infections.*

Precautions: It is essential that adequate blood studies be made during treatment with the drug. While blood studies may detect early peripheral blood changes, such as leukopenia, reticulocytopenia, or granulocytopenia, before they become irreversible, such studies cannot be relied on to detect bone marrow depression prior to development of aplastic anemia. To facilitate appropriate studies and observation during therapy, it is desirable that patients be hospitalized.

DESCRIPTION

Chloromycetin Palmitate Oral Suspension contains chloramphenicol palmitate equivalent to 150 mg chloramphenicol per 5 mL. Also contains alcohol, USP; carboxymethylcellulose sodium, USP; citric acid, USP; custard flavor, imitation; glycerin, USP; povidone, USP; propylene glycol, USP; sodium benzoate, NF; sorbitan monolaurate, NF; sucrose, NF; veegum, HV; purified water, USP.

Chloramphenicol is an antibiotic that is clinically useful for, *and should be reserved for,* serious infections caused by organisms susceptible to its antimicrobial effects when less potentially hazardous therapeutic agents are ineffective or contraindicated. Sensitivity testing is essential to determine its indicated use, but may be performed concurrently with therapy initiated on clinical impression that one of the indicated conditions exists (see Indications section).

CLINICAL PHARMACOLOGY

In vitro chloramphenicol exerts mainly a bacteriostatic effect on a wide range of gram-negative and gram-positive bacteria and is active *in vitro* against rickettsiae, the lymphogranuloma-psittacosis group and *Vibrio cholerae.* It is particularly active against *Salmonella typhi* and *Hemophilus influenzae.* The mode of action is through interference or inhibition of protein synthesis in intact cells and in cell-free systems.

Chloramphenicol administered orally is absorbed rapidly from the intestinal tract. In controlled studies in adult volunteers using the recommended dosage of 50 mg/kg/day, a dosage of 1 g every 6 hours for 8 doses was given. Using the microbiological assay method, the average peak serum level was 11.2 mcg/ml one hour after the first dose.

A cumulative effect gave a peak rise to 18.4 mcg/ml after the fifth dose of 1 g. Mean serum levels ranged from 8 to 14 mcg/ml over the 48-hour period. Total urinary excretion of chloramphenicol in these studies ranged from a low of 68% to a high of 99% over a three-day period. From 8% to 12% of the antibiotic excreted is in the form of free chloramphenicol; the remainder consists of microbiologically inactive metabolites, principally the conjugate with glucuronic acid. Since the glucuronide is excreted rapidly, most chloramphenicol detected in the blood is in the microbiologically active free form. Despite the small proportion of unchanged drug excreted in the urine, the concentration of free chloramphenicol is relatively high, amounting to several hundred mcg/ml in patients receiving divided doses of 50 mg/kg/day. Small amounts of active drug are found in bile and feces. Chloramphenicol diffuses rapidly, but its distribution is not uniform. Highest concentrations are found in liver and kidney, and lowest concentrations are found in brain and cerebrospinal fluid. Chloramphenicol enters cerebrospinal fluid even in the absence of meningeal inflammation, appearing in concentrations about half of those found in the blood. Measurable levels are also detected in pleural and in ascitic fluids, saliva, milk and in the aqueous and vitreous humors. Transport across the placental barrier occurs with somewhat lower concentration in cord blood of newborn infants than in maternal blood.

INDICATIONS AND USAGE

In accord with the concepts in the Warning Box and this Indications section, chloramphenicol must be used only in those serious infections for which less potentially dangerous drugs are ineffective or contraindicated. However, chloramphenicol may be chosen to initiate antibiotic therapy on the clinical impression that one of the conditions below is believed to be present; *in vitro* sensitivity tests should be performed concurrently so that the drug may be discontinued as soon as possible if less potentially dangerous agents are indicated by such tests. The decision to continue use of chloramphenicol rather than another antibiotic when both are suggested by *in vitro* studies to be effective against a specific pathogen should be based upon severity of the infection, susceptibility of the pathogen to the various antimicrobial drugs, efficacy of the various drugs in the infection, and the important additional concepts contained in the Warning Box above.

1. **Acute infections caused by *Salmonella typhi***
Chloramphenicol is a drug of choice.* It is not recommended for the routine treatment of the typhoid carrier state.
2. **Serious infections caused by susceptible strains in accordance with the concepts expressed above:**
   a. Salmonella species
   b. *H influenzae,* specifically meningeal infections
   c. Rickettsia
   d. Lymphogranuloma-psittacosis group
   e. Various gram-negative bacteria causing bacteremia, meningitis or other serious gram-negative infections
   f. Other susceptible organisms which have been demonstrated to be resistant to all other appropriate antimicrobial agents.
3. **Cystic fibrosis regimens**

* In the treatment of typhoid fever some authorities recommend that chloramphenicol be administered at therapeutic levels for 8 to 10 days after the patient has become afebrile to lessen the possibility of relapse.

CONTRAINDICATIONS

Chloramphenicol is contraindicated in individuals with a history of previous hypersensitivity and/or toxic reaction to it. *It must not be used in the treatment of trivial infections or where it is not indicated, as in colds, influenza, infections of the throat; or as a prophylactic agent to prevent bacterial infections.*

PRECAUTIONS

1. Baseline blood studies should be followed by periodic blood studies approximately every two days during therapy. The drug should be discontinued upon appearance of reticulocytopenia, leukopenia, thrombocytopenia, anemia, or any other blood study findings attributable to chloramphenicol. However, it should be noted that such studies do not exclude the possible later appearance of the irreversible type of bone marrow depression.
2. Repeated courses of the drug should be avoided if at all possible. Treatment should not be continued longer than required to produce a cure with little or no risk of relapse of the disease.
3. Concurrent therapy with other drugs that may cause bone marrow depression should be avoided.
4. Excessive blood levels may result from administration of the recommended dose to patients with impaired liver or kidney function, including that due to immature metabolic processes in the infant. The dosage should be adjusted accordingly or, preferably, the blood concentration should be determined at appropriate intervals.
5. There are no studies to establish the safety of this drug in pregnancy.
6. Since chloramphenicol readily crosses the placental barrier, caution in use of the drug is particularly important during pregnancy at term or during labor because of potential toxic effects on the fetus (gray syndrome).
7. Precaution should be used in therapy of premature and full-term infants to avoid "gray syndrome" toxicity. (See "Adverse Reactions.") Serum drug levels should be carefully followed during therapy of the newborn infant.
8. Precaution should be used in therapy during lactation because of the possibility of toxic effects on the nursing infant.
9. The use of this antibiotic, as with other antibiotics, may result in an overgrowth of nonsusceptible organisms, including fungi. If infections caused by nonsusceptible organisms appear during therapy, appropriate measures should be taken.

ADVERSE REACTIONS

1. **Blood Dyscrasias**
The most serious adverse effect of chloramphenicol is bone marrow depression. Serious and fatal blood dyscrasias (aplastic anemia, hypoplastic anemia, thrombocytopenia, and granulocytopenia) are known to occur after the administration of chloramphenicol. An irreversible type of marrow depression leading to aplastic anemia with a high rate of mortality is characterized by the appearance weeks or months after therapy of bone marrow aplasia or hypoplasia. Peripherally, pancytopenia is most often observed, but in a small number of cases only one or two of the three major cell types (erythrocytes, leukocytes, platelets) may be depressed.

A reversible type of bone marrow depression, which is dose related, may occur. This type of marrow depression is characterized by vacuolization of the erythroid cells, reduction of reticulocytes and leukopenia, and responds promptly to the withdrawal of chloramphenicol.

An exact determination of the risk of serious and fatal blood dyscrasias is not possible because of lack of accurate information regarding 1) the size of the population at risk, 2) the total number of drug-associated dyscrasias, and 3) the total number of nondrug associated dyscrasias.

In a report to the California State Assembly by the California Medical Association and the State Department of Public Health in January 1967, the risk of fatal aplastic anemia was estimated at 1:24,200 to 1:40,500 based on two dosage levels. There have been reports of aplastic anemia attributed to chloramphenicol which later terminated in leukemia. Paroxysmal nocturnal hemoglobinuria has also been reported.

2. **Gastrointestinal Reactions**
Nausea, vomiting, glossitis and stomatitis, diarrhea and enterocolitis may occur in low incidence.
3. **Neurotoxic Reactions**
Headache, mild depression, mental confusion and delirium have been described in patients receiving chloramphenicol. Optic and peripheral neuritis have been reported, usually following long-term therapy. If this occurs, the drug should be promptly withdrawn.
4. **Hypersensitivity Reactions**
Fever, macular and vesicular rashes, angioedema, urticaria and anaphylaxis may occur. Herxheimer reactions have occurred during therapy for typhoid fever.
5. **"Gray Syndrome"**
Toxic reactions including fatalities have occurred in the premature and newborn, the signs and symptoms associated with these reactions have been referred to as the gray syndrome. One case of gray syndrome has been reported in an infant born to a mother having received chloramphenicol during labor. One case has been reported in a 3-month-old infant. The following summarizes the clinical and laboratory studies that have been made on these patients.
   (a) In most cases therapy with chloramphenicol had been instituted within the first 48 hours of life.
   (b) Symptoms first appeared after 3 to 4 days of continued treatment with high doses of chloramphenicol
   (c) The symptoms appeared in the following order:
      1) abdominal distention with or without emesis;
      2) progressive pallid cyanosis;
      3) vasomotor collapse, frequently accompanied by irregular respiration;
      4) death within a few hours of onset of these symptoms.
   (d) The progression of symptoms from onset to exitus was accelerated with higher dose schedules.
   (e) Preliminary blood serum level studies revealed unusually high concentrations of chloramphenicol (over 90 mcg/ml after repeated doses).
   (f) Termination of therapy upon early evidence of the associated symptomatology frequently reversed the process with complete recovery.

DOSAGE AND ADMINISTRATION

Dosage Recommendations
The majority of microorganisms susceptible to chloramphenicol will respond to a concentration between 5 and 20 mcg/ml. The desired concentration of active drug in blood should fall within this range over most of the treatment period. Dosage of 50 mg/kg/day divided into 4 doses at intervals of 6 hours will usually achieve and sustain levels of this magnitude.

Except in certain circumstances (eg. premature and newborn infants and individuals with impairment of hepatic or renal function) lower doses may not achieve these concentrations. Chloramphenicol, like other potent drugs, should be prescribed at recommended doses known to have therapeutic activity. Close observation of the patient should be maintained and in the event of any adverse reactions, dosage should be reduced or the drug discontinued, if other factors in the clinical situation permit.

Adults
Adults should receive 50 mg/kg/day in divided doses at 6-hour intervals. In exceptional cases patients with infections due to moderately resistant organisms may require increased dosage up to 100 mg/kg/day to achieve blood levels inhibiting the pathogen, but these high doses should be decreased as soon as possible. Adults with impairment of hepatic or renal function or both may have reduced ability to metabolize and excrete the drug. In instances of impaired metabolic processes, dosages should be adjusted accordingly.

Continued on next page

This product information was prepared in August, 1989. On these and other Parke-Davis Products, information may be obtained by addressing PARKE-DAVIS, Division of Warner-Lambert Company, Morris Plains, New Jersey 07950.

Parke-Davis—Cont.

(See discussion under Newborn Infants.) Precise control of concentration of the drug in the blood should be carefully followed in patients with impaired metabolic processes by the available microtechniques (information available on request).

Children

Dosage of 50 mg/kg/day divided into 4 doses at 6-hour intervals yields blood levels in the range effective against most susceptible organisms. Severe infections (eg. bacteremia or meningitis), especially when adequate cerebrospinal fluid concentrations are desired, may require dosage up to 100 mg/kg/day; however, it is recommended that dosage be reduced to 50 mg/kg/day as soon as possible. Children with impaired liver or kidney function may retain excessive amounts of the drug.

Newborn Infants

(See section titled "Gray Syndrome" under Adverse Reactions.)

A total of 25 mg/kg/day in 4 equal doses at 6-hour intervals usually produces and maintains concentrations in blood and tissues adequate to control most infections for which the drug is indicated. Increased dosage in these individuals, demanded by severe infections, should be given only to maintain the blood concentration within a therapeutically effective range. After the first two weeks of life, full-term infants ordinarily may receive up to a total of 50 mg/kg/day equally divided into 4 doses at 6-hour intervals. *These dosage recommendations are extremely important because blood concentration in all premature infants and full-term infants under two weeks of age differs from that of other infants.* This difference is due to variations in the maturity of the metabolic functions of the liver and the kidneys.

When these functions are immature (or seriously impaired in adults), high concentrations of the drug are found which tend to increase with succeeding doses.

Infants and Children with Immature Metabolic Processes

In young infants and other children in whom immature metabolic functions are suspected, a dose of 25 mg/kg/day will usually produce therapeutic concentrations of the drug in the blood. In this group particularly, the concentration of the drug in the blood should be carefully followed by microtechniques. (Information available on request.)

HOW SUPPLIED

N 0071-2310-15

Oral Suspension Chloromycetin Palmitate (Chloramphenicol Palmitate Oral Suspension, USP), each 5 ml contains chloramphenicol palmitate equivalent to 150 mg chloramphenicol with 0.5% sodium benzoate as preservative, in bottles of 60 ml.

Chloramphenicol Palmitate is hydrolyzed to chloramphenicol before absorption. Resulting blood concentration is similar to that produced by the oral administration of chloramphenicol.

Chloromycetin, brand of chloramphenicol. Reg. US Pat Off
                               2310G042

Caution—Federal law prohibits dispensing without prescription.

CHLOROMYCETIN®   ℞

[chlō"rō-my-cē"tĭn sŭc'cĭ-nāte"]

SODIUM SUCCINATE
(sterile chloramphenicol
sodium succinate, USP)
FOR INTRAVENOUS ADMINISTRATION

WARNING

Serious and fatal blood dyscrasias (aplastic anemia, hypoplastic anemia, thrombocytopenia, and granulocytopenia) are known to occur after the administration of chloramphenicol. In addition, there have been reports of aplastic anemia attributed to chloramphenicol which later terminated in leukemia. Blood dyscrasias have occurred after both short-term and prolonged therapy with this drug. Chloramphenicol must not be used when less potentially dangerous agents will be effective, as described in the Indications section. *It must not be used in the treatment of trivial infections or where it is not indicated, as in colds, influenza, infections of the throat; or as a prophylactic agent to prevent bacterial infections.*

Precautions: It is essential that adequate blood studies be made during treatment with the drug. While blood studies may detect early peripheral blood changes, such as leukopenia, reticulocytopenia, or granulocytopenia, before they become irreversible, such studies cannot be relied on to detect bone marrow depression prior to development of aplastic anemia. To facilitate appropriate

---

studies and observation during therapy, it is desirable that patients be hospitalized.

IMPORTANT CONSIDERATIONS IN PRESCRIBING INJECTABLE CHLORAMPHENICOL SODIUM SUCCINATE CHLORAMPHENICOL SODIUM SUCCINATE IS INTENDED FOR INTRAVENOUS USE ONLY. IT HAS BEEN DEMONSTRATED TO BE INEFFECTIVE WHEN GIVEN INTRAMUSCULARLY.

1. Chloramphenicol sodium succinate must be hydrolyzed to its microbiologically active form and there is a lag in achieving adequate blood levels compared with the base given intravenously.

2. The oral form of chloramphenicol is readily absorbed and adequate blood levels are achieved and maintained on the recommended dosage.

3. Patients started on intravenous chloramphenicol sodium succinate should be changed to the oral form as soon as practicable.

DESCRIPTION

Chloramphenicol is an antibiotic that is clinically useful for, *and should be reserved for,* serious infections caused by organisms susceptible to its antimicrobial effects when less potentially hazardous therapeutic agents are ineffective or contraindicated. Sensitivity testing is essential to determine its indicated use, but may be performed concurrently with therapy initiated on clinical impression that one of the indicated conditions exists (see Indications section).

Each gram (10 ml of a 10% solution) of chloramphenicol sodium succinate contains approximately 52 mg (2.25 mEq) of sodium.

ACTIONS AND PHARMACOLOGY

In vitro chloramphenicol exerts mainly a bacteriostatic effect on a wide range of gram-negative and gram-positive bacteria and is active *in vitro* against rickettsiae, the lymphogranuloma-psittacosis group, and *Vibrio cholerae.* It is particularly active against *Salmonella typhi* and *Hemophilus influenzae.* The mode of action is through interference or inhibition of protein synthesis in intact cells and in cell-free systems.

Chloramphenicol administered orally is absorbed rapidly from the intestinal tract. In controlled studies in adult volunteers using the recommended dosage of 50 mg/kg/day, a dosage of 1 g every 6 hours for 8 doses was given. Using the microbiological assay method, the average peak serum level was 11.2 mcg/ml one hour after the first dose. A cumulative effect gave a peak rise to 18.4 mcg/ml after the fifth dose of 1 g. Mean serum levels ranged from 8 to 14 mcg/ml over the 48-hour period. Total urinary excretion of chloramphenicol in these studies ranged from a low of 68% to a high of 99% over a three-day period. From 8 to 12% of the antibiotic excreted is in the form of free chloramphenicol; the remainder consists of microbiologically inactive metabolites, principally the conjugate with glucuronic acid. Since the glucuronide is excreted rapidly, most chloramphenicol detected in the blood is in the microbiologically active free form. Despite the small proportion of unchanged drug excreted in the urine, the concentration of free chloramphenicol is relatively high, amounting to several hundred mcg/ml in patients receiving divided doses of 50 mg/kg/day. Small amounts of active drug are found in bile and feces. Chloramphenicol diffuses rapidly, but its distribution is not uniform. Highest concentrations are found in liver and kidney, and lowest concentrations are found in brain and cerebrospinal fluid. Chloramphenicol enters cerebrospinal fluid even in the absence of meningeal inflammation, appearing in concentrations about half of those found in the blood. Measurable levels are also detected in pleural and in ascitic fluids, saliva, milk, and in the aqueous and vitreous humors. Transport across the placental barrier occurs with somewhat lower concentration in cord blood of newborn infants than in maternal blood.

INDICATIONS

In accord with the concepts in the warning box and this Indications section, chloramphenicol must be used only in those serious infections for which less potentially dangerous drugs are ineffective or contraindicated. However, chloramphenicol may be chosen to initiate antibiotic therapy on the clinical impression that one of the conditions below is believed to be present; in vitro sensitivity tests should be performed concurrently so that the drug may be discontinued as soon as possible if less potentially dangerous agents are indicated by such tests. The decision to continue use of chloramphenicol rather than another antibiotic when both are suggested by in vitro studies to be effective against a specific pathogen should be based upon severity of the infection, susceptibility of the pathogen to the various antimicrobial drugs, efficacy of the various drugs in the infection, and the important additional concepts contained in the Warning Box above:

1. Acute infections caused by *S typhi**

It is not recommended for the routine treatment of the typhoid carrier state.

---

2. Serious infections caused by susceptible strains in accordance with the concepts expressed above:
   a. *Salmonella* species
   b. *H influenzae,* specifically meningeal infections
   c. Rickettsia
   d. Lymphogranuloma-psittacosis group
   e. Various gram-negative bacteria causing bacteremia, meningitis, or other serious gram-negative infections
   f. Other susceptible organisms which have been demonstrated to be resistant to all other appropriate antimicrobial agents.

3. **Cystic fibrosis regimens**

---

*In the treatment of typhoid fever, some authorities recommend that chloramphenicol be administered at therapeutic levels for 8 to 10 days after the patient has become afebrile to lessen the possibility of relapse.

CONTRAINDICATIONS

Chloramphenicol is contraindicated in individuals with a history of previous hypersensitivity and/or toxic reaction to it. *It must not be used in the treatment of trivial infections or where it is not indicated, as in colds, influenza, infections of the throat; or as a prophylactic agent to prevent bacterial infection.*

PRECAUTIONS

1. Baseline blood studies should be followed by periodic blood studies approximately every two days during therapy. The drug should be discontinued upon appearance of reticulocytopenia, leukopenia, thrombocytopenia, anemia, or any other blood study findings attributable to chloramphenicol. However, it should be noted that such studies do not exclude the possible later appearance of the irreversible type of bone marrow depression.

2. Repeated courses of the drug should be avoided if at all possible. Treatment should not be continued longer than required to produce a cure with little or no risk of relapse of the disease.

3. Concurrent therapy with other drugs that may cause bone marrow depression should be avoided.

4. Excessive blood levels may result from administration of the recommended dosage to patients with impaired liver or kidney function, including that due to immature metabolic processes in the infant. The dosage should be adjusted accordingly or, preferably, the blood concentration should be determined at appropriate intervals.

5. There are no studies to establish the safety of this drug in pregnancy.

6. Since chloramphenicol readily crosses the placental barrier, caution in use of the drug is particularly important during pregnancy at term or during labor because of potential toxic effects on the fetus (gray syndrome).

7. Precaution should be used in therapy of premature and full-term infants to avoid gray syndrome toxicity (see Adverse Reactions). Serum drug levels should be carefully followed during therapy of the newborn infant.

8. Precaution should be used in therapy during lactation because of the possibility of toxic effects on the nursing infant.

9. The use of this antibiotic, as with other antibiotics, may result in an overgrowth of nonsusceptible organisms, including fungi. If infections caused by nonsusceptible organisms appear during therapy, appropriate measures should be taken.

ADVERSE REACTIONS

1. Blood Dyscrasias

The most serious adverse effect of chloramphenicol is bone marrow depression. Serious and fatal blood dyscrasias (aplastic anemia, hypoplastic anemia, thrombocytopenia, and granulocytopenia) are known to occur after the administration of chloramphenicol. An irreversible type of marrow depression leading to aplastic anemia with a high rate of mortality is characterized by the appearance weeks or months after therapy of bone marrow aplasia or hypoplasia. Peripherally, pancytopenia is most often observed, but in a small number of cases only one or two of the three major cell types (erythrocytes, leukocytes, platelets) may be depressed. A reversible type of bone marrow depression, which is dose-related, may occur. This type of marrow depression is characterized by vacuolization of the erythroid cells, reduction of reticulocytes, and leukopenia, and responds promptly to the withdrawal of chloramphenicol.

An exact determination of the risk of serious and fatal blood dyscrasias is not possible because of lack of accurate information regarding (1) the size of the population at risk, (2) the total number of drug-associated dyscrasias, and (3) the total number of nondrug-associated dyscrasias.

In a report to the California State Assembly by the California Medical Association and the State Department of Public Health in January 1967, the risk of fatal aplastic anemia was estimated at 1:24,200 to 1:40,500 based on two dosage levels. There have been reports of aplastic anemia attributed to chloramphenicol which later terminated in leukemia.

Paroxysmal nocturnal hemoglobinuria has also been reported.

2. Gastrointestinal Reactions

Nausea, vomiting, glossitis and stomatitis, diarrhea, and enterocolitis may occur in low incidence.

3. Neurotoxic Reactions

Headache, mild depression, mental confusion, and delirium have been described in patients receiving chloramphenicol. Optic and peripheral neuritis have been reported, usually following long-term therapy. If this occurs, the drug should be promptly withdrawn.

4. Hypersensitivity Reactions

Fever, macular and vesicular rashes, angio- edema, urticaria, and anaphylaxis may occur. Herxheimer reactions have occurred during therapy for typhoid fever.

5. "Gray Syndrome"

Toxic reactions including fatalities have occurred in the premature and newborn; the signs and symptoms associated with these reactions have been referred to as the gray syndrome. One case of gray syndrome has been reported in an infant born to a mother having received chloramphenicol during labor. One case has been reported in a 3-month-old infant. The following summarizes the clinical and laboratory studies that have been made on these patients:

a) In most cases, therapy with chloramphenicol had been instituted within the first 48 hours of life.

b) Symptoms first appeared after 3 to 4 days of continued treatment with high doses of chloramphenicol.

c) The symptoms appeared in the following order:
   (1) abdominal distention with or without emesis;
   (2) progressive pallid cyanosis;
   (3) vasomotor collapse, frequently accompanied by irregular respiration;
   (4) death within a few hours of onset of these symptoms.

d) The progression of symptoms from onset to exitus was accelerated with higher dose schedules.

e) Preliminary blood serum level studies revealed unusually high concentrations of chloramphenicol (over 90 mcg/ml after repeated doses).

f) Termination of therapy upon early evidence of the associated symptomatology frequently reversed the process with complete recovery.

ADMINISTRATION

Chloramphenicol, like other potent drugs, should be prescribed at recommended doses known to have therapeutic activity. Administration of 50 mg/kg/day in divided doses will produce blood levels of the magnitude to which the majority of susceptible microorganisms will respond.

As soon as feasible, an oral dosage form of chloramphenicol should be substituted for the intravenous form because adequate blood levels are achieved with chloramphenicol by mouth.

The following method of administration is recommended: Intravenously as a 10% (100 mg/ml) solution to be injected over at least a one-minute interval. This is prepared by the addition of 10 ml of an aqueous diluent, such as water for injection or 5% dextrose injection.

DOSAGE

Adults

Adults should receive 50 mg/kg/day in divided doses at 6-hour intervals. In exceptional cases, patients with infections due to moderately resistant organisms may require increased dosage up to 100 mg/kg/day to achieve blood levels inhibiting the pathogen, but these high doses should be decreased as soon as possible. Adults with impairment of hepatic or renal function or both may have reduced ability to metabolize and excrete the drug. In instances of impaired metabolic processes, dosages should be adjusted accordingly. (See discussion under Newborn Infants.) Precise control of concentration of the drug in the blood should be carefully followed in patients with impaired metabolic processes by the available microtechniques (information available on request).

Children

Dosage of 50 mg/kg/day divided into 4 doses at 6-hour intervals yields blood levels in the range effective against most susceptible organisms. Severe infections (eg, bacteremia or meningitis), especially when adequate cerebrospinal fluid concentrations are desired, may require dosage up to 100 mg/kg/day; however, it is recommended that dosage be reduced to 50 mg/kg/day as soon as possible. Children with impaired liver or kidney function may retain excessive amounts of the drug.

Newborn Infants

(See section titled Gray Syndrome under Adverse Reactions.)

A total of 25 mg/kg/day in 4 equal doses at 6-hour intervals usually produces and maintains concentrations in blood and tissues adequate to control most infections for which the drug is indicated. Increased dosage in these individuals, demanded by severe infections, should be given only to maintain the blood concentration within a therapeutically effective range. After the first two weeks of life, full-term infants ordinarily may receive up to a total of 50 mg/kg/day equally divided into 4 doses at 6-hour intervals. *These dosage recommendations are extremely important because blood concentration in all premature infants and full-term infants under two weeks of age differs from that of other infants.* This difference is due to variations in the maturity of the metabolic functions of the liver and the kidneys.

When these functions are immature (or seriously impaired in adults), high concentrations of the drug are found which tend to increase with succeeding doses.

Infants and Children with Immature Metabolic Processes

In young infants and other children in whom immature metabolic functions are suspected, a dose of 25 mg/kg/day will usually produce therapeutic concentrations of the drug in the blood. In this group particularly, the concentration of the drug in the blood should be carefully followed by microtechniques. (Information available on request.)

HOW SUPPLIED

N 0071-4057-03—(Steri-Vial® No. 57) Chloromycetin Sodium Succinate (Chloramphenicol Sodium Succinate for Injection, USP) is freeze-dried in the vial and supplied in Steri-Vials (rubber diaphragm-capped vials). When reconstituted as directed, each vial contains a sterile solution equivalent to 100 mg of chloramphenicol per milliliter (1 g/10 ml). Available in packages of 10 vials.

Chloromycetin, brand of chloramphenicol, Reg US Pat Off

AHFS 8:12.08   **4057G020**

CHOLEDYL®   ℞

[clō'lĕ-dyl"]

Elixir

(oxtriphylline, USP)

DESCRIPTION

Choledyl (oxtriphylline) is the choline salt of theophylline. Theophylline is a bronchodilator structurally classified as a xanthine derivative. It occurs as a white, odorless, crystalline powder having a bitter taste. Theophylline anhydrous has the chemical name $1H$-Purine-2, 6-dione, 3,7-dihydro-1,3-dimethyl-. The molecular weight of oxtriphylline is 283.33; the empirical formula is $C_{12}H_{21}N_5O_3$.

Each 5 mL teaspoonful of elixir contains 100 mg oxtriphylline; alcohol 20%. Also contains citric acid, USP; D&C green No. 5; D&C yellow No. 10; FD&C red No. 40; flavor; glycerin, USP, saccharin sodium, USP; sodium chloride, USP; sodium citrate, USP; sorbitol solution, USP; sucrose NF; and purified water, USP. Note: 100 mg oxtriphylline is equivalent to 64 mg anhydrous theophylline.

CLINICAL PHARMACOLOGY

Theophylline directly relaxes the smooth muscle of the bronchial airways and pulmonary blood vessels, thus acting mainly as a bronchodilator and smooth muscle relaxant. It has also been demonstrated that aminophylline has a potent effect on diaphragmatic contractility in normal persons and may then be capable of reducing fatigability and thereby improve contractility in patients with chronic obstructive airways disease. The exact mode of action remains unsettled. Although theophylline does cause inhibition of phosphodiesterase with a resultant increase in intracellular cyclic AMP, other agents similarly inhibit the enzyme producing a rise of cyclic AMP but are unassociated with any demonstrable bronchodilation. Other mechanisms proposed include an effect on translocation of intracellular calcium; prostaglandin antagonism; stimulation of catecholamines endogenously; inhibition of cyclic guanosine monophosphate metabolism and adenosine receptor antagonism. None of these mechanisms has been proved, however.

In vitro, theophylline has been shown to act synergistically with beta agonists and there are now available data which do demonstrate an additive effect in vivo with combined use.

Pharmacokinetics:

The half-life of theophylline is influenced by a number of known variables. It may be prolonged in chronic alcoholics, particularly those with liver disease (cirrhosis or alcoholic liver disease), in patients with congestive heart failure, and in those patients taking certain other drugs (see PRECAUTIONS, Drug Interactions). Newborns and neonates have extremely slow clearance rates compared to older infants and children, ie, those over 1 year. Older children have rapid clearance rates while most nonsmoking adults have clearance rates between these two extremes. In premature neonates the decreased clearance is related to oxidative pathways that have yet to be established.

Theophylline Elimination Characteristics

	Half-Life (in hours)	
	Range	Mean
Children	1–9	3.7
Adults	3–15	7.7

In cigarette smokers (1–2 packs/day) the mean half-life is 4–5 hours, much shorter than in nonsmokers. The increase in clearance associated with smoking is presumably due to stimulation of the hepatic metabolic pathway by components of cigarette smoke. The duration of this effect after cessation of smoking is unknown but may require 6 months to 2 years before the rate approaches that of the nonsmoker.

INDICATIONS AND USAGE

Choledyl (oxtriphylline) is indicated for relief and/or prevention of symptoms from asthma and reversible bronchospasm associated with chronic bronchitis and emphysema.

CONTRAINDICATIONS

Choledyl is contraindicated in individuals who have shown hypersensitivity to its components. It is also contraindicated in patients with active peptic ulcer disease, and in individuals with underlying seizure disorders (unless receiving appropriate anticonvulsant medication).

WARNINGS

Serum levels above 20 mcg/mL are rarely found after appropriate administration of the recommended doses. However, in individuals in whom theophylline plasma clearance is reduced for any reason, even conventional doses may result in increased serum levels and potential toxicity. Reduced theophylline clearance has been documented in the following readily identifiable groups: 1) patients with impaired liver function; 2) patients over 55 years of age, particularly males and those with chronic lung disease; 3) those with cardiac failure from any cause; 4) patients with sustained high fever; 5) neonates and infants under 1 year of age; and 6) those patients taking certain drugs (see PRECAUTIONS, Drug Interactions). Frequently, such patients have markedly prolonged theophylline serum levels following discontinuation of the drug.

Reduction of dosage and laboratory monitoring is especially appropriate in the above individuals.

Serious side effects such as ventricular arrhythmias, convulsions or even death may appear as the first sign of toxicity without any previous warning. Less serious signs of theophylline toxicity (ie, nausea and restlessness) may occur frequently when initiating therapy, but are usually transient; when such signs are persistent during maintenance therapy, they are often associated with serum concentrations above 20 mcg/mL. Stated differently; serious toxicity is not reliably preceded by less severe side effects. A serum concentration measurement is the only reliable method of predicting potentially life-threatening toxicity.

Many patients who require theophylline exhibit tachycardia due to their underlying disease process so that the cause/effect relationship to elevated serum theophylline concentrations may not be appreciated.

Theophylline products may cause dysrhythmia and/or worsen preexisting arrhythmias and any significant change in rate and/or rhythm warrants monitoring and further investigation.

Studies in laboratory animals (minipigs, rodents, and dogs) recorded the occurrence of cardiac arrhythmias and sudden death (with histologic evidence of myocardial necrosis) when beta-agonists and methylxanthines were administered concurrently. The significance of these findings when applied to humans is currently unknown.

PRECAUTIONS

General:

On the average, theophylline half-life is shorter in cigarette and marijuana smokers than in nonsmokers, but smokers can have half-lives as long as nonsmokers. Theophylline should not be administered concurrently with other xanthines. Use with caution in patients with hypoxemia, hypertension, or those with history of peptic ulcer. Theophylline may occasionally act as a local irritant to the GI tract although gastrointestinal symptoms are more commonly centrally mediated and associated with serum drug concentrations over 20 mcg/mL.

Information for Patients:

The importance of taking only the prescribed dose and time interval between doses should be reinforced.

Laboratory Tests:

Serum levels should be monitored periodically to determine the theophylline level associated with observed clinical response and as the method of predicting toxicity. For such measurements, the serum sample should be obtained at the time of peak concentration, 1 to 2 hours after administration for immediate release products. It is important that the patient will not have missed or taken additional doses during the previous 48 hours and that dosing intervals will have been reasonably equally spaced. DOSAGE ADJUSTMENT BASED ON SERUM THEOPHYLLINE MEASUREMENTS WHEN THESE INSTRUCTIONS HAVE NOT BEEN FOL-

Continued on next page

This product information was prepared in August, 1989. On these and other Parke-Davis Products, information may be obtained by addressing PARKE-DAVIS, Division of Warner-Lambert Company, Morris Plains, New Jersey 07950.

Parke-Davis—Cont.

LOWED MAY RESULT IN RECOMMENDATIONS THAT PRESENT RISK OF TOXICITY TO THE PATIENT.

Drug Interactions:

Toxic synergism with ephedrine has been documented and may occur with other sympathomimetic bronchodilators. In addition, the following drug interactions have been demonstrated:

Theophylline with:

Allopurinol (high-dose)	Increased serum theophylline levels
Cimetidine	Increased serum theophylline levels
Erythromycin, Troleandomycin	Increased serum theophylline levels
Lithium Carbonate	Increased renal excretion of lithium
Oral Contraceptives	Increased serum theophylline levels
Phenytoin	Decreased theophylline and phenytoin serum levels
Rifampin	Decreased serum theophylline levels

Drug-Laboratory Test Interactions:

Currently available analytical methods, including high pressure liquid chromatography and immunoassay techniques, for measuring serum theophylline levels are specific. Metabolites and other drugs generally do not affect the results. Other new analytic methods are also now in use. The physician should be aware of the laboratory method used and whether other drugs will interfere with the assay for theophylline.

Carcinogenesis, Mutagenesis, and Impairment of Fertility:

Long-term carcinogenicity studies have not been performed with theophylline.

Chromosome-breaking activity was detected in human cell cultures at concentrations of theophylline up to 50 times the therapeutic serum concentration in humans. Theophylline was not mutagenic in the dominant lethal assay in male mice given theophylline intraperitoneally in doses up to 30 times the maximum daily oral dose.

Studies to determine the effect on fertility have not been performed with theophylline.

Pregnancy:

Category C—Animal reproduction studies have not been conducted with oxtriphylline. It is not known whether theophylline can cause fetal harm when administered to a pregnant woman or can affect reproduction capacity. Oxtriphylline should be given to a pregnant woman only if clearly needed.

Nursing Mothers:

Theophylline is distributed into breast milk and may cause irritability or other signs of toxicity in nursing infants. Because of the potential for serious adverse reactions in nursing infants from theophylline, a decision should be made whether to discontinue nursing or to discontinue the drug, taking into account the importance of the drug to the mother.

Pediatric Use:

Sufficient numbers of infants under the age of 1 year have not been studied in clinical trials to support use in this age group; however there is evidence recorded that the use of dosage recommendations for older infants and young children (16 mg/kg/24 hours) may result in the development of toxic serum levels. Such findings very probably reflect differences in the metabolic handling of the drug related to absent or undeveloped enzyme systems. Consequently, the use of the drug in this age group should carefully consider the associated benefits and risks. If used, the maintenance dose must be conservative and in accord with the following guidelines:

Initial Theophylline Maintenance Dosage:

Premature Infants:

Up to 24 days postnatal age—1 mg/kg q 12h

Beyond 24 days postnatal age—1.5 mg/kg q 12h

Infants 6 to 52 Weeks:

$[(0.2 \times \text{age in weeks}) + 5.0] \times \text{kg body wt} = 24$ hour dose in mg.

Up to 26 weeks, divided into q8h dosing intervals.

From 26–52 weeks, divide into q6h dosing intervals.

Final dosage should be guided by serum concentration after a steady state (no further accumulation of drug) has been achieved.

ADVERSE REACTIONS

The following adverse reactions have been observed, but there has not been enough systematic collection of data to support an estimate of their frequency. The most consistent adverse reactions are usually due to overdosage.

1. **Gastrointestinal:** nausea, vomiting, epigastric pain, hematemesis, diarrhea.
2. **Central nervous system:** headaches, irritability, restlessness, insomnia, reflex hyperexcitability, muscle twitching, clonic and tonic generalized convulsions.
3. **Cardiovascular:** palpitation, tachycardia, extrasystoles, flushing, hypotension, circulatory failure, ventricular arrhythmias.
4. **Respiratory:** tachypnea.
5. **Renal:** potentiation of diuresis.
6. **Others:** alopecia, hyperglycemia, inappropriate ADH syndrome, rash.

OVERDOSAGE

Management: It is suggested that the management principles (consistent with the clinical status of the patient when first seen) outlined below be instituted and that simultaneous contact with a Regional Poison Control Center be established. In this way both updated information and individualization regarding required therapy may be provided.

1. **When potential oral overdose is established and seizure has not occurred:**
   a) If patient is alert and seen within the early hours after ingestion, induction of emesis may be of value. Gastric lavage has been demonstrated to be of no value in influencing outcome in patients who present more than 1 hour after ingestion.
   b) Administer a cathartic. Sorbitol solution is reported to be of value.
   c) Administer repeated doses of activated charcoal and monitor theophylline serum levels.
   d) Prophylactic administration of phenobarbital has been shown to increase the seizure threshold in laboratory animals, and administration of this drug can be considered.
2. **If patient presents with a seizure:**
   a) Establish an airway.
   b) Administer oxygen.
   c) Treat the seizure with intravenous diazepam, 0.1 to 0.3 mg/kg up to 10 mg. If seizures cannot be controlled, the use of general anesthesia should be considered.
   d) Monitor vital signs, maintain blood pressure and provide adequate hydration.
3. **If postseizure coma is present:**
   a) Maintain airway and oxygenation.
   b) If a result of oral medication, follow above recommendations to prevent absorption of the drug, but intubation and lavage will have to be performed instead of inducing emesis, and the cathartic and charcoal will need to be introduced via a large bore gastric lavage tube.
   c) Continue to provide full supportive care and adequate hydration until the drug is metabolized. In general, drug metabolism is sufficiently rapid so as not to warrant dialysis. If repeated oral activated charcoal is ineffective (as noted by stable or rising serum levels), charcoal hemoperfusion may be indicated.

DOSAGE AND ADMINISTRATION

Effective use of theophylline (ie, the concentration of drug in the serum associated with optimal benefit and minimal risk of toxicity) is considered to occur when the theophylline concentration is maintained from 10 to 20 mcg/mL. The early studies from which these levels were derived were carried out in patients immediately or shortly after recovery from acute exacerbations of their disease (some hospitalized with status asthmaticus).

Although the 20 mcg/mL level remains appropriate as a critical value (above which toxicity is more likely to occur) for safety purposes, additional data are now available which indicate that the serum theophylline concentrations required to produce maximum physiologic benefit may, in fact, fluctuate with the degree of bronchospasm present and are variable. Therefore, the physician should individualize the range appropriate to the patient's requirements, based on both symptomatic response and improvement in pulmonary function. It should be stressed that serum theophylline concentrations maintained at the upper level of the 10 to 20 mcg/mL range may be associated with potential toxicity when factors known to reduce theophylline clearance are operative. (See WARNINGS.)

If it is not possible to obtain serum level determinations, restriction of the daily dose (in otherwise healthy adults) to not greater than 13 mg/kg/day (of anhydrous theophylline), to a maximum of 900 mg, in divided doses will result in relatively few patients exceeding serum levels of 20 mcg/mL and the resultant greater risk of toxicity.

Caution should be exercised for younger children who cannot complain of minor side effects. Older adults, those with cor pulmonale, congestive heart failure, and/or liver disease may have unusually low dosage requirements and thus may experience toxicity at the maximal dosage recommended below.

Theophylline does not distribute into fatty tissue. Dosage should be calculated on the basis of lean (ideal) body weight where mg/kg doses are presented.

Frequency of Dosing: When immediate release products with rapid absorption are used, dosing to maintain serum levels generally requires administration every 6 hours. This is particularly true in children, but dosing intervals up to 8 hours may be satisfactory in adults since they eliminate the drug at a slower rate. Some children, and adults requiring higher than average doses (those having rapid rates of clearance, eg, half-lives of under 6 hours) may benefit and be more effectively controlled during chronic therapy when given products with sustained release characteristics since these provide longer dosing intervals and/or less fluctuation in serum concentration between dosing.

Dosage guidelines are approximations only and the wide range of theophylline clearance between individuals (particularly those with concomitant disease) makes indiscriminate usage hazardous.

Dosage Guidelines: The following dosage information relates to initiation and titration of daily dosage requirements utilizing a nonsustained action form of Choledyl (eg, Choledyl Tabs, Elixir).

I. Acute symptoms of bronchospasm requiring rapid attainment of theophylline serum levels for bronchodilation.

NOTE: Status asthmaticus should be considered a medical emergency and is defined as that degree of bronchospasm which is not rapidly responsive to usual doses of conventional bronchodilators. Optimal therapy for such patients frequently requires both additional medication, parenterally administered, and close monitoring, preferably in an intensive care setting.

A. Patients not currently receiving theophylline products. [See table left].

B. Patients currently receiving theophylline products: Determine, where possible, the time, amount, dosage form, and route of administration of the last dose the patient received.

The loading dose for theophylline will be based on the principle that each 0.8 mg/kg oxtriphylline (equivalent to 0.5 mg/kg of theophylline) administered as a loading dose will result in a 1 mcg/mL increase in serum theophylline concentration. Ideally, the loading dose should be deferred if a serum theophylline concentration can be obtained rapidly. If this is not possible, the clinician must exercise judgment in selecting a dose based on the potential for benefit and risk. When there is sufficient respiratory distress to warrant a

	Choledyl Dosage		
	Oral Loading		**Maintenance**
Children age 1 to 9 years	7.8 mg/kg *(5 mg/kg)		6.2 mg/kg q 6 hours *(4 mg/kg q 6 hours)
Children age 9 to 16 years and smokers	7.8 mg/kg *(5 mg/kg)		4.7 mg/kg q 6 hours *(3 mg/kg q 6 hours)
Otherwise healthy nonsmoking adults	7.8 mg/kg *(5 mg/kg)		4.7 mg/kg q 8 hours *(3 mg/kg q 8 hours)
Older patients and patients with cor pulmonale	7.8 mg/kg *(5 mg/kg)		3.1 mg/kg q 8 hours *(2 mg/kg q 8 hours)
Patients with congestive heart failure	7.8 mg/kg *(5 mg/kg)		1.6–3.1 mg/kg q 12 hours *(1–2 mg/kg q 12 hours)

* Anhydrous theophylline included in ( ).

small risk, then 4 mg/kg of oxtriphylline (equivalent to 2.5 mg/kg of theophylline) administered in rapidly absorbed form is likely to increase the serum concentration by approximately 5 mcg/mL. If the patient is not experiencing theophylline toxicity, this is unlikely to result in dangerous adverse effects.

Subsequent to the decision regarding use of a loading dose for this group of patients, the maintenance dosage recommendations are the same as those described above.

II. Chronic Therapy

Theophylline is a treatment for the management of reversible bronchospasm (asthma, chronic bronchitis and emphysema) to prevent symptoms and maintain patent airways. A dosage form which allows small incremental doses is desirable for initiating therapy. A liquid preparation should be considered for children to permit both greater ease of and more accurate dosage adjustment. Slow clinical titration is generally preferred to assure acceptance and safety of the medication, and to allow the patient to develop tolerance to transient caffeine-like side effects.

Initial Dose: 25mg*/kg/24 hours or 625 mg/24 hours (whichever is less) of oxtriphylline in divided doses at 6 or 8 hour intervals.

*25 mg oxtriphylline = 16 mg anhydrous theophylline.

Increasing Dose: The above dosage may be increased in approximately 25 percent increments at 3 day intervals so long as the drug is tolerated; until clinical response is satisfactory or the maximum dose as indicated in section III (below) is reached. The serum concentration may be checked at these intervals, but at a minimum, should be determined at the end of this adjustment period.

It is important that no patient be maintained on any dosage that is not tolerated. When instructing patients to increase dosage according to the schedule above, they should be told not to take a subsequent dose if apparent side effects occur and to resume therapy at a lower dose once adverse effects have disappeared.

III. Maximum Dose of Choledyl (Oxtriphylline) Where the Serum Concentration is Not Measured

WARNING: DO NOT ATTEMPT TO MAINTAIN ANY DOSE THAT IS NOT TOLERATED.

Not to exceed the following: [or 1400 mg** (900 mg) whichever is less]

Age 1–9 years	37.5 mg/kg/day	**(24 mg/kg/day)
Age 9–12 years	31 mg/kg/day	**(20 mg/kg/day)
Age 12–16 years	28 mg/kg/day	**(18 mg/kg/day)
Age 16 years and older	20 mg/kg/day	**(13 mg/kg/day)

**Anhydrous theophylline indicated in ().

IV. Measurement of Serum Theophylline Concentrations During Chronic Therapy.

If the above maximum doses are to be maintained or exceeded, serum theophylline measurement is essential (see PRECAUTIONS, Laboratory Tests, for guidance).

V. Final Adjustment of Dosage

Dosage adjustment after serum theophylline measurement

If serum theophylline is:		Directions:
Within desired range		Maintain dosage if tolerated.
Too high	20 to 25 mcg/mL	Decrease doses by about 10% and recheck serum level after 3 days.
	25 to 30 mcg/mL	Skip the next dose and decrease subsequent doses by about 25% Recheck serum level after 3 days.
	Over 30 mcg/mL	Skip next 2 doses and decrease subsequent doses by 50%. Recheck serum level after 3 days.
Too low		Increase dosage by 25% at 3 day intervals until either the desired serum concentration and/or clinical response is achieved. The total daily dose may need to be administered at more frequent intervals if symptoms occur repeatedly at the end of a dosing interval.

The serum concentration may be rechecked at appropriate intervals, but at least at the end of any adjustment period. When the patient's condition is otherwise clinically stable and none of the recognized factors which alter elimination are present, measurement of serum levels need be repeated only every 6 to 12 months.

HOW SUPPLIED

Choledyl Elixir—sherry-flavored, each 5 mL contains 100 mg oxtriphylline; 20% alcohol. Available in bottles of 16 fl oz (474 mL) N 0071-2215-23.

Store between 15°–30°C (59°–86°F).

Caution—Federal law prohibits dispensing without prescription.

2215G030

CHOLEDYL® ℞
[clō′lĕ-dyl″]
(oxtriphylline, USP)
Delayed-release Tablets, USP

DESCRIPTION

Choledyl (oxtriphylline) is the choline salt of theophylline. Theophylline is a bronchodilator structurally classified as a xanthine derivative. It occurs as a white, odorless, crystalline powder having a bitter taste. Theophylline anhydrous has the chemical name $1H$-Purine-2,6-dione, 3,7-dihydro-1,3-dimethyl-.

The molecular formula is $C_{12}H_{21}N_5O_3$. The molecular weight is 283.33.

Choledyl tablets are available as enteric, sugar-coated tablets intended for oral administration, containing 100 mg or 200 mg oxtriphylline (64 mg and 127 mg of theophylline anhydrous, respectively). Each tablet also contains acacia, NF; precipitated calcium carbonate, USP; tribasic calcium phosphate, NF; carnauba wax; confectioner's sugar, NF; gelatin, NF; kaolin, USP; magnesium stearate, NF; pharmaceutical glaze; starch, NF; sucrose, NF; talc, USP; titanium dioxide, USP; tragacanth, NF; and white wax, NF. The 100-mg tablet also contains D&C red No. 7 Lake and FD&C yellow No. 6 Lake. The 200-mg tablet also contains D&C yellow No. 10.

CLINICAL PHARMACOLOGY

Theophylline directly relaxes the smooth muscle of the bronchial airways and pulmonary blood vessels, thus acting mainly as a bronchodilator and smooth muscle relaxant. It has also been demonstrated that aminophylline has a potent effect on diaphragmatic contractility in normal persons and may then be capable of reducing fatigability and thereby improve contractility in patients with chronic obstructive airways disease. The exact mode of action remains unsettled. Although theophylline does cause inhibition of phosphodiesterase with a resultant increase in intracellular cyclic AMP, other agents similarly inhibit the enzyme producing a rise of cyclic AMP but are unassociated with any demonstrable bronchodilation. Other mechanisms proposed include an effect on translocation of intracellular calcium; prostaglandin antagonism; stimulation of catecholamines endogenously; inhibition of cyclic guanosine monophosphate metabolism and adenosine receptor antagonism. None of these mechanisms has been proved, however,

In vitro, theophylline has been shown to act synergistically with beta agonists, and there are now available data which do demonstrate an additive effect in vivo with combined use.

Pharmacokinetics:

The half-life of theophylline is influenced by a number of known variables. It may be prolonged in chronic alcoholics, particularly those with liver disease (cirrhosis or alcoholic liver disease), in patients with congestive heart failure, and in those patients taking certain other drugs (see PRECAUTIONS, Drug Interactions). Newborns and neonates have extremely slow clearance rates compared to older infants and children, ie, those over 1 year. Older children have rapid clearance rates while most nonsmoking adults have clearance rates between these two extremes. In premature neonates, the decreased clearance is related to oxidative pathways that have yet to be established.

Theophylline Elimination Characteristics

		Half-Life (in hours)
	Range	Mean
Children	1–9	3.7
Adults	3–15	7.7

In cigarette smokers (1–2 packs/day) the mean half-life is 4–5 hours, much shorter than in nonsmokers. The increase in clearance associated with smoking is presumably due to stimulation of the hepatic metabolic pathway by components of cigarette smoke. The duration of this effect after cessation of smoking is unknown but may require 6 months to 2 years before the rate approaches that of the nonsmoker.

INDICATIONS AND USAGE

Choledyl (oxtriphylline) is indicated for relief and/or prevention of symptoms from asthma and reversible bronchospasm associated with chronic bronchitis and emphysema.

CONTRAINDICATIONS

Choledyl is contraindicated in individuals who have shown hypersensitivity to its components. It is also contraindicated

in patients with active peptic ulcer disease, and in individuals with underlying seizure disorders (unless receiving appropriate anticonvulsant medication).

WARNINGS

Serum levels above 20 mcg/mL are rarely found after appropriate administration of the recommended doses. However, in individuals in whom theophylline plasma clearance is reduced *for any reason*, even conventional doses may result in increased serum levels and potential toxicity. Reduced theophylline clearance has been documented in the following readily identifiable groups: 1) patients with impaired liver function; 2) patients over 55 years of age, particularly males and those with chronic lung disease; 3) those with cardiac failure from any cause; 4) patients with sustained high fever; 5) neonates and infants under 1 year of age; and 6) those patients taking certain drugs (see PRECAUTIONS, Drug Interactions). Frequently, such patients have markedly prolonged theophylline serum levels following discontinuation of the drug.

Reduction of dosage and laboratory monitoring is especially appropriate in the above individuals.

Serious side effects such as ventricular arrhythmias, convulsions or even death may appear as the first sign of toxicity without any previous warning. Less serious signs of theophylline toxicity (ie, nausea and restlessness) may occur frequently when initiating therapy, but are usually transient; when such signs are persistent during maintenance therapy, they are often associated with serum concentrations above 20 mcg/mL. Stated differently; *serious toxicity is not reliably preceded by less severe side effects*. A serum concentration measurement is the only reliable method of predicting potentially life-threatening toxicity.

Many patients who require theophylline exhibit tachycardia due to their underlying disease process so that the cause/effect relationship to elevated serum theophylline concentrations may not be appreciated.

Theophylline products may cause dysrhythmia and/or worsen preexisting arrhythmias and any significant change in rate and/or rhythm warrants monitoring and further investigation.

Studies in laboratory animals (minipigs, rodents, and dogs) recorded the occurrence of cardiac arrhythmias and sudden death (with histologic evidence of myocardial necrosis) when beta-agonists and methylxanthines were administered concurrently. The significance of these findings when applied to humans is currently unknown.

PRECAUTIONS

General:
On the average, theophylline half-life is shorter in cigarette and marijuana smokers than in nonsmokers, but smokers can have half-lives as long as nonsmokers. Theophylline should not be administered concurrently with other xanthines. Use with caution in patients with hypoxemia, hypertension, or those with history of peptic ulcer. Theophylline may occasionally act as a local irritant to the GI tract although gastrointestinal symptoms are more commonly centrally mediated and associated with serum drug concentrations over 20 mcg/mL.

Information for Patients:
The importance of taking only the prescribed dose and time interval between doses should be reinforced.

Laboratory Tests:
Serum levels should be monitored periodically to determine the theophylline level associated with observed clinical response and as the method of predicting toxicity. For such measurements, the serum sample should be obtained at the time of peak concentration, 1 to 2 hours after administration for immediate release products. It is important that the patient will not have missed or taken additional doses during the previous 48 hours and that dosing intervals will have been reasonably equally spaced. DOSAGE ADJUSTMENT BASED ON SERUM THEOPHYLLINE MEASUREMENTS WHEN THESE INSTRUCTIONS HAVE NOT BEEN FOLLOWED MAY RESULT IN RECOMMENDATIONS THAT PRESENT RISK OF TOXICITY TO THE PATIENT.

Drug Interactions:
Toxic synergism with ephedrine has been documented and may occur with other sympathomimetic bronchodilators. In

Continued on next page

This product information was prepared in August, 1989. On these and other Parke-Davis Products, information may be obtained by addressing PARKE-DAVIS, Division of Warner-Lambert Company, Morris Plains, New Jersey 07950.

Parke-Davis—Cont.

addition, the following drug interactions have been demonstrated:
Theophylline with:

Allopurinol (high-dose)	Increased serum theophylline levels
Cimetidine	Increased serum theophylline levels
Erythromycin, Troleandomycin	Increased serum theophylline levels
Lithium Carbonate	Increased renal excretion of lithium
Oral Contraceptives	Increased serum theophylline levels
Phenytoin	Decreased theophylline and phenytoin serum levels
Rifampin	Decreased serum theophylline levels

Drug-Laboratory Test Interactions:
Currently available analytical methods, including high pressure liquid chromatography and immunoassay techniques, for measuring serum theophylline levels are specific. Metabolites and other drugs generally do not affect the results. Other new analytic methods are also now in use. The physician should be aware of the laboratory method used and whether other drugs will interfere with the assay for theophylline.

Carcinogenesis, Mutagenesis, and Impairment of Fertility:
Long-term carcinogenicity studies have not been performed with theophylline.
Chromosome-breaking activity was detected in human cell cultures at concentrations of theophylline up to 50 times the therapeutic serum concentration in humans. Theophylline was not mutagenic in the dominant lethal assay in male mice given theophylline intraperitoneally in doses up to 30 times the maximum daily oral dose.
Studies to determine the effect on fertility have not been performed with theophylline.

Pregnancy:
Category C—Animal reproduction studies have not been conducted with oxtriphylline. It is not known whether theophylline can cause fetal harm when administered to a pregnant woman or can affect reproduction capacity. Oxtriphylline should be given to a pregnant woman only if clearly needed.

Nursing Mothers:
Theophylline is distributed into breast milk and may cause irritability or other signs of toxicity in nursing infants. Because of the potential for serious adverse reactions in nursing infants from theophylline, a decision should be made whether to discontinue nursing or to discontinue the drug, taking into account the importance of the drug to the mother.

Pediatric Use:
Sufficient numbers of infants under the age of 1 year have not been studied in clinical trials to support use in this age group; however, there is evidence recorded that the use of dosage recomendations for older infants and young children (16 mg/kg/24 hours) may result in the development of toxic serum levels. Such findings very probably reflect differences in the metabolic handling of the drug related to absent or undeveloped enzyme systems. Consequently, the use of the drug in this age group should carefully consider the associated benefits and risks. If used, the maintenance dose must be conservative and in accord with the following guidelines:

Initial Theophylline Maintenance Dosage:
Premature Infants:
Up to 24 days postnatal age—1.0 mg/kg q 12h
Beyond 24 days postnatal age—1.5 mg/kg q 12h
Infants 6 to 52 Weeks:
$[(0.2 \times \text{age in weeks}) + 5.0] \times \text{kg body wt} = 24 \text{ hour dose in mg.}$
Up to 26 weeks, divide into q 8h dosing intervals.
From 26–52 weeks, divide into q 6h dosing intervals.
Final dosage should be guided by serum concentration after a steady state (no further accumulation of drug) has been achieved.

ADVERSE REACTIONS

The following adverse reactions have been observed, but there has not been enough systematic collection of data to support an estimate of their frequency. The most consistent adverse reactions are usually due to overdosage.

1. **Gastrointestinal:** nausea, vomiting, epigastric pain, hematemesis, diarrhea.
2. **Central nervous system:** headaches, irritability, restlessness, insomnia, reflex hyperexcitability, muscle twitching, clonic and tonic generalized convulsions.
3. **Cardiovascular:** palpitation, tachycardia, extrasystoles, flushing, hypotension, circulatory failure, ventricular arrhythmias.
4. **Respiratory:** tachypnea.
5. **Renal:** potentiation of diuresis.
6. **Others:** alopecia, hyperglycemia, inappropriate ADH syndrome, rash.

OVERDOSAGE

Management:
It is suggested that the management principles (consistent with the clinical status of the patient when first seen) outlined below be instituted and that simultaneous contact with a Regional Poison Control Center be established. In this way both updated information and individualization regarding required therapy may be provided.

1. When potential oral overdose is established and seizure has not occurred:
   a. If patient is alert and seen within the early hours after ingestion, induction of emesis may be of value. Gastric lavage has been demonstrated to be of no value in influencing outcome in patients who present more than 1 hour after ingestion.
   b. Administer a cathartic. Sorbitol solution is reported to be of value.
   c. Administer repeated doses of activated charcoal and monitor theophylline serum levels.
   d. Prophylactic administration of phenobarbital has been shown to increase the seizure threshold in laboratory animals, and administration of this drug can be considered.
2. If patient presents with a seizure:
   a. Establish an airway.
   b. Administer oxygen.
   c. Treat the seizure with intravenous diazepam, 0.1 to 0.3 mg/kg up to 10 mg. If seizures cannot be controlled, the use of general anesthesia should be considered.
   d. Monitor vital signs, maintain blood pressure and provide adequate hydration.
3. If postseizure coma is present:
   a. Maintain airway and oxygenation.
   b. If a result of oral medication, follow above recommendations to prevent absorption of the drug, but intubation and lavage will have to be performed instead of inducing emesis, and the cathartic and charcoal will need to be introduced via large bore gastric lavage tube.
   c. Continue to provide full supportive care and adequate hydration until the drug is metabolized. In general, drug metabolism is sufficiently rapid so as not to warrant dialysis. If repeated oral activated charcoal is ineffective (as noted by stable or rising serum levels), charcoal hemoperfusion may be indicated.

DOSAGE AND ADMINISTRATION

Effective use of theophylline (ie, the concentration of drug in the serum associated with optimal benefit and minimal risk of toxicity) is considered to occur when the theophylline concentration is maintained from 10 to 20 mcg/mL. The early studies from which these levels were derived were carried out in patients immediately or shortly after recovery from acute exacerbations of their disease (some hospitalized with status asthmaticus).
Although the 20 mcg/mL level remains appropriate as a critical value (above which toxicity is more likely to occur) for safety purposes, additional data are now available which indicate that the serum theophylline concentrations required to produce maximum physiologic benefit may, in fact, fluctuate with the degree of bronchospasm present and are variable. Therefore, the physician should individualize the range appropriate to the patient's requirements, based on both symptomatic response and improvement in pulmonary function. It should be stressed that serum theophylline concentrations maintained at the upper level of the 10 to 20 mcg/mL range may be associated with potential toxicity when factors known to reduce theophylline clearance are operative. (See WARNINGS).
If it is not possible to obtain serum level determinations, restriction of the daily dose (in otherwise healthy adults) to not greater than 13 mg/kg/day (of anhydrous theophylline), to a maximum of 900 mg, in divided doses will result in relatively few patients exceeding serum levels of 20 mcg/mL and the resultant greater risk of toxicity.
Caution should be exercised for younger children who cannot complain of minor side effects. Older adults, those with cor pulmonale, congestive heart failure, and/or liver disease may have unusually low dosage requirements and thus may experience toxicity at the maximal dosage recommended below.
Theophylline does not distribute into fatty tissue. Dosage should be calculated on the basis of lean (ideal) body weight where mg/kg doses are presented.

Frequency of Dosing:
When immediate release products with rapid absorption are used, dosing to maintain serum levels generally requires administration every 6 hours. This is particularly true in children, but dosing intervals up to 8 hours may be satisfactory in adults since they eliminate the drug at a slower rate. Some children and adults requiring higher than average doses (those having rapid rates of clearance, eg, half-lives of under 6 hours) may benefit and be more effectively controlled during chronic therapy when given products with sustained release characteristics since these provide longer dosing intervals and/or less fluctuation in serum concentration between dosing.
Dosage guidelines are approximations only and the wide range of theophylline clearance between individuals (particularly those with concomitant disease) make indiscriminate usage hazardous.

Dosage Guidelines:
The following dosage information relates to initiation and titration of daily dosage requirements utilizing a nonsustained action form of Choledyl (eg, Choledyl Tabs, Elixir).
I. Acute symptoms of bronchospasm requiring rapid attainment of theophylline serum levels for bronchodilation.
NOTE: Status asthmaticus should be considered a medical emergency and is defined as that degree of bronchospasm which is not rapidly responsive to usual doses of conventional bronchodilators. Optimal therapy for such patients frequently requires both *additional medication*, parenterally administered, and *close monitoring*, preferably in an intensive care setting.
A. Patients not currently receiving theophylline products. [See table left].
B. Patients currently receiving theophylline products:
Determine, where possible, the time, amount, dosage form, and route of administration of the last dose the patient received.
The loading dose for theophylline will be based on the principle that each 0.8 mg/kg oxtriphylline (equivalent to 0.5 mg/kg of theophylline) administered as a loading dose will result in a 1.0 mcg/mL increase in serum theophylline concentration. Ideally, the loading dose should be deferred if a serum theophylline concentration can be obtained rapidly. If this is not possible, the clinician must exercise judgment in selecting a dose based on the potential for benefit and risk. When there is sufficient respiratory distress to warrant a small risk, then 4 mg/kg of oxtriphylline (equivalent to 2.5 mg/kg of theophylline) administered in rapidly absorbed form is likely to increase the serum concentration by approximately 5 mcg/mL. If the patient is not experiencing theophylline toxicity, this is unlikely to result in dangerous adverse effects.
Subsequent to the decision regarding use of a loading dose for this group of patients, the maintenance dosage recommendations are the same as those described above.
II. Chronic Therapy
Theophylline is a treatment for the management of reversible bronchospasm (asthma, chronic bronchitis and emphy-

Choledyl Dosage

	Oral Loading	Maintenance
Children age 1 to 9 years	7.8 mg/kg *(5 mg/kg)	6.2 mg/kg q 6 hours *(4 mg/kg q 6 hours)
Children age 9 to 16 years and smokers	7.8 mg/kg *(5 mg/kg)	4.7 mg/kg q 6 hours *(3 mg/kg q 6 hours)
Otherwise healthy nonsmoking adults	7.8 mg/kg *(5 mg/kg)	4.7 mg/kg q 8 hours *(3 mg/kg q 8 hours)
Older patients and patients with cor pulmonale	7.8 mg/kg *(5 mg/kg)	3.1 mg/kg q 8 hours *(2 mg/kg q 8 hours)
Patients with congestive heart failure	7.8 mg/kg *(5 mg/kg)	1.6–3.1 mg/kg q 12 hours *(1–2 mg/kg q 12 hours)

* Anhydrous theophylline included in ( ).

sema) to prevent symptoms and maintain patent airways. A dosage form which allows small incremental doses is desirable for initiating therapy. A liquid preparation should be considered for children to permit both greater ease of and more accurate dosage adjustment. Slow clinical titration is generally preferred to assure acceptance and safety of the medication, and to allow the patient to develop tolerance to transient caffeine-like side effects.

Initial Dose: 25 mg*/kg/24 hours or 625 mg/24 hours (whichever is less) of oxtriphylline in divided doses at 6- or 8-hour intervals.

* 25 mg oxtriphylline = 16 mg anhydrous theophylline.

Increasing Dose: The above dosage may be increased in approximately 25-percent increments at 3-day intervals as long as the drug is tolerated; until clinical response is satisfactory or the maximum dose as indicated in section III (below) is reached. The serum concentration may be checked at these intervals, but at a minimum, should be determined at the end of this adjustment period.

It is important that no patient be maintained on any dosage that is not tolerated. When instructing patients to increase dosage according to the schedule above, they should be told not to take a subsequent dose if apparent side effects occur and to resume therapy at a lower dose once adverse effects have disappeared.

III. Maximum Dose of Choledyl (oxtriphylline) Where the Serum Concentration is Not Measured

WARNING: DO NOT ATTEMPT TO MAINTAIN ANY DOSE THAT IS NOT TOLERATED.

Not to exceed the following: [or 1400 mg** (900 mg) whichever is less]

Age 1–9 years	37.5 mg/kg/day	**(24 mg/kg/day)
Age 9–12 years	31 mg/kg/day	**(20 mg/kg/day)
Age 12–16 years	28 mg/kg/day	**(18 mg/kg/day)
Age 16 years and older	20 mg/kg/day	**(13 mg/kg/day)

    **Anhydrous theophylline indicated in ( ).

IV. Measurement of Serum Theophylline Concentrations During Chronic Therapy.

If the above maximum doses are to be maintained or exceeded, serum theophylline measurement is essential (see PRECAUTIONS, Laboratory Tests, for guidance).

V. Final Adjustment of Dosage

Dosage adjustment after serum theophylline measurement:

If serum theophylline is:		Directions:
Within desired range		Maintain dosage if tolerated.
Too high	20 to 25 mcg/mL	Decrease doses by about 10% and recheck serum level after 3 days.
	25 to 30 mcg/mL	Skip the next dose and decrease subsequent doses by about 25%. Recheck serum level after 3 days.
	Over 30 mcg/mL	Skip next 2 doses and decrease subsequent doses by 50%. Recheck serum level after 3 days.
Too low		Increase dosage by 25% at 3-day intervals until either the desired serum concentration and/or clinical response is achieved. The total daily dose may need to be administered at more frequent intervals if symptoms occur repeatedly at the end of a dosing interval.

The serum concentration may be rechecked at appropriate intervals, but at least at the end of any adjustment period. When the patient's condition is otherwise clinically stable and none of the recognized factors which alter elimination are present, measurement of serum levels need be repeated only every 6 to 12 months.

HOW SUPPLIED

Choledyl (oxtriphylline) 100 mg is supplied as round, red, enteric, sugar-coated tablets, coded PD 210, in bottles of 100 (N 0071-0210-24).

Choledyl (oxtriphylline) 200 mg is supplied as round, yellow, enteric, sugar-coated tablets, coded PD 211, in bottles of 100 (N 0071-0211-24), 1000 (N 0071-0211-32) and Unit Dose—10 × 10 strips (N 0071-0211-40).

Store between 15°–30°C (59°–86°F).

Caution—Federal law prohibits dispensing without prescription.

0210G053

Shown in Product Identification Section, page 421

CHOLEDYL® SA   ℞

[*chō 'lĕ-dyl ''*]
(Oxtriphylline)
Sustained Action

DESCRIPTION

Choledyl (oxtriphylline) is a xanthine bronchodilator—the choline salt of theophylline.

Each film-coated Choledyl SA tablet contains 400 mg or 600 mg oxtriphylline (equivalent to 254 mg or 382 mg anhydrous theophylline, respectively). Each tablet also contains, candelilla wax, confectioner's sugar, NF; magnesium stearate, NF; Opaseal pharmaceutical sealant; talc, USP and other ingredients. The 400-mg tablet also contains Opaspray pink and triethyl citrate. The 600-mg tablet also contains Opaspray tan.

Each tablet of Choledyl SA contains oxtriphylline in a tablet matrix specially designed for the prolonged release of the drug in the gastrointestinal tract. Following release of the drug, the expended wax tablet matrix, which is not absorbed, may be detected in the stool.

CLINICAL PHARMACOLOGY

Choledyl (oxtriphylline), the choline salt of theophylline, effects significant improvement in pulmonary function parameters which have been impaired by bronchospasm. It is more soluble than either aminophylline or theophylline. Film-coated Choledyl SA tablets are less irritating to the gastric mucosa than aminophylline.

Choledyl SA tablets have been formulated to provide therapeutic serum levels when administered every 12 hours and minimize the peaks and valleys of serum levels commonly found with shorter acting theophylline products.

The sustained action characteristic of Choledyl SA tablets has been demonstrated in studies in human subjects. Single and multiple dose studies have shown equivalent steady-state theophylline plasma levels of Choledyl SA tablets given every 12 hours when compared with an equal total daily dose of (the nonsustained action) Choledyl Elixir given every six hours.

Theophylline directly relaxes the smooth muscle of the bronchial airways and pulmonary blood vessels, thus acting mainly as a bronchodilator, pulmonary vasodilator and smooth muscle relaxant. The drug also possesses other actions typical of the xanthine derivatives: coronary vasodilator, diuretic, cardiac stimulant, cerebral stimulant and skeletal muscle stimulant. The actions of theophylline may be mediated through inhibition of phosphodiesterase and a resultant increase in intracellular cyclic AMP which could mediate smooth muscle relaxation. At concentrations higher than attained *in vivo*, theophylline also inhibits the release of histamine by mast cells.

Theophylline has been shown to react synergistically with beta agonists that increase intracellular cyclic AMP through the stimulation of adenyl cyclase (isoproterenol).

Apparently, the development of tolerance does not occur with chronic use of theophylline.

The half-life is shortened with cigarette smoking. The half-life is prolonged in alcoholism, reduced hepatic or renal function, congestive heart failure, and in patients receiving antibiotics such as TAO (troleandomycin), erythromycin and clindamycin. High fever for prolonged periods may decrease theophylline elimination.

Theophylline Elimination Characteristics

	Theophylline Clearance Rates (mean ± S.D.)	Half-Life Average (mean ± S.D.)
Children (over 6 months of age)	1.45 ± .58 ml/kg/min	3.7 ± 1.1 hours
Adult nonsmokers with uncomplicated asthma	.65 ± .19 ml/kg/min	8.7 ± 2.2 hours

Newborn infants have extremely slow clearance and half-lives exceeding 24 hours, which approach those seen for older children after about 3–6 months.

Older adults with chronic obstructive pulmonary disease, and patients with cor pulmonale or other causes of heart failure, and patients with liver pathology may have much lower clearances with half-lives that may exceed 24 hours. The half-life of theophylline is prolonged in patients with congestive heart failure, in those with reduced hepatic or renal function, and in alcoholism. The half-life of theophylline may also be prolonged by concurrent use of various drugs such as phenobarbital, and certain antibiotics, including troleandomycin, erythromycin, and lincomycin.

Theophylline half-life is shortened in cigarette smokers (1 to 2 packs/day) as compared to nonsmokers. The increase in theophylline clearance caused by smoking is probably the result of induction of drug metabolizing enzymes that do not readily normalize after cessation of smoking. It appears that between 3 months and 2 years may be necessary for normal-

---

ization of the effect of smoking on theophylline pharmacokinetics.

INDICATIONS

Choledyl (oxtriphylline) is indicated for relief of acute and chronic bronchial asthma and for reversible bronchospasm associated with chronic bronchitis and emphysema.

CONTRAINDICATIONS

Choledyl is contraindicated in individuals who have shown hypersensitivity to theophylline or to Choledyl (oxtriphylline) or any of its components.

WARNINGS

Status asthmaticus is a medical emergency. Optimal therapy frequently requires additional medication including corticosteroids when the patient is not rapidly responsive to bronchodilators.

Excessive theophylline doses may be associated with toxicity, and serum theophylline levels are recommended to assure maximal benefit without excessive risk; incidence of toxicity increases at levels greater than 20 mcg theophylline/ml. Morphine, curare, and stilbamidine should be used with caution in patients with airflow obstruction since they stimulate histamine release and can induce asthmatic attacks. These drugs may also suppress respiration leading to respiratory failure. Alternative drugs should be chosen whenever possible.

There is an excellent correlation between high blood levels of theophylline resulting from conventional doses and associated clinical manifestations of toxicity in patients with liver dysfunction or chronic obstructive lung disease.

There is excellent correlation between high serum levels of theophylline (over 20 mcg/ml) and the clinical manifestations of toxicity. Careful reduction of dosage and monitoring of serum levels are especially important in patients manifesting a decrease in total body theophylline clearance rate, including those with generalized debility, acute hypoxia, cardiac decompensation, hepatic dysfunction, or renal failure. Dosage reduction may also be necessary in patients who are older than 55 years of age, particularly males.

Serious toxic effects may occur suddenly and are not invariably preceded by minor adverse effects such as nausea, vomiting, and restlessness. Convulsions, tachycardia, or ventricular arrhythmias may be the first sign of toxicity.

Children have a marked sensitivity to the CNS stimulant action of theophylline. Serious toxic effects, including fatalities have been reported in children as well as adults. Theophylline products may worsen pre-existing arrhythmias.

USAGE IN PREGNANCY

Safe use of Choledyl (oxtriphylline) in pregnancy and lactation has not been established relative to possible adverse effects on fetal or neonatal development. Therefore Choledyl (oxtriphylline) should not be used in patients who are pregnant or who may become pregnant, or during lactation unless, in the judgment of the physician, the potential benefits outweigh the possible hazards.

PRECAUTIONS

Mean half-life in smokers is shorter than nonsmokers, therefore, smokers may require larger doses of theophylline. Theophylline should not be administered concurrently with other xanthine medications or with xanthine-containing beverages or foods. Use with caution in patients with severe cardiac disease, severe hypoxemia, hypertension, hyperthyroidism, acute myocardial injury, cor pulmonale, congestive heart failure, or liver disease, and in the elderly (especially males) and in neonates. Great caution should especially be used in giving theophylline to patients in congestive heart failure. Such patients have shown markedly prolonged theophylline blood level curves with theophylline persisting in serum for long periods following discontinuation of the drug. Use theophylline cautiously in patients with a history of peptic ulcer. Theophylline may occasionally act as a local irritant to the GI tract although gastrointestinal symptoms are more commonly central and associated with serum theophylline concentrations over 20 mcg/ml.

ADVERSE REACTIONS

The most consistent adverse reactions are usually due to overdose and are:

1. Gastrointestinal: nausea, vomiting, epigastric pain, hematemesis, diarrhea.

2. Central nervous system: headaches, irritability, restlessness, insomnia, reflex hyperexcitability, muscle twitching, clonic and tonic generalized convulsions.

Continued on next page

This product information was prepared in August, 1989. On these and other Parke-Davis Products, information may be obtained by addressing PARKE-DAVIS, Division of Warner-Lambert Company, Morris Plains, New Jersey 07950.

Parke-Davis—Cont.

3. Cardiovascular: palpitation, tachycardia, extrasystoles, flushing, hypotension, circulatory failure, life-threatening ventricular arrhythmias.

4. Respiratory: tachypnea.

5. Renal: albuminuria, increased excretion of renal tubular cells and red blood cells, diuresis.

6. Others: hyperglycemia and inappropriate antidiuretic hormone (ADH) syndrome.

Drug Interactions: Theophylline-containing preparations have exhibited interaction with the following drugs:

Drug	Effect
Lithium carbonate	Increased excretion of lithium carbonate.
Propranolol	Antagonism of propranolol effect.
Furosemide	Increased furosemide diuresis.
Hexamethonium	Decreased hexamethonium-induced chronotropic effect
Reserpine	Reserpine-induced tachycardia.
Chlordiazepoxide	Chlordiazepoxide-induced fatty acid mobilization.
Troleandomycin, erythromycin or lincomycin	Increased theophylline plasma levels.

DOSAGE AND ADMINISTRATION

Therapy should be initiated and daily dosage requirements established utilizing a nonsustained-action form of Choledyl (oxtriphylline) (eg, Choledyl Tablets, Elixir).

If the total daily maintenance dosage requirement of the Choledyl (oxtriphylline) nonsustained preparation is established at approximately 1200 mg, Choledyl SA 600 mg Sustained Action Tablets, one every 12 hours, may be substituted to provide smoother steady-state theophylline levels and the convenience of bid dosage. Similarly, if the total daily maintenance dosage is established at approximately 800 mg, Choledyl SA 400 mg Sustained Action Tablets, one every 12 hours, may be substituted.

Therapeutic serum levels associated with optimal likelihood of benefit and minimal risk of toxicity are considered to be between 10 mcg/ml and 20 mcg/ml. Levels above 20 mcg/ml may produce toxic effects.

There is great variation from patient to patient in dosage needed in order to achieve a therapeutic blood level because of variable rates of elimination. Because of this wide variation from patient to patient and the relatively narrow therapeutic blood level range, dosage must be individualized; monitoring of theophylline serum levels is highly recommended. Dosage should be calculated on the basis of lean (ideal) body weight—mg/kg. Theophylline does not distribute into fatty tissue.

Choledyl (oxtriphylline)

Initial dose:	25 mg*/kg/day or 625 mg/day (whichever is lower) in 3 to 4 divided doses at 6–8 hour intervals.
Increased dose:	The above dosage may be increased in approximately 25 percent increments at 2 to 3 day intervals so long as no intolerance is observed until the maximum indicated below is reached.

*25 mg Choledyl = 16 mg anhydrous theophylline

Giving Choledyl (oxtriphylline) with food may prevent the rare case of stomach irritation, and although absorption may be slower, it is still complete.

When rapidly absorbed products such as solutions are used, dosing to maintain "around the clock" blood levels generally requires administration every 6 hours to obtain the greatest efficacy for use in children, dosing intervals up to 8 hours may be satisfactory for adults because of their slower elimination. Children and adults requiring higher than average doses may benefit from products with slower absorption. This may allow longer dosing intervals and/or less fluctuation in serum concentration over a dosing interval during chronic therapy. In patients receiving concurrent bronchodilator therapy, eg, beta agonists, downward adjustment of Choledyl (oxtriphylline) dosage is necessary.

The following dosage information relates to initiation and titration of daily dosage requirements utilizing a nonsustained action form of Choledyl (eg Choledyl Tabs, Elixir).
[See table below].

II. *Those currently receiving theophylline products:*
Determine where possible, the time, amount, route of administration and form of the patient's last dose.

The loading dose for theophylline will be based on the principle that each 0.8 mg/kg of Choledyl (oxtriphylline) (0.5 mg/kg of theophylline) administered as a loading dose will result in a 1 mcg/ml increase in serum theophylline concentration. Ideally, then, the loading dose should be deferred if a serum theophylline concentration can be rapidly obtained. If this is not possible, the clinician must exercise his judgment in selecting a dose based on the potential for benefit and risk. When there is sufficient respiratory distress to warrant a small risk, 4 mg/kg Choledyl (oxtriphylline) (2.5 mg/kg of theophylline) is likely to increase the serum concentration when administered as a loading dose in rapidly absorbed form by only about 5 mcg/ml. If the patient is not already experiencing theophylline toxicity, this is unlikely to result in dangerous adverse effect.

Following the decision regarding loading dose in this group of patients, the subsequent maintenance dosage recommendations are the same as those described above.

To achieve optimal therapeutic theophylline dosage, monitoring of serum theophylline concentrations is recommended. However, it is not always possible or practical to obtain a serum theophylline level.

Patients should be closely monitored for signs of toxicity. The present data suggests that the above dosage recommendations will achieve therapeutic serum concentrations with minimal risk of toxicity for most patients. However, some risk of toxic serum concentrations is still present. Adverse reactions to theophylline often occur when serum theophylline levels exceed 20 mcg/ml.

Chronic Asthma
Theophyllinization is a treatment of first choice for the management of chronic asthma (to prevent symptoms and maintain patent airways). Slow clinical titration is generally preferred to assure acceptance and safety of the medication.
[See table above].

Maximum dose of Choledyl (oxtriphylline) without measurement of serum theophylline concentration:
Not to exceed the following: (WARNING: DO NOT ATTEMPT TO MAINTAIN ANY DOSE THAT IS NOT TOLERATED)

Age <9 years	—37.5 mg/kg/day **(24 mg/kg/day)
Age 9–12 years	—31 mg/kg/day **(20 mg/kg/day)
Age 12–16 years	—28 mg/kg/day **(18 mg/kg/day)
Age >16 years	—20 mg/kg/day or 1400 mg/day (WHICHEVER IS LESS) **(13 mg/kg/day or 900 mg/day) (WHICHEVER IS LESS)

Note: Use ideal body weight for obese patients.
**anhydrous theophylline indicated in ( )

If the total daily maintenance dosage requirement of the Choledyl (oxtriphylline) nonsustained preparation is established at approximately 1200 mg, Choledyl SA 600 mg Sustained Action Tablets, one every 12 hours, may be substituted to provide smoother steady-state theophylline levels and the convenience of bid dosage. Similarly, if the total daily maintenance dosage is established at approximately 800 mg, Choledyl SA 400 mg Sustained Action Tablets, one every 12 hours, may be substituted.

Measurement of serum theophylline concentration during chronic therapy
If the above maximum dosages are to be maintained or exceeded, serum theophylline measurement is recommended. This should be obtained at the approximate time of peak absorption (1 to 2 hours after dosing) during chronic therapy. It is important that the patient will have missed *no* doses during the previous 48 hours and that dosing intervals will have been reasonably typical, with no added doses during that period of time.

DOSAGE ADJUSTMENT BASED ON SERUM THEOPHYLLINE MEASUREMENTS IF THE ABOVE INSTRUCTIONS HAVE NOT BEEN FOLLOWED MAY RESULT IN RISK OF TOXICITY TO THE PATIENT.

Caution should be exercised for younger children who cannot complain of minor side effects. Older adults, those with cor pulmonale, congestive heart failure, and/or liver disease, may have unusually low dosage requirements and thus may experience toxicity at the maximal dosage recommended above.

It is important that no patient be maintained on any dosage that he is not tolerating. In instructing patients to increase dosage according to the schedule above, they should be instructed to not take a subsequent dose if apparent side effects occur and to resume therapy at a lower dose once adverse effects have disappeared.

OVERDOSAGE

Serious toxic effects due to overdosage may occur suddenly and are not invariably preceded by minor adverse effects. Therefore, careful observation of the patient and prompt institution of appropriate therapeutic measures are essential in all cases of overdosage. All patients suspected of overdosage should be hospitalized.

Signs and symptoms of overdosage are related primarily to the cardiovascular, gastrointestinal, and central nervous systems.

Cardiovascular symptoms include precordial pain, tachycardia, ventricular and other arrhythmias; also varying degrees of hypotension including, in extreme cases, severe shock, cardiovascular collapse and death.

Gastrointestinal symptoms include abdominal pain, nausea, persistent vomiting, and hematemesis.

Central nervous system symptoms include headache, dizziness, restlessness, irritability, tremors, hyperactivity, and agitation followed, in severe cases, by convulsions, drowsiness, coma and death.

Treatment of overdosage should be directed toward minimizing absorption and supporting vital functions.

In the alert patient emesis should be induced, followed by appropriate additional measures, as listed below.

In the obtunded patient, the airway should be secured immediately by means of an endotracheal tube with cuff inflated. After the airway has been secured, lavage should be carried out, and activated charcoal slurry and a cathartic should be administered.

CNS stimulation may be controlled with diazepam, 0.1–0.3 mg/kg intravenously in children, and 10 mg intravenously in adults. Respiration should be supported by appropriate means. Hypotension and shock should be treated with appropriate fluid replacement, avoiding the use of vasopressors, if

---

CHOLEDYL (OXTRIPHYLLINE) DOSAGE FOR PATIENT POPULATION

Acute Symptoms of Asthma Requiring Rapid Theophyllinization:
1. *Not currently receiving theophylline products:*

GROUP	ORAL LOADING DOSE CHOLEDYL	MAINTENANCE DOSE FOR NEXT 12 HOURS CHOLEDYL	MAINTENANCE DOSE BEYOND 12 HOURS CHOLEDYL
1. Children 6 months to 9 years	9.4 mg/kg *(6 mg/kg)	6.2 mg/kg q4 hrs *(4 mg/kg q4 hrs)	6.2 mg/kg q6 hrs *(4 mg/kg q6 hrs)
2. Children age 9–16 and young adult smokers	9.4 mg/kg *(6 mg/kg)	4.7 mg/kg q4 hrs *(3 mg/kg q4 hrs)	4.7 mg/kg q6 hrs *(3 mg/kg q6 hrs)
3. Otherwise healthy nonsmoking adults	9.4 mg/kg *(6 mg/kg)	4.7 mg/kg q6 hrs *(3 mg/kg q6 hrs)	4.7 mg/kg q8 hrs *3 mg/kg q8 hrs)
4. Older patients and patients with cor pulmonale	9.4 mg/kg *(6 mg/kg)	3.1 mg/kg q6 hrs *(2 mg/kg q6 hrs)	3.1 mg/kg q8 hrs *(2 mg/kg q8 hrs)
5. Patients with congestive heart failure, liver failure	9.4 mg/kg *(6 mg/kg)	3.1 mg/kg q8 hrs *(2 mg/kg q8 hrs)	1.6–3.1 mg/kg q12 hrs *(1–2 mg/kg q12 hrs)

*Anhydrous theophylline indicated in ( )

possible. Additional supportive measures should be carried out as required.

Serial serum theophylline levels are of value in following the patient's course and in guiding further management.

Forced diuresis is of no value because of the small amount of theophylline excreted unchanged by the kidney. There has been a single report of survival with the use of an activated charcoal column (hemoperfusion) in massive theophylline overdosage.

HOW SUPPLIED

Choledyl SA 400 mg—each sustained action tablet contains 400 mg oxtriphylline. Available as pink film-coated tablets in bottles of 100 (N 0071-0214-24), and unit-dose 100's (N 0071-0214-40).

Choledyl SA 600 mg—each sustained action tablet contains 600 mg oxtriphylline. Available as tan film-coated tablets in bottles of 100 (N 0071-0221-24), and unit-dose 100's (N 0071-0221-40).

0214G092

Shown in Product Identification Section, page 421

CHOLYBAR®   ℞

[kō'lĭbăr]

(Cholestyramine Resin Bar)

DESCRIPTION

Cholybar (cholestyramine resin bar), the chloride salt of a basic anion exchange resin, a cholesterol-lowering agent, is intended for oral administration. Cholestyramine resin is quite hydrophilic, but insoluble in water. The cholestyramine resin is not absorbed from the digestive tract. It is represented by the following structural formula:

Representation of structure of main polymeric groups

Cholybar is available as chewable, caramel-flavored or raspberry-flavored bars, each containing 4 grams of anhydrous cholestyramine resin, USP. Both flavors of Cholybar contain fructose, sorbitol, flavors, and other ingredients. In addition, the caramel-flavored bars contain caramel color, and the raspberry-flavored bars contain FD&C Red No. 40 and FD&C Blue No. 1.

CLINICAL PHARMACOLOGY

Cholesterol is probably the sole precursor of bile acids. During normal digestion, bile acids are secreted into the intestines. A major portion of the bile acids is absorbed from the intestinal tract and returned to the liver via the enterohepatic circulation. Only very small amounts of bile acids are found in normal serum.

Cholestyramine resin adsorbs and combines with the bile acids in the intestine to form an insoluble complex which is excreted in the feces. This results in a partial removal of bile acids from the enterohepatic circulation by preventing their absorption.

The increased fecal loss of bile acids due to cholestyramine resin administration leads to an increased oxidation of cholesterol to bile acids, a decrease in beta lipoprotein or low density lipoprotein plasma levels and a decrease in serum cholesterol levels. Although in man cholestyramine resin produces an increase in hepatic synthesis of cholesterol, plasma cholesterol levels fall.

In patients with partial biliary obstruction, the reduction of serum bile acid levels by cholestyramine resin reduces excess bile acids deposited in the dermal tissue with resultant decrease in pruritus.

INDICATIONS AND USAGE

1. Cholybar is indicated as adjunctive therapy to diet for the reduction of elevated serum cholesterol in patients with primary hypercholesterolemia (elevated low density lipoprotein [LDL] cholesterol) who do not respond adequately to diet. Cholestyramine resin may be useful to lower LDL cholesterol in patients who also have hypertriglyceridemia, but it is not indicated where hypertriglyceridemia is the abnormality of most concern.

In a large, placebo-controlled, multiclinic study, the LRC-CPPT,* hypercholesterolemic subjects treated with cholestyramine resin had significant reductions in total and low-density lipoprotein cholesterol (LDL-C). Over the seven-year study period the cholestyramine resin group experienced a 19% reduction in the combined rate of coronary heart disease death plus nonfatal myocardial infarction (cumulative incidences of 7% cholestyramine resin and 8.6% placebo). The subjects included in the study were middle-aged men (age 35–59) with serum cholesterol levels above 265 mg/dL and no previous history of heart disease. It is not clear to what extent these findings can be extrapolated to other segments of the hypercholesterolemic population not studied.

Dietary therapy specific for the type of hyperlipoproteinemia is the initial treatment of choice. Excess body weight may be an important factor and caloric restriction for weight normalization should be addressed prior to drug therapy in the overweight. The use of drugs should be considered only when reasonable attempts have been made to obtain satisfactory results with nondrug methods. If the decision ultimately is to use drugs, the patient should be instructed that this does not reduce the importance of adhering to diet.

2. Cholestyramine resin is indicated for the relief of pruritus associated with partial biliary obstruction. Cholestyramine resin has been shown to have a variable effect on serum cholesterol in these patients. Patients with primary biliary cirrhosis may exhibit an elevated cholesterol level as part of their disease.

CONTRAINDICATIONS

Cholybar is contraindicated in patients with complete biliary obstruction where bile is not secreted into the intestine and in those individuals who have shown hypersensitivity to any of its components.

PRECAUTIONS

General: Before instituting therapy with Cholybar, diseases contributing to increased blood cholesterol such as hypothyroidism, diabetes mellitus, nephrotic syndrome, dysproteinemias and obstructive liver disease should be looked for and specifically treated. A favorable trend in cholesterol reduction should occur during the first month of cholestyramine resin therapy. The therapy should be continued to sustain cholesterol reduction. If adequate cholesterol reduction is not attained, cholestyramine resin therapy should be discontinued.

Chronic use of cholestyramine resin may be associated with increased bleeding tendency due to hypoprothrombinemia associated with Vitamin K deficiency. This will usually respond promptly to parenteral Vitamin K$_1$, and recurrences can be prevented by oral administration of Vitamin K$_1$. Reduction of serum or red cell folate has been reported over long term administration of cholestyramine resin. Supplementation with folic acid should be considered in these cases. There is a possibility that prolonged use of cholestyramine resin, since it is a chloride form of anion exchange resin, may produce hyperchloremic acidosis. This would especially be true in younger and smaller patients where the relative dosage may be higher.

Cholestyramine resin may produce or worsen preexisting constipation. Dosage should be reduced or discontinued in such cases. Fecal impaction and aggravation of hemorrhoids may occur. Every effort should be made to avert severe constipation and its inherent problems in those patients with clinically symptomatic coronary artery disease.

> **Information for Patients:**
> 1. Inform your physician if you are pregnant or plan to become pregnant or are breast feeding.
> 2. Cholestyramine resin may bind other drugs. Therefore, take other drugs at least one hour before or 4–6 hours after Cholybar (or at as great an interval as possible) to avoid impeding their absorption.
> 3. Chew each bar thoroughly.
> 4. Drink plenty of fluids.

Laboratory Tests: Serum cholesterol levels should be determined frequently during the first few months of therapy and periodically thereafter. Serum triglyceride levels should be measured periodically to detect whether significant changes have occurred.

The LRC-CPPT showed a dose-related increase in serum triglycerides of 10.7–17.1% in the cholestyramine-treated group, compared with an increase of 7.0–11.7% in the placebo group. Based on the mean values and adjusting for the placebo group, the cholestyramine-treated group showed an increase of 5% over pre-entry levels the first year of the study and an increase of 4.3% the seventh year.

Drug Interactions: Cholestyramine resin may delay or reduce the absorption of concomitant oral medication such as phenylbutazone, warfarin, chlorothiazide (acidic), as well as tetracycline, penicillin G, phenobarbital, thyroid and thyroxine preparations, and digitalis. The discontinuation of cholestyramine resin could pose a hazard to health if a potentially toxic drug such as digitalis has been titrated to a maintenance level while the patient was taking cholestyramine resin.

Because cholestyramine binds bile acids, cholestyramine resin may interfere with normal fat digestion and absorption and thus may prevent absorption of fat soluble vitamins such as A, D, and K. When Cholybar is given for long periods of time, concomitant supplementation with water-miscible (or parenteral) forms of vitamins A and D should be considered.

SINCE CHOLESTYRAMINE RESIN MAY BIND OTHER DRUGS GIVEN CONCURRENTLY, PATIENTS SHOULD TAKE OTHER DRUGS AT LEAST ONE HOUR BEFORE OR 4–6 HOURS AFTER CHOLYBAR (OR AT AS GREAT AN INTERVAL AS POSSIBLE) TO AVOID IMPEDING THEIR ABSORPTION.

Carcinogenesis, Mutagenesis and Impairment of Fertility: In studies conducted in rats in which cholestyramine resin was used as a tool to investigate the role of various intestinal factors, such as fat, bile salts and microbial flora, in the development of intestinal tumors induced by potent carcinogens, the incidence of such tumors was observed to be greater in cholestyramine resin treated rats than in control rats. The relevance of this laboratory observation from studies in rats to the clinical use of cholestyramine is not known. In the LRC-CPPT study referred to above, the total incidence of fatal and nonfatal neoplasms was similar in both treatment groups. When the many different catagories of tumors are examined, various alimentary system cancers were somewhat more prevalent in the cholestyramine group. The small numbers and the multiple categories prevent conclusions from being drawn. However, in view of the fact that cholestyramine resin is confined to the GI tract and not absorbed, and in light of the animal experiments referred to above, further follow-up of the LRC-CPPT participants is planned for cause-specific mortality and cancer morbidity.

Pregnancy: Since cholestyramine resin is not absorbed systemically, it is not expected to cause fetal harm when administered during pregnancy in recommended dosages. There are, however, no adequate and well controlled studies in pregnant women and the known interference with absorption of fat soluble vitamins may be detrimental even in the presence of supplementation.

Nursing Mothers: Caution should be exercised when Cholybar is administered to a nursing mother. The possible lack of proper vitamin absorption described in the "Pregnancy" section may have an effect on nursing infants.

Pediatric Use: As experience in infants and children is limited, a practical dosage schedule has not been established. The effects of long term drug administration, as well as its effect in maintaining lowered cholesterol levels in pediatric patients, are unknown.

ADVERSE REACTIONS

The most common adverse reaction is constipation. When used as a cholesterol-lowering agent, predisposing factors for most complaints of constipation are high dose and increased age (more than 60 years old). Most instances of constipation are mild, transient, and controlled with conventional therapy. Some patients require a temporary decrease in dosage or discontinuation of therapy.

Less Frequent Adverse Reactions: Abdominal discomfort, flatulence, nausea, vomiting, diarrhea, heartburn, anorexia, indigestive feeling and steatorrhea, bleeding tendencies due to hypoprothrombinemia (Vitamin K deficiency) as well as Vitamin A (one case of night blindness reported) and D deficiencies, hyperchloremic acidosis in children, osteoporosis, rash and irritation of the skin, tongue and perianal area. One ten-month-old baby with biliary atresia had an impaction presumed to be due to cholestyramine resin after three days administration of 9 grams daily. She developed acute intestinal sepsis and died.

Occasional calcified material has been observed in the biliary tree, including calcification of the gallbladder, in patients to whom cholestyramine resin has been given. However, this may be a manifestation of the liver disease and not drug related.

One patient experienced biliary colic on each of three occasions on which he took cholestyramine resin. One patient diagnosed as acute abdominal symptom complex was found to have a "pasty mass" in the transverse colon on x-ray. Other events (not necessarily drug-related) reported in patients taking cholestyramine resin include:

Gastrointestinal—GI-rectal bleeding, black stools, hemorrhoidal bleeding, bleeding from known duodenal ulcer, dysphagia, hiccups, ulcer attack, sour taste, pancreatitis, rectal pain, diverticulitis.

Hematologic—Prolonged prothrombin time, ecchymosis, anemia.

Hypersensitivity—Urticaria, asthma, wheezing, shortness of breath.

Musculoskeletal—Backache, muscle and joint pains, arthritis.

Neurologic—Headache, anxiety, vertigo, dizziness, fatigue, tinnitus, syncope, drowsiness, femoral nerve pain, paresthesia.

Continued on next page

This product information was prepared in August, 1989. On these and other Parke-Davis Products, information may be obtained by addressing PARKE-DAVIS, Division of Warner-Lambert Company, Morris Plains, New Jersey 07950.

Parke-Davis—Cont.

Eye—Uveitis.
Renal—Hematuria, dysuria, burnt odor to urine, diuresis.
Miscellaneous—Weight loss, weight gain, increased libido, swollen glands, edema, dental bleeding.

OVERDOSAGE

Overdosage of cholestyramine resin has not been reported. Should overdosage occur, however, the chief potential harm would be obstruction of the gastrointestinal tract. The location of such potential obstruction, the degree of obstruction, and the presence or absence of normal gut motility would determine treatment.

DOSAGE AND ADMINISTRATION

The recommended adult dose is one bar, which contains 4 grams of anhydrous cholestyramine resin, one to six times daily. Each bar should be chewed thoroughly. Dosage may be adjusted as required to meet the patient's needs.

HOW SUPPLIED

Cholybar is available in the following flavors in cartons of 25 bars, each containing 4 grams of anhydrous cholestyramine resin, USP;

N 0071-0895-13	Caramel-flavored (individually wrapped, light-caramel-colored, chewable bars; 50 calories/bar; 7 g fructose/bar)
N 0071-0896-13	Raspberry-flavored (individually wrapped, red, chewable bars; 60 calories/bar; 9.5 g fructose/bar)

Storage: Store below 30°C (86°F).

CLINICAL STUDIES

The NIH has concluded a 10-year randomized double-blind placebo-controlled study* in 12 lipid research clinics on the effect of lowering plasma cholesterol on coronary heart disease (CHD) risk (the risk of either coronary death or nonfatal myocardial infarction). Plasma cholesterol was lowered by a combination of a modest cholesterol-lowering diet and cholestyramine resin. The dose response relationship between the amount of cholestyramine resin ingested daily, the lowering of total plasma cholesterol, and the reduction in CHD risk is summarized below:

RELATION OF REDUCTION IN CHOLESTEROL TO REDUCTION IN CORONARY HEART DISEASE RISK

Dose (No. of 4-gram Packages)	No.	Total Cholesterol Lowering	Reduction in CHD Risk
0–2	439	4.4%	10.9%
2–5	496	11.5%	26.1%
5–6	965	19.0%	39.3%

Reference:
* Anon: The Lipid Research Clinics Coronary Primary Prevention Trial Results: (I) Reduction in Incidence of Coronary Heart Disease; (II) The Relationship of Reduction in Incidence of Coronary Heart Disease to Cholesterol Lowering. *JAMA* 1984; 251:351–374.
Caution—Federal law prohibits dispensing without prescription.
Revised December 1988
Patent 4,778,676
© Copyright 1987. Warner-Lambert Co

0895G013
Shown in Product Identification Section, page 421

COLY-MYCIN® M PARENTERAL   ℞
[cŏ″ly-my′cĭn pă″rĕn′tĕr-ăl]
(sterile colistimethate sodium, USP)
for intramuscular and intravenous use

DESCRIPTION

Coly-Mycin M Parenteral (sterile colistimethate sodium) contains the sodium salt of colistimethate. Colistimethate sodium is a polypeptide antibiotic with an approximate molecular weight of 1750; the empirical formula is $C_{58}H_{105}N_{16}Na_5O_{28}S_5$.

CLINICAL PHARMACOLOGY

Microbiology
Coly-Mycin M Parenteral has bactericidal activity against the following gram-negative bacilli: *Enterobacter aerogenes, Escherichia coli, Klebsiella pneumoniae,* and *Pseudomonas aeruginosa.*

Human Pharmacology
Typical serum and urine levels following a single 150 mg dose of Coly-Mycin M Parenteral IM or IV in normal adult subjects are shown in Figure 1.

Figure 1

Figure 1. Urine and serum values in adults following parenteral (IM or IV) administration of Coly-Mycin M Parenteral Higher serum levels were obtained at 10 minutes following IV administration. Serum concentration declined with a half-life of 2-3 hours following either intravenous or intramuscular administration in adults and children, including premature infants.

Colistimethate sodium is transferred across the placental barrier, and blood levels of about 1 mcg/ml are obtained in the fetus following intravenous administration to the mother.

Average urine levels ranged from about 270 mcg/ml at 2 hours to about 15 mcg/ml at 8 hours after intravenous administration and from about 200 to about 25 mcg/ml during a similar period following intramuscular administration.

INDICATIONS AND USAGE

Coly-Mycin M Parenteral (sterile colistimethate sodium) is indicated for the treatment of acute or chronic infections due to sensitive strains of certain gram-negative bacilli. It is particularly indicated when the infection is caused by sensitive strains of *Pseudomonas aeruginosa.* This antibiotic is not indicated for infections due to *Proteus* or *Neisseria.* Coly-Mycin M Parenteral has proven clinically effective in treatment of infections due to the following gram-negative organisms: *Enterobacter aerogenes, Escherichia coli, Klebsiella pneumoniae,* and *Pseudomonas aeruginosa.*

Pending results of appropriate bacteriologic cultures and sensitivity tests, Coly-Mycin M Parenteral may be used to initiate therapy in serious infections that are suspected to be due to gram-negative organisms.

CONTRAINDICATIONS

The use of Coly-Mycin M Parenteral is contraindicated for patients with a history of sensitivity to the drug.

WARNING

Maximum daily dose should not exceed 5 mg/kg/day (2.3 mg/lb) with normal renal function.

Transient neurological disturbances may occur. These include circumoral paresthesias or numbness, tingling or formication of the extremities, generalized pruritus, vertigo, dizziness, and slurring of speech. For these reasons, patients should be warned not to drive vehicles or use hazardous machinery while on therapy. Reduction of dosage may alleviate symptoms. Therapy need not be discontinued, but such patients should be observed with particular care. Overdosage can result in renal insufficiency, muscle weakness and apnea. See PRECAUTIONS for use concomitantly with curariform drugs, and DOSAGE and ADMINISTRATION Section for use in renal impairment.

PRECAUTIONS

Since Coly-Mycin M Parenteral (sterile colistimethate sodium) is eliminated mainly by renal excretion, it should be used with caution when the possibility of impaired renal function exists. The decline in renal function with advanced age should be considered.

When actual renal impairment is present, Coly-Mycin M Parenteral may be used, but the greatest caution should be exercised and the dosage should be reduced in proportion to the extent of the impairment. Administration of amounts of Coly-Mycin M Parenteral in excess of renal excretory capacity will lead to high serum levels and can result in further impairment of renal function, initiating a cycle which, if not recognized, can lead to acute renal insufficiency, renal shutdown and further concentration of the antibiotic to toxic levels in the body. At this point, interference of nerve transmission at neuromuscular junctions may occur and result in muscle weakness and apnea.

Easily recognized signs indicating the development of impaired renal function are diminishing urine output, rising BUN and serum creatinine. If present, therapy with Coly-Mycin M Parenteral (sterile colistimethate sodium) should be discontinued immediately.

If a life-threatening situation exists, therapy may be reinstated at a lower dosage after blood levels have fallen. Certain other antibiotics (kanamycin, streptomycin, dihydrostreptomycin, polymyxin, neomycin) have also been reported to interfere with the nerve transmission at the neuro-

---

muscular junction. Based on this reported activity, they should not be given concomitantly with Coly-Mycin M Parenteral except with the greatest caution. The antibiotics with a gram-positive antimicrobial spectrum, e.g., penicillin, tetracycline, sodium cephalothin, have not been reported to interfere with nerve transmission and, accordingly, would not be expected to potentiate this activity of Coly-Mycin M Parenteral.

Other drugs, including curariform muscle relaxants (ether, tubocurarine, succinylcholine, gallamine, decamethonium and sodium citrate), potentiate the neuromuscular blocking effect and should be used with extreme caution in patients being treated with Coly-Mycin M Parenteral.

If apnea occurs, it may be treated with assisted respiration, oxygen, and calcium chloride injections.

USE IN PREGNANCY

The safety of colistimethate sodium during human pregnancy has not been established.

ADVERSE REACTIONS

Respiratory arrest has been reported following intramuscular administration of colistimethate sodium. Impaired renal function increases the possibility of apnea and neuromuscular blockade following administration of colistimethate sodium. This has been generally due to failure to follow recommended guidelines, usually overdosage, failure to reduce dose commensurate with degree of renal impairment, and/or concomitant use of other antibiotics or drugs with neuromuscular blocking potential.

A decrease in urine output or increase in blood urea nitrogen or serum creatinine can be interpreted as signs of nephrotoxicity, which is probably a dose-dependent effect of colistimethate sodium. These manifestations of nephrotoxicity are reversible following discontinuation of the antibiotic.

Increases of blood urea nitrogen have been reported for patients receiving Coly-Mycin M Parenteral (sterile colistimethate sodium) at dose levels of 1.6-5 mg/kg per day. The BUN values returned to normal following cessation of Coly-Mycin M Parenteral administration.

Paresthesia, tingling of the extremities or tingling of the tongue and generalized itching or urticaria have been reported by patients who received Coly-Mycin M Parenteral by intravenous or intramuscular injection. In addition, the following adverse reactions have been reported for colistimethate sodium: drug fever and gastrointestinal upset, vertigo, and slurring of speech. The subjective symptoms reported by the adult may not be manifest in infants or young children, thus requiring close attention to renal function.

DOSAGE AND ADMINISTRATION

Important: Coly-Mycin M Parenteral (sterile colistimethate sodium) is supplied in vials containing colistimethate sodium equivalent to 150 mg colistin base activity per vial.
Reconstitution: The *150-mg* vial should be reconstituted with *2.0 ml* Sterile Water for Injection USP. The reconstituted solution provides colistimethate sodium at a concentration of 75 mg/ml.
During reconstitution swirl *gently* to avoid frothing.

DOSAGE

Adults and children—intravenous or intramuscular administration—Coly-Mycin M Parenteral should be given in 2 to 4 divided doses at dose levels of 2.5 to 5 mg/kg per day for patients with normal renal function, depending on the severity of the infection.

The daily dose should be reduced in the presence of any renal impairment, which can often be anticipated from the history.

Modifications of dosage in the presence of renal impairment are presented in Table 1.
[See table on top next page].

INTRAVENOUS ADMINISTRATION
1.   Direct Intermittent Administration — slowly inject one-half of the total daily dose over a period of 3 to 5 minutes every 12 hours.
2.   Continuous Infusion — slowly inject one-half the total daily dose over 3 to 5 minutes. Add the remaining half of the total daily dose of Coly-Mycin M Parenteral to one of the following: 0.9% NaCl; 5% dextrose in 0.9% NaCl; 5% dextrose in water; 5% dextrose in 0.45% NaCl; 5% dextrose in 0.225% NaCl; lactated Ringer's solution, or 10% invert sugar solution. There are not sufficient data to recommend usage of Coly-Mycin M Parenteral with other drugs or with other than the above listed infusion solutions.
Administer by slow intravenous infusion starting 1 to 2 hours after the initial dose at a rate of 5-6 mg/hr in the presence of normal renal function. In the presence of impaired renal function, reduce the infusion rate depending on the degree of renal impairment.
The choice of intravenous solution and the volume to be employed are dictated by the requirements of fluid and electrolyte management.

> Any infusion solution containing colistimethate sodium should be freshly prepared and used for no longer than 24 hours.

HOW SUPPLIED

Coly-Mycin M Parenteral (sterile colistimethate sodium) is supplied in vials containing colistimethate sodium (150 mg colistin base equivalent per vial) as a white to slightly yellow lyophilized cake and is available as one vial per carton (N 0071-4145-01) or as 50 vials per carton (N 0071-4145-47). **STORE AT CONTROLLED ROOM TEMPERATURE (15° to 30°C) (59° to 86°F).**

STORE RECONSTITUTED SOLUTION IN REFRIGERATOR (2° to 8°C) (36° to 46°F) OR AT CONTROLLED ROOM TEMPERATURE (15° to 30°C) (59° to 86°F), and use within 7 days.

Toxicology and Animal Pharmacology:

Acute Toxicity: The intravenous LD_{50} was 41.5 mg/kg in the dog and 739 mg/kg in the mouse; intramuscular toxicity was 42 mg/kg in the dog and 267 mg/kg in the mouse.

Subacute Toxicity: In albino rabbits and beagle dogs, IV doses of 5, 10 and 20 mg/kg/day for 28 days resulted in elevated blood urea nitrogen in the dog (10 mg/kg/day dose group) and in both 20 mg/kg dose groups.

Clinical Studies: Clinically, Coly-Mycin M Parenteral (sterile colistimethate sodium) has been of particular therapeutic value in acute and chronic urinary tract infections caused by sensitive strains of *Pseudomonas aeruginosa*. Colistimethate sodium is clinically effective in the treatment of infections due to other sensitive gram-negative pathogenic bacilli that have become resistant to broad-spectrum antibiotics. Colistimethate sodium has been used to treat bacteriuria and overt urinary infections in pregnant women during the third trimester. However, in view of the evidence of possible embryotoxic and teratogenic effects of colistimethate sodium in pregnant rabbits, caution should be exercised in use of this drug in women of childbearing potential.

4145G014

COLY-MYCIN® S FOR ORAL SUSPENSION   ℞
[cŏ "ly-my 'cĭn]
(colistin sulfate for oral suspension, USP)
FOR ORAL USE ONLY

DESCRIPTION

Coly-Mycin S For Oral Suspension (colistin sulfate for oral suspension) contains the sulfate salt of colistin, a polypeptide antibiotic with a molecular weight of approximately 1170. The empirical formula of colistin is $C_{53}H_{100}N_{16}O_{13}$.

Each 5 mL of Coly-Mycin S Suspension contains the equivalent of 25 mg colistin base. Also contains citric acid, USP; cocoa, NF; dried low fat milk solids; guar gum, NF; imitation chocolate flavor; imitation vanilla bean flavor; magnesium stearate, NF; menthol, USP; methylparaben, NF; propylparaben, NF; saccharin sodium, USP; sodium chloride, USP; sorbitol, NF; sucrose, NF.

CLINICAL PHARMACOLOGY

Colistin sulfate has *in vitro* bactericidal activity against most gram-negative enteric pathogens, especially enteropathogenic *E. coli* and *Shigella* (but not *Proteus*). In infants and children, it has effectively controlled acute infections of the intestinal tract due to these pathogens. Susceptible strains of *E. coli* and *Shigella in vitro* or *in vivo* rarely develop resistance to colistin sulfate. Cross resistance to polymyxin B sulfate does exist, but cross resistance to broad spectrum antibiotics has not been encountered.

INDICATIONS AND USAGE

Diarrhea in infants and children, caused by susceptible strains of enteropathogenic *E. coli.*
Gastroenteritis due to *Shigella* organisms. Clinical response may vary due to the absence of tissue levels in the bowel wall.

CONTRAINDICATIONS

Known hypersensitivity to the drug.

WARNINGS

Although colistin sulfate is not absorbed systemically in measurable amounts, it is assumed that slight absorption may occur. Therefore, in the presence of azotemia or, if dosages above the recommended range are used, a potential for possible renal toxicity exists.

With prolonged usage, suppression of intestinal bacterial flora may occur. There may be a resultant overgrowth of organisms (such as *Proteus*); appropriate therapy should be initiated immediately.

PRECAUTIONS

Renal function should be assessed prior to initiation of therapy.

Table 1

SUGGESTED MODIFICATION OF DOSAGE SCHEDULES OF COLY-MYCIN M PARENTERAL (STERILE COLISTIMETHATE SODIUM) FOR ADULTS WITH IMPAIRED RENAL FUNCTION

RENAL FUNCTION	Normal	DEGREE OF IMPAIRMENT		
		Mild	Moderate	Considerable
Plasma creatinine, (mg/100 ml)	0.7–1.2	1.3–1.5	1.6–2.5	2.6–4.0
Urea clearance, % of normal	80–100	40–70	25–40	10–25
DOSAGE				
Unit dose of Coly-Mycin M, mg	100–150	75–115	66–150	100–150
Frequency, times/day	4 to 2	2	2 or 1	every 36 hr
Total daily dose, mg	300	150–230	133–150	100
Approximate daily dose, mg/kg/day	5.0	2.5–3.8	2.5	1.5

NOTE

The suggested unit dose is 2.5–5 mg/kg; however, the time INTERVAL between injections should be increased in the presence of impaired renal function.

ADVERSE REACTIONS

Within the recommended dosage range, none reported.

DOSAGE AND ADMINISTRATION

The usual dosage of colistin base (supplied as the sulfate) is 5–15 mg/kg/day (2.3–6.8 mg/pound/day) given in three divided doses. Higher doses may be necessary. Each 5 ml of suspension contains the equivalent of 25 mg colistin base. A 10-pound infant would require a total daily dose of 23–68 mg colistin base, given in divided doses (approximately ⅓ to 1 teaspoonful three times a day). A 50-pound patient would require a total daily dose of 115–340 mg colistin base, given in divided doses (approximately 1½–4½ teaspoonfuls three times a day).

PREPARATION

Coly-Mycin S For Oral Suspension (colistin sulfate for oral suspension) is a dry powder which is reconstituted with 37 ml of distilled water. To reconstitute, slowly add one half of the diluent, replace the cap and shake well. Add the remaining diluent and repeat shaking. Volume after reconstitution is 60 ml. When reconstituted, Coly-Mycin S Oral Suspension is a chocolate-flavored mixture, each 5 ml teaspoonful containing the equivalent of 25 mg of colistin base. Reconstituted Coly-Mycin S Oral Suspension is stable for two weeks when kept below 15°C (59°F).

SUPPLIED

Bottles containing colistin sulfate equivalent to 300 mg colistin base (N 0071-2142-15).
Before reconstitution store between 15° and 30°C.

2142G013

Caution—Federal law prohibits dispensing without prescription.

COLY-MYCIN® S OTIC   ℞
[cŏ "ly-my 'cĭn s ŏ 'tĭc]
with Neomycin and Hydrocortisone
(colistin sulfate—neomycin sulfate—thonzonium bromide—hydrocortisone acetate otic suspension)

DESCRIPTION

Coly-Mycin S Otic with Neomycin and Hydrocortisone (colistin sulfate-neomycin sulfate-thonzonium bromide-hydrocortisone acetate otic suspension) is a sterile aqueous suspension containing in each ml: Colistin base activity, 3 mg (as the sulfate); Neomycin base activity, 3.3 mg (as the sulfate); Hydrocortisone acetate, 10 mg (1%); Thonzonium bromide, 0.5 mg (0.05%); Polysorbate 80, acetic acid, and sodium acetate in a buffered aqueous vehicle. Thimerosal (mercury derivative), 0.002%, added as a preservative. It is a nonviscous liquid, buffered at pH 5, for instillation into the canal of the external ear or direct application to the affected aural skin.

CLINICAL PHARMACOLOGY

1. Colistin sulfate—an antibiotic with bactericidal action against most gram-negative organisms, notably *Pseudomonas aeruginosa, E. coli.,* and *Klebsiella-Aerobacter.*
2. Neomycin sulfate—a broad-spectrum antibiotic, bactericidal to many pathogens, notably *Staph aureus* and *Proteus* sp.

3. Hydrocortisone acetate—a corticosteroid that controls inflammation, edema, pruritus and other dermal reactions.
4. Thonzonium bromide—a surface-active agent that promotes tissue contact by dispersion and penetration of the cellular debris and exudate.

INDICATIONS AND USAGE

For the treatment of superficial bacterial infections of the external auditory canal, caused by organisms susceptible to the action of the antibiotics; and for the treatment of infections of mastoidectomy and fenestration cavities, caused by organisms susceptible to the antibiotics.

CONTRAINDICATIONS

This product is contraindicated in those individuals who have shown hypersensitivity to any of its components, and in herpes simplex, vaccinia and varicella.

WARNINGS

As with other antibiotic preparations, prolonged treatment may result in overgrowth of nonsusceptible organisms and fungi.

If the infection is not improved after one week, cultures and susceptibility tests should be repeated to verify the identity of the organism and to determine whether therapy should be changed.

Patients who prefer to warm the medication before using should be cautioned against heating the solution above body temperature, in order to avoid loss of potency.

PRECAUTIONS

General: If sensitization or irritation occurs, medication should be discontinued promptly.

This drug should be used with care in cases of perforated eardrum and in longstanding cases of chronic otitis media because of the possibility of ototoxicity caused by neomycin. Treatment should not be continued for longer than ten days. Allergic cross-reactions may occur which could prevent the use of any or all of the following antibiotics for the treatment of future infections: kanamycin, paromomycin, streptomycin, and possibly gentamicin.

ADVERSE REACTIONS

Neomycin is a not uncommon cutaneous sensitizer. There are articles in the current literature that indicate an increase in the prevalence of persons sensitive to neomycin.

DOSAGE AND ADMINISTRATION

The external auditory canal should be thoroughly cleansed and dried with a sterile cotton applicator.

When using the calibrated dropper:

For adults, 5 drops of the suspension should be instilled into the affected ear 3 or 4 times daily. For infants and children, 4 drops are suggested because of the smaller capacity of the ear canal.

This dosage correlates to the 4 drops (for adults) and 3 drops (for children) recommended when using the dropper-bottle container for this product.

Continued on next page

This product information was prepared in August, 1989. On these and other Parke-Davis Products, information may be obtained by addressing PARKE-DAVIS, Division of Warner-Lambert Company, Morris Plains, New Jersey 07950.

Parke-Davis—Cont.

The patient should lie with the affected ear upward and then the drops should be instilled. This position should be maintained for 5 minutes to facilitate penetration of the drops into the ear canal. Repeat, if necessary, for the opposite ear. If preferred, a cotton wick may be inserted into the canal and then the cotton may be saturated with the solution. This wick should be kept moist by adding further solution every 4 hours. The wick should be replaced at least once every 24 hours.

HOW SUPPLIED

Coly-Mycin S Otic is supplied as:

N 0071-3141-35—5-mL bottle with dropper
N 0071-3141-36—10-mL bottle with dropper
Each ml contains: Colistin sulfate equivalent to 3 mg of colistin base, Neomycin sulfate equivalent to 3.3 mg neomycin base, Hydrocortisone acetate 10 mg (1%), Thonzonium bromide 0.5 mg (0.05%), and Polysorbate 80 in an aqueous vehicle buffered with acetic acid and sodium acetate. Thimerosal (mercury derivative) 0.002% added as a preservative.
Shake well before using.
Store at controlled room temperature 15°–30°C (59°–86°F). Stable for 18 months at room temperature; prolonged exposure to higher temperatures should be avoided.

                                   3141G033

Caution—Federal law prohibits dispensing without prescription.

KAPSEALS®
DILANTIN®   ℞
[dī-lăn ′tĭn ″]
(Extended Phenytoin Sodium Capsules, USP)

DESCRIPTION

Phenytoin Sodium is an antiepileptic drug. Phenytoin sodium is related to the barbiturates in chemical structure, but has a five-membered ring. The chemical name is sodium 5,5-diphenyl-2,4-imidazolidinedione.

Each Dilantin—*Extended Phenytoin Sodium Capsule* USP contains 30 mg or 100 mg phenytoin sodium USP. Also contains lactose, NF; sucrose, NF; talc, USP; and other ingredients. The capsule shell and band contain colloidal silicon dioxide, NF; FD&C red No. 3; gelatin, NF; glyceryl monooleate; sodium lauryl sulfate, NF. The Dilantin 30-mg capsule shell and band also contain citric acid, USP; FD&C blue No. 1; sodium benzoate, NF; titanium dioxide, USP. The Dilantin 100-mg capsule shell and band also contain FD&C yellow No. 6; hydrogen peroxide 3%; polyethylene glycol 200. Product *in vivo* performance is characterized by a slow and extended rate of absorption with peak blood concentrations expected in 4 to 12 hours as contrasted to *Prompt Phenytoin Sodium Capsules* USP with a rapid rate of absorption with peak blood concentration expected in 1½ to 3 hours.

CLINICAL PHARMACOLOGY

Phenytoin is an antiepileptic drug which can be useful in the treatment of epilepsy. The primary site of action appears to be *the motor cortex* where spread of seizure activity is inhibited. Possibly by promoting sodium efflux from neurons, phenytoin tends to *stabilize* the threshold against hyperexcitability caused by excessive stimulation or environmental changes capable of reducing membrane sodium gradient. This includes the reduction of posttetanic potentiation at synapses. Loss of posttetanic potentiation prevents cortical seizure foci from detonating adjacent cortical areas. Phenytoin reduces the maximal activity of brain stem centers responsible for the tonic phase of tonic-clonic (grand mal) seizures.

The plasma half-life in man after oral administration of phenytoin averages 22 hours, with a range of 7 to 42 hours. Steady-state therapeutic levels are achieved 7 to 10 days after initiation of therapy with recommended doses of 300 mg/day.

When serum level determinations are necessary, they should be obtained at least 5-7 half-lives after treatment initiation, dosage change, or addition or subtraction of another drug to the regimen so that equilibrium or steady-state will have been achieved. Trough levels provide information about clinically effective serum level range and confirm patient compliance and are obtained just prior to the patient's next scheduled dose. Peak levels indicate an individual's threshold for emergence of dose-related side effects and are obtained at the time of expected peak concentration. For Dilantin Kapseals peak serum levels occur 4-12 hours after administration.

Optimum control without clinical signs of toxicity occurs more often with serum levels between 10 and 20 mcg/ml, although some mild cases of tonic-clonic (grand mal) epilepsy may be controlled with lower-serum levels of phenytoin.

In most patients maintained at a steady dosage, stable phenytoin serum levels are achieved. There may be wide interpatient variability in phenytoin serum levels with equivalent dosages. Patients with unusually low levels may be noncompliant or hypermetabolizers of phenytoin. Unusually high levels result from liver disease, congenital enzyme deficiency or drug interactions which result in metabolic interference. The patient with large variations in phenytoin plasma levels, despite standard doses, presents a difficult clinical problem. Serum level determinations in such patients may be particularly helpful.

Most of the drug is excreted in the bile as inactive metabolites which are then reabsorbed from the intestinal tract and excreted in the urine. Urinary excretion of phenytoin and its metabolites occurs partly with glomerular filtration but more importantly, by tubular secretion. Because phenytoin is hydroxylated in the liver by an enzyme system which is saturable, small incremental doses may produce very substantial increases in serum levels, when these are in the upper range. The steady-state level may be disproportionately increased, with resultant intoxication, from an increase in dosage of 10% or more.

INDICATIONS AND USAGE

Dilantin is indicated for the control of tonic-clonic and psychomotor (grand mal and temporal lobe) seizures and prevention and treatment of seizures occurring during or following neurosurgery.

Phenytoin serum level determinations may be necessary for optimal dosage adjustments (see Dosage and Administration).

CONTRAINDICATIONS

Phenytoin is contraindicated in those patients who are hypersensitive to phenytoin or other hydantoins.

WARNINGS

Abrupt withdrawal of phenytoin in epileptic patients may precipitate status epilepticus. When, in the judgment of the clinician, the need for dosage reduction, discontinuation, or substitution of alternative antiepileptic medication arises, this should be done gradually. However, in the event of an allergic or hypersensitivity reaction, rapid substitution of alternative therapy may be necessary. In this case, alternative therapy should be an antiepileptic drug not belonging to the hydantoin chemical class.

There have been a number of reports suggesting a relationship between phenytoin and the development of lymphadenopathy (local or generalized) including benign lymph node hyperplasia, pseudolymphoma, lymphoma, and Hodgkin's Disease.

Although a cause and effect relationship has not been established, the occurrence of lymphadenopathy indicates the need to differentiate such a condition from other types of lymph node pathology. Lymph node involvement may occur with or without symptoms and signs resembling serum sickness eg, fever, rash and liver involvement.

In all cases of lymphadenopathy, follow-up observation for an extended period is indicated and every effort should be made to achieve seizure control using alternative antiepileptic drugs.

Acute alcoholic intake may increase phenytoin serum levels while chronic alcoholic use may decrease serum levels.

Usage in Pregnancy:

A number of reports suggests an association between the use of antiepileptic drugs by women with epilepsy and a higher incidence of birth defects in children born to these women. Data are more extensive with respect to phenytoin and phenobarbital, but these are also the most commonly prescribed antiepileptic drugs; less systematic or anecdotal reports suggest a possible similar association with the use of all known antiepileptic drugs.

The reports suggesting a higher incidence of birth defects in children of drug-treated epileptic women cannot be regarded as adequate to prove a definite cause and effect relationship. There are intrinsic methodologic problems in obtaining adequate data on drug teratogenicity in humans; genetic factors or the epileptic condition itself may be more important than drug therapy in leading to birth defects. The great majority of the mothers on antiepileptic medication deliver normal infants. It is important to note that antiepileptic drugs should not be discontinued in patients in whom the drug is administered to prevent major seizures, because of the strong possibility of precipitating status epilepticus with attendant hypoxia and threat to life. In individual cases where the severity and frequency of the seizure disorder are such that the removal of medication does not pose a serious threat to the patient, discontinuation of the drug may be considered prior to and during pregnancy, although it cannot be said with any confidence that even minor seizures do not pose some hazards to the developing embryo or fetus. The prescribing physician will wish to weigh these considerations in treating and counseling epileptic women of childbearing potential.

In addition to the reports of increased incidence of congenital malformation, such as cleft lip/palate and heart malformations in children of women receiving phenytoin and other antiepileptic drugs, there have more recently been reports of a fetal hydantoin syndrome. This consists of prenatal growth deficiency, microcephaly and mental deficiency in children born to mothers who have received phenytoin, barbiturates, alcohol, or trimethadione. However, these features are all interrelated and are frequently associated with intrauterine growth retardation from other causes.

There have been isolated reports of malignancies, including neuroblastoma, in children whose mothers received phenytoin during pregnancy.

An increase in seizure frequency during pregnancy occurs in a high proportion of patients, because of altered phenytoin absorption or metabolism. Periodic measurement of serum phenytoin levels is particularly valuable in the management of a pregnant epileptic patient as a guide to an appropriate adjustment of dosage. However, postpartum restoration of the original dosage will probably be indicated.

Neonatal coagulation defects have been reported within the first 24 hours in babies born to epileptic mothers receiving phenobarbital and/or phenytoin. Vitamin K_1 has been shown to prevent or correct this defect and has been recommended to be given to the mother before delivery and the neonate after birth.

PRECAUTIONS

General:

The liver is the chief site of biotransformation of phenytoin; patients with impaired liver function, elderly patients, or those who are gravely ill may show early signs of toxicity.

A small percentage of individuals who have been treated with phenytoin have been shown to metabolize the drug slowly. Slow metabolism may be due to limited enzyme availability and lack of induction; it appears to be genetically determined.

Phenytoin should be discontinued if a skin rash appears (see "Warnings" section regarding drug discontinuation). If the rash is exfoliative, purpuric, or bullous or if lupus erythematosus or Stevens-Johnson syndrome or toxic epidermal necrolysis is suspected, use of the drug should not be resumed. (See Adverse Reactions.) If the rash is of a milder type (measles-like or scarlatiniform), therapy may be resumed after the rash has completely disappeared. If the rash recurs upon reinstitution of therapy, further phenytoin medication is contraindicated.

Hyperglycemia, resulting from the drug's inhibitory effects on insulin release, has been reported. Phenytoin may also raise the serum glucose level in diabetic patients.

Osteomalacia has been associated with phenytoin therapy and is considered to be due to phenytoin's interference with Vitamin D metabolism.

Phenytoin is not indicated for seizures due to hypoglycemic or other causes. Appropriate diagnostic procedures should be performed as indicated.

Phenytoin is not effective for absence (petit mal) seizures. If tonic-clonic (grand-mal) and absence (petit mal) seizures are present, combined drug therapy is needed.

Serum levels of phenytoin sustained above the optimal range may produce confusional states referred to as "delirium," "psychosis," or "encephalopathy," or rarely irreversible cerebellar dysfunction. Accordingly, at the first sign of acute toxicity, plasma levels are recommended. Dose reduction of phenytoin therapy is indicated if plasma levels are excessive; if symptoms persist, termination is recommended. (See Warnings.)

Information for Patients:

Patients taking phenytoin should be advised of the importance of adhering strictly to the prescribed dosage regimen, and of informing the physician of any clinical condition in which it is not possible to take the drug orally as prescribed, eg, surgery, etc.

Patients should also be cautioned on the use of other drugs or alcoholic beverages without first seeking the physician's advice.

Patients should be instructed to call their physician if skin rash develops.

The importance of good dental hygiene should be stressed in order to minimize the development of gingival hyperplasia and its complications.

Laboratory Tests:

Phenytoin serum level determinations may be necessary to achieve optimal dosage adjustments.

Drug Interactions:

There are many drugs which may increase or decrease phenytoin levels or which phenytoin may affect. The most commonly occurring drug interactions are listed below:

1. Drugs which may increase phenytoin serum levels include: chloramphenicol, dicumarol, disulfiram, tolbutamide, isoniazid, phenylbutazone, acute alcohol intake, salicylates, chlordiazepoxide, phenothiazines, diazepam, estrogens, ethosuximide, halothane, methylphenidate, sulfonamides, cimetidine, trazodone.
2. Drugs which may decrease phenytoin levels include: carbamazepine, chronic alcohol abuse, reserpine. Moban® brand of Molindone Hydrochloride contains calcium ions which interfere with the absorption of phenytoin. Ingestion times of phenytoin and antacid preparations containing calcium should be staggered in patients with low serum phenytoin levels to prevent absorption problems.

3. Drugs which may either increase or decrease phenytoin serum levels include: phenobarbital, valproic acid, and sodium valproate. Similarly, the effect of phenytoin on phenobarbital, valproic acid and sodium valproate serum levels is unpredictable.

4. Although not a true drug interaction, tricyclic antidepressants may precipitate seizures in susceptible patients and phenytoin dosage may need to be adjusted.

5. Drugs whose efficacy is impaired by phenytoin include: corticosteroids, coumarin anticoagulants, oral contraceptives, quinidine, vitamin D, digitoxin, rifampin, doxycycline, estrogens, furosemide.

Serum level determinations are especially helpful when possible drug interactions are suspected.

Drug/Laboratory Test Interactions:
Phenytoin may cause decreased serum levels of protein-bound iodine (PBI). It may also produce lower than normal values for dexamethasone or metyrapone tests. Phenytoin may cause raised serum levels of glucose, alkaline phosphatase, and gamma glutamyl transpeptidase (GGT).

Carcinogenesis:
See 'Warnings' section for information on carcinogenesis.

Pregnancy:
See Warnings

Nursing Mothers:
Infant breast feeding is not recommended for women taking this drug because phenytoin appears to be secreted in low concentrations in human milk.

ADVERSE REACTIONS

Central Nervous System: The most common manifestations encountered with phenytoin therapy are referable to this system and are usually dose-related. These include nystagmus, ataxia, slurred speech, and mental confusion. Dizziness, insomnia, transient nervousness, motor twitchings, and headaches have also been observed. There have also been rare reports of phenytoin induced dyskinesias, including chorea, dystonia, tremor and asterixis, similar to those induced by phenothiazine and other neuroleptic drugs.

A predominantly sensory peripheral polyneuropathy has been observed in patients receiving long-term phenytoin therapy.

Gastrointestinal System: Nausea, vomiting and constipation.

Integumentary System: Dermatological manifestations sometimes accompanied by fever have included scarlatiniform or morbilliform rashes. A morbilliform rash (measles-like) is the most common; other types of dermatitis are seen more rarely. Other more serious forms which may be fatal have included bullous, exfoliative or purpuric dermatitis, lupus erythematosus, Stevens-Johnson syndrome, and toxic epidermal necrolysis (see Precautions).

Hemopoietic System: Hemopoietic complications, some fatal, have occasionally been reported in association with administration of phenytoin. These have included thrombocytopenia, leukopenia, granulocytopenia, agranulocytosis, and pancytopenia. While macrocytosis and megaloblastic anemia have occurred, these conditions usually respond to folic acid therapy. Lymphadenopathy including benign lymph node hyperplasia, pseudolymphoma, lymphoma, and Hodgkin's Disease have been reported (see Warnings).

Connective Tissue System: Coarsening of the facial features, enlargement of the lips, gingival hyperplasia, hirsutism, and Peyronie's Disease.

Other: Systemic lupus erythematosus, periarteritis nodosa, toxic hepatitis, liver damage, and immunoglobulin abnormalities may occur.

OVERDOSAGE

The lethal dose in children is not known. The lethal dose in adults is estimated to be 2 to 5 grams. The initial symptoms are nystagmus, ataxia, and dysarthria. Other signs are tremor, hyperflexia, lethargy, slurred speech, nausea, vomiting. The patient may become comatose and hypotensive. Death is due to respiratory and circulatory depression.

There are marked variations among individuals with respect to phenytoin plasma levels where toxicity may occur. Nystagmus, on lateral gaze, usually appears at 20 mcg/ml, ataxia at 30 mcg/ml, dysarthria and lethargy appear when the plasma concentration is over 40 mcg/ml, but as high a concentration as 50 mcg/ml has been reported without evidence of toxicity. As much as 25 times the therapeutic dose has been taken to result in a serum concentration over 100 mcg/ml with complete recovery.

Treatment:
Treatment is nonspecific since there is no known antidote. The adequacy of the respiratory and circulatory systems should be carefully observed and appropriate supportive measures employed. Hemodialysis can be considered since phenytoin is not completely bound to plasma proteins. Total exchange transfusion has been used in the treatment of severe intoxication in children.

In acute overdosage the possibility of other CNS depressants, including alcohol, should be borne in mind.

DOSAGE AND ADMINISTRATION

Serum concentrations should be monitored in changing from extended Phenytoin Sodium Capsules USP (Dilantin) to Prompt Phenytoin sodium capsules USP, and from the sodium salt to the free acid form.

Dilantin® Kapseals,® Dilantin Parenteral, and Dilantin with Phenobarbital are formulated with the sodium salt of phenytoin. The free acid form of phenytoin is used in Dilantin-30 Pediatric and Dilantin-125 Suspensions and Dilantin Infatabs. Because there is approximately an 8% increase in drug content with the free acid form than the sodium salt, dosage adjustments and serum level monitoring may be necessary when switching from a product formulated with the free acid to a product formulated with the sodium salt and vice versa.

General:
Dosage should be individualized to provide maximum benefit. In some cases serum blood level determinations may be necessary for optimal dosage adjustments—the clinically effective serum level is usually 10-20 mcg/ml. With recommended dosage, a period of seven to ten days may be required to achieve steady-state blood levels with phenytoin and changes in dosage (increase or decrease) should not be carried out at intervals shorter than seven to ten days.

Adult Dosage:

Divided Daily Dosage
Patients who have received no previous treatment may be started on one 100 mg Dilantin (Extended Phenytoin Sodium Capsule) three times daily and the dosage then adjusted to suit individual requirements. For most adults, the satisfactory maintenance dosage will be one capsule three to four times a day. An increase up to two capsules three times a day may be made, if necessary.

Once-a-Day Dosage:
In adults, if seizure control is established with divided doses of three 100 mg Dilantin capsules daily, once-a-day dosage with 300 mg of extended phenytoin sodium capsules may be considered. Studies comparing divided doses of 300 mg with a single daily dose of this quantity indicated absorption, peak plasma levels, biologic half-life, difference between peak and minimum values, and urinary recovery were equivalent. Once-a-day dosage offers a convenience to the individual patient or to nursing personnel for institutionalized patients and is intended to be used only for patients requiring this amount of drug daily. A major problem in motivating non-compliant patients may also be lessened when the patient can take this drug once a day. However, patients should be cautioned not to miss a dose, inadvertently.

Only extended phenytoin sodium capsules are recommended for once-a-day dosing. Inherent differences in dissolution characteristics and resultant absorption rates of phenytoin due to different manufacturing procedures and/or dosage forms preclude such recommendation for other phenytoin products. When a change in the dosage form or brand is prescribed, careful monitoring of phenytoin serum levels should be carried out.

Loading Dose:
Some authorities have advocated use of an oral loading dose of phenytoin in adults who require rapid steady-state serum levels and where intravenous administration is not desirable. This dosing regimen should be reserved for patients in a clinic or hospital setting where phenytoin serum levels can be closely monitored. Patients with a history of renal or liver disease should not receive the oral loading regimen.

Initially, one gram of phenytoin capsules is divided into 3 doses (400 mg, 300 mg, 300 mg) and administered at two-hourly intervals. Normal maintenance dosage is then instituted 24 hours after the loading dose, with frequent serum level determinations.

Pediatric Dosage:
Initially, 5 mg/kg/day in two or three equally divided doses, with subsequent dosage individualized to a maximum of 300 mg daily. A recommended daily maintenance dosage is usually 4 to 8 mg/kg. Children over 6 years old may require the minimum adult dose (300 mg/day).

HOW SUPPLIED

N 0071-0362 (Kapseal 362, transparent #3 capsule with an orange band)—Dilantin 100 mg; in 100's, 1,000's, and unit dose 100's and in a Memo Pack containing 84 unit dose capsules (28 days dosage regimen).

N 0071-0365 (Kapseal 365, transparent #4 capsule with a pink band)—Dilantin 30 mg; in 100's, 1,000's and unit dose 100's.

Store below 30°C (86°F). Protect from light and moisture.
Shown in Product Identification Section, page 421

Also available as:
N 0071-2214—Dilantin-125® Suspension 125 mg phenytoin/5 ml with a maximum alcohol content not greater than 0.6 percent, available in 8-oz bottles and individual unit dose foil pouches which deliver 5 ml (125 mg phenytoin). The minimum sales unit is 100 pouches.

N 0071-2315—Dilantin-30® Pediatric Suspension 30 mg phenytoin/5 ml with a maximum alcohol content not greater than 0.6 percent; available in 8-oz bottles and individual unit

dose foil pouches which deliver 5 ml (30 mg phenytoin). The minimum sales unit is 100 pouches.

N 0071-0375 (Kapseal 375)—Dilantin with Phenobarbital each contain 100 mg phenytoin sodium with 16 mg (¼ gr) phenobarbital; in 100's and 1,000's.

N 0071-0531 (Kapseal 531)—Dilantin with Phenobarbital each contain 100 mg phenytoin sodium with 32 mg (½ gr) phenobarbital; in 100's, 1,000's and unit dose 100's.

N 0071-0007 (Tablet 7)—Dilantin Infatabs® each contain 50 mg phenytoin, 100's and unit dose 100's.

For Parenteral Use:
N 0071-4488-05 (Ampoule 1488)—Dilantin ready-mixed solution containing 50 mg phenytoin sodium per milliliter is supplied in 2-ml ampoules. Packages of ten.

N 0071-4488-41 (Steri-Dose® 4488)—Dilantin ready-mixed solution containing 50 mg phenytoin sodium per milliliter is supplied in a 2-ml sterile disposable syringe (22 gauge × 1¼ inch needle). Packages of ten individually cartoned syringes.

N 0071-4475-35 (Ampoule 1475)—Dilantin ready-mixed solution containing 50 mg phenytoin sodium per milliliter is supplied in 5-ml ampoules with one 6-ml sterile disposable syringe (22 gauge × 1¼ inch needle). Packages of ten.

N 0071-4475-08 (Ampoule 1475)—Dilantin ready-mixed solution containing 50 mg phenytoin sodium per milliliter is supplied in packages of ten 5-ml ampoules without syringes.

N 0071-4488-45 Dilantin ready-mixed solution containing 50 mg phenytoin sodium per milliliter is supplied in 2-mL Steri-Vials.® Packages of twenty-five.

N 0071-4475-45 Dilantin ready-mixed solution containing 50 mg phenytoin sodium per milliliter is supplied in 5-mL Steri-Vials.® Packages of twenty-five.

Store below 30°C (86°F). Protect from light and moisture.
0362G027

INFATABS®
DILANTIN®   ℞
[dī-lăn'tĭn " ĭn 'fă-tăbs "]
(Phenytoin Tablets, USP)

NOT FOR ONCE A DAY DOSING

DESCRIPTION

Dilantin is an antiepileptic drug.

Dilantin (phenytoin) is related to the barbiturates in chemical structure, but has a five-membered ring. The chemical name is 5,5-diphenyl-2,4-imidazolidinedione.

Each Dilantin Infatab, for oral administration, contains 50 mg phenytoin, USP. Also contains: D&C yellow No. 10, Al lake; FD&C yellow No. 6, Al lake flavor; saccharin sodium, USP; sucrose, NF; talc, USP; and other ingredients.

CLINICAL PHARMACOLOGY

Phenytoin is an antiepileptic drug which can be useful in the treatment of epilepsy. The primary site of action appears to be the motor cortex where spread of seizure activity is inhibited. Possibly by promoting sodium efflux from neurons, phenytoin tends to stabilize the threshold against hyperexcitability caused by excessive stimulation or environmental changes capable of reducing membrane sodium gradient. This includes the reduction of posttetanic potentiation at synapses. Loss of posttetanic potentiation prevents cortical seizure foci from detonating adjacent cortical areas. Phenytoin reduces the maximal activity of brain stem centers responsible for the tonic phase of tonic-clonic (grand mal) seizures.

Clinical studies using Dilantin Infatabs have shown an average plasma half-life of 14 hours with a range of 7 to 29 hours. Steady-state therapeutic levels are achieved at least 7 to 10 days (5-7 half-lives) after initiation of therapy with recommended doses of 300 mg/day.

When serum level determinations are necessary, they should be obtained at least 5-7 half-lives after treatment initiation, dosage change, or addition or subtraction of another drug to the regimen so that equilibrium or steady-state will have been achieved. Trough levels provide information about clinically effective serum level range and confirm patient compliance and are obtained just prior to the patient's next scheduled dose. Peak levels indicate an individual's threshold for emergence of dose-related side effects and are obtained at the time of expected peak concentration. For Dilantin Infatabs peak levels occur 1½-3 hours after administration.

Optimum control without clinical signs of toxicity occurs more often with serum levels between 10 and 20 mcg/ml, although some mild cases of tonic-clonic (grand mal) epilepsy may be controlled with lower-serum levels of phenytoin.

Continued on next page

This product information was prepared in August, 1989. On these and other Parke-Davis Products, information may be obtained by addressing PARKE-DAVIS, Division of Warner-Lambert Company, Morris Plains, New Jersey 07950.

Parke-Davis—Cont.

In most patients maintained at a steady dosage, stable phenytoin serum levels are achieved. There may be wide interpatient variability in phenytoin serum levels with equivalent dosages. Patients with unusually low levels may be noncompliant or hypermetabolizers of phenytoin. Unusually high levels result from liver disease, congenital enzyme deficiency or drug interactions which result in metabolic interference. The patient with large variations in phenytoin plasma levels, despite standard doses, presents a difficult clinical problem. Serum level determinations in such patients may be particularly helpful.

Most of the drug is excreted in the bile as inactive metabolites which are then reabsorbed from the intestinal tract and excreted in the urine. Urinary excretion of phenytoin and its metabolites occurs partly with glomerular filtration but more importantly, by tubular secretion. Because phenytoin is hydroxylated in the liver by an enzyme system which is saturable at <u>high plasma levels</u> small incremental doses may increase the half-life and produce very substantial increases in serum levels, when these are in the upper range. The steady-state level may be disproportionately increased, with resultant intoxication, from an increase in dosage of 10% or more.

Clinical studies show that chewed and unchewed Dilantin Infatabs are bioequivalent, yield approximately equivalent plasma levels, and are more rapidly absorbed than 100-mg Dilantin Kapseals.®

INDICATIONS AND USAGE

Dilantin Infatabs (Phenytoin Tablets, USP) are indicated for the control of generalized tonic-clonic (grand mal) and complex partial (psychomotor, temporal lobe) seizures and prevention and treatment of seizures occurring during or following neurosurgery. Phenytoin serum level determinations may be necessary for optimal dosage adjustments (see Dosage and Administration and Clinical Pharmacology).

CONTRAINDICATIONS

Phenytoin is contraindicated in those patients who are hypersensitive to phenytoin or other hydantoins.

WARNINGS

Abrupt withdrawal of phenytoin in epileptic patients may precipitate status epilepticus. When, in the judgment of the clinician, the need for dosage reduction, discontinuation, or substitution of alternative antiepileptic medication arises, this should be done gradually. However, in the event of an allergic or hypersensitivity reaction, rapid substitution of alternative therapy may be necessary. In this case, alternative therapy should be an antiepileptic drug not belonging to the hydantoin chemical class.

There have been a number of reports suggesting a relationship between phenytoin and the development of lymphadenopathy (local or generalized) including benign lymph node hyperplasia, pseudolymphoma, lymphoma, and Hodgkin's Disease. Although a cause and effect relationship has not been established, the occurrence of lymphadenopathy indicates the need to differentiate such a condition from other types of lymph node pathology. Lymph node involvement may occur with or without symptoms and signs resembling serum sickness eg, fever, rash and liver involvement. In all cases of lymphadenopathy, follow-up observation for an extended period is indicated and every effort should be made to achieve seizure control using alternative antiepileptic drugs. Acute alcoholic intake may increase phenytoin serum levels while chronic alcoholic use may decrease serum levels.

Usage in Pregnancy

A number of reports suggest an association between the use of antiepileptic drugs by women with epilepsy and a higher incidence of birth defects in children born to these women. Data are more extensive with respect to phenytoin and phenobarbital, but these are also the most commonly prescribed antiepileptic drugs; less systematic or anecdotal reports suggest a possible similar association with the use of all known antiepileptic drugs.

The reports suggesting a higher incidence of birth defects in children of drug-treated epileptic women cannot be regarded as adequate to prove a definite cause and effect relationship. There are intrinsic methodologic problems in obtaining adequate data on drug teratogenicity in humans: genetic factors or the epileptic condition itself, may be more important than drug therapy in leading to birth defects. The great majority of mothers on antiepileptic medication deliver normal infants. It is important to note that antiepileptic drugs should not be discontinued in patients in whom the drug is administered to prevent major seizures, because of the strong possibility of precipitating status epilepticus with attendant hypoxia and threat to life. In individual cases where the severity and frequency of the seizure disorder are such that the removal of medication does not pose a serious threat to the patient, discontinuation of the drug may be considered prior to and during pregnancy, although it cannot be said with any confidence that even minor seizures do not pose some hazard to the developing embryo or fetus. The prescribing physician

will wish to weigh these considerations in treating or counseling epileptic women of childbearing potential.

In addition to the reports of increased incidence of congenital malformations, such as cleft lip/palate and heart malformations in children of women receiving phenytoin and other antiepileptic drugs, there have more recently been reports of a fetal hydantoin syndrome. This consists of prenatal growth deficiency, microcephaly and mental deficiency in children born to mothers who have received phenytoin, barbiturates, alcohol, or trimethadione. However, these features are all interrelated and are frequently associated with intrauterine growth retardation from other causes.

There have been isolated reports of malignancies, including neuroblastoma, in children whose mothers received phenytoin during pregnancy.

An increase in seizure frequency during pregnancy occurs in a high proportion of patients, because of altered phenytoin absorption or metabolism. Periodic measurement of serum phenytoin levels is particularly valuable in the management of a pregnant epileptic patient as a guide to an appropriate adjustment of dosage. However, postpartum restoration of the original dosage will probably be indicated.

Neonatal coagulation defects have been reported within the first 24 hours in babies born to epileptic mothers receiving phenobarbital and/or phenytoin. Vitamin K has been shown to prevent or correct this defect and has been recommended to be given to the mother before delivery and to the neonate after birth.

PRECAUTIONS

General

The liver is the chief site of biotransformation of phenytoin; patients with impaired liver function, elderly patients, or those who are gravely ill may show early signs of toxicity.

A small percentage of individuals who have been treated with phenytoin have been shown to metabolize the drug slowly. Slow metabolism may be due to limited enzyme availability and lack of induction; it appears to be genetically determined.

Phenytoin should be discontinued if a skin rash appears (see "Warnings" section regarding drug discontinuation). If the rash is exfoliative, purpuric, or bullous or if lupus erythematosus, Stevens-Johnson syndrome, or toxic epidermal necrolysis is suspected, use of the drug should not be resumed, and alternative therapy should be considered (see Adverse Reactions). If the rash is of a milder type (measles-like or scarlatiniform), therapy may be resumed after the rash has completely disappeared. If the rash recurs upon reinstitution of therapy, further phenytoin medication is contraindicated.

Hyperglycemia, resulting from the drug's inhibitory effects on insulin release, has been reported. Phenytoin may also raise the serum glucose level in diabetic patients.

Osteomalacia has been associated with phenytoin therapy and is considered to be due to phenytoin's interference with Vitamin D metabolism.

Phenytoin is not indicated for seizures due to hypoglycemic or other metabolic causes. Appropriate diagnostic procedures should be performed as indicated.

Phenytoin is not effective for absence (petit mal) seizures. If tonic-clonic (grand-mal) and absence (petit mal) seizures are present, combined drug therapy is needed.

Serum levels of phenytoin sustained above the optimal range may produce confusional states referred to as "delirium," "psychosis," or "encephalopathy," or rarely irreversible cerebellar dysfunction. Accordingly, at the first sign of acute toxicity, plasma levels are recommended. Dose reduction of phenytoin therapy is indicated if plasma levels are excessive; if symptoms persist, termination is recommended. (See Warnings).

Information for Patients

Patients taking phenytoin should be advised of the importance of adhering strictly to the prescribed dosage regimen, and of informing the physician of any clinical condition in which it is not possible to take the drug orally as prescribed, eg, surgery, etc.

Patients should also be cautioned on the use of other drugs or alcoholic beverages without first seeking the physician's advice.

Patients should be instructed to call their physician if skin rash develops.

The importance of good dental hygiene should be stressed in order to minimize the development of gingival hyperplasia and its complications.

Laboratory Tests

Phenytoin serum level determinations may be necessary to achieve optimal dosage adjustments.

Drug Interactions

There are many drugs which may increase or decrease phenytoin levels or which phenytoin may affect. The most commonly occurring drug interactions are listed below:

1. Drugs which may increase phenytoin serum levels include: chloramphenicol, dicumarol, disulfiram, tolbutamide, isoniazid, phenylbutazone, acute alcohol intake, salicylates, chlordiazepoxide, phenothiazines, diazepam, estrogens, ethosuximide, halothane, methylphenidate, sulfonamides, cimetidine, trazodone.

2. Drugs which may decrease phenytoin serum levels include: carbamazepine, chronic alcohol abuse, reserpine. Moban® brand of Molindone Hydrochloride contains calcium ions which interfere with the absorption of phenytoin. Ingestion times of phenytoin and antacid preparations containing calcium should be staggered in patients with low serum phenytoin levels to prevent absorption problems.

3. Drugs which may either increase or decrease phenytoin serum levels include: Phenobarbital, valproic acid, and sodium valproate. Similarly, the effect of phenytoin on phenobarbital, valproic acid and sodium valproate serum levels is unpredictable.

4. Although not a true drug interaction, tricyclic antidepressants may precipitate seizures in susceptible patients and phenytoin dosage may need to be adjusted.

5. Drugs whose efficacy is impaired by phenytoin include: corticosteroids, coumarin anticoagulants, oral contraceptives, quinidine, vitamin D, digitoxin, rifampin, doxycycline, estrogens, furosemide.

Serum level determinations are especially helpful when possible drug interactions are suspected.

Drug/Laboratory Test Interactions

Phenytoin may cause decreased serum levels of protein-bound iodine (PBI). It may also produce lower than normal values for dexamethasone or metyrapone tests. Phenytoin may cause increased serum levels of glucose, alkaline phosphatase, and gamma glutamyl transpeptidase (GGT).

Carcinogenesis

See 'Warnings' section for information on carcinogenesis.

Pregnancy

See Warnings

Nursing Mothers

Infant breast-feeding is not recommended for women taking this drug because phenytoin appears to be secreted in low concentrations in human milk.

ADVERSE REACTIONS

Central Nervous System: The most common manifestations encountered with phenytoin therapy are referable to this system and are usually dose-related. These include nystagmus, ataxia, slurred speech, decreased coordination and mental confusion. Dizziness, insomnia, transient nervousness, motor twitchings, and headache have also been observed.

There have also been rare reports of phenytoin induced dyskinesias, including chorea, dystonia, tremor and asterixis, similar to those induced by phenothiazine and other neuroleptic drugs.

A predominantly sensory peripheral polyneuropathy has been observed in patients receiving long-term phenytoin therapy.

Gastrointestinal System: Nausea, vomiting, and constipation.

Integumentary System: Dermatological manifestations sometimes accompanied by fever have included scarlatiniform or morbilliform rashes. A morbilliform rash (measles-like) is the most common; other types of dermatitis are seen more rarely. Other more serious forms which may be fatal have included bullous, exfoliative or purpuric dermatitis, lupus erythematosus, Stevens-Johnson syndrome, and toxic epidermal necrolysis (see Precautions).

Hemopoietic System: Hemopoietic complications, some fatal, have occasionally been reported in association with administration of phenytoin. These have included thrombocytopenia, leukopenia, granulocytopenia, agranulocytosis, and pancytopenia with or without bone marrow suppression. While macrocytosis and megaloblastic anemia have occurred, these conditions usually respond to folic acid therapy. Lymphadenopathy including benign lymph node hyperplasia, pseudolymphoma, lymphoma, and Hodgkin's Disease have been reported (see Warnings).

Connective Tissue System: Coarsening of the facial features, enlargement of the lips, gingival hyperplasia, hypertrichosis, and Peyronie's Disease.

Other: Systemic lupus erythematosus, periarteritis nodosa, toxic hepatitis, liver damage, and immunoglobulin abnormalities may occur.

OVERDOSAGE

The lethal dose in children is not known. The lethal dose in adults is estimated to be 2 to 5 grams. The initial symptoms are nystagmus, ataxia, and dysarthria. Other signs are tremor, hyperflexia, lethargy, slurred speech, nausea, vomiting. The patient may become comatose and hypertensive. Death is due to respiratory and circulatory depression.

There are marked variations among individuals with respect to phenytoin plasma levels where toxicity may occur. Nystagmus on lateral gaze usually appears at 20 mcg/ml, ataxia at 30 mcg/ml, dysarthria and lethargy appear when the plasma concentration is over 40 mcg/ml, but as high a concentration as 50 mcg/ml has been reported without evidence of toxicity. As much as 25 times the therapeutic dose has been taken to result in a serum concentration over 100 mcg/ml with complete recovery.

Treatment

Treatment is nonspecific since there is no known antidote. The adequacy of the respiratory and circulatory systems should be carefully observed and appropriate supportive measures employed. Hemodialysis can be considered since phenytoin is not completely bound to plasma proteins. Total exchange transfusion has been used in the treatment of severe intoxication in children.

In acute overdosage the possibility of other CNS depressants, including alcohol, should be borne in mind.

DOSAGE AND ADMINISTRATION

When given in equal doses, Dilantin Infatabs yield higher plasma levels than Dilantin Kapseals.® For this reason serum concentrations should be monitored and care should be taken when switching a patient from the sodium salt to the free acid form.

Dilantin® Kapseals,® Dilantin Parenteral, and Dilantin with Phenobarbital are formulated with the sodium salt of phenytoin. The free acid form of phenytoin is used in Dilantin-30 Pediatric and Dilantin-125 Suspensions and Dilantin Infatabs. Because there is approximately an 8% increase in drug content with the free acid form over that of the sodium salt, dosage adjustments and serum level monitoring may be necessary when switching from a product formulated with the free acid to a product formulated with the sodium salt and vice versa.

General

Not for once a day dosing.

Dosage should be individualized to provide maximum benefit. In some cases, serum blood level determinations may be necessary for optimal dosage adjustments—the clinically effective serum level is usually 10–20 mcg/ml. With recommended dosage, a period of seven to ten days may be required to achieve steady-state blood levels with phenytoin and changes in dosage (increase or decrease) should not be carried out at intervals shorter than seven to ten days.

Dilantin Infatabs can be either chewed thoroughly before being swallowed or swallowed whole.

Adult Dosage

Patients who have received no previous treatment may be started on two Infatabs three times daily, and the dose is then adjusted to suit individual requirements. For most adults, the satisfactory maintenance dosage will be six to eight Infatabs daily; an increase to twelve Infatabs daily may be made, if necessary.

Pediatric Dosage

Initially, 5 mg/kg/day in two or three equally divided doses, with subsequent dosage individualized to a maximum of 300 mg daily. A recommended daily maintenance dosage is usually 4 to 8 mg/kg. Children over 6 years old may require the minimum adult dose (300 mg/day). If the daily dosage cannot be divided equally, the larger dose should be given before retiring.

HOW SUPPLIED

Dilantin Infatabs are supplied as:

N 0071-0007-24—Bottle of 100.
N 0071-0007-40—Unit dose (10/10's).

Each tablet contains 50 mg phenytoin in a yellow triangular scored chewable tablet.

Shown in Product Identification Section, page 421
Store at controlled room temperature (59°–86°F).
Protect from moisture.
Dilantin is also supplied in the following forms:

N 0071-0362-24—Bottle of 100.
N 0071-0362-32—Bottle of 1000.
N 0071-0362-40—Unit dose (10/10's).
N 0071-0362-41–Memo Pack containing 84 unit-dose capsules (28 day dosage regimen).
Each capsule contains 100 mg phenytoin sodium.
N 0071-0365-24—Bottle of 100.
N 0071-0365-32—Bottle of 1000.
N 0071-0365-40—Unit dose (10/10's).
Each capsule contains 30 mg phenytoin sodium.
N 0071-2214-20—8 oz bottle.
N 0071-2214-40—Unit dose pouches (5 ml × 100).
Each 5 ml of suspension contains 125 mg phenytoin with a maximum alcohol content not greater than 0.6 percent.
N 0071-2315-20—8 oz bottle.
N 0071-2315-40—Unit dose pouches (5 ml × 100).
Each 5 ml of suspension contains 30 mg phenytoin with a maximum alcohol content not greater than 0.6 percent.
N 0071-0375-24—Bottle of 100.
N 0071-0375-32—Bottle of 1000.
Each capsule contains phenytoin sodium 100 mg and phenobarbital 16 mg (¼ gr).
N 0071-0531-24—Bottle of 100.
N 0071-0531-32—Bottle of 1000.
N 0071-0531-40—Unit dose (10/10's).
Each capsule contains phenytoin sodium 100 mg and phenobarbital 32 mg (½ gr).
N 0071-4488-05—2-ml ampoules.
A sterile solution for parenteral use containing 50 mg phenytoin sodium per ml. Supplied in packages of ten.

N 0071-4488-41—2-ml prefilled syringes.
A sterile solution for parenteral use containing 50 mg phenytoin sodium per ml in an individually cartoned disposable syringe (22 gauge × 1 ¼ inch needle). Supplied in packages of ten.
N 0071-4475-35—5-ml ampoules with syringes.
A sterile solution for parenteral use containing 50 mg phenytoin sodium per ml. One 6-ml sterile disposable syringe (22 gauge × 1 ¼ inch needle). Supplied in packages of ten.
N 0071-4475-08—5-ml ampoules.
A sterile solution for parenteral use containing 50 mg phenytoin sodium per ml. Supplied in packages of ten.
N 0071-4488-45 Dilantin ready-mixed solution containing 50 mg phenytoin sodium per milliliter is supplied in 2-mL Steri-Vials.® Packages of twenty-five.
N 0071-4475-45 Dilantin ready-mixed solution containing 50 mg phenytoin sodium per milliliter is supplied in 5 mL Steri-Vials.® Packages of twenty-five.

0007G045

Parenteral
DILANTIN®   ℞
[dī-lăn' tĭn"]
(Phenytoin Sodium Injection, USP)

> **IMPORTANT NOTE**
> This drug must be administered slowly. In adults do not exceed 50 mg per minute intravenously. In neonates, the drug should be administered at a rate not exceeding 1–3 mg/kg/min.

DESCRIPTION

Dilantin (phenytoin sodium injection, USP) is a ready-mixed solution of phenytoin sodium in a vehicle containing 40% propylene glycol and 10% alcohol in water for injection, adjusted to pH 12 with sodium hydroxide. Phenytoin sodium is related to the barbiturates in chemical structure, but has a five-membered ring. The chemical name is sodium 5,5-diphenyl-2,4-imidazolidinedione.

CLINICAL PHARMACOLOGY

Phenytoin is an anticonvulsant which may be useful in the treatment of status epilepticus of the grand mal type. The primary site of action appears to be the motor cortex where spread of seizure activity is inhibited. Possibly by promoting sodium efflux from neurons, phenytoin tends to stabilize the threshold against hyperexcitability caused by excessive stimulation or environmental changes capable of reducing membrane sodium gradient. This includes the reduction of posttetanic potentiation at synapses. Loss of posttetanic potentiation prevents cortical seizure foci from detonating adjacent cortical areas. Phenytoin reduces the maximal activity of brain stem centers responsible for the tonic phase of grand mal seizures.

The plasma half-life in man after intravenous administration ranges from 10 to 15 hours. Optimum control without clinical signs of toxicity occurs most often with serum levels between 10 and 20 mcg/ml.

A fall in plasma levels may occur when patients are changed from oral to intramuscular administration. The drop is caused by slower absorption, as compared to oral administration, due to the poor water solubility of phenytoin. Intravenous administration is the preferred route for producing rapid therapeutic serum levels.

There are occasions when intramuscular administration may be required, ie, postoperatively, in comatose patients, for GI upsets. During these periods, a sufficient dose must be administered intramuscularly to maintain the plasma level within the therapeutic range. Where oral dosage is resumed following intramuscular usage, the oral dose should be properly adjusted to compensate for the slow, continuing IM absorption to avoid toxic symptoms.

Patients stabilized on a daily oral regimen of Dilantin experience a drop in peak blood levels to 50–60 percent of stable levels if crossed over to an equal dose administered intramuscularly. However, the intramuscular depot of poorly soluble material is eventually absorbed, as determined by urinary excretion of 5-(p-hydroxyphenyl)-5-phenylhydantoin (HPPH), the principal metabolite, as well as the total amount of drug eventually appearing in the blood.

A short-term (one week) study indicates that patients do not experience the expected drop in blood levels when crossed over to the intramuscular route if the Dilantin IM dose is increased by 50 percent over the previously established oral dose. To avoid drug cumulation due to absorption from the muscle depots, it is recommended that for the first week back on oral Dilantin, the dose be reduced to half of the original oral dose (one third of the IM dose). Experience for periods greater than one week is lacking and blood level monitoring is recommended. For administration of Dilantin in patients who cannot take oral medication for periods greater than a week, gastric intubation may be considered.

INDICATIONS

Parenteral Dilantin is indicated for the control of status epilepticus of the grand mal type, and prevention and treatment of seizures occurring during neurosurgery.

CONTRAINDICATIONS

Phenytoin is contraindicated in patients with a history of hypersensitivity to hydantoin products.

Because of its effect on ventricular automaticity, phenytoin is contraindicated in sinus bradycardia, sino-atrial block, second and third degree A-V block, and patients with Adams-Stokes syndrome.

WARNINGS

Intravenous administration should not exceed 50 mg per minute in adults. In neonates, the drug should be administered at a rate not exceeding 1–3mg/kg/min.

Severe cardiotoxic reactions and fatalities have been reported with atrial and ventricular conduction depression and ventricular fibrillation. Severe complications are most commonly encountered in elderly or gravely ill patients. Phenytoin should be used with caution in patients with hypotension and severe myocardial insufficiency.

Hypotension usually occurs when the drug is administered rapidly by the intravenous route.

The intramuscular route is not recommended for the treatment of status epilepticus since blood levels of phenytoin in the therapeutic range cannot be readily achieved with doses and methods of administration ordinarily employed.

There have been a number of reports suggesting a relationship between phenytoin and the development of lymphadenopathy (local or generalized) including benign lymph node hyperplasia, pseudolymphoma, lymphoma, and Hodgkin's Disease. Although a cause and effect relationship has not been established, the occurrence of lymphadenopathy indicates the need to differentiate such a condition from other types of lymph node pathology. Lymph node involvement may occur with or without symptoms and signs resembling serum sickness eg, fever, rash and liver involvement.

In all cases of lymphadenopathy, follow-up observation for an extended period is indicated and every effort should be made to achieve seizure control using alternative antiepileptic drugs.

Acute alcoholic intake may increase phenytoin serum levels while chronic alcoholic use may decrease serum levels.

Usage in Pregnancy: A number of reports suggests an association between the use of antiepileptic drugs by women with epilepsy and a higher incidence of birth defects in children born to these women. Data are more extensive with respect to phenytoin and phenobarbital, but these are also the most commonly prescribed antiepileptic drugs; less systematic or anecdotal reports suggest a possible similar association with the use of all known antiepileptic drugs.

The reports suggesting a higher incidence of birth defects in children of drug-treated epileptic women cannot be regarded as adequate to prove a definite cause and effect relationship. There are intrinsic methodologic problems in obtaining adequate data on drug teratogenicity in humans; genetic factors or the epileptic condition itself may be more important than drug therapy in leading to birth defects. The great majority of mothers on antiepileptic medication deliver normal infants. It is important to note that antiepileptic drugs should not be discontinued in patients in whom the drug is administered to prevent major seizures, because of the strong possibility of precipitating status epilepticus with attendant hypoxia and threat to life. In individual cases where the severity and frequency of the seizure disorder are such that the removal of medication does not pose a serious threat to the patient, discontinuation of the drug may be considered prior to and during pregnancy, although it cannot be said with any confidence that even minor seizures do not pose some hazard to the developing embryo or fetus. The prescribing physician will wish to weigh these considerations in treating or counseling epileptic women of childbearing potential.

In addition to the reports of increased incidence of congenital malformation, such as cleft lip/palate and heart malformations in children of women receiving phenytoin and other antiepileptic drugs, there have more recently been reports of a fetal hydantoin syndrome. This consists of prenatal growth deficiency, microcephaly and mental deficiency in children born to mothers who have received phenytoin, barbiturates, alcohol, or trimethadione. However, these features are all interrelated and are frequently associated with intrauterine growth retardation from other causes.

There have been isolated reports of malignancies, including neuroblastoma, in children whose mothers received phenytoin during pregnancy.

Continued on next page

This product information was prepared in August, 1989. On these and other Parke-Davis Products, information may be obtained by addressing PARKE-DAVIS, Division of Warner-Lambert Company, Morris Plains, New Jersey 07950.

Parke-Davis—Cont.

An increase in seizure frequency during pregnancy occurs in a high proportion of patients, because of altered phenytoin absorption or metabolism. Periodic measurement of serum phenytoin levels is particularly valuable in the management of a pregnant epileptic patient as a guide to an appropriate adjustment of dosage. However, postpartum restoration of the original dosage will probably be indicated.

Neonatal coagulation defects have been reported within the first 24 hours in babies born to epileptic mothers receiving phenobarbital and/or phenytoin. Vitamin K has been shown to prevent or correct this defect and has been recommended to be given to the mother before delivery and the neonate after birth.

PRECAUTIONS

General: The addition of Dilantin solution to intravenous infusion is not recommended due to lack of solubility and resultant precipitation.

Parenteral Dilantin should be injected slowly (not exceeding 50 mg per minute in adults), directly into a large vein through a large-gauge needle or intravenous catheter. Each injection of intravenous Dilantin should be followed by an injection of sterile saline through the same needle or intravenous catheter to avoid local venous irritation due to the alkalinity of the solution. Continuous infusion should be avoided.

Soft tissue irritation and inflammation has occurred at the site of injection with and without extravasation of intravenous phenytoin. Soft tissue irritation may vary from slight tenderness to extensive necrosis, sloughing, and in rare instances has led to amputation. Improper administration including subcutaneous or perivascular injection should be avoided to help prevent possibility of the above.

The liver is the site of biotransformation. Patients with impaired liver function, elderly patients, or those who are gravely ill may show early toxicity.

A small percentage of individuals who have been treated with phenytoin have been shown to metabolize the drug slowly. Slow metabolism may be due to limited enzyme availability and lack of induction; it appears to be genetically determined.

Phenytoin should be discontinued if a skin rash appears (see "Warnings" section regarding drug discontinuation). If the rash is exfoliative, purpuric, or bullous or if lupus erythematosus, Stevens-Johnson syndrome, or toxic epidermal necrolysis is suspected, use of this drug should not be resumed and alternative therapy should be considered. (See Adverse Reactions.) If the rash is of a milder type (measles-like or scarlatiniform), therapy may be resumed after the rash has completely disappeared. If the rash recurs upon reinstitution of therapy, further phenytoin medication is contraindicated.

Hyperglycemia, resulting from the drug's inhibitory effects on insulin release, has been reported. Phenytoin may also raise the serum glucose level in diabetic patients.

Phenytoin is not indicated for seizures due to hypoglycemic or other metabolic causes. Appropriate diagnostic procedures should be performed as indicated.

Phenytoin is not effective for absence (petit mal) seizures. If tonic-clonic (grand-mal) and absence (petit mal) seizures are present, combined drug therapy is needed.

Serum levels of phenytoin sustained above the optimal range may produce confusional states referred to as "delirium," "psychosis," or "encephalopathy," or rarely irreversible cerebellar dysfunction. Accordingly, at the first sign of acute toxicity, plasma levels are recommended. Dose reduction of phenytoin therapy is indicated if plasma levels are excessive; if symptoms persist, termination is recommended. (See Warnings)

Laboratory Tests: Phenytoin serum level determinations may be necessary to achieve optimal dosage adjustments.

Drug Interactions: There are many drugs which may increase or decrease phenytoin levels or which phenytoin may affect. The most commonly occurring drug interactions are listed below:

1. Drugs which may increase phenytoin serum levels include: chloramphenicol, dicumarol, disulfiram, tolbutamide, isoniazid, phenylbutazone, acute alcohol intake, salicylates, chlordiazepoxide, phenothiazines, diazepam, estrogens, ethosuximide, halothane, methylphenidate, sulfonamides, cimetidine, trazodone.
2. Drugs which may decrease phenytoin levels include: carbamazepine, chronic alcohol abuse, reserpine. Moban* brand of Molindone Hydrochloride contains calcium ions which interfere with the absorption of phenytoin. Ingestion times of phenytoin and antacid preparations containing calcium should be staggered in patients with low serum phenytoin levels to prevent absorption problems.
3. Drugs which may either increase or decrease phenytoin serum levels include: phenobarbital, valproic acid, and sodium valproate. Similarly, the effect of phenytoin on phenobarbital, valproic acid and sodium valproate serum levels is unpredictable.
4. Although not a true drug interaction, tricyclic antidepressants may precipitate seizures in susceptible patients and phenytoin dosage may need to be adjusted.
5. Drugs whose efficacy is impaired by phenytoin include: corticosteroids, coumarin anticoagulants, oral contraceptives, quinidine, vitamin D, digitoxin, rifampin, doxycycline, estrogens, furosemide.

Serum level determinations are especially helpful when possible drug interactions are suspected.

Drug/Laboratory Test Interactions: Phenytoin may cause decreased serum levels of protein-bound iodine (PBI). It may also produce lower than normal values for dexamethasone or metyrapone tests. Phenytoin may cause increased serum levels of glucose, alkaline phosphatase, and gamma glutamyl transpeptidase (GGT).

Carcinogenesis: See 'Warnings' section for information on carcinogenesis.

Pregnancy: See Warnings

Nursing Mothers: Infant breast feeding is not recommended for women taking this drug because phenytoin appears to be secreted in low concentrations in human milk.

ADVERSE REACTIONS

The most notable signs of toxicity associated with the intravenous use of this drug are cardiovascular collapse and/or central nervous system depression. Hypotension does occur when the drug is administered rapidly by the intravenous route. The *rate* of administration is very important; it should not exceed 50 mg per minute in adults, and 1–3 mg/kg/min in neonates. At this rate, toxicity should be minimized.

Cardiovascular: Severe cardiotoxic reactions and fatalities have been reported with atrial and ventricular conduction depression and ventricular fibrillation. Severe complications are most commonly encountered in elderly or gravely ill patients.

Central Nervous System: The most common manifestations encountered with phenytoin therapy are referable to this system and are usually dose-related. These include nystagmus, ataxia, slurred speech, decreased coordination and mental confusion. Dizziness, insomnia, transient nervousness, motor twitchings, and headaches have also been observed. There have also been rare reports of phenytoin induced dyskinesias, including chorea, dystonia, tremor and asterixis, similar to those induced by phenothiazine and other neuroleptic drugs.

A predominantly sensory peripheral polyneuropathy has been observed in patients receiving long-term phenytoin therapy.

Gastrointestinal System: Nausea, vomiting, and constipation.

Integumentary System: Dermatological manifestations sometimes accompanied by fever have included scarlatiniform or morbilliform rashes. A morbilliform rash (measles-like) is the most common; other types of dermatitis are seen more rarely. Other more serious forms which may be fatal have included bullous, exfoliative or purpuric dermatitis, lupus erythematosus, Stevens-Johnson syndrome, and toxic epidermal necrolysis (see Precautions).

Hemopoietic System: Hemopoietic complications, some fatal, have occasionally been reported in association with administration of phenytoin. These have included thrombocytopenia, leukopenia, granulocytopenia, agranulocytosis, and pancytopenia with or without bone marrow suppression. While macrocytosis and megaloblastic anemia have occurred, these conditions usually respond to folic acid therapy. Lymphadenopathy including benign lymph node hyperplasia, pseudolymphoma, lymphoma, and Hodgkin's Disease have been reported (see Warnings).

Connective Tissue System: Coarsening of the facial features, enlargement of the lips, gingival hyperplasia, hypertrichosis, and Peyronie's Disease.

Injection Site: Local irritation, inflammation, tenderness, necrosis, and sloughing have been reported with or without extravasation of intravenous phenytoin.

Other: Systemic lupus erythematosus, periarteritis nodosa, toxic hepatitis, liver damage, and immunoglobulin abnormalities may occur.

OVERDOSAGE

The lethal dose in children is not known. The lethal dose in adults is estimated to be 2 to 5 grams. The initial symptoms are nystagmus, ataxia and dysarthria. Other signs are tremor, hyperflexia, lethargy, slurred speech, nausea, vomiting. The patient may become comatose and hypertensive. Death is due to respiratory and circulatory depression.

There are marked variations among individuals with respect to phenytoin plasma levels where toxicity may occur. Nystagmus, on lateral gaze, usually appears at 20 mcg/mL, ataxia at 30 mcg/mL, dysarthria and lethargy appear when the plasma concentration is over 40 mcg/mL, but as high a concentration as 50 mcg/mL has been reported without evidence of toxicity. As much as 25 times the therapeutic dose has been taken to result in a serum concentration over 100 mcg/mL with complete recovery.

Treatment: Treatment is nonspecific since there is no known antidote.

The adequacy of the respiratory and circulatory systems should be carefully observed and appropriate supportive measures employed. Hemodialysis can be considered since phenytoin is not completely bound to plasma proteins. Total exchange transfusion has been used in the treatment of severe intoxication in children.

In acute overdosage the possibility of other CNS depressants, including alcohol, should be borne in mind.

DOSAGE AND ADMINISTRATION

The addition of Dilantin solution to intravenous infusion is not recommended due to lack of solubility and resultant precipitation.

Not to exceed 50 mg per minute, intravenously in adults, and not exceeding 1–3 mg/kg/min in neonates There is a relatively small margin between full therapeutic effect and minimally toxic doses of this drug.

The solution is suitable for use as long as it remains free of haziness and precipitate. Upon refrigeration or freezing, a precipitate might form; this will dissolve again after the solution is allowed to stand at room temperature. The product is still suitable for use. Only a clear solution should be used. A faint yellow coloration may develop; however, this has no effect on the potency of the solution.

In the treatment of status epilepticus, the intravenous route is preferred because of the delay in absorption of phenytoin when administered intramuscularly.

Serum concentrations should be monitored and care should be taken when switching a patient from the sodium salt to the free acid form.

Dilantin® Kapseals®, Dilantin Parenteral, and Dilantin with Phenobarbital are formulated with the sodium salt of phenytoin. The free acid form of phenytoin is used in Dilantin-30 Pediatric and Dilantin-125 Suspensions and Dilantin Infatabs. Because there is approximately an 8% increase in drug content with the free acid form over that of the sodium salt, dosage adjustments and serum level monitoring may be necessary when switching from a product formulated with the free acid to a product formulated with the sodium salt and vice versa.

Status Epilepticus: In adults, a loading dose of 10 to 15 mg/kg should be administered slowly intravenously, at a rate not exceeding 50 mg per minute (this will require approximately 20 minutes in a 70-kg patient). The loading dose should be followed by maintenance doses of 100 mg orally or intravenously every 6–8 hours.

Recent work in neonates and children has shown that absorption of phenytoin is unreliable after oral administration, but a loading dose of 15–20 mg/kg of Dilantin intravenously will usually produce plasma concentrations of phenytoin within the generally accepted therapeutic range (10–20 mcg/mL). The drug should be injected slowly intravenously at a rate not exceeding 1–3 mg/kg/min.

Parenteral Dilantin should be injected *slowly* and directly into a large vein through a large-gauge needle or intravenous catheter. Each injection of intravenous Dilantin should be followed by an injection of sterile saline through the same needle or catheter to avoid local venous irritation due to alkalinity of the solution. Continuous infusion should be avoided; the addition of Parenteral Dilantin to intravenous infusion fluids is not recommended because of the likelihood of precipitation.

Continuous monitoring of the electrocardiogram and blood pressure is essential. The patient should be observed for signs of respiratory depression. Determination of phenytoin plasma levels is advised when using Dilantin in the management of status epilepticus and in the subsequent establishment of maintenance dosage.

Other measures, including concomitant administration of an intravenous benzodiazepine such as diazepam, or an intravenous short-acting barbiturate, will usually be necessary for rapid control of seizures because of the required slow rate of administration of Dilantin.

If administration of Parenteral Dilantin does not terminate seizures, the use of other anticonvulsants, intravenous barbiturates, general anesthesia, and other appropriate measures should be considered.

Intramuscular administration should not be used in the treatment of status epilepticus because the attainment of peak plasma levels may require up to 24 hours.

Neurosurgery: Prophylactic dosage—100 to 200 mg (2 to 4 mL) intramuscularly at approximately 4-hour intervals during surgery and continued during the postoperative period.

When intramuscular administration is required for a patient previously stabilized orally, compensating dosage adjustments are necessary to maintain therapeutic plasma levels. An intramuscular dose 50% greater than the oral dose is necessary to maintain these levels. When returned to oral administration, the dose should be reduced by 50% of the original oral dose for one week to prevent excessive plasma levels due to sustained release from intramuscular tissue sites.

If the patient requires more than a week of IM Dilantin, alternative routes should be explored, such as gastric intubation. For time periods less than one week, the patient shifted back from IM administration should receive one half the original oral dose for the same period of time the patient received IM Dilantin. Monitoring plasma levels would help prevent a fall into the subtherapeutic range. Serum blood level determinations are especially helpful when possible drug interactions are suspected.

HOW SUPPLIED

N 0071-4488-05 (Ampoule 1488) Dilantin ready-mixed solution containing 50 mg phenytoin sodium per milliliter is supplied in 2-mL ampoules. Packages of ten.

N 0071-4488-41 (Steri-Dose® 4488) Dilantin ready-mixed solution containing 50 mg phenytoin sodium per milliliter is supplied in a 2-mL sterile disposable syringe (22 gauge × 1¼ inch needle). Packages of ten individually cartoned syringes.

N 0071-4475-35 (Ampoule 1475) Dilantin ready-mixed solution containing 50 mg phenytoin sodium per milliliter is supplied in 5-mL ampoules with one 6-mL sterile disposable syringe (22 gauge × 1¼ inch needle). Packages of ten.

N 0071-4475-08 (Ampoule 1475) Dilantin ready-mixed solution contaning 50 mg phenytoin sodium per milliliter is supplied in packages of ten 5-mL ampoules without syringes.

N 0071-4488-45 Dilantin ready-mixed solution containing 50 mg phenytoin sodium per milliliter is supplied in 2-mL sterivials. Packages of twenty-five.

N 0071-4475-45 Dilantin ready-mixed solution containing 50 mg phenytoin sodium per milliliter is supplied in 5-mL sterivials. Packages of twenty-five.

Caution—Federal law prohibits dispensing without prescription.

4475G025

DILANTIN–30® PEDIATRIC/ DILANTIN–125®   ℞
[dī-lăn 'tĭn]
(Phenytoin Oral
Suspension, USP)

DESCRIPTION

Dilantin (phenytoin) is related to the barbiturates in chemical structure, but has a five-membered ring. The chemical name is 5.5-diphenyl-2,4 imidazolidinedione.

Each teaspoonful of suspension contains 30 mg or 125 mg of phenytoin, USP with a maximum alcohol content not greater than 0.6 percent. Also contains carboxymethylcellulose sodium, USP; citric acid; anhydrous, USP; flavors; glycerin, USP; magnesium aluminum silicate, NF; polysorbate 40, NF; purified water, USP; sodium benzoate, NF; sucrose, NF; vanillin NF. The 30 mg per teaspoonful suspension also contains D&C red No. 33; FD&C red No. 40. The 125 mg per teaspoonful suspension also contains FD&C yellow No. 6.

CLINICAL PHARMACOLOGY

Phenytoin is an antiepileptic drug which can be useful in the treatment of epilepsy. The primary site of action appears to be *the motor cortex* where spread of seizure activity is inhibited. Possibly by promoting sodium efflux from neurons, phenytoin tends to *stabilize* the threshold against hyperexcitability caused by excessive stimulation or environmental changes capable of reducing membrane sodium gradient. This includes the reduction of posttetanic potentiation at synapses. Loss of posttetanic potentiation prevents cortical seizure foci from detonating adjacent cortical areas. Phenytoin reduces the maximal activity of brain stem centers responsible for the tonic phase of tonic-clonic (grand mal) seizures.

The plasma half-life in man after oral administration of phenytoin averages 22 hours, with a range of 7 to 42 hours. Steady-state therapeutic levels are achieved at least 7 to 10 days (5–7 half-lives) after initiation of therapy with recommended doses of 300 mg/day.

When serum level determinations are necessary, they should be obtained at least 5–7 half-lives after treatment initiation, dosage change, or addition or subtraction of another drug to the regimen so that equilibrium or steady-state will have been achieved. Trough levels provide information about clinically effective serum level range and confirm patient compliance and are obtained just prior to the patient's next scheduled dose. Peak levels indicate an individual's threshold for emergence of dose-related side effects and are obtained at the time of expected peak concentration. For Dilantin-30 Pediatric and Dilantin-125 Suspensions peak levels occur 1½–3 hours after administration.

Optimum control without clinical signs of toxicity occurs more often with serum levels between 10 and 20 mcg/mL, although some mild cases of tonic-clonic (grand mal) epilepsy may be controlled with lower serum levels of phenytoin.

In most patients maintained at a steady dosage, stable phenytoin serum levels are achieved. There may be wide interpatient variability in phenytoin serum levels with equivalent dosages. Patients with unusually low levels may be noncompliant or hypermetabolizers of phenytoin. Unusally high levels result from liver disease, congenital enzyme deficiency or drug interactions which result in metabolic interference. The patient with large variations in phenytoin plasma lev-

els, despite standard doses, presents a difficult clinical problem. Serum level determinations in such patients may be particularly helpful.

Most of the drug is excreted in the bile as inactive metabolites which are then reabsorbed from the intestinal tract and excreted in the urine. Urinary excretion of phenytoin and its metabolites occurs partly with glomerular filtration but more importantly, by tubular secretion. Because phenytoin is hydroxylated in the liver by an enzyme system which is saturable at high plasma levels small incremental doses may increase the half-life and produce very substantial increases in serum levels, when these are in the upper range. The steady-state level may be disproportionately increased, with resultant intoxication, from an increase in dosage of 10% or more.

INDICATIONS AND USAGE

Dilantin (phenytoin) is indicated for the control of tonic-clonic (grand mal) and psychomotor (temporal lobe) seizures. Phenytoin serum level determinations may be necessary for optimal dosage adjustments (see Dosage and Administration and Clinical Pharmacology)

CONTRAINDICATIONS

Dilantin is contraindicated in those patients with a history of hypersensitivity to hydantoin products.

WARNINGS

Abrupt withdrawal of phenytoin in epileptic patients may precipitate status epilepticus. When in the judgment of the clinician the need for dosage reduction, discontinuation, or substitution of alternative anticonvulsant medication arises, this should be done gradually. In the event of an allergic or hypersensitivity reaction, more rapid substitution of alternative therapy may be necessary. In this case, alternative therapy should be an anticonvulsant not belonging to the hydantion chemical class.

There have been a number of reports suggesting a relationship between phenytoin and the development of lymphadenopathy (local or generalized) including benign lymph node hyperplasia, pseudolymphoma, lymphoma, and Hodgkin's Disease. Although a cause and effect relationship has not been established, the occurrence of lymphadenopathy indicates the need to differentiate such a condition from other types of lymph node pathology. Lymph node involvement may occur with or without symptoms and signs resembling serum sickness eg, fever, rash and liver involvement.

In all cases of lymphadenopathy, follow-up observation for an extended period is indicated and every effort should be made to achieve seizure control using alternative antiepileptic drugs. Acute alcoholic intake may increase phenytoin serum levels while chronic alcoholic use may decrease serum levels.

Usage in Pregnancy: A number of reports suggests an association between the use of antiepileptic drugs by women with epilepsy and a higher incidence of birth defects in children born to these women. Data are more extensive with respect to phenytoin and phenobarbital, but these are also the most commonly prescribed antiepileptic drugs; less systematic or anecdotal reports suggest a possible similar association with the use of all known antiepileptic drugs.

The reports suggesting a higher incidence of birth defects in children of drug-treated epileptic women cannot be regarded as adequate to prove a definite cause and effect relationship. There are intrinsic methodologic problems in obtaining adequate data on drug teratogenicity in humans; genetic factors or the epileptic condition itself may be more important than drug therapy in leading to birth defects. The great majority of mothers on antiepileptic medication deliver normal infants. It is important to note that antiepileptic drugs should not be discontinued in patients in whom the drug is administered to prevent major seizures, because of the strong possibility of precipitating status epilepticus with attendant hypoxia and threat to life. In individual cases where the severity and frequency of the seizure disorder are such that the removal of medication does not pose a serious threat to the patient, discontinuation of the drug may be considered prior to and during pregnancy, although it cannot be said with any confidence that even minor seizures do not pose some hazards to the developing embryo or fetus. The prescribing physician will wish to weigh these considerations in treating and counseling epileptic women of childbearing potential.

In addition to the reports of increased incidence of congenital malformation, such as cleft lip/palate and heart malformations in children of women receiving phenytoin and other antiepileptic drugs, there have more recently been reports of a fetal hydantoin syndrome. This consists of prenatal growth deficiency, microcephaly and mental deficiency in children born to mothers who have received phenytoin, barbiturates, alcohol, or trimethadione. However, these features are all interrelated and are frequently associated with intrauterine growth retardation from other causes.

There have been isolated reports of malignancies, including neuroblastoma, in children whose mothers received phenytoin during pregnancy.

An increase in seizure frequency during pregnancy occurs in a high proportion of patients, because of altered phenytoin

absorption or metabolism. Periodic measurement of serum phenytoin levels is particularly valuable in the management of a pregnant epileptic patient as a guide to an appropriate adjustment of dosage. However, postpartum restoration of the original dosage will probably be indicated.

Neonatal coagulation defects have been reported within the first 24 hours in babies born to epileptic mothers receiving phenobarbital and/or phenytoin. Vitamin K has been shown to prevent or correct this defect and has been recommended to be given to the mother before delivery and the neonate after birth.

PRECAUTIONS

General: The liver is the chief site of biotransformation of phenytoin; patients wth impaired liver function, elderly patients, or those who are gravely ill may show early signs of toxicity.

A small percentage of individuals who have been treated with phenytoin have been shown to metabolize the drug slowly. Slow metabolism may be due to limited enzyme availability and lack of induction; it appears to be genetically determined.

Phenytoin should be discontinued if a skin rash appears (see "Warnings" section regarding drug discontinuation). If the rash is exfoliative, purpuric, or bullous or if lupus erythematosus, Stevens-Johnson syndrome, or toxic epidermal necrolysis is suspected, use of this drug should not be resumed and alternative therapy should be considered. (See Adverse Reactions). If the rash is of a milder type (measles-like or scarlatiniform), therapy may be resumed after the rash has completely disappeared. If the rash recurs upon reinstitution of therapy, further phenytoin medication is contraindicated.

Hyperglycemia, resulting from the drug's inhibitory effects on insulin release, has been reported. Phenytoin may also raise the serum glucose level in diabetic patients.

Osteomalacia has been associated with phenytoin therapy and is considered to be due to phenytoin's interference with Vitamin D metabolism.

Phenytoin is not indicated for seizures due to hypoglycemic or other metabolic causes. Appropriate diagnostic procedures should be performed as indicated.

Phenytoin is not effective for absence (petit mal) seizures. If tonic-clonic (grand mal) and absence (petit mal) seizures are present, combined drug therapy is needed.

Serum levels of phenytoin sustained above the optimal range may produce confusional states referred to as "delirium," "psychosis" or "encephalopathy," or rarely irreversible cerebellar dysfunction. Accordingly, at the first sign of acute toxicity, plasma levels are recommended. Dose reduction of phenytoin therapy is indicated if plasma levels are excessive; if symptoms persist, termination is recommended. (See Warnings).

Information for Patients: Patients taking phenytoin should be advised of the importance of adhering strictly to the prescribed dosage regimen, and of informing the physician of any clinical condition in which it is not possible to take the drug orally as prescribed, eg, surgery, etc.

Patients should also be cautioned on the use of other drugs or alcoholic beverages without first seeking the physician's advice.

Patients should be instructed to call their physician if skin rash develops.

The importance of good dental hygiene should be stressed in order to minimize the development of gingival hyperplasia and its complications.

Laboratory Tests: Phenytoin serum level determinations may be necessary to achieve optimal dosage adjustments.

Drug Interactions: There are many drugs which may increase or decrease phenytoin levels or which phenytoin may affect. The most commonly occurring drug interactions are listed below:

1. Drugs which may increase phenytoin serum levels include: chloramphenicol, dicumarol, disulfiram, tolbutamide, isoniazid, phenylbutazone, acute alcohol intake, salicylates, chlordiazepoxide, phenothiazines, diazepam, estrogens, ethosuximide, halothane, methylphenidate, sulfonamides, cimetidine, trazodone.

2. Drugs which may decrease phenytoin levels include: carbamazepine, chronic alcohol abuse, reserpine. Moban® brand of Molindone Hydrochloride contains calcium ions which interfere with the absorption of phenytoin. Ingestion times of phenytoin and antacid preparations containing calcium should be staggered in patients with low serum phenytoin levels to prevent absorption problems.

3. Drugs which may either increase or decrease phenytoin serum levels include; phenobarbital, valproic acid, and sodium valproate. Similarly, the effect of phenytoin on

Continued on next page

This product information was prepared in August, 1989. On these and other Parke-Davis Products, information may be obtained by addressing PARKE-DAVIS, Division of Warner-Lambert Company, Morris Plains, New Jersey 07950.

Parke-Davis—Cont.

phenobarbital, valproic acid, and sodium valproate serum levels is unpredictable.

4. Although not a true drug interaction, tricyclic antidepressants may precipitate seizures in susceptible patients and phenytoin dosage may need to be adjusted.

5. Drugs whose efficacy is impaired by phenytoin include: corticosteroids, coumarin anticoagulants, oral contraceptives, quinidine, vitamin D, digitoxin, rifampin, doxycycline, estrogens, furosemide.

Serum level determinations are especially helpful when possible drug interactions are suspected.

Drug/Laboratory Test Interactions: Phenytoin may cause decreased serum levels of protein-bound iodine (PBI). It may also produce lower than normal values for dexamethasone or metyrapone tests. Phenytoin may cause increased serum levels of glucose, alkaline phosphatase, and gamma glutamyl transpeptidase (GGT).

Carcinogenesis: See 'Warnings' section for information on carcinogenesis.

Pregnancy: See Warnings

Nursing Mothers: Infant breast feeding is not recommended for women taking this drug because phenytoin appears to be secreted in low concentrations in human milk.

ADVERSE REACTIONS

Central Nervous System: The most common manifestations encountered with phenytoin therapy are referable to this system and are usually dose-related. These include nystagmus, ataxia, slurred speech, decreased coordination, and mental confusion. Dizziness, insomnia, transient nervousness, motor twitchings, and headaches have also been observed. There have also been rare reports of phenytoin induced dyskinesias, including chorea, dystonia, tremor and asterixis, similar to those induced by phenothiazine and other neuroleptic drugs.

A predominantly sensory peripheral polyneuropathy has been observed in patients receiving long-term phenytoin therapy.

Gastrointestinal System: Nausea, vomiting, and constipation.

Integumentary System: Dermatological manifestations sometimes accompanied by fever have included scarlatiniform or morbilliform rashes. A morbilliform rash (measles-like) is the most common; other types of dermatitis are seen more rarely. Other more serious forms which may be fatal have included bullous, exfoliative or purpuric dermatitis, lupus erythematosus, Stevens-Johnson syndrome, and toxic epidermal necrolysis (see Precautions).

Hemopoietic System: Hemopoietic complications, some fatal, have occasionally been reported in association with administration of phenytoin. These have included thrombocytopenia, leukopenia, granulocytopenia, agranulocytosis, and pancytopenia with or without bone marrow suppression. While macrocytosis and megaloblastic anemia have occurred, these conditions usually respond to folic acid therapy. Lymphadenopathy including benign lymph node hyperplasia, pseudolymphoma, lymphoma, and Hodgkin's Disease have been reported (see Warnings).

Connective Tissue System: Coarsening of the facial features, enlargement of the lips, gingival hyperplasia, hypertrichosis, and Peyronie's Disease.

Other: Systemic lupus erythematosus, periarteritis nodosa, toxic hepatitis, liver damage, and immunoglobulin abnormalities may occur.

OVERDOSAGE

The lethal dose in children is not known. The lethal dose in adults is estimated to be 2 to 5 grams. The initial symptoms are nystagmus, ataxia, and dysarthria. Other signs are tremor, hyperflexia, lethargy, slurred speech, nausea, vomiting. The patient may become comatose and hypotensive. Death is due to respiratory and circulatory depression.

There are marked variations among individuals with respect to phenytoin plasma levels where toxicity may occur. Nystagmus, on lateral gaze, usually appears at 20 mcg/mL, ataxia at 30 mcg/mL, dysarthria and lethargy appear when the plasma concentration is over 40 mcg/mL, but as high a concentration as 50 mcg/mL has been reported without evidence of toxicity. As much as 25 times the therapeutic dose has been taken to result in a serum concentration over 100 mcg/mL with complete recovery.

Treatment: Treatment is nonspecific since there is no known antidote.

The adequacy of the respiratory and circulatory systems should be carefully observed and appropriate supportive measures employed. Hemodialysis can be considered since phenytoin is not completely bound to plasma proteins. Total exchange transfusion has been used in the treatment of severe intoxication in children.

In acute overdosage the possibility of other CNS depressants, including alcohol, should be borne in mind.

DOSAGE AND ADMINISTRATION

Serum concentrations should be monitored and care should be taken when switching a patient from the sodium salt to the free acid form.

Dilantin® Kapseals® , Dilantin Parenteral, and Dilantin with Phenobarbital are formulated with the sodium salt of phenytoin. The free acid form of phenytoin is used in Dilantin-30 Pediatric and Dilantin-125 Suspensions and Dilantin Infatabs. Because there is approximately an 8% increase in drug content with the free acid form over that of the sodium salt, dosage adjustments and serum level monitoring may be necessary when switching from a product formulated with the free acid to a product formulated with the sodium salt and vice versa.

General: Dosage should be individualized to provide maximum benefit. In some cases serum blood level determinations may be necessary for optimal dosage adjustments—the clinically effective serum level is usually 10–20 mcg/mL. With recommended dosage, a period of seven to ten days may be required to achieve steady-state blood levels with phenytoin and changes in dosage (increase or decrease) should not be carried out at intervals shorter than seven to ten days.

Adult Dose: Patients who have received no previous treatment may be started on one teaspoonful (5 mL) of Dilantin-125 Suspension three times daily, and the dose is then adjusted to suit individual requirements. An increase to five teaspoonfuls daily may be made, if necessary.

Pediatric Dose: Initially, 5 mg/kg/day in two or three equally divided doses, with subsequent dosage individualized to a maximum of 300 mg daily. A recommended daily maintenance dosage is usually 4 to 8 mg/kg. Children over 6 years may require the minimum adult dose (300 mg/day).

HOW SUPPLIED

N 0071-2214—Dilantin-125® Suspension (phenytoin oral suspension, USP), 125 mg phenytoin/5 mL with a maximum alcohol content not greater than 0.6 percent, an orange suspension with an orange-vanilla flavor; available in 8-oz bottles and individual unit dose foil pouches which deliver 5 mL (125 mg phenytoin). The minimum sales unit is 100 pouches.

N 0071-2315—Dilantin-30® Pediatric Suspension (phenytoin oral suspension, USP), 30 mg phenytoin/5 mL with a maximum alcohol content not greater than 0.6 percent, a red suspension with a banana-orange-vanilla flavor; available in 8-oz bottles and individual unit dose foil pouches which deliver 5 mL (30 mg phenytoin). The minimum sales unit is 100 pouches.

Store below 30°C (86°F). Protect from freezing and light.

Also available as:

N 0071-0362 (Kapseal® 362)—Dilantin (extended phenytoin sodium capsules, USP) 100 mg; in 100's, 1000's, unit dose 100's and in a Memo Pack containing 84 unit-dose capsules (28 days dosage regimen).

N 0071-0365 (Kapseal 365)—Dilantin (extended phenytoin sodium capsules, USP) 30 mg; in 100's, 1000's and unit dose 100's .

N 0071-0375 (Kapseal 375)—Dilantin with Phenobarbital each contain 100 mg phenytoin sodium with 16 mg ($^1\!/_4$ gr) phenobarbital; in 100's and 1000's .

N 0071-0531 (Kapseal 531)—Dilantin with Phenobarbital each contain 100 mg phenytoin sodium with 32 mg ($^1\!/_2$ gr) phenobarbital; in 100's, 1000's and unit dose 100's.

N 0071-0007 (Tablet 7)—Dilantin Infatabs® (phenytoin tablets, USP) each contain 50 mg phenytoin; 100's and unit dose 100's.

For Parenteral Use:

N 0071-4488-05 (Ampoule 1488)—Dilantin ready-mixed solution containing 50 mg phenytoin sodium per milliliter is supplied in 2-mL ampoules. Packages of ten.

N 0071-4475-35 (Ampoule 1475)—Dilantin (phenytoin sodium injection) ready-mixed solution containing 50 mg phenytoin sodium per milliliter is supplied in 5-mL ampoules with one 6-mL sterile disposable syringe (22 gauge × 1$^1\!/_4$ inch needle). Packages of ten.

N 0071-4475-08 (Ampoule 1475)—Dilantin ready-mixed solution containing 50 mg phenytoin sodium per milliliter is supplied in packages of ten 5-mL ampoules without syringes.

N 0071-4488-41 (Steri-Dose® 4488)—Dilantin ready-mixed solution containing 50 mg phenytoin sodium per milliliter is supplied in a 2-mL sterile disposable syringe (22 gauge × 1$^1\!/_4$ inch needle). Packages of ten individually cartoned syringes.

N 0071-4488-45 Dilantin ready-mixed solution containing 50 mg phenytoin sodium per milliliter is supplied in 2 mL Steri-Vials.® Packages of twenty-five.

N 0071-4475-45 Dilantin ready-mixed solution containing 50 mg phenytoin sodium per milliliter is supplied in 5 mL Steri-Vials.® Packages of twenty-five.

Caution—Federal law prohibits dispensing without prescription.

2214G107

KAPSEALS®
DILANTIN®   ℞
[di-lăn´tĭn]
(Phenytoin Sodium) with
Phenobarbital

DESCRIPTION

Dilantin (phenytoin sodium) is related to the barbiturates in chemical structure, but has a five-membered ring. The chemical name is sodium 5,5-diphenyl-2,4-imidazolidinedione. Phenobarbital is a derivative of barbituric acid and is chemically described as 5-ethyl-5-phenylbarbituric acid.

Each Dilantin® with $^1\!/_4$ gr Phenobarbital Kapseal® contains:

Dilantin (phenytoin sodium) .... 100 mg
Phenobarbital .... 16 mg ($^1\!/_4$ gr)
(Warning—May be habit forming)

Each Dilantin with $^1\!/_2$ gr Phenobarbital Kapseal contains:

Dilantin (phenytoin sodium) .... 100 mg
Phenobarbital .... 32 mg ($^1\!/_2$ gr)
(Warning—May be habit forming)

Also contains confectioner's sugar NF, magnesium stearate, NF; talc, USP. The capsule shell and band contain citric acid, USP; colloidal silicon dioxide, NF; FD&C blue No. 1; FD&C red No. 40; gelatin NF; glyceryl monooleate; polyethylene glycol 200; sodium benzoate, NF; sodium lauryl sulfate, NF. The Dilantin with Phenobarbital $^1\!/_4$ gr capsule shell and band also contain FD&C red No. 3; hydrogen peroxide 3%. The Dilantin with Phenobarbital $^1\!/_2$ gr capsule shell and band also contain FD&C yellow No. 6.

CLINICAL PHARMACOLOGY

Phenytoin—Phenytoin is an antiepileptic drug which can be useful in the treatment of epilepsy. The primary site of action appears to be the *motor cortex* where spread of seizure activity is inhibited. Possibly by promoting sodium efflux from neurons, phenytoin tends to *stabilize* the threshold against hyperexcitability caused by excessive stimulation or environmental changes capable of reducing membrane sodium gradient. This includes the reduction of posttetanic potentiation at synapses. Loss of posttetanic potentiation prevents cortical seizure foci from detonating adjacent cortical areas. Phenytoin reduces the maximal activity of brain stem centers responsible for the tonic phase of tonic-clonic (grand mal) seizures.

The plasma half-life in man after oral administration of phenytoin averages 22 hours, with a range of 7 to 42 hours. Steady-state therapeutic levels are achieved at least 7 to 10 days (5–7 half-lives) after initiation of therapy with recommended doses of 300 mg/day.

When serum level determinations are necessary, they should be obtained at least 5–7 half-lives after treatment initiation, dosage change, or addition or subtraction of another drug to the regimen so that equilibrium or steady-state will have been achieved. Trough levels provide information about clinically effective serum level range and confirm patient compliance and are obtained just prior to the patient's next scheduled dose. Peak levels indicate an individual's threshold for emergence of dose-related side effects and are obtained at the time of expected peak concentration. For Dilantin with Phenobarbital Kapseals peak serum levels occur 1$^1\!/_2$–3 hours after administration.

Optimum control without clinical signs of toxicity occurs more often with serum levels between 10 and 20 mcg/mL, although some mild cases of tonic-clonic (grand mal) epilepsy may be controlled with lower serum levels of phenytoin.

In most patients maintained at a steady dosage, stable phenytoin serum levels are achieved. There may be wide interpatient variability in phenytoin serum levels with equivalent dosages. Patients with unusually low levels may be noncompliant or hypermetabolizers of phenytoin. Unusually high levels result from liver disease, congenital enzyme deficiency or drug interactions which result in metabolic interference. The patient with large variations in phenytoin plasma levels, despite standard doses, presents a difficult clinical problem. Serum level determinations in such patients may be particularly helpful.

Most of the drug is excreted in the bile as inactive metabolites which are then reabsorbed from the intestinal tract and excreted in the urine. Urinary excretion of phenytoin and its metabolites occurs partly with glomerular filtration, but more importantly, by tubular secretion. Because phenytoin is hydroxylated in the liver by an enzyme system which is saturable at high plasma levels small incremental doses may increase the half-life and produce very substantial increases in serum levels, when these are in the upper range. The steady-state level may be disproportionately increased, with resultant intoxication, from an increase in dosage of 10% or more.

Phenobarbital—Phenobarbital produces its anticonvulsant effect by depressing the motor cortex and raising the seizure threshold.

Phenobarbital is absorbed completely, although slowly, following oral administration and undergoes partial biotransformation in the liver by hydroxylation. Phenobarbital is excreted via the kidneys, 10% to 25% as free drug and the reminder primarily as the inactive para-hydroxyphenyl metabolite. The plasma half-life is long, approximately two to six days in adults, and shorter and more variable in children. In adults, the oral anticonvulsant dose of 1 to 3 mg/kg will produce therapeutic concentrations of 10 to 30 mcg/mL in the serum, the levels usually necessary for seizure control. At this dose, approximately three weeks may be required for the serum levels to achieve steady-state.

High serum levels occur when liver disease, diminished urinary flow, acidosis, or obesity is present. Low serum levels in adults may be due to poor patient compliance.

When used as an anticonvulsant, the clinical phenomenon of breakthrough seizures has been seen. Whether this is a case of true pharmacologic tolerance or some form of spontaneous variation is not known. Physical dependence does develop and may produce accentuation of seizures in epileptics when the drug is abruptly withdrawn.

INDICATIONS AND USAGE

Dilantin with Phenobarbital is indicated for the control of generalized tonic-clonic (grand mal) and complex partial (psychomotor, temporal lobe) seizures, only in those patients who require both drugs for seizure control and who previously have had their daily anticonvulsant requirements determined by the administration of the two drugs separately. Combinations should not be used to initiate anticonvulsant therapy and are provided as a convenience for epileptic patients.

Phenytoin serum level determinations may be necessary for optimal dosage adjustments (see Dosage and Administration and Clinical Pharmacology).

CONTRAINDICATIONS

Phenytoin is contraindicated in those patients with a history of hypersensitivity to hydantoin products.

Phenobarbital is contraindicated in the following conditions: latent or manifest porphyria or familial history of intermittent porphyria, history of confusion or restlessness from hypnotics, history of abnormal reaction or known hypersensitivity to barbital and its derivatives, including phenobarbital, or a known previous addiction to sedative-hypnotics. Other contraindications include renal and hepatic impairment and severe pulmonary insufficiency.

WARNINGS

Warning—Phenobarbital may be habit forming. Abrupt withdrawal of phenytoin in epileptic patients may precipitate status epilepticus. When, in the judgment of the clinician, the need for dosage reduction, discontinuation, or substitution of alternative anticonvulsant medication arises, this should be done gradually. In the event of an allergic or hypersensitivity reaction, more rapid substitution of alternative therapy may be necessary. In this case, alternative therapy should be an anticonvulsant not belonging to the hydantoin chemical class.

There have been a number of reports suggesting a relationship between phenytoin and the development of lymphadenopathy (local or generalized) including benign lymph node hyperplasia, pseudolymphoma, lymphoma, and Hodgkin's Disease. Although a cause and effect relationship has not been established, the occurrence of lymphadenopathy indicates the need to differentiate such a condition from other types of lymph node pathology. Lymph node involvement may occur with or without symptoms and signs resembling serum sickness eg, fever, rash and liver involvement.

In all cases of lymphadenopathy, follow-up observation for an extended period is indicated and every effort should be made to achieve seizure control using alternative antiepileptic drugs.

Acute alcoholic intake may increase phenytoin serum levels while chronic alcoholic use may decrease serum levels.

Usage in Pregnancy: A number of reports suggests an association between the use of antiepileptic drugs by women with epilepsy and a higher incidence of birth defects in children born to these women. Data are more extensive with respect to phenytoin and phenobarbital, but these are also the most commonly prescribed antiepileptic drugs; less systematic or anecdotal reports suggest a possible similar association with the use of all known antiepileptic drugs.

The reports suggesting a higher incidence of birth defects in children of drug-treated epileptic women cannot be regarded as adequate to prove a definite cause and effect relationship. There are intrinsic methodologic problems in obtaining adequate data on drug teratogenicity in humans; genetic factors or the epileptic condition itself may be more important than drug therapy in leading to birth defects. The great majority of mothers on antiepileptic medication deliver normal infants. It is important to note that antiepileptic drugs should not be discontinued in patients in whom the drug is administered to prevent major seizures, because of the strong possibility of precipitating status epilepticus with attendant hypoxia and threat to life. In individual cases where the severity and frequency of the seizure disorder are such that the removal of medication does not pose a serious threat to the patient, discontinuation of the drug may be considered prior to and during pregnancy, although it cannot be said with any

confidence that even minor seizures do not pose some hazards to the developing embryo or fetus. The prescribing physician will wish to weigh these considerations in treating and counseling epileptic women of childbearing potential. In addition to the reports of increased incidence of congenital malformation, such as cleft lip/palate and heart malformations in children of women receiving phenytoin and other antiepileptic drugs, there have more recently been reports of a fetal hydantoin syndrome. This consists of prenatal growth deficiency, microcephaly and mental deficiency in children born to mothers who have received phenytoin, barbiturates, alcohol, or trimethadione. However, these features are all interrelated and are frequently associated with intrauterine growth retardation from other causes.

There have been isolated reports of malignancies, including neuroblastoma, in children whose mothers received phenytoin during pregnancy.

An increase in seizure frequency during pregnancy occurs in a high proportion of patients, because of altered phenytoin absorption or metabolism. Periodic measurement of serum phenytoin levels is particularly valuable in the management of a pregnant epileptic patient as a guide to an appropriate adjustment of dosage. However, postpartum restoration of the original dosage will probably be indicated.

Neonatal coagulation defects have been reported within the first 24 hours in babies born to epileptic mothers receiving phenobarbital and/or phenytoin. Vitamin K has been shown to prevent or correct this defect and has been recommended to be given to the mother before delivery and the neonate after birth.

PRECAUTIONS

Phenytoin

General: The liver is the chief site of biotransformation of phenytoin; patients with impaired liver function may show early signs of toxicity. Elderly patients or those who are gravely ill may show early signs of toxicity.

A small percentage of indiviuals who have been treated with phenytoin have been shown to metabolize the drug slowly. Slow metabolism may be due to limited enzyme availability and lack of induction; it appears to be genetically determined.

Phenytoin should be discontinued if a skin rash appears (see "Warnings" section regarding drug discontinuation). If the rash is exfoliative, purpuric, or bullous or if lupus erythematosus, Stevens-Johnson syndrome, or toxic epidermal necrolysis is suspected, use of this drug should not be resumed and alternative therapy should be considered. (See Adverse Reactions.) If the rash is of a milder type (measles-like or scarlatiniform), therapy may be resumed after the rash has completely disappeared. If the rash recurs upon reinstitution of therapy, further phenytoin medication is contraindicated.

Hyperglycemia, resulting from the drug's inhibitory effects on insulin release, has been reported. Phenytoin may also raise the serum glucose level in diabetic patients.

Osteomalacia has been associated with phenytoin therapy and is considered to be due to phenytoin's interference with Vitamin D metabolism.

Phenytoin is not indicated for seizures due to hypoglycemic or other metabolic causes. Appropriate diagnostic procedures should be performed as indicated.

Phenytoin is not effective for absence (petit mal) seizures. If tonic-clonic (grand mal) and absence (petit mal) seizures are present, combined drug therapy is needed.

Serum levels of phenytoin sustained above the optimal range may produce confusional states referred to as "delirium," "psychosis," or "encephalopathy," or rarely irreversible cerebellar dysfunction. Accordingly, at the first sign of acute toxicity, plasma levels are recommended. Dose reduction of phenytoin therapy is indicated if plasma levels are excessive; if symptoms persist termination is recommended. (See Warnings)

Information for Patients: Patients taking phenytoin should be advised of the importance of adhering strictly to the prescribed dosage regimen, and of informing the physician of any clinical condition in which it is not possible to take the drug orally as prescribed, eg, surgery, etc.

Patients should also be cautioned on the use of other drugs or alcoholic beverages without first seeking the physician's advice.

Patients should be instructed to call their physician if skin rash develops.

The importance of good dental hygiene should be stressed in order to minimize the development of gingival hyperplasia and its complications.

Laboratory Tests: Phenytoin serum level determinations may be necessary to achieve optimal dosage adjustments.

Drug Interactions: There are many drugs which may increase or decrease phenytoin levels or which phenytoin may affect. The most commonly occurring drug interactions are listed below:

1. Drugs which may increase phenytoin serum levels include: chloramphenicol, dicumarol, disulfiram, tolbutamide, isoniazid, phenylbutazone, acute alcohol intake, salicylates, chlordiazepoxide, phenothiazines, diazepam,

estrogens, ethosuximide, halothane, methylphenidate, sulfonamides, cimetidine, trazodone.

2. Drugs which may decrease phenytoin levels include: carbamazepine, chronic alcohol abuse, reserpine. Moban® brand of Molindone Hydrochloride contains calcium ions which interfere with the absorption of phenytoin. Ingestion times of phenytoin and antacid preparations containing calcium should be staggered in patients with low serum phenytoin levels to prevent absorption problems.

3. Drugs which may either increase or decrease phenytoin serum levels include: phenobarbital, valproic acid, and sodium valproate. Similarly, the effect of phenytoin on phenobarbital, valproic acid and sodium valproate serum levels is unpredictable.

4. Although not a true drug interaction, tricyclic antidepressants may precipitate seizures in susceptible patients and phenytoin dosage may need to be adjusted.

5. Drugs whose efficacy is impaired by phenytoin include: corticosteroids, coumarin anticoagulants, oral contraceptives, quinidine, vitamin D, digitoxin, rifampin, doxycycline, estrogens, furosemide. Serum level determinations are especially helpful when possible drug interactions are suspected.

Drug/Laboratory Test Interactions: Phenytoin may cause decreased serum levels of protein-bound iodine (PBI). It may also produce lower than normal values for dexamethasone or metyrapone tests. Phenytoin may cause increased serum levels of glucose, alkaline phosphatase, and gamma glutamyl transpeptidase (GGT).

Carcinogenesis: See 'Warnings' section for information on carcinogenesis.

Pregnancy: See Warnings.

Nursing Mothers: Infant breast-feeding is not recommended for women taking this drug because phenytoin appears to be secreted in low concentrations in human milk.

Phenobarbital

Withdrawal symptoms, including convulsions and delirium, may occur upon discontinuance of phenobarbital in patients with chronic intoxication. Analgesics, if used with phenobarbital, should be prescribed with caution because of possible additive effects. Caution should be exercised in prescribing this drug to patients with suicidal tendencies or with a predilection to abusive use of barbiturates.

Phenobarbital should be used with caution in debilitating and pulmonary diseases.

Phenobarbital should be used with caution in patients with severely impaired liver function, severe anemia, congestive heart failure, fever, neuroses, hyperthyroidism, diabetes mellitus, and any conditions in which respiratory depression may be characteristic. Marked excitement rather than depression may occur in aged or debilitated patients, particularly those with cerebral arteriosclerosis.

Confusion or euphoria may result from use of this drug. Symptoms in mentally ill, phobic, and emotionally disturbed patients may be accentuated. Prolonged usage may produce psychological habituation. Sudden discontinuation or radical reduction of dosage may precipitate withdrawal symptoms in patients who have taken the drug for prolonged periods; dosage should be gradually reduced to the point of complete discontinuation.

Barbiturates should be prescribed with extreme caution for persons known or suspected of routinely or periodically consuming large quantities of alcoholic beverages. Potentiation of effect, even to the extent of causing death, may result from consumption of barbiturates by patients with a high serum alcohol level.

Information for Patients: Phenobarbital may impair the mental and/or physical abilities required for the performance of potentially hazardous tasks, such as driving a motor vehicle or other such activity requiring alertness; therefore, the patient should be cautioned accordingly.

Drug Interactions: The effects of phenobarbital may be increased by many drugs, including antihistamines, tranquilizers, corticosteroids, monoamine oxidase inhibitors, narcotic analgesics, amitriptyline, imipramine, and rauwolfia alkaloids.

Pregnancy

See WARNINGS

Nursing Mothers: Evidence that phenobarbital is secreted in human milk is inadequate. The drug appears to be secreted in low concentrations which are unlikely to affect the infant. If the mother is receiving large doses of phenobarbital, however, the drug concentration in milk might increase. For this reason, artificial feeding of the infant is recommended for women taking this drug.

Continued on next page

This product information was prepared in August, 1989. On these and other Parke-Davis Products, information may be obtained by addressing PARKE-DAVIS, Division of Warner-Lambert Company, Morris Plains, New Jersey 07950.

Parke-Davis—Cont.

Labor and Delivery: Barbiturates readily cross the placental barrier and, if administered during labor, may have a depressant effect on the fetus; infants born of mothers receiving barbiturates may have difficulty breathing spontaneously.

ADVERSE REACTIONS

Phenytoin

Central Nervous System: The most common manifestations encountered with phenytoin therapy are referable to this system and are usually dose-related. These include nystagmus, ataxia, slurred speech, decreased coordination and mental confusion. Dizziness, insomnia, transient nervousness, motor twitchings, and headaches have also been observed. There have also been rare reports of phenytoin induced dyskinesias, including chorea, dystonia, tremor and asterixis, similar to those induced by phenothiazine and other neuroleptic drugs.

A predominantly sensory peripheral polyneuropathy has been observed in patients receiving long-term phenytoin therapy.

Gastrointestinal System: Nausea, vomiting, and constipation.

Integumentary System: Dermatological manifestations sometimes accompanied by fever have included scarlatiniform or morbilliform rashes. A morbilliform rash (measles-like) is the most common; other types of dermatitis are seen more rarely. Other more serious forms which may be fatal have included bullous, exfoliative, or purpuric dermatitis, lupus erythematosus, Stevens-Johnson syndrome, and toxic epidermal necrolysis (see Precautions).

Hemopoietic System: Hemopoietic complications, some fatal, have occasionally been reported in association with administration of phenytoin. These have included thrombocytopenia, leukopenia, granulocytopenia, agranulocytosis, and pancytopenia with or without bone marrow suppression. While macrocytosis and megaloblastic anemia have occurred, these conditions usually respond to folic acid therapy. Lymphadenopathy including benign lymph node hyperplasia, pseudolymphoma, lymphoma, and Hodgkin's Disease have been reported (see Warnings).

Connective Tissue System: Coarsening of the facial features, enlargement of the lips, gingival hyperplasia, hypertrichosis, and Peyronie's Disease.

Other: Systemic lupus erythematosus, periarteritis nodosa, toxic hepatitis, liver damage, and immunoglobulin abnormalities may occur.

Phenobarbital

Central Nervous System: With larger doses, the most common manifestations relate to this system. These include drowsiness, vertigo, ataxia, hebetude, headache, delirium and stupor.

Gastrointestinal System: Phenobarbital may cause gastrointestinal discomfort and nausea.

Integumentary System: Hypersensitivity reactions are rare. Cutaneous eruptions are principally due to idiosyncrasy. Fatalities from exfoliative dermatitis and cutaneous eruptions have been reported. There are two syndromes associated with phenobarbital administration: Stevens-Johnson and a phenobarbital sensitivity syndrome. The phenobarbital sensitivity syndrome, which has resulted in fatalities, is characterized by an erythematous rash, high fever, jaundice, mental confusion, and toxic damage of "parenchymatous organs."

Hemopoietic System: Megaloblastic anemia has been reported; this condition usually responds to folic acid therapy.

OVERDOSAGE

The therapeutic ranges for phenytoin and phenobarbital in adults are 10 to 20 mcg/mL and 10 to 30 mcg/mL, respectively. Following acute overdosage of this combination, the patient at steady-state may experience evidence of phenytoin toxicity ahead of phenobarbital toxicity because phenytoin plasma levels rise more rapidly than phenobarbital levels. Phenytoin also has a narrower margin between therapeutic and toxic levels than does phenobarbital.

Phenytoin

The lethal dose in children is not known. The lethal dose in adults is estimated to be 2 to 5 grams. The initial symptoms are nystagmus, ataxia, and dysarthria. Other signs are tremor, hyperflexia, lethargy, slurred speech, nausea, vomiting. The patient may become comatose and hypertensive. Death is due to respiratory and circulatory depression. There are marked variations among individuals with respect to phenytoin plasma levels where toxicity may occur. Nystagmus, on lateral gaze, usually appears at 20 mcg/mL, ataxia at 30 mcg/mL, dysarthria and lethargy appear when the plasma concentration is over 40 mcg/mL, but as high a concentration as 50 mcg/mL has been reported without evidence of toxicity. As much as 25 times the therapeutic dose has been taken to result in a serum concentration over 100 mcg/mL with complete recovery.

Treatment is nonspecific since there is no known antidote. The adequacy of the respiratory and circulatory systems should be carefully observed and appropriate supportive measures employed. Hemodialysis can be considered since phenytoin is not completely bound to plasma proteins. Total exchange transfusion has been used in the treatment of severe intoxication in children.

In acute overdosage the possibility of other CNS depressants, including alcohol, should be borne in mind.

Phenobarbital

The lethal dose of phenobarbital is believed to be 5 grams. The highest known blood level from which a patient recovered was 580 mcg/mL. An overdose of phenobarbital will include the classical picture of progressive central nervous system depression. In its severest form this syndrome leads to respiratory arrest as a result of general reflex paralysis. The milder forms of this syndrome may mimic any stage of clinical anesthesia. Except for a rapid (and weak) pulse, vital signs are characteristically reduced. In addition to direct inhibition of the cardiac contractile mechanism with consequent hypotension, circulatory insufficiency may be aggravated by hypoxia from inadequate pulmonary ventilation. Early deaths are usually due to respiratory arrest, but delayed fatalities may arise from one or any combination of the following complications: hypostatic pneumonia, bronchopneumonia, lung abscess, pulmonary edema, cerebral edema, circulatory collapse, and irreversible renal shutdown. The treatment of barbiturate poisoning consists in removing any unabsorbed drug from the stomach, supporting the respiration and circulation, and expediting elimination of the drug which has been absorbed.

DOSAGE AND ADMINISTRATION

Serum concentrations should be monitored and care should be taken when switching a patient from the sodium salt to the free acid form.

Dilantin® Kapseals®, Dilantin Parenteral, and Dilantin with Phenobarbital are formulated with the sodium salt of phenytoin. The free acid form of phenytoin is used in Dilantin-30 Pediatric and Dilantin-125 Suspensions and Dilantin Infatabs. Because there is approximately an 8% increase in drug content with the free acid form over that of the sodium salt, dosage adjustments and serum level monitoring may be necessary when switching from a product formulated with the free acid to a product formulated with the sodium salt and vice versa.

The combination of Dilantin with Phenobarbital Kapseals is provided as a convenience for epileptic patients who require both drugs for seizure control. Anticonvulsant therapy should be initiated with either phenytoin or phenobarbital and, if indicated, the other drug can then be added. If the total daily doses of the two drugs used separately are within those given below, the combination of Dilantin with Phenobarbital Kapseals can then be substituted in equivalent amounts. When plasma level determinations are necessary for optimal dosage adjustments, the clinically effective level of Dilantin is usually 10 to 20 mcg/mL and for phenobarbital 10 to 30 mcg/mL in adults. Serum blood level determinations are especially helpful when possible drug interactions are suspected.

If either the phenytoin or phenobarbital dosage requires adjustment, this should be done by switching the patient to separate phenytoin and phenobarbital dosage forms in order to enable subsequent dosage adjustment of either or both drugs.

The recommended starting phenobarbital dose for children is 2 to 3 mg/kg/day in two or three equally divided doses. The recommended starting Dilantin dose for children is 5 mg/kg/day in two or three equally divided doses.

Adult Dosage: For maintenance (see above)—usually three or four capsules daily. An increase to six capsules daily may be made, if necessary.

Pediatric Dosage: For maintenance (see above)—individualized to a maximum of 300 mg Dilantin daily.

HOW SUPPLIED

N 0071-0375 (Kapseal 375, transparent #3 capsule with a garnet band)—Dilantin with Phenobarbital each contain 100 mg phenytoin sodium with 16 mg (¼ gr) phenobarbital; in 100's and 1000's.

N 0071-0531 (Kapseal 531, transparent #3 capsule with a black band)—Dilantin with Phenobarbital each contain 100 mg phenytoin sodium with 32 mg (½ gr) phenobarbital in 100's, 1000's and unit dose 100's.

Store at room temperature below 30°C (86°F).

Protect from moisture and light.

Also Available As:

N 0071-0362 (Kapseal 362)—Dilantin (phenytoin sodium) 100 mg; in 100's, 1000's, unit dose 100's and in a Memo Pack containing 84 unit-dose capsules (28 day dosage regimen).

N 0071-0365 (Kapseal 365)—Dilantin (phenytoin sodium) 30 mg in 100's, 1000's, and unit dose 100's.

N 0071-0007 (Tablet 7)—Dilantin Infatabs® each contain 50 mg phenytoin; 100's, and unit dose 100's.

N 0071-2214—Dilantin-125® Suspension (phenytoin oral suspension USP.) 125 mg phenytoin/5 mL with a maximum

alcohol content not greater than 0.6 percent; available in 8-oz bottles and individual dose foil pouches which deliver 5 mL (125 mg phenytoin). The minimum sales unit is 100 pouches.

N 0071-2315—Dilantin-30® Pediatric Suspension (phenytoin oral suspension, USP.) 30 mg phenytoin/5 mL with a maximum alcohol content not greater than 0.6 percent; available in 8-oz bottles and individual unit dose foil pouches which deliver 5 mL (30 mg phenytoin). The minimum sales unit is 100 pouches.

For Parenteral Use:

N 0071-4488-05 (Ampoule 1488)—Dilantin ready-mixed solution containing 50 mg phenytoin sodium per milliliter is supplied in 2-mL ampoules. Packages of ten.

N 0071-4488-41 (Steri-Dose® 4488)—Dilantin ready-mixed solution containing 50 mg phenytoin sodium per milliliter is supplied in a 2-mL sterile disposable syringe (22 gauge × 1¼ inch needle).

Packages of ten individually cartoned syringes.

N 0071-4475-35 (Ampoule 1475)—Dilantin ready-mixed solution containing 50 mg phenytoin sodium per milliliter is supplied in 5-mL ampoules with one 6-mL sterile disposable syringe (22 gauge × 1¼ inch needle). Packages of ten.

N 0071-4475-08 (Ampoule 1475)—Dilantin ready-mixed solution containing 50 mg phenytoin sodium per milliliter is supplied in packages of ten 5-mL ampoules without syringes.

N 0071-4488-45 Dilantin ready-mixed solution containing 50 mg phenytoin sodium per milliliter is supplied in 2-mL Steri-Vials.® Packages of twenty-five.

N 0071-4475-45 Dilantin ready-mixed solution containing 50 mg phenytoin sodium per milliliter is supplied in 5-mL Steri-Vials.® Packages of twenty-five.

REFERENCES

1. Woodbury, DM and Fingl, E. "Drugs Effective in the Therapy of the Epilepsies," in Goodman, LS and Gilman, A(eds): The Pharmacological Basis of Therapeutics ed 5. New York, Macmillan Publishing Co, Inc, 1975, pp 201–226.
2. Henn, K. "Diphenylhydantoin: Relation of Plasma Levels to Clinical Control," in Woodbury, DM, Penry, JK, and Schmidt, RP, (eds): Antiepileptic Drugs, New York, Raven Press, Publishers, 1972, pp 211–218.

Caution—Federal law prohibits dispensing without prescription.

0375G016

Shown in Product Identification Section, page 421

DORYX®   ℞
(Coated Doxycycline Hyclate Pellets)

DESCRIPTION

DORYX® Capsules contain specially coated pellets of doxycycline hyclate for oral administration. Also contains lactose, NF; microcrystalline cellulose, NF; povidone, USP. The capsule shell and/or band contains FD and C blue No. 1; FD and C yellow No. 6; D and C yellow No. 10; gelatin, NF; silicon dioxide; sodium lauryl sulfate, NF; titanium dioxide, USP. Doxycycline is a broad-spectrum antibiotic synthetically derived from oxytetracycline and available as doxycycline hyclate. The chemical designation of this light-yellow crystalline powder is alpha-6-desoxy-5-oxytetracycline. Doxycycline has a high degree of lipoid solubility and a low affinity for calcium binding. It is highly stable in normal human serum. Doxycycline will not degrade into an epianhydro form.

CLINICAL PHARMACOLOGY

Tetracyclines are readily absorbed and are bound to plasma proteins in varying degree. They are concentrated by the liver in the bile, and excreted in the urine and feces at high concentrations and in a biologically active form.

Doxycycline is virtually completely absorbed after oral administration. Following a 200 mg dose, normal adult volunteers averaged peak serum levels of 2.6 mcg/mL of doxycycline at 2 hours decreasing to 145 mcg/mL at 24 hours. Excretion of doxycycline by the kidney is about 40%/72 hours in individuals with normal function (creatinine clearance about 75 mL/min). This percentage excretion may fall as low as 1–5%/72 hours in individuals with severe renal insufficiency (creatinine clearance below 10 mL/min). Studies have shown no significant difference in serum half-life of doxycycline (range 18–22 hours) in individuals with normal and severely impaired renal function.

Hemodialysis does not alter serum half-life.

Microbiology: Doxycycline is primarily bacteriostatic and is thought to exert its antimicrobial effect by the inhibition of protein synthesis. Doxycycline is active against a wide range of gram-positive and gram-negative organisms. The drugs in the tetracycline class have closely similar antimicrobial spectra and cross resistance among them is common.

Susceptibility Tests: Diffusion Techniques: The use of antibiotic disc susceptibility test methods which measure zone diameter gives an accurate estimation of susceptibility of organisms to DORYX: One such standard procedure[1] has been recommended for use with discs for testing antimicrobials. Doxycycline 30 mcg discs should be used for the determination of the susceptibility of organisms to doxycycline. With this type of procedure, a report of "susceptible" from the laboratory indicates that the infecting organism is likely to respond to therapy. A report of "intermediate susceptibility" suggests that the organism would be susceptible if high dosage is used or if the infection is confined to tissue and fluids (e.g., urine) in which high antibiotic levels are obtained. A report of "resistant" indicates that the infecting organism is not likely to respond to therapy. With the doxycycline disc, a zone of 16 mm or greater indicates susceptibility, zone sizes of 12 mm or less indicate resistance, and zone sizes of 13 to 15 mm indicate intermediate susceptibility.

Standardized procedures require the use of laboratory control organisms. The 30 mcg tetracycline disc should give zone diameters between 19 and 28 mm for *S.aureus* ATCC 25923 and between 18 and 25 mm for *E.coli* ATCC 25922. The 30 mcg doxycycline disc should give zone diameters between 23 and 29 mm for *S.aureus* ATCC 25923, and between 18 and 24 mm for *E.coli* ATCC 25922.

Dilution Techniques: A bacterial isolate may be considered susceptible if the MIC (minimal inhibitory concentration) value for doxycycline is less than 4 mcg/mL. Organisms are considered resistant if the MIC is greater than 12.5 mcg/mL. MICs greater than 4.0 mcg/mL and less than 12.5 mcg/mL indicate intermediate susceptibility.

As with standard diffusion methods, dilution procedures require the use of laboratory control mechanisms. Standard doxycycline powder should give MIC values in the range of 0.25 mcg/mL and 1.0 mcg/mL for *S.aureus* ATCC 25923. For *E.coli* ATCC 25922 the MIC range should be between 1.0 mcg/mL and 4.0 mcg/mL.

INDICATIONS AND USAGE

Doxycycline is indicated in infections caused by the following microorganisms:

Rickettsiae (Rocky Mountain spotted fever, typhus fever and the typhus group, Q fever, rickettsialpox and tick fevers).

Mycoplasma pneumoniae (PPLO, Eaton's agent).

Agents of psittacosis and ornithosis.

Agents of lymphogranuloma venereum and granuloma inguinale.

The following gram-negative microorganisms:

Haemophilus ducreyi (chancroid)
Yersinia pestis (formerly *Pasteurella pestis*)
Francisella tularensis (formerly *Pasteurella tularensis*)
Bartonella bacilliformis
Bacteroides species
Vibrio cholerae (formerly *Vibrio comma*)
Campylobacter fetus (formerly *Vibrio fetus*)
Brucella species (in conjunction with streptomycin)

Because many strains of the following groups of microorganisms have been shown to be resistant to tetracyclines, culture and susceptibility testing are recommended.

Doxycycline is indicated for treatment of infections caused by the following gram-negative microorganisms, when bacteriological testing indicates appropriate susceptibility to the drug:

Escherichia coli
Enterobacter aerogenes (formerly *Aerobacter aerogenes*)
Shigella species
Mima species and *Herellea* species
Haemophilus influenzae (respiratory infections)
Klebsiella species (respiratory and urinary infections)

Doxycycline is indicated for treatment of infections caused by the following gram-positive microorganisms when bacteriological testing indicates appropriate susceptibility to the drug:

Streptococcus species:

Up to 44 percent of strains of *Streptococcus pyogenes* and 74 percent of *Streptococcus faecalis* have been found to be resistant to tetracycline drugs. Therefore, tetracyclines should not be used for streptococcal disease unless the organism has been demonstrated to be susceptible.

For upper respiratory infections due to group A beta-hemolytic streptococci, penicillin is the usual drug of choice, including prophylaxis of rheumatic fever.

Diplococcus pneumoniae.

Staphylococcus aureus, (respiratory, skin and soft-tissue infections). Tetracyclines are not the drug of choice in the treatment of any type of staphylococcal infection.

When penicillin is contraindicated, doxycycline is an alternative drug in the treatment of infections due to:

Treponema pallidum and *Treponema pertenue* (syphilis and yaws)
Listeria monocytogenes
Clostridium species
Bacillus anthracis
Fusobacterium fusiforme (Vincent's infection)
Actinomyces species

In acute intestinal amebiasis doxycycline may be a useful adjunct to amebicides.

In severe acne doxycycline may be useful adjunctive therapy.

Doxycycline is indicated in the treatment of trachoma, although the infectious agent is not always eliminated, as judged by immunofluorescence.

Inclusion conjunctivitis may be treated with oral doxycycline alone, or with a combination of topical agents.

Doxycycline is indicated for the treatment of uncomplicated urethral, endocervical or rectal infections in adults caused by *Chlamydia trachomatis.*[2]

Doxycycline is indicated for the treatment of nongonococcal urethritis caused by *Chlamydia trachomatis* and *Ureaplasma urealyticum* and for the treatment of acute epididymo-orchitis caused by *Chlamydia trachomatis.*[2]

Doxycycline is indicated for the treatment of uncomplicated gonococcal infections in adults (except for anorectal infections in men), the gonococcal arthritis-dermatitis syndrome and acute epididymo-orchitis caused by *N. gonorrhoeae.*[2]

CONTRAINDICATIONS

The drug is contraindicated in persons who have shown hypersensitivity to any of the tetracyclines.

WARNINGS

THE USE OF DRUGS OF THE TETRACYCLINE CLASS DURING TOOTH DEVELOPMENT (LAST HALF OF PREGNANCY, INFANCY AND CHILDHOOD TO THE AGE OF 8 YEARS) MAY CAUSE PERMANENT DISCOLORATION OF THE TEETH (YELLOW-GRAY-BROWN). This adverse reaction is more common during long term use of the drugs but has been observed following repeated short term courses. Enamel hypoplasia has also been reported. TETRACYCLINE DRUGS, THEREFORE, SHOULD NOT BE USED IN THIS AGE GROUP UNLESS OTHER DRUGS ARE NOT LIKELY TO BE EFFECTIVE OR ARE CONTRAINDICATED.

Results of animal studies indicate that tetracyclines cross the placenta, are found in fetal tissues and can have toxic effects on the developing fetus (often related to retardation of skeletal development). Evidence of embryotoxicity has been noted in animals treated early in pregnancy. If any tetracycline is used during pregnancy or if the patient becomes pregnant while taking these drugs, the patient should be apprised of potential hazard to the fetus.

As with other tetracyclines, doxycycline forms a stable calcium complex in any bone-forming tissue. A decrease in the fibula growth rate has been observed in prematures given oral tetracycline in doses of 25 mg/kg every six hours. This reaction was shown to be reversible when the drug was discontinued.

Photosensitivity manifested by an exaggerated sunburn reaction has been observed in some individuals taking tetracyclines. Patients apt to be exposed to direct sunlight or ultraviolet light should be advised that this reaction can occur with tetracycline drugs, and treatment should be discontinued at the first evidence of skin erythema.

The antianabolic action of the tetracyclines may cause an increase in BUN. Studies to date indicate that this does not occur with the use of doxycycline in patients with impaired renal function.

PRECAUTIONS

As with other antibiotic preparations, use of this drug may result in overgrowth of nonsusceptible organisms, including fungi. If superinfection occurs, the antibiotic should be discontinued and appropriate therapy instituted.

All infections due to group A beta-hemolytic streptococci should be treated for at least 10 days.

Laboratory tests: In venereal disease when coexistent syphilis is suspected, dark-field examination should be done before treatment is started and the blood serology repeated monthly for at least 4 months.

In long term therapy, periodic laboratory evaluation of organ systems, including hematopoietic, renal and hepatic studies should be performed.

Drug interactions: Because tetracyclines have been shown to depress plasma prothrombin activity, patients who are on anticoagulant therapy may require downward adjustment of their anticoagulant dosage.

Since bacteriostatic drugs may interfere with the bactericidal action of penicillin, it is advisable to avoid giving tetracyclines in conjunction with penicillin.

For concomitant therapy with antacids or iron-containing preparations and food see "Dosage and Administration" section.

Carcinogenesis, mutagenesis, impairment of fertility: Long term studies are currently being conducted to determine whether tetracyclines have carcinogenic potential. Animal studies conducted in rats and mice have not provided conclusive evidence that tetracyclines may be carcinogenic or that they impair fertility. In two mammalian cell assays (L51784 mouse lymphoma and Chinese hamster lung cells *in vitro*) positive responses for mutagenicity occurred at concentrations of 60 and 10 mcg/mL respectively. In humans no association between tetracyclines and these effects has been made.

Pregnancy: Pregnancy Category D (See Warnings section).

Nursing mothers: Tetracyclines are present in the milk of lactating women who are taking a drug in this class. Because

of the potential for serious adverse reactions in nursing infants from the tetracyclines, a decision should be made whether to discontinue nursing or discontinue the drug, taking into account the importance of the drug to the mother (see Warnings section).

Pediatric use: See Warnings and Dosage and Administration sections.

ADVERSE REACTIONS

Due to oral doxycycline's virtually complete absorption, side effects to the lower bowel, particularly diarrhea, have been infrequent. The following adverse reactions have been observed in patients receiving tetracyclines:

Gastrointestinal: Anorexia, nausea, vomiting, diarrhea, glossitis, dysphagia, enterocolitis, and inflammatory lesions (with monilial overgrowth) in the anogenital region. These reactions have been caused by both the oral and parenteral administration of tetracyclines. Rare instances of esophagitis and esophageal ulcerations have been reported in patients receiving capsule and tablet forms of drugs in the tetracycline class. Most of these patients took medications immediately before going to bed. (See Dosage and Administration).

Skin: Maculopapular and erythematous rashes. Exfoliative dermatitis has been reported but is uncommon. Photosensitivity is discussed above (see Warnings).

Renal toxicity: Rise in BUN has been reported and is apparently dose related. (See Warnings).

Hypersensitivity reactions: Urticaria, angioneurotic edema, anaphylaxis, anaphylactoid purpura, pericarditis, and exacerbation of systemic lupus erythematosus.

Bulging fontanels in infants and benign intracranial hypertension in adults have been reported in individuals receiving tetracyclines. These conditions disappeared when the drug was discontinued.

Blood: Hemolytic anemia, thrombocytopenia, neutropenia, and eosinophilis have been reported with tetracyclines.

When given over prolonged periods, tetracyclines have been reported to produce brown-black microscopic discoloration of thyroid glands. No abnormalities of thyroid function are known to occur.

DOSAGE AND ADMINISTRATION

THE USUAL DOSAGE AND FREQUENCY OF ADMINISTRATION OF DOXYCYCLINE DIFFERS FROM THAT OF THE OTHER TETRACYCLINES. EXCEEDING THE RECOMMENDED DOSAGE MAY RESULT IN AN INCREASED INCIDENCE OF SIDE EFFECTS.

Adults: The usual dose of oral doxycycline is 200 mg on the first day of treatment (administered 100 mg every 12 hours) followed by a maintenance dose of 100 mg/day. The maintenance dose may be administered as a single dose or as 50 mg every 12 hours. In the management of more severe infections (particularly chronic infections of the urinary tract), 100 mg every 12 hours is recommended.

For children above eight years of age: The recommended dosage schedule for children weighing 100 pounds or less is 2 mg/lb of body weight divided into two doses on the first day of treatment, followed by 1 mg/lb of body weight given as a single daily dose or divided into two doses on subsequent days. For more severe infections up to 2 mg/lb of body weight may be used. For children over 100 pounds, the usual adult dose should be used.

Uncomplicated gonococcal infections in adults (except anorectal infections in men): 100 mg, by mouth, twice-a-day for 7 days.[2] As an alternate single visit dose, administer 300 mg stat followed in one hour by a second 300 mg dose. The dose may be administered with food, including milk or carbonated beverage, as required.

Acute epididymo-orchitis caused by *N. gonorrhoeae:* 100 mg, by mouth, twice-a-day for at least 10 days.[2]

Primary and secondary syphilis: 300 mg a day in divided doses for at least 10 days.

Uncomplicated urethral, endocervical, or rectal infection in adults caused by *Chlamydia trachomatis:* 100 mg by mouth, twice-a-day for at least 7 days.[2]

Nongonococcal urethritis caused by *C. trachomatis* and *U. urealyticum:* 100 mg, by mouth, twice-a-day for at least 7 days.[2]

Acute epididymo-orchitis caused by *C. trachomatis:* 100 mg, by mouth, twice-a-day for at least 10 days.[2]

The therapeutic antibacterial serum activity will usually persist for 24 hours following recommended dosage.

When used in streptococcal infections, therapy should be continued for 10 days.

Administration of adequate amounts of fluid along with capsule and tablet forms of drugs in the tetracycline class is

Continued on next page

This product information was prepared in August, 1989. On these and other Parke-Davis Products, information may be obtained by addressing PARKE-DAVIS, Division of Warner-Lambert Company, Morris Plains, New Jersey 07950.

Parke-Davis—Cont.

recommended to wash down the drugs and reduce the risk of esophageal irritation and ulceration (see Adverse Reactions). If gastric irritation occurs, it is recommended that doxycycline be given with food or milk. The absorption of doxycycline is not markedly influenced by simultaneous ingestion of food or milk.

Concomitant therapy: Antacids containing aluminum, calcium or magnesium, sodium bicarbonate, and iron-containing preparations should not be given to patients taking oral tetracyclines.

Studies to date have indicated that administration of doxycycline at the usual recommended doses does not lead to excessive accumulation of the antibiotic in patients with renal impairment.

HOW SUPPLIED

DORYX® Capsules have a yellow transparent body with light blue opaque cap; the capsule bearing the inscription "DORYX" in white. Pellets are colored yellow. Each capsule contains specially coated pellets of doxycycline hyclate equivalent to 100 mg of doxycycline, supplied in:
Bottles of 50 capsules ....N 0071-0838-19

STORAGE CONDITIONS

Store at controlled room temperature below 25° C (77° F).
References:
1. NCCLS Approved Standard:
   M2-A3, Vol. 4, Performance Standards for Antimicrobial Disk Susceptibility Tests, Third Edition: available from the National Committee for Clinical Laboratory Standards, 771 East Lancaster Avenue, Villanova, Pa. 19085
2. CDC Sexually Transmitted Diseases Treatment Guidelines 1982

Caution—Federal law prohibits dispensing without prescription.
Manufactured by
Faulding International
129 Dew Street,
Thebarton, South Australia, 5031
Distributed by
PARKE-DAVIS
Div of Warner-Lambert Co
Morris Plains, NJ 07950 USA

                                     0838G021
Shown in Product Identification Section, page 421

EASPRIN®   ℞
[ēas´prĭn″]
(Aspirin Delayed-release Tablets, USP)
Enteric Coated Tablets

Caution—Federal law prohibits dispensing without prescription.

DESCRIPTION

Easprin (Aspirin Delayed-release Tablets, USP) enteric coated tablets contain 15 grains (975 mg) aspirin for oral administration. Also contains: candelilla wax; colloidal silicon dioxide, NF; corn starch 1500; dusty rose Opaspray; hydroxypropyl methylcellulose, USP (15 cps); methylparaben, NF; microcrystalline cellulose, NF; mistron spray talc; polyethylene glycol 3350, NF; propylparaben, NF; stearic acid powder; vanillin, NF; zinc stearate, USP. The enteric coating is designed to prevent the release of aspirin in the stomach and thereby reduce gastric irritation and total occult blood loss. The pharmacologic effects of aspirin include analgesia, antipyresis, antiinflammatory activity, and antirheumatic activity.

CLINICAL PHARMACOLOGY

Aspirin is a salicylate that has demonstrated antiinflammatory, analgesic, antipyretic, and antirheumatic activity.
Aspirin's mode of action as an antiinflammatory and antirheumatic agent may be due to inhibition of synthesis and release of prostaglandins.
Aspirin appears to produce analgesia by virtue of both a peripheral and CNS effect. Peripherally, aspirin acts by inhibiting the synthesis and release of prostaglandins. Acting centrally, it would appear to produce analgesia at a hypothalamic site in the brain, although the mode of action is not known.
Aspirin also acts on the hypothalamus to produce antipyresis; heat dissipation is increased as a result of vasodilation and increased peripheral blood flow. Aspirin's antipyretic activity may also be related to inhibition of synthesis and release of prostaglandins.
In a crossover study, Easprin at a dose of one tablet (15 grains) three times a day produced an average fecal blood loss of 1.54 ml per day. Uncoated aspirin at a dosage of three 5 grain tablets given three times a day caused an average fecal blood loss of 4.33 ml per day.
Easprin Tablets are enteric coated. This coating acts to prevent the release of aspirin in the stomach but permits the tablet to dissolve with resultant absorption in the upper por-

tion of the small intestine. This reduces any gastric irritation that may occur with uncoated aspirin but does delay the onset of action. Aspirin is rapidly hydrolyzed primarily in the liver to salicylic acid, which is conjugated with glycine (forming salicyluric acid) and glucuronic acid and excreted largely in the urine. As a result of the rapid hydrolysis, plasma concentrations of aspirin are always low and rarely exceed 20 mcg/ml at ordinary therapeutic doses. The peak salicylate level for uncoated aspirin occurs in about 2 hours; however with enteric coated aspirin tablets this is delayed. A direct correlation between salicylate plasma levels and clinical analgesic effectiveness has not been definitely established, but effective analgesia is usually achieved at plasma levels of 15 to 30 mg per 100 ml. Effective antiinflammatory activity is usually achieved at salicylate plasma levels of 20 to 30 mg per 100 ml. There is also poor correlation between toxic symptoms and plasma salicylate concentrations, but most patients exhibit symptoms of salicylism at plasma salicylate levels of 35 mg per 100 ml. The plasma half-life for aspirin is approximately 15 minutes; that for salicylate lengthens as the dose increases: Doses of 300 to 650 mg have a half-life of 3.1 to 3.2 hours; with doses of 1 gram, the half-life is increased to 5 hours and with 2 grams it is increased to about 9 hours.
Salicylates are excreted mainly by the kidney. Studies in man indicate that salicylate is excreted in the urine as free salicylic acid (10%), salicyluric acid (75%), salicylic phenolic (10%), and acyl (5%) glucuronides and gentisic acid.

INDICATIONS AND USAGE

Easprin is indicated in patients who need the higher 15 grain dose of aspirin in the long-term palliative treatment of mild to moderate pain and inflammation of arthritic and other inflammatory conditions.

CONTRAINDICATIONS

Easprin should not be used in patients who have previously exhibited hypersensitivity to aspirin and/or nonsteroidal antiinflammatory agents.
Easprin should not be given to patients with a recent history of gastrointestinal bleeding or in patients with bleeding disorders (eg, hemophilia).

WARNINGS

Easprin Tablets should be used with caution when anticoagulants are prescribed concurrently, for aspirin may depress the concentration of prothrombin in plasma and thereby increase bleeding time. Large doses of salicylates have a hypoglycemic action and may enhance the effect of the oral hypoglycemics. Consequently, they should not be given concomitantly; if however, this is necessary, the dosage of the hypoglycemic agent must be reduced while the salicylate is given. This hypoglycemic action may also affect the insulin requirements of diabetics.
Although salicylates in large doses are uricosuric agents, smaller amounts may decrease the uricosuric effects of probenecid, sulfinpyrazone, and phenylbutazone.

PRECAUTIONS

General: Easprin Tablets should be administered with caution to patients with asthma, nasal polyps, or nasal allergies. In patients receiving large doses of aspirin and/or prolonged therapy, mild salicylate intoxication (salicylism) may develop that may be reversed by reduction in dosage.
Although the fecal blood loss with Easprin is less than that with uncoated aspirin tablets, Easprin Tablets should be administered with caution to patients with a history of gastric distress, ulcer, or bleeding problems. Occult gastrointestinal bleeding occurs in many patients but is not correlated with gastric distress. The amount of blood lost is usually insignificant clinically, but with prolonged administration, it may result in iron deficiency anemia.
Sodium excretion produced by spironolactone may be decreased in the presence of salicylates.
Salicylates can produce changes in thyroid function tests. Salicylates should be used with caution in patients with severe hepatic damage, preexisting hypoprothrombinemia, or Vitamin K deficiency, and in those undergoing surgery.

DRUG INTERACTIONS

Anticoagulants: See Warnings.
Hypoglycemic Agents: See Warnings.
Uricosuric Agents: Aspirin may decrease the effects of probenecid, sulfinpyrazone, and phenylbutazone.
Spironolactone: See general precautions above.
Alcohol: Has a synergistic effect with aspirin in causing gastrointestinal bleeding.
Corticosteroids: Concomitant administration with aspirin may increase the risk of gastrointestinal ulceration.
Pyrazolone Derivatives (phenylbutazone, oxyphenbutazone, and possibly dipyrone): Concomitant administration with aspirin may increase the risk of gastrointestinal ulceration.
Nonsteroidal Antiinflammatory Agents: Aspirin is contraindicated in patients who are hypersensitive to nonsteroidal antiinflammatory agents.
Urinary Alkalinizers: Decrease aspirin effectiveness by increasing the rate of salicylate renal excretion.

Phenobarbital: Decreases aspirin effectiveness by enzyme induction.
Propranolol: May decrease aspirin's antiinflammatory action by competing for the same receptors.
Antacids: Easprin should not be given concurrently with antacids, since an increase in the pH of the stomach may affect the enteric coating of the tablets.
Usage in Pregnancy: Aspirin does not appear to have any teratogenic effects. However, it has been reported that adverse effects were increased in the mother and fetus following chronic ingestion of aspirin. Prolonged pregnancy and labor with increased bleeding before and after delivery, as well as decreased birth weight and increased rate of stillbirth were correlated with high blood salicylate levels. Because of possible adverse effects on the neonate and the potential for increased maternal blood loss, aspirin should be avoided during the last three months of pregnancy.

ADVERSE REACTIONS

Gastrointestinal: Dyspepsia, nausea, vomiting, diarrhea, gastrointestinal bleeding, and/or ulceration.
Ear: Tinnitus, vertigo, reversible hearing loss.
Hematologic: Prolongation of bleeding time, leukopenia, thrombocytopenia, purpura, decreased plasma iron concentration and shortened erythrocyte survival time.
Dermatologic and Hypersensitivity: Urticaria, angioedema, pruritus, various skin eruptions, asthma, and anaphylaxis.
Miscellaneous: Acute reversible hepatotoxicity, mental confusion, drowsiness, sweating, dizziness, headache, fever, thirst, and dimness of vision.

OVERDOSAGE

Overdosage of 200 to 500 mg/kg is in the fatal range. Early symptoms are CNS stimulation with vomiting, hyperpnea, hyperactivity, and possibly convulsions. This progresses quickly to depression, coma, respiratory failure, and collapse. These symptoms are accompanied by severe electrolyte disturbances.
In the treatment of salicylate overdosage, intensive supportive therapy should be instituted immediately. Plasma salicylate levels should be measured in order to determine the severity of the poisoning and to provide a guide for therapy. Emptying of the stomach should be accomplished as soon as possible with ipecac syrup unless the patient is depressed. In depressed patients use airway protected gastric lavage. Delay absorption with activated charcoal and give a saline cathartic. Proceed according to Standard Reference Procedures for Salicylate Intoxication.

DOSAGE AND ADMINISTRATION

Usual Adult Dosage: One tablet 3 to 4 times daily.
Patients who have displayed no significant adverse effects on a long term qid regimen and who receive a total daily dosage of aspirin no greater than 3.9 grams may be considered for a bid regimen (2 tablets of Easprin twice daily). Patients on the bid Easprin regimen should be closely monitored for serum salicylate levels, increased incidence of CNS-related adverse effects, increased fecal blood loss, or any other signs or symptoms suggestive of significant blood loss.
If necessary, dosage may be increased until relief is obtained, but dosage should be maintained slightly below that which produces tinnitus. Plasma salicylate levels may also be helpful in determining proper dosage (see Clinical Pharmacology section).

HOW SUPPLIED

Easprin enteric coated tablets each containing 15 grains (975 mg) aspirin are available:
N 0071-0490-24—Bottles of 100
Storage: Store at controlled room temperature 15° to 30°C (59° to 86°F).
AHFS Category 28:08   **0490G015**
Shown in Product Identification Section, page 421

ELASE®   ℞
[ē´lāse″]
(fibrinolysin and desoxyribonuclease, combined [bovine])
ELASE OINTMENT   ℞
(fibrinolysin and desoxyribonuclease, combined [bovine], ointment)
ELASE–CHLOROMYCETIN®   ℞
OINTMENT
(fibrinolysin and desoxyribonuclease, combined [bovine], with chloramphenicol ointment)

DESCRIPTION

Elase is a combination of two lytic enzymes, fibrinolysin and desoxyribonuclease, supplied as a lyophilized powder and in an ointment base of liquid petrolatum and polyethylene. The fibrinolysin component is derived from bovine plasma and the desoxyribonuclease is isolated in a purified form from bovine pancreas. The fibrinolysin used in the combination is activated by chloroform.

Elase-Chloromycetin Ointment: Elase-Chloromycetin Ointment contains two lytic enzymes, fibrinolysin and desoxyribonuclease, combined with chloramphenicol in an ointment base.

Chloramphenicol is a broad-spectrum antibiotic originally isolated from *Streptomyces venezuelae.* It is therapeutically active against a wide variety of susceptible organisms, both gram-positive and gram-negative. Chemically, chloramphenicol may be identified as D(-)- *threo*-1-*p*- nitrophenyl -2 - dichloroacetamido- 1, 3-propanediol.

ACTION

Combination of these two enzymes is based on the observation that purulent exudates consist largely of fibrinous material and nucleoprotein. Desoxyribonuclease attacks the desoxyribonucleic acid (DNA) and fibrinolysin attacks principally fibrin of blood clots and fibrinous exudates.

The activity of desoxyribonuclease is limited principally to the production of large polynucleotides, which are less likely to be absorbed than the more diffusible protein fractions liberated by certain enzyme preparations obtained from bacteria. The fibrinolytic action of Elase and of the enzymes in Elase Ointment and Elase-Chloromycetin Ointment is directed mainly against denatured proteins, such as those found in devitalized tissue, while protein elements of living cells remain relatively unaffected.

Elase, Elase Ointment, and Elase-Chloromycetin Ointment are combinations of active enzymes. This is an important consideration in treating patients suffering from lesions resulting from impaired circulation.

The enzymatic action of Elase helps to produce clean surfaces and thus supports healing in a variety of exudative lesions.

Elase-Chloromycetin Ointment:

Chloramphenicol is a broad-spectrum antibiotic that is primarily bacteriostatic and acts by inhibition of protein synthesis by interfering with the transfer of activated amino acids from soluble RNA to ribosomes. Development of resistance to chloramphenicol can be regarded as minimal for staphylococci and many other species of bacteria.

The action of Elase-Chloromycetin helps to produce clean surfaces and thus supports healing in a variety of exudative lesions.

INDICATIONS

Elase and Elase Ointment are indicated for topical use as debriding agents in a variety of inflammatory and infected lesions. These include: (1) general surgical wounds; (2) ulcerative lesions—trophic, decubitus, stasis, arteriosclerotic; (3) second- and third-degree burns; (4) circumcision and episiotomy. Elase and Elase Ointment are used intravaginally in: (1) cervicitis—benign, postpartum, and postconization, and (2) vaginitis. Elase is used as an irrigating agent in the following conditions: (1) infected wounds—abscesses, fistulae, and sinus tracts; (2) otorhinolaryngologic wounds; (3) superficial hematomas (except when the hematoma is adjacent to or within adipose tissue).

Elase-Chloromycetin Ointment:

Elase-Chloromycetin Ointment is indicated for use in the treatment of infected lesions, such as burns, ulcers, and wounds where the actions of both a debriding agent and a topical antibiotic are desired. This dual-purpose approach is especially useful in the treatment of infections caused by organisms that utilize a process of fibrin deposition as protective device (ie, coagulase and the staphylococcus). Appropriate measures should be taken to determine the susceptibility of the pathogen to chloramphenicol.

CONTRAINDICATIONS

These products (Elase, Elase Ointment, Elase-Chloromycetin Ointment) are contraindicated in individuals with a history of hypersensitivity reactions to any of their components. Elase is not recommended for parenteral use because the bovine fibrinolysin may be antigenic.

WARNINGS

Elase-Chloromycetin Ointment:

Bone marrow hypoplasia, including aplastic anemia and death, has been reported following the local application of chloramphenicol.

PRECAUTIONS

Elase-Chloromycetin Ointment: The prolonged use of antibiotics may occasionally result in overgrowth of nonsusceptible organisms, including fungi. If new infections appear during medication, the drug should be discontinued and appropriate measures should be taken.

In all except very superficial infections, the topical use of chloramphenicol should be supplemented by appropriate systemic medication.

Elase, Elase Ointment, Elase-Chloromycetin Ointment: The usual precautions against allergic reactions should be observed, particularly in persons with a history of sensitivity to materials of bovine origin or to mercury compounds.

Elase: To be maximally effective, Elase solutions must be freshly prepared before use. The loss in activity is reduced by refrigeration; however, even when stored in a refrigerator,

the solution should not be used 24 hours or more after reconstitution.

ADVERSE REACTIONS

Side effects attributable to the enzymes have not been a problem at the dose and for the indications recommended herein. With higher concentrations, side effects have been minimal, consisting of local hyperemia.

Chills and fever attributable to antigenic action of profibrinolysin activators of bacterial origin are not a problem with Elase, Elase Ointment, or Elase-Chloromycetin Ointment.

Elase-Chloromycetin Ointment: Signs of local irritation, with subjective symptoms of itching or burning, angioneurotic edema, urticaria, vesicular and maculopapular dermatitis have been reported in patients sensitive to chloramphenicol and are causes for discontinuing the medication. Similar sensitivity reactions to other materials in topical preparations may also occur. Blood dyscrasias have been associated with the use of chloramphenicol.

Preparation of Elase Solution: The contents of each vial may be reconstituted with 10 ml of isotonic sodium chloride solution. Higher or lower concentrations can be prepared if desired by varying the amount of the diluent.

DOSAGE AND ADMINISTRATION

Since the conditions for which Elase and Elase Ointment and Elase-Chloromycetin Ointment are helpful vary considerably in severity, dosage must be adjusted to the individual case; however, the following general recommendations can be made.

Successful use of enzymatic debridement depends on several factors: (1) dense, dry eschar, if present, should be removed surgically before enzymatic debridement is attempted; (2) the enzyme must be in constant contact with the substrate; (3) accumulated necrotic debris must be periodically removed; (4) the enzyme must be replenished at least once daily; and (5) secondary closure or skin grafting must be employed as soon as possible after optimal debridement has been attained. It is further essential that wound-dressing techniques be performed carefully under aseptic conditions and that appropriate systemically acting antibiotics be administered concomitantly if, in the opinion of the physician, they are indicated.

General Topical Uses: Elase Ointment: Local application should be repeated at intervals for as long as enzyme action is desired. After application Elase Ointment becomes rapidly and progressively less active and is probably exhausted for practical purposes at the end of 24 hours. A recommended procedure for application of Elase Ointment follows.

1. Clean the wound with water, peroxide, or normal saline and dry area gently. If there is a dense, dry eschar present, it should be removed surgically before applying Elase.
2. Apply a *thin* layer of Elase Ointment.
3. Cover with petrolatum gauze or another type of nonadhering dressing.
4. Change the dressing at least ONCE a day, preferably two or three times daily. Frequency of application is more important than the amount of Elase used. Flush away the necrotic debris and fibrinous exudates with saline, peroxide, or warm water so that newly applied ointment can be in direct contact with the substrate.

Elase: Local application should be repeated at intervals for as long as enzyme action is desired. Elase solution may be applied topically as a liquid, spray, or wet dressing. Application of a gentle spray of the solution can be accomplished by using a conventional atomizer. After application, Elase, especially in solution, becomes rapidly and progressively less active and is probably exhausted for practical purposes at the end of 24 hours. The dry material for solution is stable at room temperature through the expiration date printed on the package. A recommended procedure for application of a solution of Elase using a Wet-to-Dry method follows.

1. Mix one vial of Elase powder with 10 to 50 ml of saline and saturate strips of fine-mesh gauze or an unfolded sterile gauze sponge with the Elase solution.
2. Pack ulcerated area with the Elase-saturated gauze, making sure the gauze remains in contact with the necrotic substrate (if the lesion is covered with a heavy eschar, it must be removed surgically before wet-to-dry debridement is begun).
3. ALLOW GAUZE TO DRY IN CONTACT WITH THE ULCERATED LESION (approximately six to eight hours). As the gauze dries, the necrotic tissues slough and become enmeshed in the gauze.
4. Remove dried gauze. This mechanically debrides the area. Repeat wet-to-dry procedure three or four times daily, since frequent dressing changes greatly enhance results. After two, three, or four days, the area becomes clean and starts to fill in with granulation tissue.

Intravaginal use: Elase Ointment: In mild to moderate vaginitis and cervicitis, 5 ml of Elase Ointment should be deposited deep in the vagina once nightly at bedtime for approximately five applications, or until the entire contents of one 30-g tube has been used. The patient should be checked by her physician to determine possible need for further therapy. In more severe cervicitis and vaginitis, some physicians

prefer to initiate therapy with an application of Elase (fibrinolysin and desoxyribonuclease, combined, [bovine]) in solution. See Elase package insert.

Elase: In severe cervicitis and vaginitis, the physician may instill 10 ml of the solution intravaginally, wait one or two minutes for the enzyme to disperse and then insert a cotton tampon in the vaginal canal. The tampon should be removed the next day. Continuing therapy should then be instituted with Elase Ointment (fibrinolysin and desoxyribonuclease, combined [bovine] ointment). See Elase Ointment package insert.

Abscesses, empyema cavities, fistulae, sinus tracts or subcutaneous hematomas: Despite the contraindication against parenteral use, Elase has been used in irrigating these specific conditions. The Elase solution should be drained and replaced at intervals of six to ten hours to reduce the amount of by-product accumulation and minimize loss of enzyme activity. Traces of blood in the discharge usually indicate active filling in of the cavity.

HOW SUPPLIED

ELASE (fibrinolysin and desoxyribonuclease, combined [bovine])

N 0071-4256-01 Elase—lyophilized powder for solution Elase is supplied in rubber diaphragm-capped vials of 30-ml capacity containing 25 units (Loomis) of fibrinolysin and 15,000 units (modified Christensen method) of desoxyribonuclease.

This product also contains sodium chloride and sucrose as incidental ingredients.

Shown in Product Identification Section, page 421

4256G042

ELASE OINTMENT (fibrinolysin and desoxyribonuclease, combined [bovine], ointment)

N 0071-4279-10 Elase Ointment, 10 g.

The 10-g tube contains 10 units of fibrinolysin and 6,666 units of desoxyribonuclease with 0.04 mg thimerosal (mercury derivative) in a special ointment base of liquid petrolatum and polyethylene.

N 0071-4279-13 Elase Ointment, 30 g.

The 30-g tube contains 30 units of fibrinolysin and 20,000 units of desoxyribonuclease with 0.12 mg thimerosal (mercury derivative) in a special ointment base of liquid petrolatum and polyethylene.

These products also contain sodium chloride and sucrose as incidental ingredients.

Shown in Product Identification Section, page 421

4279G021

ELASE-CHLOROMYCETIN OINTMENT (fibrinolysin and desoxyribonuclease, combined [bovine], with chloramphenicol ointment)

Elase-Chloromycetin (fibrinolysin-desoxyribo-nuclease-chloramphenicol) is supplied in 30-g and 10-g ointment tubes. The 10-g tubes have an elongated nozzle to facilitate the application to surface lesions.

N 0071-4281-13 Elase-Chloromycetin Ointment, 30-gram

The 30-g tubes contain 30 units (Loomis) of fibrinolysin (bovine) and 20,000 units** of desoxyribonuclease and 0.3 g† chloramphenicol in a special ointment base of liquid petrolatum and polyethylene.

N 0071-4281-10 Elase-Chloromycetin Ointment, 10-gram

The 10-g tubes contain 10 units (Loomis) of fibrinolysin (bovine) and 6,666 units** of desoxyribonuclease and 0.1 g† chloramphenicol in a special ointment base of liquid petrolatum and polyethylene.

The ointment contains sodium chloride and sucrose used in its manufacture.

*Trademark

**Modified Christensen method.

†10 mg chloramphenicol per gram, or 1%.

Shown in Product Identification Section, page 421

4281G021

ERGOSTAT® ℞
(Ergotamine Tartrate Tablets) SUBLINGUAL

DESCRIPTION

Each sublingual tablet contains 2 mg ergotamine tartrate. Also contains hydroxypropyl cellulose, NF; FD&C yellow No. 6 Al lake; lactose, NF; magnesium stearate, NF; mannitol, USP; artificial peppermint flavor; pregelatinized starch, NF; saccharin, NF; saccharin sodium, USP; and corn starch, NF. **Pharmacological Category:** Vasoconstrictor, uterine stimulant, alpha adrenoreceptor antagonist.

Continued on next page

This product information was prepared in August, 1989. On these and other Parke-Davis Products, information may be obtained by addressing PARKE-DAVIS, Division of Warner-Lambert Company, Morris Plains, New Jersey 07950.

Parke-Davis—Cont.

Therapeutic Class: Antimigraine.
Chemical Name: Ergotaman-3′,6′,18-trione,12′-hydroxy-2′-methyl-5′-(phenylmethyl)-,(5′α)-,[R-(R*, R*)]-2,3-dihydroxybutanedioate (2:1) salt.

CLINICAL PHARMACOLOGY

The pharmacological properties of ergotamine are extremely complex; some of its actions are unrelated to each other, and even mutually antagonistic. The drug has partial agonist and/or antagonist activity against tryptaminergic, dopaminergic and alpha adrenergic receptors depending upon their site, and it is a highly active uterine stimulant. It causes constriction of peripheral and cranial blood vessels and produces depression of central vasomotor centers. The pain of a migraine attack is believed to be due to greatly increased amplitude of pulsations in the cranial arteries, especially the meningeal branches of the external carotid artery. Ergotamine reduces extracranial blood flow, causes a decline in the amplitude of pulsation in the cranial arteries, and decreases hyperperfusion of the territory of the basilar artery. It does not reduce cerebral hemispheric blood flow. Long-term usage has established the fact that ergotamine tartrate is effective in controlling up to 70% of acute migraine attacks, so that it is now considered specific for the treatment of this headache syndrome. Ergotamine produces constriction of both arteries and veins. In doses used in the treatment of vascular headaches, ergotamine usually produces only small increases in blood pressure, but it does increase peripheral resistance and decrease blood flow in various organs. Small doses of the drug increase the force and frequency of uterine contraction; larger doses increase the resting tone of the uterus also. The gravid uterus is particularly sensitive to these effects of ergotamine. Although specific teratogenic effects attributable to ergotamine have not been found, the fetus suffers if ergotamine is given to the mother. Retarded fetal growth and an increase in intrauterine death and resorption have been seen in animals. These are thought to result from ergotamine-induced increases in uterine motility and vasoconstriction in the placental vascular bed.

The bioavailability of sublingually administered ergotamine has not been determined.

Ergotamine is metabolized in the liver by largely undefined pathways, and 90% of the metabolites are excreted in the bile. The unmetabolized drug is erratically secreted in the saliva, and only traces of unmetabolized drug appear in the urine and feces. Ergotamine is secreted into breast milk. The elimination half-life of ergotamine from plasma is about 2 hours, but the drug may be stored in some tissues, which would account for its long-lasting therapeutic and toxic actions.

INDICATIONS AND USAGE

Ergotamine tartrate is indicated as therapy to abort or prevent vascular headache, e.g., migraine, migraine variants, or so called "histaminic cephalalgia".

CONTRAINDICATIONS

Ergotamine is contraindicated in peripheral vascular disease (thromboangiitis obliterans, luetic arteritis, severe arteriosclerosis, thrombophlebitis, Raynaud's disease), coronary heart disease, hypertension, impaired hepatic or renal function, severe pruritus, and sepsis. It is also contraindicated in patients who are hypersensitive to any of its components. Ergotamine may cause fetal harm when administered to a pregnant woman by virtue of its powerful uterine stimulant actions. It is contraindicated in women who are, or may become, pregnant.

PRECAUTIONS

General: Although signs and symptoms of ergotism rarely develop even after long-term intermittent use of ergotamine, care should be exercised to remain within the limits of recommended dosage.

Drug Interactions: The effects of ergotamine tartrate may be potentiated by triacetyloleandomycin which inhibits the metabolism of ergotamine. The pressor effects of ergotamine and other vasoconstrictor drugs can combine to cause dangerous hypertension.

Carcinogenesis: No studies have been performed to investigate ergotamine tartrate for carcinogenic effects.

Pregnancy: Pregnancy Category X—See CONTRAINDICATIONS.

Nursing Mothers: Ergotamine is secreted into human milk. It can reach the breast-fed infant by this route and exert pharmacologic effects in it. Caution should be exercised when ergotamine is administered to a nursing woman. Excessive dosing or prolonged administration of ergotamine may inhibit lactation.

ADVERSE REACTIONS

Nausea and vomiting occur in up to 10% of patients after ingestion of therapeutic doses of ergotamine. Weakness of the legs and pain in limb muscles are also frequent complaints. Numbness and tingling of the fingers and toes, precordial pain, transient changes in heart rate and localized edema and itching may also occur, particularly in patients who are sensitive to the drug.

DRUG ABUSE AND DEPENDENCE

Patients who take ergotamine for extended periods of time may become dependent upon it and require progressively increasing doses for relief of vascular headaches, and for prevention of dysphoric effects which follow withdrawal of the drug.

OVERDOSAGE

Overdosage with ergotamine causes nausea, vomiting, weakness of the legs, pain in limb muscles, numbness and tingling of the fingers and toes, precordial pain, tachycardia or bradycardia, hypertension or hypotension and localized edema and itching together with signs and symptoms of ischemia due to vasoconstriction of peripheral arteries and arterioles. The feet and hands become cold, pale and numb. Muscle pain occurs while walking and later at rest also. Gangrene may ensue. Confusion, depression, drowsiness, and convulsions are occasional signs of ergotamine toxicity. Overdosage is particularly likely to occur in patients with sepsis or impaired renal or hepatic function. Patients with peripheral vascular disease are especially at risk of developing peripheral ischemia following treatment with ergotamine. Some cases of ergotamine poisoning have been reported in patients who have taken less than 5 mg of the drug. Usually, however, toxicity is seen at doses of ergotamine tartrate in excess of about 15 mg in 24 hours or 40 mg in a few days.

Treatment of ergotamine overdosage consists of the withdrawal of the drug followed by symptomatic measures including attempts to maintain an adequate circulation in the affected parts. Anticoagulant drugs, low molecular weight dextran and potent vasodilator drugs may all be beneficial. Intravenous infusion of sodium nitroprusside has also been reported to be successful. Vasodilators must be used with special care in the presence of hypotension.

Nausea and vomiting may be relieved by atropine or antiemetic compounds of the phenothiazine group. Ergotamine is dialyzable.

DOSAGE AND ADMINISTRATION

All efforts should be made to initiate therapy as soon as possible after the first symptoms of the attack are noted, because success is proportional to rapidity of treatment, and lower dosages will be effective. At the first sign of an attack or to relieve the symptoms of the full-blown attack, one sublingual tablet (2 mg) is placed under the tongue. Another sublingual tablet (2 mg) should be placed under the tongue at half-hourly intervals thereafter, if necessary, for a total of three tablets (6 mg). Dosage must not exceed three tablets (6 mg) in any 24-hour period. Limit dosage to not more than five tablets (10 mg) in any one week.

HOW SUPPLIED

Ergostat (Ergotamine Tartrate Tablets) sublingual, 2 mg (round, orange, coded P-D 111), is supplied as follows:
N 0071-0111-13 Packages of 24 unit-dose tablets.
Store at controlled room temperature 15°–30°C (59°–86°F).
AHFS Category 12:16   0111G016
Shown in Product Identification Section, page 421

ERYC®   ℞
[ĕ′ryc]
(Erythromycin Delayed-Release Capsules, USP)

DESCRIPTION

ERYC Capsules contain enteric-coated pellets of erythromycin base for oral administration. Erythromycin is produced by a strain of *Streptomyces erythraeus* and belongs to the macrolide group of antibiotics. It is basic and readily forms salts with acids, but it is the base which is microbiologically active. Each ERYC Capsule contains 250 milligrams of erythromycin base. Also contains: lactose NF; povidone USP; FD&C Yellow #6. The capsule shell contains gelatin NF; titanium dioxide USP; FD&C Yellow #6. Erythromycin base is $(3R*, 4S*, 5S*, 6R*, 7R*, 9R*, 11R*, 12R*, 13S*, 14R*)$-4-[(2,6-Dideoxy-3-C-methyl-3-O-methyl-α-L-ribo-hexopyranosyl)-oxy]-14-ethyl-7, 12, 13-trihydroxy-3, 5, 7, 9, 11, 13-hexamethyl-6-[[3, 4, 6-trideoxy-3-(dimethylamino)-β-D-xylo-hexopyranosyl]oxy]oxacyclotetradecane-2, 10-dione.

CLINICAL PHARMACOLOGY

Orally administered erythromycin base and its salts are readily absorbed in the microbiologically active form. Interindividual variations in the absorption of erythromycin are, however, observed, and some patients do not achieve acceptable serum levels. Erythromycin is largely bound to plasma proteins, and the freely dissociating bound fraction after administration of erythromycin base represents 90% of the total erythromycin present. After absorption erythromycin diffuses readily into most body fluids. In the absence of meningeal inflammation, low concentrations are normally achieved in the spinal fluid but the passage of the drug across the blood-brain barrier increases in meningitis. Erythromycin is excreted in breast milk. The drug crosses the placental barrier but fetal plasma levels are low.

In the presence of normal hepatic function erythromycin is concentrated in the liver and is excreted in the bile; the effect of hepatic dysfunction on biliary excretion of erythromycin is not known. After oral administration less than 5% of the administered dose can be recovered in the active form in the urine.

The enteric coating of pellets in ERYC Capsules protects the erythromycin base from inactivation by gastric acidity. Because of their small size and enteric coating, the pellets readily pass intact from the stomach to the small intestine and dissolve efficiently to allow absorption of erythromycin in a uniform manner. After administration of a single dose of a 250 mg ERYC capsule, peak serum levels in the range of 1.13 to 1.68 mcg/ml are attained in approximately 3 hours and decline to 0.30-0.42 mcg/ml in 6 hours. Optimal conditions for stability in the presence of gastric secretion and for complete absorption are attained when ERYC is taken on an empty stomach.

Microbiology Erythromycin acts by inhibition of protein synthesis by binding 50 S ribosomal subunits of susceptible organisms. It does not affect nucleic acid synthesis. Antagonism has been demonstrated between clindamycin and erythromycin. Resistance to erythromycin by some strains of *Haemophilus influenzae* and staphylococci has been demonstrated. Specimens should be obtained for culture and susceptibility testing.

Erythromycin is usually active against the following organisms in *vitro* and in clinical infections:
Streptococcus pyogenes
Alpha hemolytic streptococci (viridans group)
Staphylococcus aureus (Resistant organisms may emerge during treatment.)
Streptococcus pneumoniae
Mycoplasma pneumoniae (Eaton's Agent)
Haemophilus influenzae (Many strains are resistant to erythromycin alone, but are susceptible to erythromycin and sulfonamides together.)
Treponema pallidum
Corynebacterium diphtheriae
Corynebacterium minutissimum
Entamoeba histolytica
Listeria monocytogenes
Neisseria gonorrhoeae
Bordetella pertussis
Legionella pneumophila (agent of Legionnaires' Disease)

Susceptibility Testing Quantitative methods that require measurement of zone diameters give the most precise estimates of antibiotic susceptibility. One such standardized single disc procedure has been recommended for use with discs to test susceptibility to erythromycin.[1] Interpretation involves correlation of the zone diameters obtained in the disc test with minimum inhibitory concentration (MIC) values for erythromycin.

Reports from the laboratory giving results of the standardized single-disc susceptibility test using a 15 mcg erythromycin disc should be interpreted according to the following criteria:

Susceptible organisms produce zones of 18 mm or greater indicating that the tested organism is likely to respond to therapy.

Resistant organisms produce zones of 13 mm or less, indicating that other therapy should be selected.

Organisms of intermediate susceptibility produce zones of 14 to 17 mm. The "intermediate" category provides a "buffer zone" which should prevent small uncontrolled technical factors from causing major discrepancies in interpretations, thus when a zone diameter falls within the "intermediate" range, the results may be considered equivocal. If alternate drugs are not available, confirmation by dilution tests may be indicated.

A bacterial isolate may be considered susceptible if the MIC value[2] (minimal inhibitory concentration) for erythromycin is not more than 2 mcg/ml. Organisms are considered resistant if the MIC is 8 mcg/ml or higher.

INDICATIONS AND USAGE

ERYC is indicated in children and adults for the treatment of the following conditions:

Upper respiratory tract infections of mild to moderate degree caused by *Streptococcus pyogenes* (group A beta hemolytic streptococci); *Streptococcus pneumoniae (Diplococcus pneumoniae): Haemophilus influenzae* (when used concomitantly with adequate doses of sulfonamides, since not all strains of *H influenzae* are susceptible at the erythromycin concentrations ordinarily achieved). (See appropriate sulfonamide labeling for prescribing information.)

Lower respiratory tract infections of mild to moderate severity caused by *Streptococcus pyogenes* (group A beta hemolytic streptococci): *Streptococcus pneumoniae (Diplococcus pneumoniae).*

Respiratory tract infections due to *Mycoplasma pneumoniae (Eaton's agent).*

Pertussis (whooping cough) caused by *Bordetella pertussis.* Erythromycin is effective in eliminating the organism from the nasopharynx of infected individuals, rendering them noninfectious. Some clinical studies suggest that erythromycin may be helpful in the prophylaxis of pertussis in exposed susceptible individuals.

Diphtheria—As an adjunct to antitoxin in infections due to *Corynebacterium diphtheriae*, to prevent establishment of carriers and to eradicate the organism in carriers.

Erythrasma—In the treatment of infections due to *Coryne-bacterium minutissimum*.

Intestinal amebiasis caused by *Entamoeba histolytica* (oral erythromycins only). Extraenteric amebiasis requires treatment with other agents.

Infections due to *Listeria monocytogenes*.

Skin and soft tissue infections of mild to moderate severity caused by *Streptococcus pyogenes* and *Staphylococcus aureus* (Resistant staphylococci may emerge during treatment.)

Primary syphilis caused by *Treponema pallidum*. Erythromycin (oral forms only) is an alternate choice of treatment for primary syphilis in patients allergic to the penicillins. In treatment of primary syphilis, spinal fluid should be examined before treatment and as part of the follow-up after therapy. The use of erythromycin for the treatment of *in utero* syphilis is not recommended (See CLINICAL PHARMACOLOGY).

Erythromycins are indicated for treatment of the following infections caused by *Chlamydia trachomatis*: conjunctivitis of the newborn, pneumonia of infancy, urogenital infections during pregnancy. When tetracyclines are contraindicated or not tolerated, erythromycin is indicated for the treatment of uncomplicated urethral, endocervical, or rectal infections in adults due to *Chlamydia trachomatis* [4].

Legionnaires' disease caused by *Legionella pneumophila*. Although no controlled clinical efficacy studies have been conducted, *in vitro* and limited preliminary clinical data suggest that erythromycin may be effective in treating Legionnaires' disease.

Therapy with erythromycin should be monitored by bacteriological studies and by clinical response (See CLINICAL PHARMACOLOGY—Microbiology).

Injectable benzathine penicillin G is considered by the American Heart Association to be the drug of choice in the treatment and prevention of streptococcal pharyngitis and in long-term prophylaxis of rheumatic fever. When oral medication is preferred for treatment of the above conditions, penicillin G, V, or erythromycin are alternate drugs of choice.

Although no controlled clinical efficacy trials have been conducted, erythromycin has been suggested by the American Heart Association and the American Dental Association for use in a regimen for prophylaxis against bacterial endocarditis in patients allergic to penicillin who have congenital and/or rheumatic or other acquired valvular heart disease when they undergo dental procedures and surgical procedures of the upper respiratory tract.[3] (Erythromycin is not suitable prior to genitourinary surgery where the organisms likely to lead to bacteremia are gram-negative bacilli or the enterococcal group of streptococci).

NOTE: When selecting antibiotics for the prevention of bacterial endocarditis the physician or dentist should read the full joint 1984 statement of the American Heart Association and the American Dental Association.[3]

CONTRAINDICATION

ERYC is contraindicated in patients with known hypersensitivity to this antibiotic.

WARNING

There have been a few reports of hepatic dysfunction, with or without jaundice, occurring in patients receiving erythromycin ethylsuccinate, base, and stearate products.

PRECAUTIONS

General: Erythromycin is principally excreted by the liver. Caution should be exercised when erythromycin is administered to patients with impaired hepatic function. (See CLINICAL PHARMACOLOGY and WARNING sections).

Prolonged or repeated use of erythromycin may result in an overgrowth of nonsusceptible bacteria or fungi. If superinfection occurs, erythromycin should be discontinued and appropriate therapy instituted.

When indicated, incision and drainage or other surgical procedures should be performed in conjunction with antibiotic therapy.

Laboratory Tests: Erythromycin interfers with the fluorometric determination of urinary catecholamines.

Drug Interactions: Recent data from studies of erythromycin reveal that its use in patients who are receiving high doses of theophylline may be associated with an increase of serum theophylline levels and potential theophylline toxicity. In cases of theophylline toxicity and/or elevated serum theophylline levels, the dose of theophylline should be reduced while the patient is receiving concomitant erythromycin therapy.

Erythromycin administration in children receiving carbamazepine has been reported to cause increased blood levels of carbamazepine with subsequent development of signs of carbamazepine toxicity (ataxia, dizziness, vomiting).

Erythromycin has been reported to decrease the clearance of triazolam and thus may increase pharmacologic effect of triazolam. Erythromycin has been reported to decrease the clearance of cyclosporine causing elevated cyclosporine levels and associated increased serum creatinine. Renal function as well as serum concentration of cyclosporine should be closely monitored when both drugs are administered concomitantly. An interaction between erythromycin and ergotamine has been reported to increase the vasospasm associated with ergotamine.

Concomitant administration of erythromycin and digoxin has been reported to result in elevated digoxin serum levels. There have been reports of increased anticoagulant effects when erythromycin and oral anticoagulants were used concomitantly.

Carcinogenesis, Mutagenesis and Impairment of Fertility: Long-term (2-year) oral studies conducted in rats with erythromycin base did not provide evidence of tumorigenicity. Mutagenicity studies have not been conducted. There was no apparent effect on male or female fertility in rats fed erythromycin (base) at levels up to 0.25 percent of diet.

Pregnancy: Pregnancy Category B: There is no evidence of teratogenicity or any other adverse effect on reproduction in female rats fed erythromycin base (up to 0.25 percent of diet) prior to and during mating, during gestation, and through weaning of two successive litters. There are, however, no adequate and well-controlled studies in pregnant women. Because animal reproduction studies are not always predictive of human response, this drug should be used during pregnancy only if clearly needed. Erythromycin has been reported to cross the placental barrier in humans, but fetal plasma levels are generally low.

Labor and Delivery: The effect of erythromycin on labor and delivery is unknown.

Nursing Mothers: Erythromycin is excreted in breast milk, therefore, caution should be exercised when erythromycin is administered to a nursing woman.

Pediatric Use: See INDICATIONS AND USAGE and DOSAGE AND ADMINISTRATION sections.

ADVERSE REACTIONS

The most frequent side effects of oral erythromycin preparations are gastrointestinal and are dose-related. They include nausea, vomiting, abdominal pain, diarrhea and anorexia. Symptoms of hepatic dysfunction and/or abnormal liver function test results may occur (see WARNING).

Mild allergic reactions such as rashes with or without pruritus, urticaria, bullous fixed eruptions, and eczema have been reported with erythromycin. Serious allergic reactions, including anaphylaxis have been reported.

A few cases of transient deafness have been reported with high doses of erythromycin.

DOSAGE AND ADMINISTRATION

Administration of a dose of ERYC in the presence of food lowers the blood levels of systemically available erythromycin. Although the blood levels obtained upon administration of enteric-coated erythromycin products in the presence of food are still above minimum inhibitory concentrations (MICs) of most organisms for which erythromycin is indicated, optimum blood levels are obtained on a fasting stomach (administration of at least ½ hour and preferably two hours before or after a meal).

ADULTS: The usual dose is 250 mg every 6 hours taken one hour before meals. If twice-a-day dosage is desired, the recommended dose is 500 mg every 12 hours. Dosage may be increased up to 4 grams per day, according to the severity of infection. Twice-a-day dosing is not recommended when doses larger than 1 gram daily are administered.

CHILDREN: Age, weight, and severity of the infection are important factors in determining the proper dosage. The usual dosage is 30 to 50 mg/kg/day in divided doses. For the treatment of more severe infections, this dose may be doubled.

Streptococcal infections: A therapeutic dosage of oral erythromycin should be administered for at least 10 days. For continuous prophylaxis against recurrences of streptococcal infections in persons with a history of rheumatic heart disease, the dose is 250 mg twice a day.

For the prevention of bacterial endocarditis in penicillin-allergic patients with valvular heart disease who are to undergo dental procedures or surgical procedures of the upper respiratory tract, the adult dose is 1 gram orally (20 mg/kg for children) one hour prior to the procedure and then 500 mg (10 mg/kg for children) orally 6 hours later.[3] (See Indications and Usage).

Primary syphilis: 30-40 grams given in divided doses over a period of 10-15 days.

Intestinal amebiasis: 250 mg four times daily for 10 to 14 days for adults; 30 to 50 mg/kg/day in divided doses for 10 to 14 days for children.

Legionnaires' Disease: Although optimal doses have not been established, doses utilized in reported clinical data were those recommended above (1 to 4 grams daily in divided doses).

Urogenital infections during pregnancy due to *Chlamydia trachomatis*: Although the optimal dose and duration of therapy have not been established, the suggested treatment is erythromycin 500 mg, by mouth, 4 times a day on an empty stomach for at least 7 days. For women who cannot tolerate this regimen, a decreased dose of 250 mg, by mouth, 4 times a day should be used for at least 14 days[4].

For adults with uncomplicated urethral, endocervical, or rectal infections caused by *Chlamydia trachomatis* in whom tetracyclines are contraindicated or not tolerated: 500 mg. by mouth, 4 times a day for at least 7 days[4].

Pertussis: Although optimum dosage and duration of therapy have not been established, doses of erythromycin utilized in reported clinical studies were 40-50 mg/kg/day, given in divided doses for 5 to 14 days.

HOW SUPPLIED

ERYC (Capsule 696), clear and orange opaque capsules, each containing 250 mg erythromycin as enteric coated pellets, are available as follows:

N 0071-0696-16 Bottles of 40
N 0071-0696-24 Bottles of 100
N 0071-0696-30 Bottles of 500
N 0071-0696-40 Unit dose package of 100 (10 strips of 10 capsules each).

Storage Conditions: Store at a room temperature below 30°C (86°F). Protect from moisture and light.

REFERENCES

1. Approved Standard ASM-2 "Performance Standards for Anti-microbial Disc Susceptibility Test." National Committee for Clinical Laboratory Standards. 771 East Lancaster Avenue, Villanova. PA 19085.
2. Ericson, H.M. and Sherris, J.C.: "Antibiotic Sensitivity Testing Report of an International Collaborative Study." *Acta Pathologica et Microbiologica Scandinavica*. Section B. Supp. 217, 1971, pp. 1-90.
3. Am. Heart Assoc. and Am. Dental Assoc. "Prevention of Bacterial Endocarditis." *Circulation*: Vol. 70, No. 6, December, 1984, 1123A-1127A.
4. CDC Sexually Transmitted Diseases Treatment Guidelines 1982.

Shown in Product Identification Section, page 421

0696G184

ESTROVIS®   ℞

[ĕs-trō'vĭs"]
(Quinestrol tablets, USP)

WARNING

1. Estrogens Have Been Reported to Increase the Risk of Endometrial Carcinoma.

Three independent case control studies have shown an increased risk of endometrial cancer in postmenopausal women exposed to exogenous estrogens for prolonged periods.[1-3] This risk was independent of the other known risk factors for endometrial cancer. These studies are further supported by the finding that incidence rates of endometrial cancer have increased sharply since 1969 in eight different areas of the United States with population-based cancer reporting systems, an increase which may be related to the rapidly expanding use of estrogens during the last decade.[4]

The three case control studies reported that the risk of endometrial cancer in estrogen users was about 4.5 to 13.9 times greater than in nonusers. The risk appears to depend on both duration of treatment[1] and on estrogen dose.[3] In view of these findings, when estrogens are used for the treatment of menopausal symptoms, the lowest dose that will control symptoms should be utilized and medication should be discontinued as soon as possible. When prolonged treatment is medically indicated, the patient should be reassessed on at least a semiannual basis to determine the need for continued therapy. Although the evidence must be considered preliminary, one study suggests that cyclic administration of low doses of estrogen may carry less risk than continuous administration.[3] Therefore, while it appears prudent to utilize such a regimen with other orally administered estrogens, Estrovis may be administered, following a seven-day priming schedule, on a once weekly mainte-

---

Continued on next page

This product information was prepared in August, 1989. On these and other Parke-Davis Products, information may be obtained by addressing PARKE-DAVIS, Division of Warner-Lambert Company, Morris Plains, New Jersey 07950.

Parke-Davis—Cont.

nance dosage beginning two weeks after the start of treatment.

Close clinical surveillance of all women taking estrogens is important. In all cases of undiagnosed persistent or recurring abnormal vaginal bleeding, adequate diagnostic measures should be undertaken to rule out malignancy.

There is no evidence at present that "natural" estrogens are more or less hazardous than "synthetic" estrogens at equiestrogenic doses.

2. Estrogens Should not be Used During Pregnancy. The use of female sex hormones, both estrogens and progestogens, during early pregnancy may seriously damage the offspring. It has been shown that females exposed *in utero* to diethylstilbestrol, a nonsteroidal estrogen, have an increased risk of developing in later life a form of vaginal or cervical cancer that is ordinarily extremely rare.[5-6] This risk has been estimated as not greater than 4 per 1,000 exposures.[7] Furthermore, a high percentage of such exposed women (from 30 to 90%) have been found to have vaginal adenosis,[8-12] epithelial changes of the vagina and cervix. Although these changes are histologically benign, it is not known whether they are precursors of malignancy. Although similar data are not available with the use of other estrogens, it cannot be presumed they would not induce similar changes.

Several reports suggest an association between intrauterine exposure to female sex hormones and congenital anomalies, including congenital heart defects and limb- reduction defects.[13-16] One case control study[16] estimated a 4.7-fold increased risk of limb-reduction defects in infants exposed *in utero* to sex hormones (oral contraceptives, hormone withdrawal tests for pregnancy, or attempted treatment for threatened abortion). Some of these exposures were very short and involved only a few days of treatment. The data suggest that the risk of limb-reduction defects in exposed fetuses is somewhat less than 1 per 1,000.

In the past, female sex hormones have been used during pregnancy in an attempt to treat threatened or habitual abortion. There is considerable evidence that estrogens are ineffective for these indications, and there is no evidence from well-controlled studies that progestogens are effective for these uses.

If Estrovis (quinestrol) is used during pregnancy, or if the patient becomes pregnant while taking this drug, she should be apprised of the potential risks to the fetus and the advisability of pregnancy continuation.

DESCRIPTION

Estrovis is the 3-cyclopentylether of ethinyl estradiol. It is an estrogenic agent for oral administration. Each tablet contains 100 mcg quinestrol, USP. Estrovis also contains: FD&C blue No. 1 Al lake; lactose, NF; and magnesium stearate, NF. The chemical name is 3-cyclopentyloxy-17α-ethynylestra-1,3,5(10)-trien-17β-ol.

It is a white, essentially odorless powder, insoluble in water and soluble in alcohol, chloroform, and ether.

CLINICAL PHARMACOLOGY

Estrovis (quinestrol) is an orally effective estrogen as judged by conventional assay procedures employing vagina and uterine end-points in mice, rats and rabbits.

The estrogenic effects of Estrovis have been demonstrated in clinical studies by its effects on the endometrium, maturation of the vaginal epithelium, thinning of cervical mucus, suppression of pituitary gonadotropin, inhibition of ovulation, and prevention of postpartum breast discomfort.

INDICATIONS

Estrovis (quinestrol) is indicated in the treatment of:
1. Moderate to severe vasomotor symptoms associated with the menopause. (There is no evidence that estrogens are effective for nervous symptoms or depression which might occur during menopause, and they should not be used to treat these conditions.)
2. Atrophic vaginitis
3. Kraurosis vulvae
4. Female hypogonadism
5. Female castration
6. Primary ovarian failure

Estrovis (Quinestrol) Has Not Been Shown to be Effective for any Purpose during Pregnancy and Its Use May Cause Severe Harm to the Fetus (See Boxed Warning).

CONTRAINDICATIONS

Estrogens should not be used in women (or men) with any of the following conditions:
1. Known or suspected cancer of the breast except in appropriately selected patients being treated for metastatic disease

2. Known or suspected estrogen-dependent neoplasia
3. Known or suspected pregnancy (See Boxed Warning)
4. Undiagnosed abnormal genital bleeding
5. Active thrombophlebitis or thromboembolic disorders
6. A past history of thrombophlebitis, thrombosis, or thromboembolic disorders associated with previous estrogen use (except when used in treatment of breast or prostatic malignancy)

WARNINGS

1. *Induction of malignant neoplasms.* Long-term continuous administration of natural and synthetic estrogens in certain animal species increases the frequency of carcinomas of the breast, cervix, vagina, and liver. There is now evidence that estrogens increase the risk of carcinoma of the endometrium in humans. (See Boxed Warning.)

At the present time, there is no satisfactory evidence that estrogens given to postmenopausal women increase the risk of cancer of the breast,[18] although a recent long-term follow up of a single physician's practice has raised this possibility.[18a] Because of the animal data, there is a need for caution in prescribing estrogens for women with a strong family history of breast cancer or who have breast nodules, fibrocystic disease, or abnormal mammograms.

2. *Gallbladder disease.* A recent study has reported a 2- to 3-fold increase in the risk of surgically confirmed gallbladder disease in women receiving postmenopausal estrogens,[18] similar to the 2-fold increase previously noted in users of oral contraceptives.[19-24] In the case of oral contraceptives, the increased risk appeared after two years of use.[24]

3. *Effects similar to those caused by estrogen-progestogen oral contraceptives.* There are several serious adverse effects of oral contraceptives, most of which have not, up to now, been documented as consequences of postmenopausal estrogen therapy. This may reflect the comparatively low doses of estrogen used in postmenopausal women. It would be expected that the larger doses of estrogen used to treat prostatic or breast cancer or postpartum breast engorgement are more likely to result in these adverse effects, and, in fact, it has been shown that there is an increased risk of thrombosis in men receiving estrogens for prostatic cancer and women for postpartum breast engorgement.[20-23]

a. *Thromboembolic disease.* It is now well established that users of oral contraceptives have an increased risk of various thromboembolic and thrombotic vascular diseases, such as thrombophlebitis, pulmonary embolism, stroke, and myocardial infarction.[24-31] Cases of retinal thrombosis, mesenteric thrombosis, and optic neuritis have been reported in oral contraceptive users. There is evidence that the risk of several of these adverse reactions is related to the dose of the drug.[32,33] An increased risk of postsurgery thromboembolic complications has also been reported in users of oral contraceptives.[34,35] If feasible, estrogen should be discontinued at least 4 weeks before surgery of the type associated with an increased risk of thromboembolism, or during periods of prolonged immobilization.

While an increased rate of thromboembolic and thrombotic disease in postmenopausal users of estrogens has not been found,[18,36] this does not rule out the possibility that such an increase may be present or that subgroups of women who have underlying risk factors or who are receiving relatively large doses of estrogens may have increased risk. Therefore, estrogens should not be used in persons with active thrombophlebitis or thromboembolic disorders, and they should not be used (except in treatment of malignancy) in persons with a history of such disorders in association with estrogen use. They should be used with caution in patients with cerebral vascular or coronary artery disease and only for those in whom estrogens are clearly needed.

Large doses of estrogen (5 mg conjugated estrogens per day), comparable to those used to treat cancer of the prostate and breast, have been shown in a large prospective clinical trial in men[37] to increase the risk of nonfatal myocardial infarction, pulmonary embolism, and thrombophlebitis. When estrogen doses of this size are used, any of the thromboembolic and thrombotic adverse effects associated with oral contraceptive use should be considered a clear risk.

b. *Hepatic adenoma.* Benign hepatic adenomas appear to be associated with the use of oral contraceptives.[38-40] Although benign, and rare, these may rupture and may cause death through intra-abdominal hemorrhage. Such lesions have not yet been reported in association with other estrogen or progestogen preparations but should be considered in estrogen users having abdominal pain and tenderness, abdominal mass, or hypovolemic shock. Hepatocellular carcinoma has also been reported in women taking estrogen-containing oral contraceptives.[39] The relationship of this malignancy to these drugs is not known at this time.

c. *Elevated blood pressure.* Increased blood pressure is not uncommon in women using oral contraceptives. There is now a report that this may occur with use of estrogens in the menopause[11] and blood pressure should be monitored with estrogen use, especially if high doses are used.

d. *Glucose tolerance.* A worsening of glucose tolerance has been observed in a significant percentage of patients on estrogen-containing oral contraceptives. For this reason, dia-

betic patients should be carefully observed while receiving estrogen.

4. *Hypercalcemia.* Administration of estrogens may lead to severe hypercalcemia in patients with breast cancer and bone metastases. If this occurs, the drug should be stopped and appropriate measures taken to reduce the serum calcium level.

PRECAUTIONS

A. General Precautions

1. A complete medical and family history should be taken prior to the initiation of any estrogen therapy. The pretreatment and periodic physical examinations should include special reference to blood pressure, abdomen, and pelvic organs, and should include a Papanicolaou smear. As a general rule, estrogen should not be prescribed for longer than one year without another physical examination being performed.

2. Fluid retention—Because estrogens may cause some degree of fluid retention, conditions which might be influenced by this factor, such as epilepsy, migraine, and cardiac or renal dysfunction, require careful observation.

3. Certain patients may develop undesirable manifestations of excessive estrogenic stimulation, such as abnormal or excessive uterine bleeding, mastodynia, etc.

4. Oral contraceptives appear to be associated with an increased incidence of mental depression.[24] Although it is not clear whether this is due to the estrogenic or progestogenic component of the contraceptive, patients with a history of depression should be carefully observed.

5. Preexisting uterine leiomyomata may increase in size during estrogen use.

6. The pathologist should be advised of estrogen therapy when relevant specimens are submitted.

7. Patients with a past history of jaundice during pregnancy have an increased risk of recurrence of jaundice while receiving estrogen-containing oral contraceptive therapy. If jaundice develops in any patient receiving estrogen, the medication should be discontinued while the cause is investigated.

8. Estrogens may be poorly metabolized in patients with impaired liver function and they should be administered with caution in such patients.

9. Because estrogens influence the metabolism of calcium and phosphorus, they should be used with caution in patients with metabolic bone diseases that are associated with hypercalcemia or in patients with renal insufficiency.

10. Because of the effects of estrogens on epiphyseal closure, they should be used judiciously in young patients in whom bone growth is not complete.

11. Certain endocrine and liver function tests may be affected by estrogen-containing oral contraceptives. The following similar changes may be expected with larger doses of estrogen:
a. Increased sulfobromophthalein retention.
b. Increased prothrombin and factors VII, VIII, IX, and X; decreased antithrombin 3; increased norepinephrine-induced platelet aggregability.
c. Increased thyroid binding globulin (TBG) leading to increased circulating total thyroid hormone, as measured by PHI, T4 by column, or T4 by radioimmunoassay. Free T3 resin uptake is decreased, reflecting the elevated TBG; free T4 concentration is unaltered.
d. Impaired glucose tolerance.
e. Decreased pregnanediol excretion.
f. Reduced response to metyrapone test.
g. Reduced serum folate concentration.
h. Increased serum triglyceride and phospholipid concentration.

B. Concomitant Progestin Use

The lowest effective dose appropriate for the specific indication should be utilized. Studies of the addition of a progestin for seven or more days of a cycle of estrogen administration have reported a lowered incidence of endometrial hyperplasia. Morphological and biochemical studies of endometrium suggest that 10 to 13 days of progestin are needed to provide maximal maturation of the endometrium and to eliminate any hyperplastic changes. Whether this will provide protection from endometrial carcinoma has not been clearly established. There are possible additional risks which may be associated with the inclusion of progestin in estrogen replacement regimens. The potential risks include adverse effects on carbohydrate and lipid metabolism. The choice of progestin and dosage may be important in minimizing these adverse effects.

C. Information for the patient. See text of Patient Package Insert.

D. Pregnancy. See Contraindications and Boxed Warning.

E. Nursing Mothers. As a general principle, the administration of any drug to nursing mothers should be done only when clearly necessary because many drugs are excreted in human milk.

ADVERSE REACTIONS

(See Warnings regarding induction of neoplasia, adverse effects on the fetus, increased incidence of gallbladder disease, and adverse effects similar to those of oral contraceptives, including thromboembolism.) The following additional adverse reactions have been reported with estrogenic therapy, including oral contraceptives:

1. *Genitourinary system.*
Breakthrough bleeding, spotting, change in menstrual flow
Dysmenorrhea
Premenstrual-like syndrome
Amenorrhea during and after treatment
Increase in size of uterine fibromyomata
Vaginal candidiasis
Change in cervical eversion and in degree of cervical secretion
Cystitis-like syndrome
2. *Breasts.*
Tenderness, enlargement, secretion
3. *Gastrointestinal.*
Nausea, vomiting
Abdominal cramps, bloating
Cholestatic jaundice
4. *Skin.*
Chloasma or melasma which may persist when drug is discontinued
Erythema multiforme
Erythema nodosum
Hemorrhagic eruption
Loss of scalp hair
Hirsutism
5. *Eyes.*
Steepening of corneal curvature
Intolerance to contact lenses
6. *CNS.*
Headache, migraine, dizziness
Mental depression
Chorea
7. *Miscellaneous.*
Increase or decrease in weight
Reduced carbohydrate tolerance
Aggravation of porphyria
Edema
Changes in libido

ACUTE OVERDOSAGE
Numerous reports of ingestion of large doses of estrogen-containing oral contraceptives by young children indicate that serious ill effects do not occur. Overdosage of estrogen may cause nausea, and withdrawal bleeding may occur in females.

DOSAGE AND ADMINISTRATION
For treatment of moderate to severe vasomotor symptoms associated with the menopause, and for atrophic vaginitis, kraurosis vulvae, female hypogonadism, female castration, and primary ovarian failure.
One Estrovis (quinestrol) 100-mcg tablet once daily for seven days, followed by one 100-mcg tablet weekly as a maintenance schedule, commencing two weeks after inception of treatment. The dosage may be increased to 200 mcg weekly if the therapeutic response is not that which may be desirable or considered optimal.
The lowest maintenance dose that will control symptoms should be chosen and medication should be discontinued as promptly as possible.
Attempts to discontinue or taper medication should be made at three- to six-month intervals.
Treated patients with an intact uterus should be monitored closely for signs of endometrial cancer and appropriate diagnostic measures should be taken to rule out malignancy in the event of persistent or recurring abnormal vaginal bleeding.

HOW SUPPLIED
N 0071-0437-24 (P-D 437) Estrovis (quinestrol) 100-mcg tablets are supplied in bottles of 100.

PHYSICIAN REFERENCES
1. Ziel, H.K. and W.D. Finkle, "Increased Risk of Endometrial Carcinoma Among Users of Conjugated Estrogens." *New England Journal of Medicine,* 293:1167–1170, 1975.
2. Smith, D.C., R. Prentic, D.J. Thompson, and W.L. Hermann, "Association of Exogenous Estrogen and Endometrial Carcinoma." *New England Journal of Medicine,* 293:1164–1167, 1975.
3. Mack, T.M., M.C. Pike, B.E. Henderson, R.I. Pfeffer, V.R. Gerkins, M. Arthur, and S.E. Brown, "Estrogens and Endometrial Cancer in a Retirement Community." *New England Journal of Medicine,* 294:1262–1267, 1976.
4. Weiss, N.D., D.R. Szekely and D.F. Austin, "Increasing Incidence of Endometrial Cancer in the United States." *New England Journal of Medicine,* 294:1259–1262, 1976.
5. Herbst, A.L., H. Ulfelder and D.C. Poskanzer, "Adenocarcinoma of Vagina." *New England Journal of Medicine,* 284:878–881, 1971.
6. Greenwald, P., J. Barlow, P. Nasca, and W. Burnett, "Vaginal Cancer after Maternal Treatment with Synthetic Estrogens." *New England Journal of Medicine,* 285:390–392, 1971.

7. Lanier, A., K. Noller, D. Decker, L. Elveback, and L. Kurland, "Cancer and Stilbestrol, A Follow-Up of 1719 Persons Exposed to Estrogens in *Utero* and Born 1943–1959." *Mayo Clinic Proceedings,* 48:793–799, 1973.
8. Herbst, A., R. Kurman, and R. Scully, "Vaginal and Cervical Abnormalities After Exposure to Stilbestrol in Utero." *Obstetrics and Gynecology,* 40:287–298, 1972.
9. Herbst, A., S. Robboy, G. Macdonald, and R. Scully, "The Effects of Local Progesterone on Stilbestrol-Associated Vaginal Adenosis." *American Journal of Obstetrics and Gynecology,* 118:607–615, 1974.
10. Herbst, A., D. Poskanzer, S. Robboy, L. Friedlander, and R. Scully, "Prenatal Exposure to Stilbestrol, A Prospective Comparison of Exposed Female Offspring with Unexpected Controls." *New England Journal of Medicine,* 292:334–339, 1975.
11. Stafl, A., R. Mattingly, D. Foley, and W. Fetherston, "Clinical Diagnosis of Vaginal Adenosis." *Obstetrics and Gynecology,* 43:118–128, 1974.
12. Sherman, A.I., M. Goldrath, A. Berlin, V. Vakhariya, F. Banooni, W. Michaels, P. Goodman, S. Brown, "Cervical-Vaginal Adenosis After *In Utero* Exposure to Synthetic Estrogens," *Obstetrics and Gynecology,* 44:531–545, 1974.
13. Gal, I., B. Kirman, and J. Stern, "Hormone Pregnancy Tests and Congenital Malformation," *Nature,* 216:83, 1967.
14. Levy, E.P., A. Cohen, and F.C. Fraser, "Hormone Treatment During Pregnancy and Congenital Heart Defects," *Lancet,* 1:611, 1973.
15. Nora, J. and A. Nora, "Birth Defects and Oral Contraceptives," *Lancet,* 1:941–942, 1973.
16. Janerich, D.T., J.M. Piper, and D.M. Glebatis, "Oral Contraceptives and Congenital Limb-Reduction Defects," *New England Journal of Medicine,* 291:697–700, 1974.
17. "Estrogens for Oral or Parenteral Use," *Federal Register,* 40:8212, 1975.
18. Boston Collaborative Drug Surveillance Program "Surgically Confirmed Gallbladder Disease, Venous Thromboembolism and Breast Tumors in Relation to Post-Menopausal Estrogen Therapy," *New England Journal of Medicine,* 210:15–19, 1974.
18a. Hoover, R., L.A. Gray, Sr., P. Cole, and B. MacMahon, "Menopausal Estrogens and Breast Cancer." *New England Journal of Medicine,* 295:401–405, 1976.
19. Boston Collaborative Drug Surveillance Program, "Oral Contraceptives and Venous Thromboembolic Disease, Surgically Confirmed Gallbladder Disease, and Breast Tumors," *Lancet,* 1:1399–1404, 1973.
20. Daniel, D.G., H. Campbell, and A.C. Turnbull, "Puerperal Thromboembolism and Suppression of Lactation." *Lancet,* 2:287–289, 1967.
21. The Veterans Administration Cooperative Urological Research Group, "Carcinoma of the Prostate: Treatment Comparisons," *Journal of Urology,* 98:516–522, 1967.
22. Ballar, J.C., "Thromboembolism and Oestrogen Therapy," *Lancet,* 2, 560. 1967.
23. Blackard, C., R. Doe, G. Mellinger, and D. Byar, "Incidence of Cardiovascular Disease and Death in Patients Receiving Diethylstilbestrol for Carcinoma of the Prostate," *Cancer,* 26:249–256, 1970.
24. Royal College of General Practitioners, "Oral Contraception and Thromboembolic Disease," *Journal of the Royal College of General Practitioners,* 13, 267–279, 1967.
25. Inman, W.H.W. and M.P. Vessey, "Investigation of Deaths from Pulmonary, Coronary, and Cerebral Thrombosis and Embolism in Women of Child-Bearing Age." *British Medical Journal,* 2:193–199, 1968.
26. Vessey, M.P. and R. Doll, "Investigation of Relation Between Use of Oral Contraceptives and Thromboembolic Disease, A Further Report," *British Medical Journal,* 2:651–657, 1969.
27. Sartwell, P.E., A.T. Masi, F.G. Arthes, G.R. Greene and H.E. Smith, "Thromboembolism and Oral Contraceptives: An Epidemiological Case Control Study." *American Journal of Epidemiology,* 90:365–380, 1969.
28. Collaborative Group for the Study of Stroke in Young Women, "Oral Contraception and Increased Risk of Cerebral Ischemia or Thrombosis," *New England Journal of Medicine,* 288:871–878, 1973.
29. Collaborative Group for the Study of Stroke in Young Women: "Oral Contraceptives and Stroke in Young Women: Associated Risk Factors," 231:718–722, 1975. *Journal of the American Medical Assoc.* 231:718–722, 1975.
30. Mann, J.I. and W.H.W. Inman, "Oral Contraceptives and Death from Myocardial Infarction," *British Medical Journal,* 2:245–248, 1975.
31. Mann, J.I., M.P. Vessey, M. Thorogood, and R. Doll, "Myocardial Infarction in Young Women with Special Reference to Oral Contraceptive Practice," *British Medical Journal,* 2:241–245, 1975.
32. Inman, W.H.W., M.P. Vessey, B. Westerholm, and A. Engelund, "Thromboembolic Disease and the Steroidal Content of Oral Contraceptives," *British Medical Journal,* 2:203–209, 1970.
33. Stolley, P.D., J.A. Tonascia, M.S. Tockman, P.E. Sartwell, A.H. Rutledge, and M.P. Jacobs, "Thrombosis with

Low-Estrogen Oral Contraceptives," *American Journal of Epidemiology,* 102:197–208, 1975.
34. Vessey, M.P., R. Doll, A.S. Fairbairn, and G. Glober, "Post-Operative Thromboembolism and the use of the Oral Contraceptives," *British Medical Journal,* 3:123–126, 1970.
35. Greene, G.R. and P.E. Sartwell, "Oral Contraceptive Use in Patients with Thromboembolism Following Surgery, Trauma or Infection," *American Journal of Public Health,* 62:680–685, 1972.
36. Rosenberg, L., M.B. Armstrong and H. Jick "Myocardial Infarction and Estrogen Therapy in Post-menopausal Women," *New England Journal of Medicine,* 294:1256–1259, 1976.
37. Coronary Drug Project Research Group, "The Coronary Drug Project: Initial Findings Leading to Modifications of Its Research Protocol," *Journal of the American Medical Association,* 214:1303–1313, 1970.
38. Baum, J., F. Holtz, J.J. Bookstein, and E.W. Klein, "Possible Association between Benign Hepatomas and Oral Contraceptives," *Lancet,* 2:926–928, 1973.
39. Mays, E.T., W.M. Christopherson, M.M. Mahr, and H.C. Williams, "Hepatic Changes in Young Women Ingesting Contraceptive Steroids, Hepatic Hemorrhage and Primary Hepatic Tumors," *Journal of the American Medical Association,* 235:780–782, 1976.
40. Edmondson, H.A., B. Henderson, and B. Benton, "Liver Cell Adenomas Association with the Use of Oral Contraceptives," *New England Journal of Medicine,* 294:470–472, 1976.
41. Pfeffer, A.I. and S. Van Den Noore, "Estrogen use and Stroke Risk in Post-menopausal Women," *American Journal of Epidemiology,* 103:545–546, 1976.

Patient Labeling for Estrogens

WHAT YOU SHOULD KNOW ABOUT ESTROGENS
Estrogens are female hormones produced by the ovaries. The ovaries make several different kinds of estrogens. In addition, scientists have been able to make a variety of synthetic estrogens. As far as we know, all these estrogens have similar properties and, therefore, much the same usefulness, side effects, and risks. This leaflet is intended to help you understand what estrogens are used for, the risks involved in their use, and how to use them as safely as possible.
This leaflet includes the most important information about estrogens, but not all the information. If you want to know more, you can ask your doctor or pharmacist to let you read the package insert prepared for the doctor.

USES OF ESTROGEN
Estrogens are prescribed by doctors for a number of purposes, including the following:
1. To provide estrogen during a period of adjustment when a woman's ovaries no longer produce estrogen, in order to prevent certain uncomfortable symptoms of estrogen deficiency. (All women normally stop producing estrogens, generally between the ages of 45 and 55; this is called the menopause.)
2. To prevent symptoms of estrogen deficiency when a woman's ovaries have been removed surgically before the natural menopause.
3. To prevent pregnancy. (Estrogens are given along with a progestogen, another female hormone; these combinations are called oral contraceptives or birth control pills. Patient labeling is available to women taking oral contraceptives and they will not be discussed in this leaflet.)
4. To treat certain cancers in women and men.
5. To prevent painful swelling of the breasts after pregnancy in women who choose not to nurse their babies.
THERE IS NO PROPER USE OF ESTROGENS IN A PREGNANT WOMAN.

ESTROGENS IN THE MENOPAUSE
In the natural course of their lives, all women eventually experience a decrease in estrogen production. This usually occurs between ages 45 and 55 but may occur earlier or later. Sometimes the ovaries may need to be removed before natural menopause by an operation, producing a "surgical menopause."
When the amount of estrogen in the blood begins to decrease, many women may develop typical symptoms: feelings of warmth in the face, neck, and chest; or sudden intense episodes of heat and sweating throughout the body (called "hot flashes" or "hot flushes"). These symptoms are sometimes very uncomfortable. A few women eventually develop changes in the vagina (called "atrophic vaginitis") which cause discomfort, especially during and after intercourse. Estrogens can be prescribed to treat these symptoms of the menopause. It is estimated that considerably more than half of all women undergoing the menopause have only mild

Continued on next page

This product information was prepared in August, 1989. On these and other Parke-Davis Products, information may be obtained by addressing PARKE-DAVIS, Division of Warner-Lambert Company, Morris Plains, New Jersey 07950.

Parke-Davis—Cont.

symptoms or no symptoms at all and, therefore, do not need estrogens. Other women may need estrogens for a few months, while their bodies adjust to lower estrogen levels. Sometimes the need will be for periods longer than six months. In an attempt to avoid overstimulation of the uterus (womb), estrogens are usually given cyclically during each month of use, that is, three weeks of pills followed by one week without pills. However, Estrovis (quinestrol tablets, USP) is given once daily for seven days, followed by once weekly use beginning two weeks after the start of treatment. Sometimes, women experience nervous symptoms or depression during menopause. There is no evidence that estrogens are effective for such symptoms and they should not be used to treat them, although other treatment may be needed. You may have heard that taking estrogens for long periods (years) after the menopause will keep your skin soft and supple and keep you feeling young. There is no evidence that this is so, however, and such long-term treatment carries important risks.

THE DANGERS OF ESTROGEN

1. *Cancer of the uterus.* If estrogens are used in the postmenopausal period for more than a year, there is an increased risk of *endometrial cancer* (cancer of the uterus). Women taking estrogens have roughly 5 to 10 times as great a chance of getting this cancer as women who take no estrogens. To put this another way, while a postmenopausal woman not taking estrogens has 1 chance in 1,000 each year of getting cancer of the uterus, a woman taking estrogens has 5 to 10 chances in 1,000 each year. For this reason *it is important to take estrogens only when you really need them.*
The risk of this cancer is greater the longer estrogens are used and also seems to be greater when larger doses are taken. For this reason *it is important to take the lowest dosage of estrogens that will control symptoms and to take it only as long as it is needed.* If estrogens are needed for longer periods of time, your doctor will want to reevaluate your need for estrogens at least every six months.
Women using estrogens should report any irregular vaginal bleeding to their doctors; although such bleeding may be of no importance, it can be an early warning of cancer of the uterus. If you have undiagnosed vaginal bleeding, you should not use estrogens until a diagnosis is made and you are certain there is no cancer of the uterus.
If you have had your uterus completely removed (total hysterectomy), there is no danger of developing cancer of the uterus.
2. *Other possible cancers.* Estrogens can cause development of other tumors in animals, such as tumors of the breast, cervix, vagina, or liver, when given for a long time. At present, there is no good evidence that women using estrogen in the menopause have an increased risk of such tumors, but there is no way yet to be sure they do not. One study raises the possibility that use of estrogen in the menopause may increase the risk of breast cancer many years later. This is a further reason to use estrogens only when clearly needed. While you are taking estrogens, it is important that you go to your doctor at least once a year for a physical examination. Also, if members of your family have had breast cancer or if you have breast nodules or abnormal mammograms (breast x-rays), your doctor may wish to carry out more frequent examinations of your breasts.
3. *Gallbladder disease.* Women who use estrogens after menopause are more likely to develop gallbladder disease requiring surgery than women who do not use estrogens. Birth control pills have a similar effect.
4. *Abnormal blood clotting.* Oral contraceptives increase the risk of blood clotting in various parts of the body. This can result in a stroke (if the clot is in the brain), a heart attack (a clot in a blood vessel of the heart), or a pulmonary embolus (a clot which forms in the legs or pelvis, then breaks off and travels to the lungs.) Any of these can be fatal.
At this time use of estrogens in the menopause is not known to cause such blood clotting, but this has not been fully studied and there could still prove to be such a risk. It is recommended that if you have had clotting in the legs or lungs or a heart attack or stroke while you were using estrogens or birth control pills, you should not use estrogens (unless they are being used to treat cancer of the breast or prostate.) If you have had a stroke or heart attack or if you have angina pectoris, estrogens should be used with great caution and only if clearly needed (for example, if you have severe symptoms of the menopause).
The larger dosages of estrogen used to prevent swelling of the breasts after pregnancy have been reported to cause clotting in the legs and lungs.

SPECIAL WARNING ABOUT PREGNANCY

You should not receive estrogen if you are pregnant. If this should occur, there is a greater than usual chance that the developing child will be born with a birth defect, although the possibility remains fairly small. A female child may have an increased risk of developing cancer of the vagina or cervix

later in life (in the teens or twenties). Every possible effort should be made to avoid exposure to estrogens during pregnancy. If exposure occurs, see your doctor.

OTHER EFFECTS OF ESTROGENS

In addition to the serious known risks of estrogens previously described, estrogens have the following side effects and potential risks:
1. *Nausea and vomiting.* The most common side effect of estrogen therapy is nausea. Vomiting is less common.
2. *Effects on the breasts.* Estrogens may cause breast tenderness or enlargement and may cause the breasts to secrete a liquid. These effects are not dangerous.
3. *Effects on the uterus.* Estrogens may cause benign fibroid tumors of the uterus to enlarge.
Some women will have menstrual bleeding when estrogens are stopped. However, if the bleeding occurs on days you are still taking estrogens, you should report this to your doctor.
4. *Effects on the liver.* On rare occasions, women taking oral contraceptives develop a tumor of the liver which can rupture and bleed into the abdomen. So far, these tumors have not been reported in women using estrogens in the menopause, but you should report to your doctor immediately any swelling or unusual pain or tenderness in the abdomen. Women with a past history of jaundice (yellowing of the skin and white parts of the eyes) may get jaundice again during estrogen use. If this occurs, stop taking estrogens and see your doctor.
5. *Other effects.* Estrogens may cause excess fluid to be retained in the body. This may make some conditions worse, such as epilepsy, migraine, heart disease, or kidney disease.

SUMMARY

Estrogens have important uses, but they have serious risks as well. You must decide, with your doctor, whether the risks are acceptable to you in view of the benefits of treatment. Except where your doctor has prescribed estrogens for use in special cases of cancer of the breast or prostate, you should not use estrogens if you have cancer of the breast or uterus, are pregnant, have undiagnosed abnormal vaginal bleeding, clotting in the legs or lungs, or have had a stroke, heart attack or angina, or clotting in the legs or lungs in the past while you were taking estrogens.
You can use estrogens as safely as possible by understanding that your doctor will require regular physical examinations while you are taking them and will try to use the smallest dosage possible and discontinue the drug as soon as possible. Be alert for signs of trouble including:
1. Abnormal bleeding from the vagina
2. Pains in the calves or chest or sudden shortness of breath, or coughing blood (indicating possible clots in the legs, heart, or lungs)
3. Severe headache, dizziness, faintness, or changes in vision (indicating possible developing clots in the brain or eye)
4. Breast lumps (you should ask you doctor how to examine your own breasts)
5. Jaundice (yellowing of the skin)
6. Mental depression
Based on his or her assessment of your medical needs, your doctor has prescribed this drug for you. Do not give this drug to anyone else.
Storage—Store between 15°–30°C (59°–86°F).
Caution—Federal law prohibits dispensing without prescription

Shown in Product Identification Section, page 421
0437G026

EUTHROID®   ℞
[*ūth 'roid*]
(Liotrix Tablets, USP)

DESCRIPTION

Euthroid (Liotrix Tablets, USP) is synthetic microcrystalline levothyroxine sodium (T_4) USP and synthetic microcrystalline liothyronine sodium (T_3) USP combined in a constant 4:1 ratio. Each Euthroid-1 tablet contains 60 mcg levothyroxine (T_4) and 15 mcg liothyronine (T_3).
Each Euthroid-1 tablet will give a dose benefit approximately equivalent to 1 grain of desiccated thryoid, 100 mcg T_4 (levothyroxine sodium), 25 mcg T_3 (liothyronine sodium), or 60 mcg T_4/15 mcg T_3 (liotrix). See Conversion Table at end of insert.
Euthroid tablets also contain calcium phosphate, USP; cellulose, NF; corn starch, NF; hydrogenated vegetable oil, NF; magnesium stearate, NF; mannitol, USP; and silicon dioxide, NF. In addition, Euthroid-½ contains D&C red No. 30 lake and FD&C yellow No 5 lake. Euthroid-1 and Euthroid-3 contain D&C red No. 30 lake, FD&C blue No. 2 lake, and FD&C yellow No. 5 lake. Euthroid-2 contains D&C red No. 30 lake and FD&C blue No. 2 lake.
Thyroid hormone drugs are natural or synthetic preparations containing tetraiodothyronine (T_4 levothyroxine) sodium or triiodothyronine (T_3, liothyronine) sodium or both. T_4 and T_3 are produced in the human thyroid gland by the iodination and coupling of the amino acid tyrosine. T_4 con-

tains four iodine atoms and is formed by the coupling of two molecules of diiodotyrosine (DIT). T_3 contains three atoms of iodine and is formed by the coupling of one molecule of DIT with one molecule of monoiodotyrosine (MIT). Both hormones are stored in the thyroid colloid as thyroglobulin.
Thyroid hormone preparations belong to two categories: (1) natural hormonal preparations derived from animal thyroid, and (2) synthetic preparations. Natural preparations include desiccated thyroid and thyroglobulin. Desiccated thyroid is derived from domesticated animals that are used for food by man (either beef or hog thyroid), and thyroglobulin is derived from thyroid glands of the hog.
There are five (5) preparations in the USP. They are: (1) Thyroid Tablets, (2) Thyroglobulin Tablets, (3) Levothyroxine Sodium Tablets, (4) Liothyronine Sodium Tablets, and (5) Liotrix Tablets (a ratio, by weight, of 4 to 1, of the sodium salts of T_4 and T_3, respectively).

CLINICAL PHARMACOLOGY

The steps in the synthesis of the thyroid hormones are controlled by thyrotropin (Thyroid Stimulating Hormone, TSH) secreted by the anterior pituitary. This hormone's secretion is in turn controlled by a feedback mechanism effected by the thyroid hormones themselves and by thyrotropin releasing hormone (TRH), a tripeptide of hypothalamic origin. Endogenous thyroid hormone secretion is suppressed when exogenous thyroid hormones are administered to euthyroid individuals in excess of the normal gland's secretion.
The mechanisms by which thyroid hormones exert their physiologic action are not well understood. These hormones enhance oxygen consumption by most tissues of the body, increase the basal metabolic rate, and the metabolism of carbohydrates, lipids, and proteins. Thus, they exert a profound influence on every organ system in the body and are of particular importance in the development of the central nervous system.
The normal thyroid gland contains approximately 200 mcg of levothyroxine (T_4) per gram of gland, and 15 mcg of triiodothyronine (T_3) per gram. The ratio of these two hormones in the circulation does not represent the ratio in the thyroid gland, since about 80 percent of peripheral triiodothyronine comes from monodeiodination of levothyroxine. Peripheral monodeiodination of levothyroxine at the 5 position (inner ring) also results in the formation of reverse triiodothyronine (rT_3), which is calorigenically inactive. These facts would seem to advocate levothyroxine as the treatment of choice for the hypothyroid patient and to militate against the administration of hormone combinations, which while normalizing thyroxine levels may produce triiodothyronine levels in the thyrotoxic range.
Triiodothyronine (T_3) level is low in the fetus and newborn, in old age, in chronic caloric deprivation, hepatic cirrhosis, renal failure, surgical stress, and chronic illnesses representing what has been called the "low triiodothyronine syndrome."
Pharmacokinetics: Animal studies have shown that T_4 is only partially absorbed from the gastrointestinal tract. The degree of absorption is dependent on the vehicle used for its administration and by the character of the intestinal contents, the intestinal flora, including plasma protein, soluble dietary factors, all of which bind thyroid and thereby make it unavailable for diffusion. Only 41 percent is absorbed when given in a gelatin capsule as opposed to a 74 percent absorption when given with an albumin carrier.
Depending on other factors, absorption has varied from 48 to 79 percent of the administered dose. Fasting increases absorption. Malabsorption syndromes, as well as dietary factors (children's soybean formula, concomitant use of anionic exchange resins such as cholestyramine), cause excessive fecal loss. T_3 is almost totally absorbed, 95 percent in 4 hours. The hormones contained in the natural preparations are absorbed in a manner similar to the synthetic hormones. More than 99 percent of circulating hormones are bound to serum proteins, including thyroid-binding globulin (TB_g), thyroid-binding prealbumin (TBPA), and albumin (TB_a), whose capacities and affinities vary for the hormones. The higher affinity of levothyroxine (T_4) for both TB_g and TBPA as compared to triiodothyronine (T_3) partially explains the higher serum levels and longer half-life of the former hormone. Both protein-bound hormones exist in reverse equilibrium with minute amounts of free hormone, the latter accounting for the metabolic activity.
Deiodination of levothyroxine (T_4) occurs at a number of sites, including liver, kidney, and other tissues. The conjugated hormone, in the form of glucuronide or sulfate, is found in the bile and gut where it may complete an enterohepatic circulation. Eighty-five percent of levothyroxine (T_4) metabolized daily is deiodinated.

INDICATIONS AND USAGE

Thyroid hormone drugs are indicated:
As replacement or supplemental therapy in patients with hypothyroidism of any etiology, except transient hypothyroidism during the recovery phase of subacute thyroiditis. This category includes cretinism, myxedema, and ordinary hypothyroidism in patients of any age (children, adults, the

elderly), or state (including pregnancy); primary hypothyroidism resulting from functional deficiency, primary atrophy, partial or total absence of thyroid gland, or the effects of surgery, radiation, or drugs, with or without the presence of goiter; and secondary (pituitary) or tertiary (hypothalamic) hypothyroidism (See WARNINGS).

CONTRAINDICATIONS

Thyroid hormone preparations are generally contraindicated in patients with diagnosed but as yet uncorrected adrenal cortical insufficiency, untreated thyrotoxicosis, and apparent hypersensitivity to any of their active or extraneous constituents. There is no well documented evidence from the literature, however, of true allergic or idiosyncratic reactions to thyroid hormone.

WARNINGS

> Drugs with thyroid hormone activity, alone or together with other therapeutic agents, have been used for the treatment of obesity. In euthyroid patients, doses within the range of daily hormonal requirements are ineffective for weight reduction. Larger doses may produce serious or even life-threatening manifestations of toxicity, particularly when given in association with sympathomimetic amines such as those used for their anorectic effects.

The use of thyroid hormones in the therapy of obesity, alone or combined with other drugs, is unjustified and has been shown to be ineffective. Neither is their use justified for the treatment of male or female infertility unless this condition is accompanied by hypothyroidism.

PRECAUTIONS

General: Thyroid hormones should be used with great caution in a number of circumstances where the integrity of the cardiovascular system, particularly the coronary arteries, is suspect. These include patients with angina pectoris or the elderly, in whom there is a greater likelihood of occult cardiac disease. In these patients, therapy should be initiated with low doses, ie, 25–50 mcg levothyroxine (T_4) or its isocaloric equivalents (see Conversion Table at end of insert). When, in such patients, a euthyroid state can only be reached at the expense of an aggravation of the cardiovascular disease, thyroid hormone dosage should be reduced.

Thyroid hormone therapy in patients with concomitant diabetes mellitus or insipidus or adrenal cortical insufficiency aggravates the intensity of their symptoms. Appropriate adjustments of the various therapeutic measures directed at these concomitant endocrine diseases are required. The therapy of myxedema coma requires simultaneous administration of glucocorticoids (See DOSAGE AND ADMINISTRATION).

Hypothyroidism decreases and hyperthyroidism increases the sensitivity to oral anticoagulants. Prothrombin time should be closely monitored in thyroid-treated patients on oral anticoagulants and dosage of the latter agents adjusted on the basis of frequent prothrombin time determination. In infants, excessive doses of thyroid hormone preparations may produce craniosynostosis.

Euthroid-½, -1, -3 contains FD&C Yellow No 5 (tartrazine) which may cause allergic-type reactions (including bronchial asthma) in certain susceptible individuals. Although the overall incidence of FD&C Yellow No 5 (tartrazine) sensitivity in the population is low, it is frequently seen in patients who also have aspirin hypersensitivity.

Information for the Patient: Patients on thyroid hormone preparations and parents of children on thyroid therapy should be informed that:

1. Replacement therapy is to be taken essentially for life, with the exception of cases of transient hypothyroidism, usually associated with thyroiditis, and in those patients receiving a therapeutic trial of the drug.

2. They should immediately report during the course of therapy any signs or symptoms of thyroid hormone toxicity, eg, chest pain, increased pulse rate, palpitations, excessive sweating, heat intolerance, nervousness, or any other unusual event.

3. In case of concomitant diabetes mellitus, the daily dosage of antidiabetic medication may need readjustment as thyroid hormone replacement is achieved. If thyroid medication is stopped, a downward readjustment of the dosage of insulin or oral hypoglycemic agent may be necessary to avoid hypoglycemia. At all times, close monitoring of urinary glucose levels is mandatory in such patients.

4. In case of concomitant oral anticoagulant therapy, the prothrombin time should be measured frequently to determine if the dosage of oral anticoagulants is to be readjusted.

5. Partial loss of hair may be experienced by children in the first few months of thyroid therapy, but this is usually a transient phenomenon and later recovery is usually the rule.

Laboratory Tests: Treatment of patients with thyroid hormones requires the periodic assessment of thyroid status by means of appropriate laboratory tests besides the full clinical evaluation. The TSH suppression test can be used to test the effectiveness of any thyroid preparation, bearing in mind the relative insensitivity of the infant pituitary to the negative feedback effect of thyroid hormones. Serum T_4 levels can be used to test the effectiveness of all thyroid medications except T_3. When the total serum T_4 is low but TSH is normal, a test specific to assess unbound (free) T_4 levels is warranted. Specific measurements of T_4 and T_3 by competitive protein binding or radioimmunoassay are not influenced by blood levels of organic or inorganic iodine and have essentially replaced older tests of thyroid hormone measurements, ie, PBI, BEI, and T_4 by column.

Drug Interactions: Oral Anticoagulants—Thyroid hormones appear to increase catabolism of vitamin K-dependent clotting factors. If oral anticoagulants are also being given, compensatory increases in clotting factor synthesis are impaired. Patients stabilized on oral anticoagulants who are found to require thyroid replacement therapy should be watched very closely when thyroid is started. If a patient is truly hypothyroid, it is likely that a reduction in anticoagulant dosage will be required. No special precautions appear to be necessary when oral anticoagulant therapy is begun in a patient already stabilized on maintenance thyroid replacement therapy.

Insulin or Oral Hypoglycemics—Initiating thyroid replacement therapy may cause increases in insulin or oral hypoglycemic requirements. The effects seen are poorly understood and depend upon a variety of factors such as dosage and type of thyroid preparations and endocrine status of the patient. Patients receiving insulin or oral hypoglycemics should be closely watched during initiation of thyroid replacement therapy.

Cholestyramine—Cholestyramine binds both T_4 and T_3 in the intestine, thus impairing absorption of these thyroid hormones. *In vitro* studies indicate that the binding is not easily removed. Therefore, four to five hours should elapse between administration of cholestyramine or similar resins, such as colestipol, and thyroid hormones.

Estrogen, Oral Contraceptives—Estrogens tend to increase serum thyroxine-binding globulin (TB_g). In a patient with a nonfunctioning thyroid gland who is receiving thyroid replacement therapy, free levothyroxine may be decreased when estrogens are started thus increasing thyroid requirements. However, if the patient's thyroid gland has sufficient function, the decreased free thyroxine will result in a compensatory increase in thyroxine output by the thyroid. Therefore, patients without a functioning thyroid gland who are on thyroid replacement therapy may need to increase their thyroid dose if estrogens or estrogen-containing oral contraceptives are given.

Drug/Laboratory Test Interactions: The following drugs or moieties are known to interfere with laboratory tests performed in patients on thyroid hormone therapy: androgens, corticosteroids, estrogens, oral contraceptives containing estrogens, iodine-containing preparations, and the numerous preparations containing salicylates.

1. Changes in TB_g concentration should be taken into consideration in the interpretation of T_4 and T_3 values. In such cases, the unbound (free) hormone should be measured. Pregnancy, estrogens, and estrogen-containing oral contraceptives increase TB_g concentrations. TB_g may also be increased during infectious hepatitis. Decreases in TB_g concentrations are observed in nephrosis, acromegaly, and after androgen or corticosteroid therapy. Familial hyper- or hypo-thyroxine binding globulinemias have been described. The incidence of TB_g deficiency approximates 1 in 9000. The binding of thyroxine by TBPA is inhibited by salicylates.

2. Medicinal or dietary iodine interferes with all *in vivo* tests of radioiodine uptake, producing low uptakes which may not be reflective of a true decrease in hormone synthesis.

3. The persistence of clinical and laboratory evidence of hypothyroidism in spite of adequate dosage replacement indicates poor patient compliance, poor absorption, excessive fecal loss, or inactivity of the preparation. Intracellular resistance to thyroid hormone is quite rare.

Carcinogenesis, Mutagenesis, and Impairment of Fertility: A reportedly apparent association between prolonged thyroid therapy and breast cancer has not been confirmed and patients on thyroid for established indications should not discontinue therapy. No confirmatory long-term studies in animals have been performed to evaluate carcinogenic potential, mutagenicity, or impairment of fertility in either males or females.

Pregnancy—Category A: Thyroid hormones do not readily cross the placental barrier. The clinical experience to date does not indicate any adverse effect on fetuses when thyroid hormones are administered to pregnant women. On the basis of current knowledge, thyroid replacement therapy to hypothyroid women should not be discontinued during pregnancy.

Nursing Mothers: Minimal amounts of thyroid hormones are excreted in human milk. Thyroid is not associated with serious adverse reactions and does not have a known tumorigenic potential. However, caution should be exercised when thyroid is administered to a nursing woman.

Pediatric Use: Pregnant mothers provide little or no thyroid hormone to the fetus. The incidence of congenital hypothyroidism is relatively high (1:4,000) and the hypothyroid fetus would not derive any benefit from the small amounts of hormone crossing the placental barrier. Routine determinations of serum T_4 and/or TSH are strongly advised in neonates in view of the deleterious effects of thyroid deficiency on growth and development.

Treatment should be initiated immediately upon diagnosis and maintained for life, unless transient hypothyroidism is suspected; in which case, therapy may be interrupted for 2 to 8 weeks after the age of 3 years to reassess the condition. Cessation of therapy is justified in patients who have maintained a normal TSH during those 2 to 8 weeks.

ADVERSE REACTIONS

Adverse reactions other than those indicative of hyperthyroidism because of therapeutic overdosage, either initially or during the maintenance period, are rare (See OVERDOSAGE).

OVERDOSAGE

Signs and Symptoms: Excessive doses of thyroid result in a hypermetabolic state resembling in every respect the condition of endogenous origin. The condition may be self-induced.

Treatment of Overdosage: Dosage should be reduced or therapy temporarily discontinued if signs and symptoms of overdosage appear. Treatment may be reinstituted at a lower dosage. In normal individuals, normal hypothalamic-pituitary-thyroid axis function is restored in 6 to 8 weeks after thyroid suppression.

Treatment of acute massive thyroid hormone overdosage is aimed at reducing gastrointestinal absorption of the drugs and counteracting central and peripheral effects, mainly those of increased sympathetic activity. Vomiting may be induced initially if further gastrointestinal absorption can reasonably be prevented and barring contraindications such as coma, convulsions, or loss of the gagging reflex. Treatment is symptomatic and supportive. Oxygen may be administered and ventilation maintained. Cardiac glycosides may be indicated if congestive heart failure develops. Measures to control fever, hypoglycemia, or fluid loss should be instituted if needed. Antiadrenergic agents, particularly propranolol, have been used advantageously in the treatment of increased sympathetic activity. Propranolol may be administered intravenously at a dosage of 1 to 3 mg over a 10 minute period or orally, 80 to 160 mg/day initially, especially when no contraindications exist for its use.

DOSAGE AND ADMINISTRATION

The dosage of thyroid hormones is determined by the indication and must in every case be individualized according to patient response and laboratory findings.

Thyroid hormones are given orally. In acute, emergency conditions, injectable sodium levothyroxine may be given intravenously when oral administration is not feasible or desirable, as in the treatment of myxedema coma, or during total parenteral nutrition. Injectable sodium liothyronine is also available upon request from the manufacturer, under investigational status, for the treatment of myxedema coma. Intramuscular administration of these two preparations is not advisable because of reported poor absorption.

Hypothyroidism: Therapy is usually instituted using low doses, with increments that depend on the cardiovascular status of the patient. The usual starting dose is 50 mcg of levothyroxine (T_4) or its isocaloric equivalent (Euthroid-½), with increments of 25 mcg every 2 to 3 weeks. A lower starting dosage, 25 mcg/day of levothyroxine (T_4) or its isocaloric equivalent, is recommended in patients with longstanding myxedema, particularly if cardiovascular impairment is suspected, in which case extreme caution is recommended. The appearance of angina is an indication for a reduction in dosage. The 200 to 400 mcg levothyroxine (T_4) recommended in the early trials are now considered excessive and most patients require 100 to 200 mcg/day or the caloric equivalent. Failure to respond to doses of 300 mcg suggests lack of compliance or malabsorption. Maintenance dosages of 100–200 mcg/day (Euthroid-1 or Euthroid-2) usually result in normal serum levothyroxine (T_4) and triiodothyronine (T_3) levels. Adequate therapy usually results in normal TSH and T_4 levels after 2 to 3 weeks of therapy.

Readjustment of thyroid hormone dosage should be made within the first four weeks of therapy, after proper clinical and laboratory evaluations, including serum levels of T_4, bound and free, and TSH.

The rapid onset and dissipation of action of sodium liothyronine (T_3), as compared with sodium levothyroxine (T_4), has led some clinicians to prefer its use in patients who might be

Continued on next page

This product information was prepared in August, 1989. On these and other Parke-Davis Products, information may be obtained by addressing PARKE-DAVIS, Division of Warner-Lambert Company, Morris Plains, New Jersey 07950.

Parke-Davis—Cont.

more susceptible to the untoward effects of thyroid medication. However, the wide swings in serum T_3 levels that follow its administration and the possibility of more pronounced cardiovascular side effects tend to counterbalance the stated advantages. Many physicians continue to use thyroid tablets, USP, a T_3/T_4 combination, or a newer synthetic combination.

T_3 may be used in preference to levothyroxine (T_4) during radioisotope scanning procedures, since induction of hypothyroidism in those cases is more abrupt and can be of shorter duration. It may also be preferred when impairment of peripheral conversion of T_4 and T_3 is suspected.

Myxedema Coma: Myxedema coma is usually precipitated in the hypothyroid patient of long standing by intercurrent illness or drugs such as sedatives and anesthetics and should be considered a medical emergency. Therapy should be directed to the correction of electrolyte disturbances and possible infection besides the administration of thyroid hormones.

Corticosteroids should be administered routinely. T_4 and T_3 may be administered via nasogastric tube, but the preferred route of administration of both hormones is intravenous.

Sodium levothyroxine (T_4) is given at a starting dose of 400 mcg (100 mcg/mL) given rapidly and is usually well tolerated, even in the elderly. This initial dose is followed by daily supplements of 100 to 200 mcg given IV. Normal T_4 levels are achieved in 24 hours followed in 3 days by threefold elevation of T_3. Triiodothyronine (T_3) (which is obtained only by special request from the manufacturer) is given at doses of 200 mcg IV followed by 25 mcg supplements at 8-hour intervals. Oral therapy with either hormone would be resumed as soon as the clinical situation has been stabilized and the patient is able to take oral medication.

Thyroid Cancer: Exogenous thyroid hormone may produce regression of metastases from follicular and papillary carcinoma of the thyroid and is used as ancillary therapy of these conditions with radioactive iodine. TSH should be suppressed to low or undetectable levels. Therefore, larger amounts of thyroid hormone than those used for replacement therapy are required. Medullary carcinoma of the thyroid is usually unresponsive to this therapy.

Thyroid Suppression Therapy: Administration of thyroid hormone in doses higher than those produced physiologically by the gland results in suppression of the production of endogenous hormone. This is the basis for the thyroid suppression test and is used as an aid in the diagnosis of patients with signs of mild hyperthyroidism in whom baseline laboratory tests appear normal or to demonstrate thyroid gland autonomy in patients with Graves' ophthalmopathy. 131_1 uptake is determined before and after the administration of the exogenous hormone. A fifty percent or greater suppression of uptake indicates a normal thyroid-pituitary axis and thus rules out thyroid gland autonomy.

For adults, the usual suppressive dose of levothyroxine (T_4) is 2.6 mcg/kg of body weight per day given for 7 to 10 days. These doses usually yield normal serum T_4 and T_3 levels and lack of response to TSH.

T_3 is given in doses of 75–100 mcg/day for 7 days and radioactive iodine uptake is determined before and after administration of the hormone. If thyroid function is under normal control, the radioiodine uptake will drop significantly after treatment with either hormone.

Either hormone or combination therapy should be administered cautiously to patients in whom there is a strong suspicion of thyroid gland autonomy, in view of the fact that the exogenous hormone effects will be additive to the endogenous source.

Pediatric Dosage: Pediatric dosage should follow the recommendations summarized in Table 1. In infants with congenital hypothyroidism, therapy with full doses should be instituted as soon as the diagnosis has been made.

Table 1 Recommended Pediatric Dosage for Congenital Hypothyroidism

Age	Tetraiodothyronine (T_4, levothyroxine) sodium	
	Dose per day	Daily dose per kg of body weight
0–6 mos	25–50 mcg	8–10 mcg
6–12 mos	50–75 mcg	6– 8 mcg
1–5 yrs	75–100 mcg	5– 6 mcg
6–12 yrs	100–150 mcg	4– 5 mcg
over 12 yrs	over 150 mcg	2– 3 mcg

[See table below].

HOW SUPPLIED

Square monogrammed scored tablets of four potencies, each identified by a different color (see Table 2).
Euthroid-½ is supplied as: N 0071-0260-24—Bottles of 100.
Euthroid-1 is supplied as: N 0071-0261-24—Bottles of 100.
Euthroid-2 is supplied as: N 0071-0262-24—Bottles of 100.
Euthroid-3 is supplied as: N 0071-0263-24—Bottles of 100.
Store between 15°-30°C (59°-86°F).
Licensed under US Patent 2,823,164
Caution—Federal law prohibits dispensing without prescription.   **0260G023**

Shown in Product Identification Section, page 421

FLUOGEN®   ℞
[flŭ 'ō-jĕn ']
(influenza virus vaccine)

The formulation of influenza virus vaccine for use during each season is established by the Office of Biologics, Food and Drug Administration, Public Health Service. For information regarding the current formulation, please refer to the product package insert, contact your Parke-Davis representative, or call (201) 540-2000.

KETALAR®   ℞
[kē 'tă-lăr ']
(Ketamine Hydrochloride Injection, USP)

SPECIAL NOTE
EMERGENCE REACTIONS HAVE OCCURRED IN APPROXIMATELY 12 PERCENT OF PATIENTS.
THE PSYCHOLOGICAL MANIFESTATIONS VARY IN SEVERITY BETWEEN PLEASANT DREAM-LIKE STATES, VIVID IMAGERY, HALLUCINATIONS, AND EMERGENCE DELIRIUM. IN SOME CASES THESE STATES HAVE BEEN ACCOMPANIED BY CONFUSION, EXCITEMENT, AND IRRATIONAL BEHAVIOR WHICH A FEW PATIENTS RECALL AS AN UNPLEASANT EXPERIENCE. THE DURATION ORDINARILY IS NO MORE THAN A FEW HOURS; IN A FEW CASES, HOWEVER, RECURRENCES HAVE TAKEN PLACE UP TO 24 HOURS POSTOPERATIVELY. NO RESIDUAL PSYCHOLOGICAL EFFECTS ARE KNOWN TO HAVE RESULTED FROM USE OF KETALAR.
THE INCIDENCE OF THESE EMERGENCE PHENOMENA IS LEAST IN THE YOUNG (15 YEARS OF AGE OR LESS) AND ELDERLY (OVER 65 YEARS OF AGE) PATIENT. ALSO, THEY ARE LESS FREQUENT WHEN THE DRUG IS GIVEN INTRAMUSCULARLY AND THE INCIDENCE IS REDUCED AS EXPERIENCE WITH THE DRUG IS GAINED.
THE INCIDENCE OF PSYCHOLOGICAL MANIFESTATIONS DURING EMERGENCE, PARTICULARLY DREAM-LIKE OBSERVATIONS AND EMERGENCE DELIRIUM, MAY BE REDUCED BY USING LOWER RECOMMENDED DOSAGES OF KETALAR IN CONJUNCTION WITH INTRAVENOUS DIAZEPAM DURING INDUCTION AND MAINTENANCE OF ANESTHESIA. (See Dosage and Administration.) ALSO, THESE REACTIONS MAY BE REDUCED IF VERBAL, TACTILE AND VISUAL STIMULATION OF THE PATIENT IS MINIMIZED DURING THE RECOVERY PERIOD. THIS DOES NOT PRECLUDE THE MONITORING OF VITAL SIGNS.
IN ORDER TO TERMINATE A SEVERE EMERGENCE REACTION THE USE OF A SMALL HYPNOTIC DOSE OF A SHORT-ACTING OR ULTRASHORT-ACTING BARBITURATE MAY BE REQUIRED.
WHEN KETALAR IS USED ON AN OUTPATIENT BASIS, THE PATIENT SHOULD NOT BE RELEASED UNTIL RECOVERY FROM ANESTHESIA IS COMPLETE AND THEN SHOULD BE ACCOMPANIED BY A RESPONSIBLE ADULT.

DESCRIPTION
Ketalar is a nonbarbiturate anesthetic, chemically designated dl 2-(o-chlorophenyl)-2-(methylamino) cyclohexanone hy- drochloride. It is formulated as a slightly acid (pH 3.5-5.5) sterile solution for intravenous or intramuscular injection in concentrations containing the equivalent of either 10, 50 or 100 mg ketamine base per milliliter and contains not more than 0.1 mg/ml Phemerol® (benzethonium chloride) added as a preservative. The 10 mg/ml solution has been made isotonic with sodium chloride.

CLINICAL PHARMACOLOGY
Ketalar is a rapid-acting general anesthetic producing an anesthetic state characterized by profound analgesia, normal pharyngeal-laryngeal reflexes, normal or slightly enhanced skeletal muscle tone, cardiovascular and respiratory stimulation, and occasionally a transient and minimal respiratory depression.
A patent airway is maintained partly by virtue of unimpaired pharyngeal and laryngeal reflexes. (See Warnings and Precautions.)
The biotransformation of Ketalar includes N-dealkylation (metabolite I), hydroxylation of the cyclohexone ring (metabolites III and IV), conjugation with glucuronic acid and dehydration of the hydroxylated metabolites to form the cyclohexene derivative (metabolite II).
Following intravenous administration, the ketamine concentration has an initial slope (alpha phase) lasting about 45 minutes with a half-life of 10 to 15 minutes. This first phase corresponds clinically to the anesthetic effect of the drug. The anesthetic action is terminated by a combination of redistribution from the CNS to slower equilibrating peripheral tissues and by hepatic biotransformation to metabolite I. This metabolite is about $\frac{1}{3}$ as active as ketamine in reducing halothane requirements (MAC) of the rat. The later half-life of ketamine (beta phase) is 2.5 hours.
The anesthetic state produced by Ketalar has been termed "dissociative anesthesia" in that it appears to selectively interrupt association pathways of the brain before producing somesthetic sensory blockade. It may selectively depress the thalamoneocortical system before significantly obtunding the more ancient cerebral centers and pathways (reticular-activating and limbic systems).
Elevation of blood pressure begins shortly after injection, reaches a maximum within a few minutes and usually returns to preanesthetic values within 15 minutes after injection. In the majority of cases, the systolic and diastolic blood pressure peaks from 10% to 50% above preanesthetic levels shortly after induction of anesthesia, but the elevation can be higher or longer in individual cases (see Contraindications).
Ketamine has a wide margin of safety; several instances of unintentional administration of overdoses of Ketalar (up to ten times that usually required) have been followed by prolonged but complete recovery.
Ketalar has been studied in over 12,000 operative and diagnostic procedures, involving over 10,000 patients from 105 separate studies. During the course of these studies Ketalar was administered as the sole agent, as induction for other general agents, or to supplement low-potency agents.
Specific areas of application have included the following:
1. debridement, painful dressings, and skin grafting in burn patients, as well as other superficial surgical procedures.
2. neurodiagnostic procedures such as pneumoencephalograms, ventriculograms, myelograms, and lumbar punctures. See also Precaution concerning increased intracranial pressure.
3. diagnostic and operative procedures of the eye, ear, nose, and mouth, including dental extractions.
4. diagnostic and operative procedures of the pharynx, larynx, or bronchial tree. NOTE: Muscle relaxants, with proper attention to respiration, may be required (see Precautions).
5. sigmoidoscopy and minor surgery of the anus and rectum, and circumcision.
6. extraperitoneal procedures used in gynecology such as dilatation and curettage.
7. orthopedic procedures such as closed reductions, manipulations, femoral pinning, amputations, and biopsies.
8. as an anesthetic in poor-risk patients with depression of vital functions.
9. in procedures where the intramuscular route of administration is preferred.
10. in cardiac catheterization procedures.
In these studies, the anesthesia was rated either "excellent" or "good" by the anesthesiologist and the surgeon at 90% and 93%, respectively; rated "fair" at 6% and 4%, respectively; and rated "poor" at 4% and 3%, respectively. In a second method of evaluation, the anesthesia was rated "adequate" in at least 90%, and "inadequate" in 10% or less of the procedures.

Table 2   Conversion Table

Euthroid (liotrix tablets, USP)			Natural	Synthetic	
Tablet	T_4*/T_3** mcg	Color	Thyroid USP	T_4*	T_3**
Euthroid-½	(30/7.5)	pale orange	½ grain	0.05 mg	12.5 mcg
Euthroid-1	(60/15)	light brown	1 grain	0.1 mg	25.0 mcg
Euthroid-2	(120/30)	violet	2 grains	0.2 mg	50.0 mcg
Euthroid-3	(180/45)	gray	3 grains	0.3 mg	75.0 mcg

*T_4= levothyroxine sodium (l-thyroxine)   **T_3= liothyronine sodium (l-triiodothyronine)

INDICATIONS AND USAGE

Ketalar is indicated as the sole anesthetic agent for diagnostic and surgical procedures that do not require skeletal muscle relaxation. Ketalar is best suited for short procedures but it can be used, with additional doses, for longer procedures.

Ketalar is indicated for the induction of anesthesia prior to the administration of other general anesthetic agents.

Ketalar is indicated to supplement low-potency agents, such as nitrous oxide.

Specific areas of application are described in the Clinical Pharmacology section.

CONTRAINDICATIONS

Ketamine hydrochloride is contraindicated in those in whom a significant elevation of blood pressure would constitute a serious hazard and in those who have shown hypersensitivity to the drug.

WARNINGS

Cardiac function should be continually monitored during the procedure in patients found to have hypertension or cardiac decompensation.

Postoperative confusional states may occur during the recovery period. (See Special Note.)

Respiratory depression may occur with overdosage or too rapid a rate of administration of Ketalar, in which case supportive ventilation should be employed. Mechanical support of respiration is preferred to administration of analeptics.

PRECAUTIONS

General

Ketalar should be used by or under the direction of physicians experienced in administering general anesthetics and in maintenance of an airway and in the control of respiration.

Because pharyngeal and laryngeal reflexes are usually active, Ketalar should not be used alone in surgery or diagnostic procedures of the pharynx, larynx, or bronchial tree. Mechanical stimulation of the pharynx should be avoided, whenever possible, if Ketalar is used alone. Muscle relaxants, with proper attention to respiration, may be required in both of these instances.

Resuscitative equipment should be ready for use.

The incidence of emergence reactions may be reduced if verbal and tactile stimulation of the patient is minimized during the recovery period. This does not preclude the monitoring of vital signs (see Special Note).

The intravenous dose should be administered over a period of 60 seconds. More rapid administration may result in respiratory depression or apnea and enhanced pressor response.

In surgical procedures involving visceral pain pathways, Ketalar should be supplemented with an agent which obtunds visceral pain.

Use with caution in the chronic alcoholic and the acutely alcohol-intoxicated patient.

An increase in cerebrospinal fluid pressure has been reported following administration of ketamine hydrochloride. Use with extreme caution in patients with preanesthetic elevated cerebrospinal fluid pressure.

Information for Patients

As appropriate, especially in cases where early discharge is possible, the duration of Ketalar and other drugs employed during the conduct of anesthesia should be considered. The patients should be cautioned that driving an automobile, operating hazardous machinery or engaging in hazardous activities should not be undertaken for 24 hours or more (depending upon the dosage of Ketalar and consideration of other drugs employed) after anesthesia.

Drug Interactions

Prolonged recovery time may occur if barbiturates and/or narcotics are used concurrently with Ketalar.

Ketalar is clinically compatible with the commonly used general and local anesthetic agents when an adequate respiratory exchange is maintained.

Usage in Pregnancy

Since the safe use in pregnancy, including obstetrics (either vaginal or abdominal delivery), has not been established, such use is not recommended (see Animal Reproduction).

ADVERSE REACTIONS

Cardiovascular: Blood pressure and pulse rate are frequently elevated following administration of Ketalar alone. However, hypotension and bradycardia have been observed. Arrhythmia has also occurred.

Respiration: Although respiration is frequently stimulated, severe depression of respiration or apnea may occur following rapid intravenous administration of high doses of Ketalar. Laryngospasms and other forms of airway obstruction have occurred during Ketalar anesthesia.

Eye: Diplopia and nystagmus have been noted following Ketalar administration.

It also may cause a slight elevation in intraocular pressure measurement.

Psychological: (See Special Note).

Neurological: In some patients, enhanced skeletal muscle tone may be manifested by tonic and clonic movements sometimes resembling seizures (see Dosage and Administration).

Gastrointestinal: Anorexia, nausea and vomiting have been observed; however this is not usually severe and allows the great majority of patients to take liquids by mouth shortly after regaining consciousness (see Dosage and Administration).

General: Local pain and exanthema at the injection site have infrequently been reported. Transient erythema and/or morbilliform rash have also been reported.

OVERDOSAGE

Respiratory depression may occur with overdosage or too rapid a rate of administration of Ketalar, in which case supportive ventilation should be employed. Mechanical support of respiration is preferred to administration of analeptics.

DOSAGE AND ADMINISTRATION

Note: Barbiturates and Ketalar, being chemically incompatible because of precipitate formation, *should not* be injected from the same syringe.

If the Ketalar dose is augmented with diazepam, the two drugs must be given separately. Do not mix Ketalar and diazepam in syringe or infusion flask. For additional information on the use of diazepam, refer to the Warnings and Dosage and Administration Sections of the diazepam insert.

Preoperative Preparations:

1. While vomiting has been reported following Ketalar administration, some airway protection may be afforded because of active laryngeal-pharyngeal reflexes. However, since aspiration may occur with Ketalar and since protective reflexes may also be diminished by supplementary anesthetics and muscle relaxants, the possibility of aspiration must be considered. Ketalar is recommended for use in the patient whose stomach is not empty when, in the judgment of the practitioner, the benefits of the drug outweigh the possible risks.

2. Atropine, scopolamine, or another drying agent should be given at an appropriate interval prior to induction.

Onset and Duration:

Because of rapid induction following the initial intravenous injection, the patient should be in a supported position during administration.

The onset of action of Ketalar is rapid; an intravenous dose of 2 mg/kg (1 mg/lb) of body weight usually produces surgical anesthesia within 30 seconds after injection, with the anesthetic effect usually lasting five to ten minutes. If a longer effect is desired, additional increments can be administered intravenously or intramuscularly to maintain anesthesia without producing significant cumulative effects.

Intramuscular doses, from experience primarily in children, in a range of 9 to 13 mg/kg (4 to 6 mg/lb) usually produce surgical anesthesia within 3 to 4 minutes following injection, with the anesthetic effect usually lasting 12 to 25 minutes.

Dosage:

As with other general anesthetic agents, the individual response to Ketalar is somewhat varied depending on the dose, route of administration, and age of patient, so that dosage recommendation cannot be absolutely fixed. The drug should be titrated against the patient's requirements.

Induction:

Intravenous Route: The initial dose of Ketalar administered intravenously may range from 1 mg/kg to 4.5 mg/kg (0.5 to 2 mg/lb). The average amount required to produce five to ten minutes of surgical anesthesia has been 2 mg/kg (1 mg/lb).

Alternatively, in adult patients an induction dose of 1.0 mg to 2.0 mg/kg intravenous ketamine at a rate of 0.5 mg/kg/min may be used for induction of anesthesia. In addition, diazepam in 2 mg to 5 mg doses, administered in a separate syringe over 60 seconds, may be used. In most cases, 15.0 mg of intravenous diazepam *or less* will suffice. The incidence of psychological manifestations during emergence, particularly dream-like observations and emergence delirium, may be reduced by this induction dosage program.

Note: The 100 mg/ml concentration of Ketalar *should not* be injected intravenously without proper dilution. It is recommended the drug be diluted with an equal volume of either Sterile Water for Injection, USP, Normal Saline, or 5% Dextrose in Water.

Rate of Administration: It is recommended that Ketalar be administered slowly (over a period of 60 seconds). More rapid administration may result in respiratory depression and enhanced pressor response.

Intramuscular Route: The initial dose of Ketalar administered intramuscularly may range from 6.5 to 13 mg/kg (3 to 6 mg/lb). A dose of 10 mg/kg (5 mg/lb) will usually produce 12 to 25 minutes of surgical anesthesia.

Maintenance of Anesthesia:

The maintenance dose should be adjusted according to the patient's anesthetic needs and whether an additional anesthetic agent is employed.

Increments of one-half to the full induction dose may be repeated as needed for maintenance of anesthesia. However, it should be noted that purposeless and tonic-clonic movements of extremities may occur during the course of anesthesia.

These movements do not imply a light plane and are not indicative of the need for additional doses of the anesthetic. It should be recognized that the larger the total dose of Ketalar administered, the longer will be the time to complete recovery.

Adult patients induced with Ketalar augmented with intravenous diazepam may be maintained on Ketalar given by slow microdrip infusion technique at a dose of 0.1 to 0.5 mg/minute, augmented with diazepam 2 to 5 mg administered intravenously as needed. In many cases 20 mg *or less* of intravenous diazepam total for combined induction and maintenance will suffice. However, slightly more diazepam may be required depending on the nature and duration of the operation, physical status of the patient, and other factors. The incidence of psychological manifestations during emergence, particularly dream-like observations and emergence delirium, may be reduced by this maintenance dosage program.

Dilution: To prepare a dilute solution containing 1 mg of ketamine per ml, aseptically transfer 10 ml (50 mg per ml Steri-Vial) or 5 ml (100 mg per ml Steri-Vial) to 500 ml of 5% Dextrose Injection, USP or Sodium Chloride (0.9%) Injection, USP (Normal Saline) and mix well. The resultant solution will contain 1 mg of ketamine per ml.

The fluid requirements of the patient and duration of anesthesia must be considered when selecting the appropriate dilution of Ketalar. If fluid restriction is required, Ketalar can be added to a 250 ml infusion as described above to provide a Ketalar concentration of 2 mg/ml.

Ketalar Steri-Vials, 10 mg/ml are not recommended for dilution.

Supplementary Agents:

Ketalar is clinically compatible with the commonly used general and local anesthetic agents when an adequate respiratory exchange is maintained.

The regimen of a reduced dose of Ketalar supplemented with diazepam can be used to produce balanced anesthesia by combination with other agents such as nitrous oxide and oxygen.

HOW SUPPLIED

Ketalar is supplied as the hydrochloride in concentrations equivalent to ketamine base.

N 0071-4581-15—Each 50-ml vial contains 10 mg/ml. Supplied in cartons of 10.

N 0071-4581-13—Each 25-ml vial contains 10 mg/ml. Supplied in cartons of 10.

N 0071-4581-12—Each 20-ml vial contains 10 mg/ml. Supplied in cartons of 10.

N 0071-4582-10—Each 10-ml vial contains 50 mg/ml. Supplied in cartons of 10.

N 0071-4585-08—Each 5-ml vial contains 100 mg/ml. Supplied in cartons of 10.

Animal Pharmacology and Toxicology:

Toxicity: The acute toxicity of Ketalar has been studied in several species. In mature mice and rats, the intraperitoneal LD_{50} values are approximately 100 times the average human intravenous dose and approximately 20 times the average human intramuscular dose. A slightly higher acute toxicity observed in neonatal rats was not sufficiently elevated to suggest an increased hazard when used in children. Daily intravenous injections in rats of five times the average human intravenous dose and intramuscular injections in dogs at four times the average human intramuscular dose demonstrated excellent tolerance for as long as 6 weeks. Similarly, twice weekly anesthetic sessions of one, three, or six hours' duration in monkeys over a four-to six-week period were well tolerated.

Interaction With Other Drugs Commonly Used For Preanesthetic Medication: Large doses (three or more times the equivalent effective human dose) of morphine, meperidine, and atropine increased the depth and prolonged the duration of anesthesia produced by a standard anesthetizing dose of Ketalar in Rhesus monkeys. The prolonged duration was not of sufficient magnitude to contraindicate the use of these drugs for preanesthetic medication in human clinical trials.

Blood Pressure: Blood pressure responses to Ketalar vary with the laboratory species and experimental conditions. Blood pressure is increased in normotensive and renal hypertensive rats with and without adrenalectomy and under pentobarbital anesthesia.

Intravenous Ketalar produces a fall in arterial blood pressure in the Rhesus monkey and a rise in arterial blood pressure in the dog. In this respect the dog mimics the cardiovascular effect observed in man. The pressor response to Ketalar injected into intact, unanesthetized dogs is accompanied by a tachycardia, rise in cardiac output and a fall in total

Continued on next page

This product information was prepared in August, 1989. On these and other Parke-Davis Products, information may be obtained by addressing PARKE-DAVIS, Division of Warner-Lambert Company, Morris Plains, New Jersey 07950.

Parke-Davis—Cont.

peripheral resistance. It causes a fall in perfusion pressure following a large dose injected into an artificially perfused vascular bed (dog hindquarters), and it has little or no potentiating effect upon vasoconstriction responses of epinephrine or norepinephrine. The pressor response to Ketalar is reduced or blocked by chlorpromazine (central depressant and peripheral α-adrenergic blockade), by β-adrenergic blockade, and by ganglionic blockade. The tachycardia and increase in myocardial contractile force seen in intact animals does not appear in isolated hearts (Langendorff) at a concentration of 0.1 mg of Ketalar nor in Starling dog heart-lung preparations at a Ketalar concentration of 50 mg/kg of HLP. These observations support the hypothesis that the hypertension produced by Ketalar is due to selective activation of central cardiac stimulating mechanisms leading to an increase in cardiac output. The dog myocardium is not sensitized to epinephrine and Ketalar appears to have a weak antiarrhythmic activity.

Metabolic Disposition: Ketalar is rapidly absorbed following parenteral administration. Animal experiments indicated that Ketalar was rapidly distributed into body tissues, with relatively high concentrations appearing in body fat, liver, lung, and brain; lower concentrations were found in the heart, skeletal muscle, and blood plasma. Placental transfer of the drug was found to occur in pregnant dogs and monkeys. No significant degree of binding to serum albumin was found with Ketalar.

Balance studies in rats, dogs, and monkeys resulted in the recovery of 85% to 95% of the dose in the urine, mainly in the form of degradation products. Small amounts of drug were also excreted in the bile and feces. Balance studies with tritium-labeled Ketalar in human subjects (1 mg/lb given intravenously) resulted in the mean recovery of 91% of the dose in the urine and 3% in the feces. Peak plasma levels averaged about 0.75 μg/ml, and CSF levels were about 0.2 μg/ml, 1 hour after dosing.

Ketalar undergoes N-demethylation and hydroxylation of the cyclohexanone ring, with the formation of water-soluble conjugates which are excreted in the urine. Further oxidation also occurs with the formation of a cyclohexanone derivative. The unconjugated N-demethylated metabolite was found to be less than one-sixth as potent as Ketalar. The unconjugated demethyl cyclohexanone derivative was found to be less than one-tenth as potent as Ketalar. Repeated doses of Ketalar administered to animals did not produce any detectable increase in microsomal enzyme activity.

Reproduction: Male and female rats, when given five times the average human intravenous dose of Ketalar for three consecutive days about one week before mating, had a reproductive performance equivalent to that of saline-injected controls. When given to pregnant rats and rabbits intramuscularly at twice the average human intramuscular dose during the respective periods of organogenesis, the litter characteristics were equivalent to those of saline-injected controls. A small group of rabbits was given a single large dose (six times the average human dose) of Ketalar on Day 6 of pregnancy to simulate the effect of an excessive clinical dose around the period of nidation. The outcome of pregnancy was equivalent in control and treated groups.

To determine the effect of Ketalar on the perinatal and postnatal period, pregnant rats were given twice the average human intramuscular dose during Days 18 to 21 of pregnancy. Litter characteristics at birth and through the weaning period were equivalent to those of the control animals. There was a slight increase in incidence of delayed parturition by one day in treated dams of this group. Three groups each of mated beagle bitches were given 2.5 times the average human intramuscular dose twice weekly for the three weeks of the first, second, and third trimesters of pregnancy, respectively, without the development of adverse effects in the pups.

4581G030

LOESTRIN® 21   ℞
(Norethindrone Acetate and Ethinyl Estradiol Tablets, USP)

LOESTRIN® 21 1/20   ℞
(Each white tablet contains 1 mg norethindrone acetate and 20 mcg ethinyl estradiol.)

LOESTRIN® 21 1.5/30   ℞
(Each green tablet contains 1.5 mg norethindrone acetate and 30 mcg ethinyl estradiol.)

LOESTRIN® Fe   ℞
(Norethindrone Acetate and Ethinyl Estradiol Tablets, USP and Ferrous Fumarate Tablets, USP)

LOESTRIN® Fe 1/20   ℞
(Each white tablet contains 1 mg norethindrone acetate and 20 mcg ethinyl estradiol. Each brown tablet contains 75 mg ferrous fumarate, USP)

LOESTRIN® Fe 1.5/30   ℞
(Each green tablet contains 1.5 mg norethindrone acetate and 30 mcg ethinyl estradiol. Each brown tablet contains 75 mg ferrous fumarate)

Each white tablet contains norethindrone acetate (17 alpha-ethinyl-19-nortestosterone acetate), 1 mg; ethinyl estradiol (17 alpha-ethinyl-1,3,5(10)-estratriene-3,17 beta-diol), 20 mcg. Also contains acacia, NF; lactose, NF; magnesium stearate, NF; starch, NF; confectioner's sugar, NF; talc, USP. Each green tablet contains norethindrone acetate (17 alpha-ethinyl-19-nortestosterone acetate), 1.5 mg; ethinyl estradiol (17 alpha-ethinyl-1,3,5(10)-estratriene-3, 17 beta-diol), 30 mcg. Also contains acacia, NF; lactose, NF; magnesium stearate, NF; starch, NF; confectioner's sugar, NF; talc, USP; D&C yellow No. 10; D&C yellow No. 6; FD&C yellow No. 6; FD&C blue No. 1. Each brown tablet contains microcrystalline cellulose, NF; ferrous fumarate, USP; magnesium stearate, NF; povidone, USP; sodium starch glycolate, NF; sucrose with modified dextrins.

DESCRIPTION

Loestrin **21** and Loestrin **Fe** are progestogen-estrogen combinations.

Loestrin **Fe** 1/20 and 1.5/30: Each provides a continuous dosage regimen consisting of 21 oral contraceptive tablets

and seven ferrous fumarate tablets. The ferrous fumarate tablets are present to facilitate ease of drug administration via a 28-day regimen and are not intended to serve any therapeutic purpose.

CLINICAL PHARMACOLOGY

Combination oral contraceptives act by suppression of gonadotropins. Although the primary mechanism of this action is inhibition of ovulation, other alterations include changes in the cervical mucus (which increase the difficulty of sperm entry into the uterus) and the endometrium (which reduce the likelihood of implantation).

INDICATIONS AND USAGE

Loestrin **21** and Loestrin **Fe** are indicated for the prevention of pregnancy in women who elect to use oral contraceptives as a method of contraception.

Oral contraceptives are highly effective. Table I lists the typical accidental pregnancy rates for users of combination oral contraceptives and other methods of contraception. The efficacy of these contraceptive methods, except sterilization, depends upon the reliability with which they are used. Correct and consistent use of methods can result in lower failure rates.

[See table below].

CONTRAINDICATIONS

Oral contraceptives should not be used in women who currently have the following conditions:

- Thrombophlebitis or thromboembolic disorders
- A past history of deep vein thrombophlebitis or thromboembolic disorders
- Cerebral vascular or coronary artery disease
- Known or suspected carcinoma of the breast
- Carcinoma of the endometrium or other known or suspected estrogen-dependent neoplasia
- Undiagnosed abnormal genital bleeding
- Cholestatic jaundice of pregnancy or jaundice with prior pill use
- Hepatic adenomas or carcinomas
- Known or suspected pregnancy

WARNINGS

> Cigarette smoking increases the risk of serious cardiovascular side effects from oral contraceptive use. This risk increases with age and with heavy smoking (15 or more cigarettes per day) and is quite marked in women over 35 years of age. Women who use oral contraceptives should be strongly advised not to smoke.

The use of oral contraceptives is associated with increased risks of several serious conditions including myocardial infarction, thromboembolism, stroke, hepatic neoplasia, and gallbladder disease, although the risk of serious morbidity or mortality is very small in healthy women without underlying risk factors. The risk of morbidity and mortality increases significantly in the presence of other underlying risk factors such as hypertension, hyperlipidemias, obesity and diabetes.

Practitioners prescribing oral contraceptives should be familiar with the following information relating to these risks. The information contained in this package insert is principally based on studies carried out in patients who used oral contraceptives with higher formulations of estrogens and progestogens than those in common use today. The effect of long-term use of the oral contraceptives with lower formulations of both estrogens and progestogens remains to be determined.

Throughout this labeling, epidemiological studies reported are of two types: retrospective or case control studies and prospective or cohort studies. Case control studies provide a measure of the relative risk of a disease, namely, a *ratio* of the incidence of a disease among oral contraceptive users to that among nonusers. The relative risk does not provide information on the actual clinical occurrence of a disease. Cohort studies provide a measure of attributable risk, which is the *difference* in the incidence of disease between oral contraceptive users and nonusers. The attributable risk does provide information about the actual occurrence of a disease in the population (adapted from refs. 2 and 3 with the author's permission). For further information, the reader is referred to a text on epidemiological methods.

1. Thromboembolic Disorders And Other Vascular Problems.

a. Myocardial infarction

An increased risk of myocardial infarction has been attributed to oral contraceptive use. This risk is primarily in smokers or women with other underlying risk factors for coronary artery disease such as hypertension, hypercholesterolemia, morbid obesity, and diabetes. The relative risk of heart attack for current oral contraceptive users has been estimated to be two to six (4–10). The risk is very low under the age of 30.

Smoking in combination with oral contraceptive use has been shown to contribute substantially to the incidence of myocardial infarctions in women in their mid-thirties or

---

TABLE I
LOWEST EXPECTED AND TYPICAL FAILURE RATES DURING THE FIRST YEAR OF CONTINUOUS USE OF A METHOD
% of Women Experiencing an Accidental Pregnancy in the First Year of Continuous Use

Method	Lowest Expected*	Typical**
(No contraception)	(89)	(89)
Oral contraceptives		3
combined	0.1	N/A***
progestin only	0.5	N/A***
Diaphragm with spermicidal cream or jelly	3	18
Spermicides alone (foam, creams, jellies and vaginal suppositories)	3	21
Vaginal sponge		
nulliparous	5	18
multiparous	>8	>28
IUD (medicated)	1	6†
Condom without spermicides	2	12
Periodic abstinence (all methods)	2–10	20
Female sterilization	0.2	0.4
Male sterilization	0.1	0.15

Adapted from J. Trussell and K. Kost, Table 11, ref. #1.

* The authors' best guess of the percentage of women expected to experience an accidental pregnancy among couples who initiate a method (not necessarily for the first time) and who use it consistently and correctly during the f irst year if they do not stop for any other reason.

** This term represents "typical" couples who initiate use of a method (not necessarily for the first time), who experience an accidental pregnancy during the first year if they do not stop use for any other reason.

*** N/A—Data not available

† Combined typical rate for both medicated and non-medicated IUD. The rate for medicated IUD alone is not available.

older with smoking accounting for the majority of excess cases (11). Mortality rates associated with circulatory disease have been shown to increase substantially in smokers over the age of 35 and nonsmokers over the age of 40 (Table II) among women who use oral contraceptives. [See table above].

Oral contraceptives may compound the effects of well-known risk factors, such as hypertension, diabetes, hyperlipidemias, age and obesity (13). In particular, some progestogens are known to decrease HDL cholesterol and cause glucose intolerance, while estrogens may create a state of hyperinsulinism (14–18). Oral contraceptives have been shown to increase blood pressure among users (see section 9 in WARNINGS). Similar effects on risk factors have been associated with an increased risk of heart disease. Oral contraceptives must be used with caution in women with cardiovascular disease risk factors.

b. Thromboembolism
An increased risk of thromboembolic and thrombotic disease associated with the use of oral contraceptives is well established. Case control studies have found the relative risk of users compared to non-users to be 3 for the first episode of superficial venous thrombosis, 4 to 11 for deep vein thrombosis or pulmonary embolism, and 1.5 to 6 for women with predisposing conditions for venous thromboembolic disease (2,3,19–24). Cohort studies have shown the relative risk to be somewhat lower, about 3 for new cases and about 4.5 for new cases requiring hospitalization (25). The risk of thromboembolic disease due to oral contraceptives is not related to length of use and disappears after pill use is stopped (2). A two- to four-fold increase in relative risk of postoperative thromboembolic complications has been reported with the use of oral contraceptives (9,26). The relative risk of venous thrombosis in women who have predisposing conditions is twice that of women without such medical conditions (9,26). If feasible, oral contraceptives should be discontinued at least four weeks prior to and for two weeks after elective surgery of a type associated with an increase in risk of thromboembolism and during and following prolonged immobilization. Since the immediate post partum period is also associated with an increased risk of thromboembolism, oral contraceptives should be started no earlier than four to six weeks after delivery in women who elect not to breast feed.

c. Cerebrovascular diseases
Oral contraceptives have been shown to increase both the relative and attributable risks of cerebrovascular events (thrombotic and hemorrhagic strokes), although, in general, the risk is greatest among older (> 35 years), hypertensive women who also smoke. Hypertension was found to be a risk factor for both users and non-users, for both types of strokes, while smoking interacted to increase the risk for hemorrhagic strokes (27–29).

In a large study, the relative risk of thrombotic strokes has been shown to range from 3 for normotensive users to 14 for users with severe hypertension (30). The relative risk of hemorrhagic stroke is reported to be 1.2 for non-smokers who used oral contraceptives, 2.6 for smokers who did not use oral contraceptives, 7.6 for smokers who used oral contraceptives, 1.8 for normotensive users and 25.7 for users with severe hypertension (30). The attributable risk is also greater in older women (3).

d. Dose-related risk of vascular disease from oral contraceptives
A positive association has been observed between the amount of estrogen and progestogen in oral contraceptives and the risk of vascular disease. (31–33). A decline in serum high density lipoproteins (HDL) has been reported with many progestational agents (14–16). A decline in serum high density lipoproteins has been associated with an increased incidence of ischemic heart disease. Because estrogens increase HDL cholesterol, the net effect of an oral contraceptive depends on a balance achieved between doses of estrogen and progestogen and the nature and absolute amount of progestogens used in the contraceptives. The amount of both hormones should be considered in the choice of an oral contraceptive.

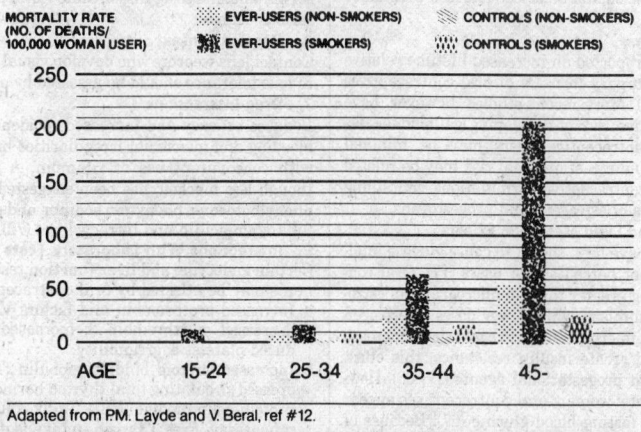

TABLE II
CIRCULATORY DISEASE MORTALITY RATES PER 100,000
WOMAN YEARS BY AGE, SMOKING STATUS AND ORAL CONTRACEPTIVE USE

MORTALITY RATE (NO. OF DEATHS/ 100,000 WOMAN USER)

EVER-USERS (NON-SMOKERS)   CONTROLS (NON-SMOKERS)
EVER-USERS (SMOKERS)   CONTROLS (SMOKERS)

AGE   15-24   25-34   35-44   45-

Adapted from P.M. Layde and V. Beral, ref #12.

Minimizing exposure to estrogen and progestogen is in keeping with good principles of therapeutics. For any particular estrogen/progestogen combination, the dosage regimen prescribed should be one which contains the least amount of estrogen and progestogen that is compatible with a low failure rate and the needs of the individual patient. New acceptors of oral contraceptive agents should be started on preparations containing the lowest dose of estrogen which produces satisfactory results for the patient.

e. Persistence of risk of vascular disease
There are two studies which have shown persistence of risk of vascular disease for ever users of oral contraceptives. In a study in the United States, the risk of developing myocardial infarction after discontinuing oral contraceptives persists for at least 9 years for women 40–49 years who had used oral contraceptives for 5 or more years, but this increased risk was not demonstrated in other age groups (8). In another study in Great Britain, the risk of developing cerebrovascular disease persisted for at least 6 years after discontinuation of oral contraceptives, although excess risk was very small (34). However, both studies were performed with oral contraceptive formulations containing 50 micrograms or higher of estrogens.

2. Estimates Of Mortality From Contraceptive Use
One study gathered data from a variety of sources which have estimated the mortality rate associated with different methods of contraception at different ages (Table III). These estimates include the combined risk of death associated with contraceptive methods plus the risk attributable to pregnancy in the event of method failure. Each method of contraception has its specific benefits and risks. The study concluded that with the exception of oral contraceptive users 35 and older who smoke and 40 and older who do not smoke, mortality associated with all methods of birth control is low and below that associated with childbirth. However, smokers 35 and older and non-smokers 40 and older who use oral contraceptives have an increase in mortality higher than those using other methods of birth control. These facts must be weighed in conjunction with failure rates for other methods and the risk associated with subsequent pregnancy.

[See Table I preceding page]

3. Carcinoma Of The Reproductive Organs
Numerous epidemiological studies have been performed on the incidence of breast, endometrial, ovarian and cervical cancer in women using oral contraceptives. The overwhelming evidence in the literature suggests that use of oral contraceptives is not associated with an increase in the risk of

developing breast cancer, regardless of the age and parity of first use or with most of the marketed brands and doses (36, 38). The Cancer and Steroid Hormone (CASH) study (36) also showed no latent effect on the risk of breast cancer for at least a decade following long-term use. A few studies have shown a slightly increased relative risk of developing breast cancer (37, 39–41), although the methodology of these studies, which included differences in examination of users and nonusers and differences in age at start of use, has been questioned (41–43).

Some studies suggest that oral contraceptive use has been associated with an increase in the risk of cervical intraepithelial neoplasia in some populations of women (45–48). However, there continues to be controversy about the extent to which such findings may be due to differences in sexual behavior and other factors.

In spite of many studies of the relationship between oral contraceptive use and breast and cervical cancers, a cause and effect relationship has not been established.

4. Hepatic Neoplasia
Benign hepatic adenomas are associated with oral contraceptive use, although the incidence of benign tumors is rare in the United States. Indirect calculations have estimated the attributable risk to be in the range of 3.3 cases/100,000 for users, a risk that increases after four or more years of use (49). Rupture of rare, benign, hepatic adenomas may cause death through intra-abdominal hemorrhage (50,51).

Studies from Britain have shown an increased risk of developing hepatocellular carcinoma (52–54) in long-term (> 8 years) oral contraceptive users. However, these cancers are extremely rare in the U.S., and the attributable risk (the excess incidence) of liver cancers in oral contraceptive users approaches less than one per million users.

5. Ocular Lesions
There have been clinical case reports of retinal thrombosis associated with the use of oral contraceptives. Oral contraceptives should be discontinued if there is unexplained partial or complete loss of vision; onset of proptosis or diplopia; papilledema; or retinal vascular lesions. Appropriate diagnostic and therapeutic measures should be undertaken immediately.

6. Oral Contraceptive Use Before Or During Early Pregnancy: Risk Of Birth Defects
Extensive epidemiological studies have revealed no increased risk of birth defects in women who have used oral contraceptives prior to pregnancy (55–57). Studies also do not suggest a teratogenic effect, particularly insofar as cardiac anomalies and limb reduction defects are concerned (55,56,58,59), when taken inadvertently during early pregnancy.

The administration of oral contraceptives to induce withdrawal bleeding should not be used as a test for pregnancy. Oral contraceptives should not be used during pregnancy to treat threatened or habitual abortion.

It is recommended that for any patient who has missed two consecutive periods, pregnancy should be ruled out before continuing oral contraceptive use. If the patient has not adhered to the prescribed schedule, the possibility of pregnancy

Continued on next page

TABLE III
ANNUAL NUMBER OF BIRTH-RELATED OR METHOD-RELATED DEATHS
ASSOCIATED WITH CONTROL OF FERTILITY PER 100,000 NONSTERILE
WOMEN, BY FERTILITY CONTROL METHOD ACCORDING TO AGE

Method of control and outcome	15–19	20–24	25–29	30–34	35–39	40–44
No fertility control methods*	7.0	7.4	9.1	14.8	25.7	28.2
Oral contraceptives non-smoker**	0.3	0.5	0.9	1.9	13.8	31.6
Oral contraceptives smoker**	2.2	3.4	6.6	13.5	51.1	117.2
IUD**	0.8	0.8	1.0	1.0	1.4	1.4
Condom*	1.1	1.6	0.7	0.2	0.3	0.4
Diaphragm/spermicide*	1.9	1.2	1.2	1.3	2.2	2.8
Periodic abstinence*	2.5	1.6	1.6	1.7	2.9	3.6

* Deaths are birth related
** Deaths are method related

Adapted from HW Ory, ref. #35.

This product information was prepared in August, 1989. On these and other Parke-Davis Products, information may be obtained by addressing PARKE-DAVIS, Division of Warner-Lambert Company, Morris Plains, New Jersey 07950.

Parke-Davis—Cont.

should be considered at the time of the first missed period. Oral contraceptive use should be discontinued if pregnancy is confirmed.

7. Gallbladder Disease

Earlier studies have reported an increased lifetime relative risk of gallbladder surgery in users of oral contraceptives and estrogens (60,61). More recent studies, however, have shown that the relative risk of developing gallbladder disease among oral contraceptive users may be minimal (62–64). The recent findings of minimal risk may be related to the use of oral contraceptive formulations containing lower hormonal doses of estrogens and progestogens.

8. Carbohydrate And Lipid Metabolic Effects

Oral contraceptives have been shown to cause glucose intolerance in a significant percentage of users (17). Oral contraceptives containing greater than 75 micrograms of estrogens cause hyperinsulinism, while lower doses of estrogen cause less glucose intolerance (65). Progestogens increase insulin secretion and create insulin resistance, this effect varying with different progestational agents (17, 66). However, in the non-diabetic woman, oral contraceptives appear to have no effect on fasting blood glucose (67). Because of these demonstrated effects, prediabetic and diabetic women should be carefully observed while taking oral contraceptives.

A small proportion of women will have persistent hypertriglyceridemia while on the pill. As discussed earlier (see WARNINGS 1a. and 1d.), changes in serum triglycerides and lipoprotein levels have been reported in oral contraceptive users.

9. Elevated Blood Pressure

An increase in blood pressure has been reported in women taking oral contraceptives (68) and this increase is more likely in older oral contraceptive users (69) and with continued use (68). Data from the Royal College of General Practitioners (12) and subsequent randomized trials have shown that the incidence of hypertension increases with increasing concentrations of progestogens.

Women with a history of hypertension or hypertension-related diseases, or renal disease (70) should be encouraged to use another method of contraception. If women elect to use oral contraceptives, they should be monitored closely and if significant elevation of blood pressure occurs, oral contraceptives should be discontinued. For most women, elevated blood pressure will return to normal after stopping oral contraceptives (69), and there is no difference in the occurrence of hypertension among ever and never users (68,70,71).

10. Headache

The onset or exacerbation of migraine or development of headache of a new pattern which is recurrent, persistent or severe requires discontinuation of oral contraceptives and evaluation of the cause.

11. Bleeding Irregularities

Breakthrough bleeding and spotting are sometimes encountered in patients on oral contraceptives, especially during the first three months of use. Non-hormonal causes should be considered and adequate diagnostic measures taken to rule out malignancy or pregnancy in the event of breakthrough bleeding, as in the case of any abnormal vaginal bleeding. If pathology has been excluded, time or a change to another formulation may solve the problem. In the event of amenorrhea, pregnancy should be ruled out.

Some women may encounter post-pill amenorrhea or oligomenorrhea, especially when such a condition was preexistent.

PRECAUTIONS

1. Physical Examination And Follow Up

A complete medical history and physical examination should be taken prior to the initiation or reinstitution of oral contraceptives and at least annually during use of oral contraceptives. These physical examinations should include special reference to blood pressure, breasts, abdomen and pelvic organs, including cervical cytology, and relevant laboratory tests. In case of undiagnosed, persistent or recurrent abnormal vaginal bleeding, appropriate diagnostic measures should be conducted to rule out malignancy. Women with a strong family history of breast cancer or who have breast nodules should be monitored with particular care.

2. Lipid Disorders

Women who are being treated for hyperlipidemias should be followed closely if they elect to use oral contraceptives. Some progestogens may elevate LDL levels and may render the control of hyperlipidemias more difficult.

3. Liver Function

If jaundice develops in any woman receiving such drugs, the medication should be discontinued. Steroid hormones may be poorly metabolized in patients with impaired liver function.

4. Fluid Retention

Oral contraceptives may cause some degree of fluid retention. They should be prescribed with caution, and only with careful monitoring, in patients with conditions which might be aggravated by fluid retention.

5. Emotional Disorders

Women with a history of depression should be carefully observed and the drug discontinued if depression recurs to a serious degree.

6. Contact Lenses

Contact lens wearers who develop visual changes or changes in lens tolerance should be assessed by an ophthalmologist.

7. Drug Interactions

Reduced efficacy and increased incidence of breakthrough bleeding and menstrual irregularities have been associated with concomitant use of rifampin. A similar association though less marked, has been suggested with barbiturates, phenylbutazone, phenytoin sodium, and possibly with griseofulvin, ampicillin and tetracyclines (72).

8. Interactions With Laboratory Tests

Certain endocrine and liver function tests and blood components may be affected by oral contraceptives:

a. Increased prothrombin and factors VII, VIII, IX, and X; decreased antithrombin 3; increased norepinephrine-induced platelet aggregability.

b. Increased thyroid binding globulin (TBG) leading to increased circulating total thyroid hormone, as measured by protein-bound iodine (PBI), T4 by column, or by radioimmunoassay. Free T3 resin uptake is decreased, reflecting the elevated TBG; free T4 concentration is unaltered.

c. Other binding proteins may be elevated in serum.

d. Sex-binding globulins are increased and result in elevated levels of total circulating sex steroids and corticoids; however, free or biologically active levels remain unchanged.

e. Triglycerides may be increased.

f. Glucose tolerance may be decreased.

g. Serum folate levels may be depressed by oral contraceptive therapy. This may be of clinical significance if a woman becomes pregnant shortly after discontinuing oral contraceptives.

9. Carcinogenesis

See WARNINGS section.

10. Pregnancy

Pregnancy Category X. See CONTRAINDICATIONS and WARNINGS sections.

11. Nursing Mothers

Small amounts of oral contraceptive steroids have been identified in the milk of nursing mothers and a few adverse effects on the child have been reported, including jaundice and breast enlargement. In addition, oral contraceptives given in the postpartum period may interfere with lactation by decreasing the quantity and quality of breast milk. If possible, the nursing mother should be advised not to use oral contraceptives but to use other forms of contraception until she has completely weaned her child.

INFORMATION FOR THE PATIENT

See patient labeling printed below.

ADVERSE REACTIONS

An increased risk of the following serious adverse reactions has been associated with the use of oral contraceptives (see WARNINGS section).

- Thrombophlebitis
- Arterial thromboembolism
- Pulmonary embolism
- Myocardial infarction
- Cerebral hemorrhage
- Cerebral thrombosis
- Hypertension
- Gallbladder disease
- Hepatic adenomas or benign liver tumors

There is evidence of an association between the following conditions and the use of oral contraceptives, although additional confirmatory studies are needed:

- Mesenteric thrombosis
- Retinal thrombosis

The following adverse reactions have been reported in patients receiving oral contraceptives and are believed to be drug related:

- Nausea
- Vomiting
- Gastrointestinal symptoms (such as abdominal cramps and bloating)
- Breakthrough bleeding
- Spotting
- Change in menstrual flow
- Amenorrhea
- Temporary infertility after discontinuation of treatment
- Edema
- Melasma which may persist
- Breast changes: tenderness, enlargement, secretion
- Change in weight (increase or decrease)
- Change in cervical erosion and secretion
- Diminution in lactation when given immediately postpartum
- Cholestatic jaundice
- Migraine
- Rash (allergic)

- Mental depression
- Reduced tolerance to carbohydrates
- Vaginal candidiasis
- Change in corneal curvature (steepening)
- Intolerance to contact lenses

The following adverse reactions have been reported in users of oral contraceptives and the association has been neither confirmed nor refuted:

- Pre-menstrual syndrome
- Cataracts
- Changes in appetite
- Cystitis-like syndrome
- Headache
- Nervousness
- Dizziness
- Hirsutism
- Loss of scalp hair
- Erythema multiforme
- Erythema nodosum
- Hemorrhagic eruption
- Vaginitis
- Porphyria
- Impaired renal function
- Hemolytic uremic syndrome
- Budd-Chiari syndrome
- Acne
- Changes in libido
- Colitis

While the following adverse reactions or conditions have been reported to be associated with the use of oral contraceptives, no causal relationship has been established:

- Congenital anomalies
- Raynaud's disease
- Sickle cell disease
- Mitral valve prolapse
- Increased risk of developing venous thromboembolic disease among women with blood types A, B, or AB, as opposed to women with blood type O.

OVERDOSAGE

Serious ill effects have not been reported following acute ingestion of large doses of oral contraceptives by young children. Overdosage may cause nausea, and withdrawal bleeding may occur in females.

NON-CONTRACEPTIVE HEALTH BENEFITS

The following non-contraceptive health benefits related to the use of oral contraceptives are supported by epidemiological studies which largely utilized oral contraceptive formulations containing estrogen doses exceeding 0.05 mg of estrogen (73–78).

Effects on menses:
- Increased menstrual cycle regularity
- Decreased blood loss and decreased incidence of iron deficiency anemia
- Decreased incidence of dysmenorrhea

Effects related to inhibition of ovulation:
- Decreased incidence of functional ovarian cysts
- Decreased incidence of ectopic pregnancies

Effects from long-term use:
- Decreased incidence of fibroadenomas and fibrocystic disease of the breast
- Decreased incidence of acute pelvic inflammatory disease
- Decreased incidence of endometrial cancer
- Decreased incidence of ovarian cancer

DOSAGE AND ADMINISTRATION

The tablet dispenser has been designed to make oral contraceptive dosing as easy and as convenient as possible. The tablets are arranged in either three or four rows of seven tablets each, with the days of the week appearing on the tablet dispenser above the first row of tablets.

Important Notes: The patient should be instructed to use an additional method of protection until after the first week of administration in the initial cycle if utilizing the Sunday-Start Regimen.

The possibility of ovulation and conception prior to initiation of use should be considered.

Dosage And Administration For 21-Day Dosage Regimen

To achieve maximum contraceptive effectiveness, Loestrin 21 must be taken exactly as directed and at intervals not exceeding 24 hours. Loestrin 21 provides the patient with a convenient tablet schedule of "3 weeks on—1 week off." Two dosage regimens are described, one of which may be more convenient or suitable than the other for an individual patient. For the initial cycle of therapy, the patient begins her tablets according to the Day-5 or Sunday-Start Regimen. With either regimen, the patient takes one tablet daily for 21 consecutive days followed by one week of no tablets.

A. Sunday-Start Regimen: The patient begins taking tablets from the top row on the first Sunday after menstrual flow begins. When menstrual flow begins on Sunday, the first tablet is taken on the same day. The last tablet in the dispenser will then be taken on a Saturday, followed by no tablets for a week (7 days). For all subsequent cycles the patient then begins a new 21-tablet regimen on the eighth day, Sunday, after taking her last tablet. Following this regimen, of 21 days on—7 days off, the patient will start all subsequent cycles on a Sunday.

B. Day-5 Regimen: The first day of menstrual flow is Day 1. On Day 5 of her menstrual flow, the patient starts taking 1 tablet daily, beginning with the tablet in the top row that corresponds to Day 5 of her flow. After the last tablet (Saturday) has been taken, if any tablets remain in the top row, the patient completes her 21-tablet regimen starting with the Sunday tablet in the top row, followed by no tablets for a week (7 days). For all subsequent cycles, the patient begins a new 21 tablet regimen on the eighth day after taking her last tablet, again beginning on the same day of the week on which she began her first course. Following this regimen of 21 days on—7 days off, the patient will start all subsequent cycles on the same day of the week as the first course. Likewise, the interval of no tablets will always start on the same day of the week.

Whether utilizing the Sunday-Start or Day-5 Regimen, all tablets should be taken regularly with a meal or at bedtime. It should be stressed that efficacy of medication depends on strict adherence to the dosage schedule.

Special Notes on Administration
Menstruation usually begins two or three days, but may begin as late as the fourth or fifth day, after discontinuing medication. Because of the relatively low estrogenic content, Loestrin 21 is not a good cyclic regulator. There are patients whose inherent hormone balance will require larger amounts of estrogen to achieve cyclic regularity than that contained in Loestrin 21. These patients experience altered bleeding patterns, which do not conform to treatment schedules, while taking Loestrin 21 tablets. However, it is important that patients adhere to the dosage schedule regardless of when bleeding occurs.

The occurrence of altered bleeding is highest in Cycle 1. The majority of patients will have seven days or less of total bleeding during the 28-day cycle (including both withdrawal bleeding and breakthrough bleeding and spotting). Should irregular bleeding occur, patients should be reassured and instructed to continue taking the tablets as directed. If by the third cycle the irregular patterns are unacceptable, consideration should be given to changing the medication to a product with a higher estrogen content (Norlestrin* 21 1/50 or Norlestrin 21 2.5/50). The physician should be alert to the fact that the irregular bleeding patterns could mask an organic cause, and appropriate diagnostic measures should be taken if the bleeding persists or continues after changing to a higher estrogen-content product.

If a patient forgets to take one or more tablets, the following is suggested: If one tablet is missed, take it as soon as remembered, or take two tablets the next day. If two consecutive tablets are missed, take two tablets daily for the next two days, then resume the regular schedule. While there is little likelihood of pregnancy occurring if the patient misses only one or two tablets, the possibility of pregnancy increases with each successive day that tablets are missed. *However if the patient is taking Loestrin 21 1/20, in addition to taking two white tablets a day for two days, the patient should use an additional means of contraception for seven consecutive days.* If three consecutive tablets are missed, the patient starts a new course of tablets in the following manner: If the patient is on the Sunday-Start Regimen, a new course of tablets is started on the first Sunday following the last missed tablet, whether or not she is still menstruating. If the patient is on the Day 5-Regimen, a new course of tablets is started on the eighth day after the last tablet was taken. For example, if the patient took her last tablet on Monday, she should start her new course of tablets the following Monday. The patient should also use an additional method of birth control during the seven days without tablets, and until she has taken a tablet daily for seven consecutive days.

The possibility of ovulation occurring increases with each successive day that scheduled tablets are missed. While there is little likelihood of ovulation occurring if only one tablet is missed, the possibility of spotting or bleeding is increased. This is particularly likely to occur if two or more consecutive tablets are missed.

---

*Norlestrin (Norethindrone Acetate and Ethinyl Estradiol Tablets, USP)

Dosage And Administration For 28-Day Dosage Regimen
To achieve maximum contraceptive effectiveness, Loestrin Fe must be taken exactly as directed and at intervals not exceeding 24 hours.

Loestrin Fe provides a continuous administration regimen consisting of 21 light-colored (white or green) tablets of Loestrin and 7 brown tablets of ferrous fumarate. The ferrous fumarate tablets are present to facilitate ease of drug administration via a 28-day regimen and do not serve any therapeutic purpose. There is no need for the patient to count days between cycles because there are no "off-tablet days."

The patient begins taking light-colored tablets from the top row on the first Sunday after menstrual flow begins. When menstrual flow begins on Sunday, the first light-colored tablet is taken on the same day. The patient takes one light-colored tablet daily for 21 days. The last light-colored tablet taken is the Saturday tablet. Upon completion of all 21 tab-

lets, and without interruption, the patient takes one *brown* tablet daily for 7 days. Upon completion of this first course of tablets, the patient begins a second course of 28 tablets without interruption, the next day, Sunday, starting with the Sunday *light-colored* tablet in the top row. Adhering to this regimen, of one *light-colored* tablet daily for 21 days, followed without interruption by one *brown* tablet daily for seven days, the patient will start all subsequent cycles on a Sunday.

Tablets should be taken regularly with a meal or at bedtime. It should be stressed that efficacy of medication depends on strict adherence to the dosage schedule.

Special Notes on Administration
Menstruation usually begins two or three days, but may begin as late as the fourth or fifth day, after the *brown* tablets have been started. Because of the relatively low estrogenic content, Loestrin Fe is not a good cyclic regulator. There are patients whose inherent hormone balance will require larger amounts of estrogen to achieve cyclic regularity than that contained in Loestrin Fe. These patients experience altered bleeding patterns, which do not conform to treatment schedules, while taking the *light-colored* Loestrin Fe tablets. However, it is important that patients adhere to the dosage schedule regardless of when bleeding occurs.

The occurrence of altered bleeding is highest in Cycle 1. The majority of patients will have seven days or less of total bleeding during the 28-day cycle (including both withdrawal bleeding and breakthrough bleeding and spotting). Should irregular bleeding occur, patients should be reassured and instructed to continue taking the tablets as directed. If by the third cycle the irregular patterns are unacceptable, consideration should be given to changing the medication to a product with a higher estrogen content (Norlestrin* Fe 1/50 or Norlestrin Fe 2.5/50). The physician should be alert to the fact that the irregular bleeding patterns could mask bleeding from organic causes, and appropriate diagnostic measures should be taken if the bleeding persists or continues after changing to a higher estrogen-content product.

If a patient forgets to take one or more *light-colored* tablets, the following is suggested. If one *light-colored* tablet is missed, take it as soon as remembered, or take two *light-colored* tablets the next day. If two consecutive *light-colored* tablets are missed, take two *light-colored* tablets daily for the next two days, then resume the regular schedule. While there is little likelihood of pregnancy occurring if the patient misses only one or two *light-colored* tablets, the possibility of pregnancy increases with each successive day that *light-colored* tablets are missed. *However, if the patient is taking Loestrin Fe 1/20, in addition to taking two white tablets a day for two days, the patient should use an additional means of contraception for seven consecutive days.* If three consecutive *light-colored* tablets are missed, the patient starts a new course of tablets the first Sunday following the last missed tablet, whether or not she is still menstruating. The patient should also use an additional method of birth control during the days without tablets, and until she has taken a tablet for seven consecutive days.

The possibility of ovulation occurring increases with each successive day that scheduled *light-colored* tablets are missed. While there is little likelihood of ovulation occurring if only one *light-colored* tablet is missed, the possibility of spotting or bleeding is increased. This is particularly likely to occur if two or more consecutive *light-colored* tablets are missed.

If one or more *brown* tablets are missed, the *light-colored* tablets should be started no later than the eighth day after the last *light-colored* tablet was taken. The possibility of conception occurring is not increased if *brown* tablets are missed.

---

*Norlestrin (Norethindrone Acetate and Ethinyl Estradiol Tablets, USP)

Use Of Oral Contraceptives In The Event Of A Missed Menstrual Period
1. If the patient has not adhered to the prescribed dosage regimen, the possibility of pregnancy should be considered after the first missed period and oral contraceptives should be withheld until pregnancy has been ruled out.
2. If the patient has adhered to the prescribed regimen and misses two consecutive periods, pregnancy should be ruled out before continuing the contraceptive regimen.

After several months on treatment, bleeding may be reduced to a point of virtual absence. This reduced flow may occur as a result of medication, in which event it is not indicative of pregnancy.

HOW SUPPLIED
Loestrin 21 1/20 is available in dispensers each containing 21 tablets. Each tablet contains 1 mg of norethindrone acetate and 20 mcg of ethinyl estradiol. Available in packages of five dispensers.

Loestrin Fe 1/20 is available in dispensers each containing 21 white tablets and 7 brown tablets. Each white tablet contains 1 mg of norethindrone acetate and 20 mcg of ethinyl estradiol. Each brown tablet contains 75 mg ferrous fumarate. Available in packages of five dispensers.

Loestrin 21 1.5/30 is available in dispensers each containing 21 tablets. Each tablet contains 1.5 mg of norethindrone acetate and 30 mcg of ethinyl estradiol. Available in packages of five dispensers.

Loestrin Fe 1.5/30 is available in dispensers each containing 21 green tablets and 7 brown tablets. Each green tablet contains 1.5 mg of norethindrone acetate and 30 mcg of ethinyl estradiol. Each brown tablet contains 75 mg ferrous fumarate. Available in packages of five dispensers.

REFERENCES
1. Reproduced with permission of the Population Council from J. Trussell and K. Kost: Contraceptive failure in the United States: A critical review of the literature. *Studies in Family Planning*, 18 (5), September–October 1987.
2. Stadel, BV: Oral contraceptives and cardiovascular disease. (Pt. 1). *New England Journal of Medicine*, 305:612–618, 1981.
3. Stadel, B.V.: Oral contraceptives and cardiovascular disease. (Pt. 2.). *New England Journal of Medicine*, 305:672–677, 1981.
4. Adam, S.A., and M. Thorogood: Oral contraception and myocardial infarction revisited: The effects of new preparations and prescribing patterns. *Brit. J. Obstet. and Gynec.*, 88:838–845, 1981.
5. Mann, J.I., and W.H. Inman: Oral contraceptives and death from myocardial infarction. *Brit. Med. J.*, 2(5965): 245–248, 1975.
6. Mann, J.I., M.P. Vessey, M. Thorogood, and R. Doll: Myocardial infarction in young women with special reference to oral contraceptive practice. *Brit. Med. J.*, 2(5956):241–245, 1975.
7. Royal College of General Practitioners' Oral Contraception Study: Further analyses of mortality in oral contraceptive users.———1:541–546, 1981.
8. Slone, D., S. Shapiro, D.W. Kaufman, L. Rosenberg, O.S. Miettinen, and P.D. Stolley: Risk of myocardial infarction in relation to current and discontinued use of oral contraceptives. *N.E.J.M.*, 305:420–424, 1981.
9. Vessey, M.P.: Female hormones and vascular disease: An epidemiological overview, *Brit. J. Fam. Plann.*, 6:1–12, 1980.
10. Russell-Brief, R.G., T.M. Ezzati, R. Fulwood, J.A. Perlman, and R.S. Murphy: Cardiovascular risk status and oral contraceptive use, United States, 1976–80. *Preventive Medicine*, 15:352–362, 1986.
11. Goldbaum, G.M., J.S. Kendrick, G.C. Hogelin, and E.M. Gentry: The relative impact of smoking and oral contraceptive use on women in the United States. *J.A.M.A.*, 258:1339–1342, 1987.
12. Layde, P.M., and V. Beral: Further analyses of mortality in oral contraceptive users: Royal College General Practitioners' Oral Contraception Study. (Table 5) *Lancet*, 1:541–546, 1981.
13. Knopp, R.H.: Arteriosclerosis risk: The roles of oral contraceptives and postmenopausal estrogens. *J. of Reprod. Med.*, 31(9)(Supplement): 913–921, 1986.
14. Krauss, R.M., S. Roy, D.R. Mishell, J. Casagrande, and M.C. Pike: Effects of two low-dose oral contraceptives on serum lipids and lipoproteins: Differential changes in high-density lipoproteins subclasses. *Am. J. Obstet. Gyn.*, 145:446–452, 1983.
15. Wahl, P., C. Walden, R. Knopp, J. Hoover, R. Wallace, G. Heiss, and B. Rifkind: Effect of estrogen/progestin potency on lipid/lipoprotein cholesterol, *N.E.J.M.*, 308:862–867, 1983.
16. Wynn, V., and R. Niththyananthan: The effect of progestin in combined oral contraceptives on serum lipids with special reference to high-density lipoproteins. *Am. J. Obstet. and Gyn.*, 142:766–771, 1982.
17. Wynn, V., and I. Godsland: Effects of oral contraceptives on carbohydrate metabolism. *J. Reprod. Medicine*, 31(9)(Supplement): 892–897, 1986.
18. LaRosa, J.C.: Atherosclerotic risk factors in cardiovascular disease. *J. Reprod. Med.*, 31(9)(Supplement): 906–912, 1986.
19. Inman, W.H., and M.P. Vessey: Investigations of death from pulmonary, coronary, and cerebral thrombosis and embolism in women of child-bearing age. *Brit. Med. J.*, 2(5599): 193–199, 1968.
20. Maguire, M.G., J. Tonascia, P.E. Sartwell, P.D. Stolley, and M.S. Tockman: Increased risk of thrombosis due to oral contraceptives: A further report. *Am. J. Epidemiology*, 110(2):188–195, 1979.
21. Pettiti, D.B., J. Wingerd, F. Pellegrin, and S. Ramacharan: Risk of vascular disease in women: Smoking, oral

Continued on next page

This product information was prepared in August, 1989. On these and other Parke-Davis Products, information may be obtained by addressing PARKE-DAVIS, Division of Warner-Lambert Company, Morris Plains, New Jersey 07950.

Parke-Davis—Cont.

contraceptives, noncontraceptive estrogens, and other factors, *J.A.M.A.*, 242:1150–1154, 1979.

22. Vessey, M.P., and R. Doll: Investigation of relation between use of oral contraceptives and thromboembolic disease. *Brit. Med. J.*, 2(5599): 199–205, 1968.

23. Vessey, M.P., and R. Doll: Investigation of relation between use of oral contraceptives and thromboembolic disease: A further report. *Brit. Med. J.*, 2(5658): 651–657, 1969.

24. Porter, J.B., J.R. Hunter, D.A. Danielson, H. Jick, and A. Stergachis: Oral contraceptives and non-fatal vascular disease: Recent experience. *Obstet. and Gyn.*, 59(3):299–302, 1982.

25. Vessey, M., R. Doll, R. Peto, B. Johnson, and P. Wiggins: A long-term follow-up study of women using different methods of contraception: An interim report. *J. Biosocial. Sci.*, 8:375–427, 1976.

26. Royal College of General Practitioners: Oral contraceptives, venous thrombosis, and varicose veins. *J. of Royal College of General Practitioners*, 28:393–399, 1978.

27. Collaborative Group for the study of stroke in young women: Oral contraception and increased risk of cerebral ischemia or thrombosis. *N.E.J.M.*, 288:871–878, 1973.

28. Petitti, D.B., and J. Wingerd: Use of oral contraceptives, cigarette smoking, and risk of subarachnoid hemorrhage. *Lancet*, 2:234–236, 1978.

29. Inman, W.H.: Oral contraceptives and fatal subarachnoid hemorrhage. *Brit. Med. J.*, 2(6203): 1468–70, 1979.

30. Collaborative Group for the study of stroke in young women: Oral contraceptives and stroke in young women: Associated risk factors. *J.A.M.A.*, 231:718–722, 1975.

31. Inman, W.H., M.P. Vessey, B. Westerholm, and A. Engelund: Thromboembolic disease and the steroidal content of oral contraceptives. A report to the Committee on Safety of Drugs. *Brit. Med. J.*, 2:203–209, 1970.

32. Meade, T.W., G. Greenberg, and S.G. Thompson: Progestogens and cardiovascular reactions associated with oral contraceptives and a comparison of the safety of 50- and 35-mcg oestrogen preparations. *Brit. Med. J.*, 280(6224): 1157–1161, 1980.

33. Kay, C.R.: Progestogens and arterial disease: Evidence from the Royal College of General Practitioners' study. *Amer. J. Obstet. Gyn.*, 142:762–765, 1982.

34. Royal College of General Practitioners: Incidence of arterial disease among oral contraceptive users. *J. Coll. Gen. Pract.*, 33:75–82, 1983.

35. Ory, H.W.: Mortality associated with fertility and fertility control: 1983. *Family Planning Perspectives*, 15:50–56, 1983.

36. The Cancer and Steroid Hormone Study of the Centers for Disease Control and the National Institute of Child Health and Human Development: Oral-contraceptive use and the risk of breast cancer. *N.E.J.M.*, 315:405–411, 1986.

37. Pike, M.C., B.E. Henderson, M.D. Krailo, A. Duke, and S. Roy: Breast cancer in young women and use of oral contraceptives: Possible modifying effect of formulation and age at use. *Lancet*, 2:926–929. 1983.

38. Paul, C., D.G. Skegg, G.F.S. Spears, and J.M. Kaldor: Oral contraceptives and breast cancer: A national study. *Brit. Med. J.*, 293:723–725, 1986.

39. Miller, D.R., L. Rosenberg, D.W. Kaufman, D. Schottenfeld, P.D. Stolley, and S. Shapiro: Breast cancer risk in relation to early oral contraceptive use. *Obstet. Gynec.*, 68:863–868, 1986.

40. Olson, H., K.L. Olson, T.R. Moller, J. Ranstam, P. Holm: Oral contraceptive use and breast cancer in young women in Sweden (letter). *Lancet*, 2:748–749, 1985.

41. McPherson, K., M. Vessey, A. Neil, R. Doll, L. Jones, and M. Roberts: Early contraceptive use and breast cancer: Results of another case-control study. *Brit. J. Cancer*, 56: 653–660, 1987.

42. Huggins, G.R., and P.F. Zucker: Oral contraceptives and neoplasia: 1987 update. *Fertil. Steril.*, 47:733–761, 1987.

43. McPherson, K., and J.O. Drife: The pill and breast cancer: Why the uncertainty? *Brit. Med. J.*, 293:709–710, 1986.

44. Shapiro, S.: Oral contraceptives: Time to take stock. *N.E.J.M.*, 315:450–451, 1987.

45. Ory, I.I., Z. Naib, S.B. Conger, R.A. Hatcher, and C.W. Tyler: Contraceptive choice and prevalence of cervical dysplasia and carcinoma in situ. *Am. J. Obstet. Gynec.*, 124:573–577, 1976.

46. Vessey, M.P., M. Lawless, K. McPherson, D. Yeates: Neoplasia of the cervix uteri and contraception: A possible adverse effect of the pill. *Lancet*, 2:930, 1983.

47. Brinton, L.A., G.R. Huggins, H.F. Lehman, K. Malli, D.A. Savitz, E. Trapido, J. Rosenthal, and R. Hoover: Long-term use of oral contraceptives and risk of invasive cervical cancer. *Int. J. Cancer*, 38:339–344, 1986.

48. WHO Collaborative Study of Neoplasia and Steroid Contraceptives: Invasive cervical cancer and combined oral contraceptives. *Brit. Med. J.*, 290:961–965, 1985.

49. Rooks, J.B., H.W. Ory, K.G. Ishak, L.T. Strauss, J.R. Greenspan, A.P. Hill, and C.W. Tyler: Epidemiology of hepatocellular adenoma: The role of oral contraceptive use. *J.A.M.A.*, 242:644–648, 1979.

50. Bein, N.N., and H.S. Goldsmith: Recurrent massive hemorrhage from benign hepatic tumors secondary to oral contraceptives. *Brit. J. Surg.*, 64:433–435, 1977.

51. Klatskin, G.: Hepatic tumors: Possible relationship to use of oral contraceptives. *Gastroenterology*, 73:386–394, 1977.

52. Henderson, B.E., S. Preston-Martin, H.A. Edmondson, R.L. Peters, and M.C. Pike: Hepatocellular carcinoma and oral contraceptives. *Brit. J. Cancer*, 48:437–440, 1983.

53. Neuberger, J., D. Forman, R. Doll, and R. Williams: Oral contraceptives and hepatocellular carcinoma, *Brit. Med. J.*, 292:1355–1357, 1986.

54. Forman, D., T.J. Vincent, and R. Doll: Cancer of the liver and oral contraceptives. *Brit. Med. J.*, 292:1357–1361, 1986.

55. Harlap, S., and J. Eldor: Births following oral contraceptive failures. *Obstet. Gynec.*, 55:447–452, 1980.

56. Savolainen, E., E. Saksela, and L. Saxen: Teratogenic hazards of oral contraceptives analyzed in a national malformation register. *Amer. J. Obstet. Gynec.*, 140:521–524, 1981.

57. Janerich, D.T., J.M. Piper, and D.M. Glebatis: Oral contraceptives and birth defects. *Am. J. Epidemiology*, 112:73–79, 1980.

58. Ferencz, C., G.M. Matanoski, P.D. Wilson, J.D. Rubin, C.A. Neill, and R. Gutberlet: Maternal hormone therapy and congenital heart disease. *Teratology*, 21:225–239, 1980.

59. Rothman, K.J., D.C. Fyler, A. Goldbatt, and M.B. Kreidberg: Exogenous hormones and other drug exposures of children with congenital heart disease. *Am. J. Epidemiology*, 109:433–439, 1979.

60. Boston Collaborative Drug Surveillance Program: Oral contraceptives and venous thromboembolic disease, surgically confirmed gallbladder disease, and breast tumors. *Lancet*, 1:1399–1404, 1973.

61. Royal College of General Practitioners: *Oral Contraceptives and Health.* New York, Pittman, 1974, 100p.

62. Layde, P.M., M.P. Vessey, and D. Yeates: Risk of gallbladder disease: A cohort study of young women attending family planning clinics. *J. of Epidemiol. and Comm. Health*, 36: 274–278, 1982.

63. Rome Group for the Epidemiology and Prevention of Cholelithiasis (GREPCO): Prevalence of gallstone disease in an Italian adult female population, *Am. J. Epidemiol.*, 119:796–805, 1984.

64. Strom, B.L., R.T. Tamragouri, M.L. Morse, E.L. Lazar, S.L. West, P.D. Stolley, and J.K. Jones: Oral contraceptives and other risk factors for gallbladder disease. *Clin. Pharmacol. Ther.*, 39:335–341, 1986.

65. Wynn, V., P.W. Adams, I.F. Godsland, J. Melrose, R. Niththyananthan, N.W. Oakley, and A. Seedj: Comparison of effects of different combined oral-contraceptive formulations on carbohydrate and lipid metabolism. *Lancet*, 1:1045–1049, 1979.

66. Wynn, V.: Effect of progesterone and progestins on carbohydrate metabolism. In Progesterone and Progestin. Edited by C.W. Bardin, E. Milgrom, P. Mauvis-Jarvis. New York, Raven Press, pp. 395–410, 1983.

67. Perlman, J.A., R.G. Roussell-Briefel, T.M. Ezzati, and G. Lieberknecht: Oral glucose tolerance and the potency of oral contraceptive progestogens. *J. Chronic Dis.*, 38:857–864, 1985.

68. Royal College of General Practitioners' Oral Contraception Study: Effect on hypertension and benign breast disease of progestogen component in combined oral contraceptives. *Lancet*, 1:624, 1977.

69. Fisch, I.R., and J. Frank. Oral contraceptives and blood pressure. *J.A.M.A.* 237:2499–2503, 1977.

70. Laragh, A.J.: Oral contraceptive induced hypertension: Nine years later. *Amer. J. Obstet. Gynecol.*, 126:141–147, 1976.

71. Ramcharan, S., E. Peritz, F.A. Pellegrin, and W.T. Williams: Incidence of hypertension in the Walnut Creek Contraceptive Drug Study cohort. In Pharmacology of Steroid Contraceptive Drugs. Edited by S. Garattini and H.W. Berendes, New York, *Raven Press*, pp. 277–288, 1977. (Monographs of the Mario Negri Institute for Pharmacological Research, Milan).

72. Stockley, I.: Interactions with oral contraceptives. *Pharm. J.* 216:140–143, 1976.

73. The Cancer and Steroid Hormone Study of the Centers for Disease Control and the National Institute of Child Health and Human Development: Oral contraceptive use and the risk of ovarian cancer. *J.A.M.A.*, 249:1596–1599, 1983.

74. The Cancer and Steroid Hormone Study of the Centers for Disease Control and the National Institute of Child Health and Human Development: Combination oral contraceptive use and the risk of endometrial cancer. *J.A.M.A.*, 257:796–800, 1987.

75. Ory, H.W.: Functional ovarian cysts and oral contraceptives: Negative association confirmed surgically. *J.A.M.A.*, 228:68–69, 1974.

76. Ory, H.W., P. Cole, B. Macmahon, and R. Hoover: Oral contraceptives and reduced risk of benign breast disease. *N.E.J.M.*, 294:41–422, 1976.

77. Ory, H.W.: The noncontraceptive health benefits from oral contraceptive use. *Fam. Plann. Perspectives*, 14:182–184, 1982.

78. Ory, H.W., J.D. Forrest, and R. Lincoln: Making Choices: Evaluating the health risks and benefits of birth control methods. New York, The Alan Guttmacher Institute, p.1, 1983.

The patient labeling for oral contraceptive drug products is set forth below:

BRIEF SUMMARY PATIENT PACKAGE INSERT

Oral contraceptives, also known as "birth control pills" or "the pill," are taken to prevent pregnancy and when taken correctly, have a failure rate of about 1% per year when used without missing any pills. The typical failure rate of large numbers of pill users is less than 3% per year when women who miss pills are included. For most women oral contraceptives are also free of serious or unpleasant side effects. However, forgetting to take pills considerably increases the chances of pregnancy.

For the majority of women, oral contraceptives can be taken safely. But there are some women who are at high risk of developing certain serious diseases that can be life-threatening or may cause temporary or permanent disability. The risks associated with taking oral contraceptives increase significantly if you:

- Smoke
- Are over the age of 40
- Have high blood pressure, diabetes, high cholesterol
- Have or have had clotting disorders, heart attack, stroke, angina pectoris, cancer of the breast or sex organs, jaundice or malignant or benign liver tumors.

You should not take the pill if you suspect you are pregnant or have unexplained vaginal bleeding.

> Cigarette smoking increases the risk of serious cardiovascular side effects from oral contraceptive use. This risk increases with age and with heavy smoking (15 or more cigarettes per day) and is quite marked in women over 35 years of age. Women who use oral contraceptives are strongly advised not to smoke.

Most side effects of the pill are not serious. The most common side effects are nausea, vomiting, bleeding between menstrual periods, weight gain, and breast tenderness, and difficulty wearing contact lenses. These side effects, especially nausea and vomiting, may subside within the first three months of use.

The serious side effects of the pill occur very infrequently, especially if you are in good health and are young. However, you should know that the following medical conditions have been associated with or made worse by the pill:

1. Blood clots in the legs (thrombophlebitis), lungs (pulmonary embolism), stoppage or rupture of a blood vessel in the brain (stroke), blockage of blood vessels in the heart (heart attack or angina pectoris) or other organs of the body. As mentioned above, smoking increases the risk of heart attacks and strokes and subsequent serious medical consequences.

2. Liver tumors, which may rupture and cause severe bleeding. A possible but not definite association has been found with the pill and liver cancer. However, liver cancers are extremely rare. The chance of developing liver cancer from using the pill is thus even rarer.

3. High blood pressure, although blood pressure usually returns to normal when the pill is stopped.

The symptoms associated with these serious side effects are discussed in the detailed leaflet given to you with your supply of pills. Notify your doctor or health care provider if you notice any unusual physical disturbances while taking the pill. In addition, drugs such as rifampin, as well as some anticonvulsants and some antibiotics may decrease oral contraceptive effectiveness.

Studies to date of women taking the pill have not shown an increase in the incidence of cancer of the breast or cervix. There is, however, insufficient evidence to rule out the possibility that pills may cause such cancers.

Taking the pill provides some important non-contraceptive benefits. These include less painful menstruation, less menstrual blood loss and anemia, fewer pelvic infections, and fewer cancers of the ovary and the lining of the uterus.

Be sure to discuss any medical condition you may have with your health care provider. Your health care provider will take a medical and family history and examine you before prescribing oral contraceptives. You should be reexamined at least once a year while taking oral contraceptives. The detailed patient information leaflet gives you further information which you should read and discuss with your health care provider.

Caution: Oral contraceptives are of no value in the prevention or treatment of venereal disease.

INSTRUCTIONS TO PATIENTS
TABLET DISPENSER

The tablet dispenser has been designed to make oral contraceptive dosing as easy and as convenient as possible. The tablets are arranged in either three or four rows of seven tablets each, with the days of the week appearing on the tablet dispenser above the first row of tablets.

If your tablet dispenser contains:	You are taking:
21 white tablets	LOESTRIN 21 1/20
21 green tablets	LOESTRIN 21 1.5/30
21 white tablets and 7 brown tablets	LOESTRIN Fe 1/20
21 green tablets and 7 brown tablets	LOESTRIN Fe 1.5/30

Each *white* tablet contains 1 mg norethindrone acetate and 20 mcg ethinyl estradiol.
Each *green* tablet contains 1.5 mg norethindrone acetate and 30 mcg ethinyl estradiol.
Each *brown* tablet contains 75 mg ferrous fumarate, and is intended to help you remember to take the tablets correctly. These brown tablets are not intended to have any health benefit.

To remove a tablet, press down on it with your thumb or finger. The tablet will drop through the back of the tablet dispenser. Do not press on the tablet with your thumbnail or fingernail or any other sharp object.

LOESTRIN 21-DAY DOSAGE REGIMEN

If your tablet dispenser contains 21 tablets (3 rows of 7), you are on a 21-day regimen and should follow either the Sunday-Start or Day-5 Start directions.

A. Sunday-Start Regimen

1. Unless your physician or health care provider has instructed you differently, begin taking tablets on the first Sunday after your menstrual period begins whether or not you are still bleeding. If your period begins on Sunday, take your first tablet that very same day. START WITH THE SUNDAY TABLET IN THE TOP ROW.
Note: During the first cycle, it is important that you use another method of birth control until you have taken a tablet daily for seven consecutive days.
2. Take all the tablets in the top row first, followed by the second row. Continue to take one tablet every day until you finish all 21 tablets. Your last tablet should be on Saturday.
3. After you have taken all 21 tablets, stop, and don't take any tablets for the next seven days. You should have a menstrual period one to three days after you stop taking tablets; sometimes it may take a day or so longer.
4. After the seven days during which you take no tablets, obtain a new course of tablets. Begin the new course of 21 tablets on Sunday, the 8th day after you took your last tablet, starting with the Sunday tablet in the top row.
5. Continue to take one tablet daily until you finish all 21 tablets. If you follow the schedule properly, you will always take the last tablet in the dispenser on a Saturday, and always start each new course of 21 tablets 8 days later, on the following Sunday.
6. If, in any cycle, you start your tablets later than the proper day, you should also use another method of birth control until you have taken seven consecutive tablets.

B. Day 5 Regimen

If your physician or health care provider has directed you to begin taking your first cycle of tablets using the Day-5 Regimen, you should start taking your tablets on Day 5 after the start of your period.

1. The first day of your period is Day 1. On the 5th day (Day 5), start taking one tablet daily, beginning with the tablet in the top row that corresponds to Day 5 after your flow began.

If your period begins on:	Start taking tablets in the top row on:
Sunday	Thursday
Monday	Friday
Tuesday	Saturday
Wednesday	Sunday
Thursday	Monday
Friday	Tuesday
Saturday	Wednesday

Note: During the first cycle, if you start taking tablets later than Day 5 of your menstrual period, you should use another method of birth control until you have taken a tablet daily for seven consecutive days.
2. Continue to take one tablet daily. After the last Saturday tablet has been taken, if any tablets remain in the first row, complete your 21-day regimen by taking one tablet daily starting with the Sunday tablet in the top row.
3. After you have taken all 21 tablets, stop and don't take any tablets for the next seven days. You should have a menstrual period one to three days after you stop taking tablets, sometimes it may take a day or so longer.
4. After the seven days during which you take no tablets, obtain a new course of 21-day tablets. Begin a new course of 21-day tablets, the 8th day after you took your last tablet, starting with the tablet in the top row that corresponds to that day.
5. Continue to take one tablet daily until you finish all 21 tablets. If you follow the schedule properly, you will always take the last tablet in the dispenser on the same day of the week, and always start each new course of 21 tablets the same day of the week on which you began the previous cycle of tablets.
6. If, in any cycle, you start your tablets later than the proper day, you should also use another method of birth control until you have taken seven consecutive tablets.

Whether you started your tablets using the Sunday-Start or Day-5 Regimen, the following directions apply:

1. Continue taking your tablets whether or not your period has occurred or is still in progress. Your period will usually occur during the time you are taking no tablets.
2. If spotting should occur at an unexpected time, continue to take your tablets as directed. Spotting is usually temporary and without significance. However, if bleeding should occur at an unexpected time, consult your physician or health care provider. Call your physician or health care provider regarding any problem or change in your general health that may concern you.

LOESTRIN 28-DAY DOSAGE REGIMEN

If your tablet dispenser contains 28 tablets (3 rows of 7 *light-colored* (white or green) tablets and 1 row of 7 *brown* tablets), you are on a 28-day regimen and should follow these directions. Each *brown* tablet contains 75 mg ferrous fumarate and is intended to help you remember to take the tablets correctly. These brown tablets are not intended to have any health benefits.

Sunday-Start Regimen:

1. Begin taking tablets on the first Sunday after your menstrual period begins whether or not you are still bleeding. If your period begins on Sunday, take your first tablet that very same day. START WITH THE SUNDAY TABLET IN THE TOP ROW.
Note: During the first cycle, it is important that you use another method of birth control until you have taken a *light-colored* tablet daily for seven consecutive days.

2. Take all the tablets in the top row first, followed by the second row and so on.
3. Continue to take one tablet every day until you finish all 21 *light-colored* tablets. On the day after taking the last *light-colored* tablet, begin taking one *brown* tablet daily until all the tablets have been taken.
4. When the last tablet has been taken, obtain a new course of tablets and, without interruption, begin a new course of 28-day tablets, the next day, starting with the Sunday tablet in the top row. There should never be a day when you are not taking a tablet.
5. If, in any cycle, you start your tablets later than the proper day, you should also use another method of birth control until you have taken seven *light-colored* tablets.
6. Continue taking *light-colored* tablets without interruption whether or not your period has occurred or is still in progress. Your period will usually occur during the time you are taking *brown* tablets.
7. If spotting should occur at an unexpected time, continue to take your tablets as directed. Spotting is usually temporary and without significance. However, if bleeding should occur at an unexpected time, consult your physician or health care provider. Call your physician or health care provider regarding any problem or change in your general health that may concern you.

In Case You Forget (21-Day and 28-Day Regimens)
The following instructions apply only to missing the white 1/20 tablets or the green 1.5/30 tablets.
If you forget to take one tablet, take it as soon as you remember, even if it is the next day. Then take the next scheduled tablet at the usual time. If you miss two consecutive tablets, take two tablets daily for the next two days. Then resume the regular schedule. While there is little likelihood of pregnancy occurring if you miss only one or two tablets, the possibility of pregnancy increases with each successive day that tablets are missed.

If you are taking Loestrin 21 1/20 or Loestrin Fe 1/20, in addition to taking two *white* tablets a day for two days, you should use an additional means of contraception until you've taken a *white* tablet every day for seven days.

21-Day Regimen: If you miss three consecutive tablets, discard any tablets remaining in the tablet dispenser and follow these instructions.

If you are on the Sunday-Start Regimen, start a new course of tablets the first Sunday following the last missed tablet, whether or not you are still menstruating.

If you are on the Day-5 Regimen, begin a new course of tablets on the 8th day after the last tablet was taken. For example, if you took your last tablet on a Monday, you should begin your new course of tablets the following Monday.

During the seven days without tablets, and until you have taken a tablet daily for seven consecutive days from your course of tablets, you should also use another method of birth control.

28-Day Regimen: If you miss three consecutive *light-colored* tablets, discard any tablets remaining in the tablet dispenser and begin a new course of tablets the first Sunday following the last missed tablet, whether or not you are still menstruating. During the days without tablets and until you have taken a tablet daily for seven consecutive days from your new course of tablets, you should also use another method of birth control.

If you miss one or more *brown* tablets discard the remainder and begin a new course of tablets on the next Sunday (which should be the 8th day after you took your last *light-colored* tablet). Start with the *light-colored* tablets in the top row. Skipping one or more *brown* tablets contained in the 28-day regimen products won't increase the risk of pregnancy. They are there to help keep you on a schedule and to eliminate the need for counting days. *Under no circumstances* should you substitute a *brown* tablet for a *light-colored* tablet nor should a *brown* tablet be taken until you have finished all the *light-colored* tablets, unless your physician or health care provider advises you to do so.

Remembering to take tablets according to schedule is stressed because of its importance in providing you the greatest degree of protection.

MISSED MENSTRUAL PERIODS FOR BOTH DOSAGE REGIMENS

At times there may be no menstrual period after a cycle of pills. Therefore, if you miss one menstrual period but have taken the pills *exactly as your were supposed to*, continue as usual into the next cycle. If you have not taken the pills correctly and miss a menstrual period, *you may be pregnant* and should stop taking oral contraceptives until your doctor or

Continued on next page

This product information was prepared in August, 1989. On these and other Parke-Davis Products, information may be obtained by addressing PARKE-DAVIS, Division of Warner-Lambert Company, Morris Plains, New Jersey 07950.

ANNUAL NUMBER OF BIRTH-RELATED OR METHOD-RELATED DEATHS ASSOCIATED WITH CONTROL OF FERTILITY PER 100,000 NONSTERILE WOMEN, BY FERTILITY CONTROL METHOD ACCORDING TO AGE

Method of control and outcome	15–19	20–24	25–29	30–34	35–39	40–44
No fertility control methods*	7.0	7.4	9.1	14.8	25.7	28.2
Oral contraceptives non-smoker**	0.3	0.5	0.9	1.9	13.8	31.6
Oral contraceptives smoker**	2.2	3.4	6.6	13.5	51.1	117.2
IUD**	0.8	0.8	1.0	1.0	1.4	1.4
Condom*	1.1	1.6	0.7	0.2	0.3	0.4
Diaphragm/spermicide*	1.9	1.2	1.2	1.3	2.2	2.8
Periodic abstinence*	2.5	1.6	1.6	1.7	2.9	3.6

* Deaths are birth related
** Deaths are method related

Parke-Davis—Cont.

health care provider determines whether or not you are pregnant. Until you can get to your doctor or health care provider, use another form of contraception. If two consecutive menstrual periods are missed, you should stop taking pills until it is determined whether or not you are pregnant. Although there does not appear to be any increase in birth defects in newborn babies if you become pregnant while using oral contraceptives, if you do become pregnant, you should discuss the situation with your doctor or health care provider.

Periodic Examination

Your doctor or health care provider will take a complete medical and family history before prescribing oral contraceptives. At that time and about once a year thereafter, he will generally examine your blood pressure, breasts, abdomen, and pelvic organs (including a Papanicolaou smear, ie, test for cancer).

SUMMARY

Oral contraceptives are the most effective method, except sterilization, for preventing pregnancy. Other methods, when used conscientiously, are also very effective and have fewer risks. Although the serious risks of oral contraceptives are uncommon, some of the risks may persist after you stop using the pill. On the other hand, the "pill" is a very convenient method of preventing pregnancy.

If you have certain conditions or have had these conditions in the past, you should not use oral contraceptives because the risk is too great. These conditions are listed in this leaflet. If you do not have these conditions, and decide to use the "pill," please read this leaflet carefully so that you can use the "pill" most safely and effectively.

Based on his or her assessment of your medical needs, your doctor or health care provider has prescribed this drug for you. Do not give this drug to anyone else.

Keep this and all drugs out of the reach of children.

Caution—Federal law prohibits dispensing without prescription.

DETAILED PATIENT PACKAGE INSERT

What You Should Know About Oral Contraceptives

Any woman who considers using oral contraceptives (the "birth control pill" or the "pill") should understand the benefits and risks of using this form of birth control. This leaflet will give you much of the information you will need to make this decision and will also help you determine if you are at risk of developing any of the serious side effects of the pill. It will tell you how to use the pill properly so that it will be as effective as possible. However, this leaflet is not a replacement for a careful discussion between you and your health care provider. You should discuss the information provided in this leaflet with him or her, both when you first start taking the pill and during your revisits. You should also follow your health care provider's advice with regard to regular check-ups while you are on the pill.

EFFECTIVENESS OF ORAL CONTRACEPTIVES

Oral contraceptives or "birth control pills" or "the pill" are used to prevent pregnancy and are more effective than other non-surgical methods of birth control. When they are taken correctly, the chance of becoming pregnant is less than 1% (1 pregnancy per 100 women per year of use) when used perfectly, without missing pills. Typical failure rates are actually 3% per year. The chance of becoming pregnant increases with each missed pill during a menstrual cycle.

In comparison, typical failure rates for other methods of birth control during the first year of use are as follows:

IUD: 6%
Diaphragm with spermicides: 18%
Spermicides alone: 21%
Vaginal sponge: 18 to 30%
Condom alone: 12%
Periodic abstinence: 20%
No method: 89%.

WHO SHOULD NOT TAKE ORAL CONTRACEPTIVES

Cigarette smoking increases the risk of serious cardiovascular side effects from oral contraceptives use. This risk increases with age and with heavy smoking (15 or more cigarettes per day) and is quite marked in women over 35 years of age. Women who use oral contraceptives are strongly advised not to smoke.

Some women should not use the pill. For example, you should not take the pill if you are pregnant or think you may be pregnant. You should also not use the pill if you have any of the following conditions:

- A history of heart attack or stroke
- Blood clots in the legs (thrombophlebitis), lungs (pulmonary embolism), or eyes
- A history of blood clots in the deep veins of your legs

- Chest pain (angina pectoris)
- Known or suspected breast cancer or cancer of the lining of the uterus, cervix or vagina
- Unexplained vaginal bleeding (until a diagnosis is reached by your doctor)
- Yellowing of the whites of the eyes or of the skin (jaundice) during pregnancy or during previous use of the pill
- Liver tumor (benign or cancerous)
- Known or suspected pregnancy

Tell your health care provider if you have ever had any of these conditions. Your health care provider can recommend a safer method of birth control.

OTHER CONSIDERATIONS BEFORE TAKING ORAL CONTRACEPTIVES

Tell your health care provider if you have:

- Breast nodules, fibrocystic disease of the breast, an abnormal breast x-ray or mammogram
- Diabetes
- Elevated cholesterol or triglycerides
- High blood pressure
- Migraine or other headaches or epilepsy
- Mental depression
- Gallbladder, heart or kidney disease
- History of scanty or irregular menstrual periods

Women with any of these conditions should be checked often by their health care provider if they choose to use oral contraceptives.

Also, be sure to inform your doctor or health care provider if you smoke or are on any medications.

RISKS OF TAKING ORAL CONTRACEPTIVES

1. Risk Of Developing Blood Clots

Blood clots and blockage of blood vessels are the most serious side effects of taking oral contraceptives. In particular, a clot in the legs can cause thrombophlebitis and a clot that travels to the lungs can cause a sudden blocking of the vessel carrying blood to the lungs. Rarely, clots occur in the blood vessels of the eye and may cause blindness, double vision, or impaired vision.

If you take oral contraceptives and need elective surgery, need to stay in bed for a prolonged illness or have recently delivered a baby, you may be at risk of developing blood clots. You should consult your doctor or health care provider about stopping oral contraceptives three to four weeks before surgery and not taking oral contraceptives for two weeks after surgery or during bed rest. You should also not take oral contraceptives soon after delivery of a baby. It is advisable to wait for at least four weeks after delivery if you are not breast feeding. If you are breast feeding, you should wait until you have weaned your child before using the pill. (See also the section on Breast Feeding in GENERAL PRECAUTIONS.)

2. Heart Attacks And Strokes

Oral contraceptives may increase the tendency to develop strokes (stoppage or rupture of blood vessels in the brain) and angina pectoris and heart attacks (blockage of blood vessels in the heart). Any of these conditions can cause death or disability.

Smoking greatly increases the possibility of suffering heart attacks and strokes. Furthermore, smoking and the use of oral contraceptives greatly increase the chances of developing and dying of heart disease.

3. Gallbladder Disease

Oral contraceptive users probably have a greater risk than nonusers of having gallbladder disease, although this risk may be related to pills containing high doses of estrogens.

4. Liver Tumors

In rare cases, oral contraceptives can cause benign but dangerous liver tumors. These benign liver tumors can rupture and cause fatal internal bleeding. In addition, a possible but not definite association has been found with the pill and liver cancers in two studies, in which a few women who developed these very rare cancers were found to have used oral contraceptives for long periods. However, liver cancers are extremely rare. The chance of developing liver cancer from using the pill is thus even rarer.

5. Cancer Of The Reproductive Organs

There is, at present, no confirmed evidence that oral contraceptives increase the risk of cancer of the reproductive organs in human studies. Several studies have found no overall increase in the risk of developing breast cancer. However, women who use oral contraceptives and have a strong family history of breast cancer or who have breast nodules or abnormal mammograms should be closely followed by their doctors.

Some studies have found an increase in the incidence of cancer of the cervix in women who use oral contraceptives. However, this finding may be related to factors other than the use of oral contraceptives.

ESTIMATED RISK OF DEATH FROM A BIRTH CONTROL METHOD OR PREGNANCY

All methods of birth control and pregnancy are associated with a risk of developing certain diseases which may lead to disability or death. An estimate of the number of deaths asso-

ciated with different methods of birth control and pregnancy has been calculated and is shown in the following table. [See table preceding page].

In the above table, the risk of death from any birth control method is less than the risk of childbirth, except for oral contraceptive users over the age of 35 who smoke and pill users over the age of 40 even if they do not smoke. It can be seen in the table that for women aged 15 to 39, the risk of death was highest with pregnancy (7–26 deaths per 100,000 women, depending on age). Among pill users who do not smoke, the risk of death was always lower than that associated with pregnancy for any age group, although over the age of 40, the risk increases to 32 deaths per 100,000 women, compared to 28 associated with pregnancy at that age. However, for pill users who smoke and are over the age of 35, the estimated number of deaths exceeds those for other methods of birth control. If a woman is over the age of 40 and smokes, her estimated risk of death is four times higher (117/100,000 women) than the estimated risk associated with pregnancy (28/100,000 women) in that age group.

Moreover, if you do not smoke and are under the age of 35, the possible risk of death from oral contraceptive use is extremely low when you consider the failure rate associated with other methods of contraception such as the condom or diaphragm and the resulting pregnancy-associated risk.

WARNING SIGNALS

If any of these adverse effects occur while you are taking oral contraceptives, call your doctor immediately:

- Sharp chest pain, coughing of blood, or sudden shortness of breath (indicating a possible clot in the lung)
- Pain in the calf (indicating a possible clot in the leg)
- Crushing chest pain or heaviness in the chest (indicating a possible heart attack)
- Sudden severe headache or vomiting, dizziness or fainting, disturbances of vision or speech, weakness, or numbness in an arm or leg (indicating a possible stroke)
- Sudden partial or complete loss of vision (indicating a possible clot in the eye)
- Breast lumps (indicating possible breast cancer or fibrocystic disease of the breast; ask your doctor and health care provider to show you how to examine your breasts)
- Severe pain or tenderness in the stomach area (indicating a possibly ruptured liver tumor)
- Difficulty in sleeping, weakness, lack of energy, fatigue, or change in mood (possibly indicating severe depression)
- Jaundice or a yellowing of the skin or eyeballs, accompanied frequently by fever, fatigue, loss of appetite, dark colored urine, or light colored bowel movements (indicating possible liver problems)

SIDE EFFECTS OF ORAL CONTRACEPTIVES

1. Vaginal Bleeding

Irregular vaginal bleeding or spotting may occur while you are taking the pills. Irregular bleeding may vary from slight staining between menstrual periods to breakthrough bleeding which is a flow much like a regular period. Irregular bleeding occurs most often during the first few months of oral contraceptive use, but may also occur after you have been taking the pill for some time. Such bleeding may be temporary and usually does not indicate any serious problems. It is important to continue taking your pills on schedule. If the bleeding occurs in more than one cycle or lasts for more than a few days, talk to your doctor or health care provider.

2. Contact Lenses

If you wear contact lenses and notice a change in vision or an inability to wear your lenses, contact your doctor or health care provider.

3. Fluid Retention

Oral contraceptives may cause edema (fluid retention) with swelling of the fingers or ankles and may raise your blood pressure. If you experience fluid retention, contact your doctor or health care provider.

4. Melasma

A spotty darkening of the skin is possible, particularly on the face.

5. Other Side Effects

Other side effects include change in appetite, headache, nervousness, depression, dizziness, loss of scalp hair, rash, and vaginal infections.

If any of these side effects bother you, call your doctor or health care provider.

GENERAL PRECAUTIONS

1. Missed Periods And Use Of Oral Contraceptives Before Or During Early Pregnancy

There may be times when you may not menstruate regularly after you have completed taking a cycle of pills. If you have taken your pills regularly and miss one menstrual period, continue taking your pills for the next cycle but be sure to inform your health care provider before doing so. If you have not taken the pills daily as instructed and missed a menstrual period, or if you missed two consecutive menstrual periods, you may be pregnant. Check with your health care provider immediately to determine whether you are pregnant. Do not continue to take oral contraceptives until you are sure you are not pregnant, but continue to use another method of contraception.

There is no conclusive evidence that oral contraceptive use is associated with an increase in birth defects, when taken inadvertently during early pregnancy. Previously, a few studies had reported that oral contraceptives might be associated with birth defects, but these studies have not been confirmed. Nevertheless, oral contraceptives or any other drugs should not be used during pregnancy unless clearly necessary and prescribed by your doctor. You should check with your doctor about risks to your unborn child of any medication taken during pregnancy.

2. While Breast Feeding

If you are breast feeding consult your doctor before starting oral contraceptives. Some of the drug will be passed on to the child in the milk. A few adverse effects on the child have been reported, including yellowing of the skin (jaundice) and breast enlargement. In addition, oral contraceptives may decrease the amount and quality of your milk. If possible, do not use oral contraceptives while breast feeding. You should use another method of contraception since breast feeding provides only partial protection from becoming pregnant and this partial protection decreases significantly as you breast feed for longer periods of time. You should consider starting oral contraceptives only after you have weaned your child completely.

3. Laboratory Tests

If you are scheduled for any laboratory tests, tell your doctor you are taking birth control pills. Certain blood tests may be affected by birth control pills.

4. Drug Interactions

Certain drugs may interact with birth control pills to make them less effective in preventing pregnancy or cause an increase in breakthrough bleeding. Such drugs include rifampin, drugs used for epilepsy such as barbiturates (for example, phenobarbital) and phenytoin (Dilantin® is one brand of this drug), phenylbutazone (Butazolidin® is one brand) and possibly certain antibiotics. You may need to use additional contraception when you take drugs which can make oral contraceptives less effective.

HOW TO TAKE ORAL CONTRACEPTIVES

1. General Instructions

You must take your pill every day according to the instructions. Oral contraceptives are most effective if taken no more than 24 hours apart. Take your pill at the same time every day so that you are less likely to forget to take it. You will then maintain an effective dose of oral contraceptive in your body.

If your doctor has scheduled you for surgery, or you need prolonged bed rest, he or she may suggest that you stop taking the pill four weeks before surgery to avoid an increased risk of blood clots. It is also advisable not to start oral contraceptives sooner than four weeks after delivery of a baby.

2. If You Forget To Take Your Pill

If you miss only one pill in a cycle, the chance of becoming pregnant is small. Take the missed pill as soon as you realize that you have forgotten it. Since the risk of pregnancy increases with each additional pill you skip, it is very important that you take one pill a day.

3. Pregnancy Due To Pill Failure

The incidence of pill failure resulting in pregnancy is approximately 1% (i.e., one pregnancy per 100 women per year) if taken every day as directed, but more typical failure rates are about 3%. If failure does occur, the risk to the fetus is minimal.

4. Pregnancy After Stopping The Pill

There may be some delay in becoming pregnant after you stop using oral contraceptives, especially if you had irregular menstrual cycles before you used oral contraceptives. It may be advisable to postpone conception until you begin menstruating regularly once you have stopped taking the pill and desire pregnancy.

5. Overdosage

Serious ill effects have not been reported following ingestion of large doses of oral contraceptives by young children. Overdosage may cause nausea and withdrawal bleeding in females. In case of overdosage, contact your health care provider or pharmacist.

6. Other Information

Your health care provider will take a medical and family history and examine you before prescribing oral contraceptives. You should be reexamined at least once a year. Be sure to inform your health care provider if there is a family history of any of the conditions listed previously in this leaflet. Be sure to keep all appointments with your health care provider, because this is a time to determine if there are early signs of side effects of oral contraceptive use.

Do not use the drug for any condition other than the one for which it was prescribed. This drug has been prescribed specifically for you; do not give it to others who may want birth control pills.

HEALTH BENEFITS FROM ORAL CONTRACEPTIVES

In addition to preventing pregnancy, use of oral contraceptives may provide certain benefits.

They are:
- Menstrual cycles may become more regular
- Blood flow during menstruation may be lighter and less iron may be lost. Therefore, anemia due to iron deficiency is less likely to occur
- Pain or other symptoms during menstruation may be encountered less frequently
- Ectopic (tubal) pregnancy may occur less frequently
- Noncancerous cysts or lumps in the breast may occur less frequently
- Acute pelvic inflammatory disease may occur less frequently
- Oral contraceptive use may provide some protection against developing two forms of cancer: cancer of the ovaries and cancer of the lining of the uterus.

If you want more information about birth control pills, ask your doctor or pharmacist. They have a more technical leaflet called the "Physician Insert," which you may wish to read.

INSTRUCTIONS TO PATIENT

TABLET DISPENSER

The tablet dispenser has been designed to make oral contraceptive dosing as easy and as convenient as possible. The tablets are arranged in either three or four rows of seven tablets each, with the days of the week appearing on the tablet dispenser above the first row of tablets.

If your tablet dispenser contains:	You are taking:
21 white tablets	LOESTRIN 21 1/20
21 green tablets	LOESTRIN 21 1.5/30
21 white tablets and 7 brown tablets	LOESTRIN Fe 1/20
21 green tablets and 7 brown tablets	LOESTRIN Fe 1.5/30

Each *white* tablet contains 1 mg norethindrone acetate and 20 mcg ethinyl estradiol.

Each *green* tablet contains 1.5 mg norethindrone acetate and 30 mcg ethinyl estradiol.

Each *brown* tablet contains 75 mg ferrous fumarate, and is intended to help you remember to take the tablets correctly. These brown tablets are not intended to have any health benefit.

To remove a tablet, press down on it with your thumb or finger. The tablet will drop through the back of the tablet dispenser. Do not press on the tablet with your thumbnail or fingernail or any other sharp object.

LOESTRIN 21-DAY DOSAGE REGIMEN

If your tablet dispenser contains 21 tablets (3 rows of 7), you are on a 21-day regimen and should follow either the Sunday-Start or Day-5 Start directions.

A. Sunday-Start Regimen

1. Unless your physician or health care provider has instructed you differently, begin taking tablets on the first Sunday after your menstrual period begins whether or not you are still bleeding. If your period begins on Sunday, take your first tablet that very same day. START WITH THE SUNDAY TABLET IN THE TOP ROW.

Note: During the first cycle, it is important that you use another method of birth control until you have taken a tablet daily for seven consecutive days.

2. Take all the tablets in the top row first, followed by the second row. Continue to take one tablet every day until you finish all 21 tablets. Your last tablet should be on Saturday.

3. After you have taken all 21 tablets, stop, and don't take any tablets for the next seven days. You should have a menstrual period one to three days after you stop taking tablets; sometimes it may take a day or so longer.

4. After the seven days during which you take no tablets, obtain a new course of tablets. Begin the new course of 21 day tablets on Sunday, the 8th day after you took your last tablet, starting with the Sunday tablet in the top row.

5. Continue to take one tablet daily until you finish all 21 tablets. If you follow the schedule properly, you will always take the last tablet in the dispenser on a Saturday, and always start each new course of 21 tablets 8 days later, on the following Sunday.

6. If, in any cycle, you start your tablets later than the proper day, you should also use another method of birth control until you have taken seven consecutive tablets.

B. Day-5 Regimen

If your physician or health care provider has directed you to begin taking your first cycle of tablets using the Day-5 Regimen, you should start taking your tablets on Day 5 after the start of your period:

1. The first day of your period is Day 1. On the 5th day (Day 5), start taking one tablet daily, beginning with the tablet in the top row that corresponds to Day 5 after your flow began.

If your period begins on:	Start taking tablets in the top row on:
Sunday	Thursday
Monday	Friday
Tuesday	Saturday
Wednesday	Sunday
Thursday	Monday
Friday	Tuesday
Saturday	Wednesday

Note: During the first cycle, if you start taking tablets later than Day 5 of your menstrual period, you should use another method of birth control until you have taken a tablet daily for seven consecutive days.

2. Continue to take one tablet daily. After the last Saturday tablet has been taken, if any tablets remain in the first row, complete your 21-day regimen by taking one tablet daily starting with the Sunday tablet in the top row.

3. After you have taken all 21 tablets, stop, and don't take any tablets for the next seven days. You should have a menstrual period one to three days after you stop taking tablets; sometimes it may take a day or so longer.

4. After the seven days during which you take no tablets, obtain a new course of tablets. Begin a new course of 21-day tablets, the 8th day after you took your last tablet, starting with the tablet in the top row that corresponds to that day.

5. Continue to take one tablet daily until you finish all 21 tablets. If you follow the schedule properly, you will always take the last tablet in the dispenser on the same day of the week, and always start each new course of 21 tablets the same day of the week on which you began the previous cycle of tablets.

6. If, in any cycle, you start your tablets later than the proper day, you should also use another method of birth control until you have taken seven consecutive tablets.

Whether you started your tablets using the Sunday-Start or Day-5 Regimen, the following directions apply:

1. Continue taking your tablets whether or not your period has occurred or is still in progress. Your period will usually occur during the seven days you are taking no tablets.

2. If spotting should occur at an unexpected time, continue to take your tablets as directed. Spotting is usually temporary and without significance. However, if bleeding should occur at an unexpected time, consult your physician or health care provider. Call your physician or health care provider regarding any problem or change in your general health that may concern you.

LOESTRIN 28-DAY DOSAGE REGIMEN

If your tablet dispenser contains 28 tablets (3 rows of 7 *light-colored* (white or green) tablets and 1 row of 7 *brown* tablets), you are on a 28-day regimen and should follow these directions.

Sunday-Start Regimen:

1. Begin taking tablets on the first Sunday after your menstrual period begins whether or not you are still bleeding. If your period begins on Sunday, take your first tablet that very same day. START WITH THE SUNDAY TABLET IN THE TOP ROW.

Note: During the first cycle, it is important that you use another method of birth control until you have taken a *light-colored* tablet daily for seven consecutive days.

2. Take all the tablets in the top row first, followed by the second row and so on.

3. Continue to take one tablet every day until you finish all 21 *light-colored* tablets. On the day after taking the last *light-colored* tablet, begin taking one *brown* tablet daily until all the tablets have been taken.

4. When the last tablet has been taken, obtain a new course of tablets and, without interruption, begin a new course of 28-day tablets, the next day, starting with the Sunday tablet in the top row. There should never be a day when you are not taking a tablet.

Continued on next page

This product information was prepared in August, 1989. On these and other Parke-Davis Products, information may be obtained by addressing PARKE-DAVIS, Division of Warner-Lambert Company, Morris Plains, New Jersey 07950.

Parke-Davis—Cont.

5. If, in any cycle, you start your tablets later than the proper day, you should also use another method of birth control until you have taken seven *light-colored* tablets.

6. Continue taking *light-colored* tablets without interruption whether or not your period has occurred or is still in progress. Your period will usually occur during the time you are taking *brown* tablets.

7. If spotting should occur at an unexpected time, continue to take your tablets as directed. Spotting is usually temporary and without significance. However, if bleeding should occur at an unexpected time, consult your physician or health care provider. Call your physician regarding any problem or change in your general health that may concern you.

In Case You Forget (21-Day and 28-Day Regimens)

The following instructions apply only to missing the white 1/20 tablets or the green 1.5/30 tablets.

If you forget to take one tablet, take it as soon as you remember, even if it is the next day. Then take the next scheduled tablet at the usual time. If you miss two consecutive tablets, take two tablets daily for the next two days. Then resume the regular schedule. While there is little likelihood of pregnancy occurring if you miss only one or two tablets, the possibility of pregnancy increases with each successive day that tablets are missed.

If you are taking Loestrin **21** 1/20 or Loestrin Fe 1/20, in addition to taking two <u>white</u> tablets a day for two days, you should use an additional means of contraception until you've taken a <u>white</u> tablet every day for seven days.

21-Day Regimen: If you miss three consecutive tablets, discard any tablets remaining in the tablet dispenser and follow these instructions.

If you are on the Sunday-Start Regimen, start a new course of tablets the first Sunday following the last missed tablet, whether or not you are still menstruating.

If you are on the Day-5 Regimen, begin a new course of tablets on the 8th day after the last tablet was taken. For example, if you took your last tablet on a Monday, you should begin your new course of tablets the following Monday.

During the seven days without tablets, and until you have taken a tablet daily for seven consecutive days from your course of tablets, you should also use another method of birth control.

28-Day Regimen: If you miss three consecutive *light-colored* tablets, discard any tablets remaining in the tablet dispenser and begin a new course of tablets the first Sunday following the last missed tablet, whether or not you are still menstruating. During the days without tablets and until you have taken a tablet daily for seven consecutive days from your new course of tablets, you should also use another method of birth control.

If you miss one or more *brown* tablets discard the remainder and begin a new course of tablets on the next Sunday (which should be the 8th day after you took your last *light-colored* tablet). Start with the *light-colored* tablets in the top row. Skipping one or more *brown* tablets contained in the 28-day regimen products won't increase the risk of pregnancy. They are there to help keep you on schedule and to eliminate the need for counting days. *Under no circumstances* should you substitute a *brown* tablet for a *light-colored* tablet nor should a *brown* tablet be taken until you have finished all the *light-colored* tablets, unless your physician or health care provider advises you to do so.

Remembering to take tablets according to schedule is stressed because of its importance in providing you the greatest degree of protection.

MISSED MENSTRUAL PERIODS FOR BOTH DOSAGE REGIMENS

At times there may be no menstrual period after a cycle of pills. Therefore, if you miss one menstrual period but have taken the pills *exactly as you were supposed to,* continue as usual into the next cycle. If you have not taken the pills correctly and miss a menstrual period, *you may be pregnant* and should stop taking oral contraceptives until your doctor or health care provider determines whether or not you are pregnant. Until you can get to your doctor or health care provider, use another form of contraception. If two consecutive menstrual periods are missed, you should stop taking pills until it is determined whether or not you are pregnant. Although there does not appear to be any increase in birth defects in newborn babies if you become pregnant while using oral contraceptives, if you do become pregnant, you should discuss the situation with your doctor or health care provider.

Periodic Examination

Your doctor will take a complete medical and family history before prescribing oral contraceptives. At that time and about once a year thereafter, he will generally examine your blood pressure, breasts, abdomen, and pelvic organs (including a Papanicolaou smear, ie, test for cancer).

SUMMARY

Oral contraceptives are the most effective method, except sterilization, for preventing pregnancy. Other methods, when used conscientiously, are also very effective and have fewer risks. Although the serious risks of oral contraceptives are uncommon, some of the risks may persist after you stop using the pill. On the other hand, the "pill" is a very convenient method of preventing pregnancy.

If you have certain conditions or have had these conditions in the past, you should not use oral contraceptives because the risk is too great. These conditions are listed in this leaflet. If you do not have these conditions, and decide to use the "pill," please read this leaflet carefully so that you can use the "pill" most safely and effectively.

Based on his or her assessment of your medical needs, your doctor or health care provider has prescribed this drug for you. Do not give this drug to anyone else.

Keep this and all drugs out of the reach of children.

Caution—Federal law prohibits dispensing without prescription.

June 1988   **0913G155**

Shown in Product Identification Section, page 421

LOPID®   ℞
[lō′pĭd]
(Gemfibrozil)

DESCRIPTION

Lopid (gemfibrozil capsules and tablets) is a lipid regulating agent. It is available as capsules or tablets for oral administration. Each capsule contains 300 mg gemfibrozil. Each also contains polysorbate 80, NF; starch, NF; silica gel. The capsule shell contains gelatin, NF; colloidal silicon dioxide, NF; sodium lauryl sulfate, NF; titanium dioxide, USP; FD&C Red No. 3; FD&C Blue No. 1. Each tablet contains 600 mg gemfibrozil. Each also contains calcium stearate, NF; candelilla wax FCC; microcrystalline cellulose, NF; hydroxypropyl cellulose, NF; hydroxypropyl methylcellulose, USP; methylparaben, NF; Opaspray white; polyethylene glycol, NF; polysorbate 80, NF; propylparaben, NF; colloidal silicon dioxide, NF; pregelatinized starch, NF. The chemical name is 5-(2,5-dimethylphenoxy)-2,2-dimethylpentanoic acid.

The empirical formula is $C_{15}H_{22}O_3$ and the molecular weight is 250.35; the solubility in water and acid is 0.0019% and in dilute base it is greater than 1%. The melting point is 58°–61°C. Gemfibrozil is a white solid which is stable under ordinary conditions.

CLINICAL PHARMACOLOGY

Lopid (gemfibrozil capsules and tablets) is a lipid regulating agent which decreases serum triglycerides and very low density lipoprotein (VLDL) cholesterol, and increases high density lipoprotein (HDL) cholesterol. While modest decreases in total and low density lipoprotein (LDL) cholesterol may be observed with Lopid therapy, treatment of patients with elevated triglycerides due to Type IV hyperlipoproteinemia often results in a rise in LDL-cholesterol. LDL-cholesterol levels in Type IIb patients with elevations of both serum LDL-cholesterol and triglycerides are, in general, minimally affected by Lopid treatment; however, Lopid usually raises HDL-cholesterol significantly in this group. Lopid increases levels of high density lipoprotein (HDL) subfractions HDL_2 and HDL_3, as well as apolipoproteins AI and AII. Epidemiological studies have shown that both low HDL-cholesterol and high LDL-cholesterol are independent risk factors for coronary heart disease.

In the Helsinki Heart Study, a large, randomized, double-blind, placebo-controlled, primary prevention trial in 4081 male patients between the ages of 40 and 55, Lopid therapy was associated with significant reductions in total plasma triglycerides and a significant increase in high density lipoprotein cholesterol. Moderate reductions in total plasma cholesterol and low density lipoprotein cholesterol were observed for the Lopid treatment group as a whole, but the lipid response was heterogeneous, especially among different Fredrickson Types. The study involved subjects with serum non-HDL-cholesterol of over 200 mg/dL and no previous history of coronary heart disease. Over the five-year study period, the Lopid group experienced a 34% reduction in serious coronary events (sudden cardiac deaths plus fatal and nonfatal myocardial infarctions) compared to placebo. There was a 37% reduction in nonfatal myocardial infarction.

The greatest reduction in the incidence of serious coronary events occurred in Type IIb patients who had elevations of both LDL-cholesterol and total plasma triglycerides. This subgroup of Type IIb gemfibrozil group patients had a lower mean HDL-cholesterol level at baseline than the Type IIa subgroup that had elevations of LDL-cholesterol and normal plasma triglycerides. The mean increase in HDL-cholesterol among the Type IIb patients in this study was 12.6% compared to placebo. It is not clear to what extent the findings of the Helsinki Heart Study can be extrapolated to other segments of the dyslipidemic population not studied or to other lipid-altering drugs.

The mechanism of action has not been definitely established. In man, Lopid has been shown to inhibit peripheral lipolysis and to decrease the hepatic extraction of free fatty acids, thus reducing hepatic triglyceride production. Lopid inhibits synthesis and increases clearance of VLDL carrier apolipoprotein B, leading to a decrease in VLDL production.

Animal studies suggest that Lopid may, in addition to elevating HDL-cholesterol, reduce incorporation of long-chain fatty acids into newly formed triglycerides, accelerate turnover and removal of cholesterol from the liver, and increase excretion of cholesterol in the feces.

Lopid is well absorbed from the gastrointestinal tract after oral administration. Peak plasma levels occur in one to two hours with a plasma half-life of 1.5 hours following multiple doses. Plasma levels appear proportional to dose and do not demonstrate accumulation across time following multiple doses.

Lopid mainly undergoes oxidation of a ring methyl group to successively form a hydroxymethyl and a carboxyl metabolite. Approximately seventy percent of the administered human dose is excreted in the urine, mostly as the glucuronide conjugate, with less than 2% excreted as unchanged gemfibrozil. Six percent of the dose is accounted for in the feces.

INDICATIONS AND USAGE

Lopid (gemfibrozil capsules and tablets) is indicated as adjunctive therapy to diet for:

1. Treatment of adult patients with very high elevations of serum triglyceride levels (Types IV and V hyperlipidemia) who present a risk of pancreatitis and who do not respond adequately to a determined dietary effort to control them. Patients who present such risk typically have serum triglycerides over 2000 mg/dL and have elevations of VLDL-cholesterol as well as fasting chylomicrons (Type V hyperlipidemia). Subjects who consistently have total serum or plasma triglycerides below 1000 mg/dL are unlikely to present a risk of pancreatitis. Lopid therapy may be considered for those subjects with triglyceride elevations between 1000 and 2000 mg/dL who have a history of pancreatitis or of recurrent abdominal pain typical of pancreatitis. It is recognized that some Type IV patients with triglycerides under 1000 mg/dL may, through dietary or alcoholic indiscretion, convert to a Type V pattern with massive triglyceride elevations accompanying fasting chylomicronemia, but the influence of Lopid therapy on the risk of pancreatitis in such situations has not been adequately studied. Drug therapy is not indicated for patients with Type I hyperlipoproteinemia, who have elevations of chylomicrons and plasma triglycerides, but who have normal levels of very low density lipoprotein (VLDL). Inspection of plasma refrigerated for 14 hours is helpful in distinguishing Types I, IV, and V hyperlipoproteinemia (ref. 3).

2. Reducing the risk of coronary heart disease, but consideration should first be given to bile acid sequestrants and nicotinic acid. Lopid therapy may be considered in those Type IIb patients who have low HDL-cholesterol levels in addition to elevated LDL-cholesterol and elevated triglycerides and who have had an inadequate response to weight loss, dietary therapy, exercise, and other pharmacologic agents, such as bile acid sequestrants and nicotinic acid, known to reduce LDL- and raise HDL-cholesterol (See WARNINGS, PRECAUTIONS, and CLINICAL PHARMACOLOGY). The National Cholesterol Education Program has defined a serum HDL-cholesterol value that is consistently below 35 mg/dL as constituting an independent risk factor for coronary heart disease. Patients with significantly elevated triglycerides should be closely observed when treated with gemfibrozil. In some patients with high triglyceride levels, treatment with gemfibrozil is associated with a significant increase in LDL-cholesterol. **Because of potential toxicity such as malignancy, gallbladder disease, abdominal pain leading to appendectomy and other abdominal surgeries, an increased incidence in noncoronary mortality, and the 29% increase in all-cause mortality seen with the chemically and pharmacologically related drug, clofibrate, the potential benefit of gemfibrozil in treating Type IIa patients with elevations of LDL-cholesterol only is not likely to outweigh the risks.** In a subgroup analysis of patients in the Helsinki Heart Study with above-median HDL-cholesterol values at baseline (greater than 46.4 mg/dL), the incidence of serious coronary events was similar for gemfibrozil and placebo subgroups.

The initial treatment for dyslipidemia is dietary therapy specific for the type of lipoprotein abnormality. Excess body weight and excess alcohol intake may be important factors in hypertriglyceridemia and should be managed prior to any drug therapy. Physical exercise can be an important ancillary measure, and has been associated with rises in HDL-cholesterol. Diseases contributory to hyperlipidemia such as hypothyroidism or diabetes mellitus should be looked for and adequately treated. Estrogen therapy is sometimes associated with massive rises in plasma triglycerides, especially in subjects with familial hypertriglyceridemia. In such cases, discontinuation of estrogen therapy may obviate the need for specific drug therapy of hypertriglyceridemia.

The use of drugs should be considered only when reasonable attempts have been made to obtain satisfactory results with nondrug methods. If the decision is made to use drugs, the patient should be instructed that this does not reduce the importance of adhering to diet.

CONTRAINDICATIONS

1. Hepatic or severe renal dysfunction, including primary biliary cirrhosis.
2. Preexisting gallbladder disease (See WARNINGS).
3. Hypersensitivity to gemfibrozil.

WARNINGS

1. Because of chemical, pharmacological, and clinical similarities between gemfibrozil and clofibrate, the adverse findings with clofibrate in two large clinical studies may also apply to gemfibrozil. In the first of those studies, the Coronary Drug Project, 1000 subjects with previous myocardial infarction were treated for five years with clofibrate. There was no difference in mortality between the clofibrate-treated subjects and 3000 placebo-treated subjects, but twice as many clofibrate-treated subjects developed cholelithiasis and cholecystitis requiring surgery. In the other study, conducted by the World Health Organization (WHO), 5000 subjects without known coronary heart disease were treated with clofibrate for five years and followed one year beyond. There was a statistically significant, 29%, higher total mortality in the clofibrate-treated than in a comparable placebo-treated control group. The excess mortality was due to a 33% increase in noncardiovascular causes, including malignancy, post-cholecystectomy complications, and pancreatitis. The higher risk of clofibrate-treated subjects for gallbladder disease was confirmed.

   During the Helsinski Heart Study and in the 1½ year follow-up period since the trial was completed, mortality from any cause was 59 (2.9%) in the Lopid group and 55 (2.7%) in the placebo group. Mortality from any cause during the double-blind portion of the study was 44 deaths in the Lopid group and 43 in the placebo group. Because of the more limited size of the Helsinki Heart Study, this result is not statistically-significantly different from the 29% excess mortality seen in the clofibrate group in the separate WHO study. Noncoronary heart disease related mortality showed a 58% greater trend in the Lopid group (43 vs 27 patients in the placebo group, p=0.056).

   In the Helsinki Heart Study, the incidence of total malignancies discovered during the trial and in the 1½ years since the trial was completed was 39 in the Lopid group and 29 in the placebo group (difference not statistically significant). This includes 5 basal cell carcinomas in the Lopid group and none in the placebo group (p=0.06; historical data predicted an expected 4.7 cases in the placebo group). GI malignancies and deaths from malignancies were not statistically different between Lopid and placebo subgroups. Follow-up of the Helsinki Heart Study participants will provide further information on cause-specific mortality and cancer morbidity.

2. A gallstone prevalence substudy of 450 Helsinki Heart Study participants showed a trend toward a greater prevalence of gallstones during the study within the Lopid treatment group (7.5% vs 4.9% for the placebo group, a 55% excess for the gemfibrozil group). A trend toward a greater incidence of gallbladder surgery was observed for the Lopid group (17 vs 11 subjects, a 54% excess). This result did not differ statistically from the increased incidence of cholecystectomy observed in the WHO study in the group treated with clofibrate. Both clofibrate and gemfibrozil may increase cholesterol excretion into the bile leading to cholelithiasis. If cholelithiasis is suspected, gallbladder studies are indicated. Lopid therapy should be discontinued if gallstones are found.

3. Since a reduction of mortality from coronary artery disease has not been demonstrated and because liver and interstitial cell testicular tumors were increased in rats, Lopid should be administered only to those patients described in the INDICATIONS AND USAGE section. If a significant serum lipid response is not obtained, Lopid should be discontinued.

4. Concomitant Anticoagulants—Caution should be exercised when anticoagulants are given in conjunction with Lopid. The dosage of the anticoagulant should be reduced to maintain the prothrombin time at the desired level to prevent bleeding complications. Frequent prothrombin determinations are advisable until it has been definitely determined that the prothrombin level has stabilized.

5. Concomitant therapy with Lopid and Mevacor® (lovastatin) has been associated with rhabdomyolysis, markedly elevated creatine kinase (CK) levels and myoglobinuria, leading in a high proportion of cases to acute renal failure. In most subjects who have had an unsatisfactory lipid response to either drug alone, the possible benefit of combined therapy with lovastatin and gemfibrozil does not outweigh the risks of severe myopathy, rhabdomyolysis, and acute renal failure (See Drug Interactions). The use of fibrates alone, including Lopid, may occasionally be associated with myositis. Patients receiving Lopid and complaining of muscle pain, tenderness, or weakness should have prompt medical evaluation for myositis, including serum creatine kinase level determination. If myositis is suspected or diagnosed, Lopid therapy should be withdrawn.

6. Cataracts—Subcapsular bilateral cataracts occurred in 10%, and unilateral in 6.3% of male rats treated with gemfibrozil at 10 times the human dose.

PRECAUTIONS

1. **Initial Therapy**—Laboratory studies should be done to ascertain that the lipid levels are consistently abnormal. Before instituting Lopid therapy, every attempt should be made to control serum lipids with appropriate diet, exercise, weight loss in obese patients, and control of any medical problems such as diabetes mellitus and hypothryroidism that are contributing to the lipid abnormalities.

2. **Continued Therapy**—Periodic determination of serum lipids should be obtained, and the drug withdrawn if lipid response is inadequate after 3 months of therapy.

3. **Drug Interactions**—(A) **Lovastatin**: Rhabdomyolysis has occurred with combined gemfibrozil and lovastatin therapy. It may be seen as early as 3 weeks after initiation of combined therapy or after several months. In most subjects who have had an unsatisfactory lipid response to either drug alone, the possible benefit of combined therapy with lovastatin and gemfibrozil does not outweigh the risks of severe myopathy, rhabdomyolysis, and acute renal failure. There is no assurance that periodic monitoring of creatine kinase will prevent the occurrence of severe myopathy and kidney damage.

   (B) **Anticoagulants**: CAUTION SHOULD BE EXERCISED WHEN ANTICOAGULANTS ARE GIVEN IN CONJUNCTION WITH LOPID. THE DOSAGE OF THE ANTICOAGULANT SHOULD BE REDUCED TO MAINTAIN THE PROTHROMBIN TIME AT THE DESIRED LEVEL TO PREVENT BLEEDING COMPLICATIONS. FREQUENT PROTHROMBIN DETERMINATIONS ARE ADVISABLE UNTIL IT HAS BEEN DEFINITELY DETERMINED THAT THE PROTHROMBIN LEVEL HAS STABILIZED.

4. **Carcinogenesis, Mutagenesis, Impairment of Fertility**—Long-term studies have been conducted in rats and mice at one and ten times the human dose. The incidence of benign liver nodules and liver carcinomas was significantly increased in high dose male rats. The incidence of liver carcinomas increased also in low dose males, but this increase was not statistically significant (p=0.1). In high dose female rats, there was a significant increase in the combined incidence of benign, and malignant liver neoplasms. In male and female mice, there were no statistically significant differences from controls in the incidence of liver tumors, but the doses tested were lower than those shown to be carcinogenic with other fibrates.

   Male rats had a dose-related and statistically significant increase of benign Leydig cell tumors at 1 and 10 times the human dose.

   Electron microscopy studies have demonstrated a florid hepatic peroxisome proliferation following Lopid administration to the male rat. An adequate study to test for peroxisome proliferation has not been done in humans but changes in peroxisome morphology have been observed. Peroxisome proliferation has been shown to occur in humans with either of two other drugs of the fibrate class when liver biopsies were compared before and after treatment in the same individual.

   Administration of approximately three or ten times the human dose to male rats for 10 weeks resulted in a dose-related decrease of fertility. Subsequent studies demonstrated that this effect was reversed after a drug-free period of about eight weeks, and it was not transmitted to the offspring.

5. **Pregnancy Category B**—Reproduction studies have been performed in the rat at doses 3 and 9 times the human dose, and in the rabbit at 2 and 6.7 times the human dose. These studies have revealed no evidence of impaired fertility in females or harm to the fetus due to Lopid. Minor fetotoxicity was manifested by reduced birth rates observed at the high dose levels. No significant malformations were found among almost 400 offspring from 36 litters of rats and 100 fetuses from 22 litters of rabbits. There are no studies in pregnant women. In view of the fact that Lopid is tumorigenic in male and female rats, the use of Lopid in pregnancy should be reserved for those patients where the benefit clearly outweighs the possible risk to the patient or fetus.

6. **Nursing Mothers**—Because of the potential for tumorigenicity shown for gemfibrozil in rats, a decision should be made whether to discontinue nursing or discontinue the drug, taking into account the importance of the drug to the mother.

7. **Hematologic Changes**—Mild hemoglobin, hematocrit and white blood cell decreases have been observed in occasional patients following initiation of Lopid therapy. However, these levels stabilize during long-term administration. Rarely, severe anemia, leukopenia, thrombocytopenia, and bone marrow hypoplasia have been reported. Therefore, periodic blood counts are recommended during the first 12 months of Lopid administration.

8. **Liver Function**—Abnormal liver function tests have been observed occasionally during Lopid administration, including elevations of AST (SGOT), ALT (SGPT), LDH, bilirubin, and alkaline phosphatase. These are usually reversible when Lopid is discontinued. Therefore periodic liver function studies are recommended and Lopid therapy should be terminated if abnormalities persist.

9. **Use in Children**—Safety and efficacy in children have not been established.

ADVERSE REACTIONS

In the double-blind controlled phase of the Helsinki Heart Study, 2046 patients received Lopid for up to 5 years. In that study, the following adverse reactions were statistically more frequent in subjects in the Lopid group:

	LOPID (N=2046)	PLACEBO (N=2035)
	Frequency in percent of subjects	
Gastrointestinal reactions	34.2	23.8
Dyspepsia	19.6	11.9
Abdominal pain	9.8	5.6
Acute appendicitis	1.2	0.6
(histologically confirmed in most cases where data were available)		
Atrial fibrillation	0.7	0.1

Adverse events reported by more than 1% of subjects, but without a significant difference between groups:

Diarrhea	7.2	6.5
Fatigue	3.8	3.5
Nausea/Vomiting	2.5	2.1
Eczema	1.9	1.2
Rash	1.7	1.3
Vertigo	1.5	1.3
Constipation	1.4	1.3
Headache	1.2	1.1

Gallbladder surgery was performed in 0.9% of Lopid and 0.5% of placebo subjects, a 64% excess, which is not statistically different from the excess of gallbladder surgery observed in the clofibrate compared to the placebo group of the WHO study.

Nervous system and special senses adverse reactions were more common in the Lopid group. These included hypesthesia, paresthesias, and taste perversion. Other adverse reactions that were more common among Lopid treatment group subjects but where a causal relationship was not established include cataracts, peripheral vascular disease, and intracerebral hemorrhage.

From other studies it seems probable that Lopid is causally related to the occurrence of **musculoskeletal symptoms** (See WARNINGS), and to **abnormal liver function tests** and **hematologic changes** (See PRECAUTIONS).

Reports of viral and bacterial infections (common cold, cough, urinary tract infections) were more common in gemfibrozil treated patients in other controlled clinical trials of 805 patients.

Additional adverse reactions that have been reported for gemfibrozil are listed below by system. These are categorized according to whether a causal relationship to treatment with Lopid is probable or not established:
[See table on top next page].

DOSAGE AND ADMINISTRATION

The recommended dose for adults is 1200 mg administered in two divided doses 30 minutes before the morning and evening meal.

MANAGEMENT OF OVERDOSE

While there has been no reported case of overdosage, symptomatic supportive measures should be taken should it occur.

HOW SUPPLIED

Lopid (Capsule 669), white and maroon opaque capsules, each containing 300 mg gemfibrozil, are available as follows:

Continued on next page

This product information was prepared in August, 1989. On these and other Parke-Davis Products, information may be obtained by addressing PARKE-DAVIS, Division of Warner-Lambert Company, Morris Plains, New Jersey 07950.

Parke-Davis—Cont.

	CAUSAL RELATIONSHIP PROBABLE	CAUSAL RELATIONSHIP NOT ESTABLISHED
General:		weight loss
Cardiac:	—	extrasystoles
Gastrointestinal:	cholestatic jaundice	pancreatitis
		hepatoma
		colitis
Central Nervous System:	dizziness	confusion
	somnolence	convulsions
	paresthesia	syncope
	peripheral neuritis	
	decreased libido	
	depression	
	headache	
Eye:	blurred vision	retinal edema
Genitourinary:	impotence	decreased male fertility
Musculoskeletal:	myopathy	
	myasthenia	
	myalgia	
	painful extremities	
	arthralgia	
	synovitis	
	rhabdomyolysis (see WARNINGS and Drug Interactions under PRECAUTIONS)	
Clinical Laboratory:	increased creatine phosphokinase	positive antinuclear antibody
	increased bilirubin	
	increased liver transaminases (AST [SGOT], ALT [SGPT])	
	increased alkaline phosphatase	
Hematopoietic:	anemia	thrombocytopenia
	leukopenia	
	bone marrow hypoplasia	
	eosinophilia	
Immunologic:	angioedema	anaphylaxis
	laryngeal edema	Lupus-like syndrome
	urticaria	vasculitis
Integumentary:	exfoliative dermatitis	alopecia
	rash	
	dermatitis	
	pruritus	

N 0071-0669-24 — Bottles of 100
N 0071-0669-30 — Bottles of 500
Parcode® No. 669
Lopid (Tablet 737), white, elliptical, film-coated, scored tablets, each containing 600 mg gemfibrozil, are available as follows:
N 0071-0737-20 — Bottles of 60
N 0071-0737-30 — Bottles of 500
Parcode No. 737
Storage: Store below 30°C (86°F).
References: 1. Frick MH, Elo O, Haapa K, et al: Helsinki Heart Study: Primary prevention trial with gemfibrozil in middle-aged men with dyslipidemia. N Engl J Med 1987; 317:1237-1245.
2. Manninen V, Elo O, Frick MH, et al: Lipid alterations and decline in the incidence of coronary heart disease in the Helsinki Heart Study. JAMA 1988; 260:641-651.
3. Nikkila EA: Familial lipoprotein lipase deficiency and related disorders of chylomicron metabolism. In Stanbury J.B. et al. (eds.): *The Metabolic Basis of Inherited Disease,* 5th ed., McGraw-Hill, 1983, Chap. 30, pp. 622-642.
Caution—Federal law prohibits dispensing without prescription.

0737G012
Shown in Product Identification Section, page 421

MANDELAMINE® TABLETS ℞
[măn "dĕ 'lă-mĭne]
(methenamine mandelate tablets, USP)

MANDELAMINE SUSPENSION FORTE, ℞
500 mg/5ml

MANDELAMINE SUSPENSION, ℞
250 mg/5ml
(methenamine mandelate oral suspension, USP)

MANDELAMINE GRANULES ℞
(methenamine mandelate)

DESCRIPTION
Mandelamine (methenamine mandelate, USP), a urinary antibacterial agent, is the chemical combination of mandelic acid with methenamine. Mandelamine is available for oral use as film-coated tablets, suspension, and granules.

Each tablet contains 0.5 g or 1 g of methenamine mandelate, USP; and also contains calcium stearate, NF; candelilla wax; colloidal silicon dioxide, NF; croscarmellose sodium, NF; hydroxypropylmethylcellulose; Opaspray brown (0.5 g tablet) or Opaspray purple (1 g tablet); povidone, USP; propylene glycol, USP; and silica gel.
Each teaspoonful of suspension contains 250 mg or 500 mg of methenamine mandelate, USP; and also contains flavors; propylparaben, NF; saccharin sodium, USP; sesame oil, NF and thixcin. The 500 mg per teaspoonful suspension also contains D&C red No. 6 Ba Lake.
Each packet of granules contains 0.5 g or 1 g of methenamine mandelate, USP; and also contains colloidal silicon dioxide, NF; D&C yellow No. 10; FD&C yellow No. 6 (sunset yellow); flavors; povidone, USP; saccharin sodium, USP; and sucrose, NF.

CLINICAL PHARMACOLOGY
Mandelamine is readily absorbed but remains essentially inactive until it is excreted by the kidney and concentrated in the urine. An acid urine is essential for antibacterial action, with maximum efficacy occurring at pH 5.5 or less. In an acid urine, mandelic acid exerts its antibacterial action and also contributes to the acidification of the urine. Mandelic acid is excreted by both glomerular filtration and tubular excretion. The methenamine component, in an acid urine, is hydrolyzed to ammonia and to the bactericidal agent formaldehyde. There is equally effective antibacterial activity against both gram-positive and gram-negative organisms, since the antibacterial action of mandelic acid and formaldehyde is nonspecific. There are reports that Mandelamine is ineffective in some infections with *Proteus vulgaris* and urea-splitting strains of *Pseudomonas aeruginosa* and *A aerogenes*. Since urea-splitting strains may raise the pH of the urine, particular attention to supplementary acidification is required. However, results in any single case will depend to a large extent on the underlying pathology and the overall management.

INDICATIONS AND USAGE
Mandelamine is indicated for the suppression or elimination of bacteriuria associated with pyelonephritis, cystitis, and other chronic urinary tract infections; also for infected residual urine sometimes accompanying neurologic diseases. When used as recommended, Mandelamine is particularly suitable for long-term therapy because of its safety and because resistance to the nonspecific bactericidal action of formaldehyde does not develop. Pathogens resistant to other antibacterial agents may respond to Mandelamine because of the non-specific effect of formaldehyde formed in an acid urine.

Prophylactic use rationale: Urine is a good culture medium for many urinary pathogens. Inoculation by a few organisms (relapse or reinfection) may lead to bacteriuria in susceptible individuals. Thus, the rationale of management in recurring urinary tract infection (bacteriuria) is to change the urine from a growth-supporting to a growth-inhibiting medium. There is a growing body of evidence that long-term administration of Mandelamine can prevent the recurrence of bacteriuria in patients with chronic pyelonephritis.

Therapeutic use rationale: Mandelamine helps to sterilize the urine, and in some situations in which underlying pathologic conditions prevent sterilization by any means, it can help to suppress the bacteriuria. Mandelamine should not be used alone for acute infections with parenchymal involvement causing systemic symptoms such as chills and fever. A thorough diagnostic investigation as a part of the overall management of the urinary tract infection should accompany the use of Mandelamine.

CONTRAINDICATIONS
Contraindicated in renal insufficiency.
Mandelamine should not be used in patients who have previously exhibited hypersensitivity to it.

PRECAUTIONS
General: Dysuria may occur (usually at higher than recommended dosage). This can be controlled by reducing the dosage and the acidification. When urine acidification is contraindicated or unattainable (as with some urea-splitting bacteria), the drug is not recommended.
To avoid inducing lipid pneumonia, administer Mandelamine Suspension Forte and Mandelamine Suspension with care to elderly, debilitated or otherwise susceptible patients.
Drug Interactions: Formaldehyde and sulfamethizole form an insoluble precipitate in acid urine; therefore, Mandelamine should not be administered concurrently with sulfamethizole.
Drug/Laboratory Test Interactions: Formaldehyde interferes with fluorometric procedures for determination of urinary catecholamines and vanilmandelic acid (VMA) causing erroneously high results. Formaldehyde also causes falsely decreased urine estriol levels by reacting with estriol when acid hydrolysis techniques are used; estriol determinations which use enzymatic hydrolysis are unaffected by formaldehyde. Formaldehyde causes falsely elevated 17-hydroxy-corticosteroid levels when the Porter-Silber method is used and falsely decreased 5-hydroxy-indoleacetic acid (5HIAA) levels by inhibiting color development when nitrosonaphthol methods are used.
Pregnancy Category C. Animal reproduction studies have not been conducted with Mandelamine. It is also not known whether Mandelamine can cause fetal harm when administered to a pregnant woman or can affect reproduction capacity. Mandelamine should be given to a pregnant woman only if clearly needed.
Since introduction, published reports on the use of Mandelamine in pregnant women have not shown an increased risk of fetal abnormalities from use during pregnancy.

ADVERSE REACTIONS
An occasional patient may experience gastrointestinal disturbance or a generalized skin rash. Microscopic and rarely gross hematuria have been described.

DOSAGE AND ADMINISTRATION
Directions for using Granules: dissolve contents of packet in 2–4 oz of water immediately before using. Solution formed may remain turbid.
Suspensions: Shake well before using.
The average adult dosage is 4 grams daily given as 1 gram after each meal and at bedtime. Children 6 to 12 should receive half the adult dose and children under 6 years of age should receive 250 mg per 30 lb body weight, four times daily. (See chart.) Since an acid urine is essential for antibacterial activity, with maximum efficacy occurring at pH 5.5 or below, restriction of alkalinizing foods and medication is thus desirable. If testing of urine pH reveals the need, supplemental acidification should be given.

DOSAGES

Dosage	Adults	Children
Tablets and Granules		
1 gram	1 tablet qid	—
	1 packet qid	—

0.5 gram	2 tablets qid	(Ages 6–12) 1 tablet qid	
	—	(Ages 6–12) 1 packet qid	
Suspension Forte 500 mg/ 5 ml teasp.	2 teaspoonfuls (10 ml) qid	(Ages 6–12) 1 teaspoonful (5 ml) qid	
Suspension 250 mg/5 ml teasp.	—	(Age under 6) 1 teaspoonful (5 ml) per 30 lb body weight qid	

HOW SUPPLIED

Mandelamine Tablets are supplied as:
N 0071-0166-24 0.5 g—Bottles of 100
N 0071-0166-32 0.5 g—Bottles of 1000
N 0071-0166-40 0.5 g—Unit dose packages of 100 (10 × 10 strips)
Each tablet is film coated, brown, and bears the P-D 166 monogram.
N 0071-0167-24 1 g—Bottles of 100
N 0071-0167-30 1 g—Bottles of 500
N 0071-0167-40 1 g—Unit dose packages of 100 (10 × 10 strips)
Each tablet is film coated, and bears the P-D 167 monogram.
Mandelamine Granules are supplied as:
N 0071-2176-03 1 g—Cartons of 56 individual packets.
Granules are orange flavored.
Mandelamine Suspension is supplied as:
N 0071-2173-23 250 mg/5 ml—Bottles of 16 fl oz
Suspension is cream colored, coconut flavored, and in vegetable oil.
Mandelamine Suspension Forte is supplied as:
N 0071-2174-20 500 mg/5 ml—Bottles of 8 fl oz
N 0071-2174-23 500 mg/5 ml—Bottles of 16 fl oz
Suspension is rosy pink, cherry flavored, and in vegetable oil.
Store between 15°–30°C (59°–86°F).

0166G036

Shown in Product Identification Section, page 421

MECLOMEN® ℞
[mĕ'clō"mĕn]
(Meclofenamate Sodium Capsules, USP)

DESCRIPTION

Meclomen (meclofenamate sodium) is N-(2, 6-dichloro-m-tolyl) anthranilic acid, sodium salt, monohydrate. It is an antiinflammatory drug for oral administration. Meclomen capsules contain 50 mg or 100 mg meclofenamic acid as the sodium salt. Also contain lactose, NF, magnesium stearate, NF; silica gel, NF; sodium lauryl sulfate, NF. The capsule shell contains colloidal silicon dioxide, NF, FD&C yellow No. 6, gelatin, NF, sodium lauryl sulfate, NF, titanium dioxide, USP.
It is a white powder with melting point 287° to 291°C, molecular weight 336.15, and water solubility greater than 250 mg/ml.

CLINICAL PHARMACOLOGY

Meclomen is a nonsteroidal agent which has demonstrated antiinflammatory, analgesic, and antipyretic activity in laboratory animals. The mode of action, like that of other nonsteroidal antiinflammatory agents, is not known. Therapeutic action does not result from pituitary-adrenal stimulation. In animal studies, Meclomen was found to inhibit prostaglandin synthesis and to compete for binding at the prostaglandin receptor site. These properties may be responsible for the antiinflammatory action of Meclomen. There is no evidence that Meclomen alters the course of the underlying disease.
Following a single oral dose to normal human volunteers, peak plasma levels occurred in 0.5 to 1 hr, with a half-life of 2 hr (3.3 hr following multiple doses). Plasma levels are proportional to dose. There is no evidence of accumulation of drug. Urinary and fecel excretion of tritium-labeled Meclomen account for 80% to 102% of the total dose, with about two thirds appearing in urine and one third in feces. Most of the urinary excretion occurs as the glucuronide conjugates of the metabolites, with only small amounts of free drug recovered.
In several human isotope studies, Meclomen, at a dosage of 300 mg/day, produced a fecal blood loss of 1 to 2 ml per day, and 2 to 3 ml per day at 400 mg/day. Aspirin, at a dosage of 3.6 g/day, caused a fecal blood loss of 6 ml per day.
In a multiple-dose, one-week study in normal human volunteers, Meclomen had little or no effect on collagen-induced platelet aggregation, platelet count, or bleeding time. In comparison, aspirin suppressed collagen-induced platelet aggregation and increased bleeding time. The concomitant administration of antacids (aluminum and magnesium hydroxides) does not interfere with absorption of Meclomen. Controlled clinical trials comparing Meclomen with aspirin demonstrated comparable efficacy in rheumatoid arthritis. The Meclomen-treated patients had fewer reactions involving the special senses, specifically tinnitus, but more gastrointestinal reactions, specifically diarrhea.
The incidence of patients who discontinued therapy due to adverse reactions was similar for both the Meclomen and aspirin-treated groups.
The improvement with Meclomen reported by patients and the reduction of the disease activity as evaluated by both physicians and patients with rheumatoid arthritis are associated with a significant reduction in number of tender joints, severity of tenderness, and duration of morning stiffness.
The improvement reported by patients and as evaluated by physicians in patients treated with Meclomen for osteoarthritis is associated with a significant reduction in night pain, pain on walking, degree of starting pain, and pain on passive motion. The function of knee joints also improved significantly.
Meclomen has been used in combination with gold salts or corticosteroids in patients with rheumatoid arthritis. Studies have demonstrated that Meclomen contributes to the improvement of patients' conditions while maintained on gold salts or corticosteroids. Data are inadequate to demonstrate that Meclomen in combination with salicylates produces greater improvement than that achieved with Meclomen alone.
In controlled clinical trials of patients with mild to moderate pain, Meclomen 50 mg provided significant pain relief. In these studies of episiotomy and dental pain, Meclomen 100 mg demonstrated additional benefit in some patients. The onset of analgesic effect was generally within one hour and the duration of action was 4 to 6 hours.

INDICATIONS AND USAGE

Meclomen is indicated for the relief of mild to moderate pain. Meclomen is also indicated for relief of the signs and symptoms of acute and chronic rheumatoid arthritis and osteoarthritis. As with all nonsteroidal antiinflammatory drugs, selection of Meclomen requires a careful assessment of the benefit/risk ratio. (See Warnings, Precautions and Adverse Reactions sections.)
The safety and effectiveness of Meclomen have not been established in those patients with rheumatism arthritis who are designated by the American Rheumatism Association as Functional Class IV (incapacitated, largely or wholly bedridden, or confined to a wheelchair, little or no self-care).
Meclomen is not recommended in children because adequate studies to demonstrate safety and efficacy have not been carried out.

CONTRAINDICATIONS

Meclomen should not be used in patients who have previously exhibited hypersensitivity to it.
Because the potential exists for cross sensitivity to aspirin or other nonsteroidal antiinflammatory drugs, Meclomen should not be given to patients in whom these drugs induce symptoms of bronchospasm, allergic rhinitis, or urticaria.

WARNINGS

Risk of GI Ulceration, Bleeding and Perforation with NSAID Therapy:
Serious gastrointestinal toxicity such as bleeding, ulceration, and perforation, can occur at any time, with or without warning symptoms, in patients treated chronically with NSAID therapy. Although minor upper gastrointestinal problems, such as dyspepsia, are common, usually developing early in therapy, physicians should remain alert for ulceration and bleeding in patients treated chronically with NSAIDs even in the absence of previous GI tract symptoms. In patients observed in clinical trials of several months to two years duration, symptomatic upper GI ulcers, gross bleeding or perforation appear to occur in approximately 1% of patients treated for 3–6 months, and in about 2–4% of patients treated for one year. Physicians should inform patients about the signs and/or symptoms of serious GI toxicity and what steps to take if they occur.
Studies to date have not identified any subset of patients not at risk of developing peptic ulceration and bleeding. Except for a prior history of serious GI events and other risk factors known to be associated with peptic ulcer disease, such as alcoholism, smoking, etc., no risk factors (e.g., age, sex) have been associated with increased risk. Elderly or debilitated patients seem to tolerate ulceration or bleeding less well than other individuals and most spontaneous reports of fatal GI events are in this population. Studies to date are inconclusive concerning the relative risk of various NSAIDs in causing such reactions. High doses of any NSAID probably carry a greater risk of these reactions, although controlled clinical trials showing this do not exist in most cases. In considering the use of relatively large doses (within the recommended dosage range), sufficient benefit should be anticipated to offset the potential increased risk of GI toxicity.

PRECAUTIONS

General: Patients receiving nonsteroidal antiinflammatory agents, such as Meclomen, should be evaluated periodically to insure that the drug is still necessary and well tolerated. (See other Precautions, Warnings, and Adverse Reactions.) Diarrhea, gastrointestinal irritation and abdominal pain may be associated with Meclomen therapy. Dosage reduction or temporarily stopping the drug have generally controlled these symptoms. (See Adverse Reactions and Dosage and Administration sections).
Decreases in hemoglobin and/or hematocrit levels have occurred in approximately 1 of 6 patients, but rarely required discontinuation of Meclomen therapy. The clinical data revealed no evidence of increased chronic blood loss, bone-marrow suppression, or hemolysis to account for the decreases in hemoglobin or hematocrit levels. Patients who are receiving long-term Meclomen therapy should have hemoglobin and hematocrit values determined if anemia is suspected on clinical grounds.
If a patient develops visual symptoms (see Adverse Reactions) during Meclomen therapy, the drug should be discontinued and the patient should have a complete ophthalmologic examination.
When Meclomen is used in combination with steroid therapy, any reduction in steroid dosage should be gradual to avoid the possible complications of sudden steroid withdrawal.
Adverse effects are seen more commonly in the elderly, therefore a lower starting dose and careful follow-up are advised.
As with other nonsteroidal antiinflammatory drugs, borderline evalutions of one or more liver tests may occur in some patients. These abnormalities may progress, may remain essentially unchanged, or may be transient with continued therapy. The SGPT (ALT) test is probably the most sensitive indicator of liver dysfunction. Meaningful (3 times the upper limit of normal) elevations of SGPT or SGOT (AST) occurred in controlled clinical trials in less than 1% of patients. A patient with symptoms and/or signs suggesting liver dysfunction, or in whom an abnormal liver test has occurred, should be evaluated for evidence of the development of more severe hepatic reaction while on therapy with Meclomen. Severe hepatic reactions, including jaundice and cases of fatal hepatitis, have been reported with other nonsteroidal antiinflammatory drugs. Although such reactions are rare, if abnormal liver tests persist or worsen, if clinical signs and symptoms consistent with liver disease develop, or if systemic manifestations occur (eg, eosinophilia, rash), Meclomen should be discontinued.
Renal Effects: As with other nonsteroidal antiinflammatory drugs, long-term administration of meclofenamate sodium to animals has resulted in renal papillary necrosis and other abnormal renal pathology. In humans, there have been reports of acute interstitial nephritis with hematuria, proteinuria, and occasionally nephrotic syndrome.
A second form of renal toxicity has been seen in patients with prerenal conditions leading to a reduction in renal blood flow or blood volume, where the renal prostaglandins have a supportive role in the maintenance of renal perfusion. In these patients administration of an NSAID may cause a dose-dependent reduction in prostaglandin formation and may precipitate overt renal decompensation. Patients at greatest risk of this reaction are those with impaired renal function, heart failure, liver dysfunction, those taking diuretics, and the elderly. Discontinuation of NSAID therapy is typically followed by recovery to the pretreatment state. Since Meclomen is eliminated primarily by the kidneys, patients with significantly impaired renal function should be closely monitored; a lower daily dosage should be anticipated to avoid excessive drug accumulation.
Information for Patients: Patients should be advised that nausea, vomiting, diarrhea, and abdominal pain have been associated with the use of Meclomen. The patient should be made aware of a possible drug connection and accordingly should consider discontinuing the drug and contacting his or her physician if any of these conditions are severe.
Meclomen may be taken with meals or milk to control gastrointestinal complaints. Concomitant administration of an antacid (specifically, aluminum and magnesium hydroxides) does not interfere with the absorption of the drug.
Meclomen, like other drugs of its class, is not free of side effects. The side effects of these drugs can cause discomfort and, rarely, there are more serious side effects, such as gas-

Continued on next page

This product information was prepared in August, 1989. On these and other Parke-Davis Products, information may be obtained by addressing PARKE-DAVIS, Division of Warner-Lambert Company, Morris Plains, New Jersey 07950.

Parke-Davis—Cont.

trointestinal bleeding, which may result in hospitalization and even fatal outcomes.

NSAIDs (nonsteroidal antiinflammatory drugs) are often essential agents in the management of arthritis and have a major role in the treatment of pain, but they also may be commonly employed for conditions which are less serious. Physicians may wish to discuss with their patients the potential risks (see WARNINGS, PRECAUTIONS, and ADVERSE REACTIONS sections) and likely benefits of NSAID treatment, particularly when the drugs are used for less serious conditions where treatment without NSAIDs may represent an acceptable alternative to both the patient and physician.
Laboratory Tests: Patients receiving long-term Meclomen therapy should have hemoglobin and hematocrit values determined if signs or symptoms of anemia occur.
Low white blood cell counts were rarely observed in clinical trials. These low counts were transient and usually returned to normal while the patient continued on Meclomen therapy. Persistent leukopenia, granulocytopenia, or thrombocytopenia warrant further clinical evaluation and may require discontinuation of the drug.
When abnormal blood chemistry values are obtained, follow-up studies are indicated.
Elevations of serum transaminase levels and of alkaline phosphatase levels occurred in approximately 4% of patients. An occasional patient had elevations of serum creatinine or BUN levels.
Because serious GI tract ulceration and bleeding can occur without warning symptoms, physicians should follow chronically treated patients for the signs and symptoms of ulceration and bleeding and should inform them of the importance of this follow-up (see Risk of GI Ulcerations, Bleeding and Perforation with NSAID Therapy).

DRUG INTERACTIONS
1.**Warfarin:** Meclomen enhances the effect of warfarin. Therefore, when Meclomen is given to a patient receiving warfarin, the dosage of warfarin should be reduced to prevent excessive prolongation of the prothrombin time.
2.**Aspirin:** Concurrent administration of aspirin may lower Meclomen plasma levels, possibly by competing for protein-binding sites. The urinary excretion of Meclomen is unaffected by aspirin, indicating no change in Meclomen absorption. Meclomen does not affect serum salicylate levels. Greater fecal blood loss results from concomitant administration of both drugs than from either drug alone.
3.**Propoxyphene:** The concurrent administration of propoxyphene hydrochloride does not affect the bioavailability of Meclomen.
4.**Antacids:** Concomitant administration of aluminum and magnesium hydroxides does not interfere with absorption of Meclomen.
Carcinogenesis: An 18-month study in rats revealed no evidence of carcinogenicity.
Usage in Pregnancy: Meclomen like aspirin and other nonsteroidal antiinflammatory drugs causes fetotoxicity, minor skeletal malformations, eg, supernumerary ribs, and delayed ossification in rodent reproduction trials, but no major teratogenicity. Similarly, it prolongs gestation and interferes with parturition and with normal development of young before weaning. Meclomen is not recommended for use during pregnancy, particularly in the 1st and 3rd trimesters based on these animal findings. There are, however, no adequate and well-controlled studies in pregnant women.
Usage in Nursing Mothers: It is not known whether Meclomen is excreted in human milk. Because of the effects on suckling rodents and the fact that many drugs are excreted in human milk, Meclomen is not recommended for nursing women.
Pediatric Use: Safety and effectiveness in children below the age of 14 have not been established.

ADVERSE REACTIONS
Incidence Greater than 1%
The following adverse reactions were observed in clinical trials and included observations from more than 2,700 patients, 594 of whom were treated for one year and 248 for at least two years.
Gastrointestinal: The most frequently reported adverse reactions associated with Meclomen involve the gastrointestinal system. In controlled studies of up to six months duration, these disturbances occurred in the following decreasing order of frequency with the approximate incidences in parentheses: diarrhea (10–33%), nausea with or without vomiting (11%), other gastrointestinal disorders (10%), and abdominal pain.* In long-term uncontrolled studies of up to four years duration, one third of the patients had at least one episode of diarrhea some time during Meclomen therapy. In approximately 4% of the patients in controlled studies, diarrhea was severe enough to require discontinuation of Meclomen. The occurrence of diarrhea is dose related, generally subsides with dose reduction, and clears with termination of therapy. The incidence of diarrhea in patients with

osteoarthritis is generally lower than that reported in patients with rheumatoid arthritis.
Other reactions less frequently reported were pyrosis,* flatulence,* anorexia, constipation, stomatitis, and peptic ulcer. The majority of the patients with peptic ulcer had either a history of ulcer disease or were receiving concomitant antiinflammatory drugs, including corticosteroids which are known to produce peptic ulceration.
Cardiovascular: edema
Dermatologic: rash,* urticaria, pruritus
Central Nervous System: headache,* dizziness*
Special Senses: tinnitus
*Incidence between 3% and 9%. Those reactions occurring in 1% to 3% of patients are not marked with an asterisk.
Incidence Less than 1%.
Probably Causally Related
The following adverse reactions were reported less frequently than 1% during controlled clinical trials and through voluntary reports since marketing. The probability of a causal relationship exists between the drug and these adverse reactions.
Gastrointestinal: Bleeding and/or perforation with or without obvious ulcer formation, colitis, cholestatic jaundice
Renal: Renal failure.
Hematologic: Neutropenia, thrombocytopenic purpura, leukopenia, agranulocytosis, hemolytic anemia, eosinophilia, decrease in hemoglobin and /or hematocrit
Dermatologic: Erythema multiforme, Stevens-Johnson syndrome, exfoliative dermatitis
Hepatic: Alteration of liver function tests
Allergic: Lupus and serum sickness-like symptoms
Incidence Less than 1%
Causal Relationship Unknown
Other reactions have been reported but under conditions where a causal relationship could not be established. However, in these rarely reported events, that possibility cannot be excluded. Therefore, these observations are listed to alert physicians.
Cardiovascular: palpitations
Central Nervous System: malaise, fatigue, paresthesia, insomnia, depression
Special Senses: blurred vision, taste disturbances, decreased visual acuity, temporary loss of vision, reversible loss of color vision, retinal changes including macular fibrosis, macular and perimacular edema, conjunctivitis, iritis
Renal: nocturia
Gastrointestinal: paralytic ileus
Dermatologic: erythema nodosum, hair loss

OVERDOSAGE
The following is based on the little information available concerning overdose with Melcomen and related compounds. After a massive overdose, CNS stimulation may be manifested by irrational behavior, marked agitation and generalized seizures. Following this phase, renal toxicity (falling urine output, rising creatinine, abnormal urinary cellular elements) may be noted with possible oliguria or anuria and azotemia. One patient was anuric for about a week before diuresis and recovery occurred.
Management consists of emptying the stomach by emesis or lavage and instilling an ample dose of activated charcoal into the stomach. There is some evidence that charcoal will actively absorb Meclomen, but dialysis or hemoperfusion may be less effective because of plasma protein binding. The seizures should be controlled by an appropriate anticonvulsant regimen. Attention should be directed throughout, by careful monitoring, to the preservation of vital functions and fluid-electrolyte balance. Dialysis may be required to correct serious azotemia or electrolyte imbalance.

DOSAGE AND ADMINISTRATION
Usual Dosage: *For mild to moderate pain,* the recommended dose is 50 mg every 4 to 6 hours. Doses of 100 mg may be needed in some patients for optimal pain relief. (See CLINICAL PHARMACOLOGY section.) However, the daily dose should not exceed 400 mg. (See ADVERSE REACTIONS section.)
For rheumatoid arthritis and osteoarthritis, including acute exacerbations of chronic disease, the dosage is 200 to 400 mg per day, administered in three or four equal doses. Therapy should be initiated at the lower dosage, then increased as necessary to improve clinical response. The dosage should be individually adjusted for each patient depending on the severity of the symptoms and the clinical response. The daily dosage should not exceed 400 mg per day. The smallest dosage of Meclomen that yields clinical control should be employed.
Although improvement may be seen in some patients in a few days, two to three weeks of treatment may be required to obtain the optimum therapeutic benefit.
After a satisfactory response has been achieved, the dosage should be adjusted as required. A lower dosage may suffice for long-term administration.
If gastrointestinal complaints occur, see Warnings and Precautions. Meclomen may be administered with meals or with milk. If intolerance occurs, the dosage may need to be re-

duced. Therapy should be terminated if any severe adverse reactions occur.

HOW SUPPLIED
(Capsule 268) Meclomen Capsules, each containing meclofenamate sodium monohydrate equivalent to 50 mg meclofenamic acid, are available:
N 0071-0268-24—bottles of 100
N 0071-0268-40—Uni/Use® 100's (10×10)
(Capsule 269) Meclomen Capsules, each containing meclofenamate sodium monohydrate equivalent to 100 mg meclofenamic acid, are available:
N 0071-0269-24—bottles of 100
N 0071-0269-30—bottles of 500
N 0071-0269-40—Uni/Use 100's (10×10)
Storage: Store at room temperature below 30°C (86°F). Protect from moisture and light.

0268G311

Shown in Product Identification Section, page 421

MILONTIN® ℞
[mĭ"lŏn'tĭn]
(phensuximide, USP)

DESCRIPTION
Milontin (phensuximide) is an anticonvulsant succinimide, chemically designated as N-methyl-2-phenylsuccinimide. Each Milontin capsule contains 500 mg phensuximide USP. The capsule and band contain citric acid, USP; colloidal silicon dioxide, NF; D&C yellow No. 10, FD&C red No. 3, FD&C yellow No. 6, gelatin, NF; glyceryl monooleate, polyethylene glycol 200, sodium benzoate, NF; sodium lauryl sulfate, NF.

ACTION
Phensuximide suppresses the paroxysmal three-cycle-per-second spike and wave activity associated with lapses of consciousness which is common in absence (petit mal) seizures. The frequency of epileptiform attacks is reduced, apparently by depression of the motor cortex and elevation of the threshold of the central nervous system to convulsive stimuli.

INDICATION
Milontin is indicated for the control of absence (petit mal) seizures.

CONTRAINDICATION
Phensuximide should not be used in patients with a history of hypersensitivity to succinimides.

WARNINGS
Blood dyscrasias, including some with fatal outcome, have been reported to be associated with the use of succinimides; therefore, periodic blood counts should be performed.
It has been reported that succinimides have produced morphological and functional changes in animal liver. For this reason, phensuximide should be administered with extreme caution to patients with known liver or renal diseases. Periodic urinalysis and liver function studies are advised for all patients receiving the drug.
Cases of systemic lupus erythematosus have been reported with the use of succinimides. The physician should be alert to this possibility.
Usage in pregnancy: The effects of Milontin in human pregnancy and nursing infants are unknown.
Recent reports suggest an association between the use of anticonvulsant drugs by women with epilepsy and an elevated incidence of birth defects in children born to these women. Data is more extensive with respect to phenytoin and phenobarbital, but these are also the most commonly prescribed anticonvulsants; less systematic or anecdotal reports suggest a possible similar association with the use of all known anticonvulsant drugs.
The reports suggesting an elevated incidence of birth defects in children of drug-treated epileptic women cannot be regarded as adequate to prove a definite cause-and-effect relationship. There are intrinsic methodologic problems in obtaining adequate data on drug teratogenicity in humans; the possibility also exists that other factors, eg, genetic factors or the epileptic condition itself, may be more important than drug therapy in leading to birth defects. The great majority of mothers on anticonvulsant medication deliver normal infants. It is important to note that anticonvulsant drugs should not be discontinued in patients in whom the drug is administered to prevent major seizures because of the strong possibility of precipitating status epilepticus with attendant hypoxia and threat to life. In individual cases where the severity and frequency of the seizure disorder are such that the removal of medication does not pose a serious threat to the patient, discontinuation of the drug may be considered prior to and during pregnancy, although it cannot be said with any confidence that even minor seizures do not pose some hazard to the developing embryo or fetus.
The prescribing physician will wish to weigh these considerations in treating or counseling epileptic women of childbearing potential.
Hazardous activities: Phensuximide may impair the mental and/or physical abilities required for the performance of

potentially hazardous tasks, such as driving a motor vehicle or other such activity requiring alertness; therefore, the patient should be cautioned accordingly.

PRECAUTIONS

Phensuximide, when used alone in mixed types of epilepsy, may increase the frequency of grand mal seizures in some patients.

As with other anticonvulsants, it is important to proceed slowly when increasing or decreasing dosage, as well as when adding or eliminating other medication. Abrupt withdrawal of anticonvulsant medication may precipitate absence (petit mal) status.

ADVERSE REACTIONS

Gastrointestinal System: Gastrointestinal symptoms, such as nausea, vomiting, and anorexia, occur frequently, but may be the result of overdosage.

Nervous System: Neurologic and sensory reactions reported during therapy with phensuximide have included drowsiness, dizziness, ataxia, headache, dreamlike state, and lethargy. Side effects, such as drowsiness and dizziness, may be relieved by a reduction in total dosage.

Integumentary System: Dermatologic manifestations reported to be associated with the administration of phensuximide have included pruritus, skin eruptions, erythema multiforme, and erythematous rashes.

Genitourinary System: Genitourinary complications which have been reported include urinary frequency, renal damage, and hematuria.

Hemopoietic System: Hemopoietic complications associated with the administration of phensuximide include granulocytopenia, transient leukopenia, and pancytopenia.

Other: Miscellaneous reactions reported have been alopecia and muscular weakness.

DOSAGE AND ADMINISTRATION

Milontin (phensuximide capsules, USP) is administered by the oral route in doses of 500 mg to 1 g two or three times daily. As with other anticonvulsant medication, the dosage should be adjusted to suit individual requirements. The total dosage, irrespective of age, may, therefore, vary between 1 and 3 g per day, the average being 1.5 g.

Milontin may be administered in combination with other anticonvulsants when other forms of epilepsy coexist with absence (petit mal).

HOW SUPPLIED

N 0071-0393-24 (Kapseal® 393)—Milontin Kapseals, each containing 0.5 g phensuximide; bottles of 100.

0393G012

Shown in Product Identification Section, page 421

NARDIL® ℞

[när´dĭl″]

(Phenelzine Sulfate Tablets, USP)

DESCRIPTION

Nardil (phenelzine sulfate) is a potent inhibitor of monoamine oxidase (MAO). Chemically, it is a hydrazine derivative. Each tablet contains phenelzine sulfate equivalent to 15 mg of phenelzine base. Also contains acacia, NF; calcium carbonate, carnauba wax, NF; corn starch, NF; FD and C yellow No. 6; gelatin, NF; kaolin, USP; magnesium stearate, NF; mannitol, USP; pharmaceutical glaze, NF; povidone, USP; sucrose, NF; talc, USP; white wax, NF; white wheat flour.

ACTIONS

Monoamine oxidase is a complex enzyme system, widely distributed throughout the body. Drugs that inhibit monoamine oxidase in the laboratory are associated with a number of clinical effects. Thus, it is unknown whether MAO inhibition *per se*, other pharmacologic actions, or an interaction of both is responsible for the clinical effects observed. Therefore, the physician should become familiar with all the effects produced by drugs of this class.

INDICATIONS

Nardil has been found to be effective in depressed patients clinically characterized as "atypical," "nonendogenous," or "neurotic." These patients often have mixed anxiety and depression and phobic or hypochondriacal features. There is less conclusive evidence of its usefulness with severely depressed patients with endogenous features.

Nardil should rarely be the first antidepressant drug used. Rather, it is more suitable for use with patients who have failed to respond to the drugs more commonly used for these conditions.

CONTRAINDICATIONS

Nardil is contraindicated in patients with known sensitivity to the drug, pheochromocytoma, congestive heart failure, a history of liver disease, or abnormal liver function tests. The potentiation of sympathomimetic substances and related compounds by MAO inhibitors may result in hypertensive crises (See WARNINGS). Therefore, patients being treated with Nardil should not take sympathomimetic drugs

(including amphetamines, cocaine, methylphenidate, dopamine, epinephrine and norepinephrine) or related compounds (including methyldopa, L-dopa, L-tryptophan, L-tyrosine, and phenylalanine). Hypertensive crises during Nardil therapy may also be caused by the ingestion of foods with a high concentration of tyramine or dopamine. Therefore, patients being treated with Nardil should avoid high protein food that has undergone protein breakdown by aging, fermentation, pickling, smoking, or bacterial contamination; patients should also avoid cheeses (especially aged varieties), pickled herring, beer, wine, liver, yeast extract (including brewer's yeast in large quantities), dry sausage (including Genoa salami, hard salami, pepperoni, and Lebanon bologna), pods of broad beans (Fava beans), and yogurt. Excessive amounts of caffeine and chocolate may also cause hypertensive reactions.

Nardil should not be used in combination with CNS depressants such as alcohol and certain narcotics. Excitation, seizures, delirium, hyperpyrexia, circulatory collapse, coma, and death have been reported in patients receiving MAOI therapy who have been given a single dose of meperidine. Nardil should not be administered together with or in rapid succession to other MAO inhibitors because HYPERTENSIVE CRISES and convulsive seizures, fever, marked sweating, excitation, delirium, tremor, coma, and circulatory collapse may occur.

List of MAO Inhibitors

Generic Name	Trademark
pargyline hydrochloride	Eutonyl® (Abbott Laboratories)
pargyline hydrochloride and methyclothiazide	Eutron® (Abbott Laboratories)
furazolidone	Furoxone® (Eaton Laboratories)
isocarboxazid	Marplan® (Roche)
procarbazine	Matulane® (Roche)
tranylcypromine	Parnate® (Smith Kline & French Laboratories)

Nardil should also not be used in combination with buspirone HCl, since several cases of elevated blood pressure have been reported in patients taking MAO inhibitors who were then given buspirone HCl. At least 10 days should elapse between the discontinuation of Nardil and the institution of another antidepressant or buspirone HCl, or the discontinuation of another MAO inhibitor and the institution of Nardil.

Patients taking Nardil should not undergo elective surgery requiring general anesthesia. Also, they should not be given cocaine or local anesthesia containing sympathomimetic vasoconstrictors. The possible combined hypotensive effects of Nardil and spinal anesthesia should be kept in mind. Nardil should be discontinued at least 10 days prior to elective surgery.

IMPORTANT

Warnings: The most serious reactions to Nardil involve changes in blood pressure.

Hypertensive Crises: The most important reaction associated with Nardil administration is the occurrence of hypertensive crises, which have sometimes been fatal.

These crises are characterized by some or all of the following symptoms: occipital headache which may radiate frontally, palpitation, neck stiffness or soreness, nausea, vomiting, sweating (sometimes with fever and sometimes with cold, clammy skin), dilated pupils, and photophobia. Either tachycardia or bradycardia may be present and can be associated with constricting chest pain.

NOTE: Intracranial bleeding has been reported in association with the increase in blood pressure.

Blood pressure should be observed frequently to detect evidence of any pressor response in all patients receiving Nardil. Therapy should be discontinued immediately upon the occurrence of palpitation or frequent headaches during therapy.

Recommended treatment in hypertensive crisis: If a hypertensive crisis occurs, Nardil should be discontinued immediately and therapy to lower blood pressure should be instituted immediately. On the basis of present evidence, phentolamine is recommended. (The dosage reported for phentolamine is 5 mg intravenously.) Care should be taken to administer this drug slowly in order to avoid producing an excessive hypotensive effect. Fever should be managed by means of external cooling.

Warning to the patient: All patients should be warned that the following foods, beverages and medications must be avoided while taking Nardil, and for two weeks after discontinuing use.

Foods and Beverages To Avoid
Meat and Fish
Pickled herring
Liver
Dry sausage (including Genoa salami, hard salami, pepperoni, and Lebanon bologna)

Vegetables
Broad bean pods (fava bean pods)
Dairy Products
Cheese (cottage cheese and cream cheese are allowed)
Yogurt
Beverages
Beer and wine
Alcohol-free and reduced-alcohol beer and wine products
Miscellaneous
Yeast extract (including brewer's yeast in large quantities)
Excessive amounts of chocolate and caffeine
Also, any spoiled or improperly refrigerated, handled or stored protein-rich foods such as meats, fish, and dairy products, including foods that may have undergone protein changes by aging, pickling, fermentation, or smoking to improve flavor should be avoided.

OTC Medications To Avoid
Cold and cough preparations (including those containing dextromethorphan)
Nasal decongestants (tablets, drops or spray)
Hay-fever medications
Sinus medications
Asthma inhalant medications
Antiappetite medicines
Weight-reducing preparations
"Pep" pills
L-tryptophan containing preparations
Also, certain prescription drugs should be avoided. Therefore, patients under the care of another physician or dentist, should inform him/her they are taking Nardil.

Patients should be warned that the use of the above foods, beverages or medications may cause a reaction characterized by headache and other serious symptoms due to a rise in blood pressure.

Patients should be instructed to report promptly the occurrence of headache or other unusual symptoms.

Concomitant Use with Dibenzazepine Derivative Drugs
If the decision is made to administer Nardil concurrently with other antidepressant drugs, or within less than 10 days after discontinuation of antidepressant therapy, the patient should be cautioned by the physician regarding the possibility of adverse drug interaction.

List of Dibenzazepine Derivative Drugs

Generic Name	Trademark
nortriptyline hydrochloride	Aventyl® (Eli Lilly & Co.)
amitriptyline hydrochloride	Elavil® (Merck Sharp & Dohme)
amitriptyline hydrochloride	Endep® (Roche)
perphenazine and amitriptyline hydrochloride	Etrafon® (Schering Corporation)
perphenazine and amitriptyline hydrochloride	Triavil® (Merck Sharp & Dohme)
clomipramine hydrochloride	Anafranil® (CIBA-Geigy)
desipramine hydrochloride	Norpramin® (Merrell-National)
desipramine hydrochloride	Pertofrane® (USV)
imipramine hydrochloride	Tofranil® (Geigy)
doxepin	Adapin® (Pennwalt)
doxepin	Sinequan® (Pfizer)
carbamazepine	Tegretol® (Geigy)
cyclobenzaprine HCl	Flexeril® (Merck Sharp & Dohme)
amoxapine	Asendin® (Lederle)
maprotiline HCl	Ludiomil® (CIBA)
trimipramine maleate	Surmontil® (Wyeth)
protriptyline HCl	Vivactil® (Merck Sharp & Dohme)

Nardil should be used with caution in combination with antihypertensive drugs, including thiazide diuretics and β-blockers, since exaggerated hypotensive effects may result. MAO inhibitors including Nardil are contraindicated in patients receiving guanethidine.

Use in Pregnancy: The safe use of Nardil during pregnancy or lactation has not been established. The potential benefit of this drug, if used during pregnancy, lactation, or in women of

Continued on next page

This product information was prepared in August, 1989. On these and other Parke-Davis Products, information may be obtained by addressing PARKE-DAVIS, Division of Warner-Lambert Company, Morris Plains, New Jersey 07950.

Parke-Davis—Cont.

childbearing age, should be weighed against the possible hazard to the mother or fetus.

Doses of Nardil in pregnant mice well exceeding the maximum recommended human dose have caused a significant decrease in the number of viable offspring per mouse. In addition, the growth of young dogs and rats has been retarded by doses exceeding the maximum human dose.

Use in Children: Nardil is not recommended for patients under 16 years of age since there are no controlled studies of safety in this age group.

Nardil, as with other hydrazine derivatives, has been reported to induce pulmonary and vascular tumors in an uncontrolled lifetime study in mice.

PRECAUTIONS

In depressed patients, the possibility of suicide should always be considered and adequate precautions taken. It is recommended that careful observations of patients undergoing Nardil treatment be maintained until control of depression is achieved. If necessary, additional measures (ECT, hospitalization, etc.) should be instituted.

All patients undergoing treatment with Nardil should be closely followed for symptoms of postural hypotension. Hypotensive side effects have occurred in hypertensive as well as normal and hypotensive patients. Blood pressure usually returns to pretreatment levels rapidly when the drug is discontinued or the dosage is reduced.

Because the effect of Nardil on the convulsive threshold may be variable, adequate precautions should be taken when treating epileptic patients.

Of the more severe side effects that have been reported with any consistency, hypomania has been the most common. This reaction has been largely limited to patients in whom disorders characterized by hyperkinetic symptoms coexist with, but are obscured by, depressive affect; hypomania usually appeared as depression improved. If agitation is present, it may be increased with Nardil. Hypomania and agitation have also been reported at higher than recommended doses, or following long-term therapy.

Nardil may cause excessive stimulation in schizophrenic patients; in manic-depressive states it may result in a swing from a depressive to a manic phase.

MAO inhibitors, including Nardil potentiate hexobarbital hypnosis in animals. Therefore, barbiturates should be given at a reduced dose with Nardil.

MAO inhibitors inhibit the destruction of serotonin and norepinephrine, which are believed to be released from tissue stores by rauwolfia alkaloids. Accordingly, caution should be exercised when rauwolfia is used concomitantly with an MAO inhibitor, including Nardil.

There is conflicting evidence as to whether or not MAO inhibitors affect glucose metabolism or potentiate hypoglycemic agents. This should be kept in mind if Nardil is administered to diabetics.

ADVERSE REACTIONS

Nardil is a potent inhibitor of monoamine oxidase. Because this enzyme is widely distributed throughout the body, diverse pharmacologic effects can be expected to occur. When they occur, such effects tend to be mild or moderate in severity (see below), often subside as treatment continues, and can be minimized by adjusting dosage; rarely is it necessary to institute counteracting measures or to discontinue Nardil.

Common side effects include:

Nervous System —Dizziness, headache, drowsiness, sleep disturbances (including insomnia and hypersomnia), fatigue, weakness, tremors, twitching, hyperreflexia.

Gastrointestinal —Constipation, dry mouth, gastrointestinal disturbances, elevated serum transaminases (without accompanying signs and symptoms).

Metabolic —Weight gain.

Cardiovascular —Postural hypotension, edema.

Genitourinary —Sexual disturbances, ie, anorgasmia and ejaculatory disturbances.

Less common mild to moderate side effects (some of which have been reported in a single patient or by a single physician) include:

Nervous System —Jitteriness, palilalia, euphoria, nystagmus, paresthesias.

Genitourinary —Urinary retention.

Metabolic —Hypernatremia.

Dermatologic —Skin rash, sweating.

Special senses —Blurred vision, glaucoma.

Although reported less frequently, and sometimes only once, additional severe side effects include:

Nervous System —Ataxia, shock-like coma, toxic delirium, manic reaction, acute anxiety reaction, precipitation of schizophrenia, transient respiratory and cardiovascular depression following ECT.

Gastrointestinal —To date, fatal progressive necrotizing hepatocellular damage has been reported in a very few patients. Reversible jaundice.

Hematologic —Leukopenia.

Other —Hypermetabolic syndrome (which may resemble an overdose), edema of the glottis.

An uncommon withdrawal syndrome following abrupt withdrawal of Nardil has been infrequently reported. Signs and symptoms of this syndrome generally commence 24 to 72 hours after drug discontinuation and may range from vivid nightmares with agitation to frank psychosis. This syndrome generally responds to reinstitution of low-dose Nardil therapy followed by cautious downward titration and discontinuation.

DOSAGE AND ADMINISTRATION

Initial dose: the usual starting dose of Nardil is one tablet (15 mg) three times a day.

Early phase treatment: dosage should be increased to at least 60 mg per day at a fairly rapid pace consistent with patient tolerance. It may be necessary to increase dosage up to 90 mg per day to obtain sufficient MAO inhibition. Many patients do not show a clinical response until treatment at 60 mg has been continued for at least 4 weeks.

Maintenance dose: after maximum benefit from Nardil is achieved, dosage should be reduced slowly over several weeks. Maintenance dose may be as low as 1 tablet, 15 mg, a day or every other day, and should be continued for as long as is required.

OVERDOSAGE

Note—For management of *hypertensive crises* see Warnings. Accidental or intentional overdosage may be more common in patients who are depressed. It should be remembered that multiple drugs and/or alcohol may have been ingested.

Depending on the amount of overdosage with Nardil, a varying and mixed clinical picture may develop, involving signs and symptoms of central nervous system and cardiovascular stimulation and/or depression. Signs and symptoms may be absent or minimal during the initial 12-hour period following ingestion and may develop slowly thereafter, reaching a maximum in 24–48 hours. Death has been reported following overdosage. Therefore, immediate hospitalization, with continuous patient observation and monitoring throughout this period, is essential.

Signs and symptoms of overdosage may include, alone or in combination, any of the following: drowsiness, dizziness, faintness, irritability, hyperactivity, agitation, severe headache, hallucinations, trismus, opisthotonus, convulsions and coma; rapid and irregular pulse, hypertension, hypotension and vascular collapse; precordial pain, respiratory depression and failure, hyperpyrexia, diaphoresis, and cool, clammy skin.

Intensive symptomatic and supportive treatment may be required. Induction of emesis or gastric lavage with instillation of charcoal slurry may be helpful in early poisoning, provided the airway has been protected against aspiration. Signs and symptoms of central nervous system stimulation, including convulsions, should be treated with diazepam, given slowly intravenously. Phenothiazine derivatives and central nervous system stimulants should be avoided. Hypotension and vascular collapse should be treated with intravenous fluids and, if necessary, blood pressure titration with an intravenous infusion of dilute pressor agent. It should be noted that adrenergic agents may produce a markedly increased pressor response.

Respiration should be supported by appropriate measures, including management of the airway, use of supplemental oxygen, and mechanical ventilatory assistance, as required. Body temperature should be monitored closely. Intensive management of hyperpyrexia may be required. Maintenance of fluid and electrolyte balance is essential.

There are no data on the lethal dose in man. The pathophysiologic effects of massive overdosage may persist for several days, since the drug acts by inhibiting physiologic enzyme systems. With symptomatic and supportive measures, recovery from *mild* overdosage may be expected within 3 to 4 days.

Hemodialysis, peritoneal dialysis, and charcoal hemoperfusion may be of value in massive overdosage, but sufficient data are not available to recommend their routine use in these cases.

Toxic blood levels of phenelzine have not been established, and assay methods are not practical for clinical or toxicological use.

HOW SUPPLIED

Tablets—each orange-coated tablet bears the P-D 270 monogram and contains phenelzine sulfate equivalent to 15 mg of phenelzine base; bottles of 100 (N 0071-0270-24). Store between 15°–30°C (59°–86°F).

US Patent 3,314,855

Shown in Product Identification Section, page 421

0270G029

NITROGARD®   ℞

[ni'trō-gärd]

(Transmucosal Controlled Release Nitroglycerin Tablets)

DESCRIPTION

Nitroglycerin, an organic nitrate, is a vasodilator which has effects on both arteries and veins. Nitrogard buccal tablets is a controlled-release nitroglycerin preparation, formulated in an inert polymer base, which delivers nitroglycerin through the oral mucosa over a sustained period of time. The Nitrogard buccal tablet, when placed under the lip or in the buccal pouch, adheres to the mucosa. As the tablet gradually dissolves it releases nitroglycerin to the systemic circulation over a 3 to 5 hour period. The chemical name for nitroglycerin is 1,2,3-Propanetriol trinitrate. The compound has a molecular weight of 227.09.

CLINICAL PHARMACOLOGY

The principal pharmacological action of nitroglycerin is relaxation of vascular smooth muscle, producing a vasodilator effect on both peripheral arteries and veins with more prominent effects on the latter. Dilation of the postcapillary vessels, including large veins, promotes peripheral pooling of blood and decreases venous return to the heart, thereby reducing left ventricular end-diastolic pressure (preload). Arteriolar relaxation reduces systemic vascular resistance and arterial pressure (afterload).

The mechanism by which nitroglycerin relieves angina pectoris is not fully understood. Myocardial oxygen consumption or demand (as measured by the pressure-rate product, tension-time index and stroke-work index) for a given level of external exercise is decreased by both the arterial and venous effects of nitroglycerin and, presumably, a more favorable supply-demand ratio is achieved. While the large epicardial coronary arteries are also dilated by nitroglycerin, the extent to which this action contributes to relief of exertional angina is unclear.

Nitroglycerin is rapidly metabolized, principally by a liver reductase to form glycerol nitrate metabolites and inorganic nitrate. Two active major metabolites, the 1,2 and 1,3 dinitroglycerols, the products of hydrolysis, appear to be less potent than nitroglycerin as vasodilators but have longer plasma half-lives. The dinitrates are further metabolized to mononitrates (biologically inactive with respect to cardiovascular effects) and ultimately glycerol and carbon dioxide. There is extensive first-pass deactivation by the liver of swallowed nitroglycerin following gastrointestinal absorption. Adequate studies defining the pharmacokinetics of Nitrogard have not been reported. The clinical relevance of nitroglycerin blood levels has not been established, since therapeutic levels of the drug and metabolites have not been defined.

Therapeutic doses of buccal nitroglycerin have been shown to reduce systolic and mean arterial blood pressures for up to two hours, and pressure is most reduced when the patient assumes upright posture. The fall in blood pressure is seen 1–2 minutes after buccal administration. Buccal nitroglycerin may reduce abnormally elevated left ventricular end-diastolic pressure (LVEDP), a hemodynamic occurrence during acute episodes of angina pectoris and this effect can be seen about one minute after dosing. Pulmonary artery pressures can be reduced for up to 3 hours.

INDICATIONS AND USAGE

Nitrogard is indicated for the treatment and prevention of angina pectoris due to coronary artery disease. Controlled clinical trials have demonstrated that single doses of this form of nitroglycerin are effective in improving exercise tolerance in patients with exertional angina pectoris. Double-blind, placebo-controlled trials have shown significant improvement in bicycle exercise time until chest pain for 3–4 hours after administration of titrated doses (1–5mg; to give 10 mmHg drop in resting systolic blood pressure or a 10 beat/min increase in heart rate) of buccal nitroglycerin. Duration of antianginal effect relates directly to time to tablet dissolution. A significant antianginal effect can persist for about 5 hours in patients in whom the tablet has not completely dissolved by this time.

Because of the relatively rapid absorption of nitroglycerin from the oral mucosa, Nitrogard may be used for acute prophylaxis, by administration a few minutes before a situation likely to provoke anginal attacks.

Controlled clinical trials have shown that therapeutically equivalent doses of buccal nitroglycerin and sublingual nitroglycerin produce similar hemodynamic effects in angina pectoris patients during the first 3 minutes after dosing. Nitrogard may therefore be tried for aborting an acute attack of angina pectoris.

CONTRAINDICATIONS

Nitroglycerin is contraindicated in patients who have shown purported hypersensitivity or idiosyncrasy to it or other nitrates or nitrites.

WARNINGS

Benefits of Nitrogard during the early days of acute myocardial infarction have not been established. If one elects to use nitrates in early infarction, careful clinical assessment and hemodynamic monitoring should be instituted because of the potential deleterious effects of hypotension.

PRECAUTIONS

Severe hypotensive response, particularly with upright posture, may occur even with small doses of nitroglycerin. The drug therefore should be used with caution in subjects who may have volume depletion from diuretic therapy or in patients who have low systolic blood pressure (e.g. below 90 mmHg). Paradoxical bradycardia and increased angina pectoris may accompany nitroglycerin-induced hypotension. Nitrate therapy may aggravate the angina caused by hypertrophic cardiomyopathy.

Tolerance to this drug and cross-tolerance to other nitrates and nitrites may occur. Tolerance to the vascular and antianginal effects of nitrates has been demonstrated in clinical trials, in experience through occupational exposure, and in isolated tissue experiments. The importance of tolerance to the appropriate use of buccal nitroglycerin in the management of patients with angina pectoris has not been determined in controlled clinical trials in angina pectoris patients, sustained therapy with some nitrate preparations has resulted in significantly less improvement and shorter duration of improvement in exercise time than had been seen when therapy was initiated. However, a controlled study of 2 weeks of repetitive doses of buccal nitroglycerin showed no significant tolerance as measured by treadmill performance. In industrial workers continuously exposed to nitroglycerin, tolerance clearly occurs. Moreover, physical dependence also occurs since chest pain, acute myocardial infarction, and even sudden death have occurred during temporary withdrawal of nitroglycerin from the workers. In clinical trials in angina patients, there are reports of anginal attacks being more easily provoked and of rebound in the hemodynamic effects soon after nitrate withdrawal. The relative importance of these observations to the routine, clinical use of Nitrogard is not known, but is seems prudent to gradually withdraw patients from nitroglycerin when the therapy is being terminated, rather than stopping the drug abruptly.

Information for Patients

Nitrogard should be placed under the upper lip or in a buccal pouch and permitted to dissolve slowly over a 3–5 hour period. It should not be chewed or swallowed. The tablet should not be placed under the tongue. Nitrogard begins to release medication immediately upon contact with the mucosa and will continue to release nitroglycerin until it dissolves. The time to dissolution of Nitrogard increases as patients familiarize themselves with its presence. The rate of dissolution of the tablet may be increased by touching the tablet with the tongue or drinking hot liquids.

Headache may occur during initial therapy with nitroglycerin. Headache is usually relieved by the use of standard headache remedies, or by lowering the dose, and tends to disappear after the first week or two of use.

Drug Interactions

Alcohol may enhance sensitivity to the hypotensive effects of nitrates. Nitroglycerin acts directly on vascular muscle. Therefore any other agent that directly or indirectly acts on vascular smooth muscle can be expected to have decreased or increased effect depending upon the agent.

Marked symptomatic, orthostatic hypotension has been reported when calcium channel blockers and organic nitrates were used in combination. Dose adjustments of either class of agents may be necessary.

Carcinogenesis, Mutagenesis, Impairment of Fertility

No long-term studies in animals have been performed to evaluate carcinogenic potential of Nitrogard: neither has its mutagenic potential been studied. It is also not known whether nitroglycerin can affect reproduction capacity.

Pregnancy

Pregnancy Category C. Animal reproduction studies have not been conducted with Nitrogard. It is also not known whether nitroglycerin can cause fetal harm when administered to a pregnant woman. Nitroglycerin should be given to a pregnant woman only if clearly needed.

Nursing Mothers

It is not known whether nitroglycerin is excreted in human milk. Because many drugs are excreted in human milk, caution should be exercised when Nitrogard is administered to a nursing woman.

Pediatric Use

Safety and effectiveness in children have not been established.

ADVERSE REACTIONS

Adverse reactions to Nitrogard, particularly headache and hypotension are generally dose-related. In clinical trials at various doses of nitroglycerin, the following adverse effects have been observed.

Headache, which may be severe and persistent, is the most commonly reported side effect of nitroglycerin, with an incidence in the order of 50% in some studies. Cutaneous vasodilation with flushing may occur. Transient episodes of dizziness and weakness, as well as other signs of cerebral ischemia associated with postural hypotension may occasionally develop. An occasional individual may exhibit marked sensitivity to the hypotensive effects of nitrates and severe responses (nausea, vomiting, weakness, restlessness, pallor, perspiration and collapse) may occur even with the therapeutic doses of nitrates. Drug rash and/or exfoliative dermatitis have been reported in patients receiving nitrate therapy. Nausea and vomiting can occur, but appear to be uncommon. Clinical trials of one to several months duration have not shown evidence of significant injury to the oral mucosa with repetitive use of Nitrogard.

OVERDOSAGE

Signs and Symptoms

Nitrate overdosage may result in severe hypotension, persistent throbbing headache, vertigo, palpitation, visual disturbance, flushing, and perspiring skin (later becoming cold and cyanotic), nausea and vomiting (possibly with colic and even bloody diarrhea), syncope (especially in the upright posture), methemoglobinemia with cyanosis and anorexia, initial hyperpnea, dyspnea and slow breathing, slow pulse (dicrotic and intermittent), heart block, increased intracranial pressure with cerebral symptoms of confusion and moderate fever, paralysis and coma followed by clonic convulsions and possibly death due to circulatory collapse.

Treatment of Overdosage

Remove any residue of the buccal Nitrogard tablet and wipe the gum clean at the site of insertion. Keep the patient recumbent in a shock position and comfortably warm. Gastric lavage may be of use if the medication has only recently been swallowed. Passive movement of the extremities may aid venous return. Administer oxygen and artificial ventilation if necessary. If methemoglobinemia is present, administration of methylene blue (1% solution), 1–2 mg/kg intravenously, may be required.

Methemoglobin

Case reports of clinically significant methemoglobinemia are rare at conventional doses of organic nitrates. The formation of methemoglobin is dose-related and in the case of genetic abnormalities of hemoglobin that favor methemoglobin formation, even conventional doses of organic nitrates could produce harmful concentrations of methemoglobin.

WARNINGS

Epinephrine is ineffective in reversing the severe hypotensive events associated with overdose. It and related compounds are contraindicated in this situation.

DOSAGE AND ADMINISTRATION

The usual starting dose for Nitrogard is 1.0 mg, placed on the oral mucosa between the lip and gum above the upper incisors or between the cheek and gum. The tablet should be allowed to dissolve undisturbed. Nitrogard should be incrementally titrated upward unitl a dose effective in controlling angina is determined or until side effects limit the dose. In ambulatory patients the magnitude of incremental dose should be guided by measurements of standing blood pressure. In the event Nitrogard does not afford prompt relief of an acute anginal attack, sublingual nitroglycerin is recommended.

The interval between doses of Nitrogard for prophylactic therapy in angina pectoris is generally 3 to 5 hours. The physical presence of the tablet, as it dissolves, may serve as an indicator of continued nitrate coverage. Bedtime usage of Nitrogard is not recommended because of the risk of aspiration.

It is recommended that for prophylaxis of angina attacks, patients be started on 1.0 mg Nitrogard every 5 hours (e.g. 8 a.m., 1 p.m., and 6 p.m.), during waking hours, and their response to treatment assessed over the following 4 to 5 days. If angina occurs while the tablet is in place, the dosage should be increased to the next tablet strength. If angina occurs after the tablet has dissolved, the frequency of dosing should be increased (e.g. every 4 hours).

Clinical experience indicates that patients are able to talk, eat, and drink while using Nitrogard. Hot drinks may increase the rate of dissolution of the tablet. A single controlled clinical trial demonstrating the effectiveness of maintenance therapy with Nitrogard for 2 weeks has been reported.

HOW SUPPLIED

Nitrogard (transmucosal controlled release nitroglycerin tablets) are supplied in three strengths as follows:

Nitrogard 1.0 mg (off-white, round standard concave, imprint: 1) is supplied as follows:
N 0071-0151-24   Bottles of 100
N 0071-0151-40   Unit-dose packages of 100 (10 strips of 10 tablets each)
Nitrogard 2.0 mg (off-white, round standard concave, imprint: 2) is supplied as follows:
N 0071-0152-24   Bottles of 100
N 0071-0152-40   Unit-dose packages of 100 (10 strips of 10 tablets each)
Nitrogard 3.0 mg (off-white, round standard concave, imprint: 3) is supplied as follows:
N 0071-0153-24   Bottles of 100
N 0071-0153-40   Unit-dose packages of 100 (10 strips of 10 tablets each)

STORAGE

Store at controlled room temperature 15°–30°C (59°–86°F). Dispense only in the original unopened container.
Caution—Federal law prohibits dispensing without prescription.

0151G011

Manufactured by
Forest Laboratories, Inc.
Inwood, New York 11696, USA
Distributed by
PARKE-DAVIS
Div of Warner-Lambert Co
Morris Plains, NJ 07950 USA
Shown in Product Identification Section, page 421

NITROSTAT® Ointment 2%   ℞
[nī'trō "stăt]
(Nitroglycerin)

DESCRIPTION

Nitroglycerin, an organic nitrate, is a vasodilator which has effects on both arteries and veins. The chemical name for nitroglycerin is 1,2,3-Propanetriol, trinitrate. The compound has a molecular weight of 227.09.

Nitrostat Ointment contains 2% nitroglycerin ointment and lactose in a lanolin and white petrolatum base. Each inch, as squeezed from the tube, contains approximately 15 mg nitroglycerin.

CLINICAL PHARMACOLOGY

The principal pharmacological action of nitroglycerin is relaxation of vascular smooth muscle, producing a vasodilator effect on both peripheral arteries and veins with more prominent effects on the latter. Dilation of the postcapillary vessels, including large veins, promotes peripheral pooling of blood and decreases venous return to the heart, thereby reducing left ventricular end-diastolic pressure (preload). Arteriolar relaxation reduces systemic vascular resistance and arterial pressure (afterload).

The mechanism by which nitroglycerin relieves angina pectoris is not fully understood. Myocardial oxygen consumption or demand (as measured by the pressure-rate product, tension-time index and stroke work index) for a given level of external exercise is decreased by both the arterial and venous effects of nitroglycerin and, presumably, a more favorable supply-demand ratio is achieved. While the large epicardial coronary arteries are also dilated by nitroglycerin, the extent to which this action contributes to relief of exertional angina is unclear.

Nitroglycerin is rapidly metabolized, principally by a liver reductase to form gylcerol nitrate metabolites and inorganic nitrate. Two active major metabolites, the 1,2 and 1,3 dinitroglycerols, the products of hydrolysis, appear to be less potent than nitroglycerin as vasodilators but have longer plasma half-lives.

The dinitrates are further metabolized to mononitrates (biologically inactive with respect to cardiovascular effects) and ultimately glycerol and carbon dioxide. There is extensive first-pass deactivation by the liver of nitroglycerin following gastrointestinal absorption.

Adequate studies defining the pharmacokinetics of Nitrostat Ointment have not been reported. The clinical relevance of nitroglycerin blood levels has not been established, since the therapeutic levels of the drug and metabolites have been defined. In general, it appears that blood levels are proportional to surface covered, but they are also related to location (chest placement gives higher levels than extremities) and to the thickness of the applied paste. Duration of effect would be expected to depend on the total amount of nitroglycerin (thickness of paste) per unit of surface area, but this has not been well studied.

Therapeutic doses of nitroglycerin have been shown to reduce systolic and mean arterial blood pressures, especially when the patient assumes upright posture, for as long as 7 hours after a single application. Nitroglycerin Ointment reduces abnormally elevated left ventricular end-diastolic pressure (LVEDP), a hemodynamic concomitant of acute

Continued on next page

This product information was prepared in August, 1989. On these and other Parke-Davis Products, information may be obtained by addressing PARKE-DAVIS, Division of Warner-Lambert Company, Morris Plains, New Jersey 07950.

Parke-Davis—Cont.

episodes of angina pectoris. The onset of hemodynamic effects of nitroglycerin ointment is not sufficiently rapid to be of use in aborting an acute episode of angina pectoris.

INDICATIONS AND USAGE

Nitrostat Ointment is indicated for the treatment and prevention of angina pectoris due to coronary artery disease. Controlled clinical trials have demonstrated that this form of nitroglycerin is effective in improving exercise tolerance in patients with exertional angina pectoris. Double-blind, placebo-controlled trials have shown significant improvement in exercise time until chest pain for up to 6 hours after single application of various doses of nitroglycerin ointment (mean doses ranged from 5 to 36 mg) to a 36 inches^2 area of trunk.

CONTRAINDICATIONS

Nitroglycerin is contraindicated in patients who have shown purported hypersensitivity or idiosyncracy to it or other nitrates or nitrites.

WARNINGS

The benefits of nitroglycerin ointment during the early days of acute myocardial infarction have not been established. If one elects to use organic nitrates in early infarction, careful assessment and hemodynamic monitoring should be used because of the potential deleterious effects of hypotension.

PRECAUTIONS

General:
Severe hypotensive response, particularly with upright posture, may occur even with small doses of nitroglycerin. The drug therefore should be used with caution in patients who may have volume depletion from diuretic therapy or in patients who have low systolic blood pressure (e.g. below 90 mm Hg). Paradoxical bradycardia and increased angina pectoris may accompany nitroglycerin-induced hypotension.
Nitrate therapy may aggravate the angina caused by hypertrophic cardiomyopathy.
Tolerance to this drug and cross-tolerance to other nitrates and nitrites may occur. Tolerance to the vascular and antianginal effects of nitrates has been demonstrated in clinical trials, in experience through occupational exposure and in isolated tissue experiments. The importance of tolerance to the appropriate use of nitroglycerin ointment in the management of patients with angina pectoris has not been determined. In controlled clinical trials in angina pectoris patients, sustained therapy with some nitrate preparations has resulted in significantly less improvement and a shorter duration of improvement in exercise time than had been seen when therapy was initiated. Sustained improvement in exercise tolerance has been reported in patients with angina pectoris who applied nitroglycerin ointment three times daily for 8-12 weeks in open studies, but there have been no controlled clinical studies involving exercise testing that have examined the efficacy of repetitive doses of Nitrostat Ointment for the long-term treatment of angina pectoris.
In industrial workers continuously exposed to nitroglycerin, tolerance clearly occurs. Moreover, physical dependence also occurs since chest pain, acute myocardial infarction and even sudden death have occurred during temporary withdrawal of nitroglycerin from the workers. In clinical trials in angina patients, there are reports of anginal attacks being more easily provoked and of rebound in the hemodynamic effects soon after nitrate withdrawal. The relative importance of these observations to the routine, clinical use of nitroglycerin is not known, but is seems prudent to gradually withdraw patients from nitroglycerin when the therapy is being terminated, rather than stopping the drug abruptly.

Drug Interactions:
Alcohol may enhance sensitivity to the hypotensive effects of nitrates.
Nitroglycerin acts directly on vascular muscle. Therefore, any other agent that directly or indirectly acts on vascular smooth muscle may have decreased or increased effect depending upon the agent.
Marked symptomatic orthostatic hypotension has been reported when calcium channel blockers and organic nitrates were used in combination. Dose adjustments of either class of agents may be necessary.

Carcinogenesis, Mutagenesis, Impairment of Fertility:
No long-term studies in animals have been performed to evaluate the carcinogenic potential of Nitrostat Ointment; neither has its mutagenic potential been studied. It is also not known whether nitroglycerin can affect reproduction capacity.

Pregnancy:
Pregnancy Category C. Animal reproduction studies have not been conducted with Nitrostat Ointment. It is also not known whether nitroglycerin can cause fetal harm when administered to a pregnant woman. Nitroglycerin should be given to a pregnant woman only if clearly needed.

Nursing Mothers:
It is not known whether nitroglycerin is excreted in human milk. Because many drugs are excreted in human milk, caution should be exercised when Nitrostat Ointment is administered to a nursing woman.

Pediatric Use:
Safety and effectiveness in children have not been established.

ADVERSE REACTIONS

Adverse reactions to Nitrostat Ointment, particularly headache and hypotension, are generally dose-related. In clinical trials at various doses of nitroglycerin, the following adverse effects have been observed.
Headache, which may be severe and persistent, is the most commonly reported side effect of nitroglycerin, with an incidence in the order of 50% in some studies. Cutaneous vasodilation with flushing may occur. Transient episodes of dizziness and weakness, as well as other signs of cerebral ischemia associated with postural hypotension may occasionally develop. An occasional individual may exhibit marked sensitivity to the hypotensive effects of nitrates and severe responses (nausea, vomiting, weakness, restlessness, pallor, perspiration and collapse) may occur even with therapeutic doses of nitrates. Drug rash and/or exfoliative dermatitis have been reported in patients receiving nitrate therapy. Nausea and vomiting can occur, but appear to be uncommon.

OVERDOSAGE

Signs and Symptoms:
Nitrate overdosage may result in: severe hypotension, persistent throbbing headache, vertigo, palpitation, visual disturbance, flushing and perspiring skin (later becoming cold and cyanotic), nausea and vomiting (possibly with colic and even bloody diarrhea), syncope (especially in the upright posture), methemoglobinemia with cyanosis and anorexia, initial hyperpnea, dyspnea and slow breathing, slow pulse (dicrotic and intermittent), heart block, increased intracranial pressure with cerebral symptoms of confusion and moderate fever, paralysis and coma followed by clonic convulsions and possibly death due to circulatory collapse.

Treatment of Overdosage:
Keep the patient recumbent in a shock position and comfortably warm. Wipe the skin clean of the nitroglycerin ointment. Passive movement of the extremities may aid venous return. Administer oxygen and artificial ventilation if necessary. If methemoglobinemia is present, administration of methylene blue (1% solution), 1-2 mg/kg intravenously, may be required.

Methemoglobin:
Case reports of clinically significant methemoglobinemia are rare at conventional doses of organic nitrates. The formation of methemoglobin is dose-related, and in the case of genetic abnormalities of hemoglobin that favor methemoglobin formation, even conventional doses of organic nitrates could produce harmful concentrations of methemoglobin.

WARNINGS

Epinephrine is ineffective in reversing the severe hypotensive events associated with overdose. It and related compounds are contraindicated in this situation.

DOSAGE AND ADMINISTRATION

When applying the ointment, place the dose determining applicator supplied with the package printed-side down and squeeze the necessary amount of ointment from the tube onto the applicator. Then place the applicator with the ointment-side down onto the desired area of skin, usually the chest or back. Several studies suggest that absorption of nitroglycerin through the skin varies with the site of application of the drug. Application of the drug to the skin of the chest is reported to give higher blood levels of nitroglycerin and greater hemodynamic effects than application to the extremities.
The amount of nitroglycerin entering the circulation varies directly with the size of skin area exposed to the drug and the amount of ointment applied. Although in major clinical trials the dose of nitroglycerin was often applied to a 6×6 inch (150×150 mm) area of skin, in clinical practice the dose is usually applied to a smaller area. The ointment should be applied in a thin uniform layer and the dose-to-area ratio kept reasonably constant. For example: 1 inch on a 2×3 inch area; 2 inches on a 3×4 inch area; 3 inches on a 4×5 inch area. When doubling the dose, the surface area over which the ointment is placed should also be doubled.
As with all nitrates, clinical studies suggest that clinical response is variable. A suggested starting dose for Nitrostat Ointment is ½ inch (7.5 mg) applied to a 1×3 inch area every 8 hours. Response to treatment should be assessed over the next several days. If angina occurs while the ointment is in place, the dose should be increased, for example to 1 inch on a 2×3 inch area. Nitrostat Ointment should be titrated upward until a dose effective in controlling angina is determined or until side effects limit the dose. If angina occurs after the ointment has been in place for several hours, the frequency of dosing should be increased (e.g. every 6 hours). Administer the smallest effective dose 3 to 4 times daily, unless clinical response suggests a different regimen. At

initiation of therapy or change in dosage, blood pressure (patient standing) should be monitored. Controlled trials have been carried out for up to 7 hours after dosing, therefore, it is not known whether the drug is effective in prevention of exertional angina beyond 7 hours after dosing. The effectiveness of repetitive applications of nitroglycerin ointment for the chronic management of angina pectoris has not been established.
Nitrostat Ointment is not intended for immediate relief of anginal attacks.
Keep the tube tightly closed and store at controlled room temperature 15°–30°C (59°–86°F). Avoid excessive heat.

PATIENT INSTRUCTIONS FOR APPLICATION

Information furnished with dose-measuring applicators.

HOW SUPPLIED

Nitrostat Ointment 2% is supplied as:
N 0071-3001-13–30-gram tube
N 0071-3001-15–60-gram tube
Each gram of ointment contains 20 mg of nitroglycerin.
Caution—Federal law prohibits dispensing without prescription.

3001G033

Shown in Product Identification Section, page 421

NITROSTAT® ℞

[ni′trō ″stăt]
(nitroglycerin tablets, USP)

DESCRIPTION

Nitrostat is a stabilized sublingual nitroglycerin tablet manufactured by a patented process* which prevents the migration of nitroglycerin by adding the nonvolatile fixing agent polyethylene glycol 3350. This stabilized formulation has been shown to be more stable and more uniform than conventional molded tablets. Nitrostat tablets contain 0.15 mg (1/400 grain), 0.3 mg (1/200 grain), 0.4 mg (1/150 grain) and 0.6 mg (1/100 grain) nitroglycerin. Also contains lactose, NF; polyethylene glycol 3350, NF; sucrose, NF.
Nitroglycerin, an organic nitrate, is a vasodilating agent. The chemical name for nitroglycerin is 1,2,3 propanetriol trinitrate.

CLINICAL PHARMACOLOGY

Relaxation of vascular smooth muscle is the principal pharmacologic action of nitroglycerin. The mechanism by which nitroglycerin produces relaxation of smooth muscle is unknown. Although venous effects predominate, nitroglycerin produces, in a dose-related manner, dilation of both arterial and venous beds. Dilation of the postcapillary vessels, including large veins, promotes peripheral pooling of blood and decreases venous return to the heart, reducing left ventricular end-diastolic pressure (preload). Arteriolar relaxation reduces systemic vascular resistance and arterial pressure (afterload). Myocardial oxygen consumption or demand (as measured by the pressure-rate product, tension-time index and stroke-work index) is decreased by both the arterial and venous effects of nitroglycerin, and a more favorable supply-demand ratio can be achieved.
Therapeutic doses of nitroglycerin may reduce systolic, diastolic and mean arterial blood pressure. Effective coronary perfusion pressure is usually maintained, but can be compromised if blood pressure falls excessively or increased heart rate decreases diastolic filling time.
Elevated central venous and pulmonary capillary wedge pressures, pulmonary vascular resistance and systemic vascular resistance are also reduced by nitroglycerin therapy. Heart rate is usually slightly increased, presumably a reflex response to the fall in blood pressure. Cardiac index may be increased, decreased, or unchanged. Patients with elevated left ventricular filling pressure and systemic vascular resistance values in conjunction with a depressed cardiac index are likely to experience an improvement in cardiac index. On the other hand, when filling pressures and cardiac index are normal, cardiac index may be slightly reduced by intravenous nitroglycerin.
Nitroglycerin is rapidly absorbed following sublingual administration. Its onset of action is approximately one to three minutes. Significant pharmacologic effects are present for 30 to 60 minutes following administration by the above route.
Nitroglycerin is rapidly metabolized to dinitrates and mononitrates, with a short half-life, estimated at 1 to 4 minutes. At plasma concentrations of between 50 and 500 ng/ml, the binding of nitroglycerin to plasma proteins is approximately 60%, while that of 1,2 dinitroglycerin and 1,3 dinitroglycerin is 60% and 30% respectively. The activity and half-life of 1,2 dinitroglycerin and 1,3 dinitroglycerin are not well characterized. The mononitrate is not active.

INDICATIONS AND USAGE

Nitroglycerin is indicated for the prophylaxis, treatment and management of patients with angina pectoris.

CONTRAINDICATIONS

Sublingual nitroglycerin therapy is contraindicated in patients with early myocardial infarction, severe anemia, increased intracranial pressure, and those with a known hypersensitivity to nitroglycerin.

PRECAUTIONS

General: Only the smallest dose required for effective relief of the acute anginal attack should be used. Excessive use may lead to the development of tolerance. Nitrostat tablets are intended for sublingual or buccal administration and should not be swallowed. The drug should be discontinued if blurring of vision or drying of the mouth occurs. Excessive dosage of nitroglycerin may produce severe headaches.

Information for Patients: If possible, patients should sit down when taking Nitrostat tablets. This eliminates the possibility of falling due to lightheadedness or dizziness.

Drug Interactions: Concomitant use of nitrates and alcohol may cause hypotension. Patients receiving antihypertensive drugs, beta-adrenergic blockers, or phenothiazines and nitrates should be observed for possible additive hypotensive effects.

Drug/Laboratory Test Interactions: Nitrates may interfere with the Zlatkis-Zak color reaction causing a false report of decreased serum cholesterol.

Carcinogenesis, Mutagenesis, Impairment of Fertility: No long-term studies in animals were performed to evaluate the carcinogenic potential of nitroglycerin.

Pregnancy Category C: Animal reproduction studies have not been conducted with nitroglycerin. It is also not known whether nitroglycerin can cause fetal harm when administered to a pregnant woman or can affect reproduction capacity. Nitroglycerin should be given to a pregnant woman only if clearly needed.

Nursing Mother: It is not known whether nitroglycerin is excreted in human milk. Because many drugs are excreted in human milk, caution should be exercised when intravenous nitroglycerin is administered to a nursing woman.

Pediatric Use: The safety and effectiveness of nitroglycerin in children have not been established.

ADVERSE REACTIONS

Transient headache may occur immediately after use. Vertigo, weakness, palpitation, and other manifestations of postural hypotension may develop occasionally, particularly in erect, immobile patients. Syncope due to nitrate vasodilation has been reported.

DOSAGE AND ADMINISTRATION

One tablet should be dissolved under the tongue or in the buccal pouch at the first sign of an acute anginal attack. The dose may be repeated approximately every five minutes until relief is obtained. If the pain persists after a total of 3 tablets in a 15-minute period, the physician should be notified. Nitrostat may be used prophylactically five to ten minutes prior to engaging in activities which might precipitate an acute attack.

HOW SUPPLIED

Nitrostat is supplied in four strengths in bottles containing 100 tablets each, with color-coded labels, and in color-coded Patient Convenience Packages of four bottles of 25 tablets each.

0.15 mg (1/400 grain):
N 0071-0568-24—Bottle of 100 tablets
N 0071-0568-13—Convenience Package
0.3 mg (1/200 grain):
N 0071-0569-24—Bottle of 100 tablets
N 0071-0569-13—Convenience Package
0.4 mg (1/150 grain):
N 0071-0570-24—Bottle of 100 tablets
N 0071-0570-13—Convenience Package
0.6 mg (1/100 grain):
N 0071-0571-24—Bottle of 100 tablets
N 0071-0571-13—Convenience Package
**Store at controlled room temperature 15°-30°C (59°-86°F).
Protect from moisture.**
*US Patent No. 3,789,119

0568G063

Shown in Product Identification Section, page 421

NITROSTAT® IV   ℞
[nī′trō″stăt]
(Nitroglycerin Injection, USP)
FOR INTRAVENOUS USE ONLY

NOT FOR DIRECT INTRAVENOUS INJECTION. NITROSTAT IV IS A CONCENTRATED, POTENT DRUG WHICH MUST BE DILUTED IN DEXTROSE (5%) INJECTION, USP OR SODIUM CHLORIDE (0.9%) INJECTION, USP PRIOR TO ITS INFUSION. THE CONTAINER AND ADMINISTRATION SET USED FOR INFUSION MAY AFFECT THE AMOUNT OF INTRAVENOUS NITROGLYCERIN DELIVERED TO THE PATIENT. (SEE WARNINGS AND DOSAGE AND ADMINISTRATION SECTIONS.)

CAUTION: SEVERAL PREPARATIONS OF NITROGLYCERIN INJECTION ARE AVAILABLE. THEY DIFFER IN CONCENTRATION AND/OR VOLUME PER VIAL. WHEN SWITCHING FROM ONE PRODUCT TO ANOTHER, ATTENTION MUST BE PAID TO THE DILUTION AND DOSAGE AND ADMINISTRATION INSTRUCTIONS.

DESCRIPTION

Nitrostat IV is a clear, practically colorless additive solution for intravenous infusion after dilution. Nitrostat IV is available in three strengths, an 8 mg per ampoule, a 50 mg per ampoule or vial, and a 100 mg per ampoule or vial. Each milliliter of Nitrostat IV 8 mg per ampoule contains 0.8 mg nitroglycerin, with citric acid, USP, anhydrous and sodium citrate, USP, hydrous as buffers, and 5% alcohol in Water for Injection, USP. Each milliliter of Nitrostat IV 50 mg per ampoule or vial contains 5 mg nitroglycerin, 30% propylene glycol, USP and 30% alcohol, USP (28.5% alcohol) in Water for Injection, USP. Each milliliter of Nitrostat IV 100 mg per ampoule or vial contains 10 mg of nitroglycerin in 50% propylene glycol, USP and 50% alcohol. The solutions are sterile, nonpyrogenic, and nonexplosive. Intravenous nitroglycerin, an organic nitrate, is a vasodilator. The chemical name for nitroglycerin is 1,2,3 propanetriol trinitrate and its chemical structure is:

$$H_2C-O-NO_2$$
$$|$$
$$HC-O-NO_2$$
$$|$$
$$H_2C-O-NO_2$$

$C_3H_5N_3O_9$ MOL WT 227.09

CLINICAL PHARMACOLOGY

Relaxation of vascular smooth muscle is the principal pharmacologic action of intravenous nitroglycerin. Although venous effects predominate, nitroglycerin produces, in a dose-related manner, dilation of both arterial and venous beds. Dilation of the postcapillary vessels, including large veins, promotes peripheral pooling of blood and decreases venous return to the heart, reducing left ventricular end-diastolic pressure (preload). Arteriolar relaxation reduces systemic vascular resistance and arterial pressure (afterload). Myocardial oxygen consumption or demand (as measured by the pressure-rate product, tension-time index and stroke-work index) is decreased by both the arterial and venous effects of nitroglycerin, and a more favorable supply-demand ratio can be achieved.

Therapeutic doses of intravenous nitroglycerin reduce systolic, diastolic and mean arterial blood pressure. Effective coronary perfusion pressure is usually maintained, but can be compromised if blood pressure falls excessively or increased heart rate decreases diastolic filling time.

Elevated central venous and pulmonary capillary wedge pressures, pulmonary vascular resistance and systemic vascular resistance are also reduced by nitroglycerin therapy. Heart rate is usually slightly increased, presumably a reflex response to the fall in blood pressure. Cardiac index may be increased, decreased, or unchanged. Patients with elevated left ventricular filling pressure and systemic vascular resistance values in conjunction with a depressed cardiac index are likely to experience an improvement in cardiac index. On the other hand, when filling pressures and cardiac index are normal, cardiac index may be slightly reduced by intravenous nitroglycerin.

Nitroglycerin is widely distributed in the body with an apparent volume of distribution of approximately 200 liters in adult male subjects, and is rapidly metabolized to dinitrates and mononitrates with a short half-life, estimated at 1 to 4 minutes. This results in a low plasma concentration after intravenous infusion. At plasma concentrations of between 50 and 500 mg/mL, the binding of nitroglycerin to plasma proteins is approximately 60%, while that of 1,2 dinitroglycerin and 1,3 dinitroglycerin is 60% and 30% respectively. The activity and half-life of 1,2 dinitroglycerin and 1,3 dinitroglycerin are not well characterized. The mononitrate is not active.

INDICATIONS AND USAGE

Nitrostat IV is indicated for:

1. *Control of blood pressure in perioperative hypertension,* ie, hypertension associated with surgical procedures, especially cardiovascular procedures, such as the hypertension seen during intratracheal intubation, anesthesia, skin incision, sternotomy, cardiac bypass, and in the immediate postsurgical period.

2. *Congestive heart failure associated with acute myocardial infarction.*

3. *Treatment of angina pectoris* in patients who have not responded to recommended doses of organic nitrates and/or a beta blocker.

4. *Production of controlled hypotension during surgical procedures.*

CONTRAINDICATIONS

Nitrostat IV should not be administered to individuals with:

1. A known hypersensitivity to nitroglycerin or a known idiosyncratic reaction to organic nitrates.
2. Hypotension or uncorrected hypovolemia, as the use of Nitrostat IV in such states could produce severe hypotension or shock.
3. Increased intracranial pressure (eg, head trauma or cerebral hemorrhage).
4. Constrictive pericarditis and pericardial tamponade.
5. Inadequate cerebral circulation.

WARNINGS

1. Nitroglycerin readily migrates into many plastics. To avoid absorption of nitroglycerin into plastic parenteral solution containers, the dilution and storage of nitroglycerin injection should be made only in glass parenteral solution bottles.
2. Some filters also absorb nitroglycerin; they should be avoided.
3. Forty to 80% of the total amount of nitroglycerin in the final diluted solution for infusion is absorbed by the polyvinyl chloride (PVC) tubing of the intravenous administration sets currently in general use. The higher rates of absorption occur when flow rates are low, nitroglycerin concentrations are high, and tubing is long. Although the rate of loss is highest during the early phase of administration (when flow rates are lowest), the loss is neither constant nor self-limiting; consequently no simple calculation or correction can be performed to convert the theoretical infusion rate (based on the concentration of the infusion solution) to the actual delivery rate.

   Because of this problem, Parke-Davis, Division of Warner-Lambert Company, has developed a nonabsorbing infusion set, Nitrostat IV intravenous infusion set, in which the loss of nitroglycerin is minimal (less than 5%). The Nitrostat IV intravenous infusion set or a similar infusion set is recommended for infusions of intravenous nitroglycerin. *Dosage instructions must be followed with care. It should be noted that when these infusion sets are used, the calculated dose will be delivered to the patient because the loss of nitroglycerin due to absorption in standard PVC tubing will be kept to a minimum. Note that the dosages commonly used in published studies utilized general-use PVC infusion sets and recommended doses based on this experience are too high if the new infusion sets are used.*
4. A potential safety problem exists with the combined use of some infusion pumps and some nonPVC infusion sets. Because the special tubing required to prevent the absorption of nitroglycerin tends to be less pliable than the conventional PVC tubing normally used with such infusion pumps, the pumps may fail to occlude the infusion sets completely. The results may be excessive flow at low infusion rate settings, causing alarms, or unregulated gravity flow when the infusion pump is stopped; this could lead to over-infusion of nitroglycerin. All infusion pumps should be tested with the infusion sets to ensure their ability to deliver nitroglycerin accurately at low flow rates, and to occlude the infusion sets properly when the infusion is stopped.

PRECAUTIONS

Nitrostat IV should be used with caution in patients who have severe hepatic or renal disease.

Excessive hypotension, especially for prolonged periods of time, must be avoided because of possible deleterious effects on the brain, heart, liver and kidney from poor perfusion and the attendant risk of ischemia, thrombosis, and altered function of these organs. Paradoxical bradycardia and increased angina pectoris may accompany nitroglycerin-induced hypotension. Patients with normal or low pulmonary capillary wedge pressure are especially sensitive to the hypotensive effects of intravenous nitroglycerin. If pulmonary capillary wedge pressure is being monitored, it will be noted that a fall in wedge pressure precedes the onset of arterial hypotension, and the pulmonary capillary wedge pressure is thus a useful guide to safe titration of the drug.

NITROSTAT IV CONTAINS ALCOHOL. SAFETY FOR INTRACORONARY INJECTION HAS NOT BEEN SHOWN.

Carcinogenesis, Mutagenesis, Impairment of Fertility: No long-term studies in animals were performed to evaluate the carcinogenic potential of nitroglycerin.

Pregnancy:
Category C: Animal reproduction studies have not been conducted with nitroglycerin. It is also not known whether nitroglycerin can cause fetal harm when administered to a

Continued on next page

This product information was prepared in August, 1989. On these and other Parke-Davis Products, information may be obtained by addressing PARKE-DAVIS, Division of Warner-Lambert Company, Morris Plains, New Jersey 07950.

Parke-Davis—Cont.

pregnant woman or can affect reproduction capacity. Nitroglycerin should be given to a pregnant woman only if clearly needed.

Nursing Mother:

It is not known whether nitroglycerin is excreted in human milk. Because many drugs are excreted in human milk, caution should be exercised when intravenous nitroglycerin is administered to a nursing woman.

Pediatric Use:

The safety and effectiveness of nitroglycerin in children have not been established.

ADVERSE REACTIONS

The most frequent adverse reaction in patients treated with nitroglycerin is headache, which occurs in approximately 2% of patients. Other adverse reactions occurring in less than 1% of patients are the following: tachycardia, nausea, vomiting, apprehension, restlessness, muscle twitching, retrosternal discomfort, palpitations, dizziness and abdominal pain.

The following additional adverse reactions have been reported with the oral and/or topical use of nitroglycerin: cutaneous flushing, weakness, and occasionally drug rash or exfoliative dermatitis.

OVERDOSAGE

Accidental overdosage of nitroglycerin may result in severe hypotension and reflex tachycardia which can be treated by elevating the legs and decreasing or temporarily terminating the infusion until the patient's condition stabilizes. Since the duration of the hemodynamic effects following nitroglycerin administration is quite short, additional corrective measures are usually not required. However, if further therapy is indicated, administration of an intravenous alpha adrenergic agonist (eg, methoxamine or phenylephrine) should be considered.

DOSAGE AND ADMINISTRATION

NOT FOR DIRECT INTRAVENOUS INJECTION
NITROSTAT IV IS A CONCENTRATED, POTENT DRUG WHICH MUST BE DILUTED IN DEXTROSE (5%) INJECTION, USP OR SODIUM CHLORIDE (0.9%) INJECTION, USP PRIOR TO ITS INFUSION.
NITROSTAT IV SHOULD NOT BE ADMIXED WITH OTHER DRUGS.

Parenteral drug products should be inspected visually for particulate matter and discoloration prior to administration, whenever solution and container permit.
[See tables below].

Dilution: Aseptically transfer the desired amount of Nitrostat IV (as noted in the preceding tables) into a glass IV bottle containing the stated volume of 5% Dextrose Injection,

USP or 0.9% Sodium Chloride Injection, USP and mix well. The resultant solution is stable for at least 96 hours at controlled room temperature (15°–30°C) or under refrigeration. It is important to consider the fluid requirements of the patient as well as the expected duration of infusion in selecting the appropriate dilution of nitroglycerin. The preceding tables give the nitroglycerin concentrations at various dilutions.

After the initial dosage titration, the concentration of the admixture may be increased, if necessary, to limit fluids given to the patient. The concentration of the infusion solution should not exceed 400 mcg/mL of nitroglycerin.

NOTE: If the concentration is adjusted, it is imperative to flush or replace the Nitrostat IV infusion set before a new concentration is utilized. The dead space of the set is approximately 20 mL and, depending on the flow rate, it could take from 6 minutes to 13 hours for the new concentration to reach the patient if the set were not flushed or replaced.

Dosage: *IMPORTANT NOTICE:* Dosage is affected by the type of container used as well as the type of infusion set used (See Warnings). Although the usual starting adult dose range reported in clinical studies was 25 mcg/min or more, those studies used *PVC TUBING. The use of nonabsorbing tubing will result in the need to use reduced doses.*

The recommended dosage when using the nonabsorbing Nitrostat IV Intravenous Infusion Set should initially be 5 mcg/min delivered through an infusion pump capable of exact and constant delivery of the drug. Subsequent titration must be adjusted to the clinical situation, with dose increments becoming more cautious as partial response is seen. Initial titration should be 5 mcg/min increments, with increases every 3 to 5 minutes until some response is noted. If no response is seen at 20 mcg/min, increments of 10 and later 20 mcg/min can be used. Once a partial blood pressure response is observed, the dose increase should be reduced and the interval between increments should be lengthened. Patients with normal or low left ventricular filling pressure or pulmonary capillary wedge pressure (eg, angina patients without other complications) may be hypersensitive to the effects of nitroglycerin and may respond fully to doses as small as 5 mcg/min. These patients require especially careful titration and monitoring.

There is no fixed optimum dose of nitroglycerin. Due to variations in the responsiveness of individual patients to the drug, each patient must be titrated to the desired level of hemodynamic function. Therefore, continuous monitoring of physiologic parameters (blood pressure and heart rate in all patients, other measurements such as pulmonary capillary wedge pressure, as appropriate) MUST BE PERFORMED to achieve the correct dose. Adequate systemic blood pressure and coronary perfusion pressure must be maintained.

DILUTION AND ADMINISTRATION TABLES
(60 microdrops = 1 milliliter)

Nitrostat IV 8 mg per ampoule

Concentration	1 amp in 250 mL approx 30 mcg/mL	2 amp in 250 mL approx 60 mcg/mL	3 amp in 250 mL approx 85 mcg/mL
Dose (mcg/min)	Flow Rate mL/hour (microdrops/minute)		
5	10	5	3
10	20	10	7
15	30	15	10
20	40	20	14
30	60	30	21
40	80	40	28
50	100	50	35
60	120	60	42
80	160	80	56
100	200	100	71

Nitrostat IV 50 mg per ampoule or vial

Concentration	1 amp/vial in 500 mL approx 100 mcg/mL	2 amp/vial in 500 mL approx 200 mcg/mL
Dose (mcg/min)	Flow Rate mL/hour (microdrops/minute)	
5	3	1.5
10	6	3
15	9	4.5
20	12	6
30	18	9
40	24	12
50	30	15
60	36	18
80	48	24
100	60	30
120	72	36
160	96	48
200	120	60

Nitrostat IV 100 mg per ampoule or vial

Concentration	1 amp/vial in 500 mL approx 200 mcg/mL	2 amp/vial in 500 mL approx 400 mcg/mL
Dose (mcg/min)	Flow Rate mL/hour (microdrops/minute)	
5	1.5	0.75
10	3	1.5
15	4.5	2.25
20	6	3
30	9	4.5
40	12	6
50	15	7.5
60	18	9
80	24	12
100	30	15
120	36	18
160	48	24
200	60	30

DIRECTIONS FOR PREPARING NITROSTAT IV INFUSION SET

Caution—The fluid path and areas under the protectors of the intravenous infusion set are sterile. Do not use if damaged or if end protectors are not in place.

1. Position control clamp 6 to 8 inches from the Male Luer Lock connector, then close clamp. (To close clamp, rotate screw stem clockwise.)

2. Remove plastic protector from each Luer Lock end and connect the Luer Lock attachment.
3. With IV solution bottle in the upright position.
  a) remove plastic protector from the piercing device;
  b) THRUST the piercing device STRAIGHT DOWN through the CENTER of the target area in the rubber stopper (push straight down, do not twist).
  c) squeeze drip chamber and hold.
4. Invert the bottle and suspend from suitable stand.
5. Release pressure from drip chamber.
6. Remove needle adapter protector by pulling straight off (do not twist off). If required, place needle on needle adapter. Hold this end of the tubing above the level of the nitroglycerin solution in the bottle. Loosen the control clamp and allow the solution to run in and fill the tubing and needle. Displace the air in the entire injection set by raising or lowering the intravenous needle end of tubing until all the air bubbles are expelled.
(NOTE: Drip chamber should not be completely filled.)
7. Attach the infusion set to a suitable mechanical infusion control device.
8. Tighten control clamp and proceed with venipuncture or connect to needle.
9. Adjust control device for precise measurement of flow rate.

NOTE: Only glass IV bottles should be used in preparing the Nitrostat IV admixture. The resulting solution should be administered using the intravenous infusion set supplied in the Nitrostat IV infusion kit.
If a Volumetric infusion pump is used: Follow step 1, then aseptically remove plastic protector from each Luer Lock end and attach both Luer Lock ends to the cassette of the infusion pump. Install cassette and close door of pump. Follow steps 3, 4, and 5. Remove needle adapter protector, prime set, and purge out air. Set rate and volume and start infusion.

Spike-Adapter

Directions for using the Spike-Adapter (use with McGaw LVP bottles): Remove the plastic protector from the piercing device on the drip chamber. Aseptically insert the piercing device on the drip chamber into the spike adapter tubing coupler as far as it will go. Remove the end plastic protector from the spike adapter and proceed with the above directions for preparing the infusion set depending on what pump/controller is used.

HOW SUPPLIED
N0071-4572-36 Nitrostat IV Infusion Kit containing one 10-mL ampoule of Nitrostat IV, 8 mg (0.8 mg/mL) and one disposable intravenous infusion set.
N0071-4572-10 Carton of 10 x 10-mL ampoules of Nitrostat IV, 8 mg (0.8 mg/mL).
N0071-4575-36 Nitrostat IV Infusion Kit containing one 10-mL vial of Nitrostat IV, 50 mg (5 mg/mL) and one disposable intravenous infusion set.
N0071-4575-10 Carton of 10 x 10-mL ampoules of Nitrostat IV, 50 mg (5 mg/mL).
N0071-4575-45 Carton of 10 x 10-mL vials of Nitrostat IV, 50 mg (5 mg/mL).
N0071-4579-35 Nitrostat IV Infusion Kit containing one 10-mL vial of Nitrostat IV, 100 mg (10 mg/mL) and one disposable intravenous infusion set.
N0071-4579-45 Carton of 10 x 10-mL vials of Nitrostat IV, 100 mg (10 mg/mL).

Store at controlled room temperature 15°–30°C (59°–86°F).
Caution—Federal law prohibits dispensing without prescription.
                         4572G026
Shown in Product Identification Section, page 421

TABLE I
LOWEST EXPECTED AND TYPICAL FAILURE RATES DURING THE FIRST YEAR OF CONTINUOUS USE OF A METHOD
% of Women Experiencing an Accidental Pregnancy in the First Year of Continuous Use

Method	Lowest Expected*	Typical**
(No contraception)	(89)	(89)
Oral contraceptives		3
combined	0.1	N/A***
progestin only	0.5	N/A***
Diaphragm with spermicidal cream or jelly	3	18
Spermicides alone (foam, creams, jellies and vaginal suppositories)	3	21
Vaginal sponge		
nulliparous	5	18
multiparous	>8	>28
IUD (medicated)	1	6†
Condom without spermicides	2	12
Periodic abstinence (all methods)	2–10	20
Female sterilization	0.2	0.4
Male sterilization	0.1	0.15

Adapted from J. Trussell and K. Kost, Table 11, ref #1.
 * The authors' best guess of the percentage of women expected to experience an accidental pregnancy among couples who initiate a method (not necessarily for the first time) and who use it consistently and correctly during the first year if they do not stop for any other reason.
 ** This term represents "typical" couples who initiate use of a method (not necessarily for the first time), who experience an accidental pregnancy during the first year if they do not stop use for any other reason.
 *** N/A—Data not available
 † Combined typical rate for both medicated and non-medicated IUD. The rate for medicated IUD alone is not available.

NORLESTRIN® 21   ℞
(Norethindrone Acetate and Ethinyl Estradiol Tablets, USP)

NORLESTRIN® ㉑ 1/50   ℞
(Each tablet contains 1 mg norethindrone acetate and 50 mcg ethinyl estradiol.)

NORLESTRIN® ㉑ 2.5/50   ℞
(Each tablet contains 2.5 mg norethindrone acetate and 50 mcg ethinyl estradiol.)

NORLESTRIN® Fe   ℞
(Norethindrone Acetate and Ethinyl Estradiol Tablets, USP and Ferrous Fumarate Tablets.)

NORLESTRIN® Fe 1/50   ℞
(Each yellow tablet contains 1 mg norethindrone acetate and 50 mcg ethinyl estradiol. Each brown tablet contains 75 mg ferrous fumarate.)

NORLESTRIN® Fe 2.5/50   ℞
(Each pink tablet contains 2.5 mg norethindrone acetate and 50 mcg ethinyl estradiol. Each brown tablet contains 75 mg ferrous fumarate.)

NORLESTRIN® 28   ℞
(Norethindrone Acetate and Ethinyl Estradiol Tablets, USP)

NORLESTRIN® ㉘ 1/50   ℞
(Each yellow tablet contains 1 mg norethindrone acetate and 50 mcg ethinyl estradiol. Each white tablet is inert.)

Each yellow tablet contains norethindrone acetate (17 alpha-ethinyl-19-nortestosterone acetate), 1 mg; ethinyl estradiol (17 alpha-ethinyl-1,3,5(10)-estratriene-3, 17 beta-diol), 50 mcg. Also contains acacia, NF; lactose, NF; magnesium stearate, NF; starch, NF; confectioner's sugar, NF; talc, USP; D&C yellow No. 10; FD&C yellow No. 6.
Each pink tablet contains norethindrone acetate (17 alpha-ethinyl-19-nortestosterone acetate), 2.5 mg; ethinyl estradiol (17 alpha-ethinyl-1,3,5(10)-estratriene-3, 17 beta-diol), 50 mcg. Also contains acacia, NF; lactose, NF; magnesium stearate, NF; starch, NF; confectioner's sugar, NF; talc, USP; FD&C red No. 40.
Each brown tablet contains microcrystalline cellulose, NF; ferrous fumarate, USP; magnesium stearate, NF; povidone, USP; sodium starch glycolate, NF; sucrose with modified dextrins.
Each white tablet contains magnesium stearate, NF and sucrose with modified dextrins.

DESCRIPTION
Norlestrin **21**, Norlestrin **Fe**, and Norlestrin **28** are progestogen-estrogen combinations.
Norlestrin Fe 1/50 and 2.5/50 provide a continuous dosage regimen consisting of 21 oral contraceptive tablets and seven ferrous fumarate tablets. The ferrous fumarate tablets are present to facilitate ease of drug administration via a 28-day regimen and are not intended to serve any therapeutic purpose.

Norlestrin **28** 1/50 provides a continuous dosage regimen consisting of 21 oral contraceptive tablets and 7 inert tablets.

CLINICAL PHARMACOLOGY
Combination oral contraceptives act by suppression of gonadotropins. Although the primary mechanism of this action is inhibition of ovulation, other alterations include changes in the cervical mucus (which increase the difficulty of sperm entry into the uterus) and the endometrium (which reduce the likelihood of implantation).

INDICATIONS AND USAGE
Norlestrin **21**, Norlestrin **Fe**, and Norlestrin **28** are indicated for the prevention of pregnancy in women who elect to use oral contraceptives as a method of contraception.
Oral contraceptives are highly effective. Table I lists the typical accidental pregnancy rates for users of combination oral contraceptives and other methods of contraception. The efficacy of these contraceptive methods, except sterilization, depends upon the reliability with which they are used. Correct and consistent use of methods can result in lower failure rates.
[See table above].

CONTRAINDICATIONS
Oral contraceptives should not be used in women who currently have the following conditions:
● Thrombophlebitis or thromboembolic disorders
● A past history of deep vein thrombophlebitis or thromboembolic disorders
● Cerebral vascular or coronary artery disease
● Known or suspected carcinoma of the breast
● Carcinoma of the endometrium or other known or suspected estrogen-dependent neoplasia
● Undiagnosed abnormal genital bleeding
● Cholestatic jaundice of pregnancy or jaundice with prior pill use
● Hepatic adenomas or carcinomas
● Known or suspected pregnancy

WARNINGS

> Cigarette smoking increases the risk of serious cardiovascular side effects from oral contraceptive use. This risk increases with age and with heavy smoking (15 or more cigarettes per day) and is quite marked in women over 35 years of age. Women who use oral contraceptives should be strongly advised not to smoke.

The use of oral contraceptives is associated with increased risks of several serious conditions including myocardial infarction, thromboembolism, stroke, hepatic neoplasia, and gallbladder disease, although the risk of serious morbidity or mortality is very small in healthy women without underly-

Continued on next page

This product information was prepared in August, 1989. On these and other Parke-Davis Products, information may be obtained by addressing PARKE-DAVIS, Division of Warner-Lambert Company, Morris Plains, New Jersey 07950.

Parke-Davis—Cont.

ing risk factors. The risk of morbidity and mortality increases significantly in the presence of other underlying risk factors such as hypertension, hyperlipidemias, obesity and diabetes.

Practitioners prescribing oral contraceptives should be familiar with the following information relating to these risks. The information contained in this package insert is principally based on studies carried out in patients who used oral contraceptives with higher formulations of estrogens and progestogens than those in common use today. The effect of long-term use of the oral contraceptives with lower formulations of both estrogens and progestogens remains to be determined.

Throughout this labeling, epidemiological studies reported are of two types: retrospective or case control studies and prospective or cohort studies. Case control studies provide a measure of the relative risk of a disease, namely, a *ratio* of the incidence of a disease among oral contraceptive users to that among nonusers. The relative risk does not provide information on the actual clinical occurrence of a disease. Cohort studies provide a measure of attributable risk, which is the *difference* in the incidence of disease between oral contraceptive users and nonusers. The attributable risk does provide information about the actual occurrence of a disease in the population (adapted from refs. 2 and 3 with the author's permission). For further information, the reader is referred to a text on epidemiological methods.

1. Thromboembolic Disorders And Other Vascular Problems.

a. Myocardial infarction

An increased risk of myocardial infarction has been attributed to oral contraceptive use. This risk is primarily in smokers or women with other underlying risk factors for coronary artery disease such as hypertension, hypercholesterolemia, morbid obesity, and diabetes. The relative risk of heart attack for current oral contraceptive users has been estimated to be two to six (4–10). The risk is very low under the age of 30.

Smoking in combination with oral contraceptive use has been shown to contribute substantially to the incidence of myocardial infarctions in women in their mid-thirties or older with smoking accounting for the majority of excess cases (11). Mortality rates associated with circulatory disease have been shown to increase substantially in smokers over the age of 35 and nonsmokers over the age of 40 (Table II) among women who use oral contraceptives.

[See table below].

Oral contraceptives may compound the effects of well-known risk factors, such as hypertension, diabetes, hyperlipidemias, age and obesity (13). In particular, some progestogens are known to decrease HDL cholesterol and cause glucose intolerance, while estrogens may create a state of hyperinsulinism (14–18). Oral contraceptives have been shown to increase blood pressure among users (see section 9 in WARNINGS). Similar effects on risk factors have been associated with an increased risk of heart disease. Oral contraceptives must be used with caution in women with cardiovascular disease risk factors.

b. Thromboembolism

An increased risk of thromboembolic and thrombotic disease associated with the use of oral contraceptives is well established. Case control studies have found the relative risk of users compared to non-users to be 3 for the first episode of superficial venous thrombosis, 4 to 11 for deep vein thrombo-

sis or pulmonary embolism, and 1.5 to 6 for women with predisposing conditions for venous thromboembolic disease (2,3,19–24). Cohort studies have shown the relative risk to be somewhat lower, about 3 for new cases and about 4.5 for new cases requiring hospitalization (25). The risk of thromboembolic disease due to oral contraceptives is not related to length of use and disappears after pill use is stopped (2).

A two- to four-fold increase in relative risk of postoperative thromboembolic complications has been reported with the use of oral contraceptives (9,26). The relative risk of venous thrombosis in women who have predisposing conditions is twice that of women without such medical conditions (9,26). If feasible, oral contraceptives should be discontinued at least four weeks prior to and for two weeks after elective surgery of a type associated with an increase in risk of thromboembolism and during and following prolonged immobilization. Since the immediate post partum period is also associated with an increased risk of thromboembolism, oral contraceptives should be started no earlier than four to six weeks after delivery in women who elect not to breast feed.

c. Cerebrovascular diseases

Oral contraceptives have been shown to increase both the relative and attributable risks of cerebrovascular events (thrombotic and hemorrhagic strokes), although, in general, the risk is greatest among older (> 35 years), hypertensive women who also smoke. Hypertension was found to be a risk factor for both users and non-users, for both types of strokes, while smoking interacted to increase the risk for hemorrhagic strokes (27–29).

In a large study, the relative risk of thrombotic strokes has been shown to range from 3 for normotensive users to 14 for users with severe hypertension (30). The relative risk of hemorrhagic stroke is reported to be 1.2 for non-smokers who used oral contraceptives, 2.6 for smokers who did not use oral contraceptives, 7.6 for smokers who used oral contraceptives, 1.8 for normotensive users and 25.7 for users with severe hypertension (30). The attributable risk is also greater in older women (3).

d. Dose-related risk of vascular disease from oral contraceptives

A positive association has been observed between the amount of estrogen and progestogen in oral contraceptives and the risk of vascular disease. (31–33). A decline in serum high density lipoproteins (HDL) has been reported with many progestational agents (14–16). A decline in serum high density lipoproteins has been associated with an increased incidence of ischemic heart disease. Because estrogens increase HDL cholesterol, the net effect of an oral contracep-

tive depends on a balance achieved between doses of estrogen and progestogen and the nature and absolute amount of progestogens used in the contraceptives. The amount of both hormones should be considered in the choice of an oral contraceptive.

Minimizing exposure to estrogen and progestogen is in keeping with good principles of therapeutics. For any particular estrogen/progestogen combination, the dosage regimen prescribed should be one which contains the least amount of estrogen and progestogen that is compatible with a low failure rate and the needs of the individual patient. New acceptors of oral contraceptive agents should be started on preparations containing the lowest dose of estrogen which produces satisfactory results for the patient.

e. Persistence of risk of vascular disease

There are two studies which have shown persistence of risk of vascular disease for ever users of oral contraceptives. In a study in the United States, the risk of developing myocardial infarction after discontinuing oral contraceptives persists for at least 9 years for women 40–49 years who had used oral contraceptives for 5 or more years, but this increased risk was not demonstrated in other age groups (8). In another study in Great Britain, the risk of developing cerebrovascular disease persisted for at least 6 years after discontinuation of oral contraceptives, although excess risk was very small (34). However, both studies were performed with oral contraceptive formulations containing 50 micrograms or higher of estrogens.

2. Estimates Of Mortality From Contraceptive Use

One study gathered data from a variety of sources which have estimated the mortality rate associated with different methods of contraception at different ages (Table III). These estimates include the combined risk of death associated with contraceptive methods plus the risk attributable to pregnancy in the event of method failure. Each method of contraception has its specific benefits and risks. The study concluded that with the exception of oral contraceptive users 35 and older who smoke and 40 and older who do not smoke, mortality associated with all methods of birth control is low and below that associated with childbirth. However, smokers 35 and older and non-smokers 40 and older who use oral contraceptives have an increase in mortality higher than those using other methods of birth control. These facts must be weighed in conjunction with failure rates for different methods and the risk associated with subsequent pregnancy. (See Table I.)

[See table above].

3. Carcinoma Of The Reproductive Organs

Numerous epidemiological studies have been performed on the incidence of breast, endometrial, ovarian and cervical cancer in women using oral contraceptives. The overwhelming evidence in the literature suggests that use of oral contraceptives is not associated with an increase in the risk of developing breast cancer, regardless of the age and parity of first use or with most of the marketed brands and doses (36, 38). The Cancer and Steroid Hormone (CASH) study (36) also showed no latent effect on the risk of breast cancer for at least a decade following long-term use. A few studies have shown a slightly increased relative risk of developing breast cancer (37, 39–41), although the methodology of these studies, which included differences in examination of users and nonusers and differences in age at start of use, has been questioned (41–43).

Some studies suggest that oral contraceptive use has been associated with an increase in the risk of cervical intraepithelial neoplasia in some populations of women (45–48). However, there continues to be controversy about the extent to which such findings may be due to differences in sexual behavior and other factors.

In spite of many studies of the relationship between oral contraceptive use and breast and cervical cancers, a cause and effect relationship has not been established.

4. Hepatic Neoplasia

Benign hepatic adenomas are associated with oral contraceptive use, although the incidence of benign tumors is rare in the United States. Indirect calculations have estimated the

TABLE III
ANNUAL NUMBER OF BIRTH-RELATED OR METHOD-RELATED DEATHS ASSOCIATED WITH CONTROL OF FERTILITY PER 100,000 NONSTERILE WOMEN, BY FERTILITY CONTROL METHOD ACCORDING TO AGE

Method of control and outcome	15–19	20–24	25–29	30–34	35–39	40–44
No fertility control methods*	7.0	7.4	9.1	14.8	25.7	28.2
Oral contraceptives non-smoker**	0.3	0.5	0.9	1.9	13.8	31.6
Oral contraceptives smoker**	2.2	3.4	6.6	13.5	51.1	117.2
IUD**	0.8	0.8	1.0	1.0	1.4	1.4
Condom*	1.1	1.6	0.7	0.2	0.3	0.4
Diaphragm/spermicide*	1.9	1.2	1.2	1.3	2.2	2.8
Periodic abstinence*	2.5	1.6	1.6	1.7	2.9	3.6

* Deaths are birth related
** Deaths are method related

Adapted from HW Ory, ref. #35.

TABLE II
CIRCULATORY DISEASE MORTALITY RATES PER 100,000 WOMAN YEARS BY AGE, SMOKING STATUS AND ORAL CONTRACEPTIVE USE

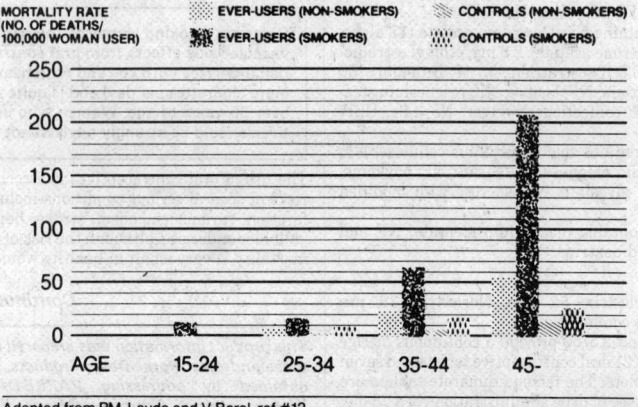

Adapted from P.M. Layde and V. Beral, ref #12.

attributable risk to be in the range of 3.3 cases/100,000 for users, a risk that increases after four or more years of use (49). Rupture of rare, benign, hepatic adenomas may cause death through intra-abdominal hemorrhage (50,51).

Studies from Britain have shown an increased risk of developing hepatocellular carcinoma (52–54) in long-term (>8 years) oral contraceptive users. However, these cancers are extremely rare in the U.S., and the attributable risk (the excess incidence) of liver cancers in oral contraceptive users approaches less than one per million users.

5. Ocular Lesions
There have been clinical case reports of retinal thrombosis associated with the use of oral contraceptives. Oral contraceptives should be discontinued if there is unexplained partial or complete loss of vision; onset of proptosis or diplopia; papilledema; or retinal vascular lesions. Appropriate diagnostic and therapeutic measures should be undertaken immediately.

6. Oral Contraceptive Use Before Or During Early Pregnancy: Risk Of Birth Defects
Extensive epidemiological studies have revealed no increased risk of birth defects in women who have used oral contraceptives prior to pregnancy (55–57). Studies also do not suggest a teratogenic effect, particularly insofar as cardiac anomalies and limb reduction defects are concerned (55,56,58,59), when taken inadvertently during early pregnancy.

The administration of oral contraceptives to induce withdrawal bleeding should not be used as a test for pregnancy. Oral contraceptives should not be used during pregnancy to treat threatened or habitual abortion.

It is recommended that for any patient who has missed two consecutive periods, pregnancy should be ruled out before continuing oral contraceptive use. If the patient has not adhered to the prescribed schedule, the possibility of pregnancy should be considered at the time of the first missed period. Oral contraceptive use should be discontinued if pregnancy is confirmed.

7. Gallbladder Disease
Earlier studies have reported an increased lifetime relative risk of gallbladder surgery in users of oral contraceptives and estrogens (60,61). More recent studies, however, have shown that the relative risk of developing gallbladder disease among oral contraceptive users may be minimal (62–64). The recent findings of minimal risk may be related to the use of oral contraceptive formulations containing lower hormonal doses of estrogens and progestogens.

8. Carbohydrate And Lipid Metabolic Effects
Oral contraceptives have been shown to cause glucose intolerance in a significant percentage of users (17). Oral contraceptives containing greater than 75 micrograms of estrogens cause hyperinsulinism, while lower doses of estrogen cause less glucose intolerance (65). Progestogens increase insulin secretion and create insulin resistance, this effect varying with different progestational agents (17, 66). However, in the non-diabetic woman, oral contraceptives appear to have no effect on fasting blood glucose (67). Because of these demonstrated effects, prediabetic and diabetic women should be carefully observed while taking oral contraceptives.

A small proportion of women will have persistent hypertriglyceridemia while on the pill. As discussed earlier (see WARNINGS 1a. and 1d.), changes in serum triglycerides and lipoprotein levels have been reported in oral contraceptive users.

9. Elevated Blood Pressure
An increase in blood pressure has been reported in women taking oral contraceptives (68) and this increase is more likely in older oral contraceptive users (69) and with continued use (68). Data from the Royal College of General Practitioners (12) and subsequent randomized trials have shown that the incidence of hypertension increases with increasing concentrations of progestogens.

Women with a history of hypertension or hypertension-related diseases, or renal disease (70) should be encouraged to use another method of contraception. If women elect to use oral contraceptives, they should be monitored closely and if significant elevation of blood pressure occurs, oral contraceptives should be discontinued. For most women, elevated blood pressure will return to normal after stopping oral contraceptives (69), and there is no difference in the occurrence of hypertension among ever and never users (68,70,71).

10. Headache
The onset or exacerbation of migraine or development of headache of a new pattern which is recurrent, persistent or severe requires discontinuation of oral contraceptives and evaluation of the cause.

11. Bleeding Irregularities
Breakthrough bleeding and spotting are sometimes encountered in patients on oral contraceptives, especially during the first three months of use. Non-hormonal causes should be considered and adequate diagnostic measures taken to rule out malignancy or pregnancy in the event of breakthrough bleeding, as in the case of any abnormal vaginal bleeding. If pathology has been excluded, time or a change to

another formulation may solve the problem. In the event of amenorrhea, pregnancy should be ruled out.

Some women may encounter post-pill amenorrhea or oligomenorrhea, especially when such a condition was preexistent.

PRECAUTIONS
1. Physical Examination And Follow Up
A complete medical history and physical examination should be taken prior to the initiation or reinstitution of oral contraceptives and at least annually during use of oral contraceptives. These physical examinations should include special reference to blood pressure, breasts, abdomen and pelvic organs, including cervical cytology, and relevant laboratory tests. In case of undiagnosed, persistent or recurrent abnormal vaginal bleeding, appropriate diagnostic measures should be conducted to rule out malignancy. Women with a strong family history of breast cancer or who have breast nodules should be monitored with particular care.

2. Lipid Disorders
Women who are being treated for hyperlipidemias should be followed closely if they elect to use oral contraceptives. Some progestogens may elevate LDL levels and may render the control of hyperlipidemias more difficult.

3. Liver Function
If jaundice develops in any woman receiving such drugs, the medication should be discontinued. Steroid hormones may be poorly metabolized in patients with impaired liver function.

4. Fluid Retention
Oral contraceptives may cause some degree of fluid retention. They should be prescribed with caution, and only with careful monitoring, in patients with conditions which might be aggravated by fluid retention.

5. Emotional Disorders
Women with a history of depression should be carefully observed and the drug discontinued if depression recurs to a serious degree.

6. Contact Lenses
Contact lens wearers who develop visual changes or changes in lens tolerance should be assessed by an ophthalmologist.

7. Drug Interactions
Reduced efficacy and increased incidence of breakthrough bleeding and menstrual irregularities have been associated with concomitant use of rifampin. A similar association though less marked, has been suggested with barbiturates, phenylbutazone, phenytoin sodium, and possibly with griseofulvin, ampicillin and tetracyclines (72).

8. Interactions With Laboratory Tests
Certain endocrine and liver function tests and blood components may be affected by oral contraceptives:
a. Increased prothrombin and factors VII, VIII, IX, and X; decreased antithrombin 3; increased norepinephrine-induced platelet aggregability.
b. Increased thyroid binding globulin (TBG) leading to increased circulating total thyroid hormone, as measured by protein-bound iodine (PBI), T4 by column, or by radioimmunoassay. Free T3 resin uptake is decreased, reflecting the elevated TBG; free T4 concentration is unaltered.
c. Other binding proteins may be elevated in serum.
d. Sex-binding globulins are increased and result in elevated levels of total circulating sex steroids and corticoids; however, free or biologically active levels remain unchanged.
e. Triglycerides may be increased.
f. Glucose tolerance may be decreased.
g. Serum folate levels may be depressed by oral contraceptive therapy. This may be of clinical significance if a woman becomes pregnant shortly after discontinuing oral contraceptives.

9. Carcinogenesis
See **WARNINGS** section.

10. Pregnancy
Pregnancy Category X. See **CONTRAINDICATIONS** and **WARNINGS** sections.

11. Nursing Mothers
Small amounts of oral contraceptive steroids have been identified in the milk of nursing mothers and a few adverse effects on the child have been reported, including jaundice and breast enlargement. In addition, oral contraceptives given in the postpartum period may interfere with lactation by decreasing the quantity and quality of breast milk. If possible, the nursing mother should be advised not to use oral contraceptives but to use other forms of contraception until she has completely weaned her child.

INFORMATION FOR THE PATIENT
See patient labeling printed below.

ADVERSE REACTIONS
An increased risk of the following serious adverse reactions has been associated with the use of oral contraceptives (see WARNINGS section).
• Thrombophlebitis
• Arterial thromboembolism
• Pulmonary embolism
• Myocardial infarction
• Cerebral hemorrhage

• Cerebral thrombosis
• Hypertension
• Gallbladder disease
• Hepatic adenomas or benign liver tumors
There is evidence of an association between the following conditions and the use of oral contraceptives, although additional confirmatory studies are needed:
• Mesenteric thrombosis
• Retinal thrombosis
The following adverse reactions have been reported in patients receiving oral contraceptives and are believed to be drug related:
• Nausea
• Vomiting
• Gastrointestinal symptoms (such as abdominal cramps and bloating)
• Breakthrough bleeding
• Spotting
• Change in menstrual flow
• Amenorrhea
• Temporary infertility after discontinuation of treatment
• Edema
• Melasma which may persist
• Breast changes: tenderness, enlargement, secretion
• Change in weight (increase or decrease)
• Change in cervical erosion and secretion
• Diminution in lactation when given immediately postpartum
• Cholestatic jaundice
• Migraine
• Rash (allergic)
• Mental depression
• Reduced tolerance to carbohydrates
• Vaginal candidiasis
• Change in corneal curvature (steepening)
• Intolerance to contact lenses
The following adverse reactions have been reported in users of oral contraceptives and the association has been neither confirmed nor refuted:
• Pre-menstrual syndrome
• Cataracts
• Changes in appetite
• Cystitis-like syndrome
• Headache
• Nervousness
• Dizziness
• Hirsutism
• Loss of scalp hair
• Erythema multiforme
• Erythema nodosum
• Hemorrhagic eruption
• Vaginitis
• Porphyria
• Impaired renal function
• Hemolytic uremic syndrome
• Budd-Chiari syndrome
• Acne
• Changes in libido
• Colitis
While the following adverse reactions or conditions have been reported to be associated with the use of oral contraceptives, no causal relationship has been established:
• Congenital anomalies
• Raynaud's disease
• Sickle cell disease
• Mitral valve prolapse
• Increased risk of developing venous thromboembolic disease among women with blood types A, B, or AB, as opposed to women with blood type O.

OVERDOSAGE
Serious ill effects have not been reported following acute ingestion of large doses of oral contraceptives by young children. Overdosage may cause nausea, and withdrawal bleeding may occur in females.

NON-CONTRACEPTIVE HEALTH BENEFITS
The following non-contraceptive health benefits related to the use of oral contraceptives are supported by epidemiological studies which largely utilized oral contraceptive formulations containing estrogen doses exceeding 0.05 mg of estrogen (73–78).
Effects on menses:
• Increased menstrual cycle regularity
• Decreased blood loss and decreased incidence of iron deficiency anemia

Continued on next page

This product information was prepared in August, 1989. On these and other Parke-Davis Products, information may be obtained by addressing PARKE-DAVIS, Division of Warner-Lambert Company, Morris Plains, New Jersey 07950.

Parke-Davis—Cont.

- Decreased incidence of dysmenorrhea

Effects related to inhibition of ovulation:
- Decreased incidence of functional ovarian cysts
- Decreased incidence of ectopic pregnancies

Effects from long-term use:
- Decreased incidence of fibroadenomas and fibrocystic disease of the breast
- Decreased incidence of acute pelvic inflammatory disease
- Decreased incidence of endometrial cancer
- Decreased incidence of ovarian cancer

DOSAGE AND ADMINISTRATION

The tablet dispenser has been designed to make oral contraceptive dosing as easy and as convenient as possible. The tablets are arranged in either three or four rows of seven tablets each, with the days of the week appearing on the tablet dispenser above the first row of tablets.

Important Notes: The patient should be instructed to use an additional method of protection until after the first week of administration in the initial cycle if utilizing the Sunday-Start Regimen.

The possibility of ovulation and conception prior to initiation of use should be considered.

Dosage And Administration For 21-Day Dosage Regimen

To achieve maximum contraceptive effectiveness, Norlestrin **21** must be taken exactly as directed and at intervals not exceeding 24 hours. Norlestrin **21** provides the patient with a convenient tablet schedule of "3 weeks on—1 week off." Two dosage regimens are described, one of which may be more convenient or suitable than the other for an individual patient. For the initial cycle of therapy, the patient begins her tablets according to the Day-5 or Sunday-Start Regimen. With either regimen, the patient takes one tablet daily for 21 consecutive days followed by one week of no tablets.

A. Sunday-Start Regimen: The patient begins taking tablets from the top row on the first Sunday after menstrual flow begins. When menstrual flow begins on Sunday, the first tablet is taken on the same day. The last tablet in the dispenser will then be taken on a Saturday, followed by no tablets for a week (7 days). For all subsequent cycles the patient then begins a new 21-tablet regimen on the eighth day, Sunday, after taking her last tablet. Following this regimen, of 21 days on—7 days off, the patient will start all subsequent cycles on a Sunday.

B. Day-5 Regimen: The first day of menstrual flow is Day 1. On Day 5 of her menstrual flow, the patient starts taking 1 tablet daily, beginning with the tablet in the top row that corresponds to Day 5 of her flow. After the last tablet (Saturday) has been taken, if any tablets remain in the top row, the patient completes her 21-tablet regimen starting with the Sunday tablet in the top row, followed by no tablets for a week (7 days). For all subsequent cycles, the patient begins a new 21 tablet regimen on the eighth day after taking her last tablet, again beginning on the same day of the week on which she began her first course. Following this regimen of 21 days on—7 days off, the patient will start all subsequent cycles on the same day of the week as the first course. Likewise, the interval of no tablets will always start on the same day of the week.

Whether utilizing the Sunday-Start or Day-5 Regimen, all tablets should be taken regularly with a meal or at bedtime. It should be stressed that efficacy of medication depends on strict adherence to the dosage schedule.

Special Notes on Administration

Menstruation usually begins two or three days, but may begin as late as the fourth or fifth day, after discontinuing medication. If spotting occurs while on the usual regimen of one tablet daily, the patient should continue medication without interruption.

If a patient forgets to take one or more tablets, the following is suggested: If one tablet is missed, take it as soon as remembered, or take two tablets the next day. If two consecutive tablets are missed, take two tablets daily for the next two days, then resume the regular schedule. While there is little likelihood of pregnancy occurring if the patient misses only one or two tablets, the possibility of pregnancy increases with each successive day that tablets are missed. If three consecutive tablets are missed, the patient starts a new course of tablets in the following manner: If the patient is on the Sunday-Start Regimen, a new course of tablets is started on the first Sunday following the last missed tablet, whether or not she is still menstruating. If the patient is on the Day-5 Regimen, a new course of tablets is started on the eighth day after the last tablet was taken. For example, if the patient took her last tablet on Monday, she should start her new course of tablets the following Monday. The patient should also use an additional method of birth control during the seven days without tablets, and until she has taken a tablet daily for seven consecutive days.

The possibility of ovulation occurring increases with each successive day that scheduled tablets are missed. While there is little likelihood of ovulation occurring if only one tablet is missed, the possibility of spotting or bleeding is in-

creased. This is particularly likely to occur if two or more consecutive tablets are missed.

In the rare case of bleeding which resembles menstruation, the patients should be advised to discontinue medication and then begin taking tablets from a dispenser on the next Sunday or the fifth day (Day 5) depending on their regimen. Persistent bleeding which is not controlled by this method indicates the need for reexamination of the patient at which time nonfunctional causes should be borne in mind.

Dosage And Administration For 28-Day Dosage Regimen

To achieve maximum contraceptive effectiveness, Norlestrin **Fe** and **28** must be taken exactly as directed and at intervals not exceeding 24 hours.

Norlestrin **Fe** and **28** provide a continuous administration regimen consisting of 21 *light-colored* (yellow or pink) tablets of Norlestrin and 7 *brown* tablets of ferrous fumarate or 7 *white* inert tablets. There is no need for the patient to count days between cycles because there are no "off-tablet days." The patient begins taking *light-colored* tablets from the top row on the first Sunday after menstrual flow begins. When menstrual flow begins on Sunday, the first *light-colored* tablet is taken on the same day. The patient takes one *light-colored* tablet daily for 21 days. The last *light-colored* tablet taken is the Saturday tablet. Upon completion of all 21 tablets, and without interruption, the patient takes one *brown* tablet daily for 7 days. Upon completion of this first course of tablets, the patient begins a second course of 28 tablets without interruption, the next day, Sunday, starting with the Sunday *light-colored* tablet in the top row. Adhering to this regimen, of one *light-colored* tablet daily for 21 days, followed without interruption by one *brown* or *white* tablet daily for seven days, the patient will start all subsequent cycles on a Sunday.

Tablets should be taken regularly with a meal or at bedtime. It should be stressed that efficacy of medication depends on strict adherence to the dosage schedule.

Special Notes on Administration

Menstruation usually begins two or three days, but may begin as late as the fourth or fifth day, after the *brown* or *white* tablets have been started. In any event, the next course of tablets should be started without interruption. There should never be a day when the patient is not taking a tablet.

If spotting occurs while the patient is taking *light-colored* tablets, continue medication without interruption.

If a patient forgets to take one or more *light-colored* tablets, the following is suggested: If one *light-colored* tablet is missed, take it as soon as remembered, or take two *light-colored* tablets the next day. If two consecutive *light-colored* tablets are missed, take two *light-colored* tablets daily for the next two days, then resume the regular schedule. While there is little likelihood of pregnancy occurring if the patient misses only one or two *light-colored* tablets, the possibility of pregnancy increases with each successive day that *light-colored* tablets are missed. If three consecutive tablets are missed, the patient starts a new course of tablets the first Sunday following the last missed tablet, whether or not she is still menstruating. The patient should also use an additional method of birth control during the days without tablets, and until she has taken a tablet for seven consecutive days.

The possibility of ovulation occurring increases with each successive day that scheduled *light-colored* tablets are missed. While there is little likelihood of ovulation occurring if only one *light-colored* tablet is missed, the possibility of spotting or bleeding is increased. This is particularly likely to occur if two or more consecutive *light-colored* tablets are missed.

If one or more *brown* tablets are missed, the *light-colored* tablets should be started no later than the eighth day after the last *light-colored* tablet was taken. The possibility of conception occurring is not increased if *brown* or *white* tablets are missed.

In the rare case of bleeding which resembles menstruation, the patient should be advised to discontinue medication and then begin taking tablets from a new dispenser on the next Sunday. Persistent bleeding which is not controlled by this method indicates the need for reexamination of the patient, at which time nonfunctional causes should be borne in mind.

Use Of Oral Contraceptives In The Event Of A Missed Menstrual Period

1. If the patient has not adhered to the prescribed dosage regimen, the possibility of pregnancy should be considered after the first missed period and oral contraceptives should be withheld until pregnancy has been ruled out.
2. If the patient has adhered to the prescribed regimen and misses two consecutive periods, pregnancy should be ruled out before continuing the contraceptive regimen.

After several months on treatment, bleeding may be reduced to a point of virtual absence.

This reduced flow may occur as a result of medication, in which event it is not indicative of pregnancy.

HOW SUPPLIED

Norlestrin **21** 1/50 is available in dispensers each containing 21 tablets. Each tablet contains 1 mg of norethindrone ace-

tate and 50 mcg of ethinyl estradiol. Available in packages of five dispensers.

Norlestrin **21** 2.5/50 is available in dispensers each containing 21 tablets. Each tablet contains 2.5 mg of norethindrone acetate and 50 mcg of ethinyl estradiol. Available in packages of five dispensers.

Norlestrin **Fe** 1/50 is available in dispensers each containing 21 yellow tablets and 7 brown tablets. Each yellow tablet contains 1 mg of norethindrone acetate and 50 mcg of ethinyl estradiol. Each brown tablet contains 75 mg ferrous fumarate. Available in packages of five dispensers.

Norlestrin **Fe** 2.5/50 is available in dispensers each containing 21 pink tablets and 7 brown tablets. Each pink tablet contains 2.5 mg of norethindrone acetate and 50 mcg of ethinyl estradiol. Each brown tablet contains 75 mg ferrous fumarate. Available in packages of five dispensers.

Norlestrin **28** 1/50 is available in dispensers each containing 21 yellow tablets and 7 white inert tablets. Each yellow tablet contains 1 mg of norethindrone acetate and 50 mcg of ethinyl estradiol. Available in packages of five dispensers.

REFERENCES

1. Reproduced with permission of the Population Council from J. Trussell and K. Kost: Contraceptive failure in the United States: A critical review of the literature. *Studies in Family Planning*, 18 (5), September–October 1987.
2. Stadel, BV: Oral contraceptives and cardiovascular disease. (Pt. 1). *New England Journal of Medicine*, 305:612–618, 1981.
3. Stadel, B.V.: Oral contraceptives and cardiovascular disease. (Pt. 2.). *New England Journal of Medicine*, 305:672–677, 1981.
4. Adam, S.A., and M. Thorogood: Oral contraception and myocardial infarction revisited: The effects of new preparations and prescribing patterns. *Brit. J. Obstet. and Gynec.*, 88:838–845, 1981.
5. Mann, J.I., and W.H. Inman: Oral contraceptives and death from myocardial infarction. *Brit. Med. J.*, 2(5965): 245–248, 1975.
6. Mann, J.I., M.P. Vessey, M. Thorogood, and R. Doll: Myocardial infarction in young women with special reference to oral contraceptive practice. *Brit. Med. J.*, 2(5956):241–245, 1975.
7. Royal College of General Practitioners' Oral Contraception Study: Further analyses of mortality in oral contraceptive users. *Lancet*, 1:541–546, 1981.
8. Slone, D., S. Shapiro, DW. Kaufman, L. Rosenberg, O.S. Miettinen, and P.D. Stolley: Risk of myocardial infarction in relation to current and discontinued use of oral contraceptives. *N.E.J.M.*, 305:420–424, 1981.
9. Vessey, M.P.: Female hormones and vascular disease: an epidemiological overview, *Brit. J. Fam. Plann.*, 6:1–12, 1980.
10. Russell-Briefel, R.G., T.M. Ezzati, R. Fulwood, J.A. Perlman, and R.S. Murphy: Cardiovascular risk status and oral contraceptive use, United States, 1976–80. *Preventive Medicine*, 15:352–362, 1986.
11. Goldbaum, G.M., J.S. Kendrick, G.C. Hogelin, and E.M. Gentry: The relative impact of smoking and oral contraceptive use on women in the United States. *J.A.M.A.*, 258:1339–1342, 1987.
12. Layde, P.M., and V. Beral: Further analyses of mortality in oral contraceptive users: Royal College General Practitioners' Oral Contraception Study. (Table 5) *Lancet*, 1:541–546, 1981.
13. Knopp, R.H.: Arteriosclerosis risk: the roles of oral contraceptives and postmenopausal estrogens. *J. of Reprod. Med.*, 31(9)(Supplement): 913–921, 1986.
14. Krauss, R.M., S. Roy, D.R. Mishell, J. Casagrande, and M.C. Pike: Effects of two low-dose oral contraceptives on serum lipids and lipoproteins: Differential changes in high-density lipoproteins subclasses. *Am. J. Obstet. Gyn.*, 145:446–452, 1983.
15. Wahl, P., C. Walden, R. Knopp, J. Hoover, R. Wallace, G. Heiss, and B. Rifkind: Effect of estrogen/progestin potency on lipid/lipoprotein cholesterol, *N.E.J.M.*, 308:862–867, 1983.
16. Wynn, V., and R. Niththyananthan: The effect of progestin in combined oral contraceptives on serum lipids with special reference to high-density lipoproteins. *Am. J. Obstet. and Gyn.*, 142:766–771, 1982.
17. Wynn, V., and I. Godsland: Effects of oral contraceptives on carbohydrate metabolism. *J. Reprod. Medicine*, 31(9)(Supplement): 892–897, 1986.
18. LaRosa, J.C.: Atherosclerotic risk factors in cardiovascular disease. *J. Reprod. Med.*, 31(9)(Supplement): 906–912, 1986.
19. Inman, W.H., and M.P. Vessey: Investigations of death from pulmonary, coronary, and cerebral thrombosis and embolism in women of child-bearing age. *Brit. Med. J.*, 2(5599): 193–199, 1968.
20. Maguire, M.G., J. Tonascia, P.E. Sartwell, P.D. Stolley, and M.S. Tockman: Increased risk of thrombosis due to oral contraceptives: A further report. *Am. J. Epidemiology*, 110(2):188–195, 1979.

21. Pettiti, D.B., J. Wingerd, F. Pellegrin, and S. Ramacharan: Risk of vascular disease in women: smoking, oral contraceptives, noncontraceptive estrogens, and other factors, *J.A.M.A.*, 242:1150–1154, 1979.

22. Vessey, M.P., and R. Doll: Investigation of relation between use of oral contraceptives and thromboembolic disease. *Brit. Med. J.*, 2(5599): 199–205, 1968.

23. Vessey, M.P., and R. Doll: Investigation of relation between use of oral contraceptives and thromboembolic disease: A further report. *Brit. Med. J.*, 2(5658): 651–657, 1969.

24. Porter, J.B., J.R. Hunter, D.A. Danielson, H. Jick, and A. Stergachis: Oral contraceptives and non-fatal vascular disease: Recent experience. *Obstet. and Gyn.*, 59(3):299–302, 1982.

25. Vessey, M., R. Doll, R. Peto, B. Johnson, and P. Wiggins: A long-term follow-up study of women using different methods of contraception: An interim report. *J. Biosocial. Sci.*, 8:375–427, 1976.

26. Royal College of General Practitioners: Oral contraceptives, venous thrombosis, and varicose veins. *J. of Royal College of General Practitioners*, 28:393–399, 1978.

27. Collaborative Group for the study of stroke in young women: Oral contraception and increased risk of cerebral ischemia or thrombosis. *N.E.J.M.*, 288:871–878, 1973.

28. Petitti, D.B., and J. Wingerd: Use of oral contraceptives, cigarette smoking, and risk of subarachnoid hemorrhage. *Lancet*, 2:234–236, 1978.

29. Inman, W.H.: Oral contraceptives and fatal subarachnoid hemorrhage. *Brit. Med. J.*, 2(6203): 1468–70, 1979.

30. Collaborative Group for the study of stroke in young women: Oral contraceptives and stroke in young women: associated risk factors. *J.A.M.A.*, 231:718–722, 1975.

31. Inman, W.H., M.P. Vessey, B. Westerholm, and A. Engelund: Thromboembolic disease and the steroidal content of oral contraceptives. A report to the Committee on Safety of Drugs. *Brit. Med. J.*, 2:203–209, 1970.

32. Meade, T.W., G. Greenberg, and S.G. Thompson: Progestogens and cardiovascular reactions associated with oral contraceptives and a comparison of the safety of 50- and 35-mcg oestrogen preparations. *Brit. Med. J.*, 280(6244): 1157–1161, 1980.

33. Kay, C.R.: Progestogens and arterial disease-evidence from the Royal College of General Practitioners' study. *Amer. J. Obstet. Gyn.*, 142:762–765, 1982.

34. Royal College of General Practitioners: Incidence of arterial disease among oral contraceptive users. *J. Coll. Gen. Pract.*, 33:75–82, 1983.

35. Ory, H.W.: Mortality associated with fertility and fertility control: 1983. *Family Planning Perspectives*, 15:50–56, 1983.

36. The Cancer and Steroid Hormone Study of the Centers for Disease Control and the National Institute of Child Health and Human Development: Oral-contraceptive use and the risk of breast cancer. *N.E.J.M.*, 315:405–411, 1986.

37. Pike, M.C., B.E. Henderson, M.D. Krailo, A. Duke, and S. Roy: Breast cancer in young women and use of oral contraceptives: possible modifying effect of formulation and age at use. *Lancet*, 2:926–929. 1983.

38. Paul, C., D.G. Skegg, G.F.S. Spears, and J.M. Kaldor: Oral contraceptives and breast cancer: A national study. *Brit. Med. J.*, 293:723–725, 1986.

39. Miller, D.R., L. Rosenberg, D.W. Kaufman, D. Schottenfeld, P.D. Stolley, and S. Shapiro: Breast cancer risk in relation to early oral contraceptive use. *Obstet. Gynec.*, 68:863–868, 1986.

40. Olson, H., K.L. Olson, T.R. Moller, J. Ranstam, P. Holm: Oral contraceptive use and breast cancer in young women in Sweden (letter). *Lancet*, 2:748–749, 1985.

41. McPherson, K., M. Vessey, A. Neil, R. Doll, L. Jones, and M. Roberts: Early contraceptive use and breast cancer: Results of another case-control study. *Brit. J. Cancer*, 56: 653–660, 1987.

42. Huggins, G.R., and P.F. Zucker: Oral contraceptives and neoplasia: 1987 update. *Fertil. Steril.*, 47:733–761, 1987.

43. McPherson, K., and J.O. Drife: The pill and breast cancer: why the uncertainty? *Brit. Med. J.*, 293:709–710, 1986.

44. Shapiro, S.: Oral contraceptives: time to take stock. *N.E.J.M.*, 315:450–451, 1987.

45. Ory, H., Z. Naib, S.B. Conger, R.A. Hatcher, and C.W. Tyler: Contraceptive choice and prevalence of cervical dysplasia and carcinoma in situ. *Am. J. Obstet. Gynec.*, 124:573–577, 1976.

46. Vessey, M.P., M. Lawless, K. McPherson, D. Yeates: Neoplasia of the cervix uteri and contraception: a possible adverse effect of the pill. *Lancet*, 2:930, 1983.

47. Brinton, L.A., G.R. Huggins, H.F. Lehman, K. Malli, D.A. Savitz, E. Trapido, J. Rosenthal, and R. Hoover: Long term use of oral contraceptives and risk of invasive cervical cancer. *Int. J. Cancer*, 38:339–344, 1986.

48. WHO Collaborative Study of Neoplasia and Steroid Contraceptives: Invasive cervical cancer and combined oral contraceptives. *Brit. Med. J.*, 290:961–965, 1985.

49. Rooks, J.B., H.W. Ory, K.G. Ishak, L.T. Strauss, J.R. Greenspan, A.P. Hill, and C.W. Tyler: Epidemiology of hepatocellular adenoma: The role of oral contraceptive use. *J.A.M.A.*, 242:644–648, 1979.

50. Bein, N.N., and H.S. Goldsmith: Recurrent massive hemorrhage from benign hepatic tumors secondary to oral contraceptives. *Brit. J. Surg.*, 64:433–435, 1977.

51. Klatskin, G.: Hepatic tumors: possible relationship to use of oral contraceptives. *Gastroenterology*, 73:386–394, 1977.

52. Henderson, B.E., S. Preston-Martin, H.A. Edmondson, R.L. Peters, and M.C. Pike: Hepatocellular carcinoma and oral contraceptives. *Brit. J. Cancer*, 48:437–440, 1983.

53. Neuberger, J., D. Forman, R. Doll, and R. Williams: Oral contraceptives and hepatocellular carcinoma, *Brit. Med. J.*, 292:1355–1357, 1986.

54. Forman, D., T.J. Vincent, and R. Doll: Cancer of the liver and oral contraceptives. *Brit. Med. J.*, 292:1357–1361, 1986.

55. Harlap, S., and J. Eldor: Births following oral contraceptive failures. *Obstet. Gynec.*, 55:447–452, 1980.

56. Savolainen, E., E. Saksela, and L. Saxen: Teratogenic hazards of oral contraceptives analyzed in a national malformation register. *Amer. J. Obstet. Gynec.*, 140:521–524, 1981.

57. Janerich, D.T., J.M. Piper, and D.M. Glebatis: Oral contraceptives and birth defects. *Am. J. Epidemiology*, 112:73–79, 1980.

58. Ferencz, C., G.M. Matanoski, P.D. Wilson, J.D. Rubin, C.A. Neill, and R. Gutberlet: Maternal hormone therapy and congenital heart disease. *Teratology*, 21:225–239, 1980.

59. Rothman, K.J., D.C. Fyler, A. Goldbatt, and M.B. Kreidberg: Exogenous hormones and other drug exposures of children with congenital heart disease. *Am. J. Epidemiology*, 109:433–439, 1979.

60. Boston Collaborative Drug Surveillance Program: Oral contraceptives and venous thromboembolic disease, surgically confirmed gallbladder disease, and breast tumors. *Lancet*, 1:1399–1404, 1973.

61. Royal College of General Practitioners: *Oral contraceptives and health.* New York, Pittman, 1974, 100p.

62. Layde, P.M., M.P. Vessey, and D. Yeates: Risk of gallbladder disease: a cohort study of young women attending family planning clinics. *J. of Epidemiol. and Comm. Health*, 36: 274–278, 1982.

63. Rome Group for the Epidemiology and Prevention of Cholelithiasis (GREPCO): Prevalence of gallstone disease in an Italian adult female population, *Am. J. Epidemiol.*, 119:796–805, 1984.

64. Strom, B.L., R.T. Tamragouri, M.L. Morse, E.L. Lazar, S.L. West, P.D. Stolley, and J.K. Jones: Oral contraceptives and other risk factors for gallbladder disease. *Clin. Pharmacol. Ther.*, 39:335–341, 1986.

65. Wynn, V., P.W. Adams, I.F. Godsland, J. Melrose, R. Niththyananthan, N.W. Oakley, and A. Seedj: Comparison of effects of different combined oral-contraceptive formulations on carbohydrate and lipid metabolism. *Lancet*, 1:1045–1049, 1979.

66. Wynn, V.: Effect of progesterone and progestins on carbohydrate metabolism. In Progesterone and Progestin. Edited by C.W. Bardin, E. Milgrom, P. Mauvis-Jarvis. New York, Raven Press, pp. 395–410, 1983.

67. Perlman, J.A., R.G. Roussell-Briefel, T.M. Ezzati, and G. Lieberknecht: Oral glucose tolerance and the potency of oral contraceptive progestogens. *J. Chronic Dis.*, 38:857–864, 1985.

68. Royal College of General Practitioners' Oral Contraception Study: Effect on hypertension and benign breast disease of progestogen component in combined oral contraceptives. *Lancet*, 1:624, 1977.

69. Fisch, I.R., and J. Frank: Oral contraceptives and blood pressure. *J.A.M.A.* 237:2499–2503, 1977.

70. Laragh, A.J.: Oral contraceptive induced hypertension: Nine years later. *Amer. J. Obstet. Gynecol.*, 126:141–147, 1976.

71. Ramcharan, S., E. Peritz, F.A. Pellegrin, and W.T. Williams: Incidence of hypertension in the Walnut Creek Contraceptive Drug Study cohort. In Pharmacology of Steroid Contraceptive Drugs. Edited by S. Garattini and H.W. Berendes, New York. Raven Press, pp. 277–288, 1977. (Monographs of the Mario Negri Institute for Pharmacological Research, Milan).

72. Stockley, I.: Interactions with oral contraceptives. *Pharm. J.* 216:140–143, 1976.

73. The Cancer and Steroid Hormone Study of the Centers for Disease Control and the National Institute of Child Health and Human Development: Oral contraceptive use and the risk of ovarian cancer. *J.A.M.A.*, 249:1596–1599, 1983.

74. The Cancer and Steroid Hormone Study of the Centers for Disease Control and the National Institute of Child Health and Human Development: Combination oral contraceptive use and the risk of endometrial cancer. *J.A.M.A.*, 257:796–800, 1987.

75. Ory, H.W.: Functional ovarian cysts and oral contraceptives: negative association confirmed surgically. *J.A.M.A.*, 228:68–69, 1974.

76. Ory, H.W., P. Cole, B. Macmahon, and R. Hoover: Oral contraceptives and reduced risk of benign breast disease. *N.E.J.M.*, 294:41–422, 1976.

77. Ory, H.W.: The noncontraceptive health benefits from oral contraceptive use. *Fam. Plann. Perspectives*, 14:182–184, 1982.

78. Ory, H.W., J.D. Forrest, and R. Lincoln: Making Choices: Evaluating the health risks and benefits of birth control methods. New York, The Alan Guttmacher Institute, p.1, 1983.

The patient labeling for oral contraceptive drug products is set forth below:

BRIEF SUMMARY PATIENT PACKAGE INSERT

Oral contraceptives, also known as "birth control pills" or "the pill," are taken to prevent pregnancy and when taken correctly, have a failure rate of about 1% per year when used without missing any pills. The typical failure rate of large numbers of pill users is less than 3% per year when women who miss pills are included. For most women oral contraceptives are also free of serious or unpleasant side effects. However, forgetting to take pills considerably increases the chances of pregnancy.

For the majority of women, oral contraceptives can be taken safely. But there are some women who are at high risk of developing certain serious diseases that can be life-threatening or may cause temporary or permanent disability. The risks associated with taking oral contraceptives increase significantly if you:

- Smoke
- Are over the age of 40
- Have high blood pressure, diabetes, high cholesterol
- Have or have had clotting disorders, heart attack, stroke, angina pectoris, cancer of the breast or sex organs, jaundice or malignant or benign liver tumors.

You should not take the pill if you suspect you are pregnant or have unexplained vaginal bleeding.

> Cigarette smoking increases the risk of serious cardiovascular side effects from oral contraceptive use. This risk increases with age and with heavy smoking (15 or more cigarettes per day) and is quite marked in women over 35 years of age. Women who use oral contraceptives are strongly advised not to smoke.

Most side effects of the pill are not serious. The most common side effects are nausea, vomiting, bleeding between menstrual periods, weight gain, and breast tenderness, and difficulty wearing contact lenses. These side effects, especially nausea and vomiting, may subside within the first three months of use.

The serious side effects of the pill occur very infrequently, especially if you are in good health and are young. However, you should know that the following medical conditions have been associated with or made worse by the pill:

1. Blood clots in the legs (thrombophlebitis), lungs (pulmonary embolism), stoppage or rupture of a blood vessel in the brain (stroke), blockage of blood vessels in the heart (heart attack or angina pectoris) or other organs of the body. As mentioned above, smoking increases the risk of heart attacks and strokes and subsequent serious medical consequences.

2. Liver tumors, which may rupture and cause severe bleeding. A possible but not definite association has been found with the pill and liver cancer. However, liver cancers are extremely rare. The chance of developing liver cancer from using the pill is thus even rarer.

3. High blood pressure, although blood pressure usually returns to normal when the pill is stopped.

The symptoms associated with these serious side effects are discussed in the detailed leaflet given to you with your supply of pills. Notify your doctor or health care provider if you notice any unusual physical disturbances while taking the pill. In addition, drugs such as rifampin, as well as some anticonvulsants and some antibiotics may decrease oral contraceptive effectiveness.

Studies to date of women taking the pill have not shown an increase in the incidence of cancer of the breast or cervix. There is, however, insufficient evidence to rule out the possibility that pills may cause such cancers.

Taking the pill provides some important non-contraceptive benefits. These include less painful menstruation, less men-

Continued on next page

This product information was prepared in August, 1989. On these and other Parke-Davis Products, information may be obtained by addressing PARKE-DAVIS, Division of Warner-Lambert Company, Morris Plains, New Jersey 07950.

Parke-Davis—Cont.

strual blood loss and anemia, fewer pelvic infections, and fewer cancers of the ovary and the lining of the uterus.

Be sure to discuss any medical condition you may have with your health care provider. Your health care provider will take a medical and family history and examine you before prescribing oral contraceptives. You should be reexamined at least once a year while taking oral contraceptives. The detailed patient information leaflet gives you further information which you should read and discuss with your health care provider.

Caution: Oral contraceptives are of no value in the prevention or treatment of venereal disease.

INSTRUCTIONS TO PATIENTS

TABLET DISPENSER

The tablet dispenser has been designed to make oral contraceptive dosing as easy and as convenient as possible. The tablets are arranged in either three or four rows of seven tablets each, with the days of the week appearing on the tablet dispenser above the first row of tablets.

If your tablet dispenser contains:	You are taking:
21 yellow tablets	NORLESTRIN 21 1/50
21 pink tablets	NORLESTRIN 21 2.5/50
21 yellow tablets and 7 brown tablets	NORLESTRIN Fe 1/50
21 pink tablets and 7 brown tablets	NORLESTRIN Fe 2.5/50
21 yellow tablets and 7 white tablets	NORLESTRIN 28/1.50

Each *yellow* tablet contains 1 mg norethindrone acetate and 50 mcg ethinyl estradiol.

Each *pink* tablet contains 2.5 mg norethindrone acetate and 50 mcg ethinyl estradiol.

Each *brown* tablet contains 75 mg ferrous fumarate, and is intended to help you remember to take the tablets correctly. These brown tablets are not intended to have any health benefit.

Each *white* tablet is inert.

To remove a tablet, press down on it with your thumb or finger. The tablet will drop through the back of the tablet dispenser. Do not press on the tablet with your thumbnail or fingernail or any other sharp object.

NORLESTRIN 21-DAY DOSAGE REGIMEN

If your tablet dispenser contains 21 tablets (3 rows of 7), you are on a 21-day regimen and should follow either the Sunday-Start or Day-5 Start directions.

A. Sunday-Start Regimen

1. Unless your physician or health care provider has instructed you differently, begin taking tablets on the first Sunday after your menstrual period begins whether or not you are still bleeding. If your period begins on Sunday, take your first tablet that very same day. START WITH THE SUNDAY TABLET IN THE TOP ROW.

Note: During the first cycle, it is important that you use another method of birth control until you have taken a tablet daily for seven consecutive days.

2. Take all the tablets in the top row first, followed by the second row. Continue to take one tablet every day until you finish all 21 tablets. Your last tablet should be on Saturday.

3. After you have taken all 21 tablets, stop, and don't take any tablets for the next seven days. You should have a menstrual period one to three days after you stop taking tablets; sometimes it may take a day or so longer.

4. After the seven days during which you take no tablets, obtain a new course of tablets. Begin the new course of 21 tablets on Sunday, the 8th day after you took your last tablet, starting with the Sunday tablet in the top row.

5. Continue to take one tablet daily until you finish all 21 tablets. If you follow the schedule properly, you will always take the last tablet in the dispenser on a Saturday, and always start each new course of 21 tablets 8 days later, on the following Sunday.

6. If, in any cycle, you start your tablets later than the proper day, you should also use another method of birth control until you have taken seven consecutive tablets.

B. Day-5 Regimen

If your physician or health care provider has directed you to begin taking your first cycle of tablets using the Day-5 Regimen, you should start taking your tablets on Day 5 after the start of your period.

1. The first day of your period is Day 1. On the 5th day (Day 5), start taking one tablet daily, beginning with the tablet

---

in the top row that corresponds to Day 5 after your flow began.

If your period begins on:	Start taking tablets in the top row on:
Sunday	Thursday
Monday	Friday
Tuesday	Saturday
Wednesday	Sunday
Thursday	Monday
Friday	Tuesday
Saturday	Wednesday

Note: During the first cycle, if you start taking tablets later than Day 5 of your menstrual period, you should use another method of birth control until you have taken a tablet daily for seven consecutive days.

2. Continue to take one tablet daily. After the last Saturday tablet has been taken, if any tablets remain in the first row, complete your 21-day regimen by taking one tablet daily starting with the Sunday tablet in the top row.

3. After you have taken all 21 tablets, stop, and don't take any tablets for the next seven days. You should have a menstrual period one to three days after you stop taking tablets; sometimes it may take a day or so longer.

4. After the seven days during which you take no tablets, obtain a new course of tablets. Begin a new course of 21-day tablets, the 8th day after you took your last tablet, starting with the tablet in the top row that corresponds to that day.

5. Continue to take one tablet daily until you finish all 21 tablets. If you follow the schedule properly, you will always take the last tablet in the dispenser on the same day of the week, and always start each new course of 21 tablets the same day of the week on which you began the previous cycle of tablets.

6. If, in any cycle, you start your tablets later than the proper day, you should also use another method of birth control until you have taken seven consecutive tablets.

Whether you started your tablets using the Sunday-Start or Day-5 Regimen, the following directions apply:

1. Continue taking your tablets whether or not your period has occurred or is still in progress. Your period will usually occur during the seven days you are taking no tablets.

2. If spotting should occur at an unexpected time, continue to take your tablets as directed. Spotting is usually temporary and without significance. However, if bleeding should occur at an unexpected time, consult your physician or health care provider. Call your physician or health care provider regarding any problem or change in your general health that may concern you.

NORLESTRIN 28-DAY DOSAGE REGIMEN

If your tablet dispenser contains 28 tablets (3 rows of 7 *light-colored* (yellow or pink) tablets and 1 row of 7 *brown* or *white* tablets), you are on a 28-day regimen and should follow these directions. Each *brown* tablet contains 75 mg ferrous fumarate and is intended to help you remember to take the tablets correctly. These brown tablets are not intended to have any health benefit.

Sunday-Start Regimen:

1. Begin taking tablets on the first Sunday after your menstrual period begins whether or not you are still bleeding. If your period begins on Sunday, take your first tablet that very same day. START WITH THE SUNDAY TABLET IN THE TOP ROW.

Note: During the first cycle, it is important that you use another method of birth control until you have taken a *light-colored* tablet daily for seven consecutive days.

2. Take all the tablets in the top row first, followed by the second row and so on.

3. Continue to take one tablet every day until you finish all 21 *light-colored* tablets. On the day after taking the last *light-colored* tablet, begin taking one *brown* or *white* tablet daily until all the tablets have been taken.

4. When the last tablet has been taken, obtain a new course of tablets and, without interruption, begin a new course of 28-day tablets, the next day, starting with the Sunday tablet in the top row. There should never be a day when you are not taking a tablet.

5. If, in any cycle, you start your tablets later than the proper day, you should also use another method of birth control until you have taken seven *light-colored* tablets.

6. Continue taking *light-colored* tablets without interruption whether or not your period has occurred or is still in progress. Your period will usually occur during the time you are taking *brown* or *white* tablets.

---

7. If spotting should occur at an unexpected time, continue to take your tablets as directed. Spotting is usually temporary and without significance. However, if bleeding should occur at an unexpected time, consult your physician or health care provider. Call your physician or health care provider regarding any problem or change in your general health that may concern you.

In Case You Forget (21-Day and 28-Day Regimens)

The following instructions apply only to missing the yellow1/50 tablets or the pink 2.5/50 tablets.

If you forget to take one tablet, take it as soon as you remember, even if it is the next day. Then take the next scheduled tablet at the usual time. If you miss two consecutive tablets, take two tablets daily for the next two days. Then resume the regular schedule. While there is little likelihood of pregnancy occurring if you miss only one or two tablets, the possibility of pregnancy increases with each successive day that tablets are missed.

21-Day Regimen: If you miss three consecutive tablets, discard any tablets remaining in the tablet dispenser and follow these instructions.

If you are on the Sunday-Start Regimen, start a new course of tablets the first Sunday following the last missed tablet, whether or not you are still menstruating.

If you are on the Day-5 Regimen, begin a new course of tablets on the 8th day after the last tablet was taken. For example, if you took your last tablet on a Monday, you should begin your new course of tablets the following Monday.

During the seven days without tablets, and until you have taken a tablet daily for seven consecutive days from your new course of tablets, you should also use another method of birth control.

28-Day Regimen: If you miss three consecutive *light-colored* tablets, discard any tablets remaining in the tablet dispenser and begin a new course of tablets the first Sunday following the last missed tablet, whether or not you are still menstruating. During the days without tablets and until you have taken a tablet daily for seven consecutive days from your new course of tablets, you should also use another method of birth control.

If you miss one or more *brown* or *white* tablets discard the remainder and begin a new course of tablets on the next Sunday (which should be the 8th day after you took your last *light-colored* tablet). Start with the *light-colored* tablets in the top row. Skipping one or more *brown* or *white* tablets contained in the 28-day regimen products won't increase the risk of pregnancy. They are there to help keep you on a schedule and to eliminate the need for counting days. *Under no circumstances* should you substitute a *brown* or *white* tablet for a *light-colored* tablet nor should a *brown* or *white* tablet be taken until you have finished all the *light-colored* tablets, unless your physician or health care provider advises you to do so.

Remembering to take tablets according to schedule is stressed because of its importance in providing you the greatest degree of protection.

MISSED MENSTRUAL PERIODS FOR BOTH DOSAGE REGIMENS

At times there may be no menstrual period after a cycle of pills. Therefore, if you miss one menstrual period but have taken the pills *exactly as you were supposed to*, continue as usual into the next cycle. If you have not taken the pills correctly and miss a menstrual period, *you may be pregnant* and should stop taking oral contraceptives until your doctor or health care provider determines whether or not you are pregnant. Until you can get to your doctor or health care provider, use another form of contraception. If two consecutive menstrual periods are missed, you should stop taking pills until it is determined whether or not you are pregnant. Although there does not appear to be any increase in birth defects in newborn babies if you become pregnant while using oral contraceptives, if you do become pregnant, you should discuss the situation with your doctor or health care provider.

Periodic Examination

Your doctor or health care provider will take a complete medical and family history before prescribing oral contraceptives. At that time and about once a year thereafter, he will generally examine your blood pressure, breasts, abdomen, and pelvic organs (including a Papanicolaou smear, ie, test for cancer).

SUMMARY

Oral contraceptives are the most effective method, except sterilization, for preventing pregnancy. Other methods, when used conscientiously, are also very effective and have fewer risks. Although the serious risks of oral contraceptives are uncommon, some of the risks may persist after you stop using the pill. On the other hand, the "pill" is a very convenient method of preventing pregnancy.

If you have certain conditions or have had these conditions in the past, you should not use oral contraceptives because the risk is too great. These conditions are listed in this leaflet. If you do not have these conditions, and decide to use the "pill," please read this leaflet carefully so that you can use the "pill" most safely and effectively.

Based on his or her assessment of your medical needs, your doctor or health care provider has prescribed this drug for you. Do not give this drug to anyone else.

Keep this and all drugs out of the reach of children.

Caution—Federal law prohibits dispensing without prescription.

DETAILED PATIENT PACKAGE INSERT

What You Should Know About Oral Contraceptives

Any woman who considers using oral contraceptives (the "birth control pill" or the "pill") should understand the benefits and risks of using this form of birth control. This leaflet will give you much of the information you will need to make this decision and will also help you determine if you are at risk of developing any of the serious side effects of the pill. It will tell you how to use the pill properly so that it will be as effective as possible. However, this leaflet is not a replacement for a careful discussion between you and your health care provider. You should discuss the information provided in this leaflet with him or her, both when you first start taking the pill and during your revisits. You should also follow your health care provider's advice with regard to regular check-ups while you are on the pill.

EFFECTIVENESS OF ORAL CONTRACEPTIVES

Oral contraceptives or "birth control pills" or "the pill" are used to prevent pregnancy and are more effective than other non-surgical methods of birth control. When they are taken correctly, the chance of becoming pregnant is less than 1% (1 pregnancy per 100 women per year of use) when used perfectly, without missing pills. Typical failure rates are actually 3% per year. The chance of becoming pregnant increases with each missed pill during a menstrual cycle.

In comparison, typical failure rates for other methods of birth control during the first year of use are as follows:

IUD: 6%
Diaphragm with spermicides: 18%
Spermicides alone: 21%
Vaginal sponge: 18 to 30%
Condom alone: 12%
Periodic abstinence: 20%
No method: 89%

WHO SHOULD NOT TAKE ORAL CONTRACEPTIVES

> Cigarettes smoking increases the risk of serious cardiovascular side effects from oral contraceptives use. This risk increases with age and with heavy smoking (15 or more cigarettes per day) and is quite marked in women over 35 years of age. Women who use oral contraceptives are strongly advised not to smoke.

Some women should not use the pill. For example, you should not take the pill if you are pregnant or think you may be pregnant. You should also not use the pill if you have any of the following conditions:

- A history of heart attack or stroke
- Blood clots in the legs (thrombophlebitis), lungs (pulmonary embolism), or eyes
- A history of blood clots in the deep veins of your legs
- Chest pain (angina pectoris)
- Known or suspected breast cancer or cancer of the lining of the uterus, cervix or vagina
- Unexplained vaginal bleeding (until a diagnosis is reached by your doctor)
- Yellowing of the whites of the eyes or of the skin (jaundice) during pregnancy or during previous use of the pill
- Liver tumor (benign or cancerous)
- Known or suspected pregnancy

Tell your health care provider if you have ever had any of these conditions. Your health care provider can recommend a safer method of birth control.

OTHER CONSIDERATIONS BEFORE TAKING ORAL CONTRACEPTIVES

Tell your health care provider if your have:

- Breast nodules, fibrocystic disease of the breast, an abnormal breast x-ray or mammogram
- Diabetes
- Elevated cholesterol or triglycerides
- High blood pressure
- Migraine or other headaches or epilepsy
- Mental depression
- Gallbladder, heart or kidney disease
- History of scanty or irregular menstrual periods

Women with any of these conditions should be checked often by their health care provider if they choose to use oral contraceptives.

Also, be sure to inform your doctor or health care provider if you smoke or are on any medications.

RISKS OF TAKING ORAL CONTRACEPTIVES

1. Risk Of Developing Blood Clots

Blood clots and blockage of blood vessels are the most serious side effects of taking oral contraceptives. In particular, a clot in the legs can cause thrombophlebitis and a clot that travels to the lungs can cause a sudden blocking of the vessel carrying blood to the lungs. Rarely, clots occur in the blood vessels of the eye and may cause blindness, double vision, or impaired vision.

If you take oral contraceptives and need elective surgery, need to stay in bed for a prolonged illness or have recently delivered a baby, you may be at risk of developing blood clots. You should consult your doctor about stopping oral contraceptives three to four weeks before surgery and not taking oral contraceptives for two weeks after surgery or during bed rest. You should also not take oral contraceptives soon after delivery of a baby. It is advisable to wait for at least four weeks after delivery if you are not breast feeding. If you are breast feeding, you should wait until you have weaned your child before using the pill. (See also the section on Breast Feeding in GENERAL PRECAUTIONS.)

2. Heart Attacks And Strokes

Oral contraceptives may increase the tendency to develop strokes (stoppage or rupture of blood vessels in the brain) and angina pectoris and heart attacks (blockage of blood vessels in the heart). Any of these conditions can cause death or disability.

Smoking greatly increases the possibility of suffering heart attacks and strokes. Furthermore, smoking and the use of oral contraceptives greatly increase the chances of developing and dying of heart disease.

3. Gallbladder Disease

Oral contraceptive users probably have a greater risk than nonusers of having gallbladder disease, although this risk may be related to pills containing high doses of estrogens.

4. Liver Tumors

In rare cases, oral contraceptives can cause benign but dangerous liver tumors. These benign liver tumors can rupture and cause fatal internal bleeding. In addition, a possible but not definite association has been found with the pill and liver cancers in two studies, in which a few women who developed these very rare cancers were found to have used oral contraceptives for long periods. However, liver cancers are extremely rare. The chance of developing liver cancer from using the pill is thus even rarer.

5. Cancer Of The Reproductive Organs

There is, at present, no confirmed evidence that oral contraceptives increase the risk of cancer of the reproductive organs in human studies. Several studies have found no overall increase in the risk of developing breast cancer. However, women who use oral contraceptives and have a strong family history of breast cancer or who have breast nodules or abnormal mammograms should be closely followed by their doctors.

Some studies have found an increase in the incidence of cancer of the cervix in women who use oral contraceptives. However, this finding may be related to factors other than the use of oral contraceptives.

ESTIMATED RISK OF DEATH FROM A BIRTH CONTROL METHOD OR PREGNANCY

All methods of birth control and pregnancy are associated with a risk of developing certain diseases which may lead to disability or death. An estimate of the number of deaths associated with different methods of birth control and pregnancy has been calculated and is shown in the following table. [See table above].

In the above table, the risk of death from any birth control method is less than the risk of childbirth, except for oral contraceptive users over the age of 35 who smoke and pill users over the age of 40 even if they do not smoke. It can be seen in the table that for women aged 15 to 39, the risk of death was highest with pregnancy (7–26 deaths per 100,000 women, depending on age). Among pill users who do not smoke, the risk of death was always lower than that associated with pregnancy for any age group, although over the age of 40, the risk increases to 32 deaths per 100,000 women, compared to 28 associated with pregnancy at that age. However, for pill users who smoke and are over the age of 35, the estimated number of deaths exceeds those for other methods of birth control. If a woman is over the age of 40 and smokes, her estimated risk of death is four times higher (117/100,000

women) than the estimated risk associated with pregnancy (28/100,000 women) in that age group.

Moreover, if you do not smoke and are under the age of 35, the possible risk of death from oral contraceptive use is extremely low when you consider the failure rate associated with other methods of contraception such as the condom or diaphragm and the resulting pregnancy-associated risk.

WARNING SIGNALS

If any of these adverse effects occur while you are taking oral contraceptives, call your doctor immediately:

- Sharp chest pain, coughing of blood, or sudden shortness of breath (indicating a possible clot in the lung)
- Pain in the calf (indicating a possible clot in the leg)
- Crushing chest pain or heaviness in the chest (indicating a possible heart attack)
- Sudden severe headache or vomiting, dizziness or fainting, disturbances of vision or speech, weakness, or numbness in an arm or leg (indicating a possible stroke)
- Sudden partial or complete loss of vision (indicating a possible clot in the eye)
- Breast lumps (indicating possible breast cancer or fibrocystic disease of the breast; ask your doctor or health care provider to show you how to examine your breasts)
- Severe pain or tenderness in the stomach area (indicating a possibly ruptured liver tumor)
- Difficulty in sleeping, weakness, lack of energy, fatigue, or change in mood (possibly indicating severe depression)
- Jaundice or a yellowing of the skin or eyeballs, accompanied frequently by fever, fatigue, loss of appetite, dark colored urine, or light colored bowel movements (indicating possible liver problems)

SIDE EFFECTS OF ORAL CONTRACEPTIVES

1. Vaginal Bleeding

Irregular vaginal bleeding or spotting may occur while you are taking the pills. Irregular bleeding may vary from slight staining between menstrual periods to breakthrough bleeding which is a flow much like a regular period. Irregular bleeding occurs most often during the first few months of oral contraceptive use, but may also occur after you have been taking the pill for some time. Such bleeding may be temporary and usually does not indicate any serious problems. It is important to continue taking your pills on schedule. If the bleeding occurs in more than one cycle or lasts for more than a few days, talk to your doctor or health care provider.

2. Contact Lenses

If you wear contact lenses and notice a change in vision or an inability to wear your lenses, contact your doctor or health care provider.

3. Fluid Retention

Oral contraceptives may cause edema (fluid retention) with swelling of the fingers or ankles and may raise your blood pressure. If you experience fluid retention, contact your doctor or health care provider.

4. Melasma

A spotty darkening of the skin is possible, particularly on the face.

5. Other Side Effects

Other side effects include change in appetite, headache, nervousness, depression, dizziness, loss of scalp hair, rash, and vaginal infections.

If any of these side effects bother you, call your doctor or health care provider.

GENERAL PRECAUTIONS

1. Missed Periods And Use Of Oral Contraceptives Before Or During Early Pregnancy

There may be times when you may not menstruate regularly

Continued on next page

This product information was prepared in August, 1989. On these and other Parke-Davis Products, information may be obtained by addressing PARKE-DAVIS, Division of Warner-Lambert Company, Morris Plains, New Jersey 07950.

ANNUAL NUMBER OF BIRTH-RELATED OR METHOD-RELATED DEATHS ASSOCIATED WITH CONTROL OF FERTILITY PER 100,000 NONSTERILE WOMEN, BY FERTILITY CONTROL METHOD ACCORDING TO AGE

Method of control and outcome	15–19	20–24	25–29	30–34	35–39	40–44
No fertility control methods*	7.0	7.4	9.1	14.8	25.7	28.2
Oral contraceptives non-smoker**	0.3	0.5	0.9	1.9	13.8	31.6
Oral contraceptives smoker**	2.2	3.4	6.6	13.5	51.1	117.2
IUD**	0.8	0.8	1.0	1.0	1.4	1.4
Condom*	1.1	1.6	0.7	0.2	0.3	0.4
Diaphragm/spermicide*	1.9	1.2	1.2	1.3	2.2	2.8
Periodic abstinence*	2.5	1.6	1.6	1.7	2.9	3.6

* Deaths are birth related
** Deaths are method related

Parke-Davis—Cont.

after you have completed taking a cycle of pills. If you have taken your pills regularly and miss one menstrual period, continue taking your pills for the next cycle but be sure to inform your health care provider before doing so. If you have not taken the pills daily as instructed and missed a menstrual period, or if you missed two consecutive menstrual periods, you may be pregnant. Check with your health care provider immediately to determine whether you are pregnant. Do not continue to take oral contraceptives until you are sure you are not pregnant, but continue to use another method of contraception.

There is no conclusive evidence that oral contraceptive use is associated with an increase in birth defects, when taken inadvertently during early pregnancy. Previously, a few studies had reported that oral contraceptives might be associated with birth defects, but these studies have not been confirmed. Nevertheless, oral contraceptives or any other drugs should not be used during pregnancy unless clearly necessary and prescribed by your doctor. You should check with your doctor about risks to your unborn child of any medication taken during pregnancy.

2. While Breast Feeding

If you are breast feeding consult your doctor before starting oral contraceptives. Some of the drug will be passed on to the child in the milk. A few adverse effects on the child have been reported, including yellowing of the skin (jaundice) and breast enlargement. In addition, oral contraceptives may decrease the amount and quality of your milk. If possible, do not use oral contraceptives while breast feeding. You should use another method of contraception since breast feeding provides only partial protection from becoming pregnant and this partial protection decreases significantly as you breast feed for longer periods of time. You should consider starting oral contraceptives only after you have weaned your child completely.

3. Laboratory Tests

If you are scheduled for any laboratory tests, tell your doctor you are taking birth control pills. Certain blood tests may be affected by birth control pills.

4. Drug Interactions

Certain drugs may interact with birth control pills to make them less effective in preventing pregnancy or cause an increase in breakthrough bleeding. Such drugs include rifampin, drugs used for epilepsy such as barbiturates (for example, phenobarbital) and phenytoin (Dilantin® is one brand of this drug), phenylbutazone (Butazolidin® is one brand) and possibly certain antibiotics. You may need to use additional contraception when you take drugs which can make oral contraceptives less effective.

HOW TO TAKE ORAL CONTRACEPTIVES

1. General Instructions

You must take your pill every day according to the instructions. Oral contraceptives are most effective if taken no more than 24 hours apart. Take your pill at the same time every day so that you are less likely to forget to take it. You will then maintain an effective dose of oral contraceptive in your body.

If your doctor has scheduled you for surgery, or you need prolonged bed rest, he or she may suggest that you stop taking the pill four weeks before surgery to avoid an increased risk of blood clots. It is also advisable not to start oral contraceptives sooner than four weeks after delivery of a baby.

2. If You Forget To Take Your Pill

If you miss only one pill in a cycle, the chance of becoming pregnant is small. Take the missed pill as soon as you realize that you have forgotten it. Since the risk of pregnancy increases with each additional pill you skip, it is very important that you take one pill a day.

3. Pregnancy Due To Pill Failure

The incidence of pill failure resulting in pregnancy is approximately 1% (i.e., one pregnancy per 100 women per year) if taken every day as directed, but more typical failure rates are about 3%. If failure does occur, the risk to the fetus is minimal.

4. Pregnancy After Stopping The Pill

There may be some delay in becoming pregnant after you stop using oral contraceptives, especially if you had irregular menstrual cycles before you used oral contraceptives. It may be advisable to postpone conception until you begin menstruating regularly once you have stopped taking the pill and desire pregnancy.

5. Overdosage

Serious ill effects have not been reported following ingestion of large doses of oral contraceptives by young children. Overdosage may cause nausea and withdrawal bleeding in females. In case of overdosage, contact your health care provider or pharmacist.

6. Other Information

Your health care provider will take a medical and family history and examine you before prescribing oral contraceptives. You should be reexamined at least once a year. Be sure

to inform your health care provider if there is a family history of any of the conditions listed previously in this leaflet. Be sure to keep all appointments with your health care provider, because this is a time to determine if there are early signs of side effects of oral contraceptive use.

Do not use the drug for any condition other than the one for which it was prescribed. This drug has been prescribed specifically for you; do not give it to others who may want birth control pills.

HEALTH BENEFITS FROM ORAL CONTRACEPTIVES

In addition to preventing pregnancy, use of oral contraceptives may provide certain benefits.

They are:

- Menstrual cycles may become more regular
- Blood flow during menstruation may be lighter and less iron may be lost. Therefore, anemia due to iron deficiency is less likely to occur
- Pain or other symptoms during menstruation may be encountered less frequently
- Ectopic (tubal) pregnancy may occur less frequently
- Noncancerous cysts or lumps in the breast may occur less frequently
- Acute pelvic inflammatory disease may occur less frequently
- Oral contraceptive use may provide some protection against developing two forms of cancer: cancer of the ovaries and cancer of the lining of the uterus.

If you want more information about birth control pills, ask your doctor or pharmacist. They have a more technical leaflet called the "Physician Insert," which you may wish to read.

INSTRUCTIONS TO PATIENTS

TABLET DISPENSER

The tablet dispenser has been designed to make oral contraceptive dosing as easy and as convenient as possible. The tablets are arranged in either three or four rows of seven tablets each, with the days of the week appearing on the tablet dispenser above the first row of tablets.

If your tablet dispenser contains:	You are taking:
21 yellow tablets	NORLESTRIN 21 1/50
21 pink tablets	NORLESTRIN 21 2.5/50
21 yellow tablets and 7 brown tablets	NORLESTRIN Fe 1/50
21 pink tablets and 7 brown tablets	NORLESTRIN Fe 2.5/50
21 yellow tablets and 7 white tablets	NORLESTRIN 28 1/50

Each *yellow* tablet contains 1 mg norethindrone acetate and 50 mcg ethinyl estradiol.

Each *pink* tablet contains 2.5 mg norethindrone acetate and 50 mcg ethinyl estradiol.

Each *brown* tablet contains 75 mg ferrous fumarate and is intended to help you remember to take the tablets correctly. These brown tablets are not intended to have any health benefit.

Each *white* tablet is inert.

To remove a tablet, press down on it with your thumb or finger. The tablet will drop through the back of the tablet dispenser. Do not press on the tablet with your thumbnail or fingernail or any other sharp object.

NORLESTRIN 21-DAY DOSAGE REGIMEN

If your tablet dispenser contains 21 tablets (3 rows of 7), you are on a 21-day regimen and should follow either the Sunday-Start or Day-5 Start directions.

A. Sunday-Start Regimen

1. Unless your physician or health care provider has instructed you differently, begin taking tablets on the first Sunday after your menstrual period begins whether or not you are still bleeding. If your period begins on Sunday, take your first tablet that very same day. START WITH THE SUNDAY TABLET IN THE TOP ROW.

Note: During the first cycle, it is important that you use another method of birth control until you have taken a tablet daily for seven consecutive days.

2. Take all the tablets in the top row first, followed by the second row. Continue to take one tablet every day until you finish all 21 tablets. Your last tablet should be on Saturday.

3. After you have taken all 21 tablets, stop, and don't take any tablets for the next seven days. You should have a menstrual period one to three days after you stop taking tablets; sometimes it may take a day or so longer.

4. After the seven days during which you take no tablets, obtain a new course of tablets. Begin the new course of 21

day tablets on Sunday, the 8th day after you took your last tablet, starting with the Sunday tablet in the top row.

5. Continue to take one tablet daily until you finish all 21 tablets. If you follow the schedule properly, you will always take the last tablet in the dispenser on a Saturday, and always start each new course of 21 tablets 8 days later, on the following Sunday.

6. If, in any cycle, you start your tablets later than the proper day, you should also use another method of birth control until you have taken seven consecutive tablets.

B. Day-5 Regimen

If your physician or health care provider has directed you to begin taking your first cycle of tablets using the Day-5 Regimen, you should start taking your tablets on Day 5 after the start of your period.

1. The first day of your period is Day 1. On the 5th day (Day 5), start taking one tablet daily, beginning with the tablet in the top row that corresponds to Day 5 after your flow began.

If your period begins on:	Start taking tablets in the top row on:
Sunday	Thursday
Monday	Friday
Tuesday	Saturday
Wednesday	Sunday
Thursday	Monday
Friday	Tuesday
Saturday	Wednesday

Note: During the first cycle, if you start taking tablets later than Day 5 of your menstrual period, you should use another method of birth control until you have taken a tablet daily for seven consecutive days.

2. Continue to take one tablet daily. After the last Saturday tablet has been taken, if any tablets remain in the first row, complete your 21-day regimen by taking one tablet daily starting with the Sunday tablet in the top row.

3. After you have taken all 21 tablets, stop, and don't take any tablets for the next seven days. You should have a menstrual period one to three days after you stop taking tablets; sometimes it may take a day or so longer.

4. After the seven days during which you take no tablets, obtain a new course of tablets. Begin a new course of 21-day tablets, the 8th day after you took your last tablet, starting with the tablet in the top row that corresponds to that day.

5. Continue to take one tablet daily until you finish all 21 tablets. If you follow the schedule properly, you will always take the last tablet in the dispenser on the same day of the week, and always start each new course of 21 tablets the same day of the week on which you began the previous cycle of tablets.

6. If, in any cycle, you start your tablets later than the proper day, you should also use another method of birth control until you have taken seven consecutive tablets.

Whether you started your tablets using the Sunday-Start or Day-5 Regimen, the following directions apply:

1. Continue taking your tablets whether or not your period has occurred or is still in progress. Your period will usually occur during the seven days you are taking no tablets.

2. If spotting should occur at an unexpected time, continue to take your tablets as directed. Spotting is usually temporary and without significance. However, if bleeding should occur at an unexpected time, consult your physician or health care provider. Call your physician or health care provider regarding any problem or change in your general health that may concern you.

NORLESTRIN 28-DAY DOSAGE REGIMEN

If your tablet dispenser contains 28 tablets (3 rows of 7 *light-colored* (yellow or pink) tablets and 1 row of 7 *brown* or *white* tablets), you are on a 28-day regimen and should follow these directions.

Sunday-Start Regimen:

1. Begin taking tablets on the first Sunday after your menstrual period begins whether or not you are still bleeding. If your period begins on Sunday, take your first tablet that very same day. START WITH THE SUNDAY TABLET IN THE TOP ROW.

Note: During the first cycle, it is important that you use another method of birth control until you have taken a *light-colored* tablet daily for seven consecutive days.

2. Take all the tablets in the top row first, followed by the second row and so on.

3. Continue to take one tablet every day until you finish all 21 *light-colored* tablets. On the day after taking the last

light-colored tablet, begin taking one *brown* or *white* tablet daily until all the tablets have been taken.

4. When the last tablet has been taken, obtain a new course of tablets and, without interruption, begin a new course of 28-day tablets, the next day, starting with the Sunday tablet in the top row. There should never be a day when you are not taking a tablet.

5. If, in any cycle, you start your tablets later than the proper day, you should also use another method of birth control until you have taken seven *light-colored* tablets.

6. Continue taking *light-colored* tablets without interruption whether or not your period has occurred or is still in progress. Your period will usually occur during the time you are taking *brown* or *white* tablets.

7. If spotting should occur at an unexpected time, continue to take your tablets as directed. Spotting is usually temporary and without significance. However, if bleeding should occur at an unexpected time, consult your physician or health care provider. Call your physician or health care provider regarding any problem or change in your general health that may concern you.

In Case You Forget (21-Day And 28-Day Regimens)
The following instructions apply only to missing the yellow 1/50 tablets or the pink 2.5/50 tablets.

If you forget to take one tablet, take it as soon as you remember, even if it is the next day. Then take the next scheduled tablet at the usual time. If you miss two consecutive tablets, take two tablets daily for the next two days. Then resume the regular schedule. While there is little likelihood of pregnancy occurring if you miss only one or two tablets, the possibility of pregnancy increases with each successive day that tablets are missed.

21-Day Regimen: If you miss three consecutive tablets, discard any tablets remaining in the tablet dispenser and follow these instructions.

If you are on the Sunday-Start Regimen, start a new course of tablets the first Sunday following the last missed tablet, whether or not you are still menstruating.

If you are on the Day-5 Regimen, begin a new course of tablets on the 8th day after the last tablet was taken. For example, if you took your last tablet on a Monday, you should begin your new course of tablets the following Monday.

During the seven days without tablets, and until you have taken a tablet daily for seven consecutive days from your new course of tablets, you should also use another method of birth control.

28-Day Regimen: If you miss three consecutive *light-colored* tablets, discard any tablets remaining in the tablet dispenser and begin a new course of tablets the first Sunday following the last missed tablet, whether or not you are still menstruating. During the days without tablets and until you have taken a tablet daily for seven consecutive days from your new course of tablets, you should also use another method of birth control.

If you miss one or more *brown* or *white* tablets discard the remainder and begin a new course of tablets on the next Sunday (which should be the 8th day after you took your last *light-colored* tablet). Start with the *light-colored* tablets in the top row. Skipping one or more *brown* or *white* tablets contained in the 28-day regimen products won't increase the risk of pregnancy. They are there to help keep you on schedule and to eliminate the need for counting days. *Under no circumstances* should you substitute a *brown* or *white* tablet for a *light-colored* tablet nor should a *brown* or *white* tablet be taken until you have finished all the *light-colored* tablets, unless your physician or health care provider advises you to do so.

Remembering to take tablets according to schedule is stressed because of its importance in providing you the greatest degree of protection.

MISSED MENSTRUAL PERIODS FOR BOTH DOSAGE REGIMENS
At times there may be no menstrual period after a cycle of pills. Therefore, if you miss one menstrual period but have taken the pills *exactly as you were supposed to*, continue as usual into the next cycle. If you have not taken the pills correctly and miss a menstrual period, *you may be pregnant* and should stop taking oral contraceptives until your doctor or health care provider determines whether or not you are pregnant. Until you can get to your doctor, use another form of contraception. If two consecutive menstrual periods are missed, you should stop taking pills until it is determined whether or not you are pregnant. Although there does not appear to be any increase in birth defects in newborn babies if you become pregnant while using oral contraceptives, if you do become pregnant, you should discuss the situation with your doctor or health care provider.

Periodic Examination
Your doctor or health care provider will take a complete medical and family history before prescribing oral contraceptives. At that time and about once a year thereafter, he will generally examine your blood pressure, breasts, abdomen, and pelvic organs (including a Papanicolaou smear, ie, test for cancer).

SUMMARY
Oral contraceptives are the most effective method, except sterilization, for preventing pregnancy. Other methods, when used conscientiously, are also very effective and have fewer risks. Although the serious risks of oral contraceptives are uncommon, some of the risks may persist after you stop using the pill. On the other hand, the "pill" is a very convenient method of preventing pregnancy.

If you have certain conditions or have had these conditions in the past, you should not use oral contraceptives because the risk is too great. These conditions are listed in this leaflet. If you do not have these conditions, and decide to use the "pill," please read this leaflet carefully so that you can use the "pill" most safely and effectively.

Based on his or her assessment of your medical needs, your doctor or health care provider has prescribed this drug for you. Do not give this drug to anyone else.

Keep this and all drugs out of the reach of children.

Caution—Federal law prohibits dispensing without prescription.

0901G135
Shown in Product Identification Section, page 422

NORLUTATE®   ℞
[*nŏr"lū'tāte*]
(norethindrone acetate tablets, USP)

WARNING

THE USE OF NORETHINDRONE ACETATE DURING THE FIRST FOUR MONTHS OF PREGNANCY IS NOT RECOMMENDED.

Progestational agents have been used beginning with the first trimester of pregnancy in an attempt to prevent habitual abortion. There is no adequate evidence that such use is effective when such drugs are given during the first four months of pregnancy. Furthermore, in the vast majority of women, the cause of abortion is a defective ovum, which progestational agents could not be expected to influence. In addition, the use of progestational agents, with their uterine-relaxant properties, in patients with fertilized defective ova may cause a delay in spontaneous abortion. Therefore, the use of such drugs during the first four months of pregnancy is not recommended.

Several reports suggest an association between intrauterine exposure to progestational drugs in the first trimester of pregnancy and genital abnormalities in male and female fetuses. The risk of hypospadias, 5 to 8 per 1,000 male births in the general population, may be approximately doubled when exposed to these drugs. There are insufficient data to quantify the risk to exposed female fetuses, but insofar as some of these drugs induce mild virilization of the external genitalia of the female fetus, and because of the increased association of hypospadias in the male fetus, it is prudent to avoid the use of these drugs during the first trimester of pregnancy.

If the patient is exposed to Norlutate during the first four months of pregnancy or if she becomes pregnant while taking this drug, she should be apprised of the potential risks to the fetus.

DESCRIPTION
Norlutate is the acetic acid ester of norethindrone, which is the 17 alpha-ethinyl derivative of 19-nortestosterone. It is a progestational agent for oral administration. Each tablet contains 5 mg of norethindrone acetate, USP. Norlutate also contains: acacia, NF; confectioner's sugar, NF; D&C red No. 30 Al lake; FD&C yellow No. 6 Al lake; lactose, NF; light mineral oil, NF; magnesium stearate, NF; corn starch, NF; and talc, USP. The chemical name is 17-Hydroxy-19-nor-17α-pregn-4-en-20-yn-3-one acetate.

CLINICAL PHARMACOLOGY
Transforms proliferative endometrium into secretory endometrium. Inhibits (at the usual dose range) the secretion of pituitary gonadotropins, which in turn prevents follicular maturation and ovulation.

May also demonstrate some estrogenic, anabolic or androgenic activity but should not be relied upon.

INDICATIONS AND USAGE
Norlutate is indicated in amenorrhea; in abnormal uterine bleeding due to hormonal imbalance in the absence of organic pathology, such as submucous fibroids or uterine cancer; and in endometriosis.

CONTRAINDICATIONS
1. Thrombophlebitis, thromboembolic disorders, cerebral apoplexy or patients with a past history of these conditions
2. Known or suspected carcinoma of the breast
3. Undiagnosed vaginal bleeding
4. Missed abortion
5. As a diagnostic test for pregnancy

WARNINGS
1. Discontinue medication pending examination if there is a sudden partial or complete loss of vision, or if there is a sudden onset of proptosis, diplopia or migraine. If examination reveals papilledema or retinal vascular lesions, medication should be withdrawn.
2. Detectable amounts of progestogens have been identified in the milk of mothers receiving them. The effect of this on the nursing infant has not been determined.
3. Because of the occasional occurrence of thrombophlebitis and pulmonary embolism in patients taking progestogens, the physician should be alert to the earliest manifestations of the disease.
4. Masculinization of the female fetus has occurred when progestogens have been used in pregnant women.
5. Some beagle dogs treated with medroxyprogesterone acetate developed mammary nodules. Although nodules occasionally appeared in control animals they were intermittent in nature, whereas nodules in treated animals were larger and more numerous, and they persisted. There is no general agreement as to whether the nodules are benign or malignant. Their significance with respect to humans has not been established.

PRECAUTIONS
General
1. The pretreatment physical examination should include special reference to breasts and pelvic organs, as well as a Papanicolaou smear.
2. Because this drug may cause some degree of fluid retention, conditions which might be influenced by this factor, such as epilepsy, migraine, asthma, cardiac or renal dysfunction, require careful observation.
3. In cases of breakthrough bleeding, as in all cases of irregular bleeding *per vaginam*, nonfunctional causes should be borne in mind. In cases of undiagnosed vaginal bleeding, adequate diagnostic measures are indicated.
4. Patients who have a history of psychic depression should be carefully observed and the drug discontinued if the depression recurs to a serious degree.
5. Any possible influence of prolonged progestogen therapy on pituitary, ovarian, adrenal, hepatic or uterine functions awaits further study.
6. A decrease in glucose tolerance has been observed in a small percentage of patients on estrogen-progestogen combination drugs. The mechanism of this decrease is obscure. For this reason, diabetic patients should be carefully observed while receiving progestogen therapy.
7. The age of the patient constitutes no absolute limiting factor although treatment with progestogens may mask the onset of the climacteric.
8. The pathologist should be advised of progestogen therapy when relevant specimens are submitted.
9. Steroid hormones are metabolized in the liver and should be administered with caution in patients with impaired liver function.

Concomitant Estrogen Use
Studies of the addition of a progestin product to an estrogen replacement regimen for seven or more days of a cycle of estrogen administration have reported a lowered incidence of endometrial hyperplasia. Morphological and biochemical studies of endometrium suggest that 10 to 13 days of a progestin are needed to provide maximal maturation of the endometrium and to eliminate any hyperplastic changes. Whether this will provide protection from endometrial carcinoma has not been clearly established. There are possible additional risks which may be associated with the inclusion of progestin in estrogen replacement regimens. The potential risks include adverse effects on carbohydrate and lipid metabolism. The dosage used may be important in minimizing these adverse effects.

Information for the Patient
See patient labeling printed below.

Laboratory Tests
The following laboratory result may be altered by the use of progestogens: Pregnanediol determination.
In addition, the following laboratory results may be altered by the concomitant use of estrogens with progestogens:
1. Hepatic function
2. Coagulation tests; increase in prothrombin, Factors VII, VIII, IX, and X

Continued on next page

This product information was prepared in August, 1989. On these and other Parke-Davis Products, information may be obtained by addressing PARKE-DAVIS, Division of Warner-Lambert Company, Morris Plains, New Jersey 07950.

Parke-Davis—Cont.

3. Increase in PBI, BEI and a decrease in T^3 uptake
4. Metyrapone test

Drug Interactions

Reduced efficacy and increased incidence of breakthrough bleeding have been associated with concomitant use of rifampin.

Carcinogenesis, Mutagenesis, Impairment of Fertility

See Warnings.

Pregnancy

Pregnancy category X. See Boxed Warning.

Nursing Mothers

Detectable amounts of progestogens have been identified in the milk of mothers receiving them. Because of the potential for serious adverse reactions in nursing infants from Norlutate, a decision should be made whether to discontinue nursing or to discontinue the drug, taking into account the importance of the drug to the mother.

ADVERSE REACTIONS

The following adverse reactions have been observed in women taking progestogens:
1. breakthrough bleeding
2. spotting
3. change in menstrual flow
4. amenorrhea
5. edema
6. changes in weight (increase or decrease)
7. changes in cervical erosion and cervical secretions
8. cholestatic jaundice
9. rash (allergic) with and without pruritus*
10. melasma or chloasma
11. mental depression

A statistically significant association has been demonstrated between use of estrogen-progestogen combination drugs and the following serious adverse reactions: thrombophlebitis; pulmonary embolism and cerebral thrombosis and embolism. For this reason patients on progestogen therapy should be carefully observed.

Although available evidence is suggestive of an association, such a relationship has been neither confirmed nor refuted for the following serious adverse reactions:

Neuro-ocular lesions, eg, retinal thrombosis and optic neuritis.

The following adverse reactions have been observed in patients receiving estrogen-progestogen combination drugs:
1. rise in blood pressure in susceptible individuals
2. premenstrual-like syndrome
3. changes in libido
4. changes in appetite
5. cystitis-like syndrome
6. headache
7. nervousness
8. dizziness
9. fatigue
10. backache
11. hirsutism
12. loss of scalp hair
13. erythema multiforme
14. erythema nodosum
15. hemorrhagic eruption
16. itching

In view of these observations, patients on progestogen therapy should be carefully observed for their occurrence.

OVERDOSAGE

Not known.

DOSAGE AND ADMINISTRATION

Therapy with Norlutate must be adapted to the specific indications and therapeutic response of the individual patient.

This dosage schedule assumes the interval between menses to be 28 days.

Amenorrhea, abnormal uterine bleeding due to hormonal imbalance in the absence of organic pathology: 2.5 to 10 mg Norlutate starting with the fifth day of the menstrual cycle and ending on the 25th day.

Endometriosis: Initial daily dose of 5 mg Norlutate for two weeks with increments of 2.5 mg per day of Norlutate every two weeks until 15 mg per day of Norlutate is reached. Therapy may be held at this level for from six to nine months or until annoying breakthrough bleeding demands temporary termination.

HOW SUPPLIED

N 0071-0918-19—Norlutate is supplied as 5-mg pink, scored, cup-shaped tablets, debossed with P-D 918 in bottles of 50.

REFERENCES

1. Gal IB, et al: Hormonal pregnancy tests and congenital malformation. *Nature* 216:83, 1967.
2. Levy EP, et al: Hormone treatment during pregnancy and congenital heart defects. *Lancet* 1:611, 1973.
3. Nora J, Nora A: Birth defects and oral contraceptives. *Lancet* 1:941, 1973.
4. Janerich DT, et al: Oral contraceptives and congenital limb reduction defects. *N Engl J Med* 291:697, 1974.
5. Heinonen OP, et al: Cardiovascular birth defects and antenatal exposure to female sex hormones. *N Engl J Med* 296:67, 1977.

PATIENT LABELING FOR NORLUTATE WARNING FOR WOMEN

Progesterone or progesterone-like drugs have been used to prevent miscarriage in the first few months of pregnancy. No adequate evidence is available to show that they are effective for this purpose. Furthermore, most cases of early miscarriage are due to causes which could not be helped by these drugs.

There is an increased risk of minor birth defects in children whose mothers take this drug during the first 4 months of pregnancy. Several reports suggest an association between mothers who take these drugs in the first trimester of pregnancy and genital abnormalities in male and female babies. The risk to the male baby is the possibility of being born with a condition in which the opening of the penis is on the underside rather than the tip of the penis (hypospadias). Hypospadias occurs in about 5 to 8 per 1,000 male births and is about doubled with exposure to these drugs. There is not enough information to quantify the risk to exposed female fetuses, but enlargement of the clitoris and fusion of the labia may occur, although rarely.

Therefore, since drugs of this type may induce mild masculinization of the external genitalia of the female fetus, as well as hypospadias in the male fetus, it is wise to avoid using the drug during the first trimester of pregnancy.

These drugs have been used as a test for pregnancy but such use is no longer considered safe because of possible damage to a developing baby. Also, more rapid methods for testing for pregnancy are now available.

If you take Norlutate and later find you were pregnant when you took it, be sure to discuss this with your doctor as soon as possible.

Storage—Store below 30°C (86°F).

Caution—Federal law prohibits dispensing without prescription.

0918G036

Shown in Product Identification Section, page 422

NORLUTIN® ℞
[nōr"lū'tin]
(norethindrone tablets, USP)

> **WARNING**
> THE USE OF NORETHINDRONE DURING THE FIRST FOUR MONTHS OF PREGNANCY IS NOT RECOMMENDED.
> Progestational agents have been used beginning with the first trimester of pregnancy in an attempt to prevent habitual abortion. There is no adequate evidence that such use is effective when such drugs are given during the first four months of pregnancy. Furthermore, in the vast majority of women, the cause of abortion is a defective ovum, which progestational agents could not be expected to influence. In addition, the use of progestational agents, with their uterine-relaxant properties, in patients with fertilized defective ova may cause a delay in spontaneous abortion. Therefore, the use of such drugs during the first four months of pregnancy is not recommended.
> Several reports suggest an association between intrauterine exposure to progestational drugs in the first trimester of pregnancy and genital abnormalities in male and female fetuses. The risk of hypospadias, 5 to 8 per 1,000 males births in the general population, may be approximately doubled with exposure to these drugs. There are insufficient data to quantify the risk to exposed female fetuses, but insofar as some of these drugs induce mild virilization of the external genitalia of the female fetus, and because of the increased association of hypospadias in the male fetus, it is prudent to avoid the use of these drugs during the first trimester of pregnancy.
> If the patient is exposed to Norlutin during the first four months of pregnancy or if she becomes pregnant while taking this drug, she should be apprised of the potential risks to the fetus.

DESCRIPTION

Norlutin is the 17 alpha-ethinyl derivative of 19-nortestosterone. It is a progestational agent for oral administration. Each tablet contains 5 mg of norethindrone, USP. Norlutin also contains: acacia, NF; confectioner's sugar, NF; lactose, NF; magnesium stearate, NF; starch potato, NF; and talc, USP. The chemical name is 17-Hydroxy-19-nor-17α-pregn-4-en-20-yn-3-one.

CLINICAL PHARMACOLOGY

Transforms proliferative endometrium into secretory endometrium.

Inhibits (at the usual dosage range) the secretion of pituitary gonadotropins, which in turn prevents follicular maturation and ovulation.

May also demonstrate some estrogenic, anabolic, or androgenic activity but should not be relied upon.

INDICATIONS AND USAGE

Norlutin is indicated in amenorrhea; in abnormal uterine bleeding due to hormonal imbalance in the absence of organic pathology, such as submucous fibroids or uterine cancer; and in endometriosis.

CONTRAINDICATIONS

1. Thrombophlebitis, thromboembolic disorders, cerebral apoplexy, or patients with a past history of these conditions
2. Known or suspected carcinoma of the breast
3. Undiagnosed vaginal bleeding
4. Missed abortion
5. As a diagnostic test for pregnancy

WARNINGS

1. Discontinue medication pending examination if there is a sudden partial or complete loss of vision, or if there is sudden onset of proptosis, diplopia, or migraine. If examination reveals papilledema or retinal vascular lesions, medication should be withdrawn.
2. Detectable amounts of progestogens have been identified in the milk of mothers receiving them. The effect of this on the nursing infant has not been determined.
3. Because of the occasional occurrence of thrombophlebitis and pulmonary embolism in patients taking progestogens, the physician should be alert to the earliest manifestations of the disease.
4. Masculinization of the female fetus has occurred when progestogens have been used in pregnant women.
5. Some beagle dogs treated with medroxyprogesterone acetate developed mammary nodules. Although nodules occasionally appeared in control animals, they were intermittent in nature, whereas nodules in treated animals were larger and more numerous, and they persisted. There is no general agreement as to whether the nodules are benign or malignant. Their significance with respect to humans has not been established.

PRECAUTIONS

General

1. The pretreatment physical examination should include special reference to breasts and pelvic organs, as well as a Papanicolaou smear.
2. Because this drug may cause some degree of fluid retention, conditions which might be influenced by this factor, such as epilepsy, migraine, asthma, cardiac or renal dysfunction, require careful observation.
3. In cases of breakthrough bleeding, as in all cases of irregular bleeding per vaginam, nonfunctional causes should be borne in mind. In cases of undiagnosed vaginal bleeding, adequate diagnostic measures are indicated.
4. Patients who have a history of psychic depression should be carefully observed and the drug discontinued if the depression recurs to a serious degree.
5. Any possible influence of prolonged progestogen therapy on pituitary, ovarian, adrenal, hepatic, or uterine functions awaits further study.
6. A decrease in glucose tolerance has been observed in a small percentage of patients on estrogen-progestogen combination drugs. The mechanism of this decrease is obscure. For this reason, diabetic patients should be carefully observed while receiving progestogen therapy.
7. The age of the patient constitutes no absolute limiting factor, although treatment with progestogens may mask the onset of the climacteric.
8. The pathologist should be advised of progestogen therapy when relevant specimens are submitted.
9. Steroid hormones are metabolized by the liver, therefore, these drugs should be administered with caution in patients with impaired liver function.

Concomitant Estrogen Use

Studies of the addition of a progestin product to an estrogen replacement regimen for seven or more days of a cycle of estrogen administration have reported a lowered incidence of endometrial hyperplasia. Morphological and biochemical studies of endometrium suggest that 10 to 13 days of a progestin are needed to provide maximal maturation of the endometrium and to eliminate any hyperplastic changes. Whether this will provide protection from endometrial carcinoma has not been clearly established. There are possible additional risks which may be associated with the inclusion of progestin in estrogen replacement regimens. The potential risks include adverse effects on carbohydrate and lipid metabolism. The dosage used may be important in minimizing these adverse effects.

Information for the Patient.
See patient labeling printed below.

Laboratory Tests
The following laboratory result may be altered by the use of progestogens: Pregnanediol determination
In addition, the following laboratory results may be altered by the concomitant use of estrogens with progestogens:
1. Hepatic function
2. Coagulation tests; increase in prothrombin, Factors VII, VIII, IX, and X
3. Increase in PBI, BEI and a decrease in T^3 uptake
4. Metyrapone test

Drug Interactions
Reduced efficacy and increased incidence of breakthrough bleeding have been associated with concomitant use of rifampin.

Carcinogenseis, Mutagenesis, Impairment of Fertility
See Warnings.

Pregnancy
Pregnancy category X. See Boxed Warning.

Nursing Mothers
Detectable amounts of progestogens have been identified in the milk of mothers receiving them. Because of the potential for serious adverse reactions in nursing infants from Norlutin, a decision should be made whether to discontinue nursing or to discontinue the drug, taking into account the importance of the drug to the mother.

ADVERSE REACTIONS
The following adverse reactions have been observed in women taking progestogens:
1. breakthrough bleeding
2. spotting
3. change in menstrual flow
4. amenorrhea
5. edema
6. changes in weight (increase or decrease)
7. changes in cervical erosion and cervical secretions
8. cholestatic jaundice
9. rash (allergic) with and without pruritus
10. melasma or chloasma
11. mental depression

A statistically significant association has been demonstrated between use of estrogen-progestogen combination drugs and the following serious adverse reactions: thrombophlebitis; pulmonary embolism; and cerebral thrombosis and embolism. For this reason patients on progestogen therapy should be carefully observed.

Although available evidence is suggestive of an association, such a relationship has been neither confirmed nor refuted for the following serious adverse reactions:

Neuro-ocular lesions, eg, retinal thrombosis and optic neuritis.

The following adverse reactions have been observed in patients receiving estrogen-progestogen combination drugs:
1. rise in blood pressure in susceptible individuals
2. premenstrual-like syndrome
3. changes in libido
4. changes in appetite
5. cystitis-like syndrome
6. headache
7. nervousness
8. dizziness
9. fatigue
10. backache
11. hirsutism
12. loss of scalp hair
13. erythema multiforme
14. erythema nodosum
15. hemorrhagic eruption
16. itching

In view of these observations, patients on progestogen therapy should be carefully observed for their occurrence.

OVERDOSAGE
Not known.

DOSAGE AND ADMINISTRATION
Therapy with Norlutin must be adapted to the specific indications and therapeutic response of the individual patient.
This dosage schedule assumes the interval between menses to be 28 days.

Amenorrhea, abnormal uterine bleeding due to hormonal imbalance in the absence of organic pathology: 5 to 20 mg Norlutin starting with the fifth day of the menstrual cycle and ending on the 25th day.

Endometriosis: Initial daily dose of 10 mg Norlutin for two weeks with increments of 5 mg per day of Norlutin every two weeks until 30 mg per day of Norlutin is reached. Therapy may be held at this level for from six to nine months or until annoying breakthrough bleeding demands temporary termination.

HOW SUPPLIED
N 0071-0882-19—Norlutin is supplied as 5-mg white, scored, cup-shaped tablets, debossed with P-D 882 in bottles of 50.

REFERENCES
1. Gal IB, et al: Hormonal pregnancy tests and congenital malformation.
   Nature 216:83, 1967.
2. Levy EP, et al: Hormone treatment during pregnancy and congenital heart defects.
   Lancet 1:611, 1973.
3. Nora J, Nora A: Birth defects and oral contraceptives.
   Lancet 1:941, 1973.
4. Janerich DT, et al: Oral contraceptives and congenital limb-reduction defects.
   N Engl J Med 291:697, 1974.
5. Heinonen OP, et al: Cardiovascular birth defects and antenatal exposure to female sex hormones.
   N Engl J Med 296:67, 1977.

PATIENT LABELING FOR NORLUTIN WARNING FOR WOMEN
Progesterone or progesterone-like drugs have been used to prevent miscarriage in the first few months of pregnancy. No adequate evidence is available to show that they are effective for this purpose. Furthermore, most cases of early miscarriage are due to causes which could not be helped by these drugs.

There is an increased risk of minor birth defects in children whose mothers take this drug during the first 4 months of pregnancy. Several reports suggest an association between mothers who take these drugs in the first trimester of pregnancy and genital abnormalities in male and female babies. The risk to the male baby is the possibility of being born with a condition in which the opening of the penis is on the underside rather than the tip of the penis (hypospadias). Hypospadias occurs in about 5 to 8 per 1,000 male births and is about doubled with exposure to these drugs. There is not enough information to quantify the risk to exposed female fetuses, but enlargement of the clitoris and fusion of the labia may occur, although rarely.

Therefore, since drugs of this type may induce mild masculinization of the external genitalia of the female fetus, as well as hypospadias in the male fetus, it is wise to avoid using the drug during the first trimester of pregnancy.

These drugs have been used as a test for pregnancy but such use is no longer considered safe because of possible damage to a developing baby. Also, more rapid methods for testing for pregnancy are now available.

If you take Norlutin and later find you were pregnant when you took it, be sure to discuss this with your doctor as soon as possible.

Storage—Store below 30°C (86°F).

Caution—Federal law prohibits dispensing without prescription.

0882G014

Shown in Product Identification Section, page 422

PERITRATE® SA   ℞
[pĕ′rĭ-trāte″]
(pentaerythritol tetranitrate tablets)
Sustained Action*

PERITRATE®   ℞
(pentaerythritol tetranitrate tablets, USP)

DESCRIPTION
Each tablet of Peritrate 40 mg contains pentaerythritol tetranitrate 40 mg.
Each tablet of Peritrate 20 mg contains pentaerythritol tetranitrate 20 mg.
Each tablet of Peritrate 10 mg contains pentaerythritol tetranitrate 10 mg.
Pentaerythritol tetranitrate is a nitric acid ester of a tetrahydric alcohol (pentaerythritol).
Peritrate 10 mg and 20 mg contain alginic acid, NF; D&C yellow No. 10; FD&C blue No. 1; gelatin, NF; lactose, NF; methylcellulose, USP; propylparaben, NF; corn starch, NF; stearic acid, NF; and may also contain magnesium stearate, NF. Peritrate 40 mg contains D&C yellow No. 10 Al lake; D&C red No. 30 Al lake; lactose, NF; povidone, USP; silicon dioxide, NF; corn starch, NF; stearic acid, NF; and confectioner's sugar, NF.
Each tablet of Peritrate SA Sustained Action contains: pentaerythritol tetranitrate 80 mg (20 mg in immediate release layer and 60 mg in sustained release base). Pentaerythritol tetranitrate is a nitric acid ester of a tetrahydric alcohol (pentaerythritol).
Peritrate SA 80 mg also contains D&C yellow No. 10; FD&C blue No. 1; lactose, NF; magnesium stearate, NF; silicon dioxide, NF; confectioner's sugar, NF; and other ingredients.

CLINICAL PHARMACOLOGY
The exact cause of angina pectoris (that is, the pain associated with coronary artery disease) remains obscure, despite the numerous and often conflicting hypotheses concerning its pathophysiology. Therapy at the present time, therefore, remains essentially empirical. Customarily, clinical improvement has been measured by: reduction in (1) number, intensity and duration of angina pectoris attacks and (2) necessity for glyceryl trinitrate intake for prevention or relief of anginal attacks. Peritrate (pentaerythritol tetranitrate) Sustained Action and Peritrate (pentaerythritol tetranitrate) have been reported in clinical usage to reduce in number and severity the incidence of angina pectoris attacks, with concomitant reduction in glyceryl trinitrate intake.

In the evaluation of Peritrate and Peritrate SA in angina pectoris, clinical improvement has been customarily measured subjectively by: reduction in number and severity of attacks and necessity for glyceryl trinitrate intake for prevention or abortion of anginal attacks. Individual patterns of angina pectoris differ widely as does the symptomatic response to antianginal agents such as pentaerythritol tetranitrate. The published literature contains both favorable and unfavorable clinical reports. In conjunction with total management of the patient with angina pectoris, Peritrate and Peritrate SA have been accepted as safe for prolonged administration and widely regarded as useful.

INDICATIONS AND USAGE
Based on a review of this drug by the National Academy of Sciences—National Research Council and/or other information, FDA has classified the indications as follows:
"Possibly" effective: Peritrate is indicated for the relief of angina pectoris (pain associated with coronary artery disease). It is not intended to abort the acute anginal episode but is widely regarded as useful in the prophylactic treatment of angina pectoris.
Final classification of the less-than-effective indications requires further investigation.

CONTRAINDICATIONS
Peritrate SA and Peritrate are contraindicated in patients who have a history of sensitivity to the drug.

WARNINGS
Data supporting the use of Peritrate or Peritrate SA during the early days of the acute phase of myocardial infarction (the period during which clinical and laboratory findings are unstable) are insufficient to establish safety.
This drug can act as a physiological antagonist to norepinephrine, acetylcholine, histamine, and many other agents.

PRECAUTIONS
Should be used with caution in patients who have glaucoma. Tolerance to this drug and cross-tolerance to other nitrites and nitrates may occur.

ADVERSE REACTIONS
Side effects reported to date have been predominantly related to rash (which requires discontinuation of medication) and headache and gastrointestinal distress, which are usually mild and transient with continuation of medication. In some cases severe persistent headaches may occur. In addition, the following adverse reactions to nitrates such as pentaerythritol tetranitrate have been reported in the literature:
(a)   Cutaneous vasodilatation with flushing.
(b)   Transient episodes of dizziness and weakness, as well as other signs of cerebral ischemia associated with postural hypotension, may occasionally develop.
(c)   An occasional individual exhibits marked sensitivity to the hypotensive effects of nitrite and severe responses (nausea, vomiting, weakness, restlessness, pallor, perspiration and collapse) can occur, even with the usual therapeutic doses. Alcohol may enhance this effect.

DOSAGE AND ADMINISTRATION
Peritrate may be administered in individualized doses up to 160 mg a day. Dosage can be initiated at one 10 mg or 20 mg tablet q.i.d. and titrated upward to 40 mg (two 20 mg tablets or one 40 mg tablet) q.i.d. one-half hour before or one hour after meals and at bedtime. Tablets can be chewed or swallowed whole. Alternatively, Peritrate SA can be administered on a convenient b.i.d. (on an empty stomach) dosage schedule. One tablet immediately on arising and 1 tablet 12 hours later. Tablets should not be chewed.

HOW SUPPLIED
Peritrate SA double layer, biconvex, dark green/light green tablets in bottles of 100 (N 0071-0004-24) and 1000 (N 0071-0004-32). Also in unit dose—package of 10 × 10 strips (N 0071-0004-40).

Continued on next page

This product information was prepared in August, 1989. On these and other Parke-Davis Products, information may be obtained by addressing PARKE-DAVIS, Division of Warner-Lambert Company, Morris Plains, New Jersey 07950.

Parke-Davis—Cont.

Also supplied as:

Peritrate 40 mg—coral, scored tablets in bottles of 100 (N 0071-0008-24).

Peritrate 20 mg—light green, scored tablets in bottles of 100 (N 0071-0001-24) and 1000 (N 0071-0001-32). Also unit dose, package of 10 × 10 strips (N 0071-0001-40).

Peritrate 10 mg—light green, unscored tablets in bottles of 100 (N 0071-0013-24) and 1000 (N 0071-0013-32.) For full prescribing information, see specific package insert.

ANIMAL PHARMACOLOGY

In a series of carefully designed studies in pigs, Peritrate was administered for 48 hours before an artificially induced occlusion of a major coronary artery and for seven days thereafter. The pigs were sacrificed at various intervals for periods up to six weeks. The result showed a significantly larger number of survivors in the drug-treated group. Damage to myocardial tissue in the drug-treated survivors was less extensive than in the untreated group. Studies in dogs subjected to oligemic shock through progressive bleeding have demonstrated that Peritrate is vasoactive at the postarteriolar level, producing increased blood flow and better tissue perfusion. These animal experiments cannot be translated to the drug's actions in humans.

0004G012/0001G012

Shown in Product Identification Section, page 422

PITOCIN®   ℞

[pĭ″tō′cĭn]

(oxytocin injection, USP) synthetic

DESCRIPTION

Pitocin (oxytocin injection, USP) is a sterile, clear, colorless aqueous solution of synthetic oxytocin, for intravenous infusion or intramuscular injection. Pitocin is a nonapeptide found in pituitary extracts from mammals. It is standardized to contain 10 units of oxytocic hormone/mL and contains 0.5% Chloretone® (chlorobutanol, a chloroform derivative) as a preservative, with the pH adjusted with acetic acid. The hormone is prepared synthetically to avoid possible contamination with vasopressin (ADH) and other small polypeptides with biologic activity. Pitocin has the empirical formula $C_{43}H_{66}N_{12}O_{12}S_2$ (molecular weight 1007.19). The structural formula is as follows:

$$H-Cys-Tyr-Ile-Glu(NH_2)-Asp(NH_2)-Cys-Pro-Leu-Gly-NH_2$$
$$1 \quad 2 \quad 3 \quad 4 \qquad 5 \qquad 6 \quad 7 \quad 8 \quad 9$$

CLINICAL PHARMACOLOGY

Uterine motility depends on the formation of the contractile protein actomyosin under the influence of the Ca^{2+}-dependent phosphorylating enzyme myosin light-chain kinase. Oxytocin promotes contractions by increasing the intracellular Ca^{2+}. Oxytocin has specific receptors in the myometrium and the receptor concentraton increases greatly during pregnancy, reaching a maximum in early labor at term. The response to a given dose of oxytocin depends on the sensitivity of the uterus, which is determined by the oxytocin receptor concentration. However, the physician should be aware of the fact that oxytocin even in its pure form has inherent pressor and antidiuretic properties which may become manifest when large doses are administered. These properties are thought to be due to the fact that oxytocin and vasopressin differ in regard to only two of the eight amino acids. (See PRECAUTIONS)

Oxytocin is distributed throughout the extracellular fluid. Small amounts of the drug probably reach the fetal circulation. Oxytocin has a plasma half-life of about 1 to 6 minutes which is decreased in late pregnancy and during lactation. Following intravenous administration of oxytocin, uterine response occurs almost immediately and subsides within 1 hour. Following intramuscular injection of the drug, uterine response occurs within 3 to 5 minutes and persists for 2 to 3 hours. Its rapid removal from plasma is accomplished largely by the kidney and the liver. Only small amounts are excreted in urine unchanged.

INDICATIONS AND USAGE

IMPORTANT NOTICE

Elective induction of labor is defined as the initiation of labor in a pregnant individual who has no medical indications for induction. Since the available data are inadequate to evaluate the benefits-to-risks considerations, Pitocin is not indicated for elective induction of labor.

Antepartum: Pitocin is indicated for the initiation or improvement of uterine contractions, where this is desirable and considered suitable for reasons of fetal or maternal concern, in order to achieve early vaginal delivery. It is indicated for (1) induction of labor in patients with a medical indication for the initiation of labor, such as Rh problems, maternal diabetes, preeclampsia at or near term, when delivery is in the best interest of mother and fetus or when membranes are prematurely ruptured and delivery is indicated; (2) stimulation or reinforcement of labor, as in selected cases of uterine inertia; (3) as adjunctive therapy in the management of incomplete or inevitable abortion. In the first trimester curettage is generally considered primary therapy. In second trimester abortion, oxytocin infusion will often be successful in emptying the uterus. Other means of therapy, however, may be required in such cases.

Postpartum: Pitocin is indicated to produce uterine contractions during the third stage of labor and to control postpartum bleeding or hemorrhage.

CONTRAINDICATIONS

Antepartum use of Pitocin is contraindicated in any of the following circumstances:

1. Where there is significant cephalopelvic disproportion;
2. In unfavorable fetal positions or presentations, such as transverse lies, which are undeliverable without conversion prior to delivery;
3. In obstetrical emergencies where the benefit-to-risk ratio for either the fetus or the mother favors surgical intervention;
4. In fetal distress where delivery is not imminent;
5. Where adequate uterine activity fails to achieve satisfactory progress;
6. Where the uterus is already hyperactive or hypertonic;
7. In cases where vaginal delivery is contraindicated, such as invasive cervical carcinoma, active herpes genitalis, total placenta previa, vasa previa, and cord presentation or prolapse of the cord;
8. In patients with hypersensitivity to the drug.

WARNINGS

Pitocin, when given for induction of labor or augmentation of uterine activity, should be administered only by the intravenous route and with adequate medical supervision in a hospital.

PRECAUTIONS

General

1. All patients receiving intravenous oxytocin must be under continuous observation by trained personnel who have a thorough knowledge of the drug and are qualified to identify complications. A physician qualified to manage any complications should be immediately available. Electronic fetal monitoring provides the best means for early detection of overdosage. However, it must be borne in mind that only intrauterine pressure recording can accurately measure the intrauterine pressure during contractions. A fetal scalp electrode provides a more dependable recording of the fetal heart rate than any external monitoring system.

2. When properly administered, oxytocin should stimulate uterine contractions comparable to those seen in normal labor. Overstimulation of the uterus by improper administration can be hazardous to both mother and fetus. Even with proper administration and adequate supervision, hypertonic contractions can occur in patients whose uteri are hypersensitive to oxytocin. This fact must be considered by the physician in exercising his judgment regarding patient selection.

3. Except in unusual circumstances, oxytocin should not be administered in the following conditions: fetal distress, partial placenta previa, prematurity, borderline cephalopelvic disproportion, and any condition in which there is a predisposition for uterine rupture, such as previous major surgery on the cervix or uterus including cesarean section, overdistention of the uterus, grand multiparity, or past history of uterine sepsis or of traumatic delivery. Because of the variability of the combinations of factors which may be present in the conditions listed above, the definition of "unusual circumstances" must be left to the judgment of the physician. The decision can be made only by carefully weighing the potential benefits which oxytocin can provide in a given case against rare but definite potential for the drug to produce hypertonicity or tetanic spasm.

4. Maternal deaths due to hypertensive episodes, subarachnoid hemorrhage, rupture of the uterus, and fetal deaths due to various causes have been reported associated with the use of parenteral oxytocic drugs for induction of labor or for augmentation in the first and second stages of labor.

5. Oxytocin has been shown to have an intrinsic antidiuretic effect, acting to increase water reabsorption from the glomerular filtrate. Consideration should, therefore, be given to the possibility of water intoxication, particularly when oxytocin is administered continuously by infusion and the patient is receiving fluids by mouth.

6. When oxytocin is used for induction or reinforcement of already existent labor, patients should be carefully selected. Pelvic adequacy must be considered and maternal and fetal conditions evaluated before use of the drug.

Drug Interactions

Severe hypertension has been reported when oxytocin was given three to four hours following prophylactic administration of a vasoconstrictor in conjunction with caudal block anesthesia. Cyclopropane anesthesia may modify oxytocin's cardiovascular effects, so as to produce unexpected results such as hypotension. Maternal sinus bradycardia with abnormal atrioventricular rhythms has also been noted when oxytocin was used concomitantly with cyclopropane anesthesia.

Carcinogenesis, Mutagenesis, Impairment of Fertility

There are no animal or human studies on the carcinogenicity and mutagenicity of this drug, nor is there any information on its effect on fertility.

Pregnancy

Teratogenic Effects

Animal reproduction studies have not been conducted with oxytocin. There are no known indications for use in the first trimester of pregnancy other than in relation to spontaneous or induced abortion. Based on the wide experience with this drug and its chemical structure and pharmacological properties, it would not be expected to present a risk of fetal abnormalities when used as indicated.

Nonteratogenic Effects

See ADVERSE REACTIONS in the fetus or infant.

Labor and Delivery

See "INDICATIONS AND USAGE"

ADVERSE REACTIONS

The following adverse reactions have been reported in the mother:

Anaphylactic reaction
Postpartum hemorrhage
Cardiac arrhythmia
Fatal afibrinogenemia
Nausea
Vomiting
Premature ventricular contractions
Pelvic hematoma

Excessive dosage or hypersensitivity to the drug may result in uterine hypertonicity, spasm, tetanic contraction, or rupture of the uterus.

The possibility of increased blood loss and afibrinogenemia should be kept in mind when administering the drug.

Severe water intoxication with convulsions and coma has occurred, associated with a slow oxytocin infusion over a 24-hour period. Maternal death due to oxytocin-induced water intoxication has been reported.

The following adverse reactions have been reported in the fetus or infant:

Due to induced uterine motility:
Bradycardia
Premature ventricular contractions and other arrhythmias
Permanent CNS or brain damage
Fetal death

Due to use of oxytocin in the mother:
Low Apgar scores at five minutes
Neonatal jaundice
Neonatal retinal hemorrhage

OVERDOSAGE

Overdosage with oxytocin depends essentially on uterine hyperactivity whether or not due to hypersensitivity to this agent. Hyperstimulation with strong (hypertonic) or prolonged (tetanic) contractions, or a resting tone of 15 to 20 mmH2O or more between contractions can lead to tumultuous labor, uterine rupture, cervical and vaginal lacerations, postpartum hemorrhage, uteroplacental hypoperfusion, and variable deceleration of fetal heart, fetal hypoxia, hypercapnia or death. Water intoxication with convulsions, which is caused by the inherent antidiuretic effect of oxytocin is a serious complication that may occur if large doses (40 to 50 milliunits/minute) are infused for long periods. Management consists of immediate discontinuation of oxytocin and symptomatic and supportive therapy.

DOSAGE AND ADMINISTRATION

Parenteral drug products should be inspected visually for particulate matter and discoloration prior to administration whenever solution and container permit.

The dosage of oxytocin is determined by the uterine response and must therefore be individualized and initiated at a very low level. The following dosage information is based upon various regimens and indications in general use.

1. Induction or Stimulation of Labor

Intravenous infusion (drip method) is the only acceptable method of parenteral administration of Pitocin for the induction or stimulation of labor. Accurate control of the rate of infusion is essential and is best accomplished by an infusion pump. It is convenient to piggyback the Pitocin infusion on a physiologic electrolyte solution, permitting the Pitocin infusion to be stopped abruptly without interrupting the electrolyte infusion. This is done in the following way:

Preparation

a. The standard solution for infusion of Pitocin is prepared by adding the contents of one 1-mL ampoule containing 10 units of oxytocin to 1,000 mL of 0.9% aqueous sodium chloride or Ringer's lactate. The combined solution containing 10 milliunits (mU) of oxytocin/mL is rotated in the infusion bottle for thorough mixing. The same concentration can be obtained by mixing the contents of one 0.5-mL ampoule, containing 5 units of oxytocin, with 500 mL of electrolyte solution.

b. Establish the infusion with a separate bottle of physiologic electrolyte solution not containing Pitocin.

c. Attach (piggyback) the Pitocin-containing bottle with the infusion pump to the infusion line as close to the infusion site as possible.

Administration

d. For the initial dose, do not exceed 1 mU/min (equal to 6 mL of the dilute oxytocin solution per hour).

e. Increase the infusion rate with the pump in steps of 1 mU/min every 15 minutes until a response is observed. From this threshold dose, further increase may be needed to achieve a satisfactory uterine activity, but the increments should be kept to 1–2 mU/min and the intervals between increments extended toward 30 minutes, until a pattern comparable to spontaneous labor can be observed.

Studies of the concentrations of oxytocin in the maternal plasma during Pitocin infusion have shown that infusion rates up to 6 mU/min give the same oxytocin levels that are found in spontaneous labor. At term, higher infusion rates should be given with great care, and rates exceeding 9-10 mU/min are rarely required. Before term, when the sensitivity of the uterus is lower because of a lower concentration of oxytocin receptors, a higher infusion rate may be required.

Monitoring

f. Electronically monitor the uterine activity and the fetal heart rate throughout the infusion of Pitocin. Attention should be given to tonus, amplitude and frequency of contractions and to the fetal heart rate in relation to uterine contractions. If uterine contractions become too powerful, the infusion can be abruptly stopped, and oxytocic stimulation of the uterine musculature will soon wane.

g. Discontinue the infusion of Pitocin immediately in the event of uterine hyperactivity and/or fetal distress. Administer oxygen to the mother, who preferably should be put in a lateral position. The condition of mother and fetus should immediately be evaluated by the responsible physician and appropriate steps taken.

2. Control of Postpartum Uterine Bleeding

a. **Intravenous infusion (drip method).** If the patient has an intravenous infusion running, 10 to 40 units of oxytocin may be added to the bottle, depending on the amount of electrolyte or dextrose solution remaining (maximum 40 units to 1000 mL). Adjust the infusion rate to sustain uterine contraction and control uterine atony.

b. **Intramuscular administration.** (One mL) Ten (10) units of Pitocin can be given after the delivery of the placenta.

3. Treatment of Incomplete, Inevitable or Elective Abortion

Intravenous infusion of 10 units of Pitocin added to 500 mL of a physiologic saline solution or 5% dextrose-in-water solution may help the uterus contract after a suction or sharp curettage for an incomplete, inevitable or elective abortion. Subsequent to intra-amniotic injection of hypertonic saline, prostaglandins, urea, etc, for midtrimester elective abortion, the injection-to-abortion time may be shortened by infusion of Pitocin at the rate of 10 to 20 milliunits (20 to 40 drops) per minute. The total dose should not exceed 30 units in a 12-hour period due to the risk of water intoxication.

HOW SUPPLIED

Pitocin (Oxytocin Injection, USP) Synthetic is available as follows:

N 0071-4160-02 Packages of ten 0.5-mL ampoules, each containing 5 units of oxytocin.

N 0071-4160-03 Packages of ten 1-mL ampoules, each containing 10 units of oxytocin.

N 0071-4160-10 A 10-mL multiple-dose vial containing 10 units of oxytocin per mL (total = 100 units of oxytocin).

N 0071-4160-40 Packages of ten sterile disposable 1-mL syringes, each containing 10 units of oxytocin.

N 0071-4160-45 Packages of twenty-five oversized 1-mL Steri-Vials®, each containing 10 units of oxytocin.

STORAGE

Store at controlled room temperature, 15°–30° C (59°–86°F). Protect from freezing.

REFERENCES

1. Seitchik J, Castillo M: Oxytocin augmentation of dysfunctional labor. I. Clinical data. *Am J Obstet Gynecol* 1982; 144:899–905.
2. Seitchik J, Castillo M: Oxytocin augmentation of dysfunctional labor. II. Multiparous patients. *Am J Obstet Gynecol* 1983, 145 777–780.
3. Fuchs A, Goeschen K, Husslein P, et al: Oxytocin and the initiation of human parturition. III. Plasma concentrations of oxytocin and 13, 14-dihydro-15-keto-prostaglandin $F_{2\alpha}$ in spontaneous and oxytocin-induced labor at term. *Am J Obstet Gynecol* 1983; 145:497–502.

Caution—Federal law prohibits dispensing without prescription.

                                             4160G063

PITRESSIN®   ℞

[pĭ″trĕ′ssĭn]

(vasopressin injection, USP)

synthetic

DESCRIPTION

Pitressin (Vasopressin Injection, USP) Synthetic is a sterile, aqueous solution of synthetic vasopressin (8-Arginine vasopressin) of the posterior pituitary gland. It is substantially free from the oxytocic principle and is standardized to contain 20 pressor units/ml. The solution contains 0.5% Chloretone (chlorobutanol) (chloroform derivative) as a preservative. The acidity of the solution is adjusted with acetic acid.

CLINICAL PHARMACOLOGY

The antidiuretic action of vasopressin is ascribed to increasing reabsorption of water by the renal tubules.

Vasopressin can cause contraction of smooth muscle of the gastrointestinal tract and of all parts of the vascular bed, especially the capillaries, small arterioles and venules with less effect on the smooth musculature of the large veins. The direct effect on the contractile elements is neither antagonized by adrenergic blocking agents nor prevented by vascular denervation.

Following subcutaneous or intramuscular administration of vasopressin injection, the duration of antidiuretic activity is variable but effects are usually maintained for 2–8 hours. The majority of a dose of vasopressin is metabolized and rapidly destroyed in the liver and kidneys. Vasopressin has a plasma half-life of about 10 to 20 minutes. Approximately 5% of a subcutaneous dose of vasopressin is excreted in urine unchanged after four hours.

CONTRAINDICATION

Anaphylaxis or hypersensitivity to the drug or its components.

INDICATIONS AND USAGE

Pitressin is indicated for prevention and treatment of postoperative abdominal distention, in abdominal roentgenography to dispel interfering gas shadows, and in diabetes insipidus.

WARNINGS

This drug should not be used in patients with vascular disease, especially disease of the coronary arteries, except with extreme caution. In such patients, even small doses may precipitate anginal pain, and with larger doses, the possibility of myocardial infarction should be considered.

Vasopressin may produce water intoxication. The early signs of drowsiness, listlessness, and headaches should be recognized to prevent terminal coma and convulsions.

PRECAUTIONS

General:

Vasopressin should be used cautiously in the presence of epilepsy, migraine, asthma, heart failure or any state in which a rapid addition to extracellular water may produce hazard for an already overburdened system.

Chronic nephritis with nitrogen retention contraindicates the use of vasopressin until reasonable nitrogen blood levels have been attained.

Information for Patients: Side effects such as blanching of skin, abdominal cramps, and nausea may be reduced by taking 1 or 2 glasses of water at the time of vasopressin administration. These side effects are usually not serious and probably will disappear within a few minutes.

Laboratory Tests: Electrocardiograms (ECG) and fluid and electrolyte status determinations are recommended at periodic intervals during therapy.

Drug Interactions: 1) The following drugs may potentiate the antidiuretic effect of vasopressin when used concurrently: carbamazepine; chlorpropamide; clofibrate; urea; fludrocortisone; tricyclic antidepressants. 2) The following drugs may decrease the antidiuretic effect of vasopressin when used concurrently: demeclocycline; norepinephrine; lithium; heparin; alcohol. 3) Ganglionic blocking agents may produce a marked increase in sensitivity to the pressor effects of vasopressin.

Pregnancy Category C: Animal reproduction studies have not been conducted with Pitressin. It is also not known whether Pitressin can cause fetal harm when administered to a pregnant woman or can affect reproduction capacity. Pitressin should be given to a pregnant woman only if clearly needed.

Labor and Delivery: Doses of vasopressin sufficient for an antidiuretic effect are not likely to produce tonic uterine contractions that could be deleterious to the fetus or threaten the continuation of the pregnancy.

Nursing Mothers: Caution should be exercised when Pitressin is administered to a nursing woman.

ADVERSE REACTIONS

Local or systemic allergic reactions may occur in hypersensitive individuals. The following side effects have been reported following the administration of vasopressin:

Body as a Whole: anaphylaxis (cardiac arrest and/or shock) have been observed shortly after injection of vasopressin.

Cardiovascular: cardiac arrest, circumoral pallor.

Gastrointestinal: abdominal cramps, nausea, vomiting, passage of gas.

Nervous System: tremor, vertigo, "pounding" in head.

Respiratory: bronchial constriction.

Skin and Appendages: sweating, urticaria.

Overdosage:

Water intoxication may be treated with water restriction and temporary withdrawal of vasopressin until polyuria occurs. Severe water intoxication may require osmotic diuresis with mannitol, hypertonic dextrose, or urea alone or with furosemide.

DOSAGE AND ADMINISTRATION

Pitressin may be administered subcutaneously or intramuscularly.

Ten units of Pitressin (0.5 mL) will usually elicit full physiologic response in adult patients; 5 units will be adequate in many cases. Pitressin should be given intramuscularly at three- or four-hour intervals as needed. The dosage should be proportionally reduced for children. (For an additional discussin of dosage, consult the sections below.)

When determining the dose of Pitressin for a given case, the following should be kept in mind:

It is particularly desirable to give a dose not much larger than is just sufficient to elicit the desired physiologic response. Excessive doses may cause undesirable side effects—blanching of the skin, abdominal cramps, nausea—which, though not serious, may be alarming to the patient. Spontaneous recovery from such side effects occurs in a few minutes. It has been found that one or two glasses of water given at the time Pitressin is administered reduce such symptoms.

Abdominal Distention: In the average postoperative adult patient, give 5 units (0.25 mL) initially, increase to 10 units (0.5 mL) at subsequent injections if necessary. It is recommended that Pitressin be given intramuscularly and that injections be repeated at three- or four-hour intervals as required. Dosage to be reduced proportionally for children. Pitressin used in this manner will frequently prevent or relieve postoperative distention. These recommendations apply also to distention complicating pneumonia or other acute toxemias.

Abdominal Roentgenography: For the average case two injections of 10 units each (0.5 mL) are suggested. These should be given two hours and one-half hour, respectively, before films are exposed. Many roentgenologists advise giving an enema prior to the first dose of Pitressin.

Diabetes Insipidus: Pitressin may be given by injection or administered intranasally on cotton pledgets, by nasal spray, or by dropper. The dose by injection is 5 to 10 units (0.25 to 0.5 mL) repeated two or three times daily as needed. When Pitressin is administered intranasally by spray or on pledgets, the dosage and interval between treatments must be determined for each patient.

HOW SUPPLIED

Pitressin (Vasopressin Injection, USP) Synthetic is supplied in ampoules and vials as follows:

N 0071-4200-02
0.5 mL ampoule (10 pressor units). Packages of 10 ampoules.

N 0071-4200-03
1 mL ampoule (20 pressor units). Packages of 10 ampoules.

N 0071-4200-45
0.5 mL vial (10 pressor units). Packages of 25 vials.

N 0071-4200-46
1 mL vial (20 pressor units). Packages of 25 vials.

Caution—Federal law prohibits dispensing without a prescription.

                                     4200G140

PITRESSIN® TANNATE IN OIL   ℞

[pĭ″trĕ′ssĭn tă′nāte]

(vasopressin tannate)

FOR INTRAMUSCULAR USE ONLY

DESCRIPTION

Pitressin Tannate in Oil (Sterile Vasopressin Tannate Suspension) is a water insoluble chemical compound of vasopressin, the pressor fraction of the posterior lobe of the pituitary gland, and tannic acid. It has antidiuretic activity. It is available as a sterile suspension for intramuscular administration. Vasopressin tannate is substantially free from the oxy-

Continued on next page

This product information was prepared in August, 1989. On these and other Parke-Davis Products, information may be obtained by addressing PARKE-DAVIS, Division of Warner-Lambert Company, Morris Plains, New Jersey 07950.

Parke-Davis—Cont.

tocic principle and is standardized to contain 5 pressor units per mL in peanut oil.

CLINICAL PHARMACOLOGY

The antidiuretic action of vasopressin tannate is ascribed to increasing reabsorption of water by the renal tubules. Vasopressin can cause contraction of smooth muscle of the gastrointestinal tract and of all parts of the vascular bed, especially the capillaries, small arterioles, and venules with less effect on the smooth musculature of the large veins. These effects are ordinarily not seen to a significant degree with recommended antidiuretic doses of vasopressin tannate. The direct effect on the contractile elements is neither antagonized by adrenergic blocking agents nor prevented by vascular denervation.

Absorption of vasopressin tannate in oil following intramuscular administration may be erratic. Vasopressin tannate in oil is more slowly absorbed than the aqueous preparation and has a longer duration of action. When administered intramuscularly, vasopressin tannate in oil usually has a duration of action of 48 to 96 hours.

The majority of a dose of vasopressin is metabolized and rapidly destroyed in the liver and kidneys. Vasopressin has a plasma half-life of about 10 to 20 minutes.

INDICATIONS AND USAGE

Pitressin Tannate in Oil is indicated for the control or prevention of the symptoms and complications of diabetes insipidus due to a deficiency of endogenous posterior pituitary antidiuretic hormone.

CONTRAINDICATIONS

Anaphylaxis or hypersensitivity to the drug or its components.

WARNINGS

This preparation should never be administered intravenously.

This drug should not be used in patients with vascular disease, especially disease of the coronary arteries, except with extreme caution. In such patients, even small doses may precipitate anginal pain.

Vasopressin may produce water intoxication. The early signs of drowsiness, listlessness, and headaches should be recognized to prevent terminal coma and convulsions.

PRECAUTIONS

General: Vasopressin should be used cautiously in the presence of epilepsy, migraine, asthma, heart failure or any state in which a rapid addition to extracellular water may produce hazard for an already overburdened system.

Chronic nephritis with nitrogen retention contraindicates the use of vasopressin until reasonable nitrogen blood levels have been attained.

Information for patients: Side effects such as blanching of skin, abdominal cramps, and nausea may be reduced by taking 1 or 2 glasses of water at the time of vasopressin administration. These side effects are usually not serious and probably will disappear within a few minutes.

Laboratory tests: Electrocardiograms (ECG) and fluid and electrolyte status determinations are recommended at periodic intervals during therapy.

Drug interactions: 1) The following drugs may potentiate the antidiuretic effect of vasopressin when used concurrently: carbamazepine, chlorpropamide, clofibrate, urea, fludrocortisone; tricyclic antidepressants. 2) The following drugs may decrease the antidiuretic effect of vasopressin when used concurrently: demeclocycline; norepinephrine; lithium; heparin; alcohol. 3) Ganglionic blocking agents may produce a marked increase in sensitivity to the pressor effects of vasopressin.

Pregnancy category C: Animal reproduction studies have not been conducted with Pitressin Tannate in Oil. It is also not known whether Pitressin Tannate in Oil can cause fetal harm when administered to a pregnant woman or can affect reproduction capacity. Pitressin Tannate in Oil should be given to a pregnant woman only if clearly needed.

Labor and delivery: Doses of vasopressin sufficient for an antidiuretic effect are not likely to produce tonic uterine contractions that could be deleterious to the fetus or threaten the continuation of the pregnancy.

Nursing mothers: Caution should be exercised when Pitressin Tannate in Oil is administered to a nursing woman.

ADVERSE REACTIONS

Local or systemic allergic reactions may occur in hypersensitive individuals. The following side effects have been reported following the administration of vasopressin:

Body as a whole: anaphylaxis
Cardiovascular: cardiac arrest, circumoral pallor
Gastrointestinal: abdominal cramps, nausea, vomiting, passage of gas

Nervous system: tremor, vertigo, "pounding" in head
Respiratory: bronchial constriction
Skin and appendages: sweating, urticaria

OVERDOSAGE

Water intoxication may be treated with water restriction and temporary withdrawal of vasopressin until polyuria occurs. Severe water intoxication may require osmotic diuresis with mannitol, hypertonic dextrose, or urea alone or with furosemide.

DOSAGE AND ADMINISTRATION

Intramuscular Administration 0.3 to 1 mL (1.5 to 5 pressor units) repeated as required. The duration of action varies with the patient and condition, and may be as prolonged as 48 to 96 hours.

Shake ampoule thoroughly before use to obtain a uniform suspension. Contents of the ampoules may show a cloudiness, or colorless crystals, of solid fats from the peanut oil vehicle. If this occurs, warm the ampoules to dissolve the solid fats. Warming of the ampoules will also facilitate transfer of product from ampoule to syringe.

HOW SUPPLIED

N 0071-4302-03

Pitressin Tannate in Oil (Sterile Vasopressin Tannate Suspension) is supplied in 1-mL ampoules containing 5 pressor units per mL in peanut oil. Packages of 10.

Store at controlled room temperature 15°–30°C (59°–86°F).
Caution—Federal law prohibits dispensing without prescription.

4302G042

PONSTEL® ℞
[pŏn´stĕl″]
(mefenamic acid)

DESCRIPTION

Ponstel (mefenamic acid) is N-(2,3-xylyl)-anthranilic acid. It is an analgesic agent for oral administration. Ponstel is available in capsules containing 250 mg of mefenamic acid. Each capsule also contains lactose, NF. The capsule shell and/or band contains citric acid, USP; D&C yellow No. 10; FD&C blue No. 1; FD&C red No. 3; FD&C yellow No. 6; gelatin, NF; glycerol monooleate; silicon dioxide, NF; sodium benzoate, NF; sodium lauryl sulfate, NF; titanium dioxide, USP.

It is a white powder with a melting point of 230–231° C, molecular weight 241.28, and water solubility of 0.004% at pH 7.1.

CLINICAL PHARMACOLOGY

Ponstel is a nonsteroidal agent with demonstrated antiinflammatory, analgesic, and antipyretic activity in laboratory animals.[1,2] The mode of action is not known. In animal studies, Ponstel was found to inhibit prostaglandin synthesis and to compete for binding at the prostaglandin receptor site.[3]

Pharmacologic studies show Ponstel did not relieve morphine abstinence signs in abstinent, morphine-habituated monkeys.[1]

Following a single 1-gram oral dose, peak plasma levels of 10 μg/ml occurred in 2 to 4 hours with a half-life of 2 hours. Following multiple doses, plasma levels are proportional to dose with no evidence of drug accumulation. One gram of Ponstel given four times daily produces peak blood levels of 20 μg/ml by the second day of administration.[4]

Following a single dose, sixty-seven percent of the total dose is excreted in the urine as unchanged drug or as one of two metabolites. Twenty to twenty-five percent of the dose is excreted in the feces during the first three days.[4]

In controlled, double-blind, clinical trials, Ponstel was evaluated for the treatment of primary spasmodic dysmenorrhea. The parameters used in determining efficacy included pain assessment by both patient and investigator; the need for concurrent analgesic medication; and evaluation of change in frequency and severity of symptoms characteristic of spasmodic dysmenorrhea. Patients received either Ponstel, 500 mg (2 capsules) as an initial dose and 250 mg every 6 hours, or placebo at onset of bleeding or of pain, whichever began first. After three menstrual cycles, patients were crossed over to the alternate treatment for an additional three cycles. Ponstel was significantly superior to placebo in all parameters, and both treatments (drug and placebo) were equally tolerated.

INDICATIONS AND USAGE

Ponstel is indicated for the relief of moderate pain[5] when therapy will not exceed one week. Ponstel is also indicated for the treatment of primary dysmenorrhea.[5,6]

Studies in children under 14 years of age have been inadequate to evaluate the safety and effectiveness of Ponstel.

CONTRAINDICATIONS

Ponstel should not be used in patients who have previously exhibited hypersensitivity to it.

Because the potential exists for cross-sensitivity to aspirin or other nonsteroidal antiinflammatory drugs, Ponstel should

not be given to patients in whom these drugs induce symptoms of bronchospasm, allergic rhinitis, or urticaria.

Ponstel is contraindicated in patients with active ulceration or chronic inflammation of either the upper or lower gastrointestinal tract.

Ponstel should be avoided in patients with preexisting renal disease.

WARNINGS

If diarrhea occurs, the dosage should be reduced or temporarily suspended (see Adverse Reactions and Dosage and Administration). Certain patients who develop diarrhea may be unable to tolerate the drug because of recurrence of the symptoms on subsequent exposure.

Risk of GI Ulceration, Bleeding and Perforation with NSAID Therapy: Serious gastrointestinal toxicity such as bleeding, ulceration, and perforation, can occur at any time, with or without warning symptoms, in patients treated chronically with NSAID therapy. Although minor upper gastrointestinal problems, such as dyspepsia, are common, usually developing early in therapy, physicians should remain alert for ulceration and bleeding in patients treated chronically with NSAIDs even in the absence of previous GI tract symptoms. In patients observed in clinical trials of several months to two years duration, symptomatic upper GI ulcers, gross bleeding or perforation appear to occur in approximately 1% of patients treated for 3–6 months, and in about 2–4% of patients treated for one year. Physicians should inform patients about the signs and/or symptoms of serious GI toxicity and what steps to take if they occur.

Studies to date have not identified any subset of patients not at risk of developing peptic ulceration and bleeding. Except for a prior history of serious GI events and other risk factors known to be associated with peptic ulcer disease, such as alcoholism, smoking, etc., no risk factors (eg, age, sex) have been associated with increased risk. Elderly or debilitated patients seem to tolerate ulceration or bleeding less well than other individuals and most spontaneous reports of fatal GI events are in this population. Studies to date are inconclusive concerning the relative risk of various NSAIDs in causing such reactions. High doses of any NSAID probably carry a greater risk of these reactions, although controlled clinical trials showing this do not exist in most cases. In considering the use of relatively large doses (within the recommended dosage range), sufficient benefit should be anticipated to offset the potential increased risk of GI toxicity.

PRECAUTIONS

If rash occurs, administration of the drug should be stopped. A false-positive reaction for urinary bile, using the diazo tablet test, may result after mefenamic acid administration. If biliuria is suspected, other diagnostic procedures, such as the Harrison spot test, should be performed.

Renal Effects: As with other nonsteroidal antiinflammatory drugs, long-term administration of mefenamic acid to animals has resulted in renal papillary necrosis and other abnormal renal pathology. In humans, there have been reports of acute interstitial nephritis with hematuria, proteinuria and occasionally nephrotic syndrome.

A second form of renal toxicity has been seen in patients with prerenal conditions leading to a reduction in renal blood flow or blood volume, where the renal prostaglandins have a supportive role in the maintenance of renal perfusion. In these patients administration of an NSAID may cause a dose-dependent reduction in prostaglandin formation and may precipitate overt renal decompensation. Patients at greatest risk of this reaction are those with impaired renal function, heart failure, liver dysfunction, those taking diuretics, and the elderly Discontinuation of NSAID therapy is typically followed by recovery to the pretreatment state. Since Ponstel is eliminated primarily by the kidneys, the drug should not be administered to patients with significantly impaired renal functions.

As with other nonsteroidal antiinflammatory drugs, borderline elevations of one or more liver tests may occur in some patients. These abnormalities may progress, may remain essentially unchanged, or may be transient with continued therapy. The SGPT (ALT) test is probably the most sensitive indicator of liver dysfunction. Meaningful (3 times the upper limit of normal) elevations of SGPT or SGOT (AST) occurred in controlled clinical trials in less than 1% of patients. A patient with symptoms and/or signs suggesting liver dysfunction, or in whom an abnormal liver test has occurred, should be evaluated for evidence of the development of more severe hepatic reaction while on therapy with Ponstel. Severe hepatic reactions, including jaundice and cases of fatal hepatitis, have been reported with other nonsteroidal antiinflammatory drugs. Although such reactions are rare, if abnormal liver tests persist or worsen, if clinical signs and symptoms consistent with liver disease develop, or if systemic manifestations occur (eg eosinophilia, rash, etc), Ponstel should be discontinued.

Information for Patients: Patients should be advised that if rash, diarrhea or other digestive problems arise, they should stop the drug and consult their physician.

Patients in whom aspirin or other nonsteroidal antiinflammatory drugs induce symptoms of bronchospasm, allergic rhinitis, or urticaria should be made aware that the potential exists for cross-sensitivity to Ponstel.

The long-term effects, if any, of intermittent Ponstel therapy for dysmenorrhea are not known. Women on such therapy should consult their physician if they should decide to become pregnant.

Ponstel, like other drugs of its class, is not free of side effects. The side effects of these drugs can cause discomfort and, rarely, there are more serious side effects, such as gastrointestinal bleeding, which may result in hospitalization and even fatal outcomes.

NSAIDs (nonsteroidal antiinflammatory drugs) are often essential agents in the management of arthritis and have a major role in the treatment of pain, but they also may be commonly employed for conditions which are less serious. Physicians may wish to discuss with their patients the potential risks (see WARNINGS, PRECAUTIONS, and ADVERSE REACTIONS sections) and likely benefits of NSAID treatment, particularly when the drugs are used for less serious conditions where treatment without NSAIDs may represent an acceptable alternative to both the patient and physician.

Laboratory Tests: Because serious GI tract ulceration and bleeding can occur without warning symptoms, physicians should follow chronically treated patients for the signs and symptoms of ulceration and bleeding and should inform them of the importance of this follow-up (see Risk of GI Ulcerations, Bleeding and Perforation with NSAID Therapy).

Drug Interactions: Ponstel may prolong prothrombin time.[5] Therefore, when the drug is administered to patients receiving oral anticoagulant drugs, frequent monitoring of prothrombin time is necessary.

Use in Pregnancy: Pregnancy Category C. Reproduction studies have been performed in rats, rabbits and dogs. Rats given up to 10 times the human dose showed decreased fertility, delay in parturition, and a decreased rate of survival to weaning. Rabbits at 2.5 times the human dose showed an increase in the number of resorptions. There were no fetal anomalies observed in these studies nor in dogs at up to 10 times the human dose.[5]

There are no adequate and well-controlled studies in pregnant women. Because animal reproduction studies are not always predictive of human response, this drug should be used only if clearly needed.

The use of Ponstel in late pregnancy is not recommended because of the effects on the fetal cardiovascular system of drugs of this class.

Nursing Mothers: Trace amounts of Ponstel may be present in breast milk and transmitted to the nursing infant[7]; thus Ponstel should not be taken by the nursing mother because of the effects on the infant cardiovascular system of drugs of this class.

Use in Children: Safety and effectiveness in children below the age of 14 have not been established.

ADVERSE REACTIONS

Gastrointestinal: The most frequently reported adverse reactions associated with the use of Ponstel involve the gastrointestinal tract. In controlled studies for up to eight months, the following disturbances were reported in decreasing order of frequency: diarrhea (approximately 5% of patients), nausea with or without vomiting, other gastrointestinal symptoms, and abdominal pain.

In certain patients, the diarrhea was of sufficient severity to require discontinuation of medication. The occurrence of the diarrhea is usually dose related, generally subsides on reduction of dosage, and rapidly disappears on termination of therapy.

Other gastrointestinal reactions less frequently reported were anorexia, pyrosis, flatulence, and constipation. Gastrointestinal ulceration with and without hemorrhage has been reported.

Hematopoietic: Cases of autoimmune hemolytic anemia have been associated with the continuous administration of Ponstel for 12 months or longer. In such cases the Coombs test results are positive with evidence of both accelerated RBC production and RBC destruction. The process is reversible upon termination of Ponstel administration.

Decreases in hematocrit have been noted in 2–5% of patients and primarily in those who have received prolonged therapy. Leukopenia, eosinophilia, thrombocytopenic purpura, agranulocytosis, pancytopenia, and bone marrow hypoplasia have also been reported on occasion.

Nervous System: Drowsiness, dizziness, nervousness, headache, blurred vision, and insomnia have occurred.

Integumentary: Urticaria, rash, and facial edema have been reported.

Renal: As with other nonsteroidal antiinflammatory agents, renal failure, including papillary necrosis, has been reported. In elderly patients renal failure has occurred after taking Ponstel for 2–6 weeks. The renal damage may not be completely reversible. Hematuria and dysuria have also been reported with Ponstel.

Other: Eye irritation, ear pain, perspiration, mild hepatic toxicity, and increased need for insulin in a diabetic have

been reported. There have been rare reports of palpitation, dyspnea, and reversible loss of color vision.

OVERDOSAGE

Although doses up to 6000 mg/day have been given, no specific information is available on the management of acute massive overdosage.

Should accidental overdosage occur, the stomach should be emptied by inducing emesis or by careful gastric lavage followed by the administration of activated charcoal.[8] Laboratory studies indicate that Ponstel should be adsorbed from the gastrointestinal tract by activated charcoal.[4] Vital functions should be monitored and supported. Because mefenamic acid and its metabolites are firmly bound to plasma proteins, hemodialysis and peritoneal dialysis may be of little value.[4]

DOSAGE AND ADMINISTRATION

Administration is by the oral route, preferably with food. The recommended regimen in acute pain for adults and children over 14 years of age is 500 mg as an initial dose followed by 250 mg every six hours as needed, usually not to exceed one week.[5]

For the treatment of primary dysmenorrhea, the recommended dosage is 500 mg as an initial dose followed by 250 mg every 6 hours, starting with the onset of bleeding and associated symptoms. Clinical studies indicate that effective treatment can be initiated with the start of menses and should not be necessary for more than 2 to 3 days.[6]

HOW SUPPLIED

N 0071-0540-24 (P-D 540) Ponstel (mefenamic acid) is available as 250 mg capsules in bottles of 100.

References:
1. Winder CV, et al: Antiinflammatory, antipyretic and antinociceptive properties of N-(2,3-xylyl) anthranilic acid (mefenamic acid). *J Pharmacol Exp Ther* 138: 405–413, 1962.
2. Wax J, et al: Comparative activities, tolerances and safety of nonsteroidal antiinflammatory agents in rats. *J Pharmacol Exp Ther* 192: 172–178, 1975.
3. Ferreira SH, Vane JR: Aspirin and prostaglandins, in *The Prostaglandins,* Ramwell PW Ed, Plenum Press, NY, vol. 2, 1974, pp 1–47.
4. Glazko AJ: Experimental observations of flufenamic, mefenamic, and meclofenamic acids. Part III. Metabolic disposition, in *Fenamates in Medicine.* A Symposium, London 1966; *Annals of Physical Medicine,* supplement, pp 23–36, 1967.
5. Data on file, Medical Affairs Dept, Parke-Davis.
6. Budoff PW: Use of mefenamic acid in the treatment of primary dysmenorrhea. *JAMA* 241: 2713–2716, 1979.
7. Buchanan RA, et al: The breast milk excretion of mefenamic acid. *Curr Ther Res* 10:592, 1968.
8. Corby DG, Decker WJ: Management of acute poisoning with activated charcoal. *Pediatrics* 54:324, 1974.

0540G019

Caution—Federal law prohibits dispensing without prescription.

Shown in Product Identification Section, page 422

PROCAN® SR   ℞
[prō'căn ″]
(procainamide hydrochloride tablets)
SUSTAINED RELEASE

> **WARNING**
> Positive ANA Titer: The prolonged administration of procainamide often leads to the development of a positive antinuclear antibody (ANA) test, with or without symptoms of a lupus erythematosus-like syndrome. If a positive ANA titer develops, the benefits versus risks of continued procainamide therapy should be assessed.

DESCRIPTION

Procan SR (procainamide hydrochloride), a Group 1A cardiac antiarrhythmic drug, is p-amino-N(2-(diethylamino)ethyl)-benzamide monohydrochloride, molecular weight 271.79.

Procainamide hydrochloride differs from procaine which is the p-aminobenzoyl ester of 2-(diethylamino)-ethanol. Procainamide as the free base has a pk_a of 9.23; the monohydrochloride is very soluble in water.

Procan SR (Procainamide Hydrochloride Tablets) Sustained Release is available for oral administration as green, film-coated tablets containing 250 mg procainamide hydrochloride; as yellow, scored, film-coated tablets containing 500 mg procainamide hydrochloride; as orange, scored, film-coated tablets containing 750 mg procainamide hydrochloride; and as red, scored, film-coated tablets containing 1000 mg procainamide hydrochloride.

All strengths of Procan SR contain candelilla wax, FCC; colloidal silicon dioxide, NF; magnesium stearate, NF; titanium

dioxide; vanillin, NF; and other ingredients. The individual strengths contain additional ingredients as follows:
250 mg: D&C yellow No. 10 Al lake; FD&C blue No. 1 Al lake; FD&C yellow No. 6 Al lake; lactose, NF; may also contain methylparaben, NF; and propylparaben, NF; or simethicone emulsion and polysorbate 80, NF.
500 mg: D&C yellow No. 10 Al lake; FD&C blue No. 2 Al lake; FD&C yellow No. 6 Al lake; sucrose, NF; may also contain methylparaben, NF; and propylparaben, NF; or simethicone emulsion and polysorbate 80, NF.
750 mg: FD&C yellow No. 6 Al lake; may also contain propylene glycol, USP; or simethicone emulsion and polysorbate 80, NF.
1000 mg: FD&C red No. 3 Al lake; FD&C yellow No. 6 Al lake; propylene glycol, USP.

CLINICAL PHARMACOLOGY

Procainamide (PA) increases the effective refractory period of the atria, and to a lesser extent the bundle of His-Purkinje system and ventricles of the heart. It reduces impulse conduction velocity in the atria, His-Purkinje fibers, and ventricular muscle, but has variable effects on the atrioventricular (A-V) node, a direct slowing action and a weaker vagolytic effect which may speed A-V conduction slightly. Myocardial excitability is reduced in the atria, Purkinje fibers, papillary muscles, and ventricles by an increase in the threshold for excitation, combined with inhibition of ectopic pacemaker activity by retardation of the slow phase of diastolic depolarization, thus decreasing automaticity especially in ectopic sites. Contractility of the undamaged heart is usually not affected by therapeutic concentrations, although slight reduction of cardiac output may occur, and may be significant in the presence of myocardial damage. Therapeutic levels of PA may exert vagolytic effects and produce slight acceleration of heart rate, while high or toxic concentrations may prolong A-V conduction time or induce A-V block, or even cause abnormal automaticity and spontaneous firing, by unknown mechanisms.

Procainamide hydrochloride sustained-release tablets are designed to provide the biopharmaceutic characteristics of a sustained and relatively constant rate of release and absorption, independent of dose, primarily from the small intestine. The electrocardiogram may reflect these effects by showing slight sinus tachycardia (due to the anticholinergic action) and widened QRS complexes and, less regularly, prolonged Q-T and P-R intervals (due to longer systole and slower conduction), as well as some decrease in QRS and T wave amplitude. These direct effects of PA on electrical activity, conduction, responsiveness, excitability and automaticity are characteristic of a Group 1A antiarrhythmic agent, the prototype for which is quinidine; PA effects are very similar. However, PA has weaker vagal blocking action than does quinidine, does not induce alpha-adrenergic blockade, and is less depressing to cardiac contractility.

Ingested PA is resistant to digestive hydrolysis, and the drug is well absorbed from the entire small intestinal surface, but individual patients vary in their completeness of absorption of PA. Following oral administration every six hours procainamide hydrochloride sustained-release tablets achieve a mean steady state of procainamide (as well as procainamide N-acetylprocainamide) serum concentrations approximately equivalent to those from a comparable dose of an immediate-release dosage form given every three hours. Procainamide hydrochloride sustained-release tablets have a half-life which is significantly longer than that of procainamide immediate-release dosage forms. About 15 to 20 percent of PA is reversibly bound to plasma proteins, and considerable amounts are more slowly and reversibly bound to tissues of the heart, liver, lung, and kidney. The apparent volume of distribution eventually reaches about 2 liters per kilogram body weight with a half-time of approximately five minutes. While PA has been shown in the dog to cross the blood-brain barrier, it did not concentrate in the brain at levels higher than in plasma. It is not known if PA crosses the placenta. Plasma esterases are far less active in hydrolysis of PA than of procaine. The half-time for elimination is three to four hours in patients with normal renal function, but reduced creatinine clearance and advancing age each prolong the half-time of elimination of PA.

A significant fraction of the circulating PA may be metabolized in hepatocytes of N-acetylprocainamide (NAPA), ranging from 16 to 21 percent of an administered dose in "slow acetylators" to 24 to 33 percent in "fast acetylators." Since NAPA also has significant antiarrhythmic activity and somewhat slower renal clearance than PA, both hepatic acetylation rate capability and renal function, as well as age, have significant effects on the effective biologic half-time of

Continued on next page

This product information was prepared in August, 1989. On these and other Parke-Davis Products, information may be obtained by addressing PARKE-DAVIS, Division of Warner-Lambert Company, Morris Plains, New Jersey 07950.

Parke-Davis—Cont.

therapeutic action of administered PA and the NAPA derivative. Trace amounts may be excreted in the urine as free and conjugated p-aminobenzoic acid, 30 to 60 percent as unchanged PA, and 6 to 52 percent as the NAPA derivative. Both PA and NAPA are eliminated by active tubular secretion as well as by glomerular filtration. Action of PA on the central nervous system is not prominent, but high plasma concentrations may cause tremors. While therapeutic plasma levels for PA have been reported to be 3 to 10 μg/mL certain patients such as those with sustained ventricular tachycardia, may need higher levels for adequate control. This may justify the increased risk of toxicity (see OVERDOSAGE). Where programmed ventricular stimulation has been used to evaluate efficacy of PA in preventing recurrent ventricular tachyarrhythmias, higher plasma levels (mean, 13.6 μg/mL) of PA were found necessary for adequate control.

INDICATIONS AND USAGE

Procan SR tablets are indicated for the treatment of life-threatening ventricular arrhythmias.

Procan SR is also indicated for the treatment of some patients with less severe symptomatic ventricular arrhythmias, including unifocal or multifocal couplets and nonsustained ventricular tachycardia. Because procainamide hydrochloride has the potential to produce serious hematological disorders (0.5 percent), particularly leukopenia or agranulocytosis (sometimes fatal), the use of procainamide hydrochloride should be reserved for patients in whom, in the opinion of the physician, the benefits of treatment clearly outweigh the risks. (See WARNINGS and Boxed Warnings.) For less serious arrhythmias, alternative therapies with less severe toxicity should be considered.

Like all other antiarrhythmics, procainamide hydrochloride has not been shown to prevent sudden death in patients with serious ventricular ectopic activity, and also, like all other antiarrhythmics, procainamide hydrochloride has potentially serious adverse effects, including the ability to worsen arrhythmias. It is, therefore, essential that each patient given procainamide hydrochloride be evaluated electrocardiographically and clinically prior to, and during, procainamide hydrochloride therapy to determine whether the response to the drug supports continued treatment.

CONTRAINDICATIONS

Complete heart block: Procainamide should not be administered to patients with complete heart block because of its effects in suppressing nodal or ventricular pacemakers and the hazard of asystole. It may be difficult to recognize complete heart block in patients with ventricular tachycardia, but if significant slowing of ventricular rate occurs during PA treatment without evidence of A-V conduction appearing; PA should be stopped. In cases of second degree A-V block or various types of hemiblock, PA should be avoided or discontinued because of the possibility of increased severity of block, unless the ventricular rate is controlled by an electrical pacemaker.

Idiosyncratic hypersensitivity: In patients sensitive to procaine or other ester-type local anesthetics, cross sensitivity to PA is unlikely; however, it should be borne in mind, and PA should not be used if it produces acute allergic dermatitis, asthma, or anaphylactic symptoms.

Lupus Erythematosus: An established diagnosis of systemic lupus erythematosus is a contraindication to PA therapy, since aggravation of symptoms is highly likely.

Torsades de Pointes: In the unusual ventricular arrhythmia called "les torsades de pointes" (twisting of the points), characterized by alternation of one or more ventricular premature beats in the directions of the QRS complexes on ECG in persons with prolonged Q-T and often enhanced U waves, Group 1A antiarrhythmic drugs are contraindicated. Administration of PA in such cases may aggravate this special type of ventricular extrasystole or tachycardia instead of suppressing it.

WARNINGS

Blood Dyscrasias: Agranulocytosis, bone marrow depression, neutropenia, hypoplastic anemia and thrombocytopenia have been reported in patients receiving procainamide hydrochloride. Most of these patients received procainamide hydrochloride within the recommended dosage range. Fatalities have occurred (with approximately 20-25 percent mortality in reported cases of agranulocytosis). Since most of these events have been noted during the first 12 weeks of therapy, it is recommended that complete blood counts including white cell, differential and platelet counts be performed at weekly intervals for the first three months of therapy; and periodically thereafter. Complete blood counts should be performed promptly if the patient develops any signs of infection (such as fever, chills, sore throat, or stomatitis), bruising, or bleeding. If any of these he-

matologic disorders are identified, procainamide hydrochloride should be discontinued. Blood counts usually return to normal within one month of discontinuation. Caution should be used in patients with preexisting marrow failure or cytopenia of any type (see ADVERSE REACTIONS).

Digitalis Intoxication: Caution should be exercised in the use of procainamide in arrhythmias associated with digitalis intoxication. Procainamide can suppress digitalis-induced arrhythmias; however, if there is concomitant marked disturbance of atrioventricular conduction, additional depression of conduction and ventricular asystole or fibrillation may result. Therefore, use of procainamide should be considered only if discontinuation of digitalis, and therapy with potassium, lidocaine, or phenytoin are ineffective.

First Degree Heart Block: Caution should be exercised also if the patient exhibits or develops first degree heart block while taking PA, and dosage reduction is advised in such cases. If the block persists despite dosage reduction, continuation of PA administration must be evaluated on the basis of current benefit versus risk of increased heart block.

Predigitalization for Atrial Flutter or Fibrillation: Patients with atrial flutter or fibrillation should be cardioverted or digitalized prior to PA administration to avoid enhancement of A-V conduction which may result in ventricular rate acceleration beyond tolerable limits. Adequate digitalization reduces but does not eliminate the possibility of sudden increase in ventricular rate as the atrial rate is slowed by PA in these arrhythmias.

Congestive Heart Failure: For patients in congestive heart failure, and those with acute ischemic heart disease or cardiomyopathy, caution should be used in PA therapy, since even slight depression of myocardial contractility may further reduce the cardiac output of the damaged heart.

Concurrent Other Antiarrhythmic Agents: Concurrent use of PA with other Group 1A antiarrhythmic agents such as quinidine or disopyramide may produce enhanced prolongation of conduction or depression of contractility and hypotension, especially in patients with cardiac decompensation. Such use should be reserved for patients with serious arrhythmias unresponsive to a single drug and employed only if close observation is possible.

Renal Insufficiency: Renal insufficiency may lead to accumulation of high plasma levels from conventional oral doses of PA, with effects similar to those of overdosage (see OVERDOSAGE), unless dosage is adjusted for the individual patient.

Myasthenia Gravis: Patients with myasthenia gravis may show worsening of symptoms from PA due to its procaine-like effect on diminishing acetylcholine release at skeletal muscle motor nerve endings, so that PA administration may be hazardous without optimal adjustment of anticholinesterase medications or other precautions.

PRECAUTIONS

General: Immediately after initiation of PA therapy, patients should be closely observed for possible hypersensitivity reactions, especially if procaine or local anesthetic sensitivity is suspected, and for muscular weakness if myasthenia gravis is a possibility.

In conversion of arterial fibrillation to normal sinus rhythm by any means, dislodgment of mural thrombi may lead to embolization, which should be kept in mind.

After approximately two days, steady state plasma PA levels are produced following regular oral administration of a given dose of Procan SR tablets at set intervals. After achieving and maintaining therapeutic plasma concentrations and satisfactory electrocardiographic and clinical responses, continued frequent periodic monitoring of vital signs and electrocardiograms is advised. If evidence of QRS widening of more than 25 percent or marked prolongation of the Q-T interval occurs, concern for overdosage is appropriate, and reduction in dosage is advisable if a 50 percent increase occurs. Elevated serum creatinine or urea nitrogen, reduced creatinine clearance, or history of renal insufficiency, as well as use in older patients (over age 50), provide grounds to anticipate that less than the usual dosage and longer time intervals between doses may suffice, since the urinary elimination of PA and NAPA may be reduced, leading to gradual accumulation beyond normally predicted amounts. If facilities are available for measurement of plasma PA and NAPA, or acetylation capability, individual dose adjustment for optimal therapeutic levels may be easier, but close observation of clinical effectiveness is the most important criterion. In the longer term, period complete blood counts are useful to detect possible idiosyncratic hematologic effects of PA on neutrophil, platelet or red cell homeostasis; agranulocytosis has been reported to occur occasionally in patients on long-term PA therapy. A rising titer of serum ANA may precede clinical symptoms of the lupoid syndrome (see Boxed Warnings and ADVERSE REACTIONS). If the lupus erythematosus-like syndrome develops in a patient with recurrent life-threatening arrhythmias not controlled by other agents, corticosteroid suppressive therapy may be used concomitantly with PA. Since the PA-induced lupoid syndrome

rarely includes the dangerous pathologic renal changes, PA therapy may not necessarily have to be stopped unless the symptoms of serositis and the possibility of further lupoid effects are of greater risk than the benefit of PA in controlling arrhythmias. Patients with rapid acetylation capability are less likely to develop the lupoid syndrome after prolonged PA therapy.

Information for Patients: The physician is advised to explain to the patient that the close cooperation in adhering to the prescribed dosage schedule is of great importance in controlling the cardiac arrhythmia safely. The patient should understand clearly that more medication is not necessarily better and may be dangerous, that skipping doses or increasing intervals between doses to suit personal convenience may lead to loss of control of the heart problem, and that "making up" missed doses by doubling up later may be hazardous.

The patient should be encouraged to disclose any past history of drug sensitivity, especially to procaine or other local anesthetic agents, or aspirin, and to report any history of kidney disease, congestive heart failure, myasthenia gravis, liver disease, or lupus erythematosus.

The patient should be counseled to report promptly any symptoms of arthralgia, myalgia, fever, chills, skin rash, easy bruising, sore throat or sore mouth, infections, dark urine or icterus, wheezing, muscular weakness, chest or abdominal pain, palpitations, nausea, vomiting, anorexia, diarrhea, hallucinations, dizziness, or depression.

The patient should be advised not to break or chew the tablet as this would interfere with designed dissolution characteristics. The tablet matrix of Procan SR may be seen in the stool since it does not disintegrate following release of procainamine.

Laboratory Tests: Laboratory tests such as complete blood count (CBC), electrocardiogram, and serum creatinine or urea nitrogen may be indicated, depending on the clinical situation, and periodic rechecking of the CBC and ANA may be helpful in early detection of untoward reactions.

Drug Interactions: If other antiarrhythmic drugs are being used, additive effects on the heart may occur with PA administration, and dosage reduction may be necessary (see WARNINGS).

Anticholinergic drugs administered concurrently with PA may produce additive antivagal effects on A-V nodal conduction, although this is not as well documented for PA as for quinidine.

Patients taking PA who require neuromuscular blocking agents such as succinylcholine may require less than usual doses of the latter, due to PA effects of reducing acetylcholine release.

Of 10,867 patients treated with mexiletine in a compassionate use program, six cases of agranulocytosis were reported. Five of the six cases involved patients who were concomitantly receiving PA.

Drug/Laboratory Test Interactions: Suprapharmacologic concentrations of lidocaine and meprobamate may inhibit fluorescence of PA and NAPA and propranolol shows a native fluorescence close to the PA/NAPA peak wavelengths, so that tests which depend on fluorescence measurement may be affected.

Carcinogenesis, Mutagenesis, Impairment of Fertility: Long term studies in animals have not been performed.

Teratogenic Effects: Pregnancy Category C: Animal reproduction studies have not been conducted with PA. It also is not known whether PA can cause fetal harm when administered to a pregnant woman or can affect reproduction capacity. PA should be given to a pregnant woman only if clearly needed.

Nursing Mothers: Both PA and NAPA are excreted in human milk, and absorbed by the nursing infant. Because of the potential for serious adverse reactions in nursing infants, a decision to discontinue nursing or the drug should be made, taking into account the importance of the drug to the mother.

Pediatric Use: Safety and effectiveness in children have not been established.

ADVERSE REACTIONS

Cardiovascular System: Hypotension following oral PA administration is rare. Hypotension and serious disturbances of cardiorhythm such as ventricular asystole or fibrillation are more common after intravenous administration (see OVERDOSAGE, WARNINGS). Second degree heart block has been reported in 2 of almost 500 patients taking PA orally.

Multisystem Effects: A lupus erythematosus-like syndrome of arthralgia, pleural or abdominal pain, and sometime arthritis, pleural effusion, pericarditis, fever, chills, myalgia, and possibly related hematologic or skin lesions (see below) is fairly common after prolonged PA administration, perhaps more often in patients who are slow acetylators (See Boxed Warnings and PRECAUTIONS). While some series have reported less than 1 in 500, others have reported the syndrome in up to 30 percent of long term oral PA therapy. If discontinuation of PA does not reverse the lupoid symptoms, corticosteroid treatment may be effective.

Hematologic System: Neutropenia, thrombocytopenia, or hemolytic anemia may rarely be encountered. Agranulocytosis has occurred after repeated use of PA, and deaths have been reported (see WARNINGS and Boxed Warnings).

Skin: Angioneurotic edema, urticaria, pruritus, flushing, and maculopapular rash have also occurred occasionally.

Gastrointestinal System: Anorexia, nausea, vomiting, abdominal pain, bitter taste, or diarrhea may occur in 3 to 4 percent of patients taking oral procainamide. Hepatomegaly with increased serum aminotransferase activity has been reported after a single oral dose.

Nervous System: Dizziness or giddiness, weakness, mental depression, and psychosis with hallucinations have been reported occasionally.

OVERDOSAGE

Progressive widening of the QRS complex, prolonged Q-T and P-R intervals, lowering of the R and T waves, as well as increasing A-V block, may be seen with doses which are excessive for a given patient, increased ventricular extrasystoles, or even ventricular tachycardia or fibrillation may occur. After intravenous administration but seldom after oral therapy, transient high plasma levels of PA may induce hypotension, affecting systolic more than diastolic pressures, especially in hypertensive patients. Such high levels may also produce central nervous depression, tremor, and even respiratory depression.

Plasma levels above 10 μg/mL are increasingly associated with toxic findings, which are seen occasionally in the 10 to 12 μg/mL range, more often in the 12 to 15 μg/mL range, and commonly in patients with plasma levels greater than 15 μg/mL. A single oral dose of 2 g may produce overdosage symptoms, while 3 g may be dangerous, especially if the patient is a slow acetylator, has decreased renal function, or underlying organic heart disease.

Treatment of overdosage or toxic manifestations includes general supportive measures, close observation, monitoring of vital signs and possibly intravenous pressor agents and mechanical cardiorespiratory support. If available, PA and NAPA plasma levels may be helpful in assessing the potential degree of toxicity and response to therapy. Both PA and NAPA are removed from the circulation by hemodialysis but not peritoneal dialysis. No specific antidote for PA is known.

DOSAGE AND ADMINISTRATION

The oral dose and interval of administration should be adjusted for the individual patient, based on clinical assessment of the degree of underlying myocardial disease, the patient's age, and renal function.

As a general guide, for younger patients with normal renal function, an initial total daily oral dose of up to 50 mg/kg of body weight of Procan SR Tablets may be used, given in divided doses, every six hours, to maintain therapeutic blood levels. For older patients, especially those over 50 years of age, or for patients with renal, hepatic or cardiac insufficiency, lesser amounts or longer intervals may produce adequate blood levels, and decrease the probability of occurrence of dose related adverse reactions.

To provide up to 50 mg per kg of body weight per day* Patients weighing	
88–110 (40–50 kg)	500mg q6 hrs
132–154 (60–70 kg)	750 mg q6 hrs
176–198 (80–90 kg)	1 g q6 hrs
> 220 lb (> 100 kg)	1.25 g q6 hrs

*Initial dosage schedule guide only, to be adjusted for each patient individually, based on age, cardiorenal function, blood level (if available), and clinical response.

HOW SUPPLIED

Procan SR 250 mg (elliptical, green, scored, film-coated, coded PD 202) is a sustained-release tablet that contains 250 mg of procainamide hydrochloride. It is supplied as follows:

N 0071-0202-24	Bottles of 100
N 0071-0202-25	Bottles of 120
N 0071-0202-30	Bottles of 500
N 0071-0202-40	Unit-dose packages of 100 (10 strips of 10 tablets each)

Procan SR 500 mg (elliptical, yellow, scored, film-coated, coded PD 204) is a sustained-release tablet that contains 500 mg of procainamide hydrochloride. It is supplied as follows:

N 0071-0204-24	Bottles of 100
N 0071-0204-25	Bottles of 120
N 0071-0204-30	Bottles of 500
N 0071-0204-40	Unit-dose packages of 100 (10 strips of 10 tablets each)

Procan SR 750 mg (elliptical, orange, scored, film-coated, coded PD 205) is a sustained-release tablet that contains 750 mg of procainamide hydrochloride. It is supplied as follows:

N 0071-0205-24	Bottles of 100
N 0071-0205-25	Bottles of 120
N 0071-0205-30	Bottles of 500
N 0071-0205-40	Unit-dose packages of 100 (10 strips of 10 tablets each)

Procan SR 1000 mg (elliptical, red, scored, film-coated, coded PD 207) is a sustained-release tablet that contains 1000 mg of procainamide hydrochloride. It is supplied as follows:

N 0071-0207-24	Bottle of 100
N 0071-0207-25	Bottle of 120
N 0071-0207-40	Unit-dose packages of 100 (10 strips of 10 tablets each)

Storage Conditions:
Protect from moisture.
Store bottles below 30°C (86°F).
Store unit-dose packages at controlled room temperature, 15°–30°C (59°–86°F).
Caution—Federal law prohibits dispensing without prescription.

0207G074

Shown in Product Identification Section, page 422

PROLOID® ℞
[prō′loid]
(Thyroglobulin Tablets, USP)

DESCRIPTION

Proloid (Thyroglobulin Tablets, USP) is a natural hormonal preparation obtained from a purified extract of hog thyroid and contains the known calorigenically active compounds, levothyroxine (T_4) and liothyronine (T_3). Each 1 grain Proloid tablet contains 60 mcg levothyroxine (T_4) and 15 mcg liothyronine (T_3).

Each 1 grain Proloid tablet will give a dose benefit approximately equivalent to 1 grain of desiccated thyroid, 100 mcg T_4 (levothyroxine sodium), 25 mcg T_3 (liothyronine sodium), or 50–60 mcg T_4/12.5–15 mcg T_3 (liotrix). See Conversion Table at end of insert.

Proloid tablets also contain gelatin, NF; lactose, NF; methylcellulose, USP; and stearic acid, NF. In addition, the 1 grain, 1 ½ grain, 2 grain, and 3 grain strengths also contain alginic acid, NF and tribasic calcium phosphate, NF.

Thyroid hormone drugs are natural or synthetic preparations containing tetraiodothyronine (T_4, levothyroxine) sodium or triiodothyronine (T_3, liothyronine) sodium or both. T_4 and T_3 are produced in the human thyroid gland by the iodination and coupling of the amino acid tyrosine. T_4 contains four iodine atoms and is formed by the coupling of two molecules of diiodotyrosine (DIT). T_3 contains three atoms of iodine and is formed by the coupling of one molecule of DIT with one molecule of monoiodotyrosine (MIT). Both hormones are stored in the thyroid colloid as thyroglobulin.

Thyroid hormone preparations belong to two categories: (1) natural hormonal preparations derived from animal thyroid, and (2) synthetic preparations. Natural preparations include desiccated thyroid and thyroglobulin. Desiccated thyroid is derived from domesticated animals that are used for food by man (either beef or hog thyroid), and thyroglobulin is derived from thyroid glands of the hog.

There are five (5) preparations in the USP. They are: (1) Thyroid Tablets, (2) Thyroglobulin Tablets, (3) Levothyroxine Sodium Tablets, (4) Liothyronine Sodium Tablets, and (5) Liotrix Tablets (a ratio, by weight, of 4 to 1, of the sodium salts of T_4 and T_3, respectively).

CLINICAL PHARMACOLOGY

The steps in the synthesis of the thyroid hormones are controlled by thyrotropin (Thyroid Stimulating Hormone, TSH) secreted by the anterior pituitary. This hormone's secretion is in turn controlled by a feedback mechanism effected by the thyroid hormones themselves and by the thyrotropin releasing hormone (TRH), a tripeptide of hypothalamic origin. Endogenous thyroid hormone secretion is suppressed when exogenous thyroid hormones are administered to euthyroid individuals in excess of the normal gland's secretion.

The mechanisms by which thyroid hormones exert their physiologic action are not well understood. These hormones enhance oxygen consumption by most tissues of the body, increase the basal metabolic rate, and the metabolism of carbohydrates, lipids, and proteins. Thus, they exert a profound influence on every organ system in the body and are of particular importance in the development of the central nervous system.

The normal thyroid gland contains approximately 200 mcg of levothyroxine (T_4) per gram of gland, and 15 mcg of triiodothyronine (T_3) per gram. The ratio of these two hormones in the circulation does not represent the ratio in the thyroid gland, since about 80 percent of peripheral triiodothyronine comes from monodeiodination of levothyroxine. Peripheral monodeiodination of levothyroxine at the 5 position (inner ring) also results in the formation of reverse triiodothyronine (r T_3), which is calorigenically inactive. These facts would seem to advocate levothyroxine as the treatment of choice for the hypothyroid patient and to militate against the administration of hormone combinations, which while normalizing thyroxine levels may produce triiodothyronine levels in the thyrotoxic range.

Triiodothyronine (T_3) level is low in the fetus and newborn, in old age, in chronic caloric deprivation, hepatic cirrhosis, renal failure, surgical stress, and chronic illnesses representing what has been called the "low triiodothyronine syndrome."

Pharmacokinetics: Animal studies have shown that T_4 is only partially absorbed from the gastrointestinal tract. The degree of absorption is dependent on the vehicle used for its administration and by the character of the intestinal contents, the intestinal flora, including plasma protein, soluble dietary factors, all of which bind thyroid and thereby make it unavailable for diffusion. Only 41 percent is absorbed when given in a gelatin capsule as opposed to a 74 percent absorption when given with an albumin carrier.

Depending on other factors, absorption has varied from 48 to 79 percent of the administered dose.

Fasting increases absorption. Malabsorption syndromes, as well as dietary factors (children's soybean formula, concomitant use of anionic exchange resins such as cholestyramine), cause excessive fecal loss. T_3 is almost totally absorbed, 95 percent in 4 hours. The hormones contained in the natural preparations are absorbed in a manner similar to the synthetic hormones.

More than 99 percent of circulating hormones are bound to serum proteins, including thyroid-binding globulin (TB$_g$), thyroid-binding prealbumin (TBPA), and albumin (TBa), whose capacities and affinities vary for the hormones. The higher affinity of levothyroxine (T_4) for both TBg and TBPA as compared to triiodothyronine (T_3) partially explains the higher serum levels and longer half-life of the former hormone. Both protein-bound hormones exist in reverse equilibrium with minute amounts of free hormone, the latter accounting for the metabolic acitivity.

Deiodination of levothyroxine (T_4) occurs at a number of sites, including liver, kidney, and other tissues. The conjugated hormone, in the form of glucuronide or sulfate, is found in the bile and gut where it may complete an enterohepatic circulation. Eighty-five percent of levothyroxine (T_4) metabolized daily is deiodinated.

INDICATIONS AND USAGE

Thyroid hormone drugs are indicated:
As replacement or supplemental therapy in patients with hypothyroidism of any etiology, except transient hypothyroidism during the recovery phase of subacute thyroiditis. This category includes cretinism, myxedema, and ordinary hypothyroidism in patients of any age (children, adults, the elderly), or state (including pregnancy), primary hypothyroidism resulting from functional deficiency, primary atrophy, partial or total absence of thyroid gland, or the effects of surgery, radiation, or drugs, with or without the presence of goiter; and secondary (pituitary) or tertiary (hypothalamic) hypothyroidism (See WARNINGS).

CONTRAINDICATIONS

Thyroid hormone preparations are generally contraindicated in patients with diagnosed but as yet uncorrected adrenal cortical insufficiency, untreated thyrotoxicosis, and apparent hypersensitivity to any of their active or extraneous constituents. There is no well documented evidence from the literature, however, of true allergic or idiosyncratic reactions to thyroid hormone.

WARNINGS

> Drugs with thyroid hormone activity, alone or together with other therapeutic agents, have been used for the treatment of obesity. In euthyroid patients, doses within the range of daily hormonal requirements are ineffective for weight reduction. Larger doses may produce serious or even life-threatening manifestations of toxicity, particularly when given in association with sympathomimetic amines such as those used for their anorectic effects.

The use of thyroid hormones in the therapy of obesity, alone or combined with other drugs, is unjustified and has been shown to be ineffective. Neither is their use justified for the treatment of male or female infertility unless this condition is accompanied by hypothyroidism.

PRECAUTIONS

General: Thyroid hormones should be used with great caution in a number of circumstances where the integrity of the cardiovascular system, particularly the coronary arteries, is suspect. These include patients with angina pectoris or the elderly, in whom there is a greater likelihood of occult cardiac disease. In these patients, therapy should be initiated with low doses, ie, 25–50 mcg levothyroxine (T_4) or its isocaloric equivalents (16–32 mg, or 0.25–0.5 grain of Proloid).

Continued on next page

This product information was prepared in August, 1989. On these and other Parke-Davis Products, information may be obtained by addressing PARKE-DAVIS, Division of Warner-Lambert Company, Morris Plains, New Jersey 07950.

Parke-Davis—Cont.

When, in such patients, a euthyroid state can only be reached at the expense of an aggravation of the cardiovascular disease, thyroid hormone dosage should be reduced.

Thyroid hormone therapy in patients with concomitant diabetes mellitus or insipidus or adrenal cortical insufficiency aggravates the intensity of their symptoms. Appropriate adjustments of the various therapeutic measures directed at these concomitant endocrine diseases are required. The therapy of myxedema coma requires simultaneous administration of glucocorticoids (See DOSAGE AND ADMINISTRATION).

Hypothyroidism decreases and hyperthyroidism increases the sensitivity to oral anticoagulants. Prothrombin time should be closely monitored in thyroid-treated patients on oral anticoagulants and dosage of the latter agents adjusted on the basis of frequent prothrombin time determination. In infants, excessive doses of thyroid hormone preparations may produce craniosynostosis.

Information for the Patient: Patients on thyroid hormone preparations and parents of children on thyroid therapy should be informed that:

1. Replacement therapy is to be taken essentially for life, with the exception of cases of transient hypothyroidism, usually associated with thyroiditis, and in those patients receiving a therapeutic trial of the drug.
2. They should immediately report during the course of therapy any signs or symptoms of thyroid hormone toxicity, eg, chest pain, increased pulse rate, palpitations, excessive sweating, heat intolerance, nervousness, or any other unusual event.
3. In case of concomitant diabetes mellitus, the daily dosage of antidiabetic medication may need readjustment as thyroid hormone replacement is achieved. If thyroid medication is stopped, a downward readjustment of the dosage of insulin or oral hypoglycemic agent may be necessary to avoid hypoglycemia. At all times, close monitoring of urinary glucose levels is mandatory in such patients.
4. In case of concomitant oral anticoagulant therapy, the prothrombin time should be measured frequently to determine if the dosage of oral anticoagulants is to be readjusted.
5. Partial loss of hair may be experienced by children in the first few months of thyroid therapy, but this is usually a transient phenomenon and later recovery is usually the rule.

Laboratory Tests: Treatment of patients with thyroid hormones requires the periodic assessment of thyroid status by means of appropriate laboratory tests besides the full clinical evaluation. The TSH suppression test can be used to test the effectiveness of any thyroid preparation, bearing in mind the relative insensitivity of the infant pituitary to the negative feedback effect of thyroid hormones. Serum T_4 levels can be used to test the effectiveness of all thyroid medications except T_3.

When the total serum T_4 is low but TSH is normal, a test specific to assess unbound (free) T_4 levels is warranted. Specific measurements of T_4 and T_3 by competitive protein binding or radioimmunoassay are not influenced by blood levels or organic or inorganic iodine and have essentially replaced older tests of thyroid hormone measurements, ie, PBI, BEI, and T_4 by column.

Drug Interactions—Oral Anticoagulants: Thyroid hormones appear to increase catabolism of vitamin K-dependent clotting factors. If oral anticoagulants are also being given, compensatory increases in clotting factor synthesis are impaired. Patients stabilized on oral anticoagulants who are found to require thyroid replacement therapy should be watched very closely when thyroid is started. If a patient is truly hypothyroid, it is likely that a reduction in anticoagulant dosage will be required. No special precautions appear to be necessary when oral anticoagulant therapy is begun in a patient already stabilized on maintenance thyroid replacement therapy.

Insulin or Oral Hypoglycemics: Initiating thyroid replacement therapy may cause increases in insulin or oral hypoglycemic requirements.The effects seen are poorly understood and depend upon a variety of factors such as dosage and type of thyroid preparations and endocrine status of the patient. Patients receiving insulin or oral hypoglycemics should be closely watched during initiation of thyroid replacement therapy.

Cholestyramine: Cholestyramine binds both T_4 and T_3 in the intestine, thus impairing absorption of these thyroid hormones. In vitro studies indicate that the binding is not easily removed. Therefore, four to five hours should elapse between administration of cholestyramine or similar resins, such as colestipol, and thyroid hormones.

Estrogen, Oral Contraceptives: Estrogens tend to increase serum thyroxine-binding globulin (TBg). In a patient with a nonfunctioning thyroid gland who is receiving thyroid replacement therapy, free levothyroxine may be decreased when estrogens are started thus increasing thyroid require-

ments. However, if the patient's thyroid gland has sufficient function, the decreased free thyroxine will result in a compensatory increase in thyroxine output by the thyroid. Therefore, patients without a functioning thyroid gland who are on thyroid replacement therapy may need to increase their thyroid dose if estrogens or estrogen-containing oral contraceptives are given.

Drug/Laboratory Test Interactions: The following drugs or moieties are known to interfere with laboratory tests performed in patients on thyroid hormone therapy: androgens, corticosteroids, estrogens, oral contraceptives containing estrogens, iodine-containing preparations, and the numerous preparations containing salicylates.

1. Changes in TBg concentration should be taken into consideration in the interpretation of T_4 and T_3 values. In such cases, the unbound (free) hormone should be measured. Pregnancy, estrogens, and estrogen-containing oral contraceptives increase TBg concentrations. TBg may also be increased during infectious hepatitis. Decreases in TBg concentrations are observed in nephrosis, acromegaly, and after androgen or corticosteroid therapy. Familial hyper or hypothyroxine-binding-globulinemias have been described. The incidence of TBg deficiency approximates 1 in 9000. The binding of thyroxine by TBPA is inhibited by salicylates.
2. Medicinal or dietary iodine interferes with all in vivo tests of radioiodine uptake, producing low uptakes which may not be reflective of a true decrease in hormone synthesis.
3. The persistence of clinical and laboratory evidence of hypothyroidism in spite of adequate dosage replacement indicates poor patient compliance, poor absorption, excessive fecal loss, or inactivity of the preparation. Intracellular resistance to thyroid hormone is quite rare.

Carcinogenesis, Mutagenesis, and Impairment of Fertility: A reportedly apparent association between prolonged thyroid therapy and breast cancer has not been confirmed and patients on thyroid for established indications should not discontinue therapy. No confirmatory long-term studies in animals have been performed to evaluate carcinogenic potential, mutagenicity, or impairment of fertility in either males or females.

Pregnancy Category A: Thyroid hormones do not readily cross the placental barrier. The clinical experience to date does not indicate any adverse effect on fetuses when the thyroid hormones are administered to pregnant women. On the basis of current knowledge, thyroid replacement therapy to hypothyroid women should not be discontinued during pregnancy.

Nursing Mothers: Minimal amounts of thyroid hormones are excreted in human milk. Thyroid is not associated with serious adverse reactions and does not have a known tumorigenic potential. However, caution should be exercised when thyroid is administered to a nursing woman.

Pediatric Use: Pregnant mothers provide little or no thyroid hormone to the fetus. The incidence of congenital hypothyroidism is relatively high (1:4,000) and the hypothyroid fetus would not derive any benefit from the small amounts of hormone crossing the placental barrier. Routine determinations of serum (T_4) and/or TSH are strongly advised in neonates in view of the deleterious effects of thyroid deficiency on growth and development.

Treatment should be initiated immediately upon diagnosis and maintained for life, unless transient hypothyroidism is suspected; in which case, therapy may be interrupted for 2 to 8 weeks after the age of 3 years to reassess the condition. Cessation of therapy is justified in patients who have maintained a normal TSH during those 2 to 8 weeks.

ADVERSE REACTIONS

Adverse reactions other than those indicative of hyperthyroidism because of therapeutic overdosage, either initially or during the maintenance period, are rare (See OVERDOSAGE).

OVERDOSAGE

Signs and Symptoms: Excessive doses of thyroid result in a hypermetabolic state resembling in every respect the condition of endogenous origin. The condition may be self-induced.

Treatment of Overdosage: Dosage should be reduced or therapy temporarily discontinued if signs and symptoms of overdosage appear. Treatment may be reinstituted at a lower dosage. In normal individuals, normal hypothalamic-pituitary-thyroid axis function is restored in 6 to 8 weeks after thyroid suppression.

Treatment of acute massive thyroid hormone overdosage is aimed at reducing gastrointestinal absorption of the drugs and counteracting central and peripheral effects, mainly those of increased sympathetic activity. Vomiting may be induced initially if further gastrointestinal absorption can reasonably be prevented and barring contraindications such as coma, convulsions, or loss of the gagging reflex. Treatment is symptomatic and supportive. Oxygen may be administered and ventilation maintained. Cardiac glycosides may be indicated if congestive heart failure develops. Measures to control fever, hypoglycemia, or fluid loss should be instituted if needed. Antiadrenergic agents, particularly propranolol, have been used advantageously in the treatment of in-

creased sympathetic activity. Propranolol may be administered intravenously at a dosage of 1 to 3 mg over a 10-minute period or orally, 80 to 160 mg/day initially, especially when no contraindications exist for its use.

DOSAGE AND ADMINISTRATION

The dosage of thyroid hormones is determined by the indication and must in every case be individualized according to patient response and laboratory findings.

Thyroid hormones are given orally. In acute, emergency conditions, injectable sodium levothyroxine may be given intravenously when oral administration is not feasible or desirable, as in the treatment of myxedema coma, or during total parenteral nutrition. Injectable sodium liothyronine is also available upon request from the manufacturer, under investigational status, for the treatment of myxedema coma. Intramuscular administration of these two preparations is not advisable because of reported poor absorption.

Hypothyroidism: Therapy is usually instituted using low doses, with increments which depend on the cardiovascular status of the patient. The usual starting dose is 50 mcg of levothyroxine (T_4) or its isocaloric equivalent (32 mg, or 0.5 grain of Proloid), with increments of 25 mcg every 2 to 3 weeks. A lower starting dosage, 25 mcg/day, is recommended in patients with longstanding myxedema, particularly if cardiovascular impairment is suspected, in which case extreme caution is recommended. The appearance of angina is an indication for a reduction in dosage. The 200 to 400 mcg levothyroxine (T_4) recommended in the early trials are now considered excessive and most patients require 100 to 200 mcg/day or the caloric equivalent. Failure to respond to doses of 300 mcg suggests lack of compliance or malabsorption. Maintenance dosages of 100–200 mcg/day usually result in normal serum levothyroxine (T_4) and triiodothyronine (T_3) levels. Adequate therapy usually results in normal TSH and T_4 levels after 2 to 3 weeks of therapy.

Readjustment of thyroid hormone dosage should be made within the first four weeks of therapy, after proper clinical and laboratory evaluations, including serum levels of T_4, bound and free, and TSH.

The rapid onset and dissipation of action of sodium liothyronine (T_3), as compared with sodium levothyroxine (T_4), has led some clinicians to prefer its use in patients who might be more susceptible to the untoward effects of thyroid medication. However, the wide swings in serum T_3 levels that follow its administration and the possibility of more pronounced cardiovascular side effects tend to counterbalance the stated advantages. Many physicians continue to use thyroid tablets, USP, a T_3/T_4 combination, or a newer synthetic combination.

T_3 may be used in preference to levothyroxine (T_4) during radioisotope scanning procedures, since induction of hypothyroidism in those cases is more abrupt and can be of shorter duration. It may also be preferred when impairment of peripheral conversion of T_4 and T_4 is suspected.

Myxedema Coma: Myxedema coma is usually precipitated in the hypothyroid patient of long-standing by intercurrent illness or drugs such as sedatives and anesthetics and should be considered a medical emergency. Therapy should be directed at the correction of electrolyte disturbances and possible infection besides the administration of thyroid hormones. Corticosteroids should be administered routinely. T_4 and T_3 may be administered via a nasogastric tube, but the preferred route of administration of both hormones is intravenous. Sodium levothyroxine (T_4) is given at a starting dose of 400mcg (100 mcg/mL) given rapidly and is usually well tolerated, even in the elderly. This initial dose is followed by daily supplements of 100 to 200 mcg given IV. Normal T_4 levels are achieved in 24 hours followed in 3 days by threefold elevation of T_3. Triiodothyronine (T_3) (which is obtained only by special request from the manufacturer) is given at doses of 200 mcg IV followed by 25 mcg supplements at 8-hour intervals. Oral therapy with either hormone would be resumed as soon as the clinical situation has been stabilized and the patient is able to take oral medication.

Thyroid Cancer: Exogenous thyroid hormone may produce regression of metastases from follicular and papillary carcinoma of the thyroid and is used as ancillary therapy of these conditions with radioactive iodine. TSH should be suppressed to low or undetectable levels. Therefore, larger amounts of thyroid hormone than those used for replacement therapy are required. Medullary carcinoma of the thyroid is usually unresponsive to this therapy.

Thyroid Suppression Therapy: Administration of thyroid hormone in doses higher than those produced physiologically by the gland results in suppression of the production of endogenous hormone. This is the basis for the thyroid suppression test and is used as an aid in the diagnosis of patients with signs of mild hyperthyroidism in whom baseline laboratory tests appear normal or to demonstrate thyroid gland autonomy in patients with Graves' ophthalmopathy. 131_I uptake is determined before and after the administration of the exogenous hormone. A 50 percent or greater suppression of uptake indicates a normal thyroid-pituitary axis and thus rules out thyroid gland autonomy.

For adults, the usual suppressive dose of levothyroxine (T_4) is 2.6 mcg/kg of body weight per day given for 7 to 10 days. These doses usually yield normal serum T_4 and T_3 levels and lack of response to TSH.

T_3 is given in doses of 75–100 mcg/day for 7 days and radioactive iodine uptake is determined before and after administration of the hormone. If thyroid function is under normal control, the radioiodine uptake will drop significantly after treatment with either hormone.

The use of Proloid for suppression therapy is not advisable. Either hormone or combination therapy should be administered cautiously to patients in whom there is a strong suspicion of thyroid gland autonomy, in view of the fact that the exogenous hormone effects will be additive to the endogenous source.

Pediatric Dosage: Pediatric dosage should follow the recommendations summarized in Table 1. In infants with congenital hypothyroidism, therapy with full doses should be instituted as soon as the diagnosis has been made.

Table 1 Recommended Pediatric Dosage for Congenital Hypothyroidism

Age	Tetraiodothyronine (T_4, levothyroxine) sodium	
	Dose per day	Daily dose per kg of body weight
0–6 mos	25–50 mcg	8–10 mcg
6–12 mos	50–75 mcg	6–8 mcg
1–5 yrs	75–100 mcg	5–6 mcg
6–12 yrs	100–150 mcg	4–5 mcg
over 12 yrs	over 150 mcg	2–3 mcg

Instructions for Use
The following conversion table lists the approximate equivalents of other thyroid preparations to Proloid when changing medication from desiccated thyroid T_3 (levothyroxine sodium). T_3 (liothyronine sodium), or T_4/T_3 (liotrix). [See table above].

HOW SUPPLIED
Proloid tablets are supplied:

N 0071-0251-24	½ grain (32 mg)		Bottles of 100
N 0071-0252-24	1 grain (65 mg)	Scored	Bottles of 100
N 0071-0252-32	1 grain (65 mg)	Scored	Bottles of 1000
N 0071-0253-24	1½ grain (100 mg)		Bottles of 100
N 0071-0257-24	2 grain (130 mg)	Scored	Bottles of 100
N 0071-0254-24	3 grain (200 mg)		Bottles of 100

Tablets are gray and uncoated.
Store at controlled room temperature 15°–30°C (59°–86°F).
Caution—Federal law prohibits dispensing without prescription.

0250G015
Shown in Product Identification Section, page 422

PYRIDIUM®   ℞
[py″ri′di-ŭm]
(Phenazopyridine Hydrochloride Tablets, USP)

DESCRIPTION
Pyridium (phenazopyridine hydrochloride) is chemically designated 2,6-Pyridinediamine, 3-(phenylazo), monohydrochloride. It is a urinary tract analgesic agent for oral administration. Pyridium tablets contain 100 mg or 200 mg phenazopyridine hydrochloride. Also contains carnauba wax, NF; corn starch, NF; D and C red No. 7; FD and C blue No. 2; FD and C yellow No. 6; gelatin, NF; lactose, NF; magnesium stearate, NF; methylcellulose, USP; sodium starch glycolate, NF; sucrose, NF; titanium dioxide, USP; white wax. NF.

CLINICAL PHARMACOLOGY
Pyridium is excreted in the urine where it exerts a topical analgesic effect on the mucosa of the urinary tract. This action helps to relieve pain, burning, urgency and frequency. The precise mechanism of action is not known.
The pharmacokinetic properties of Pyridium have not been determined. Phenazopyridine is rapidly excreted by the kidneys, with as much as 65% of an oral dose being excreted unchanged in the urine.

INDICATIONS AND USAGE
Pyridium is indicated for the symptomatic relief of pain, burning, urgency, frequency, and other discomforts arising from irritation of the lower urinary tract mucosa caused by infection, trauma, surgery, endoscopic procedures, or the passage of sounds or catheters. The use of Pyridium for relief of symptoms should not delay definitive diagnosis and treatment of causative conditions. Because it provides only symp-

Conversion Table

Dose of Proloid (thyroglobulin) grain	mg	Dose of Desiccated Thyroid grain	Dose of T_4 (levothyroxine sodium) mg	Dose of T_3 (liothyronine sodium) mcg	Dose of liotrix (T_4/T_3)
0.5	(32)	0.5	0.05	12.5	#½(30 mcg/7.5 mcg)
1	(65)	1	0.1	25	#1(60 mcg/15 mcg)
2	(130)	2	0.2	50	#2(120 mcg/30 mcg)
3	(200)	3	0.3	75	#3(180 mcg/45 mcg)
4	(260)	4	0.4	100	
5	(325)	5	0.5	125	

In changing from Thyroid USP to Proloid, substitute the equivalent dose of Proloid. Each patient may still require fine adjustment of dosage because the equivalents are only estimates.

tomatic relief, prompt appropriate treatment of the cause of pain must be instituted and Pyridium should be discontinued when symptoms are controlled.
The analgesic action may reduce or eliminate the need for systemic analgesics or narcotics. It is, however, compatible with antibacterial therapy and can help to relieve pain and discomfort during the interval before antibacterial therapy controls the infection. Treatment of a urinary tract infection with Pyridium should not exceed 2 days because there is a lack of evidence that the combined administration of Pyridium and an antibacterial provides greater benefit than administration of the antibacterial alone after 2 days. (See DOSAGE AND ADMINISTRATION Section.)

CONTRAINDICATIONS
Pyridium should not be used in patients who have previously exhibited hypersensitivity to it. The use of Pyridium is contraindicated in patients with renal insufficiency.

PRECAUTIONS
General: A yellowish tinge of the skin or sclera may indicate accumulation due to impaired renal excretion and the need to discontinue therapy.
The decline in renal function associated with advanced age should be kept in mind.
Information for Patients: Pyridium produces an orange to red color in the urine and may stain fabric. Staining of contact lenses has been reported.
Laboratory Test Interactions: Due to its properties as an azo dye, Pyridium may interfere with urinalysis based on spectrometry or color reactions.
Carcinogenesis, Mutagenesis, Impairment of Fertility: Longterm administration of phenazopyridine hydrochloride has induced neoplasia in rats (large intestine) and mice (liver). Although no association between phenazopyridine hydrochloride and human neoplasia has been reported, adequate epidemiological studies along these lines have not been conducted.
Pregnancy Category B: Reproduction studies have been performed in rats at doses up to 50 mg/kg/day and have revealed no evidence of impaired fertility or harm to the fetus due to Pyridium. There are, however, no adequate and well controlled studies in pregnant women. Because animal reproduction studies are not always predictive of human response, this drug should be used during pregnancy only if clearly needed.
Nursing Mothers: No information is available on the appearance of Pyridium or its metabolites in human milk.

ADVERSE REACTIONS
Headache, rash, pruritus and occasional gastrointestinal disturbance. An anaphylactoid-like reaction has been described. Methemoglobinemia, hemolytic anemia, renal and hepatic toxicity have been described, usually at overdose levels (see Overdosage section). Staining of contact lenses has been reported.

OVERDOSAGE
Exceeding the recommended dose in patients with good renal function or administering the usual dose to patients with impaired renal function (common in elderly patients), may lead to increased serum levels and toxic reactions. Methemoglobinemia generally follows a massive, acute overdose. Methylene blue, 1 to 2 mg/kg body weight intravenously, or ascorbic acid 100 to 200 mg given orally should cause prompt reduction of the methemoglobinemia and disappearance of the cyanosis which is an aid in diagnosis. Oxidative Heinz body hemolytic anemia may also occur, and "bite cells" (degmacytes) may be present in a chronic overdosage situation. Red blood cell G-6-PD deficiency may predispose to hemolysis. Renal and hepatic impairment and occasional failure, usually due to hypersensitivity, may also occur.

DOSAGE AND ADMINISTRATION
100 mg tablets: Adult dosage is two tablets 3 times a day after meals. 200 mg tablets: Adult dosage is one tablet 3 times a day after meals.
When used concomitantly with an antibacterial agent for the treatment of a urinary tract infection, the administration of Pyridium should not exceed 2 days.

HOW SUPPLIED
N 0071-0180-24   100 mg tablets
     Bottles of 100
N 0071-0180-32   100 mg tablets
     Bottles of 1000
N 0071-0180-40   100 mg tablets Unit dose packages of 100
     (10 strips of 10)
Tablets are dark maroon, coated, round and coded P-D 180.
N 0071-0181-24   200 mg tablets
     Bottles of 100
N 0071-0181-32   200 mg tablets
     Bottles of 1000
N 0071-0181-40   200 mg tablets Unit dose packages of 100
     (10 strips of 10)
Tablets are dark maroon, coated, round and coded P-D 181.
Store at controlled room temperature 15° to 30° C (59° to 86° F).
AHFS Category 84:08   **0180G015**
Shown in Product Identification Section, page 422

PYRIDIUM® PLUS Tablets   ℞
[py″ri′di-ŭm]

DESCRIPTION
Each Pyridium Plus tablet contains:
150 mg phenazopyridine hydrochloride (Pyridium®)
0.3 mg hyoscyamine hydrobromide
15 mg butabarbital
Also contains: carnauba wax, NF; corn starch, NF; D&C Red No. 7 Lake; FD&C Blue No. 2 Lake; FD&C Yellow No. 8 Lake; gelatin, NF; lactose, NF; magnesium stearate, NF; sodium starch glycolate, NF; sucrose, NF; titanium dioxide, USP; white wax, NF.

CLINICAL PHARMACOLOGY
Pyridium Plus relieves lower urinary symptoms of pain, frequency, urgency, burning and dysuria arising from inflammation of the urothelium, the mucosal lining of the lower urinary tract.
Lower urinary tract pain can cause reflex spasm of the detrusor. Pain and spasm are often aggravated by apprehension to promote a pain-spasm-apprehension cycle. Each of the three pharmacologic components of Pyridium Plus acts against a phase of this cycle.
Phenazopyridine hydrochloride (Pyridium), excreted in the urine, is a topical analgesic to relieve pain and discomfort. Hyoscyamine hydrobromide, a parasympatholytic, acts to relieve detrusor muscle spasm. Butabarbital, a short-to-intermediate-acting sedative, helps to allay associated anxiety and apprehension.

INDICATIONS AND USAGE
Pyridium Plus is indicated for the symptomatic relief of pain, burning, frequency, urgency, and dysuria, particularly when accompanied by detrusor muscle spasm and apprehension.
These symptoms may arise from infection, trauma, surgery, endoscopic procedures, or passage of sounds or catheters. Therapy with Pyridium Plus does not interfere with antibacterial therapy and can help to relieve symptoms of pain and discomfort before definitive treatment is effective. The use of Pyridium Plus for symptomatic relief should not delay definitive diagnosis and treatment. Treatment of a urinary tract infection with Pyridium Plus should not exceed 2 days because there is a lack of evidence that the combined administration of phenazopyridine hydrochloride and an antibacterial provides greater benefit than administration of the anti-

Continued on next page

This product information was prepared in August, 1989. On these and other Parke-Davis Products, information may be obtained by addressing PARKE-DAVIS, Division of Warner-Lambert Company, Morris Plains, New Jersey 07950.

Parke-Davis—Cont.

bacterial alone after 2 days. (See DOSAGE and ADMINIS-TRATION Section.)

In the absence of infection, Pyridium Plus may be the only medication required.

CONTRAINDICATIONS

Pyridium Plus should not be used in patients who have previously exhibited hypersensitivity to any component. The use of Pyridium Plus is contraindicated in patients with renal or hepatic insufficiency, glaucoma, bladder neck obstruction, porphyria.

WARNING

BUTABARBITAL MAY BE HABIT-FORMING. Drowsiness or dizziness may occur. Patients should be instructed to use caution in driving or operating machinery.

PRECAUTIONS

General: A yellowish tinge of the skin or sclera may indicate accumulation due to impaired renal excretion of phenazopyridine (Pyridium) and the need to discontinue therapy.

The decline in renal function asssociated with advanced age should be kept in mind.

Information for Patients: Phenazopyridine hydrochloride produces an orange to red color in the urine and may stain fabric. Staining of contact lenses has been reported. Butabarbital may cause drowsiness or dizziness, patients should be instructed to use caution in driving or operating machinery.

Laboratory Test Interactions: Due to its properties as an azo dye, phenazopyridine hydrochloride may interfere with urinalysis based on spectrometry or color reactions.

Carcinogenesis, Mutagenesis, Impairment of Fertility: Pyridium Plus has not undergone adequate studies relating to carcinogenesis, mutagenesis, or impairment of fertility; however, the component phenazopyridine hydrochloride has induced neoplasia in rats (large intestine) and mice (liver). Although no association between phenazopyridine hydrochloride and human neoplasia has been reported, adequate epidemiological studies along these lines have not been conducted.

Pregnancy Category C: Animal reproduction studies have not been conducted with Pyridium Plus. It is also not known whether Pyridium Plus can cause fetal harm when administered to a pregnant woman or can affect reproduction capacity. Pyridium Plus should be given to a pregnant woman only if clearly needed.

Nursing Mothers: No information is available on the appearance of the components of Pyridium Plus in human milk.

ADVERSE REACTIONS

Methemoglobinemia, hemolytic anemia, and renal and hepatic toxicity have been described for phenazopyridine, usually at overdosage levels (see Overdosage Section). Headache, rash, pruritus and occasional gastrointestinal disturbance. An anaphylactoid-like reaction has been described.

Hyoscyamine hydrobromide is an atropinic drug that may produce adverse effects characteristic of this class of drugs. Dry mouth, drowsiness, or dizziness is noted in more than one third of patients (and may occur in half of the patients of older age groups). Other atropine-like effects, such as blurred vision, may occur. There may be occasional gastrointestinal disturbances.

Butabarbital is a short- to intermediate-acting barbiturate which has the potential for adverse reactions attributable to barbiturates.

OVERDOSAGE

Pyridium Plus is a combination of three active drugs, and overdosage can be expected to show the effects related to each ingredient. Management includes the usual measures to empty the stomach by emesis or lavage, administration of a charcoal slurry, and supportive measures as needed.

Toxicity and management suggestions relating to the individual ingredients are as follows:

Phenazopyridine Hydrochloride (Pyridium): Exceeding the recommended dose in patients with good renal function or administering the usual dose to patients with impaired renal function (common in elderly patients), may lead to increased serum levels and toxic reactions. Methemoglobinemia generally follows a massive, acute overdose. Methylene blue, 1 to 2 mg/kg body weight intravenously or ascorbic acid 100 to 200 mg given orally should cause prompt reduction of the methemoglobinemia and disappearance of cyanosis which is an aid

in diagnosis. Oxidative Heinz body hemolytic anemia may also occur, and "bite cells" (degmacytes) may be present in a chronic overdosage situation. Red blood cell G-6-PD deficiency may predispose to hemolysis. Renal and hepatic impairment and occasional failure, usually due to hypersensitivity, may also occur.

Hyoscyamine Hydrobromide: Overdosage of hyoscyamine, a form of atropine, will cause dilated pupils, blurred vision, rapid pulse, increased intraocular tension, hot, dry, red skin, dry mouth, disorientation, delirium, fever, convulsions, and coma. As an antidote, physostigmine salicylate may be given IV slowly. Dilute 1 mg in 5 ml of saline and use 1 ml of this dilution in children. Repeat every five minutes as needed up to a total of 2 mg in children, or 6 mg in adults every 30 minutes.

Butabarbital: This drug may produce sedation and respiratory depression progressing to coma, depending on the amount ingested. General and supportive measures should be instituted.

DOSAGE AND ADMINISTRATION

Adult Dosage: One tablet four times a day (after meals and at bedtime).

When used concomitantly with an antibacterial agent for the treatment of a urinary tract infection, the administration of Pyridium Plus should not exceed 2 days.

HOW SUPPLIED

N 0071-0182-24 Bottles of 100. Tablets are dark maroon, coated, square and coded P-D 182.

Store at controlled room temperature 15° to 30°C (59° to 86°F).

AHFS Category 8:12.24   0182G065

Shown in Product Identification Section, page 422

SURITAL®   ©℞
[sŭ 'rĭ-tăl "]
(thiamylal sodium for injection, USP)

DESCRIPTION

Surital (thiamylal sodium for injection, USP) is sodium-5-allyl-5-(1-methylbutyl)-2-thiobarbiturate.

ACTIONS

Thiamylal sodium is a rapid, ultra-short-acting barbiturate, intravenous, anesthetic agent.

INDICATIONS

Surital is indicated for induction of anesthesia, for supplementing other anesthetic agents, as intravenous anesthesia for short surgical procedures with minimal painful stimuli, or as an agent for inducing a hypnotic state.

CONTRAINDICATIONS

Thiamylal sodium is contraindicated when general anesthesia is contraindicated, in patients with latent or manifest porphyria, or in patients with a known hypersensitivity to barbiturates.

WARNINGS

RESUSCITATIVE EQUIPMENT AND DRUGS SHOULD BE IMMEDIATELY AVAILABLE. This drug should be administered by persons qualified in the use of intravenous anesthetics.

Repeated and continuous infusion may cause cumulative effects resulting in prolonged somnolence, and respiratory and circulatory depression.

Usage in pregnancy: Safe use of thiamylal sodium has not been established with respect to adverse effects upon fetal development. Therefore, thiamylal sodium should not be used in women of childbearing potential, and particularly during early pregnancy, unless, in the judgment of the physician, the expected benefits outweigh the potential hazards.

PRECAUTIONS

Respiratory depression, apnea, or hypotension may occur due to variations in tolerance from individual to individual or to physical status of patient. Caution should be exercised in debilitated patients, or those with impaired function of respiratory, circulatory, renal, hepatic, and endocrine systems.

Thiamylal sodium should be used with extreme caution in patients in status asthmaticus.

Extravascular injection may cause pain, swelling, ulceration, and necrosis. Intra-arterial injection is dangerous and may produce gangrene of an extremity.

ADVERSE REACTIONS

The following adverse reactions have been reported: circulatory depression, thrombophlebitis, pain at injection site, and respiratory depression, including apnea, laryngospasm, bronchospasm, salivation, hiccups, emergence delirium, headache, injury to nerves adjacent to injection site, skin rashes, urticaria, nausea, and emesis.

DOSAGE AND ADMINISTRATION

The dosage is individualized according to the patient's response.

A 2.5% solution is recommended for induction of anesthesia as well as for maintenance by intermittent intravenous injection. A dilute solution (0.3%) may be used by continuous drip for maintenance. The rate of injection during induction should be approximately 1 ml of 2.5% solution every five seconds; an initial injection of 3 to 6 ml of 2.5% solution is generally sufficient to produce short periods of surgical anesthesia.

Sterile Water for Injection is the preferred solvent for preparing Surital (thiamylal sodium for injection, USP) solutions. Initially, Surital solutions are clear, but they may become cloudy on aging. Thiamylal sodium cannot be reconstituted with Ringer's Solution or solutions containing bacteriostatic or buffer agents, because they may tend to cause precipitation. In preparing dilute solutions for continuous drip maintenance, either 5% dextrose or isotonic sodium chloride should be used instead of sterile water for injection to avoid extreme hypotonicity. Dextrose solutions are occasionally sufficiently acid, however, to cause precipitation. Injection of air into the solution should be avoided because this may hasten the development of cloudiness.

Solutions of atropine sulfate, d-tubocurarine, or succinylcholine may be given concurrently with Surital, but they should not be mixed prior to administration.

Thiamylal sodium solutions should be prepared under aseptic conditions. Solutions cannot be heated for sterilization. The solutions should be stored in a refrigerator and used within six days. If kept at room temperature, the solution should be used within 24 hours. Only clear solutions should be used; discard if cloudiness or precipitate form. Refrigeration of the reconstituted Surital contributes to the maintenance of a clear solution.

[See table below].

HOW SUPPLIED

Surital is supplied as follows.

N 0071-4064-03 (35-64-25)
1 g, in packages of 25 (Steri-Vial® 64)
N 0071-4122-08 (35-122-10)
5 g, in packages of 10 (Steri-Vial 122)
N 0071-4123-10 (35-123-10)
10 g, in packages of 10 (Steri-Vial 123)

AHFS 28:24   4064G020

TEDRAL®SA   ℞
[tĕd 'ral]

DESCRIPTION

Tedral SA: Each tablet contains 180 mg anhydrous theophylline (90 mg in the immediate release layer and 90 mg in the sustained release layer); 48 mg ephedrine hydrochloride (16 mg in the immediate release layer and 32 mg in the sustained release layer); 25 mg phenobarbital in the immediate release layer.

Also contains: D&C red No. 30 and yellow No. 10 Lake; lactose, NF; magnesium stearate, NF; starch; sucrose and other ingredients.

ACTIONS

Tedral SA combines theophylline and ephedrine—widely accepted oral bronchodilators with differing modes of action. From experimental evidence,[1] it appears that a combination of a sympathomimetic and methylxanthine is more effective than either drug alone in inhibiting the release of bronchoconstricting mediators (histamine and slow-reacting substance of anaphylaxis) produced by antigen-antibody (IgE) interaction on sensitive cells. Th β-adrenergic stimulation by the sympathomimetics produces cyclic $3'5'$-adenosine monophosphate (cAMP), and the degradation of cAMP by the specific enzyme, phosphodiesterase, is inhibited by methylxanthines. Thus, at present, the principal action of Tedral SA in the relief or prevention of bronchoconstriction appears to be involved with the cAMP system.

Phenobarbital is incorporated into Tedral SA to counteract possible stimulation by ephedrine and to provide a mild, long-acting sedative for the apprehensive asthmatic patient. Tedral SA provides sustained as well as immediate bronchodilatation for the asthmatic patient, with the convenience of bid dosage.

INDICATIONS

Tedral SA is indicated for the symptomatic relief of bronchial asthma, asthmatic bronchitis, and other bronchospastic disorders. It may also be used prophylactically to abort or

---

PREPARING *SURITAL* SOLUTIONS

Surital (g)	Amount of solvent required (in ml) for percentage solutions shown								
	0.2%	0.3%	0.4%	2%	2.5%	3%	4%	5%	10%
1	500	333	250	50	40	33.3	25	20	10
5	2,500	1,670	1,250	250	200	167	125	100	50
10	5,000	3,333	2,500	500	400	333	250	200	100

minimize asthmatic attacks and is of value in managing occasional, seasonal, or perennial asthma.

Tedral SA (Sustained Action) offers the convenience of bid dosage.

This Tedral formulation is an adjunct in the total management of the asthmatic patient. Acute or severe asthmatic attacks may necessitate supplemental therapy with other drugs by inhalation or other parenteral routes.

CONTRAINDICATIONS

Sensitivity to any of the ingredients; porphyria.

WARNINGS

Drowsiness may occur. Phenobarbital may be habit forming.

PRECAUTIONS

Use with caution in the presence of cardiovascular disease, severe hypertension, hyperthyroidism, prostatic hypertrophy, or glaucoma.

ADVERSE REACTIONS

Mild epigastric distress, palpitation, tremulousness, insomnia, difficulty of micturition, and CNS stimulation have been reported.

DOSAGE AND ADMINISTRATION

Adults—one tablet on arising and one tablet 12 hours later. Tablets should not be chewed.

Children—not established for children under 12.

HOW SUPPLIED

Tedral SA is supplied as double-layered, uncoated, coral/mottled white tablets in bottles of 100 (N 0071-0231-24) and 1000 (N 0071-0231-32).

Store between 15°-30°C (59°-86°F).

Reference: 1. Koopman WJ, Orange RP, Austen KF. *J Immunol* 105:1096, November 1970.

0231G113

THROMBOSTAT®   ℞
(Thrombin, USP) Bovine Origin

Thrombostat must not be injected! Apply on the surface of bleeding tissue as a solution or powder.

DESCRIPTION

Thrombostat (Thrombin, USP) is a protein substance produced through a conversion reaction in which prothrombin of bovine origin is activated by tissue thromboplastin in the presence of calcium chloride. It is supplied as a sterile powder that has been freeze-dried in the final container. Also contained in this preparation are calcium chloride, sodium chloride, and aminoacetic acid (glycine) as follows: calcium chloride—5 mg per 5000 unit vial, 10 mg per 10,000 unit vial, and 21 mg per 20,000 unit vial; sodium chloride—8 mg per 5000 unit vial, 15 mg per 10,000 unit vial, and 30 mg per 20,000 unit vial; aminoacetic acid—39 mg per 5000 unit vial, 78 mg per 10,000 unit vial, and 156 mg per 20,000 unit vial. Glycine is included to make the dried product friable and more readily soluble.

A 5 mL, 10 mL, or 20 mL vial of Isotonic Saline is enclosed to be used as a diluent with the 5 mL, 5000 unit; 10 mL, 10,000 unit; or 20 mL, 20,000 unit vial, respectively, of Thrombostat. Isotonic Saline is a sterile, isotonic solution of sodium chloride in Water For Injection, USP. It contains Phemerol® (benzethonium chloride) 0.02 mg per mL as a preservative. (See Dosage and Administration for additional information on diluents which may be used.)

This product is prepared under rigid assay control. A unit is defined as the amount required to clot 1 mL of standardized fibrinogen solution in 15 seconds.

Approximately 2 units are required to clot 1 mL of oxalated human plasma in the same period of time.

CLINICAL PHARMACOLOGY

Thrombostat requires no intermediate physiological agent for its action. It clots the fibrinogen of the blood directly. Failure to clot blood occurs in the rare case where the primary clotting defect is the absence of fibrinogen itself. The speed with which thrombin clots blood is dependent upon its concentration. For example, the contents of a 5000 unit vial of Thrombostat dissolved in 5 mL of saline diluent is capable of clotting an equal volume of blood in less than a second, or 1000 mL in less than a minute.

INDICATIONS AND USAGE

Thrombostat (Thrombin, USP) is indicated as an aid in hemostasis wherever oozing blood from capillaries and small venules is accessible.

In various types of surgery solutions of Thrombostat may be used in conjunction with Absorbable Gelatin Sponge, USP for hemostasis.

CONTRAINDICATIONS

Thrombostat is contraindicated in persons known to be sensitive to any of its components and/or to material of bovine origin.

WARNING

Because of its action in the clotting mechanism, Thrombostat must not be injected or otherwise allowed to enter large blood vessels. Extensive intravascular clotting and even death may result. Thrombostat is an antigenic substance and has caused sensitivity and allergic reactions when injected into animals.

PRECAUTIONS

General: Consult the absorbable gelatin sponge product labeling for complete information for use prior to utilizing the thrombin-saturated sponge procedure.

Pregnancy—

Teratogenic effects: Pregnancy Category C. Animal reproduction studies have not been conducted with Thrombin, USP. It is also not known whether Thrombin, USP can cause fetal harm when administered to a pregnant woman or can affect reproduction capacity. Thrombin, Topical (Bovine) should be given to a pregnant woman only if clearly indicated.

Pediatric Use: Safety and effectiveness in children have not been established.

ADVERSE REACTIONS

An allergic type reaction following the use of Thrombostat for treatment of epistaxis has been reported. Febrile reactions have also been observed following the use of Thrombostat in certain surgical procedures but no cause-effect relationship has been established.

DOSAGE AND ADMINISTRATION

General: Solutions of Thrombostat may be prepared in sterile distilled water or isotonic saline. The intended use determines the strength of the solution to prepare. For general use in plastic surgery, dental extractions, skin grafting, neurosurgery, etc, solutions containing approximately 100 units per mL are frequently used. For this, an appropriate dilution of Thrombostat should be prepared to yield a concentration of 100 units per mL. Where bleeding is profuse, as from cut surfaces of liver and spleen, concentrations as high as 1000 to 2000 units per mL may be required. For this the 5000 unit vial dissolved in 5 mL or 2.5 mL, respectively, of the diluent supplied in the package is convenient. Intermediate strengths to suit the needs of the case may be prepared by selecting the proper strength package and dissolving the contents in an appropriate volume of diluent. In many situations, it may be advantageous to use Thrombostat in dry form on oozing surfaces.

Caution:

Solutions should be used immediately upon reconstitution. If necessary, refrigerate the solution and use within 3 hours of reconstitution.

The following techniques are suggested for the topical application of Thrombostat.

1. The recipient surface should be sponged (not wiped) free of blood before Thrombostat is applied.

2. A spray may be used or the surface may be flooded using a sterile syringe and small gauge needle. The most effective hemostasis results when the Thrombostat mixes freely with the blood as soon as it reaches the surface.

3. In instances where Thrombostat in dry form is needed, the vial is opened by removing the metal ring by flipping up the plastic cap and tearing counterclockwise. The rubber-diaphragm cap may be easily removed and the dried Thrombostat is then broken up into a powder by means of a sterile glass rod or other suitable sterile instrument.

4. Sponging of treated surfaces should be avoided in order that the clot remain securely in place.

Thrombostat may be used in conjunction with Absorbable Gelatin Sponge, USP as follows:

1. Prepare Thrombostat solution of the desired strength.

2. Immerse sponge strips of the desired size in the Thrombostat solution. Knead the sponge strips vigorously with moistened gloved fingers to remove trapped air, thereby facilitating saturation of the sponge.

3. Apply saturated sponge to bleeding area. Hold in place for 10 to 15 seconds with a pledget of cotton or a small gauze sponge.

Sterile Packages

Thrombostat Sterile Packages are available in two strengths, 5000 units and 10,000 units. A Sterile Package contains one sterile vial of Thrombostat, one sterile vial of Isotonic Saline Diluent, and one sterile transfer device. The Sterile Package may be used as follows:

1. Remove the Tyvek® blister lid by pulling up at the indicated corner. The sterile inner tray can be lifted out or introduced into the operating field.

2. The cover to the sterile inner tray is removed by pulling up on the finger tab, exposing the sterile contents.

3. Thrombostat solution of the desired strength is prepared using the transfer device.

4. Alternatively, when Thrombostat in dry form is needed, the vial is opened as described above and the dried Thrombostat broken up into a powder by means of a sterile glass rod or other suitable sterile instrument.

Kits

Thrombostat Kits are available in two strengths, 10,000 units and 20,000 units. The 10,000 unit kit contains one sterile 10,000 unit vial of Thrombostat, one sterile vial of Isotonic Saline Diluent, one sterile transfer device, and one sterile pump sprayer cap. The 20,000 unit kit contains one sterile 20,000 unit vial of Thrombostat, one sterile vial of Isotonic Saline Diluent, one sterile transfer device, and one sterile pump sprayer cap. The kit may be used as follows:

1. Remove the Tyvek® blister lid by pulling up at the indicated corner. The sterile inner tray can be lifted out or introduced into the operating field.

2. The cover to the sterile inner tray is removed by pulling up on the finger tab, exposing the sterile contents.

3. Thrombostat solution of the desired strength is prepared using the transfer device. See directions above. After reconstitution, the pump sprayer cap is inserted and seated on the Thrombostat solution vial. Note: Several strokes of the pump sprayer will be required before the Thrombostat solution is expelled.

4. Alternatively, when Thrombostat in dry form is needed, the vial is opened as described above and the dried Thrombostat broken up into a powder by means of a sterile glass rod or other suitable sterile instrument.

HOW SUPPLIED

Thrombostat is supplied as:

N 0071-4173-35—Package contains one 5000 unit vial of Thrombostat and one 5 mL vial of Isotonic Saline Diluent with Phemerol, 0.02 mg per mL, as a preservative.

N 0071-4176-35—Package contains one 10,000 unit vial of Thrombostat and one 10 mL vial of Isotonic Saline Diluent with Phemerol, 0.02 mg per mL, as a preservative.

N 0071-4180-35—Package contains one 20,000 unit vial of Thrombostat and one 20 mL vial of Isotonic Saline Diluent with Phemerol, 0.02 mg per mL, as a preservative.

N 0071-4173-36—Sterile Package contains one sterile 5000 unit vial of Thrombostat, one sterile 5 mL vial of Isotonic Saline Diluent with Phemerol, 0.02 mg per mL, as a preservative, and one sterile transfer device in a sterile tray with a Tyvek lid.

N 0071-4176-36—Sterile Package contains one sterile 10,000 unit vial of Thrombostat, one sterile 10 mL vial of Isotonic Saline Diluent with Phemerol, 0.02 mg per mL, as a preservative, and one sterile transfer device in a sterile tray with a Tyvek lid.

N 0071-4176-37—Kit contains one sterile 10,000 unit vial of Thrombostat, one sterile 10 mL vial of Isotonic Saline Diluent with Phemerol, 0.02 mg per mL, as a preservative, one sterile transfer device, and one sterile pump sprayer cap in a sterile tray with a Tyvek lid.

N 0071-4180-36—Kit contains one sterile 20,000 unit vial of Thrombostat, one sterile 20 mL vial of Isotonic Saline Diluent with Phemerol, 0.02 mg per mL, as a preservative, one sterile transfer device, and one sterile pump sprayer cap in a sterile tray with a Tyvek lid.

STORAGE

Store at room temperature 15 to 30°C (59 to 86°F).

Caution—Federal law prohibits dispensing without prescription.

Tyvek is a registered trademark of E. I. du Pont de Nemours & Co.

4173G200

VIRA-A®   ℞
[vĭ"rä ā']
(vidarabine concentrate for injection, USP)

DESCRIPTION

Vira-A is the trade name for vidarabine (also known as adenine arabinoside and Ara-A), an antiviral drug. Vira-A is a purine nucleoside obtained from fermentation cultures of *Streptomyces antibioticus*. Each milliliter of sterile suspension contains 200 milligrams of vidarabine monohydrate equivalent to 187.4 milligrams of vidarabine. Each milliliter contains 0.1 milligrams Phemerol® (benzethonium chloride) as a preservative; sodium phosphate, USP, 1.8 milligrams, and sodium biphosphate, USP, 4.8 milligrams as buffering agents. Hydrochloric acid may have been added to adjust pH. Vira-A is a white, crystalline solid with this empirical formula: $C_{10}H_{13}N_5O_4 \cdot H_2O$. The molecular weight is 285.2; the solubility is 0.45 mg/ml at 25°C; and the melting point ranges from 260° to 270°C. The chemical name is 9-β-D-arabinofuranosyladenine monohydrate.

Continued on next page

This product information was prepared in August, 1989. On these and other Parke-Davis Products, information may be obtained by addressing PARKE-DAVIS, Division of Warner-Lambert Company, Morris Plains, New Jersey 07950.

Parke-Davis—Cont.

CLINICAL PHARMACOLOGY

Following intravenous administration, Vira-A is rapidly deaminated into arabinosylhypoxanthine (Ara-Hx), the principal metabolite, which is promptly distributed into the tissues. In adults peak Ara-Hx and vidarabine plasma levels ranging from 3 to 6 µg/ml and 0.2 to 0.4 µg/ml, respectively, are attained after slow intravenous infusion of Vira-A doses of 10 mg/kg of body weight. These levels reflect the rate of infusion and show no accumulation across time. The mean half-life of Ara-Hx is 3.3 hours. Ara-Hx penetrates into the cerebrospinal fluid (CSF) to give a CSF/plasma ratio of approximately 1:3.

Excretion of Vira-A is principally via the kidneys. Urinary excretion is constant over 24 hours. Forty-one percent to 53% of the daily dose is recovered in the urine as Ara-Hx with 1% to 3% appearing as the parent compound. There is no evidence of fecal excretion of drug or metabolites. In patients with impaired renal function Ara-Hx may accumulate in the plasma and reach levels several-fold higher than those described above.

Vira-A possesses *in vitro* and *in vivo* antiviral activity against Herpes simplex virus types 1 and 2 (HSV-1 and HSV-2), and *in vitro* activity against varicella-zoster virus (VZV). The antiviral mechanism of action has not yet been established. Vidarabine is converted into nucleotides which inhibit viral DNA polymerase. In KB cells infected with Herpes simplex virus type 1, Vira-A inhibits viral DNA synthesis. Vira-A is rapidly deaminated to Ara-Hx, the principal metabolite, in cell cultures, laboratory animals, and humans.

Ara-Hx also possesses *in vitro* antiviral activity but this activity is significantly less than the activity of Vira-A.

INDICATIONS AND USAGE

Herpes Simplex Virus Encephalitis—Vira-A is indicated for the treatment of Herpes simplex virus encephalitis. Controlled studies indicated that Vira-A therapy will reduce the mortality caused by Herpes simplex virus encephalitis from 70 to 28% 30 days following onset. In a larger uncontrolled study of 75 patients with biopsy-proven herpes simplex encephalitis, the mortality 6 months from onset was 39%, similar to 44% in the initial controlled study at 6 months.

Morbidity from both studies one year after onset was: normal 53%, moderately debilitated 29%, and severely damaged 18%. Vira-A does not appear to alter morbidity and resulting serious neurological sequelae in the comatose patient. Therefore early diagnosis and treatment are essential. Herpes simplex virus encephalitis should be suspected in patients with a history of an acute febrile encephalopathy associated with disordered mentation, altered level of consciousness and focal cerebral signs.

Studies which may support the suspected diagnosis include examination of cerebrospinal fluid and localization of an intra-cerebral lesion by brain scan, electroencephalography or computerized axial tomography (CAT).

Brain biopsy is required in order to confirm the etiological diagnosis by means of viral isolation in cell cultures. Detection of Herpes simplex virus in the biopsied brain tissue can also be reliably done by specific fluorescent antibody techniques. Detection of Herpes virus-like particles by electron microscopy or detection of intranuclear inclusions by histopathologic techniques only provides a presumptive diagnosis.

Neonatal Herpes Simplex Virus Infections—Vira-A is also indicated for the treatment of Herpes simplex infections in the newborn, including disseminated infection with visceral involvement, encephalitis, and infections of the skin, eyes and mouth. Controlled studies indicated that Vira-A therapy reduced mortality in encephalitis and disseminated infection from 74% to 38%. Following Vira-A therapy the incidence of neurological abnormalities at one year of age was 44% in infants with localized CNS infection and 67% in infants with disseminated infection. Therefore, early diagnosis and treatment are essential to reduce both mortality and morbidity.

Herpes simplex virus infections should be suspected in babies born to mothers with a history of genital or nongenital Herpes simplex virus infections during gestation or prior to the onset of labor or to mothers with a sexual partner with a history of genital Herpes simplex virus infections. A sick newborn suspected of having a herpes virus infection may present with fever, lethargy, poor feeding or seizures. Most of the infected newborns will develop skin vesicles (about 70%) with or without signs and symptoms of CNS infection or visceral dissemination (hepatitis, pneumonitis, intravascular coagulopathy). The etiological diagnosis is established by isolation of HSV from skin vesicles, mouth, conjunctivae, cerebrospinal fluid, blood, or brain biopsy.

Herpes zoster—Vira-A is indicated for the treatment of herpes zoster (shingles) due to reactivated varicella-zoster virus infections in immunosuppressed patients. Placebo-controlled studies have shown that Vira-A significantly reduced

the severity of acute pain, new vesicle formation, time to pustulation and scabbing, cutaneous dissemination inside and outside the primary dermatome(s), and the overall frequency of visceral complications (uveitis or keratitis, hepatitis, encephalitis and peripheral neuropathy). To be effective, Vira-A therapy should be initiated as early as possible, within 72 hours after the appearance of vesicular lesions. Herpes zoster is recognized by the formation of clear skin vesicles progressing to pustules and scabs along a sensory nerve distribution. The appearance of vesicles may be preceded by fever, local pain and erythema. Varicella-zoster virus can be isolated from vesicular lesions or detected by fluorescent antibody techniques.

CONTRAINDICATIONS

Vira-A is contraindicated in patients who develop hypersensitivity reactions to it.

WARNINGS

Vira-A should not be administered by the intramuscular or subcutaneous route because of its low solubility and poor absorption.

There are no reports available to indicate that Vira-A for infusion is effective in the management of encephalitis due to varicella-zoster or vaccinia viruses. Vira-A is not effective against infections caused by adenovirus or RNA viruses. It is also not effective against bacterial or fungal infections. There are no data to support efficacy of Vira-A against cytomegalovirus, vaccinia virus, or smallpox virus.

PRECAUTIONS

General—Treatment should be discontinued in adult or pediatric patients with a clinical diagnosis of suspected encephalitis if the brain biopsy specimen is negative for Herpes simplex virus in cell cultures.

Special care should be exercised when administering Vira-A to patients susceptible to fluid overloading or cerebral edema. Examples are patients with CNS infections and impaired renal function.

Patients with impaired renal function, such as post-operative renal transplant recipients, may have a slower rate of renal excretion of Ara-Hx. Therefore, the dose of Vira-A may need to be adjusted according to the severity of impairment. These patients should be carefully monitored.

Patients with impaired liver function should also be observed for possible adverse effects.

Patients with Herpes simplex encephalitis or newborns with Herpes simplex infections should be managed by physicians skilled in the treatment of these diseases.

Although clear evidence of adverse experience in humans from simultaneous Vira-A and allopurinol administration has not been reported, laboratory studies indicate that allopurinol may interfere with Vira-A metabolism. Therefore, caution is recommended when administering Vira-A to patients receiving allopurinol.

Laboratory Tests—Appropriate hematologic tests are recommended during Vira-A administration since hemoglobin, hematocrit, white blood cells, and platelets may be depressed during therapy.

Some degree of immunocompetence must be present in order for Vira-A to achieve clinical response.

Carcinogenesis—Chronic parenteral (IM) studies of vidarabine have been conducted in mice and rats.

In the mouse study, there was a statistically significant increase in liver tumor incidence among the vidarabine-treated females. In the same study, some vidarabine-treated male mice developed kidney neoplasia. No renal tumors were found in the vehicle-treated control mice or the vidarabine-treated female mice.

In the rat study, intestinal, testicular, and thyroid neoplasia occurred with greater frequency among the vidarabine-treated animals than in the vehicle-treated controls. The increases in thyroid adenoma incidence in the high-dose (50 mg/kg) males and the low-dose (30 mg/kg) females were statistically significant.

Hepatic megalocytosis, associated with vidarabine treatment, has been found in short- and long-term rodent (rat and mouse) studies. It is not clear whether or not this represents a preneoplastic change.

In the Balb/3T3 *in vitro* neoplastic transformation assay, used to provide preliminary assessment of potential oncogenicity, vidarabine induced a significant and dose-related increase in transformed foci over the concentration range of 0.5–3.0 µg/ml.

Mutagenesis—Results of *in vitro* experiments indicate that vidarabine can be incorporated into mammalian DNA and can induce mutation in mammalian cells (mouse L5178Y cell line). In the Ames/Salmonella/microsome plate assay, vidarabine elicited a positive response for mutagenicity in *Salmonella typhimurium*, strain TA 1537, at high doses (2500 µg/plate). Thus far, *in vivo* studies have not been as conclusive, but there is some evidence (dominant lethal assay in mice) that vidarabine may be capable of producing mutagenic effects in male germ cells.

It has also been reported that vidarabine causes chromosome breaks and gaps when added to human leukocytes *in vitro*. Vidarabine also induced significant dose-related increases in

chromosome aberrations (breaks and exchange aberrations) in Chinese hamster ovary cells *in vitro*. While the significance of these effects in terms of mutagenicity is not fully understood, there is a well-known correlation between the ability of various agents to produce such effects and their ability to produce heritable genetic damage.

Pregnancy Category C—Vira-A given parenterally is teratogenic in rats and rabbits. Doses of 5 mg/kg or higher given intramuscularly to pregnant rabbits during organogenesis induced fetal abnormalities. Doses of 3 mg/kg or less did not induce teratogenic changes in pregnant rabbits. Vira-A doses ranging from 30 to 250 mg/kg were given intramuscularly to pregnant rats during organogenesis; signs of maternal toxicity were induced at doses of 100 mg/kg or higher and frank fetal anomalies were found at doses of 150 to 250 mg/kg.

A safe dose for the human embryo or fetus has not been established.

There are no adequate and well controlled studies in pregnant women. Vira-A should be used during pregnancy only if the potential benefit justifies the potential risk to the fetus.

Nursing Mothers—It is not known whether Vira-A is excreted in human milk. Because many drugs are excreted in human milk and because of the potential tumorigenicity shown for Vira-A in animal studies, a decision should be made whether to discontinue nursing or to discontinue the drug, taking into account the importance of the drug to the mother.

ADVERSE REACTIONS

The principal adverse reactions in adults involve the gastrointestinal tract and are anorexia, nausea, vomiting, and diarrhea. These reactions are mild to moderate, and seldom require termination of Vira-A therapy.

CNS disturbances have been reported at therapeutic doses. These are tremor, dizziness, hallucinations, confusion, psychosis, ataxia, headache and encephalopathy. These adverse drug reactions have occurred mostly in patients with impaired hepatic or renal function.

Hematologic clinical laboratory changes noted in controlled and uncontrolled studies were a decrease in hemoglobin or hematocrit, white blood cell count, and platelet count. Elevations of aspartate aminotransferase (SGOT) were also observed. Other changes occasionally observed were decreases in reticulocyte count and elevated total bilirubin. In newborns with HSV infections, no clear evidence of hematologic, renal, or hepatic toxicity was noted at the recommended doses.

Other symptoms which have been reported are weight loss, malaise, pruritus, rash, hematemesis, and pain at the injection site.

OVERDOSAGE

Acute massive overdose of the intravenous form has been reported without any serious evidence of adverse effect. Because of the low solubility of Vira-A, acute water overloading would pose a greater threat to the patient than Vira-A. Doses of Vira-A over 20 mg/kg/day can produce bone marrow depression with concomitant thrombocytopenia and leukopenia. If a massive overdose of the intravenous form occurs, hematologic, liver, and renal functions should be carefully monitored.

DOSAGE AND ADMINISTRATION

CAUTION—1) THE CONTENTS OF THE VIAL MUST BE DILUTED IN AN APPROPRIATE INTRAVENOUS SOLUTION PRIOR TO ADMINISTRATION. RAPID OR BOLUS INJECTION MUST BE AVOIDED. THE DOSE DEPENDS ON THE DISEASE BEING TREATED.
2) SEE SPECIAL INSTRUCTIONS FOR PREPARATION OF VIRA-A FOR ADMINISTRATION TO NEWBORNS.

Dosage—Herpes simplex virus encephalitis—15 mg/kg/day for 10 days.

    Neonatal Herpes simplex virus infections—15 mg/kg/day for 10 days.

    Herpes zoster—10 mg/kg/day for 5 days.

Method of Preparation—Each 5-ml vial contains 1 gram of Vira-A (200 mg per ml of suspension). The solubility of Vira-A in intravenous infusion fluids is limited. Each one mg of Vira-A requires 2.22 ml of intravenous infusion fluid for complete solubilization. Therefore, each one liter of intravenous infusion fluid will solubilize a maximum of 450 mg of Vira-A.

Any appropriate intravenous solution is suitable for use as a diluent *EXCEPT* biologic or colloidal fluids (e.g., blood products, protein solutions, etc.).

Shake the Vira-A vial well to obtain a homogeneous suspension before measuring and transferring.

Prepare the Vira-A solution for intravenous administration by aseptically transferring the proper dose of Vira-A into an appropriate intravenous infusion fluid. The intravenous infusion fluid used to prepare the Vira-A solution should be prewarmed to 35° to 40°C (95° to 100°F) to facilitate solution of the drug following its transference. Depending on the dose to be given, more than one liter of intravenous infusion fluid may be required. Thoroughly agitate the prepared admixture until *completely* clear. Complete solubilization of the drug, as indicated by a completely clear solution, is ascertained by careful visual inspection. Final filtration with an in-line membrane filter (0.45 μ pore size or smaller) is necessary.

Dilution should be made just prior to administration and used at least within 48 hours. Subsequent agitation, shaking, or inversion of the bottle is unnecessary once the drug is completely in solution. DO NOT REFRIGERATE THE DILUTION.

Administration—Using aseptic technique, slowly infuse the total daily dose by intravenous infusion (prepared as discussed above) at a constant rate over a 12- to 24-hour period.
Administration to Newborns—Due to the small quantity required by the infant, 1 ml of Vira-A (200 mg per ml of suspension) should be aseptically added to 9 ml of sterile normal saline or sterile water for injection to provide a suspension of 20 mg per ml. Then prepare the Vira-A solution for intravenous infusion, as described above, by transferring the proper dose to the MINIMUM VOLUME of an appropriate intravenous fluid required to assure complete solubilization of the drug. Each 1 mg of Vira-A requires 2.22 ml of intravenous infusion fluid for complete solubilization. EXTREME CARE MUST BE EXERCISED TO MAKE CERTAIN THAT THE DRUG SOLUTION IS ADMINISTERED SLOWLY.

HOW SUPPLIED

N 0071-4150-08 (Steri-Vial® 4150) Vira-A (Vidarabine Concentrate for Injection, USP), a sterile suspension containing 200 mg/ml, is supplied in 5 ml Steri-Vials; packages of 10.

ANIMAL PHARMACOLOGY AND ANIMAL TOXICITY

Acute Toxicity: The intraperitoneal LD_{50} for Vira-A ranged from 3,890 to 4,500 mg/kg in mice, and from 2,239 to 2,512 mg/kg in rats, suggesting a low order of toxicity to a single parenteral dose. Hepatic megalocytosis was observed in rats after single, intraperitoneal injections at doses near and exceeding the LD_{50} value. The hepatic megalocytosis appeared to regress completely over several months. Acute intravenous LD_{50} values could not be obtained because of the limited solubility of Vira-A.
Subacute Toxicity: Rats, dogs, and monkeys have been given daily intramuscular injections of Vira-A as a 20% suspension for 28 days. These animal species showed dose related decreases in hemoglobin, hematocrit, and lymphocytes. Bone marrow depression was also observed in monkeys. Except for localized, injection-site injury and weight gain inhibition or loss, rats tolerated daily doses up to 150 mg/kg, and dogs tolerated daily doses up to 50 mg/kg. Megalocytosis was not seen in the rats dosed by the intramuscular route for 28 days. Rhesus monkeys were particularly sensitive to Vira-A. Daily intramuscular doses of 15 mg/kg were tolerable, but doses of 25 mg/kg or higher induced progressively severe clinical signs of CNS toxicity. Three monkeys given slow intravenous infusions of Vira-A in solution at a dose of 15 mg/kg daily for 28 days had no significant adverse reactions.

4150G022

VIRA-A®   ℞
[vĭ"ră ā']
(vidarabine ophthalmic ointment, USP), 3%

DESCRIPTION

VIRA-A is the trade name for vidarabine (also known as adenine arabinoside and Ara-A), an antiviral drug for the topical treatment of epithelial keratitis caused by Herpes simplex virus. The chemical name is 9-β-D-arabinofuranosyladenine. Each gram of the ophthalmic ointment contains 30 mg of vidarabine monohydrate equivalent to 28.11 mg of vidarabine in a sterile, inert, petrolatum base.

CLINICAL PHARMACOLOGY

Vira-A is a purine nucleoside obtained from fermentation cultures of *Streptomyces antibioticus*. Vira-A possesses *in vitro* and *in vivo* antiviral activity against Herpes simplex types 1 and 2, Varicella-Zoster, and Vaccinia viruses. Except for Rhabdovirus and Oncornavirus, Vira-A does not display *in vitro* antiviral activity against other RNA or DNA viruses, including Adenovirus.
The antiviral mechanism of action has not been established. Vira-A appears to interfere with the early steps of viral DNA synthesis. Vira-A is rapidly deaminated to arabinosyl-hypoxanthine (Ara-Hx), the principal metabolite. Ara-Hx also possesses *in vitro* antiviral activity but this activity is less than that of Vira-A. Because of the low solubility of Vira-A, trace amounts of both Vira-A and Ara-Hx can be detected in the aqueous humor only if there is an epithelial defect in the cornea. If the cornea is normal, only trace amounts of Ara-Hx can be recovered from the aqueous humor.
Systemic absorption of Vira-A should not be expected to occur following ocular administration and swallowing lacrimal secretions. In laboratory animals, Vira-A is rapidly deaminated in the gastrointestinal tract to Ara-Hx.
In contrast to topical idoxuridine, Vira-A demonstrated less cellular toxicity in the regenerating corneal epithelium in the rabbit.

INDICATIONS AND USAGE

Vira-A Ophthalmic Ointment, 3%, is indicated for the treatment of acute keratoconjunctivitis and recurrent epithelial keratitis due to Herpes simplex virus types 1 and 2. It is also effective in superficial keratitis caused by Herpes simplex virus which has not responded to topical idoxuridine or when toxic or hypersensitivity reactions to idoxuridine have occurred. The effectiveness of Vira-A Ophthalmic Ointment, 3%, against stromal keratitis and uveitis due to Herpes simplex virus has not been established.
The clinical diagnosis of keratitis caused by Herpes simplex virus is usually established by the presence of typical dendritic or geographic lesions on slit-lamp examination.
In controlled and uncontrolled clinical trials, an average of seven and nine days of continuous Vira-A Ophthalmic Ointment, 3%, therapy was required to achieve corneal re-epithelialization. In the controlled trials, 70 of 81 subjects (86%) re-epithelialized at the end of three weeks of therapy. In the uncontrolled trials, 101 of 142 subjects (71%) re-epithelialized at the end of three weeks. Seventy-five percent of the subjects in these uncontrolled trials had either not healed previously or had developed hypersensitivity to topical idoxuridine therapy.
The following topical antibiotics: gentamicin, erythromycin, and chloramphenicol; or topical steroids: prednisolone or dexamethasone, have been administered concurrently with Vira-A Ophthalmic Ointment, 3%, without an increase in adverse reactions.

CONTRAINDICATION

Vira-A Ophthalmic Ointment, 3%, is contraindicated in patients who develop hypersensitivity reactions to it.

WARNINGS

Normally, corticosteroids alone are contraindicated in Herpes simplex virus infections of the eye. If Vira-A Ophthalmic Ointment, 3%, is administered concurrently with topical corticosteroid therapy, corticosteroid-induced ocular side effects must be considered. These include corticosteroid-induced glaucoma or cataract formation and progression of a bacterial or viral infection.
Vira-A is not effective against RNA virus or adenoviral ocular infections. It is also not effective against bacterial, fungal, or chlamydial infections of the cornea or nonviral trophic ulcers.
Although viral resistance to VIRA-A has not been observed, this possibility may exist.

PRECAUTIONS

General—The diagnosis of keratoconjunctivitis due to Herpes simplex virus should be established clinically prior to prescribing VIRA-A Ophthalmic Ointment, 3%.
Patients should be forewarned that VIRA-A Ophthalmic Ointment, 3%, like any ophthalmic ointment, may produce a temporary visual haze.
Carcinogenesis—Chronic parenteral (IM) studies of vidarabine have been conducted in mice and rats.
In the mouse study, there was a statistically significant increase in liver tumor incidence among the vidarabine-treated females. In the same study some vidarabine-treated male mice developed kidney neoplasia. No renal tumors were found in the vehicle-treated control mice or the vidarabine-treated female mice.
In the rat study, intestinal, testicular, and thyroid neoplasia occurred with greater frequency among the vidarabine-treated animals than in the vehicle-treated controls. The increases in thyroid adenoma incidence in the high dose (50 mg/kg) males and the low dose (30 mg/kg) females were statistically significant.
Hepatic megalocytosis, associated with vidarabine treatment, has been found in short- and long-term rodent (rat and mouse) studies. It is not clear whether or not this represents a preneoplastic change.
The recommended frequency and duration of administration should not be exceeded (See Dosage and Administration).
Mutagenesis—Results of *in vitro* experiments indicate that vidarabine can be incorporated into mammalian DNA and can induce mutation in mammalian cells (mouse L5178Y cell line). Thus far, *in vivo* studies have not been as conclusive, but there is some evidence (dominant lethal assay in mice) that vidarabine may be capable of producing mutagenic effects in male germ cells.
It has also been reported that vidarabine causes chromosome breaks and gaps when added to human leukocytes *in vitro*. While the significance of these effects in terms of mutagenicity is not fully understood, there is a well-known correlation between the ability of various agents to produce such effects and their ability to produce heritable genetic damage.
Pregnancy Category C—VIRA-A parenterally is teratogenic in rats and rabbits. Ten percent VIRA-A ointment applied to 10% of the body surface during organogenesis induced fetal abnormalities in rabbits. When 10% VIRA-A ointment was applied to 2% to 3% of the body surface of rabbits, no fetal abnormalities were found. This dose greatly exceeds the total recommended ophthalmic dose in humans. The possibility of embryonic or fetal damage in pregnant women receiv-

ing VIRA-A Ophthalmic Ointment, 3%, is remote. The topical ophthalmic dose is small, and the drug relatively insoluble. Its ocular penetration is very low. However, a safe dose for a human embryo or fetus has not been established. There are no adequate and well controlled studies in pregnant women. VIRA-A should be used during pregnancy only if the potential benefit justifies the potential risk to the fetus.
Nursing Mothers—It is not known whether VIRA-A is secreted in human milk. Because many drugs are excreted in human milk and because of the potential for tumorigenicity shown for VIRA-A in animal studies, a decision should be made whether to discontinue nursing or to discontinue the drug, taking into account the importance of the drug to the mother. However, breast milk excretion is unlikely because VIRA-A is rapidly deaminated in the gastrointestinal tract.

ADVERSE REACTIONS

Lacrimation, foreign body sensation, conjunctival injection, burning, irritation, superficial punctate keratitis, pain, photophobia, punctal occlusion, and sensitivity have been reported with VIRA-A Ophthalmic Ointment, 3%. The following have also been reported but appear disease-related: uveitis, stromal edema, secondary glaucoma, trophic defects, corneal vascularization, and hyphema.

OVERDOSAGE

Acute massive overdosage by oral ingestion of the ophthalmic ointment has not occurred. However, the rapid deamination to arabinosylhypoxanthine should preclude any difficulty. The oral LD_{50} for vidarabine is greater than 5020 mg/kg in mice and rats. No untoward effects should result from ingestion of the entire contents of a tube.
Overdosage by ocular instillation is unlikely because any excess should be quickly expelled from the conjunctival sac. Too frequent administration should be avoided.

DOSAGE AND ADMINISTRATION

Administer approximately one half inch of VIRA-A Ophthalmic Ointment, 3%, into the lower conjunctival sac five times daily at three-hour intervals.
If there are no signs of improvement after 7 days, or complete re-epithelialization has not occurred by 21 days, other forms of therapy should be considered. Some severe cases may require longer treatment.
After re-epithelialization has occurred, treatment for an additional seven days at a reduced dosage (such as twice daily) is recommended in order to prevent recurrence.

HOW SUPPLIED

N 0071-3677-07 (Stock 18-1677-139)
VIRA-A Ophthalmic Ointment, 3%, is supplied sterile in ophthalmic ointment tubes of 3.5 g. The base is a 60:40 mixture of solid and liquid petrolatum.

3677G020

ZARONTIN®   ℞
[ză"rŏn'tĭn]
(ethosuximide, USP)
Capsules

DESCRIPTION

Zarontin (ethosuximide) is an anticonvulsant succinimide, chemically designated as alpha-ethyl-alpha-methyl-succinimide.
Each Zarontin capsule contains 250 mg ethosuximide, USP. Also contains: polyethylene glycol 400, NF. The capsule contains D&C yellow No. 10; FD&C red No. 3; gelatin, NF; glycerin, USP; and sorbitol.

ACTION

Ethosuximide suppresses the paroxysmal three-cycle-per-second spike and wave activity associated with lapses of consciousness which is common in absence (petit mal) seizures. The frequency of epileptiform attacks is reduced, apparently by depression of the motor cortex and elevation of the threshold of the central nervous system to convulsive stimuli.

INDICATION

Zarontin is indicated for the control of absence (petit mal) epilepsy.

CONTRAINDICATION

Ethosuximide should not be used in patients with a history of hypersensitivity to succinimides.

WARNINGS

Blood dyscrasias, including some with fatal outcome, have been reported to be associated with the use of ethosuximide; therefore, periodic blood counts should be performed.

Continued on next page

This product information was prepared in August, 1989. On these and other Parke-Davis Products, information may be obtained by addressing PARKE-DAVIS, Division of Warner-Lambert Company, Morris Plains, New Jersey 07950.

Parke-Davis—Cont.

Ethosuximide is capable of producing morphological and functional changes in the animal liver. In humans, abnormal liver and renal function studies have been reported. Ethosuximide should be administered with extreme caution to patients with known liver or renal diseases. Periodic urinalysis and liver function studies are advised for all patients receiving the drug.

Cases of systemic lupus erythematosus have been reported with the use of ethosuximide. The physician should be alert to this possibility.

Usage in Pregnancy: The effects of Zarontin in human pregnancy and nursing infants are unknown.

Recent reports suggest an association between the use of anticonvulsant drugs by women with epilepsy and an elevated incidence of birth defects in children born to these women. Data are more extensive with respect to phenytoin and phenobarbital, but these are also the most commonly prescribed anticonvulsants. Less systematic or anecdotal reports suggest a possible similar association with the use of all known anticonvulsant drugs.

The reports suggesting an elevated incidence of birth defects in children of drug-treated epileptic women cannot be regarded as adequate to prove a definite cause-and-effect relationship. There are intrinsic methodologic problems in obtaining adequate data on drug teratogenicity in humans. The possibility also exists that other factors, eg, genetic factors or the epileptic condition itself, may be more important than drug therapy in leading to birth defects. The great majority of mothers on anticonvulsant medication deliver normal infants. It is important to note that anticonvulsant drugs should not be discontinued in patients in whom the drug is administered to prevent major seizures because of the strong possibility of precipitating status epilepticus with attendant hypoxia and threat to life. In individual cases where the severity and frequency of the seizure disorder are such that the removal of medication does not pose a serious threat to the patient, discontinuation of the drug may be considered prior to and during pregnancy, although it cannot be said with any confidence that even minor seizures do not pose some hazard to the developing embryo or fetus.

The prescribing physician will wish to weigh these considerations in treating or counseling epileptic women of childbearing potential.

Hazardous Activities: Ethosuximide may impair the mental and/or physical abilities required for the performance of potentially hazardous tasks, such as driving a motor vehicle or other such activity requiring alertness; therefore, the patient should be cautioned accordingly.

PRECAUTIONS

Ethosuximide, when used alone in mixed types of epilepsy, may increase the frequency of grand mal seizures in some patients.

As with other anticonvulsants, it is important to proceed slowly when increasing or decreasing dosage, as well as when adding or eliminating other medication. Abrupt withdrawal of anticonvulsant medication may precipitate absence (petit mal) status.

ADVERSE REACTIONS

Gastrointestinal System: Gastrointestinal symptoms occur frequently and include anorexia, vague gastric upset, nausea and vomiting, cramps, epigastric and abdominal pain, weight loss, and diarrhea.

Hemopoietic System: Hemopoietic complications associated with the administration of ethosuximide have included leukopenia, agranulocytosis, pancytopenia, aplastic anemia, and eosinophilia.

Nervous System: Neurologic and sensory reactions reported during therapy with ethosuximide have included drowsiness, headache, dizziness, euphoria, hiccups, irritability, hyperactivity, lethargy, fatigue, and ataxia. Psychiatric or psychological aberrations associated with ethosuximide administration have included disturbances of sleep, night terrors, inability to concentrate, and aggressiveness. These effects may be noted particularly in patients who have previously exhibited psychological abnormalities. There have been rare reports of paranoid psychosis, increased libido, and increased state of depression with overt suicidal intentions.

Integumentary System: Dermatologic manifestations which have occurred with the administration of ethosuximide have included urticaria, Stevens-Johnson syndrome, systemic lupus erythematosus, and pruritic erythematous rashes.

Miscellaneous: Other reactions reported have included myopia, vaginal bleeding, swelling of the tongue, gum hypertrophy, and hirsutism.

DOSAGE AND ADMINISTRATION

<u>Zarontin Capsules</u> (ethosuximide capsules, USP): Zarontin is administered by the oral route. The initial dose for patients 3 to 6 years of age is one capsule (250 mg) per day; for patients 6 years of age and older, 2 capsules (500 mg) per day. The dose thereafter must be individualized according to the pa-

tient's response. Dosage should be increased by small increments. One useful method is to increase the daily dose by 250 mg every four to seven days until control is achieved with minimal side effects. Dosages exceeding 1.5 g daily, in divided doses, should be administered only under the strictest supervision of the physician. The *optimal* dose for most children is 20 mg/kg/day. This dose has given average plasma levels within the accepted therapeutic range of 40 to 100 mcg/ml. Subsequent dose schedules can be based on effectiveness and plasma level determinations.

Zarontin may be administered in combination with other anticonvulsants when other forms of epilepsy coexist with absence (petit mal). The *optimal* dosage for most children is 20 mg/kg/day.

HOW SUPPLIED

N 0071-0237-24 Bottle of 100. Each capsule contains 250 mg ethosuximide.

0237G022

Shown in Product Identification Section, page 422

ZARONTIN®   ℞
[ză "rŏn 'tĭn]
(ethosuximide)
Syrup

DESCRIPTION

Zarontin (ethosuximide) is an anticonvulsant succinimide, chemically designated as alpha-ethyl-alpha-methyl-succinimide.

Each teaspoonful (5 ml), for oral administration, contains 250 mg ethosuximide, USP. Also contains citric acid; anhydrous, USP; FD&C red No. 40; FD&C yellow No. 6; flavor; glycerin, USP; purified water, USP; saccharin sodium, USP; sodium benzoate, NF; sodium citrate, USP; sucrose, NF.

CLINICAL PHARMACOLOGY

Ethosuximide suppresses the paroxysmal three cycle per second spike and wave activity associated with lapses of consciousness which is common in absence (petit mal) seizures. The frequency of epileptiform attacks is reduced, apparently by depression of the motor cortex and elevation of the threshold of the central nervous system to convulsive stimuli.

INDICATION AND USAGE

Zarontin is indicated for the control of absence (petit mal) epilepsy.

CONTRAINDICATION

Ethosuximide should not be used in patients with a history of hypersensitivity to succinimides.

WARNINGS

Blood dyscrasias, including some with fatal outcome, have been reported to be associated with the use of ethosuximide; therefore, periodic blood counts should be performed. Ethosuximide is capable of producing morphological and functional changes in the animal liver. In humans, abnormal liver and renal function studies have been reported.

Ethosuximide should be administered with extreme caution to patients with known liver or renal disease. Periodic urinalysis and liver function studies are advised for all patients receiving the drug.

Cases of systemic lupus erythematosus have been reported with the use of ethosuximide. The physician should be alert to this possibility.

Hazardous Activities: Ethosuximide may impair the mental and/or physical abilities required for the performance of potentially hazardous tasks, such as driving a motor vehicle or other such activity requiring alertness; therefore, the patient should be cautioned accordingly.

Usage in Pregnancy: The effects of Zarontin in human pregnancy and nursing infants are unknown.

Recent reports suggest an association between the use of anticonvulsant drugs by women with epilepsy and an elevated incidence of birth defects in children born to these women. Data are more extensive with respect to phenytoin and phenobarbital, but these are also the most commonly prescribed anticonvulsants; less systematic or anecdotal reports suggest a possible similar association with the use of all known anticonvulsant drugs.

The reports suggesting an elevated incidence of birth defects in children of drug-treated epileptic women cannot be regarded as adequate to prove a definite cause and effect relationship. There are intrinsic methodologic problems in obtaining adequate data on drug teratogenicity in humans; the possibility also exists that other factors, eg. genetic factors or the epileptic condition itself, may be more important than drug therapy in leading to birth defects. The great majority of mothers on anticonvulsant medication deliver normal infants. It is important to note that anticonvulsant drugs should not be discontinued in patients in whom the drug is administered to prevent major seizures because of the strong possibility of precipitating status epilepticus with attendant hypoxia and threat to life. In individual cases where the severity and frequency of the seizure disorder are such that the removal of medication does not pose a serious threat to the

patient, discontinuation of the drug may be considered prior to and during pregnancy, although it cannot be said with any confidence that even minor seizures do not pose some hazard to the developing embryo or fetus.

The prescribing physician will wish to weigh these considerations in treating or counseling epileptic women of childbearing potential.

PRECAUTIONS

General: Ethosuximide, when used alone in mixed types of epilepsy, may increase the frequency of grand mal seizures in some patients.

As with other anticonvulsants, it is important to proceed slowly when increasing or decreasing dosage, as well as when adding or eliminating other medication. Abrupt withdrawal of anticonvulsant medication may precipitate absence (petit mal) status.

Information for Patient: Ethosuximide may impair the mental and/or physical abilities required for the performance of potentially hazardous tasks such as driving a motor vehicle or other such activity requiring alertness; therefore, the patient should be cautioned accordingly.

Pregnancy: See WARNINGS

ADVERSE REACTIONS

Gastrointestinal System: Gastrointestinal symptoms occur frequently and include anorexia, vague gastric upset, nausea and vomiting, cramps, epigastric and abdominal pain, weight loss, and diarrhea.

Hemopoietic System: Hemopoietic complications associated with the administration of ethosuximide have included leukopenia, agranulocytosis, pancytopenia, aplastic anemia, and eosinophilia.

Nervous System: Neurologic and sensory reactions reported during therapy with ethosuximide have included drowsiness, headache, dizziness, euphoria, hiccups, irritability, hyperactivity, lethargy, fatigue, and ataxia.

Psychiatric or psychological aberrations associated with ethosuximide administration have included disturbances of sleep, night terrors, inability to concentrate, and aggressiveness. These effects may be noted particularly in patients who have previously exhibited psychological abnormalities. There have been rare reports of paranoid psychosis, increased libido, and increased state of depression with overt suicidal intentions.

Integumentary System: Dermatologic manifestations which have occurred with the administration of ethosuximide have included urticaria, Stevens-Johnson syndrome, systemic lupus erythematosus, and pruritic erythematous rashes.

Miscellaneous: Other reactions reported have included myopia, vaginal bleeding, swelling of the tongue, gum hypertrophy, and hirsutism.

DOSAGE AND ADMINISTRATION

Zarontin is administered by the oral route. The *initial* dose for patients 3 to 6 years of age is one teaspoonful (250 mg) per day; for patients 6 years of age and older, 2 teaspoonfuls (500 mg) per day. The dose thereafter must be individualized according to the patient's response. Dosage should be increased by small increments. One useful method is to increase the daily dose by 250 mg every four to seven days until control is achieved with minimal side effects. Dosages exceeding 1.5 g daily, in divided doses, should be administered only under the strictest supervision of the physician. The *optimal* dose for most children is 20 mg/kg/day. This dose has given average plasma levels within the accepted therapeutic range of 40 to 100 mcg/ml. Subsequent dose schedules can be based on effectiveness and plasma level determinations.

Zarontin may be administered in combination with other anticonvulsants when other forms of epilepsy coexist with absence (petit mal). The optimal dose for most children is 20 mg/kg/day.

HOW SUPPLIED

Zarontin is supplied as:
N0071-2418-23–1 pint bottles. Each 5 ml of syrup contains 250 mg ethosuximide in a raspberry flavored base. Store below 30°C (86°F). Protect from freezing and light.

Zarontin is also supplied in the following form:
N0071-0237-24–Bottle of 100. Each capsule contains 250 mg ethosuximide. Store below 30°C (86°F).

2418G022

Products are cross-indexed by
generic and chemical names
in the
YELLOW SECTION

Pedinol Pharmacal Inc.
30 BANFI PLAZA NORTH
FARMINGDALE, N.Y. 11735

BREEZEE MIST FOOT POWDER   OTC

COMPOSITION
Aluminum Chlorhydrate, Menthol, Undecylenic Acid, contains no Fluorocarbons.

INDICATIONS
Topical treatment for hyperhidrosis, bromidrosis and tinea pedis (athlete's foot).

HOW SUPPLIED
4 oz. aerosol can.

CASTELLANI PAINT   R
CASTELLANI PAINT-Colorless   R

COMPOSITION
Basic Fuchsin, Phenol, Resorcinol, Acetone, Alcohol. **Colorless—without Basic Fuchsin.**

INDICATIONS
Topical antifungal agent for macerations and ulcerations.

CAUTION
Federal law prohibits dispensing without prescription.

PRECAUTIONS
If irritation or sensitivity develops, discontinue treatment and consult podiatrist or physician.

ADMINISTRATION
Apply to affected areas once or twice a day.

HOW SUPPLIED
1 oz. and 1 pt. plastic bottle.

FUNGOID CREME and SOLUTION   R

COMPOSITION
Cetyl Pyridinium Chloride, Triacetin, Chloroxylenol, Vanishing Creme Base and Oil Base Solution.

INDICATIONS
Topical treatment for fungus, yeast and bacterial infections of the skin.

CAUTION
Federal law prohibits dispensing without prescription.

PRECAUTIONS
If irritation or sensitivity develops, discontinue treatment and consult podiatrist or physician.

ADMINISTRATION
Apply to affected areas twice a day.

HOW SUPPLIED
1 oz. plastic tube; 15cc plastic bottle with controlled dropper.

FUNGOID HC CREME   R

COMPOSITION
Hydrocortisone 0.5%, Cetyl Pyridinium Chloride, Triacetin, Chloroxylenol, Vanishing Creme Base

INDICATIONS
Topical treatment for fungus, yeast, bacterial infections of the skin and anti-inflammatory.

CAUTION
Federal law prohibits dispensing without prescription.

CONTRAINDICATIONS
Do not use on patients known to be sensitive to any ingredients in Fungoid HC Creme.

PRECAUTION
If irritation or sensitivity develops, discontinue treatment and consult your PODIATRIST, DERMATOLOGIST, or PHYSICIAN. Keep out of the reach of children. For External Use Only. Not for Ophthalmic use.

ADMINISTRATION
Apply to affected areas twice a day.

HOW SUPPLIED
Available in 1 oz. plastic tubes.

FUNGOID TINCTURE   R

COMPOSITION
Cetyl Pyridinium Chloride, Triacetin, Chloroxylenol, Sodium Propionate, Benzalkonium Chloride, Glacial Acetic Acid.

INDICATIONS
Topical treatment for fungus infections of the nails, tinea unguium (onychomycosis).

CAUTION
Federal law prohibits dispensing without prescription.

PRECAUTIONS
If irritation or sensitivity develops, discontinue treatment and consult podiatrist or physician.

ADMINISTRATION
Apply to affected nails twice a day.

HOW SUPPLIED
1 oz. bottle with brush applicator, 1 pt. bottle.

G-MYTICIN CREME and   R
OINTMENT 0.1%
(gentamicin sulfate 0.1%)

COMPOSITION
Creme and ointment—each gram contains gentamicin sulfate equivalent to 1 mg. of gentamicin base.

INDICATIONS
Topical wide-spectrum antibiotic provides highly effective treatment in primary and secondary bacterial infections of the skin. *NOTE:* G-myticin Creme/Ointment is not effective against viruses or fungal skin infections.

ADVERSE REACTIONS
In patients with dermatoses treated with G-myticin erythema and pruritis that did not usually require discontinuance of treatment has been reported in a small percentage of cases.

CONTRAINDICATIONS
G-myticin creme/ointment, is contraindicated in those patients with a history of hypersensitivity to any of the components of this preparation.

CAUTION
Federal law prohibits dispensing without prescription.

PRECAUTIONS
The overgrowth of nonsusceptible organisms, including fungi, occasionally occurs with the use of topical antibiotics. If this occurs, or if irritation, sensitization, or superinfection develops, treatment with G-myticin should be discontinued and consult podiatrist or physician.

ADMINISTRATION
Apply 3 to 4 times daily.

HOW SUPPLIED
G-myticin Creme/Ointment—15 grm tubes.

HYDRISALIC GEL   R

COMPOSITION
Salicyclic Acid 6%, Isopropanol, Propylene Glycol, Hydroxypropyl Cellulose.

INDICATIONS
Topical treatment for hyperkeratotic skin.

CAUTION
Federal law prohibits dispensing without prescription.

PRECAUTIONS
Use should be limited in children under 12 years of age. If irritation or sensitivity develops, discontinue treatment and consult podiatrist or physician. For External Use Only.

ADMINISTRATION
Apply to affected area in the evening. Wash hands thoroughly following application. The medication is washed off the following morning.

HOW SUPPLIED
1 oz. plastic tubes.

HYDRISINOL CREME and LOTION   OTC

COMPOSITION
Sulfonated Hydrogenated Castor Oil, N.F. IX, Hydrogenated Vegetable Oil.

INDICATIONS
Topical emollient to soften dry, cracked, calloused skin.

ADMINISTRATION
Apply as needed.

HOW SUPPLIED
4 oz. and 1 lb. jars;
8 oz. plastic bottle.

LAZER CREME   OTC

COMPOSITION
Vitamin E, 3,500 u/oz., Vitamin A, 100,000 u/oz.

INDICATIONS
To enhance post surgical regeneration of skin, revitalize lasered tissue, healing aid for post surgical lesions, keratosis and dryness of the skin.

CAUTION
FOR EXTERNAL USE ONLY. Keep out of reach of children. Keep in cool place.

ADMINISTRATION
Apply topically to affected area as often as needed or as directed by your podiatrist or physician.

HOW SUPPLIED
Available in 2 oz. plastic jar.

LAZERFORMALYDE SOLUTION   R

COMPOSITION
Formaldehyde 10%, Polysorbate 20, Mint Fragrance, Hydroxyethyl Cellulose, Water.

INDICATIONS
Drying Agent for pre and post surgical removal of warts or for non-surgical laser treatment of warts. Anti-perspirant for treatment of hyperhidrosis and bromidosis of the feet.

CONTRAINDICATIONS
Do not use in patients known to be sensitive to any ingredients in LazerFormalyde Solution.

PRECAUTION
Check skin for sensitivity to Formaldehyde prior to application since it may be irritating and sensitizing to the skin of some patients.
If redness or irritation persists, consult your podiatrist or physician.

CAUTION
FEDERAL LAW PROHIBITS DISPENSING WITHOUT PRESCRIPTION. Keep out of reach of children. For external use only. Avoid contact with eyes or mucous membranes.

ADMINISTRATION
Apply with **roll-on** applicator once a day to affected areas or as directed by your podiatrist or physician.

HOW SUPPLIED
Available in 3 oz. plastic bottle with **roll-on** applicator.

LAZERSPORIN-C SOLUTION   R

COMPOSITION
Neomycin Sulfate equivalent to 3.5 mg., Polymyxin B Sulfate 10,000 U, Hydrocortisone 1%.

INDICATIONS AND USAGE
For the treatment of superficial bacterial infections of the external auditory canal caused by organisms susceptible to the action of the antibiotics.

CONTRAINDICATIONS
Do not use in patients known to be sensitive to any ingredients in LazerSporin-C Solution.

WARNINGS
As with other antibiotic preparations, prolonged treatment may result in overgrowth of nonsusceptible organisms and fungi. If the infection is not improved after one week, cultures and susceptibility test should be repeated to verify the identity of the organism and to determine whether therapy should be changed.

PRECAUTION
If redness, irritation or pain and swelling persist, discontinue use and consult your physician.

CAUTION
FEDERAL LAW PROHIBITS DISPENSING WITHOUT A PRESCRIPTION. Keep out of reach of children. For external use only.

ADMINISTRATION
Apply to affected area 3 or 4 times a day or as directed by your physician.

HOW SUPPLIED
10cc bottle with sterile dropper.

Continued on next page

Pedinol—Cont.

OSTI–DERM LOTION   OTC

COMPOSITION

Purified water, magnesium carbonate, zinc oxide, isopropyl myristate, cetearyl alcohol, ceteareth-20, glyceryl stearate SE, PEG 8, glycerine, aluminum acetate (Burow's Solution), Bentonite, liquid phenol 1%, calcium carbonate, camphor, methyl paraben, silica, imidazolidinyl urea.

INDICATIONS

Topical treatment for bromidrosis, hyperhidrosis, decubitus ulcers, blisters, itching, poison ivy and dermatitis.

PRECAUTIONS

Check skin sensitivity to phenol. If irritation or sensitivity develops, discontinue treatment and consult podiatrist or physician. For External Use Only.

ADMINISTRATION

Apply 2–3 times a day.

HOW SUPPLIED

45cc plastic tube.

PEDI–BORO SOAK PAKS   OTC

COMPOSITION

Aluminum Sulfate, Calcium Acetate, Coloring Agent.

ACTIONS

A soothing astringent wet dressing of a modified Burow's Solution, buffered.

DOSAGE AND ADMINISTRATION

Dissolve 1 or 2 paks in a pint of water. Prepare fresh daily.

HOW SUPPLIED

Box of 12 and Box of 100.

PEDI–DRI FOOT POWDER   ℞

COMPOSITION

Aluminum Chlorhydroxide, Menthol, Zinc Undecylenate, Formaldehyde.

INDICATIONS

Topical treatment for hyperhidrosis, bromidrosis and tinea pedis (athlete's foot).

CAUTION

Federal law prohibits dispensing without prescription.

PRECAUTIONS

External use only. Keep out of reach of children. Check for skin sensitivity to formaldehyde. If irritation or sensitivity develops, discontinue treatment and consult podiatrist or physician.

ADMINISTRATION

Apply twice a day.

HOW SUPPLIED

2 oz. plastic bottle.

PEDI–PRO FOOT POWDER   OTC

COMPOSITION

Aluminum Chlorhydroxide, Chloroxylenol, Zinc Undecylenate, Menthol, Micro-Kaolin, Starch.

INDICATIONS

Athlete's Foot: Aids in temporary relief of burning, itching and cracking skin in athlete's foot.

CAUTION

External use only. Do not use near eyes or mucous membranes. Keep out of reach of children. Persons with impaired circulation, including diabetes, should consult a podiatrist or physician before using medication. If symptoms persist consult your podiatrist or physician.

CONTRAINDICATIONS

Do not use in patients known to be sensitive to any ingredients in Pedi-Pro Foot Powder.

ADMINISTRATION

Apply twice a day as needed.

HOW SUPPLIED

2 oz. plastic bottle.

PEDI–VIT A CREME   OTC

COMPOSITION

Vitamin A, 100,000 u/oz.

INDICATIONS

Topical treatment for irritated, dry, sensitive skin.

ADMINISTRATION

Apply daily as needed.

HOW SUPPLIED

2 oz. jar and 1 lb. jar.

SAL–ACID PLASTERS   OTC

INGREDIENTS

Salicylic Acid 50%

ACTION

Medicated plaster for quick removal of warts, corns or callouses, presents a perfect chemical combination treatment to effectively avoid dermatitis. The specialized felt ring relieves painful pressure, while the Sal-Acid Plaster remedies the wart, corn or callous.

DIRECTIONS

After soaking foot in warm water, dry well and apply the Sal-Acid Plaster directly over the wart, corn or callous. Two or three days later, the softened wart, corn or callous can be easily removed by soaking foot in warm water. Sal-Acid Plaster treatment can be repeated in stubborn cases. If inflammation or symptoms perist, consult your Podiatrist or Physician.

CONTRAINDICATIONS

Do not use if patient is diabetic, has inpaired blood circulation or is sensitive to ingredients. Do not use on moles, birthmarks or unusual warts with hair growing from them or corns located between toes.

PRECAUTION

Use of Salicylic Acid in children under 12 years of age should be limited. Do not use or allow to come in contact with eyes or mucous membranes. For external use only. Keep out of the reach of children. Accidental ingestion — contact poison control center. If redness or irritation persists, consult your PODIATRIST or PHYSICIAN

HOW SUPPLIED

Available in package of 8's, 24 × 8's. NDC 0884-4387-08

SALACTIC FILM   ℞

COMPOSITION

Salicyclic Acid 16.7% U.S.P., Lactic Acid 16.7% U.S.P., Flexible Collodion U.S.P., Coloring Agent.

INDICATIONS

Topical treatment as a keratolytic agent for removal of verrucae.

CONTRAINDICATIONS

Diabetics or patients with impaired blood circulation. Do not use on moles, birthmarks or warts with hair growing from them or in patients known to be sensitive to any ingredients in Salactic Film.

CAUTION

Federal law prohibits dispensing without prescription.

PRECAUTIONS

Highly flammable. Keep bottle tightly capped when not in use. If irritation or sensitivity develops, discontinue treatment and consult podiatrist or physician. For External Use Only.

ADMINISTRATION

Apply once daily as directed.

HOW SUPPLIED

½ oz. bottle with brush applicator.

UREACIN–10 LOTION   OTC
UREACIN–20 CREME   OTC
UREACIN–40 CREME   ℞

COMPOSITION

Urea 10%, Urea 20% and 40%, Vegetable Oil Base.

INDICATIONS

Ureacin-10 Lotion, Ureacin-20 Creme is a topical treatment for rough, dry, cracked, calloused skin. Ureacin-40 Creme is indicated for the treatment of nail destruction and dissolution.

CONTRAINDICATIONS

Do not use on patients known to be sensitive to any ingredients in Ureacin-10, -20, or -40.

CAUTION

For Ureacin-40 Creme—Federal law prohibits dispensing without prescription.

PRECAUTIONS

If irritation or sensitivity develops, discontinue treatment and consult podiatrist or physician. For External Use Only.

ADMINISTRATION

Rub in gently two or three times a day to affected area. **Ureacin-40 Creme to be applied to diseased nail surface by podiatrist or physician only.**

HOW SUPPLIED

8 oz. plastic bottle, 2½ oz. plastic jar, 1 oz. plastic jar.

For further product information please contact Pedinol Pharmacal Inc.

Pennwalt Corp.
See FISONS CORPORATION

Persōn & Covey, Inc.
616 ALLEN AVENUE
GLENDALE, CA 91201

AQUANIL™ LOTION
Lipid-free cleanser for sensitive skin
Non-comedogenic

DIRECTIONS

Apply a generous amount of Aquanil to the skin and gently rub, resulting in a lather. Remove the excess with a soft tissue or cloth.

CONTAINS

Purified Water, U.S.P., Glycerin, Cetyl Alcohol, Stearyl Alcohol, Benzyl Alcohol, Sodium Laureth Sulfate, Xanthan Gum.

INDICATIONS

AQUANIL™ provides gentle, complete cleansing for sensitive skin which cannot tolerate the irritating action of soaps. Aquanil is specially formulated to be free of oils and is particularly useful in such conditions as atopic dermatitis, atopic eczema, diaper dermatitis and other eczemas. Aquanil, with its emollient effect, provides a softening action to sensitive, traumatized skin, as it cleanses. Aquanil contains no fats of any type.

HOW SUPPLIED

Plastic bottles, 8 and 16 fl oz. (NDC 0096-0724-08, 0096-0724-16).

DHS™ HAIR CARE PRODUCTS

Formulated for the therapeutic needs of the dermatologist.

DHS™ Conditioning Rinse*†
Helps make hair easier to comb and manage, while adding lustre and body.

DIRECTIONS

Shampoo and rinse well (We suggest DHS™ Shampoo). Apply a generous amount of DHS™ Conditioning Rinse and work evenly through the hair for 60 seconds. Rinse with warm water for 30 seconds.

CONTAINS

Purified water, U.S.P., glyceryl stearate, quaternium-31, panthenol, cetyl alcohol, dimethicone copolyol, fragrance, FD&C Yellow #6.

HOW SUPPLIED

Plastic bottle, 8 fl. oz. (NDC 0096-0726-08).

DHS™ Shampoo*†
For routine daily hair and scalp cleansing.

DIRECTIONS

Wet hair thoroughly; apply a liberal supply of DHS™ Shampoo, and massage into a lather. Rinse thoroughly and repeat application. Repeat as necessary, or as directed by your physician.

CONTAINS

Purified water, U.S.P., TEA-lauryl sulfate, sodium chloride, PEG-8 distearate, cocamide DEA, cocamide MEA, fragrance and FD&C yellow #6.

HOW SUPPLIED

Plastic bottles, 8 and 16 fl. oz. (NDC 0096-0727-08 and 0096-0727-16).

DHS™ Clear Shampoo* †

A fragrance-free and color-free shampoo designed for routine, gentle, daily hair and scalp cleansing for patients with sensitive skin.

DIRECTIONS

Wet hair thoroughly; apply DHS Clear, lather and rinse. Repeat as necessary, or as directed by your physician.

CONTAINS

Purified Water, U.S.P., TEA-Lauryl Sulfate, Sodium Chloride, PEG-8 Distearate, Cocamide DEA and Cocamide MEA.

HOW SUPPLIED

Plastic bottles, 8 and 16 fl. oz. (NDC 0096-0725-08 and 0096-0725-16).

DHS™ Tar Shampoo and DHS™ Tar Gel Shampoo (Scented)*†

Aids in the control of the scaling of seborrhea (dandruff) and psoriasis of the scalp.

DIRECTIONS

Wet hair thoroughly; apply a liberal quantity of DHS™ Tar Shampoo and massage into a lather. Rinse thoroughly and repeat application. Allow lather to remain on scalp for about 5 minutes. Use DHS™ Tar Shampoo once or twice weekly, or as directed by your physician.

CONTAINS

Tar, equivalent to 0.5% Coal Tar U.S.P., TEA-lauryl sulfate, purified water, U.S.P., sodium chloride, PEG-8 distearate, cocamide DEA, cocamide MEA, citric acid. DHS™ Tar Gel Shampoo also contains: Hydroxypropyl methylcellulose and fragrance.

HOW SUPPLIED

Plastic bottles. DHS™ Tar Shampoo, 4, 8 and 16 fl. oz. (NDC 0096-0728-04, 0096-0728-08, 0096-0728-16). DHS™ Tar Gel Shampoo 8 fl. oz. (NDC 0096-0730-08).

DHS™ Zinc Dandruff Shampoo*† 2% Zinc Pyrithione

Aids in the control of dandruff/seborrheic dermatitis of the scalp.

DIRECTIONS

Shake well before using. Wet hair thoroughly; apply a liberal quantity of DHS™ Zinc Shampoo and massage into a lather. Rinse thoroughly and repeat application. Allow lather to remain on scalp for about 5 minutes. Use DHS™ Zinc Shampoo at least twice weekly for the first two weeks, then regularly thereafter, or as directed by your physician.

CONTAINS

2% zinc pyrithione, purified water, U.S.P., TEA-lauryl sulfate, PEG-8 distearate, sodium chloride, cocamide DEA, cocamide MEA, magnesium aluminum silicate, hydroxypropyl methylcellulose, fragrance and FD&C yellow #6.

HOW SUPPLIED

Plastic bottles, 6 and 12 fl. oz. (NDC 0096-0729-06, 0096-0729-12).

* Caution: Avoid contact with the eyes. In case of contact, wash out with water. If irritation occurs, discontinue use and consult physician.

† Warning: For external use only. Keep out of the reach of children.

DML™
Moisturizer and Skin Lubricant
Fragrance Free
Non-comedogenic

CONTAINS

Purified water, petrolatum, glycerin, methyl glucose sesquistearate, dimethicone, methyl gluceth-20 sesquistearate, benzyl alcohol, volatile silicone, glyceryl stearate, stearic acid, palmitic acid, cetyl alcohol, xanthan gum, magnesium aluminum silicate, carbomer 941, sodium hydroxide.

HOW SUPPLIED

Plastic bottles, 8 and 16 fl. oz.
(NDC 0096-0722-08, 0096-0722-16).

DIRECTIONS

Apply as often as needed, or as directed by physician.

CAUTION

Avoid contact with the eyes. In case of contact, wash out with water. If irritation occurs, discontinue use and consult physician.

WARNING

For external use only. Keep out of the reach of children.

DML™ FORTE Cream

A fragrance-free formulation to treat severe, recalcitrant dry skin.

DIRECTIONS

Apply as often as needed, or as directed by physician.

HOW SUPPLIED

Plastic tube, 4 oz. NDC 0096-0720-04

CONTAINS

Purified Water, U.S.P., Petrolatum U.S.P., PPG-2 Myristyl Ether Propionate; Glyceryl Stearate; Glycerin; Stearic Acid; D-Panthenol; DEA-Cetyl Phosphate; Simethicone U.S.P.; PVP Eicosene Copolymer; Benzyl Alcohol; Cetyl Alcohol; Silica; Disodium EDTA; BHA; Magnesium Aluminum Silicate; Sodium Carbomer 1342.

CAUTION

Avoid contact with the eyes. In case of contact, wash out with water. If irritation occurs, discontinue use and consult physician.

WARNING

For external use only. Keep out of the reach of children.

DRYSOL™   ℞

A Solution of:

Aluminum Chloride (Hexahydrate) 20% w/v in Anhydrous Ethyl Alcohol (S.D. Alcohol 40) 93% v/v.

INDICATION

An aid in the management of hyperhidrosis.

DIRECTIONS

Apply Drysol™ to the affected area once a day, **only at bedtime.** To help prevent irritation, the area should be completely dry prior to application. Do not apply Drysol to broken, irritated or recently shaved skin.

FOR MAXIMUM EFFECT

Your doctor may instruct you to cover the treated area with saran wrap held in place by a snug fitting "T" or body shirt, mitten or sock. (Never hold saran in place with tape.) Wash the treated area the following morning. Excessive sweating may be stopped after two or more treatments. Thereafter, apply Drysol™ once or twice weekly or as needed.

NOTICE

Drysol™ may produce a burning or prickling sensation. Keep cap tightly closed when not in use to prevent evaporation.

WARNING

For external use only. Keep out of the reach of children. Avoid contact with the eyes. If irritation or sensitization occurs, discontinue use or consult with a physician. Drysol™ may be harmful to certain metals and fabrics. Keep away from open flame.

HOW SUPPLIED

37.5 cc polyethylene bottle (NDC 0096-0707-37) and 35 cc bottle with Dab-O-Matic applicator head (NDC 0096-0707-35).

SOLBAR® SPF 15 SUNSCREENS

SOLBAR® SPF 15 Sunscreens are specially formulated to provide maximum protection from the sun's burning and tanning rays. Provides substantial broad spectrum protection from UVA and UVB light for sun sensitive and fair skinned persons. Fragrance-free formula. Liberal and regular use of these products over the years may help reduce the chance of premature aging of the skin and skin cancer.

SOLBAR® PF 15 LIQUID†*+

CONTAINS

Octyl methoxycinnamate 7.5%, Oxybenzone USP 6%, SD alcohol 40, 76%.

HOW SUPPLIED

Plastic bottle, 4 oz. (NDC 0096-0684-04).

WARNING

Keep away from open flame.

SOLBAR® PF 15 CREAM†*+

CONTAINS

Octyl methoxycinnamate 7.5%, Oxybenzone USP 5%.

HOW SUPPLIED

Plastic tube, 2.5 oz. (NDC 0096-0682-75)

SOLBAR® PLUS 15 CREAM†*+

CONTAINS

Oxybenzone USP 4%, Dioxybenzone USP 2%, Octyl dimethyl PABA 6%.

HOW SUPPLIED

Plastic tube, 4 oz. (NDC 0096-0681-04)

† Directions: Apply liberally on all exposed skin. To ensure maximum protection, reapply after swimming or exercise.

* Caution: If irritation or sensitization occurs, discontinue use and consult a physician. Avoid contact with the eyes.

+ Warning: For external use only. Keep out of the reach of children.

SOLBAR® PF ULTRA CREAM SPF 50
Ultra protection sunscreen
Broad Spectrum UVA and UVB protection

DIRECTIONS

Apply liberally to all exposed areas before sun exposure. Massage in gently. Reapply to dry skin after prolonged sunning, swimming, excessive perspiration or towel drying. Repeated applications during prolonged sun exposure are recommended.

CONTAINS

Oxybenzone USP, Octyl Methoxycinnamate, Octocrylene

INDICATIONS

SOLBAR® PF 50 Cream is specially formulated for ultra protection from the sun's burning and tanning rays. Oxybenzone enhances protection from UVA and UVB light which is particularly important to photosensitive or photoallergic people. Waterproof formula maintains sunburn protection up to 80 minutes in water. Liberal and regular use of this product over the years may help reduce the chance of premature aging of the skin and skin cancer.

CAUTION

For external use only, not to be swallowed. If irritation or sensitization occurs, discontinue use and consult a physician. Avoid contact with the eyes. In case of contact, rinse eyes with water. Keep this and all drugs out of reach of children.

HOW SUPPLIED

Plastic bottle, 4oz. (NDC 0096-0686-04).

XERAC™ AC   ℞
Aluminum Chloride Hexahydrate in
Anhydrous Ethyl Alcohol

DESCRIPTION

A solution of Aluminum Chloride (Hexahydrate) 6.25% (w/v) in Anhydrous Ethyl Alcohol (S.D. Alcohol 40) 96% (v/v).

INDICATION

For topical application as an antiperspirant (anhidrotic).

DIRECTIONS

Apply Xerac™ AC to the axillae at bedtime or as directed by physician. To help prevent irritation, the area should be completely dry prior to application. Do not apply Xerac AC to broken or irritated skin. Keep container tightly closed.

ADVERSE REACTIONS

Transient stinging or itching may occur. It is not evidence of contact sensitivity and may be prevented or reduced by applying Xerac™ AC only to skin which is completely dry or by removing the solution with soap and water.

WARNING

For External Use Only. Some users of this product will experience skin irritation. If this occurs, discontinue use. Avoid contact with the eyes. This product may be harmful to certain metals and fabrics. Keep the container tightly closed when not in use to prevent evaporation. Keep this and all medication out of the reach of children. Do not use near open flame.

HOW SUPPLIED

In bottles with Dab-O-Matic applicator head. 35 cc (NDC 0096-0709-35) and 60 cc (NDC 0096-0709-60).

XERAC™ BP5 XERAC™ BP10
(benzoyl peroxide water gel)

For the treatment of acne. XERAC™ BP5 and XERAC™ BP10 help dry and clear acne blemishes, reduce blackheads and prevent the development of new acne lesions.

XERAC™ BP5†*+

CONTAINS

5% benzoyl peroxide, laureth-4, carbomer-934, triethanolamine, disodium EDTA.

HOW SUPPLIED

Plastic tubes, 1½ oz. and 3 oz. (NDC 0096-0790-45 and 0096-0790-90)

XERAC™ BP10†*+

CONTAINS

10% benzoyl peroxide, laureth-4, carbomer-934, triethanolamine, disodium EDTA.

Continued on next page

Persōn & Covey—Cont.

HOW SUPPLIED

Plastic tubes, 1½ oz. and 3 oz. (NDC 0096-0791-45 and 0096-0791-90).

† Directions: Cleanse the skin thoroughly before applying medication. Cover the entire affected area with a thin layer one to three times daily. Because excessive drying of the skin may occur, start with one application daily, then gradually increase to two or three times daily, or as directed by a physician.

* Caution: Persons with very sensitive skin, or known allergy to benzoyl peroxide should not use this medication. If uncomfortable irritation, or excessive dryness and/or peeling occurs, reduce frequency of use. If excessive itching, redness, burning or swelling occurs, discontinue use and consult a physician. Keep away from eyes, lips and other mucous membranes. May bleach hair or dyed fabrics.

+ Warning: For external use only. Keep out of the reach of children.

Pfizer Laboratories Division

PFIZER INC.
235 EAST 42ND STREET
NEW YORK, NY 10017

Full prescribing information for all Pfizer Laboratories products is available from your Pfizer Laboratories representative.

Product Identification Codes

To provide quick and positive identification of Pfizer Laboratories Division products, we have imprinted the product identification number of the National Drug Code on all tablets and capsules.

In order that you may quickly identify a product by its code number, we have compiled below a numerical list of code numbers with their corresponding product names. We are also listing the code numbers by alphabetical order of products.

NUMERICAL PRODUCT INDEX

ALPHABETICAL PRODUCT INDEX

CORTRIL®   ℞

[kor'tril]
(hydrocortisone)
TOPICAL OINTMENT
1.0%
Not For Ophthalmic Use

DESCRIPTION

Cortril Topical Ointment contains 1.0% (10 mg/g) hydrocortisone in a washable base. Chemically hydrocortisone is Pregn-4-ene-3,20-dione, 11,17,21-trihydroxy-, (11β)-. The empirical formula is $C_{21}H_{30}O_5$ and the molecular weight is 362.47.

The base of the ointment contains sodium lauryl sulfate, propylene glycol, stearyl alcohol, cetyl alcohol, cholesterol, white petrolatum, mineral oil, and water. Methylparaben and propylparaben are added as preservatives.

CLINICAL PHARMACOLOGY

Topical corticosteroids share anti-inflammatory, antipruritic and vasoconstrictive actions.

The mechanism of anti-inflammatory activity of the topical corticosteroids is unclear. Various laboratory methods, including vasoconstrictor assays, are used to compare and predict potencies and/or clinical efficacies of the topical corticosteroids. There is some evidence to suggest that a recogniz-able correlation exists between vasoconstrictor potency and therapeutic efficacy in man.

Pharmacokinetics
The extent of percutaneous absorption of topical corticosteroids is determined by many factors including the vehicle, the integrity of the epidermal barrier, and the use of occlusive dressings.

Topical corticosteroids can be absorbed from normal intact skin. Inflammation and/or other disease processes in the skin increase percutaneous absorption. Occlusive dressings substantially increase the percutaneous absorption of topical corticosteroids. Thus, occlusive dressings may be a valuable therapeutic adjunct for treatment of resistant dermatoses. (See *DOSAGE AND ADMINISTRATION*.)

Once absorbed through the skin, topical corticosteroids are handled through pharmacokinetic pathways similar to systemically administered corticosteroids. Corticosteroids are bound to plasma proteins in varying degrees. Corticosteroids are metabolized primarily in the liver and are then excreted by the kidneys. Some of the topical corticosteroids and their metabolites are also excreted into the bile.

INDICATIONS AND USAGE

Topical corticosteroids are indicated for the relief of the inflammatory and pruritic manifestations of corticosteroid-responsive dermatoses.

CONTRAINDICATIONS

Topical corticosteroids are contraindicated in those patients with a history of hypersensitivity to any of the components of the preparation.

PRECAUTIONS

General
Systemic absorption of topical corticosteroids has produced reversible hypothalamic-pituitary-adrenal (HPA) axis suppression, manifestations of Cushing's syndrome, hyperglycemia, and glucosuria in some patients.

Conditions which augment systemic absorption include the application of the more potent steroids, use over large surface areas, prolonged use, and the addition of occlusive dressings.

Therefore, patients receiving a large dose of a potent topical steroid applied to a large surface area or under an occlusive dressing should be evaluated periodically for evidence of HPA axis suppression by using the urinary free cortisol and ACTH stimulation tests. If HPA axis suppression is noted, an attempt should be made to withdraw the drug, to reduce the frequency of application, or to substitute a less potent steroid.

Recovery of HPA axis function is generally prompt and complete upon discontinuation of the drug. Infrequently, signs and symptoms of steroid withdrawal may occur, requiring supplemental systemic corticosteroids.

Children may absorb proportionally larger amounts of topical corticosteroids and thus be more susceptible to systemic toxicity. (See *PRECAUTIONS—Pediatric Use.*)

If irritation develops, topical corticosteroids should be discontinued and appropriate therapy instituted.

In the presence of dermatological infections, the use of an appropriate antifungal or antibacterial agent should be instituted. If a favorable response does not occur promptly, the corticosteroid should be discontinued until the infection has been adequately controlled.

Information for the Patient
Patients using topical corticosteroids should receive the following information and instructions:

1. This medication is to be used as directed by the physician. It is for external use only. Avoid contact with the eyes.
2. Patients should be advised not to use this medication for any disorder other than that for which it was prescribed.
3. The treated skin area should not be bandaged or otherwise covered or wrapped as to be occlusive unless directed by the physician.
4. Patients should report any signs of local adverse reactions especially under occlusive dressing.
5. Parents of pediatric patients should be advised not to use tight-fitting diapers or plastic pants on a child being treated in the diaper area, as these garments may constitute occlusive dressings.

Laboratory Tests
The following tests may be helpful in evaluating the HPA axis suppression:
Urinary free cortisol test
ACTH stimulation test
Carcinogenesis, Mutagenesis, and Impairment of Fertility
Long term animal studies have not been performed to evaluate the carcinogenic potential or the effect on fertility of topical corticosteroids.

Studies to determine mutagenicity with prednisolone and hydrocortisone have revealed negative results.

Pregnancy Category C
Corticosteroids are generally teratogenic in laboratory animals when administered systemically at relatively low dosage levels. The more potent corticosteroids have been shown to be teratogenic after dermal application in laboratory animals. There are no adequate and well controlled studies in

pregnant women on teratogenic effects from topically applied corticosteroids. Therefore, topical corticosteroids should be used during pregnancy only if the potential benefit justifies the potential risk to the fetus. Drugs of this class should not be used extensively on pregnant patients, in large amounts, or for prolonged periods of time.

Nursing Mothers

It is not known whether topical administration of corticosteroids could result in sufficient systemic absorption to produce detectable quantities in breast milk. Systemically administered corticosteroids are secreted into breast milk in quantities *not* likely to have a deleterious effect on the infant. Nevertheless, caution should be exercised when topical corticosteroids are administered to a nursing woman.

Pediatric Use

Pediatric patients may demonstrate greater susceptibility to topical corticosteroid-induced HPA axis suppression and Cushing's syndrome than mature patients because of a larger skin surface area to body weight ratio.

Hypothalamic-pituitary-adrenal (HPA) axis suppression, Cushing's syndrome, and intracranial hypertension have been reported in children receiving topical corticosteroids. Manifestations of adrenal suppression in children include linear growth retardation, delayed weight gain, low plasma cortisol levels, and absence of response to ACTH stimulation. Manifestations of intracranial hypertension include bulging fontanelles, headaches, and bilateral papilledema.

Administration of topical corticosteroids to children should be limited to the least amount compatible with an effective therapeutic regimen. Chronic corticosteroid therapy may interfere with the growth and development of children.

ADVERSE REACTIONS

The following local adverse reactions are reported infrequently with topical corticosteroids, but may occur more frequently with the use of occlusive dressings. These reactions are listed in an approximate decreasing order of occurrence:

Burning	Perioral dermatitis
Itching	Allergic contact dermatitis
Irritation	Maceration of the skin
Dryness	Secondary infection
Folliculitis	Skin atrophy
Hypertrichosis	Striae
Acneiform eruptions	Miliaria
Hypopigmentation	

OVERDOSAGE

Topically applied corticosteroids can be absorbed in sufficient amounts to produce systemic effects. (See *PRECAUTIONS*.)

DOSAGE AND ADMINISTRATION

Topical corticosteroids are generally applied to the affected area as a thin film from three to four times daily depending on the severity of the condition.

Occlusive dressings may be used for the management of psoriasis or recalcitrant conditions.

If an infection develops, the use of occlusive dressings should be discontinued and appropriate antimicrobial therapy instituted.

HOW SUPPLIED

Cortril (hydrocortisone) Topical Ointment 1.0%: ½ oz (14.2g) tube containing 10 mg/g of hydrocortisone (NDC 0069-3260-13).

23-2434-00-5   Revised Aug. 1987

DIABINESE®   ℞

[dī-ab'in-ees]
(chlorpropamide)
Tablets, USP
For Oral Use

DESCRIPTION

DIABINESE (chlorpropamide), is an oral blood-glucose-lowering drug of the sulfonylurea class. Chlorpropamide is 1-[(p-Chlorophenyl) sulfonyl]-3-propylurea, $C_{10}H_{13}ClN_2O_3S$. Chlorpropamide is a white crystalline powder, that has a slight odor. It is practically insoluble in water at pH 7.3 (solubility at pH 6 is 2.2 mg/ml). It is soluble in alcohol and moderately soluble in chloroform. The molecular weight of chlorpropamide is 276.74. DIABINESE is available as 100 mg and 250 mg tablets.

Inert ingredients are: alginic acid; Blue 1 Lake; hydroxypropyl cellulose; magnesium stearate; precipitated calcium carbonate; sodium lauryl sulfate; starch.

CLINICAL PHARMACOLOGY

DIABINESE appears to lower the blood glucose acutely by stimulating the release of insulin from the pancreas, an effect dependent upon functioning beta cells in the pancreatic islets. The mechanism by which DIABINESE lowers blood glucose during long-term administration has not been clearly established. Extra-pancreatic effects may play a part in the mechanism of action of oral sulfonylurea hypoglyce-

mic drugs. While chlorpropamide is a sulfonamide derivative, it is devoid of antibacterial activity.

DIABINESE may also prove effective in controlling certain patients who have experienced primary or secondary failure to other sulfonylurea agents.

A method developed which permits easy measurement of the drug in blood is available on request.

Chlorpropamide does not interfere with the usual tests to detect albumin in the urine.

DIABINESE is absorbed rapidly from the gastrointestinal tract. Within one hour after a single oral dose, it is readily detectable in the blood, and the level reaches a maximum within two to four hours. It undergoes metabolism in humans and it is excreted in the urine as unchanged drug and as hydroxylated or hydrolyzed metabolites. The biological half-life of chlorpropamide averages about 36 hours. Within 96 hours, 80–90% of a single oral dose is excreted in the urine. However, long-term administration of therapeutic doses does not result in undue accumulation in the blood, since absorption and excretion rates become stabilized in about 5 to 7 days after the initiation of therapy.

DIABINESE exerts a hypoglycemic effect in normal humans within one hour, becoming maximal at 3 to 6 hours and persisting for at least 24 hours. The potency of chlorpropamide is approximately six times that of tolbutamide. Some experimental results suggest that its increased duration of action may be the result of slower excretion and absence of significant deactivation.

INDICATIONS AND USAGE

DIABINESE is indicated as an adjunct to diet to lower the blood glucose in patients with non-insulin-dependent diabetes mellitus (type II) whose hyperglycemia cannot be controlled by diet alone.

In initiating treatment for non-insulin-dependent diabetes, diet should be emphasized as the primary form of treatment. Caloric restriction and weight loss are essential in the obese diabetic patient. Proper dietary management alone may be effective in controlling the blood glucose and symptoms of hyperglycemia. The importance of regular physical activity should also be stressed, and cardiovascular risk factors should be identified and corrective measures taken where possible.

If this treatment program fails to reduce symptoms and/or blood glucose, the use of an oral sulfonylurea or insulin should be considered. Use of DIABINESE must be viewed by both the physician and patient as a treatment in addition to diet, and not as a substitute for diet or as a convenient mechanism for avoiding dietary restraint. Furthermore, loss of blood glucose control on diet alone may be transient, thus requiring only short-term administration of DIABINESE. During maintenance programs, DIABINESE should be discontinued if satisfactory lowering of blood glucose is no longer achieved. Judgments should be based on regular clinical and laboratory evaluations.

In considering the use of DIABINESE in asymptomatic patients, it should be recognized that controlling the blood glucose in non-insulin-dependent diabetes, has not been definitely established to be effective in preventing the long-term cardiovascular or neural complications of diabetes.

CONTRAINDICATIONS

DIABINESE is contraindicated in patients with:
1. Known hypersensitivity to the drug.
2. Diabetic ketoacidosis, with or without coma. This condition should be treated with insulin.

WARNINGS

SPECIAL WARNING ON INCREASED RISK OF CARDIOVASCULAR MORTALITY

The administration of oral hypoglycemic drugs has been reported to be associated with increased cardiovascular mortality as compared to treatment with diet alone or diet plus insulin. This warning is based on the study conducted by the University Group Diabetes Program (UGDP), a long-term prospective clinical trial designed to evaluate the effectiveness of glucose-lowering drugs in preventing or delaying vascular complications in patients with non-insulin-dependent diabetes. The study involved 823 patients who were randomly assigned to one of four treatment groups (*Diabetes,* 19 (supp. 2): 747–830, 1970.)

UGDP reported that patients treated for 5 to 8 years with diet plus a fixed dose of tolbutamide (1.5 grams per day) had a rate of cardiovascular mortality approximately 2½ times that of patients treated with diet alone. A significant increase in total mortality was not observed, but the use of tolbutamide was discontinued based on the increase in cardiovascular mortality, thus limiting the opportunity for the study to show an increase in over-all mortality. Despite controversy regarding the interpretation of these results, the findings of the UGDP study provide an adequate basis for this warning. The patient should be informed of the potential risks and advantages of DIABINESE and of alternative modes of therapy.

Although only one drug in the sulfonylurea class (tolbutamide) was included in this study, it is prudent from a safety standpoint to consider that this warning may also apply to

other oral hypoglycemic drugs in this class, in view of their close similarities in mode of action and chemical structure.

PRECAUTIONS

General

Hypoglycemia: All sulfonylurea drugs are capable of producing severe hypoglycemia. Proper patient selection, dosage, and instructions are important to avoid hypoglycemic episodes. Renal or hepatic insufficiency may cause elevated blood levels of DIABINESE and the latter may also diminish gluconeogenic capacity, both of which increase the risk of serious hypoglycemic reactions. Elderly, debilitated or malnourished patients, and those with adrenal or pituitary insufficiency are particularly susceptible to the hypoglycemic action of glucose-lowering drugs. Hypoglycemia may be difficult to recognize in the elderly, and in people who are taking beta-adrenergic blocking drugs. Hypoglycemia is more likely to occur when caloric intake is deficient, after severe or prolonged exercise, when alcohol is ingested, or when more than one glucose-lowering drug is used.

Because of the long half-life of chlorpropamide, patients who become hypoglycemic during therapy require careful supervision of the dose and frequent feedings for at least 3 to 5 days. Hospitalization and intravenous glucose may be necessary.

Loss of control of blood glucose: When a patient stabilized on any diabetic regimen is exposed to stress such as fever, trauma, infection, or surgery, a loss of control may occur. At such times, it may be necessary to discontinue DIABINESE and administer insulin.

The effectiveness of any oral hypoglycemic drug, including DIABINESE, in lowering blood glucose to a desired level decreases in many patients over a period of time, which may be due to progression of the severity of the diabetes or to diminished responsiveness to the drug. This phenomenon is known as secondary failure, to distinguish it from primary failure in which the drug is ineffective in an individual patient when first given.

INFORMATION FOR PATIENTS

Patients should be informed of the potential risks and advantages of DIABINESE and of alternative modes of therapy. They should also be informed about the importance of adherence to dietary instructions, of a regular exercise program, and of regular testing of urine and/or blood glucose.

The risks of hypoglycemia, its symptoms and treatment, and conditions that predispose to its development should be explained to patients and responsible family members. Primary and secondary failure should also be explained.

Patients should be instructed to contact their physician promptly if they experience symptoms of hypoglycemia or other adverse reactions.

LABORATORY TESTS

Blood and urine glucose should be monitored periodically. Measurement of glycosylated hemoglobin may be useful.

DRUG INTERACTIONS

The hypoglycemic action of sulfonylurea may be potentiated by certain drugs including nonsteroidal anti-inflammatory agents and other drugs that are highly protein bound, salicylates, sulfonamides, chloramphenicol, probenecid, coumarins, monoamine oxidase inhibitors, and beta-adrenergic blocking agents. When such drugs are administered to a patient receiving DIABINESE, the patient should be observed closely for hypoglycemia. When such drugs are withdrawn from a patient receiving DIABINESE, the patient should be observed closely for loss of control.

Certain drugs tend to produce hyperglycemia and may lead to loss of control. These drugs include the thiazides and other diuretics, corticosteroids, phenothiazines, thyroid products, estrogens, oral contraceptives, phenytoin, nicotinic acid, sympathomimetics, calcium channel blocking drugs, and isoniazid. When such drugs are administered to a patient receiving DIABINESE, the patient should be closely observed for loss of control. When such drugs are withdrawn from a patient receiving DIABINESE, the patient should be observed closely for hypoglycemia.

Since animal studies suggest that the action of barbiturates may be prolonged by therapy with chlorpropamide, barbiturates should be employed with caution. In some patients, a disulfiram-like reaction may be produced by the ingestion of alcohol.

A potential interaction between oral miconazole and oral hypoglycemic agents leading to severe hypoglycemia has been reported. Whether this interaction also occurs with the intravenous, topical, or vaginal preparations of miconazole is not known.

Carcinogenesis, Mutagenesis, Impairment of Fertility: Chronic toxicity studies have been carried out in dogs and rats. Dogs treated for 6, 13, or 20 months with doses of DIABINESE greater than 20 times the human dose, have not shown any gross histological or pathological abnormalities. After treatment with 100 mg/kg of DIABINESE for 20 months, a dog showed no histopathological liver changes.

Continued on next page

Pfizer—Cont.

Rats treated with continuous DIABINESE therapy for 6 to 12 months showed varying degrees of suppression of spermatogenesis at higher dosage levels (up to 125 mg/kg). The extent of suppression seemed to follow that of growth retardation associated with chronic administration of high-dose DIABINESE in rats.

Pregnancy
Teratogenic Effects:
Pregnancy Category C. Animal reproductive studies have not been conducted with DIABINESE. It is also not known whether DIABINESE can cause fetal harm when administered to a pregnant woman or can affect reproduction capacity. DIABINESE should be given to a pregnant woman only if clearly needed.

Because recent information suggests that abnormal blood glucose levels during pregnancy are associated with a higher incidence of congenital abnormalities, many experts recommend that insulin be used during pregnancy to maintain blood glucose levels as close to normal as possible.

Nonteratogenic Effects:
Prolonged severe hypoglycemia (4 to 10 days) has been reported in neonates born to mothers who were receiving a sulfonylurea drug at the time of delivery. This has been reported more frequently with the use of agents with prolonged half-lives. If DIABINESE is used during pregnancy, it should be discontinued at least one month before the expected delivery date.

Nursing Mothers: An analysis of a composite of two samples of human breast milk, each taken five hours after ingestion of 500 mg of chlorpropamide by a patient, revealed a concentration of 5 mcg/ml. For reference, the normal peak blood level of chlorpropamide after a single 250 mg dose is 30 mcg/ml. Therefore, it is not recommended that a woman breast feed while taking this medication.

Use in Children: Safety and effectiveness in children have not been established.

ADVERSE REACTIONS
Hypoglycemia: See PRECAUTIONS and OVERDOSAGE sections.

Gastrointestinal Reactions: Cholestatic jaundice may occur rarely; DIABINESE should be discontinued if this occurs. Gastrointestinal disturbances are the most common reactions; nausea has been reported in less than 5% of patients, and diarrhea, vomiting, anorexia, and hunger in less than 2%. Other gastrointestinal disturbances have occurred in less than 1% of patients including proctocolitis. They tend to be dose related and may disappear when dosage is reduced.

Dermatologic Reactions: Pruritus has been reported in less than 3% of patients. Other allergic skin reactions, e.g., urticaria and maculopapular eruptions, have been reported in approximately 1% or less of patients. These may be transient and may disappear despite continued use of DIABINESE; if skin reactions persist the drug should be discontinued.

Porphyria cutanea tarda and photosensitivity reactions have been reported with sulfonylureas.

Skin eruptions rarely progressing to erythema multiforme and exfoliative dermatitis have also been reported.

Hematologic Reactions: Leukopenia, agranulocytosis, thrombocytopenia, hemolytic anemia, aplastic anemia, pancytopenia, and eosinophilia have been reported with sulfonylureas.

Metabolic Reactions: Hepatic porphyria and disulfiram-like reactions have been reported with DIABINESE. See DRUG INTERACTIONS section.

Endocrine Reactions: On rare occasions, chlorpropamide has caused a reaction identical to the syndrome of inappropriate antidiuretic hormone (ADH) secretion. The features of this syndrome result from excessive water retention and include hyponatremia, low serum osmolality, and high urine osmolality. This reaction has also been reported for other sulfonylureas.

OVERDOSAGE
Overdose of sulfonylureas including DIABINESE can produce hypoglycemia. Mild hypoglycemic symptoms without loss of consciousness or neurologic findings should be treated aggressively with oral glucose and adjustments in drug dosage and/or meal patterns. Close monitoring should continue until the physician is assured that the patient is out of danger. Severe hypoglycemic reactions with coma, seizure, or other neurological impairment occur infrequently, but constitute medical emergencies requiring immediate hospitalization. If hypoglycemic coma is diagnosed or suspected, the patient should be given a rapid intravenous injection of concentrated (50%) glucose solution. This should be followed by a continuous infusion of a more dilute (10%) glucose solution at a rate that will maintain the blood glucose at a level above 100 mg/dL. Patients should be closely monitored for a minimum of 24 to 48 hours since hypoglycemia may recur after apparent clinical recovery.

DOSAGE AND ADMINISTRATION
There is no fixed dosage regimen for the management of diabetes mellitus with DIABINESE or any other hypoglycemic agent. In addition to the usual monitoring of urinary glucose, the patient's blood glucose must also be monitored periodically to determine the minimum effective dose for the patient; to detect primary failure, i.e., inadequate lowering of blood glucose at the maximum recommended dose of medication; and to detect secondary failure, i.e., loss of an adequate blood glucose lowering response after an initial period of effectiveness. Glycosylated hemoglobin levels may also be of value in monitoring the patient's response to therapy.

Short-term administration of DIABINESE may be sufficient during periods of transient loss of control in patients usually controlled well on diet.

The total daily dosage is generally taken at a single time each morning with breakfast. Occasionally cases of gastrointestinal intolerance may be relieved by dividing the daily dosage. A LOADING OR PRIMING DOSE IS NOT NECESSARY AND SHOULD NOT BE USED.

Initial Therapy: 1. The mild to moderately severe, middle-aged, non-insulin-dependent diabetic patient should be started on 250 mg daily. In elderly patients, debilitated or malnourished patients, and patients with impaired renal or hepatic function, the initial and maintenance dosing should be conservative to avoid hypoglycemic reactions (see PRECAUTIONS section). Older patients should be started on smaller amounts of DIABINESE, in the range of 100 to 125 mg daily.

2. No transition period is necessary when transferring patients from other oral hypoglycemic agents to DIABINESE. The other agent may be discontinued abruptly and chlorpropamide started at once. In prescribing chlorpropamide, due consideration must be given to its greater potency.

Many mild to moderately severe, middle-aged, stable non-insulin-dependent diabetic patients receiving insulin can be placed directly on the oral drug and their insulin abruptly discontinued. For patients requiring more than 40 units of insulin daily, therapy with DIABINESE may be initiated with a 50 per cent reduction in insulin for the first few days, with subsequent further reductions dependent upon the response.

During the initial period of therapy with chlorpropamide, hypoglycemic reactions may occasionally occur, particularly during the transition from insulin to the oral drug. Hypoglycemia within 24 hours after withdrawal of the intermediate or long-acting types of insulin will usually prove to be the result of insulin carry-over and not primarily due to the effect of chlorpropamide.

During the insulin withdrawal period, the patient should test his urine for sugar and ketone bodies at least three times daily and report the results frequently to his physician. If they are abnormal, the physician should be notified immediately. In some cases, it may be advisable to consider hospitalization during the transition period.

Five to seven days after the initial therapy, the blood level of chlorpropamide reaches a plateau. Dosage may subsequently be adjusted upward or downward by increments of not more than 50 to 125 mg at intervals of three to five days to obtain optimal control. More frequent adjustments are usually undesirable.

Maintenance Therapy: Most moderately severe, middle-aged, stable non-insulin-dependent diabetic patients are controlled by approximately 250 mg daily. Many investigators have found that some milder diabetics do well on daily doses of 100 mg or less. Many of the more severe diabetics may require 500 mg daily for adequate control. PATIENTS WHO DO NOT RESPOND COMPLETELY TO 500 MG DAILY WILL USUALLY NOT RESPOND TO HIGHER DOSES. MAINTENANCE DOSES ABOVE 750 mg DAILY SHOULD BE AVOIDED.

HOW SUPPLIED
[See table below].

RECOMMENDED STORAGE
Store below 86°F (30°C).

CAUTION
Federal law prohibits dispensing without prescription.
69-2141-37-0   Revised Dec. 1986
Literature Available: Yes.
Shown in Product Identification Section, page 422

FELDENE®   ℞
[fĕl 'deen]
(piroxicam)
CAPSULES
For Oral Use

DESCRIPTION
FELDENE (piroxicam) is 4-Hydroxy-2-methyl-*N*-2-pyridinyl-2*H*-1,2-benzothiazine-3-carboxamide 1,1-dioxide, an oxicam. Members of the oxicam family are not carboxylic acids, but they are acidic by virtue of the enolic 4-hydroxy substituent. FELDENE occurs as a white crystalline solid, sparingly soluble in water, dilute acid and most organic solvents. It is slightly soluble in alcohols and in aqueous alkaline solution. It exhibits a weakly acidic 4-hydroxy proton (pKa 5.1) and a weakly basic pyridyl nitrogen (pKa 1.8). Inert ingredients in the formulations are: hard gelatin capsules (which may contain Blue 1, Red 3, and other inert ingredients); lactose; magnesium stearate; sodium lauryl sulfate; starch.

CLINICAL PHARMACOLOGY
FELDENE has shown anti-inflammatory, analgesic and antipyretic properties in animals. Edema, erythema, tissue proliferation, fever, and pain can all be inhibited in laboratory animals by the administration of FELDENE. It is effective regardless of the etiology of the inflammation. The mode of action of FELDENE is not fully established at this time. However, a common mechanism for the above effects may exist in the ability of FELDENE to inhibit the biosynthesis of prostaglandins, known mediators of inflammation.

It is established that FELDENE does not act by stimulating the pituitary-adrenal axis.

FELDENE is well absorbed following oral administration. Drug plasma concentrations are proportional for 10 and 20 mg doses, generally peak within three to five hours after medication, and subsequently decline with a mean half-life of 50 hours (range of 30 to 86 hours; although values outside of this range have been encountered).

This prolonged half-life results in the maintenance of relatively stable plasma concentrations throughout the day on once daily doses and to significant drug accumulation upon multiple dosing. A single 20 mg dose generally produces peak piroxicam plasma levels of 1.5 to 2 mcg/ml, while maximum drug plasma concentrations, after repeated daily ingestion of 20 mg FELDENE, usually stabilize at 3–8 mcg/ml. Most patients approximate steady state plasma levels within 7 to 12 days. Higher levels, which approximate steady state at two to three weeks, have been observed in patients in whom longer plasma half-lives of piroxicam occurred.

FELDENE and its biotransformation products are excreted in urine and feces, with about twice as much appearing in the urine as the feces. Metabolism occurs by hydroxylation at the 5 position of the pyridyl side chain and conjugation of this product; by cyclodehydration; and by a sequence of reactions involving hydrolysis of the amide linkage, decarboxylation, ring contraction, and N-demethylation. Less than 5% of the daily dose is excreted unchanged.

Concurrent administration of aspirin (3900 mg/day) and FELDENE (20 mg/day), resulted in a reduction of plasma levels of piroxicam to about 80% of their normal values. The use of FELDENE in conjunction with aspirin is not recommended because data are inadequate to demonstrate that the combination produces greater improvement than that achieved with aspirin alone and the potential for adverse reactions is increased. Concomitant administration of antacids had no effect on FELDENE plasma levels. The effects of impaired renal function or hepatic disease on plasma levels have not been established.

FELDENE, like salicylates and other nonsteroidal anti-inflammatory agents, is associated with symptoms of gastrointestinal tract irritation (see ADVERSE REACTIONS). However, in a study utilizing ^{51}Cr-tagged red blood cells, 20 mg of FELDENE administered as a single dose for four days did not result in a significant increase in fecal blood loss and did not detectably affect the gastric mucosa. In the same study a total daily dose of 3900 mg of aspirin, i.e., 972 mg q.i.d., caused a significant increase in fecal blood loss and mucosal lesions as demonstrated by gastroscopy.

Strength	Tablet Description	Tablet Code	NDC	Package Size
DIABINESE (chlorpropamide) 100 mg	Blue, D-shaped, scored	393	0663-3930-66	100's
			0663-3930-73	500's
			0663-3930-41	100 (10 × 10) unit dose
DIABINESE (chlorpropamide) 250 mg	Blue, D-shaped, scored	394	0663-3940-66	100's
			0663-3940-71	250's
			0663-3940-82	1000's
			0663-3940-41	100 (10 × 10) unit dose

In controlled clinical trials, the effectiveness of FELDENE (piroxicam) has been established for both acute exacerbations and long-term management of rheumatoid arthritis and osteoarthritis.

The therapeutic effects of FELDENE are evident early in the treatment of both diseases with a progressive increase in response over several (8–12) weeks. Efficacy is seen in terms of pain relief and, when present, subsidence of inflammation. Doses of 20 mg/day FELDENE display a therapeutic effect comparable to therapeutic doses of aspirin, with a lower incidence of minor gastrointestinal effects and tinnitus.

FELDENE has been administered concomitantly with fixed doses of gold and corticosteroids. The existence of a "steroid-sparing" effect has not been adequately studied to date.

INDICATIONS AND USAGE

FELDENE is indicated for acute or long-term use in the relief of signs and symptoms of the following:
1. osteoarthritis
2. rheumatoid arthritis

Dosage recommendations for use in children have not been established.

CONTRAINDICATIONS

FELDENE should not be used in patients who have previously exhibited hypersensitivity to it, or in individuals with the syndrome comprised of bronchospasm, nasal polyps, and angioedema precipitated by aspirin or other nonsteroidal anti-inflammatory drugs.

WARNINGS

Risk of GI Ulceration, Bleeding and Perforation with NSAID Therapy

Serious gastrointestinal toxicity such as bleeding, ulceration, and perforation can occur at any time, with or without warning symptoms, in patients treated chronically with NSAID therapy. Although minor upper gastrointestinal problems, such as dyspepsia, are common, usually developing early in therapy, physician should remain alert for ulceration and bleeding in patients treated chronically with NSAIDs even in the absence of previous GI tract symptoms. In patients observed in clinical trials of several months to two years duration, symptomatic upper GI ulcers, gross bleeding or perforation appear to occur in approximately 1% of patients treated for 3–6 months, and in about 2–4% of patients treated for one year. Physicians should inform patients about the signs and/or symptoms of serious GI toxicity and what steps to take if they occur.

Studies to date have not identified any subset of patients not at risk of developing peptic ulceration and bleeding. Except for a prior history of serious GI events and other risk factors known to be associated with peptic ulcer disease, such as alcoholism, smoking, etc., no risk factors (e.g., age, sex) have been associated with inreased risk. Elderly or debilitated patients seem to tolerate ulceration or bleeding less well than other individuals and most spontaneous reports of fatal GI events are in this population. Studies to date are inconclusive concerning the relative risk of various NSAIDs in causing such reactions. High doses of any NSAID probably carry a greater risk of these reactions, although controlled clinical trials showing this do not exist in most cases. In considering the use of relatively large doses (within the recommended dosage range), sufficient benefit should be anticipated to offset the potential increased risk of GI toxicity.

PRECAUTIONS

Renal Effects: As with other nonsteroidal anti-inflammatory drugs, long-term administration of piroxicam to animals has resulted in renal papillary necrosis and other abnormal renal pathology. In humans, there have been reports of acute interstitial nephritis with hematuria, proteinuria, and occasionally, nephrotic syndrome.

A second form of renal toxicity has been seen in patients with prerenal conditions leading to a reduction in renal blood flow or blood volume, where the renal prostaglandins have a supportive role in the maintenance of renal perfusion. In these patients administration of an NSAID may cause a dose-dependent reduction in prostaglandin formation and may precipitate overt renal decompensation. Patients at greatest risk of this reaction are those with impaired renal function, heart failure, liver dysfunction, those taking diuretics, and the elderly. Discontinuation of NSAID therapy is typically followed by recovery to the pretreatment state.

Because of extensive renal excretion of piroxicam and its biotransformation products (less than 5% of the daily dose excreted unchanged, see CLINICAL PHARMACOLOGY), lower doses of piroxicam should be anticipated in patients with impaired renal function, and they should be carefully monitored.

Although other nonsteroidal anti-inflammatory drugs do not have the same direct effects on platelets that aspirin does, all drugs inhibiting prostaglandin biosynthesis do interfere with platelet function to some degree; therefore, patients who may be adversely affected by such an action should be carefully observed when FELDENE is administered.

Because of reports of adverse eye findings with nonsteroidal anti-inflammatory agents, it is recommended that patients who develop visual complaints during treatment with FELDENE have ophthalmic evaluation.

As with other nonsteroidal anti-inflammatory drugs, borderline elevations of one or more liver tests may occur in up to 15% of patients. These abnormalities may progress, may remain essentially unchanged, or may be transient with continued therapy. The SGPT (ALT) test is probably the most sensitive indicator of liver dysfunction. Meaningful (3 times the upper limit of normal) elevations of SGPT or SGOT (AST) occurred in controlled clinical trials in less than 1% of patients. A patient with symptoms and/or signs suggesting liver dysfunction, or in whom an abnormal liver test has occurred, should be evaluated for evidence of the development of more severe hepatic reaction while on therapy with FELDENE. Severe hepatic reactions, including jaundice and cases of fatal hepatitis, have been reported with FELDENE. Although such reactions are rare, if abnormal liver tests persist or worsen, if clinical signs and symptoms consistent with liver disease develop, or if systemic manifestations occur (e.g. eosinophilia, rash, etc.), FELDENE should be discontinued. (See also ADVERSE REACTIONS.)

Although at the recommended dose of 20 mg/day of FELDENE increased fecal blood loss due to gastrointestinal irritation did not occur (see CLINICAL PHARMACOLOGY), in about 4% of the patients treated with FELDENE alone or concomitantly with aspirin, reductions in hemoglobin and hematocrit values were observed. Therefore, these values should be determined if signs or symptoms of anemia occur. Peripheral edema has been observed in approximately 2% of the patients treated with FELDENE. Therefore, as with other nonsteroidal anti-inflammatory drugs, FELDENE should be used with caution in patients with heart failure, hypertension or other conditions predisposing to fluid retention, since its usage may be associated with a worsening of these conditions.

A combination of dermatological and/or allergic signs and symptoms suggestive of serum sickness have occasionally occurred in conjunction with the use of FELDENE. These include arthralgias, pruritus, fever, fatigue, and rash including vesiculo bullous reactions and exfoliative dermatitis.

Information for Patients

FELDENE, like other drugs of its class, is not free of side effects. The side effects of these drugs can cause discomfort and, rarely, there are more serious side effects, such as gastrointestinal bleeding, which may result in hospitalization and even fatal outcomes.

NSAIDs (Nonsteroidal Anti-Inflammatory Drugs) are often essential agents in the management of arthritis, but they also may be commonly employed for conditions which are less serious.

Physicians may wish to discuss with their patients the potential risks (see WARNINGS, PRECAUTIONS, and ADVERSE REACTIONS sections) and likely benefits of NSAID treatment, particularly when the drugs are used for less serious conditions where treatment without NSAIDs may represent an acceptable alternative to both the patient and physician.

Laboratory Tests

Because serious GI tract ulceration and bleeding can occur without warning symptoms, physicians should follow chronically treated patients for the signs and symptoms of ulceration and bleeding and should inform them of the importance of this follow-up (see Risk of GI Ulceration, Bleeding and Perforation with NSAID Therapy).

Drug Interactions

FELDENE is highly protein bound, and, therefore, might be expected to displace other protein-bound drugs. Although this has not occurred in *in vitro* studies with coumarin-type anticoagulants, interactions with coumarin-type anticoagulants have been reported with FELDENE since marketing, therefore, physicians should closely monitor patients for a change in dosage requirements when administering FELDENE to patients in coumarin-type anticoagulants and other highly protein-bound drugs.

Plasma levels of piroxicam are depressed to approximately 80% of their normal values when FELDENE is given in conjunction with aspirin (3900 mg/day), but concomitant administration of antacids has no effect on piroxicam plasma levels (see CLINICAL PHARMACOLOGY).

Nonsteroidal anti-inflammatory agents, including FELDENE, have been reported to increase steady state plasma lithium levels. It is recommended that plasma lithium levels be monitored when initiating, adjusting and discontinuing FELDENE.

Carcinogenesis, Chronic Animal Toxicity and Impairment of Fertility

Subacute and chronic toxicity studies have been carried out in rats, mice, dogs, and monkeys.

The pathology most often seen was that characteristically associated with the animal toxicology of anti-inflammatory agents: renal papillary necrosis (see PRECAUTIONS) and gastrointestinal lesions.

In classical studies in laboratory animals piroxicam did not show any teratogenic potential.

Reproductive studies revealed no impairment of fertility in animals.

Pregnancy and Nursing Mothers

Like other drugs which inhibit the synthesis and release of prostaglandins, piroxicam increased the incidence of dystocia and delayed parturition in pregnant animals when piroxicam administration was continued late into pregnancy. Gastrointestinal tract toxicity was increased in pregnant females in the last trimester of pregnancy compared to nonpregnant females or females in earlier trimesters of pregnancy.

FELDENE is not recommended for use in nursing mothers or in pregnant women because of the animal findings and since safety for such use has not been established in humans.

Use in Children

Dosage recommendations and indications for use in children have not been established.

ADVERSE REACTIONS

The incidence of adverse reactions to piroxicam is based on clinical trials involving approximately 2300 patients, about 400 of whom were treated for more than one year and 170 for more than two years. About 30% of all patients receiving daily doses of 20 mg of FELDENE experienced side effects. Gastrointestinal symptoms were the most prominent side effects—occurring in approximately 20% of the patients, which in most instances did not interfere with the course of therapy. Of the patients experiencing gastrointestinal side effects, approximately 5% discontinued therapy with an overall incidence of peptic ulceration of about 1%.

Other than the gastrointestinal symptoms, edema, dizziness, headache, changes in hematological parameters, and rash have been reported in a small percentage of patients. Routine ophthalmoscopy and slit-lamp examinations have revealed no evidence of ocular changes in 205 patients followed from 3 to 24 months while on therapy.

Incidence Greater Than 1%. The following adverse reactions occurred more frequently than 1 in 100.

Gastrointestinal: stomatitis, anorexia, epigastric distress*, nausea*, constipation, abdominal discomfort, flatulence, diarrhea, abdominal pain, indigestion

Hematological: decreases in hemoglobin* and hematocrit* (see PRECAUTIONS), anemia, leucopenia, eosinophia

Dermatologic: pruritus, rash

Central Nervous System: dizziness, somnolence, vertigo

Urogenital: BUN and creatinine elevations (see PRECAUTIONS)

Body as a Whole: headache, malaise

Special Senses: tinnitus

Cardiovascular/Respiratory: edema (see PRECAUTIONS)

*Reactions occurring in 3% to 9% of patients treated with FELDENE. Reactions occurring in 1–3% of patients are unmarked.

Incidence Less Than 1% (Causal Relationship Probable)

The following adverse reactions occurred less frequently than 1 in 100. The probability exists that there is a causal relationship between FELDENE and these reactions.

Gastrointestinal: liver function abnormalities, jaundice, hepatitis (see PRECAUTIONS), vomiting, hematemesis, melena, gastrointestinal bleeding, perforation and ulceration (see WARNINGS), dry mouth

Hematological: thrombocytopenia, petechial rash, ecchymosis, bone marrow depression including aplastic anemia, epistaxis

Dermatologic: sweating, erythema, bruising, desquamation, exfoliative dermatitis, erythema multiforme, toxic epidermal necrolysis, Stevens-Johnson syndrome, vesiculo bullous reaction, photoallergic skin reactions

Central Nervous System: depression, insomnia, nervousness

Urogenital: hematuria, proteinuria, interstitial nephritis, renal failure, hyperkalemia, glomerulitis, papillary necrosis, nephrotic syndrome (see PRECAUTIONS)

Body as a Whole: pain (colic), fever, flu-like syndrome (see PRECAUTIONS)

Special Senses: swollen eyes, blurred vision, eye irritations

Cardiovascular/Respiratory: hypertension, worsening of congestive heart failure (see PRECAUTIONS), exacerbation of angina

Metabolic: hypoglycemia, hyperglycemia, weight increase, weight decrease

Hypersensitivity: anaphylaxis, bronchospasm, urticaria/angioedema, vasculitis, "serum sickness" (see PRECAUTIONS)

Incidence Less Than 1% (Causal Relationship Unknown)

Other adverse reactions were reported with a frequency of less than 1 in 100, but a causal relationship between FELDENE and the reaction could not be determined.

Gastrointestinal: pancreatitis

Dermatologic: onycholysis, loss of hair

Central Nervous System: akathisia, hallucinations, mood alterations, dream abnormalities, mental confusion, paresthesias

Urogenital System: dysuria

Body as a Whole: weakness

Cardiovascular/Respiratory: palpitations, dyspnea

Hypersensitivity: positive ANA

Continued on next page

Pfizer—Cont.

Special Senses: transient hearing loss
Hematological: hemolytic anemia

OVERDOSAGE

In the event treatment for overdosage is required the long plasma half-life (see CLINICAL PHARMACOLOGY) of piroxicam should be considered. The absence of experience with acute overdosage precludes characterization of sequelae and recommendation of specific antidotal efficacy at this time. It is reasonable to assume, however, that the standard measures of gastric evacuation and general supportive therapy would apply. In addition to supportive measures, the use of activated charcoal may effectively reduce the absorption and reabsorption of piroxicam. Experiments in dogs have demonstrated that the use of multiple-dose treatments with activated charcoal could reduce the half-life of piroxicam elimination from 27 hours (without charcoal) to 11 hours and reduce the systemic bioavailability of piroxicam by as much as 37% when activated charcoal is given as late as 6 hours after administration of piroxicam.

ADMINISTRATION AND DOSAGE

Rheumatoid Arthritis, Osteoarthritis
It is recommended that FELDENE therapy be initiated and maintained at a single daily dose of 20 mg. If desired the daily dose may be divided. Because of the long half-life of FELDENE, steady-state blood levels are not reached for 7–12 days. Therefore although the therapeutic effects of FELDENE are evident early in treatment, there is a progressive increase in response over several weeks and the effect of therapy should not be assessed for two weeks.
Dosage recommendations and indications for use in children have not been established.

HOW SUPPLIED

FELDENE Capsules for oral administration
Bottles of 100: 10 mg (NDC 0663-3220-66) maroon and blue #322
20 mg (NDC 0663-3230-66), and (NDC 0069-3230-66) maroon #323
Bottles of 500: 20 mg (NDC 0663-3230-73) maroon #323
Unit dose packages of 100: 20 mg (NDC 0663-3230-41) maroon #323

© **1982 PFIZER INC**
Revised Oct. 1988

65-4100-00-2

LITERATURE AVAILABLE

Yes.
Shown in Product Identification Section, page 422

MINIPRESS® CAPSULES   ℞
[mĭn ′ē-prĕs]
(prazosin hydrochloride)
For Oral Use

DESCRIPTION

MINIPRESS (prazosin hydrochloride), a quinazoline derivative, is the first of a new chemical class of antihypertensives. It is the hydrochloride salt of 1-(4-amino-6,7-dimethoxy-2-quinazolinyl)-4-(2-furoyl) piperazine.
It is a white, crystalline substance, slightly soluble in water and isotonic saline, and has a molecular weight of 419.87.
Each 1 mg capsule of MINIPRESS for oral use contains drug equivalent to 1 mg free base.
Inert ingredients in the formulations are: hard gelatin capsules (which may contain Blue 1, Red 3, Red 28, Red 40, and other inert ingredients); magnesium stearate; sodium lauryl sulfate; starch; sucrose.

CLINICAL PHARMACOLOGY

The exact mechanism of the hypotensive action of prazosin is unknown. Prazosin causes a decrease in total peripheral resistance and was originally thought to have a direct relaxant action on vascular smooth muscle. Recent animal studies, however, have suggested that the vasodilator effect of prazosin is also related to blockade of postsynaptic *alpha*-adrenoceptors. The results of dog forelimb experiments demonstrate that the peripheral vasodilator effect of prazosin is confined mainly to the level of the resistance vessels (arterioles). Unlike conventional *alpha*-blockers, the antihypertensive action of prazosin is usually not accompanied by a reflex tachycardia. Tolerance has not been observed to develop in long term therapy.
Hemodynamic studies have been carried out in man following acute single dose administration and during the course of long term maintenance therapy. The results confirm that the therapeutic effect is a fall in blood pressure unaccompanied by a clinically significant change in cardiac output, heart rate, renal blood flow and glomerular filtration rate. There is no measurable negative chronotropic effect.
In clinical studies to date, MINIPRESS (prazosin hydrochloride) has not increased plasma renin activity.

In man, blood pressure is lowered in both the supine and standing positions. This effect is most pronounced on the diastolic blood pressure.
Following oral administration, human plasma concentrations reach a peak at about three hours with a plasma half-life of two to three hours. The drug is highly bound to plasma protein. Bioavailability studies have demonstrated that the total absorption relative to the drug in a 20% alcoholic solution is 90%, resulting in peak levels approximately 65% of that of the drug in solution. Animal studies indicate that MINIPRESS (prazosin hydrochloride) is extensively metabolized, primarily by demethylation and conjugation, and excreted mainly via bile and feces. Less extensive human studies suggest similar metabolism and excretion in man.
In clinical studies in which lipid profiles were followed, there were generally no adverse changes noted between pre- and post-treatment lipid levels.

INDICATIONS AND USAGE

MINIPRESS (prazosin hydrochloride) is indicated in the treatment of hypertension. It can be used alone or in combination with other antihypertensive drugs such as diuretics or beta-adrenergic blocking agents.

CONTRAINDICATIONS

None known.

WARNINGS

MINIPRESS (prazosin hydrochloride) may cause syncope with sudden loss of consciousness. In most cases this is believed to be due to an excessive postural hypotensive effect, although occasionally the syncopal episode has been preceded by a bout of severe tachycardia with heart rates of 120–160 beats per minute. Syncopal episodes have usually occurred within 30 to 90 minutes of the initial dose of the drug; occasionally they have been reported in association with rapid dosage increases or the introduction of another antihypertensive drug into the regimen of a patient taking high doses of MINIPRESS (prazosin hydrochloride). The incidence of syncopal episodes is approximately 1% in patients given an initial dose of 2 mg or greater. Clinical trials conducted during the investigational phase of this drug suggest that syncopal episodes can be minimized by limiting the initial dose of the drug to 1 mg, by subsequently increasing the dosage slowly, and by introducing any additional antihypertensive drugs into the patient's regimen with caution (see DOSAGE AND ADMINISTRATION). Hypotension may develop in patients given MINIPRESS who are also receiving a beta-blocker such as propranolol.
If syncope occurs, the patient should be placed in the recumbent position and treated supportively as necessary. This adverse effect is self-limiting and in most cases does not recur after the initial period of therapy or during subsequent dose titration.
Patients should always be started on the 1 mg capsules of MINIPRESS (prazosin hydrochloride). The 2 and 5 mg capsules are not indicated for initial therapy.
More common than loss of consciousness are the symptoms often associated with lowering of the blood pressure, namely, dizziness and lightheadedness. The patient should be cautioned about these possible adverse effects and advised what measures to take should they develop. The patient should also be cautioned to avoid situations where injury could result should syncope occur during the initiation of MINIPRESS (prazosin hydrochloride) therapy.

PRECAUTIONS

Information for Patients: Dizziness or drowsiness may occur after the first dose of this medicine. Avoid driving or performing hazardous tasks for the first 24 hours after taking this medicine or when the dose is increased. Dizziness, lightheadedness or fainting may occur, especially when rising from a lying or sitting position. Getting up slowly may help lessen the problem. These effects may also occur if you drink alcohol, stand for long periods of time, exercise, or if the weather is hot. While taking MINIPRESS, be careful in the amount of alcohol you drink. Also, use extra care during exercise or hot weather, or if standing for long periods. Check with your physician if you have any questions.
Drug Interactions
MINIPRESS (prazosin hydrochloride) has been administered without any adverse drug interaction in limited clinical experience to date with the following: (1) cardiac glycosides—digitalis and digoxin; (2) hypoglycemics—insulin, chlorpropamide, phenformin, tolazamide, and tolbutamide; (3) tranquilizers and sedatives—chlordiazepoxide, diazepam, and phenobarbital; (4) antigout—allopurinol, colchicine, and probenecid; (5) antiarrhythmics—procainamide, propranolol (see WARNINGS however), and quinidine; and (6) analgesics, antipyretics and anti-inflammatories—propoxyphene, aspirin, indomethacin and phenylbutazone.
Addition of a diuretic or other antihypertensive agent to MINIPRESS has been shown to cause an additive hypotensive effect. This effect can be minimized by reducing the MINIPRESS dose to 1 to 2 mg three times a day, by introducing additional antihypertensive drugs cautiously and then by retitrating MINIPRESS based on clinical response.

Drug/Laboratory Test Interactions
In a study on five patients given from 12 to 24 mg of prazosin per day for 10 to 14 days, there was an average increase of 42% in the urinary metabolite of norepinephrine and an average increase in urinary VMA of 17%. Therefore, false positive results may occur in screening tests for pheochromocytoma in patients who are being treated with prazosin. If an elevated VMA is found, prazosin should be discontinued and the patient retested after a month.
Laboratory Tests
In clinical studies in which lipid profiles were followed, there were generally no adverse changes noted between pre- and post-treatment lipid levels.
Carcinogenesis, Mutagenesis, Impairment of Fertility: No carcinogenic potential was demonstrated in an 18 month study in rats with MINIPRESS at dose levels more than 225 times the usual maximum recommended human dose of 20 mg per day. MINIPRESS was not mutagenic in *in vivo* genetic toxicology studies. In a fertility and general reproductive performance study in rats, both males and females, treated with 75 mg/kg (225 times the usual maximum recommended human dose), demonstrated decreased fertility while those treated with 25 mg/kg (75 times the usual maximum recommended human dose) did not.
In chronic studies (one year or more) of MINIPRESS in rats and dogs, testicular changes consisting of atrophy and necrosis occurred at 25 mg/kg/day (75 times the usual maximum recommended human dose). No testicular changes were seen in rats or dogs at 10 mg/kg/day (30 times the usual maximum recommended human dose). In view of the testicular changes observed in animals, 105 patients on long term MINIPRESS therapy were monitored for 17-ketosteroid excretion and no changes indicating a drug effect were observed. In addition, 27 males on MINIPRESS for up to 51 months did not have changes in sperm morphology suggestive of drug effect.
Usage in Pregnancy: Pregnancy Category C. MINIPRESS has been shown to be associated with decreased litter size at birth, 1, 4, and 21 days of age in rats when given doses more than 225 times the usual maximum recommended human dose. No evidence of drug-related external, visceral, or skeletal fetal abnormalities was observed. No drug-related external, visceral, or skeletal abnormalities were observed in fetuses of pregnant rabbits and pregnant monkeys at doses more than 225 times and 12 times the usual maximum recommended human dose respectively.
The use of prazosin and a beta-blocker for the control of severe hypertension in 44 pregnant women revealed no drug-related fetal abnormalities or adverse effects. Therapy with prazosin was continued for as long as 14 weeks.[1]
Prazosin has also been used alone or in combination with other hypotensive agents in severe hypertension of pregnancy by other investigators. No fetal or neonatal abnormalities have been reported with the use of prazosin.[2]
There are no adequate and well controlled studies which establish the safety of MINIPRESS (prazosin HCl) in pregnant women. MINIPRESS should be used during pregnancy only if the potential benefit justifies the potential risk to the mother and fetus.
Nursing Mothers: MINIPRESS has been shown to be excreted in small amounts in human milk. Caution should be exercised when MINIPRESS is administered to a nursing woman.
Usage in Children: Safety and effectiveness in children have not been established.

ADVERSE REACTIONS

Clinical trials were conducted on more than 900 patients. During these trials and subsequent marketing experience, the most frequent reactions associated with MINIPRESS therapy are: dizziness 10.3%, headache 7.8%, drowsiness 7.6%, lack of energy 6.9%, weakness 6.5%, palpitations 5.3%, and nausea 4.9%. In most instances side effects have disappeared with continued therapy or have been tolerated with no decrease in dose of drug.
Less frequent adverse reactions which are reported to occur in 1–4% of patients are:
Gastrointestinal: vomiting, diarrhea, constipation.
Cardiovascular: edema, orthostatic hypotension, dyspnea, syncope.
Central Nervous System: vertigo, depression, nervousness.
Dermatologic: rash.
Genitourinary: urinary frequency.
EENT: blurred vision, reddened sclera, epistaxis, dry mouth, nasal congestion.
In addition, fewer than 1% of patients have reported the following (in some instances, exact causal relationships have not been established):
Gastrointestinal: abdominal discomfort and/or pain, liver function abnormalities, pancreatitis.
Cardiovascular: tachycardia.
Central Nervous System: paresthesia, hallucinations.
Dermatologic: pruritus, alopecia, lichen planus.
Genitourinary: incontinence, impotence, priapism.

EENT: tinnitus.

Other: diaphoresis, fever, positive ANA titer, arthralgia. Single reports of pigmentary mottling and serous retinopathy, and a few reports of cataract development or disappearance have been reported. In these instances, the exact causal relationship has not been established because the baseline observations were frequently inadequate.

In more specific slit-lamp and funduscopic studies, which included adequate baseline examinations, no drug-related abnormal ophthalmological findings have been reported. Literature reports exist associating MINIPRESS therapy with a worsening of pre-existing narcolepsy. A causal relationship is uncertain in these cases.

OVERDOSAGE

Accidental ingestion of at least 50 mg of MINIPRESS (prazosin hydrochloride) in a two year old child resulted in profound drowsiness and depressed reflexes. No decrease in blood pressure was noted. Recovery was uneventful.

Should overdosage lead to hypotension, support of the cardiovascular system is of first importance. Restoration of blood pressure and normalization of heart rate may be accomplished by keeping the patient in the supine position. If this measure is inadequate, shock should first be treated with volume expanders. If necessary, vasopressors should then be used. Renal function should be monitored and supported as needed. Laboratory data indicate MINIPRESS is not dialysable because it is protein bound.

DOSAGE AND ADMINISTRATION

The dose of MINIPRESS should be adjusted according to the patient's individual blood pressure response. The following is a guide to its administration:

Initial Dose

1 mg two or three times a day. (See WARNINGS)

Maintenance Dose

Dosage may be slowly increased to a total daily dose of 20 mg given in divided doses. The therapeutic dosages most commonly employed have ranged from 6 mg to 15 mg daily given in divided doses. Doses higher than 20 mg usually do not increase efficacy, however a few patients may benefit from further increases up to a daily dose of 40 mg given in divided doses. After initial titration some patients can be maintained adequately on a twice daily dosage regimen.

Use With Other Drugs

When adding a diuretic or other antihypertensive agent, the dose of MINIPRESS should be reduced to 1 mg or 2 mg three times a day and retitration then carried out.

HOW SUPPLIED

[See table above].

References

1. Lubbe, WF, and Hodge, JV: *New Zealand Med J* **94** (691) 169–172, 1981.
2. Davey, DA, and Dommisse, J: *S.A. Med J,* Oct 4, 1980 (551–556).

77-2318-00-1   Revised Dec. 1988

Shown in Product Identification Section, page 422

MINIZIDE® CAPSULES   ℞

[mĭn 'ē-zīd]

(prazosin hydrochloride and polythiazide)

FOR ORAL ADMINISTRATION

This fixed combination drug is not indicated for initial therapy of hypertension. Hypertension requires therapy titrated to the individual patient. If the fixed combination represents the dose so determined, its use may be more convenient in patient management. The treatment of hypertension is not static, but must be re-evaluated as conditions in each patient warrant.

DESCRIPTION

MINIZIDE is a combination of MINIPRESS® (prazosin hydrochloride) plus RENESE® (polythiazide).

MINIPRESS (prazosin hydrochloride), a quinazoline derivative, is the first of a new chemical class of antihypertensives.

Strength	Capsule Color	Capsule Code	NDC	Package Size
MINIPRESS 1 mg	White	431	0663-4310-71	250's
			0069-4310-71	250's
			0663-4310-82	1000's
			0663-4310-41	100 (10×10) Unit Dose
MINIPRESS 2 mg	Pink and White	437	0663-4370-71	250's
			0663-4370-82	1000's
			0663-4370-41	100 (10×10) Unit Dose
MINIPRESS 5 mg	Blue and White	438	0663-4380-71	250's
			0663-4380-73	500's
			0663-4380-41	100 (10×10) Unit Dose

It is the hydrochloride salt of 1-(4-amino-6,7-dimethoxy-2-quinazolinyl)-4-(2-furoyl) piperazine.

It is a white, crystalline substance, slightly soluble in water and isotonic saline, and has a molecular weight of 419.87. Each 1 mg capsule of MINIPRESS (prazosin hydrochloride) contains drug equivalent to 1 mg free base.

RENESE (polythiazide) is an orally effective, nonmercurial diuretic, saluretic, and antihypertensive agent.

It is designated chemically as $2H$- 1,2,4-Benzothiadiazine-7-sulfonamide, 6-chloro-3, 4-dihydro-2-methyl-3-[[(2,2,2-trifluoroethyl)thio]methyl]-,1,1-dioxide.

It is a white, crystalline substance insoluble in water, but readily soluble in alkaline solution.

Inert ingredients in the formulations are: hard gelatin capsules (which may contain Blue 1, Green 3, Red 3 and other inert ingredients); magnesium stearate; sodium lauryl sulfate; starch; sucrose.

[See table below].

CLINICAL PHARMACOLOGY

MINIZIDE (prazosin hydrochloride/polythiazide)

Minizide produces a more pronounced antihypertensive response than occurs after either prazosin hydrochloride or polythiazide alone in equivalent doses.

MINIPRESS (prazosin hydrochloride)

The exact mechanism of the hypotensive action of prazosin is unknown. Prazosin causes a decrease in total peripheral resistance and was originally thought to have a direct relaxant action on vascular smooth muscle. Recent animal studies, however, have suggested that the vasodilator effect of prazosin is also related to blockade of postsynaptic *alpha* -adrenoceptors. The results of dog forelimb experiments demonstrate that the peripheral vasodilator effect of prazosin is confined mainly to the level of the resistance vessels (arterioles). Unlike conventional *alpha* -blockers, the antihypertensive action of prazosin is usually not accompanied by a reflex tachycardia. Tolerance has not been observed to develop in long term therapy.

Hemodynamic studies have been carried out in man following acute single dose administration and during the course of long term maintenance therapy. The results confirm that the therapeutic effect is a fall in blood pressure unaccompanied by a clinically significant change in cardiac output, heart rate, renal blood flow, and glomerular filtration rate. There is no measurable negative chronotropic effect.

In clinical studies to date, MINIPRESS has not increased plasma renin activity.

In man, blood pressure is lowered in both the supine and standing positions. This effect is most pronounced on the diastolic blood pressure.

Following oral administration, human plasma concentrations reach a peak at about three hours with a plasma half-life of two to three hours. The drug is highly bound to plasma protein. Bioavailability studies have demonstrated that the total absorption relative to the drug in a 20% alcoholic solution is 90%, resulting in peak levels approximately 65% of that of the drug in solution. Animal studies indicate that MINIPRESS is extensively metabolized, primarily by demethylation and conjugation, and excreted mainly via bile and feces. Less extensive human studies suggest similar metabolism and excretion in man.

MINIPRESS has been administered without any adverse drug interaction in limited clinical experience to date with the following: (1) cardiac glycosides—digitalis and digoxin; (2) hypoglycemics—insulin, chlorpropamide, phenformin, tolazamide, and tolbutamide; (3) tranquilizers and sedatives—chlordiazepoxide, diazepam, and phenobarbital; (4) antigout—allopurinol, colchicine, and probenecid; (5) antiarrhythmics—procainamide, propranolol (see WARNINGS however), and quinidine; and (6) analgesics, antipyretics and anti-inflammatories—propoxyphene, aspirin, indomethacin, and phenylbutazone.

RENESE (polythiazide)

RENESE is a member of the benzothiadiazine (thiazide) family of diuretic/antihypertensive agents. Its mechanism of action results in an interference with the renal tubular mechanism of electrolyte reabsorption. At maximal therapeutic dosage all thiazides are approximately equal in their diuretic potency. The mechanism whereby thiazides function in the control of hypertension is unknown. Renese is well absorbed, giving peak human plasma concentrations about 5 hours after oral administration. Drug is removed slowly thereafter with a plasma elimination half-life of approximately 27 hours. One fifth of the drug is recovered unchanged in human urine; the remainder is cleared via feces and as metabolites. Animal studies indicate metabolism occurs by rupture of the thiadiazine ring and loss of the side chain.

INDICATIONS AND USAGE

MINIZIDE is indicated in the treatment of hypertension. (See box warning.)

CONTRAINDICATIONS

RENESE (polythiazide) is contraindicated in patients with anuria, and in patients known to be sensitive to thiazides or to other sulfonamide derivatives.

WARNINGS

MINIPRESS (prazosin hydrochloride)

MINIPRESS may cause syncope with sudden loss of consciousness. In most cases this is believed to be due to an excessive postural hypotensive effect, although occasionally the syncopal episode has been preceded by a bout of severe tachycardia with heart rates of 120–160 beats per minute. Syncopal episodes have usually occurred within 30 to 90 minutes of the initial dose of the drug; occasionally they have been reported in association with rapid dosage increases or the introduction of another antihypertensive drug into the regimen of a patient taking high doses of MINIPRESS. The incidence of syncopal episodes is approximately 1% in patients given an initial dose of 2 mg or greater. Clinical trials conducted during the investigational phase of this drug suggest that syncopal episodes can be minimized by limiting the initial dose of the drug to 1 mg, by subsequently increasing the dosage slowly, and by introducing any additional antihypertensive drugs into the patient's regimen with caution (see DOSAGE AND ADMINISTRATION). Hypotension may develop in patients given MINIPRESS who are also receiving a beta-blocker such as propranolol.

If syncope occurs, the patient should be placed in the recumbent position and treated supportively as necessary. This adverse effect is self-limiting and in most cases does not recur after the initial period of therapy or during subsequent dose titration.

Patients should always be started on the 1 mg capsules of MINIPRESS (prazosin hydrochloride). The 2 and 5 mg capsules are not indicated for initial therapy.

More common than loss of consciousness are the symptoms often associated with lowering of the blood pressure, namely, dizziness and lightheadedness. The patient should be cautioned about these possible adverse effects and advised what measures to take should they develop. The patient should also be cautioned to avoid situations where injury could re-

HOW SUPPLIED

STRENGTH	COMPONENTS	COLOR	CAPSULE CODE	PKG. SIZE
MINIZIDE 1	1 mg prazosin + 0.5 mg polythiazide (NDC 0663-4300-66)	Blue-Green	430	100's
MINIZIDE 2	2 mg prazosin + 0.5 mg polythiazide (NDC 0663-4320-66)	Blue-Green/Pink	432	100's
MINIZIDE 5	5 mg prazosin + 0.5 mg polythiazide (NDC 0663-4360-66)	Blue-Green/Blue	436	100's

Continued on next page

Pfizer—Cont.

sult should syncope occur during the initiation of MINIPRESS therapy.

RENESE (polythiazide)

RENESE should be used with caution in severe renal disease. In patients with renal disease, thiazides may precipitate azotemia. Cumulative effects of the drug may develop in patients with impaired renal function.

Thiazides should be used with caution in patients with impaired hepatic function or progressive liver disease, since minor alterations of fluid and electrolyte balance may precipitate hepatic coma.

Sensitivity reactions may occur in patients with a history of allergy or bronchial asthma.

The possibility of exacerbation or activation of systemic lupus erythematosus has been reported.

Thiazides may be additive or potentiative of the action of other antihypertensive drugs.

Potentiation occurs with ganglionic or peripheral adrenergic blocking drugs.

Periodic determinations of serum electrolytes to detect possible electrolyte imbalance should be performed at appropriate intervals.

All patients receiving thiazide therapy should be observed for clinical signs of fluid or electrolyte imbalance, namely, hyponatremia, hypochloremic alkalosis, and hypokalemia. Serum and urine electrolyte determinations are particularly important when the patient is vomiting excessively or receiving parenteral fluids. Medications such as digitalis may also influence serum electrolytes. Warning signs, irrespective of cause, are: dryness of mouth, thirst, weakness, lethargy, drowsiness, restlessness, muscle pains or cramps, muscular fatigue, hypotension, oliguria, tachycardia, and gastrointestinal disturbances such as nausea and vomiting.

Hypokalemia may develop with thiazides as with any potent diuretic, especially with brisk diuresis, when severe cirrhosis is present, or during concomitant use of corticosteroids or ACTH.

Interference with adequate oral electrolyte intake will also contribute to hypokalemia. Digitalis therapy may exaggerate the metabolic effects of hypokalemia, especially with reference to myocardial activity.

Any chloride deficit is generally mild and usually does not require specific treatment except under extraordinary circumstances (as in hepatic or renal disease). Dilutional hyponatremia may occur in edematous patients in hot weather; appropriate therapy is water restriction rather than administration of salt, except in rare instances when the hyponatremia is life-threatening. In actual salt depletion, appropriate replacement is the therapy of choice.

Hyperuricemia may occur or frank gout may be precipitated in certain patients receiving thiazide therapy.

Insulin requirements in diabetic patients may be either increased, decreased, or unchanged. Latent diabetes mellitus may become manifest during thiazide administration.

Thiazide drugs may increase responsiveness to tubocurarine. The antihypertensive effects of the drug may be enhanced in the post-sympathectomy patient.

Thiazides may decrease arterial responsiveness to norepinephrine. This diminution is not sufficient to preclude effectiveness of the pressor agent for therapeutic use.

If progressive renal impairment becomes evident, as indicated by a rising nonprotein nitrogen or blood urea nitrogen, a careful reappraisal of therapy is necessary with consideration given to withholding or discontinuing diuretic therapy. Thiazides may decrease serum protein-bound iodine levels without signs of thyroid disturbance.

PRECAUTIONS

Drug/Laboratory Test Interactions: In a study on five patients given from 12 to 24 mg of prazosin per day for 10 to 14 days, there was an average increase of 42% in the urinary metabolite of norepinephrine and an average increase in urinary VMA of 17%. Therefore, false positive results may occur in screening tests for pheochromocytoma in patients who are being treated with prazosin. If an elevated VMA is found, prazosin should be discontinued and the patient retested after a month.

Carcinogenesis, Mutagenesis, Impairment of Fertility: No carcinogenic or mutagenic studies have been conducted with MINIZIDE. However, no carcinogenic potential was demonstrated in 18 month studies in rats with either MINIPRESS or RENESE at dose levels more than 100 times the usual maximum human doses. MINIPRESS was not mutagenic in *in vivo* genetic toxicology studies.

MINIZIDE produced no impairment of fertility in male or female rats at 50 and 25 mg/kg/day of MINIPRESS and RENESE respectively. In chronic studies (one year or more) of MINIPRESS in rats and dogs, testicular changes consisting of atrophy and necrosis occurred at 25 mg/kg/day (60 times the usual maximum recommended human dose). No testicular changes were seen in rats or dogs at 10 mg/kg/day (24 times the usual maximum recommended human dose). In view of the testicular changes observed in animals, 105 pa-

tients on long term MINIPRESS therapy were monitored for 17-ketosteroid excretion and no changes indicating a drug effect were observed. In addition, 27 males on MINIPRESS alone for up to 51 months did not have changes in sperm morphology suggestive of drug effect.

Use in Pregnancy: Pregnancy Category C. MINIZIDE was not teratogenic in either rats or rabbits when administered in oral doses more than 100 times the usual maximum human dose. Studies in rats indicated that the combination of RENESE (40 times the usual maximum recommended human dose) and MINIPRESS (8 times the usual maximum recommended human dose) caused a greater number of stillbirths, a more prolonged gestation, and a decreased survival of pups to weaning than that caused by MINIPRESS alone. There are no adequate and well controlled studies in pregnant women. Therefore, MINIZIDE should be used in pregnancy only if the potential benefit justifies the potential risk to the fetus.

Nursing Mothers: It is not known whether MINIPRESS or RENESE is excreted in human milk. Thiazides appear in breast milk. Thus, if use of the drug is deemed essential the patient should stop nursing.

Pediatric Use: Safety and effectiveness in children has not been established.

ADVERSE REACTIONS

MINIPRESS (prazosin hydrochloride)

The most common reactions associated with MINIPRESS therapy are: dizziness 10.3%, headache 7.8%, drowsiness 7.6%, lack of energy 6.9%, weakness 6.5%, palpitations 5.3%, and nausea 4.9%. In most instances side effects have disappeared with continued therapy or have been tolerated with no decrease in dose of drug.

The following reactions have been associated with MINIPRESS, some of them rarely. (In some instances exact causal relationships have not been established.)

    Gastrointestinal: vomiting, diarrhea, constipation, abdominal discomfort and/or pain, liver function abnormalities, pancreatitis.

    Cardiovascular: edema, dyspnea, syncope, tachycardia.

    Central Nervous System: nervousness, vertigo, depression, paresthesia, hallucinations.

    Dermatologic: rash, pruritus, alopecia, lichen planus.

    Genitourinary: urinary frequency, incontinence, impotence, priapism.

    EENT: blurred vision, reddened sclera, epistaxis, tinnitus, dry mouth, nasal congestion.

    Other: diaphoresis, fever.

Single reports of pigmentary mottling and serous retinopathy, and a few reports of cataract development or disappearance have been reported. In these instances, the exact causal relationship has not been established because the baseline observations were frequently inadequate.

In more specific slit-lamp and funduscopic studies, which included adequate baseline examinations, no drug-related abnormal ophthalmological findings have been reported.

RENESE (polythiazide)

    Gastrointestinal: anorexia, gastric irritation, nausea, vomiting, cramping, diarrhea, constipation, jaundice (intrahepatic cholestatic jaundice), pancreatitis.

    Central Nervous System: dizziness, vertigo, paresthesia, headache, xanthopsia.

    Hematologic: leukopenia, agranulocytosis, thrombocytopenia, aplastic anemia.

    Dermatologic: purpura, photosensitivity, rash, urticaria, necrotizing angiitis, (vasculitis) (cutaneous vasculitis).

    Cardiovascular: Orthostatic hypotension may occur and be aggravated by alcohol, barbiturates, or narcotics.

    Other: hyperglycemia, glycosuria, hyperuricemia, muscle spasm, weakness, restlessness.

OVERDOSAGE

MINIPRESS (prazosin hydrochloride)

Accidental ingestion of at least 50 mg of MINIPRESS in a two year old child resulted in profound drowsiness and depressed reflexes. No decrease in blood pressure was noted. Recovery was uneventful.

Should overdosage lead to hypotension, support of the cardiovascular system is of first importance. Restoration of blood pressure and normalization of heart rate may be accomplished by keeping the patient in the supine position. If this measure is inadequate, shock should first be treated with volume expanders. If necessary, vasopressors should then be used. Renal function should be monitored and supported as needed. Laboratory data indicate that MINIPRESS is not dialyzable because it is protein bound.

RENESE (polythiazide)

Should overdosage with RENESE occur, electrolyte balance and adequate hydration should be maintained. Gastric lavage is recommended, followed by supportive treatment. Where necessary, this may include intravenous dextrose and saline with potassium and other electrolyte therapy, administered with caution as indicated by laboratory testing at appropriate intervals.

DOSAGE AND ADMINISTRATION

MINIZIDE (prazosin hydrochloride/polythiazide)

Dosage: as determined by individual titration of MINIPRESS (prazosin hydrochloride) and RENESE (polythiazide). (See box warning.)

Usual MINIZIDE dosage is one capsule two or three times daily, the strength depending upon individual requirement following titration.

The following is a general guide to the administration of the individual components of MINIZIDE:

MINIPRESS (prazosin hydrochloride)

Initial Dose: 1 mg two or three times a day. (See Warnings.)

Maintenance Dose: Dosage may be slowly increased to a total daily dose of 20 mg given in divided doses. The therapeutic dosages most commonly employed have ranged from 6 mg to 15 mg daily given in divided doses. Doses higher than 20 mg usually do not increase efficacy, however a few patients may benefit from further increases up to a daily dose of 40 mg given in divided doses. After initial titration some patients can be maintained adequately on a twice daily dosage regimen.

Use With Other Drugs: When adding a diuretic or other antihypertensive agent, the dose of MINIPRESS should be reduced to 1 mg or 2 mg three times a day and retitration then carried out.

RENESE (polythiazide)

The usual dose of RENESE for antihypertensive therapy is 2 to 4 mg daily.

MINIZIDE CAPSULES

prazosin HCl/polythiazide

[See table preceding page]

69-2463-37-5   Revised December 1986

Literature Available

Yes.

Shown in Product Identification Section, page 422

MODERIL®   ℞

[mō′dĕr-ĭl]

(rescinnamine)

TABLETS

DESCRIPTION

Rescinnamine is a pure crystalline alkaloid that has been identified chemically as the 3,4,5-trimethoxycinnamic acid ester of methyl reserpate. Pure rescinnamine occurs as white, needle-shaped crystals that are readily absorbed when ingested.

Moderil is available as oval, scored salmon tablets providing 0.5 mg of crystalline rescinnamine or as oval, scored yellow tablets providing 0.25 mg of crystalline rescinnamine.

Inert ingredients are: ascorbyl palmitate; dibasic calcium phosphate; Yellow 6; lactose; magnesium stearate; polyethylene glycol; starch. The 0.25 mg tablets also contain Yellow 10.

ACTIONS

Rescinnamine probably produces its antihypertensive effects through depletion of tissue stores of catecholamines (epinephrine and norepinephrine) from peripheral sites. By contrast, its sedative and tranquilizing properties are thought to be related to depletion of 5-hydroxytryptamine from the brain.

Rescinnamine is characterized by slow onset of action and sustained effect. Both its cardiovascular and central nervous system effects may persist following withdrawal of the drug.

INDICATIONS

Indicated in the treatment of mild essential hypertension.

CONTRAINDICATIONS

Do not use in patients with known hypersensitivity, mental depression—especially with suicidal tendencies, active peptic ulcer, and ulcerative colitis. It is also contraindicated in patients receiving electroconvulsive therapy.

WARNINGS

Extreme caution should be exercised in treating patients with a history of mental depression. Discontinue the drug at the first sign of despondency, early morning insomnia, loss of appetite, impotence, or self-depreciation. Drug-induced depression may persist for several months after drug withdrawal and may be severe enough to result in suicide.

Usage in Pregnancy: The safety of rescinnamine for use during pregnancy or lactation has not been established. Therefore, the drug should be used in pregnant patients or in women of child-bearing potential only when, in the judgment of the physician, its use is deemed essential to the welfare of the patient. Increased respiratory secretions, nasal congestion, cyanosis, and anorexia may occur in infants born to rescinnamine-treated mothers, since this preparation is known to cross the placental barrier, appearing in cord blood and breast milk.

PRECAUTIONS

Because Rauwolfia preparations increase gastrointestinal motility and secretion, this drug should be used cautiously in patients with a history of peptic ulcer, ulcerative colitis, or gallstones where biliary colic may be precipitated.

Caution should be exercised when treating hypertensive patients with renal insufficiency since they adjust poorly to lowered blood pressure levels.

Use rescinnamine cautiously with digitalis and quinidine since cardiac arrhythmias have occurred with Rauwolfia preparations.

Preoperative withdrawal of rescinnamine does not assure that circulatory instability will not occur. It is important that the anesthesiologist be aware of the patient's drug intake and consider this in the over-all management, since hypotension has occurred in patients receiving Rauwolfia preparations. Anticholinergic and/or adrenergic drugs (metaraminol, norepinephrine) have been employed to treat adverse vagocirculatory effects.

ADVERSE REACTIONS

Rauwolfia preparations have caused gastrointestinal reactions including hypersecretion, nausea and vomiting, anorexia, and diarrhea; cardiovascular reactions including angina-like symptoms, arrhythmias, particularly when used concurrently with digitalis or quinidine, and bradycardia; and central nervous system reactions including drowsiness, depression, nervousness, paradoxical anxiety, nightmares, rare parkinsonian syndrome, CNS sensitization manifested by dull sensorium, deafness, glaucoma, uveitis, and optic atrophy. Nasal congestion is a frequent complaint; and pruritus, rash, dryness of mouth, dizziness, headache, dyspnea, purpura, impotence or decreased libido, dysuria, muscular aches, conjunctival injection, and weight gain have been reported. Extrapyramidal tract symptoms have also occurred. These reactions are usually reversible and disappear when the drug is discontinued.

Water retention with edema in patients with hypertensive vascular disease may occur rarely, but the condition generally clears with cessation of therapy, or with the administration of a diuretic agent.

DOSAGE AND ADMINISTRATION

For adults the average initial dose is 0.5 mg orally, twice daily. Increase dosage gradually, if necessary. Maintenance doses may vary from 0.25 mg to 0.5 mg daily. Higher doses should be used cautiously because serious mental depression and other side effects may be increased considerably.

Concomitant use of rescinnamine and ganglionic blocking agents, guanethidine, veratrum, hydralazine, methyldopa, chlorthalidone, or thiazides necessitates careful titration of dosage with each agent.

SUPPLY

0.25 mg tablets, oval, scored, yellow: bottles of 100 (NDC 0069-4410-66).

0.5 mg tablets, oval, scored, salmon: bottles of 100 (NDC 0069-4420-66).

70-0695-00-8   Revised Nov. 1986

Shown in Product Identification Section, page 422

PROCARDIA®   ℞

[pro-car'dē-ă]

(nifedipine)

CAPSULES

For Oral Use

DESCRIPTION

PROCARDIA (nifedipine) is an antianginal drug belonging to a new class of pharmacological agents, the calcium channel blockers. Nifedipine is 3,5-pyridinedicarboxylic acid, 1,4-dihydro-2,6-dimethyl-4-(2-nitrophenyl)-, dimethyl ester, $C_{17}H_{18}N_2O_6$.

Nifedipine is a yellow crystalline substance, practically insoluble in water but soluble in ethanol. It has a molecular weight of 346.3. PROCARDIA CAPSULES are formulated as soft gelatin capsules for oral administration each containing 10 mg or 20 mg nifedipine.

Inert ingredients in the formulations are: glycerin; peppermint oil; polyethylene glycol; soft gelatin capsules (which contain Yellow 6, and may contain Red Ferric Oxide and other inert ingredients), and water. The 10 mg capsules also contain saccharin sodium.

CLINICAL PHARMACOLOGY

PROCARDIA is a calcium ion influx inhibitor (slow channel blocker or calcium ion antagonist) and inhibits the transmembrane influx of calcium ions into cardiac muscle and smooth muscle. The contractile processes of cardiac muscle and vascular smooth muscle are dependent upon the movement of extracellular calcium ions into these cells through specific ion channels. PROCARDIA selectively inhibits calcium ion influx across the cell membrane of cardiac muscle and vascular smooth muscle without changing serum calcium concentrations.

Mechanism of Action

The precise means by which this inhibition relieves angina has not been fully determined, but includes at least the following two mechanisms:

1) Relaxation and prevention of coronary artery spasm

PROCARDIA dilates the main coronary arteries and coro-

---

nary arterioles, both in normal and ischemic regions, and is a potent inhibitor of coronary artery spasm, whether spontaneous or ergonovine-induced. This property increases myocardial oxygen delivery in patients with coronary artery spasm, and is responsible for the effectiveness of PROCARDIA in vasospastic (Prinzmetal's or variant) angina. Whether this effect plays any role in classical angina is not clear, but studies of exercise tolerance have not shown an increase in the maximum exercise rate-pressure product, a widely accepted measure of oxygen utilization. This suggests that, in general, relief of spasm or dilation of coronary arteries is not an important factor in classical angina.

2) Reduction of oxygen utilization

PROCARDIA regularly reduces arterial pressure at rest and at a given level of exercise by dilating peripheral arterioles and reducing the total peripheral resistance (afterload) against which the heart works. This unloading of the heart reduces myocardial energy consumption and oxygen requirements and probably accounts for the effectiveness of PROCARDIA in chronic stable angina.

Pharmacokinetics and Metabolism

PROCARDIA is rapidly and fully absorbed after oral administration. The drug is detectable in serum 10 minutes after oral administration, and peak blood levels occur in approximately 30 minutes. Bioavailability is proportional to dose from 10 to 30 mg; half-life does not change significantly with dose. There is little difference in relative bioavailability when PROCARDIA capsules are given orally and either swallowed whole; bitten and swallowed; or, bitten and held sublingually. However, biting through the capsule prior to swallowing does result in slightly earlier plasma concentrations (27 ng/ml 10 minutes after 10 mg) than if capsules are swallowed intact. It is highly bound by serum proteins. PROCARDIA is extensively converted to inactive metabolites and approximately 80 percent of PROCARDIA and metabolites are eliminated via the kidneys. The half-life of nifedipine in plasma is approximately two hours. There is no information on the effects of renal or hepatic impairment on excretion or metabolism of PROCARDIA.

Hemodynamics

Like other slow channel blockers, PROCARDIA exerts a negative inotropic effect on isolated myocardial tissue. This is rarely, if ever, seen in intact animals or man, probably because of reflex responses to its vasodilating effects. In man, PROCARDIA causes decreased peripheral vascular resistance and a fall in systolic and diastolic pressure, usually modest (5–10mm Hg systolic), but sometimes larger. There is usually a small increase in heart rate, a reflex response to vasodilation. Measurements of cardiac function in patients with normal ventricular function have generally found a small increase in cardiac index without major effects on ejection fraction, left ventricular end diastolic pressure (LVEDP) or volume (LVEDV). In patients with impaired ventricular function, most acute studies have shown some increase in ejection fraction and reduction in left ventricular filling pressure.

Electrophysiologic Effects

Although like other members of its class, PROCARDIA decreases sinoatrial node function and atrioventricular conduction in isolated myocardial preparations, such effects have not been seen in studies in intact animals or in man. In formal electrophysiologic studies, predominantly in patients with normal conduction systems, PROCARDIA has had no tendency to prolong atrioventricular conduction, prolong sinus node recovery time, or slow sinus rate.

INDICATIONS AND USAGE

I. Vasospastic Angina

PROCARDIA (nifedipine) is indicated for the management of vasospastic angina confirmed by any of the following criteria: 1) classical pattern of angina at rest accompanied by ST segment elevation, 2) angina or coronary artery spasm provoked by ergonovine, or 3) angiographically demonstrated coronary artery spasm. In those patients who have had angiography, the presence of significant fixed obstructive disease is not incompatible with the diagnosis of vasospastic angina, provided that the above criteria are satisfied. PROCARDIA may also be used where the clinical presentation suggests a possible vasospastic component but where vasospasm has not been confirmed, e.g., where pain has a variable threshold on exertion or in unstable angina where electrocardiographic findings are compatible with intermittent vasospasm, or when angina is refractory to nitrates and/or adequate doses of beta blockers.

II. Chronic Stable Angina (Classical Effort-Associated Angina)

PROCARDIA is indicated for the management of chronic stable angina (effort-associated angina) without evidence of vasospasm in patients who remain symptomatic despite adequate doses of beta blockers and/or organic nitrates or who cannot tolerate those agents.

In chronic stable angina (effort-associated angina) PROCARDIA has been effective in controlled trials of up to eight weeks duration in reducing angina frequency and increasing exercise tolerance, but confirmation of sustained effectiveness and evaluation of long term safety in these

---

patients are incomplete.

Controlled studies in small numbers of patients suggest concomitant use of PROCARDIA and beta blocking agents may be beneficial in patients with chronic stable angina, but available information is not sufficient to predict with confidence the effects of concurrent treatment, especially in patients with compromised left ventricular function or cardiac conduction abnormalities. When introducing such concomitant therapy, care must be taken to monitor blood pressure closely since severe hypotension can occur from the combined effects of the drugs. (See WARNINGS.)

CONTRAINDICATIONS

Known hypersensitivity reaction to PROCARDIA.

WARNINGS

Excessive Hypotension

Although in most patients, the hypotensive effect of PROCARDIA is modest and well tolerated, occasional patients have had excessive and poorly tolerated hypotension. These responses have usually occurred during initial titration or at the time of subsequent upward dosage adjustment, and may be more likely in patients on concomitant beta blockers.

Severe hypotension and/or increased fluid volume requirements have been reported in patients receiving PROCARDIA together with a beta blocking agent who underwent coronary artery bypass surgery using high dose fentanyl anesthesia. The interaction with high dose fentanyl appears to be due to the combination of PROCARDIA and a beta blocker, but the possibility that it may occur with PROCARDIA alone, with low doses of fentanyl, in other surgical procedures, or with other narcotic analgesics cannot be ruled out. In PROCARDIA treated patients where surgery using high dose fentanyl anesthesia is contemplated, the physician should be aware of these potential problems and, if the patient's condition permits, sufficient time (at least 36 hours) should be allowed for PROCARDIA to be washed out of the body prior to surgery.

Increased Angina and/or Myocardial Infarction

Rarely, patients, particularly those who have severe obstructive coronary artery disease, have developed well documented increased frequency, duration and/or severity of angina or acute myocardial infarction on starting PROCARDIA or at the time of dosage increase. The mechanism of this effect is not established.

Beta Blocker Withdrawal

Patients recently withdrawn from beta blockers may develop a withdrawal syndrome with increased angina, probably related to increased sensitivity to catecholamines. Initiation of PROCARDIA treatment will not prevent this occurrence and might be expected to exacerbate it by provoking reflex catecholamine release. There have been occasional reports of increased angina in a setting of beta blocker withdrawal and PROCARDIA initiation. It is important to taper beta blockers if possible, rather than stopping them abruptly before beginning PROCARDIA.

Congestive Heart Failure

Rarely, patients, usually receiving a beta blocker, have developed heart failure after beginning PROCARDIA. Patients with tight aortic stenosis may be at greater risk for such an event, as the unloading effect of PROCARDIA would be expected to be of less benefit to these patients, owing to their fixed impedance to flow across the aortic valve.

PRECAUTIONS

General: Hypotension: Because PROCARDIA decreases peripheral vascular resistance, careful monitoring of blood pressure during the initial administration and titration of PROCARDIA is suggested. Close observation is especially recommended for patients already taking medications that are known to lower blood pressure. (See WARNINGS.)

Peripheral edema: Mild to moderate peripheral edema, typically associated with arterial vasodilation and not due to left ventricular dysfunction, occurs in about one in ten patients treated with PROCARDIA. This edema occurs primarily in the lower extremities and usually responds to diuretic therapy. With patients whose angina is complicated by congestive heart failure, care should be taken to differentiate this peripheral edema from the effects of increasing left ventricular dysfunction.

Laboratory tests: Rare, usually transient, but occasionally significant elevations of enzymes such as alkaline phosphatase, CPK, LDH, SGOT and SGPT have been noted. The relationship to PROCARDIA therapy is uncertain in most cases, but probable in some. These laboratory abnormalities have rarely been associated with clinical symptoms, however, cholestasis with or without jaundice has been reported. Rare instances of allergic hepatitis have been reported.

PROCARDIA, like other calcium channel blockers, decreases platelet aggregation *in vitro*. Limited clinical studies have demonstrated a moderate but statistically significant decrease in platelet aggregation and increase in bleeding time in some PROCARDIA patients. This is thought to be a function of inhibition of calcium transport across the plate-

Continued on next page

Pfizer—Cont.

let membrane. No clinical significance for these findings has been demonstrated.

Positive direct Coombs test with/without hemolytic anemia has been reported.

Although PROCARDIA has been used safely in patients with renal dysfunction and has been reported to exert a beneficial effect in certain cases, rare, reversible elevations in BUN and serum creatinine have been reported in patients with pre-existing chronic renal insufficiency. The relationship to PROCARDIA therapy is uncertain in most cases but probable in some.

Drug interactions: Beta-adrenergic blocking agents: (See INDICATIONS and WARNINGS.) Experience in over 1400 patients in a non-comparative clinical trial has shown that concomitant administration of PROCARDIA and beta-blocking agents is usually well tolerated, but there have been occasional literature reports suggesting that the combination may increase the likelihood of congestive heart failure, severe hypotension or exacerbation of angina.

Long acting nitrates: PROCARDIA may be safely co-administered with nitrates, but there have been no controlled studies to evaluate the antianginal effectiveness of this combination.

Digitalis: Administration of PROCARDIA with digoxin increased digoxin levels in nine of twelve normal volunteers. The average increase was 45%. Another investigator found no increase in digoxin levels in thirteen patients with coronary artery disease. In an uncontrolled study of over two hundred patients with congestive heart failure during which digoxin blood levels were not measured, digitalis toxicity was not observed. Since there have been isolated reports of patients with elevated digoxin levels, it is recommended that digoxin levels be monitored when initiating, adjusting, and discontinuing PROCARDIA to avoid possible over- or under-digitalization.

Coumarin anticoagulants: There have been rare reports of increased prothrombin time in patients taking coumarin anticoagulants to whom PROCARDIA was administered. However, the relationship to PROCARDIA therapy is uncertain.

Cimetidine: A study in six healthy volunteers has shown a significant increase in peak nifedipine plasma levels (80%) and area-under-the-curve (74%) after a one week course of cimetidine at 1000 mg per day and nifedipine at 40 mg per day. Ranitidine produced smaller, non-significant increases. The effect may be mediated by the known inhibition of cimetidine on hepatic cytochrome P-450, the enzyme system probably responsible for the first-pass metabolism of nifedipine. If nifedipine therapy is initiated in a patient currently receiving cimetidine, cautious titration is advised.

Carcinogenesis, mutagenesis, impairment of fertility: Nifedipine was administered orally to rats for two years and was not shown to be carcinogenic. When given to rats prior to mating, nifedipine caused reduced fertility at a dose approximately 30 times the maximum recommended human dose. *In vivo* mutagenicity studies were negative.

Pregnancy: Pregnancy category C. Nifedipine has been shown to be teratogenic in rats when given in doses 30 times the maximum recommended human dose. Nifedipine was embryotoxic (increased fetal resorptions, decreased fetal weight, increased stunted forms, increased fetal deaths, decreased neonatal survival) in rats, mice and rabbits at doses of from 3 to 10 times the maximum recommended human dose. In pregnant monkeys, doses $\frac{2}{3}$ and twice the maximum recommended human dose resulted in small placentas and underdeveloped chorionic villi. In rats, doses three times maximum human dose and higher caused prolongation of pregnancy. There are no adequate and well controlled studies in pregnant women. PROCARDIA should be used during pregnancy only if the potential benefit justifies the potential risk to the fetus.

ADVERSE REACTIONS

In multiple-dose U.S. and foreign controlled studies in which adverse reactions were reported spontaneously, adverse effects were frequent but generally not serious and rarely required discontinuation of therapy or dosage adjustment. Most were expected consequences of the vasodilator effects of PROCARDIA.

Adverse Effect	PROCARDIA (%) (N = 226)	Placebo (%) (N = 235)
Dizziness, lightheadedness, giddiness	27	15
Flushing, heat sensation	25	8
Headache	23	20
Weakness	12	10
Nausea, heartburn	11	8
Muscle cramps, tremor	8	3
Peripheral edema	7	1
Nervousness, mood changes	7	4
Palpitation	7	5
Dyspnea, cough, wheezing	6	3
Nasal congestion, sore throat	6	8

There is also a large uncontrolled experience in over 2100 patients in the United States. Most of the patients had vasospastic or resistant angina pectoris, and about half had concomitant treatment with beta-adrenergic blocking agents. The most common adverse events were:

Incidence Approximately 10% *Cardiovascular:* peripheral edema
  Central Nervous System: dizziness or lightheadedness
  Gastrointestinal: nausea
  Systemic: headache and flushing, weakness

Incidence Approximately 5% *Cardiovascular:* transient hypotension

Incidence 2% or Less *Cardiovascular:* palpitation
  Respiratory: nasal and chest congestion, shortness of breath
  Gastrointestinal: diarrhea, constipation, cramps, flatulence
  Musculoskeletal: inflammation, joint stiffness, muscle cramps
  Central Nervous System: shakiness, nervousness, jitteriness, sleep disturbances, blurred vision, difficulties in balance
  Other: dermatitis, pruritus, urticaria, fever, sweating, chills, sexual difficulties.

Incidence Approximately 0.5% *Cardiovascular:* syncope. Syncopal episodes did not recur with reduction in the dose of PROCARDIA or concomitant antianginal medication.

Incidence Less Than 0.5% *Hematologic:* thrombocytopenia, anemia, leukopenia, purpura
  Gastrointestinal: allergic hepatitis
  Oral: gingival hyperplasia
  CNS: depression, paranoid syndrome
  Special Senses: transient blindness at the peak of plasma level
  Other: erythromelalgia, arthritis with ANA (+).

Several of these side effects appear to be dose related. Peripheral edema occurred in about one in 25 patients at doses less than 60 mg per day and in about one patient in eight at 120 mg per day or more. Transient hypotension, generally of mild to moderate severity and seldom requiring discontinuation of therapy, occurred in one of 50 patients at less than 60 mg per day and in one of 20 patients at 120 mg per day or more. Very rarely, introduction of PROCARDIA therapy was associated with an increase in anginal pain, possibly due to associated hypotension.

In addition, more serious adverse events were observed, not readily distinguishable from the natural history of the disease in these patients. It remains possible, however, that some or many of these events were drug related. Myocardial infarction occurred in about 4% of patients and congestive heart failure or pulmonary edema in about 2%. Ventricular arrhythmias or conduction disturbances each occurred in fewer than 0.5% of patients.

In a subgroup of over 1000 patients receiving PROCARDIA with concomitant beta blocker therapy, the pattern and incidence of adverse experiences was not different from that of the entire group of PROCARDIA treated patients. (See PRECAUTIONS.)

In a subgroup of approximately 250 patients with a diagnosis of congestive heart failure as well as angina, dizziness or lightheadedness, peripheral edema, headache or flushing each occurred in one in eight patients. Hypotension occurred in about one in 20 patients. Syncope occurred in approximately one patient in 250. Myocardial infarction or symptoms of congestive heart failure each occurred in about one patient in 15. Atrial or ventricular dysrhythmias each occurred in about one patient in 150.

OVERDOSAGE

Although there is no well documented experience with PROCARDIA overdosage, available data suggest that gross overdosage could result in excessive peripheral vasodilation with subsequent marked and probably prolonged systemic hypotension. Clinically significant hypotension due to PROCARDIA overdosage calls for active cardiovascular support including monitoring of cardiac and respiratory function, elevation of extremities, and attention to circulating fluid volume and urine output. A vasoconstrictor (such as norepinephrine) may be helpful in restoring vascular tone and blood pressure, provided that there is no contraindication to its use. Clearance of PROCARDIA would be expected to be prolonged in patients with impaired liver function. Since PROCARDIA is highly protein-bound, dialysis is not likely to be of benefit.

DOSAGE AND ADMINISTRATION

The dosage of PROCARDIA needed to suppress angina and that can be tolerated by the patient must be established by titration. Excessive doses can result in hypotension.

Therapy should be initiated with the 10 mg capsule. The starting dose is one 10 mg capsule, swallowed whole, 3 times/day. The usual effective dose range is 10–20 mg three times daily. Some patients, especially those with evidence of coronary artery spasm, respond only to higher doses, more frequent administration, or both. In such patients, doses of 20–30 mg three or four times daily may be

effective. Doses above 120 mg daily are rarely necessary. More than 180 mg per day is not recommended.

In most cases, PROCARDIA titration should proceed over a 7–14 day period so that the physician can assess the response to each dose level and monitor the blood pressure before proceeding to higher doses.

If symptoms so warrant, titration may proceed more rapidly provided that the patient is assessed frequently. Based on the patient's physical activity level, attack frequency, and sublingual nitroglycerin consumption, the dose of PROCARDIA may be increased from 10 mg t.i.d to 20 mg t.i.d and then to 30 mg t.i.d over a three-day period.

In hospitalized patients under close observation, the dose may be increased in 10 mg increments over four to six-hour periods as required to control pain and arrhythmias due to ischemia. A single dose should rarely exceed 30 mg.

No "rebound effect" has been observed upon discontinuation of PROCARDIA. However, if discontinuation of PROCARDIA is necessary, sound clinical practice suggests that the dosage should be decreased gradually with close physician supervision.

Co-Administration with Other Antianginal Drugs

Sublingual nitroglycerin may be taken as required for the control of acute manifestations of angina, particularly during PROCARDIA titration. See **Precautions, Drug Interactions,** for information on co-administration of PROCARDIA with beta blockers or long acting nitrates.

HOW SUPPLIED

PROCARDIA soft gelatin capsules are supplied in:
Bottles of 100: 10 mg (NDC 0069-2600-66) orange #260; 20 mg (NDC 0069-2610-66) orange and light brown #261
Bottles of 300: 10 mg (NDC 0069-2600-72) orange #260; 20 mg (NDC 0069-2610-72) orange and light brown #261
Unit dose packages of 100: 10 mg (NDC 0069-2600-41) orange #260; 20 mg (NDC 0069-2610-41) orange and light brown #261

The capsules should be protected from light and moisture and stored at controlled room temperature 59° to 77°F (15° to 25°C) in the manufacturer's original container.

© 1982, Pfizer Inc.

69-4052-00-0   Revised July 1987

LITERATURE AVAILABLE
Yes

Shown in Product Identification Section, page 422

RENESE®   ℞
[rĕ-nēs´]
(polythiazide)
TABLETS
For Oral Administration

DESCRIPTION

Renese is designated generically as polythiazide, and chemically as $2H$-1,2,4-Benzothiadiazine-7-sulfonamide, 6-chloro-3,4-dihydro-2-methyl-3-[[(2, 2, 2-trifluoroethyl)thio]methyl]-, 1, 1-dioxide. It is a white crystalline substance, insoluble in water but readily soluble in alkaline solution.

Inert Ingredients: dibasic calcium phosphate; lactose; magnesium stearate; polyethylene glycol; sodium lauryl sulfate; starch; vanillin. The 2 mg tablets also contain: Yellow 6; Yellow 10.

ACTION

The mechanism of action results in an interference with the renal tubular mechanism of electrolyte reabsorption. At maximal therapeutic dosage all thiazides are approximately equal in their diuretic potency. The mechanism whereby thiazides function in the control of hypertension is unknown.

INDICATIONS

Renese is indicated as adjunctive therapy in edema associated with congestive heart failure, hepatic cirrhosis, and corticosteroid and estrogen therapy.

Renese has also been found useful in edema due to various forms of renal dysfunction as: Nephrotic syndrome; Acute glomerulonephritis; and Chronic renal failure.

Renese is indicated in the management of hypertension either as the sole therapeutic agent or to enhance the effectiveness of other antihypertensive drugs in the more severe forms of hypertension.

Usage in Pregnancy: The routine use of diuretics in an otherwise healthy woman is inappropriate and exposes mother and fetus to unnecessary hazard. Diuretics do not prevent development of toxemia of pregnancy, and there is no satisfactory evidence that they are useful in the treatment of developed toxemia.

Edema during pregnancy may arise from pathological causes or from the physiologic and mechanical consequences of pregnancy. Thiazides are indicated in pregnancy when edema is due to pathologic causes, just as they are in the absence of pregnancy (however, see Warnings, below). Dependent edema in pregnancy, resulting from restriction of venous return by the expanded uterus, is properly treated through elevation of the lower extremities and use of support hose; use of diuretics to lower intravascular volume in this case is illogical and unnecessary. There is hypervolemia during normal pregnancy which is harmful to neither the fetus nor the mother (in the absence of cardiovascular disease), but which is associated with edema, including generalized edema, in the majority of pregnant women. If this edema produces discomfort, increased recumbency will often provide relief. In rare instances, this edema may cause extreme discomfort which is not relieved by rest. In these cases, a short course of diuretics may provide relief and may be appropriate.

CONTRAINDICATIONS

Anuria. Hypersensitivity to this or other sulfonamide derived drugs.

WARNINGS

Thiazides should be used with caution in severe renal disease. In patients with renal disease, thiazides may precipitate azotemia. Cumulative effects of the drug may develop in patients with impaired renal function.

Thiazides should be used with caution in patients with impaired hepatic function or progressive liver disease, since minor alterations of fluid and electrolyte balance may precipitate hepatic coma.

Thiazides may add to or potentiate the action of other antihypertensive drugs. Potentiation occurs with ganglionic or peripheral adrenergic blocking drugs.

Sensitivity reactions may occur in patients with a history of allergy or bronchial asthma.

The possibility of exacerbation or activation of systemic lupus erythematosus has been reported.

Usage in Pregnancy. Thiazides cross the placental barrier and appear in cord blood. The use of thiazides in pregnant women requires that the anticipated benefit be weighed against possible hazards to the fetus. These hazards include fetal or neonatal jaundice, thrombocytopenia, and possibly other adverse reactions which have occurred in the adult.

Nursing Mothers. Thiazides appear in breast milk. If use of the drug is deemed essential, the patient should stop nursing.

PRECAUTIONS

Periodic determination of serum electrolytes to detect possible electrolyte imbalance should be performed at appropriate intervals.

All patients receiving thiazide therapy should be observed for clinical signs of fluid or electrolyte imbalance; namely, hyponatremia, hypochloremic alkalosis, and hypokalemia. Serum and urine electrolyte determinations are particularly important when the patient is vomiting excessively or receiving parenteral fluids. Medication such as digitalis may also influence serum electrolytes. Warning signs, irrespective of cause, are: dryness of mouth, thirst, weakness, lethargy, drowsiness, restlessness, muscle pains or cramps, muscular fatigue, hypotension, oliguria, tachycardia, and gastrointestinal disturbances such as nausea and vomiting.

Hypokalemia may develop with thiazides as with any other potent diuretic, especially with brisk diuresis, when severe cirrhosis is present, or during concomitant use of corticosteroids or ACTH.

Interference with adequate oral electrolyte intake will also contribute to hypokalemia. Digitalis therapy may exaggerate metabolic effects of hypokalemia especially with reference to myocardial activity.

Any chloride deficit is generally mild and usually does not require specific treatment except under extraordinary circumstances (as in liver disease or renal disease). Dilutional hyponatremia may occur in edematous patients in hot weather; appropriate therapy is water restriction, rather than administration of salt except in rare instances when the hyponatremia is life threatening. In actual salt depletion, appropriate replacement is the therapy of choice.

Hyperuricemia may occur or frank gout may be precipitated in certain patients receiving thiazide therapy.

Insulin requirements in diabetic patients may be increased, decreased, or unchanged. Latent diabetes mellitus may become manifest during thiazide administration.

Thiazide drugs may increase the responsiveness to tubocurarine.

The antihypertensive effects of the drug may be enhanced in the postsympathectomy patient.

Thiazides may decrease arterial responsiveness to norepinephrine. This diminution is not sufficient to preclude effectiveness of the pressor agent for therapeutic use.

If progressive renal impairment becomes evident, as indicated by a rising nonprotein nitrogen or blood urea nitrogen, a careful reappraisal of therapy is necessary with consideration given to withholding or discontinuing diuretic therapy. Thiazides may decrease serum PBI levels without signs of thyroid disturbance.

ADVERSE REACTIONS

A. GASTROINTESTINAL SYSTEM REACTIONS
1. anorexia
2. gastric irritation
3. nausea
4. vomiting
5. cramping
6. diarrhea
7. constipation
8. jaundice (intrahepatic cholestatic jaundice)
9. pancreatitis

B. CENTRAL NERVOUS SYSTEM REACTIONS
1. dizziness
2. vertigo
3. paresthesias
4. headache
5. xanthopsia

C. HEMATOLOGIC REACTIONS
1. leukopenia
2. agranulocytosis
3. thrombocytopenia
4. aplastic anemia

D. DERMATOLOGIC–HYPERSENSITIVITY REACTIONS
1. purpura
2. photosensitivity
3. rash
4. urticaria
5. necrotizing angiitis (vasculitis) (cutaneous vasculitis)

E. CARDIOVASCULAR REACTION
Orthostatic hypotension may occur and may be aggravated by alcohol, barbiturates or narcotics.

F. OTHER
1. hyperglycemia
2. glycosuria
3. hyperuricemia
4. muscle spasm
5. weakness
6. restlessness

Whenever adverse reactions are moderate or severe, thiazide dosage should be reduced or therapy withdrawn.

DOSAGE AND ADMINISTRATION

Therapy should be individualized according to patient response. This therapy should be titrated to gain maximal therapeutic response as well as the minimal dose possible to maintain that therapeutic response. The usual dosage of Renese tablets for diuretic therapy is 1 to 4 mg daily, and for antihypertensive therapy is 2 to 4 mg daily.

HOW SUPPLIED

RENESE (polythiazide) Tablets are available as:

1 mg white, scored tablets in bottles of 100 (NDC 0995-3750-66) and 1000 (NDC 0069-3750-82);

2 mg yellow, scored tablets in bottles of 100 (NDC 0995-3760-66) and 1000 (NDC 0069-3760-82);

4 mg white, scored tablets in bottles of 100 (NDC 0995-3770-66) and 1000 (NDC 0069-3770-82).

69-1116-00-4   Revised Jan. 1987

LITERATURE AVAILABLE

Yes.

Shown in Product Identification Section, page 422

RENESE®-R   ℞
[rĕ-nēs′]
(polythiazide and reserpine)

WARNING

This fixed combination drug is not indicated for initial therapy of hypertension. Hypertension requires therapy titrated to the individual patient. If the fixed combination represents the dosage so determined, its use may be more convenient in patient management. The treatment of hypertension is not static, but must be reevaluated as conditions in each patient warrant.

RENESE-R tablets combine polythiazide and reserpine, two antihypertensive agents with complementary properties. Each blue, scored tablet of RENESE-R provides:

Renese (polythiazide)...2.0 mg
Reserpine...0.25 mg

Inert Ingredients: Blue 1; dibasic calcium phosphate; lactose; magnesium stearate; polyethylene glycol; sodium lauryl sulfate; starch; vanillin.

ACTIONS

RENESE (polythiazide) is a member of the benzothiadiazine (thiazide) family of diuretic/antihypertensive agents. RENESE (polythiazide) alone has demonstrated clinical effectiveness in lowering elevated blood pressure in patients without visible edema as well as in edematous hypertensive patients. This antihypertensive action probably comes about through depletion of sodium and fluid accumulation in the blood vessel wall.

RENESE (polythiazide) is 2H-1,2,4-Benzothiadiazine-7-sulfonamide, 6-chloro-3,4-dihydro-2-methyl-3-[[(2,2,2-trifluoroethyl)thio]methyl]-, 1, 1-dioxide.

Reserpine, an alkaloid of Rauwolfia serpentina, has several complementary actions of benefit to the hypertensive patient, including a calming effect and a slowing of the pulse rate. Its ultimate effect in lowering blood pressure is thought to be due to vasodilatation unaccompanied by reduction in cardiac performance, probably as a result of depletion of norepinephrine from tissue receptor sites.

Since polythiazide reduces or eliminates the sodium and fluid retention frequently associated with hypertension, it enhances the efficacy of reserpine in lowering elevated blood pressure. RENESE-R often has been found to be more effective than equivalent doses of either agent alone. Both the cardiovascular and central nervous system effects may persist following withdrawal of the drug.

INDICATIONS

Hypertension (see box warning).

CONTRAINDICATIONS

A. Related to polythiazide:
1. Advanced renal or hepatic failure.
2. Hypersensitivity to this or other sulfonamide derivatives.

B. Related to reserpine:
1. Demonstrated hypersensitivity.
2. Mental depression.
3. Demonstrated peptic ulcer or ulcerative colitis.

WARNINGS

Serum electrolyte determinations are especially indicated for patients with severe derangement of metabolic processes, e.g., surgery, vomiting, or parenteral fluid therapy. Electrolyte imbalance may be caused by certain diseases such as cirrhosis, or it may result from drug therapy, such as therapy with corticosteroids. Patients with cirrhosis who are continually receiving RENESE-R should be observed carefully for the development of hepatic precoma or coma. Indications of impending hepatic failure are tremor, confusion, drowsiness, and hepatic fetor.

Thiazides may precipitate kidney failure and uremia in patients with pre-existing renal pathology and impaired renal function.

Available information tends to implicate all oral dosage forms of potassium salts ingested in solid form with or without thiazides in the etiology of nonspecific, small bowel lesions consisting of ulceration with or without stenosis, causing obstruction, hemorrhage and perforation, and frequently requiring surgery. Deaths due to these complications have been reported. All oral dosage forms of potassium salts ingested in solid form should be used only when adequate dietary supplementation is not practical and should be discontinued immediately if abdominal pain, distention, nausea, vomiting or gastrointestinal bleeding occur.

RENESE-R does not itself contain enteric-coated potassium. Electroshock therapy should not be given within one week of cessation of reserpine.

Usage in Pregnancy and the Childbearing Age.

Since thiazides appear in breast milk, the usage of polythiazide is contraindicated in nursing mothers. Thiazides cross the placental barrier and appear in cord blood. The safety of reserpine for use during pregnancy or lactation has not been established. When polythiazide and reserpine are used in women of childbearing age, the potential benefits of this drug combination should be weighed against the possible hazards to the fetus. The hazards include fetal or neonatal jaundice, thrombocytopenia, and possibly other adverse reactions which have occurred in the adult.

PRECAUTIONS

Since all diuretic agents may reduce serum levels of sodium, chloride, and potassium, especially with brisk diuresis or when used concurrently with steroids, patients should be observed regularly for early signs of fluid or electrolyte imbalance and serum electrolyte studies should be performed periodically. Warning signs of possible electrolyte imbalance irrespective of cause include fatigue, muscle cramps, gastrointestinal disturbances, lethargy, oliguria, and tachycardia. In extreme cases, hypotension, shock, and coma may develop. Frequently, serum electrolyte levels do not correlate with signs or symptoms of electrolyte imbalance. Unduly restricted salt intake as well as concurrent administration of digitalis may exaggerate metabolic effects of hypokalemia. A favorable ratio of potassium to sodium excretion lessens the possibility of hypokalemia. However, should this occur or be suspected, foods with a high potassium content (bananas, apricots, citrus fruits, prune juice, etc.) should be given. When necessary, oral potassium supplements may be administered. If other antihypertensive agents are used concurrently, lower than usual doses of RENESE-R and of the other agents should be considered.

Like other thiazide diuretics, polythiazide may cause a rise in serum uric acid levels with or without overt symptoms of gout. Thiazides are known to disturb glucose tolerance in some individuals, even when there is no history of glucose intolerance or diabetes in the individual or his family. Likewise, thiazides may decrease PBI levels without signs of thyroid disturbances.

Thiazide drugs may augment the paralyzing actions of tubocurarine, and may decrease the arterial responsiveness to norepinephrine. Extra precautions may be necessary in patients who may require these drugs or their derivatives, as in surgery. The antihypertensive effects of the drug may be enhanced in the postsympathectomy patient.

Continued on next page

Pfizer—Cont.

Reserpine: Since reserpine may increase gastric acid secretion, it should be used cautiously in patients with a history of peptic ulcer or ulcerative colitis. Extreme caution is needed in patients with a history of mental depression, and reserpine should be discontinued at the first sign of depressive symptoms. Parkinsonism and confusion have been encountered, particularly in psychiatric patients, and constitute an indication for withdrawal of the drug. Caution should be exercised when treating patients with impairment of renal function, as lowered blood pressure may result in further decompensation and embarrassment of function. Reserpine should be used cautiously with digitalis or quinidine as the concurrent use may enhance the appearance of arrhythmias. Discontinue the drug one to two weeks prior to elective surgery since an unexpected degree of hypotension and bradycardia have been reported in patients receiving anesthetic agents concurrently with reserpine, probably due to a reduced responsiveness to norepinephrine. For emergency surgical procedures vagal blocking agents may be given parenterally to prevent or reverse hypotension and/or bradycardia. Reserpine may cause increased appetite and weight gain in some patients.

Animal tumorigenicity: Rodent studies have shown that reserpine is an animal tumorigen, causing an increased incidence of mammary fibroadenomas in female mice, malignant tumors of the seminal vesicles in male mice, and malignant adrenal medullary tumors in male rats. These findings arose in 2 year studies in which the drug was administered in the feed at concentrations of 5 and 10 ppm—about 100 to 300 times the usual human dose. The breast neoplasms are thought to be related to reserpine's prolactin-elevating effect. Several other prolactin-elevating drugs have also been associated with an increased incidence of mammary neoplasia in rodents.

The extent to which these findings indicate a risk to humans is uncertain. Tissue culture experiments show that about one-third of human breast tumors are prolactin-dependent *in vitro*, a factor of considerable importance if the use of the drug is contemplated in a patient with previously detected breast cancer. The possibility of an increased risk of breast cancer in reserpine users has been studied extensively; however, no firm conclusion has emerged. Although a few epidemiologic studies have suggested a slightly increased risk (less than twofold in all studies except one) in women who have used reserpine, other studies of generally similar design have not confirmed this. Epidemiologic studies conducted using other drugs (neuroleptic agents) that, like reserpine, increase prolactin levels and therefore would be considered rodent mammary carcinogens, have not shown an association between chronic administration of the drug and human mammary tumorigenesis. While long-term clinical observation has not suggested such an association, the available evidence is considered too limited to be conclusive at this time. An association of reserpine intake with pheochromocytoma or tumors of the seminal vesicles has not been explored.

ADVERSE REACTIONS

Polythiazide: Side effects such as nausea, vertigo, weakness, paresthesias, and fatigue occur but seldom require cessation of therapy. Most of these can be overcome by reducing the dose or taking measures to improve electrolyte imbalance. Maculopapular skin rash has been reported, as has reversible cholestatic jaundice. Leukopenia (neutropenia) and purpura, with or without thrombocytopenia, have been reported rarely, and agranulocytosis and aplastic anemia have been reported with the older thiazides but not as yet with the newer compounds such as polythiazide. Pancreatitis, photosensitivity reactions, gastrointestinal disturbances, headache, xanthopsia, necrotizing angiitis, orthostatic hypotension, and dizziness have all been reported following the use of the benzothiadiazine class of diuretics.

Reserpine: Gastrointestinal reactions include hypersecretion, nausea and vomiting, anorexia, and diarrhea. Cardiovascular reactions reported include angina-like symptoms, arrhythmias—particularly when used concurrently with digitalis or quinidine, flushing of the skin, and bradycardia. Central nervous system reactions range from drowsiness, depression, nervousness, paradoxical anxiety, nightmares, and a rare Parkinsonian syndrome to C.N.S. sensitization manifested by deafness, glaucoma, uveitis, and optic atrophy. Nasal congestion is a frequent complaint, and pruritus, rash, dryness of mouth, dizziness, headache, purpura, impotence or decreased libido, and miosis have been reported with use of this drug. These reactions are usually reversible and disappear when the drug is discontinued.

DOSAGE

As determined by individual titration (see box warning).

Initial dosages of the combination should conform to those dosages of the individual components established during titration.

Maintenance dosages range from ½ tablet to 2 tablets daily.

Dosage of other antihypertensive agents, particularly gan-

glionic blockers, that are used concomitantly should be reduced.

SUPPLY

RENESE-R tablets (2 mg polythiazide-0.25 mg reserpine) are available as blue, scored tablets (imprinted with code number 446) in bottles of 100 (NDC 0069-4460-66) and 1,000 (NDC 0069-4460-82).

(69-1200-00-1)   Revised Jan. 1988

Literature Available: Yes.

Shown in Product Identification Section, page 422

TERRAMYCIN®   ℞

[*tĕra-my'sĭn*]
Capsules
(oxytetracycline HCl)
Film–coated Tablets
(oxytetracycline)

DESCRIPTION

Oxytetracycline is a product of the metabolism of *Streptomyces rimosus* and is one of the family of tetracycline antibiotics.

Oxytetracycline diffuses readily through the placenta into the fetal circulation, into the pleural fluid and, under some circumstances, into the cerebrospinal fluid. It appears to be concentrated in the hepatic system and excreted in the bile, so that it appears in the feces, as well as in the urine, in a biologically active form.

ACTIONS

Oxytetracycline is primarily bacteriostatic and is thought to exert its antimicrobial effect by the inhibition of protein synthesis. Oxytetracycline is active against a wide range of gram-negative and gram-positive organisms. The drugs in the tetracycline class have closely similar antimicrobial spectra, and cross-resistance among them is common. Microorganisms may be considered susceptible if the M.I.C. (minimum inhibitory concentration) is not more than 4.0 mcg/ml and intermediate if the M.I.C. is 4.0 to 12.5 mcg/ml.

Susceptibility plate testing: A tetracycline disc may be used to determine microbial susceptiblity to drugs in the tetracycline class. If the Kirby-Bauer method of disc susceptibility testing is used, a 30 mcg tetracycline disc should give a zone of at least 19 mm when tested against a tetracycline-susceptible bacterial strain.

Tetracyclines are readily absorbed and are bound to plasma proteins in varying degree. They are concentrated by the liver in the bile and excreted in the urine and feces at high concentrations and in a biologically active form.

INDICATIONS

Oxytetracycline is indicated in infections caused by the following microorganisms:

Rickettsiae (Rocky Mountain spotted fever, typhus fever and the typhus group, Q fever, rickettsialpox and tick fevers),

Mycoplasma pneumoniae (PPLO, Eaton Agent), Agents of psittacosis and ornithosis,

Agents of lymphogranuloma venereum and granuloma inguinale,

The spirochetal agent of relapsing fever *(Borrelia recurrentis)*.

The following gram-negative microorganisms:

Haemophilus ducreyi (chancroid),

Pasteurella pestis and *Pasteurella tularensis,*

Bartonella bacilliformis,

Bacteroides species,

Vibrio comma and *Vibrio fetus,*

Brucella species (in conjunction with streptomycin).

Because many strains of the following groups of microorganisms have been shown to be resistant to tetracyclines, culture and susceptibility testing are recommended.

Oxytetracycline is indicated for treatment of infections caused by the following gram- negative microorganisms, when bacteriologic testing indicates appropriate susceptibility to the drug:

Escherichia coli,

Enterobacter aerogenes (formerly *Aerobacter aerogenes*),

Shigella species,

Mima species and *Herellea* species,

Haemophilus influenzae (respiratory infections),

Klebsiella species (respiratory and urinary infections).

Oxytetracycline is indicated for treatment of infections caused by the following gram-positive microorganisms when bacteriologic testing indicates appropriate susceptibility to the drug:

Streptococcus species:

Up to 44 percent of strains of *Streptococcus pyogenes* and 74 percent of *Streptococcus faecalis* have been found to be resistant to tetracycline drugs. Therefore, tetracyclines should not be used for streptococcal disease unless the organism has been demonstrated to be sensitive.

For upper respiratory infections due to Group A beta-hemolytic streptococci, penicillin is the usual drug of choice, including prophylaxis of rheumatic fever.

Diplococcus pneumoniae,

Staphylococcus aureus, skin and soft tissue infections. Oxytetracycline is not the drug of choice in the treatment of any type of staphylococcal infections.

When penicillin is contraindicated, tetracyclines are alternative drugs in the treatment of infections due to:

Neisseria gonorrhoeae

In acute intestinal amebiasis, the tetracyclines may be a useful adjunct to amebicides.

In severe acne, the tetracyclines may be useful adjunctive therapy. (This indication is for the oral use only, not for I.M. or I.V.)

Tetracyclines are indicated in the treatment of trachoma, although the infectious agent is not always eliminated, as judged by immunofluorescence.

Inclusion conjunctivitis may be treated with oral tetracyclines or with a combination of oral and topical agents.

CONTRAINDICATIONS

This drug is contraindicated in persons who have shown hypersensitivity to any of the tetracyclines.

WARNINGS

THE USE OF DRUGS OF THE TETRACYCLINE CLASS DURING TOOTH DEVELOPMENT (LAST HALF OF PREGNANCY, INFANCY, AND CHILDHOOD TO THE AGE OF 8 YEARS) MAY CAUSE PERMANENT DISCOLORATION OF THE TEETH (YELLOW-GRAY-BROWN). This adverse reaction is more common during long term use of the drugs but has been observed following repeated short term courses. Enamel hypoplasia has also been reported. *TETRACYCLINE DRUGS, THEREFORE, SHOULD NOT BE USED IN THIS AGE GROUP UNLESS OTHER DRUGS ARE NOT LIKELY TO BE EFFECTIVE OR ARE CONTRAINDICATED.*

When the need for intensive treatment outweighs its potential dangers (mostly during pregnancy or in individuals with known or suspected renal or liver impairment), it is advisable to perform renal and liver function tests before and during therapy. Also, tetracycline serum concentrations should be followed. If renal impairment exists, even usual oral or parenteral doses may lead to excessive systemic accumulation of the drug and possible liver toxicity. Under such conditions, lower than usual total doses are indicated, and if therapy is prolonged, serum level determinations of the drug may be advisable. This hazard is of particular importance in the parenteral administration of tetracyclines to pregnant or postpartum patients with pyelonephritis.

When used under these circumstances, the blood level should not exceed 15 mcg/ml and liver function tests should be made at frequent intervals. Other potentially hepatotoxic drugs should not be prescribed concomitantly.

Photosensitivity manifested by an exaggerated sunburn reaction has been observed in some individuals taking tetracyclines. Patients apt to be exposed to direct sunlight or ultraviolet light should be advised that this reaction can occur with tetracycline drugs, and treatment should be discontinued at the first evidence of skin erythema.

The antianabolic action of the tetracyclines may cause an increase in BUN. While this is not a problem in those with normal renal function, in patients with significantly impaired function, higher serum levels of tetracycline may lead to azotemia, hyperphosphatemia, and acidosis.

Usage in pregnancy. (See above "Warnings" about use during tooth development.)

Results of animal studies indicate that tetracyclines cross the placenta, are found in fetal tissues and can have toxic effects on the developing fetus (often related to retardation of skeletal development). Evidence of embryotoxicity has also been noted in animals treated early in pregnancy.

Usage in newborns, infants, and children. (See above "Warnings" about use during tooth development.)

All tetracyclines form a stable calcium complex in any bone forming tissue. A decrease in the fibula growth rate has been observed in prematures given oral tetracycline in doses of 25 mg/kg every 6 hours. This reaction was shown to be reversible when the drug was discontinued.

Tetracyclines are present in the milk of lactating women who are taking a drug in this class.

PRECAUTIONS

As with other antibiotic preparations, use of this drug may result in overgrowth of nonsusceptible organisms, including fungi. If superinfection occurs, the antibiotic should be discontinued and appropriate therapy instituted.

In venereal diseases when coexistent syphilis is suspected, a dark field examination should be done before treatment is started and the blood serology repeated monthly for at least 4 months.

Because tetracyclines have been shown to depress plasma prothrombin activity, patients who are on anticoagulant therapy may require downward adjustment of their anticoagulant dosage.

In long term therapy, periodic laboratory evaluation of organ systems, including hematopoietic, renal and hepatic studies should be performed.

All infections due to Group A beta-hemolytic streptococci should be treated for at least 10 days.

Since bacteriostatic drugs may interfere with the bactericidal action of penicillin, it is advisable to avoid giving tetracycline in conjunction with penicillin.

ADVERSE REACTIONS

Gastrointestinal: anorexia, nausea, vomiting, diarrhea, glossitis, dysphagia, enterocolitis, and inflammatory lesions (with monilial overgrowth) in the anogenital region. These reactions have been caused by both the oral and parenteral administration of tetracyclines. Rare instances of esophagitis and esophageal ulcerations have been reported in patients receiving capsule and tablet forms of drugs in the tetracycline class. Most of these patients took medications immediately before going to bed. (See Dosage and Administration.)

Skin: maculopapular and erythematous rashes. Exfoliative dermatitis has been reported but is uncommon. Photosensitivity is discussed above. (See "Warnings.")

Renal toxicity: Rise in BUN has been reported and is apparently dose related. (See "Warnings.")

Hypersensitivity reactions: Urticaria, angioneurotic edema, anaphylaxis, anaphylactoid purpura, pericarditis and exacerbation of systemic lupus erythematosus.

Bulging fontanels in infants and benign intracranial hypertension in adults have been reported in individuals receiving full therapeutic dosages. These conditions disappeared rapidly when the drug was discontinued.

Blood: Hemolytic anemia, thrombocytopenia, neutropenia and eosinophilia have been reported.

When given over prolonged periods, tetracyclines have been reported to produce brown-black microscopic discoloration of thyroid glands. No abnormalities of thyroid function studies are known to occur.

DOSAGE AND ADMINISTRATION

Oral: Capsules:

Adults: Usual daily dose, 1–2 g divided in four equal doses, depending on the severity of the infection.

Film-coated Tablets only:

Adults: A dosage schedule providing 2 tablets initially, then 1 tablet every six hours, is the usual average dose. In severe infections a larger dose (2 to 4 grams daily) may be indicated.

The total daily dose should be administered in four equal portions given at six hour intervals.

All Oral Forms:

For children above eight years of age: Usual daily dose, 10–20 mg per pound (25–50 mg/kg) of body weight divided in four equal doses.

Therapy should be continued for at least 24–48 hours after symptoms and fever have subsided. For treatment of brucellosis, 500 mg oxytetracycline four times daily for 3 weeks should be accompanied by streptomycin, 1 gram intramuscularly twice daily the first week, and once daily the second week.

For treatment of uncomplicated gonorrhea, when penicillin is contraindicated, tetracycline may be used for the treatment of both males and females in the following divided dosage schedule: 1.5 grams initially followed by 0.5 gram q.i.d. for a total of 9.0 grams.

For treatment of syphilis, a total of 30–40 grams in equally divided doses over a period of 10–15 days should be given. Close follow-up, including laboratory tests, is recommended.

Administration of adequate amounts of fluid along with capsule and tablet forms of drugs in the tetracycline class is recommended to wash down the drugs and reduce the risk of esophageal irritation and ulceration. (See Adverse Reactions.)

Concomitant therapy: Antacids containing aluminum, calcium, or magnesium impair absorption and should not be given to patients taking oral tetracyclines.

Food and some dairy products also interfere with absorption. Oral forms of tetracyclines should be given 1 hour before or 2 hours after meals. Pediatric oral dosage forms should not be given with milk formulas and should be given at least 1 hour prior to feeding.

In patients with renal impairment: (See "Warnings.") Total dosage should be decreased by reduction of recommended individual doses and/or by extending time intervals between doses.

In the treatment of streptococcal infections, a therapeutic dose of oxytetracycline should be administered for at least 10 days.

HOW SUPPLIED

Oral: Terramycin (oxytetracycline HCl) Capsules are available as opaque, yellow, hard gelatin capsules which contain oxytetracycline HCl equivalent to 250 mg of oxytetracycline, and glucosamine hydrochloride (imprinted with code number 073): bottles of 16, 100, and 500 and unit dose pack of 100 (10 × 10's).

60-0755-00-6   Revised Sept. 1981

Capsule Shown in Product Identification Section, page 422 (Tablets: Discontinued)

LITERATURE AVAILABLE

Yes

VANSIL™   ℞

[van'sil]

(Brand of Oxamniquine)

(Capsules of 250 mg)

DESCRIPTION

VANSIL (brand of oxamniquine) is a tetrahydroquinoline derivative for the oral treatment of *Schistosoma mansoni* infections. It is 1, 2, 3, 4,-tetrahydro-2-[[(1- methylethyl) amino]methyl]-7-nitro-6-quinolinemethanol.

Oxamniquine is a yellow-orange crystalline solid which is sparingly soluble in water, but soluble in methanol, acetone, and chloroform.

VANSIL (oxamniquine) capsules contain 250 mg of oxamniquine.

CLINICAL PHARMACOLOGY

Oxamniquine is well absorbed when administered orally. Human plasma concentrations reach a peak at 1 to 1.5 hours after oral administration of therapeutic doses, with a plasma half-life of 1 to 2.5 hours. It is extensively metabolized to inactive acidic metabolites which are largely excreted in the urine.

Male schistosomes are more susceptible than females, but after treatment with oxamniquine the residual female schistosomes cease to lay eggs thus losing the parasitological aspect of their pathological significance. Animal studies with immature *S. mansoni* infections have demonstrated oxamniquine to be highly active in the immediate post-infection phase. Oxamniquine significantly reduces the egg load of *S. mansoni*.

INDICATIONS

Oxamniquine is indicated for all stages of *S. mansoni* infection, including the acute phase and the chronic phase with hepatosplenic involvement.

CONTRAINDICATIONS

At present, there are no known contraindications to the administration of oxamniquine.

WARNINGS

In rare instances epileptiform convulsions have been observed within the first few hours after ingestion of oxamniquine. When a convulsion occurred, it was mostly in a patient with a previous history of a convulsive condition. Oxamniquine should be used with care in such individuals and they should remain under medical supervision with facilities available to treat a convulsion should it occur.

PRECAUTIONS

Pregnancy Cateogry C: Oxamniquine has been shown to have an embryocidal effect in rabbits and mice when given in doses 10 times the human dose.

There are no adequate and well controlled studies in pregnant women. Oxamniquine should be used during pregnancy only if the potential benefit justifies the potential risk to the fetus.

Nursing Mothers: It is not known whether this drug is excreted in human milk.

Because many drugs are excreted in human milk, caution should be exercised when oxamniquine is administered to a nursing mother.

ADVERSE EFFECTS

Oxamniquine is generally well tolerated and toleration is improved if the doses are given after food. Transitory dizziness/drowsiness occurred in approximately one-third of the patients assessed. Other effects observed to a lesser degree are headache, nausea, vomiting, abdominal pain and anorexia. Urticaria has also been reported. In rare instances epileptiform convulsions have been observed (see WARNINGS).

Minor and transient abnormalities in laboratory data have been observed after treatment with oxamniquine which were not considered to be drug-related and were of no clinical significance. They included rare instances of mild to moderate liver enzyme elevations but there was no evidence of hepatotoxicity even in patients with severe hepatosplenic involvement. There was evidence, however, of liver abnormalities in animals with the female rat being uniquely sensitive to relatively low doses.

DOSAGE AND ADMINISTRATION

Adults

The recommended doage is 12 to 15 mg per kilogram of body weight given as a single oral dose in patients with Western Hemisphere strains of *S. mansoni*. The recommended capsule dosage according to body weight is as follows:

Body Weight (kg)	No. of Capsules (250 mg)
30– 40	2
41– 60	3
61– 80	4
81–100	5

Children

The recommended dosage for children under 30 kg in weight is 20 mg/kg of body weight given in two divided doses of 10 mg/kg in one day with an interval of 2 to 8 hours between doses. Toleration is improved if the doses are given after food.

HOW SUPPLIED

VANSIL (brand of oxamniquine) is supplied as #1 capsules of 250 mg in dark green opaque (cap) and rich yellow opaque (body), in bottles of 24 each.

68-4058-00-0   Issued June 1980

Literature Available: Yes

Shown in Product Identification Section, page 422

VIBRAMYCIN® Hyclate   ℞

[vĭ"bra-mĭ"sĭn]

(doxycycline hyclate)

CAPSULES

VIBRA–TABS®

[vĭ"bra-tabs']

(doxycycline hyclate)

FILM COATED TABLETS

VIBRAMYCIN® Calcium

(doxycycline calcium oral suspension)

SYRUP

VIBRAMYCIN® Monohydrate

(doxycycline monohydrate)

FOR ORAL SUSPENSION

DESCRIPTION

Vibramycin is a broad-spectrum antibiotic synthetically derived from oxytetracycline, and is available as Vibramycin Monohydrate (doxycycline monohydrate), Vibramycin Hyclate and Vibra-Tabs (doxycycline hydrochloride hemiethanolate hemihydrate), and Vibramycin Calcium (doxycycline calcium). The chemical designation of this light-yellow crystalline powder is alpha-6-deoxy-5-oxytetracycline. Doxycycline has a high degree of lipoid solubility and a low affinity for calcium binding. It is highly stable in normal human serum. Doxycycline will not degrade into an epianhydro form.

Inert ingredients in the syrup formulation are: apple flavor; butylparaben; calcium chloride; carmine; glycerin; hydrochloric acid; magnesium aluminum silicate; povidone; propylene glycol; propylparaben; raspberry flavor; simethicone emulsion; sodium hydroxide; sodium metabisulfite; sorbitol solution; water.

Inert ingredients in the capsule formulations are: hard gelatin capsules (which may contain Blue 1 and other inert ingredients); magnesium stearate; microcrystalline cellulose; sodium lauryl sulfate.

Inert ingredients for the oral suspension formulation are: carboxymethylcellulose sodium; Blue 1; methylparaben; microcrystalline cellulose; propylparaben; raspberry flavor; Red 28; simethicone emulsion; sucrose.

Inert ingredients for the tablet formulation are: ethylcellulose; hydroxypropyl methylcellulose; magnesium stearate; microcrystalline cellulose; propylene glycol; sodium lauryl sulfate; talc; titanium dioxide; Yellow 6 Lake.

ACTIONS

Doxycycline is primarily bacteriostatic and is thought to exert its antimicrobial effect by the inhibition of protein synthesis. Doxycycline is active against a wide range of gram-positive and gram-negative organisms.

The drugs in the tetracycline class have closely similar antimicrobial spectra, and cross resistance among them is common. Microorganisms may be considered susceptible if the M.I.C. (minimum inhibitory concentration) is less than 4.0 mcg/ml and intermediate if the M.I.C. is 4.0 to 12.5 mcg/ml.

Susceptibility plate testing: If the Kirby-Bauer method of disc susceptibility testing is used, a 30 mcg doxycycline disc should give a zone of at least 16 mm when tested against a doxycycline-susceptible bacterial strain. A tetracycline disc may be used to determine microbial susceptibility. If the Kirby-Bauer method of disc susceptibility testing is used, a 30 mcg tetracycline disc should give a zone of at least 19 mm when tested against a tetracycline-susceptible bacterial strain.

Tetracyclines are readily absorbed and are bound to plasma proteins in varying degree. They are concentrated by the liver in the bile, and excreted in the urine and feces at high concentrations and in a biologically active form. Doxycycline is virtually completely absorbed after oral administration. Following a 200 mg dose, normal adult volunteers averaged peak serum levels of 2.6 mcg/ml of doxycycline at 2 hours decreasing to 1.45 mcg/ml at 24 hours. Excretion of doxycy-

Continued on next page

Pfizer—Cont.

cline by the kidney is about 40%/72 hours in individuals with normal function (creatinine clearance about 75 ml/min.). This percentage excretion may fall as low as 1–5%/72 hours in individuals with severe renal insufficiency (creatinine clearance below 10 ml/min.). Studies have shown no significant difference in serum half-life of doxycycline (range 18–22 hours) in individuals with normal and severely impaired renal function.

Hemodialysis does not alter serum half-life.

INDICATIONS

Doxycycline is indicated in infections caused by the following microorganisms:

Rickettsiae: Rocky Mountain spotted fever, typhus fever and the typhus group, Q. fever, rickettsialpox, and tick fevers.

Mycoplasma pneumoniae (PPLO, Eaton agent),

Agents of psittacosis and ornithosis,

Agents of lymphogranuloma venereum and granuloma inguinale,

The spirochetal agent of relapsing fever (*Borrelia recurrentis*).

The following gram-negative microorganisms:

Haemophilus ducreyi (chancroid),

Pasteurella pestis, and *Pasteurella tularensis,*

Bartonella bacilliformis,

Bacteroides species,

Vibrio comma and *Vibrio fetus,*

Brucella species (in conjunction with streptomycin).

Because many strains of the following groups of microorganisms have been shown to be resistant to tetracyclines, culture and susceptibility testing are recommended.

Doxycycline is indicated for treatment of infections caused by the following gram-negative microorganisms, when bacteriologic testing indicates appropriate susceptibility to the drug:

Escherichia coli,

Enterobacter aerogenes (formerly *Aerobacter aerogenes*),

Shigella species,

Mima species and *Herellea* species,

Haemophilus influenzae (respiratory infections),

Klebsiella species (respiratory and urinary infections).

Doxycycline is indicated for treatment of infections caused by the following gram-positive microorganisms when bacteriologic testing indicates appropriate susceptibility to the drug:

Streptococcus species:

Up to 44 percent of strains of *Streptococcus pyogenes* and 74 percent of *Streptococcus faecalis* have been found to be resistant to tetracycline drugs. Therefore, tetracyclines should not be used for streptococcal disease unless the organism has been demonstrated to be sensitive.

For upper respiratory infections due to group A beta-hemolytic streptococci, penicillin is the usual drug of choice, including prophylaxis of rheumatic fever.

Diplococcus pneumoniae,

Staphylococcus aureus, respiratory, skin and soft-tissue infections. Tetracyclines are not the drug of choice in the treatment of any type of staphylococcal infection.

When penicillin is contraindicated, doxycycline is an alternative drug in the treatment of infections due to:

Neisseria gonorrhoeae,

Treponema pallidum and *Treponema pertenue* (syphilis and yaws),

Listeria monocytogenes,

Clostridium species,

Bacillus anthracis,

Fusobacterium fusiforme (Vincent's infection),

Actinomyces species.

In acute intestinal amebiasis doxycycline may be a useful adjunct to amebicides.

In severe acne doxycycline may be useful adjunctive therapy.

Doxycycline is indicated in the treatment of trachoma, although the infectious agent is not always eliminated, as judged by immunofluorescence.

Inclusion conjunctivitis may be treated with oral doxycycline alone, or with a combination of topical agents.

Doxycycline is indicated for the treatment of uncomplicated urethral, endocervical, or rectal infections in adults caused by *Chlamydia trachomatis.*[1]

Doxycycline is indicated for the treatment of nongonococcal urethritis caused by *Chlamydia trachomatis* and *Ureaplasma urealyticum* and for the treatment of acute epididymo-orchitis caused by *Chlamydia trachomatis.*[1]

Doxycycline is indicated for the treatment of uncomplicated gonococcal infections in adults (except for anorectal infections in men) and acute epididymo-orchitis caused by *N. gonorrhoeae.*[1]

CONTRAINDICATIONS

This drug is contraindicated in persons who have shown hypersensitivity to any of the tetracyclines.

WARNINGS

THE USE OF DRUGS OF THE TETRACYCLINE CLASS DURING TOOTH DEVELOPMENT (LAST HALF OF PREGNANCY, INFANCY AND CHILDHOOD TO THE AGE OF 8 YEARS) MAY CAUSE PERMANENT DISCOLORATION OF THE TEETH (YELLOW-GRAY-BROWN). This adverse reaction is more common during long term use of the drugs but has been observed following repeated short term courses. Enamel hypoplasia has also been reported. *TETRACYCLINE DRUGS, THEREFORE, SHOULD NOT BE USED IN THIS AGE GROUP UNLESS OTHER DRUGS ARE NOT LIKELY TO BE EFFECTIVE OR ARE CONTRAINDICATED.*

Photosensitivity manifested by an exaggerated sunburn reaction has been observed in some individuals taking tetracyclines. Patients apt to be exposed to direct sunlight or ultraviolet light should be advised that this reaction can occur with tetracycline drugs, and treatment should be discontinued at the first evidence of skin erythema.

The antianabolic action of the tetracyclines may cause an increase in BUN. Studies to date indicate that this does not occur with the use of doxycycline in patients with impaired renal function.

Vibramycin Syrup contains sodium metabisulfite, a sulfite that may cause allergic-type reactions including anaphylactic symptoms and life-threatening or less severe asthmatic episodes in certain susceptible people. The over-all prevalence of sulfite sensitivity in the general population is unknown and probably low. Sulfite sensitivity is seen more frequently in asthmatic than in non-asthmatic people.

USAGE IN PREGNANCY

(See above "Warnings" about use during tooth development.) Results of animal studies indicate that tetracyclines cross the placenta, are found in fetal tissues, and can have toxic effects on the developing fetus (often related to retardation of skeletal development). Evidence of embryotoxicity has also been noted in animals treated early in pregnancy.

USAGE IN NEWBORNS, INFANTS, AND CHILDREN:

(See above "Warnings" about use during tooth development.) As with other tetracyclines, doxycycline forms a stable calcium complex in any bone-forming tissue. A decrease in the fibula growth rate has been observed in prematures given oral tetracycline in doses of 25 mg/kg every six hours. This reaction was shown to be reversible when the drug was discontinued.

Tetracyclines are present in the milk of lactating women who are taking a drug in this class.

PRECAUTIONS

As with other antibiotic preparations, use of this drug may result in overgrowth of nonsusceptible organisms, including fungi. If superinfection occurs, the antibiotic should be discontinued and appropriate therapy should be instituted.

In venereal disease when coexistent syphilis is suspected, a dark field examination should be done before treatment is started and the blood serology repeated monthly for at least four months.

Because the tetracyclines have been shown to depress plasma prothrombin activity, patients who are on anticoagulant therapy may require downward adjustment of their anticoagulant dosage.

In long term therapy, periodic laboratory evaluation of organ systems, including hematopoietic, renal, and hepatic studies should be performed.

All infections due to group A beta-hemolytic streptococci should be treated for at least 10 days.

Since bacteriostatic drugs may interfere with the bactericidal action of penicillin, it is advisable to avoid giving tetracycline in conjunction with penicillin.

ADVERSE REACTIONS

Due to oral doxycycline's virtually complete absorption, side effects of the lower bowel, particularly diarrhea, have been infrequent. The following adverse reactions have been observed in patients receiving tetracyclines:

Gastrointestinal: anorexia, nausea, vomiting, diarrhea, glossitis, dysphagia, enterocolitis, and inflammatory lesions (with monilial overgrowth) in the anogenital region. These reactions have been caused by both the oral and parenteral administration of tetracyclines. Rare instances of esophagitis and esophageal ulcerations have been reported in patients receiving capsule and tablet forms of drugs in the tetracycline class. Most of these patients took medications immediately before going to bed. (See Dosage and Administration.)

Skin: maculopapular and erythematous rashes. Exfoliative dermatitis has been reported but is uncommon. Photosensitivity is discussed above (see "Warnings").

Renal toxicity: Rise in BUN has been reported and is apparently dose related. (See "Warnings.")

Hypersensitivity reactions: urticaria, angioneurotic edema, anaphylaxis, anaphylactoid purpura, pericarditis, and exacerbation of systemic lupus erythematosus.

Bulging fontanels in infants and benign intracranial hypertension in adults have been reported in individuals receiving full therapeutic dosages. These conditions disappeared rapidly when the drug was discontinued.

Blood: Hemolytic anemia, thrombocytopenia, neutropenia, and eosinophilia have been reported with tetracyclines.

When given over prolonged periods, tetracyclines have been reported to produce brown-black microscopic discoloration of thyroid glands. No abnormalities of thyroid function studies are known to occur.

DOSAGE AND ADMINISTRATION

THE USUAL DOSAGE AND FREQUENCY OF ADMINISTRATION OF DOXYCYCLINE DIFFERS FROM THAT OF THE OTHER TETRACYCLINES. EXCEEDING THE RECOMMENDED DOSAGE MAY RESULT IN AN INCREASED INCIDENCE OF SIDE EFFECTS.

Adults: The usual dose of oral doxycycline is 200 mg on the first day of treatment (administered 100 mg every 12 hours) followed by a maintenance dose of 100 mg/day. The maintenance dose may be administered as a single dose or as 50 mg every 12 hours. In the management of more severe infections (particularly chronic infections of the urinary tract), 100 mg every 12 hours is recommended.

For children above eight years of age: The recommended dosage schedule for children weighing 100 pounds or less is 2 mg/lb. of body weight divided into two doses on the first day of treatment, followed by 1 mg/lb. of body weight given as a single daily dose or divided into two doses, on subsequent days. For more severe infections up to 2 mg/lb. of body weight may be used. For children over 100 lbs. the usual adult dose should be used.

Uncomplicated gonococcal infections in adults (except anorectal infections in men): 100 mg, by mouth, twice a day for 7 days.[1]

As an alternate single visit dose, administer 300 mg stat followed in one hour by a second 300 mg dose. The dose may be administered with food, including milk or carbonated beverage, as required.

Acute epididymo-orchitis caused by *N. gonorrhoeae:* 100 mg, by mouth, twice a day for at least 10 days.[1]

Primary and secondary syphilis: 300 mg a day in divided doses for at least 10 days.

The therapeutic antibacterial serum activity will usually persist for 24 hours following recommended dosage.

When used in streptococcal infections, therapy should be continued for 10 days.

Administration of adequate amounts of fluid along with capsule and tablet forms of drugs in the tetracycline class is recommended to wash down the drugs and reduce the risk of esophageal irritation and ulceration. (See Adverse Reactions.)

If gastric irritation occurs, it is recommended that doxycycline be given with food or milk. The absorption of doxycycline is not markedly influenced by simultaneous ingestion of food or milk.

Uncomplicated urethral, endocervical, or rectal infection in adults caused by *Chlamydia trachomatis:* 100 mg, by mouth, twice a day for at least 7 days.[1]

Nongonococcal urethritis caused by *C. trachomatis* and *U. urealyticum:* 100 mg, by mouth, twice a day for at least 7 days.[1]

Acute epididymo-orchitis caused by *C. trachomatis:* 100 mg, by mouth, twice a day for at least 10 days.[1]

Concomitant therapy: Antacids containing aluminum, calcium, or magnesium impair absorption and should not be given to patients taking oral doxycycline.

Studies to date have indicated that administration of doxycycline at the usual recommended doses does not lead to excessive accumulation of the antibiotic in patients with renal impairment.

HOW SUPPLIED

Vibramycin Hyclate (doxycycline hyclate) is available in capsules containing doxycycline hyclate equivalent to:

50 mg doxycycline (imprinted with code number 094)

bottles of 50 (NDC 0069-0940-50)

unit-dose pack of 100 (10 x 10's) (NDC 0069-0940-41)

100 mg doxycycline (imprinted with code number 095) bottles of 50 (NDC 0069-0950-50) and 500 (NDC 0069-0950-73)

unit-dose pack of 100 (10 x 10's) (NDC 0069-0950-41)

Vibra-Tabs (doxycycline hyclate) is available in film coated tablets (imprinted with code number 099) containing doxycycline hyclate equivalent to:

100 mg of doxycycline

bottles of 50 (NDC 0069-0990-50) and 500 (NDC 0069-0990-73)

unit-dose pack of 100 (10 x 10's) (NDC 0069-0990-41)

Vibramycin Calcium Syrup (doxycycline calcium oral suspension) is available as a raspberry-apple flavored oral suspension. Each teaspoonful (5 ml) contains doxycycline calcium equivalent to 50 mg of doxycycline: bottles of 1 oz. (30 ml) (NDC 0069-0971-51) and 1 Pint (473 ml) (NDC 0069-0971-93).

Vibramycin Monohydrate (doxycycline monohydrate) for Oral Suspension is available as a pleasant tasting, raspberry flavored, dry powder for oral suspension. When reconstituted, each teaspoonful (5 ml) contains doxycycline monohydrate equivalent to 25 mg of doxycycline: 2 oz. (60 ml) bottles (NDC 0069-0970-65).

Reference:
1. CDC Sexually Transmitted Diseases Treatment Guidelines 1982.

65-1680-00-9   Revised Jan. 1988

LITERATURE AVAILABLE

Yes.

Shown in Product Identification Section, page 422

VISTARIL®   ℞

[vĭs 'tăr-ĭl]
(hydroxyzine pamoate)
Capsules and Oral Suspension

DESCRIPTION

Hydroxyzine pamoate is designated chemically as 1-(p-chlorobenzhydryl) 4-[2-(2-hydroxyethoxy) ethyl] diethylenediamine salt of 1,1'-methylene bis (2 hydroxy-3-naphthalene carboxylic acid).

Inert ingredients for the capsule formulations are: hard gelatin capsules (which may contain Yellow 10, Green 3, Yellow 6, Red 33, and other inert ingredients); magnesium stearate; sodium lauryl sulfate; starch; sucrose.

Inert ingredients for the oral suspension formulation are: carboxymethylcellulose sodium; lemon flavor; propylene glycol; sorbic acid; sorbitol solution; water.

CLINICAL PHARMACOLOGY

Vistaril (hydroxyzine pamoate) is unrelated chemically to the phenothiazines, reserpine, meprobamate, or the benzodiazepines.

Vistaril is not a cortical depressant, but its action may be due to a suppression of activity in certain key regions of the subcortical area of the central nervous system. Primary skeletal muscle relaxation has been demonstrated experimentally. Bronchodilator activity, and antihistaminic and analgesic effects have been demonstrated experimentally and confirmed clinically. An antiemetic effect, both by the apomorphine test and the veriloid test, has been demonstrated. Pharmacological and clinical studies indicate that hydroxyzine in therapeutic dosage does not increase gastric secretion or acidity and in most cases has mild antisecretory activity. Hydroxyzine is rapidly absorbed from the gastrointestinal tract and Vistaril's clinical effects are usually noted within 15 to 30 minutes after oral administration.

INDICATIONS

For symptomatic relief of anxiety and tension associated with psychoneurosis and as an adjunct in organic disease states in which anxiety is manifested.

Useful in the management of pruritus due to allergic conditions such as chronic urticaria and atopic and contact dermatoses, and in histamine-mediated pruritus.

As a sedative when used as premedication and following general anesthesia, **Hydroxyzine may potentiate meperidine (Demerol®) and barbiturates,** so their use in pre-anesthetic adjunctive therapy should be modified on an individual basis. Atropine and other belladonna alkaloids are not affected by the drug. Hydroxyzine is not known to interfere with the action of digitalis in any way and it may be used concurrently with this agent.

The effectiveness of hydroxyzine as an antianxiety agent for long term use, that is more than 4 months, has not been assessed by systematic clinical studies. The physician should reassess periodically the usefulness of the drug for the individual patient.

CONTRAINDICATIONS

Hydroxyzine, when administered to the pregnant mouse, rat, and rabbit, induced fetal abnormalities in the rat and mouse at doses substantially above the human therapeutic range. Clinical data in human beings are inadequate to establish safety in early pregnancy. Until such data are available, hydroxyzine is contraindicated in early pregnancy. Hydroxyzine pamoate is contraindicated for patients who have shown a previous hypersensitivity to it.

WARNINGS

Nursing Mothers: It is not known whether this drug is excreted in human milk. Since many drugs are so excreted, hydroxyzine should not be given to nursing mothers.

PRECAUTIONS

THE POTENTIATING ACTION OF HYDROXYZINE MUST BE CONSIDERED WHEN THE DRUG IS USED IN CONJUNCTION WITH CENTRAL NERVOUS SYSTEM DEPRESSANTS SUCH AS NARCOTICS, NON-NARCOTIC ANALGESICS AND BARBITURATES. Therefore, when central nervous system depressants are administered concomitantly with hydroxyzine their dosage should be reduced. Since drowsiness may occur with use of the drug, patients

should be warned of this possibility and cautioned against driving a car or operating dangerous machinery while taking Vistaril (hydroxyzine pamoate). Patients should be advised against the simultaneous use of other CNS depressant drugs, and cautioned that the effect of alcohol may be increased.

ADVERSE REACTIONS

Side effects reported with the administration of Vistaril are usually mild and transitory in nature.

Anticholinergic: Dry mouth.

Central Nervous System: Drowsiness is usually transitory and may disappear in a few days of continued therapy or upon reduction of the dose. Involuntary motor activity including rare instances of tremor and convulsions has been reported, usually with doses considerably higher than those recommended. Clinically significant respiratory depression has not been reported at recommended doses.

OVERDOSAGE

The most common manifestation of overdosage of Vistaril is hypersedation. As in the management of overdosage with any drug, it should be borne in mind that multiple agents may have been taken.

If vomiting has not occurred spontaneously, it should be induced. Immediate gastric lavage is also recommended. General supportive care, including frequent monitoring of the vital signs and close observation of the patient, is indicated. Hypotension, though unlikely, may be controlled with intravenous fluids and Levophed® (levarterenol) or Aramine® (metaraminol). Do not use epinephrine as Vistaril counteracts its pressor action. Caffeine and Sodium Benzoate Injection, U.S.P., may be used to counteract central nervous system depressant effects.

There is no specific antidote. It is doubtful that hemodialysis would be of any value in the treatment of overdosage with hydroxyzine. However, if other agents such as barbiturates have been ingested concomitantly, hemodialysis may be indicated. There is no practical method to quantitate hydroxyzine in body fluids or tissue after its ingestion or administration.

DOSAGE

For symptomatic relief of anxiety and tension associated with psychoneurosis and as an adjunct in organic disease states in which anxiety is manifested: in adults, 50–100 mg q.i.d.; children under 6 years, 50 mg daily in divided doses and over 6 years, 50–100 mg daily in divided doses.

For use in the management of pruritus due to allergic conditions such as chronic urticaria and atopic and contact dermatoses, and in histamine-mediated pruritus: in adults, 25 mg t.i.d. or q.i.d.; children under 6 years, 50 mg daily in divided doses and over 6 years, 50–100 mg daily in divided doses.

As a sedative when used as a premedication and following general anesthesia: 50–100 mg in adults, and 0.6 mg/kg in children.

When treatment is initiated by the intramuscular route of administration, subsequent doses may be administered orally.

As with all medications, the dosage should be adjusted according to the patient's response to therapy.

SUPPLY

Vistaril Capsules (hydroxyzine pamoate equivalent to hydroxyzine hydrochloride)

25 mg: 100's (NDC 0069-5410-66), 500's (NDC 0069-5410-73), and Unit Dose (10 × 10's) (NDC 0069-5410-41) two-tone green capsules

50 mg: 100's (NDC 0069-5420-66), 500's (NDC 0069-5420-73), and Unit Dose (10 × 10's) (NDC 0069-5420-41) green and white capsules

100 mg: 100's (NDC 0069-5430-66), 500's (NDC 0069-5430-73), and Unit Dose (10 × 10's) (NDC 0069-5430-41) green and gray capsules

Vistaril Oral Suspension (hydroxyzine pamoate equivalent to 25 mg hydroxyzine hydrochloride per teaspoonful-5 ml): 1 pint bottles (NDC 0069-5440-93) and 4 ounce (120 ml) bottles (NDC 0069-5440-97) in packages of 4.

BIBLIOGRAPHY

Available on request.

69-0846-00-0   Revised November 1986

Shown in Product Identification Section, page 422

EDUCATIONAL MATERIAL

Booklets—free

The *Learning to Live With. . . .* series of patient information booklets on the symptoms of specific diseases, preventive measures, techniques for changing lifestyle habits, adherence to diet and drug regimens. This ongoing series includes booklets on angina, osteoarthritis, hypertension and diabetes.

Address requests to:
Communications Program Coordination
Pfizer Pharmaceuticals
235 East 42nd Street
New York, N.Y. 10017

Vibramycin:
Booklet:
MMWR Supplement: 1985 STD Treatment Guidelines, Centers for Disease Control, United States Department of Health and Human Services, Vol. 34, No. 4S, October 18, 1985.

A comprehensive overview of the major sexually transmitted diseases (STD) is presented in this reprint of the *1985 STD Treatment Guidelines.* The booklet presents a description of major STD pathologies, such as AIDS, *Chlamydia trachomatis* infection and PID, and their approved CDC treatments. This booklet is available free to physicians, pharmacists, and allied health practitioners.

Address requests to:
Pfizer Laboratories Medical Department
Professional Services
235 East 42nd Street
New York, N.Y. 10017

Pharmacia Inc.
800 CENTENNIAL AVENUE
P.O. BOX 1327
PISCATAWAY, NJ 08855-1327

AZULFIDINE EN-tabs®   ℞
(sulfasalazine, tablets USP)
(enteric-coated tablets)
AZULFIDINE® (sulfasalazine, USP)   ℞
[ă-zul 'fĭ-dĕn "]
Oral Suspension
AZULFIDINE® Tablets   ℞
(sulfasalazine tablets, USP)

DESCRIPTION

Azulfidine EN-tabs®, 500 mg enteric-coated tablets for Oral Administration

Azulfidine EN-tabs are film coated with cellulose acetate phthalate to prevent disintegration of the tablet in the stomach and thus reduce possible irritation of the gastric mucosa.

Azulfidine® Oral Suspension, 250 mg/5ml for Oral Administration

Azulfidine® Tablets, 500 mg for Oral Administration

Therapeutic classification: Anti-inflammatory agent.

Chemical designation: 5-([p-(2-Pyridylsulfamoyl) phenyl] azo) salicylic acid.

Chemical structure:

$$C_{18}H_{14}N_4O_5S$$

CLINICAL PHARMACOLOGY

After oral administration, AZULFIDINE is partially absorbed and extensively metabolized as described below.

About one-third of a given dose of sulfasalazine (SS) is absorbed from the small intestine. The remaining two-thirds pass to the colon where the compound is split (presumably by intestinal bacteria) into its components, 5-aminosalicylic acid (5-ASA) and sulfapyridine (SP). Most of the SP thus liberated is absorbed whereas only about one-third of the 5-ASA is absorbed, the remainder being excreted in the feces. The distribution metabolism and excretion of SS and its two components are as follows:

AZULFIDINE EN-tabs (enteric-coated tablets)

Sulfasalazine (SS): Detectable serum concentrations of SS have been found in healthy subjects within 90 minutes after the ingestion of a single 2 g dose of AZULFIDINE EN-tabs. Maximum concentrations of SS occur between 3 and 12 hours, with the mean peak concentration (6 mcg/ml) occurring at 6 hours. Small amounts of SS are excreted unchanged in the urine.

Sulfapyridine (SP): Following absorption and distribution, SP is acetylated and hydroxylated in the liver, and then conjugated with glucuronic acid. After ingestion of a single 2 g dose of AZULFIDINE EN-tabs by healthy subjects, peak concentrations of SP and its various metabolites appear in the serum between 12 and 24 hours, with the peak concentration (13 mcg/ml) occurring at 12 and lasting until 24 hours. The total recovery of SS and its SP metabolites from the urine of healthy subjects 3 days after the administration of a single 2 g dose of AZULFIDINE EN-tabs averaged 81%.

Continued on next page

Pharmacia—Cont.

5-Aminosalicylic Acid (5-ASA): The serum concentration of 5-ASA in patients with ulcerative colitis was found to range from 0 to 4 mcg/ml, and to exist mainly in the form of free 5-ASA. The urinary recovery of this compound was mostly in the acetylated form.

AZULFIDINE Oral Suspension

Sulfasalazine (SS): Detectable serum concentrations of SS have been found in healthy subjects within 90 minutes after the injestion of a single 2 g dose of AZULFIDINE Oral Suspension. Maximum concentrations of SS occur between 1.5 and 6 hours, with the mean peak concentration (20 mcg/ml) occurring at 3 hours. Small amounts of SS are excreted unchanged in the urine.

Sulfapyridine (SP): Following absorption and distribution, SP is acetylated and hydroxylated in the liver, and then conjugated with glucuronic acid. After ingestion of a single 2 g dose of AZULFIDINE Oral Suspension by healthy subjects, SP and its various metabolites appear in the serum within 3 to 6 hours. Maximum concentrations of total SP occur between 9 and 24 hours with the mean peak concentration (19 mcg/ml) occurring at 12 hours. The total recovery of SS and its SP metabolites from the urine of healthy subjects 3 days after the administration of a single 2 g dose of AZULFIDINE Oral Suspension averaged 75%.

5-Aminosalicylic Acid (5-ASA): The serum concentrations of 5-ASA in patients with ulcerative colitis was found to range from 0 to 4 mcg/ml, and to exist mainly in the form of free 5-ASA. The urinary recovery of this compound was mostly in the acetylated form.

AZULFIDINE Tablets:

Sulfasalazine (SS): Detectable serum concentrations of SS have been found in healthy subjects within 90 minutes after the ingestion of a single 2 g dose of AZULFIDINE Tablets. Maximum concentrations of SS occur between 1.5 and 6 hours, with the mean peak concentration (14 mcg/ml) occurring at 3 hours. Small amounts of SS are excreted unchanged in the urine.

Sulfapyridine (SP): Following absorption and distribution, SP is acetylated and hydroxylated in the liver, and then conjugated with glucuronic acid. After ingestion of a single 2 g dose of AZULFIDINE Tablets by healthy subjects, SP and its various metabolites appear in the serum within 3 to 6 hours. Maximum concentrations of total SP occur between 6 and 24 hours, with the mean peak concentration (21 mcg/ml) occurring at 12 hours. The total recovery of SS and its SP metabolites from the urine of healthy subjects 3 days after the administration of a single 2 g dose of AZULFIDINE Tablets averaged 91%.

5-Aminosalicylic Acid (5-ASA): The serum concentration of 5-ASA in patients with ulcerative colitis was found to range from 0 to 4 mcg/ml, and to exist mainly in the form of free 5-ASA. The urinary recovery of this compound was mostly in the acetylated form.

Mean serum concentrations of total SP, i.e. SP and its metabolites, tend to be significantly greater in patients with a slow acetylator phenotype than in those with a fast acetylator phenotype. Total serum sulfapyridine concentrations greater than 50 mcg/ml appear to be associated with an increased incidence of adverse reactions.

The mode of action of AZULFIDINE is still under investigation. It may be related to the immunosuppressant properties that have been observed in animal and **in vitro** models, to its affinity for connective tissue, and/or to the relatively high concentration it reaches in serous fluids, the liver and intestinal walls, as demonstrated in autoradiographic studies in animals. AZULFIDINE has also been described as a highly efficient vehicle for carrying its principal metabolites, SP and 5-ASA, to the colon, where a local action for both of them has been postulated. Recent clinical studies utilizing rectal administration of SS, SP, and 5-ASA have indicated that the major therapeutic action may reside in the 5-ASA moiety.

INDICATIONS AND USAGE

AZULFIDINE is indicated:

a. in the treatment of mild to moderate ulcerative colitis, and as adjunctive therapy in severe ulcerative colitis.

b. for the prolongation of the remission period between acute attacks of ulcerative colitis.

AZULFIDINE EN-tabs are particularly indicated in patients who cannot take the regular AZULFIDINE tablet because of gastrointestinal intolerance, and in whom there is evidence that this intolerance is not primarily due to high blood levels of sulfapyridine and its metabolites, e.g. patients experiencing nausea, vomiting, etc., when taking the first few doses of the drug or patients in whom a reduction in dosage does not alleviate the gastrointestinal side effects.

CONTRAINDICATIONS

Hypersensitivity to sulfasalazine, its metabolites, sulfonamides or salicylates. In infants under 2 years of age. Intestinal and urinary obstruction. Patients with porphyria should not receive sulfonamides as these drugs have been reported to precipitate an acute attack.

WARNINGS

Only after critical appraisal should AZULFIDINE be used in patients with hepatic or renal damage or blood dyscrasias. Deaths associated with the administration of AZULFIDINE have been reported from hypersensitivity reactions, agranulocytosis, aplastic anemia, other blood dyscrasias, renal and liver damage, irreversible neuromuscular and CNS changes, and fibrosing alveolitis. The presence of clinical signs such as sore throat, fever, pallor, purpura, or jaundice may be indications of serious blood disorders. Complete blood counts as well as urinalysis with careful microscopic examination should be done frequently in patients receiving AZULFIDINE. Oligospermia and infertility have been observed in men treated with AZULFIDINE. Withdrawal of the drug appears to reverse these effects.

PRECAUTIONS

General: AZULFIDINE should be given with caution to patients with severe allergy or bronchial asthma. Adequate fluid intake must be maintained in order to prevent crystalluria and stone formation. Patients with glucose-6-phosphate dehydrogenase deficiency should be observed closely for signs of hemolytic anemia. This reaction is frequently dose related. If toxic or hypersensitivity reactions occur, the drug should be discontinued immediately.

Isolated instances have been reported when AZULFIDINE EN-tabs have passed undisintegrated. This may be due to a lack of intestinal esterases in the patient. If this is observed, the administration of AZULFIDINE EN-tabs should be discontinued immediately.

Information for Patients: Patients should be informed of the possibility of adverse reactions and of the need for careful medical supervision. They should also be made aware that ulcerative colitis rarely remits completely, and that the risk of relapse can be substantially reduced by continued administration of AZULFIDINE (at a maintenance dosage). Diabetic patients should be advised that AZULFIDINE Oral Suspension contains sucrose.

Patients should be instructed to take AZULFIDINE in evenly divided doses preferably after meals. Additionally, patients should be advised that AZULFIDINE may produce an orange-yellow discoloration of the urine or skin.

Laboratory Tests: The progress of the disease during treatment can be evaluated by clinical criteria, including the presence of fever, weight changes, degree and frequency of diarrhea and bleeding as well as by sigmoidoscopy and the evaluation of biopsy samples. The determination of serum sulfapyridine levels may be useful since concentrations greater than 50 mcg/ml appear to be associated with an increased incidence of adverse reactions. Complete blood counts, as well as a urinalysis with careful microscopic examination should be done frequently in patients receiving AZULFIDINE.

Drug Interactions: Reduced absorption of folic acid and digoxin have been reported when administered concomitantly with AZULFIDINE.

Drug/Laboratory Test Interactions: The presence of AZULFIDINE or its metabolites in body fluids has not been reported to interfere with laboratory test procedures.

Carcinogenesis, Mutagenesis, Impairment of Fertility: There have been no long-term studies of the carcinogenic or mutagenic potential of AZULFIDINE. Impairment of male fertility was observed in reproductive studies performed in rats and rabbits at doses up to six times the human dose. Oligospermia and infertility have been described in men treated with AZULFIDINE. Withdrawal of the drug appears to reverse these effects (see "**WARNINGS**").

Pregnancy:

Teratogenic Effects:

Pregnancy Category B: Reproduction studies have been performed in rats and rabbits at doses up to 6 times the human dose and have revealed no evidence of impaired female fertility or harm to the fetus due to AZULFIDINE.

There are, however, no adequate and well-controlled studies in pregnant women. Because animal reproduction studies are not always predictive of human response, this drug should be used during pregnancy only if clearly needed. A national survey evaluated the outcome of pregnancies associated with inflammatory bowel disease (IBD). In a group of 186 women treated with AZULFIDINE alone or AZULFIDINE and concomitant steroid therapy, the incidence of fetal morbidity and mortality was comparable to that for 245 untreated IBD pregnancies as well as to population data from the National Center for Health Statistics[1]. Another study of 1,445 pregnancies associated with exposure to sulfonamides in which AZULFIDINE was included indicated that this group of drugs appeared to be devoid of any association with fetal malformation[2]. A review of the medical literature covering 1,155 pregnancies which occurred in women having ulcerative colitis suggested that the outcome was similar to what was expected in the general population[3]. No clinical studies have been performed which indicate the effect of AZULFIDINE on the later growth development and functional maturation of children whose mothers received the drug during pregnancy.

Nonteratogenic Effects: AZULFIDINE and sulfapyridine pass the placental barrier. Although sulfapyridine has been shown to have a poor bilirubin displacing capacity, the potential for kernicterus in newborns should be kept in mind.

Nursing Mothers: Caution should be exercised when AZULFIDINE is administered to a nursing woman. Sulfonamides are excreted in the milk. In the newborn, they compete with bilirubin for binding sites on the plasma proteins and may thus cause kernicterus. Insignificant amounts of uncleaved sulfasalazine have been found in milk, whereas the sulfapyridine levels in milk are about 30–60 per cent of those in the serum. Sulfapyridine has been shown to have a poor bilirubin displacing capacity.

Pediatric Use: Safety and effectiveness in children below the age of two years have not been established.

ADVERSE REACTIONS

The most common adverse reactions associated with AZULFIDINE are anorexia, headache, nausea, vomiting, gastric distress and apparently reversible oligospermia. These occur in about one-third of the patients. Less frequent adverse reactions are skin rash, pruritus, urticaria, fever, Heinz body anemia, hemolytic anemia and cyanosis which may occur at a frequency of one in every thirty patients or less. Experience suggests that with a daily dosage of 4 g or more, or total serum sulfapyridine levels above 50 mcg/ml, the incidence of adverse reactions tends to increase.

Although the listing which follows includes a few adverse reactions which have not been reported with this specific drug, the pharmacological similarities among the sulfonamides require that each of these reactions be considered when AZULFIDINE is administered.

Other adverse reactions which occur rarely, in approximately 1 in 1000 patients or less are:

Blood dyscrasias: aplastic anemia, agranulocytosis, leukopenia, megaloblastic (macrocytic) anemia, purpura, thrombocytopenia, hypoprothrombinemia and methemoglobinemia.

Hypersensitivity reactions: erythema multiforme (Stevens Johnson syndrome), exfoliative dermatitis, epidermal necrolysis (Lyell's syndrome) with corneal damage, anaphylaxis, serum sickness syndrome, transient pulmonary changes with eosinophilia and decreased pulmonary function, allergic myocarditis, polyartenitis nodosa, L.E. syndrome, hepatitis with immune complexes, parapsoriasis varioliformis acuta (Mucha Haberman syndrome), photosensitization, arthralgia, periorbital edema, conjuctival and scleral injection and alopecia.

Gastrointestinal reactions: hepatitis, pancreatitis, bloody diarrhea, impaired folic acid absorption, impaired digoxin absorption, stomatitis, diarrhea and abdominal pains.

CNS reactions: transverse myelitis, convulsions, transient lesions of the posterior spinal column, peripheral neuropathy, mental depression, vertigo, hearing loss, insomnia, ataxia, hallucinations, tinnitus and drowsiness.

Renal reactions: toxic nephrosis with oliguria and anuria, nephrotic syndrome, hematuria, crystalluria and proteinuria.

Other reactions: urine discoloration and skin discoloration. The sulfonamides bear certain chemical similarities to some goitrogens, diuretics, (acetazolamide and the thiazides), and oral hypoglycemic agents. Goiter production, diuresis, and hypoglycemia have occurred rarely in patients receiving sulfonamides. Cross-sensitivity may exist with these agents. Rats appear to be especially susceptible to the goitrogenic effects of sulfonamides and long-term administration has produced thyroid malignancies in this species.

DRUG ABUSE AND DEPENDENCE

None reported.

Overdosage: There is evidence that the incidence and severity of toxicity are directly related to the total serum sulfapyridine concentration. Symptoms of overdosage may include nausea, vomiting, gastric distress and abdominal pains. In more advanced cases, CNS symptoms such as drowsiness, convulsions, etc. may be observed. Serum sulfapyridine concentrations may be used to monitor the progress of recovery from overdosage.

Experience suggests that with a daily dosage of 4 g or more or total serum sulfapyridine levels above 50 mcg/ml the incidence of adverse reactions tends to increase. There are no documented reports of deaths due to ingestion of large single doses of AZULFIDINE.

It has not been possible to determine the oral LD_{50} in laboratory animals such as mice, since the highest daily oral dose which can be given (12 g/kg) is not lethal. Doses of AZULFIDINE of 16 g per day have been given to patients without mortality.

Instructions for overdosage: Gastric lavage or emesis plus catharsis as indicated. Alkalinize urine. If kidney function is normal, force fluids. If anuria is present, restrict fluids and salt, and treat appropriately. Catheterization of the ureters may be indicated for complete renal blockage by crystals. The low molecular weight of AZULFIDINE and its metabolites may facilitate their removal by dialysis. For agranulocytosis, discontinue the drug immediately, hospitalize the patient and institute appropriate therapy.

For hypersensitivity reactions, discontinue treatment immediately. Such reactions may be controlled with antihistamines and, if necessary, systemic corticosteroids.

When in the physician's opinion, reinstitution of AZULFIDINE is warranted, regimens modeled upon desensitization procedures may be attempted approximately two weeks after AZULFIDINE has been discontinued and symptoms have disappeared (see "**Dosage and Administration**").

DOSAGE AND ADMINISTRATION

Dosage should be adjusted to each individual's response and tolerance. The drug should be given in evenly divided doses over each 24-hour period; intervals between nighttime doses should not exceed 8 hours, with administration after meals recommended when feasible. Experience suggests that with daily dosages of 4 g or more, the incidence of adverse reactions tends to increase; hence, patients receiving these dosages should be instructed about and carefully observed for the appearance of adverse effects.

Various desensitization-like regimens have been reported to be effective in 34 of 53 patients[4], 7 of 8 patients[5] and 19 of 20 patients[6]. Upon reinstituting AZULFIDINE, such regimens comprise a total daily dose of 50 to 250 mg which, every 4 to 7 days thereafter, is doubled until the desired therapeutic level is achieved. Administration of small desensitization doses of AZULFIDINE are achieved most easily through the use of AZULFIDINE Oral Suspension (250 mg/5 ml). If the symptoms of sensitivity recur, AZULFIDINE should be discontinued. Desensitization should not be attempted in patients who have a history of agranulocytosis or who have experienced an anaphylactoid reaction while on a previous course of AZULFIDINE therapy.

USUAL DOSAGE

AZULFIDINE Tablets and AZULFIDINE EN-tabs (enteric-coated tablets)

Initial therapy: ADULTS: 3-4 g daily in evenly divided doses. In some cases it is advisable to initiate therapy with a small dosage, e.g. 1-2 g daily, to lessen adverse gastrointestinal effects. If daily doses exceeding 4 g are required to achieve desired effects, the increased risk of toxicity should be kept in mind. CHILDREN TWO YEARS OF AGE AND OLDER: 40-60 mg per kg body weight in each 24-hour period, divided into 3-6 doses.

Maintenance therapy: ADULTS: 2 g daily. CHILDREN TWO YEARS OF AGE AND OLDER: 30 mg per kg body weight in each 24-hour period, divided into 4 doses.

AZULFIDINE Oral Suspension

[Each 5 ml (one teaspoonful) contains 250 mg of sulfasalazine.]

Initial Therapy:

Adults: 3-4 g daily in evenly divided doses. In some cases it is advisable to initiate therapy with a smaller dosage, e.g. 1-2 g daily, to lessen adverse gastrointestinal effects. If daily doses up to 4 g are required to achieve desired effects, the increased risk of toxicity should be kept in mind.

Children two years of age and older: 40-60 mg per kg body weight in each 24-hour period, divided into 3-6 doses.

Maintenance Therapy:

Adults: 2 g daily.

Children two years of age and older: 30 mg per kg body weight in each 24-hour period, divided into 4 doses.

Response to therapy and adjustment of dosage should be determined by periodic examination. It is often necessary to continue medication, even when clinical symptoms, including diarrhea, have been controlled. When endoscopic examination confirms satisfactory improvement, dosage is reduced to a maintenance level. If symptoms of gastric intolerance (anorexia, nausea, vomiting, etc.) occur after the first few doses of AZULFIDINE, they are probably due to mucosal irritation and may be alleviated by distributing the total daily dose more evenly over the day or by giving enteric-coated EN-tabs. If diarrhea recurs, dosage should be increased to previous effective levels. If such symptoms occur after the first few days of treatment with AZULFIDINE, they are probably due to increased serum levels of total sulfapyridine, and may be alleviated by halving the dose and subsequently increasing it gradually over several days. If symptoms continue, the drug should be stopped for 5–7 days, then reinstituted at a lower daily dose.

HOW SUPPLIED

AZULFIDINE Tablets are round, gold-colored, scored tablets, monogrammed "101" in the following package sizes:

AZULFIDINE Tablets 500 mg 100's — NDC No. 0016-0101-01

AZULFIDINE Tablets 500 mg 500's — NDC No. 0016-0101-05

AZULFIDINE Unit Dose Tablets

  500 mg 100's — NDC No. 0016-0101-11

AZULFIDINE Unit Dose Tablets

  500 mg 10 × 100's — NDC No. 0016-0101-10

AZULFIDINE EN-tabs are eliptical, gold colored, film enteric coated tablets, monogrammed "102" in the following package sizes.

AZULFIDINE EN-tabs 500 mg 100's — NDC No. 0016-0102-01

AZULFIDINE EN-tabs 500 mg 500's — NDC No. 0016-0102-05

Storage: Room temperature (15–30°C/59–86°F).

AZULFIDINE Oral Suspension is an orange-yellow, flavored suspension in the following package size.

AZULFIDINE Oral Suspension 250 mg/5 ml — 1 Pint (473 ml) — NDC No. 0016-0103-06

Storage: Room temperature (15–30°C/59–86°F)

             Avoid Freezing.

             Shake Well Before Use

References:

1. Mogadam M, et al: Pregnancy in inflammatory bowel disease: Effect of sulfasalazine and corticosteroids on fetal outcome *Gastroenterol* 80:72–76, 1981.
2. Kaufman D W (ed): *Birth Defects and Drugs in Pregnancy.* Littleton, MA, Publishing Sciences Group, Inc. 1977, pp 296–313.
3. Jarnerot G: Fertility, sterility and pregnancy in chronic inflammatory bowel disease. *Scand J Gastroenterol* 17:1–4, 1982.
4. Korelitz BI, et al: *Gastroenterol* 82:1104, 1982.
5. Holdsworth C G: *Brit Med J* 282:110, 1981.
6. Taffet S L, Das K M: *Amer J Med* 73:520–524, 1982.

CAUTION

Federal law prohibits dispensing without prescription.
Pharmacia Inc.
800 Centennial Avenue
P.O. Box 1327
Piscataway, New Jersey 08855-1327
© 1984, Pharmacia Inc.; Revised June 1989
Shown in Product Identification Section, page 422

EMCYT®   ℞

[em 'sit]
(estramustine phosphate sodium/Pharmacia)
CAPSULES

DESCRIPTION

Estramustine phosphate sodium, an antineoplastic agent, is an off-white powder readily soluble in water. Emcyt is available as white opaque capsules, each containing estramustine phosphate sodium as the disodium salt monohydrate equivalent to 140 mg estramustine phosphate, for oral administration. Each capsule also contains magnesium stearate, silicon dioxide, sodium lauryl sulfate and talc. Gelatin capsule shells contain the following pigment: titanium dioxide.

Chemically, estramustine phosphate sodium is estra-1,3,5(10)-triene-3,17-diol(17β)-,3-[bis(2-chloroethyl) carbamate] 17-dihydrogen phosphate), disodium salt, monohydrate. It is also referred to as estradiol 3-[bis(2-chloroethyl) carbamate 17-(dihydrogen phosphate), disodium salt, monohydrate. Estramustine phosphate sodium has an empiric formula of $C_{23}H_{30}Cl_2NNa_2O_6P \cdot H_2O$ and a calculated molecular weight of 582.4.

CLINICAL PHARMACOLOGY

Estramustine phosphate is a molecule combining estradiol and nornitrogen mustard by a carbamate link. The molecule is phosphorylated to make it water soluble.

Estramustine phosphate taken orally is readily dephosphorylated during absorption, and the major metabolites in plasma are estramustine, the estrone analog, estradiol and estrone.

Prolonged treatment with estramustine phosphate produces elevated total plasma concentrations of estradiol that fall within ranges similar to the elevated estradiol levels found in prostatic cancer patients given conventional estradiol therapy. Estrogenic effects, as demonstrated by changes in circulating levels of steroids and pituitary hormones, are similar in patients treated with either estramustine phosphate or conventional estradiol.

The metabolic urinary patterns of the estradiol moiety of estramustine phosphate and estradiol itself are very similar, although the metabolites derived from estramustine phosphate are excreted at a slower rate.

INDICATIONS AND USAGE

Emcyt is indicated in the palliative treatment of patients with metastatic and/or progressive carcinoma of the prostate.

CONTRAINDICATIONS

Emcyt should not be used in patients with any of the following conditions:

1) Known hypersensitivity to either estradiol or to nitrogen mustard.

2) Active thrombophlebitis or thromboembolic disorders, except in those cases where the actual tumor mass is the cause of the thromboembolic phenomenon and the physician feels the benefits of therapy may outweigh the risks.

WARNINGS

It has been shown that there is an increased risk of thrombosis, including nonfatal myocardial infarction, in men receiving estrogens for prostatic cancer. Emcyt should be used with caution in patients with a history of thrombophlebitis, thrombosis or thromboembolic disorders, especially if they were associated with estrogen therapy. Caution should also be used in patients with cerebral vascular or coronary artery disease.

Glucose Tolerance—Because glucose tolerance may be decreased, diabetic patients should be carefully observed while receiving Emcyt.

Elevated Blood Pressure—Because hypertension may occur, blood pressure should be monitored periodically.

PRECAUTIONS

General: Fluid Retention—Exacerbation of preexisting or incipient peripheral edema or congestive heart disease has been seen in some patients receiving Emcyt therapy. Other conditions which might be influenced by fluid retention, such as epilepsy, migraine or renal dysfunction, require careful observation.

Emcyt may be poorly metabolized in patients with impaired liver function and should be administered with caution in such patients.

Because Emcyt may influence the metabolism of calcium and phosphorus, it should be used with caution in patients with metabolic bone diseases that are associated with hypercalcemia or in patients with renal insufficiency.

Information for the Patient: Because of the possibility of mutagenic effects, patients should be advised to use contraceptive measures.

Laboratory Tests: Certain endocrine and liver function tests may be affected by estrogen-containing drugs. Abnormalities of hepatic enzymes and of bilirubin have occurred in patients receiving Emcyt, but have seldom been severe enough to require cessation of therapy. Such tests should be done at appropriate intervals during therapy and repeated after the drug has been withdrawn for two months.

Food/Drug Interaction: Milk, milk products and calcium-rich foods or drugs may impair the absorption of Emcyt.

Carcinogenesis, Mutagenesis, Impairment of Fertility: Long-term continuous administration of estrogen in certain animal species increases the frequency of carcinomas of the breast and liver. Compounds structurally similar to Emcyt are carcinogenic in mice. Carcinogenic studies of Emcyt have not been conducted in man. Although testing by the Ames method failed to demonstrate mutagenicity for estramustine phosphate sodium, it is known that both estradiol and nitrogen mustard are mutagenic. For this reason and because some patients who had been impotent while on estrogen therapy have regained potency while taking Emcyt, the patient should be advised to use contraceptive measures.

ADVERSE REACTIONS

In a randomized, double-blind trial comparing therapy with Emcyt in 93 patients (11.5 to 15.9 mg/kg/day) or diethylstilbestrol (DES) in 93 patients (3.0 mg/day), the following adverse effects were reported:

	EMCYT n=93	DES n=93
CARDIOVASCULAR–		
RESPIRATORY		
Cardiac Arrest	0	2
Cerebrovascular Accident	2	0
Myocardial Infarction	3	1
Thrombophlebitis	3	7
Pulmonary Emboli	2	5
Congestive Heart Failure	3	2
Edema	19	17
Dyspnea	11	3
Leg Cramps	8	11
Upper Respiratory Discharge	1	1
Hoarseness	1	0
GASTROINTESTINAL		
Nausea	15	8
Diarrhea	12	11
Minor Gastrointestinal		
Upset	11	6
Anorexia	4	3
Flatulence	2	0
Vomiting	1	1
Gastrointestinal Bleeding	1	0
Burning Throat	1	0
Thirst	1	0
INTEGUMENTARY		
Rash	1	4
Pruritus	2	2
Dry Skin	2	0
Pigment Changes	0	3
Easy Bruising	3	0
Flushing	1	0
Night Sweats	0	1
Fingertip—Peeling Skin	1	0
Thinning Hair	1	1

Continued on next page

Pharmacia—Cont.

BREAST CHANGES		
Tenderness	66	64
Enlargement		
Mild	60	54
Moderate	10	16
Marked	0	5
MISCELLANEOUS		
Lethargy Alone	4	3
Depression	0	2
Emotional Lability	2	0
Insomnia	3	0
Headache	1	1
Anxiety	1	0
Chest Pain	1	1
Hot Flashes	0	1
Pain in Eyes	0	1
Tearing of Eyes	1	1
Tinnitus	0	1
LABORATORY ABNORMALITIES		
Hematologic		
Leukopenia	4	2
Thrombopenia	1	2
Hepatic		
Bilirubin Alone	1	5
Bilirubin and LDH	0	1
Bilirubin and SGOT	2	1
Bilirubin, LDH and SGOT	2	0
LDH and/or SGOT	31	28
Miscellaneous		
Hypercalcemia—Transient	0	1

OVERDOSAGE

Although there has been no experience with overdosage to date, it is reasonable to expect that such episodes may produce pronounced manifestations of the known adverse reactions. In the event of overdosage, the gastric contents should be evacuated by gastric lavage and symptomatic therapy should be initiated. Hematologic and hepatic parameters should be monitored for at least six weeks after overdosage of Emcyt.

DOSAGE AND ADMINISTRATION

The recommended daily dose is 14 mg per kg of body weight (*i.e.*, one 140 mg capsule for each 10 kg or 22 lb of body weight), given in 3 or 4 divided doses. Most patients in studies in the United States have been treated at a dosage range of 10 to 16 mg per kg per day.

Patients should be instructed to take Emcyt at least one hour before or two hours after meals. Emcyt should be swallowed with water. Milk, milk products and calcium-rich foods or drugs (such as calcium-containing antacids) must not be taken simultaneously with Emcyt.

Patients should be treated for 30 to 90 days before the physician determines the possible benefits of continued therapy. Therapy should be continued as long as the favorable response lasts. Some patients have been maintained on therapy for more than three years at doses ranging from 10 to 16 mg per kg of body weight per day.

Procedures for proper handling and disposal of anticancer drugs should be considered. Several guidelines on this subject have been published.[1-6] There is no general agreement that all of the procedures recommended in the guidelines are necessary or appropriate.

HOW SUPPLIED

White opaque capsules, each containing estramustine phosphate sodium as the disodium salt monohydrate equivalent to 140 mg estramustine phosphate—bottles of 100 (NDC 0016-0132-02).

Note: Emcyt should be stored in the refrigerator at 36° to 46°F (2° to 8°C).

REFERENCES

1. Recommendations for the safe handling of parenteral antineoplastic drugs. Washington, DC, U.S. Government Printing Office (NIH Publication No. 83-2621). 2. AMA Council Report. Guidelines for handling parenteral antineoplastics. *JAMA* 253:1590–1592, Mar. 15, 1985. 3. National Study Commission on Cytotoxic Exposure: Recommendations for handling cytotoxic agents. Available from Louis P. Jeffrey, ScD, Director of Pharmacy Services, Rhode Island Hospital, 593 Eddy Street, Providence, Rhode Island 02902. 4. Clinical Oncological Society of Australia: Guidelines and recommendations for safe handling of antineoplastic agents. *Med J Aust 1* :426–428, Apr. 30, 1983. 5. Jones RB, Frank R, Mass T: Safe handling of chemotherapeutic agents: a report from the Mount Sinai Medical Center, *CA 33* :258–263, Sept-Oct 1983. 6. ASHP technical assistance bulletin on handling cytotoxic drugs in hospitals. *Am J Hosp Pharm 42* :131–137, Jan 1985.

© 1988, Pharmacia Inc. text issued January 1988

Shown in Product Identification Section, page 422

HYSKON® Hysteroscopy Fluid ℞
[*his 'kon*]
32% (W/V) dextran-70 in dextrose

DESCRIPTION

HYSKON® Hysteroscopy Fluid is a clear, viscid, sterile, non-pyrogenic solution of dextran-70 (32% W/V) in dextrose (10% W/V). Dextran-70 is that fraction of dextran, a branched polysaccharide composed of glucose units, having a weight average molecular weight of 70,000. The fluid is electrolyte-free and non-conductive. At room temperature HYSKON® Hysteroscopy Fluid has a viscosity of 220 cS.

HYSKON® has a tendency to crystalize when subjected to temperature variations or when stored for long periods. If flakes of dextran are present, heat at 100°–110° C until complete dissolution is achieved.

INDICATIONS

HYSKON® Hysteroscopy Fluid is indicated for use with the hysteroscope as an aid in distending the uterine cavity and in irrigating and visualizing its surfaces.

CONTRAINDICATIONS

HYSKON® Hysteroscopy Fluid should not be instilled in patients known to be hypersensitive to dextran. All other contraindications are those related to the hysteroscopic procedure itself, such as pregnancy, endometrial carcinoma, etc.

WARNINGS

It is possible that during hysteroscopy dextran may leak into the peritoneal cavity, the precise amount depending on the volume of HYSKON® used and the infusion pressure. Slow absorption from the peritoneal cavity (peak blood levels are reached in 3–4 days) (1) may result in systemic effects varying from simple plasma volume expansion or a transient prolongation of the bleeding time, to severe, fatal anaphylactic reactions. It is also reported that dextran may enter the pleural cavity through a pathway that has yet to be defined (2). When HYSKON® is employed during diagnostic hysteroscopy adverse effects are rare. In hysteroscopic surgery greater volumes of HYSKON® are infused over a longer period of time and the exposed blood vessels of the freshly traumatized endometrium allow the dextran direct access to the systemic circulation.

There is, therefore, the potential for these patients to rapidly develop adverse systemic effects, in particular pulmonary edema (3). Patients are considered at increased risk of developing pulmonary edema if:
1. They undergo a surgical procedure lasting more than 45 minutes when HYSKON® is being used to distend the uterus.
2. Greater than 500 ml of HYSKON® are infused.
3. Large areas of endometrium are traumatized during surgery.

ADVERSE REACTIONS

The following adverse reactions, although rare, have been reported for HYSKON®: fatal anaphylactic reaction, generalized itching, macular rash, urticaria, nasal congestion, flushing, hypotension, dyspnea, tightness of chest, cyanosis, wheezing, coughing, peripheral edema, pulmonary edema, pleural effusion, ascites, nausea, vomiting, fever, joint pains, oliguria, convulsions and increased clotting time.

DOSAGE AND ADMINISTRATION

The amount of HYSKON® Hysteroscopy Fluid required depends on a number of factors, including the type and length of the procedure and whether manipulation or surgery is performed. Usually, the amount of HYSKON® instilled into the uterus will be between 50 ml and 100 ml. HYSKON® should be introduced into the uterine cavity through the cannula of a hysteroscope under low pressure (approximately 100 mm Hg) until the uterus is sufficiently distended to permit adequate visualization. During the hysteroscopic examination, HYSKON® should be infused at a rate that keeps the cavity suitably distended. To avoid injection of the fluid into the tissues of the uterus and parametria and to prevent unnecessary amounts of the fluid leaking into the peritoneal cavity and backwards along the side of the hysteroscope, infusion pressures should not exceed 150 mm Hg.

HOW SUPPLIED

Non-pyrogenic HYSKON® Hysteroscopy Fluid (32% W/V dextran-70 in 10% W/V dextrose) is available as a sterile, nonpyrogenic solution in 100 ml bottles packed 12 to a carton.

(NDC No. 0016-0231-61.)

and 250 ml bottles packed 6 to a carton

(NDC No. 0016-0231-62)

Store at 20–25°C (68–77°F). Protect from cold.

CAUTION

Federal law restricts this device to sale by or on the order of a physician.

REFERENCES

1. Cleary R.E., Howard T., diZerega G.S.: Plasma dextran levels after abdominal instillation of 32% dextran 70: Evidence for prolonged intraperitoneal retention. Submitted for publication, 1984.
2. Adoni A., Adatto-Levy R., Mogle P., Palti Z.: Post-operative pleural effusion caused by dextran. Int J Gyn Obs 18:243, 1980.
3. Flores E., Neuwirth R.S.: Acute pulmonary edema occurring after a hysteroscopic surgical procedure using HYSKON® as the distending medium. Submitted for publication, 1984.
Revised August 1985

MACRODEX® ℞
[*mak 'ro-dex*]
(Plasma Volume Expander)

6% Dextran 70 in 5% Dextrose Injection. 500 ml.
6% Dextran 70 in 0.9% Sodium Chloride Injection. 500 ml.

RHEOMACRODEX® ℞
[*re "o-mak 'ro-dex*]
(Plasma Volume Expander)

10% Dextran 40 in 5% Dextrose Injection. 500 ml.
10% Dextran 40 in 0.9% Sodium Chloride Injection. 500 ml.

Pharmafair, Inc.
205C KELSEY LANE
TAMPA, FL 33619

NDC 24208		TOPICALS	
-430-53		**BENZOYL PEROXIDE GEL 5%**	OTC
		1.5 oz. plastic tube	
-435-53		**BENZOYL PEROXIDE GEL 10%**	OTC
		1.5 oz. plastic tube	
-410-		**BETAMETHASONE VALERATE 0.1% CREAM**	℞
	-89	15 gm	
	-56	45 gm	
-460-67		**BETAMETHASONE VALERATE 0.1% LOTION**	℞
		60 ml	
-440-		**BETAMETHASONE VALERATE 0.1% OINTMENT**	℞
	-89	15 gm	
	-56	45 gm	
-515-		**CORTIFAIR 1% CREAM** (Hydrocortisone Cream 1% USP)	℞
	-02	15 gm	
	-88	120 gm	
	-18	425 gm	
	-04	30 gm	
-510-		**CORTIFAIR 0.5% CREAM** (Hydrocortisone 0.5% Cream)	OTC
	-82	15 gm	
	-84	30 gm	
	-88	120 gm	
	-90	425 gm	
-551-67		**ERYTHROMYCIN 2% TOPICAL SOLUTION**	℞
		60 ml bottles	
-450-		**FLUOCINOLONE ACETONIDE 0.01% CREAM**	℞
	-89	15 gm	
	-93	30 gm	
	-92	60 gm	
	-97	425 gm	
-445-		**FLUOCINOLONE ACETONIDE 0.025% CREAM**	℞
	-89	15 gm	
	-93	30 gm	
	-92	60 gm	
	-97	425 gm	
-455-		**FLUOCINOLONE ACETONIDE 0.025% OINTMENT**	℞
	-89	15 gm	
	-93	30 gm	
	-92	60 gm	
-465-		**FLUOCINOLONE ACETONIDE 0.01% SOLUTION**	℞
	-63	20 ml	
	-67	60 ml	
-470-89		**GENTAFAIR CREAM** (Gentamicin Sulfate Cream USP 0.1%) 15 gram tube	℞
-475-89		**GENTAFAIR OINTMENT** (Gentamicin Sulfate Ointment USP 0.1%) 15 gram tube	℞

-525-83	**IODO-CORTIFAIR CREAM** (Iodochlorhydroxyquin 3% w/ Hydrocortisone 1%) 20 gm	℞
-566-	**NYSTATIN & TRIAMCINOLONE** **ACETONIDE CREAM**	℞
-89	15 gm	
-93	30 gm	
-571-	**NYSTATIN & TRIAMCINOLONE** **ACETONIDE OINTMENT**	℞
-89	15 gm	
-93	30 gm	
-985-62	**TOLNAFTATE 1% CREAM** 15 gm	OTC
-506-62	**TOLNAFTATE 1% SOLUTION** 10 ml bottles	OTC
-530-	**TOPISPORIN** (Neomycin and Polymyxin B Sulfates and Baci- tracin Zinc Ointment)	OTC
-02	15 gm	
-04	30 gm	
-650-	**TRIAMCINAIR CREAM 0.025%** (Triamcinolone Acetonide 0.025% Cream)	℞
-02	15 gm	
-04	30 gm	
-54	80 gm	
-08	1 lb.	
-98	5 lb.	
-655-	**TRIAMCINAIR 0.1% CREAM** (Triamcinolone Acetonide 0.1% Cream)	℞
-02	15 gm	
-04	30 gm	
-54	80 gm	
-08	1 lb.	
-98	5 lb.	
-660-	**TRIAMCINAIR 0.5% CREAM** (Triamcinolone Acetonide 0.5% Cream)	℞
-02	15 gm	
-04	30 gm	
-08	1 lb.	

OTICS

-561-64	**AURAFAIR OTIC SOLUTION** (Antipyrine and Benzocaine) 15 ml	℞
-615-77	**BOROFAIR OTIC** (Acetic Acid 2% in a modified Burow's Solution Sterile) 60 mL	℞
-531-73	**EAR DROPS** (Carbamide Peroxide 6.5%) 15 ml	OTC
-630-04	**OCTICAIR® OTIC SOLUTION** (Neomycin Sulfate and Polymyxin B Sulfate and Hydrocortisone Otic Solution-Sterile) 10 ml	℞
-635-62	**OCTICAIR® OTIC SUSPENSION** (Neomycin Sulfate and Polymyxin B Sulfate and Hydrocortisone Otic Suspension-Sterile) 10 ml	℞
-556-62	**OTOFAIR-B BUFFERED OTIC** **SUSPENSION** 10 ml	℞

ORAL PREPARATIONS

-001-	**ACETAMINOPHEN 300 mg.** **W/CODEINE 30 mg.**	Ⓒ III
-01	100	
-10	1000	
-11	Unit Dose	
-003-	**BUTALBITAL 50 mg.** **W/AC TABLETS**	Ⓒ III
-01	100	
-10	1000	
-11	Unit Dose	
-330-	**CHLORPHENIRAMINE MALEATE 4 mg.**	℞
-01	100	
-10	1000	
-11	Unit Dose	
-005-	**DIPHENOXYLATE HCl 2.5 mg.** **W/ATROPINE SULFATE .25 mg.**	Ⓒ V
-01	100	

-10	1000	
-11	Unit dose	
-965-	**ERYTHROMYCIN ETHYLSUCCINATE** **ORAL SUSPENSION** 200 mg/5 ml	℞
-64	473 ml (pint)	
-39	100 ml bottles	
-970-	**ERYTHROMYCIN ETHYLSUCCINATE** **ORAL SUSPENSION** 400 mg/5 ml	℞
-64	473 ml (pint)	
-39	100 ml bottles	
-145-	**HYDROCHLOROTHIAZIDE 25 mg.**	℞
-01	100	
-10	1000	
-11	Unit Dose	
-150-	**HYDROCHLOROTHIAZIDE 50 mg.**	℞
-01	100	
-10	1000	
-11	Unit Dose	
-075-	**MECLIZINE HCl** **CHEWABLE TABLETS 25 mg.**	℞
-01	100	
-10	1000	
-11	Unit Dose	
-008-	**MEPROBAMATE 400 mg.**	℞
-01	100	
-10	1000	
-11	Unit Dose	
-250-	**METHOCARBAMOL 500 mg.**	℞
-01	100	
-05	500	
-11	Unit Dose	
-255-	**METHOCARBAMOL 750 mg.**	℞
-01	100	
-05	500	
-11	Unit Dose	
-960-	**NYSTATIN ORAL SUSPENSION, USP** 100,000 units per ml	℞
-67	60 ml (with calibrated dropper)	
-60	5 ml (single use)	
-94	pint	
-076-	**SODIUM FLUORIDE 2.2 mg.**	℞
-10	1000	
-11	Unit Dose	
-280-	**SULFISOXAZOLE 500 mg.**	℞
-01	100	
-10	1000	
-11	Unit Dose	

IRRIGATING SOLUTIONS

-605-	**BALANCED SALT SOLUTION**	℞
-64	15 ml plastic bottle	
-66	30 ml plastic bottle	
-46	300 ml glass bottle	
-99	500 ml glass bottle	

Please see **PDR FOR OPHTHALMOLOGY** for a complete list of our ophthalmic products

---

Porton Products, Ltd.
6625 VALJEAN AVENUE
VAN NUYS, CA 91406

ANTIHEMOPHILIC FACTOR (PORCINE)   ℞
HYATE:C®
[hī'āt]

WARNING
THIS IS A POTENT DRUG WITH POTENTIAL HAZARDS. FOR MAXIMAL SAFETY AND EFFICACY CAREFULLY READ AND FOLLOW DIRECTIONS BELOW.

DESCRIPTION
Antihemophilic Factor (Porcine)—Hyate:C is a highly purified sterile freeze-dried concentrate of porcine antihemophilic factor (Factor VIII:C) in the form of a white lyophilized powder for reconstitution with 20 ml Sterile Water for Injection, U.S.P. Each vial contains between 400 and 700 porcine units of Factor VIII:C. The assayed amount of activity is stated on the label, but may vary depending on the type of assay and hemophilic substrate plasma used. The Factor VIII specific activity for each vial is greater than 15 porcine units/mg of protein. The level of platelet aggregating factor (porcine von Willebrand factor) is 1 unit to 5 or more porcine units of Factor VIII:C. The sodium ion concentration is not more than 200 millimoles per liter and the citrate ion con-

centration not more than 55 millimoles per liter. Antihemophilic Factor (Porcine) is administered intravenously. The preparation contains no preservative.

CLINICAL PHARMACOLOGY
Porcine Factor VIII:C can replace human Factor VIII:C in the human blood coagulation cascade, and has been shown to be effective in controlling bleeding in patients with congenital Factor VIII:C deficiency (Hemophilia A).[1,2] Circulating antibodies to Factor VIII:C occur in 10—15% of severe hemophiliacs,[3] and may also arise in non-hemophiliacs who consequently develop a state of acquired hemophilia. These antibodies generally show a weaker neutralizing activity against porcine Factor VIII:C than against human Factor VIII:C and Antihemophilic Factor (Porcine)—Hyate:C can thus be used to produce a hemostatic level of Factor VIII:C in patients whose antibody level precludes treatment with human Factor VIII concentrates[4,5].

The activity of a patient's antibody against Antihemophilic Factor (Porcine)—Hyate:C can be determined in the laboratory using a modification of the Bethesda assay[6] and this value used as a guide to the likely effectiveness of Antihemophilic Factor (Porcine)—Hyate:C in the individual patient. (See Indications and Usage).

After infusion of Antihemophilic Factor (Porcine)—Hyate:C, the level in the circulation can be monitored by measurement of Factor VIII:C in the patient's plasma. Recovery and half-life of Hyate:C will vary, being dependent on both the level and the kinetics of the patient's antibody, and it is thus desirable to monitor pre- and post-infusion Factor VIII:C levels for each dose of Hyate:C. This information will assist in determination of dose size and frequency (see Dosage and Administration).

Recovery of Factor VIII:C has been reported to improve with successive doses of Antihemophilic Factor (Porcine)—Hyate:C, possibly as a result of saturation of circulating antibody[5].

No evidence of human viral infection has been reported with the use of Antihemophilic Factor (Porcine)—Hyate:C.

INDICATIONS AND USAGE
Antihemophilic Factor (Porcine)—Hyate:C is intended for the treatment of congenital hemophiliacs with antibodies to Factor VIII:C and also for previously nonhemophilic patients with spontaneously acquired inhibitors to human Factor VIII:C.

Use of Antihemophilic Factor (Porcine)—Hyate:C is indicated for patients with inhibitors who are bleeding or who are to undergo surgery.

Antihemophilic Factor (Porcine)—Hyate:C has not been known to transmit hepatitis or human immuno-deficiency virus (HIV).[7] It may therefore be justified to consider Antihemophilic Factor (Porcine)—Hyate:C as a primary treatment option in acquired inhibitor patients.

Antihemophilic Factor (Porcine)—Hyate:C treatment is not normally indicated in patients with an antibody titer of less than 5 Bethesda units/ml (BU/ml) against human Factor VIII:C and is likely to be ineffective in patients with an antibody titer of greater than 50 BU/ml against human Factor VIII. If a patient has an antibody titer of greater than 50 BU/ml against human Factor VIII:C the activity of the antibody against porcine Factor VIII should be determined. An antibody titer of less than 15–20 BU/ml against porcine Factor VIII:C indicates suitability for treatment with Antihemophilic Factor (Porcine)—Hyate:C.

CONTRAINDICATIONS
Antihemophilic Factor (Porcine)—Hyate:C should not be used to treat patients who have previously suffered acute allergic reaction to Antihemophilic Factor (Porcine).

WARNINGS
Acute Infusion Reactions On rare occasions Antihemophilic Factor (Porcine)—Hyate:C administration has been associated with anaphylaxis. Adrenaline, hydrocortisone and facilities for cardiopulmonary resuscitation should be available in case such a reaction occurs.

PRECAUTIONS
Immune Response to Hyate:C Infusion of Antihemophilic Factor (Porcine)—Hyate:C may be followed by a rise in plasma levels of antibody to both human and porcine Factor VIII:C[8,9]. Inhibitor levels should therefore be monitored both during and after treatment.

General Hydrocortisone and/or antihistamine may help to prevent or alleviate side effects to Antihemophilic Factor (Porcine)—Hyate:C and may thus be prescribed as a precautionary measure.

Following reconstitution Antihemophilic Factor (Porcine)—Hyate:C must not be frozen. Any dose not used within 3 hours of reconstitution should be discarded.

Antihemophilic Factor (Porcine) is for administration by intravenous route only.

Antihemophilic Factor (Porcine) is not recommended for use in home treatment programs.

Continued on next page

Porton—Cont.

Laboratory Tests The activity of the patient's antibody against Hyate:C can be determined using a modification of the Bethesda assay[6] in which Antihemophilic Factor (Porcine)—Hyate:C is diluted to 1 porcine U/ml in hemophilic plasma and used as substrate for the assay.

Carcinogenesis, Mutagenesis, Impairment of Fertility Long term studies have not been conducted with Antihemophilic Factor (Porcine)—Hyate:C.

Pregnancy Category C, Antihemophilic Factor (Porcine)—Hyate:C. Animal reproduction studies have not been conducted with Hyate:C. It is also not known whether Hyate:C can cause fetal harm when administered to a pregnant woman or can affect reproduction capacity. Hyate:C should be given to a pregnant woman only if clearly needed.

ADVERSE REACTIONS

Mild Infusion Reactions Antihemophilic Factor (Porcine)—Hyate:C may give rise to reactions such as fever, chills, headache, nausea, vomiting and skin rashes. Such reactions have been reported to occur after approximately 10% of infusions[4] and are more common after the first infusion in a course of treatment. Reactions tend to lessen in frequency and severity as further infusions are given.

Thrombocytopenia Acute thrombocytopenia has been reported to occur on rare occasions[5]. Monitoring of the platelet count during the treatment period is thus recommended.

DOSAGE AND ADMINISTRATION

The dosage of Antihemophilic Factor (Porcine)—Hyate:C required for control of bleeding varies for individual patients, but is dependent upon the patient's weight, the level of circulating antibody and the type of hemorrhage and desired plasma Factor VIII level.

It is commonly observed that recovery of Factor VIII:C increases during a course of treatment, possibly as a result of saturation of circulating antibody. It is therefore desirable to monitor pre- and post-infusion levels of Factor VIII:C for each dose. This is of particular importance during long courses of treatment when variation in the patient's antibody level may give rise to considerable variation in the recovery of Factor VIII:C in the plasma.

Initial Dose

Because of the variation in patient response and the possible variation in the assayed unitage (see Description) each patient should be monitored closely. Rather than relying upon a particular laboratory value for recovery of Factor VIII:C, clinical response should be used to assess efficacy. In view of the difficulty in managing hemophiliacs with inhibitors close consultation with a regional comprehensive hemophilia center is advised.

1. If the patient's anti-human Factor VIII:C antibody level is less than 50 BU/ml an initial dose of 100 to 150 porcine units per Kg body weight is recommended.
2. If the patient's antibody titer to human Factor VIII:C is greater than 50 BU/ml the activity of the antibody against Antihemophilic Factor (Porcine)—Hyate:C should be determined. An anti-porcine Factor VIII:C antibody level of more than 20 Bethesda units indicates that the patient is unlikely to benefit from treatment with Antihemophilic Factor (Porcine)—Hyate:C. For lower titers, a dose of 100 to 150 porcine U/Kg is recommended.
3. If a patient has previously been treated with Antihemophilic Factor (Porcine)—Hyate:C this may provide a guide as to his likely response and therefore assist in estimation of the preliminary dose.

Subsequent Doses Following administration of the initial dose, if the recovery of Factor VIII:C in the patient's plasma is not sufficient, a further higher dose should be administered. If recovery after the second dose is still insufficient, a third and higher dose may prove effective. As previously noted, the recovery of Factor VIII:C tends to improve with successive doses.

Determination of the Activity of the Inhibitor Against Hyate:C A modification of the Bethesda assay[6] is recommended. Antihemophilic Factor (Porcine)—Hyate:C should be diluted to 1 porcine unit per ml in hemophilic plasma and used as a substrate in the Bethesda assay.

Reconstitution and Administration

1. Warm the unopened vials of Antihemophilic Factor (Porcine)—Hyate:C to between 20°C and 37°C.
2. Clean the exposed central portion of the rubber stopper with antiseptic immediately prior to piercing.
3. Using a sterile needle and a syringe slowly inject 20 ml of Sterile Water for Injection U.S.P. into the vial.
4. Withdraw the needle and shake the vial gently avoiding frothing, until the powder is completely dissolved. This usually takes less than 5 minutes.
5. Parenteral drug products should be inspected visually for particulate matter and discoloration prior to administration, whenever solution and container permit.

6. Withdraw the solution into a syringe using a filter needle.
7. Replace the filter needle with a sterile injection needle and administer intravenously at a rate of not more than 2–5 ml per minute.
8. Following reconstitution Antihemophilic Factor (Porcine)—Hyate:C must not be stored. Any dose not used within 3 hours of reconstitution should be discarded.

HOW SUPPLIED

Antihemophilic Factor (Porcine)—Hyate:C is supplied in vials containing between 400–700 porcine units of Factor VIII:C, to be reconstituted with 20 ml Sterile Water for Injection U.S.P. (not supplied).

STORAGE

Antihemophilic Factor (Porcine)—Hyate:C should be stored at a temperature of minus 15°C to minus 20°C and should be used before the expiration date stated on the package. Reconstituted Antihemophilic Factor (Porcine)—Hyate:C must not be stored, and should be used within 3 hours.

REFERENCES

[1]Macfarlane R. G., Mallam P. C., Witts L. J., Bidwell E., Biggs R., Fraenkel G. J., Honey G. E., Taylor K. B.: Surgery in haemophilia. The use of animal antihaemophilic globulin and human plasma in thirteen cases. Lancet 2:251 (1957).
[2]Biggs R., Macfarlane R. G. (eds): Treatment of Haemophilia and other Coagulation Disorders. Oxford, Blackwell Scientific (1966).
[3]Shapiro S. S., Hultin M.: Acquired inhibitors to the blood coagulation factors. Semin. Thromb. Hemostas. 1:336 (1975).
[4]Kernoff P. B.A., Thomas N. D., Lilley P. A., Matthews K. B., Goldman E., Tuddenham E. G. D.: Clinical Experience with Polyelectrolyte–Fractionated Porcine Factor VIII Concentrate in the Treatment of Haemophiliacs with Antibodies to Factor VIII. Blood 63:31 (1984).
[5]Gatti L., Mannucci P. M.: Use of Porcine Factor VIII in the Management of Seventeen Patients with Factor VIII Antibodies. Thromb. Haemostas. 51:379 (1984).
[6]Kasper C. K., Aledort L. M., Counts R. B., Edson J. R., Frantantoni J., Green D., Hampton J. W., Hilgartner M. W., Lazerson J., Levine P. H., McMillan C. W., Pool J. G., Shapiro S. S.: Thombos. Diathes. Haemorrh. 34:869 (1975).
[7]Lusher J. M.: Factor VIII Inhibitors—Etiology, Characterization, Natural History and Management. Annals of the New York Academy of Sciences 509:96 (1987).
[8]Hewitt P., Mackie I. J., Machin S. J.: Highly purified Factor VIII in haemophilia A. Lancet 1:741 (1982).
[9]Verroust F., Allain J. P.: Immune response induced by porcine Factor VIII in severe hemophiliacs with antibody to Factor VIII. Thromb. Haemostas. 48:238 (1982).

Manufactured by:
Porton Speywood Limited
Ash Road, Wrexham Industrial Estate
Wrexham, Clwyd LL13 9UF
United Kingdom
Tel: (0978) 661181
Distributed by:
Porton Products, Ltd.
6625 Valjean Avenue
Van Nuys, CA 91406 U.S.A.
Tel: (818) 989-5356
FAX (818) 989-4533
LR-9031805   Issued April 1989
©1989 Porton Products, Ltd.

Poythress Laboratories, Inc.

16 N. 22nd ST.
POST OFFICE BOX 26946
RICHMOND, VA 23261

NDC 0095	PRODUCT	
-0040	ANTROCOL TABLETS and	℞
-0041	ANTROCOL CAPSULES	℞
	(Atropine Sulfate, 0.195 mg; Phenobarbital, 16 mg)	
-0042	ANTROCOL ELIXIR	℞
	(Each ml/ Atropine Sulfate, 0.039 mg; Phenobarbital, 3 mg; Alcohol, 20%)	
-0015	BENSULFOID TABLETS	℞
	(Bensulfoid, 130 mg [33% Colloidal Sulfur])	
-0050	MUDRANE TABLETS	℞
	(Potassium Iodide, 195 mg; Aminophylline [Anhyd.], 130 mg; Phenobarbital, 8 mg; Ephedrine HCl, 16 mg)	
-0051	MUDRANE GG TABLETS	℞
	(Guaifenesin, 100 mg; Aminophylline [Anhyd.], 130 mg; Phenobarbital, 8 mg; Ephedrine HCl, 16 mg)	
-0032	MUDRANE-2 TABLETS	℞
	(Potassium Iodide, 195 mg; Aminophylline [Anhyd.], 130 mg)	
-0033	MUDRANE GG-2 TABLETS	℞
	(Guaifenesin, 100 mg; Aminophylline [Anhyd.], 130 mg)	
-0053	MUDRANE GG ELIXIR	℞
	(Each 5 ml/ Guaifenesin, 26 mg; Theophylline, 20 mg; Phenobarbital, 2.5 mg; Ephedrine HCl, 4 mg; Alcohol, 20%)	
-0023	SOLFOTON TABLETS and	Ⓒⱽ
-0025	SOLFOTON CAPSULES	Ⓒⱽ
	(Phenobarbital, 16 mg)	
-0031	URO-PHOSPHATE TABLETS	℞
	(Methenamine, 300 mg; Sodium Biphosphate, 500 mg)	

Princeton Pharmaceutical Products

(A Squibb Company)
P. O. BOX 4500
PRINCETON, NJ 08543-4500

UNILOG®
(Tablet and Capsule Identification Code)
NUMERICAL INDEX

CORGARD®   ℞
[kor 'gard]
Nadolol Tablets USP

DESCRIPTION

CORGARD (nadolol) is a synthetic nonselective beta-adrenergic receptor blocking agent designated chemically as 1-(tert -butylamino) -3- [(5,6,7,8-tetrahydro-cis -6,7-dihydroxy-1-naphthyl)oxy]-2-propanol.

Nadolol is a white crystalline powder. It is freely soluble in ethanol, soluble in hydrochloric acid, slightly soluble in water and in chloroform, and very slightly soluble in sodium hydroxide.

CORGARD (nadolol) is available for oral administration as 20 mg, 40 mg, 80 mg, 120 mg, and 160 mg tablets. Inactive ingredients: microcrystalline cellulose, colorant (FD&C Blue No. 2), corn starch, magnesium stearate, povidone (except 20 mg and 40 mg), and other ingredients.

CLINICAL PHARMACOLOGY

CORGARD (nadolol) is a nonselective beta-adrenergic receptor blocking agent. Clinical pharmacology studies have demonstrated beta-blocking activity by showing (1) reduction in heart rate and cardiac output at rest and on exercise, (2) reduction of systolic and diastolic blood pressure at rest and on exercise, (3) inhibition of isoproterenol-induced tachycardia, and (4) reduction of reflex orthostatic tachycardia.

CORGARD (nadolol) specifically competes with beta-adrenergic receptor agonists for available beta receptor sites; it inhibits both the beta$_1$ receptors located chiefly in cardiac muscle and the beta$_2$ receptors located chiefly in the bronchial and vascular musculature, inhibiting the chronotropic, inotropic, and vasodilator responses to beta-adrenergic stimulation proportionately. CORGARD (nadolol) has no intrinsic sympathomimetic activity and, unlike some other beta-adrenergic blocking agents, nadolol has little direct myocardial depressant activity and does not have an anesthetic-like membrane-stabilizing action. Animal and human studies show that CORGARD (nadolol) slows the sinus rate and depresses AV conduction. In dogs, only minimal amounts of nadolol were detected in the brain relative to amounts in blood and other organs and tissues. CORGARD has low lipophilicity as determined by octanol/water partition coefficient, a characteristic of certain beta-blocking agents that has been correlated with the limited extent to which these agents cross the blood-brain barrier, their low concentration in the brain, and low incidence of CNS-related side effects. In controlled clinical studies, CORGARD (nadolol) at doses of 40 to 320 mg/day has been shown to decrease both standing and supine blood pressure, the effect persisting for approximately 24 hours after dosing.

The mechanism of the antihypertensive effects of beta-adrenergic receptor blocking agents has not been established; however, factors that may be involved include (1) competitive antagonism of catecholamines at peripheral (non-CNS) adrenergic neuron sites (especially cardiac) leading to decreased cardiac output, (2) a central effect leading to reduced tonic-sympathetic nerve outflow to the periphery, and (3) suppression of renin secretion by blockade of the beta-adrenergic receptors responsible for renin release from the kidneys.

While cardiac output and arterial pressure are reduced by nadolol therapy, renal hemodynamics are stable, with preservation of renal blood flow and glomerular filtration rate. By blocking catecholamine-induced increases in heart rate, velocity and extent of myocardial contraction, and blood pressure, CORGARD (nadolol) generally reduces the oxygen requirements of the heart at any given level of effort, making it useful for many patients in the long-term management of angina pectoris. On the other hand, nadolol can increase oxygen requirements by increasing left ventricular fiber length and end diastolic pressure, particularly in patients with heart failure.

Although beta-adrenergic receptor blockade is useful in treatment of angina and hypertension, there are also situations in which sympathetic stimulation is vital. For example, in patients with severely damaged hearts, adequate ventricular function may depend on sympathetic drive. Beta-adrenergic blockade may worsen AV block by preventing the necessary facilitating effects of sympathetic activity on conduction. Beta$_2$-adrenergic blockade results in passive bronchial constriction by interfering with endogenous adrenergic bronchodilator activity in patients subject to bronchospasm and may also interfere with exogenous bronchodilators in such patients.

Absorption of nadolol after oral dosing is variable, averaging about 30 percent. Peak serum concentrations of nadolol usually occur in three to four hours after oral administration and the presence of food in the gastrointestinal tract does not affect the rate or extent of nadolol absorption. Approximately 30 percent of the nadolol present in serum is reversibly bound to plasma protein.

Unlike many other beta-adrenergic blocking agents, nadolol is not metabolized by the liver and is excreted unchanged, principally by the kidneys.

The half-life of therapeutic doses of nadolol is about 20 to 24 hours, permitting once-daily dosage. Because nadolol is excreted predominantly in the urine, its half-life increases in renal failure (see PRECAUTIONS and DOSAGE AND ADMINISTRATION). Steady-state serum concentrations of nadolol are attained in six to nine days with once-daily dosage in persons with normal renal function. Because of variable absorption and different individual responsiveness, the proper dosage must be determined by titration.

Exacerbation of angina and, in some cases, myocardial infarction and ventricular dysrhythmias have been reported after abrupt discontinuation of therapy with beta-adrenergic blocking agents in patients with coronary artery disease. Abrupt withdrawal of these agents in patients without coronary artery disease has resulted in transient symptoms, including tremulousness, sweating, palpitation, headache, and malaise. Several mechanisms have been proposed to explain these phenomena, among them increased sensitivity to catecholamines because of increased numbers of beta receptors.

INDICATIONS AND USAGE

Angina Pectoris—CORGARD (nadolol) is indicated for the long-term management of patients with angina pectoris.

Hypertension—CORGARD (nadolol) is indicated in the management of hypertension; it may be used alone or in combination with other antihypertensive agents, especially thiazide-type diuretics.

CONTRAINDICATIONS

Nadolol is contraindicated in bronchial asthma, sinus bradycardia and greater than first degree conduction block, cardiogenic shock, and overt cardiac failure (see WARNINGS).

WARNINGS

Cardiac Failure—Sympathetic stimulation may be a vital component supporting circulatory function in patients with congestive heart failure, and its inhibition by beta-blockade may precipitate more severe failure. Although beta-blockers should be avoided in overt congestive heart failure, if necessary, they can be used with caution in patients with a history of failure who are well-compensated, usually with digitalis and diuretics. Beta-adrenergic blocking agents do not abolish the inotropic action of digitalis on heart muscle.

IN PATIENTS WITHOUT A HISTORY OF HEART FAILURE, continued use of beta-blockers can, in some cases, lead to cardiac failure. Therefore, at the first sign or symptom of heart failure, the patient should be digitalized and/or treated with diuretics, and the response observed closely, or nadolol should be discontinued (gradually, if possible).

Exacerbation of Ischemic Heart Disease Following Abrupt Withdrawal—Hypersensitivity to catecholamines has been observed in patients withdrawn from beta-blocker therapy; exacerbation of angina and, in some cases, myocardial infarction have occurred after *abrupt* discontinuation of such therapy. When discontinuing chronically administered nadolol, particularly in patients with ischemic heart disease, the dosage should be gradually reduced over a period of one to two weeks and the patient should be carefully monitored. If angina markedly worsens or acute coronary insufficiency develops, nadolol administration should be reinstituted promptly, at least temporarily, and other measures appropriate for the management of unstable angina should be taken. Patients should be warned against interruption or discontinuation of therapy without the physician's advice. Because coronary artery disease is common and may be unrecognized, it may be prudent not to discontinue nadolol therapy abruptly even in patients treated only for hypertension.

Nonallergic Bronchospasm (e.g., chronic bronchitis, emphysema)—PATIENTS WITH BRONCHOSPASTIC DISEASES SHOULD IN GENERAL NOT RECEIVE BETA-BLOCKERS. Nadolol should be administered with caution since it may block bronchodilation produced by endogenous or exogenous catecholamine stimulation of beta$_2$ receptors.

Major Surgery—Because beta-blockade impairs the ability of the heart to respond to reflex stimuli and may increase the risks of general anesthesia and surgical procedures, resulting in protracted hypotension or low cardiac output, it has generally been suggested that such therapy should be withdrawn several days prior to surgery. Recognition of the increased sensitivity to catecholamines of patients recently withdrawn from beta-blocker therapy, however, has made this recommendation controversial. If possible, beta-blockers should be withdrawn well before surgery takes place. In the event of emergency surgery, the anesthesiologist should be informed that the patient is on beta-blocker therapy. The effects of nadolol can be reversed by administration of beta-receptor agonists such as isoproterenol, dopamine, dobutamine, or levarterenol. Difficulty in restarting and maintaining the heart beat has also been reported with beta-adrenergic receptor blocking agents.

Diabetes and Hypoglycemia—Beta-adrenergic blockade may prevent the appearance of premonitory signs and symptoms (e.g., tachycardia and blood pressure changes) of acute hypoglycemia. This is especially important with labile diabetics. Beta-blockade also reduces the release of insulin in response to hyperglycemia; therefore, it may be necessary to adjust the dose of antidiabetic drugs.

Thyrotoxicosis—Beta-adrenergic blockade may mask certain clinical signs (e.g., tachycardia) of hyperthyroidism. Patients suspected of developing thyrotoxicosis should be managed carefully to avoid abrupt withdrawal of beta-adrenergic blockade which might precipitate a thyroid storm.

PRECAUTIONS

Impaired Renal Function—Nadolol should be used with caution in patients with impaired renal function (see DOSAGE AND ADMINISTRATION).

Information for Patients

Patients, especially those with evidence of coronary artery insufficiency, should be warned against interruption or discontinuation of nadolol therapy without the physician's advice. Although cardiac failure rarely occurs in properly selected patients, patients being treated with beta-adrenergic blocking agents should be advised to consult the physician at the first sign or symptom of impending failure. The patient should also be advised of a proper course in the event of an inadvertently missed dose.

Drug Interactions

When administered concurrently, the following drugs may interact with beta-adrenergic receptor blocking agents:

Anesthetics, general—exaggeration of the hypotension induced by general anesthetics (see WARNINGS, Major Surgery).

Antidiabetic drugs (oral agents and insulin)—hypoglycemia or hyperglycemia; adjust dosage of antidiabetic drug accordingly (see WARNINGS, Diabetes and Hypoglycemia).

Catecholamine-depleting drugs (e.g., reserpine)—additive effect; monitor closely for evidence of hypotension and/or excessive bradycardia (e.g., vertigo, syncope, postural hypotension).

Carcinogenesis, Mutagenesis, Impairment of Fertility

In chronic oral toxicologic studies (one to two years) in mice, rats, and dogs, nadolol did not produce any significant toxic effects. In two-year oral carcinogenic studies in rats and mice, nadolol did not produce any neoplastic, preneoplastic, or nonneoplastic pathologic lesions. In fertility and general reproductive performance studies in rats, nadolol caused no adverse effects.

Pregnancy Category C

In animal reproduction studies with nadolol, evidence of embryo- and fetotoxicity was found in rabbits, but not in rats or hamsters, at doses 5 to 10 times greater (on a mg/kg basis) than the maximum indicated human dose. No teratogenic potential was observed in any of these species.

There are no adequate and well-controlled studies in pregnant women. Nadolol should be used during pregnancy only if the potential benefit justifies the potential risk to the fetus. Neonates whose mothers are receiving nadolol at parturition have exhibited bradycardia, hypoglycemia, and associated symptoms.

Nursing Mothers

Nadolol is excreted in human milk. Because of the potential for adverse effects in nursing infants, a decision should be made whether to discontinue nursing or to discontinue therapy taking into account the importance of CORGARD (nadolol) to the mother.

Pediatric Use

Safety and effectiveness in children have not been established.

ADVERSE REACTIONS

Most adverse effects have been mild and transient and have rarely required withdrawal of therapy.

Cardiovascular—Bradycardia with heart rates of less than 60 beats per minute occurs commonly, and heart rates below 40 beats per minute and/or symptomatic bradycardia were seen in about 2 of 100 patients. Symptoms of peripheral vascular insufficiency, usually of the Raynaud type, have occurred in approximately 2 of 100 patients. Cardiac failure, hypotension, and rhythm/conduction disturbances have each occurred in about 1 of 100 patients. Single instances of first degree and third degree heart block have been reported; intensification of AV block is a known effect of beta-blockers (see also CONTRAINDICATIONS, WARNINGS, and PRECAUTIONS).

Central Nervous System—Dizziness or fatigue has been reported in approximately 2 of 100 patients; paresthesias, sedation, and change in behavior have each been reported in approximately 6 of 1000 patients.

Respiratory—Bronchospasm has been reported in approximately 1 of 1000 patients (see CONTRAINDICATIONS and WARNINGS).

Gastrointestinal—Nausea, diarrhea, abdominal discomfort, constipation, vomiting, indigestion, anorexia, bloating, and flatulence have been reported in 1 to 5 of 1000 patients.

Miscellaneous—Each of the following has been reported in 1 to 5 of 1000 patients: rash; pruritus; headache; dry mouth, eyes, or skin; impotence or decreased libido; facial swelling; weight gain; slurred speech; cough; nasal stuffiness; sweating; tinnitus; blurred vision. Reversible alopecia has been reported infrequently.

The following adverse reactions have been reported in patients taking nadolol and/or other beta-adrenergic blocking agents, but no causal relationship to nadolol has been established.

Central Nervous System—Reversible mental depression progressing to catatonia; visual disturbances; hallucinations; an acute reversible syndrome characterized by disorientation for time and place, short-term memory loss, emotional lability with slightly clouded sensorium, and decreased performance on neuropsychometrics.

Gastrointestinal—Mesenteric arterial thrombosis; ischemic colitis; elevated liver enzymes.

Hematologic—Agranulocytosis; thrombocytopenic or nonthrombocytopenic purpura.

Continued on next page

Princeton—Cont.

Allergic—Fever combined with aching and sore throat; laryngospasm; respiratory distress.

Miscellaneous—Pemphigoid rash; hypertensive reaction in patients with pheochromocytoma; sleep disturbances; Peyronie's disease.

The oculomucocutaneous syndrome associated with the beta-blocker practolol has not been reported with nadolol.

OVERDOSAGE

Nadolol can be removed from the general circulation by hemodialysis.

In addition to gastric lavage, the following measures should be employed, as appropriate. In determining the duration of corrective therapy, note must be taken of the long duration of the effect of nadolol.

Excessive Bradycardia—Administer atropine (0.25 to 1.0 mg). If there is no response to vagal blockade, administer isoproterenol cautiously.

Cardiac Failure—Administer a digitalis glycoside and diuretic. It has been reported that glucagon may also be useful in this situation.

Hypotension—Administer vasopressors, e.g., epinephrine or levarterenol. (There is evidence that epinephrine may be the drug of choice.)

Bronchospasm—Administer a beta$_2$-stimulating agent and /or a theophylline derivative.

DOSAGE AND ADMINISTRATION

DOSAGE MUST BE INDIVIDUALIZED. CORGARD (NADOLOL) MAY BE ADMINISTERED WITHOUT REGARD TO MEALS.

Angina Pectoris—The usual initial dose is 40 mg CORGARD (nadolol) once daily. Dosage may be gradually increased in 40 to 80 mg increments at 3 to 7 day intervals until optimum clinical response is obtained or there is pronounced slowing of the heart rate. The usual maintenance dose is 40 or 80 mg administered once daily. Doses up to 160 or 240 mg administered once daily may be needed.

The usefulness and safety in angina pectoris of dosage exceeding 240 mg per day have not been established. If treatment is to be discontinued, reduce the dosage gradually over a period of one to two weeks (see WARNINGS).

Hypertension—The usual initial dose is 40 mg CORGARD (nadolol) once daily, whether it is used alone or in addition to diuretic therapy. Dosage may be gradually increased in 40 to 80 mg increments until optimum blood pressure reduction is achieved. The usual maintenance dose is 40 or 80 mg administered once daily. Doses up to 240 or 320 mg administered once daily may be needed.

Dosage Adjustment in Renal Failure—Absorbed nadolol is excreted principally by the kidneys and, although nonrenal elimination does occur, dosage adjustments are necessary in patients with renal impairment. The following dose intervals are recommended:

Creatinine Clearance (mL/min/1.73m^2)	Dosage Interval (hours)
>50	24
31–50	24–36
10–30	24–48
<10	40–60

HOW SUPPLIED

CORGARD Tablets (Nadolol Tablets USP)

20 mg tablets in bottles of 100 (NDC 0003-0232-50), **40 mg tablets** in bottles of 100 (NDC 0003-0207-50) and 1000 (NDC 0003-0207-76), **80 mg tablets** in bottles of 100 (NDC 0003-0241-50) and 1000 (NDC 0003-0241-76), **120 mg tablets** in bottles of 100 (NDC 0003-0208-50) and 1000 (NDC 0003-0208-76), and **160 mg tablets** in bottles of 100 (NDC 0003-0246-49). Unimatic® unit-dose packs containing 100 tablets: **20 mg** (NDC 0003-0232-51); **40 mg** (NDC 0003-0207-53); **80 mg** (NDC 0003-0241-55).

All tablets are scored (bisect bar) and easy to break. Tablet identification numbers: 20 mg, **232**; 40 mg, **207**; 80 mg, **241**; 120 mg, **208**; and 160 mg, **246**.

Storage

Store at room temperature; avoid excessive heat. Protect from light. Keep bottle tightly closed. Dispense in tight, light-resistant containers.

(J4-156)

Shown in Product Identification Section, page 422

CORZIDE® 40/5   ℞
CORZIDE® 80/5

[*kor'zīd*]

Nadolol and Bendroflumethiazide Tablets

DESCRIPTION

CORZIDE (Nadolol and Bendroflumethiazide Tablets) for oral administration combines two antihypertensive agents: CORGARD® (nadolol), a nonselective beta-adrenergic blocking agent, and NATURETIN® (bendroflumethiazide), a thiazide diuretic-antihypertensive. Formulations: 40 mg and 80 mg nadolol per tablet combined with 5 mg bendroflumethiazide. Inactive ingredients: cellulose, colorant (FD&C Blue No. 2), lactose, magnesium stearate, povidone, sodium starch glycolate, and starch.

Nadolol

Nadolol is a white crystalline powder. It is freely soluble in ethanol, soluble in hydrochloric acid, slightly soluble in water and in chloroform, and very slightly soluble in sodium hydroxide.

Nadolol is designated chemically as 1-(*tert*-butylamino) -3- [(5,6,7,8-tetrahydro-*cis* -6,7,-dihydroxy-1-naphthyl)oxy]-2-propanol.

Bendroflumethiazide

Bendroflumethiazide is a white crystalline powder. It is soluble in alcohol and in sodium hydroxide, and insoluble in hydrochloric acid, water, and chloroform.

Bendroflumethiazide is designated chemically as 3-benzyl-3,4-dihydro-6-(trifluoromethyl)-2H-1,2,4- benzothiadiazine-7-sulfonamide 1,1-dioxide.

CLINICAL PHARMACOLOGY

Nadolol

Nadolol is a nonselective beta-adrenergic receptor blocking agent. Clinical pharmacology studies have demonstrated beta-blocking activity by showing (1) reduction in heart rate and cardiac output at rest and on exercise, (2) reduction of systolic and diastolic blood pressure at rest and on exercise, (3) inhibition of isoproterenol-induced tachycardia, and (4) reduction of reflex orthostatic tachycardia.

Nadolol specifically competes with beta-adrenergic receptor agonists for available beta receptor sites; it inhibits both the beta$_1$ receptors located chiefly in cardiac muscle and the beta$_2$ receptors located chiefly in the bronchial and vascular musculature, inhibiting the chronotropic, inotropic, and vasodilator responses to beta-adrenergic stimulation proportionately. Nadolol has no intrinsic sympathomimetic activity and, unlike some other beta-adrenergic blocking agents, nadolol has little direct myocardial depressant activity and does not have an anesthetic-like membrane-stabilizing action. Animal and human studies show that nadolol slows the sinus rate and depresses AV conduction. In dogs, only minimal amounts of nadolol were detected in the brain relative to amounts in blood and other organs and tissues. Nadolol has low lipophilicity as determined by octanol/water partition coefficient, a characteristic of certain beta-blocking agents that has been correlated with the limited extent to which these agents cross the blood-brain barrier, their low concentration in the brain, and low incidence of CNS-related side effects.

In controlled clinical studies, nadolol at doses of 40 to 320 mg/day has been shown to decrease both standing and supine blood pressure, the effect persisting for approximately 24 hours after dosing.

The mechanism of the antihypertensive effects of beta-adrenergic receptor blocking agents has not been established; however, factors that may be involved include (1) competitive antagonism of catecholamines at peripheral (non-CNS) adrenergic neuron sites (especially cardiac) leading to decreased cardiac output, (2) a central effect leading to reduced tonic-sympathetic nerve outflow to the periphery, and (3) suppression of renin secretion by blockade of the beta-adrenergic receptors responsible for renin release from the kidneys.

While cardiac output and arterial pressure are reduced by nadolol therapy, renal hemodynamics are stable, with preservation of renal blood flow and glomerular filtration rate. By blocking catecholamine-induced increases in heart rate, velocity and extent of myocardial contraction, and blood pressure, nadolol generally reduces the oxygen requirements of the heart at any given level of effort, making it useful for many patients in the long-term management of angina pectoris. On the other hand, nadolol can increase oxygen requirements by increasing left ventricular fiber length and end diastolic pressure, particularly in patients with heart failure.

Although beta-adrenergic receptor blockade is useful in treatment of angina and hypertension, there are also situations in which sympathetic stimulation is vital. For example, in patients with severely damaged hearts, adequate ventricular function may depend on sympathetic drive. Beta-adrenergic blockade may worsen AV block by preventing the necessary facilitating effects of sympathetic activity on conduction. Beta$_2$-adrenergic blockade results in passive bronchial constriction by interfering with endogenous adrenergic bronchodilator activity in patients subject to bronchospasm and may also interfere with exogenous bronchodilators in such patients.

Absorption of nadolol after oral dosing is variable, averaging about 30 percent. Peak serum concentrations of nadolol usually occur in three to four hours after oral administration and the presence of food in the gastrointestinal tract does not affect the rate or extent of nadolol absorption. Approximately 30 percent of the nadolol present in serum is reversibly bound to plasma protein.

Unlike many other beta-adrenergic blocking agents, nadolol is not metabolized by the liver and is excreted unchanged, principally by the kidneys.

The half-life of therapeutic doses of nadolol is about 20 to 24 hours, permitting once-daily dosage. Because nadolol is excreted predominantly in the urine, its half-life increases in renal failure (see PRECAUTIONS, *General*, and DOSAGE AND ADMINISTRATION). Steady state serum concentrations of nadolol are attained in six to nine days with once-daily dosage in persons with normal renal function. Because of variable absorption and different individual responsiveness, the proper dosage must be determined by titration. Exacerbation of angina and, in some cases, myocardial infarction and ventricular dysrhythmias have been reported after abrupt discontinuation of therapy with beta-adrenergic blocking agents in patients with coronary artery disease. Abrupt withdrawal of these agents in patients without coronary artery disease has resulted in transient symptoms, including tremulousness, sweating, palpitation, headache, and malaise. Several mechanisms have been proposed to explain these phenomena, among them increased sensitivity to catecholamines because of increased numbers of beta receptors.

Bendroflumethiazide

The mechanism of action of bendroflumethiazide results in an interference with the renal tubular mechanism of electrolyte reabsorption. At maximal therapeutic dosage all thiazides are approximately equal in their diuretic potency. The mechanism whereby thiazides function in the control of hypertension is unknown.

INDICATIONS

CORZIDE (Nadolol and Bendroflumethiazide Tablets) is indicated in the management of hypertension.

This fixed combination drug is not indicated for initial therapy of hypertension. If the fixed combination represents the dose titrated to the individual patient's needs, it may be more convenient than the separate components.

CONTRAINDICATIONS

Nadolol

Nadolol is contraindicated in bronchial asthma, sinus bradycardia and greater than first degree conduction block, cardiogenic shock, and overt cardiac failure (see WARNINGS).

Bendroflumethiazide

Bendroflumethiazide is contraindicated in anuria. It is also contraindicated in patients who have previously demonstrated hypersensitivity to bendroflumethiazide or other sulfonamide-derived drugs.

WARNINGS

Nadolol

Cardiac Failure—Sympathetic stimulation may be a vital component supporting circulatory function in patients with congestive heart failure, and its inhibition by beta-blockade may precipitate more severe failure. Although beta-blockers should be avoided in overt congestive heart failure, if necessary, they can be used with caution in patients with a history of failure who are well compensated, usually with digitalis and diuretics. Beta-adrenergic blocking agents do not abolish the inotropic action of digitalis on heart muscle.

IN PATIENTS WITHOUT A HISTORY OF HEART FAILURE, continued use of beta-blockers can, in some cases, lead to cardiac failure. Therefore, at the first sign or symptom of heart failure, the patient should be digitalized and/or treated with diuretics, and the response observed closely, or nadolol should be discontinued (gradually, if possible).

Exacerbation of Ischemic Heart Disease Following Abrupt Withdrawal—Hypersensitivity to catecholamines has been observed in patients withdrawn from beta-blocker therapy; exacerbation of angina and, in some cases, myocardial infarction have occurred after *abrupt* discontinuation of such therapy. When discontinuing chronically administered nadolol, particularly in patients with ischemic heart disease, the dosage should be gradually reduced over a period of one to two weeks and the patient should be carefully monitored. If angina markedly worsens or acute coronary insufficiency develops, nadolol administration should be reinstituted promptly, at least temporarily, and other measures appropriate for the management of unstable angina should be taken. Patients should be warned against interruption or discontinuation of therapy without the physician's advice. Because coronary artery disease is common and may be unrecognized, it may be prudent not to discontinue nadolol therapy abruptly even in patients treated only for hypertension.

Nonallergic Bronchospasm (e.g., chronic bronchitis, emphysema)—PATIENTS WITH BRONCHOSPASTIC DISEASES SHOULD IN GENERAL NOT RECEIVE BETA-BLOCKERS. Nadolol should be administered with caution since it may block bronchodilation produced by endogenous or exogenous catecholamine stimulation of beta$_2$ receptors.

Major Surgery—Because beta blockade impairs the ability of the heart to respond to reflex stimuli and may increase the risks of general anesthesia and surgical procedures, resulting in protracted hypotension or low cardiac output, it has generally been suggested that such therapy should be withdrawn several days prior to surgery. Recognition of the increased sensitivity to catecholamines of patients recently withdrawn from beta-blocker therapy, however, has made this recommendation controversial. If possible, beta-blockers should be withdrawn well before surgery takes place. In the event of emergency surgery, the anesthesiologist should be informed that the patient is on beta-blocker therapy. The effects of nadolol can be reversed by administration of beta-receptor agonists such as isoproterenol, dopamine, dobutamine, or levarterenol. Difficulty in restarting and maintaining the heart beat has also been reported with beta-adrenergic receptor blocking agents.

Diabetes and Hypoglycemia—Beta-adrenergic blockade may prevent the appearance of premonitory signs and syptoms (e.g., tachycardia and blood pressure changes) of acute hypoglycemia. This is especially important in labile diabetics. Beta-blockade also reduces the release of insulin in response to hyperglycemia; therefore, it may be necessary to adjust the dose of antidiabetic drugs.

Thyrotoxicosis—Beta-adrenergic blockage may mask certain clinical signs (e.g., tachycardia) of hyperthyroidism. Patients suspected of developing thyrotoxicosis should be managed carefully to avoid abrupt withdrawal of beta-adrenergic blockade which might precipitate a thyroid storm.

Bendroflumethiazide

Thiazides should be used with caution in severe renal disease. In patients with renal disease, thiazides may precipitate azotemia. Cumulative effects of the drug may develop in patients with impaired renal function.

Thiazides should be used with caution in patients with impaired hepatic function or progressive liver disease, since minor alterations of fluid and electrolyte balance may precipitate hepatic coma.

Sensitivity reactions may occur in patients with a history of allergy or bronchial asthma.

The possibility of exacerbation or activation of systemic lupus erythematosus has been reported.

PRECAUTIONS

General

Nadolol

Nadolol should be used with caution in patients with impaired renal function (see DOSAGE AND ADMINISTRATION).

Bendroflumethiazide

All patients receiving thiazide therapy should be observed for clinical signs of fluid or electrolyte imbalance, namely, hyponatremia, hypochloremic alkalosis, and hypokalemia. Serum and urine electrolyte determinations are particularly important when the patient is vomiting excessively or receiving parenteral fluids. Medication such as digitalis may also influence serum electrolytes. Warning signs, irrespective of cause, are: dryness of the mouth, thirst, weakness, lethargy, drowsiness, restlessess, muscle pains or cramps, muscular fatigue, hypotension, oliguria, tachycardia, and gastrointestinal disturbances, such as nausea and vomiting. Hypokalemia may develop with thiazides as with any other potent diuretic, especially with brisk diuresis, when severe cirrhosis is present.

Interference with adequate oral electrolyte intake will also contribute to hypokalemia. Hypokalemia can sensitize or exaggerate the response of the heart to the toxic effects of digitalis (e.g., increased ventricular irritability). Hypokalemia may be avoided or treated by use of potassium supplements such as foods with a high potassium content.

Any chloride deficit is generally mild and usually does not require specific treatment except under extraordinary circumstances (as in liver disease or renal disease). Dilutional hyponatremia may occur in edematous patients in hot weather; appropriate therapy is water restriction, rather than administration of salt except in rare instances when the hyponatremia is life threatening. In actual salt depletion, appropriate replacement is the therapy of choice.

Hyperuricemia may occur or frank gout may be precipitated in certain patients receiving thiazide therapy.

Latent diabetes mellitus may become manifest during thiazide administration.

The antihypertensive effects of the drug may be enhanced in the post-sympathectomy patient.

If progressive renal impairment becomes evident, as indicated by rising nonprotein nitrogen or blood urea nitrogen, a careful reappraisal of therapy is necessary with consideration given to withholding or discontinuing diuretic therapy.

Thiazides may decrease serum PBI levels without signs of thyroid disturbance.

Calcium excretion is decreased by thiazides. Pathologic changes in the parathyroid gland with hypercalcemia and hypophosphatemia have been observed in a few patients on prolonged thiazide therapy. The common complications of hyperparathyroidism have not been seen.

Information for Patients

Patients, especially those with evidence of coronary artery insufficiency, should be warned against interruption or discontinuation of therapy without the physician's advice. Although cardiac failure rarely occurs in properly selected patients, patients being treated with beta-adrenergic blocking agents should be advised to consult the physician at the first sign or symptom of impending failure.

The patient should also be advised of a proper course in the event of an inadvertently missed dose.

Laboratory Tests

Serum and urine electrolyte levels should be regularly monitored (see WARNINGS, *Bendroflumethiazide*, also PRECAUTIONS, *General, Bendroflumethiazide*).

Drug Interactions

Nadolol

When administered concurrently the following drugs may interact with beta-adrenergic receptor blocking agents:

Anesthetics, general—exaggeration of the hypotension induced by general anesthetics (see WARNINGS, *Nadolol, Major Surgery*).

Antidiabetic drugs (oral agents and insulin)—hypoglycemia or hyperglycemia; adjust dosage of antidiabetic drug accordingly (see WARNINGS, *Nadolol, Diabetes and Hypoglycemia*).

Catecholamine-depleting drugs (e.g., reserpine)—additive effect; monitor closely for evidence of hypotension and/or excessive bradycardia (e.g., vertigo, syncope, postural hypotension).

Bendroflumethiazide

When administered concurrently the following drugs may interact with thiazide diuretics:

Alcohol, barbiturates, or narcotics—potentiation of orthostatic hypotension may occur.

Antidiabetic drugs (oral agents and insulin)—hyperglycemia induced by thiazide may require dosage adjustment of antidiabetic drug.

Other antihypertensive drugs—additive effect or potentiation of other antihypertensive drugs.

Corticosteroids, ACTH—intensified electrolyte depletion, particularly hypokalemia.

Ganglionic or peripheral adrenergic blocking drugs—potentiated effect of ganglionic or peripheral adrenergic blocking drugs.

Preanesthetic and anesthetic agents—effects of preanesthetic and anesthetic agents may be potentiated; adjust dosage of these agents accordingly.

Pressor amines (e.g., norepinephrine)—possible decreased response to pressor amines but not sufficient to preclude their use.

Skeletal muscle relaxants, nondepolarizing (e.g., tubocurarine)—possible increased responsiveness to the muscle relaxant.

Drug/Laboratory Test Interactions

Thiazides should be discontinued before carrying out tests for parathyroid function (see PRECAUTIONS, *General, Bendroflumethiazide*).

Carcinogenesis, Mutagenesis, Impairment of Fertility

Nadolol

In chronic oral toxicologic studies (one to two years) in mice, rats, and dogs, nadolol did not produce any significant toxic effects. In two-year oral carcinogenicity studies in rats and mice, nadolol did not produce any neoplastic, preneoplastic, or nonneoplastic pathologic lesions. In fertility and general reproductive performance studies in rats, nadolol caused no adverse effect.

Bendroflumethiazide

Long-term studies in animals have not been performed to evaluate carcinogenic potential, mutagenesis, or whether this drug affects fertility in males or females.

Pregnancy—Teratogenic Effects

Nadolol

Category C. In animal reproduction studies with nadolol, evidence of embryo- and fetotoxicity was found in rabbits, but not in rats or hamsters, at doses 5 to 10 times greater (on a mg/kg basis) than the maximum indicated human dose. No teratogenic potential was observed in any of these species. There are no adequate and well-controlled studies in pregnant women. Nadolol should be used during pregnancy only if the potential benefit justifies the potential risk to the fetus. Neonates whose mothers are receiving nadolol at parturition have exhibited bradycardia, hypoglycemia, and associated symptoms.

Bendroflumethiazide

Category C. Animal reproduction studies have not been conducted with bendroflumethiazide. It is also not known whether this drug can cause fetal harm when administered to a pregnant woman or can affect reproduction capacity. Bendroflumethiazide should be given to a pregnant woman only if clearly needed.

Pregnancy—Nonteratogenic Effects

Thiazides cross the placental barrier and appear in cord blood. The use of thiazides in pregnant women requires that the anticipated benefit be weighed against possible hazards to the fetus. These hazards include fetal or neonatal jaun-

dice, thrombocytopenia, and possibly other adverse reactions which have occurred in the adult.

Nursing Mothers

Both nadolol and bendroflumethiazide are excreted in human milk. Because of the potential for serious adverse reactions in nursing infants from both drugs, a decision should be made whether to discontinue nursing or to discontinue therapy taking into account the importance of CORZIDE (Nadolol and Bendroflumethiazide Tablets) to the mother.

Pediatric Use

Safety and effectiveness in children have not been established.

ADVERSE REACTIONS

Nadolol

Most adverse effects have been mild and transient and have rarely required withdrawal of therapy.

Cardiovascular—Bradycardia with heart rates of less than 60 beats per minute occurs commonly, and heart rates below 40 beats per minute and/or symptomatic bradycardia were seen in about 2 of 100 patients. Symptoms of peripheral vascular insufficiency, usually of the Raynaud type, have occurred in approximately 2 of 100 patients. Cardiac failure, hypotension, and rhythm/conduction disturbances have each occurred in about 1 of 100 patients. Single instances of first degree and third degree heart block have been reported; intensification of AV block is a known effect of beta-blockers (see also CONTRAINDICATIONS, WARNINGS, and PRECAUTIONS).

Central Nervous System—Dizziness or fatigue has been reported in approximately 2 of 100 patients; paresthesias, sedation, and change in behavior have each been reported in approximately 6 of 1000 patients.

Respiratory—Bronchospasm has been reported in approximately 1 of 1000 patients (see CONTRAINDICATIONS and WARNINGS).

Gastrointestinal—Nausea, diarrhea, abdominal discomfort, constipation, vomiting, indigestion, anorexia, bloating, and flatulence have been reported in 1 to 5 of 1000 patients.

Miscellaneous—Each of the following has been reported in 1 to 5 of 1000 patients: rash; pruritus; headache; dry mouth, eyes, or skin; impotence or decreased libido; facial swelling; weight gain; slurred speech; cough; nasal stuffiness; sweating; tinnitus; blurred vision. Reversible alopecia has been reported infrequently.

The following adverse reactions have been reported in patients taking nadolol and/or other beta-adrenergic blocking agents, but no causal relationship to nadolol has been established.

Central Nervous System—Reversible mental depression progressing to catatonia; visual disturbances; hallucinations; an acute reversible syndrome characterized by disorientation for time and place, short-term memory loss, emotional lability with slightly clouded sensorium, and decreased performance on neuropsychometrics.

Gastrointestinal—Mesenteric arterial thrombosis; ischemic colitis; elevated liver enzymes.

Hematologic—Agranulocytosis; thrombocytopenic or nonthrombocytopenic purpura.

Allergic—Fever combined with aching and sore throat; laryngospasm; respiratory distress.

Miscellaneous—Pemphigoid rash; hypertensive reaction in patients with pheochromocytoma; sleep disturbances; Peyronie's disease.

The oculomucocutaneous syndrome associated with the beta-blocker practolol has not been reported with nadolol.

Bendroflumethiazide

Gastrointestinal System—anorexia, gastric irritation, nausea, vomiting, cramping, diarrhea, constipation, jaundice (intrahepatic cholestatic jaundice), and pancreatitis.

Central Nervous System—dizziness, vertigo, paresthesia, headache, and xanthopsia.

Hematologic—leukopenia, agranulocytosis, thrombocytopenia, and aplastic anemia.

Dermatologic-Hypersensitivity — purpura, photosensitivity, rash, urticaria, and necrotizing angiitis (vasculitis, cutaneous vasculitis).

Cardiovascular—Orthostatic hypotension may occur.

Other—hyperglycemia, glycosuria, occasional metabolic acidosis in diabetic patients, hyperuricemia, allergic glomerulonephritis, muscle spasm, weakness, and restlessness. Whenever adverse reactions are moderate or severe, thiazide dosage should be reduced or therapy withdrawn.

OVERDOSAGE

In the event of overdosage, nadolol may cause excessive bradycardia, cardiac failure, hypotension, or bronchospasm. In addition to the expected diuresis, overdosage of thiazides may produce varying degrees of lethargy which may progress to coma within a few hours, with minimal depression of respiration and cardiovascular function and without evidence of serum electrolyte changes or dehydration. The mechanism of thiazide-induced CNS depression is unknown. Gastrointestinal irritation and hypermotility may occur.

Continued on next page

Princeton—Cont.

Transitory increase in BUN has been reported, and serum electrolyte changes may occur, especially in patients with impaired renal function.

Treatment

Nadolol can be removed from the general circulation by hemodialysis. In determining the duration of corrective therapy, note must be taken of the long duration of the effect of nadolol. In addition to gastric lavage, the following measures should be employed, as appropriate.

Excessive Bradycardia—Administer atropine (0.25 to 1.0 mg). If there is no response to vagal blockade, administer isoproterenol cautiously.

Cardiac Failure—Administer a digitalis glycoside and diuretic. It has been reported that glucagon may also be useful in this situation.

Hypotension—Administer vasopressors, e.g., epinephrine or levarterenol. (There is evidence that epinephrine may be the drug of choice.)

Bronchospasm—Administer a beta₂-stimulating agent and/or a theophylline derivative.

Stupor or Coma—Supportive therapy as warranted.

Gastrointestinal Effects—Symptomatic treatment as needed.

BUN and/or Serum Electrolyte Abnormalities—Institute supportive measures as required to maintain hydration, electrolyte balance, respiration, and cardiovascular and renal function.

DOSAGE AND ADMINISTRATION

DOSAGE MUST BE INDIVIDUALIZED (SEE INDICATIONS). CORZIDE MAY BE ADMINISTERED WITHOUT REGARD TO MEALS.

Bendroflumethiazide is usually given at a dose of 5 mg daily. The usual initial dose of nadolol is 40 mg once daily whether used alone or in combination with a diuretic. Bendroflumethiazide in CORZIDE is 30 percent more bioavailable than that of 5 mg NATURETIN tablets. Conversion from 5 mg NATURETIN to CORZIDE represents a 30 percent increase in dose of bendroflumethiazide.

The initial dose of CORZIDE (Nadolol and Bendroflumethiazide Tablets) may therefore be the 40 mg/5 mg tablet once daily. When the antihypertensive response is not satisfactory, the dose may be increased by administering the 80 mg/5 mg tablet once daily.

When necessary, another antihypertensive agent may be added gradually beginning with 50 percent of the usual recommended starting dose to avoid an excessive fall in blood pressure.

Dosage Adjustment in Renal Failure—Absorbed nadolol is excreted principally by the kidneys and, although nonrenal elimination does occur, dosage adjustments are necessary in patients with renal impairment. The following dose intervals are recommended:

Creatinine Clearance (ml/min/1.73m²)	Dosage Interval (hours)
>50	24
31-50	24-36
10-30	24-48
<10	40-60

HOW SUPPLIED

CORZIDE (Nadolol and Bendroflumethiazide Tablets)
- **40 mg nadolol combined with 5 mg bendroflumethiazide** in bottles of 100 tablets (NDC 0003-0283-50).
- **80 mg nadolol combined with 5 mg bendroflumethiazide** in bottles of 100 tablets (NDC 0003-0284-50).

Round, biconvex tablets are white to bluish white with dark blue specks. Each tablet has a full bisect bar. Tablet identification numbers: 40 mg/5 mg combination, **283**; 80 mg/5 mg combination, **284**.

Storage

Keep bottle tightly closed. Store at room temperature; avoid excessive heat.

(J4-117)

Shown in Product Identification Section, page 422

HALOG CREAMS   ℞
Halcinonide Cream USP 0.025% and 0.1%
HALOG Ointment   ℞
Halcinonide Ointment USP 0.1%
HALOG Solution   ℞
Halcinonide Topical Solution USP 0.1%
HALOG-E Cream   ℞
Halcinonide Cream USP 0.1%

DESCRIPTION

The topical corticosteroids constitute a class of primarily synthetic steroids used as anti-inflammatory and antipruritic agents. The steroids in this class include halcinonide. Halcinonide is designated chemically as 21-Chloro-9-fluoro-11β, 16α, 17-trihydroxypregn-4-ene-3,20-dione cyclic 16,17-acetal with acetone.

Each gram of 0.025% HALOG Cream (Halcinonide Cream) contains 0.25 mg halcinonide in a specially formulated cream base consisting of glyceryl monostearate NF XII, cetyl alcohol, cetyl esters wax, polysorbate 60, propylene glycol, dimethicone 350, and purified water. Each gram of 0.1% HALOG Cream (Halcinonide Cream) contains 1 mg halcinonide in a specially formulated cream base consisting of glyceryl monostearate NF XII, cetyl alcohol, isopropyl palmitate, dimethicone 350, polysorbate 60, titanium dioxide, propylene glycol, and purified water.

Each gram of 0.1% HALOG Ointment (Halcinonide Ointment) contains 1 mg halcinonide in Plastibase® (Plasticized Hydrocarbon Gel), a polyethylene and mineral oil gel base with polyethylene glycol 400, polyethylene glycol 6000 distearate, polyethylene glycol 300, polyethylene glycol 1450, and butylated hydroxytoluene as an antioxidant.

Each mL of 0.1% HALOG Solution (Halcinonide Topical Solution) contains 1 mg halcinonide with edetate disodium, polyethylene glycol 300, purified water, and butylated hydroxytoluene as an antioxidant.

Each gram of 0.1% HALOG-E Cream (Halcinonide Cream) contains 1 mg halcinonide in a hydrophilic vanishing cream base consisting of propylene glycol, dimethicone 350, castor oil, cetearyl alcohol (and) ceteareth-20, propylene glycol stearate, white petrolatum, and purified water. This formulation is water-washable, greaseless, and nonstaining, with moisturizing and emollient properties.

CLINICAL PHARMACOLOGY

Topical corticosteroids share anti-inflammatory, antipruritic and vasoconstrictive actions.

The mechanism of anti-inflammatory activity of the topical corticosteroids is unclear. Various laboratory methods, including vasoconstrictor assays, are used to compare and predict potencies and/or clinical efficacies of the topical corticosteroids. There is some evidence to suggest that a recognizable correlation exists between vasoconstrictor potency and therapeutic efficacy in man.

PHARMACOKINETICS

The extent of percutaneous absorption of topical corticosteroids is determined by many factors including the vehicle, the integrity of the epidermal barrier, and the use of occlusive dressings.

Topical corticosteroids can be absorbed from normal intact skin. Inflammation and/or other disease processes in the skin increase percutaneous absorption. Occlusive dressings substantially increase the percutaneous absorption of topical corticosteroids. Thus, occlusive dressings may be a valuable therapeutic adjunct for treatment of resistant dermatoses (see DOSAGE AND ADMINISTRATION).

Once absorbed through the skin, topical corticosteroids are handled through pharmacokinetic pathways similar to systemically administered corticosteroids. Corticosteroids are bound to plasma proteins in varying degrees. Corticosteroids are metabolized primarily in the liver and are then excreted by the kidneys. Some of the topical corticosteroids and their metabolites are also excreted into the bile.

INDICATIONS AND USAGE

HALOG (Halcinonide) preparations are indicated for the relief of the inflammatory and pruritic manifestations of corticosteroid-responsive dermatoses.

CONTRAINDICATIONS

Topical corticosteroids are contraindicated in those patients with a history of hypersensitivity to any of the components of the preparations.

PRECAUTIONS

General

Systemic absorption of topical corticosteroids has produced reversible hypothalamic-pituitary-adrenal (HPA) axis suppression, manifestations of Cushing's syndrome, hyperglycemia, and glucosuria in some patients.

Conditions which augment systemic absorption include the application of the more potent steroids, use over large surface areas, prolonged use, and the addition of occlusive dressings.

Therefore, patients receiving a large dose of any potent topical steroid applied to a large surface area or under an occlusive dressing should be evaluated periodically for evidence of HPA axis suppression by using the urinary free cortisol and ACTH stimulation tests, and for impairment of thermal homeostasis. If HPA axis suppression or elevation of the body temperature occurs, an attempt should be made to withdraw the drug, to reduce the frequency of application, substitute a less potent steroid, or use a sequential approach when utilizing the occlusive technique.

Recovery of HPA axis function and thermal homeostasis are generally prompt and complete upon discontinuation of the drug. Infrequently, signs and symptoms of steroid withdrawal may occur, requiring supplemental systemic corticosteroids. Occasionally, a patient may develop a sensitivity reaction to a particular occlusive dressing material or adhesive and a substitute material may be necessary.

Children may absorb proportionally larger amounts of topical corticosteroids and thus be more susceptible to systemic toxicity (see PRECAUTIONS, Pediatric Use).

If irritation develops, topical corticosteroids should be discontinued and appropriate therapy instituted.

In the presence of dermatological infections, the use of an appropriate antifungal or antibacterial agent should be instituted. If a favorable response does not occur promptly, the corticosteroid should be discontinued until the infection has been adequately controlled.

These preparations are not for ophthalmic use.

Information for the Patient

Patients using topical corticosteroids should receive the following information and instructions:

1. These medications are to be used as directed by the physician. They are for dermatologic use only. Avoid contact with the eyes.
2. Patients should be advised not to use these medications for any disorder other than for which it was prescribed.
3. The treated skin area should not be bandaged or otherwise covered or wrapped as to be occlusive unless directed by the physician.
4. Patients should report any signs of local adverse reactions especially under occlusive dressing.
5. Parents of pediatric patients should be advised not to use tight-fitting diapers or plastic pants on a child being treated in the diaper area, as these garments may constitute occlusive dressings.

Laboratory Tests

A urinary free cortisol test and ACTH stimulation test may be helpful in evaluating HPA axis suppression.

Carcinogenesis, Mutagenesis, and Impairment of Fertility

Long-term animal studies have not been performed to evaluate the carcinogenic potential or the effect on fertility of topical corticosteroids. Studies to determine mutagenicity with prednisolone and hydrocortisone showed negative results.

Pregnancy: Teratogenic Effects

Category C. Corticosteroids are generally teratogenic in laboratory animals when administered systemically at relatively low dosage levels. The more potent corticosteroids have been shown to be teratogenic after dermal application in laboratory animals. There are no adequate and well-controlled studies in pregnant women on teratogenic effects from topically applied corticosteroids. Therefore, topical corticosteroids should be used during pregnancy only if the potential benefit justifies the potential risk to the fetus. Drugs of this class should not be used extensively on pregnant patients, in large amounts, or for prolonged periods of time.

Nursing Mothers

It is not known whether topical administration of corticosteroids could result in sufficient systemic absorption to produce detectable quantities in breast milk. Systemically administered corticosteroids are secreted into breast milk in quantities **not** likely to have a deleterious effect on the infant. Nevertheless, caution should be exercised when topical corticosteroids are administered to a nursing woman.

Pediatric Use

Pediatric patients may demonstrate greater susceptibility to topical corticosteroid-induced HPA axis suppression and Cushing's syndrome than mature patients because of a larger skin surface area to body weight ratio.

HPA axis suppression, Cushing's syndrome, and intracranial hypertension have been reported in children receiving topical corticosteroids. Manifestations of adrenal suppression in children include linear growth retardation, delayed weight gain, low plasma cortisol levels, and absence of response to ACTH stimulation. Manifestations of intracranial hypertension include bulging fontanelles, headaches, and bilateral papilledema.

Administration of topical corticosteroids to children should be limited to the least amount compatible with an effective therapeutic regimen. Chronic corticosteroid therapy may interfere with the growth and development of children.

ADVERSE REACTIONS

The following local adverse reactions are reported infrequently with topical corticosteroids, but may occur more frequently with the use of occlusive dressings (reactions are listed in an approximate decreasing order of occurrence): burning, itching, irritation, dryness, folliculitis, hypertrichosis, acneiform eruptions, hypopigmentation, perioral dermatitis, allergic contact dermatitis, maceration of the skin, secondary infection, skin atrophy, striae, and miliaria.

OVERDOSAGE

Topically applied corticosteroids can be absorbed in sufficient amounts to produce systemic effects (see PRECAUTIONS, General).

DOSAGE AND ADMINISTRATION

HALOG Creams (Halcinonide Cream): Apply the 0.025% or the 0.1% HALOG Cream (Halcinonide Cream) to the affected area two to three times daily. Rub in gently.

HALOG Ointment (Halcinonide Ointment): Apply a thin film of 0.1% HALOG Ointment (Halcinonide Ointment) to the affected area two to three times daily.

HALOG Solution (Halcinonide Topical Solution): Apply HALOG Solution (Halcinonide Topical Solution) 0.1% to the affected area two to three times daily.

HALOG-E Cream (Halcinonide Cream): Apply HALOG-E Cream (Halcinonide Cream) 0.1% to the affected area one to three times daily. Rub in gently.

Occlusive Dressing Technique

Occlusive dressings may be used for the management of psoriasis or other recalcitrant conditions.

HALOG Creams (Halcinonide Cream) 0.025% and 0.1% and HALOG-E Cream (Halcinonide Cream) 0.1%: Gently rub a small amount of the cream into the lesion until it disappears. Reapply the preparation leaving a thin coating on the lesion, cover with a pliable nonporous film, and seal the edges. If needed, additional moisture may be provided by covering the lesion with a dampened clean cotton cloth before the nonporous film is applied or by briefly wetting the affected area with water immediately prior to applying the medication. The frequency of changing dressings is best determined on an individual basis. It may be convenient to apply HALOG/HALOG-E Cream under an occlusive dressing in the evening and to remove the dressing in the morning (i.e., 12-hour occlusion). When utilizing the 12-hour occlusion regimen, additional cream should be applied, without occlusion, during the day. Reapplication is essential at each dressing change.

If an infection develops, the use of occlusive dressings should be discontinued and appropriate antimicrobial therapy instituted.

HALOG Ointment (Halcinonide Ointment) 0.1%: Apply a thin film of the ointment to the lesion, cover with a pliable nonporous film, and seal the edges. If needed, additional moisture may be provided by covering the lesion with a dampened clean cotton cloth before the nonporous film is applied or by briefly wetting the affected area with water immediately prior to applying the medication. The frequency of changing dressings is best determined on an individual basis. It may be convenient to apply HALOG Ointment under an occlusive dressing in the evening and to remove the dressing in the morning (i.e., 12-hour occlusion). When utilizing the 12-hour occlusion regimen, additional ointment should be applied, without occlusion, during the day. Reapplication is essential at each dressing change.

If an infection develops, the use of occlusive dressings should be discontinued and appropriate antimicrobial therapy instituted.

HALOG Solution (Halcinonide Topical Solution) 0.1%: Apply the solution to the lesion, cover with a pliable nonporous film, and seal the edges. If needed, additional moisture may be provided by covering the lesion with a dampened clean cotton cloth before the nonporous film is applied or by briefly wetting the affected area with water immediately prior to applying the medication. The frequency of changing dressings is best determined on an individual basis. It may be convenient to apply HALOG solution under an occlusive dressing in the evening and to remove the dressing in the morning (i.e., 12-hour occlusion). When utilizing the 12-hour occlusion regimen, additional solution should be applied, without occlusion, during the day. Reapplication is essential at each dressing change.

If an infection develops, the use of occlusive dressings should be discontinued and appropriate antimicrobial therapy instituted.

HOW SUPPLIED

HALOG Creams (Halcinonide Cream USP)

0.025%: tubes containing 15 g (NDC 0003-0296-15), and 60 g (NDC 0003-0296-30) of cream.

0.1%: tubes containing 15 g (NDC 0003-1482-15), 30 g (NDC 0003-1482-20), 60 g (NDC 0003-1482-30); and jars containing 240 g (NDC 0003-1482-40) of cream.

HALOG Ointment (Halcinonide Ointment USP)

0.1%: tubes containing 15 g (NDC 0003-0248-15), 30 g (NDC 0003-0248-20), and 60 g (NDC 0003-0248-30); and jars containing 240 g (NDC 0003-0248-40) of ointment.

HALOG Solution (Halcinonide Topical Solution USP)

0.1%: plastic squeeze bottles containing 20 mL (NDC 0003-0249-15) and 60 mL (NDC 0003-0249-20) of solution.

HALOG-E Cream (Halcinonide Cream USP)

0.1%: tubes containing 15 g (NDC 0003-1494-14), 30 g (NDC 0003-1494-21), and 60 g (NDC 0003-1494-31) of cream.

Storage

HALOG Creams (Halcinonide Cream USP)

Store at room temperature; avoid excessive heat (104°F).

HALOG Ointment (Halcinonide Ointment USP)

Store at room temperature; avoid excessive heat (104°F).

HALOG Solution (Halcinonide Topical Solution USP)

Store at room temperature; avoid freezing and temperatures above 104°F.

HALOG-E Cream (Halcinonide Cream USP)

Store at room temperature; avoid freezing and refrigeration.

(J4-127/105/115/102)

NATURETIN®   ℞

[na "chūr-ē'tin]

Bendroflumethiazide Tablets USP

DESCRIPTION

NATURETIN (Bendroflumethiazide Tablets USP) is a benzothiadiazine derivative containing a benzyl and a trifluoromethyl group. It is a potent oral diuretic and antihypertensive agent. Bendroflumethiazide is designated chemically as 3-benzyl-3,4-dihydro-6-(trifluoromethyl)-2H-1, 2, 4-benzothiadiazine-7-sulfonamide 1,1-dioxide.

It is available as compressed tablets providing 5 or 10 mg bendroflumethiazide. Inactive ingredients: microcrystalline cellulose, colorants [D&C Yellow No. 10; FD&C Blue No. 1 for 5 mg only, and FD&C Yellow No. 6 for 10 mg only], lactose, magnesium stearate, sodium starch glycolate, and pregelatinized starch.

CLINICAL PHARMACOLOGY

Thiazides affect the renal tubular mechanism of electrolyte reabsorption. At maximal therapeutic dosage all thiazides are approximately equal in their diuretic potency.

Thiazides increase excretion of sodium and chloride in approximately equivalent amounts. Natriuresis causes a secondary loss of potassium and bicarbonate.

The mechanism of the antihypertensive effect of thiazides is unknown. Thiazides do not affect normal blood pressure. Onset of action of thiazides occurs in two hours and the peak effect at about four hours. Duration of action persists for approximately six to 12 hours. Thiazides are eliminated rapidly by the kidney.

INDICATIONS AND USAGE

NATURETIN is indicated as adjunctive therapy in edema associated with congestive heart failure, hepatic cirrhosis, and corticosteroid and estrogen therapy.

NATURETIN has also been found useful in edema due to various forms of renal dysfunction such as: nephrotic syndrome, acute glomerulonephritis, and chronic renal failure.

NATURETIN tablets are indicated in the management of hypertension either as the sole therapeutic agent or to enhance the effectiveness of other antihypertensive drugs in the more severe forms of hypertension.

Usage in Pregnancy. The routine use of diuretics in an otherwise healthy woman is inappropriate and exposes mother and fetus to unnecessary hazard. Diuretics do not prevent development of toxemia of pregnancy, and there is no satisfactory evidence that they are useful in the treatment of developed toxemia.

Edema during pregnancy may arise from pathological causes or from the physiologic and mechanical consequences of pregnancy. Thiazides are indicated in pregnancy when edema is due to pathologic causes, just as they are in the absence of pregnancy (however, see PRECAUTIONS, Pregnancy: Nonteratogenic effects below). Dependent edema in pregnancy, resulting from restriction of venous return by the expanded uterus, is properly treated through elevation of the lower extremities and use of support hose; use of diuretics to lower intravascular volume in this case is illogical and unnecessary. There is hypervolemia during normal pregnancy which is harmful to neither the fetus nor the mother (in the absence of cardiovascular disease), but which is associated with edema, including generalized edema, in the majority of pregnant women. If this edema produces discomfort, increased recumbency will often provide relief. In rare instances, this edema may cause extreme discomfort which is not relieved by rest. In these cases, a short course of diuretics may provide relief and may be appropriate.

CONTRAINDICATIONS

Bendroflumethiazide is contraindicated in anuria.

It is also contraindicated in patients who have previously demonstrated hypersensitivity to it or other sulfonamide-derived drugs.

WARNINGS

Thiazides should be used with caution in severe renal disease. In patients with renal disease, thiazides may precipitate azotemia. Cumulative effects of the drug may develop in patients with impaired renal function.

Thiazides should be used with caution in patients with impaired hepatic function or progressive liver disease, since minor alterations of fluid and electrolyte balance may precipitate hepatic coma.

Sensitivity reactions may occur in patients with or without a history of allergy or bronchial asthma.

The possibility of exacerbation or activation of systemic lupus erythematosus has been reported.

Lithium generally should not be given with diuretics; diuretic agents reduce the renal clearance of lithium and add a high risk of lithium toxicity. Refer to the package insert for lithium preparations before use of such concomitant therapy.

PRECAUTIONS

General

Periodic determination of serum electrolytes to detect possible electrolyte imbalance should be performed at appropriate intervals.

All patients receiving thiazide therapy should be observed for clinical signs of fluid or electrolyte imbalance, namely: hyponatremia, hypochloremic alkalosis, and hypokalemia. Serum and urine electrolyte determinations are particularly important when the patient is vomiting excessively or receiving parenteral fluids. Warning signs or symptoms of fluid and electrolyte imbalance include: dryness of the mouth, thirst, weakness, lethargy, drowsiness, restlessness, muscle pains or cramps, muscular fatigue, hypotension, oliguria, tachycardia, and gastrointestinal disturbances such as nausea and vomiting.

Hypokalemia may develop, especially with brisk diuresis, or when severe cirrhosis is present.

Interference with adequate oral electrolyte intake will also contribute to hypokalemia. Hypokalemia can sensitize or exaggerate the response of the heart to the toxic effects of digitalis (e.g., increased ventricular irritability). Concurrent administration of a potassium-sparing diuretic or potassium supplements may be indicated in these patients.

Any chloride deficit is generally mild and usually does not require specific treatment except under extraordinary circumstances (as in liver disease or renal disease). Dilutional hyponatremia may occur in edematous patients in hot weather; appropriate therapy is water restriction, rather than administration of salt, except in rare instances when the hyponatremia is life threatening. In actual salt depletion, appropriate replacement is the therapy of choice.

Hyperuricemia may occur or frank gout may be precipitated in certain patients receiving thiazide therapy.

Latent diabetes mellitus may become manifest during thiazide administration.

Thiazide drugs may increase the responsiveness to tubocurarine.

The antihypertensive effects of the drug may be enhanced in the postsympathectomy patient.

If progressive renal impairment becomes evident, as indicated by a rising nonprotein nitrogen or blood urea nitrogen, a careful reappraisal of therapy is necessary with consideration given to withholding or discontinuing diuretic therapy. Calcium excretion is decreased by thiazides. Pathological changes in the parathyroid gland with hypercalcemia and hypophosphatemia have been observed in a few patients on prolonged thiazide therapy. The common complications of hyperparathyroidism such as renal lithiasis, bone resorption, and peptic ulceration have not been seen. Thiazides should be discontinued before carrying out tests for parathyroid function.

Thiazides have been shown to increase the urinary excretion of magnesium; this may result in hypomagnesemia.

ADVERSE REACTIONS

Gastrointestinal: nausea, vomiting, cramping and anorexia are not uncommon; diarrhea, constipation, gastric irritation, abdominal bloating, jaundice (intrahepatic cholestatic jaundice), hepatitis, and sialadenitis occasionally occur; and pancreatitis has been reported.

Central nervous system: dizziness, vertigo, headache, and xanthopsia occasionally occur.

Hematologic: leukopenia, agranulocytosis, thrombocytopenia, hemolytic anemia, and aplastic anemia have been reported.

Dermatologic-Hypersensitivity: purpura, exfoliative dermatitis, pruritus, ecchymosis, urticaria, necrotizing angiitis (vasculitis, cutaneous vasculitis), respiratory distress including pneumonitis, fever, and anaphylactic reactions occasionally occur; photosensitivity and rash have been reported.

Cardiovascular: orthostatic hypotension may occur and may be potentiated by coadministration with certain other drugs (e.g., alcohol, barbiturates, narcotics, other antihypertensive medications, etc.; see PRECAUTIONS, Drug Interactions).

Other: muscle spasm, weakness, or restlessness is not uncommon; hyperglycemia, glycosuria, metabolic acidosis in diabetic patients, hyperuricemia, allergic glomerulonephritis, and transient blurred vision occasionally occur.

Whenever adverse reactions are moderate or severe, thiazide dosage should be reduced or therapy withdrawn.

Information for Patients

The patient should be advised to take the medication at the same time each day as prescribed to minimize the inconvenience of diuresis, warned against interruption or discontinuation of medication even though he may feel well, and advised about a proper course in the event of an inadvertent missed dose.

The patient should be informed of symptoms that would suggest potential adverse effects and told to report them promptly.

Continued on next page

Princeton—Cont.

Laboratory Tests
During long-term therapy, the patient's serum electrolyte levels should be regularly monitored (see PRECAUTIONS, General, and also WARNINGS).

Drug Interactions
When administered concurrently, the following drugs may interact with bendroflumethiazide:

Alcohol, barbiturates, or narcotics —potentiation of orthostatic hypotension may occur.

Amphotericin B, corticosteroids, or corticotropin (ACTH) —may intensify electrolyte imbalance, particularly hypokalemia. Monitor potassium levels; use potassium replacements if necessary.

Anticoagulants (oral) —dosage adjustments of anticoagulant medication may be necessary since bendroflumethiazide may decrease their effects.

Antigout medications —dosage adjustments of antigout medication may be necessary since bendroflumethiazide may raise the level of blood uric acid.

Other antihypertensive medications (e.g., ganglionic or peripheral adrenergic blocking agents) —dosage adjustments may be necessary since bendroflumethiazide may potentiate their effects.

Antidiabetic drugs (oral agents and insulin) —since thiazides may elevate blood glucose levels, dosage adjustments of antidiabetic agents may be necessary.

Calcium salts —increased serum calcium levels due to decreased excretion. If calcium must be prescribed monitor serum calcium levels and adjust calcium dosage accordingly.

Cardiac glycosides —enhanced possibility of digitalis toxicity associated with hypokalemia. Monitor potassium levels; use potassium replacement if necessary.

Cholestyramine resin and colestipol HCL —may delay or decrease absorption of bendroflumethiazide. Sulfonamide diuretics should be taken at least one hour before or four to six hours after these medications.

Diazoxide —enhanced hyperglycemic, hyperuricemic, and antihypertensive effects. Be cognizant of possible interaction; monitor blood glycose and serum uric acid levels.

Lithium salts —may enhance lithium toxicity due to reduced renal clearance. Avoid concurrent use; if lithium must be prescribed monitor serum lithium levels and adjust lithium dosage accordingly.

MAO inhibitors —dosage adjustments of one or both agents may be necessary since hypotensive effects are enhanced.

Nondepolarizing muscle relaxants, preanesthetics and anesthetics used in surgery (e.g. tubocurarine chloride and gallamine triethiodide)—increased responsiveness to muscle relaxants. Be cognizant of interaction; monitor and correct any electrolyte imbalances prior to surgery if feasible.

Nonsteroidal anti-inflammatory agents —In some patients, the administration of a nonsteroidal anti-inflammatory agent can reduce the diuretic, natriuretic, and antihypertensive effects of loop, potassium-sparing and thiazide diuretics. Therefore, when bendroflumethiazide and nonsteroidal anti-inflammatory agents are used concomitantly, the patient should be observed closely to determine if the desired effect of the diuretic is obtained.

Methenamine —possible decreased effectiveness due to alkalinization of the urine.

Pressor amines (e.g. norepinephrine)—decreased arterial responsiveness, but not sufficient to preclude effectiveness of the pressor agent for therapeutic use. Use caution in patients taking both medications who undergo surgery. Administer pre-anesthetic and anesthetic agents in reduced dosage, and if possible, discontinue bendroflumethiazide one week prior to surgery.

Probenecid or sulfinpyrazone —increased dosage of these agents may be necessary since bendroflumethiazide may exhibit increased hyperuricemic effects.

Drug/Laboratory Test Interactions
Bendroflumethiazide may produce false-negative results with the phentolamine and tyramine tests; may interfere with the phenosulfonphthalein test due to decreased excretion; and it may cause diagnostic interference of serum electrolyte levels, blood and urine glucose levels, and a decrease in serum PBI levels without signs of thyroid disturbance.

Carcinogenesis, Mutagenesis, Impairment of Fertility
Studies have not been performed to evaluate the carcinogenic or mutagenic potential of bendroflumethiazide or the potential of this medication to adversely affect fertility in males or females.

Pregnancy: Teratogenic Effects
Category C. Animal reproduction studies have not been conducted with bendroflumethiazide. It is also not known whether bendroflumethiazide can cause fetal harm when administered to a pregnant woman or can affect reproduction capacity. Bendroflumethiazide should be given to a pregnant women only if clearly needed (see INDICATIONS).

Pregnancy: Nonteratogenic Effects
Thiazides cross the placental barrier and appear in cord blood. The use of thiazides in pregnant women requires that the anticipated benefit be weighed against possible hazards to the fetus. These hazards include fetal or neonatal jaundice, thrombocytopenia, and possibly other adverse reactions which have occurred in the adult.

Nursing Mothers
Because of the potential for serious adverse reactions in nursing infants from bendroflumethiazide, a decision should be made whether to discontinue nursing or to discontinue the drug, taking into account the importance of the drug to the mother.

Pediatric Use
Safety and effectiveness in children have not been established.

OVERDOSAGE

Symptoms of overdosage may be manifested in several ways: temporary elevation of BUN; gastrointestinal irritation; and lethargy progressing to coma with minimal depression of respiration and cardiovascular function and without significant serum electrolyte changes or dehydration. Serum electrolyte changes may occur, especially in patients with impaired renal function. The mechanism of thiazide-induced central nervous system depression is unknown.

Treatment is essentially supportive. Evacuation of gastric contents may be useful provided aspiration is avoided in unconscious patients. In conscious patients, induced vomiting using Ipecac Syrup USP is helpful in removing the drug from the stomach. Cathartics should be avoided since they tend to enhance the loss of fluid and electrolytes. Electrolyte levels and renal function should be monitored, and supportive measures instituted to maintain hydration, electrolyte balance, respiration, and cardiovascular-renal function as required. Gastrointestinal irritation is usually of short duration and may be treated symptomatically.

DOSAGE AND ADMINISTRATION

Therapy should be individualized according to patient response and titrated to obtain maximal therapeutic response as well as the lowest dose possible to maintain that therapeutic response and minimize side effects.

Diuretic: The usual dose is 5 mg once daily, preferably given in the morning. To initiate therapy, doses up to 20 mg may be given once daily or divided into two doses. A single daily dose of 2.5 to 5 mg should suffice for maintenance.

Alternatively, intermittent therapy may be advantageous in many patients. By administering the preparation every other day or on a three to five day per week schedule, electrolyte imbalance is less likely to occur; however, the possibility still exists.

In general, the lowest dosage that achieves the therapeutic response should be employed.

Antihypertensive: The suggested initial dosage is 5 to 20 mg daily. Maintenance dosage may range from 2.5 to 15 mg per day depending on the individual response of the patient. When the diuretic is used with other antihypertensive agents, lower maintenance doses for each drug are usually sufficient.

HOW SUPPLIED

NATURETIN (Bendroflumethiazide Tablets USP)

5 mg/tablet: bottles of 100 (NDC 0003-0606-50) and 1000 (NDC 0003-0606-80).

Each green, round, biconvex tablet with bisect bar is imprinted with identification number **606**.

10 mg/tablet: bottles of 100 (NDC0003-0618-50).

Each orange, round, biconvex tablet with bisect bar is imprinted with identification number **618**.

STORAGE

Dispense in tight containers. Store at room temperature; avoid excessive heat.

(J4-265B)

Shown in Product Identification Section, page 422

PROLIXIN® INJECTION   ℞
Fluphenazine Hydrochloride Injection USP
FOR INTRAMUSCULAR USE ONLY

DESCRIPTION

PROLIXIN Injection (Fluphenazine Hydrochloride Injection) is a trifluoromethyl phenothiazine derivative intended for the management of schizophrenia. PROLIXIN Injection is available in multiple dose vials providing 2.5 mg fluphenazine hydrochloride per mL. The preparation also includes sodium chloride for isotonicity, sodium hydroxide or hydrochloric acid to adjust the pH to 4.8–5.2, and 0.1% methylparaben and 0.01% propylparaben as preservatives. At the time of manufacture, the air in the vials is replaced by nitrogen.

CLINICAL PHARMACOLOGY

PROLIXIN has activity at all levels of the central nervous system as well as on multiple organ systems. The mechanism whereby its therapeutic action is exerted is unknown.

INDICATIONS AND USAGE

PROLIXIN Injection is indicated in the management of manifestations of psychotic disorders.

PROLIXIN has not been shown effective in the management of behavorial complications in patients with mental retardation.

CONTRAINDICATIONS

Phenothiazines are contraindicated in patients with suspected or established subcortical brain damage, in patients receiving large doses of hypnotics, and in comatose or severely depressed states. The presence of blood dyscrasia or liver damage precludes the use of fluphenazine hydrochloride. PROLIXIN (fluphenazine hydrochloride) is contraindicated in patients who have shown hypersensitivity to fluphenazine; cross-sensitivity to phenothiazine derivatives may occur.

WARNINGS

Tardive Dyskinesia
Tardive dyskinesia, a syndrome consisting of potentially irreversible, involuntary, dyskinetic movements may develop in patients treated with neuroleptic (antipsychotic) drugs. Although the prevalence of the syndrome appears to be highest among the elderly, especially elderly women, it is impossible to rely upon prevalence estimates to predict, at the inception of neuroleptic treatment, which patients are likely to develop the syndrome. Whether neuroleptic drug products differ in their potential to cause tardive dyskinesia is unknown.

Both the risk of developing the syndrome and the likelihood that it will become irreversible are believed to increase as the duration of treatment and the total cumulative dose of neuroleptic drugs administered to the patient increase. However, the syndrome can develop, although much less commonly, after relatively brief treatment periods at low doses.

There is no known treatment for established cases of tardive dyskinesia, although the syndrome may remit, partially or completely, if neuroleptic treatment is withdrawn. Neuroleptic treatment, itself, however, may suppress (or partially suppress) the signs and symptoms of the syndrome and thereby may possibly mask the underlying disease process. The effect that symptomatic suppression has upon the long-term course of the syndrome is unknown.

Given these considerations, neuroleptics should be prescribed in a manner that is most likely to minimize the occurrence of tardive dyskinesia. Chronic neuroleptic treatment should generally be reserved for patients who suffer from a chronic illness that, 1) is known to respond to neuroleptic drugs, and, 2) for whom alternative, equally effective, but potentially less harmful treatments are *not* available or appropriate. In patients who do require chronic treatment, the smallest dose and the shortest duration of treatment producing a satisfactory clinical response should be sought. The need for continued treatment should be reassessed periodically.

If signs and symptoms of tardive dyskinesia appear in a patient on neuroleptics, drug discontinuation should be considered. However, some patients may require treatment despite the presence of the syndrome.

(For further information about the description of tardive dyskinesia and its clinical detection, please refer to the sections on PRECAUTIONS, Information for Patients and ADVERSE REACTIONS, Tardive Dyskinesia.)

Neuroleptic Malignant Syndrome (NMS)
A potentially fatal symptom complex somtimes referred to as Neuroleptic Malignant Syndrome (NMS) has been reported in association with antipsychotic drugs. Clinical manifestations of NMS are hyperpyrexia, muscle rigidity, altered mental status and evidence of autonomic instability (irregular pulse or blood pressure, tachycardia, diaphoresis, and cardiac dysrhythmias).

The diagnostic evaluation of patients with this syndrome is complicated. In arriving at a diagnosis, it is important to identify cases where the clinical presentation includes both serious medical illness (e.g., pneumonia, systemic infection, etc.) and untreated or inadequately treated extrapyramidal signs and symptoms (EPS). Other important considerations in the differential diagnosis include central anticholinergic toxicity, heat stroke, drug fever and primary central nervous system (CNS) pathology.

The management of NMS should include: 1) immediate discontinuation of antipsychotic drugs and other drugs not essential to concurrent therapy; 2) intensive symptomatic treatment and medical monitoring; and 3) treatment of any concomitant serious medical problems for which specific treatments are available. There is no general agreement about specific pharmacological treatment regimens for uncomplicated NMS.

If a patient requires antipsychotic drug treatment after recovery from NMS, the potential reintroduction of drug therapy should be carefully considered. The patient should be carefully monitored, since recurrences of NMS have been reported.

The use of this drug may impair the mental and physical abilities required for driving a car or operating heavy machinery.

Potentiation of the effects of alcohol may occur with the use of this drug.

Since there is no adequate experience in children who have received this drug, safety and efficacy in children have not been established.

Usage in Pregnancy

The safety for the use of this drug during pregnancy has not been established; therefore, the possible hazards should be weighed against the potential benefits when administering this drug to pregnant patients.

PRECAUTIONS

General

Because of the possibility of cross-sensitivity, fluphenazine hydrochloride should be used cautiously in patients who have developed cholestatic jaundice, dermatoses or other allergic reactions to phenothiazine derivatives.

Psychotic patients on large doses of a phenothiazine drug who are undergoing surgery should be watched carefully for possible hypotensive phenomena. Moreover, it should be remembered that reduced amounts of anesthetics or central nervous system depressants may be necessary.

The effects of atropine may be potentiated in some patients receiving fluphenazine because of added anticholinergic effects.

Fluphenazine hydrochloride should be used cautiously in patients exposed to extreme heat or phosphorus insecticides; in patients with a history of convulsive disorders, since grand mal convulsions have been known to occur; and in patients with special medical disorders, such as mitral insufficiency or other cardiovascular diseases and pheochromocytoma.

The possibility of liver damage, pigmentary retinopathy, lenticular and corneal deposits, and development of irreversible dyskinesia should be remembered when patients are on prolonged therapy.

Neuroleptic drugs elevate prolactin levels; the elevation persists during chronic administration. Tissue culture experiments indicate that approximately one-third of human breast cancers are prolactin dependent *in vitro*, a factor of potential importance if the prescription of these drugs is contemplated in a patient with a previously detected breast cancer. Although disturbances such as galactorrhea, amenorrhea, gynecomastia, and impotence have been reported, the clinical significance of elevated serum prolactin levels is unknown for most patients. An increase in mammary neoplasms has been found in rodents after chronic administration of neuroleptic drugs. Neither clinical studies nor epidemiologic studies conducted to date, however, have shown an association between chronic administration of these drugs and mammary tumorigenesis; the available evidence is considered too limited to be conclusive at this time.

Information for Patients

Given the likelihood that some patients exposed chronically to neuroleptics will develop tardive dyskinesia, it is advised that all patients in whom chronic use is contemplated be given, if possible, full information about this risk. The decision to inform patients and/or their guardians must obviously take into account the clinical circumstances and the competency of the patient to understand the information provided.

Abrupt Withdrawal

In general, phenothiazines do not produce psychic dependence; however, gastritis, nausea and vomiting, dizziness, and tremulousness have been reported following abrupt cessation of high dose therapy. Reports suggest that these symptoms can be reduced if concomitant antiparkinsonian agents are continued for several weeks after the phenothiazine is withdrawn.

Facilities should be available for periodic checking of hepatic function, renal function and the blood picture. Renal function of patients on long-term therapy should be monitored; if BUN (blood urea nitrogen) becomes abnormal, treatment should be discontinued.

As with any phenothiazine, the physician should be alert to the possible development of "silent pneumonias" in patients under treatment with fluphenazine hydrochloride.

ADVERSE REACTIONS

Central Nervous System: The side effects most frequently reported with phenothiazine compounds are extrapyramidal symptoms including pseudoparkinsonism, dystonia, dyskinesia, akathisia, oculogyric crises, opisthotonos, and hyperreflexia. Most often these extrapyramidal symptoms are reversible; however, they may be persistent (see below). With any given phenothiazine derivative, the incidence and severity of such reactions depend more on individual patient sensitivity than on other factors, but dosage level and patient age are also determinants.

Extrapyramidal reactions may be alarming, and the patient should be forewarned and reassured. These reactions can usually be controlled by administration of antiparkinsonian drugs such as Benztropine Mesylate or intravenous Caffeine and Sodium Benzoate Injection, and by subsequent reductions in dosage.

Tardive Dyskinesia: See WARNINGS. The syndrome is characterized by involuntary choreoathetoid movements which variously involve the tongue, face, mouth, lips, or jaw (e.g., protrusion of the tongue, puffing of cheeks, puckering of the mouth, chewing movements), trunk and extremities. The severity of the syndrome and the degree of impairment produced vary widely.

The syndrome may become clinically recognizable either during treatment, upon dosage reduction, or upon withdrawal of treatment. Early detection of tardive dyskinesia is important. To increase the likelihood of detecting the syndrome at the earliest possible time, the dosage of neuroleptic drug should be reduced periodically (if clinically possible) and the patient observed for signs of the disorder. This maneuver is critical, since neuroleptic drugs may mask the signs of the syndrome.

Other CNS Effects: Occurrences of neuroleptic malignant syndrome (NMS) have been reported in patients on neuroleptic therapy (see WARNINGS, Neuroleptic Malignant Syndrome). Leukocytosis, elevated CPK, liver function abnormalities, and acute renal failure may also occur with NMS. Drowsiness or lethargy, if they occur, may necessitate a reduction in dosage; the induction of a catatonic-like state has been known to occur with dosages of fluphenazine far in excess of the recommended amounts. As with other phenothiazine compounds, reactivation or aggravation of psychotic processes may be encountered.

Phenothiazine derivatives have been known to cause, in some patients, restlessness, excitement, or bizarre dreams.

Autonomic Nervous System: Hypertension and fluctuations in blood pressure have been reported with fluphenazine hydrochloride.

Hypotension has rarely presented a problem with fluphenazine. However, patients with pheochromocytoma, cerebral vascular or renal insufficiency, or a severe cardiac reserve deficiency (such as mitral insufficiency) appear to be particularly prone to hypotensive reactions with phenothiazine compounds, and should therefore be observed closely when the drug is administered. If severe hypotension should occur, supportive measures including the use of intravenous vasopressor drugs should be instituted immediately. Levarterenol Bitartrate Injection is the most suitable drug for this purpose; *epinephrine should not be used* since phenothiazine derivatives have been found to reverse its action, resulting in a further lowering of blood pressure.

Autonomic reactions including nausea and loss of appetite, salivation, polyuria, perspiration, dry mouth, headache, and constipation may occur. Autonomic effects can usually be controlled by reducing or temporarily discontinuing dosage. In some patients, phenothiazine derivatives have caused blurred vision, glaucoma, bladder paralysis, fecal impaction, paralytic ileus, tachycardia, or nasal congestion.

Metabolic and Endocrine: Weight change, peripheral edema, abnormal lactation, gynecomastia, menstrual irregularities, false results on pregnancy tests, impotency in men and increased libido in women have all been known to occur in some patients on phenothiazine therapy.

Allergic Reactions: Skin disorders such as itching, erythema, urticaria, seborrhea, photosensitivity, eczema and even exfoliative dermatitis have been reported with phenothiazine derivatives. The possibility of anaphylactoid reactions occurring in some patients should be borne in mind.

Hematologic: Routine blood counts are advisable during therapy since blood dyscrasias including leukopenia, agranulocytosis, thrombocytopenic or nonthrombocytopenic purpura, eosinophilia, and pancytopenia have been observed with phenothiazine derivatives. Furthermore, if any soreness of the mouth, gums, or throat, or any symptoms of upper respiratory infection occur and confirmatory leukocyte count indicates cellular depression, therapy should be discontinued and other appropriate measures instituted immediately.

Hepatic: Liver damage as manifested by cholestatic jaundice may be encountered, particularly during the first months of therapy; treatment should be discontinued if this occurs. An increase in cephalin flocculation, sometimes accompanied by alterations in other liver function tests, have been reported in patients receiving fluphenazine hydrochloride who have had no clinical evidence of liver damage.

Others: Sudden, unexpected and unexplained deaths have been reported in hospitalized psychotic patients receiving phenothiazines. Previous brain damage or seizures may be predisposing factors; high doses should be avoided in known seizure patients. Several patients have shown sudden flareups of psychotic behavior patterns shortly before death. Autopsy findings have usually revealed acute fulminating pneumonia or pneumonitis, aspiration of gastric contents, or intramyocardial lesions.

Although this is not a general feature of fluphenazine, potentiation of central nervous system depressants (opiates, analgesics, antihistamines, barbiturates, alcohol) may occur.

The following adverse reactions have also occurred with phenothiazine derivatives: systemic lupus erythematosus-like syndrome, hypotension severe enough to cause fatal cardiac arrest, altered electrocardiographic and electroencephalographic tracings, altered cerebrospinal fluid proteins, cerebral edema, asthma, laryngeal edema and angioneurotic edema; with long-term use—skin pigmentation, and lenticular and corneal opacities.

DOSAGE AND ADMINISTRATION

The average well-tolerated starting dose for adult psychotic patients is 1.25 mg (0.5 mL) intramuscularly. Depending on the severity and duration of symptoms, initial total daily dosage may range from 2.5 to 10.0 mg and should be divided and given at six- to eight-hour intervals.

The smallest amount that will produce the desired results must be carefully determined for each individual, since optimal dosage levels of this potent derivative vary from patient to patient. In general, the parenteral dose for fluphenazine has been found to be approximately ⅓ to ½ the oral dose. Treatment may be instituted with a *low initial dosage*, which may be increased, if necessary, until the desired clinical effects are achieved. Dosages exceeding 10.0 mg daily should be used with caution.

When symptoms are controlled, oral maintenance therapy can generally be instituted, often with single daily doses. Continued treatment, by the oral route if possible, is needed to achieve maximum therapeutic benefits; further adjustments in dosage may be necessary during the course of therapy to meet the patient's requirements.

HOW SUPPLIED

PROLIXIN Injection (Fluphenazine Hydrochloride Injection USP) is available in multiple dose vials as a sterile, aqueous solution providing 2.5 mg fluphenazine hydrochloride per mL. The drug is also available for oral administration as sugar-coated tablets, a flavored elixir, and an oral solution concentrate.

Storage

Solutions should be protected from exposure to light. Parenteral solutions may vary in color from essentially colorless to light amber. If a solution has become any darker than light amber or is discolored in any other way it should not be used. Store at room temperature; avoid freezing.

(J4-153A)

PROLIXIN® ORAL CONCENTRATE ℞
Fluphenazine Hydrochloride Oral Solution USP

DESCRIPTION

PROLIXIN (fluphenazine hydrochloride) is a trifluoromethyl phenothiazine derivative intended for the management of schizophrenia. PROLIXIN Oral Concentrate (Fluphenazine Hydrochloride Oral Solution) contains 5 mg fluphenazine hydrochloride per mL. Inactive ingredients: alcohol 14%, glycerin, purified water, and sodium benzoate.

CLINICAL PHARMACOLOGY

PROLIXIN has activity at all levels of the central nervous system as well as on multiple organ systems. The mechanism whereby its therapeutic action is exerted is unknown.

INDICATIONS AND USAGE

PROLIXIN is indicated in the management of manifestations of psychotic disorders.

PROLIXIN has not been shown effective in the management of behavorial complications in patients with mental retardation.

CONTRAINDICATIONS

Phenothiazines are contraindicated in patients with suspected or established subcortical brain damage, in patients receiving large doses of hypnotics, and in comatose or severely depressed states. The presence of blood dyscrasia or liver damage precludes the use of fluphenazine hydrochloride. PROLIXIN (fluphenazine hydrochloride) is contraindicated in patients who have shown hypersensitivity to fluphenazine; cross-sensitivity to phenothiazine derivatives may occur.

WARNINGS

Tardive Dyskinesia

Tardive dyskinesia, a syndrome consisting of potentially irreversible, involuntary, dyskinetic movements may develop in patients treated with neuroleptic (antipsychotic) drugs. Although the prevalence of the syndrome appears to be highest among the elderly, especially elderly women, it is impossible to rely upon prevalence estimates to predict, at the inception of neuroleptic treatment, which patients are likely to develop the syndrome. Whether neuroleptic drug products differ in their potential to cause tardive dyskinesia is unknown.

Both the risk of developing the syndrome and the likelihood that it will become irreversible are believed to increase as the duration of treatment and the total cumulative dose of neuroleptic drugs administered to the patient increase. However, the syndrome can develop, although much less commonly, after relatively brief treatment periods at low doses. There is no known treatment for established cases of tardive dyskinesia, although the syndrome may remit, partially or completely, if neuroleptic treatment is withdrawn. Neuroleptic treatment, itself, however, may suppress (or partially suppress) the signs and symptoms of the syndrome and

Continued on next page

Princeton—Cont.

thereby may possibly mask the underlying disease process. The effect that symptomatic suppression has upon the long-term course of the syndrome is unknown.

Given these considerations, neuroleptics should be prescribed in a manner that is most likely to minimize the occurrence of tardive dyskinesia. Chronic neuroleptic treatment should generally be reserved for patients who suffer from a chronic illness that, 1) is known to respond to neuroleptic drugs, and, 2) for whom alternative, equally effective, but potentially less harmful treatments are *not* available or appropriate. In patients who do require chronic treatment, the smallest dose and the shortest duration of treatment producing a satisfactory clinical response should be sought. The need for continued treatment should be reassessed periodically.

If signs and symptoms of tardive dyskinesia appear in a patient on neuroleptics, drug discontinuation should be considered. However, some patients may require treatment despite the presence of the syndrome.

(For further information about the description of tardive dyskinesia and its clinical detection, please refer to the sections on PRECAUTIONS, Information for Patients and ADVERSE REACTIONS, Tardive Dyskinesia.)

Neuroleptic Malignant Syndrome (NMS)

A potentially fatal symptom complex somtimes referred to as Neuroleptic Malignant Syndrome (NMS) has been reported in association with antipsychotic drugs. Clinical manifestations of NMS are hyperpyrexia, muscle rigidity, altered mental status and evidence of autonomic instability (irregular pulse or blood pressure, tachycardia, diaphoresis, and cardiac dysrhythmias).

The diagnostic evaluation of patients with this syndrome is complicated. In arriving at a diagnosis, it is important to identify cases where the clinical presentation includes both serious medical illness (e.g., pneumonia, systemic infection, etc.) and untreated or inadequately treated extrapyramidal signs and symptoms (EPS). Other important considerations in the differential diagnosis include central anticholinergic toxicity, heat stroke, drug fever and primary central nervous system (CNS) pathology.

The management of NMS should include: 1) immediate discontinuation of antipsychotic drugs and other drugs not essential to concurrent therapy; 2) intensive symptomatic treatment and medical monitoring; and 3) treatment of any concomitant serious medical problems for which specific treatments are available. There is no general agreement about specific pharmacological treatment regimens for uncomplicated NMS.

If a patient requires antipsychotic drug treatment after recovery from NMS, the potential reintroduction of drug therapy should be carefully considered. The patient should be carefully monitored, since recurrences of NMS have been reported.

The use of this drug may impair the mental and physical abilities required for driving a car or operating heavy machinery.

Potentiation of the effects of alcohol may occur with the use of this drug.

Since there is no adequate experience in children who have received this drug, safety and efficacy in children have not been established.

Usage In Pregnancy

The safety for the use of this drug during pregnancy has not been established; therefore, the possible hazards should be weighed against the potential benefits when administering this drug to pregnant patients.

PRECAUTIONS

General

Because of the possibility of cross-sensitivity, fluphenazine hydrochloride should be used cautiously in patients who have developed cholestatic jaundice, dermatoses or other allergic reactions to phenothiazine derivatives.

Psychotic patients on large doses of a phenothiazine drug who are undergoing surgery should be watched carefully for possible hypotensive phenomena. Moreover, it should be remembered that reduced amounts of anesthetics or central nervous system depressants may be necessary.

The effects of atropine may be potentiated in some patients receiving fluphenazine because of added anticholinergic effects.

Fluphenazine hydrochloride should be used cautiously in patients exposed to extreme heat or phosphorus insecticides; in patients with a history of convulsive disorders, since grand mal convulsions have been known to occur; and in patients with special medical disorders, such as mitral insufficiency or other cardiovascular diseases and pheochromocytoma.

The possibility of liver damage, pigmentary retinopathy, lenticular and corneal deposits, and development of irreversible dyskinesia should be remembered when patients are on prolonged therapy.

Neuroleptic drugs elevate prolactin levels; the elevation persists during chronic administration. Tissue culture experiments indicate that approximately one-third of human breast cancers are prolactin dependent *in vitro*, a factor of potential importance if the prescription of these drugs is contemplated in a patient with a previously detected breast cancer. Although disturbances such as galactorrhea, amenorrhea, gynecomastia, and impotence have been reported, the clinical significance of elevated serum prolactin levels is unknown for most patients. An increase in mammary neoplasms has been found in rodents after chronic administration of neuroleptic drugs. Neither clinical studies nor epidemiologic studies conducted to date, however, have shown an association between chronic administration of these drugs and mammary tumorigenesis; the available evidence is considered too limited to be conclusive at this time.

Information for Patients

Given the likelihood that some patients exposed chronically to neuroleptics will develop tardive dyskinesia, it is advised that all patients in whom chronic use is contemplated be given, if possible, full information about this risk. The decision to inform patients and/or their guardians must obviously take into account the clinical circumstances and the competency of the patient to understand the information provided.

Abrupt Withdrawal

In general, phenothiazines do not produce psychic dependence; however, gastritis, nausea and vomiting, dizziness, and tremulousness have been reported following abrupt cessation of high dose therapy. Reports suggest that these symptoms can be reduced if concomitant antiparkinsonian agents are continued for several weeks after the phenothiazine is withdrawn.

Facilities should be available for periodic checking of hepatic function, renal function and the blood picture. Renal function of patients on long-term therapy should be monitored; if BUN (blood urea nitrogen) becomes abnormal, treatment should be discontinued.

As with any phenothiazine, the physician should be alert to the possible development of "silent pneumonias" in patients under treatment with fluphenazine hydrochloride.

ADVERSE REACTIONS

Central Nervous System: The side effects most frequently reported with phenothiazine compounds are extrapyramidal symptoms including pseudoparkinsonism, dystonia, dyskinesia, akathisia, oculogyric crises, opisthotonos, and hyperreflexia. Most often these extrapyramidal symptoms are reversible; however, they may be persistent (see below). With any given phenothiazine derivative, the incidence and severity of such reactions depend more on individual patient sensitivity than on other factors, but dosage level and patient age are also determinants.

Extrapyramidal reactions may be alarming, and the patient should be forewarned and reassured. These reactions can usually be controlled by administration of antiparkinsonian drugs such as Benztropine Mesylate or intravenous Caffeine and Sodium Benzoate Injection, and by subsequent reduction in dosage.

Tardive Dyskinesia: See WARNINGS. The syndrome is characterized by involuntary choreoathetoid movements which variously involve the tongue, face, mouth, lips, or jaw (e.g., protrusion of the tongue, puffing of cheeks, puckering of the mouth, chewing movements), trunk and extremities. The severity of the syndrome and the degree of impairment produced vary widely.

The syndrome may become clinically recognizable either during treatment, upon dosage reduction, or upon withdrawal of treatment. Early detection of tardive dyskinesia is important. To increase the likelihood of detecting the syndrome at the earliest possible time, the dosage of neuroleptic drug should be reduced periodically (if clinically possible) and the patient observed for signs of the disorder. This maneuver is critical, since neuroleptic drugs may mask the signs of the syndrome.

Other CNS Effects: Occurrences of neuroleptic malignant syndrome (NMS) have been reported in patients on neuroleptic therapy (see WARNINGS, Neuroleptic Malignant Syndrome). Leukocytosis, elevated CPK, liver function abnormalities, and acute renal failure may also occur with NMS. Drowsiness or lethargy, if they occur, may necessitate a reduction in dosage; the induction of a catatonic-like state has been known to occur with dosages of fluphenazine far in excess of the recommended amounts. As with other phenothiazine compounds, reactivation or aggravation of psychotic processes may be encountered.

Phenothiazine derivatives have been known to cause, in some patients, restlessness, excitement, or bizarre dreams.

Autonomic Nervous System: Hypertension and fluctuation in blood pressure have been reported with fluphenazine hydrochloride.

Hypotension has rarely presented a problem with fluphenazine. However, patients with pheochromocytoma, cerebral vascular or renal insufficiency, or a severe cardiac reserve deficiency (such as mitral insufficiency) appear to be particularly prone to hypotensive reactions with phenothiazine

compounds, and should therefore be observed closely when the drug is administered. If severe hypotension should occur, supportive measures including the use of intravenous vasopressor drugs should be instituted immediately. Levarterenol Bitartrate Injection is the most suitable drug for this purpose; *epinephrine should not be used* since phenothiazine derivatives have been found to reverse its action, resulting in a further lowering of blood pressure.

Autonomic reactions including nausea and loss of appetite, salivation, polyuria, perspiration, dry mouth, headache, and constipation may occur. Autonomic effects can usually be controlled by reducing or temporarily discontinuing dosage. In some patients, phenothiazine derivatives have caused blurred vision, glaucoma, bladder paralysis, fecal impaction, paralytic ileus, tachycardia, or nasal congestion.

Metabolic and Endocrine: Weight change, peripheral edema, abnormal lactation, gynecomastia, menstrual irregularities, false results on pregnancy tests, impotency in men and increased libido in women have all been known to occur in some patients on phenothiazine therapy.

Allergic Reactions: Skin disorders such as itching, erythema, urticaria, seborrhea, photosensitivity, eczema and even exfoliative dermatitis have been reported with phenothiazine derivatives. The possibility of anaphylactoid reactions occurring in some patients should be borne in mind.

Hematologic: Routine blood counts are advisable during therapy since blood dyscrasias including leukopenia, agranulocytosis, thrombocytopenic or nonthrombocytopenic purpura, eosinophilia, and pancytopenia have been observed with phenothiazine derivatives. Furthermore, if any soreness of the mouth, gums, or throat, or any symptoms of upper respiratory infection occur and confirmatory leukocyte count indicates cellular depression, therapy should be discontinued and other appropriate measures instituted immediately.

Hepatic: Liver damage as manifested by cholestatic jaundice may be encountered, particularly during the first months of therapy; treatment should be discontinued if this occurs. An increase in cephalin flocculation, sometimes accompanied by alterations in other liver function tests, have been reported in patients receiving fluphenazine hydrochloride who have had no clinical evidence of liver damage.

Others: Sudden, unexpected and unexplained deaths have been reported in hospitalized psychotic patients receiving phenothiazines. Previous brain damage or seizures may be predisposing factors; high doses should be avoided in known seizure patients. Several patients have shown sudden flareups of psychotic behavior patterns shortly before death. Autopsy findings have usually revealed acute fulminating pneumonia or pneumonitis, aspiration of gastric contents, or intramyocardial lesions.

Although this is not a general feature of fluphenazine, potentiation of central nervous system depressants (opiates, analgesics, antihistamines, barbiturates, alcohol) may occur.

The following adverse reactions have also occurred with phenothiazine derivatives: systemic lupus erythematosus-like syndrome, hypotension severe enough to cause fatal cardiac arrest, altered electrocardiographic and electroencephalographic tracings, altered cerebrospinal fluid proteins, cerebral edema, asthma, laryngeal edema, and angioneurotic edema; with long-term use—skin pigmentation, and lenticular and corneal opacities.

DOSAGE AND ADMINISTRATION

Depending on the severity and duration of symptoms, total daily dosage for *adult* psychotic patients may range initally from 2.5 to 10.0 mg and should be divided and given at six- to eight-hour intervals.

The smallest amount that will produce the desired results must be carefully determined for each individual, since optimal dosage levels of this potent drug vary from patient to patient. In general, the oral dose has been found to be approximately two to three times the parenteral dose of fluphenazine. Treatment is best instituted with a *low initial dosage*, which may be increased, if necessary, until the desired clinical effects are achieved. Therapeutic effect is often achieved with doses under 20 mg daily. Patients remaining severely disturbed or inadequately controlled may require upward titration of dosage. Daily doses up to 40 mg may be necessary; controlled clinical studies have not been performed to demonstrate safety of prolonged administration of such doses.

When symptoms are controlled, dosage can generally be reduced gradually to daily maintenance doses of 1.0 or 5.0 mg, often given as a single daily dose. Continued treatment is needed to achieve maximum therapeutic benefits; further adjustments in dosage may be necessary during the course of therapy to meet the patient's requirements.

For psychotic patients who have been stabilized on a fixed daily dosage of orally administered PROLIXIN (fluphenazine hydrochloride) dosage forms, conversion to the long-acting injectable PROLIXIN DECANOATE may be indicated [see package insert for PROLIXIN DECANOATE (Fluphenazine Decanoate Injection) for conversion information].

For *geriatric* patients, the suggested starting dose is 1.0 to 2.5 mg daily, adjusted according to the response of the patient.

When the Oral Concentrate dosage form is to be used, the desired dose (measured by calibrated device only) should be added to at least 60 mL (2 fl oz) of a suitable diluent *just prior to administration* to insure palatability and stability. Suggested diluents include tomato or fruit juice, milk, and uncaffeinated soft drinks. The Oral Concentrate should not be mixed with beverages containing caffeine (coffee, cola), tannics (tea), or pectinates (apple juice) because of potential incompatibility.

PROLIXIN Injection (Fluphenazine Hydrochloride Injection USP) is useful when psychotic patients are unable or unwilling to take oral therapy.

HOW SUPPLIED

120 mL bottle with a 1 mL safety-cap dropper calibrated at 0.1 mL and in 0.2 mL increments. 5 mg fluphenazine hydrochloride per mL. NDC 0003-0801-10.

PROLIXIN (fluphenazine hydrochloride) is also available as a sterile aqueous solution for intramuscular use, plus tablets and elixir for oral administration. See specific package insert for complete information.

Storage

Store at room temperature; avoid freezing. Protect from light. Keeep tightly closed.

(J4-147B)

PROLIXIN® TABLETS   ℞
Fluphenazine Hydrochloride Tablets USP
PROLIXIN® ELIXIR   ℞
Fluphenazine Hydrochloride Elixir USP

DESCRIPTION

PROLIXIN is a trifluoromethyl phenothiazine derivative intended for the management of schizophrenia.
PROLIXIN Tablets (Fluphenazine Hydrochloride Tablets) contain 1, 2.5, 5, and 10 mg fluphenazine hydrochloride per tablet. Inactive ingredients: acacia; carnauba wax for 1 and 2.5 mg only; castor oil; colorants [D&C Yellow No. 10 for 5 and 10 mg only; FD&C Blue No. 1 for 5 and 10 mg only; FD&C Blue No. 2 for 2.5 mg only; FD&C Red No. 3 for 1 and 10 mg only; and FD&C Yellow No. 5 (tartrazine) for 2.5, 5, and 10 mg only]; corn starch; ethylcellulose; gelatin; lactose; magnesium carbonate; magnesium stearate; pharmaceutical glaze; polyethylene glycol for 1 and 2.5 mg only; povidone for 1 and 2.5 mg only; precipitated calcium carbonate; sodium benzoate for 1, 2.5, and 5 mg only; sucrose; synthetic iron oxide; talc; titanium dioxide; white wax for 1 and 2.5 mg only; and other ingredients.
PROLIXIN Elixir (Fluphenazine Hydrochloride Elixir) contains 0.5 mg fluphenazine hydrochloride per mL. Inactive ingredients: alcohol [14% (v/v)], colorant (FD&C Yellow No. 6), flavors, glycerin, polysorbate 40, purified water, sodium benzoate, and sucrose.

CLINICAL PHARMACOLOGY

PROLIXIN has activity at all levels of the central nervous system as well as on multiple organ systems. The mechanism whereby its therapeutic action is exerted is unknown.

INDICATIONS AND USAGE

PROLIXIN is indicated in the management of manifestations of psychotic disorders.
PROLIXIN has not been shown effective in the management of behavioral complications in patients with mental retardation.

CONTRAINDICATIONS

Phenothiazines are contraindicated in patients with suspected or established subcortical brain damage, in patients receiving large doses of hypnotics, and in comatose or severely depressed states. The presence of blood dyscrasia or liver damage precludes the use of fluphenazine hydrochloride. PROLIXIN (fluphenazine hydrochloride) is contraindicated in patients who have shown hypersensitivity to fluphenazine; cross-sensitivity to phenothiazine derivatives may occur.

WARNINGS

Tardive Dyskinesia

Tardive dyskinesia, a syndrome consisting of potentially irreversible, involuntary, dyskinetic movements may develop in patients treated with neuroleptic (antipsychotic) drugs. Although the prevalence of the syndrome appears to be highest among the elderly, especially elderly women, it is impossible to rely upon prevalence estimates to predict, at the inception of neuroleptic treatment, which patients are likely to develop the syndrome. Whether neuroleptic drug products differ in their potential to cause tardive dyskinesia is unknown.

Both the risk of developing the syndrome and the likelihood that it will become irreversible are believed to increase as the duration of treatment and the total cumulative dose of neuroleptic drugs administered to the patient increase. However, the syndrome can develop, although much less commonly, after relatively brief treatment periods at low doses. There is no known treatment for established cases of tardive dyskinesia, although the syndrome may remit, partially or completely, if neuroleptic treatment is withdrawn. Neuroleptic treatment, itself, however, may suppress (or partially suppress) the signs and symptoms of the syndrome and thereby may possibly mask the underlying disease process. The effect that symptomatic suppression has upon the long-term course of the syndrome is unknown.

Given these considerations, neuroleptics should be prescribed in a manner that is most likely to minimize the occurrence of tardive dyskinesia. Chronic neuroleptic treatment should generally be reserved for patients who suffer from a chronic illness that, 1) is known to respond to neuroleptic drugs, and, 2) for whom alternative, equally effective, but potentially less harmful treatments are *not* available or appropriate. In patients who do require chronic treatment, the smallest dose and the shortest duration of treatment producing a satisfactory clinical response should be sought. The need for continued treatment should be reassessed periodically.

If signs and symptoms of tardive dyskinesia appear in a patient on neuroleptics, drug discontinuation should be considered. However, some patients may require treatment despite the presence of the syndrome.

(For further information about the description of tardive dyskinesia and its clinical detection, please refer to the sections on PRECAUTIONS, Information for Patients and ADVERSE REACTIONS, Tardive Dyskinesia.)

Neuroleptic Malignant Syndrome (NMS)

A potentially fatal symptom complex somtimes referred to as Neuroleptic Malignant Syndrome (NMS) has been reported in association with antipsychotic drugs. Clinical manifestations of NMS are hyperpyrexia, muscle rigidity, altered mental status and evidence of autonomic instability (irregular pulse or blood pressure, tachycardia, diaphoresis, and cardiac dysrhythmias).

The diagnostic evaluation of patients with this syndrome is complicated. In arriving at a diagnosis, it is important to identify cases where the clinical presentation includes both serious medical illness (e.g., pneumonia, systemic infection, etc.) and untreated or inadequately treated extrapyramidal signs and symptoms. Other important considerations in the differential diagnosis include central anticholinergic toxicity, heat stroke, drug fever and primary central nervous system pathology.

The management of NMS should include: 1) immediate discontinuation of antipsychotic drugs and other drugs not essential to concurrent therapy; 2) intensive symptomatic treatment and medical monitoring; and 3) treatment of any concomitant serious medical problems for which specific treatments are available. There is no general agreement about specific pharmacological treatment regimens for uncomplicated NMS.

If a patient requires antipsychotic drug treatment after recovery from NMS, the potential reintroduction of drug therapy should be carefully considered. The patient should be carefully monitored, since recurrences of NMS have been reported.

The use of this drug may impair the mental and physical abilities required for driving or operating heavy machinery. Potentiation of the effects of alcohol may occur with the use of this drug.

Since there is no adequate experience in children who have received this drug, safety and efficacy in children have not been established.

Usage in Pregnancy

The safety for the use of this drug during pregnancy has not been established; therefore, the possible hazards should be weighed against the potential benefits when administering this drug to pregnant patients.

PRECAUTIONS

General

Because of the possibility of cross-sensitivity, fluphenazine hydrochloride should be used cautiously in patients who have developed cholestatic jaundice, dermatoses or other allergic reactions to phenothiazine derivatives.

PROLIXIN Tablets (Fluphenazine Hydrochloride Tablets) 2.5, 5, and 10 mg contain FD&C Yellow No. 5 (tartrazine) which may cause allergic-type reactions (including bronchial asthma) in certain susceptible individuals. Although the overall incidence of FD&C Yellow No. 5 (tartrazine) sensitivity in the general population is low, it is frequently seen in patients who also have aspirin hypersensitivity.

Psychotic patients on large doses of a phenothiazine drug who are undergoing surgery should be watched carefully for possible hypotensive phenomena. Moreover, it should be remembered that reduced amounts of anesthetics or central nervous system depressants may be necessary.

The effects of atropine may be potentiated in some patients receiving fluphenazine because of added anticholinergic effects.

Fluphenazine hydrochloride should be used cautiously in patients exposed to extreme heat or phosphorus insecticides; in patients with a history of convulsive disorders, since grand mal convulsions have been known to occur; and in patients with special medical disorders, such as mitral insuf-

ficiency or other cardiovascular diseases and pheochromocytoma.

The possibility of liver damage, pigmentary retinopathy, lenticular and corneal deposits, and development of irreversible dyskinesia should be remembered when patients are on prolonged therapy.

Neuroleptic drugs elevate prolactin levels; the elevation persists during chronic administration. Tissue culture experiments indicate that approximately one-third of human breast cancers are prolactin dependent *in vitro*, a factor of potential importance if the prescription of these drugs is contemplated in a patient with a previously detected breast cancer. Although disturbances such as galactorrhea, amenorrhea, gynecomastia, and impotence have been reported, the clinical significance of elevated serum prolactin levels is unknown for most patients. An increase in mammary neoplasms has been found in rodents after chronic administration of neuroleptic drugs. Neither clinical studies nor epidemiologic studies conducted to date, however, have shown an association between chronic administration of these drugs and mammary tumorigenesis; the available evidence is considered too limited to be conclusive at this time.

Information for Patients

Given the likelihood that some patients exposed chronically to neuroleptics will develop tardive dyskinesia, it is advised that all patients in whom chronic use is contemplated be given, if possible, full information about this risk. The decision to inform patients and/or their guardians must obviously take into account the clinical circumstances and the competency of the patient to understand the information provided.

Abrupt Withdrawal

In general, phenothiazines do not produce psychic dependence; however, gastritis, nausea and vomiting, dizziness, and tremulousness have been reported following abrupt cessation of high dose therapy. Reports suggest that these symptoms can be reduced if concomitant antiparkinsonian agents are continued for several weeks after the phenothiazine is withdrawn.

Facilities should be available for periodic checking of hepatic function, renal function and the blood picture. Renal function of patients on long-term therapy should be monitored; if BUN (blood urea nitrogen) becomes abnormal, treatment should be discontinued.

As with any phenothiazine, the physician should be alert to the possible development of "silent pneumonias" in patients under treatment with fluphenazine hydrochloride.

ADVERSE REACTIONS

Central Nervous System: The side effects most frequently reported with phenothiazine compounds are extrapyramidal symptoms including pseudoparkinsonism, dystonia, dyskinesia, akathisia, oculogyric crises, opisthotonos, and hyperreflexia. Most often these extrapyramidal symptoms are reversible; however, they may be persistent (see below). With any given phenothiazine derivative, the incidence and severity of such reactions depend more on individual patient sensitivity than on other factors, but dosage level and patient age are also determinants.

Extrapyramidal reactions may be alarming, and the patient should be forewarned and reassured. These reactions can usually be controlled by administration of antiparkinsonian drugs such as Benztropine Mesylate or intravenous Caffeine and Sodium Benzoate Injection, and by subsequent reduction in dosage.

Tardive Dyskinesia: See WARNINGS. The syndrome is characterized by involuntary choreoathetoid movements which variously involve the tongue, face, mouth, lips, or jaw (e.g., protrusion of the tongue, puffing of cheeks, puckering of the mouth, chewing movements), trunk and extremities. The severity of the syndrome and the degree of impairment produced vary widely.

The syndrome may become clinically recognizable either during treatment, upon dosage reduction, or upon withdrawal of treatment. Early detection of tardive dyskinesia is important. To increase the likelihood of detecting the syndrome at the earliest possible time, the dosage of neuroleptic drug should be reduced periodically (if clinically possible) and the patient observed for signs of the disorder. This maneuver is critical, since neuroleptic drugs may mask the signs of the syndrome.

Other CNS Effects: Occurrences of neuroleptic malignant syndrome (NMS) have been reported in patients on neuroleptic therapy (see WARNINGS, Neuroleptic Malignant Syndrome). Leukocytosis, elevated CPK, liver function abnormalities, and acute renal failure may also occur with NMS.

Drowsiness or lethargy, if they occur, may necessitate a reduction in dosage; the induction of a catatonic-like state has been known to occur with dosages of fluphenazine far in excess of the recommended amounts. As with other phenothiazine compounds, reactivation or aggravation of psychotic processes may be encountered.

Phenothiazine derivatives have been known to cause, in some patients, restlessness, excitement, or bizarre dreams.

Continued on next page

Princeton—Cont.

Autonomic Nervous System: Hypertension and fluctuations in blood pressure have been reported with fluphenazine hydrochloride.

Hypotension has rarely presented a problem with fluphenazine. However, patients with pheochromocytoma, cerebral vascular or renal insufficiency, or a severe cardiac reserve deficiency (such as mitral insufficiency) appear to be particularly prone to hypotensive reactions with phenothiazine compounds, and should therefore be observed closely when the drug is administered. If severe hypotension should occur, supportive measures including the use of intravenous vasopressor drugs should be instituted immediately. Levarterenol Bitartrate Injection is the most suitable drug for this purpose; *epinephrine should not be used* since phenothiazine derivatives have been found to reverse its action, resulting in a further lowering of blood pressure.

Autonomic reactions including nausea and loss of appetite, salivation, polyuria, perspiration, dry mouth, headache, and constipation may occur. Autonomic effects can usually be controlled by reducing or temporarily discontinuing dosage. In some patients, phenothiazine derivatives have caused blurred vision, glaucoma, bladder paralysis, fecal impaction, paralytic ileus, tachycardia, or nasal congestion.

Metabolic and Endocrine: Weight change, peripheral edema, abnormal lactation, gynecomastia, menstrual irregularities, false results on pregnancy tests, impotency in men and increased libido in women have all been known to occur in some patients on phenothiazine therapy.

Allergic Reactions: Skin disorders such as itching, erythema, urticaria, seborrhea, photosensitivity, eczema and even exfoliative dermatitis have been reported with phenothiazine derivatives. The possibility of anaphylactoid reactions occurring in some patients should be borne in mind.

Hematologic: Routine blood counts are advisable during therapy since blood dyscrasias including leukopenia, agranulocytosis, thrombocytopenic or nonthrombocytopenic purpura, eosinophilia, and pancytopenia have been observed with phenothiazine derivatives. Furthermore, if any soreness of the mouth, gums, or throat, or any symptoms of upper respiratory infection occur and confirmatory leukocyte count indicates cellular depression, therapy should be discontinued and other appropriate measures instituted immediately.

Hepatic: Liver damage as manifested by cholestatic jaundice may be encountered, particularly during the first months of therapy; treatment should be discontinued if this occurs. An increase in cephalin flocculation, sometimes accompanied by alterations in other liver function tests, has been reported in patients receiving fluphenazine hydrochloride who have had no clinical evidence of liver damage.

Others: Sudden, unexpected and unexplained deaths have been reported in hospitalized psychotic patients receiving phenothiazines. Previous brain damage or seizures may be predisposing factors; high doses should be avoided in known seizure patients. Several patients have shown sudden flareups of psychotic behavior patterns shortly before death. Autopsy findings have usually revealed acute fulminating pneumonia or pneumonitis, aspiration of gastric contents, or intramyocardial lesions.

Although this is not a general feature of fluphenazine, potentiation of central nervous system depressants (opiates, analgesics, antihistamines, barbiturates, alcohol) may occur.

The following adverse reactions have also occurred with phenothiazine derivatives: systemic lupus erythematosuslike syndrome, hypotension severe enough to cause fatal cardiac arrest, altered electrocardiographic and electroencephalographic tracings, altered cerebrospinal fluid proteins, cerebral edema, asthma, laryngeal edema and angioneurotic edema; with long-term use—skin pigmentation, and lenticular and corneal opacities.

DOSAGE AND ADMINISTRATION

Depending on the severity and duration of symptoms, total daily oral dosage for *adult* psychotic patients may range initially from 2.5 to 10.0 mg and should be divided and given at six- to eight-hour intervals.

The smallest amount that will produce the desired results must be carefully determined for each individual, since optimal dosage levels of this potent drug vary from patient to patient. In general, the oral dose has been found to be approximately two to three times the parenteral dose of fluphenazine. Treatment is best instituted with a *low initial dosage*, which may be increased, if necessary, until the desired clinical effects are achieved. Therapeutic effect is often achieved with doses under 20 mg daily. Patients remaining severely disturbed or inadequately controlled may require upward titration of dosage. Daily doses up to 40 mg may be necessary; controlled clinical studies have not been performed to demonstrate safety of prolonged administration of such doses.

When symptoms are controlled, dosage can generally be reduced gradually to daily maintenance doses of 1.0 or 5.0 mg, often given as a single daily dose. Continued treatment is needed to achieve maximum therapeutic benefits; further adjustments in dosage may be necessary during the course of therapy to meet the patient's requirements.

For psychotic patients who have been stabilized on a fixed daily dosage of orally administered PROLIXIN (fluphenazine hydrochloride) dosage forms, conversion to the long-acting injectable PROLIXIN DECANOATE may be indicated [see package insert for PROLIXIN DECANOATE (Fluphenazine Decanoate Injection) for conversion information]. For *geriatric* patients, the suggested starting dose is 1.0 to 2.5 mg daily, adjusted according to the response of the patient. PROLIXIN Injection (Fluphenazine Hydrochloride Injection USP) is useful when psychotic patients are unable or unwilling to take oral therapy.

HOW SUPPLIED

PROLIXIN Tablets

(Fluphenazine Hydrochloride Tablets USP)

1 mg: bottles of 50 (NDC 0003-0863-40), 100 (NDC 0003-0863-50), and 500 (NDC 0003-0863-70)

2.5 mg: bottles of 50 (NDC 0003-0864-40), 100 (NDC 0003-0864-50), and 500 (NDC 0003-0864-70)

5 mg: bottles of 50 (NDC 0003-0877-40), 100 (NDC 0003-0877-50), and 500 (NDC 0003-0877-70)

10 mg: bottles of 50 (NDC 0003-0956-40), 100 (NDC 0003-0956-50), and 500 (NDC 0003-0956-70)

Unimatic® single dose

(tablets individually sealed) packages

1 mg: 100 (NDC 0003-0863-55)

2.5 mg: 100 (NDC 0003-0864 52)

5 mg: 100 (NDC 0003-0877-52)

10 mg: 100 (NDC 0003-0956-52)

Identification Numbers on Tablets: 1 mg, **863**; 2.5 mg, **864**; 5 mg **877**; 10 mg, **956.**

PROLIXIN Elixir

(Fluphenazine Hydrochloride Elixir USP)

0.5 mg/mL (2.5 mg per 5 mL teaspoonful)

60 mL bottle with calibrated dropper: NDC 0003-0820-30

473 mL bottle: NDC 0003-0820-50

PROLIXIN (fluphenazine hydrochloride) is also available as an oral solution concentrate and a sterile aqueous solution for intramuscular use. See specific package inserts for complete information.

Storage

Store tablets and elixir at room temperature. Protect from light. Keep tightly closed.

Tablets: Avoid excessive heat.

Elixir: Avoid freezing.

(J4-120C)

Shown in Product Identification Section, page 422

PROLIXIN DECANOATE®   ℞

[pro "lik 'sin dek "ah-nō 'āt]

Fluphenazine Decanoate Injection

DESCRIPTION

PROLIXIN DECANOATE is the decanoate ester of a trifluoromethyl phenothiazine derivative. It is a highly potent behavior modifier with a markedly extended duration of effect. PROLIXIN DECANOATE is available for intramuscular or subcutaneous administration, providing 25 mg fluphenazine decanoate per mL in a sesame oil vehicle with 1.2% (w/v) benzyl alcohol as a preservative. At the time of manufacture, the air in the vials is replaced by nitrogen.

CLINICAL PHARMACOLOGY

The basic effects of fluphenazine decanoate appear to be no different from those of fluphenazine hydrochloride, with the exception of duration of action. The esterification of fluphenazine markedly prolongs the drug's duration of effect without unduly attenuating its beneficial action.

PROLIXIN DECANOATE has activity at all levels of the central nervous system as well as on multiple organ systems. The mechanism whereby its therapeutic action is exerted is unknown.

Fluphenazine differs from other phenothiazine derivatives in several respects: it is more potent on a milligram basis, it has less potentiating effect on central nervous system depressants and anesthetics than do some of the phenothiazines and appears to be less sedating, and it is less likely than some of the older phenothiazines to produce hypotension (nevertheless, appropriate cautions should be observed—see sections on PRECAUTIONS and ADVERSE REACTIONS).

INDICATIONS AND USAGE

PROLIXIN DECANOATE (Fluphenazine Decanoate Injection) is a long-acting parenteral antipsychotic drug intended for use in the management of patients requiring prolonged parenteral neuroleptic therapy (e.g., chronic schizophrenics).

PROLIXIN DECANOATE has not been shown effective in the management of behavioral complications in patients with mental retardation.

CONTRAINDICATIONS

Phenothiazines are contraindicated in patients with suspected or established subcortical brain damage.

Phenothiazine compounds should not be used in patients receiving large doses of hypnotics.

PROLIXIN DECANOATE (Fluphenazine Decanoate Injection is contraindicated in comatose or severely depressed states.

The presence of blood dyscrasia or liver damage precludes the use of fluphenazine decanoate.

Fluphenazine decanoate is not intended for use in children under 12 years of age.

PROLIXIN DECANOATE is contraindicated in patients who have shown hypersensitivity to fluphenazine; crosssensitivity to phenothiazine derivatives may occur.

Warnings

Tardive Dyskinesia

Tardive dyskinesia, a syndrome consisting of potentially irreversible, involuntary, dyskinetic movements may develop in patients treated with neuroleptic (antipsychotic) drugs. Although the prevalence of the syndrome appears to be highest among the elderly, especially elderly women, it is impossible to rely upon prevalence estimates to predict, at the inception of neuroleptic treatment, which patients are likely to develop the syndrome. Whether neuroleptic drug products differ in their potential to cause tardive dyskinesia is unknown.

Both the risk of developing the syndrome and the likelihood that it will become irreversible are believed to increase as the duration of treatment and the total cumulative dose of neuroleptic drugs administered to the patient increase. However, the syndrome can develop, although much less commonly, after relatively brief treatment periods at low doses. There is no known treatment for established cases of tardive dyskinesia, although the syndrome may remit, partially or completely, if neuroleptic treatment is withdrawn. Neuroleptic treatment, itself, however, may suppress (or partially suppress) the signs and symptoms of the syndrome and thereby may possibly mask the underlying disease process. The effect that symptomatic suppression has upon the long-term course of the syndrome is unknown.

Given these considerations, neuroleptics should be prescribed in a manner that is most likely to minimize the occurrence of tardive dyskinesia. Chronic neuroleptic treatment should generally be reserved for patients who suffer from a chronic illness that, 1) is known to respond to neuroleptic drugs, and, 2) for whom alternative, equally effective, but potentially less harmful treatments are *not* available or appropriate. In patients who do require chronic treatment, the smallest dose and the shortest duration of treatment producing a satisfactory clinical response should be sought. The need for continued treatment should be reassessed periodically.

If signs and symptoms of tardive dyskinesia appear in a patient on neuroleptics, drug discontinuation should be considered. However, some patients may require treatment despite the presence of the syndrome.

(For further information about the description of tardive dyskinesia and its clinical detection, please refer to the sections on PRECAUTIONS, Information for Patients and ADVERSE REACTIONS, Tardive Dyskinesia.)

Neuroleptic Malignant Syndrome (NMS)

A potentially fatal symptom complex sometimes referred to as Neuroleptic Malignant Syndrome (NMS) has been reported in association with antipsychotic drugs. Clinical manifestations of NMS are hyperpyrexia, muscle rigidity, altered mental status and evidence of autonomic instability (irregular pulse or blood pressure, tachycardia, diaphoresis, and cardiac dysrhythmias).

The diagnostic evaluation of patients with this syndrome is complicated. In arriving at a diagnosis, it is important to identify cases where the clinical presentation includes both serious medical illness (e.g., pneumonia, systemic infection, etc.) and untreated or inadequately treated extrapyramidal signs and symptoms (EPS). Other important considerations in the differential diagnosis include central anticholinergic toxicity, heat stroke, drug fever and primary central nervous system (CNS) pathology.

The management of NMS should include: 1) immediate discontinuation of antipsychotic drugs and other drugs not essential to concurrent therapy; 2) intensive symptomatic treatment and medical monitoring; and 3) treatment of any concomitant serious medical problems for which specific treatments are available. There is no general agreement about specific pharmacological treatment regimens for uncomplicated NMS.

If a patient requires antipsychotic drug treatment after recovery from NMS, the potential reintroduction of drug therapy should be carefully considered. The patient should be carefully monitored, since recurrences of NMS have been reported.

The use of this drug may impair the mental and physical abilities required for driving a car or operating heavy machinery.

Physicians should be alert to the possibility that severe adverse reactions may occur which require immediate medical attention.

Potentiation of the effects of alcohol may occur with the use of this drug.

Since there is no adequate experience in children who have received this drug, safety and efficacy in children have not been established.

Usage in Pregnancy

The safety for the use of this drug during pregnancy has not been established; therefore, the possible hazards should be weighed against the potential benefits when administering this drug to pregnant patients.

PRECAUTIONS

General

Because of the possibility of cross-sensitivity, fluphenazine decanoate should be used cautiously in patients who have developed cholestatic jaundice, dermatoses, or other allergic reactions to phenothiazine derivatives.

Psychotic patients on large doses of a phenothiazine drug who are undergoing surgery should be watched carefully for possible hypotensive phenomena. Moreover, it should be remembered that reduced amounts of anesthetics or central nervous system depressants may be necessary.

The effects of atropine may be potentiated in some patients receiving fluphenazine because of added anticholinergic effects.

Fluphenazine decanoate should be used cautiously in patients exposed to extreme heat or phosphorus insecticides. The preparation should be used with caution in patients with a history of convulsive disorders, since grand mal convulsions have been known to occur.

Use with caution in patients with special medical disorders such as mitral insufficiency or other cardiovascular diseases and pheochromocytoma.

The possibility of liver damage, pigmentary retinopathy, lenticular and corneal deposits, and development of irreversible dyskinesia should be remembered when patients are on prolonged therapy.

Outside state hospitals or other psychiatric institutions, fluphenazine decanoate should be administered under the direction of a physician experienced in the clinical use of psychotropic drugs, particularly phenothiazine derivatives. Furthermore, facilities should be available for periodic checking of hepatic function, renal function, and the blood picture. Renal function of patients on long-term therapy should be monitored; if BUN (blood urea nitrogen) becomes abnormal, treatment should be discontinued.

As with any phenothiazine, the physician should be alert to the possible development of "silent pneumonias" in patients under treatment with fluphenazine decanoate.

Neuroleptic drugs elevate prolactin levels; the elevation persists during chronic administration. Tissue culture experiments indicate that approximately one-third of human breast cancers are prolactin dependent *in vitro*, a factor of potential importance if the prescription of these drugs is contemplated in a patient with a previously detected breast cancer. Although disturbances such as galactorrhea, amenorrhea, gynecomastia, and impotence have been reported, the clinical significance of elevated serum prolactin levels is unknown for most patients. An increase in mammary neoplasms has been found in rodents after chronic administration of neuroleptic drugs. Neither clinical studies nor epidemiologic studies conducted to date, however, have shown an association between chronic administration of these drugs and mammary tumorigenesis; the available evidence is considered too limited to be conclusive at this time.

Information for Patients

Given the likelihood that a substantial proportion of patients exposed chronically to neuroleptics will develop tardive dyskinesia, it is advised that all patients in whom chronic use is contemplated be given, if possible, full information about this risk. The decision to inform patients and/or their guardians must obviously take into account the clinical circumstances and the competency of the patient to understand the information provided.

ADVERSE REACTIONS

Central Nervous System: The side effects most frequently reported with phenothiazine compounds are extrapyramidal symptoms including pseudoparkinsonism, dystonia, dyskinesia, akathisia, oculogyric crises, opisthotonos, and hyperreflexia. Muscle rigidity sometimes accompanied by hyperthermia has been reported following use of fluphenazine decanoate. Most often these extrapyramidal symptoms are reversible; however, they may be persistent (see below). The frequency of such reactions is related in part to chemical structure: one can expect a higher incidence with fluphenazine decanoate than with less potent piperazine derivatives or with straight-chain phenothiazines such as chlorpromazine. With any given phenothiazine derivative, the incidence and severity of such reactions depend more on individual patient sensitivity than on other factors, but dosage level and patient age are also determinants.

Extrapyramidal reactions may be alarming, and the patient should be forewarned and reassured. These reactions can usually be controlled by administration of antiparkinsonian drugs such as Benztropine Mesylate or intravenous Caffeine and Sodium Benzoate Injection, and by subsequent reduction in dosage.

Tardive Dyskinesia: See WARNINGS. The syndrome is characterized by involuntary choreoathetoid movements which variously involve the tongue, face, mouth, lips, or jaw (e.g., protrusion of the tongue, puffing of cheeks, puckering of the mouth, chewing movements), trunk and extremities. The severity of the syndrome and the degree of impairment produced vary widely.

The syndrome may become clinically recognizable either during treatment, upon dosage reduction, or upon withdrawal of treatment. Early detection of tardive dyskinesia is important. To increase the likelihood of detecting the syndrome at the earliest possible time, the dosage of neuroleptic drug should be reduced periodically (if clinically possible) and the patient observed for signs of the disorder. This maneuver is critical, since neuroleptic drugs may mask the signs of the syndrome.

Other CNS Effects: Occurrences of neuroleptic malignant syndrome (NMS) have been reported in patients on neuroleptic therapy (see WARNINGS, Neuroleptic Malignant Syndrome). Leukocytosis, elevated CPK, liver function abnormalities, and acute renal failure may also occur with NMS. Drowsiness or lethargy, if they occur, may necessitate a reduction in dosage; the induction of a catatonic-like state has been known to occur with dosages of fluphenazine far in excess of the recommended amounts. As with other phenothiazine compounds, reactivation or aggravation of psychotic processes may be encountered.

Phenothiazine derivatives have been known to cause, in some patients, restlessness, excitement, or bizarre dreams.

Autonomic Nervous System: Hypertension and fluctuations in blood pressure have been reported with fluphenazine.

Hypotension has rarely presented a problem with fluphenazine. However, patients with pheochromocytoma, cerebral vascular or renal insufficiency, or a severe cardiac reserve deficiency (such as mitral insufficiency) appear to be particularly prone to hypotensive reactions with phenothiazine compounds, and should therefore be observed closely when the drug is administered. If severe hypotension should occur, supportive measures including the use of intravenous vasopressor drugs should be instituted immediately. Levarterenol Bitartrate Injection is the most suitable drug for this purpose; *epinephrine should not be used* since phenothiazine derivatives have been found to reverse its action, resulting in a further lowering of blood pressure.

Autonomic reactions including nausea and loss of appetite, salivation, polyuria, perspiration, dry mouth, headache, and constipation may occur. Autonomic effects can usually be controlled by reducing or temporarily discontinuing dosage. In some patients, phenothiazine derivatives have caused blurred vision, glaucoma, bladder paralysis, fecal impaction, paralytic ileus, tachycardia, or nasal congestion.

Metabolic and Endocrine: Weight change, peripheral edema, abnormal lactation, gynecomastia, menstrual irregularities, false results on pregnancy tests, impotency in men and increased libido in women have all been known to occur in some patients on phenothiazine therapy.

Allergic Reactions: Skin disorders such as itching, erythema, urticaria, seborrhea, photosensitivity, eczema and even exfoliative dermatitis have been reported with phenothiazine derivatives. The possibility of anaphylactoid reactions occurring in some patients should be borne in mind.

Hematologic: Routine blood counts are advisable during therapy since blood dyscrasias including leukopenia, agranulocytosis, thrombocytopenic or nonthrombocytopenic purpura, eosinophilia, and pancytopenia have been observed with phenothiazine derivatives. Furthermore, if any soreness of the mouth, gums, or throat, or any symptoms of upper respiratory infection occur and confirmatory leukocyte count indicates cellular depression, therapy should be discontinued and other appropriate measures instituted immediately.

Hepatic: Liver damage as manifested by cholestatic jaundice may be encountered, particularly during the first months of therapy; treatment should be discontinued if this occurs. An increase in cephalin flocculation, sometimes accompanied by alterations in other liver function tests, has been reported in patients receiving the enanthate ester of fluphenazine (a closely related compound) who have had no clinical evidence of liver damage.

Others —Sudden, unexpected and unexplained deaths have been reported in hospitalized psychotic patients receiving phenothiazines. Previous brain damage or seizures may be predisposing factors: high doses should be avoided in known seizure patients. Several patients have shown sudden flare-ups of psychotic behavior patterns shortly before death. Autopsy findings have usually revealed acute fulminating pneumonia or pneumonitis, aspiration of gastric contents, or intramyocardial lesions.

Although this is not a general feature of fluphenazine, potentiation of central nervous system depressants (opiates, analgesics, antihistamines, barbiturates, alcohol) may occur.

The following adverse reactions have also occurred with phenothiazine derivatives: systemic lupus erythematosus-like syndrome, hypotension severe enough to cause fatal cardiac arrest, altered electrocardiographic and electroencephalographic tracings, altered cerebrospinal fluid proteins, cerebral edema, asthma, laryngeal edema, and angioneurotic edema; with long-term use—skin pigmentation, and lenticular and corneal opacities.

Injections of fluphenazine decanoate are extremely well tolerated, local tissue reactions occurring only rarely.

DOSAGE AND ADMINISTRATION

Parenteral drug products should be inspected visually for particulate matter and discoloration prior to administration, whenever solution and container permit.

PROLIXIN DECANOATE (Fluphenazine Decanoate Injection) may be given intramuscularly or subcutaneously. A dry syringe and needle of at least 21 gauge should be used. Use of a wet needle or syringe may cause the solution to become cloudy.

To begin therapy with PROLIXIN DECANOATE the following regimens are suggested:

For *most patients,* a dose of 12.5 to 25 mg (0.5 to 1 mL) may be given to initiate therapy. The onset of action generally appears between 24 and 72 hours after injection and the effects of the drug on psychotic symptoms becomes significant within 48 to 96 hours. Subsequent injections and the dosage interval are determined in accordance with the patient's response. When administered as maintenance therapy, a single injection may be effective in controlling schizophrenic symptoms up to four weeks or longer. The response to a single dose has been found to last as long as six weeks in a few patients on maintenance therapy.

It may be advisable that patients who have no history of taking phenothiazines should be treated initially with a shorter-acting form of fluphenazine (see HOW SUPPLIED section for the availability of the shorter-acting fluphenazine hydrochloride dosage forms) before administering the decanoate to determine the patient's response to fluphenazine and to establish appropriate dosage. For psychotic patients who have been stabilized on a fixed daily dosage of PROLIXIN Tablets (Fluphenazine Hydrochloride Tablets USP), PROLIXIN Elixir (Fluphenazine Hydrochloride Elixir USP), or PROLIXIN Oral Concentrate (Fluphenazine Hydrochloride Oral Solution), conversion of therapy from these short-acting oral forms to the long-acting injectable PROLIXIN DECANOATE may be indicated.

Appropriate dosage of PROLIXIN DECANOATE (Fluphenazine Decanoate Injection) should be individualized for each patient and responses carefully monitored. No precise formula can be given to convert to use of PROLIXIN DECANOATE; however, a controlled multicentered study,* in patients receiving oral doses from 5 to 60 mg fluphenazine hydrochloride daily, showed that 20 mg fluphenazine hydrochloride daily was equivalent to 25 mg (1 mL) PROLIXIN DECANOATE every three weeks. This represents an approximate conversion ratio of 0.5 mL (12.5 mg) of decanoate every three weeks for every 10 mg of fluphenazine hydrochloride daily.

Once conversion to PROLIXIN DECANOATE is made, careful clinical monitoring of the patient and appropriate dosage adjustment should be made at the time of each injection.

Severely agitated patients may be treated initially with a rapid-acting phenothiazine compound such as PROLIXIN Injection (Fluphenazine Hydrochloride Injection USP—see package insert accompanying that product for complete information). When acute symptoms have subsided, 25 mg (1 mL) of PROLIXIN DECANOATE may be administered; subsequent dosage is adjusted as necessary.

"Poor risk" patients (those with known hypersensitivity to phenothiazines, or with disorders that predispose to undue reactions): Therapy may be initiated cautiously with oral or parenteral fluphenazine hydrochloride (see package inserts accompanying these products for complete information). When the pharmacologic effects and an appropriate dosage are apparent, an equivalent dose of PROLIXIN DECANOATE may be administered. Subsequent dosage adjustments are made in accordance with the response of the patient.

The optimal amount of the drug and the frequency of administration must be determined for each patient, since dosage requirements have been found to vary with clinical circumstances as well as with individual response to the drug.

Dosage should not exceed 100 mg. If doses greater than 50 mg are deemed necessary, the next dose and succeeding doses should be increased cautiously in increments of 12.5 mg.

HOW SUPPLIED

PROLIXIN DECANOATE (Fluphenazine Decanoate Injection) is available in Unimatic® single dose preassembled

Continued on next page

Princeton—Cont.

syringes, and vials, providing 25 mg fluphenazine decanoate per mL. PROLIXIN (fluphenazine) is also available for oral administration as PROLIXIN® Tablets (Fluphenazine Hydrochloride Tablets USP) providing 1, 2.5, 5, and 10 mg fluphenazine hydrochloride per tablet, PROLIXIN® Elixir (Fluphenazine Hydrochloride Elixir USP) providing 0.5 mg fluphenazine hydrochloride per mL (2.5 mg per 5 mL teaspoonful), and PROLIXIN® Oral Concentrate (Fluphenazine Hydrochloride Oral Solution) providing 5 mg fluphenazine hydrochloride per mL.

Storage
Store at room temperature; avoid freezing and excessive heat. Protect from light.

*The Initiation of Long-Term Pharmacotherapy in Schizophrenia: Dosage and Side Effect Comparisons Between Oral and Depot Fluphenazine; N.R. Schooler; Pharmakopsych. 9:159-169, 1976.
(J4-150A)

PROLIXIN ENANTHATE®   ℞
Fluphenazine Enanthate Injection USP

DESCRIPTION
PROLIXIN ENANTHATE (Fluphenazine Enanthate Injection) is an esterified trifluoromethyl phenothiazine derivative, chemically designated as 2-[4-[3-[2-(Trifluoromethyl)-phenothiazine-10-yl]propyl]-1-piperazinyl]ethyl heptanoate. It is a highly potent behavior modifier with a markedly extended duration of effect. PROLIXIN ENANTHATE is available for intramuscular or subcutaneous administration, providing 25 mg fluphenazine enanthate per mL in a sesame oil vehicle with 1.5% (w/v) benzyl alcohol as a preservative. At the time of manufacture, the air in the vials is replaced by nitrogen.

CLINICAL PHARMACOLOGY
The basic effects of fluphenazine enanthate appear to be no different from those of fluphenazine hydrochloride, with the exception of duration of action. The esterification of fluphenazine markedly prolongs the drug's duration of effect without unduly attenuating its beneficial action. The onset of action generally appears between 24 to 72 hours after injection, and the effects of the drug on psychotic symptoms become significant within 48 to 96 hours. Amelioration of symptoms then continues for one to three weeks or longer, with an average duration of effect of about two weeks.

Prolixin has activity at all levels of the central nervous system as well as on multiple organ systems. The mechanism whereby its therapeutic action is exerted is unknown.

Fluphenazine differs from other phenothiazine derivatives in several respects: it is more potent on a milligram basis, it has less potentiating effect on central nervous system depressants and anesthetics that do some of the phenothiazines and appears to be less sedating, and it is less likely than some of the older phenothiazines to produce hypotension (nevertheless, appropriate cautions should be observed—see sections on PRECAUTIONS and ADVERSE REACTIONS).

INDICATIONS AND USAGE
PROLIXIN ENANTHATE is a long-acting parenteral antipsychotic drug intended for use in the management of patients requiring prolonged parenteral neuroleptic therapy (e.g., chronic schizophrenics).

PROLIXIN ENANTHATE (Fluphenazine Enanthate Injection) has not been shown effective in the management of behavioral complications in patients with mental retardation.

CONTRAINDICATIONS
Phenothiazines are contraindicated in patients with suspected or established subcortical brain damage.

Phenothiazine compounds should not be used in patients receiving large doses of hypnotics.

PROLIXIN ENANTHATE is contraindicated in comatose or severely depressed states.

The presence of blood dyscrasia or liver damage precludes the use of fluphenazine enanthate.

Fluphenazine enanthate is not intended for use in children under 12 years of age.

PROLIXIN ENANTHATE is contraindicated in patients who have shown hypersensitivity to fluphenazine; cross-sensitivity to phenothiazine derivatives may occur.

WARNINGS
Tardive Dyskinesia
Tardive dyskinesia, a syndrome consisting of potentially irreversible, involuntary, dyskinetic movements may develop in patients treated with neuroleptic (antipsychotic) drugs. Although the prevalence of the syndrome appears to be highest among the elderly, especially elderly women, it is impossible to rely upon prevalence estimates to predict, at the inception of neuroleptic treatment, which patients are

likely to develop the syndrome. Whether neuroleptic drug products differ in their potential to cause tardive dyskinesia is unknown.

Both the risk of developing the syndrome and the likelihood that it will become irreversible are believed to increase as the duration of treatment and the total cumulative dose of neuroleptic drugs administered to the patient increase. However, the syndrome can develop, although much less commonly, after relatively brief treatment periods at low doses.

There is no known treatment for established cases of tardive dyskinesia, although the syndrome may remit, partially or completely, if neuroleptic treatment is withdrawn. Neuroleptic treatment, itself, however, may suppress (or partially suppress) the signs and symptoms of the syndrome and thereby may possibly mask the underlying disease process. The effect that symptomatic suppression has upon the long-term course of the syndrome is unknown.

Given these considerations, neuroleptics should be prescribed in a manner that is most likely to minimize the occurrence of tardive dyskinesia. Chronic neuroleptic treatment should generally be reserved for patients who suffer from a chronic illness that, 1) is known to respond to neuroleptic drugs, and, 2) for whom alternative, equally effective, but potentially less harmful treatments are *not* available or appropriate. In patients who do require chronic treatment, the smallest dose and the shortest duration of treatment producing a satisfactory clinical response should be sought. The need for continued treatment should be reassessed periodically.

If signs and symptoms of tardive dyskinesia appear in a patient on neuroleptics, drug discontinuation should be considered. However, some patients may require treatment despite the presence of the syndrome.

(For further information about the description of tardive dyskinesia and its clinical detection, please refer to the sections on PRECAUTIONS, Information for Patients and ADVERSE REACTIONS, Tardive Dyskinesia.)

Neuroleptic Malignant Syndrome (NMS)
A potentially fatal symptom complex sometimes referred to as Neuroleptic Malignant Syndrome (NMS) has been reported in association with antipsychotic drugs. Clinical manifestations of NMS are hyperpyrexia, muscle rigidity, altered mental status and evidence of autonomic instability (irregular pulse or blood pressure, tachycardia, diaphoresis, and cardiac dysrhythmias).

The diagnostic evaluation of patients with this syndrome is complicated. In arriving at a diagnosis, it is important to identify cases where the clinical presentation includes both serious medical illness (e.g., pneumonia, systemic infection, etc.) and untreated or inadequately treated extrapyramidal signs and symptoms (EPS). Other important considerations in the differential diagnosis include central anticholinergic toxicity, heat stroke, drug fever and primary central nervous system (CNS) pathology.

The management of NMS should include: 1) immediate discontinuation of antipsychotic drugs and other drugs not essential to concurrent therapy; 2) intensive symptomatic treatment and medical monitoring; and 3) treatment of any concomitant serious medical problems for which specific treatments are available. There is no general agreement about specific pharmacological treatment regimens for uncomplicated NMS.

If a patient requires antipsychotic drug treatment after recovery from NMS, the potential reintroduction of drug therapy should be carefully considered. The patient should be carefully monitored, since recurrences of NMS have been reported.

The use of this drug may impair the mental and physical abilities required for driving a car or operating heavy machinery.

Physicians should be alert to the possibility that severe adverse reactions may occur which require immediate medical attention.

Potentiation of the effects of alcohol may occur with the use of this drug. Since there is no adequate experience in children who have received this drug, safety and efficacy in children have not been established.

Usage in Pregnancy
The safety for the use of this drug during pregnancy has not been established; therefore, the possible hazards should be weighed against the potential benefits when administering the drug to pregnant patients.

PRECAUTIONS
General
Because of the possibility of cross-sensitivity, fluphenazine enanthate should be used cautiously in patients who have developed cholestatic jaundice, dermatoses, or other allergic reactions to phenothiazine derivatives.

Psychotic patients on large doses of a phenothiazine drug who are undergoing surgery should be watched carefully for possible hypotensive phenomena. Moreover, it should be remembered that reduced amounts of anesthetics or central nervous system depressants may be necessary.

The effects of atropine may be potentiated in some patients receiving fluphenazine because of added anticholinergic effects.

Fluphenazine enanthate should be used cautiously in patients exposed to extreme heat or phosphorus insecticides. The preparation should be used with caution in patients with a history of convulsive disorders, since grand mal convulsions have been known to occur.

Use with caution in patients with special medical disorders such as mitral insufficiency or other cardiovascular diseases and pheochromocytoma.

The possibility of liver damage, pigmentary retinopathy, lenticular and corneal deposits, and development of irreversible dyskinesia should be remembered when patients are on prolonged therapy.

Outside state hospitals or other psychiatric institutions, fluphenazine enanthate should be administered under the direction of a physician experienced in the clinical use of psychotropic drugs, particularly phenothiazine derivatives. Furthermore, facilities should be available for periodic checking of hepatic function, renal function, and the blood picture. Renal function of patients on long-term therapy should be monitored; if BUN (blood urea nitrogen) becomes abnormal, treatment should be discontinued.

As with any phenothiazine, the physician should be alert to the possible development of "silent pneumonias" in patients under treatment with fluphenazine enanthate.

Neuroleptic drugs elevate prolactin levels; the elevation persists during chronic administration. Tissue culture experiments indicate that approximately one-third of human breast cancers are prolactin dependent *in vitro*, a factor of potential importance if the prescription of these drugs is contemplated in a patient with a previously detected breast cancer. Although disturbances such as galactorrhea, amenorrhea, gynecomastia, and impotence have been reported, the clinical significance of elevated serum prolactin levels is unknown for most patients. An increase in mammary neoplasms has been found in rodents after chronic administration of neuroleptic drugs. Neither clinical studies nor epidemiologic studies conducted to date, however, have shown an association between chronic administration of these drugs and mammary tumorigenesis; the available evidence is considered too limited to be conclusive at this time.

Information for Patients
Given the likelihood that some patients exposed chronically to neuroleptics will develop tardive dyskinesia, it is advised that all patients in whom chronic use is contemplated be given, if possible, full information about this risk. The decision to inform patients and/or their guardians must obviously take into account the clinical circumstances and the competency of the patient to understand the information provided.

ADVERSE REACTIONS
Central Nervous System: The side effects most frequently reported with phenothiazine compounds are extrapyramidal symptoms including pseudoparkinsonism, dystonia, dyskinesia, akathisia, oculogyric crises, opisthotonos, and hyperreflexia. Most often these extrapyramidal symptoms are reversible; however, they may be persistent (see below). The frequency of such reactions is related in part to chemical structure: one can expect a higher incidence with fluphenazine enanthate than with less potent piperazine derivatives or with straight-chain phenothiazines such as chlorpromazine. With any given phenothiazine derivative, the incidence and severity of such reactions depend more on individual patient sensitivity than on other factors, but dosage level and patient age are also determinants.

Extrapyramidal reactions may be alarming, and the patient should be forewarned and reassured. These reactions can usually be controlled by administration of antiparkinsonian drugs such as Benztropine Mesylate or intravenous Caffeine and Sodium Benzoate Injection, and by subsequent reduction in dosage.

Tardive Dyskinesia: See WARNINGS. The syndrome is characterized by involuntary choreoathetoid movements which variously involve the tongue, face, mouth, lips, or jaw (e.g., protrusion of the tongue, puffing of cheeks, puckering of the mouth, chewing movements), trunk and extremities. The severity of the syndrome and the degree of impairment produced vary widely.

The syndrome may become clinically recognizable either during treatment, upon dosage reduction, or upon withdrawal of treatment. Early detection of tardive dyskinesia is important. To increase the likelihood of detecting the syndrome at the earliest possible time, the dosage of neuroleptic drug should be reduced periodically (if clinically possible) and the patient observed for signs of the disorder. This maneuver is critical, since neuroleptic drugs may mask the signs of the syndrome.

Other CNS Effects: Occurrences of neuroleptic malignant syndrome (NMS) have been reported in patients on neuroleptic therapy (see WARNINGS, Neuroleptic Malignant Syndrome). Leukocytosis, elevated CPK, liver function abnormalities, and acute renal failure may also occur with NMS.

Drowsiness or lethargy, if they occur, may necessitate a reduction in dosage; the induction of a catatonic-like state has been known to occur with dosages of fluphenazine far in excess of the recommended amounts. As with other phenothiazine compounds, reactivation or aggravation of psychotic processes may be encountered.

Phenothiazine derivatives have been known to cause, in some patients, restlessness, excitement, or bizarre dreams.

Autonomic Nervous System: Hypertension and fluctuations in blood pressure have been reported with fluphenazine enanthate.

Hypotension has rarely presented a problem with fluphenazine. However, patients with pheochromocytoma, cerebral vascular or renal insufficiency, or a severe cardiac reserve deficiency (such as mitral insufficiency) appear to be particularly prone to hypotensive reactions with phenothiazine compounds, and should therefore be observed closely when the drug is administered. If severe hypotension should occur, supportive measures including the use of intravenous vasopressor drugs should be instituted immediately. Levarterenol Bitartrate Injection is the most suitable drug for this purpose; *epinephrine should not be used* since phenothiazine derivatives have been found to reverse its action, resulting in a further lowering of blood pressure.

Autonomic reactions including nausea and loss of appetite, salivation, polyuria, perspiration, dry mouth, headache, and constipation may occur. Autonomic effects can usually be controlled by reducing or temporarily discontinuing dosage. In some patients, phenothiazine derivatives have caused blurred vision, glaucoma, bladder paralysis, fecal impaction, paralytic ileus, tachycardia, or nasal congestion.

Metabolic and Endocrine: Weight change, peripheral edema, abnormal lactation, gynecomastia, menstrual irregularities, false results on pregnancy tests, impotency in men and increased libido in women have all been known to occur in some patients on phenothiazine therapy.

Allergic Reactions: Skin disorders such as itching, erythema, urticaria, seborrhea, photosensitivity, eczema and even exfoliative dermatitis have been reported with phenothiazine derivatives. The possibility of anaphylactoid reactions occurring in some patients should be borne in mind.

Hematologic: Routine blood counts are advisable during therapy since blood dyscrasias including leukopenia, agranulocytosis, thrombocytopenic or nonthrombocytopenic purpura, eosinophilia, and pancytopenia have been observed with phenothiazine derivatives. Furthermore, if any soreness of the mouth, gums, or throat, or any symptoms of upper respiratory infection occur and confirmatory leukocyte count indicates cellular depression, therapy should be discontinued and other appropriate measures instituted immediately.

Hepatic: Liver damage as manifested by cholestatic jaundice may be encountered, particularly during the first months of therapy; treatment should be discontinued if this occurs. An increase in cephalin flocculation, sometimes accompanied by alterations in other liver function tests, has been reported in patients receiving fluphenazine enanthate who have had no clinical evidence of liver damage.

Others: Sudden, unexpected and unexplained deaths have been reported in hospitalized psychotic patients receiving phenothiazines. Previous brain damage or seizures may be predisposing factors; high doses should be avoided in known seizure patients. Several patients have shown sudden flare-ups of psychotic behavior patterns shortly before death. Autopsy findings have usually revealed acute fulminating pneumonia or pneumonitis, aspiration of gastric contents, or intramyocardial lesions.

Although this is not a general feature of fluphenazine, potentiation of central nervous system depressants (opiates, analgesics, antihistamines, barbiturates, alcohol) may occur.

The following adverse reactions have also occurred with phenothiazine derivatives: systemic lupus erythematosus-like syndrome, hypotension severe enough to cause fatal cardiac arrest, altered electrocardiographic and electroencephalographic tracings, altered cerebrospinal fluid proteins, cerebral edema, asthma, laryngeal edema, and angioneurotic edema; with long-term use—skin pigmentation, and lenticular and corneal opacities.

Injections of fluphenazine enanthate are extremely well tolerated, local tissue reactions occurring only rarely.

DOSAGE AND ADMINISTRATION

PROLIXIN ENANTHATE (Fluphenazine Enanthate Injection USP) may be given intramuscularly or subcutaneously. A dry syringe and needle of at least 21 gauge should be used. Use of a wet needle or syringe may cause the solution to become cloudy.

To begin therapy with PROLIXIN ENANTHATE the following regimens are suggested:

For most patients a dose of 25 mg (1 mL) every two weeks should prove to be adequate, and therapy may be started on that basis. Subsequent adjustments in the amount and the dosage interval may be made, if necessary, in accordance with the patient's response.

It may be advisable that patients who have no history of taking phenothiazines should be treated initially with a shorter-acting form of fluphenazine before administering the enanthate to determine the patient's response to fluphenazine and to establish appropriate dosage. Since the dosage comparability of the shorter-acting forms of fluphenazine to the longer-acting enanthate is not known, special caution should be exercised when switching from the shorter-acting forms to the enanthate.

Severely agitated patients may be treated initially with a rapid-acting phenothiazine compound such as Prolixin Injection (Fluphenazine Hydrochloride Injection USP—see package insert accompanying that product for complete information). When acute symptoms have subsided, 25 mg (1 mL) of PROLIXIN ENANTHATE may be administered; subsequent dosage is adjusted as necessary.

"Poor risk" patients (those with known hypersensitivity to phenothiazines, or with disorders that predispose to undue reactions): Therapy may be initiated cautiously with oral or parenteral fluphenazine hydrochloride. (See package inserts accompanying these products for complete information.) When the pharmacologic effects and an appropriate dosage are apparent, an equivalent dose of PROLIXIN ENANTHATE may be administered. Subsequent dosage adjustments are made in accordance with the response of the patient.

The optimal amount of the drug and the frequency of administration must be determined for each patient, since dosage requirements have been found to vary with clinical circumstances as well as with individual response to the drug. Although in a large series of patients the optimal dose was usually 25 mg every two weeks, the amount required ranged from 12.5 to 100 mg (0.5 to 4 mL). The interval between doses ranged from one to three weeks in most instances. The response to a single dose was found to last as long as six weeks in a few patients on maintenance therapy.

Dosage should not exceed 100 mg. If doses greater than 50 mg are deemed necessary, the next dose and succeeding doses should be increased cautiously in increments of 12.5 mg.

HOW SUPPLIED

PROLIXIN ENANTHATE (Fluphenazine Enanthate Injection USP) is available in vials providing 25 mg fluphenazine enanthate per mL.

Storage

Store at room temperature; avoid freezing and excessive heat. Protect from light.

(J4-135B)

PRONESTYL® INJECTION   ℞
Procainamide Hydrochloride Injection USP

WARNING

The prolonged administration of procainamide often leads to the development of a positive anti-nuclear antibody (ANA) test, with or without symptoms of a lupus erythematosus-like syndrome. If a positive ANA titer develops, the benefits versus risks of continued procainamide therapy should be assessed.

DESCRIPTION

PRONESTYL (procainamide hydrochloride), a Group 1A cardiac antiarrhythmic drug, is p-amino-N-[2-(diethylamino)ethyl]-benzamide monohydrochloride, molecular weight 271.79.

It differs from procaine which is the p-aminobenzoyl *ester* of 2-(diethylamino)-ethanol. Procainamide as the free base has a pK_a of 9.23; the monohydrochloride is very soluable in water. PRONESTYL Injection is a sterile, aqueous solution for intramuscular or intravenous use providing 100 mg or 500 mg procainamide hydrochloride per mL. The 100 mg/mL potency contains 9 mg/mL of benzyl alcohol and not more than 0.9 mg/mL sodium bisulfite as preservatives; the 500 mg/mL potency contains 1 mg/mL methylparaben and not more than 2 mg/mL sodium bisulfite as preservatives. In both formulations, the pH has been adjusted between 4.0 and 6.0 with hydrochloric acid and/or sodium hydroxide. At the time of manufacture, the air in the containers is replaced by nitrogen.

CLINICAL PHARMACOLOGY

Procainamide (PA) increases the effective refractory period of the atria, and to a lesser extent the bundle of His-Purkinje system and ventricles of the heart. It reduces impulse conduction velocity in the atria, His-Purkinje fibers, and ventricular muscle, but has variable effects on the atrioventricular (A-V) node, a direct slowing action and a weaker vagolytic effect which may speed A-V conduction slightly. Myocardial excitability is reduced in the atria, Purkinje fibers, papillary muscles, and ventricles by an increase in the threshold for excitation, combined with inhibition of ectopic pacemaker activity by retardation of the slow phase of diastolic depolarization, thus decreasing automaticity especially in ectopic sites. Contractility of the undamaged heart is usually not affected by therapeutic concentrations, although slight reduction of cardiac output may occur, and may be significant in the presence of myocardial damage. Therapeutic levels of PA may exert vagolytic effects and produce slight acceleration of heart rate, while high or toxic concentrations may prolong A-V conduction time or induce A-V block, or even cause abnormal automaticity and spontaneous firing, by unknown mechanisms.

The electrocardiogram may reflect these effects by showing slight sinus tachycardia (due to the anticholinergic action) and widened QRS complexes and, less regularly, prolonged Q-T and P-R intervals (due to longer systole and slower conduction), as well as some decreases in QRS and T wave amplitude. These direct effects of PA on electrical activity, conduction, responsiveness, excitability and automaticity are characteristic of a Group 1A antiarrhythmic agent, the prototype for which is quinidine; PA effects are very similar. However, PA has weaker vagal blocking action than does quinidine, does not induce alpha-adrenergic blockade, and is less depressing to cardiac contractility.

Following intramuscular injection, PRONESTYL is rapidly absorbed into the bloodstream, and plasma levels peak in 15 to 60 minutes, considerably faster than orally administered PRONESTYL Tablets (Procainamide Hydrochloride Tablets) or PRONESTYL Capsules (Procainamide Hydrochloride Capsules USP) which produce peak plasma levels in 90 to 120 minutes. Intravenous administration of PRONESTYL can produce therapeutic procainamide levels within minutes after infusion is started. About 15 to 20 percent of PA is reversibly bound to plasma proteins, and considerable amounts are more slowly and reversibly bound to tissues of the heart, liver, lung, and kidney. The apparent volume of distribution eventually reaches about 2 liters per kilogram body weight with a half-time of approximately five minutes. While PA has been shown in the dog to cross the blood-brain barrier, it did not concentrate in the brain at levels higher than in plasma. It is not known if PA crosses the placenta. Plasma esterases are far less active in hydrolysis of PA than of procaine. The half-time for elimination of PA is three to four hours in patients with normal renal function, but reduced creatinine clearance and advancing age each prolong the half-time of elimination of PA.

A significant fraction of the circulating PA may be metabolized in hepatocytes to N-acetylprocainamide (NAPA), ranging from 16 to 21 percent of an administered dose in "slow acetylators" to 24 to 33 percent in "fast-acetylators". Since NAPA also has significant antiarrhythmic activity and somewhat slower renal clearance than PA, both hepatic acetylation rate capability and renal function, as well as age, have significant effects on the effective biological half-time of therapeutic action of administered PA and the NAPA derivative. Trace amounts may be excreted in the urine as free and conjugated p-aminobenzoic acid, 30 to 60 percent as unchanged PA, and 6 to 52 percent as the NAPA derivative. Both PA and NAPA are eliminated by active tubular secretion as well as by glomerular filtration. Action of PA on the central nervous system is not prominent, but high plasma concentrations may cause tremors. While therapeutic plasma levels for PA have been reported to be 3 to 10 μg/mL, certain patients such as those with sustained ventricular tachycardia may need higher levels for adequate control. This may justify the increased risk of toxicity (see OVERDOSAGE). Where programmed ventricular stimulation has been used to evaluate efficacy of PA in preventing recurrent ventricular tachyarrhythmias, higher plasma levels (mean, 13.6 μg/mL) of PA were found necessary for adequate control.

INDICATIONS AND USAGE

PRONESTYL (procainamide hydrochloride) is indicated for the treatment of life-threatening ventricular arrhythmias. PRONESTYL (procainamide hydrochloride) is also indicated for the treatment of some patients with less severe, symptomatic ventricular arrhythmias, including unifocal or multifocal couplets and nonsustained ventricular tachycardia. Because procainamide has the potential to produce serious hematological disorders (0.5 percent) particularly leukopenia or agranulocytosis (sometimes fatal), its use should be reserved for patients in whom, in the opinion of the physician, the benefits of treament clearly outweigh the risks. (See WARNINGS and Boxed Warning.) For less serious arrhythmias, alternative therapies with less severe toxicity, such as certain beta-adrenergic blockers (see specific product labeling), should be considered.

Like all other antiarrhythmics, procainamide has not been shown to prevent sudden death in patients with serious ventricular ectopic activity, and, as with all other antiarrhythmics, procainamide has potentially serious adverse effects, including the ability to worsen arrhythmias. It is therefore essential that each patient be evaluated electrocardiographically and clinically prior to, and during, procainamide therapy to determine whether the response to the drug supports continued treatment.

Continued on next page

Princeton—Cont.

CONTRAINDICATIONS

Complete heart block: Procainamide should not be administered to patients with complete heart block because of its effects in suppressing nodal or ventricular pacemakers and the hazard of asystole. It may be difficult to recognize complete heart block in patients with ventricular tachycardia, but if significant slowing of ventricular rate occurs during PA treatment without evidence of A-V conduction appearing, PA should be stopped. In cases of second degree A-V block or various types of hemiblock, PA should be avoided or discontinued because of the possibility of increased severity of block, unless the ventricular rate is controlled by an electrical pacemaker.

Idiosyncratic hypersensitivity: In patients sensitive to procaine or other ester-type local anesthetics, cross sensitivity to PA is unlikely. However, it should be borne in mind, and PA should not be used if it produces acute allergic dermatitis, asthma, or anaphylactic symptoms.

Lupus Erythematosus: An established diagnosis of systemic lupus erythematosus is a contraindication to PA therapy, since aggravation of symptoms is highly likely.

Torsades de Pointes: In the unusual ventricular arrhythmia called "les torsades de pointes" (twistings of the points), characterized by alternation of one or more ventricular premature beats in the directions of the QRS complexes on ECG in persons with prolonged Q-T and often enhanced U waves, Group 1A antiarrhythmic drugs are contraindicated. Administration of PA in such cases may aggravate this special type of ventricular extrasystole or tachycardia instead of suppressing it.

WARNINGS

> **Blood Dyscrasias:** Agranulocytosis, bone marrow depression, neutropenia, hypoplastic anemia and thrombocytopenia in patients receiving procainamide hydrochloride have been reported at a rate of approximately 0.5 percent. Most of these patients received procainamide within the recommended dosage range. Fatalities have occurred (with approximately 20–25 percent mortality in reported cases of agranulocytosis). Since most of these events have been noted during the first 12 weeks of therapy, it is recommended that complete blood counts including white cell, differential and platelet counts be performed at weekly intervals for the first three months of therapy, and periodically thereafter. Complete blood counts should be performed promptly if the patient develops any signs of infection (such as fever, chills, sore throat or stomatitis), bruising or bleeding. If any of these hematologic disorders are identified, procainamide therapy should be discontinued. Blood counts usually return to normal within one month of discontinuation. Caution should be used in patients with pre-existing marrow failure or cytopenia of any type (see ADVERSE REACTIONS).

Digitalis intoxication

Caution should be exercised in the use of procainamide in arrhythmias associated with digitalis intoxication. Procainamide can suppress digitalis-induced arrhythmias; however, if there is concomitant marked disturbance of atrioventricular conduction, additional depression of conduction and ventricular asystole or fibrillation may result. Therefore, use of procainamide should be considered only if discontinuation of digitalis, and therapy with potassium, lidocaine, or phenytoin are ineffective.

First degree heart block

Caution should be exercised also if the patient exhibits or develops first degree heart block while taking PA, and dosage reduction is advised in such cases. If the block persists despite dosage reduction, continuation of PA administration must be evaluated on the basis of current benefit versus risk of increased heart block.

Predigitalization for atrial flutter or fibrillation

Patients with atrial flutter or fibrillation should be cardioverted or digitalized prior to PA administration to avoid enhancement of A-V conduction which may result in ventricular rate acceleration beyond tolerable limits. Adequate digitalization reduces but does not eliminate the possibility of sudden increase in ventricular rate as the atrial rate is slowed by PA in these arrhythmias.

Congestive heart failure

For patients in congestive heart failure, and those with acute ischemic heart disease or cardiomyopathy, caution should be used in PA therapy, since even slight depression of myocardial contractility may further reduce cardiac output of the damaged heart.

Concurrent other antiarrhythmic agents

Concurrent use of PA with other Group 1A antiarrhythmic agents such as quinidine or disopyramide may produce enhanced prolongation of conduction or depression of contractility and hypotension, especially in patients with cardiac decompensation. Such use should be reserved for patients with serious arrhythmias unresponsive to a single drug and employed only if close observation is possible.

Renal insufficiency

Renal insufficiency may lead to accumulation of high plasma levels from conventional doses of PA, with effects similar to those of overdosage (see OVERDOSAGE), unless dosage is adjusted for the individual patient.

Myasthenia gravis

Patients with myasthenia gravis may show worsening of symptoms from PA due to its procaine-like effect on diminishing acetylcholine release at skeletal muscle motor nerve endings, so that PA administration may be hazardous without optimal adjustment of anticholinesterase medications and other precautions.

Sulfite sensitivity

PRONESTYL Injection (Procainamide Hydrochloride Injection) contains sodium bisulfite, a sulfite that may cause allergic-type reactions including anaphylactic symptoms and life-threatening or less severe asthmatic episodes in certain susceptible people. The overall prevalence of sulfite sensitivity in the general population is unknown and probably low. Sulfite sensitivity is seen more frequently in asthmatic than in nonasthmatic people.

PRECAUTIONS

Blood-pressure and ECG monitoring

Blood pressure should be monitored with the patient supine during parenteral, especially intravenous, administration of PA (see DOSAGE AND ADMINISTRATION). There is a possibility that relatively high although transient plasma levels of PA may be attained and cause hypotension before the PA can be distributed from the plasma volume to its full apparent volume of distribution which is approximately 50 times greater. Therefore, caution should be exercised to avoid overly rapid administration of PA. If the blood pressure falls 15 mm Hg or more, PA administration should be temporarily discontinued. Electrocardiographic (ECG) monitoring is advisable as well, both for observation of the progress and response of the arrhythmia under treatment, and for early detection of any tendency to excessive widening of the QRS complex, prolongation of the P-R interval, or any signs of heart block (see OVERDOSAGE). Parenteral therapy with PA should be limited to use in hospitals in which monitoring and intensive supportive care are available, or to emergency situations in which equivalent observation and treatment can be provided.

General

Immediately after initiation of PA therapy, patients should be closely observed for possible hypersensitivity reactions. In conversion of atrial fibrillation to normal sinus rhythm by any means, dislodgement of mural thrombi may lead to embolization, which should be kept in mind.

After achieving and maintaining therapeutic plasma concentrations and satisfactory electrocardiographic and clinical responses, continued frequent periodic monitoring of vital signs and electrocardiograms is advised. If evidence of QRS widening of more than 25 percent or marked prolongation of the Q-T interval occurs, concern for overdosage is appropriate, and interruption of the PA infusion is advisable if a 50 percent increase occurs. Elevated serum creatinine or urea nitrogen, reduced creatinine clearance or history of renal insufficiency, as well as use in older patients (over age 50), provide grounds to anticipate that less than the usual dosage or infusion rate may suffice, since the urinary elimination of PA and NAPA may be reduced, leading to gradual accumulation beyond normally-predicted amounts. If facilities are available for measurement of plasma PA and NAPA, or acetylation capability, individual dose adjustment for optimal therapeutic levels may be easier, but close observation of clinical effectiveness is the most important criterion.

Information for Patients

The patient should be encouraged to disclose any past history of drug sensitivity, especially to procaine or other local anesthetic agents, or aspirin, and to report any history of kidney disease, congestive heart failure, myasthenia gravis, liver disease, or lupus erythematosus.

The patient should be counseled to report any symptoms of arthralgia, myalgia, fever, chills, skin rash, easy bruising, sore throat or sore mouth, infections, dark urine or icterus, wheezing, muscular weakness, chest or abdominal pain, palpitations, nausea, vomiting, anorexia, diarrhea, hallucinations, dizziness, or depression.

Laboratory Tests

Laboratory tests such as complete blood count (CBC), electrocardiogram, and serum creatinine or urea nitrogen may be indicated depending on the clinical situation, and periodic rechecking of the CBC and ANA may be helpful in early detection of untoward reactions.

Drug Interactions

If other antiarrhythmic drugs are being used, additive effects on the heart may occur with PA administration, and dosage reduction may be necessary (see WARNINGS). Anticholinergic drugs administered concurrently with PA may produce additive antivagal effects on A-V nodal conduction, although this is not as well documented for PA as for quinidine.

Patients taking PA who require neuromuscular blocking agents such as succinylcholine may require less than usual doses of the latter, due to PA effects on reducing acetylcholine release.

Drug/Laboratory Test Interactions

Suprapharmacologic concentrations of lidocaine and meprobamate may inhibit fluorescence of PA and NAPA, and propranolol shows a native fluorescence close to the PA/NAPA peak wavelengths, so that tests which depend on fluorescence measurement may be affected.

Carcinogenesis, Mutagenesis, Impairment of Fertility

Long term studies in animals have not been performed.

Teratogenic Effects: Pregnancy Category C

Animal reproduction studies have not been conducted with PA. It also is not known whether PA can cause fetal harm when administered to a pregnant woman or can affect reproduction capacity. PA should be given to a pregnant woman only if clearly needed.

Nursing Mothers

Both PA and NAPA are excreted in human milk, and absorbed by the nursing infant. Because of the potential for serious adverse reactions in nursing infants, a decision to discontinue nursing or the drug should be made, taking into account the importance of the drug to the mother.

Pediatric Use

Safety and effectiveness in children have not been established.

ADVERSE REACTIONS

Cardiovascular system: Hypotension and serious disturbances of cardiac rhythm such as ventricular asystole or fibrillation are more common with intravenous administration of PA than with intramuscular administration. Because PA is a peripheral vasodilator in concentrations higher than the usual therapeutic range, transient high plasma levels which may occur especially during intravenous administration may produce temporary but at times severe lowering of blood pressure (see OVERDOSAGE and PRECAUTIONS).

Multisystem: A lupus erythematosus-like syndrome of arthralgia, pleural or abdominal pain, and sometimes arthritis, pleural effusion, pericarditis, fever, chills, myalgia, and possibly related hematologic or skin lesions (see below) is fairly common after prolonged PA administration, perhaps more often in patients who are slow acetylators (see BOXED WARNINGS and PRECAUTIONS). While some series have reported less than 1 in 500, others have reported the syndrome in up to 30 percent of patients on long term oral PA therapy. If discontinuation of PA does not reverse the lupoid symptoms, corticosteroid treatment may be effective.

Hematologic: Neutropenia, thrombocytopenia, or hemolytic anemia may rarely be encountered. Agranulocytosis has occurred after repeated use of PA, and deaths have been reported. (See Boxed Warning, WARNINGS section.)

Skin: Angioneurotic edema, urticaria, pruritus, flushing, and maculopapular rash have also occurred.

Gastrointestinal system: Anorexia, nausea, vomiting, abdominal pain, diarrhea, bitter taste, and hepatomegaly with increased serum aminotransferase activity have been reported following single doses of PA.

Nervous system: Dizziness or giddiness, weakness, mental depression and psychosis with hallucinations have been reported.

OVERDOSAGE

Progressive widening of the QRS complex, prolonged Q-T and P-R intervals, lowering of the R and T waves, as well as increasing A-V block, may be seen with doses which are excessive for a given patient. Increased ventricular extrasystoles, or even ventricular tachycardia or fibrillation may occur. After intravenous administration but seldom after oral therapy, transient high plasma levels of PA may induce hypotension, affecting systolic more than diastolic pressures, especially in hypertensive patients. Such high levels may also produce central nervous depression, tremor, and even respiratory depression.

Plasma levels above 10 μg /mL are increasingly associated with toxic findings, which are seen occasionally in the 10 to 12 μg/mL range, more often in the 12 to 15 μg/mL range, and commonly in patients with plasma levels greater than 15 μg/mL.

Treatment of overdosage or toxic manifestations includes general supportive measures, close observation, monitoring of vital signs and possibly intravenous pressor agents and mechanical cardiorespiratory support. If available, PA and NAPA plasma levels may be helpful in assessing the potential degree of toxicity and response to therapy. Both PA and NAPA are removed from the circulation by hemodialysis but not peritoneal dialysis. No specific antidote for PA is known.

DOSAGE AND ADMINISTRATION

PRONESTYL Injection (Procainamide Hydrochloride Injection) is useful for arrhythmias which require immediate suppression and for maintenance of arrhythmia control. Intravenous therapy allows most rapid control of serious arrhythmias, including those following myocardial infarction; it should be carried out in circumstances where close observation and monitoring of the patient are possible, such as in hospital or emergency facilities. Intramuscular administration is less apt to produce temporary high plasma levels but therapeutic plasma levels are not obtained as rapidly as with intravenous administration. Oral procainamide dosage forms are preferable for less urgent arrhythmias as well as for long-term maintenance after initial parenteral PA therapy.

Intramuscular administration may be used as an alternative to the oral route for patients with less threatening arrhythmias but who are nauseated or vomiting, who are ordered to receive nothing by mouth preoperatively, or who may have malabsorptive problems. An initial daily dose of 50 mg per kg body weight may be estimated. This amount should be divided into fractional doses of one eighth to one quarter to be injected intramuscularly every three to six hours until oral therapy is possible. If more than three injections are given, the physician may wish to assess patient factors such as age and renal function (see below), clinical response and, if available, blood levels of PA and NAPA in adjusting further doses for that individual. For treatment of arrhythmias associated with anesthesia or surgical operation, the suggested dose is 100 to 500 mg by intramuscular injection.

[See table above].

Intravenous administration of PRONESTYL Injection should be done cautiously to avoid a possible hypotensive response (see PRECAUTIONS and OVERDOSAGE). Initial arrhythmia control, under blood pressure and ECG monitoring, may usually be accomplished safely within a half-hour by either of the two methods which follow:

a) Direct injection into a vein or into tubing of an established infusion line should be done slowly at a rate not to exceed 50 mg per minute. It is advisable to dilute either the 100 mg/mL or the 500 mg/mL concentrations of PRONESTYL Injection prior to intravenous injection to facilitate control of dosage rate. Doses of 100 mg may be administered every 5 minutes at this rate until the arrhythmia is suppressed or until 500 mg has been administered, after which it is advisable to wait 10 minutes or longer to allow for more distribution into tissues before resuming.

b) Alternatively, a loading infusion containing 20 mg of PRONESTYL per mL (1 g diluted to 50 mL with 5% Dextrose Injection USP) may be administered at a constant rate of 1 mL per minute for 25 to 30 minutes to deliver 500 to 600 mg of PA. Some effects may be seen after infusion of the first 100 or 200 mg; it is unusual to require more than 600 mg to achieve satisfactory antiarrhythmic effects.

The maximum advisable dosage to be given either by repeated bolus injections or such loading infusion is 1 g.

To maintain therapeutic levels, a more dilute intravenous infusion at a concentration of 2 mg/mL is convenient (1 g PRONESTYL in 500 mL of 5% Dextrose Injection USP), and may be administered at 1 to 3 mL/minute. If daily total fluid intake must be limited, a 4 mg/mL concentration (1 g of PRONESTYL Injection [Procainamide Hydrochloride Injection] in 250 mL of 5% Dextrose Injection USP) administered at 0.5 to 1.5 mL/minute will deliver an equivalent 2 to 6 mg per minute. The amount needed in a given patient to maintain the therapeutic level should be assessed principally from the clinical response, and will depend upon the patient's weight and age, renal elimination, hepatic acetylation rate, and cardiac status, but should be adjusted for each patient based upon close observation. A maintenance infusion rate of 50 μg/min/kg body weight to a person with a normal renal PA elimination half-time of three hours may be expected to produce a plasma level of approximately 6.5 μg/mL.

Since the principal route for elimination of PA and NAPA is renal excretion, reduced excretion will prolong the half-life of elimination and lower the dose rate needed to maintain therapeutic levels. Advancing age reduces the renal excretion of PA and NAPA independently of reductions in creatinine clearance; compared to normal young adults, there is approximately 25 percent reduction at age 50 and 50 percent at age 75.

Intravenous therapy should be terminated if persistent conduction disturbances or hypotension develop. As soon as the patient's basic cardiac rhythm appears to be stabilized, oral antiarrhythmic maintenance therapy is preferable, if indicated and possible. A period of about three to four hours (one half-time for renal elimination, ordinarily) should elapse after the last intravenous dose before administering the first dose of PRONESTYL Tablets or Capsules.

Parenteral drug products should be examined visually for particulate matter and discoloration (see HOW SUPPLIED) prior to administration.

HOW SUPPLIED

PRONESTYL Injection (Procainamide Hydrochloride Injection USP) is available as a sterile, aqueous solution in either 10 mL vials containing 100 mg procainamide hydrochloride per mL or 2 mL vials containing 500 mg procainamide hydrochloride per mL.

DILUTIONS AND RATES FOR INTRAVENOUS INFUSIONS*
PRONESTYL INJECTION (PROCAINAMIDE HYDROCHLORIDE INJECTION)

	Final Concentration	Infusion Volume†	PRONESTYL To Be Added	Infusion Rate
Initial Loading Infusion	20 mg/mL	50 mL	1000 mg	1 mL/min (for up to 25–30 min*)
Maintenance infusion	2 mg/mL	500 mL	1000 mg	1 to 3 mL/min
	or			
	4 mg/mL	250 mL	1000 mg	0.5 to 1.5 mL/min

The maintenance infusion rates are calculated to deliver 2 to 6 mg per minute, depending on body weight, renal elimination rate, and steady-state plasma level needed to maintain control of the arrhythmia*. The 4 mg/mL maintenance concentration may be preferred if total infused volume must be limited.

† (All infusions should be made up to final volume with 5% Dextrose Injection USP.)

* Please see text under DOSAGE AND ADMINISTRATION for further details. The flow rate of any intravenous procainamide infusion must be monitored closely to avoid transiently high plasma levels and possible hypotension (see PRECAUTIONS).

The solutions, which are clear and colorless initially, may develop a slight yellow color in time. This does not indicate a change which should preclude its use, but a solution any darker than light amber or otherwise discolored should not be used.

PRONESTYL is also available for oral administration as PRONESTYL Tablets (Procainamide Hydrochloride Tablets) and PRONESTYL Capsules (Procainamide Hydrochloride Capsules USP) providing 250, 375, and 500 mg procainamide hydrochloride (see package insert accompanying those products for further information).

STORAGE

Store PRONESTYL Injection between 50° and 80°F (10° and 27°C).

(J4-126D)

PRONESTYL® TABLETS   ℞
Procainamide Hydrochloride Tablets
PRONESTYL® CAPSULES   ℞
Procainamide Hydrochloride Capsules USP

WARNING

The prolonged administration of procainamide often leads to the development of a positive anti-nuclear antibody (ANA) test, with or without symptoms of a lupus erythematosus-like syndrome. If a positive ANA titer develops, the benefits versus risks of continued procainamide therapy should be assessed.

DESCRIPTION

PRONESTYL (procainamide hydrochloride), a Group 1A cardiac antiarrhythmic drug, is p-amino-N-[2-(diethylamino)ethyl]-benzamide monohydrochloride, molecular weight 271.79.

It differs from procaine which is the p-aminobenzoyl *ester* of 2-(diethylamino)-ethanol. Procainamide as the free base has a pK_a of 9.23; the monohydrochloride is very soluble in water. PRONESTYL (procainamide hydrochloride) is supplied for oral administration as capsules and tablets in potencies of 250, 375, and 500 mg.

Inactive ingredients: Tablets—calcium silicate, microcrystalline cellulose, colorants [FD&C Yellow No. 5 (tartrazine) and Yellow No. 6], flavor, povidone, starch, stearic acid, and other ingredients.

Capsules—colorants (D&C Yellow No. 10, except 375 mg; FD&C Yellow No. 6), gelatin, lactose (except 500 mg), magnesium stearate, talc, and titanium dioxide.

CLINICAL PHARMACOLOGY

Procainamide (PA) increases the effective refractory period of the atria, and to a lesser extent the bundle of His-Purkinje system and ventricles of the heart. It reduces impulse conduction velocity in the atria, His-Purkinje fibers, and ventricular muscle, but has variable effects on the atrioventricular (A-V) node, a direct slowing action and a weaker vagolytic effect which may speed A-V conduction slightly. Myocardial excitability is reduced in the atria, Purkinje fibers, papillary muscles, and ventricles by an increase in the threshold for excitation, combined with inhibition of ectopic pacemaker activity by retardation of the slow phase of diastolic depolarization, thus decreasing automaticity especially in ectopic sites. Contractility of the undamaged heart is usually not affected by therapeutic concentrations, although slight reduction of cardiac output may occur, and may be significant in the presence of myocardial damage. Therapeutic levels of PA may exert vagolytic effects and produce slight acceleration of heart rate, while high or toxic concentrations may prolong A-V conduction time or induce A-V block, or even cause abnormal automaticity and spontaneous firing, by unknown mechanisms.

The electrocardiogram may reflect these effects by showing slight sinus tachycardia (due to the anticholinergic action) and widened QRS complexes and, less regularly, prolonged Q-T and P-R intervals (due to longer systole and slower conduction), as well as some decrease in QRS and T wave amplitude. These direct effects of PA on electrical activity, conduction, responsiveness, excitability and automaticity are characteristic of a Group 1A antiarrhythmic agent, the prototype for which is quinidine; PA effects are very similar. However, PA has weaker vagal blocking action than does quinidine, does not induce alpha-adrenergic blockade, and is less depressing to cardiac contractility.

Ingested PA is resistant to digestive hydrolysis, and the drug is well absorbed from the entire small intestinal surface, but individual patients vary in their completeness of absorption of PA. Following oral administration of PRONESTYL, plasma PA levels reach about 50 percent of peak in 30 minutes, 90 percent at an hour, and peak at about 90 to 120 minutes. About 15 to 20 percent of PA is reversibly bound to plasma proteins, and considerable amounts are more slowly and reversibly bound to tissues of the heart, liver, lung, and kidney. The apparent volume of distribution eventually reaches about 2 liters per kilogram body weight with a half-time of approximately five minutes. While PA has been shown in the dog to cross the blood-brain barrier, it did not concentrate in the brain at levels higher than in plasma. It is now known if PA crosses the placenta. Plasma esterases are far less active in hydrolysis of PA than of procaine. The half-time for elimination of PA is three to four hours in patients with normal renal function, but reduced creatinine clearance and advancing age each prolong the half-time of elimination of PA.

A significant fraction of the circulating PA may be metabolized in hepatocytes to N-acetylprocainamide (NAPA), ranging from 16 to 21 percent of an administered dose in "slow acetylators" to 24 to 33 percent in "fast-acetylators". Since NAPA also has significant antiarrhythmic activity and somewhat slower renal clearance than PA, both hepatic acetylation rate capability and renal function, as well as age, have significant effects on the effective biological half-time of therapeutic action of adminstered PA and the NAPA derivative. Trace amounts may be excreted in the urine as free and conjugated p-aminobenzoic acid, 30 to 60 percent as unchanged PA, and 6 to 52 percent as the NAPA derivative. Both PA and NAPA are eliminated by active tubular secretion as well as by glomerular filtration. Action of PA on the central nervous system is not prominent, but high plasma concentrations may cause tremors. While therapeutic plasma levels for PA have been reported to be 3 to 10 μg/mL, certain patients such as those with sustained ventricular tachycardia may need higher levels for adequate control. This may justify the increased risk of toxicity (see OVERDOSAGE). Where programmed ventricular stimulation has been used to evaluate efficacy of PA in preventing recurrent ventricular tachyarrhythmias, higher plasma levels (mean, 13.6 μg/mL) of PA were found necessary for adequate control.

INDICATIONS AND USAGE

PRONESTYL (procainamide hydrochloride) is indicated for the treatment of life-threatening ventricular arrhythmias. PRONESTYL (procainamide hydrochloride) is also indicated for the treatment of some patients with less severe, symptomatic ventricular arrhythmias, including unifocal or multifocal couplets and nonsustained ventricular tachycardia. Because procainamide has the potential to produce serious hematological disorders (0.5 percent) particularly leukopenia or agranulocytosis (sometimes fatal), its use should be reserved for patients in whom, in the opinion of the physician, the benefits of treament clearly outweigh the risks. (See WARNINGS and Boxed Warning.) For less serious arrhythmias, alternative therapies with less severe toxicity, such as certain beta-adrenergic blockers (see specific product labeling), should be considered.

Like all other antiarrhythmics, procainamide has not been shown to prevent sudden death in patients with serious ven-

Continued on next page

Princeton—Cont.

tricular ectopic activity, and, as with all other antiarrhythmics, procainamide has potentially serious adverse effects, including the ability to worsen arrhythmias. It is therefore essential that each patient be evaluated electrocardiographically and clinically prior to, and during, procainamide therapy to determine whether the response to the drug supports continued treatment.

CONTRAINDICATIONS

Complete heart block: Procainamide should not be administered to patients with complete heart block because of its effects in suppressing nodal or ventricular pacemakers and the hazard of asystole. It may be difficult to recognize complete heart block in patients with ventricular tachycardia, but if significant slowing of ventricular rate occurs during PA treatment without eivdence of A-V conduction appearing, PA should be stopped. In cases of second degree A-V block or various types of hemiblock, PA should be avoided or discontinued because of the possibility of increased severity of block, unless the ventricular rate is controlled by an electrical pacemaker.

Idiosyncratic hypersensitivity: In patients sensitive to procaine or other ester-type local anesthetics, cross sensitivity to PA is unlikely; however, it should be borne in mind, and PA should not be used if it produces acute allergic dermatitis, asthma, or anaphylactic symptoms.

Lupus Erythematosus: An established diagnosis of systemic lupus erythematosus is a contraindication to PA therapy, since aggravation of symptoms is highly likely.

Torsades de Pointes: In the unusual ventricular arrhythmia called "les torsades de pointes" (twistings of the points), characterized by alternation of one or more ventricular premature beats in the directions of the QRS complexes on ECG in persons with prolonged Q-T and often enhanced U waves, Group 1A antiarrhythmic drugs are contraindicated. Administration of PA in such cases may aggravate this special type of ventricular extrasystole or tachycardia instead of suppressing it.

WARNINGS

> **Blood Dyscrasias:** Agranulocytosis, bone marrow depression, neutropenia, hypoplastic anemia and thrombocytopenia in patients receiving procainamide hydrochloride have been reported at a rate of approximately 0.5 percent. Most of these patients received procainamide within the recommended dosage range. Fatalities have occurred (with approximately 20-25 percent mortality in reported cases of agranulocytosis). Since most of these events have been noted during the first 12 weeks of therapy, it is recommended that complete blood counts including white cell, differential and platelet counts be performed at weekly intervals for the first three months of therapy, and periodically thereafter. Complete blood counts should be performed promptly if the patient develops any signs of infection (such as fever, chills, sore throat or stomatitis), bruising or bleeding. If any of these hematologic disorders are identified, procainamide therapy should be discontinued. Blood counts usually return to normal within one month of discontinuation. Caution should be used in patients with pre-existing marrow failure or cytopenia of any type (see ADVERSE REACTIONS).

Digitalis intoxication

Caution should be exercised in the use of procainamide in arrhythmias associated with digitalis intoxication. Procainamide can suppress digitalis-induced arrhythmias; however, if there is concomitant marked disturbance of atrioventricular conduction, additional depression of conduction and ventricular asystole or fibrillation may result. Therefore, use of procainamide should be considered only if discontinuation of digitalis, and therapy with potassium, lidocaine, or phenytoin are ineffective.

First degree heart block

Caution should be exercised also if the patient exhibits or develops first degree heart block while taking PA, and dosage reduction is advised in such cases. If the block persists despite dosage reduction, continuation of PA administration must be evaluated on the basis of current benefit versus risk of increased heart block.

Predigitalization for atrial flutter or fibrillation

Patients with atrial flutter or fibrillation should be cardioverted or digitalized prior to PA administration to avoid enhancement of A-V conduction which may result in ventricular rate acceleration beyond tolerable limits. Adequate digitalization reduces but does not eliminate the possibility of sudden increase in ventricular rate as the atrial rate is slowed by PA in these arrhythmias.

Congestive heart failure

For patients in congestive heart failure, and those with acute ischemic heart disease or cardiomyopathy, caution should be used in PA therapy, since even slight depression of myocar-

dial contractility may further reduce cardiac output of the damaged heart.

Concurrent other antiarrhythmic agents

Concurrent use of PA with other Group 1A antiarrhythmic agents such as quinidine or disopyramide may produce enhanced prolongation of conduction or depression of contractility and hypotension, especially in patients with cardiac decompensation. Such use should be reserved for patients with serious arrhythmias unresponsive to a single drug and employed only if close observation is possible.

Renal insufficiency

Renal insufficiency may lead to accumulation of high plasma levels from conventional oral doses of PA, with effects similar to those of overdosage (see OVERDOSAGE), unless dosage is adjusted for the individual patient.

Myasthenia gravis

Patients with myasthenia gravis may show worsening of symptoms from PA due to its procaine-like effect on diminishing acetylcholine release at skeletal muscle motor nerve endings, so that PA administration may be hazardous without optimal adjustment of anticholinesterase medications and other precautions.

PRECAUTIONS

General

Immediately after initiation of PA therapy, patients should be closely observed for possible hypersensitivity reactions, especially if procaine or local anesthetic sensitivity is suspected, and for muscular weakness if myasthenia gravis is a possibility.

In conversion of atrial fibrillation to normal sinus rhythm by any means, dislodgement of mural thrombi may lead to embolization, which should be kept in mind.

After a day or so, steady state plasma PA levels are produced following regular oral administration of a given dose of PRONESTYL (Procainamide Hydrochloride Tablets; Procainamide Hydrochloride Capsules) at set intervals, with peak plasma concentrations at about 90 to 120 minutes after each dose. After achieving and maintaining therapeutic plasma concentrations and satisfactory electrocardiographic and clinical responses, continued frequent periodic monitoring of vital signs and electrocardiograms is advised. If evidence of QRS widening of more than 25 percent or marked prolongation of the Q-T interval occurs, concern for overdosage is appropriate, and reduction in dosage is advisable if a 50 percent increase occurs. Elevated serum creatinine or urea nitrogen, reduced creatinine clearance, or history of renal insufficiency, as well as use in older patients (over age 50), provide grounds to anticipate that less than the usual dosage and longer time intervals between doses may suffice, since the urinary elimination of PA and NAPA may be reduced, leading to gradual accumulation beyond normally-predicted amounts. If facilities are available for measurement of plasma PA and NAPA, or acetylation capability, individual dose adjustment for optimal therapeutic levels may be easier, but close observation of clinical effectiveness is the most important criterion.

In the longer term, periodic complete blood counts are useful to detect possible idiosyncratic hematologic effects of PA on neutrophil, platelet or red cell homeostasis; agranulocytosis has been reported to occur occasionally in patients on long-term PA therapy. A rising titer of serum ANA may precede clinical symptoms of the lupus syndrome (see Boxed Warnings and ADVERSE REACTIONS). If the lupus erythematosus-like syndrome develops in a patient with recurrent life-threatening arrhythmias not controlled by other agents, corticosteroid suppressive therapy may be used concomitantly with PA. Since the PA-induced lupoid syndrome rarely includes the dangerous pathologic renal changes, PA therapy may not necessarily have to be stopped unless the symptoms of serositis and the possibility of further lupoid effects are of greater risk than the benefit of PA in controlling arrhythmias. Patients with rapid acetylation capability are less likely to develop the lupoid syndrome after prolonged PA therapy.

PRONESTYL Tablets (Procainamide Hydrochloride Tablets) contain FD&C Yellow No. 5 (tartrazine) which may cause allergic-type reactions (including bronchial asthma) in certain susceptible individuals. Although the overall incidence of FD&C Yellow No. 5 (tartrazine) sensitivity in the general population is low, it is frequently seen in patients who also have aspirin hypersensitivity.

Information for Patients

The physician is advised to explain to the patient that close cooperation in adhering to the prescribed dosage schedule is of great importance in controlling the cardiac arrhythmia safely. The patient should understand clearly that more medication is not necessarily better and may be dangerous, that skipping doses or increasing intervals between doses to suit personal convenience may lead to loss of control of the heart problem, and that "making up" missed doses by doubling up later may be hazardous.

The patient should be encouraged to disclose any past history of drug sensitivity, especially to procaine or other local anesthetic agents, or aspirin, and to report any history of

kidney disease, congestive heart failure, myasthenia gravis, liver disease, or lupus erythematosus.

The patient should be counseled to report promptly any symtoms of arthralgia, myalgia, fever, chills, skin rash, easy bruising, sore throat or sore mouth, infections, dark urine or icterus, wheezing, muscular weakness, chest or abdominal pain, palpitations, nausea, vomiting, anorexia, diarrhea, hallucinations, dizziness, or depression.

Laboratory Tests

Laboratory tests such as complete blood count (CBC), electrocardiogram, and serum creatinine or urea nitrogen may be indicated, depending on the clinical situation, and periodic rechecking of the CBC and ANA may be helpful in early detection of untoward reactions.

Drug Interactions

If other antiarrhythmic drugs are being used, additive effects on the heart may occur with PA administration, and dosage reduction may be necessary (see WARNINGS). Anticholinergic drugs administered concurrently with PA may produce additive antivagal effects on A-V nodal conduction, although this is not as well documented for PA as for quinidine.

Patients taking PA who require neuromuscular blocking agents such as succinylcholine may require less than usual doses of the latter, due to PA effects on reducing acetylcholine release.

Drug/Laboratory Test Interactions

Suprapharmacologic concentrations of lidocaine and meprobamate may inhibit fluorescence of PA and NAPA, and propranolol shows a native fluorescence close to the PA/NAPA peak wavelengths, so that tests which depend on fluorescence measurement may be affected.

Carcinogenesis, Mutagenesis, Impairment of Fertility

Long term studies in animals have not been performed.

Teratogenic Effects: Pregnancy Category C

Animal reproduction studies have not been conducted with PA. It also is not known whether PA can cause fetal harm when administered to a pregnant woman or can affect reproduction capacity. PA should be given to a pregnant woman only if clearly needed.

Nursing Mothers

Both PA and NAPA are excreted in human milk, and absorbed by the nursing infant. Because of the potential for serious adverse reactions in nursing infants, a decision to discontinue nursing or the drug should be made, taking into account the importance of the drug to the mother.

Pediatric Use

Safety and effectiveness in children have not been established.

ADVERSE REACTIONS

Cardiovascular: Hypotension following oral PA administration is rare. Hypotension and serious disturbances of cardiorhythm such as ventricular asystole or fibrillation are more common after intravenous administration (see OVERDOSAGE, WARNINGS). Second degree heart block has been reported in 2 of almost 500 patients taking PA orally.

Multisystem: A lupus erythematosus-like syndrome of arthralgia, pleural or abdominal pain, and sometimes arthritis, pleural effusion, pericarditis, fever, chills, myalgia, and possibly related hematologic or skin lesions (see below) is fairly common after prolonged PA administration, perhaps more often in patients who are slow acetylators (see Boxed Warnings and PRECAUTIONS). While some series have reported less than 1 in 500, others have reported the syndrome in up to 30 percent of patients on long term oral PA therapy. If discontinuation of PA does not reverse the lupoid symptoms, corticosteroid treatment may be effective.

Hematologic: Neutropenia, thrombocytopenia, or hemolytic anemia may rarely be encountered. Agranulocytosis has occurred after repeated use of PA, and deaths have been reported. (See Boxed Warning, WARNINGS section.)

Skin: Angioneurotic edema, urticaria, pruritus, flushing, and maculopapular rash have also occurred occasionally.

Gastrointestinal: Anorexia, nausea, vomiting, abdominal pain, bitter taste, or diarrhea may occur in 3 to 4 percent of patients taking oral procainamide. Hepatomegaly with increased serum aminotransferase activity have been reported after a single oral dose.

Nervous System: Dizziness or giddiness, weakness, mental depression, and psychosis with hallucinations have been reported occasionally.

OVERDOSAGE

Progressive widening of the QRS complex, prolonged Q-T and P-R intervals, lowering of the R and T waves, as well as increasing A-V block, may be seen with doses which are excessive for a given patient. Increased ventricular extrasystoles, or even ventricular tachycardia or fibrillation may occur. After intravenous administration but seldom after oral therapy, transient high plasma levels of PA may induce hypotension, affecting systolic more than diastolic pressures, especially in hypertensive patients. Such high levels may also produce central nervous depression, tremor, and even respiratory depression.

Plasma levels above 10 μg/mL are increasingly associated with toxic findings, which are seen occasionally in the 10 to 12 μg/mL range, more often in the 12 to 15 μg/mL range, and commonly in patients with plasma levels greater than 15 μg/mL. Overdosage symptoms may result following a single 2 g dose; while 3 g may be dangerous, especially if the patient is a slow acetylator, has decreased renal function, or underlying organic heart disease.

Treatment of overdosage or toxic manifestations includes general supportive measures, close observation, monitoring of vital signs and possibly intravenous pressor agents and mechanical cardiorespiratory support. If available, PA and NAPA plasma levels may be helpful in assessing the potential degree of toxicity and response to therapy. Both PA and NAPA are removed from the circulation by hemodialysis but not peritoneal dialysis. No specific antidote for PA is known.

DOSAGE AND ADMINISTRATION

The oral dose and interval of administration should be adjusted for the individual patient, based on clinical assessment of the degree of underlying myocardial disease, the patient's age, and renal function.

As a general guide, for younger adult patients with normal renal function, an initial total daily oral dose of up to 50 mg/kg of body weight of PRONESTYL Capsules or Tablets may be used, given in divided doses, every three hours, to maintain therapeutic blood levels. For older patients, especially those over 50 years of age, or for patients with renal, hepatic, or cardiac insufficiency, lesser amounts or longer intervals may produce adequate blood levels, and decrease the probability of occurrence of dose related adverse reactions. The total daily dose should be administered in divided doses at three, four, or six hour intervals and adjusted according to the patient's response.

To provide up to 50 mg per kg of body weight per day:* Patients weighing:		
lb	**Kg**	
88–110	40–50	250 mg q3 hrs to 500 mg q6 hrs
132–154	60–70	375 mg q3 hrs to 750 mg q6 hrs
176–198	80–90	500 mg q3 hrs to 1 g q6 hrs
>220	>100	625 mg q3 hrs to 1.25 g q6 hrs

*Initial dosage schedule guide only, to be adjusted for each patient individually, based on age, cardiorenal function, blood level (if available), and clinical response.

HOW SUPPLIED

*PRONESTYL Capsules (Procainamide Hydrochloride Capsules USP)

Two-piece gelatin capsules: 250 mg in bottles of 100 (NDC 0003-0758-50) and 1000 (NDC 0003-0758-80), **375 mg** in bottles of 100 (NDC 0003-0756-50), and **500 mg** in bottles of 100 (NDC 0003-0757-50) and 1000 (NDC 0003-0757-80).

Unimatic® unit-dose packs containing 100 capsules are also available for each potency: **250 mg** (NDC 0003-0758-53), **375 mg** (NDC 0003-0756-53), and **500 mg** (NDC 0003-0757-53).

Capsule color and identification numbers: **250 mg** yellow, **758; 375 mg** white and orange, **756; 500 mg** yellow and orange, **757.**

*PRONESTYL Tablets (Procainamide Hydrochloride Tablets)

FILMLOK®* tablets: **250 mg** in bottles of 100 (NDC 0003-0431-50), **375 mg** in bottles of 100 (NDC 0003-0434-50), and **500 mg** in bottles of 100 (NDC 0003-0438-50).

Tablet color and identification numbers: **250 mg** yellow, **431; 375 mg** orange, **434; 500 mg** red, **438.**

Also Available

PRONESTYL is available for parenteral administration as PRONESTYL Injection (Procainamide Hydrochloride Injection USP) in 10 mL vials of 100 mg per mL or 2 mL vials of 500 mg per mL of procainamide hydrochloride (see the package insert accompanying those products for further information).

STORAGE

Store at room temperature; avoid excessive heat (104° F); protect from moisture.

*FILMLOK is a Squibb trademark for veneer-coated tablets. (J4-141C)

Shown in Product Identification Section, pages 422 & 423

PRONESTYL-SR® TABLETS ℞
[pro"nest'tl es-ahr]
Procainamide Hydrochloride Sustained-Release Tablets

WARNING
The prolonged administration of procainamide often leads to the development of a positive anti-nuclear antibody (ANA) test, with or without symptoms of a lupus erythematosus-like syndrome. If a positive ANA titer develops, the benefits versus risks of continued procainamide therapy should be assessed.

DESCRIPTION

PRONESTYL (procainamide hydrochloride), a Group 1A cardiac antiarrhythmic drug, is p-amino-N-[2-(diethylamino)ethyl]-benzamide monohydrochloride, molecular weight 271.79.

It differs from procaine which is the p-aminobenzoyl *ester* of 2-(diethylamino)ethanol. Procainamide as the free base has a pKa of 9.23; the monohydrochloride is very soluble in water.

PRONESTYL-SR Tablets (Procainamide Hydrochloride Sustained-Release Tablets) for oral administration contain 500 mg procainamide hydrochloride. Inactive ingredients: microcrystalline cellulose, colorants (D&C Yellow No. 10; FD&C Blue No. 2), silicon dioxide, stearic acid, and other ingredients.

CLINICAL PHARMACOLOGY

Procainamide (PA) increases the effective refractory period of the atria, and to a lesser extent the bundle of His-Purkinje system and ventricles of the heart. It reduces impulse conduction velocity in the atria, His-Purkinje fibers, and ventricular muscle, but has variable effects on the atrioventricular (A-V) node, a direct slowing action and a weaker vagolytic effect which may speed A-V conduction slightly. Myocardial excitability is reduced in the atria, Purkinje fibers, papillary muscles, and ventricles by an increase in the threshold for excitation, combined with inhibition of ectopic pacemaker activity by retardation of the slow phase of diastolic depolarization, thus decreasing automaticity especially in ectopic sites. Contractility of the undamaged heart is usually not affected by therapeutic concentrations, although slight reduction of cardiac output may occur, and may be significant in the presence of myocardial damage. Therapeutic levels of PA may exert vagolytic effects and produce slight acceleration of heart rate, while high or toxic concentrations may prolong A-V conduction time or induce A-V block, or even cause abnormal automaticity and spontaneous firing, by unknown mechanisms.

Procainamide hydrochloride sustained-release tablets are designed to provide the biopharmaceutic characteristics of a sustained and relatively constant rate of release and absorption, independent of dose, primarily from the small intestine. The electrocardiogram may reflect these effects by showing slight sinus tachycardia (due to the anticholinergic action) and widened QRS complexes and, less regularly, prolonged Q-T and P-R intervals (due to longer systole and slower conduction), as well as some decrease in QRS and T wave amplitude. These direct effects of PA on electrical activity, conduction, responsiveness, excitability and automaticity are characteristic of a Group 1A antiarrhythmic agent, the prototype for which is quinidine; PA effects are very similar. However, PA has weaker vagal blocking action than does quinidine, does not induce alpha-adrenergic blockade, and is less depressing to cardiac contractility.

Ingested PA is resistant to digestive hydrolysis, and the drug is well absorbed from the entire small intestinal surface, but individual patients vary in their completeness of absorption of PA. Following oral administration q6h, procainamide hydrochloride sustained-release tablets achieve a mean steady state of procainamide (as well as procainamide plus N-acetylprocainamide) serum concentrations approximately equivalent to those from a comparable dose of an immediate-release (conventional) dosage form given q3h. Procainamide hydrochloride sustained-release tablets result in a significantly later time to peak plasma concentration when compared to immediate-release dosage forms. About 15 to 20 percent of PA is reversibly bound to plasma proteins, and considerable amounts are more slowly and reversibly bound to tissues of the heart, liver, lung, and kidney. The apparent volume of distribution eventually reaches about 2 liters per kilogram body weight with a half-time of approximately five minutes. While PA has been shown in the dog to cross the blood-brain barrier, it did not concentrate in the brain at levels higher than in plasma. It is not known if PA crosses the placenta. Plasma esterases are far less active in hydrolysis of PA than of procaine. The half-time for elimination of PA is three to four hours in patients with normal renal function, but reduced creatinine clearance and advancing age each prolong the half-time of elimination of PA.

A significant fraction of the circulating PA may be metabolized in hepatocytes to N-acetylprocainamide (NAPA), ranging from 16 to 21 percent of an administered dose in "slow acetylators" to 24 to 33 percent in "fast-acetylators". Since NAPA also has significant antiarrhythmic activity and somewhat slower renal clearance than PA, both hepatic acetylation rate capability and renal function, as well as age, have significant effects on the effective biologic half-time of therapeutic action of administered PA and the NAPA derivative. Trace amounts may be excreted in the urine as free and conjugated p-aminobenzoic acid, 30 to 60 percent as unchanged PA, and 6 to 52 percent as the NAPA derivative. Both PA and NAPA are eliminated by active tubular secretion as well as by glomerular filtration. Action of PA on the central nervous system is not prominent, but high plasma concentrations may cause tremors. While therapeutic plasma levels for PA have been reported to be 3 to 10 μg/mL certain patients such as those with sustained ventricular tachycardia, may need higher levels for adequate control. This may justify the increased risk of toxicity (see OVERDOSAGE). Where programmed ventricular stimulation has been used to evaluate efficacy of PA in preventing recurrent ventricular tachyarrhythmias, higher plasma levels (mean, 13.6 μg/mL) of PA were found necessary for adequate control.

INDICATIONS AND USAGE

PRONESTYL-SR Tablets (Procainamide Hydrochloride Sustained-Release Tablets) are indicated for the treatment of life-threatening ventricular arrhythmias.

PRONESTYL-SR Tablets are also indicated for the treatment of some patients with less severe, symptomatic ventricular arrhythmias, including unifocal or multifocal couplets and non-sustained ventricular tachycardia.

Because procainamide has the potential to produce serious hematological disorders (0.5 percent) particularly leukopenia or agranulocytosis (sometimes fatal), its use should be reserved for patients in whom, in the opinion of the physician, the benefits of treatment clearly outweigh the risks. (See WARNINGS and Boxed Warning.) For less serious arrhythmias, alternative therapies with less severe toxicity, such as certain beta-adrenergic blockers (see specific product labeling), should be considered.

Like all other antiarrhythmics, procainamide has not been shown to prevent sudden death in patients with serious ventricular ectopic activity, and, as with all other antiarrhythmics, procainamide has potentially serious adverse effects, including the ability to worsen arrhythmias. It is therefore essential that each patient be evaluated electrocardiographically and clinically prior to, and during, procainamide therapy to determine whether the response to the drug supports continued treatment.

CONTRAINDICATIONS

Complete heart block: Procainamide should not be administered to patients with complete heart block because of its effects in suppressing nodal or ventricular pacemakers and the hazard of asystole. It may be difficult to recognize complete heart block in patients with ventricular tachycardia, but if significant slowing of ventricular rate occurs during PA treatment without evidence of A-V conduction appearing, PA should be stopped. In cases of second degree A-V block or various types of hemiblock, PA should be avoided or discontinued because of the possibility of increased severity of block, unless the ventricular rate is controlled by an electrical pacemaker.

Idiosyncratic hypersensitivity: In patients sensitive to procaine or other ester-type local anesthetics, cross sensitivity to PA is unlikely; however, it should be borne in mind, and PA should not be used if it produces acute allergic dermatitis, asthma, or anaphylactic symptoms.

Lupus Erythematosus: An established diagnosis of systemic lupus erythematosus is a contraindication to PA therapy, since aggravation of symptoms is highly likely.

Torsades de Pointes: In the unusual ventricular arrhythmia called "les torsades de pointes" (Twistings of the points), characterized by alternation of one or more ventricular premature beats in the directions of the QRS complexes on ECG in persons with prolonged Q-T and often enhanced U waves, Group 1A antiarrhythmic drugs are contraindicated. Administration of PA in such cases may aggravate this special type of ventricular extrasystole or tachycardia instead of suppressing it.

WARNINGS

Blood Dyscrasias: Agranulocytosis, bone marrow depression, neutropenia, hypoplastic anemia and thrombocytopenia have been reported in patients receiving procainamide at a rate of approximately 0.5 percent. Most of these patients received procainamide within the recommended dosage range. Fatalities have occurred (with approximately 20-25 percent mortality in reported cases of agranulocytosis). Since most of these events have been noted during the first 12 weeks of therapy, it is recommended that complete blood counts including white cell, differential and platelet counts be performed at weekly intervals for the first three months of therapy, and periodically thereafter. Complete blood counts should be performed promptly if the patient develops any signs of infection (such as fever, chills, sore throat or stomatitis), bruising or bleeding. If any of these hematologic disorders are identified, procainamide therapy should be discontinued. Blood counts usually return to normal within one month of discontinua-

Continued on next page

Princeton—Cont.

tion. Caution should be used in patients with pre-existing marrow failure or cytopenia of any type. (See ADVERSE REACTIONS.)

Digitalis intoxication

Caution should be exercised in the use of procainamide in arrhythmias associated with digitalis intoxication. Procainamide can suppress digitalis-induced arrhythmias; however, if there is concomitant marked disturbance of atrioventricular conduction, additional depression of conduction and ventricular asystole or fibrillation may result. Therefore, use of procainamide should be considered only if discontinuation of digitalis, and therapy with potassium, lidocaine, or phenytoin are ineffective.

First degree heart block

Caution should be exercised also if the patient exhibits or develops first degree heart block while taking PA, and dosage reduction is advised in such cases. If the block persists despite dosage reduction, continuation of PA administration must be evaluated on the basis of current benefit versus risk of increased heart block.

Predigitalization for atrial flutter or fibrillation

Patients with atrial flutter or fibrillation should be cardioverted or digitalized prior to PA administration to avoid enhancement of A-V conduction which may result in ventricular rate acceleration beyond tolerable limits. Adequate digitalization reduces but does not eliminate the possiblity of sudden increase in ventricular rate as the atrial rate is slowed by PA in these arrhythmias.

Congestive heart failure

For patients in congestive heart failure, and those with acute ischemic heart disease or cardiomyopathy, caution should be used in PA therapy, since even slight depression of myocardial contractility may further reduce cardiac output of the damaged heart.

Concurrent other antiarrhythmic agents

Concurrent use of PA with other Group 1A antiarrhythmic agents such as quinidine or disopyramide may produce enhanced prolongation of conduction or depression of contractility and hypotension, especially in patients with cardiac decompensation. Such use should be reserved for patients with serious arrhythmias unresponsive to a single drug and employed only if close observation is possible.

Renal insufficiency

Renal insufficiency may lead to accumulation of high plasma levels from conventional oral doses of PA, with effects similar to those of overdosage (see OVERDOSAGE), unless dosage is adjusted for the individual patient.

Myasthenia gravis

Patients with myasthenia gravis may show worsening of symptoms from PA due to its procaine-like effect on diminishing acetylcholine release at skeletal muscle motor nerve endings, so that PA administration may be hazardous without optimal adjustment of anticholinesterase medications and other precautions.

PRECAUTIONS

General

Patients should be closely observed for possible hypersensitivity reactions, especially if procaine or local anesthetic sensitivity is suspected, and for muscular weakness if myasthenia gravis is a possibility.

In conversion of atrial fibrillation to normal sinus rhythm by any means, dislodgement of mural thrombi may lead to embolization, which should be kept in mind.

After approximately two days, steady state plasma PA levels are produced following regular oral administration of a given dose of PRONESTYL-SR Tablets (Procainamide Hydrochloride Sustained-Release Tablets) at set intervals. After achieving and maintaining therapeutic plasma concentrations and satisfactory electrocardiographic and clinical responses, continued frequent periodic monitoring of vital signs and electrocardiograms is advised. If evidence of QRS widening of more than 25 percent or marked prolongation of the Q-T interval occurs, concern for overdosage is appropriate, and reduction in dosage is advisable if a 50 percent increase occurs. Elevated serum creatinine or urea nitrogen, reduced creatinine clearance, or history of renal insufficiency, as well as use in older patients (over age 50), provide grounds to anticipate that less than the usual dosage and longer time intervals between doses may suffice, since the urinary elimination of PA and NAPA may be reduced, leading to gradual accumulation beyond normally predicted amounts. If facilities are available for measurement of plasma PA and NAPA, or acetylation capability, individual dose adjustment for optimal therapeutic levels may be easier, but close observation of clinical effectiveness is the most important criterion.

In the longer term, periodic blood counts are useful to detect possible idiosyncratic hematologic effects of PA on neutrophil, platelet or red cell homeostasis; agranulocytosis has been reported to occur occasionally in patients on long-term PA therapy. A rising titer of serum ANA may precede clinical symptoms of the lupoid syndrome (see BOX WARNING and ADVERSE REACTIONS). If the lupus erythematosus-like syndrome develops in a patient with recurrent life-threatening arrhythmias not controlled by other agents, corticosteroid suppressive therapy may be used concomitantly with PA. Since the PA-induced lupoid syndrome rarely includes the dangerous pathologic renal changes, PA therapy may not necessarily have to be stopped unless the symptoms of serositis and the possibility of further lupoid effects are of greater risk than the benefit of PA in controlling arrhythmias. Patients with rapid acetylation capability are less likely to develop the lupoid syndrome after prolonged PA therapy.

Information for Patients

The physician is advised to explain to the patient that close cooperation in adhering to the prescribed dosage schedule is of great importance in controlling the cardiac arrhythmia safely. The patient should understand clearly that more medication is not necessarily better and may be dangerous, that skipping doses or increasing intervals between doses to suit personal convenience may lead to loss of control of the heart problem, and that "making up" missed doses by doubling up later may be hazardous.

The patient should be encouraged to disclose any past history of drug sensitivity, especially to procaine or other local anesthetic agents, or aspirin, and to report any history of kidney disease, congestive heart failure, myasthenia gravis, liver disease, or lupus erythematosus.

The patient should be counseled to report promptly any symptoms of arthralgia, myalgia, fever, chills, skin rash, easy bruising, sore throat or sore mouth, infections, dark urine or icterus, wheezing, muscular weakness, chest or abdominal pain, palpitations, nausea, vomiting, anorexia, diarrhea, hallucinations, dizziness, or depression.

The patient should be advised not to break or chew the tablet, as this would interfere with designed dissolution characteristics. The tablet matrix may be seen in the stool since it does not disintegrate following release of procainamide.

Laboratory Tests

Laboratory tests such as complete blood count (CBC), electrocardiogram, and serum creatinine or urea nitrogen may be indicated, depending on the clinical situation, and periodic rechecking of the CBC and ANA may be helpful in early detection of untoward reactions.

Drug Interactions

If other antiarrhythmic drugs are being used, additive effects on the heart may occur with PA administration, and dosage reduction may be necessary (see WARNINGS).

Anticholinergic drugs administered concurrently with PA may produce additive antivagal effects on A-V nodal conduction, although this is not as well documented for PA as for quinidine.

Patients taking PA who require neuromuscular blocking agents such as succinylcholine may require less than usual doses of the latter, due to PA effects on reducing acetylcholine release.

Drug/Laboratory Test Interactions

Suprapharmacologic concentrations of lidocaine and meprobamate may inhibit fluorescence of PA and NAPA, and propranolol shows a native fluorescence close to the PA/NAPA peak wavelengths, so that tests which depend on fluorescence measurement may be affected.

Carcinogenesis, Mutagenesis, Impairment of Fertility

Long term studies in animals have not been performed.

Teratogenic Effects: Pregnancy Category C

Animal reproduction studies have not been conducted with PA. It also is not known whether PA can cause fetal harm when administered to a pregnant woman or can affect reproduction capacity. PA should be given to a pregnant woman only if clearly needed.

Nursing Mothers

Both PA and NAPA are excreted in human milk, and absorbed by the nursing infant. Because of the potential for serious adverse reactions in nursing infants, a decision to discontinue nursing or the drug should be made, taking into account the importance of the drug to the mother.

Pediatric Use

Safety and effectiveness in children have not been established.

ADVERSE REACTIONS

Cardiovascular: Hypotension following oral PA administration is rare. Hypotension and serious disturbances of cardiorhythm such as ventricular asystole or fibrillation are more common after intravenous administration (see OVERDOSAGE, WARNINGS). Second degree heart block has been reported in 2 of almost 500 patients taking PA orally.

Multisystem: A lupus erythematosus-like syndrome of arthralgia, pleural or abdominal pain, and sometimes arthritis, pleural effusion, pericarditis, fever, chills, myalgia, and possibly related hematologic or skin lesions (see below) is fairly common after prolonged PA administration, perhaps more often in patients who are slow acetylators (see BOX WARNING and PRECAUTIONS). While some series have reported less than 1 in 500, others have reported the syndrome in up to 30 percent of patients on long term oral PA therapy. If discontinuation of PA does not reverse the lupoid symptoms, corticosteroid treatment may be effective.

Hematologic: Neutropenia, thrombocytopenia, or hemolytic anemia may rarely be encountered. Agranulocytosis has occurred after repeated use of PA, and deaths have been reported. (See Boxed Warning, WARNINGS section.)

Skin: Angioneurotic edema, urticaria, pruritus, flushing, and maculopapular rash have also occurred occasionally.

Gastrointestinal: Anorexia, nausea, vomiting, abdominal pain, bitter taste, or diarrhea may occur in 3 to 4 percent of patients taking oral procainamide. Hepatomegaly with increased serum aminotransferase activity have been reported after a single oral dose.

Nervous System: Dizziness or giddiness, weakness, mental depression, and psychosis with hallucinations have been reported occasionally.

OVERDOSAGE

Progressive widening of the QRS complex, prolonged Q-T and P-R intervals, lowering of the R and T waves, as well as increasing A-V block, may be seen with doses which are excessive for a given patient. Increased ventricular extrasystoles, or even ventricular tachycardia or fibrillation may occur. After intravenous administration but seldom after oral therapy, transient high plasma levels of PA may induce hypotension, affecting systolic more than diastolic pressures, especially in hypertensive patients. Such high levels may also produce central nervous depression, tremor, and even respiratory depression.

Plasma levels above 10 $\mu g/mL$ are increasingly associated with toxic findings, which are seen occasionally in the 10 to 12 $\mu g/mL$ range, more often in the 12 to 15 $\mu g/mL$ range, and commonly in patients with plasma levels greater than 15 $\mu g/mL$. Overdosage symptoms may result following a single 2 g dose of conventionally formulated oral procainamide; 3 g may be dangerous, especially if the patient is a slow acetylator, has decreased renal function, or underlying organic heart disease.

Treatment of overdosage or toxic manifestations includes general supportive measures, close observation, monitoring of vital signs and possibly intravenous pressor agents and mechanical cardiorespiratory support. If available, PA and NAPA plasma levels may be helpful in assessing the potential degree of toxicity and response to therapy. Both PA and NAPA are removed from the circulation by hemodialysis but not peritoneal dialysis. No specific antidote for PA is known.

DOSAGE AND ADMINISTRATION

The oral dose and interval of administration should be adjusted for the individual patient, based on clinical assessment of the degree of underlying myocardial disease, the patient's age, and renal function.

As a general guide, for younger adult patients with normal renal function, an initial total daily oral dose of up to 50 mg/kg of body weight of PRONESTYL-SR Tablets (Procainamide Hydrochloride Sustained-Release Tablets) may be used, given in divided doses, every six hours to maintain therapeutic blood levels.

To provide approximately 50 mg per kg of body weight per day:* Patients weighing		
lb	kg	
88–110	40–50	500 mg q6h
132–154	60–70	750 mg q6h
176–198	80–90	1 g q6h
>220	>100	1.25 g q6h

* Initial dosage schedule guide only, to be adjusted for each patient individually, based on age, cardiorenal function, blood level (if available), and clinical response.

For older patients, especially those over 50 years of age, or for patients with renal, hepatic, or cardiac insufficiency, lesser amounts or longer intervals may produce adequate blood levels, and decrease the probability of occurrence of dose-related adverse reactions.

HOW SUPPLIED

PRONESTYL-SR Tablets (Procainamide Hydrochloride Sustained-Release Tablets) are available as FILMLOK®* tablets containing 500 mg procainamide hydrochloride in bottles of 100 (NDC 0003-0775-50) and in Unimatic® unit-dose packs (NDC 0003-0775-51) of 100 individually packaged tablets. Tablets are unscored, biconvex, greenish-yellow elongated ovals. Tablet identification number **775.**

Also Available: For initial therapy, available oral dosage forms include PRONESTYL Capsules (Procainamide Hydrochloride Capsules USP) and conventionally formulated capsule-shaped FILMLOK PRONESTYL Tablets (Procainamide Hydrochloride Tablets); tablets and capsules are available in potencies of 250 mg, 375 mg, and 500 mg procainamide hydrochloride. Consult the common package insert provided with these formulations for complete information.

PRONESTYL is also available for parenteral use as PRONESTYL Injection (Procainamide Hydrochloride Injection USP) sterile aqueous solutions in 10 mL vials providing

100 mg procainamide hydrochloride per mL or 2 mL vials providing 500 mg procainamide hydrochloride per mL. Consult the package insert provided with this product for complete information.

STORAGE

Store at room temperature; avoid excessive heat (104°F). Keep tightly closed; protect from moisture.

---

* FILMLOK is a Squibb trademark for veneer-coated tablets. (J4-104C)

Shown in Product Identification Section, page 423

RAUDIXIN®   ℞

[raw″dik′sin]
Rauwolfia Serpentina Tablets USP
Whole Root—Biologically Standardized

DESCRIPTION

RAUDIXIN (Rauwolfia Serpentina Tablets) contains powdered rauwolfia serpentina, an antihypertensive agent for oral administration, prepared from the powdered whole root of *Rauwolfia serpentina* Benth.

Each tablet contains 50 mg or 100 mg powdered rauwolfia serpentina composed of not less than 0.15 percent and not more than 0.2 percent of reserpine-rescinnamine group alkaloids, calculated as reserpine. Inactive ingredients: acacia, precipitated calcium carbonate, carnauba wax, castor oil, color additives [FD&C Red No. 3, FD&C Yellow No. 5 (tartrazine), FD&C Yellow No. 6], corn starch, ethylcellulose, flavor, gelatin, lactose, magnesium carbonate, mineral oil, shellac, stearic acid, sucrose, talc, titanium dioxide, and white wax.

Reserpine is a white to slightly yellow, crystalline powder, insoluble in water, very slightly soluble in ether and alcohol, slightly soluble in benzene, and freely soluble in acetic acid and chloroform. It is designated chemically as methyl 18β-hydroxy-11,17α-dimethoxy-3β, 20α-yohimban-16β-carboxylate 3,4,5-trimethoxybenzoate (ester).

CLINICAL PHARMACOLOGY

The rauwolfia alkaloids probably exert their antihypertensive effects through depletion of tissue stores of catecholamines (epinephrine and norepinephrine) from peripheral sites. By contrast, their sedative and tranquilizing properties are thought to be related to depletion of catecholamines and serotonin (5-hydroxytryptamine) from the brain.

Following absorption from the gastrointestinal tract, rauwolfia alkaloids concentrate in tissues with high lipid content. The drug crosses the blood-brain barrier and the placenta.

The rauwolfia alkaloids are characterized by slow onset of action and sustained effect. Both its cardiovascular and central nervous system effects may persist following withdrawal of the drug. The rauwolfia alkaloids are metabolized in the liver to inactive compounds that are excreted primarily in the urine. Unchanged alkaloids are excreted primarily in the feces.

INDICATIONS AND USAGE

RAUDIXIN (Rauwolfia Serpentina Tablets) is indicated in the treatment of mild essential hypertension. It is also useful as adjunctive therapy with other antihypertensive agents in the more severe forms of hypertension.

RAUDIXIN is also indicated for the relief of symptoms in agitated psychotic states (e.g., schizophrenia), primarily in those individuals unable to tolerate phenothiazine derivatives or those who also require antihypertensive medication.

CONTRAINDICATIONS

The preparation is contraindicated in patients who have previously demonstrated hypersensitivity to rauwolfia. It is also contraindicated in patients with a history of mental depression (especially with suicidal tendencies); active peptic ulcer; ulcerative colitis; and in patients receiving electroconvulsive therapy.

WARNINGS

Reserpine may cause mental depression. Recognition of depression may be difficult because this condition may often be disguised by somatic complaints (Masked Depression). The drug should be discontinued at first signs of depression such as despondency, early morning insomnia, loss of appetite, impotence, or self-deprecation. Drug-induced depression may persist for several months after drug withdrawal and may be severe enough to result in suicide.

Sensitivity reactions may occur in patients with or without a history of allergy or bronchial asthma.

The use of this drug may impair the mental and physical abilities required for the performance of tasks requiring alertness, such as driving or operating heavy machinery.

PRECAUTIONS

General

Because rauwolfia preparations increase gastrointestinal motility and secretion, this drug should be used cautiously in patients with a history of peptic ulcer, ulcerative colitis, or gallstones where biliary colic may be precipitated. Patients on high dosage should be observed carefully at regular intervals to detect possible reactivation of peptic ulcer.

Chronic administration of rauwolfia alkaloids may increase serum prolactin levels and decrease urinary catecholamine and vanilmandelic acid (VMA) excretion. Therefore, any diagnostic tests performed for these determinations should be interpreted with caution.

Caution should be exercised when treating hypertensive patients with renal insufficiency since they adjust poorly to lowered blood pressure levels.

Preoperative withdrawal of rauwolfia serpentina does not insure that circulatory instability will not occur. It is important that the anesthesiologist be aware of the patient's drug intake and consider this in the overall management since hypotension has occurred in patients receiving rauwolfia preparations. Anticholinergic and/or adrenergic drugs (metaraminol, norepinephrine) have been employed to treat adverse vagocirculatory effects.

This product contains FD&C Yellow No. 5 (tartrazine) which may cause allergic-type reactions (including bronchial asthma) in certain susceptible individuals. Although the overall incidence of FD&C Yellow No. 5 (tartrazine) sensitivity in the general population is low, it is frequently seen in patients who also have aspirin hypersensitivity.

Information for the Patient

Patients should be advised to report any symptoms of potential adverse effects.

Patients should be warned against taking this medication for any disorder other than for which it was prescribed, or discontinuing medication unless instructed by the physician. Caution patients that the drug may impair mental and/or physical abilities required for performance of hazardous tasks, such as operating machinery or driving a motor vehicle.

Drug Interactions

When administered concurrently, the following drugs may interact with rauwolfia alkaloids:

Alcohol/CNS Depressants —may increase the CNS depressant effects of these drugs or the rauwolfia alkaloids.

Other Antihypertensives/Diuretics —antihypertensive effects may be potentiated.

Digitalis Glycosides/Quinidine —may result in cardiac arrhythmias.

Levodopa —effects of levodopa may be inhibited.

Methotrimeprazine —may result in increased orthostatic hypotension.

Monamine Oxidase (MAO) Inhibitors —may result in excessive excitation, hypertension, and sympathetic response.

Sympathomimetics (Direct-acting) —rauwolfia alkaloids may prolong their effects; (Indirect-acting)—rauwolfia alkaloids may inhibit their action.

Tricycylic Antidepressants —the antidepressant effects of these drugs and the antihypertensive effects of rauwolfia alkaloids may be decreased.

Drug/Laboratory Test Interactions

Since rauwolfia alkaloids slightly decrease absorbance readings obtained on urinary steroid colorimetric determinations (e.g., modified Glenn-Nelson technique or Holtorff Koch modification of Zimmerman reaction), false low results may be reported.

Carcinogenesis, Mutagenesis, Impairment of Fertility

Animal carcinogenicity studies using reserpine at dosages of 25 to 50 times and 50 to 100 times the average human dose were conducted with rats and mice, respectively. Carcinogenic effects associated with the administration of reserpine were increased incidence of adrenal medullary pheochromocytomas in male rats, undifferentiated carcinomas of the seminal vesicles in male mice, and mammary cancer in female mice; carcinogenic effects were not seen in female rats.

Bacteriological studies to determine mutagenicity using reserpine showed negative results.

Long-term animal studies have not been performed with rauwolfia alkaloids to determine any impairment of fertility in males or females.

Animal tumorigenicity: rodent studies have shown that reserpine is an animal tumorigen, causing an increased incidence of mammary fibroadenomas in female mice, malignant tumors of the seminal vesicles in male mice, and malignant adrenal medullary tumors in male rats. These findings arose in two year studies in which the drug was administered in the feed at concentrations of 5 and 10 ppm—about 100 to 300 times the usual human dose. The breast neoplasms are thought to be related to reserpine's prolactin-elevating effect. Several other prolactin-elevating drugs have also been associated with an increased incidence of mammary neoplasia in rodents.

The extent to which these findings indicate a risk to humans is uncertain. Tissue culture experiments show that about one-third of human breast tumors are prolactin-dependent *in vitro,* a factor of considerable importance if the use of the drug is contemplated in a patient with previously detected breast cancer. The possibility of an increased risk of breast cancer in reserpine users has been studied extensively; however, no firm conclusion has emerged. Although a few epide-

miologic studies have suggested a slightly increased risk (less than twofold in all studies except one) in women who have used reserpine, other studies of generally similar design have not confirmed this. Epidemiologic studies conducted using other drugs (neuroleptic agents) that, like reserpine, increase prolactin levels and therefore would be considered rodent mammary carcinogens, have not shown an association between chronic administration of the drug and human mammary tumorigenesis. While long-term clinical observation has not suggested such an association, the available evidence is considered too limited to be conclusive at this time. An association of reserpine intake with pheochromocytoma or tumors of the seminal vesicles has not been explored.

Pregnancy: Teratogenic Effects

Category C. Animal reproduction studies have not been conducted with rauwolfia alkaloids. There are no adequte and well-controlled studies in pregnant women. Since rauwolfia alkaloids cross the placental barrier and appear in cord blood, drugs of this class should be used during pregnancy only if the potential benefit justifies the potential risk to the fetus.

Pregnancy: Nonteratogenic Effects

Increased respiratory secretions, nasal congestion, cyanosis and hypothermia, and anorexia are potential hazards in neonates of rauwolfia alkaloid-treated mothers.

Nursing Mothers

Rauwolfia alkaloids are excreted in human milk. Because of the potential for serious adverse reactions in nursing infants from rauwolfia alkaloids, a decision should be made whether to continue nursing or to discontinue therapy taking into account the importance of the drug to the mother.

Pediatric Use

Safety and effectiveness in children have not been established.

ADVERSE REACTIONS

The following adverse reactions (categorized by organ system in decreasing order of severity) have been observed, but there are insufficient data to support an estimate of their frequency. The reactions are usually reversible and disappear when the drug is discontinued.

Cardiovascular: Bradycardia; arrhythmias, particularly when used concurrently with digitalis or quinidine (see PRECAUTIONS, Drug Interactions); angina-like symptoms. Water retention with edema in patients with hypertensive vascular disease may occur rarely, but the condition generally clears with cessation of therapy, or the administration of a diuretic agent.

Central Nervous System: CNS sensitization manifested by optic atrophy, glaucoma, uveitis, deafness, and dull sensorium; extrapyramidal tract symptoms, rare Parkinsonian disease; depression; paradoxical anxiety; nightmares; nervousness; headache; dizziness; drowsiness.

Gastrointestinal: Gastrointestinal bleeding; hypersecretion and increased intestinal motility; diarrhea; vomiting; nausea; anorexia; dryness of mouth.

Respiratory: Dyspnea; epistaxis; nasal congestion.

Hypersensitivity: Purpura; pruritus; rash.

Other: Conjunctival injection; dysuria; muscular aches; weight gain; breast engorgement; pseudolactation; impotence or decreased libido; gynecomastia.

OVERDOSAGE

Signs and symptoms of overdosage include CNS depression ranging from drowsiness to coma, flushing of the skin, bradycardia, hypotension, conjunctival congestion, and pupillary constriction. Hypothermia, central respiratory depression, mental depression, diarrhea, vomiting, ptosis, miosis, and extrapyramidal signs such as stiffness, leg pain, and tremors may also occur.

Treatment is symptomatic. Provided the patient is not comatose or convulsing, evacuation of stomach contents by emesis or gastric lavage is recommended; precautions should be taken to preclude aspiration of contents by the patient, and to protect the airway. An activated charcoal slurry or saline cathartic may then be administered. Bradycardia and parasympathetic effects may be relieved with appropriate anticholinergic medication. Hypotension and coma usually respond to conservative supportive therapy. In cases of severe hypotension, treatment with a vasopressor having direct action upon vascular smooth muscle or a direct-acting sympathomimetic (see PRECAUTIONS, Drug Interactions), is recommended. Rapid infusion of IV solutions intended to raise arterial blood pressure should be avoided, since cardiac status in rauwolfia poisoning is uncertain. Because the effects of rauwolfia alkaloids are long acting, patients should be carefully observed for at least 72 hours.

DOSAGE AND ADMINISTRATION

For adults, the average oral dose is 200 to 400 mg daily, given in divided doses in the morning and evening. Higher doses should be used cautiously because serious mental depression and other side effects may be considerably increased. (Orally, 200 to 300 mg of powdered whole root is equivalent to 0.5 mg

Continued on next page

Princeton—Cont.

of reserpine.) Maintenance doses may vary from 50 to 300 mg per day given as a single dose or as two divided doses. Concomitant use of rauwolfia serpentina and ganglionic blocking agents, guanethidine, veratrum, hydralazine, methyldopa, chlorthalidone, or thiazides necessitates careful titration of dosage with each agent in order to obtain maximal therapeutic response as well as the lowest dose necessary to maintain that therapeutic response and minimize side effects.

Elderly and severely debilitated patients may require dosage lower than the usual adult dosage.

HOW SUPPLIED

RAUDIXIN (Rauwolfia Serpentina Tablets USP)
50 mg/tablet: bottles of 100 (NDC 0003-0713-50) and 1000 (NDC 0003-0713-80).
100 mg/tablet: bottles of 100 (NDC 0003-0776-50).
Each round, biconvex, red tablet is imprinted with the following identification numbers: 50 mg, **713**; 100 mg, **776**.

Storage
Keep and dispense in tightly closed, light-resistant containers. Store at room temperature; avoid excessive heat. (J4-151B)

Shown in Product Identification Section, page 423

RAUZIDE® ℞
Powdered Rauwolfia Serpentina
with Bendroflumethiazide Tablets

> **WARNING**
> This fixed combination drug is not indicated for initial therapy of hypertension. Hypertension requires therapy titrated to the individual patient. If the fixed combination represents the dosage so determined, its use may be more convenient in patient management. The treatment of hypertension is not static, but must be reevaluated as conditions in each patient warrant.

DESCRIPTION

RAUZIDE (Powdered Rauwolfia Serpentina with Bendroflumethiazide Tablets) is an antihypertensive agent for oral administration.

Each tablet contains 50 mg powdered rauwolfia serpentina composed of not less than 0.15 percent and not more than 0.2 percent of reserpine-rescinnamine group alkaloids calculated as reserpine, combined with 4 mg bendroflumethiazide. Inactive ingredients: acacia, precipitated calcium carbonate, castor oil, microcrystalline cellulose, color additives [FD&C Blue No. 1, FD&C Yellow No. 5 (tartrazine)], corn starch, ethylcellulose, gelatin, lactose, magnesium carbonate, shellac, stearic acid, sucrose, talc, and titanium dioxide.

Reserpine is a white to slightly yellow crystalline powder, insoluble in water, very slightly soluble in ether and alcohol, slightly soluble in benzene, and freely soluble in acetic acid and chloroform. It is designated chemically as methyl 18β-hydroxy-11, 17α-dimethoxy-3β, 20α-yohimban-16β-carboxylate 3,4,5-trimethoxybenzoate (ester). Bendroflumethiazide is a white to cream crystalline powder, practically insoluble in water, and freely soluble in acetone and alcohol. It is designated chemically as 3-benzyl-3,4-dihydro-6-(trifluoromethyl)-2H-1, 2, 4-benzothiadiazine-7-sulfonamide 1,1-dioxide.

CLINICAL PHARMACOLOGY

Either of the components of RAUZIDE (Powdered Rauwolfia Serpentine with Bendroflumethiazide Tablets), when administered alone, may produce a reduction of blood pressure in hypertension. When the two agents are administered simultaneously, the action of the one appears to supplement that of the other so that a hypotensive effect may be produced which is greater than that produced by either agent alone. Thus, hypertension which does not adequately respond to either drug alone may frequently respond to the combination of both drugs.

Rauwolfia Serpentina
Rauwolfia serpentina probably exerts its antihypertensive effects through depletion of tissue stores of catecholamines (epinephrine and norepinephrine) from peripheral sites. By contrast, its sedative and tranquilizing properties are thought to be related to depletion of catecholamines and serotonin (5-hydroxytryptamine) from the brain.

Following absorption from the gastrointestinal tract, rauwolfia alkaloids concentrate in tissues with high lipid content. The drug crosses the blood-brain barrier and the placenta.

The rauwolfia alkaloids are characterized by slow onset of action and sustained effect. Cardiovascular and central nervous system effects may persist following discontinuation of therapy. The rauwolfia alkaloids are metabolized in the liver to inactive compounds that are excreted primarily in the urine. Unchanged alkaloids are excreted primarily in the feces.

Bendroflumethiazide
Bendroflumethiazide interferes with the renal tubular mechanism of electrolyte reabsorption. At maximal therapeutic dosage all thiazides are approximately equal in their diuretic potency. Thiazides produce less alteration in the extracellular fluid composition than other diuretic agents. The mechanism whereby thiazides function in the control of hypertension has not been completely elucidated.

Thiazides increase the excretion of sodium and chloride in approximately equivalent amounts. Natriuresis may be accompanied by some loss of potassium, bicarbonate, and other electrolytes. The thiazides are absorbed from the gastrointestinal tract in varying degrees and exhibit a high degree of binding to plasma proteins. They are distributed in the extracellular space and cross the placenta. It has been reported that the diuretic effect of bendroflumethiazide is apparent within one to two hours, the peak effect occurs within 6 to 12 hours, and its diuretic activity persists for approximately 18 to 24 hours. Thiazides are excreted principally by tubular secretion, primarily in unchanged form.

INDICATIONS AND USAGE

RAUZIDE (Powdered Rauwolfia Serpentina with Bendroflumethiazide Tablets) is indicated for hypertension (see boxed WARNING).

Usage in Pregnancy. The routine use of diuretics in an otherwise healthy woman is inappropriate and exposes mother and fetus to unnecessary hazard. Diuretics do not prevent development of toxemia of pregnancy, and there is no satisfactory evidence that they are useful in the treatment of developed toxemia.

Edema during pregnancy may arise from pathological causes or from the physiologic and mechanical consequences of pregnancy. Thiazides are indicated in pregnancy when edema is due to pathologic causes, just as they are in the absence of pregnancy (however, see PRECAUTIONS below). Dependent edema in pregnancy, resulting from restriction of venous return by the expanded uterus, is properly treated through elevation of the lower extremities and use of support hose; use of diuretics to lower intravascular volume in this case is illogical and unnecessary. There is hypervolemia during normal pregnancy which is harmful to neither the fetus nor the mother (in the absence of cardiovascular disease), but which is associated with edema, including generalized edema, in the majority of pregnant women. If this edema produces discomfort, increased recumbency will often provide relief. In rare instances, this edema may cause extreme discomfort which is not relieved by rest. In these cases, a short course of diuretics may provide relief and may be appropriate.

CONTRAINDICATIONS

Rauwolfia Serpentina
Rauwolfia serpentina is contraindicated in patients who have previously demonstrated hypersensitivity to this agent; those with a history of mental depression (especially with suicidal tendencies); active peptic ulcer; ulcerative colitis; and in patients receiving electroconvulsive therapy.

Bendroflumethiazide
Bendroflumethiazide is contraindicated in anuria and in patients who have previously demonstrated hypersensitivity to thiazides or other sulfonamide-derived drugs.

WARNINGS

Sensitivity reactions may occur in patients with or without a history of allergy or bronchial asthma.

Lithium generally should not be given with diuretics; diuretic agents reduce the renal clearance of lithium and add a high risk of lithium toxicity. Refer to the package insert for lithium preparations before use of such concomitant therapy.

Rauwolfia Serpentina
Reserpine may cause mental depression. Recognition of depression may be difficult because this condition may often be disguised by somatic complaints (Masked Depression). The drug should be discontinued at first signs of depression such as despondency, early morning insomnia, loss of appetite, impotence, or self-deprecation. Drug-induced depression may persist for several months after drug withdrawal and may be severe enough to result in suicide.

Rauwolfia serpentina may impair the mental and physical abilities required for the performance of tasks requiring alertness, such as driving or operating heavy machinery.

Bendroflumethiazide
In patients with renal disease, thiazides may precipitate azotemia. Cumulative effects of the drug may develop in patients with impaired renal function.

Thiazides should be used with caution in patients with impaired hepatic function or progressive liver disease, since minor alterations of fluid and electrolyte balance may precipitate hepatic coma.

The possibility of exacerbation or activation of systemic lupus erythematosus has been reported.

PRECAUTIONS

General
This product contains FD&C Yellow No. 5 (tartrazine) which may cause allergic-type reactions (including bronchial asthma) in certain susceptible individuals. Although the overall incidence of FD&C Yellow No. 5 (tartrazine) sensitivity in the general population is low, it is frequently seen in patients who also have aspirin hypersensitivity.

Rauwolfia Serpentina
Because rauwolfia preparations increase gastrointestinal motility and secretion, this drug should be used cautiously in patients with a history of peptic ulcer, ulcerative colitis, or gallstones where biliary colic may be precipitated. Patients on high dosage should be observed carefully at regular intervals to detect possible reactivation of peptic ulcer.

Chronic administration of rauwolfia alkaloids may increase serum prolactin levels and decrease urinary catecholamine and vanilmandelic acid (VMA) excretion. Therefore, any diagnostic tests performed for these determinations should be interpreted with caution.

Caution should be exercised when treating hypertensive patients with renal insufficiency since they adjust poorly to lowered blood pressure levels.

Preoperative withdrawal of rauwolfia serpentina does not insure that circulatory instability will not occur. It is important that the anesthesiologist be aware of the patient's drug intake and consider this in the overall management since hypotension has occurred in patients receiving rauwolfia preparations. Anticholinergic and/or adrenergic drugs (metaraminol, norepinephrine) have been employed to treat adverse vagocirculatory effects.

Animal tumorigenicity: Rodent studies have shown that reserpine is an animal tumorigen, causing an increased incidence of mammary fibroadenomas in female mice, and malignant tumors of the seminal vesicles in male mice, and malignant adrenal medullary tumors in male rats. These findings arose in two year studies in which the drug was administered in the feed at concentrations of 5 and 10 ppm—about 100 to 300 times the usual human dose. The breast neoplasms are thought to be related to reserpine's prolactin-elevating effect. Several other prolactin-elevating drugs have also been associated with an increased incidence of mammary neoplasia in rodents.

The extent to which these findings indicate a risk to humans is uncertain. Tissue culture experiments show that about one-third of human breast tumors are prolactin-dependent *in vitro*, a factor of considerable importance if the use of the drug is contemplated in a patient with previously detected breast cancer. The possibility of an increased risk of breast cancer in reserpine users has been studied extensively; however, no firm conclusion has emerged. Although a few epidemiologic studies have suggested a slightly increased risk (less than twofold in all studies except one) in women who have used reserpine, other studies of generally similar design have not confirmed this. Epidemiologic studies conducted using other drugs (neuroleptic agents) that, like reserpine, increase prolactin levels and therefore would be considered rodent mammary cancinogens, have not shown an association between chronic administration of the drug and human mammary tumorigenesis. While long-term clinical observation has not suggested such an association, the available evidence is considered too limited to be conclusive at this time. An association of reserpine intake with pheochromocytoma or tumors of the seminal vesicles has not been explored.

Bendroflumethiazide
All patients receiving thiazide therapy should be observed for clinical signs of fluid or electrolyte imbalance; namely, hyponatremia, hypochloremic alkalosis, and hypokalemia. Serum and urine electrolyte determinations are particularly important when the patient is vomiting excessively or receiving parenteral fluids. Warning signs or symptoms of fluid and electrolyte imbalance include: dryness of the mouth, thirst, weakness, lethargy, drowsiness, restlessness, muscle pains or cramps, muscular fatigue, hypotension, oliguria, tachycardia, and gastrointestinal disturbances such as nausea and vomiting.

Hypokalemia may develop with thiazides as with any other potent diuretic, especially with brisk diuresis, when severe cirrhosis is present, or during concomitant use of corticosteroids, ACTH, digitalis, or after prolonged thiazide therapy. Interference with adequate oral electrolyte intake will also contribute to hypokalemia. Hypokalemia can sensitize or exaggerate the response of the heart to the toxic effects of digitalis (e.g., increased ventricular irritability). Concurrent administration of a potassium-sparing diuretic or potassium supplements may be indicated in these patients.

Any chloride deficit is generally mild and usually does not require specific treatment except under extraordinary circumstances (as in liver disease or renal disease). Dilutional hyponatremia may occur in edematous patients in hot weather; appropriate therapy is water restriction, rather than administration of salt except in rare instances when the hyponatremia is life threatening. In actual salt depletion appropriate replacement is the therapy of choice.

Calcium excretion is decreased by thiazides. Pathological changes in the parathyroid gland with hypophosphatemia have been observed in a few patients on prolonged thiazide therapy. The common complications of hyperparathyroidism such as renal lithiasis, bone resorption, and peptic ulceration have not been seen. Thiazides should be discontinued before carrying out tests for parathyroid function.

Hyperuricemia may occur or frank gout may be precipitated in certain patients receiving thiazide therapy.

Latent diabetes mellitus may become manifest during thiazide administration.

The antihypertensive effects of the drug may be enhanced in the postsympathectomy patient.

If progressive renal impairment becomes evident, as indicated by a rising nonprotein nitrogen or blood urea nitrogen, a careful reappraisal of therapy is necessary with consideration given to withholding or discontinuing diuretic therapy.

Information for the Patient

Patients should be advised to report any symptoms of potential adverse effects.

Patients should be warned against taking this medication for any disorder other than for which it was prescribed, or discontinuing medication unless instructed by the physician. Caution patients that the drug may impair mental and/or physical abilities required for performance of hazardous tasks, such as operating machinery or driving a motor vehicle.

Laboratory Tests

Serum and urine electrolyte levels should be regularly monitored (see WARNINGS, Bendroflumethiazide, also PRECAUTIONS, General, Bendroflumethiazide).

Drug Interactions

Rauwolfia Serpentina

When administered concurrently, the following drugs may interact with rauwolfia alkaloids:

Alcohol/CNS Depressants —may increase the CNS depressant effects of these drugs or the rauwolfia alkaloids.

Other Antihypertensives/Diuretics —antihypertensive effects may be potentiated.

Digitalis Glycosides/Quinidine —may result in cardiac arrhythmias.

Levodopa —effects of levodopa may be inhibited.

Methotrimeprazine —may result in increased orthostatic hypotension.

Monamine Oxidase (MAO) Inhibitors—may result in excessive excitation, hypertension, and sympathetic response.

Sympathomimetics (Direct-acting) —rauwolfia alkaloids may prolong their effects; *(Indirect-acting)* —rauwolfia alkaloids may inhibit their action.

Tricyclic Antidepressants —the antidepressant effects of these drugs and the antihypertensive effects of rauwolfia alkaloids may be decreased.

Bendroflumethiazide

When administered concurrently, the following drugs may interact with thiazide diuretics:

Alcohol, Barbiturates, or Narcotics —aggravation of orthostatic hypotension may occur.

Amphotericin B, Corticosteroids, or Corticotropin (ACTH) —may intensify electrolyte imbalance, particularly hypokalemia.

Anticoagulants (oral) —dosage adjustments of anticoagulant medication may be necessary since bendroflumethiazide may decrease their effects.

Antigout medications —dosage adjustments of antigout medication may be necessary since bendroflumethiazide may raise the level of blood uric acid.

Other Antihypertensive medications (e.g., ganglionic or peripheral adrenergic blocking agents) —dosage adjustments may be necessary since bendroflumethiazide may potentiate their effects.

Antidiabetic drugs (oral agents and insulin) —dosage adjustments of antidiabetic agents may be necessary due to the possible hyperglycemic effect of bendroflumethiazide.

Calcium —increased serum calcium levels due to decreased excretion.

Cardiac Glycosides —increased possibility of digitalis toxicity associated with hypokalemia.

Cholestyramine Resin and Colestipol HCL —may delay or decrease absorption of bendroflumethiazide. Sulfonamide diuretics should be taken at least one hour before or four to six hours after these medications.

Diazoxide —possible hyperglycemic, hyperuricemic, and antihypertensive effects.

Lithium —possible lithium toxicity due to reduced renal clearance (see WARNINGS, Bendroflumethiazide).

MAO Inhibitors —dosage adjustments of MAO Inhibitors and/or thiazides may be necessary since hypotensive effects are increased.

Nondepolarizing muscle relaxants, Preanesthetics and Anesthetics used in surgery (e.g., tubocurarine chloride and gallamine triethiodide)—increased responsiveness to muscle relaxants; *Pressor amines* (e.g., norepinephrine)—decreased arterial responsiveness to pressor amines, but not sufficient to preclude effectiveness of the pressor agent for therapeutic use.

Use caution in patients taking any of these medications who undergo surgery. Administer preanesthetic and anesthetic agents in reduced dosage, and if possible, discontinue bendroflumethiazide one week prior to surgery.

Methenamine —possible decreased effectiveness of methenamine due to possible increased alkalinization of the urine from thiazide therapy.

Probenecid or Sulfinpyrazone —increased dosage of these agents may be necessary since bendroflumethiazide may exhibit increased hyperuricemic effects.

Drug/Laboratory Test Interactions

Rauwolfia Serpentina

Since rauwolfia alkaloids slightly decrease absorbance readings obtained on urinary steroid colorimetric determinations (e.g., modified Glenn-Nelson technique or Holtorff Koch modification of Zimmerman reaction), false low results may be obtained.

Bendroflumethiazide

Thiazides may produce false-negative results with the phentolamine and tyramine tests, and may interfere with the phenosulfonphthalein (PSP) test due to decreased excretion of PSP.

Thiazides may decrease serum PBI levels without signs of thyroid disturbance.

Carcinogenesis, Mutagenesis, Impairment of Fertility

Rauwolfia Serpentina

Animal carcinogenicity studies using reserpine at dosages of 25 to 50 times and 50 to 100 times the average human dose were conducted with rats and mice, respectively. Carcinogenic effects associated with the administration of reserpine were increased incidence of adrenal medullary pheochromocytomas in male rats, undifferentiated carcinomas of the seminal vesicles in male mice, and mammary cancer in female mice; carcinogenic effects were not seen in female rats.

Bacteriological studies to determine mutagenicity using reserpine showed negative results.

Long-term studies in animals have not been performed to evaluate mutagenicity, or possible impairment of fertility in males or females.

Bendroflumethiazide

Long-term studies in animals have not been performed to evaluate carcinogenic or mutagenic potential, or possible impairment of fertility in males or females.

Pregnancy: Teratogenic Effects

Category C. Animal reproduction studies have not been conducted with rauwolfia alkaloids or bendroflumethiazide. There are no adequate and well-controlled studies in pregnant women. Since rauwolfia alkaloids and thiazides cross the placental barrier and appear in cord blood, drugs in these classes should be used during pregnancy only if the potential benefit justifies the potential risk to the fetus.

Pregnancy: Nonteratogenic Effects

Rauwolfia Serpentina

Increased respiratory secretions, nasal congestion, cyanosis and hypothermia, and anorexia are potential hazards in neonates of rauwolfia alkaloid-treated mothers.

Bendroflumethiazide

Fetal or neonatal jaundice, thrombocytopenia, and possibly other adverse reactions which have occurred in the adult are potential hazards in fetuses and neonates of thiazide-treated mothers.

Nursing Mothers

Both rauwolfia serpentina and bendroflumethiazide are excreted in human milk. Because of the potential for serious adverse reactions in nursing infants from both drugs, a decision should be made whether to continue nursing or to discontinue therapy taking into account the importance of this preparation to the mother.

Pediatric Use

Safety and effectiveness in children have not been established.

ADVERSE REACTIONS

The following adverse reactions (categorized by organ system in decreasing order of severity) have been observed with bendroflumethiazide and rauwolfia serpentina; there is, however, insufficient data to support an estimate of their frequency.

Rauwolfia Serpentina

Cardiovascular: Bradycardia; arrhythmias, particularly when used concurrently with digitalis or quinidine (see PRECAUTIONS, Drug Interactions); angina-like symptoms.

Central Nervous System: CNS sensitization manifested by optic atrophy, glaucoma, uveitis, deafness, and dull sensorium; extrapyramidal tract symptoms; rare parkinsonian disease; depression, paradoxical anxiety; nightmares, nervousness; drowsiness.

Gastrointestinal: Gastrointestinal bleeding; hypersecretion and increased intestinal motility; dryness of mouth.

Respiratory: Dyspnea; epistaxis; nasal congestion.

Other: Conjunctival injection; dysuria; muscular aches; weight gain; breast engorgement; pseudolactation; impotence or decreased libido; gynecomastia.

These reactions are usually reversible and disappear when the drug is discontinued.

Bendroflumethiazide

Central Nervous System: Vertigo; paresthesias; xanthopsia; lightheadedness.

Hematologic: Leukopenia (agranulocytopenia); agranulocytosis; thrombocytopenia; aplastic anemia; hemolytic anemia.

Cardiovascular: Orthostatic hypotension (may be aggravated by alcohol, barbiturates, or narcotics—see PRECAUTIONS, Drug Interactions, Bendroflumethiazide).

Gastrointestinal: Gastric irritation; abdominal cramps or bloating; constipation; pancreatitis; sialadenitis.

Hepatic: Jaundice (intrahepatic cholestatic jaundice).

Renal: Allergic glomerulonephritis.

Hypersensitivity: Ecchymosis; skin photosensitivity; exfoliative dermatitis; urticaria; necrotizing angiitis (vasculitis, cutaneous vasculitis); fever; respiratory distress including pneumonitis; anaphylactic reactions.

Other: Hyperglycemia; glycosuria; occasional metabolic acidosis in diabetic patients; hyperuricemia; muscle spasm or cramps; weakness; restlessness; transient blurred vision. Whenever adverse reactions are moderate or severe, thiazide dosage should be reduced or therapy withdrawn.

Common to Bendroflumethiazide and Rauwolfia Serpentina

Gastrointestinal: Anorexia; nausea; vomiting; diarrhea.

Central Nervous System: Headache; dizziness.

Hypersensitivity: Purpura; pruritus; rash.

OVERDOSAGE

Rauwolfia Serpentina

In the event of overdosage, rauwolfia serpentina may cause CNS depression ranging from drowsiness to coma, flushing of the skin, bradycardia, hypotension, conjunctival congestion, and pupillary constriction. Hypothermia, central respiratory depression, mental depression, diarrhea, vomiting, ptosis, miosis, and extrapyramidal signs such as stiffness, leg pain, and tremors may also occur.

Treatment is symptomatic. Provided the patient is not comatose or convulsing, evacuation of stomach contents by emesis or gastric lavage is recommended; precautions should be taken to preclude aspiration of contents by the patient, and to protect the airway. An activated charcoal slurry may then be administered. Bradycardia and parasympathetic effects may be relieved with appropriate anticholinergic medication. Hypotension and coma usually respond to conservative supportive therapy. In cases of severe hypotension, treatment with a vasopressor having direct action upon vascular smooth muscle or a direct-acting sympathomimetic (see PRECAUTIONS, Drug Interactions) is recommended. Rapid infusion of IV solutions intended to raise arterial blood pressure should be avoided, since cardiac status in rauwolfia poisoning is uncertain. Because the effects of rauwolfia alkaloids are long acting, patients should be carefully observed for at least 72 hours.

Bendroflumethiazide

In addition to the expected diuresis, overdosage of thiazides may produce varying degrees of lethargy which may progress to coma within a few hours, with minimal depression of respiration and cardiovascular function and without evidence of serum electrolyte changes or dehydration. The mechanism of thiazide-induced CNS depression is unknown. Gastrointestinal irritation and hypermotility may occur. Transitory increase in BUN has been reported, and serum electrolyte changes may occur, especially in patients with impaired renal function.

In addition to gastric lavage and supportive therapy for stupor or coma, symptomatic treatment of gastrointestinal effects may be needed. Cathartics should be avoided since they tend to enhance the loss of fluid and electrolytes. Measures as required to maintain hydration, electrolyte balance, respiration, and cardiovascular and renal function should be instituted.

DOSAGE AND ADMINISTRATION

As determined by individual titration (see boxed WARNING). Usual dosage may range from one to four tablets daily.

HOW SUPPLIED

RAUZIDE (Powdered Rauwolfia Serpentina with Bendroflumethiazide Tablets)

Tablets providing 50 mg powdered rauwolfia serpentina with 4 mg bendroflumethiazide are available in bottles of 100 (NDC 0003-0769-51) and 1000 (NDC 0003-0769-80). Each dark green, discoid-shaped tablet is imprinted with identification number **769**.

Storage

Keep and dispense in tightly closed containers. Store at room temperature; avoid excessive heat.

(J4-144A)

Shown in Product Identification Section, page 423

Products are cross-indexed by
generic and chemical names in the
YELLOW SECTION

Procter & Gamble
P. O. BOX 171
CINCINNATI, OH 45201

HEAD & SHOULDERS®
Antidandruff Shampoo

Head & Shoulders Shampoo offers effective dandruff control and beautiful hair in a formula that is pleasant to use. Independently conducted clinical testing (double-blind and dermatologist-graded) has proved that Head & Shoulders reduces dandruff flaking. Head & Shoulders is also gentle enough to use every day for clean, manageable hair.

ACTIVE INGREDIENT
1.0% pyrithione zinc suspended in an anionic detergent system. Cosmetic ingredients are also included.

INDICATIONS
For effective control of dandruff and seborrheic dermatitis of the scalp.

ACTIONS
Pyrithione zinc is substantive to the scalp and remains after rinsing. Its mechanism of action has not been fully established, but it is believed to control the microorganisms associated with dandruff flaking and itching.

PRECAUTIONS
Not to be taken internally. Keep out of children's reach. Avoid getting shampoo in eyes— if this happens, rinse eyes with water.

DOSAGE AND ADMINISTRATION
For best results in controlling dandruff, Head & Shoulders should be used regularly. It is gentle enough to use for every shampoo. In treating seborrheic dermatitis, a minimum of four shampooings are needed to achieve full effectiveness.

COMPOSITION
Lotion—Normal to Oily Formula: Pyrithione zinc in a shampoo base of water, ammonium laureth sulfate, ammonium lauryl sulfate, cocamide MEA, glycol distearate, ammonium xylene sulfonate, fragrance, citric acid, methylchloroisothiazolinone, methylisothiazolinone, and FD&C Blue No. 1. Lotion—Normal to Dry Formula: Pyrithione zinc in a shampoo base of water, ammonium laureth sulfate, ammonium lauryl sulfate, cocamide MEA, glycol distearate, ammonium xylene sulfonate, propylene glycol, fragrance, citric acid, methylchloroisothiazolinone, methylisothiazolinone, and FD&C Blue No. 1. Lotion—Dry Scalp Regular Formula: Pyrithione zinc in a shampoo base of water, ammonium laureth sulfate, ammonium lauryl sulfate, cocamide MEA, glycol distearate, dimethicone, ammonium xylene sulfonate, fragrance, tricetylomonium chloride, cetyl alcohol, stearyl alcohol, DMDM hydantoin, sodium chloride, FD&C blue no. 1. Lotion—Dry Scalp Conditioning Formula: Pyrithione zinc in a shampoo base of water, ammonium laureth sulfate, ammonium lauryl sulfate, cocamide MEA, glycol distearate, dimethicone, ammonium xylene sulfonate, fragrance, tricetylmonium chloride, cetyl alcohol, stearyl alcohol, DMDM hydantoin, sodium chloride, FD&C blue no. 1. Cream—Normal to Oily Formula: Pyrithione zinc in a shampoo base of water, sodium cocoglyceryl ether sulfonate, sodium chloride, sodium lauroyl sarcosinate, cocamide DEA, cocoyl sarcosine, fragrance, and FD&C Blue No. 1. Cream—Normal to Dry Formula: Pyrithione zinc in a shampoo base of water, sodium cocoglyceryl ether sulfonate, sodium chloride, sodium lauroyl sarcosinate, cocamide DEA, propylene glycol, cocoyl sarcosine, fragrance, and FD&C Blue No. 1.

HOW SUPPLIED
Lotion available in 4.0, 7.0, 11.0, and 15.0 fl. oz. unbreakable plastic bottles, dry scalp available in 7.0, 11.0, and 15.0 oz. Concentrate cream available in 5.5 oz. tube. Both lotion and concentrate are available in formulas for "Normal to Oily" and "Normal to Dry" hair, dry scalp formula is available in "regular" and "conditioning".

Shown in Product Identification Section, page 423

Regular Flavor
METAMUCIL® Powder
(psyllium hydrophilic mucilloid)

PRODUCT OVERVIEW

KEY FACTS
Regular Flavor Metamucil is a bulk forming natural fiber used to relieve constipation and to restore and maintain regularity. It contains psyllium hydrophilic mucilloid, a concentrated source of soluble fiber. Metamucil contains no chemical stimulants and is non-addictive.

MAJOR USES
Metamucil is used in the management of chronic constipation, as adjunctive therapy in constipation associated with other conditions such as diverticular disease and pregnancy, and to ease passage of stools in patients with anorectal disorders.

SAFETY INFORMATION
Contraindicated in patients with intestinal obstruction or fecal impaction. This product may cause allergic reaction in people sensitive to inhaled or ingested psyllium powder.

PRESCRIBING INFORMATION
Regular Flavor
METAMUCIL® Powder
[met "uh-mū 'sil]
(psyllium hydrophilic mucilloid)

DESCRIPTION
Regular Flavor Metamucil contains hydrophilic mucilloid, a highly efficient dietary fiber derived from the husk of the psyllium seed (*Plantago ovata*). Each dose contains approximately 3.4 g of psyllium hydrophilic mucilloid. Inactive ingredients include dextrose, a carbohydrate. Each dose contains less than 10 mg of sodium, 31 mg of potassium, and 14 calories. Carbohydrate content is approximately 3.5 g.

ACTIONS
Metamucil provides bulk that promotes normal elimination. The product is uniform, instantly miscible, palatable, and nonirritative in the gastrointestinal tract.

INDICATIONS
Metamucil is indicated in the management of chronic constipation, in irritable bowel syndrome, as adjunctive therapy in the constipation of diverticular disease, in the bowel management of patients with hemorrhoids, and for constipation during pregnancy, convalescence, and senility.

CONTRAINDICATIONS
Intestinal obstruction, fecal impaction.

PRECAUTION
May cause allergic reaction in people sensitive to inhaled or ingested psyllium powder.

DOSAGE AND ADMINISTRATION
The usual adult dosage is one rounded teaspoonful (7 g) stirred into a standard 8-oz glass of cool water, fruit juice, milk or other beverage. It can be taken orally one to three times a day, depending on the need and response. It may require continued use for 2 or 3 days to provide optimal benefit. An additional glass of liquid after each dose is helpful. For children (6 to 12 years old), use ½ the adult dose in 8 oz. of liquid, 1 to 3 times daily.
New Users: Medical research shows that high fiber intake is important for good digestive health. To help the body adjust and avoid the minor gas and bloating sometimes associated with high fiber intake, it may be necessary to increase fiber intake gradually. Initial dose: one teaspoonful of Metamucil per day. If minor gas or bloating occurs, reduce the amount for several days. Gradually increase to 3 teaspoonfuls per day if needed.

HOW SUPPLIED
Powder, containers of 7 oz, 14 oz, 21 oz, and 32 oz. (OTC); also available in cartons of 30 single-dose (7g) packets (OTC) and 100 single-dose (7g) packets (Professional).

IS THIS PRODUCT OTC
Yes. See also PDR For Nonprescription Drugs.

Sugar Free Regular Flavor
METAMUCIL® Powder
(psyllium hydrophilic mucilloid)

PRODUCT OVERVIEW

KEY FACTS
Sugar Free Regular Flavor Metamucil is a bulk forming natural fiber used to relieve constipation and to restore and maintain regularity. It contains psyllium hydrophilic mucilloid, a concentrated source of soluble fiber. Metamucil contains no chemical stimulants and is non-addictive.

MAJOR USES
Metamucil is used in the management of chronic constipation, as adjunctive therapy in constipation associated with other conditions such as diverticular disease and pregnancy, and to ease passage of stools in patients with anorectal disorders.

SAFETY INFORMATION
Contraindicated in patients with intestinal obstruction or fecal impaction. This product may cause allergic reaction in people sensitive to inhaled or ingested psyllium powder. Phenylketonurics should be aware that Sugar Free Metamucil contains phenylalanine.

PRESCRIBING INFORMATION
Sugar Free Regular Flavor
METAMUCIL® Powder
[met "uh-mū 'sil]
(psyllium hydrophilic mucilloid)

DESCRIPTION
Sugar Free Regular Flavor Metamucil contains hydrophilic mucilloid, a highly efficient dietary fiber derived from the husk of the psyllium seed (*Plantago ovata*), which has been sweetened with NutraSweet®* brand sweetener (aspartame). It contains no sugar. Each dose contains approximately 3.4 g of psyllium hydrophilic mucilloid. Inactive ingredients include aspartame and maltodextrin. Each dose contains about 1 calorie, less than 10 mg. of sodium, 31 mg of potassium and 6 mg of phenylalanine. Carbohydrate content is 0.3 grams.

ACTIONS
Metamucil provides bulk that promotes normal elimination. The product is uniform, instantly miscible, palatable, and nonirritative in the gastrointestinal tract.

INDICATIONS
Metamucil is indicated in the management of chronic constipation, in irritable bowel syndrome, as adjunctive therapy in the constipation of diverticular disease, in the bowel management of patients with hemorrhoids, and for constipation during pregnancy, convalescence, and senility.

CONTRAINDICATIONS
Intestinal obstruction, fecal impaction.

WARNING
Phenylketonurics should be aware that Sugar Free Metamucil contains phenylalanine.

PRECAUTION
May cause allergic reaction in people sensitive to inhaled or ingested psyllium powder.

DOSAGE AND ADMINISTRATION
The usual adult dosage is one rounded teaspoonful (3.7 g) stirred into a standard 8-oz glass of cool water, fruit juice, milk or other beverage. It can be taken orally one to three times a day, depending on the need and response. It may require continued use for 2 or 3 days to provide optimal benefit. An additional glass of liquid after each dose is helpful. For children (6–12 years old), use ½ the adult dose in 8 oz. of liquid, 1 to 3 times daily.
New User: Medical research shows that high fiber intake is important for good digestive health. To help the body adjust and avoid the minor gas and bloating sometimes associated with high fiber intake, it may be necessary to increase fiber intake gradually. Initial dose: one teaspoonful of Metamucil per day. If minor gas or bloating occurs, reduce the amount for several days. Gradually increase to 3 teaspoonfuls per day if needed.

HOW SUPPLIED
Powder, containers of 3.7 oz, 7.4 oz, 11.1 oz, and 16.9 oz. (OTC); also available in cartons of 100 single-dose (3.7 g) packets (Professional).

IS THIS PRODUCT OTC
Yes. See also PDR For Nonprescription Drugs.

_____

* NutraSweet is a registered trademark of the NutraSweet Company.

Orange Flavor
METAMUCIL® Powder
(psyllium hydrophilic mucilloid)

PRODUCT OVERVIEW

KEY FACTS
Orange Flavor Metamucil is a bulk forming natural fiber used to relieve constipation and to restore and maintain regularity. It contains psyllium hydrophilic mucilloid, a concentrated source of soluble fiber. Metamucil contains no chemical stimulants and is non-addictive.

MAJOR USES
Metamucil is used in the management of chronic constipation, as adjunctive therapy in constipation associated with other conditions such as diverticular disease and pregnancy, and to ease passage of stools in patients with anorectal disorders.

SAFETY INFORMATION
Contraindicated in patients with intestinal obstruction or fecal impaction. The product may cause allergic reaction in people sensitive to inhaled or ingested psyllium powder.

PRESCRIBING INFORMATION
Orange Flavor METAMUCIL® Powder
[met "uh-mū 'sil]
(psyllium hydrophilic mucilloid)

DESCRIPTION
Orange Flavor Metamucil contains hydrophilic mucilloid, a highly efficient dietary fiber derived from the husk of the psyllium seed (*Plantago ovata).* Each dose contains approxi-

mately 3.4 g of psyllium hydrophilic mucilloid. Inactive ingredients include citric acid, FD&C Yellow No. 6, flavoring, and sucrose (a carbohydrate). Each dose contains less than 10 mg. of sodium, 31 mg of potassium, and 30 calories. Carbohydrate content is approximately 7.1 g.

ACTIONS
Metamucil provides bulk that promotes normal elimination. The product is uniform, instantly miscible, palatable, and nonirritative in the gastrointestinal tract.

INDICATIONS
Metamucil is indicated in the management of chronic constipation, in irritable bowel syndrome, as adjunctive therapy in the constipation of diverticular disease, in the bowel management of patients with hemorrhoids, and for constipation during pregnancy, convalescence, and senility.

CONTRAINDICATIONS
Intestinal obstruction, fecal impaction.

PRECAUTION
May cause allergic reaction in people sensitive to inhaled or ingested psyllium powder.

DOSAGE AND ADMINISTRATION
The usual adult dose is one rounded tablespoonful (11 g) stirred into a standard 8-oz glass of cool water, fruit juice, milk or other beverage. It can be taken orally one to three times a day, depending on the need and response. It may require continued use for 2 or 3 days to provide optimal benefit. An additional glass of liquid after each dose is helpful. For children (6 to 12 years old), use ½ the adult dose in 8 oz. of liquid, 1 to 3 times daily.
New Users: Medical research shows that high fiber intake is important for good digestive health. To help the body adjust and avoid the minor gas and bloating sometimes associated with high fiber intake, it may be necessary to increase fiber intake gradually. Initial dose: one tablespoonful of Metamucil per day. If minor gas or bloating occurs, reduce the amount for several days. Gradually increase to 3 tablespoonfuls per day if needed.

HOW SUPPLIED
Powder, containers of 7 oz, 14 oz, 21 oz, and 32 oz. (OTC)

IS THIS PRODUCT OTC
Yes. See also PDR For Nonprescription Drugs.

Sugar Free Orange Flavor
METAMUCIL® Powder
(psyllium hydrophilic mucilloid)

PRODUCT OVERVIEW
KEY FACTS
Sugar Free Orange Flavor Metamucil is a bulk forming natural fiber used to relieve constipation and to restore and maintain regularity. It contains psyllium hydrophilic mucilloid, a concentrated source of soluble fiber. Metamucil contains no chemical stimulants and is non-addictive.

MAJOR USES
Metamucil is used in the management of chronic constipation, as adjunctive therapy in constipation associated with other conditions such as diverticular disease and pregnancy, and to ease passage of stools in patients with anorectal disorders.

SAFETY INFORMATION
Contraindicated in patients with intestinal obstruction or fecal impaction. This product may cause allergic reaction in people sensitive to inhaled or ingested psyllium powder. Phenylketonurics should be aware that Sugar Free Metamucil contains phenylalanine.

PRESCRIBING INFORMATION
Sugar Free Orange Flavor
METAMUCIL® Powder
[met "uh-mū 'sil]
(psyllium hydrophilic mucilloid)

DESCRIPTION
Sugar Free Orange Flavor Metamucil contains hydrophilic mucilloid, a highly efficient dietary fiber derived from the husk of the psyllium seed (Plantago ovata), which has been sweetened with NutraSweet®* brand sweetener (aspartame). It contains no sugar. Each dose contains approximately 3.4 g of psyllium hydrophilic mucilloid. Inactive ingredients include aspartame, citric acid, FD&C Yellow No. 6, flavoring, and maltodextrin, and silicon dioxide. Each dose contains about 5 calories, less than 10 mg. of sodium, 31 mg of potassium, and 30 mg of phenylalanine. Carbohydrate content is approximately 1.4 grams.

ACTIONS
Metamucil provides bulk that promotes normal elimination. The product is uniform, instantly miscible, palatable, and nonirritative in the gastrointestinal tract.

INDICATIONS
Metamucil is indicated in the management of chronic constipation, in irritable bowel syndrome, as adjunctive therapy in the constipation of diverticular disease, in the bowel management of patients with hemorrhoids, and for constipation during pregnancy, convalescence, and senility.

CONTRAINDICATIONS
Intestinal obstruction, fecal impaction.

WARNING
Phenylketonurics should be aware that Sugar Free Metamucil contains phenylalanine.

PRECAUTIONS
May cause allergic reaction in people sensitive to inhaled or ingested psyllium powder.

DOSAGE AND ADMINISTRATION
The usual adult dosage is one rounded teaspoonful (5.2 g) stirred into a standard 8-oz glass of cool water, fruit juice, milk or other beverage. It can be taken orally one to three times a day, depending on the need and response. It may require continued use for 2 or 3 days to provide optimal benefit. An additional glass of liquid after each dose is helpful. For children (6–12 years old), use ½ the adult dose in 8 oz. of liquid, 1 to 3 times daily.
New Users: Medical research shows that high fiber intake is important for good digestive health. To help the body adjust and avoid the minor gas and bloating sometimes associated with high fiber intake, it may be necessary to increase fiber intake gradually. Initial dose: one teaspoonful of Metamucil per day. If minor gas or bloating occurs, reduce the amount for several days. Gradually increase to 3 teaspoonfuls per day if needed.

HOW SUPPLIED
Powder, containers of 4.7 oz, 8.7 oz, 12.9, and 20.7 oz (OTC).

IS THIS PRODUCT OTC
Yes. See also PDR For Nonprescription Drugs.

---

* NutraSweet is a registered trademark of the NutraSweet Company.

Strawberry Flavor METAMUCIL® Powder
(psyllium hydrophilic mucilloid)

PRODUCT OVERVIEW
KEY FACTS
Strawberry Flavor Metamucil is a bulk forming natural fiber used to relieve constipation and to restore and maintain regularity. It contains psyllium hydrophilic mucilloid, a concentrated source of soluble fiber. Metamucil contains no chemical stimulants and is non-addictive.

MAJOR USES
Metamucil is used in the management of chronic constipation, as adjunctive therapy in constipation associated with other conditions such as diverticular disease and pregnancy, and to ease passage of stools in patients with anorectal disorders.

SAFETY INFORMATION
Contraindicated in patients with intestinal obstruction or fecal impaction. This product may cause allergic reaction in people sensitive to inhaled or ingested psyllium powder.

PRESCRIBING INFORMATION
Strawberry Flavor METAMUCIL® Powder
[met "uh-mū 'sil]
(psyllium hydrophilic mucilloid)

DESCRIPTION
Strawberry Flavor Metamucil contains hydrophilic mucilloid, a highly efficient dietary fiber derived from the husk of the psyllium seed (Plantago ovata). Each dose contains approximately 3.4 g of psyllium hydrophilic mucilloid. Inactive ingredients include citric acid, FD&C Red No. 40, flavoring, and sucrose (a carbohydrate). Each dose contains less than 10 mg. of sodium, 31 mg of potassium, and 30 calories. Carbohydrate content is approximately 7.1 g.

ACTIONS
Metamucil provides bulk that promotes normal elimination. The product is uniform, instantly miscible, palatable, and nonirritative in the gastrointestinal tract.

INDICATIONS
Metamucil is indicated in the management of chronic constipation, in irritable bowel syndrome, as adjunctive therapy in the constipation of diverticular disease, in the bowel management of patients with hemorrhoids, and for constipation during pregnancy, convalescence, and senility.

CONTRAINDICATIONS
Intestinal obstruction, fecal impaction.

PRECAUTION
May cause allergic reaction in people sensitive to inhaled or ingested psyllium powder.

DOSAGE AND ADMINISTRATION
The usual adult dose is one rounded tablespoonful (11 g) stirred into a standard 8-oz glass of cool water, fruit juice, milk or other beverage. It can be taken orally one to three times a day, depending on the need and response. It may require continued use for 2 or 3 days to provide optimal benefit. An additional glass of liquid after each dose is helpful. For children (6–12 years old), use ½ tablespoonful in 8 oz. of liquid, 1 to 3 times daily.
New Users: Medical research shows that high fiber intake is important for good digestive health. To help the body adjust and avoid the minor gas and bloating sometimes associated with high fiber intake, it may be necessary to increase fiber intake gradually. Initial dose: one tablespoonful of Metamucil per day. If minor gas or bloating occurs, reduce the amount for several days. Gradually increase to 3 tablespoonfuls per day if needed.

HOW SUPPLIED
Powder, containers of 7 oz, 14 oz, and 21 oz. (OTC)

IS THIS PRODUCT OTC
Yes. See also PDR For Nonprescription Drugs.

Sugar Free Lemon-Lime Flavor
EFFERVESCENT METAMUCIL®
(psyllium hydrophilic mucilloid)

PRODUCT OVERVIEW
KEY FACTS
Sugar Free Lemon-Lime Flavor Effervescent Metamucil is a bulk forming natural fiber used to relieve constipation and to restore and maintain regularity. It contains psyllium hydrophilic mucilloid, a concentrated source of soluble fiber. Metamucil contains no chemical stimulants and is non-addictive.

MAJOR USES
Metamucil is used in the management of chronic constipation, as adjunctive therapy in constipation associated with other conditions such as diverticular disease and pregnancy, and to ease passage of stools in patients with anorectal disorders.

SAFETY INFORMATION
Contraindicated in patients with intestinal obstruction or fecal impaction. This product may cause allergic reaction in people sensitive to inhaled or ingested psyllium powder. Phenylketonurics should be aware that Sugar Free Metamucil contains phenylalanine.

PRESCRIBING INFORMATION
Sugar Free Lemon-Lime Flavor
EFFERVESCENT METAMUCIL®
[met "uh-mū 'sil]
(psyllium hydrophilic mucilloid)

DESCRIPTION
Sugar Free Lemon-Lime Flavor Effervescent Metamucil contains hydrophilic mucilloid, a highly efficient dietary fiber derived from the husk of the psyllium seed (Plantago ovata), which has been sweetened with NutraSweet®* brand sweetener (aspartame). It contains no sugar. Each dose contains approximately 3.4 g of psyllium hydrophilic mucilloid. Inactive ingredients include aspartame, calcium carbonate, citric acid, flavoring, potassium bicarbonate, silicon dioxide, and sodium bicarbonate. Each packet contains less than 1 calorie, 290 mg of potassium, less than 10 mg. of sodium, and 30 mg phenylalanine.

ACTIONS
Effervescent Metamucil provides bulk that promotes normal elimination. The product is effervescent and requires no stirring. It is uniform, instantly miscible, palatable, and nonirritative in the gastrointestinal tract.

INDICATIONS
Effervescent Metamucil is indicated in the management of chronic constipation, in irritable bowel syndrome, as adjunctive therapy in the constipation of diverticular disease, in the bowel management of patients with hemorrhoids, and for constipation during pregnancy, convalescence, and senility.

CONTRAINDICATIONS
Intestinal obstruction, fecal impaction.

WARNING
Phenylketonurics should be aware that Sugar Free Effervescent Metamucil contains phenylalanine.

Continued on next page

Procter & Gamble—Cont.

PRECAUTION
May cause allergic reaction in people sensitive to inhaled or ingested psyllium powder.

DOSAGE AND ADMINISTRATION
The usual adult dosage is the contents of one packet (0.19 oz.). The entire contents of a packet are poured into a standard 8-oz glass. The glass is slowly filled with cool water, fruit juice, milk or beverage. Drink promptly. An additional glass of liquid after each dose is helpful. The product can be taken orally one to three times a day, depending on the need and the response. It may require continued use for two or three days to provide optimal benefit.

New Users: Medical research shows that high hiber intake is important for good digestive health. To help the body adjust and avoid the minor gas and bloating sometimes associated with high fiber intake, it may be necessary to increase fiber intake gradually. Initial dose: one packet of Metamucil per day. If minor gas or bloating occurs, reduce the amount for several days. Gradually increase to 3 packets per day if needed.

HOW SUPPLIED
Cartons of 30 single-dose (0.19 oz.) packets (OTC); also available in cartons of 100 single-dose (0.19 oz.) packets (Professional).

IS THIS PRODUCT OTC
Yes. See also PDR For Nonprescription Drugs.

---

* NutraSweet is a registered trademark of the NutraSweet Company.

Sugar Free Orange Flavor
EFFERVESCENT METAMUCIL®
(psyllium hydrophilic mucilloid)

PRODUCT OVERVIEW
KEY FACTS
Sugar Free Orange Flavor Effervescent Metamucil is a bulk forming natural fiber used to relieve constipation and to restore and maintain regularity. It contains psyllium hydrophilic mucilloid, a concentrated source of soluble fiber. Metamucil contains no chemical stimulants and is non-addictive.

MAJOR USES
Metamucil is used in the management of chronic constipation, as adjunctive therapy in constipation associated with other conditions such as diverticular disease and pregnancy, and to ease passage of stools in patients with anorectal disorders.

SAFETY INFORMATION
Contraindicated in patients with intestinal obstruction or fecal impaction. This product may cause allergic reaction in people sensitive to inhaled or ingested psyllium powder. Phenylketonurics should be aware that Sugar Free Metamucil contains phenylalanine.

PRESCRIBING INFORMATION
Sugar Free Orange Flavor
EFFERVESCENT METAMUCIL®
[met "uh-mū'sil]
(psyllium hydrophilic mucilloid)

DESCRIPTION
Sugar Free Orange Flavor Effervescent Metamucil contains hydrophilic mucilloid, a highly efficient dietary fiber derived from the husk of the psyllium seed (Plantago ovata), which has been sweetened with NutraSweet®* brand sweetener (aspartame). It contains no sugar. Each dose contains approximately 3.4 g of psyllium hydrophilic mucilloid. Inactive ingredients include aspartame, citric acid, FD&C Yellow No. 6, flavoring, potassium bicarbonate, silicon dioxide, and sodium bicarbonate. Each packet contains less than 1 calorie, 310 mg of potassium, less than 10 mg. of sodium, and 30 mg phenylalanine.

ACTIONS
Effervescent Metamucil provides bulk that promotes normal elimination. It is effervescent and requires no stirring. The product is uniform, instantly miscible, palatable, and nonirritative in the gastrointestinal tract.

INDICATIONS
Effervescent Metamucil is indicated in the management of chronic constipation, in irritable bowel syndrome, as adjunctive therapy in the constipation of diverticular disease, in the bowel management of patients with hemorrhoids, and for constipation during pregnancy, convalescence, and senility.

CONTRAINDICATIONS
Intestinal obstruction, fecal impaction.

WARNING
Phenylketonurics should be aware that Sugar Free Effervescent Metamucil contains phenylalanine.

PRECAUTION
May cause allergic reaction in people sensitive to inhaled or ingested psyllium powder.

DOSAGE AND ADMINISTRATION
The usual adult dosage is the contents of one packet (0.18 oz.) The entire contents of a packet are poured into a standard 8-oz. glass. The glass is slowly filled with cool water, fruit juice, milk or beverage. Drink promptly. An additional glass of liquid after each dose is helpful. The product can be taken orally one to three times a day, depending on the need and the response. It may require continued use for two or three days to provide optimal benefit.

New Users: Medical research shows that high fiber intake is important for good digestive health. To help the body adjust and avoid the minor gas and bloating sometimes associated with high fiber intake, it may be necessary to increase fiber intake gradually. Initial dose: one packet of Metamucil per day. If minor gas or bloating occurs, reduce the amount for several days. Gradually increase to 3 packets per day if needed.

HOW SUPPLIED
Cartons of 30 single-dose (0.18 oz.) packets (OTC)

IS THIS PRODUCT OTC
Yes. See also PDR For Nonprescription Drugs.

---

* NutraSweet is a registered trademark of the NutraSweet Company.

PEPTO-BISMOL®
LIQUID AND TABLETS
For diarrhea, heartburn, indigestion, upset stomach and nausea.

DESCRIPTION
Each Pepto-Bismol Tablet contains 262 mg bismuth subsalicylate and each tablespoonful (15 ml) of Pepto-Bismol Liquid contains 262 mg bismuth subsalicylate. Each tablet contains 102 mg salicylate and each tablespoonful of liquid contains 130 mg salicylate. Liquid and tablets contain no sugar. Tablets are sodium-free (less than 2 mg/tablet) and Liquid is low in sodium (5 mg/tablespoonful). Inactive ingredients include (Tablets): calcium carbonate, FD&C Red. No. 27, flavor, magnesium stearate, mannitol, povidone, saccharin sodium and talc; (Liquid): FD&C Red No. 3, FD&C Red No 40, flavor, magnesium aluminum silicate, methylcellulose, saccharin sodium, salicylic acid, sodium salicylate and water.

INDICATIONS
Pepto-Bismol controls diarrhea within 24 hours, relieving associated abdominal cramps; soothes heartburn and indigestion without constipating; and relieves nausea and upset stomach.

CAUTION
This product contains salicylates. If taken with aspirin and ringing of the ears occurs, discontinue use. This product does not contain aspirin, but should not be administered to those patients who have a known allergy to aspirin or salicylates. Caution is advised in the administration to patients taking medication for anticoagulation, diabetes and gout.

WARNING
Caution is advised in the administration to children, including teenagers, during or after recovery from chicken pox or flu. As with any drug, caution is advised in the administration to pregnant or nursing women.
Note: This medication may cause a temporary and harmless darkening of the tongue and/or stool. Stool darkening should not be confused with melena.

DOSAGE AND ADMINISTRATION
Tablets:
Adults—Two tablets
Children (according to age)—

9–12 yrs.	1 tablet
6–9 yrs.	⅔ tablet
3–6 yrs.	⅓ tablet

Chew or dissolve in mouth. Repeat every ½ to 1 hour as needed, to a maximum of 8 doses in a 24-hour period.
Liquid: Shake well before using.
Adults—2 tablespoonfuls
Children (according to age)—

9–12 yrs.	1 tablespoonful
6–9 yrs.	2 teaspoonfuls
3–6 yrs.	1 teaspoonful

Repeat dosage every ½ to 1 hour, if needed, to a maximum of 8 doses in a 24-hour period.

For children under 3 years, dose according to weight.

28+ lbs.	1 teaspoonful
14–18 lbs.	½ teaspoonful

Repeat every 4 hours, if needed, to a maximum of 6 doses in a 24-hour period.

HOW SUPPLIED
Pepto-Bismol Liquid is available in:

NDC 37000-032-01	4 fl. oz. bottle
NDC 37000-032-02	8 fl. oz. bottle
NDC 37000-032-03	12 fl. oz. bottle
NDC 37000-032-04	16 fl. oz. bottle

Pepto-Bismol Tablets are pink triangular chewable tablets imprinted with "Pepto-Bismol" on one side. Tablets are available in:

NDC 37000-033-03	box of 24
NDC 37000-033-04	box of 42

MAXIMUM STRENGTH
PEPTO-BISMOL®
LIQUID
For diarrhea, heartburn, indigestion, upset stomach and nausea.

DESCRIPTION
Each tablespoonful (15 ml) of Maximum Strength Pepto-Bismol Liquid contains 525 mg bismuth subsalicylate. (230 mg salicylate). Maximum Strength Pepto-Bismol Liquid contains no sugar and is low in sodium (less than 5 mg/tablespoonful). Inactive ingredients include: FD&C Red No. 3, FD&C Red No. 40, flavor, magnesium aluminum silicate, methylcellulose, saccharin sodium, salicylic acid, sodium salicylate, and water.

INDICATIONS
Maximum Strength Pepto-Bismol controls diarrhea within 24 hours, relieving associated abdominal cramps; soothes heartburn and indigestion without constipating; and relieves nausea and upset stomach.

CAUTION
This product contains salicylates. If taken with aspirin and ringing of the ears occurs, discontinue use. This product does not contain aspirin, but should not be administered to those patients who have a known allergy to aspirin or salicylates. Caution is advised in the administration to patients taking medication for anticoagulation, diabetes, and gout.

WARNING
Caution is advised in the administration to children, including teenagers, during or after recovery from chicken pox or flu. As with any drug, caution is advised in the administration to pregnant or nursing women.
Note: This medication may cause a temporary and harmless darkening of the tongue and/or stool. Stool darkening should not be confused with melena.

DOSAGE AND ADMINISTRATION
Shake well before using.
Adults—2 tablespoonfuls
Children (according to age)—

9–12 yrs.	1 tablespoonful
6–9 yrs.	2 teaspoonfuls
3–6 yrs.	1 teaspoonful

Repeat dosage every hour, if needed, to a maximum of 4 doses in a 24 hour period.

HOW SUPPLIED
Maximum Strength Pepto-Bismol is available in:

NDC 37000-019-01	4 fl. oz. bottle
NDC 37000-019-02	8 fl. oz. bottle
NDC 37000-019-03	12 fl. oz. bottle

PERIDEX®   ℞
[per-i-dex]
(chlorhexidine gluconate)
Oral Rinse

PRODUCT OVERVIEW
KEY FACTS
Peridex is an antimicrobial oral rinse containing 0.12% chlorhexidine gluconate. Peridex has been shown to achieve significant reductions in plaque, gingival inflammation, and associated bleeding. Approximately 30% of the active ingredient, is retained in the oral cavity following a single rinsing. This retained active ingredient is slowly released into the oral fluids.

MAJOR USES
Peridex has proved to be clinically effective for use between dental visits as part of a professional program for the treatment of gingivitis as characterized by redness, swelling of the gingivae and gingival bleeding. Therapy should be initiated directly following an oral prophylaxis. Patients using Peridex should be reevaluated and given a thorough prophylaxis at intervals no longer than six months. Recommended

use is a 30-second rinse of ½ fluid ounce (marked in cap) twice daily.

SAFETY INFORMATION

The most common side effects associated with chlorhexidine oral rinses are (1) an increase in staining of teeth and other oral surfaces on certain individuals, (2) an increase in supragingival calculus formation, and (3) an alteration in taste perception. Not all patients will experience a visually significant increase in tooth staining. No serious systemic adverse reactions associated with use of Peridex were observed in clinical testing.

PRESCRIBING INFORMATION

PERIDEX® ℞
(chlorhexidine gluconate)
Oral Rinse

DESCRIPTION

Peridex is an oral rinse containing 0.12% chlorhexidine gluconate (1, 1′ -hexamethylene bis [5-(p-chlorophenyl) biguanide] di-D-gluconate) in a base containing water, 11.6% alcohol, glycerin, PEG-40 sorbitan diisostearate, flavor, sodium saccharin, and FD&C Blue No. 1. Peridex is a near-neutral solution (pH range 5–7). Chlorhexidine gluconate is a salt of chlorhexidine and gluconic acid. Its chemical structure is:

CLINICAL PHARMACOLOGY

Peridex provides microbicidal activity during oral rinsing. The clinical significance of Peridex's antimicrobial activities is not clear. Microbiological sampling of plaque has shown a general reduction of counts of certain assayed bacteria, both aerobic and anaerobic, ranging from 54–97% through six months' use.

Use of Peridex in a six-month clinical study did not result in any significant changes in bacterial resistance, overgrowth of potentially opportunistic organisms or other adverse changes in the oral microbial ecosystem. Three months after Peridex use was discontinued the number of bacteria in plaque had returned to baseline levels and resistance of plaque bacteria to chlorhexidine gluconate was equal to that at baseline.

PHARMACOKINETICS

Pharmacokinetic studies with Peridex indicate approximately 30% of the active ingredient, chlorhexidine gluconate, is retained in the oral cavity following rinsing. This retained drug is slowly released into the oral fluids.

Studies conducted on human subjects and animals demonstrate that any ingested chlorhexidine gluconate is poorly absorbed from the gastrointestinal tract. The mean plasma level of chlorhexidine gluconate reached a peak of 0.206 ug/g in humans 30 minutes after they ingested a 300-mg dose of the drug. Detectable levels of chlorhexidine gluconate were not present in the plasma of these subjects 12 hours after the compound was administered. Excretion of chlorhexidine gluconate occurred primarily through the feces (~90%). Less than 1% of the chlorhexidine gluconate ingested by these subjects was excreted in the urine.

INDICATION

Peridex is indicated for use between dental visits as part of a professional program for the treatment of gingivitis as characterized by redness and swelling of the gingivae, including gingival bleeding upon probing. Peridex has not been tested among patients with acute necrotizing ulcerative gingivitis (ANUG). For patients having coexisting gingivitis and periodontitis, see PRECAUTIONS.

CONTRAINDICATIONS

Peridex should not be used by persons who are known to be hypersensitive to chlorhexidine gluconate.

WARNINGS

The effect of Peridex on periodontitis has not been determined. An increase in supragingival calculus was noted in clinical testing in Peridex users compared with control users. It is not known if Peridex use results in an increase in subgingival calculus. Calculus deposits should be removed by a dental prophylaxis at intervals no greater than six months. Rare hypersensitivity and generalized allergic reactions have also been reported. Peridex should not be used by persons who have a sensitivity to it or its components.

PRECAUTIONS
GENERAL:
1. For patients having coexisting gingivitis and periodontitis, the presence or absence of gingival inflammation following treatment with Peridex should not be used as a major indicator of underlying periodontitis.
2. Peridex can cause staining of oral surfaces, such as tooth surfaces, restorations, and the dorsum of the tongue. Not all patients will experience a visually significant increase

in toothstaining. In clinical testing, 56% of Peridex users exhibited a measurable increase in facial anterior stain, compared to 35% of control users after six months; 15% of Peridex users developed what was judged to be heavy stain, compared to 1% of control users after six months. Stain will be more pronounced in patients who have heavier accumulations of unremoved plaque.

Stain resulting from use of Peridex does not adversely affect health of the gingivae or other oral tissues. Stain can be removed from most tooth surfaces by conventional professional prophylactic techniques. Additional time may be required to complete the prophylaxis.

Discretion should be used when prescribing to patients with anterior facial restorations with rough surfaces or margins. If natural stain cannot be removed from these surfaces by a dental prophylaxis, patients should be excluded from Peridex treatment if permanent discoloration is unacceptable. Stain in these areas may be difficult to remove by dental prophylaxis and on rare occasions may necessitate replacement of these restorations.
3. Some patients may experience an alteration in taste perception while undergoing treatment with Peridex. Most patients accommodate to this effect with continued use of Peridex. No instances of permanent taste alteration due to Peridex have been reported.

USAGE IN PREGNANCY: Pregnancy Category B. Reproduction and fertility studies with chlorhexidine gluconate have been conducted. No evidence of impaired fertility was observed in rats at doses up to 100 mg/kg/day, and no evidence of harm to the fetus was observed in rats and rabbits at doses up to 300 mg/kg/day and 40 mg/kg/day, respectively. These doses are approximately 100, 300, and 40 times that which would result from a person's ingesting 30 ml (2 capfuls) of Peridex per day. Since controlled studies in pregnant women have not been conducted, the benefits of the drug in pregnant women should be weighed against possible risk to the fetus.

NURSING MOTHERS: It is not known whether this drug is excreted in human milk. Because many drugs are excreted in human milk, caution should be exercised when Peridex is administered to a nursing woman.

In parturition and lactation studies with rats, no evidence of impaired parturition or of toxic effects to suckling pups was observed when chlorhexidine gluconate was administered to dams at doses that were over 100 times greater than that which would result from a person's ingesting 30 ml (2 capfuls) of Peridex per day.

PEDIATRIC USE: Clinical effectiveness and safety of Peridex have not been established in children under the age of 18.

CARCINOGENESIS, MUTAGENESIS: In a drinking water study in rats, carcinogenesis was not observed. The highest dose of chlorhexidine gluconate used in this study, 38 mg/kg/day, is at least 500 times the amount that would be ingested from the recommended daily dose of Peridex.

In two mammalian *in vivo* mutagenic studies with chlorhexidine gluconate, mutagenesis was not observed. The highest dose of chlorhexidine gluconate used in a mouse dominant lethal assay was 1000 mg/kg/day and in a hamster cytogenetics test was 250 mg/kg/day, i.e. > 3200 times the amount that would be ingested from the recommended daily dose of Peridex.

ADVERSE REACTIONS

The most common side effects associated with chlorhexidine gluconate oral rinses are (1) an increase in staining of teeth and other oral surfaces, (2) an increase in calculus formation, and (3) an alteration in taste perception; see WARNINGS and PRECAUTIONS. No serious systemic adverse reactions associated with use of Peridex were observed in clinical testing.

Minor irritation and superficial desquamation of the oral mucosa have been noted in patients using Peridex, particularly among children.

Although there have been no reports of parotitis (inflammation or swelling of salivary glands) among Peridex users in controlled clinical studies, transient parotitis has been reported in research studies with chlorhexidine-containing mouthrinses.

OVERDOSAGE

Ingestion of 1 or 2 ounces of Peridex by a small child (~10 kg body weight) might result in gastric distress, including nausea, or signs of alcohol intoxication. Medical attention should be sought if more than 4 ounces of Peridex is ingested by a small child or if signs of alcohol intoxication develop.

DOSAGE AND ADMINISTRATION

Peridex therapy should be initiated directly following a dental prophylaxis and periodontal examination. Patients using Peridex should be reevaluated and given a thorough prophylaxis at intervals no longer than six months.

Recommended use is twice daily oral rinsing for 30 seconds, morning and evening after toothbrushing. Usual dosage is ½ fl. oz. (marked in cap) of undiluted Peridex. Peridex is not intended for ingestion and should be expectorated after rinsing.

HOW SUPPLIED

Peridex is supplied as a blue liquid in dispenser packs of three 1-pint amber plastic bottles with child-resistant dispensing closures. Store above freezing (32°F).
NDC 37000-007- 01
Military-6505-01-253-8138

The Purdue Frederick Company
**100 CONNECTICUT AVENUE
NORWALK, CT 06856**

BETADINE® Microbicides
[bā′tăh-dīn″]
(povidone-iodine)

BETADINE Microbicides (povidone-iodine) are available in 24 product forms—more than any other antiseptic agent. Formulated for topical, vaginal, perineal and oral application, BETADINE Microbicides are designed especially to meet the varied antiseptic needs of physicians, nurses and patients in the hospital, office and home. Of all antiseptic preparations, only povidone-iodine, as in BETADINE Microbicides, is capable of killing all classes of pathogens encountered in nosocomial infections: gram-positive bacteria and gram-negative bacteria (including antibiotic-resistant strains and mycobacteria), fungi/yeasts, viruses, and protozoa. It is the only microbicide with this broad spectrum of activity.

Other advantages: Most bacteria are killed in 15 to 30 seconds. Resistance has not been reported. Microbicidal activity is retained in the presence of moderate quantities of blood, pus, mucosal secretions, and soap and water. More frequent application of BETADINE Microbicides is indicated in the presence of excessive amount of blood, pus, or mucosal secretions. When used as a surgical scrub, the effect lasts 6 to 8 hours. Virtually nonirritating when used as directed; washes easily off skin and natural fabrics. BETADINE® Solution and BETADINE® Aerosol Spray are film-forming and may be applied with or without bandages. BETADINE® Cream, BETADINE® Ointment and BETADINE® Hēlafoam Solution may be bandaged or covered with gauze.

Note: BETADINE Microbicides should not be heated prior to application. Patients with iodine sensitivity should not use BETADINE preparations. Avoid pooling of BETADINE® Solution in preoperative prepping.

BETADINE® Microbicides are available for hospital use and home healthcare.
BETADINE® Aerosol Spray (povidone-iodine, 10%)
BETADINE® Antiseptic Gauze Pad (povidone-iodine, 10%)
BETADINE® Antiseptic Lubricating Gel (povidone-iodine, 1%)
BETADINE® Cream (povidone-iodine, 5%)
BETADINE® Hēlafoam Solution (povidone-iodine, 10%)
BETADINE® Medicated Disposable Douche (povidone-iodine, 10%)
BETADINE® Medicated Douche (povidone-iodine, 10%)
BETADINE® Medicated Douche Kit (povidone-iodine, 10%)
BETADINE® Medicated Gel (povidone-iodine, 10%)
BETADINE® Medicated Vaginal Suppositories (povidone-iodine, 10%)
BETADINE® Mouthwash/Gargle (povidone-iodine, 0.5%)
BETADINE® Ointment (povidone-iodine, 10%)
BETADINE® Perineal Wash Concentrate Kit (povidone-iodine, 10%)
BETADINE® Pre-Mixed Medicated Disposable Douche (povidone-iodine, .30%)
BETADINE® Shampoo (povidone-iodine, 7.5%)
BETADINE® Skin Cleanser (povidone-iodine, 7.5%)
BETADINE® Skin Cleanser Foam (povidone-iodine, 7.5%)
BETADINE® Solution (povidone-iodine, 10%)
BETADINE® Solution Swab Aid® (povidone-iodine, 10%)
BETADINE® Solution Swabsticks (povidone-iodine, 10%)
BETADINE® Surgical Scrub (povidone-iodine, 7.5%)
BETADINE® Surgi-Prep Sponge-Brush (povidone-iodine, 7.5%)
BETADINE® Viscous Formula Antiseptic Gauze Pad (povidone-iodine, 10%)
BETADINE® Whirlpool Concentrate (povidone-iodine, 10%)

BETADINE® CREAM
[bā′tăh-dīn″]
(povidone-iodine, 5%)

ACTION AND USES

BETADINE Cream is a topical antiseptic containing 5% povidone-iodine (PVP-I) in an oil-in-water emulsion. It combines the essential microbicidal properties of povidone-io-

Continued on next page

Purdue Frederick—Cont.

dine with the ease of application and comfort of a cream formulation. BETADINE Cream is non-irritating and does not burn or sting when applied to open cuts, burns, or scrapes. BETADINE Cream kills most bacteria and other pathogens virtually on contact. It enhances wound healing by controlling infection and has a very broad spectrum of microbicidal activity.

BETADINE Cream is easy to apply and remove. Oil-in-water creams mix with exudates and are particularly suitable for weeping or wounded surfaces. BETADINE Cream has shown no phototoxic or contact sensitizing potential and has exhibited no photocontact allergenicity when tested on humans. BETADINE Cream is preservative-free and therefore presents no risk of allergic reaction to the patient from preservative additives.

ADMINISTRATION

Apply directly to affected area as needed. May be bandaged. For external use only.

CAUTION

In case of deep or puncture wounds or serious burns, consult physician. If redness, irritation, swelling or pain persists or increases, or if infection occurs, discontinue use and consult physician.

SUPPLIED

½ oz. plastic tube, with an applicator tip for easy and economical application.

BETADINE® Medicated Gel
[bā′tăh-dīn″]
(povidone-iodine, 10%)

ACTION AND USES

BETADINE Medicated Gel provides prompt, soothing, symptomatic relief of minor vaginal irritation, itching and soreness associated with vaginitis due to *Candida albicans*, *Trichomonas vaginalis*, and *Gardnerella vaginalis*. Its active ingredient—the broad-spectrum microbicide povidone-iodine—significantly and rapidly reduces the aerobic and anaerobic count. Offers comfort on contact from annoying vaginal symptoms and odor. May also be used as part of a preoperative degerming regimen.

ADVANTAGES

Its gel formulation offers the advantage of prolonged contact with irritated vaginal tissue to help provide long-lasting relief. BETADINE Medicated Gel is gentle and virtually nonirritating to delicate vaginal tissue. It is nongreasy and nonsticky.

DIRECTIONS FOR USE

Insert one applicatorful of BETADINE Medicated Gel. A sanitary napkin should be worn. When external irritation is present, BETADINE Medicated Gel may be applied manually to the affected area. Treatment should be continued for seven days.

WARNING

Do not use during pregnancy or while nursing except with the approval of your physician. If symptoms persist after seven days of treatment, or redness, pain or swelling develops, discontinue use and consult physician. Women with iodine sensitivity should not use this product.

HOW SUPPLIED

18 g tubes (approximately 1 use) and 3 oz. tubes (approximately 14 uses), each packaged with a convenient, easy-to-use vaginal applicator.

BETADINE® MEDICATED DOUCHE
[bā′tăh-dīn″]
(povidone-iodine, 10%)

A pleasantly scented solution, BETADINE Medicated Douche is indicated for the prompt symptomatic relief of minor vaginal irritation, itching, and soreness associated with vaginitis due to *Candida albicans*, *Trichomonas vaginalis*, and *Gardnerella vaginalis*. May be used as a cleansing douche.

ADVANTAGES

Low surface tension, with uniform wetting action to assist penetration into vaginal crypts and crevices. Microbicidal activity is retained in the presence of moderate quantities of blood, pus, mucosal secretions, and soap and water. Virtually nonirritating to vaginal mucosa. Will not stain skin or natural fabrics.

DIRECTIONS FOR USE

Professional Labeling
Suggested Regimen For Therapeutic Use: In the office, swab the cervix and vulvovaginal area with BETADINE Solution.
Prescribe BETADINE Medicated Douche: Two tablespoon-

fuls of BETADINE Douche Concentrate or two ½ fl. oz. packets to a quart of lukewarm water once daily for five days. If further therapy is warranted, douching should be continued through the next cycle. The patient may be instructed to return for an office visit following two weeks of therapy.
As a Routine Cleansing Douche: One (1) tablespoonful of BETADINE Douche Concentrate to a quart of lukewarm water once or twice per week.
As a douche for prompt symptomatic relief of minor vaginal irritation and itching: One (1) tablespoonful of BETADINE Douche Concentrate to a quart of lukewarm water once daily for five days. Treatment should continue for the full five days, even if symptoms are relieved earlier.

WARNING

Douching does not prevent pregnancy.
Do not use during pregnancy or while nursing except with the approval of your physician. If symptoms persist after seven days of treatment, or redness, pain or swelling develops, discontinue use and consult physician. Women with iodine sensitivity should not use this product.

HOW SUPPLIED

1 oz. (approximately 2 uses), 4 oz. (approximately 8 uses), and 8 oz. (approximately 16 uses) plastic bottles. Disposable ½ oz. (1 tablespoonful) packets. Also available: BETADINE Medicated Douche Kit 8 oz. (approximately 40 uses), BETADINE Medicated Disposable Douche (single- and twin-pack) and BETADINE Pre-Mixed Medicated Douche, which requires no measuring or mixing (single- and twin-pack).

BETADINE® OINTMENT
[bā′tăh-dīn″]
(povidone-iodine, 10%)

ACTION

BETADINE Ointment, in a water-soluble base, is a topical microbicide active against organisms commonly encountered in skin and wound infections.

INDICATIONS

Therapeutically, BETADINE Ointment may be used as an adjunct to systemic therapy where indicated; for primary or secondary topical infections, infected surgical incisions, infected decubitus or stasis ulcers, pyodermas, secondarily infected dermatoses, and infected traumatic lesions.
Prophylactically: BETADINE Ointment may be used to prevent microbial contamination in burns, incisions and other topical lesions; for degerming skin in hyperalimentation, catheter care, the umbilical area or circumcision. The use of BETADINE Ointment for abrasions, minor cuts, and wounds, may prevent the development of infections and permit wound healing.

ADMINISTRATION

Apply directly to affected area as needed. May be bandaged.

CAUTION

In case of deep or puncture wounds or serious burns, consult physician. If redness, irritation, swelling or pain persists or increases, or if infection occurs, discontinue use and consult physician.

SUPPLIED

1/32 oz. and ⅛ oz. packettes; 1 oz. tubes; 16 oz. (1 lb.) and 5 lbs.

BETADINE® SKIN CLEANSER
[bā′tăh-dīn″]
(povidone-iodine, 7.5%)

BETADINE Skin Cleanser is a sudsing, antiseptic bactericidal, virucidal liquid cleanser which forms a rich, golden lather.

INDICATIONS

BETADINE Skin Cleanser aids in degerming the skin of patients with common pathogens, including *Staphylococcus aureus*. To help prevent the recurrence of acute inflammatory skin infections caused by iodine-susceptible pyogenic bacteria. In pyodermas, as a topical adjunct to systemic antimicrobial therapy. To help prevent spread of infection in acne pimples. Also kills three organisms often associated with acne vulgaris: *Staph. epidermidis*, *Corynebacterium acnes* and Pityrosporon. To clean superficial wounds. Aids in removal of foreign material such as dirt and debris.

DIRECTIONS FOR USE

Wet the skin and apply a sufficient amount of Skin Cleanser to work up a rich golden lather. Allow lather to remain about 3 minutes. Then rinse thoroughly with water. Repeat 2–3 times a day or as needed.

CAUTION

In case of deep or puncture wounds or serious burns, consult physician. If redness, irritation, swelling or pain persists or

increases, or if infection occurs, discontinue use and consult physician.

HOW SUPPLIED

1 fl. oz. and 4 fl. oz. plastic bottles.

NOTE

Blue stains on starched linen will wash off with soap and water.

BETADINE® SOLUTION
[bā′tăh-dīn″]
(povidone-iodine, 10%)
Topical Antiseptic Bactericide/Virucide

ACTION AND USES

For preoperative prepping of operative site, including the vagina, and as a general topical bactericide/virucide for: disinfection of wounds; emergency treatment of lacerations and abrasions; second- and third-degree burns; as a prophylactic anti-infective agent in hospital and office procedures, including postoperative application to incisions to help prevent infection; oral moniliasis (thrush); bacterial and mycotic skin infections; decubitus and stasis ulcers; as a preoperative swab in the mouth and throat.

ADMINISTRATION

Apply full strength as often as needed as a paint, spray, or wet soak. May be bandaged.

CAUTION

In preoperative prepping, avoid "pooling" beneath the patient. Prolonged exposure to unabsorbed, wet solution may cause irritation. Do not heat prior to application. In case of deep or puncture wounds or serious burns, consult physician. If redness, irritation, swelling or pain persists or increases, or if infection occurs, discontinue use and consult physician.

INFORMATION FOR PATIENTS

For external use only. This product is not for use on wild or domestic animal bites. If you have an animal bite, consult your physician immediately. Do not use this product for more than 10 days. If the infection worsens or persists, see your physician.

HOW SUPPLIED

½ oz., 4 oz., 8 oz., 16 oz. (1 pt.), 32 oz. (1 qt.) and 1 gal. plastic bottles and 1 oz. packettes.

ALSO AVAILABLE

BETADINE® Solution Swab Aid® Pads for degerming small areas of skin or mucous membranes prior to injections, aspirations, catheterization and surgery; boxes of 100 packettes. Also: disposable BETADINE® Solution Swabsticks, in packettes of 1's and 3's.

BETADINE® SURGICAL SCRUB
[bā′tăh-dīn″]
(povidone-iodine, 7.5%)
Topical Antiseptic Bactericide/Virucide

ACTION AND USES

A broad-spectrum antiseptic, bactericidal, virucidal sudsing skin cleanser for pre- and postoperative scrubbing or washing by hospital operating room personnel; for preoperative use on patients; and general use as an antiseptic microbicide in physician's office. Forms rich, golden lather.

DIRECTIONS FOR USE

A.   **For Preoperative Washing by Operating Personnel**
     1.   Wet hands and forearms with water. Pour about 5 cc. (1 teaspoonful) of BETADINE Surgical Scrub on the palm of the hand and spread over both hands and forearms. Without adding more water, rub the Scrub thoroughly over all areas for about five minutes. Use a brush if desired. Clean thoroughly under fingernails. Add a little water and develop copious suds. Rinse thoroughly under running water.
     2.   Complete the wash by scrubbing with another 5 cc. of BETADINE Surgical Scrub in the same way.
B.   **For Preoperative Use on Patients**
After the skin area is shaved, wet it with water. Apply BETADINE Surgical Scrub (1 cc. is sufficient to cover an area of 20-30 square inches), develop lather and scrub thoroughly for about five minutes. Rinse off by aid of sterile gauze saturated with water. The area may then be painted with BETADINE Solution or sprayed with BETADINE Aerosol Spray and allowed to dry.
C.   **For Use in the Physician's Office**
Use for washing whenever a bactericidal/virucidal detergent is required. For maximum degerming of the hands proceed as under (A). To prepare the patient's skin proceed as under (B).
Note: Blue stains on starched linen will wash off with soap and water.

CAUTION

In case of deep or puncture wounds or serious burns, consult physician. If redness, irritation, swelling or pain persists or increases, or if infection occurs, discontinue use and consult physician.

SUPPLIED

16 oz. (1 pint) plastic bottle with and without pump, 32 oz. (1 quart) and 1 gal. plastic bottles, and ½ oz. packettes.

BETADINE® Medicated Vaginal Suppositories
[bā'tăh-dĭn"]
(povidone-iodine, 10%)

ACTION AND USES

BETADINE Medicated Vaginal Suppositories provide prompt symptomatic relief of minor vaginal irritation, itching and soreness associated with vaginitis due to Candida albicans, Trichomonas vaginalis, and Gardnerella vaginalis. Its active ingredient—the broad-spectrum microbicide povidone-iodine—significantly and rapidly reduces the aerobic and anaerobic count. Offers soothing relief from annoying vaginal symptoms and odor.

ADVANTAGES

Each measured-dose BETADINE Medicated Vaginal Suppository is easily and quickly inserted to provide prolonged contact with irritated vaginal tissue to help provide long-lasting relief. BETADINE Medicated Vaginal Suppositories are gentle and virtually nonirritating to delicate vaginal tissue. Nonstaining to skin and natural fabrics, color can be washed off with soap and water.

DIRECTIONS FOR USE

Unwrap a suppository and gently insert its smaller end into the applicator. Insert the applicator into the vagina and release the suppository. A sanitary napkin should be worn. Treatment should be continued for seven days.

WARNING

Women with iodine sensitivity should not use this product. Do not use during pregnancy or while nursing except with the approval of your physician. If symptoms persist after seven days of treatment, or redness, pain or swelling develops, discontinue use and consult your physician.

HOW SUPPLIED

7 Suppositories packaged with a convenient, easy-to-use applicator and patient instruction booklet.

CARDIOQUIN® TABLETS   ℞
[car'dē"ō-quin]
(quinidine polygalacturonate)
275 mg
In the treatment of cardiac arrhythmias
Purdue Frederick

DESCRIPTION

CARDIOQUIN Tablets, for oral administration, contain 275 mg quinidine polygalacturonate equivalent in content to 200 mg (3 grains) of quinidine sulfate.

Chemically, quinidine polygalacturonate is $C_{20}H_{24}N_2O_2C_6H_{10}O_7H_2O$ and has the following structural formula:

Inactive components include: Corn starch, Lactose, Magnesium stearate, Povidone and Talc.

ACTIONS

The quinidine component slows conduction time, prolongs the refractory period, and depresses the excitability of heart muscle. Polygalacturonate slows ionization of the drug and protects the gastrointestinal tract by its demulcent effect.

INDICATIONS

CARDIOQUIN Tablets are indicated as maintenance therapy after spontaneous and electrical conversion of atrial tachycardia, flutter or fibrillation and in the treatment of:
- Premature atrial and ventricular contractions.
- Paroxysmal atrial tachycardia.
- Paroxymal A-V junctional rhythm.
- Atrial flutter.
- Paroxysmal atrial fibrillation.
- Established atrial fibrillation when therapy is appropriate.
- Paroxysmal ventricular tachycardia when not associated with complete heartblock.

CONTRAINDICATIONS

1. History of hypersensitivity to quinidine manifested by thrombocytopenia, skin eruptions, febrile reactions, etc.
2. Complete A-V block.
3. Complete bundle branch block or other severe intraventricular conduction defects exhibiting marked QRS widening or bizarre complexes.
4. Myasthenia gravis.
5. Arrhythmias associated with digitalis toxicity.

WARNINGS

1. In the treatment of atrial fibrillation with rapid ventricular response, ventricular rate should be controlled with digitalis glycosides <u>prior</u> to administration of quinidine.
2. In the treatment of atrial flutter with quinidine, reversion to sinus rhythm may be preceded by progressive reduction in the degree of A-V block to a 1:1 ratio resulting in an extremely high ventricular rate. This potential hazard may be reduced by digitalization prior to administration of quinidine.

   Recent reports have described increased, potentially toxic, digoxin plasma levels when quinidine is administered concurrently. When concurrent use is necessary, digoxin dosage should be reduced and plasma concentration should be monitored and patients observed closely for digitalis intoxication.
3. Quinidine cardiotoxicity may be manifested by increased P-R and Q-T intervals, 50% widening of QRS, and/or ventricular ectopic beats or tachycardia. Appearance of these toxic signs during quinidine administration mandates immediate discontinuation of the drug, and/or close clinical and electrocardiographic monitoring. Note: Quinidine effect is enhanced by potassium and reduced in the presence of hypokalemia.
4. Quinidine syncope may occur as a complication of long-term therapy. It is manifested by sudden loss of consciousness and by ventricular arrhythmias with bizarre QRS complexes. This syndrome does not appear to be related to dose or plasma levels, but occurs more often with prolonged Q-T intervals.
5. Because quinidine antagonizes the effect of vagal excitation upon the atrium and the A-V node, the administration of parasympathomimetic drugs (choline esters) or the use of any other procedure to enhance vagal activity may fail to terminate paroxysmal supraventricular tachycardia in patients receiving quinidine.
6. Quinidine should be used with extreme caution in:
   a) The presence of incomplete A-V block, since a complete block and asystole may result.
   b) Quinidine may cause unpredictable abnormalities of rhythm in digitalized hearts. Therefore, it should be used with caution in the presence of digitalis intoxication (see 2 above).
   c) Partial bundle branch block.
   d) Severe congestive heart failure and hypotensive states due to the depressant effects of quinidine on myocardial contractility and arterial pressure.
   e) Poor renal function, especially renal tubular acidosis, because of the potential accumulation of quinidine in plasma leading to toxic concentrations.

PRECAUTIONS

1. **Test Dose**—A preliminary test dose of a single tablet of quinidine *sulfate* should be administered prior to the initiation of treatment with CARDIOQUIN Tablets to determine whether the patient has an idiosyncrasy to the quinidine molecule.
2. **Hypersensitivity**—During the first weeks of therapy, hypersensitivity to quinidine, although rare, should be considered (e.g., angioedema, purpura, acute asthmatic episode, vascular collapse).
3. **Long-Term Therapy**—Periodic blood counts and liver and kidney function tests should be performed during long-term therapy, and the drug should be discontinued if blood dyscrasias or signs of hepatic or renal disorders occur.
4. **Large Doses**—ECG monitoring and determination of plasma quinidine levels are recommended when doses greater than 2.5 g/day are administered.
5. **Usage in Pregnancy**—The use of quinidine in pregnancy should be reserved only for those cases where the benefits outweigh the possible hazards to the patient and fetus.
6. **Nursing Mothers**—The drug should be used with extreme caution in nursing mothers because the drug is excreted in breast milk.
7. **General**—In patients exhibiting asthma, muscle weakness and infection with fever *prior* to quinidine administration, hypersensitivity reactions to the drug may be masked.

DRUG INTERACTIONS

1. Caution should be used when quinidine and its analogs are administered concurrently with coumarin anticoagulants. This combination may reduce prothrombin levels and cause bleeding.
2. Quinidine, a weak base, may have its half-life prolonged in patients who are concurrently taking drugs that can alkalize the urine, such as thiazide diuretics, sodium bicarbonate, and carbonic anhydrase inhibitors. Quinidine and drugs which alkalize the urine should be used together cautiously.
3. Quinidine exhibits a distinct anticholinergic activity in the myocardial tissues. An additive vagolytic effect may be seen when quinidine and drugs having anticholinergic blocking activity are used together. Drugs having cholinergic activity may be antagonized by quinidine.
4. Quinidine and other antiarrhythmic agents may produce additive cardiac depressant effects when administered together.
5. Quinidine interaction with cardiac glycosides (digoxin). See **WARNINGS**.
6. Antacids may delay absorption of quinidine but appear unlikely to cause incomplete absorption.
7. Phenobarbital and phenytoin may reduce plasma half-life of quinidine by 50%.
8. Quinidine may potentiate the neuromuscular blocking effect in ventilatory depression of patients receiving decamethonium, tubocurare or succinylcholine.

ADVERSE REACTIONS

Symptoms of cinchonism (ringing in the ears, headache, disturbed vision) may appear in sensitive patients after a single dose of the drug.

Gastrointestinal:
The most common side effects encountered with quinidine are referable to this system. Diarrhea frequently occurs, but it rarely necessitates withdrawal of the drug. Nausea, vomiting and abdominal pain also occur. Some of these effects may be minimized by administering the drug with meals.

Cardiovascular:
Widening of QRS complex, cardiac asystole, ventricular ectopic beats, idioventricular rhythms including ventricular tachycardia and fibrillation; paradoxical tachycardia, arterial embolism, and hypotension.

Hematologic:
Acute hemolytic anemia, hypoprothrombinemia, thrombocytopenic purpura, agranulocytosis.

CNS:
Headache, fever, vertigo, apprehension, excitement, confusion, delirium, and syncope, disturbed hearing (tinnitus, decreased auditory acuity), disturbed vision (mydriasis, blurred vision, disturbed color perception, photophobia, diplopia, night blindness, scotomata), optic neuritis.

Dermatologic:
Cutaneous flushing with intense pruritus.

Hypersensitivity Reactions:
Angioedema, acute asthmatic episode, vascular collapse, respiratory arrest, hepatic dysfunction.

DOSAGE AND ADMINISTRATION

Each CARDIOQUIN Tablet contains 275 mg quinidine polygalacturonate, equivalent to a 3-grain tablet of quinidine sulfate. Dosage must be adjusted to individual patient's needs, both for conversion and maintenance. An initial dose of 1 to 3 tablets may be used to terminate arrhythmia, and may be repeated in 3–4 hours. If normal sinus rhythm is not restored after 3 or 4 equal doses, the dose may be increased by ½ to 1 tablet (137.5 to 275 mg) and administered three to four times before any further dosage increase. For maintenance, one tablet may be used two or three times a day; generally, one tablet morning and night will be adequate.

OVERDOSAGE

Cardiotoxic effects of quinidine may be reversed in part by molar sodium lactate; the hypotension may be reversed by vasoconstrictors and by catecholamines (since vasodilation is partly due to alpha-adrenergic blockage).

HOW SUPPLIED

CARDIOQUIN (quinidine polygalacturonate) 275 mg scored, uncoated Tablets are supplied in white-opaque plastic bottles containing 100 tablets (NDC #0034-5470-80) and 500 tablets (NDC #0034-5470-90). Each round tablet bears the symbol "PF" on one side and is marked "C275" on the other.
Store tablets at controlled room temperature 15° to 30°C (59°–86°F).

CAUTION

Federal law prohibits dispensing without prescription.

REFERENCES

1. Schwartz, G.: *Angiology* 10:115 (Apr.) 1959.
2. Tricot, R., Nogrette, P.: *Presse med.* 68:1085 (June 4) 1960.
3. Shaftel, N., Halpern, A.: *Am. J. Med. Sci.* 236:184 (Aug.) 1958.
June 30, 1989   I8038
Shown in Product Identification Section, page 423

Continued on next page

Purdue Frederick—Cont.

CERUMENEX® DROPS   ℞
[sĕ-rū'mĕn-ĕx"]
(triethanolamine polypeptide oleate-condensate)

A Unique Cerumenolytic Agent for Effective and Easy Removal of Earwax

DESCRIPTION
CERUMENEX Drops contain Triethanolamine polypeptide oleate-condensate (10.0%) in propylene glycol with chlorbutanol (0.5%), for effective and convenient cerumenolytic action and easy removal of earwax. Among its properties are:
1. Aqueous-miscible solution—low surface tension and optimal viscosity.
2. Slightly acid pH range to approximate surface of normal ear canal.
3. Hygroscopic—helps absorb aqueous transudates.
4. Antiseptic protection against contamination.

ACTION
CERUMENEX Drops are specifically designed as a cerumenolytic agent, to emulsify and disperse excess or impacted earwax for easier removal without painful instrumentation. They are usually effective with a single 15–30 minutes treatment, and are simple and easy to administer. (see Dosage and Administration)

INDICATIONS
- REMOVAL OF CERUMEN
- REMOVAL OF IMPACTED CERUMEN PRIOR TO EAR EXAMINATION
- REMOVAL OF IMPACTED CERUMEN PRIOR TO OTOLOGIC THERAPY
- REMOVAL OF IMPACTED CERUMEN PRIOR TO AUDIOMETRY

CONTRAINDICATIONS
- Perforated tympanic membrane or otitis media is considered a contraindication to the use of any medication in the external ear canal.
- A history of a previous untoward reaction to CERUMENEX Drops.
- A positive patch test (see Precautions).

WARNINGS
Discontinue promptly if sensitization or irritation occurs.

PRECAUTIONS
It is recommended that the following precautions be observed in prescribing and administration of this agent:
1. Extreme caution is indicated in patients with demonstrable dermatologic idiosyncrasies or with history of allergic reactions in general.
2. In case of doubt, a patch test should be performed by placing a drop of CERUMENEX Drops on the flexor surface of the arm or forearm and covering it with a small Band-Aid strip. The results are read and interpreted after 24 hours. Positive reaction indicates the probability of an allergic reaction following instillation in the ear.
3. Exposure of the ear canal to the CERUMENEX Drops should be limited to 15–30 minutes.
4. Patients must be instructed not to exceed the time of exposure, nor to use the medication more frequently than directed by the physician.
5. When administering CERUMENEX Drops, care must be taken to avoid undue exposure of the periaural skin during the instillation and the flushing out of the medication. If the medication comes in contact with the skin, the area should be washed with soap and water. Use of proper technique (see Dosage and Administration) will help avoid such undue exposure.
6. Although introduction of CERUMENEX Drops (triethanolamine polypeptide oleate-condensate) into the middle ear of animals with surgically perforated drums or into patients with ruptured drums has been accomplished without untoward reactions, the use of this medication should be avoided in the presence of underlying disease in the middle ear (otitis media, perforated drum) and it should be used only with caution in certain types of external otitis.
7. Patients should be advised to discontinue the use of the medication in case of a possible reaction and to consult their physician promptly.

ADVERSE REACTIONS
Clinical Reactions of Possible Allergic Origin.
Localized dermatitis reactions were reported in about 1% of 2,700 patients treated, ranging from a very mild erythema and pruritus of the external canal to a severe eczematoid reaction involving the external ear and periauricular tissue, generally with duration of 2–10 days. In all cases, complete and uneventful resolution occurred without residual sequelae, sometimes without supplemental therapy. Such therapy may consist of only symptomatic relief in mild cases and may include anti-inflammatory agents when indicated. Thus,

while reactions of a possible allergic origin may occur, their incidence is minimal and usually not disproportionate to other commonly used dermatologic agents.

DOSAGE AND ADMINISTRATION
1. Fill ear canal with CERUMENEX Drops with the patient's head tilted at a 45° angle.
2. Insert cotton plug and allow to remain 15–30 minutes.
3. Then gently flush ear with lukewarm water, using soft rubber syringe (avoid excessive pressure). Avoid undue exposure of large skin areas to the drug. If a second application is necessary in unusually hard impactions, the procedure may be repeated.

CAUTION: Federal Law Prohibits Dispensing Without a Prescription

HOW SUPPLIED
6 ml and 12 ml bottles with cellophane-wrapped dropper. Store at Controlled Room Temperature 15°–30°C (59°–86°F)

FIBERMED®
[fĭ'bĕr-mĕd"]
High–Fiber Supplements
Fruit Flavor/Original Flavor
Also Fruit Flavor Miniatures

DESCRIPTION
FIBERMED High-Fiber Supplements provide a measured quantity of natural dietary fiber in a palatable, ready-to-eat form. FIBERMED Supplements are standardized to provide concentrated dietary fiber in precise amounts—10 grams in two delicious biscuits. Original-Flavor FIBERMED contain natural dietary fiber from corn, wheat and oats. Fruit-Flavor FIBERMED contain natural dietary fiber from six sources: corn, oats, wheat, soy, apples and currants.
Lack of fiber in the diet is a recognized cause of constipation, irritable bowel syndrome, diverticulosis and hemorrhoids. Two FIBERMED High-Fiber Biscuits a day help provide the supplementary bulk that patients may need in their diet to avoid constipation.
FIBERMED also helps curb appetite and may help in weight control programs. Fiber produces feelings of satiety and fullness, and can reduce one's desire for food.
FIBERMED Supplements are superior to other fiber sources because of their uniform high-fiber content, convenience and good taste, qualities which encourage good compliance.
Ready-to-eat FIBERMED Supplements can be eaten any time, any place. Unlike most high-fiber foods or powdered bulks, FIBERMED requires no preparation and no mixing. They can be eaten with milk, coffee, tea, juice, soup or fruit; or dunked in a beverage.

INGREDIENTS
FIBERMED Supplements Original Flavor contain: Corn Bran, Brown Sugar, Corn Starch, Wheat Flour, Wheat Bran, Vegetable Shortening (Partially Hydrogenated Soybean Oil), Sodium Bicarbonate, Vanilla, Ammonium Bicarbonate, Baking Acid, Salt, Cinnamon, Citric Acid, Nutmeg and Ginger.
FIBERMED Supplements Fruit Flavor contain: Corn Bran, Brown Sugar, Whole Rolled Oats, Vegetable Shortening (Partially Hydrogenated Soybean Oil), Textured Soy Flour, Currants, Wheat Bran, Wheat Flour, Corn Starch, Dried Apple, Baking Soda, Ammonium Bicarbonate, Vanilla, Fumaric Acid, Salt, Baking Acid, Cinnamon.

USAGE
FIBERMED Supplements are indicated for those conditions, including constipation, in which it is desirable to regulate gastrointestinal transit time, increase stool weight and make elimination easier. Because of their taste and convenience, FIBERMED Supplements are the product of choice to significantly increase intake of dietary fiber in uniform amounts. Two FIBERMED Supplements a day provide a high level of dietary fiber—10 grams—more dietary fiber than a serving of high-fiber cereal.

DIRECTIONS
Two FIBERMED Biscuits per day provide the extra fiber required by most people. As with any healthful diet, adequate fluid intake is important.

SUPPLIED
FIBERMED Supplements Fruit Flavor, and Original Flavor Biscuits are each supplied in boxes of 14. For most individuals, 14 is a week's supply.

ALSO AVAILABLE
Fruit Flavor FIBERMED® High-Fiber MINIATURES. Four bite-size FIBERMED MINIATURES provide 5 grams of concentrated natural dietary fiber. Supplied in 8.75 oz. boxes.

MS CONTIN® 30 mg Tablets   ℃
MS CONTIN® 60 mg Tablets   ℃
[em es"kŏn'tĕn]
Morphine Sulfate Controlled Release
WARNING: May be habit forming.

DESCRIPTION
Chemically, morphine sulfate is 7,8-didehydro-4,5α-epoxy-17-methylmorphinan-3,6 α-diol sulfate (2:1) (salt) pentahydrate and has the following structural formula:

Each MS CONTIN 30 mg Controlled Release Tablet contains: 30 mg Morphine Sulfate U.S.P. Inactive ingredients: Cetostearyl Alcohol, FD&C Blue No. 1, FD&C Red No. 3, FD&C Yellow No. 6, Hydroxyethyl Cellulose, Hydroxypropyl Methylcellulose, Lactose, Magnesium Stearate, Talc, Titanium Dioxide, and other ingredients.
Each MS CONTIN 60 mg Controlled Release Tablet contains: 60 mg Morphine Sulfate U.S.P. Inactive ingredients: Cetostearyl Alcohol, D&C Red No. 30, D&C Yellow No. 10, Hydroxyethyl Cellulose, Hydroxypropyl Methylcellulose, Lactose, Magnesium Stearate, Talc, Titanium dioxide, and other ingredients.

CLINICAL PHARMACOLOGY
Metabolism and Pharmacokinetics
MS CONTIN is a controlled release tablet containing morphine sulfate. Following oral administration of a given dose of morphine, the amount ultimately absorbed is essentially the same whether the source is MS CONTIN or a conventional formulation. Morphine is released from MS CONTIN somewhat more slowly than from conventional oral preparations. Because of pre-systemic elimination (i.e., metabolism in the gut wall and liver) only about 40% of the administered dose reaches the central compartment.
Once absorbed, morphine is distributed to skeletal muscle, kidneys, liver, intestinal tract, lungs, spleen and brain. Morphine also crosses the placental membranes and has been found in breast milk.
Although a small fraction (less than 5%) of morphine is demethylated, for all practical purposes, virtually all morphine is converted to glucuronide metabolites; among these, morphine-3-glucuronide is present in the highest plasma concentration following oral administration.
The glucuronide system has a very high capacity and is not easily saturated even in disease. Therefore, rate of delivery of morphine to the gut and liver should not influence the total and, probably, the relative quantities of the various metabolites formed. Moreover, even if rate affected the relative amounts of each metabolite formed, it should be unimportant clinically because morphine's metabolites are ordinarily inactive.
The following pharmacokinetic parameters show considerable inter-subject variation but are representative of average values reported in the literature. The volume of distribution (Vd) for morphine is 4 liters per kilogram, and its terminal elimination half-life is normally 2 to 4 hours.
Following the administration of conventional oral morphine products, approximately fifty percent of the morphine that will reach the central compartment intact, reaches it within 30 minutes. Following the administration of an equal amount of MS CONTIN to normal volunteers, however, this extent of absorption occurs, on average, after 1.5 hours.
The possible effect of food upon the systemic bioavailability of MS CONTIN has not been evaluated.
Variation in the physical/mechanical properties of a formulation of an oral morphine drug product can affect both its absolute bioavailability and its absorption rate constant (k_a). The formulation employed in MS CONTIN does not affect morphine's oral bioavailability, but does decrease its apparent k_a. Other basic pharmacokinetic parameters (e.g., volume of distribution [Vd], elimination rate constant [k_e], clearance [Cl]), are unchanged as they are fundamental properties of morphine in the organism. However, in chronic use, the possibility that shifts in metabolite to parent drug ratios may occur cannot be excluded.
When immediate release oral morphine or MS CONTIN is given on a fixed dosing regimen, steady state is achieved in about a day.
For a given dose and dosing interval, the AUC and average blood concentration of morphine at steady state (Css) will be independent of the specific type of oral formulation administered so long as the formulations have the same absolute bioavailability. The absorption rate of a formulation will,

however, affect the maximum (Cmax) and minimum (Cmin) blood levels and the times of their occurrence.

While there is no predictable relationship between morphine blood levels and analgesic response, effective analgesia will not occur below some minimum blood level in a given patient. The minimum effective blood level for analgesia will, of course, vary among patients, especially among patients who have been previously treated with potent mu agonist opioids. Similarly, there is no predictable relationship between blood morphine concentration and untoward clinical responses; again, however, higher concentrations are more likely to be toxic than lower ones.

For any fixed dose and dosing interval, MS CONTIN will have at steady state, a lower Cmax and a higher Cmin than conventional morphine. This is a potential advantage; a reduced fluctuation in morphine concentration during the dosing interval should keep morphine blood levels more centered within the theoretical "therapeutic window." (Fluctuation for a dosing interval is defined as [Cmax-Cmin]/[Css-average].) On the other hand, the degree of fluctuation in serum morphine concentration might conceivably affect other phenomena. For example, reduced fluctuations in blood morphine concentrations might influence the rate of tolerance induction.

The elimination of morphine occurs primarily as renal excretion of 3-morphine glucuronide. A small amount of the glucuronide conjugate is excreted in the bile, and there is some minor enterohepatic recycling. Because morphine is primarily metabolized to inactive metabolites, the effects of renal disease on morphine's elimination are not likely to be pronounced. However, as with any drug, caution should be taken to guard against unanticipated accumulation if renal and/or hepatic function is seriously impaired.

PHARMACODYNAMICS

The effects described below are common to all morphine-containing products.

Central Nervous System

The principal actions of therapeutic value of morphine are analgesia and sedation (i.e., sleepiness and anxiolysis).

The precise mechanism of the analgesic action is unknown. However, specific CNS opiate receptors and endogenous compounds with morphine-like activity have been identified throughout the brain and spinal cord and are likely to play a role in the expression of analgesic effects.

Morphine produces respiratory depression by direct action on brain stem respiratory centers. The mechanism of respiratory depression involves a reduction in the responsiveness of the brain stem respiratory centers to increases in carbon dioxide tension, and to electrical stimulation.

Morphine depresses the cough reflex by direct effect on the cough center in the medulla. Antitussive effects may occur with doses lower than those usually required for analgesia. Morphine causes miosis, even in total darkness. Pinpoint pupils are a sign of narcotic overdose but are not pathognomonic (e.g., pontine lesions of hemorrhagic or ischemic origins may produce similar findings). Marked mydriasis rather than miosis may be seen with worsening hypoxia.

Gastrointestinal Tract and Other Smooth Muscle

Gastric, biliary and pancreatic secretions are decreased by morphine. Morphine causes a reduction in motility associated with an increase in tone in the antrum of the stomach and duodenum. Digestion of food in the small intestine is delayed and propulsive contractions are decreased. Propulsive peristaltic waves in the colon are decreased, while tone is increased to the point of spasm. The end result is constipation. Morphine can cause a marked increase in biliary tract pressure as a result of spasm of sphincter of Oddi.

Cardiovascular System

Morphine produces peripheral vasodilation which may result in orthostatic hypotension. Release of histamine can occur and may contribute to narcotic-induced hypotension. Manifestations of histamine release and/or peripheral vasodilation may include pruritus, flushing, red eyes and sweating.

INDICATIONS AND USAGE

MS CONTIN is a controlled release oral morphine formulation indicated for the relief of moderate to severe pain. It is intended for use in patients who require repeated dosing with potent opioid analgesics over periods of more than a few days.

CONTRAINDICATIONS

MS CONTIN is contraindicated in patients with known hypersensitivity to the drug, in patients with respiratory depression in the absence of resuscitative equipment, and in patients with acute or severe bronchial asthma.

WARNINGS

(See also: CLINICAL PHARMACOLOGY)

Impaired Respiration

Respiratory depression is the chief hazard of all morphine preparations. Respiratory depression occurs most frequently in the elderly and debilitated patients, as well as in those suffering from conditions accompanied by hypoxia or hyper-

capnia when even moderate therapeutic doses may dangerously decrease pulmonary ventilation.

Morphine should be used with extreme caution in patients with chronic obstructive pulmonary disease or cor pulmonale, and in patients having a substantially decreased respiratory reserve, hypoxia, hypercapnia, or preexisting respiratory depression. In such patients, even usual therapeutic doses of morphine may decrease respiratory drive while simultaneously increasing airway resistance to the point of apnea.

Head Injury and Increased Intracranial Pressure

The respiratory depressant effects of morphine with carbon dioxide retention and secondary elevation of cerebrospinal fluid pressure may be markedly exaggerated in the presence of head injury, other intracranial lesions, or preexisting increase in intracranial pressure. Morphine produces effects which may obscure neurologic signs of further increases in pressure in patients with head injuries.

Hypotensive Effect

MS CONTIN, like all opioid analgesics, may cause severe hypotension in an individual whose ability to maintain his blood pressure has already been compromised by a depleted blood volume, or a concurrent administration of drugs such as phenothiazines or general anesthetics. (See also: PRECAUTIONS: Drug Interactions.) MS CONTIN may produce orthostatic hypotension in ambulatory patients.

MS CONTIN, like all opioid analgesics, should be administered with caution to patients in circulatory shock, since vasodilation produced by the drug may further reduce cardiac output and blood pressure.

Interactions with other CNS Depressants

MS CONTIN, like all opioid analgesics, should be used with great caution and in reduced dosage in patients who are concurrently receiving other central nervous system depressants including sedatives or hypnotics, general anesthetics, phenothiazines, other tranquilizers and alcohol because respiratory depression, hypotension and profound sedation or coma may result.

Interactions with Mixed Agonist/Antagonist Opioid Analgesics

From a theoretical perspective, agonist/antagonist analgesics (i.e., pentazocine, nalbuphine, butorphanol and buprenorphine) should NOT be administered to a patient who has received or is receiving a course of therapy with a pure opioid agonist analgesic. In these patients, mixed agonist/antagonist analgesics may reduce the analgesic effect or may precipitate withdrawal symptoms.

Drug Dependence

Morphine can produce drug dependence and has a potential for being abused. Tolerance, psychological and physical dependence may develop upon repeated administration. Physical dependence, however, is not of paramount importance in the management of terminally ill patients or any patients in severe pain. Abrupt cessation or a sudden reduction in dose after prolonged use may result in withdrawal symptoms. After prolonged exposure to opioid analgesics, if withdrawal is necessary, it must be undertaken gradually. (See DRUG ABUSE AND DEPENDENCE.)

Infants born to mothers physically dependent on opioid analgesics may also be physically dependent and exhibit respiratory depression and withdrawal symptoms. (See DRUG ABUSE AND DEPENDENCE.)

PRECAUTIONS

(See also: CLINICAL PHARMACOLOGY)

General

MS CONTIN is intended for use in patients who require more than several days continuous treatment with a potent opioid analgesic. The controlled release nature of the formulation allows it to be administered on a more convenient schedule than conventional immediate release oral morphine products. (See CLINICAL PHARMACOLOGY: "Metabolism and Pharmacokinetics".) However, MS CONTIN does not release morphine continuously over the course of a dosing interval. The administration of single doses of MS CONTIN on a q12 hour dosing schedule will result in higher peak and lower trough plasma levels than those that occur when an identical daily dose of morphine is administered using conventional oral formulations on a q4h regimen. The clinical significance of greater fluctuations in morphine plasma level has not been systematically evaluated. (See DOSAGE AND ADMINISTRATION)

As with any potent opioid, it is critical to adjust the dosing regimen for each patient individually, taking into account the patient's prior analgesic treatment experience. Although it is clearly impossible to enumerate every consideration that is important to the selection of the initial dose and dosing interval of MS CONTIN, attention should be given to 1) the daily dose, potency, and characteristics of the opioid the patient has been taking previously (e.g., whether it is a pure agonist or mixed agonist/antagonist), 2) the reliability of the relative potency estimate used to calculate the dose of morphine needed [N.B. potency estimates may vary with the route of administration], 3) the degree of opioid tolerance, if any, and 4) the general condition and medical status of the patient.

Selection of patients for treatment with MS CONTIN should be governed by the same principles that apply to the use of morphine or other potent opioid analgesics. Specifically, the increased risks associated with its use in the following populations should be considered: the elderly or debilitated and those with severe impairment of hepatic, pulmonary or renal function; myxedema or hypothyroidism; adrenocortical insufficiency (e.g., Addison's Disease); CNS depression or coma; toxic psychosis; prostatic hypertrophy or urethral stricture; acute alcoholism; delirium tremens; kyphoscoliosis, or inability to swallow.

The administration of morphine, like all opioid analgesics, may obscure the diagnosis or clinical course in patients with acute abdominal conditions.

Morphine may aggravate preexisting convulsions in patients with convulsive disorders.

Morphine should be used with caution in patients about to undergo surgery of the biliary tract since it may cause spasm of the sphincter of Oddi. Similarly, morphine should be used with caution in patients with acute pancreatitis secondary to biliary tract disease.

Information for Patients

If clinically advisable, patients receiving MS CONTIN should be given the following instructions by the physician:

1. Morphine may produce psychological and/or physical dependence. For this reason, the dose of the drug should not be adjusted without consulting a physician.

2. Morphine may impair mental and/or physical ability required for the performance of potentially hazardous tasks (e.g., driving, operating machinery).

3. Morphine should not be taken with alcohol or other CNS depressants (sleep aids, tranquilizers) because additive effects including CNS depression may occur. A physician should be consulted if other prescription medications are currently being used or are prescribed for future use.

4. For women of childbearing potential who become or are planning to become pregnant, a physician should be consulted regarding analgesics and other drug use.

Drug Interactions (See WARNINGS)

The concomitant use of other central nervous system depressants including sedatives or hypnotics, general anesthetics, phenothiazines, tranquilizers and alcohol may produce additive depressant effects. Respiratory depression, hypotension and profound sedation or coma may occur. When such combined therapy is contemplated, the dose of one or both agents should be reduced. Opioid analgesics, including MS CONTIN, may enhance the neuromuscular blocking action of skeletal muscle relaxants and produce an increased degree of respiratory depression.

Carcinogenicity/Mutagenicity/Impairment of Fertility

Studies of morphine sulfate in animals to evaluate the drug's carcinogenic and mutagenic potential or the effect on fertility have not been conducted.

Pregnancy

Teratogenic effects—CATEGORY C: Adequate animal studies on reproduction have not been performed to determine whether morphine affects fertility in males or females. There are no well-controlled studies in women, but marketing experience does not include any evidence of adverse effects on the fetus following routine (short-term) clinical use of morphine sulfate products. Although there is no clearly defined risk, such experience can not exclude the possibility of infrequent or subtle damage to the human fetus.

MS CONTIN should be used in pregnant women only when clearly needed. (See also: PRECAUTIONS: Labor and Delivery, and DRUG ABUSE AND DEPENDENCE.)

Nonteratogenic effects: Infants born from mothers who have been taking morphine chronically may exhibit withdrawal symptoms.

Labor and Delivery

MS CONTIN is not recommended for use in women during and immediately prior to labor. Occasionally, opioid analgesics may prolong labor through actions which temporarily reduce the strength, duration and frequency of uterine contractions. However, this effect is not consistent and may be offset by an increased rate of cervical dilatation which tends to shorten labor.

Neonates whose mothers received opioid analgesics during labor should be observed closely for signs of respiratory depression. A specific narcotic antagonist, naloxone, should be available for reversal of narcotic-induced respiratory depression in the neonate.

Nursing Mothers

Low levels of morphine sulfate have been detected in human milk. Withdrawal symptoms can occur in breast-feeding infants when maternal administration of morphine sulfate is stopped. Ordinarily, nursing should not be undertaken while a patient is receiving MS CONTIN since morphine may be excreted in the milk.

Pediatric Use

MS CONTIN has not been evaluated systematically in children.

Continued on next page

Purdue Frederick—Cont.

ADVERSE REACTIONS

The adverse reactions caused by morphine are essentially those observed with other opioid analgesics. They include the following major hazards: respiratory depression, apnea, and to a lesser degree, circulatory depression; respiratory arrest, shock and cardiac arrest.

Most Frequently Observed

Constipation, lightheadedness, dizziness, sedation, nausea, vomiting, sweating, dysphoria and euphoria.

Some of these effects seem to be more prominent in ambulatory patients and in those not experiencing severe pain. Some adverse reactions in ambulatory patients may be alleviated if the patient lies down.

Less Frequently Observed Reactions

Central Nervous System: Weakness, headache, agitation, tremor, uncoordinated muscle movements, seizure, alterations of mood (nervousness, apprehension, depression, floating feelings), dreams, muscle rigidity, transient hallucinations and disorientation, visual disturbances, insomnia and increased intracranial pressure.

Gastrointestinal: Dry mouth, constipation, biliary tract spasm, laryngospasm, anorexia, diarrhea, cramps and taste alterations.

Cardiovascular: Flushing of the face, chills, tachycardia, bradycardia, palpitation, faintness, syncope, hypotension and hypertension.

Genitourinary: Urine retention or hesitance, reduced libido and/or potency.

Dermatologic: Pruritis, urticaria, other skin rashes, edema and diaphoresis.

Other: Antidiuretic effect, paresthesia, muscle tremor, blurred vision, nystagmus, diplopia and miosis.

DRUG ABUSE AND DEPENDENCE

Opioid analgesics may cause psychological and physical dependence (see WARNINGS). Physical dependence results in withdrawal symptoms in patients who abruptly discontinue the drug or may be precipitated through the administration of drugs with narcotic antagonist activity, e.g., naloxone or mixed agonist/antagonist analgesics (pentazocine, etc.; See also OVERDOSAGE). Physical dependence usually does not occur to a clinically significant degree until after several weeks of continued narcotic usage. Tolerance, in which increasingly large doses are required in order to produce the same degree of analgesia, is initially manifested by a shortened duration of analgesic effect, and, subsequently, by decreases in the intensity of analgesia.

In chronic pain patients, and in narcotic-tolerant cancer patients, the administration of MS CONTIN should be guided by the degree of tolerance manifested. Physical dependence, per se, is not ordinarily a concern when one is dealing with opioid-tolerant patients whose pain and suffering is associated with an irreversible illness.

If MS CONTIN is abruptly discontinued, a moderate to severe abstinence syndrome may occur. The opioid agonist abstinence syndrome is characterized by some or all of the following: restlessness, lacrimation, rhinorrhea, yawning, perspiration, gooseflesh, restless sleep or "yen" and mydriasis during the first 24 hours. These symptoms often increase in severity and over the next 72 hours may be accompanied by increasing irritability, anxiety, weakness, twitching and spasms of muscles; kicking movements; severe backache, abdominal and leg pains; abdominal and muscle cramps; hot and cold flashes, insomnia; nausea, anorexia, vomiting, intestinal spasm, diarrhea; coryza and repetitive sneezing; increase in body temperature, blood pressure, respiratory rate and heart rate. Because of excessive loss of fluids through sweating, vomiting and diarrhea, there is usually marked weight loss, dehydration, ketosis, and disturbances in acid-base balance. Cardiovascular collapse can occur. Without treatment most observable symptoms disappear in 5–14 days; however, there appears to be a phase of secondary or chronic abstinence which may last for 2–6 months characterized by insomnia, irritability, and muscular aches.

If treatment of physical dependence of patients on MS CONTIN is necessary, the patient may be detoxified by gradual reduction of the dosage. Gastrointestinal disturbances or dehydration should be treated accordingly.

OVERDOSAGE

Acute overdosage with morphine is manifested by respiratory depression, somnolence progressing to stupor or coma, skeletal muscle flaccidity, cold and clammy skin, constricted pupils, and, sometimes, bradycardia and hypotension.

In the treatment of overdosage, primary attention should be given to the re-establishment of a patent airway and institution of assisted or controlled ventilation. The pure opioid antagonist, naloxone, is a specific antidote against respiratory depression which results from opioid overdose. Naloxone (usually 0.4 to 2.0 mg) should be administered intravenously; however, because its duration of action is relatively short, the patient must be carefully monitored until spontaneous respiration is reliably re-established. If the response to

naloxone is suboptimal or not sustained, additional naloxone may be re-administered, as needed, or given by continuous infusion to maintain alertness and respiratory function; however, there is no information available about the cumulative dose of naloxone that may be safely administered. Naloxone should not be administered in the absence of clinically significant respiratory or circulatory depression secondary to morphine overdose. Naloxone should be administered cautiously to persons who are known, or suspected to be physically dependent on MS CONTIN. In such cases, an abrupt or complete reversal of narcotic effects may precipitate an acute abstinence syndrome.

Note: In an individual physically dependent on opioids, administration of the usual dose of the antagonist will precipitate an acute withdrawal syndrome. The severity of the withdrawal syndrome produced will depend on the degree of physical dependence and the dose of the antagonist administered. Use of a narcotic antagonist in such a person should be avoided. If necessary to treat serious respiratory depression in the physically dependent patient, the antagonist should be administered with extreme care and by titration with smaller than usual doses of the antagonist.

Supportive measures (including oxygen, vasopressors) should be employed in the management of circulatory shock and pulmonary edema accompanying overdose as indicated. Cardiac arrest or arrhythmias may require cardiac massage or defibrillation.

DOSAGE AND ADMINISTRATION

(See also: CLINICAL PHARMACOLOGY, WARNINGS AND PRECAUTIONS sections)

MS CONTIN TABLETS ARE TO BE TAKEN WHOLE, AND ARE NOT TO BE BROKEN, CHEWED OR CRUSHED.

MS CONTIN is intended for use in patients who require more than several days continuous treatment with a potent opioid analgesic. The controlled release nature of the formulation allows it to be administered on a more convenient schedule than conventional immediate-release oral morphine products. (See CLINICAL PHARMACOLOGY: "Metabolism and Pharmacokinetics".) However, MS CONTIN does not release morphine continuously over the course of the dosing interval. The administration of single doses of MS CONTIN on a q12h dosing schedule will result in higher peak and lower trough plasma levels than those that occur when an identical daily dose of morphine is administered using conventional oral formulations on a q4h regimen. The clinical significance of greater fluctuations in morphine plasma level has not been systematically evaluated.

As with any potent opioid drug product, it is critical to adjust the dosing regimen for each patient individually, taking into account the patient's prior analgesic treatment experience. Although it is clearly impossible to enumerate every consideration that is important to the selection of initial dose and dosing interval of MS CONTIN, attention should be given to 1) the daily dose, potency and precise characteristics of the opioid the patient has been taking previously (e.g., whether it is a pure agonist or mixed agonist/antagonist), 2) the reliability of the relative potency estimate used to calculate the dose of morphine needed [N.B. potency estimates may vary with the route of administration], 3) the degree of opioid tolerance, if any, and 4) the general condition and medical status of the patient.

The following dosing recommendations, therefore, can only be considered suggested approaches to what is actually a series of clinical decisions in the management of the pain of an individual patient.

Conversion from Conventional Oral Morphine to MS CONTIN

A patient's daily morphine requirement is established using immediate release oral morphine (dosing every 4 to 6 hours). The patient is then converted to MS CONTIN in either of two ways: 1) by administering one-half of the patient's 24 hour requirement as MS CONTIN on an every 12 hour schedule; or, 2) by administering one-third of the patient's daily requirement as MS CONTIN on an every eight hour schedule. With either method, dose and dosing interval is then adjusted as needed (See discussion below.) For initial conversion, the 30 mg tablet strength is recommended for patients with a daily morphine requirement of 120 mg or less.

Conversion from Parenteral Morphine or Other Opioids (Parenteral or Oral) to MS CONTIN

MS CONTIN can be administered as the initial oral morphine drug product; in this case, however, particular care must be exercised in the conversion process. Because of uncertainty about and intersubject variation in relative estimates of opioid potency and cross tolerance, initial dosing regimens should be conservative; that is, an underestimation of the 24 hour oral morphine requirement is preferred to an overestimate. To this end, initial individual doses of MS CONTIN should be estimated conservatively. In patients whose daily morphine requirements are expected to be less than or equal to 120 mg per day, the 30 mg tablet strength is recommended for the initial titration period. Once a stable dose regimen is reached, the patient can be converted to the 60 mg tablet strength, if desired.

Estimates of the relative potency of opioids are only approximate and are influenced by route of administration, individual patient differences, and possibly, by an individual's medical condition. Consequently, it is difficult to recommend any fixed rule for converting a patient to MS CONTIN directly. The following general points should be considered, however.

1. *Parenteral to oral morphine ratio:* Estimates of the oral to parenteral potency of morphine vary. Some authorities suggest that a dose of oral morphine only three times the daily parenteral morphine requirement may be sufficient in chronic use settings.

2. Other parenteral or oral opioids to oral morphine: Because there is lack of systemic evidence bearing on these types of analgesic substitutions, specific recommendations are not possible. Physicians are advised to refer to published relative potency data, keeping in mind that such ratios are only approximate. In general, it is safer to underestimate the daily dose of MS CONTIN required and rely upon ad hoc supplementation to deal with inadequate analgesia. (See discussion which follows.)

Use of MS CONTIN as the First Opioid Analgesic

There has been no systematic evaluation of MS CONTIN as an initial opioid analgesic in the management of pain. Because it may be more difficult to titrate a patient using a controlled release morphine, it is ordinarily advisable to begin treatment using an immediate release formulation.

Considerations in the Adjustment of Dosing Regimens

Whatever the approach, if signs of excessive opioid effects are observed early in a dosing interval, the next dose should be reduced. If this adjustment leads to inadequate analgesia, that is, 'breakthrough' pain occurs late in the dosing interval, the dosing interval should be shortened. Alternatively, a supplemental dose of a short-acting analgesic may be given. As experience is gained, adjustments can be made to obtain an appropriate balance between pain relief, opioid side effects, and the convenience of the dosing schedule.

In adjusting dosing requirements, it is recommended that the dosing interval **never** be extended beyond 12 hours because the administration of very large single doses may lead to acute overdose. (N.B. MS CONTIN is a controlled release formulation; it does not release morphine continuously over the dosing interval.)

For patients with low daily morphine requirements, precise titration may be difficult because the smallest available tablet of MS CONTIN contains 30 mg of morphine. In this regard, adjustment in dose should NOT be attempted by breaking or crushing the tablets. MS CONTIN tablets are intended to be swallowed whole.

Conversion from MS CONTIN to parenteral opioids:

When converting a patient from MS CONTIN to parenteral opioids, it is best to assume that the parenteral to oral potency is high. NOTE THAT THIS IS THE CONVERSE OF THE STRATEGY USED WHEN THE DIRECTION OF CONVERSION IS FROM THE PARENTERAL TO ORAL FORMULATIONS. IN BOTH CASES, HOWEVER, THE AIM IS TO ESTIMATE THE NEW DOSE CONSERVATIVELY. For example, to estimate the required 24 hour dose of morphine for IM use, one could employ a conversion of 1 mg of morphine IM for every 6 mg of morphine as MS CONTIN. Of course, the IM 24-hour dose would have to be divided by six and administered on a q4h regimen. This approach is recommended because it is least likely to cause overdose.

HOW SUPPLIED

NDC 0034-0515-50: MS CONTIN (morphine sulfate controlled release tablets) 30 mg are supplied in opaque plastic bottles containing 50 tablets.

NDC 0034-0515-10: MS CONTIN (morphine sulfate controlled release tablets) 30 mg are supplied in opaque plastic bottles containing 100 tablets.

NDC 0034-0515-45: MS CONTIN (morphine sulfate controlled release tablets) 30 mg are supplied in opaque plastic bottles containing 250 tablets.

NDC 0034-0515-90: MS CONTIN (morphine sulfate controlled release tablets) 30 mg are supplied in opaque plastic bottles containing 500 tablets.

NDC 0034-0515-25: MS CONTIN (morphine sulfate controlled release tablets) 30 mg supplied in unit dose packaging with 25 individually-numbered tablets per card (numbered in descending order for easier counting) and shrink-wrapped in inner packs of 100 tablets (4 cards of 25 tablets per card). One shipper contains 300 tablets (3 inner packs of 100 tablets each). Each individual tablet-unit is labeled "MS CONTIN."

NDC 0034-0516-10: MS CONTIN (morphine sulfate controlled release tablets) 60 mg are supplied in opaque plastic bottles containing 100 tablets.

NDC 0034-0516-25: MS CONTIN (morphine sulfate controlled release tablets) 60 mg supplied in unit dose packaging with 25 individually numbered tablets per card (numbered in descending order for easier counting) and shrink-wrapped in inner packs of 100 tablets (4 cards of 25 tablets per card). One shipper contains 300 tablets (3 inner packs of 100 tablets each). Each individual tablet-unit is labeled "MS CONTIN CII, 60 mg".

30 mg: Each round, lavender-colored tablet bears the symbol PF on one side and M30 on the other side.

60 mg: Each round, orange-colored tablet bears the symbol PF on one side and M60 on the other side.

Store tablets at controlled room temperature 15° to 30℃ (59°–86°F).

Dispense in tight, light-resistant container.

CAUTION
DEA Order Form Required.

Federal law prohibits dispensing without prescription.
April, 1988   K1609

Shown in Product Identification Section, page 423

MSIR® Oral Solution   Ⓒ
[em ′es ī″ahr]
(morphine sulfate)
   (WARNING: May be habit forming)
MSIR® Oral Solution Concentrate   Ⓒ
(morphine sulfate)
   (WARNING: May be habit forming)
MSIR® Immediate Release Oral Tablets   Ⓒ
(morphine sulfate)
   (WARNING: May be habit forming)

DESCRIPTION
Chemically, morphine sulfate is 7,8 didehydro-4,5 α-epoxy-17 methyl-morphinian-3,6 α-diol sulfate (2:1) (salt) pentahydrate and has the following structural formula:

Each 5 ml of MSIR Oral Solution contains:
Morphine Sulfate .... 10 or 20 mg
Inactive Ingredients: Edetate disodium, FD&C Red. No. 40, Glycerin, Invert Sugar, Sodium benzoate, Sodium chloride, Sucrose, Artificial & Natural Flavors, and other ingredients.
Each 1 ml of MSIR Oral Solution Concentrate contains:
Morphine Sulfate .... 20 mg
Inactive Ingredients: Edetate disodium, Sodium benzoate, and other ingredients.
Each MSIR Tablet for oral administration contains:
Morphine Sulfate .... 15 or 30 mg
Inactive Ingredients: Corn starch, Lactose, Magnesium stearate, and Talc.
   (WARNING: May be habit forming)

CLINICAL PHARMACOLOGY

Metabolism and Pharmacokinetics
MSIR Solutions and Tablets containing morphine sulfate are for oral administration and are conventional immediate release products. Only about 40% of the administered dose reaches the central compartment because of pre-systemic elimination (i.e., metabolism in the gut wall and liver).

Once absorbed, morphine is distributed in skeletal muscle, kidneys, liver, intestinal tract, lungs, spleen and brain. Morphine also crosses the placental membranes and has been found in breast milk.

Although a small fraction (less than 5%) of morphine is demethylated, for all practical purposes, virtually all morphine is converted to glucuronide metabolites; among these, morphine-3-glucuronide is present in the highest plasma concentration following oral administration.

The glucuronide system has a very high capacity and is not easily saturated even in disease. Therefore, the rate of delivery of morphine to the gut and liver does not influence the total and/or the relative quantities of the various metabolites formed.

The following pharmacokinetic parameters show considerable inter-subject variation but are representative of average values reported in the literature. The volume of distribution (Vd) for morphine is 4 liters per kilogram, and the terminal elimination half-life is approximately 2 to 4 hours. Fifty percent of the morphine that will reach the central compartment intact, reaches it within 30 minutes following the administration of conventional oral morphine products.

Variation in the physical/mechanical properties of a formulation of an oral morphine drug product can affect both its absolute bioavailability and its absorption rate constant (k_a). The basic pharmacokinetic parameters (e.g., volume of distribution [Vd], elimination rate constant [k_e], clearance [Cl]) are fundamental properties of morphine in the organism. While there is no predictable relationship between morphine blood levels and analgesic response, effective analgesia probably will not occur below some minimum blood level in a given patient. The minimum effective blood level for analgesia will vary among patients, especially among patients who have or have not been previously treated with potent mu (μ) agonist opioids. Similarly, there is no predictable relationship between blood morphine concentration and untoward clinical responses; but higher concentrations are more likely to be toxic.

The elimination of morphine occurs primarily as renal excretion of 3-morphine glucuronide. A small amount of the glucuronide conjugate is excreted in the bile, and there is some minor enterohepatic recycling.

The elimination half-life of morphine is reported to vary between 2 and 4 hours. Thus, steady state is probably achieved on most regimens within a day. Because morphine is primarily metabolized to inactive metabolites, the effects of renal disease on morphine's elimination are not likely to be pronounced. However, as with any drug, caution should be taken to guard against unanticipated accumulation if renal and/or hepatic function is seriously impaired.

Individual differences in the metabolism of morphine suggest that MSIR Oral Solutions and Tablets be dosed conservatively according to the dosing initiation and titration recommendations in the Dosage and Administration section.

PHARMACODYNAMICS
The effects described below are common to all morphine-containing products.

Central Nervous System
The principal actions of therapeutic value of morphine are analgesia and sedation.

The precise mechanism of analgesic action is unknown. However, specific CNS opiate receptors and endogenous compounds with morphine-like activity have been identified throughout the brain and spinal cord and are likely to play a role in the expression of analgesic effects.

Morphine produces respiratory depression by direct action on brain stem respiratory centers. The mechanism of respiratory depression involves a reduction in the responsiveness of the brain stem respiratory centers to increases in carbon dioxide tension, and to electrical stimulation.

Morphine depresses the cough reflex by direct effect on the cough center in the medulla. Antitussive effects may occur with doses lower than those usually required for analgesia. Morphine causes miosis, even in total darkness. Pinpoint pupils are a sign of narcotic overdose but are not pathognomonic (e.g., pontine lesions hemorrhagic or ischemic origins may produce similar findings). Marked mydriasis rather than miosis may be seen with worsening hypoxia.

Gastrointestinal Tract and Other Smooth Muscle
Gastric, biliary and pancreatic secretions are decreased by morphine. Morphine causes a reduction in motility associated with an increase in tone in the antrum of the stomach and duodenum. Digestion of food in the small intestine is delayed and propulsive contractions are decreased. In addition propulsive peristaltic waves in the colon are decreased, while tone is increased to the point of spasm. The end result is constipation. Morphine can cause a marked increase in biliary tract pressure as a result of spasm of the sphincter of Oddi.

Cardiovascular System
Morphine produces peripheral vasodilation which may result in orthostatic hypotension. Release of histamine can occur and may contribute to narcotic-induced hypotension. Manifestations of histamine release and/or peripheral vasodilation may include pruritus, flushing, red eyes and sweating.

INDICATIONS AND USAGE
MSIR Oral Solutions and Tablets are indicated for the relief of moderate to severe pain.

CONTRAINDICATIONS
MSIR Oral Solutions and Tablets are contraindicated in patients with known hypersensitivity to the drug, in patients with respiratory depression in the absence of resuscitative equipment, and in patients with acute or severe bronchial asthma.

WARNINGS
(see also: **CLINICAL PHARMACOLOGY**)

Impaired Respiration
Respiratory depression is the chief hazard of all morphine preparations although mitigated in the presence of pain. Respiratory depression occurs most frequently in elderly and debilitated patients, and those suffering from conditions accompanied by hypoxia or hypercapnia when even moderate therapeutic doses may dangerously decrease pulmonary ventilation.

Morphine should be used with extreme caution in patients with chronic obstructive pulmonary disease or cor pulmonale, and in patients having a substantially decreased respiratory reserve, hypoxia, hypercapnia, or preexisting respiratory depression. In such patients, even usual therapeutic doses of morphine may decrease respiratory drive while simultaneously increasing airway resistance to the point of apnea.

Head Injury and Increased Intracranial Pressure
The respiratory depressant effects of morphine with carbon dioxide retention and secondary elevation of cerebrospinal fluid pressure may be markedly exaggerated in the presence of head injury, other intracranial lesions, or preexisting increase in intracranial pressure. Morphine produces effects which may obscure neurologic signs of further increase in pressure in patients with head injuries.

Hypotensive Effects
MSIR Oral Solutions and Tablets, like all opioid analgesics, may cause severe hypotension in an individual whose ability to maintain his blood pressure has already been compromised by a depleted blood volume, or a concurrent administration of drugs such as phenothiazines, or general anesthetics. (see also: PRECAUTIONS: Drug Interactions.) MSIR Oral Solutions and Tablets may produce orthostatic hypotension in ambulatory patients.

MSIR Oral Solutions and Tablets, like all opioid analgesics, should be administered with caution to patients in circulatory shock, since vasodilation produced by the drug may further reduce cardiac output and blood pressure.

Interactions with Other CNS Depressants
MSIR Oral Solutions and Tablets, like all opioid analgesics, should be used with great caution and in reduced dosage in patients who are concurrently receiving other central nervous system depressants including sedatives or hypnotics, general anesthetics, phenothiazines, other tranquilizers and alcohol, because respiratory depression, hypotension and profound sedation or coma may result.

Interactions with Mixed Agonist/Antagonist Opioid Analgesics
From a theoretical perspective, agonist/antagonist analgesics (i.e., pentazocine, nalbuphine, butorphanol and buprenorphine) should NOT be administered to a patient who has received or is receiving a course of therapy with a pure agonist opioid analgesic. In these patients, mixed agonist-antagonist analgesics may reduce the analgesic effect or may precipitate withdrawal symptoms.

Drug Dependence
Morphine can produce drug dependence and has a potential for being abused. Tolerance and psychological and physical dependence may develop upon repeated administration. Physical dependence, however, is not of paramount importance in the management of any patient in severe pain. Abrupt cessation or a sudden reduction in dose after prolonged use may result in withdrawal symptoms. After prolonged exposure to opioid analgesics, if withdrawal is necessary, it must be undertaken gradually. (See DRUG ABUSE AND DEPENDENCE.)

Infants born to mothers physically dependent on opioid analgesics may also be physically dependent and exhibit respiratory depression and withdrawal symptoms. (See **DRUG ABUSE AND DEPENDENCE.**)

The development of psychological dependence is relatively rare when morphine is used under medically supervised conditions.

PRECAUTIONS
(See also: **CLINICAL PHARMACOLOGY**)

General
MSIR Oral Solutions and Tablets are intended for use in patients who require a potent opioid analgesic for relief of moderate to severe pain.

Selection of patients for treatment with MSIR Oral Solutions and Tablets should be governed by the same principles that apply to the use of morphine and other potent opioid analgesics which take into account: the elderly or debilitated and those with the following—severe impairment of hepatic, pulmonary or renal function; myxedema or hypothyroidism; adrenocortical insufficiency (e.g., Addison's Disease); CNS depression or coma; toxic psychoses; prostatic hypertrophy or urethral stricture; acute alcoholism; delirium tremens; kyphoscoliosis.

The administration of morphine, like all opioid analgesics, may obscure the diagnosis or clinical course in patients with acute abdominal conditions.

Morphine may aggravate preexisting convulsions in patients with convulsive disorders.

Morphine should be used with caution in patients about to undergo surgery of the biliary tract, since it may cause spasm of the sphincter of Oddi. Similarly, morphine should be used with caution in patients with acute pancreatitis secondary to biliary tract disease.

Information for Patients
If clinically advisable, patients receiving MSIR Oral Solutions and Tablets should be given the following instructions by the physician.

1. Morphine may produce physical dependence and may be associated with the development of psychological dependence. For this reason, the dose of the drug should not be adjusted without consulting a physician.
2. Morphine may impair mental and/or physical ability required for the performance of potentially hazardous tasks (e.g., driving, operating machinery).
3. Morphine should not be taken with alcohol or other CNS depressants (sleep aids, tranquilizers) because additive effects including CNS depression may occur. A physician should be consulted if other prescription medications are currently being used or are prescribed for future use.

Continued on next page

Purdue Frederick—Cont.

4. For women of childbearing potential who become or are planning to become pregnant, a physician should be consulted regarding analgesics and other drug use.

Drug Interactions (See also **WARNINGS**)

The concomitant use of other central nervous system depressants including sedatives or hypnotics, general anesthetics, phenothiazines, tranquilizers and alcohol may produce additive depressant effects. Respiratory depression, hypotension and profound sedation or coma may occur. When such combined therapy is contemplated, the dose of one or both agents should be reduced. Opioid analgesics, including MSIR Oral Solutions and Tablets, may enhance the neuromuscular blocking action of skeletal muscle relaxants and produce an increased degree of respiratory depression.

Carcinogenicity/Mutagenicity/Impairment of Fertility

Studies of morphine sulfate in animals to evaluate the drug's carcinogenic and mutagenic potential or the effect on fertility have not been conducted.

Pregnancy

Teratogenic effects—CATEGORY C: There are no well-controlled studies in women, but marketing experience does not include any evidence of adverse effects on the fetus following routine (short-term) clinical use of morphine sulfate products. Although there is no clearly defined risk, such experience cannot exclude the possibility of infrequent or subtle damage to the human fetus. MSIR Oral Solutions and Tablets should be used in pregnant women only when clearly needed. (See also: **PRECAUTIONS: Labor and Delivery, and DRUG ABUSE AND DEPENDENCE.**)

Nonteratogenic effects: Infants born from mothers who have been taking morphine chronically may exhibit withdrawal symptoms.

Labor and Delivery

MSIR Oral Solutions and Tablets are not recommended for use in women during and immediately prior to labor. Occasionally, opioid analgesics may prolong labor through actions which temporarily reduce the strength, duration and frequency of uterine contractions. However, this effect is not consistent and may be offset by an increased rate of cervical dilatation which tends to shorten labor.

Neonates whose mothers received opioid analgesics during labor should be observed closely for signs of respiratory depression. A specific narcotic antagonist, naloxone, should be available for reversal of narcotic-induced respiratory depression in the neonate.

Nursing Mothers

Low levels of morphine sulfate have been detected in human milk. Withdrawal symptoms can occur in breast-feeding infants when maternal administration of morphine sulfate is stopped. Nursing should not be undertaken while a patient is receiving MSIR Oral Solutions and Tablets since morphine may be excreted in the milk.

ADVERSE REACTIONS

The adverse reactions caused by morphine are essentially the same as those observed with other opioid analgesics. They include the following major hazards: respiratory depression, apnea, and to a lesser degree, circulatory depression; respiratory arrest, shock, and cardiac arrest.

Most Frequently Observed

Constipation, lightheadedness, dizziness, sedation, nausea, vomiting, and sweating.

Some of these effects seem to be more prominent in ambulatory patients and in those not experiencing severe pain. Some adverse reactions in ambulatory patients may be alleviated if the patient lies down.

Less Frequently Observed Reactions

Central Nervous System: Weakness, headache, agitation, tremor, uncoordinated muscle movements, seizure, alterations of mood (dysphoria, euphoria, nervousness, apprehension, depression, floating feelings), dreams, muscle rigidity, transient hallucinations and disorientation, visual disturbances, insomnia and increased intracranial pressure.

Gastrointestinal: Dry mouth, biliary tract spasm, anorexia, diarrhea, cramps and taste alterations.

Cardiovascular: Flushing of the face, chills, tachycardia, bradycardia, palpitation, faintness, syncope, hypotension and hypertension.

Genitourinary: Urinary retention or hesitance, reduced libido, and/or impotence.

Dermatologic: Pruritus, urticaria, other skin rashes, and edema.

Other: Antidiuretic effect, paresthesia, muscle tremor, blurred vision, nystagmus, diplopia, miosis and laryngospasm.

DRUG ABUSE AND DEPENDENCE

Opioid analgesics may cause physical dependence and be associated with the development of psychological dependence. (See WARNINGS.) Physical dependence results in withdrawal symptoms in patients who abruptly discontinue the drug or may be precipitated through the administration of drugs with narcotic antagonist activity, e.g., naloxone or

mixed agonist/antagonist analgesics (pentazocine, etc.; see also OVERDOSE). Physical dependence usually does not occur to a clinically significant degree until after several weeks of continued narcotic usage. Tolerance, in which increasingly large doses are required in order to produce the same degree of analgesia, is initially manifested by a shortened duration of analgesic effect, and, subsequently, by decreases in the intensity of analgesia. In chronic-pain patients and in narcotic-tolerant cancer patients, the administration of MSIR Oral Solutions and Tablets should be guided by the degree of tolerance manifested. Physical dependence, per se, is not a concern when one is dealing with the cancer patient with moderate to severe pain. The primary objective in this situation is to relieve the patient's pain.

If MSIR Oral Solutions and Tablets are abruptly discontinued, a moderate to severe abstinence syndrome may occur. The opioid agonist abstinence syndrome is characterized by some or all of the following: restlessness, lacrimation, rhinorrhea, yawning, perspiration, cutis anserina, restless sleep known as the "yen" and mydriasis during the first 24 hours. These symptoms often increase in severity and over the next 72 hours may be accompanied by increasing irritability, anxiety, weakness, twitching and spasms of muscles; kicking movements; severe backache, abdominal and leg pains; abdominal and muscle cramps; hot and cold flashes; insomnia; nausea, anorexia, vomiting, intestinal spasm, diarrhea; coryza and repetitive sneezing; and increase in body temperature, blood pressure, respiratory rate and heart rate. Because of excessive loss of fluids through sweating, vomiting and diarrhea, there is usually marked weight loss, dehydration, ketosis, and disturbances in acid-base balance. Cardiovascular collapse can occur. Without treatment, most observable symptoms disappear in 5–14 days; however, there appears to be a phase of secondary or chronic abstinence which may last for 2–6 months, characterized by insomnia, irritability, and muscular aches.

If treatment of physical dependence on MSIR Oral Solutions and Tablets is necessary, the patient may be detoxified by gradual reduction of the dosage. If abstinence symptoms become severe, the patient may be given methadone. Temporary administration of tranquilizers and sedatives may aid in reducing patient anxiety and narcotic craving. Gastrointestinal disturbances or dehydration should be treated accordingly.

OVERDOSE

Acute overdosage with morphine is manifested by respiratory depression, somnolence progressing to stupor or coma, skeletal muscle flaccidity, cold and clammy skin, constricted pupils, and, sometimes, bradycardia and hypotension.

In the treatment of overdosage, primary attention should be given to the re-establishment of a patent airway and institution of assisted or controlled ventilation. The pure opioid antagonist, naloxone, is a specific antidote against respiratory depression which results from opioid overdose. Naloxone (usually 0.4 to 2.0 mg) should be administered intravenously; however, because its duration of action is relatively short, the patient must be carefully monitored until spontaneous respiration is reliably reestablished. If the response to naloxone is suboptimal or not sustained, additional naloxone may be re-administered, as needed, or given by continuous infusion to maintain alertness and respiratory function; however, there is no information available about the cumulative dose of naloxone that may be safely administered.

Naloxone should not be administered in the absence of clinically significant respiratory or circulatory depression secondary to morphine overdose. Naloxone should be administered cautiously to persons who are known or suspected to be physically dependent on morphine. In such cases, an abrupt or complete reversal of narcotic effects may precipitate an acute abstinence syndrome.

Note: In an individual physically dependent on opioids, administration of the usual dose of the antagonist will precipitate an acute withdrawal syndrome. The severity of the withdrawal syndrome produced will depend on the degree of physical dependence and the dose of the antagonist administered. Use of a narcotic antagonist in such a person should be avoided. If necessary to treat serious respiratory depression in the physically dependent patient, the antagonist should be administered with extreme care and by titration with smaller than usual doses of the antagonist.

Supportive measures (including oxygen, vasopressors) should be employed in the management of circulatory shock and pulmonary edema accompanying overdose as indicated. Cardiac arrest or arrhythmias may require cardiac massage or defibrillation.

CAUTION

DEA Order Form Required.

Federal law prohibits dispensing without prescription.

DOSAGE AND ADMINISTRATION: (See also: **CLINICAL PHARMACOLOGY, WARNINGS AND PRECAUTIONS** sections)

Dosage of morphine is a patient-dependent variable, which must be individualized according to patient metabolism, age

and disease state and also response to morphine. Each patient should be maintained at the lowest dosage level that will produce acceptable analgesia. As the patient's well-being improves after successful relief of moderate to severe pain, periodic reduction of dosage and/or extension of dosing interval should be attempted to minimize exposure to morphine.

Usual Adult Oral Dose: 5 to 30 mg every four (4) hours or as directed by physician administered either as MSIR Oral Solutions or MSIR Oral Tablets. For control of pain in terminal illness, it is recommended that the appropriate dose of MSIR Oral Solutions or MSIR Oral Tablets be given on a regularly scheduled basis every four hours at the minimum dose to achieve acceptable analgesia. If converting a patient from another narcotic to morphine sulfate on the basis of standard equivalence tables, a 1 to 3 ratio of parenteral to oral morphine equivalence is suggested. This ratio is conservative and may underestimate the amount of morphine required. If this is the case, the dose of MSIR Oral Solutions or MSIR Oral Tablets should be gradually increased to achieve acceptable analgesia and tolerable side effects.

HOW SUPPLIED

MSIR (morphine sulfate) Oral Solution:
(pleasantly flavored)
10 mg per 5 ml.
NDC 0034-0521-01: 5 ml polypropylene unit dose cups, 10 cups per single tray, ten trays per shipper carton.
NDC 0034-0521-02: high density polyethylene plastic metered dose dispenser bottle of 120 ml with child-resistant closure.
NDC 0034-0521-03: high density polyethylene plastic metered dose dispenser bottle of 500 ml with child-resistant closure.
20 mg per 5 ml.
NDC 0034-0522-01: 5 ml polypropylene unit dose cups, 10 cups per single tray, ten trays per shipper carton.
NDC 0034-0522-02: high density polyethylene plastic metered dose dispenser bottle of 120 ml with child-resistant closure.
NDC 0034-0522-03: high density polyethylene plastic metered dose dispenser bottle of 500 ml with child-resistant closure.

MSIR (morphine sulfate) Oral Solution Concentrate:
(unflavored)
20 mg per 1 ml.
NDC 0034-0523-01: high density polyethylene plastic, child-resistant closure bottle with child-resistant dropper in 30 ml size.
NDC 0034-0523-02: high density polyethylene plastic, child-resistant closure bottle with child-resistant dropper in 120 ml size.
Discard opened bottle of Oral Solution after 90 days. Protect from light.

MSIR (morphine sulfate) Tablets:
15 mg round, white scored tablets
NDC 0034-0518-15: opaque plastic bottle, containing 50 tablets. Each tablet bears the symbol *PF* on the scored side and *MI 15* on the other side.
30 mg capsule-shaped, white scored tablets
NDC 0034-0519-30: opaque plastic bottle containing 50 tablets. Each tablet bears the symbol *PF* on the scored side and *MI 30* on the other side.

Store Oral Solutions and Tablets at controlled room temperature 15°to 30°C (59°–86°F).

Shown in Product Identification Section, page 423

NORZINE®   ℞

[nōr¹-zēēn]
(thiethylperazine maleate)
tablets USP
(thiethylperazine malate)
injection USP
(for intramuscular use only)
(thiethylperazine maleate)
suppositories USP

Prescribing Information

Caution: Federal law prohibits dispensing without a prescription.

DESCRIPTION

Norzine (thiethylperazine USP) is a phenothiazine. Thiethylperazine is characterized by a substituted thioethyl group at position 2 in the phenothiazine nucleus, and a piperazine moiety in the side chain. The chemical designation is: 2-ethyl- mercapto-10-[3'-(1''-methyl-piperazinyl-4'')-propyl-1'] phenothiazine. Thiethylperazine has the following structural formula:

[See Chemical Formula at top of next page]

Tablets, 10 mg, for oral administration.
ACTIVE INGREDIENT: thiethylperazine maleate USP 10 mg. *INACTIVE INGREDIENTS:* acacia, carnauba wax, FD&C Yellow No. 5 aluminum lake (tartrazine), FD&C Yellow No. 6 aluminum lake, gelatin, lactose, magnesium stearate, povidone, sodium benzoate, sorbitol, starch, stearic acid, sucrose, talc, titanium dioxide.
Ampul, 2 ml, for intramuscular administration.
ACTIVE INGREDIENT: thiethylperazine malate USP 10 mg per 2 ml. *INACTIVE INGREDIENTS:* sodium metabisulfite NF, 0.5 mg; ascorbic acid USP, 2.0 mg; sorbitol NF, 40 mg; carbon dioxide gas q.s.; water for injection USP, q.s. to 2 ml.
Suppository, 10 mg, for rectal administration.
ACTIVE INGREDIENT: thiethylperazine maleate USP 10 mg. *INACTIVE INGREDIENT:* cocoa butter, NF.

ACTIONS
The pharmacodynamic action of Norzine (thiethylperazine USP) in humans is unknown. However, a direct action of Norzine (thiethylperazne USP) on both the CTZ and the vomiting center may be concluded from induced vomiting experiments in animals.

INDICATIONS
Norzine (thiethylperazine USP) is indicated for the relief of nausea and vomiting.

CONTRAINDICATIONS
Severe central nervous system (CNS) depression and comatose states. In patients who have demonstrated a hypersensitivity reaction (e.g., blood dyscrasias, jaundice) to phenothiazines.
Because severe hypotension has been reported after the intravenous administration of phenothiazines, this route of administration is contraindicated.
Usage in Pregnancy: Norzine (thiethylperazine USP) is contraindicated in pregnancy.

WARNINGS
Norzine (thiethylperazine USP) for intramuscular injection contains sodium metabisulfite, a sulfite that may cause allergic-type reactions including anaphylactic symptoms and life-threatening or less severe asthmatic episodes in certain susceptible people. The overall prevalence of sulfite sensitivity in the general population is unknown and probably low. Sulfite sensitivity is seen more frequently in asthmatic than in nonasthmatic people.
Phenothiazines are capable of potentiating CNS depressants (e.g., anesthetics, opiates, alcohol, etc.) as well as atropine and phosphorous insecticides.
Since Norzine (thiethylperazine USP) may impair mental and/or physical ability required in the peformance of potentially hazardous tasks such as driving a car or operating machinery, it is recommended that patients be warned acccordingly.
Postoperative Nausea and Vomiting: With the use of this drug to control postoperative nausea and vomiting occurring in patients undergoing elective surgical procedures, restlessness and postoperative CNS depression during anesthesia recovery may occur. Possible postoperative complications of a severe degree of any of the known reactions of this class of drug must be considered. Postural hypotension may occur after an initial injection, rarely with the tablet or suppository.
The administration of epinephrine should be avoided in the treatment of drug-induced hypotension in view of the fact that phenothiazines may induce a reversed epinephrine effect on occasion.
Should a vasoconstrictive agent be required, the most suitable are norepinephrine bitartrate and phenylephrine.
The use of this drug has not been studied following intracardiac and intracranial surgery.
Usage in Pediatrics: The safety and efficacy of Norzine (thiethylperazine USP) in children under 12 years of age has not been established.
Nursing Mothers: Information is not available concerning the secretion of Norzine (thiethylperazine USP) in the milk of nursing mothers. As a general rule, nursing should not be undertaken while a patient is on a drug, since many drugs are secreted in human milk.

PRECAUTIONS
Abnormal movements such as extrapyramidal symptoms (EPS) (e.g., dystonia, torticollis, dysphasia, oculogyric crises, akathisia) have occurred. Convulsions have also been reported. The varied symptom complex is more likely to occur in young adults and children. Extrapyramidal effects must be treated by reduction of dosage or cessation of medication. Norzine (thiethylperazine USP) tablets contain FD&C Yellow No. 5 (tartrazine) which may cause allergic-type reactions (including bronchial asthma) in certain susceptible individuals. Although the overall incidence of FD&C Yellow No. 5 (tartrazine) sensitivity in the general population is low, it is frequently seen in patients who also have aspirin hypersensitivity.
Postoperative Nausea and Vomiting: When used in the treatment of the nausea and/or vomiting associated with anesthesia and surgery, it is recommended that Norzine (thiethylperazine USP) should be administered by deep intramuscular injection at or shortly before termination of anesthesia.

ADVERSE REACTIONS
Central Nervous System: Serious: Convulsions have been reported. Extrapyramidal symptoms (EPS) may occur, such as dystonia, torticollis, oculogyric crises, akathisia, and gait disturbances. Others: Occasional cases of dizziness, headache, fever and restlessness have been reported.
Drowsiness may occur on occasion, following an initial injection. Generally, this effect tends to subside with continued therapy or is usually alleviated by a reduction in dosage.
Autonomic Nervous System: Dryness of the mouth and nose, blurred vision, tinnitus. An occasional case of sialorrhea together with altered gustatory sensation has been observed.
Endocrine System: Peripheral edema of the arms, hands and face.
Hepatotoxicity: An occasional case of cholestatic jaundice has been observed.
Other: An occasional case of cerebral vascular spasm and trigeminal neuralgia has been reported.
Phenothiazine Derivatives: The physician should be aware that the following have occurred with one or more phenothiazines and should be considered whenever one of these drugs is used:
Blood Dyscrasias: Serious—Agranulocytosis, leukopenia, thrombocytopenia, aplastic anemia, pancytopenia. Others: Eosinophilia, leukocytosis.
Autonomic Reactions: Miosis, obstipation, anorexia, paralytic ileus.
Cutaneous Reactions: Serious—Erythema, exfoliative dermatitis, contact dermatitis.
Hepatotoxicity: Serious—Jaundice, biliary stasis.
Cardiovascular Effects: Serious—Hypotension, rarely leading to cardiac arrest; electrocardiographic (ECG) changes.
Extrapyramidal Symptoms: Serious—Akathisia, agitation, motor restlessness, dystonic reactions, trismus, torticollis, opisthotonos, oculogyric crises, tremor, muscular rigidity, akinesia—some of which have persisted for several months or years especially in patients of advanced age with brain damage.
Endocrine Disturbances: Menstrual irregularities, altered libido, gynecomastia, weight gain. False positive pregnancy tests have been reported.
Urinary Disturbances: Retention, incontinence.
Allergic Reactions: Serious—Fever, laryngeal edema, angioneurotic edema, asthma.
Others: Hyperpyrexia. Behavioral effects suggestive of a paradoxical reaction have been reported. These include excitement, bizarre dreams, aggravation of psychoses and toxic confusional states. While there is no evidence at present that ECG changes observed in patients receiving phenothiazines are in any way precursors of any significant disturbance of cardiac rhythm, it should be noted that sudden and unexpected deaths apparently due to cardiac arrest have been reported in a few instances in hospitalized psychotic patients previously showing characteristic ECG changes. A peculiar skin-eye syndrome has also been recognized as a side effect following long-term treatment with certain phenothiazines. This reaction is marked by progressive pigmentation of areas of the skin or conjuctiva and/or accompanied by discoloration of the exposed sclera and cornea. Opacities of the anterior lens and cornea described as irregular or stellate in shape have also been reported.
Drug Interactions: Phenothiazines are capable of potentiating CNS depressants (e.g., anesthetics, opiates, alcohol, etc.) as well as atropine and phosphorous insecticides.
Phenothiazines may induce a reversed epinephrine effect on occasion.

DOSAGE AND ADMINISTRATION
Adult: Usual daily dose range is 10 mg to 30 mg. *ORAL:* One tablet, one to three times daily. *INTRAMUSCULAR:* 2 ml IM, one to three times daily. (See Precautions.) *SUPPOSITORY:* Insert one suppository, one to three times daily.
Children: Appropriate dosage of Norzine (thiethylperazine USP) has not been determined in children.

HOW SUPPLIED
Tablets: Each tablet contains 10 mg thiethylperazine maleate USP. Bottles of 100 (NDC 0034-5100-80).

Ampuls: Each 2 ml ampul contains in aqueous solution 10 mg thiethylperazine malate USP. Box of 20 (NDC 0034-5110-20).
Storage: Below 86°F (30°C); light-resistant container. Administer only if clear and colorless.
Suppositories: Each suppository contains 10 mg thiethylperazine maleate USP. Packages of 12 (NDC 0034-5120-12).
Storage: Below 77°F (25°C); tight container (sealed foil).
Manufactured by:
Sandoz Pharmaceuticals Corporation
East Hanover, NJ 07936
Distributed by:
The Purdue Frederick Company
Norwalk, CT 06856   1/89 A2843
Shown in Product Identification Section, page 423

SENOKOT® TABLETS/GRANULES
[sen 'o-kot]
SENOKOTXTRA® TABLETS
(standardized senna concentrate)

ACTION AND USES
Indicated for relief of functional constipation (chronic or occasional). SENOKOT Tablets/Granules and Double-Strength SenokotXTRA Tablets contain a natural vegetable derivative, purified and standardized for uniform action. Each Double-Strength SenokotXTRA Tablet contains twice the active ingredient in one SENOKOT Tablet; patients may take one Double-Strength SenokotXTRA Tablet instead of two SENOKOT Tablets.
Senokot Laxatives provide a virtually colon-specific action which is gentle, effective and predictable, usually inducing comfortable evacuation of well-formed stool within 8–10 hours. SENOKOT has been found to be effective even in many previously intractable cases of functional constipation. SENOKOT preparations may aid in rehabilitation of the constipated patient by facilitating regular elimination. At proper dosage levels, SENOKOT preparations are virtually free of adverse reactions (such as loose stools or abdominal discomfort) and enjoy high patient acceptance. Numerous and extensive clinical studies show their high degree of effectiveness in several types of functional constipation: chronic, geriatric, antepartum and postpartum, drug-induced, pediatric, as well as in functional constipation concurrent with heart disease or anorectal surgery.

ADMINISTRATION AND DOSAGE
Preferably at bedtime. GRANULES (deliciously cocoa-flavored): Adults: 1 level tsp. (maximum—2 level tsp. twice in a day). For older, debilitated, and OB/GYN patients, the physician may consider prescribing ½ the initial adult dose. Children above 60 lb.: ½ level tsp. (maximum—1 level tsp. twice in a day).
SENOKOT TABLETS: Adults: 2 tablets (maximum—4 tablets twice in a day). For older, debilitated, and OB/GYN patients, the physician may consider prescribing ½ the initial dose. Children above 60 lb.: 1 tablet (maximum—2 tablets twice in a day). To meet individual requirements, if comfortable bowel movement is not achieved by the second day, decrease or increase daily dose by ½ level tsp. or 1 tablet (up to maximum) until optimal dose for evacuation is established.
Double-Strength SenokotXTRA TABLETS: Recommended Adult Dose (preferably at bedtime): One tablet (maximum: 2 tablets twice in a day). For older, debilitated, and OB/GYN patients, the physician may consider prescribing ½ the initial adult dose. [Note: One Double-Strength SenokotXTRA Tablet is equal to two SENOKOT Tablets.]

WARNING
Do not use when abdominal pain, nausea or vomiting are present. Frequent or prolonged use of laxatives may result in dependence on laxatives. If constipation persists, consult your physician.

HOW SUPPLIED
Granules: 2, 6, and 12 oz. plastic canisters. Tablets: Box of 20, bottles of 50, 100 and 1000. Unit Strip Packs in boxes of 100 tablets; each tablet individually sealed in see-through packets. Double-Strength SenokotXTRA Tablets: Boxes of 12.

ALSO AVAILABLE
SENOKOT Syrup (standardized extract of senna fruit) in bottles of 2 and 8 fl. oz.

ADMINISTRATION AND DOSAGE
Preferably at bedtime. Adults: 2 to 3 tsp. (maximum—3 tsp. twice in a day). For older, debilitated, and OB/GYN patients, the physician may consider prescribing ½ the initial adult dose. Children 5–15 years: 1 to 2 tsp. (maximum—2 tsp. twice in a day). 1–5 years: ½ to 1 tsp. (maximum—1 tsp. twice in a day). 1 month to 1 year: ¼ to ½ tsp. (maximum—½ tsp. twice in a day).

Continued on next page

Purdue Frederick—Cont.

SENOKOT-S® Tablets
[sĕn′ō-kŏt-ĕs″]
(standardized senna concentrate and docusate sodium)
Natural Laxative/Stool Softener Combination

ACTION AND USES

SENOKOT-S Tablets are designed to relieve both aspects of functional constipation—bowel inertia and hard, dry stools. They provide a natural neuroperistaltic stimulant combined with a classic stool softener: standardized senna concentrate gently stimulates the colon while docusate sodium softens the stool for smoother and easier evacuation. This coordinated dual action of the two ingredients results in colon-specific, predictable laxative effect, usually in 8–10 hours. Administering the tablets at bedtime allows the patient an uninterrupted night's sleep, with a comfortable evacuation in the morning. Flexibility of dosage permits fine adjustment to individual requirements. At proper dosage levels, SENOKOT-S Tablets are virtually free from side effects. SENOKOT-S Tablets are highly suitable for relief of postsurgical and postpartum constipation, and effectively counteract drug-induced constipation. They facilitate regular elimination in impaction-prone and elderly patients, and are indicated in the presence of cardiovascular disease where straining must be avoided, as well as in the presence of hemorrhoids and anorectal disease.

ADMINISTRATION AND DOSAGE

(Preferably at bedtime). Recommended Initial Dosage: ADULTS—2 tablets (maximum dosage—4 tablets twice in a day); CHILDREN (above 60 lbs.)—1 tablet (maximum dosage—2 tablets twice in a day). For older or debilitated patients, the physician may consider prescribing half the initial adult dose. To meet individual requirements, if comfortable bowel movement is not achieved by the second day, dosage may be decreased or increased by 1 tablet, up to maximum, until the most effective dose is established.

WARNING

Do not use when abdominal pain, nausea or vomiting are present. Frequent or prolonged use of laxatives may result in dependence on laxatives. If constipation persists, consult your physician.

SUPPLIED

Bottles of 30, 60 and 1000 Tablets.

T–PHYL® Tablets (Formerly UNIPHYL) ℞
[t-fĭl]
(theophylline)
200 mg
UNICONTIN®
Controlled-Release System

DESCRIPTION

Uniphyl Tablets contain 200 mg anhydrous theophylline in a controlled-release system. Inactive Ingredients: Cetostearyl alcohol, Hydroxyethyl cellulose, Magnesium stearate, Povidone, Talc, and other ingredients. The tablets are scored to facilitate dosage adjustment.

Theophylline anhydrous, a xanthine bronchodilator, is a white, odorless, crystalline powder having a bitter taste. Theophylline has a molecular weight of 180.18, represented by $C_7H_8N_4O_2$ and depicted as:

CLINICAL PHARMACOLOGY

Theophylline directly relaxes the smooth muscle of the bronchial airways and pulmonary blood vessels. The drug also produces other actions typical of the xanthine derivatives: coronary vasodilation, cardiac stimulation, diuresis, cerebral stimulation, and skeletal muscle stimulation. These actions may be mediated through inhibition of phosphodiesterase with a resultant increase in intracellular cyclic AMP. *In vitro*, theophylline has been shown to act synergistically with beta agonists that increase intracellular cyclic AMP through the stimulation of adenyl cyclase; but synergism has not been demonstrated in patient studies. More data are needed to determine if theophylline and beta agonists have a clinically important additive effect *in vivo*.

Pharmacokinetics: A single dose randomized crossover bioavailability study in healthy male volunteers compared 200 mg Uniphyl Tablets with an approved controlled-release BID theophylline product. Uniphyl 200 mg tablets were found to be interchangeable on a mg basis according to average AUC (area under curve), C-max (maximum theophylline concentration), T-max (time to maximum concentration), absorption rate and apparent elimination half-life.

In a multiple dose, steady-state study with Uniphyl Tablets, a single 400 mg dose produced a peak average serum level of 10.0 mcg/ml within 4 hours. The average trough level was 7.8 mcg/ml during steady-state indicating little fluctuation between C-max and C-min.

Newborns and neonates have extremely slow clearance rates compared to older infants (over 6 months) and children, and may also have a theophylline half-life of over 24 hours.

The half-life of theophylline in smokers averages 4 to 5 hours contrasted with 7 to 11 hours in non-smokers. Following the cessation of smoking, the effects on theophylline pharmacokinetics may persist for 3 months to 2 years.

Theophylline	Elimination	Characteristics
	Theophylline Clearance Rates (mean ± S.D.)	Half-Life Average (mean ± S.D.)
Children (over 6 months of age)	1.45 ± 0.58 ml/kg/min	3.7 ± 1.1 hr
Adult non-smokers with uncomplicated asthma	0.65 ± 0.19 ml/kg/min	8.7 ± 2.2 hr

INDICATIONS

Uniphyl Tablets are indicated for relief and/or prevention of symptoms of asthma and reversible bronchospasm associated with chronic bronchitis and emphysema.

CONTRAINDICATIONS

This product is contraindicated in individuals who have shown hypersensitivity to theophylline.

WARNINGS

Status asthmaticus should be considered a medical emergency and is defined as that degree of bronchospasm which is not rapidly reponsive to usual doses of conventional bronchodilators. Optimal therapy for such patients frequently requires both *additional medication*, parenterally administered, and *close monitoring*, preferably in an intensive care setting.

Excessive theophylline doses may be associated with toxicity. Determination of serum theophylline levels is recommended to assure maximum therapeutic benefit without excessive risk. The incidence of toxicity increases at serum levels greater than 20 mcg/ml.

Optimum therapeutic response occurs in most patients when the serum theophylline concentration is 10 to 20 mcg/ml. In other patients satisfactory results (as determined by both relief of symptoms and improvement in pulmonary function) may be obtained at lower levels. In still others, adequate response may require higher levels. The physician should adjust the desired serum concentration range to the patients' requirements, keeping in mind that *an increased probability of toxicity exists when levels exceed 20 mcg/ml.* Therefore, in order to assure maximum benefit without excessive risk, measurement of serum levels is highly recommended.

Reduced theophylline clearance may result in increased serum levels and potential toxicity in the following patient groups: those with impaired renal or liver function, (2) those over 55 years of age, particularly males and those with chronic lung disease, (3) those with cardiac failure, (4) those receiving macrolide antibiotics or cimetidine, and (5) neonates. Decreased theophylline clearance may occur following immunization for influenza, with active influenza and also with high fever for prolonged periods.

Less serious signs of theophylline toxicity, i.e. nausea and restlessness, may appear. Serious side effects such as ventricular arrhythmias, convulsions or even death may appear as the first sign of toxicity without any previous warning. *Serious toxicity is not reliably preceded by less severe side effects.*

Patients who require theophylline may exhibit tachycardia due to their underlying disease. The possible relationship of elevated serum theophylline concentration to tachycardia may not be recognized.

Theophylline products may cause arrhythmia and/or worsen pre-existing arrhythmia. Any significant change in rate and/or rhythm warrants monitoring and further investigation.

PRECAUTIONS

General: Use with caution in patients with severe cardiac disease, severe hypoxemia, hypertension, hyperthyroidism, acute myocardial injury, cor pulmonale, liver disease, in the elderly (especially males) and in neonates. Particular caution should be used in giving theophylline to patients with congestive heart failure. Frequently, such patients have markedly prolonged theophylline serum levels with theophylline persisting in serum for long periods following discontinuation of the drug.

Caution should be exercised in patients concurrently receiving other xanthine medications.

Some patients who are rapid metabolizers of theophylline, such as the young, smokers and some nonsmoking adults, may not be suitable candidates for once daily dosing. Dividing the total daily dose into two doses may be indicated for these patients, who may exhibit symptoms of bronchospasm repeatedly, especially near the end of a 24-hour dosing interval. Also, such individuals may have wider peak-to-trough differences than desired.

Theophylline half-life is shorter in smokers than in non-smokers. Therefore, smokers may require larger or more frequent doses.

Use theophylline cautiously in patients with history of peptic ulcer. Theophylline may occasionally act as a local irritant to the G.I. tract although gastrointestinal symptoms are more commonly centrally mediated and associated with serum drug concentrations over 20 mcg/ml.

Caution must also be exercised in children with a history of febrile convulsions, petit or grand mal seizures, or who are receiving anticonvulsant medications.

Information for Patients: The physician should reinforce the importance of taking only the prescribed dose and observing the time interval between doses. All patients should be asked to report side effects which occur at any time, or recurrence of symptoms, especially toward the end of a dosing interval. Uniphyl Tablets are not to be chewed or crushed.

Drug Interactions: Toxic synergism with ephedrine has been documented and may occur with other sympathomimetic bronchodilators. Concomitant administration of theophylline with cimetidine, troleandomycin or erythromycin may lead to higher serum theophylline levels. Theophylline may increase the excretion of lithium carbonate and antagonize the effects of propranolol.

Drug-Laboratory Test Interactions: When plasma levels of theophylline are measured by spectrophotometric methods, coffee, tea, cola beverages, chocolate and acetaminophen contribute to falsely high values.

Carcinogenesis, Mutagenesis, and Impairment of Fertility: Long-term animal studies have not been performed to evaluate the carcinogenic potential, mutagenic potential or the effect on fertility of xanthine compounds.

Pregnancy: Category C—Animal reproduction studies have not been conducted with theophylline. It is not known whether theophylline can cause fetal harm when administered to a pregnant woman or can effect reproduction capacity. Xanthines should be given to a pregnant woman only if clearly needed.

Nursing Mothers: It has been reported that theophylline distributes readily into breast milk and may cause adverse effects in the infant. Caution must be used when prescribing xanthines to a mother who is nursing, taking into account the risk-benefit of this therapy.

Pediatric Use: Safety and effectiveness in children under six (6) years of age have not been established with 200 mg Uniphyl Tablets.

ADVERSE REACTIONS

The most consistent adverse reactions are usually due to overdose and are:

1. *Gastrointestinal:* nausea, vomiting, epigastric pain, hematemesis, diarrhea.
2. *Central Nervous System:* headaches, irritability, restlessness, insomnia, reflex hyperexcitability, muscle twitching, clonic and tonic generalized convulsions.
3. *Cardiovascular:* palpitation, tachycardia, extrasystole, flushing, hypotension, circulatory failure, ventricular arrhythmia.
4. *Respiratory:* tachypnea.
5. *Renal:* albuminuria, microhematuria, potentiation of diuresis.
6. *Others:* hyperglycemia; inappropriate ADH syndrome; rash.

OVERDOSAGE

Management: If potential oral overdose is established and seizure has not occurred:
A. Induce vomiting.
B. Administer a cathartic. This is particularly important with sustained-release drugs.
C. Administer activated charcoal.
If patient is having a seizure:
A. Establish an airway.
B. Administer oxygen.
C. Treat the seizure with intravenous diazepam, 0.1 to 0.3 mg/kg up to 10 mg.
D. Monitor vital signs, maintain blood pressure and provide adequate hydration.
Post Seizure Coma:
A. Maintain airway and oxygenation.
B. If a result of oral medication, follow above recommendations to prevent absorption of the drug, but intubation

and lavage will have to be performed instead of inducing emesis, and the cathartic and charcoal will need to be introduced via a large bore gastric lavage tube.

C. Continue to provide full supportive care and adequate hydration while waiting for drug to be metabolized. In general, the drug is metabolized sufficiently rapidly so as not to warrant consideration of dialysis. However, if serum levels exceed 50 mcg/ml, charcoal hemoperfusion may be indicated.

DOSAGE AND ADMINISTRATION

In chronic therapy, theophylline, as found in Uniphyl Tablets is a treatment of first choice for the management of chronic asthma and other reversible obstructive pulmonary diseases to prevent and/or relieve symptoms and maintain patent airways.

Monitoring of clinical response and determining serum theophylline concentration is appropriate to guide dosing and minimize risk of toxicity due to overdosing. A serum level of 20 mcg/ml is an important safety reference point to reduce the possibility of toxicity.

There is considerable variation from patient to patient in the dosage required to achieve and maintain therapeutic and safe levels, primarily due to variable rates of elimination and the degree of bronchospasm present. Therefore, it is essential that dosage be individualized to the patient's clinical response and that serum levels be monitored before and after transfer to any sustained-release product.

Uniphyl, like other controlled-release theophylline products, is intended for patients with relatively continuous or recurring symptoms who have a need to maintain therapeutic serum levels of theophylline. It is not intended for patients experiencing an acute episode of bronchospasm (associated with asthma, chronic bronchitis, or emphysema). Such patients require rapid relief of symptoms and should be treated with an immediate-release or intravenous theophylline preparation (or other bronchodilators) and not with controlled-release products.

Effective use of theophylline (i.e., the concentration of drug in the serum associated with optimal benefit and minimal risk of toxicity) is considered to occur when the theophylline concentration is maintained from 10 to 20 mcg/ml. The early studies from which these levels were derived were carried out in patients immediately after or shortly after recovery from acute exacerbations of their disease (some hospitalized with status asthmaticus).

Although the 20 mcg/ml level remains appropriate as a critical value (above which toxicity is more likely to occur) for safety purposes, additional data are now available which indicate that the serum theophylline concentrations required to produce maximum physiologic benefit may, in fact, fluctuate with the degree of bronchospasm present and are variable. Therefore, the physician should individualize the range appropriate to the patient's requirements, based on both symptomatic response and improvement in pulmonary function. It should be stressed that serum theophylline concentrations maintained at the upper level of the 10 to 20 mcg/ml range may be associated with potential toxicity when factors known to reduce theophylline clearance become operative. (See PRECAUTIONS, including *Drug Interactions.*)

Dosage guidelines are approximations only and the wide range of theophylline clearance between individuals (particularly those with concomitant disease) makes indiscriminate usage hazardous. Each patient should be titrated to establish the appropriate dosage, and serum theophylline levels used for any dosage adjustment after transfer to Uniphyl Tablets. As a practical consideration, it is not always possible to obtain serum level determinations. Under such conditions, restriction of the daily dose of Uniphyl Tablets (in otherwise healthy adults) to approximately 13 mg/kg/day (or up to 900 mg) will result in relatively few patients exceeding serum levels of 20 mcg/ml and the associated risk of toxicity.

DOSAGE GUIDELINES

When appropriate, dosage should be calculated on the basis of lean body weight where mg/kg doses are to be prescribed, since theophylline does not distribute into fatty tissue.

I INITIATION OF THERAPY WITH UNIPHYL TABLETS

a. *Stabilized Patients*

Individuals who are taking an immediate-release or controlled-release theophylline product may be transferred to twice-daily administration of 200 mg Uniphyl Tablets on a mg-for-mg basis. For example, a patient stabilized on 400 mg twice daily (800 mg total daily dose) should be given two 200 mg Uniphyl Tablets q12h.

It must be recognized that the peak and trough serum theophylline levels produced by the twice-daily dosing may vary from those produced by the previous product and/or regimen.

b. *Initiation of Theophylline Dosing*

Patients not currently receiving theophylline may be initiated on Uniphyl 200 mg Tablets as follows:

THE AVERAGE INITIAL ADULT AND CHILDREN'S (over 25 KG) DOSE IS ONE UNIPHYL 200 MG TABLET q12h.

c. *Children Less Than 25 kg*

Children weighing 15–25 kg should have daily theophylline therapy established with a liquid preparation administered on a four hourly basis until appropriate serum theophylline levels are reached or to a well-tolerated dose with a satisfactory clinical response. The use of an oral liquid preparation permits careful dose titration. The patient may then be converted to Uniphyl 200 mg Tablets based upon the total daily dose achieved but on q12h basis. Some children may require dosing q8h but with the same total daily theophylline dose.

If the desired response is not achieved with the above AVERAGE INITIAL DOSAGE recommendations, the dose may be adjusted as is described below:

II. TITRATION AND DOSE ADJUSTMENT

a. *When Serum Levels Are Measured*

After 4 days therapy with Uniphyl Tablets, steady-state should have been achieved, and peak serum theophylline concentration should be determined from blood samples obtained 8 to 12 hours after the morning dose. Trough concentration should be taken just prior to the administration of the next dose. It is important that the patient not have missed or added any dose during the previous 72 hours, and that the dosing intervals remain relatively constant. DOSAGE ADJUSTMENT BASED ON THE MEASUREMENTS WHEN THESE INSTRUCTIONS HAVE NOT BEEN FOLLOWED MAY RESULT IN TOXICITY.

Peak and trough theophylline serum concentration values allow: 1) maintaining the established dosage schedule if values are within the desired range and the dose is tolerated, 2) increasing the dose, or 3) decreasing the dose.

b. *When Serum Levels Are Not Measured*

In the absence of laboratory facilities for determining serum theophylline concentration levels, clinical judgment should be followed.

- The original total twice-daily dose should continue if it is well-tolerated and the clinical response is satisfactory.
- Minimal improvement with the initial dose usually requires increasing the dose as described below.
- If adverse reactions occur, decrease the dose as stated below.

c. *Increasing the Dose of Uniphyl Tablets*

If patient response with Uniphyl Tablets is unsatisfactory and/or the observed serum theophylline concentration range is too low, the dosage may be increased at recommended intervals as follows:

Serum Theophylline (mcg/ml)	Directions
7.5 to 10	Increase dose by about 25%* and recheck serum concentrations in 3 days.
5 to 7.5	Increase dose by about 25% to the nearest dose increment and recheck serum theophylline for guidance in further dosage adjustment (another increase will probably be needed, but this provides a safety check).

d. *Decreasing the Dose of Uniphyl Tablets*

Serum theophylline values above 20 mcg/ml require decreasing the daily dose unless such dose is required to maintain the patient and is well-tolerated. Dosage may be reduced by adjustments as are described below. Peak and trough measurements should be taken 3 days after each decrease in dosage.

Serum Theophylline (mcg/ml)	Directions
20 to 25	Decrease dose by about 10%.*
25 to 30	Skip next dose and decrease subsequent doses by about 25%.
Over 30	Skip next 2 doses and decrease subsequent doses by 50%.

*Dividing the daily dose into 3 doses administered at 8-hour intervals may be indicated if symptoms occur repeatedly at the end of a dosing interval.

Finer adjustments in dosage may be needed for some patients.

III. MAINTENANCE THERAPY

Careful clinical titration is important to assure patient acceptance and safety of the medication. Patients when stabilized as established by serum theophylline concentration or respiratory function usually remain controlled without further dosage adjustment. It should be borne in mind, however, that for reasons stated in the Precautions and Warnings sections, dosage adjustments may be necessary. Serum theophylline levels should be measured periodically (at 6- to 12-month intervals) even in clinically controlled patients. As with all sustained-release theophylline products, Uniphyl Tablets are for chronic or long-term use only and are not

intended for initial treatment in a patient with acute symptoms.

Caution should be exercised for younger children who cannot complain of minor side effects. The elderly as well as patients with congestive heart failure, cor pulmonale, and/or liver disease may have unusually low dosage requirements and thus may experience toxicity even at the dosages recommended above.

It is important that no patient be maintained on any dosage that is not tolerated. In instructing patients to increase dosage according to the schedule above, they should be instructed not to take a subsequent dose if apparent side effects occur and to resume therapy at a lower dose once adverse effects have disappeared.

WARNING: DO NOT MAINTAIN ANY DOSE THAT IS NOT TOLERATED.

CAUTION

Federal law prohibits dispensing without prescription.

HOW SUPPLIED

Uniphyl (theophylline, anhydrous) 200 mg scored Controlled-Release Tablets are supplied in white-opaque plastic bottles, containing 100 tablets [NDC 0034-7002-80]. Each round, white tablet bears the symbol PF on one side and is marked U200 on the other side.

Store tablets at controlled room temperature 15° to 30°C (59°–86°F).

U.S. Patent Numbers 3965256 and 4235870

2-7-87   G1494

Shown in Product Identification Section, page 423

TRILISATE® TABLETS/LIQUID ℞
[trī'ĭ-sāt"]
(choline magnesium trisalicylate)
500 mg. 750 mg or 1000 mg
salicylate content

DESCRIPTION

TRILISATE Tablets/Liquid are nonsteroidal, anti-inflammatory preparations combining choline salicylate and magnesium salicylate in mixtures which are freely soluble in water.

TRILISATE Tablets are available in scored, pale pink 500 mg tablets; in scored, white, film-coated 750 mg tablets, and in scored, red film-coated 1000 mg tablets. Trilisate Liquid is a cherry cordial-flavored liquid providing 500 mg salicylate content per teaspoonful (5 ml) for oral administration.

Each 500 mg tablet contains 293 mg of choline salicylate combined with 362 mg of magnesium salicylate to provide 500 mg salicylate content. Each 750 mg tablet contains 440 mg of choline salicylate combined with 544 mg of magnesium salicylate to provide 750 mg salicylate content. Each 1000 mg tablet contains 587 mg of choline salicylate combined with 725 mg of magnesium salicylate to provide 1000 mg salicylate content. TRILISATE Liquid contains 293 mg of choline salicylate combined with 362 mg of magnesium salicylate to provide 500 mg salicylate per teaspoonful (5 ml) in a clear amber, cherry cordial-flavored vehicle.

INACTIVE INGREDIENTS

Each 500 mg tablet contains Carboxymethylcellulose sodium, Edetate disodium, FD&C Yellow No. 6, Povidone, Pregelatinized starch, Stearic acid, and other ingredients. Each 750 mg tablet contains Carboxymethylcellulose sodium, Edetate disodium, Polyethylene glycol, Polysorbate 20, Stearic acid, Talc, Titanium dioxide, and other ingredients.

Each 1000 mg tablet contains Carboxymethylcellulose sodium, Edetate disodium, FD&C Red No. 40, FD&C Yellow No. 6, FD&C Blue No. 2, Polyethylene glycol, Polysorbate 20, Stearic acid, Talc, and other ingredients.

Each teaspoonful (5 ml) of Liquid contains: Caramel, Carboxymethylcellulose sodium. Edetate disodium, FD&C Yellow No. 6, Glycerin, High fructose corn syrup, Potassium sorbate, Water, Artificial flavors, and other ingredients.

CLINICAL PHARMACOLOGY

TRILISATE Tablets/Liquid contain salicylate with anti-inflammatory, analgesia and antipyretic action. On ingestion of TRILISATE Tablets/Liquid, the salicylate moiety is absorbed rapidly and reaches peak blood levels within an average of one to two hours after single doses of the tablets or liquid. The primary route of excretion is renal: the excretion products are chiefly the glycine and glucuronide conjugates. At higher serum salicylate concentrations, the glycine conjugation pathway becomes rapidly saturated. Thus, the slower glucuronide conjugation pathway becomes the rate limiting step for salicylate excretion. In addition, salicylate excreted in the bile as glucuronide conjugate may be reabsorbed. These factors account for the prolongation of salicylate half life and the nonlinear increase in plasma salicylate level as the salicylate dose is increased. TRILISATE preparations differ from other non-steroidal anti-arthritic agents

Continued on next page

Purdue Frederick—Cont.

and from aspirin in having a more selective action on the prostaglandin pathway.

The bioequivalence of TRILISATE Liquid and Tablets 500 mg/750 mg/1000 mg has been established. With the tablets, a steady-state condition is usually reached after 4 to 5 doses, and the half-life of elimination, on repeated administration of the tablets, is 9 to 17 hours. This permits a maintenance dosage schedule of once or twice daily. Unlike aspirin and certain other non-steroidal anti-inflammatory agents, such as arylpropionic acid derivatives and arylacetic acid derivatives, choline magnesium trisalicylate, at therapeutic dosage levels, does not affect platelet aggregation, as shown in in-vitro and in-vivo studies.

INDICATIONS AND USAGE

Osteoarthritis, Rheumatoid Arthritis and Acute Painful Shoulder: Salicylates are considered the base therapy of choice in the arthritides; and TRILISATE preparations are indicated for the relief of the signs and symptoms of rheumatoid arthritis, osteoarthritis and other arthritides. TRILISATE Tablets or Liquid are indicated in the long-term management of these diseases and especially in the acute flare of rheumatoid arthritis. TRILISATE Tablets or Liquid are also indicated for the treatment of acute painful shoulder.

TRILISATE preparations are effective and generally well tolerated, and are logical choices whenever salicylate treatment is indicated. They are particularly suitable when a once-a-day or b.i.d. dosage regimen is important to patient compliance, when gastrointestinal intolerance to aspirin is encountered; when gastrointestinal microbleeding or hematologic effects of aspirin are considered a patient hazard; and when interference (or the risk of interference) with normal platelet function by aspirin or by propionic acid derivatives is considered to be clinically undesirable. Use of TRILISATE Liquid is appropriate when a liquid dosage form is preferred, as in the elderly patient.

The efficacy of TRILISATE preparations has not been studied in those patients who are designated by the American Rheumatism Association as belonging in Functional Class IV (incapacitated, largely or wholly bedridden or confined to a wheelchair, with little or no self-care). Analgesic and Antipyretic Action: TRILISATE Tablets/Liquid are also indicated for the relief of mild to moderate pain and for antipyresis. In children, TRILISATE preparations are indicated for conditions requiring anti-inflammatory, analgesic or antipyretic action—such as juvenile rheumatoid arthritis and other appropriate conditions. Used concomitantly with antibiotics, TRILISATE preparations are useful for analgesia and antipyresis in many bacterial or viral infections.

CONTRAINDICATIONS

Patients who are hypersensitive to non-acetylated salicylates should not take TRILISATE Tablets or Liquid.

WARNING

Reye's Syndrome is a rare but serious disease which may develop in children and teenagers who have chicken pox, influenza, or flu symptoms. While the cause of Reye's Syndrome is unknown, some studies suggest a possible association between the development of Reye's Syndrome and the use of medicines containing acetylated salicylates or aspirin. TRILISATE Tablets and Liquid are a combination of choline and magnesium salicylate which are nonacetylated salicylates, and there has been no reported cases associating TRILISATE with Reye's Syndrome. Nevertheless, physicians should exercise caution in the use of any salicylate-containing product and make a risk benefit assessment before prescribing this product for use in children and teenagers with chicken pox, influenza or flu symptoms.

PRECAUTIONS

Like other salicylates, TRILISATE preparations should be used with caution in patients with chronic renal insufficiency, with acute or chronic hepatic dysfunction or with active erosive gastritis or peptic ulcer.

Reports indicate that when acetylated salicylates are given with steroids, the butazones, or alcohol, the risk of gastrointestinal ulceration is increased. Caution should be exercised in patients requiring coumarin or indandione anticoagulants, or heparin.

While salicylates are not known to be associated with teratogenic potential in man, the usual care should be exercised in the administration of any drug during pregnancy. Because of the possible inhibition of prostaglandin with high doses of salicylates, the use of TRILISATE (choline magnesium trisalicylate) preparations immediately prior to the onset of labor is not recommended.

ADVERSE REACTIONS

Choline magnesium trisalicylate is generally well-tolerated at recommended dosage ranges, and has been shown to be particularly well-tolerated by the gastrointestinal system. Salicylism and/or salicylate intoxication may occur with large doses or with extended therapy. Common symptoms of salicylism include headache, vertigo, tinnitus, confusion, drowsiness, sweating, vomiting, diarrhea, and hyperventilation. Tinnitus may be regarded as a therapeutic guide. Should it develop, reduction of daily dosage is recommended until the tinnitus is resolved.

DOSAGE

ADULTS: In rheumatoid arthritis, osteoarthritis, the more severe arthritides, and acute painful shoulder, the recommended daily dosage is 3000 mg given once a day (h.s.) or 1500 mg b.i.d. In the elderly patient, a daily dosage of 2250 mg given as 750 mg t.i.d. may be efficacious and well tolerated. Dosage should be adjusted in accordance with the patient's response.

For mild to moderate pain or for antipyresis, the usual dosage is 2000 mg to 3000 mg daily in divided doses (b.i.d.). Based on patient response or salicylate blood levels, dosage may be adjusted to achieve optimum therapeutic effect. Salicylate blood levels should be in the range of 15 to 30 mg/100 ml for anti-inflammatory effect and 5 to 15 mg/100 ml for analgesia and antipyresis.

Each 500 mg tablet or teaspoonful is equivalent in salicylate content to 10 gr of aspirin; each 750 mg tablet, to 15 gr of aspirin; and each 1000 mg tablet, to 20 gr of aspirin.

If the physician prefers, the recommended daily dosage may be administered on a t.i.d. schedule.

As with other therapeutic agents, individual dosage adjustment is advisable, and a number of patients may require higher or lower dosages than those recommended. Certain patients require 2 to 3 weeks of therapy for optimal effect.

CHILDREN: *Usual total daily dose for children* for anti-inflammatory, analgesic and antipyretic action:

TRILISATE 500 mg Tablets/Liquid and TRILISATE 750 mg and 1000 mg Tablets, 50 mg/kg/day.

Weight (kg)	Total daily dose
12–13	500 mg
14–17	750 mg
18–22	1000 mg
23–27	1250 mg
28–32	1500 mg
33–37	1750 mg

Total daily doses should be administered in divided doses (b.i.d.). Doses of TRILISATE preparations are calculated as the total daily dose of 50 mg/kg/day for children of 37 kg body weight or less and 2250 mg/day for heavier children. TRILISATE Liquid is available for greater convenience in treating younger patients. TRILISATE Liquid may be mixed with fruit juices just before drinking.

CAUTION

Federal law prohibits dispensing without a prescription.

HOW SUPPLIED

NDC 0034-0500-80: TRILISATE 500 mg Tablets (pale pink, scored) supplied in bottles of 100 tablets.

NDC 0034-0500-50: TRILISATE 500 mg Tablets (pale pink, scored) supplied in bottles of 500 tablets.

NDC 0034-0500-10: TRILISATE 500 mg Tablets (pale pink, scored) supplied in unit dose packaging with 10 tablets per card. Ten cards are packed in each carton; 10 cartons are packed in each shipper.

NDC 0034-0505-80: TRILISATE 750 mg Tablets (scored, white, film-coated) in bottles of 100 tablets.

NDC 0034-0505-50: TRILISATE 750 mg Tablets (scored, white, film-coated) in bottles of 500 tablets.

NDC 0034-0505-10: TRILISATE 750 mg Tablets (scored, white film-coated) supplied in unit dose packaging with 10 tablets per card. Ten cards are packed in each carton; 10 cartons are packed in each shipper.

NDC 0034-0510-60: TRILISATE 1000 mg Tablets (scored, red, film-coated) in bottles of 60 tablets.

NDC 0034-0510-80: TRILISATE 1000 mg Tablets (scored, red, film-coated) in bottles of 100 tablets.

NDC 0034-0520-80: TRILISATE Liquid in bottles of 8 fl. oz. (237 ml).

Store at controlled room temperature 59° to 86°F (15° to 30°C).
Copyright 1982, 1988. The Purdue Frederick Company
U.S. Patent Numbers 3759980 and 4067974

Shown in Product Identification Section, page 423

UNIPHYL® Tablets   ℞
[ū'nĭ-fĭl]
(theophylline)
400 mg

UNICONTIN®
Controlled-Release System

DESCRIPTION

Uniphyl Tablets for oral administration contain 400 mg anhydrous theophylline in a controlled-release system which allows a 24-hour dosing interval for appropriate patients. Theophylline anhydrous, a xanthine bronchodilator, is a white, odorless crystalline powder having a bitter taste. Theophylline has a molecular weight of 180.18, represented by $C_7H_8N_4O_2$ and is depicted as:

Inactive Ingredients: Cetostearyl alcohol, Hydroxyethyl cellulose, Magnesium stearate, Povidone, Talc, and other ingredients.

CLINICAL PHARMACOLOGY

Theophylline directly relaxes the smooth muscle of the bronchial airways and pulmonary blood vessels, thus acting mainly as a bronchodilator and smooth muscle relaxant. It has also been demonstrated that aminophylline has a potent effect on diaphragmatic contractility in normal persons and may then be capable of reducing fatigability and thereby improve contractility in patients with chronic obstructive airways disease. The exact mode of action remains unsettled. Although theophylline does cause inhibition of phosphodiesterase with a resultant increase in intracellular cyclic AMP, other agents similarly inhibit the enzyme producing a rise of cyclic AMP but are unassociated with any demonstrable bronchodilation. Other mechanisms proposed included an effect on translocation of intracellular calcium; prostaglandin antagonism; stimulation of catecholamines endogenously; inhibition of cyclic guanosine monophosphate metabolism and adenosine receptor antagonism. None of these mechanisms have been proven, however.

In vitro, theophylline has been shown to act synergistically with beta agonists and there are now available data which do demonstrate an additive effect *in vivo* with combined use. *Pharmacokinetics:* The half-life of theophylline is influenced by a number of known variables. It may be prolonged in chronic alcoholics, partcularly those with liver disease (cirrhosis or alcoholic liver disease), in patients with congestive heart failure, and in those patients taking certain other drugs (see PRECAUTIONS, Drug Interactions). Newborns and neonates have extremely slow clearance rates compared to older infants and children, i.e., those over 1 year. Older children have rapid clearance rates while most non-smoking adults have clearance rates between these two extremes. In premature neonates the decreased clearance is related to oxidative pathways that have yet to be established.

Conventional Theophylline
Immediate-Release
Elimination Characteristics
Half-Life (in hours)

	Range	Mean
Children	1–9	3.7
Adults	3–15	7.7

In cigarette smokers (1–2 packs/day) the mean half-life is 4–5 hours, much shorter than in non-smokers. The increase in clearance associated with smoking is presumably due to stimulation of the hepatic metabolic pathways by components of cigarette smoke. The duration of this effect after cessation of smoking is unknown but may require 6 months to 2 years before the rate approaches that of a non-smoker. A single-dose study in 15 normal fasting male volunteers whose theophylline inherent mean elimination half-life was verified by a liquid theophylline product to be 6.9 ± 2.5 (S.D.) hours were administered two or three 400 mg Uniphyl Tablets. The relative bioavailability of Uniphyl given in the fasting state in comparison to an immediate-release product was 59%. Peak serum theophylline levels occurred at 6.9 ± 5.2 (S.D.) hours, with a normalized (to 800 mg) peak level being 6.2 ± 2.1 (S.D.). The apparent elimination half-life for the 400 mg Uniphyl Tablets was 17.2 ± 5.8 (S.D.) hours.

Steady-state pharmacokinetics were determined in a study in 12 fasted patients with chronic reversible obstructive pulmonary disease. All were dosed with two 400 mg Uniphyl Tablets given once-daily in the morning and a widely-used approved controlled-release BID product administered as two 200 mg tablets given 12 hours apart. The pharmacokinetic parameters obtained for Uniphyl Tablets given at doses of 800 mg once-daily in the morning were virtually identical to the corresponding parameters for the reference drug when given as 400 mg BID. In particular, the AUC, Cmax and Cmin values obtained in this study were as follows:

	Uniphyl Tablets 800 mg O 24 h ± S.D.	Reference Drug 400 mg O 12 h ± S.D.
AUC, (0–24 hours), mcg hr/ml	288.9 ± 21.5	283.5 ± 38.4
Cmax, mcg/ml	15.7 ± 2.8	15.2 ± 2.1
Cmin, mcg/ml	7.9 ± 1.6	7.8 ± 1.7
Cmax-Cmin diff.	7.7 ± 1.5	7.4 ± 1.5

Bioavailability was calculated to be 104 ± 18% (S.D.) for the 24-hour period with Uniphyl Tablets once-daily as compared with the reference drug given twice daily, as shown above.

In a single-dose crossover study, two 400 mg Uniphyl Tablets were administered to 19 normal volunteers in the morning or evening immediately following the same standardized meal (769 calories consisting of 97 grams carbohydrates, 33 grams protein and 27 grams fat). There was no evidence of dose dumping nor were there any significant differences in pharmacokinetic parameters attributable to time of drug administration. On the morning arm, the pharmacokinetic parameters were AUC = 241.9 ± 83.0 mcg hr/ml, Cmax = 9.3 ± 2.0 mcg/ml, Tmax = 12.8 ± 4.2 hours. On the evening arm, the pharmacokinetic parameters were AUC = 219.7 ± 83.0 mcg hr/ml, Cmax = 9.2 ± 2.0 mcg/ml, Tmax = 12.5 ± 4.2 hours.

A study in which Uniphyl was administered to 17 fed adult asthmatics produced similar theophylline level-time curves when administered in the morning or evening. Serum levels were generally higher in the evening regimen but there were no statistically significant differences between the two regimens.

	MORNING	EVENING
AUC (0–24 hrs) (mcg hr/ml)	236.0 ± 76.7	256.0 ± 80.4
Cmax (mcg/ml)	14.5 ± 4.1	16.3 ± 4.5
Cmin (mcg/ml)	5.5 ± 2.9	5.0 ± 2.5
Tmax (hours)	8.1 ± 3.7	10.1 ± 4.1

The absorption characteristics of Uniphyl Tablets (theophylline, anhydrous) have been extensively studied. A steady-state crossover bioavailability study in 22 normal males compared two Uniphyl 400 mg Tablets administered O24h at 8 a.m. immediately after breakfast with a reference controlled-release theophylline product administered BID in fed subjects at 8 a.m. immediately after breakfast and 8 p.m. immediately after dinner (769 calories, consisting of 97 grams carbohydrates, 33 grams protein and 27 grams fat).

The pharmacokinetic parameters for Uniphyl 400 mg Tablets under these steady-state conditions were AUC = 203.3 ± 87.1 mcg hr/ml, Cmax = 12.1 ± 3.8 mcg/ml, Cmin = 4.50 ± 3.6, Tmax = 8.8 ± 4.6 hours. For the reference BID product, the pharmacokinetic parameters were AUC = 219.2 ± 88.4 mcg hr/ml, Cmax = 11.0 ± 4.1 mcg/ml, Cmin = 7.28 ± 3.5, Tmax = 6.9 ± 3.4 hours. The mean percent fluctuation [(Cmax-Cmin/Cmin) ×100] = 169% for the once-daily regimen and 51% for the reference product BID regimen.

Single-dose studies in which subjects were fasted for twelve (12) hours prior and an additional four (4) hours following dosing, demonstrated reduced bioavailability as compared to dosing with food. One single-dose study in 20 normal volunteers dosed with two 400 mg tablets in the morning, compared dosing under these fasting conditions with dosing immediately prior to a standardized breakfast (769 calories, consisting of 97 grams carbohydrates, 33 grams protein and 27 grams fat). Under fed conditions, the pharmacokinetic parameters were: AUC = 231.7 ± 92.4 mcg hr/ml, Cmax = 8.4 ± 2.6 mcg/ml, Tmax = 17.3 ± 6.7 hours. Under fasting conditions, these parameters were AUC = 141.2 ± 65.3 mcg hr/ml, Cmax = 5.5 ± 1.5 mcg/ml, Tmax = 6.5 ± 2.1 hours. Another single-dose study in 21 normal male volunteers, dosed in the evening, compared fasting to a standardized high calorie, high fat meal (870–1,020 calories, consisting of 33 grams protein, 55–75 grams fat, 58 grams carbohydrates). In the fasting arm subjects received one Uniphyl 400 mg Tablet at 8 p.m. after an eight hour fast followed by a further four hour fast. In the fed arm, subjects were again dosed with one 400 mg Uniphyl Tablet, but at 8 p.m. immediately after the high fat content standardized meal cited above. The pharmacokinetic parameters (normalized to 800 mg) fed were AUC = 221.8 ± 40.9 mcg hr/ml, Cmax = 10.9 ± 1.7 mcg/ml, Tmax = 11.8 ± 2.2 hours. In the fasting arm, the pharmacokinetic parameters (normalized to 800 mg) were AUC = 146.4 ± 40.9 mcg hr/ml, Cmax = 6.7 ± 1.7 mcg/ml, Tmax = 7.3 ± 2.2 hours.

Thus, it has been established that while there is reduced bioavailability with fasting there is no failure of the delivery system leading to a sudden and unexpected release of a large quantity of theophylline with Uniphyl Tablets even when they are administered with a high fat, high calorie meal. These studies demonstrate that as long as subjects were either consistently fed or consistently fasted, there is similar bioavailability with once-daily administration of Uniphyl Tablets, whether dosed in the morning or evening.

The AUC and Cmax are dose-dependent and will increase by upward dosage adjustment with Uniphyl Tablets. Patients who are fast theophylline metabolizers (clearance-greater than 5 L/hr) may not be suitable candidates for once-daily dosing. Those patients who are not well-maintained on recommended once-a-day therapy are likely to be better controlled when theophylline is administered in divided doses.

INDICATIONS AND USAGE

For relief and/or prevention of symptoms from asthma and reversible bronchospasm associated with chronic bronchitis and emphysema.

CONTRAINDICATIONS

This product is contraindicated in individuals who have shown hypersensitivity to its components. It is also contraindicated in patients with active peptic ulcer disease, and in individuals with underlying seizure disorders (unless receiving appropriate anticonvulsant medication).

WARNINGS

Serum levels above 20 mcg/ml are rarely found after appropriate administration of the recommended doses. However, in individuals in whom theophylline plasma clearance is reduced for any reason, even conventional doses may result in increased serum levels and potential toxicity. Reduced theophylline clearance has been documented in the following readily identifiable groups: 1) patients with impaired liver function; 2) patients over 55 years of age, particularly males and those with chronic lung disease; 3) those with cardiac failure from any cause; 4) patients with sustained high fever; 5) neonates and infants under 1 year of age; and 6) those patients taking certain drugs (see PRECAUTIONS, Drug Interactions). Frequently, such patients have markedly prolonged theophylline serum following discontinuation of the drug.

Reduction of dosage and laboratory monitoring are especially appropriate in the above individuals.

Serious side effects such as ventricular arrhythmias, convulsions or even death may appear as the first sign of toxicity without any previous warning. Less serious signs of theophylline toxicity (i.e., nausea and restlessness) may occur frequently when initiating therapy, but are usually transient; when such signs are persistent during maintenance therapy, they are often associated with serum concentrations above 20 mcg/ml. Stated differently: *serious toxicity is not reliably preceded by less severe side effects.* A serum concentration measurement is the only reliable method of predicting potentially life-threatening toxicity.

Many patients who require theophylline exhibit tachycardia due to their underlying disease process so that the cause/effect relationship to elevated serum theophylline concentrations may not be appreciated.

Theophylline products may cause dysrhythmia and/or worsen pre-existing arrhythmias and any significant change in rate and/or rhythm warrants monitoring and further investigation.

Studies in laboratory animals (minipigs, rodents and dogs) recorded the occurrence of cardiac arrhythmias and sudden death (with histologic evidence of myocardial necrosis) when beta-agonists and methylxanthines were administered concurrently. The significance of these findings when applied to humans is currently unknown.

PRECAUTIONS

General: On the average, theophylline half-life is shorter in cigarette and marijuana smokers than in non-smokers, but smokers can have half-lives as long as non-smokers. Theophylline should not be administered concurrently with other xanthines. Use with caution in patients with hypoxemia, hypertension, or those with history of peptic ulcer. Theophylline may occasionally act as a local irritant to G.I. tract although gastrointestinal symptoms are more commonly centrally mediated and associated with serum drug concentrations over 20 mcg/ml.

Information for Patients: The physician should reinforce the importance of taking only the prescribed dose and observing the time interval between doses. Information relating to taking Uniphyl in relation to meals or fasting should be provided. All patients should be asked to report side effects which occur at any time or recurrence of symptoms, especially toward the end of a 24-hour dosing interval. Uniphyl Tablets are not to be chewed or crushed.

Laboratory Tests: Serum levels should be monitored periodically to determine the theophylline level associated with observed clinical response and as the method of predicting toxicity. For such measurements, the serum sample should be obtained at the approximate time of the expected peak concentration, i.e., about 9 hours after administration in the morning or about 12 hours after administration in the evening. It is important that the patient will not have missed or taken additional doses during the previous 48 hours and that dosing intervals will have been reasonably equally spaced. DOSAGE ADJUSTMENT BASED ON SERUM THEOPHYLLINE MEASUREMENTS WHEN THESE INSTRUCTIONS HAVE NOT BEEN FOLLOWED MAY RESULT IN RECOMMENDATIONS THAT PRESENT RISK OF TOXICITY TO THE PATIENT.

Drug Interactions: Toxic synergism with ephedrine has been documented and may occur with other sympathomimetic bronchodilators. In addition, the following drug interactions have been demonstrated:

Theophylline with:

Allopurinol (high-dose)	Increased serum theophylline levels
Cimetidine	Increased serum theophylline levels
Ciprofloxacin	Increased serum theophylline levels
Erythromycin, Troleandomycin	Increased serum theophylline levels
Lithium carbonate	Increased renal excretion of lithium
Oral Contraceptives	Increased serum theophylline levels
Phenytoin	Decreased theophylline and phenytoin serum levels
Rifampin	Decreased serum theophylline levels

Drug-Food Interactions: The absorption characteristics of Uniphyl® Tablets (theophylline, anydrous) have been studied and are enhanced by co-administration with food. In two single-dose studies in which subjects were given Uniphyl with either a standardized breakfast or a high fat content meal, bioavailability under the fasting conditions were 61% and 66% respectively in comparison to under the fed condition. (SEE CLINICAL PHARMACOLOGY, Pharmacokinetics).

A drug-free effect, if any, would likely have its greatest clinical significance when high theophylline serum levels are being maintained and/or when large single doses (greater than 13 mg/kg or 900 mg) of a controlled-release theophylline product are given.

Drug-Laboratory Test Interactions: Currently available analytical methods, including high pressure liquid chromatography and immunoassay techniques, for measuring serum theophylline levels are specific. Metabolites and other drugs generally do not affect the results. Other new analytic methods are also now in use. The physician should be aware of the laboratory method used and whether other drugs will interfere with the assay for theophylline.

Carcinogenesis, Mutagenesis, and Impairment of Fertility: Long-term carcinogenicity studies have not been performed with theophylline.

Chromosome-breaking activity was detected in human cell cultures at concentrations of theophylline up to 50 times the therapeutic serum concentrations in humans. Theophylline was not mutagenic in the dominant lethal assay in male mice given theophylline intraperitoneally in doses up to 30 times the maximum daily human oral dose.

Studies to determine the effect on fertility have not been performed with theophylline.

Pregnancy: Category C—Animal reproduction studies have not been conducted with theophylline. It is also not known whether theophylline can cause fetal harm when administered to a pregnant woman or can affect reproduction capacity. Xanthines should be given to a pregnant woman only if clearly needed.

Nursing Mothers: Theophylline is distributed into breast milk and may cause irritability or other signs of toxicity in nursing infants. Because of the potential for serious adverse reactions in nursing infants from theophylline, a decision should be made whether to discontinue nursing or to discontinue the drug, taking into account the importance of the drug to the mother.

Pediatric Use: Safety and effectiveness in children under 12 years of age have not been established with 400 mg Uniphyl Tablets.

ADVERSE REACTIONS

The following adverse reactions have been observed, but there has not been enough systematic collection of data to support an estimate of their frequency. The most consistent adverse reactions are usually due to overdosage.

1. *Gastrointestinal:* nausea, vomiting, epigastric pain, hematemesis, diarrhea.
2. *Central nervous system:* headaches, irritability, restlessness, insomnia, reflex hyperexcitability, muscle twitching, clonic and tonic generalized convulsions.
3. *Cardiovascular:* palpitation, tachycardia, extrasystoles, flushing, hypotension, circulatory failure, ventricular arrhythmias.
4. *Respiratory:* tachypnea.
5. *Renal:* potentiation of diuresis.
6. *Others:* alopecia, hyperglycemia, inappropriate ADH syndrome, rash.

OVERDOSAGE

Management: It is suggested that the management principles (consistent with the clinical status of the patient when first seen) outlined below be instituted and that simultaneous contact with a Regional Poison Control Center be established. In this way, both updated information and individualization regarding required therapy may be provided.

1. When potential oral overdose is established and seizure has not occurred:

   a) If patient is alert and seen within the early hours after ingestion, induction of emesis may be of value. Gastric lavage has been demonstrated to be of no value in influencing outcome in patients who present more than 1 hour after ingestion.

Continued on next page

Purdue Frederick—Cont.

b) Administer a cathartic. Sorbitol solution is reported to be of value.

c) Administer repeated doses of activated charcoal and monitor theophylline serum levels.

d) Prophylactic administration of phenobarbital has been shown to increase the seizure threshold in laboratory animals, and administration of this drug can be considered.

2. If patient presents with a seizure:

a) Establish an airway.

b) Administer oxygen.

c) Treat the seizure with intravenous diazepam, 0.1 to 0.3 mg/kg up to 10 mg. If seizure cannot be controlled, the use of general anesthesia should be considered.

d) Monitor vital signs, maintain blood pressure and provide adequate hydration.

3. If post-seizure coma is present:

a) Maintain airway and oxygenation.

b) If post-seizure coma is a result of oral medication, follow above recommendations to prevent absorption of the drug, but intubation and lavage will have to be performed instead of inducing emesis, and the cathartic and charcoal will need to be introduced via a large bore gastric lavage tube.

c) Continue to provide full supportive care and adequate hydration until the drug is metabolized. In general, drug metabolism is sufficiently rapid so as not to warrant dialysis. If repeated oral activated charcoal is ineffective (as noted by stable or rising serum levels) charcoal hemoperfusion may be indicated.

DOSAGE AND ADMINISTRATION

Uniphyl 400 mg Tablets can be taken once a day in the morning or evening. Until further data are available, evening dosing is limited to patients whose daily dose is 800 mg or less. It is recommended that Uniphyl be taken with meals. Patients should be advised that if they choose to take Uniphyl with food it should be taken consistently with food and if they take it in a fasted condition it should routinely be taken fasted. It is important that the product whenever dosed be dosed consistently with or without food.

Effective use of theophylline (i.e., the concentration of drug in the serum associated with optimal benefit and minimal risk of toxicity) is considered to occur when the theophylline concentration is maintained from 10 to 20 mcg/ml. The early studies from which these levels were derived were carried out in patients immediately or shortly after recovery from acute exacerbations of their disease (some hospitalized with status asthmaticus).

Although the 20 mcg/ml level remains appropriate as a critical value (above which toxicity is more likely to occur) for safety purposes, additional data are now available which indicate that the serum theophylline concentrations required to produce maximum physiologic benefit may, in fact, fluctuate with the degree of bronchospasm present and are variable. Therefore, the physician should individualize the range appropriate to the patient's requirements, based on both symptomatic response and improvement in pulmonary function.

As with all sustained-release theophylline products, Uniphyl Tablets are for chronic or long-term use and are not intended for initial treatment in a patient with acute symptoms.

If it is not possible to obtain serum level determinations, restriction of the daily dose (in otherwise healthy adults) to not greater than 13 mg/kg/day, to a maximum of 900 mg, in divided doses will result in relatively few patients exceeding serum levels of 20 mcg/ml and the resultant greater risk of toxicity.

Caution should be exercised in younger children who cannot complain of minor side effects. Older adults, those with cor pulmonale, congestive heart failure, and/or liver disease may have unusually low dosage requirements and thus may experience toxicity at the maximal dosage recommended below.

Theophylline does not distribute to fatty tissue. Dosage should be calculated on the basis of lean (ideal) body weight where mg/kg doses are presented.

Frequency of Dosing: Patients who clear theophylline normally or relatively slowly, e.g., non-smokers, may be reasonable candidates for taking Uniphyl Tablets once-daily. However, certain patients, such as the young, smokers and some non-smoking adults are likely to metabolize theophylline more rapidly and may require dosing at 12 hour intervals. Such patients may experience symptoms of bronchospasm toward the end of a once-daily dosing interval and/or require a high daily dose (higher than those recommended in labeling) and are more likely to experience relatively wide peak to trough differences in serum theophylline concentrations.

Dosage Guidelines: WARNING: DO NOT ATTEMPT TO MAINTAIN ANY DOSE THAT IS NOT WELL TOLERATED. Dosage guidelines are approximations only, and the wide range of clearance of theophylline among individuals (particularly those with concomitant disease) makes indiscriminate usage hazardous. When appropriate, dosage should be calculated on the basis of lean body weight where mg/kg doses are to be prescribed since theophylline does not distribute into fatty tissue.

I. *Initiation of Therapy with Uniphyl Tablets*

a. *Stabilized Patients (12 years of age or older)*

Individuals who are taking an immediate-release or controlled-release theophylline product may be transferred to once-daily administration of 400 mg Uniphyl Tablets on a mg-for-mg basis. For example, a patient stabilized on 400 mg twice daily (800 mg total daily dose) should be given two 400 mg Uniphyl Tablets as a single daily dose of 800 mg in either the morning or the evening. However, until further data are available, evening dosing is limited to patients whose total daily dose is 800 mg or less.

It must be recognized that the peak and trough serum theophylline levels produced by the once-daily dosage may vary from those produced by the previous product and/or regimen.

b. *Initiation of Theophylline Dosing*

Adult patients and children 12 years of age and over not currently receiving theophylline may be titrated using an immediate or sustained-release theophylline product, which can be adjusted in small dosage increments. Patients titrated to a total daily dose of approximately 400, 600, 800, 1,000 or 1,200 mg may be transferred to once-daily dosage with 400 mg Uniphyl Tablets as is described in (a) above. However, until further data are available, evening dosing is limited to patients whose total daily dose is 800 mg or less.

II. *Titration and Dose Adjustment*

a. *When Serum Levels Are Measured*

After 4 days therapy with Uniphyl Tablets, steady-state should have been achieved, and approximate peak serum theophylline concentration samples should be determined from blood samples obtained about 9 hours after administration in the morning or about 12 hours after administration in the evening. When taken in the evening with supper it may not be possible to get blood levels within 12 hours following the daily dose. Under these circumstances blood levels should be measured as early in the morning as practical, recognizing that such levels may be somewhat lower than the actual peak achieved. Trough concentration should be taken just prior to the administration of the next dose. It is important that the patient not have missed or added any dose during the previous 72 hours, and that the dosing intervals remain relatively constant. DOSAGE ADJUSTMENT BASED ON MEASUREMENTS WHEN THESE INSTRUCTIONS HAVE NOT BEEN FOLLOWED RESULT IN TOXICITY.

b. *When Serum Levels Are Not Measured*

In the absence of laboratory facilities for determining serum theophylline concentration levels, clinical judgment should be followed. The original total once-daily dose should continue if it is well tolerated and the clinical response is satisfactory.

If adverse reactions occur, decrease the dose as stated below.

If a patient is better controlled on another regimen than on a once-daily regimen, the patient should be maintained on the more effective regimen.

c. *Increasing the Dose of Uniphyl Tablets*

If patient response with Uniphyl Tablets is unsatisfactory and/or the observed serum theophylline concentration range is too low, the patient should be transferred to an immediate or controlled-release (BID) theophylline schedule and dosage increased at recommended intervals as follows:

Serum Theophylline (mcg/ml)	Directions
Too low	Increase dosage at 3 day intervals by 25%. The serum concentration may be re-checked at appropriate intervals, but at least at the end of the adjustment period.*

When the patient's condition is otherwise clinically stable and none of the recognized factors which alter elimination are present, measurement of serum levels need be repeated only every 6 to 12 months.

* The total daily dose may need to be administered at more frequent intervals if symptoms occur repeatedly at the end of a dosing interval.

d. *Decreasing the Dose of Uniphyl Tablets*

Serum theophylline values above 20 mcg/ml require decreasing the daily dose unless such dose is required to maintain the present and is well-tolerated. Dosage may be reduced by transferring the patient to an immediate or controlled-release (BID) theophylline product and making adjustments. Peak

and trough measurements should be taken 3 days after each decrease in dosage.

Serum Theophylline (mcg/ml)	Directions
20 to 25	Decrease dose by about 10%
25 to 30	Skip next dose and decrease subsequent doses by about 25%
Over 30	Skip next 2 doses and decrease subsequent doses by 50%

Finer adjustments in dosage may be needed for some patients.

III. *Maintenance Therapy*

Careful clinical titration is important to assure patient acceptance and safety of the medication. Patients, when stabilized as established by serum theophylline concentration or respiratory function, usually remain controlled without further dosage adjustment. It should be borne in mind, however, that for reasons stated in the PRECAUTIONS and WARNINGS sections, dosage adjustments may be necessary. Serum theophylline levels should be measured periodically (at 6 to 12-month intervals) even in clinically controlled patients.

The elderly as well as patients with congestive heart failure, cor pulmonale, and/or liver disease may have unusually low dosage requirements and thus may experience toxicity even at the dosages recommended above.

WARNING

DO NOT MAINTAIN ANY DOSE THAT IS NOT TOLERATED

HOW SUPPLIED

Uniphyl (theophylline, anhydrous) 400 mg scored Controlled-Release Tablets are supplied in white-opaque plastic bottles, containing 100 tablets [NDC #0034-7004-80] or 500 tablets [NDC #0034-7004-70] or in unit dose packaging with 10 tablets per card [NDC #0034-7004-10]; ten cards are packed in each carton; 10 cartons are packed in each shipper. Each round, white tablet bears the symbols PF on one side and is marked U400 on the other side.

Store tablets at controlled room temperature 15° to 30°C (59–86°F).

CAUTION

Federal law prohibits dispensing without prescription.

The Purdue Frederick Company

Norwalk, CT 06856

U.S. Patent Numbers 3965256 and 4235870

February, 1989

Shown in Product Identification Section, page 423

EDUCATIONAL MATERIAL

Audio Visuals—Booklets—Samples

"Fiber and Your Health" Booklets (Fibermed)

"How You Can Relieve Constipation Naturally" (Senokot-S)

Cancer Pain Management Videotape Program (MS Contin)

Pain Assessment Program medical forms and patient booklets (MS Contin)

Cancer Pain Management Slide Program (MS Contin)

"Up-To-Date Answers About Pain Medications" booklet for patient education. (MS Contin)

"Home Care of the Hospice Patient"—Guide to caring for cancer patients. (MS Contin)

"Protect Your Family From Germs" patient aid booklet (English and Spanish). (Betadine)

"Your Betadine Antiseptics Guide to First Aid" patient aid booklet.

Samples of Betadine First Aid and Betadine Feminine Hygiene Products.

"Fem-Facts®" booklets (Facts about Vaginitis Symptoms for Patients)

"Betadine Microbicides and the AIDS Virus" brochures
Arthritis Exercise Pads (Trilisate)
Osteoarthritis Exercise card boxes with refills (Trilisate)

Quad Pharmaceuticals, Inc.
Pharmaceutical Products Division
Oncology Products Division
6340 LAPAS TRAIL
INDIANAPOLIS, IN 46268 USA

NDC # 51309-	PRODUCT	VIAL SIZE
	Acetazolamide Sodium sterile, USP	
611-10	500 mg SDV	10 mL
	Acetylcysteine solution, USP	
935-04	10% (100 mg/mL) vial	4 mL
935-10	10% (100 mg/mL) vial	10 mL
935-30	10% (100 mg/mL) vial	30 mL
936-04	20% (200 mg/mL) vial	4 mL
936-10	20% (200 mg/mL) vial	10 mL
936-30	20% (200 mg/mL) vial	30 mL
	Aminocaproic Acid INJ., USP	
901-20A	250 mg/mL MultiDose Vial	20 mL
901-98	250 mg/mL Pharmacy Bulk Pack	96 mL
	Aminohippurate Sodium Injection, USP	
620-10	20% (2 grams/10 mL)	10 mL Single Dose Vial
	Azathioprine Sodium FOR INJ. USP	
227-20	100 mg SDV	20 mL
801-01	**B C G Vaccine, USP** For Intradermal Use Only Freeze Dried	1 mL
	Bacitracin Sterile, USP (Lyophilized)	
309-20	10,000 units/vial	20 mL
310-50	50,000 units/vial	30 mL
	Bethanechol Chloride Injection, USP	
948-02	5 mg (5 mg/mL)	1 mL Single Dose Vial
518-02	**Caffeine Sodium Benzoate INJ., USP** .5 g Single Dose (Ampule)	2 mL
	Chorionic Gonadotropin FOR INJ., USP (Lyophilized)	
411-10	10,000 USP units 10 mL MultiDose with diluent (two vial set)	10 mL
	Clindamycin Phosphate Injection, USP	
327-02	300 mg (150 mg/mL)	2 mL SDV
327-05	600 mg (150 mg/mL)	4 mL SDV
327-10	900 mg (150 mg/mL)	6 mL SDV
327-60	9 g (150 mg/mL)	60 mL Bulk Pack
	Cyanide antidote package	
821-00	1 package	
	L-Cysteine Hydrochloride INJ., USP I.V. Additive (Low in Aluminium Content)	
109-10	50 mg/mL SingleDose Vial (Preservative Free)	10 mL
	Cytarabine FOR INJ., USP (Lyophilized)	
219-10	100 mg/vial	10 mL
220-15	500 mg/vial	15 mL
	Dacarbazine FOR INJ., USP (Lyophilized)	
204-20	100 mg/vial	20 mL
205-30	200 mg/vial	30 mL
254-50	500 mg SDV	50 mL
	Dexamethasone Sodium Phosphate INJ., USP	
405-05	4 mg/mL MultiDose Vial	5 mL
405-30	4 mg/mL MultiDose Vial	30 mL
406-10	10 mg/mL MultiDose Vial	10 mL
407-05	20 mg/mL MultiDose Vial	5 mL
408-05	24 mg/mL MultiDose Vial	5 mL
616-20	**Diazoxide injection, USP** 300 mg (15 mg/mL) SDV	20 mL
	Droperidol injection, USP	
508-02	5 mg/2 mL Preservative Free SDV	2 mL
508-05	12.5 mg/5 mL Preservative Free SDV	5 mL
510-10	2.5 mg/mL Preserved MDV	10 mL
	Estradiol Cypionate INJ., USP	
417-10	5mg/mL MultiDose Vial	10 mL
	Floxuridine injection	
232-10	500 mg (100 mg/mL)	5 mL
	Floxuridine Sterile, USP (Lyophilized)	
231-10	500 mg/vial	10 mL
	Fluorouracil INJ., USP (Preservative Free)	
217-20	500 mg (50 mg/mL) SingleDose Vial	10 mL
217-50	2.5 g (50 mg/mL) (Pharmacy Bulk Pack)	50 mL in 100 n

217-98	5 g (50 mg/mL) (Pharmacy Bulk Pack)	100 mL
	Fluphenazine Decanoate INJ.	
907-05	25 mg/mL MultiDose Vial	5 mL
	Fluphenazine Hydrochloride Injection, USP	
941-10	2.5 mg/mL	10 mL Multi Dose Vial
	Glucagon FOR INJ., USP (Lyophilized)	
435-03	1 Unit (1 mg)/Vial with Diluent	3 mL
	Glycopyrrolate INJ., USP	
506-01	0.2 mg/mL SDV	1 mL
506-02	0.2 mg/mL SDV	2 mL
506-05	0.2 mg/mL MultiDose Vial	5 mL
506-20	0.2 mg/mL MultiDose Vial	20 mL
	Gold Sodium Thiomalate INJ., USP	
923-02	50mg/mL Single Dose Vial	1 mL
923-10	50mg/mL Multi Dose Vial	10 mL
	Haloperidol (as Lactate) INJ., USP	
513-02	5mg/mL Multi Dose Vial	1 mL
513-10	5mg/mL Multi Dose Vial	10 mL
	Hydrocortisone Sodium Phosphate injection, USP	
442-02	50 mg MDV	2 mL
442-10	50 mg MDV	10 mL
	Hydroxyprogesterone Caproate INJ., USP	
421-10	125mg/mL Multi Dose Vial	10 mL
422-05	250mg/mL Multi Dose Vial	5 mL
	Isoniazid Injection, USP	
947-10	100 mg/mL	10 mL Multi Dose Vial
	Kanamycin Sulfate INJ., USP	
303-02	75 mg/2 mL (Pediatric) SingleDose Vial	2 mL
304-02	500 mg/2 mL SingleDose Vial	2 mL
305-05	1 g/3 mL SingleDose Vial	3 mL
	Ketamine Hydrochloride injection, USP	
514-20	10 mg/mL MDV	20 mL
514-30	10 mg/mL MDV	25 mL
515-10	50 mg/mL MDV	10 mL
516-05	100 mg/mL MDV	5 mL
	Leucovorin Calcium Tablets	
741-30	5 mg, bottle of 30	
741-91	5 mg, bottle of 100	
742-25	25 mg, bottle of 25	
	Leucovorin Calcium INJ. USP Ready to use solution:	
234-05	25mg (5 mg/mL) SDV	5 mL
	Lyophilized Powder:	
241-10	50mg/vial (Preservative Free)	10 mL
242-20	100 mg/vial (Preservative Free)	20mL
	Levothyroxine Sodium FOR INJ. (Lyophilized) (Preservative Free)	
438-07	200mcg/vial	6 mL
439-07	500mcg/vial	6 mL
	Megestrol Acetate Tablets	
746-91	20 mg, Bottle of 100	
747-91	40 mg, Bottle of 100	
	Metaproterenol Sulfate Inhalation Solution, USP	
829-05	0.4%, 2.5 mL Unit Dose	2.5 mL UD
830-05	0.6%, 2.5 mL Unit Dose	2.5 mL UD
	Methotrexate Sodium for injection	
206-10	100 mg (25 mg/mL) MDV	4 mL in 10 mL
206-15	200 mg (25 mg/mL) MDV	8 mL in 15 mL
207-20	250 mg (25 mg/mL) SDV	10 mL in 25 mL
	Methotrexate Sodium FOR INJ., USP Lyophilized Powder: Ready to use Solution (Preserved):	
206-05	50 mg (25 mg/mL) MultiDose Vial	2 mL in 5 mL
	Ready to use Solution (Preservative Free):	
207-05	50 mg (25 mg/mL) SingleDose Vial	2 mL in 5 mL
207-15	200 mg (25 mg/mL) SingleDose Vial	8 mL in 15 mL
	Methyldopate Hydrochloride INJ., USP	
610-05	250 mg (50 mg/mL) Single Dose Vial	5 mL
610-10	500 mg (50 mg/mL) Single Dose Vial	10 mL
	Metoclopramide Hydrochloride INJ., USP	
235-02	10 mg (5 mg/mL) SingleDose Vial	2 mL
	Metocurine Iodide injection, USP	
512-20	2 mg/mL MDV	20 mL
	Morrhuate Sodium injection, USP	
946-30	5% MDV	30 mL
	Nalbuphine Hydrochloride INJ.	
504-02	10 mg/mL MultiDose Vial	1 mL
504-10	10 mg/mL MultiDose Vial	10 mL
505-02	20 mg/mL MultiDose Vial	1 mL
505-10	20 mg/mL MultiDose Vial	10 mL
	Naloxone Hydrochloride INJ., USP	
502-02	0.02mg/mL Single Dose Vial (Preservative Free) Neonatal	2 mL
501-02	0.4 mg/mL SDV	1 mL
501-10	0.4 mg/mL MultiDose Vial	10 mL
503-02	1 mg/mL SDV	2 mL

	Neostigmine Methylsulfate Injection, USP	
532-10	1:1000 (1 mg/mL) MDV	10 mL
533-10	1:2000 (0.5 mg/mL) MDV	10 mL
	Nitroglycerin Injection, USP	
608-05	25 mg (5 mg/mL) SDV	5 mL
608-10	50 mg (5 mg/mL) SDV	10 mL
609-05	50 mg (10 mg/mL) SDV	5 mL
609-10	100 mg (10 mg/mL) SDV	10 mL
	Pancuronium Bromide Injection	
524-02	2 mg/mL SDV	2 mL
524-05	2 mg/mL MDV	5 mL
525-10	1 mg/mL MDV	10 mL
	Phenylephrine Hydrochloride Injection, USP	
626-02	10 mg (10 mg/mL) (1%)	1 mL SDV
	Physostigmine Salicylate	
943-02	1 mg/mL Ampule	2 mL
	Procainamide Hydrochloride INJ., USP	
904-10	1 g (100 mg/mL) MultiDose Vial	10 mL
905-03	1 g (500 mg/mL) MultiDose Vial	2 mL
	Prochlorperazine Edisylate injection	
938-02	5 mg/mL SDV (Preserved)	2 mL
939-10	5 mg/mL MDV	10 mL
	Protamine Sulfate FOR INJ., USP Lyophilized (Refrigeration Required):	
604-10	50 mg/vial	10 mL
	Ready to Use Solution (Refrigeration Required):	
605-05	50 mg/5 mL Single Dose Vial (Preservative Free)	5 mL
605-30	250 mg/25 mL Single Dose Vial (Preservative Free)	25 mL
	Ritodrine Hydrochloride INJ., USP	
902-05	10 mg/mL Single Dose Vial (Preservative Free)	5 mL
903-10	15 mg/mL Single Dose Vial (Preservative Free)	10 mL
	Sodium Iodide Injection	
828-10	1 gram	10 mL Single Dose Vial
	Sodium Thiosulfate INJ., USP (Non-Returnable)	
915-10	10% (1g) Single Dose Vial	10 mL
916-50	25% (12.5g) Single Dose Vial	50 mL
	Sterile Pralidoxime Chloride, USP	
944-20	1 gram	20 mL Single Dose Vial
	Sulfamethoxazole and Trimethoprim Concentrate for injection, USP	
312-05	80 mg/mL SMX & 16 mg/mL TMP	5 mL vial
312-10	80 mg/mL SMX & 16 mg/mL TMP	10 mL MDV
312-30	80 mg/mL SMX & 16 mg/mL TMP	30 mL MDV
312-50	80 mg/mL SMX & 16 mg/mL TMP	50 mL MDV
	Testosterone Enanthate INJ., USP	
428-10	100mg/mL Multi Dose Vial	10 mL
429-10	200mg/mL Multi Dose Vial	10 mL
	Trifluoperazine Hydrochloride Injection, USP	
951-10	2 mg/mL	10 mL Multi Dose Vial
	Tubocurarine Chloride Injection, USP	
511-10	3 mg/mL MDV	10 mL
	Vancomycin Hydrochloride Sterile	
329-10	500 mg/vial	10 mL
330-20	1000 mg/vial	20 mL
	Vasopressin INJ., USP Synthetic	
930-01	10 Units/Vial Multi Dose Vial	0.5 mL
930-02	20 Units/Vial Multi Dose Vial	1 mL
	Verapamil Hydrochloride INJ.	
603-02	5 mg/2 mL Single Dose Vial	2 mL
603-04	10 mg/4 mL Single Dose Vial	4 mL
	Vinblastine Sulfate Injection	
202-30	25 mg (1 mg/mL) MDV	25 mL
	Vinblastine Sulfate Injection Ready to Use Solution (Refrigerate):	
202-20	10 mg (1 mg/mL) Multi Dose Vial	10 mL in 20 mL
	Vincristine Sulfate Injection	
200-05	5 mg MDV (pres. w/o Manitol)	5 mL
	Vincristine Sulfate INJ., USP Ready to use Solution: (Preservative Free)	
201-02	1 mg Single Dose Vial	1 mL in 2 mL
201-05	2 mg Single Dose Vial	2 mL in 5 mL

Products are
listed alphabetically
in the
PINK SECTION.

RAM Laboratories Corp.
P. O. BOX 559071
MIAMI, FL 33255

ALGISIN Capsules ℞
(chlorzoxazone 250 mg. + acetaminophen 300 mg.)

SUPPLIED
Bottles of 60 capsules.

APETIL Liquid
(Therapeutic Vitamins–Minerals)

SUPPLIED
Bottles 8 ounces.

DIGEPEPSIN
Enteric coated digestant tablets
(pepsin 250 mg. + pancreatin 300 mg. + bile salts 150 mg.)

SUPPLIED
Bottles of 60 tablets.

GEROTON FORTE
Supplement—Stimulant tonic

SUPPLIED
Bottles of 1 pint.

HEPACOLIN Capsules
Hepatotropic-Lipotropic

SUPPLIED
Bottles 60 capsules

NEUROCHOL Capsules
Phosphatidylcholine, phosphatidylethanolamine and inositol phosphatides

SUPPLIED
Bottles of 60 capsules.

OTISAN Drops ℞
Otic solution

SUPPLIED
10 ml. plastic dropper.

PASMOL Tablets ℞
(Ethaverine Hydrochloride 100 mg.)

SUPPLIED
Bottles 30 scored tablets.

TRICOL Softgels
Natural fish oil concentrate
(eicosapentaenoic acid 180 mg. +
docosahexaenoic acid 120 mg.)

SUPPLIED
Bottles 60 softgels.

TUSIBRON
(Guaifenesin 100 mg.)

SUPPLIED
Bottles of 4 ounces.

TUSIBRON–DM
(Guaifenesin w/D-Methorphan Hydrobromide)

SUPPLIED
Bottles of 4 ounces.

ZINCVIT Capsules ℞
Multivitamin and Multimineral Formula
with 1 mg. folic acid and 120 mg. Zinc

SUPPLIED
Bottles 60 capsules.

Reed & Carnrick
1 NEW ENGLAND AVENUE
PISCATAWAY, NJ 08855

COLYTE® ℞
[kō 'lĭt]
PEG-3350 & Electrolytes For Oral Solution

DESCRIPTION
Colyte® is an orally administered colon electrolyte lavage preparation delivered in the form of water-soluble components for reconstitution. Each Colyte® preparation contains the following, in grams per liter of water on a delivered basis:

Polyethylene glycol
3350 ....60 grams
Sodium chloride ....1.46 grams
Potassium chloride ....0.745 grams
Sodium bicarbonate ....1.68 grams
Sodium sulfate
(anhydrous) ....5.68 grams

When reconstituted with water, final solution contains 125 mEq/L sodium, 10 mEq/L potassium, 20 mEg/L bicarbonate, 80 mEq/L sulfate, 35 mEq/L chloride amd 18 mEq/L polyethylene glycol 3350.
It is an isotonic (with respect to colon contents) and isosmotic solution.

CLINICAL PHARMACOLOGY
When administered orally, it cleanses the bowel rapidly by inducing diarrhea. Because the Polyethylene glycol 3350 acts as an osmotic agent, there is virtually no net ion absorption or loss. Water and electrolyte balances do not change significantly when large volumes of Colyte® are ingested.

INDICATIONS AND USAGE
Colyte® is indicated for cleansing the bowel by means of total gut perfusion and whole bowel irrigation in preparation for gastrointestinal examination.

CONTRAINDICATIONS
Colyte® is contraindicated for patients with ileus, gastric retention, gastrointestinal obstruction, bowel perforation, toxic colitis and toxic megacolon.

WARNINGS
No additional ingredients, e.g. flavoring, should be added to the solution. Colyte® should be used with caution in patients with severe ulcerative colitis.

PRECAUTIONS
General: Patients with impaired gag reflex, unconscious or semiconscious patients and patients prone to regurgitation or aspiration should be observed during the administration of Colyte, especially if it is administered via nasogastric tube.
If gastrointestinal obstruction or perforation is suspected appropriate studies should be performed to rule out these conditions before administration of Colyte®.

DRUG INTERACTIONS
Oral medication administered within one hour of the start of administration of Colyte® may be flushed from the gastrointestinal tract and not be absorbed.

CARCINOGENESIS, MUTAGENESIS, IMPAIRMENT OF FERTILITY
Studies to evaluate carcinogenic or mutagenic potential or potential to adversely affect male or female fertility have not been performed.

PREGNANCY
Category C. Animal reproduction studies have not been conducted with Colyte® , and it is not known whether Colyte® can affect reproductive capacity or harm the fetus when administered to a pregnant patient. Colyte® should be given to a pregnant patient only if clearly needed.
Safety and effectiveness in children has not been established.

ADVERSE REACTIONS
The most frequent adverse reactions to Colyte® are nausea and bloating. Less frequent adverse reactions include vomiting and rectal irritation. These adverse reactions are temporary and generally disappear rapidly. Isolated cases of urticaria, rhinorrhea and dermatitis have been reported which may represent allergic reactions.

DOSAGE AND ADMINISTRATION
Preparation of Solution: The preparation is made by dissolving the contents in a sufficient quantity of water to produce the final volume according to package directions. Mix well.
Usual Dosage: Colyte® can be ingested orally or administered via nasogastric intubation. Lavage is complete when fecal discharge is clear. The typical dosage per patient is 4 liters or one gallon (3.785 liters).
Peroral: Drink 200 ml to 300 ml every 10 minutes (7 to 10 ounces).
Recommended ingestion rate ranges from 1.2 liters per hour to 1.8 liters per hour.

Nasogastric intubation: Infuse at a rate of 20 ml per minute to 30 ml per minute.
If possible, patients should fast for three or four hours before ingestion begins. Patients should never be given solid food less than two hours prior to administration. Only clear liquids are permitted during the interval between Colyte® ingestion and examination.

PREPARATION OF COLYTE® SOLUTION
4 Liter: Add tap water to FILL line. Replace cap tightly and mix or shake well until all ingredients have dissolved. (No additional ingredients, e.g., flavoring, should be added to the solution.)
One Gallon: The preparation is made by dissolving the contents of either the packets or of the bottle in a food-grade container, in a sufficient quantity of water to produce the final volume according to package directions. Mix well.

HOW SUPPLIED
In powdered form, for oral administration as a solution.
Each 18 Oz. bottle contains the following to prepare one gallon of solution:
One gallon, (NDC 0021-4401-49): polyethylene glycol 3350 227.1 g. sodium chloride 5.53 g. potassium chloride 2.82 g. sodium bicarbonate 6.36 g. sodium sulfate 21.5 g. in a bottle.
Also available as five separately packaged components to prepare one gallon of solution for oral administration:
One gallon (NDC 0021-0001-02): polyethylene glycol 3350 227.1 g. sodium chloride 5.53 g. potassium chloride 2.82 g. sodium bicarbonate 6.36 g. sodium sulfate 21.5 g.
Also available in a jug containing the following:
Four liter, (NDC 0021-4401-23): polyethylene glycol 3350 240 g. sodium chloride 5.84 g. potassium chloride 2.98 g. sodium bicarbonate 6.72 g. sodium sulfate 22.72 g.

CAUTION
Federal law prohibits dispensing without a prescription.
KEEP RECONSTITUTED SOLUTION REFRIGERATED.
USE WITHIN 48 HOURS. DISCARD UNUSED PORTION.
June 1988
Shown in Product Identification Section, page 423

CORTIFOAM® ℞
(hydrocortisone acetate) 10%

DESCRIPTION
Contains hydrocortisone acetate 10% as the sole active ingredient in 20 g of a foam containing propylene glycol, emulsifying wax, polyoxyethylene-10-stearyl ether, cetyl alcohol, methylparaben and propylparaben, trolamine, purified water and inert propellants, dichlorodifluoromethane and dichlorotetrafluoroethane.
Each application delivers approximately 900 mg of foam containing 80 mg of hydrocortisone (90 mg of hydrocortisone acetate).

CLINICAL PHARMACOLOGY
CORTIFOAM provides effective topical administration of an anti-inflammatory corticosteroid as adjunctive therapy of ulcerative proctitis.

INDICATIONS
CORTIFOAM is indicated as adjunctive therapy in the topical treatment of ulcerative proctitis of the distal portion of the rectum in patients who cannot retain hydrocortisone or other corticosteroid enemas. Direct observations of methylene blue-containing foam have shown staining about 10 centimeters into the rectum.

CONTRAINDICATIONS
Local contraindications to the use of intrarectal steroids include obstruction, abscess, perforation, peritonitis, fresh intestinal anastomoses, extensive fistulas and sinus tracts. Tuberculosis (active, latent or questionably healed), ocular herpes simplex and acute psychosis are usually considered absolute contraindications to the use of corticosteroids. Relative contraindications include active peptic ulcer, acute glomerulonephritis, myasthenia gravis, osteoporosis, diverticulitis, thrombophlebitis, psychic disturbances, pregnancy, diabetes, hyperthyroidism, acute coronary disease, hypertension, limited cardiac reserve, and local or systemic infections, including fungal or exanthematous diseases. Where these conditions exist, the expected benefits from steroid therapy must be weighed against the risks involved in its use. Pregnancy is a relative contraindication to corticosteroids, particularly during third trimester. If corticosteroids must be administered in pregnancy, watch newborn infant closely for signs of hypoadrenalism, and administer appropriate therapy if needed.

WARNING
Do not insert any part of the aerosol container into the anus. Contents of the container are under pressure, but not flammable. Do not burn or puncture the aerosol container. Store at room temperature but not over 120˚ F. Because CORTIFOAM is not expelled, systemic hydrocortisone absorption may be greater from CORTIFOAM than from corticosteroid

enema formulations. If there is no evidence of clinical or proctologic improvement within two or three weeks after starting CORTIFOAM therapy, or if the patient's condition worsens, discontinue the drug.

PRECAUTIONS

Steroid therapy should be administered with caution in patients with severe ulcerative disease because these patients are predisposed to perforation of the bowel wall. Where surgery is imminent, it is hazardous to wait more than a few days for a satisfactory response to medical treatment. General precautions common to all corticosteroid therapy should be observed during treatment with CORTIFOAM. These include gradual withdrawal of therapy to allow for possible adrenal insufficiency and awareness to possible growth suppression in children. Patients should be kept under close observation, for, as with all drugs, rare individuals may react unfavorably under certain conditions. If severe reactions or idiosyncrasies occur, steroids should be discontinued immediately and appropriate measures instituted. Do not employ in immediate or early postoperative period following ileorectostomy.

ADVERSE REACTIONS

Corticosteroid therapy may produce side effects which include moon face, fluid retention, excessive appetite and weight gain, abnormal fat deposits, mental symptoms, hypertrichosis, acne, ecchymosis, increased sweating, pigmentation, dry scaly skin, thinning scalp hair, thrombophlebitis, decreased resistance to infection, negative nitrogen balance with delayed bone and wound healing, menstrual disorders, neuropathy, peptic ulcer, decreased glucose tolerance, hypopotassemia, adrenal insufficiency, necrotizing angiitis, hypertension, pancreatitis and increased intraocular pressure. In children, suppression of growth may occur. Increased intracranial pressure may occur and possibly account for headache, insomnia and fatigue. Subcapsular cataracts may result from prolonged usage. Long-term use of all corticosteroids results in catabolic effects characterized by negative protein and calcium balance. Osteoporosis, spontaneous fractures and aseptic necrosis of the hip and humerus may occur as part of this catabolic phenomenon. Where hypopotassemia and other symptoms associated with fluid and electrolyte imbalance call for potassium supplementation and salt poor or salt-free diets, these may be instituted and are compatible with diet requirements for ulcerative proctitis.

ADMINISTRATION AND DOSAGE

Usual dose is one applicatorful once or twice daily for two or three weeks, and every second day thereafter, administered rectally. The patient directions packaged with the applicator describe how to use the aerosol container and applicator. Satisfactory response usually occurs within five to seven days marked by a decrease in symptoms. Symptomatic improvement in ulcerative proctitis should not be used as the sole criterion for evaluating efficacy. Sigmoidoscopy is also recommended to judge dosage adjustment, duration of therapy and rate of improvement.

Directions For Use:

1. Shake foam container vigorously for 5–10 seconds. Do not remove cap.
2. Withdraw applicator plunger past the fill line until it stops.
3. Place foam container upright on level surface, insert tip of cap into tip of applicator.
   To fill applicator:
   - Depress cap on foam container-RELEASE.
   - Pause, a few seconds, allowing foam to enter and expand in applicator barrel.
   - Repeat until foam rises to fill applicator to Fill Line.
4. Hold applicator by barrel and gently insert tip into anus. Once in place, push plunger to expel foam, then withdraw applicator.
   Note: Pull applicator apart and wash thoroughly with warm water.

HOW SUPPLIED

CORTIFOAM (NDC 0021-0695-20) is supplied in an aerosol container with a special rectal applicator. Each applicator delivers approximately 900 mg of foam containing approximately 80 mg of hydrocortisone as 90 mg of hydrocortisone acetate. When used correctly the aerosol container will deliver a minimum of 14 applications.
Revised February 1989

LITERATURE AVAILABLE

Patient information available on request.

Shown in Product Identification Section, page 423

DILATRATE®-SR   ℞
[dī'lă-trāt]
(Isosorbide Dinitrate)
Sustained Release Capsules
40 mg

DESCRIPTION

Isosorbide dinitrate, an organic nitrate, is a vasodilator with effects on both arteries and veins. Isosorbide dinitrate is available as a 40 mg sustained release capsule. The chemical name for isosorbide dinitrate is D-Glucitol, 1,4:3,6-dianhydro-dinitrate, and the compound has the following structural formula:

$$\begin{array}{c} CH_2 \\ HCONO_2 \\ CH \\ HC \\ HCONO_2 \\ CH_2 \end{array}$$

$C_6H_8N_2O_8$
Molecular Weight: 236.14
Isosorbide dinitrate is a white, crystalline, odorless compound which is stable in air and in solution, has a melting point of 70°C and has an optical rotation of $+134°$ (c=1.0, alcohol, 20°C). Isosorbide dinitrate is freely soluble in organic solvents such as acetone, alcohol, and ether, but is only sparingly soluble in water.

CLINICAL PHARMACOLOGY

The principal pharmacological action of isosorbide dinitrate is relaxation of vascular smooth muscle, producing a vasodilatory effect on both peripheral arteries and veins, with predominant effects on the latter. Dilation of the post-capillary vessels, including large veins, promotes peripheral pooling of blood and decreases venous return to the heart, thereby reducing left-ventricular end-diastolic pressure (preload). Arteriolar relaxation reduces systemic vascular resistance and arterial pressure (after-load).

The mechanism by which isosorbide dinitrate relieves angina pectoris is not fully understood. Myocardial oxygen consumption or demand (as measured by the pressure-rate product, tension-time index, and stroke work index) is decreased by both the arterial and venous effects of isosorbide dinitrate and, presumably, a more favorable supply-demand ratio is achieved. While the large epicardial coronary arteries are also dilated by isosorbide dinitrate, the extent to which this contributes to relief of exertional angina is unclear.

Therapeutic doses of isosorbide dinitrate may reduce systolic, diastolic, and mean arterial blood pressures, especially in the upright posture. Effective coronary perfusion is usually maintained. The decrease in systemic blood pressure may result in reflex tachycardia, an effect which results in an unfavorable influence on myocardial oxygen demand. Hemodynamic studies indicate that isosorbide dinitrate may reduce the abnormally elevated left ventricular end-diastolic and pulmonary capillary wedge pressures that occur during an acute episode of angina pectoris.

Isosorbide dinitrate is metabolized by enzymatic denitration to the intermediate products isosorbide-2-mononitrate and isosorbide-5-mononitrate. Both metabolites have biological activity, especially the 5-mononitrate which is also the principal metabolite. The liver is a principal site of metabolism and isosorbide dinitrate is subject to a large first pass effect. The systemic clearance of the drug following intravenous infusion is about 3.4 liters/min. Since the clearance exceeds hepatic blood flow, considerable extra hepatic metabolism must also occur.

The average bioavailability of isosorbide dinitrate is 59 and 22 percent following sublingual and oral administration, respectively. The terminal half-life is about 20 minutes, 60 minutes, and 4 hours following IV, sublingual, and oral administration, respectively. The dependence of half-life on the route of administration is not understood. Over limited ranges of IV dosing, the pharmacokinetics of isosorbide dinitrate appear linear. However, both the 2- and 5-mononitrate metabolites have been shown to decrease the rate of disappearance of the dinitrate from the blood and the half-lives of isosorbide-5-mononitrate and isosorbide-2-mononitrate range from 4.0–5.6 and 1.5–3.1 hours, respectively.

The pharmacokinetics and/or bioavailability of isosorbide dinitrate during multiple dosing have not been well-studied. Because the metabolites influence the clearance of isosorbide dinitrate, prediction of blood levels of parent compound or metabolites from single-dose studies is uncertain.

INDICATIONS AND USAGE

Isosorbide dinitrate is indicated for the treatment and prevention of angina pectoris. Controlled clinical trials have demonstrated that the sublingual, chewable, immediate release, and controlled-release oral dosage forms of isosorbide dinitrate are effective in improving exercise tolerance in patients with angina pectoris. When single sublingual or chewable doses (5mg) of isosorbide dinitrate were administered prophylactically to patients with angina pectoris in various clinical studies, duration of exercise until chest pain or fatigue was significantly improved for at least 45 minutes (and as long as 2 hours in some studies) following dosing. Similar studies after single oral (15 to 120 mg) and oral controlled-released (40 to 80 mg) doses of isosorbide dinitrate have shown significant improvement in exercise tolerance for up to 8 hours following dosing. The exercise electrocardiographic evidence suggests that improved exercise tolerance with isosorbide dinitrate is not at the expense of greater myocardial ischemia. All dosage forms of isosorbide dinitrate may therefore be used prophylactically to decrease frequency and severity of anginal attacks and can be expected to decrease the need for sublingual nitroglycerin.

The sublingual and chewable forms of the drug are indicated for acute prophylaxis of angina pectoris when taken a few minutes before situations likely to provoke anginal attacks. Because of a slower onset of effect, the oral forms of isosorbide dinitrate are not indicated for acute prophylaxis.

In controlled clinical trials chewable and sublingual isosorbide dinitrate were effective in relieving an acute attack of angina pectoris. Relief occurred with a mean time of 2.9 and 3.4 minutes (chewable and sublingual respectively) compared to relief of angina with a mean time of 1.9 minutes following sublingual nitroglycerin. Because of the more rapid relief of chest pain with sublingual nitroglycerin, the use of sublingual or chewable isosorbide dinitrate for aborting an acute anginal attack should be limited to patients intolerant or unresponsive to sublingual nitroglycerin.

CONTRAINDICATIONS

Isosorbide dinitrate is contraindicated in patients who have shown purported hypersensitivity or idiosyncrasy to it or other nitrates or nitrites.

WARNINGS

The benefits of isosorbide dinitrate during the early days of an acute myocardial infarction have not been established. If one elects to use organic nitrates in early infarction hemodynamic monitoring and frequent clinical assessment should be used because of the potential deleterious effects of hypotension.

PRECAUTIONS

General: Severe hypotensive response, particularly with upright posture, may occur with even small doses of isosorbide dinitrate. The drug should therefore be used with caution in subjects who may have blood volume depletion from diuretic therapy or in subjects who have low systolic blood pressure (e.g., below 90 mm Hg). Paradoxical bradycardia and increased angina pectoris may accompany nitrate-induced hypotension.

Nitrate therapy may aggravate the angina caused by hypertrophic cardiomyopathy. Tolerance to this drug and cross-tolerance to other nitrates and nitrites may occur.

Marked symptomatic, orthostatic hypotension has been reported when calcium channel blockers and organic nitrates were used in combination. Dose adjustment of either class of agents may be necessary.

Tolerance to the vascular and antianginal effects of isosorbide dinitrate or nitroglycerin has been demonstrated in clinical trials, experience through occupational exposure, and in isolated tissue experiments in the laboratory. The importance of tolerance to the appropriate use of isosorbide dinitrate in the management of patients with angina pectoris has not been determined. However, one clinical trial using treadmill exercise tolerance (as an endpoint) found an 8 hour duration of action of oral isosorbide dinitrate following the first dose (after a 2 week placebo washout) and only a 2 hour duration of effect of the same dose after 1 week of repetitive dosing a conventional dosing intervals. On the other hand, several trials have been able to differentiate isosorbide dinitrate from placebo after 4 weeks of therapy, and in open trials an effect seems detectable for as long as several months.

Tolerance clearly occurs in industrial workers continuously exposed to nitroglycerin. Moreover, physical dependence also occurs since chest pain, acute myocardial infarction, and even sudden death have occurred during temporary withdrawal of nitroglycerin from the workers. In clinical trials in angina patients, there are reports of anginal attacks being more easily provoked and of rebound in the hemodynamic effects soon after nitrate withdrawal. The relative importance of these observations to the routine, clinical use of isosorbide dinitrate is not known. However, it seems prudent to gradually withdraw patients from isosorbide dinitrate when the therapy is being terminated, rather than stopping the drug abruptly.

Information for Patients: Headache may occur during initial therapy with isosorbide dinitrate. Headache is usually relieved by the use of standard headache remedies, or by lowering the dose, and tends to disappear after the first week or two of use.

Continued on next page

Reed & Carnrick—Cont.

Drug Interactions: Alcohol may enhance any marked sensitivity to the hypotensive effect of nitrates. Isosorbide dinitrate acts directly on vascular smooth muscle; therefore, any other agent that depends on vascular smooth muscle as the final common path can be expected to have decreased or increased effect depending on the agent.

Carcinogenesis, Mutagenesis, Impairment of Fertility: No long-term studies in animals have been performed to evaluate the carcinogenic potential of this drug. A modified two-litter reproduction study in rats fed isosorbide dinitrate at 25 or 100 mg/kg/day did not reveal any effects on fertility or gestation or any remarkable growth pathology in any parent or offspring fed isosorbide dinitrate as compared with rats fed a basal controlled diet.

Pregnancy Category C: Isosorbide dinitrate has been shown to cause a dose-related increase in embryotoxicity (increase in mummified pups) in rabbits at oral doses 35 and 150 times the maximum recommended human daily dose. There are no adequate and well-controlled studies in pregnant women. Isosorbide dinitrate should be used during pregnancy only if the potential benefit justifies the potential risk to the fetus.

Nursing Mothers: It is not known whether this drug is excreted in human milk. Because many drugs are excreted in human milk, caution should be exercised when isosorbide dinitrate is administered to a nursing woman.

Pediatric Use: The safety and effectiveness of isosorbide dinitrate in children has not been established.

ADVERSE REACTIONS

Adverse reactions, particularly headache and hypotension, are dose related. In clinical trials at various doses, the following have been observed.

Headache is the most common (reported incidence varies widely, apparently being dose related, with an average occurrence of about 25%) adverse reaction and may be severe and persistent. Cutaneous vasodilation wth flushing may occur. Transient episodes of dizziness and weakness, as well as other signs of cerebral ischemia associated with postural hypotension, may occasionally develop (the incidence of reported symptomatic hypotension ranges from 2% to 36%). An occasional individual will exhibit marked sensitivity to the hypotensive effects of nitrates and severe responses (nausea, vomiting, weakness, restlessness, pallor, perspiration, and collapse) may occur even with the usual therapeutic dose. Drug rash and/or exfoliative dermatitis may occasionally occur. Nausea and vomiting appear to be uncommon.

OVERDOSAGE

Signs and Symptoms: These may include the following: a prompt fall in blood pressure, persistent and throbbing headache, vertigo, palpitation, visual disturbances, flushed and perspiring skin (later becoming cold and cyanotic), nausea and vomiting (possibly with colic and even bloody diarrhea), syncope (especially in the upright position), methemoglobinemia with cyanosis and anoxia, initial hyperpnea, dyspnea and slow breathing, slow pulse (dicrotic and intermittent), heart block, increased intracranial pressure with cerebral symptoms of confusion and moderate fever, paralysis and coma followed by clonic convulsions and possibly death due to circulatory collapse.

It is not known what dose of the drug is associated with symptoms of overdosing or what dose of the drug would be life-threatening. The acute oral LD50 of isosorbide dinitrate in rats was found to be approximately 1100 mg/kg of body weight. These animal experiments indicate that approximately 500 times the usual therapeutic dose would be required to produce such toxic symptoms in humans. It is not known whether the drug is dialyzable.

Treatment of Overdosage: Prompt removal of the ingested material by gastric lavage is reasonable but not documented to be useful. Keep the patient recumbent in a shock position and comfortably warm. Passive movements of the extremities may aid venous return. Administer oxygen and artificial respiration if necessary. If methemoglobinemia is present, administer methylene blue (1% solution), 1 to 2 mg/kg intravenously.

Methemoglobin: Case reports of clinically significant methemoglobinemia are rare at conventional doses of organic nitrates. The formation of methemoglobin is dose related and in the case of genetic abnormalities of hemoglobin that favor methemoglobin formation, even conventional doses of organic nitrate could produce harmful concentrations of methemoglobin.

WARNING

Epinephrine is ineffective in reversing the severe hypotensive events associated with overdose. It and related compounds are contraindicated in this situation.

DOSAGE AND ADMINISTRATION

Because of a slower onset of effect, the oral forms of isosorbide dinitrate are not indicated for acute prophylaxis or for the treatment of acute anginal attacks.

Isosorbide dinitrate should be titrated upward until angina is relieved or side effects limit the dose. In ambulatory patients, the magnitude of the incremental dose increase should be guided by measurements of standing blood pressure.

For the treatment of chronic stable angina pectoris, the usual starting dose for controlled-release forms, 40 mg. For maintenance therapy, oral controlled-release doses of 40 to 80 mg given every 8 to 12 hours is generally recommended. The extent to which development of tolerance should modify the dosage program has not been defined. The oral controlled release forms of isosorbide dinitrate should not be chewed.

HOW SUPPLIED

Bottles of 100 and unit dose 100's (opaque pink and colorless body) capsules.

STORAGE

Store at controlled room temperature 15-30°C (59-86°F) in a dry place.

WARNING

KEEP OUT OF REACH OF CHILDREN.

CAUTION

Federal law prohibits dispensing without prescription.
Manufactured for
Reed & Carnrick
Piscataway, N.J. 08855
by Vitarine Pharmaceuticals, Inc.
Springfield Gardens, N.Y. 11413

Date of Revision
May 1989
Shown in Product Identification Section, page 423

EPIFOAM®   ℞
[ĕp'ē-fōm]
**(hydrocortisone acetate 1% and
pramoxine hydrochloride 1% topical aerosol)**

DESCRIPTION

A topical corticosteroid aerosol foam containing hydrocortisone acetate 1% and pramoxine hydrochloride 1% in a base containing: propylene glycol, cetyl alcohol, glyceryl stearate, PEG-100 stearate, laureth-23, polyoxyl-40 stearate, methylparaben, propylparaben, trolamine or hydrochloric acid to adjust pH, purified water and propellants (inert): butane and propane.

EPIFOAM contains a synthetic steroid used as an anti-inflammatory and anti-pruritic agent, and a local anesthetic. Molecular weight: Hydrocortisone acetate 404.51. Solubility of hydrocortisone acetate in water: 1 mg/100 ml. Chemical name: Pregn-4-ene, 3,20-dione, 21-(acetyloxy)-11, 17-dihydroxy-, (11B).

Pramoxine Hydrochloride

CLINICAL PHARMACOLOGY

Topical corticosteroids share anti-inflammatory, anti-pruritic and vasoconstrictive actions.

The mechanism of anti-inflammatory activity of the topical corticosteroids is unclear. Various laboratory methods, including vasoconstrictor assays, are used to compare and predict potencies clinical efficacies of the topical corticosteroids. There is some evidence to suggest that a recognizable correlation exists between vasoconstrictor potency and therapeutic efficacy in man.

Pramoxine Hydrochloride: A surface or local anesthetic which is not chemically related to the "caine" types of local anesthetics. Its unique chemical structure is likely to minimize the danger of cross-sensitivity reactions in patients allergic to other local anesthetics.

Pharmacokinetics: The extent of percutaneous absorption of topical corticosteroids is determined by many factors including the vehicle, the integrity of the epidermal barrier, and the use of occlusive dressings.

Topical corticosteroids can be absorbed from normal intact skin. Inflammation and/or other disease processes in the skin increase the percutaneous absorption of topical corticosteroids. Occlusive dressings substantially increase the per-

cutaneous absorption of topical corticosteroids. Thus, occlusive dressings may be a valuable therapeutic adjunct for treatment of resistant dermatoses. (See DOSAGE AND ADMINISTRATION.)

Once absorbed through the skin, topical corticosteroids are handled through pharmacokinetic pathways similar to systemically administered corticosteroids. Corticosteroids are bound to plasma proteins in varying degrees. Corticosteroids are metabolized primarily in the liver and are then excreted by the kidneys. Some of the topical corticosteroids and their metabolites are also excreted in the bile.

INDICATIONS AND USAGE

Topical corticosteroids are indicated for the relief of the inflammatory and pruritic manifestations of corticosteroid-responsive dermatoses.

CONTRAINDICATIONS

Topical corticosteroid products are contraindicated in those patients with a history of hypersensitivity to any of the components of the preparation.

WARNING

Not for prolonged use. If redness, pain, irritation or swelling persists, discontinue use and consult a physician. Contents of the container are under pressure, but not flammable. Do not burn or puncture the aerosol container. Store at temperatures below 120°F. Keep this and all medicines out of the reach of children.

PRECAUTIONS

General: Systemic absorption of topical corticosteroids has produced reversible hypothalamic-pituitary-adrenal (HPA) axis suppression, manifestations of Cushing's syndrome, hyperglycemia and glucosuria in some patients.

Conditions which augment systemic absorption include the application of the more potent steroids, use over large surface areas, prolonged use and the addition of occlusive dressings.

Therefore, patients receiving a large dose of a potent topical steroid applied to a large surface area or under an occlusive dressing should be evaluated periodically for evidence of HPA axis suppression by using the urinary hydrocortisone and ACTH stimulation tests. If HPA axis suppression is noted, an attempt should be made to withdraw the drug, to reduce the frequency of application, or to substitute a less potent steroid.

Recovery of HPA axis function is generally prompt and complete upon discontinuation of the drug. Infrequently, signs and symptoms of steroid withdrawal may occur, requiring supplemental systemic corticosteroids.

In children absorption may result in higher blood levels and thus more susceptibility to systemic toxicity. (See PRECAUTIONS—Pediatric Use.)

If irritation develops, topical corticosteroids should be discontinued and appropriate therapy instituted.

In the presence of dermatological infections, the use of an appropriate antifungal or antibacterial agent should be instituted. If a favorable response does not occur promptly, the corticosteroid should be discontinued until the infection has been adequately controlled.

Information for the Patient: Patients using topical corticosteroids should receive the following information and instructions:

1. This medication is to be used as directed by the physician. It is for external use only. Avoid contact with the eyes.
2. Do not use this medication for any disorder other than for which it was prescribed.
3. The treated skin area should not be bandaged or otherwise covered or wrapped as to be occlusive unless directed by physician.
4. Report any signs of local adverse reactions especially under occlusive dressings.
5. Do not use tight fitting diapers or plastic pants on a child being treated in the diaper area, as these garments may constitute occlusive dressings.

Laboratory Tests: The following test may be helpful in evaluating the HPA axis suppression:
Urinary hydrocortisone test
ACTH stimulation test

Carcinogenesis, Mutagenesis, and Impairment of Fertility: Long-term animal studies have not been performed to evaluate the carcinogenic potential or the effect on fertility of topical corticosteroids.

Studies to determine mutagenicity with prednisolone and hydrocortisone have revealed negative results.

Pregnancy Category C: Corticosteroids are generally teratogenic in laboratory animals when administered systemically at relatively low dosage levels. The more potent corticosteroids have been shown to be teratogenic after dermal application in laboratory animals. There are no adequate and well-controlled studies in pregnant women of teratogenic effects from topically applied corticosteroids. Therefore, topical corticosteroids should be used during pregnancy only if the potential benefit justifies the potential risk to the fetus. Drugs of this class should not be used extensively on pregnant patients, in large amounts, or for prolonged periods of time.

Nursing Mothers: It is not known whether topical administration of corticosteroids could result in sufficient systemic absorption to produce detectable quantities in breast milk. Systemically administered corticosteroids are secreted into breast milk in quantities not likely to have a deleterious effect on the infant. Caution should be exercised when any topical corticosteroids are administered to a nursing woman.

Pediatric Use: Pediatric patients may demonstrate greater susceptibility to topical corticosteroid-induced HPA axis suppression and Cushing's syndrome than mature patients because of a larger skin surface area to body weight ratio. Hypothalamic-pituitary-adrenal (HPA) axis suppression, Cushing's syndrome and intracranial hypertension have been reported in children receiving topical corticosteroids. Manifestations of adrenal suppression in children include linear growth retardation, delayed weight gain, low plasma cortisone levels and absence of response to ACTH stimulation. Manifestations of intracranial hypertension include bulging fontanelles, headaches and bilateral papilledema. Administration of topical corticosteroids to children should be limited to the least amount compatible with an effective therapeutic regimen. Chronic corticosteroid therapy may interfere with the growth and development of children.

ADVERSE REACTIONS

The following local adverse reactions are reported infrequently with topical corticosteroids, but may occur more frequently with the use of occlusive dressings. These reactions are listed in an approximately decreasing order of occurrence:

Burning
Itching
Irritation
Dryness
Folliculitis
Hypopigmentation
Perioral dermatitis
Allergic contact dermatitis
Maceration of the skin
Secondary infection
Skin atrophy
Striae
Miliaria

OVERDOSAGE

Topically applied corticosteroids can be absorbed in sufficient amounts to produce systemic effects. (See PRECAUTIONS.)

DOSAGE AND ADMINISTRATION

Apply to affected area 3 or 4 times daily.
(NOTE: Refer to the enclosed Directions for Use.):

DIRECTIONS FOR USE

1. Shake foam container vigorously before use.
2. Hold container upright and dispense medication onto a pad by depressing the container cap several times. A small amount of foam is all that is needed on the pad. Apply to affected areas.
   Alternatively, the foam may be applied directly to affected areas.
3. The container and cap should be disassembled and rinsed with warm water after use.

NOTE: The aerosol container should never be inserted into the vagina or anus.

HOW SUPPLIED

EPIFOAM (NDC-0021-0740-10) available in 10g pressurized cans.

CAUTION

FEDERAL LAW PROHIBITS DISPENSING WITHOUT PRESCRIPTION.
Reed & Carnrick
1 New England Avenue
Piscataway, NJ 08855

Revised May 1989
Shown in Product Identification Section, page 423

KWELL® Cream   ℞
[*kwel*]
(lindane) 1%

DESCRIPTION

KWELL Cream (lindane) 1% is an ectoparasiticide and ovicide effective against Sarcoptes scabiei (scabies) and their ova. Inert ingredients: 99% in a pleasantly scented water dispersible cream containing stearic acid, glycerin, lanolin, 2-amino-2-methyl-1-propanol, perfume and purified water. Lindane, which is the highly purified gamma isomer of 1, 2, 3, 4, 5, 6, hexachlorocyclohexane, has the following chemical structure.
[See Chemical Formula at top of next column].

CLINICAL PHARMACOLOGY

KWELL Cream exerts its parasiticidal action by being directly absorbed into the parasites and their ova. Feldmann and Maibach[1] reported approximately 10% absorption of a lindane acetone solution applied to the forearm and left in place to 24 hours. Dale, et al[2] reported a blood level of 290ng/ml associated with convulsions following the accidental ingestion of a lindane containing product. Ginsburg[3] found a mean peak blood level of 28ng/ml 6 hours after total body application of KWELL Lotion to scabietic infants and children. The half-life was determined to be 18 hours.

INDICATIONS AND USAGE

KWELL Cream is indicated for the treatment of patients infested with Sarcoptes scabiei (scabies).

CONTRAINDICATIONS

KWELL Cream is contraindicated for premature neonates because their skin may be more permeable than full term infants and their liver enzymes may not be sufficiently developed. It is also contraindicated for patients with known seizure disorders and for individuals with a known sensitivity to the product or any of its components.

WARNINGS

LINDANE PENETRATES HUMAN SKIN AND HAS THE POTENTIAL FOR CNS TOXICITY (SEE CLINICAL PHARMACOLOGY SECTION). KWELL CREAM SHOULD BE USED ACCORDING TO RECOMMENDED DOSAGE (SEE DIRECTIONS FOR USE) ESPECIALLY ON INFANTS, PREGNANT WOMEN AND NURSING MOTHERS. ANIMAL STUDIES INDICATE THAT POTENTIAL TOXIC EFFECTS OF TOPICALLY APPLIED LINDANE ARE GREATER IN THE YOUNG. Seizures have been reported after excessive use or oral ingestion of lindane. No residual effects of KWELL treatment have been demonstrated, therefore, this product should not be used to ward off a possible infestation. If accidental ingestion occurs prompt gastric lavage is indicated. Because oils may enhance absorption, saline rather than oily cathartics should be used. Central nervous excitation can be controlled by the administration of pentobarbital, phenobarbital or diazepam.

PRECAUTIONS

General
Care should be taken to avoid contact with the eyes. If such contact occurs, eyes should be immediately flushed with water. If irritation or sensitization occurs, the patient should be advised to consult a physician.
Information to Patients
Patients should be instructed on the proper use of the medication. Directions for Use should accompany the prescription.

LABORATORY TESTS

No laboratory tests are needed for the proper use of this medication.

DRUG INTERACTIONS

Oils may enhance absorption, therefore, simultaneous use of creams, ointments or oils should be avoided.

CARCINOGENESIS

Although no studies have been conducted with KWELL Cream, numerous long term feeding studies have been conducted in mice and rats to evaluate the carcinogenic potential of the technical grade of hexachlorocyclohexane (BHC) as well as the alpha, beta, gamma lindane) and delta isomers. Both oral and topical applications have been evaluated. Nagasaki[4], Goto[5] and Hanada[6] found varying amounts of benign and malignant hepatomas associated with BHC and the alpha, delta and epsilon isomers. None reported a carcinogenic potential for lindane. Tumors were found only in the animals which had received the alpha isomer. Weisse and Herbst[7] also evaluated the carcinogenic potential of lindane in mice but could find no evidence of lindane in mice but could find no evidnece of lindane carcinogenicity. The National Cancer Institute[8] also found no evidence of carcinogenicity.
Thorpe and Walker[9] compared beta BHC with lindane, dieldrin, DDT and hexabarbital in mice. Despite the unusually high incidence of tumors in the control group, they concluded that 600 ppm of lindane was associated with a significant increase in the incidence of hepatoma and thus considered it a tumorigen.
Orr[10] and Kashyap, et al[11] evaluated the carcinogenic potential in mice of topically applied BHC. In neither study was there any evidence of a tumorigenic or carcinogenic potential associated with topical application of BHC.

Mutagenicity tests have been used as predictive information about the carcinogenicity of various chemical compounds. Numerous types of mutagenicity tests have been performed with lindane. The results of these tests do not indicate that lindane is mutagenic.

PREGNANCY

Teratogenic Effects
Pregnancy category B: Reproduction, including multigeneration, studies have been performed in mice, rats, rabbits, pigs, and dogs at doses up to 10 times the human dose and have revealed no evidence of impaired fertility or harm to the fetus due to administered lindane. There are, however, no adequate and well controlled studies in pregnant women. Because animal reproduction studies are not always predictive of human response, the recommended dosage should not be exceeded on pregnant women. They should be treated no more than twice during a pregnancy.

NURSING MOTHERS

Lindane is secreted in human milk in low concentrations. Studies conducted in the United States as well as Europe and South America found levels of lindane in human milk ranging from 0 to 113 ppb, as the result of ingestion of foods which had been treated with lindane. There appeared to be no difference in concentrations between country and urban dwellers. Although the levels of lindane found in blood after topical application with KWELL Cream make it unlikely that amounts of lindane sufficient to cause serious adverse reactions will be excreted in the milk of nursing mothers who have used KWELL Cream, if there is any concern, an alternate method of feeding may be used for 2 days.

PEDIATRIC USE

Refer to the Contraindications and Warnings sections.

ADVERSE REACTIONS

Lindane has been reported to cause central nervous stimulation ranging from dizziness to convulsions. Cases of convulsions have been reported in connection with KWELL Cream therapy. However, these incidents were almost always associated with accidental oral ingestion or misuse of the product. Eczematous eruptions due to irritation from this product have also been reported. Incidence of these adverse reactions is relatively infrequent, occurring in less than 1 in 100,000 patients.

DRUG ABUSE AND DEPENDENCE

KWELL Cream is not subject to abuse, nor is there any dependence on the drug.

OVERDOSAGE

Overdosage or oral ingestion of KWELL Cream can cause central nervous system excitation and, if taken in sufficient quantities, convulsions may occur.
If accidental ingestion occurs, prompt gastric lavage should be instituted. However, since oils favor absorption, saline cathartics for intestinal evacuation should be given rather than oil laxatives. If central nervous system manifestations occur they can be antagonized by the administration of pentobarbital, phenobarbital or diazepam.

DOSAGE AND ADMINISTRATION

CAUTION: USE ONLY AS DIRECTED. DO NOT EXCEED RECOMENDED DOSAGE
No residual effects of KWELL treatment have been demonstrated therefore, this product should not be used to ward off a possible infestation.
       NOTE: PLEASE READ CAREFULLY.

DIRECTIONS FOR USE

Scabies (sarcoptes scabiei)—The cream should be applied to dry skin in a thin layer and rubbed in thoroughly. If crusted lesions are present, a tepid bath preceding the medication is helpful. If a bath is used, allow the skin to dry before applying the cream. Usually two ounces are sufficient for an adult. A total body application should be made from the neck down including the soles of the feet. Scabies rarely affects the head of children or adults but may occur in infants.
The cream should be left on for 8–12 hours and should then be removed by thorough washing. ONE APPLICATION IS USUALLY CURATIVE.
Sexual contacts should be treated simultaneously.
Avoid unnecessary skin contact. Particularly when applying to more than one patient, those assisting in lindane therapy (especially pregnant and/or nursing women) should wear rubber gloves.
Avoid use on open cuts and extensive excoriations.
Many patients exhibit persistent pruritus after treatment; this is rarely a sign of treatment failure and is not an indication for retreatment unless living mites can be demonstrated.

CAUTION

Federal law prohibits dispensing without prescription.

HOW SUPPLIED

KWELL Cream in tubes of 2 oz (57 g).

Continued on next page

Reed & Carnrick—Cont.

REFERENCES

1. Feldmann, R.J. and Maibach, H.I., *Toxicol. Applied. Pharmacol.*, 28:126, 1974.
2. Dale, W.E., Curly, A. and Cueto, C. *Life Sci* 5:47, 1966.
3. Ginsburg, C.M., et al., *J. Pediatr.* 91:6, 998–1000, 1977.
4. Nagasaki, T., Tomii, S., Mepa, T., Marugami, M. and Ito, *N. Gann* (Cancer) 63(3):393, 1972.
5. Goto, M. Hattori, M., Miyagawa, T. and Enomoto, M., *Chemosphere* 6:279, 1972.
6. Hanada, M., Yatani, C., Miyaji, T., *Gann* 64:511, 1973.
7. Weisse, I, and Herbst, M., *Toxicol.* 7:233, 1977.
8. Technical Report Series, NCI-CG-TR-14, *HEW PUBLICATIONS*, No. (NIH) 77–814.
9. Thorpe, E., and Walker, A.I.T., *Food Cosmetic Toxicol.* 11:433, 1973.
10. Orr, J.W., *Nature* 162:189, 1948.
11. Kashyap, S.K. et al., *J. Environ, Sci. Health* 14:305–318, 1979.

MANUFACTURED FOR
REED & CARNRICK
Piscataway, NJ 08855
By Reedco Inc., Humacao, PR 00661

Date of Revision
May 1989
Shown in Product Identification Section, page 423

KWELL® Lotion   ℞
[*kwel*]
(lindane) 1%

DESCRIPTION

KWELL Lotion (lindane) 1% is an ectoparasiticide and ovicide effective against Sarcoptes scabiei (scabies). In addition to the active ingredient, lindane, it contains glycerol monostearate, cetyl alcohol, stearic acid, trolamine, 2-amino-2-methyl-1 propanol, methyl p-hydroxybenzoate, butyl p-hydroxybenzoate, carrageenan perfume and purified water to form a non-greasy lotion. Lindane, which is the highly purified gamma isomer of 1, 2, 3, 4, 5, 6, hexachlorocyclohexane, has the following chemical structure.

CLINICAL PHARMACOLOGY

KWELL Lotion exerts its parasiticidal action by being directly absorbed into the parasites and their ova. Feldmann and Maibach[1] reported approximately 10% absorption of a lindane acetone solution applied to the forearm and left in place to 24 hours. Dale, et al[2] reported a blood level of 290ng/ml associated with convulsions following the accidental ingestion of a lindane containing product. Ginsburg[3] found a mean peak blood level of 28ng/ml 6 hours after total body application of KWELL Lotion to scabietic infants and children. The half-life was determined to be 18 hours.

INDICATIONS AND USAGE

KWELL Lotin is indicated for the treatment of patients infested with Sarcoptes scabiei (scabies).

CONTRAINDICATIONS

KWELL Lotion is contraindicated for premature neonates because their skin may be more permeable than full term infants and their liver enzymes may not be sufficiently developed. It is also contraindicated for patients with known seizure disorders and for individuals with a known sensitivity to the product or any of its components.

WARNINGS

LINDANE PENETRATES HUMAN SKIN AND HAS THE POTENTIAL FOR CNS TOXICITY (SEE CLINICAL PHARMACOLOGY SECTION). KWELL CREAM SHOULD BE USED ACCORDING TO RECOMMENDED DOSAGE (SEE DIRECTIONS FOR USE) ESPECIALLY ON INFANTS, PREGNANT WOMEN AND NURSING MOTHERS. ANIMAL STUDIES INDICATE THAT POTENTIAL TOXIC EFFECTS OF TOPICALLY APPLIED LINDANE ARE GREATER IN THE YOUNG. Seizures have been reported after excessive use or oral ingestion of lindane. No residual effects of KWELL treatment have been demonstrated, therefore, this product should not be used to ward off a possible infestation. If accidental ingestion occurs prompt gastric lavage is indicated. Because oils may enhance absorption, saline rather than oily cathartics should be used. Central nervous excitation can be controlled by the administration of pentobarbital, phenobarbital or diazepam.

PRECAUTIONS
General

Care should be taken to avoid contact with the eyes. If such contact occurs, eyes should be immediately flushed with water. If irritation or sensitization occurs, the patient should be advised to consult a physician.
Information to Patients

Patients should be instructed on the proper use of the medication. Directions for Use should accompany the prescription.

LABORATORY TESTS

No laboratory tests are needed for the proper use of this medication.

DRUG INTERACTIONS

Oils may enhance absorption, therefore, simultaneous use of creams, ointments or oils should be avoided.

CARCINOGENESIS

Although no studies have been conducted with KWELL Lotion, numerous long term feeding studies have been conducted in mice and rats to evaluate the carcinogenic potential of the technical grade of hexachlorocyclohexane (BHC) as well as the alpha, beta, gamma lindane) and delta isomers. Both oral and topical applications have been evaluated. Nagasaki[4], Goto[5] and Hanada[6] found varying amounts of benign and malignant hepatomas associated with BHC and the alpha, delta and epsilon isomers. None reported a carcinogenic potential for lindane. Tumors were found only in the animals which had received the alpha isomer. Weisse and Herbst[7] also evaluated the carcinogenic potential of lindane in mice but could find no evidence of lindane in mice but could find no evidnece of lindane carcinogenicity. The National Cancer Institute[8] also found no evidence of carcinogenicity.
Thorpe and Walker[9] compared beta BHC with lindane, dieldrin, DDT and hexabarbital in mice. Despite the unusually high incidence of tumors in the control group, they concluded that 600 ppm of lindane was associated with a significant increase in the incidence of hepatoma and thus considered it a tumorigen.
Orr[10] and Kashyap, et al[11] evaluated the carcinogenic potential in mice of topically applied BHC. In neither study was there any evidence of a tumorigenic or carcinogenic potential associated with topical application of BHC.
Mutagenicity tests have been used as predictive information about the carcinogenicity of various chemical compounds. Numerous types of mutagenicity tests have been performed with lindane. The results of these tests do not indicate that lindane is mutagenic.

PREGNANCY
Teratogenic Effects

Pregnancy category B: Reproduction, including multigeneration, studies have been performed in mice, rats, rabbits, pigs, and dogs at doses up to 10 times the human dose and have revealed no evidence of impaired fertility or harm to the fetus due to administered lindane. There are, however, no adequate and well controlled studies in pregnant women. Because animal reproduction studies are not always predictive of human response, the recommended dosage should not be exceeded on pregnant women. They should be treated no more than twice during a pregnancy.

NURSING MOTHERS

Lindane is secreted in human milk in low concentrations. Studies conducted in the United States as well as Europe and South America found levels of lindane in human milk ranging from 0 to 113 ppb, as the result of ingestion of foods which had been treated with lindane. There appeared to be no difference in concentrations between country and urban dwellers. Although the levels of lindane found in blood after topical application with KWELL Lotion make it unlikely that amounts of lindane sufficient to cause serious adverse reactions will be excreted in the milk of nursing mothers who have used KWELL Lotion, if there is any concern, an alternate method of feeding may be used for 2 days.

PEDIATRIC USE

Refer to the Contraindications and Warnings sections.

ADVERSE REACTIONS

Lindane has been reported to cause central nervous stimulation ranging from dizziness to convulsions. Cases of convulsions have been reported in connection with KWELL Lotion therapy. However, these incidents were almost always associated with accidental oral ingestion or misuse of the product. Eczematous eruptions due to irritation from this product have also been reported. Incidence of these adverse reactions is relatively infrequent, occurring in less than 1 in 100,000 patients.

DRUG ABUSE AND DEPENDENCE

KWELL Lotion is not subject to abuse, nor is there any dependence on the drug.

OVERDOSAGE

Overdosage or oral ingestion of KWELL Lotion can cause central nervous system excitation and, if taken in sufficient quantities, convulsions may occur.
If accidental ingestion occurs, prompt gastric lavage should be instituted. However, since oils favor absorption, saline cathartics for intestinal evacuation should be given rather than oil laxatives. If central nervous system manifestations occur they can be antagonized by the administration of pentobarbital, phenobarbital or diazepam.

DOSAGE AND ADMINISTRATION

CAUTION: USE ONLY AS DIRECTED. DO NOT EXCEED RECOMENDED DOSAGE
No residual effects of KWELL treatment have been demonstrated therefore, this product should not be used to ward off a possible infestation.
    NOTE: PLEASE READ CAREFULLY.

DIRECTIONS FOR USE

Scabies (sarcoptes scabiei)—The lotion should be applied to dry skin in a thin layer and rubbed in thoroughly. If crusted lesions are present, a tepid bath preceding the medication is helpful. If a bath is used, allow the skin to dry before applying the lotion. Usually two ounces are sufficient for an adult. A total body application should be made from the neck down including the soles of the feet. Scabies rarely affects the head of children or adults but may occur in infants. The lotion should be left on for 8–12 hours and should then be removed by thorough washing. ONE APPLICATION IS USUALLY CURATIVE.
Sexual contacts should be treated simultaneously.
Avoid unnecessary skin contact. Particularly when applying to more than one patient, those assisting in lindane therapy (especially pregnant and/or nursing women) should wear rubber gloves.
Avoid use on open cuts and extensive excoriations.
Many patients exhibit persistent pruritus after treatment; this is rarely a sign of treatment failure and is not an indication for retreatment unless living mites can be demonstrated.

CAUTION

Federal law prohibits dispensing without prescription.

HOW SUPPLIED

KWELL Lotion in in bottles of 59 ml (2 fl. oz.) and 472 ml (16 fl. oz.) and 3.8 liters (1 gallon).

REFERENCES

1. Feldmann, R.J. and Maibach, H.I., *Toxicol. Applied. Pharmacol.*, 28:126, 1974.
2. Dale, W.E., Curly, A. and Cueto, C. *Life Sci* 5:47, 1966.
3. Ginsburg, C.M., et al., *J. Pediatr.* 91:6, 998–1000, 1977.
4. Nagasaki, T., Tomii, S., Mepa, T., Marugami, M. and Ito, *N. Gann* (Cancer) 63(3):393, 1972.
5. Goto, M. Hattori, M., Miyagawa, T. and Enomoto, M., *Chemosphere* 6:279, 1972.
6. Hanada, M., Yatani, C., Miyaji, T., *Gann* 64:511, 1973.
7. Weisse, I, and Herbst, M., *Toxicol.* 7:233, 1977.
8. Technical Report Series, NCI-CG-TR-14, *HEW PUBLICATIONS*, No. (NIH) 77–814.
9. Thorpe, E., and Walker, A.I.T., *Food Cosmetic Toxicol.* 11:433, 1973.
10. Orr, J.W., *Nature* 162:189, 1948.
11. Kashyap, S.K. et al., *J. Environ, Sci. Health* 14:305–318, 1979.

MANUFACTURED FOR
REED & CARNRICK
Piscataway, NJ 08855
By Reedco Inc., Humacao, PR 00661

Date of Revision
May 1989
Shown in Product Identification Section, page 423

KWELL® Shampoo   ℞
[*kwel*]
(lindane) 1%

DESCRIPTION

KWELL Shampoo (lindane) 1% is an ectoparasiticide and ovicide effective against Pediculosis capitis (head lice), Pediculosis pubis (crab lice) and their ova. In addition to the active ingredient, lindane, it contains Trolamine Lauryl Sulfate, Polysorbate 60, acetone and purified water to form a cosmetically pleasant shampoo. Lindane, which is the highly purified gamma isomer of 1, 2, 3, 4, 5, 6, hexachlorocyclohexane, has the following chemical structure:

CLINICAL PHARMACOLOGY

KWELL Shampoo exerts its parasiticidal action by being directly absorbed into the parasites and their ova. Dale et al.[1] reported a blood level of 290ng/ml associated with convulsions following the accidental ingestion of a lindane containing product. Analysis of blood taken from subjects before and after the use of KWELL Shampoo showed a mean peak blood level of only 3ng/ml which appeared at six hours and disappeared at eight hours after the shampoo was applied.[2].

INDICATIONS AND USAGE

KWELL Shampoo is indicated for the treatment of patients infested with Pediculus capitis (head lice), Pediculus pubis (crab lice) and their ova.

CONTRAINDICATIONS

KWELL Shampoo is contraindicated for premature neonates because their skin may be more permeable than full term infants and their liver enzymes may not be sufficiently developed. It is also contraindicated for patients with known seizure disorders and for individuals with a known sensitivity to the product or any of its components.

WARNINGS

LINDANE PENETRATES HUMAN SKIN AND HAS THE POTENTIAL FOR CNS TOXICITY (SEE CLINICAL PHARMACOLOGY SECTION). KWELL SHAMPOO SHOULD BE USED ACCORDING TO RECOMMENDED DOSAGE (SEE DIRECTIONS FOR USE) ESPECIALLY ON INFANTS, PREGNANT WOMEN AND NURSING MOTHERS. ANIMAL STUDIES INDICATE THAT POTENTIAL TOXIC EFFECTS OF TOPICALLY APPLIED LINDANE ARE GREATER IN THE YOUNG. Seizures have been reported after excessive use or oral ingestion of lindane. No residual effects of KWELL treatment have been demonstrated, therefore, this product should not be used to ward off a possible infestation.

If accidental ingestion occurs prompt gastric lavage is indicated. Because oils may enhance absorption, saline rather than oily cathartics should be used. Central nervous excitation can be controlled by the administration of pentobarbital, phenobarbital or diazepam.

PRECAUTIONS

General

Care should be taken to avoid contact with the eyes. If such contact occurs, eyes should be immediately flushed with water. If irritation or sensitization occurs, the patient should be advised to consult a physician.

Information to Patients

Patients should be instructed on the proper use of the medication. Directions for use should accompany the prescription.

LABORATORY TESTS

No laboratory tests are needed for the proper use of this medication.

DRUG INTERACTIONS

Oils may enhance absorption, therefore, if an oil-based hair dressing is used, it is recommended that the hair be shampooed, rinsed and dried before application of KWELL Shampoo.

CARCINOGENESIS

Although no studies have been conducted with KWELL Shampoo, numerous long term feeding studies have been conducted in mice and rats to evaluate the carcinogenic potential of the technical grade of hexachlorocyclohexane (BHC) as well as the alpha, beta, gamma (lindane) and delta isomers. Both oral and topical applications have been evaluated. Nagasaki[3], Goto[4] and Hanada[5] found varying amounts of benign and malignant hepatomas associated with BHC and the alpha, delta and epsilon isomers. None reported a carcinogenic potential for lindane. Tumors were found only in the animals which had received the alpha isomer. Weisse and Herbst[6] also evaluated the carcinogenic potential of lindane in mice but could find no evidence of lindane carcinogenicity. The National Cancer Institute[7] had also found no evidence of carcinogenicity.

Thorpe and Walker[8] compared beta BHC with lindane, dieldrin, DDT and hexabarbital in mice. Despite the unusually high incidence of tumors in the control group, they concluded that 600 ppm of lindane was associated with a significant increase in the incidence of hepatoma and thus, considered it a tumorigen.

Orr[9] and Kashyap, et al[10] evaluated the carcinogenic potential in mice of topically applied BHC. In neither study was there any evidence of a tumorigenic or carcinogenic potential associated with topical application of BHC.

Mutagenicity tests have been used as predictive information about the carcinogenicity of various chemical compounds. Numerous types of mutagenicity tests have been performed with lindane. The results of these tests do not indicate that lindane is mutapenic.

PREGNANCY

Teratogenic Effects

Pregnancy category B: Reproduction, including multigeneration, studies have been performed in mice, rats, rabbits, pigs, and dogs at doses up to 10 times the human dose and have revealed no evidence of impaired fertility or harm to the fetus due to orally administered lindane. There are, however, no adequate and well controlled studies in pregnant women. Because animal reproduction studies are not always predictive of human response, the recommended dosage should not be exceeded on pregnant women. They should be treated no more than twice during a pregnancy.

NURSING MOTHERS

Lindane is secreted in human milk in low concentrations. Studies conducted in the United States as well as Europe and South America found levels of lindane in human milk ranging from 0 to 113 ppb, as the result of ingestion of foods which had been treated with lindane. There appeared to be no difference in concentrations between country and urban dwellers. Although the levels of lindane found in blood after topical application with KWELL Shampoo make it unlikely that amounts of lindane sufficient to cause serious adverse reactions will be excreted in the milk of nursing mothers who have used KWELL Shampoo, if there is any concern, an alternate method of feeding may be used for 2 days.

PEDIATRIC USE

Refer to the Contraindications and Warnings sections.

ADVERSE REACTIONS

Lindane has been reported to cause central nervous stimulation ranging from dizziness to convulsions. Cases of convulsions have been reported in connection with KWELL Shampoo therapy. However, these incidents were almost always associated with accidental oral ingestion or misuse of the product. Eczematous eruptions due to irritation from this product have also been reported. Incidence of these adverse reactions is relatively infrequent, occurring in less than 1 in 100,000 patients.

DRUG ABUSE AND DEPENDENCE

KWELL Shampoo is not subject to abuse nor is there any dependence on the drug.

OVERDOSAGE

Overdosage or oral ingestion of KWELL Shampoo can cause central nervous system excitation and, if taken in sufficient quantities, convulsions may occur.

If accidental ingestion occurs, prompt gastric lavage should be instituted. However, since oils favor absorption, saline cathartics for intestinal evacuation should be given rather than oil laxatives. If central nervous system manifestations occur, they can be antagonized by the administration of pentobarbital, phenobarbital or diazepam.

DOSAGE AND ADMINISTRATION

CAUTION: USE ONLY AS DIRECTED. DO NOT EXCEED RECOMMENDED DOSAGE.

No residual effects of KWELL treatment have been demonstrated, therefore, this product should not be used to ward off a possible infestation.

NOTE: PLEASE READ CAREFULLY

DIRECTIONS FOR USE

Pediculosis capitis (head lice)—1) Apply a sufficient quantity of the shampoo to the dry hair. Approximately 1 oz. (30ml) for short, 1.5 oz. (45 ml) for medium and 2 oz. (60 ml) for long hair. 2) Work thoroughly into the hair and allow to remain in place four minutes. 3) Add small quantities of water until a good lather forms. 4) Rinse thoroughly. Towel briskly. Nits should be removed using a nit comb or tweezers.

Pediculosis pubis (crab lice)—1) Apply a sufficient quantity of the shampoo to the dry hair. 2) Work thoroughly into the hair and allow to remain in place four minutes. 3) Add small quantities of water until a good lather forms. 4) Rinse thoroughly. Towel briskly. Nits should be removed using a nit comb or tweezers.

Retreatment is usually not necessary. Demonstrable living organisms after 7 days indicate that retreatment is necessary.

NOTE

1. If person to be treated uses an oil-based hair dressing, it is recommended that their hair be shampooed and dried before applying KWELL Shampoo.
2. Avoid unnecessary skin contact. Particularly when applying to more than one patient, those assisting in lindane therapy (especially pregnant and/or nursing women) should wear rubber gloves.
3. Avoid use on open cuts and extensive excoriations. Sexual contacts should be treated simultaneously.

CAUTION

Federal law prohibits dispensing without prescription.

HOW SUPPLIED

KWELL Shampoo in bottles of 59 ml (2 fl. oz.) and 472 ml (16 fl. oz.) and 3.8 liters (1 gallon).

REFERENCES

1. Dale, W.E., Curly, A. and Cueto, C. *Life Sci* 5:47, 1966.
2. Data on File at Reed & Carnrick.
3. Nagasaki, T., Tomii, S., Mega, T., Marugami, M. and Ito, N. *Gann* (Cancer) 63(3):373, 1972.
4. Goto, M., Hattori, M., Miyagawa, T. and Enomoto, M., *Chemosphere* 6:279, 1972.
5. Hanada, M., Yatani, C., Miyaji, T., *Gann* 64:511, 1973.
6. Weisse, I. and Herbst, M., *Toxicol.* 7:233, 1977.
7. Technical Report Series, NCI-CG-TR-14, *HEW PUBLICATIONS*, No. (NIH) 77–814.
8. Thorpe, E., and Walker, A.I.T., *Food Cosmetic Toxicol.* 11:433, 1973.
9. Orr, J.W., *Nature* 162:189, 1948.
10. Kashyap, S.K., et al, *J. Environ. Sci. Health* 14:305–318, 1979.

MANUFACTURED FOR
REED & CARNRICK
Piscataway, NJ 08855
By Reedco Inc., Humacao, P.R. 00661

Date of Revision
May 1989
Shown in Product Identification Section, page 423

LEVATOL®   ℞
[lev'a-tol]
(penbutolol sulfate)
TABLETS

Levatol® (penbutolol sulfate) is a synthetic β-receptor antagonist for oral administration. The chemical name of penbutolol sulfate is (S)-1-tert-Butylamino-3-(o-cyclopentylphenoxy)-2-propanol sulfate. It is provided as the levorotatory isomer. The empirical formula for penbutolol sulfate is $C_{36}H_{60}N_2O_8S$. Its molecular weight is 680.94. A dose of 20 mg is equivalent to 29.4 μmol. The structural formula is as follows:

Penbutolol is a white, odorless, crystalline powder. Levatol is available as tablets for oral administration. Each tablet contains 20 mg of penbutolol sulfate. It also contains corn starch, D&C Yellow No. 10, lactose, magnesium stearate, povidone, silicon dioxide, talc, titanium dioxide, and other inactive ingredients.

CLINICAL PHARMACOLOGY

Penbutolol is a β-1, β-2 (nonselective) adrenergic receptor antagonist. Experimental studies showed a dose-dependent increase in heart rate in reserpinized (norepinephrine-depleted) rats given penbutolol intravenously at doses of 0.25 to 1.0 mg/kg, suggesting that penbutolol has some intrinsic sympathomimetic activity. In human studies, however, heart rate decreases have been similar to those seen with propranolol.

Penbutolol antagonizes the heart rate effects of exercise and infused isoproterenol. The β-blocking potency of penbutolol is approximately 4 times that of propranolol. An oral dose of less than 10 mg will reduce exercise-induced tachycardia to one-half its usual level; maximum antagonism follows doses of 10 to 20 mg. The peak effect is between 1.5 and 3 hours after oral administration. The duration of effect exceeds 20 hours during a once-daily dosing regimen. During chronic administration of penbutolol, the duration of antihypertensive effects permits a once-daily dosage schedule.

Acute hemodynamic effects of penbutolol have been studied following single intravenous doses between 0.1 and 4 mg. The cardiovascular responses included significant reductions in heart rate, left ventricular maximum dP/dt, cardiac output, stroke volume index, stroke work, and stroke work index. Systolic pressure and mean arterial pressure were reduced, and total peripheral resistance was increased.

Chronic administration of penbutolol to hypertensive patients results in the hemodynamic pattern typical of β-adrenergic blocking drugs: a reduction in cardiac index, heart rate, systolic and diastolic blood pressures, and the product of heart rate and mean arterial pressure both at rest and with all levels of exercise, without significant change in total peripheral resistance. Penbutolol causes a reduction in left ventricular contractility. Penbutolol decreases glomerular filtration rate, but not significantly.

In clinical trial doses of 10 to 80 mg per day in single daily doses have reduced supine and standing systolic and diastolic blood pressures. In most studies, effects were small, generally a change in blood pressure 5 to 8/3 to 5 mm Hg

Continued on next page

Reed & Carnrick—Cont.

greater than seen with a placebo measured 24 hours after dosing. It is not clear whether this relatively small effect reflects a characteristic of penbutolol or the particular population studied (the population had relatively mild hypertension but did not appear unusual in others respects). In a direct comparison of penbutolol with adequate doses of twice daily propranolol, no difference in blood pressure effect was seen. In a comparison of placebo and 10-, 20- and 40 mg single daily doses of penbutolol, no significant dose-related difference was seen in response to active drug at 6 weeks, but compared to the 10 mg dose, the two larger doses showed greater effects at 2 and 4 weeks and reached their maximum effect at 2 weeks. In several studies, dose increases from 40 to 80 mg were without additional effect on blood pressure. Response rates to penbutolol are unaffected by sex or age but are greater in caucasians than blacks.

Penbutolol decreases plasma renin activity in normal subjects and in patients with essential and renovascular hypertension. The mechanisms of the antihypertensive actions of β-receptor antagonists have not been established. However, factors that may be involved are: (1) competitive antagonism of catecholamines at peripheral adrenergic receptor sites (especially cardiac) that leads to decreased cardiac output; (2) a central-nervous-system (CNS) action that results in a decrease in tonic sympathetic neural outflow to the periphery; and (3) a reduction of renin secretion through blockade of β-receptors involved in release of renin from the kidneys.

Penbutolol dose dependently increases the RR and QT intervals. There is no influence on the PR, QRS or QT (corrected) intervals.

Pharmacokinetics—Following oral administration, penbutolol is rapidly and completely absorbed. Peak plasma concentrations of penbutolol occur between 2 and 3 hours after oral administration and are proportional to single and multiple doses between 10 and 40 mg once a day. The average plasma elimination half-life of penbutolol is approximately 5 hours in normal subjects. There is no significant difference in the plasma half-life of penbutolol in healthy elderly persons or patients on renal dialysis. Twelve to 24 hours after oral administration of doses up to 120 mg, plasma concentrations of parent drug are 0% to 10% of the peak level. No accumulation of penbutolol is observed in hypertensive patients after 8 days of therapy at doses of 40 mg daily or 20 mg twice a day. Penbutolol is approximately 80% to 98% bound to plasma proteins.

The metabolism of penbutolol in humans involves conjugation and oxidation. The metabolites are excreted principally in the urine. When radiolabeled penbutolol was administered to humans, approximately 90% of the radioactivity was excreted in the urine. Approximately $\frac{1}{6}$ of the dose of penbutolol was recovered as penbutolol conjugate, while the remaining fraction was not identified. Conjugated penbutolol has a plasma elimination half-life of approximately 20 hours in healthy persons, 25 hours in healthy elderly persons and 100 hours in patients on renal dialysis. Thus, accumulation of penbutolol conjugate may be expected upon multiple-dosing in renal insufficiency. An alternative metabolite of penbutolol, 4-hydroxypenbutolol, has been identified in small quantities in plasma and urine. It is $\frac{1}{8}$ to $\frac{1}{15}$ times as active as the parent compound in blocking isoproterenol-induced β-adrenergic receptor responses in isolated guinea-pig trachea and is $\frac{1}{8}$ to 1 times as potent in anesthetized dogs.

INDICATIONS AND USAGE

Levatol is indicated in the treatment of mild to moderate arterial hypertension. It may be used alone or in combination with other antihypertensive agents, especially thiazide-type diuretics.

CONTRAINDICATIONS

Levatol is contraindicated in patients with cardiogenic shock, sinus bradycardia, second and third degree atrioventricular conduction block, bronchial asthma, and those with known hypersensitivity to this product (see WARNINGS).

WARNINGS

Cardiac Failure—Sympathetic stimulation may be essential for supporting circulatory function in patients with heart failure, and its inhibition by β-adrenergic receptor blockade may precipitate more severe failure. Although β-blockers should be avoided in overt congestive heart failure, Levatol can, if necessary, be used with caution in patients with a history of cardiac failure who are well compensated, on treatment with vasodilators, digitalis and/or diuretics. Both digitalis and penbutolol slow AV conduction. Beta-adrenergic receptor antagonists do not inhibit the inotropic action of digitalis on heart muscle. If cardiac failure persists, treatment with Levatol should be discontinued.

Patients Without History of Cardiac Failure—Continued depression of the myocardium with β-blocking agents over a period of time can, in some cases, lead to cardiac failure. At the first evidence of heart failure, patients receiving Levatol should be given appropriate treatment, and the response

should be closely observed. If cardiac failure continues despite adequate intervention with appropriate drugs, Levatol should be withdrawn (gradually, if possible).

Exacerbation of Ischemic Heart Disease Following Abrupt Withdrawal—Hypersensitivity to catecholamines has been observed in patients who were withdrawn from therapy with β-blocking agents; exacerbation of angina, and, in some cases, myocardial infarction have occurred after abrupt discontinuation of such therapy. When discontinuing Levatol, particularly in patients with ischemic heart disease, the dosage should be reduced gradually over a period of 1 to 2 weeks and the patient should be monitored carefully. If angina becomes more pronounced or acute coronary insufficiency develops, administration of Levatol should be reinstated promptly, at least on a temporary basis, and appropriate measures should be taken for the management of unstable angina. Patients should be warned against interruption or discontinuation of therapy without the physician's advice. Because coronary artery disease is common and may not be recognized, it may not be prudent to discontinue Levatol abruptly, even in patients who are being treated only for hypertension.

Nonallergic Bronchospasm (e.g., chronic bronchitis, emphysema)—Levatol is contraindicated in bronchial asthma. In general, patients with bronchospastic diseases should not receive β-blockers. Levatol should be administered with caution because it may block bronchodilation produced by endogenous catecholamine stimulation of β-2 receptors.

Anesthesia and Major Surgery—The necessity, or desirability, of withdrawal of a β-blocking therapy prior to major surgery is controversial. Beta-adrenergic receptor blockade impairs the ability of the heart to respond to β-adrenergically mediated reflex stimuli. Although this might be of benefit in preventing arrhythmic response, the risk of excessive myocardial depression during general anesthesia may be enhanced and difficulty in restarting and maintaining the heartbeat has been reported with β-blockers. If treatment is continued, particular care should be taken when using anesthetic agents that depress the myocardium, such as ether, cyclopropane, and trichloroethylene, and it is prudent to use the lowest possible dose of Levatol. Levatol like other β-blockers, is a competitive inhibitor β-receptor agonists, and its effect on the heart can be reversed by cautious administration of such agents (e.g., dobutamine or isoproterenol—see Overdose). Manifestations of excessive vagal tone (e.g., profound bradycardia, hypotension) may be corrected with atropine 1 to 3 mg IV in divided doses.

Diabetes Mellitus and Hypoglycemia—Beta-adrenergic receptor blockade may prevent the appearance of signs and symptoms of acute hypoglycemia, such as tachycardia and blood pressure changes. This is especially important in patients with labile diabetes. Beta-blockade also reduces the release of insulin in response to hyperglycemia; therefore, it may be necessary to adjust the dose of hypoglycemic drugs. Beta-adrenergic blockade may also impair the homeostatic response to hypoglycemia; in that event, the spontaneous recovery from hypoglycemia may be delayed during treatment with β-adrenergic receptor antagonists.

Thyrotoxicosis—Beta-adrenergic blockade may mask certain clinical signs (e.g., tachycardia) of hyperthyrodism. Patients suspected of developing thyrotoxicosis should be managed carefully to avoid abrupt withdrawal of β-adrenergic receptor blockers that might precipitate a thyroid storm.

PRECAUTIONS

Information for Patients—Patients, especially those with evidence of coronary artery insufficiency, should be warned against interruption or discontinuation of Levatol without the physician's advice. Although cardiac failure rarely occurs in properly selected patients, those being treated with β-adrenergic receptor antagonists should be advised of the symptoms of heart failure and to report such symptoms immediately, should they develop.

Drug Interactions—Levatol has been used in combination with hydrochlorothiazide in at least 100 patients without unexpected adverse reactions.

In one study, the combination of penbutolol and alcohol increased the number of errors in the eye-hand psychomotor function test.

Penbutolol increases the volume of distribution of lidocaine in normal subjects. This could result in a requirement for higher loading doses of lidocaine.

Cimetidine has no effect on the clearance of penbutolol. The major metabolite of penbutolol is a glucuronide, and it has been shown that cimetidine does not inhibit glucoronidation. Synergistic hypotensive effects, bradycardia, and arrhythmias have been reported in some patients receiving β-adrenergic blocking agents when an oral calcium antagonist was added to the treatment regimen.

Generally, Levatol should not be used in patients receiving catecholamine-depleting drugs.

Carcinogenesis, Mutagenesis, and Impairment of Fertility—There was no evidence of carcinogenicity observed in a 21-month study in mice or a 2-year study in rats. Mice were given penbutolol in the diet for 18 months at doses up to 395 mg/kg/day (about 500 times the maximum recommended

dose of 40 mg in a 50 kg person). Rats were given 141 mg/kg/day for the same length of time. Mice were observed for 3 months and rats for 5.5 to 7 months after termination of treatment before necropsy was performed.

No evidence of mutagenic activity of penbutolol was seen in the *Salmonella* mutagenicity test (Ames test), the point mutation induction test (*Saccharomyces*) and the micronucleus test.

Penbutolol had no adverse effects on fertility or general reproductive performance in mice and rats at oral doses up to 172 mg/kg/day.

Pregnancy—Teratogenic Effects: Pregnancy Category C—Teratology studies in rats and rabbits revealed no teratogenic effects related to treatment with penbutolol at oral doses up to 200 mg/kg/day (250 times the maximum recommended human dose). In rabbits, a slight increase in the intrauterine fetal mortality and a reduced 24-hour offspring survival rate were observed in the groups treated with 125 mg/kg/day (156 times the maximum recommended dose) but not in the groups treated with 0.2 and 5 mg (0.25 to 6 times the maximum recommended dose).

There are no adequate and well-controlled studies in pregnant women. Levatol should be used during pregnancy only if the potential benefit justifies the potential risk to the fetus.

Nonteratogenic Effects—In a perinatal and postnatal study in rats, the pup body weight and pup survival rate were reduced at the highest dose level of 160 mg/kg/day (200 times the maximum recommended dose).

Nursing Mothers—It is not known whether Levatol is excreted in human milk. Because many drugs are excreted in human milk, caution should be exercised when Levatol is administered to a nursing woman.

Usage in Children—Safety and effectiveness of Levatol in children have not been established.

ADVERSE REACTIONS

Levatol is usually well tolerated in properly selected patients. Most adverse effects observed during clinical trials have been mild and reversible.

Table 1 lists the adverse reactions reported from 4 controlled studies conducted in the United States involving once-a-day administration of Levatol (at doses ranging from 10 to 120 mg) as monotherapy or in combination with hydrochlorothiazide. Levatol doses above 40 mg/day are not, however, recommended. The table includes only those events where the prevalence rate in the Levatol group was at least 1.5%, or where the reaction is of particular interest.

Over a dose range from 10 to 40 mg, once a day, fatigue, nausea, and sexual impotence occurred at a greater frequency as the dose was increased.

[See table on top next page].

In a double-blind clinical trial comparing Levatol (40 mg and greater once a day) and propranolol (40 mg or more twice a day), heart rates of less than 60 beats/min were recorded at least once in 25% of the patients in the group receiving Levatol and in 37% of the patients in the propranolol group. Corresponding figures for heart rates of less than 50 beats/min were 1.2% and 6%, respectively. No symptoms associated with bradycardia were reported.

Discontinuations of Levatol because of adverse reactions has ranged between 2.4% and 6.9% of patients in double-blind, parallel, controlled clinical trials, as compared to 1.8% to 4.1% in the corresponding control groups that were given placebo. The frequency and severity of adverse reactions have not increased during long-term administration of Levatol. The prevalence of adverse reactions reported from 4 controlled clinical trials (referred to in Table 1) as reasons for discontinuation of therapy by ≥ 0.5% of the Levatol group is listed in Table 2.

[See table on bottom next page].

Potential Adverse Effects—In addition, certain adverse effects not listed above have been reported with other β-blocking agents and should also be considered as potential adverse effects of Levatol.

Central Nervous System—Reversible mental depression progressing to catatonia (an acute syndrome characterized by disorientation for time and place), short-term memory loss, emotional lability, slightly clouded sensorium, and decreased performance (neuropsychometrics).

Cardiovascular—Intensification of AV block (seeCONTRAINDICATIONS).

Allergic—Erythematous rash, fever combined with aching and sore throat, laryngospasm, and respiratory distress.

Hematologic—Agranulocytosis, nonthrombocytopenic and thrombocytopenic purpura.

Gastrointestinal—Mesenteric arterial thrombosis and ischemic colitis.

Miscellaneous—Reversible alopecia and Peyronie's disease. The oculomucocutaneous syndrome associated with the β-blocker practolol has not been reported with Levatol during investigational use and extensive foreign clinical experience.

OVERDOSAGE

There is no actual experience with Levatol overdose. The signs and symptoms that would be expected with overdosage

Table 1.
ADVERSE REACTIONS DURING CONTROLLED U.S. STUDIES

Body System Experience	Penbutolol (N = 628) %	Placebo (N = 212) %	Propranolol (N = 266) %
Body as a Whole			
Asthenia	1.6	0.9	4.9
Pain, chest	2.4	2.8	2.3
Pain, limb	2.4	1.4	1.5
Digestive System			
Diarrhea	3.3	1.9	2.6
Nausea	4.3	0.9	2.3
Dyspepsia	2.7	1.4	5.3
Nervous System			
Dizziness	4.9	2.4	4.2
Fatigue	4.4	1.9	2.6
Headache	7.8	6.1	7.5
Insomnia	1.9	0.9	2.6
Respiratory System			
Cough	2.1	0.5	1.1
Dyspnea	2.1	1.4	3.4
Upper respiratory infection	2.5	3.3	4.9
Skin and Appendages			
Sweating, excessive	1.6	0.5	2.3
Urogenital System			
Impotency, sexual	0.5	0.0	0.8

of β-adrenergic receptor antagonists are symptomatic bradycardia, hypotension, bronchospasm, and acute cardiac failure. In addition to discontinuation of Levatol, gastric emptying, and close observatioin of the patient, the following measures might be considered as appropriate:

Excessive Bradycardia —Administer atropine sulfate to induce vagal blockade. If bradycardia persists, intravenous isoproterenol hydrochloride may be administered cautiously; larger than usual doses may be needed. In refractory cases, the use of a transvenous cardiac pacemaker may be necessary.

Hypotension —Sympathomimetic drug therapy, such as dopamine, dobutamine, or levarterenol, may be considered if hypotension persists despite correction of bradycardia. In refractory cases, administration of glucagon hydrochloride has been reported to be useful.

Bronchospasm —A β-2-agonist or isoproterenol hydrochloride may be administered. Additional therapy with aminophylline may be considered.

Acute Cardiac Failure —Institute conventional therapy immediately. Intravenous administration of dobutamine and glucagon hydrochloride has been reported to be useful.

Heart Block (Second or Third Degree) —Isoproterenol hydrochloride or a transvenous cardiac pacemaker may be used.

DOSAGE AND ADMINISTRATION
The usual starting and maintenance dose of Levatol, used alone or in combination with other antihypertensive agents, such as thiazide-type diuretics is 20 mg given once daily. Doses of 40 mg and 80 mg have been well-tolerated but have not been shown to give a greater antihypertensive effect. The full effect of a 20- or 40-mg dose is seen by the end of 2 weeks. A dose of 10 mg also lowers blood pressure, but the full effect is not seen for 4 to 6 weeks.

HOW SUPPLIED
Tablets, yellow, scored capsule-shaped, engraved RC 22 20 mg—(100s) NDC 0021-4500-15.
Store at controlled room temperature 15–30°C (59–86°F) Keep tightly closed and protect from light.

ANIMAL TOXICOLOGY
Studies in rats indicated that the combination of penbutolol, triamterene, and hydrochlorothiazide (up to 40, 50 and 25 mg/kg respectively) increased the incidence and severity of renal tubular dilation and regeneration when compared to that in rats treated only with triamterene and hydrochlorothiazide. Dogs administered the same doses of triamterene and hydrochlorothiazide alone and in combination with penbutolol had an increase in serum alklaine phosphatase and serum alanine transferase, but there were no gross or microscopic abnormalities observed. No significant toxicologic findings were observed in rats and dogs treated with a combination of penbutolol and hydrochlorothiazide.

Date of last revision September 22, 1988

Manufactured for
REED & CARNRICK
Piscataway, NJ 08855
by ELI LILLY AND COMPANY
Indianapolis, IN 46285 USA   LV 281 G88
Shown in Product Identification Section, page 423

PHAZYME®   OTC
[*fā'zīm*]

DESCRIPTION
A two-phase tablet. Contains specially-activated simethicone, both in the outer layer for release in the stomach and in the inner enteric-coated core for release in the small intestine.
CONTAINS: ACTIVE INGREDIENTS: Specially-activated simethicone, both in the outer layer for release in the stomach and in the inner enteric-coated core for release in the small intestine, a total of 60 mg.
INACTIVE INGREDIENTS: Acacia, Calcium sulfate, Carnauba Wax, Crospovidone, D&C Red No. 7 Lake, FD&C Blue No. 1 Lake, Gelatin, Lactose, Microcrystalline Cellulose, Polyoxyl-40 Stearate, Polyvinyl Acetate Phthalate, Povidone, Pregelatinized Starch, Rice Starch, Sodium Benzoate, Sucrose, Titanium Dioxide.

ACTIONS/CLINICAL PHARMACOLOGY
PHAZYME is the only dual approach to the problem of gastrointestinal gas. Simethicone minimizes gas formation and relieves gas entrapment in both the stomach and lower G.I. tract. This action helps combat discomfort, due to gastrointestinal gas. Also, for relief of gas distress associated with other functional or organic conditions such as: diverticulitis, spastic colitis, hyperacidity, postcholecystectomy syndrome and chronic cholecystitis.

INDICATIONS AND USAGE
PHAZYME is indicated for the relief of occasional or chronic discomfort caused by gas entrapped in the stomach or in the lower gastrointestinal tract—resulting from aerophagia, post-operative distention, dyspepsia and food intolerance.

CONTRAINDICATIONS
A known sensitivity to any ingredient.

DOSAGE AND ADMINISTRATION
One or two tablets with each meal and at bedtime, or as directed by a physician.

HOW SUPPLIED
Pink coated two-phase tablet in bottles of 50, 100 and 1,000.
Revision Date May 1989
Shown in Product Identification Section, page 423

PHAZYME®–95 Tablets
[*fā'zīm*]

DESCRIPTION
CONTAINS: ACTIVE INGREDIENT: Specially-activated simethicone, both in the outer layer for release in the stomach and in the inner enteric-coated core for release in the small intestine, a total of 95 mg.
INACTIVE INGREDIENT: Acacia, Calcium Sulfate, Carnauba Wax, Crospovidone, FD&C Yellow No. 6 Lake, FD&C Red No. 40 Lake, Gelatin, Lactose, Microcrystalline Cellulose, Polyoxyl-40 Stearate, Polyvinyl Acetate Phthalate, Povidone, Pregelatinized Starch, Rice Starch, Sodium Benzoate, Sucrose, Titanium Dioxide.

ACTIONS/CLINICAL PHARMACOLOGY
SEE PHAZYME

INDICATIONS AND USAGE
SEE PHAZYME

DOSAGE AND ADMINISTRATION
One tablet with each meal and at bedtime, or as directed by a physician.

HOW SUPPLIED
Red coated two-phase tablet in 10 pack, bottles of 50, 100 and 500.
Revision Date Oct 1985
Shown in Product Identification Section, page 423

PHAZYME®–125 Softgels
[*fā'zīm*]

DESCRIPTION
A red capsule containing the highest dose of simethicone available in a single softgel.
ACTIVE INGREDIENTS: Simethicone 125 mg.
INACTIVE INGREDIENTS: Soybean oil, gelatin, glycerin, vegetable shortening, polysorbate 80, purified water, hydrogenated soybean oil, yellow wax, lecithin, titanium dioxide, FD&C Red #40, methylparaben, propylparaben.

ACTIONS/CLINICAL PHARMACOLOGY
SEE PHAZYME

INDICATIONS AND USAGE
SEE PHAZYME

DOSAGE AND ADMINISTRATION
One capsule with each meal and at bedtime, or as directed by a physician.

HOW SUPPLIED
Red capsule in 10 pack and bottle of 50.
Revision Date Oct 1985
Shown in Product Identification Section, page 423

PROCTOCREAM™–HC   ℞
[*prŏc'tō-krēm*]
(Hydrocortisone acetate 1% and Pramoxine hydrochloride 1%)

DESCRIPTION
PROCTO CREAM-HC™ is a topical preparation containing Hydrocortisone acetate 1.0% and Pramoxine hydrochloride 1.0% in a hydrophilic cream base containing stearic acid, cetyl alcohol, aquaphor, isopropylpalmitate, polyoxyl-40 stearate, propylene glycol, potassium sorbate 0.1%, sorbic acid 0.1%, triethanolamine lauryl sulfate and water.
Topical corticosteroids are anti-inflammatory and anti-pruritic agents. The chemical structural formula for the active ingredients are presented below.

Hydrocortisone acetate
(Pregn-4-ene-3,20-dione, 21-(acetyloxy)-11, 17-dihydroxy-, (11β-.)

Continued on next page

Table 2.
DISCONTINUATIONS DURING CONTROLLED U.S. STUDIES

Body System Experience	Penbutolol (N = 628) %	Placebo (N = 212) %	Propranolol (N = 266) %
Body as a Whole			
Asthenia	0.6	0.0	0.4
Pain, chest	0.6	1.4	0.4
Digestive System			
Nausea	0.8	0.0	0.8
Nervous System			
Depression	0.6	0.5	0.8
Dizziness	0.6	0.0	0.4
Fatigue	0.5	0.5	0.0
Headache	0.6	0.5	0.4

Reed & Carnrick—Cont.

$$CH_3CH_2CH_2CH_2O-\bigcirc-OCH_2CH_2CH_2N\bigcirc O.HCl$$

Pramoxine hydrochloride
(4-(3-(p-butoxyphenoxy)propyl)morpholine
hydrochloride)

CLINICAL PHARMACOLOGY

Topical corticosteroids share anti-inflammatory, anti-pruritic and vasoconstrictive actions.

The mechanism of anti-inflammatory activity of the topical corticosteroids is unclear. Various laboratory methods, including vasoconstrictor assays, are used to compare and predict potencies and/or clinical efficacies of the topical corticosteroids. There is some evidence to suggest that a recognizable correlation exists between vasoconstrictor potency and therapeutic efficacy in man.

Pramoxine hydrochloride is a topical anesthetic agent which provides temporary relief from itching and pain. It acts by stabilizing the neuronal membrane of nerve endings with which it comes into contact.

PHARMACOKINETICS

The extent of percutaneous absorption of topical corticosteroids is determined by many factors including the vehicle, the integrity of the epidermal barrier, and the use of occlusive dressings.

Topical corticosteroids can be absorbed from normal intact skin. Inflammation and/or other disease processes in the skin increase the percutaneous absorption. Occlusive dressings substantially increase the percutaneous absorption of topical corticosteroids. Thus, occlusive dressings may be valuable therapeutic adjunct for treatment of resistant dermatoses. (See DOSAGE AND ADMINISTRATION.)

Once absorbed through the skin, topical corticosteroids are handled through pharmacokinetic pathways similar to systemically administered corticosteroids. Corticosteroids are bound to plasma proteins in varying degress. Corticosteroids are metabolized primarily in the liver and are then excreted by the kidneys. Some of the topical corticosteroids and their metabolites are also excreted into the bile.

INDICATIONS AND USAGE

Topical corticosteroids are indicated for the relief of the inflammatory and pruritic manifestations of corticosteroid-responsive dermatoses.

CONTRAINDICATIONS

Topical corticosteroids are contraindicated in those patients with a history of hypersensitivity to any of the components of the preparation.

PRECAUTIONS

General: Systemic absorption of topical corticosteroids has produced reversible hypothalamic-pituitary-adrenal (HPA) axis suppression, manifestations of Cushing's syndrome, hyperglycemia, and glucosuria in some patients.

Conditions which augment systematic absorption include the applications of the more potent steroids, use over large surface areas, prolonged use, and the addition of occlusive dressings.

Therefore patients receiving a large dose of a potent topical steroid applied to a large surface area and under an occlusive dressing should be evaluated periodically for evidence of HPA axis suppression by using the urinary free cortisol and ACTH stimulation tests. If HPA axis suppression is noted, an attempt should be made to withdraw the drug, to reduce the frequency of application, or to substitute a less potent steroid.

Recovery of HPA axis function is generally prompt and complete upon discontinuation of the drug. Infrequently, signs and symptoms of steroid withdrawal may occur, requiring supplemental systemic corticosteroids.

Children may absorb proportionally larger amounts of topical corticosteroids and thus be more susceptible to systemic toxicity. (See PRECAUTIONS—Pediatric Use.)

If irritation develops, topical corticosteroids should be discontinued and appropriate therapy instituted.

In the presence of dermatological infections, the use of an appropriate antifungal or antibacterial agent should be instituted. If a favorable response does not occur promptly, the corticosteroid should be discontinued until the infection has been adequately controlled.

Information for the Patient: Patients using topical corticosteroids should receive the following information and instructions.

1. The medication is to be used as directed by the physician. It is for external use only. Avoid contact with the eyes.
2. Patients should be advised not to use this medication for any disorder other than for which it was prescribed.

3. The treated skin area should not be bandaged or otherwise covered or wrapped as to be occlusive unless directed by the physician.
4. Patients should report any signs of local adverse reactions especially under occlusive dressing.
5. Parents of pediatric patients should be advised not to use tight-fitting diapers or plastic pants on a child being treated in the diaper area, as these garments may constitute occlusive dressings.

Laboratory Tests: The following tests may be helpful in evaluating the HPA axis suppression:

Urinary free cortisol test
ACTH stimulation test

Carcinogenesis, Mutagenesis, and Impairment of Fertility: Long-term animal studies have not been performed to evaluate the carcinogenic potential or the effect on fertility of topical corticosteroids.

Studies to determine mutagenicity with prednisolone and hydrocortisone have revealed negative results.

Pregnancy Category C: Corticosteroids are genrally teratogenic in laboratory animals when administered systemically at relatively low dosage levels. The more potent corticosteroids have been shown to be teratogenic after dermal application in laboratory animals. There are no adequate and well-controlled studies in pregnant women on teratogenic effects from topically applied corticosteroids. Therefore, topical corticosteroids should be used during pregnancy only if the potential benefit justifies the potential risk to the fetus. Drugs of this class should not be used extensively on pregnant patients, in large amounts, or for prolonged periods of time.

Nursing Mothers: It is not known whether topical administration of corticosteroids could result in sufficient systemic absorption to produce detectable amounts in breast milk. Systemically administered corticosteroids are secreted into breast milk in quantities NOT likely to have a deleterious effect on the infant. Nevertheless, caution should be exercised when topical corticosteroids are administered to a nursing woman.

Pediatric Use: Pediatric patients may demonstrate greater susceptibility to topical corticosteroid-induced HPA axis suppression and Cushing's syndrome than mature patients because of a large skin surface area to body weight ratio.

Hypothalamic-pituitary-adrenal (HPA) axis suppression, Cushing's syndrome, and intracranial hypertension have been reported in children receiving topical corticosteroids. Manifestations of adrenal suppression in children include linear growth retardation, delayed weight gain, low plasma cortisol levels, and absence of response of ACTH stimulation. Manifestations of intracranial hypertension include bulging fontanelles, headaches, and bilateral papilledema.

Administration of topical corticosteroids to children should be limited to the least amount compatible with an effective therapeutic regimen. Chronic corticosteroid therapy may interfere with the growth and development of children.

ADVERSE REACTIONS

The following local adverse reactions are reported infrequently with topical corticosteroids, but may occur more frequently with the use of occlusive dressings. These reactions are listed in an approximate decreasing order of occurrence:

Burning	Perioral dermatitis
Itching	Allergic contact
Irritation	dermatitis
Dryness	Maceration of the skin
Folliculitis	Secondary infection
Hypertrichosis	Skin Atrophy
Acneiform eruptions	Striae
Hypopigmentation	Miliaria

OVERDOSAGE

Topically applied corticosteroids can be absorbed in sufficient amounts to produce systemic effects (See PRECAUTIONS).

DOSAGE AND ADMINISTRATION

Topical corticosteroids are generally applied to the affected area as a thin film three or four times daily depending on the severity of the condition.

Occlusive dressings may be used for the management of psoriasis or recalcitrant conditions.

If an infection develops, the use of occlusive dressings should be discontinued and appropriate antimicrobial therapy instituted.

HOW SUPPLIED

1 oz. tube.

CAUTION

Federal law prohibits dispensing without prescription.
Manufactured for
REED & CARNRICK
Piscataway, NJ 08855
By FERNDALE LABORATORIES, INC.
Ferndale, Michigan 48220
APRIL 1988   PTC281L87

Shown in Product Identification Section, page 423

PROCTOFOAM®-HC   ℞

[prŏc'tō-fōm]
(hydrocortisone acetate) 1%
(and pramoxine hydrochloride 1%
topical aerosol)

DESCRIPTION

A topical corticosteroid aerosol foam for anal use containing hydrocortisone acetate 1% and pramoxine hydrochloride 1% in a hydrophilic base of: propylene glycol, ethoxylated cetyl and stearyl alcohols, steareth-10, cetyl alcohol, methylparaben, propylparaben, trolamine, purified water and propellants (inert): dichlorodifluoromethane and dichlortetrafluoroethane.

PROTOFOAM®-HC contains a synthetic steroid used as an anti-inflammatory and anti-pruritic agent, and a local anesthetic.

Molecular weight: Hydrocortisone acetate 404.51. Solubility of hydrocortisone acetate in water: 1 mg/100ml.

Chemical name: Pregn-4-ene, 3,20-dione, 21-(acetyloxy)-11, 17-dihydroxy- (11β).

$$CH_2O\overset{O}{\overset{\|}{C}}-CH_3$$

Pramoxine Hydrochloride

$$CH_3CH_2CH_2CH_2O-\bigcirc-OCH_2CH_2CH_2-N\bigcirc O\cdot HCl$$

CLINICAL PHARMACOLOGY

Topical corticosteroids share anti-inflammatory, anti-pruritic and vasoconstrictive actions.

The mechanism of anti-inflammatory activity of the topical corticosteroids is unclear. Various laboratory methods, including vasoconstrictor assays, are used to compare and predict potencies and/or clinical efficacies of the topical corticosteroids. There is some evidence to suggest that a recognizable correlation exists between vasoconstrictor potency and therapeutic efficacy in man.

Pramoxine Hydrochloride: A surface or local anesthetic which is not chemically related to the "caine" types of local anesthetics. Its unique chemical structure is likely to minimize the danger of cross-sensitivity reactions in patients allergic to other local anesthetics.

Pharmacokinetics: The extent of percutaneous absorption of topical corticosteroids is determined by many factors including the vehicle, the integrity of the epidermal barrier, and the use of occlusive dressings.

Topical corticosteroids can be absorbed from normal intact skin. Inflammation and/or other disease processes in the skin increase the percutaneous absorption of topical corticosteroids. Occlusive dressings substantially increase the percutaenous absorption of topical corticosteroids. Thus, occlusive dressings may be a valuable therapeutic adjunct for treatment of resistant dermatoses. (See DOSAGE AND ADMINISTRATION.)

Once absorbed through the skin, topical corticosteroids are handled through pharmacokinetic pathways similar to systemically administered corticosteroids. Corticosteroids are bound to plasma proteins in varying doegrees. Corticosteroids are metabolized primarily in the liver and are then excreted by the kidneys. Some of the topical corticosteroids and their metabolites are also excreted in the bile.

INDICATIONS AND USAGE

Topical corticosteroids are indicated for the relief of the inflammatory and pruritic manifestations of corticosteroid-responsive dermatoses of the anal region.

CONTRAINDICATIONS

Topical corticosteroid products are contraindicated in those patients with a history of hypersensitivity to any of the components of the preparation.

WARNINGS

Do not insert any part of the aerosol container into the anus. Contents of the container are under pressure. Do not burn or puncture the aerosol container. Store at temperatures below 120°F. If there is no evidence of clinical or proctologic improvement within two or three weeks after therapy, or if the patient's condition worsens, discontinue the drug. Keep this and all medicines out of the reach of children.

PRECAUTIONS

General: Systemic absorption of topical corticosteroids has produced reversible hypothalamic-pituitary-adrenal (HPA) axis suppression, manifestations of Cushing's syndrome, hyperglycemia and glucosuria in some patients. Conditions which augment systemic absorption include the application of the more potent steroids, use over large surface areas, prolonged use and the addition of occlusive dressings.

Therefore, patients receiving a large dose of a potent topical steroid applied to a large surface area or under an occlusive dressing should be evaluated periodically for evidence of HPA axis suppression by using the urinary hydrocortisone and ACTH stimulation tests. If HPA axis suppression is noted, an attempt should be made to withdraw the drug, to reduce the frequency of application, or to substitute a less potent steroid.

Recovery of HPA axis function is generally prompt and complete upon discontinuation of the drug. Infrequently, signs and symptoms of steroid withdrawal may occur, requiring supplemental systemic corticosteroids.

In children absorption may result in higher blood levels and thus more susceptibility to systemic toxicity. (See PRECAUTIONS—Pediatric Use.)

If irritation develops, topical corticosteroids should be discontinued and appropriate therapy instituted.

In the presence of dermatological infections, the use of an appropriate antifungal or antibacterial agent should be instituted. If a favorable response does not occur promptly, the corticosteroid should be discontinued until the infection has been adequately controlled.

Information for the Patient
Patients using topical corticosteroids should receive the following information and instructions.

1. This medication is to be used as directed by the physician. It is for anal or parianal use only. Avoid contact with the eyes.
2. Be advised not to use this medication for any disorder other than for which it has been prescribed.
3. Report any signs of adverse reactions.

Laboratory Tests
The following tests may be helpful in evaluating the HPA axis suppression:
    Urinary hydrocortisone test
    ACTH stimulation test

Carcinogenesis, Mutagenesis, and Impairment of Fertility
Long-term animal studies have not been performed to evaluate carcinogenic potential or the effect on fertility of topical corticosteroids.

Studies to determine mutagenicity with prednisolone and hydrocortisone have revealed negative results.

Pregnancy Category C
Corticosteroids are generally teratogenic in laboratory animals when administered systemically at relatively low dosage levels. The more potent corticosteroids have been shown to be teratogenic after dermal application in laboratory animals. There are no adequate and well-controlled studies in pregnant women of teratogenic effects from topically applied corticosteroids. Therefore, topical corticosteroids should be used during pregnancy only if the potential benefit justifies the potential risk to the fetus. Drugs of this class should not be used extensively on pregnant patients, in large amounts, or for prolonged periods of time.

Nursing Mothers
It is not known whether topical administration of corticosteroids could result in sufficient systemic absorption to produce detectable quantities in breast milk. Systemically administered corticosteroids are secreted into breast milk in quantities not likely to have a deleterious effect on the infant. Caution should be exercised when any topical corticosteroids are administered to a nursing woman.

Pediatric Use
Pediatric patients may demonstrate greater susceptibility to topical corticosteroid-induced HPA axis suppression and Cushing's syndrome than mature patients because of a larger skin surface area to body weight ratio.

Hypothalamic-pituitary-adrenal (HPA) axis suppression. Cushing's syndrome and intracranial hypertension have been reported in children receiving topical corticosteroids. Manifestations of adrenal suppression in children include linear growth retardation, delayed weight gain, low plasma cortisone levels and absense of response to ACTH stimulation. Manifestations of intracranial hypertension include bulging fontanelles, headaches and bilateral papilledema.

Administration of topical corticosteroids to children should be limited to the least amount compatible with an effective therapeutic regimen. Chronic corticosteroid therapy may interfere with the growth and development of children.

ADVERSE REACTIONS

The following local adverse reactions are reported infrequently with topical corticosteroids, but may occur more frequently with the use of occlusive dressings. These reactions are listed in an approximate decreasing order of occurrence.

Burning	Perioral dermatitis
Itching	Allergic contact
Irritation	dermatitis
Dryness	Maceration of the skin
Folliculitis	Secondary infection
Hypertrichosis	Skin atrophy
Acneiform eruptions	Striae
Hypopigmentation	Miliaria

OVERDOSAGE

Topically applied corticosteroids can be absorbed in sufficient amounts to produce systemic effects. (See PRECAUTIONS.)

DOSAGE AND ADMINISTRATION
(NOTE: SEE INNER PACKAGE FOR FULL DIRECTIONS FOR USE.)

Apply to affected areas 3 or 4 times daily. Use the applicator supplied for rectal application. For perianal use, transfer a small quantity to a tissue and rub in gently.

1. Shake foam container vigorously before use. Hold container upright and insert into opening of the tip of the applicator. Be sure applicator plunger is drawn all the way out. **CONTAINER MUST BE HELD UPRIGHT TO OBTAIN PROPER FLOW OF MEDICATION.**
2. To fill, press down slowly on container cap. Repeat until foam reaches **fill line** in the applicator. CAUTION: The aerosol container should never be inserted directly into the anus.
3. Remove applicator from container. Allow some foam to remain on the applicator tip. Hold applicator by barrel and gently insert tip into the anus. With applicator in place, push plunger in order to expel foam, then withdraw applicator. (Applicator parts should be pulled apart for thorough cleaning with warm water.)

HOW SUPPLIED

PROCTOFOAM®-HC (NDC 0021-0690-10) is supplied in 10 gram aerosol container with a special rectal applicator. When used correctly the aerosol container will deliver a minimum of 14 applications.

CAUTION

FEDERAL LAW PROHIBITS DISPENSING WITHOUT PRESCRIPTION.

Revised May 1989
Shown in Product Identification Section, page 423

Reid-Rowell
901 SAWYER ROAD
MARIETTA, GA 30062

BALNEOL®
[băl ′nē-ŏl]
Perianal cleansing lotion

(See PDR For Nonprescription Drugs)

CHENIX®   ℞
[kē ′nix]
Chenodiol Tablets 250 mg

SPECIAL NOTE
Because of the potential hepatotoxicity of chenodiol, poor response rates to some subgroups of chenodiol-treated patients, and an increased rate of a need for cholecystectomy in other chenodiol-treated subgroups, chenodiol is not an appropriate treatment for many patients with gallstones. Chenodiol should be reserved for carefully selected patients and treatment must be accompanied by systematic monitoring for liver function alterations. Aspects of patient selection, response rates and risks versus benefits are given in the insert.

DESCRIPTION
CHENIX is chenodiol, the nonproprietary name for chenodeoxycholic acid, a naturally occurring human bile acid. It is a bitter tasting white powder consisting of crystalline and amorphous particles freely soluble in methanol, acetone and acetic acid and practically insoluble in water. Its chemical name is 3α, 7α-dihydroxy-5β-cholan-24-oic acid ($C_{24}H_{40}O_4$), it has a molecular weight of 392.58, and its structure is shown below.

CHENIX film-coated tablets for oral administration contain 250 mg of chenodiol.
Inactive ingredients: Magnesium stearate, pregelatinized starch, silicon dioxide and sodium starch glycolate. In addition, the tablet film-coating contains carnauba wax, hydroxypropyl methylcellulose, cetyl alcohol, dibutyl sebacate, polyethylene glycol and sodium lauryl sulfate.

CLINICAL PHARMACOLOGY

At therapeutic doses, chenodiol suppresses hepatic synthesis of both cholesterol and cholic acid, gradually replacing the latter and its metabolite, deoxycholic acid, in an expanded bile acid pool. These actions contribute to biliary cholesterol desaturation and gradual dissolution of radiolucent cholesterol gallstones in the presence of a gallbladder visualized by oral cholecystography. Chenodiol has no effects on radiopaque (calcified) gallstones or on radiolucent bile pigment stones.

Chenodiol is well absorbed from the small intestine and taken up by the liver, where it is converted to its taurine and glycine conjugates and secreted in bile. Owing to 60% to 80% first-pass hepatic clearance, the body pool of chenodiol resides mainly in the enterohepatic circulation, serum and urinary bile acid levels are not significantly affected during chenodiol therapy.

At steady-state, an amount of chenodiol near the daily dose escapes to the colon and is converted by bacterial action to lithocholic acid. About 80% of the lithocholate is excreted in the feces; the remainder is absorbed and converted in the liver to its poorly absorbed sulfolithocholyl conjugates. During chenodiol therapy there is only a minor increase in biliary lithocholate, while fecal bile acids are increased three- to fourfold.

Chenodiol is unequivocally hepatotoxic in many animal species, including sub-human primates at doses close to the human dose. Although the theoretical cause is the metabolite, lithocholic acid, an established hepatotoxin, and man has an efficient mechanism for sulfating and eliminating this substance, there is some evidence that the demonstrated hepatotoxicity is partly due to chenodiol *per se*. The hepatotoxicity of lithocholic acid is characterized biochemically and morphologically as cholestatic.

Man has the capacity to form sulfate conjugates of lithocholic acid. Variation in this capacity among individuals has not been well established and a recent published report suggests that patients who develop chenodiol-induced serum aminotransferase elevations are poor sulfators of lithocholic acid (see **WARNINGS** and **ADVERSE REACTIONS**).

General Clinical Results: Both the desaturation of bile and the clinical dissolution of cholesterol gallstones are dose-related. In the National Cooperative Gallstone Study (NCGS) involving 305 patients in each treatment group, placebo and chenodiol dosages of 375 mg and 750 mg per day were associated with complete stone dissolution in 0.8%, 5.2% and 13.5%, respectively, of enrolled subjects over 24 months of treatment. Uncontrolled clinical trials using higher doses than those used in the NCGS have shown complete dissolution rates of 28 to 38% of enrolled patients receiving body weight doses of from 13 to 16 mg/kg/day for up to 24 months. In a prospective trial using 15 mg/kg/day, 31% enrolled surgical-risk patients treated more than six months (n = 86) achieved complete confirmed dissolutions. Observed stone dissolution rates achieved with chenodiol treatment are higher in subgroups having certain pretreatment characteristics. In the NCGS, patients with small (less than 15 mm in diameter) radiolucent stones, the observed rate of complete dissolution was approximately 20% on 750 mg/day. In the uncontrolled trials using 13 to 16 mg/kg/day doses of chenodiol, the rates of complete dissolution for small radiolucent stones ranged from 42% to 60%. Even higher dissolution rates have been observed in patients with small floatable stones. (See **Floatable versus Nonfloatable Stones,** below). Some obese patients and occasional normal weight patients fail to achieve bile desaturation even with doses of chenodiol up to 19 mg/kg/day for unknown reasons.

Although dissolution is generally higher with increased dosage of chenodiol, doses that are too low are associated with increased cholecystectomy rates (see **ADVERSE REACTIONS**).

Stones have recurred within five years in about 50% of patients following complete confirmed dissolutions. Although retreatment with chenodiol has proven successful in dissolving some newly formed stones, the indications for and safety of retreatment are not well defined. Serum aminotransferase elevations and diarrhea have been notable in all clinical trials and are dose-related (refer to **ADVERSE REACTIONS** and **WARNING** sections for full information).

Floatable versus Nonfloatable Stones: A major finding in clinical trials was a difference between floatable and nonfloatable stones, with respect to both natural history and response to chenodiol. Over the two-year course of the National Cooperative Gallstone Study (NCGS), placebo-treated patients with floatable stones (n = 47) had significantly higher rates of biliary pain and cholecystectomy than patients with nonfloatable stones (n = 258) (47% versus 27% and 19% versus 4%, respectively). Chenodiol treatment (750 mg/day) compared to placebo was associated with a significant reduction in both biliary pain and the cholecystectomy rate in the group with floatable stones (27% versus 47% and 1.5% versus 19%, respectively). In an uncontrolled clinical trial using 15 mg/kg/day, 70% of the patients with small

Continued on next page

Reid-Rowell—Cont.

(less than 15 mm) floatable stones (n = 10) had complete confirmed dissolutions.

In the NCGS in patients with nonfloatable stones, chenodiol produced no reduction in biliary pain and showed a tendency to increase the cholecystectomy rate (8% versus 4%). This finding was more pronounced with doses of chenodiol below 10 mg/kg. The subgroup of patients with nonfloatable stones and a history of biliary pain had the highest rates of cholecystectomy and aminotransferase elevations during chenodiol treatment. Except for the NCGS subgroup with pretreatment biliary pain, dose-related aminotransferase elevations and diarrhea have occurred with equal frequency in patients with floatable or nonfloatable stones. In the uncontrolled clinical trial mentioned above, 27% of the patients with nonfloatable stones (n = 59) had complete confirmed dissolutions, including 35% with small (less than 15 mm) (n = 40) and only 11% with large, nonfloatable stones (n = 19).

Of 916 patients enrolled in NCGS, 17.8% had stones seen in upright films (horizontal X-ray beam) to float in the dyeladen bile during oral cholecystography using iopanoic acid. Other investigators report similar findings. Floatable stones are not detected by ultrasonography in the absence of dye. Chemical analysis has shown floatable stones to be essentially pure cholesterol.

Other Radiographic and Laboratory Features: Radiolucent stones may have rims or centers of opacity representing calcification. Pigment stones and partially calcified radiolucent stones do not respond to chenodiol. Subtle calcification can sometimes be detected in flat film X-rays, if not obvious in the oral cholecystogram. Among nonfloatable stones, cholesterol stones are more apt than pigment stones to be smoothsurfaced, less than 0.6 cm in diameter, and to occur in numbers less than 10. As stone size, number and volume increase, the probability of dissolution within 24 months decreases. Hemolytic disorders, chronic alcoholism, biliary cirrhosis and bacterial invasion of the biliary system predispose to pigment gallstone formation. Pigment stones of primary biliary cirrhosis should be suspected in patients with elevated alkaline phosphatase, especially if positive antimitochondrial antibodies are present. The presence of microscopic cholesterol crystals in aspirated gallbladder bile, and demonstration of cholesterol supersaturation by bile lipid analysis, increase the likelihood that the stones are cholesterol stones.

PATIENT SELECTION

Evaluation of Surgical Risk: Surgery offers the advantage of immediate and permanent stone removal, but carries a fairly high risk in some patients. About 5% of cholecystectomized patients have residual symptoms or retained common duct stones. The spectrum to surgical risk varies as a function of age and the presence of disease other than cholelithiasis. Selected tabulation of results from the National Halothane Study (**JAMA, 1966, 197:775–778**) is shown below; the study included 27,600 cholecystectomies.

Mortality per Operation
(Smoothed rates with denominators adjusted to one death.)

		Cholecystectomy	Cholecystectomy & Common Duct Exploration
Low Risk Patients*			
Women	0–49 yrs	1/1851	1/469
	50–69 yrs	1/357	1/99
Men	0–49 yrs	1/961	1/243
	50–69 yrs	1/185	1/52
High Risk Patients**			
Women	0–49 yrs	1/79	1/21
	50–69 yrs	1/58	1/17
Men	0–49 yrs	1/41	1/11
	50–69 yrs	1/30	1/9

*Includes those with good health or moderate systemic disease, with or without emergency surgery.
**Severe or extreme systemic disease, with or without emergency surgery.

Women in good health, or having only moderate systemic disease, under 49 years of age have the lowest rate (0.054%), men in all categories have a surgical mortality rate twice that of women; common duct exploration quadruples the rates in all categories; the rates rise with each decade of life and increase tenfold or more in all categories with severe or extreme systemic disease.

Relatively young patients requiring treatment might be better treated by surgery than with CHENIX, because treatment with chenodiol, even if successful, is associated with a high rate of recurrence. The long-term consequences of repeated courses of chenodiol in terms of liver toxicity, neoplasia and elevated cholesterol levels are not known.

Watchful waiting has the advantage that no therapy may ever be required. For patients with silent or minimally symptomatic stones, the rate of moderate to severe symptoms or gallstone complications is estimated to be between 2% and 6% per year, leading to a cumulative rate of 7% and 27% in five years. Presumably the rate is higher for patients already having symptoms.

INDICATIONS AND USAGE

CHENIX is indicated for patients with radiolucent stones in well-opacifying gallbladders, in whom effective surgery would be undertaken except for the presence of increased surgical risk due to systemic disease or age. The likelihood of successful dissolution is far greater if the stones are floatable or small. For patients with nonfloatable stones, dissolution is less likely and added weight should be given to the risk that more emergent surgery might result from a delay due to unsuccessful treatment. Safety of use beyond 24 months is not established. CHENIX will not dissolve calcified (radiopaque) or radiolucent bile pigment stones.

CONTRAINDICATIONS

Chenodiol is contraindicated in the presence of known hepatocyte dysfunction or bile ductal abnormalities such as intrahepatic cholestasis, primary biliary cirrhosis or sclerosing cholangitis (see **Warnings**); a gallbladder confirmed as nonvisualizing after two consecutive single doses of dye; radiopaque stones; or gallstone complications or compelling reasons for gallbladder surgery including unremitting acute cholecystitis, cholangitis, biliary obstruction, gallstone pancreatitis, or biliary gastrointestinal fistula.

Pregnancy Category X:
Chenodiol may cause fetal harm when administered to a pregnant woman. Serious hepatic, renal and adrenal lesions occurred in fetuses of female Rhesus monkeys given 60 to 90 mg/kg/day (4 to 6 times the maximum recommended human dose, MRHD) from day 21 to day 45 of pregnancy. Hepatic lesions also occurred in neonatal baboons whose mothers had received 18 to 38 mg/kg (1 to 2 times the MRHD), all during pregnancy. Fetal malformations were not observed. Neither fetal liver damage nor fetal abnormalities occurred in reproduction studies in rats and hamsters. No human data are available at this time. Chenodiol is contraindicated in women who are or may become pregnant. If this drug is used during pregnancy, or if the patient becomes pregnant while taking this drug, the patient should be apprised of the potential hazard to the fetus.

WARNINGS

Safe use of chenodiol depends upon selection of patients without preexisting liver disease and upon faithful monitoring of serum aminotransferase levels to detect drug-induced liver toxicity. Aminotransferase elevations over three times the upper limit of normal have required discontinuation of chenodiol in 2% to 3% of patients. Although clinical and biopsy studies have not shown fulminant lesions, the possibility remains that an occasional patient may develop serious hepatic disease.

Three patients with biochemical and histologic pictures of chronic active hepatitis while on chenodiol, 375 mg/day or 750 mg/day, have been reorted. The biochemical abnormalities returned spontaneously to normal in two of the patients within 13 and 17 months; and after 17 months' treatment with prednisone in the third. Followup biopsies were not done, and the causal relationship of the drug could not be determined. Another biopsied patient was terminated from therapy because of elevated aminotransferase levels and a liver biopsy was interpreted as showing active drug hepatitis.

One patient with sclerosing cholangitis, biliary cirrhosis and a history of jaundice died during chenodiol treatment for hepatic duct stones. Before treatment, serum aminotransferase and alkaline phosphatase levels were over twice the upper limit of normal, within one month they rose to over 10 times normal. Chenodiol was discontinued at seven weeks when the patient was hospitalized with advanced hepatic failure and E. coli peritonitis; death ensued at the eighth week. A contribution of chenodiol to the fatal outcome could not be ruled out.

Epidemiologic studies suggest that bile acids might contribute to human colon cancer, but direct evidence is lacking. Bile acids, including chenodiol and lithocholic acid, have no carcinogenic potential in animal models, but have been shown to increase the number of tumors when administered with certain known carcinogens. The possibility that chenodiol therapy might contribute to colon cancer in otherwise susceptible individuals cannot be ruled out.

PRECAUTIONS

Information for Patients: Patients should be counseled on the importance of periodic visits for liver function tests and oral cholecystograms (or ultrasonograms) for monitoring stone dissolution; they should be made aware of the symptoms of gallstone complications and be warned to report immediately symptoms to the physician. Patients should be instructed on ways to facilitate faithful compliance with the dosage regimen throughout the usual long term of therapy, and on temporary dose reduction if episodes of diarrhea occur.

Drug Interactions: Bile acid sequestering agents, such as cholestyramine and colestipol, may interfere with the action of CHENIX by reducing its absorption. Aluminum-based antacids have been shown to adsorb bile acids *in vitro* and may be expected to interfere with CHENIX in the same manner as the sequestering agents. Estrogens, oral contraceptives and clofibrate (and perhaps other lipid-lowering drugs) increase biliary cholesterol secretion, and the incidence of cholesterol gallstones hence may counteract the effectiveness of CHENIX.

Carcinogenesis, Mutagenesis, and Impairment of Fertility: A two-year oral study of chenodiol in rats failed to show a carcinogenic potential at the tested levels of 15 to 60 mg/kg/day (1 to 4 times the maximum recommended human dose, MRHD). It has been reported that chenodiol given in long-term studies at oral doses up to 600 mg/kg/day (40 times the MRHD) to rats and 1000 mg/kg/day (65 times the MRHD) to mice induced benign and malignant liver tumors in female rats and cholangiomata in female rats and male mice. Two-year studies of lithocholic acid (a major metabolite of chenodiol) in mice (125 to 250 mg/kg/day) and rats (250 and 500 mg/kg/day) found it not to be carcinogenic. The dietary administration of lithocholic acid to chickens is reported to cause hepatic adenomatous hyperplasia.

Pregnancy Category X: See **CONTRAINDICATIONS**.

Nursing Mothers: It is not known whether chenodiol is excreted in human milk. Because many drugs are excreted in human milk, caution should be exercised when chenodiol is administered to a nursing mother.

Pediatric Use: The safety and effectiveness of chenodiol in children have not been established.

ADVERSE REACTIONS

Hepatobiliary: Dose-related serum aminotransferase (mainly SGPT) elevations, usually not accompanied by rises in alkaline phosphatase or bilirubin, occurred in 30% or more of patients treated with the recommended dose of CHENIX. In most cases, these elevations were minor (1½ to 3 times the upper limit of laboratory normal) and transient, returning to within the normal range within six months despite continued administration of the drug. In 2% to 3% of patients, SGPT levels rose to over three times the upper limit of laboratory normal, recurred on rechallenge with the drug, and required discontinuation of chenodiol treatment. Enzyme levels have returned to normal following withdrawal of chenodiol (see **WARNINGS** section).

Morphologic studies of liver biopsies taken before and after 9 and 24 months' treatment with chenodiol have shown that 63% of the patients prior to chenodiol treatment had evidence of intrahepatic cholestasis. Almost all pretreatment patients had electron microscopic abnormalities. By the ninth month of treatment, reexamination of two-thirds of the patients showed an 89% incidence of the signs of intrahepatic cholestasis. Two of 89 patients at the ninth month had lithocholate-like lesions in the canalicular membrane, although there were no clinical enzyme abnormalities in the face of continued treatment and no change in Type 2 light microscopic parameters.

Increased Cholecystectomy Rate: NCGS patients with a history of biliary pain prior to treatment had higher cholecystectomy rates during the study if assigned to low dosage chenodiol (375 mg/day) than if assigned to either placebo or high dosage chenodiol (750 mg/day). The association with low dosage chenodiol though not clearly a causal one, suggests that patients unable to take higher doses of chenodiol may be at greater risk of cholecystectomy.

Gastrointestinal: Dose-related diarrhea has been encountered in 30% to 40% of chenodiol-treated patients and may occur at any time during treatment, but is most commonly encountered when treatment is initiated. Usually, the diarrhea is mild, transient, well-tolerated and does not interfere with therapy. Dose reduction has been required in 10% to 15% of patients, and in a controlled trial about half of these required a permanent reduction in dose. Anti-diarrheal agents have proven useful in some patients. Discontinuation of chenodiol because of failure to control diarrhea is to be expected in approximately 3% of patients treated. Steady epigastric pain with nausea typical of lithiasis (biliary colic) usually is easily distinguishable from the crampy abdominal pain of drug-induced diarrhea.

Other, less frequent, gastrointestinal side effects reported included urgency, cramps, heartburn, constipation, nausea and vomiting, anorexia, epigastric distress, dyspepsia, flatulence and nonspecific abdominal pain.

Serum Lipids: Serum total cholesterol and low-density lipoprotein (LDL) cholesterol may rise 10% or more during administration of chenodiol; no change has been seen in the high-density lipoprotein (HDL) fraction; small decreases in serum triglyceride levels for females have been reported.

Hematologic: Decreases in white cell count, never below 3000, have been noted in a few patients treated with chenodiol; the drug was continued in all patients without incident.

OVERDOSAGE

Accidental or intentional overdoses of chenodiol have not been reported. One patient tolerated 4 gm/day (58 mg/kg/day) for six months without incident.

DOSAGE AND ADMINISTRATION

The recommended dose range for CHENIX is 13 to 16 mg/kg/day in two divided doses, morning and night, starting with 250 mg b.i.d. the first two weeks and increasing by 250 mg/day each week thereafter until the recommended or maximum tolerated dose is reached. If diarrhea occurs during dosage buildup or later in treatment, it usually can be controlled by temporary dosage adjustment until symptoms abate, after which the previous dose usually is tolerated. Dosage less than 10 mg/kg usually is ineffective and may be associated with increased risk of cholecystectomy, so is not recommended.

Weight/Dosage Guide

Body Weight		Recommended	Dose Range
lb	kg	Tablets/Day	mg/kg
100–130	45–58	3	17–13
131–165	59–75	4	17–13
166–200	76–90	5	16–14
201–235	91–107	6	16–14
236–275	108–125	7	16–14

The optimal frequency of monitoring liver function tests is not known. It is suggested that serum aminotransferase levels should be monitored monthly for the first three months and every three months thereafter during CHENIX administration. Under NCGS guidelines, if a minor, usually transient, elevation (1½ to 3 times the upper limit of normal) persisted longer than three to six months, chenodiol was discontinued and resumed only after the aminotransferase level returned to normal; however, allowing the elevations to persist over such an interval is not known to be safe. Elevations over three times the upper limit of normal require immediate discontinuation of CHENIX, and usually reoccur on challenge.

Serum cholesterol should be monitored at six-month intervals. It may be advisable to discontinue CHENIX if cholesterol rises above the acceptable age-adjusted limit for a given patient.

Oral cholecystograms or ultrasonograms are recommended at six- to nine-month intervals to monitor response. Complete dissolutions should be confirmed by a repeat test after one to three months' continued CHENIX administration. Most patients who eventually achieve complete dissolution will show partial (or complete) dissolution at the first on-treatment test. If partial dissolution is not seen by nine to 12 months, the likelihood of success of treating longer is greatly reduced; CHENIX should be discontinued if there is no response by 18 months. Safety of use beyond 24 months is not established.

Stone recurrence can be expected within five years in 50% of cases. After confirmed dissolution, treatment generally should be stopped. Serial cholecystograms or ultrasonograms are recommended to monitor for recurrence, keeping in mind that radiolucency and gallbladder function should be established before starting another course of CHENIX. A prophylactic dose is not established; reduced doses cannot be recommended; stones have recurred on 500 mg/day. Low cholesterol or carbohydrate diets, and dietary bran, have been reported to reduce biliary cholesterol; maintenance of reduced weight is recommended to forestall stone recurrence.

CAUTION

Federal law prohibits dispensing without prescription.

HOW SUPPLIED

CHENIX brand chenodiol is available as white, film-coated 250 mg tablets imprinted "RR 7720" in bottles of 100. NDC 0032-7720-01.

Store at controlled room temperature, 15°–30° C (59°–86° F).
Revised: 8/88
Shown in Product Identification Section, page 423

CORTENEMA® ℞

[kort ″en′a-ma]
(Hydrocortisone Retention Enema)
Disposable Unit for Rectal Use Only

Each disposable unit (60 mL) contains:
Hydrocortisone, 100 mg in an aqueous solution containing carboxypolymethylene, polysorbate 80, and methylparaben, 0.18% as a preservative.

DESCRIPTION

CORTENEMA is a convenient disposable single-dose hydrocortisone enema designed for ease of self-administration. Hydrocortisone is a naturally occurring glucocorticoid (adrenal corticosteroid), which similarly as its acetate and sodium hemisuccinate derivatives, is partially absorbed following rectal administration. Absorption studies in ulcerative colitis patients have shown up to 50% absorption of hydrocortisone administered as CORTENEMA and up to 30% of hydrocortisone acetate administered in an identical vehicle.

ACTIONS

CORTENEMA provides the potent anti-inflammatory effect of hydrocortisone. Because this drug is absorbed from the colon, it acts both topically and systemically. Although rectal hydrocortisone, used as recommended for CORTENEMA, has a low incidence of reported adverse reactions, prolonged use presumably may cause systemic reactions associated with oral dosage forms.

INDICATIONS

CORTENEMA is indicated as adjunctive therapy in the treatment of ulcerative colitis, especially distal forms, including ulcerative proctitis, ulcerative proctosigmoiditis, and left-sided ulcerative colitis. It has proved useful also in some cases involving the transverse and ascending colons.

CONTRAINDICATIONS

Systemic fungal infections; and ileocolostomy during the immediate or early postoperative period.

WARNINGS

In severe ulcerative colitis, it is hazardous to delay needed surgery while awaiting response to medical treatment.

Damage to the rectal wall can result from careless or improper insertion of an enema tip.

In patients on corticosteroid therapy subjected to unusual stress, increased dosage of rapidly acting corticosteroids before, during, and after the stressful situation is indicated.

Corticosteroids may mask some signs of infection, and new infections may appear during their use. There may be decreased resistance and inability to localize infection when corticosteroids are used.

Prolonged use of corticosteroids may produce posterior subcapsular cataracts, glaucoma with possible damage to the optic nerves, and may enhance the establishment of secondary ocular infections due to fungi or viruses.

Usage in pregnancy: Since adequate human reproduction studies have not been done with corticosteroids, the use of these drugs in pregnancy, nursing mothers or women of childbearing potential requires that the possible benefits of the drug be weighed against the potential hazards to the mother and embryo or fetus. Infants born of mothers who have received substantial doses of corticosteroids during pregnancy, should be carefully observed for signs of hypoadrenalism.

Average and large doses of hydrocortisone or cortisone can cause elevation of blood pressure, salt and water retention, and increased excretion of potassium. These effects are less likely to occur with the synthetic derivatives except when used in large doses. Dietary salt restriction and potassium supplementation may be necessary. All corticosteroids increase calcium excretion.

While on corticosteroid therapy patients should not be vaccinated against smallpox. Other immunization procedures should not be undertaken in patients who are on corticosteroids, especially on high dose, because of possible hazards of neurological complications and a lack of antibody response. If corticosteroids are indicated in patients with latent tuberculosis or tuberculin reactivity, close observation is necessary as reactivation of the disease may occur. During prolonged corticosteroid therapy, these patients should receive chemoprophylaxis.

PRECAUTIONS

CORTENEMA Hydrocortisone Retention Enema should be used with caution where there is a probability of impending perforation, abscess or other pyogenic infection; fresh intestinal anastomoses; obstruction; or extensive fistulas and sinus tracts. Use with caution in presence of active or latent peptic ulcer; diverticulitis; renal insufficiency; hypertension; osteoporosis; and myasthenia gravis.

Steroid therapy might impair prognosis in surgery by increasing the hazard of infection. If infection is suspected, appropriate antibiotic therapy must be administered, usually in larger than ordinary doses.

Drug-induced secondary adrenocortical insufficiency may occur with prolonged CORTENEMA therapy. This is minimized by gradual reduction of dosage. This type of relative insufficiency may persist for months after discontinuation of therapy; therefore, in any situation of stress occurring during that period, hormone therapy should be reinstituted. Since mineralocorticoid secretion may be impaired, salt and/or a mineralocorticoid should be administered concurrently.

There is an enhanced effect of corticosteroids on patients with hypothyroidism and in those with cirrhosis.

Corticosteroids should be used cautiously in patients with ocular herpes simplex because of possible corneal perforation.

The lowest possible dose of corticosteroid should be used to control the condition under treatment, and when reduction in dosage is possible, the reduction should be gradual.

Psychic derangement may appear when corticosteroids are used, ranging from euphoria, insomnia, mood swings, personality changes, and severe depression to frank psychotic manifestations. Also, existing emotional instability or psychotic tendencies may be aggravated by corticosteroids.

Aspirin should be used cautiously in conjunction with corticosteroids in hypoprothrombinemia.

Growth and development of infants and children on prolonged corticosteroid therapy should be carefully observed.

ADVERSE REACTIONS

Local pain or burning, and rectal bleeding attributed to CORTENEMA have been reported rarely. Apparent exacerbations or sensitivity reactions also occur rarely. The following adverse reactions should be kept in mind when ever corticosteroids are given by rectal administration.

Fluid and Electrolyte Disturbances: Sodium retention; fluid retention; congestive heart failure in susceptible patients; potassium loss; hypokalemic alkalosis; hypertension. Musculoskeletal: Muscle Weakness; steroid myopathy; loss of muscle mass; osteoporosis; vertebral compression fractures; aseptic necrosis of femoral and humeral heads; pathologic fracture of long bones. Gastrointestinal: Peptic ulcer with possible perforation and hemorrhage; pancreatitis; abdominal distention; ulcerative esophagitis. Dermatologic: Impaired wound healing; thin fragile skin; petechiae and ecchymoses; facial erythema; increased sweating; may suppress reactions to skin tests. Neurological: Convulsions; increased intracranial pressure with papilledema (pseudo-tumor cerebri) usually after treatment; vertigo; headache. Endocrine: Menstrual irregularities; development of Cushingoid state; suppression of growth in children; secondary adrenocortical and pituitary unresponsiveness, particularly in times of stress, as in trauma, surgery or illness; decreased carbohydrate tolerance; manifestations of latent diabetes mellitus; increased requirements for insulin or oral hypoglycemic agents in diabetics. Ophthalmic: Posterior subcapsular cataracts; increased intraocular pressure; glaucoma; exophthalmos. Metabolic: Negative nitrogen balance due to protein catabolism.

DOSAGE AND ADMINISTRATION

The use of CORTENEMA Hydrocortisone Retention Enema is predicated upon the concomitant use of modern supportive measures such as rational dietary control, sedatives, antidiarrheal agents, antibacterial therapy, blood replacement if necessary, etc.

The usual course of therapy is one CORTENEMA nightly for 21 days, or until the patient comes into remission both clinically and proctologically. Clinical symptoms usually subside promptly within 3 to 5 days. Improvement in the appearance of the mucosa, as seen by sigmoidoscopic examination, may lag somewhat behind clinical improvement. Difficult cases may require as long as 2 or 3 months of CORTENEMA treatment. Where the course of therapy extends beyond 21 days, CORTENEMA should be discontinued gradually by reducing administration to every other night for 2 or 3 weeks.

If clinical or proctologic improvement fail to occur within 2 or 3 weeks after starting CORTENEMA, discontinue its use. Symptomatic improvement, evidenced by decreased diarrhea and bleeding; weight gain; improved appetite; lessened fever; and decrease in leukocytosis, may be misleading and should not be used as the sole criterion in judging efficacy. Sigmoidoscopic examination and X-ray visualization are essential for adequate monitoring of ulcerative colitis. Biopsy is useful for differential diagnosis.

Patient instructions for administering CORTENEMA are enclosed in each box of seven units. We recommend that the patient lie on his left side during administration and for 30 minutes thereafter, so that the fluid will distribute throughout the left colon. Every effort should be made to retain the enema for at least an hour and, preferably, all night. This may be facilitated by prior sedation and/or antidiarrheal medication, especially early in therapy, when the urge to evacuate is great.

HOW SUPPLIED

CORTENEMA, Hydrocortisone 100 mg Retention Enema, is supplied as disposable single-dose bottles with lubricated rectal applicator tips, in boxes of seven × 60 mL (NDC 0032-1904-82) and boxes of one × 60 mL (NDC 0032-1904-73).

CAUTION

Federal law prohibits dispensing without prescription.
Revised: 1/89
Shown in Product Identification Section, page 423

CREON® ℞

[cree ′on]
PANCREATIN, USP
HIGH LIPASE ENTERIC COATED
MICROSPHERES

DESCRIPTION

CREON Capsules contain pancreatin USP, a standardized concentrate of high lipase enteric coated microspheres of porcine pancreatic enzymes.

Continued on next page

Reid-Rowell—Cont.

Each capsule contains:
Lipase .... 8,000 USP Units
Amylase ....30,000 USP Units
Protease ....13,000 USP Units
Inactive ingredients include hydroxypropylmethylcellulose phthalate, polyethylene glycol, dibutyl phthalate, polydimethylsiloxane, liquid paraffin, gelatin, D&C Yellow #10, FD&C Red #40, black iron oxide, red iron oxide, yellow iron oxide, and titanium dioxide.

CLINICAL PHARMACOLOGY
CREON contains a pancreatic enzyme concentrate used as pancreatic enzyme replacement therapy in pancreatic exocrine insufficiency. The pancreatic enzymes in CREON are enteric coated to resist gastric destruction or inactivation. The protected enzymes are delivered to the duodenum. The pancreatic enzymes catalyze the hydrolysis of fats to glycerol and fatty acids, starch into dextrins and short chain sugars, and protein into proteoses and derived substances.
The lipase content of CREON is present at a higher level than conventional pancreatin preparations, and therefore effective in controlling steatorrhea and its consequences at lower daily dosage levels.

INDICATIONS
CREON is indicated in the treatment of pancreatic exocrine insufficiency, as is often associated with cystic fibrosis, chronic pancreatitis, and pancreatectomy.

CONTRAINDICATIONS
CREON is contraindicated in patients known to be hypersensitive to pork or enzymes. Substitution with pancreatic enzymes is contraindicated in the early stages of acute pancreatitis.

WARNINGS
Pancreatic exocrine replacement therapy should not delay or supplant treatment of the primary disorder. Should symptoms of sensitivity appear, discontinue medication and initiate symptomatic and supportive therapy if necessary.
To protect the enteric coating, microspheres should be swallowed whole, without crushing or chewing. Should microspheres be administered with liquids or soft foods, they should be swallowed quickly, without chewing, as the proteolytic action may cause irritation of the mucosa.

PRECAUTIONS
General:
TO PROTECT ENTERIC COATING, MICROSPHERES SHOULD NOT BE CRUSHED OR CHEWED.
Where swallowing of capsules is difficult, the capsules may be carefully opened and the microspheres added to a small amount (i.e., one spoonful) of liquid or soft food, such as applesauce or pudding. The soft food should be swallowed immediately without chewing, and followed with a glass of water or juice to insure complete swallowing of the microspheres. The food used should not be hot and should be soft enough to swallow without chewing. Contact of the microspheres with foods having a pH greater than 5.5 can dissolve the protective enteric coating. Any mixture of the microspheres with small quantities of food or liquids should be used immediately and not stored.
Information For Patients:
As with other pancreatic enzyme preparations, the microspheres in CREON should not be held in the mouth, as this may cause mouth irritation. To protect the enteric coating, do not crush or chew the microspheres. Where swallowing of capsules is difficult, the capsules may be opened and the microspheres taken with liquids or added to small quantities of soft foods which do not require chewing. For complete directions on this method of use, see PRECAUTIONS, General, above.
Carcinogenesis, Mutagenesis, Impairment of Fertility:
Long-term studies in animals have not been performed to evaluate carcinogenic potential.
Pregnancy Category C:
Animal reproduction studies have not been conducted with CREON. It is also not known whether CREON can cause fetal harm when administered to a pregnant woman or can affect reproduction capacity. CREON should be given to a pregnant woman only if clearly needed.
Nursing Mothers:
It is not known whether this drug is excreted in human milk. Because many drugs are excreted in human milk, caution should be exercised when CREON is administered to a nursing mother.

ADVERSE REACTIONS
Gastrointestinal effects such as nausea, cramping, and/or diarrhea may occur with excessive dosage, and are the most frequently reported reactions. Very high doses of pancreatin have been associated with hyperuricosuria and hyperuricemia. Perianal irritation could occur, and rarely, inflammation when large doses are used.

DOSAGE AND ADMINISTRATION
Usual Dosage:
Initially one or two capsules with meals or snacks, then adjust depending on individual requirements for control of steatorrhea. The daily dose of CREON can be administered in divided doses either at one- or two-hour intervals or with meals.

HOW SUPPLIED
CREON is available in opaque brown/clear yellow hard gelatin capsules imprinted in white with "REID-ROWELL" and "Creon". The capsules contain buff-colored enteric-coated microspheres of pancreatin supplied in bottles of 100 capsules (NDC 0032-1200-01) and 250 capsules (NDC 0032-1200-07).
Storage
Store at controlled room temperature, 15°–30° C (59°–86° F). PROTECT FROM MOISTURE. Do not refrigerate. Dispense in tight, light-resistant containers.
Manufactured By:
Kali-Chemie Pharma GmbH*
Hannover, West Germany
Marketed By:
REID-ROWELL*
Marietta, GA 30062
*Members of the Solvay Group

                 Rev. 1/89
Shown in Product Identification Section, page 423

CURRETAB®   ℞
[kur'e-tab]
Medroxyprogesterone Acetate Tablets, USP 10 mg

HOW SUPPLIED
Curretab 10mg Tablets are white, round, scored imprinted RR 1007, supplied in bottles of 50 tablets (NDC 0032-1007-42).
Shown in Product Identification Section, page 423

DUPHALAC®   ℞
(Lactulose Syrup, USP)
10 g/15 mL

PRODUCT OVERVIEW
KEY FACTS
Duphalac (lactulose) is a synthetic disaccharide in syrup form for oral administration. Each 15 mL of Duphalac contains: 10 g lactulose (and less than 2.2 g galactose, less than 1.2 g lactose, and 1.2 g or less of other sugars).
MAJOR USES
Duphalac is indicated for the treatment of primary constipation. Patients with constipation associated with other conditions e.g. anal fissures, hemorrhoids, post surgery, or post partum may benefit from Duphalac therapy.
SAFETY INFORMATION
Since Duphalac contains galactose (less than 2.2 g/15 mL), it is contraindicated in patients who require a low galactose diet; it should be used with caution in diabetes.

PRESCRIBING INFORMATION
DUPHALAC®   ℞
(Lactulose Syrup, USP)
10 g/15 mL

DESCRIPTION
Duphalac (lactulose) is a synthetic disaccharide in syrup form for oral administration. Each 15 mL of Duphalac contains: 10 g lactulose (and less than 2.2 g galactose, less than 1.2 g lactose, and 1.2 g or less of other sugars).
Duphalac is a colonic acidifier which promotes laxation.
The chemical name for lactulose is 4-O-β-D-galacto pyranosyl-D-fructofuranose. It has the following structural formula:

The molecular weight is 342.30. It is freely soluble in water.

CLINICAL PHARMACOLOGY
Duphalac is poorly absorbed from the gastrointestinal tract and no enzyme capable of hydrolysis of this disaccharide is present in human gastrointestinal tissue. As a result, oral doses of Duphalac reach the colon virtually unchanged. In the colon, Duphalac is broken down primarily to lactic acid, and also to small amounts of formic and acetic acids, by the action of colonic bacteria, which results in an increase in osmotic pressure and slight acidification of the colonic contents. This in turn causes an increase in stool water content and softens the stool.
Since Duphalac does not exert its effect until it reaches the colon, and since transit time through the colon may be slow, 24 to 48 hours may be required to produce the desired bowel movement.
Duphalac given orally to man and experimental animals resulted in only small amounts reaching the blood. Urinary excretion has been determined to be 3% or less and is essentially complete within 24 hours.

INDICATIONS AND USAGE
For the treatment of constipation. In patients with a history of chronic constipation, Duphalac (lactulose syrup) therapy increases the number of bowel movements per day and the number of days on which bowel movements occur.

CONTRAINDICATIONS
Since Duphalac contains galactose (less than 2.2 g/15 mL), it is contraindicated in patients who require a low galactose diet.

WARNINGS
A theoretical hazard may exist for patients being treated with lactulose syrup who may be required to undergo electrocautery procedures during proctoscopy or colonoscopy. Accumulation of H_2 gas in significant concentration in the presence of an electrical spark may result in an explosive reaction. Although this complication has not been reported with lactulose, patients on lactulose therapy undergoing such procedures should have a thorough bowel cleansing with a non-fermentable solution. Insufflation of CO_2 as an additional safeguard may be pursued but is considered to be a redundant measure.

PRECAUTIONS
General: Since Duphalac contains galactose (less than 2.2 g/15 mL) and lactose (less than 1.2 g/15 mL), it should be used with caution in diabetics.
Information for Patients: In the event that an unusual diarrheal condition occurs, contact your physician.
Laboratory Tests: Elderly, debilitated patients who receive Duphalac for more than six months should have serum electrolytes (potassium, chloride, carbon dioxide) measured periodically.
Drug Interactions: Results of preliminary studies in humans and rats suggest that nonabsorbable antacids given concurrently with lactulose may inhibit the desired lactulose-induced drop in colonic pH. Therefore, a possible lack of desired effect of treatment should be taken into consideration before such drugs are given concomitantly with Duphalac.
Carcinogenesis, Mutagenesis, Impairment of Fertility: There are no known human data on long-term potential for carcinogenicity, mutagenicity, or impairment of fertility.
There are no known animal data on long-term potential for mutagenicity.
Administration of lactulose syrup in the diet of mice for 18 months in concentrations of 3 and 10 percent (V/W) did not produce any evidence of carcinogenicity.
In studies in mice, rats and rabbits doses of lactulose syrup up to 6 or 12 mL/kg/day produced no deleterious effects in breeding, conception, or parturition.
Pregnancy:
Teratogenic Effects:
Pregnancy Category B: Reproduction studies have been performed in mice, rats, and rabbits at doses up to 3 or 6 times the usual human oral dose and have revealed no evidence of impaired fertility or harm to the fetus due to lactulose. There are, however, no adequate and well-controlled studies in pregnant women. Because animal reproduction studies are not always predictive of human response, this drug should be used during pregnancy only if clearly needed.
Nursing Mothers: It is not known whether this drug is excreted in human milk. Because many drugs are excreted in human milk, caution should be exercised when Duphalac is administered to a nursing woman.
Pediatric Use: Safety and effectiveness in children have not been established.

ADVERSE REACTIONS
Precise frequency data are not available.
Initial dosing may produce flatulence and intestinal cramps, which are usually transient. Excessive dosage can lead to diarrhea with potential complications such as loss of fluids, hypokalemia and hypernatremia.
Nausea and vomiting have been reported.

OVERDOSAGE
Signs and Symptoms: There have been no reports of accidental overdosage. In the event of overdosage, it is expected that diarrhea and abdominal cramps would be the major symptoms. Medication should be terminated.
Oral LD$_{50}$: The acute oral LD$_{50}$ of the drug is 48.8 mL/kg in mice and greater than 30 mL/kg in rats.

Dialysis: Dialysis data are not available for lactulose. Its molecular similarity to sucrose, however, would suggest that it should be dialyzable.

DOSAGE AND ADMINISTRATION

The usual dose is 1 to 2 tablespoonfuls (15 to 30 mL, containing 10 g to 20 g of lactulose) daily. The dose may be increased to 60 mL daily if necessary. Twenty-four to 48 hours may be required to produce a normal bowel movement.
Note: Some patients have found that Duphalac may be more acceptable when mixed with fruit juice, water or milk.

HOW SUPPLIED

Duphalac (lactulose syrup) is a colorless to yellow color+ syrup, that may darken on standing, for oral administration, containing 10 g/15 mL lactulose (667 mg/mL). It is available as:
NDC 0032-1602-08
8 fl oz bottles
NDC 0032-1602-78
16 fl oz bottles
NDC 0032-1602-80
32 fl oz bottles
NDC 0032-1602-84
30 mL unit dose cups in trays of 10 cups.
Store at controlled room temperature, 15°–30°C (59°–86°F). Do not freeze.
+Under recommended storage conditions, a normal darkening of color may occur. Such darkening is characteristic of sugar solutions and does not affect therapeutic action. Prolonged exposure to temperatures above 30°C (86°F) or to direct light may cause extreme darkening and turbidity which may be pharmaceutically objectionable. If this condtion develops, do not use.
Prolonged exposure to freezing temperatures may cause change to a semi-solid, too viscous to pour. Viscosity will return to normal upon warming to room temperature.

CAUTION

Federal law prohibits dispensing without prescription.
Duphalac® is a registered trademark of Duphar, B.V.
Manufactured By:
Duphar, B.V.*
Weesp, The Netherlands
Marketed By:
Reid-Rowell*
Marietta, GA 30062
*Members of the Solvay Group   Rev. 12/88
Shown in Product Identification Section, page 424

ESTRATAB®   ℞

[es'trah-tab]
Esterified Estrogens Tablets, USP
0.3 mg., 0.625 mg. 1.25 mg 2.5 mg

WARNING

1. ESTROGENS HAVE BEEN REPORTED TO INCREASE THE RISK OF ENDOMETRIAL CARCINOMA.

Three independent case control studies have reported an increased risk of endometrial cancer in postmenopausal women exposed to exogenous estrogens for prolonged periods.[1-3] This risk was independent of the other known risk factors for endometrial cancer. These studies are futher supported by the finding that incidence rates of endometrial cancer have increased sharply since 1969 in eight different areas of the United States with population-based cancer reporting systems, an increase which may be related to the rapidly expanding use of estrogens during the last decade.[4]
The three case control studies reported that the risk of endometrial cancer in estrogen users was about 4.5 to 13.9 times greater than in nonusers. The risk appears to depend on both duration of treatment[1] and on estrogen dose.[3] In view of these findings, when estrogens are used for the treatment of menopausal symptoms, the lowest dose that will control symptoms should be utilized and medication should be discontinued as soon as possible. When prolonged treatment is medically indicated, the patient should be reassessed on at least a semiannual basis to determine the need for continued therapy. Although the evidence must be considered preliminary, one study suggests that cyclic administration of low doses of estrogen may carry less risk than continuous administration;[3] it therefore appears prudent to utilize such a regimen.
Close clinical surveillance of all women taking estrogens is important. In all cases of undiagnosed persistent or recurring abnormal vaginal bleeding, adequate diagnostic measures should be undertaken to rule out malignancy.
There is no evidence at present that "natural" estrogens are more or less hazardous than "synthetic" estrogens at equiestrogenic doses.

---

2. ESTROGENS SHOULD NOT BE USED DURING PREGNANCY.

The use of female sex hormones, both estrogens and progestogens, during early pregnancy may seriously damage the offspring. It has been shown that females exposed in utero to diethylstilbestrol, a non-steroidal estrogen, have an increased risk of developing in later life a form of vaginal or cervical cancer that is ordinarily extremely rare.[5-6] This risk has been estimated as not greater than 4 per 1000 exposures.[7] Furthermore, a high percentage of such exposed women (from 30 to 90 percent) have been found to have vaginal adenosis,[8-12] epithelial changes of the vagina and cervix. Although these changes are histologically benign, it is not known whether they are precursors of malignancy. Although similar data are not available with the use of other estrogens, it cannot be presumed they would not induce similar changes.
Several reports suggest an association between intra-uterine exposure to female sex hormones and congenital anomalies, including congenital heart defects and limb reduction defects.[13-16] One case control study[16] estimated a 4.7 fold increased risk of limb reduction defects in infants exposed in utero to sex hormones (oral contraceptives, hormone withdrawal tests for pregnancy, or attempted treatment for threatened abortion). Some of these exposures were very short and involved only a few days of treatment. The data suggest that the risk of limb reduction defects in exposed fetuses is somewhat less than 1 per 1000.
In the past, female sex hormones have been used during pregnancy in an attempt to treat threatened or habitual abortion. There is considerable evidence that estrogens are ineffective for these indications, and there is no evidence from well controlled studies that progestogens are effective for these uses.
If ESTRATAB® is used during pregnancy, or if the patient becomes pregnant while taking this drug, she should be apprised of the potential risks to the fetus, and the advisability of pregnancy continuation.

DESCRIPTION

ESTRATAB® (Esterified Estrogens Tablets). Each blue, sugar coated tablet contains 0.3 mg. Each yellow, sugar coated tablet contains 0.625 mg. Each orange-red, sugar coated tablet contains 1.25 mg. Each pink, sugar coated tablet contains 2.5 mg.
Inactive Ingredients: Acacia, calcium carbonate, carnauba wax, carboxymethylcellulose sodium, citric acid, colloidal silicon dioxide, diacetylated monoglyceride, gelatin, lactose, magnesium stearate, methylparaben, microcrystalline cellulose, pharmaceutical glaze, povidone, propylparaben, shellac, sodium benzoate, sodium bicarbonate, sorbic acid, sucrose, corn starch, talc, titanium dioxide and tribasic calcium phosphate. Tablet imprinting ink contains black iron oxide. FD&C Blue #2 Lake, FD&C Red #40 Lake and FD&C Yellow #6 Lake. In addition the 0.3 mg tablet contains FD&C Blue #1 Lake; the 0.625 mg tablet contains D&C Yellow #10 Lake, FD&C Yellow #6 Lake and FD&C Blue #2 Lake; the 1.25 mg tablet contains FD&C Yellow #6 Lake and FD&C Red #3 Lake and the 2.5 mg tablet contains FD&C Red #3 Lake.
ESTRATAB® (Esterified Estrogens Tablets) for oral administration is a mixture of the sodium salts of the sulfate esters of the estrogenic substances, principally estrone, that are of the type excreted by pregnant mares. Esterified Estrogens contain not less than 75.0 percent and not more than 85.0 percent of sodium estrone sulfate, and not less than 6.0 percent and not more than 15.0 percent of sodium equilin sulfate, in such proportion that the total of these two components is not less than 90.0 percent.

CLINICAL PHARMACOLOGY

Estrogens are important in the development and maintenance of the female reproductive system and secondary sex characteristics. They promote growth and development of the vagina, uterus, and fallopian tubes, and enlargement of the breasts. Indirectly, they contribute to the shaping of the skeleton, maintenance of tone and elasticity of urogenital structures, changes in the epiphyses of the long bones that allow for the pubertal growth spurt and its termination, growth of axillary and pubic hair, and pigmentation of the nipples and genitals. Decline of estrogenic activity at the end of the menstrual cycle can bring on menstruation, although the cessation of progesterone secretion is the most important factor in the mature ovulatory cycle. However, in the preovulatory or nonovulatory cycle, estrogen is the primary determinant in the onset of menstruation. Estrogens also affect the release of pituitary gonadotropins.
The pharmacologic effects of conjugated estrogens are similar to those of endogenous estrogens. They are soluble in water and are well absorbed from the gastrointestinal tract. In responsive tissues (female genital organs, breasts, hypothalamus, pituitary) estrogens enter the cell and are trans-

---

ported into the nucleus. As a result of estrogen action, specific RNA and protein synthesis occurs.
Metabolism and inactivation occur primarily in the liver. Some estrogens are excreted into the bile; however they are reabsorbed from the intestine and returned to the liver through the portal venous system. Water soluble estrogen conjugates are strongly acidic and are ionized in body fluids, which favor excretion through the kidneys since tubular reabsorption is minimal.

INDICATIONS

ESTRATAB® is indicated in the treatment of:
1. Moderate to severe *vasomotor* symptoms associated with the menopause. (There is no evidence that estrogens are effective for nervous symptoms or depression which might occur during menopause and they should not be used to treat these conditions).
2. Atrophic vaginitis.
3. Kraurosis vulvae.
4. Female hypogonadism.
5. Female castration.
6. Primary ovarian failure.
7. Breast cancer (for palliation only) in appropriately selected women and men with metastatic disease.
8. Prostatic carcinoma—palliative therapy of advanced disease.
ESTRATAB® HAS NOT BEEN SHOWN TO BE EFFECTIVE FOR ANY PURPOSE DURING PREGNANCY AND ITS USE MAY CAUSE SEVERE HARM TO THE FETUS (SEE BOXED WARNING).
The lowest effective dose appropriate for the specific indication should be utilized. Studies of the addition of a progestin for seven or more days of a cycle of estrogen administration have reported a lowered incidence of endometrial hyperplasia. Morphological and biochemical studies of endometrium suggest that 10 to 13 days of progestin are needed to provide maximal maturation of the endometrium and to eliminate any hyperplastic changes. Whether this will provide protection from endometrial carcinoma has not been clearly established. There are possible additional risks which may be associated with the inclusion of progestin in estrogen replacement regimens. The potential risks include adverse effects on carbohydrate and lipid metabolism. The choice of progestin and dosage may be important in minimizing these adverse effects.

CONTRAINDICATIONS

Estrogens should not be used in women (or men) with any of the following conditions:
1. Known or suspected cancer of the breast except in appropriately selected patients being treated for metastatic disease.
2. Known or suspected estrogen-dependent neoplasia.
3. Known or suspected pregnancy (See Boxed Warning).
4. Undiagnosed abnormal genital bleeding.
5. Active thrombophlebitis or thromboembolic disorders.
6. A past history of thrombophlebitis, thrombosis, or thromboembolic disorders associated with previous estrogen use (except when used in treatment of breast or prostatic malignancy).

WARNINGS

1. **Induction of malignant neoplasms.** Long term continuous administration of natural and synthetic estrogens in certain animal species increases the frequency of carcinomas of the breast, cervix, vagina, and liver. There is now evidence that estrogens increase the risk of carcinoma of the endometrium in humans (See Boxed Warning).
At the present time there is no satisfactory evidence that estrogens given to postmenopausal women increase the risk of cancer of the breast,[18] although a recent long-term followup of a single physician's practice has raised this possibility.[18a] Because of the animal data, there is a need for caution in prescribing estrogens for women with a strong family history of breast cancer or who have breast nodules, fibrocystic disease, or abnormal mammograms.
2. **Gall bladder disease.** A recent study has reported a 2 to 3-fold increase in the risk of surgically confirmed gall bladder disease in women receiving postmenopausal estrogens,[18] similar to the 2-fold increase previously noted in users of oral contraceptives.[19-24] In the case of oral contraceptives the increased risk appeared after two years of use.[24]
3. **Effects similar to those caused by estrogen-progestogen oral contraceptives.** There are several serious adverse effects of oral contraceptives, most of which have not, up to now, been documented as consequences of postmenopausal estrogen therapy. This may reflect the comparatively low doses of estrogen used in postmenopausal women. It would be expected that the larger doses of estrogen used to treat prostatic or breast cancer or postpartum breast engorgement are more likely to result in these adverse effects, and, in fact, it has been shown that there is an increased risk of thrombosis in men receiving estrogens

Continued on next page

Reid-Rowell—Cont.

for prostatic cancer and women for postpartum breast engorgement.[20-23]

a. **Thromboembolic disease.** It is now well established that users of oral contraceptives have an increased risk of various thromboembolic and thrombotic vascular disease, such as thrombophlebitis, pulmonary embolism, stroke, and myocardial infarction.[24-31] Cases of retinal thrombosis, mesenteric thrombosis, and optic neuritis have been reported in oral contraceptive users. There is evidence that the risk of several of these adverse reactions is related to the dose of the drug.[32-33] An increased risk of postsurgery thromboembolic complications has also been reported in users of oral contraceptives.[34-35] If feasible, estrogen should be discontinued at least 4 weeks before surgery of the type associated with an increased risk of thromboembolism, or during periods of prolonged immobilization.

While an increased rate of thromboembolic and thrombotic disease in postmenopausal users of estrogens has not been found,[18-36] this does not rule out the possibility that such an increase may be present or that subgroups of women who have underlying risk factors or who are receiving relatively large doses of estrogens may have increased risk. Therefore estrogens should not be used in persons with active thrombophlebitis or thromboembolic disorders, and they should not be used (except in treatment of malignancy) in persons with a history of such disorders in association with estrogen use. They should be used with caution in patients with cerebral vascular or coronary artery disease and only for those in whom estrogens are clearly needed.

Large doses of estrogen (5 mg esterified estrogens per day) comparable to those used to treat cancer of the prostate and breast, have been shown in a large prospective clinical trial in men[37] to increase the risk of nonfatal myocardial infarction, pulmonary embolism and thrombophlebitis. When estrogen doses of this size are used, any of the thromboembolic and thrombotic adverse effects associated with oral contraceptive use should be considered a clear risk.

b. **Hepatic adenoma.** Benign hepatic adenomas appear to be associated with the use of oral contraceptives.[38-40] Although benign and rare, these may rupture and may cause death through intraabdominal hemorrhage. Such lesions have not yet been reported in association with other estrogen or progestogen preparations but should be considered in estrogen users having abdominal pain and tenderness, abdominal mass, or hypovolemic shock. Hepatocellular carcinoma has also been reported in women taking estrogen-containing oral contraceptives.[39] The relationship of this malignancy to these drugs is not known at this time.

c. **Elevated blood pressure.** Increased blood pressure is not uncommon in women using oral contraceptives. There is now a report that this may occur with use of estrogens in the menopause[41] and blood pressure should be monitored with estrogen use, especially if high doses are used.

d. **Glucose tolerance.** A worsening of glucose tolerance has been observed in a significant percentage of patients on estrogen-containing oral contraceptives. For this reason, diabetic patients should be carefully observed while receiving estrogens.

4. **Hypercalcemia.** Administration of estrogens may lead to severe hypercalcemia in patients with breast cancer and bone metastases. If this occurs, the drug should be stopped and appropriate measures taken to reduce the serum calcium level.

PRECAUTIONS

A. **General Precautions.**

1. A complete medical and family history should be taken prior to the initiation of any estrogen therapy. The pretreatment and periodic physical examinations should include special reference to blood pressure, breasts, abdomen, and pelvic organs, and should include a Papanicolaou smear. As a general rule, estrogen should not be prescribed for longer than one year without another physical examination being performed.

2. Fluid retention—Because estrogens may cause some degree of fluid retention, conditions which might be influenced by this factor such as epilepsy, migraine, and cardiac or renal dysfunction, require careful observation.

3. Certain patients may develop undesirable manifestations of excessive estrogenic stimulation, such as abnormal or excessive uterine bleeding, mastodynia, etc.

4. Oral contraceptives appear to be associated with an increased incidence of mental depression.[24] Although it is not clear whether this is due to the estrogenic or progestogenic component of the contraceptive, patients with a history of depression should be carefully observed.

5. Preexisting uterine leiomyomata may increase in size during estrogen use.

6. The pathologist should be advised of estrogen therapy when relevant specimens are submitted.

7. Patients with a past history of jaundice during pregnancy have an increased risk of recurrence of jaundice while receiving estrogen-containing oral contraceptive therapy. If jaundice develops in any patient receiving estrogen, the medication should be discontinued while the cause is investigated.

8. Estrogens may be poorly metabolized in patients with impaired liver function and they should be administered with caution in such patients.

9. Because estrogens influence the metabolism of calcium and phosphorus, they should be used with caution in patients with metabolic bone diseases that are associated with hypercalcemia or in patients with renal insufficiency.

10. Because of the effects of estrogens on epiphyseal closure, they should be used judiciously in young patients in whom bone growth is not complete.

11. Certain endocrine and liver function tests may be affected by estrogen-containing oral contraceptives. The following similar changes may be expected with larger doses of estrogen:

  a. Increased sulfobromophthalein retention.

  b. Increased prothrombin and factors VII, VIII, IX and X; decreased antithrombin 3, increased norepinephrine-induced platelet aggregability.

  c. Increased thyroid binding globulin (TBG) leading to increased circulating total thyroid hormone, as measured by PBI, T4 by column, or T4 by radioimmunoassay. Free T3 resin uptake is decreased, reflecting the elevated TBG; free T4 concentration is unaltered.

  d. Impaired glucose tolerance.

  e. Decreased pregnanediol excretion.

  f. Reduced response to metyrapone test.

  g. Reduced serum folate concentration.

  h. Increased serum triglyceride and phospholipid concentration.

B. **Information for the Patient.** See text of Patient Package Insert which appears after the REFERENCES.

C. **Pregnancy Category X.** See CONTRAINDICATIONS and Boxed WARNING.

D. **Nursing Mothers.** As a general principle, the administration of any drug to nursing mothers should be done only when clearly necessary since many drugs are excreted in human milk.

ADVERSE REACTIONS

(See Warnings regarding induction of neoplasia, adverse effects on the fetus, increased incidence of gall bladder disease, and adverse effects similar to those of oral contraceptives, including thromboembolism). The following additional adverse reactions have been reported with estrogenic therapy, including oral contraceptives:

1. **Genitourinary system.**
Breakthrough bleeding, spotting, change in menstrual flow.
Dysmenorrhea.
Premenstrual-like syndrome.
Amenorrhea during and after treatment.
Increase in size of uterine fibromyomata.
Vaginal candidiasis.
Change in cervical erosion and in degree of cervical secretion.
Cystitis-like syndrome.

2. **Breasts**
Tenderness, enlargement, secretion.

3. **Gastrointestinal.**
Nausea, vomiting.
Abdominal cramps, bloating.
Cholestatic jaundice.

4. **Skin.**
Chloasma or melasma which may persist when drug is discontinued.
Erythema multiforme.
Erythema nodosum.
Hemorrhagic eruption.
Loss of scalp hair.
Hirsutism.

5. **Eyes.**
Steepening of corneal curvature.
Intolerance to contact lenses.

6. **CNS.**
Headache, migraine, dizziness.
Mental depression.
Chorea.

7. **Miscellaneous.**
Increase or decrease in weight.
Reduced carbohydrate tolerance.
Aggravation of porphyria.
Edema.
Changes in libido.

OVERDOSAGE

Numerous reports of ingestion of large doses of estrogen-containing oral contraceptives by young children indicate that serious ill effects do not occur. Overdosage of estrogen may cause nausea, and withdrawal bleeding may occur in females.

DOSAGE AND ADMINISTRATION

1. **Given cyclically for short term use only:**
For treatment of moderate to severe *vasomotor* symptoms, atrophic vaginitis, or kraurosis vulvae associated with the menopause.
The lowest dose that will control symptoms should be chosen and medication should be discontinued as promptly as possible.
Administration should be cyclic (e.g., three weeks on and one week off). Attempts to discontinue or taper medication should be made at three to six month intervals.
Usual dosage ranges:
Vasomotor symptoms—1.25 mg daily. If the patient has not menstruated within the last two months or more, cyclic administration is started arbitrarily. If the patient is menstruating, cyclic administration is started on day 5 of bleeding.
Atrophic vaginitis and kraurosis vulvae—0.3 mg to 1.25 mg or more daily, depending upon the tissue response of the individual patient. Administer cyclically.

2. **Given cyclically:** Female hypogonadism; female castration; primary ovarian failure.
Usual dosage ranges:
Female hypogonadism—2.5 to 7.5 mg daily, in divided doses for 20 days, followed by a rest period of 10 days' duration. If bleeding does not occur by the end of this period, the same dosage schedule is repeated. The number of courses of estrogen therapy necessary to produce bleeding may vary depending on the responsiveness of the endometrium.
If bleeding occurs before the end of the 10 day period, begin a 20 day estrogen-progestin cyclic regimen with ESTRATAB® (Esterified Estrogens Tablets, USP), 2.5 to 7.5 mg daily in divided doses, for 20 days. During the last five days of estrogen therapy, give an oral progestin. If bleeding occurs before this regimen is concluded, therapy is discontinued and may be resumed on the fifth day of bleeding.
Female castration, and primary ovarian failure—1.25 mg daily, cyclically. Adjust dosage upward or downward according to severity of symptoms and response of the patient. For maintenance, adjust dosage to lowest level that will provide effective control.

3. **Given chronically:** Inoperable progressing prostatic cancer—1.25 to 2.5 mg three times daily. The effectiveness of therapy can be judged by phosphatase determinations as well as by symptomatic improvement of the patient.
Inoperable progressing breast cancer in appropriately selected men and postmenopausal women. (See INDICATIONS)—Suggested dosage is 10 mg three times daily for a period of at least three months.
Treated patients with an intact uterus should be monitored closely for signs of endometrial cancer and appropriate diagnostic measures should be taken to rule out malignancy in the event of persistent or recurring abnormal vaginal bleeding.

HOW SUPPLIED

ESTRATAB® (Esterified Estrogens Tablets, USP):
Each blue tablet contains 0.3 mg in bottles of 100 (NDC 0032-1014-01).
Each yellow tablet contains 0.625 mg in bottles of 100 (NDC 0032-1022-01) and 1000 (NDC 0032-1022-10).
Each orange-red tablet contains 1.25 mg in bottles of 100 (NDC 0032-1024-01) and 1000 (NDC 0032-1024-10).
Each pink tablet contains 2.5 mg in bottles of 100 (NDC 0032-1025-01).

STORAGE

Store and dispense in tight, light-resistant containers as defined in the USP. Store below 30°C (86°F).
Protect from moisture.

Revised: 1/89

REFERENCES

1. Ziel, H. K. and Finkle, W. D., "Increased Risk of Endometrial Carcinoma Among Users of Conjugated Estrogens," **New England Journal of Medicine,** 293:1167–1170, 1975.

2. Smith, D. C., Prentic, R., Thompson, D. J., and Hermann, W. L., "Association of Exogenous Estrogen and Endometrial Carcinoma," **New England Journal of Medicine,** 293:1164–1167, 1975.

3. Mack, T. M., Pike, M. C., Henderson, B. E., Pfeffer, R. I., Gerkins, V. R., Arthur, M. and Brown, S. E., "Estrogens and Endometrial Cancer in a Retirement Community," **England Journal of Medicine,** *294*:1262–1267, 1976.

4. Weiss, N.S., Szekely, D. R. and Austin, D. F., "Increasing Incidence of Endometrial Cancer in the United States," **New England Journal of Medicine,** 294:1259–1262, 1976.

5. Herbst, A. L., Ulfelder, H. and Poskanzer, D. C., "Adenocarcinoma of Vagina," **New England Journal of Medicine,** 284:878–881, 1971.

6. Greenwald, P., Barlow, J., Nasca, P. and Burnett, W., "Vaginal Cancer after Maternal Treatment with Synthetic Estrogens," **New England Journal of Medicine,** 285:390–392, 1971.

7. Lanier, A., Noller, K., Decker, D., Elveback, L. and Kurland, L., "Cancer and Stilbestrol. A Followup of 1719 Persons Exposed to Estrogens in Utero and Born 1943-1959," **Mayo Clinic Preceedings,** 48:793–799, 1973.

8. Herbst, A., Kurman, R. and Scully, R.,"Vaginal and Cervical Abnormalities After Exposure to Stilbestrol In Utero," **Obstetrics and Gynecology,** 40:287–298, 1972.

9. Herbst, A., Robboy, S., Macdonald, G. and Scully, R., "The Effects of Local Progesterone on Stilbestrol-Associated Vaginal Adenosis," **American Journal of Obsetrics and Gynecology,** 118:607–615, 1974.

10. Herbst, A., Poskanzer, D., Robboy, S., Friedlander, L. and Scully, R., "Prenatal Exposure to Stilbestrol, A Prospective Comparison of Exposed Female Offspring with Unexposed Controls," **New England Journal of Medicine,** 292:334–339, 1975.

11. Stafl, A., Mattingly, R., Foley, D. and Fetherston, W., "Clinical Diagnosis of Vaginal Adenosis," **Obstetrics and Gynecology,** 43:118–128, 1974.

12. Sherman, A. I., Goldrath, M., Berlin, A., Vakhariya, V., Banooni, F., Michaels, W., Goodman, P., Brown, S., "Cervical-Vaginal Adenosis After In Utero Exposure to Synthetic Estrogens," **Obstetrics and Gynecology,** 44:531–545, 1974.

13. Gal, I., Kirman, B. and Stern, J., "Hormone Pregnancy Tests and Congenital Malformation," **Nature,** 216:83, 1967.

14. Levy, E. P., Cohen, A. and Fraser, F. C., "Hormone Treatment During Pregnancy and Congenital Heart Defects," **Lancet,** 1:611, 1973.

15. Nora, J. and Nora, A., "Birth Defects and Oral Contraceptives," **Lancet,** 1:941–942, 1973.

16. Janerich, D. T., Piper, J. M. and Glebatis, D. M., "Oral Contraceptives and Congenital Limb-Reduction Defects," **New England Journal of Medicine,** 291:697–700, 1974.

17. "Estrogens for Oral or Parenteral Use," **Federal Register,** 40:8212, 1975.

18. Boston Collaborative Drug Surveillance Program, "Surgically Confirmed Gall Bladder Disease, Venous Thromboembolism and Breast Tumors in Relation to Post-Menopausal Estrogen Therapy," **New England Journal of Medicine,** 290:15–19, 1974.

18a.Hoover, R., Gray, Sr., L. A., Cole, P. and MacMahon, B., "Menopausal Estrogens and Breast Cancer," **New England Journal of Medicine,** 295:401–405, 1976.

19. Boston Collaborative Drug Surveillance Program, "Oral Contraceptives and Venous Thromboembolic Disease, Surgically Confirmed Gall Bladder Disease, and Breast Tumors," **Lancet** 1:1399–1404, 1973.

20. Daniel, D., Campbell, G. H. and Turnbull, A. C., "Puerperal Thromboembolism and Suppression of Lactation", **Lancet** 2:287–289, 1967.

21. The Veterans Administration Cooperative Urological Research Group, "Carcinoma of the Prostate: Treatment Comparisons," **Journal of Urology,** 98:516–522, 1967.

22. Ballar, J. C., "Thromboembolism and Oestrogen Therapy," **Lancet,** 2:560, 1967.

23. Blackard, C., Doe, R., Mellinger, G. and Byar, D., "Incidence of Cardiovascular Disease and Death in Patients Receiving Diethylstilbestrol for Carcinoma of the Prostate," **Cancer,** 26:249–256, 1970.

24. Royal College of General Practitioners, "Oral Contraception and Thromboembolic Disease," **Journal of the Royal College of General Practitioners,** 13:267–279, 1967.

25. Inman, W. H. and Vessey, FM. P., "Investigation of Deaths from Pulmonary, Coronary, and Cerebral Thrombosis and Embolism in Women of Child-Bearing Age," **British Medical Journal,** 2:193–199, 1968.

26. Vessey, M. P. and Doll, R., "Investigation of Relation Between Use of Oral Contraceptives and Thromboembolic Disease, A Further Report," **British Medical Journal,** 2:651–657, 1969.

27. Sartwell, P. E., Masi, A. T., Arthes, F. G., Greene, G. R. and Smith, H.E., "Thromboembolism and Oral Contraceptives: An Epidemiological Case Control Study," **American Journal of Epidemiology,** 90:365–380, 1969.

28. Collaborative Group for the Study of Stroke in Young Women, "Oral Contraception and Increased Risk of Cerebral Ischemia or Thrombosis," **New England Journal of Medicine,** 288:871–878, 1973.

29. Collaborative Group for the Study of Stroke in Young Women, "Oral Contraceptives and Stroke in Young Women: Associated Risk Factors," **Journal of the American Medical Association,** 231:718–722, 1975.

30. Mann, J. I. and Inman, W. H. W., "Oral Contraceptives and Death from Myocardial Infarction," **British Medical Journal,** 2:245–248, 1975.

31. Mann, J. I., Vessey, M. P., Thorogood, M. and Doll, R., "Myocardial Infarction in Young Women with Special Reference to Oral Contraceptive Practice," **British Medical Journal,** 2:241–245, 1975.

32. Inman, W. H. W., Vessey, V. P., Westerholm, B. and Engelund, A., "Thromboembolic Disease and the Steroidal Content of Oral Contraceptives," **British Medical Journal,** 2:203–209, 1970.

33. Stolley, P.D., Tonascia, J. A., Tockman, M. S., Sartwell, P. E., Rutledge, A. H. and Jacobs, M. P., "Thrombosis with Low-Estrogen Oral Contraceptives," **American Journal of Epidemiology,** 102:197–208, 1975.

34. Vessey, M. P., Doll, R., Fairbairn, A. S., and Glober, G., "Post-Operative Thromboembolism and the Use of the Oral Contraceptives," **British Medical Journal,** 3:123–126, 1970.

35. Greene, G. R. and Sartwell, P. E., "Oral Contraceptive Use in Patients with Thromboembolism Following Surgery, Trauma or Infection," **American Journal of Public Health,** 62:680–685, 1972.

36. Rosenberg, L., Armstrong, M. B. and Jick, H., "Myocardial Infarction and Estrogen Therapy in Postmenopausal Women," **New England Journal of Medicine,** 294:1256–1259, 1976.

37. Coronary Drug Project Research Group, The Coronary Drug Project: Initial Findings Leading to Modifications of Its Research Protocol, **Journal of the American Medical Association,** 214:1303–1313, 1970.

38. Baum, J., Holtz, F., Bookstein, J. J., and Klein, E. W., "Possible Association between Benign Hepatomas and Oral Contraceptives," **Lancet,** 2:926–928, 1973.

39. Mays, E. T., Christopherson, W. M., Mahr, M. M. and Williams, H. C., "Hepatic Changes in Young Women Ingesting Contraceptive Steroids, Hepatic Hemorrhage and Primary Hepatic Tumors," **Journal of the American Medical Association,** 235:730–782, 1976.

40. Edmondson, H. A., Henderson, B. and Benton, B., "Liver Cell Adenomas Associated with the Use of Oral Contraceptives," **New England Journal of Medicine,** 294:470–472, 1976.

41. Pfeffer, R. I. and Van Den Noore, S., "Estrogen Use and Stroke Risk in Postmenopausal Women," **American Journal of Epidemiology,** 103:445–456, 1976.

INFORMATION FOR THE PATIENT

WHAT YOU SHOULD KNOW ABOUT ESTROGENS: Estrogens are female hormones produced by the ovaries. The ovaries make several different kinds of estrogens. In addition, scientists have been able to make a variety of synthetic estrogens. As far as we know, all these estrogens have similar properties and therefore much the same usefulness, side effects, and risks. This leaflet is intended to help you understand what estrogens are used for, the risks involved in their use, and how to use them as safely as possible.

This leaflet includes the most important information about estrogens, but not all the information. If you want to know more, you can ask your doctor or pharmacist to let you read the package insert prepared for the doctor.

USES OF ESTROGEN: Estrogens are prescribed by doctors for a number of purposes, including:

1. To provide estrogen during a period of adjustment when a woman's ovaries no longer produce it, in order to prevent certain uncomfortable symptoms of estrogen deficiency. (All women normally stop producing estrogens, generally between the ages of 45 and 55; this is called the menopause).

2. To prevent symptoms of estrogen deficiency when a woman's ovaries have been removed surgically before the natural menopause.

3. To prevent pregnancy. (Estrogens are given along with a progestogen, another female hormone; these combinations are called oral contraceptives or birth control pills. Patient labeling is available to women taking oral contraceptives and they will not be discussed in this leaflet).

4. To treat certain cancers in women and men.

5. To prevent painful swelling of the breasts after pregnancy in women who choose not to nurse their babies.

THERE IS NO PROPER USE OF ESTROGENS IN A PREGNANT WOMAN.

ESTROGENS IN THE MENOPAUSE: In the natural course of their lives, all women eventually experience a decrease in estrogen production. This usually occurs between ages 45 and 55 but may occur earlier or later. Sometimes the ovaries may need to be removed before natural menopause by an operation, producing a "surgical menopause."

When the amount of estrogen in the blood begins to decrease, many women may develop typical symptoms: Feelings of warmth in the face, neck, and chest or sudden intense episodes of heat and sweating throughout the body (called "hot flashes" or "hot flushes"). These symptoms are sometimes very uncomfortable. A few women eventually develop changes in the vagina (called "atrophic vaginitis") which cause discomfort, especially during and after intercourse. Estrogens can be prescribed to treat these symptoms of the menopause. It is estimated that considerably more than half of all women undergoing the menopause have only mild symptoms or no symptoms at all and therefore do not need estrogens. Other women may need estrogens for a few months, while their bodies adjust to lower estrogen levels. Sometimes the need will be for periods longer than six months. In an attempt to avoid overstimulation of the uterus (womb), estrogens are usually given cyclically during each month of use, that is three weeks of pills followed by one week without pills.

Sometimes women experience nervous symptoms or depression during menopause. There is no evidence that estrogens are effective for such symptoms and they should not be used to treat them, although other treatment may be needed.

You may have heard that taking estrogens for long periods (years) after the menopause will keep your skin soft and supple and keep you feeling young. There is no evidence that this is so, however, and such long-term treatment carries important risks.

ESTROGENS TO PREVENT SWELLING OF THE BREASTS AFTER PREGNANCY: If you do not breast feed your baby after delivery, your breasts may fill up with milk and become painful and engorged. This usually begins about 3 to 4 days after delivery and may last for a few days to up to a week or more. Sometimes the discomfort is severe, but usually it is not and can be controlled by pain relieving drugs such as aspirin and by binding the breasts up tightly. Estrogens can be used to try to prevent the breasts from filling up. While this treatment is sometimes successful, in many cases the breasts fill up to some degree in spite of treatment. The dose of estrogens needed to prevent pain and swelling of the breasts is much larger than the dose needed to treat symptoms of the menopause and this may increase your chances of developing blood clots in the legs or lungs (see below). Therefore, it is important that you discuss the benefits and the risks of estrogen use with your doctor if you have decided not to breast feed your baby.

THE DANGERS OF ESTROGENS:

1. **Cancer of the uterus.** If estrogens are used in the postmenopausal period for more than a year, there is an increased risk of **endometrial cancer** (cancer of the uterus). Women taking estrogens have roughly 5 to 10 times as great a chance of getting this cancer as women who take no estrogens. To put this another way, a postmenopausal woman not taking estrogens has 1 chance in 1,000 each year of getting cancer of the uterus, a woman taking estrogens has 5 to 10 chances in 1,000 each year. For this reason **it is important to take estrogens only when you really need them.**

The risk of this cancer is greater the longer estrogens are used and also seems to be greater when larger doses are taken. For this reason **it is important to take the lowest dose of estrogen that will control symptoms and to take it only as long as it is needed.** If estrogens are needed for longer periods of time, your doctor will want to reevaluate your need for estrogens at least every six months.

Women using estrogens should report any irregular vaginal bleeding to their doctors; such bleeding may be of no importance, but it can be an early warning of cancer of the uterus. If you have undiagnosed vaginal bleeding, you should not use estrogens until a diagnosis is made and you are certain there is no cancer of the uterus.

2. **Other possible cancers.** Estrogens can cause development of other tumors in animals, such as tumors of the breast, cervix, vagina, or liver, when given for a long time. At present there is no good evidence that women using estrogen in the menopause have an increased risk of such tumors, but there is no way yet to be sure they do not; and one study raises the possibility that use of estrogens in the menopause may increase the risk of breast cancer many years later. This is a further reason to use estrogens only when clearly needed. While you are taking estrogens, it is important that you go to your doctor at least once a year for a physical examination. Also, if members of your family have had breast cancer or if you have breast nodules or abnormal mammograms (breast x-rays), your doctor may wish to carry out more frequent examinations of your breasts.

3. **Gall bladder disease.** Women who use estrogens after menopause are more likely to develop gall bladder disease needing surgery as women who do not use estrogens. Birth control pills have a similar effect.

4. **Abnormal blood clotting.** Oral contraceptives increase the risk of blood clotting in various parts of the body. This can result in a stroke (if the clot is in the brain), a heart attack (clot in a blood vessel of the heart), or pulmonary embolus (a clot which forms in the legs or pelvis, then breaks off and travels to the lungs). Any of these can be fatal.

At this time use of estrogens in the menopause is not known to cause such blood clotting, but this has not been fully studied and there could still prove to be such a risk. It is recommended that if you have had clotting in the legs or lungs or a heart attack or stroke while you were using estrogens or birth control pills, you should not use estrogens (unless they are being used to treat cancer of the breast or prostate). If you have had a stroke or heart attack or if you have angina pectoris, estrogens should be used with great caution and only if clearly needed (for example, if you have severe symptoms of the menopause).

Continued on next page

Reid-Rowell—Cont.

The larger doses of estrogen used to prevent swelling of the breasts after pregnancy have been reported to cause clotting in the legs and lungs.

SPECIAL WARNING ABOUT PREGNANCY: You should not receive estrogen if you are pregnant. If this should occur, there is a greater than usual chance that the developing child will be born with a birth defect, although the possibility remains fairly small. A female child may have an increased risk of developing cancer of the vagina or cervix later in life (in the teens or twenties). Every possible effort should be made to avoid exposure to estrogens during pregnancy. If exposure occurs, see your doctor.

OTHER EFFECTS OF ESTROGENS: In addition to the serious known risks of estrogens described above, estrogens have the following side effects and potential risks:

1. **Nausea and vomiting.** The most common side effect of estrogen therapy is nausea. Vomiting is less common.
2. **Effects on breasts.** Estrogens may cause breast tenderness or enlargement and may cause the breasts to secrete a liquid. These effects are not dangerous.
3. **Effects on the uterus.** Estrogens may cause benign fibroid tumors of the uterus to get larger.

Some women will have menstrual bleeding when estrogens are stopped. But if the bleeding occurs on days you are still taking estrogens you should report this to your doctor.

4. **Effects on liver.** Women taking oral contraceptives develop on rare occasions a benign tumor of the liver which can rupture and bleed into the abdomen. So far, these tumors have not been reported in women using estrogens in the menopause, but you should report any swelling or unusual pain or tenderness in the abdomen to your doctor immediately.

Women with a past history of jaundice (yellowing of the skin and white parts of the eyes) may get jaundice again during estrogen use. If this occurs, stop taking estrogens and see your doctor.

5. **Other effects.** Estrogens may cause excess fluid to be retained in the body. This may make some conditions worse, such as epilepsy, migraine, heart disease, or kidney disease.

SUMMARY

Estrogens have important uses, but they have serious risks as well. You must decide, with your doctor, whether the risks are acceptable to you in view of the benefits of treatment. Except where your doctor has prescribed estrogens for use in special cases of cancer of the breast or prostate, you should not use estrogens if you have cancer of the breast or uterus, are pregnant, have undiagnosed abnormal vaginal bleeding, or have had a stroke, heart attack or angina, or clotting in the legs or lungs in the past while you were taking estrogens. You can use estrogens as safely as possible by understanding that your doctor will require regular physical examinations while you are taking them and will try to discontinue the drug as soon as possible and use the smallest dose possible. Be alert for signs of trouble including:

1. Abnormal bleeding from the vagina.
2. Pains in the calves or chest or sudden shortness of breath, or coughing blood (indicating possible clots in the legs, heart, or lungs).
3. Severe headache, dizziness, faintness, or changes in vision (indicating possible developing clots in the brain or eye).
4. Breast lumps (you should ask your doctor how to examine your own breasts).
5. Jaundice (yellowing of the skin).
6. Mental depression.

Based on his or her assessment of your medical needs, your doctor has prescribed this drug for you. Do not give the drug to anyone else.

HOW SUPPLIED

ESTRATAB® (Esterified Estrogen Tablets, USP)—Tablets for oral administration.
0.3 mg/Tablet (Blue); 0.625 mg/Tablet (Yellow); 1.25 mg/Tablet (Orange-Red); and 2.5 mg/Tablet (Pink).
Reid-Rowell
Marietta, Georgia 30062   Revised: 1/89
Shown in Product Identification Section, page 424

ESTRATEST®   ℞
[es 'trah-test]
ESTRATEST® H.S. (Half-Strength)   ℞
Estrogen-Androgen Therapy

WARNING
1. ESTROGENS HAVE BEEN REPORTED TO INCREASE THE RISK OF ENDOMETRIAL CARCINOMA.
Three independent case control studies have reported an increased risk of endometrial cancer in postmeno-

---

pausal women exposed to exogenous estrogens for prolonged periods.[1–3] This risk was independent of the other known risk factors for endometrial cancer. These studies are further supported by the finding that incidence rates of endometrial cancer have increased sharply since 1969 in eight different areas of the United States with population-based cancer reporting systems, an increase which may be related to the rapidly expanding use of estrogens during the last decade.[4]

The three case control studies reported that the risk of endometrial cancer in estrogen users was about 4.5 to 13.9 times greater than in nonusers. The risk appears to depend on both duration of treatment[1] and on estrogen dose.[3] In view of these findings, when estrogens are used for the treatment of menopausal symptoms, the lowest dose that will control symptoms should be utilized and medication should be discontinued as soon as possible. When prolonged treatment is medically indicated, the patient should be reassessed on at least a semiannual basis to determine the need for continued therapy. Although the evidence must be considered preliminary, one study suggests that cyclic administration of low doses of estrogen may carry less risk than continuous administration;[3] it therefore appears prudent to utilize such a regimen.

Close clinical surveillance of all women taking estrogens is important. In all cases of undiagnosed persistent or recurring abnormal vaginal bleeding, adequate diagnostic measures should be undertaken to rule out malignancy.

There is no evidence at present that "natural" estrogens are more or less hazardous than "synthetic" estrogens at equiestrogenic doses.

2. ESTROGENS SHOULD NOT BE USED DURING PREGNANCY.

The use of female sex hormones, both estrogens and progestogens, during early pregnancy may seriously damage the offspring. It has been shown that females exposed in utero to diethylstilbestrol, a non-steroidal estrogen, have an increased risk of developing in later life a form of vaginal or cervical cancer that is ordinarily extremely rare.[5,6] This risk has been estimated as not greater than 4 per 1000 exposures.[7] Furthermore, a high percentage of such exposed women (from 30 to 90 percent) have been found to have vaginal adenosis,[8–12] epithelial changes of the vagina and cervix. Although these changes are histologically benign, it is not known whether they are precursors of malignancy. Although similar data are not available with the use of other estrogens, it cannot be presumed they would not induce similar changes.

Several reports suggest an association between intrauterine exposure to female sex hormones and congenital anomalies, including congenital heart defects and limb reduction defects.[13–16] One case control study[16] estimated a 4.7 fold increased risk of limb reduction defects in infants exposed in utero to sex hormones (oral contraceptives, hormone withdrawal tests for pregnancy, or attempted treatment for threatened abortion). Some of these exposures were very short and involved only a few days of treatment. The data suggest that the risk of limb reduction defects in exposed fetuses is somewhat less than 1 per 1000.

In the past, female sex hormones have been used during pregnancy in an attempt to treat threatened or habitual abortion. There is considerable evidence that estrogens are ineffective for these indications, and there is no evidence from well controlled studies that progestogens are effective for these uses.

If ESTRATEST® or ESTRATEST® H.S. is used during pregnancy, or if the patient becomes pregnant while taking this drug, she should be apprised of the potential risks to the fetus, and the advisability of pregnancy continuation.

DESCRIPTION

ESTRATEST®: Each dark green, capsule shaped, sugar-coated oral tablet contains: 1.25 mg of Esterified Estrogens, USP and 2.5 mg of Methyltestosterone.
ESTRATEST® H.S. (Half-Strength): Each light green, capsule shaped, sugar-coated oral tablet contains: 0.625 mg of Esterified Estrogens, USP and 1.25 mg of Methyltestosterone.
ESTERIFIED ESTROGENS: Esterified Estrogens, USP is a mixture of the sodium salts of the sulfate esters of the estrogenic substances, principally estrone, that are of the type excreted by pregnant mares. Esterified Estrogens contain not less than 75.0 percent and not more than 85.0 percent of sodium estrone sulfate, and not less than 6.0 percent and not more than 15.0 percent of sodium equilin sulfate, in such proportion that the total of these two components is not less than 90.0 percent.
Category: Estrogens
METHYLTESTOSTERONE: Methyltestosterone is an androgen.

Androgens are derivatives of cyclopentano-perhydrophenanthrene. Endogenous androgens are C-19 steriods with a side chain at C-17, and with two angular methyl groups. Testosterone is the primary endogenous androgen. Fluoxymesterone and methyltestosterone are synthetic derivatives of testosterone.

Methyltestosterone is a white to light yellow crystalline substance that is virtually insoluble in water but soluble in organic solvents. It is stable in air but decomposes in light.
Methyltestosterone structural formula:

$C_{20}H_{30}O_2$, 302.46
Androst-4-en-3-one, 17-hydroxy-17-methyl-, (17B)-
Category: Androgen

ESTRATEST® and ESTRATEST® H.S. tablets also contain the following inactive ingredients: colloidal silicon dioxide, lactose (hydrous), magnesium stearate, microcrystalline cellulose, and sodium bicarbonate.
Ingredients used in the color for ESTRATEST® tablets are: D&C Yellow #10 Lake, FD&C Yellow #6 Lake, FD&C Blue #1 Lake, Methylparaben, Povidone, Propylparaben, Sodium Benzoate, Sucrose and Titanium Dioxide.
Ingredients used in the color for ESTRATEST® H.S. tablets are: D&C Yellow #10 Lake, FD&C Blue #1 Lake, FD&C Blue #2 Lake, Methylparaben, Povidone, Propylparaben, Sodium Benzoate, Sucrose, and Titanium Dioxide.

CLINICAL PHARMACOLOGY

Estrogens: Estrogens are important in the development and maintenance of the female reproductive system and secondary sex characteristics. They promote growth and development of the vagina, uterus, and fallopian tubes, and enlargement of the breasts. Indirectly, they contribute to the shaping of the skeleton, maintenance of tone and elasticity of urogenital structures, changes in the epiphyses of the long bones that allow for the pubertal growth spurt and its termination, growth of axillary and pubic hair, and pigmentation of the nipples and genitals. Decline of estrogenic activity at the end of the menstrual cycle can bring on menstruation, although the cessation of progesterone secretion is the most important factor in the mature ovulatory cycle. However, in the preovulatory or nonovulatory cycle, estrogen is the primary determinant in the onset of menstruation. Estrogens also affect the release of pituitary gonadotropins.

The pharmacologic effects of esterified estrogens are similar to those of endogenous estrogens. They are soluble in water and are well absorbed from the gastrointestinal tract.
In responsive tissues (female genital organs, breasts, hypothalamus, pituitary) estrogens enter the cell and are transported into the nucleus. As a result of estrogen action, specific RNA and protein synthesis occurs.

Estrogen Pharmacokinetics
Metabolism and inactivation occur primarily in the liver. Some estrogens are excreted into the bile; however they are reabsorbed from the intestine and returned to the liver through the portal venous system. Water soluble esterified estrogens are strongly acidic and are ionized in body fluids, which favor excretion through the kidneys since tubular reabsorption is minimal.

Androgens Endogenous androgens are responsible for the normal growth and development of the male sex organs and for maintenance of secondary sex characteristics. These effects include the growth and maturation of prostate, seminal vesicles, penis, and scrotum, the development of male hair distribution, such as beard, pubic, chest, and axillary hair, laryngeal enlargement, vocal cord thickening, alterations in body musculature, and fat distribution. Drugs in this class also cause retention of nitrogen, sodium, potassium, phosphorus, and decreased urinary excretion of calcium. Androgens have been reported to increase protein anabolism and decrease protein catabolism. Nitrogen balance is improved only when there is sufficient intake of calories and protein. Androgens are responsible for the growth spurt of adolescence and for the eventual termination of linear growth which is brought about by fusion of the epiphyseal growth centers. In children, exogenous androgens accelerate linear growth rates, but may cause a disproportionate advancement in bone maturation. Use over long periods may result in fusion of the epiphyseal growth centers and termination of growth process. Androgens have been reported to stimulate the production of red blood cells by enhancing the production of erythropoietic stimulating factor.

Androgen Pharmacokinetics
Testosterone given orally is metabolized by the gut and 44 percent is cleared by the liver in the first pass. Oral doses as high as 400 mg per day are needed to achieve clinically effective blood levels for full replacement therapy. The synthetic androgens (methyltestosterone and fluoxymesterone) are less extensively metabolized by the liver and have longer

half-lives. They are more suitable than testosterone for oral administration.

Testosterone in plasma is 98 percent bound to a specific testosterone-estradiol binding globulin, and about 2 percent is free. Generally, the amount of this sex-hormone binding globulin in the plasma will determine the distribution of testosterone between free and bound forms, and the free testosterone concentration will determine its half-life.

About 90 percent of a dose of testosterone is excreted in the urine as glucuronic and sulfuric acid conjugates of testosterone and its metabolites; about 6 percent of a dose is excreted in the feces, mostly in the unconjugated form. Inactivation of testosterone occurs primarily in the liver. Testosterone is metabolized to various 17-keto steroids through two different pathways. There are considerable variations of the half-life of testosterone as reported in the literature, ranging from 10 to 100 minutes.

In many tissues the activity of testosterone appears to depend on reduction to dihydrotestosterone, which binds to cytosol receptor proteins. The steroid-receptor complex is transported to the nucleus where it initiates transcription events and cellular changes related to androgen action.

INDICATIONS

ESTRATEST® and ESTRATEST® H.S. are indicated in the treatment of:

Moderate to severe *vasomotor* symptoms associated with the menopause in those patients not improved by estrogens alone. (There is no evidence that estrogens are effective for nervous symptoms or depression without associated vasomotor symptoms, and they should not be used to treat such conditions.)

ESTRATEST® AND ESTRATEST® H.S. HAVE NOT BEEN SHOWN TO BE EFFECTIVE FOR ANY PURPOSE DURING PREGNANCY AND ITS USE MAY CAUSE SEVERE HARM TO THE FETUS (SEE BOXED WARNING).

CONTRAINDICATIONS

Estrogens should not be used in women with any of the following conditions:

1. Known or suspected cancer of the breast except in appropriately selected patients being treated for metastatic disease.
2. Known or suspected estrogen-dependent neoplasia.
3. Known or suspected pregnancy (See Boxed Warning).
4. Undiagnosed abnormal genital bleeding.
5. Active thrombophlebitis or thromboembolic disorders.
6. A past history of thrombophlebitis, thrombosis, or thromboembolic disorders associated with previous estrogen use (except when used in treatment of breast malignancy).

Methyltestosterone should not be used in:

1. The presence of severe liver damage.
2. Pregnancy and in breast-feeding mothers because of the possibility of masculinization of the female fetus or breast-fed infant.

WARNINGS

Associated with Estrogens:

1. **Induction of malignant neoplasms.** Long term continuous administration of natural and synthetic estrogens in certain animal species increases the frequency of carcinomas of the breast, cervix, vagina, and liver. There is now evidence that estrogens increase the risk of carcinoma of the endometrium in humans (See Boxed Warning).

   At the present time there is no satisfactory evidence that estrogens given to postmenopausal women increase the risk of cancer of the breast,[18] although a recent long-term followup of a single physician's practice has raised this possibility.[18a] Because of the animal data, there is a need for caution in prescribing estrogens for women with a strong family history of breast cancer or who have breast nodules, fibrocystic disease, or abnormal mammograms.
2. **Gallbladder disease.** A recent study has reported a 2 to 3-fold increase in the risk of surgically confirmed gall bladder disease in women receiving postmenopausal estrogens,[18] similar to the 2-fold increase previously noted in users of oral contraceptives.[19-24] In the case of oral contraceptives the increased risk appeared after two years of use.[24]
3. **Effects similar to those caused by estrogen-progestogen oral contraceptives.** There are several serious adverse effects of oral contraceptives, most of which have not, up to now, been documented as consequences of postmenopausal estrogen therapy. This may reflect the comparatively low doses of estrogen used in postmenopausal women. It would be expected that the larger doses of estrogen used to treat prostatic or breast cancer or postpartum breast engorgement are more likely to result in these adverse effects, and, in fact, it has been shown that there is an increased risk of thrombosis in men receiving estrogens for prostatic cancer and women for postpartum breast engorgement.[20-23]

   a. **Thromboembolic disease.** It is now well established that users of oral contraceptives have an increased risk of various thromboembolic and thrombotic vascular diseases, such as thrombophlebitis, pulmonary embolism, stroke, and myocardial infarction.[24-31] Cases of retinal thrombosis, mesenteric thrombosis, and optic neuritis have been reported in oral contraceptive users. There is evidence that the risk of several of these adverse reactions is related to the dose of the drug.[32,33] An increased risk of postsurgery thromboembolic complications has also been reported in users of oral contraceptives.[34,35] If feasible, estrogen should be discontinued at least 4 weeks before surgery of the type associated with an increased risk of thromboembolism, or during periods of prolonged immobilization.

   While an increased rate of thromboembolic and thrombotic disease in postmenopausal users of estrogens has not been found,[18-36] this does not rule out the possibility that such an increase may be present or that subgroups of women who have underlying risk factors or who are receiving relatively large doses of estrogens may have increased risk. Therefore estrogens should not be used in persons with active thrombophlebitis or thromboembolic disorders, and they should not be used (except in treatment of malignancy) in persons with a history of such disorders in association with estrogen use. They should be used with caution in patients with cerebral vascular or coronary artery disease and only for those in whom estrogens are clearly needed.

   Large doses of estrogen (5 mg esterified estrogens per day), comparable to those used to treat cancer of the prostate and breast, have been shown in a large prospective clinical trial in men[37] to increase the risk of nonfatal myocardial infarction, pulmonary embolism and thrombophlebitis. When estrogen doses of this size are used, any of the thromboembolic and thrombotic adverse effects associated with oral contraceptive use should be considered a clear risk.

   b. **Hepatic adenoma.** Benign hepatic adenomas appear to be associated with the use of oral contraceptives.[38-40] Although benign and rare, these may rupture and may cause death through intra-abdominal hemorrhage. Such lesions have not yet been reported in association with other estrogen or progestogen preparations but should be considered in estrogen users having abdominal pain and tenderness, abdominal mass, or hypovolemic shock. Hepatocellular carcinoma has also been reported in women taking estrogen-containing oral contraceptives.[39] The relationship of this malignancy to these drugs is not known at this time.

   c. **Elevated blood pressure.** Increased blood pressure is not uncommon in women using oral contraceptives. There is now a report that this may occur with use of estrogens in the menopause[41] and blood pressure should be monitored with estrogen use, especially if high doses are used.

   d. **Glucose tolerance.** A worsening of glucose tolerance has been observed in a significant percentage of patients on estrogen-containing oral contraceptives. For this reason, diabetic patients should be carefully observed while receiving estrogens.
4. **Hypercalcemia.** Administration of estrogens may lead to severe hypercalcemia in patients with breast cancer and bone metastases. If this occurs, the drug should be stopped and appropriate measures taken to reduce the serum calcium level.

Associated with Methyltestosterone

In patients with breast cancer, androgen therapy may cause hypercalcemia by stimulating osteolysis. In this case, the drug should be discontinued. Prolonged use of high doses of androgens has been associated with the development of peliosis hepatis and hepatic neoplasms including hepatocellular carcinoma. (See PRECAUTIONS—*Carcinogenesis*). Peliosis hepatis can be a life-threatening or fatal complication.

Cholestatic hepatitis and jaundice occur with 17-alpha-alkylandrogens at a relatively low dose. If cholestatic hepatitis with jaundice appears or if liver function tests become abnormal, the androgen should be discontinued and the etiology should be determined. Drug-induced jaundice is reversible when the medication is discontinued.

Edema with or without heart failure may be a serious complication in patients with preexisting cardiac, renal, or hepatic disease. In addition to discontinuation of the drug, diuretic therapy may be required.

PRECAUTIONS

Associated with Estrogens

A. General Precautions.

1. A complete medical and family history should be taken prior to the initiation of any estrogen therapy. The pretreatment and periodic physical examinations should include special reference to blood pressure, breasts, abdomen, and pelvic organs, and should include a Papanicolaou smear. As a general rule, estrogen should not be prescribed for longer than one year without another physical examination being performed.
2. Fluid retention—Because estrogens may cause some degree of fluid retention, conditions which might be influenced by this factor such as asthma, epilepsy, migraine, and cardiac or renal dysfunction, require careful observation.
3. Certain patients may develop undesirable manifestations of excessive estrogenic stimulation, such as abnormal or excessive uterine bleeding, mastodynia, etc.
4. Oral contraceptives appear to be associated with an increased incidence of mental depression.[24] Although it is not clear whether this is due to the estrogenic or progestogenic component of the contraceptive, patients with a history of depression should be carefully observed.
5. Preexisting uterine leiomyomata may increase in size during estrogen use.
6. The pathologist should be advised of estrogen therapy when relevant specimens are submitted.
7. Patients with a past history of jaundice during pregnancy have an increased risk of recurrence of jaundice while receiving estrogen-containing oral contraceptive therapy. If jaundice develops in any patient receiving estrogen, the medication should be discontinued while the cause is investigated.
8. Estrogens may be poorly metabolized in patients with impaired liver function and they should be administered with caution in such patients.
9. Because estrogens influence the metabolism of calcium and phosphorus, they should be used with caution in patients with metabolic bone diseases that are associated with hypercalcemia or in patients with renal insufficiency.
10. Because of the effects of estrogens on epiphyseal closure, they should be used judiciously in young patients in whom bone growth is not complete.
11. Certain endocrine and liver function tests may be affected by estrogen-containing oral contraceptives. The following similar changes may be expected with larger doses of estrogen:
    a. Increased sulfobromophthalein retention.
    b. Increased prothrombin and factors VII, VIII, IX and X; decreased antithrombin 3; increased norepinephrine-induced platelet aggregability.
    c. Increased thyroid binding globulin (TBG) leading to increased circulating total thyroid hormone, as measured by PBI, T4 by column, or T4 by radioimmunoassay. Free T3 resin uptake is decreased, reflecting the elevated TBG; free T4 concentration is unaltered.
    d. Impaired glucose tolerance.
    e. Decreased pregnanediol excretion.
    f. Reduced response to metyrapone test.
    g. Reduced serum folate concentration.
    h. Increased serum triglyceride and phospholipid concentration.

B. Information for the Patient. See text of Patient Package Insert which appears after the REFERENCES.

C. Pregnancy Category X. See CONTRAINDICATIONS and Boxed WARNING.

D. Nursing Mothers. As a general principle, the administration of any drug to nursing mothers should be done only when clearly necessary since many drugs are excreted in human milk.

Associated with Methyltestosterone:

A. General Precautions

1. Women should be observed for signs of virilization (deepening of the voice, hirsutism, acne, clitoromegaly, and menstrual irregularities). Discontinuation of drug therapy at the time of evidence of mild virilism is necessary to prevent irreversible virilization. Such virilization is usual following androgen use at high doses.
2. Prolonged dosage of androgen may result in sodium and fluid retention. This may present a problem, especially in patients with compromised cardiac reserve or renal disease.
3. Hypersensitivity may occur rarely.
4. PBI may be decreased in patients taking androgens.
5. Hypercalcemia may occur. If this does occur, the drug should be discontinued.

B. Information for the Patient

The physician should instruct patients to report any of the following side effects of androgens:

Women: Hoarseness, acne, changes in menstrual periods, or more hair on the face.

All Patients: Any nausea, vomiting, changes in skin color or ankle swelling.

C. Laboratory tests

1. Women with disseminated breast carcinoma should have frequent determination of urine and serum calcium levels during the course of androgen therapy (See WARNINGS).
2. Because of the hepatotoxicity associated with the use of 17-alpha-alkylated androgens, liver function tests should be obtained periodically.
3. Hemoglobin and hematocrit should be checked periodically for polycythemia in patients who are receiving high doses of androgens.

D. Drug Interactions

1. *Anticoagulants* C-17 substituted derivatives of testosterone, such as methandrostenolone, have been reported to

Continued on next page

Reid-Rowell—Cont.

decrease the anticoagulant requirements of patients receiving oral anticoagulants. Patients receiving oral anticoagulant therapy require close monitoring, especially when androgens are started or stopped.

2. *Oxyphenbutazone.* Concurrent administration of oxyphenbutazone and androgens may result in elevated serum levels of oxyphenbutazone.

3. *Insulin.* In diabetic patients the metabolic effects of androgens may decrease blood glucose and insulin requirements.

E. Drug/Laboratory Test Interferences

Androgens may decrease levels of thyroxine-binding globulin, resulting in decreased T_4 serum levels and increased resin uptake of T_3 and T_4. Free thyroid hormone levels remain unchanged, however, and there is no clinical evidence of thyroid dysfunction.

F. Carcinogenesis

Animal Data. Testosterone has been tested by subcutaneous injection and implantation in mice and rats. The implant induced cervical-uterine tumors in mice, which metastasized in some cases. There is suggestive evidence that injection of testosterone into some strains of female mice increases their susceptibility to hepatoma. Testosterone is also known to increase the number of tumors and decrease the degree of differentiation of chemically induced carcinomas of the liver in rats.

Human Data. There are rare reports of hepatocellular carcinoma in patients receiving long-term therapy with androgens in high doses. Withdrawal of the drugs did not lead to regression of the tumors in all cases.

Geriatric patients treated with androgens may be at an increased risk for the development of prostatic hypertrophy and prostatic carcinoma.

G. Pregnancy

Teratogenic Effects. Pregnancy Category X (see CONTRAINDICATIONS).

H. Nursing Mothers

It is not known whether androgens are excreted in human milk. Because many drugs are excreted in human milk and because of the potential for serious adverse reactions in nursing infants from androgens, a decision should be made whether to discontinue nursing or to discontinue the drug, taking into account the importance of the drug to the mother.

ADVERSE REACTIONS

Associated with Estrogens (See Warnings regarding induction of neoplasia, adverse effects on the fetus, increased incidence of gall bladder disease, and adverse effects similar to those of oral contraceptives, including thromboembolism). The following additional adverse reactions have been reported with estrogenic therapy, including oral contraceptives:

1. Genitourinary system.
Breakthrough bleeding, spotting, change in menstrual flow.
Dysmenorrhea.
Premenstrual-like syndrome.
Amenorrhea during and after treatment.
Increase in size of uterine fibromyomata.
Vaginal candidiasis.
Change in cervical erosion and in degree of cervical secretion.
Cystitis-like syndrome.

2. Breasts
Tenderness, enlargement, secretion.

3. Gastrointestinal.
Nausea, vomiting.
Abdominal cramps, bloating.
Cholestatic jaundice.

4. Skin.
Chloasma or melasma which may persist when drug is discontinued.
Erythema multiforme.
Erythema nodosum.
Hemorrhagic eruption.
Loss of scalp hair.
Hirsutism.

5. Eyes.
Steepening of corneal curvature.
Intolerance to contact lenses.

6. CNS.
Headache, migraine, dizziness.
Mental depression.
Chorea.

7. Miscellaneous.
Increase or decrease in weight.
Reduced carbohydrate tolerance.
Aggravation of porphyria.
Edema.
Changes in libido.

Associated with Methyltestosterone

A. Endocrine and Urogenital

1. *Female:* The most common side effects of androgen therapy are amenorrhea and other menstrual irregularities, inhibition of gonadotropin secretion, and virilization, including deepening of the voice and clitoral enlargement. The latter usually is not reversible after androgens are discontinued. When administered to a pregnant woman androgens cause virilization of external genitalia of the female fetus.

2. *Skin and Appendages:* Hirsutism, male pattern of baldness, and acne.

3. *Fluid and Electrolyte Disturbances:* Retention of sodium, chloride, water, potassium, calcium, and inorganic phosphates.

4. *Gastrointestinal:* Nausea, cholestatic jaundice, alterations in liver function test, rarely hepatocellular neoplasms, and peliosis hepatis (see WARNINGS).

5. *Hematologic:* Suppression of clotting factors II, V, VII, and X, bleeding in patients on concomitant anticoagulant therapy, and polycythemia.

6. *Nervous System:* Increased or decreased libido, headache, anxiety, depression, and generalized paresthesia.

7. *Metabolic:* Increased serum cholesterol.

8. *Miscellaneous:* Inflammation and pain at the site of intramuscular injection or subcutaneous implantation of testosterone containing pellets, stomatitis with buccal preparations, and rarely anaphylactoid reactions.

OVERDOSAGE

Numerous reports of ingestion of large doses of estrogen-containing oral contraceptives by young children indicate that serious ill effects do not occur. Overdosage of estrogen may cause nausea, and withdrawal bleeding may occur in females.

There have been no reports of acute overdosage with the androgens.

DOSAGE AND ADMINISTRATION

1. *Given cyclically for short-term use only:*
For treatment of moderate to severe *vasomotor* symptoms associated with the menopause in patients not improved by estrogen alone.

The lowest dose that will control symptoms should be chosen and medication should be discontinued as promptly as possible.

Administration should be cyclic (e.g., three weeks on and one week off).

Attempts to discontinue or taper medication should be made at three to six month intervals.

Usual Dosage Range: 1 or 2 tablets of ESTRATEST® or ESTRATEST® H.S. daily as recommended by the physician. Treated patients with an intact uterus should be monitored closely for signs of endometrial cancer and appropriate diagnostic measures should be taken to rule out malignancy in the event of persistent or recurring abnormal vaginal bleeding.

HOW SUPPLIED

ESTRATEST® (Imprinted RR 1026) in bottles of 100—NDC 0032-1026-01 and 1000—NDC 0032-1026-10.
ESTRATEST® (Dark green, capsule shaped, sugar-coated oral tablets) contains: 1.25 mg of Esterified Estrogens, USP and 2.5 mg of Methyltestosterone, USP.
ESTRATEST® H.S. (Imprinted RR 1023) in bottles of 100—NDC 0032-1023-01.
ESTRATEST® H.S. "Half-Strength" (Light green, capsule shaped, sugar-coated oral tablets) contains: 0.625 mg of Esterified Estrogens, USP and 1.25 mg of Methyltestosterone, USP.
Store at controlled room temperature, 15°–30°C (59°–86°F).

REFERENCES

1. Ziel, H.K., *et al.:* N. Engl. J. Med. 293:1167–1170, 1975.
2. Smith, D.C., *et al.:* N. Engl. J. Med. 293:1164–1167, 1975.
3. Mack, T.M., *et al.:* N. Engl. J. Med. 294:1262–1267, 1976.
4. Weiss, N.S., *et al.:* N. Engl. J. Med. 294:1259–1262, 1976.
5. Herbst, A.L., *et al.:* N. Engl. J. Med. 284:878–881, 1971.
6. Greenwald, P., *et al.:* N. Engl. J. Med. 285:390–392, 1971.
7. Lanier, A., *et al.:* Mayo Clin. Proc. 48:793–799, 1973.
8. Herbst, A., *et al.:* Obstet. Gynecol. 40:287–298, 1972.
9. Herbst, A., *et al.:* Am. J. Obstet. Gynecol. 118:607–615, 1974.
10. Herbst, A., *et al.:* N. Engl. J. Med. 292:334–339, 1975.
11. Stafl, A., *et al.:* Obstet. Gynecol. 43:118–128, 1974.
12. Sherman, A.I., *et al.:* Obstet. Gynecol. 44:531–545, 1974.
13. Gal, I., *et al.:* Nature 216:83, 1967.
14. Levy, E.P., *et al.:* Lancet *1*:611, 1973.
15. Nora, J., *et al.:* Lancet *1*:941–942, 1973.
16. Janerich, D.T., *et al.:* N. Engl. J. Med. 291:697–700, 1974.
17. Estrogens for Oral or Parenteral Use: Federal Register 40:8212, 1975.
18. Boston Collaborative Drug Surveillance Program: N. Engl. J. Med. 290:15–19, 1974.
18a.Hoover, R., *et al.:* N. Engl. J. Med. 295:401–405, 1976.
19. Boston Collaborative Drug Surveillance Program: Lancet *1*:1399–1404, 1973.
20. Daniel, D.G., *et al.:* Lancet 2:287–289, 1967.
21. The Veterans Administration Cooperative Urological Research Group: J. Urol. 98:516–522, 1967.
22. Bailar, J. C.: Lancet 2:560, 1967.
23. Blackard, C., *et al.:* Cancer 26:249–256, 1970.
24. Royal College of General Practitioners: J.R. Coll, Gen. Pract. 13:267–279, 1967.
25. Inman, W.H.W., *et al.:* Br. Med. J. 2:193–199, 1968.
26. Vessey, M.P., *et al.:* Br. Med. J. 2:651–657, 1969.
27. Sartwell, P.E., *et al.:* Am. J. Epidemiol, 90:365–380, 1969.
28. Collaborative Group for the Study of Stroke in Young Women: N. Engl. J. Med. 288:871–878, 1973.
29. Collaborative Group for the Study of Stroke in Young Women: J.A.M.A. 231:718–722, 1975.
30. Mann, J.I., *et al.:* Br. Med. J. 2:245–248, 1975.
31. Mann, J.I., *et al.:* Br. Med. J. 2:241–245, 1975.
32. Inman, W.H.W., *et al.:* Br. Med. J. 2:203–209, 1970.
33. Stolley, P.D., *et al.:* Am. J. Epidemiol, 102:197–208, 1975.
34. Vessey, M.P., *et al.:* Br. Med. J. 3:123–126, 1970.
35. Greene, G.R., *et al.:* Am. J. Public Health 62:680–685, 1972.
36. Rosenberg, L., *et al.:* N. Engl. J. Med. 294:1256–1259, 1976.
37. Coronary Drug Project Research Group: J.A.M.A. 214:1303–1313, 1970.
38. Baum, J., *et al.:* Lancet 2:926–928, 1973.
39. Mays, E.T., *et al.:* J.A.M.A. 235:730–732, 1976.
40. Edmondson, H.A., *et al.:* N. Engl. J. Med. 294:470–472, 1976.
41. Pfeffer, R.I., *et al.:* Am. J. Epidemiol, 103:445–456, 1976.

INFORMATION FOR THE PATIENT:

WHAT YOU SHOULD KNOW ABOUT ESTROGENS: Estrogens are female hormones produced by the ovaries. The ovaries make several different kinds of estrogens. In addition, scientists have been able to make a variety of synthetic estrogens. As far as we know, all these estrogens have similar properties and therefore much the same usefulness, side effects, and risks. This leaflet is intended to help you understand what estrogens are used for, the risks involved in their use, and how to use them as safely as possible.

This leaflet includes the most important information about estrogens, but not all the information. If you want to know more, you can ask your doctor or pharmacist to let you read the package insert prepared for the doctor.

USES OF ESTROGEN:

Estrogens are prescribed by doctors for a number of purposes, including:

1. To provide estrogen during a period of adjustment when a woman's ovaries no longer produce it, in order to prevent certain uncomfortable symptoms of estrogen deficiency. (All women normally stop producing estrogens, generally between the ages of 45 and 55; this is called the menopause).

2. To prevent symptoms of estrogen deficiency when a woman's ovaries have been removed surgically before the natural menopause.

3. To prevent pregnancy. (Estrogens are given along with a progestogen, another female hormone; these combinations are called oral contraceptives or birth controll pills. Patient labeling is available to women taking oral contraceptives and they will not be discussed in this leaflet).

4. To treat certain cancers in women and men.

5. To prevent painful swelling of the breasts after pregnancy in women who choose not to nurse their babies.

THERE IS NO PROPER USE OF ESTROGENS IN A PREGNANT WOMAN.

ESTROGENS IN THE MENOPAUSE: In the natural course of their lives, all women eventually experience a decrease in estrogen production. This usually occurs between ages 45 and 55 but may occur earlier or later. Sometimes the ovaries may need to be removed before natural menopause by an operation, producing a "surgical menopause."

When the amount of estrogen in the blood begins to decrease, many women may develop typical symptoms: Feelings of warmth in the face, neck, and chest or sudden intense episodes of heat and sweating throughout the body (called "hot flashes" or "hot flushes"). These symptoms are sometimes very uncomfortable. A few women eventually develop changes in the vagina (called "atrophic vaginitis") which cause discomfort, especially during and after intercourse.

Estrogens can be prescribed to treat these symptoms of the menopause. It is estimated that considerably more than half of all women undergoing the menopause have only mild symptoms or no symptoms at all and therefore do not need estrogens. Other women may need estrogens for a few months, while their bodies adjust to lower estrogen levels. Sometimes the need will be for periods longer than six months. In an attempt to avoid overstimulation of the uterus (womb), estrogens are usually given cyclically during each month of use, that is three weeks of pills followed by one week without pills.

Sometimes women experience nervous symptoms or depression during menopause. There is no evidence that estrogens are effective for such symptoms and they should not be used to treat them, although other treatment may be needed.

You may have heard that taking estrogens for long periods (years) after the menopause will keep your skin soft and supple and keep you feeling young.

There is no evidence that this is so, however, and such long-term treatment carries important risks.

ESTROGENS TO PREVENT SWELLING OF THE BREASTS AFTER PREGNANCY: If you do not breast feed your baby after delivery, your breasts may fill up with milk and become painful and engorged. This usually begins about 3 to 4 days after delivery and may last for a few days to up to a week or more. Sometimes the discomfort is severe, but usually it is not and can be controlled by pain relieving drugs such as aspirin and by binding the breasts up tightly. Estrogens can be used to try to prevent the breasts from filling up. While this treatment is sometimes successful, in many cases the breasts fill up to some degree in spite of treatment. The dose of estrogens needed to prevent pain and swelling of the breasts is much larger than the dose needed to treat symptoms of the menopause and this may increase your chances of developing blood clots in the legs or lungs (see below). Therefore, it is important that you discuss the benefits and the risks of estrogen use with your doctor if you have decided not to breast feed your baby.

THE DANGER OF ESTROGENS:

1. **Cancer of the uterus.** If estrogens are used in the postmenopausal period for more than a year, there is an increased risk of **endometrial cancer** (cancer of the uterus). Women taking estrogens have roughly 5 to 10 times as great a chance of getting this cancer as women who take no estrogens. To put this another way, while a postmenopausal woman not taking estrogens has 1 chance in 1,000 each year of getting cancer of the uterus, a woman taking estrogens has 5 to 10 chances in 1,000 each year. For this reason **it is important to take estrogens only when you really need them.** The risk of this cancer is greater the longer estrogens are used and also seems to be greater when larger doses are taken. For this reason **it is important to take the lowest dose of estrogen that will control symptoms and to take it only as long as it is needed.** If estrogens are needed for longer periods of time, your doctor will want to reevaluate your need for estrogens at least every six months.

   Women using estrogens should report any irregular vaginal bleeding to their doctors; such bleeding may be of no importance, but it can be an early warning of cancer of the uterus. If you have undiagnosed vaginal bleeding, you should not use estrogens until a diagnosis is made and you are certain there is no cancer of the uterus.

2. **Other possible cancers.** Estrogens can cause development of other tumors in animals, such as tumors of the breast, cervix, vagina, or liver, when given for a long time. At present there is no good evidence that women using estrogen in the menopause have an increased risk of such tumors, but there is no way yet to be sure they do not; and one study raises the possibility that use of estrogens in the menopause may increase the risk of breast cancer many years later. This is a further reason to use estrogens only when clearly needed. While you are taking estrogens, it is important that you go to your doctor at least once a year for a physical examination. Also, if members of your family have had breast cancer or if you have had breast nodules or abnormal mammograms (breast x-rays), your doctor may wish to carry out more frequent examinations of your breasts.

3. **Gall bladder disease.** Women who use estrogens after menopause are more likely to develop gall bladder disease needing surgery as women who do not use estrogens. Birth control pills have a similar effect.

4. **Abnormal blood clotting.** Oral contraceptives increase the risk of blood clotting in various parts of the body. This can result in a stroke (if the clot is in the brain), a heart attack (clot in a blood vessel of the heart), or pulmonary embolus (a clot which forms in the legs or pelvis, then breaks off and travels to the lungs). Any of these can be fatal.

   At this time use of estrogens in the menopause is not known to cause such blood clotting, but this has not been fully studied and there could still prove to be such a risk. It is recommended that if you have had clotting in the legs or lungs or a heart attack or stroke while you were using estrogens or birth control pills, you should not use estrogens (unless they are being used to treat cancer of the breast or prostate). If you have had a stroke or heart attack of if you have angina pectoris, estrogens should be used with great caution and only if clearly needed (for example, if you have severe symptoms of the menopause). The larger doses of estrogen used to prevent swelling of the breasts after pregnancy have been reported to cause clotting in the legs and lungs.

SPECIAL WARNING ABOUT PREGNANCY: You should not receive estrogen if you are pregnant. If this should occur, there is a greater than usual chance that the developing child will be born with a birth defect, although the possibility remains fairly small. A female child may have an increased risk of developing cancer of the vagina or cervix later in life (in the teens or twenties). Every possible effort should be made to avoid exposure to estrogens during pregnancy. If exposure occurs, see your doctor.

OTHER EFFECTS OF ESTROGENS: In addition to the serious known risks of estrogens described above, estrogens have the following side effects and potential risks:

1. **Nausea and vomiting.** The most common side effect of estrogen therapy is nausea. Vomiting is less common.
2. **Effects on breasts.** Estrogens may cause breast tenderness or enlargement and may cause the breasts to secrete a liquid. These effects are not dangerous.
3. **Effects on the uterus.** Estrogens may cause benign fibroid tumors of the uterus to get larger.

   Some women will have menstrual bleeding when estrogens are stopped. But if the bleeding occurs on days you are still taking esrogens you should report this to your doctor.
4. **Effect on liver.** Women taking oral contraceptives develop on rare occasions a benign tumor of the liver which can rupture and bleed into the abdomen. So far, these tumors have not been reported in women using estrogens in the menopause, but you should report any swelling or unusual pain or tenderness in the abdomen to your doctor immediately.

   Women with a past history of jaundice (yellowing of the skin and white parts of the eyes) may get jaundice again during estrogen use. If this occurs, stop taking estrogens and see your doctor.
5. **Other effects.** Estrogens may cause excess fluid to be retained in the body. This may make some conditions worse, such as epilepsy, migraine, heart disease, or kidney disease.

SUMMARY: Estrogens have important uses, but they have serious risks as well. You must decide, with your doctor, whether the risks are acceptable to you in view of the benefits of treatment. Except where your doctor has prescribed estrogens for use in special cases of cancer of the breast or prostate, you should not use estrogens if you have cancer of the breast or uterus, are pregnant, have undiagnosed abnormal vaginal bleeding, or have had a stroke, heart attack or angina, or clotting in the legs or lungs in the past while you were taking estrogens.

You can use estrogens as safely as possible by understanding that your doctor will require regular physical examinations while you are taking them and will try to discontinue the drug as soon as possible and use the smallest dose possible. Be alert for signs of trouble including:

1. Abnormal bleeding from the vagina.
2. Pains in the calves or chest or sudden shortness of breath, or coughing blood (indicating possible clots in the legs, heart, or lungs).
3. Severe headaches, dizziness, faintness, or changes in vision (indicating possible developing clots in the brain or eye).
4. Breast lumps (you should ask your doctor how to examine your own breasts).
5. Jaundice (yellowing of the skin).
6. Mental depression.

Based on his or her assessment of your medical needs, your doctor has prescribed this drug for you. Do not give the drug to anyone else.

HOW SUPPLIED

ESTRATEST® H.S. a combination of Esterified Estrogens and Methyltestosterone. Each capsule-shaped Light Green sugar coated Tablet contains: 0.625 mg of Esterified Estrogens, USP and 1.25 mg of Methyltestosterone, USP.

ESTRATEST® a combination of Esterified Estrogens and Methyltestosterone. Each capsule-shaped Dark Green Sugar Coated Tablet contains: 1.25 mg of Esterified Estrogens, USP and 2.5 mg of Methyltestosterone, USP.

REID-ROWELL
Marietta, Georgia 30062   Revised: 1/89
Shown in Product Identification Section, page 424

HYDROCIL® INSTANT
[hĭ'dro-sĭl]

(See PDR For Nonprescription Drugs)

MELFIAT®-105   ⒸⓁ ℞
UNICELLES®
[mel'fĕ-aht 105 ūn'i-sels]
(phendimetrazine tartrate)
105 mg
Sustained Release Capsules

HOW SUPPLIED

Each orange and clear sustained release capsule contains 105 mg Phendimetrazine Tartrate in bottles of 100 (NDC 0032-1082-01).

Shown in Product Identification Section, page 424

P-V-TUSSIN® SYRUP   ⒸⓁ ℞
[p-v-tŭs'in]
P-V-TUSSIN® TABLETS

DESCRIPTION

Each teaspoonful (5 mL) of P-V-Tussin Syrup contains: Hydrocodone Bitartrate 2.5 mg (WARNING: May be habit forming), Phenylephrine HCl 5 mg, Pyrilamine Maleate 6 mg, Chlorpheniramine Maleate 2 mg, Phenindamine Tartrate 5 mg, Ammonium Chloride 50 mg; Alcohol 5%.
Each scored P-V-Tussin Tablet contains: Hydrocodone Bitartrate 5 mg (WARNING: May be habit forming), Phenindamine Tartrate 25 mg, Guaifenesin 200 mg.

HOW SUPPLIED

P-V-Tussin Syrup
NDC 0032-1087-78, 16 fl oz bottles
NDC 0032-1087-79, gallon bottles
P-V-Tussin Tablets
NDC 0032-1088-01, bottles of 100 tablets
Store at controlled room temperature 15°–30°C (59°–86°F).

ROWASA®   ℞
[rōă's ă]
(mesalamine)
Rectal Suspension Enema
4.0 grams/unit (60 mL)

DESCRIPTION

The active ingredient in ROWASA® rectal suspension enema, a disposable (60 mL) unit, is mesalamine, also known as 5-amino-salicylic acid (5-ASA). Chemically, mesalamine is 5-amino-2-hydroxybenzoic acid.
The empirical formula is $C_7H_7NO_3$, representing a molecular weight of 153.14. The structural formula is:

Each rectal suspension enema unit contains 4 grams of mesalamine. In addition to mesalamine the preparation contains the inactive ingredients potassium metabisulfite, carbomer 943P, edetate disodium, potassium acetate, water and xanthan gum. Sodium benzoate is added as a preservative. The disposable unit consists of an applicator tip protected by a polyethylene cover and lubricated with USP white petrolatum. The unit has a one-way valve to prevent back flow of the dispensed product.

CLINICAL PHARMACOLOGY

Sulfasalazine is split by bacterial action in the colon into sulfapyridine (SP) and mesalamine (5-ASA). It is thought that the mesalamine component is therapeutically active in ulcerative colitis [A.K. Azad Khan et al, Lancet 2:892–895 (1977)]. The usual oral dose of sulfasalazine for active ulcerative colitis in adults is two to four grams per day in divided doses. Four grams of sulfasalazine provide 1.6 g of free mesalamine to the colon. Each ROWASA suspension enema delivers up to 4 g of mesalamine to the left side of the colon. The mechanism of action of mesalamine (and sulfasalazine) is unknown, but appears to be topical rather than systemic. Mucosal production of arachidonic acid (AA) metabolites, both through the cyclooxygenase pathways, i.e., prostanoids, and through the lipoxygenase pathways, i.e., leukotrienes (LTs) and hydroxyeicosatetraenoic acids (HETEs) is increased in patients with chronic inflammatory bowel disease, and it is possible that mesalamine diminishes inflammation by blocking cyclooxygenase and inhibiting prostaglandin (PG) production in the colon.

PRECLINICAL TOXICOLOGY

Preclinical studies have shown the kidney to be the major target organ for mesalamine toxicity. Adverse renal function changes were observed in rats after a single 600 mg/kg oral dose, but not after a 200 mg/kg dose. Gross kidney lesions, including papillary necrosis, were observed after a single oral > 900 mg/kg dose, and after i.v. doses of > 214 mg/kg. Mice responded similarly. In a 13-week oral (gavage) dose study in rats, the high dose of 640 mg/kg/day mesalamine caused deaths, probably due to renal failure, and dose-related renal lesions (papillary necrosis and/or multifocal tubular injury) were seen in most rats given the high dose (males and females) as well as in males receiving lower doses 160 mg/kg/day. Renal lesions were not observed in the 160 mg/kg/day female rats. Minimal tubular epithelial damage was seen in the 40 mg/kg/day males and was reversible. In a six-month oral study in dogs, the no-observable dose level of mesalamine was 40 mg/kg/day and doses of 80 mg/kg/day and higher caused renal pathology similar to that described

Continued on next page

Reid-Rowell—Cont.

for the rat. The oral preclinical studies were done with a highly bioavailable suspension where absorption throughout the gastrointestinal tract occurred. The human dose of 4 grams represents approximately 80 mg/kg but when mesalamine is given rectally as a suspension, absorption is poor and limited to the distal colon (see **Pharmacokinetics**). Overt renal toxicity has not been observed (see **Adverse Reactions** and **Precautions**), but the potential must be considered.

PHARMACOKINETICS

Mesalamine administered rectally as ROWASA suspension enema is poorly absorbed from the colon and is excreted principally in the feces during subsequent bowel movements. The extent of absorption is dependent upon the retention time of the drug product, and there is considerable individual variation. At steady state, approximatey 10 to 30% of the daily 4-gram dose can be recovered in cumulative 24-hour urine collections. Other than the kidney, the organ distribution and other bioavailability characteristics of absorbed mesalamine in man are not known. It is known that the compound undergoes acetylation but whether this process takes place at colonic or systemic sites has not been elucidated. Whatever the metabolic site, most of the absorbed mesalamine is excreted in the urine as the N-acetyl-5-ASA metabolite. The poor colonic absorption of rectally administered mesalamine is substantiated by the low serum concentration of 5-ASA and N-acetyl-5-ASA seen in ulcerative colitis patients after dosage with mesalamine. Under clinical conditions patients demonstrated plasma levels 10 to 12 hours post mesalamine administration of 2 ug/mL, about two-thirds of which was the N-acetyl metabolite. While the elimination half-life of mesalamine is short (0.5 to 1.5 h), the acetylated metabolite exhibits a half-life of 5 to 10 hours [U. Klotz, **Clin. Pharmacokin. 10**:285–302 (1985)]. In addition, steady state plasma levels demonstrated a lack of accumulation of either free or metabolized drug during repeated daily administrations.

EFFICACY

In a placebo-controlled, international, multicenter trial of 153 patients with active distal ulcerative colitis, proctosigmoiditis or proctitis, ROWASA suspension enema reduced the overall disease activity index (DAI) and individual components as follows:
[See table below].
Differences between ROWASA and placebo were also statistically different in subgroups of patients on concurrent sulfasalazine and in those having an upper disease boundary between 5 and 20 or 20 and 40 cm. Significant differences between ROWASA and placebo were not achieved in those subgroups of patients on concurrent prednisone or with an upper disease boundary between 40 and 50 cm.

INDICATIONS AND USAGE

ROWASA suspension enema is indicated for the treatment of active mild to moderate distal ulcerative colitis, proctosigmoiditis or proctitis.

CONTRAINDICATIONS

ROWASA suspension enema is contraindicated for patients known to have hypersensitivity to the drug or any component of this medication.

WARNINGS

ROWASA suspension enema contains potassium metabisulfite, a sulfite that may cause allergic-type reactions including anaphylactic symptoms and life-threatening or less severe asthmatic episodes in certain susceptible people. The overall prevalence of sulfite sensitivity in the general population is unknown but probably low. Sulfite sensitivity is seen more frequently in asthmatic or in atopic nonasthmatic persons.
Epinephrine is the preferred treatment for serious allergic or emergency situations even though epinephrine injection contains sodium or potassium metabisulfite with the above-mentioned potential liabilities. The alternatives to using epinephrine in a life-threatening situation may not be satisfactory. The presence of a sulfite(s) in epinephrine injection should not deter the administration of the drug for treatment of serious allergic or other emergency situations.

PRECAUTIONS

Mesalamine has been implicated in the production of an acute intolerance syndrome characterized by cramping, acute abdominal pain and bloody diarrhea, sometimes fever, headache and a rash; in such cases prompt withdrawal is required. The patient's history of sulfasalazine intolerance, if any, should be re-evaluated. If a rechallenge is performed later in order to validate the hypersensitivity it should be carried out under close supervision and only if clearly needed, giving consideration to reduced dosage. In the literature one patient previously sensitive to sulfasalazine was rechallenged with 400 mg oral mesalamine, within eight hours she experienced headache, fever, intensive abdominal colic, profuse diarrhea and was readmitted as an emergency. She responded poorly to steroid therapy and two weeks later a pancolectomy was required.
Although renal abnormalities were not noted in the clinical trials with ROWASA suspension enema, the possibility of increased absorption of mesalamine and concomitant renal tubular damage as noted in the preclinical studies must be kept in mind. Patients on ROWASA suspension enema, especially those on concurrent oral products which liberate mesalamine and those with preexisting renal disease, should be carefully monitored with urinalysis, BUN and creatinine studies.
In a clinical trial most patients who were hypersensitive to sulfasalazine were able to take mesalamine enemas without evidence of any allergic reaction. Nevertheless, caution should be exercised when mesalamine is initially used in patients known to be allergic to sulfasalazine. These patients should be instructed to discontinue therapy if signs of rash or fever become apparent.
While using ROWASA suspension enema some patients have developed pancolitis. However, extension of upper disease boundary and/or flare-ups occurred less often in the ROWASA-treated group than in the placebo-treated group.
Rare instances of pericarditis have been reported with mesalamine containing products including sulfasalazine. Cases of pericarditis have also been reported as manifestations of inflammatory bowel disease. In the cases reported with Rowasa Rectal Suspension Enema there have been positive rechallenges with mesalamine or mesalamine containing products. In one of these cases, however, a second rechallenge with sulfasalazine was negative throughout a 2 month follow-up. Chest pain or dypsnea in patients treated with Rowasa should be investigated with this information in mind. Discontinuation of Rowasa may be warranted in some cases, but rechallenge with mesalamine can be performed under careful clinical observation should the continued therapeutic need for mesalamine be present.

Carcinogenesis, Mutagenesis, Impairment of Fertility

There have been no completed long-term studies of the carcinogenic potential of ROWASA. Mesalamine is not mutagenic to Salmonella typhimurium tester strains TA98, TA100, TA1535, TA1537, TA1538. There were no reverse mutations in an assay using E. coli strain WP2UVRA. There were no effects in an in vivo mouse micronucleus assay at 600 mg/kg and in an in vivo sister chromatid exchange at doses up to 610 mg/kg. No effects on fertility were observed in rats receiving up to 320 mg/kg/day. The oligospermia and infertility in men associated with sulfasalazine have not been reported with mesalamine.

Pregnancy (Category B)

Teratologic studies have been performed in rats and rabbits at oral doses of up to five and eight times respectively, the maximum recommended human dose, and have revealed no evidence of harm to the embryo or the fetus. There are, however, no adequate and well controlled studies in pregnant women for either sulfasalazine or 5-ASA. Because animal reproduction studies are not always predictive of human response, 5-ASA should be used during pregnancy only if clearly needed.

Nursing Mothers

It is not known whether mesalamine or its metabolite(s) are excreted in human milk. As a general rule, nursing should not be undertaken while a patient is on a drug since many drugs are excreted in human milk.

Pediatric Use

Safety and effectiveness in children have not been established.

ADVERSE REACTIONS

Clinical Adverse Experience

ROWASA suspension enema is usually well tolerated. Most adverse effects have been mild and transient.

ADVERSE REACTIONS OCCURRING IN MORE THAN 0.1% OF ROWASA SUSPENSION ENEMA TREATED PATIENTS (COMPARISON TO PLACEBO)

SYMPTOM	ROWASA n=815 n	ROWASA %	PLACEBO n=128 n	PLACEBO %
Abdominal Pain/Cramps/Discomfort	66	8.10	10	7.81
Headache	53	6.50	16	12.50
Gas/Flatulence	50	6.13	5	3.91
Nausea	47	5.77	12	9.38
Flu	43	5.28	1	0.78
Tired/Weak/Malaise/Fatigue	28	3.44	8	6.25
Fever	26	3.19	0	0.00
Rash/Spots	23	2.82	4	3.12
Cold/Sore Throat	19	2.33	9	7.03
Diarrhea	17	2.09	5	3.91
Leg/Joint Pain	17	2.09	1	0.78
Dizziness	15	1.84	3	2.34
Bloating	12	1.47	2	1.56
Back Pain	11	1.35	1	0.78
Pain on Insertion of Enema Tip	11	1.35	1	0.78
Hemorrhoids	11	1.35	0	0.00
Itching	10	1.23	1	0.78
Rectal Pain	10	1.23	0	0.00
Constipation	8	0.98	4	3.12
Hair Loss	7	0.86	0	0.00
Peripheral Edema	5	0.61	11	8.59
UTI/Urinary Burning	5	0.61	4	3.12
Rectal Pain/Soreness/Burning	5	0.61	3	2.34
Asthenia	1	0.12	4	3.12
Insomnia	1	0.12	3	2.34

Hair Loss

Mild hair loss characterized by "more hair in the comb" but no withdrawal from clinical trials has been observed in seven of 815 mesalamine patients but none of the placebo-treated patients. In the literature there are at least six additional patients with mild hair loss who received either mesalamine or sulfasalazine. Retreatment is not always associated with repeated hair loss.

Overdosage

There have been no documented reports of serious toxicity in man resulting from massive overdosing with mesalamine. Under ordinary circumstances, mesalamine absorption from the colon is limited.

DOSAGE AND ADMINISTRATION

The usual dosage of ROWASA (mesalamine) suspension enema in 60 mL units is one rectal instillation (4 grams) once a day, preferably at bedtime, and retained for approximately eight hours. While the effect of ROWASA (mesalamine) may be seen within three to twenty-one days, the usual course of therapy would be from three to six weeks depending on symptoms and sigmoidoscopic findings. Studies available to date have not assessed if ROWASA suspension enema will modify relapse rates after the 6-week short-term treatment.

**EFFECT OF TREATMENT ON SEVERITY OF DISEASE
DATA FROM U.S.-CANADA TRIAL
COMBINED RESULTS OF EIGHT CENTERS
Activity Indices, mean**

		n	Base-line	Day 22	End-Point	Change Baseline to End-Point†
Overall DAI	ROWASA	76	7.42	4.05**	3.37***	−55.07%***
	Placebo	77	7.40	6.03	5.83	−21.58%
Stool Frequency	ROWASA		1.58	1.11*	1.01**	−0.57*
	Placebo		1.92	1.47	1.50	−0.41
Rectal Bleeding	ROWASA		1.82	0.59***	0.51***	−1.30***
	Placebo		1.73	1.21	1.11	−0.61
Mucosal inflammation	ROWASA		2.17	1.22**	0.96***	−1.21**
	Placebo		2.18	1.74	1.61	−0.56
Physician's Assessment of Disease Severity	ROWASA		1.86	1.13***	0.88***	−0.97***
	Placebo		1.87	1.62	1.55	−0.30

Each parameter has a 4-point scale with a numerical rating:
0 = normal, 1 = mild, 2 = moderate, 3 = severe. The four parameters are added together to produce a maximum overall DAI of 12.
† Percent change for overall DAI only (calculated by taking the average of the change for each individual patient).
  * Significant ROWASA/placebo difference. $p < 0.05$
 ** Significant ROWASA/placebo difference. $p < 0.01$
*** Significant ROWASA/placebo difference. $p < 0.001$

Patients should be instructed to shake the bottle well to make sure the suspension is homogeneous. The patient should remove the protective sheath from the applicator tip. Holding the bottle at the neck will not cause any of the medication to be discharged. The position most often used is obtained by lying on the left side (to facilitate migration into the sigmoid colon); with the lower leg extended and the upper right leg flexed forward for balance. An alternative is the knee-chest position. The applicator tip should be gently inserted in the rectum pointing toward the umbilicus. A steady squeezing of the bottle will discharge most of the preparation. The preparation should be taken at bedtime with the objective of retaining it all night. Patient instructions are included with every seven units.

HOW SUPPLIED

ROWASA suspension for rectal administration is supplied in units of seven disposable bottles, each containing 4.0 grams of mesalamine in a 60 mL aqueous suspension. Boxes of seven (NDC 0032-1924-82) for rectal use only.
Patient instructions are included.
Store at controlled room temperature 15° to 30°C (59° to 86°F).
Once the foil-wrapped unit of seven bottles is opened, individual bottles should be used as directed.

3EEH9

Shown in Product Identification Section, page 424

ZENATE®   ℞

[ze'nāt]
Prenatal Multivitamin/Mineral Supplement
Film Coated Tablets

Each tablet contains:

VITAMINS:			%RDA[1] Pregnant Women
A (as palmitate)	5,000	I.U.	100
D (as calciferol)	400	I.U.	100
E (as dl-alpha tocopheryl acetate)	30	I.U.	200
C (ascorbic acid)	80	mg	100
Folic Acid	1	mg	125
B$_1$ (as thiamine mononitrate)	3	mg	214
B$_2$ (riboflavin)	3	mg	200
Niacin (as niacinamide)	20	mg	133
B$_6$ (as pyridoxine hydrochloride)	10	mg	385
B$_{12}$ (cyanocobalamin)	12	mcg	300
MINERALS:			
Calcium (from calcium carbonate)	300	mg	25
Iodine (from potassium iodide)	175	mcg	100
Iron (from ferrous fumarate)	65	mg	+
Magnesium (from magnesium oxide)	100	mg	22
Zinc (from zinc oxide)	20	mg	100

+ The increased requirement during pregnancy cannot be met by the iron content of habitual American diets nor by the existing iron stores of many women; therefore the use of 30–60 mg of supplemental iron is recommended.[1]

[1] Recommended Dietary Allowances, National Academy of Sciences, Washington, D.C., 9th ed., 1980.

DESCRIPTION

Zenate is a prenatal film coated tablet. Zenate contains the vitamin and mineral components specified above. Zenate may also contain the following inactive ingredients: carnauba wax, cellulose, FD&C Blue No. 1 Aluminum Lake, magnesium stearate, polyethylene glycol, silicon dioxide, sodium starch glycolate, stearic acid, and titanium dioxide.

CLINICAL PHARMACOLOGY

Zenate is a phosphorous free[1] multivitamin/mineral dietary supplement specifically formulated for use during pregnancy and lactation. All ingredients covered by a warning or caution for usage in pregnancy have been formulated so as not to exceed maximum recommended strengths. The formulation includes essential vitamins and minerals, including 300 mg of elemental calcium, 65 mg of elemental iron, and 20 mg of elemental zinc. Zenate also offers 1 mg of folic acid to aid in the prevention of megaloblastic anemia.

INDICATIONS

Zenate is a vitamin-mineral dietary adjunct in nutritional stress associated with pregnancy and lactation.

CONTRAINDICATIONS

Zenate is contraindicated in those patients with known hypersensitivity to its use.

PRECAUTIONS

Folic acid in doses above 0.1 mg daily may obscure pernicious anemia in that hematologic remission can occur while neurological manifestations remain progressive. Periodic laboratory studies are considered essential and are recommended. Allergic sensitization has been reported following both oral and parenteral administration of folic acid.

DOSAGE AND ADMINISTRATION

One tablet daily before the first meal, or as directed by the physician.

HOW SUPPLIED

Zenate tablets are baby blue film coated capsule-shaped tablets embossed RR on one side and 1146 on the other and supplied in bottles of 100 tablets; (NDC 0032-1146-01). Storage: Store at controlled room temperature, 15°–30°C (59°–86°F).

CAUTION

Federal Law Prohibits Dispensing Without Prescription.

Reference 1. Pitkin, R.M.: Vitamins and Minerals in Pregnancy. Clinics in Perinatology, 2:221–223, 1975.

Rev. 10/87

Shown in Product Identification Section, page 424

Research Industries Corporation
Pharmaceutical Division
1847 WEST 2300 SOUTH
SALT LAKE CITY, UTAH 84119

RIMSO®-50   ℞

[rĭm'sō-50]
(brand of dimethyl sulfoxide)

PRODUCT OVERVIEW

KEY FACTS

The active component of Rimso®-50 is sterile and pyrogen-free dimethyl sulfoxide.

MAJOR USES

Rimso®-50 has been proved to be clinically effective for the symptomatic relief of patients with interstitial cystitis.

SAFETY INFORMATION

Intravesical instillation of Rimso®-50 may be harmful to patients with urinary tract malignancy because of dimethyl sulfoxide-induced vasodilation.
Dimethyl sulfoxide can initiate the liberation of histamine and there have been occasional hypersensitivity reactions with topical administration.
Dimethyl sulfoxide should be used during pregnancy only if the potential benefit justifies the potential risk to the fetus.

PRESCRIBING INFORMATION

RIMSO®-50   ℞

[rĭm'sō-50]
(brand of dimethyl sulfoxide)

DESCRIPTION

RIMSO®-50, brand of dimethyl sulfoxide ((DMSO)
50% w/w Aqueous Solution for intravesical instillation.
Each ml contains 0.54 gm dimethyl sulfoxide STERILE AND PYROGEN-FREE.
Intravesical instillation for the treatment of interstitial cystitis.
NOT FOR I.M. OR I.V. INJECTION

CAUTION

Federal law prohibits dispensing without a prescription.
The active component of RIMSO®-50 is dimethyl sulfoxide which has the empirical formula C_2H_6OS.
Dimethyl sulfoxide is a clear, colorless and essentially odorless liquid which is miscible with water and most organic solvents. Other physical characteristics include: molecular weight 78.13, melting point 18.4°C, and a specific gravity of 1.1014.

CLINICAL PHARMACOLOGY

Dimethyl sulfoxide is metabolized in man by oxidation to dimethyl sulfone or by reduction to dimethyl sulfide. Dimethyl sulfoxide and dimethyl sulfone are excreted in the urine and feces. Dimethyl sulfide is eliminated through the breath and skin and is responsible for the characteristic odor from patients on dimethyl sulfoxide medication. Dimethyl sulfone can persist in serum for longer than two weeks after a single intravesical instillation. No residual accumulation of dimethyl sulfoxide has occurred in man or lower animals who have received treatment for protracted periods of time. Following topical application, dimethyl sulfoxide is absorbed and generally distributed in the tissues and body fluids.

INDICATIONS AND USAGE

RIMSO®-50 (dimethyl sulfoxide) is indicated for the symptomatic relief of patients with interstitial cystitis. RIMSO®-50 has not been approved as being safe and effective for any other indication. There is no clinical evidence of effectiveness of dimethyl sulfoxide in the treatment of bacterial infections of the urinary tract.

CONTRAINDICATIONS

None known.

WARNINGS

Dimethyl sulfoxide can initiate the liberation of histamine and there has been an occasional hypersensitivity reaction with topical administration of dimethyl sulfoxide. This hypersensitivity has been reported in one patient receiving intravesical RIMSO®-50. The physician should be cognizant of this possibility in prescribing RIMSO®-50. If anaphylactoid symtoms develop, appropriate therapy should be instituted.

PRECAUTIONS

Changes in the refractive index and lens opacities have been seen in monkeys, dogs and rabbits given high doses of dimethyl sulfoxide chronically. Since lens changes were noted in animals, full eye evaluations, including slit lamp examinations are recommended prior to and periodically during treatment.
Approximately every six months patients receiving dimethyl sulfoxide should have a biochemical screening, particularly liver and renal function tests, and complete blood count. Intravesical instillation of RIMSO®-50 may be harmful to patients with urinary tract malignancy because of dimethyl sulfoxide-induced vasodilation.
Some data indicate that dimethyl sulfoxide potentiates other concomitantly administered medications.
Pregnancy Category C. Dimethyl sulfoxide caused teratogenic responses in hamsters, rats and mice when administered intraperitoneally at high doses (2.5–12 gm/kg). Oral or topical doses of dimethyl sulfoxide did not cause problems of reproduction in rats, mice and hamsters. Topical doses (5 gm/kg first two days, then 2.5 gm/kg-last eight days) produced terata in rabbits, but in another study, topical doses of 1.1 gm/kg days 3 through 16 of gestation failed to produce any abnormalities. There are not adequate and well controlled studies in pregnant women. Dimethyl sulfoxide should be used during pregnancy only if the potential benefit justifies the potential risk to the fetus. It is not known whether this drug is excreted in human milk. Because many drugs are excreted in human milk, caution should be exercised when dimethyl sulfoxide is administered to a nursing woman.
Safety and effectiveness in children have not been established.
Information available to be given to the patient is reprinted at the end of this text.

ADVERSE REACTIONS

A garlic-like taste may be noted by the patient within a few minutes after instillation of RIMSO®-50 (dimethyl sulfoxide). This taste may last several hours and because of the presence of metabolites an odor on the breath and skin may remain for 72 hours.
Transient chemical cystitis has been noted following instillation of dimethyl sulfoxide.
The patient may experience moderately severe discomfort on administration. Usually this becomes less prominent with repeated administration.

DRUG ABUSE AND DEPENDENCE

None known.

OVERDOSAGE

The oral LD$_{50}$ of dimethyl sulfoxide in the dog is greater than 10 gm/kg. It is improbable that this dosage level could be obtained with intravesical instillation of RIMSO®-50 in the patient.
In case of accidental oral ingestion, specific measures should be taken to induce emesis. Additional measures which may be considered are gastric lavage, activated charcoal and forced diuresis.

DOSAGE AND ADMINISTRATION

Instillation of 50 ml of RIMSO®-50 (dimethyl sulfoxide) directly into the bladder may be accomplished by catheter or asepto syringe and allowed to remain for 15 minutes. Application of an analgesic lubricant gel such as lidocaine jelly to the urethra is suggested prior to insertion of the catheter to avoid spasm. The medication is expelled by spontaneous voiding. It is recommended that the treatment be repeated every two weeks until maximum symptomatic relief is obtained. Thereafter, time intervals between therapy may be increased appropriately.
Administration of oral analgesic medication or suppositories containing belladonna and opium prior to the instillation of RIMSO®-50 can reduce the bladder spasm.
In patients with severe interstitial cystitis with very sensitive bladders, the initial treatment, and possibly the second and third (depending on patient response) should be done under anesthesia. (Saddle block has been suggested).

HOW SUPPLIED

Bottles contain 50 ml of sterile and pyrogen-free RIMSO®-50 (50% w/w dimethyl sulfoxide aqueous solution).
Dimethyl sulfoxide is clear and colorless
Protect from strong light
Store at room temperature (59° to 86°F) (15° to 30°C)

Continued on next page

Research Industries—Cont.

Do not autoclave
NDC #0433-0433-05
For additional information concerning RIMSO®-50, contact the Pharmaceutical Division, Research Industries Corporation. Salt Lake City, Utah
  RIMSO®-50 is manufactured by Tera Pharmaceuticals, Inc., Buena Park, California, for the Pharmaceutical Division, Research Industries Corp., Salt Lake City, Utah.

Rhone-Poulenc Pharmaceuticals
117 CAMPUS DRIVE
PRINCETON, NJ 08540

NITRONG® OINTMENT   ℞
(Nitroglycerin 2%)

DESCRIPTION
NITRONG® Ointment provides 2% nitroglycerin in an absorptive base for topical administration. Each inch, as squeezed from the tube, provides approx. 15 mg nitroglycerin in controlled-release form.

HOW SUPPLIED
30 g tube (NDC 0195-280-50); 60 g tube (NDC 0195-280-51)

NITRONG® 2.6 mg. Tablets   ℞
(nitroglycerin, oral, controlled-release)

DESCRIPTION
Each NITRONG 2.6 mg. tablet for oral administration contains 2.6 mg. nitroglycerin in controlled-release form with light green granules.

NITRONG® 6.5 mg. Tablets   ℞
(nitroglycerin, oral, controlled-release)

DESCRIPTION
Each NITRONG 6.5 mg. tablets for oral administration contains 6.5 mg. nitroglycerin in controlled-release form with light orange granules.

HOW SUPPLIED
NITRONG 2.6 mg (NDC 0195-0021-20), and 6.5 mg (NDC 0195-0274-20) in 100's.

Richardson-Vicks Inc.
ONE FAR MILL CROSSING
SHELTON, CT 06484

CHILDREN'S
CHLORASEPTIC®
LOZENGES

PRODUCT OVERVIEW

KEY FACTS
Chloraseptic Lozenges are a benzocaine-based topical anesthetic.

MAJOR USES
Chloraseptic has been clinically proven to be effective for fast, temporary relief of occassional pain and irritations of the throat, mouth, and gum.

SAFETY INFORMATION
Chloraseptic is not recommended for children under 3 years old, without the direction of a physician.

PRESCRIBING INFORMATION

CHILDREN'S
CHLORASEPTIC®
LOZENGES

ACTIVE INGREDIENTS
Benzocaine 5 mg per lozenge in a grape flavored base.

INACTIVE INGREDIENTS
Corn syrup, FD&C Blue #1, FD&C Red #4, flavor, glycerine, sucrose and water.

INDICATIONS
Chloraseptic's anesthetic and antiseptic formula is a valuable adjunct to systemic antibacterial therapy for fast, temporary relief of minor oral pain and discomfort due to the following conditions. **Medical:** oropharyngitis and throat infections; acute tonsilitis; and post-tonsillectomy soreness. **Dental:** minor irritations or injury of soft tissue of the mouth; minor oral surgery or extractions; irritations caused by dentures or orthodontic appliances; and aphthous ulcers.

DOSAGE AND ADMINISTRATION
Allow one lozenge to dissolve slowly in the mouth. Repeat hourly as needed. Do not take more than 12 lozenges per day.

WARNING
If sore throat is severe, persists for more than 2 days, is accompanied or followed by fever, headache, rash, nausea or vomiting, consult a doctor promptly. If sore mouth symptoms do not improve in 7 days, see your doctor or dentist promptly. In case of accidental overdose, seek professional assistance or contact a Poison Control Center immediately. As with any drug, if you are pregnant or nursing a baby, seek the advice of a health professional before using this product. Store below 86°F (30°C) and protect from moisture.
KEEP THIS AND ALL MEDICINES OUT OF THE REACH OF CHILDREN.

HOW SUPPLIED
Cartons of 18.

CHLORASEPTIC® LIQUID
(oral anesthetic, antiseptic)

PRODUCT OVERVIEW

KEY FACTS
Chloraseptic Liquid is a phenol-based topical anesthetic and antibacterial.

MAJOR USES
Chloraseptic has been clinically proven to be effective for fast, temporary relief of occasional pain and irritations of the throat, mouth, and gum. It is also an effective deodorizing mouthwash.

SAFETY INFORMATION
Chloraseptic is not recommended for children under 3 years old, without the direction of a physician.

PRESCRIBING INFORMATION

CHLORASEPTIC® LIQUID
(oral anesthetic, antiseptic)

ACTIVE INGREDIENTS
Liquid: Phenol and sodium phenolate (total phenol 1.4%).
Aerosol Spray: Phenol and sodium phenolate (total phenol 1.4%).

INACTIVE INGREDIENTS
Menthol Liquid: Alcohol (12.5%), Citric Acid, D&C Yellow #10, FD&C Green #3, Flavor, Glycerin, Propylene Glycol, Sodium Citrate, Sodium Saccharin, Sorbitol and Water.
Cherry Liquid: Alcohol (12.5%). Citric Acid, FD&C Red #40, Flavor, Glycerin, Propylene Glycol, Sodium Citrate, Sodium Saccharin, Sorbitol and Water.
Cherry Aerosol Spray: FD&C Red #40, Flavor, Glycerin, Saccharin Sodium and Water.
Cool Mint Liquid: Alcohol (12.5%), Citric Acid, FD&C Blue #1, Flavor, Glycerin, Menthol, Propylene Glycol, Sodium Citrate, Sodium Saccharin, Sorbitol and Water.

INDICATIONS
Chloraseptic's anesthetic and antiseptic formula is a valuable adjunct to systemic antibacterial therapy for fast, temporary relief of minor oral pain and discomfort due to the following conditions. **Medical:** oropharyngitis and throat infections; acute tonsilitis; and post-tonsillectomy soreness. **Dental:** minor irritations or injury of soft tissue of the mouth; minor oral surgery or extractions; irritations caused by dentures or orthodontic appliances; and aphthous ulcers. It is also an effective preprophy treatment and deodorizing mouthwash.

ADMINISTRATION AND DOSAGE
Chloraseptic Spray (Pump), Mouthwash and Gargle—*Irritated throat:* Spray 5 times (children 3–12 years of age, 3 times) directly on throat and swallow. Repeat every 2 hours as necessary. *After oral surgery:* Allow full-strength solution to run over affected areas for 15 seconds without swishing, then expel remainder. Repeat every 2 hours as necessary. *Adjunctive gingival therapy:* Rinse vigorously with full-strength solution for 15 seconds, working between teeth, then expel remainder. Repeat every 2 hours as necessary. *Daily deodorizing mouthwash and gargle:* Dilute with equal parts of water and rinse thoroughly, or spray full strength, then expel remainder.
Chloraseptic Aerosol Spray: *Irritated throat:* Spray throat about 2 seconds (children 3-12 years about 1 second) and swallow. Repeat every 2 hours as necessary. *After oral surgery:* Spray affected area for 1 to 2 seconds, allow solution to remain for 15 seconds without swishing, then expel remainder. Repeat every 2 hours if necessary. *Adjunctive gingival therapy:* Spray affected area for about 2 seconds, swish for 15 seconds working between teeth, then expel remainder. Repeat every 2 hours if necessary. *Daily deodorizing spray:* Spray, rinse thoroughly, and expel remainder.

WARNING
If sore throat is severe, persists for more than 2 days, is accompanied or followed by fever, headache, rash, nausea or vomiting, consult a doctor promptly. If sore mouth symptoms do not improve in 7 days, see your doctor or dentist promptly. In case of accidental overdose, seek professional assistance or contact a Poison Control Center immediately. As with any drug, if you are pregnant or nursing a baby, seek the advice of a health professional before using this product.
For 1.5 oz. Aerosol Spray—Avoid spraying in eyes. Contents under pressure. Do not puncture or incinerate. (Do not burn or throw in fire, as can will burst). Do not store at temperature above 120°F. (Such high temperatures may cause bursting.)
Store at room temperature.
KEEP THIS AND ALL MEDICINE OUT OF CHILDREN'S REACH.

HOW SUPPLIED
Available in Menthol, Cherry and Cool Mint Flavors in 6 fluid oz. plastic bottles with sprayer. Menthol and Cherry Flavors also available in 12 fluid oz. gargle and 1.5 oz. nitrogen propelled aerosol sprays.

CHLORASEPTIC® LOZENGES

PRODUCT OVERVIEW

KEY FACTS
Chloraseptic Menthol and Cherry Lozenges are a phenol-based topical anesthetic and antibacterial. Chloraseptic Cool Mint Lozenges are a benzocaine and menthol-based topical anesthetic.

MAJOR USES
Chloraseptic has been clinically proven to be effective for fast, temporary relief of occasional pain and irritations of the throat, mouth, and gum.

SAFETY INFORMATION
Chloraseptic is not recommended for children under 3 years old, without the direction of a physician.

PRESCRIBING INFORMATION

CHLORASEPTIC® LOZENGES

ACTIVE INGREDIENTS
Menthol and Cherry: Phenol and Sodium Phenolate (total phenol 32.5 mg/Lozenge).
Cool Mint: Benzocaine 6.0 mg/Lozenge, Menthol 10 mg/Lozenge.

INACTIVE INGREDIENTS
Menthol: Corn Syrup, D&C Yellow #10, FD&C Blue #1, FD&C Yellow #6, Flavor, and Sucrose.
Cherry: Corn Syrup, FD&C Blue #1, FD&C Red #40, Flavor, and Sucrose.
Cool Mint: FD&C Blue #1, Flavor, Sucrose.

INDICATIONS
Chloraseptic's anesthetic and antiseptic formula is a valuable adjunct to systemic antibacterial therapy for fast, temporary relief of minor oral pain and discomfort due to the following conditions. **Medical:** oropharyngitis and throat infections; acute tonsilitis; and post-tonsillectomy soreness. **Dental:** minor irritations or injury of soft tissue of the mouth; minor oral surgery or extractions; irritations caused by dentures or orthodontic appliances; and aphthous ulcers.

ADMINISTRATION AND DOSAGE
Adults and children over 3 years of age: Dissolve 1 lozenge in the mouth repeat every 2 hours as necessary. Children under 12 years, do not exceed 8 lozenges per day.

WARNING
If sore throat is severe, persists for more than 2 days, is accompanied or followed by fever, headache, rash, nausea, or vomiting, consult a doctor promptly. If sore mouth symptoms do not improve in 7 days, see your doctor or dentist promptly. In case of accidental overdose, seek professional assistance or contact a Poison Control Center immediately. As with any drug, if you are pregnant or nursing a baby, seek the advice of a health professional before using this product.
Menthol and Cherry: Store at room temperature.
Cool Mint: Store below 86°F (30°C) and protect from moisture.
KEEP THIS AND ALL MEDICINES OUT OF THE REACH OF CHILDREN.

HOW SUPPLIED
Available in Menthol or Cherry flavor in packages of 18 and 36.
Also available in Cool Mint flavor in packages of 18.

DRAMAMINE® Liquid
[dram 'uh-meen]
(dimenhydrinate syrup USP)
DRAMAMINE® Tablets
(dimenhydrinate USP)
DRAMAMINE® Chewable Tablets
(dimenhydrinate USP)

DESCRIPTION
Dramamine is available as an OTC drug.
Dimenhydrinate is the chlorotheophylline salt of the antihistaminic agent diphenhydramine. Dimenhydrinate contains not less than 53% and not more than 56% of diphenhydramine, and not less than 44% and not more than 47% of 8-chlorotheophylline, calculated on the dried basis.

INACTIVE INGREDIENTS
Dramamine Tablets: Acacia, Carboxymethylcellulose Sodium, Corn Starch, Magnesium Stearate, and Sodium Sulfate.
Dramamine Chewable Tablets: Aspartame, Citric Acid, FD&C Yellow No. 6, Flavor, Magnesium Stearate, Methacrylic Acid Copolymer, Sorbitol.
Dramamine Liquid: Cherry Flavor, FD&C Red #40, Ethyl Alcohol 5%, Glycerin, Methylparaben, Sucrose, and Water.

ACTIONS
While the precise mode of action of dimenhydrinate is not known, it has a depressant action on hyperstimulated labyrinthine function.

INDICATIONS
Dramamine is indicated for the prevention and treatment of the nausea, vomiting, dizziness or vertigo associated with motion sickness. Such an illness may arise from the motion of ships, planes, trains, automobiles, buses, swings, or even amusement park rides. Regardless of the cause of motion sickness, Dramamine has been found to be effective in its prevention or treatment.

WARNINGS
DRAMAMINE may cause marked drowsiness; alcohol, sedatives, and tranquilizers may increase the drowsiness effect. Avoid alcoholic beverages while taking this product. Do not take this product if you are taking sedatives or tranquilizers, without first consulting your doctor. Use caution when driving a motor vehicle or operating machinery. Do not take this product if you have asthma, glaucoma, emphysema, chronic pulmonary disease, shortness of breath, difficulty in breathing, or difficulty in urination due to enlargement of the prostate gland unless directed by a doctor. Do not give to chidren under 2 years of age unless directed by a doctor. In case of accidental overdose, seek professional assistance or contact a Poison Control Center immediately. As with any drug, if you are pregnant or nursing a baby, seek the advice of a health professional before using this product. Keep this and all medications out of the reach of children.
Dramamine Chewable: Phenylketonurics: contains Phenylalanine 1.5 mg per tablet.

DOSAGE AND ADMINISTRATION
Dramamine Tablets: To prevent motion sickness, the first dose should be taken ½ to 1 hour before starting the activity. Additional medication depends on travel conditions. *Adults and children 12 years of age and older:* 1 to 2 tablets every 4 to 6 hours, not to exceed 8 tablets in 24 hours. *Children 6 to under 12 years of age:* ½ to 1 tablet every 6 to 8 hours, not to exceed 3 tablets in 24 hours. *Children 2 to under 6 years of age:* Up to ½ tablet every 6 to 8 hours, not to exceed 1½ tablets in 24 hours. Children may also be given Dramamine cherry-flavored liquid in accordance with directions for use. Not for frequent or prolonged use except on advice of a physician. Do not exceed recommended dosage.
Dramamine Liquid: To prevent motion sickness, the first dose should be taken ½ to 1 hour before starting the activity. Additional medication depends on travel conditions. *Adults:* 4 to 8 teaspoonfuls (5 ml per teaspoonful) every 4 to 6 hours, not to exceed 32 teaspoonfuls in 24 hours. *Children 6 to 12 years:* 2 to 4 teaspoonfuls every 6 to 8 hours, not to exceed 12 teaspoonfuls in 24 hours. *Children 2 to 6 years:* 1 to 2 teaspoonfuls every 6 to 8 hours, not to exceed 6 teaspoonfuls in 24 hours. *Children under 2 years:* Only on advice of a physician.
Not for frequent or prolonged use except on advice of a physician. Do not exceed recommended dosage. Use of a measuring device is recommended for all liquid medication.

HOW SUPPLIED
Tablets —scored, white tablets containing 50 mg of dimenhydrinate. Available in packets of 12 and 36 and bottles of 100 (OTC); *Chewable Tablets* —scored, orange tablets containing 50 mg of dimenhydrinate. Available in packets of 8 and 24 (OTC); *Liquid* —12.5 mg dimenhydrinate per 5 ml, ethyl alcohol 5%, bottles of 3 fl oz (OTC).

PERCOGESIC®
[pĕr 'kō-gē-sĭk]
Analgesic Tablets

ACTIVE INGREDIENTS
Each tablet contains:
Acetaminophen ....325 mg
Phenyltoloxamine citrate ....30 mg

INACTIVE INGREDIENTS
Cellulose, FD&C Yellow #6, FD&C Yellow #6 Aluminum Lake, Flavor, Hydroxypropyl Methylcellulose, Magnesium Stearate, Polyethylene Glycol, Povidone, Silica Gel, Starch, Stearic acid, Sucrose.

INDICATIONS
For temporary relief of minor aches and pains associated with colds, headaches, toothaches, muscular aches, backaches, premenstrual and menstrual periods, minor arthritis pain and to reduce fever.

WARNING
May cause excitability especially for children. Don't take if you have asthma, glaucoma, emphysema, chronic pulmonary disease, shortness of breath, difficulty in breathing or difficulty in urination due to enlargement of the prostate gland unless directed by a doctor. May cause drowsiness: alcohol, sedatives, and tranquilizers may increase drowsiness. Avoid alcoholic beverages while taking this product. Don't use if you're taking sedatives or tranquilizers, without first consulting a doctor. Use caution when driving a motor vehicle or operating machinery. Don't take for pain for more than 10 days (adults) or 5 days (children), and don't take for fever for more than 3 days unless directed by a doctor. If pain or fever persists or worsens, new symptoms occur, or redness or swelling is present, consult a doctor as these could be signs of a serious condition. Don't give this product to children for arthritis pain unless directed by a doctor. Keep out of reach of children. In case of accidental overdose, seek professional help or contact a poison control center immediately. Prompt medical attention is critical for adults and children, even if you don't notice signs or symptoms. If pregnant or nursing a baby, seek a health professional's advice before using this product.
KEEP THIS AND ALL MEDICATION OUT OF CHILDREN'S REACH

DOSAGE AND ADMINISTRATION
  ADULTS (12 years and over)—1 or 2 tablets every four hours. Maximum daily dose—8 tablets
  CHILDREN (6-12 years)—1 tablet every 4 hours; maximum daily dose 4 tablets.
    Do not use for more than 10 days unless directed by a physician.
Store at room temperature; avoid excessive heat.

HOW SUPPLIED
Bottles of 24, 50 and 90 tablets.

VICKS® CHILDREN'S COUGH SYRUP
Expectorant, Antitussive Cough Syrup

(See PDR For Nonprescription Drugs)

VICKS CHILDREN'S NYQUIL

PRODUCT OVERVIEW
KEY FACTS
Vicks Children's NyQuil is formulated with the maximum childrens recommended dose of Dextromethorphan HBr (15 mg), Pseudoephedrine HCl (30 mg) and Chlorpheniramine Maleate (2 mg) for effective relief of cough, nasal congestion, runny nose and sneezing that keep children awake. It is analgesic and alcohol free.

MAJOR USES
For the temporary relief of coughing, nasal congestion, runny nose, and sneezing due to a cold.

SAFETY INFORMATION
For children under 6, consult a physician before using Children's NyQuil®.

PRESCRIBING INFORMATION
VICKS CHILDREN'S NYQUIL
ACTIVE INGREDIENTS
Per ½ oz dose (1 tbls): Chlorpheniramine Maleate 2 mg, Pseudoephedrine HCl 30 mg, Dextromethorphan Hydrobromide 15 mg.

INACTIVE INGREDIENTS
Citric Acid, Flavor, FD&C Red #40, Grape Juice, Potassium Sorbate, Propylene Glycol, Purified Water, Sodium Citrate, Sucrose.

INDICATIONS
For temporary relief of nasal congestion, runny nose, sneezing and cough due to a cold, to help children rest.

ADMINISTRATION AND DOSAGE

DOSAGE INSTRUCTIONS:	Take at bedtime as directed. Use medicine cup provided.

AGE	WEIGHT	DOSE
Under 6	Under 48 lbs	Consult Physician*
6–11	48–95 lbs	½ oz (1 Tbls)
12 and over	Over 95 lbs	Use NyQuil Nighttime Cold Medicine (Adult Formula) as directed.

*Suggested dose for children 2–5 yrs is ¼ oz (½ Tbls)
If cold symptoms keep your child confined to bed or at home, a total of 4 doses may be taken per day, each 6–8 hours apart.

WARNING
Do not exceed recommended dosage because at higher doses nervousness, dizziness or sleeplessness may occur. Do not give this product to children for more than 7 days. If symptoms do not improve or are accompanied by fever, consult a physician. Do not give this product to children who have heart disease, high blood pressure, diabetes or thyroid disease, unless directed by a physician. May cause excitability especially in children. Do not give this product to children who have asthma or glaucoma unless directed by a physician. May cause drowsiness. Sedatives and tranquilizers may increase the drowsiness effect. Do not give this product to children who are taking sedatives or tranquilizers without first consulting your childs doctor. Do not give this product to children under 6 years except on advice and supervision of a physician. Do not give this product for persistent or chronic cough such as occurs with asthma or if cough is accompanied by excessive mucus unless directed by a physician. A persistent cough may be a sign of a serious condition. If cough persists for more than 1 week, tends to recur, or is accompanied by fever, rash, or persistent headache, consult a physician. In case of accidental overdose, seek professional assistance or contact a poison control center immediately.

DRUG INTERACTION PRECAUTION
Do not give this product to a child who is taking a prescription drug for high blood pressure or depression, without first consulting the child's physician.
TAKE ONLY AS DIRECTED. KEEP OUT OF REACH OF CHILDREN.
Store at room temperature.

HOW SUPPLIED
4 fl. oz bottles.
Shown in Product Identification Section, page 424

VICKS® COUGH SILENCERS
Cough Drops

(See PDR For Nonprescription Drugs)

VICKS® DAYCARE® LIQUID
VICKS® DAYCARE® CAPLETS
Multi-Symptom Colds Medicine

(See PDR For Nonprescription Drugs)

VICKS® FORMULA 44® COUGH CONTROL DISCS

(See PDR For Nonprescription Drugs)

VICKS® FORMULA 44® COUGH MIXTURE

(See PDR For Nonprescription Drugs)

VICKS® FORMULA 44D
DECONGESTANT COUGH MIXTURE

(See PDR For Nonprescription Drugs)

VICKS® FORMULA 44M
Multi-Symptom Cough Mixture

(See PDR For Nonprescription Drugs)

Continued on next page

Richardson-Vicks—Cont.

VICKS® INHALER
with decongestant action

(See PDR For Nonprescription Drugs)

VICKS® NYQUIL®
[nĭ'quĭl]
Nighttime Colds Medicine
in oral liquid form.

(See PDR For Nonprescription Drugs)

VICKS® PEDIATRIC FORMULA 44® COUGH MEDICINE
VICKS® PEDIATRIC FORMULA 44® COUGH & CONGESTION MEDICINE
VICKS® PEDIATRIC FORMULA 44® COUGH & COLD MEDICINE

PRODUCT OVERVIEW
KEY FACTS
Vicks Pediatric Formula 44® is a new line of dextromethorphan-based cough medicines designed to provide children effective relief of cough and accompanying symptoms. Pediatric Formula 44® medicines are analgesic-and alcohol- free and non-narcotic.

MAJOR USES
Pediatric Formula 44® Cough Medicine provides temporary relief of coughing due to the common cold or minor throat and bronchial irritation.
Pediatric Formula 44® Cough & Congestion Medicine provides temporary relief of coughing and nasal congestion.
Pediatric Formula 44® Cough & Cold Medicine provides temporary relief of coughing, nasal congestion, runny nose and sneezing.

SAFETY INFORMATION
For children under 2, consult a physician before using Pediatric Formula 44® Cough Medicine and Pediatric Formula 44® Cough & Congestion Medicine.
For children under 6, consult a physician before using Pediatric Formula 44® Cough & Cold Medicine.

PRESCRIBING INFORMATION
VICKS® PEDIATRIC FORMULA 44® COUGH MEDICINE
ACTIVE INGREDIENTS
Per 1 TBS. (15 ml.): Dextromethorphan Hydrobromide, USP 15 mg.

INACTIVE INGREDIENTS
Carboxymethylcellulose Sodium, Cellulose, Citric Acid, FD&C Red No. 40, Flavor, Glycerin, Polysorbate 80, Potassium Sorbate, Propylene Glycol, Purified Water, Sodium Citrate, Sorbitol, Sucrose.

INDICATIONS
For the temporary relief of coughs due to the common cold or minor throat and bronchial irritation.

ADMINISTRATION AND DOSAGE
DIRECTIONS FOR USE:
(CUP INSIDE)
SHAKE WELL BEFORE USING
Squeeze bottle to accurately dispense medicine into dosage cup provided.　　1 TBS.　½ TBS.
Dosage—Choose by weight (if weight is not known, choose by age):

Age	Weight	Dose
Under 2 yrs.	Under 24 lbs.	Consult physician*
2–5 yrs.	24–47 lbs.	Fill cup to ½ Tbs.
6–11 yrs.	48–95 lbs.	Fill cup to 1 Tbs.
12 yrs. and over	96 lbs. and over	2 Tbs. or Try one of the Adult Formula 44® Medicines

Repeat every 6–8 hours as needed, not to exceed 4 doses in 24 hours.
*Suggested doses for children 0–2 are:

Age	Weight	DOSE
0–3 months	6–11 lbs.	¼ tsp.
4–11 months	12–17 lbs.	⅖ tsp.
12–23 months	18–23 lbs.	½ tsp.

WARNING
Do not exceed recommended dosage. Do not take this product for persistent or chronic cough such as occurs with smoking, asthma, or emphysema, or if cough is accompanied by excessive phlegm (mucus) unless directed by a doctor. A persistent cough may be a sign of a serious condition. If cough persists for more than 1 week, tends to recur, or is accompanied by fever, rash, or persistent headache, consult a doctor. In case of accidental overdose, seek professional assistance or contact a poison control center immediately. As with any drug, if you are pregnant or nursing a baby, seek the advice of a health professional before using this product.
KEEP OUT OF CHILDREN'S REACH.
STORE AT ROOM TEMPERATURE.
AVOID EXCESSIVE HEAT.

PRESCRIBING INFORMATION

VICKS® PEDIATRIC FORMULA 44® COUGH & CONGESTION MEDICINE

ACTIVE INGREDIENTS
Per 1 TBS. (15 ml.): Dextromethorphan Hydrobromide, USP 15 mg.
Pseudoephedrine Hydrochloride, USP 30 mg.

INACTIVE INGREDIENTS
Carboxymethylcellulose Sodium. Cellulose, Citric Acid, FD&C Red No. 40, Flavor, Glycerin, Polysorbate 80, Potassium Sorbate, Propylene Glycol, Purified Water, Sodium Citrate, Sorbitol, Sucrose.

INDICATIONS
For the temporary relief of coughs and nasal congestion due to the common cold or upper respiratory allergies.

ADMINISTRATION AND DOSAGE
DIRECTIONS FOR USE:
(CUP INSIDE)
SHAKE WELL BEFORE USING
Squeeze bottle to accurately dispense medicine into dosage cup provided　　1 TBS.　½ TBS.
Dosage—Choose by weight (if weight is not known, choose by age):

Age	Weight	Dose
Under 2 yrs.	Under 24 lbs.	Consult physician
2–5 yrs.	24–47 lbs.	Fill cup to ½Tbs.
6–11 yrs.	48–95 lbs.	Fill cup to 1 Tbs.
12 yrs. and over	96 lbs. and over	2 Tbs. or Try one of the Adult Formula 44® Medicines

Repeat every 6–8 hours as needed, not to exceed 4 doses in 24 hours.

WARNING
Do not exceed recommended dosage because at higher doses nervousness, dizziness, or sleeplessness may occur. Do not take this product for more than 7 days. If symptoms do not improve or are accompanied by fever, consult a doctor. Do not take this product if you have heart disease, diabetes, or difficulty in urination due to enlargement of the prostate gland unless directed by a doctor. Do not take this product for persistent or chronic cough such as occurs with smoking, asthma, or emphysema, or if cough is accompanied by excessive phlegm (mucus) unless directed by a doctor. A persistent cough may be a sign of a serious condition. If cough persists for more than 1 week, tends to recur, or is accompanied by fever, rash, or persistent headache, consult a doctor. In case of accidental overdose, seek professional assistance or contact a poison control center immediately. If pregnant or nursing a baby, consult a health professional before using this product.
Drug Interaction Precaution: Do not take this product if you are presently taking a prescription drug for high blood pressure or depression, without first consulting your doctor.
KEEP OUT OF CHILDREN'S REACH.
STORE AT ROOM TEMPERATURE.
AVOID EXCESSIVE HEAT.

PRESCRIBING INFORMATION
VICKS® PEDIATRIC FORMULA 44® COUGH & COLD MEDICINE
ACTIVE INGREDIENTS
Per 1 TBS. (15 ml.): Dextromethorphan Hydrobromide, USP 15 mg.
Pseudoephedrine Hydrochloride, USP 30 mg.
Chlorpheniramine Maleate, USP 2 mg.

INACTIVE INGREDIENTS
Carboxymethylcellulose Sodium, Cellulose, Citric Acid, FD&C Red No. 40, Flavor, Glycerin, Polysorbate 80, Potassium Sorbate, Propylene Glycol, Purified Water, Sodium Citrate, Sorbitol, Sucrose.

INDICATIONS
For the temporary relief of coughs, nasal congestion, runny nose and sneezing due to the common cold or upper respiratory allergies.

ADMINISTRATION AND DOSAGE
DIRECTIONS FOR USE:
(CUP INSIDE)
SHAKE WELL BEFORE USING
Squeeze bottle to accurately dispense medicine into dosage cup provided　　1 TBS.　½TBS.
Dosage—Choose by weight (if weight is not known, choose by age):

Age	Weight	Dose
Under 6 yrs.	Under 48 lbs.	Consult physician
6–11 yrs.	48–95 lbs.	Fill cup to 1 Tbs.
12 yrs. and over	96 lbs. and over	2 Tbs. or Try one of the Adult Formula 44® Medicines

Repeat every 6–8 hours as needed, not to exceed 4 doses in 24 hours.

WARNING
Do not exceed recommended dosage because at higher doses nervousness, dizziness, or sleeplessness may occur. Do not take this product for more than 7 days. If symptoms do not improve or are accompanied by fever, consult a doctor. Do not take this product if you have heart disease, thyroid disease, diabetes, or difficulty in urination due to enlargement of the prostate gland unless directed by a doctor. Do not take this product for persistent or chronic cough such as occurs with smoking, asthma, or emphysema, or if cough is accompanied by excessive phlegm (mucus) unless directed by a doctor. A persistent cough may be a sign of a serious condition. If cough persists for more than 1 week, tends to recur, or is accompanied by fever, rash, or persistent headache, consult a doctor. May cause excitability especially in children. Do not take this product if you have asthma, glaucoma, emphysema, chronic pulmonary disease, shortness of breath or difficulty in breathing unless directed by a doctor. May cause drowsiness: alcohol, sedatives, and tranquilizers may increase the drowsiness effect. Avoid alcoholic beverages while taking this product. Do not take this product if you are taking sedatives or tranquilizers without first consulting your doctor. Use caution when driving a motor vehicle or operating machinery. In case of accidental overdose, seek professional assistance or contact a poison control center immediately. If pregnant or nursing a baby, consult a health professional before using this product.
Drug Interaction Precaution: Do not take this product if you are presently taking a prescription drug for high blood pressure or depression, without first consulting your doctor.
KEEP OUT OF CHILDREN'S REACH.
STORE AT ROOM TEMPERATURE.
AVOID EXCESSIVE HEAT.

HOW SUPPLIED
4 fl. oz. squeeze bottles with Vicks AccuTip Dispenser for clean, easy, accurate dosing.
Calibrated dose cup accompanies each bottle.
Shown in Product Identification Section, page 424

VICKS® SINEX™
[sī'něx]
Decongestant Nasal Spray

(See PDR For Nonprescription Drugs)

VICKS® SINEX™ LONG–ACTING
[sī'něx]
Decongestant Nasal Spray

(See PDR For Nonprescription Drugs)

VICKS® THROAT LOZENGES

(See PDR For Nonprescription Drugs)

VICKS® VAPORUB®
Decongestant Vaporizing Ointment

(See PDR For Nonprescription Drugs)

VICKS® VAPOSTEAM®
[vā'pō"stēm]
Liquid Medication for
Hot Steam Vaporizers.

(See PDR For Nonprescription Drugs)

VICKS® VATRONOL®
[vă'trŏ"nŏl]
Nose Drops

(See PDR For Nonprescription Drugs)

Richardson-Vicks USA
Personal Care Products Division
ONE FAR MILL CROSSING
SHELTON, CT 06484

CLEARASIL® Adult Care™
(Sulfur/Resorcinol)

(See PDR For Nonprescription Drugs)

CLEARASIL® Maximum Strength Medicated
Anti-Acne Cream
(10% Benzoyl Peroxide)
Vanishing and Tinted

(See PDR For Nonprescription Drugs)

CLEARASIL® 10% Benzoyl Peroxide
Medicated Anti-Acne Lotion

(See PDR For Nonprescription Drugs)

CLEARASIL® Medicated Astringent
(Salicylic Acid 0.5%)

(See PDR For Nonprescription Drugs)

A. H. Robins Company
PHARMACEUTICAL DIVISION
1407 CUMMINGS DRIVE
RICHMOND, VA 23220

ALLBEE® WITH C CAPLETS
[all-be']

(See PDR For Nonprescription Drugs)

ALLBEE® C–800 TABLETS
ALLBEE® C–800 plus IRON TABLETS
[all-be']

(See PDR For Nonprescription Drugs)

DIMACOL® CAPLETS
[di'mă-col]

(See PDR For Nonprescription Drugs)

DIMETANE EXTENTABS®
[di'mĕ-tāne eks"tĕn'tabs]
brand of Brompheniramine Maleate, USP
8 mg and 12 mg

(See PDR For Nonprescription Drugs)

DIMETANE®
[di'mĕ-tāne]
brand of Brompheniramine Maleate, USP
Tablets—4 mg
Elixir—2 mg/5 ml
   Alcohol, 3%

(See PDR For Nonprescription Drugs)

DIMETANE® DECONGESTANT ELIXIR
[di'mĕ-tāne]
DIMETANE® DECONGESTANT
CAPLETS

(See PDR For Nonprescription Drugs)

DIMETANE®-DC   © ℞
COUGH SYRUP
[di'mĕ-tāne]

DESCRIPTION
Dimetane-DC Cough Syrup is a light bluish-pink syrup with a raspberry flavor.

Each 5 mL (1 teaspoonful) contains:
Brompheniramine Maleate, USP ....2.0 mg
Phenylpropanolamine
  Hydrochloride, USP ....12.5 mg
Codeine Phosphate, USP ....10.0 mg
  (Warning: May be habit forming)
    Alcohol 0.95 percent
In a palatable aromatic vehicle.
Inactive Ingredients: Citric Acid, FD&C Blue 1, FD&C Red 40, Flavors, Glycerin, Sodium Benzoate, Sorbitol, Water.
Antihistamine/Nasal Decongestant/Antitussive syrup for oral administration.

CLINICAL PHARMACOLOGY
Brompheniramine maleate is a histamine antagonist, specifically an H_1-receptor-blocking agent belonging to the alkylamine class of antihistamines. Antihistamines appear to compete with histamine for receptor sites on effector cells. Brompheniramine also has anticholinergic (drying) and sedative effects. Among the antihistaminic effects, it antagonizes the allergic response (vasodilatation, increased vascular permeability, increased mucus secretion) of nasal tissue. Brompheniramine is well absorbed from the gastrointestinal tract, with peak plasma concentration after a single oral dose of 4 mg reached in 5 hours; urinary excretion is the major route of elimination, mostly as products of biodegradation; the liver is assumed to be the main site of metabolic transformation.
Phenylpropanolamine hydrochloride is a sympathomimetic drug which is readily absorbed from the gastrointestinal tract and produces nasal vasoconstriction (decongestion). Phenylpropanolamine stimulates both α and β-adrenergic receptors, similar to ephedrine. Part of its peripheral action is indirect and is due to the displacement of norepinephrine from storage sites, but it also has direct effect on the adrenergic receptors.
Codeine is an opiate analgesic and antitussive. Codeine calms the cough control center.

INDICATIONS AND USAGE
For relief of coughs and upper respiratory symptoms, including nasal congestion, associated with allergy or the common cold.

CONTRAINDICATIONS
Hypersensitivity to any of the ingredients. Do not use in the newborn, in premature infants, in nursing mothers, in patients with severe hypertension or severe coronary artery disease, or in those receiving monoamine oxidase (MAO) inhibitors.
Antihistamines should not be used to treat lower respiratory tract conditions including asthma.

WARNINGS
Especially in infants and small children, antihistamines in overdosage may cause hallucinations, convulsions, death. Codeine may cause or aggravate constipation.
Antihistamines may diminish mental alertness. In the young child, they may produce excitation.

PRECAUTIONS
General: Because of its antihistamine component, Dimetane-DC Cough Syrup should be used with caution in patients with a history of bronchial asthma, narrow angle glaucoma, gastrointestinal obstruction, or urinary bladder neck obstruction. Because of its sympathomimetic component, Dimetane-DC Cough Syrup should be used with caution in patients with diabetes, hypertension, heart disease, or thyroid disease.
Information for Patients: Patients should be warned about engaging in activities requiring mental alertness, such as driving a car or operating dangerous machinery.
Drug Interactions: Antihistamines have additive effects with alcohol and other CNS depressants (hypnotics, sedatives, tranquilizers, antianxiety agents, etc.). MAO inhibitors prolong and intensify the anticholinergic (drying) effects of antihistamines. MAO inhibitors may enhance the effect of phenylpropanolamine. Sympathomimetics may reduce the effects of antihypertensive drugs.
Carcinogenesis, Mutagenesis: Long-term studies in animals to evaluate carcinogenic and mutagenic potential have not been performed.
Pregnancy Category C: Animal reproduction studies have not been conducted with Dimetane-DC Cough Syrup. It is also not known whether Dimetane-DC Cough Syrup can cause fetal harm when administered to a pregnant woman or can affect reproduction capacity. Dimetane-DC Cough Syrup should be given to a pregnant woman only if clearly needed. Reproduction studies of brompheniramine maleate (one of the components of the Dimetane formulations) in rats and mice at doses up to 16 times the maximum human dose have revealed no evidence of impaired fertility or harm to the fetus.
Nursing Mothers: Because of the higher risk of intolerance of antihistamines in small infants generally, and in newborns and prematures in particular, and the fact that codeine appears in human milk, Dimetane-DC Cough Syrup is contraindicated in nursing mothers.

ADVERSE REACTIONS
The most frequent adverse reactions to Dimetane-DC Cough Syrup are: sedation; dryness of mouth, nose and throat; thickening of bronchial secretions; dizziness. Other adverse reactions may include:
Dermatologic: Urticaria, drug rash, photosensitivity, pruritus.
Cardiovascular System: Hypotension, hypertension, cardiac arrhythmias.
CNS: Disturbed coordination, tremor, irritability, insomnia, visual disturbances, weakness, nervousness, convulsions, headache, euphoria, and dysphoria.
G. U. System: Urinary frequency, difficult urination.
G. I. System: Epigastric discomfort, anorexia, nausea, vomiting, diarrhea, constipation.
Respiratory System: Tightness of chest and wheezing, shortness of breath. At higher doses, codeine has most of the disadvantages of morphine including respiratory depression.
Hematologic System: Hemolytic anemia, thrombocytopenia, agranulocytosis.

DRUG ABUSE AND DEPENDENCE
Codeine can produce drug dependence of the morphine type, and therefore has the potential for being abused. Psychic dependence, physical dependence and tolerance may develop upon repeated administration of this drug, and it should be prescribed and administered with the same degree of caution appropriate to the use of other oral narcotic medications. Dimetane-DC Cough Syrup is subject to the Federal Controlled Substances Act (Schedule V).

OVERDOSAGE
Signs and Symptoms: Serious overdose with codeine is characterized by respiratory depression, extreme somnolence progressing to stupor or coma. In severe overdosage, apnea, circulatory collapse, cardiac arrest and death may occur. The central nervous system effects from overdosage of brompheniramine may vary from depression to stimulation. Anticholinergic effects may also occur. Overdosage of phenylpropanolamine may be associated with tachycardia, hypertension and cardiac arrhythmias.
Toxic Doses: Doses of 800 mg or more of codeine have caused partial loss of consciousness, delirium, restlessness, excitement, tremors, convulsions and collapse; or respiratory paralysis with such sequelae as mydriasis, marked vasodilatation, and finally death. A 2½-year-old child survived a dose of 300–900 mg of brompheniramine; the lethal dose of phenylpropanolamine is in the range of 50 mg/kg.
Treatment: Respiratory depression should be treated promptly. Oxygen, intravenous fluids, vasopressors and other supportive measures should be employed as indicated. If necessary, reestablishment of adequate respiratory exchange through provision of a patent airway and the institution of assisted or controlled ventilation must be provided. The narcotic antagonist, naloxone, is a specific antidote to codeine-induced respiratory depression, and should be administered by the intravenous route if appropriate (see package insert for naloxone). Since the duration of action of codeine may exceed that of the antagonist, the patient should be kept under constant surveillance.
Gastric emptying may be useful in removing unabsorbed drug, either by inducing emesis or lavage; precautions against aspiration must be taken. Stimulants or depressants should be used cautiously and only when specifically indicated. If marked excitement is present, one of the short-acting barbiturates or chloral hydrate may be used.

DOSAGE AND ADMINISTRATION
Adults and children 12 years of age and over: 2 teaspoonfuls every 4 hours. Children 6 to under 12 years: 1 teaspoonful every 4 hours. Children 2 to under 6 years: ½ teaspoonful every 4 hours. Children 6 months to under 2 years: Dosage to be established by physician.
Do not exceed 6 doses during a 24-hour period.

HOW SUPPLIED
Dimetane-DC Cough Syrup is a light bluish-pink syrup containing in each 5 mL (1 teaspoonful) brompheniramine maleate 2 mg, phenylpropanolamine HCl 12.5 mg, and codeine phosphate 10 mg; available in pints (NDC 0031-1833-25) and gallons (NDC 0031-1833-29).
Store at controlled room temperature, between 15°C and 30°C (59°F and 86°F).
Dispense in tight, light-resistant container.

Continued on next page

Prescribing information on A. H. Robins products listed here is based on official labeling in effect June 1, 1989, with Indications, Contraindications, Warnings, Precautions, Adverse Reactions, and Dosage stated in full.

Robins—Cont.

DIMETANE®–DX Cough Syrup   ℞
[di'mĕ-tāne]

DESCRIPTION
Dimetane-DX Cough Syrup is a light-red syrup with a butterscotch flavor.

Each 5 mL (1 teaspoonful) contains:
Brompheniramine Maleate, USP .... 2 mg
Pseudoephedrine Hydrochloride, USP ....30 mg
Dextromethorphan Hydrobromide, USP ....10 mg
    Alcohol 0.95 percent
in a palatable, aromatic vehicle.

Inactive Ingredients: Citric Acid, FD&C Red 40, FD&C Yellow 6, Flavors, Glycerin, Saccharin Sodium, Sodium Benzoate, Sorbitol, Water.
Antihistamine/Nasal Decongestant/Antitussive syrup for oral administration.

CLINICAL PHARMACOLOGY
Brompheniramine maleate is a histamine antagonist, specifically an H_1-receptor-blocking agent belonging to the alkylamine class of antihistamines. Antihistamines appear to compete with histamine for receptor sites on effector cells. Brompheniramine also has anticholinergic (drying) and sedative effects. Among the antihistaminic effects, it antagonizes the allergic response (vasodilatation, increased vascular permeability, increased mucus secretion) of nasal tissue. Brompheniramine is well absorbed from the gastrointestinal tract, with peak plasma concentration after single, oral dose of 4 mg reached in 5 hours; urinary excretion is the major route of elimination, mostly as products of biodegradation; the liver is assumed to be the main site of metabolic transformation.
Pseudoephedrine acts on sympathetic nerve endings and also on smooth muscle, making it useful as a nasal decongestant. The nasal decongestant effect is mediated by the action of pseudoephedrine on α-sympathetic receptors, producing vasoconstriction of the dilated nasal arterioles. Following oral administration, effects are noted within 30 minutes with peak activity occurring at approximately one hour.
Dextromethorphan acts centrally to elevate the threshold for coughing. It has no analgesic or addictive properties. The onset of antitussive action occurs in 15 to 30 minutes after administration and is of long duration.

INDICATIONS AND USAGE
For relief of coughs and upper respiratory symptoms, including nasal congestion, associated with allergy or the common cold.

CONTRAINDICATIONS
Hypersensitivity to any of the ingredients. Do not use in the newborn, in premature infants, in nursing mothers, in patients with severe hypertension or severe coronary artery disease, or in those receiving monoamine oxidase (MAO) inhibitors.
Antihistamines should not be used to treat lower respiratory tract conditions including asthma.

WARNINGS
Especially in infants and small children, antihistamines in overdosage may cause hallucinations, convulsions, and death.
Antihistamines may diminish mental alertness. In the young child, they may produce excitation.

PRECAUTIONS
General: Because of its antihistamine component, Dimetane-DX Cough Syrup should be used with caution in patients with a history of bronchial asthma, narrow angle glaucoma, gastrointestinal obstruction, or urinary bladder neck obstruction. Because of its sympathomimetic component, Dimetane-DX Cough Syrup should be used with caution in patients with diabetes, hypertension, heart disease, or thyroid disease.
Information for Patients: Patients should be warned about engaging in activities requiring mental alertness, such as driving a car or operating dangerous machinery.
Drug Interactions: Antihistamines have additive effects with alcohol and other CNS depressants (hypnotics, sedatives, tranquilizers, antianxiety agents, etc.) MAO inhibitors prolong and intensify the anticholinergic (drying) effects of antihistamines. MAO inhibitors may enhance the effect of pseudoephedrine. Sympathomimetics may reduce the effects of antihypertensive drugs.
Carcinogenesis, Mutagenesis, Impairment of Fertility
Animal studies of Dimetane-DX Cough Syrup to assess the carcinogenic and mutagenic potential or the effect on fertility have not been performed.
Pregnancy
Teratogenic Effects—Pregnancy Category C
Animal reproduction studies have not been conducted with Dimetane-DX Cough Syrup. It is also not known whether Dimetane-DX Cough Syrup can cause fetal harm when ad-ministered to a pregnant woman or can affect reproduction capacity. Dimetane-DX Cough Syrup should be given to a pregnant woman only if clearly needed.
Reproduction studies of brompheniramine maleate (a component of Dimetane-DX Cough Syrup) in rats and mice at doses up to 16 times the maximum human dose have revealed no evidence of impaired fertility or harm to the fetus.
Nursing Mothers: Because of the higher risk of intolerance of antihistamines in small infants generally, and in newborns and prematures in particular. Dimetane-DX Cough Syrup is contraindicated in nursing mothers.

ADVERSE REACTIONS
The most frequent adverse reactions to Dimetane-DX Cough Syrup are: sedation; dryness of mouth, nose and throat; thickening of bronchial secretions; dizziness. Other adverse reactions may include:
Dermatologic: Urticaria, drug rash, photosensitivity, pruritus.
Cardiovascular System: Hypotension, hypertension, cardiac arrhythmias, palpitation.
CNS: Disturbed coordination, tremor, irritability, insomnia, visual disturbances, weakness, nervousness, convulsions, headache, euphoria, and dysphoria.
G. U. System: Urinary frequency difficult urination.
G. I. System: Epigastric discomfort, anorexia, nausea, vomiting, diarrhea, constipation.
Respiratory System: Tightness of chest and wheezing, shortness of breath.
Hematologic System: Hemolytic anemia, thrombocytopenia, agranulocytosis.

OVERDOSAGE
Signs and Symptoms: Central nervous system effects from overdosage of brompheniramine may vary from depression to stimulation, especially in children. Anticholinergic effects may be noted. Toxic doses of pseudoephedrine may result in CNS stimulation, tachycardia, hypertension, and cardiac arrhythmias; signs of CNS depression may occasionally be seen. Dextromethorphan in toxic doses will cause drowsiness, ataxia, nystagmus, opisthotonos, and convulsive seizures.
Toxic Doses: Data suggest that individuals may respond in an unexpected manner to apparently small amounts of a particular drug. A 2½-year-old child survived the ingestion of 21 mg/kg of dextromethorphan exhibiting only ataxia, drowsiness, and fever, but seizures have been reported in 2 children following the ingestion of 13–17 mg/kg. Another 2½-year-old child survived a dose of 300–900 mg of brompheniramine. The toxic dose of pseudoephedrine should be less than that of ephedrine, which is estimated to be 50 mg/kg.
Treatment: Induce emesis if patient is alert and is seen prior to 6 hours following ingestion. Precautions against aspiration must be taken, especially in infants and small children. Gastric lavage may be carried out, although in some instances tracheostomy may be necessary prior to lavage. Naloxone hydrochloride 0.005 mg/kg intravenously may be of value in reversing the CNS depression that may occur from an overdose of dextromethorphan. CNS stimulants may counter CNS depression. Should CNS hyperactivity or convulsive seizures occur, intravenous short-acting barbiturates may be indicated. Hypertensive responses and/or tachycardia should be treated appropriately. Oxygen, intravenous fluids, and other supportive measures should be employed as indicated.

DOSAGE AND ADMINISTRATION
Adults and children 12 years of age and over: 2 teaspoonfuls every 4 hours. Children 6 to under 12 years: 1 teaspoonful every 4 hours. Children 2 to under 6 years: ½ teaspoonful every 4 hours. Children 6 months to under 2 years: Dosage to be established by physician.
Do not exceed 6 doses during a 24-hour period.

HOW SUPPLIED
Dimetane-DX Cough Syrup is a light-red syrup containing in each 5 mL (1 teaspoonful) brompheniramine maleate 2 mg, pseudoephedrine hydrochloride 30 mg and dextromethorphan hydrobromide 10 mg, available in pints (NDC 0031-1836-25), and gallons (NDC 0031-1836-29).
Store at controlled room temperature, between 15°C and 30°C (59°F and 86°F).
Dispense in tight, light-resistant container.

DIMETAPP® ELIXIR
[di'mĕ-tap]

(See PDR For Nonprescription Drugs)

DIMETAPP EXTENTABS®
[di'mĕ-tap eks"tĕn'tabs]

(See PDR For Nonprescription Drugs)

DIMETAPP® PLUS CAPLETS
[di'mĕ-tap]

(See PDR For Nonprescription Drugs)

DONNAGEL®
[don'nă-gel]

(See PDR For Nonprescription Drugs)

DONNAGEL®–PG   Ⓒ
[don'nă-gel]

DESCRIPTION
Each fluid ounce (2 tablespoonfuls) contains: Powdered Opium, USP or equivalent 24.0 mg. (Warning: May be habit forming), Kaolin, USP 6.0 g, Pectin, USP 142.8 mg, Hyoscyamine Sulfate, USP 0.1037 mg, Atropine Sulfate, USP 0.0194 mg, Scopolamine Hydrobromide, USP 0.0065 mg, Sodium Benzoate, NF 60.0 mg (preservative), Alcohol 5.0 per cent.
Inactive Ingredients: Citric Acid, D&C Yellow 10, Flavors, High Fructose Corn Syrup, Sodium Carboxymethylcellulose, Sodium Chloride, Water.
Donnagel-PG combines the effects of kaolin, pectin and the natural belladonna alkaloids with the efficacy of powdered opium (or equivalent). The opium content in 1 fluid ounce of Donnagel-PG is equivalent to 5 mL of paregoric.

ACTIONS
Donnagel-PG contains a paregoric equivalent for more complete symptomatic control of acute, non-specific diarrheas. This combination of drugs affords a more complete approach to stopping diarrhea and relieving tenesmus and pain. The belladonna alkaloids partly antagonize the occasional cramping effect of opium upon the colon.

INDICATIONS
Donnagel-PG is indicated for the treatment of diarrhea.

CONTRAINDICATIONS
Glaucoma, advanced renal or hepatic disease or hypersensitivity to any of the ingredients.

CAUTIONS
As with all preparations containing belladonna alkaloids, Donnagel-PG must be administered cautiously to patients with incipient glaucoma or urinary bladder neck obstruction as in prostatic hypertrophy. Caution should be exercised when prescribing this or any other medication for pregnant or nursing patients.

WARNINGS TO PATIENT
Diarrhea may be serious. Do not use for more than two days or in the presence of high fever unless prescribed by a physician. Not to be used by persons having glaucoma or excessive pressure within the eye, by elderly persons (where undiagnosed glaucoma or excessive pressure within the eye occurs most frequently), or by children under 6 years of age, unless directed by a physician. Discontinue use if blurring of vision, rapid pulse, or dizziness occurs. Do not exceed recommended dosage. Not for frequent or prolonged use. If dryness of the mouth occurs, decrease dosage. If eye pain occurs, discontinue use and see your physician immediately as this may indicate undiagnosed glaucoma.

ADVERSE REACTIONS
Blurred vision, dry mouth, difficult urination or flushing and dryness of the skin may occur at higher dosage levels, rarely at the usual dose.

DOSAGE AND ADMINISTRATION
Adults and children 12 years of age and over: two tablespoonfuls (one fl. oz.) initially, followed by 1 tablespoonful every 3 hours
Children 6 to under 12 years: two teaspoonfuls initially and 1 or 2 teaspoonfuls every 3 hours thereafter.
Pediatric Dosage Recommendations (For Physician Use Only):

Body Weight	Initial Dosage
10 lb.	½ teaspoonful (2.5 mL)
20 lb.	1 teaspoonful (5 mL)
30 lb. and over	1–2 teaspoonfuls (5–10 mL)

Do not administer more than 4 doses in any 24-hour period.

HOW SUPPLIED
Donnagel-PG (light yellow, banana-flavored suspension) in 6 fl. oz. (NDC 0031-3083-15) and pint (NDC 0031-3083-25).

DONNATAL® TABLETS   ℞
DONNATAL® CAPSULES   ℞
DONNATAL® ELIXIR   ℞
[don 'nă-tal]

PRODUCT OVERVIEW

KEY FACTS

This drug combination provides natural belladonna alkaloids in a specific, fixed ratio combined with phenobarbital to provide peripheral anticholinergic/antispasmodic action and mild sedation.

MAJOR USES

For use as adjunctive therapy in the treatment of irritable bowel syndrome and acute enterocolitis.

SAFETY INFORMATION

The signs and symptoms of overdose are headache, nausea, vomiting, blurred vision, dilated pupils, hot and dry skin, dizziness, dryness of the mouth, difficulty in swallowing, CNS stimulation.

PRESCRIBING INFORMATION

DONNATAL® TABLETS   ℞
DONNATAL® CAPSULES   ℞
DONNATAL® ELIXIR   ℞
[don 'nă-tal]

DESCRIPTION

Each Donnatal tablet, capsule or 5 mL (teaspoonful) of elixir (23% alcohol) contains:
Phenobarbital, USP ($\frac{1}{4}$ gr) ....16.2 mg
  (Warning: May be habit forming)
Hyoscyamine Sulfate, USP ....0.1037 mg
Atropine Sulfate, USP ....0.0194 mg
Scopolamine Hydrobromide, USP ....0.0065 mg
Inactive Ingredients:
TABLETS: Dibasic Calcium Phosphate, Magnesium Stearate, Microcrystalline Cellulose, Silicon Dioxide, Sodium Starch Glycolate, Stearic Acid, Sucrose. May contain Corn Starch, Dextrose, or Invert Sugar.
CAPSULES: Corn Starch, Edible Ink, D&C Yellow 10 and FD&C Green 3 or FD&C Blue 1 and FD&C Yellow 6, FD&C Blue 2 Aluminum Lake, Gelatin, Lactose, Sucrose. May contain FD&C Red 40 and Yellow 6 Aluminum Lakes.
ELIXIR: D&C Yellow 10, FD&C Blue 1, FD&C Yellow 6, Flavors, Glucose, Saccharin Sodium, Water.

ACTIONS

This drug combination provides natural belladonna alkaloids in a specific, fixed ratio combined with phenobarbital to provide peripheral anticholinergic/antispasmodic action and mild sedation.

Indications

Based on a review of this drug by the National Academy of Sciences—National Research Council and/or other information, FDA has classified the following indications as "possibly" effective:
For use as adjunctive therapy in the treatment of irritable bowel syndrome (irritable colon, spastic colon, mucous colitis) and acute enterocolitis.
May also be useful as adjunctive therapy in the treatment of duodenal ulcer. IT HAS NOT BEEN SHOWN CONCLUSIVELY WHETHER ANTICHOLINERGIC/ANTISPASMODIC DRUGS AID IN THE HEALING OF A DUODENAL ULCER, DECREASE THE RATE OF RECURRENCES OR PREVENT COMPLICATIONS.

CONTRAINDICATIONS

Glaucoma, obstructive uropathy (for example, bladder neck obstruction due to prostatic hypertrophy); obstructive disease of the gastrointestinal tract (as in achalasia, pyloroduodenal stenosis, etc.); paralytic ileus, intestinal atony of the elderly or debilitated patient; unstable cardiovascular status in acute hemorrhage; severe ulcerative colitis especially if complicated by toxic megacolon; myasthenia gravis; hiatal hernia associated with reflux esophagitis.
Donnatal is contraindicated in patients with known hypersensitivity to any of the ingredients. Phenobarbital is contraindicated in acute intermittent porphyria and in those patients in whom phenobarbital produces restlessness and/or excitement.

WARNINGS

In the presence of a high environmental temperature, heat prostration can occur with belladonna alkaloids (fever and heatstroke due to decreased sweating).
Diarrhea may be an early symptom of incomplete intestinal obstruction, especially in patients with ileostomy or colostomy. In this instance treatment with this drug would be inappropriate and possibly harmful.
Donnatal may produce drowsiness or blurred vision. The patient should be warned, should these occur, not to engage in activities requiring mental alertness, such as operating a motor vehicle or other machinery, and not to perform hazardous work.
Phenobarbital may decrease the effect of anticoagulants, and necessitate larger doses of the anticoagulant for optimal effect. When the phenobarbital is discontinued, the dose of the anticoagulant may have to be decreased.
Phenobarbital may be habit forming and should not be administered to individuals known to be addiction prone or to those with a history of physical and/or psychological dependence upon drugs.
Since barbiturates are metabolized in the liver, they should be used with caution and initial doses should be small in patients with hepatic dysfunction.

PRECAUTIONS

Use with caution in patients with: autonomic neuropathy, hepatic or renal disease, hyperthyroidism, coronary heart disease, congestive heart failure, cardiac arrhythmias, tachycardia, and hypertension.
Belladonna alkaloids may produce a delay in gastric emptying (antral stasis) which would complicate the management of gastric ulcer.
Theoretically, with overdosage, a curare-like action may occur.
Carcinogenesis, mutagenesis. Long-term studies in animals have not been performed to evaluate carcinogenic potential.
Pregnancy Category C. Animal reproduction studies have not been conducted with Donnatal. It is not known whether Donnatal can cause fetal harm when administered to a pregnant woman or can affect reproduction capacity. Donnatal should be given to a pregnant woman only if clearly needed.
Nursing mothers. It is not known whether this drug is excreted in human milk. Because many drugs are excreted in human milk, caution should be exercised when Donnatal is administered to a nursing mother.

ADVERSE REACTIONS

Adverse reactions may include xerostomia; urinary hesitancy and retention; blurred vision; tachycardia; palpitation; mydriasis; cycloplegia; increased ocular tension; loss of taste sense, headache, nervousness; drowsiness; weakness; dizziness; insomnia; nausea; vomiting; impotence; suppression of lactation; constipation; bloated feeling; musculoskeletal pain; severe allergic reaction or drug idiosyncrasies, including anaphylaxis, urticaria and other dermal manifestations; and decreased sweating. Elderly patients may react with symptoms of excitement, agitation, drowsiness, and other untoward manifestations to even small doses of the drug.
Phenobarbital may produce excitement in some patients, rather than a sedative effect. In patients habituated to barbiturates, abrupt withdrawal may produce delirium or convulsions.

DOSAGE AND ADMINISTRATION

The dosage of Donnatal should be adjusted to the needs of the individual patient to assure symptomatic control with a minimum of adverse effects.
Donnatal Tablets or Capsules. Adults: One or two Donnatal tablets or capsules three or four times a day according to condition and severity of symptoms.
Donnatal Elixir. Adults: One or two teaspoonfuls of elixir three or four times a day according to conditions and severity of symptoms.
Children (Elixir)—may be dosed every 4 or 6 hours.:

Body Weight	Starting Dosage q4h	q6h
10 lb (4.5 kg)	0.5 mL	0.75 mL
20 lb (9.1 kg)	1.0 mL	1.5 mL
30 lb (13.6 kg)	1.5 mL	2.0 mL
50 lb (22.7 kg)	$\frac{1}{2}$ tsp	$\frac{3}{4}$ tsp
75 lb (34.0 kg)	$\frac{3}{4}$ tsp	1 tsp
100 lb (45.4 kg)	1 tsp	$1\frac{1}{2}$ tsp

OVERDOSAGE

The signs and symptoms of overdose are headache, nausea, vomiting, blurred vision, dilated pupils, hot and dry skin, dizziness, dryness of the mouth, difficulty in swallowing, CNS stimulation. Treatment should consist of gastric lavage, emetics, and activated charcoal. If indicated, parenteral cholinergic agents such as physostigmine or bethanechol chloride, should be added.

HOW SUPPLIED

Donnatal Tablets. White, compressed, embossed "R" on one side, scored and engraved 4250 on the reverse side; in bottles of 100 (NDC 0031-4250-63), 1000 (NDC 0031-4250-74) and Dis-Co® Unit Dose Packs of 100 (NDC 0031-4250-64).
Donnatal Capsules. Green and white, monogrammed "AHR" and "4207"; in bottles of 100 (NDC 0031-4207-63) and 1000 (NDC 0031-4207-74).
Donnatal Elixir. Green, citrus flavored, in 4 fl. oz. (NDC 0031-4221-12), pints (NDC 0031-4221-25), gallons (NDC 0031-4221-29) and 5 mL Dis-Co® Unit Dose Packs (4 × 25s) (NDC 0031-4221-13).

Store at controlled room temperature, between 15°C and 30°C (59°F and 86°F).
Dispense in tight, light-resistant container.
Shown in Product Identification Section, page 424

DONNATAL EXTENTABS®   ℞
[don 'nă-tal ěks "těn 'tabs]

DESCRIPTION

Each Donnatal Extentabs Tablet contains:
Phenobarbital, USP ($\frac{3}{4}$gr) ....48.6 mg
  (Warning: May be habit forming)
Hyoscyamine Sulfate, USP ....0.3111 mg
Atropine Sulfate, USP ....0.0582 mg
Scopolamine Hydrobromide,
USP ....0.0195 mg
Each Donnatal Extentabs tablet contains the equivalent of three Donnatal tablets. Extentabs are designed to release the ingredients gradually to provide effects for up to twelve (12) hours.
Inactive Ingredients: Acacia, Acetylated Monoglycerides, Calcium Sulfate, Carnauba Wax, D&C Yellow 10, Edible Ink, FD&C Blue 1, FD&C Blue 2 Aluminum Lake, FD&C Yellow 6, Gelatin, Guar Gum, Magnesium Stearate, Polysorbates, Shellac, Sodium Phosphate, Sucrose, Titanium Dioxide, Wheat Flour, White Wax and other ingredients, one of which is a corn derivative. May include FD&C Red 40 and Yellow 6 Aluminum Lakes.

ACTIONS

This drug combination provides natural belladonna alkaloids in a specific, fixed ratio combined with phenobarbital to provide peripheral anticholinergic/antispasmodic action and mild sedation.

Indications

Based on a review of this drug by the National Academy of Sciences—National Research Council and/or other information, FDA has classified the following indications as "possibly" effective:
For use as adjunctive therapy in the treatment of irritable bowel syndrome (irritable colon, spastic colon, mucous colitis) and acute enterocolitis.
May also be useful as adjunctive therapy in the treatment of duodenal ulcer. IT HAS NOT BEEN SHOWN CONCLUSIVELY WHETHER ANTICHOLINERGIC/ANTISPASMODIC DRUGS AID IN THE HEALING OF A DUODENAL ULCER, DECREASE THE RATE OF RECURRENCES OR PREVENT COMPLICATIONS.

CONTRAINDICATIONS

Glaucoma, obstructive uropathy (for example, bladder neck obstruction due to prostatic hypertrophy); obstructive disease of the gastrointestinal tract (as in achalasia, pyloroduodenal stenosis, etc.); paralytic ileus, intestinal atony of the elderly or debilitated patient; unstable cardiovascular status in acute hemorrhage; severe ulcerative colitis especially if complicated by toxic megacolon; myasthenia gravis; hiatal hernia associated with reflux esophagitis.
Donnatal is contraindicated in patients with known hypersensitivity to any of the ingredients. Phenobarbital is contraindicated in acute intermittent porphyria and in those patients in whom phenobarbital produces restlessness and/or excitement.

WARNINGS

In the presence of a high environmental temperature, heat prostration can occur with belladonna alkaloids (fever and heatstroke due to decreased sweating).
Diarrhea may be an early symptom of incomplete intestinal obstruction, especially in patients with ileostomy or colostomy. In this instance treatment with this drug would be inappropriate and possibly harmful.
Donnatal may produce drowsiness or blurred vision. The patient should be warned, should these occur, not to engage in activities requiring mental alertness, such as operating a motor vehicle or other machinery, and not to perform hazardous work.
Phenobarbital may decrease the effect of anticoagulants and necessitate larger doses of the anticoagulant for optimal effect. When the phenobarbital is discontinued, the dose of the anticoagulant may have to be decreased.
Phenobarbital may be habit forming and should not be administered to individuals known to be addiction prone or to those with a history of physical and/or psychological dependence upon drugs.

Continued on next page

Prescribing information on A. H. Robins products listed here is based on official labeling in effect June 1, 1989, with Indications, Contraindications, Warnings, Precautions, Adverse Reactions, and Dosage stated in full.

Robins—Cont.

Since barbiturates are metabolized in the liver, they should be used with caution and initial doses should be small in patients with hepatic dysfunction.

PRECAUTIONS

Use with caution in patients with: autonomic neuropathy, hepatic or renal disease, hyperthyroidism, coronary heart disease, congestive heart failure, cardiac arrhythmias, tachycardia, and hypertension.

Belladonna alkaloids may produce a delay in gastric emptying (antral stasis) which would complicate the management of gastric ulcer.

Theoretically, with overdosage, a curare-like action may occur.

Carcinogenesis, mutagenesis. Long-term studies in animals have not been performed to evaluate carcinogenic potential.

Pregnancy Category C. Animal reproduction studies have not been conducted with Donnatal. It is not known whether Donnatal can cause fetal harm when administered to a pregnant woman or can affect reproduction capacity. Donnatal should be given to a pregnant woman only if clearly needed.

Nursing mothers. It is not known whether this drug is excreted in human milk. Because many drugs are excreted in human milk, caution should be exercised when Donnatal is administered to a nursing mother.

ADVERSE REACTIONS

Adverse reactions may include xerostomia; urinary hesitancy and retention; blurred vision; tachycardia; palpitation; mydriasis; cycloplegia; increased ocular tension; loss of taste sense; headache; nervousness; drowsiness; weakness; dizziness, insomnia; nausea; vomiting; impotence; suppression of lactation; constipation; bloated feeling; musculoskeletal pain; severe allergic reaction or drug idiosyncrasies, including anaphylaxis, urticaria and other dermal manifestations; and decreased sweating. Elderly patients may react with symptoms of excitement, agitation, drowsiness, and other untoward manifestations to even small doses of the drug. Phenobarbital may produce excitement in some patients, rather than a sedative effect. In patients habituated to barbiturates, abrupt withdrawal may produce delirium or convulsions.

DOSAGE AND ADMINISTRATION

The dosage of Donnatal Extentabs should be adjusted to the needs of the individual patient to assure symptomatic control with a minimum of adverse reactions. The usual dose is one tablet every twelve (12) hours. If indicated, one tablet every eight (8) hours may be given.

OVERDOSAGE

The signs and symptoms of overdose are headache, nausea, vomiting, blurred vision, dilated pupils; hot and dry skin, dizziness, dryness of the mouth, difficulty in swallowing, CNS stimulation. Treatment should consist of gastric lavage, emetics, and activated charcoal. If indicated, parenteral cholinergic agents such as physostigmine or bethanechol chloride should be added.

HOW SUPPLIED

Pale green, coated tablets, monogrammed AHR and Donnatal Extentab in bottles of 100 (NDC 0031-4235-63) and 500 (NDC 0031-4235-70); and Dis-Co® Unit Dose Packs of 100 (NDC 0031-4235-64).

Store at controlled room temperature, between 15°C and 30°C (59°F and 86°F).

Dispense in well-closed, light-resistant container.

Shown in Product Identification Section, page 424

DONNAZYME® TABLETS　　　　　　　　℞
[don ′nă″ zīm]

DESCRIPTION

Donnazyme tablets are available for oral administration. Each tablet contains:

Pancreatin, USP equivalent ....300 mg
Pepsin ....150 mg
Bile Salts ....150 mg
Hyoscyamine Sulfate, USP ....0.0518 mg
Atropine Sulfate, USP ....0.0097 mg
Scopolamine Hydrobromide,
　USP ....0.0033 mg
Phenobarbital, USP (⅛ gr) ....8.1 mg
　(Warning: may be habit forming)

Inactive Ingredients: Acacia, Acetylated Monoglycerides, Calcium Sulfate, Carnauba Wax, Cellulose Acetate Phthalate, Corn Starch, D&C Yellow 10 Aluminum Lake, Diethyl Phthalate, Edible Ink, FD&C Blue 1 Aluminum Lake, FD&C Yellow 6 Aluminum Lake, Gelatin, Methylparaben, Microcrystalline Cellulose, Polysorbates, Povidone, Propylparaben, Shellac, Sodium Benzoate, Stearic Acid, Sucrose, Tartaric Acid, Titanium Dioxide, Wheat Flour, White Wax. May contain Docusate Sodium.

The combination of anticholinergic/antispasmodic/sedative components with natural digestive enzymes plus bile salts makes it useful for symptomatic relief of functional G.I. disorders.

CLINICAL PHARMACOLOGY

The outer layer of Donnazyme tablets is gastric-soluble and contains the belladonna alkaloids, phenobarbital and pepsin. These ingredients rapidly become available for absorption as the tablet begins disintegrating in the stomach. The pepsin supplements the stomach's digestive secretions by aiding the breakdown of proteins into proteoses and peptones. Spasmolysis and sedation are produced as the belladonna alkaloids and phenobarbital are absorbed.

The core of the tablet contains pancreatin and bile salts. It is designed to disintegrate in the alkaline medium of the duodenum where it releases the active enzyme components of pancreatin (trypsin, amylase and lipase), along with the bile salts. Trypsin breaks down larger protein fractions into peptides; amylase converts starch into maltose; lipase splits fat into fatty acids and glycerin; and bile salts enhance the fat-splitting action of the lipase and aid in the emulsification of fats and the absorption of fatty acids.

INDICATIONS AND USAGE

Donnazyme is indicated for the relief of symptoms associated with "nervous indigestion" and other functional G.I. disorders in the absence of organic pathology. Some of these conditions are chronic pancreatitis, chronic gastritis, postcholecystectomy syndrome, and chronic biliary disorders. Donnazyme may prove especially useful in patients with decreased digestive enzyme secretory activity, which is frequently suspect in older patients with visceral complaints.

CONTRAINDICATIONS

Glaucoma, obstructive uropathy (for example, bladder neck obstruction due to prostatic hypertrophy); obstructive disease of the gastrointestinal tract (as in achalasia, pyloroduodenal stenosis, etc.); paralytic ileus, intestinal atony of the elderly or debilitated patient, unstable cardiovascular status in acute hemorrhage, severe ulcerative colitis especially if complicated by toxic megacolon; myasthenia gravis; hiatal hernia associated with reflux esophagitis.

Donnazyme is contraindicated in patients with known hypersensitivity to any of the ingredients. Phenobarbital is contraindicated in acute intermittent porphyria and in those patients in whom phenobarbital produces restlessness and/or excitement.

WARNINGS

In the presence of a high environmental temperature, heat prostration can occur with belladonna alkaloids (fever and heatstroke due to decreased sweating).

Diarrhea may be an early symptom of incomplete intestinal obstruction, especially in patients with ileostomy or colostomy. In this instance, treatment with this drug would be inappropriate and possibly harmful.

Donnazyme may produce drowsiness or blurred vision. The patient should be warned, should these occur, not to engage in activities requiring mental alertness, such as operating a motor vehicle or other machinery, and not to perform hazardous work.

Phenobarbital may decrease the effect of anticoagulants and necessitate larger doses of the anticoagulant for optimal effect. When the phenobarbital is discontinued, the dose of the anticoagulant may have to be decreased.

Phenobarbital may be habit forming and should not be administered to individuals known to be addiction prone or to those with a history of physical and/or psychological dependence upon drugs.

Since barbiturates are metabolized in the liver, they should be used with caution and initial small doses in patients with hepatic dysfunction.

PRECAUTIONS

General. Use with caution in patients with autonomic neuropathy, hepatic or renal disease, hyperthyroidism, coronary heart disease, congestive heart failure, cardiac arrhythmias, tachycardia, and hypertension.

Belladonna alkaloids may produce a delay in gastric emptying (antral stasis) which would complicate the management of gastric ulcer.

Theoretically, with overdosage, a curare-like action may occur.

Carcinogenesis, mutagenesis: Long-term studies in animals have not been performed to evaluate carcinogenic potential.

Pregnancy Category C. Animal reproduction studies have not been conducted with Donnazyme. It is not known whether Donnazyme can cause fetal harm when administered to a pregnant woman or can affect reproduction capacity. Donnazyme should be given to a pregnant woman only if clearly needed.

Nursing mothers: It is not known whether this drug is excreted in human milk. Because many drugs are excreted in human milk, caution should be exercised when Donnazyme is administered to a nursing mother.

Pediatric Use: Safety and effectiveness in children have not been established.

ADVERSE REACTIONS

Adverse reactions may include xerostomia; urinary hesitancy and retention; blurred vision; tachycardia; palpitation; mydriasis; cycloplegia; increased ocular tension; loss of taste sense; headache; nervousness; drowsiness; weakness; dizziness, insomnia; nausea; vomiting; impotence; suppression of lactation; constipation; bloated feeling; musculoskeletal pain; severe allergic reaction or drug idiosyncrasies, including "anaphylaxis, urticaria and other dermal manifestations; and decreased sweating." Elderly patients may react with symptoms of excitement, agitation, drowsiness, and other untoward manifestations to even small doses of the drug.

Phenobarbital may produce excitement in some patients, rather than a sedative effect. In patients habituated to barbiturates, abrupt withdrawal may produce delirium or convulsions.

OVERDOSAGE

The signs and symptoms of overdose are headache, nausea, vomiting, blurred vision, dilated pupils, hot and dry skin, dizziness, dryness of the mouth, difficulty in swallowing, CNS stimulation. Treatment should consist of gastric lavage, emetics, and activated charcoal. If indicated, parenteral cholinergic agents, such as physostigmine or bethanechol chloride, should be added.

DOSAGE AND ADMINISTRATION

Adult dosage: Two tablets after each meal.

HOW SUPPLIED

Kelly green tablets in bottles of 100 (NDC 0031-4649-63) and 500 (NDC 0031-4649-70). Store at controlled room temperature, between 15°C and 30°C (59°F and 86°F). Dispense in tight container.

Shown in Product Identification Section, page 424

DOPRAM® INJECTABLE　　　　　　　　℞
[do ′ pram]
brand of Doxapram Hydrochloride Injection, USP

PRODUCT <u>OVERVIEW</u>

KEY FACTS

Dopram Injectable is a clear, colorless, sterile, non-pyrogenic, aqueous solution for intravenous injection. The respiratory stimulant action is manifested by an increase in tidal volume associated with a slight increase in respiratory rate. Due to its benzyl alcohol (preservative) content, Dopram Injectable should not be used in newborns.

MAJOR USES

Post Anesthesia: To stimulate respiration in patients with drug-induced respiratory depression or apnea other than that due to muscle relaxant drugs. To pharmacologically stimulate deep breathing.

Drug-Induced CNS Depression: To stimulate respiration, hasten arousal, and to encourage the return of laryngopharyngeal reflexes.

Chronic Plumonary Disease Associated with Acute Hypercapnia: To aid in the prevention of elevated arterial CO_2 tension during the administration of oxygen; restricted to a short period of time (approximately 2 hours).

Doxapram Hydrochloride is compatible wiith 5% and 10% dextrose in water or normal saline. Admixture of Doxapram with alkaline solutions such as 2.5% thiopental sodium, bicarbonate, or aminophylline will result in precipitation or gas formation.

SAFETY INFORMATION

Dopram Injectable should not be used in patients with convulsive disorders, mechanical disorders of ventilation, head injury, or cardiovascular impairment. Doxapram should not be used in conjunction with mechanical ventilation.

PRESCRIBING <u>INFORMATION</u>

DOPRAM® INJECTABLE　　　　　　　　℞
[do ′pram]
brand of Doxapram Hydrochloride Injection, USP

DESCRIPTION

Dopram Injectable (Doxapram Hydrochloride Injection, USP) is a clear, colorless, sterile, non-pyrogenic, aqueous solution with pH 3.5—5.0, for intravenous administration. Each 1 mL contains:

Doxapram Hydrochloride, USP.....................20 mg.
Benzyl Alcohol, NF (as preservative).............0.9%
Water for Injection, USP...............................q.s.

Due to its benzyl alcohol content, Dopram Injectable should not be used in newborns.

Dopram Injectable is a respiratory stimulant.

Doxapram hydrochloride is a white to off-white, crystalline powder, sparingly soluble in water, alcohol and chloroform. It has the following chemical name:

1-ethyl-4-[2-(4-morpholinyl)ethyl]-3,3-diphenyl-2-pyrrolidinone monohydrochloride, monohydrate.

CLINICAL PHARMACOLOGY

Doxapram hydrochloride produces respiratory stimulation mediated through the peripheral carotid chemoreceptors. As the dosage level is increased, the central respiratory centers in the medulla are stimulated with progressive stimulation of other parts of the brain and spinal cord.

The onset of respiratory stimulation following the recommended single intravenous injection of doxapram hydrochloride usually occurs in 20–40 seconds with peak effect at 1–2 minutes. The duration of effect may vary from 5–12 minutes. The respiratory stimulant action is manifested by an increase in tidal volume associated with a slight increase in respiratory rate.

A pressor response may result following doxapram administration. Provided there is no impairment of cardiac function, the pressor effect is more marked in hypovolemic than in normovolemic states. The pressor response is due to the improved cardiac output rather than peripheral vasoconstriction. Following doxapram administration an increased release of catecholamines has been noted.

Although opiate induced respiratory depression is antagonized by doxapram, the analgesic effect is not affected.

INDICATIONS

1. *Post-anesthesia.*
   a. When the possibility of airway obstruction and/or hypoxia have been eliminated, doxapram may be used to stimulate respiration in patients with drug-induced post-anesthesia respiratory depression or apnea other than that due to muscle relaxant drugs.
   b. To pharmacologically stimulate deep breathing in the so-called "stir-up" regimen in the postoperative patient. (Simultaneous administration of oxygen is desirable.)
2. *Drug-induced central nervous system depression.*
   Exercising care to prevent vomiting and aspiration, doxapram may be used to stimulate respiration, hasten arousal, and to encourage the return of laryngopharyngeal reflexes in patients with mild to moderate respiratory and CNS depression due to drug overdosage.
3. *Chronic pulmonary disease associated with acute hypercapnia.*
   Doxaram is indicated as a temporary measure in hospitalized patients with acute respiratory insufficiency superimposed on chronic obstructive pulmonary disease. Its use should be for a short period of time (approximately 2 hours) as an aid in the prevention of elevation of arterial CO_2 tension during the administration of oxygen. It should not be used in conjuction with mechanical ventilation.

CONTRAINDICATIONS

Due to its benzyl alcohol content, Dopram Injectable should not be used in newborns.

Doxapram should not be used in patients with epilepsy or other convulsive disorders.

Doxapram is contraindicated in patients with mechanical disorders of ventilation such as mechanical obstruction, muscle paresis, flail chest, pneumothorax, acute bronchial asthma, pulmonary fibrosis or other conditions resulting in restriction of chest wall, muscles of respiration or alveolar expansion.

Doxapram is contraindicated in patients with evidence of head injury or cerebral vascular accident and in those with significant cardiovascular impairment, severe hypertension, or known hypersensitivity to the drug.

WARNINGS

1. *In postanesthetic use.*
   a. Doxapram is neither an antagonist to muscle relaxant drugs nor a specific narcotic antagonist. Adequacy of airway and oxygenation must be assured prior to doxapram administration.
   b. Doxapram should be administered with great care and only under careful supervision to patients with hypermetabolic states such as hyperthyroidism or pheochromocytoma.
   c. Since narcosis may recur after stimulation with doxapram, care should be taken to maintain close observation until the patient has been fully alert for $\frac{1}{2}$ to 1 hour.
2. *In drug-induced CNS and respiratory depression.*
   Doxapram alone may not stimulate adequate spontaneous breathing or provide sufficient arousal in patients who are **severely** depressed either due to respiratory failure or to CNS depressant drugs, but should be used as an adjunct to established supportive measures and resuscitative techniques.
3. *In chronic obstructive pulmonary disease.*
   a. Because of the associated increased work of breathing, do not increase the rate of infusion of doxapram in severely ill patients in an attempt to lower pCO$_2$.
   b. Doxapram should not be used in conjunction with mechanical ventilation.

PRECAUTIONS

1. *General.*
   a. An adequate airway is essential.
   b. Recommended dosages of doxapram should be employed and maximum total dosages should not be exceeded. In order to avoid side effects, it is advisable to use the minimum effective dosage.
   c. Monitoring of the blood pressure and deep tendon reflexes is recommended to prevent overdosage.
   d. Vascular extravasation or use of a single injection site over an extended period should be avoided since either may lead to thrombophlebitis or local skin irritation.
   e. Rapid infusion may result in hemolysis.
   f. Lowered pCO$_2$ induced by hyperventilation produces cerebral vasoconstriction and slowing of the cerebral circulation. This should be taken into consideration on an individual basis.
   g. Intravenous short-acting barbiturates, oxygen and resuscitative equipment should be readily available to manage overdosage manifested by excessive central nervous system stimulation. Slow administration of the drug, and careful observation of the patient during administration and for some time subsequently, are advisable. These precautions are to assure that the protective reflexes have been restored and to prevent possible posthyperventilation hypoventilation.
   h. Doxapram should be administered cautiously to patients receiving sympathomimetic or monoamine oxidase inhibiting drugs, since an additive pressor effect may occur.
   i. Blood pressure increases are generally modest but significant increases have been noted in some patients. Because of this doxapram is not recommended for use in severe hypertension (see Contraindications).
   j. If sudden hypotension or dyspnea develops, doxapram should be stopped.
2. *In postanesthetic use.*
   a. The same consideration to pre-existing disease states should be exercised as in non-anesthetized individuals. See Contraindications and Warnings covering use in hypertension, asthma, disturbances of respiratory mechanics including airway obstruction, CNS disorders including increased cerebrospinal fluid pressure, convulsive disorders, acute agitation, and profound metabolic disorders.
   b. See Drug Interactions.
3. *In chronic obstructive pulmonary disease.*
   a. Arrhythmias seen in some patients in acute respiratory failure secondary to chronic obstructive pulmonary disease are probably the result of hypoxia. Doxapram should be used with caution in these patients.
   b. Arterial blood gases should be drawn prior to the initiation of doxapram infusion and oxygen administration, then at least every $\frac{1}{2}$ hour. Doxapram administration does not diminish the need for careful monitoring of the patient or the need for supplemental oxygen in patients with acute respiratory failure. Doxapram should be stopped if the arterial blood gases deteriorate, and mechanical ventilation initiated.

Drug Interactions: Administration of doxapram to patients who are receiving sympathomimetic or monoamine oxidase inhibiting drugs may result in an additive pressor effect. (See Precautions).

In patients who have received muscle relaxants, doxapram may temporarily mask the residual effects of muscle relaxant drugs.

In patients who have received anesthetics known to sensitize the myocardium to catecholamines, such as halothane, cyclopropane and enflurane, initiation of doxapram therapy should be delayed for at least 10 minutes following discontinuance of anesthesia, since an increase in epinephrine release has been noted with doxapram.

Carcinogenesis, mutagenesis, impairment of fertility. No carcinogenic or mutagenic studies have been performed using doxapram. Doxapram did not adversely affect the breeding performance of rats.

Pregnancy Category B. Reproduction studies have been performed in rats at doses up to 1.6 times the human dose and have revealed no evidence of impaired fertility or harm to the fetus due to doxapram. There are, however, no adequate and well-controlled studies in pregnant women. Since the animals in the reproduction studies were dosed by the IM and oral routes and animal reproduction studies, in general, are not always predictive of human response, this drug should be used during pregnancy only if clearly needed.

Nursing mothers. It is not known whether this drug is excreted in human milk. Because many drugs are excreted in human milk, caution should be exercised when doxapram hydrochloride is administered to a nursing mother.

Pediatric. The use of the preservative benzyl alcohol in the newborn has been associated with metabolic, CNS, respiratory, circulatory, and renal dysfunction. Safety and effectiveness in children below the age of 12 years have not been established.

ADVERSE REACTIONS

The following adverse reactions have been reported:
1. *Central and autonomic nervous systems.*
   Pyrexia, flushing, sweating; pruritus and paresthesia, such as a feeling of warmth, burning, or hot sensation, especially in the area of genitalia and perineum; apprehension, disorientation, pupillary dilatation, headache, dizziness, hyperactivity, involuntary movements, muscle spasticity, increased deep tendon reflexes, clonus, bilateral Babinski, and convulsions.
2. *Respiratory*
   Dyspnea, cough, tachypnea, laryngospasm, bronchospasm, hiccough, and rebound hypoventilation.
3. *Cardiovascular.*
   Phlebitis, variations in heart rate, lowered T-waves, arrhythmias, chest pain, tightness in chest. A mild to moderate increase in blood pressure is commonly noted and may be of concern in patients with severe cardiovascular diseases.
4. *Gastrointestinal.*
   Nausea, vomiting, diarrhea, desire to defecate.
5. *Genitourinary.*
   Stimulation of urinary bladder with spontaneous voiding; urinary retention.
6. *Laboratory determinations.*
   A decrease in hemoglobin, hematocrit, or red blood cell count has been observed in postoperative patients. In the presence of pre-existing leukopenia, a further decrease in WBC has been observed following anesthesia and treatment with doxapram hydrochloride. Elevation of BUN and albuminuria have also been observed. As some of the patients cited above had received multiple drugs concomitantly, a cause and effect relationship could not be determined.

OVERDOSAGE

Signs and Symptoms. Symptoms of overdosage are extensions of the pharmacologic effects of the drug. Excessive pressor effect, tachycardia, skeletal muscle hyperactivity, and enhanced deep tendon reflexes may be early signs of overdosage. Therefore, the blood pressure, pulse rate and deep tendon reflexes should be evaluated periodically and the dosage or infusion rate adjusted accordingly.

Convulsive seizures are unlikely at recommended dosages. In unanesthetized animals, the convulsant dose is 70 times greater than the respiratory stimulant dose. Intravenous LD$_{50}$ values in the mouse and rat were approximately 75 mg/kg and in the cat and dog were 40–80 mg/kg.

Except for management of chronic obstructive pulmonary disease associated with acute hypercapnia, the maximum recommended dosage is 3 GRAMS/24 HOURS. (See Dosage and Administration.)

Management. There is no specific antidote for doxapram. Management should be symptomatic. Short-acting intravenous barbiturates, oxygen and resuscitative equipment should be used as needed for supportive treatment.

There is no evidence that doxapram is dialyzable; further, the half-life of doxapram makes it unlikely that dialysis would be appropriate in managing overdose with this drug.

DOSAGE AND ADMINISTRATION

1. Doxapram hydrochloride is compatible with 5% and 10% dextrose in water or normal saline. ADMIXTURE OF DOXAPRAM WITH ALKALINE SOLUTIONS SUCH AS 2.5% THIOPENTAL SODIUM, BICARBONATE, OR AMINOPHYLLINE WILL RESULT IN PRECIPITATION OR GAS FORMATION.

2. *In postanesthetic use.*
   a. By i.v. injection (see Table I. Dosage for postanesthetic use—I.V.) Slow administration of the drug and careful observation of the patient during administration and for some time subsequently are advisable.
   [See table on bottom next page].
   b. By infusion. The solution is prepared by adding 250 mg of doxapram (12.5 mL) to 250 mL of dextrose or saline solution. The infusion is initiated at a rate of approximately 5 mg/minute until a satisfactory respiratory response is observed, and maintained at a rate of 1–3 mg/minute. The rate of infusion should be adjusted to sustain the desired level of respiratory stimulation with a minimum of side effects. The recommended total dosage by infusion is 4 mg/kg (2.0 mg/lb), or approximately 300 mg for the average adult.

3. *In the management of drug-induced CNS depression.*
   (See Table II. Dosage for drug-induced CNS depression.)
   [See table on top next page].

Continued on next page

Prescribing information on A. H. Robins products listed here is based on official labeling in effect June 1, 1989, with Indications, Contraindications, Warnings, Precautions, Adverse Reactions, and Dosage stated in full.

Robins—Cont.

Table II. Dopram Injectable Dosage for drug-induced CNS depression.

Level of Depression	METHOD ONE Priming dose single/repeat i.v. injection		METHOD TWO Rate of intermittent i.v. infusion	
	mg/kg	mg/lb	mg/kg/hr	mg/lb/hr
Mild*	1.0	0.5	1.0–2.0	0.5–1.0
Moderate†	2.0	1.0	2.0–3.0	1.0–1.5

*Mild Depression
Class 0:   Asleep, but can be aroused and can answer questions.
Class 1:   Comatose, will withdraw from painful stimuli, reflexes intact.

†Moderate Depression
Class 2:   Comatose, will not withdraw from painful stimuli, reflexes intact.
Class 3:   Comatose, reflexes absent, no depression of circulation or respiration.

METHOD ONE

Using Single and/or Repeat Single I.V. *Injections.*

a. Give priming dose of 1.0 mg/lb (2.0 mg/kg) body weight and repeat in 5 minutes.

b. Repeat same dose q1–2h until patient wakens. Watch for relapse into unconsciousness or development of respiratory depression, since Dopram does not affect the metabolism of CNS-depressant drugs.

c. If relapse occurs, resume injections q1–2h until arousal is sustained, or total maximum daily dose (3 grams) is given. Allow patients to sleep until 24 hours have elapsed from first injection of Dopram, using assisted or automatic-respiration if necessary.

d. Repeat procedure the following day until patient breathes spontaneously and sustains desired level of consciousness, or until maximum dosage (3 grams) is given.

e. Repetitive doses should be administered only to patients who have shown response to the initial dose.

f. Failure to respond appropriately indicates the need for neurologic evaluation for a possible central nervous system source of sustained coma.

METHOD TWO

By Intermittent I.V. *Infusion.*

a. Give priming dose as in Method One.

b. If patient wakens, watch for relapse; if no response, continue general supportive treatment for 1–2 hours and repeat Dopram. If some respiratory stimulation occurs, prepare I.V. infusion by adding 250 mg of Dopram (12.5 mL) to 250 mL of saline or dextrose solution. Deliver at rate of 1–3 mg/min (60–180 mL/hr) according to size of patient and depth of coma. Discontinue Dopram if patient begins to waken or at end of 2 hours.

c. Continue supportive treatment for $\frac{1}{2}$ to 2 hours and repeat Step b.

d. Do not exceed 3 grams/day.

4. *Chronic obstructive pulmonary disease associated with acute hypercapnia.*

a. One vial of doxapram (400 mg) should be mixed with 180 mL of dextrose or saline solution (concentration of 2.0 mg/mL). The infusion should be started at 1–2 mg/minute ($\frac{1}{2}$–1 mL/minute); if indicated, increase to a maximum of 3 mg/minute. Arterial blood gases should be determined prior to the onset of doxapram's administration and at least every half hour during the two hours of infusion to insure against the insidious development of CO_2-RETENTION AND ACIDOSIS. Alteration of oxygen concentration or flow rate may necessitate adjustment in the rate of doxapram infusion.

b. Predictable blood gas patterns are more readily established with a continuous infusion of doxapram. If the blood gases show evidence of deterioration, the infusion of doxapram should be discontinued.

c. ADDITIONAL INFUSIONS BEYOND THE SINGLE MAXIMUM TWO HOUR ADMINISTRATION PERIOD ARE NOT RECOMMENDED.

Parenteral drug products should be inspected visually for particulate matter and discoloration prior to administration, whenever solution and container permit.

HOW SUPPLIED

Dopram Injectable (doxapram hydrochloride injection) is available in 20 mL multiple dose vials containing 20 mg of doxapram hydrochloride per mL. with benzyl alcohol 0.9% as the preservative (NDC 0031-4849-83).

Store at Controlled Room Temperature, Between 15°C and 30°C (59°F and 86°F).

Manufactured for Pharmaceutical Division, A. H. Robins Company, Richmond, Virginia 23220 by Elkins-Sinn, Inc., Cherry Hill, New Jersey 08003-4099, a subsidiary of A. H. Robins Co.

Shown in Product Identification Section, page 424

ENTOLASE®–HP CAPSULES   ℞
(Pancrelipase)
Enteric-Coated Microbeads
ENTOLASE® CAPSULES   ℞
(Pancrelipase)
Enteric-Coated Microbeads

DESCRIPTION

Dye-free Entolase-HP and Entolase Capsules (Pancrelipase) are pancreatic enzyme concentrates of porcine origin containing standardized lipase, protease, and amylase as well as other pancreatic enzymes. They are available as enteric-coated microbeads of pancrelipase in hard gelatin capsules for oral administration. The enzyme potencies of Entolase-HP and Entolase Capsules are no less than:

	Each Entolase-HP Capsule	Each Entolase Capsule
Lipase, USP Units	8,000	4,000
Protease, USP Units	50,000	25,000
Amylase, USP Units	40,000	20,000

Inactive Ingredients: Entolase-HP Capsules —cellulose acetate phthalate, corn starch, edible inks, gelatin, iron oxide, povidone, simethicone, sodium chloride, stearic acid, sucrose, talc, titanium dioxide.

Entolase Capsules —cellulose acetate phthalate, corn starch, edible inks, gelatin, povidone, simethicone, sodium chloride, stearic acid, sucrose, talc, titanium dioxide.

CLINICAL PHARMACOLOGY

The natural digestive enzymes in Entolase-HP and Entolase Capsules hydrolyze fats into fatty acids and glycerol, split protein into peptides and amino acids, and convert carbohydrates to dextrins and short chain sugars.

Under conditions of the USP test method (*in vitro*), the Entolase products have the following total digestive capacity:

	Each Entolase-HP Capsule	Each Entolase Capsule
Dietary Fat, grams	28	14
Dietary Protein, grams	50	25
Dietary Starch, grams	40	20

The digestive capacity of a pancreatic enzyme concentrate depends on the amount that passes through the stomach unchanged and is available at the site of action in the small intestine. The pancrelipase in Entolase-HP and Entolase Capsules is contained within enteric-coated microbeads as a safeguard against inactivation of the enzymes in the acid medium of the stomach.

INDICATIONS

Entolase (Pancrelipase) is indicated in the treatment of exocrine pancreatic insufficiency as associated with but not limited to:
- cystic fibrosis
- chronic pancreatitis
- post-pancreatectomy
- post-gastrointestinal bypass surgery (e.g., Billroth II gastroenterostomy)
- obstruction of the pancreatic ducts.

CONTRAINDICATIONS

Do not use in patients hypersensitive to pork protein.

PRECAUTIONS

General: Individuals previously sensitized to trypsin, pancreatin, or pancrelipase may have allergic manifestations to the Entolase products.

Information for Patients: Patients should be advised to avoid chewing or crushing the enteric-coated microbeads. Where swallowing of capsules is difficult, capsules may be opened and the enteric-coated microbeads sprinkled over soft food which does not require chewing (e.g., applesauce, gelatin, etc.) and swallowed immediately. Prolonged contact of microbeads with food of pH greater than 5.5 may dissolve the protective enteric coating.

Carcinogenesis, Mutagenesis, Impairment of Fertility: Long-term studies in animals have not been performed to evaluate carcinogenic potential.

Pregnancy Category C: Animal reproduction studies have not been conducted with the Entolase products. It is also not known whether these products can cause fetal harm when administered to a pregnant woman or can affect reproduction capacity. Entolase products should be given to a pregnant woman only if clearly needed.

Nusing Mothers: It is not known whether this drug is excreted in human milk. Because many drugs are excreted in human milk, caution should be exercised when Entolase products are administered to a nursing mother.

ADVERSE REACTIONS

Extremely high doses of exogenous pancreatic enzymes have been associated with hyperuricemia and hyperuricosuria. Diarrhea or transient intestinal upset may occur with pancreatic enzyme concentrate. Allergic manifestations (see Precautions).

OVERDOSAGE

Acute toxicity determinations in animals have not been possible since the maximum dose that could be given orally produced no toxic reaction.

DOSAGE AND ADMINISTRATION

The requirement for replacement digestive enzymes varies from patient to patient. To provide dosage flexibility, Entolase is available in two strengths.

Entolase-HP Capsules and Entolase Capsules: One (1) to three (3) or more capsules with meals as directed by physician depending on patient requirements.

HOW SUPPLIED

Entolase-HP Capsules, enteric-coated microbeads in brown and clear No. 00 capsules monogrammed Entolase-HP and AHR in bottles of 100 (NDC 0031-5035-63) and 250 (NDC 0031-5035-67).

Entolase Capsules, enteric-coated microbeads in white and clear No. 1 capsules, monogrammed Entolase and AHR in bottles of 100 (NDC 0031-5025-63) and 500 (NDC 0031-5025-70).

Store in a tightly closed container in a dry place at controlled room temperature between 15°C and 30°C (59°F and 86°F). Do not refrigerate.

Dispense Entolase-HP Capsules and Entolase Capsules in tight container, preferably with a desiccant.

Shown in Product Identification Section, page 424

ENTOZYME® TABLETS   ℞
[ĕn 'to-zīm]

DESCRIPTION

Entozyme tablets are available for oral administration. Each tablet contains:
Pancreatin, USP equivalent ....300 mg
Pepsin ....250 mg

Table I. Dopram Injectable Dosage for post-anesthetic use—I.V.

I.V. Administration	Recommended dosage		Maximum dose per single injection		Maximum total dose	
	mg/kg	mg/lb	mg/kg	mg/lb	mg/kg	mg/lb
Single Injection	0.5–1.0	0.25–0.5	1.5	0.70	1.5	0.70
Repeat Injections (5 min. intervals)	0.5–1.0	0.25–0.5	1.5	0.70	2.0	1.0
Infusion	0.5–1.0	0.25–0.5	—	—	4.0	2.0

Bile salts ....150 mg
Natural Digestive Enzymes
Inactive Ingredients: Acacia, Acetylated Monoglycerides, Calcium Carbonate, Calcium Sulfate, Carnauba Wax, Cellulose Acetate Phthalate, Corn Starch, Diethyl Phthalate, Edible Ink, FD&C Blue 2 Aluminum Lake, Gelatin, Microcrystalline Cellulose, Polysorbates, Shellac, Stearic Acid, Sucrose, Tartaric Acid, Titanium Dioxide, White Wax. May contain FD&C Red 40 and Yellow 6 Aluminum Lakes.

CONSTRUCTION

Entozyme is a specially constructed tablet. The outer layer dissolves in the stomach and releases pepsin. The "inner tablet" is protected by an enteric coating that disintegrates in the alkaline medium of the small intestine and releases pancreatin and bile salts, thus preserving the digestive potency of the pancreatin as it passes through the stomach.

CLINICAL PHARMACOLOGY

Entozyme should be considered a form of nutritional therapy since it is made up of naturally-occurring digestive enzymes. Entozyme enhances proteolysis by its peptic and tryptic activity, carbohydrate digestion by amylolytic activity, and fat emulsification and transport by lipolytic activity and the action of the bile salts. The components of six Entozyme tablets will digest 60 grams of fat, 48 grams of protein and 48 grams of carbohydrate, amounts of food that yield nearly 1,000 calories (one-third to one-half the daily caloric intake for many patients).

INDICATIONS AND USAGE

Entozyme is indicated for the relief of steatorrhea, pyrosis, flatulence, and belching associated with incomplete digestion of food due to a deficiency of digestive enzymes.
By effectively supplementing the patient's secretion of digestive enzymes, Entozyme promotes more complete digestion of carbohydrates, proteins and fats.

CONTRAINDICATIONS

Biliary tract obstruction or hypersensitivity to any of the ingredients.

WARNINGS

Do not administer to patients who are allergic to pork products.

PRECAUTIONS

Carcinogenesis, mutagenesis. Long-term studies in animals have not been performed to evaluate carcinogenic potential.
Pregnancy Category C. Animal reproduction studies have not been conducted with Entozyme. It is not known whether Entozyme can cause fetal harm when administered to a pregnant woman or can affect reproduction capacity. Entozyme should be given to a pregnant woman only if clearly needed.
Nursing mothers. It is not known whether this drug is excreted in human milk. Because many drugs are excreted in human milk, caution should be exercised when Entozyme is administered to a nursing woman.
Pediatric Use. Safety and effectiveness in children have not been established.

ADVERSE REACTIONS

Skin rash is the most frequently reported adverse reaction to Entozyme, and appears to be associated with hypersensitivity to pork protein in the pancreatin. At high doses, a laxative effect may occur.

OVERDOSAGE

Excessive dosage may produce a laxative effect. Systemic toxicity does not occur.

DOSAGE AND ADMINISTRATION

Two tablets with each meal and 1 or 2 tablets with each snack. The dose may be increased as necessary to achieve adequate digestion. Entozyme tablets should be swallowed whole and not crushed or chewed.

HOW SUPPLIED

White coated tablets, monogrammed "AHR" and 5049 in bottles of 100 (NDC 0031-5049-63) and 500 (NDC 0031-5049-70).
Store at controlled room temperature, between 15°C and 30°C (59°F and 86°F). Dispense in tight container.
Shown in Product Identification Section, page 424

EXNA® TABLETS   ℞
[ĕks'nă]
brand of Benzthiazide Tablets, USP

DESCRIPTION

Exna (benzthiazide) is a diuretic available in round, yellow, scored tablets engraved AHR and 5449 for oral administration. Each tablet contains 50 mg benzthiazide.
Inactive Ingredients: Corn Starch, Dibasic Calcium Phosphate, FD&C Yellow 5, Lactose, Magnesium Stearate, Polyethylene Glycol , Sodium Lauryl Sulfate.

Benzthiazide is a white, crystalline powder with a characteristic odor, freely soluble in alkaline solution.

CLINICAL PHARMACOLOGY

Exna is a diuretic and antihypertensive. It affects the renal tubular mechanism of electrolyte reabsorption. At maximal therapeutic dosage, all thiazides are approximately equal in their diuretic potency. The mechanism whereby thiazides function in the control of hypertension is unknown. Exna increases excretion of sodium and chloride in approximately equivalent amounts. Natriuresis may be accompanied by some loss of potassium and bicarbonate.
In humans, benzthiazide is excreted in the urine almost entirely unchanged. Following a single oral dose of Exna Tablets or benzthiazide solution, 1% and 4.3% of the respective doses were recovered in the urine in 24 hr. The relative bioavailability of Exna Tablets was determined to be about 25% in reference to benzthiazide solution.

INDICATIONS

Exna (benzthiazide) is indicated as adjunctive therapy in edema associated with congestive heart failure, hepatic cirrhosis and corticosteroid and estrogen therapy.
Exna has also been found useful in edema due to various forms of renal dysfunction as: nephrotic syndrome; acute glomerulonephritis; and chronic renal failure.
Exna is indicated in the management of hypertension either as the sole therapeutic agent or to enhance the effectiveness of other antihypertensive drugs in the more severe forms of hypertension.
Usage in Pregnancy. The routine use of diuretics in an otherwise healthy woman is inappropriate and exposes mother and fetus to unnecessary hazard. Diuretics do not prevent development of toxemia of pregnancy, and there is no satisfactory evidence that they are useful in the treatment of developed toxemia.
Edema during pregnancy may arise from pathological causes or from the physiologic and mechanical consequences of pregnancy. Thiazides are indicated in pregnancy when edema is due to pathologic causes, just as they are in the absence of pregnancy (however, see Warnings). Dependent edema in pregnancy, resulting from restriction of venous return by the expanded uterus, is properly treated through elevation of the lower extremities and use of support hose; use of diuretics to lower intravascular volume in this case is illogical and unnecessary. There is hypervolemia during normal pregnancy which is harmful to neither the fetus nor the mother (in the absence of cardiovascular disease), but which is associated with edema, including generalized edema, in the majority of pregnant women. If this edema produces discomfort, increased recumbency will often provide relief. In rare instances, this edema may cause extreme discomfort which is not relieved by rest. In these cases, a short course of diuretics may provide relief and may be appropriate.

CONTRAINDICATIONS

Anuria. Hypersensitivity to this or other sulfonamide derived drugs.

WARNINGS

Thiazides should be used with caution in severe renal disease. In patients with renal disease, thiazides may precipitate azotemia. Cumulative effects of the drug may develop in patients with impaired renal function.
Thiazides should be used with caution in patients with impaired hepatic function or progressive liver disease, since minor alterations of fluid and electrolyte balance may precipitate hepatic coma.
Sensitivity reactions may occur in patients with a history of allergy or bronchial asthma.
The possibility of exacerbation or activation of systemic lupus erythematosus has been reported.
Latent diabetes mellitus may become manifest during thiazide administration; hyperuricemia or frank gout may also be precipitated in certain patients. The antihypertensive effect of the drug may be enhanced in the postsympathectomy patient.

PRECAUTIONS

General: All patients receiving thiazide therapy should be observed for clinical signs of fluid or electrolyte imbalance; namely, hyponatremia, hypochloremic alkalosis, and hypokalemia.
Dilutional hyponatremia may occur in edematous patients in hot weather; appropriate therapy is water restriction, rather than administration of salt except in rare instances when hyponatremia is life threatening.
In actual salt depletion, appropriate replacement is the therapy of choice. Any chloride deficit is generally mild and usually does not require specific treatment except under extraordinary circumstances (as in liver disease or renal disease).
Hypokalemia may develop with thiazides as with any other potent diuretic especially with brisk diuresis. Inadequate oral electrolyte intake will also contribute to hypokalemia. This product contains FD&C Yellow No. 5 (tartrazine) which may cause allergic-type reactions (including bronchial

asthma) in certain susceptible individuals. Although the over-all incidence of FD&C Yellow No. 5 (tartrazine) sensitivity in the general population is low, it is frequently seen in patients who have aspirin hypersensitivity.
Information for patients: Warning signs of electrolyte imbalance are: dryness of mouth, thirst, weakness, lethargy, drowsiness, restlessness, muscle pains or cramps. muscular fatigue, hypotension, oliguria, tachycardia, and gastrointestinal disturbances such as nausea and vomiting.
Laboratory tests: Periodic determination of serum electrolytes to detect possible electrolyte imbalance should be performed at appropriate intervals. When the patient is vomiting excessively or receiving parenteral fluids, serum and urine electrolyte determinations are particularly important. In patients with renal impairment, nonprotein nitrogen or blood urea nitrogen level should be tested periodically; rising values would indicate progressive renal impairment and careful reappraisal of therapy is necessary with consideration given to withholding or discontinuing diuretic therapy.
Drug interaction: Thiazides may add to or potentiate the action of other hypotensive drugs. Potentiation occurs with ganglionic or peripheral adrenergic-blocking drugs.
Thiazides may increase the responsiveness to tubocurarine. Thiazides may decrease arterial responsiveness to norepinephrine. This diminution is not sufficient to preclude effectiveness of the pressor agent for therapeutic use.
Insulin requirement in diabetic patients may be increased, decreased, or unchanged.
Medication such as digitalis may also influence serum electrolytes. Digitalis therapy may exaggerate metabolic effects of hypokalemia especially with reference to myocardial activity.
Drug/Laboratory Test Interactions: Thiazides may decrease serum PBI levels without signs of thyroid disturbance.
Carcinogenesis, mutagenesis, impairment of fertility: No animal carcinogenicity or mutagenesis studies on benzthiazide are known.
Pregnancy-teratogenic effects: Pregnancy Category C. Benzthiazide has an embryocidal effect in rats when given in doses several hundred times the human dose. Exna (benzthiazide) can cause fetal harm when administered to a pregnant woman. Fetal or neonatal jaundice has been reported. Thrombocytopenia and possibly other adverse reactions have occurred in the adult. If this drug is used during pregnancy, or if patient becomes pregnant while taking this drug, the patient should be apprised of the potential hazard to the fetus.
Thiazides cross the placental barrier and appear in cord blood.
Nursing mothers: It is not known whether this drug is excreted in human milk. Because many drugs are excreted in human milk, caution should be exercised when Exna is administered to a nursing mother.
Pediatric use: Safety and effectiveness in children have not been established.

ADVERSE REACTIONS

The following adverse reactions have been observed, but there is not enough systematic collection of data to support an estimate of their frequency.
Gastrointestinal System: jaundice (intrahepatic cholestatic jaundice); pancreatitis; gastric irritation; vomiting; cramping; nausea; anorexia; diarrhea; constipation.
Central Nervous System: dizziness; restlessness; paresthesia; headache; xanthopsia.
Hematologic: aplastic anemia; thrombocytopenia; agranulocytosis; leukopenia.
Dermatologic-Hypersensitivity: necrotizing angiitis (vasculitis) (cutaneous vasculitis); purpura; urticaria; rash; photosensitivity.
Cardiovascular: Orthostatic hypotension may occur and may be aggravated by alcohol, barbiturates or narcotics.
Other: hyperglycemia; glycosuria; hyperuricemia; weakness; muscle spasm.
Whenever adverse reactions are moderate or severe, thiazide dosage should be reduced or therapy withdrawn.

OVERDOSAGE

Symptoms of overdosage include electrolyte imbalance and signs of potassium deficiency such as confusion, dizziness, muscular weakness, and gastrointestinal disturbances. General supportive measures including replacement of fluids and electrolytes may be indicated in treatment of overdosage.

DOSAGE AND ADMINISTRATION

Therapy should be individualized according to patient response. This therapy should be titrated to gain maximal

Continued on next page

Prescribing information on A. H. Robins products listed here is based on official labeling in effect June 1, 1989, with Indications, Contraindications, Warnings, Precautions, Adverse Reactions, and Dosage stated in full.

Robins—Cont.

therapeutic response as well as the minimal dose possible to maintain that therapeutic response.

	Diuretic	Antihypertensive
Benzthiazide	50 to 200 mg	50 to 200 mg

Edema: *Initiation of diuresis:* 50 to 200 mg daily should be used for several days, or until dry weight is attained. With 100 mg or more daily, it is generally preferable to administer benzthiazide in two doses, following morning and evening meals.
Maintenance of diuresis: 50 to 150 mg daily depending upon the patient's response. To maintain effectiveness, reduction to minimal effective dosage should be gradual.
Hypertension: *Initiation of antihypertensive therapy:* 50 to 100 mg daily is the average dose. It may be given in two doses of 25 mg or 50 mg each after breakfast and after lunch. This dosage may be continued until a therapeutic drop in blood pressure occurs.
Maintenance of antihypertensive therapy: Dosage should be adjusted according to the patient response, either upward to as much as 50 mg q.i.d., or downward to the minimal effective dosage level.

HOW SUPPLIED
Exna (benzthiazide) is supplied in 50 mg yellow, scored engraved AHR and 5449 tablets, packaged in bottles of 100 (NDC 0031-5449-63).
Store at controlled room temperature, between 15°C and 30°C (59°F and 86°F).
Dispense in tight container.
Shown in Product Identification Section, page 424

MICRO–K EXTENCAPS®   ℞
[mi 'cro "ĕks "tĕn 'caps]
MICRO–K® 10 EXTENCAPS®   ℞
brand of Potassium Chloride

PRODUCT OVERVIEW
KEY FACTS
Each particle of potassium chloride is microencapsulated with a polymeric coating which allows for the controlled release of potassium and chloride ions over an eight-to-ten hour period. The dispersibility of the microcapsules and the controlled release of ions are intended to minimize the likelihood of high localized concentration of potassium chloride and resultant mucosal ulceration within the gastrointestinal tract.

MAJOR USES
For therapeutic use in patients with hypokalemia with or without metabolic alkalosis; in digitalis intoxication and in patients with hypokalemic familial periodic paralysis.
For prevention of potassium depletion when the dietary intake of potassium is inadequate.

SAFETY INFORMATION
Potassium supplements are contraindicated in patients with hyperkalemia since a further increase in serum potassium concentration in such patients can produce cardiac arrest. The treatment of potassium depletion, particularly in the presence of cardiac disease, renal disease, or acidosis, requires careful attention to acid-base balance and appropriate monitoring of serum electrolytes, the electrocardiogram and the clinical status of the patient.

PRESCRIBING INFORMATION

MICRO-K EXTENCAPS®   ℞
MICRO-K 10 EXTENCAPS®   ℞
brand of Potassium Chloride

DESCRIPTION
Micro-K Extencaps are pale orange, hard gelatin capsules, each containing 600 mg of dispersible small crystalline particles of potassium chloride (equivalent to 8 mEq K), monogrammed Micro-K and AHR/5720
Micro-K 10 Extencaps are pale orange and opaque white, hard gelatin capsules, each containing 750 mg of dispersible, small crystalline particles of potassium chloride (equivalent to 10 mEq K) monogrammed Micro-K 10 and AHR/5730.
Each particle of potassium chloride (KCl) is microencapsulated with a polymeric coating which allows for the controlled release of potassium and chloride ions over an eight-to ten-hour period. The dispersibility of the microcapsules and the controlled release of ions are intended to minimize the likelihood of high localized concentrations of potassium chloride and resultant mucosal ulceration within the gastrointestinal tract.
The polymeric coating forming the microcapsules functions as a water-permeable membrane. Fluids pass through the membrane and gradually dissolve the potassium chloride within the microcapsules. The resulting potassium chloride solution slowly diffuses outward through the membrane.
Inactive Ingredients: Edible Ink, Ethylcellulose, FD&C Blue 2 Aluminum Lake, FD&C Yellow 6, Gelatin, Magnesium Stearate, Sodium Lauryl Sulfate, Titanium Dioxide. May contain FD&C Red 40 and Yellow 6 Aluminum Lakes.

ACTIONS
Potassium ion is the principal intracellular cation of most body tissues. Potassium ions participate in a number of essential physiological processes, including the maintenance of intracellular tonicity, the transmission of nerve impulses, the contraction of cardiac, skeletal, and smooth muscle and the maintenance of normal renal function.
Potassium depletion may occur whenever the rate of potassium loss through renal excretion and/or loss from the gastrointestinal tract exceeds the rate of potassium intake. Such depletion usually develops slowly as a consequence of prolonged therapy with oral diuretics, primary or secondary hyperaldosteronism, diabetic ketoacidosis, severe diarrhea, or inadequate replacement of potassium in patients on prolonged parenteral nutrition. Potassium depletion due to these causes is usually accompanied by a concomitant deficiency of chloride and is manifested by hypokalemia and metabolic alkalosis. Potassium depletion may produce weakness, fatigue, disturbances of cardiac rhythm (primarily ectopic beats), prominent U-waves in the electrocardiogram, and in advanced cases, flaccid paralysis and/or impaired ability to concentrate urine.
Potassium depletion associated with metabolic alkalosis is managed by correcting the fundamental causes of the deficiency whenever possible and administering supplemental potassium chloride, in the form of high potassium food or potassium chloride solution, capsules or tablets. In rare circumstances (e.g., patients with renal tubular acidosis) potassium depletion may be associated with metabolic acidosis and hyperchloremia. In such patients potassium replacement should be accomplished with potassium salts other than the chloride, such as potassium bicarbonate, potassium citrate, or potassium acetate.

INDICATIONS
BECAUSE OF REPORTS OF INTESTINAL AND GASTRIC ULCERATION AND BLEEDING WITH SLOW-RELEASE POTASSIUM CHLORIDE PREPARATIONS, THESE DRUGS SHOULD BE RESERVED FOR THOSE PATIENTS WHO CANNOT TOLERATE OR REFUSE TO TAKE LIQUID OR EFFERVESCENT POTASSIUM PREPARATIONS OR FOR PATIENTS IN WHOM THERE IS A PROBLEM OF COMPLIANCE WITH THESE PREPARATIONS.
1. For therapeutic use in patients with hypokalemia with or without metabolic alkalosis; in digitalis intoxication and in patients with hypokalemic familial periodic paralysis.
2. For prevention of potassium depletion when the dietary intake of potassium is inadequate in the following conditions: patients receiving digitalis and diuretics for congestive heart failure; hepatic cirrhosis with ascites; states of aldosterone excess with normal renal function; potassium-losing nephropathy, and certain diarrheal states.
3. The use of potassium salts in patients receiving diuretics for uncomplicated essential hypertension is often unnecessary when such patients have a normal dietary pattern. Serum potassium should be checked periodically, however, and, if hypokalemia occurs, dietary supplementation with potassium-containing foods may be adequate to control milder cases. In more severe cases, supplementation with potassium salts may be indicated.

CONTRAINDICATIONS
Potassium supplements are contraindicated in patients with hyperkalemia since a further increase in serum potassium concentration in such patients can produce cardiac arrest. Hyperkalemia may complicate any of the following conditions: chronic renal failure, systemic acidosis such as diabetic acidosis, acute dehydration, extensive tissue breakdown as in severe burns, adrenal insufficiency, or the administration of a potassium-sparing diuretic (e.g., spironolactone, triamterene).
Wax-matrix potassium chloride preparations have produced esophageal ulceration in certain cardiac patients with esophageal compression due to an enlarged left atrium.
All solid dosage forms of potassium supplements are contraindicated in any patient in whom there is cause for arrest or delay in tablet passage through the gastrointestinal tract. In these instances, potassium supplementation should be with a liquid preparation.

WARNINGS
Hyperkalemia. In patients with impaired mechanisms for excreting potassium, the administration of potassium salts can produce hyperkalemia and cardiac arrest. This occurs most commonly in patients given potassium by the intravenous route but may also occur in patients given potassium orally. Potentially fatal hyperkalemia can develop rapidly and be asymptomatic.
The use of potassium salts in patients with chronic renal disease, or any other condition which impairs potassium excretion, requires particularly careful monitoring of the serum potassium concentration and appropriate dosage adjustments.
Interaction with Potassium-Sparing Diuretics. Hypokalemia should not be treated by the concomitant administration of potassium salts and a potassium-sparing diuretic (e.g., spironolactone or triamterene), since the simultaneous administration of these agents can produce severe hyperkalemia.
Gastrointestinal lesions. Potassium chloride tablets have produced stenotic and/or ulcerative lesions of the small bowel and deaths, in addition to upper gastrointestinal bleeding. These lesions are caused by a high localized concentration of potassium ion in the region of a rapidly dissolving tablet which injures the bowel wall and thereby produces obstruction, hemorrhage, or perforation.
Micro-K Extencaps contain microcapsules which disperse upon dissolution of the hard gelatin capsule. The microcapsules are formulated to provide a controlled release of potassium chloride. The dispersibility of the microcapsules and the controlled release of ions from the microcapsules are intended to minimize the possibility of a high local concentration near the gastrointestinal mucosa and the ability of the KCl to cause stenosis or ulceration. Other means of accomplishing this (e.g., incorporation of KCl into a wax matrix) have reduced the frequency of such lesions to less than one per 100,000 patient years (compared to 40–50 per 100,000 patient years with enteric-coated KCl), but have not eliminated them. The frequency of GI lesions with Micro-K Extencaps is, at present, unknown. Micro-K Extencaps should be discontinued immediately and the possibility of bowel obstruction or perforation considered if severe vomiting, abdominal pain, distention, or gastrointestinal bleeding occurs.
Metabolic Acidosis. Hypokalemia in patients with metabolic *acidosis* should be treated with an alkalinizing potassium salt such as potassium bicarbonate, potassium citrate, or potassium acetate.

PRECAUTIONS
The diagnosis of potassium depletion is ordinarily made by demonstrating hypokalemia in a patient with a clinical history suggesting some cause for potassium depletion. In interpreting the serum potassium level, the physician should bear in mind that acute alkalosis per se can produce hypokalemia in the absence of a deficit in total body potassium, while acute acidosis per se can increase the serum potassium concentration into the normal range even in the presence of a reduced total body potassium. The treatment of potassium depletion, particularly in the presence of cardiac disease, renal disease, or acidosis, requires careful attention to acid-base balance and appropriate monitoring of serum electrolytes, the electrocardiogram, and the clinical status of the patient.

ADVERSE REACTIONS
The most common adverse reactions to oral potassium salts are nausea, vomiting, abdominal discomfort, and diarrhea. These symptoms are due to irritation of the gastrointestinal tract and may be minimized by taking the dose with meals or by reducing the dose.
Intestinal bleeding, ulceration, perforation and obstruction have been reported in patients treated with solid dosage forms of potassium salts and may occur with Micro-K Extencaps (see Contraindications and Warnings).
One of the most severe adverse effects of potassium supplementation is hyperkalemia (see Contraindications, Warnings, and Overdosage).
Skin rash has been reported rarely with potassium preparations.

OVERDOSAGE
The administration of oral potassium salts to persons with normal excretory mechanisms for potassium rarely causes serious hyperkalemia. However, if excretory mechanisms are impaired or if potassium is administered too rapidly intravenously, potentially fatal hyperkalemia can result (see Contraindications and Warnings). It is important to recognize that hyperkalemia is usually asymptomatic and may be manifested only by an increased serum potassium concentration and characteristic electrocardiogram changes (peaking of T-waves, loss of P-wave, depression of S-T segment, and prolongation of the QT interval). Late manifestations include muscle paralysis and cardiovascular collapse from cardiac arrest.
Treatment measures for hyperkalemia include the following: (1) elimination of foods and medications containing potassium and of potassium-sparing diuretics; (2) intravenous administration of 300 to 500 ml/hr of 10% dextrose solution containing 10–20 units of insulin per 1,000 ml; (3) correction of acidosis, if present, with intravenous sodium bicarbonate; (4) use of exchange resins, hemodialysis, or peritoneal dialysis.
In treating hyperkalemia, it should be recalled that in patients who have been stabilized on digitalis, too rapid a lowering of the serum potassium concentration can produce digitalis toxicity.

DOSAGE AND ADMINISTRATION

The usual dietary intake of potassium by the average adult is 40 to 80 mEq per day. Potassium depletion sufficient to cause hypokalemia usually requires the loss of 200 or more mEq of potassium from the total body store.

Dosage must be adjusted to the individual needs of each patient, but typically is around 20 mEq per day for the prevention of hypokalemia and 40 to 100 mEq per day for the treatment of potassium depletion.

	For Prevention	For Treatment
Micro-K Extencaps (8 mEq K)	2 or 3 Extencaps/day (16–24 mEq K)	5 to 12 Extencaps/day (40–96 mEq K)
Micro-K 10 Extencaps (10 mEq K)	2 Extencaps/day (20 mEq K)	4 to 10 Extencaps/day (40–100 mEq K)

If more than 2 Extencaps are prescribed per day, the total daily dosage should be divided into two or more separate doses. Those patients having difficulty swallowing the capsules may be advised to sprinkle the contents onto a spoonful [of] soft food to facilitate ingestion.

[HO]W SUPPLIED

[Micro]-K Extencaps® are pale orange capsules mono[gramm]ed Micro-K and AHR/5720, each containing 600 mg [micro]encapsulated potassium chloride (equivalent to 8 mEq [K) in bott]les of 100 (NDC 0031-5720-63), 500 (NDC 0031-5720[-]) [Uni]s-Co® unit dose packs of 100 (NDC 0031-5720-64).

[Micro-K 10] Extencaps® are pale orange and opaque white [capsules mo]nogrammed Micro-K 10 and AHR/5730, each [containing]750 mg microencapsulated potassium chloride [(equivalent t]o 10 mEq K) in bottles of 100 (NDC 0031-5730[-] [Unit] Use 100 (NDC 0031-5730-68), 500 (NDC 0031[-]) [Uni-]Dis-Co® unit dose packs of 100 (NDC 0031[-])

[Animal Toxi]cology: The ulcerogenic potential of microen[capsulated K]Cl was studied in anesthetized cats by direct [instillation o]n exteriorized gastric mucosa. The microcap[sules] [we]re found to be non-ulcerogenic and signifi[cantly less irrita]ting than wax-matrix tablets and 20% solu[tion]

[In mon]keys (up to 8 monkeys per group) receiving [oral for]mulations of potassium chloride at equivalent [dose (]2400 mg KCl) for four and one-half days, Micro-[K Extenc]aps showed no tendency to cause intestinal ulcer[ation s]imilar to liquid KCl and a wax-matrix preparation [(in contrast] to an enteric-coated KCl tablet) and minimal [gastri]c irritation (less than a wax-matrix preparation).

[Product] Shown in Product Identification Section, page 424

[M]ICRO–K® LS   ℞
[mi'cro"k]

brand of Potassium Chloride
Extended-Release Formulation
for Liquid Suspension

DESCRIPTION

Micro-K LS is an oral dosage form of microencapsulated potassium chloride. Each packet contains 1.5 g of Potassium Chloride, USP equivalent to 20 mEq of potassium. Micro-K LS is comprised of specially formulated granules. After reconstitution with 2–6 fl oz of water and 1 minute of stirring, the suspension is odorless and tasteless.

Each crystal of potassium chloride (KCl) is microencapsulated with an insoluble polymeric coating which functions as a semipermeable membrane; it allows for the controlled release of potassium and chloride ions over an eight–ten hour period. The controlled release of K^+ ions by the microcapsular membrane is intended to reduce the likelihood of a high localized concentration of potassium chloride at any point on the mucosa of the gastrointestinal tract. Fluids pass through the membrane and gradually dissolve the potassium chloride within the microcapsules. The resulting potassium chloride solution slowly diffuses outward through the membrane.

Micro-K LS is an electrolyte replenisher. The chemical name of the active ingredient is potassium chloride and the structural formula is KCl. Potassium Chloride, USP occurs as a white, granular powder or as colorless crystals. It is odorless and has a saline taste. Its solutions are neutral to litmus. It is freely soluble in water and insoluble in alcohol.

Inactive Ingredients: Docusate Sodium, Ethylcellulose, Povidone, Silicon Dioxide, Sucrose, and another ingredient.

CLINICAL PHARMACOLOGY

The potassium ion is the principal intracellular cation of most body tissues. Potassium ions participate in a number of essential physiological processes including the maintenance of intracellular tonicity, the transmission of nerve impulses, the contraction of cardiac, skeletal, and smooth muscle, and the maintenance of normal renal function.

The intracellular concentration of potassium is approximately 150 to 160 mEq per liter. The normal adult plasma concentration is 3.5 to 5 mEq per liter. An active ion transport system maintains this gradient across the plasma membrane.

Potassium is a normal dietary constituent and under steady-state conditions the amount of potassium absorbed from the gastrointestinal tract is equal to the amount excreted in the urine. The usual dietary intake of potassium is 50 to 100 mEq per day.

Potassium depletion will occur whenever the rate of potassium loss through renal excretion and/or loss from the gastrointestinal tract exceeds the rate of potassium intake. Such depletion usually develops as a consequence of therapy with diuretics, primary or secondary hyperaldosteronism, diabetic ketoacidosis, or inadequate replacement of potassium in patients on prolonged parenteral nutrition. Depletion can develop rapidly with severe diarrhea, especially if associated with vomiting. Potassium depletion due to these causes is usually accompanied by a concomitant loss of chloride and is manifested by hypokalemia and metabolic alkalosis. Potassium depletion may produce weakness, fatigue, disturbances of cardiac rhythm (primarily ectopic beats), prominent U-waves in the electrocardiogram, and, in advanced cases, flaccid paralysis and/or impaired ability to concentrate urine.

If potassium depletion associated with metabolic alkalosis cannot be managed by correcting the fundamental cause of the deficiency, e.g., where the patient requires long-term diuretic therapy, supplemental potassium in the form of high potassium food or potassium chloride may be able to restore normal potassium levels.

In rare circumstances (e.g., patients with renal tubular acidosis) potassium depletion may be associated with metabolic acidosis and hyperchloremia. In such patients potassium replacement should be accomplished with potassium salts other than the chloride, such as potassium bicarbonate, potassium citrate, potassium acetate, or potassium gluconate.

INDICATIONS AND USAGE

BECAUSE OF REPORTS OF INTESTINAL AND GASTRIC ULCERATION AND BLEEDING WITH CONTROLLED RELEASE POTASSIUM CHLORIDE PREPARATIONS, THESE DRUGS SHOULD BE RESERVED FOR THOSE PATIENTS WHO CANNOT TOLERATE OR REFUSE TO TAKE IMMEDIATE RELEASE LIQUIDS/EFFERVESCENT POTASSIUM PREPARATIONS OR FOR PATIENTS IN WHOM THERE IS A PROBLEM OF COMPLIANCE WITH THESE PREPARATIONS.

1. For the treatment of patients with hypokalemia, with or without metabolic alkalosis; in digitalis intoxication; and in patients with hypokalemic familial periodic paralysis. If hypokalemia is the result of diuretic therapy, consideration should be given to the use of a lower dose of diuretic, which may be sufficient without leading to hypokalemia.
2. For the prevention of hypokalemia in patients who would be at particular risk if hypokalemia were to develop, e.g., digitalized patients or patients with significant cardiac arrhythmias, hepatic cirrhosis with ascites, states of aldosterone excess with normal renal function, potassium losing nephropathy, and certain diarrheal states.

The use of potassium salts in patients receiving diuretics for uncomplicated essential hypertension is often unnecessary when such patients have a normal dietary pattern and when low doses of the diuretic are used. Serum potassium should be checked periodically, however, and if hypokalemia occurs, dietary supplementation with potassium-containing foods may be adequate to control milder cases. In more severe cases, and if dose adjustment of the diuretic is ineffective or unwarranted, supplementation with potassium salts may be indicated.

CONTRAINDICATIONS

Potassium supplements are contraindicated in patients with hyperkalemia since a further increase in serum potassium concentration in such patients can produce cardiac arrest. Hyperkalemia may complicate any of the following conditions: chronic renal failure, systemic acidosis such as diabetic acidosis, acute dehydration, extensive tissue breakdown as in severe burns, adrenal insufficiency, or the administration of a potassium-sparing diuretic (e.g., spironolactone, triamterene, amiloride) (see OVERDOSAGE).

Controlled release formulations of potassium chloride have produced esophageal ulceration in certain cardiac patients with esophageal compression due to an enlarged left atrium. Potassium supplementation, when indicated in such patients, should be given as an immediate release liquid preparation.

All solid oral dosage forms of potassium chloride are contraindicated in any patient in whom there is structural, pathological (e.g., diabetic gastroparesis) or pharmacologic (use of anticholinergic agents or other agents with anticholinergic properties at sufficient doses to exert anticholinergic effects) cause for arrest or delay in tablet or capsule-passage through the gastrointestinal tract.

WARNINGS

Hyperkalemia (see OVERDOSAGE). In patients with impaired mechanisms for excreting potassium, the administration of potassium salts can produce hyperkalemia and cardiac arrest. This occurs most commonly in patients given potassium by the intravenous route but may also occur in patients given potassium orally. Potentially fatal hyperkalemia can develop rapidly and be asymptomatic. The use of potassium salts in patients with chronic renal disease, or any other condition which impairs potassium excretion, requires particularly careful monitoring of the serum potassium concentration and appropriate dosage adjustment.

Interaction with Potassium-Sparing Diuretics. Hypokalemia should not be treated by the concomitant administration of potassium salts and a potassium-sparing diuretic (e.g., spironolactone, triamterene or amiloride) since the simultaneous administration of these agents can produce severe hyperkalemia.

Interaction with Angiotensin Converting Enzyme Inhibitors. Angiotensin converting enzyme (ACE) inhibitors (e.g., captopril, enalapril) will produce some potassium retention by inhibiting aldosterone production. Potassium supplements should be given to patients receiving ACE inhibitors only with close monitoring.

Gastrointestinal Lesions. Solid oral dosage forms of potassium chloride can produce ulcerative and/or stenotic lesions of the gastrointestinal tract. Based on spontaneous adverse reaction reports, enteric coated preparations of potassium chloride are associated with an increased frequency of small bowel lesions (40–50 per 100,000 patient years) compared to sustained release wax matrix formulations (less than one per 100,000 patient years). Because of the lack of extensive marketing experience with microencapsulated products, a comparison between such products and wax matrix or enteric coated products is not available. Micro-K LS is administered as a liquid suspension of microencapsulated potassium chloride formulated to provide a controlled rate of release of potassium chloride and thus to minimize the possibility of a high local concentration of potassium near the gastrointestinal wall.

Prospective trials have been conducted in normal human volunteers in which the upper gastrointestinal tract was evaluated by endoscopic inspection before and after one week of solid oral potassium chloride therapy. The ability of this model to predict events occurring in usual clinical practice is unknown. Trials which approximated usual clinical practice did not reveal any clear differences between the wax matrix and microencapsulated dosage forms. In contrast, there was a higher incidence of gastric and duodenal lesions in subjects receiving a high dose of a wax matrix controlled release formulation under conditions which did not resemble usual or recommended clinical practice (i.e., 96 mEq per day in divided doses of potassium chloride administered to fasted patients, in the presence of an anticholinergic drug to delay gastric emptying). The upper gastrointestinal lesions observed by endoscopy were asymptomatic and were not accompanied by evidence of bleeding (hemoccult testing). The relevance of these findings to the usual conditions (i.e., non-fasting, no anticholinergic agent, smaller doses) under which controlled release potassium chloride products are used is uncertain; epidemiologic studies have not identified an elevated risk, compared to microencapsulated products, for upper gastrointestinal lesions in patients receiving wax matrix formulations. Micro-K LS should be discontinued immediately and the possibility of ulceration, obstruction or perforation considered if severe vomiting, abdominal pain, distention, or gastrointestinal bleeding occurs.

Diarrhea or Dehydration. Micro-K LS contains, as a dispersing agent, docusate sodium, which also increases stool water and is used as a stool softener. Clinical studies with Micro-K LS indicate that minor changes in stool consistency may be common, although usually are well-tolerated. However, rarely patients may experience diarrhea or cramping abdominal pain. Patients with severe or chronic diarrhea or who are dehydrated ordinarily should not be prescribed Micro-K LS.

Metabolic Acidosis. Hypokalemia in patients with metabolic acidosis should be treated with an alkalinizing potassium salt such as potassium bicarbonate, potassium citrate, potassium acetate, or potassium gluconate.

PRECAUTIONS

General: The diagnosis of potassium depletion is ordinarily made by demonstrating hypokalemia in a patient with a clinical history suggesting some cause for potassium depletion. In interpreting the serum potassium level, the physician should bear in mind that acute alkalosis *per se* can produce hypokalemia in the absence of a deficit in total body potassium while acute acidosis *per se* can increase the serum potassium concentration into the normal range even in the presence of a reduced total body potassium. The treatment of potassium depletion, particularly in the presence of cardiac

Continued on next page

Prescribing information on A. H. Robins products listed here is based on official labeling in effect June 1, 1989, with Indications, Contraindications, Warnings, Precautions, Adverse Reactions, and Dosage stated in full.

Robins—Cont.

disease, renal disease, or acidosis requires careful attention to acid-base balance and appropriate monitoring of serum electrolytes, the electrocardiogram, and the clinical status of the patient.

Information for Patients: Physicians should consider reminding the patient of the following:

To take each dose with meals mixed in water or other suitable liquid.

To take this medicine following the frequency and amount prescribed by the physician. This is especially important if the patient is also taking diuretics and/or digitalis preparations.

To inform patients that this product contains as a dispersing agent the stool softener, docusate sodium, which may change stool consistency, or rarely produce diarrhea or cramps.

To check with the physician at once if tarry stools or other evidence of gastrointestinal bleeding is noticed.

Laboratory Tests: Regular serum potassium determinations are recommended, especially in patients with renal insufficiency or diabetic nephropathy.

When blood is drawn for analysis of plasma potassium, it is important to recognize that artifactual elevations can occur after improper venipuncture technique or as a result of *in vitro* hemolysis of the sample.

Drug Interactions: Potassium-sparing diuretics, angiotensin converting enzyme inhibitors: see WARNINGS.

Carcinogenesis, Mutagenesis, Impairment of Fertility: Carcinogenicity, mutagenicity, and fertility studies in animals have not been performed. Potassium is a normal dietary constituent.

Pregnancy Category C. Animal reproduction studies have not been conducted with Micro-K LS. It is unlikely that potassium supplementation that does not lead to hyperkalemia would have an adverse effect on the fetus or would affect reproductive capacity.

Nursing Mothers: The normal potassium ion content of human milk is about 13 mEq per liter. Since oral potassium becomes part of the body potassium pool, so long as body potassium is not excessive, the contribution of potassium chloride supplementation should have little or no effect on the level in human milk.

Pediatric Use: Safety and effectiveness in children have not been established.

ADVERSE REACTIONS

One of the most severe adverse effects is hyperkalemia (see CONTRAINDICATIONS, WARNINGS, AND OVERDOSAGE).

Gastrointestinal bleeding and ulceration have been reported in patients treated with microencapsulated KCl (see WARNINGS).

In addition to bleeding and ulceration, perforation and obstruction have been reported in patients treated with solid KCl dosage forms, and may occur with Micro-K LS.

The most common adverse reactions to the oral potassium salts are nausea, vomiting, flatulence, abdominal pain/discomfort, and diarrhea. These symptoms are due to irritation of the gastrointestinal tract and are best managed by taking the dose with meals, or reducing the amount taken at one time.

Skin rash has been reported rarely with potassium preparations.

In a controlled clinical study Micro-K LS was associated with an increased frequency of gastrointestinal intolerance (e.g., diarrhea, loose stools, abdominal pain, etc.) compared to equal doses (100 mEq/day) of Micro-K Extencaps (see WARNINGS, Diarrhea or Dehydration). This finding was attributed to an inactive ingredient used in the Micro-K LS formulation that is not present in the Micro-K Extencaps formulation.

OVERDOSAGE

The administration of oral potassium salts to persons with normal excretory mechanisms for potassium rarely causes serious hyperkalemia. However, if excretory mechanisms are impaired, or if potassium is administered too rapidly intravenously, potentially fatal hyperkalemia can result (see CONTRAINDICATIONS and WARNINGS). It is important to recognize that hyperkalemia is usually asymptomatic and may be manifested only by an increased serum potassium concentration (6.5–8.0 mEq/L) and characteristic electrocardiographic changes (peaking of T-waves, loss of P-wave, depression of S-T segment, and prolongation of the QT interval). Late manifestations include muscle paralysis and cardiovascular collapse from cardiac arrest (9–12 mEq/L).

Treatment measures for hyperkalemia include the following:

1. Elimination of foods and medications containing potassium and of any agents with potassium-sparing properties;
2. Intravenous administration of 300 to 500 mL/hr of 10% dextrose solution containing 10–20 units of crystalline insulin per 1,000 mL;
3. Correction of acidosis, if present, with intravenous sodium bicarbonate;
4. Use of exchange resins, hemodialysis, or peritoneal dialysis.

In treating hyperkalemia, it should be recalled that in patients who have been stabilized on digitalis, too rapid a lowering of the serum potassium concentration can produce digitalis toxicity.

DOSAGE AND ADMINISTRATION

The usual dietary potassium intake by the average adult is 50 to 100 mEq per day. Potassium depletion sufficient to cause hypokalemia usually requires the loss of 200 or more mEq of potassium from the total body store.

Dosage must be adjusted to the individual needs of each patient. The dose for the prevention of hypokalemia is typically in the range of 20 mEq per day. Doses of 40–100 mEq per day or more are used for the treatment of potassium depletion. Dosage should be divided if more than 20 mEq per day are given such that no more than 20 mEq is given in a single dose.

Usual Adult dose—One Micro-K LS 20 mEq packet 1 to 5 times daily, depending on the requirements of the patient. This product must be suspended in a liquid, preferably water, or sprinkled on food prior to ingestion.

Suspension in Water: Pour contents of packet slowly into approximately 2–6 fluid ounces ($\frac{1}{4}$–$\frac{3}{4}$ glassful) of water. Stir thoroughly for approximately 1 minute until slightly thickened, then drink. The entire contents of the packet must be used immediately and not stored for future use. Any microcapsule/water mixture should be used immediately and not stored for future use.

Suspension in Liquids other than Water: Studies conducted using orange juice, tomato juice, apple juice and milk as the suspending liquid have shown that the quantity of fluid used to suspend one Micro-K LS packet MUST be limited to *2 fluid ounces* ($\frac{1}{4}$ *glassful*). The use of volumes greater than 2 fluid ounces substantially reduces the dose of potassium chloride delivered. If a liquid other than water is used to suspend Micro-K LS then the contents of the packet should be slowly poured into *2 fluid ounces* ($\frac{1}{4}$ *glassful*) of liquid. Stir thoroughly for approximately 1 minute, then drink. The entire contents of the packet must be used immediately and not stored for future use. Any microcapsule/liquid mixture should be used immediately and not stored for future use.

Sprinkling Contents on Food: Micro-K LS may be given on soft food that may be swallowed easily without chewing, such as applesauce or pudding. After sprinkling the contents of the packet on the food, it should be swallowed immediately without chewing and followed with a glass of cool water, milk, or juice to ensure complete swallowing of all the microcapsules. Do not store microcapsule/food mixture for future use.

HOW SUPPLIED

Micro-K LS containing 1.5 g microencapsulated potassium chloride (equivalent to 20 mEq K) per packet in cartons of 30 (NDC 0031-5760-56) and 100 packets (NDC 0031-5760-63).

Store at controlled room temprature, between 15°C and 30°C (59°F and 86°F).

CAUTION: Federal law prohibits dispensing without prescription.

MITROLAN® TABLETS

[mǐ'tro"lan]
brand of Calcium Polycarbophil

Each chewable tablet contains:
Calcium Polycarbophil (equivalent to 500 mg Polycarbophil, USP)

Inactive Ingredients: Aminoacetic Acid, Corn Starch, D&C Yellow 10 Aluminum Lake, Flavors, Magnesium Stearate, Mannitol, Povidone, Sucrose.

ACTIONS

Mitrolan (calcium polycarbophil) is a hydrophilic agent. As a bulk laxative, Mitrolan retains free water within the lumen of the intestine, and indirectly opposes dehydrating forces of the bowel, promoting well-formed stools. In diarrhea, when the intestinal mucosa is incapable of absorbing water at normal rates, Mitrolan absorbs free fecal water, forming a gel and producing formed stools. Thus, in both diarrhea and constipation, the drug works by restoring a more normal moisture level and providing bulk in the patient's intestinal tract.

INDICATIONS

For the treatment of constipation or diarrhea, associated with conditions such as irritable bowel syndrome and diverticulosis. Also for the treatment of acute non-specific diarrhea. Restores normal stool consistency by regulating its water and bulk content.

CONTRAINDICATIONS

As with all hydrophilic bulking agents, calcium polycarbophil should not be used in patients with signs of gastrointestinal obstruction.

WARNINGS

As with any drug, if you are pregnant or nursing a baby, seek the advice of a health professional before using this product.

ADVERSE REACTIONS

Abdominal fullness may be noted occasionally. An adjustment of the dosage schedule with smaller doses given more frequently but spaced evenly throughout the day may provide relief of this symptom during continued use of Mitrolan.

DRUG INTERACTION

Antacids containing aluminum, calcium or magnesium impair absorption of tetracycline. Although Mitrolan is not an antacid, it releases free calcium after ingestion and should not be used by any patient who is taking a prescription antibiotic drug containing any form of tetracycline.

Directions of Use:
CHEW TABLETS BEFORE SWALLOWING.
Recommended dosage for OTC use: Adults— Chew and swallow 2 tablets 4 times a day, or as needed. Do not exceed 12 tablets in a 24-hour period. Children (6 to under 12 years)— Chew and swallow 1 tablet 3 times a day, or as needed. Do exceed 6 tablets in a 24-hour period. Children (3 to und years)—Chew and swallow 1 tablet 2 times a day, needed. Do not exceed 3 tablets in a 24-hour period.
For episodes of severe diarrhea, the dose may be r every $\frac{1}{2}$ hour, but do not exceed the maximum daily
Dosage may be adjusted according to individual r
When using as a laxative, patient should drink a fu fl. oz.) of water or other liquid with each dose.
Sodium Content: Less than 0.02 mEq (0.46 mg)

HOW SUPPLIED

Chewable Tablets—cartons of 36 individual blister units (NDC 0031-1535-57) and bottles 0031-1535-63).
Shown in Product Identification Section, p

PABALATE® TABLETS

[pǎb'ah"lāt]

DESCRIPTION

Pabalate® tablets are intended for oral admini
Each enteric-coated tablet contains:
Sodium Salicylate, USP ....
Sodium Aminobenzoate ....
Inactive Ingredients: Acacia, Acetylated Monoglyce
Calcium Carbonate, Calcium Sulfate, Carnauba Wax, C
lose Acetate Phthalate, D&C Yellow 10, Diethyl Phthala
Edible Ink, FD&C Blue 2 Aluminum Lake, FD&C Yellow
Gelatin, Magnesium Stearate, Polysorbates, Shellac, Stear
Acid, Sucrose, Talc, Titanium Dioxide, Wheat Flour, Whit
Wax. May contain FD&C Red 40 and Yellow 6 Aluminum
Lakes.
Sodium content per tablet: 88.4 mg (3.8 mEq)

CLINICAL PHARMACOLOGY

Sodium salicylate is a mild analgesic with antiinflammatory and antipyretic activity. Compared to aspirin, sodium salicylate has substantially less effect on platelet adhesiveness. In large doses, however, it has a hypoprothrombinemic effect. Sodium salicylate in conventional dosage form dissolves in the stomach and is absorbed as un-ionized salicylic acid. However, in Pabalate, the enteric coating delays release of the salicylate until the tablet reaches the alkaline medium of the intestine. After absorption, salicylic acid is extensively bound to plasma protein, and the bound portion is in equilibrium with the free salicylate in the plasma. The action of sodium aminobenzoate in this formulation has not been established.

INDICATIONS

For the temporary relief of occasional minor aches, pains and headache and for the reduction of fever.

CONTRAINDICATIONS

Hypersensitivity to any of the ingredients. Presence of an active ulcer, hypoprothrombinemia, Vitamin K deficiency, severe hepatic or renal damage, or hemophilia. This product is not recommended for persons on a sodium-restricted diet.

WARNINGS

Children and teenagers should not use this medicine for chicken pox or flu symptoms before a doctor is consulted about Reye syndrome, a rare but serious illness.

PRECAUTIONS

General: Treatment with salicylates may interfere with blood clotting; therefore, salicylate therapy should be stopped at least one week prior to surgery.

Drug Interaction: This product contains sodium aminobenzoate, the aminobenzoic acid portion of which inhibits the bacteriostatic action of sulfonamides when the two are present concurrently.

Carcinogenesis, mutagenesis: Long-term studies in animals have not been performed to evaluate carcinogenic potential.

Pregnancy Category C: Animal reproduction studies have not been conducted with Pabalate.

Safe use of Pabalate has not been established with regard to possible adverse effects upon fetal development. Therefore, Pabalate should not be used in women who are or may become pregnant and particularly during early pregnancy unless in the judgment of the physician the potential benefits outweigh the possible hazards.

Nursing Mothers: Salicylates appear in human milk in moderate amounts. They can produce a bleeding tendency by decreasing the amount of prothrombin in the infant's blood. As a general rule, nursing should not be undertaken while a patient is on this drug.

Pediatric Use: Safety and effectiveness in children below the age of 12 years have not been established.

ADVERSE REACTIONS

The most frequent adverse reactions to products such as Pabalate which contain salicylates are nausea and gastrointestinal upset. Fine rash with or without pruritus and urticaria occurs less frequently. The occasional occurrence of mild salicylism (diarrhea, tinnitus, dizziness) may require an adjustment in dosage.

Overdosage: Mild chronic overdosage, termed salicylism, may cause symptoms such as tinnitus, nausea, headache, hyperventilation, dizziness, drowsiness, mental confusion, dimness of vision, sweating, thirst and occasionally diarrhea. Withdrawal of salicylates and supportive therapy may be sufficient treatment.

A more severe degree of salicylate intoxication may occur with acute massive overdosage or the chronic administration of more moderate overdoses, especially in infants and children. CNS effects are more pronounced and may progress to delirium, hallucinations, generalized convulsions and coma. A variety of cutaneous lesions may be observed.

A most important feature of salicylate intoxication is a disturbance of acid-base balance and plasma electrolytes. Careful monitoring of these laboratory parameters along with plasma glucose concentration is essential. The type and quantity of repair solutions used will depend upon interpretation of the laboratory data. Bicarbonate solution should be administered IV in order to produce alkaline diuresis. Correction of hypoglycemia and ketosis by the administration of glucose is essential.

Since hyperthermia and dehydration are immediate threats to life, external sponging and the administration of adequate quantities of IV fluids are important first steps to correct these conditions and maintain adequate renal function.

If hemorrhagic phenomena (petechiae, thrombocytopenia) occur, whole blood transfusions and vitamin K may be necessary.

The gastrointestinal tract should be emptied either by emesis or purging to remove undissolved tablets in cases of acute ingestion of a large single dose. Since enteric coated tablets do not disintegrate in the stomach, they cannot be removed by lavage.

Rapid and immediate removal of salicylate from the body by alkaline diuresis is essential. In more severe cases, extrarenal measures such as peritoneal dialysis, hemodialysis, hemoperfusion or exchange transfusion may be required.

DOSAGE AND ADMINISTRATION

Adults and children 12 years of age and over: For pain—2 tablets ever 4 hours while symptoms persist, not to exceed 12 tablets in 24 hours for not more than 10 days or as directed by a doctor. For fever—2 tablets every 4 hours while fever persists, not to exceed 12 tablets in 24 hours for not more than 3 days or as directed by a doctor. Due to the enteric coating, tablets should not be taken within one hour of ingesting milk or antacids.

HOW SUPPLIED

Yellow, enteric-coated tablets, monogrammed AHR and 5816 in bottles of 100 (NDC 0031-5816-63) and 500 (NDC 0031-5816-70).

Store at Controlled Room Temperature, Between 15℃ and 30℃ (59℉ and 86℉).

Shown in Product Identification Section, page 424

PABALATE®-SF TABLETS   ℞
[păb'ah "lāt]
Pabalate-Sodium Free

DESCRIPTION

Pabalate®-SF tablets are intended for oral administration. Each enteric-coated tablet contains:

Potassium Salicylate ....0.3 g
Potassium Aminobenzoate ....0.3 g
Potassium content per tablet:
131.5 mg (3.4 mEq)

Inactive Ingredients: Acacia, Acetylated Monoglycerides, Calcium Carbonate, Calcium Sulfate, Carnauba Wax, Cellulose Acetate Phthalate, Diethyl Phthalate, Docusate Sodium, Edible Ink, FD&C Blue 1 Aluminum Lake, FD&C Blue 2 Aluminum Lake, FD&C Red 3 Aluminum Lake, Gelatin, Magnesium Stearate, Polysorbates, Shellac, Stearic Acid,

Sucrose, Talc, Titanium Dioxide, Wheat Flour, White Wax. May contain FD&C Red 40 and Yellow 6 Aluminum Lakes. Analgesic Drug Product

CLINICAL PHARMACOLOGY

Potassium salicylate is a mild analgesic with antiinflammatory and antipyretic activity. Compared to aspirin, potassium salicylate has substantially less effect on platelet adhesiveness. In large doses, however, it has a hypoprothrombinemic effect. Potassium salicylate in conventional dosage form dissolves in the stomach and is absorbed as un-ionized salicylic acid. However, in Pabalate-SF, the enteric coating delays release of the salicylate until the tablet reaches the alkaline medium of the intestine. After absorption, salicylic acid is extensively bound to plasma protein, and the bound portion is in equilibrium with the free salicylate in the plasma. The action of potassium aminobenzoate in this formulation has not been established.

INDICATIONS

Pabalate-SF tablets are indicated for the temporary relief of mild to moderate pain complicated by conditions in which the restriction of sodium intake may be desirable, such as: congestive heart failure, essential hypertension and glomerulonephritis.

CONTRAINDICATIONS

Hypersensitivity to any of the ingredients. Presence of an active ulcer, hypoprothrombinemia, Vitamin K deficiency, severe hepatic or renal damage, hemophilia, or hyperkalemia. Do not administer to patients who are receiving a potassium-sparing diuretic.

WARNINGS

Salicylates have been reported to be associated with the development of Reye syndrome in children and teenagers with chicken pox, influenza, and influenza-like infections. There have been several reports, published and unpublished, concerning non-specific small bowel lesions consisting of stenosis with or without ulceration, associated with the administration of enteric-coated thiazides with potassium salts. These lesions may occur with enteric-coated potassium tablets alone or when they are used with nonenteric-coated thiazides, or certain other oral diuretics.

These small bowel lesions have caused obstruction, hemorrhage, and perforation. Surgery was frequently required and deaths have occurred.

Based on a large survey of physicians and hospitals, both American and foreign, the incidence of these lesions is low, and a causal relationship in man has not been definitely established.

Available information tends to implicate enteric-coated potassium salts although lesions of this type also occur spontaneously. Therefore, coated potassium-containing formulations should be administered only when indicated, and should be discontinued immediately if abdominal pain, distension, nausea, vomiting, or gastrointestinal bleeding occur.

When prescribing Pabalate-SF for patients who are receiving concurrent potassium supplementation (e.g., to replace potassium excreted during thiazide therapy), it should be kept in mind that each Pabalate-SF tablet contains 131.5 mg (3.4 mEq) of potassium. A decrease in supplemental potassium dosage should be considered in order to avoid hyperkalemia.

The use of potassium salts in patients with chronic renal disease, or any other condition which impairs potassium excretion, requires particularly careful monitoring of the serum potassium concentration and appropriate dosage adjustment.

PRECAUTIONS

General: Treatment with salicylates may interfere with blood clotting; therefore, salicylate therapy should be stopped at least one week prior to surgery.

Drug Interaction: This product contains aminobenzoic acid which inhibits the bacteriostatic action of sulfonamides when the two are administered concurrently.

Carcinogenesis, mutagenesis: Long-term studies in animals have not been performed to evaluate carcinogenic potential.

Pregnancy Category C: Animal reproduction studies have not been conducted with Pabalate-SF.

Safe use of Pabalate-SF has not been established with regard to possible adverse effects upon fetal development. Therefore, Pabalate-SF should not be used in women who are or may become pregnant and particularly during early pregnancy unless in the judgment of the physician the potential benefits outweigh the possible hazards.

Nursing Mothers: Salicylates appear in human milk in moderate amounts. They can produce a bleeding tendency by decreasing the amount of prothrombin in the infant's blood. As a general rule, nursing should not be undertaken while a patient is on this drug.

Pediatric Use: Safety and effectiveness in children below the age of 12 have not been established.

ADVERSE REACTIONS

Hyperkalemia is a potential adverse effect (see Contraindications and Warnings). The most frequent adverse reactions to products such as Pabalate-SF which contain potassium and/or salicylates are nausea and gastrointestinal upset. Fine rash with or without pruritus and urticaria occur less frequently. The occasional occurrence of mild salicylism may require adjustment in dosage.

OVERDOSAGE

Overdose may cause symptoms of hyperkalemia and/or salicylate intoxication. Mild chronic overdosage, termed salicylism, may cause symptoms such as tinnitus, nausea, headache, hyperventilation, dizziness, drowsiness, mental confusion, dimness of vision, sweating, thirst, and occasionally diarrhea. Withdrawal of salicylates and supportive therapy may be sufficient treatment.

A more severe degree of salicylate intoxication may occur with acute massive overdosage or the chronic administration of more moderate overdoses, especially in infants and children. CNS effects are more pronounced and may progress to delirium, hallucinations, generalized convulsions and coma. A variety of cutaneous lesions may be observed.

A most important feature of salicylate intoxication is a disturbance of acid-base balance and plasma electrolytes. Careful monitoring of these laboratory parameters along with plasma glucose concentration is essential. The type and quantity of repair solutions used will depend upon interpretation of the laboratory data. Bicarbonate solution should be administered IV in order to produce alkaline diuresis. Correction of hypoglycemia and ketosis by the administration of glucose is essential.

Since hyperthermia and dehydration are immediate threats to life, external sponging and the administration of adequate quantities of IV fluids are important first steps to correct these conditions and maintain adequate renal function.

If hemorrhagic phenomena (petechiae, thrombocytopenia) occur, whole blood transfusions and vitamin K may be necessary.

The gastrointestinal tract should be emptied either by emesis or purging to remove undissolved tablets in cases of acute ingestion of a large single dose. Since enteric-coated tablets do not disintegrate in the stomach, they cannot be removed by lavage.

Rapid and immediate removal of salicylate from the body by alkaline diuresis is essential. In more severe cases, extrarenal measures such as peritoneal dialysis, hemodialysis, hemoperfusion or exchange transfusion may be required.

DOSAGE AND ADMINISTRATION

The average adult dose is two tablets every 4 hours. Due to the enteric coating, tablets should not be taken within one hour of ingesting milk or antacids. For Chicken Pox or Flu, see Warnings.

HOW SUPPLIED

Persian rose, enteric-coated tablets, monogrammed AHR and 5883 in bottles of 100 (NDC 0031-5883-63) and 500 (NDC 0031-5883-70).

Store at Controlled Room Temperature, Between 15℃ and 30℃ (59℉ and 86℉).

Dispense in well-closed container.

Shown in Product Identification Section, page 424

PHENAPHEN®   ℞ ©
WITH CODEINE NO. 2
PHENAPHEN®   ℞ ©
WITH CODEINE NO. 3
PHENAPHEN®   ℞ ©
WITH CODEINE NO. 4
(Acetaminophen and Codeine Phosphate Capsules)
[fen'ah-fen "]

DESCRIPTION

Each Phenaphen® with Codeine No. 2 capsule contains:
Acetaminophen, USP ....325 mg
Codeine Phosphate, USP ....15 mg
   (Warning: May be habit forming)

Inactive Ingredients: Corn Starch, D&C Yellow 10, Edible Ink, FD&C Blue 1, FD&C Red 3 or 40, FD&C Yellow 6, Gelatin, Magnesium Stearate, Sodium Starch Glycolate, Stearic Acid.

Continued on next page

Prescribing information on A. H. Robins products listed here is based on official labeling in effect June 1, 1989, with Indications, Contraindications, Warnings, Precautions, Adverse Reactions, and Dosage stated in full.

Robins—Cont.

Each Phenaphen® with Codeine No. 3 capsule contains:
Acetaminophen, USP ....325 mg
Codeine Phosphate, USP ....30 mg
  (Warning: May be habit forming)
Inactive Ingredients: D&C Yellow 10, Edible Ink, FD&C Blue 1, (FD&C Green 3 *and* Red 40) or Red 3, FD&C Yellow 6, Gelatin, Magnesium Stearate, Sodium Starch Glycolate, Stearic Acid.
Each Phenaphen® with Codeine No. 4 capsule contains:
Acetaminophen, USP ....325 mg
Codeine Phosphate, USP ....60 mg
  (Warning: May be habit forming)
Inactive Ingredients: Corn Starch, D&C Yellow 10, Edible Ink, FD&C Green 3 or Blue 1, FD&C Yellow 6, Gelatin, Lactose, Magnesium Stereate, Sodium Starch Glycolate, Stearic Acid.

Acetaminophen, 4'-hydroxyacetanilide, is a non-opiate, non-salicylate analgesic and antipyretic which occurs as a white, odorless, crystalline powder, possessing a slightly bitter taste.
Codeine is an alkaloid, obtained from opium or prepared from morphine by methylation. Codeine phosphate occurs as fine, white, needle-shaped crystals, or white, crystalline powder. It is affected by light. Its chemical name is: 7,8-didehydro-4, 5α-epoxy-3-methoxy-17-methylmorphinan-6α-ol phosphate (1:1) (salt) hemihydrate.

CLINICAL PHARMACOLOGY

Phenaphen with Codeine capsules combine the analgesic effects of a centrally acting analgesic, codeine, with a peripherally acting analgesic, acetaminophen. Both ingredients are well absorbed orally. The plasma elimination half-life ranges from 1 to 4 hours for acetaminophen, and from 2.5 to 3 hours for codeine.
Codeine retains at least one-half of its analgesic activity when administered orally. A reduced first-pass metabolism of codeine by the liver accounts for the greater oral efficacy of codeine when compared to most other morphine-like narcotics. Following absorption, codeine is metabolized by the liver and metabolic products are excreted in the urine.
Approximately 10 percent of the administered codeine is demethylated to morphine, which may account for its analgesic activity.
Acetaminophen is distributed throughout most fluids of the body and is metabolized primarily in the liver. Little unchanged drug is excreted in the urine, but most metabolic products appear in the urine within 24 hours.

INDICATIONS AND USAGE

Phenaphen with Codeine capsules are indicated for the relief of mild to moderately severe pain.

CONTRAINDICATIONS

Acetaminophen and codeine phosphate should not be administered to patients who have previously exhibited hypersensitivity to codeine or acetaminophen.

PRECAUTIONS

General
Head Injury and Increased Intracranial Pressure: The respiratory depressant effects of narcotics and their capacity to elevate cerebrospinal fluid pressure may be markedly exaggerated in the presence of head injury, other intracranial lesions or a pre-existing increase in intracranial pressure. Furthermore, narcotics produce adverse reactions which may obscure the clinical course of patients with head injuries.
Acute Abdominal Conditions: The administration of this product or other narcotics may obscure the diagnosis or clinical course of patients with acute abdominal conditions.
Special risk patients: This drug should be given with caution to certain patients such as the elderly or debilitated, and those with severe impairment of hepatic or renal function, hypothyroidism, Addison's disease, and prostatic hypertrophy or urethral structure.
Information for Patients: Codeine may impair the mental and/or physical abilities required for the performance of potentially hazardous tasks such as driving a car or operating machinery. The patient using this drug should be cautioned accordingly.
The patient should understand the single-dose and 24-hour dose limits and the time interval between doses.
Drug Interactions: Patients receiving other narcotic analgesics, antipsychotics, antianxiety agents, or other CNS depressants (including alcohol) concomitantly with this drug may exhibit an additive CNS depression. When such combined therapy is contemplated, the dose of one or both agents should be reduced.
The use of MAO inhibitors or tricyclic antidepressants with codeine preparations may increase the effect of either the antidepressant or codeine.
The concurrent use of anticholinergics with codeine may produce paralytic ileus.

Carcinogenesis, Mutagenesis, Impairment of Fertility: No long-term studies in animals have been performed with acetaminophen or codeine to determine carcinogenic potential or effects on fertility.
Acetaminophen and codeine have been found to have no mutagenic potential using the Ames Salmonella-Microsomal Activation test, the Basc test on Drosophila germ cells, and the Micronucleus test on mouse bone marrow.
Pregnancy:
Teratogenic Effects: Pregnancy Category C.
Codeine: A study in rats and rabbits reported no teratogenic effect of codeine administered during the period of organogenesis in doses ranging from 5 to 120 mg/kg. In the rat, doses at the 120 mg/kg level, in the toxic range for the adult animal, were associated with an increase in embryo resorption at the time of implantation. In another study a single 100 mg/kg dose of codeine administered in pregnant mice reportedly resulted in delayed ossification in the offspring.
There are no studies in humans, and the significance of these findings to humans, if any, is not known.
Acetaminophen and codeine phosphate should be used during pregnancy only if the potential benefit justifies the potential risk to the fetus.
Nonteratogenic Effects: Dependence has been reported in newborns whose mothers took opiates regularly during pregnancy. Withdrawal signs include irritability, excessive crying, tremors, hyperreflexia, fever, vomiting, and diarrhea. Signs usually appear during the first few days of life.
Labor and Delivery: Narcotic analgesics cross the placental barrier. The closer to delivery and the larger the dose used, the greater the possibility of respiratory depression in the newborn. Narcotic analgesics should be avoided during labor if delivery of a premature infant is anticipated. If the mother has received narcotic analgesics during labor, newborn infants should be observed closely for signs of respiratory depression. Resuscitation may be required (see "Overdosage"). The effect of codeine, if any, on the later growth, development, and functional maturation of the child is unknown.
Nursing Mothers: Some studies, but not others, have reported detectable amounts of codeine in breast milk. The levels are probably not clinically significant after usual therapeutic dosage. The possibility of clinically important amounts being excreted in breast milk in individuals abusing codeine should be considered.

ADVERSE REACTIONS

The most frequently observed adverse reactions include lightheadedness, dizziness, sedation, shortness of breath, nausea and vomiting. These effects seem to be more prominent in ambulatory than in non-ambulatory patients, and some of these adverse reactions may be alleviated if the patient lies down. Other adverse reactions include allergic reactions, euphoria, dysphoria, constipation, abdominal pain and pruritus.
At higher doses, codeine has most of the disadvantages of morphine including respiratory depression.

DRUG ABUSE AND DEPENDENCE

Acetaminophen and Codeine Phosphate capsules are a Schedule III controlled substance.
Codeine can produce drug dependence of the morphine type, and therefore has the potential for being abused. Psychic dependence, physical dependence and tolerance may develop upon repeated administration of this drug, and it should be prescribed and administered with the same degree of caution appropriate in the use of other oral narcotic-containing medications.

OVERDOSAGE

Acetaminophen:
Signs and Symptoms: In acute acetaminophen overdosage, dose-dependent, potentially fatal hepatic necrosis is the most serious adverse effect. Renal tubular necrosis, hypoglycemic coma and thrombocytopenia may also occur.
In adults, hepatic toxicity has rarely been reported with acute overdoses of less than 10 grams and fatalities with less than 15 grams. Importantly, young children seem to be more resistant than adults to the hepatotoxic effect of an acetaminophen overdose. Despite this, the measures outlined below should be initiated in any adult or child suspected of having ingested an acetaminophen overdose.
Early symptoms following a potentially hepatotoxic overdose may include: nausea, vomiting, diaphoresis and general malaise. Clinical and laboratory evidence of hepatic toxicity may not be apparent until 48 to 72 hours post-ingestion.
Treatment: Stomach should be emptied promptly by lavage or by induction of emesis with syrup of ipecac. Patients' estimates of the quantity of a drug ingested are notoriously unreliable. Therefore, if an acetaminophen overdose is suspected, a serum acetaminophen assay should be obtained as early as possible, but no sooner than four hours following ingestion. Liver function studies should be obtained initially and repeated at 24-hour intervals.
The antidote, N-acetylcysteine, should be administered as early as possible, preferably within 16 hours of the overdose ingestion for optimal results, but in any case, within 24

hours. Following recovery, there are no residual, structural or functional hepatic abnormalities.
Codeine:
Signs and Symptoms: Serious overdose with codeine is characterized by respiratory depression (a decrease in respiratory rate and/or tidal volume, Cheyne-Stokes respiration, cyanosis), extreme somnolence progressing to stupor or coma, skeletal muscle flaccidity, cold and clammy skin, and sometimes bradycardia and hypotension. In severe overdosage, apnea, circulatory collapse, cardiac arrest and death may occur.
Treatment: Primary attention should be given to the reestablishment of adequate respiratory exchange through provision of a patent airway and the institution of assisted or controlled ventilation. The narcotic antagonist naloxone is a specific antidote against respiratory depression which may result from overdosage or unusual sensitivity to narcotics, including codeine. Therefore, an appropriate dose of naloxone hydrochloride (see package insert) should be administered, preferably by the intravenous route, and simultaneously with efforts at respiratory resuscitation. Since the duration of action of codeine may exceed that of the antagonist, the patient should be kept under continued surveillance and repeated doses of the antagonist should be administered as needed to maintain adequate respiration.
An antagonist should not be administered in the absence of clinically significant respiratory or cardiovascular depression. Oxygen, intravenous fluids, vasopressors and other supportive measures should be employed as indicated.
Gastric emptying may be useful in removing unabsorbed drug.

DOSAGE AND ADMINISTRATION

Dosage should be adjusted according to severity of pain and response of the patient.
The usual adult dosage is:

	Single Doses (Range)	Maximum 24 Hour Dose
Codeine Phosphate	15 mg–60 mg	360 mg
Acetaminophen	300 mg–1000 mg	4000 mg

Doses may be repeated up to every 4 hours.
The prescriber must determine the number of capsules per dose, and the maximum number of capsules per 24 hours, based upon the above dosage guidance. This information should be conveyed in the prescription.
For children, the single dose of codeine phosphate is 0.5 mg/kg.
This dose may be repeated up to every four hours.
It should be kept in mind, however, that tolerance to codeine can develop with continued use and that the incidence of untoward effects is dose related. Adult doses of codeine higher than 60 mg fail to give commensurate relief of pain but merely prolong analgesia and are associated with an appreciably increased incidence of undesirable side effects. Equivalently high doses in children would have similar effects.

HOW SUPPLIED

Phenaphen with Codeine No. 2, black and yellow capsules in bottles of 100 (NDC 0031-6242-63).
Phenaphen with Codeine No. 3, black and green capsules in bottles of 100 (NDC 0031-6257-63) and 500 (NDC 0031-6257-70) and Dis-Co® Unit Dose Packs (4×25's) (6257-61).
Phenaphen with Codeine No. 4, green and white capsules in bottles of 100 (NDC 0031-6274-63) and 500 (NDC 0031-6274-70).
Store at controlled room temperature, between 15°C and 30°C (59°F and 86°F).
Dispense capsules in tight, light-resistant container.
Shown in Product Identification Section, page 424

PHENAPHEN®-650   ℞ Ⓒ
WITH CODEINE TABLETS
[*fen'ah-fen"*]
(Acetaminophen and Codeine Phosphate Tablets)

DESCRIPTION

Each Phenaphen®-650 with Codeine tablet contains:
Acetaminophen, USP ....650 mg
Codeine Phosphate, USP ....30 mg
  (Warning: May be habit forming)
Inactive Ingredients: Calcium Sulfate, Corn Starch, Microcrystalline Cellulose, Polyethylene Glycol, Povidone, Colloidal Silicon Dioxide, Sodium Starch Glycolate, Stearic Acid.
Acetaminophen, 4'-hydroxyacetanilide, is a non-opiate, nonsalicylate analgesic and antipyretic which occurs as a white, odorless, crystalline powder, possessing a slightly bitter taste.
Codeine is an alkaloid, obtained from opium or prepared from morphine by methylation. Codeine phosphate occurs as fine, white, needle-shaped crystals, or white, crystalline powder. It is affected by light. Its chemical name is: 7,8-didehydro-4, 5α-epoxy-3-methoxy-17-methylmorphinan-6α-ol phosphate (1:1) (salt) hemihydrate.

Clinical Pharmacology

Phenaphen-650 with Codeine combines the analgesic effects of a centrally acting analgesic, codeine, with a peripherally acting analgesic, acetaminophen. Both ingredients are well absorbed orally. The plasma elimination half-life ranges from 1 to 4 hours for acetaminophen, and from 2.5 to 3 hours for codeine.

Codeine retains at least one-half of its analgesic activity when administered orally. A reduced first-pass metabolism of codeine by the liver accounts for the greater oral efficacy of codeine when compared to most other morphine-like narcotics. Following absorption, codeine is metabolized by the liver and metabolic products are excreted in the urine. Approximately 10 percent of the administered codeine is demethylated to morphine, which may account for its analgesic activity.

Acetaminophen is distributed throughout most fluids of the body, and is metabolized primarily in the liver. Little unchanged drug is excreted in the urine, but most metabolic products appear in the urine within 24 hours.

INDICATIONS AND USAGE

Phenaphen-650 with Codeine tablets are indicated for the relief of mild to moderately severe pain.

CONTRAINDICATIONS

Acetaminophen and codeine phosphate should not be administered to patients who have previously exhibited hypersensitivity to codeine or acetaminophen.

PRECAUTIONS

General:

Head Injury and increased intracranial pressure. The respiratory depressant effects of narcotics and their capacity to elevate cerebrospinal fluid pressure may be markedly exaggerated in the presence of head injury, other intracranial lesions or a pre-existing increase in intracranial pressure. Furthermore, narcotics produce adverse reactions which may obscure the clinical course of patients with head injuries.

Acute abdominal conditions. The administration of this product or other narcotics may obscure the diagnosis or clinical course in patients with acute abdominal conditions.

Special risk patients. This drug should be given with caution to certain patients such as the elderly or debilitated, and those with severe impairment of hepatic or renal function, hypothyroidism, Addison's disease, and prostatic hypertrophy or, urethral stricture.

Information for Patients. Codeine may impair the mental and/or physical abilities required for the performance of potentially hazardous tasks such as driving a car or operating machinery. The patient using this drug should be cautioned accordingly.

The patient should understand the single-dose and 24 hour dose limits and the time interval between doses.

Drug Interactions. Patients receiving other narcotic analgesics, antipsychotics, antianxiety agents, or other CNS depressants (including alcohol) concomitantly with this drug may exhibit additive CNS depression. When such combined therapy is contemplated, the dose of one or both agents should be reduced.

The use of monoamine oxidase inhibitors or tricyclic antidepressants with codeine preparations may increase the effect of either the antidepressant or codeine.

The concurrent use of anticholinergics with codeine may produce paralytic ileus.

Carcinogenesis, Mutagenesis, Impairment of Fertility: No long-term studies in animals have been performed with acetaminophen or codeine to determine carcinogenic potential or effects on fertility.

Acetaminophen and codeine have been found to have no mutagenic potential using the Ames Salmonella-Microsomal Activation test, the Basc test on Drosophila germ cells, and the Micronucleus test on mouse bone marrow.

Pregnancy:

Teratogenic Effects: Pregnancy Category C.

Codeine: A study in rats and rabbits reported no teratogenic effect of codeine administered during the period of organogenesis in doses ranging from 5 to 120 mg/kg. In the rat, doses at the 120 mg/kg level, in the toxic range for the adult animal, were associated with an increase in embryo resorption at the time of implantation. In another study a single 100 mg/kg dose of codeine administered to pregnant mice reportedly resulted in delayed ossification in the offspring.

There are no studies in humans, and the significance of these findings to humans, if any, is not known.

Acetaminophen and codeine phosphate should be used during pregnancy only if the potential benefit justifies the potential risk to the fetus.

Nonteratogenic Effects: Dependence has been reported in newborns whose mothers took opiates regularly during pregnancy. Withdrawal signs include irritability, excessive crying, tremors, hyperreflexia, fever, vomiting, and diarrhea. Signs usually appear during the first days of life.

Labor and Delivery: Narcotic analgesics cross the placental barrier. The closer to delivery and the larger the dose used,

the greater the possibility of respiratory depression in the newborn. Narcotic analgesics should be avoided during labor if delivery of a premature infant is anticipated. If the mother has received narcotic analgesics during labor, newborn infants should be observed closely for signs of respiratory depression. Resuscitation may be required (see "Overdosage"). The effect of codeine, if any, on the later growth, development, and functional maturation of the child is unknown.

Nursing Mothers: Some studies, but not others, have reported detectable amounts of codeine in breast milk. The levels are probably not clinically significant after usual therapeutic dosage. The possibility of clinically important amounts being excreted in breast milk in individuals abusing codeine should be considered.

ADVERSE REACTIONS

The most frequently observed adverse reactions include lightheadedness, dizziness, sedation; shortness of breath, nausea and vomiting. These effects seem to be more prominent in ambulatory than nonambulatory patients, and some of these adverse reactions may be alleviated if the patient lies down.

Other adverse reactions include allergic reactions, euphoria, dysphoria, constipation, abdominal pain and pruritus.

At higher doses, codeine has most of the disadvantages of morphine including respiratory depression.

Drug Abuse and Dependence

Acetaminophen and Codeine Phosphate Tablets are a Schedule III controlled substance.

Codeine can produce drug dependence of the morphine type, and, therefore, has the potential for being abused. Psychic dependence, physical dependence and tolerance may develop upon repeated administration of this drug and it should be prescribed and administered with the same degree of caution appropriate to the use of other oral narcotic medications.

OVERDOSAGE

Acetaminophen:

Signs and Symptoms: In acute acetaminophen overdosage, dose-dependent, potentially fatal hepatic necrosis is the most serious adverse effect. Renal tubular necrosis, hypoglycemic coma and thrombocytopenia may also occur.

In adults, hepatic toxicity has rarely been reported with acute overdoses of less than 10 grams and fatalities with less than 15 grams. Importantly, young children seem to be more resistant than adults to the hepatotoxic effect of an acetaminophen overdose. Despite this, the measures outlined below should be initiated in any adult or child suspected of having ingested an acetaminophen overdose.

Early symptoms following a potentially hepatotoxic overdose may include: nausea, vomiting, diaphoresis and general malaise. Clinical and laboratory evidence of hepatic toxicity may not be apparent until 48 to 72 hours post-ingestion.

Treatment: The stomach should be emptied promptly by lavage or by induction of emesis with syrup of ipecac. Patient's estimates of the quantity of a drug ingested are notoriously unreliable. Therefore, if an acetaminophen overdose is suspected, a serum acetaminophen assay should be obtained as early as possible, but no sooner than four hours following ingestion. Liver function studies should be obtained initially and repeated at 24-hour intervals.

The antidote, N-acetylcysteine, should be administered as early as possible, preferably within 16 hours of the overdose ingestion for optimal results but in any case, within 24 hours. Following recovery, there are no residual, structural or functional hepatic abnormalities.

Codeine:

Signs and Symptoms: Serious overdose with codeine is characterized by respiratory depression (a decrease in respiratory rate and/or tidal volume, Cheyne-Stokes respiration, cyanosis), extreme somnolence progressing to stupor or coma, skeletal muscle flaccidity, cold and clammy skin, and sometimes bradycardia and hypotension. In severe overdosage, apnea, circulatory collapse, cardiac arrest and death may occur.

Treatment: Primary attention should be given to the reestablishment of adequate respiratory exchange through provision of a patent airway and the institution of assisted or controlled ventilation. The narcotic antagonist naloxone is a specific antidote against respiratory depression which may result from overdosage or unusual sensitivity to narcotics, including codeine. Therefore, an appropriate dose of naloxone (see package insert) should be administered, preferably by the intravenous route, and simultaneously with efforts at respiratory resuscitation. Since the duration of action of codeine may exceed that of the antagonist, the patient should be kept under continued surveillance and repeated doses of the antagonist should be administered as needed to maintain adequate respiration.

An antagonist should not be administered in the absence of clinically significant respiratory or cardiovascular depression. Oxygen, intravenous fluids, vasopressors and other supportive measures should be employed as indicated.

Gastric emptying may be useful in removing unabsorbed drug.

DOSAGE AND ADMINISTRATION

Dosage should be adjusted according to severity of pain and response of the patient.

The usual adult dosage is:

	Single-Doses (Range)	Maximum 24-Hour Dose
Codeine Phosphate	15 mg–60 mg	360 mg
Acetaminophen	300 mg–1000 mg	4000 mg

Doses may be repeated up to every 4 hours.

The prescriber must determine the number of tablets per dose, and the maximum number of tablets per 24 hours, based upon the above dosage guidance. This information should be conveyed in the prescription.

For children, the single dose of codeine phosphate is 0.5 mg/kg.

This dose may be repeated up to every four hours.

It should be kept in mind, however, that tolerance to codeine can develop with continued use and that the incidence of untoward effects is dose related. Adult doses of codeine higher than 60 mg fail to give commensurate relief of pain but merely prolong analgesia and are associated with an appreciably increased incidence of undesirable side effects. Equivalently high doses in children would have similar effects.

HOW SUPPLIED

Phenaphen-650 with Codeine is available as a scored, white, capsule-shaped compressed tablet, engraved AHR and 6251 in bottles of 50 (NDC 0031-6251-60).

Store at controlled room temperature, between 15°C and 30°C (59°F and 86°F).

Dispense tablets in tight, light-resistant container.

Shown in Product Identification Section, page 424

PONDIMIN® TABLETS   R̆ ℂ̆
[pŏn′dĭ-min]
brand of fenfluramine hydrochloride
Tablets—20 mg

DESCRIPTION

Pondimin (fenfluramine hydrochloride) is an anorectic drug for oral administration. Immediate release tablets containing 20 mg fenfluramine hydrochloride are orange, scored, compressed tablets engraved AHR and 6447.

Inactive Ingredients: Corn Starch, FD&C Yellow 6, Magnesium Stearate, Microcrystalline Cellulose, Silicon Dioxide, Sodium Lauryl Sulfate.

Pondimin has the chemical name, N-ethyl-α-methyl-3-(trifluoromethyl) benzeneethanamine hydrochloride.

CLINICAL PHARMACOLOGY

Fenfluramine is a sympathomimetic amine, the pharmacologic activity of which differs somewhat from that of the prototype drugs of this class used in obesity, the amphetamines, in appearing to produce more central nervous system depression than stimulation.

The mechanism of action of Pondimin is unclear but may be related to brain levels (or turnover rates) of serotonin or to increased glucose utilization. The antiappetite effects of Pondimin are suppressed by serotonin-blocking drugs and by drugs that lower brain levels of the amine. Furthermore, decreased serotonin levels produced by selective brain lesions suppress the action of Pondimin.

In a study of 20 normal males, fenfluramine increased glucose utilization, resulting in decreased blood glucose levels. Experimental work in animals suggested that increased glucose utilization activated the satiety center and decreased the activity of the feeding center. Perhaps by this mechanism Pondimin inhibits appetite. The relationship between glucose utilization and serotonin has not been clarified.

Fenfluramine is well-absorbed from the gastrointestinal tract, and a maximal anorectic effect is generally seen after 2 to 4 hours. In man, fenfluramine is de-ethylated to norfenfluramine which is subsequently oxidized to m-trifluoromethyl benzoic acid and excreted as the glycine conjugate, m-trifluoromethylhippuric acid. Other compounds found in the urine include unchanged fenfluramine and norfenfluramine.

The rate of excretion of fenfluramine is pH dependent, with much smaller amounts appearing in an alkaline than in an acid urine.

The half-life of fenfluramine is said to be about 20 hours, compared with 5 hours for amphetamines; however, if urinary excretion is rapid and the pH maintained in the acidic range (below pH 5), half-life can be reduced to 11 hours. Fenfluramine and norfenfluramine reach steady state concen-

Continued on next page

Robins—Cont.

trations in plasma within 3 to 4 days following chronic dosage.

The greatest weight loss is seen in those patients who maintain the highest levels of Pondimin. A 2-to-3-kg weight loss over 6 weeks is associated with a plasma level of 0.1 mcg/mL (or 10 mcg/100 mL).

Fenfluramine is widely distributed in almost all body tissues. It is soluble in lipids and crosses the blood-brain barrier. Fenfluramine crosses the placenta readily in monkeys.

INDICATIONS AND USAGE

Pondimin is indicated in the management of exogenous obesity as a short-term (a few weeks) adjunct in a regimen of weight reduction based on caloric restriction.

Drugs of this class used in obesity are commonly known as "anorectics" or "anorexigenics." It has not been established, however, that the action of such drug in treating obesity is primarily one of appetite suppression. Other central nervous system actions or metabolic effects may be involved.

Adult obese subjects instructed in dietary management and treated with "anorectic" drugs, lose more weight on the average than those treated with placebo and diet, as determined in relatively short-term trials.

The average magnitude of increased weight loss of drug-treated patients over placebo-treated is only a fraction of a pound a week. The rate of weight loss is greatest in the first weeks of therapy for both drug and placebo subjects and tends to decrease in succeeding weeks. The possible origins of the increased weight loss due to the various drug effects are not established. The average amount of weight loss associated with the use of an "anorectic" drug varies from trial to trial, and the increased weight loss appears to be related in part to variables other than the drug prescribed such as the physician-investigator, the population treated and the diet prescribed. Studies do not permit conclusions as to the relative importance of the drug and non-drug factors on weight loss.

The natural history of obesity is measured in years, whereas the studies cited are restricted to a few weeks duration; thus, the total impact of drug-induced weight loss over that of diet alone must be considered clinically limited.

CONTRAINDICATIONS

Fenfluramine is contraindicated in patients with glaucoma or with hypersensitivity to fenfluramine or other sympathomimetic amines. Do not administer fenfluramine during or within 14 days following the administration of monoamine oxidase inhibitors, since hypertensive crises may result. Patients with a history of drug abuse should not receive the drug.

Do not administer fenfluramine to patients with alcoholism since psychiatric symptoms (paranoia, depression, psychosis) have been reported in a few such patients who had been administered this drug.

Fenfluramine should also generally be avoided in patients with psychotic illness. There have been reports of schizophrenic patients who have become agitated, delusional, and assaultive.

A fatal cardiac arrest has been reported shortly after the induction of anesthesia in a patient who had been taking fenfluramine prior to surgery. Fenfluramine may have a catecholamine-depleting effect when administered for prolonged periods of time; therefore, potent anesthetic agents should be administered with caution to patients taking fenfluramine. If general anesthesia cannot be avoided, full cardiac monitoring and facilities for instant resuscitative measures are a minimum necessity.

WARNINGS

When tolerance to the "anorectic" effect develops, the maximum recommended dose should not be exceeded in an attempt to increase the effect; rather, the drug should be discontinued.

PRECAUTIONS

General. Fenfluramine differs in its pharmacological profile from other "anorectic" drugs with which the prescribing practitioner may be familiar. Correspondingly, there are possible adverse effects not associated with other "anorectics"; such effects include those of diarrhea, sedation, and depression. The possibility of these effects should be weighed against the possible advantage of decreased central nervous system stimulation and/or abuse potential.

There have been four causes of pulmonary hypertension reported in association with fenfluramine use. Two cases were apparently reversible after discontinuation of fenfluramine, but evidence of pulmonary hypertension recurred in one of these patients upon rechallenge with fenfluramine. A third patient was initially improved with nifedipine treatment, but was noted to have increased pulmonary arterial pressure again at a four month follow up visit. Finally, an irreversible and fatal case of pulmonary hypertension has been reported in a patient who had seven 1-month courses of fenfluramine in the twelve years prior to death. Patients

taking fenfluramine should be advised to report immediately any deterioration in exercise tolerance.

Use only with caution in hypertension, with monitoring of blood pressure, since evidence is insufficient to rule out a possible adverse effect on blood pressure in some hypertensive patients. The drug is not recommended in severely hypertensive patients. The drug is not recommended for patients with symptomatic cardiovascular disease including arrhythmias.

Caution should be exercised in prescribing fenfluramine for patients with a history of mental depression. Further depression of mood may become evident while the patient is on fenfluramine or following withdrawal of fenfluramine. Symptoms of depression occurring immediately following abrupt withdrawal can be readily controlled by reinstituting Pondimin, followed by a gradual tapering off of the daily dose.

Information for Patients. Fenfluramine may impair the ability of the patient to engage in potentially hazardous activities such as operating machinery or driving a motor vehicle (see "Adverse Reactions"); the patient should be cautioned accordingly. Patient should also be advised to avoid alcoholic beverages while taking Pondimin.

Drug Interactions. Fenfluramine may increase slightly the effect of antihypertensive drugs, e.g., guanethidine, methyldopa, reserpine.

Other CNS depressant drugs should be used with caution in patients taking fenfluramine, since the effects may be additive.

Carcinogenesis, Mutagenesis. No carcinogenic studies or mutagenic studies have been undertaken with this drug.

Pregnancy Category C. Pondimin was shown to produce a questionable embryotoxic effect in rats and a reduced conception rate when given in a dose of 20 times the human dose. However, additional reproduction studies in rats, rabbits, mice, and monkeys at doses up to, respectively, 5 times, 20 times, 1 time, and 5 times the human dose yielded negative results.

There are no adequate and well-controlled studies in pregnant women. Pondimin should be used during pregnancy only if the potential benefit justifies the potential risk to the fetus.

Labor and Delivery. The effect of fenfluramine during labor or delivery on the mother and the fetus is unknown. The effect on later growth, development, and functional maturation of the child is unknown.

Nursing Mothers. It is not known whether this drug is excreted in human milk. Because many drugs are excreted in human milk, caution should be exercised when fenfluramine is administered to a nursing mother.

Pediatric Use. Safety and effectiveness in children below the age of 12 years have not been established.

ADVERSE REACTIONS

The most common adverse reactions of fenfluramine are drowsiness, diarrhea, and dry mouth. Less frequent adverse reactions reported in association with fenfluramine are:

Central nervous system. Dizziness; confusion; incoordination; headache; elevated mood; depression; anxiety, nervousness, or tension; insomnia; weakness or fatigue; increased or decreased libido; agitation, dysarthria.

Gastrointestinal. Constipation; abdominal pain; nausea.
Autonomic. Sweating; chills; blurred vision.
Genitourinary. Dysuria; urinary frequency.
Cardiovascular. Palpitation; hypotension; hypertension; fainting; pulmonary hypertension.
Skin. Rash; urticaria; burning sensation.
Miscellaneous. Eye irritation; myalgia; fever; chest pain; bad taste.

DRUG ABUSE AND DEPENDENCE

Pondimin (fenfluramine hydrochloride) is a controlled substance in Schedule IV. Fenfluramine is related chemically to the amphetamines, although it differs somewhat pharmacologically. The amphetamines and related stimulant drugs have been extensively abused and can produce tolerance and severe psychological dependence, as well as other adverse organic and mental changes. In this regard, there has been a report of abuse of fenfluramine by subjects with a history of abuse of other drugs. Abuse of 80 to 400 milligrams of the drug has been reported to be associated with euphoria, derealization, and perceptual changes. Fenfluramine did not produce signs of dependence in animals and appears to produce sedation more often than CNS stimulation at therapeutic doses. Its abuse potential appears qualitatively different from that of amphetamines. The possibility that fenfluramine may induce dependence should be kept in mind when evaluating the desirability of including the drug in the weight reduction programs of individual patients.

OVERDOSAGE

Signs and Symptoms: Only limited data have been reported concerning clinical effects and management of overdosage of fenfluramine.

Agitation and drowsiness, confusion, flushing, tremor (or shivering), fever, sweating, abdominal pain, hyperventilation, and dilated non-reactive pupils seem frequent in fenfluramine overdosage. Reflexes may be either exaggerated

or depressed and some patients may have rotary nystagmus. Tachycardia may be present, but blood pressure may be normal or only slightly elevated. Convulsions, coma, and ventricular extrasystoles, culminating in ventricular fibrillation, and cardiac arrest, may occur at higher dosages.

Human Toxicity. Less than 5 mg/kg are toxic to humans. Five-ten mg/kg may produce coma and convulsions. Reported single overdoses have ranged from 300 to 2000 mg; the lowest reported fatal dose was a few hundred mg in a small child, and the highest reported nonfatal dose was 1800 mg in an adult. Most deaths were apparently due to respiratory failure and cardiac arrest.

Toxic effects will appear within 30 to 60 minutes and may progress rapidly to potentially fatal complications in 90 to 240 minutes. Symptoms may persist for extended periods depending upon the dose ingested.

Management. After overdosage, only a small percentage of the drug is excreted in the urine. Forced acid diuresis has been recommended only in extreme cases in which the patient survives the early hours of intoxication but fails to show decisive improvement from other measures. Hemodialysis and peritoneal dialysis are of theoretical advantage but have not been used clinically.

Reportedly the treatment of fenfluramine intoxication should include:

- *Gastric lavage* (but not drug-induced emesis because the patient may become unconscious at a very early stage.)
- In the event that gastric lavage is not feasible due to trismus, consult an anesthesiologist for endotracheal intubation after administration of muscle relaxants; only then gastric evacuation should be tried.
- Administration of activated charcoal after emesis or lavage may reduce absorption of drug.
- *Monitoring of vital functions.* If necessary, mechanical respiration, defibrillation, or "cardioversion" should be instituted.
- *Drug therapy.* Diazepam or phenobarbital for convulsions or muscular hyperactivity. In the presence of extreme tachycardia; propranolol; in the presence of ventricular extrasystoles; lidocaine; in the presence of hyperpyrexia; chlorpromazine.

Since fenfluramine has been shown to have a slight lowering effect on blood sugar in some patients, the theoretical possibility of hypoglycemia should be borne in mind although this effect has not been reported in cases of clinical overdosage.

DOSAGE AND ADMINISTRATION

The usual dose is one 20 mg tablet three times daily before meals. Depending on the degree of effectiveness and side effects, the dosage may be increased at weekly intervals by one tablet (20 mg) daily until a maximum dosage of two tablets three times daily is attained. Total dosage of fenfluramine should not exceed 120 mg per day.

HOW SUPPLIED

Pondimin is available in 20 mg orange, scored, compressed tablets monogrammed AHR and 6447, in bottles of 100 (NDC 0031-6447-63) and 500 (NDC 0031-6447-70).

Store at controlled room temperature, between 15°C and 30°C (59°F and 86°F).

Dispense in well-closed container.

Shown in Product Identification Section, page 424

QUINIDEX EXTENTABS®   ℞
[kwĭn 'ĭ "dĕks ĕks "tĕn 'tabs]
brand of Quinidine Sulfate Extended-release Tablets, USP

PRODUCT OVERVIEW

KEY FACTS

Quinidex Extentabs (300 mg), a long acting form of quinidine sulfate, are constructed to release one-third of their alkaloidal salt, quinidine sulfate (100 mg), on reaching the stomach. The remaining two-thirds (200 mg) is evenly distributed throughout a homogeneous core which slowly dissolves as it moves along the intestinal tract, releasing quinidine sulfate for continuous absorption over an 8–12 hour period.

MAJOR USES

Quinidex Extentabs are indicated in the treatment of atrial and ventricular arrhythmias and may be administered on a BID or TID dosage regimen. G-I symptoms can be minimized by giving the drug with food.

SAFETY INFORMATION

Quinidex Extentabs are contraindicated in patients with intraventricular conduction defects, A-V block, idiosyncrasy or hypersensitivity.

All precautions applying to regular quinidine therapy apply to Quinidex Extentabs.

PRESCRIBING INFORMATION

QUINIDEX EXTENTABS®   ℞
[kwĭn 'ĭ "dĕks ĕks "tĕn 'tabs]
brand of Quinidine Sulfate Extended-release Tablets, USP
300 mg in each Quinidex Extentabs tablet.

DESCRIPTION

Quinidex Extentabs (quinidine sulfate extended-release tablets) are constructed to release one-third of their alkaloidal salt, quinidine sulfate (100 mg), on reaching the stomach, to begin absorption in the upper intestinal tract. The remaining two-thirds of the active drug (200 mg) is evenly distributed throughout a homogeneous core which slowly dissolves as it moves along the intestinal tract, releasing the quinidine sulfate for continuous absorption over an 8–12 hour period. Each Quinidex Extentabs tablet contains 300 mg of quinidine sulfate, the equivalent of 248.6 mg of the anhydrous quinidine alkaloid.

Chemically, quinidine sulfate is cinchonan-9-ol,6'-methoxy-,(9s)-sulfate(2:1) (salt) dihydrate.

Inactive Ingredients: Acacia, Acetylated Monoglycerides, Calcium Sulfate, Carnauba Wax, Edible Ink, FD&C Blue 2, Gelatin, Guar Gum, Magnesium Oxide, Magnesium Stearate, Polysorbates, Shellac, Sucrose, Titanium Dioxide, White Wax and other ingredients, one of which is a corn derivative. May contain FD&C Red 40 and FD&C Yellow 6 Aluminum Lakes.

ACTION

The action of quinidine in preventing aberrant cardiac rhythms of atrial and ventricular origin resides in its ability to (a) depress excitability of cardiac muscle, (b) slow the rate of spontaneous rhythm, (c) decrease vagal tone, and (d) prolong conduction and effective refractory period.

INDICATIONS AND USAGE

Quinidex Extentabs are indicated for the treatment of:
Premature atrial and ventricular contractions.
Paroxysmal atrial tachycardia.
Paroxysmal A-V junctional rhythm.
Atrial flutter.
Paroxysmal atrial fibrillation.
Established atrial fibrillation when therapy is appropriate.
Paroxysmal ventricular tachycardia when not associated with complete heartblock.
Maintenance therapy after electrical conversion of atrial fibrillation and/or flutter.

CONTRAINDICATIONS

Intraventricular conduction defects. Complete A-V block. A-V conduction disorders caused by digitalis intoxication. Aberrant impulses and abnormal rhythms due to escape mechanisms. Idiosyncrasy or hypersensitivity to quinidine or related cinchona derivatives. Myasthenia gravis.

WARNINGS

In the treatment of atrial flutter, reversion to sinus rhythm may be preceded by a progressive reduction in the degree of A-V block to a 1:1 ratio, resulting in an extremely rapid ventricular rate. This possible hazard may be reduced by digitalization prior to administration of quinidine.

Reports in the literature indicate that serum concentrations of digoxin may increase and may even double when quinidine is administered concurrently. Patients on concomitant therapy should be carefully monitored for digitalis toxicity. Reduction of digoxin dosage may have to be considered.

Manifestations of quinidine cardiotoxicity such as excessive prolongation of the QT interval, widening of the QRS complex and ventricular tachyarrhythmias mandate immediate discontinuation of the drug and/or close clinical and electrocardiographic monitoring.

In susceptible individuals, such as those with marginally compensated cardiovascular disease, quinidine may produce clinically important depression of cardiac function manifested by hypotension, bradycardia, or heartblock. Quinidine therapy should be carefully monitored in such individuals.

Quinidine should be used with extreme caution in patients with incomplete AV block since complete AV block and asystole may be produced. Quinidine may cause abnormalities of cardiac rhythm in digitalized patients and therefore should be used with caution in the presence of digitalis intoxication.

Quinidine should be used with caution in patients exhibiting renal, cardiac or hepatic insufficiency because of potential accumulation of quinidine in serum, leading to toxicity.

Patients taking quinidine occasionally have syncopal episodes which usually result from ventricular tachycardia or fibrillation. This syndrome has not been shown to be related to dose or serum levels. Syncopal episodes frequently terminate spontaneously or in response to treatment, but sometimes are fatal.

Cases of hepatotoxicity, including granulomatous hepatitis, due to quinidine hypersensitivity have been reported. Unexplained fever and/or elevation of hepatic enzymes, particularly in the early stages of therapy, warrant consideration of possible hepatotoxicity. Monitoring liver function during the first 4–8 weeks should be considered. Cessation of quinidine in these cases usually results in the disappearance of toxicity.

PRECAUTIONS

General—All the precautions applying to regular quinidine therapy apply to this product. Hypersensitivity or anaphy-

lactoid reactions to quinidine, although rare, should be considered, especially during the first weeks of therapy. Hospitalization for close clinical observation, electrocardiographic monitoring, and determination of serum quinidine levels are indicated when large doses of quinidine are used or with patients who present an increased risk.

Information for Patients—As with all solid dosage medications, Quinidex Extentabs should be taken with an adequate amount of fluid, preferably with the patient in an upright position to facilitate swallowing. They should be swallowed whole in order to preserve the controlled-release mechanism.

Laboratory Tests—Periodic blood counts and liver and kidney function tests should be performed during long-term therapy; the drug should be discontinued if blood dyscrasias or evidence of hepatic or renal dysfunction occurs.

Drug Interactions

Drug	Effect
Quinidine with anticholinergic drugs	Additive vagolytic effect
Quinidine with cholinergic drugs	Antagonism of cholinergic effects
Quinidine with carbonic anhydrase inhibitors, sodium bicarbonate, thiazide diuretics	Alkalinization of urine resulting in decreased excretion of quinidine
Quinidine with coumarin anticoagulants	Reduction of clotting factor concentrations
Quinidine with tubocurare, succinylcholine and decamethonium	Potentiation of neuro-muscular blockade
Quinidine with phenothiazines and reserpine	Additive cardiac depressive effects
Quinidine with hepatic enzyme-inducing drugs (phenobarbital, phenytoin, rifampin)	Decreased plasma half-life of quinidine
Quinidine with digoxin	Increased serum concentration of digoxin (See Warnings)
Quinidine with amiodarone	Increased serum concentration of quinidine
Quinidine with cimetidine	Prolonged quinidine half-life and an increase in serum quinidine level
Quinidine with ranitidine	Premature ventricular contractions and/or bigeminy
Quinidine with verapamil	Increased quinidine half-life and an increase in serum quinidine level; potential hypotensive reactions
Quinidine with nifedipine	Decreased serum concentrations of quinidine

Carcinogenesis: Studies in animals have not been performed to evaluate the carcinogenic potential of quinidine.

Pregnancy, Teratogenic Effects: Pregnancy Category C. Animal reproduction studies have not been conducted with quinidine. There are no adequate and well-controlled studies in pregnant women. Quinidex Extentabs should be administered to a pregnant woman only if clearly indicated.

Nonteratogenic Effects: Like quinine, quinidine has been reported to have oxytocic properties. The significance of this property in the clinical setting has not been established.

Labor and Delivery—There is no known use for Quinidex Extentabs in labor and delivery. However, quinidine has been reported to have oxytocic properties. The significance of this property in the clinical setting has not been established.

Nursing Mothers—Because of passage of the drug into breast milk, caustion should be exercised when Quinidex Extentabs are administered to a nursing woman.

Pediatric Use—There are no adequate and well-controlled studies establishing the safety and effectiveness of Quinidex Extentabs in children.

ADVERSE REACTIONS

Symptoms of cinchonism, such as ringing in the ears, loss of hearing, dizziness, lightheadedness, headache, nausea, and/or disturbed vision may appear in sensitive patients after a single dose of the drug. The most frequently encountered side effects to quinidine are gastrointestinal.

Gastrointestinal—Nausea, vomiting, abdominal pain, diarrhea, anorexia, granulomatous hepatitis (which may be preceded by fever), esophagitis.

Cardiovascular—Ventricular extrasystoles occurring at a rate of one or more every 6 normal beats; widening of the QRS complex and prolonged QT interval; complete A-V block; ventricular tachycardia and fibrillation; ventricular flutter; torsade de pointes; arterial embolism; hypotension; syncope.

Central Nervous System—Headache, vertigo, apprehension, excitement, confusion, delirium, dementia, ataxia, depression.

Ophthalmologic and Otologic—Disturbed hearing (tinnitus, decreased auditory acuity), disturbed vision (mydriasis, blurred vision, disturbed color perception, photophobia, diplopia, night blindness, scotomata), optic neuritis, reduced visual field.

Dermatologic—Cutaneous flushing with intense pruritus, photosensitivity, urticaria, rash, eczema, exfoliative eruptions, psoriasis, abnormalities of pigmentation.

Hypersensitivity—Angioedema, acute asthmatic episode, vascular collapse, respiratory arrest, hepatotoxicity, granulomatous hepatitis (See Warnings), purpura, vasculitis.

Hematologic—Thrombocytopenia, thrombocytopenic purpura, agranulocytosis, acute hemolytic anemia, hypoprothrombinemia, leukocytosis, shift to left in WBC differential, neutropenia.

Immunologic—Systemic lupus erythematosus, lupus nephritis.

Miscellaneous—Fever, increase in serum skeletal muscle creatine phosphokinase, arthralgia, myalgia.

OVERDOSAGE

Symptoms—Overdosage of quinidine can lead to accelerated idioventricular rhythm, change in the morphologic appearance of QRS complexes, prolonged QT intervals, intermittent sinus capture beats, paroxysms of tachycardia, ventricular arrhythmias, hypotension, oliguria, respiratory depression, pulmonary edema, acidosis, seizures, and coma.

Treatment—Early treatment to empty the stomach using syrup of ipecac and/or gastric lavage is recommended. Since Quinidex Extentabs cannot be removed through a nasogastric tube, gastric lavage should be followed by saline cathartics. Administration of activated charcoal may reduce absorption. Other general supportive measures should be employed as indicated by patient response. In severe cases, circulation should be stabilized and measurements of pulmonary capillary wedge pressure should be performed to assure adequate left ventricular filling pressure. Electrolyte and blood gas abnormalities should be corrected. In quinidine-induced vasodilation, catecholamines and other alpha-adrenergic agonists may be tried. Arrhythmias may be treated with lidocaine, pacing, and cardioversion. Administration of sodium lactate reportedly reduces the cardiotoxicity of quinidine; however, sodium lactate is contraindicated in the presence of alkalosis as increased urinary pH can lead to an increase in the renal tubular absorption of quinidine. Acidification of the urine may enhance the urinary excretion of quinidine.

DOSAGE AND ADMINISTRATION

One or two Quinidex Extentabs tablets every 8 to 12 hours as may be required to achieve the desired therapeutic effect.

HOW SUPPLIED

White sugar-coated Extentabs tablets monogrammed Quinidex and AHR in bottles of 100 (NDC 0031-6649-63), 250 (NDC 0031-6649-67), and Dis-Co® unit dose packs of 100 (NDC 0031-6649-64).

Store at controlled room temperature, between 15℃ and 30℃ (59℉ and 86℉).

Dispense tablets in well-closed light-resistant container.

Shown in Product Identification Section, page 424

REGLAN®   ℞
[rĕg'lan]
(Metoclopramide Hydrochloride)
Tablets, Syrup and Injectable

PRODUCT OVERVIEW

KEY FACTS

Reglan increases LES pressure and the rate of gastric emptying, providing the pharmacological basis for its use in gastroesophageal reflux and gastric stasis. Its effects on motility in the upper gastrointestinal tract appear to be mediated by sensitizing tissues to acetylcholine and/or antagonizing dopamine. Dopamine antagonism within the chemoreceptor trigger zone may also contribute to the antiemetic activity of Reglan. Reglan is not indicated for long-term use.

MAJOR USES

Reglan tablets are indicated as short-term (4 to 12 weeks) therapy for adults with symptomatic, documented gastroesophageal reflux who fail to respond to conventional therapy. If symptoms are confined to particular situations, such as following the evening meal, use of single doses of Reglan prior to the provocative situation should be considered, rather than continuous therapy. In higher dosages, Reglan Injectable is effective in preventing vomiting associated with emetogenic cancer chemotherapy, especially cisplatin.

Continued on next page

Prescribing information on A. H. Robins products listed here is based on official labeling in effect June 1, 1989, with Indications, Contraindications, Warnings, Precautions, Adverse Reactions, and Dosage stated in full.

Robins—Cont.

SAFETY INFORMATION

The most common side effects are restlessness, drowsiness, fatigue, and lassitude, which occur in approximately 10 percent of patients receiving the most commonly prescribed dosage of 10 mg qid. Extrapyramidal symptoms may occur in approximately 1 in 500 patients; usually these are manifested as dystonic reactions, but rarely may present as parkinsonism or tardive dyskinesia.

PRESCRIBING INFORMATION

REGLAN®   ℞

[rĕg'lan]

(Metoclopramide Hydrochloride)
Tablets, Syrup And Injectable

DESCRIPTION

For oral administration, **Reglan Tablets** (metoclopramide hydrochloride) **10 mg** are pink, scored, capsule-shaped tablets engraved Reglan on one side and AHR 10 on the opposite side.

Each tablet contains:

Metoclopramide base   **10 mg**
  (as the monohydrochloride monohydrate)

Inactive Ingredients: FD&C Red 3 Aluminum Lake, FD&C Yellow 6 Aluminum Lake, Magnesium Stearate, Mannitol, Microcrystalline Cellulose, Stearic Acid.

Reglan Tablets (metoclopramide hydrochloride) **5 mg** are green, elliptical-shaped tablets engraved Reglan 5 on one side and AHR on the opposite side.

Each tablet contains:

Metoclopramide base   **5 mg**
  (as the monohydrochloride monohydrate)

Inactive Ingredients: Corn Starch, D&C Yellow 10 Lake, FD&C Blue 1 Aluminum Lake, Lactose, Microcrystalline Cellulose, Silicon Dioxide, Stearic Acid.

Reglan Syrup (metoclopramide hydrochloride) is an orange-colored, palatable, aromatic, sugar-free liquid.

Each 5 mL (1 teaspoonful) contains:

Metoclopramide base   **5 mg**
  (as the monohydrochloride monohydrate)

Inactive Ingredients: Citric Acid, FD&C Yellow 6, Flavors, Glycerin, Methylparaben, Propylparaben, Sorbitol, Water.
For parenteral administration, **Reglan Injectable** (metoclopramide hydrochloride) is a clear, colorless, sterile solution with a pH of 4.5–6.5 for intravenous or intramuscular administration.

CONTAIN NO PRESERVATIVE.

2 mL and 10 mL **single dose** vials/ampuls; 30 mL **single dose** vial

Each **1** mL contains:

Metoclopramide base   **5 mg**
  (as the monohydrochloride monohydrate)

Sodium Chloride, USP 8.5 mg, Water for Injection, USP q.s. pH adjusted, when necessary, with hydrochloric acid and/or sodium hydroxide.

Metoclopramide hydrochloride is a white crystalline, odorless substance, freely soluble in water. Chemically, it is 4-amino-5-chloro-N-[2-(diethylamino)ethyl]-2-methoxy benzamide monohydrochloride monohydrate. Molecular weight: 354.3.

CLINICAL PHARMACOLOGY

Metoclopramide stimulates motility of the upper gastrointestinal tract without stimulating gastric, biliary, or pancreatic secretions. Its mode of action is unclear. It seems to sensitize tissues to the action of acetylcholine. The effect of metoclopramide on motility is not dependent on intact vagal innervation, but it can be abolished by anticholinergic drugs. Metoclopramide increases the tone and amplitude of gastric (especially antral) contractions, relaxes the pyloric sphincter and the duodenal bulb, and increases peristalsis of the duodenum and jejunum resulting in accelerated gastric emptying and intestinal transit. It increases the resting tone of the lower esophageal sphincter. It has little, if any effect on the motility of the colon or gallbladder.

In patients with gastroesophageal reflux and low LESP (lower esophageal sphincter pressure), single oral doses of metoclopramide produce dose-related increases in LESP. Effects begin at about 5 mg and increase through 20 mg (the largest dose tested). The increase in LESP from a 5 mg dose lasts about 45 minutes and that of 20 mg lasts between 2 and 3 hours. Increased rate of stomach emptying has been observed with single oral doses of 10 mg.

The antiemetic properties of metoclopramide appear to be a result of its antagonism of central and peripheral dopamine receptors. Dopamine produces nausea and vomiting by stimulation of the medullary chemoreceptor trigger zone (CTZ), and metoclopramide blocks stimulation of the CTZ by agents like l-dopa or apomorphine which are known to increase dopamine levels or to possess dopamine-like effects. Metoclopramide also abolishes the slowing of gastric emptying caused by apomorphine.

Like the phenothiazines and related drugs, which are also dopamine antagonists, metoclopramide produces sedation and may produce extrapyramidal reactions, although these are comparatively rare (See Warnings). Metoclopramide inhibits the central and peripheral effects of apomorphine, induces release of prolactin and causes a transient increase in circulating aldosterone levels, which may be associated with transient fluid retention.

The onset of pharmacological action of metoclopramide is 1 to 3 minutes following an intravenous dose, 10 to 15 minutes following intramuscular administration, and 30 to 60 minutes following an oral dose; pharmacological effects persist for 1 to 2 hours.

Pharmacokinetics: Metoclopramide is rapidly and well absorbed. Relative to an intravenous dose of 20 mg, the absolute oral bioavailability of metoclopramide is 80% ± 15.5% as demonstrated in a crossover study of 18 subjects. Peak plasma concentrations occur at about 1–2 hr after a single oral dose. Similar time to peak is observed after individual doses at steady state.

In a single dose study of 12 subjects the area under the drug concentration-time curve increases linearly with doses from 20 to 100 mg. Peak concentrations increase linearly with dose; time to peak concentrations remains the same; whole body clearance is unchanged; and the elimination rate remains the same. The average elimination half-life in individuals with normal renal function is 5–6 hr. Linear kinetic processes adequately describe the absorption and elimination of metoclopramide.

Approximately 85% of the radioactivity of an orally administered dose appears in the urine within 72 hr. Of the 85% eliminated in the urine, about half is present as free or conjugated metoclopramide.

The drug is not extensively bound to plasma proteins (about 30%). The whole body volume of distribution is high (about 3.5 L/kg) which suggests extensive distribution of drug to the tissues.

Renal impairment affects the clearance of metoclopramide. In a study with patients with varying degrees of renal impairment, a reduction in creatinine clearance was correlated with a reduction in plasma clearance, renal clearance, non-renal clearance, and increase in elimination half-life. The kinetics of metoclopramide in the presence of renal impairment remained linear however. The reduction in clearance as a result of renal impairment suggests that adjustment downward of maintenance dosage should be done to avoid drug cumulation.

INDICATIONS AND USAGE

Symptomatic gastroesophageal reflux: Reglan Tablets and Syrup are indicated as short-term (4 to 12 weeks) therapy for adults with symptomatic, documented gastroesophageal reflux who fail to respond to conventional therapy.

The principal effect of metoclopramide is on symptoms of postprandial and daytime heartburn with less observed effect on nocturnal symptoms. If symptoms are confined to particular situations, such as following the evening meal, use of metoclopramide as single doses prior to the provocative situation should be considered, rather than using the drug throughout the day. Healing of esophageal ulcers and erosions has been endoscopically demonstrated at the end of a 12-week trial using doses of 15 mg q.i.d. As there is no documented correlation between symptoms and healing of esophageal lesions, patients with documented lesions should be monitored endoscopically.

Diabetic gastroparesis (diabetic gastric stasis). Reglan (metoclopramide hydrochloride) is indicated for the relief of symptoms associated with acute and recurrent diabetic gastric stasis. The usual manifestations of delayed gastric emptying (e.g., nausea, vomiting, heartburn, persistent fullness after meals and anorexia) appear to respond to Reglan within different time intervals. Significant relief of nausea occurs early and continues to improve over a three-week period. Relief of vomiting and anorexia may precede the relief of abdominal fullness by one week or more.

The prevention of nausea and vomiting associated with emetogenic cancer chemotherapy. Reglan Injectable is indicated for the prophylaxis of vomiting associated with emetogenic cancer chemotherapy.

The prevention of postoperative nausea and vomiting. Reglan Injectable is indicated for the prophylaxis of postoperative nausea and vomiting in those circumstances where nasogastric suction is undesirable.

Small bowel intubation. Reglan Injectable may be used to facilitate small bowel intubation in adults and children in whom the tube does not pass the pylorus with conventional maneuvers.

Radiological examination. Reglan Injectable may be used to stimulate gastric emptying and intestinal transit of barium in cases where delayed emptying interferes with radiological examination of the stomach and/or small intestine.

CONTRAINDICATIONS

Metoclopramide should not be used whenever stimulation of gastrointestinal motility might be dangerous, e.g., in the presence of gastrointestinal hemorrhage, mechanical obstruction, or perforation.

Metoclopramide is contraindicated in patients with pheochromocytoma because the drug may cause a hypertensive crisis, probably due to release of catecholamines from the tumor. Such hypertensive crises may be controlled by phentolamine.

Metoclopramide is contraindicated in patients with known sensitivity or intolerance to the drug.

Metoclopramide should not be used in epileptics or patients receiving other drugs which are likely to cause extrapyramidal reactions, since the frequency and severity of seizures or extrapyramidal reactions may be increased.

WARNINGS

Mental depression has occurred in patients with and without prior history of depression. Symptoms have ranged from mild to severe and have included suicidal ideation and suicide. Metoclopramide should be given to patients with a prior history of depression only if the expected benefits outweigh the potential risks.

Extrapyramidal symptoms, manifested primarily as acute dystonic reactions, occur in approximately 1 in 500 patients treated with the usual adult dosages of 30–40 mg/day of metoclopramide. These usually are seen during the first 24–48 hours of treatment with metoclopramide, occur more frequently in children and young adults, and are even more frequent at the higher doses used in prophylaxis of vomiting due to cancer chemotherapy. These symptoms may include involuntary movements of limbs and facial grimacing, torticollis, oculogyric crisis, rhythmic protrusion of tongue, bulbar type of speech, trismus, or dystonic reactions resembling tetanus. Rarely, dystonic reactions may present as stridor and dyspnea, possibly due to laryngospasm. If these symptoms should occur, inject 50 mg Benadryl® (diphenhydramine hydrochloride) intramuscularly, and they usually will subside. Cogentin® (benztropine mesylate), 1 to 2 mg intramuscularly, may also be used to reverse these reactions.

Parkinsonian-like symptoms have occurred, more commonly within the first 6 months after beginning treatment with metoclopramide, but occasionally after longer periods. These symptoms generally subside within 2–3 months following discontinuance of metoclopramide. Patients with preexisting Parkinson's disease should be given metoclopramide cautiously, if at all, since such patients may experience exacerbation of parkinsonian symptoms when taking metoclopramide.

Tardive Dyskinesia: Tardive dyskinesia, a syndrome consisting of potentially irreversible, involuntary, dyskinetic movements may develop in patients treated with metoclopramide. Although the prevalence of the syndrome appears to be highest among the elderly, especially elderly women, it is impossible to predict which patients are likely to develop the syndrome. Both the risk of developing the syndrome and the likelihood that it will become irreversible are believed to increase with the duration of treatment and the total cumulative dose.

Less commonly, the syndrome can develop after relatively brief treatment periods at low doses; in these cases, symptoms appear more likely to be reversible.

There is no known treatment for established cases of tardive dyskinesia although the syndrome may remit, partially or completely, within several weeks-to-months after metoclopramide is withdrawn. Metoclopramide itself, however, may suppress (or partially suppress) the signs of tardive dyskinesia, thereby masking the underlying disease process. The effect of this symptomatic suppression upon the long-term course of the syndrome is unknown. Therefore, the use of metoclopramide for the symptomatic control of tardive dyskinesia is not recommended.

PRECAUTIONS

General. In one study in hypertensive patients, intravenously administered metoclopramide was shown to release catecholamines; hence, caution should be exercised when metoclopramide is used in patients with hypertension.

Intravenous injections of undiluted metoclopramide should be made slowly allowing 1- to 2-minutes for 10 mg since a transient but intense feeling of anxiety and restlessness, followed by drowsiness, may occur with rapid administration.

Intravenous administration of Reglan Injectable diluted in a parenteral solution should be made slowly over a period of not less than 15 minutes.

Giving a promotility drug such as metoclopramide theoretically could put increased pressure on suture lines following a gut anastomosis or closure. Although adverse events related to this possibility have not been reported to date, the possibility should be considered and weighed when deciding whether to use metoclopramide or nasogastric suction in the prevention of postoperative nausea and vomiting.

Information for patients: Metoclopramide may impair the mental and/or physical abilities required for the performance of hazardous tasks such as operating machinery or driving a motor vehicle. The ambulatory patient should be cautioned accordingly.

Drug Interactions. The effects of metoclopramide on gastrointestinal motility are antagonized by anticholinergic drugs and narcotic analgesics. Additive sedative effects can occur when metoclopramide is given with alcohol, sedatives, hypnotics, narcotics or tranquilizers.

The finding that metoclopramide releases catecholamines in patients with essential hypertension suggests that it should be used cautiously, if at all, in patients receiving monoamine oxidase inhibitors.

Absorption of drugs from the stomach may be diminished (e.g., digoxin) by metoclopramide, whereas absorption of drugs from the small bowel may be accelerated (e.g., acetaminophen, tetracycline, levodopa, ethanol).

Gastroparesis (gastric stasis) may be responsible for poor diabetic control in some patients. Exogenously administered insulin may begin to act before food has left the stomach and lead to hypoglycemia. Because the action of metoclopramide will influence the delivery of food to the intestines and thus the rate of absorption, insulin dosage or timing of dosage may require adjustment.

Carcinogenesis, Mutagenesis, Impairment of Fertility: A 77-week study was conducted in rats in oral doses up to about 40 times the maximum recommended human daily dose. Metoclopramide elevates prolactin levels and the elevation persists during chronic administration. Tissue culture experiments indicate that approximately one-third of human breast cancers are prolactin-dependent *in vitro*, a factor of potential importance if the prescription of metoclopramide is contemplated in a patient with previously detected breast cancer. Although disturbances such as galactorrhea, amenorrhea, gynecomastia, and impotence have been reported with prolactin-elevating drugs, the clinical significance of elevated serum prolactin levels is unknown for most patients. An increase in mammary neoplasms has been found in rodents after chronic administration of prolactin-stimulating neuroleptic drugs and metoclopramide. Neither clinical studies nor epidemiologic studies conducted to date, however, have shown an association between chronic administration of these drugs and mammary tumorigenesis; the available evidence is too limited to be conclusive at this time. An Ames mutagenicity test performed on metoclopramide was negative.

Pregnancy Category B. Reproduction studies performed in rats, mice, and rabbits by the i.v., i.m., s.c. and oral routes at maximum levels ranging from 12 to 250 times the human dose have demonstrated no impairment of fertility or significant harm to the fetus due to metoclopramide. There are, however, no adequate and well-controlled studies in pregnant women. Because animal reproduction studies are not always predictive of human response, this drug should be used during pregnancy only if clearly needed.

Nursing Mothers. Metoclopramide is excreted in human milk. Caution should be exercised when metoclopramide is administered to a nursing mother.

ADVERSE REACTIONS

In general, the incidence of adverse reactions correlates with the dose and duration of metoclopramide administration. The following reactions have been reported, although in most instances, data do not permit an estimate of frequency.

CNS Effects. Restlessness, drowsiness, fatigue and lassitude occur in approximately 10% of patients receiving the most commonly prescribed dosage of 10 mg q.i.d. (see Precautions). Insomnia, headache, confusion, dizziness or mental depression with suicidal ideation (see Warnings) occur less frequently. In cancer chemotherapy patients being treated with 1–2 mg/kg per dose, incidence of drowsiness is about 70%. There are isolated reports of convulsive seizures without clearcut relationship to metoclopramide. Rarely, hallucinations have been reported.

Extrapyramidal Reactions (EPS). Acute dystonic reactions, the most common type of EPS associated with metoclopramide, occur in approximately 0.2% of patients (1 in 500) treated with 30 to 40 mg of metoclopramide per day. In cancer chemotherapy patients receiving 1–2 mg/kg per dose, the incidence is 2% in patients over the ages of 30–35, and 25% or higher in children and young adults who have not had prophylactic administration of diphenhydramine. Symptoms include involuntary movements of limbs, facial grimacing, torticollis, oculogyric crisis, rhythmic protrusion of tongue, bulbar type of speech, trismus, opisthotonus (tetanus-like reactions) and rarely, stridor and dyspnea possibly due to laryngospasm; ordinarily these symptoms are readily reversed by diphenhydramine (see Warnings).

Parkinsonian-like symptoms may include bradykinesia, tremor, cogwheel rigidity, mask-like facies (see Warnings). Tardive dyskinesia most frequently is characterized by involuntary movements of the tongue, face, mouth or jaw, and sometimes by involuntary movements of the trunk and/or extremities (see Warnings).

Motor restlessness (akathisia) may consist of feelings of anxiety, agitation, jitteriness, and insomnia, as well as inability to sit still, pacing, foot-tapping. These symptoms may disappear spontaneously or respond to a reduction in dosage.

Endocrine Disturbances. Galactorrhea, amenorrhea, gynecomastia, impotence secondary to hyperprolactinemia (see Precautions). Fluid retention secondary to transient elevation of aldosterone (see Clinical Pharmacology).

Cardiovascular. Hypotension, hypertension and a single instance of supraventricular tachycardia (see Contraindications, Precautions).

Gastrointestinal. Nausea and bowel disturbances, primarily diarrhea.

Hepatic. Rarely, cases of hepatotoxicity, characterized by such findings as jaundice and altered liver function tests, when metoclopramide was administered with other drugs with known hepatotoxic potential.

Renal. Urinary frequency and incontinence.

Hematologic. A few cases of neutropenia, leukopenia, or agranulocytosis, generally without clearcut relationship to metoclopramide. Methemoglobinemia, especially with overdosage in neonates (see Overdosage).

Allergic Reactions. A few cases of rash, urticaria, or bronchospasm, especially in patients with a history of asthma. Rarely, angioneurotic edema, including glossal or laryngeal edema.

Miscellaneous. Visual disturbances. Porphyria. Rare occurrences of neuroleptic malignant syndrome (NMS) have been reported. This potentially fatal syndrome is comprised of the symptom complex of hyperthermia, altered consciousness, muscular rigidity and autonomic dysfunction.

Transient flushing of the face and upper body, without alterations in vital signs, following high doses intravenously.

OVERDOSAGE

Symptoms of overdosage may include drowsiness, disorientation and extrapyramidal reactions. Anticholinergic or antiparkinson drugs or antihistamines with anticholinergic properties may be helpful in controlling the extrapyramidal reactions. Symptoms are self-limiting and usually disappear within 24 hours.

Hemodialysis removes relatively little metoclopramide, probably because of the small amount of the drug in blood relative to tissues. Similarly, continuous ambulatory peritoneal dialysis does not remove significant amounts of drug. It is unlikely that dosage would need to be adjusted to compensate for losses through dialysis. Dialysis is not likely to be an effective method of drug removal in overdose situations.

Methemoglobinemia has occurred in premature and full-term neonates who were given overdoses of metoclopramide (1–4 mg/kg/day orally, intramuscularly or intravenously for 1–3 or more days). Methemoglobinemia has not been reported in neonates treated with 0.5 mg/kg/day in divided doses. Methemoglobinemia can be reversed by the intravenous administration of methylene blue.

DOSAGE AND ADMINISTRATION

For the relief of symptomatic gastroesophageal reflux: Administer from 10 mg to 15 mg Reglan orally up to q.i.d. 30 minutes before each meal and at bedtime, depending upon symptoms being treated and clinical response (see Clinical Pharmacology and Indications). If symptoms occur only intermittently or at specific times of the day, use of metoclopramide in single doses up to 20 mg prior to the provoking situation may be preferred rather than continuous treatment. Occasionally, patients (such as elderly patients) who are more sensitive to the therapeutic or adverse effects of metoclopramide will require only 5 mg per dose.

Experience with esophageal erosions and ulcerations is limited, but healing has thus far been documented in one controlled trial using q.i.d. therapy at 15 mg/dose, and this regimen should be used when lesions are present, so long as it is tolerated (see Adverse Reactions). Because of the poor correlation between symptoms and endoscopic appearance of the esophagus, therapy directed at esophageal lesions is best guided by endoscopic evaluation.

Therapy longer than 12 weeks has not been evaluated and cannot be recommended.

For the relief of symptoms associated with diabetic gastroparesis (diabetic gastric stasis): Administer 10 mg of metoclopramide 30 minutes before each meal and at bedtime for two to eight weeks, depending upon response and the likelihood of continued well-being upon drug discontinuation.

The initial route of administration should be determined by the severity of the presenting symptoms. If only the earliest manifestations of diabetic gastric stasis are present, oral administration of Reglan may be initiated. However, if severe symptoms are present, therapy should begin with Reglan Injectable (I.M. or I.V.). Doses of 10 mg may be administered slowly by the intravenous route over a 1-to-2 minute period.

Administration of Reglan Injectable up to 10 days may be required before symptoms subside, at which time oral administration may be instituted. Since diabetic gastric stasis is frequently recurrent, Reglan therapy should be reinstituted at the earliest manifestation.

For the prevention of nausea and vomiting associated with emetogenic cancer chemotherapy: For doses in excess of 10 mg, Reglan Injectable should be diluted in 50 mL of a parenteral solution.

The preferred parenteral solution is Sodium Chloride Injection (normal saline), which when combined with Reglan Injectable, can be stored frozen for up to 4 weeks. Reglan Injectable is degraded when admixed and frozen with Dex-

trose-5% in Water. Reglan Injectable diluted in Sodium Chloride Injection, Dextrose-5% in Water, Dextrose-5% in 0.45% Sodium Chloride, Ringer's Injection or Lactated Ringer's Injection may be stored up to 48 hours (without freezing) after preparation if protected from light. All dilutions may be stored unprotected from light under normal light conditions up to 24 hours after preparation.

Intravenous infusions should be made slowly over a period of not less than 15 minutes, 30 minutes before beginning cancer chemotherapy and repeated every 2 hours for two doses, then every 3 hours for three doses.

The initial two doses should be 2 mg/kg if highly emetogenic drugs such as cisplatin or dacarbazine are used alone or in combination. For less emetogenic regimens, 1 mg/kg per dose may be adequate.

If extrapyramidal symptoms should occur, inject 50 mg Benadryl® (diphenhydramine hydrochloride) intramuscularly, and EPS usually will subside.

For the prevention of postoperative nausea and vomiting: Reglan Injectable should be given intramuscularly near the end of surgery. The usual adult dose is 10 mg; however, doses of 20 mg may be used.

To facilitate small bowel intubation: If the tube has not passed the pylorus with conventional maneuvers in 10 minutes, a single dose (undiluted) may be administered slowly by the intravenous route over a 1- to 2-minute period.

The recommended single dose is: Adults—10 mg metoclopramide base. Children (6–14 years of age)—2.5 to 5 mg metoclopramide base; (under 6 years of age)—0.1 mg/kg metoclopramide base.

To aid in radiological examinations: In patients where delayed gastric emptying interferes with radiological examination of the stomach and/or small intestine, a single dose may be administered slowly by the intravenous route over a 1- to 2-minute period.

For dosage, see intubation, above.

Use in Patients with Renal or Hepatic Impairment: Since metoclopramide is excreted principally through the kidneys, in those patients whose creatinine clearance is below 40 mL/min, therapy should be initiated at approximately one-half the recommended dosage. Depending upon clinical efficacy and safety considerations, the dosage may be increased or decreased as appropriate.

See Overdosage section for information regarding dialysis. Metoclopramide undergoes minimal hepatic metabolism, except for simple conjugation. Its safe use has been described in patients with advanced liver disease whose renal function was normal.

NOTE: Parenteral drug products should be inspected visually for particulate matter and discoloration prior to administration, whenever solution and container permit.

Admixture Compatibilities. Reglan (metoclopramide hydrochloride) Injectable is compatible for mixing and injection with the following dosage forms to the extent indicated below:

Physically and Chemically Compatible up to 48 hours. Cimetidine Hydrochloride (SK&F), Mannitol, USP (Abbott), Potassium Acetate, USP (Invenex), Potassium Chloride, USP (ESI), Potassium Phosphate, USP (Invenex).

Physically Compatible up to 48 hours. Ascorbic Acid, USP (Abbott), Benztropine Mesylate, USP (MS&D), Cytarabine, USP (Upjohn), Dexamethasone Sodium Phosphate, USP (ESI, MS&D), Diphenhydramine Hydrochloride, USP (Parke-Davis), Doxorubicin Hydrochloride, USP (Adria), Heparin Sodium, USP (ESI), Hydrocortisone Sodium Phosphate (MS&D), Lidocaine Hydrochloride, USP (ESI), Magnesium Sulfate, USP (ESI), Multi-Vitamin Infusion (must be refrigerated-USV), Vitamin B Complex with Ascorbic Acid (Roche).

Physically Compatible up to 24 hours (Do not use if precipitation occurs). Aminophylline, USP (ESI), Clindamycin Phosphate, USP (Upjohn), Cyclophosphamide, USP (Mead-Johnson), Insulin, USP (Lilly), Methylprednisolone Sodium Succinate, USP (ESI).

Conditionally Compatible (Use within one hour after mixing or may be infused directly into the same running IV line). Ampicillin Sodium, USP (Bristol), Calcium Gluconate, USP (ESI), Cisplatin (Bristol), Erythromycin Lactobionate, USP (Abbott), Methotrexate Sodium, USP (Lederle), Penicillin G Potassium, USP (Squibb), Tetracycline Hydrochloride, USP (Lederle).

Incompatible (Do Not Mix). Cephalothin Sodium, USP (Lilly), Chloramphenicol Sodium, USP (Parke-Davis), Sodium Bicarbonate, USP (Abbott).

HOW SUPPLIED

Each pink, capsule-shaped, scored Reglan® Tablet contains 10 mg metoclopramide base (as the monohydrochloride mon-

Continued on next page

Robins—Cont.

Container	Total Contents #	Concen- tration #	Administration
2 mL single dose vial/ampul	10 mg	5 mg/mL	FOR IV or IM ADMINISTRATION
10 mL single dose vial/ampul	50 mg	5 mg/mL	FOR IV INFUSION ONLY; DILUTE BEFORE USING
30 mL single dose vial	150 mg	5 mg/mL	FOR IV INFUSION ONLY; DILUTE BEFORE USING

\# Metoclopramide base (as the monohydrochloride monohydrate)

ohydrate). Available in bottles of 100 (NDC 0031-6701-63), and 500 tablets (NDC 0031-6701-70) and Dis-Co® Unit Dose Packs of 100 tablets (NDC 0031-6701-64).

Each green, elliptical-shaped Reglan® Tablet contains 5 mg metoclopramide base (as the monohydrochloride monohydrate). Available in bottles of 100 (NDC 0031-6705-63) and Dis-Co® Unit Dose Packs of 100 tablets (NDC 0031-6705-64). Dispense in tight, light-resistant container.

Reglan® Syrup, 5 mg metoclopramide base (as the monohydrochloride monohydrate) per 5 mL, available in pints (NDC 0031-6706-25) and 10 mL Dis-Co® Unit Dose Packs (10 × 10s) (NDC 0031-6706-26). Dispense syrup in tight, light-resistant container.

Preservative-free:
Reglan® Injectable, **5 mg** metoclopramide base (as the monohydrochloride monohydrate) **per mL;** available in 2 mL single dose vials in cartons of 25 (NDC 0031-6709-72), 10 mL single dose vials in cartons of 25 (NDC 0031-6709-78); 30 mL single dose vials in cartons of 6 (NDC 0031-6709-85) and in cartons of 25 (NDC 0031-6709-24); 2 mL ampuls in cartons of 5 (NDC 0031-6709-90) and 25 (NDC 0031-6709-95); 10 mL ampuls in cartons of 25 (NDC 0031-6709-94).
[See table above.]

Store vials and ampuls in carton until used. Do not store open single dose vials or ampuls for later use, as they contain no preservative.

Dilutions may be stored unprotected from light under normal light conditions up to 24 hours after preparation.
TABLETS, SYRUP AND INJECTABLE SHOULD BE STORED AT CONTROLLED ROOM TEMPERATURE BETWEEN 15°C and 30°C (59°F and 86°F).
Reglan Injectable is manufactured for Pharmaceutical Division, A. H. Robins Company, Richmond, Virginia 23220 by Elkins-Sinn, Inc., Cherry Hill, NJ 08003, a subsidiary of A. H. Robins.

Tablets Shown in Product Identification Section, page 424

ROBAXIN® INJECTABLE   ℞
[ro "baks 'in]
brand of Methocarbamol Injection, USP

PRODUCT OVERVIEW

KEY FACTS
Robaxin Injectable is a parenteral dosage form containing 100 mg of methocarbamol per mL, for intravenous and intramuscular use.

MAJOR USE
The injectable form of methocarbamol is indicated as an adjunct to rest, physical therapy and other measures for the relief of discomfort associated with acute painful musculoskeletal conditions.

SAFETY INFORMATION
Robaxin Injectable is contraindicated in patients hypersensitive to any of the ingredients. Patients should be cautioned about the combined effects with alcohol and other CNS depressants. Administration to patients with epilepsy is not recommended. The rate of injection should not exceed 3 mL per minute. Vascular extravasation must be avoided.

PRESCRIBING INFORMATION

ROBAXIN® INJECTABLE   ℞
[ro "baks 'in]
brand of Methocarbamol Injection, USP

DESCRIPTION
Robaxin Injectable is a parenteral dosage form.
Each mL contains:
Methocarbamol, USP **100 mg;** Polyethylene Glycol 300, NF 0.5 mL; Water for Injection, USP q.s. pH adjusted, when necessary, with hydrochloric acid and/or sodium hydroxide.
AFTER MIXING WITH I.V. INFUSION FLUIDS, **DO NOT REFRIGERATE.**

ACTIONS
The mechanism of action of methocarbamol in humans has not been established, but may be due to general central nervous system depression. It has no direct action on the contractile mechanism of striated muscle, the motor end plate or the nerve fiber.

INDICATIONS
The injectable form of methocarbamol is indicated as an adjunct to rest, physical therapy, and other measures for the relief of discomfort associated with acute, painful musculoskeletal conditions. The mode of action of this drug has not been clearly identified, but may be related to its sedative properties. Methocarbamol does not directly relax tense skeletal muscles in man.

CONTRAINDICATIONS
Robaxin Injectable should not be administered to patients with known or suspected renal pathology. This caution is necessary because of the presence of polyethylene glycol 300 in the vehicle.
A much larger amount of polyethylene glycol 300 than is present in recommended doses of Robaxin Injectable is known to have increased pre-existing acidosis and urea retention in patients with renal impairment. Although the amount present in this preparation is well within the limits of safety, caution dictates this contraindication.
Robaxin Injectable is contraindicated in patients hypersensitive to any of the ingredients.

WARNINGS
Since methocarbamol may possess a general central nervous system depressant effect, patients receiving Robaxin Injectable (methocarbamol injection) should be cautioned about combined effects with alcohol and other CNS depressants. Safe use of Robaxin Injectable has not been established with regard to possible adverse effects upon fetal development. Therefore, Robaxin Injectable should not be used in women who are or may become pregnant and particularly during early pregnancy unless in the judgment of the physician the potential benefits outweigh the possible hazards.

PRECAUTIONS
As with other agents administered either intravenously or intramuscularly, careful supervision of dose and rate of injection should be observed. Rate of injection should not exceed 3 mL per minute—i.e., one 10 mL vial in approximately three minutes. Since Robaxin Injectable is hypertonic, vascular extravasation must be avoided. A recumbent position will reduce the likelihood of side reactions.
Blood aspirated into the syringe does not mix with the hypertonic solution. This phenomenon occurs with many other intravenous preparations. The blood may be safely injected with the methocarbamol, or the injection may be stopped when the plunger reaches the blood, whichever the physician prefers.
The total dosage should not exceed 30 mL (three vials) a day for more than three consecutive days except in the treatment of tetanus.
Caution should be observed in using the injectable form in suspected or known epileptic patients.
Safety and effectiveness in children below the age of 12 years have not been established except in tetanus. See special directions for use in tetanus.
It is not known whether this drug is secreted in human milk. As a general rule, nursing should not be undertaken while a patient is on a drug since many drugs are excreted in human milk.
Methocarbamol may cause a color interference in certain screening tests for 5-hydroxyindoleacetic acid (5-HIAA) and vanillylmandelic acid (VMA).

ADVERSE REACTIONS
Dizziness, lightheadedness, drowsiness, vertigo, fainting, syncope, hypotension, gastrointestinal upset, metallic taste, thrombophlebitis, sloughing at the site of injection, pain at the site of injection, anaphylactic reaction, urticaria, pruritus, rash, conjunctivitis with nasal congestion, flushing, nystagmus, diplopia, mild muscular incoordination, bradycardia, blurred vision, headache, fever. In most cases of syncope there was spontaneous recovery. In others, epinephrine, injectable steroids and/or injectable antihistamines were employed to hasten recovery. Certain of these complaints may have been due to any overly rapid rate of intravenous injection.
The onset of convulsive seizures during intravenous administration has been reported, including instances in known epileptics. The psychic trauma of the procedure may have been a contributing factor. Although several observers have reported success in terminating epileptiform seizures with Robaxin Injectable, its administration to patients with epilepsy is not recommended.

DOSAGE AND ADMINISTRATION
For Intravenous and Intramuscular Use Only. Total adult dosage should not exceed 30 mL (3 vials) a day for more than 3 consecutive days except in the treatment of tetanus. A like course may be repeated after a lapse of 48 hours if the condition persists. Dosage and frequency of injection should be based on the severity of the condition being treated and therapeutic response noted.
For the relief of symptoms of moderate degree, 10 mL (one vial) may be adequate. Ordinarily this injection need not be repeated, as the administration of the oral form will usually sustain the relief initiated by the injection. For the severest cases or in postoperative conditions in which oral administration is not feasible, 20 to 30 mL (two to three vials) may be required.
Directions for Intravenous Use. Robaxin Injectable may be administered undiluted directly into the vein at a *maximum rate of three mL per minute.* It may also be added to an intravenous drip of Sodium Chloride Injection (Sterile Isotonic Sodium Chloride Solution for Parenteral Use) or five per cent Dextrose Injection (Sterile 5 per cent Dextrose Solution); one vial given as a single dose should not be diluted to more than 250 mL for I. V. infusion. Care should be exercised to avoid vascular extravasation of this hypertonic solution which may result in thrombophlebitis. It is preferable that the patient be in a recumbent position during and for at least 10 to 15 minutes following the injection.
Directions for Intramuscular Use. When the intramuscular route is indicated, not more than five mL (one-half vial) should be injected into each gluteal region. The injections may be repeated at eight hour intervals, if necessary. When satisfactory relief of symptoms is achieved, it can usually be maintained with tablets.
Not Recommended for Subcutaneous Administration.
Special Directions for Use in Tetanus: There is clinical evidence which suggests that methocarbamol may have a beneficial effect in the control of the neuromuscular manifestations of tetanus. It does not, however, replace the usual procedure of debridement, tetanus antitoxin, penicillin, tracheotomy, attention to fluid balance, and supportive care. Robaxin Injectable should be added to the regimen as soon as possible.
For adults: Inject one or two vials directly into the tubing of a previously inserted indwelling needle. An additional 10 mL or 20 mL may be added to the infusion bottle so that a total of up to 30 mL (three vials) is given as the initial dose (note Precautions). This procedure should be repeated every six hours until conditions allow for the insertion of a nasogastric tube. Crushed Robaxin (methocarbamol) tablets suspended in water or saline may then be given through this tube. Total daily oral doses up to 24 grams may be required as judged by patient response.
For children: A minimum initial dose of 15 mg/kg is recommended. This dosage may be repeated every six hours as indicated. The maintenance dosage may be given by injection into the tubing or by I.V. infusion with an appropriate quantity of fluid. See directions for I.V. use.

HOW SUPPLIED
Robaxin Injectable—10 mL single dose vials in packages of 5 (NDC 0031-7409-87) and 25 (NDC 0031-7409-94).
Manufactured for PHARMACEUTICAL DIVISION, A. H. ROBINS CO., Richmond, VA 23220, by ELKINS-SINN, INC. Cherry Hill, NJ 08003-4099 a subsidiary of A. H. Robins.
Shown in Product Identification Section, page 424

ROBAXIN® TABLETS   ℞
[ro "baks 'in]
brand of Methocarbamol Tablets, USP
500 mg per tablet
ROBAXIN®–750 TABLETS
brand of Methocarbamol Tablets, USP   ℞
750 mg per tablet

PRODUCT OVERVIEW

KEY FACTS
Robaxin/Robaxin-750 tablets contain 500 mg and 750 mg of methocarbamol, respectively.

MAJOR USE
Robaxin (methocarbamol) is indicated as an adjunct to rest, physical therapy, and other measures for the relief of discomforts associated with acute, painful musculoskeletal conditions.

SAFETY INFORMATION
Robaxin (methocarbamol) is contraindicated in patients hypersensitive to any of the ingredients. Patients should be cautioned about combined effects with alcohol and other CNS depressants.

PRESCRIBING INFORMATION

ROBAXIN® TABLETS   ℞
[ro "baks 'in]
brand of Methocarbamol Tablets, USP
500 mg per tablet

ROBAXIN®–750 TABLETS ℞
brand of Methocarbamol Tablets, USP
750 mg per tablet

DESCRIPTION
Inactive Ingredients: ROBAXIN—Corn Starch, FD&C Yellow 6 Aluminum Lake, Hydroxypropyl Cellulose, Hydroxypropyl Methylcellulose, Magnesium Stearate, Polysorbate 20, Povidone, Propylene Glycol, Saccharin Sodium, Sodium Lauryl Sulfate, Sodium Starch Glycolate, Stearic Acid, Titanium Dioxide.
ROBAXIN-750—Corn Starch, D&C Yellow 10 Aluminum Lake, FD&C Yellow 6 Aluminum Lake, Hydroxypropyl Cellulose, Hydroxypropyl Methylcellulose, Magnesium Stearate, Polysorbate 20, Povidone, Propylene Glycol, Saccharin Sodium, Sodium Lauryl Sulfate, Sodium Starch Glycolate, Stearic Acid, Titanium Dioxide.

ACTIONS
The mechanism of action of methocarbamol in humans has not been established, but may be due to general central nervous system depression. It has no direct action on the contractile mechanism of striated muscle, the motor end plate or the nerve fiber.

INDICATIONS
Robaxin (methocarbamol) is indicated as an adjunct to rest, physical therapy, and other measures for the relief of discomforts associated with acute, painful musculoskeletal conditions. The mode of action of this drug has not been clearly identified, but may be related to its sedative properties. Methocarbamol does not directly relax tense skeletal muscles in man.

CONTRAINDICATIONS
Robaxin is contraindicated in patients hypersensitive to any of the ingredients.

WARNINGS
Since methocarbamol may possess a general central nervous system depressant effect, patients receiving Robaxin/Robaxin-750 (methocarbamol tablets) should be cautioned about combined effects with alcohol and other CNS depressants. Safe use of methocarbamol has not been established with regard to possible adverse effects upon fetal development. Therefore, methocarbamol tablets should not be used in women who are or may become pregnant and particularly during early pregnancy unless in the judgment of the physician the potential benefits outweigh the possible hazards.

PRECAUTIONS
Safety and effectiveness in children below the age of 12 years have not been established.
It is not known whether this drug is secreted in human milk. As a general rule, nursing should not be undertaken while a patient is on a drug since many drugs are excreted in human milk.
Methocarbamol may cause a color interference in certain screening tests for 5-hydroxyindoleacetic acid (5-HIAA) and vanilmandelic acid (VMA).

ADVERSE REACTIONS
Lightheadedness, dizziness, drowsiness, nausea, allergic manifestations such as urticaria, pruritus, rash, conjunctivitis with nasal congestion, blurred vision, headache, fever.

DOSAGE AND ADMINISTRATION
Robaxin (methocarbamol), 500 mg—Adults: initial dosage, 3 tablets q.i.d.; maintenance dosage, 2 tablets q.i.d.
Robaxin-750 (methocarbamol), 750 mg — Adults: initial dosage, 2 tablets q.i.d.; maintenance dosage, 1 tablet q.4h. or 2 tablets t.i.d.
Six grams a day are recommended for the first 48 to 72 hours of treatment. (For severe conditions 8 grams a day may be administered.) Thereafter, the dosage can usually be reduced to approximately 4 grams a day.

HOW SUPPLIED
Robaxin—light orange, round, film-coated tablets monogrammed Robaxin and AHR in bottles of 100 (NDC 0031-7429-63), 500 (NDC 0031-7429-70) and Dis-Co® unit dose packs of 100 (NDC 0031-7429-64).
Robaxin-750—orange, capsule-shaped, film-coated tablets monogrammed Robaxin-750 and AHR in bottles of 100 (NDC 0031-7449-63), 500 (NDC 0031-7449-70) and Dis-Co® unit dose packs of 100 (NDC 0031-7449-64).
Store at Controlled Room Temperature. Between 15°C and 30°C (59°F and 86°F).
Dispense in tight container.
Shown in Product Identification Section, page 424

ROBAXISAL® TABLETS ℞
[ro"baks'ĭ-sal"]

PRODUCT OVERVIEW
KEY FACTS
Robaxisal is available as a pink and white laminated tablet containing 400 mg of methocarbamol and 325 mg of aspirin. Robaxisal provides a double approach to the management of discomforts associated with musculoskeletal disorders.

MAJOR USE
Robaxisal is indicated as an adjunct to rest, physical therapy, and other measures for the relief of discomfort associated with acute, painful musculoskeletal conditions.

SAFETY INFORMATION
Robaxisal is contraindicated in patients hypersensitive to aspirin or methocarbamol. Patients should be cautioned about combined effects with alcohol and other CNS depressants.

PRESCRIBING INFORMATION
ROBAXISAL® TABLETS ℞
[ro"baks'ĭ-sal"]

DESCRIPTION
For oral administration, Robaxisal is available as a pink and white laminated tablet containing:
Methocarbamol, USP ....400 mg
Aspirin, USP...325 mg
Inactive Ingredients: Corn Starch, FD&C Red 3, Magnesium Stearate, Povidone, Sodium Lauryl Sulfate, Sodium Starch Glycolate, Stearic Acid.

ACTIONS
Robaxisal provides a double approach to the management of discomforts associated with musculoskeletal disorders.
Methocarbamol. The mechanism of action of methocarbamol in humans has not been established, but may be due to general central nervous system depression. It has no direct action on the contractile mechanism of striated muscle, the motor end plate or the nerve fiber.
Aspirin. Aspirin is a mild analgesic with anti-inflammatory and antipyretic activity.

INDICATIONS
Robaxisal is indicated as an adjunct to rest, physical therapy, and other measures for the relief of discomfort associated with acute, painful musculoskeletal conditions. The mode of action of methocarbamol has not been clearly identified but may be related to its sedative properties. Methocarbamol does not directly relax tense skeletal muscles in man.

CONTRAINDICATIONS
Hypersensitivity to methocarbamol or aspirin.

WARNINGS
Salicylates have been reported to be associated with the development of Reye syndrome in children and teenagers with chicken pox, influenza, and influenza-like infections. Since methocarbamol may possess a general central nervous system depressant effect, patients receiving Robaxisal should be cautioned about combined effects with alcohol and other CNS depressants.

PRECAUTIONS
Products containing aspirin should be administered with caution to patients with gastritis or peptic ulceration, or those receiving hypoprothrombinemic anticoagulants.
Methocarbamol may cause a color interference in certain screening tests for 5-hydroxyindoleacetic acid (5-HIAA) and vanilmandelic acid (VMA).
Pregnancy. Safe use of Robaxisal has not been established with regard to possible adverse effects upon fetal development. Therefore, Robaxisal should not be used in women who are or may become pregnant and particularly during early pregnancy unless in the judgment of the physician the potential benefits outweigh the possible hazards.
Nursing Mothers. It is not known whether methocarbamol is secreted in human milk; however, aspirin does appear in human milk in moderate amounts. It can produce a bleeding tendency either by interfering with the function of the infant's platelets or by decreasing the amount of prothrombin in the blood. The risk is minimal if the mother takes the aspirin just after nursing and if the infant has an adequate store of vitamin K. As a general rule, nursing should not be undertaken while a patient is on a drug.
Pediatric Use. Safety and effectiveness in children 12 years of age and below have not been established.
Use in Activities Requiring Mental Alertness. Robaxisal may rarely cause drowsiness. Until the patient's response has been determined, he should be cautioned against the operation of motor vehicles or dangerous machinery.

ADVERSE REACTIONS
The most frequent adverse reaction to methocarbamol is dizziness or lightheadedness and nausea. This occurs in about one in 20–25 patients. Less frequent reactions are drowsiness, blurred vision, headache, fever, allergic manifestations such as urticaria, pruritus, and rash.
Adverse reactions that have been associated with the use of aspirin include: nausea and other gastrointestinal discomfort, gastritis, gastric erosion, vomiting, constipation, diarrhea, angio-edema, asthma, rash, pruritus, urticaria. Gastrointestinal discomfort may be minimized by taking Robaxisal with food.

DOSAGE AND ADMINISTRATION
Adults and children over 12 years of age: Two tablets four times daily. Three tablets four times daily may be used in severe conditions for one to three days in patients who are able to tolerate salicylates. These dosage recommendations provide respectively 3.2 and 4.8 grams of methocarbamol per day. For Chicken Pox or Flu, see Warnings.

OVERDOSAGE
Toxicity due to overdosage of methocarbamol is unlikely; however, acute overdosage of aspirin may cause symptoms of salicylate intoxication.
Treatment of Overdosage. Supportive therapy for 24 hours, as methocarbamol is excreted within that time. If salicylate intoxication occurs, especially in children, the hyperpnea may be controlled with sodium bicarbonate. Judicious use of 5% CO_2 with 95% O_2 may be of benefit. Abnormal electrolyte patterns should be corrected with appropriate fluid therapy.

HOW SUPPLIED
Robaxisal® is supplied as pink and white laminated, compressed tablets monogrammed AHR and Robaxisal in bottles of 100 (NDC 0031-7469-63), 500 (NDC 0031-7469-70) and Dis-Co® Unit Dose Packs of 100 (NDC 0031-7469-64).
Store at controlled room temperature, between 15°C and 30°C (59°F and 86°F).
Dispense in well-closed container.
Shown in Product Identification Section, page 424

ROBINUL® TABLETS ℞
[ro'bĭ-nul]
ROBINUL® FORTE TABLETS ℞
brand of Glycopyrrolate Tablets, USP

DESCRIPTION
Robinul and Robinul Forte tablets contain the synthetic anticholinergic, glycopyrrolate. Glycopyrrolate is a quaternary ammonium compound with the following chemical name: 3-[(cyclopentylhydroxyphenylacetyl)oxy]-1,1-dimethylpyrrolidinium bromide.
Robinul tablets are scored, compressed pink tablets engraved AHR and 7824. Each tablet contains:
Glycopyrrolate, USP..1 mg
Robinul Forte tablets are scored, compressed pink tablets engraved $\frac{AHR}{2}$ on one side and 7840 on the reverse side.
Each tablet contains:
Glycopyrrolate, USP..2 mg
Inactive Ingredients: Dibasic Calcium Phosphate, FD&C Red 3 Aluminum Lake, Lactose, Magnesium Stearate, Povidone, Sodium Starch Glycolate.

ACTIONS
Glycopyrrolate, like other anticholinergic (antimuscarinic) agents, inhibits the action of acetylcholine on structures innervated by postganglionic cholinergic nerves and on smooth muscles that respond to acetylcholine but lack cholinergic innervation. These peripheral cholinergic receptors are present in the autonomic effector cells of smooth muscle, cardiac muscle, the sino-atrial node, the atrioventricular node, exocrine glands, and, to a limited degree, in the autonomic ganglia. Thus, it diminishes the volume and free acidity of gastric secretions and controls excessive pharyngeal, tracheal, and bronchial secretions.
Glycopyrrolate antagonizes muscarinic symptoms (e.g., bronchorrhea, bronchospasm, bradycardia, and intestinal hypermotility) induced by cholinergic drugs such as the anticholinesterases.
The highly polar quaternary ammonium group of glycopyrrolate limits its passage across lipid membranes, such as the blood-brain barrier, in contrast to atropine sulfate and scopolamine hydrobromide, which are non-polar tertiary amines which penetrate lipid barriers easily.

INDICATIONS
For use as adjunctive therapy in the treatment of peptic ulcer.

Continued on next page

Prescribing information on A. H. Robins products listed here is based on official labeling in effect June 1, 1989, with Indications, Contraindications, Warnings, Precautions, Adverse Reactions, and Dosage stated in full.

Robins—Cont.

CONTRAINDICATIONS

Glaucoma; obstructive uropathy (for example, bladder neck obstruction due to prostatic hypertrophy); obstructive disease of the gastrointestinal tract (as in achalasia, pyloroduodenal stenosis, etc.); paralytic ileus; intestinal atony of the elderly or debilitated patient; unstable cardiovascular status in acute hemorrhage; severe ulcerative colitis; toxic megacolon complicating ulcerative colitis; myasthenia gravis. Robinul (glycopyrrolate) tablets are contraindicated in those patients with a hypersensitivity to glycopyrrolate.

WARNINGS

In the presence of a high environmental temperature, heat prostration (fever and heat stroke due to decreased sweating) can occur with use of Robinul.

Diarrhea may be an early symptom of incomplete intestinal obstruction, especially in patients with ileostomy or colostomy. In this instance treatment with this drug would be inappropriate and possibly harmful.

Robinul (glycopyrrolate) may produce drowsiness or blurred vision. In this event, the patient should be warned not to engage in activities requiring mental alertness such as operating a motor vehicle or other machinery, or performing hazardous work while taking this drug.

Theoretically, with overdosage a curare-like action may occur, i.e., neuromuscular blockade leading to muscular weakness and possible paralysis.

Pregnancy. The safety of this drug during pregnancy has not been established. The use of any drug during pregnancy requires that the potential benefits of the drug be weighed against possible hazards to mother and child. Reproduction studies in rats revealed no teratogenic effects from glycopyrrolate; however, the potent anticholinergic action of this agent resulted in diminished rates of conception and of survival at weaning, in a dose-related manner. Other studies in dogs suggest that this may be due to diminished seminal secretion which is evident at high doses of glycopyrrolate. Information on possible adverse effects in the pregnant female is limited to uncontrolled data derived from marketing experience. Such experience has revealed no reports of teratogenic or other fetus-damaging potential. No controlled studies to establish the safety of the drug in pregnancy have been performed.

Nursing Mothers. It is not known whether this drug is secreted in human milk. As a general rule, nursing should not be undertaken while a patient is on a drug since many drugs are excreted in human milk.

Pediatric Use. Since there is no adequate experience in children who have received this drug, safety and efficacy in children have not been established.

PRECAUTIONS

Use Robinul with caution in the elderly and in all patients with:
- Autonomic neuropathy.
- Hepatic or renal disease.
- Ulcerative colitis—large doses may suppress intestinal motility to the point of producing a paralytic ileus and for this reason may precipitate or aggravate "toxic megacolon," a serious complication of the disease.
- Hyperthyroidism, coronary heart disease, congestive heart failure, cardiac tachyarrhythmias, tachycardia, hypertension and prostatic hypertrophy.
- Hiatal hernia associated with reflux esophagitis, since anticholinergic drugs may aggravate this condition.

ADVERSE REACTIONS

Anticholinergics produce certain effects, most of which are extensions of their fundamental pharmacological actions. Adverse reactions to anticholinergics in general may include xerostomia; decreased sweating; urinary hesitancy and retention; blurred vision; tachycardia; palpitations; dilatation of the pupil; cycloplegia; increased ocular tension; loss of taste; headaches; nervousness; mental confusion; drowsiness; weakness; dizziness; insomnia; nausea; vomiting; constipation; bloated feeling; impotence; suppression of lactation; severe allergic reaction or drug idiosyncrasies including anaphylaxis; urticaria and other dermal manifestations.

Robinul (glycopyrrolate) is chemically a quaternary ammonium compound; hence, its passage across lipid membranes, such as the blood-brain barrier, is limited in contrast to atropine sulfate and scopolamine hydrobromide. For this reason the occurrence of CNS related side effects is lower, in comparison to their incidence following administration of anticholinergics which are chemically tertiary amines that can cross this barrier readily.

OVERDOSAGE

The symptoms of overdosage of glycopyrrolate are peripheral in nature rather than central.

1. To guard against further absorption of the drug—use gastric lavage, cathartics and/or enemas.

2. To combat peripheral anticholinergic effects (residual mydriasis, dry mouth, etc.)—utilize a quaternary ammo-

nium anticholinesterase, such as neostigmine methylsulfate.

3. To combat hypotension—use pressor amines (norepinephrine, metaraminol) i.v.; and supportive care.

4. To combat respiratory depression—administer oxygen; utilize a respiratory stimulant such as Dopram® i.v.; artificial respiration.

DOSAGE AND ADMINISTRATION

The dosage of Robinul or Robinul Forte should be adjusted to the needs of the individual patient to assure symptomatic control with a minimum of adverse reactions. The presently recommended maximum daily dosage of glycopyrrolate is 8 mg.

Robinul (glycopyrrolate, 1 mg) tablets. The recommended initial dosage of Robinul for adults is one tablet three times daily (in the morning, early afternoon, and at bedtime). Some patients may require two tablets at bedtime to assure overnight control of symptoms. For maintenance, a dosage of one tablet twice a day is frequently adequate.

Robinul Forte (glycopyrrolate, 2 mg) tablets. The recommended dosage of Robinul Forte for adults is one tablet two or three times daily at equally spaced intervals.

Robinul tablets are not recommended for use in children under the age of 12 years.

DRUG INTERACTIONS

There are no known drug interactions.

HOW SUPPLIED

Robinul (glycopyrrolate, 1 mg) tablets in bottles of 100 (NDC 0031-7824-63) and 500 (NDC 0031-7824-70).

Robinul Forte (glycopyrrolate, 2 mg) tablets in bottles of 100 (NDC 0031-7840-63).

Shown in Product Identification Section, page 424

ROBINUL® INJECTABLE   ℞
[ro'bĭ-nul]
brand of Glycopyrrolate Injection, USP

PRODUCT OVERVIEW

KEY FACTS

Robinul is a synthetic anticholinergic agent for intramuscular or intravenous administration. The highly polar quaternary ammonium moiety of glycopyrrolate limits its passage across lipid membranes, such as the blood-brain or placental barriers.

MAJOR USES

Robinul Injectable is indicated as a preoperative antimuscarinic to reduce salivary, tracheobronchial and pharyngeal secretions; intraoperatively to counteract drug-induced or vagal traction reflexes with the associated arrhythmias. Postoperatively, Robinul protects against the peripheral muscarinic effects of cholinergic agents given to reverse the neuromuscular blockade due to nondepolarizing muscle relaxants.

SAFETY INFORMATION

Robinul Injectable is contraindicated in patients hypersensitive to glycopyrrolate. It should be used with great caution, if at all, in patients with glaucoma or asthma. Robinul may produce drowsiness or blurred vision.

PRESCRIBING INFORMATION

ROBINUL® INJECTABLE   ℞
[ro'bĭ-nul]
brand of Glycopyrrolate Injection, USP

DESCRIPTION

Robinul (glycopyrrolate) is a synthetic anticholinergic agent. Each 1 mL contains:

Glycopyrrolate, USP ....0.2 mg
Water for Injection, USP ....q.s.
Benzyl Alcohol, NF (preservative) 0.9%

pH adjusted, when necessary, with hydrochloric acid and/or sodium hydroxide.

For Intramuscular or Intravenous administration.

Glycopyrrolate is a quaternary ammonium compound with the following chemical name:

3[(cyclopentylhydroxyphenylacetyl) oxy]- 1, 1-dimethyl pyrrolidinium bromide.

Unlike atropine, glycopyrrolate is completely ionized at physiological pH values.

Robinul Injectable is a clear, colorless, sterile liquid; pH 2.0–3.0.

CLINICAL PHARMACOLOGY

Glycopyrrolate, like other anticholinergic (antimuscarinic) agents, inhibits the action of acetylcholine on structures innervated by postganglionic cholinergic nerves and on smooth muscles that respond to acetylcholine but lack cholinergic innervation. These peripheral cholinergic receptors are present in the autonomic effector cells of smooth muscle, cardiac muscle, the sinoatrial node, the atrioventricular node, exocrine glands and, to a limited degree, in the autonomic ganglia. Thus, it diminishes the volume and free acid-

ity of gastric secretions and controls excessive pharyngeal, tracheal, and bronchial secretions.

Glycopyrrolate antagonizes muscarinic symptoms (e.g., bronchorrhea, bronchospasm, bradycardia, and intestinal hypermotility) induced by cholinergic drugs such as the anticholinesterases.

The highly polar quaternary ammonium group of glycopyrrolate limits its passage across lipid membranes, such as the blood-brain barrier, in contrast to atropine sulfate and scopolamine hydrobromide, which are non-polar tertiary amines which penetrate lipid barriers easily.

Peak effects occur approximately 30 to 45 minutes after intramuscular administration. The vagal blocking effects persist for 2 to 3 hours and the antisialagogue effects persist up to 7 hours, periods longer than for atropine. With intravenous injection, the onset of action is generally evident within one minute.

INDICATIONS AND USAGE

In Anesthesia: Robinul (glycopyrrolate) Injectable is indicated for use as a preoperative antimuscarinic to reduce salivary, tracheobronchial, and pharyngeal secretions; to reduce the volume and free acidity of gastric secretions; and, to block cardiac vagal inhibitory reflexes during induction of anesthesia and intubation. When indicated, Robinul Injectable may be used intraoperatively to counteract drug-induced or vagal traction reflexes with the associated arrhythmias. Glycopyrrolate protects against the peripheral muscarinic effects (e.g., bradycardia and excessive secretions) of cholinergic agents such as neostigmine and pyridostigmine given to reverse the neuromuscular blockade due to nondepolarizing muscle relaxants.

In Peptic Ulcer: For use in adults as adjunctive therapy for the treatment of peptic ulcer when rapid anticholinergic effect is desired or when oral medication is not tolerated.

CONTRAINDICATIONS

Known hypersensitivity to glycopyrrolate.

Due to its benzyl alcohol content, Robinul Injectable should not be used in newborns (children less than 1 month of age). In addition, in the management of *peptic ulcer* patients, because of the longer duration of therapy, Robinul Injectable may be contraindicated in patients with concurrent glaucoma; obstructive uropathy (for example, bladder neck obstruction due to prostatic hypertrophy); obstructive disease of the gastrointestinal tract (as in achalasia, pyloroduodenal stenosis, etc.); paralytic ileus, intestinal atony of the elderly or debilitated patient; unstable cardiovascular status in acute hemorrhage; severe ulcerative colitis; toxic megacolon complicating ulcerative colitis; myasthenia gravis.

WARNINGS

This drug should be used with great caution, if at all, in patients with glaucoma or asthma.

In the ambulatory patient. Robinul (glycopyrrolate) may produce drowsiness or blurred vision. The patient should be cautioned regarding activities requiring mental alertness such as operating a motor vehicle or other machinery or performing hazardous work while taking this drug.

In addition, in the presence of a high environmental temperature, heat prostration (fever and heat stroke due to decreased sweating) can occur with use of Robinul (glycopyrrolate).

Diarrhea may be an early symptom of incomplete intestinal obstruction, especially in patients with ileostomy or colostomy. In this instance treatment with Robinul (glycopyrrolate) would be inappropriate and possibly harmful.

PRECAUTIONS

General.

Investigate any tachycardia before giving glycopyrrolate since an increase in the heart rate may occur.

Use with caution in patients with: coronary artery disease; congestive heart failure; cardiac arrhythmias; hypertension; hyperthyroidism.

In managing ulcer patients, use Robinul with caution in the elderly and in all patients with autonomic neuropathy, hepatic or renal disease, ulcerative colitis or hiatal hernia, since anticholinergic drugs may aggravate these conditions. With overdosage, a curare-like action may occur.

Drug Interactions. The intravenous administration of any anticholinergic in the presence of cyclopropane anesthesia can result in ventricular arrhythmias; therefore, caution should be observed if Robinul (glycopyrrolate) Injectable is used during cyclopropane anesthesia. If the drug is given in small incremental doses of 0.1 mg or less, the likelihood of producing ventricular arrhythmias is reduced.

Carcinogenesis, mutagenesis, impairment of fertility. Long-term studies in animals have not been performed to evaluate carcinogenic potential. In the teratology studies, diminished rates of conception and of survival at weaning were observed in rats, in a dose-related manner. Studies in dogs suggest that this may be due to diminished seminal secretion which is evident at high doses of glycopyrrolate.

Pregnancy Category B. Reproduction studies have been performed in rats and rabbits up to 1000 times the human dose and have revealed no teratogenic effects from glycopyr-

rolate. There are, however, no adequate and well-controlled studies in pregnant women. Because animal reproduction studies are not always predictive of human response, this drug should be used during pregnancy only if clearly needed.
Nursing Mothers. It is not known whether this drug is excreted in human milk. Because many drugs are excreted in human milk, caution should be exercised when Robinul is administered to a nursing woman.
Pediatric Use. Safety and effectiveness in children below the age of 12 years have not been established for the management of peptic ulcer.

ADVERSE REACTIONS

Anticholinergics produce certain effects, most of which are extensions of their pharmacologic actions. Adverse reactions to anticholinergics in general may include dry mouth; urinary hesitancy and retention; blurred vision due to mydriasis; increased ocular tension; tachycardia; palpitation; decreased sweating; loss of taste; headache; nervousness; drowsiness; weakness; dizziness; insomnia; nausea; vomiting; impotence; suppression of lactation; constipation; bloated feeling; severe allergic reaction or drug idiosyncrasies incuding anaphylaxis; urticaria and other dermal manifestations; some degree of mental confusion and/or excitement, especially in elderly persons.
Robinul is chemically a quaternary ammonium compound; hence, its passage across lipid membranes, such as the blood-brain barrier is limited in contrast to atropine sulfate and scopolamine hydrobromide. For this reason the occurrence of CNS related side effects is lower, in comparison to their incidence following administration of anticholinergics which are chemically tertiary amines that can cross this barrier readily.

OVERDOSAGE

To combat peripheral anticholinergic effects, a quaternary ammonium anticholinesterase such as neostigmine methylsulfate (which does not cross the blood-brain barrier) may be given intravenously in increments of 0.25 mg in adults. This dosage may be repeated every five to ten minutes until anticholinergic over-activity is reversed or up to a maximum of 2.5 mg. Proportionately smaller doses should be used in children. Indication for repetitive doses of neostigmine should be based on close monitoring of the decrease in heart rate and the return of bowel sounds.
In the unlikely event that CNS symptoms (excitement, restlessness, convulsions, psychotic behavior) occur, physostigmine (which does cross the blood-brain barrier) should be used. Physostigmine 0.5 to 2 mg should be slowly administered intravenously and repeated as necessary up to a total of 5 mg in adults. Proportionately smaller doses should be used in children.
Fever should be treated symptomatically. In the event of a curare-like effect on respiratory muscles, artificial respiration should be instituted and maintained until effective respiratory action returns.

DOSAGE AND ADMINISTRATION

Robinul (glycopyrrolate) Injectable may be administered intramuscularly, or intravenously, without dilution, in the following indications:
Adults: *Preanesthetic Medication.* The recommended dose of Robinul (glycopyrrolate) Injectable is 0.002 mg (0.01 mL) per pound of body weight by intramuscular injection, given 30 to 60 minutes prior to the anticipated time of induction of anesthesia or at the time the preanesthetic narcotic and/or sedative are administered.
Intraoperative Medication. Robinul (glycopyrrolate) Injectable may be used during surgery to counteract drug induced or vagal traction reflexes with the associated arrhythmias (e.g., bradycardia). It should be administered intravenously as single doses of 0.1 mg (0.5 mL) and repeated, as needed, at intervals of 2–3 minutes. The usual attempts should be made to determine the etiology of the arrhythmia, and the surgical or anesthetic manipulations necessary to correct parasympathetic imbalance should be performed.
Reversal of Neuromuscular Blockade. The recommended dose of Robinul (glycopyrrolate) Injectable is 0.2 mg (1.0 mL) for each 1.0 mg of neostigmine or 5.0 mg of pyridostigmine. In order to minimize the appearance of cardiac side effects, the drugs may be administered simultaneously by intravenous injection and may be mixed in the same syringe.
Children: (Read Contraindications) *Preanesthetic Medication.* The recommended dose of Robinul (glycopyrrolate) Injectable in children 1 month to 12 years of age is 0.002 mg (0.01 mL) per pound of body weight intramuscularly, given 30 to 60 minutes prior to the anticipated time of induction of anesthesia or at the time the preanesthetic narcotic and/or sedative are administered.
Children 1 month to 2 years of age may require up to 0.004 mg (0.02 mL) per pound of body weight.
Intraoperative Medication. Because of the long duration of action of Robinul (glycopyrrolate) if used as preanesthetic medication, additional Robinul (glycopyrrolate) Injectable for anticholinergic effect intraoperatively is rarely needed; in the event it is required the recommended pediatric dose is 0.002 mg (0.01 mL) per pound of body weight intravenously,

not to exceed 0.1 mg (0.5 mL) in a single dose which may be repeated, as needed, at intervals of 2–3 minutes. The usual attempts should be made to determine the etiology of the arrhythmia, and the surgical or anesthetic manipulations necessary to correct parasympathetic imbalance should be performed.
Reversal of Neuromuscular Blockade. The recommended pediatric dose of Robinul (glycopyrrolate) Injectable is 0.2 mg (1.0 mL) for each 1.0 mg of neostigmine or 5.0 mg of pyridostigmine. In order to minimize the appearance of cardiac side effects, the drugs may be administered simultaneously by intravenous injection and may be mixed in the same syringe.
Adults: *Peptic Ulcer.* The usual recommended dose of Robinul Injectable is 0.1 mg (0.5 mL) administered at 4-hour intervals, 3 or 4 times daily intravenously or intramuscularly. Where more profound effect is required, 0.2 mg (1.0 mL) may be given. Some patients may need only a single dose, and frequency of administration should be dictated by patient response up to a maximum of four times daily.
Robinul Injectable is not recommended for peptic ulcers in children under 12 years of age. (See Precautions.)
NOTE: Parenteral drug products should be inspected visually for particulate matter and discoloration prior to administration whenever solution and container permit.
Admixture Compatibilities. Robinul (glycopyrrolate) Injectable is compatible for mixing and injection with the following injectable dosage forms: 5% and 10% glucose in water or saline; atropine sulfate, USP; Antilirium® (physostigmine salicylate); Benadryl® (diphenhydramine HCl); codeine phosphate, USP; Emete-Con® (benzquinamide HCl); hydromorphone HCl, USP; Inapsine® (droperidol); Innovar® (droperidol and fentanyl citrate); Largon® (propiomazine HCl); Levo-Dromoran® (levorphanol tartrate); lidocaine, USP; Mepergan® (meperidine and promethazine HCls); meperidine HCl, USP; Mestinon® /Regonol® (pyridostigmine bromide); morphine sulfate, USP; Nisentil® (alphaprodine HCl); Nubain® (nalbuphine HCl); Numorphan® (oxymorphone HCl); Pantopon® (opium alkaloids HCls); procaine HCl, USP; promethazine HCl, USP; Prostigmin® (neostigmine methylsulfate, USP); scopolamine HBr, USP; Sparine® (promazine HCl); Stadol® (butorphanol tartrate); Sublimaze® (fentanyl citrate); Talwin® (pentazocine lactate); Tigan® (trimethobenzamide HCl); Vesprin® (triflupromazine HCl); and Vistaril® (hydroxyzine HCl). Robinul Injectable may be administered via the tubing of a running infusion of physiological saline or lactated Ringer's solution.
Since the stability of glycopyrrolate is questionable above a pH of 6.0, do *not* combine Robinul Injectable in the same syringe with Brevital® (methohexital Na); Chloromycetin® (chloramphenicol Na succinate); Dramamine® (dimenhydrinate); Nembutal® (pentobarbital Na); Pentothal® (thiopental Na); Seconal® (secobarbital Na); sodium bicarbonate (Abbott); or Valium® (diazepam). A gas will evolve or a precipitate may form. Mixing with Decadron® (dexamethasone Na phosphate) or a buffered solution of lactated Ringer's solution will result in a pH higher than 6.0. Mixing chlorpromazine HCl, USP, or Compazine® (prochlorperazine) with other agents in a syringe is not recommended by the manufacturer, although the mixture with Robinul Injectable is physically compatible.

HOW SUPPLIED

Robinul (glycopyrrolate) Injectable, 0.2 mg/mL, is available in 1 mL single dose vials packaged in 5's (NDC 0031-7890-87), and 25's (NDC 0031-7890-11), 2 mL single dose vials packaged in 25's (NDC 0031-7890-95), 5 mL multiple dose vials packaged individually (NDC 0031-7890-93) and in 25's (NDC 0031-7890-06), and 20 mL (NDC 0031-7890-83) multiple dose vials. Store at controlled room temperature, between 15°C and 30°C (59°F and 86°F).
Manufactured for Pharmaceutical Division, A. H. Robins Company, Richmond, Virginia 23220 by Elkins-Sinn, Inc., Cherry Hill, NJ 08003-4099, a subsidiary of A. H. Robins Co.
Shown in Product Identification Section, page 424

ROBITUSSIN®
[ro " bĭ-tuss ' ĭn]
ROBITUSSIN–CF®
ROBITUSSIN–DM®
ROBITUSSIN–PE®

(See PDR For Nonprescription Drugs)

ROBITUSSIN A–C®   ℂ
[ro " bĭ-tuss ' ĭn]

PRODUCT OVERVIEW
KEY FACTS
Guaifenesin enhances the output of lower respiratory tract fluid. Codeine phosphate is favored for its antitussive efficacy in low dosage. As a result, dry, unproductive coughs become more productive and less frequent.

MAJOR USES
Temporarily controls cough due to minor throat and bronchial irritation as may occur with the common cold or inhaled irritants. Helps loosen phlegm (mucus) and thin bronchial secretions to make coughs more productive.

SAFETY INFORMATION
Use this product with caution in children under six years or in children taking another drug. Prescribe cautiously for patients with persistent or chronic cough.

PRESCRIBING INFORMATION

ROBITUSSIN A–C®   ℂ
[ro " bĭ-tuss ' ĭn]

Robitussin and codeine.
Each 5 mL (1 teaspoonful) contains:
Guaifenesin, USP ....100 mg
Codeine Phosphate, USP ....10 mg
  (Warning: May be habit forming)
Alcohol 3.5 per cent
In a palatable, aromatic syrup
Inactive Ingredients: Caramel, Citric Acid, FD&C Red 40, Flavors, Glycerin, Saccharin Sodium, Sodium Benzoate, Sorbitol, Water.

ACTIONS
Robitussin A-C combines the expectorant, guaifenesin, with the cough suppressant, codeine. Guaifenesin enhances the output of lower respiratory tract fluid (RTF). The enhanced flow of less viscid secretions promotes and facilitates the removal of mucus.
Codeine is a centrally acting agent which elevates the threshold for cough. As a result, dry, unproductive coughs become more productive and less frequent.
Under Federal law, Robitussin A-C is available without a prescription. Certain state laws may differ. The container label contains the following indications, warnings and drug interaction precaution statements and directions:

INDICATIONS
Temporarily controls cough due to minor throat and bronchial irritation as may occur with the common cold or inhaled irritants. Helps loosen phlegm (mucus) and thin bronchial secretions to make coughs more productive.

WARNINGS
A persistent cough may be a sign of a serious condition. If cough persists for more than 1 week, tends to recur, or is accompanied by fever, rash, or persistent headache, consult a doctor. Do not take this product for persistent or chronic cough such as occurs with smoking, asthma, chronic bronchitis, emphysema, or if cough is accompanied by excessive phlegm (mucus) unless directed by a doctor. Adults and children who have a chronic pulmonary disease or shortness of breath, or children who are taking other drugs, should not take this product unless directed by a doctor. May cause or aggravate constipation. As with any drug, if you are pregnant or nursing a baby, seek the advice of a health professional before using this product.
PROFESSIONAL NOTE: Guaifenesin has been shown to produce a color interference with certain clinical laboratory determinations of 5-hydroxyindoleacetic acid (5-HIAA) and vanillylmandelic acid (VMA).

DRUG INTERACTION PRECAUTION
Caution should be used when taking this product with sedatives, tranquilizers and drugs used for depression, especially monoamine oxidase inhibitors (MAOIs). These combinations may cause greater sedation (drowsiness) than is caused by the products used alone.

DIRECTIONS
Take orally as stated below or use as directed by a doctor. Adults and children 12 years of age and over: 2 teaspoonfuls every 4 hours, not to exceed 12 teaspoonfuls in a 24-hour period; children 6 to under 12 years: 1 teaspoonful every 4 hours, not to exceed 6 teaspoonfuls in a 24-hour period; children under 6 years: consult a doctor. A special measuring device should be used to give an accurate dose of this product to children under 6 years of age. Giving a higher dose than recommended by a doctor could result in serious side effects for a child. Use of codeine-containing preparations is not recommended for children under 2 years of age. Do not exceed recommended dosage.

HOW SUPPLIED
Bottles of 2 fl. ounces (NDC 0031-8674-05), 4 fl. ounces (NDC 0031-8674-12), one pint (NDC 0031-8674-25), and one gallon (NDC 0031-8674-29).

Continued on next page

Prescribing information on A. H. Robins products listed here is based on official labeling in effect June 1, 1989, with Indications, Contraindications, Warnings, Precautions, Adverse Reactions, and Dosage stated in full.

Robins—Cont.

ROBITUSSIN® –DAC   ℂ
[ro "bĭ-tuss 'ĭn]

PRODUCT OVERVIEW

KEY FACTS
The expectorant, guaifenesin, relieves irritated membranes in the respiratory passages; the nasal decongestant, pseudoephedrine, reduces the swelling of nasal passages; the antitussive, codeine, calms the cough control center and relieves coughing.

MAJOR USES
Temporarily relieves nasal congestion and controls cough due to minor throat and bronchial irritation as may occur with the common cold or inhaled irritants. Temporarily restores freer breathing through the nose. Helps loosen phlegm (mucus) and thin bronchial secretions to make coughs more productive.

SAFETY INFORMATION
Use this product with caution in children under six years of age or in children taking another drug. Do not exceed recommended dosage since nervousness, dizziness, or sleeplessness may occur. Prescribe cautiously for patients with persistent or chronic cough.

PRESCRIBING INFORMATION

ROBITUSSIN® –DAC   ℂ
[ro "bĭ-tuss 'ĭn]

Each 5 mL (1 teaspoonful) contains:
Guaifenesin, USP ....100 mg
Pseudoephedrine
  Hydrochloride, USP .... 30 mg
Codeine Phosphate, USP .... 10 mg
  (Warning: May be habit forming)
In a palatable, aromatic syrup
Alcohol 1.9 per cent
Inactive Ingredients: Caramel, Citric Acid, FD&C Red 40, Flavors, Glycerin, Saccharin Sodium, Sodium Benzoate, Sorbitol, Water.

ACTIONS
Robitussin-DAC combines the expectorant, guaifenesin, the nasal decongestant, pseudoephedrine, and the cough suppressant, codeine. Guaifenesin enhances the output of lower respiratory tract fluid. The enhanced flow of less viscid secretions promotes and facilitates the removal of mucus. Codeine is a centrally acting agent which elevates the threshold for cough. As a result, dry, unproductive coughs become more productive and less frequent. The nasal decongestant, pseudoephedrine, reduces the swelling of nasal passages.
Under Federal law, Robitussin-DAC is available without a prescription. Certain state laws may differ, The container label contains the following indications, warnings and drug interaction precaution statements and directions:

INDICATIONS
Temporarily relieves nasal congestion and controls cough due to minor throat and bronchial irritation as may occur with the common cold or inhaled irritants. Temporarily restores freer breathing through the nose. Helps loosen phlegm (mucus) and thin bronchial secretions to make coughs more productive.

WARNINGS
A persistent cough may be a sign of a serious condition. If cough persists for more than 1 week, tends to recur, or is accompanied by fever, rash, or persistent headache, consult a doctor. Do not take this product for persistent or chronic cough such as occurs with smoking, asthma, chronic bronchitis, emphysema, or if cough is accompanied by excessive phlegm (mucus) unless directed by a doctor. Adults and children who have a chronic pulmonary disease or shortness of breath, or children who are taking other drugs, should not take this product unless directed by a doctor. Do not take this product if you have high blood pressure, heart disease, diabetes or thyroid disease, except under the advice and supervision of a doctor. Do not exceed recommended dosage because at higher doses nervousness, dizziness or sleeplessness may occur. May cause or aggravate constipation. As with any drug, if you are pregnant or nursing a baby, seek the advice of a health professional before using this product.

PROFESSIONAL NOTE: Guaifenesin has been shown to produce a color interference with certain clinical laboratory determinations of 5-hydroxyindoleacetic acid (5-HIAA) and vanillymandelic acid (VMA).

DRUG INTERACTION PRECAUTION
Do not take this product if you are presently taking a prescription drug for high blood pressure or depression, especially monoamine oxidase inhibitors (MAOIs), without first consulting your doctor.

DIRECTIONS
Take orally as stated below or use as directed by a doctor. Adults and children 12 years of age and over: 2 teaspoonfuls every 4 hours, not to exceed 8 teaspoonfuls in a 24-hour period; children 6 to under 12 years: 1 teaspoonful every 4 hours, not to exceed 4 teaspoonfuls in a 24-hour period; children under 6 years: consult a doctor. A special measuring device should be used to give an accurate dose of this product to children under 6 years of age. Giving a higher dose than recommended by a doctor could result in serious side effects for a child. Use of codeine-containing preparations is not recommended for children under 2 years of age. Do not exceed recommended dosage.

HOW SUPPLIED
Bottles of one pint (NDC 0031-8680-25).

TENEX®   ℞
[ten 'ex]
(Guanfacine Hydrochloride)
1 mg Tablets

PRODUCT OVERVIEW

KEY FACTS
Tenex is a centrally acting antihypertensive with α_2-adrenoceptor agonist properties. Controlled clinical trials in patients with mild to moderate hypertension who were receiving a thiazide-type diuretic have shown that the blood pressure response to guanfacine can persist for 24 hours after a single dose. Doses of 1, 2, and 3 mg. resulted in decreased blood pressure in the sitting position. While most of the effectiveness of guanfacine was present at 1 mg., adverse reactions at this dose were not clearly distinguishable from those associated with placebo. Adverse reactions were clearly present at 2 and 3 mg.

MAJOR USES
Tenex is indicated in the management of hypertension. Since dosing information has been established in the presence of a thiazide-type diuretic, Tenex should, therefore, be used in patients who are already receiving a thiazide-type diuretic.

SAFETY INFORMATION
Like other antihypertensive agents, Tenex should be used with caution in patients with severe coronary insufficiency, recent myocardial infarction, cerebrovascular disease or chronic renal or hepatic failure. Patients who receive Tenex should be advised to exercise caution when operating dangerous machinery or driving motor vehicles until it is determined that they do not become drowsy or dizzy from the medication. Patients should be warned that their tolerance for alcohol and other CNS depressants may be diminished. Patients should be advised not to discontinue therapy abruptly.

PRESCRIBING INFORMATION

TENEX®   ℞
[ten 'ex]
(Guanfacine Hydrochloride)
1 mg Tablets

DESCRIPTION
Tenex (guanfacine hydrochloride) is a centrally acting antihypertensive with α_2-adrenoceptor agonist properties. It is supplied as a light pink diamond shaped tablet for oral administration embossed with a 1 and engraved AHR on one side and engraved TENEX on the other side. Each tablet contains guanfacine base 1 mg (as the hydrochloride salt). The chemical name of Tenex (guanfacine hydrochloride) is N-amidino-2-(2,6-dichlorophenyl) acetamide hydrochloride and its molecular weight is 282.56.
Guanfacine hydrochloride is a white to off-white powder; sparingly soluble in water and alcohol and slightly soluble in acetone. The tablets contain the following inactive ingredients: FD&C Red No. 40 aluminum lake, Lactose, Microcrystalline cellulose, Povidone, Stearic Acid.

CLINICAL PHARMACOLOGY
Tenex (guanfacine hydrochloride) is an orally active antihypertensive agent whose principal mechanism of action appears to be stimulation of central α_2-adrenergic receptors. By stimulating these receptors, guanfacine reduces sympathetic nerve impulses from the vasomotor center to the heart and blood vessels. This results in a decrease in peripheral vascular resistance and a reduction in heart rate.
Controlled clinical trials in patients with mild to moderate hypertension who were receiving a thiazide-type diuretic have defined the dose-response relationship for blood pressure response and adverse reactions of guanfacine given at bedtime and have shown that the blood pressure response to guanfacine can persist for 24 hours after a single dose. In the dose-response study, patients were randomized to placebo or to doses of 0.5, 1, 2, and 3 mg of guanfacine, each given at bedtime. The observed mean changes from baseline, tabulated below, indicate the similarity of response for placebo and the 0.5 mg dose. Doses of 1, 2, and 3 mg resulted in decreased blood pressure in the sitting position with no real differences among the three doses. In the standing position there was some increase in response with dose.
[See table below].
While most of the effectiveness of guanfacine was present at 1 mg, adverse reactions at this dose were not clearly distinguishable from those associated with placebo. Adverse reactions were clearly present at 2 and 3 mg (see Adverse Reactions).
In a placebo-controlled study of Tenex (guanfacine hydrochloride) a significant decrease in blood pressure was maintained for a full 24 hours after dosing. While there was no significant difference between the 12 and 24 hour blood pressure readings, the fall in blood pressure at 24 hours was numerically smaller, suggesting possible escape of blood pressure in some patients and the need for individualization of therapy.
In a double-blind, randomized trial, either guanfacine or clonidine was given at recommended doses with 25 mg chlorthalidone for 24 weeks and then abruptly discontinued. Results showed equal degrees of blood pressure reduction with the two drugs and there was no tendency for blood pressures to increase despite maintenance of the same daily dose of the two drugs. Signs and symptoms of rebound phenomena were infrequent upon discontinuation of either drug. Abrupt withdrawal of clonidine produced a rapid return of diastolic and especially, systolic blood pressure to approximately pretreatment levels, with occasional values significantly greater than baseline, whereas guanfacine withdrawal produced a more gradual increase to pre-treatment levels, but also with occasional values significantly greater than baseline.
Pharmacodynamics: Hemodynamic studies in man showed that the decrease in blood pressure observed after single-dose or long-term oral treatment with guanfacine was accompanied by a significant decrease in peripheral resistance and a slight reduction in heart rate (5 beats/min). Cardiac output under conditions of rest or exercise was not altered by guanfacine.
Tenex (guanfacine hydrochloride) lowered elevated plasma renin activity and plasma catecholamine levels in hypertensive patients, but this does not correlate with individual blood-pressure responses.
Growth hormone secretion was stimulated with single oral doses of 2 and 4 mg of guanfacine. Long-term use of Tenex had no effect on growth hormone levels.
Guanfacine had no effect on plasma aldosterone. A slight but insignificant decrease in plasma volume occurred after one month of guanfacine therapy. There were no changes in mean body weight or electrolytes.
Pharmacokinetics: Relative to an intravenous dose of 3 mg, the absolute oral bioavailability of guanfacine is about 80%. Peak plasma concentrations occur from 1 to 4 hours with an average of 2.6 hours after single oral doses or at steady state. The area under the concentration-time curve (AUC) increases linearly with the dose.
In individuals with normal renal function, the average elimination half-life is approximately 17 hr (range 10–30 hr). Younger patients tend to have shorter elimination half-lives (13–14 hr) while older patients tend to have half-lives at the upper end of the range. Steady state blood levels were attained within 4 days in most subjects.
In individuals with normal renal function, guanfacine and its metabolites are excreted primarily in the urine. Approximately 50% (40–75%) of the dose is eliminated in the urine as unchanged drug; the remainder is eliminated mostly as conjugates of metabolites produced by oxidative metabolism of the aromatic ring.
The guanfacine-to-creatinine clearance ratio is greater than 1.0, which would suggest that tubular secretion of drug occurs.
The drug is approximately 70% bound to plasma proteins, independent of drug concentration.
The whole body volume of distribution is high (a mean of 6.3 L/kg), which suggests a high distribution of drug to the tissues.

	Mean Decrease in Seated and Standing Blood Pressure (BP) by Guanfacine Dosage Group				
Vital Sign	Placebo	0.5 mg	1 mg	2 mg	3 mg
n =	63	63	64	58	59
Change in Systolic BP (seated)	–5	–5	–14	–12	–16
Change in Diastolic BP (seated)	–7	–6	–13	–13	–13
Change in Systolic BP (standing)	–3	–5	–11	– 9	–15
Change in Diastolic BP (standing)	–5	–4	– 9	–10	–12

The clearance of guanfacine in patients with varying degrees of renal insufficiency is reduced, but plasma levels of drug are only slightly increased compared to patients with normal renal function. When prescribing for patients with renal impairment, the low end of the dosing range should be used. Patients on dialysis also can be given usual doses of guanfacine hydrochloride as the drug is poorly dialyzed.

INDICATIONS AND USAGE

Tenex (guanfacine hydrochloride) is indicated in the management of hypertension. Since dosing information (see Dosage and Administration) has been established in the presence of a thiazide-type diuretic; Tenex should, therefore, be used in patients who are already receiving a thiazide-type diuretic.

CONTRAINDICATIONS

Tenex is contraindicated in patients with known hypersensitivity to guanfacine hydrochloride.

PRECAUTIONS

General. Like other antihypertensive agents, Tenex (guanfacine hydrochloride) should be used with caution in patients with severe coronary insufficiency, recent myocardial infarction, cerebrovascular disease or chronic renal or hepatic failure.

Sedation. Tenex, like other orally active central alpha-2-adrenergic agonists, causes sedation or drowsiness, especially when beginning therapy. These symptoms are dose-related (see Adverse Reactions). When Tenex is used with other centrally active depressants (such as phenothiazines, barbiturates, or benzodiazepines), the potential for additive sedative effects should be considered.

Rebound. Abrupt cessation of therapy with orally active central alpha-2 adrenergic agonists may be associated with increases (from depressed on-therapy levels) in plasma and urinary catecholamines, symptoms of "nervousness and anxiety" and, less commonly, increases in blood pressure to levels significantly greater than those prior to therapy.

Information for Patients. Patients who receive Tenex should be advised to exercise caution when operating dangerous machinery or driving motor vehicles until it is determined that they do not become drowsy or dizzy from the medication. Patients should be warned that their tolerance for alcohol and other CNS depressants may be diminished. Patients should be advised not to discontinue therapy abruptly.

Laboratory Tests. In clinical trials, no clinically relevant laboratory test abnormalities were identified as causally related to drug during short-term treatment with Tenex (guanfacine hydrochloride).

Drug Interactions. No specific adverse drug interactions have been identified, but the potential for increased sedation when Tenex is given with other CNS-depressant drugs should be appreciated.

Anticoagulants. Ten patients who were stabilized on oral anticoagulants were given guanfacine, 1–2 mg/day, for 4 weeks. No changes were observed in the degree of anticoagulation.

In several well-controlled studies, guanfacine was administered together with diuretics with no drug interactions reported. In the long-term safety studies, Tenex was given concomitantly with many drugs without evidence of any interactions. The principal drugs given (number of patients in parentheses) were: cardiac glycosides (115), sedatives and hypnotics (103), coronary vasodilators (52), oral hypoglycemics (45), cough and cold preparations (45), NSAIDs (38), antihyperlipidemics (29), antigout drugs (24), oral contraceptives (18), bronchodilators (13), insulin (10), and beta blockers (10).

Drug/Laboratory Test Interactions. No laboratory test abnormalities related to the use of Tenex (guanfacine hydrochloride) have been identified.

Carcinogenesis, Mutagenesis, Impairment of Fertility. No carcinogenic effect was observed in studies of 78 weeks in mice at doses more than 150 times the maximum recommended human dose and 102 weeks in rats at doses more than 100 times the maximum recommended human dose. In a variety of test models guanfacine was not mutagenic. No adverse effects were observed in fertility studies in male and female rats.

Pregnancy Category B. Administration of guanfacine to rats at 70 times the maximum recommended human dose and rabbits at 20 times the maximum recommended human dose resulted in no evidence of impaired fertility or harm to the fetus. Higher doses (100 and 200 times the maximum recommended human dose in rabbits and rats respectively) were associated with reduced fetal survival and maternal toxicity. Rat experiments have shown that guanfacine crosses the placenta.

There are, however, no adequate and well-controlled studies in pregnant women. Because animal reproduction studies are not always predictive of human response, this drug should be used during pregnancy only if clearly needed.

Labor and Delivery. Tenex (guanfacine hydrochloride) is not recommended in the treatment of acute hypertension associated with toxemia of pregnancy. There is no informa-

Adverse Reaction	Assigned Treatment Group									
	Placebo		0.5 mg		1.0 mg		2.0 mg		3.0 mg	
n=	73		72		72		72		72	
Dry Mouth	5	(7%)	4	(5%)	6	(8%)	8	(11%)	20	(28%)
Somnolence	1	(1%)	3	(4%)	0	(0%)	1	(1%)	10	(14%)
Asthenia	0	(0%)	2	(3%)	0	(0%)	2	(2%)	7	(10%)
Dizziness	2	(2%)	1	(1%)	3	(4%)	6	(8%)	3	(4%)
Headache	3	(4%)	4	(3%)	3	(4%)	1	(1%)	2	(2%)
Impotence	1	(1%)	1	(1%)	0	(0%)	1	(1%)	3	(4%)
Constipation	0	(0%)	0	(0%)	0	(0%)	1	(1%)	1	(1%)
Fatigue	3	(3%)	2	(3%)	2	(3%)	5	(6%)	3	(4%)

tion available on the effects of guanfacine on the course of labor and delivery.

Nursing Mothers. It is not known whether Tenex (guanfacine hydrochloride) is excreted in human milk. Because many drugs are excreted in human milk, caution should be exercised when Tenex is administered to a nursing woman. Experiments with rats have shown that guanfacine is excreted in the milk.

Pediatric Use. Safety and effectiveness in children under 12 years of age have not been demonstrated. Therefore, the use of Tenex in this age group is not recommended.

ADVERSE REACTIONS

Adverse reactions noted with Tenex (guanfacine hydrochloride) are similar to those of other drugs of the central α–2 adrenoreceptor agonist class; dry mouth, sedation (somnolence), weakness (asthenia), dizziness, constipation, and impotence. While the reactions are common, most are mild and tend to disappear on continued dosing.

Skin rash with exfoliation has been reported in a few cases; although clear cause and effect relationships to Tenex could not be established, should a rash occur, Tenex should be discontinued and the patient monitored appropriately.

In a 12-week placebo-controlled, dose-response study the frequency of the most commonly observed adverse reactions showed a clear dose relationship from 0.5 to 3 mg, as follows: [See table above].

There were 41 premature terminations because of adverse reactions in this study. The percent of patients who terminated and the dose at which they terminated were as follows:

Dose:	Placebo	0.5 mg	1 mg	2 mg	3 mg
Terminated:	6.9%	4.2%	3.2%	6.9%	8.3%

Reasons for dropouts among patients who received guanfacine were: somnolence, headache, weakness, dry mouth, dizziness, impotence, insomnia, constipation, syncope, urinary incontinence, conjunctivitis, paresthesia, and dermatitis.

In a second placebo-controlled study in which the dose could be adjusted upward to 3 mg per day in 1-mg increments at 3-week intervals, i.e., a setting more similar to ordinary clinical use, the most commonly recorded reactions were: dry mouth 47%, constipation 16%, fatigue 12%, somnolence 10%, asthenia 6%, dizziness 6%, headache 4%, and insomnia 4%.

Reasons for dropouts among patients who received guanfacine were: somnolence, dry mouth, dizziness, impotence, constipation, confusion, depression, and palpitations.

In the clonidine/guanfacine comparison described in Clinical Pharmacology, the most common adverse reactions noted were:

	Guanfacine (n = 279)	Clonidine (n = 278)
Dry mouth	30%	37%
Somnolence	21%	35%
Dizziness	11%	8%
Constipation	10%	5%
Fatigue	9%	8%
Headache	4%	4%
Insomnia	4%	3%

Adverse reactions occurring in 3% or less of patients in the three controlled trials were:

Cardiovascular— bradycardia, palpitations, substernal pain
Gastrointestinal— abdominal pain, diarrhea, dyspepsia, dysphagia, nausea
CNS— amnesia, confusion, depression, insomnia, libido decrease
ENT disorders— rhinitis, taste perversion, tinnitus
Eye disorders— conjunctivitis, iritis, vision disturbance
Musculoskeletal— leg cramps, hypokinesia
Respiratory— dyspnea
Dermatologic— dermatitis, pruritus, purpura, sweating
Urogenital— testicular disorder, urinary incontinence
Other— malaise, paresthesia, paresis

Adverse reaction reports tend to decrease over time. In an open-label trial of one year's duration, 580 hypertensive subjects were given guanfacine, titrated to achieve goal blood pressure, alone (51%), with diuretic (38%), with beta blocker (3%), with diuretic plus beta blocker (6%), or with diuretic

plus vasodilator (2%). The mean daily dose of guanfacine reached was 4.7 mg.

Adverse Reactions	Incidence of adverse reactions at any time during the study	Incidence of adverse reactions at the end of one year
	N=580	N=580
Dry mouth	60%	15%
Drowsiness	33%	6%
Dizziness	15%	1%
Constipation	14%	3%
Weakness	5%	1%
Headache	4%	0.2%
Insomnia	5%	0%

There were 52 (8.9%) dropouts due to adverse effects in this 1-year trial. The causes were: dry mouth (n = 20), weakness (n = 12), constipation (n = 7), somnolence (n = 3), nausea (n = 3), orthostatic hypotension (n = 2), insomnia (n = 1), rash (n = 1), nightmares (n = 1), headache (n = 1), and depression (n = 1).

DRUG ABUSE AND DEPENDENCE

No reported abuse or dependence has been associated with the administration of Tenex (guanfacine hydrochloride).

OVERDOSAGE

Signs and Symptoms. One case of guanfacine overdose has been reported. A 25-year-old female intentionally ingested 60 mg. She presented with severe drowsiness and bradycardia of 45 beats/minute. Gastric lavage was performed and an infusion of isoproterenol (0.8 mg in 12 hours) was administered. She recovered quickly and without sequelae.

Treatment of Overdosage. Gastric lavage and infusion of isoproterenol, as appropriate.

Guanfacine is not dialyzable in clinically significant amounts (2.4%).

DOSAGE AND ADMINISTRATION

The recommended dose of Tenex (guanfacine hydrochloride) is 1 mg daily given at bedtime to minimize somnolence. Patients should already be receiving a thiazide type diuretic. If after 3 to 4 weeks of therapy, 1 mg does not give a satisfactory result, doses of 2 and then subsequently 3 mg may be given, although most of the effect of Tenex is seen at 1 mg (see Clinical Pharmacology). Some patients may show a rise in pressure toward the end of the dosing interval; in this event a divided dose may be utilized.

Higher daily doses (rarely up to 40 mg/day, in divided doses) have been used, but adverse reactions increase significantly with doses above 3 mg/day and there is no evidence of increased efficacy. No studies have established an appropriate dose or dosing interval when Tenex (guanfacine hydrochloride) is given as the sole antihypertensive agent.

The frequency of rebound hypertension is low, but rebound can occur. When rebound occurs, it does so after 2–4 days, which is delayed compared with clonidine hydrochloride. This is consistent with the longer half-life of guanfacine. In most cases, after abrupt withdrawal of guanfacine, blood pressure returns to pretreatment levels slowly (within 2–4 days) without ill effects.

HOW SUPPLIED

Tenex tablets containing 1 mg guanfacine (as the hydrochloride salt) are available in bottles of 100 (NDC 0031-8901-63) and 500 (NDC 0031-8901-70) and in Dis-Co® Unit Dose Packs of 100 (NDC 0031-8901-64).

Store at controlled room temperature, between 15°C and 30°C (59°F and 86°F). Dispense in tight, light-resistant container.

Shown in Product Identification Section, page 424

Continued on next page

Robins—Cont.

VIOKASE® ℞
[vi 'o-kās]
(Pancrelipase, USP)
Tablets
Powder

DESCRIPTION

Viokase (Pancrelipase, USP) is a pancreatic enzyme concentrate of porcine origin containing standardized lipase, protease, and amylase as well as other pancreatic enzymes. Viokase is available in tablet and powder dosage form for oral administration.

The enzyme potencies of the tablets and powder are:

	Each Tablet	Each 0.7g powder (1/4 teaspoonful)
Lipase, USP Units	8,000	16,800
Protease, USP Units	30,000	70,000
Amylase, USP Units	30,000	70,000

Inactive Ingredients:
TABLETS—Lactose, Magnesium Stearate, Sodium Chloride, Stearic Acid.
POWDER—Lactose, Sodium Chloride

CLINICAL PHARMACOLOGY

The natural digestive enzymes in Viokase hydrolyze fats into fatty acids and glycerol, split protein into amino acids, and convert carbohydrates to dextrins and short chain sugars. Under conditions of the USP test method (in vitro) Viokase has the following total digestive capacity:

	Each Tablet	Each 0.7g powder
Dietary Fat, grams	28	59
Dietary Protein, grams	30	70
Dietary Starch, grams	30	70

Viokase Tablets are not enteric coated.
The digestive capacity of a pancreatic enzyme concentrate depends on the amount that passes through the stomach unchanged and is available at the site of action in the small intestine.

INDICATIONS

Viokase (Pancrelipase, USP) is indicated as a digestive aid in the treatment of exocrine pancreatic insufficiency as associated with but not limited to cystic fibrosis, chronic pancreatitis, pancreatectomy, or obstruction of the pancreas ducts.

CONTRAINDICATIONS

Do not use in patients hypersensitive to pork protein.

PRECAUTIONS

General: Individuals previously sensitized to trypsin, pancreatin or pancrelipase may have allergic manifestations.
Information for patients: Viokase should not be held in the mouth as the proteolytic action may cause irritation of the mucosa.
Avoid inhalation of the powder when administering Viokase.
Carcinogenesis, Mutagenesis, Impairment of fertility: - Long-term studies in animals have not been performed to evaluate carcinogenic potential.
Pregnancy Category C. Animal reproduction studies have not been conducted with Viokase. It is also not known whether Viokase can cause fetal harm when administered to a pregnant woman or can affect reproduction capacity. Viokase should be given to a pregnant woman only if clearly needed.
Nursing Mothers: It is not known whether this drug is excreted in human milk. Because many drugs are excreted in human milk, caution should be exercised when Viokase is administered to a nursing mother.

ADVERSE REACTIONS

The dust or finely powdered pancreatic enzyme concentrate is irritating to the nasal mucosa and the respiratory tract. It has been documented that inhalation of the airborne powder can precipitate an asthma attack. The literature also contains several references to asthma due to inhalation in patients sensitized to pancreatic enzyme concentrates. Extremely high doses of exogenous pancreatic enzymes have been associated with hyperuricemia and hyperuricosuria. Overdosage of pancreatic enzyme concentrate may cause diarrhea or transient intestinal upset.

OVERDOSAGE

Acute toxicity determinations in animals have not been possible since the maximum dose that could be given orally produced no toxic reaction. In chronic feeding tests. rats developed swollen salivary glands. This is believed due to the proteolytic activity and the mucosal irritation caused by tissue digestion.

No acute toxic reactions have been reported.

DOSAGE AND ADMINISTRATION

Powder: Dosage for patients with cystic fibrosis—1/4 teaspoonful (0.7 grams) with meals.
Tablets: Dosage for patients with cystic fibrosis or chronic pancreatitis—1 to 3 tablets with meals or as directed by physician. As a digestive aid in patients with pancreatectomy or obstruction of pancreatic ducts—1 to 2 tablets taken at 2-hour intervals or as directed by physician.

HOW SUPPLIED

Tablets —Tan, round, compressed tablets engraved Viokase/AHR on one side and 9111 on the other side in bottles of 100 (NDC 0031-9111-63) and 500 (NDC 0031-9111-70). *Powder* —Tan powder in bottles of 4 oz. (113.5 grams) (NDC 0031-9115-12) and 8 oz. (227 grams) (NDC 0031-9115-25).
Store in tightly closed container in a dry place at a temperature not exceeding 25°C (77°F).
Dispense tablets and powder in tight container, preferably with a desiccant.

CLINICAL STUDIES

The effectiveness of Viokase as a digestive aid in the treatment of patients with exocrine pancreatic insufficiency has been documented in the literature as follows:
1. Regan, PT, Malagelada J-R, DiMagno EP, Glanzman SL, Go VLW: Comparative effects of antacids, cimetidine and enteric coating on the therapeutic response to oral enzymes in severe pancreatic insufficiency. N. Engl. J. Med. 297:854-8, 1977.
2. Graham DY: Enzyme replacement therapy of exocrine pancreatic insufficiency in man. N. Engl. J. Med. 296:1314-7, 1977.

Shown in Product Identification Section, page 424

Z–BEC®
[zē 'běk]

(See PDR For Nonprescription Drugs)

Roche Dermatologics
Division of Hoffmann-La Roche Inc.
NUTLEY, NJ 07110

ACCUTANE® ℞
[acc 'u-tane]
(isotretinoin/Roche)
CAPSULES

The following text is complete prescribing information based on official labeling in effect June 1, 1989.

Avoid Pregnancy

CONTRAINDICATION AND WARNING

Accutane must not be used by females who are pregnant or who may become pregnant while undergoing treatment. There is an extremely high risk that a deformed infant will result if pregnancy occurs while taking Accutane in any amount even for short periods. Potentially all exposed fetuses can be affected.

Accutane is contraindicated in women of childbearing potential unless the <u>patient meets all of</u> the following conditions:

- **has severe disfiguring cystic acne that is recalcitrant to standard therapies**
- **is reliable in understanding and carrying out instructions**
- **is capable of complying with the mandatory contraceptive measures**
- **has received both oral and written warnings of the hazards of taking Accutane during pregnancy and the risk of possible contraception failure and has acknowledged her understanding of these warnings in writing**
- **has had a negative <u>serum</u> pregnancy test within two weeks prior to beginning therapy (It is also recommended that pregnancy testing and contraception counseling be repeated on a monthly basis.)**
- **will begin therapy only on the second or third day of the next normal menstrual period**

Major human fetal abnormalities related to Accutane administration have been documented, including hydro-

cephalus, microcephalus, abnormalities of the external ear (micropinna, small or absent external auditory canals), microphthalmia, cardiovascular abnormalities, facial dysmorphia, thymus gland abnormalities, parathyroid hormone deficiency and cerebellar malformation. There is also an increased risk of spontaneous abortion.

Effective contraception must be used for at least one month before beginning Accutane therapy, during therapy and for one month following discontinuation of therapy. It is recommended that two reliable forms of contraception be used simultaneously unless abstinence is the chosen method.

If pregnancy does occur during treatment, the physician and patient should discuss the desirability of continuing the pregnancy.

Accutane should be prescribed only by physicians who have special competence in the diagnosis and treatment of severe recalcitrant cystic acne, are experienced in the use of systemic retinoids and understand the risk of teratogenicity if Accutane is used during pregnancy.

DESCRIPTION

Accutane (isotretinoin/Roche), a retinoid which inhibits sebaceous gland function and keratinization, is available in 10-mg, 20-mg and 40-mg soft gelatin capsules for oral administration. Each capsule also contains beeswax, butylated hydroxyanisole, edetate disodium, hydrogenated soybean oil flakes, hydrogenated vegetable oil and soybean oil. Gelatin capsules contain glycerin and parabens (methyl and propyl), with the following dye systems: 10 mg—iron oxide (red) and titanium dioxide; 20 mg—FD&C Red No. 3, FD&C Blue No. 1 and titanium dioxide; 40 mg—FD&C Yellow No. 6, D&C Yellow No. 10 and titanium dioxide.

Chemically, isotretinoin is 13-*cis* -retinoic acid and is related to both retinoic acid and retinol (vitamin A). It is a yellow-orange to orange crystalline powder with a molecular weight of 300.44.

CLINICAL PHARMACOLOGY

The exact mechanism of action of Accutane is unknown.
Cystic Acne: Clinical improvement in cystic acne patients occurs in association with a reduction in sebum secretion. The decrease in sebum secretion is temporary and is related to the dose and duration of treatment with Accutane, and reflects a reduction in sebaceous gland size and an inhibition of sebaceous gland differentiation.[1]
Clinical Pharmacokinetics: The pharmacokinetic profile of isotretinoin is predictable and can be described using linear pharmacokinetic theory.
After oral administration of 80 mg (two 40-mg capsules), peak blood concentrations ranged from 167 to 459 ng/mL (mean 256 ng/mL) and mean time to peak was 3.2 hours in normal volunteers, while in acne patients peak concentrations ranged from 98 to 535 ng/mL (mean 262 ng/mL) with a mean time to peak of 2.9 hours. The drug is 99.9% bound in human plasma almost exclusively to albumin. The terminal elimination half-life of isotretinoin ranged from 10 to 20 hours in volunteers and patients. Following an 80-mg liquid suspension oral dose of ^{14}C-isotretinoin, ^{14}C-activity in blood declined with a half-life of 90 hours. Relatively equal amounts of radioactivity were recovered in the urine and feces with 65% to 83% of the dose recovered.
The major identified metabolite in blood is 4-*oxo* -isotretinoin. Tretinoin and 4-*oxo* -tretinoin were also observed. The terminal elimination of 4-*oxo* -isotretinoin is formation rate limited and therefore the apparent half-life of the 4-*oxo* metabolite is similar to isotretinoin following Accutane administration. After two 40-mg capsules of isotretinoin, maximum concentrations of the metabolite of 87 to 399 ng/mL occurred at 6 to 20 hours. The blood concentration of the major metabolite generally exceeded that of isotretinoin after six hours.
The mean ± SD minimum steady-state blood concentration of isotretinoin was 160 ± 19 ng/mL in ten patients receiving 40-mg *b.i.d.* doses. After single and multiple doses, the mean ratio of areas under the blood concentration:time curves of 4-*oxo* -isotretinoin to isotretinoin was 3 to 3.5.
Tissue Distribution in Animals: Tissue distribution of ^{14}C-isotretinoin in rats after oral dosing revealed high concentrations of radioactivity in many tissues after 15 minutes, with a maximum in one hour, and declining to nondetectable levels by 24 hours in most tissues. After seven days, however, low levels of radioactivity were detected in the liver, ureter, adrenal, ovary and lacrimal gland.

INDICATIONS AND USAGE

Cystic Acne: Accutane is indicated for the treatment of severe recalcitrant cystic acne, and a single course of therapy has been shown to result in complete and prolonged remission of disease in many patients.[1-3] If a second course of therapy is needed, it should not be initiated until at least eight weeks after completion of the first course, since experience has shown that patients may continue to improve while off drug.

Because of significant adverse effects associated with its use, Accutane should be reserved for patients with severe cystic acne who are unresponsive to conventional therapy, including systemic antibiotics.

CONTRAINDICATIONS

Pregnancy: Category X. See boxed CONTRAINDICATION and WARNING.

Accutane should not be given to patients who are sensitive to parabens, which are used as preservatives in the gelatin capsule.

WARNINGS

> *Pseudotumor cerebri:* Accutane use has been associated with a number of cases of pseudotumor cerebri (benign intracranial hypertension). Early signs and symptoms of pseudotumor cerebri include papilledema, headache, nausea and vomiting, and visual disturbances. Patients with these symptoms should be screened for papilledema and, if present, they should be told to discontinue Accutane immediately and be referred to a neurologist for further diagnosis and care.

Decreased Night Vision: A number of cases of decreased night vision have occurred during Accutane therapy. Because the onset in some patients is sudden, patients should be advised of this potential problem and warned to be cautious when driving or operating any vehicle at night. Visual problems should be carefully monitored.

Corneal opacities: Corneal opacities have occurred in patients receiving Accutane for acne and more frequently when higher drug dosages were used in patients with disorders of keratinization. All Accutane patients experiencing visual difficulties should discontinue the drug and have an ophthalmological examination. The corneal opacities that have been observed in patients treated with Accutane have either completely resolved or were resolving at follow-up six to seven weeks after discontinuation of the drug. See ADVERSE REACTIONS.

Inflammatory Bowel Disease: Accutane has been temporally associated with inflammatory bowel disease (including regional ileitis) in patients without a prior history of intestinal disorders. Patients experiencing abdominal pain, rectal bleeding or severe diarrhea should discontinue Accutane immediately.

Lipids: Blood lipid determinations should be performed before Accutane is given and then at intervals until the lipid response to Accutane is established, which usually occurs within four weeks. See PRECAUTIONS.

Approximately 25% of patients receiving Accutane experienced an elevation in plasma triglycerides. Approximately 15% developed a decrease in high density lipoproteins and about 7% showed an increase in cholesterol levels. These effects on triglycerides, HDL and cholesterol were reversible upon cessation of Accutane therapy.

Patients with increased tendency to develop hypertriglyceridemia include those with diabetes mellitus, obesity, increased alcohol intake and familial history.

The cardiovascular consequences of hypertriglyceridemia are not well understood, but may increase the patient's risk status. In addition, elevation of serum triglycerides in excess of 800 mg/dL has been associated with acute pancreatitis. Therefore, every attempt should be made to control significant triglyceride elevation.

Some patients have been able to reverse triglyceride elevation by reduction in weight, restriction of dietary fat and alcohol, and reduction in dose while continuing Accutane.[4] An obese male patient with Darier's disease developed elevated triglycerides and subsequent eruptive xanthomas.[5]

Hyperostosis: In clinical trials of disorders of keratinization with a mean dose of 2.24 mg/kg/day, a high prevalence of skeletal hyperostosis was noted. Two children showed x-ray findings suggestive of premature closure of the epiphysis. Additionally, skeletal hyperostosis was noted in six of eight patients in a prospective study of disorders of keratinization.[6] Minimal skeletal hyperostosis has also been observed by x-rays in prospective studies of cystic acne patients treated with a single course of therapy at recommended doses.

Hepatotoxicity: Several cases of clinical hepatitis have been noted which are considered to be possibly or probably related to Accutane therapy. Additionally, mild to moderate elevations of liver enzymes have been observed in approximately 15% of individuals treated during clinical trials, some of which normalized with dosage reduction or continued administration of the drug. If normalization does not readily occur or if hepatitis is suspected during treatment with Accutane, the drug should be discontinued and the etiology further investigated.

Animal Studies: In rats given 32 or 8 mg/kg/day of isotretinoin for 18 months or longer, the incidences of focal calcification, fibrosis and inflammation of the myocardium, calcification of coronary, pulmonary and mesenteric arteries and metastatic calcification of the gastric mucosa were greater than in control rats of similar age. Focal endocardial and myocardial calcifications associated with calcification of the coronary arteries were observed in two dogs after approximately six to seven months of treatment with isotretinoin at a dosage of 60 to 120 mg/kg/day.

In dogs given isotretinoin chronically at a dosage of 60 mg/kg/day, corneal ulcers and corneal opacities were encountered at a higher incidence than in control dogs. In general, these ocular changes tended to revert toward normal when treatment with isotretinoin was stopped, but did not completely clear during the observation period.

In rats given isotretinoin at a dosage of 32 mg/kg/day for approximately 15 weeks, long bone fracture has been observed.

PRECAUTIONS

Information for Patients: **Women of childbearing potential should be instructed that they must not be pregnant when Accutane therapy is initiated, and that they should use effective contraception while taking Accutane and for one month after Accutane has been stopped. They should also sign a consent form prior to beginning Accutane therapy. See boxed CONTRAINDICATION AND WARNING.**

Because of the relationship of Accutane to vitamin A, patients should be advised against taking vitamin supplements containing vitamin A to avoid additive toxic effects.

Patients should be informed that transient exacerbation of acne has been seen, generally during the initial period of therapy.

Patients should be informed that they may experience decreased tolerance to contact lenses during and after therapy.

Laboratory Tests: The incidence of hypertriglyceridemia is 1 patient in 4 on Accutane therapy. Pretreatment and follow-up blood lipids should be obtained under fasting conditions. After consumption of alcohol at least 36 hours should elapse before these determinations are made. It is recommended that these tests be performed at weekly or biweekly intervals until the lipid response to Accutane is established. Certain patients receiving Accutane have experienced problems in the control of their blood sugar. In addition, new cases of diabetes have been diagnosed during Accutane therapy, although no causal relationship has been established. Some patients undergoing vigorous physical activity while on Accutane therapy have experienced elevated CPK levels; however, the clinical significance is unknown.

Carcinogenesis, Mutagenesis, Impairment of Fertility: In Fischer 344 rats given isotretinoin at dosages of 32 or 8 mg/kg/day for greater than 18 months, there was an increased incidence of pheochromocytoma. The incidence of adrenal medullary hyperplasia was also increased at the higher dosage. The relatively high level of spontaneous pheochromocytomas occurring in the Fischer 344 rat makes it a poor model for study of this tumor, since the increase in adrenal medullary proliferative lesions following chronic treatment with relatively high dosages of isotretinoin may be an accentuation of a genetic predisposition in the Fischer 344 rat, and its relevance to the human population is not clear. In addition, a decreased incidence of liver adenomas, liver angiomas and leukemia was noted at the dose levels of 8 and 32 mg/kg/day.

The Ames test was conducted in two laboratories. The results of the tests in one laboratory were completely negative, while in the second laboratory a weakly positive (less than 1.6 x background) was seen with S. typhimurium TA100. No dose-response effect was seen and all other strains were negative. Additionally, other mutagenicity tests (Chinese hamster cells, mouse micronucleus test and S. cerevisiae) were also negative.

No adverse effects on gonadal function, fertility, conception rate, gestation or parturition were observed at dose levels of 2, 8 or 32 mg/kg/day in male and female rats.

In dogs, testicular atrophy was noted after treatment with isotretinoin for approximately 30 weeks at dosages of 60 or 20 mg/kg/day. In general, there was microscopic evidence for appreciable depression of spermatogenesis but some sperm were observed in all testes examined and in no instance were completely atrophic tubules seen. In studies in 66 human males, 30 of whom were patients with cystic acne, no significant changes were noted in the count or motility of spermatozoa in the ejaculate. In a study of 50 men (ages 17–32 years) receiving Accutane therapy for cystic acne, no significant effects were seen on ejaculate volume, sperm count, total sperm motility, morphology or seminal plasma fructose.

Pregnancy: **Category X. See boxed CONTRAINDICATION AND WARNING.**

Nursing Mothers: It is not known whether this drug is excreted in human milk. Because of the potential for adverse effects, nursing mothers should not receive Accutane.

ADVERSE REACTIONS

Clinical: Many of the side effects and adverse reactions seen or expected in patients receiving Accutane are similar to those described in patients taking high doses of vitamin A. The percentages of adverse reactions listed below reflect the total experience in Accutane studies, including investigational studies of disorders of keratinization, with the exception of those pertaining to dry skin and mucous membranes. These latter reflect the experience only in patients with cystic acne because reactions relating to dryness are more commonly recognized as adverse reactions in this disease. Included in this category are dry skin, skin fragility, pruritus, epistaxis, dry nose and dry mouth, which may be seen in up to 80% of cystic acne patients.

The most frequent adverse reaction to Accutane is cheilitis, which occurs in over 90% of patients. A less frequent reaction was conjunctivitis (about two patients in five).

Skeletal hyperostosis has been observed on x-rays of patients treated with Accutane. See WARNINGS. Other types of bone abnormalities have also been reported; however, no causal relationship has been established.

Approximately 16% of patients treated with Accutane developed musculoskeletal symptoms (including arthralgia) during treatment. In general, these were mild to moderate and have occasionally required discontinuation of drug. Less frequently, transient pain in the chest has also been reported. These symptoms generally cleared rapidly after discontinuation of Accutane but in rare cases have persisted.

In less than one patient in ten—rash (including erythema); thinning of hair, which in rare cases has persisted.

In approximately one patient in twenty—peeling of palms and soles, skin infections, nonspecific urogenital findings, nonspecific gastrointestinal symptoms, fatigue, headache and increased susceptibility to sunburn.

Accutane has been associated with a number of cases of pseudotumor cerebri, some of which involved concomitant use of tetracyclines. See WARNINGS.

The following CNS reactions have been reported and may bear no relationship to therapy—seizures, emotional instability, dizziness, nervousness, drowsiness, malaise, weakness, insomnia, lethargy and paresthesias.

Depression has been reported in some patients on Accutane therapy. In some of these patients, this has subsided with discontinuation of therapy and recurred with reinstitution of therapy.

The following reactions have been reported in less than 1% of patients and may bear no relationship to therapy—changes in skin pigment (hypo- and hyperpigmentation), flushing, urticaria, bruising, disseminated herpes simplex, edema, hair problems (other than thinning), hirsutism, respiratory infections, weight loss, erythema nodosum, paronychia, nail dystrophy, bleeding and inflammation of the gums, abnormal menses, optic neuritis, photophobia, eye lid inflammation, arthritis, anemia, palpitation, tachycardia and lymphadenopathy.

A few isolated reports of vasculitis, including Wegener's granulomatosis have been received, but no causal relationship to Accutane therapy has been established.

In Accutane studies to date, of 72 patients who had normal pretreatment ophthalmological examinations, five developed corneal opacities while on Accutane (all five patients had a disorder of keratinization). Corneal opacities have also been reported in cystic acne patients treated with Accutane. See WARNINGS. Dry eyes and decrease in night vision have been reported and in rare instances have persisted. See WARNINGS. Cataracts and visual disturbances have also been reported.

Accutane has been temporally associated with inflammatory bowel disease. See WARNINGS.

As may be seen with healing cystic acne lesions, an occasional exaggerated healing response, manifested by exuberant granulation tissue with crusting, has also been reported in patients receiving therapy with Accutane. Pyogenic granuloma has also been diagnosed in a number of cases.

Laboratory: Accutane therapy induces change in serum lipids in a significant number of treated subjects. Approximately 25% of patients had elevation of plasma triglycerides. Five out of 135 patients treated for cystic acne and 32 out of 298 total subjects treated for all diagnoses showed an elevation of triglycerides above 500 mg percent. About 16% of patients showed a mild to moderate decrease in serum high density lipoprotein (HDL) levels while receiving treatment with Accutane and about 7% of patients experienced minimal elevations of serum cholesterol during treatment. Abnormalities of serum triglycerides, HDL and cholesterol were reversible upon cessation of Accutane therapy.

Approximately 40% of patients receiving Accutane developed elevated sedimentation rates, often from elevated baseline values.

From one in ten to one in five patients showed decreases in red blood cell parameters and white blood cell counts, elevated platelet counts, white cells in the urine, increased alkaline phosphatase, SGOT, SGPT, GGTP or LDH. See WARNINGS: Hepatotoxicity.

Less than one in ten patients showed proteinuria, microscopic or gross hematuria, elevated fasting blood sugar, elevated CPK or hyperuricemia.

Dose Relationship and Duration: Cheilitis and hypertriglyceridemia are usually dose-related.

Continued on next page

Roche Derm.—Cont.

Most adverse reactions were reversible when therapy was discontinued; however, some have persisted after cessation of therapy. (See WARNINGS and ADVERSE REACTIONS.)

Overdosage: The oral LD_{50} of isotretinoin is greater than 4000 mg/kg in rats and mice and is approximately 1960 mg/kg in rabbits. Overdose has been associated with transient headache, vomiting, facial flushing, cheilosis, abdominal pain, headache, dizziness and ataxia. All symptoms quickly resolved without apparent residual effects.

DOSAGE AND ADMINISTRATION

The recommended dosage range for Accutane is 0.5 to 2 mg/kg given in two divided doses daily for 15 to 20 weeks. In studies comparing 0.1, 0.5 and 1 mg/kg/day,[7] it was found that all doses provided initial clearing of disease but there was a greater need for retreatment with the lower dose(s).

It is recommended that for most patients the initial dose of Accutane be 0.5 to 1 mg/kg/day. Patients whose disease is very severe or is primarily manifest on the body may require up to the maximum recommended dose, 2 mg/kg/day. During treatment, the dose may be adjusted according to response of the disease and/or the appearance of clinical side effects—some of which may be dose-related.

If the total cyst count has been reduced by more than 70 percent prior to completing 15 to 20 weeks of treatment, the drug may be discontinued. After a period of two months or more off therapy, and if warranted by persistent or recurring severe cystic acne, a second course of therapy may be initiated.

ACCUTANE DOSING BY BODY WEIGHT

Body Weight		Total Mg/Day		
kilograms	pounds	0.5 mg/kg	1 mg/kg	2 mg/kg
40	88	20	40	80
50	110	25	50	100
60	132	30	60	120
70	154	35	70	140
80	176	40	80	160
90	198	45	90	180
100	220	50	100	200

HOW SUPPLIED

Soft gelatin capsules, 10 mg (light pink), imprinted ACCUTANE 10 ROCHE. Boxes of 100 containing 10 Prescription Paks of 10 capsules (NDC 0004-0155-49).

Soft gelatin capsules, 20 mg (maroon), imprinted ACCUTANE 20 ROCHE. Boxes of 100 containing 10 Prescription Paks of 10 capsules (NDC 0004-0169-49).

Soft gelatin capsules, 40 mg (yellow), imprinted ACCUTANE 40 ROCHE. Boxes of 100 containing 10 Prescription Paks of 10 capsules (NDC 0004-0156-49).

REFERENCES

1. Peck GL, Olsen TG, Yoder FW, Strauss JS, Downing DT, Pandya M, Butkus D, Arnaud-Battandier J: Prolonged remissions of cystic and conglobate acne with 13-*cis*-retinoic acid. *N Engl J Med 300*:329–333, 1979. 2. Farrell LN, Strauss JS, Stranieri AM: The treatment of severe cystic acne with 13-*cis*-retinoic acid. Evaluation of sebum production and the clinical response in a multiple-dose trial. *J Am Acad Dermatol 3*:602–611, 1980. 3. Jones H, Blanc D, Cunliffe WJ: 13-*cis*-retinoic acid and acne. *Lancet 2*:1048–1049, 1980. 4. Katz RA, Jorgensen H, Nigra TP: Elevation of serum triglyceride levels from oral isotretinoin in disorders of keratinization. *Arch Dermatol 116*:1369–1372, 1980. 5. Dicken CH, Connolly SM: Eruptive xanthomas associated with isotretinoin (13-*cis*-retinoic acid). *Arch Dermatol 116*:951–952, 1980. 6. Ellis CN, Madison KC, Pennes DR, Martel W, Voorhees JJ: Isotretinoin therapy is associated with early skeletal radiographic changes. *J Am Acad Dermatol 10*:1024–1029, 1984. 7. Strauss JS, Rapini RP, Shalita AR, Konecky E, Pochi PE, Comite H, Exner JH: Isotretinoin therapy for acne: Results of a multicenter dose-response study. *J Am Acad Dermatol 10*:490–496, 1984.

PATIENT INFORMATION/CONSENT

Accutane must not be used by females who are pregnant or who may become pregnant while undergoing treatment.

IMPORTANT INFORMATION AND WARNING: Accutane can cause severe birth defects if it is taken when a woman is pregnant. There is an extremely high risk that you will have a severely deformed baby if:

- you are pregnant when you start taking Accutane,
- you become pregnant while you are taking Accutane,
- you do not wait at least one month after you stop taking Accutane before becoming pregnant.

It is recommended that you and your doctor schedule an appointment every month to repeat the pregnancy test and check your body's response to Accutane. For your health and well-being, be sure to keep your appointments as scheduled.

THE CONSENT

My treatment with Accutane has been personally explained to me by Dr. _____ .

The following points of information, among others, have been specifically discussed and made clear:

1. I, _____ ,
   (Patient's Name)
   understand that Accutane is a very powerful medicine used to treat severe cystic acne that did not get better with other treatments including oral antibiotics.
   INITIALS: _____
2. I understand that I must not take Accutane if I am or may become pregnant during treatment.
   INITIALS: _____
3. I understand that severe birth defects have occurred in babies of women who took Accutane during pregnancy. I have been warned by my doctor that there is an extremely high risk of severe damage to my unborn baby if I am or become pregnant while I am taking Accutane.
   INITIALS: _____
4. I have been told by my doctor that effective birth control (contraception) must be used for at least one month before starting Accutane, all during Accutane therapy and for at least one month after Accutane treatment has stopped. My doctor has recommended that I either abstain from sexual intercourse or use two reliable kinds of birth control at the same time. I have also been told that any method of birth control can fail.
   INITIALS: _____
5. I know that I must have a blood test that shows I am not pregnant within two weeks before starting Accutane, and I understand that I must wait until the second or third day of my next normal menstrual period before starting Accutane. INITIALS: _____
6. My doctor has told me that I can participate in the "Patient Referral" program for an initial free pregnancy test and birth control counseling session by a consulting physician.
   INITIALS: _____
7. I also know that I must immediately stop taking Accutane if I become pregnant while taking the drug and immediately contact my doctor to discuss the desirability of continuing the pregnancy. INITIALS: _____
8. I have carefully read the Accutane patient brochure, "Important information concerning your treatment with Accutane," given to me by my doctor. I understand all of its contents and have talked over any questions I have with my doctor. INITIALS: _____
9. I am not now pregnant, nor do I plan to become pregnant for at least 30 days after I have completely finished taking Accutane. INITIALS: _____
10. My doctor has told me that I can participate in a survey concerning Accutane use in women by completing an additional form. INITIALS: _____

I now authorize Dr. _____ to begin my treatment with Accutane.

_____
Patient, Parent or Guardian   Date

Address _____

_____

_____

Telephone Number

I have fully explained to the patient, _____ , the nature and purpose of the treatment described above and the risks to women of childbearing potential. I have asked the patient if she has any questions regarding the treatment with Accutane and have answered those questions to the best of my ability.

_____
Physician   Date

P.I. 0688

Shown in Product Identification Section, page 424

EFUDEX®   ℞
[*ef'u-dex*]
(fluorouracil/Roche)

The following text is complete prescribing information based on official labeling in effect June 1, 1989.

DESCRIPTION

Efudex solutions and cream are topical preparations containing the fluorinated pyrimidine 5-fluorouracil, an antineoplastic antimetabolite.

Efudex Solution consists of 2% or 5% fluorouracil/Roche on a weight/weight basis, compounded with propylene glycol, tris(hydroxymethyl) aminomethane, hydroxypropyl cellulose, parabens (methyl and propyl) and disodium edetate.

Efudex Cream contains 5% fluorouracil/Roche in a vanishing cream base consisting of white petrolatum, stearyl alcohol, propylene glycol, polysorbate 60 and parabens (methyl and propyl).

ACTIONS

There is evidence that the metabolism of fluorouracil in the anabolic pathway blocks the methylation reaction of deoxyuridylic acid to thymidylic acid. In this fashion fluorouracil interferes with the synthesis of deoxyribonucleic acid (DNA) and to a lesser extent inhibits the formation of ribonucleic acid (RNA). Since DNA and RNA are essential for cell division and growth, the effect of fluorouracil may be to create a thymine deficiency which provokes unbalanced growth and death of the cell. The effects of DNA and RNA deprivation are most marked on those cells which grow more rapidly and which take up fluorouracil at a more rapid pace. The catabolic metabolism of fluorouracil results in degradative products (e.g., CO_2, urea, α-fluoro-β-alanine) which are inactive. Studies in man with topical application of ^{14}C-labeled Efudex demonstrated insignificant absorption as measured by ^{14}C content of plasma, urine and respiratory CO_2.

INDICATIONS

Efudex is recommended for the topical treatment of multiple actinic or solar keratoses. In the 5% strength it is also useful in the treatment of superficial basal cell carcinomas, when conventional methods are impractical, such as with multiple lesions or difficult treatment sites. The diagnosis should be established prior to treatment, since this new method has not been proven effective in other types of basal cell carcinomas. With isolated, easily accessible lesions, conventional techniques are preferred since success with such lesions is almost 100% with these methods. The success rate with Efudex cream and solution is approximately 93%. This 93% success rate is based on 113 lesions in 54 patients. Twenty-five lesions treated with the solution produced one failure and 88 lesions treated with the cream produced 7 failures.

CONTRAINDICATIONS

Efudex is contraindicated in patients with known hypersensitivity to any of its components.

WARNINGS

If an occlusive dressing is used, there may be an increase in the incidence of inflammatory reactions in the adjacent normal skin. A porous gauze dressing may be applied for cosmetic reasons without increase in reaction.

Prolonged exposure to ultraviolet rays should be avoided while under treatment with Efudex because the intensity of the reaction may be increased.

Usage in Pregnancy: Safety for use in pregnancy has not been established.

PRECAUTIONS

If Efudex is applied with the fingers, the hands should be washed immediately afterward. Efudex should be applied with care near the eyes, nose and mouth. Solar keratoses which do not respond should be biopsied to confirm the diagnosis. Patients should be forewarned that the reaction in the treated areas may be unsightly during therapy, and, in some cases, for several weeks following cessation of therapy. Follow-up biopsies should be performed as indicated in the management of superficial basal cell carcinoma.

ADVERSE REACTIONS

The most frequently encountered local reactions are pain, pruritus, hyperpigmentation and burning at the site of application. Other local reactions include allergic contact dermatitis, scarring, soreness, tenderness, suppuration, scaling and swelling.

Also reported are alopecia, insomnia, stomatitis, irritability, medicinal taste, photosensitivity, lacrimation, telangiectasia and urticaria, although a causal relationship is remote.

Laboratory abnormalities reported are leukocytosis, thrombocytopenia, toxic granulation and eosinophilia.

DOSAGE AND ADMINISTRATION

When Efudex is applied to a lesion, a response occurs with the following sequence: erythema, usually followed by vesiculation, erosion, ulceration, necrosis and epithelization.

Actinic or solar keratosis: Apply cream or solution twice daily in an amount sufficient to cover the lesions. Medication should be continued until the inflammatory response reaches the erosion, necrosis and ulceration stage, at which time use of the drug should be terminated. The usual duration of therapy is from two to four weeks. Complete healing of the lesions may not be evident for one to two months following cessation of Efudex therapy.

Superficial basal cell carcinomas: **Only the 5% strength is recommended.** Apply cream or solution twice daily in an amount sufficient to cover the lesions. Treatment should be continued for at least three to six weeks. Therapy may be required for as long as 10 to 12 weeks before the lesions are obliterated. As in any neoplastic condition, the patient should be followed for a reasonable period of time to determine if a cure has been obtained.

HOW SUPPLIED

Efudex Solution, 10-ml drop dispensers—containing 2% or 5% fluorouracil/Roche on a weight/weight basis, compounded with propylene glycol, tris(hydroxymethyl)-

aminomethane, hydroxypropyl cellulose, parabens (methyl and propyl) and disodium edetate.

Efudex Cream, 25-Gm tubes—containing 5% fluorouracil/Roche in a vanishing cream base consisting of white petrolatum, stearyl alcohol, propylene glycol, polysorbate 60 and parabens (methyl and propyl).

P.I. 1181

SOLATENE®   ℞
[sol 'a-teen]
(beta-carotene/Roche)
capsules

The following text is complete prescribing information based on official labeling in effect June 1, 1989.

DESCRIPTION
Solatene (beta-carotene) is available in capsules for oral administration. Each capsule is composed of beadlets containing 30 mg beta-carotene, ascorbyl palmitate, corn starch, dl-α-tocopherol, gelatin, peanut oil and sucrose. Gelatin capsule shells may contain parabens (methyl and propyl), potassium sorbate, FD&C Blue No. 1, D&C Yellow No. 10, FD&C Red No. 3, FD&C Green No. 3 and titanium dioxide.

Beta-carotene, precursor of vitamin A, is a carotenoid pigment occurring naturally in green and yellow vegetables. Chemically, beta-carotene has the empirical formula $C_{40}H_{56}$ and a calculated molecular weight of 536.85. Trans-beta-carotene is a red, crystalline compound which is insoluble in water.

CLINICAL PHARMACOLOGY
Beta-carotene, a provitamin A, belongs to the class of carotenoid pigments. In terms of its vitamin activity, 6 μg of dietary beta-carotene is considered equivalent to 1 μg of vitamin A (retinol). Bioavailability of beta-carotene depends on the presence of fat in the diet to act as a carrier, and bile in the intestinal tract for its absorption. Beta-carotene is metabolized, primarily in the intestine, to vitamin A at a rate of approximately 50% to 60% of normal dietary intake and falls off rapidly as intake goes up. In humans, an appreciable amount of unchanged beta-carotene is absorbed and stored in various tissues, especially the depot fat. Small amounts may be converted to vitamin A in the liver. The vitamin A derived from beta-carotene follows the same metabolic pathway as that from dietary sources. The major route of elimination is fecal excretion. Excessive ingestion of carotenes is not harmful, but it may cause yellow coloration of the skin, which disappears upon reduction or cessation of intake.

INDICATIONS AND USAGE
Solatene is used to reduce the severity of photosensitivity reactions in patients with erythropoietic protoporphyria (EPP).

CONTRAINDICATIONS
Solatene is contraindicated in patients with known hypersensitivity to the drug.

WARNINGS
Solatene has not been shown to be effective as a sunscreen.

PRECAUTIONS
General: Solatene should be used with caution in patients with impaired renal or hepatic function because safe use in the presence of these conditions has not been established.
Information for Patients: Patients receiving Solatene should be advised against taking supplementary vitamin A since Solatene administration will fulfill normal vitamin A requirements. They should be cautioned to continue sun protection, and forewarned that their skin may appear slightly yellow while receiving Solatene.
Carcinogenesis, Mutagenesis, Impairment of Fertility: Long-term studies in animals to determine carcinogenesis have not been completed. *In vitro* and *in vivo* studies to evaluate mutagenic potential were negative. No effects on fertility in male rats were observed at doses as high as 500 mg/kg/day (100 times the recommended human dose).
Pregnancy: Teratogenic Effects: Pregnancy Category C. Beta-carotene has been shown to be fetotoxic (i.e., cause an increase in resorption rate), but not teratogenic when given to rats at doses 300 to 400 times the maximum recommended human dose. No such fetotoxicity was observed at 75 times the maximum recommended human dose or less. A three-generation reproduction study in rats receiving beta-carotene at a dietary concentration of 0.1% (1000 ppm) has revealed no evidence of impaired fertility or effect on the fetus. There are no adequate and well-controlled studies in pregnant women. Solatene should be used during pregnancy only if the potential benefit justifies the potential risk to the fetus.
Nursing Mothers: It is not known whether this drug is excreted in human milk. Because many drugs are excreted in human milk, caution should be exercised when Solatene is administered to a nursing mother.

ADVERSE REACTIONS
Some patients may have occasional loose stools while taking Solatene. This reaction is sporadic and may not require discontinuance of medication. Other reactions which have been reported rarely are ecchymoses and arthralgia.

OVERDOSAGE
There are no reported cases of overdosage. The oral LD_{50} of beta-carotene (suspended in 5% gum acacia solution) in mice and rats is greater than 20,000 mg/kg. No lethality was observed in mice following administration of 30-mg beadlet capsules (ground and suspended in 5% gum acacia) at a dose of 1200 mg/kg beta-carotene.

DOSAGE AND ADMINISTRATION
Solatene may be administered either as a single daily dose or in divided doses, preferably with meals.
Usage in Children: The usual dosage for children under 14 is 30 to 150 mg (1 to 5 capsules) per day. Capsules may be opened and the contents mixed in orange juice or tomato juice to aid administration.
Usage in Adults: The usual adult dosage is 30 to 300 mg (1 to 10 capsules) per day.
Dosage should be adjusted depending on the severity of the symptoms and the response of the patient. Several weeks of therapy are necessary to accumulate enough Solatene in the skin to exert its effect. Patients should be instructed not to increase exposure to sunlight until they appear carotenemic (first seen as yellowness of palms and soles). This usually occurs after two to six weeks of therapy. Exposure to the sun may then be increased gradually. The protective effect is not total and each patient should establish his or her own limits of exposure.

HOW SUPPLIED
Solatene is available in blue and green capsules, each containing 30 mg of beta-carotene—bottles of 100 (NDC 0004-0115-01). Imprint on capsules: SOLATENE ROCHE.
P.I. 0489
     Shown in Product Identification Section, page 425

TEGISON®   ℞
[teg 'is-on]
etretinate/Roche
CAPSULES

The following text is complete prescribing information based on official labeling in effect June 1, 1989.

CONTRAINDICATION
Tegison must not be used by females who are pregnant, who intend to become pregnant, or who are unreliable or may not use reliable contraception while undergoing treatment. The period of time during which pregnancy must be avoided after treatment is concluded has not been determined. Tegison blood levels of 0.5 to 12 ng/mL have been reported in 5 of 47 patients in the range of 2.1 to 2.9 years after treatment was concluded. The length of time necessary to wait after discontinuation of treatment to assure that no drug will be detectable in the blood has not been determined. The significance of undetectable blood levels relative to the risk of teratogenicity is unknown.

Major human fetal abnormalities related to Tegison administration have been reported, including meningomyelocoele, meningoencephalocoele, multiple synostoses, facial dysmorphia, syndactylies, absence of terminal phalanges, malformations of hip, ankle and forearm, low set ears, high palate, decreased cranial volume, and alterations of the skull and cervical vertebrae on x-ray.

Women of childbearing potential must not be given Tegison until pregnancy is excluded. It is strongly recommended that a pregnancy test be performed within two weeks prior to initiating Tegison therapy. Tegison therapy should start on the second or third day of the next normal menstrual period. An effective form of contraception must be used for at least one month before Tegison therapy, during therapy and following discontinuation of Tegison therapy for an indefinite period of time.

Females should be fully counseled on the serious risks to the fetus should they become pregnant while undergoing treatment or after discontinuation of therapy. If pregnancy does occur, the physician and patient should discuss the desirability of continuing the pregnancy.

DESCRIPTION
Tegison (brand of etretinate/Roche), a retinoid, is available in 10-mg and 25-mg gelatin capsules for oral administration. Each capsule also contains corn starch, lactose and talc. Gelatin capsule shells contain parabens (methyl and propyl) and potassium sorbate, with the following dye systems: 10 mg—iron oxide (yellow, black and red). FD&C Blue No. 2 and tita-

nium dioxide; 25 mg—iron oxide (yellow, black and red) and titanium dioxide.

Chemically, etretinate is ethyl (all-E)-9-(4-methoxy-2,3,6-trimethylphenyl)-3,7-dimethyl-2,4,6,8-nonate traenoate and is related to both retinoic acid and retinol (vitamin A). It is a greenish-yellow to yellow powder with a calculated molecular weight of 354.5.

CLINICAL PHARMACOLOGY
The mechanism of action of Tegison is unknown.
Clinical: Improvement in psoriatic patients occurs in association with a decrease in scale, erythema and thickness of lesions, as well as histological evidence of normalization of epidermal differentiation, decreased stratum corneum thickness and decreased inflammation in the epidermis and dermis.
Pharmacokinetics: The pharmacokinetic profile of etretinate is predictable and is linear following single and multiple doses. Etretinate is extensively metabolized following oral dosing, with significant first-pass metabolism to the acid form, which also has the all-*trans* structure and is pharmacologically active. Subsequent metabolism results in the 13-*cis* acid form, chain-shortened breakdown products and conjugates that are ultimately excreted in the bile and urine.
After a six-month course of therapy with doses ranging from 25 mg once daily to 25 mg four times daily, Cmax values ranged from 102 to 389 ng/mL and occurred at Tmax values of two to six hours. In one study the apparent terminal half-life after six months of therapy was approximately 120 days. In another study of 47 patients treated chronically with etretinate, 5 had detectable serum drug levels (in the range of 0.5 to 12 ng/mL) 2.1 to 2.9 years after therapy was discontinued. The long half-life appears to be due to storage of etretinate in adipose tissue.
Etretinate is more than 99% bound to plasma proteins, predominantly lipoproteins, whereas its active metabolite, the all-*trans* acid form, is predominantly bound to albumin. Concentrations of etretinate in blister fluid after six weeks of dosing were approximately one-tenth of those observed in plasma. Concentrations of etretinate and its all-*trans* acid metabolite in epidermal specimens obtained after 1 to 36 months of therapy were a function of location; subcutis > > serum > epidermis > dermis. Similarly, liver concentrations of etretinate in patients receiving therapy for six months were generally higher than concomitant plasma concentrations and tended to be higher in livers with a higher degree of fatty infiltration.
Studies in normal volunteers indicated that, when compared with the fasting state, the absorption of etretinate was increased by whole milk or a high-lipid diet.

INDICATIONS AND USAGE
Tegison is indicated for the treatment of severe recalcitrant psoriasis, including the erythrodermic and generalized pustular types. Because of significant adverse effects associated with its use, Tegison should be prescribed only by physicians knowledgeable in the systemic use of retinoids and reserved for patients with severe recalcitrant psoriasis who are unresponsive to or intolerant of standard therapies; topical tar plus UVB light; psoralens plus UVA light; systemic corticosteroids; and methotrexate.
The use of Tegison resulted in clinical improvement in the majority of patients treated. Complete clearing of the disease was observed after four to nine months of therapy in 13% of all patients treated for severe psoriasis. This included complete clearing in 16% of patients with erythrodermic psoriasis and 37% of patients with generalized pustular psoriasis.
After discontinuation of Tegison the majority of patients experience some degree of relapse by the end of two months. After relapse, subsequent four- to nine-month courses of Tegison therapy resulted in approximately the same clinical response as experienced during the initial course of therapy.

CONTRAINDICATIONS
Pregnancy: Category X. See boxed CONTRAINDICATION.

WARNINGS

Pseudotumor cerebri: Tegison and other retinoids have been associated with cases of pseudotumor cerebri (benign intracranial hypertension). Early signs and symptoms of pseudotumor cerebri include papilledema, headache, nausea and vomiting, and visual disturbances. Patients with these symptoms should be examined for papilledema and, if present, they should discontinue Tegison immediately and be referred for neurologic diagnosis and care.
Hepatoxicity: Of the 652 patients treated in U.S. clinical trials, ten had clinical or histologic hepatitis considered possibly or probably related to Tegison treatment. Liver function tests returned to normal in eight of these patients after Tegison was discontinued; one patient had histologic changes resembling chronic active hepatitis six months off therapy, and one patient had no fol-

---

Continued on next page

Roche Derm.—Cont.

low-up available. There have been four reports of hepatitis-related deaths worldwide; two of these patients had received etretinate for a month or less before presenting with hepatic symptoms. Elevations of AST (SGOT), ALT (SGPT) or LDH have occurred in 18%, 23% and 15%, respectively, of individuals treated with Tegison. Cases with pathology findings of hepatic fibrosis, necrosis and/or cirrhosis which may be related to Tegison therapy have been reported. If hepatotoxicity is suspected during treatment with Tegison, the drug should be discontinued and the etiology further investigated.

Ophthalmic effects: Corneal erosion, abrasion, irregularity and punctate staining have occurred in patients treated with Tegison, although these effects were absent or improved after therapy was stopped in those patients who had follow-up examinations. Corneal opacities have occurred in patients receiving isotretinoin; they had either completely resolved or were resolving at follow-up six to seven weeks after discontinuation of the drug. Other ophthalmic effects that have occurred in Tegison patients include decreased visual acuity and blurring of vision, minimal posterior subcapsular cataract, iritis, blot retinal hemorrhage, scotoma and photophobia. A number of cases of decreased night vision have occurred during Tegison therapy. Because the onset in some patients was sudden, patients should be advised of this potential problem and warned to be cautious when driving or operating any vehicle at night. Any Tegison patient experiencing visual difficulties should discontinue the drug and have an ophthalmological examination.

Hyperostosis: There is a very high likelihood of the development of hyperostosis with Tegison therapy. In one clinical trial, 45 patients with a mean age of 40 years were retrospectively evaluated for evidence of hyperostosis. They had received etretinate at a mean dose of 0.8 mg/kg for a mean duration of 33 months at the time of x-ray. Eleven patients had psoriasis, while 34 patients had a disorder of keratinization. Of these, 38 patients who continued to receive etretinate at an average dose of 0.8 mg/kg for an average duration of 60 months, 32 (84%) had radiographic evidence of extraspinal tendon and ligament calcification. The most common sites of involvement were the ankles (76%), pelvis (53%) and knees (42%); spinal changes were uncommon. Involvement tended to be bilateral and multifocal. There were no bone or joint symptoms at the sites of radiographic abnormalities in 47% of the affected patients.

Lipids: Blood lipid determinations should be performed before Tegison is administered and then at intervals of one or two weeks until the lipid response to Tegison is established; this usually occurs within four to eight weeks. Approximately 45% of patients receiving Tegison during clinical trials experienced an elevation of plasma triglycerides. Approximately 37% developed a decrease in high density lipoproteins and about 16% showed an increase in cholesterol levels. These effects on triglycerides, HDL and cholesterol were reversible after cessation of Tegison therapy. Patients with an increased tendency to develop hypertriglyceridemia include those with diabetes mellitus, obesity, increased alcohol intake or a familial history of these conditions.

Hypertriglyceridemia, hypercholesterolemia and lowered HDL may increase a patient's cardiovascular risk status. In addition, elevation of serum triglycerides in excess of 800 mg/dL has been associated with acute pancreatitis. Therefore, every attempt should be made to control significant elevations of triglycerides or cholesterol or significant decreases in HDL. Some patients have been able to reverse triglyceride and cholesterol elevations or HDL decrease by reduction in weight or restriction of dietary fat and alcohol while continuing Tegison therapy.

Cardiovascular effects: During clinical trials of 652 patients, 21 significant cardiovascular adverse incidents were reported, all in patients who had a strong history of cardiovascular risk. These incidents were not considered related to Tegison therapy except for two cases of myocardial infarction: one which was considered possibly related to Tegison therapy and one for which a relationship was not specified.

Animal studies: In general, the signs of etretinate toxicity in rats, mice and dogs are dose-related with respect to incidence, onset and severity. In rodents, the most striking manifestations of this toxicity are bone fractures; no evidence of fractures was observed in a one-year dog study. Other dose-related changes in some animals treated with etretinate in subchronic or chronic toxicity studies include alopecia, erythema, reductions in body weight and food consumption, stiffness, altered gait, hematologic changes, elevations in serum alkaline phosphatase and testicular atrophy with microscopic evidence of reduced spermatogenesis.

PRECAUTIONS

Information for Patients: Women of childbearing potential should be advised that they must not be pregnant when Tegison therapy is initiated, and that they should use an effective form of contraception for one month prior to Tegison therapy, while taking Tegison and after Tegison has been discontinued. Tegison has been found in the blood of some patients two to three years after the drug was discontinued. See boxed CONTRAINDICATION.

Because of the relationship of Tegison to vitamin A, patients should be advised against taking vitamin A supplements to avoid possible additive toxic effects.

Patients should be advised that transient exacerbation of psoriasis is commonly seen during the initial period of therapy.

Patients should be informed that they may experience decreased tolerance to contact lenses during and after therapy.

Laboratory Tests: See WARNINGS section. In clinical studies, the incidence of hypertriglyceridemia was one patient in two, that of hypercholesterolemia one patient in six, and that of decreased HDL one patient in three during Tegison therapy. Pretreatment and follow-up blood lipids should be obtained under fasting conditions. If alcohol has been consumed, at least 36 hours should elapse before these determinations are made. It is recommended that these tests be performed at weekly or biweekly intervals until the lipid response to Tegison is established.

Elevations of AST (SGOT), ALT (SGPT) or LDH have occurred in 18%, 23% and 15%, respectively, of individuals treated with Tegison. It is recommended that these tests be performed prior to initiation of Tegison therapy, at one to two week intervals for the first one to two months of therapy and thereafter at intervals of one to three months, depending on the response to Tegison administration.

Drug Interactions: Little information is available on drug interactions with Tegison; however, concomitant consumption of milk increases the absorption of etretinate. See *Pharmacokinetics* and DOSAGE AND ADMINISTRATION sections.

Carcinogenesis, Mutagenesis, Impairment of Fertility:
Carcinogenesis: In a two-year study, male or female Sprague-Dawley rats given etretinate by dietary admixture at doses up to 3 mg/kg/day (two times the maximum recommended human therapeutic dose) had no increase in tumor incidence. In an 80-week study, Crl:CD-1 (ICR) BR mice were given etretinate by dietary admixture at doses of 1 to 5 mg/kg/day. An increased incidence of blood vessel tumors (hemangiomas and hemangiosarcomas in several different tissue sites) was noted in the high-dose male group (4 to 5 mg/kg/day) but not in the female group.

Mutagenesis: Etretinate was evaluated by the Ames test in a host-mediated assay, in the micronucleus test, and in a "treat and plate" test using the diploid yeast strain *S. cerevisiae* D7. Except for a weakly positive response in the Ames test using the tester strain TA 100, there was no evidence of genotoxicity. No differences in the rate of sister chromatid exchange (SCE) were noted in lymphocytes of patients before and after four weeks of treatment with therapeutic doses of etretinate.

Impairment of Fertility: In a study of fertility and general reproductive performance in rats, no etretinate-related effects were observed at doses up to 2.5 mg/kg/day. At a dose of 5 mg/kg/day (approximately three times the maximum recommended human therapeutic dose) the readiness of the treated animals to copulate was reduced but the pregnancy rate was unaffected. The number of viable young at birth and their postnatal weight gain and survival were adversely affected at the high dose. The pregnancy rate of the untreated first generation animals and postnatal weight gain of the untreated second generation animals were also reduced. No adverse effects on sperm production were noted in 12 psoriatic patients given 75 mg/day of etretinate for one month and 50 mg/day for an additional two months. However, testicular atrophy was noted in subchronic and chronic rat studies and in a chronic dog study, in some cases at doses approaching those recommended for use in humans. Decreased sperm counts were reported in a 13-week dog study at doses as low as 3 mg/kg/day (approximately twice the maximum recommended human dose). Spermatogenic arrest also was reported with chronic administration of the all-*trans* metabolite to dogs.

Pregnancy: Category X. See boxed CONTRAINDICATION. The following limited preliminary data must not be read or understood to diminish the serious risk of teratogenicity set forth in the boxed pregnancy CONTRAINDICATION.

Thirty women worldwide have been reported as having taken one or more doses of Tegison during pregnancy. In 29 cases in which information was available, there were a total of ten congenital abnormalities. The occurrence of congenital abnormalities was four of 20 among delivered infants, two of two among spontaneously aborted fetuses, and four of seven among induced abortions.

A further 38 women are reported to have become pregnant within 24 months after discontinuing Tegison therapy. Because congenital abnormalities have been reported in these pregnancies, it cannot be stated that there is a "safe" time to become pregnant after Tegison therapy. In 37 cases in which information was available, there were a total of three congenital abnormalities. The occurrence of congential abnormalities was two of 29 among delivered infants, zero of one among spontaneously aborted fetuses, and one of five among induced abortions. Two stillbirths with no apparent congenital abnormalities were attributed to other causes.

Nonteratogenic Effects: No adverse effects on various parameters of late gestation and lactation were observed in rats at doses of etretinate up to 4 mg/kg/day (approximately three times the maximum human recommended dose). At doses of 8 mg/kg/day (approximately five times the maximum human recommended dose) of etretinate, the rate of stillbirths was increased and neonatal weight gain and survival rate were markedly reduced.

Nursing Mothers: Studies have shown that etretinate is excreted in the milk of lactating rats; however, it is not known whether this drug is excreted in human milk. Because of the potential for adverse effects, nursing mothers should not receive Tegison.

Pediatric Use: No clinical studies have been conducted in the U. S. using Tegison in children. Ossification of interosseous ligaments and tendons of the extremities has been reported. Two children showed x-ray changes suggestive of premature epiphyseal closure during treatment with Tegison. Skeletal hyperostosis has also been reported after treatment with isotretinoin. It is not known if any of these effects occur more commonly in children, but concern should be

---

TABLE I
ADVERSE EVENTS FREQUENTLY REPORTED DURING CLINICAL TRIALS
PERCENT OF PATIENTS REPORTING

BODY SYSTEM	>75%	50–75%	25–50%	10–25%
Mucocutaneous	Dry nose Chapped lips	Excessive thirst Sore mouth	Nosebleed	Cheilitis Sore tongue
Dermatologic	Loss of hair Palm/sole/ fingertip peeling	Dry skin Itching Rash Red scaly face Skin fragility	Bruising Sunburn	Nail disorder Skin peeling
Musculoskeletal	Hyperostosis*	Bone/joint pain	Muscle cramps	
Central Nervous		Fatigue	Headache	Fever
Special Senses		Irritation of eyes	Eyeball pain Eyelid abnormalities	Abnormalities of: —conjunctiva —cornea —lens —retina Conjunctivitis Decrease in visual acuity Double vision
Gastrointestinal			Abdominal pain Changes in appetite	Nausea

*In a retrospective study of 45 patients, 38 of whom received long-term etretinate therapy, 32 (84%) had radiographic evidence of hyperotosis. See WARNINGS.

TABLE II
LESS FREQUENT ADVERSE EVENTS REPORTED DURING CLINICAL TRIALS
(SOME OF WHICH MAY BEAR NO RELATIONSHIP TO THERAPY)
PERCENT OF PATIENTS REPORTING

BODY SYSTEM	1–10%	<1%
Mucocutaneous	Dry eyes Mucous membrane abnormalities Dry mouth Gingival bleeding/inflammation	Decreased mucous secretion Rhinorrhea
Dermatologic	Hair abnormalities Bullous eruption Cold/clammy skin Onycholysis Paronychia Pyogenic granuloma Changes in perspiration	Abnormal skin odor Granulation tissue Healing impairment Herpes simplex Hirsutism Increased pore size Sensory skin changes Skin atrophy Skin fissures Skin infection Skin nodule Skin ulceration Urticaria
Musculoskeletal	Myalgia	Gout Hyperkinesia Hypertonia
Central Nervous System	Dizziness Lethargy Changes in sensation Pain Rigors	Abnormal thinking Amnesia Anxiety Depression Pseudotumor cerebri Emotional lability Faint feeling Flu-like symptoms
Special Senses	Abnormal lacrimation Abnormal vision Abnormalities of: —Extraocular musculature —Ocular tension —Pupil —Vitreous Earache Otitis externa	Change in equilibrium Ear drainage Ear infection Hearing change Night vision decrease Photophobia Visual change Scotoma
Gastrointestinal	Hepatitis	Constipation Diarrhea Melena Flatulence Weight loss Oral ulcers Taste perversion Tooth caries
Cardiovascular	Cardiovascular thrombotic or obstructive events Edema	Atrial fibrillation Chest pain Coagulation disorder Phlebitis Postural hypotension Syncope
Respiratory	Dyspnea	Coughing Increased sputum Dysphonia Pharyngitis
Renal		Kidney stones
Urogenital		Abnormal menses Atrophic vaginitis Dysuria Polyuria Urinary retention
Other	Malignant neoplasms	

greater because of the growth process. Pretreatment x-rays for bone age including x-rays of the knees, followed by yearly monitoring, are advised. In addition, pain or limitation of motion should be evaluated with appropriate radiological examination. Because of the lack of data on the use of etretinate in children and the possibility of their being more sensitive to effects of the drug, this product should be used only when all alternative therapies have been exhausted.

ADVERSE EVENTS

Clinical: Hepatitis was observed in about 1.5% of patients treated with Tegison in clinical trials. Pathology findings of hepatic fibrosis, necrosis and/or cirrhosis have been reported. See WARNINGS section.

Tegison has been associated with pseudotumor cerebri. See WARNINGS section.

Hypervitaminosis A produces a wide spectrum of signs and symptoms of primarily the mucocutaneous, musculoskeletal, hepatic and central nervous systems. Nearly all of the clinical adverse events reported to date with Tegison administration resemble those of the hypervitaminosis A syndrome. Table I lists the adverse events frequently reported during clinical trials in which 652 patients were treated either for psoriasis (591 patients) or a disorder of keratinization (61 patients). Table II lists less frequently reported adverse events in these same patients. However the number of patients evaluated for each adverse event was not 652 in every case.

[See table I on preceding page].

[See table II left].

Laboratory: Tegison therapy induces change in serum lipids in a significant number of treated patients. Approximately 45% of patients experienced elevation in serum triglycerides, 37% a decrease in high density lipoproteins and 16% an increase in cholesterol levels.

Approximately 46% of patients has elevations of triglycerides above 250 mg/dL, 54% had decreases of HDL below 36 mg%, and 19% had elevations of cholesrerol above 300 mg%. One case of eruptive xanthomas associated with triglyceride levels greater than 1000 mg% has been reported. Elevations of AST (SGOT), ALT (SGPT) or LDH were experienced by 18%, 23% and 15%, respectively, of individuals treated with Tegison. In most of the patients, the elevations were slight to moderate and became normal either during therapy or after cessation of treatment. See WARNINGS section.

Table III list the laboratory abnormalities reported during clinical trials. Data for patients who received intermittent courses of therapy for periods up to five years are included. Any instance of two consecutive values outside the range of normal, or an abnormal value with no follow-up during therapy, was considered to be possibly related to Tegison.

[See table III on next page].

OVERDOSAGE

There has been no experience with acute overdosage in humans.

The acute oral and intraperitoneal toxicities (LD_{50}) of etretinate capsules in mice and rats were greater than 4000 mg/kg. The acute oral toxicity (LD_{50}) of etretinate substance in 4% solution was 2300 mg/kg in mice and 1300 mg/kg in rats.

DOSAGE AND ADMINISTRATION

There is intersubject variation in the absorption and the rate of metabolism of Tegison. Individualization of dosage is required to achieve the maximal therapeutic response with a tolerable degree of side effects. Therapy with Tegison should generally be initiated at a dosage of 0.75 to 1 mg/kg of body weight/day taken in divided doses. A maximum dose of 1.5 mg/kg/day should not be exceeded. Erythrodermic psoriasis may respond to lower initial doses of 0.25 mg/kg/day increased by 0.25 mg/kg/day each week until optimal initial response is attained.

Maintenance doses of 0.5 to 0.75 mg/kg/day may be initiated after initial response, generally after 8 to 16 weeks of therapy. In general, therapy should be terminated in patients whose lesions have sufficiently resolved. Relapses may be treated as outlined for initial therapy.

Tegison should be administered with food.

HOW SUPPLIED

Brown and green capsules, 10 mg, imprinted TEGISON 10 ROCHE; Prescription Paks of 30 (NDC 0004-0177-57).
Brown and caramel capsules, 25 mg, imprinted TEGISON 25 ROCHE; Prescription Paks of 30 (NDC 0004-0179-57).
STORE AT 59° TO 86°F; 15° TO 30°C. PROTECT FROM LIGHT.
P.I. 1286

Shown in Product Identification Section, page 425

Continued on next page

Roche Derm.—Cont.

TABLE III
LABORATORY ABNORMALITIES REPORTED DURING CLINICAL TRIALS
PERCENT OF PATIENTS REPORTING

BODY SYSTEM	25–50%	10–25%	1–10%

Hematologic	Increased:
	—MCHC (60%)
	—MCH
	—Reticulocytes
	—PTT
	—ESR
		Decreased:
		—Hemoglobin/HCT
		—RBC
		—MCV
		Increased platelets
		Increased or
		  decreased:
		—WBC and compo-
		  nents
		—Prothrombin time
			Decreased:
			—Platelets
			—MCH
			—MCHC
			—PTT
			Increased:
			—Hemoglobin/HCT
			—RBC

Urinary		WBC in urine	Proteinuria Glycosuria Microscopic hematuria Casts in urine Acetonuria Hemoglobinuria

Hepatic	Increased
	  triglycerides
		Increased:
		—AST (SGOT)
		—ALT (SGPT)
		—Alkaline
		  phosphatase
		—GGTP
		—Globulin
		—Cholesterol
			Increased bilirubin
			Increased or
			  decreased:
			—Total protein
			—Albumin

Renal			Increased: —BUN —Creatinine

Electrolytes	Increased or
	  decreased potassium
		Increased or
		  decreased:
		—Venous CO_2
		—Sodium
		—Chloride	

Miscellaneous	Increased or decreased: —Calcium —Phosphorus	Increased or decreased FBS	Increased CPK

Roche Laboratories
Division of Hoffmann-La Roche Inc.
NUTLEY, NJ 07110

ALURATE® ELIXIR   ℞
[al'u-rate]
(aprobarbital/Roche)

The following text is complete prescribing information based on official labeling in effect June 1, 1989.

The following sections contain information specifically applicable to Alurate as well as information pertinent to other barbiturates. The information pertinent to other barbiturates should be considered when administering Alurate.

DESCRIPTION
Alurate (aprobarbital/Roche) is an intermediate-acting barbiturate which is used as a sedative-hypnotic. As with other barbiturates, it acts as a CNS depressant. Alurate is available for oral administration as a red elixir providing 40 mg of aprobarbital per teaspoonful (5 ml) in a vehicle containing 20 percent alcohol, dextrose, saccharin, sorbitol, sucrose, FD&C Yellow No. 6, FD&C Red No. 40, flavors and water. Chemically, aprobarbital is 5-allyl-5-isopropylbarbituric acid. It is a bitter, white crystalline powder with an empirical formula of $C_{10}H_{14}N_2O_3$ and a molecular weight of 210.23.

CLINICAL PHARMACOLOGY
Barbiturates are capable of producing all levels of CNS mood alteration from excitation to mild sedation, hypnosis and deep coma. Overdosage can produce death. In high enough therapeutic doses, barbiturates induce anesthesia.

Barbiturates depress the sensory cortex, decrease motor activity, alter cerebellar function and produce drowsiness, sedation and hypnosis.

Barbiturate-induced sleep differs from physiological sleep. Sleep laboratory studies have demonstrated that barbiturates reduce the amount of time spent in the rapid eye movement (REM) phase of sleep or dreaming stage. Also, Stages III and IV sleep are decreased. Patients may experience markedly increased dreaming, nightmares and/or insomnia if barbiturates are prescribed for a period of time and then abruptly withdrawn. It is recommended that dosage be reduced gradually over a period of 5 or 6 days to lessen REM rebound and disturbed sleep (for example, decrease the dose from 3 to 2 doses a day for 1 week).

In studies, secobarbital sodium and pentobarbital sodium have been found to lose most of their effectiveness for both inducing and maintaining sleep by the end of 2 weeks of continued drug administration, even with the use of multiple doses. Other barbiturates might also be expected to lose their effectiveness for inducing and maintaining sleep after about 2 weeks. Therefore, as sleep medications, the barbiturates are of limited value beyond short-term use.

Barbiturates have little analgesic action at subanesthetic doses. Rather, they may increase the reaction to painful stimuli. All barbiturates exhibit anticonvulsant activity in anesthetic doses; however, only phenobarbital, mephobarbital and metharbital are effective as oral anticonvulsants in subhypnotic doses.

Barbiturates are respiratory depressants; the degree of depression is dose-dependent. With hypnotic doses, respiratory depression produced by barbiturates is similar to that which occurs during physiologic sleep. Hypnotic doses also cause a slight decrease in blood pressure and heart rate.

Studies in laboratory animals have shown that barbiturates cause reduction in the tone and contractility of the uterus, ureters and urinary bladder. However, concentrations of the drugs required to produce this effect in humans are not reached with sedative-hypnotic doses.

Barbiturates do not impair normal hepatic function, but have been shown to induce liver microsomal enzymes, thus altering the metabolism of certain other drugs. (See Precautions — Drug Interactions section.)

Pharmacokinetics: Barbiturates are absorbed in varying degrees following oral administration. The onset of action for oral barbiturate administration varies from 20 to 60 minutes. Duration of action, which is related to the rate at which the barbiturates are redistributed throughout the body, varies among persons and in the same person from time to time. Aprobarbital, which is an intermediate-acting barbiturate, has a duration of action ranging from 6 to 8 hours.

Barbiturates are weak acids that are absorbed and rapidly distributed to all tissues and fluids, with high concentrations in the brain, liver and kidneys. Lipid solubility of the barbiturates is the dominant factor in their distribution throughout the body. Barbiturates are bound to plasma and tissue proteins to a varying degree, with the degree of binding increasing directly as a function of lipid solubility. Aprobarbital is approximately 20 percent plasma protein-bound. The half-life of aprobarbital ranges from 14 to 34 hours with a mean half-life of 24 hours.

Barbiturates are metabolized primarily by the hepatic microsomal enzyme system; the metabolic products are excreted in the urine and, less commonly, in the feces. Approximately 13 to 24 percent of aprobarbital is eliminated unchanged in the urine. The inactive metabolites of the barbiturates are excreted as conjugates of glucuronic acid.

INDICATIONS AND USAGE
Alurate is indicated for sedation and induction of sleep, on a short-term basis, in conditions requiring a sedative-hypnotic.

CONTRAINDICATIONS
Barbiturates are contraindicated in patients with known barbiturate sensitivity. Barbiturates are also contraindicated in patients with a history of manifest or latent porphyria.

WARNINGS
Habit forming: Barbiturates may be habit forming. Tolerance and psychological and physical dependence may occur with continued use. (See Drug Abuse and Dependence section.) Patients who have a psychological dependence on barbiturates may increase the dosage or decrease the dosage interval without consulting a physician and may subsequently develop a physical dependence. To minimize the possibility of overdosage or the development of dependence, the quantity of sedative-hypnotic barbiturates prescribed or dispensed should be limited to the amount required between appointments. Abrupt cessation after prolonged use may result in withdrawal symptoms, including delirium, convulsions and possibly death.

Barbiturates should be withdrawn gradually from any patient known to be taking excessive doses over long periods of time.

Acute or chronic pain: Caution should be exercised when barbiturates are administered to patients with acute or chronic pain, because paradoxical excitement may be induced or important symptoms may be masked.

Use in pregnancy: Barbiturates can cause fetal damage when administered to a pregnant woman. Retrospective case-controlled studies have suggested a connection between maternal consumption of barbiturates and a higher than expected incidence of fetal abnormalities. Following oral administration, barbiturates readily cross the placental barrier and are distributed throughout the placenta and fetal tissues, with highest concentrations found in the liver and brain.

Withdrawal symptoms occur in infants born to mothers who receive barbiturates throughout the last trimester of pregnancy. (See Drug Abuse and Dependence section.) If this drug is used during pregnancy, or if the patient becomes pregnant while taking this drug, the patient should be apprised of the potential hazard to the fetus.

Synergistic effects: The concomitant use of alcohol or other CNS depressants may produce additive CNS-depressant effects.

PRECAUTIONS
General: Barbiturates may be habit forming. Tolerance and psychological and physical dependence may occur with continued use. (See Drug Abuse and Dependence section.) Barbiturates should be administered with caution, if at all, to patients who are mentally depressed, have suicidal tendencies, or a history of drug abuse. Elderly or debilitated patients may react to barbiturates with marked excitement, depression and confusion. In some persons, barbiturates repeatedly produce excitement rather than depression. In patients with hepatic damage, barbiturates should be administered with caution, and initially in reduced doses. Barbiturates should not be administered to patients showing the premonitory signs of hepatic coma.

Information for Patients: The use of barbiturates carries with it an associated risk of psychological and/or physical dependence. The patient should be warned against increasing the dose of the drug without consulting a physician.

Barbiturates may impair mental and/or physical abilities required for the performance of potentially hazardous tasks, such as driving a car or operating machinery.

Alcohol should not be consumed while taking barbiturates. Concurrent use of barbiturates with other CNS depressants (e.g., alcohol, narcotics, tranquilizers, antihistamines) may result in additional CNS depressant effects.

Laboratory Tests: Prolonged therapy with barbiturates should be accompanied by periodic laboratory evaluation of organ systems, including hematopoietic, renal and hepatic systems.

Drug Interactions: Most reports of clinically significant drug interactions occurring with the barbiturates have involved phenobarbital. However, the application of these data to other barbiturates appears valid and warrants serial blood level determinations of the relevant drugs when there are multiple therapies.

1. *Anticoagulants.* Phenobarbital lowers the plasma levels of dicumarol (name previously used: bishydroxycoumarin) and causes a decrease in anticoagulant activity as measured by the prothrombin time. Barbiturates can induce hepatic microsomal enzymes resulting in increased metabolism of and decreased anticoagulant response to oral anticoagulants (e.g., warfarin, acenocoumarol, dicumarol and phenprocoumon). Patients stabilized on anticoagulant therapy may require dosage adjustments if barbiturates are added to or withdrawn from their dosage regimen.

2. *Corticosteroids.* Barbiturates appear to enhance the metabolism of exogenous corticosteroids, probably through the induction of hepatic microsomal enzymes. Patients stabilized on corticosteroid therapy may require dosage adjustments if barbiturates are added to or withdrawn from their dosage regimen.

3. *Griseofulvin.* Phenobarbital appears to interfere with the absorption of orally administered griseofulvin, thus decreasing its blood level. This effect on therapeutic response has not been established; however, it would be preferable to avoid concomitant administration of these drugs.

4. *Doxycycline.* Phenobarbital has been shown to shorten the half-life of doxycycline for as long as two weeks after discontinuance of the barbiturate therapy. This action is probably the result of induction of hepatic microsomal enzymes that metabolize the antibiotic. If phenobarbital and doxycycline are administered concurrently, the clinical response to doxycycline should be monitored closely.

5. *Phenytoin, sodium valproate, valproic acid.* The effect of barbiturates on the metabolism of phenytoin appears to be variable. Some investigators report an accelerating effect, while others report no effect. Because the effect is not predictable, phenytoin and barbiturate blood levels should be monitored more frequently if these drugs are given concurrently. Sodium valproate and valproic acid appear to decrease barbiturate metabolism; therefore, barbiturate blood levels should be monitored and appropriate dosage adjustments made.

6. *Central nervous system depressants.* The concomitant use of other central nervous system depressants, including other sedatives or hypnotics, antihistamines, tranquilizers or alcohol, may produce additive effects.

7. *Monoamine oxidase inhibitors (MAOI).* MAOI prolong the effects of barbiturates, probably because metabolism of the barbiturates is inhibited.

8. *Estradiol, estrone, progesterone and other steroidal hormones.* Pretreatment with or concurrent administration of phenobarbital may decrease the effect of estradiol by increasing its metabolism. There have been reports of patients treated with antiepileptic drugs (e.g., phenobarbital) who became pregnant while taking oral contraceptives. An alternate contraceptive method might be suggested to women taking phenobarbital.

Carcinogenesis: 1. Animal data. Phenobarbital sodium is carcinogenic in mice and rats after lifetime administration. In mice, it produced benign and malignant liver cell tumors. In rats, benign liver cell tumors were observed very late in life.

2. Human data. In a 29-year epidemiological study of 9136 patients who were treated on an anticonvulsant protocol which included phenobarbital sodium, results indicated a higher than normal incidence of hepatic carcinoma. Previously, some of these patients were treated with Thorotrast, a drug which is known to produce hepatic carcinomas. Thus, this study did not provide sufficient evidence that phenobarbital sodium is carcinogenic in humans.

A retrospective study of 84 children with brain tumors matched to 73 normal controls and 78 cancer controls (malignant disease other than brain tumors) suggested an association between exposure to barbiturates prenatally and an increased incidence of brain tumors.

Pregnancy: 1. Teratogenic Effects. Pregnancy Category D. See Warnings section.

2. Nonteratogenic Effects. Reports of infants suffering from long-term barbiturate exposure *in utero* include the acute withdrawal syndrome of seizures and hyperirritability from birth. A delayed onset of the symptoms may be seen for up to 14 days. (See Drug Abuse and Dependence section.)

Labor and Delivery: Hypnotic doses of barbiturates do not appear to significantly impair uterine activity during labor. Full anesthetic doses of barbiturates decrease the force and frequency of uterine contractions. Administration of sedative-hypnotic barbiturates to the mother during labor may result in respiratory depression in the newborn.

Premature infants are particularly susceptible to the depressant effects of barbiturates. If barbiturates are used during labor and delivery, resuscitation equipment should be available.

Data are not currently available to evaluate the effect of these barbiturates when forceps delivery or other intervention is necessary. Also, data are not available to determine the effect of these barbiturates on the later growth, development and functional maturation of the child.

Nursing mothers: Small amounts of barbiturates are excreted in the human milk. Because of the potential for serious adverse reactions in nursing infants from barbiturates, a decision should be made whether to discontinue nursing or to discontinue the drug, taking into account the importance of the drug to the mother.

Pediatric use: Safety and effectiveness in children have not been established.

ADVERSE REACTIONS

The following adverse reactions have been reported following the use of Alurate in an incidence of less than 1 in 100 patients.

Nervous system: Dizziness, nervousness.

Digestive system: Nausea and vomiting.

Other reported reactions: Headache, hypersensitivity reactions (skin rashes) and purpura.

Although the following adverse reactions have not been reported with Alurate, they have been compiled from surveillance of thousands of hospitalized patients receiving barbiturates and should be considered when administering Alurate:

More than 1 in 100 patients. The most common adverse reaction estimated to occur at a rate of 1 to 3 patients per 100 is:

Nervous system: Somnolence.

Less than 1 in 100 patients. Adverse reactions estimated to occur at a rate of less than 1 in 100 patients are listed below, grouped by organ system and by decreasing order of occurrence:

Nervous system: Agitation, confusion, hyperkinesia, ataxia, CNS depression, nightmares, psychiatric disturbances, hallucinations, insomnia, anxiety, thinking abnormality.

Respiratory system: Hypoventilation, apnea.

Cardiovascular system: Bradycardia, hypotension, syncope.

Digestive system: Constipation.

Other reported reactions: Hypersensitivity reactions (angioedema, exfoliative dermatitis), fever, liver damage, megaloblastic anemia following chronic phenobarbital use.

DRUG ABUSE AND DEPENDENCE

Alurate is subject to Class III control under the Federal Controlled Substances Act.

Barbiturates may be habit forming. Tolerance, psychological dependence and physical dependence may occur especially following prolonged use of high doses of barbiturates. Daily administration in excess of 400 mg of pentobarbital or secobarbital for approximately 90 days is likely to produce some degree of physical dependence. A dosage of from 600 to 800 mg taken for at least 35 days is sufficient to produce withdrawal seizures. The average daily dose for the barbiturate addict is usually about 1.5 grams. As tolerance to barbiturates develops, the amount needed to maintain the same level of intoxication increases; tolerance to fatal dosage, however, does not increase more than twofold. As this occurs, the margin between an intoxicating dosage and fatal dosage becomes smaller.

Symptoms of acute intoxication with barbiturates include unsteady gait, slurred speech and sustained nystagmus. Mental signs of chronic intoxication include confusion, poor judgment, irritability, insomnia and somatic complaints.

Symptoms of barbiturate dependence are similar to those of chronic alcoholism. If an individual appears to be intoxicated with alcohol to a degree that is radically disproportionate to the amount of alcohol in his or her blood, the use of barbiturates should be suspected. The lethal dose of a barbiturate is far less if alcohol is also ingested.

The symptoms of barbiturate withdrawal can be severe and may cause death. Minor withdrawal symptoms may appear 8 to 12 hours after the last dose of a barbiturate. These symptoms usually appear in the following order: anxiety, muscle twitching, tremor of hands or fingers, progressive weakness, dizziness, distortion in visual perception, nausea, vomiting, insomnia and orthostatic hypotension. Major withdrawal symptoms (convulsions and delirium) may occur within 16 hours and last up to 5 days after abrupt cessation of these drugs. Intensity of withdrawal symptoms gradually declines over a period of approximately 15 days. Individuals susceptible to barbiturate abuse and dependence include alcoholics and opiate abusers, as well as other sedative-hypnotic and amphetamine abusers.

Drug dependence to barbiturates arises from repeated administration of a barbiturate or an agent with barbiturate-like effect on a continuous basis, generally in amounts exceeding therapeutic dosage levels. The characteristics of drug dependence to barbiturates include: (a) a strong desire or need to continue taking the drug; (b) a tendency to increase the dose; (c) a psychic dependence on the effects of the drug related to subjective and individual appreciation of those effects; and (d) a physical dependence on the effects of the drug requiring its presence for maintenance of homeostasis and resulting in a definite, characteristic and self-limited abstinence syndrome when the drug is withdrawn.

Treatment of barbiturate dependence consists of cautious and gradual withdrawal of the drug. Barbiturate-dependent patients can be withdrawn by using a number of different withdrawal regimens. In all cases withdrawal takes an extended period of time. One method involves substituting 30 mg of phenobarbital for each 100 mg of the short-acting barbiturate which the patient has been taking. The total daily amount of phenobarbital is then administered in 4 divided doses, not to exceed 600 mg daily. Should signs of withdrawal occur on the first day of treatment, a loading dose of 200 mg of phenobarbital may be administered IM, and the daily oral dosage increased. After stabilization with phenobarbital is achieved, the total daily dose of phenobarbital is decreased by 30 mg a day as long as withdrawal is proceeding smoothly. An alternative method of treatment is to decrease the daily dosage of the barbiturate which the patient has been taking by 10 percent/day, if tolerated by the patient.

Infants physically dependent on barbiturates may be given phenobarbital 3 to 10 mg/kg/day. After withdrawal symptoms (hyperactivity, disturbed sleep, tremors, hyperreflexia) are relieved, the dosage of phenobarbital should be gradually decreased and completely withdrawn over a 2-week period.

OVERDOSAGE

The toxic dose of barbiturates varies considerably. In general, an oral dose of 1 gram of most barbiturates produces serious poisoning in an adult. Death commonly occurs after ingestion of 2 to 10 grams of barbiturate. Barbiturate intoxication may be confused with alcoholism, bromide intoxication and with various neurological disorders.

Acute overdosage with barbiturates is manifested by CNS and respiratory depression which may progress to Cheyne-Stokes respiration, areflexia, constriction of the pupils to a slight degree (though in severe poisoning they may show paralytic dilation), oliguria, tachycardia, hypotension, lowered body temperature and coma. Typical shock syndrome (apnea, circulatory collapse, respiratory arrest and death) may occur.

In extreme overdose, all electrical activity in the brain may cease, in which case the EEG may be "flat," which does not necessarily indicate clinical death. This effect is fully reversible unless hypoxic damage occurs. Consideration should be given to the possibility of barbiturate intoxication even in situations that appear to involve trauma.

Complications such as pneumonia, pulmonary edema, cardiac arrhythmias, congestive heart failure and renal failure may occur. Uremia may increase CNS sensitivity to barbiturates if renal function is impaired. Differential diagnosis should include hypoglycemia, head trauma, cerebrovascular accidents, convulsive states and diabetic coma. Blood levels from acute overdosage for some barbiturates are listed in the accompanying table.

[See table on next page].

Treatment of overdosage is mainly supportive and consists of the following:

1. Maintenance of an adequate airway, with assisted respiration and oxygen administration as necessary.

2. Monitoring of vital signs and fluid balance.

3. If the patient is conscious and has not lost the gag reflex, emesis may be induced with ipecac. Care should be taken to prevent pulmonary aspiration of vomitus. After completion of vomiting, 30 grams activated charcoal, in a glass of water, may be administered.

4. If emesis is contraindicated, gastric lavage may be performed with a cuffed endotracheal tube in place with the patient in the face down position. Activated charcoal may be left in the emptied stomach and a saline cathartic administered.

5. Fluid therapy and other standard treatment for shock, if needed.

6. If renal function is normal, forced diuresis may aid in the elimination of the barbiturate. *Alkalinization of the urine increases renal excretion of some barbiturates, especially* phenobarbital, *aprobarbital* and mephobarbital (which is metabolized to phenobarbital).

7. Although not recommended as a routine procedure, hemodialysis may be used in severe barbiturate intoxication or if the patient is anuric or in shock.

8. Patient should be rolled from side to side every 30 minutes.

9. Antibiotics should be given if pneumonia is suspected.

Continued on next page

Roche Labs.—Cont.

Concentration of Barbiturate in the Blood Versus Degree of CNS Depression

Barbiturate	Onset/ duration	Degree of depression in nontolerant persons*				
		1	2	3	4	5
		Barbiturate blood levels in ppm (mcg/ml)				
Pentobarbital	Fast/short	≤ 2	0.5 to 3	10 to 15	12 to 25	15 to 40
Secobarbital	Fast/short	≤ 2	0.5 to 5	10 to 15	15 to 25	15 to 40
Amobarbital	Intermediate/ intermediate	≤ 3	2 to 10	30 to 40	30 to 60	40 to 80
Butabarbital	Intermediate/ intermediate	≤ 5	3 to 25	40 to 60	50 to 80	60 to 100
Phenobarbital	Slow/long	≤ 10	5 to 40	50 to 80	70 to 120	100 to 200

*Categories of degree of depression in nontolerant persons:
1. Under the influence and appreciably impaired for purposes of driving a motor vehicle or performing tasks requiring alertness and unimpaired judgment and reaction time.
2. Sedated, therapeutic range, calm, relaxed, and easily aroused.
3. Comatose, difficult to arouse, significant depression of respiration.
4. Compatible with death in aged or ill persons or in presence of obstructed airway, other toxic agents, or exposure to cold.
5. Usual lethal level, the upper end of the range includes those who received some supportive treatment.

10. Appropriate nursing care to prevent hypostatic pneumonia, decubiti, aspiration and other complications in patients with altered states of consciousness.

DOSAGE AND ADMINISTRATION

Usual Adult Dosage: As a sedative, one 5-ml teaspoonful (40 mg) three times daily; for mild insomnia, one to two 5-ml teaspoonfuls before retiring; for pronounced insomnia, two to four 5-ml teaspoonfuls before retiring.
Special Patient Population: Dosage should be reduced in the elderly or debilitated because these patients may be more sensitive to barbiturates. Dosage should be reduced for patients with impaired renal function or hepatic disease.

HOW SUPPLIED

Elixir (red) providing 40 mg of aprobarbital/Roche per 5 ml in a vehicle containing 20 percent alcohol — bottles of 16 oz (1 pint) (NDC 0004-1000-28).
P.I. 0385

ANCOBON®
[an 'co-bon]
(flucytosine/Roche)

℞

The following text is complete prescribing information based on official labeling in effect June 1, 1989.

> **WARNING**
>
> Use with extreme caution in patients with impaired renal function. Close monitoring of hematologic, renal and hepatic status of all patients is essential. These instructions should be thoroughly reviewed before administration of Ancobon.

DESCRIPTION

Ancobon (flucytosine/Roche), an antifungal agent, is available as 250-mg and 500-mg capsules for oral administration. Each capsule also contains corn starch, lactose and talc. Gelatin capsule shells contain parabens (butyl, methyl, propyl) and sodium propionate, with the following dye systems: 250-mg capsules—black iron oxide, FD&C Blue No. 1, FD&C Yellow No. 6, D&C Yellow No. 10 and titanium dioxide; 500-mg capsules—black iron oxide and titanium dioxide. Chemically, flucytosine is 5-fluorocytosine, a fluorinated pyrimidine which is related to fluorouracil and floxuridine. It is a white to off-white crystalline powder with a molecular weight of 129.09.

CLINICAL PHARMACOLOGY

Flucytosine is rapidly and virtually completely absorbed following oral administration. Bioavailability estimated by comparing the area under the curve of serum concentrations after oral and intravenous administration showed 78% to 89% absorption of the oral dose. Peak blood concentrations of 30 to 40 mcg/mL were reached within two hours of administration of a 2-Gm oral dose to normal subjects. The mean blood concentrations were approximately 70 to 80 mcg/mL one to two hours after a dose in patients with normal renal function who received a six-week regimen of flucytosine (150 mg/kg/day given in divided doses every 6 hours) in combination with amphotericin B. The half-life in the majority of normal subjects ranged between 2.4 and 4.8 hours. Flucytosine is excreted via the kidneys by means of glomerular filtration without significant tubular reabsorption. More than 90% of the total radioactivity after oral administration was recovered in the urine as intact drug. Approximately 1% of

the dose is present in the urine as the α-fluoro-β-ureido-propionic acid metabolite. A small portion of the dose is excreted in the feces.
The half-life of flucytosine is prolonged in patients with renal insufficiency; the average half-life in nephrectomized or anuric patients was 85 hours (range: 29.9 to 250 hours). A linear correlation was found between the elimination rate constant of flucytosine and creatinine clearance.
In vitro studies have shown that 2.9% to 4% of flucytosine is protein-bound over the range of therapeutic concentrations found in the blood. Flucytosine readily penetrates the blood-brain barrier, achieving clinically significant concentrations in cerebrospinal fluid. Studies in pregnant rats have shown that flucytosine injected intraperitoneally crosses the placental barrier (see PRECAUTIONS).

MICROBIOLOGY

Flucytosine has *in vitro* and *in vivo* activity against Candida and Cryptococcus. Although the exact mode of action is unknown, it has been proposed that flucytosine acts directly on fungal organisms by competitive inhibition of purine and pyrimidine uptake and indirectly by intracellular metabolism to 5-fluorouracil. Flucytosine enters the fungal cell via cytosine permease; thus, flucytosine is metabolized to 5-fluorouracil within in fungal organisms. The 5-fluorouracil is extensively incorporated into fungal RNA and inhibits synthesis of both DNA and RNA. The result is unbalanced growth and death of the fungal organism. Antifungal synergism between Ancobon and polyene antibiotics, particularly amphotericin B, has been reported.

ACTIONS

Flucytosine has *in vitro* and *in vivo* activity against Candida and Cryptococcus. The exact mode of action against these fungi is not known. Ancobon is not metabolized significantly when given orally to man.

SUSCEPTIBILITY

Cryptococcus: Most strains initially isolated from clinical material have shown flucytosine minimal inhibitory concentrations (MIC's) ranging from .46 to 7.8 mcg/mL. Any isolate with an MIC greater than 12.5 mcg/mL is considered resistant. In vitro resistance has developed in originally susceptible strains during therapy. It is recommended that clinical cultures for susceptibility testing be taken initially and at weekly intervals during therapy. The initial culture should be reserved as a reference in susceptibilty testing of subsequent isolates.
Candida: As high as 40 to 50 percent of the pretreatment clinical isolates of Candida have been reported to be resistant to flucytosine. It is recommended that susceptibility studies be performed as early as possible and be repeated during therapy. An MIC value greater than 100 mcg/mL is considered resistant.
Interference with *in vitro* activity of flucytosine occurs in complex or semisynthetic media. In order to rely upon the recommended *in vitro* interpretations of susceptibility, it is essential that the broth medium and the testing procedure used be that described by Shadomy.[1]

INDICATIONS AND USAGE

Ancobon is indicated only in the treatment of serious infections caused by susceptible strains of Candida and/or Cryptococcus. *Candida:* Septicemia, endocarditis and urinary system infections have been effectively treated with flucytosine. Limited trials in pulmonary infections justify the use of flucytosine. *Cryptococcus:* Meningitis and pulmonary infections have been treated effectively. Studies in septicemias and urinary tract infections are limited, but good responses have been reported.

CONTRAINDICATIONS

Ancobon should not be used in patients with a known hypersensitivity to the drug.

WARNINGS

Ancobon must be given with extreme caution to patients with impaired renal function. Since Ancobon is excreted primarily by the kidneys, renal impairment may lead to accumulation of the drug. Ancobon blood concentrations should be monitored to determine the adequacy of renal excretion in such patients.[1] Dosage adjustments should be made in patients with renal insufficiency to prevent progressive accumulation of active drug.
Ancobon must be given with extreme caution to patients with bone marrow depression. Patients may be more prone to depression of bone marrow function if they: 1) have a hematologic disease, 2) are being treated with radiation or drugs which depress bone marrow, or 3) have a history of treatment with such drugs or radiation. Frequent monitoring of hepatic function and of the hematopoietic system is indicated during therapy.

PRECAUTIONS

General: Before therapy with Ancobon is instituted, electrolytes (because of hypokalemia) and the hematologic and renal status of the patient should be determined (see WARNINGS). Close monitoring of the patient during therapy is essential.
Laboratory tests: Since renal impairment can cause progressive accumulation of the drug, blood concentrations and kidney function should be monitored during therapy. Hematologic status (leucocyte and thrombocyte count) and liver function (alkaline phosphatase, SGOT and SGPT) should be determined at frequent intervals during treatment as indicated.
Drug interactions: Cytosine arabinoside, a cytostatic agent, has been reported to inactivate the antifungal activity of Ancobon by competitive inhibition. Drugs which impair glomerular filtration may prolong the biological half-life of flucytosine. Antifungal synergism between Ancobon and polyene antibiotics, particularly amphotericin B, has been reported.
Drug/laboratory test interactions: Measurement of serum creatinine levels should be determined by the Jaffe method, since Ancobon does not interfere with the determination of creatinine values by this method, as it does when the dry-slide enzymatic method with the Kodak Ektachem analyzer is used.
Carcinogenesis, mutagenesis, impairment of fertility: Ancobon has not undergone adequate animal testing to evaluate carcinogenic potential. The mutagenic potential of Ancobon was evaluated in Ames-type studies with five different mutants of *S. typhimurium* and no mutagenicity was detected in the presence or absence of activating enzymes. Ancobon was nonmutagenic in three different repair assay systems.
There have been no adequate trials in animals on the effects of Ancobon on fertility or reproductive performance. The fertility and reproductive performance of the offspring (F_1 generation) of mice treated with 100, 200 or 400 mg/kg/day of flucytosine on days 7 to 13 of gestation was studied; the *in utero* treatment had no adverse effect on the fertility or reproductive performance of the offspring.
Pregnancy: Teratogenic effects. Pregnancy Category C. Ancobon has been shown to be teratogenic in the rat and mouse at doses of 40 mg/kg/day (*i.e.,* 0.27 times the maximum recommended human dose). There are no adequate and well-controlled studies in pregnant women. Ancobon should be used during pregnancy only if the potential benefit justifies the potential risk to the fetus.
The teratogenicity of Ancobon is apparently species-related. Although there is confirmation of rat teratogenicity in the published literature, three studies in the mouse and studies in the rabbit and monkey have failed to reveal a teratogenic liability.
Nursing mothers: It is not known whether this drug is excreted in human milk. Because many drugs are excreted in human milk and because of the potential for serious adverse reactions in nursing infants from Ancobon, a decision should be made whether to discontinue nursing or to discontinue the drug, taking into account the importance of the drug to the mother.
Pediatric use: Safety and effectiveness in children have not been established.

ADVERSE REACTIONS

The adverse reactions which have occurred during treatment with Ancobon are grouped according to organ system affected.
Cardiovascular: Cardiac arrest.
Respiratory: Respiratory arrest, chest pain, dyspnea.
Dermatologic: Rash, pruritus, urticaria, photosensitivity.
Gastrointestinal: Nausea, emesis, abdominal pain, diarrhea, anorexia, dry mouth, duodenal ulcer, gastrointestinal hemorrhage, hepatic dysfunction, jaundice, ulcerative colitis, bilirubin elevation.

Genitourinary: Azotemia, creatinine and BUN elevation, crystalluria, renal failure.
Hematologic: Anemia, agranulocytosis, aplastic anemia, eosinophilia, leukopenia, pancytopenia, thrombocytopenia.
Neurologic: Ataxia, hearing loss, headache, paresthesia, parkinsonism, peripheral neuropathy, pyrexia, vertigo, sedation.
Psychiatric: Confusion, hallucinations, psychosis.
Miscellaneous: Fatigue, hypoglycemia, hypokalemia, weakness.

OVERDOSAGE

There is no experience with intentional overdosage. It is reasonable to expect that overdosage may produce pronounced manifestations of the known clinical adverse reactions. Prolonged serum concentrations in excess of 100 mcg/mL may be associated with an increased incidence of toxicity, especially gastrointestinal (diarrhea, nausea, vomiting), hematologic (leukopenia, thrombocytopenia) and hepatic (hepatitis).

In the management of overdosage, prompt gastric lavage or the use of an emetic is recommended. Adequate fluid intake should be maintained, by the intravenous route if necessary, since Ancobon is excreted unchanged via the renal tract. The hematologic parameters should be monitored frequently; liver and kidney function should be carefully monitored. Should any abnormalities appear in any of these parameters, appropriate therapeutic measures should be instituted. Since hemodialysis has been shown to rapidly reduce serum concentrations in anuric patients, this method may be considered in the management of overdosage.

DOSAGE AND ADMINISTRATION

The usual dosage of Ancobon is 50 to 150 mg/kg/day administered in divided doses at 6-hour intervals. Nausea or vomiting may be reduced or avoided if the capsules are given a few at a time over a 15-minute period. If the BUN or the serum creatinine is elevated, or if there are other signs of renal impairment, the initial dose should be at the lower level (see WARNINGS).

HOW SUPPLIED

Capsules, 250 mg (gray and green), imprinted ANCOBON® 250 ROCHE; bottles of 100 (NDC 0004-0077-01). *Capsules,* 500 mg (gray and white), imprinted ANCOBON® 500 ROCHE, bottles of 100 (NDC 0004-0079-01).

REFERENCE

1. Shadomy S: *Appl Microbiol* 17: 871–877, June 1969.

P.I. 1187

Shown in Product Identification Section, page 424

ARFONAD®

[ar'fo-nad]
(trimethaphan camsylate/Roche)
Ampuls

The following text is complete prescribing information based on official labeling in effect June 1, 1989.

DESCRIPTION

Arfonad (trimethaphan camsylate/Roche) Injection, a vasodepressor agent, is available as a sterile solution to be used only for intravenous infusion. Each 10-mL ampul contains 500 mg trimethaphan camsylate compounded with 0.013% sodium acetate and hydrochloric acid to adjust pH to approximately 5.2.
Trimethaphan camsylate is a sulfonium derivative. The chemical name is (+)-1,3-dibenzyldecahydro-2-oxoimidazo[4,5-*c*]thieno[1,2-*a*]-thiolium 2-oxo-10-bornanesulfonate (1:1). It occurs as white crystals or a white, crystalline powder which is freely soluble in water and alcohol. It has a molecular weight of 596.80.

CLINICAL PHARMACOLOGY

Trimethaphan camsylate is primarily a ganglionic blocking agent. It blocks transmission in autonomic ganglia without producing any preceding or concomitant change in the membrane potentials of the ganglion cells. It does not modify the conduction of impulses in the preganglionic or postganglionic neurons and does not prevent the release of acetylcholine by preganglionic impulses. Trimethaphan camsylate produces ganglionic blockade by occupying receptor sites on the ganglion cells and by stabilizing the postsynaptic membranes against the action of acetylcholine liberated from the presynaptic nerve endings.
In addition to ganglionic blocking, trimethaphan camsylate may also exert a direct peripheral vasodilator effect. By inducing vasodilation, it causes pooling of blood in the dependent periphery and the splanchnic system. The vasodilation results in a lowering of the blood pressure. Trimethaphan camsylate liberates histamine.
Trimethaphan crosses the placenta. Other pharmacokinetic data are unavailable because there is no acceptable assay procedure for the determination of trimethaphan in biological specimens.

INDICATIONS AND USAGE

Arfonad is indicated for the production of controlled hypotension during surgery; for the short term (acute) control of blood pressure in hypertensive emergencies; and in the emergency treatment of pulmonary edema in patients with pulmonary hypertension associated with systemic hypertension.

CONTRAINDICATIONS

Arfonad is contraindicated in those conditions where hypotension may subject the patient to undue risk, *e.g.,* uncorrected anemia, hypovolemia, shock (both incipient and frank), asphyxia or uncorrected respiratory insufficiency. Inadequate availability of fluids and inability to replace blood for technical reasons may also constitute contraindications.

WARNINGS

Arfonad is a powerful hypotensive drug and should always be diluted before use.

It is recommended that the use of Arfonad to produce hypotension in surgical or medical indications be limited to physicians with proper training in this technique. Adequate facilities, equipment and personnel should be available for vigilant monitoring of the circulation since Arfonad is an extremely potent hypotensive agent. Adequate oxygenation must be assured throughout the treatment period, especially in regard to coronary and cerebral circulation.

Arfonad should be used with extreme caution in patients with arteriosclerosis, cardiac disease, hepatic or renal disease, degenerative disease of the central nervous system, Addison's disease or diabetes, and in patients who are under treatment with steroids.

Usage in Pregnancy: **Arfonad can cause fetal harm when administered to a pregnant woman. Trimethaphan camsylate crosses the placenta, decreasing fetal gastrointestinal motility and resulting in meconium ileus. In addition, Arfonad-induced hypotension may have other serious adverse effects on the fetus. If Arfonad is used during pregnancy, or if the patient becomes pregnant while taking Arfonad, the patient should be apprised of the potential hazard to the fetus.**

PRECAUTIONS

General: Arfonad should be used with extreme caution in the elderly or debilitated. Because Arfonad liberates histamine, it should be used with caution in patients with a history of allergies.
Respiratory depression and arrest have occurred during Arfonad administration, although a causal relationship has not been firmly established. The patient's respiratory status must be monitored closely, particularly if large doses of Arfonad are used.
Occasionally, patients may fail to show an adequate hypotensive response to Arfonad administration. When this is observed, administration should be discontinued and other methods to control hypertension instituted. Tachyphylaxis has also been reported.
NOTE: Because Arfonad causes mydriasis, pupillary dilation does not necessarily indicate anoxia or the depth of anesthesia.
Drug interactions: Arfonad should be used with care in patients who have been receiving antihypertensive drugs, since an additive hypotensive effect may occur. Arfonad may also have an additive hypotensive effect when administered with anesthetic agents, especially spinal anesthetics. Procainamide also has an additive hypotensive effect with Arfonad. Diuretic agents may markedly enhance the responses evoked by ganglionic-blocking drugs. Arfonad may also prolong the effects of neuromuscular blocking agents such as tubocurarine chloride or succinylcholine chloride, especially when large doses of Arfonad are administered.
Concomitant therapy with other drugs can considerably modify the dose of Arfonad necessary to achieve the desired response. In general, the deeper the plane of anesthesia, the smaller the dose of Arfonad that is required to produce hypotension; conversely, less anesthetic is required after hypotension has been induced by Arfonad.
Carcinogenesis, mutagenesis and impairment of fertility: Arfonad has not undergone adequate animal testing to evaluate its carcinogenic potential. The mutagenicity of Arfonad has not been studied nor has the drug been evaluated for effects on fertility.
Pregnancy: Teratogenic effects—Pregnancy Category D. See WARNINGS section.
Nonteratogenic effects—See WARNINGS section.
Nursing mothers: It is not known whether Arfonad is excreted in human milk. Because of the potential for serious adverse reactions from Arfonad in nursing infants, mothers who require Arfonad should be advised not to nurse.
Pediatric use: Safety and effectiveness in children have not been established.

ADVERSE REACTIONS

The adverse reactions produced by Arfonad are primarily due to its nonselective blockade of the autonomic nervous system. The following adverse reactions have been observed,

but there is not enough systematic collection of data to support an estimate of their frequency.
Cardiovascular: Tachycardia, precipitation of angina, syncope which may occur without warning. *Respiratory:* Respiratory depression and arrest have occurred during Arfonad administration, although a causal relationship has not been firmly established. *Gastrointestinal:* Paralytic ileus, dry mouth, constipation, occasional diarrhea, abdominal discomfort, anorexia, heartburn, nausea, vomiting, eructation. *Genitourinary:* Urinary hesitancy, decreased potentia. *Ophthalmic:* Cycloplegia, mydriasis, difficulty in accommodation, conjunctival suffusion. *Miscellaneous:* Subjective chilliness, weakness, restlessness, urticaria, itching. Arfonad prevents surgically-induced elevation of blood glucose and decreases serum potassium slightly.
Generally, side effects are decreased when dosage is reduced or the drug is temporarily discontinued.

OVERDOSAGE

Vasopressor agents may be used to correct excessive hypotension during surgery or to effect a more rapid return to normotensive levels. Phenylephrine HCl or mephentermine sulfate should be tried initially and norepinephrine should be reserved for refractory cases.
The acute intravenous toxicity of trimethaphan camsylate is as follows:

Species	LD$_{50}$ mg/kg
mouse	21
rat	21
rabbit	23
dog	0.75
guinea pig	13
monkey	> 8

DOSAGE AND ADMINISTRATION

Arfonad must always be diluted and administered by intravenous infusion. Solutions should be freshly prepared and any unused portions discarded. For this purpose a 0.1 percent (1 mg/mL) concentration of Arfonad in 5% Dextrose Injection USP, normal saline solution, or Ringer's Injection USP should be employed. Arfonad is stable in these diluents for at least 24 hours at room temperature. Use of other diluents is not recommended, since experience with them has not been reported.
Arfonad is physically incompatible with thiopental, gallamine triethiodide, tubocurarine chloride, iodides, bromides and strongly alkaline solutions. **Therefore, the infusion fluid used for administration of Arfonad should not be employed as a vehicle for the simultaneous administration of any other drugs.**
One (1) ampul of Arfonad—10 mL, 50 mg/mL—should be diluted to 500 mL. Since individual response varies, the rate of administration must be adjusted to the requirements of each patient.
When Arfonad is given, the patient should be positioned so as to avoid cerebral anoxia. During surgery, adequate anesthesia should be established. Intravenous drip with Arfonad is started at an average rate of 3 mL to 4 mL (3 mg to 4 mg) per minute (see chart below). The rate of administration is then adjusted to maintain the desired level of hypotension. Since there is a marked variation of individual response, **frequent blood pressure determinations are essential to maintain proper control.** Rates from as low as 0.3 mL (0.3 mg) per minute to rates exceeding 6 mL (6 mg) per minute have been found necessary, based upon clinical experience.

0.1% (1 mg/mL) CONCENTRATION OF ARFONAD

Delivery System Drops/mL	Drops/Min to Obtain 3–4 mL (3–4 mg) Arfonad
10	30–40
15	45–60
60	180–240

During surgery, administration of Arfonad should be stopped prior to wound closure in order to permit blood pressure to return to normal. A systolic pressure of 100 mm will usually be attained within 10 minutes after stopping Arfonad.
Parenteral drug products should be inspected visually for particulate matter and discoloration prior to administration, whenever solution and container permit.

HOW SUPPLIED

10 mL Ampuls (500 mg trimethaphan camsylate/10 mL)—boxes of 10 (NDC 0004-1900-06).
Arfonad is stable under refrigeration (36° to 46°F or 2° to 8°C). Arfonad should not be frozen as ampul breakage may result from ice formation.
P.I. 0288

Continued on next page

Roche Labs.—Cont.

AZO GANTANOL®   ℞
[a "zo gan 'tan-ol]

The following text is complete prescribing information based on official labeling in effect June 1, 1989.

DESCRIPTION
Azo Gantanol combines the antibacterial effectiveness of sulfamethoxazole (Gantanol®) with the local urinary analgesic activity of phenazopyridine hydrochloride. Each tablet contains 0.5 Gm sulfamethoxazole/Roche and 100 mg phenazopyridine hydrochloride. Each tablet also contains carnauba wax, castor oil, corn starch, docusate sodium, magnesium stearate, polyvinyl acetate, polyvinyl alcohol, pregelatinized starch, shellac and FD&C Red No. 3, and may contain red and brown synthetic iron oxides.
Gantanol (sulfamethoxazole/Roche) is an intermediate-dosage sulfonamide. Sulfamethoxazole is an almost white, odorless, tasteless compound. Chemically, it is N^1-(5-methyl-3-isoxazolyl) sulfanilamide.
Phenazopyridine hydrochloride is a urinary analgesic. Chemically, it is 3-phenylazo-2,6- diaminopyridine hydrochloride.
Sulfonamides exist in the blood as free, conjugated (acetylated and possibly other forms) and protein-bound forms. The "free" form is considered to be the therapeutically active form. It has been shown that approximately 70 per cent of Gantanol is protein bound in the blood;[1] of the unbound portion 80 to 90 per cent is in the nonacetylated form.[2,3] Excretion of sulfonamides is chiefly by the kidneys with glomerular filtration as the primary mechanism.

ACTIONS
The systemic sulfonamides are bacteriostatic agents. The spectrum of activity is similar for all. Sulfonamides competitively inhibit bacterial synthesis of folic acid (pteroylglutamic acid) from para-aminobenzoic acid. Resistant strains are capable of utilizing folic acid precursors or preformed folic acid.
Phenazopyridine hydrochloride has a specific analgesic effect in the urinary tract, promptly relieving pain and burning.

INDICATIONS
For the initial treatment of uncomplicated urinary tract infections caused by susceptible strains of the following microorganisms: *Escherichia coli, Klebsiella* species, *Enterobacter* species, *Proteus mirabilis, Proteus vulgaris* and *Staphylococcus aureus* when relief of symptoms of pain, burning or urgency is needed during the first 2 days of therapy. Treatment with Azo Gantanol should not exceed 2 days. There is a lack of evidence that the combination of sulfamethoxazole and phenazopyridine hydrochloride provides greater benefit than sulfamethoxazole alone after 2 days. Treatment beyond 2 days should only be continued with Gantanol (sulfamethoxazole/Roche). (See DOSAGE AND ADMINISTRATION section.)
Important note. In vitro sulfonamide sensitivity tests are not always reliable. The test must be carefully coordinated with bacteriologic and clinical response. When the patient is already taking sulfonamides, follow-up cultures should have aminobenzoic acid added to the culture media.
Currently, the increasing frequency of resistant organisms is a limitation of the usefulness of antibacterial agents including the sulfonamides.
Wide variation in blood levels may result with identical doses. Blood levels should be measured in patients receiving sulfonamides for serious infections. Free sulfonamide blood levels of 5 to 15 mg per 100 ml may be considered therapeutically effective for most infections, with blood levels of 12 to 15 mg per 100 ml optimal for serious infections; 20 mg per 100 ml should be the maximum total sulfonamide level, as adverse reactions occur more frequently above this level.

CONTRAINDICATIONS
Children below age 12. Hypersensitivity to sulfonamides. Pregnancy at term and during the nursing period, because sulfonamides pass the placenta and are excreted in the milk and may cause kernicterus.
Because Azo Gantanol contains phenazopyridine hydrochloride it is contraindicated in glomerulonephritis, severe hepatitis, uremia, and pyelonephritis of pregnancy with gastrointestinal disturbances.

WARNINGS
Usage in Pregnancy: The safe use of sulfonamides in pregnancy has not been established. The teratogenicity potential of most sulfonamides has not been thoroughly investigated in either animals or humans. However, a significant increase in the incidence of cleft palate and other bony abnormalities of offspring has been observed when certain sulfonamides of the short, intermediate and long-acting types were given to pregnant rats and mice at high oral doses (7 to 25 times the human therapeutic dose).

Deaths associated with the administration of sulfonamides have been reported from hypersensitivity reactions, hepatocellular necrosis, agranulocytosis, aplastic anemia and other blood dyscrasias.
The presence of clinical signs such as sore throat, fever, arthralgia, cough, shortness of breath, pallor, purpura or jaundice may be early indications of serious reactions, including serious blood disorders. Complete blood counts should be done frequently in patients receiving sulfonamides.
The frequency of renal complications is considerably lower in patients receiving the more soluble sulfonamides. Urinalysis with careful microscopic examination should be obtained frequently in patients receiving sulfonamides.

PRECAUTIONS
Sulfonamides should be given with caution to patients with impaired renal or hepatic function and to those with severe allergy or bronchial asthma. In glucose-6-phosphate dehydrogenase-deficient individuals, hemolysis may occur. This reaction is frequently dose-related. Adequate fluid intake must be maintained in order to prevent crystalluria and stone formation.
Carcinogenesis: Azo Gantanol has not undergone adequate trials relating to carcinogenicity; each component, however, has been evaluated separately. Rats appear to be especially susceptible to the goitrogenic effects of sulfonamides, and long-term administration of sulfonamides has resulted in thyroid malignancies in this species. Long-term administration of phenazopyridine hydrochloride has induced neoplasia in rats (large intestine) and mice (liver). Although no association between phenazopyridine hydrochloride and human neoplasia has been reported, adequate epidemiological studies have not been conducted.

ADVERSE REACTIONS
Blood dyscrasias: Agranulocytosis, aplastic anemia, thrombocytopenia, leukopenia, hemolytic anemia, purpura, hypoprothrombinemia, methemoglobinemia, and eosinophilia.
Allergic reactions: Erythema multiforme (Stevens-Johnson syndrome), generalized skin eruptions, epidermal necrolysis, urticaria, serum sickness, pruritus, exfoliative dermatitis, anaphylactoid reactions, periorbital edema, conjunctival and scleral injection, photosensitization, arthralgia and allergic myocarditis.
Gastrointestinal reactions: Nausea, emesis, abdominal pains, hepatitis, hepatocellular necrosis, diarrhea, anorexia, pancreatitis and stomatitis.
C.N.S. reactions: Headache, peripheral neuritis, mental depression, convulsions, ataxia, hallucinations, tinnitus, vertigo and insomnia.
Miscellaneous reactions: Drug fever, chills, and toxic nephrosis with oliguria and anuria. Polyarteritis nodosa and L.E. phenomenon have occurred.
Respiratory reactions: Pulmonary infiltrates.
The sulfonamides bear certain chemical similarities to some goitrogens, diuretics (acetazolamide and the thiazides) and oral hypoglycemic agents. Goiter production, diuresis and hypoglycemia have occurred rarely in patients receiving sulfonamides. Cross-sensitivity may exist with these agents.

DOSAGE AND ADMINISTRATION
Azo Gantanol is intended for the acute, painful phase of urinary tract infections. The usual dosage in adults is 4 tablets initially followed by 2 tablets morning and evening for up to 2 days. Treatment with Azo Gantanol should not exceed 2 days. Treatment beyond 2 days should only be continued with Gantanol (sulfamethoxazole/Roche).
NOTE: Patients should be told that the orange-red dye (phenazopyridine HCl) will color the urine soon after ingestion of the medication.

HOW SUPPLIED
Tablets, red, film-coated, each containing 0.5 Gm sulfamethoxazole/Roche and 100 mg phenazopyridine HCl—bottles of 100.

REFERENCES
1.   Struller, T.: *Antibiot. Chemother., 14:* 179, 1968.
2.   Boger, W. P., and Gavin, J. J.: *Antibiotics and Chemother., 10 :*572, 1960.
3.   Brandman, O., and Engelberg, R.: *Curr. Therap. Res., 2 :*364, 1960.
P.I. 0788
Shown in Product Identification Section, page 424

AZO GANTRISIN®   ℞
[a "zo gan 'tris-in]

The following text is complete prescribing information based on official labeling in effect June 1, 1989.

DESCRIPTION
Azo Gantrisin is a combination containing 0.5 Gm of the antibacterial sulfisoxazole/Roche and 50 mg of the urinary analgesic phenazopyridine hydrochloride per tablet for oral administration. Each tablet also contains carnauba wax, castor oil, docusate sodium, hydrogenated cottonseed oil, magnesium stearate, pregelatinized starch, shellac, FD&C Red No. 3 and D&C Red No. 28.
Gantrisin® (sulfisoxazole/Roche), a rapid-acting sulfamide, is N^1-(3,4-dimethyl-5-isoxazolyl) sulfanilamide. It is a white to slightly yellowish, odorless, slighty-bitter, crystalline powder which is soluble in alcohol and very slightly soluble in water. Sulfisoxazole has an empirical formula of $C_{11}H_{13}N_3O_3S$, and a molecular weight of 267.30.
Phenazopyridine hydrochloride, a local urinary analgesic, is 2,6-diamino-3-(phenylazo)-pyridine monohydrochloride. It is a light or dark red to dark violet, odorless, slightly bitter, crystalline powder with an empirical formula of $C_{11}H_{11}N_5 \cdot HCl$, and a molecular weight of 249.70.

CLINICAL PHARMACOLOGY
An oral dose of sulfisoxazole is rapidly and completely absorbed. Sulfonamides are present in the blood as free, conjugated (acetylated and possibly other forms) and protein-bound forms. The amount present as "free" drug is considered to be the therapeutically active form. Approximately 85% of a dose of sulfisoxazole is bound to plasma proteins. Following a single 2.0-Gm dose of sulfisoxazole, the mean time of peak plasma concentration was 2.5 hours; the mean peak plasma concentration was 169 µg/ml, ranging from 127 to 211 µg/ml. Of the 97% of the original dose excreted in the urine within 0 to 48 hours, 52% was free sulfisoxazole and 45% was the metabolite N^4-acetyl sulfisoxazole. The mean elimination half-life was 5.8 hours, ranging from 4.6 to 7.8 hours.
Sulfonamides are excreted primarily by the kidneys through glomerular filtration. The drug diffuses across the placenta into the fetus and crosses the blood-brain barrier.
Phenazopyridine hydrochloride has a specific local analgesic effect in the urinary tract, promptly relieving pain and burning. No pharmacokinetic data are available on this drug.
Microbiology: The systemic sulfonamides are bacteriostatic agents. The spectrum of activity is similar for all. Sulfonamides competitively inhibit bacterial synthesis of folic acid (pteroylglutamic acid) from *para*-aminobenzoic acid. Resistant strains are capable of utilizing folic acid precursors or preformed folic acid.

INDICATIONS
For the initial treatment of uncomplicated urinary tract infections caused by susceptible strains of the following microorganisms: *Escherichia coli, Klebsiella* species, *Enterobacter* species, *Proteus mirabilis, Proteus vulgaris* and *Staphylococcus aureus* when relief of symptoms of pain, burning or urgency is needed during the first 2 days of therapy. Treatment with Azo Gantrisin should not exceed 2 days. There is a lack of evidence that the combination of sulfisoxazole and phenazopyridine hydrochloride provides greater benefit than sulfisoxazole alone after 2 days. Treatment beyond 2 days should only be continued with Gantrisin (sulfisoxazole/Roche). (See DOSAGE AND ADMINISTRATION section.)
Important Note: In vitro sensitivity tests for sulfonamides are not always reliable, and must be carefully coordinated with bacteriologic and clinical response. When the patient is already taking sulfonamides, follow-up cultures should have aminobenzoic acid added to the culture media.
Currently, the increasing frequency of resistant organisms is a limitation of the usefulness of antibacterial agents, including the sulfonamides.
Wide variation in blood levels may result with identical doses of a sulfonamide. Blood levels should be measured in patients receiving these drugs for serious infections. Free sulfonamide blood levels of 5 to 15 mg/100 ml may be considered therapeutically effective for most infections, with blood levels of 12 to 15 mg/100 ml being optimal for serious infections. The maximum sulfonamide level should be 20 mg/100 ml, since adverse reactions occur more frequently above this concentration.

CONTRAINDICATIONS
Azo Gantrisin is contraindicated in patients with a known sensitivity to either of its components; in children younger than 12 years; and in pregnancy *at term* and during the nursing period, because sulfonamides pass the placenta and are excreted in the milk and may cause kernicterus.
Azo Gantrisin, because it contains phenazopyridine hydrochloride, is also contraindicated in glomerulonephritis, severe hepatitis, uremia, and pyelonephritis of pregnancy with gastrointestinal disturbances.

WARNINGS
Sulfonamides are bacteriostatic and resistance is frequent in organisms responsible for common infections. Sulfa drugs will not eradicate group A streptococci and have not been demonstrated, in these infections, to prevent sequelae such as rheumatic fever and glomerulonephritis.
Deaths associated with the administration of sulfonamides have been reported from hypersensitivity reactions, hepatocellular necrosis, agranulocytosis, aplastic anemia and other blood dyscrasias.
The presence of clinical signs such as sore throat, fever, arthralgia, cough, shortness of breath, pallor, purpura or jaun-

dice may be early indications of serious reactions, including serious blood disorders. Blood counts and renal function tests are recommended during treatment.

PRECAUTIONS

General: Sulfonamides should be given with caution to patients with impaired renal or hepatic function and to those with severe allergy or bronchial asthma. In glucose-6-phosphate dehydrogenase-deficient individuals, hemolysis may occur; this reaction is frequently dose-related.

The frequency of renal complications is considerably lower in patients receiving the more soluble sulfonamides. Adequate fluid intake must be maintained in order to prevent crystalluria and stone formation.

Information for Patients: Patients should maintain an adequate fluid intake. Patients should also be told that soon after ingestion of this medication, the phenazopyridine HCl component will produce reddish-orange discoloration of the urine.

Laboratory Tests: Urinalysis with careful microscopic examination should be performed at least once a week for patients receiving sulfonamides. Blood counts should be performed regularly in patients receiving sulfonamide therapy for longer than two weeks. Blood levels of a sulfonamide should be measured in patients receiving these drugs for serious infection (see INDICATIONS section).

Drug Interactions: It has been reported that some sulfonamides may displace oral anticoagulants from plasma protein binding sites and thereby increase the anticoagulant effect. Sulfonamides can also displace methotrexate from plasma protein binding sites.

Drug/Laboratory Test Interactions: Both components of Azo Gantrisin have been reported to affect results of liver function tests in isolated cases of hepatitis.

Carcinogenesis, Mutagenesis, Impairment of Fertility:
Carcinogenesis: Azo Gantrisin has not undergone adequate trials relating to carcinogenicity; each component, however, has been evaluated separately. Rats appear to be especially susceptible to the goitrogenic effects of sulfonamides, and long-term administration of sulfonamides has resulted in thyroid malignancies in this species. Long-term administration of phenazopyridine hydrochloride has induced neoplasia in rats (large intestine) and mice (liver). Although no association between phenazopyridine hydrochloride and human neoplasia has been reported, adequate epidemiological studies have not been conducted.

Mutagenesis: There are no studies available that evaluate the mutagenic potential of Azo Gantrisin or either of its components.

Impairment of Fertility: Azo Gantrisin has not undergone adequate trials relating to impairment of fertility; each component, however, has been studied in laboratory animals. In a reproduction study of rats given 800 mg/kg/day sulfisoxazole, no effects were observed regarding mating behavior, conception rate or fertility index (percent pregnant). No effects on fertility were demonstrated in a two-litter reproduction study of rats given 50 mg/kg/day phenazopyridine.

Pregnancy:
Teratogenic Effects: Pregnancy Category C. Each component of Azo Gantrisin has been evaluated in reproduction studies in laboratory animals. At dosages of 800 mg/kg/day, sulfisoxazole was not teratogenic in either rats or rabbits, and had no perinatal or postnatal effects in rats. However, in two other teratogenicity studies, cleft palates developed in both rats and mice after administration of 500 to 1000 mg/kg/day sulfisoxazole (8 to 16 times the therapeutic dose for an individual weighing 143 lbs). In regard to phenazopyridine, no congenital malformations developed in rats given 50 mg/kg/day.

There are no adequate or well-controlled studies of Azo Gantrisin in either laboratory animals or in pregnant women. It is not known whether Azo Gantrisin can cause fetal harm when administered to a pregnant woman or can affect reproduction capacity. Azo Gantrisin should be used during pregnancy only if the potential benefit justifies the potential risk to the fetus.

Nonteratogenic Effects: See **Contraindications** section.
Nursing Mothers: See **Contraindications** section.
Pediatric Use: See **Contraindications** section.

ADVERSE REACTIONS

Included in the listing that follows are adverse reactions that have not been reported with this specific drug; however, the pharmacologic similarities among the sulfonamides require that each of the reactions be considered with Azo Gantrisin administration.

Allergic: Anaphylaxis, generalized allergic reactions, angioneurotic edema, arteritis and vasculitis, myocarditis, serum sickness, conjunctival and scleral injection. In addition, periarteritis nodosa and systemic lupus erythematosus have been reported.

Cardiovascular: Tachycardia, palpitations, syncope and cyanosis.

Dermatologic: Rash, urticaria, pruritus, erythema multiforme, Stevens-Johnson syndrome, toxic epidermal necrolysis, exfoliative dermatitis and photosensitivity.

Endocrine: The sulfonamides bear certain chemical similarities to some goitrogens, diuretics (acetazolamide and the thiazides) and oral hypoglycemic agents. Cross-sensitivity may exist with these agents. Goiter production, diuresis and hypoglycemia have occurred rarely in patients receiving sulfonamides.

Gastrointestinal: Nausea, emesis, abdominal pain, anorexia, diarrhea, glossitis, stomatitis, flatulence, salivary gland enlargement, G.I. hemorrhage, pseudomembranous enterocolitis, melena and pancreatitis. Hepatic dysfunction, jaundice and hepatocellular necrosis have also been reported following the use of sulfonamides.

Genitourinary: Crystalluria, hematuria, BUN and creatinine elevation, nephritis and toxic nephrosis with oliguria and anuria. Acute renal failure and urinary retention have also been reported.

Hematologic: Leukopenia, agranulocytosis, aplastic anemia, thrombocytopenia, purpura, hemolytic anemia, anemia, eosinophilia, clotting disorders including hypoprothrombinemia and hypofibrinogenemia, sulfhemoglobinemia and methemoglobinemia.

Musculoskeletal: Arthralgia, chest pain and myalgia.

Neurologic: Headache, dizziness, peripheral neuritis, paresthesia, convulsions, tinnitus, vertigo, ataxia and intracranial hypertension.

Psychiatric: Psychosis, hallucinations, disorientation, depression and anxiety.

Respiratory: Pulmonary infiltrates.

Miscellaneous: Edema (including periorbital), pyrexia, drowsiness, weakness, fatigue, lassitude, rigors, flushing, hearing loss, insomnia and pneumonitis.

OVERDOSAGE

Signs and symptoms of overdosage with Azo Gantrisin include anorexia, colic, nausea, vomiting, dizziness, drowsiness, and even unconsciousness. Pyrexia, hematuria and crystalluria may be noted. Blood dyscrasias and jaundice are potential late manifestations of overdosage.

General principles of treatment include instituting gastric lavage or emesis; forcing oral fluids; and administering intravenous fluids if urine output is low and renal function is normal. The patient should be monitored with blood counts and appropriate blood chemistries, including electrolytes. If the patient becomes cyanotic, the possibility of methemoglobinemia should be considered and, if present, the condition should be treated appropriately with intravenous 1% methylene blue. If a significant blood dyscrasia or jaundice occurs, specific therapy should be instituted for these complications. The oral LD_{50} of Azo Gantrisin in mice is 4317 mg/kg.

DOSAGE AND ADMINISTRATION

Azo Gantrisin is intended for the acute, painful phase of urinary tract infections. The recommended dosage in adults is 4 to 6 tablets initially, followed by 2 tablets four times daily for up to 2 days. Treatment with Azo Gantrisin should not exceed 2 days. Treatment beyond 2 days should only be continued with Gantrisin (sulfisoxazole/Roche).

HOW SUPPLIED

Each red, film-coated tablet contains 0.5 Gm sulfisoxazole/ Roche and 50 mg phenazopyridine HCl. Azo Gantrisin is available in bottles of 100 tablets (NDC-0004-0012-01) and 500 tablets (NDC-0004-0012-14).

Imprint on tablets: AZO GANTRISIN® ROCHE.
P.I. 0587

Shown in Product Identification Section, page 424

BACTRIM™ I.V. INFUSION   ℞

[*bac 'trim*]
(trimethoprim and sulfamethoxazole/Roche)

The following text is complete prescribing information based on official labeling in effect June 1, 1989.

DESCRIPTION

Bactrim (trimethoprim and sulfamethoxazole) I.V. Infusion, a sterile solution for intravenous infusion only, is a synthetic antibacterial combination product. Each 5 ml contains 80 mg trimethoprim (16 mg/ml) and 400 mg sulfamethoxazole (80 mg/ml) compounded with 40% propylene glycol, 10% ethyl alcohol and 0.3% diethanolamine; 1% benzyl alcohol and 0.1% sodium metabisulfite added as preservatives, water for injection, and pH adjusted to approximately 10 with sodium hydroxide.

Trimethoprim is 2,4-diamino-5-(3,4,5-trimethoxybenzyl) pyrimidine. It is a white to light yellow, odorless, bitter compound with a molecular weight of 290.3.

Sulfamethoxazole is N^1-(5-methyl-3-isoxazolyl)sulfanilamide. It is an almost white, odorless, tasteless compound with a molecular weight of 253.28.

CLINICAL PHARMACOLOGY

Following a one-hour intravenous infusion of a single dose of 160 mg trimethoprim and 800 mg sulfamethoxazole to 11 patients whose weight ranged from 105 lbs to 165 lbs (mean, 143 lbs), the peak plasma concentrations of trimethoprim and sulfamethoxazole were 3.4 ± 0.3 μg/ml and 46.3 ± 2.7

μg/ml, respectively. Following repeated intravenous administration of the same dose at eight-hour intervals, the mean plasma concentrations just prior to and immediately after each infusion at steady state were 5.6 ± 0.6 μg/ml and 8.8 ± 0.9 μg/ml for trimethoprim and 70.6 ± 7.3 μg/ml and 105.6 ± 10.9 μg/ml for sulfamethoxazole. The mean plasma half-life was 11.3 ± 0.7 hours for trimethoprim and 12.8 ± 1.8 hours for sulfamethoxazole. All of these 11 patients had normal renal function, and their ages ranged from 17 to 78 years (median, 60 years).[1]

Pharmacokinetic studies in children and adults suggest an age-dependent half-life of trimethoprim, as indicated in the following table.[2]

Age (years)	No. of Patients	Mean TMP Half-life (hours)
<1	2	7.67
1–10	9	5.49
10–20	5	8.19
20–63	6	12.82

Patients with severely impaired renal function exhibit an increase in the half-lives of both components, requiring dosage regimen adjustment (See DOSAGE AND ADMINISTRATION section).

Both trimethoprim and sulfamethoxazole exist in the blood as unbound, protein-bound and metabolized forms; sulfamethaxazole also exists as the conjugated form. The metabolism of sulfamethoxazole occurs predominately by N_4-acetylation, although the glucuronide conjugate has been identified. The principal metabolites of trimethoprim are the 1- and 3-oxides and the 3'- and 4'-hydroxy derivatives. The free forms of trimethoprim and sulfamethoxazole are considered to be the therapeutically active forms. Approximately 44% of trimethoprim and 70% of sulfamethoxazole are bound to plasma proteins. The presence of 10 mg percent sulfamethoxazole in plasma decreases the protein binding of trimethoprim by an insignificant degree; trimethoprim does not influence the protein binding of sulfamethoxazole.

Excretion of trimethoprim and sulfamethoxazole is primarily by the kidneys through both glomerular filtration and tubular secretion. Urine concentrations of both trimethoprim and sulfamethoxazole are considerably higher than are the concentrations in the blood. The percent of dose excreted in urine over a 12-hour period following the intravenous administration of the first dose of 240 mg of trimethoprim and 1200 mg of sulfamethoxazole on day 1 ranged from 17% to 42.4% as free trimethoprim; 7% to 12.7% as free sulfamethoxazole; and 36.7% to 56% as total (free plus the N_4-acetylated metabolite) sulfamethoxazole. When administered together as Bactrim, neither trimethoprim nor sulfamethoxazole affects the urinary excretion pattern of the other. Both trimethoprim and sulfamethoxazole distribute to sputum and vaginal fluid; trimethoprim also distributes to bronchial secretions, and both pass the placental barrier and are excreted in breast milk.

Microbiology: Sulfamethoxazole inhibits bacterial synthesis of dihydrofolic acid by competing with *para*-aminobenzoic acid (PABA). Trimethoprim blocks the production of tetrahydrofolic acid from dihydrofolic acid by binding to and reversibly inhibiting the required enzyme, dihydrofolate reductase. Thus, Bactrim blocks two consecutive steps in the biosynthesis of nucleic acids and proteins essential to many bacteria.

In vitro studies have shown that bacterial resistance develops more slowly with Bactrim than with either trimethoprim or sulfamethoxazole alone.

In vitro serial dilution tests have shown that the spectrum of antibacterial activity of Bactrim includes common bacterial pathogens with the exception of *Pseudomonas aeruginosa*. The following organisms are usually susceptible: *Escherichia coli, Klebsiella* species, *Enterobacter* species, *Morganella morganii, Proteus mirabilis*, indole-positive *Proteus* species including *Proteus vulgaris, Haemophilus influenzae* (including ampicillin-resistant strains), *Streptococcus pneumoniae, Shigella flexneri* and *Shigella sonnei*. It should be noted, however, that there are little clinical data on the use of Bactrim I.V. Infusion in serious systemic infections due to *Haemophilus influenzae* and *Streptococcus pneumoniae*.
[See table on next page].

The recommended quantitative disc susceptibility method may be used for estimating the susceptibility of bacteria to Bactrim.[3,4] With this procedure, a report from the laboratory of "Susceptible to trimethoprim and sulfamethoxazole" indicates that the infection is likely to respond to therapy with Bactrim. If the infection is confined to the urine, a report of "Intermediate susceptibility to trimethoprim and sulfamethoxazole" also indicates that the infection is likely to respond. A report of "Resistant to trimethoprim and sulfamethoxazole" indicates that the infection is unlikely to respond to therapy with Bactrim.

Continued on next page

Roche Labs.—Cont.

INDICATIONS AND USAGE

PNEUMOCYSTIS CARINII PNEUMONIA: Bactrim I.V. Infusion is indicated in the treatment of *Pneumocystis carinii* pneumonia in children and adults.

SHIGELLOSIS: Bactrim I.V. Infusion is indicated in the treatment of enteritis caused by susceptible strains of *Shigella flexneri* and *Shigella sonnei* in children and adults.

URINARY TRACT INFECTIONS: Bactrim I.V. Infusion is indicated in the treatment of severe or complicated urinary tract infections due to susceptible strains of *Escherichia coli, Klebsiella* species, *Enterobacter* species, *Morganella morganii* and *Proteus* species when oral administration of Bactrim is not feasible and when the organism is not susceptible to single agent antibacterials effective in the urinary tract.

Although appropriate culture and susceptibility studies should be performed, therapy may be started while awaiting the results of these studies.

CONTRAINDICATIONS

Hypersensitivity to trimethoprim or sulfonamides. Patients with documented megaloblastic anemia due to folate deficiency. Pregnancy at term and during the nursing period, because sulfonamides pass the placenta and are excreted in the milk and may cause kernicterus. Infants less than two months of age.

WARNINGS

FATALITIES ASSOCIATED WITH THE ADMINISTRATION OF SULFONAMIDES, ALTHOUGH RARE, HAVE OCCURRED DUE TO SEVERE REACTIONS, INCLUDING STEVENS-JOHNSON SYNDROME, TOXIC EPIDERMAL NECROLYSIS, FULMINANT HEPATIC NECROSIS, AGRANULOCYTOSIS, APLASTIC ANEMIA AND OTHER BLOOD DYSCRASIAS.

BACTRIM SHOULD BE DISCONTINUED AT THE FIRST APPEARANCE OF SKIN RASH OR ANY SIGN OF ADVERSE REACTION. Clinical signs, such as rash, sore throat, fever, arthralgia, cough, shortness of breath, pallor, purpura or jaundice may be early indications of serious reactions. In rare instances a skin rash may be followed by more severe reactions, such as Stevens-Johnson syndrome, toxic epidermal necrolysis, hepatic necrosis or serious blood disorder. Complete blood counts should be done frequently in patients receiving sulfonamides.

BACTRIM SHOULD NOT BE USED IN THE TREATMENT OF STREPTOCOCCAL PHARYNGITIS. Clinical studies have documented that patients with group A β-hemolytic streptococcal tonsillopharyngitis have a greater incidence of bacteriologic failure when treated with Bactrim than do those patients treated with penicillin, as evidenced by failure to eradicate this organism from the tonsillopharyngeal area. Bactrim I.V. Infusion contains sodium metabisulfite, a sulfite that may cause allergic-type reactions, including anaphylactic symptoms and life-threatening or less severe asthmatic episodes in certain susceptible people. The overall prevalence of sulfite sensitivity in the general population is unknown and probably low. Sulfite sensitivity is seen more frequently in asthmatic than in nonasthmatic people.

PRECAUTIONS

General: Bactrim should be given with caution to patients with impaired renal or hepatic function, to those with possible folate deficiency (*e.g.*, the elderly, chronic alcoholics, patients receiving anticonvulsant therapy, patients with malabsorption syndrome, and patients in malnutrition states) and to those with severe allergies or bronchial asthma. In glucose-6-phosphate dehydrogenase deficient individuals, hemolysis may occur. This reaction is frequently dose-related.

Local irritation and inflammation due to extravascular infiltration of the infusion have been observed with Bactrim I.V.

Infusion. If these occur, the infusion should be discontinued and restarted at another site.

Use in the Elderly: There may be an increased risk of severe adverse reactions in elderly patients, particularly when complicating conditions exist, *e.g.*, impaired kidney and/or liver function, or concomitant use of other drugs. Severe skin reactions, generalized bone marrow suppression (see WARNINGS and ADVERSE REACTIONS sections) or a specific decrease in platelets (with or without purpura) are the most frequently reported severe adverse reactions in elderly patients. In those concurrently receiving certain diuretics, primarily thiazides, an increased incidence of thrombocytopenia with purpura has been reported. Appropriate dosage adjustments should be made for patients with impaired kidney function (see DOSAGE AND ADMINISTRATION section).

Use in the Treatment of Pneumocystis Carinii Pneumonia in Patients with Acquired Immunodeficiency Syndrome (AIDS): AIDS patients may not tolerate or respond to Bactrim in the same manner as non-AIDS patients. The incidence of side effects, particularly rash, fever, leukopenia, and elevated aminotransferase (transaminase) values, with Bactrim therapy in AIDS patients who are being treated for *Pneumocystis carinii* pneumonia has been reported to be greatly increased compared with the incidence normally associated with the use of Bactrim in non-AIDS patients.

Laboratory Tests: Appropriate culture and susceptibility studies should be performed before and throughout treatment. Complete blood counts should be done frequently in patients receiving Bactrim; if a significant reduction in the count of any formed blood element is noted, Bactrim should be discontinued. Urinalyses with careful microscopic examination and renal function tests should be performed during therapy, particularly for those patients with impaired renal function.

Drug Interactions: In elderly patients concurrently receiving certain diuretics, primarily thiazides, an increased incidence of thrombocytopenia with purpura has been reported. It has been reported that Bactrim may prolong the prothrombin time in patients who are receiving the anticoagulant warfarin. This interaction should be kept in mind when Bactrim is given to patients already on anticoagulant therapy, and the coagulation time should be reassessed.

Bactrim may inhibit the hepatic metabolism of phenytoin. Bactrim, given at a common clinical dosage, increased the phenytoin half-life by 39% and decreased the phenytoin metabolic clearance rate by 27%. When administering these drugs concurrently, one should be alert for possible excessive phenytoin effect.

Sulfonamides can also displace methotrexate from plasma protein binding sites, thus increasing free methotrexate concentrations.

Drug/Laboratory Test Interactions: Bactrim, specifically the trimethoprim component, can interfere with a serum methotrexate assay as determined by the competitive binding protein technique (CBPA) when a bacterial dihydrofolate reductase is used as the binding protein. No interference occurs, however, if methotrexate is measured by a radioimmunoassay (RIA).

The presence of trimethoprim and sulfamethoxazole may also interfere with the Jaffé alkaline picrate reaction assay for creatinine, resulting in overestimations of about 10% in the range of normal values.

Carcinogenesis, Mutagenesis, Impairment of Fertility:
Carcinogenesis: Long-term studies in animals to evaluate carcinogenic potential have not been conducted with Bactrim I.V. Infusion.

Mutagenesis: Bacterial mutagenic studies have not been performed with sulfamethoxazole and trimethoprim in combination. Trimethoprim was demonstrated to be nonmutagenic in the Ames assay. No chromosomal damage was observed in human leukocytes cultured *in vitro* with sulfamethoxazole and trimethoprim alone or in combination; the concentrations used exceeded blood levels of these com-

pounds following therapy with Bactrim. Observations of leukocytes obtained from patients treated with Bactrim revealed no chromosomal abnormalities.

Impairment of Fertility: Bactrim I.V. Infusion has not been studied in animals for evidence of impairment of fertility. However, studies in rats at oral dosages as high as 70 mg/kg trimethoprim plus 350 mg/kg sulfamethoxazole daily showed no adverse effects on fertility or general reproductive performance.

Pregnancy: Teratogenic Effects: Pregnancy Category C. In rats, oral doses of 533 mg/kg sulfamethoxazole or 200 mg/kg trimethoprim produced teratological effects manifested mainly as cleft palates.

The highest dose which did not cause cleft palates in rats was 512 mg/kg sulfamethoxazole or 192 mg/kg trimethoprim when administered separately. In two studies in rats, no teratology was observed when 512 mg/kg of sulfamethoxazole was used in combination with 128 mg/kg of trimethoprim. In one study, however, cleft palates were observed in one litter out of nine when 355 mg/kg of sulfamethoxazole was used in combination with 88 mg/kg of trimethoprim. In some rabbit studies, an overall increase in fetal loss (dead and resorbed and malformed conceptuses) was associated with doses of trimethoprim six times the human therapeutic dose.

While there are no large, well-controlled studies on the use of trimethoprim and sulfamethoxazole in pregnant women, Brumfitt and Pursell,[5] in a retrospective study, reported the outcome of 186 pregnancies during which the mother received either placebo or oral trimethoprim and sulfamethoxazole. The incidence of congenital abnormalities was 4.5% (3 of 66) in those who received placebo and 3.3% (4 of 120) in those receiving trimethoprim and sulfamethoxazole. There were no abnormalities in the 10 children whose mothers received the drug during the first trimester. In a separate survey, Brumfitt and Pursell also found no congenital abnormalities in 35 children whose mothers had received oral trimethoprim and sulfamethoxazole at the time of conception or shortly thereafter.

Because trimethoprim and sulfamethoxazole may interfere with folic acid metabolism, Bactrim I.V. Infusion should be used during pregnancy only if the potential benefit justifies the potential risk to the fetus.

Nonteratogenic Effects: See CONTRAINDICATIONS section.

Nursing Mothers: See CONTRAINDICATIONS section.

Pediatric Use: Bactrim I.V. Infusion is not recommended for infants younger than two months of age (see CONTRAINDICATIONS section).

ADVERSE REACTIONS

The most common adverse effects are gastrointestinal disturbances (nausea, vomiting, anorexia) and allergic skin reactions (such as rash and urticaria). **FATALITIES ASSOCIATED WITH THE ADMINISTRATION OF SULFONAMIDES, ALTHOUGH RARE, HAVE OCCURRED DUE TO SEVERE REACTIONS, INCLUDING STEVENS-JOHNSON SYNDROME, TOXIC EPIDERMAL NECROLYSIS, FULMINANT HEPATIC NECROSIS, AGRANULOCYTOSIS, APLASTIC ANEMIA AND OTHER BLOOD DYSCRASIAS (SEE WARNINGS SECTION).** Local reaction, pain and slight irritation on I.V. administration are infrequent. Thrombophlebitis has rarely been observed.

Hematologic: Agranulocytosis, aplastic anemia, thrombocytopenia, leukopenia, neutropenia, hemolytic anemia, megaloblastic anemia, hypoprothrombinemia, methemoglobinemia, eosinophilia.

Allergic Reactions: Stevens-Johnson syndrome, toxic epidermal necrolysis, anaphylaxis, allergic myocarditis, erythema multiforme, exfoliative dermatitis, angioedema, drug fever, chills, Henoch-Schoenlein purpura, serum sickness-like syndrome, generalized allergic reactions, generalized skin eruptions, conjunctival and scleral injection, photosensitivity, pruritus, urticaria and rash. In addition, periarteritis nodosa and systemic lupus erythematosus have been reported.

Gastrointestinal: Hepatitis (including cholestatic jaundice and hepatic necrosis), elevation of serum transaminase and bilirubin, pseudomembraneous enterocolitis, pancreatitis, stomatitis, glossitis, nausea, emesis, abdominal pain, diarrhea, anorexia.

Genitourinary: Renal failure, interstitial nephritis, BUN and serum creatinine elevation, toxic nephrosis with oliguria and anuria, and crystalluria.

Neurologic: Aseptic meningitis, convulsions, peripheral neuritis, ataxia, vertigo, tinnitus, headache.

Psychiatric: Hallucinations, depression, apathy, nervousness.

Endocrine: The sulfonamides bear certain chemical similarities to some goitrogens, diuretics (acetazolamide and the thiazides) and oral hypoglycemic agents. Cross-sensitivity may exist with these agents. Diuresis and hypoglycemia have occurred rarely in patients receiving sulfonamides.

REPRESENTATIVE MINIMUM INHIBITORY CONCENTRATION VALUES FOR BACTRIM-SUSCEPTIBLE ORGANISMS (MIC—µg/ml)

Bacteria	TMP alone	SMX alone	TMP/SMX (1:20) TMP	TMP/SMX (1:20) SMX
Escherichia coli	0.05–1.5	1.0–245	0.05–0.5	0.95–9.5
Proteus species (indole positive)	0.5–5.0	7.35–300	0.05–1.5	0.95–28.5
Morganella morganii	0.5–5.0	7.35–300	0.05–1.5	0.95–28.5
Proteus mirabilis	0.5–1.5	7.35–30	0.05–0.15	0.95–2.85
Klebsiella species	0.15–5.0	2.45–245	0.05–1.5	0.95–28.5
Enterobacter species	0.15–5.0	2.45–245	0.05–1.5	0.95–28.5
Haemophilus influenzae	0.15–1.5	2.85–95	0.015–0.15	0.285–2.85
Streptococcus pneumoniae	0.15–1.5	7.35–24.5	0.05–0.15	0.95–2.85
*Shigella flexneri**	<0.01–0.04	<0.16–>320	<0.002–0.03	0.04–0.625
*Shigella sonnei**	0.02–0.08	0.625–>320	0.004–0.06	0.08–1.25

TMP = trimethoprim

SMX = sulfamethoxazole

*Rudoy RC, Nelson JD, Haltalin KC: *Antimicrob Agents Chemother* 5:439–443, May 1974.

Musculoskeletal: Arthralgia and myalgia.
Respiratory: Pulmonary infiltrates.
Miscellaneous: Weakness, fatigue, insomnia.

OVERDOSAGE

Acute: Since there has been no extensive experience in humans with single doses of Bactrim I.V. Infusion in excess of 25 ml (400 mg trimethoprim and 2000 mg sulfamethoxazole), the maximum tolerated dose in humans is unknown. Signs and symptoms of overdosage reported with sulfonamides include anorexia, colic, nausea, vomiting, dizziness, headache, drowsiness and unconsciousness. Pyrexia, hematuria and crystalluria may be noted. Blood dyscrasias and jaundice are potential late manifestations of overdosage. Signs of acute overdosage with trimethoprim include nausea, vomiting, dizziness, headache, mental depression, confusion and bone marrow depression.

General principles of treatment include the administration of intravenous fluids if urine output is low and renal function is normal. Acidification of the urine will increase renal elimination of trimethoprim. The patient should be monitored with blood counts and appropriate blood chemistries, including electrolytes. If a significant blood dyscrasia or jaundice occurs, specific therapy should be instituted for these complications. Peritoneal dialysis is not effective and hemodialysis is only moderately effective in eliminating trimethoprim and sulfamethoxazole.

Chronic: Use of Bactrim I.V. Infusion at high doses and/or for extended periods of time may cause bone marrow depression manifested as thrombocytopenia, leukopenia and/or megaloblastic anemia. If signs of bone marrow depression occur, the patient should be given leucovorin 5 to 15 mg daily until normal hematopoiesis is restored.

Animal Toxicity: The LD_{50} of Bactrim I.V. Infusion in mice is 700 mg/kg or 7.3 ml/kg; in rats and rabbits the LD_{50} is >500 mg/kg or >5.2 ml/kg. The vehicle produced the same LD_{50} in each of these species as the active drug.

The signs and symptoms noted in mice, rats and rabbits with Bactrim I.V. Infusion or its vehicle at the high I.V. doses used in acute toxicity studies included ataxia, decreased motor activity, loss of righting reflex, tremors or convulsions, and/or respiratory depression.

DOSAGE AND ADMINISTRATION

CONTRAINDICATED IN INFANTS LESS THAN TWO MONTHS OF AGE. CAUTION—BACTRIM I.V. INFUSION MUST BE DILUTED IN 5% DEXTROSE IN WATER SOLUTION PRIOR TO ADMINISTRATION. DO NOT MIX BACTRIM I.V. INFUSION WITH OTHER DRUGS OR SOLUTIONS. RAPID INFUSION OR BOLUS INJECTION MUST BE AVOIDED.

Dosage:

Children and Adults:
PNEUMOCYSTIS CARINII PNEUMONIA: Total daily dose is 15 to 20 mg/kg (based on the trimethoprim component) given in three or four equally divided doses every 6 to 8 hours for up to 14 days. One investigator noted that a total daily dose of 10 to 15 mg/kg was sufficient in ten adult patients with normal renal function.[6]

SEVERE URINARY TRACT INFECTIONS AND SHIGELLOSIS: Total daily dose is 8 to 10 mg/kg (based on the trimethoprim component) given in two to four equally divided doses every 6, 8 or 12 hours for up to 14 days for severe urinary tract infections and five days for shigellosis. The maximum recommended daily dose is 60 ml per day.

For Patients with Impaired Renal Function: When renal function is impaired, a reduced dosage should be employed using the following table:

Creatinine Clearance (ml/min)	Recommended Dosage Regimen
Above 30	Usual standard regimen
15–30	½ the usual regimen
Below 15	Use not recommended

Method of Preparation: Bactrim I.V. Infusion must be diluted. EACH 5 ML SHOULD BE ADDED TO 125 ML OF 5% DEXTROSE IN WATER. After diluting with 5% dextrose in water, the solution should not be refrigerated and should be used within six hours. If a dilution of 5 ml per 100 ml of 5% dextrose in water is desired, it should be used within 4 hours. If upon visual inspection there is cloudiness or evidence of crystallization after mixing, the solution should be discarded and a fresh solution prepared.

Multidose Vials: After initial entry into the vial, the remaining contents must be used within 48 hours.

The following infusion systems have been tested and found satisfactory: unit-dose glass containers; unit-dose polyvinyl chloride and polyolefin containers. No other systems have been tested and therefore no others can be recommended.

Dilution: EACH 5 ML OF BACTRIM I.V. INFUSION SHOULD BE ADDED TO 125 ML OF 5% DEXTROSE IN WATER.

NOTE: *In those instances where fluid restriction is desirable,* each 5 ml may be added to 75 ml of 5% dextrose in water. Under these circumstances the solution should be mixed just prior to use and should be administered within two (2) hours. If upon visual inspection there is cloudiness or evidence of crystallization after mixing, the solution should be discarded and a fresh solution prepared.

DO NOT MIX BACTRIM I.V. INFUSION—5% DEXTROSE IN WATER WITH DRUGS OR SOLUTIONS IN THE SAME CONTAINER.

Administration: The solution should be given by intravenous infusion over a period of 60 to 90 minutes. Rapid infusion or bolus injection must be avoided. Bactrim I.V. Infusion should not be given intramuscularly.

HOW SUPPLIED

5-ml *ampuls,* containing 80 mg trimethoprim (16 mg/ml) and 400 mg sulfamethoxazole (80 mg/ml) for infusion with 5% dextrose in water. Boxes of 10 (NDC 0004-1943-06).

5-ml *vials,* containing 80 mg trimethoprim (16 mg/ml) and 400 mg sulfamethoxazole (80 mg/ml) for infusion with 5% dextrose in water. Boxes of 10 (NDC 0004-1956-01).

10-ml *vials,* containing 160 mg trimethoprim (16 mg/ml) and 800 mg sulfamethoxazole (80 mg/ml) for infusion with 5% dextrose in water. Boxes of 10 (NDC 0004-1955-01).

30-ml *multidose vials,* each 5 ml containing 80 mg trimethoprim (16 mg/ml) and 400 mg sulfamethoxazole (80 mg/ml) for infusion with 5% dextrose in water. Boxes of 1 (NDC 0004-1958-01).

50-ml *multidose vials,* each 5 ml containing 80 mg trimethoprim (16 mg/ml) and 400 mg sulfamethoxazole (80 mg/ml) for infusion with 5% dextrose in water. Boxes of 1 (NDC 0004-1958-02).

STORE AT ROOM TEMPERATURE (15°–30°C or 59°–86°F). DO NOT REFRIGERATE.

Bactrim is also available as *DS (double strength) Tablets* (white, notched, capsule shaped), containing 160 mg trimethoprim and 800 mg sulfamethoxazole—bottles of 100 (NDC 0004-0117-01), 250 (NDC 0004-0117-04) and 500 (NDC 0004-0117-14); Tel-E-Dose® packages of 100 (NDC 0004-0117-49); Prescription Paks of 20 (NDC 0004-0117-54). Imprint on tablets: (front) BACTRIM-DS; (back) ROCHE.

Tablets (light green, scored, capsule shaped), containing 80 mg trimethoprim and 400 mg sulfamethoxazole—bottles of 100 (NDC 0004-0050-01) and 500 (NDC 0004-0050-14); Tel-E-Dose® packages of 100 (NDC 0004-0050-49); Prescription Paks of 40 (NDC 0004-0050-34). Imprint on tablets: (front) BACTRIM; (back) ROCHE.

Pediatric Suspension (pink, cherry flavored), containing 40 mg trimethoprim and 200 mg sulfamethoxazole per teaspoonful (5 ml)—bottles of 100 ml (NDC 0004-1033-01) and 16 oz (1 pint) (NDC 0004-1033-28).

Suspension (pink, fruit-licorice flavored), containing 40 mg trimethoprim and 200 mg sulfamethoxazole per teaspoonful (5 ml)—bottles of 16 oz (1 pint) (NDC 0004-1015-28).

REFERENCES

1. Grose WE, Bodey GP, Loo TL: Clinical Pharmacology of Intravenously Administered Trimethoprim-Sulfamethoxazole. *Antimicrob Agents Chemother* 15 :447-451, Mar 1979. 2. Siber GR, Gorham C, Durbin W, Lesko L, Levin MJ: Pharmacology of Intravenous Trimethoprim-Sulfamethoxazole in Children and Adults. *Current Chemotherapy and Infectious Diseases,* American Society for Microbiology, Washington, D.C., 1980, Vol. 1, pp. 691-692. 3. Bauer AW, Kirby WMM, Sherris JC, Turck M: Antibiotic Susceptibility Testing by a Standardized Single Disk Method. *Am J Clin Pathol* 45 :493-496, Apr 1966. 4. Approved Standard ASM-2 Performance Standards for Antimicrobial Disc Susceptibility Test: National Committee for Clinical Laboratory Standards, 771 East Lancaster Avenue, Villanova, Pennsylvania 19085. 5. Brumfitt W, Pursell R: Trimethoprim/Sulfamethoxazole in the Treatment of Bacteriuria in Women. *J Infect Dis* 128 (Suppl): S657-S663, Nov 1973. 6. Winston DJ, Lau WK, Gale RP, Young LS: Trimethoprim-Sulfamethoxazole for the Treatment of *Pneumocystis carinii* pneumonia. *Ann Intern Med* 92 :762-769, June 1980.
P.I. 0288

BACTRIM™   ℞

[*bac 'trim*]
(trimethoprim and sulfamethoxazole/Roche)
DS (double strength) Tablets
Tablets
Suspension
and
Pediatric Suspension

The following text is complete prescribing information based on official labeling in effect June 1, 1989.

DESCRIPTION

Bactrim (trimethoprim and sulfamethoxazole) is a synthetic antibacterial combination product available in DS (double strength) tablets, tablets, pediatric suspension and suspension for oral administration. Each DS tablet contains 160 mg trimethoprim and 800 mg sulfamethoxazole plus magnesium stearate, pregelatinized starch and sodium starch glycolate. Each tablet contains 80 mg trimethoprim and 400 mg sulfamethoxazole plus magnesium stearate, pregelatinized starch, sodium starch glycolate, FD&C Blue No. 1 lake, FD&C Yellow No. 6 lake and D&C Yellow No. 10 lake. Each teaspoonful (5 ml) of the pediatric suspension or suspension contains 40 mg trimethoprim and 200 mg sulfamethoxazole in a vehicle containing 0.3 percent alcohol, edetate disodium, glycerin, microcrystalline cellulose, parabens (methyl and propyl), polysorbate 80, saccharin sodium, simethicone, sorbitol, sucrose, FD&C Yellow No. 6, FD&C Red No. 40, flavors and water.

Trimethoprim is 2,4-diamino-5-(3,4,5-trimethoxybenzyl) pyrimidine. It is a white to light yellow, odorless, bitter compound with a molecular weight of 290.3.

Sulfamethoxazole is N^1-(5-methyl-3-isoxazolyl) sulfanilamide. It is an almost white, odorless, tasteless compound with a molecular weight of 253.28.

CLINICAL PHARMACOLOGY

Bactrim is rapidly absorbed following oral administration. Both sulfamethoxazole and trimethoprim exist in the blood as unbound, protein-bound and metabolized forms; sulfamethoxazole also exists as the conjugated form. The metabolism of sulfamethoxazole occurs predominately by N_4-acetylation, although the glucuronide conjugate has been identified. The principal metabolites of trimethoprim are the 1- and 3-oxides and the 3'- and 4'-hydroxy derivatives. The free forms of sulfamethoxazole and trimethoprim are considered to be the therapeutically active forms. Approximately 44% of trimethoprim and 70% of sulfamethoxazole are bound to plasma proteins. The presence of 10 mg percent sulfamethoxazole in plasma decreases the protein binding of trimethoprim by an insignificant degree; trimethoprim does not influence the protein binding of sulfamethoxazole.

Peak blood levels for the individual components occur 1 to 4 hours after oral administration. The mean serum half-lives of sulfamethoxazole and trimethoprim are 10 and 8 to 10 hours, respectively. However, patients with severely impaired renal function exhibit an increase in the half-lives of both components, requiring dosage regimen adjustment (see DOSAGE AND ADMINISTRATION section). Detectable amounts of trimethoprim and sulfamethoxazole are present in the blood 24 hours after drug administration. During administration of 160 mg trimethoprim and 800 mg sulfamethoxazole *b.i.d.,* the mean steady-state plasma concentration of trimethoprim was 1.72 µg/ml. The steady-state mean plasma levels of free and total sulfamethoxazole were 57.4 µg/ml and 68.0 µg/ml, respectively. These steady-state levels were achieved after three days of drug administration.[1] Excretion of sulfamethoxazole and trimethoprim is primarily by the kidneys through both glomerular filtration and tubular secretion. Urine concentrations of both sulfamethoxazole and trimethoprim are considerably higher than are the concentrations in the blood. The average percentage of the dose recovered in urine from 0 to 72 hours after a single oral dose of Bactrim is 84.5% for total sulfonamide and 66.8% for free trimethoprim. Thirty percent of the total sulfonamide is excreted as free sulfamethoxazole, with the remaining as N_4-acetylated metabolite.[2] When administered together as Bactrim, neither sulfamethoxazole nor trimethoprim affects the urinary excretion pattern of the other.

Both trimethoprim and sulfamethoxazole distribute to sputum, vaginal fluid and middle ear fluid; trimethoprim also distributes to bronchial secretion, and both pass the placental barrier and are excreted in breast milk.

Microbiology: Sulfamethoxazole inhibits bacterial synthesis of dihydrofolic acid by competing with *para* -aminobenzoic acid (PABA). Trimethoprim blocks the production of tetrahydrofolic acid from dihydrofolic acid by binding to and reversibly inhibiting the required enzyme, dihydrofolate reductase. Thus, Bactrim blocks two consecutive steps in the biosynthesis of nucleic acids and proteins essential to many bacteria.

In vitro studies have shown that bacterial resistance develops more slowly with Bactrim than with either trimethoprim or sulfamethoxazole alone.

In vitro serial dilution tests have shown that the spectrum of antibacterial activity of Bactrim includes the common urinary tract pathogens with the exception of *Pseudomonas aeruginosa.* The following organisms are usually susceptible: *Escherichia coli, Klebsiella* species, *Enterobacter* species, *Morganella morganii, Proteus mirabilis,* and indole-positive *Proteus* species including *Proteus vulgaris.* The usual spectrum of antimicrobial activity of Bactrim includes the following bacterial pathogens isolated from middle ear exudate and from bronchial secretions: *Haemophilus influenzae,* including ampicillin-resistant strains, and *Streptococcus pneumoniae. Shigella flexneri* and *Shigella sonnei* are usually susceptible.

[See table on next page].

The recommended quantitative disc susceptibility method may be used for estimating the susceptibility of bacteria to Bactrim.[3,4] With this procedure, a report from the laboratory of "Susceptible to trimethoprim and sulfamethoxazole" indicates that the infection is likely to respond to therapy with

Continued on next page

Roche Labs.—Cont.

Bactrim. If the infection is confined to the urine, a report of "Intermediate susceptibility to trimethoprim and sulfamethoxazole" also indicates that the infection is likely to respond. A report of "Resistant to trimethoprim and sulfamethoxazole" indicates that the infection is unlikely to respond to therapy with Bactrim.

INDICATIONS AND USAGE

URINARY TRACT INFECTIONS: For the treatment of urinary tract infections due to susceptible strains of the following organisms: *Escherichia coli, Klebsiella* species, *Enterobacter* species, *Morganella morganii, Proteus mirabilis* and *Proteus vulgaris.* It is recommended that initial episodes of uncomplicated urinary tract infections be treated with a single effective antibacterial agent rather than the combination.

ACUTE OTITIS MEDIA: For the treatment of acute otitis media in children due to susceptible strains of *Streptococcus pneumoniae* or *Haemophilus influenzae* when in the judgment of the physician Bactrim offers some advantage over the use of other antimicrobial agents. To date, there are limited data on the safety of repeated use of Bactrim in children under two years of age. Bactrim is not indicated for prophylactic or prolonged administration in otitis media at any age.

ACUTE EXACERBATIONS OF CHRONIC BRONCHITIS IN ADULTS: For the treatment of acute exacerbations of chronic bronchitis due to susceptible strains of *Streptococcus pneumoniae* or *Haemophilus influenzae* when in the judgment of the physician Bactrim offers some advantage over the use of a single antimicrobial agent.

SHIGELLOSIS: For the treatment of enteritis caused by susceptible strains of *Shigella flexneri* and *Shigella sonnei* when antibacterial therapy is indicated.

PNEUMOCYSTIS CARINII PNEUMONIA: For the treatment of documented *Pneumocystis carinii* pneumonia.

CONTRAINDICATIONS

Hypersensitivity to trimethoprim or sulfonamides. Patients with documented megaloblastic anemia due to folate deficiency. Pregnancy at term and during the nursing period, because sulfonamides pass the placenta and are excreted in the milk and may cause kernicterus. Infants less than two months of age.

WARNINGS

FATALITIES ASSOCIATED WITH THE ADMINISTRATION OF SULFONAMIDES, ALTHOUGH RARE, HAVE OCCURRED DUE TO SEVERE REACTIONS, INCLUDING STEVENS-JOHNSON SYNDROME, TOXIC EPIDERMAL NECROLYSIS, FULMINANT HEPATIC NECROSIS, AGRANULOCYTOSIS, APLASTIC ANEMIA AND OTHER BLOOD DYSCRASIAS.
BACTRIM SHOULD BE DISCONTINUED AT THE FIRST APPEARANCE OF SKIN RASH OR ANY SIGN OF ADVERSE REACTION. Clinical signs, such as rash, sore throat, fever, arthralgia, cough, shortness of breath, pallor, purpura or jaundice may be early indications of serious reactions. In rare instances a skin rash may be followed by more severe reactions, such as Stevens-Johnson syndrome, toxic epidermal necrolysis, hepatic necrosis or serious blood disorder. Complete blood counts should be done frequently in patients receiving sulfonamides.
BACTRIM SHOULD NOT BE USED IN THE TREATMENT OF STREPTOCOCCAL PHARYNGITIS. Clinical studies have demonstrated that patients with group A β-hemolytic streptococcal tonsillopharyngitis have a greater incidence of bacteriologic failure when treated with Bactrim than do those patients treated with penicillin, as evidenced by failure to eradicate this organism from the tonsillopharyngeal area.

PRECAUTIONS

General: Bactrim should be given with caution to patients with impaired renal or hepatic function, to those with possible folate deficiency (*e.g.,* the elderly, chronic alcoholics, patients receiving anticonvulsant therapy, patients with malabsorption syndrome, and patients in malnutrition states) and to those with severe allergies or bronchial asthma. In glucose-6-phosphate dehydrogenase deficient individuals, hemolysis may occur. This reaction is frequently dose-related.

Use in the Elderly: There may be an increased risk of severe adverse reactions in elderly patients, particularly when complicating conditions exist, *e.g.,* impaired kidney and/or liver function, or concomitant use of other drugs. Severe skin reactions, generalized bone marrow suppression (see WARNINGS and ADVERSE REACTIONS sections) or a specific decrease in platelets (with or without purpura) are the most frequently reported severe adverse reactions in elderly patients. In those concurrently receiving certain diuretics, primarily thiazides, an increased incidence of thrombocytopenia with purpura has been reported. Appropriate dosage adjustments should be made for patients with impaired kidney function (see DOSAGE AND ADMINISTRATION section).

Use in the Treatment of Pneumocystis Carinii Pneumonia in Patients with Acquired Immunodeficiency Syndrome (AIDS): AIDS patients may not tolerate or respond to Bactrim in the same manner as non-AIDS patients. The incidence of side effects, particularly rash, fever, leukopenia, and elevated aminotransferase (transaminase) values, with Bactrim therapy in AIDS patients who are being treated for *Pneumocystis carinii* pneumonia has been reported to be greatly increased compared with the incidence normally associated with the use of Bactrim in non-AIDS patients.

Information for Patients: Patients should be instructed to maintain an adequate fluid intake in order to prevent crystalluria and stone formation.

Laboratory Tests: Complete blood counts should be done frequently in patients receiving Bactrim; if a significant reduction in the count of any formed blood element is noted, Bactrim should be discontinued. Urinalyses with careful microscopic examination and renal function tests should be performed during therapy, particularly for those patients with impaired renal function.

Drug Interactions: In elderly patients concurrently receiving certain diuretics, primarily thiazides, an increased incidence of thrombocytopenia with purpura has been reported. It has been reported that Bactrim may prolong the prothrombin time in patients who are receiving the anticoagulant warfarin. This interaction should be kept in mind when Bactrim is given to patients already on anticoagulant therapy, and the coagulation time should be reassessed.

Bactrim may inhibit the hepatic metabolism of phenytoin. Bactrim, given at a common clinical dosage, increased the phenytoin half-life by 39% and decreased the phenytoin metabolic clearance rate by 27%. When administering these drugs concurrently, one should be alert for possible excessive phenytoin effect.

Sulfonamides can also displace methotrexate from plasma protein binding sites, thus increasing free methotrexate concentrations.

Drug/Laboratory Test Interactions: Bactrim, specifically the trimethoprim component, can interfere with a serum methotrexate assay as determined by the competitive binding protein technique (CBPA) when a bacterial dihydrofolate reductase is used as the binding protein. No interference occurs, however, if methotrexate is measured by a radioimmunoassay (RIA).

The presence of trimethoprim and sulfamethoxazole may also interfere with the Jaffé alkaline picrate reaction assay for creatinine, resulting in overestimations of about 10% in the range of normal values.

Carcinogenesis, Mutagenesis, Impairment of Fertility:
Carcinogenesis: Long-term studies in animals to evaluate carcinogenic potential have not been conducted with Bactrim.

Mutagenesis: Bacterial mutagenic studies have not been performed with sulfamethoxazole and trimethoprim in combination. Trimethoprim was demonstrated to be nonmutagenic in the Ames assay. No chromosomal damage was observed in human leukocytes *in vitro* with sulfamethoxazole and trimethoprim alone or in combination; the concentrations used exceeded blood levels of these compounds following therapy with Bactrim. Observations of leukocytes obtained from patients treated with Bactrim revealed no chromosomal abnormalities.

Impairment of Fertility: No adverse effects on fertility or general reproductive performance were observed in rats given oral dosages as high as 70 mg/kg/day trimethoprim plus 350 mg/kg/day sulfamethoxazole.

Pregnancy: Teratogenic Effects: Pregnancy Category C. In rats, oral doses of 533 mg/kg sulfamethoxazole or 200 mg/kg trimethoprim produced teratologic effects manifested mainly as cleft palates.

The highest dose which did not cause cleft palates in rats was 512 mg/kg sulfamethoxazole or 192 mg/kg trimethoprim when administered separately. In two studies in rats, no teratology was observed when 512 mg/kg of sulfamethoxazole was used in combination with 128 mg/kg of trimethoprim. In one study, however, cleft palates were observed in one litter out of 9 when 355 mg/kg of sulfamethoxazole was used in combination with 88 mg/kg of trimethoprim.

In some rabbit studies, an overall increase in fetal loss (dead and resorbed and malformed conceptuses) was associated with doses of trimethoprim 6 times the human therapeutic dose.

While there are no large, well-controlled studies on the use of trimethoprim and sulfamethoxazole in pregnant women, Brumfitt and Pursell,[5] in a retrospective study, reported the outcome of 186 pregnancies during which the mother received either placebo or trimethoprim and sulfamethoxazole. The incidence of congenital abnormalities was 4.5% (3 of 66) in those who received placebo and 3.3% (4 of 120) in those receiving trimethoprim and sulfamethoxazole. There were no abnormalities in the 10 children whose mothers received the drug during the first trimester. In a separate survey, Brumfitt and Pursell also found no congenital abnormalities in 35 children whose mothers had received oral trimethoprim and sulfamethoxazole at the time of conception or shortly thereafter.

Because trimethoprim and sulfamethoxazole may interfere with folic acid metabolism, Bactrim should be used during pregnancy only if the potential benefit justifies the potential risk to the fetus.

Nonteratogenic Effects: See CONTRAINDICATIONS section.

Nursing Mothers: See CONTRAINDICATIONS section.

Pediatric Use: Bactrim is not recommended for infants younger than two months of age (see INDICATIONS and CONTRAINDICATIONS sections).

ADVERSE REACTIONS

The most common adverse effects are gastrointestinal disturbances (nausea, vomiting, anorexia) and allergic skin reactions (such as rash and urticaria). **FATALITIES ASSOCIATED WITH THE ADMINISTRATION OF SULFONAMIDES, ALTHOUGH RARE, HAVE OCCURRED DUE TO SEVERE REACTIONS, INCLUDING STEVENS-JOHNSON SYNDROME, TOXIC EPIDERMAL NECROLYSIS, FULMINANT HEPATIC NECROSIS, AGRANULOCYTOSIS, APLASTIC ANEMIA AND OTHER BLOOD DYSCRASIAS (SEE WARNINGS SECTION).**

Hematologic: Agranulocytosis, aplastic anemia, thrombocytopenia, leukopenia, neutropenia, hemolytic anemia, megaloblastic anemia, hypoprothrombinemia, methemoglobinemia, eosinophilia.

Allergic Reactions: Stevens-Johnson syndrome, toxic epidermal necrolysis, anaphylaxis, allergic myocarditis, erythema multiforme, exfoliative dermatitis, angioedema, drug fever, chills, Henoch-Schoenlein purpura, serum sickness-like syndrome, generalized allergic reactions, generalized skin eruptions, photosensitivity, conjunctival and scleral injection, pruritus, urticaria and rash. In addition, periarteritis nodosa and systemic lupus erythematosus have been reported.

Gastrointestinal: Hepatitis (including cholestatic jaundice and hepatic necrosis), elevation of serum transaminase and bilirubin, pseudomembranous enterocolitis, pancreatitis, stomatitis, glossitis, nausea, emesis, abdominal pain, diarrhea, anorexia.

Genitourinary: Renal failure, interstitial nephritis, BUN and serum creatinine elevation, toxic nephrosis with oliguria and anuria, and crystalluria.

Neurologic: Aseptic meningitis, convulsions, peripheral neuritis, ataxia, vertigo, tinnitus, headache.

Psychiatric: Hallucinations, depression, apathy, nervousness.

REPRESENTATIVE MINIMUM INHIBITORY CONCENTRATION VALUES FOR BACTRIM-SUSCEPTIBLE ORGANISMS
(MIC—µg/ml)

Bacteria	TMP alone	SMX alone	TMP/SMX (1:20) TMP	TMP/SMX (1:20) SMX
Escherichia coli	0.05–1.5	1.0–245	0.05–0.5	0.95–9.5
Proteus species				
(indole positive)	0.5–5.0	7.35–300	0.05–1.5	0.95–28.5
Morganella morganii	0.5–5.0	7.35–300	0.05–1.5	0.95–28.5
Proteus mirabilis	0.5–1.5	7.35–30	0.05–0.15	0.95–2.85
Klebsiella species	0.15–5.0	2.45–245	0.05–1.5	0.95–28.5
Enterobacter species	0.15–5.0	2.45–245	0.05–1.5	0.95–28.5
Haemophilus influenzae	0.15–1.5	2.85–95	0.015–0.15	0.285–2.85
Streptococcus pneumoniae	0.15–1.5	7.35–24.5	0.05–0.15	0.95–2.85
*Shigella flexneri**	<0.01–0.04	<0.16–>320	<0.002–0.03	0.04–0.625
*Shigella sonnei**	0.02–0.08	0.625–>320	0.004–0.06	0.08–1.25

TMP = trimethoprim   SMX = sulfamethoxazole

*Rudoy RC, Nelson JD, Haltalin KC: *Antimicrob Agents Chemother 5:* 439–443, May 1974.

Endocrine: The sulfonamides bear certain chemical similarities to some goitrogens, diuretics (acetazolamide and the thiazides) and oral hypoglycemic agents. Cross-sensitivity may exist with these agents. Diuresis and hypoglycemia have occurred rarely in patients receiving sulfonamides.
Musculoskeletal: Arthralgia and myalgia.
Respiratory: Pulmonary infiltrates.
Miscellaneous: Weakness, fatigue, insomnia.

OVERDOSAGE

Acute: The amount of a single dose of Bactrim that is either associated with symptoms of overdosage or is likely to be life-threatening has not been reported. Signs and symptoms of overdosage reported with sulfonamides include anorexia, colic, nausea, vomiting, dizziness, headache, drowsiness and unconsciousness. Pyrexia, hematuria and crystalluria may be noted. Blood dyscrasias and jaundice are potential late manifestations of overdosage.
Signs of acute overdosage with trimethoprim include nausea, vomiting, dizziness, headache, mental depression, confusion and bone marrow depression.
General principals of treatment include the institution of gastric lavage or emesis, forcing oral fluids, and the administration of intravenous fluids if urine output is low and renal function is normal. Acidification of the urine will increase renal elimination of trimethoprim. The patient should be monitored with blood counts and appropriate blood chemistries, including electrolytes. If a significant blood dyscrasia or jaundice occurs, specific therapy should be instituted for these complications. Peritoneal dialysis is not effective and hemodialysis is only moderately effective in eliminating trimethoprim and sulfamethoxazole.
Chronic: Use of Bactrim at high doses and/or for extended periods of time may cause bone marrow depression manifested as thrombocytopenia, leukopenia and/or megaloblastic anemia. If signs of bone marrow depression occur, the patient should be given leucovorin 5 to 15 mg daily until normal hematopoiesis is restored.

DOSAGE AND ADMINISTRATION

Not recommended for use in infants less than two months of age.
URINARY TRACT INFECTIONS AND SHIGELLOSIS IN ADULTS AND CHILDREN, AND ACUTE OTITIS MEDIA IN CHILDREN:
Adults: The usual adult dosage in the treatment of urinary tract infections is one Bactrium DS (double strength) tablet, two Bactrim tablets or four teaspoonfuls (20 ml) of Bactrim Pediatric Suspension or Bactrim Suspension every 12 hours for 10 to 14 days. An identical daily dosage is used for 5 days in the treatment of shigellosis.
Children: The recommended dose for children with urinary tract infections or acute otitis media is 8 mg/kg trimethoprim and 40 mg/kg sulfamethoxazole per 24 hours, given in two divided doses every 12 hours for 10 days. An identical daily dosage is used for 5 days in the treatment of shigellosis. The following table is a guideline for the attainment of this dosage:
Children two months of age or older:

Weight		Dose—every 12 hours	
lb	kg	Teaspoonfuls	Tablets
22	10	1 teasp. (5 ml)	—
44	20	2 teasp. (10 ml)	1 tablet
66	30	3 teasp. (15 ml)	1½ tablets
88	40	4 teasp. (20 ml)	2 tablets or 1 DS tablet

For Patients with Impaired Renal Function: When renal function is impaired, a reduced dosage should be employed using the following table:

Creatinine Clearance (ml/min)	Recommended Dosage Regimen
Above 30	Usual standard regimen
15–30	½ the usual regimen
Below 15	Use not recommended

ACUTE EXACERBATIONS OF CHRONIC BRONCHITIS IN ADULTS:
The usual adult dosage in the treatment of acute exacerbations of chronic bronchitis is one Bactrim DS (double strength) tablet, two Bactrim tablets or four teaspoonfuls (20 ml) of Bactrim Pediatric Suspension or Bactrim Suspension every 12 hours for 14 days.
PNEUMOCYSTIS CARINII PNEUMONIA:
The recommended dosage for patients with documented *Pneumocystis carinii* pneumonia is 20 mg/kg trimethoprim and 100 mg/kg sulfamethoxazole per 24 hours given in equally divided doses every 6 hours for 14 days. The following table is a guideline for the attainment of this dosage in children:

Weight		Dose—every six hours	
lb	kg	Teaspoonfuls	Tablets
18	8	1 teasp. (5 ml)	—
35	16	2 teasp. (10 ml)	1 tablet
53	24	3 teasp. (15 ml)	1½ tablets
70	32	4 teasp. (20 ml)	2 tablets or 1 DS tablet

HOW SUPPLIED

DS (double strength) Tablets (white, notched, capsule shaped), containing 160 mg trimethoprim and 800 mg sulfamethoxazole—bottles of 100 (NDC 0004-0117-01), 250 (NDC 0004-0117-04) and 500 (NDC 0004-0117-14); Tel-E-Dose® packages of 100 (NDC 0004-0117-49); Prescription Paks of 20 (NDC 0004-0117-54). Imprint on tablets: (front) BACTRIM-DS; (back) ROCHE.
Tablets (light green, scored, capsule shaped), containing 80 mg trimethoprim and 400 mg sulfamethoxazole—bottles of 100 (NDC 0004-0050-01) and 500 (NDC 0004-0050-14); Tel-E-Dose® packages of 100 (NDC 0004-0050-49); Prescription Paks of 40 (NDC 0004-0050-34). Imprint on tablets: (front) BACTRIM; (back) ROCHE.
Pediatric Suspension (pink, cherry flavored), containing 40 mg trimethoprim and 200 mg sulfamethoxazole per teaspoonful (5 ml)—bottles of 100 ml (NDC 0004-1033-01) and 16 oz (1 pint) (NDC 0004-1033-28).
Suspension (pink, fruit-licorice flavored), containing 40 mg trimethoprim and 200 mg sulfamethoxazole per teaspoonful (5 ml)—bottles of 16 oz (1 pint) (NDC 0004-1015-28).
TABLETS SHOULD BE STORED AT 15°–30°C (59°–86°F) IN A DRY PLACE AND PROTECTED FROM LIGHT.
SUSPENSIONS SHOULD BE STORED AT 15°–30°C (59°–86°F) AND PROTECTED FROM LIGHT.

REFERENCES

1. Kremers P, Duvivier J, Heusghem C: Pharmacokinetic Studies of Co-Trimoxazole in Man after Single and Repeated Doses. *J Clin Pharmacol 14:* 112–117, Feb-Mar 1974. 2. Kaplan SA, *et al:* Pharmacokinetic Profile of Trimethoprim-Sulfamethoxazole in Man. *J Infect Dis 128* (Suppl): S547–S555, Nov 1973. 3. *Federal Register 37:* 20527–20529, 1972. 4. Bauer AW, Kirby WMM, Sherris JC, Turck M: Antibiotic Susceptibility Testing by a Standardized Single Disk Method. *Am J Clin Path 45:* 493–496, Apr 1966. 5. Brumfitt W, Pursell R: Trimethoprim/Sulfamethoxazole in the Treatment of Bacteriuria in Women. *J Infect Dis 128* (Suppl): S657–S663, Nov 1973.
P.I. 0288

Shown in Product Identification Section, page 424

BEROCCA®   ℞
[ber-o'ka]
PARENTERAL NUTRITION
Injectable
Vitamins for Addition to Intravenous Fluids

The following text is complete prescribing information based on official labeling in effect June 1, 1989.

DESCRIPTION

Berocca Parenteral Nutrition is a sterile injectable solution of nine water-soluble and three fat-soluble vitamins for addition to intravenous fluids. Each duplex package contains Solution 1 and Solution 2 in either ampuls or vials. When the contents of both containers are combined, 2 ml of the resulting parenteral multivitamin solution will provide eight B-complex vitamins and vitamins C, A, D and E at levels recommended by the American Medical Association.*
* *Multivitamin Preparations for Parenteral Use: A Statement by the Nutrition Advisory Group.* American Medical Association Department of Foods and Nutrition, 1975. *JPEN 3:*258–269, Jul-Aug 1979.
Each ml of Berocca Parenteral Nutrition Solution 1 provides:

Thiamine hydrochloride (B₁)	3	mg
d-Biotin	60	mcg
Riboflavin (as riboflavin 5'-phosphate sodium) (B₂)	3.6	mg
Niacinamide	40	mg
Pyridoxine hydrochloride (B₆)	4	mg
Dexpanthenol	15	mg
Ascorbic Acid (C)	100	mg

compounded with propylene glycol 40%, gentisic acid ethanolamide 2%, disodium edetate 0.01% and benzyl alcohol 1% as stabilizers and preservatives; and sodium hydroxide to adjust pH to approximately 5.

Each ml of Berocca Parenteral Nutrition Solution 2 provides:

Vitamin A palmitate	3300	USP units
Vitamin E (dl-alpha tocopherol)	10	USP units
Vitamin D₂ (ergocalciferol)	200	USP units
Folic acid	400	mcg
Cyanocobalamin (B₁₂)	5	mcg

compounded with polyoxyethylated vegetable oil 10% as solubilizer for vitamins A, D, E; propylene glycol 10%, ethyl alcohol 10%, gentisic acid ethanolamine 2%, sodium citrate 1.7%, benzyl alcohol 1%, and disodium edetate 0.01% as stabilizers and preservatives; and sodium hydroxide and citric acid to adjust pH to approximately 6.5.

CLINICAL PHARMACOLOGY

Vitamins are essential for maintenance of normal metabolic functions including hematopoiesis: The water-soluble vitamins play vital roles in the conversion of carbohydrate, protein and fat into tissue and energy. *Thiamine (B₁)* acts as a coenzyme in carbohydrate metabolism. *Riboflavin (B₂)* functions as a coenzyme in the electron transport system associated with conversion of tissue oxidations into usable energy. *Niacin* serves as a coenzyme in oxidation-reduction reactions in tissue respiration. *Pyridoxine hydrochloride (B₆)* is essential for the metabolism of amino acids. *Pantothenic acid* functions as a coenzyme in various metabolic acetylation reactions and *biotin* in specific carboxylation reactions in lipid metabolism. *Folic acid* and *cyanocobalamin (B₁₂)* are metabolically interrelated. They are essential to nucleic acid synthesis and normal maturation of red blood cells. *Ascorbic acid (C)* performs a vital function in the process of cellular respiration, and is involved in both carbohydrate and amino acid metabolism. It is essential for collagen formation and tissue repair.
Vitamin A is necessary for proper functioning of the retina; it appears to be essential to the integrity of epithelial cells. *Vitamin D* is necessary for the absorption of calcium and for the maintenance of bone structure. *Vitamin E* is an antioxidant which preserves essential cellular constituents, including those of the red blood cell. It also serves as protection against lipid peroxidation.
Berocca Parenteral Nutrition provides, in a 2 ml dose, the daily requirements of twelve essential vitamins for nutritional rehabilitation and maintenance of optimal nutritional status in conditions for which parenteral vitamin nutrition is indicated.

INDICATIONS

Berocca Parenteral Nutrition is indicated as daily multivitamin maintenance dosage for adults and children age 11 and above receiving parenteral nutrition. It is also indicated in other situations where administration by the intravenous route is required. Such situations include surgery, excessive burns, fractures and other trauma, severe infectious diseases and comatose states, which may provoke a "stress" situation with profound alterations in the body's metabolic demands and consequent tissue depletion of nutrients.
The physician should not await the development of clinical signs of vitamin deficiency before initiating vitamin therapy. The use of a multivitamin product obviates the need to speculate on the status of individual vitamin nutriture.
Berocca Parenteral Nutrition (administered in intravenous fluids under proper dilution) contributes vitamins, except vitamin K, necessary for maintaining the body's normal resistance and repair processes.
Patients with multiple vitamin deficiencies or with markedly increased requirements may be given multiples of the daily dosage for two or more days as indicated by the clinical status. Berocca Parenteral Nutrition does not contain vitamin K, which may have to be administered separately. Clinical testing indicates that some patients do not maintain adequate levels of certain vitamins when Berocca Parenteral Nutrition in recommended amounts is the sole source of vitamins. No vitamin deficiencies were clinically evident, but blood levels of vitamins A, C, D, E and folic acid declined in a number of subjects who received Berocca Parenteral Nutrition as the only vitamin source for 4 to 6 months. Therefore, in patients for whom total parenteral nutrition will be continued for long periods of time, these vitamins should be monitored. If deficiencies appear to be developing, multiples of the formulation (1.5 to 3 times) may be needed for a period of time. When multiples of the formulation are used for more than a few weeks, vitamins A, D and E should be monitored occasionally to be certain that an excess accumulation of these vitamins is not occurring.

CONTRAINDICATIONS

Berocca Parenteral Nutrition is contraindicated in patients known to be hypersensitive to any of its components and in those with a preexisting hypervitaminosis.

WARNINGS

The solubilizer used in Berocca Parenteral Nutrition has been associated with anaphylaxis or anaphylactoid reactions.
Allergic reactions, including anaphylaxis, may occur in patients hypersensitive to thiamine or other components of the product.

Continued on next page

Roche Labs.—Cont.

Patients who have early Leber's disease (hereditary optic nerve atrophy) have been found to suffer severe, acute optic atrophy when treated with vitamin B_{12}. Pyridoxine can decrease the efficacy of levodopa in the treatment of patients with parkinsonism. Folic acid may alter patient response to methotrexate therapy. These facts should be considered before prescribing Berocca Parenteral Nutrition for such patients.

Folic acid in doses above 0.1 mg daily may obscure pernicious anemia. Berocca Parenteral Nutrition is not intended for treatment of pernicious anemia or other megaloblastic anemias where vitamin B_{12} is deficient. Neurologic involvement may develop or progress, despite temporary remission of anemia, in patients with vitamin B_{12} deficiency who receive supplemental folic acid and who are inadequately treated with B_{12}. This product should not be used as primary treatment for specific vitamin deficiencies such as beriberi, pellagra, scurvy, and riboflavin or pyridoxine deficiency.

PRECAUTIONS

Because fat-soluble vitamins can accumulate in the body, toxicity from vitamins A and D is possible, especially if patients are inadvertently administered oral vitamin supplementation in addition to the parenteral regimen.

Berocca Parenteral Nutrition does not contain vitamin K. Supplements of vitamin K may be necessary to meet patients' individual requirements. Patients routinely receiving fat emulsion as part of the total parenteral regimen may have increased requirements for vitamin E.

Most antibiotics, methotrexate and pyrimethamine invalidate diagnostic microbiological blood assays for folic acid and cyanocobalamin.

Safety and effectiveness in children under the age of 11 have not been established.

ADVERSE REACTIONS

Allergic sensitization has been reported following parenteral administration of folic acid and thiamine. Hepatomegaly, leukopenia and projectile vomiting have been reported in the literature as vitamin A toxicity symptoms; elevated serum calcium and multiple areas of tissue calcification have been reported with hypervitaminosis D.

DOSAGE AND ADMINISTRATION

For addition to intravenous fluids. I.V. administration should always be done slowly. Initial administration should only be done when facilities are available to cope with anaphylactic events, if they should occur.

In a recent dog study, histamine-like reactions were induced with infusions given over a two-hour period, at dosages approximately five times the therapeutic human dose.

The recommended daily dose is 2 ml of Berocca Parenteral Nutrition (1 ml of Solution 1 and 1 ml of Solution 2) added to intravenous infusion fluids. **Berocca Parenteral Nutrition should be infused over a period of at least two hours.**

IMPORTANT: DIRECTIONS FOR RECONSTITUTION, ADDITION TO INTRAVENOUS INFUSION SOLUTIONS AND STORAGE:

Ampuls: To prepare solution for single dose administration, mix 1 ml of Berocca Parenteral Nutrition Solution 1 with 1 ml of Berocca Parenteral Nutrition Solution 2. The reconstituted product is ready for addition to intravenous infusion fluids. Or, add the contents of each ampul directly to the intravenous infusion fluid. *Multiple dose vials:* To prepare solution for 10 doses, add 10 ml of Berocca Parenteral Nutrition Solution 2 to 10 ml of Berocca Parenteral Nutrition Solution 1 (20 ml vial, 10 ml fill). To administer single doses, add 2 ml of the reconstituted product to intravenous infusion fluids. Or, add 1 ml of Solution 1 and 1 ml of Solution 2 directly to the intravenous infusion fluid.

BEROCCA PARENTERAL NUTRITION CAN BE USED WITH COMPATIBLE INTRAVENOUS INFUSION SOLUTIONS: 0.9% sterile saline, 5% or 10% sterile glucose or dextrose, lactated Ringer's solution. Two ml of Berocca Parenteral Nutrition (1 ml of Solution 1 and 1 ml of Solution 2) should be added to at least 250 ml of the intravenous infusion solution. Either glass or plastic containers can be used.

Berocca Parenteral Nutrition, like other parenteral vitamins, should not be added to I.V. fluids containing sodium bisulfite as this causes rapid degradation of vitamin B_1 (thiamine). If Berocca Parenteral Nutrition is added to I.V. fluids which do contain the preservative sodium bisulfite, a separate supplemental injection of thiamine should be administered.

Store unreconstituted product in refrigerator (2°– 8°C, 36°–46°F). PROTECT FROM LIGHT. DO NOT STORE AT ROOM TEMPERATURE.

Store reconstituted (mixed) product for no longer than 14 days in refrigerator (2°–8°C, 36°–46°F). PROTECT FROM LIGHT.

Store intravenous fluids with added Berocca Parenteral Nutrition in refrigerator (2°–8°C, 36°–46°F) for no longer than 24 hours. PROTECT FROM LIGHT.

Note: Berocca Parenteral Nutrition contains a soluble form of riboflavin which permits use of a large dose and minimizes pain on injection. This form of riboflavin may result in darkening of the solution and the color change is intensified on prolonged storage. However, the darkening of the solution in no way affects the safety and therapeutic efficacy of the preparation.

Parenteral drug products should be inspected visually for particulate matter prior to administration, whenever solution and container permit.

HOW SUPPLIED

Vials: Duplex packages, each containing a 20-ml vial (10-ml fill) of Solution 1 and a 10-ml vial (10-ml fill) of Solution 2; boxes of 1.

P.I. 0589

BEROCCA® TABLETS   ℞

[*ber-o'ka*]

The following text is complete prescribing information based on official labeling in effect June 1, 1989.

[See table below].

Each tablet also contains acacia, calcium sulfate, carnauba wax, hydrogenated vegetable oil, magnesium oxide, magnesium stearate, povidone, shellac, sodium benzoate, sugar and talc with the following dyes: FD&C Blue No. 1, FD&C Yellow No. 6, D&C Yellow No. 10 and titanium dioxide.

DESCRIPTION

Berocca is a prescription-only oral multivitamin tablet specially formulated for prophylactic or therapeutic nutritional supplementation in conditions requiring water-soluble vitamins.

Berocca tablets supply *therapeutic* levels of ascorbic acid, vitamins B_1, B_2, B_6, niacin and pantothenic acid and a *supplemental* level of vitamin B_{12}. Berocca tablets also supply a supplemental level of folic acid for pregnant or lactating women and a therapeutic level for adults and children four or more years of age.

CLINICAL PHARMACOLOGY

Vitamins are essential for normal metabolic functions including hematopoiesis. The B-complex vitamins are necessary for the conversion of carbohydrate, protein and fat into tissue and energy.

Ascorbic acid (C) is involved in collagen formation and tissue repair.

The water-soluble vitamins (B-complex and C) are not significantly stored by the body; excess quantities are excreted in the urine. They must be replenished regularly through diet or other means to maintain essential tissue levels. Thus, these vitamins are rapidly depleted in conditions interfering with their intake or absorption.

INDICATIONS AND USAGE

Berocca is indicated for supportive nutritional supplementation in conditions in which water-soluble vitamins are required prophylactically or therapeutically. These include:

Conditions causing depletion, or reduced absorption or bioavailability of water-soluble vitamins—

Gastrointestinal disorders, chronic alcoholism, febrile illnesses, prolonged or wasting diseases, hyperthyroidism or poorly controlled diabetes.

Conditions resulting in increased needs for water-soluble vitamins—

Pregnancy, severe burns, recovery from surgery.

CONTRAINDICATIONS

Berocca is contraindicated in patients known to be hypersensitive to any of its components.

WARNINGS

Berocca is not intended for treatment of pernicious anemia or other megaloblastic anemias where vitamin B_{12} is deficient. Neurologic involvement may develop or progress, despite temporary remission of anemia, in patients with vitamin B_{12} deficiency who receive supplemental folic acid and who are inadequately treated with B_{12}.

PRECAUTIONS

General: Certain conditions listed above may require additional nutritional supplementation. During pregnancy, for instance, supplementation with fat-soluble vitamins and minerals may be required according to the dietary habits of the individual. Berocca is not intended for treatment of severe specific deficiencies.

Information for the Patient: Because toxic reactions have been reported with injudicious use of certain vitamins, urge patients to follow your specific instructions regarding dosage regimen. As with any medication, advise patients to keep Berocca out of reach of children.

Drug and Treatment Interactions: As little as 5 mg pyridoxine daily can decrease the efficacy of levodopa in the treatment of parkinsonism. Therefore, Berocca is not recommended for patients undergoing such therapy.

ADVERSE REACTIONS

Adverse reactions have been reported with specific vitamins, but generally at levels substantially higher than those in Berocca. However, allergic and idiosyncratic reactions are possible at lower levels.

DOSAGE AND ADMINISTRATION

Usual adult dosage: one tablet daily.

Berocca is available on prescription only.

HOW SUPPLIED

Light green, capsule-shaped tablets—bottles of 100 (NDC 0004-0020-01) and 500 (NDC 0004-0020-14).

Imprint on tablets: BEROCCA®
                     ROCHE

P.I. 1185

Shown in Product Identification Section, page 424

BEROCCA® PLUS TABLETS   ℞

[*ber-o'ka*]

The following text is complete prescribing information based on official labeling in effect June 1, 1988.

[See table on next page].

DESCRIPTION

Berocca Plus is a prescription-only oral multivitamin/mineral tablet specially formulated for prophylactic or therapeutic nutritional supplementation in physiologically stressful conditions.

Berocca Plus supplies: *therapeutic* levels of water-soluble vitamins (ascorbic acid and all B-complex vitamins except biotin); *supplemental* levels of biotin, fat-soluble vitamins (A and E) and minerals (iron, chromium, manganese, copper and zinc); plus magnesium.

CLINICAL PHARMACOLOGY

Vitamins and minerals are essential for normal metabolic functions including hematopoiesis. The B-complex vitamins are necessary for the conversion of carbohydrate, protein and fat into tissue and energy. Ascorbic acid is involved in tissue repair and collagen formation. Vitamin A is necessary for proper functioning of the retina; it appears to be essential to the integrity of epithelial cells. Vitamin E is an antioxidant which preserves essential cellular constituents. Magnesium is a structural component of body tissues; iron, chromium, manganese, copper and zinc serve as catalysts in enzyme systems which perform vital cellular functions.

Water-soluble vitamins (B-complex and C) are not significantly stored by the body and must be replaced continually to maintain essential tissue levels; excess quantities are excreted in urine. These vitamins are rapidly depleted in conditions interfering with their intake or absorption. Berocca Plus supplies therapeutic levels of vitamin C and all B-complex vitamins (except biotin).

Fat-soluble vitamins and several trace minerals, however, can accumulate in the body and do not need replacement as frequently. Therefore, Berocca Plus supplies more conservative levels of vitamins A and E and various essential minerals.

Specifically, Berocca Plus contains an adequate level of vitamin B_6 (25 mg) to normalize the tryptophan metabolism disturbance which has been associated with the use of estrogenic oral contraceptives or other estrogen therapy. It provides zinc (22.5 mg) which facilitates wound healing, the

Each **Berocca®** tablet contains:	Quantity	U.S. RDA— Adults and children 4 or more years of age	U.S. RDA— Pregnant or lactating women
Vitamin C (ascorbic acid)	500 mg	60 mg	60 mg
Vitamin B_1 (as thiamine mononitrate)	15 mg	1.5 mg	1.7 mg
Vitamin B_2 (riboflavin)	15 mg	1.7 mg	2 mg
Niacin (as niacinamide)	100 mg	20 mg	20 mg
Vitamin B_6 (as pyridoxine HCl)	4 mg	2 mg	2.5 mg
Pantothenic acid (as calcium *d*-pantothenate)	18 mg	10 mg	10 mg
Folic acid	0.5 mg	0.4 mg	0.8 mg
Vitamin B_{12} (cyanocobalamin)	5 mcg	6 mcg	8 mcg

Each Berocca® Plus tablet contains:	Quantity	U.S. RDA— Adults and children 4 or more years of age	U.S. RDA— Pregnant or lactating women
Fat-Soluble Vitamins			
Vitamin A (as vitamin A acetate)	5000 IU	5000 IU	8000 IU
Vitamin E	30 IU	30 IU	30 IU
(as *dl*-alpha tocopheryl acetate)			
Water-Soluble Vitamins			
Vitamin C (ascorbic acid)	500 mg	60 mg	60 mg
Vitamin B$_1$ (as thiamine mononitrate)	20 mg	1.5 mg	1.7 mg
Vitamin B$_2$ (riboflavin)	20 mg	1.7 mg	2 mg
Niacin (as niacinamide)	100 mg	20 mg	20 mg
Vitamin B$_6$ (as pyridoxine HCl)	25 mg	2 mg	2.5 mg
Biotin	0.15 mg	0.30 mg	0.30 mg
Pantothenic acid	25 mg	10 mg	10 mg
(as calcium pantothenate)			
Folic acid	0.8 mg	0.4 mg	0.8 mg
Vitamin B$_{12}$ (cyanocobalamin)	50 mcg	6 mcg	8 mcg
Minerals			
Iron (as ferrous fumarate)	27 mg	18 mg	18 mg
Chromium (as chromium nitrate)	0.1 mg	0.05–0.2 mg *	
Magnesium (as magnesium oxide)	50 mg	400 mg	450 mg
Manganese (as manganese dioxide)	5 mg	2.5–5 mg *	
Copper (as cupric oxide)	3 mg	2 mg	2 mg
Zinc (as zinc oxide)	22.5 mg	15 mg	15 mg

Each tablet also contains carnauba wax, ethylcellulose, ethyl vanillin, hydroxypropyl methylcellulose, magnesium stearate, povidone, silicon dioxide, stearic acid, triacetin and flavor with the following dyes: yellow iron oxide and titanium dioxide.
*Not established. Estimated by NAS/NRC as safe and adequate daily dietary intake for adults.

level of folic acid (0.8 mg) recommended during pregnancy, and ascorbic acid (500 mg) which has been demonstrated to improve the absorption of inorganic iron.

INDICATIONS

Berocca Plus is indicated for prophylactic or therapeutic nutritional supplementation in physiologically stressful conditions. These include:

Conditions causing depletion, or reduced absorption or bioavailability of essential vitamins and minerals—
Inadequate intake due to highly restricted or unbalanced diets such as those frequently associated with anorexic conditions and other states of severe malnutrition.
Gastrointestinal disorders, chronic alcoholism, chronic or acute infections (especially those involving febrile illness), prolonged or wasting disease, congestive heart failure, hyperthyroidism, poorly controlled diabetes or other physiologic stress.
Also, patients on estrogenic oral contraceptives or other estrogen therapy, antibacterials which affect intestinal microflora, or other interfering drugs.
Certain conditions resulting from severe B-vitamin or ascorbic acid deficiency—
Cheilosis, gingivitis, stomatitis and certain other classic water-soluble vitamin deficiency syndromes.
Conditions resulting in increased needs for essential vitamins and minerals—
Recovery from surgery or trauma involving severe burns, fractures or other extensive tissue damage.
Also, pregnant women and those with heavy menstrual bleeding.

CONTRAINDICATIONS

Berocca Plus is contraindicated in patients hypersensitive to any of its components.

WARNINGS

Not intended for treatment of pernicious anemia or other megaloblastic anemias where vitamin B$_{12}$ is deficient. Neurologic involvement may develop or progress, despite temporary remission of anemia, in patients with vitamin B$_{12}$ deficiency who receive supplemental folic acid and who are inadequately treated with B$_{12}$.

PRECAUTIONS

General: Certain conditions listed above may require additional nutritional supplementation. During pregnancy, for instance, supplementation with vitamin D and calcium may be required according to the dietary habits of the individual. Berocca Plus is not intended for treatment of severe specific deficiencies.
Information for the Patient: Because toxic reactions have been reported with injudicious use of certain vitamins and minerals, urge patients to follow your specific instructions regarding dosage regimen. Advise patients to keep Berocca Plus out of reach of children.
Drug and Treatment Interactions: As litte as 5 mg pyridoxine daily can decrease the efficacy of levodopa in the treatment of parkinsonism. Therefore, Berocca Plus is not recommended for patients undergoing such therapy.

ADVERSE REACTIONS

Adverse reactions have been reported with specific vitamins and minerals, but generally at levels substantially higher than those in Berocca Plus. However, allergic and idiosyncratic reactions are possible at lower levels. Iron, even at the usual recommended levels, has been associated with gastrointestinal intolerance in some patients.

DOSAGE AND ADMINISTRATION

Usual adult dosage: one tablet daily. Not recommended for children. *Berocca Plus is available on prescription only.*

HOW SUPPLIED

Golden yellow, capsule-shaped tablets—bottles of 100.
Imprint on tablets: (front) BEROCCA PLUS; (back) ROCHE. P.I. 1185
Shown in Product Identification Section, page 424

BUMEX® ℞

[*bu'mex*]
(bumetanide/Roche)
TABLETS
INJECTION

The following text is complete prescribing information based on official labeling in effect June 1, 1989.

WARNING

Bumex (bumetanide/Roche) is a potent diuretic which, if given in excessive amounts, can lead to a profound diuresis with water and electrolyte depletion. Therefore, careful medical supervision is required, and dose and dosage schedule have to be adjusted to the individual patient's needs. (See DOSAGE AND ADMINISTRATION.)

DESCRIPTION

Bumex® (bumetanide/Roche) is a loop diuretic, available as scored tablets, 0.5 mg (light green), 1 mg (yellow) and 2 mg (peach) for oral administration; each tablet also contains lactose, magnesium stearate, microcrystalline cellulose, corn starch and talc, with the following dye systems: 0.5 mg—D&C Yellow No. 10 and FD&C Blue No. 1; 1 mg—D&C Yellow No. 10; 2 mg—red iron oxide. Also as 2-ml ampuls, 2-ml vials, 4-ml vials and 10-ml vials (0.25 mg/ml) for intravenous or intramuscular injection as a sterile solution, each 2 ml of which contains 0.5 mg (0.25 mg/ml) bumetanide compounded with 0.85% sodium chloride and 0.4% ammonium acetate as buffers; 0.01% disodium edetate; 1% benzyl alcohol as preservative, and pH adjusted to approximately 7 with sodium hydroxide.
Chemically, bumetanide is 3-(butylamino)-4-phenoxy-5-sulfamoylbenzoic acid. It is a practically white powder having a calculated molecular weight of 364.41.

CLINICAL PHARMACOLOGY

Bumex is a loop diuretic with a rapid onset and short duration of action. Pharmacological and clinical studies have shown that 1 mg Bumex has a diuretic potency equivalent to approximately 40 mg furosemide. The major site of Bumex action is the ascending limb of the loop of Henle.
The mode of action has been determined through various clearance studies in both humans and experimental animals. Bumex inhibits sodium reabsorption in the ascending limb of the loop of Henle, as shown by marked reduction of free-water clearance (^CH_2O) during hydration and tubular free-water reabsorption (T^CH_2O) during hydropenia. Reabsorption of chloride in the ascending limb is also blocked by Bumex, and Bumex is somewhat more chloruretic than natriuretic.
Potassium excretion is also increased by Bumex, in a dose-related fashion.
Bumex may have an additional action in the proximal tubule. Since phosphate reabsorption takes place largely in the proximal tubule, phosphaturia during Bumex-induced diuresis is indicative of this additional action. This is further supported by the reduction in the renal clearance of Bumex by probenecid, associated with diminution in the natriuretic response. This proximal tubular activity does not seem to be related to an inhibition of carbonic anhydrase. Bumex does not appear to have a noticeable action on the distal tubule. Bumex decreases uric acid excretion and increases serum uric acid. Following oral administration of Bumex the onset of diuresis occurs in 30 to 60 minutes. Peak activity is reached between 1 and 2 hours. At usual doses (1 to 2 mg) diuresis is largely complete within 4 hours; with higher doses, the diuretic action lasts for 4 to 6 hours. Diuresis starts within minutes following an intravenous injection and reaches maximum levels within 15 to 30 minutes.
Several pharmacokinetic studies have shown that Bumex, administered orally or parenterally, is eliminated rapidly in humans, with a half-life of between 1 and 1½ hours. Plasma protein-binding is in the range of 94% to 96%.
Oral administration of carbon-14 labeled Bumex to human volunteers revealed that 81% of the administered radioactivity was excreted in the urine, 45% of it as unchanged drug. Urinary and biliary metabolites identified in this study were formed by oxidation of the N-butyl side chain. Biliary excretion of Bumex amounted to only 2% of the administered dose.

INDICATIONS AND USAGE

Bumex is indicated for the treatment of edema associated with congestive heart failure, hepatic and renal disease, including the nephrotic syndrome.
Almost equal diuretic response occurs after oral and parenteral administration of Bumex. Therefore, if impaired gastrointestinal absorption is suspected or oral administration is not practical, Bumex should be given by the intramuscular or intravenous route.
Successful treatment with Bumex following instances of allergic reactions to furosemide suggests a lack of cross-sensitivity.

CONTRAINDICATIONS

Bumex is contraindicated in anuria. Although Bumex can be used to induce diuresis in renal insufficiency, any marked increase in blood urea nitrogen or creatinine, or the development of oliguria during therapy of patients with progressive renal disease, is an indication for discontinuation of treatment with Bumex. Bumex is also contraindicated in patients in hepatic coma or in states of severe electrolyte depletion until the condition is improved or corrected. Bumex is contraindicated in patients hypersensitive to this drug.

WARNINGS

1. Volume and electrolyte depletion. The dose of Bumex should be adjusted to the patient's need. Excessive doses or too frequent administration can lead to profound water loss, electrolyte depletion, dehydration, reduction in blood volume and circulatory collapse with the possibility of vascular thrombosis and embolism, particularly in elderly patients.
2. Hypokalemia. Hypokalemia can occur as a consequence of Bumex administration. Prevention of hypokalemia requires particular attention in the following conditions: patients receiving digitalis and diuretics for congestive heart failure, hepatic cirrhosis and ascites, states of aldosterone excess with normal renal function, potassium-losing nephropathy, certain diarrheal states, or other states where hypokalemia is thought to represent particular added risks to the patient, *i.e.*, history of ventricular arrhythmias.
In patients with hepatic cirrhosis and ascites, sudden alterations of electrolyte balance may precipitate hepatic encephalopathy and coma. Treatment in such patients is best initiated in the hospital with small doses and careful monitoring of the patient's clinical status and electrolyte balance. Supplemental potassium and/or spironolactone may prevent hypokalemia and metabolic alkalosis in these patients.
3. Ototoxicity. In cats, dogs and guinea pigs, Bumex has been shown to produce ototoxicity. In these test animals Bumex was 5 to 6 times more potent than furosemide and, since the diuretic potency of Bumex is about 40 to 60 times furosemide, it is anticipated that blood levels necessary to produce ototoxicity will rarely be achieved. The potential exists, however, and must be considered a risk of intravenous therapy, especially at high doses, repeated frequently in the face of renal excretory function impairment. Potentiation of aminoglycoside ototoxicity has not been tested for Bumex. Like other members of this class of diuretics, Bumex probably shares this risk.
4. Allergy to sulfonamides. Patients allergic to sulfonamides may show hypersensitivity to Bumex.

Continued on next page

Roche Labs.—Cont.

PRECAUTIONS

General: Serum potassium should be measured periodically and potassium supplements or potassium-sparing diuretics added if necessary. Periodic determinations of other electrolytes are advised in patients treated with high doses or for prolonged periods, particularly in those on low salt diets. Hyperuricemia may occur; it has been asymptomatic in cases reported to date. Reversible elevations of the BUN and creatinine may also occur, especially in association with dehydration and particularly in patients with renal insufficiency. Bumex may increase urinary calcium excretion with resultant hypocalcemia.

Laboratory Tests: Studies in normal subjects receiving Bumex revealed no adverse effects on glucose tolerance, plasma insulin, glucagon and growth hormone levels, but the possibility of an effect on glucose metabolism exists. Periodic determinations of blood sugar should be done, particularly in patients with diabetes or suspected latent diabetes.

Patients under treatment should be observed regularly for possible occurrence of blood dyscrasias, liver damage or idiosyncratic reactions, which have been reported occasionally in foreign marketing experience. The relationship of these occurrences to Bumex use is not certain.

Drug Interactions:

1. Drugs with ototoxic potential (see WARNINGS): Especially in the presence of impaired renal function, the use of parenterally administered Bumex in patients to whom aminoglycoside antibiotics are also being given should be avoided, except in life-threatening conditions.

2. Drugs with nephrotoxic potential: There has been no experience on the concurrent use of Bumex with drugs known to have a nephrotoxic potential. Therefore, the simultaneous administration of these drugs should be avoided.

3. Lithium: Lithium should generally not be given with diuretics (such as Bumex) because they reduce its renal clearance and add a high risk of lithium toxicity.

4. Probenecid: Pretreatment with probenecid reduces both the natriuresis and hyperreninemia produced by Bumex. This antagonistic effect of probenecid on Bumex natriuresis is not due to a direct action on sodium excretion but is probably secondary to its inhibitory effect on renal tubular secretion of bumetanide. Thus, probenecid should not be administered concurrently with Bumex.

5. Indomethacin: Indomethacin blunts the increases in urine volume and sodium excretion seen during Bumex treatment and inhibits the bumetanide-induced increase in plasma renin activity. Concurrent therapy with Bumex is thus not recommended.

6. Antihypertensives: Bumex may potentiate the effect of various antihypertensive drugs, necessitating a reduction in the dosage of these drugs.

7. Digoxin: Interaction studies in humans have shown no effect on digoxin blood levels.

8. Anticoagulants: Interaction studies in humans have shown Bumex to have no effect on warfarin metabolism or on plasma prothrombin activity.

Carcinogenesis, Mutagenesis, Impairment of Fertility: Bumex was devoid of mutagenic activity in various strains of *Salmonella typhimurium* when tested in the presence or absence of an *in vitro* metabolic activation system. An 18-month study showed an increase in mammary adenomas of questionable significance in female rats receiving oral doses of 60 mg/kg/day (2000 times a 2-mg human dose). A repeat study at the same doses failed to duplicate this finding.

Reproduction studies were performed to evaluate general reproductive performance and fertility in rats at oral dose levels of 10, 30, 60 or 100 mg/kg/day. The pregnancy rate was slightly decreased in the treated animals; however, the differences were small and not statistically significant.

Pregnancy: Teratogenic Effects: Pregnancy Category C. Bumex is neither teratogenic nor embryocidal in mice when given in doses up to 3400 times the maximum human therapeutic dose.

Bumex has been shown to be nonteratogenic, but it has a slight embryocidal effect in rats when given in doses of 3400 times the maximum human therapeutic dose and in rabbits at doses of 3.4 times the maximum human therapeutic dose. In one study, moderate growth retardation and increased incidence of delayed ossification of sternebrae were observed in rats at oral doses of 100 mg/kg/day, 3400 times the maximum human therapeutic dose. These effects were associated with maternal weight reductions noted during dosing. No such adverse effects were observed at 30 mg/kg/day (1000 times the maximum human therapeutic dose). No fetotoxicity was observed at 1000 to 2000 times the human therapeutic dose.

In rabbits, a dose-related decrease in litter size and an increase in resorption rate were noted at oral doses of 0.1 and 0.3 mg/kg/day (3.4 and 10 times the maximum human therapeutic dose). A slightly increased incidence of delayed ossification of sternebrae occurred at 0.3 mg/kg/day; however, no such adverse effects were observed at the dose of 0.03

mg/kg/day. The sensitivity of the rabbit to Bumex parallels the marked pharmacologic and toxicologic effects of the drug in this species.

Bumex was not teratogenic in the hamster at an oral dose of 0.5 mg/kg/day (17 times the maximum human therapeutic dose). Bumex was not teratogenic when given intravenously to mice and rats at doses up to 140 times the maximum human therapeutic dose.

There are no adequate and well-controlled studies in pregnant women. A small investigational experience in the United States and marketing experience in other countries to date have not indicated any evidence of adverse effects on the fetus, but these data do not rule out the possibility of harmful effects. Bumex should be given to a pregnant woman only if the potential benefit justifies the potential risk to the fetus.

Nursing Mothers: It is not known whether this drug is excreted in human milk. As a general rule, nursing should not be undertaken while the patient is on Bumex since it may be excreted in human milk.

Pediatric Use: Safety and effectiveness in children below the age of 18 have not been established.

ADVERSE REACTIONS

The most frequent clinical adverse reactions considered probably or possibly related to Bumex are muscle cramps (seen in 1.1% of treated patients), dizziness (1.1%), hypotension (0.8%), headache (0.6%), nausea (0.6%), and encephalopathy (in patients with preexisting liver disease) (0.6%). One or more of these adverse reactions have been reported in approximately 4.1% of Bumex-treated patients.

Less frequent clinical adverse reactions to Bumex are impaired hearing (0.5%), pruritus (0.4%), electrocardiogram changes (0.4%), weakness (0.2%), hives (0.2%), abdominal pain (0.2%), arthritic pain (0.2%), musculoskeletal pain (0.2%), rash (0.2%) and vomiting (0.2%). One or more of these adverse reactions have been reported in approximately 2.9% of Bumex-treated patients.

Other clinical adverse reactions, which have each occurred in approximately 0.1% of patients, are vertigo, chest pain, ear discomfort, fatigue, dehydration, sweating, hyperventilation, dry mouth, upset stomach, renal failure, asterixis, itching, nipple tenderness, diarrhea, premature ejaculation and difficulty maintaining an erection.

Laboratory abnormalities reported have included hyperuricemia (in 18.4% of patients tested), hypochloremia (14.9%), hypokalemia (14.7%), azotemia (10.6%), hyponatremia (9.2%), increased serum creatinine (7.4%), hyperglycemia (6.6%), and variations in phosphorus (4.5%), CO_2 content (4.3%), bicarbonate (3.1%) and calcium (2.4%). Although manifestations of the pharmacologic action of Bumex, these conditions may become more pronounced by intensive therapy.

Also reported have been thrombocytopenia (0.2%) and deviations in hemoglobin (0.8%), prothrombin time (0.8%), hematocrit (0.6%), WBC (0.3%) and differential counts (0.1%). There have been rare spontaneous reports of thrombocytopenia from postmarketing experience.

Diuresis induced by Bumex may also rarely be accompanied by changes in LDH (1.0%), total serum bilirubin (0.8%), serum proteins (0.7%), SGOT (0.6%), SGPT (0.5%), alkaline phosphatase (0.4%), cholesterol (0.4%) and creatinine clearance (0.3%). Increases in urinary glucose (0.7%) and urinary protein (0.3%) have also been seen.

OVERDOSAGE

Overdosage can lead to acute profound water loss, volume and electrolyte depletion, dehydration, reduction of blood volume and circulatory collapse with a possibility of vascular thrombosis and embolism. Electrolyte depletion may be manifested by weakness, dizziness, mental confusion, anorexia, lethargy, vomiting and cramps. Treatment consists of replacement of fluid and electrolyte losses by careful monitoring of the urine and electrolyte output and serum electrolyte levels.

DOSAGE AND ADMINISTRATION

Dosage should be individualized with careful monitoring of patient response.

Oral Administration: The usual total daily dosage of Bumex is 0.5 to 2.0 mg and in most patients is given as a single dose.

If the diuretic response to an initial dose of Bumex is not adequate, in view of its rapid onset and short duration of action, a second or third dose may be given at 4- to 5-hour intervals up to a maximum daily dose of 10 mg. An intermittent dose schedule, whereby Bumex is given on alternate days or for 3 to 4 days with rest periods of 1 to 2 days in between, is recommended as the safest and most effective method for the continued control of edema. In patients with hepatic failure, the dosage should be kept to a minimum, and if necessary, dosage increased very carefully.

Because cross-sensitivity with furosemide has rarely been observed, Bumex can be substituted at approximately a 1:40 ratio of Bumex to furosemide in patients allergic to furosemide.

Parenteral Administration: Bumex may be administered parenterally (IV or IM) to patients in whom gastrointestinal absorption may be impaired or in whom oral administration is not practical.

Parenteral treatment should be terminated and oral treatment instituted as soon as possible.

The usual initial dose is 0.5 to 1.0 mg intravenously or intramuscularly. Intravenous administration should be given over a period of 1 to 2 minutes. If the response to an initial dose is deemed insufficient, a second or third dose may be given at intervals of 2 to 3 hours, but should not exceed a daily dosage of 10 mg.

Miscibility and Parenteral Solutions: The compatibility tests of Bumex injection (0.25 mg/ml, 2-ml ampuls) with 5% dextrose in water, 0.9% sodium chloride, and lactated Ringer's solution in both glass and plasticized PVC (Viaflex) containers have shown no significant absorption effect with either containers, nor a measurable loss of potency due to degradation of the drug. However, solutions should be freshly prepared and used within 24 hours.

Parenteral drug products should be inspected visually for particulate matter and discoloration prior to administration whenever solution and container permit.

HOW SUPPLIED

Tablets: 0.5 mg (light green), bottles of 100 (NDC 0004-0125-01) and 500 (NDC 0004-0125-14); Tel-E-Dose® packages of 100 (NDC 0004-0125-49). 1 mg (yellow), bottles of 100 (NDC 0004-0121-01) and 500 (NDC 0004-0121-14); Tel-E-Dose® packages of 100 (NDC 0004-0121-49). 2 mg (peach), bottles of 100 (NDC 0004-0162-01); Tel-E-Dose® packages of 100 (NDC 0004-0162-07).

Imprint on tablets: 0.5 mg—ROCHE BUMEX 0.5; 1 mg—ROCHE BUMEX 1; 2 mg—ROCHE BUMEX 2.

Ampuls (0.25 mg/ml), 2 ml, boxes of 10 (NDC 0004-1944-06). *Vials* (0.25 mg/ml), 2 ml, boxes of 10 (NDC 0004-1968-01); 4 ml, boxes of 10 (NDC 0004-1969-01); 10 ml, boxes of 10 (NDC 0004-1970-01).

Store all tablets, vials and ampuls at 59° to 86° F.

P.I. 0688

Shown in Product Identification Section, page 425

FANSIDAR®   ℞

[fan 'sid-ar]

(sulfadoxine and pyrimethamine/Roche)

TABLETS

The following text is complete prescribing information based on official labeling in effect June 1, 1989.

> **WARNING: FATALITIES ASSOCIATED WITH THE ADMINISTRATION OF FANSIDAR HAVE OCCURRED DUE TO SEVERE REACTIONS, INCLUDING STEVENS-JOHNSON SYNDROME AND TOXIC EPIDERMAL NECROLYSIS. FANSIDAR PROPHYLAXIS SHOULD BE DISCONTINUED AT THE FIRST APPEARANCE OF SKIN RASH, IF A SIGNIFICANT REDUCTION IN THE COUNT OF ANY FORMED BLOOD ELEMENTS IS NOTED, OR UPON THE OCCURRENCE OF ACTIVE BACTERIAL OR FUNGAL INFECTIONS.**

DESCRIPTION

Fansidar is an antimalarial agent, each tablet containing 500 mg N^1-(5,6-dimethoxy-4-pyrimidinyl) sulfanilamide (sulfadoxine) and 25 mg 2,4-diamino-5-(p-chlorophenyl)-6-ethylpyrimidine (pyrimethamine). Each tablet also contains corn starch, gelatin, lactose, magnesium stearate and talc.

CLINICAL PHARMACOLOGY

Fansidar is an antimalarial agent which acts by reciprocal potentiation of its two components, achieved by a sequential blockade of two enzymes involved in the biosynthesis of folinic acid within the parasites. Fansidar is effective against certain strains of *Plasmodium falciparum* that are resistant to chloroquine.

Both the sulfadoxine and the pyrimethamine of Fansidar are absorbed orally and are excreted mainly by the kidney. Following a single tablet administration, sulfadoxine peak plasma concentrations of 51 to 76 mcg/ml were achieved in 2.5 to 6 hours and the pyrimethamine peak plasma concentrations of 0.13 to 0.4 mcg/ml were achieved in 1.5 to 8 hours. The apparent half-life of elimination of sulfadoxine ranged from 100 to 231 hours with a mean of 169 hours, whereas pyrimethamine half-lives ranged from 54 to 148 hours with a mean of 111 hours. Both drugs appear in breast milk of nursing mothers.

INDICATIONS AND USAGE

Fansidar is indicated for the treatment of *P. falciparum* malaria for those patients in whom chloroquine resistance is suspected. Malaria prophylaxis with Fansidar is indicated for travelers to areas where chloroquine-resistant *P. falciparum* malaria is endemic. However, strains of *P. falciparum* may be encountered which have developed resistance to Fansidar.

CONTRAINDICATIONS

Prophylactic (repeated) use of Fansidar is contraindicated in patients with severe renal insufficiency, marked liver parenchymal damage or blood dyscrasias. Hypersensitivity to pyrimethamine or sulfonamides. Patients with documented megaloblastic anemia due to folate deficiency. Infants less than two months of age. Pregnancy at term and during the nursing period because sulfonamides pass the placenta and are excreted in the milk and may cause kernicterus.

WARNINGS

> FATALITIES ASSOCIATED WITH THE ADMINISTRATION OF FANSIDAR HAVE OCCURRED DUE TO SEVERE REACTIONS, INCLUDING STEVENS-JOHNSON SYNDROME AND TOXIC EPIDERMAL NECROLYSIS. FANSIDAR PROPHYLAXIS SHOULD BE DISCONTINUED AT THE FIRST APPEARANCE OF SKIN RASH, IF A SIGNIFICANT REDUCTION IN THE COUNT OF ANY FORMED BLOOD ELEMENTS IS NOTED, OR UPON THE OCCURRENCE OF ACTIVE BACTERIAL OR FUNGAL INFECTIONS.

Fatalities associated with the administration of sulfonamides, although rare, have occurred due to severe reactions, including fulminant hepatic necrosis, agranulocytosis, aplastic anemia and other blood dyscrasias. Fansidar prophylactic regimen has been reported to cause leukopenia during a treatment of two months or longer. This leukopenia is generally mild and reversible.

PRECAUTIONS

1. *General:* Fansidar should be given with caution to patients with impaired renal or hepatic function, to those with possible folate deficiency and to those with severe allergy or bronchial asthma. As with some sulfonamide drugs, in glucose-6-phosphate dehydrogenase-deficient individuals, hemolysis may occur. Urinalysis with microscopic examination and renal function tests should be performed during therapy of those patients who have impaired renal function.

2. *Information for the patient:* Patients should be warned that at the first appearance of a skin rash, they should stop use of Fansidar and seek medical attention immediately. Adequate fluid intake must be maintained in order to prevent crystalluria and stone formation.

Patients should also be warned that the appearance of sore throat, fever, arthralgia, cough, shortness of breath, pallor, purpura, jaundice or glossitis may be early indications of serious disorders which require prophylactic treatment to be stopped and medical treatment to be sought.

Females should be cautioned against becoming pregnant and should not breast feed their infants during Fansidar therapy or prophylactic treatment.

Patients should be warned to keep Fansidar out of reach of children.

3. *Laboratory tests:* Periodic blood counts and analysis of urine for crystalluria are desirable during prolonged prophylaxis.

4. *Drug interactions:* There have been reports which may indicate an increase in incidence and severity of adverse reactions when chloroquine is used with Fansidar as compared to the use of Fansidar alone. Fansidar is compatible with quinine and with antibiotics. However, antifolic drugs such as sulfonamides or trimethoprim-sulfamethoxazole combinations should not be used while the patient is receiving Fansidar for antimalarial prophylaxis. Fansidar has not been reported to interfere with antidiabetic agents.

If signs of folic acid deficiency develop, Fansidar should be discontinued. Folinic acid (leucovorin) may be administered in doses of 5 mg to 15 mg intramuscularly daily, for 3 days or longer, for depressed platelet or white blood cell counts in patients with drug-induced folic acid deficiency when recovery is too slow.

5. *Carcinogenesis, mutagenesis, impairment of fertility:* Pyrimethamine was not found carcinogenic in female mice or in male and female rats. The carcinogenic potential of pyrimethamine in male mice could not be assessed from the study because of markedly reduced life-span. Pyrimethamine was found to be mutagenic in laboratory animals and also in human bone marrow following 3 or 4 consecutive daily doses totaling 200 mg to 300 mg. Pyrimethamine was not found mutagenic in the Ames test. Testicular changes have been observed in rats treated with 105 mg/kg/day of Fansidar and with 15 mg/kg/day of pyrimethamine alone. Fertility of male rats and the ability of male or female rats to mate were not adversely affected at dosages of up to 210 mg/kg/day of Fansidar. The pregnancy rate of female rats was not affected following their treatment with 10.5 mg/kg/day, but was significantly reduced at dosages of 31.5 mg/kg/day or higher, a dosage approximately 30 times the weekly human prophylactic dose or higher.

6. *Pregnancy:* Teratogenic effects: Pregnancy Category C. Fansidar has been shown to be teratogenic in rats when given in weekly doses approximately 12 times the weekly human prophylactic dose. Teratology studies with pyrimeth-

amine plus sulfadoxine (1:20) in rats showed the minimum oral teratogenic dose to be approximately 0.9 mg/kg pyrimethamine plus 18 mg/kg sulfadoxine. In rabbits, no teratogenic effects were noted at oral doses as high as 20 mg/kg pyrimethamine plus 400 mg/kg sulfadoxine.

There are no adequate and well-controlled studies in pregnant women. However, due to the teratogenic effect shown in animals and because pyrimethamine plus sulfadoxine may interfere with folic acid metabolism, Fansidar therapy should be used during pregnancy only if the potential benefit justifies the potential risk to the fetus. Women of childbearing potential who are traveling to areas where malaria is endemic should be warned against becoming pregnant.

Nonteratogenic effects: See "CONTRAINDICATIONS" section.

7. *Nursing mothers:* See "CONTRAINDICATIONS" section.

8. *Pediatric use:* Fansidar should not be given to infants less than two months of age because of inadequate development of the glucuronide-forming enzyme system.

ADVERSE REACTIONS

For completeness, all major reactions to sulfonamides and to pyrimethamine are included below, even though they may not have been reported with Fansidar. See "WARNINGS" and "PRECAUTIONS" (Information for the Patient) sections.

Blood dyscrasias: Agranulocytosis, aplastic anemia, megaloblastic anemia, thrombopenia, leukopenia, hemolytic anemia, purpura, hypoprothrombinemia, methemoglobinemia and eosinophilia.

Allergic reactions: Erythema multiforme, Stevens-Johnson syndrome, generalized skin eruptions, toxic epidermal necrolysis, urticaria, serum sickness, pruritus, exfoliative dermatitis, anaphylactoid reactions, periorbital edema, conjunctival and scleral injection, photosensitization, arthralgia and allergic myocarditis.

Gastrointestinal reactions: Glossitis, stomatitis, nausea, emesis, abdominal pains, hepatitis, hepatocellular necrosis, diarrhea and pancreatitis.

C.N.S. reactions: Headache, peripheral neuritis, mental depression, convulsions, ataxia, hallucinations, tinnitus, vertigo, insomnia, apathy, fatigue, muscle weakness and nervousness.

Respiratory reactions: Pulmonary infiltrates.

Miscellaneous reactions: Drug fever, chills, and toxic nephrosis with oliguria and anuria. Periarteritis nodosa and L. E. phenomenon have occurred.

The sulfonamides bear certain chemical similarities to some goitrogens, diuretics (acetazolamide and the thiazides) and oral hypoglycemic agents. Diuresis and hypoglycemia have occurred rarely in patients receiving sulfonamides. Cross-sensitivity may exist with these agents. Rats appear to be especially susceptible to the goitrogenic effects of sulfonamides, and long-term administration has produced thyroid malignancies in the species.

OVERDOSAGE

Acute intoxication may be manifested by anorexia, vomiting and central nervous system stimulation (including convulsions), followed by megaloblastic anemia, leukopenia, thrombocytopenia, glossitis and crystalluria. In acute intoxication, emesis and gastric lavage followed by purges may be of benefit. The patient should be adequately hydrated to prevent renal damage. The renal and hematopoietic systems should be monitored for at least one month after an overdosage. If the patient is having convulsions, the use of a parenteral barbiturate is indicated. For depressed platelet or white blood cell counts, folinic acid (leucovorin) should be administered in a dosage of 5 mg to 15 mg intramuscularly daily for 3 days or longer.

DOSAGE AND ADMINISTRATION

(See Indications and Usage Section):

(a) *Treatment of acute attack of malaria*

A single dose of the following number of Fansidar Tablets is used in sequence with quinine or alone:

Adults	2 to 3 tablets
9 to 14 years	2 tablets
4 to 8 years	1 tablet
Under 4 years	½ tablet

(b) *Malaria prophylaxis*

The first dose of Fansidar should be taken one or two days before departure to an endemic area; administration should be continued during the stay and for four to six weeks after return.

	Once Weekly	Once Every Two Weeks
Adults	1 tablet	2 tablets
9 to 14 years	¾ tablet	1½ tablets
4 to 8 years	½ tablet	1 tablet
Under 4 years	¼ tablet	½ tablet

HOW SUPPLIED

Scored tablets, containing 500 mg sulfadoxine and 25 mg pyrimethamine—boxes of 25 (NDC-0004-0161-03).

P.I. 0587

Shown in Product Identification Section, page 425

FLUOROURACIL   ℞

[*flu "ro-u 'ra-sil*]

INJECTION

The following text is complete prescribing information based on official labeling in effect June 1, 1989.

> **WARNING**
>
> It is recommended that FLUOROURACIL be given only by or under the supervision of a qualified physician who is experienced in cancer chemotherapy and who is well versed in the use of potent antimetabolites. Because of the possibility of severe toxic reactions, it is recommended that patients be hospitalized at least during the initial course of therapy.

DESCRIPTION

FLUOROURACIL INJECTION/Roche, an antineoplastic antimetabolite, is a sterile, nonpyrogenic injectable solution for intravenous administration. Each 10-mL contains 500 mg fluorouracil; pH is adjusted to approximately 9.2 with sodium hydroxide.

Chemically, fluorouracil, a fluorinated pyrimidine, is 5-fluoro-2,4 (1H,3H)-pyrimidinedione. It is a white to practically white crystalline powder which is sparingly soluble in water. The molecular weight of fluorouracil is 130.08.

CLINICAL PHARMACOLOGY

There is evidence that the metabolism of fluorouracil in the anabolic pathway blocks the methylation reaction of deoxyuridylic acid to thymidylic acid. In this manner, fluorouracil interferes with the synthesis of deoxyribonucleic acid (DNA) and to a lesser extent inhibits the formation of ribonucleic acid (RNA). Since DNA and RNA are essential for cell division and growth, the effect of fluorouracil may be to create a thymine deficiency which provokes unbalanced growth and death of the cell. The effects of DNA and RNA deprivation are most marked on those cells which grow more rapidly and which take up fluorouracil at a more rapid rate.

Following intravenous injection, fluorouracil distributes into tumors, intestinal mucosa, bone marrow, liver and other tissues throughout the body. In spite of its limited lipid solubility, fluorouracil diffuses readily across the blood-brain barrier and distributes into cerebrospinal fluid and brain tissue.

Seven to twenty percent of the parent drug is excreted unchanged in the urine in six hours; of this over 90% is excreted in the first hour. The remaining percentage of the administered dose is metabolized, primarily in the liver. The catabolic metabolism of fluorouracil results in degradation products (*e.g.*, CO_2, urea and α-fluoro-β-alanine) which are inactive. The inactive metabolites are excreted in the urine over the next 3 to 4 hours. When fluorouracil is labeled in the six carbon position, thus preventing the ^{14}C metabolism to CO_2, approximately 90% of the total radioactivity is excreted in the urine. When fluorouracil is labeled in the two carbon position approximately 90% of the total radioactivity is excreted in expired CO_2. Ninety percent of the dose is accounted for during the first 24 hours following intravenous administration.

Following intravenous administration of fluorouracil, the mean half-life of elimination from plasma is approximately 16 minutes, with a range of 8 to 20 minutes, and is dose dependent. No intact drug can be detected in the plasma three hours after an intravenous injection.

INDICATIONS AND USAGE

Fluorouracil is effective in the palliative management of carcinoma of the colon, rectum, breast, stomach and pancreas.

CONTRAINDICATIONS

Fluorouracil therapy is contraindicated for patients in a poor nutritional state, those with depressed bone marrow function, those with potentially serious infections or those with a known hypersensitivity to Fluorouracil.

WARNINGS

THE DAILY DOSE OF FLUOROURACIL IS NOT TO EXCEED 800 MG. IT IS RECOMMENDED THAT PATIENTS BE HOSPITALIZED DURING THEIR FIRST COURSE OF TREATMENT.

Fluorouracil should be used with extreme caution in poor risk patients with a history of high-dose pelvic irradiation or previous use of alkylating agents, those who have a widespread involvement of bone marrow by metastatic tumors or those with impaired hepatic or renal function.

Pregnancy: Teratogenic effects: Pregnancy category D. Fluorouracil may cause fetal harm when administered to a pregnant woman. Fluorouracil has been shown to be terato-

Continued on next page

Roche Labs.—Cont.

genic in laboratory animals. Fluorouracil exhibited maximum teratogenicity when given to mice as single intraperitoneal injections of 10 to 40 mg/kg on day 10 or 12 of gestation. Similarly, intraperitoneal doses of 12 to 37 mg/kg given to rats between days 9 and 12 of gestation and intramuscular doses of 3 to 9 mg given to hamsters between days 8 and 11 of gestation were teratogenic. Malformations included cleft palates, skeletal defects and deformed appendages, paws and tails. The dosages which were teratogenic in animals are 1 to 3 times the maximum recommended human therapeutic dose. In monkeys, divided doses of 40 mg/kg given between days 20 and 24 of gestation were not teratogenic.

There are no adequate and well-controlled studies with Fluorouracil in pregnant women. While there is no evidence of teratogenicity in humans due to Fluorouracil, it should be kept in mind that other drugs which inhibit DNA synthesis (e.g., methotrexate and aminopterin) have been reported to be teratogenic in humans. Women of childbearing potential should be advised to avoid becoming pregnant. If the drug is used during pregnancy, or if the patient becomes pregnant while taking the drug, the patient should be told of the potential hazard to the fetus. Fluorouracil should be used during pregnancy only if the potential benefit justifies the potential risk to the fetus.

Combination Therapy: Any form of therapy which adds to the stress of the patient, interferes with nutrition or depresses bone marrow function will increase the toxicity of Fluorouracil.

PRECAUTIONS

General: Fluorouracil is a highly toxic drug with a narrow margin of safety. Therefore, patients should be carefully supervised, since therapeutic response is unlikely to occur without some evidence of toxicity. Severe hematological toxicity, gastrointestinal hemorrhage and even death may result from the use of Fluorouracil despite meticulous selection of patients and careful adjustment of dosage. Although severe toxicity is more likely in poor risk patients, fatalities may be encountered occasionally even in patients in relatively good condition.

Therapy is to be discontinued promptly whenever one of the following signs of toxicity appears:

Stomatitis or esophagopharyngitis, at the first visible sign.

Leukopenia (WBC under 3500) or a rapidly falling white blood count.

Vomiting, intractable.

Diarrhea, frequent bowel movements or watery stools.

Gastrointestinal ulceration and bleeding.

Thrombocytopenia (platelets under 100,000).

Hemorrhage from an site.

Information for Patients: Patients should be informed of expected toxic effects, particularly oral manifestations. Patients should be alerted to the possibility of alopecia as a result of therapy and should be informed that it is usually a transient effect.

Laboratory Tests: White blood counts with differential are recommended before each dose.

Drug Interactions: Leucovorin calcium may enhance the toxicity of fluorouracil.

Also see WARNINGS section.

Carcinogenesis, Mutagenesis, Impairment of Fertility: Carcinogenesis: Long-term studies in animals to evaluate the carcinogenic potential of fluorouracil have not been conducted. However, there was no evidence of carcinogenicity in small groups of rats given fluorouracil orally at doses of 0.01, 0.3, 1 or 3 mg per rat 5 days per week for 52 weeks, followed by a six-month observation period. Also, in other studies, 33 mg/kg of flourouracil was administered intravenously to male rats once a week for 52 weeks followed by observation for the remainder of their lifetimes with no evidence of carcinogenicity. Female mice were given 1 mg of fluorouracil intravenously once a week for 16 weeks with no effect on the incidence of lung adenomas. On the basis of the available data, no evaluation can be made of the carcinogenic risk of fluorouracil to humans.

Mutagenesis: Oncogenic transformation of fibroblasts from mouse embryo has been induced *in vitro* by fluorouracil, but the relationship between oncogenicity and mutagenicity is not clear. Fluorouracil has been shown to be mutagenic to several strain of *Salmonella typhimurium*, including TA 1535, TA 1537 and TA 1538, and to *Saccharomyces cerevisiae*, although no evidence of mutagenicity was found with *Salmonella typhimurium* strains TA 92, TA 98 and TA 100. In addition, a positive effect was observed in the micronucleus test on bone marrow cells of the mouse, and fluorouracil at very high concentrations produced chromosomal breaks in hamster fibroblasts *in vitro*.

Impairment of fertility: Fluorouracil has not been adequately studied in animals to permit an evaluation of its effects on fertility and general reproductive performance. However, doses of 125 or 250 mg/kg, administered intraperitoneally, have been shown to induce chromosomal aberrations and changes in chromosomal organization of spermatogonia in rats. Spermatogonial differentiation was also inhibited by fluorouracil, resulting in transient infertility. However, in studies with a strain of mouse which is sensitive to the induction of sperm head abnormalities after exposure to a range of chemical mutagens and carcinogens, fluorouracil did not produce any abnormalities at oral doses of up to 80 mg/kg/day. In female rats, fluorouracil, administered intraperitoneally at weekly doses of 25 or 50 mg/kg for three weeks during the pre-ovulatory phases of oogenesis, significantly reduced the incidence of fertile matings, delayed the development of pre- and postimplantation embryos, increased the incidence of pre-implantation lethality and induced chromosomal anomalies in these embryos. In a limited study in rabbits, a single 25 mg/kg dose of fluorouracil or 5 daily doses of 5 mg/kg had no effect on ovulation, appeared not to affect implantation and had only a limited effect in producing zygote destruction. Compounds such as fluorouracil, which interfere with DNA, RNA and protein synthesis, might be expected to have adverse effects on gametogenesis.

Pregnancy: Pregnancy Category D. See WARNINGS section.

Nonteratogenic effect: Fluorouracil has not been studied in animals for its effects on peri- and postnatal development. However, fluorouracil has been shown to cross the placenta and enter into fetal circulation in the rat. Administration of fluorouracil has resulted in increased resorptions and embryolethality in rats. In monkeys, maternal doses higher than 40 mg/kg resulted in abortion of all embryos exposed to fluorouracil. Compounds which inhibit DNA, RNA and protein synthesis might be expected to have adverse effects on peri- and postnatal development.

Nursing Mothers: It is not known whether fluorouracil is excreted in human milk. Because fluorouracil inhibits DNA, RNA and protein synthesis, mothers should not nurse while receiving this drug.

Pediatric Use: Safety and effectiveness in children have not been established.

ADVERSE REACTIONS

Stomatitis and esophagopharyngitis (which made lead to sloughing and ulceration), diarrhea, anorexia, nausea and emesis are commonly seen during therapy.

Leukopenia usually follows every course of adequate therapy with Fluorouracil. The lowest white blood cell counts are commonly observed between the 9th and 14th days after the first course of treatment, although uncommonly the maximal depression may be delayed for as long as 20 days. By the 30th day the count has usually returned to the normal range. Alopecia and dermatitis may be seen in a substantial number of cases. The dermatitis most often seen is a pruritic maculopapular rash usually appearing on the extremities and less frequently on the trunk. It is generally reversible and usually responsive to symptomatic treatment.

Other adverse reactions are:

Hematologic: pancytopenia, thrombocytopenia, agranulocytosis, anemia.

Cardiovascular: myocardial ischemia, angina.

Gastrointestinal: gastrointestinal ulceration and bleeding.

Allergic reactions: anaphylaxis and generalized allergic reactions.

Neurologic: acute cerebellar syndrome (which may pesist following discontinuance of treatment), nystagmus, headache.

Dermatologic: dry skin; fissuring; photosensitivity, as manifested by erythema or increased pigmentation of the skin; vein pigmentation.

Ophthalmic: lacrimal duct stenosis, visual changes, lacrimation, photophobia.

Psychiatric: disorientation, confusion, euphoria.

Miscellaneous: thrombophlebitis, epistaxis, nail changes (including loss of nails).

OVERDOSAGE

The possibility of overdosage with Fluorouracil is unlikely in view of the mode of administration. Nevertheless, the anticipated manifestations would be nausea, vomiting, diarrhea, gastrointestinal ulceration and bleeding, bone marrow depression (including thrombocytopenia, leukopenia and agranulocytosis). No specific antidotal therapy exists. Patients who have been exposed to an overdose of Fluorouracil should be monitored hematologically for at least four weeks. Should abnormalities appear, appropriate therapy should be utilized.

The acute intravenous toxicity of fluorouracil is as follows:

Species	LD_{50} (mg/kg±S.E.)
Mouse	340±17
Rat	165±26
Rabbit	27±5.1
Dog	31.5±3.8

DOSAGE AND ADMINISTRATION

General Instructions: Fluorouracil Injection should be administered only intravenously, using care to avoid extravasation. No dilution is required.

All dosages are based on the patient's actual weight. However, the estimated lean body mass (dry weight) is used if the patient is obese or if there has been a spurious weight gain due to edema, ascites or other forms of abnormal fluid retention.

It is recommended that prior to treatment each patient be carefully evaluated in order to estimate as accurately as possible the optimum initial dosage of Fluorouracil.

Dosage: Twelve mg/kg are given intravenously once daily for four successive days. The daily dose should not exceed 800 mg. *If no toxicity is observed,* 6 mg/kg are given on the 6th, 8th, 10th and 12th days *unless toxicity occurs.* No therapy is given on the 5th, 7th, 9th or 11th days. *Therapy is to be discontinued at the end of the 12th day, even if no toxicity has become apparent.* (See WARNINGS and PRECAUTIONS sections.)

Poor risk patients or those who are not in an adequate nutritional state (see CONTRAINDICATIONS and WARNINGS sections) should receive 6 mg/kg/day for three days. *If no toxicity is observed,* 3 mg/kg may be given on the 5th, 7th and 9th days *unless toxicity occurs.* No therapy is given on the 4th, 6th or 8th days. The daily dose should not exceed 400 mg. A sequence of injections on either schedule constitutes a "course of therapy."

Maintenance Therapy: In instances where toxicity has not been a problem, it is recommended that therapy be continued using either of the following schedules:

1. Repeat dosage of first course every 30 days after the last day of the previous course of treatment.

2. When toxic signs resulting from the initial course of therapy have subsided, administer a maintenance dosage of 10 to 15 mg/kg/week as a single dose. Do not exceed 1 Gm per week.

The patient's reaction to the previous course of therapy should be taken into account in determining the amount of the drug to be used, and the dosage should be adjusted accordingly. Some patients have received from 9 to 45 courses of treatment during periods which ranged from 12 to 60 months.

Procedures for proper handling and disposal of anticancer drugs should be considered. Several guidelines on this subject have been published.[1-6] There is no general agreement that all of the procedures recommended in the guidelines are necessary or appropriate.

Note: Parenteral drug products should be inspected visually for particulate matter and discoloration prior to administration, whenever solution and container permit. Although the Fluorouracil solution may discolor slightly during storage, the potency and safety are not adversely affected. If a precipitate occurs due to exposure to low temperatures, resolubilize by heating to 140°F and shaking vigorously; allow to cool to body temperature before using.

HOW SUPPLIED

For intravenous use—10-mL single-use vials, boxes of 10 (NDC 0004-1977-01). Each 10 mL contains 500 mg fluorouracil in a colorless to faint yellow aqueous solution, with pH adjusted to approximately 9.2 with sodium hydroxide.

Store at room temperature (59° to 86°F; 15° to 30°C). Protect from light.

REFERENCES

1. Recommendations for the safe handling of parenteral antineoplastic drugs. Washington, DC, U.S. Government Printing Office (NIH Publication No. 83-2621).
2. AMA Council Report. Guidelines for handling parenteral antineoplastics. *JAMA 253:* 1590–1592, Mar 15, 1985.
3. National Study Commission on Cytotoxic Exposure: Recommendations for handling cytotoxic agents. Available from Louis P. Jeffrey, ScD, Director of Pharmacy Services, Rhode Island Hospital, 593 Eddy Street, Providence, Rhode Island 02902.
4. Clinical Oncological Society of Australia: Guidelines and recommendations for safe handling of antineoplastic agents. *Med J Aust 1:* 426–428, Apr 30, 1983.
5. Jones RB, Frank R, Mass T: Safe handling of chemotherapeutic agents: a report from the Mount Sinai Medical Center. *CA 33:* 258–263, Sept–Oct 1983.
6. ASHP technical assistance bulletin on handling cytotoxic drugs in hospitals. *Am J Hosp Pharm 42:* 131–137, Jan 1985.

P.I. 0788

FUDR   ℞

[ef-u-dee-are]
(floxuridine/Roche)

The following text is complete prescribing information based on official labeling in effect June 1, 1989.

FOR INTRA-ARTERIAL INFUSION ONLY

WARNING

It is recommended that FUDR be given only by or under the supervision of a qualified physician who is experienced in cancer chemotherapy and intra-arterial drug therapy and is well versed in the use of potent antimetabolites.

> Because of the possibility of severe toxic reactions, all patients should be hospitalized for initiation of the first course of therapy.

DESCRIPTION

FUDR (floxuridine/Roche), an antineoplastic antimetabolite, is available as a sterile lyophilized powder for reconstitution. Each vial contains 500 mg of floxuridine which is to be reconstituted with 5 mL of sterile water for injection. An appropriate amount of reconstituted solution is then diluted with a parenteral solution for intra-arterial infusion (see DOSAGE AND ADMINISTRATION section).

Floxuridine is a fluorinated pyrimidine. Chemically, floxuridine is 2'-deoxy-5-fluorouridine. It is a white to off-white odorless solid which is freely soluble in water.

The 2% aqueous solution has a pH of between 4.0 to 5.5. The molecular weight of floxuridine is 246.19.

CLINICAL PHARMACOLOGY

When FUDR is given by rapid intra-arterial injection it is apparently rapidly catabolized to 5-fluorouracil. Thus, rapid injection of FUDR produces the same toxic and antimetabolic effects as does 5-fluorouracil. The primary effect is to interfere with the synthesis of deoxyribonucleic acid (DNA) and to a lesser extent inhibit the formation of ribonucleic acid (RNA). However, when FUDR is given by continuous intra-arterial infusion its direct anabolism to FUDR-monophosphate is enhanced, thus increasing the inhibition of DNA.

Floxuridine is metabolized in the liver. The drug is excreted intact and as urea, fluorouracil, α-fluoro-β-ureidopropionic acid, dihydrofluorouracil, α-fluoro-β-guanidopropionic acid and α-fluoro-β-alanine in the urine; it is also expired as respiratory carbon dioxide. Pharmacokinetic data on intra-arterial infusion of FUDR are not available.

INDICATIONS AND USAGE

FUDR is effective in the palliative management of gastrointestinal adenocarcinoma metastatic to the liver, when given by continuous regional intra-arterial infusion in carefully selected patients who are considered incurable by surgery or other means. Patients with known disease extending beyond an area capable of infusion via a single artery should, except in unusual circumstances, be considered for systemic therapy with other chemotherapeutic agents.

CONTRAINDICATIONS

FUDR therapy is contraindicated for patients in a poor nutritional state, those with depressed bone marrow function or those with potentially serious infections.

WARNINGS

BECAUSE OF THE POSSIBILITY OF SEVERE TOXIC REACTIONS, ALL PATIENTS SHOULD BE HOSPITALIZED FOR THE FIRST COURSE OF THERAPY.

FUDR should be used with extreme caution in poor risk patients with impaired hepatic or renal function or a history of high-dose pelvic irradiation or previous use of alkylating agents. The drug is not intended as an adjuvant to surgery.

FUDR may cause fetal harm when administered to a pregnant woman. It has been shown to be teratogenic in the chick embryo, mouse (at doses of 2.5 to 100 mg/kg) and rat (at doses of 75 to 150 mg/kg). Malformations included cleft palates; skeletal defects; and deformed appendages, paws and tails. The dosages which were teratogenic in animals are 4.2 to 125 times the recommended human therapeutic dose.

There are no adequate and well-controlled studies in pregnant women. If this drug is used during pregnancy or if the patient becomes pregnant while taking (receiving) this drug, the patient should be apprised of the potential hazard to the fetus. Women of childbearing potential should be advised to avoid becoming pregnant.

Combination therapy: Any form of therapy which adds to the stress of the patient, interferes with nutrition or depresses bone marrow function will increase the toxicity of FUDR.

PRECAUTIONS

General: FUDR is a highly toxic drug with a narrow margin of safety. Therefore, patients should be carefully supervised since therapeutic response is unlikely to occur without some evidence of toxicity. Severe hematological toxicity, gastrointestinal hemorrhage and even death may result from the use of FUDR despite meticulous selection of patients and careful adjustment of dosage. Although severe toxicity is more likely in poor risk patients, fatalities may be encountered occasionally even in patients in relatively good condition. Therapy is to be discontinued promptly whenever one of the following signs of toxicity appears:

Myocardial ischemia

Stomatitis or esophagopharyngitis, at the first visible sign

Leukopenia (WBC under 3500) or a rapidly falling white blood count

Vomiting, intractable

Diarrhea, frequent bowel movements or watery stools

Gastrointestinal ulceration and bleeding

Thrombocytopenia (platelets under 100,000)

Hemorrhage from any site

Information for patients: Patients should be informed of expected toxic effects, particularly oral manifestations. Patients should be alerted to the possibility of alopecia as a result of therapy and should be informed that it is usually a transient effect.

Laboratory tests: Careful monitoring of the white blood count and platelet count is recommended.

Drug interactions: See WARNINGS section.

Carcinogenesis, mutagenesis, impairment of fertility:

Carcinogenesis: Long-term studies in animals to evaluate the carcinogenic potential of floxuridine have not been conducted. On the basis of the available data, no evaluation can be made of the carcinogenic risk of FUDR to humans.

Mutagenesis: Oncogenic transformation of fibroblasts from mouse embryo has been induced *in vitro* by FUDR, but the relationship between oncogenicity and mutagenicity is not clear. Floxuridine has also been shown to be mutagenic in human leukocytes *in vitro* and in the *Drosophila* test system. In addition, 5-fluorouracil, to which floxuridine is catabolized when given by intra-arterial injection, has been shown to be mutagenic in *in vitro* tests.

Impairment of fertility: The effects of floxuridine on fertility and general reproductive performance have not been studied in animals. However, because floxuridine is catabolized to 5-fluorouracil, it should be noted that 5-fluorouracil has been shown to induce chromosomal aberrations and changes in chromosome organization of spermatogonia in rats at doses of 125 or 250 mg/kg, administered intraperitoneally.

Spermatogonial differentiation was also inhibited by fluorouracil, resulting in transient infertility. In female rats, fluorouracil, administered intraperitoneally at doses of 25 or 50 mg/kg during the preovulatory phase of oogenesis, significantly reduced the incidence of fertile matings, delayed the development of pre- and post-implantation embryos, increased the incidence of preimplantation lethality and induced chromosomal anomalies in these embryos. Compounds such as FUDR, which interfere with DNA, RNA and protein synthesis, might be expected to have adverse effects on gametogenesis.

Pregnancy: Teratogenic effects: Pregnancy category D. See WARNINGS section. Floxuridine has been shown to be teratogenic in the chick embryo, mouse (at doses of 2.5 to 100 mg/kg) and rat (at doses of 75 to 150 mg/kg). Malformations included cleft palates, skeletal defects and deformed appendages, paws and tails. The dosages which were teratogenic in animals are 4.2 to 125 times the recommended human therapeutic dose.

There are no adequate and well-controlled studies with FUDR in pregnant women. While there is no evidence of teratogenicity in humans due to FUDR, it should be kept in mind that other drugs which inhibit DNA synthesis (*e.g.*, methotrexate and aminopterin) have been reported to be teratogenic in humans. FUDR should be used during pregnancy only if the potential benefit justifies the potential risk to the fetus.

Nonteratogenic effects: Floxuridine has not been studied in animals for its effects on peri- and postnatal development. However, compounds which inhibit DNA, RNA and protein synthesis might be expected to have adverse effects on peri- and postnatal development.

Nursing mothers: It is not known whether FUDR is excreted in human milk. Because FUDR inhibits DNA and RNA synthesis, mothers should not nurse while receiving this drug.

Pediatric use: Safety and effectiveness in children have not been established.

ADVERSE REACTIONS

Adverse reactions to the arterial infusion of FUDR are generally related to the procedural complications of regional arterial infusion.

The more common adverse reactions to the drug are nausea, vomiting, diarrhea, enteritis, stomatitis and localized erythema. The more common laboratory abnormalities are anemia, leukopenia, thrombocytopenia and elevations of alkaline phosphatase, serum transaminase, serum bilirubin and lactic dehydrogenase.

Other adverse reactions are:

Gastrointestinal: duodenal ulcer, duodenitis, gastritis, bleeding, gastroenteritis, glossitis, pharyngitis, anorexia, cramps, abdominal pain; possible intra- and extrahepatic biliary sclerosis, as well as acalculous cholecystitis.

Dermatologic: alopecia, dermatitis, nonspecific skin toxicity, rash.

Cardiovascular: myocardial ischemia.

Miscellaneous clinical reactions: fever, lethargy, malaise, weakness.

Laboratory abnormalities: BSP, prothrombin, total proteins, sedimentation rate and thrombopenia.

Procedural complications of regional arterial infusion: arterial aneurysm; arterial ischemia; arterial thrombosis; embolism; fibromyositis; thrombophlebitis; hepatic necrosis; abscesses; infection at catheter site; bleeding at catheter site; catheter blocked, displaced or leaking.

The following adverse reactions have not been reported with FUDR but have been noted following the administration of 5-fluorouracil. While the possibility of these occurring following FUDR therapy is remote because of its regional administration, one should be alert for these reactions following the administration of FUDR because of the pharmacological similarity of these two drugs: pancytopenia, agranulocytosis, myocardial ischemia, angina, anaphylaxis, generalized allergic reactions, acute cerebellar syndrome, nystagmus, headache, dry skin, fissuring, photosensitivity, pruritic maculopapular rash, increased pigmentation of the skin, vein pigmentation, lacrimal duct stenosis, visual changes, lacrimation, photophobia, disorientation, confusion, euphoria, epistaxis and nail changes, including loss of nails.

OVERDOSAGE

The possibility of overdosage with FUDR is unlikely in view of the mode of administration. Nevertheless, the anticipated manifestations would be nausea, vomiting, diarrhea, gastrointestinal ulceration and bleeding, bone marrow depression (including thrombocytopenia, leukopenia and agranulocytosis).

No specific antidotal therapy exists. Patients who have been exposed to an overdosage of FUDR should be monitored hematologically for at least four weeks. Should abnormalities appear, appropriate therapy should be utilized.

The acute intravenous toxicity of floxuridine is as follows:

Species	LD_{50} (mg/kg ± S.E.)
Mouse	880 ± 51
Rat	670 ± 73
Rabbit	94 ± 19.6
Dog	157 ± 46

DOSAGE AND ADMINISTRATION

Each vial must be reconstituted with 5 mL of sterile water for injection to yield a solution containing approximately 100 mg of floxuridine/mL. The calculated daily dose(s) of the drug is then diluted with 5% dextrose or 0.9% sodium chloride injection to a volume appropriate for the infusion apparatus to be used. The administration of FUDR is best achieved with the use of an appropriate pump to overcome pressure in large arteries and to ensure a uniform rate of infusion.

Parenteral drug products should be inspected visually for particulate matter and discoloration prior to administration whenever solution and container permit.

The recommended therapeutic dose schedule of FUDR by continuous arterial infusion is 0.1 to 0.6 mg/kg/day. The higher dosage ranges (0.4 to 0.6 mg) are usually employed for hepatic artery infusion because the liver metabolizes the drug, thus reducing the potential for systemic toxicity. Therapy can be given until adverse reactions appear. (See PRECAUTIONS section.) When these side effects have subsided, therapy may be resumed. The patient should be maintained on therapy as long as response to FUDR continues.

Procedures for proper handling and disposal of anticancer drugs should be considered. Several guidelines on this subject have been published.[1-6] There is no general agreement that all of the procedures recommended in the guidelines are necessary or appropriate.

HOW SUPPLIED

500 mg FUDR (floxuridine) sterile powder in a 5-mL vial (NDC 0004-1935-08). This is to be reconstituted with 5 mL sterile water for injection.

Reconstituted vials should be stored under refrigeration (36° to 46°F, 2° to 8°C) for not more than two weeks.

REFERENCES

1. Recommendations for the safe handling of parenteral antineoplastic drugs. Washington, DC, U.S. Government Printing Office (NIH Publication No. 83-2621).
2. AMA Council Report. Guidelines for handling parenteral antineoplastics. *JAMA 253:* 1590–1592, Mar 15, 1985.
3. National Study Commission on Cytotoxic Exposure: Recommendations for handling cytotoxic agents. Available from Louis P. Jeffrey, ScD, Director of Pharmacy Services, Rhode Island Hospital, 593 Eddy Street, Providence, Rhode Island 02902.
4. Clinical Oncological Society of Australia: Guidelines and recommendations for safe handling of antineoplastic agents. *Med J Aust 1:* 426–428, Apr 30, 1983.
5. Jones RB, Frank R, Mass T: Safe handling of chemotherapeutic agents: a report from the Mount Sinai Medical Center. *CA 33:* 258–263, Sept–Oct 1983.
6. ASHP technical assistance bulletin on handling cytotoxic drugs in hospitals. *Am J Hosp Pharm 42:* 131–137, Jan 1985.

P.I. 1288

Continued on next page

Roche Labs.—Cont.

GANTANOL®   ℞
[gan'tan-ol]
sulfamethoxazole/Roche
TABLETS ● SUSPENSION

The following text is complete prescribing information based on official labeling in effect June 1, 1989.

DESCRIPTION
Gantanol® (brand of sulfamethoxazole/Roche) is an intermediate-dosage antibacterial sulfonamide available in tablets and suspension. Each tablet contains 0.5 Gm sulfamethoxazole plus corn starch, polyvinyl acetate, polyvinyl alcohol, magnesium stearate, FD&C Blue No. 1 Lake, FD&C Yellow No. 6 Lake and D&C Yellow No. 10 Lake. Each teaspoonful (5 mL) of the suspension contains 0.5 Gm sulfamethoxazole in a vehicle containing carboxyvinyl polymer, citric acid, edetate disodium, methylcellulose, saccharin, saccharin sodium, simethicone, sodium benzoate, sodium citrate, sodium hydroxide, sodium lauryl sulfate, sorbitol, sucrose, FD&C Red. No. 40, flavors and water.
Sulfamethoxazole is N^1-(5-methyl-3-isoxazolyl) sulfanilamide. It is an almost white, odorless, tasteless compound with a molecular weight of 253.28.

CLINICAL PHARMACOLOGY
Sulfamethoxazole is rapidly absorbed following oral administration. It exists in the blood as unbound, protein-bound, metabolized and conjugated forms. The metabolism of sulfamethoxazole occurs predominately by N_4-acetylation, although the glucuronide conjugate has been identified. The free form is considered to be the therapeutically active form. Approximately 70% of sulfamethoxazole is bound to plasma proteins; of the unbound portion, 80% to 90% is in the nonacetylated form.
Following a single 1-Gm oral dose in 12 volunteer male subjects, the mean peak plasma concentration of 38 mcg/mL of intact sulfamethoxazole was achieved by 2 hours. The mean half-life of sulfamethoxazole is approximately 10 hours. However, patients with severely impaired renal function, as shown by a creatinine clearance of less than 30 mL/minute, exhibit an increase of the half-life of sulfamethoxazole, requiring dosage regimen adjustment.
Sulfamethoxazole is excreted primarily by the kidneys chiefly through glomerular filtration but also through tubular secretion. Urine concentrations of sulfamethoxazole are considerably higher than are the concentrations in blood. Eighty percent to 100 percent of the dose is excreted in the urine as total sulfamethoxazole, of which 30% is intact drug with the remaining as the N_4-acetylated metabolite.
Sulfamethoxazole diffuses into cerebrospinal fluid, with peak concentrations occurring at 8 hours and reaching approximately 14% of simultaneous plasma concentrations. The drug has also been shown to distribute to aqueous humor, vaginal fluid and middle ear fluid; it also passes the placental barrier and is excreted in breast milk.
Microbiology: The systemic sulfonamides are bacteriostatic agents and the spectrum of activity is similar for all. Sulfonamides inhibit bacterial synthesis of dihydrofolic acid by competing with *para*-aminobenzoic acid (PABA). Resistant strains are capable of utilizing folic acid precursors or preformed folic acid.

INDICATIONS AND USAGE
Acute, recurrent or chronic urinary tract infections (primarily pyelonephritis, pyelitis and cystitis) due to susceptible organisms (usually *E. coli, Klebsiella-Enterobacter,* staphylococcus, *Proteus mirabilis* and, less frequently, *Proteus vulgaris*) in the absence of obstructive uropathy or foreign bodies.
Meningococcal meningitis prophylaxis when sulfonamide-sensitive group A strains are known to prevail in family groups or larger closed populations. (The prophylactic usefulness of sulfonamides when group B or C infections are prevalent has not been proven and in closed population groups may be harmful.)
Acute otitis media due to *Haemophilus influenzae* when used concomitantly with adequate doses of penicillin.
Trachoma, Inclusion conjunctivitis, Nocardiosis, Chancroid.
Toxoplasmosis as adjunctive therapy with pyrimethamine.
Malaria due to chloroquine-resistant strains of *Plasmodium falciparum,* when used as adjunctive therapy.
Important note: In vitro sulfonamide susceptibility tests are not always reliable. The test must be carefully coordinated with bacteriologic and clinical response. When the patient is already taking sulfonamides, follow-up cultures should have aminobenzoic acid added to the culture media. Currently, the increasing frequency of resistant organisms is a limitation of the usefulness of antibacterial agents including the sulfonamides, especially in the treatment of chronic and recurrent urinary tract infections.
Wide variation in blood concentrations may result with identical doses. Blood concentrations should be measured in patients receiving sulfonamides for serious infections. Free sulfonamide blood concentrations of 5 to 15 mg/100 mL may

be considered therapeutically effective for most infections, with blood concentrations of 12 to 15 mg/100 mL optimal for serious infections; 20 mg/100 mL should be the maximum total sulfonamide concentration, since adverse reactions occur more frequently above this concentration.

CONTRAINDICATIONS
Hypersensitivity to sulfonamides. Infants less than 2 months of age (except in the treatment of congenital toxoplasmosis as adjunctive therapy with pyrimethamine). Pregnancy at term and during the nursing period because sulfonamides pass the placenta and are excreted in the milk and may cause kernicterus.

WARNINGS
The sulfonamides should not be used for the treatment of group A beta-hemolytic streptococcal infections. In an established infection, they will not eradicate the streptococcus, and therefore will not prevent sequelae such as rheumatic fever and glomerulonephritis.
Deaths associated with the administration of sulfonamides have been reported from hypersensitivity reactions, hepatocellular necrosis, agranulocytosis, aplastic anemia and other blood dyscrasias.
The presence of clinical signs such as sore throat, fever, arthralgia, cough, shortness of breath, pallor, purpura or jaundice may be early indications of serious reactions, including serious blood disorders.

PRECAUTIONS
General: Sulfonamides should be given with caution to patients with impaired renal or hepatic function and to those with severe allergy or bronchial asthma. In glucose-6-phosphate dehydrogenase-deficient individuals, hemolysis may occur. This reaction is frequently dose-related.
Information for patients: Patients should be instructed to maintain an adequate fluid intake in order to prevent crystalluria and stone formation.
Laboratory tests: Complete blood counts should be done frequently in patients receiving sulfonamides. If a significant reduction in the count of any formed blood element is noted, Gantanol should be discontinued. Urinalyses with careful microscopic examination and renal function tests should be performed during therapy, particularly for those patients with impaired renal function.
Drug interactions: In elderly patients concurrently receiving certain diuretics, primarily thiazides, an increased incidence of thrombopenia with purpura has been reported.
It has been reported that sulfamethoxazole may prolong the prothrombin time in patients who are receiving the anticoagulant warfarin. This interaction should be kept in mind when Gantanol is given to patients already on anticoagulant therapy, and the coagulation time should be reassessed.
Sulfamethoxazole may inhibit the hepatic metabolism of phenytoin. At a 1.6 Gm dose, sulfamethoxazole produced a slight but significant increase in the half-life of phenytoin but did not produce a corresponding decrease in the metabolic clearance rate. When administering these drugs concurrently, one should be alert for possible excessive phenytoin effect.
Sulfonamides can also displace methotrexate from plasma protein-binding sites, thus increasing free methotrexate concentrations.
The presence of sulfamethoxazole may interfere with the Jaffé alkaline picrate reaction assay for creatinine, resulting in overestimations of about 10% in the range of normal values.
Carcinogenesis, mutagenesis, impairment of fertility: Carcinogenesis: Sulfamethoxazole has not been adequately tested in animals to permit an evaluation of its carcinogenic potential. Mutagenesis: Bacterial mutagenic studies have not been performed with sulfamethoxazole. No chromosomal damage was observed in human leukocytes cultured *in vitro* with sulfamethoxazole; the concentrations used exceeded blood levels of sulfamethoxazole following therapy with Gantanol. Impairment of fertility: No adverse effects on fertility or general reproductive performance were observed in rats given sulfamethoxazole in oral dosages as high as 350 mg/kg/day.
Pregnancy: Teratogenic Effects: Pregnancy Category C. In rats, oral doses of 533 mg/kg of sulfamethoxazole produced teratologic effects manifested mainly as cleft palates. The highest dose which did not cause cleft palates in rats was 512 mg/kg of sulfamethoxazole. In rabbits, 150 to 350 mg/kg/day increased maternal mortality but had no deleterious effects on fetal development.
There are no adequate and well-controlled studies of Gantanol in pregnant women. Gantanol should be used during pregnancy only if the potential benefit justifies the potential risk to the fetus.
Nonteratogenic effects: See CONTRAINDICATIONS section.
Nursing mothers: See CONTRAINDICATIONS section.
Pediatric Use: Gantanol is not recommended in infants under 2 months of age, except in the treatment of congenital toxoplasmosis as adjunctive therapy with pyrimethamine. (See CONTRAINDICATIONS section.) At the present time

there are insufficient clinical data on prolonged or recurrent therapy in chronic renal diseases of children under 6 years of age.

ADVERSE REACTIONS
Included in the listing that follows are adverse reactions that have not been reported with this specific drug; however, the pharmacologic similarities among the sulfonamides require that each of the reactions be considered with Gantanol administration.
Hematologic: Agranulocytosis, aplastic anemia, thrombocytopenia, leukopenia, hemolytic anemia, purpura, hypoprothrombinemia, methemoglobinemia, neutropenia, eosinophilia.
Allergic Reactions: Anaphylaxis, allergic myocarditis, serum sickness, conjunctival and scleral injection, generalized allergic reactions. In addition, periarteritis nodosa and systemic lupus erythematosus have been reported.
Dermatologic: Stevens-Johnson syndrome, epidermal necrolysis, erythema multiforme, exfoliative dermatitis, photosensitivity, pruritus, urticaria, rash, generalized skin eruptions.
Gastrointestinal: Hepatitis, hepatocellular necrosis, pseudomembranous enterocolitis, pancreatitis, stomatitis, glossitis, nausea, emesis, abdominal pain, diarrhea, anorexia.
Genitourinary: Creatinine elevation, toxic nephrosis with oliguria and anuria. The frequency of renal complications is considerably lower in patients receiving the more soluble sulfonamides.
Neurologic: Convulsions, peripheral neuritis, ataxia, vertigo, tinnitus, headache.
Psychiatric: Hallucinations, depression, apathy.
Endocrine: The sulfonamides bear certain chemical similarities to some goitrogens, diuretics (acetazolamide and the thiazides) and oral hypoglycemic agents. Cross-sensitivity may exist with these agents. Diuresis and hypoglycemia have occurred rarely in patients receiving sulfonamides.
Musculoskeletal: Arthralgia, myalgia.
Respiratory: Pulmonary infiltrates.
Miscellaneous: Edema (including periorbital), pyrexia, chills, weakness, fatigue, insomnia.

OVERDOSAGE
Acute: The amount of a single dose of sulfamethoxazole that is either associated with symptoms of overdosage or is likely to be life-threatening has not been reported. Signs and symptoms of overdosage reported with sulfonamides include anorexia, colic, nausea, vomiting, dizziness, headache, drowsiness and unconsciousness. Pyrexia, hematuria and crystalluria may be noted. Blood dyscrasias and jaundice are potential late manifestations of overdosage.
General principles of treatment include the institution of gastric lavage or emesis; forcing oral fluids; and the administration of intravenous fluids if urine output is low and renal function is normal. The patient should be monitored with blood counts and appropriate blood chemistries, including electrolytes. If a significant blood dyscrasia or jaundice occurs, specific therapy should be instituted for these complications. Peritoneal dialysis is not effective and hemodialysis is only moderately effective in eliminating sulfamethoxazole.
Chronic: Use of sulfamethoxazole at high doses and/or for extended periods of time may cause bone marrow depression manifested as thrombocytopenia, leukopenia and/or megaloblastic anemia. If signs of bone marrow depression occur, the patient should be given leucovorin 3 to 6 mg intramuscularly daily for three days, or as required to restore normal hematopoiesis.
Animal Toxicity: The oral LD_{50} of sulfamethoxazole is 2300 mg/kg in mice, 3000 mg/kg in rats and >2000 mg/kg in rabbits.

DOSAGE AND ADMINISTRATION
Systemic sulfonamides are contraindicated in infants under 2 months of age, except in the treatment of congenital toxoplasmosis as adjunctive therapy with pyrimethamine.
The usual dosage schedules are as follows:

Children Infants (2 Months or Older) and Children	Initial Dose (50–60 mg/kg)	Dose Morning and Evening Daily Thereafter (25–30 mg/kg)
20 lbs	1 tablet or 1 teasp. (0.5 Gm)	½ tablet or ½ teasp. (0.25 Gm)
40 lbs	2 tablets or 2 teasp. (1 Gm)	1 tablet or 1 teasp. (0.5 Gm)
60 lbs	3 tablets or 3 teasp. (1.5 Gm)	1½ tablets or 1½ teasp. (0.75 Gm)
80 lbs	4 tablets or 4 teasp. (2 Gm)	2 tablets or 2 teasp. (1 Gm)

The maximum dose for children should not exceed 75 mg/kg/24 hours.

Adults

Mild to Moderate Infections	4 tablets or 4 teasp. (2 Gm)	2 tablets or 2 teasp. (1 Gm)

Note: One teaspoonful equals 5 ml.

Severe Infections: 4 tablets or 4 teaspoonfuls (2 Gm) initially, followed by 2 tablets or 2 teaspoonfuls (1 Gm) three times daily thereafter.

Patients with impaired renal function (creatinine clearance below 20 to 30 mL/min) require decreased dosage adjustment.

HOW SUPPLIED

Tablets (pale green, scored), containing 0.5 Gm sulfamethoxazole—bottles of 100 (NDC 0004-0010-01); Tel-E-Dose® packages of 100 (NDC 0004-0010-49). Imprint on tablets: GANTANOL® ROCHE.

Suspension, 10%, containing 0.5 Gm sulfamethoxazole per teaspoonful (5 mL); cherry-flavored—bottles of 1 pint (473 mL) (NDC 0004-1002-28).

P.I. 0788

Shown in Product Identification Section, page 425

GANTRISIN® ℞
[gan 'tris-in]
(sulfisoxazole diolamine/Roche)
OPHTHALMIC SOLUTION
OPHTHALMIC OINTMENT

The following text is complete prescribing information based on official labeling in effect June 1, 1989.

DESCRIPTION

Gantrisin (sulfisoxazole diolamine/Roche) Ophthalmic Solution and Ointment are antibacterial sulfonamide preparations specifically intended for topical ophthalmic use. The solution is a sterile, isotonic preparation containing 4% (40 mg/ml) sulfisoxazole in the form of the diolamine salt, and phenylmercuric nitrate 1:100,000 as a preservative. The solution has a physiologic pH, and does not cause significant stinging or burning on application. The ointment is a sterile preparation containing 4% sulfisoxazole in the form of the diolamine salt, compounded with white petrolatum, mineral oil and phenylmercuric nitrate 1:50,000 as a preservative. Chemically, sulfisoxazole diolamine is N^1-(3,4-dimethyl-5-isoxazolyl)sulfanilamide compound with 2,2'-iminodiethanol (1:1). It is a white to off-white, odorless, crystalline powder that is freely soluble in water and soluble in alcohol. Sulfisoxazole diolamine has a molecular weight of 372.44.

CLINICAL PHARMACOLOGY

Sulfonamides do not appear to be appreciably absorbed from mucous membranes.
Microbiology: Sulfonamides exert a bacteriostatic effect against a wide range of gram-positive and gram-negative microorganisms. Sulfonamides inhibit bacterial synthesis of dihydrofolic acid by competing with *para*-aminobenzoic acid (PABA). Resistant strains are capable of utilizing folic acid precursors or preformed folic acid. Currently, the increasing frequency of resistant organisms is a limitation of the usefulness of antibacterial agents, including the sulfonamides.

INDICATIONS

For the treatment of conjunctivitis, corneal ulcers and other superficial ocular infections due to susceptible microorganisms, and as an adjunct in systemic sulfonamide therapy of trachoma.

CONTRAINDICATIONS

Hypersensitivity to sulfonamides or to other ingredients in the formulation. Infants less than 2 months of age. Pregnancy at term and during the nursing period because sulfonamides pass the placenta and are excreted in the milk and may cause kernicterus.

PRECAUTIONS

General: Ophthalmic ointments may retard corneal healing. Nonsusceptible organisms, including fungi, may proliferate with the use of these preparations. Sulfonamides are inactivated by the *para*-aminobenzoic acid present in purulent exudates. Should undesirable reactions occur, discontinue Gantrisin immediately.
Information for patients: Patients using Gantrisin Ophthalmic Solution should be instructed not to touch the dropper tip to any surface, since contamination of the solution may result.
Drug Interactions: Gantrisin Ophthalmic Solution and Ointment are incompatible with preparations containing silver. In vitro antagonism with sulfisoxazole diolamine and gentamicin sulfate (Garamycin) has been reported.
Carcinogenesis, mutagenesis, impairment of fertility: Carcinogenesis: Carcinogenic studies have not been performed with ophthalmic preparations of sulfisoxazole. Sulfisoxazole was not carcinogenic in either sex when administered by gavage for 103 weeks at dosages up to 2000 mg/kg/day in mice or 400 mg/kg/day in rats.
Mutagenesis: Bacterial mutagenic studies have not been performed with sulfisoxazole. However, Gantrisin was not

observed to be mutagenic in *E. coli* Sd-4-73 when tested in the absence of a metabolic activating system.
Impairment of fertility: Fertility studies have not been performed with ophthalmic preparations of sulfisoxazole. No effects on mating behavior, conception rate or fertility index (percent pregnant) were observed in a reproduction study in rats given oral dosages of 800 mg/kg/day sulfisoxazole.
Pregnancy: Teratogenic effects: Pregnancy Category C. Teratogenic studies of ophthalmic preparations of sulfisoxazole have not been performed in laboratory animals. Sulfisoxazole was not teratogenic in either rats or rabbits at oral dosages of 800 mg/kg/day. However, in another teratogenicity study, cleft palates developed in both rats and mice after oral administration of 1000 mg/kg/day sulfisoxazole; skeletal defects were also observed in rats. This dose is 9 to 18 times the usual adult dosage for oral Gantrisin.
There are not adequate and well-controlled studies of Gantrisin in pregnant women. Gantrisin Ophthalmic Solution and Ointment should be used during pregnancy only if the potential benefit justifies the potential risk to the fetus.
Nursing mothers: See CONTRAINDICATIONS section.
Pediatric use: Gantrisin Ophthalmic Solution is not recommended for use in infants younger than 2 months of age.

ADVERSE REACTIONS

Topical application of the sulfonamides may produce sensitization and preclude later systemic use of these drugs. In addition, patients who have been sensitized by systemic sulfonamide administration may exhibit hypersensitivity reactions following topical application of the drugs.
Ophthalmic: Ocular irritation, chemosis, itching.
Included in the listing that follows are adverse reactions that have not been reported with these dosage forms but have been reported for the systemically absorbed sulfonamides.
Hematologic: Agranulocytosis, aplastic anemia, thrombocytopenia, leukopenia, hemolytic anemia, purpura, hypoprothrombinemia and methemoglobinemia.
Allergic reactions: Erythema multiforme (Stevens-Johnson syndrome), generalized skin eruptions, epidermal necrolysis, urticaria, serum sickness, pruritus, exfoliative dermatitis, anaphylactoid reactions, periorbital edema, conjunctival and scleral injection, photosensitization, arthralgia and allergic myocarditis.
Gastrointestinal reactions: Nausea, emesis, abdominal pains, hepatitis, hepatocellular necrosis, diarrhea, anorexia, pancreatitis and stomatitis.
C.N.S. reactions: Headache, peripheral neuritis, mental depression, convulsions, ataxia, hallucinations, tinnitus, vertigo and insomnia.
Miscellaneous reactions: Drug fever, chills, and toxic nephrosis with oliguria and anuria. Periarteritis, nodosa and L.E. phenomenon have occurred.
Endocrine: The sulfonamides bear certain chemical similarities to some goitrogens, diuretics (acetazolamide and the thiazides) and oral hypoglycemic agents. Goiter production, diuresis and hypoglycemia have occurred rarely in patients receiving sulfonamides. Cross sensitivity may exist with these agents.

DOSAGE AND ADMINISTRATION

Solution: Instill two or three drops in the eye three or more times daily. Care should be taken not to touch dropper tip to any surface, since contamination of the solution may result.
Ointment: Instill small amount in the lower conjunctival sac one to three times daily and at bedtime.

HOW SUPPLIED

Gantrisin Ophthalmic Solution, containing 4% (40 mg/ml) sulfisoxazole in the form of the diolamine salt—½ oz bottles with dropper (NDC 0004-1702-39).
Gantrisin Ophthalmic Ointment, containing 4% sulfisoxazole in the form of the diolamine salt—⅛ oz tubes (NDC 0004-1501-41).
Both dosage forms are stable at room temperature and do not require refrigeration.
P.I. 0885

GANTRISIN® ℞
[gan 'tris-in]
sulfisoxazole/Roche Tablets
GANTRISIN® ℞
acetyl sulfisoxazole/Roche
Pediatric Suspension and Syrup

The following text is complete prescribing information based on official labeling in effect June 1, 1989.

DESCRIPTION

Gantrisin (brand of sulfisoxazole/Roche) is an antibacterial sulfonamide available in tablets, pediatric suspension and syrup for oral administration. Each tablet contains 0.5 Gm sulfisoxazole with corn starch, gelatin, lactose and magnesium stearate. Each teaspoonful (5 mL) of the pediatric suspension contains the equivalent of approximately 0.5 Gm sulfisoxazole in the form of acetyl sulfisoxazole in a vehicle containing 0.3 percent alcohol, carboxymethylcellulose (sodium), citric acid, methylcellulose, parabens (methyl and

propyl), partial invert sugar, sodium citrate, sorbitan monolaurate, sucrose, flavors and water. Each teaspoonful (5 mL) of the syrup contains the equivalent of approximately 0.5 Gm sulfisoxazole in the form of acetyl sulfisoxazole in a vehicle containing 0.9 percent alcohol, benzoic acid, carrageenan, citric acid, cocoa, sodium citrate, sorbitan monolaurate, sucrose, flavors and water.
Sulfisoxazole is N^1-(3,4-dimethyl-5-isoxazoly)sulfanilamide. It is a white to slightly yellowish, odorless, slightly bitter, crystalline powder that is soluble in alcohol and very slightly soluble in water. Sulfisoxazole has a molecular weight of 267.30.
Acetyl sulfisoxazole, the tasteless form of sulfisoxazole, is N^1-acetyl sulfisoxazole and must be distinguished from N^4-acetyl sulfisoxazole, which is a metabolite of sulfisoxazole. Acetyl sulfisoxazole is a white or slightly yellow, crystalline powder that is slightly soluble in alcohol and practically insoluble in water. Acetyl sulfisoxazole has a molecular weight of 309.34.

CLINICAL PHARMACOLOGY

Following oral administration, sulfisoxazole is rapidly and completely absorbed; the small intestine is the major site of absorption, but some of the drug is absorbed from the stomach. Sulfisoxazole exists in the blood as unbound, protein-bound and conjugated forms. Sulfisoxazole is metabolized primarily by acetylation and oxidation in the liver. The free form is considered to be the therapeutically active form. Approximately 85% of sulfisoxazole is bound to plasma proteins, primarily to albumin; of the unbound portion, 65% to 72% is in the nonacetylated form.
Maximum plasma concentrations of intact sulfisoxazole following a single 2-Gm oral dose of sulfisoxazole to healthy adult volunteers ranged from 127 to 211 mcg/mL (mean, 169 mcg/mL) and the time of peak plasma concentration ranged from 1 to 4 hours (mean, 2.5 hours). The half-life of elimination of sulfisoxazole ranged from 4.6 to 7.8 hours after oral administration. The elimination of sulfisoxazole has been shown to be slower in elderly subjects (63 to 75 years) with diminished renal function (creatinine clearance, 37 to 68 mL/min).[1] After multiple dose oral administration of 500 mg Q.I.D. to healthy volunteers, the average steady-state plasma concentrations of intact sulfisoxazole ranged from 49.9 to 88.8 mcg/mL (mean, 63.4 mcg/mL).[2]
N^1-acetyl sulfisoxazole is metabolized to sulfisoxazole by digestive enzymes in the gastrointestinal tract and is absorbed as sulfisoxazole. This enzymatic splitting is presumed to be responsible for slower absorption and lower peak blood concentrations than are attained following administration of an equal oral dose of sulfisoxazole. With continued administration of acetyl sulfisoxazole, blood concentrations approximate those of sulfisoxazole. Following a single 4-Gm dose of acetyl sulfisoxazole to healthy volunteers, maximum plasma concentrations of sulfisoxazole ranged from 122 to 282 mcg/mL (mean, 181 mcg/mL) for the pediatric suspension and from 101 to 202 mcg/mL (mean, 144 mcg/mL) for the syrup, and occurred between 2 and 6 hours postadministration. The half-lives of elimination from plasma ranged from 5.4 to 7.4 and from 5.9 to 8.5 hours, respectively.
Sulfisoxazole and acetylated metabolites are excreted primarily by the kidneys through glomerular filtration. Urine concentrations of sulfisoxazole are considerably higher than are the concentrations in blood. The mean urinary excretion recovery following oral administration of sulfisoxazole is 97% within 48 hours, of which 52% is intact drug, with the remaining as the N^4-acetylated metabolite. Following administration of acetyl sulfisoxazole syrup or suspension, approximately 58% is excreted in the urine as total drug within 72 hours.
Sulfisoxazole is distributed only in extracellular body water. It readily crosses the placental barrier and enters into fetal circulation; it is also secreted in breast milk. It also crosses the blood-brain barrier. In healthy subjects, cerebrospinal fluid concentrations of sulfisoxazole vary; in patients with meningitis, however, concentrations of free drug as high as 94 mcg/mL have been reported.
Microbiology: The systemic sulfonamides are bacteriostatic agents. The spectrum of activity is similar for all. Sulfonamides inhibit bacterial synthesis of dihydrofolic acid by competing with *para*-aminobenzoic acid (PABA). Resistant strains are capable of utilizing folic acid precursors or preformed folic acid.

INDICATIONS AND USAGE

Acute, recurrent or chronic urinary tract infections (primarily pyelonephritis, pyelitis and cystitis) due to susceptible organisms (usually *Escherichia coli, Klebsiella-Enterobacter*, staphylococcus, *Proteus mirabilis* and, less frequently, *Proteus vulgaris*) in the absence of obstructive uropathy or foreign bodies.
Meningococcal meningitis where the organism has been demonstrated to be susceptible. *Haemophilus influenzae* meningitis as adjunctive therapy with parenteral streptomycin.

Continued on next page

Roche Labs.—Cont.

Meningococcal meningitis prophylaxis when sulfonamide-sensitive group A strains are known to prevail in family groups or larger closed populations. (The prophylactic usefulness of sulfonamides when group B or C infections are prevalent has not been proven and in closed population groups may be harmful.)

Acute otitis media due to *Haemophilus influenzae* when used concomitantly with adequate doses of penicillin or erythromycin (see appropriate labeling for prescribing information). Trachoma. Inclusion conjunctivitis. Nocardiosis. Chancroid. Toxoplasmosis as adjunctive therapy with pyrimethamine. Malaria due to chloroquine-resistant strains of *Plasmodium falciparum*, when used as adjunctive therapy.

Important Note: In vitro sulfonamide susceptibility tests are not always reliable. The test must be carefully coordinated with bacteriologic and clinical response. When the patient is already taking sulfonamides, follow-up cultures should have aminobenzoic acid added to the culture media.

Currently, the increasing frequency of resistant organisms is a limitation of the usefulness of antibacterial agents including the sulfonamides, especially in the treatment of chronic and recurrent urinary tract infections.

Wide variation in blood concentrations may result with identical doses. Blood concentrations should be measured in patients receiving sulfonamides for serious infections. Free sulfonamide blood concentrations of 5 to 15 mg/100 mL may be considered therapeutically effective for most infections, with blood concentrations of 12 to 15 mg/100 mL optimal for serious infections; 20 mg/100 mL should be the maximum total sulfonamide concentration, since adverse reactions occur more frequently above this concentration.

CONTRAINDICATIONS

Hypersensitivity to sulfonamides. Infants less than 2 months of age (except in the treatment of congenital toxoplasmosis as adjunctive therapy with pyrimethamine). Pregnancy at term and during the nursing period, because sulfonamides pass the placenta and are excreted in the milk and may cause kernicterus.

WARNINGS

The sulfonamides should not be used for the treatment of group A beta-hemolytic streptococcal infections. In an established infection, they will not eradicate the streptococcus, and therefore will not prevent sequelae such as rheumatic fever and glomerulonephritis.

Deaths associated with the administration of sulfonamides have been reported from hypersensitivity reactions, hepatocellular necrosis, agranulocytosis, aplastic anemia and other blood dyscrasias.

The presence of clinical signs such as sore throat, fever, arthralgia, cough, shortness of breath, pallor, purpura or jaundice may be early indications of serious reactions, including serious blood disorders.

PRECAUTIONS

General: Sulfonamides should be given with caution to patients with impaired renal or hepatic function and to those with severe allergy or bronchial asthma. In glucose-6-phosphate dehydrogenase-deficient individuals, hemolysis may occur. This reaction is frequently dose-related. Patients should be instructed to maintain an adequate fluid intake in order to prevent crystalluria and stone formation.

Laboratory tests: Complete blood counts should be done frequently in patients receiving sulfonamides. If a significant reduction in the count of any formed blood element is noted, Gantrisin should be discontinued. Urinalyses with careful microscopic examination and renal function tests should be performed during therapy, particularly for those patients with impaired renal function.

Drug interactions: It has been reported that sulfisoxazole may prolong the prothrombin time in patients who are receiving the anticoagulant warfarin. This interaction should be kept in mind when Gantrisin is given to patients already on anticoagulant therapy, and the coagulation time should be reassessed.

It has been proposed that sulfisoxazole competes with thiopental for plasma protein binding. In one study involving 48 patients, intravenous sulfisoxazole reduced the amount of thiopental required for anesthesia and shortened the awakening time. It is not known whether chronic oral doses of sulfisoxazole would have a similar effect. Until more is known about this interaction, physicians should be aware that patients receiving sulfisoxazole might require less thiopental for anesthesia.

Sulfonamides can displace methotrexate from plasma protein-binding sites, thus increasing free methotrexate concentrations. Studies in man have shown sulfisoxazole infusions to decrease plasma protein-bound methotrexate by one-fourth.

Sulfisoxazole can also potentiate the blood sugar lowering activity of sulfonylureas.

Carcinogenesis, mutagenesis, impairment of fertility: Carcinogenesis: Sulfisoxazole was not carcinogenic in either sex

when administered by gavage for 103 weeks at dosages up to 2000 mg/kg/day to mice or 400 mg/kg/day to rats.

Mutagenesis: Bacterial mutagenic studies have not been performed with sulfisoxazole. However, Gantrisin was not observed to be mutagenic in *E. coli* Sd-4-73 when tested in the absence of a metabolic activating system.

Impairment of fertility: No effects on mating behavior, conception rate or fertility index (percent pregnant) were observed in a reproduction study in rats given 800 mg/kg/day sulfisoxazole.

Pregnancy: Teratogenic effects: Pregnancy Category C. Sulfisoxazole was not teratogenic in either rats or rabbits at dosages of 800 mg/kg/day. However, in another teratogenicity study, cleft palates developed in both rats and mice after administration of 1000 mg/kg/day sulfisoxazole; skeletal defects were also observed in rats. This dose is 9 to 18 times the usual adult dosage for Gantrisin.

There are no adequate and well-controlled studies of Gantrisin in pregnant women. Gantrisin should be used during pregnancy only if the potential benefit justifies the potential risk to the fetus.

Nonteratogenic effects: See CONTRAINDICATIONS section.

Nursing mothers: See CONTRAINDICATIONS section.

Pediatric use: Gantrisin is not recommended for use in infants younger than 2 months of age except in the treatment of congenital toxoplasmosis as adjunctive therapy with pyrimethamine. (See CONTRAINDICATIONS section.)

ADVERSE REACTIONS

Included in the listing that follows are adverse reactions that have not been reported with this specific drug; however, the pharmacologic similarities among the sulfonamides require that each of the reactions be considered with the administration of any of the Gantrisin dosage forms.

Hematologic: Agranulocytosis, aplastic anemia, thrombocytopenia, leukopenia, hemolytic anemia, purpura, hypoprothrombinemia, methemoglobinemia, eosinophilia.

Allergic reactions: Anaphylaxis, allergic myocarditis, serum sickness, conjunctival and scleral injection, generalized allergic reactions. In addition, periarteritis nodosa and systemic lupus erythematosus have been reported.

Dermatologic: Stevens-Johnson syndrome, epidermal necrolysis, erythema multiforme, exfoliative dermatitis, photosensitivity, pruritus, urticaria, rash, generalized skin eruptions.

Gastrointestinal: Hepatitis, hepatocellular necrosis, pseudomembranous enterocolitis, pancreatitis, stomatitis, glossitis, nausea, emesis, abdominal pain, diarrhea, anorexia.

Genitourinary: Creatinine elevation, toxic nephrosis with oliguria and anuria. The frequency of renal complications is considerably lower in patients receiving the more soluble sulfonamides.

Neurologic: Convulsions, peripheral neuritis, ataxia, vertigo, tinnitus, headache.

Psychiatric: Hallucinations, depression, apathy.

Endocrine: The sulfonamides bear certain chemical similarities to some goitrogens, diuretics (acetazolamide and the thiazides) and oral hypoglycemic agents. Cross-sensitivity may exist with these agents. Diuresis and hypoglycemia have occurred rarely in patients receiving sulfonamides.

Musculoskeletal: Arthralgia, myalgia.

Respiratory: Pulmonary infiltrates.

Miscellaneous: Edema (including periorbital), pyrexia, chills, weakness, fatigue, insomnia.

OVERDOSAGE

The amount of a single dose of sulfisoxazole that is either associated with symptoms of overdosage or is likely to be life-threatening has not been reported. Signs and symptoms of overdosage reported with sulfonamides include anorexia, colic, nausea, vomiting, dizziness, headache, drowsiness and unconsciousness. Pyrexia, hematuria and crystalluria may be noted. Blood dyscrasias and jaundice are potential late manifestations of overdosage.

General principles of treatment include the immediate discontinuation of the drug; institution of gastric lavage or emesis; forcing oral fluids; and the administration of intravenous fluids if urine output is low and renal function is normal. The patient should be monitored with blood counts and appropriate blood chemistries, including electrolytes. If a significant blood dyscrasia or jaundice occurs, specific therapy should be instituted for these complications. Peritoneal dialysis is not effective and hemodialysis is only moderately effective in eliminating sulfonamides.

The acute toxicity of sulfisoxazole in animals is as follows:

Species	$LD_{50} \pm S.E.$ (mg/kg)
mouse	5700 ± 235
rats	$> 10,000$
rabbits	> 2000

DOSAGE AND ADMINISTRATION

Systemic sulfonamides are contraindicated in infants under 2 months of age, except in the treatment of congenital toxoplasmosis as adjunctive therapy with pyrimethamine.

Usual dose for infants over 2 months of age and children: Initial dose: One-half of the 24-hour dose. Maintenance dose: 150 mg/kg/24 hours or 4 Gm/M²/24 hours—dose to be divided into 4 to 6 doses/24 hours. The maximum dose should not exceed 6 Gm/24 hours.

Usual adult dose: Initial dose: 2 to 4 Gm. Maintenance dose: 4 to 8 Gm/24 hours, divided in 4 to 6 doses/24 hours.

HOW SUPPLIED

Tablets (white, scored), containing 0.5 Gm sulfisoxazole—bottles of 100 (NDC 0004-0009-01) and 500 (NDC 0004-0009-14); Tel-E-Dose® packages of 100 (NDC 0004-0009-49). Imprint on tablets: ROCHE GANTRISIN®.

Pediatric Suspension (raspberry flavored), containing acetyl sulfisoxazole equivalent to approximately 0.5 Gm sulfisoxazole per teaspoonful (5 mL)—bottles of 4 oz (NDC 0004-1003-30) and 16 oz (1 pint) (NDC 0004-1003-28).

Syrup (chocolate flavored), containing acetyl sulfisoxazole equivalent to approximately 0.5 Gm sulfisoxazole per teaspoonful (5 mL)—bottles of 16 oz (1 pint) (NDC 0004-1004-28).

REFERENCES

1. Boisvert A, Barbeau G, Belanger PM: Pharmacokinetics of sulfisoxazole in young and elderly subjects. *Gerontology 30:* 125–131, 1984
2. Oie S, Gambertoglio JG, Fleckenstein L: Comparison of the disposition of total and unbound sulfisoxazole after single and multiple dosing. *J Pharmacokinet Biopharm 10:* 157–172, 1982
P.I. 0788

Shown in Product Identification Section, page 425

KLONOPIN® ℞

[*klon'o-pin*]
(clonazepam/Roche)
(formerly known as Clonopin®)

The following text is complete prescribing information based on official labeling in effect June 1, 1989.

DESCRIPTION

Klonopin is available as scored tablets containing 0.5 mg, 1 mg or 2 mg clonazepam/Roche. Each tablet also contains lactose, magnesium stearate, microcrystalline cellulose and corn starch, with the following dye systems: 0.5 mg—FD&C Yellow No. 6; 1 mg—FD&C Blue No. 1 and FD&C Blue No. 2. Chemically, clonazepam is 5-(2-chlorophenyl)-1,3-dihydro-7-nitro-2H-1,4-benzodiazepin-2-one. It is a light yellow crystalline powder. It has a molecular weight of 315.7.

ACTIONS

In laboratory animals, Klonopin exhibits several pharmacologic properties which are characteristic of the benzodiazepine class of drugs. Convulsions produced in rodents by pentylenetetrazol or electrical stimulation are antagonized, as are convulsions produced by photic stimulation in susceptible baboons. A taming effect in aggressive primates, muscle weakness and hypnosis are likewise produced by Klonopin. In humans it is capable of suppressing the spike and wave discharge in absence seizures (petit mal) and decreasing the frequency, amplitude, duration and spread of discharge in minor motor seizures.

Single oral dose administration of Klonopin to humans gave maximum blood levels of drug, in most cases, within one to two hours. The half-life of the parent compound varied from approximately 18 to 50 hours, and the major route of excretion was in the urine. In humans, five metabolites have been identified. In general, the biotransformation of clonazepam followed two pathways: oxidative hydroxylation at the C-3 position and reduction of the 7-nitro function to form 7-amino and/or 7-acetyl-amino derivatives.

INDICATIONS

Klonopin is useful alone or as an adjunct in the treatment of the Lennox-Gastaut syndrome (petit mal variant), akinetic and myoclonic seizures. In patients with absence seizures (petit mal) who have failed to respond to succinimides, Klonopin may be useful.

In some studies, up to 30% of patients have shown a loss of anticonvulsant activity, often within three months of administration. In some cases, dosage adjustment may reestablish efficacy.

CONTRAINDICATIONS

Klonopin should not be used in patients with a history of sensitivity to benzodiazepines, nor in patients with clinical or biochemical evidence of significant liver disease. It may be used in patients with open angle glaucoma who are receiving appropriate therapy, but is contraindicated in acute narrow angle glaucoma.

WARNINGS

Since Klonopin produces CNS depression, patients receiving this drug should be cautioned against engaging in hazardous occupations requiring mental alertness, such as operating machinery or driving a motor vehicle. They should also be warned about the concomitant use of alcohol or other CNS-depressant drugs during Klonopin therapy (see Drug Interactions).

Usage in Pregnancy: The effects of Klonopin in human pregnancy and nursing infants are unknown.

Recent reports suggest an association between the use of anticonvulsant drugs by women with epilepsy and an elevated incidence of birth defects in children born to these women. Data are more extensive with respect to diphenylhydantoin and phenobarbital, but these are also the most commonly prescribed anticonvulsants; less systematic or anecdotal reports suggest a possible similar association with the use of all known anticonvulsant drugs.

The reports suggesting an elevated incidence of birth defects in children of drug-treated epileptic women cannot be regarded as adequate to prove a definite cause and effect relationship. There are intrinsic methodologic problems in obtaining adequate data on drug teratogenicity in humans; the possibility also exists that other factors, *e.g.*, genetic factors or the epileptic condition itself, may be more important than drug therapy in leading to birth defects. The great majority of mothers on anticonvulsant medication deliver normal infants. It is important to note that anticonvulsant drugs should not be discontinued in patients in whom the drug is administered to prevent seizures because of the strong possibility of precipitating status epilepticus with attendant hypoxia and threat to life. In individual cases where the severity and frequency of the seizure disorder are such that the removal of medication does not pose a serious threat to the patient, discontinuation of the drug may be considered prior to and during pregnancy, although it cannot be said with any confidence that even mild seizures do not pose some hazards to the developing embryo or fetus.

These considerations should be weighed in treating or counseling epileptic women of childbearing potential.

Use of Klonopin in women of childbearing potential should be considered only when the clinical situation warrants the risk. Mothers receiving Klonopin should not breast feed their infants.

In a two-generation reproduction study with Klonopin given orally to rats at 10 or 100 mg/kg/day, there was a decrease in the number of pregnancies and a decrease in the number of offspring surviving until weaning. When Klonopin was administered orally to pregnant rabbits at 0.2, 1.0, 5.0 or 10.0 mg/kg/day, a nondose-related incidence of cleft palates, open eyelids, fused sternebrae and limb defects was observed at the 0.2 and 5.0 mg/kg/day levels. Nearly all of the malformations were seen from one dam in each of the affected dosages.

Usage in Children: Because of the possibility that adverse effects on physical or mental development could become apparent only after many years, a benefit-risk consideration of the long-term use of Klonopin is important in pediatric patients.

Physical and Psychological Dependence: Withdrawal symptoms similar in character to those noted with barbiturates and alcohol have occurred following abrupt discontinuance of benzodiazepine drugs. These symptoms include convulsions, tremor, abdominal and muscle cramps, vomiting and sweating. Addiction-prone individuals, such as drug addicts or alcoholics, should be under careful surveillance when receiving benzodiazepines because of the predisposition of such patients to habituation and dependence.

PRECAUTIONS

When used in patients in whom several different types of seizure disorders coexist, Klonopin may increase the incidence or precipitate the onset of generalized tonic-clonic seizures (grand mal). This may require the addition of appropriate anticonvulsants or an increase in their dosages. The concomitant use of valproic acid and clonazepam may produce absence status.

Periodic blood counts and liver function tests are advisable during long-term therapy with Klonopin.

The abrupt withdrawal of Klonopin, particularly in those patients on long-term, high-dose therapy, may precipitate status epilepticus. Therefore, when discontinuing Klonopin, gradual withdrawal is essential. While Klonopin is being gradually withdrawn, the simultaneous substitution of another anticonvulsant may be indicated. Metabolites of Klonopin are excreted by the kidneys; to avoid their excess accumulation, caution should be exercised in the administration of the drug to patients with impaired renal function. Klonopin may produce an increase in salivation. This should be considered before giving the drug to patients who have difficulty handling secretions. Because of this and the possibility of respiratory depression, Klonopin should be used with caution in patients with chronic respiratory diseases.

ADVERSE REACTIONS

The most frequently occurring side effects of Klonopin are referable to CNS depression. Experience to date has shown that drowsiness has occurred in approximately 50% of patients and ataxia in approximately 30%. In some cases, these may diminish with time; behavior problems have been noted in approximately 25% of patients. Others, listed by system, are:

Neurologic: Abnormal eye movements, aphonia, choreiform movements, coma, diplopia, dysarthria, dysdiadochokinesis, "glassy-eyed" appearance, headache, hemiparesis, hypotonia, nystagmus, respiratory depression, slurred speech, tremor, vertigo.

Psychiatric: Confusion, depression, forgetfulness, hallucinations, hysteria, increased libido, insomnia, psychosis, suicidal attempt (the behavior effects are more likely to occur in patients with a history of psychiatric disturbances).

Respiratory: Chest congestion, rhinorrhea, shortness of breath, hypersecretion in upper respiratory passages.

Cardiovascular: Palpitations.

Dermatologic: Hair loss, hirsutism, skin rash, ankle and facial edema.

Gastrointestinal: Anorexia, coated tongue, constipation, diarrhea, dry mouth, encopresis, gastritis, hepatomegaly, increased appetite, nausea, sore gums.

Genitourinary: Dysuria, enuresis, nocturia, urinary retention.

Musculoskeletal: Muscle weakness, pains.

Miscellaneous: Dehydration, general deterioration, fever, lymphadenopathy, weight loss or gain.

Hematopoietic: Anemia, leukopenia, thrombocytopenia, eosinophilia.

Hepatic: Transient elevations of serum transaminases and alkaline phosphatase.

DRUG INTERACTIONS

The CNS-depressant action of the benzodiazepine class of drugs may be potentiated by alcohol, narcotics, barbiturates, nonbarbiturate hypnotics, antianxiety agents, the phenothiazines, thioxanthene and butyrophenone classes of antipsychotic agents, monoamine oxidase inhibitors and the tricyclic antidepressants, and by other anticonvulsant drugs.

OVERDOSAGE

Symptoms of Klonopin overdosage, like those produced by other CNS depressants, include somnolence, confusion, coma and diminished reflexes. Treatment includes monitoring of respiration, pulse and blood pressure, general supportive measures and immediate gastric lavage. Intravenous fluids should be administered and an adequate airway maintained. Hypotension may be combated by the use of levarterenol or metaraminol. Methylphenidate or caffeine and sodium benzoate may be given to combat CNS depression. Dialysis is of no known value.

DOSAGE AND ADMINISTRATION

Infants and Children: Klonopin is administered orally. In order to minimize drowsiness, the initial dose for infants and children (up to 10 years of age or 30 kg of body weight) should be between 0.01 and 0.03 mg/kg/day but not to exceed 0.05 mg/kg/day given in two or three divided doses. Dosage should be increased by no more than 0.25 to 0.5 mg every third day until a daily maintenance dose of 0.1 to 0.2 mg/kg of body weight has been reached unless seizures are controlled or side effects preclude further increase. Whenever possible, the daily dose should be divided into three equal doses. If doses are not equally divided, the largest dose should be given before retiring.

Adults: The initial dose for adults should not exceed 1.5 mg/day divided into three doses. Dosage may be increased in increments of 0.5 to 1 mg every three days until seizures are adequately controlled or until side effects preclude any further increase. Maintenance dosage must be individualized for each patient depending upon response. Maximum recommended daily dose is 20 mg.

The use of multiple anticonvulsants may result in an increase of depressant adverse effects. This should be considered before adding Klonopin to an existing anticonvulsant regimen.

HOW SUPPLIED

Scored tablets—0.5 mg, orange; 1 mg, blue; 2 mg, white—Prescription Paks of 100.

P.I. 1085

     Shown in Product Identification Section, page 425

KONAKION®   ℞
[ko-nak 'e-on]
(phytonadione/Roche)
INJECTABLE

The following text is complete prescribing information based on official labeling in effect June 1, 1989.

DESCRIPTION

Konakion (phytonadione/Roche) Injectable, a prothrombogenic vitamin, is an essentially clear, sterile, aqueous dispersion of vitamin K_1. It is intended for intramuscular administration only. Konakion Injectable is available in the following concentrations:

0.5-mL Ampuls —each 0.5 mL contains 1 mg phytonadione (vitamin K_1) compounded with 10 mg polysorbate 80, 0.45% phenol as preservative, 10.4 mg propylene glycol, 0.17 mg sodium acetate and 0.00002 mL glacial acetic acid.

1-mL Ampuls —each mL contains 10 mg phytonadione (vitamine K_1) compounded with 40 mg polysorbate 80, 20.7 mg propylene glycol, 0.8 mg sodium acetate and 0.00006 mL glacial acetic acid.

Phytonadione is a fat-soluble naphthoquinone derivative which is identical to naturally occurring vitamin K_1. Chemically, phytonadione is 1,4-naphthalenedione, 2-methyl-3-(3,7,11,15-tetramethyl-2-hexadecenyl)-[R-[R*, R*-(E)]]. It is a clear, yellow to amber, very viscous liquid and is insoluble in water and slightly soluble in alcohol. It has a molecular weight of 450.70.

CLINICAL PHARMACOLOGY

Phytonadione possesses the same type and degree of activity as does naturally occurring vitamin K, which is necessary for the synthesis in the liver of blood coagulation factors prothrombin (factor II), proconvertin (factor VII), plasma thromboplastin component (factor IX) and Stuart factor (factor X). The prothrombin test is sensitive to the concentrations of factors II, VII and X. The mechanism by which vitamin K_1 promotes formation of these clotting factors in the liver is not known, but animal data suggest that it acts as an enzyme or catalyst upon a substrate within the liver or combines with an apoenzyme (AE) to form an active enzyme (AEK) which is then involved in prothrombin synthesis. Following intramuscular injection, phytonadione is readily absorbed, almost entirely by way of the lymph. After absorption, phytonadione is initially concentrated in the liver, but the concentration declines rapidly. Very little vitamin K accumulates in tissues. There is considerable evidence that the synthesis of prothrombin and the related vitamin K-dependent blood clotting factors are linked to a metabolic cycle in which vitamin K_1 is oxidized and reduced to its inactive 2,3 epoxide metabolite. This vitamin K epoxide cycle is mediated by at least two enzymes which have been partially characterized as phytonadione epoxidase and phytonadione epoxide reductase. Phytonadione is known to cross the placenta.

Following intravenous administration of tritiated vitamin K_1, the half-life of elimination of phytonadione ranged from two to four hours. The lipid-soluble radioactivity in the plasma, which is assumed to represent the injected phytonadione, was rapidly cleared and resembles the clearance of orally administered phytonadione.

The action of the aqueous dispersion when administered parenterally is generally detectable within an hour or two, and hemorrhage is usually controlled within three to six hours. A normal prothrombin level may often be obtained in 12 to 14 hours.

INDICATIONS AND USAGE

Konakion is indicated for:
- anticoagulant-induced prothrombin deficiency;
- prophylaxis and therapy of hemorrhagic disease of the newborn, and it may also be given to the mother before delivery;
- hypoprothrombinemia due to oral antibacterial therapy;
- hypoprothrombinemia secondary to factors limiting absorption or synthesis of vitamin K, *e.g.*, obstructive jaundice, biliary fistula, sprue, ulcerative colitis, celiac disease, intestinal resection, cystic fibrosis of the pancreas and regional enteritis;
- other drug-induced hypoprothrombinemia (such as that due to salicylates) when it is definitely shown that the result is due to interference with vitamin K metabolism.

In the prophylaxis and treatment of hemorrhagic disease of the newborn, Konakion has demonstrated a greater margin of safety than that of the water-soluble vitamin K analogs.

CONTRAINDICATIONS

Konakion is contraindicated in patients with known hypersensitivity to the drug.

WARNINGS

Konakion does not directly counteract the effects of oral anticoagulants, but it promotes the synthesis of prothrombin by the liver, usually within two hours. Fresh plasma or blood transfusions may be required for severe blood loss or lack of response to vitamin K. Phytonadione will not counteract the anticoagulant action of heparin.

When vitamin K_1 is used to correct excessive anticoagulant-induced hypoprothrombinemia but anticoagulant therapy is still indicated, the patient is again faced with the clotting hazards existing prior to starting the anticoagulant therapy. Phytonadione is not a clotting agent, but overzealous therapy with vitamin K may restore conditions which originally permitted thromboembolic phenomena. Dosage, therefore, should be kept as low as possible, and prothrombin time should be checked regularly as clinical conditions indicate.

PRECAUTIONS

General: Temporary resistance to prothrombin-depressing anticoagulants may result, especially when larger doses of phytonadione are used. If relatively large doses have been employed, it may be necessary when reinstituting anticoagulant therapy to use somewhat larger doses of the prothrom-

Continued on next page

Roche Labs.—Cont.

bin-depressing anticoagulant or one which has a different mode of action, such as heparin.

Since the liver is the site of metabolic synthesis of prothrombin, hypoprothrombinemia resulting from hepatocellular damage is not corrected by administration of vitamin K. Repeated large doses of vitamin K are not warranted in liver disease if the response to initial use of the vitamin is unsatisfactory (Koller test).

Failure to respond to vitamin K may indicate that a coagulation defect is present or that the condition being treated is unresponsive to vitamin K.

Laboratory tests: The dose and frequency of administration and duration of treatment depend on the severity of the prothrombin deficiency and should be regulated by repeated determinations of prothrombin time.

Drug interactions: Because vitamin K_1 is a pharmacologic antagonist to coumarin and indanedione derivatives, patients being treated with these anticoagulants should not receive Konakion except for the treatment of excessive hypoprothrombinemia.

Carcinogenesis, mutagenesis, impairment of fertility: Konakion has not undergone adequate animal testing to evaluate carcinogenic or mutagenic potential, or impairment of fertility.

Pregnancy: Teratogenic effects: Pregnancy Category C. Animal reproduction studies have not been conducted with phytonadione. When menaquinone (vitamin K_2), which is structurally similar to phytonadione, was administered to mice and rats on gestation days 7 through 14 at maximum doses of 1000 mg/kg/day (p.o.) and 100 mg/kg/day (i.p.), no teratogenicity was observed. It is not known whether Konakion can cause fetal harm when administered to pregnant women or can affect reproductive capacity. Konakion should be given to pregnant women only if clearly needed.

Nonteratogenic effects: Retardation of skeletal ossification has been reported in mice with vitamin K_2 (menaquinone).

Nursing mothers: A study has shown that vitamin K is excreted in human milk. This should be considered if it is necessary to administer Konakion to a nursing mother.

Pediatric use: Hemolysis and jaundice in newborns, particularly in premature infants, may be related to the dose of Konakion. Therefore, the recommended dose should not be exceeded (see ADVERSE REACTIONS and DOSAGE AND ADMINISTRATION sections).

ADVERSE REACTIONS

Allergic reactions: The possibility of allergic reactions, including an anaphylactoid reaction, should be kept in mind.

Miscellaneous: Pain, swelling and tenderness at the injection site have occurred rarely.

Although Konakion has a greater margin of safety than the water-soluble vitamin K analogs, hyperbillirubinemia has been reported in the newborn, particularly in prematures when used at 5 to 10 times the recommended dosage. This effect, with the possibility of attendant kernicterus, should be considered if such dosages are deemed necessary.

In patients with severe hepatic disease, large doses of phytonadione may further depress liver function. Paradoxically, the administration of excessive doses of vitamin K or its analogs in an attempt to correct the hypoprothrombinemia associated with severe hepatitis or cirrhosis may actually result in a further depression of the concentration of prothrombin (also see PRECAUTIONS: *General* section).

OVERDOSAGE

There are no data available on overdosage of Konakion in man. Phytonadione is nontoxic to animals, even when given in huge amounts. The acute toxicity of vitamin K_1 is as follows:

Species	Route	LD_{50}
Mouse	p.o.	> 25 Gm/kg
Mouse	i.p.	> 25 Gm/kg
Mouse*	i.v.	57 (48–112) mg/kg

* Konakion formulation used

If anticoagulation is needed following overdosage of phytonadione, heparin may be used.

DOSAGE AND ADMINISTRATION

The U.S. Recommended Daily Allowances for vitamin K in humans have not been established officially. The adequate daily dietary intake of vitamin K for adults has been estimated to be 70 to 140 mcg; for infants 10 to 20 mcg; for children and adolescents 15 to 100 mcg. The dietary abundance of vitamin K normally satisfies the requirements except for the neonatal period of 5 to 8 days.

INFANTS	ADULTS
Neonatal hemorrhage due to hypoprothrombinemia: 0.5 to 1 mg I.M. immediately after birth, which may be repeated if the mother	hypoprothrombinemia due to: ●*Anticoagulant therapy* (except of heparin type)—5 to 10 mg I.M. initially; up to 20 mg, if neces-

has received anticoagulant or anticonvulsant drug therapy, or if the infant develops bleeding tendencies. 1 to 5 mg I.M. may be given to the mother 12 to 24 hours before delivery.

sary.
●*Antibacterial therapy*—5 to 20 mg I.M.
●*Factors limiting absorption or synthesis*—2 to 20 mg I.M.
●*Other drugs* (e.g., salicylates) 2 to 20 mg I.M.

In older children and adults, injection of Konakion should be in the upper outer quadrant of the buttocks. In infants and young children, the anterolateral aspect of the thighs or the deltoid region is preferred so that danger of sciatic nerve injury is avoided.

It is recommended that Konakion be injected by itself, since phytonadione injection has been reported to be incompatible with many drugs in admixtures.

Parenteral drug products should be inspected visually for particulate matter and discoloration prior to administration, whenever solution and container permit. Slight opalescence may occur with Konakion ampuls, but this does not affect the safety or potency of the product.

Konakion is stable in the air, but it is photosensitive, decomposing with loss of potency on exposure to light. Therefore, it should be stored in a dark place and protected from light at all times. Konakion need not be refrigerated.

HOW SUPPLIED

0.5-mL Ampuls (1 mg phytonadione/0.5 mL)—boxes of 10 (NDC 0004-1907-06).

1-mL Ampuls (10 mg phytonadione/mL)—boxes of 10 (NDC 0004-1908-06).

STORE AT ROOM TEMPERATURE (15° to 30°C; 59° to 86°F). DO NOT FREEZE. PROTECT FROM LIGHT AT ALL TIMES.

P.I. 0288

LAROBEC® TABLETS　　　　　　　　　　℞
[lar 'o-bek]

The following text is complete prescribing information based on official labeling in effect June 1, 1989.

Each Larobec® tablet contains:	Quantity	U.S. RDA— Adults and children 4 or more years of age
Water-Soluble Vitamins		
Vitamin C (ascorbic acid)	500 mg	60 mg
Vitamin B_1 (as thiamine mononitrate)	15 mg	1.5 mg
Vitamin B_2 (riboflavin)	15 mg	1.7 mg
Niacin (as niacinamide)	100 mg	20 mg
Pantothenic acid (as calcium *d*-pantothenate)	18 mg	10 mg
Folic acid	0.5 mg	0.4 mg
Vitamin B_{12} (cyanocobalamin)	5 mcg	6 mcg

Each tablet also contains acacia, calcium sulfate, carnauba wax, hydrogenated vegetable oil, magnesium oxide, magnesium stearate, povidone, shellac, sodium benzoate, sugar and talc with the following dyes: FD&C Yellow No. 6, D&C Yellow No. 10 and titanium dioxide.

DESCRIPTION

Larobec is a prescription-only oral multivitamin tablet specially formulated for patients who require prophylactic or therapeutic nutritional supplementation of water-soluble vitamins and are receiving levodopa therapy for Parkinson's disease and syndrome. Larobec provides *therapeutic* levels of ascorbic acid, vitamins B_1, B_2, niacin, pantothenic acid and folic acid and a *supplemental* level of vitamin B_{12} *without* pyridoxine (vitamin B_6), which has been reported to reduce the clinical benefits of levodopa therapy.

CLINICAL PHARMACOLOGY

Vitamins are essential for maintenance of normal metabolic functions including hematopoiesis. The water-soluble vitamins play vital roles in the conversion of carbohydrate, protein and fat into tissue and energy. *Thiamine (B_1)* acts as a coenzyme in carbohydrate metabolism. *Riboflavin (B_2)* functions as a coenzyme in the electron transport system associated with conversion of tissue oxidations into usable energy. *Niacin* serves as a coenzyme in oxidation-reduction reactions in tissue respiration. *Pantothenic acid* functions as a coenzyme in various metabolic acetylation reactions. *Folic acid* and *cyanocobalamin (B_{12})* are metabolically interrelated. They are essential to nucleic acid synthesis and normal maturation of red blood cells. *Ascorbic acid (C)* performs a vital function in the process of cellular respiration, and is involved in both carbohydrate and amino acid metabolism. It is essential for collagen formation and tissue repair.

The water-soluble vitamins (B-complex and C) are not significantly stored by the body; excess quantities are excreted in the urine. They must be replenished regularly through diet or other means to maintain essential tissue levels. Thus these vitamins are rapidly depleted in conditions interfering with their intake or absorption.

INDICATIONS AND USAGE

Larobec is indicated for supportive nutritional supplementation when a water-soluble vitamin formulation (without pyridoxine) is required prophylactically or therapeutically in patients who are undergoing treatment with levodopa.

CONTRAINDICATIONS

Larobec is contraindicated in patients known to be hypersensitive to any of its components.

WARNINGS

Administration of vitamin B_6 may be required if signs of pyridoxine deficiency develop. Folic acid in doses above 0.1 mg daily may obscure pernicious anemia. Larobec is not intended for treatment of pernicious anemia or other megaloblastic anemias where vitamin B_{12} is deficient. Neurologic involvement may develop or progress, despite temporary remission of anemia, in patients with vitamin B_{12} deficiency who receive supplemental folic acid and who are inadequately treated with B_{12}.

PRECAUTIONS

General: Certain patients may require additional nutritional supplementation with fat-soluble vitamins and minerals according to the dietary habits of the individual. Larobec is not intended for treatment of severe specific vitamin deficiencies.

Information for the Patient: Because toxic reactions have been reported with injudicious use of certain vitamins, urge patients to follow your specific instructions regarding dosage regimen. As with any medication, advise patients to keep Larobec out of reach of children.

ADVERSE REACTIONS

Adverse reactions have been reported with specific vitamins, but generally at levels substantially higher than those in Larobec. However, allergic and idiosyncratic reactions are possible at lower levels.

DOSAGE AND ADMINISTRATION

Usual adult dosage: one tablet daily.
Larobec is available on prescription only.

HOW SUPPLIED

Orange-colored, capsule-shaped tablets—bottles of 100 (NDC 0004-0073-01).
Imprint on tablets: LAROBEC® ROCHE
P.I. 1185
Shown in Product Identification Section, page 425

LARODOPA®　　　　　　　　　　℞
[lar ''o-do 'pa]
(levodopa/Roche)

The following text is complete prescribing information based on official labeling in effect June 1, 1989.

> In order to reduce the high incidence of adverse reactions, it is necessary to individualize the therapy and to gradually increase the dosage to the desired therapeutic level.

DESCRIPTION

Larodopa is available as tablets and capsules containing 0.1 Gm, 0.25 Gm or 0.5 Gm levodopa. Each tablet also contains corn starch, magnesium stearate, microcrystalline cellulose, povidone, talc and D&C Red No. 7 lake dye. Each capsule also contains corn starch and talc. Gelatin capsule shells have the following dye systems: 100 mg—FD&C Blue No. 1, FD&C Red No. 3, D&C Red No. 33, FD&C Yellow No. 6 and D&C Yellow No. 10; 250 mg—FD&C Blue No. 1, D&C Red No. 33, FD&C Yellow No. 6; 500 mg—D&C Red No. 33, FD&C Yellow No. 6.

Chemically, levodopa is (−)-3-(3,4-dihydroxyphenyl)-*L*-alanine. It is a colorless, crystalline compound, slightly soluble in water and insoluble in alcohol, with a molecular weight of 197.2.

ACTIONS

Evidence indicates that the symptoms of Parkinson's disease are related to depletion of striatal dopamine. Since dopamine apparently does not cross the blood-brain barrier, its administration is ineffective in the treatment of Parkinson's disease. However, levodopa, the levo-rotatory isomer of dihydroxyphenylalanine (dopa) which is the metabolic precursor of dopamine, does cross the blood-brain barrier. Presumably it is converted into dopamine in the basal ganglia. This is generally thought to be the mechanism whereby oral levodopa acts in relieving the symptoms of Parkinson's disease.

The major urinary metabolites of levodopa in man appear to be dopamine and homovanillic acid (HVA). In 24-hour urine samples, HVA accounts for 13 to 42 percent of the ingested dose of levodopa.

INDICATIONS

Larodopa is indicated in the treatment of idiopathic Parkinson's disease (Paralysis Agitans), postencephalitic parkinsonism, symptomatic parkinsonism which may follow injury to the nervous system by carbon monoxide intoxication, and manganese intoxication. It is indicated in those elderly patients believed to develop parkinsonism in association with cerebral arteriosclerosis.

CONTRAINDICATIONS

Monoamine oxidase (MAO) inhibitors and Larodopa should not be given concomitantly and these inhibitors must be discontinued two weeks prior to initiating therapy with Larodopa. Larodopa is contraindicated in patients with known hypersensitivity to the drug and in narrow angle glaucoma.

Because levodopa may activate a malignant melanoma, it should not be used in patients with suspicious, undiagnosed skin lesions or a history of melanoma.

WARNINGS

Larodopa should be administered cautiously to patients with severe cardiovascular or pulmonary disease, bronchial asthma, renal, hepatic or endocrine disease.

Care should be exercised in administering Larodopa to patients with a history of myocardial infarction who have residual atrial, nodal or ventricular arrhythmias. If Larodopa is necessary in this type of patient, it should be used in a facility with a coronary care unit or an intensive care unit.

One must be on the alert for the possibility of upper gastrointestinal hemorrhage in those patients with a past history of active peptic ulcer disease.

All patients should be carefully observed for the development of depression with concomitant suicidal tendencies. Psychotic patients should be treated with caution.

Pyridoxine hydrochloride (vitamin B_6) in oral doses of 10 to 25 mg rapidly reverses the toxic and therapeutic effects of Larodopa. This should be considered before recommending vitamin preparations containing pyridoxine hydrochloride (vitamin B_6).

Usage in Pregnancy: The safety of Larodopa in women who are or who may become pregnant has not been established; hence it should be given only when the potential benefits have been weighed against possible hazards to mother and child. Studies in rodents have shown that levodopa at dosages in excess of 200 mg/kg/day has an adverse effect on fetal and postnatal growth and viability.

Larodopa should not be used in nursing mothers.

Usage in Children: The safety of Larodopa under the age of 12 has not been established.

PRECAUTIONS

Periodic evaluations of hepatic, hematopoietic, cardiovascular and renal function are recommended during extended therapy in all patients.

Patients with chronic wide angle glaucoma may be treated cautiously with Larodopa, provided the intraocular pressure is well controlled and the patient monitored carefully for changes in intraocular pressure during therapy.

Postural hypotension episodes have been reported as adverse reactions. Therefore, Larodopa should be administered to patients on antihypertensive drug cautiously (for patients receiving pargyline, see note on MAO inhibitors contraindications), and it may be necessary to adjust the dosage of the antihypertensive drugs.

ADVERSE REACTIONS

The most serious adverse reactions associated with the administration of Larodopa having frequent occurrences are: adventitious movements such as choreiform and/or dystonic movements. Other serious adverse reactions with a lower incidence are: cardiac irregularities and/or palpitations, orthostatic hypotensive episodes, bradykinetic episodes (the "on-off" phenomena), mental changes including paranoid ideation and psychotic episodes, depression with or without the development of suicidal tendencies, dementia, and urinary retention.

Rarely, gastrointestinal bleeding, development of duodenal ulcer, hypertension, phlebitis, hemolytic anemia, agranulocytosis, and convulsions have been observed. (The causal relationship between convulsions and Larodopa has not been established.)

Adverse reactions of a less serious nature having a relatively frequent occurrence are the following: anorexia, nausea and vomiting with or without abdominal pain and distress, dry mouth, dysphagia, sialorrhea, ataxia, increased hand tremor, headache, dizziness, numbness, weakness and faintness, bruxism, confusion, insomnia, nightmares, hallucinations and delusions, agitation and anxiety, malaise, fatigue and euphoria. Occurring with a lesser order of frequency are the following: muscle twitching and blepharospasm (which may be taken as an early sign of overdosage; consideration of dosage reduction may be made at this time), trismus, burn-

ing sensation of the tongue, bitter taste, diarrhea, constipation, flatulence, flushing, skin rash, increased sweating, bizarre breathing patterns, urinary incontinence, diplopia, blurred vision, dilated pupils, hot flashes, weight gain or loss, dark sweat and/or urine.

Rarely, oculogyric crises, sense of stimulation, hiccups, development of edema, loss of hair, hoarseness, priapism and activation of latent Horner's syndrome have been observed. Elevations of blood urea nitrogen, SGOT, SGPT, LDH, bilirubin, alkaline phosphatase or protein-bound iodine have been reported; and the significance of this is not known. Occasional reductions in WBC, hemoglobin, and hematocrit have been noted.

Leukopenia has occurred and requires cessation, at least temporarily, of Larodopa administration. The Coombs test has occasionally become positive during extended therapy. Elevations of uric acid have been noted when colorimetric method was used but not when uricase method was used.

OVERDOSAGE

For acute overdosage general supportive measures should be employed, along with immediate gastric lavage. Intravenous fluids should be administered judiciously and an adequate airway maintained.

Electrocardiographic monitoring should be instituted and the patient carefully observed for the possible development of arrhythmias; if required, appropriate antiarrhythmic therapy should be given. Consideration should be given to the possibility of multiple drug ingestion by the patient. To date, no experience has been reported with dialysis; hence its value in Larodopa overdosage is not known. Although pyridoxine hydrochloride (vitamin B_6) has been reported to reverse the antiparkinson effects of Larodopa, its usefulness in the management of acute overdosage has not been established.

DOSAGE AND ADMINISTRATION

The optimal daily dose of Larodopa, *i.e.,* the dose producing maximal improvement with tolerated side effects, must be determined and *carefully titrated for each individual patient.* The usual initial dosage is 0.5 to 1 Gm daily, divided in two or more doses with food.

The total daily dosage is then increased gradually in increments not more than 0.75 Gm every three to seven days as tolerated. The usual optimal therapeutic *dosage should not exceed 8 Gm.* The exceptional patient may carefully be given more than 8 Gms as required. In some patients, a significant therapeutic response may not be obtained until six months of treatment.

In the event general anesthesia is required, Larodopa therapy may be continued as long as the patient is able to take fluids and medication by mouth. If therapy is temporarily interrupted, the usual daily dosage may be administered as soon as the patient is able to take oral medication. Whenever therapy has been interrupted for longer periods, dosage should again be adjusted gradually; however, in many cases the patient can be rapidly titrated to his previous therapeutic dosage.

HOW SUPPLIED

Tablets, pink, scored, each containing levodopa/Roche 0.1 Gm, bottles of 100; 0.25 Gm or 0.5 Gm—bottles of 100 and 500.

Capsules, each containing levodopa/Roche 0.1 Gm (pink and scarlet)—bottles of 100; 0.25 Gm (pink and beige) or 0.5 Gm (pink)—bottles of 100 and 500.

P.I. 0985

Shown in Product Identification Section, page 425

LEVO-DROMORAN®   Ⓒ
[*lee "vo dro 'mo-ran*]
(levorphanol tartrate/Roche)
Ampuls ● Vials ● Tablets

The following text is complete prescribing information based on official labeling in effect June 1, 1989.

DESCRIPTION

Levo-Dromoran is available as 1-ml ampuls containing 2 mg levorphanol tartrate compounded with 0.2% parabens (methyl and propyl) as preservatives and sodium hydroxide to adjust pH to approximately 4.3; as 10-ml vials containing 2 mg levorphanol tartrate per ml, compounded with 0.45% phenol as preservative and sodium hydroxide to adjust pH to approximately 4.3; and as scored tablets, each containing 2 mg levorphanol tartrate plus lactose, corn starch, stearic acid and talc.

Levo-Dromoran is a highly potent synthetic analgesic with properties and actions similar to those of morphine. It produces a degree of analgesia at least equal to that of morphine and greater than that of meperidine at far smaller doses than either. It is longer acting than either; from 6 to 8 hours of pain relief can be expected with Levo-Dromoran whether given orally or by injection. It is almost as effective orally as it is parenterally. Its safety margin is about equal to that of morphine, but it is less likely to produce nausea, vomiting and constipation.

INDICATIONS

Levo-Dromoran is recommended whenever a narcotic-analgesic is required. It is recommended for the relief of pain whether moderate or severe. For example, it may be used in alleviating pain due to biliary and renal colic, myocardial infarction, and severe trauma; intractable pain due to cancer and other tumors; and for postoperative pain relief. Used preoperatively, it allays apprehension, provides prolonged analgesia, reduces thiopental requirements and shortens recovery-room time. Levo-Dromoran is compatible with a wide range of anesthetic agents. It is a useful supplement to nitrous oxide-oxygen anesthesia. It has been given by slow intravenous injection for special indications.

CONTRAINDICATIONS

As with the use of morphine, Levo-Dromoran is contraindicated in acute alcoholism, bronchial asthma, increased intracranial pressure, respiratory depression and anoxia.

WARNING

May be habit forming. Levo-Dromoran is a narcotic with an addiction liability similar to that of morphine, and for this reason the same precautions should be taken in administering the drug as with morphine. As with all narcotics, Levo-Dromoran should be used in early pregnancy only when expected benefits outweigh risks.

PRECAUTIONS

To counteract narcotic-induced respiratory depression, a narcotic antagonist, such as Narcan (naloxone hydrochloride), is recommended and should be readily available whenever Levo-Dromoran is used by parenteral administration.

ADVERSE REACTIONS

As is true with the use of any narcotic-analgesic, nausea, emesis and dizziness are not uncommon in the ambulatory patient. Respiratory depression, hypotension, urinary retention and various cardiac arrhythmias have been infrequently reported following the use of Levo-Dromoran, primarily in surgical patients. Occasional allergic reactions in the form of skin rash or urticaria have been reported. Pruritus or sweating are rarely observed.

DOSAGE AND ADMINISTRATION

Good medical practice dictates that the dose of any narcotic-analgesic be appropriate to the degree of pain to be relieved. This is especially important during the postoperative period because (a) residual CNS-depressant effects of anesthetic agents may still be present, and (b) later, gradual lessening of pain may not warrant full narcotizing doses. The average adult dose is 2 mg orally or subcutaneously. The dosage may be increased to 3 mg, if necessary.

ANTIDOTE FOR OVERDOSAGE

In the event of overdosage of Levo-Dromoran, an appropriate dose of a narcotic antagonist, such as Narcan (naloxone HCl), should be administered; consult the prescribing information of the specific narcotic antagonist for details about use.

HOW SUPPLIED

Ampuls, 1 ml (boxes of 10). Each ml of solution contains 2 mg levorphanol tartrate/Roche (WARNING: May be habit forming).

Multiple Dose Vials, 10 ml, 2 mg/ml (boxes of 1). Each ml of solution contains 2 mg levorphanol tartrate/Roche (WARNING: May be habit forming).

Oral Tablets, 2 mg, scored (bottles of 100). Each tablet contains 2 mg levorphanol tartrate/Roche (WARNING: May be habit forming).

Narcotic order required.

P.I. 0985

Shown in Product Identification Section, page 425

MARPLAN® TABLETS   ℞
[*mar 'plan*]
(isocarboxazid/Roche)

The following text is complete prescribing information based on official labeling in effect June 1, 1989.

DESCRIPTION

Marplan (isocarboxazid/Roche), an amine-oxidase inhibitor, is available for oral administration in 10-mg tablets. Each tablet also contains gelatin, lactose, magnesium stearate, corn starch, talc, FD&C Red No. 3 and FD&C Yellow No. 6. Chemically, isocarboxazid is 5-methyl-3-isoxazolecarboxylic acid 2-benzylhydrazide.

Isocarboxazid is a colorless, crystalline substance with very little taste.

ACTIONS

Isocarboxazid, a potent inhibitor of amine-oxidase, exhibits antidepressant activity. *In vivo* and *in vitro* studies demonstrated inhibition of amine-oxidase in the brain, heart and liver.

The oral LD_{50} in mice was 171 mg/kg and in rats, 270 mg/kg. In rats administered 120 mg/kg daily for 6 weeks, isocarbox-

Continued on next page

Roche Labs.—Cont.

azid produced a reduction of growth rate and appetite. In chronic tolerance studies of 24 weeks duration, hyperexcitability and depression of growth rate occurred in male rats given oral doses of 5 mg/kg/day and in both sexes of this species given 10 mg/kg/day orally. The relevance of these findings to the clinical use of Marplan is not known. No hematologic changes were observed.

Dogs given 15 mg/kg/day for 2 weeks showed emetic effects and a slight lowering of hemoglobin and hematocrit. No adverse effects were noted, however, at doses of 10 mg/kg/day for 6 weeks. Given as successively increasing daily oral doses to a dog, isocarboxazid was tolerated up to 40 mg/kg.

Monkeys given 20 mg/kg/day orally for 2 weeks tolerated the drug with no apparent adverse effects.

Reproduction studies were carried out in rats given 0.5 and 5 mg/kg/day of isocarboxazid as a dietary mixture for 10 weeks prior to mating and continuing through two mating cycles to the weaning of the second litter. The parent animals remained in good condition throughout the test period. Litters of the treated groups compared favorably with those of the controls. No evidence of teratogenic effects was seen in any of the young.

INDICATIONS: Based on a review of this drug by the National Academy of Sciences—National Research Council and/or other information, FDA has classified the indications as follows:

"Probably" effective for the treatment of depressed patients who are refractory to tricyclic antidepressants or electroconvulsive therapy and depressed patients in whom tricyclic antidepressants are contraindicated.

Final classification of the less-than-effective indications requires further investigation.

Careful selection of candidates for Marplan—with due regard to the symptomatology of the patient and to the properties of the compound—will result in more effective therapy. Complete review of the package insert is advised before initiating treatment.

CONTRAINDICATIONS

Marplan is contraindicated in patients with known hypersensitivity to the drug, severe impairment of liver or renal function, congestive heart failure or pheochromocytoma.

The potentiation of sympathomimetic substances by MAO inhibitors may result in *hypertensive crisis;* therefore, patients taking Marplan should not be given *sympathomimetic drugs* (including amphetamines, methyldopa, levodopa, dopamine, and tryptophan as well as epinephrine and norepinephrine) nor *foods with a high concentration of tryptophan* (broad beans) or *tyramine* (cheese, beers, wines, alcohol-free and reduced-alcohol beer and wine products, pickled herring, chicken livers, yeast extract). Excessive amounts of caffeine can also cause hypertensive reactions.

These hypertensive crises can be fatal, due to circulatory collapse or intracranial bleeding. Hypertensive crises are characterized by some or all of the following symptoms: occipital headache which may radiate frontally, neck stiffness or soreness, nausea, vomiting, photophobia, dilated pupils, sweating (sometimes with fever and sometimes with cold, clammy skin) and palpitations. Either tachycardia or bradycardia may be present, and can be associated with constricting chest pain. These crises usually occur within several hours after the ingestion of a contraindicated substance. Marplan should be discontinued immediately upon the occurrence of palpitations or frequent headaches.

Recommended treatment in hypertensive crisis: Marplan should be discontinued and therapy to lower blood pressure should be started immediately. A successful method of treatment is with an alpha-adrenergic blocking agent such as phentolamine, 5 mg, I.V., or pentolinium, 3 mg, subcutaneously. These drugs should be administered slowly to avoid excessive hypotension. Fever should be managed by external cooling.

Marplan should not be administered together with or immediately following other MAO inhibitors or dibenzazepines. Such combinations can produce hypertensive crisis, fever, marked sweating, excitation, delirium, tremor, twitching, convulsions, coma, and circulatory collapse. Marplan should also not be used in combination with buspirone, since several cases of elevated blood pressure have been reported in patients taking MAO inhibitors who were then given buspirone. At least 10 days should elapse between the discontinuation of Marplan and the institution of another antidepressant or buspirone, or the discontinuation of another MAO inhibitor and the institution of Marplan.

Some other amine-oxidase inhibitors commonly used in this country include pargyline HCl, phenelzine sulfate and tranylcypromine.

Some dibenzazepine-related compounds are antidepressants commonly used in this country, including amitriptyline HCl, amoxapine, desipramine HCl, doxepin HCl, imipramine HCl, maprotiline HCl, nortriptyline HCl, protriptyline HCl, and trimipramine maleate. Carbamazepine and cyclobenzaprine HCl are also dibenzazepines.

MAO inhibitors, including Marplan, are contraindicated in patients receiving clomipramine hydrochloride (Anafranil®).

Patients taking Marplan should not undergo elective surgery requiring general anesthesia. Should spinal anesthesia be essential, consideration should be given to possible combined hypotensive effects of Marplan and the blocking agent. Also, they should not be given cocaine or local anesthetic solutions containing sympathomimetic vasoconstrictors. Marplan should be discontinued at least 10 days prior to elective surgery.

Marplan should not be used in combination with CNS depressants such as narcotics and ethanol (see PRECAUTIONS for barbiturates). Circulatory collapse and death have been reported from the combination of amine-oxidase inhibitors and a single dose of meperidine. In addition, serious hyperpyrexia can occur following administration of this combination. It is thought that this latter reaction may be mediated by release of 5-hydroxytryptamine, as it does not occur in experimental animals pretreated with inhibitors of 5-HT synthesis.

The combination of MAO inhibitors and dextromethorphan has been reported to cause brief episodes of psychosis or bizarre behavior.

The combination of MAO inhibitors and tryptophan has been reported to cause behavioral and neurologic syndromes, including disorientation, confusion, amnesia, delirium, agitation, hypomanic signs, ataxia, myoclonus, hyperreflexia, shivering, ocular oscillations and Babinski signs.

WARNINGS

Because the most serious reactions to Marplan relate to effects on blood pressure, it is not advisable to use this drug in elderly or debilitated patients or in the presence of hypertension, cardiovascular or cerebrovascular disease. Patients with severe or frequent headaches should not be considered as candidates for therapy with Marplan because headaches during therapy may be the first symptom of a hypertensive reaction to the drug.

Marplan should be used with caution in combination with antihypertensive drugs including thiazide diuretics since hypotension may result.

In patients who may be suicidal risks, no single form of treatment, such as Marplan, electroshock or other therapy, should be relied on as a sole therapeutic measure. The strictest supervision, and preferably hospitalization, are advised.

Warning to patient: All patients taking Marplan should be warned against self-medication with proprietary cold, hay fever or reducing preparations, since most of these contain sympathomimetic agents. They should be warned against eating the foods previously mentioned that contain high concentrations of tyramine or tryptophan. Beverages containing caffeine should be used in moderation. Patients should be instructed to report promptly the occurrence of headache or other unusual symptoms.

Use in Children: Marplan is not recommended for use in patients under 16 years of age since there are no controlled studies of safety or efficacy in this group.

Use in Pregnancy: Safe use of Marplan during pregnancy or lactation has not yet been established. Before prescribing Marplan in pregnancy, lactation, or in women of childbearing age, the potential benefit of the drug should be weighed against its possible hazard to mother and child. (See ACTIONS.)

PRECAUTIONS

Concomitant use of Marplan and other psychotropic agents is not recommended because of possible potentiating effects and decreased margin of safety. This is especially true in patients who may subject themselves to an overdosage of drugs. If combination therapy is indicated, careful consideration should be given to the pharmacology of all agents to be employed. The effects of Marplan may persist for a substantial period after discontinuation of the drug, and this should be borne in mind when another drug is prescribed following Marplan. To avoid potentiation, the physician wishing to terminate treatment with Marplan and begin therapy with another agent should allow for an interval of 10 days.

Marplan should be used cautiously in hyperactive or agitated patients, as well as schizophrenic patients, because it may cause excessive stimulation. Characteristically, in manic-depressive states there may be a tendency for patients to swing from a depressive to a manic phase. If such a swing should occur during Marplan therapy, brief discontinuation of the drug, followed by resumption of therapy at a reduced dosage, is advised.

Clinical evidence indicates only a low incidence of altered liver function or jaundice in patients treated with Marplan. It is difficult to differentiate most cases of drug-induced hepatocellular jaundice from viral hepatitis since they are histopathologically and biochemically indistinguishable. Moreover, many of the clinical signs and symptoms are identical. While some of the few cases of jaundice reported during Mar-

plan therapy may have been drug-induced, the reaction is rare. Nevertheless, Marplan is an amine-oxidase inhibitor and, as with the use of all these agents, it is advisable to watch for hepatic complications. It is suggested that periodic liver function tests, such as bilirubins, alkaline phosphatase or transaminases, be performed during Marplan therapy; use of the drug should be discontinued at the first sign of hepatic dysfunction or jaundice. In patients with impaired renal function, Marplan should be used cautiously to prevent accumulation.

Marplan appears to have varying effects in epileptic patients; while some have a decrease in frequency of seizures, others have more seizures. Appropriate consideration must be given to the latter possibility if Marplan is prescribed for such patients.

All patients taking Marplan should be watched for symptoms of postural hypotension. If such hypotension occurs, the dose should be reduced or the drug discontinued.

Since the MAO inhibitors, including Marplan, potentiate hexobarbital hypnosis in animals, the dose of barbiturates if given concomitantly should be reduced.

Since the MAO inhibitors inhibit the destruction of serotonin, which is believed to be released from tissue stores by rauwolfia alkaloids, caution should be exercised when these drugs are used together.

There is conflicting evidence as to whether MAO inhibitors affect glucose metabolism or potentiate hypoglycemic agents. This should be considered if Marplan is used in diabetics.

ADVERSE REACTIONS

Marplan is a potent therapeutic agent with a relatively low incidence of adverse reactions. Since Marplan affects many enzyme systems of the body, a variety of side effects may be anticipated. The most frequently noted have been orthostatic hypotension, associated in some patients with falling, disturbances in cardiac rate and rhythm, complaints of dizziness and vertigo, constipation, headache, overactivity, hyperreflexia, tremors and muscle twitching, mania, hypomania, jitteriness, confusion and memory impairment, insomnia, peripheral edema, weakness, fatigue, dryness of the mouth, blurred vision, hyperhidrosis, anorexia and body weight changes, gastrointestinal disturbances, and minor sensitivity reactions such as skin rashes. Isolated cases of akathisia, ataxia, black tongue, coma, dysuria, euphoria, hematologic changes, incontinence, neuritis, photosensitivity, sexual disturbances, spider telangiectases and urinary retention have been reported. These side effects sometimes necessitate discontinuation of therapy. In rare instances, hallucinations have been reported with high dosages, but they have disappeared upon reduction of dosage or discontinuation of therapy. Toxic amblyopia was reported in one psychiatric patient who had received isocarboxazid for about a year; no causal relationship to isocarboxazid was established. Impaired water excretion compatible with the syndrome of inappropriate secretion of antidiuretic hormone (SIADH) has been reported.

DOSAGE AND ADMINISTRATION

As with other potent drugs, for maximum therapeutic effect the dosage of Marplan must be individually adjusted on the basis of careful observation of the patient. The usual starting dose is 30 mg daily, to be given in single or divided doses. Marplan has a cumulative effect; therefore, as soon as clinical improvement is observed, the dosage should be reduced to a maintenance level of 10 to 20 mg daily (or less). Since daily doses larger than 30 mg may cause an increase in the incidence or severity of side effects, it is recommended that this dosage generally not be exceeded. Many patients may show a favorable response to Marplan therapy within a week or less; however, since Marplan acts by directly affecting enzyme metabolism, a beneficial effect may not be seen in some patients for three or four weeks. If no response is obtained by then, continued administration is unlikely to help.

MANAGEMENT OF OVERDOSAGE

The lethal dose of Marplan in man is not known. There has been one report of a fatality in a patient who ingested 400 mg of Marplan together with an unspecified amount of another drug. Major overdosage may be evidenced by symptoms such as tachycardia, hypotension, coma, convulsions, respiratory depression, sluggish reflexes, pyrexia and diaphoresis; these signs may persist for 8 to 14 days. General supportive measures should be employed, along with immediate gastric lavage or emetics. If the latter are given, the danger of aspiration must be borne in mind. An adequate airway should be maintained, with supplemental oxygen if necessary. The mechanism by which amine-oxidase inhibitors produce hypotension is not fully understood, but there is evidence that these agents block the vascular bed response. Thus it is suggested that plasma may be of value in the management of this hypotension. Administration of pressor amines such as Levophed® (levarterenol bitartrate) may be of limited value (note that their effects may be potentiated by Marplan). Continue treatment for several days until homeostasis is restored. Liver function studies are recommended during the 4 to 6 weeks after recovery, as well as at the time of overdosage. As with the management of intentional overdosage with any drug, it should be borne in mind that multiple agents may have been ingested.

HOW SUPPLIED

Tablets, 10 mg isocarboxazid/Roche each, peach-colored, scored—bottles of 100.
P.I. 0389

Shown in Product Identification Section, page 425

MATULANE®   ℞
[*mat'u-lane*]
procarbazine hydrochloride/Roche
CAPSULES

The following text is complete prescribing information based on official labeling in effect June 1, 1989.

WARNING

It is recommended that MATULANE be given only by or under the supervision of a physician experienced in the use of potent antineoplastic drugs. Adequate clinical and laboratory facilities should be available to patients for proper monitoring of treatment.

DESCRIPTION

Matulane (procarbazine hydrochloride/Roche), a hydrazine derivative antineoplastic agent, is available as capsules containing the equivalent of 50 mg procarbazine as the hydrochloride. Each capsule also contains corn starch, mannitol and talc. Gelatin capsule shells contain parabens (methyl and propyl), potassium sorbate, titanium dioxide, F D & C Yellow No. 6 and D & C Yellow No. 10.

Chemically, procarbazine hydrochloride is N-isopropyl-α-(2-methylhydrazino)-p-toluamide monohydrochloride. It is a white to pale yellow crystalline powder which is soluble but unstable in water or aqueous solutions. The molecular weight of procarbazine hydrochloride is 257.76.

CLINICAL PHARMACOLOGY

The precise mode of cytotoxic action of procarbazine has not been clearly defined. There is evidence that the drug may act by inhibition of protein, RNA and DNA synthesis. Studies have suggested that procarbazine may inhibit transmethylation of methyl groups of methionine into t-RNA. The absence of functional t-RNA could cause the cessation of protein synthesis and consequently DNA and RNA synthesis. In addition, procarbazine may directly damage DNA. Hydrogen peroxide, formed during the auto-oxidation of the drug, may attack protein sulfhydryl groups contained in residual protein which is tightly bound to DNA.

Procarbazine is metabolized primarily in the liver and kidneys. The drug appears to be auto-oxidized to the azo derivative with the release of hydrogen peroxide. The azo derivative isomerizes to the hydrazone, and following hydrolysis splits into a benzyladehyde derivative and methylhydrazine. The methylhydrazine is further degraded to CO_2 and CH_4 and possibly hydrazine, whereas the aldehyde is oxidized to N-isopropylterphthalamic acid, which is excreted in the urine.

Procarbazine is rapidly and completely absorbed. Following oral administration of 30 mg of ^{14}C-labeled procarbazine, maximum peak plasma radioactive concentrations were reached within 60 minutes.

After intravenous injection, the plasma half-life of procarbazine is approximately 10 minutes. Approximately 70% of the radioactivity is excreted in the urine as N-isopropylterphthalamic acid within 24 hours following both oral and intravenous administration of ^{14}C-labeled procarbazine.

Procarbazine crosses the blood-brain barrier and rapidly equilibrates between plasma and cerebrospinal fluid after oral administration.

INDICATIONS AND USAGE

Matulane is indicated for use in combination with other anticancer drugs for the treatment of Stage III and IV Hodgkin's disease. Matulane is used as part of the MOPP (nitrogen mustard, vincristine, procarbazine, prednisone) regimen.

CONTRAINDICATIONS

Matulane is contraindicated in patients with known hypersensitivity to the drug or inadequate marrow reserve as demonstrated by bone marrow aspiration. Due consideration of this possible state should be given to each patient who has leukopenia, thrombocytopenia or anemia.

WARNINGS

To minimize CNS depression and possible potentiation, barbiturates, antihistamines, narcotics, hypotensive agents or phenothiazines should be used with caution. Ethyl alcohol should not be used since there may be an Antabuse (disulfiram)-like reaction. Because Matulane exhibits some monoamine oxidase inhibitory activity, sympathomimetic drugs, tricyclic antidepressant drugs (*e.g.*, amitriptyline HCl, imipramine HCl) and other drugs and foods with known high tyramine content, such as wine, yogurt, ripe cheese and

bananas, should be avoided. A further phenomenon of toxicity common to many hydrazine derivatives is hemolysis and the appearance of Heinz-Ehrlich inclusion bodies in erythrocytes.

Pregnancy: Teratogenic effects: Pregnancy Category D. Procarbazine hydrochloride can cause fetal harm when administered to a pregnant woman. While there are no adequate and well-controlled studies with procarbazine hydrochloride in pregnant women, there are case reports of malformations in the offspring of women who were exposed to procarbazine hydrochloride in combination with other antineoplastic agents during pregnancy. Matulane should be used during pregnancy only if the potential benefit justifies the potential risk to the fetus. If this drug is used during pregnancy, or if the patient becomes pregnant while taking this drug, the patient should be apprised of the potential hazard to the fetus. Women of childbearing potential should be advised to avoid becoming pregnant. Procarbazine hydrochloride is teratogenic in the rat when given at doses approximately 4 to 13 times the maximum recommended human therapeutic dose of 6 mg/kg/day.

Nonteratogenic effects: Procarbazine hydrochloride has not been adequately studied in animals for its effects on peri- and postnatal development. However, neurogenic tumors were noted in the offspring of rats given intravenous injections of 125 mg/kg of procarbazine hydrochloride on day 22 of gestation. Compounds which inhibit DNA, RNA and protein synthesis might be expected to have adverse effects on peri- and postnatal development.

Carcinogenesis, mutagenesis and impairment of fertility:

Carcinogenesis: The carcinogenicity of procarbazine hydrochloride in mice, rats and monkeys has been reported in a considerable number of studies. Instances of a second nonlymphoid malignancy, including acute myelocytic leukemia, have been reported in patients with Hodgkin's disease treated with procarbazine in combination with other chemotherapy and/or radiation. The International Agency for Research on Cancer (IARC) considers that there is "sufficient evidence" for the human carcinogenicity of procarbazine hydrochloride when it is given in intensive regimens which include other antineoplastic agents but that there is inadequate evidence of carcinogenicity in humans given procarbazine hydrochloride alone.

Mutagenesis: Procarbazine hydrochloride has been shown to be mutagenic in a variety of bacterial and mammalian test systems.

Impairment of fertility: Azoospermia and antifertility effects associated with procarbazine hydrochloride administration in combination with other chemotherapeutic agents for treating Hodgkin's disease have been reported in human clinical studies. Since these patients received multicombination therapy, it is difficult to determine to what extent procarbazine hydrochloride alone was involved in the male germ-cell damage. The usual Segment 1 fertility/reproduction studies in laboratory animals have not been carried out with procarbazine hydrochloride. However, compounds which inhibit DNA, RNA and/or protein synthesis might be expected to have adverse effects on gametogenesis. Unscheduled DNA synthesis in the testis of rabbits and decreased fertility in male mice treated with procarbazine hydrochloride have been reported.

PRECAUTIONS

General: Undue toxicity may occur if Matulane is used in patients with impairment of renal and/or hepatic function. When appropriate, hospitalization for the initial course of treatment should be considered.

If radiation or a chemotherapeutic agent known to have marrow-depressant activity has been used, an interval of one month or longer without such therapy is recommended before starting treatment with Matulane. The length of this interval may also be determined by evidence of bone marrow recovery based on successive bone marrow studies.

Prompt cessation of therapy is recommended if any one of the following occurs:

Central nervous system signs or symptoms such as paresthesias, neuropathies or confusion.
Leukopenia (white blood count under 4000).
Thrombocytopenia (platelets under 100,000).
Hypersensitivity reaction.
Stomatitis—The first small ulceration or persistent spot soreness around the oral cavity is a signal for cessation of therapy.
Diarrhea—Frequent bowel movements or watery stools.
Hemorrhage or bleeding tendencies.

Bone marrow depression often occurs 2 to 8 weeks after the start of treatment. If leukopenia occurs, hospitalization of the patient may be needed for appropriate treatment to prevent systemic infection.

Information for patients: Patients should be warned not to drink alcoholic beverages while on Matulane therapy since there may be an Antabuse (disulfiram)-like reaction. They should also be cautioned to avoid foods with known high tyramine content such as wine, yogurt, ripe cheese and bananas. Over-the-counter drug preparations which contain antihistamines or sympathomimetic drugs should also be

avoided. Patients taking Matulane should also be warned against the use of prescription drugs without the knowledge and consent of their physician.

Laboratory tests: Baseline laboratory data should be obtained prior to initiation of therapy. The hematologic status as indicated by hemoglobin, hematocrit, white blood count (WBC), differential, reticulocytes and platelets should be monitored closely—at least every 3 or 4 days.

Hepatic and renal evaluation are indicated prior to beginning therapy. Urinalysis, transaminase, alkaline phosphatase and blood urea nitrogen tests should be repeated at least weekly.

Drug interactions: See WARNINGS section.

No cross-resistance with other chemotherapeutic agents, radiotherapy or steroids has been demonstrated.

Carcinogenesis, mutagenesis and impairment of fertility: See WARNINGS section.

Pregnancy: Pregnancy Category D. See WARNINGS section.

Nursing mothers: It is not known whether Matulane is excreted in human milk. Because of the potential for tumorigenicity shown for procarbazine hydrochloride in animal studies, mothers should not nurse while receiving this drug.

ADVERSE REACTIONS

Leukopenia, anemia and thrombopenia occur frequently. Nausea and vomiting are the most commonly reported side effects.

Other adverse reactions are:

Hematologic: Pancytopenia; eosinophilia; hemolytic anemia; bleeding tendencies such as petechiae, purpura, epistaxis and hemoptysis.

Gastrointestinal: Hepatic dysfunction, jaundice, stomatitis, hematemesis, melena, diarrhea, dysphagia, anorexia, abdominal pain, constipation, dry mouth.

Neurologic: Coma, convulsions, neuropathy, ataxia, paresthesia, nystagmus, diminished reflexes, falling, foot drop, headache, dizziness, unsteadiness.

Cardiovascular: Hypotension, tachycardia, syncope.

Ophthalmic: Retinal hemorrhage, papilledema, photophobia, diplopia, inability to focus.

Respiratory: Pneumonitis, pleural effusion, cough.

Dermatologic: Herpes, dermatitis, pruritus, alopecia, hyperpigmentation, rash, urticaria, flushing.

Allergic: Generalized allergic reactions.

Genitourinary: Hematuria, urinary frequency, nocturia.

Musculoskeletal: Pain, including myalgia and arthralgia; tremors.

Psychiatric: Hallucinations, depression, apprehension, nervousness, confusion, nightmares.

Endocrine: Gynecomastia in prepubertal and early pubertal boys.

Miscellaneous: Intercurrent infections, hearing loss, pyrexia, diaphoresis, lethargy, weakness, fatigue, edema, chills, insomnia, slurred speech, hoarseness, drowsiness.

Second nonlymphoid malignancies, including acute myelocytic leukemia and malignant myelosclerosis, and azoospermia have been reported in patients with Hodgkin's disease treated with procarbazine in combination with other chemotherapy and/or radiation.

OVERDOSAGE

The major manifestations of overdosage with Matulane would be anticipated to be nausea, vomiting, enteritis, diarrhea, hypotension, tremors, convulsions and coma. Treatment should consist of either the administration of an emetic or gastric lavage. General supportive measures such as intravenous fluids are advised. Since the major toxicity of procarbazine hydrochloride is hematologic and hepatic, patients should have frequent complete blood counts and liver function tests throughout their period of recovery and for a minimum of two weeks thereafter. Should abnormalities appear in any of these determinations, appropriate measures for correction and stabilization should be immediately undertaken.

The estimated mean lethal dose of procarbazine hydrochloride in laboratory animals varied from approximately 150 mg/kg in rabbits to 1300 mg/kg in mice.

DOSAGE AND ADMINISTRATION

The following doses are for administration of the drug as a single agent. When used in combination with other anticancer drugs, the Matulane dose should be appropriately reduced, *e.g.*, in the MOPP regimen, the Matulane dose is 100 mg/m^2 daily for 14 days. All dosages are based on the patient's actual weight. However, the estimated lean body mass (dry weight) is used if the patient is obese or if there has been a spurious weight gain due to edema, ascites or other forms of abnormal fluid retention.

Adults—To minimize the nausea and vomiting experienced by a high percentage of patients beginning Matulane therapy, single or divided doses of 2 to 4 mg/kg/day for the first week are recommended. Daily dosage should then be maintained at 4 to 6 mg/kg/day until maximum response is obtained or until the white blood count falls below 4000/cmm

Continued on next page

Roche Labs.—Cont.

or the platelets fall below 100,000/cmm. When maximum response is obtained, the dose may be maintained at 1 to 2 mg/kg/day. Upon evidence of hematologic or other toxicity (see PRECAUTIONS section), the drug should be discontinued until there has been satisfactory recovery. After toxic side effects have subsided, therapy may then be resumed at the discretion of the physician, based on clinical evaluation and appropriate laboratory studies, at a dosage of 1 to 2 mg/kg/day.

Children—Very close clinical monitoring is mandatory. Undue toxicity, evidenced by tremors, coma and convulsions, has occurred in a few cases. Dosage, therefore, should be individualized. The following dosage schedule is provided as a guideline only.

Fifty (50) mg per square meter of body surface per day is recommended for the first week. Dosage should then be maintained at 100 mg per square meter of body surface per day until maximum response is obtained or until leukopenia or thrombocytopenia occurs. When maximum response is attained, the dose may be maintained at 50 mg per square meter of body surface per day. Upon evidence of hematologic or other toxicity (see PRECAUTIONS section), the drug should be discontinued until there has been satisfactory recovery, based on clinical evaluation and appropriate laboratory tests. After toxic side effects have subsided, therapy may then be resumed.

Procedures for proper handling and disposal of anticancer drugs should be considered. Several guidelines on this subject have been published.[1-6] There is no general agreement that all of the procedures recommended in the guidelines are necessary or appropriate.

HOW SUPPLIED

Capsules, ivory, containing the equivalent of 50 mg procarbazine as the hydrochloride; bottles of 100 (NDC 0004-0053-01). Imprint on capsules; MATULANE® ROCHE.

REFERENCES

1. Recommendations for the safe handling of parenteral antineoplastic drugs. Washington, DC, U.S. Government Printing Office (NIH Publication No. 83-2621).
2. AMA Council Report. Guidelines for handling parenteral antineoplastics. *JAMA* 253:1590–1592, Mar 15, 1985.
3. National Study Commission on Cytotoxic Exposure: Recommendations for handling cytotoxic agents. Available from Louis P. Jeffrey, ScD, Director of Pharmacy Services, Rhode Island Hospital, 593 Eddy Street, Providence, Rhode Island 02902.
4. Clinical Oncological Society of Australia: Guidelines and recommendations for safe handling of antineoplastic agents. *Med. J. Aust 1*:426–428, Apr 30, 1983.
5. Jones RB, Frank R. Mass T: Safe handling of chemotherapeutic agents: a report from the Mount Sinai Medical Center. *CA 33*:258–263, Sept–Oct 1983.
6. ASHP technical assistance bulletin on handling cytotoxic drugs in hospitals. *Am J Hosp Pharm 42*:131–137, Jan 1985.

P.I. 0187

Shown in Product Identification Section, page 425

NIPRIDE® ℞

[ny′pryde]

(sodium nitroprusside/Roche)

The following text is complete prescribing information based on official labeling in effect June 1, 1989.

> Nipride is to be used only as an infusion with sterile 5% dextrose in water. Not for direct injection.
>
> Nipride should be used only when the necessary facilities and equipment for continuous monitoring of blood pressure are available.
>
> If at infusion rates of up to 10 mcg/kg/minute, an adequate reduction of blood pressure is not obtained within 10 minutes, administration of Nipride should be terminated.
>
> As metabolic acidosis is the earliest and most reliable evidence of cyanide toxicty, blood pH and acid base balance should be determined frequently in all patients and, particularly, if there is increased tolerance to the drug.
>
> The instructions herein should be reviewed thoroughly before administration of Nipride.

DESCRIPTION

Nipride (sodium nitroprusside/Roche), a hypotensive agent, is available as a sterile powder for reconstitution and dilution in sterile 5% dextrose in water to be used only for intravenous infusion. Each 5-ml vial contains the equivalent of 50 mg of sodium nitroprusside dihydrate. Chemically, sodium nitroprusside is disodium pentacyanonitrosylferrate(2-) dihydrate. It is a reddish-brown powder which is soluble in water. In aqueous solution, it is photosensitive and should be protected from light. It has a molecular weight of 297.95.

CLINICAL PHARMACOLOGY

Nipride is a potent immediate-acting, intravenous hypotensive agent. The active component of sodium nitroprusside is the free nitroso (NO) group, not its metabolites. The onset of Nipride's hypotensive activity is observed within 0.5 to 5 minutes of initiation of intravenous infusion. The intensity of the pharmacodynamic response is related to the infusion rate; whereas the duration of action continues only as long as the infusion is maintained. Blood pressure returns to pretreatment levels within one to ten minutes after cessation of the infusion.

It has been demonstrated in animals that sodium nitroprusside acts on the excitation-contraction coupling of vascular smooth muscle by interfering with both influx and the intracellular activation of calcium without affecting cAMP, ATP or the contractile proteins. No relaxation is seen in the smooth muscle of the uterus or duodenum *in situ* in animals. Nitroprusside is rapidly metabolized to cyanide and thiocyanate through a reaction with hemoglobin, yielding methemoglobin and an unstable intermediate which dissociates, releasing cyanide. The major elimination pathway of cyanide is by conversion in the liver and kidney to thiocyanate which requires the enzyme rhodanase. Other pathways include the formulation of biologically inert cyanmethemoglobin and cyanocobalamin. Cyanocobalamin is formed by the complexing of cyanide with hydroxocobalamin. The rate of conversion from cyanide to thiocyanate is dependent on the availability of sulfur, usually thiosulfate.

Because of its rapid decomposition in the presence of red blood cells, plasma concentrations of nitroprusside cannot be determined. Nitroprusside is not excreted intact. Animal studies indicate that some metabolites are excreted in urine, some are exhaled and others may be present in the feces since the thiocyanate ion can be detected in saliva and gastric juice. Thiocyanate, the major metabolite of sodium nitroprusside, is largely excreted through the kidneys.

The passage of nitroprusside through the blood-brain or placental barriers or excretion in breast milk have not been determined.

Sodium nitroprusside administered by infusion to hypertensive and normotensive patients produced a marked lowering of arterial blood pressure, slight increase in heart rate, a mild decrease in cardiac output and a moderate diminution in calculated total peripheral vascular resistance.

The decrease in calculated total peripheral vascular resistance suggests arteriolar vasodilatation. The decreases in cardiac and stroke index noted may be due to peripheral vascular pooling of blood.

In hypertensive patients, moderate depressor doses induce renal vasodilatation roughly equivalent to the decrease in pressure without an appreciable increase in renal blood flow or a decrease in glomerular filtration.

In normotensive subjects, acute reduction of mean arterial pressure to 60 to 75 mmHg by infusion of sodium nitroprusside caused a significant increase in renin activity of renal venous plasma in correlation with the degree of reduction in pressure. Renal response to reduction in pressure was more striking in renovascular hypertensive patients with significant increase in renin release occurring from the involved kidney at mean arterial pressures ranging from 90 to 137 mmHg. Furthermore, the magnitude of renin release from the involved kidney was significantly greater when compared with that in normotensive subjects, while in the contralateral, uninvolved kidney, no significant release of renin was detected during the reduction of pressure.

INDICATIONS AND USAGE

Nipride is indicated for the immediate reduction of blood pressure of patients in hypertensive crises. Concomitant oral antihypertensive medication should be started while the hypertensive emergency is being brought under control with Nipride. There is no contraindication in using Nipride simultaneously with oral antihypertensive medications.

Nipride is also indicated for producing controlled hypotension during anesthesia in order to reduce bleeding in surgical procedures when the surgeon and anesthesiologist deem it appropriate.

CONTRAINDICATIONS

Nipride should not be used in the treatment of compensatory hypertension, *e.g.*, arteriovenous shunt or coarctation of the aorta.

The use of Nipride to produce controlled hypotension during surgery is contraindicated in patients with known inadequate cerebral circulation. Nipride is not intended for use during emergency surgery in moribund patients (A.S.A. Class 5E).

WARNINGS

> If excessive amounts of Nipride are used and/or sulfur—usually thiosulfate—supplies are depleted, cyanide toxicity can occur. See OVERDOSAGE section.

> If sodium nitroprusside infusion is to be extended, particularly if renal impairment is present, close attention should be given to not exceeding the recommended maximum infusion rate of 10 mcg/kg/minute. If in the course of therapy increased tolerance to the drug (as shown by the need for a higher infusion rate) develops, it is essential to monitor blood acid-base balance, as metabolic acidosis is the earliest and most reliable evidence of cyanide toxicity. If signs of metabolic acidosis appear, Nipride should be discontinued and an alternate drug administered.
>
> Plasma thiocyanate concentrations do not reflect cyanide toxicity (see subsequent Warning concerning thiocyanate toxicity).

Some patients may fail to respond to adequate Nipride administration. Since failure to respond to Nipride may represent associated increase in free cyanide, appearance of increased tolerance to the drug constitutes reason for discontinuing Nipride and promptly instituting alternate therapy. Prolonged use of sodium nitroprusside may result in excessive thiocyanate formation. Thiocyanate accumulation and toxicity can manifest itself as tinnitus, blurred vision, mental confusion, psychotic behavior, convulsions, delirium, lactic acidosis, bone marrow depression, and hypothyroidism. Plasma thiocyanate concentrations should be monitored daily in any patient receiving therapy for longer than 48 hours, especially in patients with renal or hepatic impairment. Plasma thiocyanate levels above 10 mg/100 ml have been considered toxic and levels of 20 mg/100 ml have been judged fatal.

Since cyanide is converted into thiocyanate through the mediation of a hepatic enzyme, rhodanase, Nipride should be used with caution in patients with hepatic insufficiency.

Since thiocyanate inhibits both the uptake and binding of iodine, caution should be exercised in using Nipride in patients with hypothyroidism or severe renal impairment.

Hypertensive patients are more sensitive to the intravenous effect of sodium nitroprusside than are normotensive subjects. Patients who are receiving concomitant antihypertensive medications are more sensitive to the hypotensive effect of sodium nitroprusside and the dosage of Nipride should be adjusted accordingly.

The following warnings apply to the use of Nipride for controlled hypotension during anesthesia:

1. Tolerance to blood loss, anemia and hypovolemia may be diminished. If possible, prexisting anemia and hypovolemia should be corrected prior to employing controlled hypotension.
2. Hypotensive anesthetic techniques may alter pulmonary ventilation perfusion ratio. Patients intolerant of additional dead air space at ordinary oxygen partial pressure may benefit from higher oxygen partial pressure.
3. Extreme caution should be exercised in patients who are especially poor surgical risks (A.S.A. Class 4 and 4E).

Nipride is to be used only as an infusion with sterile 5% dextrose in water. Not for direct injection.

Infusion rates greater than 10 mcg/kg/minute are rarely required. If, at this rate, an adequate reduction in blood pressure is not obtained within 10 minutes, administration of Nipride should be stopped. Tachyphylaxis has been reported during Nipride usage, particularly when used in dosages higher than 10 mcg/kg/minute. Should this occur, immediately discontinue the administration of Nipride.

PRECAUTIONS

General: Adequate facilities, equipment and personnel should be available for frequent and vigilant monitoring of blood pressure, since the hypotensive effect of Nipride occurs rapidly. When the infusion is slowed or stopped, blood pressure usually begins to rise immediately and returns to pretreatment levels within one to ten minutes. It should be used with caution and initially in low doses in elderly patients since they may be more sensitive to the hypotensive effects of the drug. Young, vigorous males may require somewhat larger than ordinary doses of sodium nitroprusside for hypotensive anesthesia; however, the infusion rate of 10 mcg/kg/minute should not be exceeded. Deepening of anesthesia, if indicated, might permit satisfactory conditions to exist within the recommended dosage range.

Because of the rapid onset of action and potency of Nipride, it should preferably be administered with the use of an infusion pump, micro-drip regulator, or any similar device that would allow precise measurement of the flow rate.

Laboratory tests: See WARNINGS section.

Drug interactions: Patients receiving other antihypertensive medications appear to be more sensitive to the effects of sodium nitroprusside and may require lower doses of Nipride.

The hypotensive effect of Nipride is augmented by ganglionic blocking agents, volatile liquid anesthetics (such as halothane and enflurane) and by most other circulatory depressants.

Carcinogenesis, mutagenesis, impairment of fertility: Nipride has not undergone adequate carcinogenicity testing in animals. The mutagenic potential of Nipride has not been assessed. Nipride has not been tested for effects on fertility.

Pregnancy: Teratogenic effects: Pregnancy Category C. There are no adequate or well-controlled studies of Nipride in either laboratory animals or pregnant women. It is not known whether Nipride can cause fetal harm when administered to a pregnant woman or can affect reproductive capacity. Nipride should be given to a pregnant woman only if clearly needed.

Nonteratogenic effects: In three studies in pregnant ewes, nitroprusside was shown to cross the placental barrier. Fetal cyanide levels were shown to be dose-related to maternal levels of nitroprusside. The metabolic transformation of sodium nitroprusside given to pregnant ewes led to fatal levels of cyanide in the fetuses. The infusion of 25 mcg/kg/minute of sodium nitroprusside for one hour in pregnant ewes resulted in the death of all fetuses. Pregnant ewes infused with 1 mcg/kg/minute of sodium nitroprusside for one hour delivered normal lambs.

Nursing mothers: It is not known whether Nipride is excreted in human milk. Because of the potential for serious adverse reactions from Nipride in nursing infants, mothers who require Nipride should not nurse.

ADVERSE REACTIONS

Nausea, retching, diaphoresis, apprehension, headache, restlessness, muscle twitching, retrosternal discomfort, palpitations, dizziness and abdominal pain have been noted when the blood pressure was too rapidly reduced. The symptoms quickly disappeared when the rate of infusion was slowed or the infusion was temporarily discontinued and did not reappear with a continued slower rate of administration.

Other adverse reactions reported are:

Cardiovascular: Bradycardia, electrocardiographic changes, tachycardia.

Dermatologic: Rash.

Hematologic: Methemoglobinemia.

Neurologic: Raised intracranial pressure.

Miscellaneous: Flushing, venous streaking, irritation at the infusion site.

One case of hypothyroidism following prolonged therapy with intravenous sodium nitroprusside has been reported. A patient with severe hypertension with uremia received 3900 mg of sodium nitroprusside intravenously over a period of 21 days. This is one of the longest reported intravenous uses of this agent. There was no tachyphylaxis, but the patient developed evidence of hypothyrodism, together with retention of thiocyanate (9.5 mg/100 ml). With peritoneal dialysis the thiocyanate level diminished and the signs of hypothyroidism subsided.

OVERDOSAGE

The first signs of sodium nitroprusside overdosage are those of profound hypotension. As with instances of depletion of thiosulfate supplies, overdosage may lead to cyanide toxicity. Metabolic acidosis and increasing tolerance to the drug are early indications of overdosage. These may be associated with or followed by dyspnea, headache, vomiting, dizziness, ataxia and loss of consciousness. Sodium nitroprusside should be immediately discontinued. Other signs of cyanide poisoning are coma, imperceptible pulse, absent reflexes, widely dilated pupils, pink color, distant heart sounds and shallow breathing. Oxygen alone will not provide relief. Nitrites should be administered to induce methemoglobin formation. Methemoglobin, in turn, combines with cyanide bound to cytochrome oxidase to liberate cytochrome oxidase and form a nontoxic complex, cyanmethemoglobin. Cyanide then gradually dissociates from the latter and is converted by administration of thiosulfate to sodium thiocyanate in the presence of rhodanase.

Treatment of overdosage: In cases of massive overdosage when signs of cyanide toxicity are present use the following regimen:

1. Discontinue administration of Nipride.
2. Administer amyl nitrite inhalations for 15 to 30 seconds per each minute until a 3% sodium nitrite solution can be prepared for I.V. administration.
3. Inject sodium nitrite 3% solution intravenously at a rate not to exceed 2.5 to 5.0 ml/minute, up to a total dose of 10 to 15 ml. Carefully monitor the blood pressure.
4. Next, inject sodium thiosulfate intravenously, 12.5 gm in 50 ml of 5% dextrose in water, over a ten-minute period.
5. Since signs of overdosage may reappear, the patient must be observed for several hours.
6. If signs of overdosage reappear, repeat sodium nitrite and sodium thiosulfate injections at one-half of the above doses.
7. During the administration of nitrites and later when thiocyanate formation is taking place, blood pressure may drop, but it can be corrected with vasopressor agents.

The acute toxicity of Nipride is as follows:

Species	Route	LD$_{50}$± S.E. (mg/kg)
Mouse	I.V.	8.4 ± 0.3
Rat	I.V.	11.2 ± 1.1
Rabbit	I.V.	2.8 ± 1.1
Dog	I.V.	~5

DOSAGE AND ADMINISTRATION

The contents of a 50-mg Nipride vial should be dissolved in 2 to 3 ml of dextrose in water. No other diluent should be used. Depending on the desired concentration, all of the prepared stock solution should be diluted in 250 to 1000 ml of 5% dextrose in water. Once it is dissolved in solution, Nipride tends to deteriorate in the presence of light. Therefore, the container of the prepared solution should be promptly wrapped with aluminum foil or other opaque material affording protection from light. Both the stock solution and the infusion solution should be freshly prepared and any unused portion discarded. The freshly prepared solution for infusion has a very faint brownish tint. Nipride in aqueous solution yields the nitroprusside ion which reacts with even minute quantities of a wide variety of inorganic and organic substances to form usually highly colored reaction products (blue, green or dark red). If this occurs, the infusion should be replaced. *Once prepared, the solution should not be kept or used for longer than twenty-four hours, while protected from light. The infusion fluid used for the administration of Nipride should not be employed as a vehicle for simultaneous administraion of any other drug.*

In patients who are not receiving antihypertensive drugs, the average dose of Nipride for both adults and children is 3 mcg/kg/minute (range of 0.5 to 10 mcg/kg/minute). Usually, at 3 mcg/kg/minute, blood pressure can be lowered by about 30 to 40 percent below the pretreatment diastolic levels and maintained. In hypertensive patients receiving concomitant antihypertensive medications, smaller doses are required. In order to avoid excessive levels of thiocyanate and lessen the possibility of a precipitous drop in blood pressure, infusion rates greater than 10 mcg/kg/minute should rarely be used. If, at this rate, an adequate reduction of blood pressure is not obtained within 10 minutes, administraion of Nipride should be stopped.

1 Vial (50 mg) Nipride in 1000 ml 5% DW (50 mcg/ml)
1 Vial (50 mg) Nipride in 500 ml 5% DW (100 mcg/ml)
1 Vial (50 mg) Nipride in 250 ml 5% DW (200 mcg/ml)

Dose	mcg/kg/minute
Average	3
Range	0.5 to 10

The intravenous infusion of Nipride should be administered by an infusion pump, micro-drip regulator or any similar device that will allow precise measurement of the flow rate. Care should be taken to avoid extravasation. The rate of administration should be adjusted to maintain the desired antihypertensive or hypotensive effect, as determined by frequent blood pressure determinations. It is recommended that the blood pressure should not be allowed to drop at too rapid a rate and that the systolic pressure should not be allowed to drop below 60 mmHg. In hypertensive emergencies, Nipride infusion may be continued until the patient can safely be treated with oral antihypertensive medications alone.

Parenteral drug products should be inspected visually for particulate matter and discoloration prior to administration, whenever solution and container permit. (See above.)

HOW SUPPLIED

Nipride is supplied in 5-ml amber-colored vials containing the equivalent of 50 mg sodium nitroprusside dihydrate for reconstitution with dextrose in water—boxes of 1 (NDC 0004-1938-08).

P.I. 0785

NOLUDAR® 300   Ⓒ
[nol 'u-dar]
(methyprylon/Roche)
CAPSULES
NOLUDAR® 200   Ⓒ
(methyprylon/Roche)
TABLETS

The following text is complete prescribing information based on official labeling in effect June 1, 1989.

DESCRIPTION

Noludar (methyprylon/Roche), a hypnotic, is available for oral use as capsules and tablets. Each capsule contains 300 mg methyprylon plus aluminum hydroxide and calcium carbonate coprecipitate and magnesium stearate; gelatin capsule shells contain methyl and propyl parabens, potassium sorbate, FD&C Blue No. 1 and FD&C Red No. 3. Each tablet contains 200 mg methyprylon with aluminum hydroxide and calcium carbonate coprecipitate, corn starch, magnesium stearate and talc.

Chemically, methyprylon, a piperidine derivative, is 3,3-diethyl-5-methyl-2,4-piperidinedione. Methyprylon is a white crystalline powder, freely soluble in water, with a molecular weight of 183.25.

CLINICAL PHARMACOLOGY

In animal studies, methyprylon has been shown to increase the threshold of the arousal centers in the brainstem. In humans, when taken at bedtime, Noludar usually induces sleep within 45 minutes and provides sleep for 5 to 8 hours. Methyprylon is rapidly absorbed following oral administration and is approximately 60% bound to plasma proteins. Mean peak plasma concentrations of methyprylon in six subjects following a single 650-mg dose occurred at one to two hours postadministration at concentrations of 5.7 to 10.0 mcg/mL. The concentrations declined to 3.3 to 7.9 mcg/mL at 4 hours. Trace amounts of the dihydro-metabolite were detected in the one- to four-hour plasma specimens. Following administration of 400 mg of Noludar, less than 1% of the dose was recovered as intact drug and approximately 23% as identified metabolites in the 0- to 72-hour urine specimens. Identified metabolites include the dihydro-metabolite, the 6-oxo, the 5-hydroxymethyl and the 5-carboxyl derivatives. Methyprylon is metabolized by two pathways: dehydrogenation with subsequent oxidation to form the alcohol and corresponding acid, and oxidation to form 6-oxymethyprylon. Therapeutic blood concentrations are approximately 1 mg%. Serum concentrations in excess of 30 mg/L are generally consistent with unconsciousness in the acutely poisoned patient.

INDICATIONS AND USAGE

Noludar is indicated for use as a hypnotic. In the sleep laboratory it has been objectively determined that Noludar is effective for at least 7 consecutive nights of drug administration. Since insomnia is often transient and intermittent, the prolonged use of hypnotics is usually not indicated and should only be undertaken concomitantly with appropriate evaluation of the patient.

CONTRAINDICATIONS

Noludar is contraindicated in patients with known hypersensitivity to the drug.

WARNINGS

Synergistic effects: The concomitant use of alcohol or other CNS depressants may produce additive CNS depressant effects.

PRECAUTIONS

General: Total daily intake should not exceed 400 mg, as greater amounts do not significantly increase hypnotic effects. Caution should be exercised in treating patients with impaired renal or hepatic function. In view of isolated reports associating methyprylon with exacerbation of porphyria, caution should be exercised in prescribing methyprylon to patients suffering from this disease.

Information for patients: Patients receiving Noludar should be cautioned about possible combined effects with alcohol and other CNS depressants. Since Noludar is an effective hypnotic agent, patients should also be cautioned against engaging in hazardous occupations requiring complete mental alertness, such as operating machinery or driving a motor vehicle shortly after ingesting the drug.

Laboratory tests: If Noludar is used repeatedly or over prolonged periods of time, periodic blood counts should be made.

Drug interactions: Noludar stimulates the hepatic microsomal enzyme system. (Also see WARNINGS section.)

Carcinogenesis, mutagenesis, impairment of fertility: Studies sufficient to evaluate the carcinogenic or mutagenic potential of Noludar have not been performed. Noludar had no adverse effects on the reproductive process in rats when administered at dose levels of 5 and 50 mg/kg/day.

Pregnancy: Teratogenic effects: Pregnancy Category B. Reproduction studies have been performed in rats and in rabbits at doses up to approximately 9 times the maximum recommended human dose and have revealed no evidence of teratogenic effects on the fetus due to Noludar. There are, however, no adequate or well-controlled studies in pregnant women. Because animal reproduction studies are not always predictive of human response, this drug should be used in pregnancy only if clearly needed.

Nonteratogenic effects: At a dose of 50 mg/kg/day, Noludar caused an increased incidence of resorptions in the rabbit.

Nursing mothers: It is not known whether this drug is excreted in human milk. Because many drugs are excreted in human milk, caution should be exercised when Noludar is administered to a nursing woman.

Pediatric use: Safety and effectiveness in children below the age of 12 have not been established.

ADVERSE REACTIONS

Neurologic: Convulsions, hallucinations, ataxia, EEG changes, pyrexia, morning drowsiness, headache, dizziness, vertigo.

Psychiatric: Acute brain syndrome and confusion (particularly in elderly patients), paradoxical excitation, anxiety, depression, nightmares, dreaming.

Hematologic: Aplastic anemia, thrombocytopenic purpura, neutropenia.

Continued on next page

Roche Labs.—Cont.

Cardiovascular: Hypotension, syncope.
Ophthalmic: Diplopia, blurred vision.
Gastrointestinal: Esophagitis, vomiting, nausea, diarrhea, constipation.
Allergic: Generalized allergic reactions.
Dermatologic: Pruritus, rash.
Miscellaneous: Hangover effect.

DRUG ABUSE AND DEPENDENCE
Noludar is subject to Schedule III control under the Federal Controlled Substances Act of 1970. Physical and psychological dependence have been reported in patients receiving Noludar therapy. Withdrawal symptoms, when they occur, tend to resemble those associated with the withdrawal of barbiturates and should be treated in a similar fashion. Caution must be exercised in administering Noludar to individuals known to be addiction-prone or to those whose history suggests that they may increase the dosage on their own initiative. As with all hypnotic agents, good medical practice suggests the desirability of limiting repeated prescriptions without adequate medical supervision.

OVERDOSAGE
Manifestations of Noludar overdosage include somnolence, confusion, coma, shock, constricted pupils, respiratory depression, hypotension, tachycardia, edema and hepatic dysfunction. Blood concentrations of methyprylon associated with serious toxic symptoms in humans have been reported to range from 3 to 6 mg%. Blood concentrations of methyprylon that have been reported to cause death range from 5.3 to 114 mg%. A fatality occurred after ingestion of 6 grams of the drug. Respiration, pulse and blood pressure should be monitored, as in all cases of drug overdosage. General supportive measures should be employed, along with immediate gastric lavage with precautions to prevent pulmonary aspiration. Appropriate intravenous fluids should be administered and an adequate airway maintained. Hypotension may be combated by the use of Levophed® (norepinephrine bitartrate), Aramine (metaraminol bitartrate) or other accepted antihypotensive measures. Several reports clearly indicate that hemodialysis is of value. Therefore, its use should be considered, especially in those cases where supportive measures are failing and adequate urinary output cannot be maintained. There have been occasional reports of excitation and convulsions in patients following methyprylon overdosage, almost invariably during the recovery phase. Should these occur, barbiturates may be used, but only with great caution. As with the management of intentional overdosage of any drug, it should be borne in mind that multiple agents may have been ingested.

The acute toxicity of Noludar is as follows:

Species	Route	$LD_{50} \pm S.E.$ (mg/kg)
Mouse	P.O.	1000 ± 45
Rat	P.O.	400 ± 32
Rabbit	P.O.	340 ± 78

DOSAGE AND ADMINISTRATION
The dosage should be individualized for maximum beneficial effects. The usual adult dosage is one capsule (300 mg) or one or two tablets of 200 mg (200 or 400 mg) before retiring. Noludar is not recommended for use in children under 12 years of age. In children over 12 years, the effective dosage of Noludar varies greatly and, therefore, should also be individualized.

HOW SUPPLIED
Noludar is available as amethyst and white 300-mg capsules in bottles of 100 (NDC 0004-0019-01) and in bottles of 500 (NDC 0004-0019-14); and as 200-mg white, scored tablets in bottles of 100 (NDC 0004-0017-01). Imprints are as follows: Noludar 300—NOLUDAR® 300 Roche; Noludar 200-mg tablets—(front) NOLUDAR 200, (back) ROCHE.
P.I. 1188

Shown in Product Identification Section, page 425

PANTOPON®   Ⓒ
[*pan'to-pon*]
(hydrochlorides of opium alkaloids/Roche)

The following text is complete prescribing information based on official labeling in effect June 1, 1989.

DESCRIPTION
Pantopon (hydrochlorides of opium alkaloids), a narcotic analgesic, is a sterile injectable preparation for intramuscular and subcutaneous administration. It contains all the alkaloids of opium in a highly purified form free from inert matter and in approximately the same proportions as they occur in nature.
Hydrochlorides of opium alkaloids is a yellowish-gray powder which is freely soluble in water. The approximate composition of Pantopon is as follows: anhydrous morphine — 50 percent, and bases of secondary opium alkaloids — 29.9 to

34.2 percent. One part of Pantopon is equivalent to five parts of opium, U.S.P.
One ml of Pantopon contains 20 mg hydrochlorides of opium alkaloids compounded with 6% alcohol, 136 mg glycerin, 0.2% parabens (methyl and propyl) as preservatives, and either acetic acid, sodium hydroxide, or both, as necessary to adjust pH to approximately 3.3.

CLINICAL PHARMACOLOGY
The action of Pantopon is essentially that of opium. Pantopon, therefore, exhibits not only the action of morphine but also the actions of codeine, papaverine and other alkaloids present in opium. The other alkaloids in Pantopon enhance the sedative and analgesic effects of morphine and tend to minimize its undesirable side effects. Pharmacokinetic data on Pantopon are not available; however, data are available on morphine, the major component of Pantopon.
Morphine acts as an agonist interacting with stereospecific receptors in the brain and other tissues; the receptor sites are distributed throughout the CNS and are present in highest concentrations in the limbic system, thalamus, striatum, hypothalamus, midbrain and spinal cord. Morphine is well absorbed after subcutaneous and intramuscular administration. When therapeutic concentrations of morphine are present in plasma, approximately one-third of the drug is protein bound. Unbound morphine accumulates in parenchyma tissues (such as lung, liver, kidney and spleen) and skeletal muscle; however, 24 hours following the last dose, concentrations of the drug in these tissues are quite low.
The half-life of morphine in plasma is about 2.5 to 3 hours in young adults; in older patients, the half-life may be more prolonged. The major metabolic pathway for the drug is conjugation with glucuronic acid and the major route of elimination is through glomerular filtration. Ninety percent of the total excretion takes place during the first 24 hours after administration, although traces of the drug are detectable in the urine for well over 48 hours. About 7 to 10% of administered morphine eventually appears in the feces.

INDICATIONS AND USAGE
Pantopon is indicated in conditions in which the analgesic, sedative-hypnotic or narcotic effect of an opiate is needed. It is recommended for the relief of severe pain in place of morphine.

CONTRAINDICATIONS
Pantopon is contraindicated in patients with a known hypersensitivity to this drug or to other opiates.

WARNINGS
Drug Dependence. Pantopon may be habit forming. Pantopon can produce drug dependence of the morphine type and has the potential for being abused. Psychological and physical dependence and tolerance may develop upon repeated administration of Pantopon; it should be prescribed and administered with the same degree of caution appropriate to the use of morphine.
Intravenous Use: Pantopon should not be administered intravenously. Rapid intravenous injection of narcotic analgesics increases the incidence of adverse reactions; severe respiratory depression, apnea, hypotension, peripheral circulatory collapse and cardiac arrest have occurred.
Interaction with Other Central Nervous System Depressants: Pantopon should be used with great caution and in reduced dosage in patients who are concurrently receiving other narcotic analgesics, general anesthetics, tranquilizers (including phenothiazines), sedative-hypnotics (including barbiturates), tricyclic antidepressants, MAO inhibitors and other CNS depressants, including alcohol. Respiratory depression, hypotension and profound sedation or coma may result.
Hypotensive Effects: The administration of Pantopon may result in severe hypotension in the postoperative patient or in any individual whose ability to maintain blood pressure has been compromised by a depleted blood volume or by the administration of drugs, such as phenothiazines or certain anesthetics.
Head Injury: The respiratory depressant effects of Pantopon may be markedly exaggerated in the presence of head injury or other intracranial lesions. Furthermore, narcotics produce adverse reactions which may obscure the clinical course of patients with head injuries. In such patients Pantopon must be used with extreme caution and only if its use is deemed essential.
Asthma and Other Respiratory Conditions: Pantopon should be used with extreme caution in patients with bronchial asthma, chronic obstructive pulmonary disease or *cor pulmonale.* Similarly, it should be used with extreme caution in patients having a decreased respiratory reserve or with pre-existing respiratory depression, hypoxia or hypercapnia. In such patients, usual therapeutic doses of narcotics may decrease respiratory drive while simultaneously increasing airway resistance to the point of apnea.

PRECAUTIONS
General: The administration of Pantopon or other narcotics may obscure the diagnosis or clinical course in patients with acute abdominal conditions. Pantopon should be administered with caution and the initial dose should be reduced in

patients who are elderly or debilitated and in those patients with severe impairment of hepatic or renal function, hypothyroidism, Addison's disease, toxic psychosis, and prostatic hypertrophy or urethral stricture.
Information for Patients: In the unlikely event that Pantopon would be administered to ambulatory patients, they should be cautioned that Pantopon may impair the mental and/or physical abilities required for the performance of potentially hazardous tasks such as driving a car or operating machinery.
Drug Interactions: See WARNINGS section.
Carcinogenesis, mutagenesis, impairment of fertility: There have been no studies performed with Pantopon to permit an evaluation of its carcinogenic or mutagenic potential. Studies have not been performed to determine the effect of Pantopon on fertility and reproduction.
Pregnancy:
Teratogenic Effects. Pregnancy Category C. Animal studies have demonstrated the teratogenicity of morphine, the major component of Pantopon, in rats, mice and hamsters. There are no adequate or well-controlled studies of Pantopon in either laboratory animals or in pregnant women. It is also not known whether Pantopon can cause fetal harm when administered to a pregnant woman or if it can affect reproductive capacity. Pantopon should be used during pregnancy only if the potential benefit justifies the potential risk to the fetus.
Nursing Mothers: It has been reported that morphine is excreted in human milk in microgram amounts. Because of the potential for serious adverse reactions from Pantopon in nursing infants, a decision should be made whether to discontinue nursing or to discontinue the drug, taking into account the importance of the drug to the mother.
Pediatric Use: Safety and effectiveness in children have not been established.

ADVERSE REACTIONS
Note: Included in this listing are adverse reactions which have not been reported with this specific drug; however, the pharmacologic similarities among the narcotics require that each of the reactions be considered with Pantopon administration.
Neurologic: Respiratory depression and arrest, pinpoint pupils, visual disturbances, coma, sedation, dizziness, headache, tremors, uncoordinated muscle movements. Inadvertent injection in close proximity to a nerve may result in a sensory-motor paralysis which is usually, though not always, transitory.
Psychiatric: Delirium, euphoria, dysphoria, weakness, agitation, hallucinations.
Cardiovascular: Hypotension, collapse, tachycardia, bradycardia, palpitation.
Dermatologic: Rash, urticaria (local and generalized), pruritus.
Gastrointestinal: Nausea, emesis, constipation, dry mouth, biliary tract spasm.
Genitourinary: Urinary retention.
Miscellaneous: Diaphoresis, flushing, pain at the site of injection, anaphylactoid reactions.

DRUG ABUSE AND DEPENDENCE
Pantopon is subject to Schedule II control under the Federal Controlled Substances Act of 1970. This drug can produce drug dependence of the morphine type and, therefore, has the potential for being abused. Psychological and physical dependence and tolerance may develop upon repeated administration of Pantopon, and consequently the same precautions should be taken in administering the drug as with morphine. A narcotic order is required.

OVERDOSAGE
Serious overdosage with Pantopon is characterized by respiratory depression (a decrease in respiratory rate and/or tidal volume, Cheyne-Stokes respiration, cyanosis), extreme somnolence progressing to stupor or coma, skeletal muscle flaccidity, cold and clammy skin, and sometimes bradycardia and hypotension. In severe overdosage, apnea, circulatory collapse, cardiac arrest and death may occur. The triad of coma, pinpoint pupils and depressed respiration strongly suggests opioid poisoning.
Primary attention should be given to the reestablishment of adequate respiratory exchange through provision of a patent airway and through the institution of assisted or controlled ventilation. The narcotic antagonist, naloxone hydrochloride (Narcan), is a specific antidote against respiratory depression resulting from narcotic overdosage or unusual sensitivity to narcotics. An appropriate dose of this antagonist should be administered, preferably by the intravenous route, simultaneously with efforts at respiratory resuscitation.
An antagonist should not be administered in the absence of clinically significant respiratory or cardiovascular depression.
Oxygen, intravenous fluids, vasopressors and other supportive measures should be employed if needed.

NOTE

The administration of the usual dose of a narcotic antagonist will precipitate an acute withdrawal syndrome in patients physically dependent on narcotics. The severity of this syndrome will depend on the degree of physical dependence and the dose of the antagonist administered. The use of narcotic antagonists in such patients should be avoided if possible. If a narcotic antagonist must be used in physically dependent patients to treat serious respiratory depression, the antagonist should be administered with extreme care using only one-fifth to one-tenth the usual initial dose.

The intravenous LD_{50} of Pantopon in mice is 96 to 99 mg/kg.

DOSAGE AND ADMINISTRATION

One-third grain (20 mg) of Pantopon with a morphine content of $\frac{1}{6}$ grain (10 mg) is therapeutically equivalent to and is usually administered where $\frac{1}{4}$ grain (15 mg) of morphine is indicated.

Usual Adult Dosage:
5 to 20 mg ($\frac{1}{12}$ to $\frac{1}{3}$ grain) approximately every 4 to 5 hours according to the individual needs and severity of pain. Administer only by intramuscular or subcutaneous injection. Parenteral drug products should be inspected visually for particulate matter and discoloration prior to administration, whenever solution and container permit.

HOW SUPPLIED

Pantopon is supplied in 1-ml ampuls each containing 20 mg (1/3 grain) hydrochlorides of opium alkaloids/Roche — boxes of 10 (NDC 0004-1918-06).
P.I. 0585

PROVOCHOLINE®   ℞
[pro"vo-kol 'leen]
(methacholine Cl/Roche)

The following text is complete prescribing information based on official labeling in effect June 1, 1989.

> PROVOCHOLINE IS A BRONCHOCONSTRICTOR AGENT FOR DIAGNOSTIC PURPOSES ONLY AND SHOULD NOT BE USED AS A THERAPEUTIC AGENT. PROVOCHOLINE INHALATION CHALLENGE SHOULD BE PERFORMED ONLY UNDER THE SUPERVISION OF A PHYSICIAN TRAINED IN AND THOROUGHLY FAMILIAR WITH ALL ASPECTS OF THE TECHNIQUE OF METHACHOLINE CHALLENGE, ALL CONTRAINDICATIONS, WARNINGS AND PRECAUTIONS, AND THE MANAGEMENT OF RESPIRATORY DISTRESS.
>
> EMERGENCY EQUIPMENT AND MEDICATION SHOULD BE IMMEDIATELY AVAILABLE TO TREAT ACUTE RESPIRATORY DISTRESS.
>
> PROVOCHOLINE SHOULD BE ADMINISTERED ONLY BY INHALATION. SEVERE BRONCHOCONSTRICTION AND REDUCTION IN RESPIRATORY FUNCTION CAN RESULT FROM THE ADMINISTRATION OF PROVOCHOLINE. PATIENTS WITH SEVERE HYPERREACTIVITY OF THE AIRWAYS CAN EXPERIENCE BROCHOCONSTRICTION AT A DOSAGE AS LOW AS 0.025 MG/ML (0.125 CUMULATIVE UNITS). IF SEVERE BRONCHOCONSTRICTION OCCURS, IT SHOULD BE REVERSED IMMEDIATELY BY THE ADMINISTRATION OF A RAPID-ACTING INHALED BRONCHODILATOR AGENT (BETA AGONIST). BECAUSE OF THE POTENTIAL FOR SEVERE BRONCHOCONSTRICTION, PROVOCHOLINE CHALLENGE SHOULD NOT BE PERFORMED IN ANY PATIENT WITH CLINICALLY APPARENT ASTHMA, WHEEZING, OR VERY LOW BASELINE PULMONARY FUNCTION TESTS (E.G., FEV, LESS THAN 1 TO 1.5 LITER OR LESS THAN 70% OF THE PREDICTED VALUES). PLEASE CONSULT STANDARD NOMOGRAMS FOR PREDICTED VALUES.[1]

DESCRIPTION

Provocholine (brand of methacholine chloride/Roche) is a parasympathomimetic (cholinergic) bronchoconstrictor agent to be administered in solution only, by inhalation, for diagnostic purposes. Each 5-mL vial contains 100 mg of methacholine Cl powder which is to be reconstituted with 0.9% sodium chloride injection containing 0.4% phenol (pH 7.0). See DOSAGE AND ADMINISTRATION for dilution procedures, concentrations and schedule of administration. Chemically, methacholine Cl (the active ingredient) is 1-propanaminium, 2-(acetyloxy)-*N,N,N*,-trimethyl,-chloride. It is a white to practically white deliquescent compound, soluble in water. Methacholine Cl has an empirical formula of $C_8H_{18}ClNO_2$ and a calculated molecular weight of 195.69.

CLINICAL PHARMACOLOGY

Methacholine Cl is the β-methyl homolog of acetylcholine and differs from the latter primarily in its greater duration and selectivity of action. Bronchial smooth muscle contains significant parasympathetic (cholinergic) innervation. Bron-

choconstriction occurs when the vagus nerve is stimulated and acetylcholine is released from the nerve endings. Muscle constriction is essentially confined to the local site of release because acetylcholine is rapidly inactivated by acetylcholinesterase.

Compared with acetylcholine, methacholine Cl is more slowly hydrolyzed by acetylcholinesterase and is almost totally resistant to inactivation by nonspecific cholinesterase or pseudocholinesterase.

When a sodium chloride solution containing methacholine Cl is inhaled, subjects with asthma are markedly more sensitive to methacholine-induced bronchoconstriction than are healthy subjects. This difference in response is the pharmacologic basis for the Provocholine inhalation diagnostic challenge. However, it should be recognized that methacholine challenge may occasionally be positive after influenza, upper respiratory infections or immunizations, in very young or very old patients, or in patients with chronic lung disease (cystic fibrosis, sarcoidosis, tuberculosis, chronic obstructive pulmonary disease). The challenge may also be positive in patients with allergic rhinitis without asthma, in smokers, in patients after exposure to air pollutants, or in patients who have had or will in the future develop asthma.

There are no metabolic and pharmacokinetic data available on methacholine Cl.

INDICATIONS AND USAGE

Provocholine is indicated for the diagnosis of bronchial airway hyperreactivity in subjects who do not have clinically apparent asthma.

CONTRAINDICATIONS

Provocholine is contraindicated in patients with known hypersensitivity to this drug or to other parasympathomimetic agents.

Repeated administration of Provocholine by inhalation other than on the day that a patient undergoes challenge with increasing doses is contraindicated.

Inhalation challenge should not be performed in patients receiving any beta-adrenergic blocking agent because in such patients responses to methacholine Cl can be exaggerated or prolonged, and may not respond as readily to accepted modalities of treatment (see WARNINGS box).

PRECAUTIONS

General: Administration of Provocholine to patients with epilepsy, cardiovascular disease accompanied by bradycardia, vagotonia, peptic ulcer disease, thyroid disease, urinary tract obstruction or other condition that could be adversely affected by a cholinergic agent should be undertaken only if the physician feels benefit to the individual outweighs the potential risks.

Information for Patients: To assure the safe and effective use of Provocholine inhalation challenge, the following instructions and information should be given to patients:
1. Patients should be instructed regarding symptoms that may occur as a result of the test and how such symptoms can be managed.
2. A female patient should inform her physician if she is pregnant, or the date of her last onset of menses, or the date and result of her last pregnancy test. (See PRECAUTIONS: *Pregnancy*.)

Carcinogenesis, Mutagenesis, Impairment of Fertility: There have been no studies with methacholine Cl that would permit an evaluation of its carcinogenic or mutagenic potential or of its effect on fertility.

Pregnancy: Teratogenic Effects: Pregnancy Category C. Animal reproduction studies have not been conducted with methacholine Cl. It is not known whether methacholine Cl can cause fetal harm when administered to a pregnant patient or affect reproductive capacity. Methacholine Cl should be given to a pregnant woman only if clearly needed.

IN FEMALES OF CHILDBEARING POTENTIAL, PROVOCHOLINE INHALATION CHALLENGE SHOULD BE PERFORMED EITHER WITHIN TEN DAYS FOLLOWING THE ONSET OF MENSES OR WITHIN TWO WEEKS OF A NEGATIVE PREGNANCY TEST.

Nursing Mothers: Provocholine inhalation challenge should not be administered to a nursing mother since it is not known whether methacholine Cl when inhaled is excreted in breast milk.

Pediatric Use: The safety and efficacy of Provocholine inhalation challenge have not been established in children below the age of 5 years.

ADVERSE REACTIONS

Adverse reactions associated with 153 inhaled methacholine Cl challenges include one occurrence each of headache, throat irritation, lightheadedness and itching.

Provocholine is to be administered only by inhalation. When administered orally or by injection, methacholine Cl is reported to be associated with nausea and vomiting, substernal pain or pressure, hypotension, fainting and transient complete heart block. (See OVERDOSAGE.)

OVERDOSAGE

Provocholine is to be administered only by inhalation. When administered orally or by injection, overdosage with metha-

choline Cl can result in a syncopal reaction, with cardiac arrest and loss of consciousness. Serious toxic reactions should be treated with 0.5 mg to 1 mg of atropine sulfate, administered IM or IV.

The acute (24-hour) oral LD_{50} of methacholine Cl and related compounds is 1100 mg/kg in the mouse and 750 mg/kg in the rat.

Cynomolgus monkeys were exposed to a 2% (20 mg/mL) aerosol of methacholine Cl in acute (10-minute) and subchronic (7-day) inhalation toxicity studies. In the former study, animals exposed to the aerosol for up to 10 minutes demonstrated an increase in respiratory rate and decrease in tidal volume after 30 seconds. These changes peaked at 2 minutes and were followed by a rise in pulmonary resistance and a decrease in compliance. Pulmonary function returned to normal 20 to 25 minutes after exposure ended. In the 7-day study, monkeys were given daily inhalations equivalent to the maximum and roughly five times the maximum standard human dose. Although the typical pulmonary response/recovery sequence was observed, distinct changes in airway resistance were noted at the end of the study. These changes were not rapidly reversed in the maximum equivalent standard-dose group, which was observed for 9 weeks.

DOSAGE AND ADMINISTRATION

Before Provocholine inhalation challenge is begun, baseline pulmonary function tests must be performed. A subject to be challenged must have an FEV_1 of at least 70% of the predicted value.

The target level for a positive challenge is a 20% reduction in the FEV_1 compared with the baseline value after inhalation of the control sodium chloride solution. This target value should be calculated and recorded before Provocholine challenge is started.

Dilutions: (Note: Do not inhale powder. Do not handle this material if you have asthma or hay fever.) All dilutions should be made with 0.9% sodium chloride injection containing 0.4% phenol (pH 7.0). After adding the sodium chloride solution, shake each vial to obtain a clear solution.

Vial A.	Add 4 mL of 0.9% sodium chloride injection containing 0.4% phenol (pH 7.0) to the 5-ML vial containing 100 mg of Provocholine. This is *vial A,* which contains a concentration of 25 mg/mL.
Vial B.	Remove 3 mL from vial A (25 mg/mL), transfer to another vial and add 4.5 mL of 0.9% sodium chloride injection containing 0.4% phenol (pH 7.0). This is *vial B,* which contains a concentration of 10 mg/mL. An alternative method of preparing vial B is to remove 1 mL from vial A and add 1.5 mL of 0.9% sodium chloride injection containing 0.4% phenol (pH 7.0).
Vial C.	Remove 1 mL from vial A (25 mg/mL), transfer to another vial and add 9 mL of 0.9% sodium chloride injection containing 0.4% phenol (pH 7.0). This is *vial C,* which contains a concentration of 2.5 mg/mL. (This step depletes the contents of vial A if the first dilution method under Vial B directions is used.)
Vial D.	Remove 1 mL from vial C (2.5 mg/mL), transfer to another vial and add 9 mL of 0.9% sodium chloride injection containing 0.4% phenol (pH 7.0). This is *vial D,* which contains a concentration of 0.25 mg/mL.
Vial E.	Remove 1 mL from vial D (0.25 mg/mL), transfer to another vial and add 9 mL of 0.9% sodium chloride injection containing 0.4% phenol (pH 7.0). This is *vial E,* which contains a concentration of 0.025 mg/mL.

Dilutions A through D should be stored at 36° to 46°F in a refrigerator and can be stored for up to two weeks. (The unreconstituted powder should be stored at 59° to 86°F.) After this time, discard the vials and prepare new dilutions. Freezing does not affect the stability of dilutions A through D. Vial E must be prepared on the day of challenge. A bacterial-retentive filter (porosity 0.22μ) should be used when transferring a solution from each vial to a nebulizer.

Procedure: A standardized procedure for inhalation has been developed.

The challenge is performed by giving a subject ascending serial concentrations of Provocholine. At each concentration, five breaths are administered by a nebulizer that permits intermittent delivery time of 0.6 seconds by either a Y-tube or a breath-actuated timing device (dosimeter).

At each of five inhalations of a serial concentration, the subject begins at functional residual capacity (FRC) and slowly and completely inhales the dose delivered. Within five minutes, FEV_1 values are determined. The procedure ends either when there is a 20% or greater reduction in the FEV_1 compared with the baseline sodium chloride solution value (*i.e.,* a positive response) or if 188.88 total cumulative units has been administered (see table below) and the FEV_1 has been reduced by 14% or less (*i.e.,* a negative response). If there is a reduction of 15% to 19% in the FEV_1 compared with baseline, either the challenge may be repeated at that

Continued on next page

Roche Labs.—Cont.

concentration or a higher concentration may be given as long as the dosage administered does not result in total cumulative units exceeding 188.88.

The following is a suggested schedule for the administration of Provocholine challenge. Cumulative units are calculated by multiplying the number of breaths by the concentration administered.

Total cumulative units is the sum of cumulative units for each concentration administered.

[See table below].

An inhaled beta-agonist may be administered after Provocholine challenge to expedite the return of the FEV_1 to baseline and to relieve the discomfort of the subject. Most patients revert to normal pulmonary function within 5 minutes following bronchodilators or within 30 to 45 minutes without any bronchodilator.

HOW SUPPLIED

5 mL vials containing 100 mg of methacholine chloride powder which is to be reconstituted with 0.9% sodium chloride injection containing 0.4% phenol (pH 7.0)—boxes of 1 (NDC 0004-6102-01). Store the powder at 59° to 86°F. Refrigerate the reconstituted solutions at 36° to 46°F.

REFERENCE

1. Morris JF, Koski WA, Johnson LC: Spirometric standards for healthy nonsmoking adults. *Am Rev Resp Dis* 103 :57–67, Jan 1971.

P.I. 0288

ROCALTROL®   ℞
[ro-cal'trol]
(calcitriol/Roche)
CAPSULES

The following text is complete prescribing information based on official labeling in effect June 1, 1989.

DESCRIPTION

Rocaltrol (calcitriol/Roche) is a synthetic vitamin D analog which is active in the regulation of the absorption of calcium from the gastrointestinal tract and its utilization in the body. It is available in capsules containing 0.25 mcg or 0.5 mcg calcitriol/Roche. Each capsule also contains butylated hydroxyanisole (BHA), butylated hydroxytoluene (BHT) and fractionated triglyceride of coconut oil. Gelatin capsule shells contain glycerin, parabens (methyl and propyl) and sorbitol, with the following dye systems: 0.25 mcg—FD&C Yellow No. 6 and titanium dioxide; 0.5 mcg—FD&C Red No. 3, FD&C Yellow No. 6 and titanium dioxide.

Calcitriol is a colorless, crystalline compound which occurs naturally in humans. It has a calculated molecular weight of 416.65 and is soluble in organic solvents but relatively insoluble in water. Chemically, calcitriol is 9,10-seco(5Z,7E)-5,7,10(19)-cholestatriene-1α, 3β, 25-triol.

The other names frequently used for calcitriol are 1α,25-dihydroxycholecalciferol, 1,25-dihydroxyvitamin D_3, 1,25-DHCC, 1,25$(OH)_2D_3$ and 1,25-diOHC.

CLINICAL PHARMACOLOGY

Man's natural supply of vitamin D depends mainly on exposure to the ultraviolet rays of the sun for conversion of 7-dehydrocholesterol in the skin to vitamin D_3 (cholecalciferol). Vitamin D_3 must be metabolically activated in the liver and the kidney before it is fully active as a regulator of calcium and phosphorus metabolism at target tissues. The initial transformation of vitamin D_3 is catalyzed by a vitamin D_3-25-hydroxylase enzyme (25-OHase) present in the liver, and the product of this reaction is 25-hydroxyvitamin D_3 [25-$(OH)D_3$]. Hydroxylation of 25-$(OH)D_3$ occurs in the mitochondria of kidney tissue, activated by the renal 25-hydroxyvitamin D_3-1 alpha-hydroxylase (alpha-OHase), to produce 1,25-$(OH)_2D_3$ (calcitriol), the active form of vitamin D_3. Several metabolites of calcitriol have been identified which include:

1α, 25, $(OH)_2$-24-oxo-D_3
1α, 23,25$(OH)_3$-24-oxo-D_3
1α, 24R,25$(OH)_3D_3$
1α, 25R$(OH)_2$-26-23S-lactone D_3
1α, 25S,26$(OH)_3D_3$
1α, 25$(OH)_2$-23-oxo-D_3

1α, 25R,26$(OH)_3$-23-oxo-D_3
1α, (OH)24,25,26,27-tetranor-COOH-D_3

The two known sites of action of calcitriol are intestine and bone. A calcitriol receptor-binding protein appears to exist in the mucosa of human intestine. Additional evidence suggests that calcitriol may also act on the kidney and the parathyroid glands. Calcitriol is the most active known form of vitamin D_3 in stimulating intestinal calcium transport. In acutely uremic rats calcitriol has been shown to stimulate intestinal calcium absorption. The kidneys of uremic patients cannot adequately synthesize calcitriol, the active hormone formed from precursor vitamin D. Resultant hypocalcemia and secondary hyperparathyroidism are a major cause of the metabolic bone disease of renal failure. However, other bone-toxic substances which accumulate in uremia (*e.g.*, aluminum) may also contribute.

The beneficial effect of Rocaltrol in renal osteodystrophy appears to result from correction of hypocalcemia and secondary hyperparathyroidism. It is uncertain whether Rocaltrol produces other independent beneficial effects.

Calcitriol is rapidly absorbed from the intestine. Peak serum concentrations (above basal values) were reached within 3 to 6 hours following oral administration of single doses of 0.25 to 1.0 mcg of Rocaltrol. The half-life of calcitriol elimination from serum was found to range from 3 to 6 hours. Following a single oral dose of 0.5 mcg, mean serum concentrations of calcitriol rose from a baseline value of 40.0 ± 4.4 (S.D.) pg/ml to 60.0 ± 4.4 pg/ml at 2 hours, and declined to 53.0 ± 6.9 at 4 hours, 50 ± 7.0 at 8 hours, 44 ± 4.6 at 12 hours and 41.5 ± 5.1 at 24 hours. The duration of pharmacologic activity of a single dose of calcitriol is about 3 to 5 days.

Calcitriol and other vitamin D metabolites are transported in blood, bound to specific plasma proteins. Enterohepatic recycling and biliary excretion of calcitriol occurs. Following intravenous administration of radiolabeled calcitriol in normal subjects, approximately 27% and 7% of the radioactivity appeared in the feces and urine, respectively, within 24 hours. When a 1-mcg oral dose of radiolabeled calcitriol was administered to normals, approximately 10% of the total radioactivity appeared in urine within 24 hours. Cumulative excretion of radioactivity on the sixth day following intravenous administration of radiolabeled calcitriol averaged 16% in urine and 49% in feces.

There is evidence that maternal calcitriol may enter the fetal circulation. It is not known if calcitriol is excreted in human milk.

INDICATIONS AND USAGE

Rocaltrol is indicated in the management of hypocalcemia and the resultant metabolic bone disease in patients undergoing chronic renal dialysis. In these patients, Rocaltrol administration enhances calcium absorption, reduces serum alkaline phosphatase levels and may reduce elevated parathyroid hormone levels and the histological manifestations of osteitis fibrosa cystica and defective mineralization.

Rocaltrol is also indicated in the management of hypocalcemia and its clinical manifestations in patients with postsurgical hypoparathyroidism, idiopathic hypoparathyroidism, and pseudohypoparathyroidism.

CONTRAINDICATIONS

Rocaltrol should not be given to patients with hypercalcemia or evidence of vitamin D toxicity.

WARNINGS

Since Rocaltrol is the most potent metabolite of vitamin D available, pharmacologic doses of vitamin D and its derivatives should be withheld during Rocaltrol treatment to avoid possible additive effects and hypercalcemia.

Both appropriate oral phosphate-binders and a low phosphate diet should be used to control serum phosphate levels in patients undergoing dialysis.

Magnesium-containing antacids and Rocaltrol should not be used concomitantly in patients on chronic renal dialysis because such use may lead to the development of hypermagnesemia.

Overdosage of any form of vitamin D is dangerous (see also OVERDOSAGE). Progressive hypercalcemia due to overdosage of vitamin D and its metabolites may be so severe as to require emergency attention. Chronic hypercalcemia can lead to generalized vascular calcification, nephrocalcinosis and other soft-tissue calcification. **The serum calcium times phospate (Ca × P) product should not be allowed to exceed 70.** Radiographic evaluation of suspect anatomical regions may be useful in the early detection of this condition.

PRECAUTIONS

General: Excessive dosage of Rocaltrol induces hypercalcemia and in some instances hypercalciuria; therefore, early in treatment during dosage adjustment, serum calcium should be determined twice weekly. In dialysis patients, a fall in serum alkaline phosphatase levels usually antedates the appearance of hypercalcemia and may be an indication of impending hypercalcemia. Should hypercalcemia develop, the drug should be discontinued immediately. Rocaltrol should be given cautiously to patients on digitalis, because hypercalcemia in such patients may precipitate cardiac arrhythmias.

In patients with normal renal function, chronic hypercalcemia may be associated with an increase in serum creatinine. While this is usually reversible, it is important in such patients to pay careful attention to those factors which may lead to hypercalcemia. Rocaltrol therapy should always be started at the lowest possible dose and should not be increased without careful monitoring of the serum calcium. An estimate of daily dietary calcium intake should be made and the intake adjusted when indicated.

Patients with normal renal function taking Rocaltrol should avoid dehydration. Adequate fluid intake should be maintained.

Information for the patient: The patient and his or her parents or spouse should be informed about compliance with dosage instructions, adherence to instructions about diet and calcium supplementation and avoidance of the use of unapproved nonprescription drugs. Patients should also be carefully informed about the symptoms of hypercalcemia (see ADVERSE REACTIONS section).

Laboratory tests: For dialysis patients, serum calcium, phosphorus, magnesium and alkaline phosphatase should be determined periodically. For hypoparathyroid patients, serum calcium, phosphorus and 24-hour urinary calcium should be determined periodically.

Drug interactions: Cholestyramine has been reported to reduce intestinal absorption of fat-soluble vitamins; as such it may impair intestinal absorption of Rocaltrol. (Also see WARNINGS and PRECAUTIONS [General] sections.)

Carcinogenesis, mutagenesis, impairment of fertility: Long-term studies in animals have not been conducted to evaluate the carcinogenic potential of Rocaltrol. There was no evidence of mutagenicity as studied by the Ames method. No significant effects of Rocaltrol on fertility and/or general reproductive performances were reported.

Pregnancy: Teratogenic effects: Pregnancy Category C. Rocaltrol has been found to be teratogenic in rabbits when given in doses 4 and 15 times the dose recommended for human use. All 15 fetuses in 3 litters at these doses showed external and skeletal abnormalities. However, none of the other 23 litters (156 fetuses) showed significant abnormalities compared with controls. Teratogenicity studies in rats showed no evidence of teratogenic potential. There are no adequate and well-controlled studies in pregnant women. Rocaltrol should be used during pregnancy only if the potential benefit justifies the potential risk to the fetus.

Nonteratogenic effects: In the rabbit, dosages of 0.3 mcg/kg/day administered on days 7 to 18 of gestation resulted in 19% maternal mortality, a decrease in mean fetal body weight and a reduced number of newborn surviving to 24 hours. A study of peri- and postnatal development in rats resulted in hypercalcemia in the offspring of dams given Rocaltrol at doses of 0.08 or 0.3 mcg/kg/day, hypercalcemia and hypophosphatemia in dams at doses of 0.08 or 0.3 mcg/kg/day, and increased serum urea nitrogen in dams given Rocaltrol at a dose of 0.3 mcg/kg/day. In another study in rats, maternal weight gain was slightly reduced at a dose of 0.3 mcg/kg/day administered on days 7 to 15 of gestation. The offspring of a woman administered 17 to 36 mcg/day of Rocaltrol (17 to 144 times the recommended dose) during pregnancy manifested mild hypercalcemia in the first two days of life which returned to normal at day 3.

Nursing mothers: It is not known whether calcitriol is excreted in human milk. Because many drugs are excreted in human milk and because of the potential for serious adverse reactions from Rocaltrol in nursing infants, a mother should not nurse while taking this drug.

Pediatric use: Safety and efficacy of Rocaltrol in children undergoing dialysis have not been established.

ADVERSE REACTIONS

Since Rocaltrol is believed to be the active hormone which exerts vitamin D activity in the body, adverse effects are, in general, similar to those encountered with excessive vitamin D intake. The early and late signs and symptoms of vitamin D intoxication associated with hypercalcemia include:

Early: Weakness, headache, somnolence, nausea, vomiting, dry mouth, constipation, muscle pain, bone pain and metallic taste.

Late: Polyuria, polydipsia, anorexia, weight loss, nocturia, conjunctivitis (calcific), pancreatitis, photophobia, rhinorrhea, pruritus, hyperthermia, decreased libido, elevated BUN, albuminuria, hypercholesterolemia, elevated SGOT

Serial Concentration		Number of Breaths	Cumulative Units per Concentration	Total Cumulative Units
0.025	mg/mL	5	0.125	0.125
0.25	mg/mL	5	1.25	1.375
2.5	mg/mL	5	12.5	13.88
10.0	mg/mL	5	50.0	63.88
25.0	mg/mL	5	125.0	188.88

and SGPT, ectopic calcification, hypertension, cardiac arrhythmias and, rarely, overt psychosis.

In clinical studies on hypoparathyroidism and pseudohypoparathyroidism, hypercalcemia was noted on at least one occasion in about 1 in 3 patients and hypercalciuria in about 1 in 7. Elevated serum creatinine levels were observed in about 1 in 6 patients (approximately one half of whom had normal levels at baseline).

One case of erythema multiforme was confirmed by rechallenge.

OVERDOSAGE

Administration of Rocaltrol to patients in excess of their daily requirements can cause hypercalcemia, hypercalciuria and hyperphosphatemia. High intake of calcium and phosphate concomitant with Rocaltrol may lead to similar abnormalities. High levels of calcium in the dialysate bath may contribute to the hypercalcemia.

Treatment of Hypercalcemia and Overdosage: General treatment of hypercalcemia (greater than 1 mg/dl above the upper limit of the normal range) consists of immediate discontinuation of Rocaltrol therapy, institution of a low calcium diet and withdrawal of calcium supplements. Serum calcium levels should be determined daily until normocalcemia ensues. Hypercalcemia frequently resolves in two to seven days. When serum calcium levels have returned to within normal limits, Rocaltrol therapy may be reinstituted at a dose of 0.25 mcg/day less than prior therapy. Serum calcium levels should be obtained at least twice weekly after all dosage changes and subsequent dosage titration. In dialysis patients, persistent or markedly elevated serum calcium levels may be corrected by dialysis against a calcium-free dialysate.

Treatment of Accidental Overdosage of Rocaltrol: The treatment of acute accidental overdosage of Rocaltrol should consist of general supportive measures. If drug ingestion is discovered within a relatively short time, induction of emesis or gastric lavage may be of benefit in preventing further absorption. If the drug has passed through the stomach, the administration of mineral oil may promote its fecal elimination. Serial serum electrolyte determinations (especially calcium), rate of urinary calcium excretion and assessment of electrocardiographic abnormalities due to hypercalcemia should be obtained. Such monitoring is critical in patients receiving digitalis. Discontinuation of supplemental calcium and a low calcium diet are also indicated in accidental overdosage. Due to the relatively short duration of the pharmacological action of calcitriol, further measures are probably unnecessary. Should, however, persistent and markedly elevated serum calcium levels occur, there are a variety of therapeutic alternatives which may be considered, depending on the patient's underlying condition. These include the use of drugs such as phosphates and corticosteroids as well as measures to induce an appropriate forced diuresis. The use of peritoneal dialysis against a calcium-free dialysate has also been reported.

The oral toxicity of calcitriol is as follows:

Species	LD$_{50}$ (mg/kg)
mouse	2.0
rat	>5.0

DOSAGE AND ADMINISTRATION

The optimal daily dose of Rocaltrol must be carefully determined for each patient.

The effectiveness of Rocaltrol therapy is predicated on the assumption that each patient is receiving an adequate daily intake of calcium. The U.S. RDA for calcium in adults is 800 to 1200 mg. To ensure that each patient receives an adequate daily intake of calcium, the physician should either prescribe a calcium supplement or instruct the patient in proper dietary measures.

Dialysis patients: The recommended initial dose of Rocaltrol is 0.25 mcg/day. If a satisfactory response in the biochemical parameters and clinical manifestations of the disease state is not observed, dosage may be increased by 0.25 mcg/day at four- to eight-week intervals. During this titration period, serum calcium levels should be obtained at least twice weekly, and if hypercalcemia is noted, the drug should be immediately discontinued until normocalcemia ensues.

Patients with normal or only slightly reduced serum calcium levels may respond to Rocaltrol doses of 0.25 mcg every other day. Most patients undergoing hemodialysis respond to doses between 0.5 and 1 mcg/day.

Oral Rocaltrol may normalize plasma ionized calcium in some uremic patients, yet fail to suppress parathyroid hyperfunction. In these individuals with autonomous parathyroid hyperfunction, oral Rocaltrol may be useful to maintain normocalcemia, but has not been shown to be adequate treatment for hyperparathyroidism.

Hypoparathyroidism: The recommended initial dose of Rocaltrol is 0.25 mcg/day given in the morning. If a satisfactory response in the biochemical parameters and clinical manifestations of the disease is not observed, the dose may be increased at two- to four-week intervals. During the dosage titration period, serum calcium levels should be obtained at least twice weekly and, if hypercalcemia is noted, Rocaltrol should be immediately discontinued until normocalcemia ensues. Careful consideration should also be given to lowering the dietary calcium intake.

Most adult patients and pediatric patients age 6 years and older have responded to dosages in the range of 0.5 to 2 mcg daily. Pediatric patients in the 1–5 year age group with hypoparathyroidism have usually been given 0.25 to 0.75 mcg daily. The number of treated patients with pseudohypoparathyroidism less than 6 years of age is too small to make dosage recommendations.

HOW SUPPLIED

0.25 mcg calcitriol/Roche in soft gelatin, light orange, oval capsules, imprinted ROCALTROL 0.25 ROCHE; bottles of 30, (NDC 0004-0143-23), and bottles of 100, (NDC 0004-0143-01).

0.5 mcg calcitriol/Roche in soft gelatin, dark orange, oblong capsules, imprinted ROCALTROL 0.5 ROCHE; bottles of 100, (NDC 0004-0144-01).

Rocaltrol should be protected from heat and light.
P.I. 0286

Shown in Product Identification Section, page 425

ROCEPHIN® ℞

[ro-sef'in]
(ceftriaxone sodium/Roche)

The following text is complete prescribing information based on official labeling in effect June 1, 1989.

DESCRIPTION

Rocephin* (ceftriaxone sodium/Roche) is a sterile, semisynthetic, broad-spectrum cephalosporin antibiotic for intravenous or intramuscular administration. Ceftriaxone sodium is 5-Thia-1-azabicyclo[4.2.0]oct-2-ene-2-carboxylic acid, 7-[[(2-amino-4-thiazolyl)(methoxyimino) acetyl]-amino]-8-oxo-3-[[(1, 2, 5, 6-tetrahydro-2-methyl-5, 6-dioxo-1, 2, 4-triazin-3-yl)thio]methyl]-, disodium salt, [6R-[6α,7β(Z)]]-.

The chemical formula of ceftriaxone sodium is $C_{18}H_{16}N_8Na_2O_7S_3$·3.5 H_2O. It has a calculated molecular weight of 661.59.

Rocephin is a white to yellowish-orange crystalline powder which is readily soluble in water, sparingly soluble in methanol and very slightly soluble in ethanol. The pH of a 1% aqueous solution is approximately 6.7. The color of Rocephin solutions ranges from light yellow to amber, depending on the length of storage, concentration and diluent used.

Rocephin contains approximately 83 mg (3.6 mEq) of sodium per gram of ceftriaxone activity.

CLINICAL PHARMACOLOGY

Average plasma concentrations of ceftriaxone following a single 30-minute intravenous (I.V.) infusion of a 0.5, 1 or 2 gm dose and intramuscular (I.M.) administration of a single 0.5 or 1 gm dose in healthy subjects are presented in Table 1. [See table above].

Ceftriaxone was completely absorbed following I.M. administration with mean maximum plasma concentrations occurring between two and three hours postdosing. Multiple I.V. or I.M. doses ranging from 0.5 to 2 gm at 12- to 24-hour intervals resulted in 15 to 36% accumulation of ceftriaxone above single dose values.

Ceftriaxone concentrations in urine are high, as shown in Table 2. [See table below].

Thirty-three to 67% of a ceftriaxone dose was excreted in the urine as unchanged drug and the remainder was secreted in the bile and ultimately found in the feces as microbiologically inactive compounds. After a 1 gm I.V. dose, average concentrations of ceftriaxone, determined from one to three hours after dosing, were 581 mcg/ml in the gallbladder bile, 788 mcg/ml in the common duct bile, 898 mcg/ml in the cystic duct bile, 78.2 mcg/gm in the gallbladder wall and 62.1 mcg/ml in the concurrent plasma.

Over a 0.15 to 3 gm dose range in healthy adult subjects, the values of elimination half-life ranged from 5.8 to 8.7 hours; apparent volume of distribution from 5.78 to 13.5 L; plasma clearance from 0.58 to 1.45 L/hour; and renal clearance from 0.32 to 0.73 L/hour. Ceftriaxone is reversibly bound to human plasma proteins, and the binding decreased from a value of 95% bound at plasma concentrations of <25 mcg/ml to a value of 85% bound at 300 mcg/ml.

The average values of maximum plasma concentration, elimination half-life, plasma clearance and volume of distribution after a 50 mg/kg I.V. dose and after a 75 mg/kg I.V. dose in pediatric patients suffering from bacterial meningitis are shown in Table 3. Ceftriaxone penetrated the inflamed meninges of infants and children; CSF concentrations after a 50 mg/kg I.V. dose and after a 75 mg/kg I.V. dose are also shown in Table 3.

TABLE 3
Average Pharmacokinetic Parameters of Ceftriaxone in Pediatric Patients with Meningitis

	50 mg/kg I.V.	75 mg/kg I.V.
Maximum Plasma Concentrations (mcg/ml)	216	275
Elimination Half-life (hr)	4.6	4.3
Plasma Clearance (ml/hr/kg)	49	60
Volume of Distribution (ml/kg)	338	373
CSF Concentration—inflamed meninges (mcg/ml)	5.6	6.4
Range (mcg/ml)	1.3–18.5	1.3–44
Time after dose (hr)	3.7 (± 1.6)	3.3 (± 1.4)

Compared to that in healthy adult subjects, the pharmacokinetics of ceftriaxone were only minimally altered in elderly subjects and in patients with renal impairment or hepatic dysfunction (Table 4); therefore, dosage adjustments are not necessary for these patients with ceftriaxone dosages up to 2 gm per day. Ceftriaxone was not removed to any significant extent from the plasma by hemodialysis. In 6 of 26 dialysis patients, the elimination rate of ceftriaxone was markedly reduced, suggesting that plasma concentrations of ceftriaxone should be monitored in these patients to determine if dosage adjustments are necessary.

[See table on next page].

MICROBIOLOGY: The bactericidal activity of ceftriaxone results from inhibition of cell wall synthesis. Ceftriaxone has a high degree of stability in the presence of beta-lactamases, both penicillinases and cephalosporinases, of gram-negative

TABLE 1
Ceftriaxone Plasma Concentrations After Single Dose Administration

Dose/Route	Average Plasma Concentrations (mcg/ml)								
	0.5 hr	1 hr	2 hr	4 hr	6 hr	8 hr	12 hr	16 hr	24 hr
0.5 gm I.V.*	82	59	48	37	29	23	15	10	5
0.5 gm I.M.	30	41	43	39	31	25	16	ND†	ND
1 gm I.V.*	151	111	88	67	53	43	28	18	9
1 gm I.M.	40	68	76	68	56	44	29	ND	ND
2 gm I.V.*	257	192	154	117	89	74	46	31	15

* I.V. doses were infused at a constant rate over 30 minutes.
† ND = Not determined.

TABLE 2
Urinary Concentrations of Ceftriaxone After Single Dose Administration

Dose/Route	Average Urinary Concentrations (mcg/ml)					
	0–2 hr	2–4 hr	4–8 hr	8–12 hr	12–24 hr	24–48 hr
0.5 gm I.V.	526	366	142	87	70	15
0.5 gm I.M.	115	425	308	127	96	28
1 gm I.V.	995	855	293	147	132	32
1 gm I.M.	504	628	418	237	ND*	ND
2 gm I.V.	2692	1976	757	274	198	40

*ND = Not determined.

Continued on next page

Roche Labs.—Cont.

and gram-positive bacteria. Ceftriaxone is usually active against the following microorganisms *in vitro* and in clinical infections (see Indications and Usage):

GRAM-NEGATIVE AEROBES: Enterobacter aerogenes, Enterobacter cloacae, Escherichia coli, Haemophilus influenzae (including ampicillin-resistant strains), *H. parainfluenzae, Klebsiella* species (including *K. pneumoniae*), *Neisseria gonorrhoeae* (including penicillinase and nonpenicillinase producing strains), *Neisseria meningitidis, Proteus mirabilis, Proteus vulgaris, Morganella morganii* and *Serratia marcescens.*

Note: Many strains of the above organisms that are multiply resistant to other antibiotics, *e.g.,* penicillins, cephalosporins and aminoglycosides, are susceptible to ceftriaxone sodium.

Ceftriaxone is also active against many strains of *Pseudomonas aeruginosa.*

GRAM-POSITIVE AEROBES: Staphylococcus aureus (including penicillinase-producing strains) and *Staphylococcus epidermidis* (Note: methicillin-resistant staphylococci are resistant to cephalosporins, including ceftriaxone), *Streptococcus pyogenes* (Group A beta-hemolytic streptococci), *Streptococci agalactiae* (Group B streptococci) and *Streptococcus pneumoniae.* (Note: Most strains of enterococci, *Streptococcus faecalis* and Group D streptococci are resistant.)

Ceftriaxone also demonstrates *in vitro* activity against the following microorganisms, although the clinical significance is unknown:

GRAM-NEGATIVE AEROBES: Citrobacter freundii, Citrobacter diversus, Providencia species (including *Providencia rettgeri*), *Salmonella* species (including *S. typhi*), *Shigella* species and *Acinetobacter calcoaceticus.*

ANAEROBES: Bacteroides species, *Clostridium* species (Note: most strains of *C. difficile* are resistant.)

SUSCEPTIBILITY TESTING: Standard susceptibility disk method. Quantitative methods that require measurement of zone diameters give the most precise estimate of antibiotic susceptibility. One such procedure (Bauer AW, Kirby WMM, Sherris JC, Turck M: Antibiotic Susceptibility Testing by a Standardized Single Disk Method, *Am J Clin Pathol 45* :493–496, 1966; Standardized Disk Susceptibility Test, *Federal Register 39* :19182–19184, 1974; National Committee for Clinical Laboratory Standards, Approved Standard: ASM-2, Performance Standards for Antimicrobial Disk Susceptibility Tests, July 1975.) has been recommended for use with disks to test susceptibility to ceftriaxone.

Laboratory results of the standardized single-disk susceptibility test using a 30-mcg ceftriaxone disk should be interpreted according to the following three criteria:

1. Susceptible organisms produce zones of 18 mm or greater, indicating that the tested organism is likely to respond to therapy.
2. Organisms that produce zones of 14 to 17 mm are expected to be susceptible if a high dosage (not to exceed 4 gm per day) is used or if the infection is confined to tissues and fluids (*e.g.,* urine), in which high antibiotic levels are attained.
3. Resistant organisms produce zones of 13 mm or less, indicating that other therapy should be selected.

Organisms should be tested with the ceftriaxone disk, since ceftriaxone has been shown by *in vitro* tests to be active against certain strains found resistant to cephalosporin class disks.

Organisms having zones of less than 18 mm around the cephalothin disk are not necessarily of intermediate susceptibility or resistant to ceftriaxone.

Standardized procedures require use of control organisms. The 30-mcg ceftriaxone disk should give zone diameters between 29 and 35 mm, 22 and 28 mm and 17 and 23 mm for the reference strains *E. coli* ATCC 25922, *S. aureus* ATCC 25923 and *P. aeruginosa* ATCC 27853, respectively.

DILUTION TECHNIQUES: Based on the pharmacokinetic profile of ceftriaxone, a bacterial isolate may be considered susceptible if the MIC value for ceftriaxone is not more than 16 mcg/ml. Organisms are considered resistant to ceftriaxone if the MIC is equal to or greater than 64 mcg/ml. Organisms having an MIC value of less than 64 mcg/ml, but greater than 16 mcg/ml, are expected to be susceptible if a high dosage (not to exceed 4 gm per day) is used or if the infection is confined to tissues and fluids (*e.g.,* urine), in which high antibiotic levels are attained.

E. coli ATCC 25922, *S. aureus* ATCC 25923 and *P. aeruginosa* ATCC 27853 are also the recommended reference strains for controlling ceftriaxone dilution tests. Greater than 95% of MICs for the *E. coli* strain should fall within the range of 0.016 to 0.5 mcg/ml. The range for the *S. aureus* strain should be 1 to 2 mcg/ml, while for the *P. aeruginosa* strain the range should be 8 to 64 mcg/ml.

INDICATIONS AND USAGE

Rocephin is indicated for the treatment of the following infections when caused by susceptible organisms.

LOWER RESPIRATORY TRACT INFECTIONS caused by *Strep. pneumoniae, Streptococcus* species (excluding enterococci), *Staph. aureus, H. influenzae, H. parainfluenzae, Klebsiella* species (including *K. pneumoniae*), *E. coli, E. aerogenes, Proteus mirabilis* and *Serratia marcescens.*

SKIN AND SKIN STRUCTURE INFECTIONS caused by *Staph. aureus, Staph. epidermidis, Streptococcus* species (excluding enterococci), *E. cloacae, Klebsiella* species (including *K. pneumoniae*), *Proteus mirabilis* and *Pseudomonas aeruginosa.*

URINARY TRACT INFECTIONS (complicated and uncomplicated) caused by *E. coli, Proteus mirabilis, Proteus vulgaris, M. morganii* and *Klebsiella* species (including *K. pneumoniae*).

UNCOMPLICATED GONORRHEA (cervical/urethral and rectal) caused by *Neisseria gonorrhoeae,* including both penicillinase and nonpenicillinase producing strains.

PELVIC INFLAMMATORY DISEASE caused by *N. gonorrhoeae.*

BACTERIAL SEPTICEMIA caused by *Staph. aureus, Strep. pneumoniae, E. coli, H. influenzae* and *K. pneumoniae.*

BONE AND JOINT INFECTIONS caused by *Staph. aureus, Strep. pneumoniae, Streptococcus* species (excluding enterococci), *E. coli, P. mirabilis, K. pneumoniae* and *Enterobacter* species.

INTRA-ABDOMINAL INFECTIONS caused by *E. coli* and *K. pneumoniae.*

MENINGITIS caused by *H. influenzae, N. meningitidis* and *Strep. pneumoniae.* Ceftriaxone has also been used successfully in a limited number of cases of meningitis and shunt infections caused by *Staph. epidermidis* and *E. coli.*

SURGICAL PROPHYLAXIS: The preoperative administration of a single 1 gm dose of Rocephin may reduce the incidence of postoperative infections in patients undergoing surgical procedures classified as contaminated or potentially contaminated (*e.g.,* vaginal or abdominal hysterectomy) and in surgical patients for whom infection at the operative site would present serious risk (*e.g.,* during coronary artery bypass surgery). Although ceftriaxone has been shown to have been as effective as cefazolin in the prevention of infection following coronary artery bypass surgery, no placebo-controlled trials have been conducted to evaluate any cephalosporin antibiotic in the prevention of infection following coronary artery bypass surgery.

When administered prior to surgical procedures for which it is indicated, a single 1 gm dose of Rocephin provides protection from most infections due to susceptible organisms throughout the course of the procedure.

SUSCEPTIBILITY TESTING: Before instituting treatment with Rocephin, appropriate specimens should be obtained for isolation of the causative organism and for determination of its susceptibility to the drug. Therapy may be instituted prior to obtaining results of susceptibility testing.

CONTRAINDICATIONS

Rocephin is contraindicated in patients with known allergy to the cephalosporin class of antibiotics.

WARNINGS

BEFORE THERAPY WITH ROCEPHIN IS INSTITUTED, CAREFUL INQUIRY SHOULD BE MADE TO DETER-MINE WHETHER THE PATIENT HAS HAD PREVIOUS HYPERSENSITIVITY REACTIONS TO CEPHALOSPORINS, PENICILLINS OR OTHER DRUGS. THIS PRODUCT SHOULD BE GIVEN CAUTIOUSLY TO PENICILLIN-SENSITIVE PATIENTS. ANTIBIOTICS SHOULD BE ADMINISTERED WITH CAUTION TO ANY PATIENT WHO HAS DEMONSTRATED SOME FORM OF ALLERGY, PARTICULARLY TO DRUGS. SERIOUS ACUTE HYPERSENSITIVITY REACTIONS MAY REQUIRE THE USE OF SUBCUTANEOUS EPINEPHRINE AND OTHER EMERGENCY MEASURES.

Pseudomembranous colitis has been reported with nearly all antibacterial agents, including ceftriaxone, and may range in severity from mild to life-treatening. Therefore, it is important to consider this diagnosis in patients who present with diarrhea subsequent to the administration of antibacterial agents.

Treatment with antibacterial agents alters the normal flora of the colon and may permit overgrowth of clostridia. Studies indicate that a toxin produced by *Clostridium difficile* is one primary cause of "antibiotic-associated colitis."

After the diagnosis of pseudomembranous colitis has been established, therapeutic measures should be initiated. Mild cases of pseudomembranous colitis usually respond to drug discontinuation alone. In moderate to severe cases, consideration should be given to management with fluids and electrolytes, protein supplementation and treatment with an oral antibacterial drug effective against *C. difficile.*

In rare cases, shadows suggesting sludge have been detected by sonograms of the gallbladder in asymptomatic and symptomatic patients. This condition appears to be reversible on discontinuation of Rocephin therapy. In a few symptomatic patients receiving higher than usual doses, who underwent surgery, sludge containing traces of ceftriaxone was recovered from surgical specimens. Rocephin therapy should be discontinued in patients who develop signs or symptoms suggestive of gallbladder disease and conservative management considered.

PRECAUTIONS

GENERAL: Although transient elevations of BUN and serum creatinine have been observed, at the recommended dosages, the nephrotoxic potential of Rocephin is similar to that of other cephalosporins.

Ceftriaxone is excreted via both biliary and renal excretion (see Clinical Pharmacology). Therefore, patients with renal failure normally require no adjustment in dosage when usual doses of Rocephin are administered, but concentrations of drug in the serum should be monitored periodically. If evidence of accumulation exists, dosage should be decreased accordingly.

Dosage adjustments should not be necessary in patients with hepatic dysfunction; however, in patients with both hepatic dysfunction and significant renal disease, Rocephin dosage should not exceed 2 gm daily without close monitoring of serum concentrations.

Alterations in prothrombin times have occurred rarely in patients treated with Rocephin. Patients with impaired vitamin K synthesis or low vitamin K stores (*e.g.,* chronic hepatic disease and malnutrition) may require monitoring of prothrombin time during Rocephin treatment. Vitamin K administration (10 mg weekly) may be necessary if the prothrombin time is prolonged before or during therapy.

Prolonged use of Rocephin may result in overgrowth of nonsusceptible organisms. Careful observation of the patient is essential. If superinfection occurs during therapy, appropriate measures should be taken.

Rocephin should be prescribed with caution in individuals with a history of gastrointestinal disease, especially colitis.

CARCINOGENESIS, MUTAGENESIS, IMPAIRMENT OF FERTILITY:

Carcinogenesis: Considering the maximum duration of treatment and the class of the compound, carcinogenicity studies with ceftriaxone in animals have not been performed. The maximum duration of animal toxicity studies was six months.

Mutagenesis: Genetic toxicity tests included the Ames test, a micronucleus test and a test for chromosomal aberrations in human lymphocytes cultured *in vitro* with ceftriaxone. Ceftriaxone showed no potential for mutagenic activity in these studies.

Impairment of Fertility: Ceftriaxone produced no impairment of fertility when given intravenously to rats at daily doses up to 586 mg/kg/day, approximately 20 times the recommended clinical dose of 2 gm/day.

PREGNANCY: Teratogenic Effects: Pregnancy Category B. Reproductive studies have been performed in mice and rats at doses up to 20 times the usual human dose and have no evidence of embryotoxicity, fetotoxicity or teratogenicity. In primates, no embryotoxicity or teratogenicity was demonstrated at a dose approximately three times the human dose. There are, however, no adequate and well-controlled studies in pregnant women. Because animal reproductive studies are not always predictive of human response, this drug should be used during pregnancy only if clearly needed.

TABLE 4
Average Pharmacokinetic Parameters of Ceftriaxone in Humans

Subject Group	Elimination Half-Life (hr)	Plasma Clearance (L/hr)	Volume of Distribution (L)
Healthy Subjects	5.8–8.7	0.58–1.45	5.8–13.5
Elderly Subjects (mean age, 70.5 yr)	8.9	0.83	10.7
Patients with renal impairment			
Hemodialysis patients			
(0–5 ml/min)*	14.7	0.65	13.7
Severe (5–15 ml/min)	15.7	0.56	12.5
Moderate (16–30 ml/min)	11.4	0.72	11.8
Mild (31–60 ml/min)	12.4	0.70	13.3
Patients with liver disease	8.8	1.1	13.6

*Creatinine clearance.

Nonteratogenic Effects: In rats, in the Segment I (fertility and general reproduction) and Segment III (perinatal and postnatal) studies with intravenously administered ceftriaxone, no adverse effects were noted on various reproductive parameters during gestation and lactation, including postnatal growth, functional behavior and reproductive ability of the offspring, at doses of 586 mg/kg/day or less.

NURSING MOTHERS: Low concentrations of ceftriaxone are excreted in human milk. Caution should be exercised when Rocephin is administered to a nursing woman.

PEDIATRIC USE: Safety and effectiveness of Rocephin in neonates, infants and children have been established for the dosages described in the Dosage and Administration section. *In vitro* studies have shown that ceftriaxone, like some other cephalosporins, can displace bilirubin from serum albumin. Rocephin should not be administered to hyperbilirubinemic neonates, especially prematures.

ADVERSE REACTIONS

Rocephin is generally well tolerated. In clinical trials, the following adverse reactions, which were considered to be related to Rocephin therapy or of uncertain etiology, were observed:

LOCAL REACTIONS—pain, induration or tenderness at the site of injection (1%). Less frequently reported (less than 1%) was phlebitis after I.V. administration.

HYPERSENSITIVITY—rash (1.7%). Less frequently reported (less than 1%) were pruritus, fever or chills.

HEMATOLOGIC—eosinophilia (6%), thrombocytosis (5.1%) and leukopenia (2.1%). Less frequently reported (less than 1%) were anemia, neutropenia, lymphopenia, thrombocytopenia and prolongation of the prothrombin time.

GASTROINTESTINAL—diarrhea (2.7%). Less frequently reported (less than 1%) were nausea or vomiting, and dysgeusia. Onset of pseudomembranous colitis symptoms may occur during or after antibiotic treatment (see WARNINGS).

HEPATIC—elevations of SGOT (3.1%) or SGPT (3.3%). Less frequently reported (less than 1%) were elevations of alkaline phosphatase and bilirubin.

RENAL—elevations of the BUN (1.2%). Less frequently reported (less than 1%) were elevations of creatinine and the presence of casts in the urine.

CENTRAL NERVOUS SYSTEM—headache or dizziness were reported occasionally (less than 1%).

GENITOURINARY—moniliasis or vaginitis were reported occasionally (less than 1%).

MISCELLANEOUS—diaphoresis and flushing were reported occasionally (less than 1%).

Other rarely observed adverse reactions (less than 0.1%) include leukocytosis, lymphocytosis, monocytosis, basophilia, a decrease in the prothrombin time, jaundice, gallbladder sludge, glycosuria, hematuria, anaphylaxis, bronchospasm, serum sickness, abdominal pain, colitis, flatulence, dyspepsia, palpitations and epistaxis.

DOSAGE AND ADMINISTRATION

Rocephin may be administered intravenously or intramuscularly. The usual adult daily dose is 1 to 2 gm given once a day (or in equally divided doses twice a day) depending on the type and severity of the infection. The total daily dose should not exceed 4 grams.

For the treatment of serious miscellaneous infections in children, other than meningitis, the recommended total daily dose is 50 to 75 mg/kg (not to exceed 2 grams), given in divided doses every 12 hours.

Generally, Rocephin therapy should be continued for at least two days after the signs and symptoms of infection have disappeared. The usual duration is 4 to 14 days; in complicated infections longer therapy may be required.

In the treatment of meningitis, a daily dose of 100 mg/kg (not to exceed 4 grams), given in divided doses every 12 hours, should be administered with or without a loading dose of 75 mg/kg.

For the treatment of uncomplicated gonococcal infections, a single intramuscular dose of 250 mg is recommended.

For preoperative use (surgical prophylaxis), a single dose of 1 gm administered ½ to 2 hours before surgery is recommended.

When treating infections caused by *Streptococcus pyogenes*, therapy should be continued for at least ten days.

No dosage adjustment is necessary for patients with impairment of renal or hepatic function; however, blood levels should be monitored in patients with severe renal impairment (*e.g.*, dialysis patients) and in patients with both renal and hepatic dysfunctions.

DIRECTIONS FOR USE

INTRAMUSCULAR ADMINISTRATION: Reconstitute Rocephin powder with the appropriate diluent (see Compatibility-Stability section).

Vial Dosage Size	Amount of Diluent to be Added
250 mg	0.9 ml
500 mg	1.8 ml
1 gm	3.6 ml
2 gm	7.2 ml

After reconstitution, each 1 ml of solution contains approximately 250 mg equivalent of ceftriaxone. If required, more dilute solutions could be utilized. As with all intramuscular preparations, Rocephin should be injected well within the body of a relatively large muscle; aspiration helps to avoid unintentional injection into a blood vessel.

INTRAVENOUS ADMINISTRATION: Rocephin should be administered intravenously by infusion over a period of 30 minutes. Concentrations between 10 mg/ml and 40 mg/ml are recommended; however, lower concentrations may be used if desired. Reconstitute vials or "piggyback" bottles with an appropriate I.V. diluent (see Compatibility-Stability section).

Vial Dosage Size	Amount of Diluent to be Added
250 mg	2.4 ml
500 mg	4.8 ml
1 gm	9.6 ml
2 gm	19.2 ml

After reconstitution, each 1 ml of solution contains approximately 100 mg equivalent of ceftriaxone. Withdraw entire contents and dilute to the desired concentration with the appropriate I.V. diluent.

Piggyback Bottle Dosage Size	Amount of Diluent to be Added
1 gm	10 ml
2 gm	20 ml

After reconstitution, further dilute to 50 ml or 100 ml volumes with the appropriate I.V. diluent.

10 gm Bulk Pharmacy Container: This dosage size is *NOT FOR DIRECT ADMINISTRATION.* Reconstitute powder with 95 ml of an appropriate I.V. diluent. Before parenteral administration, withdraw the required amount, then further dilute to the desired concentration.

COMPATIBILITY AND STABILITY

Rocephin sterile powder should be stored at room temperature—77°F (25°C)—or below and protected from light. After reconstitution, protection from normal light is not necessary. The color of solutions ranges from light yellow to amber, depending on the length of storage, concentration and diluent used.

Rocephin *intramuscular* solutions remain stable (loss of potency less than 10%) for the following time periods: [See table above].

Rocephin *intravenous* solutions, at concentrations of 10, 20 and 40 mg/ml, remain stable (loss of potency less than 10%) for the following time periods stored in glass or PVC containers: [See table below].

Similarly, Rocephin *intravenous* solutions, at concentrations of 100 mg/ml, remain stable in the I.V. piggyback glass containers for the above specified time periods.

The following *intravenous* Rocephin solutions are stable at room temperature (25°C) for 24 hours, at concentrations between 10 mg/ml and 40 mg/ml: Sodium Lactate (PVC container), 10% Invert Sugar (glass container), 5% Sodium Bicarbonate (glass container), Freamine III (glass container), Normosol-M in 5% Dextrose (glass and PVC containers), Ionosol-B in 5% Dextrose (glass container), 5% Mannitol (glass container), 10% Mannitol (glass container).

After the indicated stability time periods, unused portions of solutions should be discarded.

Rocephin reconstituted with 5% Dextrose or 0.9% Sodium Chloride solution at concentrations between 10 mg/ml and 40 mg/ml, and then stored in frozen state (−20°C) in PVC (Viaflex) or polyolefin containers, remains stable for 26 weeks.

Frozen solutions should be thawed at room temperature before use. After thawing, unused portions should be discarded. Do not refreeze.

Rocephin solutions should *not* be physically mixed with or piggybacked into solutions containing other antimicrobial drugs or into diluent solutions other than those listed above, due to possible incompatibility.

ANIMAL PHARMACOLOGY

Concretions consisting of the precipitated calcium salt of ceftriaxone have been found in the gallbladder bile of dogs and baboons treated with ceftriaxone.

These appeared as a gritty sediment in dogs that received 100 mg/kg/day for four weeks. A similar phenomenon has been observed in baboons but only after a protracted dosing period (6 months) at higher dose levels (335 mg/kg/day or more). The likelihood of this occurrence in humans is considered to be low, since ceftriaxone has a greater plasma half-life in humans, the calcium salt of ceftriaxone is more soluble in human gallbladder bile and the calcium content of human gallbladder bile is relatively low.

HOW SUPPLIED

Rocephin (ceftriaxone sodium/Roche) is supplied as a sterile crystalline powder in glass vials and piggyback bottles. The following packages are available:

Vials containing 250 mg equivalent of ceftriaxone. Boxes of 1 (NDC 0004-1962-02) and boxes of 10 (NDC 0004-1962-01).

Vials containing 500 mg equivalent of ceftriaxone. Boxes of 1 (NDC 0004-1963-02) and boxes of 10 (NDC 0004-1963-01).

Vials containing 1 gm equivalent of ceftriaxone. Boxes of 1 (NDC 0004-1964-04) and boxes of 10 (NDC 0004-1964-01).

Piggyback bottles containing 1 gm equivalent of ceftriaxone. Boxes of 10 (NDC 0004-1964-03).

Vials containing 2 gm equivalent of ceftriaxone. Boxes of 10 (NDC 0004-1965-01).

Piggyback bottles containing 2 gm equivalent of ceftriaxone. Boxes of 10 (NDC 0004-1965-03).

Bulk pharmacy containers, containing 10 gm equivalent of ceftriaxone. Boxes of 1 (NDC 0004-1971-01). NOT FOR DIRECT ADMINISTRATION.

Rocephin (ceftriaxone sodium/Roche) is also supplied as a sterile crystalline powder in ADD-Vantage®* Vials as follows:

ADD-Vantage Vials containing 1 gm equivalent of ceftriaxone. Boxes of 10 (NDC 0004-1964-05).

ADD-Vantage Vials containing 2 gm equivalent of ceftriaxone. Boxes of 10 (NDC 0004-1965-05).

*Registered trademark of Abbott Laboratories, Inc.

Rocephin (ceftriaxone sodium/Roche) injection is also supplied premixed as a frozen, iso-osmotic, sterile, nonpyrogenic solution of ceftriaxone sodium in 50 mL single dose plastic containers. The following strengths are available:

1 gm equivalent of ceftriaxone, iso-osmotic with approximately 1.9 gm Dextrose Hydrous, USP, added (NDC 0004-1995-78).

2 gm equivalent of ceftriaxone, iso-osmotic with approximately 1.2 gm Dextrose Hydrous, USP, added (NDC 0004-1996-78).

NOTE: Rocephin in the frozen state should not be stored above −20°C.

Rocephin, supplied as a frozen, iso-osmotic, sterile, nonpyrogenic solution in plastic containers, is manufactured for Roche Laboratories. Division of Hoffmann-La Roche Inc., by Travenol Laboratories, Inc., Deerfield, Illinois 60015.

P.I. 0489

Table (top right — Intravenous stability)

Diluent	Concentration mg/ml	Storage — Room Temp. (25°C)	Storage — Refrigerated (4°C)
Sterile Water for Injection	100	3 days	10 days
	250	24 hours	3 days
0.9% Sodium Chloride Solution	100	3 days	10 days
	250	24 hours	3 days
5% Dextrose Solution	100	3 days	10 days
	250	24 hours	3 days
Bacteriostatic Water + 0.9% Benzyl Alcohol	100	24 hours	10 days
	250	24 hours	3 days
1% Lidocaine Solution (without epinephrine)	100	24 hours	10 days
	250	24 hours	3 days

Table (bottom left — Intravenous stability)

Diluent	Storage — Room Temp. (25°C)	Storage — Refrigerated (4°C)
Sterile Water	3 days	10 days
0.9% Sodium Chloride Solution	3 days	10 days
5% Dextrose Solution	3 days	10 days
10% Dextrose Solution	3 days	10 days
5% Dextrose + 0.9% Sodium Chloride Solution*	3 days	Incompatible
5% Dextrose + 0.45% Sodium Chloride Solution	3 days	Incompatible

*Data available for 10–40 mg/ml concentrations in this diluent in PVC containers only.

Continued on next page

Roche Labs.—Cont.

ROFERON®-A ℞

[ro-fear'on]

(Interferon alfa-2a, recombinant/Roche)

The following text is complete prescribing information based on official labeling in effect June 1, 1989.

DESCRIPTION

Roferon®-A (Interferon alfa-2a, recombinant/Roche) is a sterile protein product for use by injection. Roferon-A is manufactured by recombinant DNA technology that employs a genetically engineered *E. coli* bacterium containing DNA that codes for the human protein. Interferon alfa-2a, recombinant/Roche is a highly purified protein containing 165 amino acids, and it has an approximate molecular weight of 19,000 daltons. The purification procedure includes affinity chromatography using a murine monoclonal antibody. Fermentation is carried out in a defined nutrient medium containing the antibiotic tetracycline hydrochloride, 5 mg/L. However, the presence of the antibiotic is not detectable in the final product. Roferon-A is supplied as an injectable solution or as a sterile powder for injection with its accompanying diluent.

Injectable Solution:

3 million IU Roferon-A per vial—The solution is colorless and each mL contains 3 million IU of Interferon alfa-2a, recombinant/Roche, 9 mg sodium chloride, 5 mg Albumin (Human) and 3 mg phenol as a preservative.

18 million IU Roferon-A per vial—The solution is colorless and each mL contains 6 million IU of Interferon alfa-2a, recombinant/Roche, 9 mg sodium chloride, 5 mg Albumin (Human) and 3 mg phenol as a preservative. Each 0.5 mL contains 3 million IU of Interferon alfa-2a, recombinant-/Roche.

36 million IU Roferon-A per vial—The solution is colorless and each mL contains 36 million IU of Interferon alfa-2a, recombinant/Roche, 9 mg sodium chloride, 5 mg Albumin (Human) and 3 mg phenol as a preservative.

Sterile Powder for Injection:

18 million IU Roferon-A per vial—The powder is white to beige and when reconstituted with Diluent for Sterile Powder for Injection each 1 mL of reconstituted solution contains 6 million IU of Interferon alfa-2a, recombinant/Roche, 9 mg sodium chloride, 5 mg Albumin (Human) and 3 mg phenol as a preservative. Each 0.5 mL contains 3 million IU of Interferon alfa-2a, recombinant/Roche.

Diluent for Sterile Powder for Injection:

3 mL per vial—Each mL contains 6 mg sodium chloride, 3.3 mg Albumin (Human) and 3 mg phenol as a preservative.

The specific activity of Interferon alfa-2a, recombinant/Roche is 2×10^8 IU/mg protein. The route of administration is subcutaneous or intramuscular.

CLINICAL PHARMACOLOGY

The mechanism by which Interferon alfa-2a, recombinant/Roche, or any other interferon, exerts antitumor activity is not clearly understood. However, it is believed that direct antiproliferative action against tumor cells and modulation of the host immune response play important roles in the antitumor activity.

The biological activities of Interferon alfa-2a, recombinant/Roche are species-restricted, *i.e.*, they are expressed in a very limited number of species other than humans. As a consequence, preclinical evaluation of Interferon alfa-2a, recombinant/Roche has involved *in vitro* experiments with human cells and some *in vivo* experiments.[1] Using human cells in culture, Interferon alfa-2a, recombinant/Roche has been shown to have antiproliferative and immunomodulatory activities that are very similar to those of the mixture of interferon alfa subtypes produced by human leukocytes. *In vivo*, Interferon alfa-2a, recombinant/Roche has been shown to inhibit the growth of several human tumors growing in immunocompromised (nude) mice. Because of its species-restricted activity, it has not been possible to demonstrate antitumor activity in immunologically intact syngeneic tumor model systems, where effects on the host immune system would be observable. However, such antitumor activity has been repeatedly demonstrated with, for example, mouse interferon-alfa in transplantable mouse tumor systems. The clinical significance of these findings is unknown.

The metabolism of Interferon alfa-2a, recombinant/Roche is consistent with that of alfa interferons in general. Alfa interferons are totally filtered through the glomeruli and undergo rapid proteolytic degradation during tubular reabsorption, rendering a negligible reappearance of intact alfa interferon in the systemic circulation. Small amounts of radiolabeled Interferon alfa-2a, recombinant/Roche appear in the urine of isolated rat kidneys, suggesting near complete reabsorption of Interferon alfa-2a, recombinant/Roche catabolites. Liver metabolism and subsequent biliary excretion are considered minor pathways of elimination for alfa interferons. In a small study, Roferon-A was shown to have an effect on specific microsomal enzyme systems.[2] The clinical relevance of these findings is unknown.

The serum concentrations of Interferon alfa-2a, recombinant/Roche reflected a large intersubject variation in both healthy volunteers and patients with disseminated cancer. In healthy people, Interferon alfa-2a, recombinant/Roche exhibited an elimination half-life of 3.7 to 8.5 hours (means 5.1 hours), volume of distribution at steady-state of 0.223 to 0.748 L/kg (mean 0.400 L/kg) and a total body clearance of 2.14 to 3.62 mL/min/kg (mean 2.79 mL/min/kg) after a 36 million IU (2.2×10^8 pg) intravenous infusion. After intramuscular and subcutaneous administrations of 36 million IU, peak serum concentrations ranged from 1500 to 2580 pg/mL (mean 2020 pg/mL) at a mean time to peak of 3.8 hours and from 1250 to 2320 pg/mL (mean 1730 pg/mL) at a mean time to peak of 7.3 hours, respectively. The apparent fraction of the dose absorbed after intramuscular injection was greater than 80%.

The pharmacokinetics of Interferon alfa-2a, recombinant/Roche after single intramuscular doses to patients with disseminated cancer were similar to those found in healthy volunteers. Dose proportional increases in serum concentrations were observed after single doses up to 198 million IU. There were no changes in the distribution or elimination of Interferon alfa-2a, recombinant/Roche during twice daily (0.5 to 36 million IU), once daily (1 to 54 million IU), or three times weekly (1 to 136 million IU) dosing regimens up to 28 days of dosing. Multiple intramuscular doses of Interferon alfa-2a, recombinant/Roche resulted in an accumulation of 2 to 4 times the single dose serum concentrations. Pharmacokinetic information in patients with hairy cell leukemia or AIDS-related Kaposi's sarcoma is presently unknown.

Serum neutralizing activity, determined by a highly sensitive enzyme immunoassay and a neutralization bioassay, was detected in approximately 25% of all patients who received Roferon-A.[3] Antibodies to human leukocyte interferon may occur spontaneously in certain clinical conditions (cancer, systemic lupus erythematosus, herpes zoster) in patients who have never received exogenous interferon.[4] The significance of the appearance of serum neutralizing activity is not known.

The acute parenteral toxicity of Interferon alfa-2a, recombinant/Roche has been studied in mice, rats, rabbits and ferrets at doses up to 30 million IU/kg intravenously, and 500 million IU/kg intramuscularly. No treatment-related mortality was noted in any species given Interferon alfa-2a, recombinant/Roche by any of the routes of administration.

EFFECTS ON HAIRY CELL LEUKEMIA: During the first one to two months of treatment of patients with hairy cell leukemia, significant depression of hematopoiesis was likely to occur. Subsequently, there was improvement in circulating blood cell counts.

Of the 75 patients who were evaluable for efficacy following at least 16 weeks of therapy, 46 (61%) achieved complete or partial response. Twenty-one patients (28%) had a minor remission, eight (11%) remained stable, and none had worsening of disease. All patients who achieved either a complete or partial response had complete or partial normalization of all peripheral blood elements including hemoglobin level, white blood cell, neutrophil, monocyte and platelet counts with a concomitant decrease in peripheral blood and bone marrow hairy cells. Responding patients also exhibited a marked reduction in red blood cell and platelet transfusion requirements, a decrease in infectious episodes and improvement in performance status. The probability of survival for two years in patients receiving Roferon-A (94%) was statistically increased compared to a historical control group (75%).

EFFECTS ON AIDS-RELATED KAPOSI'S SARCOMA: In six studies with Roferon-A, doses of 3 to 54 million IU daily were evaluated for the treatment of AIDS-related Kaposi's sarcoma in more than 350 patients. Four dosage regimens of Roferon-A were evaluated for initial induction. Thirty-nine

patients received 3 million IU daily; 99 patients received an escalating regimen of 3 million, 9 million and 18 million IU each daily for 3 days, followed by 36 million IU daily; 119 patients received 36 million IU daily; and 16 patients received doses greater than 36 million IU to a maximum of 54 million IU daily. An additional 91 patients received Roferon-A in combination with vinblastine. The best response rate associated with acceptable toxicity was observed when Roferon-A was administered as a single agent at a dose of 36 million IU daily. The escalating regimen of 3 to 36 million IU daily provided equivalent therapeutic benefit with some amelioration of acute toxicity in some patients. In AIDS-related Kaposi's sarcoma, lower doses were less effective in inducing tumor regression and doses higher than 36 million IU daily were associated with unacceptable toxicity.

As summarized in Table 1, the likelihood of response to Roferon-A varied with the clinical manifestations of human immunodeficiency virus (HIV) infection. Patients with prior opportunistic infection or B symptoms are unlikely to respond to treatment with Roferon-A.

[See table below].

In the 28 patients evaluated who had prior opportunistic infection or B symptoms, the response rate was 3.6%.

*Patients had no prior opportunistic infection or B symptoms. B symptoms include night sweats, weight loss of greater than 10% of body weight or 15 lbs., or fever greater than 100°F without an identifiable source of infection.

Patients who were otherwise asymptomatic, with no prior opportunistic infection and near-normal levels of CD₄ lymphocytes, experienced higher response rates. Responding patients with a baseline CD₄ lymphocyte count greater than 200 cells/mm³ had a distinct survival advantage over both responding patients with a baseline CD₄ lymphocyte count of 200 cells/mm³ or less and nonresponding patients regardless of their baseline CD₄ lymphocyte count. Median survival for responding patients with CD₄ lymphocyte counts of greater than 200 to 400 cells/mm³ had not been reached but was greater than 32.7 months from the initiation of therapy. For responding patients with CD₄ lymphocyte counts of greater than 400 cells/mm³, the median survival had not been reached but was greater than 29.5 months.

A classification system for staging AIDS-related Kaposi's sarcoma has been described based on location and extent of disease. In studies of Roferon-A, no difference was noted in response rates for patients with different stages of Kaposi's sarcoma. Likelihood of response was related to manifestations of HIV Infection (baseline CD₄ lymphocyte count, prior opportunistic infection or B symptons) and not to extent of tumor involvement. The median time to response was 2.7 months. The median duration of response for patients achieving a partial or complete response was 6.3 and 20.7 months, respectively. Complete and partial responses lasting in excess of three years have been observed. Therapy was discontinued because of progression of Kaposi's sarcoma, development of severe opportunistic infection or severe adverse effects. The median time to discontinuation of treatment was 12.5 months for responding patients and 2.3 months for patients who did not respond.

INDICATIONS AND USAGE

Roferon-A is indicated for use in the treatment of hairy cell leukemia and AIDS-related Kaposi's sarcoma in select patients 18 years of age or older. Studies have shown that Roferon-A can produce clinically meaningful tumor regression or disease stabilization in patients with hairy cell leukemia or in patients with AIDS-related Kaposi's sarcoma.[5–7]

FOR PATIENTS WITH HAIRY CELL LEUKEMIA: Prior to initiation of therapy, tests should be performed to quantitate peripheral blood hemoglobin, platelets, granulocytes and hairy cells and bone marrow hairy cells. These parameters should be monitored periodically (*e.g.*, monthly) during treatment to determine whether response to treatment has occurred. If a patient does not respond within six months, treatment should be discontinued. If a response to treatment does occur, treatment should be continued until no further improvement is observed and these laboratory parameters have been stable for about three months. It is not known whether continued treatment after that time is beneficial. Studies are in progress to evaluate this question.

FOR PATIENTS WITH AIDS-RELATED KAPOSI'S SARCOMA: Roferon-A is useful for the treatment of AIDS-related Kaposi's sarcoma in a select group of patients. In determining whether a patient should be treated, the physician should assess the likelihood of response based on the clinical manifestations of HIV infection and the manifestations of Kaposi's sarcoma requiring treatment. See CLINICAL PHARMACOLOGY.

Indicator lesion measurements and total lesion count should be performed before initiation of therapy. These parameters should be monitored periodically (*e.g.*, monthly) during treatment to determine whether response to treatment or disease stabilization has occurred. When disease stabilization or a response to treatment occurs, treatment should continue until there is no further evidence of tumor or until discontinuation is required because of a severe opportunistic infection or adverse effects.

Table 1

Likelihood of Response to Roferon-A in Patients with AIDS-Related Kaposi's Sarcoma

No. Pts.*	CD₄(T₄) Lymphocyte Count (cells/mm³)	Objective Response Rate (%)		
		CR	PR	Total
83	0–200	3.6	3.6	7.2
51	>200–400	15.7	11.8	27.5
33	>400	24.2	21.2	45.4

CONTRAINDICATIONS

Roferon-A is contraindicated in patients with known hypersensitivity to alfa interferon, mouse immunoglobulin or any component of the product.

WARNINGS

Roferon-A should be administered under the guidance of a qualified physician. (See DOSAGE AND ADMINISTRATION.) Appropriate management of the therapy and its complications is possible only when adequate diagnostic and treatment facilities are readily available.

Roferon-A should not be used for the treatment of visceral AIDS-related Kaposi's sarcoma associated with rapidly progressive or life-threatening disease.

Roferon-A should be used with caution in patients with severe preexisting cardiac disease, severe renal or hepatic disease, seizure disorders and/or compromised central nervous system function.

Because of the possibility of severe or even fatal adverse reactions, patients should be informed not only of the benefits of therapy but also of the risks involved.

Roferon-A should be administered with caution to patients with cardiac disease or with any history of cardiac illness. No direct cardiotoxic effect has been demonstrated, but it is likely that acute, self-limited toxicities (*i.e.*, fever, chills) frequently associated with Roferon-A administration may exacerbate preexisting cardiac conditions. Rarely, myocardial infarction has occurred in patients receiving Roferon-A. Cases of cardiomyopathy have been observed on rare occasions in patients treated with alfa-interferons.

Caution should be exercised when administering Roferon-A to patients with myelosuppression or when Roferon-A is used in combination with other agents that are known to cause myelosuppression. Syngeristic toxicity has been observed when Roferon-A is administered in combination with zidovudine (AZT).[8] The effects of Roferon-A when combined with other drugs used in the treatment of AIDS-related disease are not known.

Central nervous system adverse reactions have been reported in a number of patients. These reactions included decreased mental status, exaggerated central nervous system function, and dizziness. More severe obtundation and coma have been rarely observed. Most of these abnormalities were mild and reversible within a few days to three weeks upon dose reduction or discontinuation of Roferon-A therapy. Careful periodic neuropsychiatric monitoring of all patients is recommended.

Leukopenia and elevation of hepatic enzymes occurred frequently but were rarely dose-limiting. Thrombocytopenia occurred less frequently. Proteinuria and increased cells in urinary sediment were also seen infrequently. Rarely, significant hepatic, renal and myelosuppressive toxicities were noted.

PRECAUTIONS

General: In all instances where the use of Roferon-A is considered for chemotherapy, the physician must evaluate the need and usefulness of the drug against the risk of adverse reactions. Most adverse reactions are reversible if detected early. If severe reactions occur, the drug should be reduced in dosage or discontinued and appropriate corrective measures should be taken according to the clinical judgment of the physician. Reinstitution of Roferon-A therapy should be carried out with caution and with adequate consideration of the further need for the drug and alertness as to possible recurrence of toxicity.

The minimum effective doses of Roferon-A for treatment of hairy cell leukemia and AIDS-related Kaposi's sarcoma have not been established. Variations in dosage and adverse reactions exist among different brands of Interferon. Therefore, do not use different brands of Interferon in a single treatment regimen.

Information for Patient: Patients should be cautioned not to change brands of Interferon without medical consultation, as a change in dosage may result. Patients should be informed regarding the potential benefits and risks attendant to the use of Roferon-A. If home use is determined to be desirable by the physician, instructions on appropriate use should be given, including review of the contents of the enclosed Patient Information Sheet. Patients should be well hydrated, especially during the initial stages of treatment.

Patients should be thoroughly instructed in the importance of proper disposal procedures and cautioned against reusing syringes and needles. If home use is prescribed, a puncture resistant container for the disposal of used syringes and needles should be supplied to the patient. The full container should be disposed of according to directions provided by the physician.

Patients receiving high dose alfa-interferson should be cautioned against performing tasks that require complete mental alertness such as operating machinery or driving a motor vehicle.

Laboratory Tests: Complete blood counts and clinical chemistry tests should be performed before initiation of Roferon-A therapy and at appropriate periods during therapy. Since responses of hairy cell leukemia and AIDS-related Kaposi's

sarcoma are not generally observed for one to three months after initiation of treatment, very careful monitoring for severe depression of blood cell counts is warranted during the initial phase of treatment.

Those patients who have preexisting cardiac abnormalities and/or are in advanced stages of cancer should have electrocardiograms taken before and during the course of treatment.

Carcinogenesis, Mutagenesis and Impairment of Fertility:
Carcinogenesis: Roferon-A has not been tested for its carcinogenic potential.

Mutagenesis: A. Internal studies—Ames tests using six different tester strains, with and without metabolic activation, were performed with Roferon-A up to a concentration of 1920 µg/plate. There was no evidence of mutagenicity.

Human lymphocyte cultures were treated *in vitro* with Roferon-A at noncytotoxic concentrations. No increase in the incidence of chromosomal damage was noted.

B. Published studies—There are no published studies on the mutagenic potential of Roferon-A. However, a number of studies on the genotoxicity of human leukocyte interferon have been reported.

A chromosomal defect following the addition of human leukocyte interferon to lymphocyte cultures from a patient suffering from a lymphoproliferative disorder has been reported.

In contrast, other studies have failed to detect chromosomal abnormalities following treatment of lymphocyte cultures from healthy volunteers with human leukocyte interferon. It has also been shown that human leukocyte interferon protects primary chick embryo fibroblasts from chromosomal aberrations produced by gamma rays.

Impairment of Fertility: Roferon-A has been studied for its effect on fertility in Macaca mulatta (rhesus monkeys). Nonpregnant rhesus females treated with Roferon-A at doses of 5 and 25 milion IU/kg/day have shown menstrual cycle irregularities, including prolonged or shortened menstrual periods and erratic bleeding; these cycles were considered to be anovulatory on the basis that reduced progesterone levels were noted and that expected increases in preovulatory estrogen and luteinizing hormones were not observed. These monkeys returned to a normal menstrual rhythm following discontinuation of treatment.

Drug Interactions: Interactions between Roferon-A and other drugs have not been fully evaluated. Caution should be exercised when administering Roferon-A in combination with other potentially myelosuppressive agents. See WARNINGS.

PREGNANCY

Teratogenic Effects: Pregnancy Category C. Roferon-A has been shown to demonstrate a statistically significant increase in abortifacient activity in rhesus monkeys when given at approximately 20 to 500 times the human dose. A study in pregnant rhesus monkeys treated with 1, 5 or 25 million IU kg/day of Roferon-A in their early to midfetal period (days 22 to 70 of gestation) has failed to demonstrate teratogenic activity for Roferon-A.

There are no adequate and well-controlled studies in pregnant women.

Nonteratogenic Effects: Dose-related abortifacient activity was observed in pregnant rhesus monkeys treated with 1, 5 or 25 million IU/kg/day of Roferon-A in their early to midfetal period (days 22 to 70 of gestation). A late-fetal period study (days 79 to 100 of gestation) is in progress and as yet there have been no reports of any increased rate of abortion. *Usage in Pregnancy:* Safe use in human pregnancy has not been established. Therefore, Roferon-A should be used during pregnancy only if the potential benefit justifies the potential risk to the fetus. Information from primate studies showed dose-related menstrual irregularities and an increased incidence of spontaneous abortions. Decreases in serum estradiol and progesterone concentrations have been reported in women treated with human leukocyte interferon.[9] Therefore, fertile women should not receive Roferon-A unless they are using effective contraception during the therapy period.

Male fertility and teratologic evaluations have yielded no significant adverse effects to date.

Nursing Mothers: It is not known whether this drug is excreted in human milk. Because many drugs are excreted in human milk and because of the potential for serious adverse reactions in nursing infants from Roferon-A, a decision should be made whether to discontinue nursing or to discontinue the drug, taking into account the importance of the drug to the mother.

Pediatric Use: Safety and effectiveness in children under 18 years of age have not been established.

ADVERSE REACTIONS

The following data on adverse reactions are based on the subcutaneous or intramuscular administration of Roferon-A as a single agent. Most of the adverse reactions reported were mild to moderate and diminished in severity and number with continued therapy. More severe adverse reactions

were observed at higher doses and may require dose reduction.

FOR PATIENTS WITH HAIRY CELL LEUKEMIA:
Flu-like Symptoms—Fever (98%), fatigue (89%), myalgia (73%), headache (71%), chills (64%) and arthralgia (5%).
Gastrointestinal—Anorexia (46%), nausea (32%), diarrhea (29%) and emesis (10%).
Central and Peripheral Nervous System—Dizziness (21%), paresthesia (6%), numbness (6%) and transient impotence (6%).
Skin—Rash (18%), dry skin or pruritus (13%) and partial alopecia (8%).
Other—Dryness or inflammation of the oropharynx (16%), weight loss (14%), change in taste (13%), diaphoresis (8%) and reactivation of herpes liabialis (8%).

Rarely, (< 3%), central nervous system effects including decreased mental status, depression, visual disturbances, sleep disturbances and nervousness, as well as cardiac adverse events, including hypertension, chest pain, arrhythmias and palpitations, were reported. Adverse experiences that occurred rarely, and may have been related to underlying disease, included epistaxis, bleeding gums, ecchymosis and petechiae. Miscellaneous adverse events, such as night sweats, urticaria, conjunctivitis and inflammation at the site of injection, were also rarely observed.

FOR PATIENTS WITH AIDS-RELATED KAPOSI'S SARCOMA:
Flu-like Symptoms—Fatigue (95%), fever (74%), myalgia (69%), headache (66%), chills (41%) and arthralgia (24%).
Gastrointestinal—Anorexia (65%), nausea (51%), diarrhea (42%), emesis (17%) and abdominal pain (15%).
Central and Peripheral Nervous System—Dizziness (40%), decreased mental status (17%), depression (16%), paresthesia (8%), confusion (8%), diaphoresis (7%), visual disturbances (5%), sleep disturbances (5%) and numbness (3%).
Pulmonary and Cardiovascular—Coughing (27%), dyspnea (11%), edema (9%), chest pain (4%) and hypotension (4%).
Skin—Partial alopecia (22%), rash (11%) and dry skin or pruritus (5%).
Other—Weight loss (25%), change in taste (25%), dryness or inflammation of the oropharynx (14%), night sweats (8%) and rhinorrhea (4%).

Occasionally (< 3%) nervous system effects including anxiety, nervousness, emotional liability, vertigo and forgetfulness, as well as cardiac adverse events, including palpitations and arrhythmia, were reported. Other adverse experiences that occurred occasionally (< 3%) and may have been related to underlying disease, included sinusitis, constipation, chest congestion, urticaria, and flatulence. Adverse experiences which occurred rarely (< 1%) included ataxia, seizures, cyanosis, gastric distress, bronchospasm, pain at injection site, earache, eye irritation and rhinitis. Miscellaneous adverse experiences such as poor coordination, lethargy, muscle contractions, neuropathy, tremor, involuntary movement, syncope, aphasia, aphonia, dysarthria, amnesia, weakness, and flushing of skin were observed in less than 0.5% of patients. Cases of cardiomyopathy have been observed on rare occasions in patients treated with alfa-interferons.

In other investigational studies of Roferon-A, in addition to the adverse experiences noted above, other adverse experiences that occurred included: abdominal fullness, hypermotility, hepatitis, gait disturbance, hallucinations, encephalopathy. psychomotor retardation, coma, stroke, transient ischemic attacks, dysphasia, sedation, apathy, irritability, hyperactivity, claustrophobia, loss of libido, congestive heart failure, myocardial infarction, Raynaud's phenomenon, hot flashes, tachypnea, and excessive salivation. These adverse experiences occurred rarely (< 1%).

ABNORMAL LABORATORY TEST VALUES: The percentage of patients with hairy cell leukemia or AIDS-related Kaposi's sarcoma who experienced a significant abnormal laboratory test value (NCI grades III or IV) at least once during their treatment with Roferon-A is shown in the following table:

ABNORMAL LABORATORY TEST VALUES

	Hairy Cell Leukemia (n=63)	AIDS-Related Kaposi's Sarcoma (n=241)
Leukopenia	NA*	49%
Neutropenia	NA	52%
Thrombocytopenia	NA	35%
Decreased Hemoglobin	NA	27%
SGOT	42%	46%
Alkaline Phosphate	8%	11%
LDH	13%	10%
Bilirubin	2%	< 1%
BUN	4%	0%
Serum Creatinine	2%	< 1%
Proteinuria	0%	< 1%

*Not Applicable—Patient's initial hematologic laboratory test values were abnormal due to their underlying disease.

Continued on next page

Roche Labs.—Cont.

Increases in fasting serum glucose, serum phosphorus and serum uric acid levels and decreases in serum calcium levels were also observed in less than 5% of patients.

DOSAGE AND ADMINISTRATION

The recommended dosages of Roferon-A differ for hairy cell leukemia and AIDS-related Kaposi's sarcoma. See indication-specific dosages below.

HAIRY CELL LEUKEMIA—The induction dose of Roferon-A is 3 million IU daily for 16 to 24 weeks, administered as a subcutaneous or intramuscular injection. Subcutaneous administration is particularly suggested for, but not limited to, thrombocytopenia patients (platelet count <50,000) or for patients at risk for bleeding. The recommended maintenance dose is 3 million IU, three times per week. Dose reduction by one-half or withholding of individual doses may be needed when severe adverse reactions occur. The use of doses higher than 3 million IU is not recommended in hairy cell leukemia. The 36 million IU dosage form should not be used for the treatment of hairy cell leukemia.

Patients should be treated for approximately six months before the physician determines whether to continue therapy in patients who respond or discontinue therapy in patients who did not respond. Patients with hairy cell leukemia have been treated for up to 24 consecutive months. The optimal duration of treatment for this disease has not been determined.

AIDS-RELATED KAPOSI'S SARCOMA—The recommended induction dose of Roferon-A is 36 million IU daily for 10 to 12 weeks, administered as an intramuscular or subcutaneous injection. Subcutaneous administration is particularly suggested for, but not limited to, patients who are thrombocytopenic (platelet count <50,000) or who are at risk for bleeding. The recommended maintenance dose is 36 million IU, three times per week. Dose reductions by one-half or withholding of individual doses may be required when severe adverse reactions occur. An escalating schedule of 3 million IU, 9 million IU and 18 million IU each daily for 3 days followed by 36 million IU daily for the remainder of the 10 to 12 week induction period has also produced equivalent therapeutic benefit with some amelioration of the acute toxicity in some patients.

When disease stabilization or a response to treatment occurs, treatment should continue until there is no further evidence of tumor or until discontinuation is required because of a severe opportunistic infection or adverse effects. The optimal duration of treatment for this disease has not been determined.

If severe reactions occur, the dose should be modified (50% reduction) or therapy should be temporarily discontinued until the adverse reactions abate. The need for dose reduction should take into account the effects of prior X-ray therapy or chemotherapy that may have compromised bone marrow reserve. The minimum effective doses of Roferon-A for the treatment of hairy cell leukemia and AIDS-related Kaposi's sarcoma have not been established.

Parenteral drug products should be inspected visually for particulate matter and discoloration before administration, whenever solution and container permit.

HOW SUPPLIED

Injectable Solution:

3 million IU Roferon-A per vial—Each 1 mL contains 3 million IU of Interferon alfa-2a, recombinant/Roche, 9 mg sodium chloride, 5 mg phenol (Human) and 3 mg phenol as a preservative. Boxes of 1 (NDC 0004-1987-09).

18 million IU Roferon-A per vial—Each 1 mL contains 6 million IU of Interferon alfa-2a, recombinant/Roche, 9 mg sodium chloride, 5 mg Albumin (Human) and 3 mg phenol as a preservative. Each 0.5 mL contains 3 million IU of Interferon alfa-2a, recombinant/Roche. Boxes of 1 (NDC 0004-1988-09).

36 million IU Roferon-A per vial—Each 1 mL contains 36 million IU of Interferon alfa-2a, recombinant/Roche, 9 mg sodium chloride, 5 mg Albumin (Human) and 3 mg phenol as a preservative. This dosage form should not be used for the treatment of hairy cell leukemia. Boxes of 1 (NDC 0004-2005-09).

Sterile Powder for Injection:

18 million IU Roferon-A per vial—Reconstitute with 3 mL diluent and swirl gently to dissolve. When reconstituted with accompanying Diluent for Roferon-A, each 1 mL of reconstituted solution contains 6 million IU Interferon alfa-2a, recombinant/Roche, 9 mg sodium chloride, 5 mg Albumin (Human) and 3 mg phenol as a preservative. Each 0.5 mL contains 3 million IU of Interferon alfa-2a, recombinant/Roche. Once the powder is reconstituted, it must be used within 30 days. Boxes of 1 (NDC 0004-1993-09).

STORAGE

The sterile powder and its accompanying diluent, the reconstituted solution and the injectible solution should be stored in the refrigerator at 36° to 46°F (2° to 8°C). Do *not* freeze or shake.

REFERENCES

1. Trown PW *et al: Cancer* 57 (Suppl.): 1648–1656, 1986. 2. Williams SJ, Farrell GC: *Br J Clin Pharmacol* 22: 610–612, 1986. 3. Itri LM *et al: Cancer* 59: 668–674, 1987. 4. Jones GJ, Itri LM: *Cancer* 57 (Suppl.): 1709–1715, 1986. 5. Foon KA *et al: Blood* 64 (Suppl. 1): 164a, 1984. 6. Quesada JR *et al: Cancer* 57 (Suppl.): 1678–1680, 1986. 7. Krown SE *et al: N Engl J Med* 308: 1071–1076, 1983. 8. Krown SE *et al: Proc Am Soc Clin Oncol* 7: 1, 1988. 9. Kauppila A *et al: Int J Cancer* 29: 291–294, 1982.
P.I. 1188

SYNKAYVITE®   ℞
(menadiol sodium diphosphate/Roche)
INJECTION

The following text is complete product information based on official labeling in effect June 1, 1989.

DESCRIPTION

Synkayvite (menadiol sodium diphosphate/Roche) Injection, a synthetic water-soluble derivative of menadione (vitamin K_3), is a sterile aqueous solution intended for intramuscular, intravenous or subcutaneous administration. Synkayvite Injection is available in the following concentrations:

1-ml Ampuls, 5 mg/ml—each ml contains 5 mg menadiol sodium diphosphate compounded with 2.5 mg sodium metabisulfite, 0.45% phenol as preservative, 0.4% sodium chloride for isotonicity and sodium hydroxide to adjust pH to approximately 8.0.

1-ml Ampuls, 10 mg/ml—each ml contains 10 mg menadiol sodium diphosphate compounded with 2.5 mg sodium metabisulfite, 0.45% phenol as preservative, 0.4% sodium chloride for isotonicity and sodium hydroxide to adjust pH to approximately 8.0.

2-ml Ampuls, 75 mg/2 ml—each 2 ml contains 75 mg menadiol sodium diphosphate compounded with 5 mg sodium metabisulfite, 0.45% phenol as preservative, 0.4% sodium chloride for isotonicity and sodium hydroxide to adjust pH to approximately 8.0.

Chemically, menadiol sodium diphosphate is 2-methyl-1,4-naphthalenediol bis (dihydrogen phosphate) tetrasodium salt, hexahydrate. It is a white to pink hygroscopic powder with a characteristic odor and is very soluble in water and insoluble in alcohol. It has a molecular weight of 530.18.

CLINICAL PHARMACOLOGY

Synkayvite is converted *in vivo* to menadione (vitamin K_3). Its potency is approximately one-half that of menadione. Synkayvite is similar in activity to naturally occurring vitamin K, which is necessary for the synthesis in the liver of blood coagulation factors prothrombin (factor II), proconvertin (factor VII), thromboplastin (factor IX) and Stuart factor (factor X). The prothrombin test is sensitive to the concentrations of factors II, VII and X. The mechanism by which vitamin K_1 promotes formation of these clotting factors is not known, but animal data suggest that it acts as an enzyme or catalyst upon a substrate within the liver or combines with an apoenzyme (AE) to form an active enzyme (AE-K) which then is involved in prothrombin synthesis.

Pharmacokinetic data are unavailable because there is no acceptable assay procedure for the determination of menadiol in biological specimens. The physiochemical properties of menadiol sodium diphosphate indicate a negligible potential for absorption problems. The action of menadiol sodium diphosphate is generally detectable within one to two hours following parenteral administration; the prothrombin time often returns to normal in 8 to 24 hours. Vitamin K appears to pass through the placenta.

INDICATIONS AND USAGE

Synkayvite Injection is indicated for the treatment of hypoprothrombinemia secondary to factors limiting absorption or synthesis of vitamin K, *e.g.,* obstructive jaundice, biliary fistula, sprue, ulcerative colitis, celiac disease, intestinal resection, cystic fibrosis of the pancreas, regional enteritis and antibacterial therapy.

It is also indicated in hypoprothrombinemia secondary to administration of salicylates.

Synkayvite Injection may also be used as a liver function test, although newer methods are available.

CONTRAINDICATIONS

Vitamin K, or any of its synthetic analogs, should not be administered to the mother during the *last few weeks of pregnancy* as a prophylactic measure against physiologic hypoprothrombinemia or hemorrhagic disease of the newborn.

Synkayvite is contraindicated in patients with known hypersensitivity to the drug.

WARNINGS

Synkayvite Injection should not be used in the prophylaxis and treatment of hemorrhagic disease of the newborn, because phytonadione/Roche (Konakion®) is safer than the water-soluble vitamin K analogs.

Synkayvite and other water-soluble vitamin K analogs are ineffective in the treatment of oral anticoagulant-induced hypoprothrombinemia and, therefore, should not be used in its treatment. Synkayvite will not counteract the anticoagulant action of heparin.

Synkayvite Injection contains sodium metabisulfite, a sulfite that may cause allergic-type reactions, including anaphylactic symptoms and life-threatening or less severe asthmatic episodes in certain susceptible people. The overall prevalence of sulfite sensitivity in the general population is unknown and probably low. Sulfite sensitivity is seen more frequently in asthmatic than in nonasthmatic people.

PRECAUTIONS

General: Temporary resistance to prothrombin-depressing anticoagulants may result, especially when larger doses of Synkayvite are used. If relatively large doses have been employed, it may be necessary when reinstituting anticoagulant therapy to use somewhat larger doses of prothrombin-depressing anticoagulant or one which has a different mode of action, such as heparin.

Since the liver is the site of metabolic synthesis of prothrombin, hypoprothrombinemia resulting from hepatocellular damage is not corrected by administration of vitamin K. Repeated large doses of vitamin K are not warranted in liver disease if the response to initial use of the vitamin is unsatisfactory (Koller test).

Failure to respond to vitamin K may indicate that a coagulation defect is present or that the condition being treated is unresponsive to vitamin K.

Laboratory Tests: The dose, route and frequency of administration and duration of treatment depend on the severity of the prothrombin deficiency and should be regulated by repeated determinations of prothrombin time.

Drug Interactions: Patients being treated with coumarin and indandione derivative anticoagulants are extremely sensitive to changes in available vitamin K. Therefore, large doses of menadione or menadiol sodium diphosphate may decrease patient sensitivity to oral anticoagulants, although these vitamin K analogs are ineffective in treating anticoagulant overdosage.

Drug/Laboratory Test Interactions: Menadione has been reported to interfere with the modified Reedy, Jenkins, Thorn procedure for determining urinary 17-hydroxycorticosteroids, producing falsely elevated levels.

Carcinogenesis, Mutagenesis and Impairment of Fertility: Synkayvite has not undergone adequate animal testing to evaluate carcinogenic potential. The mutagenicity of Synkayvite has not been evaluated in the Ames test. Synkayvite has not been evaluated for effects on fertility.

Pregnancy: Teratogenic Effects: Pregnancy Category C. Segment II reproduction studies have not been conducted with menadiol. However, menadione (vitamin K_3) was nonteratogenic in rats at doses of 15 and 150 mg/day. The 150 mg/day dose in rats is approximately 872 times the maximum human therapeutic dose of 30 mg daily for the treatment of hypoprothrombinemia and 350 times the human dose of 75 mg for the liver function test. It is not known whether Synkayvite can cause fetal harm when administered to a pregnant woman or can affect reproductive capacity. Synkayvite should be given to a pregnant woman only if clearly needed.

Nonteratogenic effects: Retardation of skeletal ossification and an increase in fetal resorptions have been reported in rats with menadione (vitamin K_3).

Menadione and its derivatives have been implicated in producing hemolytic anemia, hyperbilirubinemia and kernicterus in the newborn, especially in premature infants, when administered to the mother prior to delivery or to the newborn. A marked hyperbilirubinemia has been reported in premature infants of mothers given menadione 2 to 112 hours prior to delivery. Synkayvite given parenterally during labor caused an elevation in prothrombin levels in 16 of 22 infants. (Also see **Contraindications** section.)

Nursing Mothers: A study has shown that vitamin K is excreted in human milk. This should be considered if it is necessary to administer Synkayvite to a nursing mother.

Pediatric Use: See **Warnings** section.

ADVERSE REACTIONS

In adults, bromsulfalein retention and prolongation of prothrombin time have been reported after maximum doses of vitamin K analogs. In infants (particularly premature babies), excessive doses of vitamin K analogs may cause increased bilirubinemia in the first few days of life. This, in turn, may result in kernicterus, which may lead to brain damage or even death. Immaturity is apparently an important factor in the appearance of toxic reactions to vitamin K analogs as full-term and larger premature infants demonstrate greater tolerance than smaller premature infants. (Also see **Warnings** section.)

Menadione can induce erythrocyte hemolysis in persons having a genetic deficiency of glucose-6-phosphate dehydrogenase in their red blood cells.

In patients with severe hepatic disease, large doses of menadione may further depress liver function. Paradoxically, the administration of excessive doses of vitamin K or its analogs in an attempt to correct the hypoprothrombinemia associated with severe hepatitis or cirrhosis may actually result in a further depression of the concentration of prothrombin. (Also see **Precautions,** *General,* section.)

Occasional allergic reactions, such as skin rash and urticaria, have been reported.

OVERDOSAGE

There are no data available on overdosage of Synkayvite in man. The administration of large doses of menadione and its derivatives to animals has resulted in the production of anemia, polycythemia, splenomegaly, renal and hepatic damage and death.

The acute intravenous toxicity of Synkayvite is as follows:

	$LD_{50} \pm$ S.D.
Mouse	500 $\pm$ 55 mg/kg
Rat	400 $\pm$ 65 mg/kg

DOSAGE AND ADMINISTRATION

The U.S. Recommended Daily Allowances for vitamin K in humans have not been established officially. The adequate daily dietary intake of vitamin K for adults has been estimated to be 70 to 140 mcg; for infants 10 to 20 mcg; for children and adolescents 15 to 100 mcg. The dietary abundance of vitamin K normally satisfies the requirements except for the neonatal period of 5 to 8 days.

Synkayvite may be injected subcutaneously, intramuscularly or intravenously. The response after intravenous administration may be more prompt, but more sustained action follows intramuscular or subcutaneous use.

Duration of treatment and frequency of dosage should be governed by blood prothrombin-time determination. In the absence of impaired liver function, a single dose usually corrects hypoprothrombinemia in 8 to 24 hours. Injections should be repeated in 12 hours if tests at this time show no evidence of improvement.

Following are the usual recommended dosages:

	ADULTS	CHILDREN
For treatment of hypoprothrombinemia	5 to 15 mg once or twice daily	5 to 10 mg once or twice daily
For liver function test	75 mg intravenously	

Parenteral drug products should be inspected visually for particulate matter and discoloration prior to administration, whenever solution and container permit. Synkayvite Injection is incompatible with protein hydrolysate.

HOW SUPPLIED

1-ml Ampuls (5 mg menadiol sodium diphosphate/ml) —boxes of 10 (NDC 0004-1923-06).

1-ml Ampuls (10 mg menadiol sodium diphosphate/ml) —boxes of 10 (NDC 0004-1924-06).

2-ml Ampuls (75 mg menadiol sodium diphosphate/2 ml) —boxes of 10 (NDC 0004-1925-06).

Store at room temperature (15° to 30°C or 59° to 86°F). Synkayvite need not be refrigerated.

P.I. 0287

SYNKAYVITE® ℞
(menadiol sodium diphosphate/Roche)
TABLETS

The following text is complete product information based on official labeling in effect June 1, 1989.

DESCRIPTION

Synkayvite (menadiol sodium diphosphate/Roche), a synthetic, water-soluble derivative of menadione (vitamin K_3), is available for oral administration in 5-mg tablets. Each tablet also contains gelatin, lactose, magnesium stearate, corn starch and talc. Chemically, menadiol sodium diphosphate is 2-methyl-1,4-naphthalenediol bis (dihydrogen phosphate) tetrasodium salt, hexahydrate. It is a white to pink hygroscopic powder with a characteristic odor and is very soluble in water and insoluble in alcohol. It has a molecular weight of 530.18.

CLINICAL PHARMACOLOGY

Synkayvite is converted *in vivo* to menadione (vitamin K_3). Its potency is approximately one-half that of menadione. Synkayvite is similar in activity to naturally occurring vitamin K, which is necessary for the synthesis in the liver of blood coagulation factors prothrombin (factor II), proconvertin (factor VII), thromboplastin (factor IX) and Stuart factor (factor X). The prothrombin test is sensitive to the concentrations of factors II, VII and X. The mechanism by which vitamin K_1 promotes formation of these clotting factors is not known, but animal data suggest that it acts as an enzyme or catalyst upon a substrate within the liver or combines with an apoenzyme (AE) to form an active enzyme (AE-K) which then is involved in prothrombin synthesis.

Pharmacokinetic data are unavailable because there is no acceptable assay procedure for the determination of menadiol in biological specimens. The physiochemical properties of menadiol sodium diphosphate indicate a negligible poten-

tial for absorption problems. The onset and duration of action following oral administration are not known. Vitamin K appears to pass through the placenta.

INDICATIONS AND USAGE

Synkayvite Tablets are indicated for:
—vitamin K deficiency secondary to the administration of antibacterial therapy;
—hypoprothrombinemia secondary to obstructive jaundice and biliary fistulas;
—hypoprothrombinemia secondary to administration of salicylates.

CONTRAINDICATIONS

Vitamin K, or any of its synthetic analogs, should not be administered to the mother *during the last few weeks of pregnancy* as a prophylactic measure against physiologic hypoprothrombinemia or hemorrhagic disease of the newborn. Synkayvite is contraindicated in patients with known hypersensitivity to the drug.

WARNINGS

Synkayvite and other water-soluble vitamin K analogs are ineffective in the treatment of oral anticoagulant-induced hypoprothrombinemia and should, therefore, not be used in its treatment. Synkayvite will not counteract the anticoagulant action of heparin.

PRECAUTIONS

General: Temporary resistance to prothrombin-depressing anticoagulants may result, especially when larger doses of Synkayvite are used. If relatively large doses have been employed, it may be necessary when reinstituting anticoagulant therapy to use somewhat larger doses of the prothrombin-depressing anticoagulant or one which has a different mode of action, such as heparin.

Since the liver is the site of metabolic synthesis of prothrombin, hypoprothrombinemia resulting from hepatocellular damage is not corrected by administration of vitamin K. Repeated large doses of vitamin K are not warranted in liver disease if the response to initial use of the vitamin is unsatisfactory (Koller test).

Failure to respond to vitamin K may indicate that a coagulation defect is present or that the condition being treated is unresponsive to vitamin K.

Information for Patients: To assure safe and effective use of this drug, the following information and instructions should be given to the patient:

1. Take this medication exactly as directed by your doctor. Do not increase or decrease the prescribed dosage, or take it more often, or take it for a longer period of time than instructed.
2. If you miss a dose, take it as soon as possible, and then continue with your normal dosing schedule. Do not take the missed dose if it is almost time for your next dose; continue on your normal schedule and inform your doctor about any doses that you miss. If you have any questions about this, ask your doctor or pharmacist.
3. Inform all doctors and pharmacists that you are taking this medication; other medicines may affect the way this medicine works.
4. Before starting or stopping any other medications, including nonprescription drugs such as aspirin, check with your doctor or pharmacist.
5. A blood test should be performed at regular intervals to determine how this medicine is working. This will help your doctor decide the best dosing schedule for you.
6. Inform your doctor if you are pregnant or become pregnant while using this drug, even though vitamin K has not been shown to cause birth defects or other problems. Also inform your doctor if you are nursing.

Laboratory Tests: The dose, route and frequency of administration and duration of treatment depend on the severity of the prothrombin deficiency and should be regulated by repeated determinations of prothrombin time.

Drug Interactions: Patients being treated with coumarin and indandione derviative anticoagulants are extremely sensitive to changes in available vitamin K. Therefore, large doses of menadione or menadiol sodium diphosphate may decrease patient sensitivity to oral anticoagulants, although these vitamin K analogs are ineffective in treating anticoagulant overdosage.

Drug/Laboratory Test Interactions: Menadione has been reported to interfere with the modified Reddy, Jenkins, Thorn procedure for determining urinary 17-hydroxycorticosteroids, producing falsely elevated levels.

Carcinogenesis, Mutagenesis and Impairment of Fertility: Synkayvite has not undergone adequate animal testing to evaluate carcinogenic potential. The mutagenicity of Synkayvite has not been evaluated in the Ames test. Synkayvite has not been evaluated for effects on fertility.

Pregnancy: Teratogenic Effects: Pregnancy Category C. Segment II reproduction studies have not been conducted with menadiol. However, menadione (vitamin K_3) was nonteratogenic in rats at doses of 15 and 150 mg/day. The 150 mg/day dose in rats is approximately 2640 times the maximum human therapeutic dose of 10 mg daily. It is not known

whether Synkayvite can cause fetal harm when administered to a pregnant woman or can affect reproductive capacity. Synkayvite should be given to a pregnant woman only if clearly needed.

Nonteratogenic Effects: Retardation of skeletal ossification and an increase in fetal resorptions have been reported in rats with menadione (vitamin K_3).

Menadione and its derivatives have been implicated in producing hemolytic anemia, hyperbilirubinemia and kernicterus in the newborn, especially in premature infants, when administered to the mother prior to delivery or to the newborn. A marked hyperbilirubinemia has been reported in premature infants of mothers given menadione 2 to 112 hours prior to delivery. Synkayvite given parenterally during labor caused an elevation in prothrombin levels in 16 of 22 infants. (Also see **Contraindications** section.)

Nursing Mothers: A study has shown that vitamin K is excreted in human milk. This should be considered if it is necessary to administer Synkayvite to a nursing mother.

ADVERSE REACTIONS

Bromsulfalein retention and prolongation of prothrombin time have been reported after maximum doses of vitamin K analogs.

Menadione can induce erythrocyte hemolysis in persons having a genetic deficiency of glucose-6-phosphate dehydrogenase in their red blood cells.

In patients with severe hepatic disease, large doses of menadione may further depress liver function. Paradoxically, the administration of excessive doses of vitamin K or its analogs in an attempt to correct the hypoprothrombinemia associated with severe hepatitis or cirrhosis may actually result in a further depression of the concentration of prothrombin. (Also see **Precautions,** *General,* section.)

Occasional allergic reactions, such as skin rash and urticaria, have been reported. There have also been minor instances of gastric disturbance.

OVERDOSAGE

There are no data on overdosage of Synkayvite in man. The administration of large doses of menadione and its derivatives to animals has resulted in the production of anemia, polycythemia, splenomegaly, renal and hepatic damage and death.

The acute oral toxicity of Synkayvite is as follows:

	$LD_{50} \pm$ S.D.
Mouse	6172 $\pm$ 966 mg/kg
Rat	5250 $\pm$ 740 mg/kg

DOSAGE AND ADMINISTRATION

The U.S. Recommended Daily Allowances for vitamin K in humans have not been established officially. The adequate daily dietary intake of vitamin K for adults has been estimated to be 70 to 140 mcg. The dietary abundance of vitamin K normally satisfies these requirements.

Following are the usual recommended dosages:

For hypoprothrombinemia secondary to obstructive jaundice and biliary fistulas	5 mg daily
For hypoprothrombinemia secondary to the administration of antibacterials or salicylates	5 to 10 mg daily

HOW SUPPLIED

White tablets containing 5 mg menadiol sodium diphosphate—bottls of 100 (NDC 0004-0037-01). Imprint on tablets: (front) SYNKAYVITE 5; (back) ROCHE.

Note: Slight pink discoloration of tablets does not affect the safety and efficacy of Synkayvite.

Store at room temperature (15° to 30° C or 59° to 86° F).

P.I. 0385

Shown in Product Identification Section, page 425

TARACTAN® ℞
[*tar-ac'tan*]
(chlorprothixene/Roche)
TABLETS

TARACTAN® ℞
(chlorprothixene lactate and HCl/Roche)
CONCENTRATE

TARACTAN® ℞
(chlorprothixene HCl/Roche)
AMPULS

The following text is complete prescribing information based on official labeling in effect June 1, 1989.

DESCRIPTION

Tablets—each containing 10 mg, 25 mg, 50 mg or 100 mg chlorprothixene; each tablet also contains acacia, corn starch, dibasic calcium phosphate, gelatin, magnesium stearate, shellac, sugar, talc, hydrogenated vegetable oil, wax (beeswax and carnauba) and other ingredients, with the following dye systems: 10-mg, 25-mg and 50-mg tablets—FD&C

Continued on next page

Roche Labs.—Cont.

Blue No. 2, FD&C Red No. 3, FD&C Yellow No. 5 and FD&C Yellow No. 6; 100-mg tablets—FD&C Blue No. 2, FD&C Red No. 3 and FD&C Yellow No. 5. Concentrate—100 mg/5 ml as the lactate and hydrochloride, fruit flavored; also contains benzoic acid, edetate disodium, glycerin, hydrochloric acid, lactic acid, magnesium aluminum silicate, parabens (methyl and propyl), polyoxyethylene (8) stearate, silicone emulsion, sodium hydroxide, sorbitol, sucrose, FD&C Red No. 40, FD&C Blue No. 1, FD&C Yellow No. 6, flavors and water. Ampuls—25 mg/2 ml as the hydrochloride, with 0.2% parabens (methyl and propyl) added as preservatives and pH adjusted to approximately 3.4 with HCl.

Taractan (chlorprothixene/Roche) is a thioxanthene derivative. Chemically, it is the alpha isomer of 2-chloro-*N, N*-dimethylthioxanthene-Δ⁹, γ-propylamine. In chemical structure chlorprothixene resembles the phenothiazines; however, in place of the nitrogen (N) in the phenothiazine ring, chlorprothixene carries a carbon atom with a double bond to a side chain.

ACTIONS

EEG changes following the injection of Taractan into cats suggest that it acts on the brain stem. Effects demonstrated were the synchronization of the EEG tracings during rest, a shortening of cortical activation obtained by stimulation of the reticular formation, and modifications of elicited potentials.

INDICATIONS

Taractan is indicated for the management of manifestations of psychotic disorders. Taractan has not been shown effective in the management of behavioral complications in patients with mental retardation.

CONTRAINDICATIONS

Circulatory collapse, comatose states due to central depressant drugs (alcohol, hypnotics, opiates, etc.) and known sensitivity to the drug are contraindications.

WARNINGS

Tardive Dyskinesia: Tardive dyskinesia, a syndrome consisting of potentially irreversible, involuntary, dyskinetic movements, may develop in patients treated with neuroleptic (antipsychotic) drugs. Although the prevalence of the syndrome appears to be highest among the elderly, especially elderly women, it is impossible to rely upon prevalence estimates to predict, at the inception of neuroleptic treatment, which patients are likely to develop the syndrome. Whether neuroleptic drug products differ in their potential to cause tardive dyskinesia is unknown.

Both the risk of developing the syndrome and the likelihood that it will become irreversible are believed to increase as the duration of treatment and the total cumulative dose of neuroleptic drugs increase. However, the syndrome can develop, although much less commonly, after relatively brief treatment periods at low doses.

There is no known treatment for established cases of tardive dyskinesia, although the syndrome may remit, partially or completely, if neuroleptic treatment is withdrawn. Neuroleptic treatment itself, however, may suppress (or partially suppress) the signs and symptoms of the syndrome and thereby may possibly mask the underlying disease process. The effect that symptomatic suppression has upon the long-term course of the syndrome is unknown.

Given these considerations, neuroleptics should be prescribed in a manner that is most likely to minimize the occurrence of tardive dyskinesia. Chronic neuroleptic treatment should generally be reserved for patients who suffer from a chronic illness that 1) is known to respond to neuroleptic drugs, and 2) for whom alternative, equally effective, but potentially less harmful treatments are not available or appropriate. In patients who do require chronic treatment, the smallest dose and the shortest duration of treatment producing a satisfactory clinical response should be sought. The need for continued treatment should be reassessed periodically.

If signs and symptoms of tardive dyskinesia appear in a patient on neuroleptics, drug discontinuation should be considered. However, some patients may require treatment despite the presence of the syndrome.

(For further information about the description of tardive dyskinesia and its clinical detection, please refer to the sections on Information for Patients and Adverse Reactions.)

Neuroleptic Malignant Syndrome: A potentially fatal symptom complex sometimes referred to as neuroleptic malignant syndrome (NMS) has been reported in association with antipsychotic drugs. Clinical manifestations of NMS are hyperpyrexia, muscle rigidity, altered mental status and evidence of autonomic instability (irregular pulse or blood pressure, tachycardia, diaphoresis and cardiac dysrhythmias).

The diagnostic evaluation of patients with this syndrome is complicated. In arriving at a diagnosis, it is important to identify cases where the clinical presentation includes both serious medical illness (*e.g.*, pneumonia, systemic infection,

etc.) and untreated or inadequately treated extrapyramidal signs and symptoms (EPS). Other important considerations in the differential diagnosis include central anticholinergic toxicity, heat stroke, drug fever and primary central nervous system (CNS) pathology.

The management of NMS should include 1) immediate discontinuation of antipsychotic drugs and other drugs not essential to concurrent therapy, 2) intensive symptomatic treatment and medical monitoring, and 3) treatment of any concomitant serious medical problems for which specific treatments are available. There is no general agreement about specific pharmacological treatment regimens for uncomplicated NMS.

If a patient requires antipsychotic drug treatment after recovery from NMS, the potential reintroduction of drug therapy should be carefully considered. The patient should be carefully monitored, since recurrences of NMS have been reported.

Usage in Pregnancy: The safety of Taractan during pregnancy or lactation in humans has not been established. Therefore, use of Taractan in women who may become pregnant requires weighing the drug's potential benefits against its possible hazards to mother and child. For the results of reproductive and teratogenic studies in rats and rabbits see **Animal Pharmacology and Toxicology.**

This drug may impair the mental and/or physical abilities required for the performance of hazardous tasks such as operating machinery or driving a motor vehicle; therefore, the patient should be cautioned accordingly.

As in the case of other CNS-acting drugs, patients receiving Taractan should be cautioned about possible combined effects with alcohol.

The safety and efficacy of Taractan have not been established for oral administration in children under age 6 or for parenteral use in those under age 12.

PRECAUTIONS

Because of its structural similarity to the phenothiazines, all of the precautions associated with phenothiazine therapy should be considered when patients receive Taractan. Therefore, Taractan should be used with caution in patients who:

— are receiving barbiturates or narcotics, because of additive effects of central nervous system depressants. The dosage of the narcotic or barbiturate should be reduced when given concomitantly with Taractan.

— are receiving atropine or related drugs, because of additive anticholinergic effects.

— have a history of epilepsy. When necessary, Taractan may be used concomitantly with anticonvulsant drugs. However, use of Taractan may lower the convulsive threshold; therefore, an adequate dosage of the anticonvulsant should be maintained.

— are exposed to extreme heat or phosphorous insecticides.
— have cardiovascular disease.
— have respiratory impairment due to acute pulmonary infections or chronic respiratory disorders such as severe asthma or emphysema.

The concurrent use of Taractan and electroshock treatment should be reserved for those patients for whom it is essential, but the hazards may be increased.

Taractan may augment or interfere with the absorption, metabolism or therapeutic activity of other psychotropic drugs and vice versa.

The appearance of signs of blood dyscrasias requires immediate discontinuance of the drug and the institution of appropriate therapy.

The possibility of liver damage, variations in thyroid function, pigmentary retinopathy, lenticular or corneal deposits and development of irreversible dyskinesias should be kept in mind when patients are on prolonged therapy.

When used in the treatment of agitated states accompanying depression, the usual precautions indicated with such patients are necessary, particularly the recognition that a suicidal tendency may be present and protective measures necessary.

Taractan has been demonstrated to have a prominent uricosuric effect when used at usual therapeutic doses. Consequently clinicians should be alert to the possible occurence of acute renal insufficiency after voluntary overdose of chlorprothixene or during the first days of treatment, especially in dehydrated patients.

Taractan tablets contain FD&C Yellow No. 5 (tartrazine) which may cause allergic-type reactions (including bronchial asthma) in certain susceptible individuals. Although the overall incidence of FD&C Yellow No. 5 (tartrazine) sensitivity in the general population is low, it is frequently seen in patients who also have aspirin hypersensitivity.

Information for Patients: Given the likelihood that some patients exposed chronically to neuroleptics will develop tardive dyskinesia, it is advised that all patients in whom chronic use is contemplated be given, if possible, full information about this risk. The decision to inform patients and/or their guardians must obviously take into account the clinical circumstances and the competency of the patient to understand the information provided.

Abrupt Withdrawal: Taractan is not known to produce physical dependence. However, gastritis, nausea and vomiting, dizziness and tremulousness have been reported following abrupt cessation of high-dose therapy.

Neuroleptic drugs elevate prolactin levels; the elevation persists during chronic administration. Tissue culture experiments indicate that approximately one-third of human breast cancers are prolactin-dependent *in vitro*, a factor of potential importance if the prescription of these drugs is contemplated in a patient with a previously detected breast cancer. Although disturbances such as galactorrhea, amenorrhea, gynecomastia and impotence have been reported, the clinical significance of elevated serum prolactin levels is unknown for most patients. An increase in mammary neoplasms has been found in rodents after chronic administration of neuroleptic drugs. Neither clinical studies nor epidemiologic studies conducted to date, however, have shown an association between chronic administration of these drugs and mammary tumorigenesis; the available evidence is considered too limited to be conclusive at this time.

ADVERSE REACTIONS

General Introduction: Untoward events reported in association with a drug's use can be classified into three general categories: 1) those which are more or less predictable extensions of the pharmacological activity of the drug; 2) those which are caused by the drug, but in an unpredictable and/or idiosyncratic manner (*e.g.*, jaundice, agranulocytosis, etc.); and 3) those which have occurred in circumstances where evidence of a causal link to the drug's use is inconclusive. The first section describes the neurological events that are commonly seen in association with the use of neuroleptics, regardless of mechanism. The second and third sections present events that have been reported in association with the use of Taractan and of phenothiazine derivatives, respectively.

Common Reactions Linked to the Use of Neuroleptics: Untoward Neurological Events: The following section details events that have been reported to occur in association with the use of neuroleptics or drugs which share the ability to block CNS dopamine receptors.

The common acute neurological untoward effects of neuroleptics consist of dystonia, akathisia and pseudoparkinsonism.

Chronic use of neuroleptics, including Taractan, may be associated with the development of tardive dyskinesia. The salient features of this syndrome are described below and in the WARNINGS section. Additional details about the common acute neurological impairments also follow.

Tardive Dyskinesia: Clinical picture and detection. The syndrome is characterized by involuntary choreoathetoid movements which variously involve the tongue, face, mouth, lips or jaw (*e.g.*, protrusion of the tongue, puffing of the cheeks, puckering of the mouth, chewing movements), trunk and extremities. The severity of the syndrome and the degree of impairment produced vary widely.

The syndrome may become clinically recognizable either during treatment, upon dosage reduction, or upon withdrawal of treatment. Movements may decrease in intensity and may disappear altogether if further treatment with neuroleptics is withheld. It is generally believed that reversibility is more likely after short- rather than long-term neuroleptic exposure. Consequently, early detection of tardive dyskinesia is important. To increase the likelihood of detecting the syndrome at the earliest possible time, the dosage of neuroleptic drug should be reduced periodically (if clinically possible) and the patient observed for signs of the disorder. This maneuver is critical, for neuroleptic drugs may mask the signs of the syndrome.

Neuroleptic Malignant Syndrome: See **Warnings**.

Acute Neurological Effects:

1. Dystonia. This may present as acute, reversible torticollis, opisthotonos, carpopedal spasm, trismus, dysphagia, respiratory difficulty, oculogyric crisis, and protrusion of the tongue. Treatment consists of the parenteral administration of either an anticholinergic antiparkinsonism agent or diphenhydramine.

2. Akathisia. Akathisia presents as constant motor restlessness. It is often confused with agitation and the differential diagnosis can be difficult. One feature that may permit a distinction is that the patient with akathisia often complains, *when asked*, about his or her inability to stop moving. The importance of the differential diagnosis is that akathisia should *not* be treated with an increased dose of neuroleptic. In the treatment of akathisia, the dose of antipsychotic may be lowered until the motor restlessness has subsided. The efficacy of anticholinergic treatment of this side effect is unestablished.

3. Pseudoparkinsonism. Pseudoparkinsonism refers to a drug-induced state similar to the classic syndrome. Its features include a generalized increase in muscle tone, often accompanied by "cogwheeling," tremor, and other signs and symptoms of the spontaneously occurring syndrome (*i.e.*, bradyphrenia, bradykinesia, masked facies, drooling, difficulty initiating movements, lack of associated movements, micrographia, etc.). Generally, anticho-

linergic antiparkinsonism agents (*i.e.*, benztropine, biperiden, procyclidine, or trihexyphenidyl) and amantadine are helpful in alleviating symptoms that cannot be managed by neuroleptic dose reduction. The value of prophylactic antiparkinsonism drug therapy has not been established. The need for continued use of antiparkinsonism medication should be reevaluated periodically.

Adverse Reactions Associated with Taractan: See **Warnings** and **Adverse Reactions:** *Common Reactions Linked to the Use of Neuroleptics: Untoward Neurological Events.*
Note: Sudden death has occasionally been reported in patients who have received phenothiazines. In some cases death was apparently due to cardiac arrest; in others the cause appeared to be asphyxia due to failure of the cough reflex. In some patients the cause could not be determined nor could it be established that death was due to the phenothiazine.
Taractan commonly causes sedation and hypotension.
The following adverse reactions have been reported with Taractan:
Central Nervous System: The most frequently occurring effect is initial drowsiness which usually disappears with or without dose adjustments. Hyperactivity or stimulation can occur, sometimes requiring discontinuation of the medication. Convulsions, particularly in patients with a history of EEG abnormalities, have been reported. Ataxia.
Autonomic Nervous System: Dry mouth, nasal stuffiness, visual changes and constipation have been occasionally reported. Headache. Gastric upset.
Cardiovascular System: Postural hypotension, tachycardia (especially with sudden marked increase in dosage) and dizziness have been reported. In the event that a vasoconstrictor is required, Levophed® (levarterenol) or Aramine (metaraminol) are the most suitable. Other pressor agents, including epinephrine, should not be used, as a paradoxical further lowering of the blood pressure may ensue.
EKG changes—particularly nonspecific, usually reversible Q and T wave distortions—have been observed in some patients receiving phenothiazine tranquilizers. Their relationship to myocardial damage has not been confirmed.
Skin: Dermatitis and urticarial type skin reactions have been observed infrequently. Photosensitivity is rare but undue exposure to the sun should be avoided.
Hepatotoxicity: Jaundice has been reported occasionally.
Hematological Disorders: Agranulocytosis, eosinophilia, leukopenia, hemolytic anemia, thrombocytopenic purpura and pancytopenia have been reported very rarely.
Endocrine Disorders: Galactorrhea and increased libido have been reported in isolated cases.
Other: Excessive weight gain and excessive thirst have occasionally been reported. Hyperpyrexia, paradoxical exacerbation of psychotic symptoms and ocular changes may also occur. Insomnia. Weakness.
Adverse Reactions Associated with Phenothiazine Derivatives: See **Warnings** and **Adverse Reactions:** *Common Reactions Linked to the Use of Neuroleptics: Untoward Neurological Events.*
Adverse Reactions Associated with Phenothiazine Derivatives: The following adverse reactions have not been reported specifically for Taractan nor have they been observed with every phenothiazine derivative; however, because of pharmacological similarities of Taractan to the various phenothiazine derivatives, they should be considered when administering drugs of this class.
Central Nervous System: Extrapyramidal symptoms (opisthotonos, oculogyric crisis, hyperreflexia); grand mal convulsions; altered cerebrospinal fluid proteins; cerebral edema; intensification and prolongation of the action of central nervous system depressants (opiates, analgesics, antihistamines, barbiturates, alcohol), atropine, exposure to extreme heat or organophosphorus insecticides.
Autonomic Nervous System: Obstipation; adynamic ileus; inhibition of ejaculation.
Cardiovascular System: Cardiac arrest; bradycardia; faintness.
Hepatotoxicity: Biliary stasis.
Endocrine Disorders: Lactation; gynecomastia; menstrual irregularities; moderate breast engorgement; hyperglycemia, hypoglycemia, glycosuria.
Allergic Reactions: Itching; erythema; eczema up to exfoliative dermatitis; asthma; laryngeal edema; angioneurotic edema; anaphylactoid reactions.
Other: Enlargement of the parotid gland; catatonic-like states; peripheral edema, reversed epinephrine effect; systemic lupus erythematosus-like syndrome; pigmentary retinopathy; with prolonged administration of substantial doses—skin pigmentation, epithelial keratopathy, and lenticular and corneal deposits.

DOSAGE AND ADMINISTRATION

Dosage should be individually adjusted according to diagnosis and severity of the condition. In general, small doses should be used initially, and increased to the optimal effective level as rapidly as possible based on therapeutic response. When higher dosage is required, greater sedation may be encountered; therefore, patients should be closely

supervised. Lethargy and drowsiness are readily controlled by dosage reduction. Initially, lower doses (10 to 25 mg three or four times daily) should be used for elderly or debilitated patients.
For convenience in prescribing and dispensing, all recommended dosages are expressed as strengths of the active moiety, chlorprothixene.
Taractan may be administered orally as tablets or concentrate. The concentrate, containing 100 mg of the drug per 5 ml teaspoonful, is pleasantly flavored and may be administered alone or in milk, water, fruit juices, coffee and carbonated beverages.

ORAL	AVERAGE DAILY DOSE
Adults:	Initially, 25 to 50 mg three or four times daily; to be increased as needed. Dosages exceeding 600 mg daily are rarely required.
Children (over 6 years of age):	10 to 25 mg three or four times daily.
PARENTERAL Not to be used in children under the age of 12.	25 to 50 mg I.M. up to three or four times daily.

Pain or induration at the site of injection is minimal. Since postural hypotension may occur in some patients, injection should be given with the patient seated or recumbent. If hypotension does occur, recovery is usually spontaneous; however, the patient should be observed until symptoms of weakness or dizziness pass.
As soon as the acutely agitated patient is brought under control, oral medication should be instituted. The changeover should be made gradually, with oral and parenteral doses being given alternately on the same day, then oral doses only, adjusted to the required maintenance level.

OVERDOSAGE

Taractan can be fatal in overdosage in the range of 2.5 to 4 Gm or above. Manifestations of overdosage or drowsiness, coma, respiratory depression, hypotension (which may appear after a delay of several hours and may persist for two to three days), tachycardia, pyrexia and constricted pupils. Convulsions, hyperactivity and hematuria may be seen in the recovery period.
Treatment is essentially symptomatic. Early gastric lavage is recommended, along with supportive measures such as I.V. fluids and the maintenance of an adequate airway. Severe hypotension usually responds to the use of levarterenol or metaraminol. Should coma be prolonged, caffeine and sodium benzoate, or ethamivan may be used, but the possibility must be borne in mind that these may lead to a convulsive episode. Should convulsions occur, the judicious use of sodium amytal is recommended. **Epinephrine must not be used in these patients.**

HOW SUPPLIED

Tablets — 10 mg chlorprothixene/Roche—bottles of 100; 25 mg, 50 mg or 100 mg chlorprothixene/Roche—bottles of 100 and 500.
Concentrate—containing, in each teaspoonful, chlorprothixene/Roche 100 mg base (as the lactate and hydrochloride)—bottles of 16 fluid ounces (1 pint).
Ampuls—containing chlorprothixene/Roche 25 mg/2 ml as the hydrochloride—boxes of 10.

ANIMAL PHARMACOLOGY AND TOXICOLOGY

In mice, the oral LD$_{50}$ of the two oral dosage forms of chlorprothixene were 350 ± 27 mg/kg (as the 2 per cent concentrate) and 220 ± 24 mg/kg (as the tablet form ground and suspended in 5 per cent gum acacia). For the injectable form the intramuscular LD$_{50}$ in mice was greater than 125 mg/kg.
Reproduction Studies: Reproductive and teratological studies in rats and rabbits were performed at levels of 12 and 24 mg/kg. In the rats, a decreased conception rate and an increased incidence of stillborns was noted at both levels. An increased number of resorptions was noted only at the high dose level. There was a decrease in the number of implantation sites at both doses. The number of live fetuses per litter and the mean fetal body weights were reduced slightly at 12 mg/kg and more so at 24 mg/kg. No teratological effects were observed. No deleterious effects on reproduction were seen in rabbits nor were any teratological findings noted.
P.I. 0588

Shown in Product Identification Section, page 425

TEL-E-DOSE®

Tel-E-Dose is a unit package designed by Roche for convenience in dispensing medications in the hospital and nursing home. Each unit, sealed against contamination and moisture, is clearly identified by product name and strength and carries the control number and expiration date.
Currently available in this package form are the following products: Bactrim™ (80 mg trimethoprim and 400 mg sulfamethoxazole) tablets; Bactrim™ DS (160 mg trimethoprim and 800 mg sulfamethoxazole) tablets; Bumex® (bumetanide HCl) tablets, 0.5 mg, 1 mg, 2 mg; Gantanol® (sulfamethoxazole) tablets, 0.5 Gm; Gantrisin® (sulfisoxazole) tab-

lets, 0.5 Gm; Trimpex® (trimethoprim) tablets, 100 mg.
Shown in Product Identification Section, page 425

TRIMPEX®   ℞
[*trim 'pex*]
(trimethoprim/Roche)
TABLETS

The following text is complete prescribing information based on official labeling in effect June 1, 1989.

DESCRIPTION

Trimpex (trimethoprim/Roche) is a synthetic antibacterial available as 100-mg tablets for oral administration. Each tablet also contains lactose, magnesium stearate, sodium starch glycolate and pregelatinized starch.
Trimethoprim is 2,4-diamino-5-(3,4,5-trimethoxybenzyl)pyrimidine. It is a white to light yellow, odorless, bitter compound with a molecular weight of 290.3.

CLINICAL PHARMACOLOGY

Trimethoprim is rapidly absorbed following oral administration. It exists in the blood as unbound, protein-bound and metabolized forms. Ten to twenty percent of trimethoprim is metabolized, primarily in the liver; the remainder is excreted unchanged in the urine. The principal metabolites of trimethoprim are the 1- and 3-oxides and the 3'- and 4'-hydroxy derivatives. The free form is considered to be the therapeutically active form. Approximately 44% of trimethoprim is bound to plasma proteins.
Mean peak plasma concentrations of approximately 1.0 mcg/ml occur 1 to 4 hours after oral administration of a single 100-mg dose. A single 200-mg dose will result in plasma concentrations approximately twice as high. The half-life of trimethoprim ranges from 8 to 10 hours. However, patients with severely impaired renal function exhibit an increase in the half-life of trimethoprim, which requires either dosage regimen adjustment or not using the drug in such patients (see DOSAGE AND ADMINISTRATION section). During a 13-week study of trimethoprim administered at a dosage of 50 mg *q.i.d.,* the mean minimum steady-state concentration of the drug was 1.1 mcg/ml. Steady-state concentrations were achieved within 2 to 3 days of chronic administration and were maintained throughout the experimental period.
Excretion of trimethoprim is primarily by the kidneys through glomerular filtration and tubular secretion. Urine concentrations of trimethoprim are considerably higher than are the concentrations in the blood. After a single oral dose of 100 mg, urine concentrations of trimethoprim ranged from 30 to 160 mcg/ml during the 0- to 4-hour period and declined to approximately 18 to 91 mcg/ml during the 8- to 24-hour period. A 200-mg single oral dose will result in trimethoprim urine concentrations approximately twice as high. After oral administration, 50% to 60% of trimethoprim is excreted in urine within 24 hours, approximately 80% of this being unmetabolized trimethoprim.
Since normal vaginal and fecal flora are the source of most pathogens causing urinary tract infections, it is relevant to consider the distribution of trimethoprim into these sites. Concentrations of trimethoprim in vaginal secretions are consistently greater than those found simultaneously in the serum, being typically 1.6 times the concentrations of simultaneously obtained serum samples. Sufficient trimethoprim is excreted in the feces to markedly reduce or eliminate trimethoprim-susceptible organisms from the fecal flora. The dominant non-*Enterobacteriaceae* fecal organisms, *Bacteroides* spp. and *Lactobacillus* spp., are not susceptible to trimethoprim concentrations obtained with the recommended dosage.
Trimethoprim also passes the placental barrier and is excreted in breast milk.
Microbiology: Trimpex blocks the production of tetrahydrofolic acid from dihydrofolic acid by binding to and reversibly inhibiting the required enzyme, dihydrofolate reductase. This binding is very much stronger for the bacterial enzyme than for the corresponding mammalian enzyme. Thus, Trimpex selectively interferes with bacterial biosynthesis of nucleic acids and proteins.
In vitro serial dilution tests have shown that the spectrum of antibacterial activity of Trimpex includes the common urinary tract pathogens with the exception of *Pseudomonas aeruginosa.*

Representative Minimum Inhibitory Concentrations for Trimethoprim-Susceptible Organisms	
Bacteria	Trimethoprim MIC—mcg/ml (Range)
Escherichia coli	0.05—1.5
Proteus mirabilis	0.5—1.5
Klebsiella pneumoniae	0.5—5.0
Enterobacter species	0.5—5.0
Staphylococcus species (coagulase-negative)	0.15—5.0

Continued on next page

Roche Labs.—Cont.

The recommended quantitative disc susceptibility method[1,2] may be used for estimating the susceptibility of bacteria to Trimpex. With this procedure, reports from the laboratory giving results using the 5-mcg trimethoprim disc should be interpreted according to the following criteria: Organisms producing zones of 16 mm or greater are classified as susceptible, whereas those producing zones of 11 to 15 mm are classified as having intermediate susceptibility. A report from the laboratory of "Susceptible to trimethoprim" or "Intermediate susceptibility to trimethoprim" indicates that the infection is likely to respond when, as in uncomplicated urinary tract infections, effective therapy is dependent upon the urine concentration of trimethoprim. Organisms producing zones of 10 mm or less are reported as resistant, indicating that other therapy should be selected.

Dilution methods for determining susceptibility are also used, and results are reported as the minimum drug concentration inhibiting microbial growth (MIC).[3] If the MIC is 8 mcg per ml or less, the microorganism is considered "susceptible." If the MIC is 16 mcg per ml or greater, the microorganism is considered "resistant."

INDICATIONS AND USAGE

For the treatment of initial episodes of uncomplicated urinary tract infections due to susceptible strains of the following organisms: *Escherichia coli, Proteus mirabilis, Klebsiella pneumoniae, Enterobacter* species and coagulase-negative *Staphylococcus* species, including *S. saprophyticus.*

Cultures and susceptibility tests should be performed to determine the susceptibility of the bacteria to trimethoprim. Therapy may be initiated prior to obtaining the results of these tests.

CONTRAINDICATIONS

Trimpex is contraindicated in individuals hypersensitive to trimethoprim and in those with documented megaloblastic anemia due to folate deficiency.

WARNINGS

Serious hypersensitivity reactions have been reported rarely in patients on trimethoprim therapy. Trimethoprim has been reported rarely to interfere with hematopoiesis, especially when administered in large doses and/or for prolonged periods.

The presence of clinical signs such as sore throat, fever, pallor or purpura may be early indications of serious blood disorders.

PRECAUTIONS

General: Trimethoprim should be given with caution to patients with possible folate deficiency. Folates may be administered concomitantly without interfering with the antibacterial action of trimethoprim. Trimethoprim should also be given with caution to patients with impaired renal or hepatic function. If any clinical signs of a blood disorder are noted in a patient receiving trimethoprim, a complete blood count should be obtained and the drug discontinued if a significant reduction in the count of any formed blood element is found.

Drug interactions: Trimpex may inhibit the hepatic metabolism of phenytoin. Trimethoprim, given at a common clinical dosage, increased the phenytoin half-life by 51% and decreased the phenytoin metabolic clearance rate by 30%. When administering these drugs concurrently, one should be alert for possible excessive phenytoin effect.

Drug/laboratory test interactions: Trimethoprim can interfere with a serum methotrexate assay as determined by the competitive binding protein technique (CBPA) when a bacterial dihydrofolate reductase is used as the binding protein. No interference occurs, however, if methotrexate is measured by a radioimmunoassay (RIA).

The presence of trimethoprim may also interfere with the Jaffé alkaline picrate reaction assay for creatinine resulting in overestimations of about 10% in the range of normal values.

Carcinogenesis, mutagenesis, impairment of fertility:

Carcinogenesis: Long-term studies in animals to evaluate carcinogenic potential have not been conducted with trimethoprim.

Mutagenesis: Trimethoprim was demonstrated to be nonmutagenic in the Ames assay. No chromosomal damage was observed in human leukocytes cultured *in vitro* with trimethoprim; the concentration used exceeded blood levels following therapy with Trimpex.

Impairment of fertility: No adverse effects on fertility or general reproductive performance were observed in rats given trimethoprim in oral dosages as high as 70 mg/kg/day for males and 14 mg/kg/day for females.

Pregnancy: Teratogenic effects: Pregnancy Category C. Trimethoprim has been shown to be teratogenic in the rat when given in doses 40 times the human dose. In some rabbit studies, the overall increase in fetal loss (dead and resorbed

and malformed conceptuses) was associated with doses 6 times the human therapeutic dose.

While there are no large well-controlled studies on the use of trimethoprim in pregnant women, Brumfitt and Pursell,[4] in a retrospective study, reported the outcome of 186 pregnancies during which the mother received either placebo or trimethoprim in combination wih sulfamethoxazole. The incidence of congenital abnormalities was 4.5% (3 of 66) in those who received placebo and 3.3% (4 of 120) in those receiving trimethoprim plus sulfamethoxazole. There were no abnormalities in the 10 children whose mothers received the drug during the first trimester. In a separate survey, Brumfitt and Pursell also found no congenital abnormalities in 35 children whose mothers had received trimethoprim plus sulfamethoxazole at the time of conception or shortly thereafter.

Because trimethoprim may interfere with folic acid metabolism, Trimpex should be used during pregnancy only if the potential benefit justifies the potential risk to the fetus.

Nonteratogenic effects: The oral administration of trimethoprim to rats at a dose of 70 mg/kg/day commencing with the last third of gestation and continuing through parturition and lactation caused no deleterious effects on gestation or pup growth and survival.

Nursing mothers: Trimethoprim is excreted in human milk. Because trimethoprim may interfere with folic acid metabolism, caution should be exercised when Trimpex is administered to a nursing woman.

Pediatric use: The safety of trimethoprim in infants under two months of age has not been demonstrated. The effectiveness of trimethoprim has not been established in children under 12 years of age.

ADVERSE REACTIONS

The adverse effects encountered most often with trimethoprim were rash and pruritus. Other adverse effects reported involved the gastrointestinal and hematopoietic systems.

Dermatologic: Rash, pruritus and phototoxic skin eruptions. At the recommended dosage regimens of 100 mg *b.i.d.* or 200 mg *q.d.*, each for 10 days, the incidence of rash is 2.9% to 6.7%. In clinical studies which employed high doses of Trimpex, an elevated incidence of rash was noted. These rashes were maculopapular, morbilliform, pruritic and generally mild to moderate, appearing 7 to 14 days after the initiation of therapy.

Hypersensitivity: There have been rare reports of exfoliative dermatitis, erytherma multiforme, Stevens-Johnson syndrome, Lyell syndrome, anaphylaxis and aseptic meningitis.

Gastrointestinal: Epigastric distress, nausea, vomiting and glossitis. Elevation of serum transaminase and bilirubin.

Hematologic: Thrombocytopenia, leukopenia, neutropenia, megaloblastic anemia and methemoglobinemia.

Miscellaneous: Fever, increases in BUN and serum creatinine levels.

OVERDOSAGE

Acute: Signs of acute overdosage with trimethoprim may appear following ingestion of 1 gram or more of the drug and include nausea, vomiting, dizziness, headaches, mental depression, confusion and bone marrow depression (see CHRONIC OVERDOSAGE).

Treatment consists of gastric lavage and general supportive measures. Acidification of the urine will increase renal elimination of trimethoprim. Peritoneal dialysis is not effective and hemodialysis only moderately effective in eliminating the drug.

Chronic: Use of trimethoprim at high doses and/or for extended periods of time may cause bone marrow depression manifested as thrombocytopenia, leukopenia and/or megaloblastic anemia. If signs of bone marrow depression occur, trimethoprim should be discontinued and the patient should be given leucovorin, 3 to 6 mg intramuscularly daily for three days, or as required to restore normal hematopoiesis.

DOSAGE AND ADMINISTRATION

The usual oral adult dosage is 100 mg (one tablet) every 12 hours or 200 mg (two tablets) every 24 hours, each for 10 days. The use of trimethoprim in patients with a creatinine clearance of less than 15 ml/min is not recommended. For patients with a creatinine clearance of 15 to 30 ml/min, the dose should be 50 mg every 12 hours.

The effectiveness of trimethoprim has not been established in children under 12 years of age.

HOW SUPPLIED

100-mg tablets (white, elliptical, scored)—bottles of 100 (NDC 0004-0127-01); Tel-E-Dose® packages of 100 (NDC 0004-0127-49). Imprint on tablets: TRIMPEX 100 ROCHE.

REFERENCES

1. Bauer AW, Kirby WMM, Sherris JC, Turck M: Antibiotic Susceptibility Testing by Standardized Single Disk Method, *Am J Clin Pathol* 45:493–496, 1966.
2. Approved Standard ASM-2 Performance Standards for Antimicrobial Disc Susceptibility Test; National Committee for Clinical Laboratory Standards, 771 East Lancaster Avenue, Villanova, Pennsylvania 19085.
3. Ericsson HM, Sherris JC: Antibiotic Sensitivity Testing. Report of an International Collaborative Study. *Acta Pathol Microbiol Scand* [B] (Suppl 217): 1–90, 1971.
4. Brumfitt W, Pursell R: Trimethoprim/Sulfamethoxazole in the Treatment of Bacteriuria in Women, *J Infect Dis* 128 (Suppl): S657–S663, 1973.
P.I. 0988
Shown in Product Identification Section, page 425

VALRELEASE®   ℞
[*val 're-lease*]
(diazepam/Roche)
CAPSULES
A slow-release dosage form of
Valium® (diazepam/Roche)

The following text is complete prescribing information based on official labeling in effect June 1, 1989.

DESCRIPTION

Diazepam is a benzodiazepine derivative developed through original Roche research. Chemically, diazepam is 7-chloro-1,3- dihydro-1-methyl-5-phenyl-2H-1, 4-benzodiazepin -2-one. It is a colorless crystalline compound, insoluble in water and has a molecular weight of 284.74.

Valrelease capsules provide the actions of Valium® (diazepam/Roche) in a slow-release dosage form.

Valrelease capsule shells contain the following dye system: FD&C Blue No. 1, FD&C Yellow No. 6 and D&C Yellow No. 10.

PHARMACOLOGY

In animals, diazepam appears to act on parts of the limbic system, the thalamus and hypothalamus, and induces calming effects. Diazepam, unlike chlorpromazine and reserpine, has no demonstrable peripheral autonomic blocking action, nor does it produce extrapyramidal side effects; however, animals treated with diazepam do have a transient ataxia at higher doses. Diazepam was found to have transient cardiovascular depressor effects in dogs. Long-term experiments in rats revealed no disturbances of endocrine function.

Oral LD$_{50}$ of diazepam is 720 mg/kg in mice and 1240 mg/kg in rats. Intraperitoneal administration of 400 mg/kg to a monkey resulted in death on the sixth day.

Reproduction Studies: A series of rat reproduction studies was performed with diazepam in oral doses of 1, 10, 80 and 100 mg/kg. At 100 mg/kg there was a decrease in the number of pregnancies and surviving offspring in these rats. Neonatal survival of rats at doses lower than 100 mg/kg was within normal limits. Several neonates in these rat reproduction studies showed skeletal or other defects. Further studies in rats at doses up to and including 80 mg/kg/day did not reveal teratological effects on the offspring.

In humans, measurable blood levels of diazepam were obtained in maternal and cord blood, indicating placental transfer of the drug.

The administration of one 15-mg Valrelease capsule results in blood levels of diazepam over a 24-hour period which are comparable to those of 5-mg Valium tablets given three times daily.

The mean time to maximum plasma diazepam concentrations after administration of 15-mg Valrelease capsules to eleven fasted subjects was 5.3 hours. The harmonic mean half-life of diazepam was 36 hours. The range of average minimum steady-state plasma diazepam concentrations during once daily administration of 15-mg Valrelease capsules to eleven normal subjects was 196 to 341 ng/ml.

INDICATIONS

Valrelease is indicated for the management of anxiety disorders or for the short-term relief of the symptoms of anxiety. Anxiety or tension associated with the stress of everyday life usually does not require treatment with an anxiolytic.

Valrelease is a useful adjunct for the relief of skeletal muscle spasm due to reflex spasm to local pathology (such as inflammation of the muscles or joints, or secondary to trauma); spasticity caused by upper motor neuron disorders (such as cerebral palsy and paraplegia); athetosis; and stiff-man syndrome.

The effectiveness of diazepam in long-term use, that is, more than 4 months, has not been assessed by systematic clinical studies. The physician should periodically reassess the usefulness of the drug for the individual patient.

CONTRAINDICATIONS

Valrelease is contraindicated in patients with a known hypersensitivity to this drug and, because of lack of sufficient clinical experience, in children under 6 months of age. It may be used in patients with open angle glaucoma who are receiving appropriate therapy, but is contraindicated in acute narrow angle glaucoma.

WARNINGS

Valrelease is not of value in the treatment of psychotic patients and should not be employed in lieu of appropriate treatment. As is true of most preparations containing CNS-acting drugs, patients receiving Valrelease should be cautioned against engaging in hazardous occupations requiring complete mental alertness such as operating machinery or driving a motor vehicle.

If the use of Valrelease in patients with seizure disorders results in an increase in the frequency and/or severity of grand mal seizures, there may be a need to increase the dosage of standard anticonvulsant medication.

Abrupt withdrawal of Valrelease in patients with a history of seizures may also be associated with a temporary increase in the frequency and/or severity of seizures.

Since Valrelease has a central nervous system depressant effect, patients should be advised against the simultaneous ingestion of alcohol and other CNS-depressant drugs during Valrelease therapy.

> *Usage in Pregnancy:* An increased risk of congenital malformations associated with the use of minor tranquilizers (diazepam, meprobamate and chlordiazepoxide) during the first trimester of pregnancy has been suggested in several studies. Because use of these drugs is rarely a matter of urgency, their use during this period should almost always be avoided. The possibility that a woman of childbearing potential may be pregnant at the time of institution of therapy should be considered. Patients should be advised that if they become pregnant during therapy or intend to become pregnant they should communicate with their physicians about the desirability of discontinuing the drug.

Management of Overdosage: Manifestations of diazepam overdosage include somnolence, confusion, coma and diminished reflexes. Respiration, pulse and blood pressure should be monitored, as in all cases of drug overdosage, although, in general, these effects have been minimal following overdosage. General supportive measures should be employed, along with immediate gastric lavage. Intravenous fluids should be administered and an adequate airway maintained. Hypotension may be combated by the use of Levophed® (levarterenol) or Aramine (metaraminol). Dialysis is of limited value. As with the management of intentional overdosage with any drug, it should be borne in mind that multiple agents may have been ingested.

Withdrawal symptoms of the barbiturate type have occurred after the discontinuation of benzodiazepines. (See DRUG ABUSE AND DEPENDENCE section.)

PRECAUTIONS

If Valrelease is to be combined with other psychotropic agents or anticonvulsant drugs, careful consideration should be given to the pharmacology of the agents to be employed—particularly with known compounds which may potentiate the action of diazepam, such as phenothiazines, narcotics, barbiturates, MAO inhibitors and other antidepressants. The usual precautions are indicated for severely depressed patients or those in whom there is any evidence of latent depression; particularly the recognition that suicidal tendencies may be present and protective measures may be necessary. The usual precautions in treating patients with impaired renal or hepatic function should be observed.

In elderly and debilitated patients, it is recommended that the dosage be limited to the smallest effective amount to preclude the development of ataxia or oversedation (2 mg to 2½ mg once or twice daily, initially, to be increased gradually as needed and tolerated).

NOTE: If 2 or 2½ mg is the desired dose, scored Valium® (diazepam/Roche) tablets should be used.

The clearance of Valium and certain other benzodiazepines can be delayed in association with Tagamet (cimetidine) administration. The clinical significance of this is unclear.

Information for Patients: To assure the safe and effective use of benzodiazepines, patients should be informed that, since benzodiazepines may produce psychological and physical dependence, it is advisable that they consult with their physician before either increasing the dose or abruptly discontinuing this drug.

ADVERSE REACTIONS

Side effects most commonly reported were drowsiness, fatigue and ataxia. Infrequently encountered were confusion, constipation, depression, diplopia, dysarthria, headache, hypotension, incontinence, jaundice, changes in libido, nausea, changes in salivation, skin rash, slurred speech, tremor, urinary retention, vertigo and blurred vision. Paradoxical reactions such as acute hyperexcited states, anxiety, hallucinations, increased muscle spasticity, insomnia, rage, sleep disturbances and stimulation have been reported; should these occur, use of the drug should be discontinued.

Because of isolated reports of neutropenia and jaundice, periodic blood counts and liver function tests are advisable during long-term therapy. Minor changes in EEG patterns, usually low-voltage fast activity, have been observed in patients during and after diazepam therapy and are of no known significance.

DRUG ABUSE AND DEPENDENCE

Withdrawal symptoms, similar in character to those noted with barbiturates and alcohol (convulsions, tremor, abdominal and muscle cramps, vomiting and sweating), have occurred following abrupt discontinuation of diazepam. The

more severe withdrawal symptoms have usually been limited to those patients who had received excessive doses over an extended period of time. Generally milder withdrawal symptoms (*e.g.*, dysphoria and insomnia) have been reported following abrupt discontinuance of benzodiazepines taken continuously at therapeutic levels for several months. Consequently, after extended therapy, abrupt discontinuation should generally be avoided and a gradual dosage tapering schedule followed. Addiction-prone individuals (such as drug addicts or alcoholics) should be under careful surveillance when receiving diazepam or other psychotropic agents because of the predisposition of such patients to habituation and dependence.

DOSAGE AND ADMINISTRATION

Dosage should be individualized for maximum beneficial effect. While the usual daily dosages given below will meet the needs of most patients, there will be some who may require higher doses. In such cases dosage should be increased cautiously to avoid adverse effects.

Whenever oral Valium® (diazepam/Roche), 5 mg t.i.d., would be considered the appropriate dosage, one 15-mg Valrelease capsule daily may be used.

Note: If 1 mg or 2½ mg is the desired dose, scored Valium (diazepam/Roche) tablets should be used.

Valrelease 15-mg capsules are recommended for elderly or debilitated patients and children only when it has been determined that 5 mg oral Valium t.i.d. is the optimal daily dose. Oral Valium is not recommended for children under 6 months of age.

Adults:	USUAL DAILY DOSE
Management of Anxiety Disorders and Relief of Symptoms of Anxiety.	Depending upon severity of symptoms—1 or 2 (15 to 30 mg) capsules once daily
Adjunctively for Relief of Skeletal Muscle Spasm.	1 or 2 capsules (15 to 30 mg) once daily

HOW SUPPLIED

For oral administration, Valrelease (diazepam/Roche) capsules—15 mg (yellow and blue)—bottles of 100; Prescription Paks of 30.
P.I. 0288

Shown in Product Identification Section, page 425

VERSED®   Ⓒ
[ver-sed ']
midazolam HCl/Roche
INJECTION

The following text is complete prescribing information based on official labeling in effect June 1, 1989.

> Intravenous VERSED has been associated with respiratory depression and respiratory arrest, especially when used for conscious sedation. In some cases, where this was not recognized promptly and treated effectively, death or hypoxic encephalopathy has resulted. Intravenous VERSED should be used only in hospital or ambulatory care settings, including physicians' offices, that provide for continuous monitoring of respiratory and cardiac function. Immediate availability of resuscitative drugs and equipment and personnel trained in their use should be assured. (See WARNINGS.)
>
> The initial intravenous dose for conscious sedation may be as little as 1 mg, but should not exceed 2.5 mg in a normal healthy adult. Lower doses are necessary for older (over 60 years) or debilitated patients and in patients receiving concomitant narcotics or other CNS depressants. The initial dose and all subsequent doses should never be given as a bolus; administer over at least 2 minutes and allow an additional 2 or more minutes to fully evaluate the sedative effect. The use of the 1 mg/mL formulation or dilution of the 1 mg/mL or 5 mg/mL formulation is recommended to facilitate slower injection. See DOSAGE AND ADMINISTRATION for complete dosing information.

DESCRIPTION

VERSED (brand of midazolam hydrochloride/Roche) is a water-soluble benzodiazepine available as a sterile, nonpyrogenic parenteral dosage form for intravenous or intramuscular injection. Each mL contains midazolam hydrochloride equivalent to 1 mg or 5 mg midazolam compounded with 0.8% sodium chloride and 0.01% disodium edetate, with 1% benzyl alcohol as preservative; the pH is adjusted to approximately 3 with hydrochloric acid and, if necessary, sodium hydroxide.

Midazolam is a white to light yellow crystalline compound, insoluble in water. The hydrochloride salt of midazolam, which is formed *in situ*, is soluble in aqueous solutions. Chemically, midazolam HCl is 8-chloro-6-(2-fluorophenyl)-1-methyl-4*H*-imidazo[1,5-a][1,4] benzodiazepine hydrochlo-

ride. Midazolam hydrochloride has the empirical formula $C_{18}H_{13}ClFN_3 \cdot HCl$, a calculated molecular weight of 362.25.

CLINICAL PHARMACOLOGY

VERSED is a short-acting benzodiazepine central nervous system depressant.

The effects of VERSED on the CNS are dependent on the dose administered, the route of administration, and the presence or absence of other premedications. Onset time of sedative effects after IM administration was 15 minutes, with peak sedation occurring 30 to 60 minutes following injection. In one study, when tested the following day, 73% of the patients who received VERSED intramuscularly had no recall of memory cards shown 30 minutes following drug administration; 40% had no recall of the memory cards shown 60 minutes following drug administration.

Sedation after IV injection was achieved within 3 to 5 minutes; the time of onset is affected by total dose administered and the concurrent administration of narcotic premedication. Seventy-one percent of the patients in the endoscopy studies had no recall of introduction of the endoscope; 82% of the patients had no recall of withdrawal of the endoscope. When VERSED is given intravenously as an anesthetic induction agent, induction of anesthesia occurs in approximately 1.5 minutes when narcotic premedication has been administered and in 2 to 2.5 minutes without narcotic premedication or with sedative premedication. Some impairment in a test of memory was noted in 90% of the patients studied.

VERSED, used as directed, does not delay awakening from general anesthesia. Gross tests of recovery after awakening (orientation, ability to stand and walk, suitability for discharge from the recovery room, return to baseline Trieger competency) usually indicate recovery within 2 hours but recovery may take up to 6 hours in some cases. When compared with patients who received thiopental, patients who received midazolam generally recovered at a slightly slower rate.

In patients without intracranial lesions, induction with VERSED is associated with a moderate decrease in cerebrospinal fluid pressure (lumbar puncture measurements), similar to that seen following use of thiopental. Preliminary data in intracranial surgical patients with normal intracranial pressure but decreased compliance (subarachnoid screw measurements) show comparable elevations of intracranial pressure with VERSED and with thiopental during intubation.

Usual intramuscular premedicating doses of VERSED do not depress the ventilatory response to carbon dioxide stimulation to a clinically significant extent. Induction doses of VERSED depress the ventilatory response to carbon dioxide stimulation for 15 minutes or more beyond the duration of ventilatory depression following administration of thiopental. Impairment of ventilatory response to carbon dioxide is more marked in patients with chronic obstructive pulmonary disease (COPD). Sedation with intravenous VERSED does not adversely affect the mechanics of respiration (resistance, static recoil, most lung volume measurements); total lung capacity and peak expiratory flow decrease significantly but static compliance and maximum expiratory flow at 50% of awake total lung capacity (Vmax) increase.

In cardiac hemodynamic studies, induction with VERSED was associated with a slight to moderate decrease in mean arterial pressure, cardiac output, stroke volume and systemic vascular resistance. Slow heart rates (less than 65/minute), particularly in patients taking propranolol for angina, tended to rise slightly; faster heart rates (*e.g.*, 85/minute) tended to slow slightly.

The following preliminary pharmacokinetic data for midazolam have been reported. In normal subjects and healthy patients intravenous midazolam exhibited an elimination half-life of 1.2 to 12.3 hours, a large volume of distribution (0.95 to 6.6 L/kg) and a plasma clearance of 0.15 to 0.77 L/hr/kg. Clinical effects of VERSED do not directly correlate with the blood concentrations of midazolam.

Following intravenous administration, less than 0.03% of the dose is excreted in the urine as intact midazolam. Midazolam is rapidly metabolized to 1-hydroxymethyl midazolam, which is conjugated, with subsequent excretion in the urine. Approximately 45% to 57% of the dose is excreted in the urine as the conjugate of 1-hydroxymethyl midazolam, the major metabolite of midazolam. The half-life of elimination of 1-hydroxymethyl midazolam is similar to the parent compound. The concentration of midazolam is 10- to 30-fold greater than that of 1-hydroxymethyl midazolam after single IV administration.

In a small group of patients (n = 11) with congestive heart failure, there appeared to be a 2- to 3-fold increase in the elimination half-life and volume of distribution of midazolam; however, the total body clearance of midazolam appeared to remain unchanged at a single 5-mg intravenous dose. There was no apparent change in the pharmacokinetic profile following the intravenous administration of 5 mg of midazolam to a small group of patients (n = 12) with hepatic

Continued on next page

Roche Labs.—Cont.

dysfunction. There was a 1.5- to 2-fold increase in elimination half-life, total body clearance and volume of distribution in a small group of patients (n = 15) with chronic renal failure.

In a small group (n = 12) of surgical patients, aged 49 to 60 years old, given 0.2 mg/kg midazolam intravenously, there appeared to be a small increase in the volume of distribution and elimination half-life with little change in total body clearance compared to an equal number of younger surgical patients (aged 18 to 30).

The mean absolute bioavailability of midazolam following intramuscular administration is greater than 90%. The mean time of maximum midazolam plasma concentrations following intramuscular dosing occurs within 45 minutes postadministration. Peak concentrations of midazolam as well as 1-hydroxymethyl midazolam after intramuscular administration are about one-half of those achieved after equivalent intravenous doses. The pharmacokinetic profile of elimination after intramuscularly administered midazolam is comparable to that observed following intravenous administration of the drug. Dose-linearity relationships have not been adequately defined.

Midazolam is approximately 97% plasma protein-bound in normal subjects and patients with renal failure. In animals, midazolam has been shown to cross the blood-brain barrier. In animals and in humans, midazolam has been shown to cross the placenta and enter into fetal circulation. It is not known whether midazolam is excreted in human milk.

INDICATIONS

Injectable VERSED is indicated—
- intramuscularly for preoperative sedation (induction of sleepiness or drowsiness and relief of apprehension) and to impair memory of perioperative events;
- intravenously as an agent for conscious sedation prior to short diagnostic or endoscopic procedures, such as bronchoscopy, gastroscopy, cystoscopy, coronary angiography and cardiac catheterization, either alone or with a narcotic.
- intravenously for induction of general anesthesia, before administration of other anesthetic agents. With the use of narcotic premedication, induction of anesthesia can be attained within a relatively narrow dose range and in a short period of time. Intravenous VERSED can also be used as a component of intravenous supplementation of nitrous oxide and oxygen (balanced anesthesia) *for short surgical procedures;* longer procedures have not been studied.

When used intravenously, VERSED is associated with a high incidence of partial or complete impairment of recall for the next several hours. (See CLINICAL PHARMACOLOGY.)

CONTRAINDICATIONS

Injectable VERSED is contraindicated in patients with a known hypersensitivity to the drug. Benzodiazepines are contraindicated in patients with acute narrow angle glaucoma. Benzodiazepines may be used in patients with open angle glaucoma only if they are receiving appropriate therapy. Measurements of intraocular pressure in patients without eye disease show a moderate lowering following induction with VERSED; patients with glaucoma have not been studied.

WARNINGS

VERSED must never be used without individualization of dosage. Prior to the intravenous administration of VERSED in any dose, the immediate availability of oxygen, resuscitative equipment and skilled personnel for the maintenance of a patent airway and support of ventilation should be ensured. Patients should be continuously monitored for early signs of underventilation or apnea, which can lead to hypoxia/cardiac arrest unless effective countermeasures are taken immediately. Vital signs should continue to be monitored during the recovery period. Because intravenous VERSED depresses respiration (see CLINICAL PHARMACOLOGY) and because opioid agonists and other sedatives can add to this depression, VERSED should be administered as an induction agent only by a person trained in general anesthesia and should be used for conscious sedation only in the presence of personnel skilled in early detection of underventilation, maintaining a patent airway and supporting ventilation. When used for conscious sedation, VERSED should not be administered by rapid or single bolus intravenous administration.

Serious cardiorespiratory adverse events have occurred. These have included respiratory depression, apnea, respiratory arrest and/or cardiac arrest, sometimes resulting in death. There have also been rare reports of hypotensive episodes requiring treatment during or after diagnostic or surgical manipulations in patients who have received VERSED. Hypotension occurred more frequently in the conscious sedation studies in patients premedicated with a narcotic.

Reactions such as agitation, involuntary movements (including tonic/clonic movements and muscle tremor), hyperactivity and combativeness have been reported. These reactions may be due to inadequate or excessive dosing or improper administration of VERSED; however, consideration should be given to the possibility of cerebral hypoxia or true paradoxical reactions. Should such reactions occur, the response to each dose of VERSED and all other drugs, including local anesthetics, should be evaluated before proceeding.

Concomitant use of barbiturates, alcohol or other central nervous system depressants may increase the risk of underventilation or apnea and may contribute to profound and/or prolonged drug effect. Narcotic premedication also depresses the ventilatory response to carbon dioxide stimulation.

Higher risk surgical patients, elderly patients and debilitated patients require lower dosages, whether premedicated or not. Patients with chronic obstructive pulmonary disease are unusually sensitive to the respiratory depressant effect of VERSED. Patients with chronic renal failure and patients with congestive heart failure eliminate midazolam more slowly. (See CLINICAL PHARMACOLOGY.) Because elderly patients frequently have inefficient function of one or more organ systems, and because dosage requirements have been shown to decrease with age, reduced initial dosage of VERSED is recommended and the possibility of profound and/or prolonged effect should be considered.

Injectable VERSED should not be administered to patients in shock or coma, or in acute alcohol intoxication with depression of vital signs. Particular care should be exercised in the use of intravenous VERSED in patients with uncompensated acute illnesses, such as severe fluid or electrolyte disturbances.

The hazards of intra-arterial injection of VERSED solutions in humans are unknown; therefore, precautions against unintended intra-arterial injection should be taken. Extravasation should also be avoided.

The decision as to when patients who have received injectable VERSED, particularly on an outpatient basis, may again engage in activities requiring complete mental alertness, operate hazardous machinery or drive a motor vehicle must be individualized. Gross tests of recovery from the effects of VERSED (see CLINICAL PHARMACOLOGY) cannot be relied upon alone to predict reaction time under stress. This drug is never used alone during anesthesia and the contribution of other perioperative drugs and events can vary. It is recommended that no patient operate hazardous machinery or a motor vehicle until the effects of the drug, such as drowsiness, have subsided or until the day after anesthesia and surgery, whichever is longer.

Usage in Pregnancy: An increased risk of congenital malformations associated with the use of benzodiazepine drugs (diazepam and chlordiazepoxide) has been suggested in several studies. If this drug is used during pregnancy, the patient should be apprised of the potential hazard to the fetus.

PRECAUTIONS

General: Intravenous doses of VERSED should be decreased for elderly and for debilitated patients. (See WARNINGS and DOSAGE AND ADMINISTRATION.) These patients will also probably take longer to recover completely after VERSED administration for the induction of anesthesia.

VERSED does not protect against the increase in intracranial pressure or against the heart rate rise and/or blood pressure rise associated with endotracheal intubation under light general anesthesia.

Information for patients: To assure safe and effective use of benzodiazepines, the following information and instructions should be communicated to the patient when appropriate:

1. Inform your physician about any alcohol consumption and medicine you are now taking, including drugs you buy without a prescription. Alcohol has an increased effect when consumed with benzodiazepines; therefore, caution should be exercised regarding simultaneous ingestion of alcohol during benzodiazepine treatment.
2. Inform your physician if you are pregnant or are planning to become pregnant.
3. Inform your physician if you are nursing.

Drug interactions: The sedative effect of intravenous VERSED is accentuated by premedication, particularly narcotics (*e.g.,* morphine, meperidine and fentanyl) and also secobarbital and Innovar (fentanyl and droperidol). Consequently, the dosage of VERSED should be adjusted according to the type and amount of premedication administered. (See DOSAGE AND ADMINISTRATION.)

A moderate reduction in induction dosage requirements of thiopental (about 15%) has been noted following use of intramuscular VERSED for premedication.

The intravenous administration of VERSED decreases the minimum alveolar concentration (MAC) of halothane required for general anesthesia. This decrease correlates with the dose of VERSED administered.

Although the possibility of minor interactive effects has not been fully studied, VERSED and pancuronium have been used together in patients without noting clinically significant changes in dosage, onset or duration. VERSED does not protect against the characteristic circulatory changes noted after administration of succinylcholine or pancuronium and does not protect against the increased intracranial pressure noted following administration of succinylcholine. VERSED does not cause a clinically significant change in dosage, onset or duration of a single intubating dose of succinylcholine.

No significant adverse interactions with commonly used premedications or drugs used during anesthesia and surgery (including atropine, scopolamine, glycopyrrolate, diazepam, hydroxyzine, d-tubocurarine, succinylcholine and nondepolarizing muscle relaxants) or topical local anesthetics (including lidocaine, dyclonine HCl and Cetacaine) have been observed.

Drug/laboratory test interactions: Midazolam has not been shown to interfere with results obtained in clinical laboratory tests.

Carcinogenesis, mutagenesis, impairment of fertility:

Carcinogenesis: Midazolam maleate was administered with diet in mice and rats for two years at dosages of 1, 9 and 80 mg/kg/day. In female mice in the highest dose group there was a marked increase in the incidence of hepatic tumors. In high dose male rats there was a small but statistically significant increase in benign thyroid follicular cell tumors. Dosages of 9 mg/kg/day of midazolam maleate (25 times a human dose of 0.35 mg/kg) do not increase the incidence of tumors. The pathogenesis of induction of these tumors is not known. These tumors were found after chronic administration, whereas human use will ordinarily be of single or several doses.

Mutagenesis: Midazolam did not have mutagenic activity in *Salmonella typhimurium* (5 bacterial strains), Chinese hamster lung cells (V79), human lymphocytes, or in the micronucleus test in mice.

Impairment of fertility: A reproduction study in male and female rats did not show any impairment of fertility at dosages up to ten times the human IV dose of 0.35 mg/kg.

Pregnancy: Teratogenic effects: Pregnancy Category D. See WARNINGS section.

Segment II teratology studies, performed with midazolam maleate injectable in rabbits and rats at 5 and 10 times the human dose of 0.35 mg/kg, did not show evidence of teratogenicity.

Nonteratogenic effects: Studies in rats showed no adverse effects on reproductive parameters during gestation and lactation. Dosages tested were approximately 10 times the human dose of 0.35 mg/kg.

Labor and delivery: In humans, measurable levels of midazolam were found in maternal venous serum, umbilical venous and arterial serum and amniotic fluid, indicating placental transfer of the drug. Following intramuscular administration of 0.05 mg/kg of midazolam, both the venous and the umbilical arterial serum concentrations were lower than maternal concentrations.

The use of injectable VERSED in obstetrics has not been evaluated in clinical studies. Because midazolam is transferred transplacentally and because other benzodiazepines given in the last weeks of pregnancy have resulted in neonatal CNS depression, VERSED is not recommended for obstetrical use.

Nursing mothers: It is not known whether midazolam is excreted in human milk. Because many drugs are excreted in human milk, caution should be exercised when injectable VERSED is administered to a nursing woman.

Pediatric use: Safety and effectiveness of VERSED in children below the age of 18 years have not been established.

ADVERSE REACTIONS

See WARNINGS concerning serious cardiorespiratory events and possible paradoxical reactions. Fluctuations in vital signs were the most frequently seen findings following parenteral administration of VERSED and included decreased tidal volume and/or respiratory rate decrease (23.3% of patients following IV and 10.8% of patients following IM administration) and apnea (15.4% of patients following IV administration), as well as variations in blood pressure and pulse rate.

The following additional adverse reactions were reported after intramuscular administration:

headache (1.3%)	Local effects at IM injection site
	pain (3.7%)
	induration (0.5%)
	redness (0.5%)
	muscle stiffness (0.3%)

The following additional adverse reactions were reported subsequent to intravenous administration:

hiccoughs (3.9%)	Local effects at the IV site
nausea (2.8%)	tenderness (5.6%)
vomiting (2.6%)	pain during injection (5.0%)
coughing (1.3%)	redness (2.6%)
"oversedation" (1.6%)	induration (1.7%)
headache (1.5%)	phlebitis (0.4%)
drowsiness (1.2%)	

Other adverse experiences, observed mainly following IV injection and occurring at an incidence of less than 1.0%, are as follows:

Respiratory: Laryngospasm, bronchospasm, dyspnea, hyperventilation, wheezing, shallow respirations, airway obstruction, tachypnea.

Cardiovascular: Bigeminy, premature ventricular contractions, vasovagal episode, tachycardia, nodal rhythm.

Gastrointestinal: Acid taste, excessive salivation, retching.

CNS/Neuromuscular: Retrograde amnesia, euphoria, confusion, argumentativeness, nervousness, anxiety, grogginess, restlessness, emergence delirium or agitation, prolonged emergence from anesthesia, dreaming during emergence, sleep disturbance, insomnia, nightmares, athetoid movements, ataxia, dizziness, dysphoria, slurred speech, dysphonia, paresthesia.

Special sense: Blurred vision, diplopia, nystagmus, pinpoint pupils, cyclic movements of eyelids, visual disturbance, difficulty focusing eyes, ears blocked, loss of balance, light-headedness.

Integumentary: Hives, hive-like elevation at injection site, swelling or feeling of burning, warmth or coldness at injection site, rash, pruritus.

Miscellaneous: Yawning, lethargy, chills, weakness, toothache, faint feeling, hematoma.

DRUG ABUSE AND DEPENDENCE

Midazolam is subject to Schedule IV control under the Controlled Substances Act of 1970.

Midazolam was actively self-administered in primate models used to assess the positive reinforcing effects of psychoactive drugs.

Midazolam produced physical dependence of a mild to moderate intensity in cynomolgus monkeys after 5 to 10 weeks of administration. Available data concerning the drug abuse and dependence potential of midazolam suggest that its abuse potential is at least equivalent to that of diazepam.

OVERDOSAGE

While there is insufficient human data on overdosage with VERSED, the manifestations of VERSED overdosage are expected to be similar to those observed with other benzodiazepines and include sedation, somnolence, confusion, impaired coordination, diminished reflexes, coma and untoward effects on vital signs. No evidence of specific organ toxicity from VERSED overdosage would be expected.

Treatment of overdosage: Treatment of injectable VERSED overdosage is the same as that followed for overdosage with other benzodiazepines. Respiration, pulse rate and blood pressure should be monitored and general supportive measures should be employed. Attention should be given to the maintenance of a patent airway and support of ventilation. An intravenous infusion should be started. Should hypotension develop, treatment may include intravenous fluid therapy, repositioning, judicious use of vasopressors appropriate to the clinical situation, if indicated, and other appropriate countermeasures. There is no information as to whether peritoneal dialysis, forced diuresis or hemodialysis are of any value in the treatment of midazolam overdosage.

DOSAGE AND ADMINISTRATION

VERSED is a potent sedative agent which requires slow administration and individualization of dosage. Clinical experience has shown VERSED to be 3 to 4 times as potent per mg as diazepam. BECAUSE SERIOUS AND LIFE-THREATENING CARDIORESPIRATORY ADVERSE EVENTS HAVE BEEN REPORTED, PROVISION FOR MONITORING, DETECTION AND CORRECTION OF THESE REACTIONS MUST BE MADE FOR EVERY PATIENT TO WHOM VERSED INJECTION IS ADMINISTERED, REGARDLESS OF AGE OR HEALTH STATUS. Excess doses or rapid or single bolus intravenous administration may result in respiratory depression and/or arrest. (See WARNINGS.)

Reactions such as agitation, involuntary movements, hyperactivity and combativeness have been reported. Should such reactions occur, caution should be exercised before continuing administration of VERSED. (See WARNINGS.)

Care should be taken to avoid intra-arterial injection or extravasation. (See WARNINGS.)

VERSED Injection may be mixed in the same syringe with the following frequently used premedications: morphine sulfate, meperidine, atropine sulfate or scopolamine. VERSED Injection is compatible with 5% dextrose in water, 0.9% sodium chloride and lactated Ringer's solution. Both the 1 mg/mL and 5 mg/mL formulations of VERSED may be diluted with 0.9% sodium chloride or 5% dextrose in water.

INTRAMUSCULARLY

For preoperative sedation (induction of sleepiness or drowsiness and relief of apprehension) and to impair memory of perioperative events.

For intramuscular use, VERSED should be injected deep in a large muscle mass.

USUAL ADULT DOSE

For premedication the recommended dose of VERSED is 0.07 to 0.08 mg/kg IM (approximately 5 mg IM for an average adult) approximately one hour before surgery.

Lower doses may be sufficient in elderly or debilitated patients. Onset is within 15 minutes, peaking at 30 to 60 minutes. It can be administered concomitantly with atropine sulfate or scopolamine hydrochloride and reduced doses of narcotics.

INTRAVENOUSLY

Conscious Sedation
(See INDICATIONS):
Narcotic premedication results in less variability in patient response and a reduction in dosage of VERSED. For peroral procedures, the use of an appropriate topical anesthetic is recommended. For bronchoscopic procedures, the use of narcotic premedication is recommended.

VERSED 1 mg/mL formulation is recommended for conscious sedation, to facilitate slower injection. Both the 1 mg/mL and the 5 mg/mL formulations may be diluted with 0.9% sodium chloride or 5% dextrose in water.

When used for conscious sedation, dosage must be individualized and titrated. VERSED should not be administered by rapid or single bolus intravenous administration. Individual response will vary with age, physical status and concomitant medications, but may also vary independent of these factors. (See WARNINGS concerning cardiac/respiratory arrest.)

1. *Healthy adults below the age of 60:*
Titrate *slowly* to the desired effect, *e.g.,* the initiation of slurred speech.
Some patients may respond to as little as 1 mg. No more than 2.5 mg should be given over a period of at least 2 minutes. Wait an additional 2 or more minutes to fully evaluate the sedative effect. If further titration is necessary, continue to titrate, using small increments, to the appropriate level of sedation. Wait an additional 2 or more minutes after each increment to fully evaluate the sedative effect. A total dose greater than 5 mg is not usually necessary to reach the desired endpoint.
If narcotic premedication or other CNS depressants are used, patients will require approximately 30% less VERSED than unpremedicated patients.

2. *Patients age 60 or older, and debilitated or chronically ill patients:*
Because the danger of underventilation or apnea is greater in elderly patients and those with chronic disease states or decreased pulmonary reserve, and because the peak effect may take longer in these patients, increments should be smaller and the rate of injection slower.
Titrate *slowly* to the desired effect, *e.g.,* the initiation of slurred speech. Some patients may respond to as little as 1 mg. No more than 1.5 mg should be given over a period of no less than 2 minutes. Wait an additional 2 or more minutes to fully evaluate the sedative effect. If additional titration is necessary, it should be given at a rate of no more than 1 mg over a period of 2 minutes, waiting an additional 2 or more minutes each time to fully evaluate the sedative effect. Total doses greater than 3.5 mg are not usually necessary.
If concomitant CNS depressant premedications are used in these patients, they will require at least 50% less VERSED than healthy young unpremedicated patients.

3. *Maintenance dose:*
Additional doses to maintain the desired level of sedation may be given in increments of 25% of the dose used to first reach the sedative endpoint, but again only by slow titration, especially in the elderly and chronically ill or debilitated patient. These additional doses should be given *only* after a thorough clinical evaluation clearly indicates the need for additional sedation.

Induction of Anesthesia:
For induction of general anesthesia, before administration of other anesthetic agents.

Individual response to the drug is variable, particularly when a narcotic premedication is not used. The dosage should be titrated to the desired effect according to the patient's age and clinical status.

Unpremedicated Patients:
In the absence of premedication, an average adult under the age of 55 years will usually require an initial dose of 0.3 to 0.35 mg/kg for induction, administered over 20 to 30 seconds and allowing 2 minutes for effect. If needed to complete induction, increments of approximately 25% of the patient's initial dose may be used; induction may instead be completed with volatile liquid inhalational anesthetics. In resistant cases, up to 0.6 mg/kg total dose may be used for induction, but such larger doses may prolong recovery.

Unpremedicated patients over the age of 55 years usually require less VERSED for induction; an initial dose of 0.3 mg/kg is recommended. Unpremedicated patients with severe systemic disease or other debilitation usually require less VERSED for induction. An initial dose of 0.2 to 0.25 mg/kg will usually suffice; in some cases, as little as 0.15 mg/kg may suffice.

Premedicated Patients:
When the patient has received sedative or narcotic premedication, particularly narcotic premedication, the range of recommended doses is 0.15 to 0.35 mg/kg.

In average adults below the age of 55 years, a dose of 0.25 mg/kg, administered over 20 to 30 seconds and allowing 2 minutes for effect, will usually suffice.

The initial dose of 0.2 mg/kg is recommended for good risk (ASA I & II) surgical patients over the age of 55 years.
In some patients with severe systemic disease or debilitation, as little as 0.15 mg/kg may suffice.

Narcotic premedication frequently used during clinical trials included fentanyl (1.5 to 2 µg/kg IV, administered five minutes before induction), morphine (dosage individualized, up to 0.15 mg/kg IM), meperidine (dosage individualized, up to 1 mg/kg IM) and Innovar (0.02 mL/kg IM). Sedative premedications were hydroxyzine pamoate (100 mg orally) and sodium secobarbital (200 mg orally). Except for intravenous fentanyl, administered five minutes before induction, all other premedications should be administered approximately one hour prior to the time anticipated for VERSED induction.

Continued on next page

Roche Labs.—Cont.

Injectable VERSED can also be used during maintenance of anesthesia, *for short surgical procedures,* as a component of balanced anesthesia. Effective narcotic premedication is especially recommended in such cases. Long surgical procedures have not been studied.

Incremental injections of approximately 25% of the induction dose should be given in response to signs of lightening of anesthesia and repeated as necessary.

Note: Parenteral drug products should be inspected visually for particulate matter and discoloration prior to administration, whenever solution and container permit.

HOW SUPPLIED

Package configurations containing midazolam hydrochloride equivalent to **5 mg** midazolam/mL:
1-mL vials (5 mg)—boxes of 10 (NDC 0004-1974-01);
2-mL vials (10 mg)—boxes of 10 (NDC 0004-1973-01);
5-mL vials (25 mg)—boxes of 10 (NDC 0004-1975-01);
10-mL vials (50 mg)—boxes of 10 (NDC 0004-1946-01);
2-mL Tel-E-Ject® disposable syringes (10 mg)—boxes of 10 (NDC 0004-1947-01).
Package configurations containing midazolam hydrochloride equivalent to **1 mg** midazolam/mL:
2-mL vials (2 mg)—boxes of 10 (NDC 0004-1998-06);
5-mL vials (5 mg)—boxes of 10 (NDC 0004-1999-01);
10-mL vials (10 mg)—boxes of 10 (NDC 0004-2000-06).
Store at 59° to 86°F (15° to 30°C).
P.I. 0988

EDUCATIONAL MATERIAL

Please contact your Roche representative concerning availability of educational programs and material.

Roche Products Inc.
MANATI, PUERTO RICO 00701

DALMANE®
[dal'mane]
(flurazepam hydrochloride/Roche)
Capsules

The following text is complete prescribing information based on official labeling in effect June 1, 1989.

DESCRIPTION

Dalmane is available as capsules containing 15 mg or 30 mg fluazepam hydrochloride/Roche. Each 15-mg capsule also contains corn starch, lactose, magnesium stearate and talc; gelatin capsule shells may contain methyl and propyl parabens and potassium sorbate, with the following dye system: FD&C Red No. 3, FD&C Yellow No. 6 and D&C Yellow No. 10. Each 30-mg capsule also contains corn starch, lactose and magnesium stearate; gelatin capsule shells may contain methyl and propyl parabens and potassium sorbate, with the following dye systems: FD&C Blue No. 1, FD&C Yellow No. 6, D&C Yellow No. 10 and either FD&C Red No. 3 or FD&C Red No. 40.

Flurazepam hydrochloride is chemically 7-chloro-1-[2-(diethylamino) ethyl]-5-(o -fluorophenyl) -1, 3-dihydro-2H -1, 4-benzodiazepin-2-one dihydrochloride. It is a pale yellow, crystalline compound, freely soluble in U.S.P. alcohol and very soluble in water. It has a molecular weight of 460.826.

CLINICAL PHARMACOLOGY

Flurazepam hydrochloride is rapidly absorbed from the G.I. tract. Flurazepam is rapidly metabolized and is excreted primarily in the urine. Following a single oral dose, peak flurazepam plasma concentrations ranging from 0.5 to 4.0 ng/ml occur at 30 to 60 minutes post-dosing. The harmonic mean apparent half-life of flurazepam is 2.3 hours. The blood level profile of flurazepam and its major metabolites was determined in man following the oral administration of 30 mg daily for 2 weeks. The N_1-hydroxyethyl-flurazepam was measurable only during the early hours after a 30-mg dose and was not detectable after 24 hours. The major metabolite in blood was N_1-desalkyl-flurazepam, which reached steady-state (plateau) levels after 7 to 10 days of dosing, at levels approximately five- to sixfold greater than the 24-hour levels observed on Day 1. The half-life of elimination of N_1-desalkyl-flurazepam ranged from 47 to 100 hours. The major urinary metabolite is conjugated N_1-hydroxyethyl-flurazepam which accounts for 22 to 55 percent of the dose. Less than 1% of the dose is excreted in the urine as N_1-desalkyl-flurazepam.

This pharmacokinetic profile may be responsible for the clinical observation that flurazepam is increasingly effective on the second or third night of consecutive use and that for one or two nights after the drug is discontinued both sleep latency and total wake time may still be decreased.

INDICATIONS

Dalmane is a hypnotic agent useful for the treatment of insomnia characterized by difficulty in falling asleep, frequent nocturnal awakenings, and/or early morning awakening. Dalmane can be used effectively in patients with recurring insomnia or poor sleeping habits, and in acute or chronic medical situations requiring restful sleep. Sleep laboratory studies have objectively determined that Dalmane is effective for at least 28 consecutive nights of drug administration. Since insomnia is often transient and intermittent, short-term use is usually sufficient. Prolonged use of hypnotics is usually not indicated and should only be undertaken concomitantly with appropriate evaluation of the patient.

CONTRAINDICATIONS

Dalmane is contraindicated in patients with known hypersensitivity to the drug.

Usage in Pregnancy: Benzodiazepines may cause fetal damage when administered during pregnancy. An increased risk of congenital malformations associated with the use of diazepam and chlordiazepoxide during the first trimester of pregnancy has been suggested in several studies.

Dalmane is contraindicated in pregnant women. Symptoms of neonatal depression have been reported; a neonate whose mother received 30 mg of Dalmane nightly for insomnia during the 10 days prior to delivery appeared hypotonic and inactive during the first four days of life. Serum levels of N_1-desalkyl-flurazepam in the infant indicated transplacental circulation and implicate this long-acting metabolite in this case. If there is a likelihood of the patient becoming pregnant while receiving flurazepam, she should be warned of the potential risks to the fetus. Patients should be instructed to discontinue the drug prior to becoming pregnant. The possibility that a woman of childbearing potential may be pregnant at the time of institution of therapy should be considered.

WARNINGS

Patients receiving Dalmane should be cautioned about possible combined effects with alcohol and other CNS depressants. Also, caution patients that an additive effect may occur if alcoholic beverages are consumed during the day following the use of Dalmane for nighttime sedation. The potential for this interaction continues for several days following discontinuance of flurazepam, until serum levels of psychoactive metabolites have declined.

Patients should also be cautioned about engaging in hazardous occupations requiring complete mental alertness such as operating machinery or driving a motor vehicle after ingesting the drug, including potential impairment of the performance of such activities which may occur the day following ingestion of Dalmane.

Usage in Children: Clinical investigations of Dalmane have not been carried out in children. Therefore, the drug is not currently recommended for use in persons under 15 years of age.

Withdrawal symptoms of the barbiturate type have occurred after the discontinuation of benzodiazepines. (See DRUG ABUSE AND DEPENDENCE section.)

PRECAUTIONS

Since the risk of the development of oversedation, dizziness, confusion and/or ataxia increases substantially with larger doses in elderly and debilitated patients, it is recommended that in such patients the dosage be limited to 15 mg. If Dalmane is to be combined with other drugs having known hypnotic properties or CNS-depressant effects, due consideration should be given to potential additive effects.

The usual precautions are indicated for severely depressed patients or those in whom there is any evidence of latent depression; particularly the recognition that suicidal tendencies may be present and protective measures may be necessary.

The usual precautions should be observed in patients with impaired renal or hepatic function and chronic pulmonary insufficiency.

Information for Patients: To assure the safe and effective use of benzodiazepines, patients should be informed that since benzodiazepines may produce psychological and physical dependence, it is advisable that they consult with their physician before either increasing the dose or abruptly discontinuing the drug.

ADVERSE REACTIONS

Dizziness, drowsiness, light-headedness, staggering, ataxia and falling have occurred, particularly in elderly or debilitated persons. Severe sedation, lethargy, disorientation and coma, probably indicative of drug intolerance or overdosage, have been reported.

Also reported were headache, heartburn, upset stomach, nausea, vomiting, diarrhea, constipation, gastrointestinal pain, nervousness, talkativeness, apprehension, irritability, weakness, palpitations, chest pains, body and joint pains and genitourinary complaints. There have also been rare occurrences of leukopenia, granulocytopenia, sweating, flushes, difficulty in focusing, blurred vision, burning eyes, faintness, hypotension, shortness of breath, pruritus, skin rash, dry mouth, bitter taste, excessive salivation, anorexia, euphoria, depression, slurred speech, confusion, restlessness, hallucinations, and elevated SGOT, SGPT, total and direct bilirubins, and alkaline phosphatase. Paradoxical reactions, *e.g.,* excitement, stimulation and hyperactivity, have also been reported in rare instances.

DRUG ABUSE AND DEPENDENCE

Withdrawal symptoms, similar in character to those noted with barbiturates and alcohol (convulsions, tremor, abdominal and muscle cramps, vomiting and sweating), have occurred following abrupt discontinuance of benzodiazepines. The more severe withdrawal symptoms have usually been limited to those patients who had received excessive doses over an extended period of time. Generally milder withdrawal symptoms (*e.g.,* dysphoria and insomnia) have been reported following abrupt discontinuance of benzodiazepines taken continuously at therapeutic levels for several months. Consequently, after extended therapy, abrupt discontinuation should generally be avoided and a gradual dosage tapering schedule followed. Addiction-prone individuals (such as drug addicts or alcoholics) should be under careful surveillance when receiving flurazepam or other psychotropic agents because of the predisposition of such patients to habituation and dependence.

DOSAGE AND ADMINISTRATION

Dosage should be individualized for maximal beneficial effects. The usual adult dosage is 30 mg before retiring. In some patients, 15 mg may suffice. In elderly and /or debilitated patients, 15 mg is usually sufficient for a therapeutic response and it is therefore recommended that therapy be initiated with this dosage.

OVERDOSAGE

Manifestations of Dalmane overdosage include somnolence, confusion and coma. Respiration, pulse and blood pressure should be monitored as in all cases of drug overdosage. General supportive measures should be employed, along with immediate gastric lavage. Intravenous fluids should be administered and an adequate airway maintained. Hypotension and CNS depression may be combated by judicious use of appropriate therapeutic agents. The value of dialysis has not been determined. If excitation occurs in patients following Dalmane overdosage, barbiturates should not be used. As with the management of intentional overdosage with any drug, it should be borne in mind that multiple agents may have been ingested.

HOW SUPPLIED

Dalmane (flurazepam hydrochloride/Roche) capsules—15 mg, orange and ivory; 30 mg, red and ivory—bottles of 100 and 500; Tel-E-Dose® packages of 100, available in boxes containing 10 strips of 10, in trays of 4 boxes each containing a reverse-numbered roll of 25 and in boxes of 4 reverse-numbered cards of 25.
P.I. 0788

Shown in Product Identification Section, page 425

ENDEP®
[en'dep]
(amitriptyline HCl/Roche)
TABLETS

The following text is complete prescribing information based on official labeling in effect June 1, 1989.

DESCRIPTION

Endep (amitriptyline HCl/Roche), a tricyclic antidepressant, is available as 10-mg, 25-mg, 50-mg, 75-mg, 100-mg and 150-mg tablets for oral administration. Each tablet also contains corn starch, ethylcellulose, hydroxypropyl methylcellulose, lactose, magnesium stearate, microcrystalline cellulose, povidone, talc and triacetin, with the following dye systems: 10 mg, 25 mg, 50 mg and 75 mg—FD&C Yellow No. 6 and D&C Yellow No. 10; 100 mg and 150 mg—D&C Red No. 30 and FD&C Yellow No. 6.

Amitriptyline HCl, a dibenzocycloheptadiene derivative, is a white or practically white crystalline compound that is freely soluble in water. It is designated chemically as 10, 11-dihydro-N,N-dimethyl-5H-dibenzo[a,d]cycloheptene-$\Delta^{5,\gamma}$-propylamine hydrochloride. The molecular weight is 313.87. The empirical formula is $C_{20}H_{23}N \cdot HCl$.

CLINICAL PHARMACOLOGY

Endep is an antidepressant with sedative effects. Its mechanism of action in man is not known. It is not a monoamine oxidase inhibitor, and it does not act primarily by stimulation of the central nervous system.

Amitriptyline inhibits the membrane pump mechanism responsible for uptake of norepinephrine and serotonin in adrenergic and serotonergic neurons. Pharmacologically this action may potentiate or prolong neuronal activity, since reuptake of these biogenic amines is important physiologically in terminating its transmitting activity. This interference with reuptake of norepinephrine and/or serotonin is believed by some to underlie the antidepressant activity of amitriptyline.

Amitriptyline undergoes extensive metabolism primarily through N-demethylation to nortriptyline, an active metabolite, followed by extensive hydroxylation to their respective 10-hydroxy metabolites which are eliminated as glucuronide conjugates.

Following a single oral dose of 75 mg of amitriptyline HCl, the mean maximum plasma concentrations of 39.4 ng/ml of amitriptyline and 16.1 ng/ml of nortriptyline were reached in approximately 4 and 10 hours, respectively. The average minimum steady-state plasma concentrations in patients receiving 50 mg of amitriptyline HCl, three times a day for an average of 32 days, were 81 ng/ml for amitriptyline, 71 ng/ml for nortriptyline, 12 ng/ml for 10-hydroxyamitriptyline, 91 ng/ml for conjugated 10-hydroxyamitriptyline, 82 ng/ml for 10-hydroxynortriptyline and 176 ng/ml for conjugated 10-hydroxynortriptyline. Steady-state plasma concentrations are usually reached by day 14. The mean apparent half-life of elimination of amitriptyline is 22.4 hours and the apparent half-life of elimination of nortriptyline is 26.0 hours. Amitriptyline is approximately 96% bound to plasma proteins.

Amitriptyline has been shown to cross the blood-brain barrier in cats, mice and rats. It has also been shown to pass the placental barrier and to enter fetal circulation in mice after intramuscular and intravenous administration. Amitriptyline is excreted in human breast milk.

INDICATIONS AND USAGE

Endep is indicated for the relief of symptoms of depression. Endogenous depression is more likely to be alleviated than are other depressive states.

CONTRAINDICATIONS

Endep is contraindicated in patients who have shown prior hypersensitivity to this agent; cross-sensitivity to other tricyclic antidepressants can occur.

Endep should not be given concomitantly with a monoamine oxidase inhibitor. Hyperpyretic crises, severe convulsions and deaths have occurred in patients receiving tricyclic antidepressant and monoamine oxidase inhibiting drugs simultaneously. When it is desired to replace a monoamine oxidase inhibitor with Endep, a minimum of 14 days should be allowed to elapse after the former is discontinued. Endep should then be initiated cautiously with gradual increase in dosage until optimum response is achieved.

Endep is not recommended for use during the acute recovery phase following myocardial infarction.

WARNINGS

Endep may block the antihypertensive action of guanethidine or similarly acting compounds.

Endep should be used with caution in patients with a history of seizures and, because of its atropine-like action, in patients with a history of urinary retention, angle-closure glaucoma or increased intraocular pressure. In patients with angle-closure glaucoma, even average doses may precipitate an attack.

Patients with cardiovascular disorders should be watched closely. Tricyclic antidepressant drugs, including Endep, particularly when given in high doses, have been reported to produce arrhythmias, sinus tachycardia and prolongation of the conduction time. Myocardial infarction and stroke have been reported with drugs of this class.

Close supervision is required when Endep is given to hyperthyroid patients or those receiving thyroid medication.

Amitriptyline HCl may enhance the response to alcohol and the effects of barbiturates and other CNS depressants. In patients who may use alcohol excessively, it should be borne in mind that the potentiation may increase the danger inherent in any suicide attempt or overdosage. Delirium has been reported with concurrent administration of amitriptyline HCl and disulfiram.

PRECAUTIONS

General: Schizophrenic patients may develop increased symptoms of psychosis; patients with paranoid symptomatology may have an exaggeration of such symptoms. Depressed patients, particularly those with known manic-depressive illness, may experience a shift to mania or hypomania. In these circumstances, the dose of Endep may be reduced or a major tranquilizer such as perphenazine may be administered concurrently.

The possibility of suicide in depressed patients remains during treatment and until significant remission occurs. Potentially suicidal patients should not have access to large quantities of this drug. Prescriptions should be written for the smallest amount feasible.

Concurrent administration of Endep and electroshock therapy may increase the hazards associated with such therapy. Such treatment should be limited to patients for whom it is essential.

Amitriptyline HCl should be used with caution in patients with impaired liver function.

Both elevation and lowering of blood sugar levels have been reported.

The drug should be discontinued several days before elective surgery, if possible.

Information for Patients: When being treated with amitriptyline HCl, patients should be advised as to the possible impairment of mental and/or physical abilities required for performance of hazardous tasks, such as operating machinery or driving a motor vehicle.

Patients receiving amitriptyline HCl should also be cautioned about the possible combined effects with alcohol, barbiturates and other CNS depressants.

Drug Interactions: MAO inhibitors—see CONTRAINDICATIONS section. Thyroid medications; alcohol, barbiturates and other CNS depressants; and guanethidine or similarly acting compounds—see WARNINGS section.

When Endep is given with anticholinergic agents or sympathomimetic drugs, including epinephrine combined with local anesthetics, close supervision and careful adjustment of dosages are required.

Paralytic ileus may occur in patients taking tricyclic antidepressants in combination with anticholinergic-type drugs.

Cimetidine is reported to reduce hepatic metabolism of certain tricyclic antidepressants, thereby delaying elimination and increasing steady-state concentrations of these drugs. Clinically significant effects have been reported with the tricyclic antidepressants when used concomitantly with cimetidine (Tagamet). Increases in plasma levels of tricyclic antidepressants, and in the frequency and severity of side effects, particularly anticholinergic, have been reported when cimetidine was added to the drug regimen. Discontinuation of cimetidine in well-controlled patients receiving tricyclic antidepressants and cimetidine may decrease the plasma levels and efficacy of the antidepressants.

Caution is advised if patients receive large doses of ethchlorvynol concurrently. Transient delirium has been reported in patients who were treated with one gram of ethchlorvynol and 75 to 150 mg of amitriptyline HCl.

Carcinogenesis, Mutagenesis, Impairment of Fertility: Carcinogenesis: Amitriptyline HCl has not been adequately studied in animals to permit an evaluation of its carcinogenic potential. However, in a study during which relatively small numbers of rats received amitriptyline HCl as a dietary admixture at dosages up to 100 mg/kg/day for 78 weeks, no increase in the incidence of any tumor was reported.

Mutagenesis: Amitriptyline HCl was tested in a bacterial mutagenesis assay (Ames test) in the presence and absence of activating enzymes. No evidence for mutagenicity was found using *Salmonella* tester strains TA 1535, TA 100, TA 98 and TA 1537 at concentrations up to 5000 mcg/plate.

Impairment of Fertility: Amitriptyline HCl was studied in a Segment I fertility and general reproduction study in rats at dosages up to 20 mg/kg/day. There were no adverse effects on fertility, fetal growth and development, litter size, pup survival or pup growth. Similarly, no adverse effects were reported in a rat litter test in which amitriptyline HCl was administered at dosages up to 20 mg/kg/day.

Pregnancy: Teratogenic Effects: Pregnancy Category C. Animal reproduction studies have been inconclusive, and clinical experience has been limited. Amitriptyline HCl was tested in rats and in rabbits for teratogenic potential at dosages up to 20 mg/kg/day. Although stunting and increased neonatal mortality were observed in rabbits, there was no evidence for teratogenicity in either rats or rabbits. In a brief report, amitriptyline HCl was shown to be teratogenic in the hamster at dosages up to 100 mg/kg administered intraperitoneally on day 8 of gestation. In a more detailed study, amitriptyline HCl was shown to produce malformations in the rabbit at dosages of 15 to 60 mg/day and in the mouse at dosages of 14 to 56 mg/kg/day. In another study, amitriptyline HCl was shown to be teratogenic in JBT/Jd and JBT/Ju strains of mice at dosages of 60 to 65 mg/kg, respectively; these dosages are near the litter LD$_{50}$. The dosages which were teratogenic in animals ranged from 10.5 to 70 times the maximum recommended adult maintenance dosage of 100 mg/day of Endep and from 3.5 to 23 times the maximum recommended initial dosage for hospitalized patients (300 mg/day).

There are no adequate or well-controlled studies of Endep in pregnant women. Endep should be used during pregnancy only if the potential benefit justifies the potential risk to the fetus.

Nonteratogenic Effects: Amitriptyline HCl was tested in rats in a Segment II study at dosages up to 20 mg/kg/day. No significant adverse effects were observed in the peri- or postnatal development and growth of pups.

Nursing Mothers: Amitriptyline and its metabolite, nortriptyline, are excreted in breast milk. Because of the potential for serious adverse reactions from Endep in nursing infants, a decision should be made whether to discontinue nursing or to discontinue the drug, taking into account the importance of the drug to the mother.

Pediatric Use: Safety and effectiveness in children below the age of 12 have not been established.

ADVERSE REACTIONS

Note: Included in this listing which follows are a few adverse reactions which have not been reported with this specific drug. However, pharmacological similarities among the tricyclic antidepressant drugs require that each of the reactions be considered when Endep is administered.

Cardiovascular: Hypotension, particularly orthostatic hypotension, hypertension, tachycardia, palpitation, myocardial infarction, arrhythmias, heart block, stroke.

CNS and Neuromuscular: Confusional states; disturbed concentration; disorientation; delusions; hallucinations; excitement; anxiety; restlessness; insomnia; nightmares; numbness; tingling and paresthesias of the extremities; peripheral neuropathy; incoordination; ataxia; tremors; seizures; alteration in EEG patterns; extrapyramidal symptoms; tinnitus.

Anticholinergic: Dry mouth, blurred vision, disturbance of accommodation, increased intraocular pressure, constipation, paralytic ileus, urinary retention, dilatation of urinary tract.

Allergic: Skin rash, urticaria, photosensitization, edema of face and tongue.

Hematologic: Bone marrow depression including agranulocytosis, leukopenia, eosinophilia, purpura, thrombocytopenia.

Gastrointestinal: Nausea, epigastric distress, vomiting, anorexia, stomatitis, peculiar taste, diarrhea, parotid swelling, black tongue. Rarely, hepatitis (including altered liver function and jaundice).

Endocrine: Testicular swelling and gynecomastia in the male, breast enlargement and galactorrhea in the female, increased or decreased libido, elevation and lowering of blood sugar levels, syndrome of inappropriate ADH (antidiuretic hormone) secretion.

Other: Dizziness, weakness, fatigue, headache, weight gain or loss, edema, increased perspiration, urinary frequency, mydriasis, drowsiness, alopecia, ageusia.

Withdrawal Symptoms: Abrupt cessation of treatment after prolonged administration may produce nausea, headache and malaise. Gradual dosage reduction has been reported to produce, within two weeks, transient symptoms including irritability, restlessness, and dream and sleep disturbance. These symptoms are not indicative of addiction. Rare instances have been reported of mania or hypomania occurring within 2 to 7 days following cessation of chronic therapy with tricyclic antidepressants.

OVERDOSAGE

Manifestations: High doses may cause temporary confusion, disturbed concentration or transient visual hallucinations. Overdosage may cause drowsiness; hypothermia; tachycardia and other arrhythmic abnormalities, such as bundle branch block; ECG evidence of impaired conduction; congestive heart failure; dilated pupils; disorders of ocular motility; convulsions; severe hypotension; stupor and coma. Other symptoms may be agitation, hyperactive reflexes, muscle rigidity, polyradiculoneuropathy, vomiting, hyperpyrexia or any of those listed in the ADVERSE REACTIONS section.

Treatment: **All patients suspected of having taken an overdosage should be admitted to a hospital as soon as possible.** Treatment is symptomatic and supportive. Empty the stomach as quickly as possible by emesis followed by gastric lavage upon arrival at the hospital. Following gastric lavage, activated charcoal may be administered. Twenty to 30 Gm of activated charcoal may be given every four to six hours during the first 24 to 48 hours after ingestion. An ECG should be taken and close monitoring of cardiac function instituted if there is any sign of abnormality. Maintain an open airway and adequate fluid intake; regulate body temperature.

The intravenous administration of 1 to 3 mg of physostigmine salicylate has been reported to reverse the symptoms of tricyclic antidepressant poisoning. Because physostigmine is rapidly metabolized, the dosage of physostigmine should be repeated as required, particularly if life-threatening signs such as arrhythmias, convulsions and deep coma recur or persist after the initial dosage of physostigmine. Because physostigmine itself may be toxic, it is not recommended for routine use.

Standard measures should be used to manage circulatory shock and metabolic acidosis. Cardiac arrhythmias may be treated with neostigmine, pyridostigmine or propranolol. Should cardiac failure occur, the use of digitalis should be considered. Close monitoring of cardiac function for not less than five days is advisable. Anticonvulsants may be given to control convulsions. Amitriptyline increases the CNS depressant action but not the anticonvulsant action of barbiturates; therefore, an inhalation anesthetic, diazepam or paraldehyde is recommended for control of convulsions.

Dialysis is of no value because of low plasma concentrations of the drug.

Since overdosage is often deliberate, patients may attempt suicide by other means during the recovery phase.

Deaths by deliberate or accidental overdosage have occurred with this class of drugs.

The acute oral toxicity of amitriptyline HCl is as follows:

Continued on next page

Roche Products—Cont.

Species	$LD_{50} \pm$ S.E. (mg/kg)
Mouse	260 ± 16
Rat	617 ± 50
Rabbit	446 ± 32
Dog	~ 290

DOSAGE AND ADMINISTRATION

Oral Dosage: Dosage should be initiated at a low level and increased gradually, noting carefully the clinical response and any evidence of intolerance.

Initial Dosage for Adults: Twenty-five mg 3 times a day usually is satisfactory for outpatients. If necessary, this may be increased to a total of 150 mg a day. Increases are made preferably in the late afternoon and/or bedtime doses. A sedative effect may be apparent before the antidepressant effect is noted, but an adequate therapeutic effect may take as long as 30 days to develop.

An alternative method of initiating therapy in outpatients is to begin with 50 to 100 mg amitriptyline HCl at bedtime. This may be increased by 25 to 50 mg as necessary in the bedtime dose to a total of 150 mg per day.

Hospitalized patients may require 100 mg a day initially. This can be increased gradually to 200 mg a day if necessary. A small number of hospitalized patients may need as much as 300 mg a day.

Adolescent and Elderly Patients: In general, lower dosages are recommended for these patients. Ten mg 3 times a day with 20 mg at bedtime may be satisfactory in adolescent and elderly patients who do not tolerate higher dosages.

Maintenance: The usual maintenance dosage of amitriptyline HCl is 50 to 100 mg per day. In some patients 40 mg per day is sufficient. For maintenance therapy the total daily dosage may be given in a single dose preferably at bedtime. When satisfactory improvement has been reached, dosage should be reduced to the lowest amount that will maintain relief of symptoms. It is appropriate to continue maintenance therapy 3 months or longer to lessen the possibility of relapse.

Usage in Children: In view of the lack of experience in children, this drug is not recommended at the present time for patients under 12 years of age.

Plasma Levels: Because of the wide variation in the absorption and distribution of tricyclic antidepressants in body fluids, it is difficult to directly correlate plasma levels and therapeutic effect. However, determination of plasma levels may be useful in identifying patients who appear to have toxic effects and may have excessively high levels, or those in whom lack of absorption or noncompliance is suspected. Adjustments in dosage should be made according to the patient's clinical response and not on the basis of plasma levels.

HOW SUPPLIED

10-mg tablets, orange, round, film-coated, scored—bottles of 100 (NDC 0140-0106-01). Imprint on tablets: ENDEP 10 ROCHE.

25-mg tablets, orange, round, film-coated, scored—bottles of 100 (NDC 0140-0107-01). Imprint on tablets: ENDEP 25 ROCHE.

50-mg tablets, orange, round, film-coated, scored—bottles of 100 (NDC 0140-0109-01). Imprint on tablets: ENDEP 50 ROCHE.

75-mg tablets, yellow, round, film-coated, scored—bottles of 100 (NDC 0140-0114-01). Imprint on tablets: ENDEP 75 ROCHE.

100-mg tablets, peach, round, film-coated, scored—bottles of 100 (NDC 0140-0116-01). Imprint on tablets: ENDEP 100 ROCHE.

150-mg tablets, salmon, round, film-coated, scored—bottles of 100 (NDC 0140-0124-01). Imprint on tablets: ENDEP 150 ROCHE.

P.I. 0389

Shown in Product Identification Section, page 425

LIBRAX®   ℞
[lib´rax]

The following text is complete prescribing information based on official labeling in effect June 1, 1989.

COMPOSITION

Each capsule contains 5 mg chlordiazepoxide hydrochloride (Librium®) and 2.5 mg clidinium bromide (Quarzan®).

DESCRIPTION

Librax combines in a single capsule formulation the antianxiety action of Librium (chlordiazepoxide hydrochloride/Roche) and the anticholinergic/spasmolytic effects of Quarzan (clidinium bromide/Roche), both exclusive developments of Roche research.

Each Librax capsule contains 5 mg chlordiazepoxide hydrochloride and 2.5 mg clidinium bromide. Each capsule also contains corn starch, lactose and talc. Gelatin capsule shells may contain methyl and propyl parabens and potassium sorbate, with the following dye systems: D&C Yellow No. 10 and either FD&C Blue No. 1 or FD&C Green No. 3.

Librium (chlordiazepoxide hydrochloride/Roche) is a versatile therapeutic agent of proven value for the relief of anxiety and tension. It is indicated when anxiety, tension or apprehension are significant components of the clinical profile. It is among the safer of the effective psychopharmacologic compounds.

Chlordiazepoxide hydrochloride is 7-chloro-2-methylamino-5-phenyl-3H-1, 4-benzodiazepine 4-oxide hydrochloride. A colorless, crystalline substance, it is soluble in water. It is unstable in solution and the powder must be protected from light. The molecular weight is 336.22.

Quarzan (clidinium bromide/Roche) is a synthetic anticholinergic agent which has been shown in experimental and clinical studies to have a pronounced antispasmodic and antisecretory effect on the gastrointestinal tract.

ANIMAL PHARMACOLOGY

Chlordiazepoxide hydrochloride has been studied extensively in many species of animals and these studies are suggestive of action on the limbic system of the brain,[1,2,3] which recent evidence indicates is involved in emotional responses.[4,5]

Hostile monkeys were made tame by oral drug doses which did not cause sedation. Chlordiazepoxide hydrochloride revealed a "taming" action with the elimination of fear and aggression.[6] The taming effect of chlordiazepoxide hydrochloride was further demonstrated in rats made vicious by lesions in the septal area of the brain. The drug dosage which effectively blocked the vicious reaction was well below the dose which caused sedation in these animals.[6]

The oral LD_{50} of single doses of chlordiazepoxide hydrochloride, calculated according to the method of Miller and Tainter,[7] is 720 ± 51 mg/kg as determined in mice observed over a period of five days following dosage.

Clidinium bromide is an effective anticholinergic agent with activity approximating that of atropine sulfate against acetylcholine-induced spasms in isolated intestinal strips. On oral administration in mice it proved an effective antisialagogue in preventing pilocarpine-induced salivation. Spontaneous intestinal motility in both rats and dogs is reduced following oral dosing with 0.1 to 0.25 mg/kg. Potent cholinergic ganglionic blocking effects (vagal) are produced with intravenous usage in anesthetized dogs.

Oral doses of 2.5 mg/kg to dogs produced signs of nasal dryness and slight pupillary dilation. In two other species, monkeys and rabbits, doses of 5 mg/kg, p.o., given three times daily for 5 days did not produce apparent secretory or visual changes.

The oral LD_{50} of single doses of clidinium bromide is 860 ± 57 mg/kg as determined in mice observed over a period of 5 days following dosage; the calculations were made according to the method of Miller and Tainter.[7]

Effects on Reproduction: Reproduction studies in rats fed chlordiazepoxide hydrochloride, 10, 20 and 80 mg/kg daily, and bred through one or two matings showed no congenital anomalies, nor were there adverse effects on lactation of the dams or growth of the newborn. However, in another study at 100 mg/kg daily there was noted a significant decrease in the fertilization rate and a marked decrease in the viability and body weight of offspring which may be attributable to sedative activity, thus resulting in lack of interest in mating and lessened maternal nursing and care of the young.[8,9] One neonate in each of the first and second matings in the rat reproduction study at the 100 mg/kg dose exhibited major skeletal defects. Further studies are in progress to determine the significance of these findings.

Two series of reproduction experiments with clidinium bromide were carried out in rats, employing dosages of 2.5 and 10 mg/kg daily in each experiment. In the first experiment clidinium bromide was administered for a 9-week interval prior to mating; no untoward effect on fertilization or gestation was noted. The offspring were taken by caesarean section and did not show a significant incidence of congenital anomalies when compared to control animals. In the second experiment adult animals were given clidinium bromide for ten days prior to and through two mating cycles. No significant effects were observed on fertility, gestation, viability of offspring or lactation, as compared to control animals, nor was there a significant incidence of congenital anomalies in the offspring derived from these experiments.

A reproduction study of Librax was carried out in rats through two successive matings. Oral daily doses were administered in two concentrations: 2.5 mg/kg chlordiazepoxide hydrochloride with 1.25 mg/kg clidinium bromide, or 25 mg/kg chlordiazepoxide hydrochloride with 12.5 mg/kg clidinium bromide. In the first mating no significant differences were noted between the control or the treated groups, with the exception of a slight decrease in the number of animals surviving during lactation among those receiving the highest dosage. As with all anticholinergic drugs, an inhibiting effect on lactation may occur. In the second mating similar results were obtained except for a slight decrease in the number of pregnant females and in the percentage of offspring surviving until weaning. No congenital anomalies were observed in both matings in either the control or

treated groups. Additional animal reproduction studies are in progress.

INDICATIONS

Based on a review of this drug by the National Academy of Sciences—National Research Council and/or other information, FDA has classified the indications as follows:

"Possibly" effective: as adjunctive therapy in the treatment of peptic ulcer and in the treatment of the irritable bowel syndrome (irritable colon, spastic colon, mucous colitis) and acute enterocolitis.

Final classification of the less-than-effective indications requires further investigation.

CONTRAINDICATIONS

Librax is contraindicated in the presence of glaucoma (since the anticholinergic component may produce some degree of mydriasis) and in patients with prostatic hypertrophy and benign bladder neck obstruction. It is contraindicated in patients with known hypersensitivity to chlordiazepoxide hydrochloride and/or clidinium bromide.

WARNINGS

As in the case of other preparations containing CNS-acting drugs, patients receiving Librax should be cautioned about possible combined effects with alcohol and other CNS depressants. For the same reason, they should be cautioned against hazardous occupations requiring complete mental alertness such as operating machinery or driving a motor vehicle.

Usage in Pregnancy: **An increased risk of congenital malformations associated with the use of minor tranquilizers (chlordiazepoxide, diazepam and meprobamate) during the first trimester of pregnancy has been suggested in several studies. Because use of these drugs is rarely a matter of urgency, their use during this period should almost always be avoided. The possibility that a woman of childbearing potential may be pregnant at the time of institution of therapy should be considered. Patients should be advised that if they become pregnant during therapy or intend to become pregnant they should communicate with their physicians about the desirability of discontinuing the drug.**

As with all anticholinergic drugs, an inhibiting effect on lactation may occur. (See Animal Pharmacology.)

Management of Overdosage: Manifestations of Librium (chlordiazepoxide hydrochloride/Roche) overdosage include somnolence, confusion, coma and diminished reflexes. Respiration, pulse and blood pressure should be monitored, as in all cases of drug overdosage, although, in general, these effects have been minimal following Librium overdosage.

While the signs and symptoms of Librax overdosage may be produced by either of its components, usually such symptoms will be overshadowed by the anticholinergic actions of Quarzan (clidinium bromide/Roche). The symptoms of overdosage of Quarzan are excessive dryness of mouth, blurring of vision, urinary hesitancy and constipation.

General supportive measures should be employed, along with immediate gastric lavage. Administer physostigmine (Antilirium) 0.5 to 2 mg at a rate of no more than 1 mg per minute. This may be repeated in 1 to 4 mg doses if arrhythmias, convulsions or deep coma recur. Intravenous fluids should be administered and an adequate airway maintained. Hypotension may be combated by the use of Levophed® (levarterenol) or Aramine (metaraminol). Ritalin (methylphenidate) or caffeine and sodium benzoate may be given to combat CNS-depressive effects. Dialysis is of limited value. Should excitation occur, barbiturates should not be used. As with the management of intentional overdosage with any drug, it should be borne in mind that multiple agents may have been ingested.

Withdrawal symptoms of the barbiturate type have occurred after the discontinuation of benzodiazepines. (See DRUG ABUSE AND DEPENDENCE section.)

PRECAUTIONS

In elderly and debilitated patients, it is recommended that the dosage be limited to the smallest effective amount to preclude the development of ataxia, oversedation, or confusion (not more than two Librax capsules per day initially, to be increased gradually as needed and tolerated). In general, the concomitant administration of Librax and other psychotropic agents is not recommended. If such combination therapy seems indicated, careful consideration should be given to the pharmacology of the agents to be employed—particularly when the known potentiating compounds such as the MAO inhibitors and phenothiazines are to be used. The usual precautions in treating patients with impaired renal or hepatic function should be observed.

Paradoxical reactions to chlordiazepoxide hydrochloride, e.g., excitement, stimulation and acute rage, have been reported in psychiatric patients and should be watched for during Librax therapy. The usual precautions are indicated when chlordiazepoxide hydrochloride is used in the treatment of anxiety states where there is any evidence of impending depression; it should be borne in mind that suicidal tendencies may be present and protective measures may be necessary. Although clinical studies have not established a cause and effect relationship, physicians should be aware that variable effects on blood coagulation have been reported very rarely in patients receiving oral anticoagulants and Librium (chlordiazepoxide hydrochloride).

Information for Patients: To assure the safe and effective use of benzodiazepines, patients should be informed that, since benzodiazepines may produce psychological and physical dependence, it is advisable that they consult with their physician before either increasing the dose or abruptly discontinuing this drug.

ADVERSE REACTIONS[10]

No side effects or manifestations not seen with either compound alone have been reported with the administration of Librax. However, since Librax contains chlordiazepoxide hydrochloride and clidinium bromide, the possibility of untoward effects which may be seen with either of these two compounds cannot be excluded.

When chlordiazepoxide hydrochloride has been used alone the necessity of discontinuing therapy because of undesirable effects has been rare.[11] Drowsiness,[12] ataxia[13] and confusion[9] have been reported in some patients—particularly the elderly and debilitated.[9] While these effects can be avoided in almost all instances by proper dosage adjustment, they have occasionally been observed at the lower dosage ranges. In a few instances syncope has been reported.[14]

Other adverse reactions reported during therapy with Librium (chlordiazepoxide hydrochloride/ Roche) include isolated instances of skin eruptions,[12] edema,[15] minor menstrual irregularities,[12] nausea and constipation,[16] extrapyramidal symptoms,[9] as well as increased and decreased libido. Such side effects have been infrequent and are generally controlled with reduction of dosage. Changes in EEG patterns (low-voltage fast activity) have been observed in patients during and after Librium treatment.[17]

Blood dyscrasias,[10] including agranulocytosis,[18] jaundice and hepatic dysfunction[19] have occasionally been reported during therapy with Librium. When Librium treatment is protracted, periodic blood counts and liver function tests are advisable.

Adverse effects reported with use of *Librax* are those typical of anticholinergic agents, *i.e.*, dryness of the mouth, blurring of vision, urinary hesitancy and constipation. Constipation has occurred most often when Librax therapy has been combined with other spasmolytic agents and/or a low residue diet.

DRUG ABUSE AND DEPENDENCE

Withdrawal symptoms, similar in character to those noted with barbiturates and alcohol (convulsions, tremor, abdominal and muscle cramps, vomiting and sweating), have occurred following abrupt discontinuance of chlordiazepoxide. The more severe withdrawal symptoms have usually been limited to those patients who had received excessive doses over an extended period of time. Generally milder withdrawal symptoms (*e.g.*, dysphoria and insomnia) have been reported following abrupt discontinuance of benzodiazepines taken continuously at therapeutic levels for several months. Consequently, after extended therapy, abrupt discontinuation should generally be avoided and a gradual dosage tapering schedule followed. Addiction-prone individuals (such as drug addicts or alcoholics) should be under careful surveillance when receiving chlordiazepoxide or other psychotropic agents because of the predisposition of such patients to habituation and dependence.

DOSAGE

Because of the varied individual responses to tranquilizers and anticholinergics, the optimum dosage of Librax varies with the diagnosis and response of the individual patient. The dosage, therefore, should be individualized for maximum beneficial effects. The usual maintenance dose is 1 or 2 capsules, 3 or 4 times a day administered before meals and at bedtime.

HOW SUPPLIED

Librax is available in green capsules, each containing 5 mg chlordiazepoxide hydrochloride (Librium®) and 2.5 mg clidinium bromide (Quarzan®)—bottles of 100 (NDC 0140-0007-01) and 500 (NDC 0140-0007-14); Tel-E-Dose® packages of 100 (NDC 0140-0007-49).

REFERENCES

1. Schallek, W., *et al:* Arch. Int. Pharmacodyn. *149*:467-483, 1964.
2. Himwich, H. E., *et al:* J. Neuropsych. *3* (Suppl. 1):S15-S26, August 1962.
3. Morillo, A., *et al:* Psychopharmacologia *3* (No. 5):386-394, 1962.
4. MacLean, P. D.: Psychosomatic Med. *17:* 355-366, September 1955.
5. Morgan, C. T.: Physiological Psychology, 3rd Ed.; New York, McGraw-Hill, 1965.
6. Randall, L. O. *et al:* J. Pharm. Exper. Therap. *129*:163-171, June 1960.
7. Miller, L. C. and Tainter, M. C.: Proc. Soc. Exp. Biol. & Med. *57*:261, 1944.
8. Zbinden, G., *et al:* Toxicology and Applied Pharmacology *3*:619-637, November 1961.
9. Data on file, Hoffmann-La Roche Inc., Nutley, New Jersey.
10. Bibliography and References available on request from Roche Laboratories.
11. Rickels, K. *et al:* Med. Times *93*:238-245, March 1965.
12. Tobin, J. M. *et al:* J. Amer. Med. Assoc. *174*: 1242-1249, November 1960.
13. Jenner, F. A., *et al:* J. Ment. Sci. *107*:575-582, May 1961.
14. Robinson, R. C. V.: Dis. Nerv. System *21*:43-45, March 1960.
15. Rose, J. T.: Amer. J. Psychiat. *120*:899-900, March 1964.
16. Hines, L. R.: Curr. Therap. Res. *2*:227-236, June 1960.
17. Gibbs, F. A. and Gibbs, E. L.: J. Neuropsych., 3 (Suppl. 1):S73-S78, August 1962.
18. Kaelbling, R., *et al:* J. Amer. Med. Assoc. *174*:1863-1865, December 1960.
19. Cacioppo, J., *et al:* Amer. J. Psychiat. *117*:1040-1041, May 1961.

P.I. 0288

Shown in Product Identification Section, page 425

LIBRIUM® CAPSULES
[*lib'ree-um*]
(chlordiazepoxide HCl/Roche)
LIBRITABS®
[*lib'rit-abs*]
(chlordiazepoxide/Roche)

The following text is complete prescribing information based on official labeling in effect June 1, 1989.

DESCRIPTION

Librium (the original chlordiazepoxide HCl) and Libritabs (the original chlordiazepoxide), prototypes for the benzodiazepine compounds, were synthesized and developed at Hoffmann-La Roche Inc. They are versatile therapeutic agents of proven value for the relief of anxiety, and are among the safer of the effective psychopharmacologic compounds available, as demonstrated by extensive clinical evidence.

Librium is available as capsules containing 5 mg, 10 mg or 25 mg chlordiazepoxide HCl. Each capsule also contains corn starch, lactose and talc. Gelatin capsule shells may contain methyl and propyl parabens and potassium sorbate, with the following dye systems: 5-mg capsules—FD&C Yellow No. 6 plus D&C Yellow No. 10 and either FD&C Blue No. 1 or FD&C Green No. 3. 10-mg capsules—FD&C Yellow No. 6 plus D&C Yellow No. 10 and either FD&C Blue No. 1 plus FD&C Red No. 3 or FD&C Green No. 3 plus FD&C Red No. 40. 25-mg capsules—D&C Yellow No. 10 and either FD&C Green No. 3 or FD&C Blue No. 1.

Chlordiazepoxide hydrochloride is 7-chloro-2-(methylamino)-5-phenyl-3H-1,4-benzodiazepine 4-oxide hydrochloride. A white to practically white crystalline substance, it is soluble in water. It is unstable in solution and the powder must be protected from light. The molecular weight is 336.22.

Libritabs is available as tablets containing 5 mg, 10 mg or 25 mg chlordiazepoxide. Each tablet also contains corn starch, ethylcellulose, hydroxypropyl methylcellulose, lactose, magnesium stearate, microcrystalline cellulose and triacetin; with FD&C Blue No. 1, D&C Yellow No. 10 and FD&C Yellow No. 6 dyes.

Chlordiazepoxide is 7-chloro-2-(methylamino)-5-phenyl-3H-1,4-benzodiazepine 4-oxide. A yellow crystalline substance, it is insoluble in water. The powder must be protected from light. The molecular weight is 299.76.

ACTIONS

Librium (chlordiazepoxide HCl/Roche) and Libritabs (chlordiazepoxide/Roche) have antianxiety, sedative, appetite-stimulating and weak analgesic actions. The precise mechanism of action is not known. The drugs block EEG arousal from stimulation of the brain stem reticular formation. It takes several hours for peak blood levels to be reached and the half-life of the drugs is between 24 and 48 hours. After Librium or Libritabs is discontinued plasma levels decline slowly over a period of several days. Chlordiazepoxide is excreted in the urine, with 1 to 2% unchanged and 3 to 6% as a conjugate.

Animal Pharmacology: The drug has been studied extensively in many species of animals and these studies are suggestive of action on the limbic system of the brain, which recent evidence indicates is involved in emotional responses. Hostile monkeys were made tame by oral drug doses which did not cause sedation. Chlordiazepoxide HCl revealed a "taming" action with the elimination of fear and aggression. The taming effect of chlordiazepoxide HCl was further demonstrated in rats made vicious by lesions in the septal area of the brain. The drug dosage which effectively blocked the

vicious reaction was well below the dose which caused sedation in these animals.

The LD_{50} of parenterally administered chlordiazepoxide HCl was determined in mice (72 hours) and rats (5 days), and calculated according to the method of Miller and Tainter, with the following results: mice, I.V., 123 ± 12 mg/kg; mice, I.M., 366 ± 7 mg/kg; rats, I.V., 120 ± 7 mg/kg; rats, I.M., > 160 mg/kg.

Effects on Reproduction: Reproduction studies in rats fed 10, 20 and 80 mg/kg daily and bred through one or two matings showed no congenital anomalies, nor were there adverse effects on lactation of the dams or growth of the newborn. However, in another study at 100 mg/kg daily there was noted a significant decrease in the fertilization rate and a marked decrease in the viability and body weight of offspring which may be attributable to sedative activity, thus resulting in lack of interest in mating and lessened maternal nursing and care of the young. One neonate in each of the first and second matings in the rat reproduction study at the 100 mg/kg dose exhibited major skeletal defects. Further studies are in progress to determine the significations of these findings.

INDICATIONS

Librium and Libritabs are indicated for the management of anxiety disorders or for the short-term relief of symptoms of anxiety, withdrawal symptoms of acute alcoholism, and preoperative apprehension and anxiety. Anxiety or tension associated with the stress of everyday life usually does not require treatment with an anxiolytic.

The effectiveness of Librium or Libritabs in long-term use, that is, more than 4 months, has not been assessed by systematic clinical studies. The physician should periodically reassess the usefulness of the drug for the individual patient.

CONTRAINDICATIONS

Librium and Libritabs are contraindicated in patients with known hypersensitivity to the drug.

WARNINGS

Chlordiazepoxide HCl and chlordiazepoxide may impair the mental and/or physical abilities required for the performance of potentially hazardous tasks such as driving a vehicle or operating machinery. Similarly, they may impair mental alertness in children. The concomitant use of alcohol or other central nervous system depressants may have an additive effect. PATIENTS SHOULD BE WARNED ACCORDINGLY.

Usage in Pregnancy: An increased risk of congenital malformations associated with the use of minor tranquilizers (chlordiazepoxide, diazepam and meprobamate) during the first trimester of pregnancy has been suggested in several studies. Because use of these drugs is rarely a matter of urgency, their use during this period should almost always be avoided. The possibility that a woman of childbearing potential may be pregnant at the time of institution of therapy should be considered. Patients should be advised that if they become pregnant during therapy or intend to become pregnant they should communicate with their physicians about the desirability of discontinuing the drug.

Withdrawal symptoms of the barbiturate type have occurred after the discontinuance of benzodiazepines. (See DRUG ABUSE AND DEPENDENCE section.)

PRECAUTIONS

In elderly and debilitated patients, it is recommended that the dosage be limited to the smallest effective amount to preclude the development of ataxia or oversedation (10 mg or less per day initially, to be increased gradually as needed and tolerated). In general, the concomitant administration of Librium or Libritabs and other psychotropic agents is not recommended. If such combination therapy seems indicated, careful consideration should be given to the pharmacology of the agents to be employed — particularly when the known potentiating compounds such as the MAO inhibitors and phenothiazines are to be used. The usual precautions in treating patients with impaired renal or hepatic function should be observed.

Paradoxical reactions, *e.g.*, excitement, stimulation and acute rage, have been reported in psychiatric patients and in hyperactive aggressive children, and should be watched for during Librium or Libritabs therapy. The usual precautions are indicated when Librium or Libritabs is used in the treatment of anxiety states where there is any evidence of impending depression; it should be borne in mind that suicidal tendencies may be present and protective measures may be necessary. Although clinical studies have not established a cause and effect relationship, physicians should be aware that variable effects on blood coagulation have been reported very rarely in patients receiving oral anticoagulants and Librium or Libritabs. In view of isolated reports associating chlordiazepoxide HCl and chlordiazepoxide with exacerbation of porphyria, caution should be exercised in prescribing these agents to patients suffering from this disease.

Continued on next page

Roche Products—Cont.

Information for Patients: To assure the safe and effective use of benzodiazepines, patients should be informed that, since benzodiazepines may produce psychological and physical dependence it is advisable that they consult with their physician before either increasing the dose or abruptly discontinuing this drug.

ADVERSE REACTIONS

The necessity of discontinuing therapy because of undesirable effects has been rare. Drowsiness, ataxia and confusion have been reported in some patients — particularly the elderly and debilitated. While these effects can be avoided in almost all instances by proper dosage adjustment, they have occasionally been observed at the lower dosage ranges. In a few instances syncope has been reported.

Other adverse reactions reported during therapy include isolated instances of skin eruptions, edema, minor menstrual irregularities, nausea and constipation, extrapyramidal symptoms, as well as increased and decreased libido. Such side effects have been infrequent and are generally controlled with reduction of dosage. Changes in EEG patterns (low-voltage fast activity) have been observed in patients during and after Librium or Libritabs treatment.

Blood dyscrasias (including agranulocytosis), jaundice and hepatic dysfunction have occasionally been reported during therapy. When Librium or Libritabs treatment is protracted, periodic blood counts and liver function tests are advisable.

DRUG ABUSE AND DEPENDENCE

Chlordiazepoxide hydrochloride capsules are classified by the Drug Enforcement Administration as a Schedule IV controlled substance.

Withdrawal symptoms, similar in character to those noted with barbiturates and alcohol (convulsions, tremor, abdominal and muscle cramps, vomiting and sweating), have occurred following abrupt discontinuation of chlordiazepoxide. The more severe withdrawal symptoms have usually been limited to those patients who had received excessive doses over an extended period of time. Generally milder withdrawal symptoms (*e.g.*, dysphoria and insomnia) have been reported following abrupt discontinuance of benzodiazepines taken continuously at therapeutic levels for several months. Consequently, after extended therapy, abrupt discontinuation should generally be avoided and a gradual dosage tapering schedule followed. Addiction-prone individuals (such as drug addicts or alcoholics) should be under careful surveillance when receiving chlordiazepoxide or other psychotropic agents because of the predisposition of such patients to habituation and dependence.

OVERDOSAGE

Manifestations of Librium or Libritabs overdosage include somnolence, confusion, coma and diminished reflexes. Respiration, pulse and blood pressure should be monitored, as in all cases of drug overdosage although, in general, these effects have been minimal following Librium or Libritabs overdosage. General supportive measures should be employed, along with immediate gastric lavage. Intravenous fluids should be administered and an adequate airway maintained. Hypotension may be combated by the use of Levophed® (norepinephrine) or Aramine (metaraminol). Dialysis is of limited value. There have been occasional reports of excitation in patients following chlordiazepoxide HCl or chlordiazepoxide overdosage; if this occurs barbiturates should not be used. As with the management of intentional overdosage with any drug, it should be borne in mind that multiple agents may have been ingested.

DOSAGE AND ADMINISTRATION

Because of the wide range of clinical indications for Librium and Libritabs, the optimum dosage varies with the diagnosis and response of the individual patient. The dosage, therefore, should be individualized for maximum beneficial effects.

ADULTS	Usual Daily Dose
Relief of mild and moderate anxiety disorders and symptoms of anxiety	5 mg or 10 mg, 3 or 4 times daily
Relief of severe anxiety disorders and symptoms of anxiety	20 mg or 25 mg, 3 or 4 times daily
Geriatric patients, or in the presence of debilitating disease	5 mg, 2 to 4 times daily

Preoperative apprehension and anxiety:
On days preceding surgery, 5 to 10 mg orally, 3 or 4 times daily. If used as preoperative medication, 50 to 100 mg I.M.* one hour prior to surgery.

CHILDREN	Usual Daily Dose
Because of the varied response of children to CNS-acting drugs, therapy should be initiated	5 mg, 2 to 4 times daily (may be increased in some children to 10 mg, 2 or 3 times daily)

with the lowest dose and increased as required. Since clinical experience in children under 6 years of age is limited, the use of the drug in this age group is not recommended.

For the relief of withdrawal symptoms of acute alcoholism, the parenteral form* is usually used initially. If the drug is administered orally, the suggested initial dose is 50 to 100 mg, to be followed by repeated doses as needed until agitation is controlled — up to 300 mg per day. Dosage should then be reduced to maintenance levels.

* See package insert for injectable Librium (chlordiazepoxide HCl/Roche).

HOW SUPPLIED

Librium (chlordiazepoxide HCl/Roche) capsules — 5 mg, green and yellow; 10 mg, green and black; 25 mg, green and white — bottles of 100 and 500; Tel-E-Dose® packages of 100, available in trays of 4 reverse-numbered cards of 25, and in boxes containing 10 strips of 10.

Libritabs (chlordiazepoxide/Roche) tablets — 5 mg or 10 mg— bottles of 100 and 500; 25 mg—bottles of 100.

P.I. 0788

Shown in Product Identification Section, page 425

LIBRIUM® INJECTABLE   Ⓡ
[*lib 'ree-um*]
(chlordiazepoxide HCl/Roche)

Librium Injectable is manufactured by Hoffmann-La Roche Inc., Nutley, N.J. 07110 and distributed by Roche Products Inc., Manati, P.R. 00701.

The following text is complete prescribing information based on official labeling in effect June 1, 1989.

DESCRIPTION

Librium is a versatile therapeutic agent of proven value for the relief of anxiety and tension.

Librium is the first of a new class, unrelated chemically and pharmacologically to other types of tranquilizers. Librium promptly relieves anxiety and is among the safer of the effective psychopharmacologic compounds available.

Chlordiazepoxide HCl is 7-chloro-2-methylamino-5-phenyl-3H-1,4-benzodiazepine 4-oxide hydrochloride. A colorless, crystalline substance, it is soluble in water. It is unstable in solution and the powder must be protected from light. The molecular weight is 336.22.

ANIMAL PHARMACOLOGY

The drug has been studied extensively in many species of animals and these studies are suggestive of action on the limbic system of the brain, which recent evidence indicates is involved in emotional responses.

Hostile monkeys were made tame by oral drug doses which did not cause sedation. Librium revealed a "taming" action with the elimination of fear and aggression. The taming effect of Librium was further demonstrated in rats made vicious by lesions in the septal area of the brain. The drug dosage which effectively blocked the vicious reaction was well below the dose which caused sedation in these animals.

The LD_{50} of parenterally administered chlordiazepoxide HCl was determined in mice (72 hours) and rats (5 days), and calculated according to the method of Miller and Tainter, with the following results: mice, I.V., 123 ± 12 mg/kg; mice, I.M., 366 ± 7 mg/kg; rats, I.V., 120 ± 7 mg/kg; rats, I.M., >160 mg/kg.

Effects on Reproduction: Reproduction studies in rats fed 10, 20 and 80 mg/kg daily and bred through one or two matings showed no congenital anomalies, nor were there adverse effects on lactation of the dams or growth of the newborn. However, in another study at 100 mg/kg daily there was noted a significant decrease in the fertilization rate and a marked decrease in the viability and body weight of offspring which may be attributable to sedative activity, thus resulting in lack of interest in mating and lessened maternal nursing and care of the young. One neonate in each of the first and second matings in the rat reproduction study at the 100 mg/kg dose exhibited major skeletal defects. Further studies are in progress to determine the significance of these findings.

INDICATIONS

Injectable Librium is indicated for the management of anxiety disorders or for the short-term relief of symptoms of anxiety, withdrawal symptoms of acute alcoholism, and preoperative apprehension and anxiety. Anxiety or tension associated with the stress of everyday life usually does not require treatment with an anxiolytic.

CONTRAINDICATIONS

Librium is contraindicated in patients with known hypersensitivity to the drug.

WARNINGS

As in the case of other CNS-acting drugs, patients receiving Librium should be cautioned about possible combined effects with alcohol and other CNS depressants.

As is true of all preparations containing CNS-acting drugs, patients receiving Librium should be cautioned against hazardous occupations requiring complete mental alertness such as operating machinery or driving a motor vehicle.

Usage in Pregnancy: An increased risk of congenital malformations associated with the use of minor tranquilizers (chlordiazepoxide, diazepam and meprobamate) during the first trimester of pregnancy has been suggested in several studies. Because use of these drugs is rarely a matter of urgency, their use during this period should almost always be avoided. The possibility that a woman of childbearing potential may be pregnant at the time of institution of therapy should be considered. Patients should be advised that if they become pregnant during therapy or intend to become pregnant they should communicate with their physicians about the desirability of discontinuing the drug.

Management of Overdosage: Manifestations of Librium overdosage include somnolence, confusion, coma and diminished reflexes. Respiration, pulse and blood pressure should be monitored, as in all cases of drug overdosage, although, in general, these effects have been minimal following Librium overdosage. General supportive measures should be employed, along with immediate gastric lavage. Intravenous fluids should be administered and an adequate airway maintained. Hypotension may be combated by the use of Levophed® (levarterenol) or Aramine (metaraminol). Dialysis is of limited value. There have been occasional reports of excitation in patients following Librium overdosage; if this occurs barbiturates should not be used. As with the management of intentional overdosage with any drug, it should be borne in mind that multiple agents may have been ingested.

Withdrawal symptoms of the barbiturate type have occurred after the discontinuation of benzodiazepines. (See DRUG ABUSE AND DEPENDENCE section.)

PRECAUTIONS

Injectable Librium (intramuscular or intravenous) is indicated primarily in acute states, and patients receiving this form of therapy should be kept under observation, preferably in bed, for a period of up to three hours. Ambulatory patients should not be permitted to operate a vehicle following an injection. Injectable Librium should not be given to patients in shock or comatose states. Reduced dosage (usually 25 to 50 mg) should be used for elderly or debilitated patients, and for children age twelve or older. In general, the concomitant administration of Librium and other psychotropic agents is not recommended. If such combination therapy seems indicated, careful consideration should be given to the pharmacology of the agents to be employed—particularly when the known potentiating compounds such as the MAO inhibitors and phenothiazines are to be used. The usual precautions in treating patients with impaired renal or hepatic function should be observed.

Paradoxical reactions, *e.g.*, excitement, stimulation and acute rage, have been reported in psychiatric patients and in hyperactive aggressive children, and should be watched for during Librium therapy. The usual precautions are indicated when Librium is used in the treatment of anxiety states where there is any evidence of impending depression; it should be borne in mind that suicidal tendencies may be present and protective measures may be necessary. Although clinical studies have not established a cause and effect relationship, physicians should be aware that variable effects on blood coagulation have been reported very rarely in patients receiving oral anticoagulants and Librium. In view of isolated reports associating chlordiazepoxide with exacerbation of porphyria, caution should be exercised in prescribing chlordiazepoxide to patients suffering from this disease.

ADVERSE REACTIONS

The necessity of discontinuing therapy because of undersirable effects has been rare. Drowsiness, ataxia and confusion are more commonly seen in the elderly and debilitated.

Other adverse reactions reported during therapy include isolated instances of syncope, hypotension, tachycardia, skin eruptions, edema, minor menstrual irregularities, nausea and constipation, extrapyramidal symptoms, blurred vision, as well as increased and decreased libido. Such side effects have been infrequent and are generally controlled with reduction of dosage. Similarly, hypotension associated with spinal anesthesia has occurred. Pain following intramuscular injection has been reported. Changes in EEG patterns (low-voltage fast activity) have been observed in patients during and after Librium treatment.

Blood dyscrasias (including agranulocytosis), jaundice and hepatic dysfunction, have occasionally been reported during therapy. When Librium treatment is protracted, periodic blood counts and liver function tests are advisable.

DRUG ABUSE AND DEPENDENCE

Withdrawal symptoms, similar in character to those noted with barbiturates and alcohol (convulsions, tremor, abdominal and muscle cramps, vomiting and sweating), have occurred following abrupt discontinuance of chlordiazepoxide. The more severe withdrawal symptoms have usually been limited to those patients who had received excessive doses over an extended period of time. Generally milder withdrawal symptoms (e.g., dysphoria and insomnia) have been reported following abrupt discontinuance of benzodiazepines taken continuously at therapeutic levels for several months. Consequently, after extended therapy, abrupt discontinuation should generally be avoided and a gradual dosage tapering schedule followed. Addiction-prone individuals (such as drug addicts or alcoholics) should be under careful surveillance when receiving chlordiazepoxide or other psychotropic agents because of the predisposition of such patients to habituation and dependence.

PREPARATION AND ADMINISTRATION OF SOLUTIONS

Solutions of Librium for intramuscular or intravenous use should be prepared aseptically. Sterilization by heating should not be attempted.

Intramuscular: Add 2 ml of *Special Intramuscular Diluent* to contents of 5-ml dry-filled amber ampul of Librium Sterile Powder (100 mg). Avoid excessive pressure in injecting this special diluent into the ampul containing the powder since bubbles will form on the surface of the solution. Agitate gently until completely dissolved. Solution should be prepared immediately before administration. Any unused solution should be discarded. Deep intramuscular injection should be given *slowly* into the upper outer quadrant of the gluteus muscle.

Caution: Librium solution made with the Special Intramuscular Diluent should not be given intravenously because of the air bubbles which form when the intramuscular diluent is added to the Librium powder. Do not use diluent solution if it is opalescent or hazy.

Intravenous: In most cases, intramuscular injection is the preferred route of administration of Injectable Librium since beneficial effects are usually seen within 15 to 30 minutes. When, in the judgment of the physician, even more rapid action is mandatory, Injectable Librium may be administered intravenously. A suitable solution for intravenous administration may be prepared as follows: Add 5 ml of *sterile physiological saline* or *sterile water for injection* to contents of 5-ml dry-filled amber ampul of Librium Sterile Powder (100 mg). Agitate gently until thoroughly dissolved. Solution should be prepared immediately before administration. Any unused portion should be discarded. *Intravenous injection should be given slowly over a one-minute period.*

Caution: Librium solution made with physiological saline or sterile water for injection should not be given intramuscularly because of pain on injection.

DOSAGE

Dosage should be individualized according to the diagnosis and the response of the patient. While 300 mg may be given during a 6-hour period, this dose should not be exceeded in any 24-hour period.

INDICATION	ADULT DOSAGE*
Withdrawal Symptoms of Acute Alcoholism	50 to 100 mg I.M. or I.V. initially; repeat in 2 to 4 hours, if necessary
Acute or Severe Anxiety Disorders or Symptoms of Anxiety	50 to 100 mg I.M. or I.V. initially; then 25 to 50 mg 3 or 4 times daily, if necessary
Preoperative Apprehension and Anxiety	50 to 100 mg I.M. one hour prior to surgery

* Lower doses (usually 25 to 50 mg) should be used for elderly or debilitated patients, and for older children. Since clinical experience in children under 12 years of age is limited, the use of the drug in this age group is not recommended.

In most cases, acute symptoms may be rapidly controlled by parenteral administration so that subsequent treatment, if necessary, may be given orally. (See package insert for Oral Librium.)

HOW SUPPLIED

For Parenteral Administration: Ampuls—Duplex package consisting of a 5-ml dry-filled ampul containing 100 mg chlordiazepoxide HCl in dry crystalline form, and a 2-ml ampul of Special Intramuscular Diluent (for intramuscular administration) compounded with 1.5% benzyl alcohol, 4% polysorbate 80, 20% propylene glycol, 1.6% maleic acid and sodium hydroxide to adjust pH to approximately 3.0. Boxes of 10.

CAUTION

Before preparing solution for intramuscular or intravenous administration, please read instructions for PREPARATION AND ADMINISTRATION OF SOLUTIONS.
P.I. 0288

LIMBITROL®   ℞

[*lim 'bit-roll*]
(chlordiazepoxide and amitriptyline HCl/Roche)
DS (double strength) Tablets
Tablets

The following text is complete prescribing information based on official labeling in effect June 1, 1989.

DESCRIPTION

Limbitrol combines for oral administration, chlordiazepoxide, an agent for the relief of anxiety and tension, and amitriptyline, an antidepressant. It is available in DS (double strength) white, film-coated tablets, each containing 10 mg chlordiazepoxide and 25 mg amitriptyline (as the hydrochloride salt); and in blue, film-coated tablets, each containing 5 mg chlordiazepoxide and 12.5 mg amitriptyline (as the hydrochloride salt). Each tablet also contains corn starch, ethylcellulose, hydroxypropyl methylcellulose, lactose, magnesium stearate, povidone and triacetin; Limbitrol tablets contain the following dye: FD&C Blue No. 1; Limbitrol DS tablets contain no dye.

Chlordiazepoxide is a benzodiazepine with the formula 7-chloro-2-(methylamino)-5-phenyl-$3H$-1,4-benzodiazepine 4-oxide. It is a slightly yellow crystalline material and is insoluble in water. The molecular weight is 299.76.

Amitriptyline is a dibenzocycloheptadiene derivative. The formula is 10,11-dihydro-N,N-dimethyl-5H-dibenzo [a, d] cycloheptene-$\Delta^{5,\gamma}$-propylamine hydrochloride. It is a white or practically white crystalline compound that is freely soluble in water. The molecular weight is 313.87.

ACTIONS

Both components of Limbitrol exert their action in the central nervous system. Extensive studies with chlordiazepoxide in many animal species suggest action in the limbic system. Recent evidence indicates that the limbic system is involved in emotional response. Taming action was observed in some species. The mechanism of action of amitriptyline in man is not known, but the drug appears to interfere with the reuptake of norepinephrine into adrenergic nerve endings. This action may prolong the sympathetic activity of biogenic amines.

INDICATIONS

Limbitrol is indicated for the treatment of patients with moderate to severe depression associated with moderate to severe anxiety.

The therapeutic response to Limbitrol occurs earlier and with fewer treatment failures than when either amitriptyline or chlordiazepoxide is used alone.

Symptoms likely to respond in the first week of treatment include: insomnia, feelings of guilt or worthlessness, agitation, psychic and somatic anxiety, suicidal ideation and anorexia.

CONTRAINDICATIONS

Limbitrol is contraindicated in patients with hypersensitivity to either benzodiazepines or tricyclic antidepressants. It should not be given concomitantly with a monoamine oxidase inhibitor. Hyperpyretic crises, severe convulsions and deaths have occurred in patients receiving a tricyclic antidepressant and a monoamine oxidase inhibitor simultaneously. When it is desired to replace a monoamine oxidase inhibitor with Limbitrol, a minimum of 14 days should be allowed to elapse after the former is discontinued. Limbitrol should then be initiated cautiously with gradual increase in dosage until optimum response is achieved.

This drug is contraindicated during the acute recovery phase following myocardial infarction.

WARNINGS

Because of the atropine-like action of the amitriptyline component, great care must be used in treating patients with a history of urinary retention or angle-closure glaucoma. In patients with glaucoma, even average doses may precipitate an attack. Severe constipation may occur in patients taking tricyclic antidepressants in combination with anticholinergic-type drugs.

Patients with cardiovascular disorders should be watched closely. Tricyclic antidepressant drugs, particularly when given in high doses, have been reported to produce arrhythmias, sinus tachycardia and prolongation of conduction time. Myocardial infarction and stroke have been reported in patients receiving drugs of this class.

Because of the sedative effects of Limbitrol, patients should be cautioned about combined effects with alcohol or other CNS depressants. The additive effects may produce a harmful level of sedation and CNS depression.

Patients receiving Limbitrol should be cautioned against engaging in hazardous occupations requiring complete mental alertness, such as operating machinery or driving a motor vehicle.

Usage in Pregnancy: Safe use of Limbitrol during pregnancy and lactation has not been established. Because of the chlordiazepoxide component, please note the following:

An increased risk of congenital malformations associated with the use of minor tranquilizers (chlordiazepoxide, diazepam and meprobamate) during the first trimester of pregnancy has been suggested in several studies. Because the use of these drugs is rarely a matter of urgency, their use during this period should almost always be avoided. The possibility that a woman of childbearing potential may be pregnant at the time of institution of therapy should be considered. Patients should be advised that if they become pregnant during therapy or intend to become pregnant they should communicate with their physicians about the desirability of discontinuing the drug.

Withdrawal symptoms of the barbiturate type have occurred after the discontinuation of benzodiazepines. (See DRUG ABUSE AND DEPENDENCE section.)

PRECAUTIONS

General: Use with caution in patients with a history of seizures.

Close supervision is required when Limbitrol is given to hyperthyroid patients or those on thyroid medication.

The usual precautions should be observed when treating patients with impaired renal or hepatic function.

Patients with suicidal ideation should not have easy access to large quantities of the drug. The possibility of suicide in depressed patients remains until significant remission occurs.

Essential Laboratory Tests: Patients on prolonged treatment should have periodic liver function tests and blood counts.

Drug and Treatment Interactions: Because of its amitriptyline component, Limbitrol may block the antihypertensive action of guanethidine or compounds with a similar mechanism of action.

The effects of concomitant administration of Limbitrol and other psychotropic drugs have not been evaluated. Sedative effects may be additive.

Cimetidine is reported to reduce hepatic metabolism of certain tricyclic antidepressants and benzodiazepines, thereby delaying elimination and increasing steady state concentrations of these drugs. Clinically significant effects have been reported with the tricyclic antidepressants when used concomitantly with cimetidine (Tagamet).

The drug should be discontinued several days before elective surgery.

Concurrent administration of ECT and Limbitrol should be limited to those patients for whom it is essential.

Pregnancy: See WARNINGS section.

Nursing Mothers: It is not known whether this drug is excreted in human milk. As a general rule, nursing should not be undertaken while a patient is on a drug, since many drugs are excreted in human milk.

Pediatric Use: Safety and effectiveness in children below the age of 12 years have not been established.

Elderly Patients: In elderly and debilitated patients it is recommended that dosage be limited to the smallest effective amount to preclude the development of ataxia, oversedation, confusion or anticholinergic effects.

Information for Patients: To assure the safe and effective use of benzodiazepines, patients should be informed that, since benzodiazepines may produce psychological and physical dependence, it is advisable that they consult with their physician before either increasing the dose or abruptly discontinuing this drug.

ADVERSE REACTIONS

Adverse reactions to Limbitrol are those associated with the use of either component alone. Most frequently reported were drowsiness, dry mouth, constipation, blurred vision, dizziness and bloating. Other side effects occurring less commonly included vivid dreams, impotence, tremor, confusion and nasal congestion. Many symptoms common to the depressive state, such as anorexia, fatigue, weakness, restlessness and lethargy, have been reported as side effects of treatment with both Limbitrol and amitriptyline.

Granulocytopenia, jaundice and hepatic dysfunction of uncertain etiology have also been observed rarely with Limbitrol. When treatment with Limbitrol is prolonged, periodic blood counts and liver function tests are advisable.

Note: Included in the listing which follows are adverse reactions which have not been reported with Limbitrol. However, they are included because they have been reported during therapy with one or both of the components or closely related drugs.

Cardiovascular: Hypotension, hypertension, tachycardia, palpitations, myocardial infarction, arrhythmias, heart block, stroke.

Psychiatric: Euphoria, apprehension, poor concentration, delusions, hallucinations, hypomania and increased or decreased libido.

Neurologic: Incoordination, ataxia, numbness, tingling and paresthesias of the extremities, extrapyramidal symptoms, syncope, changes in EEG patterns.

Anticholinergic: Disturbance of accommodation, paralytic ileus, urinary retention, dilatation of urinary tract.

Continued on next page

Roche Products—Cont.

Allergic: Skin rash, urticaria, photosensitization, edema of face and tongue, pruritus.

Hematologic: Bone marrow depression including agranulocytosis, eosinophilia, purpura, thrombocytopenia.

Gastrointestinal: Nausea, epigastric distress, vomiting, anorexia, stomatitis, peculiar taste, diarrhea, black tongue.

Endocrine: Testicular swelling and gynecomastia in the male, breast enlargement, galactorrhea and minor menstrual irregularities in the female, elevation and lowering of blood sugar levels, and syndrome of inappropriate ADH (antidiuretic hormone) secretion.

Other: Headache, weight gain or loss, increased perspiration, urinary frequency, mydriasis, jaundice, alopecia, parotid swelling, ageusia.

DRUG ABUSE AND DEPENDENCE

Withdrawal symptoms, similar in character to those noted with barbiturates and alcohol (convulsions, tremor, abdominal and muscle cramps, vomiting and sweating), have occurred following abrupt discontinuance of chlordiazepoxide. The more severe withdrawal symptoms have usually been limited to those patients who had received excessive doses over an extended period of time. Generally milder withdrawal symptoms (*e.g.*, dysphoria and insomnia) have been reported following abrupt discontinuance of benzodiazepines taken continuously at therapeutic levels for several months. Withdrawal symptoms (*e.g.*, nausea, headache and malaise) have also been reported in association with abrupt amitriptyline discontinuation. Consequently, after extended therapy, abrupt discontinuation should generally be avoided and a gradual dosage tapering schedule followed. Addiction-prone individuals (such as drug addicts or alcoholics) should be under careful surveillance when receiving chlordiazepoxide or other psychotropic agents because of the predisposition of such patients to habituation and dependence.

OVERDOSAGE

There has been limited experience with Limbitrol overdosage *per se*; the manifestations of overdosage and recommendations for treatment are based on clinical experience with its components. Primary concern should be with the dangers associated with amitriptyline overdosage. Deaths by deliberate or accidental overdosage have occurred with this class of drugs.

All patients suspected of having an overdosage of Limbitrol should be admitted to a hospital as soon as possible.

Manifestations: High doses may cause drowsiness, temporary confusion, disturbed concentration or transient visual hallucinations. Overdosage may cause hypothermia, tachycardia and other arrhythmias, ECG evidence of impaired conduction (such as bundle branch block), congestive heart failure, dilated pupils, convulsions, severe hypotension, stupor and coma. Other symptoms may be agitation, hyperactive reflexes, muscle rigidity, polyradiculoneuropathy, vomiting, hyperpyrexia or any of those listed under Adverse Reactions.

Treatment: Empty the stomach as quickly as possible by emesis or lavage. In the comatose patient a cuff endotracheal tube should be placed in position prior to either of these measures. The instillation of activated charcoal into the stomach also should be considered. If the patient is stuporous but responds to stimuli, only close observation and nursing care may be required. It is essential to maintain an adequate airway and fluid intake. Body temperature should be watched closely and appropriate measures taken should deviations occur.

The intramuscular or slow intravenous administration of 1 to 3 mg in adults (or 0.5 mg in children) of physostigmine salicylate (Antilirium)[1-3] has been reported to reverse the manifestations of amitriptyline overdosage. Because of its relatively short half-life, additional doses may be needed at intervals of 30 minutes to 2 hours.

Convulsions may be treated by the use of an inhalation anesthetic rather than the use of barbiturates. Cardiac monitoring is advisable, and the cautious use of digitalis or other antiarrhythmic agents should be considered if serious cardiovascular abnormalities occur. Serum potassium levels should be monitored and kept within normal limits by the use of appropriate I.V. fluids. Standard measures including oxygen, I.V. fluids, plasma expanders and corticosteroids may be used to control circulatory shock.

Dialysis is unlikely to be of value, as it has not proven useful in overdosages of either amitriptyline or chlordiazepoxide. Since many suicidal attempts involve multiple drugs including barbiturates, the possibility of dialysis being beneficial for removal of other drugs should not be overlooked.

Treatment should be continued for at least 48 hours, along with cardiac monitoring in patients who do not respond to therapy promptly. Since relapses are frequent, patients should be hospitalized until their conditions remain stable without physostigmine for at least 24 hours.

Since overdosage is often deliberate, patients may attempt suicide by other means during the recovery phase.

References:
1. Granacher RP, Baldessarini RJ: Physostigmine: Its use in acute anticholinergic syndrome with antidepressant and antiparkinson drugs. *Arch Gen Psychiatry* 32:375–380, March 1975.
2. Burks JS, Walker JE, Rumack BH, Ott JE: Tricyclic antidepressant poisoning: Reversal of coma, choreoathetosis, and myoclonus by physostigmine. *JAMA* 230:1405–1407, Dec. 9, 1974.
3. Snyder BD, Blonde L, McWhirter WR: Reversal of amitriptyline intoxication by physostigmine. *JAMA* 230:1433–1434, Dec. 9, 1974.

DOSAGE AND ADMINISTRATION

Optimum dosage varies with the severity of the symptoms and the response of the individual patient. When a satisfactory response is obtained, dosage should be reduced to the smallest amount needed to maintain the remission. The larger portion of the total daily dose may be taken at bedtime. In some patients, a single dose at bedtime may be sufficient. In general, lower dosages are recommended for elderly patients.

Limbitrol DS (double strength) Tablets are recommended in an initial dosage of three or four tablets daily in divided doses; this may be increased to six tablets daily as required. Some patients respond to smaller doses and can be maintained on two tablets daily.

Limbitrol Tablets in an initial dosage of three or four tablets daily in divided doses may be satisfactory in patients who do not tolerate higher doses.

HOW SUPPLIED

DS (double strength) Tablets, containing 10 mg chlordiazepoxide and 25 mg amitriptyline (as the hydrochloride salt)—bottles of 100 and 500; Tel-E-Dose® packages of 100; Prescription Paks of 50.

Tablets, containing 5 mg chlordiazepoxide and 12.5 mg amitriptyline (as the hydrochloride salt)—bottles of 100 and 500; Tel-E-Dose® packages of 100; Prescription Paks of 50.
P.I. 0389

Shown in Product Identification Section, page 425

MENRIUM® 5–2   ℞

[men 'ree-um]

Each tablet contains 5 mg chlordiazepoxide and 0.2 mg water-soluble esterified estrogens.

MENRIUM® 5–4

Each tablet contains 5 mg chlordiazepoxide and 0.4 mg water-soluble esterified estrogens.

MENRIUM® 10–4

Each tablet contains 10 mg chlordiazepoxide and 0.4 mg water-soluble esterified estrogens.

Menrium tablets are manufactured by Hoffmann-La Roche Inc., Nutley, N.J. 07110 and distributed by Roche Products Inc., Manati, P.R. 00701.

The following text is complete prescribing information based on official labeling in effect June 1, 1989.

Since estrogens are a component of Menrium, please note:

1. ESTROGENS HAVE BEEN REPORTED TO INCREASE THE RISK OF ENDOMETRIAL CARCINOMA.

Three independent case control studies have shown an increased risk of endometrial cancer in postmenopausal women exposed to exogenous estrogens for prolonged periods.[1-3] This risk was independent of the other known risk factors for endometrial cancer. These studies are further supported by the finding that incidence rates of endometrial cancer have increased sharply since 1969 in eight different areas of the United States with population-based cancer reporting systems, an increase which may be related to the rapidly expanding use of estrogens during the last decade.[4] The three case control studies reported that the risk of endometrial cancer in estrogen users was about 4.5 to 13.9 times greater than in nonusers. The risk appears to depend on both duration of treatment[1] and on estrogen dose.[3] In view of these findings, when estrogens are used for the treatment of menopausal symptoms, the lowest dose that will control symptoms should be utilized and medication should be discontinued as soon as possible. When prolonged treatment is medically indicated, the patient should be reassessed on at least a semiannual basis to determine the need for continued therapy. Although the evidence must be considered preliminary, one study suggests that cyclic administration of low doses of estrogen may carry less risk than continuous administration;[3] it therefore appears prudent to utilize such a regimen.

Close clinical surveillance of all women taking estrogens is important. In all cases of undiagnosed persistent or recurring abnormal vaginal bleeding, adequate diagnostic measures should be undertaken to rule out malignancy.

There is no evidence at present that "natural" estrogens are more or less hazardous than "synthetic" estrogens at equiestrogenic doses.

2. ESTROGENS SHOULD NOT BE USED DURING PREGNANCY

The use of female sex hormones, both estrogens and progestogens, during early pregnancy may seriously damage the offspring. It has been shown that females exposed in utero to diethylstilbestrol, a nonsteroidal estrogen, have an increased risk of developing, in later life, a form of vaginal or cervical cancer that is ordinarily extremely rare.[5,6] This risk has been estimated as not greater than 4 per 1000 exposures.[7] Furthermore, a high percentage of such exposed women (from 30 to 90 percent) have been found to have vaginal adenosis,[8-12] epithelial changes of the vagina and cervix. Although these changes are histologically benign, it is not known whether they are precursors of malignancy. Although similar data are not available with the use of other estrogens, it cannot be presumed they would not induce similar changes.

Several reports suggest an association between intrauterine exposure to female sex hormones and congenital anomalies, including congenital heart defects and limb reduction defects.[13-16] One case control study[16] estimated a 4.7-fold increased risk of limb reduction defects in infants exposed in utero to sex hormones (oral contraceptives, hormone withdrawal tests for pregnancy, or attempted treatment for threatened abortion). Some of these exposures were very short and involved only a few days of treatment. The data suggest that the risk of limb reduction defects in exposed fetuses is somewhat less than 1 per 1,000. In the past, female sex hormones have been used during pregnancy in an attempt to treat threatened or habitual abortion. There is considerable evidence that estrogens are ineffective for these indications, and there is no evidence from well-controlled studies that progestogens are effective for these uses.

If Menrium is used during pregnancy, or if the patient becomes pregnant while taking this drug, she should be apprised of the potential risks to the fetus, and the advisability of pregnancy continuation.

DESCRIPTION

Menrium tablets are available in three strengths: Menrium 5-2, containing 5 mg chlordiazepoxide and 0.2 mg water-soluble esterified estrogens; Menrium 5-4, containing 5 mg chlordiazepoxide and 0.4 mg water-soluble esterified estrogens; and Menrium 10-4, containing 10 mg chlordiazepoxide and 0.4 mg water-soluble esterified estrogens. Each tablet also contains acacia, calcium stearate, calcium sulfate, carnauba wax, corn starch, lactose, pregelatinized starch, sodium bicarbonate, sucrose and flavor, with the following dye systems: Menrium 5-2 and Menrium 5-4—FD&C Blue 1, FD&C Yellow No. 6 and D&C Yellow No. 10; Menrium 10-4—FD&C Blue No. 1 and FD&C Red No. 3.

Menrium affords in a single formulation the psychotropic action of Librium® (chlordiazepoxide/Roche) and hormonal replacement in the form of water-soluble esterified estrogens (expressed in terms of sodium estrone sulfate) to provide comprehensive management of the menopausal syndrome or the climacteric.

Librium (chlordiazepoxide/Roche) is a versatile therapeutic agent of proven value for the relief of anxiety and tension. It is indicated when anxiety, tension or apprehension are significant components of the clinical profile. It is among the safer of the effective psychopharmacologic compounds.

Chlordiazepoxide is 7-chloro-2-methylamino-5-phenyl-3H-1, 4-benzodiazepine 4-oxide. It is a slightly yellow, crystalline material and is insoluble in water. The molecular weight is 299.75.

Water-soluble esterified estrogens provide hormonal replacement in the menopausal patient, the need for which is widely recognized and accepted. Esterified estrogens is a mixture of the sodium salts of the sulfate esters of the estrogenic substances, principally estrone, that are of the type excreted by pregnant mares. It is a white to buff-colored, amorphous powder, odorless or having a slight, characteristic odor.

CLINICAL PHARMACOLOGY

The estrogenic component of Menrium is water-soluble esterified estrogens—steroidal compounds—which occur naturally. The action of this substance is substantially equal to the action of both conjugated estrogens, also naturally occurring, and synthetic estrogenic substances.

Menopausal changes, such as atrophic changes of the genital tract and breasts due to a slow decline in estrogen secretion, may be reversed by substitution therapy with estrogenic substances.

Estrogens are, in general, completely absorbed following oral administration. Estrogens are detoxified by the liver, and excretion occurs by way of the urine and the feces.

Librium (chlordiazepoxide HCl/Roche) has antianxiety and sedative actions. The drug has been studied extensively in many species of animals and these studies are suggestive of action on the limbic system of the brain, which recent evidence indicates is involved in emotional responses. However, the precise mechanism of action in man is not known. The drug blocks EEG arousal from stimulation of the brain stem reticular formation. The mean $\pm$S.E. plasma peak time is 1.4 ($\pm$0.3) hours, and the half-life ranges between 7.1 and 19.8 hours with a mean $\pm$S.E. half-life of 12.0 ($\pm$0.7) hours. After the drug is discontinued, plasma levels are usually at the lowest quantitatively detectable amounts by 48 to 72 hours. Chlordiazepoxide HCl is excreted in urine with 1% or less unchanged and 12 to 34% recoverable as conjugates.

INDICATIONS

Menrium is indicated in the management of the manifestations generally associated with the menopausal syndrome—anxiety and tension, vasomotor complaints and hormonal deficiency states.

MENRIUM HAS NOT BEEN SHOWN TO BE EFFECTIVE FOR ANY PURPOSE DURING PREGNANCY AND ITS USE MAY CAUSE SEVERE HARM TO THE FETUS (SEE BOXED WARNING).

CONTRAINDICATIONS

Menrium is contraindicated in patients with known hypersensitivity to chlordiazepoxide and/or esterified estrogens. Estrogens should not be used in women (or men) with any of the following conditions:
1. Known or suspected cancer of the breast except in appropriately selected patients being treated for metastatic disease.
2. Known or suspected estrogen-dependent neoplasia.
3. Known or suspected pregnancy. (See Boxed Warning.)
4. Undiagnosed abnormal genital bleeding.
5. Active thrombophlebitis or thromboembolic disorders.
6. A past history of thrombophlebitis, thrombosis, or thromboembolic disorders associated with previous estrogen use.

WARNINGS

1. *Induction of malignant neoplasms.* Long term continuous administration of natural and synthetic estrogens in certain animal species increases the frequency of carcinomas of the breast, cervix, vagina, and liver. There is now evidence that estrogens increase the risk of carcinoma of the endometrium in humans. (See Boxed Warning.)

At the present time there is no satisfactory evidence that estrogens given to postmenopausal women increase the risk of cancer of the breast,[17] although a recent long-term followup of a single physician's practice has raised this possibility.[18] Because of the animal data, there is a need for caution in prescribing estrogens for women with a strong family history of breast cancer or who have breast nodules, fibrocystic disease, or abnormal mammograms.

2. *Gall bladder disease.* A recent study has reported a 2- to 3-fold increase in the risk of surgically confirmed gall bladder disease in women receiving postmenopausal estrogens,[17] similar to the 2-fold increase previously noted in users of oral contraceptives.[19,24] In the case of oral contraceptives the increased risk appeared after two years of use.[24]

3. *Effects similar to those caused by estrogen-progestogen oral contraceptives.* There are several serious adverse effects of oral contraceptives, most of which have not, up to now, been documented as consequences of postmenopausal estrogen therapy. This may reflect the comparatively low doses of estrogen used in postmenopausal women. It would be expected that the larger doses of estrogen used to treat prostatic or breast cancer or postpartum breast engorgement are more likely to result in these adverse effects, and, in fact, it has been shown that there is an increased risk of thrombosis in men receiving estrogens for prostatic cancer and women for postpartum breast engorgement.[20-23]

a. *Thromboembolic disease.* It is now well established that users of oral contraceptives have an increased risk of various thromboembolic and thrombotic vascular diseases, such as thrombophlebitis, pulmonary embolism, stroke, and myocardial infarction.[24-31] Cases of retinal thrombosis, mesenteric thrombosis, and optic neuritis have been reported in oral contraceptive users. There is evidence that the risk of several of these adverse reactions is related to the dose of the drug.[32,33] An increased risk of postsurgery thromboembolic complications has also been reported in users of oral contraceptives.[34,35] If feasible, estrogen should be discontinued at least 4 weeks before surgery of the type associated with an increased risk of thromboembolism, or during periods of prolonged immobilization.

While an increased rate of thromboembolic and thrombotic disease in postmenopausal users of estrogens has not been found,[17,36] this does not rule out the possibility that such an increase may be present or that subgroups of women who have underlying risk factors or who are receiving relatively large doses of estrogens may have increased risk. Therefore,

estrogens should not be used in persons with active thrombophlebitis or thromboembolic disorders, and they should not be used in persons with a history of such disorders in association with estrogen use. They should be used with caution in patients with cerebral vascular or coronary artery disease and only for those in whom estrogens are clearly needed.

Large doses of estrogen (5 mg conjugated estrogens per day), comparable to those used to treat cancer of the prostate and breast, have been shown in a large prospective clinical trial in men[37] to increase the risk of nonfatal myocardial infarction, pulmonary embolism and thrombophlebitis. When estrogen doses of this size are used, any of the thromboembolic and thrombotic adverse effects associated with oral contraceptive use should be considered a clear risk.

b. *Hepatic adenoma.* Benign hepatic adenomas appear to be associated with the use of oral contraceptives.[38-40] Although benign, and rare, these may rupture and may cause death through intra-abdominal hemorrhage. Such lesions have not yet been reported in association with other estrogen or progestogen preparations but should be considered in estrogen users having abdominal pain and tenderness, abdominal mass, or hypovolemic shock. Hepatocellular carcinoma has also been reported in women taking estrogen-containing oral contraceptives.[39] The relationship of this malignancy to these drugs is not known at this time.

c. *Elevated blood pressure.* Increased blood pressure is not uncommon in women using oral contraceptives. There is now a report that this may occur with the use of estrogens in the menopause[41] and blood pressure should be monitored with estrogen use, especially if high doses are used.

d. *Glucose tolerance.* A worsening of glucose tolerance has been observed in a significant percentage of patients on estrogen-containing oral contraceptives. For this reason, diabetic patients should be carefully observed while receiving estrogen.

4. *Hypercalcemia.* Administration of estrogens may lead to severe hypercalcemia in patients with breast cancer and bone metastases. If this occurs, the drug should be stopped and appropriate measures taken to reduce the serum calcium level.

As in the case of other preparations containing CNS-acting drugs, patients receiving Menrium should be cautioned about possible combined effects with alcohol and other CNS depressants. Other causes of manifestations of the menopausal syndrome, such as pregnancy, should be excluded. As is true of all preparations containing CNS-acting drugs, patients receiving Menrium should be cautioned against hazardous occupations requiring complete mental alertness such as operating machinery or driving a motor vehicle.

Physical and Psychological Dependence: Withdrawal symptoms have not been observed in more than 1300 subjects during clinical trials with Menrium. Physical and psychological dependence have rarely been reported in persons taking recommended doses of Librium (chlordiazepoxide/ Roche). However, caution must be exercised in administering Librium to individuals known to be addiction-prone or those whose history suggests they may increase the dosage on their own initiative. Withdrawal symptoms following discontinuation of chlordiazepoxide hydrochloride have been reported. These symptoms (including convulsions) are similar to those seen with barbiturates.

PRECAUTIONS

A. General Precautions.
1. A complete medical and family history should be taken prior to the initiation of any estrogen therapy. The pretreatment and periodic physical examinations should include special reference to blood pressure, breasts, abdomen, and pelvic organs, and should include a Papanicolaou smear. As a general rule, estrogen should not be prescribed for longer than one year without another physical examination being performed.

2. Fluid retention—Because estrogens may cause some degree of fluid retention, conditions which might be influenced by this factor, such as epilepsy, migraine, and cardiac or renal dysfunction, require careful observation.

3. Certain patients may develop undesirable manifestations of excessive estrogenic stimulation, such as abnormal or excessive uterine bleeding, mastodynia, etc.

4. Oral contraceptives appear to be associated with an increased incidence of mental depression.[24] Although it is not clear whether this is due to the estrogenic or progestogenic component of the contraceptive, patients with a history of depression should be carefully observed.

5. Preexisting uterine leiomyomata may increase in size during estrogen use.

6. The lowest effective dose appropriate for the specific indication should be utilized. Studies of the addition of a progestin for seven or more days of a cycle of estrogen administration have reported a lowered incidence of endometrial hyperplasia. Morphological and biochemical studies of endometrium suggest that 10 to 13 days of progestin are needed to provide maximal maturation of the endometrium and to eliminate any hyperplastic changes. Whether this will provide protection from endometrial carcinoma has not been clearly established. There are possible additional risks which

may be associated with the inclusion of progestin in estrogen replacement regimens. The potential risks include adverse effects on carbohydrate and lipid metabolism. The choice of progestin and dosage may be important in minimizing these adverse effects.

7. The pathologist should be advised of estrogen therapy when relevant specimens are submitted.

8. Patients with a past history of jaundice during pregnancy have an increased risk of recurrence of jaundice while receiving estrogen-containing oral contraceptive therapy. If jaundice develops in any patient receiving estrogen, the medication should be discontinued while the cause is investigated.

9. Estrogens may be poorly metabolized in patients with impaired liver function and they should be administered with caution in such patients.

10. Because estrogens influence the metabolism of calcium and phosphorus, they should be used with caution in patients with metabolic bone diseases that are associated with hypercalcemia or in patients with renal insufficiency.

11. Because of the effects of estrogens on epiphyseal closure, they should be used judiciously in young patients in whom bone growth is not complete.

12. Certain endocrine and liver function tests may be affected by estrogen-containing oral contraceptives. The following similar changes may be expected with larger doses of estrogen:
a. Increased sulfobromophthalein retention.
b. Increased prothrombin and factors VII, VIII, IX, and X; decreased antithrombin 3; increased norepinephrine-induced platelet aggregability.
c. Increased thyroid binding globulin (TBG) leading to increased circulating total thyroid hormone, as measured by PBI, T4 by column, or T4 by radioimmunoassay. Free T3 resin uptake is decreased, reflecting the elevated TBG; free T4 concentration is unaltered.
d. Impaired glucose tolerance.
e. Decreased pregnanediol excretion.
f. Reduced response to metyrapone test.
g. Reduced serum folate concentration.
h. Increased serum triglyceride and phospholipid concentration.
B. Information for the Patient.
See Text of Patient Package Insert which follows below.

WHAT YOU SHOULD KNOW ABOUT ESTROGENS

Estrogens are female hormones produced by the ovaries. The ovaries make several different kinds of estrogens. In addition, scientists have been able to make a variety of synthetic estrogens. As far as we know, all these estrogens have similar properties and therefore much the same usefulness, side effects, and risks. This leaflet is intended to help you understand what estrogens are used for, the risks involved in their use, and how to use them as safely as possible.

This leaflet includes the most important information about estrogens, but not all the information. If you want to know more, you can ask your doctor or pharmacist to let you read the package insert prepared for the doctor.

USES OF ESTROGEN

Estrogens are prescribed by doctors for a number of purposes, including:
1. To provide estrogen during a period of adjustment when a woman's ovaries no longer produce it, in order to prevent certain uncomfortable symptoms of estrogen deficiency. (All women normally stop producing estrogens, generally between the ages of 45 and 55; this is called the menopause.)
2. To prevent symptoms of estrogen deficiency when a woman's ovaries have been removed surgically before the natural menopause.
3. To prevent pregnancy. (Estrogens are given along with a progestogen, another female hormone; these combinations are called oral contraceptives or birth control pills. Patient labeling is available to women taking oral contraceptives and they will not be discussed in this leaflet.)
4. To treat certain cancers in women and men.
5. To prevent painful swelling of the breasts after pregnancy in women who choose not to nurse their babies.
THERE IS NO PROPER USE OF ESTROGENS IN A PREGNANT WOMAN.

ESTROGENS IN THE MENOPAUSE

In the natural course of their lives, all women eventually experience a decrease in estrogen production. This usually occurs between ages 45 and 55 but may occur earlier or later. Sometimes the ovaries may need to be removed before natural menopause by an operation, producing a "surgical menopause."

When the amount of estrogen in the blood begins to decrease, many women may develop typical symptoms: Feelings of warmth in the face, neck, and chest or sudden intense episodes of heat and sweating throughout the body (called "hot flashes" or "hot flushes"). These symptoms are sometimes very uncomfortable. A few women eventually develop

Continued on next page

Roche Products—Cont.

changes in the vagina (called "atrophic vaginitis") which cause discomfort, especially during and after intercourse. Estrogens can be prescribed to treat these symptoms of the menopause. It is estimated that considerably more than half of all women undergoing the menopause have only mild symptoms or no symptoms at all and therefore do not need estrogens. Other woman may need estrogens for a few months, while their bodies adjust to lower estrogen levels. Sometimes the need will be for periods longer than six months. In an attempt to avoid overstimulation of the uterus (womb), estrogens are usually given cyclically during each month of use, that is three weeks of pills followed by one week without pills.

Sometimes women experience nervous symptoms or depression during menopause. There is no evidence that estrogens are effective for such symptoms and they should not be used to treat them, although other treatment may be needed.

You may have heard that taking estrogens for long periods (years) after the menopause will keep your skin soft and supple and keep you feeling young. There is no evidence that this is so, however, and such long-term treatment carries important risks.

Estrogens to Prevent Swelling of the Breasts After Pregnancy: If you do not breast feed your baby after delivery, your breasts may fill up with milk and become painful and engorged. This usually begins about 3 to 4 days after delivery and may last for a few days to up to a week or more. Sometimes the discomfort is severe, but usually it is not and can be controlled by pain relieving drugs such as aspirin and by binding the breasts up tightly. Estrogens can be used to try to prevent the breasts from filling up. While this treatment is sometimes successful, in many cases the breasts fill up to some degree in spite of treatment. The dose of estrogens needed to prevent pain and swelling of the breasts is much larger than the dose needed to treat symptoms of the menopause and this may increase your chances of developing blood clots in the legs or lungs (see below). Therefore, it is important that you discuss the benefits and the risks of estrogen use with your doctor if you have decided not to breast feed your baby.

The Dangers of Estrogens:

1. *Cancer of the uterus.* If estrogens are used in the postmenopausal period for more than a year, there is an increased risk of *endometrial cancer* (cancer of the uterus). Women taking estrogens have roughly 5 to 10 times as great a chance of getting this cancer as women who take no estrogens. To put this another way, while a postmenopausal woman not taking estrogens has 1 chance in 1,000 each year of getting cancer of the uterus, a woman taking estrogens has 5 to 10 chances in 1,000 each year. For this reason *it is important to take estrogens only when you really need them.*

The risk of this cancer is greater the longer estrogens are used and also seems to be greater when larger doses are taken. For this reason *it is important to take the lowest dose of estrogen that will control symptoms and to take it only as long as it is needed.* If estrogens are needed for longer periods of time, your doctor will want to reevaluate your need for estrogens at least every six months.

Women using estrogens should report any irregular vaginal bleeding to their doctors; such bleeding may be of no importance, but it can be an early warning of cancer of the uterus. If you have undiagnosed vaginal bleeding, you should not use estrogens until a diagnosis is made and you are certain there is no cancer of the uterus.

If you have had your uterus completely removed (total hysterectomy), there is no danger of developing cancer of the uterus.

2. *Other possible cancers.* Estrogens can cause development of other tumors in animals, such as tumors of the breast, cervix, vagina, or liver, when given for a long time. At present there is no good evidence that women using estrogen in the menopause have an increased risk of such tumors, but there is no way yet to be sure they do not; and one study raises the possibility that use of estrogens in the menopause may increase the risk of breast cancer many years later. This is a further reason to use estrogens only when clearly needed. While you are taking estrogens, it is important that you go to your doctor at least once a year for a physical examination. Also, if members of your family have had breast cancer or if you have breast nodules or abnormal mammograms (breast x-rays), your doctor may wish to carry out more frequent examinations of your breasts.

3. *Gall bladder disease.* Women who use estrogens after menopause are more likely to develop gall bladder disease needing surgery as women who do not use estrogens. Birth control pills have a similar effect.

4. *Abnormal blood clotting.* Oral contraceptives increase the risk of blood clotting in various parts of the body. This can result in a stroke (if the clot is in the brain), a heart attack (clot in a blood vessel of the heart), or a pulmonary embolus (a clot which forms in the legs or pelvis, then breaks off and travels to the lungs). Any of these can be fatal.

At this time use of estrogens in the menopause is not known to cause such blood clotting, but this has not been fully studied and there could still prove to be such a risk. It is recommended that if you have had clotting in the legs or lungs or a heart attack or stroke while you were using estrogens or birth control pills, you should not use estrogens (unless they are being used to treat cancer of the breast or prostate). If you have had a stroke or heart attack or if you have angina pectoris, estrogens should be used with great caution and only if clearly needed (for example, if you have severe symptoms of the menopause).

The larger doses of estrogen used to prevent swelling of the breasts after pregnancy have been reported to cause clotting in the legs and lungs.

Special Warning About Pregnancy: You should not receive estrogen if you are pregnant. If this should occur, there is a greater than usual chance that the developing child will be born with a birth defect, although the possibility remains fairly small. A female child may have an increased risk of developing cancer of the vagina or cervix later in life (in the teens or twenties). Every possible effort should be made to avoid exposure to estrogens during pregnancy. If exposure occurs, see your doctor.

Other Effects of Estrogens: In addition to the serious known risks of estrogens described above, estrogens have the following side effects and potential risks:

1. *Nausea and vomiting.* The most common side effect of estrogen therapy is nausea. Vomiting is less common.

2. *Effects on breasts.* Estrogens may cause breast tenderness or enlargement and may cause the breasts to secrete a liquid. These effects are not dangerous.

3. *Effects on the uterus.* Estrogens may cause benign fibroid tumors of the uterus to get larger.

Some women will have menstrual bleeding when estrogens are stopped. But if the bleeding occurs on days you are still taking estrogens you should report this to your doctor.

4. *Effects on liver.* Women taking oral contraceptives develop on rare occasions a tumor of the liver which can rupture and bleed into the abdomen. So far, these tumors have not been reported in women using estrogens in the menopause, but you should report any swelling or unusual pain or tenderness in the abdomen to your doctor immediately.

Women with a past history of jaundice (yellowing of the skin and white parts of the eyes) may get jaundice again during estrogen use. If this occurs, stop taking estrogens and see your doctor.

5. *Other effects.* Estrogens may cause excess fluid to be retained in the body. This may make some conditions worse, such as epilepsy, migraine, heart disease, or kidney disease.

SUMMARY

Estrogens have important uses, but they have serious risks as well. You must decide, with your doctor, whether the risks are acceptable to you in view of the benefits of treatment. Except where your doctor has prescribed estrogens for use in special cases of cancer of the breast or prostate, you should not use estrogens if you have cancer of the breast or uterus, are pregnant, have undiagnosed abnormal vaginal bleeding, clotting in the legs or lungs, or have had a stroke, heart attack or angina, or clotting in the legs or lungs in the past while you were taking estrogens.

You can use estrogens as safely as possible by understanding that your doctor will require regular physical examinations while you are taking them and will try to discontinue the drug as soon as possible and use the smallest dose possible. Be alert for signs of trouble including:

1. Abnormal bleeding from the vagina.

2. Pains in the calves or chest or sudden shortness of breath, or coughing blood (indicating possible clots in the legs, heart, or lungs).

3. Severe headache, dizziness, faintness, or changes in vision (indicating possible developing clots in the brain or eye).

4. Breast lumps (you should ask your doctor how to examine your own breasts).

5. Jaundice (yellowing of the skin).

6. Mental depression.

Based on his or her assessment of your medical needs, your doctor has prescribed this drug for you. Do not give the drug to anyone else.

C. Pregnancy: See Contraindications and Box Warning.

D. Nursing Mothers: As a general principle, the administration of any drug to nursing mothers should be done only when clearly necessary since many drugs are excreted in human milk.

In elderly and debilitated patients, it is recommended that the dosage be limited to the smallest effective amount to preclude the development of ataxia or oversedation (10 mg chlordiazepoxide or less per day initially, to be increased gradually as needed and tolerated). In general, the concomitant administration of Menrium and other psychotropic agents is not recommended. If such combination therapy seems indicated, careful consideration should be given to the pharmacology of the agents to be employed—particularly when the known potentiating compounds such as the MAO inhibitors and phenothiazines are to be used. The usual pre-

cautions in treating patients with impaired renal or hepatic function should be observed.

Paradoxical reactions to chlordiazepoxide, e.g., excitement, stimulation and acute rage, have been reported in psychiatric patients and should be watched for during Menrium therapy. The usual precautions are indicated when chlordiazepoxide is used in the treatment of anxiety states where there is any evidence of impending depression; it should be borne in mind that suicidal tendencies may be present and protective measures may be necessary. Although clinical studies have not established a cause and effect relationship, physicians should be aware that variable effects on blood coagulation have been reported very rarely in patients receiving oral anticoagulants and Librium (chlordiazepoxide/Roche).

ADVERSE REACTIONS

No side effects or manifestations not seen with either compound alone have been reported with the administration of Menrium. However, since Menrium contains chlordiazepoxide and water-soluble esterified estrogens, the possibility of untoward effects which may be seen with either of these two compounds cannot be excluded.

(See Warnings regarding induction of neoplasia, adverse effects on the fetus, increased incidence of gall bladder disease, and adverse effects similar to those of oral contraceptives, including thromboembolism.) The following additional adverse reactions have been reported with estrogenic therapy, including oral contraceptives:

1. *Genitourinary system.*
Breakthrough bleeding, spotting, change in menstrual flow.
Dysmenorrhea.
Premenstrual-like syndrome.
Amenorrhea during and after treatment.
Increase in size of uterine fibromyomata.
Vaginal candidiasis.
Change in cervical eversion and in degree of cervical secretion.
Cystitis-like syndrome.

2. *Breasts.*
Tenderness, enlargement, secretion.

3. *Gastrointestinal.*
Nausea, vomiting.
Abdominal cramps, bloating.
Cholestatic jaundice.

4. *Skin.*
Chloasma or melasma which may persist when drug is discontinued.
Erythema multiforme.
Erythema nodosum.
Hemorrhagic eruption.
Loss of scalp hair.
Hirsutism.

5. *Eyes.*
Steepening of corneal curvature.
Intolerance to contact lenses.

6. *CNS.*
Headache, migraine, dizziness.
Mental depression.
Chorea.

7. *Miscellaneous.*
Increase or decrease in weight.
Reduced carbohydrate tolerance.
Aggravation of porphyria.
Edema.
Changes in libido.

When chlordiazepoxide has been used alone the necessity of discontinuing therapy because of undesirable effects has been rare. Drowsiness, ataxia and confusion have been reported in some patients—particularly the elderly and debilitated. While these effects can be avoided in almost all instances by proper dosage adjustment, they have occasionally been observed at the lower dosage ranges. In a few instances syncope has been reported.

Other adverse reactions reported during therapy include isolated instances of skin eruptions, edema, minor menstrual irregularities, nausea and constipation, extrapyramidal symptoms, as well as increased and decreased libido. Such side effects have been infrequent and are generally controlled with reduction of dosage. Changes in EEG patterns (low-voltage fast activity) have been observed in patients during and after Librium (chlordiazepoxide/Roche) treatment.

Blood dyscrasias, including agranulocytosis, jaundice and hepatic dysfunction have occasionally been reported during therapy. When Librium treatment is protracted, periodic blood counts and liver function tests are advisable.

Management of Overdosage: Numerous reports of ingestion of large doses of estrogen-containing oral contraceptives by young children indicate that serious ill effects do not occur. Overdosage of estrogen may cause nausea, and withdrawal bleeding may occur in females. Manifestations of Librium (chlordiazepoxide/Roche) overdosage include somnolence, confusion, coma and diminished reflexes. Respiration, pulse and blood pressure should be monitored, as in all cases of drug overdosage, although, in general, these effects have been minimal following Librium overdosage. General supportive measures should be employed, along with immediate gastric lavage. Intravenous fluids should be administered and an adequate airway maintained. Hypotension may be combated by the use of Levophed® (levarterenol) or Aramine (metaraminol). Dialysis is of limited value. There have been occasional reports of excitation in patients following chlordiazepoxide overdosage; if this occurs barbiturates should not be used. As with the management of intentional overdosage with any drug, it should be borne in mind that multiple agents may have been ingested.

DOSAGE

The lowest dose that will control symptoms should be chosen and medication should be discontinued as promptly as possible.

MENRIUM 5-2—for the majority of patients with the menopausal syndrome or the climacteric having anxiety and tension and hormonal deficiency states requiring estrogen replacement—One tablet, t.i.d.

MENRIUM 5-4—for patients with the menopausal syndrome or the climacteric with anxiety and tension and more severe vasomotor manifestations—One tablet, t.i.d.

MENRIUM 10-4—for patients with the menopausal syndrome or the climacteric with pronounced anxiety and tension and marked vasomotor complaints—One tablet, t.i.d. Therapy should be continued for 21-day courses, followed by one-week rest periods. While these dosage schedules will prove generally satisfactory, individual adjustment of dosage is desirable, since some patients may obtain satisfactory relief with as little as one tablet daily of Menrium 5-2. Treated patients with an intact uterus should be monitored closely for signs of endometrial cancer and appropriate diagnostic measures should be taken to rule out malignancy in the event of persistent or recurring abnormal vaginal bleeding.

HOW SUPPLIED

Menrium 5-2, light green tablets; Menrium 5-4, dark green tablets; and Menrium 10-4, purple tablets—bottles of 100.

PHYSICIAN REFERENCES

1. Ziel HK, Finkel WD: *N Engl J Med* 293 :1167–1170, 1975
2. Smith DC, et al: *N Engl J Med* 293 :1164–1167, 1975
3. Mack TM, et al: *N Engl J Med* 294 :1262–1267, 1976
4. Weiss NS, Szekely DR, Austin DF: *N Engl J Med* 294 :1259–1262, 1976
5. Herbst AL, Ulfelder H, Poskanzer DC: *N Engl J Med* 284 :878–881, 1971
6. Greenwald P, et al: *N Engl J Med* 285 :390–392, 1971
7. Lanier A, et al: *Mayo Clin Proc* 48 :793–799, 1973
8. Herbst A, Kurman R, Scully R: *Obstet Gynecol* 40 :287–298, 1972
9. Herbst A, et al: *Am J Obstet Gynecol* 118 :607–615, 1974
10. Herbst, A, et al: *N Engl J Med* 292 :334–339, 1975
11. Stafl A, et al: *Obstet Gynecol* 43 :118–128, 1974
12. Sherman AI, et al: *Obstet Gynecol* 44 :531–545, 1974
13. Gal I, Kirman B, Stern J: *Nature* 216 :83, 1967
14. Levy EP, Cohen A, Fraser FC: *Lancet* 1 :611, 1973
15. Nora J, Nora A: *Lancet* 1 :941–942, 1973
16. Janerich DT, Piper JM, Glebatis DM: *N Engl J Med* 291 :697–700, 1974
17. Boston Collaborative Drug Surveillance Program: *N Engl J Med* 290 :15–19, 1974
18. Hoover R, et al: *N Engl J Med* 295 :401–405, 1976
19. Boston Collaborative Drug Surveillance Program: *Lancet* 1 :1399–1404, 1973
20. Daniel DG, Campbell H, Turnbull AC: *Lancet* 2 :287–289, 1967
21. The Veterans Administration Cooperative Urological Research Group: *J Urol* 98 :516–522, 1967
22. Bailar JC: *Lancet* 2 :560, 1967
23. Blackard C, et al: *Cancer* 26 :249–256, 1970
24. Royal College of General Practitioners: *J Coll Gen Pract* 13 :267–279, 1967
25. Inman WHW, Vessey MP: *Br Med J* 2 :193–199, 1968
26. Vessey MP, Doll R: *Br Med J* 2 :651–657, 1969
27. Sartwell PE, et al: *Am J Epidemiol* 90 :365–380, 1969
28. Collaborative Group for the Study of Stroke in Young Women: *N Engl J Med* 288 :871–878, 1973
29. Collaborative Group for the Study of Stroke in Young Women: *JAMA* 231 :718–722, 1975
30. Mann JI, Inman WHW: *Br Med J* 2 :245–248, 1975
31. Mann JI, et al: *Br Med J* 2 :241–245, 1975
32. Inman WHW, et al: *Br Med J* 2 :203–209, 1970
33. Stolley PD, et al: *Am J Epidemiol* 102 :197–208, 1975
34. Vessey MP, et al: *Br Med J* 3 :123–126, 1970
35. Greene GR, Sartwell PE: *Am J Public Health* 62 :680–685, 1972
36. Rosenberg L, Armstrong MB, Jick H: *N Engl J Med* 294 :1256–1259, 1976
37. Coronary Drug Project Research Group: *JAMA* 214 :1303–1313, 1970
38. Baum J, et al: *Lancet* 2 :926–928, 1973
39. Mays ET, et al: *JAMA* 235 :730–732, 1976
40. Edmondson HA, Henderson B, Benton B: *N Engl J Med* 294 :470–472, 1976
41. Pfeffer RI, Van Den Noort S: *Am J Epidemiol* 103 :445–456, 1976
P.I. 0787
Shown in Product Identification Section, page 425

QUARZAN®   ℞
[kwar'zan]
(clidinium bromide/Roche)
CAPSULES

The following text is complete prescribing information based on official labeling in effect June 1, 1989.

DESCRIPTION

Clidinium bromide is 3-hydroxy-1-methylquinuclidinium bromide benzilate. A white or nearly white crystalline compound, it is soluble in water and has a calculated molecular weight of 432.36.

Clidinium bromide is a quaternary ammonium compound with anticholinergic and antispasmodic activity. Quarzan is available as green and red opaque capsules each containing 2.5 mg clidinium bromide, and green and grey opaque capsules each containing 5 mg clidinium bromide. Each capsule also contains corn starch, lactose and talc. Gelatin capsule shells contain methyl and propyl parabens and potassium sorbate, with the following dye systems: 2.5-mg capsules—FD&C Blue No. 1, FD&C Green No. 3, FD&C Red No. 3, D&C Red No. 33 and D&C Yellow No. 10. 5-mg capsules—FD&C Green No. 3, D&C Red No. 33, FD&C Yellow No. 6 and D&C Yellow No. 10.

ACTIONS

Quarzan inhibits gastrointestinal motility and diminishes gastric acid secretion. Its anticholinergic activity approximates that of atropine sulfate and propantheline bromide.

INDICATIONS

Quarzan is effective as adjunctive therapy in peptic ulcer disease. **Quarzan has not been shown to be effective in contributing to the healing of peptic ulcer, decreasing the rate of recurrence or preventing complications.**

CONTRAINDICATIONS

Known hypersensitivity to clidinium bromide or to other anticholinergic drugs, glaucoma, obstructive uropathy (for example, bladder neck obstruction due to prostatic hypertrophy), obstructive disease of the gastrointestinal tract (for example, pyloroduodenal stenosis), paralytic ileus, intestinal atony of the elderly or debilitated patient, unstable cardiovascular status in acute hemorrhage, severe ulcerative colitis, toxic megacolon complicating ulcerative colitis, myasthenia gravis.

WARNINGS

Quarzan may produce drowsiness or blurred vision. The patient should be cautioned regarding activities requiring mental alertness such as operating a motor vehicle or other machinery or performing hazardous work while taking this drug. In the presence of high environmental temperature, heat prostration (fever and heat stroke) may occur with the use of anticholinergics due to decreased sweating. Diarrhea may be an early symptom of incomplete intestinal obstruction, especially in patients with ileostomy or colostomy. Use of anticholinergics in patients with suspected intestinal obstruction would be inappropriate and possibly harmful. With overdosage, a curare-like action may occur, *i.e.*, neuromuscular blockade leading to muscular weakness and possible paralysis.

Usage in Pregnancy: No controlled studies in humans have been performed to establish the safety of the drug in pregnancy. Uncontrolled data derived from clinical usage have failed to show abnormalities attributable to its use. Reproduction studies in rats have failed to show any impaired fertility or abnormality in the fetuses that might be associated with the use of Quarzan. Use of any drug in pregnancy or in women of childbearing potential requires that the pontential benefit of the drug be weighed against the possible hazards to mother and fetus.

Nursing Mothers: As with all anticholinergic drugs, Quarzan may be secreted in human milk and may inhibit lactation. As a general rule, nursing should not be undertaken while a patient is on Quarzan, or the drug should not be used by nursing mothers.

Pediatric Use: Since there is no adequate experience in children who have received this drug, safety and efficacy in children have not been established.

PRECAUTIONS

Use Quarzan with caution in the elderly and in all patients with autonomic neuropathy, hepatic or renal disease, ulcerative colitis— large doses may suppress intestinal motility to the point of producing a paralytic ileus and for this reason precipitate or aggravate "toxic megacolon," a serious complication of the disease; hyperthyroidism; coronary heart disease; congestive heart failure; cardiac tachy-arrhythmias; tachycardia; hypertension; prostatic hypertrophy; hiatal hernia associated with reflux esophagitis, since anticholinergic drugs may aggravate this condition.

ADVERSE REACTIONS

As with other anticholinergic drugs, the most frequently reported adverse effects are dryness of mouth, blurring of vision, urinary hesitancy and constipation. Other adverse effects reported with the use of anticholinergic drugs include decreased sweating, urinary retention, tachycardia, palpitations, dilatation of the pupils, cycloplegia, increased ocular tension, loss of taste, headaches, nervousness, mental confusion, drowsiness, weakness, dizziness, insomnia, nausea, vomiting, bloated feeling, impotence, suppression of lactation and severe allergic reactions or drug idiosyncrasies including anaphylaxis, urticaria and other dermal manifestations.

OVERDOSAGE

The symptoms of overdosage with Quarzan progress from an intensification of the usual side effects to CNS disturbances (from restlessness and excitement to psychotic behavior), circulatory changes (flushing, tachycardia, fall in blood pressure, circulatory failure), respiratory failure, paralysis and coma.

Treatment should consist of: *General measures* —(1) gastric lavage, (2) maintenance of adequate airway, using artificial respiration if needed, (3) administration of i.v. fluids, and (4) for fever: alcohol sponging or ice packs.

Specific measures—(1) Antidotes: physostigmine (Antilirium) 0.5 to 2 mg, i.v., repeated as needed up to a total of 5 mg; or pilocarpine, 5 mg, s.c. at intervals until mouth is moist; neostigmine may also be useful. (2) Against excitement: sodium pentothal 2% may be given i.v. or chloral hydrate (100 to 200 ml, 2% solution) *rectally*. (3) Against hypotension and circulatory collapse: levarterenol (Levophed®) or metaraminol (Aramine) infusions. (4) Against CNS depression: caffeine and sodium benzoate.
The usefulness of dialysis is not known.

DOSAGE AND ADMINISTRATION

For maximum efficacy, dosage should be individualized according to severity of symptoms and occurrence of side effects. The usual dosage is 2.5 to 5 mg three or four times daily before meals and at bedtime. Dosage in excess of 20 mg daily is usually not required to obtain maximum effectiveness. For the aged or debilitated, one 2.5-mg capsule three times daily before meals is recommended. The desired pharmacological effect of the drug is unlikely to be attained without occasional side effects.

DRUG INTERACTIONS

No specific drug interactions are known.

HOW SUPPLIED

Opaque capsules, 2.5 mg, green and red—bottles of 100 (NDC 0140-0119-01); 5 mg, green and grey—bottles of 100 (NDC 0140-0120-01).
P.I. 0186
Shown in Product Identification Section, page 425

TEL-E-DOSE®

Tel-E-Dose is a unit package designed by Roche for convenience in dispensing medications in the hospital and nursing home. Each unit, sealed against contamination and moisture, is clearly identified by product name and strength and carries the control number and expiration date.

Currently available in this package form are the following products: Dalmane® (flurazepam HCl) capsules, 15 mg, 30 mg; Librax® (5 mg chlordiazepoxide HCl and 2.5 mg clidinium Br) capsules; Librium® (chlordiazepoxide HCl) capsules, 5 mg, 10 mg, 25 mg; Limbitrol® (5 mg chlordiaxepoxide and 12.5 mg amitriptyline HCl) tablets; Limbitrol® DS (10 mg chlordiazepoxide and 25 mg amitriptyline HCl) tablets; Valium® (diazepam) tablets, 2 mg, 5 mg, 10 mg.

VALIUM® Injectable   ℞
[val 'ee-um]
(diazepam/Roche)

Valium Injectable is manufactured by Hoffmann-La Roche Inc., Nutley, N.J. 07110 and distributed by Roche Products Inc., Manati, P.R. 00701.
The following text is complete prescribing information based on official labeling in effect June 1, 1989.

DESCRIPTION

Each ml contains 5 mg diazepam/Roche compounded with 40% propylene glycol, 10% ethyl alcohol, 5% sodium benzoate and benzoic acid as buffers, and 1.5% benzyl alcohol as preservative.

Diazepam is a benzodiazepine derivative developed through original Roche research. Chemically, diazepam is 7-chloro-1, 3-dihydro-1-methyl-5-phenyl-2H-1,4-benzodiazepin-2-one. It is a colorless crystalline compound, insoluble in water and has a molecular weight of 284.74.

Continued on next page

Roche Products—Cont.

RECOMMENDED DOSAGE FOR *INJECTABLE VALIUM* ® (diazepam/Roche)

	USUAL ADULT DOSAGE	DOSAGE RANGE IN CHILDREN (I.V. administration should be made slowly)
Moderate Anxiety Disorders and Symptoms of Anxiety	2 mg to 5 mg, I.M. or I.V. Repeat in 3 to 4 hours, if necessary.	
Severe Anxiety Disorders and Symptoms of Anxiety	5 mg to 10 mg, I.M. or I.V. Repeat in 3 to 4 hours, if necessary.	
Acute Alcohol Withdrawal: As an aid in symptomatic relief of acute agitation, tremor, impending or acute delirium tremens and hallucinosis.	10 mg, I.M. or I.V. initially, then 5 mg to 10 mg in 3 to 4 hours, if necessary.	
Endoscopic Procedures: Adjunctively, if apprehension, anxiety or acute stress reactions are present prior to endoscopic procedures. Dosage of narcotics should be reduced by at least a third and in some cases may be omitted. See *Precautions* for peroral procedures.	Titrate I.V. dosage to desired sedative response, such as slurring of speech, with slow administration immediately prior to the procedure. Generally 10 mg or less is adequate, but up to 20 mg I.V. may be given, particularly when concomitant narcotics are omitted. If I.V. cannot be used, 5 mg to 10 mg I.M. approximately 30 minutes prior to the procedure.	
Muscle Spasm: Associated with local pathology, cerebral palsy, athetosis, stiff-man syndrome or tetanus.	5 mg to 10 mg, I.M. or I.V. initially, then 5 mg to 10 mg in 3 to 4 hours, if necessary. For tetanus, larger doses may be required.	For tetanus in infants over 30 days of age, 1 mg to 2 mg I.M. or I.V., slowly, repeated every 3 to 4 hours as necessary. In children 5 years or older, 5 mg to 10 mg repeated every 3 to 4 hours may be required to control tetanus spasms. Respiratory assistance should be available.
Status Epilepticus and Severe Recurrent Convulsive Seizures: In the convulsing patient, the I.V. route is by far preferred. This injection should be administered slowly. However, if I.V. administration is impossible, the I.M. route may be used.	5 mg to 10 mg initially (I.V. preferred). This injection may be repeated if necessary at 10 to 15 minute intervals up to a maximum dose of 30 mg. If necessary, therapy with Valium may be repeated in 2 to 4 hours; however, residual active metabolites may persist, and readministration should be made with this consideration. Extreme caution must be exercised with individuals with chronic lung disease or unstable cardiovascular status.	Infants over 30 days of age and children under 5 years, 0.2 mg to 0.5 mg slowly every 2 to 5 minutes up to a maximum of 5 mg (I.V. preferred). Children 5 years or older, 1 mg every 2 to 5 minutes up to a maximum of 10 mg (slow I.V. administration preferred). Repeat in 2 to 4 hours if necessary. EEG monitoring of the seizure may be helpful.
Preoperative Medication: To relieve anxiety and tension. (If atropine, scopolamine or other premedications are desired, they must be administered in separate syringes.)	10 mg, I.M. (preferred route), before surgery.	
Cardioversion: To relieve anxiety and tension and to reduce recall of procedure.	5 mg to 15 mg, IV., within 5 to 10 minutes prior to the procedure.	

ACTIONS

In animals, diazepam appears to act on parts of the limbic system, the thalamus and hypothalamus, and induces calming effects. Diazepam, unlike chlorpromazine and reserpine, has no demonstrable peripheral autonomic blocking action, nor does it produce extrapyramidal side effects; however, animals treated with diazepam do have a transient ataxia at higher doses. Diazepam was found to have transient cardiovascular depressor effects in dogs. Long-term experiments in rats revealed no disturbances of endocrine function. Injections into animals have produced localized irritation of tissue surrounding injection sites and some thickening of veins after intravenous use.

INDICATIONS

Valium is indicated for the management of anxiety disorders or for the short-term relief of the symptoms of anxiety. Anxiety or tension associated with the stress of everyday life usually does not require treatment with an anxiolytic.

In acute alcohol withdrawal, Valium may be useful in the symptomatic relief of acute agitation, tremor, impending or acute delirium tremens and hallucinosis.

As an adjunct prior to endoscopic procedures if apprehension, anxiety or acute stress reactions are present, and to diminish the patient's recall of the procedures. (See WARNINGS.)

Valium is a useful adjunct for the relief of skeletal muscle spasm due to reflex spasm to local pathology (such as inflammation of the muscles or joints, or secondary to trauma); spasticity caused by upper motor neuron disorders (such as cerebral palsy and paraplegia); athetosis; stiff-man syndrome; and tetanus.

Injectable Valium is a useful adjunct in status epilepticus and severe recurrent convulsive seizures.

Valium is a useful premedication (the I.M. route is preferred) for relief of anxiety and tension in patients who are to undergo surgical procedures. Intravenously, prior to cardioversion for the relief of anxiety and tension and to diminish the patient's recall of the procedure.

CONTRAINDICATIONS

Injectable Valium is contraindicated in patients with a known hypersensitivity to this drug; acute narrow angle glaucoma; and open angle glaucoma unless patients are receiving appropriate therapy.

WARNINGS

When used intravenously, the following procedures should be undertaken to reduce the possibility of venous thrombosis, phlebitis, local irritation, swelling, and, rarely, vascular impairment: the solution should be injected slowly, taking at least one minute for each 5 mg (1 ml) given; do not use small veins, such as those on the dorsum of the hand or wrist; extreme care should be taken to avoid intra-arterial administration or extravasation.

Do not mix or dilute Valium with other solutions or drugs in syringe or infusion flask. If it is not feasible to administer Valium directly I.V., it may be injected slowly through the infusion tubing as close as possible to the vein insertion.

Extreme care must be used in administering Injectable Valium, particularly by the I.V. route, to the elderly, to very ill patients and to those with limited pulmonary reserve because of the possibility that apnea and/or cardiac arrest may occur. Concomitant use of barbiturates, alcohol or other central nervous system depressants increases depression with increased risk of apnea. Resuscitative equipment including that necessary to support respiration should be readily available.

When Valium is used with a narcotic analgesic, the dosage of the narcotic should be reduced by at least one-third and administered in small increments. In some cases the use of a narcotic may not be necessary.

Injectable Valium should not be administered to patients in shock, coma, or in acute alcoholic intoxication with depression of vital signs. As is true of most CNS-acting drugs, patients receiving Valium should be cautioned against engaging in hazardous occupations requiring complete mental alertness, such as operating machinery or driving a motor vehicle.

Tonic status epilepticus has been precipitated in patients treated with I.V. Valium for petit mal status or petit mal variant status.

Usage in Pregnancy: **An increased risk of congenital malformations associated with the use of minor tranquilizers (diazepam, meprobamate and chlordiazepoxide) during the first trimester of pregnancy has been suggested in several studies. Because use of these drugs is rarely a matter of urgency, their use during this period should almost always be avoided. The possibility that a woman of childbearing potential may be pregnant at the time of institution of therapy should be considered. Patients should be advised that if they become pregnant during therapy or intend to become pregnant they should communicate with their physicians about the desirability of discontinuing the drug.**

In humans, measurable amounts of diazepam were found in maternal and cord blood, indicating placental transfer of the drug. Until additional information is available, Valium Injectable is not recommended for obstetrical use.

Use in Children: Efficacy and safety of parenteral Valium has not been established in the neonate (30 days or less of age).

Prolonged central nervous system depression has been observed in neonates, apparently due to inability to biotransform Valium into inactive metabolites.

In pediatric use, in order to obtain maximal clinical effect with the minimum amount of drug and thus to reduce the risk of hazardous side effects, such as apnea or prolonged periods of somnolence, it is recommended that the drug be given slowly over a three-minute period in a dosage not to exceed 0.25 mg/kg. After an interval of 15 to 30 minutes the initial dosage can be safely repeated. If, however, relief of symptoms is not obtained after a third administration, adjunctive therapy appropriate to the condition being treated is recommended.

Withdrawal symptoms of the barbiturate type have occurred after the discontinuation of benzodiazepines. (See DRUG ABUSE AND DEPENDENCE section.)

PRECAUTIONS

Although seizures may be brought under control promptly, a significant proportion of patients experience a return to seizure activity, presumably due to the short-lived effect of Valium after I.V. administration. The physician should be prepared to re-administer the drug. However, Valium is not recommended for maintenance, and once seizures are brought under control, consideration should be given to the administration of agents useful in longer term control of seizures.

If Valium is to be combined with other psychotropic agents or anticonvulsant drugs, careful consideration should be given to the pharmacology of the agents to be employed—particularly with known compounds which may potentiate the action of Valium, such as phenothiazines, narcotics, barbiturates, MAO inhibitors and other antidepressants. In highly anxious patients with evidence of accompanying depression, particularly those who may have suicidal tendencies, protective measures may be necessary. The usual precautions in treating patients with impaired hepatic function should be observed. Metabolites of Valium are excreted by the kidney; to avoid their excess accumulation, caution should be exercised in the administration to patients with compromised kidney function.

Since an increase in cough reflex and laryngospasm may occur with peroral endoscopic procedures, the use of a topical anesthetic agent and the availability of necessary countermeasures are recommended.

Until additional information is available, injectable diazepam is not recommended for obstetrical use.

Injectable Valium has produced hypotension or muscular weakness in some patients particularly when used with narcotics, barbiturates or alcohol.

Lower doses (usually 2 mg to 5 mg) should be used for elderly and debilitated patients.

The clearance of Valium and certain other benzodiazepines can be delayed in association with Tagamet (cimetidine) administration. The clinical significance of this is unclear.

ADVERSE REACTIONS

Side effects most commonly reported were drowsiness, fatigue and ataxia; venous thrombosis and phlebitis at the site of injection. Other adverse reactions less frequently reported include: *CNS:* confusion, depression, dysarthria, headache, hypoactivity, slurred speech, syncope, tremor, vertigo. *G.I.:* constipation, nausea. *G.U.:* incontinence, changes in libido, urinary retention. *Cardiovascular:* bradycardia, cardiovascular collapse, hypotension. *EENT:* blurred vision, diplopia, nystagmus. *Skin:* urticaria, skin rash. *Other:* hiccups, changes in salivation, neutropenia, jaundice. Paradoxical reactions such as acute hyperexcited states, anxiety, hallucinations, increased muscle spasticity, insomnia, rage, sleep disturbances and stimulation have been reported; should these occur, use of the drug should be discontinued. Minor changes in EEG patterns, usually low-voltage fast activity, have been observed in patients during and after Valium therapy and are of no known significance.

In peroral endoscopic procedures, coughing, depressed respiration, dyspnea, hyperventilation, laryngospasm and pain in throat or chest have been reported.

Because of isolated reports of neutropenia and jaundice, periodic blood counts and liver function tests are advisable during long-term therapy.

DRUG ABUSE AND DEPENDENCE

Withdrawal symptoms, similar in character to those noted with barbiturates and alcohol (convulsions, tremor, abdominal and muscle cramps, vomiting and sweating), have occurred following abrupt discontinuance of diazepam. The more severe withdrawal symptoms have usually been limited to those patients who had received excessive doses over an extended period of time. Generally milder withdrawal symptoms (*e.g.*, dysphoria and insomnia) have been reported following abrupt discontinuance of benzodiazepines taken continuously at therapeutic levels for several months. Consequently, after extended therapy, abrupt discontinuation should generally be avoided and a gradual dosage tapering schedule followed. Addiction-prone individuals (such as drug addicts or alcoholics) should be under careful surveillance when receiving diazepam or other psychotropic agents because of the predisposition of such patients to habituation and dependence.

DOSAGE AND ADMINISTRATION

Dosage should be individualized for maximum beneficial effect. The usual recommended dose in older children and adults ranges from 2 mg to 20 mg I.M. or I.V., depending on the indication and its severity. In some conditions, *e.g.*, tetanus, larger doses may be required. (See dosage for specific indications.) In acute conditions the injection may be repeated within one hour although an interval of 3 to 4 hours is usually satisfactory. Lower doses (usually 2 mg to 5 mg) and slow increase in dosage should be used for elderly or debilitated patients and when other sedative drugs are administered. (See WARNINGS and ADVERSE REACTIONS.)

For dosage in infants above the age of 30 days and children, see the specific indications below. When intravenous use is indicated, facilities for respiratory assistance should be readily available.

Intramuscular: Injectable Valium should be injected deeply into the muscle.

Intravenous use: (See WARNINGS, particularly for use in children.) The solution should be injected slowly, taking at least one minute for each 5 mg (1 ml) given. Do not use small veins, such as those on the dorsum of the hand or wrist. Extreme care should be taken to avoid intra-arterial administration or extravasation.

Do not mix or dilute Valium with other solutions or drugs in syringe or infusion flask. If it is not feasible to administer Valium directly I.V., it may be injected slowly through the infusion tubing as close as possible to the vein insertion. [See table on preceding page].

Once the acute symptomatology has been properly controlled with Injectable Valium, the patient may be placed on oral therapy with Valium if further treatment is required.

Management of Overdosage:

Manifestations of Valium overdosage include somnolence, confusion, coma, and diminished reflexes. Respiration, pulse and blood pressure should be monitored, as in all cases of drug overdosage, although, in general, these effects have been minimal. General supportive measures should be employed, along with intravenous fluids, and an adequate airway maintained. Hypotension may be combated by the use of Levophed® (levarterenol) or Aramine (metaraminol). Dialysis is of limited value.

HOW SUPPLIED

Ampuls, 2 ml, boxes of 10; Vials, 10 ml, boxes of 1 and 10; Tel-E-Ject® (disposable syringes), 2 ml, boxes of 10.

ANIMAL PHARMACOLOGY

Oral LD$_{50}$ of diazepam is 720 mg/kg in mice and 1240 mg/kg in rats. Intraperitoneal administration of 400 mg/kg to a monkey resulted in death on the sixth day.

Reproduction Studies: A series of rat reproduction studies was performed with diazepam in oral doses of 1, 10, 80 and 100 mg/kg given for periods ranging from 60–228 days prior to mating. At 100 mg/kg there was a decrease in the number of pregnancies and surviving offspring in these rats. These effects may be attributable to prolonged sedative activity, resulting in lack of interest in mating and lessened maternal nursing and care of the young. Neonatal survival of rats at doses lower than 100 mg/kg was within normal limits. Several neonates, both controls and experimentals, in these rat reproduction studies showed skeletal or other defects. Further studies in rats at doses up to and including 80 mg/kg/day did not reveal significant teratological effects on the offspring. Rabbits were maintained on doses of 1, 2, 5 and 8 mg/kg from day 6 through day 18 of gestation. No adverse effects on reproduction and no teratological changes were noted.

P.I. 0288

Shown in Product Identification Section, page 425

VALIUM® TABLETS   ©
[*val'ee-um*]
(diazepam/Roche)

The following text is complete prescribing information based on official labeling in effect June 1, 1989.

DESCRIPTION

Valium (brand of diazepam/Roche) is a benzodiazepine derivative developed through original Roche research. Chemically, diazepam is 7- chloro - 1,3 - dihydro - 1 - methyl - 5 - phenyl - 2H-1,4-benzodiazepin-2-one. It is a colorless crystalline compound, insoluble in water and has a molecular weight of 284.74.

Valium 5-mg tablets contain FD&C Yellow No. 6 and D&C Yellow No. 10 dyes. Valium 10-mg tablets contain FD&C Blue No. 1 dye. Valium 2-mg tablets contain no dye.

PHARMACOLOGY

In animals Valium appears to act on parts of the limbic system, the thalamus and hypothalamus, and induces calming effects. Valium, unlike chlorpromazine and reserpine, has no demonstrable peripheral autonomic blocking action, nor does it produce extrapyramidal side effects; however, animals treated with Valium do have a transient ataxia at higher doses. Valium was found to have transient cardiovascular depressor effects in dogs. Long-term experiments in rats revealed no disturbances of endocrine function.

Oral LD$_{50}$ of diazepam is 720 mg/kg in mice and 1240 mg/kg in rats. Intraperitoneal administration of 400 mg/kg to a monkey resulted in death on the sixth day.

Reproduction Studies: A series of rat reproduction studies was performed with diazepam in oral doses of 1, 10, 80 and 100 mg/kg. At 100 mg/kg there was a decrease in the number of pregnancies and surviving offspring in these rats. Neonatal survival of rats at doses lower than 100 mg/kg was within normal limits. Several neonates in these rat reproduction studies showed skeletal or other defects. Further studies in rats at doses up to and including 80 mg/kg/day did not reveal teratological effects on the offspring.

In humans, measurable blood levels of Valium were obtained in maternal and cord blood, indicating placental transfer of the drug.

INDICATIONS

Valium is indicated for the management of anxiety disorders or for the short-term relief of the symptoms of anxiety. Anxi-

ety or tension associated with the stress of everyday life usually does not require treatment with an anxiolytic.

In acute alcohol withdrawal, Valium may be useful in the symptomatic relief of acute agitation, tremor, impending or acute delirium tremens and hallucinosis.

Valium is a useful adjunct for the relief of skeletal muscle spasm due to reflex spasm to local pathology (such as inflammation of the muscles or joints, or secondary to trauma); spasticity caused by upper motor neuron disorders (such as cerebral palsy and paraplegia); athetosis; and stiff-man syndrome.

Oral Valium may be used adjunctively in convulsive disorders, although it has not proved useful as the sole therapy. The effectiveness of Valium in long-term use, that is, more than 4 months, has not been assessed by systematic clinical studies. The physician should periodically reassess the usefulness of the drug for the individual patient.

CONTRAINDICATIONS

Valium is contraindicated in patients with a known hypersensitivity to this drug and, because of lack of sufficient clinical experience, in children under 6 months of age. It may be used in patients with open angle glaucoma who are receiving appropriate therapy, but is contraindicated in acute narrow angle glaucoma.

WARNINGS

Valium is not of value in the treatment of psychotic patients and should not be employed in lieu of appropriate treatment. As is true of most preparations containing CNS-acting drugs, patients receiving Valium should be cautioned against engaging in hazardous occupations requiring complete mental alertness such as operating machinery or driving a motor vehicle.

As with other agents which have anticonvulsant activity, when Valium is used as an adjunct in treating convulsive disorders, the possibility of an increase in the frequency and/or severity of grand mal seizures may require an increase in the dosage of standard anticonvulsant medication. Abrupt withdrawal of Valium in such cases may also be associated with a temporary increase in the frequency and/or severity of seizures.

Since Valium has a central nervous system depressant effect, patients should be advised against the simultaneous ingestion of alcohol and other CNS-depressant drugs during Valium therapy.

Usage in Pregnancy: **An increased risk of congenital malformations associated with the use of minor tranquilizers (diazepam, meprobamate and chlordiazepoxide) during the first trimester of pregnancy has been suggested in several studies. Because use of these drugs is rarely a matter of urgency, their use during this period should almost always be avoided. The possibility that a woman of childbearing potential may be pregnant at the time of institution of therapy should be considered. Patients should be advised that if they become pregnant during therapy or intend to become pregnant they should communicate with their physicians about the desirability of discontinuing the drug.**

Management of Overdosage: Manifestations of Valium overdosage include somnolence, confusion, coma and diminished reflexes. Respiration, pulse and blood pressure should be monitored, as in all cases of drug overdosage, although, in general, these effects have been minimal following overdosage. General supportive measures should be employed, along with immediate gastric lavage. Intravenous fluids should be administered and an adequate airway maintained. Hypotension may be combated by the use of Levophed® (levarterenol) or Aramine (metaraminol). Dialysis is of limited value. As with the management of intentional overdosage with any drug, it should be borne in mind that multiple agents may have been ingested.

Withdrawal symptoms of the barbiturate type have occurred after the discontinuation of benzodiazepines. (See DRUG ABUSE AND DEPENDENCE section.)

PRECAUTIONS

If Valium is to be combined with other psychotropic agents or anticonvulsant drugs, careful consideration should be given to the pharmacology of the agents to be employed—particularly with known compounds which may potentiate the action of Valium, such as phenothiazines, narcotics, barbiturates, MAO inhibitors and other antidepressants. The usual precautions are indicated for severely depressed patients or those in whom there is any evidence of latent depression; particularly the recognition that suicidal tendencies may be present and protective measures may be necessary. The usual precautions in treating patients with impaired renal or hepatic function should be observed.

In elderly and debilitated patients, it is recommended that the dosage be limited to the smallest effective amount to preclude the development of ataxia or oversedation (2 mg to

Continued on next page

Roche Products—Cont.

2½ mg once or twice daily, initially, to be increased gradually as needed and tolerated).

The clearance of Valium and certain other benzodiazepines can be delayed in association with Tagamet (cimetidine) administration. The clinical significance of this is unclear.

Information for Patients: To assure the safe and effective use of benzodiazepines, patients should be informed that, since benzodiazepines may produce psychological and physical dependence, it is advisable that they consult with their physician before either increasing the dose or abruptly discontinuing this drug.

ADVERSE REACTIONS

Side effects most commonly reported were drowsiness, fatigue and ataxia. Infrequently encountered were confusion, constipation, depression, diplopia, dysarthria, headache, hypotension, incontinence, jaundice, changes in libido, nausea, changes in salivation, skin rash, slurred speech, tremor, urinary retention, vertigo and blurred vision. Paradoxical reactions such as acute hyperexcited states, anxiety, hallucinations, increased muscle spasticity, insomnia, rage, sleep disturbances and stimulation have been reported; should these occur, use of the drug should be discontinued.

Because of isolated reports of neutropenia and jaundice, periodic blood counts and liver function tests are advisable during long-term therapy. Minor changes in EEG patterns, usually low-voltage fast activity, have been observed in patients during and after Valium therapy and are of no known significance.

DRUG ABUSE AND DEPENDENCE

Withdrawal symptoms, similar in character to those noted with barbiturates and alcohol (convulsions, tremor, abdominal and muscle cramps, vomiting and sweating), have occurred following abrupt discontinuance of diazepam. The more severe withdrawal symptoms have usually been limited to those patients who had received excessive doses over an extended period of time. Generally milder withdrawal symptoms (*e.g.*, dysphoria and insomnia) have been reported following abrupt discontinuation of benzodiazepines taken continuously at therapeutic levels for several months. Consequently, after extended therapy, abrupt discontinuation should generally be avoided and a gradual dosage tapering schedule followed. Addiction-prone individuals (such as drug addicts or alcoholics) should be under careful surveillance when receiving diazepam or other psychotropic agents because of the predisposition of such patients to habituation and dependence.

DOSAGE AND ADMINISTRATION

Dosage should be individualized for maximum beneficial effect. While the usual daily dosages given below will meet the needs of most patients, there will be some who may require higher doses. In such cases dosage should be increased cautiously to avoid adverse effects.

Adults:	USUAL DAILY DOSE
Management of Anxiety Disorders and Relief of Symptoms of Anxiety	Depending upon severity of symptoms —2 mg to 10 mg, 2 to 4 times daily
Symptomatic Relief in Acute Alcohol Withdrawal.	10 mg, 3 or 4 times during the first 24 hours, reducing to 5 mg, 3 or 4 times daily as needed
Adjunctively for Relief of Skeletal Muscle Spasm.	2 mg to 10 mg, 3 or 4 times daily
Adjunctively in Convulsive Disorders.	2 mg to 10 mg, 2 to 4 times daily
Geriatric Patients, or in the presence of debilitating disease.	2 mg to 2½ mg, 1 or 2 times daily initially; increase gradually as needed and tolerated
Children: Because of varied responses to CNS-acting drugs, initiate therapy with lowest dose and increase as required. Not for use in children under 6 months.	1 mg to 2½ mg, 3 or 4 times daily initially; increase gradually as needed and tolerated

HOW SUPPLIED

For oral administration, round, scored tablets with a cut out "V" design—2 mg, white; 5 mg, yellow; 10 mg, blue—bottles of 100 and 500. Tel-E-Dose® packages of 100, available in boxes of 4 reverse-numbered cards of 25, and in boxes containing 10 strips of 10.

Imprint on tablets:

2 mg:
2 VALIUM® (front)
ROCHE (scored side)

5 mg:
5 VALIUM® (front)
ROCHE (scored side)

10 mg:
10 VALIUM® (front)
ROCHE (scored side)

P.I. 0788

Shown in Product Identification Section, page 425

Roerig
A division of Pfizer Pharmaceuticals
235 EAST 42nd STREET
NEW YORK, NY 10017

Product Identification Codes

To provide quick and positive identification of Roerig Division products, we have imprinted the product identification number of the National Drug Code on most tablets and capsules.

In order that you may quickly identify a product by its code number, we have compiled below a numerical list of code numbers with their corresponding product names. We are also listing the code numbers by alphabetical order of products.

Numerical Listing

Product Ident. Number	Product
035	Spectrobid® (bacampicillin HCl) Tablets, 400 mg., equivalent to 280 mg. ampicillin
092	Urobiotic®-250 (oxytetracycline HCl 250 mg. with sulfamethizole 250 mg. and phenazopyridine 50 mg.) Capsules
143	Geocillin® (carbenicillin indanyl sodium) Tablets, equivalent to 382 mg. carbenicillin
159	TAO® (troleandomycin) Capsules, 250 mg.
210	Antivert® (meclizine HCl) Tablets, 12.5 mg.
211	Antivert® /25 (meclizine HCl) Tablets, 25 mg.
212	Antivert® /25 (meclizine HCl) Chewable Tablets
214	Antivert® /50 (meclizine HCl) Tablets, 50 mg.
254	Marax® (ephedrine sulfate, 25 mg; theophylline, 130 mg; and Atarax® [hydroxyzine HCl], 10 mg) Tablets
411	Glucotrol® (glipizide) Tablets, 5 mg.
412	Glucotrol® (glipizide) Tablets, 10 mg.
504	Heptuna® Plus (iron plus vitamins and minerals), Capsules.
534	Sinequan® (doxepin HCl) Capsules 10 mg.
535	Sinequan® (doxepin HCl) Capsules 25 mg.
536	Sinequan® (doxepin HCl) Capsules 50 mg.
537	Sinequan® (doxepin HCl) Capsules 150 mg.
538	Sinequan® (doxepin HCl) Casules 100 mg.
539	Sinequan® (doxepin HCl) Capsules 75 mg.
560	Atarax® (hydroxyzine HCl) Tablets, 10 mg.
561	Atarax® (hydroxyzine HCl) Tablets, 25 mg.
562	Atarax® (hydroxyzine HCl) Tablets, 50 mg.
563	Atarax® (hydroxyzine HCl) Tablets, 100 mg.
571	Navane® (thiothixene) Capsules, 1 mg.
572	Navane® (thiothixene) Capsules, 2 mg.
573	Navane® (thiothixene) Capsules, 5 mg.
574	Navane® (thiothixene) Capsules, 10 mg.
577	Navane® (thiothixene) Capsules, 20 mg.

Alphabetical Listing

Prod. Ident. Number	Product
210	Antivert® (meclizine HCl) Tablets, 12.5 mg.
211	Antivert® /25 (meclizine HCl) Tablets, 25 mg.
212	Antivert® /25 (meclizine HCl) Chewable Tablets
214	Antivert® /50 (meclizine HCl) Tablets, 50 mg.
560	Atarax® (hydroxyzine HCl) Tablets, 10 mg.
561	Atarax® (hydroxyzine HCl) Tablets, 25 mg.
562	Atarax® (hydroxyzine HCl) Tablets, 50 mg.
563	Atarax® (hydroxyzine HCl) Tablets, 100 mg.
143	Geocillin® (carbenicillin indanyl sodium) Tablets equivalent to 382 mg. carbenicillin
411	Glucotrol® (glipizide) Tablets, 5 mg.
412	Glucotrol® (glipizide) Tablets, 10 mg.
504	Heptuna® Plus (iron plus vitamins and minerals), Capsules.
254	Marax® (ephedrine sulfate, 25 mg; theophylline, 130 mg; and Atarax® [hydroxyzine HCl], 10 mg) Tablets
571	Navane® (thiothixene) Capsules, 1 mg.
572	Navane® (thiothixene) Capsules, 2 mg.
573	Navane® (thiothixene) Capsules, 5 mg.
574	Navane® (thiothixene) Capsules, 10 mg.
577	Navane® (thiothixene) Capsules, 20 mg.
534	Sinequan® (doxepin HCl) Capsules 10 mg.
535	Sinequan® (doxepin HCl) Capsules 25 mg.
536	Sinequan® (doxepin HCl) Capsules 50 mg.
539	Sinequan® (doxepin HCl) Capsules 75 mg.
538	Sinequan® (doxepin HCl) Capsules 100 mg.
537	Sinequan® (doxepin HCl) Capsules 150 mg.
035	Spectrobid® (bacampicillin HCl) Tablets, 400 mg., equivalent to 280 mg. ampicillin
159	TAO® (troleandomycin) Capsules, 250 mg.
092	Urobiotic®-250 (oxytetracycline HCl 250 mg. with sulfamethizole 250 mg. and phenazopyridine 50 mg.) Capsules

ANTIVERT® TABLETS   ℞
[ăn ′tĭ-vert ″]
(12.5 mg. meclizine HCl)
ANTIVERT®/25 TABLETS   ℞
(25 mg. meclizine HCl)
ANTIVERT®/25 CHEWABLE TABLETS   ℞
(25 mg. meclizine HCl)
ANTIVERT®/50 TABLETS   ℞
(50 mg. meclizine HCl)

DESCRIPTION

Chemically, Antivert (meclizine HCl) is 1-(*p*-chloro-α-phenylbenzyl)-4-(*m*-methylbenzyl) piperazine dihydrochloride monohydrate.

Inert ingredients for the tablets are: dibasic calcium phosphate; magnesium stearate; polyethylene glycol; starch; sucrose. The 12.5 mg tablets also contain: Blue 1, The 25 mg tablets also contain: Yellow 6 Lake; Yellow 10 Lake. The 50 mg tablets also contain: Blue 1 Lake; Yellow 10 Lake.

Inert ingredients for the chewable tablets are: lactose, magnesium stearate; raspberry flavor; Red 40; saccharine sodium; siliceous earth; starch; talc.

ACTIONS

Antivert is an antihistamine which shows marked protective activity against nebulized histamine and lethal doses of intravenously injected histamine in guinea pigs. It has a marked effect in blocking the vasodepressor response to histamine, but only a slight blocking action against acetylcholine. Its activity is relatively weak in inhibiting the spasmogenic action of histamine on isolated guinea pig ileum.

INDICATIONS

Based on a review of this drug by the National Academy of Sciences-National Research Council and/or other information, FDA has classified the indications as follows:

Effective: Management of nausea and vomiting, and dizziness associated with motion sickness.

Possibly Effective: Management of vertigo associated with diseases affecting the vestibular system.

Final classification of the less than effective indications requires further investigation.

CONTRAINDICATIONS

Meclizine HCl is contraindicated in individuals who have shown a previous hypersensitivity to it.

WARNINGS

Since drowsiness may, on occasion, occur with use of this drug, patients should be warned of this possibility and cautioned against driving a car or operating dangerous machinery.

Patients should avoid alcoholic beverages while taking the drug. Due to its potential anticholinergic action, this drug should be used with caution in patients with asthma, glaucoma, or enlargement of the prostate gland.

USAGE IN CHILDREN:
Clinical studies establishing safety and effectiveness in children have not been done; therefore, usage is not recommended in children under 12 years of age.
USAGE IN PREGNANCY:
Pregnancy Category B. Reproduction studies in rats have shown cleft palates at 25–50 times the human dose. Epidemiological studies in pregnant women, however, do not indicate that meclizine increases the risk of abnormalities when administered during pregnancy. Despite the animal findings, it would appear that the possibility of fetal harm is remote. Nevertheless, meclizine, or any other medication, should be used during pregnancy only if clearly necessary.

ADVERSE REACTIONS

Drowsiness, dry mouth and, on rare occasions, blurred vision have been reported.

DOSAGE AND ADMINISTRATION

Vertigo:
For the control of vertigo associated with diseases affecting the vestibular system, the recommended dose is 25 to 100 mg. daily, in divided dosage, depending upon clinical response.
Motion Sickness:
The initial dose of 25 to 50 mg. of Antivert should be taken one hour prior to embarkation for protection against motion sickness. Thereafter, the dose may be repeated every 24 hours for the duration of the journey.

HOW SUPPLIED

Antivert—12.5 mg tablets: bottles of 100 (NDC 0662-2100-66), 1000 (NDC 0662-2100-82), and unit dose 100's (NDC 0662-2100-41).

Antivert/25—25 mg tablets: bottles of 100 (NDC 0662-2110-66), 1000 (NDC 0662-2110-82), and unit dose 100's (NDC 0662-2110-41).

Antivert/25 Chewable tablets—25 mg pink scored tablets: bottles of 100 (NDC 0662-2120-66), and 500 (NDC 0662-2120-73).

Antivert/50—50 mg tablets: bottles of 100 (NDC 0662-2140-66).

69-2148-37-7
Shown in Product Identification Section, page 425

ATARAX®   ℞
[ăt′ā-raks″]
(hydroxyzine hydrochloride)
TABLETS AND SYRUP

DESCRIPTION

Hydroxyzine hydrochloride is designated chemically as 1-(p-chlorobenzhydryl) 4-[2-(2-hydroxyethoxy)-ethyl] piperazine dihydrochloride.

Inert ingredients for the tablets are: acacia; carnauba wax; dibasic calcium phosphate; gelatin; lactose; magnesium stearate; precipitated calcium carbonate; shellac; sucrose; talc; white wax. The 10 mg tablets also contain: sodium hydroxide; starch; titanium dioxide; Yellow 6 Lake. The 25 mg tablets also contain: starch; velo dark green. The 50 mg tablets

also contain: starch; velo yellow. The 100 mg tablets also contain: alginic acid; Blue 1; polyethylene glycol; Red 3. The inert ingredients for the syrup are: alcohol; menthol; peppermint oil; sodium benzoate; spearmint oil; sucrose; water.

CLINICAL PHARMACOLOGY

Atarax is unrelated chemically to the phenothiazines, reserpine, meprobamate, or the benzodiazepines.

Atarax is not a cortical depressant, but its action may be due to a suppression of activity in certain key regions of the subcortical area of the central nervous system. Primary skeletal muscle relaxation has been demonstrated experimentally. Bronchodilator activity, and antihistaminic and analgesic effects have been demonstrated experimentally and confirmed clinically. An antiemetic effect, both by the apomorphine test and the veriloid test, has been demonstrated. Pharmacological and clinical studies indicate that hydroxyzine in therapeutic dosage does not increase gastric secretion or acidity and in most cases has mild antisecretory activity. Hydroxyzine is rapidly absorbed from the gastrointestinal tract and Atarax's clinical effects are usually noted within 15 to 30 minutes after oral administration.

INDICATIONS

For symptomatic relief of anxiety and tension associated with psychoneurosis and as an adjunct in organic disease states in which anxiety is manifested.

Useful in the management of pruritus due to allergic conditions such as chronic urticaria and atopic and contact dermatoses, and in histamine-mediated pruritus.

As a sedative when used as premedication and following general anesthesia. **Hydroxyzine may potentiate meperidine (Demerol®) and barbiturates,** so their use in pre-anesthetic adjunctive therapy should be modified on an individual basis. Atropine and other belladonna alkaloids are not affected by the drug. Hydroxyzine is not known to interfere with the action of digitalis in any way and it may be used concurrently with this agent.

The effectiveness of hydroxyzine as an antianxiety agent for long term use, that is more than 4 months, has not been assessed by systematic clinical studies. The physician should reassess periodically the usefulness of the drug for the individual patient.

CONTRAINDICATIONS

Hydroxyzine, when administered to the pregnant mouse, rat, and rabbit, induced fetal abnormalities in the rat and mouse at doses substantially above the human therapeutic range. Clinical data in human beings are inadequate to establish safety in early pregnancy. Until such data are available, hydroxyzine is contraindicated in early pregnancy.

Hydroxyzine is contraindicated for patients who have shown a previous hypersensitivity to it.

WARNINGS

Nursing Mothers: It is not known whether this drug is excreted in human milk. Since many drugs are so excreted, hydroxyzine should not be given to nursing mothers.

PRECAUTIONS

THE POTENTIATING ACTION OF HYDROXYZINE MUST BE CONSIDERED WHEN THE DRUG IS USED IN CONJUNCTION WITH CENTRAL NERVOUS SYSTEM DEPRESSANTS SUCH AS NARCOTICS, NON-NARCOTIC ANALGESICS AND BARBITURATES. Therefore when central nervous system depressants are administered concomitantly with hydroxyzine their dosage should be reduced. Since drowsiness may occur with use of this drug, patients should be warned of this possibility and cautioned against driving a car or operating dangerous machinery while taking Atarax. Patients should be advised against the simultaneous use of other CNS depressant drugs, and cautioned that the effect of alcohol may be increased.

ADVERSE REACTIONS

Side effects reported with the administration of Atarax (hydroxyzine hydrochloride) are usually mild and transitory in nature.

Anticholinergic: Dry mouth.

Central Nervous System: Drowsiness is usually transitory and may disappear in a few days of continued therapy or upon reduction of the dose. Involuntary motor activity including rare instances of tremor and convulsions have been reported, usually with doses considerably higher than those recommended. Clinically significant respiratory depression has not been reported at recommended doses.

OVERDOSAGE

The most common manifestation of Atarax overdosage is hypersedation. As in the management of overdosage with any drug, it should be borne in mind that multiple agents may have been taken.

If vomiting has not occurred spontaneously, it should be induced. Immediate gastric lavage is also recommended. General supportive care, including frequent monitoring of the vital signs and close observation of the patient, is indicated. Hypotension, though unlikely, may be controlled with intravenous fluids and Levophed® (levarterenol), or Aramine®

(metaraminol). Do not use epinephrine as Atarax counteracts its pressor action.

There is no specific antidote. It is doubtful that hemodialysis would be of any value in the treatment of overdosage with hydroxyzine. However, if other agents such as barbiturates have been ingested concomitantly, hemodialysis may be indicated. There is no practical method to quantitate hydroxyzine in body fluids or tissue after its ingestion or administration.

DOSAGE

For symptomatic relief of anxiety and tension associated with psychoneurosis and as an adjunct in organic disease states in which anxiety is manifested: in adults, 50–100 mg q.i.d.: children under 6 years, 50 mg daily in divided doses and over 6 years, 50–100 mg daily in divided doses.

For use in the management of pruritus due to allergic conditions such as chronic urticaria and atopic and contact dermatoses, and in histamine-mediated pruritus: in adults, 25 mg t.i.d. or q.i.d.; children under 6 years, 50 mg daily in divided doses and over 6 years, 50–100 mg daily in divided doses.

As a sedative when used as a premedication and following general anesthesia: 50–100 mg in adults, and 0.6 mg/kg in children.

When treatment is initiated by the intramuscular route of administration, subsequent doses may be administered orally.

As with all medications, the dosage should be adjusted according to the patient's response to therapy.

SUPPLY

Atarax Tablets
10 mg: 100's (NDC 0049-5600-66), 500's (NDC 0049-5600-73), Unit Dose 10 × 10's (NDC 0049-5600-41), and Unit of Use 40's (NDC 0049-5600-43)—orange tablets
25 mg: 100's (NDC 0049-5610-66), 500's (NDC 0049-5610-73), Unit Dose 10 × 10's (NDC 0049-5610-41), and Unit of Use 40's (NDC 0049-5610-43)—green tablets
50 mg: 100's (NDC 0049-5620-66), 500's (NDC 0049-5620-73), and Unit Dose 10 × 10's (NDC 0049-5620-41)—yellow tablets
Atarax 100 Tablets
100 mg: 100's (NDC 0049-5630-66), and Unit Dose 10 × 10's (NDC 0049-5630-41)—red tablets

Atarax Syrup
10 mg per teaspoon (5 ml): 1 pint bottles (NDC 0049-5590-93)
Alcohol Content—Ethyl Alcohol—0.5% v/v

BIBLIOGRAPHY

Available on request.

77-0618-00-4
Shown in Product Identification Section, page 426

CEFOBID®   ℞
[sĕf′ō-bĭd]
(cefoperazone sodium)
and cefoperazone sodium injection
For Intravenous or Intramuscular Use

DESCRIPTION

CEFOBID (cefoperazone sodium) is a sterile, semisynthetic, broad-spectrum, parenteral cephalosporin antibiotic for intravenous or intramuscular administration. It is the sodium salt of 7-[D(-)-α-(4-ethyl-2,3-dioxo-1-piperazinecarboxamido)-α-(4-hydroxyphenyl)acetamido]-3-[(1-methyl-1H-tetrazol-5-yl)thiomethyl]-3-cephem-4-carboxylic acid. Its chemical formula is $C_{25}H_{26}N_9NaO_8S_2$ with a molecular weight of 667.65. The structural formula is given below:

CEFOBID contains 34 mg sodium (1.5 mEq) per gram. CEFOBID is a white powder which is freely soluble in water. The pH of a 25% (w/v) freshly reconstituted solution varies between 4.5–6.5 and the solution ranges from colorless to straw yellow depending on the concentration.

CEFOBID in crystalline form is supplied in vials equivalent to 1 g or 2 g of cefoperazone and in Piggyback Units for intravenous administration equivalent to 1 g or 2 g cefoperazone. CEFOBID is also supplied premixed as a frozen, sterile, nonpyrogenic, iso-osmotic solution equivalent to 1 g or 2 g cefoperazone in plastic containers. After thawing, the solution is intended for intravenous use.

The plastic container is fabricated from specially formulated polyvinyl chloride. Solutions in contact with the plastic container can leach out certain of its chemical components in very small amounts within the expiration period, e.g., di 2-ethylhexyl phthalate (DEHP), up to 5 parts per million. However, the safety of the plastic has been confirmed in tests

Continued on next page

Roerig—Cont.

in animals according to the USP biological tests for plastic containers, as well as by tissue culture toxicity studies.

CLINICAL PHARMACOLOGY

High serum and bile levels of CEFOBID are attained after a single dose of the drug. Table 1 demonstrates the serum concentrations of CEFOBID in normal volunteers following either a single 15-minute constant rate intravenous infusion of 1, 2, 3 or 4 grams of the drug, or a single intramuscular injection of 1 or 2 grams of the drug.
[See table below].

The mean serum half-life of CEFOBID is approximately 2.0 hours, independent of the route of administration.

In vitro studies with human serum indicate that the degree of CEFOBID reversible protein binding varies with the serum concentration from 93% at 25 mcg/ml of CEFOBID to 90% at 250 mcg/ml and 82% at 500 mcg/ml.

CEFOBID achieves therapeutic concentrations in the following body tissues and fluids:

Tissue or Fluid	Dose	Concentration	
Ascitic Fluid	2 g	64	mcg/ml
Cerebrospinal Fluid (in patients with inflamed meninges)	50 mg/kg	1.8 mcg/ml to 8.0	mcg/ml
Urine	2 g	3,286	mcg/ml
Sputum	3 g	6.0	mcg/ml
Endometrium	2 g	74	mcg/g
Myometrium	2 g	54	mcg/g
Palatine Tonsil	1 g	8	mcg/g
Sinus Mucous Membrane	1 g	8	mcg/g
Umbilical Cord Blood	1 g	25	mcg/ml
Amniotic Fluid	1 g	4.8	mcg/ml
Lung	1 g	28	mcg/g
Bone	2 g	40	mcg/g

CEFOBID is excreted mainly in the bile. Maximum bile concentrations are generally obtained between one and three hours following drug administration and exceed concurrent serum concentrations by up to 100 times. Reported biliary concentrations of CEFOBID range from 66 mcg/ml at 30 minutes to as high as 6000 mcg/ml at 3 hours after an intravenous bolus injection of 2 grams.

Following a single intramuscular or intravenous dose, the urinary recovery of CEFOBID over a 12-hour period averages 20–30%. No significant quantity of metabolites has been found in the urine. Urinary concentrations greater than 2200 mcg/ml have been obtained following a 15-minute infusion of a 2 g dose. After an IM injection of 2 g, peak urine concentrations of almost 1000 mcg/ml have been obtained, and therapeutic levels are maintained for 12 hours.

Repeated administration of CEFOBID at 12-hour intervals does not result in accumulation of the drug in normal subjects. Peak serum concentrations, areas under the curve (AUC's), and serum half-lives in patients with severe renal insufficiency are not significantly different from those in normal volunteers. In patients with hepatic dysfunction, the serum half-life is prolonged and urinary excretion is increased. In patients with combined renal and hepatic insufficiencies, CEFOBID may accumulate in the serum.

CEFOBID has been used in pediatrics, but the safety and effectiveness in children have not been established. The half-life of CEFOBID in serum is 6–10 hours in low birth-weight neonates.

Microbiology

CEFOBID is active *in vitro* against a wide range of aerobic and anaerobic, gram-positive and gram-negative pathogens. The bactericidal action of CEFOBID results from the inhibition of bacterial cell wall synthesis. CEFOBID has a high degree of stability in the presence of beta-lactamases produced by most gram-negative pathogens. CEFOBID is usually active against organisms which are resistant to other beta-lactam antibiotics because of beta-lactamase production. CEFOBID is usually active against the following organisms *in vitro* and in clinical infections:

Gram-Positive Aerobes:
Staphylococcus aureus, penicillinase and non-penicillinase-producing strains
Staphylococcus epidermidis
Streptococcus pneumoniae (formerly *Diplococcus pneumoniae*)
Streptococcus pyogenes (Group A beta-hemolytic streptococci)
Streptococcus agalactiae (Group B beta-hemolytic streptococci)
Enterococcus (*Streptococcus faecalis, S. faecium* and *S. durans*)

Gram-Negative Aerobes:
Escherichia coli
Klebsiella species (including *K. pneumoniae*)
Enterobacter species
Citrobacter species
Haemophilus influenzae
Proteus mirabilis
Proteus vulgaris
Morganella morganii (formerly *Proteus morganii*)
Providencia stuartii
Providencia rettgeri (formerly *Proteus rettgeri*)
Serratia marcescens
Pseudomonas aeruginosa
Pseudomonas species
Some strains of *Acinetobacter calcoaceticus*
Neisseria gonorrhoeae

Anaerobic Organisms:
Gram-positive cocci (including *Peptococcus* and *Peptostreptococcus*)
Clostridium species
Bacteroides fragilis
Other *Bacteroides* species

CEFOBID is also active *in vitro* against a wide variety of other pathogens although the clinical significance is unknown. These organisms include: *Salmonella* and *Shigella* species, *Serratia liquefaciens, N. meningitidis, Bordetella pertussis, Yersinia enterocolitica, Clostridium difficile, Fusobacterium* species, *Eubacterium* species and beta-lactamase producing strains of *H. influenzae* and *N. gonorrhoeae.*

Susceptibility Testing:

Diffusion Technique. For the disk diffusion method of susceptibility testing, a 75 mcg CEFOBID diffusion disk should be used. Organisms should be tested with the CEFOBID 75 mcg disk since CEFOBID has been shown *in vitro* to be active against organisms which are found to be resistant to other beta-lactam antibiotics.

Tests should be interpreted by the following criteria:

Zone Diameter	Interpretation
Greater than or equal to 21 mm	Susceptible
16–20 mm	Moderately Susceptible
Less than or equal to 15 mm	Resistant

Quantitative procedures that require measurement of zone diameters give the most precise estimate of susceptibility. One such method which has been recommended for use with the CEFOBID 75 mcg disk is the NCCLS approved standard. (Performance Standards for Antimicrobic Disc Susceptibility Tests. Second Information Supplement Vol. 2 No. 2 pp. 49–69. Publisher—National Committee for Clinical Laboratory Standards, Villanova, Pennsylvania.)

A report of "susceptible" indicates that the infecting organism is likely to respond to CEFOBID therapy and a report of "resistant" indicates that the infecting organism is not likely to respond to therapy. A "moderately susceptible" report suggests that the infecting organism will be susceptible to CEFOBID if a higher than usual dosage is used or if the infection is confined to tissues and fluids (e.g., urine or bile) in which high antibiotic levels are attained.

Dilution Techniques. Broth or agar dilution methods may be used to determine the minimal inhibitory concentration (MIC) of CEFOBID. Serial twofold dilutions of CEFOBID should be prepared in either broth or agar. Broth should be inoculated to contain 5×10^5 organisms/ml and agar "spotted" with 10^4 organisms.

MIC test results should be interpreted in light of serum, tissue, and body fluid concentrations of CEFOBID. Organisms

inhibited by CEFOBID at 16 mcg/ml or less are considered susceptible, while organisms with MIC's of 17–63 mcg/ml are moderately susceptible. Organisms inhibited at CEFOBID concentrations of greater than or equal to 64 mcg/ml are considered resistant, although clinical cures have been obtained in some patients infected by such organisms.

INDICATIONS AND USAGE

CEFOBID is indicated for the treatment of the following infections when caused by susceptible organisms:

Respiratory Tract Infections caused by *S. pneumoniae, H. influenzae, S. aureus* (penicillinase and non-penicillinase producing strains), *S. pyogenes** (Group A beta-hemolytic streptococci), *P. aeruginosa, Klebsiella pneumoniae, E. coli, Proteus mirabilis,* and *Enterobacter* species.

Peritonitis and Other Intra-abdominal Infections caused by *E. coli, P. aeruginosa,** anaerobic and gram-negative bacilli (including *Bacteroides fragilis*).

Bacterial Septicemia caused by *S. pneumoniae, S. agalactiae**, *S. aureus, Pseudomonas aeruginosa**, *E. coli, Klebsiella* spp.,* Klebsiella pneumoniae* , Proteus species* (indolepositive and indole-negative), *Clostridium* spp.* and anaerobic gram-positive cocci.*

Infections of the Skin and Skin Structures caused by *S. aureus* (penicillinase and non-penicillinase producing strains), *S. pyogenes**, and *P. aeruginosa.*

Pelvic Inflammatory Disease, Endometritis, and Other Infections of the Female Genital Tract caused by *N. gonorrhoeae, S. epidermidis**, *S. agalactiae, E. coli, Clostridium* spp.,* *Bacteroides* species (including *Bacteroides fragilis*) and anaerobic gram-positive cocci.

Urinary Tract Infections caused by *Escherichia coli,* and *Pseudomonas aeruginosa.*

Enterococcal Infections: Although cefoperazone has been shown to be clinically effective in the treatment of infections caused by enterococci in cases of peritonitis and other intraabdominal infections, infections of the skin and skin structures, pelvic inflammatory disease, endometritis and other infections of the female genital tract, and urinary tract infection,* the majority of clinical isolates of enterococci tested are not susceptible to cefoperazone but fall just at or in the intermediate zone of susceptibilty, and are moderately resistant to cefoperazone. However, *in vitro* susceptibility testing may not correlate directly with *in vivo* results. Despite this, cefoperazone therapy has resulted in clinical cures of enterococcal infections, chiefly in polymicrobial infections. Cefoperazone should be used in enterococcal infections with care and at doses that achieve satisfactory serum levels of cefoperazone.

* Efficacy of this organism in this organ system was studied in fewer than 10 infections.

Susceptibility Testing

Before instituting treatment with CEFOBID, appropriate specimens should be obtained for isolation of the causative organism and for determination of its susceptibility to the drug. Treatment may be started before results of susceptibility testing are available.

Combination Therapy

Synergy between CEFOBID and aminoglycosides has been demonstrated with many gram-negative bacilli. However, such enhanced activity of these combinations is not predictable. If such therapy is considered, *in vitro* susceptibility tests should be performed to determine the activity of the drugs in combination, and renal function should be monitored carefully. (See PRECAUTIONS, and DOSAGE AND ADMINISTRATION sections).

CONTRAINDICATIONS

CEFOBID is contraindicated in patients with known allergy to the cephalosporin-class of antibiotics.

WARNINGS

BEFORE THERAPY WITH CEFOBID IS INSTITUTED, CAREFUL INQUIRY SHOULD BE MADE TO DETERMINE WHETHER THE PATIENT HAS HAD PREVIOUS HYPERSENSITIVITY REACTIONS TO CEPHALOSPORINS, PENICILLINS OR OTHER DRUGS. THIS PRODUCT SHOULD BE GIVEN CAUTIOUSLY TO PENICILLIN-SENSITIVE PATIENTS. ANTIBIOTICS SHOULD BE ADMINISTERED WITH CAUTION TO ANY PATIENT WHO HAS DEMONSTRATED SOME FORM OF ALLERGY, PARTICULARLY TO DRUGS. SERIOUS ACUTE HYPERSENSITIVITY REACTIONS MAY REQUIRE THE USE OF SUBCUTANEOUS EPINEPHRINE AND OTHER EMERGENCY MEASURES.

PSEUDOMEMBRANOUS COLITIS HAS BEEN REPORTED WITH THE USE OF CEPHALOSPORINS (AND OTHER BROAD-SPECTRUM ANTIBIOTICS); THEREFORE, IT IS IMPORTANT TO CONSIDER ITS DIAGNOSIS IN PATIENTS WHO DEVELOP DIARRHEA IN ASSOCIATION WITH ANTIBIOTIC USE.

Treatment with broad-spectrum antibiotics alters normal flora of the colon and may permit overgrowth of clostridia. Studies indicate a toxin produced by *Clostridium difficile* is one primary cause of antibiotic-associated colitis. Choles-

---

TABLE 1. Cefoperazone Serum Concentrations

	Mean Serum Concentrations (mcg/ml)						
Dose/Route	0*	0.5 hr	1 hr	2 hr	4 hr	8 hr	12 hr
1 g IV	153	114	73	38	16	4	0.5
2 g IV	252	153	114	70	32	8	2
3 g IV	340	210	142	89	41	9	2
4 g IV	506	325	251	161	71	19	6
1 g IM	32**	52	65	57	33	7	1
2 g IM	40**	69	93	97	58	14	4

* Hours post-administration, with 0 time being the end of the infusion.
** Values obtained 15 minutes post-injection.

tyramine and colestipol resins have been shown to bind the toxin *in vitro*.

Mild cases of colitis may respond to drug discontinuance alone.

Moderate to severe cases should be managed with fluid, electrolyte, and protein supplementation as indicated.

When the colitis is not relieved by drug discontinuance or when it is severe, oral vancomycin is the treatment of choice for antibiotic-associated pseudomembranous colitis produced by *C. difficile*. Other causes of colitis should also be considered.

PRECAUTIONS

Although transient elevations of the BUN and serum creatinine have been observed, CEFOBID alone does not appear to cause significant nephrotoxicity. However, concomitant administration of aminoglycosides and other cephalosporins has caused nephrotoxicity.

CEFOBID is extensively excreted in bile. The serum half-life of CEFOBID is increased 2–4 fold in patients with hepatic disease and/or biliary obstruction. In general, total daily dosage above 4 g should not be necessary in such patients. If higher dosages are used, serum concentrations should be monitored.

Because renal excretion is not the main route of elimination of CEFOBID (see CLINICAL PHARMACOLOGY), patients with renal failure require no adjustment in dosage when usual doses are administered. When high doses of CEFOBID are used, concentrations of drug in the serum should be monitored periodically. If evidence of accumulation exists, dosage should be decreased accordingly.

The half-life of CEFOBID is reduced slightly during hemodialysis. Thus, dosing should be scheduled to follow a dialysis period. In patients with both hepatic dysfunction and significant renal disease, CEFOBID dosage should not exceed 1–2 g daily without close monitoring of serum concentrations.

As with other antibiotics, vitamin K deficiency has occurred rarely in patients treated with CEFOBID. The mechanism is most probably related to the suppression of gut flora which normally synthesize this vitamin. Those at risk include patients with a poor nutritional status, malabsorption states (e.g., cystic fibrosis), alcoholism, and patients on prolonged hyper-alimentation regimens (administered either intravenously or via a naso-gastric tube). Prothrombin time should be monitored in these patients and exogenous vitamin K administered as indicated.

A disulfiram-like reaction characterized by flushing, sweating, headache, and tachycardia has been reported when alcohol (beer, wine) was ingested within 72 hours after CEFOBID administration. Patients should be cautioned about the ingestion of alcoholic beverages following the administration of CEFOBID. A similar reaction has been reported with other cephalosporins.

Prolonged use of CEFOBID may result in the overgrowth of nonsusceptible organisms. Careful observation of the patient is essential. If superinfection occurs during therapy, appropriate measures should be taken.

CEFOBID should be prescribed with caution in individuals with a history of gastrointestinal disease, particularly colitis.

Drug Laboratory Test Interactions

A false-positive reaction for glucose in the urine may occur with Benedict's or Fehling's solution.

Carcinogenesis, Mutagenesis, Impairment of Fertility

Long term studies in animals have not been performed to evaluate carcinogenic potential. The maximum duration of CEFOBID animal toxicity studies is six months. In none of the *in vivo* or *in vitro* genetic toxicology studies did CEFOBID show any mutagenic potential at either the chromosomal or subchromosomal level. CEFOBID produced no impairment of fertility and had no effects on general reproductive performance or fetal development when administered subcutaneously at daily doses up to 500 to 1000 mg/kg prior to and during mating, and to pregnant female rats during gestation. These doses are 10 to 20 times the estimated usual single clinical dose. CEFOBID had adverse effects on the testes of prepubertal rats at all doses tested. Subcutaneous administration of 1000 mg/kg per day (approximately 16 times the average adult human dose) resulted in reduced testicular weight, arrested spermatogenesis, reduced germinal cell population and vacuolation of Sertoli cell cytoplasm. The severity of lesions was dose dependent in the 100 to 1000 mg/kg per day range; the low dose caused a minor decrease in spermatocytes. This effect has not been observed in adult rats. Histologically the lesions were reversible at all but the highest dosage levels. However, these studies did not evaluate subsequent development of reproductive function in the rats. The relationship of these findings to humans is unknown.

Usage in Pregnancy

Pregnancy Category B: Reproduction studies have been performed in mice, rats, and monkeys at doses up to 10 times the human dose and have revealed no evidence of impaired fertility or harm to the fetus due to CEFOBID. There are, however, no adequate and well controlled studies in pregnant women. Because animal reproduction studies are not always predictive of human response, this drug should be used during pregnancy only if clearly needed.

Usage in Nursing Mothers

Only low concentrations of CEFOBID are excreted in human milk. Although CEFOBID passes poorly into breast milk of nursing mothers, caution should be exercised when CEFOBID is administered to a nursing woman.

Pediatric Use

Safety and effectiveness in children have not been established. For information concerning testicular changes in prepubertal rats (see Carcinogenesis, Mutagenesis, Impairment of Fertility).

ADVERSE REACTIONS

In clinical studies the following adverse effects were observed and were considered to be related to CEFOBID therapy or of uncertain etiology:

Hypersensitivity: As with all cephalosporins, hypersensitivity manifested by skin reactions (1 patient in 45), drug fever (1 in 260), or a change in Coombs' test (1 in 60) has been reported. These reactions are more likely to occur in patients with a history of allergies, particularly to penicillin.

Hematology: As with other beta-lactam antibiotics, reversible neutropenia may occur with prolonged administration. Slight decreases in neutrophil count (1 patient in 50) have been reported. Decreased hemoglobins (1 in 20) or hematocrits (1 in 20) have been reported, which is consistent with published literature on other cephalosporins. Transient eosinophilia has occurred in 1 patient in 10.

Hepatic: Of 1285 patients treated with cefoperazone in clinical trials, one patient with a history of liver disease developed significantly elevated liver function enzymes during CEFOBID therapy. Clinical signs and symptoms of nonspecific hepatitis accompanied these increases. After CEFOBID therapy was discontinued, the patient's enzymes returned to pre-treatment levels and the symptomatology resolved. As with other antibiotics that achieve high bile levels, mild transient elevations of liver function enzymes have been observed in 5–10% of the patients receiving CEFOBID therapy. The relevance of these findings, which were not accompanied by overt signs or symptoms of hepatic dysfunction, has not been established.

Gastrointestinal: Diarrhea or loose stools has been reported in 1 in 30 patients. Most of these experiences have been mild or moderate in severity and self-limiting in nature. In all cases, these symptoms responded to symptomatic therapy or ceased when cefoperazone therapy was stopped. Nausea and vomiting have been reported rarely.

Symptoms of pseudomembranous colitis can appear during or for several weeks subsequent to antibiotic therapy (see WARNINGS).

Renal Function Tests: Transient elevations of the BUN (1 in 16) and serum creatinine (1 in 48) have been noted.

Local Reactions: CEFOBID is well tolerated following intramuscular administration. Occasionally, transient pain (1 in 140) may follow administration by this route. When CEFOBID is administered by intravenous infusion some patients may develop phlebitis (1 in 120) at the infusion site.

DOSAGE AND ADMINISTRATION

The usual adult daily dose of CEFOBID is 2 to 4 grams per day administered in divided doses every 12 hours.

In severe infections or infections caused by less sensitive organisms, the total daily dose and/or frequency may be increased. Patients have been successfully treated with a total daily dosage of 6–12 grams divided into 2, 3 or 4 administrations ranging from 1.5 to 4 grams per dose.

In a pharmacokinetic study, a total daily dose of 16 grams was administered to severely immunocompromised patients by constant infusion without complications. Steady state serum concentrations were approximately 150 mcg/ml in these patients.

When treating infections caused by *Streptococcus pyogenes*, therapy should be continued for at least 10 days.

Solutions of CEFOBID and aminoglycoside should not be directly mixed, since there is a physical incompatibility between them. If combination therapy with CEFOBID and an aminoglycoside is contemplated (see INDICATIONS) this can be accomplished by sequential intermittent intravenous infusion provided that separate secondary intravenous tubing is used, and that the primary intravenous tubing is adequately irrigated with an approved diluent between doses. It is also suggested that CEFOBID be administered prior to the aminoglycoside. *In vitro* testing of the effectiveness of drug combination(s) is recommended

RECONSTITUTION

The following solutions may be used for the initial reconstitution of CEFOBID sterile powder:

Table 1. Solutions for Initial Reconstitution.

5% Dextrose Injection (USP)
5% Dextrose and 0.9% Sodium Chloride Injection (USP)
5% Dextrose and 0.2% Sodium Chloride Injection (USP)
10% Dextrose Injection (USP)
Bacteriostatic Water for Injection [Benzyl Alcohol or Parabens] (USP)*†

0.9% Sodium Chloride Injection (USP)
Normosol® M and Dextrose Injection
Normosol® R
Sterile Water for Injection*

* Not to be used as a vehicle for intravenous infusion
† Preparations containing Benzyl Alcohol should not be used in neonates.

General Reconstitution Procedures

CEFOBID sterile powder for intravenous or intramuscular use may be initially reconstituted with any compatible solution mentioned above in Table 1. Solutions should be allowed to stand after reconstitution to allow any foaming to dissipate to permit visual inspection for complete solubilization. Vigorous and prolonged agitation may be necessary to solubilize CEFOBID in higher concentrations (above 333 mg cefoperazone/ml). The maximum solubility of CEFOBID sterile powder is approximately 475 mg cefoperazone/ml of compatible diluent.

Preparation For Intravenous Use

General. CEFOBID concentrations between 2 mg/ml and 50 mg/ml are recommended for intravenous administration.

Preparation of Vials. Vials of CEFOBID sterile powder may be initially reconstituted with a minimum of 2.8 ml per gram of cefoperazone of any compatible reconstituting solution appropriate for intravenous administration listed above in Table 1. For ease of reconstitution the use of 5 ml of compatible solution per gram of CEFOBID is recommended. The entire quantity of the resulting solution should then be withdrawn for further dilution and administration using any of the following vehicles for intravenous infusion:

Table 2. Vehicles for Intravenous Infusion.

5% Dextrose Injection (USP)
5% Dextrose and Lactated Ringer's Injection
5% Dextrose and 0.9% Sodium Chloride Injection (USP)
5% Dextrose and 0.2% Sodium Chloride Injection (USP)
10% Dextrose Injection (USP)
Lactated Ringer's Injection (USP)
0.9% Sodium Chloride Injection (USP)
Normosol® M and 5% Dextrose Injection
Normosol® R

Preparation of Piggy Back Units. CEFOBID sterile powder in Piggy Back Units for intravenous use may be prepared by adding between 20 ml and 40 ml of any appropriate diluent listed in Table 2 per gram of cefoperazone. If 5% Dextrose and Lactated Ringer's Injection or Lactated Ringer's Injection (USP) is the chosen vehicle for administration the CEFOBID sterile powder should initially be reconstituted using 2.8–5 ml per gram of any compatible reconstituting solution listed in Table 1 prior to the final dilution.

The resulting intravenous solution should be administered in one of the following manners:

Intermittent Infusion: Solutions of CEFOBID should be administered over a 15–30 minute time period.

Continuous Infusion: CEFOBID can be used for continuous infusion after dilution to a final concentration of between 2 and 25 mg cefoperazone per ml.

Preparation For Intramuscular Injection

Any suitable solution listed above may be used to prepare CEFOBID sterile powder for intramuscular injection. When concentrations of 250 mg/ml or more are to be administered, a lidocaine solution should be used. These solutions should be prepared using a combination of Sterile Water for Injection and 2% Lidocaine Hydrochloride Injection (USP) that approximates a 0.5% Lidocaine Hydrochloride Solution. A two-step dilution process as follows is recommended: First, add the required amount of Sterile Water for Injection and agitate until CEFOBID powder is completely dissolved. Second, add the required amount of 2% lidocaine and mix.

[See table on bottom next page].

DIRECTIONS FOR USE OF CEFOBID (cefoperazone sodium) INJECTION IN PLASTIC CONTAINERS

CEFOBID supplied premixed as a frozen, sterile, iso-osmotic solution in plastic containers is to be administered either as continuous or intermittent infusion.

Thaw container at room temperature. After thawing, check for minute leaks by squeezing bag firmly. If leaks are found, discard solution as sterility may be impaired. Additives should not be introduced into this solution. Do not use if the solution is cloudy or precipitated or if the seal is not intact. After thawing, the solution is stable for 10 days if stored under refrigeration (5°C) and for 48 hours at room temperature. DO NOT REFREEZE. Use sterile equipment.

CAUTION: Do not use plastic container in series connections. Such use could result in air embolism due to residual air being drawn from the primary container before administration of the fluid from the secondary container is complete.

Preparation for administration

1. Suspend container from eyelet support.
2. Remove plastic protector from outlet port at bottom of container.
3. Attach administration set. Refer to complete directions accompanying set.

Continued on next page

Roerig—Cont.

Storage and Stability: CEFOBID sterile powder is to be stored at or below 25°C (77°F) and protected from light prior to reconstitution. After reconstitution, protection from light is not necessary.

The following parenteral diluents and approximate concentrations of CEFOBID provide stable solutions under the following conditions for the indicated time periods. (After the indicated time periods, unused portions of solutions should be discarded.)

[See table right].

HOW SUPPLIED

CEFOBID sterile powder is available in vials containing cefoperazone sodium equivalent to 1 gram cefoperazone × 10 (NDC 0049-1201-83), and 2 gram cefoperazone × 10 (NDC 0049-1202-83) for intramuscular and intravenous administration.

CEFOBID sterile powder is available in Piggyback Units containing cefoperazone sodium equivalent to 1 gram cefoperazone × 10 (NDC 0049-1211-83), and 2 gram cefoperazone × 10 (NDC 0049-1212-83) for intravenous administration.

CEFOBID (cefoperazone sodium) injection is supplied premixed as a frozen, sterile, nonpyrogenic, iso-osmotic solution in plastic containers. Each 50 mL unit contains cefoperazone sodium equivalent to 1 g cefoperazone with approximately 2.3 g dextrose hydrous USP added (NDC 0049-1216-18) or 2 g cefoperazone with approximately 1.8 g dextrose hydrous USP added (NDC 0049-1215-18). The solution is iso-osmotic (approximately 300 mOsmol/L), and solution pH may have been adjusted with sodium hydroxide and/or hydrochloric acid. Do not store above −20°C.

CEFOBID supplied as a frozen, sterile, nonpyrogenic, iso-osmotic solution in 50 ml plastic containers (NDC 0049-1215-18) is manufactured for Roerig Division of Pfizer Pharmaceuticals by Travenol Laboratories, Inc., Deerfield, IL 60015.

70-4169-00-3

EMETE-CON® ℞
[ă-mĕt 'ă-kŏn"]
(benzquinamide hydrochloride)
For Intramuscular and Intravenous Use

DESCRIPTION

Benzquinamide is a non-amine-depleting benzoquinolizine derivative, chemically unrelated to the phenothiazines and to other antiemetics.

Chemically, Emete-con (benzquinamide hy-drochloride) is N,N-diethyl-1,3,4,6,7,11b-hex-ahydro-2-hydroxy-9, 10-dimethoxy-2H-benzo-[a]quinolizine-3-carboxamide acetate hydrochloride. The empirical formula is $C_{22}H_{32}N_2O_5 \cdot HCl$ and the molecular weight is 441.

Emete-con for injection contains benzquinamide hydrochloride equivalent to 50 mg/vial of benzquinamide. When reconstituted with 2.2 ml of proper diluent, each vial yields 2 ml of a solution containing benzquinamide hydrochloride equivalent to 25 mg/ml of benzquinamide. When reconstituted this product maintains its potency for 14 days at room temperature.

ACTIONS

Benzquinamide HCl exhibited antiemetic, antihistaminic, mild anticholinergic and sedative action in animals. Studies conducted in dogs and human volunteers have demonstrated suppression of apomorphine-induced vomiting; however, relevance to clinical efficacy has not been established. The mechanism of action in humans is unknown. The onset of antiemetic activity in humans usually occurs within 15 minutes.

Benzquinamide metabolism has been studied in animals and in man. In both species, 5-10% of an administered dose is excreted unchanged in the urine. The remaining drug undergoes metabolic transformation in the liver by at least three pathways to a spectrum of metabolites which are excreted in the urine and in the bile, from which the more polar metabolites are not reabsorbed but are excreted in the feces.

Controlled Room Temperature (15°–25°C/59°–77°F) 24 Hours

	Approximate Concentrations
Bacteriostatic Water for Injection [Benzyl Alcohol or Parabens] (USP)	300 mg/ml
5% Dextrose Injection (USP)	2 mg to 50 mg/ml
5% Dextrose and Lactated Ringer's Injection	2 mg to 50 mg/ml
5% Dextrose and 0.9% Sodium Chloride Injection (USP)	2 mg to 50 mg/ml
5% Dextrose and 0.2% Sodium Chloride Injection (USP)	2 mg to 50 mg/ml
10% Dextrose Injection (USP)	2 mg to 50 mg/ml
Lactated Ringer's Injection (USP)	2 mg/ml
0.5% Lidocaine Hydrochloride Injection (USP)	300 mg/ml
0.9% Sodium Chloride Injection (USP)	2 mg to 300 mg/ml
Normosol® M and 5% Dextrose Injection	2 mg to 50 mg/ml
Normosol® R	2 mg to 50 mg/ml
Sterile Water for Injection	300 mg/ml

Reconstituted CEFOBID solutions may be stored in glass or plastic syringes, or in glass or flexible plastic parenteral solution containers.

Refrigerator Temperature (2°–8°C/36°–46°F) 5 Days

	Approximate Concentrations
Bacteriostatic Water for Injection [Benzyl Alcohol or Parabens] (USP)	300 mg/ml
5% Dextrose Injection (USP)	2 mg to 50 mg/ml
5% Dextrose and 0.9% Sodium Chloride Injection (USP)	2 mg to 50 mg/ml
5% Dextrose and 0.2% Sodium Chloride Injection (USP)	2 mg to 50 mg/ml
Lactated Ringer's Injection (USP)	2 mg/ml
0.5% Lidocaine Hydrochloride Injection (USP)	300 mg/ml
0.9% Sodium Chloride Injection (USP)	2 mg to 300 mg/ml
Normosol® M and 5% Dextrose Injection	2 mg to 50 mg/ml
Normosol® R	2 mg to 50 mg/ml
Sterile Water for Injection	300 mg/ml

Reconstituted CEFOBID solutions may be stored in glass or plastic syringes, or in glass or flexible plastic parenteral solution containers.

Freezer Temperature (−20° to −10°C/−4° to 14°F) 3 Weeks

	Approximate Concentrations
5% Dextrose Injection (USP)	50 mg/ml
5% Dextrose and 0.9% Sodium Chloride Injection (USP)	2 mg/ml
5% Dextrose and 0.2% Sodium Chloride Injection (USP)	2 mg/ml

5 Weeks

0.9% Sodium Chloride Injection (USP)	300 mg/ml
Sterile Water for Injection	300 mg/ml

Reconstituted CEFOBID solutions may be stored in plastic syringes, or in flexible plastic parenteral solution containers. Frozen samples should be thawed at room temperature before use. After thawing, unused portions should be discarded. Do not refreeze.

The half-life in plasma of Emete-con is about 40 minutes. More than 95% of an administered dose was excreted within 72 hours in animal studies using C14-labeled benzquinamide. In blood, benzquinamide is about 58% bound to plasma protein.

INDICATIONS

Emete-con is indicated for the prevention and treatment of nausea and vomiting associated with anesthesia and surgery.

Since the incidence of postoperative and postanesthetic vomiting has decreased with the adoption of modern techniques and agents, the prophylactic use of Emete-con should be restricted to those patients in whom emesis would endanger the results of surgery or result in harm to the patient.

CONTRAINDICATIONS

Emete-con is contraindicated in individuals who have demonstrated hypersensitivity to the drug.

WARNINGS

Use in Pregnancy
No teratogenic effects of benzquinamide were demonstrated in reproduction studies in chick embryos, mice, rats and rabbits. The relevance of these data to the human is not known. However, safe use of this drug in pregnancy has not been established and its use in pregnancy is not recommended.

Use in Children
As the data available at present are insufficient to establish proper dosage in children, the use of Emete-con in children is not recommended.

Intravenous use
Sudden increase in blood pressure and transient arrhythmias (premature ventricular and auricular contractions) have been reported following intravenous administration of benzquinamide. Until a more predictable pattern of the effect of intravenous benzquinamide has been estab-

lished, the intramuscular route of administration is considered preferable. The intravenous route of administration should be restricted to patients without cardiovascular disease and receiving no pre-anesthetic and/or concomitant cardiovascular drugs.

If patients receiving pressor agents or epinephrine-like drugs are also given benzquinamide, the latter should be given in fractions of the normal dose. Blood pressure should be monitored. Safeguards against hypertensive reactions are particularly important in hypertensive patients.

PRECAUTIONS

Benzquinamide, like other antiemetics, may mask signs of overdosage of toxic drugs or may obscure diagnosis of such conditions as intestinal obstruction and brain tumor.

ADVERSE REACTIONS

The following adverse reactions have been reported in subjects who have received benzquinamide. However, drowsiness appears to be the most common reaction. One case of pronounced allergic reaction has been encountered, characterized by pyrexia and urticaria.

System Affected

Autonomic Nervous System: Dry mouth, shivering, sweating, hiccoughs, flushing, salivation, blurred vision.

Cardiovascular System: Hypertension, hypotension, dizziness, atrial fibrillation, premature auricular and ventricular contractions.

Hypertensive episodes have occurred after IM and IV administration.

Central Nervous System: Drowsiness, insomnia, restlessness, headache, excitement, nervousness.

Gastrointestinal System: Anorexia, nausea.

Musculoskeletal System: Twitching, shaking/tremors, weakness.

Skin: Hives/rash.

Other Systems: Fatigue, shaking chills, increased temperature.

DOSAGE AND ADMINISTRATION

Intramuscular: 50 mg (0.5 mg/kg–1.0 mg/kg) First dose may be repeated in one hour with subsequent doses every 3-4 hours, as necessary. The precautions applicable to all intramuscular injections should be observed. Emete-con should be injected well within the mass of a larger muscle. The deltoid area should be used only if well developed. Injections should not be made into the lower and mid-thirds of the upper arm. Aspiration of the syringe should be carried out to avoid inadvertent intravascular injection. Therapeutic blood levels and demonstrable antiemetic activity appear within fifteen minutes of intramuscular administration. When the objective of therapy is the prevention of nausea and vomiting, intramuscular administration is recommended at least fifteen minutes prior to emergence from anesthesia.

	Final Cefoperazone Concentration	Step 1 Volume of Sterile Water	Step 2 Volume of 2% Lidocaine	Withdrawable Volume*†
1 g vial	333 mg/ml	2.0 ml	0.6 ml	3 ml
	250 mg/ml	2.8 ml	1.0 ml	4 ml
2 g vial	333 mg/ml	3.8 ml	1.2 ml	6 ml
	250 mg/ml	5.4 ml	1.8 ml	8 ml

When a diluent other than Lidocaine HCl Injection (USP) is used reconstitute as follows:

	Cefoperazone Concentration	Volume of Diluent to be Added		Withdrawable Volume*
1 g vial	333 mg/ml	2.6 ml		3 ml
	250 mg/ml	3.8 ml		4 ml
2 g vial	333 mg/ml	5.0 ml		6 ml
	250 mg/ml	7.2 ml		8 ml

* There is sufficient excess present to allow for withdrawal of the stated volume.
† Final lidocaine concentration will approximate that obtained if a 0.5% Lidocaine Hydrochloride Solution is used as diluent.

Intravenous: 25 mg (0.2 mg/kg–0.4 mg/kg as a single dose) administered slowly (1 ml per 0.5 to 1 minute). Subsequent doses should be given intramuscularly.

The intravenous route of administration should be restricted to patients without cardiovascular disease (See WARNINGS). If it is necessary to use Emete-con intravenously in elderly or debilitated patients, benzquinamide should be administered cautiously and the lower dose range is recommended.

This preparation must be initially reconstituted with 2.2 ml of Sterile Water for Injection, Bacteriostatic Water for Injection with benzyl alcohol or with methylparaben and propylparaben. This procedure yields 2 ml of a solution equivalent to 25 mg benzquinamide/ml, which maintains its potency for 14 days at room temperature.

OVERDOSAGE

Manifestations: On the basis of acute animal toxicology studies, gross Emete-con overdosage in humans might be expected to manifest itself as a combination of Central Nervous System stimulant and depressant effects. This speculation is derived from experimental studies in which intravenous doses of benzquinamide, at least 150 times the human therapeutic dose, were administered to dogs.

Treatment: There is no specific antidote for Emete-con overdosage. General supportive measures should be instituted, as indicated. Atropine may be helpful. Although there has been no direct experience with dialysis, it is not likely to be of value, since benzquinamide is extensively bound to plasma protein.

HOW SUPPLIED

Emete-con for IM/IV use is available in a vial containing benzquinamide HCl equivalent to 50 mg of benzquinamide in packages of 10 vials.

CAUTION

Federal law prohibits dispensing without prescription.

60-1787-00-4

GEOCILLIN® ℞

[gē 'ō-sil-ĭn]

(carbenicillin indanyl sodium)
TABLETS
For Oral Use

DESCRIPTION

Geocillin, a semisynthetic penicillin, is the sodium salt of the indanyl ester of Geopen® (carbenicillin disodium). The chemical name is:

1-(5-Indanyl)-N-(2-carboxy-3, 3-dimethyl-7-oxo-4-thia-I-aza-bicyclo[3.2.0] hept-6-yl)-2-phenyl-malonamate monosodium salt.

The structural formula is:

The empirical formula is: $C_{26}H_{25}N_2NaO_6S$ and mol. wt. is 516.55.

Geocillin tablets are yellow, capsule-shaped and film-coated, made of a white crystalline solid. Carbenicillin is freely soluble in water. Each Geocillin tablet contains 382 mg of carbenicillin, 118 mg of indanyl sodium ester. Each Geocillin tablet contains 23 mg of sodium.

Inert ingredients are: glycine; hydroxypropyl cellulose; hydroxypropyl methylcellulose; magnesium stearate; opaspray (which may include Blue 2 Lake, Yellow 6 Lake, Yellow 10 Lake, and other inert ingredients); sodium lauryl sulfate.

CLINICAL PHARMACOLOGY

Free carbenicillin is the predominant pharmacologically active fraction of Geocillin. Carbenicillin exerts its antibacterial activity by interference with final cell wall synthesis of susceptible bacteria.

Geocillin is acid stable, and rapidly absorbed from the small intestine following oral administration. It provides relatively low plasma concentrations of antibiotic and is primarily excreted in the urine. After absorption, Geocillin is rapidly converted to carbenicillin by hydrolysis of the ester linkage. Following ingestion of a single 500 mg tablet of Geocillin, a peak carbenicillin plasma concentration of approximately 6.5 mcg/ml is reached in 1 hour. About 30% of this dose is excreted in the urine unchanged within 12 hours, with another 6% excreted over the next 12 hours.

DRUG	DOSE	Mean Urine Concentration of Carbenicillin mcg/ml Hours After Initial Dose		
		0–3	3–6	6–24
Geocillin	1 tablet q.6 hr	1130	352	292
Geocillin	2 tablets q.6 hr	1428	789	809

Mean serum concentrations of carbenicillin in this study for these dosages are:

DRUG	DOSE	Mean Serum Concentration mcg/ml Hours After Initial Dose								
		½	1	2	4	6	24	25	26	28
Geocillin	1 tablet q.6 hr	5.1	6.5	3.2	1.9	0.0	0.4	8.8	5.4	0.4
Geocillin	2 tablets q.6 hr	6.1	9.6	7.9	2.6	0.4	0.8	13.2	12.8	3.8

In a multiple dose study utilizing volunteers with normal renal function, the following mean urine and serum levels of carbenicillin were achieved:
[See table above].

Microbiology

The antibacterial activity of Geocillin is due to its rapid conversion to carbenicillin by hydrolysis after absorption. Though Geocillin provides substantial *in vitro* activity against a variety of both gram-positive and gram-negative microorganisms, the most important aspect of its profile is in its antipseudomonal and antiproteal activity. Because of the high urine levels obtained following administration, Geocillin has demonstrated clinical efficacy in urinary infections due to susceptible strains of:

Escherichia coli
Proteus mirabilis
Proteus vulgaris
Morganella morganii (formerly *Proteus morganii*)
Pseudomonas species
Providencia rettgeri (formerly *Proteus rettgeri*)
Enterobacter species
Enterococci *(S. faecalis)*

In addition, *in vitro* data, not substantiated by clinical studies, indicate the following pathogens to be usually susceptible to Geocillin:

Staphylococcus species (nonpenicillinase producing)
Streptococcus species

Resistance

Most *Klebsiella* species are usually resistant to the action of Geocillin. Some strains of *Pseudomonas* species have developed resistance to carbenicillin.

Susceptibility Testing

Geopen (carbenicillin disodium) Susceptibility Powder or 100 ug. Geopen Susceptibility Discs may be used to determine microbial susceptibility to Geocillin using one of the following standard methods recommended by the National Committee for Clinical Laboratory Standards:

M2-A3, "Performance Standards for Antimicrobial Disk Susceptibility Tests"

M7-A, "Methods for Dilution Antimicrobial Susceptibility Tests for Bacteria that Grow Aerobically"

M11-A, "Reference Agar Dilution Procedure for Antimicrobial Susceptibility Testing of Anaerobic Bacteria"

M17-P, "Alternative Methods for Antimicrobial Susceptibility Testing of Anaerobic Bacteria"

Tests should be interpreted by the following criteria:

Organisms	Disk Diffusion Zone diameter (mm)		
	Suscept.	Intermed.	Resist.
Enterobacter	≥ 23	18–22	≤ 17
Pseudomonas sp.	≥ 17	14–16	≤ 13

Organisms	Dilution MIC (μ/ml)		
	Suscept.	Moderately Suscept.	Resist.
Enterobacter	≤ 16	32	≥ 64
Pseudomonas sp.	≤ 128	—	≥ 156

Interpretations of susceptible, intermediate, and resistant correlate zone size diameters with MIC values. A laboratory report of "susceptible" indicates that the suspected causative microorganism most likely will respond to therapy with carbenicillin. A laboratory report of "resistant" indicates that the infecting microorganism most likely will not respond to therapy. A laboratory report of "moderately susceptible" indicates that the microorganism is most likely susceptible if a high dosage of carbenicillin is used, or if the infection is such that high levels of carbenicillin may be attained as in urine. A report of "intermediate" using the disk diffusion method may be considered an equivocal result, and dilution tests may be indicated.

INDICATIONS AND USAGE

Geocillin (carbenicillin indanyl sodium) is indicated in the treatment of acute and chronic infections of the upper and lower urinary tract and in asymptomatic bacteriuria due to susceptible strains of the following organisms:

Escherichia coli
Proteus mirabilis
Morganella morganii (formerly *Proteus morganii*)
Providencia rettgeri (formerly *Proteus rettgeri*)
Proteus vulgaris
Pseudomonas
Enterobacter
Enterococci

Geocillin is also indicated in the treatment of prostatitis due to susceptible strains of the following organisms:

Escherichia coli
Enterococcus *(S. faecalis)*
Proteus mirabilis
Enterobacter sp.

WHEN HIGH AND RAPID BLOOD AND URINE LEVELS OF ANTIBIOTIC ARE INDICATED, THERAPY WITH GEOPEN (CARBENICILLIN DISODIUM) SHOULD BE INITIATED BY PARENTERAL ADMINISTRATION FOLLOWED, AT THE PHYSICIAN'S DISCRETION, BY ORAL THERAPY.

NOTE: Susceptibility testing should be performed prior to and during the course of therapy to detect the possible emergence of resistant organisms which may develop.

CONTRAINDICATIONS

Geocillin is ordinarily contraindicated in patients who have a known penicillin allergy.

WARNINGS

Serious and occasionally fatal hypersensitivity (anaphylactic) reactions have been reported in patients on oral penicillin therapy. Although anaphylaxis is more frequent following parenteral therapy, it has occurred in patients on oral penicillins. These reactions are more apt to occur in individuals with a history of penicillin hypersensitivity and/or a history of sensitivity to multiple allergens.

There have been reports of individuals with a history of penicillin hypersensitivity who have experienced severe hypersensitivity reactions when treated with a cephalosporin, and vice versa. Before initiating therapy with a penicillin, careful inquiry should be made concerning previous hypersensitivity reactions to penicillins, cephalosporins, or other allergens. If an allergic reaction occurs, the drug should be discontinued and the appropriate therapy instituted.

SERIOUS ANAPHYLACTOID REACTIONS REQUIRE IMMEDIATE EMERGENCY TREATMENT WITH EPINEPHRINE. OXYGEN, INTRAVENOUS STEROIDS AND AIRWAY MANAGEMENT, INCLUDING INTUBATION, SHOULD ALSO BE ADMINISTERED AS INDICATED.

PRECAUTIONS

General: As with any penicillin preparation, an allergic response, including anaphylaxis, may occur particularly in a hypersensitive individual.

Long term use of Geocillin may result in the overgrowth of nonsusceptible organisms. If superinfection occurs during therapy, appropriate measures should be taken.

Since carbenicillin is primarily excreted by the kidney, patients with severe renal impairment (creatinine clearance of less than 10 ml/min) will not achieve therapeutic urine levels of carbenicillin.

In patients with creatinine clearance of 10–20 ml/min it may be necessary to adjust dosage to prevent accumulation of drug.

Laboratory Tests: As with other penicillins, periodic assessment of organ system function including renal, hepatic, and hematopoietic systems is recommended during prolonged therapy.

Drug Interactions: Geocillin (carbenicillin indanyl sodium) blood levels may be increased and prolonged by concurrent administration of probenecid.

Continued on next page

Roerig—Cont.

Carcinogenesis, Mutagenesis, Impairment of Fertility: There are no long-term animal or human studies to evaluate carcinogenic potential. Rats fed 250–1000 mg/kg/day for 18 months developed mild liver pathology (e.g., bile duct hyperplasia) at all dose levels, but there was no evidence of drug-related neoplasia. Geocillin administered at daily doses ranging to 1000 mg/kg had no apparent effect on the fertility or reproductive performance of rats.

Pregnancy Category B: Reproduction studies have been performed at dose levels of 1000 or 500 mg/kg in rats, 200 mg/kg in mice, and at 500 mg/kg in monkeys with no harm to fetus due to Geocillin. There are, however, no adequate and well controlled studies in pregnant women. Because animal reproduction studies are not always predictive of human response, this drug should be used during pregnancy only if clearly needed.

Labor and Delivery: It is not known whether the use of Geocillin in humans during labor or delivery has immediate or delayed adverse effects on the fetus, prolongs the duration of labor, or increases the likelihood that forceps delivery or other obstetrical intervention or resuscitation of the newborn will be necessary.

Nursing Mothers: Carbenicillin class antibiotics are excreted in milk although the amounts excreted are unknown; therefore, caution should be exercised if administered to a nursing woman.

Pediatric Use: Since only limited clinical data is available to date in children, the safety of Geocillin administration in this age group has not yet been established.

ADVERSE REACTIONS

The following adverse reactions have been reported as possibly related to Geocillin administration in controlled studies which include 344 patients receiving Geocillin.

Gastrointestinal: The most frequent adverse reactions associated with Geocillin therapy are related to the gastrointestinal tract. Nausea, bad taste, diarrhea, vomiting, flatulence, and glossitis were reported. Abdominal cramps, dry mouth, furry tongue, rectal bleeding, anorexia, and unspecified epigastric distress were rarely reported.

Dermatologic: Hypersensitivity reactions such as skin rash, urticaria, and less frequently pruritus.

Hematologic: As with other penicillins, anemia, thrombocytopenia, leukopenia, neutropenia, and eosinophilia have infrequently been observed. The clinical significance of these abnormalities is not known.

Miscellaneous: Other reactions rarely reported were hyperthermia, headache, itchy eyes, vaginitis, and loose stools.

Abnormalities of Hepatic Function Tests: Mild SGOT elevations have been observed following Geocillin administration.

OVERDOSAGE

Geocillin is generally nontoxic. Geocillin when taken in excessive amounts may produce mild gastrointestinal irritation. The drug is rapidly excreted in the urine and symptoms are transitory. The usual symptoms of anaphylaxis may occur in hypersensitive individuals.

Carbenicillin blood levels achievable with Geocillin are very low, and toxic reactions as a function of overdosage should not occur systematically. The oral LD_{50} in mice is 3,600 mg/kg, in rats 2,000 mg/kg, and in dogs is in excess of 500 mg/kg. The lethal human dose is not known.

Although never reported, the possibility of accumulation of indanyl should be considered when large amounts of Geocillin are ingested. Free indole, which is a phenol derivative, may be potentially toxic. In general 8–15 grams of phenol, and presumably a similar amount of indole, are required orally before toxicity (peripheral vascular collapse) may occur. The metabolic by-products of indole are nontoxic. In patients with hepatic failure it may be possible for unmetabolized indole to accumulate.

The metabolic by-products of Geocillin, indanyl sulfate and glucuronide, as well as free carbenicillin, are dialyzable.

DOSAGE AND ADMINISTRATION

Geocillin is available as a coated tablet to be administered orally.

Usual Adult Dose

URINARY TRACT INFECTIONS	
Escherichia coli, Proteus species, and *Enterobacter*	1–2 tablets 4 times daily
Pseudomonas and *Enterococcus*	2 tablets 4 times daily
PROSTATITIS	
Escherichia coli, Proteus mirabilis, Enterobacter and *Enterococcus*	2 tablets 4 times daily

Organisms	Disk Diffusion Zone diameter (mm)			Dilution MIC (ug/ml)		
	Suscept.	Intermed.	Resist.	Suscept.	Moderately Suscept.	Resist.
Enterobacteriaceae	≥ 23	18–22	≤ 17	≤ 16	32	≥ 64
Pseudomonas sp.	≥ 17	14–16	≤ 13	≤ 128	—	≥ 156

HOW SUPPLIED

Geocillin is available as film-coated tablets in bottles of 100's (NDC 0049-1430-66), and unit-dose packages of 100 (10 × 10's) (NDC 0049-1430-41). Each tablet contains carbenicillin indanyl sodium equivalent to 382 mg of carbenicillin.

69-1970-00-0

Shown in Product Identification Section, page 426

GEOPEN®

[gē'ō-pen "]
sterile carbenicillin disodium
For Intramuscular and Intravenous Use

DESCRIPTION

Geopen (carbenicillin disodium) is a sterile semisynthetic injectable penicillin. Geopen is a benzyl penicillin derivative with substitution of alpha-carboxyl group in the benzyl side chain.

Chemically, carbenicillin disodium is N-(2-carboxy-3,3-dimethyl-7-oxo-4-thia-1-azabicyclo [3.2.0] hept-6-yl)-2-phenylmalonamic disodium acid. The empirical formula is $C_{17}H_{16}O_6N_2S\text{-}Na_2$, and molecular weight is 422.4.

Structural Formula

Carbenicillin Disodium

Geopen is a fine white or slightly off-white amorphous hygroscopic powder, readily soluble in water, which yields a clear solution upon reconstitution by label directions.

The normal range of pH for reconstituted Geopen is from pH 6.0 to 8.0. The pKa of Geopen is 3.3 and it is completely ionized in the blood.

Geopen contains a maximum concentration of 4% sodium benzylpenicillin. Available preparations of Geopen contain 5.3 mEq of sodium per gram, however, the actual vial content may be as high as 6.5 mEq of sodium per gram.

CLINICAL PHARMACOLOGY

Geopen interferes with final cell wall synthesis of susceptible bacteria.

Geopen (carbenicillin disodium) must be administered parenterally since it is not acid stable and is not absorbed from the gastrointestinal tract. Geopen is about 50% reversibly protein bound in plasma and its tissue distribution is similar to other penicillins.

After intravenous administration of a 2 gram Geopen dose (15 min. infusion) peak mean serum antibiotic concentrations of approximately 240.7 mcg/ml are attained at the end of the infusion. Serum carbenicillin levels of 43.7 mcg/ml and 1.2 mcg/ml are found at two and six hours. After a 6 gram Geopen dose (15 min. infusion) a mean peak serum level of 673.8 mcg/ml is obtained at the end of the infusion. Serum carbenicillin levels of 185.3 mcg/ml and 15.7 mcg/ml are found at two and six hours. In patients with normal hepatic and renal function, the serum half-life of carbenicillin is approximately one hour. The serum half-life of carbenicillin is markedly increased in patients with impaired renal function, and to an even greater extent in patients with combined hepatic dysfunction and renal failure. (See DOSAGE AND ADMINISTRATION section for guidelines on dosage adjustment.)

Geopen is excreted unchanged primarily by the kidney and about 75 to 85% of a dose is recoverable in its active form in the urine in 9 hours. After an IM dose of 0.5 to 2 grams, a urine concentration of 1,000 to 5,000 mcg/ml may be achieved. Pretreatment with oral probenecid results in

higher and more prolonged Geopen serum levels as noted in the following table.
[See table below.]

Microbiology: Though Geopen has substantial *in vitro* activity against a variety of both gram-positive and gram-negative microorganisms, the most important aspect of its profile is in its antipseudomonal and antiproteal effect.

While *in vitro* studies have demonstrated the susceptibility of most strains of the following organisms, clinical efficacy for infections other than those included in the INDICATIONS AND USAGE section has not been documented.

- *Staphylococcus aureus* (Non-penicillinase producing)
- *Staphylococcus epidermidis*
- *Streptococcus pneumoniae*
- Beta-hemolytic *Streptococci*
- *Streptococcus faecalis*
- *Proteus vulgaris*
- *Escherichia coli*
- *Salmonella* species
- *Pseudomonas aeruginosa*
- *Hemophilus influenzae*
- *Neisseria* species
- *Enterobacter* species
- *Proteus mirabilis*
- *Morganella morganii* (formerly *Proteus rettgeri*)
- *Providencia rettgeri* (formerly *Proteus rettgeri*)
- Anaerobic bacteria, including:
- *Bacteroides* species
- *Peptostreptococcus* species
- *Peptococcus* species
- *Clostridium* species
- *Fusobacterium* species

In vitro synergism between Geopen and aminoglycosides in certain strains of *Pseudomonas aeruginosa* has been demonstrated.

Some of the pathogenic strains of such microorganisms as *Herellea, Mima, Citrobacter* and *Serratia* have shown susceptibility to Geopen.

Resistance: Most *Klebsiella* species and some *Serratia* species are usually resistant to the action of Geopen. Some strains of *Pseudomonas* have developed resistance to Geopen fairly rapidly.

Geopen is not stable in the presence of penicillinase producing bacteria.

In vitro synergism between Geopen and aminoglycoside antibiotics in certain strains of *Pseudomonas aeruginosa* has been demonstrated.

Susceptibility Testing

Geopen (Carbenicillin disodium) Susceptibility Powder or 100 ug Geopen Susceptibility Discs may be used to determine microbial susceptibility to Geopen using one of the following standard methods recommended by the National Committee for Clinical Laboratory Standards:

M2-A3, "Performance Standards for Antimicrobial Disk Susceptibility Tests"

M7-A, "Methods for Dilution Antimicrobial Susceptibility Tests for Bacteria that Grow Aerobically"

M11-A, "Reference Agar Dilution Procedure for Antimicrobial Susceptibility Testing of Anaerobic Bacteria"

M17-P, "Alternative Methods for Antimicrobial Susceptibility Testing of Anaerobic Bacteria"

Tests should be interpreted by the following criteria:
[See table above.]

Interpretations of susceptible, intermediate, and resistant correlate zone size diameters with MIC values. A laboratory report of "susceptible" indicates that the suspected causative microorganism most likely will respond to therapy with carbenicillin. A laboratory report of "resistant" indicates that the infecting microorganism most likely will not respond to therapy. A laboratory report of "moderately susceptible" indicates that the microorganism is most likely susceptible if

CARBENICILLIN BLOOD LEVELS AND URINARY EXCRETION

DOSAGE	ROUTE	SERUM LEVELS mcg/ml								Urinary excretion of administered dose 0–9 hours
		¼ hr.	½ hr.	1 hr.	2 hr.	3 hr.	4 hr.	6 hr.	8 hr.	
500 mg.	IM	8	10	13	9.8	6.5	3.2	0	—	85%
1000 mg.	IM	—	13	18	15	12	7.5	1.7	0.7	74.6%*
2000 mg.	IM	26	38	47	37	25	15	5.9	1.2	79%
1000 mg.	IV	71	45	31	14	8.2	3	0	—	73%
1000 mg. + 1 g probenecid	IV Oral	72	55	40	26	17	12	6.5	2.0	74%
*0–24 hr. collection										

a high dosage of carbenicillin is used, or if the infection is such that high levels of carbenicillin may be attained as in urine. A report of "intermediate" using the disk diffusion method may be considered an equivocal result, and dilution tests may be indicated.

INDICATIONS AND USAGE

Geopen is indicated for the treatment of the following infections when caused by susceptible organisms:

Bacterial Septicemia caused by *Hemophilus influenzae*, *Streptoccus pneumoniae* and susceptible anaerobic bacteria.

Urinary Tract Infections caused by *Pseudomonas aeruginosa*, *Proteus* species (particularly indole positive strains), certain strains of *Escherichia coli*, *Neisseria gonorrhoeae*, and *Streptoccus faecalis* (enteroccus).

Respiratory Tract Infections due to susceptible isolates including susceptible anaerobic bacteria.

Skin and Skin Structure Infections due to susceptible isolates including susceptible anaerobic bacteria.

Peritonitis and Other Intra-abdominal Infections resulting from anaerobic organisms resident in the normal gastrointestinal tract.

Pelvic Inflammatory Disease, Endometritis, and Other Infections of the Female Genital Tract caused by susceptible anaerobic bacteria.

CONTRAINDICATIOS

Geopen is ordinarily contraindicated in patients who have a known penicillin allergy.

WARNINGS

Serious and occasional fatal hypersensitivity (anaphylactic) reactions have been reported in patients on penicillin therapy. These reactions are more apt to occur in individuals with a history of sensitivity to multiple allergens.

Patients with renal impairment should be observed for bleeding manifestations. Such patients should be dosed strictly according to recommendations (see Dosage and Administration section). If bleeding manifestations appear, the antibiotic should be discontinued and appropriate therapy be instituted.

There have been reports of individuals with a history of penicillin hypersensitivity reactions who have experienced severe hypersensitivity reactions when treated with a cephalosporin. Before therapy with a penicillin, careful inquiry should be made concerning previous hypersensitivity reactions to penicillins, cephalosporins, and other allergens. If an allergic reaction occurs, appropriate therapy should be instituted and discontinuance of carbenicillin therapy considered, unless, in the opinion of the physician the condition being treated is life threatening and amenable only to carbenicillin therapy. The usual agents (antihistamines, pressor amines and corticosteroids) should be readily available.

SERIOUS ANAPHYLACTOID REACTIONS REQUIRE IMMEDIATE EMERGENCY TREATMENT WITH EPINEPHRINE. OXYGEN AND INTRAVENOUS CORTICOSTEROIDS SHOULD ALSO BE ADMINISTERED AS INDICATED.

Pediatric Use: Diluents for reconstitution of Geopen containing benzyl alcohol should not be used in neonates.

PRECAUTIONS

While Geopen (carbenicillin disodium) exhibits the characteristic low toxicity of the penicillin group of antibiotics, as with any other potent agent, it is advisable to check periodically for organ system dysfunction, including renal, hepatic and hematopoietic systems, during prolonged therapy.

Emergence of resistant organisms, such as *Klebsiella* spp., and *Serratia* spp., which may cause superinfection, should be kept in mind.

Geopen is a disodium salt of carboxybenzylpenicillin and hence each gram of Geopen contains 5.3 mEq. of sodium. The actual vial content may be as high as 6.5 mEq./g of sodium. In patients where sodium restriction is necessary, such as cardiac patients, periodic electrolyte determinations and monitoring of cardiac status should be made.

In a few patients receiving high doses of Geopen, hypokalemia has been reported. Periodic serum potassium determinations should be made and corrective measures should be implemented when necessary.

As with any penicillin preparation, an allergic response, including anaphylaxis, may occur particularly in a hypersensitive individual.

Cases of gonorrhea with a suspected primary lesion of syphilis should have dark field examinations before treatment. In all other cases where concomitant syphilis is suspected, monthly serological tests should be made for a minimum of 4 months.

Drug Interactions: Geopen may be synergistic with aminoglycosides when used in combination for *Pseudomonas* infections.

Probenecid increases and prolongs carbenicillin blood levels when administered concurrently.

Laboratory Tests: Positive Coomb's tests have been reported after large IV doses of carbenicillin.

Carcinogenesis, Mutagenesis, Impairment of Fertility: Fertility studies in animals were not conducted since Geopen would usually be given over a short period of time. There are

ADULTS:

	Pseudomonas	Proteus and E. coli	Enterobacter and S. faecalis	Anaerobes	H. influenzae and S. pneumoniae
Urinary Tract Infections					
Serious	200 mg/kg/ day by I.V. drip	200 mg/kg/ day by I.V. drip	200 mg/kg/ day by I.V. drip		
Uncomplicated	1–2 g I.M. or I.V. every 6 hours	1–2 g I.M. or I.V. every 6 hours	1–2 g I.M. or I.V. every 6 hours		
Severe Systemic Infections Septicemia Respiratory Infections Soft Tissue Infections	400–500 mg/ kg/day (30–40 grams) I.V. in divided doses or continuously	300–400 mg/ kg/day (20–30 grams) I.V. in divided doses or continuously		400–500 mg/ kg/day (30–40 grams) I.V. in divided doses or continuously	
Infections complicated by renal insufficiency (Creatinine clearance less than 5 ml/min)		2 g I.V.[1] every 8–12 hours			
Meningitis				400–500 mg/kg/day (30–40 grams) I.V. in divided doses or continuously	
During peritoneal dialysis		2 g I.V. every 6 hours			
During hemodialysis		2 g I.V. every 4 hours			

(1) The serum half-life of Geopen in patients with severe renal failure is 12.5 hours. As a consequence 2 grams of Geopen administered intravenously to these patients every 8–12 hours will give Geopen serum levels of approximately 100 mcg/ml, a level notably free of any untoward effects while adequate for treatment of a majority of the infections amenable to Geopen therapy.

Treatment of gonorrhea[2]; acute uncomplicated ano-genital and urethral infections due to ***N. gonorrhoeae.***

SINGLE 4 g I.M. injection, divided between 2 sites.

(2) Probenecid in a dosage of 1 gram may be administered orally about 30 minutes prior to the I.M. treatment of acute gonorrhoeal infections. For complete information and dosage of probenecid, refer to manufacturer's product information.

---

no adequate or controlled studies in pregnant women. There are no long term animal or human studies to evaluate carcinogenic potential. Rats fed 250–1000 mg/kg/day for 18 months developed mild liver pathology (e.g., bile duct hyperplasia) at all dose levels, but there was no evidence of drug related neoplasia. Geocillin administered at daily doses ranging to 1000 mg/kg had no apparent effect on the fertility or reproductive performance of rats.

Pregnancy Category B: Reproduction studies have been performed in mice and rats at doses up to and including 500 mg/kg/day subcutaneously and have revealed no evidence of impaired fertility or harm to fetus due to Geopen. There are, however, no adequate and well controlled studies in pregnant women. Because animal reproduction studies are not always predictive of human response, this drug should be used during pregnancy only if clearly needed.

Labor and Delivery: It is not known whether the use of Geopen in humans during labor or delivery has immediate or delayed adverse effects on the fetus, prolongs the duration of labor, or increases the likelihood that forceps delivery or other obstetrical intervention or resuscitation of the newborn will be necessary.

Nursing Mothers: Carbenicillin class antibiotics are excreted in milk, therefore, caution should be exercised if administered to a nursing woman.

Pediatric Use: Guidelines for administration of this drug to pediatric patients are presented in DOSAGE AND ADMINISTRATION (also see WARNINGS).

ADVERSE REACTIONS

Adverse reactions possibly related to Geopen administration have been reported. Pain at the injection site appears to be the most common reaction after IM injection, occurring in 40–60% of both adult and pediatric patients. Some induration has been observed in approximately 6% of these cases. Phlebitis has also been reported when Geopen was employed IV without further dilution.

The following adverse reactions have been reported in controlled studies which include 205 adults and 250 children receiving parenteral Geopen:

Hypersensitivity Reactions: Rash and urticaria, pruritus, edema, drug fever, and anaphylactic reactions.

Gastrointestinal Effects: Nausea, diarrhea, gastrointestinal disturbance, vomiting in children.

Central Nervous System: As with other penicillins, convulsions or neuromuscular irritability could occur with excessively high serum levels.

Hemic and Lymphatic Systems: As with other penicillins, anemia, thrombocytopenia, leukopenia, neutropenia, and eosinophilia may possibly occur.

Laboratory Tests: As with other semisynthetic penicillins, SGOT and SGPT elevations have been observed after Geopen administration (particularly in children). In all studies to date, no clinical manifestations of hepatic or renal disorders have been demonstrated.

Serum sodium determinations will help detect hypernatremia.

Other: Several uremic patients receiving high doses (24 grams/day) have developed hemorrhagic manifestations associated with abnormalities of coagulation tests such as clotting time and prothrombin time. On withdrawal of the antibiotic, the bleeding ceased. The exact relationship of these findings to carbenicillin therapy is not clear.

OVERDOSAGE

Neurologic adverse reactions, including convulsions, may occur with attainment of high CSF levels of beta-lactams. Carbenicillin is dialyzable. In case of overdosage, discontinue medication, treat symptomatically, and institute supportive measures as required.

DOSAGE AND ADMINISTRATION

Indication: Clinical experience indicates that in serious urinary tract and systemic infections intravenous therapy in the higher doses should be used. The recommended maximum dose is 40 g per day. Intramuscular injections should not exceed 2 g per injection.

[See Adults table above].

[See Children's table on bottom next page].

Seriously ill patients should receive the higher doses. Geopen has proved to be useful in infections in which protective mechanisms are impaired, such as in acute leukemia and during therapy with immunosuppressive or oncolytic drugs.

Intramuscular Use

As with all intramuscular preparations, Geopen should be injected well within the body of a relatively large muscle. Adults: The preferred site is the upper outer quadrant of the buttock (i.e., gluteus maximus), or the mid-lateral thigh.

Children: It is recommended that intramuscular injections be given preferably in the midlateral muscles of the thigh. In infants and small children the periphery of the upper outer quadrant of the gluteal region should be used only when necessary, such as in burn patients, in order to minimize the possibility of damage to the sciatic nerve.

The deltoid area should be used only if well developed such as in certain adults and older children, and then only with caution to avoid radial nerve injury. Intramuscular injections should not be made into the lower and mid-third of the upper arm. As with all intramuscular injections, aspiration is necessary to help avoid inadvertent injection into a blood vessel.

Intravenous Use

As with all intravenous administrations, particular attention should be directed to insure that the drug is injected only into a vein (including aspiration and proper anatomical site selection) to avoid either intra-arterial injection or extravasation.

PREPARATION OF SOLUTIONS

For Intramuscular Use: The 2 g vial should be reconstituted with 4.0 ml of Sterile Water for Injection, 0.5% Lidocaine Hydrochloride (without epinephrine), or Bacteriostatic Water containing 0.9% benzyl alcohol. (Preparations containing

Continued on next page

Roerig—Cont.

benzyl alcohol should not be used in neonates.) In order to facilitate reconstitution up to 7.2 ml of diluent can be used.

Amount of Diluent to be Added to the 2 g Vial	Volume to be Withdrawn for a 1 g Dose
4.0 ml	2.5 ml
5.0 ml	3.0 ml
7.2 ml	4.0 ml

The 5 g vial should be reconstituted with 7.0 ml of Sterile Water for Injection, 0.5% Lidocaine Hydrochloride (without epinephrine), or Bacteriostatic Water containing 0.9% benzyl alcohol. (Preparations containing benzyl alcohol should not be used in neonates.) In order to facilitate reconstitution, up to 17 ml of diluent can be used.

Amount of Diluent to be Added to the 5 g Vial	Volume to be Withdrawn for a 1 g Dose
7.0 ml	2.0 ml
9.5 ml	2.5 ml
12.0 ml	3.0 ml
17.0 ml	4.0 ml

After reconstitution, no significant loss of potency occurs for up to 24 hours at room temperature, and for 72 hours if refrigerated. Any of these unused solutions should be discarded.

For Direct Intravenous Injection: Following reconstitution, each gram should be further diluted by no less than 5 ml Sterile Water for Injection or other suitable diluent listed in Table 1. In order to avoid vein irritation, the solution should be administered as slowly as possible.

For Intravenous Infusion: Following reconstitution, according to directions, Geopen (carbenicillin disodium) may be added to the desired volume of usual intravenous infusion solutions.

When Using the Bulk Pharmacy Package for Intravenous Use: As with all intravenous administrations, particular attention should be directed to insure that the drug is injected only into a vein (including aspiration and proper anatomical site selection) to avoid either intra-arterial injection or extravasation.

Bulk Pharmacy Package: The 30 gram vial should be reconstituted by adding 80 ml of any compatible diluent listed in Table 1, in two separate 40 ml aliquots. Add 40 ml, shake 25 seconds and add the last 40 ml aliquot and shake for final solution. The resulting solution will contain 300 mg/ml of carbenicillin. Transfer recommended dosage to appropriate intravenous infusion solution.

> **Reconstituted bulk solution should not be used for direct infusion.**

After reconstitution of the Bulk Pharmacy Package, no significant loss of potency occurs for 24 hours at room tempera-

ture and for 72 hours if refrigerated. Discard unused portions held longer than these time periods.

For Continuous Intravenous Infusion: After reconstitution as directed, Geopen (carbenicillin disodium) may be added to the desired volume of usual intravenous infusion solutions. Studies of Geopen at concentrations of 10 mg/ml in intravenous infusion diluents listed in Table 1 indicate no significant loss of potency when stored at room temperature and under refrigeration (5°C) for the time periods stated: [See table above].

It is recommended that Geopen and aminoglycosides not be mixed together in the same IV solution due to the gradual inactivation of aminoglycosides under these circumstances. The therapeutic effect of the two drugs remains unimpaired when administered separately.

For Intramuscular Use Only: Geopen for intramuscular injection ONLY may be diluted with one of the following:
1. 0.5% Lidocaine Hydrochloride (without epinephrine).
2. Bacteriostatic Water containing 0.9% Benzyl Alcohol. (Preparations containing benzyl alcohol should not be used in neonates.)

For reconstitution of Geopen with these diluents for intramuscular use ONLY, follow the directions for the amount of diluent in the **PREPARATION OF SOLUTION, For Intramuscular Use** section.

Geopen may be diluted with these solutions and stored for up to 24 hours at room temperature or for 72 hours when refrigerated. Discard unused solutions stored longer than these time periods.

For full product information, refer to the package insert for Lidocaine Hydrochloride (without epinephrine).

HOW SUPPLIED

Geopen is available in 2 g (NDC 0049-1417-83), and 5 g (NDC 0049-1419-83) vials for intramuscular/intravenous use.

Table 1. Solutions For Continuous Intravenous Infusion

Intravenous Solution	Stability Room Temperature	Refrigerated
Sterile water for injection	72 hours	14 days
Sodium chloride injection, USP	72 hours	14 days
Dextrose injection, USP (5%)	72 hours	14 days
Ringer's injection, USP	72 hours	14 days
Dextrose 5% with 0.255% sodium chloride	24 hours	3 days
Lactated Ringer's injection, USP	24 hours	3 days
5% dextrose with electrolyte #48	24 hours	3 days
5% Levugen (fructose) with electrolyte #75	24 hours	3 days
Invert sugar 10% in water	24 hours	3 days
Dextrose 5% and 0.45% sodium chloride, USP	24 hours	3 days
5% alcohol, 5% dextrose in water	24 hours	3 days
5% alcohol, 5% dextrose in 0.9% sodium chloride	24 hours	3 days
5% dextrose in alcohol	24 hours	3 days
Maintenance electrolyte solution (electrolyte #75)	24 hours	3 days
Pediatric maintenance electrolyte solution (electrolyte #48)	24 hours	3 days

Discard any unused solutions after the time periods outlined above.

Geopen is available in 30g (NDC 0049-1322-83) Bulk Pharmacy Package for intravenous use.

70-1856-00-9

GLUCOTROL®   ℞
[glu'kă-trōl]
(glipizide)
TABLETS
For Oral Use

DESCRIPTION

GLUCOTROL (glipizide) is an oral blood-glucose-lowering drug of the sulfonylurea class.

The Chemical Abstracts name of glipizide is 1-cyclohexyl-3-[[p-[2-(5-methylpyrazinecarboxamido)ethyl]phenyl]sulfonyl]urea. The molecular formula is $C_{21}H_{27}N_5O_4S$; the molecular weight is 445.55; the structural formula is shown below:

Glipizide is a whitish, odorless powder with a pKa of 5.9. It is insoluble in water and alcohols, but soluble in 0.1 N NaOH; it is freely soluble in dimethylformamide. GLUCOTROL tablets for oral use are available in 5 and 10 mg strengths. Inert ingredients are: colloidal silicon dioxide; lactose; microcrystalline cellulose; starch; stearic acid.

CLINICAL PHARMACOLOGY

Mechanism of Action: The primary mode of action of GLUCOTROL in experimental animals appears to be the stimulation of insulin secretion from the beta cells of pancreatic islet tissue and is thus dependent on functioning beta cells in the pancreatic islets. In humans GLUCOTROL appears to lower the blood glucose acutely by stimulating the release of insulin from the pancreas, an effect dependent upon functioning beta cells in the pancreatic islets. The mechanism by which GLUCOTROL lowers blood glucose during long-term administration has not been clearly established. In man, stimulation of insulin secretion by GLUCOTROL in response to a meal is undoubtedly of major importance. Fasting insulin levels are not elevated even on long-term GLUCOTROL administration, but the postprandial insulin response continues to be enhanced after at least 6 months of treatment. The insulinotropic response to a meal occurs within 30 minutes after an oral dose of GLUCOTROL in diabetic patients, but elevated insulin levels do not persist beyond the time of the meal challenge. Extrapancreatic effects may play a part in the mechanism of action of oral sulfonylurea hypoglycemic drugs.

Blood sugar control persists in some patients for up to 24 hours after a single dose of GLUCOTROL, even though plasma levels have declined to a small fraction of peak levels by that time (see Pharmacokinetics below).

Some patients fail to respond initially, or gradually lose their responsiveness to sulfonylurea drugs, including GLUCOTROL. Alternatively, GLUCOTROL may be effective in some patients who have not responded or have ceased to respond to other sulfonylureas.

Other Effects: It has been shown that GLUCOTROL therapy was effective in controlling blood sugar without deleterious changes in the plasma lipoprotein profiles of patients treated for NIDDM.

In a placebo-controlled, crossover study in normal volunteers, GLUCOTROL had no anti-diuretic activity and, in fact, led to a slight increase in free water clearance.

Pharmacokinetics: Gastrointestinal absorption of GLUCOTROL in man is uniform, rapid, and essentially complete.

CHILDREN:	Pseudomonas	Proteus and E. coli	Enterobacter and S. faecalis	Anaerobes	H. influenzae and S. pneumoniae
Urinary Tract Infections	50–200 mg/ kg/day in divided doses every 4–6 hours I.M. or I.V.	50–100 mg/ kg/day in divided doses every 4–6 hours I.M. or I.V.	50–200 mg/ kg/day in divided doses every 4–6 hours I.M. or I.V		
Severe Systemic Infections Septicemia Respiratory Infections Soft Tissue Infections	400–500 mg/ kg/day I.V. in divided doses or by continuous drip	300–400 mg/ kg/day I.M. or I.V. in divided doses			400–500 mg/ kg/day I.V. in divided doses or by continuous drip
Infections complicated by renal insufficiency (Creatinine clearance less than 5 ml/min)		Clinical data is insufficient to recommend an optimum dose			
Meningitis					400–500 mg/kg/day in divided doses or by continuous drip

NEONATES: In the neonate, for severe systemic infections (sepsis) due to susceptible strains of *Pseudomonas, Proteus, E. coli, H. influenzae* and *S. pneumoniae,* the following Geopen (carbenicillin disodium) dosages may be given I.M. or by fifteen (15) minute I.V. infusion:

Infants under 2000 g body weight.
  Initial dose: 100 mg/kg
    Subsequent doses during first week: 75 mg/kg/8 hrs (225 mg/kg/day)
    After 7 days of age: 100 mg/kg/6 hrs (400 mg/kg/day)
Infants over 2000 g body weight.
  Initial dose: 100 mg/kg
    Subsequent doses during first 3 days: 75 mg/kg/6 hrs (300 mg/kg/day)
    After 3 days of age: 100 mg/kg/6 hrs (400 mg/kg/day)
NOTE: This dosage schedule should give maximum serum levels of approximately 150–175 mcg/ml and minimum levels of approximately 50–75 mcg/ml of Geopen.
Gentamicin may be used concurrently with carbenicillin for initial therapy until results of culture and susceptibility studies are known.

Peak plasma concentrations occur 1–3 hours after a single oral dose. The half-life of elimination ranges from 2–4 hours in normal subjects, whether given intravenously or orally. The metabolic and excretory patterns are similar with the two routes of administration, indicating that first-pass metabolism is not significant. GLUCOTROL does not accumulate in plasma on repeated oral administration. Total absorption and disposition of an oral dose was unaffected by food in normal volunteers, but absorption was delayed by about 40 minutes. Thus GLUCOTROL was more effective when administered about 30 minutes before, rather than with, a test meal in diabetic patients. Protein binding was studied in serum from volunteers who received either oral or intravenous GLUCOTROL and found to be 98–99% one hour after either route of administration. The apparent volume of distribution of GLUCOTROL after intravenous administration was 11 liters, indicative of localization within the extracellular fluid compartment. In mice no GLUCOTROL or metabolites were detectable autoradiographically in the brain or spinal cord of males or females, nor in the fetuses of pregnant females. In another study, however, very small amounts of radioactivity were detected in the fetuses of rats given labelled drug.

The metabolism of GLUCOTROL is extensive and occurs mainly in the liver. The primary metabolites are inactive hydroxylation products and polar conjugates and are excreted mainly in the urine. Less than 10% unchanged GLUCOTROL is found in the urine.

INDICATIONS AND USAGE

GLUCOTROL is indicated as an adjunct to diet for the control of hyperglycemia and its associated symptomatology in patients with non-insulin-dependent diabetes mellitus (NIDDM; type II), formerly known as maturity-onset diabetes, after an adequate trial of dietary therapy has proved unsatisfactory.

In initiating treatment for non-insulin-dependent diabetes, diet should be emphasized as the primary form of treatment. Caloric restriction and weight loss are essential in the obese diabetic patient. Proper dietary management alone may be effective in controlling the blood glucose and symptoms of hyperglycemia. The importance of regular physical activity should also be stressed, and cardiovascular risk factors should be identified, and corrective measures taken where possible.

If this treatment program fails to reduce symptoms and/or blood glucose, the use of an oral sulfonylurea or insulin should be considered. Use of GLUCOTROL must be viewed by both the physician and patient as a treatment in addition to diet, and not as a substitute for diet or as a convenient mechanism for avoiding dietary restraint. Furthermore, loss of blood glucose control on diet alone also may be transient, thus requiring only short-term administration of GLUCOTROL.

During maintenance programs, GLUCOTROL should be discontinued if satisfactory lowering of blood glucose is no longer achieved. Judgments should be based on regular clinical and laboratory evaluations.

In considering the use of GLUCOTROL in asymptomatic patients, it should be recognized that controlling blood glucose in non-insulin-dependent diabetes has not been definitely established to be effective in preventing the long-term cardiovascular or neural complications of diabetes.

CONTRAINDICATIONS

GLUCOTROL is contraindicated in patients with:
1. Known hypersensitivity to the drug.
2. Diabetic ketoacidosis, with or without coma. This condition should be treated with insulin.

WARNINGS

SPECIAL WARNING ON INCREASED RISK OF CARDIO-VASCULAR MORTALITY: The administration of oral hypoglycemic drugs has been reported to be associated with increased cardiovascular mortality as compared to treatment with diet alone or diet plus insulin. This warning is based on the study conducted by the University Group Diabetes Program (UGDP), a long-term prospective clinical trial designed to evaluate the effectiveness of glucose-lowering drugs in preventing or delaying vascular complications in patients with non-insulin-dependent diabetes. The study involved 823 patients who were randomly assigned to one of four treatment groups (*Diabetes*, 19, supp. 2: 747–830, 1970).

UGDP reported that patients treated for 5 to 8 years with diet plus a fixed dose of tolbutamide (1.5 grams per day) had a rate of cardiovascular mortality approximately 2½ times that of patients treated with diet alone. A significant increase in total mortality was not observed, but the use of tolbutamide was discontinued based on the increase in cardiovascular mortality, thus limiting the opportunity for the study to show an increase in overall mortality. Despite controversy regarding the interpretation of these results, the findings of the UGDP study provide an adequate basis for this warning. The patient should be informed of the potential risks and advantages of GLUCOTROL and of alternative modes of therapy.

Although only one drug in the sulfonylurea class (tolbutamide) was included in this study, it is prudent from a safety standpoint to consider that this warning may also apply to other oral hypoglycemic drugs in this class, in view of their close similarities in mode of action and chemical structure.

PRECAUTIONS

General

Renal and Hepatic Disease: The metabolism and excretion of GLUCOTROL may be slowed in patients with impaired renal and/or hepatic function. If hypoglycemia should occur in such patients, it may be prolonged and appropriate management should be instituted.

Hypoglycemia: All sulfonylurea drugs are capable of producing severe hypoglycemia. Proper patient selection, dosage, and instructions are important to avoid hypoglycemic episodes. Renal or hepatic insufficiency may cause elevated blood levels of GLUCOTROL and the latter may also diminish gluconeogenic capacity, both of which increase the risk of serious hypoglycemic reactions. Elderly, debilitated or malnourished patients, and those with adrenal or pituitary insufficiency are particularly susceptible to the hypoglycemic action of glucose-lowering drugs. Hypoglycemia may be difficult to recognize in the elderly, and in people who are taking beta-adrenergic blocking drugs. Hypoglycemia is more likely to occur when caloric intake is deficient, after severe or prolonged exercise, when alcohol is ingested, or when more than one glucose-lowering drug is used.

Loss of Control of Blood Glucose: When a patient stabilized on any diabetic regimen is exposed to stress such as fever, trauma, infection, or surgery, a loss of control may occur. At such times, it may be necessary to discontinue GLUCOTROL and administer insulin.

The effectiveness of any oral hypoglycemic drug, including GLUCOTROL, in lowering blood glucose to a desired level decreases in many patients over a period of time, which may be due to progression of the severity of the diabetes or to diminished responsiveness to the drug. This phenomenon is known as secondary failure, to distinguish it from primary failure in which the drug is ineffective in an individual patient when first given.

Laboratory Tests: Blood and urine glucose should be monitored periodically. Measurement of glycosylated hemoglobin may be useful.

Information for Patients: Patients should be informed of the potential risks and advantages of GLUCOTROL and of alternative modes of therapy. They should also be informed about the importance of adhering to dietary instructions, of a regular exercise program, and of regular testing of urine and/or blood glucose.

The risks of hypoglycemia, its symptoms and treatment, and conditions that predispose to its development should be explained to patients and responsible family members. Primary and secondary failure should also be explained.

Drug Interactions: The hypoglycemic action of sulfonylureas may be potentiated by certain drugs including nonsteroidal anti-inflammatory agents and other drugs that are highly protein bound, salicylates, sulfonamides, chloramphenicol, probenecid, coumarins, monoamine oxidase inhibitors, and beta-adrenergic blocking agents. When such drugs are administered to a patient receiving GLUCOTROL, the patient should be observed closely for hypoglycemia. When such drugs are withdrawn from a patient receiving GLUCOTROL, the patient should be observed closely for loss of control. *In vitro* binding studies with human serum proteins indicate that GLUCOTROL binds differently than tolbutamide and does not interact with salicylate or dicumarol. However, caution must be exercised in extrapolating these findings to the clinical situation and in the use of GLUCOTROL with these drugs.

Certain drugs tend to produce hyperglycemia and may lead to loss of control. These drugs include the thiazides and other diuretics, corticosteroids, phenothiazines, thyroid products, estrogens, oral contraceptives, phenytoin, nicotinic acid, sympathomimetics, calcium channel blocking drugs, and isoniazid. When such drugs are administered to a patient receiving GLUCOTROL, the patient should be closely observed for loss of control. When such drugs are withdrawn from a patient receiving GLUCOTROL, the patient should be observed closely for hypoglycemia.

A potential interaction between oral miconazole and oral hypoglycemic agents leading to severe hypoglycemia has been reported. Whether this interaction also occurs with the intravenous, topical, or vaginal preparations of miconazole is not known.

Carcinogenesis, Mutagenesis, Impairment of Fertility: A twenty month study in rats and an eighteen month study in mice at doses up to 75 times the maximum human dose revealed no evidence of drug-related carcinogenicity. Bacterial and *in vivo* mutagenicity tests were uniformly negative. Studies in rats of both sexes at doses up to 75 times the human dose showed no effects on fertility.

Pregnancy: Pregnancy Category C: GLUCOTROL (glipizide) was found to be mildly fetotoxic in rat reproductive studies at all dose levels (5–50 mg/kg). This fetotoxicity has been similarly noted with other sulfonylureas, such as tolbuta-

mide and tolazamide. The effect is perinatal and believed to be directly related to the pharmacologic (hypoglycemic) action of GLUCOTROL. In studies in rats and rabbits no teratogenic effects were found. There are no adequate and well controlled studies in pregnant women. GLUCOTROL should be used during pregnancy only if the potential benefit justifies the potential risk to the fetus.

Because recent information suggests that abnormal blood glucose levels during pregnancy are associated with a higher incidence of congenital abnormalities, many experts recommend that insulin be used during pregnancy to maintain blood glucose levels as close to normal as possible.

Nonteratogenic Effects: Prolonged severe hypoglycemia (4 to 10 days) has been reported in neonates born to mothers who were receiving a sulfonylurea drug at the time of delivery. This has been reported more frequently with the use of agents with prolonged half-lives. If GLUCOTROL is used during pregnancy, it should be discontinued at least one month before the expected delivery date.

Nursing Mothers: Although it is not known whether GLUCOTROL is excreted in human milk, some sulfonylurea drugs are known to be excreted in human milk. Because the potential for hypoglycemia in nursing infants may exist, a decision should be made whether to discontinue nursing or to discontinue the drug, taking into account the importance of the drug to the mother. If the drug is discontinued and if diet alone is inadequate for controlling blood glucose, insulin therapy should be considered.

Pediatric Use: Safety and effectiveness in children have not been established.

ADVERSE REACTIONS

In U.S. and foreign controlled studies, the frequency of serious adverse reactions reported was very low. Of 702 patients, 11.8% reported adverse reactions and in only 1.5% was GLUCOTROL discontinued.

Hypoglycemia: See PRECAUTIONS and OVERDOSAGE sections.

Gastrointestinal: Gastrointestinal disturbances are the most common reactions. Gastrointestinal complaints were reported with the following approximate incidence: nausea and diarrhea, one in seventy; constipation and gastralgia, one in one hundred. They appear to be dose-related and may disappear on division or reduction of dosage. Cholestatic jaundice may occur rarely with sulfonylureas: GLUCOTROL should be discontinued if this occurs.

Dermatologic: Allergic skin reactions including erythema, morbilliform or maculopapular eruptions, urticaria, pruritus, and eczema have been reported in about one in seventy patients. These may be transient and may disappear despite continued use of GLUCOTROL; if skin reactions persist, the drug should be discontinued. Porphyria cutanea tarda and photosensitivity reactions have been reported with sulfonylureas.

Hematologic: Leukopenia, agranulocytosis, thrombocytopenia, hemolytic anemia, aplastic anemia, and pancytopenia have been reported with sulfonylureas.

Metabolic: Hepatic porphyria and disulfiram-like reactions have been reported with sulfonylureas. In the mouse, GLUCOTROL pretreatment did not cause an accumulation of acetaldehyde after ethanol administration. Clinical experience to date has shown that GLUCOTROL has an extremely low incidence of disulfiram-like alcohol reactions.

Endocrine Reactions: Cases of hyponatremia and the syndrome of inappropriate antidiuretic hormone (SIADH) secretion have been reported with this and other sulfonylureas.

Miscellaneous: Dizziness, drowsiness, and headache have each been reported in about one in fifty patients treated with GLUCOTROL. They are usually transient and seldom require discontinuance of therapy.

Laboratory Tests: The pattern of laboratory test abnormalities observed with GLUCOTROL was similar to that for other sulfonylureas. Occasional mild to moderate elevations of SGOT, LDH, alkaline phosphatase, BUN and creatinine were noted. One case of jaundice was reported. The relationship of these abnormalities to GLUCOTROL is uncertain, and they have rarely been associated with clinical symptoms.

OVERDOSAGE

There is no well documented experience with GLUCOTROL overdosage. The acute oral toxicity was extremely low in all species tested (LD$_{50}$ greater than 4 g/kg).

Overdosage of sulfonylureas including GLUCOTROL can produce hypoglycemia. Mild hypoglycemic symptoms without loss of consciousness or neurologic findings should be treated aggressively with oral glucose and adjustments in drug dosage and/or meal patterns. Close monitoring should continue until the physician is assured that the patient is out of danger. Severe hypoglycemic reactions with coma, seizure, or other neurological impairment occur infrequently, but constitute medical emergencies requiring immediate hospitalization. If hypoglycemic coma is diagnosed or suspected, the patient should be given a rapid intravenous injection of

Continued on next page

Roerig—Cont.

concentrated (50%) glucose solution. This should be followed by a continuous infusion of a more dilute (10%) glucose solution at a rate that will maintain the blood glucose at a level above 100 mg/dL. Patients should be closely monitored for a minimum of 24 to 48 hours since hypoglycemia may recur after apparent clinical recovery. Clearance of GLUCOTROL from plasma would be prolonged in persons with liver disease. Because of the extensive protein binding of GLUCOTROL, dialysis is unlikely to be of benefit.

DOSAGE AND ADMINISTRATION

There is no fixed dosage regimen for the management of diabetes mellitus with GLUCOTROL or any other hypoglycemic agent. In addition to the usual monitoring of urinary glucose, the patient's blood glucose must also be monitored periodically to determine the minimum effective dose for the patient; to detect primary failure, i.e., inadequate lowering of blood glucose at the maximum recommended dose of medication; and to detect secondary failure, i.e., loss of an adequate blood-glucose-lowering response after an initial period of effectiveness. Glycosylated hemoglobin levels may also be of value in monitoring the patient's response to therapy.

Short-term administration of GLUCOTROL may be sufficient during periods of transient loss of control in patients usually controlled well on diet.

In general, GLUCOTROL should be given approximately 30 minutes before a meal to achieve the greatest reduction in postprandial hyperglycemia.

Initial Dose: The recommended starting dose is 5 mg, given before breakfast. Geriatric patients or those with liver disease may be started on 2.5 mg.

Titration: Dosage adjustments should ordinarily be in increments of 2.5–5 mg, as determined by blood glucose response. At least several days should elapse between titration steps. If response to a single dose is not satisfactory, dividing that dose may prove effective. The maximum recommended once daily dose is 15 mg. Doses above 15 mg should ordinarily be divided and given before meals of adequate caloric content. The maximum recommended total daily dose is 40 mg.

Maintenance: Some patients may be effectively controlled on a once-a-day regimen, while others show better response with divided dosing. Total daily doses above 15 mg should ordinarily be divided. Total daily doses above 30 mg have been safely given on a b.i.d. basis to long-term patients.

In elderly patients, debilitated or malnourished patients, and patients with impaired renal or hepatic function, the initial and maintenance dosing should be conservative to avoid hypoglycemic reactions (see PRECAUTIONS section).

Patients Receiving Insulin: As with other sulfonylurea-class hypoglycemics, many stable non-insulin-dependent diabetic patients receiving insulin may be safely placed on GLUCOTROL. When transferring patients from insulin to GLUCOTROL, the following general guidelines should be considered:

For patients whose daily insulin requirement is 20 units or less, insulin may be discontinued and GLUCOTROL therapy may begin at usual dosages. Several days should elapse between GLUCOTROL titration steps.

For patients whose daily insulin requirement is greater than 20 units, the insulin dose should be reduced by 50% and GLUCOTROL therapy may begin at usual dosages. Subsequent reductions in insulin dosage should depend on individual patient response. Several days should elapse between GLUCOTROL titration steps.

During the insulin withdrawal period, the patient should test urine samples for sugar and ketone bodies at least three times daily. Patients should be instructed to contact the prescriber immediately if these tests are abnormal. In some cases, especially when patient has been receiving greater than 40 units of insulin daily, it may be advisable to consider hospitalization during the transition period.

Patients Receiving Other Oral Hypoglycemic Agents: As with other sulfonylurea-class hypoglycemics, no transition period is necessary when transferring patients to GLUCOTROL. Patients should be observed carefully (1–2 weeks) for hypoglycemia when being transferred from longer half-life sulfonylureas (e.g., chlorpropamide) to GLUCOTROL due to potential overlapping of drug effect.

HOW SUPPLIED

GLUCOTROL tablets are white, dye-free, scored, diamond-shaped, and imprinted as follows:

5 mg—Pfizer 411; 10 mg—Pfizer 412.

5 mg Bottles: 100's (NDC 0049-4110-66); (NDC 0662-4110-66); 500's (NDC 0049-4110-73); (NDC 0662-4110-73); Unit Dose 100's (NDC 0049-4110-41); (NDC 0662-4110-41)

10 mg Bottles: 100's (NDC 0049-4120-66); (NDC 0662-4120-66); 500's (NDC 0662-4120-73); Unit Dose 100's (NDC 0049-4120-41); (NDC 0662-4120-41)

Recommended Storage: Store below 86°F (30°C).

Caution: Federal law prohibits dispensing without prescription.   69-4227-37-7

Shown in Product Identification Section, page 426

HEPTUNA® PLUS   ℞
[hep-tū′na]
CAPSULES
(Hard Gelatin)
Fortified Oral Hematopoietic Formulation
Each capsule contains:

HEMATOPOIETIC FACTORS
Ferrous Sulfate, dried, U.S.P.	
(provides 100 mg of elemental iron)	311 mg
Desiccated Liver (undefatted)	50 mg
Vitamin B₁₂, cobalamin concentrate NF	
(as Stablets®)	5 mcg
With intrinsic factor concentrate	
(non-inhibitory)	25 mg

VITAMINS
B₁ (thiamine mononitrate, U.S.P.)	3.1 mg
B₂ (riboflavin, U.S.P.)	.2 mg
B₆ (pyridoxine hydrochloride, U.S.P.)	1.6 mg
Vitamin C (from sodium ascorbate)	150 mg
Niacin (niacinamide, U.S.P.)	15 mg
Pantothenic Acid (calcium	
pantothenate, U.S.P.)	0.9 mg

MINERALS
Copper (from copper sulfate)	1 mg
Molybdenum (from sodium	
molybdate)	0.2 mg
Calcium (from dibasic calcium	
phosphate)	37.4 mg
Iodine (from potassium iodide)	0.05 mg
Manganese (from manganese	
sulfate)	0.033 mg
Magnesium (from magnesium sulfate)	2 mg
Phosphorus (from dibasic calcium	
phosphate)	29 mg
Potassium (from potassium sulfate)	1.7 mg

Stablets® U.S. Pat. No. 2.830.933

Inert ingredients in the formulation are: ethylcellulose; hard gelatin capsules (which may contain Blue 1, Red 3, Red 40 and other inert ingredients); magnesium stearate; sodium lauryl sulfate; starch.

INDICATIONS

Heptuna Plus is a multicomponent preparation effective in the treatment of those anemias amenable to oral hematinic therapy. These include pernicious anemia and other megaloblastic anemias, and also iron deficiency anemia. Heptuna Plus also contains balanced amounts of vitamin B complex, vitamin C, and minerals as nutritional supplements.

CLINICAL PHARMACOLOGY

Hematopoietic Factors

Vitamin B₁₂: Exogenous sources of B₁₂ are required for normal growth and maintenance of normal erythropoiesis as well as nucleo-protein synthesis, myelin synthesis, and cell reproduction. Vitamin B₁₂ is irregularly absorbed from the intact gastrointestinal tract. Free vitamin B₁₂ is bound to intrinsic factor which is normally secreted by the gastric mucosal tissue, and acts as a carrier protein for active transport through the gastrointestinal tract. This normal active transport system is usually saturated by 1.5 to 3 mg of vitamin B₁₂. Under conditions of functional or anatomical derangements of the stomach or ileum, where secretion of intrinsic factor is abnormally low, absorption of vitamin B₁₂ will proceed poorly, if at all. Megaloblastic anemias may develop after gastrectomy, in Addinsonian pernicious anemia, and in fish tapeworm (*Diphyllobothrium latum*) infection; treatment to free the host of competing bacteria and parasites is required. Other causes of B₁₂deficiency are strict vegetarianism, surgical compromise of gastric or ileum activity, gastric atrophy due to multiple sclerosis or iron deficiency or malabsorption syndromes of various etiologies; in this last case parenteral therapy or oral therapy with massive doses of vitamin B₁₂ may be necessary for successful treatment. The megaloblastic anemias of malabsorption syndromes may be due to a deficiency of folate—which is not contained in Heptuna Plus, as well as to B₁₂ deficiency, and combined therapy may be warranted.

Desiccated Liver: Desiccated Liver is an extract of mammalian livers used in Heptuna Plus as a source of naturally occurring riboflavin, nicotinic acid, and choline as a nutritional supplement. Desiccated liver (undefatted) 50 mg. provides approximately 2.5 mcg riboflavin, 12.5 mcg nicotinic acid, and 0.5 mg choline.

Ferrous Sulfate: As compared to other sources of iron, ferrous sulfate provides the highest amounts of elemental iron for utilization in patients with hypochronic anemias. Iron is a constituent of hemoglobin and its administration usually corrects erythropoietic abnormalities, and may reverse esophageal and gastrointestinal tissue changes associated with iron deficiency.

Approximately 25% of an orally administered dose of ferrous sulfate will be utilizable iron. The primary sites of iron absorption are the duodenum, the jejunum, the stomach, and the proximal portion of the ileum. The ferrous species of iron is the most readily absorbed fraction. While the exact mechanism of absorption is not known, the absorption, metabolism, and excretion of iron appear to be related to body requirements for this mineral. The excretion of iron as ferritin is by way of epithelial cells sloughed from the skin and gastrointestinal tract. There may be trace losses in bile, and cell-free sweat.

Vitamins

Vitamin C: It is known that an acidic environment favors the maintenance of iron in the ferrous state, retards formation of insoluble complexes of iron with food or other substrates, and will thus promote gastric absorption of ferrous iron. The vitamin C content of Heptuna Plus, in addition to contributing to the overall acidic environment of gastric fluids, may also be useful as a supplement to deficiency states. Prolonged and severe vitamin C deficiency is associated with an anemia which is usually hypochronic but occasionally megaloblastic. Vitamin C is also utilized in intracellular reactions such as conversion of folic acid and carbohydrate synthesis.

Vitamin B Complex (B₁, B₂, B₆, Niacin, Pantothenic Acid): These are provided in Heptuna Plus as nutritional supplements. Vitamin B complex is essential for the metabolism of carbohydrates and protein. Administration of these water-soluble vitamins may be useful in deficiency states associated with febrile diseases, severe burns, gastrointestinal disorders interfering with absorption of these vitamins, in prolonged or wasting diseases, or in nutritional deficiency. One capsule of Heptuna Plus provides the following approximate percentage of the U.S. Recommended Adult Daily Allowances (U.S. RDA):

	% U.S. RDA
B₁	221.4
B₂	125
B₆	80
Vitamin C	333.3
Niacin	83.3
Pantothenic Acid	9

Minerals

One capsule of Heptuna Plus provides the following approximate percentages of U.S. Recommended Adult Daily Allowances (U.S. RDA):

	% U.S. RDA
Copper	50
Molybdenum	*
Calcium	4.25
Iodine	38.46
Manganese	*
Magnesium	0.57
Phosphorous	3.63
Potassium	*

*U.S. RDA not yet established.

The precise role of minerals in human nutritional maintenance has yet to be defined. However, several trace elements (including copper, molybdenum, calcium, iodine, manganese) have been identified as being essential for animal life.

Copper: Copper has been identified as a component of several amine oxidases. Copper depletion in experimental animals results in failure to utilize ferritin iron and is accompanied by increases in hepatic iron concentration sometimes with clear evidence of hemosiderosis. Copper-dependent enzyme systems may be intimately involved in tissue iron mobilization.

Molybdenum: Molybdenum has been identified as a component of xanthine oxidase (involved in purine oxidation and possibly in the release of iron from ferritin), aldehydeoxidase, and sulfite oxidase.

Calcium: In addition to this element's well known important roles in maintenance of bone, neurologic, and muscular tissue integrity, calcium may also play a role in maintaining the integrity of cell membrane structures.

Iodine: As the central element of thyroid activity, iodine intake may influence carbohydrate and cholesterol metabolism, functions of the central nervous system, catecholamine secretion, and skeletal growth and maturation. Its exact role in the hematopoietic process, if any, has not been determined.

Manganese: The main manifestations of manganese deficiency in laboratory animals are impaired growth, disturbed or depressed reproductive function, skeletal abnormalities, and nervous disorders. Its exact role in the hematopoietic process, if any, has not been determined.

Magnesium: Magnesium plays a fundamental role in most reactions that include phosphate transfer, and it is believed to be essential for the structural stabilization of nucleic acids. Magnesium depletion has been known to impair homeostasis of potassium and calcium. Deficiency of magnesium almost always occurs as a consequence of some underlying disease, including malabsorption syndromes.

Phosphorus: Hypophosphatemia may cause a marked decrease in erythrocytic concentrations of ATP and of 2,3 diphosphoglycerate. Acute hemolytic-type anemia may develop in severe deficiency states.

Potassium: Potassium is an essential mineral in electrolyte maintenance and in maintaining electrical excitability of cells and acid-base homeostasis. Its exact role in the hematopoietic process, if any, has not been determined.

CONTRAINDICATIONS

Hemachromatosis and hemosiderosis are contraindications to iron therapy. Previous hypersensitivity to any of the components of Heptuna Plus contraindicates its use.

PRECAUTIONS

Anemia is a manifestation of an underlying disease process. While Heptuna Plus provides components useful in the management of certain anemias, appropriate attention should be directed to an etiological diagnosis and treatment of the underlying causes of the anemia.

Resistance to the effects of exogenous intrinsic factor has been reported. Local intestinal antibodies which render exogenous intrinsic factor inactive have been noted to develop in approximately 50% of patients treated within one year of continuous oral therapy. If resistance develops, parenteral therapy or oral therapy with large doses of vitamin B_{12} may be necessary to circumvent normal active transport mechanisms and adequately treat the patient.

Although this product contains vitamin B_{12} (as Stablets®) with intrinsic factor concentrate (non-inhibitory) and desiccated liver, it is not as reliable as parenterally administered cyanocobalamin (vitamin B_{12}) in the management of pernicious anemia. Some patients with pernicious anemia may not respond to orally ingested cobalamin concentrate (vitamin B_{12}). There is no known way to predict which patients will respond or which patients may cease to respond.

Information for Patients: As Heptuna Plus contains substantial amounts of iron, patients should be advised that gastrointestinal reactions such as diarrhea or constipation may occur with usage. Patients should be cautioned against concomitant usage of Heptuna Plus and tetracycline, or its analogs, so as to avoid a chelation interaction which would reduce the amounts of antibiotic and iron or divalent ions available for gastrointestinal absorption.

Laboratory Tests: Periodic clinical and laboratory monitoring are considered essential to proper use of hematopoietics. The following laboratory tests may be useful in evaluating patients' response to therapy: peripheral blood smears, reticulocyte count, serum iron, iron binding capacity, serum B_{12}, serum folic acid, hemoglobin and hematocrit, mean corpuscular volume.

Drug Interactions: The following drug/drug interactions may occur with the use of Heptuna Plus.

Agent	Interaction
Tetracycline and derivatives	Complexation of antibiotic and iron or divalent ions (such as calcium) decrease availability of component for gastric absorption. This may be avoided by administration of Heptuna Plus at least one hour before tetracycline-type agent.
Levodopa	Doses of pyridoxine of approximately 5 mg (three capsules Heptuna Plus provide 4.8 mg B_6) or more per day may reduce the beneficial effects of levodopa in parkinsonian disease. This is thought to be due to increased transamination of levodopa. Patients receiving this combination should be carefully observed for unwanted variations in parkinson control.
Lithium	The presence of iodine in Heptuna Plus may enhance the hypothyroid and goiterogenic potential of these two components. Patients receiving lithium and Heptuna Plus should have baseline and periodic thyroid status checks.

Laboratory Interactions: Heptuna Plus contains iodine 0.05 mg (as potassium iodide) as an active component and the iodinated dye tetraiodofluorescein (FD and C#3) in the capsule shell. These agents may interfere with I^{131} or other diagnostic radioiodine neucleotide testing procedures. Other than changes induced from the therapeutic effects of the components of Heptuna Plus, no other interferences with laboratory testing procedures have been identified.

Carcinogenesis, Mutagenesis, Impairment of Fertility: The potential for Heptuna Plus to impair fertility or act as a carcinogen or a mutagen has not been studied *in vivo* or *in vitro*.

Use in Pregnancy

Category C: Animal reproductive studies have not been conducted with Heptuna Plus. It is also not known whether Heptuna Plus can cause fetal harm when administered to a pregnant woman or can affect reproductive capacity. Heptuna Plus should be given to a pregnant woman only if clearly needed.

Nursing Mothers: It is not known whether this drug is excreted in human milk. Because many drugs are excreted in human milk, caution should be exercised when Heptuna Plus is administered to a nursing woman.

Pediatric Use: Safety and effectiveness in children have not been established.

ADVERSE REACTIONS

Ferrous Sulfate: The most frequent adverse reactions to Heptuna Plus are those associated with oral iron therapy. An incidence of gastrointestinal discomfort in 19.5% to 27% of patients receiving "iron placebo" tablets has been reported. The gastrointestinal complaints usually noted are diarrhea, constipation, nausea, epigastric pain, ructus, vomiting, and black staining of stools. Reduction in dosage or administration with meals may minimize these effects.

In extremely rare instances, skin rash suggesting allergy has been noted following the oral administration of desiccated liver preparations.

Iodine: Allergic reactions, including angioedema, rashes, lymphadenopathy, eosinophilia, arteritis, and febrile reactions have been reported with iodine usage. Also, acne, swelling of salivary glands, iodine coryza, and stomach upsets have been reported. Iodine use may precipitate hypo- or hyperthyroid activity and goiter.

B Complex Vitamins: Adverse reactions to these water-soluble vitamins are rare:

—Thiamine; Hypersensitivity reactions are rare and have been reported mostly with parenteral administration.

—Pyridoxine; Allergic reactions have been reported, but are rare.

—Cyanocobalamine/Cobalamine; Mild forms of polycythemia, and peripheral vascular thrombosis during recovery from pernicious anemia treated with B_{12} have been observed. Use of high dose oral vitamin B_{12} has been associated with the appearance of acne.

Minerals: No adverse reactions other than those specified for iodine have been reported with orally administered minerals as supplied in Heptuna Plus.

OVERDOSAGE

Acute Toxicity: Toxicity may result from overdosage due to ingestion of ferrous sulfate. In young children 300 mg of elemental iron may be fatal. The remainder of the ingredients are essentially nontoxic (water-soluble vitamins) or present in such small amounts as to be nontoxic even with overdosage.

Symptoms: Symptoms may occur 30 to 60 minutes after ingestion. Danger may exist for 24-48 hours. Acute gastroenteritis, vomiting, diarrhea, dehydration, collapse, and coma ending in death may occur. A severe acidosis may also be present. The diarrhea may initially be watery, becoming bloody and then tarry.

Dialyzability: It is known that iron, magnesium, potassium, iodide, and phosphate are dialyzable. Dialysis may not be effective in removing vitamin B_{12} or copper. The effect of dialysis on the other components in Heptuna Plus is not certain.

Management: Management should be directed primarily at the treatment of iron toxicity. Acute toxicity may occur in young children after ingestion of 1 gram of ferrous sulfate (equivalent to 3 capsules of Heptuna Plus). In adults iron toxicity is rare and is most likely to occur only after ingestion of more than 50 grams of ferrous sulfate (equivalent to 150 capsules of Heptuna Plus). Treatment involves gastric lavage and/or use of absorbents. A 1% sodium bicarbonate lavage fluid may be useful to prevent further iron absorption. Lavage must be performed with caution after the first hour of an overdosage because of the potential for gastric necrosis and perforation. Shock and acid-base imbalances should be treated with standard methods. Serum iron levels should be monitored and deferoxamine mesylate therapy initiated if necessary. Other chelating agents should be used only if deferoxamine mesylate is not available or otherwise contraindicated, as it may form toxic complexes with iron.

DOSAGE AND ADMINISTRATION

For many patients one capsule of Heptuna Plus daily will provide sufficient amounts of hematopoietic factors for therapeutic results. If the severity and etiology of the anemia so indicate, 1 capsule three times a day (approximately every six hours) may be prescribed. Therapy with Heptuna Plus may be continued until patient response indicates discontinuation of therapy.

HOW SUPPLIED

Heptuna Plus capsules are available as red and white gelatin capsules, in bottles of 100 (NDC 0049-5040-66).

69-0331-00-8

Shown in Product Identification Section, page 426

MARAX®   ℞
[mă'rax]
(ephedrine sulfate, theophylline, hydroxyzine HCl)
TABLETS AND DF SYRUP

CONTENTS

	Each Tablet Contains:	Each Teaspoon (5 ml.) Syrup Contains:
Ephedrine Sulfate	25 mg.	6.25 mg.
Theophylline	130 mg.	32.50 mg.
Atarax® (hydroxyzine HCl)	10 mg.	2.5 mg.
Alcohol (Ethyl Alcohol)		5% v/v.

Inert ingredients for tablets are: alginic acid; magnesium stearate; precipitated calcium carbonate; sodium lauryl sulfate.

Inert ingredients for syrup are: alcohol; cherry flavor; hydrochloric acid; sodium benzoate; special flavor compound; sucrose; water.

ACTIONS

The action of ephedrine as a vasoconstrictor is well known. It is therefore of significant benefit in symptomatic relief of the congestion occurring in bronchial asthma. As a bronchodilator, it has a slower onset but longer duration of action than does epinephrine, which, in contrast to ephedrine, is not effective upon oral administration.

The diverse actions of theophylline—broncho- spasmolytic, cardiovascular, and diuretic—are well established, and make it a particularly useful drug in the treatment of bronchial asthma, both in the acute attack and in the prophylactic therapy of the disease.

Atarax (hydroxyzine HCl) modifies the central stimulatory action of ephedrine preventing excessive excitation in patients on Marax therapy.

In animal studies Atarax (hydroxyzine HCl) has demonstrated antiserotonin activity and antispasmodic potency of a nonspecific nature.

Marax-DF Syrup produces an expectorant action wherein the tenacity of the sputum is decreased and the ease of expectoration is increased.

Indications

Based on a review of this drug by the National Academy of Sciences-National Research Council and/or other information, FDA has classified the indications as follows:

"Possibly" Effective: For controlling bronchospastic disorders.

Final classification of the less than effective indication requires further investigation.

CONTRAINDICATIONS

Because of the ephedrine, Marax is contraindicated in cardiovascular disease, hyperthyroidism, and hypertension. This drug is contraindicated in individuals who have shown hypersensitivity to the drug or its components.

Hydroxyzine, when administered to the pregnant mouse, rat, and rabbit induced fetal abnormalities in the rat at doses substantially above the human therapeutic range. Clinical data in human beings are inadequate to establish safety in early pregnancy. Until such data are available, hydroxyzine is contraindicated in early pregnancy.

PRECAUTIONS

Because of the ephedrine component this drug should be used with caution in elderly males or those with known prostatic hypertrophy.

The potentiating action of hydroxyzine, although mild, must be taken into consideration when the drug is used in conjunction with central nervous system depressants; and when other central nervous system depressants are administered concomitantly with hydroxyzine their dosage should be reduced. Patients should be cautioned that hydroxyzine can increase the effect of alcohol.

Patients should be warned—because of the hydroxyzine component—of the possibility of drowsiness occurring and cautioned against driving a car or operating dangerous machinery while taking this drug.

ADVERSE REACTIONS

With large doses of ephedrine, excitation, tremulousness, insomnia, nervousness, palpitation, tachycardia, precordial pain, cardiac arrhythmias, vertigo, dryness of the nose and throat, headache, sweating, and warmth may occur. Because ephedrine is a sympathomimetic agent some patients may develop vesical sphincter spasm and resultant urinary hesitation, and occasionally acute urinary retention. This should

Continued on next page

Roerig—Cont.

be borne in mind when administering preparations containing ephedrine to elderly males or those with known prostatic hypertrophy. At the recommended dose for Marax, a side effect occasionally reported is palpitation, and this can be controlled with dosage adjustment, additional amounts of concurrently administered Atarax (hydroxyzine HCl), or discontinuation of the medication. When ephedrine is given three or more times daily patients may develop tolerance after several weeks of therapy.

Theophylline when given on an empty stomach frequently causes gastric irritation accompanied by upper abdominal discomfort, nausea, and vomiting. Administration of the medication after meals will serve to minimize this side effect. Theophylline may cause diuresis and cardiac stimulation. The amount of Atarax (hydroxyzine HCl) present in Marax has not resulted in disturbing side effects. When used alone specifically as a tranquilizer in the normal dosage range (25 to 50 mg. three or four times a day), side effects are infrequent; even at these higher doses, no serious side effects have been reported and confirmed to date. Those which do occasionally occur when Atarax (hydroxyzine HCl) is used alone are drowsiness, xerostomia and, at extremely high doses, involuntary motor activity, unsteadiness of gait, neuromuscular weakness, all of which may be controlled by reduction of the dosage or discontinuation of the medication.

With the relatively low dose of Atarax (hydroxyzine HCl) in Marax, these effects are not likely to occur. In addition, the ataractic action of Atarax (hydroxyzine HCl) may modify the cardiac stimulatory action of ephedrine, and concurrently, increasing the amount of Atarax (hydroxyzine HCl) may control or abolish this undesirable effect of ephedrine.

DOSAGE AND ADMINISTRATION

The dosage of Marax should be adjusted according to the severity of complaints, and the patient's individual toleration.

Tablets: In general, an adult dose of 1 tablet, 2 to 4 times daily, should be sufficient. Some patients are controlled adequately with ½ to 1 tablet at bedtime. The time interval between doses should not be shorter than four hours. The dosage for children over 5 years of age and for adults who are sensitive to ephedrine, is one-half the usual adult dose. Clinical experience to date has been confined to ages above 5 years.

Syrup: The dose for children over 5 years of age is 1 teaspoon (5 ml.), 3 to 4 times daily. Dosage for children 2 to 5 years of age is ½ to 1 teaspoon (2.5-5 ml.), 3 to 4 times daily. Not recommended for children under 2 years of age.

HOW SUPPLIED

Marax Tablets are available as scored, dye free, m-shaped tablets in bottles of 100 (NDC 0049-2540-66) and 500 (NDC 0049-2540-73).

Marax-DF Syrup is available in pints (NDC 0049-2550-93) and gallons (NDC 0049-2550-54) as a colorless syrup, free of all coal tar dyes, and should be dispensed in tight, light-resistant containers (USP).

69-0928-00-7
66-2265-00-4

Shown in Product Identification Section, page 426

NAVANE®   ℞
[*nah'vān*]
(thiothixene) CAPSULES
NAVANE®
(thiothixene hydrochloride) CONCENTRATE

DESCRIPTION

Navane (thiothixene) is a thioxanthene derivative. Specifically, it is the *cis* isomer of N,N-dimethyl-9-[3-(4-methyl-1-piperazinyl)-propylidene] thioxanthene-2-sulfonamide.

The thioxanthenes differ from the phenothiazines by the replacement of nitrogen in the central ring with a carbon-linked side chain fixed in space in a rigid structural configuration. An N,N-dimethyl sulfonamide functional group is bonded to the thioxanthene nucleus.

Inert ingredients for the capsule formulations are: hard gelatin capsules (which contain gelatin and titanium dioxide; may contain Yellow 10, Yellow 6, Blue 1, Green 3, Red 3, and other inert ingredients); lactose; magnesium stearate; sodium lauryl sulfate; starch.

Inert ingredients for the oral concentrate formulation are: alcohol; cherry flavor; dextrose; passion fruit flavor; sorbitol solution; water.

ACTIONS

Navane is a psychotropic agent of the thioxanthene series. Navane possesses certain chemical and pharmacological similarities to the piperazine phenothiazines and differences from the aliphatic group of phenothiazines.

INDICATIONS

Navane is effective in the management of manifestations of psychotic disorders. Navane has not been evaluated in the management of behavioral complications in patients with mental retardation.

CONTRAINDICATIONS

Navane is contraindicated in patients with circulatory collapse, comatose states, central nervous system depression due to any cause, and blood dyscrasias. Navane is contraindicated in individuals who have shown hypersensitivity to the drug. It is not known whether there is a cross sensitivity between the thioxanthenes and the phenothiazine derivatives, but this possibility should be considered.

WARNINGS

Tardive Dyskinesia—Tardive dyskinesia, a syndrome consisting of potentially irreversible, involuntary, dyskinetic movements may develop in patients treated with neuroleptic (antipsychotic) drugs. Although the prevalence of the syndrome appears to be highest among the elderly, especially elderly women, it is impossible to rely upon prevalence estimates to predict, at the inception of neuroleptic treatment, which patients are likely to develop the syndrome. Whether neuroleptic drug products differ in their potential to cause tardive dyskinesia is unknown.

Both the risk of developing the syndrome and the likelihood that it will become irreversible are believed to increase as the duration of treatment and the total cumulative dose of neuroleptic drugs administered to the patient increase. However, the syndrome can develop, although much less commonly, after relatively brief treatment periods at low doses.

There is no known treatment for established cases of tardive dyskinesia, although the syndrome may remit, partially or completely, if neuroleptic treatment is withdrawn. Neuroleptic treatment, itself, however, may suppress (or partially suppress) the signs and symptoms of the syndrome and thereby may possibly mask the underlying disease process. The effect that symptomatic suppression has upon the long-term course of the syndrome is unknown.

Given these considerations, neuroleptics should be prescribed in a manner that is most likely to minimize the occurrence of tardive dyskinesia. Chronic neuroleptic treatment should generally be reserved for patients who suffer from a chronic illness that, 1) is known to respond to neuroleptic drugs, and 2) for whom alternative, equally effective, but potentially less harmful treatments are *not* available or appropriate. In patients who do require chronic treatment, the smallest dose and the shortest duration of treatment producing a satisfactory clinical response should be sought. The need for continued treatment should be reassessed periodically.

If signs and symptoms of tardive dyskinesia appear in a patient on neuroleptics, drug discontinuation should be considered. However, some patients may require treatment despite the presence of the syndrome.

(For further information about the description of tardive dyskinesia and its clinical detection, please refer to "Information for Patients" in the PRECAUTIONS section, and to the ADVERSE REACTIONS section.)

Neuroleptic Malignant Syndrome (NMS)—A potentially fatal symptom complex sometimes referred to as Neuroleptic Malignant Syndrome (NMS) has been reported in association with antipsychotic drugs. Clinical manifestations of NMS are hyperpyrexia, muscle rigidity, altered mental status and evidence of autonomic instability (irregular pulse or blood pressure, tachycardia, diaphoresis, and cardiac dysrhythmias).

The diagnostic evaluation of patients with this syndrome is complicated. In arriving at a diagnosis, it is important to identify cases where the clinical presentation includes both serious medical illness (e.g., pneumonia, systemic infection, etc.) and untreated or inadequately treated extrapyramidal signs and symptoms (EPS). Other important considerations in the differential diagnosis include central anticholinergic toxicity, heat stroke, drug fever and primary central nervous system (CNS) pathology.

The management of NMS should include 1) immediate discontinuation of antipsychotic drugs and other drugs not essential to concurrent therapy, 2) intensive symptomatic treatment and medical monitoring, and 3) treatment of any concomitant serious medical problems for which specific treatments are available. There is no general agreement about specific pharmacological treatment regimens for uncomplicated NMS.

If a patient requires antipsychotic drug treatment after recovery from NMS, the potential reintroduction of drug therapy should be carefully considered. The patient should be carefully monitored, since recurrences of NMS have been reported.

Usage in Pregnancy—Safe use of Navane during pregnancy has not been established. Therefore, this drug should be given to pregnant patients only when, in the judgment of the physician, the expected benefits from the treatment exceed the possible risks to mother and fetus. Animal reproduction studies and clinical experience to date have not demonstrated any teratogenic effects.

In the animal reproduction studies with Navane, there was some decrease in conception rate and litter size, and an increase in resorption rate in rats and rabbits. Similar findings have been reported with other psychotropic agents. After repeated oral administration of Navane to rats (5 to 15 mg/kg/day), rabbits (3 to 50 mg/kg/day), and monkeys (1 to 3 mg/kg/day) before and during gestation, no teratogenic effects were seen.

Usage in Children—The use of Navane in children under 12 years of age is not recommended because safe conditions for its use have not been established.

As is true with many CNS drugs, Navane may impair the mental and/or physical abilities required for the performance of potentially hazardous tasks such as driving a car or operating machinery, especially during the first few days of therapy. Therefore, the patient should be cautioned accordingly.

As in the case of other CNS-acting drugs, patients receiving Navane (thiothixene) should be cautioned about the possible additive effects (which may include hypotension) with CNS depressants and with alcohol.

PRECAUTIONS

General: An antiemetic effect was observed in animal studies with Navane; since this effect may also occur in man, it is possible that Navane may mask signs of overdosage of toxic drugs and may obscure conditions such as intestinal obstruction and brain tumor.

In consideration of the known capability of Navane and certain other psychotropic drugs to precipitate convulsions, extreme caution should be used in patients with a history of convulsive disorders or those in a state of alcohol withdrawal, since it may lower the convulsive threshold. Although Navane potentiates the actions of the barbiturates, the dosage of the anticonvulsant therapy should not be reduced when Navane is administered concurrently.

Though exhibiting rather weak anticholinergic properties, Navane should be used with caution in patients who might be exposed to extreme heat or who are receiving atropine or related drugs.

Use with caution in patients with cardiovascular disease.

Caution as well as careful adjustment of the dosages is indicated when Navane is used in conjunction with other CNS depressants.

Also, careful observation should be made for pigmentary retinopathy, and lenticular pigmentation (fine lenticular pigmentation has been noted in a small number of patients treated with Navane for prolonged periods). Blood dyscrasias (agranulocytosis, pancytopenia, thrombocytopenic purpura), and liver damage (jaundice, biliary stasis), have been reported with related drugs.

Neuroleptic drugs elevate prolactin levels; the elevation persists during chronic administration. Tissue culture experiments indicate that approximately one-third of human breast cancers are prolactin dependent *in vitro*, a factor of potential importance if the prescription of these drugs is contemplated in a patient with a previously detected breast cancer. Although disturbances such as galactorrhea, amenorrhea, gynecomastia, and impotence have been reported, the clinical significance of elevated serum prolactin levels is unknown for most patients. An increase in mammary neoplasms has been found in rodents after chronic administration of neuroleptic drugs. Neither clinical studies nor epidemiologic studies conducted to date, however, have shown an association between chronic administration of these drugs and mammary tumorigenesis; the available evidence is considered too limited to be conclusive at this time.

Information for Patients: Given the likelihood that some patients exposed chronically to neuroleptics will develop tardive dyskinesia, it is advised that all patients in whom chronic use is contemplated be given, if possible, full information about this risk. The decision to inform patients and/or their guardians must obviously take into account the clinical circumstances and the competency of the patient to understand the information provided.

ADVERSE REACTIONS

NOTE: Not all of the following adverse reactions have been reported with Navane. However, since Navane has certain chemical and pharmacologic similarities to the phenothiazines, all of the known side effects and toxicity associated with phenothiazine therapy should be borne in mind when Navane is used.

Cardiovascular Effects: Tachycardia, hypotension, light-headedness, and syncope. In the event hypotension occurs, epinephrine should not be used as a pressor agent since a paradoxical further lowering of blood pressure may result.

Nonspecific EKG changes have been observed in some patients receiving Navane. These changes are usually reversible and frequently disappear on continued Navane therapy. The incidence of these changes is lower than that observed with some phenothiazines. The clinical significance of these changes is not known.

CNS Effects: Drowsiness, usually mild, may occur although it usually subsides with continuation of Navane therapy. The incidence of sedation appears similar to that of the piperazine group of phenothiazines but less than that of certain aliphatic phenothiazines. Restlessness, agitation and insomnia have been noted with Navane. Seizures and paradoxical exacerbation of psychotic symptoms have occurred with Navane infrequently.

Hyperreflexia has been reported in infants delivered from mothers having received structurally related drugs.

In addition, phenothiazine derivatives have been associated with cerebral edema and cerebrospinal fluid abnormalities. Extrapyramidal symptoms, such as pseudo-parkinsonism, akathisia and dystonia have been reported. Management of these extrapyramidal symptoms depends upon the type and severity. Rapid relief of acute symptoms may require the use of an injectable antiparkinson agent. More slowly emerging symptoms may be managed by reducing the dosage of Navane and/or administering an oral antiparkinson agent.

Persistent Tardive Dyskinesia: As with all antipsychotic agents tardive dyskinesia may appear in some patients on long term therapy or may occur after drug therapy has been discontinued. The syndrome is characterized by rhythmical involuntary movements of the tongue, face, mouth or jaw (e.g., protrusion of tongue, puffing of cheeks, puckering of mouth, chewing movements). Sometimes these may be accompanied by involuntary movements of extremities.

Since early detection of tardive dyskinesia is important, patients should be monitored on an ongoing basis. It has been reported that fine vermicular movement of the tongue may be an early sign of the syndrome. If this or any other presentation of the syndrome is observed, the clinician should consider possible discontinuation of neuroleptic medication. (See Warnings section.)

Hepatic Effects: Elevations of serum transaminase and alkaline phosphatase, usually transient, have been infrequently observed in some patients. No clinically confirmed cases of jaundice attributable to Navane have been reported.

Hematologic Effects: As is true with certain other psychotropic drugs, leukopenia and leucocytosis, which are usually transient, can occur occasionally with Navane. Other antipsychotic drugs have been associated with agranulocytosis, eosinophilia, hemolytic anemia, thrombocytopenia and pancytopenia.

Allergic Reactions: Rash, pruritus, urticaria, photosensitivity and rare cases of anaphylaxis have been reported with Navane. Undue exposure to sunlight should be avoided. Although not experienced with Navane, exfoliative dermatitis and contact dermatitis (in nursing personnel), have been reported with certain phenothiazines.

Endocrine Disorders: Lactation, moderate breast enlargement and amenorrhea have occurred in a small percentage of females receiving Navane (thiothixene). If persistent, this may necessitate a reduction in dosage or the discontinuation of therapy. Phenothiazines have been associated with false positive pregnancy tests, gynecomastia, hypoglycemia, hyperglycemia and glycosuria.

Autonomic Effects: Dry mouth, blurred vision, nasal congestion, constipation, increased sweating, increased salivation and impotence have occurred infrequently with Navane therapy. Phenothiazines have been associated with miosis, mydriasis, and adynamic ileus.

Other Adverse Reactions: Hyperpyrexia, anorexia, nausea, vomiting, diarrhea, increase in appetite and weight, weakness or fatigue, polydipsia, and peripheral edema.

Although not reported with Navane, evidence indicates there is a relationship between phenothiazine therapy and the occurrence of a systemic lupus erythematosus-like syndrome.

Neuroleptic Malignant Syndrome (NMS): Please refer to the text regarding NMS in the WARNINGS section.

NOTE: Sudden deaths have occasionally been reported in patients who have received certain phenothiazine derivatives. In some cases the cause of death was apparently cardiac arrest or asphyxia due to failure of the cough reflex. In others, the cause could not be determined nor could it be established that death was due to phenothiazine administration.

DOSAGE AND ADMINISTRATION

Dosage of Navane should be individually adjusted depending on the chronicity and severity of the condition. In general, small doses should be used initially and gradually increased to the optimal effective level, based on patient response. Some patients have been successfully maintained on once-a-day Navane therapy.

The use of Navane in children under 12 years of age is not recommended because safe conditions for its use have not been established.

In milder conditions, an initial dose of 2 mg. three times daily. If indicated, a subsequent increase to 15 mg./day total daily dose is often effective.

In more severe conditions, an initial dose of 5 mg. twice daily. The usual optimal dose is 20 to 30 mg. daily. If indicated, an increase to 60 mg./day total daily dose is often effective. Exceeding a total daily dose of 60 mg. rarely increases the beneficial response.

OVERDOSAGE

Manifestations include muscular twitching, drowsiness and dizziness. Symptoms of gross overdosage may include CNS depression, rigidity, weakness, torticollis, tremor, salivation, dysphagia, hypotension, disturbances of gait, or coma.

Treatment: Essentially symptomatic and supportive. Early gastric lavage is helpful. Keep patient under careful observation and maintain an open airway, since involvement of the extrapyramidal system may produce dysphagia and respiratory difficulty in severe overdosage. If hypotension occurs, the standard measures for managing circulatory shock should be used (I.V. fluids and/or vasoconstrictors).

If a vasoconstrictor is needed, levarterenol and phenylephrine are the most suitable drugs. Other pressor agents, including epinephrine, are not recommended, since phenothiazine derivatives may reverse the usual pressor action of these agents and cause further lowering of blood pressure. If CNS depression is marked, symptomatic treatment is indicated. Extrapyramidal symptoms may be treated with antiparkinson drugs.

There are no data on the use of peritoneal or hemodialysis, but they are known to be of little value in phenothiazine intoxication.

HOW SUPPLIED

Navane (thiothixene) Capsules
Bottles of 100's: 1 mg (NDC 0049-5710-66); 2 mg (NDC 0049-5720-66); 5 mg (NDC 0049-5730-66); 10 mg (NDC 0049-5740-66); 20 mg (NDC 0049-5770-66). 1000's: 2 mg (NDC 0049-5720-82); 5 mg (NDC 0049-5730-82); 10 mg (NDC 0049-5740-82). 500's 20 mg (NDC 0049-5770-73).
Unit Doses of: 1 mg (NDC 0049-5710-41); 2 mg (NDC 0049-5720-41); 5 mg (NDC 0049-5730-41); 10 mg (NDC 0049-5740-41); and 20 mg (NDC 0049-5770-41).
Navane (thiothixene hydrochloride) Concentrate is available in 120 ml (4 oz.) bottles (NDC 0049-5750-47) with an accompanying dropper calibrated at 2 mg, 3 mg, 4 mg, 5 mg, 6 mg, 8 mg, and 10 mg and in 30 ml (1 oz.) bottles (NDC 0049-5750-51) with an accompanying dropper calibrated at 2 mg, 3 mg, 4 mg, and 5 mg. Each ml. contains thiothixene hydrochloride equivalent to 5 mg. of thiothixene. Contains alcohol, U.S.P. 7.0% v/v. (small loss unavoidable).

70-1655-00-7

Shown in Product Identification Section, page 426

NAVANE®   ℞
[nah'vān]
(thiothixene hydrochloride)
Intramuscular
2 mg./ml. 5 mg./ml.

DESCRIPTION

Navane (thiothixene hydrochloride) is a thioxanthene derivative. Specifically, thiothixene is the *cis* isomer of N,N-dimethyl-9-[3-(4-methyl-1-piperazinyl)-propylidene] thioxanthene-2-sulfonamide.

The thioxanthenes differ from the phenothiazines by the replacement of nitrogen in the central ring with a carbon-linked side chain fixed in space in a rigid structural configuration. An N,N-dimethyl sulfonamide functional group is bonded to the thioxanthene nucleus.

thiothixene hydrochloride

Inert ingredients for the intramuscular solution formulation are: dextrose; benzyl alcohol; propyl gallate.
Inert ingredients for the intramuscular for injection formulation is: mannitol.

ACTIONS

Navane is a psychotropic agent of the thioxanthene series. Navane possesses certain chemical and pharmacological similarities to the piperazine phenothiazines and differences from the aliphatic group of phenothiazines. Navane's mode of action has not been clearly established.

INDICATIONS

Navane is effective in the management of manifestations of psychotic disorders. Navane has not been evaluated in the management of behavioral complications in patients with mental retardation.

CONTRAINDICATIONS

Navane is contraindicated in patients with circulatory collapse, comatose states, central nervous system depression due to any cause, and blood dyscrasias. Navane is contraindicated in individuals who have shown hypersensitivity to the drug. It is not known whether there is a cross sensitivity between the thioxanthenes and the phenothiazine derivatives, but this possibility should be considered.

WARNINGS

Tardive Dyskinesia—Tardive dyskinesia, a syndrome consisting of potentially irreversible, involuntary, dyskinetic movements may develop in patients treated with neuroleptic (antipsychotic) drugs. Although the prevalence of the syndrome appears to be highest among the elderly, especially elderly women, it is impossible to rely upon prevalence estimates to predict, at the inception of neuroleptic treatment, which patients are likely to develop the syndrome. Whether neuroleptic drug products differ in their potential to cause tardive dyskinesia is unknown.

Both the risk of developing the syndrome and the likelihood that it will become irreversible are believed to increase as the duration of treatment and the total cumulative dose of neuroleptic drugs administered to the patient increase. However, the syndrome can develop, although much less commonly, after relatively brief treatment periods at low doses.

There is no known treatment for established cases of tardive dyskinesia, although the syndrome may remit, partially or completely, if neuroleptic treatment is withdrawn. Neuroleptic treatment, itself, however, may suppress (or partially suppress) the signs and symptoms of the syndrome and thereby may possibly mask the underlying disease process. The effect that symptomatic suppression has upon the long-term course of the syndrome is unknown.

Given these considerations, neuroleptics should be prescribed in a manner that is most likely to minimize the occurrence of tardive dyskinesia. Chronic neuroleptic treatment should generally be reserved for patients who suffer from a chronic illness that, 1) is known to respond to neuroleptic drugs, and, 2) for whom alternative, equally effective, but potentially less harmful treatments are *not* available or appropriate. In patients who do require chronic treatment, the smallest dose and the shortest duration of treatment producing a satisfactory clinical response should be sought. The need for continued treatment should be reassessed periodically.

If signs and symptoms of tardive dyskinesia appear in a patient on neuroleptics, drug discontinuation should be considered. However, some patients may require treatment despite the presence of the syndrome.

(For further information about the description of tardive dyskinesia and its clinical detection, please refer to "Information for Patients" in the PRECAUTIONS section, and to the ADVERSE REACTIONS section.)

Neuroleptic Malignant Syndrome (NMS)—A potentially fatal symptom complex sometimes referred to as Neuroleptic Malignant Syndrome (NMS) has been reported in association with antipsychotic drugs. Clinical manifestations of NMS are hyperpyrexia, muscle rigidity, altered mental status and evidence of autonomic instability (irregular pulse or blood pressure, tachycardia, diaphoresis, and cardiac dysrhythmias).

The diagnostic evaluation of patients with this syndrome is complicated. In arriving at a diagnosis, it is important to identify cases where the clinical presentation includes both serious medical illness (e.g., pneumonia, systemic infection, etc.) and untreated or inadequately treated extrapyramidal signs and symptoms (EPS). Oher important considerations in the differential diagnosis include central anticholinergic toxicity, heat stroke, drug fever and primary central nervous system (CNS) pathology.

The management of NMS should include 1) immediate discontinuation of antipsychotic drugs and other drugs not essential to concurrent therapy, 2) intensive symptomatic treatment and medical monitoring, and 3) treatment of any concomitant serious medical problems for which specific treatments are available. There is no general agreement about specific pharmacological treatment regiments for uncomplicated NMS.

If a patient requires antipsychotic drug treatment after recovery from NMS, the potential reintroduction of drug therapy should be carefully considered. The patient should be carefully monitored, since recurrences of NMS have been reported.

Usage in Pregnancy—Safe use of Navane during pregnancy has not been established. Therefore, this drug should be given to pregnant patients only when, in the judgment of the physician, the expected benefits from treatment exceed the possible risks to mother and fetus. Animal reproductive studies and clinical experience to date have not demonstrated any teratogenic effects.

Continued on next page

Roerig—Cont.

In the animal reproduction studies with Navane, there was some decrease in conception rate and litter size, and an increase in resorption rate in rats and rabbits, changes which have been similarly reported with other psychotropic agents. After repeated oral administration of Navane to rats (5 to 15 mg./kg./day), rabbits (3 to 50 mg./kg./day), and monkeys (1 to 3 mg./kg./day) before and during gestation, no teratogenic effects were seen. (See Precautions).

Usage in Children—The use of Navane in children under 12 years of age is not recommended because safety and efficacy in the pediatric age group have not been established.

As is true with many CNS drugs, Navane may impair the mental and/or physical abilities required for the performance of potentially hazardous tasks such as driving a car or operating machinery, especially during the first few days of therapy. Therefore, the patient should be cautioned accordingly.

As in the case of other CNS-acting drugs, patients receiving Navane should be cautioned about the possible additive effects (which may include hypotension) with CNS depressants and with alcohol.

PRECAUTIONS

General: An antiemetic effect was observed in animal studies with Navane (thiothixene hydrochloride); since this effect may also occur in man, it is possible that Navane may mask signs of overdosage of toxic drugs and may obscure conditions such as intestinal obstruction and brain tumor.

In consideration of the known capability of Navane and certain other psychotropic drugs to precipitate convulsions, extreme caution should be used in patients with a history of convulsive disorders, or those in a state of alcohol withdrawal since it may lower the convulsive threshold. Although Navane potentiates the actions of the barbiturates, the dosage of the anticonvulsant therapy should not be reduced when Navane is administered concurrently.

Caution as well as careful adjustment of the dosage is indicated when Navane is used in conjunction with other CNS depressants other than anticonvulsant drugs.

Though exhibiting rather weak anticholinergic properties, Navane should be used with caution in patients who are known or suspected to have glaucoma, or who might be exposed to extreme heat, or who are receiving atropine or related drugs.

Use with caution in patients with cardiovascular disease.

Also, careful observation should be made for pigmentary retinopathy, and lenticular pigmentation (fine lenticular pigmentation has been noted in a small number of patients treated with Navane for prolonged periods). Blood dyscrasias (agranulocytosis, pancytopenia, thrombocytopenic purpura), and liver damage (jaundice, biliary stasis), have been reported with related drugs.

Undue exposure to sunlight should be avoided. Photosensitive reactions have been reported in patients on Navane.

As with all intramuscular preparations, Navane Intramuscular should be injected well within the body of a relatively large muscle. The preferred sites are the upper outer quadrant of the buttock (i.e., gluteus maximus) and the mid-lateral thigh.

The deltoid area should be used only if well developed such as in certain adults and older children, and then only with caution to avoid radial nerve injury. Intramuscular injections should not be made into the lower and mid-thirds of the upper arm. As with all intramuscular injections, aspiration is necessary to help avoid inadvertent injection into a blood vessel.

Neuroleptic drugs elevate prolactin levels; the elevation persists during chronic administration. Tissue culture experiments indicate that approximately one-third of human breast cancers are prolactin dependent *in vitro*, a factor of potential importance if the prescription of these drugs is contemplated in a patient with a previously detected breast cancer. Although disturbances such as galactorrhea, amenorrhea, gynecomastia, and impotence have been reported, the clinical significance of elevated serum prolactin levels is unknown for most patients. An increase in mammary neoplasms has been found in rodents after chronic administration of neuroleptic drugs. Neither clinical studies nor epidemiologic studies conducted to date, however, have shown an association between chronic administration of these drugs and mammary tumorigenesis; the available evidence is considered too limited to be conclusive at this time.

Information for Patients: Given the likelihood that some patients exposed chronically to neuroleptics will develop tardive dyskinesia, it is advised that all patients in whom chronic use is contemplated be given, if possible, full information about this risk. The decision to inform patients and/or their guardians must obviously take into account the clinical circumstances and the competency of the patient to understand the information provided.

ADVERSE REACTIONS

NOTE: Not all of the following adverse reactions have been reported with Navane. However, since Navane has certain chemical and pharmacologic similarities to the phenothiazines, all of the known side effects and toxicity associated with phenothiazine therapy should be borne in mind when Navane is used.

Cardiovascular Effects: Tachycardia, hypotension, lightheadedness, and syncope. In the event hypotension occurs, epinephrine should not be used as a pressor agent since a paradoxical further lowering of blood pressure may result. Nonspecific EKG changes have been observed in some patients receiving Navane. These changes are usually reversible and frequently disappear on continued Navane therapy. The clinical significance of these changes is not known.

CNS Effects: Drowsiness, usually mild, may occur although it usually subsides with continuation of Navane therapy. The incidence of sedation appears similar to that of the piperazine group of phenothiazines, but less than that of certain aliphatic phenothiazines. Restlessness, agitation and insomnia have been noted with Navane. Seizures and paradoxical exacerbation of psychotic symptoms have occurred with Navane infrequently.

Hyperreflexia has been reported in infants delivered from mothers having received structurally related drugs.

In addition, phenothiazine derivatives have been associated with cerebral edema and cerebrospinal fluid abnormalities. Extrapyramidal symptoms, such as pseudo-parkinsonism, akathisia, and dystonia have been reported. Management of these extrapyramidal symptoms depends upon the type and severity. Rapid relief of acute symptoms may require the use of an injectable antiparkinson agent. More slowly emerging symptoms may be managed by reducing the dosage of Navane and/or administering an oral antiparkinson agent.

Persistent Tardive Dyskinesia: As with all antipsychotic agents tardive dyskinesia may appear in some patients on long term therapy or may occur after drug therapy has been discontinued. The syndrome is characterized by rhythmical involuntary movements of the tongue, face, mouth or jaw (e.g., protrusion of tongue, puffing of cheeks, puckering of mouth, chewing movements). Sometimes these may be accompanied by involuntary movements of extremities.

Since early detection of tardive dyskinesia is important, patients should be monitored on an ongoing basis. It has been reported that fine vermicular movement of the tongue may be an early sign of the syndrome. If this or any other presentation of the syndrome is observed, the clinician should consider possible discontinuation of neuroleptic medication. (See Warnings section).

Hepatic Effects: Elevations of serum transaminase and alkaline phosphatase, usually transient, have been infrequently observed in some patients. No clinically confirmed cases of jaundice attributable to Navane (thiothixene hydrochloride) have been reported.

Hematologic Effects: As is true with certain other psychotropic drugs, leukopenia and leucocytosis, which are usually transient, can occur occasionally with Navane. Other antipsychotic drugs have been associated with agranulocytosis, eosinophilia, hemolytic anemia, thrombocytopenia and pancytopenia.

Allergic Reactions: Rash, pruritus, urticaria, and rare cases of anaphylaxis have been reported with Navane. Undue exposure to sunlight should be avoided. Although not experienced with Navane, exfoliative dermatitis, contact dermatitis (in nursing personnel), have been reported with certain phenothiazines.

Endocrine Disorders: Lactation, moderate breast enlargement and amenorrhea have occurred in a small percentage of females receiving Navane. If persistent, this may necessitate a reduction in dosage or the discontinuation of therapy. Phenothiazines have been associated with false positive pregnancy tests, gynecomastia, hypoglycemia, hyperglycemia, and glycosuria.

Autonomic Effects: Dry mouth, blurred vision, nasal congestion, constipation, increased sweating, increased salivation, and impotence have occurred infrequently with Navane therapy. Phenothiazines have been associated with miosis, mydriasis, and adynamic ileus.

Other Adverse Reactions: Hyperpyrexia, anorexia, nausea, vomiting, diarrhea, increase in appetite and weight, weakness or fatigue, polydipsia and peripheral edema.

Although not reported with Navane, evidence indicates there is a relationship between phenothiazine therapy and the occurrence of a systemic lupus erythematosus-like syndrome.

Neuroleptic Malignant Syndrome (NMS): Please refer to the text regarding NMS in the WARNINGS section.

NOTE: Sudden deaths have occasionally been reported in patients who have received certain phenothiazine derivatives. In some cases the cause of death was apparently cardiac arrest or asphyxia due to failure of the cough reflex. In others, the cause could not be determined nor could it be established that death was due to phenothiazine administration.

DOSAGE AND ADMINISTRATION

Preparation

Navane (thiothixene hydrochloride) Intramuscular Solution is ready for use as supplied.

Navane (thiothixene hydrochloride) Intramuscular For Injection must be reconstituted with 2.2 ml of Sterile Water for Injection.

For Intramuscular Use Only

Dosage of Navane should be individually adjusted depending on the chronicity and severity of the condition. In general, small doses should be used initially and gradually increased to the optimal effective level, based on patient response. Usage in children under 12 years of age is not recommended. Where more rapid control and treatment of acute behavior is desirable, the intramuscular form of Navane may be indicated. It is also of benefit where the very nature of the patient's symptomatology, whether acute or chronic, renders oral administration impractical or even impossible.

For treatment of acute symptomatology or in patients unable or unwilling to take oral medication, the usual dose is 4 mg. of Navane Intramuscular administered 2 to 4 times daily. Dosage may be increased or decreased depending on response. Most patients are controlled on a total daily dosage of 16 to 20 mg. The maximum recommended dosage is 30 mg./day. An oral form should supplant the injectable form as soon as possible. It may be necessary to adjust the dosage when changing from the intramuscular to oral dosage forms. Dosage recommendations for Navane Capsules and Concentrate can be found in the Navane oral package insert.

OVERDOSAGE

Manifestations include muscular twitching, drowsiness, and dizziness. Symptoms of gross overdosage may include CNS depression, rigidity, weakness, torticollis, tremor, salivation, dysphagia, hypotension, disturbances of gait, or coma.

Treatment: Essentially symptomatic and supportive. Keep patient under careful observation and maintain an open airway, since involvement of the extrapyramidal system may produce dysphagia and respiratory difficulty in severe overdosage. If hypotension occurs, the standard measures for managing circulatory shock should be used (I.V. fluids and/or vasoconstrictors).

If a vasoconstrictor is needed, levarterenol and phenylephrine are the most suitable drugs. Other pressor agents, including epinephrine, are not recommended, since phenothiazine derivatives may reverse the usual pressor elevating action of these agents and cause further lowering of blood pressure.

If CNS depression is marked, symptomatic treatment is indicated. Extrapyramidal symptoms may be treated with antiparkinson drugs.

There are no data on the use of peritoneal or hemodialysis, but they are known to be of little value in phenothiazine intoxication.

HOW SUPPLIED

Navane (thiothixene hydrochloride) Intramuscular Solution is available in a 2 ml. amber glass vial in packages of 10 vials (NDC 0049-5760-83). Each ml. contains thiothixene hydrochloride equivalent to 2 mg. of thiothixene, dextrose 5% w/v, benzyl alcohol 0.9% w/v, and propyl gallate 0.02% w/v.

Navane (thiothixene hydrochloride) Intramuscular For Injection is available in amber glass vials in packages of 10 vials (NDC 0049-5765-83). When reconstituted with 2.2 ml of STERILE WATER FOR INJECTION, each ml contains thiothixene hydrochloride equivalent to 5 mg of thiothixene, and 59.6 mg of mannitol. The reconstituted solution of Navane Intramuscular For Injection may be stored for 48 hours at room temperature before discarding.

70-1865-00-3
70-4177-00-4

Buffered
PFIZERPEN®   ℞
(penicillin G potassium)
for Injection

DESCRIPTION

Buffered Pfizerpen (penicillin G potassium) for Injection is a sterile, pyrogen-free powder for reconstitution. Buffered Pfizerpen for Injection is an antibacterial agent for intramuscular, continuous intravenous drip, intrapleural or other local infusion, and intrathecal administration.

Each million units contains approximately 6.8 milligrams of sodium (0.3 mEq) and 65.6 milligrams of potassium (1.68 mEq).

Chemically, Pfizerpen is monopotassium 3,3-dimethyl-7oxo-6-(2-phenylacetamido)-4-thia-1-azabicyclo (3.2.0) heptane-2-carboxylate. It has a molecular weight of 372.48 and the following chemical structure:

[See Chemical Formula at top of next column].

Penicillin G potassium is a colorless or white crystal, or a white crystalline powder which is odorless, or practically so,

Formula
$C_{16}H_{17}KN_2O_4S$

and moderately hygroscopic. Penicillin G potassium is very soluble in water. The pH of the reconstituted product is between 6.0–8.5.

CLINICAL PHARMACOLOGY

Aqueous penicillin G is rapidly absorbed following both intramuscular and subcutaneous injection. Initial blood levels following parenteral administration are high but transient. Penicillins bind to serum proteins, mainly albumin. Therapeutic levels of the penicillins are easily achieved under normal circumstances in extracellular fluid and most other body tissues. Penicillins are distributed in varying degrees into pleural, pericardial, peritoneal, ascitic, synovial, and interstitial fluids. Penicillins are excreted in breast milk. Penetration into the cerebrospinal fluid, eyes, and prostate is poor. Penicillins are rapidly excreted in the urine by glomerular filtration and active tubular secretion, primarily as unchanged drug. Approximately 60 percent of the total dose of 300,000 units is excreted in the urine within this 5 hour period. For this reason high and frequent doses are required to maintain the elevated serum levels desirable in treating certain severe infections in individuals with normal kidney function. In neonates and young infants, and in individuals with impaired kidney function, excretion is considerably delayed.

Microbiology

Penicillin G exerts a bactericidal action against penicillin-susceptible microorganisms during the stage of active multiplication. It acts through the inhibition of biosynthesis of cell wall mucopeptide rendering the cell wall osmotically unstable. It is not active against the penicillinase-producing bacteria, which include many strains of staphylococci. While *in vitro* studies have demonstrated the susceptibility of most strains of the following organisms, clinical efficacy for infections other than those included in the INDICATIONS AND USAGE section has not been documented. Penicillin G exerts high *in vitro* activity against staphylococci (except penicillinase-producing strains), streptococci (groups A, C, G, H, L, and M), and pneumococci. Other organisms susceptible to penicillin G are *N. gonorrhoeae, Corynebacterium diphtheriae, Bacillus anthracis,* Clostridia, *Actinomyces bovis, Streptobacillus moniliformis, Listeria monocytogenes* and Leptospira. *Treponema pallidum* is extremely sensitive to the bactericidal action of penicillin G. Some species of gram-negative bacilli are sensitive to moderate to high concentrations of the drug obtained with intravenous administration. These include most strains of *Escherichia coli;* all strains of *Proteus mirabilis,* Salmonella and Shigella; and some strains of *Aerobacter aerogenes* and *Alcaligenes faecalis.*
Penicillin acts synergistically with gentamicin or tobramycin against many strains of enterococci.

Susceptibility Testing: Penicillin G Susceptibility Powder or 10 units Penicillin G Susceptibility Discs may be used to determine microbial susceptibility to penicillin G using one of the following standard methods recommended by the National Committee for Laboratory Standards:

M2-A3, "Performance Standards for Antimicrobial Disk Susceptibility Tests"

M7-A, "Methods for Dilution Antimicrobial Susceptibility Tests for Bacteria that Grow Aerobically"

M11-A, "Reference Agar Dilution Procedure for Antimicrobial Susceptibility Testing of Anaerobic Bacteria"

M17-P, "Alternative Methods for Antimicrobial Susceptibility Testing of Anaerobic Bacteria"

Tests should be interpreted by the following criteria:

Zone Diameter, nearest whole mm			
	Susceptible	Moderately Susceptible	Resistant
Staphylococci	≥ 29	—	≤ 28
N. gonorrhoeae	≥ 20	—	≤ 19
Enterococci	—	≥ 15	≤ 14
Non-enterococcal streptococci and *L. monocytogenes*	≥ 28	20-27	≤ 19

Approximate MIC Correlates		
	Susceptible	Resistant
Staphylococci	≤ 0.2 µg/mL	β-lactamase
N. gonorrhoeae	≤ 0.1 µg/mL	β-lactamase
Enterococci		≥ 16 µg/mL
Non-enterococcal streptococci and *L. monocytogenes*	≤ 0.12 µg/mL	≥ 4 µg/mL

Interpretations of susceptible, intermediate, and resistant correlate zone size diameters with MIC values. A laboratory

report of "susceptible" indicates that the suspected causative microorganism most likely will respond to therapy with penicillin G. A laboratory report of "resistant" indicates that the infecting microorganism most likely will not respond to therapy. A laboratory report of "moderately susceptible" indicates that the microorganism is most likely susceptible if a high dosage of penicillin G is used, or if the infection is such that high levels of penicillin G may be attained, as in urine. A report of "intermediate" using the disk diffusion method may be considered an equivocal result, and dilution tests may be indicated.

Control organisms are recommended for susceptibility testing. Each time the test is performed the following organisms should be included. The range for zones of inhibition is shown below;

Control Organism	Zone of Inhibition Range
Staphylococcus aureus (ATCC 25923)	27–35

INDICATIONS AND USAGE

Aqueous penicillin G (parenteral) is indicated in the therapy of severe infections caused by penicillin G-susceptible microorganisms when rapid and high penicillin levels are required in the conditions listed below. Therapy should be guided by bacteriological studies (including susceptibility tests) and by clinical response.

The following infections will usually respond to adequate dosage of aqueous penicillin G (parenteral):

Streptococcal infections.

NOTE: Streptococci in groups A, C, H, G, L, and M are very sensitive to penicillin G. Some group D organisms are sensitive to the high serum levels obtained with aqueous penicillin G.

Aqueous penicillin (parenteral) is the penicillin dosage form of choice for bacteremia, empyema, severe pneumonia, pericarditis, endocarditis, meningitis, and other severe infections caused by sensitive strains of the gram-positive species listed above.

Pneumococcal infections.

Staphylococcal infections —penicillin G sensitive.

Other infections:

Anthrax.

Actinomycosis.

Clostridial infections (including tetanus).

Diphtheria (to prevent carrier state).

Erysipeloid (*Erysipelothrix insidiosa*) endocarditis.

Fusospirochetal infections—severe infections of the oropharynx (Vincent's), lower respiratory tract and genital area due to *Fusobacterium fusiformisans* spirochetes.

Gram-negative bacillary infections (bateremias)—(*E. coli, A. aerogenes, A. faecalis,* Salmonella, Shigella and *P. mirabilis*).

Listeria infections (*Listeria monocytogenes*).

Meningitis and endocarditis.

Pasteurella infections (*Pasteurella multocida*).

Bacteremia and meningitis.

Rat-bite fever (*Spirillum minus* or *Streptobacillus moniliformis*).

Gonorrheal endocarditis and arthritis (*N. gonorrhoeae*).

Syphilis (*T. pallidum*) including congenital syphilis.

Meningococcic meningitis.

Although no controlled clinical efficacy studies have been conducted, aqueous crystalline penicillin G for injection and penicillin G procaine suspension have been suggested by the American Heart Association and the American Dental Association for use as part of a combined parenteral-oral regimen for prophylaxis against bacterial endocarditis in patients with congenital heart disease or rheumatic, or other acquired valvular heart disease when they undergo dental procedures and surgical procedures of the upper respiratory tract.[1] Since it may happen that *alpha* hemolytic streptococci relatively resistant to penicillin may be found when patients are receiving continuous oral penicillin for secondary prevention of rheumatic fever, prophylactic agents other than penicillin may be chosen for these patients and prescribed in addition to their continuous rheumatic fever prophylactic regimen.

NOTE: When selecting antibiotics for the prevention of bacterial endocarditis the physician or dentist should read the full joint statement of the American Heart Association and the American Dental Association.[1]

CONTRAINDICATIONS

A history of a previous hypersensitivity reaction to any penicillin is a contraindication.

WARNINGS

Serious and occasionally fatal hypersensitivity (anaphylactoid) reactions have been reported in patients on penicillin therapy. These reactions are more likely to occur in individuals with a history of penicillin hypersensitivity and/or a history of sensitivity to multiple allergens. There have been reports of individuals with a history of penicillin hypersensitivity who have experienced severe reactions when treated with cephalosporins. Before initiating therapy with any penicillin, careful inquiry should be made concerning previous

hypersensitivity reactions to penicillin, cephalosporins, or other allergens. If an allergic reaction occurs, the drug should be discontinued and the appropriate therapy instituted. Serious anaphylactoid reactions require immediate emergency treatment with epinephrine. Oxygen, intravenous steroids, and airway management including incubation, should also be administered as indicated.

PRECAUTIONS

General: Penicillin should be used with caution in individuals with histories of significant allergies and/or asthma.

Intramuscular Therapy: Care should be taken to avoid intravenous or accidental intraarterial administration, or injection into or near major peripheral nerves or blood vessels, since such injections may produce neurovascular damage. Particular care should be taken with IV administration because of the possibility of thrombophlebitis.

In streptococcal infections, therapy must be sufficient to eliminate the organism (10 days minimum) otherwise the sequelae of streptococcal disease may occur. Cultures should be taken following the completion of treatment to determine whether streptococci have been eradicated.

The use of antibiotics may result in overgrowth of nonsusceptible organisms. Constant observation of the patient is essential. If new infections due to bacteria or fungi appear during therapy, the drug should be discontinued and appropriate measures taken. Whenever allergic reactions occur, penicillin should be withdrawn unless, in the opinion of the physician, the condition being treated is life threatening and amenable only to penicillin therapy.

Aqueous penicillin G by the intravenous route in high doses (above 10 million units), should be administered slowly because of the adverse effects of electrolyte imbalance from either the potassium or sodium content of the penicillin. Potassium penicillin G contains 1.7 mEq potassium and 0.3 mEq sodium per million units. The patient's renal, cardiac, and vascular status should be evaluated and if impairment of function is suspected or known to exist a reduction in the total dosage should be considered. Frequent evaluation of electrolyte balance, renal and hematopoietic function is recommended during therapy when high doses of intravenous aqueous penicillin G are used.

Laboratory Tests: In prolonged therapy with penicillin, periodic evaluation of the renal, hepatic, and hematopoietic systems is recommended for organ system dysfunction. This is particularly important in prematures, neonates and other infants, and when high doses are used.

Positive Coomb's tests have been reported after large intravenous doses.

Monitor serum potassium and implement corrective measures when necessary.

When treating gonococcal infections in which primary and secondary syphilis are suspected, proper diagnostic procedures, including dark field examinations, should be done before receiving penicillin and monthly serological tests made for at least four months. All cases of penicillin treated syphilis should receive clinical and serological examinations every six months for two to three years.

In suspected staphylococcal infections, proper laboratory studies, including susceptibility tests, should be performed.

In streptococcal infections, cultures should be taken following completion of treatment to determine whether streptococci have been eradicated. Therapy must be sufficient to eliminate the organism (a minimum of 10 days), otherwise the sequelae of streptococcal disease (e.g., endocarditis, rheumatic fever) may occur.

Drug Interactions: Concurrent administration of bacteriostatic antibiotics (e.g., erythromycin, tetracycline) may diminish the bactericidal effects of penicillins by slowing the rate of bacterial growth. Bactericidal agents work most effectively against the immature cell wall of rapidly proliferating microorganisms. This has been demonstrated *in vitro:* however, the clinical significance of this interaction is not well documented. There are few clinical situations in which the concurrent use of "static" and "cidal" antibiotics are indicated. However, in selected circumstances in which such therapy is appropriate, using adequate doses of antibacterial agents and beginning penicillin therapy first, should minimize the potential for interaction.

Penicillin blood levels may be prolonged by concurrent administration of probenecid which blocks the renal tubular secretion of penicillins.

Displacement of penicillin from plasma protein binding sites will elevate the level of free penicillin in the serum.

Carcinogenesis, Mutagenesis, Impairment of Fertility: No information on long-term studies are available on the carcinogenesis, mutagenesis, or the impairment of fertility with the use of penicillins.

Pregnancy Category B—*Teratogenic Effects:* Reproduction studies performed in the mouse, rat, and rabbit have revealed no evidence of impaired fertility or harm to the fetus due to penicillin G. Human experience with the penicillins during pregnancy has not shown any positive evidence of adverse effects on the fetus. There are, however, no adequate

Continued on next page

Roerig—Cont.

and well controlled studies in pregnant women showing conclusively that harmful effects of these drugs on the fetus can be excluded. Because animal reproduction studies are not always predictive of human response, this drug should be used during pregnancy only if clearly needed.

Nursing Mothers: Penicillins are excreted in human milk. Caution should be exercised when penicillin G is administered to a nursing woman.

Pediatric Use: Penicillins are excreted largely unchanged by the kidney. Because of incompletely developed renal function in infants, the rate of elimination will be slow. Use caution in administering to newborns and evaluate organ system function frequently.

ADVERSE REACTIONS

Penicillin is a substance of low toxicity but does have a significant index of sensitization. The following hypersensitivity reactions have been reported: skin rashes ranging from maculopapular eruptions to exfoliative dermatitis: urticaria and reactions resembling serum sickness, including chills, fever, edema, arthralgia and prostration. Severe and occasionally fatal anaphylaxis has occurred (see "Warnings").

Hemolytic anemia, leucopenia, thrombocytopenia, nephropathy, and neuropathy are rarely observed adverse reactions and are usually associated with high intravenous dosage. Patients given continuous intravenous therapy with penicillin G potassium in high dosage (10 million to 100 million units daily) may suffer severe or even fatal potassium poisoning, particularly if renal insufficiency is present. Hyperreflexia, convulsions and coma may be indicative of this syndrome.

Cardiac arrhythmias and cardiac arrest may also occur. (High dosage of penicillin G sodium may result in congestive heart failure due to high sodium intake.)

The Jarisch-Herxheimer reaction has been reported in patients treated for syphilis.

OVERDOSAGE

Neurological adverse reactions, including convulsions, may occur with the attainment of high CSF levels of beta-lactams. In case of overdosage, discontinue medication, treat symptomatically, and institute supportive measures as required. Penicillin G potassium is hemodialyzable.

DOSAGE AND ADMINISTRATION

Severe infections due to Susceptible Strains of Streptococci, Pneumococci and Staphylococci —bacteremia, pneumonia, endocarditis, pericarditis, empyema, meningitis and other severe infections—a minimum of 5 million units daily.

Syphilis —Aqueous penicillin G may be used in the treatment of acquired and congenital syphilis, but because of the necessity of frequent dosage, hospitalization is recommended. Dosage and duration of therapy will be determined by age of patient and stage of disease.

Gonorrheal endocarditis —a minimum of 5 million units daily.

Meningococcic meningitis —1–2 million units intramuscularly every 2 hours, or continuous IV drip of 20–30 million units/day.

Actinomycosis —1–6 million units/day for cervicofacial cases; 10–20 million units/day for thoracic and abdominal disease.

Clostridial infections —20 million units/day; penicillin is adjunctive therapy to antitoxin.

Fusospirochetal infections —severe infections of oropharynx, lower respiratory tract and genital area—5–10 million units/day.

Rat-bite fever (Spirillum minus or Streptobacillus moniliformis) —12–15 million units/day for 3–4 weeks.

Listeria infections (Listeria monocytogenes).
Neonates—500,000 to 1 million units/day.
Adults with meningitis—15–20 million units/day for 2 weeks.
Adults with endocarditis—15–20 million units/day for 4 weeks.

Pasteurella infections (Pasteurella multocida).
Bacteremia and meningitis—4–6 million units/day for 2 weeks.

Erysipeloid (Erysipelothrix insidiosa).
Endocarditis—2–20 million units/day for 4–6 weeks.

Gram-negative bacillary infections (E. coli, A. aerogenes, A. faecalis, Salmonella, Shigella and Proteus mirabilis).

Bacteremia—20–80 million units/day.

Diphtheria (carrier state): 300,000–400,000 units of penicillin/day in divided doses for 10–12 days.

Anthrax —A minimum of 5 million units of penicillin/day in divided doses until cure is effected.

For prophylaxis against bacterial endocarditis[1] in patients with congenital heart disease or rheumatic, or other acquired valvular heart disease when undergoing dental procedures or surgical procedures of the upper respiratory tract, use a combined parenteral-oral regimen. One million units of aqueous crystalline penicillin G (30,000 units/kg in children) intramuscularly mixed with 600,000 units procaine penicillin G (600,000 units for children) should be given one-half to one hour before the procedure. Oral penicillin V (phenoxymethyl penicillin), 500 mg for adults or 250 mg for children less than 60 lb, should be given every 6 hours for 8 doses. Doses for children should not exceed recommendations for adults for a single dose or for a 24 hour period.

Reconstitution
The following table shows the amount of solvent required for solution of various concentrations.
[See table below].

When the required volume of solvent is greater than the capacity of the vial, the penicillin can be dissolved by first injecting only a portion of the solvent into the vial, then withdrawing the resultant solution and combining it with the remainder of the solvent in a larger sterile container. Buffered Pfizerpen (penicillin G potassium) for Injection is highly water soluble. It may be dissolved in small amounts of Water for Injection, or Sterile Isotonic Sodium Chloride Solution for Parenteral Use. All solutions should be stored in a refrigerator. When refrigerated, penicillin solutions may be stored for seven days without significant loss of potency.

Buffered Pfizerpen for Injection may be given intramuscularly or by continuous intravenous drip for dosages of 500,000, 1,000,000, or 5,000,000 units. It is also suitable for intrapleural, intraarticular, and other local instillations. THE 20,000,000 UNIT DOSAGE MAY BE ADMINISTERED BY INTRAVENOUS INFUSION ONLY.

(1) Intramuscular Injection: Keep total volume of injection small. The intramuscular route is the preferred route of administration. Solutions containing up to 100,000 units of penicillin per ml of diluent may be used with a minimum of discomfort. Greater concentration of penicillin G per ml is physically possible and may be employed where therapy demands. When large dosages are required, it may be advisable to administer aqueous solutions of penicillin by means of continuous intravenous drip.

(2) Continuous Intravenous Drip: Determine the volume of fluid and rate of its administration required by the patient in a 24-hour period in the usual manner for fluid therapy, and add the appropriate daily dosage of penicillin to this fluid. For example, if an adult patient requires 2 liters of fluid in 24 hours and a daily dosage of 10 million units of penicillin, add 5 million units to 1 liter and adjust the rate of flow so that the liter will be infused in 12 hours.

(3) Intrapleural or Other Local Infusion: If fluid is aspirated, give infusion in a volume equal to $\frac{1}{4}$ or $\frac{1}{2}$ the amount of fluid aspirated, otherwise, prepare as for intramuscular injection.

(4) Intrathecal Use: The intrathecal use of penicillin in meningitis must be highly individualized. It should be employed only with full consideration of the possible irritating effects of penicillin when used by this route. The preferred route of therapy in bacterial meningitides is intravenous, supplemented by intramuscular injection.

Parenteral drug products should be inspected visually for particulate matter and discoloration prior to administration, whenever solution and container permit.

Sterile solution may be left in refrigerator for one week without significant loss of potency.

HOW SUPPLIED

Buffered Pfizerpen (penicillin G potassium) for Injection is available in vials containing respectively 1,000,000 units × 10's (NDC 0049-0510-83), 1,000,000 units × 100's (NDC 0049-0510-95), 5,000,000 units × 10's (NDC 0049-0520-83), 5,000,000 units × 100's (NDC 0049-0520-95), 20,000,000 units × 1's (NDC 0049-0530-28), and a bulk pharmacy package of 20,000,000 units × 10's (NDC 0049-0530-83) of dry powder for reconstitution; buffered with sodium citrate and citric acid to an optimum pH.

Each million units contains approximately 6.8 milligrams of sodium (0.3 mEq) and 65.6 milligrams of potassium (1.68 mEq).

Store the dry powder below 86°F (30°C).

REFERENCE

1. American Heart Association. 1977. Prevention of bacterial endocarditis. Circulation. 56:139A–143A.

70-4209-00-5

PFIZERPEN®–AS ℞
(penicillin G procaine)
in Aqueous Suspension
For Intramuscular Use Only

DESCRIPTION

Pfizerpen-AS (penicillin G procaine) is a highly potent antibacterial agent effective against a wide variety of pathogenic organisms. It is an equimolecular compound of procaine and penicillin G in aqueous suspension for intramuscular administration.

Pfizerpen-AS is supplied in 10 ml vials (3,000,000 units).

Chemically, Pfizerpen-AS is: 3,3-Dimethyl-7-oxo-6-(2-phenylacetamido)-4-thia-1-azabicyclo [3.2.0] heptane-2-carboxylic acid compound with 2-(diethylamino) ethyl-ρ-aminobenzoate (1:1) monohydrate.

It has a molecular weight of 588.72 and the following chemical structure:

Formula
$C_{16}H_{18}N_2O_4S \cdot C_{13}H_{20}N_2O_2 \cdot H_2O$

Penicillin G procaine is a white, fine crystal, or a white, very fine microcrystalline powder. Penicillin G procaine is odorless or practically so and 1 gram is soluble in 250 ml water. The pH of the aqueous suspension is between 5.0–7.5.

CLINICAL PHARMACOLOGY

Penicillin G procaine is an equimolecular compound of procaine and penicillin G administered intramuscularly as a suspension. It dissolves slowly at the site of injection, giving a plateau type of blood level at about 4 hours, which falls slowly over a period of the next 15–20 hours.

Approximately 60% of penicillin G is bound to serum protein. The drug is distributed throughout the body tissues in widely varying amounts. Highest levels are found in the kidneys with lesser amounts in the liver, skin, and intestines. Penicillin G penetrates into all other tissues to a lesser degree with a very small level found in the cerobrospinal fluid. With normal kidney function the drug is excreted rapidly by tubular excretion. In neonates and young infants, and in individuals with impaired kidney function, excretion is considerably delayed. Approximately 60%–90% of a dose of parenteral penicillin G is excreted in the urine within 24–36 hours. Penicillin G crosses the placental barrier and is found in the amniotic fluid and cord serum.

Microbiology

Penicillin G exerts a bactericidal action against penicillin-susceptible microorganisms during the stage of active multiplication. It acts through the inhibition of biosynthesis of cell wall mucopeptide. It is not active against the penicillinase-producing bacteria, which include many strains of staphylococci. While *in vitro* studies have demonstrated the susceptibility of most strains of the following organisms, clinical efficacy for infections other than those included in the INDICATIONS AND USAGE section has not been documented. Penicillin G exerts high *in vitro* activity against staphylococci (except penicillinase-producing strains), streptococci (groups A, C, G, H, L, and M), and pneumococci. Other organisms sensitive to penicillin G are *N. gonorrhoeae. Corynebacterium diphtheriae, Bacillus anthracis,* Clostridia, *Actinomyces bovis. Streptobacillus moniliformis, Listeria monocytogenes,* and Leptospira. *Treponema pallidum* is extremely sensitive to the bactericidal action of penicillin G. Penicillin acts synergistically with gentamicin or tobramycin against many strains of enterococci.

Susceptibility Testing: Penicillin G Susceptibility Powder or 10 units Penicillin G Susceptibility Discs may be used to determine microbial susceptibility to penicillin G using one of the following standard methods recommended by the National Committee for Laboratory Standards:

M2-A3, "Performance Standards for Antimicrobial Disk Susceptibility Tests"
M7-A, "Methods for Dilution Antimicrobial Susceptibility Tests for Bacteria that Grow Aerobically"
M11-A, "Reference Agar Dilution Procedure for Antimicrobial Susceptibility Testing of Anaerobic Bacteria"
M17-P, "Alternative Methods for Antimicrobial Susceptibility Testing of Anaerobic Bacteria"

Approx. Desired Concentration (units/ml)	Approx. Volume (ml) 1,000,000 units	Solvent for Vial of 5,000,000 units	Infusion Only 20,000,000 units
50,000	20.0	—	—
100,000	10.0	—	—
250,000	4.0	18.2	75.0
500,000	1.8	8.2	33.0
750,000	—	4.8	—
1,000,000	—	3.2	11.5

Tests should be interpreted by the following criteria:

	Zone Diameter, nearest whole mm		
	Susceptible	Moderately Susceptible	Resistant
Staphylococci	≥ 29	–	≥ 28
N. gonorrhoeae	≥ 20	–	≥ 19
Enterococci	–	≥ 15	≥ 14
Non-enterococcal streptococci and L. monocytogenes	≥ 28	20–27	≥ 19

	Approximate MIC Correlates	
	Susceptible	Resistant
Staphylococci	≤ 0.1 µg/mL	β-lactamase
N. gonorrhoeae	≤ 0.1 µg/mL	β-lactamase
Enterococci	–	≥ 16 µg/mL
Non-enterococcal streptococci and L. monocytogenes	≤ 0.12 µg/mL	≥ 4 µg/mL

Interpretations of susceptible, intermediate, and resistant correlate zone size diameters with MIC values. A laboratory report of "susceptible" indicates that the suspected causative microorganism most likely will respond to therapy with penicillin G. A laboratory report of "resistant" indicates that the infecting microorganism most likely will not respond to therapy. A laboratory report of "moderately susceptible" indicates that the microorganism is most likely susceptible if a high dosage of penicillin G is used, or if the infection is such that high levels of penicillin G may be attained as in urine. A report of "intermediate" using the disk diffusion method may be considered an equivocal result, and dilution tests may be indicated.

Control organisms are recommended for susceptibility testing. Each time the test is performed the following organisms should be included. The range for zones of inhibition is shown below:

Control Organism	Zone of Inhibition Range
Staphylococcus aureus (ATCC 25923)	27–35

INDICATIONS AND USAGE

Penicillin G procaine is indicated in the treatment of moderately severe infections in both adults and children due to penicillin G-susceptible microorganisms that are susceptible to the low and persistent serum levels common to this particular dosage form in the indications listed below. Therapy should be guided by bacteriological studies (including susceptibility tests) and by clinical response.

NOTE: When high sustained serum levels are required, aqueous penicillin G either IM or IV should be used.

The following infections will usually respond to adequate dosages of intramuscular penicillin G procaine.

Streptococcal infections Group A (without bacteremia). Moderately severe to severe infections of the upper respiratory tract (including middle ear infections-otitis media), skin and soft tissue infections, scarlet fever, and erysipelas.

NOTE: Streptococci in groups A, C, H, G, L, and M are very sensitive to penicillin G. Other groups, including group D (enterococcus) are resistant. Aqueous penicillin G is recommended for streptococcal infections with bacteremia.

Pneumococcal infections: Moderately severe infections of the respiratory tract (including middle ear infections-otitis media).

NOTE: Severe pneumonia, empyema, bacteremia, pericarditis, meningitis, peritonitis, and purulent or septic arthritis of pneumonococcal etiology are better treated with aqueous penicillin G during the acute stage.

Staphylococcal infections: penicillin G-sensitive. Moderately severe infections of the skin and soft tissues.

NOTE: Reports indicate an increasing number of strains of staphylococci resistant to penicillin G emphasizing the need for culture and sensitivity studies in treating suspected staphylococcal infections.

Indicated surgical procedures should be performed.

Fusospirochetosis (Vincent's gingivitis and pharyngitis). Moderately severe infections of the oropharynx respond to therapy with penicillin G procaine.

NOTE: Necessary dental care should be accomplished in infections involving the gum tissue.

Treponema pallidum (syphilis): all stages.

N. gonorrhoeae: acute and chronic (without bacteremia).

Yaws, Bejel, Pinta.

C. diphtheriae—penicillin G procaine as an adjunct to antitoxin for prevention of the carrier stage.

Anthrax.

Streptobacillus moniliformis and *Spirillum minus* infections (rat bite fever).

Erysipeloid.

Subacute bacterial endocarditis (group A streptococcus) only in extremely sensitive infections.

Prophylaxis Against Bacterial endocarditis—Although no controlled clinical efficacy studies have been conducted, aqueous crystalline penicillin G for injection and penicillin G procaine suspension have been suggested by the American Heart Association and the American Dental Association for use as part of a combined parenteral-oral regimen for prophylaxis against bacterial endocarditis in patients with congenital heart disease or rheumatic, or other acquired valvular heart disease when they undergo dental procedures and surgical procedures of the upper respiratory tract.[1] Since it may happen that *alpha* hemolytic streptococci relatively resistant to penicillin may be found when patients are receiving continuous oral penicillin for secondary prevention of rheumatic fever, prophylactic agents other than penicillin may be chosen for these patients and prescribed in addition to their continuous rheumatic fever prophylactic regimen.

NOTE: When selecting antibiotics for the prevention of bacterial endocarditis the physician or dentist should read the full joint statement of the American Heart Association and the American Dental Association.

CONTRAINDICATIONS

A previous hypersensitivity reaction to any penicillin or procaine is a contraindication.

WARNINGS

Serious and occasionally fatal hypersensitivity (anaphylactoid) reactions have been reported in patients on penicillin therapy. These reactions are more likely to occur in individuals with a history of penicillin hypersensitivity and/or a history of sensitivity to multiple allergens. There have been reports of individuals with a history of penicillin hypersensitivity who have experienced severe reactions when treated with cephalosporins. Before initiating therapy with any penicillin, careful inquiry should be made concerning previous hypersensitivity reactions to penicillin, cephalosporins, or other allergens. If an allergic reaction occurs, the drug should be discontinued and the appropriate therapy instituted. Serious anaphylactoid reactions require immediate emergency treatment with epinephrine. Oxygen, intravenous steroids, and airway management-including intubation, should be administered as indicated.

Immediate toxic reactions to procaine may occur in some individuals, particularly when a large single dose is administered in the treatment of gonorrhea (4.8 million units). These reactions may be manifested by mental disturbances including anxiety, confusion, agitation, depression, weakness, seizures, hallucinations, combativeness, and expressed "fear of impending death." The reactions noted in carefully controlled studies occurred in approximately one in 500 patients treated for gonorrhea. Reactions are transient, lasting from 15-30 minutes.

PRECAUTIONS

General: Penicillin should be used with caution in individuals with histories of significant allergies and/or asthma.

Intramuscular Therapy: Care should be taken to avoid intravenous or accidental intraarterial administration, or injection into or near major peripheral nerves or blood vessels, since such injections may produce neurovascular damage.

As with all intramuscular preparations, Pfizerpen-AS (penicillin G procaine) should be injected well within the body of a relatively large muscle, ADULTS: The preferred site is the upper quadrant of the buttock (i.e., gluteus maximus), or the mid-lateral thigh. CHILDREN: It is recommended that intramuscular injections be given preferably in the mid-lateral muscles of the thigh. In infants and small children the periphery of the upper outer quadrant of the gluteal region should only be used when necessary, such as in burn patients, in order to minimize the possibility of damage to the sciatic nerve.

The deltoid area should be used only if well developed, such as in certain adults and older children, and then only with caution to avoid radial nerve injury. Intramuscular injections should not be made into the lower and mid-third of the upper arm. As with all intramuscular injections, aspiration is necessary to help avoid inadvertent injection into a blood vessel.

In streptococcal infections, therapy must be sufficient to eliminate the organism (10 days minimum), otherwise the sequelae of streptococcal disease may occur. Cultures should be taken following completion of treatment to determine whether streptococci have been eradicated.

The use of antibiotics may result in overgrowth of nonsusceptible organisms. Constant observation of the patient is essential. If new infections due to bacteria or fungi appear during therapy, the drug should be discontinued and appropriate measures taken. Whenever allergic reactions occur, penicillin should be withdrawn unless, in the opinion of the physician, the condition being treated is life threatening and amenable only to penicillin therapy.

A small percentage of patients are sensitive to procaine. If there is a history of sensitivity make the usual test. Inject intradermally 0.1 ml of a 1 to 2 percent solution. Development of an erythema, wheal, flare, or eruption indicates procaine sensitivity. Sensitivity should be treated by the usual methods, including barbiturates, and penicillin G procaine preparations should not be used. Antihistamines appear beneficial in treatment of procaine reactions.

Laboratory Tests: In prolonged therapy with penicillin, periodic evaluation of the renal, hepatic, and hematopoietic systems is recommended. This is particularly important in prematures, neonates and other infants, and when high doses are used.

When treating gonococcal infections in which primary or secondary syphilis may be suspected, proper diagnostic procedures, including dark field examinations, should be done. In all cases in which concomitant syphilis is suspected, monthly serological tests should be made for at least four months. All cases of penicillin treated syphilis should receive clinical and serological examinations every six months for two to three years.

In suspected staphylococcal infections, proper laboratory studies, including susceptibility tests, should be performed. In streptococcal infections, cultures should be taken following completion of treatment to determine whether streptococci have been eradicated.

Drug Interactions: Concurrent administration of bacteriostatic antibiotics (e.g., erythromycin, tetracycline) may diminish the bactericidal effects of penicillins by slowing the rate of bacterial growth. Bactericidal agents work most effectively against the immature cell wall of rapidly proliferating microorganisms. This has been demonstrated *in vitro*; however, the clinical significance of this interaction is not well documented. There are few clinical situations in which the concurrent use of "static" and "cidal" antibiotics are indicated. However, in selected circumstances in which such therapy is appropriate, using adequate doses of antibacterial agents and beginning penicillin therapy first, should minimize the potential for interaction.

Penicillin blood levels may be prolonged by concurrent administration of probenecid which blocks the renal tubular secretion of penicillins.

Displacement of penicillins from plasma protein binding sites will elevate the level of free penicillin in the serum.

Carcinogenesis, Mutagenesis, Impairment of Fertility: No information or long-term studies are available on the carcinogenesis, mutagenesis, or the impairment of fertility with the use of penicillin.

Pregnancy Category B. *Teratogenic Effects:* Reproduction studies performed in the mouse, rat, and rabbit have revealed no evidence of impaired fertility or harm to the fetus due to penicillin G. Human experience with the penicillins during pregnancy has not shown any positive evidence of adverse effects on the fetus. There are, however, no adequate and well controlled studies in pregnant women showing conclusively that harmful effects of these drugs on the fetus can be excluded. Because animal reproduction studies are not always predictive of human response, this drug should be used during pregnancy only if clearly needed.

Nursing Mothers: Penicillin G procaine has been reported in milk. Caution should be exercised when penicillin G is administered to a nursing woman.

Pediatric Use: Penicillins are excreted largely unchanged by the kidney. Because of incompletely developed renal function in infants, the rate of elimination will be slow. Use caution in administering to newborns and evaluate organ system function frequently.

ADVERSE REACTIONS

Penicillin is a substance of low toxicity, but does possess a significant index of sensitization. The following hypersensitivity reactions associated with use of penicillin have been reported: skin rashes, ranging from maculopapular eruptions to exfoliative dermatitis; urticaria, serum sickness-like reactions, including chills, fever, edema, arthralgia, and prostration. Severe and often fatal anaphylaxis has been reported (see WARNINGS). As with other treatments for syphilis, the Jarisch-Herxheimer reaction has been reported. Procaine toxicity manifestations have been reported (see WARNINGS). Procaine hypersensitivity reactions have not been reported with this drug.

OVERDOSAGE

In case of overdosage, discontinue medication, treat symptomatically, and institute supportive measures as required. Convulsions have been reported in individuals receiving 4.8 million units.

Penicillin is hemodialyzable.

DOSAGE AND ADMINISTRATION

Pediatric Dosage Schedule: In children under 3 months of age, the absorption of aqueous penicillin G produces such high and sustained levels that penicillin G procaine dosage forms offer no advantages and are usually unnecessary.

In children under 12 years of age, dosage should be adjusted in accordance with the age and weight of the child, and the severity of the infection.

Under 2 years of age, the dose may be divided between the two buttocks if necessary.

Penicillin G procaine (aqueous) is for intramuscular injection only.

Continued on next page

Roerig—Cont.

Recommended Dosage for Penicillin G Procaine Aqueous

Pneumonia (pneumococcal), moderately severe (uncomplicated): 600,000–1,000,000 units daily.

Streptococcal infections (group A), moderately severe to severe tonsillitis, erysipelas, scarlet fever, upper respiratory tract, skin and soft tissue: 600,000–1,000,000 units daily for a minimum of 10 days.

Staphylococcal infections, moderately severe to severe: 600,000–1,000,000 units daily.

Bacterial endocarditis (group A streptococci), only in extremely sensitive infections: 600,000–1,000,000 units daily. For prophylaxis against bacterial endocarditis[1] in patients with congenital heart disease or rheumatic or other acquired valvular heart disease, when undergoing dental procedures or surgical procedures of the upper respiratory tract, use a combined parenteral-oral regimen. One million units of aqueous crystalline penicillin G (30,000 units/kg in children) intramuscularly, mixed with 600,000 units penicillin G (600,000 units for children) should be given one-half to one hour before the procedure. Oral penicillin V (phenoxymethyl penicillin), 500 mg for adults or 250 mg for children less than 60 lb. should be given every six hours for 8 doses. Doses for children should not exceed recommendations for adults for a single dose or for a 24 hour period.

Syphilis: Primary, secondary and latent with a negative spinal fluid in adults and children over 12 years of age: 600,000 units daily for 8 days, total 4,800,000 units.

Late (tertiary neurosyphilis and latent syphilis with positive spinal fluid examination or no spinal fluid examination): 600,000 units daily for 10–15 days, total 6–9 million units.

Congenital syphilis (early and late): 50,000 units/kg per day for a minimum of 10 days.

Yaws, Bejel, and *Pinta:* Treatment as syphilis in corresponding stage of disease.

Gonorrheal infections (uncomplicated): Men or women—4.8 million units intramuscularly divided into at least two doses and injected at different sites at one visit, together with 1 gram of oral probenecid, preferably given at least 30 minutes prior to the injection.

NOTE: Gonorrheal endocarditis should be treated intensively with aqueous penicillin G.

Diphtheria—adjunctive therapy with antitoxin: 300,000–600,000 units daily.

Diphtheria—carrier state: 300,000 units daily for 10 days.

Anthrax—cutaneous: 600,000–1,000,000 units/day.

Vincent's infection (fusospirochetosis): 600,000–1,000,000 units/day.

Erysipeloid: 600,000–1,000,000 units/day.

Streptobacillus moniliformis and *Spirillum minus* (rat bite fever): 600,000–1,000,000 units/day.

Parenteral drug products should be inspected visually for particulate matter and discoloration prior to administration, whenever solution and container permit.

HOW SUPPLIED

Pfizerpen-AS (penicillin G procaine) in Aqueous Suspension is supplied in 10 ml vials (3,000,000 units)—packages of 5 (NDC 0049-0540-77), packages of 100 (NDC 0049-0540-95). Each ml contains 300,000 units penicillin G as penicillin G procaine, and as w/v 0.8% sodium citrate, 0.15% sodium carboxymethylcellulose, 25% of sorbitol solution U.S.P., 0.6% polyvinylpyrrolidone, and 0.6% lecithin.

Preservatives: 0.103% methylparaben, 0.011% propylparaben.

The product should be stored between 2°–8°C (36°–46°F).

REFERENCE

1. American Heart Association, 1977. Prevention of Bacterial Endocarditis. Circulation 56:139A-143A.

70-0033-00-0

SINEQUAN®   ℞

[sin 'a-kwon]
(doxepin HCl)
Capsules
Oral Concentrate

DESCRIPTION

SINEQUAN (doxepin hydrochloride) is one of a class of psychotherapeutic agents known as dibenzoxepin tricyclic compounds. The molecular formula of the compound is $C_{19}H_{21}NO\cdot HCl$ having a molecular weight of 316. It is a white crystalline solid readily soluble in water, lower alcohols and chloroform.

Inert ingredients for the capsule formulations are: hard gelatin capsules (which may contain Blue 1, Red 3, Red 40, Yellow 10, and other inert ingredients); magnesium stearate; sodium lauryl sulfate; starch.

Inert ingredients for the oral concentrate formulation are: glycerin; methylparaben; peppermint oil; propylparaben; water.

CHEMISTRY

SINEQUAN (doxepin HCl) is a dibenzoxepin derivative and is the first of a family of tricyclic psychotherapeutic agents. Specifically, it is an isomeric mixture of 1-Propanamine, 3-dibenz[b,e]oxepin-11(6H)ylidene-N,N -dimethyl-, hydrochloride.

SINEQUAN (doxepin HCl)

ACTIONS

The mechanism of action of SINEQUAN (doxepin HCl) is not definitely known. It is not a central nervous system stimulant nor a monoamine oxidase inhibitor. The current hypothesis is that the clinical effects are due, at least in part, to influences on the adrenergic activity at the synapses so that deactivation of norepinephrine by reuptake into the nerve terminals is prevented. Animal studies suggest that doxepin HCl does not appreciably antagonize the antihypertensive action of guanethidine. In animal studies anticholinergic, antiserotonin and antihistamine effects on smooth muscle have been demonstrated. At higher than usual clinical doses, norepinephrine response was potentiated in animals. This effect was not demonstrated in humans.

At clinical dosages up to 150 mg per day, SINEQUAN can be given to man concomitantly with guanethidine and related compounds without blocking the antihypertensive effect. At dosages above 150 mg per day blocking of the antihypertensive effect of these compounds has been reported.

SINEQUAN is virtually devoid of euphoria as a side effect. Characteristic of this type of compound, SINEQUAN has not been demonstrated to produce the physical tolerance or psychological dependence associated with addictive compounds.

INDICATIONS

SINEQUAN is recommended for the treatment of:
1. Psychoneurotic patients with depression and/or anxiety.
2. Depression and/or anxiety associated with alcoholism (not to be taken concomitantly with alcohol).
3. Depression and/or anxiety associated with organic disease (the possibility of drug interaction should be considered if the patient is receiving other drugs concomitantly).
4. Psychotic depressive disorders with associated anxiety including involutional depression and manic-depressive disorders.

The target symptoms of psychoneurosis that respond particularly well to SINEQUAN include anxiety, tension, depression, somatic symptoms and concerns, sleep disturbances, guilt, lack of energy, fear, apprehension and worry.

Clinical experience has shown that SINEQUAN is safe and well-tolerated even in the elderly patient. Owing to lack of clinical experience in the pediatric population, SINEQUAN is not recommended for use in children under 12 years of age.

CONTRAINDICATIONS

SINEQUAN is contraindicated in individuals who have shown hypersensitivity to the drug. Possibility of cross sensitivity with other dibenzoxepines should be kept in mind. SINEQUAN is contraindicated in patients with glaucoma or a tendency to urinary retention. These disorders should be ruled out, particularly in older patients.

WARNINGS

The once-a-day dosage regimen of SINEQUAN in patients with intercurrent illness or patients taking other medications should be carefully adjusted. This is especially important in patients receiving other medications with anticholinergic effects.

Usage in Geriatrics

The use of SINEQUAN on a once-a-day dosage regimen in geriatric patients should be adjusted carefully based on the patient's condition.

Usage in Pregnancy

Reproduction studies have been performed in rats, rabbits, monkeys and dogs and there was no evidence of harm to the animal fetus. The relevance to humans is not known. Since there is no experience in pregnant women who have received this drug, safety in pregnancy has not been established. There has been a report of apnea and drowsiness occurring in a nursing infant whose mother was taking SINEQUAN.

Usage in Children

The use of SINEQUAN in children under 12 years of age is not recommended because safe conditions for its use have not been established.

DRUG INTERACTIONS

MAO Inhibitors

Serious side effects and even death have been reported following the concomitant use of certain drugs with MAO inhibitors. Therefore, MAO inhibitors should be discontinued at least two weeks prior to the cautious initiation of therapy with SINEQUAN. The exact length of time may vary and is dependent upon the particular MAO inhibitor being used, the length of time it has been administered, and the dosage involved.

Cimetidine

Cimetidine has been reported to produce clinically significant fluctuations in steady-state serum concentrations of various tricyclic antidepressants. Serious anticholinergic symptoms (i.e., severe dry mouth, urinary retention and blurred vision) have been associated with elevations in the serum levels of tricyclic antidepressant when cimetidine therapy is initiated. Additionally, higher than expected tricyclic antidepressant levels have been observed when they are begun in patients already taking cimetidine. In patients who have been reported to be well controlled on tricyclic antidepressants receiving concurrent cimetidine therapy, discontinuation of cimetidine has been reported to decrease established steady-state serum tricyclic antidepressant levels and compromise their therapeutic effects.

Alcohol

It should be borne in mind that alcohol ingestion may increase the danger inherent in any intentional or unintentional SINEQUAN overdosage. This is especially important in patients who may use alcohol excessively.

Tolazamide

A case of sever hypoglycemia has been reported in a type II diabetic patient maintained on tolazamide (1 gm/day) 11 days after the addition of doxepin (75 mg/day).

PRECAUTIONS

Since drowsiness may occur with the use of this drug, patients should be warned of the possibility and cautioned against driving a car or operating dangerous machinery while taking the drug. Patients should also be cautioned that their response to alcohol may be potentiated.

Since suicide is an inherent risk in any depressed patient and may remain so until significant improvement has occurred, patients should be closely supervised during the early course of therapy. Prescriptions should be written for the smallest feasible amount.

Should increased symptoms of psychosis or shift to manic symptomatology occur, it may be necessary to reduce dosage or add a major tranquilizer to the dosage regimen.

ADVERSE REACTIONS

NOTE: Some of the adverse reactions noted below have not been specifically reported with SINEQUAN use. However, due to the close pharmacological similarities among the tricyclics, the reactions should be considered when prescribing SINEQUAN (doxepin HCl).

Anticholinergic Effects: Dry mouth, blurred vision, constipation, and urinary retention have been reported. If they do not subside with continued therapy, or become severe, it may be necessary to reduce the dosage.

Central Nervous System Effects: Drowsiness is the most commonly noticed side effect. This tends to disappear as therapy is continued. Other infrequently reported CNS side effects are confusion, disorientation, hallucinations, numbness, paresthesias, ataxia, and extrapyramidal symptoms and seizures.

Cardiovascular: Cardiovascular effects including hypotension and tachycardia have been reported occasionally.

Allergic: Skin rash, edema, photosensitization, and pruritus have occasionally occurred.

Hematologic: Eosinophilia has been reported in a few patients. There have been occasional reports of bone marrow depression manifesting as agranulocytosis, leukopenia, thrombocytopenia, and purpura.

Gastrointestinal: Nausea, vomiting, indigestion, taste disturbances, diarrhea, anorexia, and aphthous stomatitis have been reported. (See anticholinergic effects.)

Endocrine: Raised or lowered libido, testicular swelling, gynecomastia in males, enlargement of breasts and galactorrhea in the female, raising or lowering of blood sugar levels have been reported with tricyclic administration.

Other: Dizziness, tinnitus, weight gain, sweating, chills, fatigue, weakness, flushing, jaundice, alopecia, and headache have been occasionally observed as adverse effects.

Withdrawal Symptoms: The possibility of development of withdrawal symptoms upon abrupt cessation of treatment after prolonged Sinequan administration should be borne in mind. These are not indicative of addiction and gradual withdrawal of medication should not cause these symptoms.

DOSAGE AND ADMINISTRATION

For most patients with illness of mild to moderate severity, a starting daily dose of 75 mg is recommended. Dosage may subsequently be increased or decreased at appropriate intervals and according to individual response. The usual optimum dose range is 75 mg/day to 150 mg/day.

In more severely ill patients higher doses may be required with subsequent gradual increase to 300 mg/day if necessary. Additional therapeutic effect is rarely to be obtained by exceeding a dose of 300 mg/day.

In patients with very mild symptomatology or emotional symptoms accompanying organic disease, lower doses may suffice. Some of these patients have been controlled on doses as low as 25-50 mg/day.

The total daily dosage of SINEQUAN may be given on a divided or once-a-day dosage schedule. If the once-a-day schedule is employed the maximum recommended dose is 150 mg/day. This dose may be given at bedtime. **The 150 mg capsule strength is intended for maintenance therapy only and is not recommended for initiation of treatment.**

Anti-anxiety effect is apparent before the antidepressant effect. Optimal antidepressant effect may not be evident for two to three weeks.

OVERDOSAGE

A. Signs and Symptoms
1. Mild: Drowsiness, stupor, blurred vision, excessive dryness of mouth.
2. Severe: Respiratory depression, hypotension, coma, convulsions, cardiac arrhythmias and tachycardias.

Also: urinary retention (bladder atony), decreased gastrointestinal motility (paralytic ileus), hyperthermia (or hypothermia), hypertension, dilated pupils, hyperactive reflexes.

B. Management and Treatment
1. Mild: Observation and supportive therapy is all that is usually necessary.
2. Severe: Medical management of severe SINEQUAN overdosage consists of aggressive supportive therapy. If the patient is conscious, gastric lavage, with appropriate precautions to prevent pulmonary aspiration, should be performed even though SINEQUAN is rapidly absorbed. The use of activated charcoal has been recommended, as has been continuous gastric lavage with saline for 24 hours or more. An adequate airway should be established in comatose patients and assisted ventilation used if necessary. EKG monitoring may be required for several days, since relapse after apparent recovery has been reported. Arrhythmias should be treated with the appropriate antiarrhythmic agent. It has been reported that many of the cardiovascular and CNS symptoms of tricyclic antidepressant poisoning in adults may be reversed by the slow intravenous administration of 1 mg to 3 mg of physostigmine salicylate. Because physostigmine is rapidly metabolized, the dosage should be repeated as required. Convulsions may respond to standard anticonvulsant therapy, however, barbiturates may potentiate any respiratory depression. Dialysis and forced diuresis generally are not of value in the management of overdosage due to high tissue and protein binding of SINEQUAN.

SUPPLY

SINEQUAN is available as capsules containing doxepin HCl equivalent to:
10 mg—100's (NDC 0662-5340-66), 1000's (NDC 0662-5340-82), Unit Dose 10×10's (NDC 0662-5340-41).
25 mg—100's (NDC 0662-5350-66), (NDC 0049-5350-66); 1000's (NDC 0662-5350-82), 5000's (NDC 0662-5350-94), Unit Dose 10×10's (NDC 0662-5350-41).
50 mg—100's (NDC 0662-5360-66), (NDC 0049-5360-66); 1000's (NDC 0662-5360-82), 5000's (NDC 0662-5360-94), Unit Dose 10×10's (NDC 0662-5360-41).
75 mg—100's (NDC 0662-5390-66), 1000's (NDC 0662-5390-82), Unit Dose 10×10's (NDC 0662-5390-41).
100 mg—100's (NDC 0662-5380-66), 1000's (NDC 0662-5380-82), Unit Dose 10×10's (NDC 0662-5380-41).
150 mg—50's (NDC 0662-5370-50), 500's (NDC 0662-5370-73), Unit Dose 10×10's (NDC 0662-5370-41).

SINEQUAN Oral Concentrate is available in 120 ml bottles (NDC 0662-5100-47) with an accompanying dropper calibrated at 5 mg, 10 mg, 15 mg, 20 mg and 25 mg. Each ml contains doxepin HCl equivalent to 10 mg doxepin. Just prior to administration, SINEQUAN Oral Concentrate should be diluted with approximately 120 ml of water, whole or skimmed milk, or orange, grapefruit, tomato, prune or pineapple juice. SINEQUAN Oral Concentrate is not physically compatible with a number of carbonated beverages. For those patients requiring antidepressant therapy who are on methadone maintenance, SINEQUAN Oral Concentrate and methadone syrup can be mixed together with Gatorade®, lemonade, orange juice, sugar water, Tang®, or water; but not with grape juice. Preparation and storage of bulk dilutions is not recommended.

Literature Available: Yes.

65-2135-37-7

Shown in Product Identification Section, page 426

SPECTROBID®
[spek 'trō-bid]
(bacampicillin HCl)
TABLETS and POWDER
for ORAL SUSPENSION

DESCRIPTION

SPECTROBID (bacampicillin HCl) is a member of the ampicillin class of semi-synthetic penicillins derived from the basic penicillin nucleus: 6-aminopenicillanic acid. SPECTROBID, as well as ampicillin and other ampicillin analogues, is acid resistant and suitable for oral administration. SPECTROBID is the hydrochloride salt of 1-ethoxycarbonyloxyethyl ester of ampicillin, available either as tablets or as a microencapsulated oral suspension. During the process of absorption from the gastrointestinal tract, SPECTROBID is hydrolyzed rapidly to ampicillin, a well characterized and effective antibacterial agent. Each 400 mg tablet of SPECTROBID is chemically equivalent to 280 mg of ampicillin, and 125 mg/5 ml of the oral suspension is chemically equivalent to 87.5 mg of ampicillin.

Chemically, SPECTROBID is 1'-ethoxycarbonyloxyethyl -6 - (D-α aminophenylacetamide) - penicillinate hydrochloride. It has a molecular weight of 501.96 and the following structural formula:

Inert ingredients for the tablets are: hydroxypropyl methylcellulose; lactose; magnesium stearate; microcrystalline cellulose; opaspray.

Inert ingredients for the oral suspension are: carboxymethylcellulose sodium; cherry flavor; compressible sugar; ethylcellulose; hydroxypropyl cellulose; mannitol; saccharin sodium; sodium bicarbonate; titanium dioxide; xanthan gum.

ACTIONS

Clinical Pharmacology

SPECTROBID is characterized by its more complete and more rapid absorption from the GI tract than ampicillin. SPECTROBID tablets of 400 mg, 800 mg, and 1600 mg have provided ampicillin peak serum concentrations of 7.9, 12.9, and 20.1 mcg/ml. These peak levels are approximately three times the levels obtained with administration of equivalent amounts of ampicillin. The areas-under-the-serum-concentration curves obtained during the first 6 hours were 24.8 and 12.9 mcg/ml/hr., when bacampicillin HCl 800 mg and ampicillin 500 mg were administered to adults. (See Graph 1.) Graph 2 shows the serum ampicillin curves following a 28 mg/kg dose of bacampicillin HCl and a 25 mg/kg dose of ampicillin in infants and young children. The areas-under-the-serum-concentration-curves were 28.2 and 13.1 respectively. The absorption of the SPECTROBID oral suspension was shown to be equivalent to that of the 400 mg tablet in fasting adult volunteers. A 400 mg dose of suspension gave a peak serum ampicillin concentration of 7.6 mcg/ml and the tablet gave a peak of 7.2 mcg/ml. In fasting pediatric patients a 12.5 mg/kg dose provided a peak of 8.4 mcg/ml.

After oral administration of SPECTROBID tablet or suspension, ampicillin activity in serum peaks at 0.7–0.9 hours (compared to 1.5–2.0 hours after administration of ampicillin). Serum ampicillin half-life is 1.1 hours after either SPECTROBID or ampicillin administration.

Peak tissue and body fluid ampicillin concentrations also are higher after administration of SPECTROBID. Utilizing a special skin window technique to determine ampicillin levels, therapeutic levels in the interstitial fluid were higher and more prolonged after SPECTROBID than after ampicillin administration. SPECTROBID is stable in the presence of gastric acid. SPECTROBID oral suspension absorption is affected by food. Food does not retard absorption of SPECTROBID tablets which may be given without regard to meals. SPECTROBID has been shown to be rapidly and well absorbed after oral administration, with about 75% of a given dose being recoverable in the urine as active ampicillin within 8 hours of administration. Urinary excretion can be delayed by concurrent administration of probenecid. The active moiety of SPECTROBID (i.e., ampicillin) diffuses readily into most body tissues and fluids. In serum, ampicillin is only 20% protein-bound, compared to 60–90% for other penicillins.

Microbiology

SPECTROBID per se has no *in vitro* antibacterial activity and owes its *in vivo* bactericidal activity to the parent compound, ampicillin. The ampicillin class of penicillins (including SPECTROBID) has a broad spectrum of activity against gram-negative and gram-positive bacteria. Like other penicillins, the ampicillin class of penicillins inhibits the synthesis of cell wall mucopeptide.

Ampicillin class antibiotics are inactivated by β-lactamases produced by certain strains of *Enterobacter, Citrobacter, Haemophilus influenzae,* and *Escherichia coli,* and by most strains of staphylococci and indole-positive *Proteus* spp. Ampicillin class antibiotics are not active against *Pseudomonas, Klebsiella,* or *Serratia* spp.

Susceptibility Testing:

Elution Technique: For the automated method of susceptibility testing (i.e., AutobacTM), gram-negative organisms should be tested with the 4.5 mcg ampicillin elution disk, while gram-positive organisms should be tested with the 0.22 mcg disk.

Diffusion Technique: For the Kirby-Bauer method of susceptibility testing, a 10 mcg ampicillin diffusion disk should be used. With this procedure, a laboratory report of "susceptible" indicates that the infecting organism is likely to respond to SPECTROBID therapy, and a report of "resistant" indicates that the infecting organism is not likely to respond to therapy. An "intermediate susceptibility" report suggests that the infecting organism would be susceptible to SPECTROBID if a high dosage is used or if the infection is confined to tissues and fluids (e.g., urine) in which high antibiotic levels are attained.

Dilution Techniques: Broth or agar dilution methods may be used to determine the minimal inhibitory concentration (MIC) value for susceptibility of bacterial isolates to SPECTROBID. Since SPECTROBID per se has no *in vitro* activity, ampicillin powder should be used in a twofold concentration series of the antibiotic prepared in either broth (in tubes) or agar (in petri plates). Tubes should be inoculated to contain 10^4 to 10^5 organisms/ml or plates "spotted" with 10^3 to 10^4 organisms.

INDICATIONS AND USAGE

SPECTROBID is indicated for the treatment of the following infections when caused by ampicillin-susceptible organisms:

1. Upper and Lower Respiratory Tract Infections (including acute exacerbations of chronic bronchitis) due to streptococci (β-hemolytic streptococci, *Streptococcus pyogenes*), pneumococci (*Streptococcus pneumoniae*), nonpenicillinase-producing staphylococci and *H. influenzae;*
2. Urinary Tract Infections due to *E. coli, Proteus mirabilis,* and *Streptococcus faecalis* (enterococci);
3. Skin and Skin Structure Infections due to streptococci and susceptible staphylococci;
4. Gonorrhea (acute uncomplicated urogenital infections) due to *Neisseria gonorrhoeae.*

Bacteriological studies to determine the causative organisms and their susceptibility to SPECTROBID (i.e., ampicillin) should be performed. Therapy may be instituted prior to obtaining results of susceptibility testing. Indicated surgical procedures should be performed.

CONTRAINDICATIONS

The use of ampicillin class antibiotics is contraindicated in individuals with a history of an allergic reaction to any of the penicillin antibiotics and/or cephalosporins.

WARNINGS

Serious and occasional fatal hypersensitivity (anaphylactic) reactions have been reported in patients on penicillin therapy. Although anaphylaxis is more frequent following parenteral therapy, it has occurred in patients on oral penicillins. These reactions are more apt to occur in individuals with a history of penicillin hypersensitivity and/or hypersensitivity to multiple allergens.

There have been reports of individuals with a history of penicillin hypersensitivity who have experienced severe reactions when treated with cephalosporins. Before therapy with a penicillin, careful inquiry should be made concerning previous hypersensitivity reactions to penicillins, cephalosporins, and other allergens.

IF AN ALLERGIC REACTION OCCURS, THE DRUG SHOULD BE DISCONTINUED AND THE APPROPRIATE THERAPY INSTITUTED. SERIOUS ANAPHYLACTOID REACTIONS REQUIRE IMMEDIATE EMERGENCY TREATMENT WITH EPINEPHRINE. OXYGEN, INTRAVENOUS STEROIDS, AND AIRWAY MANAGEMENT, INCLUDING INTUBATION, SHOULD ALSO BE ADMINISTERED AS INDICATED.

PRECAUTIONS

1. General: The possibility of superinfections with mycotic or bacterial pathogens should be kept in mind during therapy. If superinfections occur (usually involving *Aerobacter, Pseudomonas,* or *Candida*), the drug should be discontinued and appropriate therapy instituted.

As with any potent agent, it is advisable to check periodically for organ system dysfunction during prolonged therapy. This includes renal, hepatic, and hematopoietic systems and is particularly important in prematures, neonates, and patients with liver or renal impairments.

A high percentage of patients with mononucleosis who receive ampicillin develop a skin rash. Thus, ampicillin class

Continued on next page

Roerig—Cont.

antibiotics should not be administered to patients with mononucleosis.

2. Clinically Significant Drug Interactions: The concurrent administration of allopurinol and ampicillin increases substantially the incidence of rashes in patients receiving both drugs as compared to patients receiving ampicillin alone. It is not known whether this potentiation of ampicillin rashes is due to allopurinol or the hyperuricemia present in these patients. There are no data available on the incidence of rash in patients treated concurrently with SPECTROBID (bacampicillin HCl) and allopurinol. SPECTROBID should not be co-administered with Antabuse (disulfiram).

3. Drug and Laboratory Test Interactions: When testing for the presence of glucose in urine using Clinitest™, Benedict's Solution, or Fehling's Solution, high urine concentrations of ampicillin may result in false-positive reactions. Therefore, it is recommended that glucose tests based on enzymatic glucose oxidase reactions (such as Clinistix™ or Testape™) be used.

Following administration of ampicillin to pregnant women a transient decrease in plasma concentration of total conjugated estriol, estriol-glucuronide, conjugated estrone and estradiol, has been noted.

4. Pregnancy Category B: Reproduction studies have been performed in mice and rats at SPECTROBID doses of up to 750 mg/kg (more than 25 times the human dose) and have revealed no evidence of impaired fertility or harm to the fetus due to SPECTROBID.

There are, however, no adequate and well controlled studies in pregnant women. Because animal reproduction studies are not always predictive of human response, this drug should be used during pregnancy only if clearly needed.

5. Carcinogenesis, Mutagenesis, Impairment of Fertility: No carcinogenicity or mutagenicity studies were conducted. No impairment of fertility and no significant effect on general reproductive performance was observed in rats administered oral doses of up to 750 mg/kg of bacampicillin HCl per day prior to and during mating and gestation. In addition, bacampicillin HCl caused no drug-related effects on the reproductive organs of rats or dogs receiving daily oral doses of up to 800 and 650 mg/kg respectively for 6 months.

6. Labor and Delivery: Oral ampicillin class antibiotics are generally poorly absorbed during labor. Studies in guinea pigs showed that intravenous administration of ampicillin decreased the uterine tone, frequency of contractions, height of contractions, and duration of contractions. However, it is not known whether use of SPECTROBID in humans during labor or delivery has immediate or delayed adverse effects on the fetus, prolongs the duration of labor, or increases the likelihood that forceps delivery or other obstetrical intervention or resuscitation of the newborn will be necessary.

7. Nursing Mothers: Ampicillin class antibiotics are excreted in milk; therefore, caution should be exercised when ampicillin class antibiotics are administered to a nursing woman.

8. Pediatric Use: SPECTROBID tablets are indicated for children weighing 25 kg or more. The SPECTROBID oral suspension is indicated for children and infants weighing less than 25 kg or in those children not able to swallow a tablet.

ADVERSE REACTIONS
As with other penicillins, it may be expected that untoward reactions will be essentially limited to sensitivity phenomena. They are more likely to occur in individuals who have previously demonstrated hypersensitivity to penicillins and in those with a history of allergy, asthma, hay fever, or urticaria.

In well controlled clinical trials conducted in the U.S. the most frequent adverse reactions to SPECTROBID were epigastric upset (2%) and diarrhea (2%). Increased dosage may result in an increased incidence of diarrhea. In the same clinical trials the most frequent adverse effects for amoxicillin were diarrhea (4%) and nausea (2%).

The following adverse reactions have been reported for ampicillin.

Gastrointestinal: diarrhea, gastritis, stomatitis, nausea, vomiting, glossitis, black "hairy" tongue, enterocolitis, and pseudomembranous colitis.

Hypersensitivity Reactions: skin rashes, urticaria, erythema multiforme, and an occasional case of exfoliative dermatitis. These reactions may be controlled with antihistamines and, if necessary, systemic corticosteroids. Whenever such reactions occur, the drug should be discontinued, unless the opinion of the physician dictates otherwise.

Serious and occasional fatal hypersensitivity (anaphylactic) reactions can occur with oral penicillins. (See Warnings).

Liver: A moderate rise in serum glutamic oxaloacetic transaminase (SGOT) has been noted in some ampicillin treated patients, but the significance of this finding is unknown. In well controlled clinical trials no difference was noted between ampicillin and SPECTROBID with regard to the incidence of liver function test abnormalities.

Hemic and Lymphatic Systems: Anemia, thrombocytopenia, thrombocytopenic purpura, eosinophilia, leukopenia, and agranulocytosis have been reported during therapy with penicillins. These reactions are usually reversible on discontinuation of therapy and are believed to be hypersensitivity phenomena.

DOSAGE AND ADMINISTRATION
SPECTROBID tablets may be given without regard to meals. SPECTROBID oral suspension should be administered to fasting patients.
UPPER RESPIRATORY TRACT INFECTIONS (including otitis media) due to streptococci, pneumococci, nonpenicillinase-producing staphylococci and *H. influenzae;*
URINARY TRACT INFECTIONS due to *E. coli, Proteus mirabilis,* and *Streptococcus faecalis;*
SKIN AND SKIN STRUCTURES INFECTIONS due to streptococci and susceptible staphylococci;

Usual Dosage
Adults: 1 × 400 mg tablet every 12 hours (for patients weighing 25 kg or more).
Children: 25 mg/kg per day in 2 equally divided doses at 12 hour intervals.
IN SEVERE INFECTIONS OR THOSE CAUSED BY LESS SUSCEPTIBLE ORGANISMS:

Usual Dosage
Adults: 2 × 400 mg tablets every 12 hours (for patients weighing 25 kg or more).
Children: 50 mg/kg per day in 2 equally divided doses at 12 hour intervals.
LOWER RESPIRATORY TRACT INFECTIONS due to streptococci, pneumococci, nonpenicillinase-producing staphylococci, and *H. influenzae:*

Usual Dosage
Adults: 2 × 400 mg tablets every 12 hours (for patients weighing 25 kg or more).
Children: 50 mg/kg per day in 2 equally divided doses at 12 hour intervals.
GONORRHEA—acute uncomplicated urogenital infections due to *N. gonorrhoeae* (males and females):
1.6 grams (4 × 400 mg tablet plus 1 gram probenecid) as a single oral dose.
No pediatric dosage has been established.
Cases of gonorrhea with a suspected lesion of syphilis should have dark field examination before receiving SPECTROBID and monthly serological tests for a minimum of four months. Larger doses may be required for stubborn or severe infections.
It should be recognized that in the treatment of chronic urinary tract infections, frequent bacteriological and clinical appraisals are necessary. Smaller doses than those recommended above should not be used. In stubborn infections, therapy may be required for several weeks. It may be necessary to continue clinical and/or bacteriological follow-up for several months after cessation of therapy. Except for gonorrhea, treatment should be continued for a minimum of 48 to 72 hours beyond the time that the patient becomes asymptomatic or evidence of bacterial eradication has been obtained.
IT IS RECOMMENDED THAT THERE BE AT LEAST 10 DAYS' TREATMENT FOR ANY INFECTION CAUSED BY HEMOLYTIC STREPTOCOCCI TO PREVENT THE OCCURRENCE OF ACUTE RHEUMATIC FEVER OR GLOMERULONEPHRITIS.

Directions for Mixing Oral Suspension:
Prepare suspension at the time of dispensing as follows:
Prior to reconstitution, tap bottle to thoroughly loosen powder. Add the required amount (see table below) of water to the contents of the bottle in approximately two equally divided portions and SHAKE WELL after each addition. Let stand at least 30 minutes and SHAKE WELL just prior to administering each dose. Each level teaspoon (5 ml) will contain 125 mg of bacampicillin HCl.

Final Volume after reconstitution	Amount of Water Required for reconstitution
70 ml	53 ml
100 ml	75 ml

Reconstituted suspension *must be stored under refrigeration and discarded after 10 days.*

HOW SUPPLIED
SPECTROBID (bacampicillin HCl) Tablets
400 mg (NDC 0049-0350-66): white, film-coated, oblong, unscored are available in bottles of 100.
SPECTROBID (bacampicillin HCl) Powder for Oral Suspension.
Each 5 ml of reconstituted suspension contains 125 mg of bacampicillin HCl.
Bottles containing the following volumes are available: 70 ml (NDC 0049-0357-37), 100 ml (NDC 0049-0357-44).

GRAPH 1.
Comparison of Bacampicillin HCl 800 mg, Ampicillin 500 mg, and Amoxicillin 500 mg
*800 mg Bacampicillin HCl is chemically equivalent to 560 mg of Ampicillin

GRAPH 2.
Crossover Comparison of Bacampicillin HCl Oral Suspension (28 mg/kg)* with Ampicillin Oral Suspension (25 mg/kg) in Fasted Infants and Children (n = 7).
*equivalent to 19.5 mg/kg of Ampicillin

69-4092-00-5
Shown in Product Identification Section, page 426

STREPTOMYCIN SULFATE   ℞
Dry Powder: Vials of 1 g and 5 g

WARNING
THE RISK OF SEVERE NEUROTOXIC REACTIONS IS SHARPLY INCREASED IN PATIENTS WITH IMPAIRED KIDNEY FUNCTION OR PRERENAL AZOTEMIA. THESE INCLUDE DISBURBANCES OF THE AUDITORY NERVE, OPTIC NERVE, PERIPHERAL NEURITIS, ARACHNOIDITIS, AND ENCEPHALOPATHY. RENAL FUNCTION SHOULD BE CAREFULLY DETERMINED AND PATIENTS WITH RENAL DAMAGE AND NITROGEN RETENTION SHOULD HAVE REDUCED DOSAGE. THE PEAK SERUM CONCENTRATION IN INDIVIDUALS WITH KIDNEY DAMAGE SHOULD NOT EXCEED 20 TO 25 MCG PER MILLILITER.
THE CONCURRENT OR SEQUENTIAL USE OF OTHER NEUROTOXIC AND/OR NEPHROTOXIC DRUGS WITH STREPTOMYCIN SULFATE, PARTICULARLY NEOMYCIN, KANAMYCIN, GENTAMICIN, CEPHALORIDINE, PAROMOMYCIN, VIOMYCIN, POLYMYXIN B, COLISTIN, AND TOBRAMYCIN SHOULD BE AVOIDED.
THE NEUROTOXICITY OF STREPTOMYCIN CAN RESULT IN RESPIRATORY PARALYSIS FROM NEUROMUSCULAR BLOCKADE, ESPECIALLY WHEN THE DRUG IS GIVEN SOON AFTER ANESTHESIA AND THE USE OF MUSCLE RELAXANTS.
THE ADMINISTRATION OF STREPTOMYCIN IN PARENTERAL FORM SHOULD BE RESERVED FOR PATIENTS WHERE ADEQUATE LABORATORY FACILITIES ARE AVAILABLE AND CONSTANT SUPERVISION OF THE PATIENT IS POSSIBLE.

DESCRIPTION
Streptomycin is a water-soluble aminoglycoside derived from *Streptomyces griseus.* It is marketed as the sulfate salt of streptomycin.

ACTIONS
Streptomycin sulfate is a bactericidal antibiotic in therapeutic dosage. The mode of action is the interference with normal protein synthesis and production of "faulty proteins." Following intramuscular injection of 1 g of the drug, a peak serum level of 25 to 50 mcg per milliliter is reached within 1 hour, diminishing slowly to about 50 percent after 5 to 6 hours. Appreciable concentrations are found in all organ tissues except the brain. Significant amounts have been found in pleural fluid and tuberculous cavities. Streptomycin passes through the placenta with serum levels in the cord

blood similar to maternal levels. Small amounts are excreted in milk, saliva, and sweat.

Streptomycin is excreted rapidly in the urine by glomerular filtration. In patients with normal kidney function, between 29 and 89 percent of a single 0.6 g dose is excreted within 24 hours. Any reduction of glomerular activity results in decreased excretion of the drug and concurrent rise in serum and tissue levels.

Sensitivity plate testing: If the Kirby-Bauer method of disc sensitivity is used, a 10 mcg streptomycin disc should give a zone of over 15 millimeters when tested against a streptomycin-sensitive bacterial strain.

INDICATIONS

1. Mycobacterium tuberculosis: Streptomycin may be indicated for all forms of this infection when the infecting organisms are susceptible. It should be used only in combination with other antituberculosis drugs. The common combined drug therapy is streptomycin, PAS, and, isoniazid; this combination is effective only where the organisms are susceptible to the drugs being used in combination.

2. Nontuberculosis infections: Streptomycin should be used only in those serious nontuberculosis infections caused by organisms shown by *in vitro* sensitivity studies to be susceptible to it and when less potentially hazardous therapeutic agents are ineffective or contraindicated.

a. *Pasteurella pestis* (plague).
b. *Pasteurella tularensis* (tularemia).
c. *Brucella.*
d. *Donovanosis* (granuloma inguinale).
e. *H. ducreyi* (chancroid).
f. *H. influenzae* (in respiratory, endocardial, and meningeal infections—concomitantly with another antibacterial agent).
g. *K. pneumoniae* pneumonia (concomitantly with another antibacterial agent).
h. *E. coli, Proteus, A. aerogenes, K. pneumoniae,* and *Streptococcus faecalis* in urinary tract infections.
i. *Strep. viridans, Strep. faecalis* (in endocardial infections—concomitantly with penicillin).
j. Gram-negative bacillary bacteremia (concomitantly with another antibacterial agent).

Note: The use of streptomycin should be limited to the treatment of infections caused by bacteria which have been shown to be susceptible to the antibacterial effects of streptomycin and which are not amenable to therapy with less potentially toxic agents.

CONTRAINDICATIONS

Streptomycin is contraindicated in those individuals who have shown previous toxic or hypersensitivity reaction to it.

WARNINGS

Ototoxicity: Streptomycin may frequently affect the vestibular branch of the auditory nerve causing severe nausea, vomiting, and vertigo. The incidence is directly proportional to duration and amount of the drug administered. Advanced age and renal impairment predispose to ototoxicity. Symptoms subside and recovery is usually complete following discontinuance of the drug.

Loss of hearing has been reported following long term therapy; however, ototoxic effect on the auditory branch of the eighth nerve is infrequent and usually is preceded by vestibular symptoms. Hearing loss, when extensive, is usually permanent.

Streptomycin contains sodium bisulfite, a sulfite that may cause allergic-type reactions including anaphylactic symptoms and life-threatening or less severe asthmatic episodes in certain susceptible people. The over-all prevalance of sulfite sensitivity in the general population is unknown and probably low. Sulfite sensitivity is seen more frequently in asthmatic than in non-asthmatic people.

USAGE IN PREGNANCY: Since streptomycin readily crosses the placental barrier, caution in use of the drug is important to prevent ototoxicity in the fetus.

PRECAUTIONS

Baseline and periodic caloric stimulation tests and audiometric tests are advisable with extended streptomycin therapy. Tinnitus, roaring noises, or a sense of fullness in the ears indicates need for audiometric examination or termination of streptomycin therapy or both.

Care should be taken by individuals handling or preparing streptomycin for injection to avoid skin sensitivity reactions. As with all intramuscular preparations, Streptomycin Sulfate Injection should be injected well within the body of a relatively large muscle. ADULTS: The preferred site is the upper outer quadrant of the buttock, (i.e., gluteus maximus), or the mid-lateral thigh. CHILDREN: It is recommended that intramuscular injections be given preferably in the mid-lateral muscles of the thigh. In infants and small children the periphery of the upper outer quadrant of the gluteal region should be used only when necessary, such as in burn patients, in order to minimize the possibility of damage to the sciatic nerve.

The deltoid area should be used only if well developed such as in certain adults and older children, and then only with caution to avoid radial nerve injury. Intramuscular injections should not be made into the lower and mid-third of the upper arm. As with all intramuscular injections, aspiration is necessary to help avoid inadvertent injection into a blood vessel.

Injection sites should be alternated, and solutions of concentration greater than 500 mg/ml are not recommended.

As higher doses or more prolonged therapy with streptomycin may be indicated for more severe or fulminating infections (endocarditis, meningitis, etc.), the physician should always take adequate measures to be immediately aware of any toxic signs or symptoms occurring in the patient as a result of streptomycin therapy.

While disturbances in renal function due to streptomycin have been reported in the past, purification of the drug has minimized this side effect. In the presence of pre-existing renal insufficiency, however, extreme caution must be exercised in the administration of streptomycin. Since in severely uremic patients a single dose may produce reasonably high blood levels for several days, the cumulative effect may produce ototoxic sequelae. When streptomycin must be given for prolonged periods of time, alkalinization of the urine may minimize or prevent renal irritation.

A syndrome of apparent central nervous system depression, characterized by stupor and flaccidity, at times to the extent of coma and deep respiratory depression, has been reported in very young infants in whom streptomycin dosage had materially exceeded the recommended limits. Thus, infants should not receive streptomycin in excess of the recommended dosage.

In the treatment of venereal infections such as granuloma inguinale, and chancroid, if concomitant syphilis is suspected, suitable laboratory procedures such as a dark field examination should be performed before the start of treatment, and monthly serologic tests should be done for at least four months.

As with other antibiotics, use of this drug may result in overgrowth of nonsusceptible organisms, including fungi. If superinfection occurs, appropriate therapy should be instituted.

ADVERSE REACTIONS

The following reactions are common: ototoxicity—nausea, vomiting, and vertigo; paresthesia of face; rash; fever; urticaria; angioneurotic edema; and eosinophilia.

The following reactions are less frequent: deafness, exfoliative dermatitis, anaphylaxis, azotemia, leucopenia, thrombocytopenia, pancytopenia, hemolytic anemia, muscular weakness, and amblyopia.

Vestibular dysfunction resulting from the parenteral administration of streptomycin is cumulatively related to the total daily dose. When 1.8 to 2.0 g/day are given, symptoms are likely to develop in the large percentage of patients—especially in the elderly or patients with impaired renal function—within four weeks. Therefore, it is recommended that caloric and audiometric tests be done prior to, during, and following intensive therapy with streptomycin in order to facilitate detection of any vestibular dysfunction and/or impairment of hearing which may occur.

Vestibular symptoms generally appear early and usually are reversible with early detection and cessation of administration of the drug. After two to three months, gross vesibular symptoms usually disappear, except for the relative inability to walk in total darkness or on very rough terrain.

Clinical judgment as to termination of therapy must be exercised when side effects occur.

DOSAGE AND ADMINISTRATION

Intramuscular Route Only

1. Tuberculosis: All forms when organisms are known or believed to be drug susceptible.

Adult, combined therapy: Streptomycin—1 g daily with PAS 5 g t.i.d. and isoniazid 200 to 300 mg daily. Elderly patients should have a smaller daily dose of streptomycin, based on age, renal function, and eighth nerve function. Ultimately the streptomycin should be discontinued or reduced in dosage to 1 g 2 to 3 times weekly. Therapy with streptomycin may be terminated when toxic symptoms have appeared, when impending toxicity is feared, when organisms become resistant, or when full treatment effect has been obtained. The total period of drug treatment of tuberculosis is a minimum of 1 year; however, indications for terminating therapy with streptomycin may occur at any time as noted above.

2. Tularemia: One to 2 g daily in divided doses for 7 to 10 days until the patient is afebrile for 5 to 7 days.

3. Plague: Two to 4 g daily in divided doses until the patient is afebrile for at least 3 days.

4a. Bacterial endocarditis: In penicillin-sensitive alpha and nonhemolytic streptococcal endocarditis (penicillin sensitive to 0.1 mcg per milliliter or less), streptomycin may be used for 2-week treatment concomitantly with penicillin. Streptomycin dosage is 1 g b.i.d. for 1 week, and 0.5 g b.i.d. for the 2d week. If the patient is over 60 years of age, the dosage should be 0.5 g b.i.d. for the entire 2-week period.

b. Enterococcal endocarditis: Streptomycin in doses of 1 g b.i.d. for 2 weeks and 0.5 g b.i.d. for 4 weeks is given in combination with penicillin. Ototoxicity may require termination of the streptomycin prior to completion of the 6-week course of treatment.

5. For use concomitantly with other agents to which the infecting organism is also sensitive. Streptomycin in these conditions is considered as a drug of secondary choice: gramnegative bacillary bacteremia, meningitis, and pneumonia; brucellosis; granuloma inguinale; chancroid, and urinary tract infection.

For adults:

a. Severe fulminating infection: 2 to 4 g daily, administered intramuscularly in divided doses every 6 to 12 hours.

b. With less severe infections and with highly susceptible organisms: 1 to 2 g daily.

For children: 20 to 40 mg per kg of body weight daily (8 to 20 mg per pound) in divided doses every 6 to 12 hours. (Particular care should be taken to avoid excessive dosage in children.)

The dry powder is dissolved by adding Water for Injection, U.S.P. or Sodium Chloride Solution, U.S.P. in an amount to yield the desired concentration as indicated in the following table:

Approx. Conc. (mg/ml)	Volume (ml) of Solvent	
	1 g Vial	5 g Vial
200	4.2	—
250	3.2	—
400	1.8	9.0

Sterile reconstituted solutions should be protected from light and may be stored at room temperature for four weeks without significant loss of potency.

SUPPLY

Streptomycin Sulfate is supplied as a sterile powder in packages of 100 vials, each vial containing streptomycin sulfate equivalent to 1.0 g (NDC 0995-0620-95) and 5.0 g (NDC 0069-0630-95) of streptomycin base.

70-0072-00-6

TAO® ℞

[tā´ō]
(troleandomycin)
Capsules and Oral Suspension

DESCRIPTION

TAO (troleandomycin) is a synthetically derived acetylated ester of oleandomycin, an antibiotic elaborated by a species of *Streptomyces antibioticus*. It is a white crystalline compound, insoluble in water, but readily soluble and stable in the presence of gastric juice. The compound has a molecular weight of 814 and corresponds to the empirical formula $C_{41}H_{67}NO_{15}$.

Inert ingredients in the formulation are: hard gelatin capsules (which may contain inert ingredients); lactose; magnesium stearate; sodium lauryl sulfate; starch.

ACTIONS

TAO is an antibiotic shown to be active *in vitro* against the following gram-positive organisms:

Streptococcus pyogenes
Diplococcus pneumoniae

Susceptibility plate testing: If the Kirby-Bauer method of disc sensitivity is used, a 15 mcg. oleandomycin disc should give a zone of over 18 mm. when tested against a troleandomycin sensitive bacterial strain.

INDICATIONS

Diplococcus pneumoniae
   Pneumococcal pneumonia due to susceptible strains.
Streptococcus pyogenes
   Group A beta-hemolytic streptococcal infections of the upper respiratory tract.

Injectable benzathine penicillin G is considered by the American Heart Association to be the drug of choice in the treatment and prevention of streptococcal pharyngitis and in long term prophylaxis of rheumatic fever.

Troleandomycin is generally effective in the eradication of streptococci from the nasopharynx. However, substantial data establishing the efficacy of TAO in the subsequent prevention of rheumatic fever are not available at present.

CONTRAINDICATIONS

Troleandomycin is contraindicated in patients with known hypersensitivity to this antibiotic.

WARNINGS

Usage in Pregnancy: Safety for use in pregnancy has not been established.

The administration of troleandomycin has been associated with an allergic type of cholestatic hepatitis. Some patients receiving troleandomycin for more than two weeks or in repeated courses have shown jaundice accompanied by right upper quadrant pain, fever, nausea, vomiting, eosinophilia, and leukocytosis. The changes have been reversible on discontinuance of the drug. Liver function tests should be monitored in patients on such dosage, and the drug discontinued if abnormalities develop. Reports in the literature have sug-

Continued on next page

Roerig—Cont.

gested that the concurrent use of ergotamine-containing drugs and troleandomycin may induce ischemic reactions. Therefore, the concurrent use of ergotamine-containing drugs and troleandomycin should be avoided. Troleandomycin should be administered with caution to patients concurrently receiving estrogen containing oral contraceptives. Studies in chronic asthmatic patients have suggested that the concurrent use of theophylline and troleandomycin may result in elevated serum concentrations of theophylline. Therefore, it is recommended that patients receiving such concurrent therapy be observed for signs of theophylline toxicity, and that therapy be appropriately modified if such signs develop.

PRECAUTIONS
Troleandomycin is principally excreted by the liver.
Caution should be exercised in administering the antibiotic to patients with impaired hepatic function.

ADVERSE REACTIONS
The most frequent side effects of troleandomycin preparations are gastrointestinal, such as abdominal cramping and discomfort, and are dose related. Nausea, vomiting, and diarrhea occur infrequently with usual oral doses.
During prolonged or repeated therapy, there is a possibility of overgrowth of nonsusceptible bacteria or fungi. If such infections occur, the drug should be discontinued and appropriate therapy instituted.
Mild allergic reactions such as urticaria and other skin rashes have occurred. Serious allergic reactions, including anaphylaxis, have been reported.

DOSAGE AND ADMINISTRATION
Clinical judgment based on the type of infection and its severity should determine dosage within the below listed ranges.
Adults: 250 to 500 mg. 4 times a day
Children: 125 to 250 mg. (3-5 mg./lb. or 6.6 to 11 mg./kg.) every 6 hours
When used in streptococcal infection, therapy should be continued for ten days.

HOW SUPPLIED
TAO is supplied as:
Capsules 250 mg. Each capsule contains troleandomycin equivalent to 250 mg of oleandomycin; bottle of 100 (NDC 0049-1590-66).

69-1800-00-7
Shown in Product Identification Section, page 426

TERRA–CORTRIL®   ℞
Terramycin ® (oxytetracycline HCl)
—Cortril® (hydrocortisone acetate)
OPHTHALMIC SUSPENSION

DESCRIPTION
Terra-Cortril suspension combines the antibiotic, oxytetracycline HCl ($C_{22}H_{24}N_2O_9 \cdot HCl$) and the adrenocorticoid, hydrocortisone acetate ($C_{23}H_{32}O_6$). **Each ml of Terra-Cortril contains Terramycin (oxytetracycline HCl) equivalent to 5 mg of oxytetracycline, and 15 mg of Cortril (hydrocortisone acetate) incorporated in mineral oil with aluminum tristearate.**

For Ophthalmic Use Only.

CLINICAL PHARMACOLOGY
Corticosteroids suppress the inflammatory response to a variety of agents and they probably delay or slow healing. Since corticoids may inhibit the body's defense mechanism against infection, a concomitant antimicrobial drug may be used when this inhibition is considered to be clinically significant in a particular case.
The anti-infective component in the combination is included to provide action against specific organisms suspectible to it. Terramycin is considered active against the following microorganisms:
Rickettsiae (Rocky Mountain spotted fever, typhus fever and the typhus group, Q fever, rickettsialpox and tick fevers),
Mycoplasma pneumoniae (PPLO, Eaton Agent),
Agents of psittacosis and ornithosis,
Agents of lymphogranuloma venereum and granuloma inguinale,
The spirochetal agent of relapsing fever (*Borrelia recurrentis*).
The following gram-negative microorganisms:
Haemophilus ducreyi (chancroid),
Pasteurella pestis and *Pasteurella tularensis,*
Bartonella bascilloformis,
Bacteroides species,

Vibrio comma and *Vibrio fetus,*
Brucella species (in conjunction with streptomycin).
Because many strains of the following groups of microorganisms have been shown to be resistant to tetracyclines, culture and suspectibility testing are recommended.
Oxytetracycline is indicated for treatment of infections caused by the following gram-negative microorganisms, when bacteriologic testing indicates appropriate susceptibility to the drug:
Escherichia coli,
Enterobacter aerogenes (formerly *Aerobacter aerogenes*),
Shigella species,
Mima species and *Herellea* species,
Haemophilus influenzae (respiratory infections),
Klebsiella species (respiratory and urinary infections).
Oxytetracycline is indicated for treatment of infections caused by the following gram-positive microorganisms when bacteriologic testing indicates appropriate suspectibility to the drug:
Streptococcus species:
Up to 44 percent of strains of *Streptococcus pyogenes* and 74 percent of *Streptococcus faecalis* have been found to be resistant to tetracycline drugs. Therefore, tetracyclines should not be used for streptococcal disease unless the organism has been demonstrated to be sensitive.
For upper respiratory infections due to Group A beta-hemolytic streptococci, pencillin is the usual drug of choice, including prophylaxis of rheumatic fever.
Diplococcus pneumoniae,
Staphylococcus aureus, skin and soft tissue infections. Oxytetracycline is not the drug of choice in the treatment of any type of staphylococcus infections.
When penicillin is contraindicated, tetracyclines are alternative drugs in the treatment of infections due to:
Neisseria gonorrhoeae,
Treponema pallidum and *Treponema pertenue* (syphilis and yaws),
Listeria monocytogenes,
Clostridium species,
Bacillus anthracis,
Fusobacterium fusiforme (Vincent's infection),
Actinomyces species.
Tetracyclines are indicated in the treatment of trachoma, although the infectious agent is not always eliminated, as judged by immunofluorescence.
Inclusion conjunctivitis may be treated with oral tetracyclines or with a combination of oral and topical agents.
When a decision to administer both a corticoid and an antimicrobial is made, the administration of such drugs in combination has the advantage of greater patient compliance and convenience, with the added assurance that the appropriate dosage of both drugs is administered, plus assured compatibility of ingredients when both types of drug are in the same formulation and, particularly, that the correct volume of drug is delivered and retained.
The relative potency of corticosteroids depends on the molecular structure, concentration, and release from the vehicle.

INDICATIONS AND USAGE
For steroid-responsive inflammatory ocular conditions for which a corticosteroid is indicated and where bacterial infection or risk of bacterial ocular infection exists.
Ocular steroids are indicated in inflammatory conditions of the palpebral and bulbar conjunctiva, cornea, and anterior segment of the globe where the inherent risk of steroid use in certain infective conjunctivitides is accepted to obtain a diminution in edema and inflammation. They are also indicated in chronic anterior uveitis and corneal injury from chemical radiation, thermal burns, or penetration of foreign bodies.
The use of a combination drug with an anti-infective component is indicated where the risk of infection is high or where there is an expectation that potentially dangerous numbers of bacteria will be present in the eye.
The particular anti-infective drug in this product is active against the following common bacterial eye pathogens:
Staphylococcus aureus
Streptococci, including *Streptococcus pneumoniae*
Escherichia coli
Neisseria species
The product does not provide adequate coverage against:
Haemophilus influenzae
Klebsiella/Enterobacter species
Pseudomonas aeruginosa
Serratia marcescens

CONTRAINDICATIONS
Epithelial herpes simplex keratitis (dendritic keratitis), vaccinia, varicella, and many other viral diseases of the cornea and conjunctiva. Mycobacterial infection of the eye. Fungal diseases of ocular structures. Hypersensitivity to a component of the medication. (Hypersensitivity to the antibiotic component occurs at a higher rate than for other components.)
The use of these combinations is always contraindicated after uncomplicated removal of a corneal foreign body.

WARNINGS
Prolonged use may result in glaucoma, with damage to the optic nerve, defects in visual acuity and fields of vision, and posterior subcapsular cataract formation. Prolonged use may suppress the host response and thus increase the hazard of secondary ocular infections. In those diseases causing thinning of the cornea or sclera, perforations have been known to occur with the use of topical steroids. In acute purulent conditions of the eye, steroids may mask infection or enhance existing infection. If these products are used for 10 days or longer, intraocular pressure should be routinely monitored even though it may be difficult in children and uncooperative patients.
Employment of steroid medication in the treatment of herpes simplex requires great caution.

PRECAUTIONS
The initial prescription and renewal of the medication order beyond 20 milliliters should be made by a physician only after examination of the patient with the aid of magnification, such as slit lamp biomicroscopy and, where appropriate, fluorescein staining.
The possibility of persistent fungal infections of the cornea should be considered after prolonged steroid dosing.

ADVERSE REACTIONS
Adverse reactions have occurred with steroid/anti-infective combination drugs which can be attributed to the steroid component, the anti-infective component, or the combination. Exact incidence figures are not available since no denominator of treated patients is available.
Reactions occurring most often from the presence of the anti-infective ingredient are allergic sensitizations. The reactions due to the steroid component in decreasing order of frequency are: elevation of intraocular pressure (IOP) with possible development of glaucoma, and infrequent optic nerve damage; posterior subcapsular cataract formation; and delayed wound healing.
Secondary Infection: The development of secondary infection has occurred after use of combinations containing steroids and antimicrobials. Fungal infections of the cornea are particularly prone to develop coincidentally with long-term applications of steroid. The possibility of fungal invasion must be considered in any persistent corneal ulceration where steroid treatment has been used.
Secondary bacterial ocular infection following suppression of host responses also occurs.

DOSAGE AND ADMINISTRATION
Instill 1 or 2 drops of Terra-Cortril Ophthalmic Suspension into the affected eye three times daily.
Not more than 20 milliliters should be prescribed initially and the prescription should not be refilled without further evaluation as outlined in "Precautions" above.

HOW SUPPLIED
Terra-Cortril Ophthalmic Suspension (NDC 0049-0670-48) is supplied in 5 ml vials with separate sterile dropper.
60-2323-00-3

TERRAMYCIN®   ℞
(oxytetracycline)
INTRAMUSCULAR SOLUTION*
FOR INTRAMUSCULAR USE ONLY
contains 2% lidocaine

DESCRIPTION
Oxytetracycline is a product of the metabolism of *Streptomyces rimosus* and is one of the family of tetracycline antibiotics.
Oxytetracycline diffuses readily through the placenta into the fetal circulation, into the pleural fluid and, under some circumstances, into the cerebrospinal fluid. It appears to be concentrated in the hepatic system and excreted in the bile, so that it appears in the feces, as well as in the urine, in a biologically active form.

COMPOSITION
[See table on next page].

ACTIONS
Oxytetracycline is primarily bacteriostatic and is thought to exert its antimicrobial effect by the inhibition of protein synthesis. Oxytetracycline is active against a wide range of gram-negative and gram-positive organisms.
The drugs in the tetracycline class have closely similar antimicrobial spectra, and cross resistance among them is common. Microorganisms may be considered susceptible if the M.I.C. (minimum inhibitory concentration) is not more than 4.0 mcg/ml and intermediate if the M.I.C. is 4.0 to 12.5 mcg/ml.
Susceptibility plate testing: A tetracycline disc may be used to determine microbial susceptibility to drugs in the tetracycline class. If the Kirby-Bauer method of disc susceptibility testing is used, a 30 mcg tetracycline disc should give a zone of at least 19 mm when tested against an oxytetracycline-susceptible bacterial strain.

Tetracyclines are readily absorbed and are bound to plasma proteins in varying degree. They are concentrated by the liver in the bile and excreted in the urine and feces at high concentrations and in a biologically active form.

INDICATIONS

Oxytetracycline is indicated in infections caused by the following microorganisms:

Rickettsiae (Rocky Mountain spotted fever, typhus fever and the typhus group, Q fever, rickettsialpox and tick fevers).

Mycoplasma pneumoniae (PPLO, Eaton agent),

Agents of psittacosis and ornithosis,

Agents of lymphogranuloma venereum and granuloma inguinale,

The spirochetal agent of relapsing fever *(Borrelia recurrentis)*.

The following gram-negative microorganisms:

Haemophilus ducreyi (chancroid),

Pasteurella pestis and *Pasteurella tularensis*,

Bartonella bacilliformis,

Bacteroides species,

Vibrio comma and *Vibrio fetus*,

Brucella species (in conjunction with streptomycin).

Because many strains of the following groups of microorganisms have been shown to be resistant to tetracyclines, culture and susceptibility testing are recommended.

Oxytetracycline is indicated for treatment of infections caused by the following gram-negative microorganisms when bacteriologic testing indicates appropriate susceptibility to the drug:

Escherichia coli,

Enterobacter aerogenes (formerly *Aerobacter aerogenes)*,

Shigella species,

Mima species and *Herellea* species,

Haemophilus influenzae (respiratory infections),

Klebsiella species (respiratory and urinary infections).

Oxytetracycline is indicated for treatment of infections caused by the following gram-positive microorganisms when bacteriologic testing indicates appropriate susceptibility to the drug: Streptococcus species;

Up to 44 percent of strains of *Streptococcus pyogenes* and 74 percent of *Streptococcus faecalis* have been found to be resistant to tetracycline drugs. Therefore, tetracyclines should not be used for streptococcal disease unless the organism has been demonstrated to be sensitive.

For upper respiratory infections due to Group A beta-hemolytic streptococci, penicillin is the usual drug of choice, including prophylaxis of rheumatic fever.

Diplococcus pneumoniae,

Staphylococcus aureus, skin and soft tissue infections. Oxytetracycline is not the drug of choice in the treatment of any type of staphylococcal infections.

When penicillin is contraindicated, tetracyclines are alternative drugs in the treatment of infections due to:

Neisseria gonorrhoeae,

Treponema pallidum and *Treponema pertenue* (syphilis and yaws),

Listeria monocytogenes,

Clostridium species,

Bacillus anthracis,

Fusobacterium fusiforme (Vincent's infection),

Actinomyces species.

In acute intestinal amebiasis, the tetracyclines may be a useful adjunct to amebicides.

Tetracyclines are indicated in the treatment of trachoma, although the infectious agent is not always eliminated, as judged by immunofluorescence.

Inclusion conjunctivitis may be treated with oral tetracyclines or with a combination of oral and topical agents.

CONTRAINDICATIONS

This drug is contraindicated in persons who have shown hypersensitivity to any of the tetracyclines.

WARNINGS

THE USE OF TETRACYCLINES DURING TOOTH DEVELOPMENT (LAST HALF OF PREGNANCY, INFANCY, AND CHILDHOOD TO THE AGE OF 8 YEARS) MAY CAUSE PERMANENT DISCOLORATION OF THE TEETH (YELLOW-GRAY-BROWN).

This adverse reaction is more common during long term use of the drugs but has been observed following repeated short term courses. Enamel hypoplasia has also been reported. *TETRACYCLINES, THEREFORE, SHOULD NOT BE USED IN THIS AGE GROUP UNLESS OTHER DRUGS ARE NOT LIKELY TO BE EFFECTIVE OR ARE CONTRAINDICATED.*

If renal impairment exists, even usual oral or parenteral doses may lead to excessive systemic accumulation of the drug and possible liver toxicity. Under such conditions, lower than usual total doses are indicated and, if therapy is prolonged, serum level determinations of the drug may be advisable. This hazard is of particular importance in the parenteral administration of tetracyclines to pregnant or postpartum patients with pyelonephritis. When used under these circumstances, the blood level should not exceed 15 mcg/ml and liver function tests should be made at frequent

Terramycin Intramuscular
contents per ml (w/v)

Ingredient	2 ml Single Dose Ampules		10 ml/Vial Multidose
	100 mg/2 ml	250 mg/2 ml	50 mg/ml 10 ml (5 × 2 ml Doses)
oxytetracycline	50 mg	25 mg	50 mg
lidocaine	2.0%	2.0%	2.0%
magnesium chloride hexahydrate	2.5%	6.0%	2.5%
sodium formaldehyde sulfoxylate	0.5%	0.5%	0.3%
α-monothioglycerol	—	—	1.0%
monoethanolamine	approx. 1.7%	approx. 4.2%	approx. 2.6%
citric acid	—	—	1.0%
propyl gallate	—	—	0.02%
propylene glycol	75.2%	67.0%	74.1%
water	18.8%	16.8%	18.5%

intervals. Other potentially hepatotoxic drugs should not be prescribed concomitantly.

(In the presence of renal dysfunction, particularly in pregnancy, intravenous tetracycline therapy in daily doses exceeding 2 grams has been associated with deaths due to liver failure.)

Photosensitivity manifested by an exaggerated sunburn reaction has been observed in some individuals taking tetracyclines. Patients apt to be exposed to direct sunlight or ultraviolet light should be advised that this reaction can occur with tetracycline drugs, and treatment should be discontinued at the first evidence of skin erythema.

The antianabolic action of the tetracyclines may cause an increase in BUN. While this is not a problem in those with normal renal function, in patients with significantly impaired function, higher serum levels of this drug may lead to azotemia, hyperphosphatemia, and acidosis.

The product contains sodium formaldehyde sulfoxylate which serves as an antioxidant. Upon oxidation, this compound can form a potential sulfiting agent. Sulfiting agents may cause allergic-type reactions including anaphylactic symptoms and life-threatening or less severe asthmatic episodes in certain susceptible people. The over-all prevalence of sulfite sensitivity in the general population is unknown and probably low. Sulfite sensitivity is seen more frequently in asthmatic than in nonasthmatic people.

Usage in pregnancy. (See above "Warnings" about use during tooth development.)

Results of animal studies indicate that tetracyclines cross the placenta, are found in fetal tissues and can have toxic effects on the developing fetus (often related to retardation of skeletal development). Evidence of embryotoxicity has also been noted in animals treated early in pregnancy.

Usage in newborns, infants, and children. (See above "Warnings" about use during tooth deveopment).

All tetracyclines form a stable calcium complex in any bone-forming tissue. A decrease in the fibula growth rate has been observed in prematures given oral tetracyclne in doses of 25 mg/kg every 6 hours. This reaction was shown to be reversible when the drug was discontinued.

Tetracyclines are present in the milk of lactating women who are taking a drug in this class.

PRECAUTIONS

As with all intramuscular preparations, Terramycin (oxytetracycline) Intramuscular Solution should be injected well within the body of a relatively large muscle. ADULTS: The preferred sites are the upper outer quadrant of the buttock, (i.e., gluteus maximus), and the mid-lateral thigh. CHILDREN: It is recommended that intramuscular injections be given preferably in the mid-lateral muscles of the thigh. In infants and small children the periphery of the upper outer quadrant of the gluteal region should be used only when necessary, such as in burn patients, in order to minimize the possibility of damage to the sciatic nerve.

The deltoid area should be used only if well developed such as in certain adults and older children, and then only with caution to avoid radial nerve injury. Intramuscular injections should not be made into the lower and mid-thirds of the upper arm. As with all intramuscular injections, aspiration is necessary to help avoid inadvertent injection into a blood vessel.

As with other antibiotic preparations, use of this drug may result in overgrowth of nonsusceptible organisms, including fungi. If superinfection occurs, the antibiotic should be discontinued and appropriate therapy instituted.

In venereal diseases when coexistent syphilis is suspected, a dark field examination should be done before treatment is started and the blood serology repeated monthly for at least 4 months.

Because tetracyclines have been shown to depress plasma prothrombin activity, patients who are on anticoagulant therapy may require downward adjustment of their anticoagulant dosage.

In long term therapy, periodic laboratory evaluation of organ systems, including hematopoietic, renal and hepatic studies should be performed.

All infections due to Group A beta-hemolytic streptococci should be treated for at least 10 days.

Since bacteriostatic drugs may interfere with the bactericidal action of penicillin, it is advisable to avoid giving tetracycline in conjunction with penicillin.

ADVERSE REACTIONS

Local irritation may be present after intramuscular injection. The injection should be deep, with care taken not to injure the sciatic nerve nor inject intravascularly.

Gastrointestinal: anorexia, nausea, vomiting, diarrhea, glossitis, dyphagia, enterocolitis, and inflammatory lesions (with monilial overgrowth) in the anogenital region. These reactions have been caused by both the oral and parenteral administration of tetracyclines.

Skin: maculopapular and erythematous rashes. Exfoliative dermatitis has been reported but is uncommon. Photosensitivity is discussed above. (See "Warnings").

Renal toxicity: Rise in BUN has been reported and is apparently dose related. (See "Warnings").

Hypersensitivity reactions: Urticaria, angioneurotic edema, anaphylaxis, anaphylactoid purpura, pericarditis, and exacerbation of systemic lupus erythematosus.

Bulging fontanels in infants and benign intracranial hypertension in adults have been reported in individuals receiving full therapeutic dosages. These conditions disappeared rapidly when the drug was discontinued.

Blood: Hemolytic anemia, thrombocytopenia, neutropenia, and eosinophilia have been reported.

When given over prolonged periods, tetracyclines have been reported to produce brown-black microscopic discoloration of thyroid glands. No abnormalities of thyroid function studies are known to occur.

DOSAGE AND ADMINISTRATION

Intramuscular Administration:

Adults: The usual daily dose is 250 mg administered once every 24 hours or 300 mg given in divided doses at 8 to 12 hour intervals.

For children above eight years of age: 15–25 mg/kg body weight up to a maximum of 250 mg per single daily injection. Dosage may be divided and given at 8 to 12 hour intervals. Intramuscular therapy should be reserved for situations in which oral therapy is not feasible.

The intramuscular administration of oxytetracycline produces lower blood levels than oral administration in the recommended dosages. Patients placed on intramuscular oxytetracycline should be changed to the oral dosage form as soon as possible. If rapid, high blood levels are needed, oxytetracycline should be administered intravenously.

In patients with renal impairment: (See "Warnings") Total dosage should be decreased by reduction of recommended individual doses and/or by extending time intervals between doses.

HOW SUPPLIED

Terramycin (oxytetracycline) Intramuscular Solution is available as follows:

250 mg/2 ml—in 2 ml pre-scored glass ampules, packages of 5 (NDC 0069-0770-09).

100 mg/2 ml—in 2 ml pre-scored glass ampules, packages of 5 (NDC 0069-0760-09).

50 mg/ml—in 10 ml multiple dose vials, packages of 5 (NDC 0069-0750-77).

*U.S. Pat. Nos. 3,017,323 and 3,026,248

70-1051-00-2

Continued on next page

Roerig—Cont.

TERRAMYCIN®   ℞
(oxytetracycline HCl with polymyxin B sulfate)
OPHTHALMIC OINTMENT
STERILE

DESCRIPTION
Each gram of sterile ointment contains oxytetracycline HCl equivalent to 5 mg oxytetracycline, 10,000 units of polymyxin B sulfate, white petrolatum, and liquid petrolatum.

ACTIONS
Terramycin® is a widely used antibiotic with clinically proved activity against gram-positive and gram-negative bacteria, rickettsiae, spirochetes, large viruses, and certain protozoa.
Polymyxin B Sulfate, one of a group of related antibiotics derived from *Bacillus polymyxa*, is rapidly bactericidal. This action is exclusively against gram-negative organisms. It is particularly effective against *Pseudomonas aeruginosa (B. pyocyaneus)* and Koch-Weeks bacillus, frequently found in local infections of the eye.
There is thus made available a particularly effective antimicrobial combination of the broad-spectrum antibiotic Terramycin as well as polymyxin B sulfate against primarily causative or secondarily infecting organisms.

INDICATIONS
The sterile preparation, Terramycin with Polymyxin B Sulfate Ophthalmic Ointment, is indicated for the treatment of superficial ocular infections involving the conjunctiva and /or cornea caused by Terramycin with Polymyxin B Sulfate-susceptible organisms.
It may be administered topically alone, or as an adjunct to systemic therapy.
It is effective in infections caused by susceptible strains of staphylococci, streptococci, pneumococci, *Hemophilus influenzae*, *Pseudomonas aeruginosa*, Koch-Weeks bacillus, and *Proteus*.

CONTRAINDICATIONS
This drug is contraindicated in individuals who have shown hypersensitivity to any of its components.

PRECAUTIONS
As with all antibiotic preparations, use of this drug may result in overgrowth of nonsusceptible organisms, including fungi. If super-infection occurs, the antibiotic should be discontinued and appropriate specific therapy should be instituted.

ADVERSE REACTIONS
Terramycin with Polymyxin B Sulfate Ophthalmic Ointment is well tolerated by the epithelial membranes and other tissues of the eye. Allergic or inflammatory reactions due to individual hypersensitivity are rare.

DOSAGE AND ADMINISTRATION
Approximately ½ inch of the ointment is squeezed from the tube onto the lower lid of the affected eye two to four times daily.
The patient should be instructed to avoid contamination of the tip of the tube when applying the ointment.

HOW SUPPLIED
Terramycin with Polymyxin B Sulfate Ophthalmic Ointment is supplied in ⅛ oz., (3.5 g) tubes (NDC 0049-0801-08).
60-2324-00-1

UNASYN®   ℞
Ampicillin Sodium/Sulbactam Sodium

DESCRIPTION
UNASYN is an injectable antibacterial combination consisting of the semisynthetic antibiotic ampicillin sodium and the beta-lactamase inhibitor sulbactam sodium for intravenous and intramuscular administration.
Ampicillin sodium is derived from the penicillin nucleus, 6-aminopenicillanic acid. Chemically, it is monosodium (2S,5R,6R)-6-[(R)-2-amino-2-phenylacetamido]-3,3-dimethyl-7-oxo-4-thia-1-azabicyclo[3.2.0]heptane-2-carboxylate and has a molecular weight of 371.39. Its chemical formula is $C_{16}H_{18}N_3NaO_4S$. The structural formula is:

Sulbactam sodium is a derivative of the basic penicillin nucleus. Chemically, sulbactam sodium is sodium penicillinate sulfone; sodium (2S, 5R)-3,3-dimethyl-7-oxo-4-thia-1-azabicyclo[3.2.0]heptane-2-carboxylate 4,4-dioxide. Its chem-

ical formula is $C_8H_{10}NNaO_5S$ with a molecular weight of 255.22. The structural formula is:

UNASYN, ampicillin sodium/sulbactam sodium parenteral combination, is available as a white to off-white dry powder for reconstitution. UNASYN dry powder is freely soluble in aqueous diluents to yield pale yellow to yellow solutions containing ampicillin sodium and sulbactam sodium equivalent to 250 mg ampicillin per mL and 125 mg sulbactam per mL. The pH of the solutions is between 8.0 and 10.0.
Dilute solutions (up to 30 mg ampicillin and 15 mg sulbactam per mL) are essentially colorless to pale yellow. The pH of dilute solutions remains the same.
1.5 g of UNASYN (1 g ampicillin as the sodium salt plus 0.5 g sulbactam as the sodium salt) parenteral contains approximately 115 mg (5 mEq) of sodium.

CLINICAL PHARMACOLOGY
General: Immediately after completion of a 15-minute intravenous infusion of UNASYN, peak serum concentrations of ampicillin and sulbactam are attained. Ampicillin serum levels are similar to those produced by the administration of equivalent amounts of ampicillin alone. Peak ampicillin serum levels ranging from 109 to 150 mcg/mL are attained after administration of 2000 mg of ampicillin plus 1000 mg sulbactam and 40 to 71 mcg/mL after administration of 1000 mg ampicillin plus 500 mg sulbactam. The corresponding mean peak serum levels for sulbactam range from 48 to 88 mcg/mL and 21 to 40 mcg/mL, respectively. After an intramuscular injection of 1000 mg ampicillin plus 500 mg sulbactam, peak ampicillin serum levels ranging from 8 to 37 mcg/mL and peak sulbactam serum levels ranging from 6 to 24 mcg/mL are attained.
The mean serum half-life of both drugs is approximately 1 hour in healthy volunteers.
Approximately 75 to 85% of both ampicillin and sulbactam are excreted unchanged in the urine during the first 8 hours after administration of UNASYN to individuals with normal renal function. Somewhat higher and more prolonged serum levels of ampicillin and sulbactam can be achieved with the concurrent administration of probenecid.
In patients with impaired renal function the elimination kinetics of ampicillin and sulbactam are similarly affected, hence the ratio of one to the other will remain constant whatever the renal function. The dose of UNASYN in such patients should be administered less frequently in accordance with the usual practice for ampicillin (see Dosage and Administration).
Ampicillin has been found to be approximately 28% reversibly bound to human serum protein and sulbactam approximately 38% reversibly bound.
The following average levels of ampicillin and sulbactam were measured in the tissues and fluids listed:

TABLE A
Concentration of UNASYN in Various Body Tissues and Fluids

Fluid or Tissue	Dose (grams) Ampicillin/ Sulbactam	Concentration (mcg/mL or or mcg/g) Ampicillin/ Sulbactam
Peritoneal Fluid	0.5/0.5 IV	7/14
Blister Fluid (Cantharides)	0.5/0.5 IV	8/20
Tissue Fluid	1/0.5 IV	8/4
Intestinal Mucosa	0.5/0.5 IV	11/18
Appendix	2/1 IV	3/40

Penetration of both ampicillin and sulbactam into cerebrospinal fluid in the presence of inflamed meninges has been demonstrated after IV administration of UNASYN.

MICROBIOLOGY
Ampicillin is similar to benzyl penicillin in its bactericidal action against susceptible organisms during the stage of active multiplication. It acts through the inhibition of cell wall mucopeptide biosynthesis. Ampicillin has a broad spectrum of bactericidal activity against many gram-positive and gram-negative aerobic and anaerobic bacteria. (Ampicillin is, however, degraded by beta-lactamases and therefore the spectrum of activity does not normally include organisms which produce these enzymes.)
A wide range of beta-lactamases found in microorganisms resistant to penicillins and cephalosporins have been shown in biochemical studies with cell free bacterial systems to be irreversibly inhibited by sulbactam. Although sulbactam alone possesses little useful antibacterial activity except against the *Neisseriaciae*, whole organism studies have shown that sulbactam restores ampicillin activity against beta-lactamase producing strains. In particular, sulbactam has good inhibitory activity against the clinically important

plasmid mediated beta-lactamases most frequently responsible for transferred drug resistance. Sulbactam has no effect on the activity of ampicillin against ampicillin susceptible strains.
The presence of sulbactam in the UNASYN formulation effectively extends the antibiotic spectrum of ampicillin to include many bacteria normally resistant to it and to other beta-lactam antibiotics. Thus, UNASYN possesses the properties of a broad-spectrum antibiotic and a beta-lactamase inhibitor.
While *in vitro* studies have demonstrated the susceptibility of most strains of the following organisms, clinical efficacy for infections other than those included in the indications section has not been documented.
Gram-Positive Bacteria: *Staphylococcus aureus* (beta-lactamase and non-beta-lactamase producing), *Staphylococcus epidermidis* (beta-lactamase and non-beta-lactamase producing), *Staphylococcus saprophyticus* (beta-lactamase and non-beta-lactamase producing), *Streptococcus faecalis†* (Enterococcus), *Streptococcus pneumoniae†* (formerly *D. pneumoniae*), *Streptococcus pyogenes†*, *Streptococcus viridans†*.
Gram-Negative Bacteria: *Hemophilus influenzae* (beta-lactamase and non-beta-lactamase producing), *Branhamella catarrhalis* (formerly *Neisseria catarrhalis*) (beta-lactamase and non-beta-lactamase producing), *Escherichia coli* (beta-lactamase and non-beta-lactamase producing), *Klebsiella* species (all known strains are beta-lactamase producing), *Proteus mirabilis* (beta-lactamase and non-beta-lactamase producing), *Proteus vulgaris*, *Providencia rettgeri*, *Providencia stuartii*, *Morganella morganii*, and *Neisseria gonorrhoeae* (beta-lactamase and non-beta-lactamase producing).
Anaerobes: *Clostridium* species†, *Peptococcus* species†, *Peptostreptococcus* species, *Bacteroides* species, including *B. fragilis*.
† These are not beta-lactamase producing strains and, therefore, are susceptible to ampicillin alone.
Susceptibility Testing
Diffusion Technique: For the Kirby-Bauer method of susceptibility testing, a 20 mcg (10 mcg ampicillin + 10 mcg sulbactam) diffusion disk should be used. The method is one outlined in the NCCLS publication M 2–A 3 *. With this procedure, a report from the laboratory of "Susceptible" indicates that the infecting organism is likely to respond to UNASYN therapy and a report of "Resistant" indicates that the infecting organism is not likely to respond to therapy. An "Intermediate" susceptibility report suggests that the infecting organism would be susceptible to UNASYN if a higher dosage is used or if the infection is confined to tissues or fluids (e.g., urine) in which high antibiotic levels are attained.
Dilution Techniques: Broth or agar dilution methods may be used to determine the minimal inhibitory concentration (MIC) value for susceptibility of bacterial isolates to ampicillin/sulbactam. The method used is one outlined in the NCCLS publication M 7-A.** Tubes should be inoculated to contain 10^5 to 10^6 organisms/mL or plates "spotted" with 10^4 organisms.
The recommended dilution method employs a constant ampicillin/sulbactam ratio of 2:1 in all tubes with increasing concentrations of ampicillin. MIC's are reported in terms of ampicillin concentration in the presence of sulbactam at a constant 2 parts ampicillin to 1 part sulbactam.
[See table on next page.]
*Performance standards for Antimicrobial Disk Susceptibility Tests M2-A3, Vol. 4, No. 16, pp. 369–403, National Committee for Clinical Laboratory Standards, 771 East Lancaster Ave., Villanova, PA 19085.
**Methods for Dilution Antimicrobial Susceptibility Tests for Bacteria that Grow Aerobically M7-A, Vol. 5, No. 22, pp. 579–616, National Committee for Clinical Laboratory Standards, 771 East Lancaster Ave., Villanova, PA 19085.

INDICATIONS AND USAGE
UNASYN is indicated for the treatment of infections due to susceptible strains of the designated microorganisms in the conditions listed below.
Skin and Skin Structure Infections caused by beta-lactamase producing strains of *Staphylococcus aureus*, *Escherichia coli**, *Klebsiella* spp.* (including *K. pneumoniae**), *Proteus mirabilis**, *Bacteroides fragilis**, *Enterobacter* spp.*, and *Acinetobacter calcoaceticus**.
Intra-Abdominal Infections caused by beta-lactamase producing strains of *Escherichia coli*, *Klebsiella* spp. (including *K. pneumoniae*), *Bacteroides* spp. (including *B. fragilis*), and *Enterobacter* spp.*
Gynecological Infections caused by beta-lactamase producing strains of *Escherichia coli**, and *Bacteroides* spp.* (including *B. fragilis**).
* Efficacy for this organism in this organ system was studied in fewer than 10 infections.
While UNASYN is indicated only for the conditions listed above, infections caused by ampicillin-susceptible organisms are also amenable to treatment with UNASYN due to its ampicillin content. Therefore, mixed infections caused by ampicillin-susceptible organisms and beta-lactamase producing organisms susceptible to UNASYN should not require the addition of another antibiotic.

Appropriate culture and susceptibility tests should be performed before treatment in order to isolate and identify the organisms causing infection and to determine their susceptibility to UNASYN.

Therapy may be instituted prior to obtaining the results from bacteriological and susceptibility studies, when there is reason to believe the infection may involve any of the beta-lactamase producing organisms listed above in the indicated organ systems. Once the results are known, therapy should be adjusted if appropriate.

CONTRAINDICATIONS

The use of UNASYN is contraindicated in individuals with a history of hypersensitivity reactions to any of the penicillins.

WARNINGS

SERIOUS AND OCCASIONALLY FATAL HYPERSENSITIVITY (ANAPHYLACTIC) REACTIONS HAVE BEEN REPORTED IN PATIENTS ON PENICILLIN THERAPY. THESE REACTIONS ARE MORE APT TO OCCUR IN INDIVIDUALS WITH A HISTORY OF PENICILLIN HYPERSENSITIVITY AND/OR HYPERSENSITIVITY REACTIONS TO MULTIPLE ALLERGENS. THERE HAVE BEEN REPORTS OF INDIVIDUALS WITH A HISTORY OF PENICILLIN HYPERSENSITIVITY WHO HAVE EXPERIENCED SEVERE REACTIONS WHEN TREATED WITH CEPHALOSPORINS. BEFORE THERAPY WITH A PENICILLIN, CAREFUL INQUIRY SHOULD BE MADE CONCERNING PREVIOUS HYPERSENSITIVITY REACTIONS TO PENICILLINS, CEPHALOSPORINS, AND OTHER ALLERGENS. IF AN ALLERGIC REACTION OCCURS, UNASYN SHOULD BE DISCONTINUED AND THE APPROPRIATE THERAPY INSTITUTED.

SERIOUS ANAPHYLACTOID REACTIONS REQUIRE IMMEDIATE EMERGENCY TREATMENT WITH EPINEPHRINE. OXYGEN, INTRAVENOUS STEROIDS, AND AIRWAY MANAGEMENT, INCLUDING INTUBATION, SHOULD ALSO BE ADMINISTERED AS INDICATED.

PRECAUTIONS

General: A high percentage of patients with mononucleosis who receive ampicillin develop a skin rash. Thus, ampicillin class antibiotics should not be administered to patients with mononucleosis. In patients treated with UNASYN the possibility of superinfections with mycotic or bacterial pathogens should be kept in mind during therapy. If superinfections occur (usually involving *Pseudomonas* or *Candida*), the drug should be discontinued and/or appropriate therapy instituted.

Drug Interactions: Probenecid decreases the renal tubular secretion of ampicillin and sulbactam. Concurrent use of probenecid with UNASYN may result in increased and prolonged blood levels of ampicillin and sulbactam. The concurrent administration of allopurinol and ampicillin increases substantially the incidence of rashes in patients receiving both drugs as compared to patients receiving ampicillin alone. It is not known whether this potentiation of ampicillin rashes is due to allopurinol or the hyperuricemia present in these patients. There are no data with UNASYN and allopurinol administered concurrently. UNASYN and aminoglycosides should not be reconstituted together due to the *in vitro* inactivation of aminoglycosides by the ampicillin component of UNASYN.

Drug/Laboratory Test Interactions: Administration of UNASYN will result in high urine concentration of ampicillin. High urine concentrations of ampicillin may result in false positive reactions when testing for the presence of glucose in urine using Clinitest™, Benedict's Solution or Fehling's Solution. It is recommended that glucose tests based on enzymatic glucose oxidase reactions (such as Clinistix™ or Testape™) be used. Following administration of ampicillin to pregnant women, a transient decrease in plasma concentration of total conjugated estriol, estriol-glucuronide, conjugated estrone and estradiol has been noted. This effect may also occur with UNASYN.

Carcinogenesis, Mutagenesis, Impairment of Fertility: Long-term studies in animals have not been performed to evaluate carcinogenic or mutagenic potential.

Pregnancy

Pregnancy Category B: Reproduction studies have been performed in mice, rats, and rabbits at doses up to ten (10) times the human dose and have revealed no evidence of impaired fertility or harm to the fetus due to UNASYN. There are, however, no adequate and well controlled studies in pregnant women. Because animal reproduction studies are not always predictive of human response, this drug should be used during pregnancy only if clearly needed. (See—Drug/Laboratory Test Interactions).

Labor and Delivery: Studies in guinea pigs have shown that intravenous administration of ampicillin decreased the uterine tone, frequency of contractions, height of contractions, and duration of contractions. However, it is not known whether the use of UNASYN in humans during labor or delivery has immediate or delayed adverse effects on the fetus, prolongs the duration of labor, or increases the likelihood that forceps delivery or other obstetrical intervention or resuscitation of the newborn will be necessary.

Recommended ampicillin/sulbactam, Susceptibility Ranges[1,2,3]

	Resistant	Intermediate	Susceptible
Gram(-) and Staphylococcus			
Bauer/Kirby Zone Sizes	≤11 mm	12–13 mm	≥14 mm
MIC (mcg of ampicillin/mL)	≥32	16	≤ 8
Hemophilus influenzae			
Bauer/Kirby Zone Sizes	≤19	—	≥20
MIC (mcg of ampicillin/mL)	≥ 4	—	≤2

[1] The non-beta-lactamase producing organisms which are normally susceptible to ampicillin, such as *Streptococci*, will have similar zone sizes as for ampicillin disks.

[2] *Staphylococci* resistant to methicillin, oxacillin, or nafcillin must be considered resistant to UNASYN.

[3] The quality control cultures should have the following assigned daily ranges for ampicillin/sulbactam:

		Disks	Mode MIC (mcg/mL ampicillin/mcg/mL sulbactam)
E. coli	(ATCC 25922)	20–24 mm	2/1
S. aureus	(ATCC 25923)	29–37 mm	0.12/0.06
E. coli	(ATCC 35218)	13–19 mm	8/4

Nursing Mothers: Low concentrations of ampicillin and sulbactam are excreted in the milk; therefore, caution should be exercised when UNASYN is administered to a nursing woman.

Pediatric Use: The efficacy and safety of UNASYN have not been established in infants and children under the age of 12.

ADVERSE REACTIONS

UNASYN is generally well tolerated. The following adverse reactions have been reported.

Local Adverse Reactions

Pain at IM injection site—16%
Pain at IV injection site—3%
Thrombophlebitis—3%

Systemic Adverse Reactions

The most frequently reported adverse reactions were diarrhea in 3% of the patients and rash in less than 2% of the patients.

Additional systemic reactions reported in less than 1% of the patients were: itching, nausea, vomiting, candidiasis, fatigue, malaise, headache, chest pain, flatulence, abdominal distension, glossitis, urine retention, dysuria, edema, facial swelling, erythema, chills, tightness in throat, substernal pain, epistaxis and mucosal bleeding.

Adverse Laboratory Changes

Adverse laboratory changes without regard to drug relationship that were reported during clinical trials were:

Hepatic: Increased AST (SGOT), ALT (SGPT), alkaline phosphatase, and LDH.

Hematologic: Decreased hemoglobin, hematocrit, RBC, WBC, neutrophils, lymphocytes, platelets and increased lymphocytes, monocytes, basophils, eosinophils, and platelets.

Blood Chemistry: Decreased serum albumin and total proteins.

Renal: Increased BUN and creatinine.

Urinalysis: Presence of RBC's and hyaline casts in urine.

The following adverse reactions have been reported with ampicillin-class antibiotics and can also occur with UNASYN.

Gastrointestinal: Gastritis, stomatitis, black "hairy" tongue, enterocolitis and pseudomembranous colitis.

Hypersensitivity Reactions: Urticaria, erythema multiforme, and an occasional case of exfoliative dermatitis have been reported. These reactions may be controlled with antihistamines and, if necessary, systemic corticosteroids. Whenever such reactions occur, the drug should be discontinued, unless the opinion of the physician dictates otherwise. Serious and occasional fatal hypersensitivity (anaphylactic) reactions can occur with a penicillin (see **WARNINGS**).

Hematologic: In addition to the adverse laboratory changes listed above for UNASYN, agranulocytosis has been reported during therapy with penicillins. All of these reactions are usually reversible on discontinuation of therapy and are believed to be hypersensitivity phenomena.

OVERDOSAGE

Neurological adverse reactions, including convulsions, may occur with the attainment of high CSF levels of beta-lactams. Ampicillin may be removed from circulation by hemodialysis. The molecular weight, degree of protein binding and pharmacokinetics profile of sulbactam suggest that this compound may also be removed by hemodialysis.

DOSAGE AND ADMINISTRATION

UNASYN may be administered by either the IV or the IM routes.

For IV administration, the dose can be given by slow intravenous injection over at least 10–15 minutes or can also be delivered, in greater dilutions with 50–100 mL of a compatible diluent as an intravenous infusion over 15–30 minutes.

UNASYN may be administered by deep intramuscular injection. (See Preparation for Intramuscular Injection.)

The recommended adult dosage of UNASYN is 1.5 g (1 g ampicillin as the sodium salt plus 0.5 g sulbactam as the sodium salt) to 3 g (2 g ampicillin as the sodium salt plus 1 g sulbactam as the sodium salt) every six hours. This 1.5 to 3 g range represents the total of ampicillin content plus the sulbactam content of UNASYN, and corresponds to a range of 1 g ampicillin/0.5 sulbactam to 2 g ampicillin/1 g sulbactam. The total dose of sulbactam should not exceed 4 grams per day.

Impaired Renal Function

In patients with impairment of renal function the elimination kinetics of ampicillin and sulbactam are similarly affected, hence the ratio of one to the other will remain constant whatever the renal function. The dose of UNASYN in such patients should be administered less frequently in accordance with the usual practice for ampicillin and according to the following recommendations:

UNASYN Dosage Guide For Patients With Renal Impairment

Creatinine Clearance (mL/min 1.73m²)	Ampicillin Sulbactam Half-Life (Hours)	Recommended UNASYN Dosage
≥30	1	1.5–3.0 g q 6h–q 8h
15–29	5	1.5–3.0 g q12h
5–14	9	1.5–3.0 g q24h

When only serum creatinine is available, the following formula (based on sex, weight, and age of the patient) may be used to convert this value into creatinine clearance. The serum creatinine should represent a steady state of renal function.

Males $\dfrac{\text{weight (kg)} \times (140 - \text{age})}{72 \times \text{serum creatinine}}$

Females $0.85 \times$ above value

COMPATABILITY, RECONSTITUTION AND STABILITY

UNASYN sterile powder is to be stored at or below 30°C (86°F) prior to reconstitution.

When concomitant therapy with aminoglycosides is indicated, UNASYN and aminoglycosides should be reconstituted and administered separately, due to the *in vitro* inactivation of aminoglycosides by any of the aminopenicillins.

DIRECTIONS FOR USE

General Dissolution Procedures: UNASYN sterile powder for intravenous and intramuscular use may be reconstituted with any of the compatible diluents described in this insert. Solutions should be allowed to stand after dissolution to allow any foaming to dissipate in order to permit visual inspection for complete solubilization.

Preparation for Intravenous Use

1.5 g and 3.0 g Bottles: UNASYN sterile powder in piggyback units may be reconstituted directly to the desired concentrations using any of the following parenteral diluents. Reconstitution of UNASYN, at the specified concentrations, with these diluents provide stable solutions for the time periods indicated in the following table: (After the indicated time periods, any unused portions of solutions should be discarded.)

[See table on next page].

If piggyback bottles are unavailable, standard vials of UNASYN sterile powder may be used. Initially, the vials may be reconstituted with Sterile Water for Injection to yield solutions containing 375 mg UNASYN per mL (250 mg ampicillin/125 mg sulbactam per mL). An appropriate volume should then be immediately diluted with a suitable parenteral diluent to yield solutions containing 3 to 45 mg UNASYN per mL (2 to 30 mg ampicillin/1 to 15 mg sulbactam/per mL).

Continued on next page

Roerig—Cont.

1.5 g ADD-Vantage™ Vials: UNASYN in the ADD-Vantage™ system is intended as a single dose for intravenous administration after dilution with the ADD-Vantage™ Flexible Diluent Container containing 50 mL, 100 mL or 250 mL of 0.9% Sodium Chloride Injection, USP. UNASYN in the ADD-Vantage™ system is to be reconstituted with 0.9% Sodium Chloride Injection, USP only. See INSTRUCTIONS FOR USE OF THE ADD-Vantage™ VIAL. Reconstitution of UNASYN, at the specified concentration, with 0.9% Sodium Chloride Injection, USP provides stable solutions for the time period indicated below:

Maximum Concentration (mg/mL)

Diluent	UNASYN (Ampicillin/Sulbactam)	Use Period
0.9% Sodium Chloride Injection	30 (20/10)	8 hrs @ 25℃

In 0.9% Sodium Chloride Injection, USP
The final diluted solution of UNASYN should be completely administered *within 8 hours* in order to assure proper potency.

Preparation for Intramuscular Injection
1.5 g and 3.0 g Standard Vials: Vials for intramuscular use may be reconstituted with Sterile Water for Injection USP, 0.5% Lidocaine Hydrochloride Injection USP or 2% Lidocaine Hydrochloride Injection USP. Consult the following table for recommended volumes to be added to obtain solutions containing 375 mg UNASYN per mL (250 mg ampicillin/125 mg sulbactam per mL). Note: *Use only freshly prepared solutions and administer within one hour after preparation.*

UNASYN Vial Size	Volume of Diluent to be Added	Withdrawal Volume*
1.5 g	3.2 mL	4.0 mL
3.0 g	6.4 mL	8.0 mL

*There is sufficient excess present to allow withdrawal and administration of the stated volumes.

Animal Pharmacology: While reversible glycogenosis was observed in laboratory animals, this phenomenon was dose- and time-dependent and is not expected to develop at the therapeutic doses and corresponding plasma levels attained during the relatively short periods of combined ampicillin/sulbactam therapy in man.

HOW SUPPLIED
UNASYN (ampicillin sodium/sulbactam sodium) is supplied as a sterile off-white dry powder in glass vials and piggyback bottles. The following packages are available:
Vials containing 1.5 g (NDC 0049-0013-83) equivalent of UNASYN (1 g ampicillin as the sodium salt plus 0.5 g sulbactam as the sodium salt)
Vials containing 3 g (NDC 0049-0014-83) equivalent of UNASYN (2 g ampicillin as the sodium salt plus 1 g sulbactam as the sodium salt)
Bottles containing 1.5 g (NDC 0049-0022-83) equivalent of UNASYN (1 g ampicillin as the sodium salt plus 0.5 g sulbactam as the sodium salt)
Bottles containing 3 g (NDC 0049-0023-83) equivalent of UNASYN (2 g ampicillin as the sodium salt plus 1 g sulbactam as the sodium salt)
ADD-Vantage™ vials containing 1.5 g (NDC 0049-0031-83) equivalent of UNASYN (1 g ampicillin as the sodium salt plus 0.5 g sulbctam as the sodium salt) are distributed by Pfizer Inc.
The ADD-Vantage™ vials are only to be used with Abbott Laboratories' ADD-Vantage™ Flexible
Diluent Container containing:
0.9% Sodium Chloride Injection, USP, 50 mL, 100 mL, or 250 mL sizes.

INSTRUCTIONS FOR USE OF THE ADD-Vantage™ VIAL
To Open Diluent Container: Peel overwrap from the corner and remove container. Some opacity of the plastic due to moisture absorption during the sterilization process may be observed. This is normal and does not affect the solution quality or safety. The opacity will diminish gradually.
To Assemble Vial and Flexible Diluent Container: (Use Aseptic Technique)
1. Remove the protective covers from the top of the vial and the vial port on the diluent container as follows:
a. To remove the breakaway vial cap, swing the pull ring over the top of the vial and pull down far enough to start the opening (see Figure 1), then pull straight up to remove the cap (see Figure 2).
Note: Do not access vial with syringe.

Fig. 1   **Fig. 2**

b. To remove the vial port cover, grasp the tab on the pull ring, pull up to break the three tie strings, then pull back to remove the cover. (See Figure 3.)
2. Screw the vial into the vial port until it will go no further. THE VIAL MUST BE SCREWED IN TIGHTLY TO ASSURE A SEAL. This occurs approximately ½ turn (180°) after the first audible click. (See Figure 4.) The clicking sound does not assure a seal, the vial must be turned as far as it will go.
Note: Once vial is sealed, do not attempt to remove. (See Figure 4.)
3. Recheck the vial to assure that it is tight by trying to turn it further in the direction of assembly.
4. Label appropriately.

Fig. 3   **Fig. 4**

To Prepare Admixture
1. Squeeze the bottom of the diluent container gently to inflate the portion of the container surrounding the end of the drug vial.
2. With the other hand, push the drug vial down into the container telescoping the walls of the container. Grasp the inner cap of the vial through the walls of the container. (See Figure 5.)
3. Pull the inner cap from the drug vial. (See Figure 6.) Verify that the rubber stopper has been pulled out, allowing the drug and diluent to mix.
4. Mix container contents thoroughly and use within the specified time.

Fig. 5   **Fig. 6**

65-4361-00-5

Maximum Concentration (mg/mL)

Diluent	UNASYN (Ampicillin/Sulbactam)	Use Periods
Sterile Water for Injection	45 (30/15)	8 hrs @ 25℃
	45 (30/15)	48 hrs @ 4℃
	30 (20/10)	72 hrs @ 4℃
0.9% Sodium Chloride Injection	45 (30/15)	8 hrs @ 25℃
	45 (30/15)	48 hrs @ 4℃
	30 (20/10)	72 hrs @ 4℃
5% Dextrose Injection	30 (20/10)	2 hrs @ 25℃
	30 (20/10)	4 hrs @ 4℃
	3 (2/1)	4 hrs @ 25℃
Lactated Ringer's Injection	45 (30/15)	8 hrs @ 25℃
	45 (30/15)	24 hrs @ 4℃
M/6 Sodium Lactate Injection	45 (30/15)	8 hrs @ 25℃
	45 (30/15)	8 hrs @ 4℃
5% Dextrose in 0.45% Saline	3 (2/1)	4 hrs @ 25℃
	15 (10/5)	4 hrs @ 4℃
10% Invert Sugar	3 (2/1)	4 hrs @ 25℃
	30 (20/10)	3 hrs @ 4℃

UROBIOTIC®-250   ℞
[u″rō-bī-ot′ik]

Each capsule contains
Oxytetracycline hydrochloride equivalent to 250 mg. oxytetracycline
Sulfamethizole .... 250 mg.
Phenazopyridine hydrochloride .... 50 mg.

CAPSULES
Inert ingredients in the formulation are: hard gelatin capsules (which may contain Green 3, Yellow 6, Yellow 10 and other inert ingredients); magnesium stearate; sodium lauryl sulfate; starch.

ACTIONS
Urobiotic-250 is a product designed for use specifically in urinary tract infections. Terramycin (oxytetracycline HCl) is a widely used antibiotic with clinically proved activity against gram-positive and gram-negative bacteria, rickettsiae, spirochetes, large viruses, and certain protozoa. Terramycin is well tolerated and well absorbed after oral administration. It diffuses readily through the placenta and is present in the fetal circulation. It diffuses into the pleural fluid, and under some circumstances, into the cerebrospinal fluid. Oxytetracycline HCl appears to be concentrated in the hepatic system and is excreted in the bile. It is excreted in the urine and in the feces, in high concentrations, in a biologically active form.
Sulfamethizole is a chemotherapeutic agent active against a number of important gram-positive and gram-negative bacteria. This sulfonamide is well absorbed, has a low degree of acetylation, and is extremely soluble. Because of these features and its rapid renal excretion, sulfamethizole has a low order of toxicity and provides prompt and high concentrations of the active drug in the urinary tract.
Phenazopyridine is an orally absorbed agent which produces prompt and effective local analgesia and relief of urinary symptoms by virtue of its rapid excretion in the urinary tract. These effects are confined to the genitourinary system and are not accompanied by generalized sedation or narcosis.

Indications
Based on a review of this drug by the National Academy of Sciences-National Research Council and/or other information, FDA has classified the indications as follows:
"Lacking substantial evidence of effectiveness as a fixed combination":
Urobiotic-250 is indicated in the therapy of a number of genitourinary infections caused by susceptible organisms. These infections include the following: pyelonephritis, pyelitis, ureteritis, cystitis, prostatitis, and urethritis.
Since both Terramycin and sulfamethizole provide effective levels in blood, tissue, and urine, Urobiotic-250 provides a multiple antimicrobial approach at the site of infection. Both antibacterial components are active against the most common urinary pathogens, including *Escherichia coli, Pseudomonas aeruginosa, Aerobacter aerogenes, Streptococcus faecalis, Streptococcus hemolyticus, and Micrococcus pyogenes.* Urobiotic-250 is particularly useful in the treatment of infections caused by bacteria more sensitive to the combination than to either component alone. The combination is also of value in those cases with mixed infections, and in those instances where the causative organism is unknown pending laboratory isolation.
Final classification of the less than effective indications require further investigation. Clinical studies to substantiate the efficacy of Urobiotic-250 are ongoing. Completion of these ongoing studies will provide data for final classification of these indications.

CONTRAINDICATIONS
This drug is contraindicated in individuals who have shown hypersensitivity to any of its components.
This drug, because of the sulfonamide component, should not be used in patients with a history of sulfonamide sensitivities, and in pregnant females at term.

WARNINGS
If renal impairment exists, even usual oral or parenteral doses may lead to excessive systemic accumulation of the drug and possible liver toxicity. Under such conditions, lower than usual doses are indicated and if therapy is prolonged, tetracycline serum level determinations may be advisable.
Oxytetracycline HCl, which is one of the ingredients of Urobiotic-250, may form a stable calcium complex in any bone-forming tissue with no serious harmful effects reported thus far in humans. However, use of oxytetracycline during tooth development (last trimester of pregnancy, neonatal

period and early childhood) may cause discoloration of the teeth (yellow-grey-brownish). This effect occurs mostly during long term use of the drug but it also has been observed in usual short treatment courses.

Because of its sulfonamide content, this drug should be used only after critical appraisal in patients with liver damage, renal damage, urinary obstruction, or blood dyscrasias. Deaths have been reported from hypersensitivity reactions, agranulocytosis, aplastic anemia, and other blood dyscrasias associated with sulfonamide administration. When used intermittently, or for a prolonged period, blood counts and liver and kidney function tests should be performed.

Certain hypersensitive individuals may develop a photodynamic reaction precipitated by exposure to direct sunlight during the use of this drug. This reaction is usually of the photoallergic type which may also be produced by other tetracycline derivatives. Individuals with a history of photosensitivity reactions should be instructed to avoid exposure to direct sunlight while under treatment with this or other tetracycline drugs, and treatment should be discontinued at first evidence of skin discomfort.

NOTE: Reactions of a photoallergic nature are exceedingly rare with Terramycin (oxytetracycline HCl). Phototoxic reactions are not believed to occur with Terramycin.

PRECAUTIONS

As with all antibiotic preparations, use of this drug may result in overgrowth of nonsusceptible organisms, including fungi. If superinfection occurs, the antibiotic should be discontinued and appropriate specific therapy should be instituted. This drug should be used with caution in persons having histories of significant allergies and/or asthma.

ADVERSE REACTIONS

Glossitis, stomatitis, proctitis, nausea, diarrhea, vaginitis, and dermatitis, as well as reactions of an allergic nature, may occur during oxytetracycline HCl therapy, but are rare. If adverse reactions, individual idiosyncrasy, or allergy occur, discontinue medication. Rare instances of esophagitis and esophageal ulcerations have been reported in patients receiving capsule forms of drugs in the tetracycline class. Most of these patients took medications immediately before going to bed. (See Dosage and Administration.)

With oxytetracycline therapy bulging fontanels in infants and benign intracranial hypertension in adults have been reported in individuals receiving full therapeutic dosages. These conditions disappeared rapidly when the drug was discontinued.

As in all sulfonamide therapy, the following reactions may occur: nausea, vomiting, diarrhea, hepatitis, pancreatitis, blood dyscrasias, neuropathy, drug fever, skin rash, infection of the conjunctiva and sclera, petechiae, purpura, hematuria and crystalluria. The dosage should be decreased or the drug withdrawn, depending upon the severity of the reaction.

DOSAGE AND ADMINISTRATION

Urobiotic-250 is recommended in adults only. A dose of 1 capsule four times daily is suggested. In refractory cases 2 capsules four times a day may be used.

Therapy should be continued for a minimum of seven days or until bacteriologic cure in acute urinary tract infections.

Administration of adequate amounts of fluid along with capsule forms of drugs in the tetracycline class is recommended to wash down the drugs and reduce the risk of esophageal irritation and ulceration. (See Adverse Reactions.)

To aid absorption of the drug, it should be given at least one hour before or two hours after eating. Aluminum hydroxide gel given with antibiotics has been shown to decrease their absorption and is contraindicated.

SUPPLY

Urobiotic-250 capsules: bottles of 50 (NDC 0049-0920-50), and unit dose packages of 100 (10 × 10's) (NDC 0049-0920-41).

LITERATURE AVAILABLE

Yes.

70-1636-00-9
Shown in Product Identification Section, page 426

VIBRAMYCIN® Hyclate
[vī"bra-mĭ'sin]
(doxycycline hyclate for injection)
INTRAVENOUS
For Intravenous Use Only

℞

DESCRIPTION

Vibramycin (doxycycline hyclate for injection) Intravenous is a broad–spectrum antibiotic synthetically derived from oxytetracycline, and is available as Vibramycin Hyclate (doxycycline hydrochloride hemiethanolate hemihydrate). The chemical designation of this light-yellow crystalline powder is alpha-6-deoxy-5-oxytetracycline. Doxycycline has a high degree of lipoid solubility and a low affinity for calcium binding. It is highly stable in normal human serum.

ACTIONS

Doxycycline is primarily bacteriostatic and thought to exert its antimicrobial effect by the inhibition of protein synthesis. Doxycycline is active against a wide range of gram-positive and gram-negative organisms.

The drugs in the tetracycline class have closely similar antimicrobial spectra, and cross resistance among them is common. Microorganisms may be considered susceptible to doxycycline (likely to respond to doxycycline therapy) if the minimum inhibitory concentration (M.I.C.) is not more than 4.0 mcg/ml. Microorganisms may be considered intermediate (harboring partial resistance) if the M.I.C. is 4.0 to 12.5 mcg/ml and resistant (not likely to respond to therapy) if the M.I.C. is greater than 12.5 mcg/ml.

Susceptibility plate testing: If the Kirby-Bauer method of disc susceptibility testing is used, a 30 mcg doxycycline disc should give a zone of at least 16 mm when tested against a doxycycline-susceptible bacterial strain. A tetracycline disc may be used to determine microbial susceptibility. If the Kirby-Bauer method of disc susceptibility testing is used, a 30 mcg tetracycline disc should give a zone of at least 19 mm when tested against a tetracycline-susceptible bacterial strain.

Tetracyclines are readily absorbed and are bound to plasma proteins in varying degree. They are concentrated by the liver in the bile, and excreted in the urine and feces at high concentrations and in a biologically active form.

Following a single 100 mg dose administered in a concentration of 0.4 mg/ml in a one-hour infusion, normal adult volunteers average a peak of 2.5 mcg/ml, while 200 mg of a concentration of 0.4 mg/ml administered over two hours averaged a peak of 3.6 mcg/ml.

Excretion of doxycycline by the kidney is about 40 percent/72 hours in individuals with normal function (creatinine clearance about 75 ml/min.). This percentage excretion may fall as low as 1-5 percent/72 hours in individuals with severe renal insufficiency (creatinine clearance below 10 ml/min.). Studies have shown no significant difference in serum half-life of doxycycline (range 18-22 hours) in individuals with normal and severely impaired renal function. Hemodialysis does not alter this serum half-life of doxycycline.

INDICATIONS

Doxycycline is indicated in infections caused by the following microorganisms:

Rickettsiae (Rocky Mountain spotted fever, typhus fever, and the typhus group, Q fever, rickettsialpox and tick fevers).
Mycoplasma pneumoniae (PPLO, Eaton Agent).
Agents of psittacosis and ornithosis.
Agents of lymphogranuloma venereum and granuloma inguinale.
The spirochetal agent of relapsing fever (*Borrelia recurrentis*).

The following gram-negative microorganisms:

Haemophilus ducreyi (chancroid),
Pasteurella pestis and *Pasteurella tularensis,*
Bartonella bacilliformis,
Bacteroides species,
Vibrio comma and *Vibrio fetus,*
Brucella species (in conjunction with streptomycin).

Because many strains of the following groups of microorganisms have been shown to be resistant to tetracyclines, culture and susceptibility testing are recommended. Doxycycline is indicated for treatment of infections caused by the following gram-negative microorganisms when bacteriologic testing indicates appropriate susceptibility to the drug:

Escherichia coli,
Enterobacter aerogenes (formerly *Aerobacter aerogenes),*
Shigella species,
Mima species and *Herellea* species,
Haemophilus influenzae (respiratory infections),
Klebsiella species (respiratory and urinary infections).

Doxycycline is indicated for treatment of infections caused by the following gram-positive microorganisms when bacteriologic testing indicates appropriate susceptibility to the drug:

Streptococcus species:

Up to 44 percent of strains of *Streptococcus pyogenes* and 74 percent of *Streptococcus faecalis* have been found to be resistant to tetracycline drugs. Therefore, tetracyclines should not be used for streptococcal disease unless the organism has been demonstrated to be sensitive.

For upper respiratory infections due to group A beta-hemolytic streptococci, penicillin is the usual drug of choice, including prophylaxis of rheumatic fever.

Diplococcus pneumoniae,
Staphylococcus aureus, respiratory, skin and soft tissue infections. Tetracyclines are not the drugs of choice in the treatment of any type of staphylococcal infections.

When penicillin is contraindicated, doxycycline is an alternative drug in the treatment of infections due to:

Neisseria gonorrhoeae and *N. meningitidis,*
Treponema pallidum and *Treponema per tenue* (syphilis and yaws),
Listeria monocytogenes,
Clostridium species,
Bacillus anthracis,
Fusobacterium fusiforme (Vincent's infection),
Actinomyces species.

In acute intestinal amebiasis, doxycycline may be a useful adjunct to amebicides.

Doxycycline is indicated in the treatment of trachoma, although the infectious agent is not always eliminated, as judged by immunofluorescence.

CONTRAINDICATIONS

This drug is contraindicated in persons who have shown hypersensitivity to any of the tetracyclines.

WARNINGS

THE USE OF DRUGS OF THE TETRACYCLINE CLASS DURING TOOTH DEVELOPMENT (LAST HALF OF PREGNANCY, INFANCY AND CHILDHOOD TO THE AGE OF 8 YEARS) MAY CAUSE PERMANENT DISCOLORATION OF THE TEETH (YELLOW-GRAY-BROWN). This adverse reaction is more common during long-term use of the drugs but has been observed following repeated short-term courses. Enamel hypoplasia has also been reported. *TETRACYCLINE DRUGS, THEREFORE, SHOULD NOT BE USED IN THIS AGE GROUP UNLESS OTHER DRUGS ARE NOT LIKELY TO BE EFFECTIVE OR ARE CONTRAINDICATED.*

Photosensitivity manifested by an exaggerated sunburn reaction has been observed in some individuals taking tetracyclines. Patients apt to be exposed to direct sunlight or ultraviolet light should be advised that this reaction can occur with tetracycline drugs, and treatment should be discontinued at the first evidence of skin erythema.

The antianabolic action of the tetracyclines may cause an increase in BUN. Studies to date indicate that this does not occur with the use of doxycycline in patients with impaired renal function.

Usage in Pregnancy

(See above "Warnings" about use during tooth development.) Vibramycin Intravenous has not been studied in pregnant patients. It should not be used in pregnant women unless, in the judgment of the physician, it is essential for the welfare of the patient.

Results of animal studies indicate that tetracyclines cross the placenta, are found in fetal tissues and can have toxic effects on the developing fetus (often related to retardation of skeletal development). Evidence of embryotoxicity has also been noted in animals treated early in pregnancy.

Usage in Children

The use of Vibramycin Intravenous in children under 8 years is not recommended because safe conditions for its use have not been established.

(See above "Warnings" about use during tooth development.) As with other tetracyclines, doxycycline forms a stable calcium complex in any bone-forming tissue. A decrease in the fibula growth rate has been observed in prematures given oral tetracycline in doses of 25 mg/kg every 6 hours. This reaction was shown to be reversible when the drug was discontinued.

Tetracyclines are present in the milk of lactating women who are taking a drug in this class.

PRECAUTIONS

As with other antibiotic preparations, use of this drug may result in overgrowth of nonsusceptible organisms, including fungi. If superinfection occurs, the antibiotic should be discontinued and appropriate therapy instituted.

In venereal diseases when coexistent syphilis is suspected, a dark field examination should be done before treatment is started and the blood serology repeated monthly for at least 4 months.

Because tetracyclines have been shown to depress plasma prothrombin activity, patients who are on anticoagulant therapy may require downward adjustment of their anticoagulant dosage.

In long-term therapy, periodic laboratory evaluation of organ systems, including hematopoietic, renal, and hepatic studies should be performed.

All infections due to group A beta-hemolytic streptococci should be treated for at least 10 days.

Since bacteriostatic drugs may interfere with the bactericidal action of penicillin, it is advisable to avoid giving tetracycline in conjunction with penicillin.

ADVERSE REACTIONS

Gastrointestinal: anorexia, nausea, vomiting, diarrhea, glossitis, dysphagia, enterocolitis, and inflammatory lesions (with monilial overgrowth) in the anogenital region. These reactions have been caused by both the oral and parenteral administration of tetracyclines.

Continued on next page

Roerig—Cont.

Skin: maculopapular and erythematous rashes. Exfoliative dermatitis has been reported but is uncommon. Photosensitivity is discussed above. (See "Warnings.")

Renal toxicity: Rise in BUN has been reported and is apparently dose related. (See "Warnings.")

Hypersensitivity reactions: urticaria, angioneurotic edema, anaphylaxis, anaphylactoid purpura, pericarditis and exacerbation of systemic lupus erythematosus.

Bulging fontanels in infants and benign intracranial hypertension in adults have been reported in individuals receiving full therapeutic dosages. These conditions disappeared rapidly when the drug was discontinued.

Blood: Hemolytic anemia, thrombocytopenia, neutropenia and eosinophilia have been reported.

When given over prolonged periods, tetracyclines have been reported to produce brown-black microscopic discoloration of thyroid glands. No abnormalities of thyroid function studies are known to occur.

DOSAGE AND ADMINISTRATION

Note: Rapid administration is to be avoided. Parenteral therapy is indicated only when oral therapy is not indicated. Oral therapy should be instituted as soon as possible. If intravenous therapy is given over prolonged periods of time, thrombophlebitis may result.

THE USUAL DOSAGE AND FREQUENCY OF ADMINISTRATION OF VIBRAMYCIN I.V. (100-200 MG/DAY) DIFFERS FROM THAT OF THE OTHER TETRACYCLINES (1-2 G/DAY). EXCEEDING THE RECOMMENDED DOSAGE MAY RESULT IN AN INCREASED INCIDENCE OF SIDE EFFECTS.

Studies to date have indicated that Vibramycin at the usual recommended doses does not lead to excessive accumulation of the antibiotic in patients with renal impairment.

Adults: The usual dosage of Vibramycin I.V. is 200 mg on the first day of treatment administered in one or two infusions. Subsequent daily dosage is 100 to 200 mg depending upon the severity of infection, with 200 mg administered in one or two infusions.

In the treatment of primary and secondary syphilis, the recommended dosage is 300 mg daily for at least 10 days. For children above eight years of age: The recommended dosage schedule for children weighing 100 pounds or less is 2 mg/lb. of body weight on the first day of treatment, administered in one or two infusions. Subsequent daily dosage is 1 to 2 mg/lb. of body weight given as one or two infusions, depending on the severity of the infection. For children over 100 pounds the usual adult dose should be used. (See "Warning" Section for Usage in Children.)

General: The duration of infusion may vary with the dose (100 to 200 mg per day), but is usually one to four hours. A recommended minimum infusion time for 100 mg of a 0.5 mg/ml solution is one hour. Therapy should be continued for at least 24-48 hours after symptoms and fever have subsided. The therapeutic antibacterial serum activity will usually persist for 24 hours following recommended dosage.

Intravenous solutions should not be injected intramuscularly or subcutaneously. Caution should be taken to avoid the inadvertent introduction of the intravenous solution into the adjacent soft tissue.

PREPARATION OF SOLUTION

To prepare a solution containing 10 mg/ml, the contents of the vial should be reconstituted with 10 ml (for the 100 mg/vial container) or 20 ml (for the 200 mg/vial container) of Sterile Water for Injection or any of the ten intravenous infusion solutions listed below. Each 100 mg of Vibramycin (i.e., withdraw entire solution from the 100 mg vial) is further diluted with 100 ml to 1000 ml of the intravenous solutions listed below. Each 200 mg of Vibramycin (i.e., withdraw entire solution from the 200 mg vial) is further diluted with 200 ml to 2000 ml of the following intravenous solutions:

1. Sodium Chloride Injection, USP
2. 5% Dextrose Injection, USP
3. Ringer's Injection, USP
4. Invert Sugar, 10% in Water
5. Lactated Ringer's Injection, USP
6. Dextrose 5% in Lactated Ringer's
7. Normosol-M® in D5-W (Abbott)
8. Normosol-R® in D5-W (Abbott)
9. Plasma-Lyte® 56 in 5% Dextrose (Travenol)
10. Plasma-Lyte® 148 in 5% Dextrose (Travenol)

This will result in desired concentrations of 0.1 to 1.0 mg/ml. Concentrations lower than 0.1 mg/ml or higher than 1.0 mg/ml are not recommended.

Stability:

Vibramycin IV is stable for 48 hours in solution when diluted with Sodium Chloride Injection, USP, or 5% Dextrose Injection, USP, to concentrations between 1.0 mg/ml and 0.1

mg/ml and stored at 25°C. Vibramycin IV in these solutions is stable under fluorescent light for 48 hours, but must be protected from direct sunlight during storage and infusion. Reconstituted solutions (1.0 to 0.1 mg/ml) may be stored up to 72 hours prior to start of infusion if refrigerated and protected from sunlight and artificial light. Infusion must then be completed within 12 hours. Solutions must be used within these time periods or discarded.

Vibramycin IV, when diluted with Ringer's Injection, USP, or Invert Sugar, 10% in Water, or Normosol-M® in D5-W (Abbott), or Normosol-R® in D5-W (Abbott), or Plasma-Lyte® 56 in 5% Dextrose (Travenol), or Plasma-Lyte® 148 in 5% Dextrose (Travenol) to a concentration between 1.0 mg/ml and 0.1 mg/ml, must be completely infused within 12 hours after reconstitution to ensure adequate stability. During infusion, the solution must be protected from direct sunlight. Reconstituted solutions (1.0 to 0.1 mg/ml) may be stored up to 72 hours prior to start of infusion if refrigerated and protected from sunlight and artifical light. Infusion must then be completed within 12 hours. Solutions must be used within these time periods or discarded.

When diluted with Lactated Ringer's Injection, USP, or Dextrose 5% in Lactated Ringer's, infusion of the solution (ca. 1.0 mg/ml) or lower concentrations (not less than 0.1 mg/ml) must be completed within six hours after reconstitution to ensure adequate stability. During infusion, the solution must be protected from direct sunlight. Solutions must be used within this time period or discarded.

Solutions of Vibramycin (doxycycline hyclate for injection) at a concentration of 10 mg/ml in Sterile Water for Injection, when frozen immediately after reconstitution are stable for 8 weeks when stored at −20°C. If the product is warmed, care should be taken to avoid heating it after the thawing is complete. Once thawed the solution should not be refrozen.

HOW SUPPLIED

Vibramycin (doxycycline hyclate for injection) Intravenous is available as a sterile powder in a vial containing doxycycline hyclate equivalent to 100 mg of doxycycline with 480 mg of ascorbic acid, packages of 5 (NDC 0049-0960-77); and in individually packaged vials containing doxycycline hyclate equivalent to 200 mg of doxycycline with 960 mg of ascorbic acid (NDC 0049-0980-81).

65-1940-00-0

LITERATURE AVAILABLE

Yes.

VISTARIL®   ℞
(hydroxyzine hydrochloride)
Intramuscular Solution
For Intramuscular Use Only

CHEMISTRY

Hydroxyzine hydrochloride is designated chemically as 1-(p-chlorobenzhydryl) 4-[2-(2-hydroxyethoxy) ethyl] piperazine dihydrochloride.

ACTIONS

VISTARIL (hydroxyzine hydrochloride) is unrelated chemically to phenothiazine, reserpine, and meprobamate. Hydroxyzine has demonstrated its clinical effectiveness in the chemotherapeutic aspect of the total management of neuroses and emotional disturbances manifested by anxiety, tension, agitation, apprehension or confusion.

Hydroxyzine has been shown clinically to be a rapid-acting true ataraxic with a wide margin of safety. It induces a calming effect in anxious, tense, psychoneurotic adults and also in anxious, hyperkinetic children without impairing mental alertness. It is not a cortical depressant, but its action may be due to a suppression of activity in certain key regions of the subcortical area of the central nervous system.

Primary skeletal muscle relaxation has been demonstrated experimentally.

Hydroxyzine has been shown experimentally to have antispasmodic properties, apparently mediated through interference with the mechanism that reponds to spasmogenic agents such as serotonin, acetylcholine, and histamine.

Antihistaminic effects have been demonstrated experimentally and confirmed clinically.

An antiemetic effect, both by the apomorphine test and the veriloid test, has been demonstrated. Pharmacological and clinical studies indicate that hydroxyzine in therapeutic dosage does not increase gastric secretion or acidity and in most cases provides mild antisecretory benefits.

INDICATIONS

The total management of anxiety, tension, and psychomotor agitation in conditions of emotional stress requires in most instances a combined approach of psychotherapy and chemotherapy. Hydroxyzine has been found to be particularly useful for this latter phase of therapy in its ability to render the disturbed patient more amenable to psychotherapy in long term treatment of the psychoneurotic and psychotic, al-

though it should not be used as the sole treatment of psychosis or of clearly demonstrated cases of depression.

Hydroxyzine is also useful in alleviating the manifestations of anxiety and tension as in the preparation for dental procedures and in acute emotional problems. It has also been recommended for the management of anxiety associated with organic disturbances and as adjunctive therapy in alcoholism and allergic conditions with strong emotional overlay, such as in asthma, chronic urticaria, and pruritus.

VISTARIL (hydroxyzine hydrochloride) Intramuscular Solution is useful in treating the following types of patients when intramuscular administration is indicated:

1. The acutely disturbed or hysterical patient.
2. The acute or chronic alcoholic with anxiety withdrawal symptoms or delirium tremens.
3. As pre- and postoperative and pre- and postpartum adjunctive medication to permit reduction in narcotic dosage, allay anxiety and control emesis.

VISTARIL (hydroxyzine hydrochloride) has also demonstrated effectiveness in controlling nausea and vomiting, excluding nausea and vomiting of pregnancy. (See Contraindications.)

In prepartum states, the reduction in narcotic requirement effected by hydroxyzine is of particular benefit to both mother and neonate.

Hydroxyzine benefits the cardiac patient by its ability to allay the associated anxiety and apprehension attendant to certain types of heart disease. Hydroxyzine is not known to interfere with the action of digitalis in any way and may be used concurrently with this agent.

The effectiveness of hydroxyzine in long term use, that is, more than 4 months, has not been assessed by systematic clinical studies. The physician should reassess periodically the usefulness of the drug for the individual patient.

CONTRAINDICATIONS

Hydroxyzine hydrochloride intramuscular solution is intended only for intramuscular administration and should not, under any circumstances, be injected subcutaneously, intra-arterially, or intravenously.

This drug is contraindicated for patients who have shown a previous hypersensitivity to it.

Hydroxyzine, when administered to the pregnant mouse, rat, and rabbit, induced fetal abnormalities in the rat at doses substantially above the human therapeutic range. Clinical data in human beings are inadequate to establish safety in early pregnancy. Until such data are available, hydroxyzine is contraindicated in early pregnancy.

PRECAUTIONS

THE POTENTIATING ACTION OF HYDROXYZINE MUST BE CONSIDERED WHEN THE DRUG IS USED IN CONJUNCTION WITH CENTRAL NERVOUS SYSTEM DEPRESSANTS SUCH AS NARCOTICS, BARBITURATES, AND ALCOHOL. Therefore when central nervous system depressants are administered concomitantly with hydroxyzine their dosage should be reduced up to 50 per cent. The efficacy of hydroxyzine as adjunctive pre- and postoperative sedative medication has also been well established, especially as regards its ability to allay anxiety, control emesis, and reduce the amount of narcotic required.

HYDROXYZINE MAY POTENTIATE NARCOTICS AND BARBITURATES, so their use in preanesthetic adjunctive therapy should be modified on an individual basis. Atropine and other belladonna alkaloids are not affected by the drug. When hydroxyzine is used preoperatively or prepartum, narcotic requirements may be reduced as much as 50 per cent. Thus, when 50 mg of VISTARIL (hydroxyzine hydrochloride) Intramuscular Solution is employed, meperidine dosage may be reduced from 100 mg to 50 mg. The administration of meperidine may result in severe hypotension in the postoperative patient or any individual whose ability to maintain blood pressure has been compromised by a depleted blood volume. Meperidine should be used with great caution and in reduced dosage in patients who are receiving other pre- and/or postoperative medications and in whom there is a risk of respiratory depression, hypotension, and profound sedation or coma occurring. Before using any medications concomitant with hydroxyzine, the manufacturer's prescribing information should be read carefully.

Since drowsiness may occur with the use of this drug, patients should be warned of this possibility and cautioned against driving a car or operating dangerous machinery while taking this drug.

As with all intramuscular preparations, VISTARIL Intramuscular Solution should be injected well within the body of a relatively large muscle. Inadvertent subcutaneous injection may result in significant tissue damage.

ADULTS: The preferred site is the upper outer quadrant of the buttock, (i.e., gluteus maximus), or the mid-lateral thigh.

CHILDREN: It is recommended that intramuscular injections be given preferably in the mid-lateral muscles of the thigh. In infants and small children the periphery of the upper outer quadrant of the gluteal region should be used only when necessary, such as in burn patients, in order to minimize the possibility of damage to the sciatic nerve.

The deltoid area should be used only if well developed such as in certain adults and older children, and then only with caution to avoid radial nerve injury. Intramuscular injections should not be made into the lower and mid-third of the upper arm. As with all intramuscular injections, aspiration is necessary to help avoid inadvertent injection into a blood vessel.

ADVERSE REACTIONS

Therapeutic doses of hydroxyzine seldom produce impairment of mental alertness. However, drowsiness may occur; if so, it is usually transitory and may disappear in a few days of continued therapy or upon reduction of the dose. Dryness of the mouth may be encountered at higher doses. Extensive clinical use has substantiated the absence of toxic effects on the liver or bone marrow when administered in the recommended doses for over four years of uninterrupted therapy. The absence of adverse effects has been further demonstrated in experimental studies in which excessively high doses were administered.

Involuntary motor activity, including rare instances of tremor and convulsions, has been reported, usually with doses considerably higher than those recommended. Continuous therapy with over one gram per day has been employed in some patients without these effects having been encountered.

DOSAGE AND ADMINISTRATION

The recommended dosages for VISTARIL (hydroxyzine hydrochloride) Intramuscular Solution are:

For adult psychiatric and emotional emergencies, including acute alcoholism.	I.M.: 50–100 mg stat., and q. 4–6h., p.r.n.
Nausea and vomiting excluding nausea and vomiting of pregnancy.	Adults: 25–100 mg I.M. Children: 0.5 mg/lb. body weight I.M.
Pre- and postoperative adjunctive medication.	Adults: 25–100 mg I.M. Children: 0.5 mg/lb. body weight I.M.
Pre- and postpartum adjunctive therapy.	25–100 mg I.M.

As with all potent medications, the dosage should be adjusted according to the patient's response to therapy.

FOR ADDITIONAL INFORMATION ON THE ADMINISTRATION AND SITE OF SELECTION SEE PRECAUTIONS SECTION. NOTE: VISTARIL (hydroxyzine hydrochloride) Intramuscular Solution may be administered without further dilution.

Patients may be started on intramuscular therapy when indicated. They should be maintained on oral therapy whenever this route is practicable.

SUPPLY

VISTARIL (hydroxyzine hydrochloride) Intramuscular Solution

Multi-Dose Vials

25 mg/ml; 10 ml vials (NDC 0049-5450-74)

50 mg/ml; 10 ml vials (NDC 0049-5460-74)

Unit Dose Vials

50 mg/ml–1 ml fill; packages of 25 vials (NDC 0049-5462-76)

100 mg/2 ml–2 ml fill; packages of 25 vials (NDC 0049-5460-76)

FORMULA

Dosage Strength	25 mg/1 ml	50 mg/1 ml 100 mg/2 ml
Hydroxyzine hydrochloride	25 mg/ml	50 mg/ml
Benzyl Alcohol	0.9%	50 mg/ml
Sodium hydroxide	to adjust to optimum pH	

BIBLIOGRAPHY

Available upon request.

70-0843-00-4

ROERIG EDUCATIONAL MATERIALS

Printed Material

1. *Comprehensive Product Information* (Glucotrol)—a 50-page Roerig publication describing the chemistry, pharmacokinetics, pharmacology, clinical experience, and other important information about Glucotrol. Free to physicians.
2. *Glipizide: A Worldwide Review*—a 300-page monograph published by Excerpta Medica. Covers Glucotrol's pathology and physiology, clinical pharmacology, and clinical experience. Free to physicians.
3. *The Efficacy and Safety of Cefoperazone—A Two-Year Review*—Proceedings of a symposium reviewing two years of clinical and safety data associated with the use of cefoperazone. Free to physicians.
4. *Product Reference Monograph* (Unasyn)—A comprehensive product publication detailing the pharmacokinetics,

microbiological spectrum, clinical efficacy, and safety parameters of Unasyn. Free to physicians.

5. *The Cost of Antibiotic Therapy*—Results of a multicenter trial examining the cost components of antibiotic therapy and the impact different regimens have on length of therapy and length of hospital stay. Free to physicians and pharmacists.
6. *Discussion on Depression: Patient Perspectives*—a 14-page patient information booklet for people suffering from depression. Free to physicians and their patients.
7. *Psychiatric Reference Book*—a 123-page pocket-sized reference publication published for Roerig by C. Medica Inc. Edited by Marvin Stern, MD, this book is designed to help with the diagnosis and management of commonly encountered psychiatric disorders. Free to physicians.
8. *Patient/Family Educational Booklets on Schizophrenia and Organic Mental Disorders*—These 20-page booklets are provided free to mental health professionals for their use in consultation with their patients and/or family members.
9. *Roerig Pharmacy Management Series*—Practical tips on pharmacy management. Free to pharmacists.

Films

1. "New Perspectives in NIDDM"—30-minute film. Covers NIDDM, effect of sulfonylureas, especially 2nd-generation and glipizide. Narrated by Drs. Lebovitz and Reaven. A 7-minute edited version is also available.
2. "Risk Factors in Non-Insulin-Dependent Diabetes Mellitus"—21-minute color film. Reviews lipid metabolism, the lipid abnormalities found in the Type II diabetic patient, and the associated atherosclerotic complications. Clinical research on lipid metabolism that demonstrates the effect of GLUCOTROL (glipizide) is presented. Narrated by Drs. Castelli, Krall, and Reaven.
3. "Complications: A Diabetic's Future?"—This 20-minute film discusses the serious nature of Type II diabetes in terms of its resultant complications. Key diabetologists across the country discuss specific complications and the need to control blood sugar.
4. "You're In Control: Managing Your Diabetes"—This 11-minute videotape is available to physicians for patient education.
5. "Organ Transplantation: A Miracle Kept Waiting"—a 30-minute film describing transplantation of the heart and lung, liver transplantation, and surgical construction of a bladder for a patient faced with a lifetime of incontinence. Narrated by Drs. Cooley, Starzl, and Olsson.
6. "Update: The Management of Surgical Infection in the 1980s."—A discussion of factors contributing to infection following surgery and approaches to its management. Narrated by Harlan Stone, MD. 20 Minutes.
7. "In the Absence of Angels—A Report on the Homeless Mentally Ill"—28-minute film. Explores the plight of the homeless mentally ill in major urban centers of the U.S., and shows how community groups and mental health centers are attempting to cope with the problem. Participants are Drs. Lamb, Mills, Pepper, Stein, and Talbott.
8. "Ward 5C-4: The Prediction and Management of Violence in the Schizophrenic Patient"—22-minute film. Illustrates how violent and abusive schizophrenic patients can be maintained in a nonthreatening and supportive environment with therapeutic treatment. Narrated by Jerome Yesavage, MD.
9. "Dynamic Brain Mapping (The Psychiatric Electroencephalogram)"—13 minute film. Computerized electroencephalogram (CEEG) technology is demonstrated as a measurement of brain wave activity and as a potential means by which to further the understanding of drug actions of brain waves. Narrated by Turan Itil, MD.
10. The Negative Symptoms of Schizophrenia—Examines recent advances in the assessment, differential diagnosis, treatment, and etiology of the negative symptoms of schizophrenia. Participants are: Drs. Andreasen, Carpenter, Crow, Lewine, Stein, Weinberger, and Yesavage.
11. Displaced Americans—Poignant portrayal of clinical depression among farmers in Hills, Iowa and workers in Gary, Indiana who are confronted with radical changes in lifestyles as a result of economic and social disruption. Narrated by Drs. Schatzberg, Winokur, and Kidd.

Computer Programs (IBM Compatible)

1. "Diabetes Discovery"

Interactive Videodiscs

1. "Nephrostolithotomy—The Percutaneous Route" Free to physicians.
2. "Urodynamics in Clinical Practice" Free to physicians.
3. "Challenges in Urology". Free to physicians.

Audiotapes

1. "Diabetes Digest"
2. "Dialogues in Urology." Free to physicians.

Samples

Antivert (meclizine HCl) Tablets—25 mg

Atarax (hydroxyzine HCl) Tablets—10 mg, 25 mg

Atarax Syrup

Geocillin (carbenicillin indanyl sodium) Tablets (equivalent to 382 mg carbenicillin)

Glucotrol (glipizide) Tablets—5 mg

Navane (thiothixene) Capsules—2 mg, 5 mg, 10 mg

Sinequan (doxepin HCl) Capsules—25 mg, 50 mg, 75 mg

Rorer Consumer Pharmaceuticals
a division of
Rorer Pharmaceutical Corporation
500 VIRGINIA DRIVE
FORT WASHINGTON, PA 19034

Regular Strength
ASCRIPTIN® Tablets

(See PDR For Nonprescription Drugs)

ASCRIPTIN® A/D Caplets

(See PDR For Nonprescription Drugs)

Extra Strength
ASCRIPTIN® Caplets

(See PDR For Nonprescription Drugs)

CAMALOX® Suspension and Tablets

(See PDR For Nonprescription Drugs)

MAALOX® Suspension and Tablets

(See PDR For Nonprescription Drugs)

Extra Strength
MAALOX® Tablets

(See PDR For Nonprescription Drugs)

Extra Strength
MAALOX® PLUS Suspension

(See PDR For Nonprescription Drugs)

MAALOX® PLUS Tablets

(See PDR For Nonprescription Drugs)

Extra Strength
MAALOX® PLUS Tablets
(reformulated Extra Strength Maalox Tablets)

(See PDR For Nonprescription Drugs)

Extra Strength
MAALOX® WHIP™

(See PDR For Nonprescription Drugs)

MAALOX® TC Suspension and Tablets

(See PDR For Nonprescription Drugs)

MYOFLEX® Analgesic Creme

(See PDR For Nonprescription Drugs)

PERDIEM® Granules

(See PDR For Nonprescription Drugs)

PERDIEM® FIBER Granules

(See PDR For Nonprescription Drugs)

Continued on next page

Rorer Pharmaceuticals
a division of
Rorer Pharmaceutical Corporation
500 VIRGINIA DRIVE
FORT WASHINGTON, PA 19034

H.P. ACTHAR® GEL* ℞
[ăch pē ăk'thär jĕl]
(repository corticotropin injection)
and
ACTHAR® ℞
(corticotropin for injection)

DESCRIPTION

H.P. ACTHAR® GEL (Repository Corticotropin Injection) is a highly purified sterile preparation of the adrenocorticotropic hormone in 16% gelatin to provide a prolonged release after intramuscular or subcutaneous injection. Also contains 0.5% phenol, not more than 0.1% cysteine (added), sodium hydroxide and/or acetic acid to adjust pH, and water for injection, q.s.

ACTHAR® (Corticotropin for Injection) is a sterile lyophilized ACTH which in dry form is stable at room temperature. Each vial contains 25 or 40 Units of Corticotropin U.S.P. and approximately 9 and 14 milligrams of hydrolyzed gelatin respectively. After reconstitution, this product is administered in the intravenous, intramuscular, or subcutaneous route.

ACTH is a 39 amino acid peptide with the following chemical formula:

H-Ser-Tyr-Ser-Met-Glu-His-Phe-Arg-Trp-
1 2 3 4 5 6 7 8 9
Gly-Lys-Pro-Val-Gly-Lys-Lys-Arg-Arg-Pro-
10 11 12 13 14 15 16 17 18 19
NH_2
Val-Lys-Val-Try-Pro-Asp-Gly-Ala-Glu-Asp-
20 21 22 23 24 25 26 27 28 29
Glu-Leu-Ala-Glu-Ala-Phe-Pro-Leu-Glu-
30 31 32 33 34 35 36 37 38
Phe-OH
39

CLINICAL PHARMACOLOGY

ACTH stimulates the adrenal cortex to secrete cortisol, corticosterone, aldosterone, and a number of weakly androgenic substances. Although ACTH does stimulate secretion of aldosterone, the rate is relatively independent. Prolonged administration of large doses of ACTH induces hyperplasia and hypertrophy of the adrenal cortex and continuous high output of cortisol, corticosterone, and weak androgens. The release of ACTH is under the influence of the nervous system via the corticotropin regulatory hormone released from the hypothalamus and by a negative corticosteroid feedback mechanism. Elevated plasma cortisol suppresses ACTH release.

The trophic effects of ACTH on the adrenal cortex are not understood beyond the fact that they appear to be mediated by cyclic AMP.

ACTH rapidly disappears from the circulation following its intravenous administration; in man the plasma half-life is about 15 minutes.

The maximal effects of a trophic hormone on a target organ are achieved when optimal amounts of hormone are acting continuously. Thus, a fixed dose of ACTH will demonstrate a linear increase in adrenocortical secretion with increasing duration of the infusion.

INDICATIONS AND USAGE

ACTHAR (Corticotropin for Injection) and H.P. ACTHAR GEL (Repository Corticotropin Injection) are indicated for diagnostic testing of adrenocortical function.

ACTHAR (Corticotropin for Injection) and H.P. ACTHAR GEL (Repository Corticotropin Injection) have limited therapeutic value in those conditions responsive to corticosteroid therapy; in such cases, corticosteroid therapy is considered to be the treatment of choice. ACTHAR (Corticotropin for Injection) and H.P. ACTHAR GEL (Repository Corticotropin Injection) may be employed in the following disorders:

ENDOCRINE DISORDERS: Nonsuppurative thyroiditis; Hypercalcemia associated with cancer.

NERVOUS SYSTEM DISEASES: Acute exacerbations of multiple sclerosis.

RHEUMATIC DISORDERS: As adjunctive therapy for short-term administration (to tide the patient over an acute episode or exacerbation) in:

Psoriatic arthritis; Rheumatoid arthritis, including juvenile rheumatoid arthritis (selected cases may require low-dose maintenance therapy); Ankylosing spondylitis; Acute and subacute bursitis; Acute nonspecific tenosynovitis; Acute gouty arthritis; Post-traumatic arthritis; Synovitis of osteoarthritis; Epicondylitis.

COLLAGEN DISEASES: During an exacerbation or as maintenance therapy in selected cases of:

Systemic lupus erythematosus; Systemic dermatomyositis (polymyositis); Acute rheumatic carditis.

DERMATOLOGIC DISEASES: Pemphigus; Bullous dermatitis herpetiformis; Severe erythema multiforme (Stevens-Johnson syndrome); Exfoliative dermatitis; Severe psoriasis; Severe seborrheic dermatitis; Mycosis fungoides.

ALLERGIC STATES: Control of severe or incapacitating allergic conditions intractable to adequate trials of conventional treatment:

Seasonal or perennial allergic rhinitis; Bronchial asthma; Contact dermatitis; Atopic dermatitis; Serum sickness.

OPHTHALMIC DISEASES: Severe acute and chronic allergic and inflammatory processes involving the eye and its adnexa such as:

Allergic conjunctivitis; Keratitis; Herpes zoster ophthalmicus; Iritis and iridocyclitis; Diffuse posterior uveitis and choroiditis; Optic neuritis; Sympathetic ophthalmia; Chorioretinitis; Anterior segment inflammation; Allergic corneal marginal ulcers.

RESPIRATORY DISEASES: Symptomatic sarcoidosis; Loeffler's syndrome not manageable by other means; Berylliosis; Fulminating or disseminated pulmonary tuberculosis when used concurrently with antituberculous chemotherapy; Aspiration pneumonitis.

HEMATOLOGIC DISORDERS: Acquired (autoimmune) hemolytic anemia; Secondary thrombocytopenia in adults; Erythroblastopenia (RBC anemia); Congenital (erythroid) hypoplastic anemia.

NEOPLASTIC DISEASES: For palliative management of: Leukemias and lymphomas in adults; Acute leukemia of childhood.

EDEMATOUS STATE: To induce a diuresis or a remission of proteinuria in the nephrotic syndrome without uremia of the idiopathic type or that due to lupus erythematosus.

GASTROINTESTINAL DISEASES: To tide the patient over a critical period of the disease in: Ulcerative colitis; Regional enteritis.

MISCELLANEOUS: Tuberculous meningitis with subarachnoid block or impending block when used concurrently with appropriate anti-tuberculous chemotherapy; Trichinosis with neurologic or myocardial involvement.

CONTRAINDICATIONS

Corticotropin is contraindicated in patients with scleroderma, osteoporosis, systemic fungal infections, ocular herpes simplex, recent surgery, history of or the presence of a peptic ulcer, congestive heart failure, hypertension, or sensitivity to proteins of porcine origin.

Treatment of conditions listed within the INDICATIONS section (see above) is contraindicated when they are accompanied by primary adrenocortical insufficiency or adrenocortical hyperfunction.

Intravenous administration of corticotropin is contraindicated for treatment of conditions listed within the indications section, but Acthar is used intravenously for diagnostic purposes (see DOSAGE AND ADMINISTRATION).

WARNINGS

Chronic administration of corticotropin may lead to adverse effects which are not reversible. Corticotropin may only suppress symptoms and signs of chronic diseases without altering the natural course of the disease. Neither H.P. ACTHAR GEL (Repository Corticotropin Injection) nor ACTHAR (Corticotropin for Injection) should be administered for treatment until adrenal responsiveness has been verified with the route of administration which will be utilized during treatment, intramuscularly or subcutaneously. A rise in urinary and plasma corticosteroid values provides direct evidence of a stimulatory effect. Prolonged administration of corticotropin increases the risk of hypersensitivity reactions. Although the action of corticotropin is similar to that of exogenous adrenocortical steroids the quantity of adrenocorticoid may be variable. In patients who receive prolonged corticotropin therapy the additional use of rapidly acting corticosteroids before, during, and after an unusual stressful situation is indicated.

Prolonged use of corticotropin may produce posterior subcapsular cataracts and glaucoma with possible damage to the optic nerves.

Corticotropin may mask some signs of infection, and new infections including those of the eye due to fungi or viruses may appear during its use. There may be decreased resistance and inability to localize infection when corticotropin is used.

Corticotropin can cause elevation of blood pressure, salt and water retention, and increased excretion of potassium. Dietary salt restriction and potassium supplementation may be necessary. Corticotropin increases calcium excretion.

While on corticotropin therapy, patients should not be vaccinated against smallpox. Other immunization procedures should be undertaken with caution in patients who are receiving corticotropin, especially when high doses are administered because of the possible hazards of neurological complications and lack of antibody response.

PRECAUTIONS

1. General

Corticotropin injection should be used in the lowest dose for the shortest period of time to accomplish the therapeutic goal. Corticotropin should be used for treatment only when the disease is intractable to non-steroid treatment. There is an enhanced effect in patients with hypothyroidism and in those with cirrhosis of the liver. Sensitivity to porcine protein should be considered before starting therapy and during the course of treatment should symptoms arise.

When an infection is present, appropriate antibiotic therapy should be given. Patients with latent tuberculosis should be observed closely and if therapy is prolonged, chemoprophylaxis should be instituted.

Psychic symptoms may appear with use of corticotropin or pre-existing symptoms may be enhanced. These may range from mood alteration to a psychotic state.

Patients with a secondary disease may have that disease worsened. Caution should be used when prescribing corticotropin in patients with diabetes, renal insufficiency, diverticulitis, and myasthenia gravis.

Corticotropin often acts by suppressing symptoms without altering the course of the underlying disease. Since complications with corticotropin use are dependent on the dose and duration of treatment, a risk/benefit decision must be made in each case.

Suppression of the pituitary adrenal axis occurs following prolonged therapy which may be slow in returning to normal. Patients should be protected from the stress of trauma or surgery by the use of corticosteroids during the period of stress.

Since maximal corticotropin stimulation of the adrenals may be limited during the first few days of treatment, other drugs should be administered when an immediate therapeutic effect is desirable.

Although controlled clinical trials have shown ACTH to be effective in speeding the resolution of acute exacerbations of multiple sclerosis they do not show that it affects the ultimate outcome or natural history of the disease. The studies do show that relatively high doses of ACTH are necessary to demonstrate a significant effect. (See DOSAGE AND ADMINISTRATION section.)

Treatment of acute gouty arthritis should be limited to a few days. Since rebound attacks may occur when corticotropin is discontinued, conventional concomitant therapy should be administered during corticotropin treatment and for several days after it is stopped.

Aspirin should be used cautiously in conjunction with corticotropin in hypoprothrombinemia.

2. Drug Interactions

Corticotropin may accentuate the electrolyte loss associated with diuretic therapy.

3. Carcinogenesis, Mutagenesis, Impairment of Fertility

Adequate and well-controlled studies have not been done in animals. Human use has not been associated with an increase in malignant disease. See Pregnancy warning below.

4. Pregnancy

Pregnancy Class C. Corticotropin has been shown to have an embryocidal effect. There are no adequate and well-controlled studies in pregnant women. Corticotropin should be used during pregnancy only if the potential benefit justifies the potential risk to the fetus.

5. Nursing Mothers

It is not known whether this drug is excreted in human milk. Because many drugs are excreted in human milk and because of the potential for serious adverse reactions in nursing infants from corticotropin, a decision should be made whether to discontinue nursing or to discontinue the drug, taking into account the importance of the drug to the mother.

6. Pediatric Use

Prolonged use of corticotropin in children will inhibit skeletal growth. If use is necessary, it should be given intermittently and the child carefully observed.

ADVERSE REACTIONS

Fluid and electrolyte disturbances:
Sodium retention; fluid retention; potassium loss; hypokalemic alkalosis; calcium loss.

Musculoskeletal:
Muscle weakness; steroid myopathy; loss of muscle mass; osteoporosis; vertebral compression fractures; aseptic necrosis of femoral and humeral heads; pathologic fracture of long bones.

Gastrointestinal:
Peptic ulcer with possible perforation and hemorrhage; pancreatitis; abdominal distention; ulcerative esophagitis.

Dermatologic:
Impaired wound healing; thin fragile skin; petechiae and ecchymoses; facial erythema; increased sweating; suppression of skin test reactions; acne; hyperpigmentation.

Cardiovascular:
Hypertension, necrotizing angitis; congestive heart failure.

Neurological:
Convulsions; increased intracranial pressure with papilledema, (pseudo-tumor cerebri) usually after treatment; headache, vertigo.

Endocrine:
Menstrual irregularities; development of Cushingoid state; suppression of growth in children; secondary adrenocortical and pituitary unresponsiveness, particularly in times of stress, as in trauma, surgery or illness; decreased carbohydrate tolerance; manifestations of latent diabetes mellitus; increased requirements for insulin or oral hypoglycemic agents in diabetics; hirsutism.

Ophthalmic:
Posterior subcapsular cataracts; increased intraocular pressure; glaucoma with possible damage to optic nerve; exophthalmos.

Metabolic:
Negative nitrogen balance due to protein catabolism.

Allergic reactions:
Especially in patients with allergic responses to proteins manifesting as dizziness, nausea and vomiting, shock, skin reactions.

Miscellaneous:
Abscess: prolonged use of ACTH may result in antibodies to it and resulting loss of stimulatory effect.

Drug Abuse and Dependence:
Although drug dependence does not occur, sudden withdrawal of corticotropin after prolonged use may lead to recurrent symptoms which make it difficult to stop. It may be necessary to taper the dose and increase the injection interval to gradually discontinue the medication.

OVERDOSAGE

An acute overdose would present no different adverse reactions.

DOSAGE AND ADMINISTRATION

Standard tests for verification of adrenal responsiveness to corticotropin may utilize as much as 80 units as a single injection or one or more injections of a lesser dosage. Verification tests should be performed prior to treatment with corticotropins. The test should utilize the route(s) of administration proposed for treatment. Following verification, dosage should be individualized according to the disease under treatment and the general medical condition of each patient. Frequency and dose of the drug should be determined by considering severity of the disease, plasma and urine corticosteroid levels and the initial response of the patient. Only gradual change in dosage schedules should be attempted, after full drug effects have become apparent.

The chronic administration of more than 40 units daily may be associated with uncontrollable adverse effects.

When reduction in dosage is indicated this should be done gradually by either reducing the amount of each injection, administering injections at longer intervals, or by a combination of both of the above. During reduction of dosage careful consideration should be given to the disease being treated, the general medical conditions of the patient and the duration over which corticotropin was administered.

ACTHAR must be reconstituted at the time of use by dissolving in a convenient volume of Sterile Water for Injection or Sodium Chloride Injection in such a manner that the individual dose will be contained in 1–2 mL of solution. The reconstituted solution should be refrigerated and used within 24 hours.

H.P. ACTHAR GEL (Repository Corticotropin Injection) and ACTHAR (Corticotropin for Injection) may be administered intramuscularly or subcutaneously.

H.P. ACTHAR GEL (Repository Corticotropin Injection) is given intramuscularly or subcutaneously every 24-72 hours in doses of 40-80 units.

The usual intramuscular or subcutaneous dose for ACTHAR (Corticotropin for Injection) is 20 units four times a day.

In the treatment of acute exacerbations of multiple sclerosis daily intramuscular doses of 80–120 units for 2–3 weeks may be administered.

For diagnostic purposes, ACTHAR (Corticotropin for Injection) may be given intravenously in doses of 10-25 units dissolved in 500 mL of 5% glucose infused over an 8-hour period.

HOW SUPPLIED

H.P. ACTHAR GEL (Repository Corticotropin Injection) is available in 5-mL multiple-dose vials in strengths of 40 USP Units per mL (NDC 0053-1330-01), or 80 USP Units per mL (NDC 0053-1350-01) and in 1-mL vials in strengths of 40 USP Units per mL (NDC 0053-1330-02), or 80 USP Units per mL (NDC-0053-1350-02).

ACTHAR (Corticotropin for Injection) is available as a lyophilized powder in vials containing 25 USP Units per vial (NDC 0053-1025-01) and 40 USP Units per vial (NDC 0053-1040-01).

H.P. ACTHAR GEL (Repository Corticotropin Injection) is stable for the period indicated on the label when stored under refrigeration between 2°-8°C (36°-46°F).

ACTHAR (Corticotropin for Injection) is stable for the period indicated on the label when stored at controlled room temperature between 15°-30°C (59°-86°F).

CAUTION

Federal (U.S.A.) Law Prohibits Dispensing Without Prescription

Rev. 7/88

ARMOUR PHARMACEUTICAL COMPANY
Kankakee, Illinois 60901, U.S.A.

ARLIDIN® ℞

[ar'lǐ-dǐn"]
nylidrin HCl
6 mg tablets
12 mg tablets

DESCRIPTION

Arlidin® is an oral sympathomimetic agent and is an original compound of organic synthesis, phenyl secondary butyl norhydroxyephedrine. It is available in 6 mg and 12 mg tablets and is related chemically to the epinephrine-ephedrine series.

ACTIONS

Arlidin acts predominantly by beta-receptor stimulation. Beta stimulation with Arlidin has been demonstrated in a variety of isolated tissues from rabbits, guinea pigs, and dogs. It has been shown to dilate arterioles in skeletal muscle and to increase cardiac output in the anesthetized dog and cat and in unanesthetized man.

INDICATIONS

Based on a review of this drug by the National Academy of Sciences—National Research Council and/or other information, FDA has classified the indications as follows:

"Possibly" effective whenever an increase in blood supply is desirable in vasospastic disorders such as:

peripheral vascular disease
Arteriosclerosis Obliterans
Thromboangiitis Obliterans
Diabetic Vascular Disease
Night Leg Cramps
Raynaud's Phenomenon and Disease
Ischemic Ulcer
Frostbite
Acrocyanosis
Acroparesthesia
Thrombophlebitis
Cold Feet, Legs and Hands

circulatory disturbances of the inner ear
Primary Cochlear Cell Ischemia
Cochlear Stria Vascular Ischemia
Macular or Ampullar Ischemia and other disturbances due to labyrinthine artery spasm or obstruction

"Lacks substantial evidence of effectiveness" for the indications:

cerebrovascular disorders
Cerebral Ischemia
Cerebral Arteriosclerosis and other circulatory insufficiencies of the brain

Final classification of the less-than-effective indications requires further investigation.

CONTRAINDICATIONS

Acute myocardial infarction, paroxysmal tachycardia, progressive angina pectoris, and thyrotoxicosis.

WARNINGS

In patients with cardiac disease such as tachyarrhythmias and uncompensated congestive heart failure, the benefit/risk ratio should be weighed prior to therapy and reconsidered at intervals during treatment.

ADVERSE REACTIONS

Trembling, nervousness, weakness, dizziness (not associated with labyrinthine artery insufficiency), palpitations, nausea and vomiting may occur. Postural hypotension, while not reported, may also occur.

DOSAGE

Orally, 3 to 12 mg, three or four times a day.

HOW SUPPLIED

Arlidin Tablets are white and scored. Arlidin 6 mg are embossed with USV and 45 and are available in bottles of 100

(NDC 0075-0045-00). Arlidin 12 mg are embossed with USV and 46 and are available in bottles of 100 (NDC 0075-0046-00).

STORAGE CONDITIONS: Keep tightly closed. Store at room temperature; avoid excessive heat. Dispense in tight containers as defined in USP.

CAUTION

Federal (U.S.A.) law prohibits dispensing without prescription.

Revised: 6/88

RORER PHARMACEUTICALS
a division of
RORER PHARMACEUTICAL CORPORATION
Fort Washington, PA, U.S.A. 19034

AZMACORT™ ℞

[ăz'ma-kort]
(triamcinolone acetonide)
inhaler

FOR ORAL INHALATION ONLY

PRODUCT OVERVIEW

KEY FACTS

Azmacort™ is an anti-inflammatory steroid in a metered-dose aerosol unit containing at least 240 inhalations. Each actuation releases approximately 200 mcg triamcinolone acetonide, of which approximately 100 mcg are delivered from the unit. Azmacort provides effective local steroid activity with minimal systemic effect. Triamcinolone acetonide is a very potent derivative of triamcinolone.

MAJOR USES

Azmacort™ inhaler is indicated only for patients who require chronic treatment with corticosteroids for the control of symptoms of bronchial asthma. Azmacort™ inhaler is not to be regarded as a bronchodilator and is not indicated for rapid relief of bronchospasm.

SAFETY INFORMATION

Azmacort™ inhaler is contraindicated in the primary treatment of status asthmaticus or other acute episodes of asthma requiring intensive measures. Particular care is needed in patients transferred from systemically active corticosteroids to Azmacort™ inhaler because deaths due to adrenal insufficiency have occurred in asthmatic patients during and after such a transfer.

PRESCRIBING INFORMATION

AZMACORT™ ℞

[ăz'ma-kort]
(triamcinolone acetonide)
inhaler

For Oral Inhalation Only

DESCRIPTION

Azmacort™ (triamcinolone acetonide) is an anti-inflammatory steroid having the chemical name 9α-fluoro-11β, 21-dihydroxy-16α, 17α-isopropylidenedioxy-1, 4-pregnadiene-3, 20-dione ($C_{24}H_{31}FO_6$).

Azmacort™ inhaler is a metered-dose aerosol unit containing a microcrystalline suspension of triamcinolone acetonide in the propellant dichlorodifluoromethane and dehydrated alcohol USP 1% w/w. Each canister contains 60 mg triamcinolone acetonide. Each actuation releases approximately 200 mcg triamcinolone acetonide, of which approximately 100 mcg are delivered from the unit (in-vitro testing). There are at least 240 oral inhalations in one Azmacort™ inhaler canister. The device should not be used after 240 inhalations, since the amount delivered thereafter per actuation may be less than consistent.

CLINICAL PHARMACOLOGY

The precise mechanism of the action of the inhaled drug is unknown. However, use of the inhaler makes it possible to provide effective local steroid activity with minimal systemic effect.

Continued on next page

This product information was prepared in September, 1989. Information concerning these products may be obtained by addressing Rorer Pharmaceutical Corporation, 500 Virginia Drive, Fort Washington, PA 19034.

Rorer Pharm.—Cont.

Triamcinolone acetonide is a very potent derivative of triamcinolone. Although triamcinolone itself is 1–2 times as potent as prednisone in animal models of inflammation, triamcinolone acetonide is much more potent.

Pharmacokinetic studies with radiolabeled triamcinolone acetonide have been carried out by the oral route and intravenous route in several species. The pharmacokinetic behavior of the triamcinolone acetonide was similar in all species within each route of administration. The major portion of the dose was eliminated in the feces irrespective of route of administration with only one species (rabbit) showing significant urinary excretion of radioactivity.

The results of studies in which triamcinolone acetonide was administered as an aerosol showed rapid disappearance of radioactivity from the lungs comparable to that observed following oral administration with peak blood levels occurring in 1–2 hours. Virtually no radioactivity was present in the lung and trachea 24 hours after dosing.

Three metabolites of triamcinolone acetonide have been identified. They are: 6β-hydroxy-triamcinolone acetonide, 21-carboxytriamcinolone acetonide, and 21-carboxy-6β-hydroxytriamcinolone acetonide. There appeared to be some quantitative differences in the metabolites among species. No differences were detected in metabolic pattern related to route of administration.

INDICATIONS

Azmacort™ (triamcinolone acetonide) inhaler is indicated only for patients who require chronic treatment with corticosteroids for the control of the symptoms of bronchial asthma. Such patients would include those already receiving systemic corticosteroids and selected patients who are inadequately controlled on a non-steroid regimen and in whom steroid therapy has been withheld because of concern over potential adverse effects.

Azmacort™ inhaler is NOT indicated:

1. For relief of asthma which can be controlled by bronchodilators and other non-steroid medications.
2. In patients who require systemic corticosteroid treatment infrequently.
3. In the treatment of non-asthmatic bronchitis.

CONTRAINDICATIONS

Azmacort™ inhaler is contraindicated in the primary treatment of status asthmaticus or other acute episodes of asthma where intensive measures are required.

Hypersensitivity to any of the ingredients of this preparation contraindicates its use.

WARNINGS

Particular care is needed in patients who are transferred from systemically active corticosteroids to Azmacort™ inhaler because deaths due to adrenal insufficiency have occurred in asthmatic patients during and after transfer from systemic corticosteroids to aerosolized steroids in recommended doses. After withdrawal from systemic corticosteroids, a number of months is usually required for recovery of hypothalamic-pituitary-adrenal (HPA) function. For some patients who have received large doses of oral steroids for long periods of time before therapy with Azmacort™ inhaler is initiated, recovery may be delayed for one year or longer. During this period of HPA suppression, patients may exhibit signs and symptoms of adrenal insufficiency when exposed to trauma, surgery or infections, particularly gastroenteritis or other conditions with acute electrolyte loss. Although Azmacort™ inhaler may provide control of asthmatic symptoms during these episodes, in recommended doses it supplies only normal physiological amounts of corticosteroid systemically and does NOT provide the increased systemic steroid which is necessary for coping with these emergencies.

During periods of stress or a severe asthmatic attack, patients who have been recently withdrawn from systemic corticosteroids should be instructed to resume systemic steroids (in large doses) immediately and to contact their physician for further instruction. These patients should also be instructed to carry a warning card indicating that they may need supplementary systemic steroids during periods of stress or a severe asthma attack.

Localized infections with *Candida albicans* have occurred infrequently in the mouth and pharynx. These areas should be examined by the treating physician at each patient visit. The percentage of positive mouth and throat cultures for *Candida albicans* did not change during a year of continuous therapy. The incidence of clinically apparent infection is low (2.5%). These infections may disappear spontaneously or may require treatment with appropriate antifungal therapy or discontinuance of treatment with Azmacort™ inhaler.

Azmacort™ inhaler is not to be regarded as a bronchodilator and is not indicated for rapid relief of bronchospasm. Patients should be instructed to contact their physicians immediately when episodes of asthma which are not responsive to bronchodilators occur during the course of treatment with Azmacort™ inhaler. During such episodes, patients may require therapy with systemic corticosteroids.

There is no evidence that control of asthma can be achieved by the administration of Azmacort™ inhaler in amounts greater than the recommended doses, which appear to be the therapeutic equivalent of approximately 10 mg/day of oral prednisone.

Theoretically, the use of inhaled corticosteroids with alternate day prednisone oral therapy should be accompanied by more HPA suppression than a therapeutically equivalent regimen of either alone.

Transfer of patients from systemic steroid therapy to Azmacort™ inhaler may unmask allergic conditions previously suppressed by the systemic steroid therapy, e.g., rhinitis, conjunctivitis, and eczema.

PRECAUTIONS

During withdrawal from oral steroids, some patients may experience symptoms of systemically active steroid withdrawal, e.g., joint and/or muscular pain, lassitude and depression, despite maintenance or even improvement of respiratory function (see DOSAGE AND ADMINISTRATION for details). Although steroid withdrawal effects are usually transient and not severe, severe and even fatal exacerbation of asthma can occur if the previous daily oral corticosteroid requirement had significantly exceeded 10 mg/day of prednisone or equivalent.

In responsive patients, inhaled corticosteroids will often permit control of asthmatic symptoms with less suppression of HPA function than therapeutically equivalent oral doses of prednisone. Since triamcinolone acetonide is absorbed into the circulation and can be systemically active, the beneficial effects of Azmacort™ inhaler in minimizing or preventing HPA dysfunction may be expected only when recommended dosages are not exceeded.

Suppression of HPA function has been reported in volunteers who received 4000 mcg daily of triamcinolone acetonide. In addition, suppression of HPA function has been reported in some patients who have received recommended doses for as little as 6–12 weeks. Since the response of HPA function to inhaled corticosteroids is highly individualized, the physician should consider this information when treating patients.

Because of the possibility of systemic absorption of inhaled corticosteroids, patients treated with these drugs should be observed carefully for any evidence of systemic corticosteroid effects including suppression of growth in children. Particular care should be taken in observing patients postoperatively or during periods of stress for evidence of a decrease in adrenal function.

The long-term effects of triamcinolone acetonide inhaler in human subjects are not completely known, although patients have received Azmacort™ inhaler on a continuous basis for periods of two years or longer. While there has been no clinical evidence of adverse experiences, the local effects of the agent on developmental or immunologic processes in the mouth, pharynx, trachea and lung are also unknown. The potential effects of Azmacort™ inhaler on acute, recurrent, or chronic pulmonary infections, including active or quiescent tuberculosis, are not known. For this reason, since systemic administration of corticosteroids may mask some signs of fungal, bacterial or viral infection, the same caution should be observed when treating patients with Azmacort™ inhaler. The potential effects of long-term administration of Azmacort™ inhaler on lung or other tissues are unknown. However, pulmonary infiltrates with eosinophilia have occurred in patients receiving other inhaled corticosteroids.

Pregnancy: Pregnancy Category D. Azmacort™ (triamcinolone acetonide) has been shown to be teratogenic in rats and rabbits when given in doses comparable to the highest dose recommended for human use (approximately 0.032 mg/kg/day). Administration of aerosol inhalation to pregnant rats and rabbits produced embryotoxic and fetotoxic effects which were comparable to those produced by administration by other routes.

Teratogenic effects in both species included a low incidence of cleft palate and/or internal hydrocephaly and axial skeletal defects. These findings represent known effects of glucocorticoids in laboratory animals.

There are no well-controlled studies in pregnant women. Experience with other dosage forms of triamcinolone acetonide does not include any positive evidence of adverse effects on the fetus. However, since such experience cannot exclude possibility of fetal damage, Azmacort™ inhaler should be used during pregnancy only if the benefit clearly justifies the potential risk to the fetus. Infants born to mothers who have received substantial doses of corticosteroids during pregnancy should be carefully observed for hypoadrenalism.

Nursing mothers: It is not known whether this drug is excreted in human milk. Because of the potential for tumorigenicity shown for triamcinolone acetonide in animal studies, a

decision should be made whether to discontinue nursing or to discontinue the drug, taking into account the importance of the drug to the mother.

ADVERSE REACTIONS

A few cases of oral candidiasis have been reported (see WARNINGS). In addition, some patients receiving Azmacort™ inhaler have experienced hoarseness, dry throat, irritated throat and dry mouth. Increased wheezing and cough have been reported infrequently as has facial edema. These adverse effects have generally been mild and transient.

DOSAGE AND ADMINISTRATION

All patients should be instructed that the Azmacort™ inhaler must be used on a regular daily basis rather than prn. Reliable dosage delivery cannot be assured after 240 actuations and patients should be cautioned against longer use of individual canisters.

Good oral hygiene including rinsing of the mouth after inhalation is recommended.

Adults: The usual dosage is two inhalations (approximately 200 mcg) given three to four times a day. The maximal daily intake should not exceed 16 inhalations (1600 mcg) in adults. Higher initial doses (12–16 inhalations per day) may be advisable in patients with more severe asthma, the dosage then being adjusted downward according to the response of the patient. In some patients maintenance can be accomplished when the total daily dose is given on a twice a day schedule.

Children 6 to 12 years of age: The usual dosage is one or two inhalations (100 to 200 mcg) given three to four times a day according to the response of the patient. The maximal daily intake should not exceed 12 inhalations (1200 mcg) in children 6 to 12 years of age. Insufficient clinical data exist with respect to the administration of Azmacort™ inhaler in children below the age of 6. The long-term effects of inhaled steroids on growth are still under evaluation.

Patients receiving bronchodilators by inhalation should be advised to use the bronchodilator before Azmacort™ inhaler in order to enhance penetration of triamcinolone acetonide into the bronchial tree. After use of an aerosol bronchodilator, several minutes should elapse before use of the Azmacort™ inhaler to reduce the potential toxicity from the inhaled fluorocarbon propellants in the two aerosols.

Different considerations must be given to the following groups of patients in order to obtain the full therapeutic benefit of Azmacort™ inhaler:

Patients not receiving systemic steroids: The use of Azmacort™ inhaler is straightforward in patients who are inadequately controlled with non-steroid medications but in whom systemic steroid therapy has been withheld because of concern over potential adverse reactions. In patients who respond to Azmacort™, an improvement in pulmonary functon is usually apparent within one to two weeks after the start of Azmacort™ inhaler.

Patients receiving systemic steroids: In those patients dependent on systemic steroids, transfer to Azmacort™ inhaler and subsequent management may be more difficult because recovery from impaired adrenal function is usually slow. Such suppression has been known to last for up to 12 months or longer. Clinical studies, however, have demonstrated that Azmacort™ inhaler may be effective in the management of these asthmatic patients and may permit replacement or significant reduction in the dosage of systemic corticosteroids.

The patient's asthma should be reasonably stable before treatment with Azmacort™ inhaler is started. Initially, the inhaler should be used concurrently with the patient's usual maintenance dose of systemic steroid. After approximately one week, gradual withdrawal of the systemic steroid is started by reducing the dose. The next reduction is made after an interval of one or two weeks, depending on the response of the patient. Generally, these decrements should not exceed 2.5 mg of prednisone or its equivalent. A slow rate of withdrawal cannot be overemphasized. During withdrawal, some patients may experience symptoms of systemically active steroid withdrawal, e.g., joint and/or muscular pain, lassitude and depression, despite maintenance or even improvement of respiratory function. Such patients should be encouraged to continue with the inhaler but should be watched carefully for objective signs of adrenal insufficiency, such as hypotension and weight loss. If evidence of adrenal insufficiency occurs, the systemic steroid dose should be boosted temporarily and thereafter further withdrawal should continue more slowly. No clinical studies have been conducted evaluating Azmacort™ with alternate day prednisone regimens. However, based on the results of such a study with another inhaled corticosteroid, inhaled corticosteroids generally are not recommended for chronic use with alternate day prednisone regimens (see WARNINGS).

During periods of stress or a severe asthma attack, transfer patients will require supplementary treatment with systemic steroids. Exacerbations of asthma which occur during the course of treatment with Azmacort™ inhaler should be treated with a short course of systemic steroid which is gradually tapered as these symptoms subside. There is no evidence that control of asthma can be achieved by administration of **Azmacort**™ inhaler in amounts greater than the recommended doses.

Directions for Use: An illustrated leaflet of patient instructions for proper use accompanies each package of Azmacort™ inhaler.

Contents Under Pressure: Do not puncture. Do not use or store near heat or open flame. Exposure to temperatures above 120°F may cause bursting. Never throw container into fire or incinerator. Keep out of reach of children.

HOW SUPPLIED

Azmacort™ inhaler contains 60 mg triamcinolone acetonide in a 20 gram package which delivers at least 240 oral inhalations. It is supplied with an oral adapter and patient's leaflet of instructions: box of one.

NDC 0075-0060-37

STORE AT ROOM TEMPERATURE.

CAUTION

Federal (U.S.A.) law prohibits dispensing without prescription.

Rev. 5/89

Marketed by

RORER PHARMACEUTICALS

a division of

RORER PHARMACEUTICAL CORPORATION

Fort Washington, PA, U.S.A. 19034

Shown in Product Identification Section, page 426

CALCIMAR®   ℞

[kal'sĭmar]

(calcitonin-salmon)

INJECTION, SYNTHETIC

PRODUCT OVERVIEW

KEY FACTS

Calcimar® Injection, Synthetic is a synthetic polypeptide of 32 amino acids in the same linear sequence found in calcitonin of salmon origin. It is provided as a sterile solution in 2 mL vials containing 400 I.U. (200 I.U. per ml) for subcutaneous or intramuscular injection.

MAJOR USES

Calcimar® Injection, Synthetic is indicated for the relief of bone pain and other symptoms of Paget's disease, for the treatment of hypercalcemia, and for the treatment of postmenopausal osteoporosis (PMO) to prevent the progressive loss of bone mass. Adequate calcium and Vitamin D intake in conjunction with Calcimar is essential to prevent the progressive loss of bone mass in PMO.

SAFETY INFORMATION

Skin testing should be considered prior to treatment with calcitonin because of its protein nature. Careful instruction in sterile injection techniques should be given to the patient or other persons who may administer Calcimar.

PRESCRIBING INFORMATION

CALCIMAR®   ℞

[kal'sĭ-mar]

(calcitonin-salmon)

INJECTION, SYNTHETIC

DESCRIPTION

Calcitonin is a polypeptide hormone secreted by the parafollicular cells of the thyroid gland in mammals and by the ultimobranchial gland of birds and fish.

CALCIMAR® (calcitonin-salmon) Injection, Synthetic is a synthetic polypeptide of 32 amino acids in the same linear sequence that is found in calcitonin of salmon origin. This is shown by the following graphic formula:

Cys-	Ser-	Asn-	Leu-	Ser-	Thr-	Cys-	Val-	Leu-	Gly-	Lys-
1	2	3	4	5	6	7	8	9	10	11
Leu-	Ser-	Gln-	Glu-	Leu-	His-	Lys-	Leu-	Gln-	Thr-	Tyr-
12	13	14	15	16	17	18	19	20	21	22
Pro-	Arg-	Thr-	Asn-	Thr-	Gly-	Ser-	Gly-	Thr-	Pro-	NH_2
23	24	25	26	27	28	29	30	31	32	

It is provided in sterile solution for subcutaneous or intramuscular injection. Each milliliter contains 200 I.U. (MRC) of calcitonin-salmon, 5 mg phenol (as preservative), with sodium chloride, sodium acetate, acetic acid, and sodium hydroxide to adjust tonicity and pH.

The activity of CALCIMAR is stated in International Units (equal to MRC or Medical Research Council units) based on bio-assay in comparison with the International Reference Preparation of Calcitonin, Salmon for Bioassay, distributed by the National Institute for Biological Standards and Control, Holly Hill, London.

CLINICAL PHARMACOLOGY

Calcitonin acts primarily on bone, but direct renal effects and actions on the gastrointestinal tract are also recognized. Calcitonin-salmon appears to have actions essentially identical to calcitonins of mammalian origin, but its potency per mg is greater and it has a longer duration of action. The actions of calcitonin on bone and its role in normal human bone physiology are still incompletely understood.

Bone—Single injections of calcitonin cause a marked transient inhibition of the ongoing bone resorptive process. With prolonged use, there is a persistent, smaller decrease in the rate of bone resorption. Histologically this is associated with a decreased number of osteoclasts and an apparent decrease in their resorptive activity. Decreased osteocytic resorption may also be involved. There is some evidence that initially bone formation may be augmented by calcitonin through increased osteoblastic activity. However, calcitonin will probably not induce a long-term increase in bone formation. Animal studies indicate that endogenous calcitonin, primarily through its action on bone, participates with parathyroid hormone in the homeostatic regulation of blood calcium. Thus, high blood calcium levels cause increased secretion of calcitonin which, in turn, inhibits bone resorption. This reduces the transfer of calcium from bone to blood and tends to return blood calcium to the normal level. The importance of this process in humans has not been determined. In normal adults, who have a relatively low rate of bone resorption, the administration of exogenous calcitonin results in only a slight decrease in serum calcium. In normal children and in patients with generalized Paget's disease, bone resorption is more rapid and decreases in serum calcium are more pronounced in response to calcitonin.

Paget's Disease of Bone (osteitis deformans)—Paget's disease is a disorder of uncertain etiology characterized by abnormal and accelerated bone formation and resorption in one or more bones. In most patients only small areas of bone are involved and the disease is not symptomatic. In a small fraction of patients, however, the abnormal bone may lead to bone pain and bone deformity, cranial and spinal nerve entrapment, or spinal cord compression. The increased vascularity of the abnormal bone may lead to high output congestive heart failure.

Active Paget's disease involving a large mass of bone may increase the urinary hydroxyproline excretion (reflecting breakdown of collagen-containing bone matrix) and serum alkaline phosphatase (reflecting increased bone formation). Calcitonin-salmon, presumably by an initial blocking effect on bone resorption, causes a decreased rate of bone turnover with a resultant fall in the serum alkaline phosphatase and urinary hydroxyproline excretion in approximately $2/3$ of patients treated. These biochemical changes appear to correspond to changes toward more normal bone, as evidenced by a small number of documented examples of: 1) radiologic regression of Pagetic lesions, 2) improvement of impaired auditory nerve and other neurologic function, 3) decreases (measured) in abnormally elevated cardiac output. These improvements occur extremely rarely, if ever, spontaneously (elevated cardiac output may disappear over a period of years when the disease slowly enters a sclerotic phase; in the cases treated with calcitonin, however, the decreases were seen in less than one year).

Some patients with Paget's disease who have good biochemical and/or symptomatic responses initially, later relapse. Suggested explanations have included the formation of neutralizing antibodies and the development of secondary hyperparathyroidism, but neither suggestion appears to explain adequately the majority of relapses.

Although the parathyroid hormone levels do appear to rise transiently during each hypocalcemic response to calcitonin, most investigators have been unable to demonstrate persistent hypersecretion of parathyroid hormone in patients treated chronically with calcitonin.

Circulating antibodies to calcitonin after 2–18 months' treatment have been reported in about half of the patients with Paget's disease in whom antibody studies were done, but calcitonin treatment remained effective in many of these cases. Occasionally patients with high antibody titers are found. These patients usually will have suffered a biochemical relapse of Paget's disease and are unresponsive to the acute hypocalcemic effects of calcitonin.

Hypercalcemia—In clinical trials, CALCIMAR® (calcitonin-salmon) Injection, Synthetic has been shown to lower the elevated serum calcium of patients with carcinoma (with or without demonstrated metastases), multiple myeloma or primary hyperparathyroidism (lesser response). Patients with higher values for serum calcium tend to show greater reduction during CALCIMAR therapy. The decrease in calcium occurs about 2 hours after the first injection and lasts for about 6–8 hours. CALCIMAR given every 12 hours maintained a calcium lowering effect for about 5–8 days, the time period evaluated for most patients during the clinical studies. The average reduction of 8-hour post-injection serum calcium during this period was about 9 percent.

Kidney—Calcitonin increases the excretion of filtered phosphate, calcium, and sodium by decreasing their tubular reabsorption. In some patients the inhibition of bone resorption by calcitonin is of such magnitude that the consequent reduction of filtered calcium load more than compensates for the decrease in tubular reabsorption of calcium. The result in these patients is a decrease rather than an increase in urinary calcium.

Transient increases in sodium and water excretion may occur after the initial injection of calcitonin. In most patients these changes return to pre-treatment levels with continued therapy.

Gastrointestinal tract—Increasing evidence indicates that calcitonin has significant actions on the gastrointestinal tract. Short-term administration results in marked transient decreases in the volume and acidity of gastric juice and in the volume and the trypsin and amylase content of pancreatic juice. Whether these effects continue to be elicited after each injection of calcitonin during chronic therapy has not been investigated.

Metabolism—The metabolism of calcitonin-salmon has not yet been studied clinically. Information from animal studies with calcitonin-salmon and from clinical studies with calcitonins of porcine and human origin suggest that calcitonin-salmon is rapidly metabolized by conversion to smaller inactive fragments, primarily in the kidneys, but also in the blood and peripheral tissues. A small amount of unchanged hormone and its inactive metabolites are excreted in the urine.

It appears that calcitonin-salmon cannot cross the placental barrier and its passage to the cerebrospinal fluid or to breast milk has not been determined.

INDICATIONS AND USAGE

CALCIMAR (calcitonin-salmon) Injection, Synthetic is indicated for the treatment of symptomatic Paget's disease of bone, the treatment of hypercalcemia, and the treatment of postmenopausal osteoporosis.

Paget's Disease—At the present time effectiveness has been demonstrated principally in patients with moderate to severe disease characterized by polyostotic involvement with elevated serum alkaline phosphatase and urinary hydroxyproline excretion.

In these patients, the biochemical abnormalities were substantially improved (more than 30% reduction) in about $2/3$ of patients studied, and bone pain was improved in a similar fraction. A small number of documented instances of reversal of neurologic deficits has occurred, including improvement in the basilar compression syndrome, and improvement of spinal cord and spinal nerve lesions. At present there is too little experience to predict the likelihood of improvement of any given neurologic lesion. Hearing loss, the most common neurologic lesion of Paget's disease is improved infrequently (4 of 29 patients studied audiometrically).

Patients with increased cardiac output due to extensive Paget's disease have had measured decreases in cardiac output while receiving calcitonin. The number of treated patients in this category is still too small to predict how likely such a result will be.

The large majority of patients with localized, especially monostotic disease do not develop symptoms and most patients with mild symptoms can be managed with analgesics. There is no evidence that the prophylactic use of calcitonin is beneficial in asymptomatic patients, although treatment may be considered in exceptional circumstances in which there is extensive involvement of the skull or spinal cord with the possibility of irreversible neurologic damage. In these instances treatment would be based on the demonstrated effect of calcitonin on Pagetic bone, rather than on clinical studies in the patient population in question.

Hypercalcemia—CALCIMAR (calcitonin-salmon) Injection, Synthetic is indicated for early treatment of hypercalcemic emergencies, along with other appropriate agents, when a rapid decrease in serum calcium is required, until more specific treatment of the underlying disease can be accomplished. It may also be added to existing therapeutic regimens for hypercalcemia such as intravenous fluids and furosemide, oral phosphate or corticosteroids, or other agents.

Postmenopausal Osteoporosis—CALCIMAR is indicated for the treatment of postmenopausal osteoporosis in conjunction with an adequate calcium and vitamin D intake to prevent the progressive loss of bone mass. The evidence of efficacy was based on an increase in total body calcium. No significant differences were observed in bone density measurements of the distal radius, and the clinical studies were not designed to detect differences in fracture rates.

CONTRAINDICATIONS

Clinical allergy to synthetic calcitonin-salmon.

WARNINGS

Allergic Reactions

Because calcitonin is protein in nature, the possibility of a systemic allergic reaction exists. Administration of calcito-

Continued on next page

This product information was prepared in September, 1989. Information concerning these products may be obtained by addressing Rorer Pharmaceutical Corporation, 500 Virginia Drive, Fort Washington, PA 19034.

Rorer Pharm.—Cont.

nin-salmon has been reported in a few cases to cause serious allergic-type reaction (e.g. bronchospasm, swelling of the tongue or throat, and anaphylactic shock). The usual provisions should be made for the emergency treatment of such a reaction should it occur. Allergic reactions should be differentiated from generalized flushing and hypotension.

Skin testing should be considered prior to treatment with calcitonin, particularly for patients with suspected sensitivity to calcitonin. The following procedure is suggested: Prepare a dilution at 10 I.U. per mL by withdrawing ¹⁄₂₀ mL (0.05 mL) in a tuberculin syringe and filling it to 1.0 mL with Sodium Chloride Injection, USP. Mix well, discard 0.9 mL and inject intracutaneously 0.1 mL (approximately 1 I.U.) on the inner aspect of the forearm. Observe the injection site 15 minutes after injection. The appearance of more than mild erythema or wheal constitutes a positive response.

General.

The incidence of osteogenic sarcoma is known to be increased in Paget's disease. Pagetic lesions, with or without therapy, may appear by X-ray to progress markedly, possibly with some loss of definition of periosteal margins. Such lesions should be evaluated carefully to differentiate these from osteogenic sarcoma.

PRECAUTIONS

1. General

The administration of calcitonin possibly could lead to hypocalcemic tetany under special circumstances although no cases have yet been reported. Provisions for parenteral calcium administration should be available during the first several administrations of calcitonin.

2. Laboratory Tests

Periodic examinations of urine sediment of patients on chronic therapy are recommended.

Coarse granular casts and casts containing renal tubular epithelial cells were reported in young adult volunteers at bed rest who were given calcitonin-salmon to study the effect on immobilization osteoporosis. There was no other evidence of renal abnormality and the urine sediment became normal after calcitonin was stopped. Urine sediment abnormalities have not been reported by other investigators.

3. Instructions for the patient

Careful instruction in sterile injection technique should be given to the patient, and to other persons who may administer CALCIMAR (calcitonin-salmon) Injection, Synthetic.

4. Carcinogenesis

No long-term studies have been performed to evaluate carcinogenic potential of calcitonin-salmon.

5. Pregnancy: Teratogenic effects. Category C.

Calcitonin-salmon has been shown to cause decrease in fetal birth weights in rabbits when given in doses 14–56 times the dose recommended for human use. Since calcitonin does not cross the placental barrier, this finding may be due to metabolic effects of calcitonin on the pregnant animal. There are no adequate and well-controlled studies in pregnant women. CALCIMAR should be used during pregnancy only if the potential benefit justifies the potential risk to the fetus.

6. Nursing Mothers

It is not known whether this drug is excreted in human milk. As a general rule, nursing should not be undertaken while a patient is on this drug since many drugs are excreted in human milk. Calcitonin has been shown to inhibit lactation in animals.

7. Pediatric Use

Disorders of bone in children referred to as juvenile Paget's disease have been reported rarely. The relationship of these disorders to adult Paget's disease has not been established and experience with the use of calcitonin in these disorders is very limited. There are no adequate data to support the use of CALCIMAR in children.

ADVERSE REACTIONS

Gastrointestinal System —Nausea with or without vomiting has been noted in about 10% of patients treated with calcitonin. It is most evident when treatment is first initiated and tends to decrease or disappear with continued administration.

Dermatologic/Hypersensitivity —Local inflammatory reactions at the site of subcutaneous or intramuscular injection have been reported in about 10% of patients. Flushing of face or hands occurred in about 2% to 5% of patients. Skin rashes have been reported occasionally. Administration of calcitonin-salmon has been reported in a few cases to cause serious allergic-type reactions (e.g. bronchospasm, swelling of the tongue or throat, and anaphylactic shock). (SEE WARNINGS.)

OVERDOSAGE

A dose of 1000 I.U. subcutaneously may produce nausea and vomiting as the only adverse effects. Doses of 32 units per kg per day for one or two days demonstrate no other adverse effects.

Data on chronic high dose administration are insufficient to judge toxicity.

DOSAGE AND ADMINISTRATION

Paget 's Disease —The recommended starting dose of calcitonin in Paget's disease is 100 I.U. (0.5 mL) per day administered subcutaneously (preferred for outpatient self-administration) or intramuscularly. Drug effect should be monitored by periodic measurement of serum alkaline phosphatase and 24-hour urinary hydroxyproline (if available) and evaluation of symptoms. A decrease toward normal of the biochemical abnormalities is usually seen, if it is going to occur, within the first few months. Bone pain may also decrease during that time. Improvement of neurologic lesions, when it occurs, requires a longer period of treatment, often more than one year.

In many patients doses of 50 I.U. (0.25 mL) per day or every other day are sufficient to maintain biochemical and clinical improvement. At the present time, however, data are insufficient to determine whether this reduced dose will have the same effect as the higher dose on forming more normal bone structure. It appears preferable, therefore, to maintain the higher dose in any patient with serious deformity or neurological involvement.

In any patient with a good response initially who later relapses, either clinically or biochemically, the possibility of antibody formation should be explored. The patient may be tested for antibodies by an appropriate specialized test or evaluated for the possibility of antibody formation by critical clinical evaluation.

Patient compliance should also be assessed in the event of relapse.

In patients who relapse, whether because of antibodies or for unexplained reasons, a dosage increase beyond 100 I.U. per day does not usually appear to elicit an improved response.

Hypercalcemia —The recommended starting dose of CALCIMAR (calcitonin-salmon) Injection, Synthetic in hypercalcemia is 4 I.U./kg body weight every 12 hours by subcutaneous or intramuscular injection. If the response to this dose is not satisfactory after one or two days, the dose may be increased to 8 I.U./kg every 12 hours. If the response remains unsatisfactory after two more days, the dose may be further increased to a maximum of 8 I.U./kg every 6 hours.

Postmenopausal Osteoporosis —The recommended dose of calcitonin is 100 I.U. per day administered subcutaneously or intramuscularly. Patients also receive supplemental calcium such as calcium carbonate 1.5 g daily and an adequate vitamin D intake (400 units daily). An adequate diet is also essential.

If the volume of CALCIMAR to be injected exceeds 2 mL, intramuscular injection is preferable and multiple sites of injection should be used.

Parenteral drug products should be inspected visually for particulate matter and discoloration prior to administration whenever solution and container permit.

HOW SUPPLIED

CALCIMAR® is available as a sterile solution in 2 mL vials containing 200 I.U. per mL (NDC 0075-1306-01).

Store in Refrigerator, 36°-46°F (2°-8°C).

CAUTION: FEDERAL (U.S.A.) LAW PROHIBITS DISPENSING WITHOUT PRESCRIPTION.

Rev. June 1988

RORER PHARMACEUTICALS
a division of
RORER PHARMACEUTICAL CORPORATION
Fort Washington, PA, U.S.A. 19034

Shown in Product Identification Section, page 426

CALEL–D®

DESCRIPTION

Each tablet provides 500 mg of elemental Calcium (50% of U.S. RDA) from calcium carbonate and 200 I.U. of Vitamin D₃ (Cholecalciferol) (50% of U.S. RDA). The inactive ingredients are cornstarch, croscarmellose sodium, hydroxypropyl methylcellulose, polyethylene glycol, calcium stearate.

INDICATIONS

CALEL-D is indicated as a dietary supplement for those adults not receiving an adequate intake of calcium and Vitamin D.

USUAL DOSE

One or two tablets daily or as directed by a physician.

Store tablets at room temperature. Keep out of the reach of children.

HOW SUPPLIED

Bottles of 75 tablets.
RORER PHARMACEUTICALS
a division of
RORER PHARMACEUTICAL CORPORATION
Fort Washington, PA, U.S.A. 19034

DDAVP® Injection ℞
(desmopressin acetate)

PRODUCT OVERVIEW

KEY FACTS

DDAVP® Injection (desmopressin acetate) is an antidiuretic hormone affecting renal water conservation and is a synthetic analogue of 8-arginine vasopressin. DDAVP Injection is provided as a sterile, aqueous solution for injection only. One ml (4 mcg) of DDAVP solution has an antidiuretic activity of about 16 IU; 1 mcg of DDAVP is equivalent to 4 IU.

MAJOR USES

DDAVP Injection is indicated for patients with hemophilia A with factor VIII coagulant activity levels greater than 5%. DDAVP Injection is also indicated for patients with mild to moderate classic von Willebrand's disease (Type I) with factor VIII levels greater than 5%.

DDAVP Injection is also indicated as an antidiuretic replacement therapy in the management of central (cranial) diabetes insipidus and for the management of the temporary polyuria and polydipsia following head trauma or surgery in the pituitary region. DDAVP is ineffective for the treatment of nephrogenic diabetes insipidus. DDAVP is also available as an intranasal preparation for the treatment of central (cranial) diabetes insipidus.

SAFETY INFORMATION

Patients who do not have need of antidiuretic hormone for its antidiuretic effect, in particular those who are young or elderly, should be cautioned to ingest only enough fluid to satisfy thirst, in order to decrease the potential occurrence of water intoxication and hyponatremia.

DDAVP Injection should not be used to treat patients with Type IIB von Willebrand's disease since platelet aggregation may be induced.

PRESCRIBING INFORMATION

DDAVP® Injection ℞
(desmopressin acetate)

DESCRIPTION

DDAVP® Injection (desmopressin acetate) is an antidiuretic hormone affecting renal water conservation and is a synthetic analogue of 8-arginine vasopressin. It is chemically defined as follows:

Mol. Wt. 1183.2

Empirical Formula: $C_{48}H_{74}N_{14}O_{17}S_2$

SCH₂CH₂CO-Tyr-Phe-Gln-Asn-Cys-Pro-D-Arg-Gly-NH₂·
$\overline{|}$

$C_2H_4O_2 \cdot 3H_2O$

1-(3-mercaptopropionic acid)-8-D-arginine vasopressin monoacetate (salt) trihydrate.

DDAVP® Injection is provided as a sterile, aqueous solution for injection.

Each ml provides:	
Desmopressin acetate	4.0 mcg
Chlorobutanol	5.0 mg
Sodium chloride	9.0 mg
Hydrochloric acid to adjust pH to 3.5	

CLINICAL PHARMACOLOGY

DDAVP® Injection contains as active substance, 1-(3-mercaptopropionic acid)-8-D-arginine vasopressin, a synthetic analogue of the natural hormone arginine vasopressin. One ml (4 mcg) of DDAVP (desmopressin acetate) solution has an antidiuretic activity of about 16 IU; 1 mcg of DDAVP is equivalent to 4 IU.

DDAVP has been shown to be more potent than arginine vasopressin in increasing plasma levels of factor VIII activity in patients with hemophilia and von Willebrand's disease Type I.

Dose-response studies were performed in healthy persons, using doses of 0.1 to 0.4 mcg/kg body weight, infused over a 10-minute period. Maximal dose response occurred at 0.3 to 0.4 mcg/kg. The response to DDAVP of factor VIII activity and plasminogen activator is dose-related, with maximal plasma levels of 300 to 400 percent of initial concentrations obtained after infusion of 0.4 mcg/kg body weight. The increase is rapid and evident within 30 minutes, reaching a maximum at a point ranging from 90 minutes to two hours. The factor VIII related antigen and ristocetin cofactor activity were also increased to a smaller degree, but still dose-dependent.

1. The biphasic half-lives of DDAVP were 7.8 and 75.5 minutes for the fast and slow phases, respectively, compared with 2.5 and 14.5 minutes for lysine vasopressin, another form of the hormone. As a result, DDAVP (desmopressin acetate) provides a prompt onset of antidiuretic action with a long duration after each administration.

2. The change in structure of arginine vasopressin to DDAVP has resulted in a decreased vasopressor action and decreased actions on visceral smooth muscle relative to the enhanced antidiuretic activity, so that clinically effective antidiuretic doses are usually below threshold levels for effects on vascular or visceral smooth muscle.

3. When administered by injection, DDAVP has an antidiuretic effect about ten times that of an equivalent dose administered intranasally.

4. The bioavailability of the subcutaneous route of administration was determined qualitatively using urine output data. The exact fraction of drug absorbed by that route of administration has not been quantitatively determined.

5. The percentage increase of factor VIII levels in patients with mild hemophilia A and von Willebrand's disease was not significantly different from that observed in normal healthy individuals when treated with 0.3 mcg/kg of DDAVP infused over 10 minutes.

6. Plasminogen activator activity increases rapidly after DDAVP infusion, but there has been no clinically significant fibrinolysis in patients treated with DDAVP.

7. The effect of repeated DDAVP administration when doses were given every 12 to 24 hours has generally shown a gradual diminution of the factor VIII activity increase noted with a single dose. The initial response is reproducible in any particular patient if there are 2 or 3 days between administrations.

INDICATIONS AND USAGE

Hemophilia A

DDAVP® Injection is indicated for patients with hemophilia A with factor VIII coagulant activity levels greater than 5%.

DDAVP will often maintain hemostasis in patients with hemophilia A during surgical procedures and postoperatively when administered 30 minutes prior to scheduled procedure.

DDAVP will also stop bleeding in hemophilia A patients with episodes of spontaneous or trauma-induced injuries such as hemarthroses, intramuscular hematomas or mucosal bleeding.

DDAVP is not indicated for the treatment of hemophilia A with factor VIII coagulant activity levels equal to or less than 5%, or for the treatment of hemophilia B, or in patients who have factor VIII antibodies.

In certain clinical situations, it may be justified to try DDAVP in patients with factor VIII levels between 2%-5%; however, these patients should be carefully monitored.

von Willebrand's Disease (Type I)

DDAVP® Injection is indicated for patients with mild to moderate classic von Willebrand's disease (Type I) with factor VIII levels greater than 5%. DDAVP will often maintain hemostasis in patients with mild to moderate von Willebrand's disease during surgical procedures and postoperatively when administered 30 minutes prior to the scheduled procedure.

DDAVP will usually stop bleeding in mild to moderate von Willebrand's patients with episodes of spontaneous or trauma-induced injuries such as hemarthroses, intramuscular hematomas or mucosal bleeding.

Those von Willebrand's disease patients who are least likely to respond are those with severe homozygous von Willebrand's disease with factor VIII coagulant activity and factor VIII von Willebrand factor antigen levels less than 1%. Other patients may respond in a variable fashion depending on the type of molecular defect they have. Bleeding time and factor VIII coagulant activity, ristocetin cofactor activity, and von Willebrand factor antigen should be checked during administration of DDAVP to ensure that adequate levels are being achieved.

DDAVP is not indicated for the treatment of severe classic von Willebrand's disease (Type I) and when there is evidence of an abnormal molecular form of factor VIII antigen. See Warning.

Diabetes Insipidus

DDAVP® Injection is indicated as antidiuretic replacement therapy in the management of central (cranial) diabetes insipidus and for the management of the temporary polyuria and polydipsia following head trauma or surgery in the pituitary region. DDAVP is ineffective for the treatment of nephrogenic diabetes insipidus.

DDAVP is also available as an intranasal preparation. However, this means of delivery can be compromised by a variety of factors that can make nasal insufflation ineffective or inappropriate. These include poor intranasal absorption, nasal congestion and blockage, nasal discharge, atrophy of nasal mucosa, and severe atrophic rhinitis. Intranasal delivery may be inappropriate where there is an impaired level of consciousness. In addition, cranial surgical procedures, such as transphenoidal hypophysectomy, create situations where an alternative route of administration is needed as in cases of nasal packing or recovery from surgery.

CONTRAINDICATION

Known hypersensitivity to DDAVP.

WARNINGS

Patients who do not have need of antidiuretic hormone for its antidiuretic effect, in particular those who are young or elderly, should be cautioned to ingest only enough fluid to satisfy thirst, in order to decrease the potential occurrence of water intoxication and hyponatremia.

DDAVP should not be used to treat patients with Type IIB von Willebrand's disease since platelet aggregation may be induced.

PRECAUTIONS

GENERAL: For injection use only.

DDAVP® Injection (desmopressin acetate) has infrequently produced a slight elevation of blood pressure, which disappeared with a reduction in dosage. The drug should be used with caution in patients with coronary artery insufficiency and/or hypertensive cardiovascular disease, because of possible rise in blood pressure.

Severe allergic reactions have not been reported with DDAVP® Injection (desmopressin acetate). It is not known whether antibodies to DDAVP® Injection (desmopressin acetate) are produced after repeated injections.

Hemophilia A

Laboratory tests for assessing patient status include levels of factor VIII coagulant, factor VIII antigen and factor VIII ristocetin cofactor (von Willebrand factor) as well as activated partial thromboplastin time. Factor VIII coagulant activity should be determined before giving DDAVP for hemostasis. If factor VIII coagulant activity is present at less than 5% of normal, DDAVP should not be relied on.

von Willebrand's Disease

Laboratory tests for assessing patient status include levels of factor VIII coagulant activity, factor VIII ristocetin cofactor activity, and factor VIII von Willebrand factor antigen. The skin bleeding time may be helpful in following these patients.

Diabetes Insipidus

Laboratory tests for monitoring the patient include urine volume and osmolality. In some cases, plasma osmolality may be required.

DRUG INTERACTIONS: Although the pressor activity of DDAVP is very low compared with the antidiuretic activity, use of doses as large as 0.3 mcg/kg of DDAVP with other pressor agents should be done only with careful patient monitoring.

DDAVP has been used with epsilon aminocaproic acid without adverse effects.

CARCINOGENICITY, MUTAGENICITY, IMPAIRMENT OF FERTILITY: Teratology studies in rats have shown no abnormalities. No further data are available.

PREGNANCY CATEGORY B: Reproduction studies performed in rats and rabbits with subcutaneous doses up to 12.5 times the human dose when used for factor VIII stimulation and 125 times the human dose when used in diabetes insipidus have revealed no evidence of harm to the fetus due to DDAVP. There are several publications of management of diabetes insipidus in pregnant women with no harm to the fetus reported; however, there are no adequate and well-controlled studies in pregnant women. Published reports stress that, as opposed to preparations containing the natural hormones, DDAVP in antidiuretic doses has no uterotonic action, but the physician will have to weigh possible therapeutic advantages against possible danger in each case.

NURSING MOTHERS: It is not known whether this drug is excreted in human milk. Because many drugs are excreted in human milk, caution should be exercised when DDAVP is administered to a nursing woman.

PEDIATRIC USE: Use in infants and children will require careful fluid intake restriction to prevent possible hyponatremia and water intoxication. *DDAVP® Injection should not be used in infants younger than three months* in the treatment of hemophilia A or von Willebrand's disease; safety and effectiveness in children under 12 years of age with diabetes insipidus have not been established.

ADVERSE REACTIONS

Infrequently, DDAVP has produced transient headache, nausea, mild abdominal cramps and vulval pain. These symptoms disappeared with reduction in dosage. Occasionally, injection of DDAVP has produced local erythema, swelling or burning pain. Occasional facial flushing has been reported with the administration of DDAVP.

DDAVP has infrequently produced a slight elevation of blood pressure, which disappeared with a reduction in dosage.

See WARNING for the possibility of water intoxication and hyponatremia.

OVERDOSAGE

See ADVERSE REACTIONS above. In case of overdosage, the dosage should be reduced, frequency of administration decreased, or the drug withdrawn according to the severity of the condition.

There is no known specific antidote for DDAVP. An oral LD_{50} has not been established. An intravenous dose of 2 mg/kg in mice demonstrated no effect.

DOSAGE AND ADMINISTRATION

Hemophilia A and von Willebrand's Disease (Type I)

DDAVP® Injection is administered as an intravenous infusion at a dose of 0.3 mcg DDAVP/kg body weight diluted in sterile physiological saline and infused slowly over 15 to 30 minutes. In adults and children weighing more than 10 kg, 50 ml of diluent is used; in children weighing 10 kg or less, 10 ml of diluent is used. Blood pressure and pulse should be monitored during infusion. If DDAVP® Injection is used preoperatively, it should be administered 30 minutes prior to the scheduled procedure.

The necessity for repeat administration of DDAVP or use of any blood products for hemostasis should be determined by laboratory response as well as the clinical condition of the patient. The tendency toward tachyphylaxis (lessening of response) with repeated administration given more frequently than every 48 hours should be considered in treating each patient.

Diabetes Insipidus

This formulation is administered subcutaneously or by direct intravenous injection. DDAVP® Injection (desmopressin acetate) dosage must be determined for each patient and adjusted according to the pattern of response. Response should be estimated by two parameters: adequate duration of sleep and adequate, not excessive, water turnover.

The usual dosage range in adults is 0.5 ml (2.0 mcg) to 1 ml (4.0 mcg) daily, administered intravenously or subcutaneously, usually in two divided doses. The morning and evening doses should be separately adjusted for an adequate diurnal rhythm of water turnover. For patients who have been controlled on intranasal DDAVP and who must be switched to the injection form, either because of poor intranasal absorption or because of the need for surgery, the comparable antidiuretic dose of the injection is about one-tenth the intranasal dose.

Parenteral drug products should be inspected visually for particulate matter and discoloration prior to administration whenever solution and container permit.

HOW SUPPLIED

DDAVP® Injection (desmopressin acetate) is available as a sterile solution in cartons of ten 1 ml single-dose ampules (NDC 0075-2451-01) and in 10 ml multiple-dose vials (NDC 0075-2451-53), each containing 4.0 mcg DDAVP per ml. Keep refrigerated at about 4°C.

CAUTION: Federal (U.S.A.) law prohibits dispensing without prescription.
Rev. 6/88

Manufactured for
RORER PHARMACEUTICALS
a division of
RORER PHARMACEUTICAL CORPORATION
Fort Washington, PA. U.S.A. 19034
By Ferring Pharmaceuticals, Malmö, Sweden

DDAVP® Nasal Spray   ℞
(desmopressin acetate)

DDAVP® [Intranasal]   ℞
(desmopressin acetate)

COMBINED PRODUCT OVERVIEW

KEY FACTS

DDAVP® is an antidiuretic hormone affecting renal water conservation and is a synthetic analogue of 8-arginine vasopressin. DDAVP Nasal Spray and DDAVP [intranasal] are each provided as a sterile, aqueous solution for intranasal use only.

MAJOR USES

DDAVP is indicated as antidiuretic replacement therapy in the management of central cranial Diabetes Insipidus and for temporary polyuria and polydipsia following head trauma or surgery in the pituitary region. DDVAP is not effective for the treatment of nephrogenic diabetes insipidus.

Continued on next page

This product information was prepared in September, 1989. Information concerning these products may be obtained by addressing Rorer Pharmaceutical Corporation, 500 Virginia Drive, Fort Washington, PA 19034.

Rorer Pharm.—Cont.

SAFETY INFORMATION

Patients who do not have need of antidiuretic hormone for its antidiuretic effect (i.e. those who are young or elderly) should be cautioned to ingest only enough fluid to satisfy thirst, in order to decrease the potential occurrence of water intoxication and hyponatremia.

DDAVP® Nasal Spray
(desmopressin acetate)   ℞

DDAVP® [Intranasal]
(desmopressin acetate)   ℞
COMBINED PRESCRIBING INFORMATION

DESCRIPTION

DDAVP (desmopressin acetate) is an antidiuretic hormone affecting renal water conservation and a synthetic analogue of 8-arginine vasopressin. It is chemically defined as follows:
Mol. Wt. 1183.2
Empirical formula: $C_{48}H_{74}N_{14}O_{17}S_2$
$SCH_2CH_2CO-Tyr-Phe-Gln-Asn-Cys-Pro-D-Arg-Gly-NH_2 \cdot$

$C_2H_4O_2 \cdot 3H_2O$
1-(3-mercaptopropionic acid)-8-D-arginine vasopressin monoacetate (salt) trihydrate.
DDAVP Nasal Spray (desmopressin acetate) and DDAVP [intranasal] (desmopressin acetate) are each provided as a sterile, aqueous solution for intranasal use. Each mL contains:

Desmopressin acetate .... 0.1 mg
Chlorobutanol .... 5.0 mg
Sodium chloride .... 9.0 mg
Hydrochloric acid to adjust pH to approximately 4
The DDAVP compression pump delivers 0.1 mL (10 mcg) of DDAVP per spray.

CLINICAL PHARMACOLOGY

DDAVP contains as active substance, 1-(3-mercaptopropionic acid)-8-D-arginine vasopressin, which is a synthetic analogue of the natural hormone arginine vasopressin. One mL (0.1 mg) of DDAVP has an antidiuretic activity of about 400 IU: 10 mcg is equivalent to 40 IU.

1. The biphasic half-lives of DDAVP were 7.8 and 75.5 minutes for the fast and slow phases, compared with 2.5 and 14.5 minutes for lysine vasopressin, another form of the hormone used in this condition. As a result, DDAVP provides a prompt onset of antidiuretic action with a long duration after each administration.
2. The change in structure of arginine vasopressin to DDAVP has resulted in a decreased vasopressor action and decreased actions on visceral smooth muscle relative to the enhanced antidiuretic activity, so that clinically effective antidiuretic doses are usually below threshold levels for effects on vascular or visceral smooth muscle.
3. DDAVP administered intranasally has an antidiuretic effect about one-tenth that of an equivalent dose administered by injection.

INDICATIONS AND USAGE

DDAVP is indicated as antidiuretic replacement therapy in the management of central cranial Diabetes Insipidus and for the management of the temporary polyuria and polydipsia following head trauma or surgery in the pituitary region. DDAVP is ineffective for the treatment of nephrogenic Diabetes Insipidus.

The use of DDAVP Nasal Spray or DDAVP [intranasal] in patients with an established diagnosis will result in a reduction in urinary output with increase in urine osmolality and a decrease in plasma osmolality. This will allow the resumption of a more normal life-style with a decrease in urinary frequency and nocturia.

There are reports of an occasional change in response to DDAVP Nasal Spray or DDAVP [intranasal] with time, usually greater than 6 months. Some patients may show a decreased responsiveness, others a shortened duration of effect. There is no evidence this effect is due to the development of binding antibodies but may be due to a local inactivation of the peptide.

Patients are selected for therapy by establishing the diagnosis by means of the water deprivation test, the hypertonic saline infusion test, and/or the response to antidiuretic hormone. Continued response to DDAVP can be monitored by urine volume and osmolality.

DDAVP is also available as a solution for injection when the intranasal route may be compromised. These situations include nasal congestion and blockage, nasal discharge, atrophy of nasal mucosa, and severe atrophic rhinitis. Intranasal delivery may also be inappropriate where there is an impaired level of consciousness. In addition, cranial surgical procedures, such as transphenoidal hypophysectomy, create situations where an alternative route of administration is needed as in cases of nasal packing or recovery from surgery.

CONTRAINDICATION
Known hypersensitivity to DDAVP.

WARNINGS
1. For intranasal use only.
2. In very young and elderly patients in particular, fluid intake should be adjusted in order to decrease the potential occurrence of water intoxication and hyponatremia.

PRECAUTIONS
General: DDAVP Nasal Spray and DDAVP [intranasal] at high dosage have infrequently produced a slight elevation of blood pressure, which disappeared with a reduction in dosage. The drug should be used with caution in patients with coronary artery insufficiency and/or hypertensive cardiovascular disease, because of possible rise in blood pressure. Since DDAVP is used intranasally, changes in the nasal mucosa such as scarring, edema, or other disease may cause erratic, unreliable absorption in which case intranasal DDAVP should not be used. For such situations, DDAVP Injection should be considered.

INFORMATION FOR PATIENTS: Patients should be informed that the DDAVP Nasal Spray bottle accurately delivers 50 doses of 10 mcg each. Any solution remaining after 50 doses should be discarded since the amount delivered thereafter may be substantially less than 10 mcg of drug. No attempt should be made to transfer remaining solution to another bottle. Patients should be instructed to read accompanying directions on use of the spray pump carefully before use.

LABORATORY TESTS: Laboratory tests for following the patient include urine volume and osmolality. In some cases, plasma osmolality may be required.

DRUG INTERACTIONS: Although the pressor activity of DDAVP is very low compared to the antidiuretic activity, use of large doses of DDAVP with other pressor agents should be done only with careful patient monitoring.

CARCINOGENESIS, MUTAGENESIS, IMPAIRMENT OF FERTILITY: Teratology studies in rats have shown no abnormalities. No further information is available.

PREGNANCY CATEGORY B: Reproduction studies performed in rats and rabbits with subcutaneous doses up to 12.5 times the human intranasal dose (i.e. about 125 times the total adult human dose given systemically) have revealed no evidence of harm to the fetus due to desmopressin acetate. There are several publications of management of Diabetes Insipidus in pregnant women with no harm to the fetus reported; however, no controlled studies in pregnant women have been carried out. Published reports stress that, as opposed to preparations containing the natural hormones, DDAVP in antidiuretic doses has no uterotonic action, but the physician will have to weigh possible therapeutic advantages against possible danger in each individual case.

NURSING MOTHERS: There have been no controlled studies in nursing mothers. A single study in a post-partum woman demonstrated a marked change in plasma, but little if any change in assayable DDAVP in breast milk following an intranasal dose of 10 mcg.

PEDIATRIC USE: DDAVP Nasal Spray and DDAVP [intranasal] have been used in children with Diabetes Insipidus. Use in infants and children will require careful fluid intake restrictions to prevent possible hyponatremia and water intoxication. The dose must be individually adjusted to the patient with attention in the very young to the danger of an extreme decrease in plasma osmolality with resulting convulsions. Dose should start at 0.05 mL or less.
Since the spray cannot deliver less than 0.1 mL (10 mcg), smaller doses should be administered using the nasal tube delivery system. Do not use the nasal spray in pediatric patients requiring less than 0.1 mL (10 mcg) per dose.
There are reports of an occasional change in response to DDAVP Nasal Spray or DDAVP [intranasal] with time, usually greater than 6 months. Some patients may show a decreased responsiveness, others a shortened duration of effect. There is no evidence this effect is due to the development of binding antibodies but may be due to a local inactivation of the peptide.

ADVERSE REACTIONS
Infrequently, high dosages of DDAVP Nasal Spray or DDAVP [intranasal] have produced transient headache and nausea. Nasal congestion, rhinitis and flushing have also been reported occasionally along with mild abdominal cramps. These symptoms disappeared with reduction in dosage.

OVERDOSAGE
See ADVERSE REACTIONS above. In case of overdosage, the dose should be reduced, frequency of administration decreased, or the drug withdrawn according to the severity of the condition.

There is no known specific antidote for DDAVP.
An oral LD_{50} has not been established. An intravenous dose of 2 mg/kg in mice demonstrated no effect.

DOSAGE AND ADMINISTRATION

DDAVP dosage must be determined for each individual patient and adjusted according to the diurnal pattern of response. Response should be estimated by two parameters, adequate duration of sleep and adequate, not excessive, water turnover. Patients with nasal congestion and blockage have often responded well to DDAVP. The nasal spray pump can only deliver doses of 0.1 mL (10 mcg) or multiples of 0.1 mL. If doses other than these are required, the nasal tube delivery system may be used. DDAVP [intranasal] is administered into the nose through a soft flexible plastic nasal tube that has four graduation marks on it that measure 0.2, 0.15, 0.1, and 0.05 mL. The usual dosage range in adults is 0.1 to 0.4 mL daily, either as a single dose or divided into two or three doses. Most adults require 0.2 mL daily in two divided doses. The morning and evening doses should be separately adjusted for an adequate diurnal rhythm of water turnover. For children aged 3 months to 12 years, the usual dosage range is 0.05 to 0.3 mL daily, either as a single dose or divided into two doses. About one-quarter to one-third of patients can be controlled by a single daily dose of DDAVP administered intranasally.

HOW SUPPLIED

DDAVP Nasal Spray is available in a bottle with spray pump delivering 50 doses of 10 mcg (NDC 0075-2450-02).
DDAVP [intranasal] 2.5 mL per vial is packaged with two applicator tubes per carton (NDC 0075-2450-01). Keep refrigerated at about 36°–46°F (2°–8°C). When traveling, product will maintain stability for up to 3 weeks when stored in a closed sterile bottle at room temperature, 72°F (22°C).

CAUTION
Federal (USA) law prohibits dispensing without prescription.
DDAVP®
Manufactured for:
RORER PHARMACEUTICALS
a division of
RORER PHARMACEUTICAL CORPORATION
Fort Washington, PA, U.S.A. 19034
By: Ferring Pharmaceuticals, Malmö, Sweden
Shown in Product Identification Section, page 426

DEMI–REGROTON®   ℞
[děm "ē-rěg 'rō-tŏn]
Oral antihypertensive

See under Regroton®.
RORER PHARMACEUTICALS
a division of
RORER PHARMACEUTICAL CORPORATION
Fort Washington, PA, U.S.A. 19034
Shown in Product Identification Section, page 426

DORIDEN®   ⓒIII
[dôr 'ĭ-dĭn "]
glutethimide USP

0.5 g tablets
0.25 g tablets

PRODUCT OVERVIEW

KEY FACTS
Doriden (glutethimide), an oral hypnotic, is a piperidinedione derivative that occurs as a white, crystalline powder and is practically insoluble in water, soluble in alcohol. This drug is controlled in Schedule III.

MAJOR USE
Glutethimide has been shown to be effective as a hypnotic for three to seven days. It is not indicated for chronic administration. Should insomnia persist, a drug-free interval of one or more weeks should elapse before retreatment is considered.

SAFETY INFORMATION
The patient should be warned about the possible additive effects when glutethimide is taken concomitantly with other central nervous system depressants such as alcohol. The patient on Doriden must be warned against driving a car or operating dangerous machinery while on the drug, since glutethimide may impair the ability to perform hazardous activities requiring mental alertness or physical coordination.

PRESCRIBING INFORMATION

DORIDEN®   Ⓒ
[*dôr'ĭ-dĭn''*]
(glutethimide, USP)

0.5 g tablets
0.25 g tablets

DESCRIPTION

DORIDEN (glutethimide), an oral hypnotic, is a piperidine-dione derivative that occurs as a white, crystalline powder and is practically insoluble in water, soluble in alcohol. Its chemical name is 2-ethyl-2-phenylglutarimide with the following structural formula:

The tablets also contain starch, magnesium aluminum silicate, methylcellulose, colloidal silica, and stearic acid.

CLINICAL PHARMACOLOGY

Doriden is erratically absorbed from the gastrointestinal tract. Following single oral doses of 500 mg, wide variations in absorption of the drug were observed, and the peak plasma concentration occurred from one to six hours after administration. The average plasma half-life is 10–12 hours. Glutethimide is a racemate; both isomers are hydroxylated; the d-isomer on the piperidinedione ring and the l-isomer on the phenyl substituent. Both hydroxylates are conjugated with glucuronic acid; the glucuronides pass into the enterohepatic circulation, and thence are excreted in the urine. Less than 2% of a usual dose is excreted in the urine unchanged. About 50% of the drug is bound to plasma proteins. Glutethimide exhibits pronounced anticholinergic activity, which is manifested by mydriasis, inhibition of salivary secretions, and decreased intestinal motility.

INDICATIONS AND USAGE

Glutethimide has been shown to be effective as a hypnotic for three to seven days. It is not indicated for chronic administration. Should insomnia persist, a drug-free interval of one or more weeks should elapse before retreatment is considered. Attempts should be made to find alternative nondrug therapy in chronic insomnia.

CONTRAINDICATIONS

Glutethimide is contraindicated in patients with known hypersensitivity to the drug. It is also contraindicated in patients with porphyria.

WARNINGS

The concomitant use of alcohol or other CNS depressants may produce additive CNS depressant effects.

PRECAUTIONS

Information for Patients: The patient should be warned about the possible additive effects when glutethimide is taken concomitantly with other central nervous system depressants such as alcohol.

The patient on Doriden must be warned against driving a car or operating dangerous machinery while on the drug, since glutethimide may impair the ability to perform hazardous activities requiring mental alertness or physical coordination.

Drug Interactions: Glutethimide induces hepatic microsomal enzymes resulting in increased metabolism of coumarin anticoagulants and decreased anticoagulant response.

Carcinogenesis: No carcinogenicity studies in animals have been performed.

Pregnancy/Teratogenic Effects: *Pregnancy Category C.* Animal reproduction studies have not been conducted with glutethimide. It is also not known *whether glutethimide can cause fetal harm when administered to a pregnant woman or can affect reproduction capacity. Glutethimide should be given to a pregnant woman only if clearly needed.*

Nursing Mothers: Because of the potential for serious adverse reactions in nursing infants from glutethimide, a decision should be made whether to discontinue nursing or to discontinue the drug, taking into account the importance of the drug to the mother.

Pediatric Use: Glutethimide is not recommended for use in children, because its safety and effectiveness in the pediatric age group have not been established by clinical trials.

ADVERSE REACTIONS

In clinical studies in more than 796 patients, 8.6% exhibited skin rash, 2.7% reported nausea, 1.1% hangover, and 1% reported drowsiness. The following reactions occurred in less than 1% of the patient population: vertigo, headache, depression, dizziness, ataxia, confusion, edema, indigestion, lightheadedness, nocturnal diaphoresis, vomiting, dry mouth, euphoria, impaired memory, slurred speech, and tinnitus. Paradoxical excitation, blurred vision, acute hypersensitivity, porphyria, and blood dyscrasia such as thrombocytopenic purpura, aplastic anemia, and leukopenia are rare.

In cases in which a generalized skin rash occurs, the medication should be withdrawn. This rash usually clears spontaneously within a few days after drug withdrawal.

DRUG ABUSE AND DEPENDENCE

Controlled Substance: This drug is controlled in Schedule III.

Dependence: Both physical and psychological dependence have occurred; therefore patients should be carefully evaluated before prescribing Doriden. Ordinarily, an amount adequate for one week is sufficient. The patient should be reevaluated before represcribing, after an interval of one or more weeks. Withdrawal symptoms include nausea, abdominal discomfort, tremors, convulsions, and delirium. Newborn infants of mothers dependent on glutethimide may also exhibit withdrawal symptoms. In the presence of dependence, dosage should be reduced gradually.

OVERDOSAGE

Acute Overdosage: The single acute lethal dose of glutethimide in humans ranges from 10 g to 20 g. Although the majority of fatalities have resulted from single doses in this range, patients have died from single doses as low as 5 g and have recovered from single doses as high as 35 g. A single oral dose of 5 g usually produces severe intoxication. A plasma level of 3 mg/100 mL is indicative of severe poisoning, but the level may be higher if the patient is tolerant to the drug. However, the level may also be lower because of sequestration of the drug in body fat depots and in the gastrointestinal tract. A lower level does not preclude the possibility of severe poisoning; therefore, the extent of intoxication may not be accurately reflected by single glutethimide plasma level determinations. Serial determinations are mandatory for proper patient evaluation.

Ingestion of acutely excessive dosage of glutethimide can give rise to a life-threatening situation. The effects of glutethimide are exaggerated by concomitant ingestion of other hypnotics or sedatives such as alcohol, barbiturates, etc., and suicidal effects commonly involve multiple drugs of the sedative-hypnotic-tranquilizer types.

Signs and Symptoms: The principal signs and symptoms caused by glutethimide intoxication vary in severity in ratio to the ingested dosage, in general, and are indistinguishable from those caused by barbiturate intoxication. The degree of CNS depression often fluctuates, possibly due to irregular absorption of the drug and/or accumulation of an active toxic metabolite, 4-hydroxy-2-ethyl-2-phenyl-glutarimide (4-HG). They are: CNS depression, including coma *(profound and prolonged in severe intoxication);* hypothermia, which may be followed by fever even without apparent infection; depressed or lost deep tendon reflexes; depression or absence of corneal and pupillary reflexes; dilation of pupils; depressed or absent response to painful stimuli; inadequate ventilation (even with relatively normal respiratory rate), sometimes with cyanosis; sudden apnea, especially with manipulation such as gastric lavage or endotracheal intubation; diminished or absent peristalsis. Severe hypotension unresponsive to volume expansion, tonic muscular spasms, twitching and convulsions may occur.

Treatment: As with all forms of acute intoxication, the sooner adequate treatment is instituted, the better the prognosis. Early and vigorous cardiopulmonary supportive measures should be employed and should include:

1) Maintenance of a patent airway with assisted ventilation if necessary.

2) Monitoring of vital signs and level of consciousness.

3) Continuous electrocardiogram to detect arrhythmias.

4) Maintenance of blood pressure with plasma volume expanders and, if absolutely essential, pressor drugs.

Blood for glutethimide levels and other chemical determinations should be obtained as well as arterial blood for blood gas determinations.

Vomiting should be induced if the patient is fully conscious. Gastric lavage should be done in all cases regardless of elapsed time since drug ingestion, with due caution to prevent aspiration of gastric contents or respiratory arrest during manipulation, including prior insertion of a cuffed endotracheal tube or employment of tracheostomy. Lavage with a 1:1 mixture of castor oil and water is capable of removing larger amounts of glutethimide from the stomach than with aqueous lavage. Fifty mL of castor oil should be left in the stomach as a cathartic.

Intestinal lavage is used to remove unabsorbed Doriden (glutethimide) from the intestines (100–250 mL of 20–40% sorbitol or mannitol). If emesis or gastric lavage cannot be effected in the fully conscious patient, delay absorption of Doriden by giving one pint of water, milk or fruit juice; flour or cornstarch suspension, or activated charcoal in water. Follow up as soon as possible with production of emesis or gastric lavage.

Adequate respiratory gas exchange must be maintained and may require tracheostomy and mechanical assistance. If coma is prolonged, urine output must be monitored and maintained while preventing overhydration which might contribute to pulmonary or cerebral edema.

In *Severe Intoxication,* in addition to intensive supportive measures and symptomatic care, consideration should be given to dialysis or hemoperfusion in the following circumstances: Grade III or Grade IV coma, but the level of coma per se is not a mandatory indication for the procedure. Hemodialysis may also be required when renal shutdown or impaired renal function are manifest and in life-threatening overdose situations complicated by (a) pulmonary edema, (b) heart failure, (c) circulatory collapse, (d) significant liver disease, (e) major metabolic disturbance, (f) uremia. While aqueous hemodialysis is less effective for glutethimide than for readily water-soluble compounds that are not bound by proteins or sequestered in body fat depots, glutethimide blood levels may decline more rapidly with hemodialysis and the duration of coma may be shortened; efficacy of the procedure, however, is largely controversial. As long as significant amounts of glutethimide remain in fat depots or as an unabsorbed bolus in the intestinal tract, the fall in serum level accelerated by hemodialysis may be followed by increased absorption into the bloodstream on termination of dialysis and may require further dialysis.

Recent clinical data indicate that use of pure food-grade soybean oil as the dialysate enhances removal of glutethimide and some other lipid-soluble substances by means of hemodialysis. Peritoneal dialysis, while able to remove some glutethimide, apparently is of minimal value.

Hemoperfusion appears to be a promising technique for eliminating glutethimide from the body. Charcoal hemoperfusion utilizing acrylic hydrogel microencapsulation of activated charcoal has been reported to be simpler and more effective than hemodialysis. Similarly, a microcapsule artificial kidney has been developed utilizing activated charcoal granules encapsulated with cellulose nitrate and albumin. *Resin* hemoperfusion utilizing a column containing Amberlite XAD-2 has demonstrated exceptionally high clearance capabilities in glutethimide intoxication and has been reported to be clinically superior to hemodialysis in patients with profound life-threatening coma and potentially lethal blood concentrations of intoxicant drugs.

Drug extraction techniques should be continued for at least two hours after the patient regains consciousness. Glutethimide is highly lipid soluble and therefore, rapidly accumulated in lipoid tissue. As the drug is removed from the bloodstream by any technique, it is gradually released from fat storage depots back into the bloodstream. Even after substantial quantities of the drug have been extracted, this blood-level rebound can cause coma to persist or recur.

As in the case of any prolonged coma, appropriate antibiotic therapy is indicated if pulmonary or other infection intervenes.

Chronic Overdosage: Signs and symptoms of chronic glutethimide intoxication (and for all drugs producing barbiturate-alcohol type of dependence in chronic overdosage) include impairment of memory and ability to concentrate, impaired speech, ataxia, tremors, hyporeflexia, and slurring of speech. Abrupt discontinuance of glutethimide after prolonged overdosage will in most cases cause withdrawal reactions ranging from nervousness and anxiety to grand mal seizures, and may include abdominal cramping, chills, numbness of extremities, and dysphagia.

Treatment: Chronic glutethimide intoxication may be treated by gradual, stepwise reduction of dosage over a period of days or weeks. Watch patient carefully. If withdrawal reactions occur, they can be controlled by readministration of glutethimide, or substitution of pentobarbital, and subsequent gradual withdrawal.

DOSAGE AND ADMINISTRATION

For use as a hypnotic, dosage should be individualized. The usual adult dosage is 0.25 to 0.5 g at bedtime. For elderly or debilitated patients, the initial daily dosage should not exceed 0.5 g at bedtime, in order to avoid oversedation.

HOW SUPPLIED

DORIDEN tablets are identified as follows: 0.25 g—white, scored and imprinted with USV and 353. 0.5g—white, scored and imprinted with USV and 354. Doriden tablets (0.25 g) are available in bottles of 100 (NDC 0075-0353-00). 0.5 g are available in bottles of 100 (NDC 0075-0354-00).

Keep tightly closed. Store at room temperature; avoid excessive heat. Dispense in tight container as defined in USP.

Continued on next page

This product information was prepared in September, 1989. Information concerning these products may be obtained by addressing Rorer Pharmaceutical Corporation, 500 Virginia Drive, Fort Washington, PA 19034.

Rorer Pharm.—Cont.

CAUTION

Federal (U.S.A.) law prohibits dispensing without prescription.
Revised: 4/88
RORER PHARMACEUTICALS
a division of
RORER PHARMACEUTICAL CORPORATION
Fort Washington, PA, U.S.A. 19034

HISTASPAN-D®　　　　　　　　　　　　　℞
[hĭst'ŭ-spăn-dē"]
in sustained-release microdialysis cells

DESCRIPTION

Each Histaspan-D capsule provides 8 mg chlorpheniramine maleate, 20 mg phenylephrine hydrochloride, and 2.5 mg methscopolamine nitrate in sustained-release microdialysis cells, uniquely processed for sustained release of medication to provide prolonged therapeutic effect. Inactive ingredients: calcium silicate, cornstarch, ethylcellulose, gelatin, iron oxide, pharmaceutical glaze, povidone, sucrose, talc, titanium dioxide.

ACTIONS

Histaspan-D combines the highly effective and widely used antihistamine, chlorpheniramine maleate, with a decongestant, phenylephrine hydrochloride, and a drying agent, methscopolamine nitrate, for relief of rhinorrhea, sneezing, lacrimation, nasal congestion, and other respiratory symptoms accompanying the common cold, sinusitis, hay fever and similar allergic conditions. Prolonged therapeutic effect is obtained by sustained release of medication through the microdialysis process.

INDICATIONS

One capsule q 12 h usually provides relief of rhinorrhea, sneezing, lacrimation, itching of eyes and nose, and nasal congestion accompanying upper respiratory infections such as the common cold, sinusitis, hay fever, and similar allergic conditions.

CONTRAINDICATIONS

Hypersensitivity to any component of the drug, glaucoma, paralytic ileus, pyloric obstruction, and prostatic hypertrophy.

PRECAUTIONS

Use with caution in diabetes mellitus, hyperthyroidism, hypertension, cardiovascular disease, debilitated patients with chronic lung disease, in the aged and in children under age 12. Since blurred vision, drowsiness and dizziness may occur, patients should be cautioned about driving or operating machinery.

ADVERSE REACTIONS

May include drowsiness, dizziness, blurred vision, and excessive dryness of the nose, throat, and mouth. Other possible adverse reactions to individual components, infrequently seen, include photophobia, tachycardia, gastrointestinal symptoms, increased irritability or excitement, flushing, incoordination, headache, nervousness, weakness, and urinary disturbances.

ADMINISTRATION AND DOSAGE

Adults and children over age 12, one capsule in the morning and one at night (q 12 h).

CAUTION

Federal (U.S.A.) law prohibits dispensing without prescription.

HOW SUPPLIED

Bottles of 100 capsules (NDC 0075-0132-00).
Revised: June 1988
RORER PHARMACEUTICALS
a division of
RORER PHARMACEUTICAL CORPORATION
Fort Washington, PA, U.S.A. 19034

HISTASPAN®-PLUS　　　　　　　　　　℞
[hĭst'ŭ-spăn-plŭs"]
in sustained-release microdialysis cells

DESCRIPTION

Each Histaspan-Plus capsule provides 8 mg chlorpheniramine maleate and 20 mg phenylephrine hydrochloride in sustained-release microdialysis cells, uniquely processed for sustained release of medication to provide prolonged therapeutic effect. Inactive ingredients: calcium silicate, cornstarch, gelatin, pharmaceutical glaze, povidone, sucrose, talc, titanium dioxide, yellow 6, and other coloring agents.

INDICATIONS

Antihistaminic and decongestant for relief of nasal congestion and other respiratory symptoms accompanying the common cold, sinusitis, hay fever and similar allergic conditions.

CONTRAINDICATION

Hypersensitivity to any component of the drug.

PRECAUTIONS

Use with caution in diabetes mellitus, hyperthyroidism, hypertension and cardiovascular disease. Since blurred vision, drowsiness or dizziness may occur, patients should be cautioned about driving or operating machinery.

ADVERSE REACTIONS

May include drowsiness, dizziness, blurred vision, dry mouth, disturbed coordination, G.I. disturbance, tachycardia, headache, nervousness, weakness, and urinary disturbances.

DOSAGE

Adults and children over age 12, one capsule every 12 hours. Keep tightly closed. Store at controlled room temperature—15°–30°C (59°–86°F).
Dispense in tight containers as defined in USP.

CAUTION

Federal (U.S.A.) law prohibits dispensing without prescription.

HOW SUPPLIED

Bottles of 100.
5/86
RORER PHARMACEUTICALS
a division of
RORER PHARMACEUTICAL CORPORATION
Fort Washington, PA, U.S.A. 19034

HYGROTON®　　　　　　　　　　　　℞
[hĭ'grō-tŏn"]
(chlorthalidone, USP)
25 mg tablets
50 mg tablets
100 mg tablets
Oral antihypertensive/diuretic

DESCRIPTION

HYGROTON (chlorthalidone) is an oral antihypertensive/diuretic. It is a monosulfamyl diuretic that differs chemically from thiazide diuretics in that a double-ring system is incorporated in its structure. It is 2-chloro-5-(1-hydroxy-3-oxo-1-isoindolinyl) benzenesulfonamide, with the following structural formula:

Chlorthalidone is practically insoluble in water, in ether, and in chloroform; soluble in methanol; slightly soluble in alcohol.
HYGROTON tablets also contain colloidal silica, cornstarch, gelatin, glycerin, lactose, magnesium stearate, talc, and other ingredients. The 25 mg tablets also contain Yellow 6, methylparaben, and propylparaben. The 50 mg tablets also contain F.D.&C. Blue #1, methylparaben, and propylparaben.

CLINICAL PHARMACOLOGY

HYGROTON is an oral diuretic with prolonged action (48–72 hours) and low toxicity. The major portion of the drug is excreted unchanged by the kidneys. The diuretic effect of the drug occurs in approximately 2.6 hours and continues for up to 72 hours. The mean half-life following a 50 to 200 mg dose is 40 hours. In the first order of absorption, the elimination half-life is 53 hours following a 50 mg dose, and 60 hours following a 100 mg dose. Approximately 75 percent of the drug is bound to plasma proteins, 58 percent of the drug being bound to albumin. This is caused by an increased affinity of the drug to erythrocyte carbonic anhydrase. Nonrenal routes of elimination have yet to be clarified. Data are not available regarding percentage of dose as unchanged drug and metabolites, concentration of the drug in body fluids, degree of uptake by a particular organ or in the fetus, or passage across the blood-brain barrier.
The drug produces copious diuresis with greatly increased excretion of sodium and chloride. At maximal therapeutic dosage, chlorthalidone is approximately equal in its diuretic effect to comparable maximal therapeutic doses of benzothiadiazine diuretics. The site of action appears to be the cortical diluting segment of the ascending limb of Henle's loop of the nephron.

ANIMAL PHARMACOLOGY

Biochemical studies in animals have suggested reasons for the prolonged effect of chlorthalidone. Absorption from the gastrointestinal tract is slow, due to its low solubility. After passage to the liver, some of the drug enters the general circulation, while some is excreted in the bile, to be reabsorbed later. In the general circulation, it is distributed widely to the tissues, but is taken up in highest concentrations by the kidneys, where amounts have been found 72 hours after ingestion, long after it has disappeared from other tissues. The drug is excreted unchanged in the urine.

INDICATIONS AND USAGE

Diuretics such as HYGROTON are indicated in the management of hypertension either as the sole therapeutic agent or to enhance the effect of other antihypertensive drugs in the more severe forms of hypertension.
HYGROTON is indicated as adjunctive therapy in edema associated with congestive heart failure, hepatic cirrhosis, and corticosteroid and estrogen therapy.
HYGROTON has also been found useful in edema due to various forms of renal dysfunction such as nephrotic syndrome, acute glomerulonephritis, and chronic renal failure.
USAGE IN PREGNANCY: The routine use of diuretics in an otherwise healthy woman is inappropriate and exposes mother and fetus to unnecessary hazard. Diuretics do not prevent development of toxemia of pregnancy, and there is no satisfactory evidence that they are useful in the treatment of developed toxemia.
Edema during pregnancy may arise from pathological causes or from the physiologic and mechanical consequences of pregnancy. Chlorthalidone is indicated in pregnancy when edema is due to pathologic causes, just as it is in the absence of pregnancy (however, see Warnings, below). Dependent edema in pregnancy, resulting from restriction of venous return by the expanded uterus, is properly treated through elevation of the lower extremities and use of support hose; use of diuretics to lower intravascular volume in this case is illogical and unnecessary. There is hypervolemia during normal pregnancy that is harmful to neither the fetus nor the mother (in the absence of cardiovascular disease), but that is associated with edema, including generalized edema, in the majority of pregnant women. If this edema produces discomfort, increased recumbency will often provide relief. In rare instances, this edema may cause extreme discomfort that is not relieved by rest. In these cases, a short course of diuretics may provide relief and may be appropriate.

CONTRAINDICATIONS

Anuria.
Known hypersensitivity to chlorthalidone or other sulfonamide-derived drugs.

WARNINGS

Chlorthalidone should be used with caution in severe renal disease. In patients with renal disease, chlorthalidone or related drugs may precipitate azotemia. Cumulative effects of the drug may develop in patients with impaired renal function.
Chlorthalidone should be used with caution in patients with impaired hepatic function or progressive liver disease, because minor alterations of fluid and electrolyte balance may precipitate hepatic coma.
Sensitivity reactions may occur in patients with a history of allergy or bronchial asthma.
The possibility of exacerbation or activation of systemic lupus erythematosus has been reported with thiazide diuretics, which are structurally related to chlorthalidone. However, systemic lupus erythematosus has not been reported following chlorthalidone administration.

PRECAUTIONS

GENERAL: Hypokalemia may develop with chlorthalidone as with any other potent diuretic, especially with brisk diuresis, when severe cirrhosis is present, or during concomitant use of corticosteroids or ACTH.
Interference with adequate oral electrolyte intake will also contribute to hypokalemia. Digitalis therapy may exaggerate metabolic effects of hypokalemia especially with reference to myocardial activity.
Any chloride deficit is generally mild and usually does not require specific treatment except under extraordinary circumstances (as in liver disease or renal disease). Dilutional hyponatremia may occur in edematous patients in hot weather; appropriate therapy is water restriction, rather than administration of salt except in rare instances when the hyponatremia is life threatening. In actual salt depletion, appropriate replacement is the therapy of choice.
Hyperuricemia may occur or frank gout may be precipitated in certain patients receiving chlorthalidone.
The antihypertensive effects of the drug may be enhanced in the postsympathectomy patient.
If progressive renal impairment becomes evident, as indicated by a rising nonprotein nitrogen or blood urea nitrogen, a careful reappraisal of therapy is necessary with consideration given to withholding or discontinuing diuretic therapy.
INFORMATION FOR PATIENTS: Patients should inform their doctor if they have: 1) had an allergic reaction to HYGROTON or other diuretics or have asthma 2) kidney

disease 3) liver disease 4) gout 5) systemic lupus erythematosus, or 6) been taking other drugs such as cortisone, digitalis, lithium carbonate, or drugs for diabetes.

Patients should be cautioned to contact their physician if they experience any of the following symptoms of potassium loss: excess thirst, tiredness, drowsiness, restlessness, muscle pains or cramps, nausea, vomiting or increased heart rate or pulse.

Patients should also be cautioned that taking alcohol can increase the chance of dizziness occurring.

LABORATORY TESTS: Periodic determination of serum electrolytes to detect possible electrolyte imbalance should be performed at appropriate intervals.

All patients receiving chlorthalidone should be observed for clinical signs of fluid or electrolyte imbalance: namely, hyponatremia, hypochloremic alkalosis, and hypokalemia. Serum and urine electrolyte determinations are particularly important when the patient is vomiting excessively or receiving parenteral fluids.

DRUG INTERACTIONS: Chlorthalidone may add to or potentiate the action of other antihypertensive drugs. Potentiation occurs with ganglionic or peripheral adrenergic blocking drugs.

Medication such as digitalis may also influence serum electrolytes. Warning signs, irrespective of cause, are: Dryness of mouth, thirst, weakness, lethargy, drowsiness, restlessness, muscle pains or cramps, muscular fatigue, hypotension, oliguria, tachycardia, and gastrointestinal disturbances such as nausea and vomiting.

Insulin requirements in diabetic patients may be increased, decreased, or unchanged. Higher dosage of oral hypoglycemic agents may be required. Latent diabetes mellitus may become manifest during chlorthalidone administration.

Chlorthalidone and related drugs may increase the responsiveness to tubocurarine.

Chlorthalidone and related drugs may decrease arterial responsiveness to norepinephrine. This diminution is not sufficient to preclude effectiveness of the pressor agent for therapeutic use.

DRUG/LABORATORY TEST INTERACTIONS: Chlorthalidone and related drugs may decrease serum PBI levels without signs of thyroid disturbance.

CARCINOGENESIS, MUTAGENESIS, IMPAIRMENT OF FERTILITY: No information is available.

PREGNANCY/TERATOGENIC EFFECTS: Pregnancy Category B: Reproduction studies have been performed in the rat and the rabbit at doses up to 420 times the human dose and have revealed no evidence of impaired fertility or harm to the fetus due to chlorthalidone. There are, however, no adequate and well-controlled studies in pregnant women. Because animal reproduction studies are not always predictive of human response, this drug should be used during pregnancy only if clearly needed.

PREGNANCY/NON-TERATOGENIC EFFECTS: Thiazides cross the placental barrier and appear in cord blood. The use of chlorthalidone and related drugs in pregnant women requires that the anticipated benefits of the drug be weighed against possible hazards to the fetus. These hazards include fetal or neonatal jaundice, thrombocytopenia, and possibly other adverse reactions that have occurred in the adult.

NURSING MOTHERS: Thiazides are excreted in human milk. Because of the potential for serious adverse reactions in nursing infants from chlorthalidone, a decision should be made whether to discontinue nursing or to discontinue the drug, taking into account the importance of the drug to the mother.

PEDIATRIC USE: Safety and effectiveness in children have not been established.

ADVERSE REACTIONS

The following adverse reactions have been observed, but there is not enough systematic collection of data to support an estimate of their frequency.

Gastrointestinal System Reactions:

anorexia	diarrhea
gastric irritation	constipation
nausea	jaundice (intrahepatic
vomiting	cholestatic jaundice)
cramping	pancreatitis

Central Nervous System Reactions:

dizziness	headache
vertigo	xanthopsia
paresthesias	

Hematologic Reactions:

leukopenia	thrombocytopenia
agranulocytosis	aplastic anemia

Dermatologic-Hypersensitivity Reactions:

purpura	necrotizing angiitis
photosensitivity	(vasculitis)
rash	(cutaneous vasculitis)
urticaria	Lyell's syndrome (toxic
	epidermal necrolysis)

Cardiovascular Reaction: Orthostatic hypotension may occur and may be aggravated by alcohol, barbiturates or narcotics.

Other Adverse Reactions:

hyperglycemia	muscle spasm
glycosuria	weakness
hyperuricemia	restlessness
	impotence

Whenever adverse reactions are moderate or severe, chlorthalidone dosage should be reduced or therapy withdrawn.

OVERDOSAGE

Symptoms of acute overdosage include nausea, weakness, dizziness, and disturbances of electrolyte balance. The oral LD_{50} of the drug in the mouse and the rat is more than 25,000 mg/kg body weight. The minimum lethal dose (MLD) in humans has not been established. There is no specific antidote, but gastric lavage is recommended, followed by supportive treatment. Where necessary, this may include intravenous dextrose-saline with potassium, administered with caution.

DOSAGE AND ADMINISTRATION

Therapy should be initiated with the lowest possible dose. This dose should be titrated according to individual patient response to gain maximal therapeutic benefit while maintaining the minimal dosage possible. A single dose given in the morning with food is recommended; divided doses are unnecessary.

Hypertension: *Initiation:* Therapy, in most patients, should be initiated with a single daily dose of 25 mg. If the response is insufficient after a suitable trial, the dosage may be increased to a single daily dose of 50 mg. If additional control is required, the dosage of HYGROTON (chlorthalidone) may be increased to 100 mg once daily or a second antihypertensive drug (step-2 therapy) may be added. Dosage above 100 mg daily usually does not increase effectiveness. Increases in serum uric acid and decreases in serum potassium are dose-related over the 25–100 mg day range.

Maintenance: Maintenance doses may be lower than initial doses and should be adjusted according to individual patient response. Effectiveness is well sustained during continued use.

Edema: *Initiation:* Adults, initially 50 to 100 mg daily, or 100 mg on alternate days. Some patients may require 150 to 200 mg at these intervals, or up to 200 mg daily. Dosages above this level, however, do not usually produce a greater response.

Maintenance: Maintenance doses may often be lower than initial doses and should be adjusted according to the individual patient. Effectiveness is well sustained during continued use.

HOW SUPPLIED

HYGROTON (chlorthalidone) is available as 25 mg peach-color, uniquely-shaped* tablets in bottles of 100 (NDC 0075-0022-00), 1000 (NDC 0075-0022-99), and unit-dose blister packs, boxes of 100 (10 × 10 strips) (NDC 0075-0022-62); 50 mg aqua, uniquely-shaped* tablets in bottles of 100 (NDC 0075-0020-00), 1000 (NDC 0075-0020-99), and unit-dose blister packs, boxes of 100 (10 × 10 strips) (NDC 0075-0020-62); 100 mg white, single-scored tablets in bottles of 100 (NDC 0075-0021-00). Store at controlled room temperature, 59°-86°F (15°-30°C). Avoid excessive heat. Dispense in tight containers as defined in USP.

*The distinctive design of Hygroton Tablets is patented by Rorer Pharmaceutical Corporation. U.S. Pat. No. Des. 290,412

CAUTION:

Federal (U.S.A.) law prohibits dispensing without prescription.

RORER PHARMACEUTICALS
a division of
RORER PHARMACEUTICAL CORPORATION
Fort Washington, PA, U.S.A. 19034

Shown in Product Identification Section, page 426

LEVOTHROID® TABLETS   ℞
(Levothyroxine Sodium Tablets, U.S.P.)
for oral use

LEVOTHROID® FOR INJECTION   ℞
(Levothyroxine Sodium)
for parenteral use

DESCRIPTION

LEVOTHROID® (Levothyroxine Sodium Tablets, U.S.P.) provides crystalline sodium levothyroxine (T_4), a potent thyroid hormone, in nine different strengths to permit easy convenient dosage adjustment.

The inactive ingredients are microcrystalline cellulose, lactose, magnesium stearate and silica. The tablets also contain the following dyes: 25 mcg—F.D.&C. Red No. 40 and D.&C. Yellow No. 10; 75 mcg—F.D.&C. Blue No. 1, F.D.&C. Red No. 40 and D.&C. Yellow No. 10; 100 mcg—F.D.&C. Red No. 40 and D.&C. Yellow No. 10; 125 mcg—F.D.&C. Blue No. 1 and F.D.&C. Red No. 40; 150 mcg—F.D.&C. Blue No. 1; 175 mcg—F.D.&C. Blue No. 1, F.D.&C. Red No. 40, and D.&C. Yellow No. 10; 200 mcg—F.D.&C. Red No. 40; 300 mcg—F.D.&C. Blue No. 1, F.D.&C. Red No. 40, and D.&C. Yellow No. 10.

LEVOTHROID FOR INJECTION (Levothyroxine Sodium) is a sterile, lyophilized powder supplied in 6 mL vials containing 200 or 500 mcg of levothyroxine sodium U.S.P. with 15 mg of mannitol, U.S.P.

The structural formula for sodium levothyroxine is:

Sodium L-3, 3', 5',-tetraiodothyronine

CLINICAL PHARMACOLOGY

The major thyroid hormones are L-thyroxine (T_4) and L-triiodothyronine (T_3). The amounts of T_4 and T_3 released into the circulation from the normally functioning thyroid gland are regulated by the amount of Thyrotropin (TSH) secreted from the anterior pituitary gland. TSH secretion is in turn regulated by the levels of circulating T_4 and T_3 and by secretion of thyrotropin releasing factor (TRH) from the hypothalamus. Recognition of this complex feedback system is important in the diagnosis and treatment of thyroid dysfunction. The principal effect of exogenous thyroid hormones is to increase the metabolic rate of body tissues.

The thyroid hormones are also concerned with growth and differentiation of tissues. In deficiency states in the young there is retardation of growth and failure of maturation of the skeletal and other body systems, especially in failure of ossification in the epiphyses and in the growth and development of the brain.

The precise mechanism of action by which thyroid hormones affect thermogenesis and cellular growth and differentiation is not known. It is recognized that these physiologic effects are mediated at the cellular level primarily by T_3, a large part of which is derived from T_4 by deiodination in the peripheral tissues. Thyroxine (T_4) is the major component of normal secretions of the thyroid gland and is thus the primary determinant of normal thyroid function.

Depending on other factors, absorption of LEVOTHROID TABLETS has varied from 48 to 79 percent of the administered dose. Fasting increases absorption. Malabsorption syndromes, as well as dietary factors, (children's soybean formula, concomitant use of anionic exchange resins such as cholestyramine) cause excessive fecal loss.

More than 99 percent of circulating hormones are bound to serum proteins, including thyroid-binding globulin (TB_g), thyroid-binding prealbumin (TBPA), and albumin (TB_a), whose capacities and affinities vary for the hormones.

L-thyroxine displays greater binding affinity than L-triiodothyronine, both in the circulation and at the cellular level, which explains its longer duration of action. The half-life of T_4 in normal plasma is 6-7 days while that of T_3 is about 1 day. The plasma half-lives of T_4 and T_3 are decreased in hyperthyroidism and increased in hypothyroidism.

INDICATIONS AND USAGE

LEVOTHROID is indicated as replacement or substitution therapy for diminished or absent thyroid function (e.g., cretinism, myxedema, non-toxic goiter or hypothyroidism generally, including the hypothyroid state in children, in pregnancy and in the elderly) resulting from functional deficiency, primary atrophy, from partial or complete absence of the gland or from the effects of surgery, radiation or antithyroid agents. Therapy must be maintained continuously to control the symptoms of hypothyroidism.

It may also be used to suppress the secretion of thyrotropin (TSH) action which may be beneficial in simple nonendemic goiter and in chronic lymphocytic thyroiditis. This may cause a reduction in the goiter size.

Thyroid hormone drugs are indicated as a diagnostic agent in suppression tests to differentiate suspected mild hyperthyroidism or thyroid gland autonomy.

Thyroid hormones may also be used with antithyroid drugs to treat thyrotoxicosis. This combination has been used to prevent goitrogenesis and hypothyroidism. This may be particularly useful in the management of thyrotoxicosis during pregnancy.

CONTRAINDICATIONS

LEVOTHROID administration is contraindicated in untreated thyrotoxicosis and in acute myocardial infarction.

Continued on next page

This product information was prepared in September, 1969. Information concerning these products may be obtained by addressing Rorer Pharmaceutical Corporation, 500 Virginia Drive, Fort Washington, PA 19034.

Rorer Pharm.—Cont.

LEVOTHROID is contraindicated in the presence of uncorrected adrenal insufficiency because it increases the tissue demands for adrenocortical hormones and may cause an acute adrenal crisis in such patients. (See Precautions.) LEVOTHROID is also contraindicated in cases of hypersensitivity to any of the ingredients.

WARNINGS

> Drugs with thyroid hormone activity, alone or together with other therapeutic agents, have been used for the treatment of obesity. In euthyroid patients, doses within the range of daily hormonal requirements are ineffective for weight reduction. Larger doses may produce serious or even life-threatening manifestations of toxicity, particularly when given in association with sympathomimetic amines such as those used for their anorectic effects.

The use of thyroid hormones in the therapy of obesity, alone or combined with other drugs, is unjustified and has been shown to be ineffective. Neither is their use justified for the treatment of male or female infertility unless this condition is accompanied by hypothyroidism.

PRECAUTIONS

GENERAL—LEVOTHROID should be used with caution in patients with cardiovascular disease, including hypertension. The development of chest pain or other aggravation of cardiovascular disease will require a decrease in dosage. Thyroid hormone therapy in patients with concomitant diabetes mellitus or diabetes insipidus or adrenal cortical insufficiency aggravates the intensity of their symptoms. Appropriate adjustments of the various therapeutic measures directed at these concomitant endocrine diseases are required. The therapy of myxedema coma requires simultaneous administration of glucocorticoids. (See DOSAGE AND ADMINISTRATION.)

INFORMATION FOR THE PATIENT—Patients on thyroid preparations and parents of children on thyroid therapy should be informed that:

1. Replacement therapy is to be taken essentially for life, with the exception of cases of transient hypothyroidism, usually associated with thyroiditis, and in those patients receiving a therapeutic trial of the drug.
2. They should immediately report during the course of therapy any signs or symptoms of thyroid hormone toxicity, e.g., chest pain, increased pulse rate, palpitations, excessive sweating, heat intolerance, nervousness, or any other unusual event.
3. In case of concomitant diabetes mellitus, the daily dosage of antidiabetic medication may need readjustment as thyroid hormone replacement is achieved. If thyroid medication is stopped, a downward readjustment of the dosage of insulin or oral hypoglycemic agent may be necessary to avoid hypoglycemia. At all times, close monitoring of urinary glucose levels is mandatory in such patients.
4. In case of concomitant oral anticoagulant therapy, the prothrombin time should be measured frequently to determine if the dosage of oral anticoagulants is to be readjusted.
5. Partial loss of hair may be experienced by children in the first few months of thyroid therapy, but this is usually a transient phenomenon and later recovery is usually the rule.

LABORATORY TESTS—The patient's response to thyroid replacement therapy may be followed by laboratory tests such as serum thyroxine (T_4), serum triiodothyronine (T_3), free thyroxine index and thyroid stimulating hormone (TSH) blood levels.

DRUG INTERACTIONS—In patients with diabetes mellitus, addition of thyroid hormone therapy may cause an increase in the required dosage of insulin or oral hypoglycemic agents. Conversely, decreasing the dose of thyroid hormone may possibly cause hypoglycemic reactions if the dosage of insulin or oral hypoglycemic agents is not adjusted.

Thyroid replacement may potentiate anticoagulant effects with agents such as warfarin or bishydroxycoumarin and reduction of one-third in anticoagulant dosage should be undertaken upon initiation of LEVOTHROID therapy. Subsequent anticoagulant dosage adjustment should be made on the basis of frequent prothrombin determinations.

Injection of epinephrine in patients with coronary artery disease may precipitate an episode of coronary insufficiency. This may be enhanced in patients receiving thyroid preparations. Careful observation is required if catecholamines are administered to patients in this category.

Cholestyramine or colestipol binds both T_4 and T_3 in the intestine, thus impairing absorption of these thyroid hormones. In vitro studies indicate that the binding is not easily removed. Therefore, four to five hours should elapse between administration of cholestyramine or colestipol and thyroid hormones.

Estrogens tend to increase serum thyroxine-binding globulin (TBg). Thus during pregnancy or when using estrogen-containing drug products, the total serum thyroxine (T_4) will increase. The ratio of bound to free T_4 will increase but the available free T_4 concentration remains normal. An adjustment in the exogenous dose of T_4 should be made on the basis of free T_4 measurements.

DRUG/LABORATORY TEST INTERACTIONS—The following drugs or moieties are known to interfere with laboratory tests performed in patients on thyroid hormone therapy: androgens, corticosteroids, estrogens, oral contraceptives containing estrogens, iodine-containing preparations, and the numerous preparations containing salicylates.

1. Changes in TBg concentration should be taken into consideration in the interpretation of T_4 and T_3 values. In such cases, the unbound (free) hormone should be measured. Pregnancy, estrogens, and estrogen-containing oral contraceptives increase TBg concentrations. TBg may also be increased during infectious hepatitis. Decreases in TBg concentrations are observed in nephrosis, acromegaly, and after androgen or corticosteroid therapy. Familial hyper- or hypo-thyroxine-binding-globulinemias have been described. The incidence of TBg deficiency approximates 1 in 9000. The binding of thyroxine by thyroid-binding prealbumin (TBPA) is inhibited by salicylates.
2. Medical or dietary iodine interferes with all in vivo tests of radio-iodine uptake, producing low uptakes which may not be reflective of a true decrease in hormone synthesis.
3. The persistence of clinical and laboratory evidence of hypothyroidism in spite of adequate dosage replacement indicates either poor patient compliance, poor absorption, excessive fecal loss, or inactivity of the preparation. Intracellular resistance to thyroid hormone is quite rare.

CARCINOGENESIS, MUTAGENESIS, AND IMPAIRMENT OF FERTILITY—A reportedly apparent association between prolonged thyroid therapy and breast cancer has not been confirmed and patients on thyroid for established indications should not discontinue therapy. No confirmatory long-term studies in animals have been performed to evaluate carcinogenic potential, mutagenicity, or impairment of fertility in either males or females.

PREGNANCY-CATEGORY A—Thyroid hormones do not readily cross the placental barrier. The clinical experience to date does not indicate any adverse effect on fetuses when thyroid hormones are administered to pregnant women. On the basis of current knowledge, thyroid replacement therapy to hypothyroid women should not be discontinued during pregnancy.

NURSING MOTHERS—Minimal amounts of thyroid hormones are excreted in human milk. Thyroid is not associated with serious adverse reactions and does not have a known tumorigenic potential. However, caution should be exercised when thyroid is administered to a nursing woman.

PEDIATRIC USE—The diagnosis and institution of therapy for cretinism should be done as soon after birth as feasible to prevent developmental deficiency. Screening tests for serum T_4 and TSH will identify this group of newborn patients.

ADVERSE REACTIONS

Patients who are sensitive to lactose may show intolerance to LEVOTHROID TABLETS since this substance is used in the manufacture of the product.

Adverse reactions other than those indicative of hyperthyroidism because of therapeutic overdosage, either initially or during the maintenance period, are rare. (See OVERDOSAGE.)

OVERDOSAGE

Excessive dosage of thyroid medication may result in symptoms of hyperthyroidism. Since, however, the effects do not appear at once, the symptoms may not appear for one to three weeks after the dosage regimen is begun. The most common signs and symptoms of overdosage are weight loss, palpitation, nervousness, diarrhea or abdominal cramps, sweating, tachycardia, cardiac arrhythmias, angina pectoris, tremors, headache, insomnia, intolerance to heat and fever. If symptoms of overdosage appear, discontinue medication for several days and reinstitute treatment at a lower dosage level.

Laboratory tests such as serum T_4, serum T_3 and the free thyroxine index will be elevated during the period of overdosage.

Complications as a result of the induced hypermetabolic state may include cardiac failure and death due to arrhythmia or failure.

TREATMENT OF OVERDOSAGE—Dosage should be reduced or therapy temporarily discontinued if signs and symptoms of overdosage appear. Treatment may be reinstituted at a lower dosage. In normal individuals, normal hypothalamic-pituitary-thyroid axis function is restored in 6 to 8 weeks after thyroid suppression.

Treatment of acute massive thyroid hormone overdosage is aimed at reducing gastrointestinal absorption of the drugs and counteracting central and peripheral effects, mainly those of increased sympathetic activity. Vomiting may be induced initially if further gastrointestinal absorption can

reasonably be prevented and barring contraindications such as coma, convulsions, or loss of the gagging reflex. Treatment is symptomatic and supportive. Oxygen may be administered and ventilation maintained. Cardiac glycosides may be indicated if congestive heart failure develops. Measures to control fever, hypoglycemia, or fluid loss should be instituted if needed. Antiadrenergic agents, particularly propranolol, have been used advantageously in the treatment of increased sympathetic activity. Propranolol may be administered intravenously at a dosage of 1 to 3 mg over a 10 minute period or orally, 80 to 160 mg/day, especially when no contraindications exist for its use.

DOSAGE AND ADMINISTRATION

The goal of therapy should be the restoration of euthyroidism as judged by clinical response and confirmed by appropriate laboratory values. In adults with no complicating endocrine or cardiovascular disease, the predicted full maintenance dose may be achieved immediately with adjustments made as indicated by clinical evaluation. The usual maintenance dose of LEVOTHROID TABLETS is 100 mcg to 200 mcg daily.

In patients with known complications or in case of doubt, individual dose titration at 2 to 4 week intervals is recommended. The usual starting dose is 50 mcg with increases of 50 mcg at 2 to 4 week intervals until the patient is euthyroid or symptoms ensue which preclude further dose increase.

In adult myxedema or hypothyroid patients with angina, the starting dose should be 25 mcg with increases at 2 to 4 week intervals of 25 to 50 mcg as determined by clinical response. Myxedema coma is usually precipitated in the hypothyroid patient of long-standing by intercurrent illness or drugs such as sedatives and anesthetics and should be considered a medical emergency. Therapy should be directed at the correction of electrolyte disturbances and possible infection besides the administration of thyroid hormones. Corticosteroids should be administered routinely. T_4 and T_3 may be administered via a nasogastric tube, but the preferred route of administration of both hormones is intravenous.

In cretinism or severe hypothyroidism in children, the initial dose should be 25 to 50 mcg with increases of 50 to 100 mcg at weekly intervals until the child is clinically euthyroid and laboratory values are in the normal range. In growing children, the usual maintenance dose may be as high as 300 to 400 mcg daily. It is essential in children to reach the euthyroid state as rapidly as possible because of the importance of thyroid in growth and maturation.

LEVOTHROID® (Levothyroxine Sodium) FOR INJECTION is given at a starting dose of 200–500 mcg in patients without severe cardiac disease. This initial dose is followed in 24 hours by 100–200 mcg given intravenously. Normal T_4 levels may be achieved in 24 hours followed in 3 days by a three-fold increase in T_3. Oral therapy with Levothroid® Tablets should be resumed as soon as the clinical situation permits.

In the presence of severe cardiac disease, the risk of a rapid increase in metabolism should be weighed against the danger of prolonging the severe hypothyroid state. This may necessitate a smaller initial I.V. dose of Levothroid® for Injection.

Directions for reconstitution: using aseptic technique add 2 mL, 0.9% Sodium Chloride Injection, USP to the 200 mcg vial and 5 mL, 0.9% Sodium Chloride Injection, USP to the 500 mcg vial.

Note: Do not use Bacteriostatic Sodium Chloride Injection, USP. Shake to dissolve the contents of the vial. Use immediately and discard the unused portion.

Parenteral drug products should be inspected visually for particulate matter and discoloration prior to administration whenever solution and container permit.

HOW SUPPLIED

LEVOTHROID TABLETS (Levothyroxine Sodium Tablets, USP) are supplied as follows: 25 mcg are available in bottles of 100 (NDC 0075-2540-06). 50 mcg are available in bottles of 100 (NDC 0075-2541-06), drums of 50,000 (NDC 0075-2541-50) and unit dose cartons of 100 (NDC 0075-2541-02). 75 mcg are available in bottles of 100 (NDC 0075-2547-06). 100 mcg are available in bottles of 100 (NDC 0075-2542-06), and unit dose cartons of 100 (NDC 0075-2542-02). 125 mcg are available in bottles of 100 (NDC 0075-2548-06) and unit dose cartons of 100 (NDC 0075-2548-02). 150 mcg are available in bottles of 100 (NDC 0075-2543-06), drums of 50,000 (NDC 0075-2543-50), and unit dose cartons of 100 (NDC 0075-2543-02). 175 mcg are available in bottles of 100 (NDC 0075-2544-06). 200 mcg are available in bottles of 100 (NDC 0075-2545-06), drums of 50,000 (NDC 0075-2545-50), and unit dose cartons of 100 (NDC 0075-2545-02). 300 mcg are available in bottles of 100 (NDC 0075-2546-06), drums of 50,000 (NDC 0075-2546-50), and unit dose cartons of 100 (NDC 0075-2546-02). Each Levothroid Tablet is distinctively colored and bears identifying markings:

Strength (mcg)	Tablets Color	Markings
25	Orange	LK
50	White	LL
75	Grey	LT
100	Yellow	LM
125	Purple	LH
150	Blue	LN
175	Turquoise	LP
200	Pink	LR
300	Green	LS

Tablets should be stored at controlled room temperature—between 59°–86°F (15°–30°C) in capped bottles or unbroken plastic strip packaging.

LEVOTHROID (Levothyroxine Sodium) for Injection is supplied in 6 mL vials containing 200 (0075-2551-01) or 500 (0075-2552-01) mcg of levothyroxine sodium, USP.

The vials should be stored at controlled room temperature, between 59°–86°F (15°–30°C).

CAUTION

Federal (U.S.A.) law prohibits dispensing without prescription.

RORER PHARMACEUTICALS
a division of
RORER PHARMACEUTICAL CORPORATION
Fort Washington, PA, U.S.A. 19034
Shown in Product Identification Section, page 426

LOZOL® ℞
[lō′zôl]
(indapamide)
2.5 mg tablets

PRODUCT OVERVIEW

KEY FACTS

Lozol® (indapamide) is the first of a new class of oral antihypertensive/diuretics, the indolines. In addition to its diuretic effect, the drug decreases peripheral resistance with little or no effect on cardiac output, rate or rhythm. Chronic administration of indapamide has little or no effect on glomerular filtration rate or renal plasma flow. Mean changes in potassium, sodium, chloride and uric acid are slight.

MAJOR USES

Lozol is indicated for the treatment of hypertension, alone or in combination with other antihypertensive drugs. Lozol is also indicated for the treatment of salt and fluid retention associated with congestive heart failure. The adult starting dose for hypertension or edema of congestive heart failure is 2.5 mg as a single daily dose taken in the morning. Higher doses (5.0 mg and larger) provide little additional antihypertensive effect, yet may produce greater electrolyte shifts.

SAFETY INFORMATION

Hypokalemia occurs commonly with diuretics, and electrolyte monitoring is essential. Diuretics should not be given concomitantly with lithium. Lozol is contraindicated in anuria as well as in known hypersensitivity to indapamide or to other sulfonamide-derived drugs.

PRESCRIBING INFORMATION

LOZOL® ℞
[lō′zôl]
indapamide
2.5 mg tablets

DESCRIPTION

LOZOL (indapamide) is an oral antihypertensive/diuretic. Its molecule contains both a polar sulfamoyl chlorobenzamide moiety and a lipid-soluble methylindoline moiety. It differs chemically from the thiazides in that it does not possess the thiazide ring system and contains only one sulfonamide group. The chemical name of LOZOL is 1-(4-chloro-3-sulfamoylbenzamido)-2-methylindoline, and its molecular weight is 365.84. The compound is a weak acid, $pK_a = 8.8$, and is soluble in aqueous solutions of strong bases. It is a white to yellow-white crystalline (tetragonal) powder.

The tablets also contain microcrystalline cellulose, coloring agent, corn starch, hydroxypropyl methylcellulose, lactose, magnesium stearate, polyethylene glycol, and talc.

CLINICAL PHARMACOLOGY

Indapamide is the first of a new class of antihypertensive/diuretics, the indolines. The oral administration of 5 mg (two 2.5-mg tablets) of indapamide to healthy male subjects produced peak concentrations of approximately 260 ng/ml of the drug in the blood within two hours. A minimum of 70% of a single oral dose is eliminated by the kidneys and an additional 23% by the gastrointestinal tract, probably including the biliary route. The half-life of LOZOL in whole blood is approximately 14 hours.

LOZOL is preferentially and reversibly taken up by the erythrocytes in the peripheral blood. The whole blood/plasma ratio is approximately 6:1 at the time of peak concentration and decreases to 3.5:1 at eight hours. From 71 to 79% of the LOZOL in plasma is reversibly bound to plasma proteins.

LOZOL is extensively metabolized, unchanged drug accounting for approximately 7% of the total dose recovered in the urine during the first 48 hours after administration. The urinary elimination of ^{14}C-labeled indapamide and metabolites is biphasic with a terminal half-life of excretion of total radioactivity of 26 hours.

In parallel design, dose-ranging clinical trials in hypertension and edema, daily doses of indapamide between 0.5 and 5.0 mg produced dose-related effects. Generally, doses of 2.5 and 5.0 mg were not distinguishable from each other although each was differentiated from placebo and from 0.5 or 1.0 mg indapamide. At daily doses of 2.5 and 5.0 mg a mean decrease of serum potassium of 0.5 and 0.6 mEq/liter, respectively, was observed and uric acid increased by about 1.0 mg/100 mL.

Thus, at these doses, the effects of indapamide on blood pressure and edema are approximately equal to those obtained with conventional doses of other antihypertensive/diuretics. In hypertensive patients, daily doses of 2.5 and 5.0 mg of indapamide have no appreciable cardiac inotropic or chronotropic effect. The drug decreases peripheral resistance, with little or no effect on cardiac output, rate or rhythm. Chronic administration of indapamide to hypertensive patients has little or no effect on glomerular filtration rate or renal plasma flow.

LOZOL had an antihypertensive effect in patients with varying degrees of renal impairment, although in general, diuretic effects declined as renal function decreased.

In limited controlled studies adding LOZOL to other antihypertensive drugs such as hydralazine, propranolol, guanethidine, and methyldopa, indapamide appeared to have the additive effect typical of thiazide-type diuretics.

INDICATIONS

LOZOL is indicated for the treatment of hypertension, alone or in combination with other antihypertensive drugs.

LOZOL is also indicated for the treatment of salt and fluid retention associated with congestive heart failure.

Usage in Pregnancy: The routine use of diuretics in an otherwise healthy woman is inappropriate and exposes mother and fetus to unnecessary hazard (see PRECAUTIONS).

Diuretics do not prevent development of toxemia of pregnancy, and there is no satisfactory evidence that they are useful in the treatment of developed toxemia.

Edema during pregnancy may arise from pathological causes or from the physiologic and mechanical consequences of pregnancy. Indapamide is indicated in pregnancy when edema is due to pathologic causes, just as it is in the absence of pregnancy (however, see PRECAUTIONS). Dependent edema in pregnancy, resulting from restriction of venous return by the expanded uterus, is properly treated through elevation of the lower extremities and use of support hose; use of diuretics to lower intravascular volume in this case is illogical and unnecessary. There is hypervolemia during normal pregnancy which is not harmful to either the fetus or the mother (in the absence of cardiovascular disease), but which is associated with edema, including generalized edema in the majority of pregnant women. If this edema produces discomfort, increased recumbency will often provide relief. In rare instances, this edema may cause extreme discomfort which is not relieved by rest. In these cases, a short course of diuretics may provide relief and may be appropriate.

CONTRAINDICATIONS

Anuria. Known hypersensitivity to indapamide or to other sulfonamide-derived drugs.

WARNINGS

Hypokalemia occurs commonly with diuretics, and electrolyte monitoring is essential, particularly in patients who would be at increased risk from hypokalemia, such as those with cardiac arrhythmias or who are receiving concomitant cardiac glycosides.

In general, diuretics should not be given concomitantly with lithium because they reduce its renal clearance and add a high risk of lithium toxicity. Read prescribing information for lithium preparations before use of such concomitant therapy.

PRECAUTIONS

General:

1. *Hypokalemia and Other Fluid and Electrolyte Imbalances:* Periodic determinations of serum electrolytes should be performed at appropriate intervals. In addition, patients should be observed for clinical signs of fluid or electrolyte imbalance, such as hyponatremia, hypochloremic alkalosis, or hypokalemia. Warning signs include dry mouth, thirst, weakness, fatigue, lethargy, drowsiness, restlessness, muscle pains or cramps, hypotension, oliguria, tachycardia, and gastrointestinal disturbance. Electrolyte determinations are particularly important in patients who are vomiting excessively or receiving parenteral fluids, in patients subject to electrolyte imbalance (including those with heart failure, kidney disease, and cirrhosis), and in patients on a salt-restricted diet.

The risk of hypokalemia secondary to diuresis and natriuresis is increased when larger doses are used, when the diuresis is brisk, when severe cirrhosis is present and during concomitant use of corticosteroids or ACTH. Interference with adequate oral intake of electrolytes will also contribute to hypokalemia. Hypokalemia can sensitize or exaggerate the response of the heart to the toxic effects of digitalis, such as increased ventricular irritability.

Dilutional hyponatremia may occur in edematous patients; the appropriate treatment is restriction of water rather than administration of salt, except in rare instances when the hyponatremia is life threatening. However, in actual salt depletion, appropriate replacement is the treatment of choice. Any chloride deficit that may occur during treatment is generally mild and usually does not require specific treatment except in extraordinary circumstances as in liver or renal disease.

2. *Hyperuricemia and Gout:* Serum concentrations of uric acid increased by an average of 1.0 mg/100 mL in patients treated with indapamide, and frank gout may be precipitated in certain patients receiving indapamide (see ADVERSE REACTIONS). Serum concentrations of uric acid should therefore be monitored periodically during treatment.

3. *Renal Impairment:* Indapamide, like the thiazides, should be used with caution in patients with severe renal disease, as reduced plasma volume may exacerbate or precipitate azotemia. If progressive renal impairment is observed in a patient receiving indapamide, withholding or discontinuing diuretic therapy should be considered. Renal function tests should be performed periodically during treatment with indapamide.

4. *Impaired Hepatic Function:* Indapamide, like the thiazides, should be used with caution in patients with impaired hepatic function or progressive liver disease, since minor alterations of fluid and electrolyte balance may precipitate hepatic coma.

5. *Glucose Tolerance:* Latent diabetes may become manifest and insulin requirements in diabetic patients may be altered during thiazide administration. Serum concentrations of glucose should be monitored routinely during treatment with LOZOL.

6. *Calcium Excretion:* Calcium excretion is decreased by diuretics pharmacologically related to indapamide. In long-term studies of hypertensive patients, however, serum concentrations of calcium increased only slightly with indapamide. Prolonged treatment with drugs pharmacologically related to indapamide may in rare instances be associated with hypercalcemia and hypophosphatemia secondary to physiologic changes in the parathyroid gland; however, the common complications of hyperparathyroidism, such as renal lithiasis, bone resorption, and peptic ulcer, have not been seen. Treatment should be discontinued before tests for parathyroid function are performed. Like the thiazides, indapamide may decrease serum PBI levels without signs of thyroid disturbance.

7. *Interaction With Systemic Lupus Erythematosus:* Thiazides have exacerbated or activated systemic lupus erythematosus and this possibility should be considered with indapamide as well.

DRUG INTERACTIONS

1. *Other Antihypertensives:* LOZOL (indapamide) may add to or potentiate the action of other antihypertensive drugs. In limited controlled trials that compared the effect of indapamide combined with other antihypertensive drugs with the effect of the other drugs administered alone, there was no notable change in the nature or frequency of adverse reactions associated with the combined therapy.

2. *Lithium:* See WARNINGS.

3. *Post-Sympathectomy Patient:* The antihypertensive effect of the drug may be enhanced in the postsympathectomized patient.

4. *Norepinephrine:* Indapamide, like the thiazides, may decrease arterial responsiveness to norepinephrine, but this diminution is not sufficient to preclude effectiveness of the pressor agent for therapeutic use.

CARCINOGENESIS, MUTAGENESIS, IMPAIRMENT OF FERTILITY: Both mouse and rat lifetime carcinogenicity studies were conducted. There was no significant difference in the incidence of tumors between the indapamide-treated

Continued on next page

This product information was prepared in September, 1989. Information concerning these products may be obtained by addressing Rorer Pharmaceutical Corporation, 500 Virginia Drive, Fort Washington, PA 19034.

Rorer Pharm.—Cont.

animals and the control groups.

Pregnancy/Teratogenic Effects: Pregnancy Category B. Reproduction studies have been performed in rats, mice, and rabbits at doses up to 6,250 times the therapeutic human dose and have revealed no evidence of impaired fertility or harm to the fetus due to LOZOL. Postnatal development in rats and mice was unaffected by pretreatment of parent animals during gestation. There are, however, no adequate and well-controlled studies in pregnant women. Moreover, diuretics are known to cross the placental barrier and appear in cord blood. Because animal reproduction studies are not always predictive of human response, this drug should be used during pregnancy only if clearly needed. There may be hazards associated with this use such as fetal or neonatal jaundice, thrombocytopenia, and possibly other adverse reactions that have occurred in the adult.

Nursing Mothers: It is not known whether this drug is excreted in human milk. Because most drugs are excreted in human milk, if use of this drug is deemed essential, the patient should stop nursing.

ADVERSE REACTIONS

Most adverse effects have been mild and transient. The clinical adverse reactions listed in the following table represent data from Phase II placebo-controlled studies and long-term controlled clinical trials (426 patients given LOZOL 2.5 mg or 5.0 mg). The reactions are arranged into two groups: 1) a cumulative incidence equal to or greater than 5%; and 2) a cumulative incidence less than 5%. Reactions are counted regardless of relation to drug.

Incidence ≥ 5%	Incidence < 5%
CENTRAL NERVOUS SYSTEM/ NEUROMUSCULAR	
Headache	Lightheadedness
Dizziness	Drowsiness
Fatigue, weakness, loss	Vertigo
of energy, lethargy,	Insomnia
tiredness, or malaise	Depression
Muscle cramps or	Blurred Vision
spasm or numbness	
of the extremities	
Nervousness, tension,	
anxiety, irritability, or	
agitation	
GASTROINTESTINAL SYSTEM	
	Constipation
	Nausea
	Vomiting
	Diarrhea
	Gastric irritation
	Abdominal pain or
	cramps
	Anorexia
CARDIOVASCULAR SYSTEM	
	Orthostatic hypotension
	Premature ventricular
	contractions
	Irregular heart beat
	Palpitations
GENITOURINARY SYSTEM	
	Frequency of urination
	Nocturia
	Polyuria
DERMATOLOGIC/HYPERSENSITIVITY	
	Rash
	Hives
	Pruritus
	Vasculitis
OTHER	Impotence or reduced
	libido
	Rhinorrhea
	Flushing
	Hyperuricemia
	Hyperglycemia
	Hyponatremia
	Hypochloremia
	Increase in serum urea
	nitrogen (BUN) or creatinine
	Glycosuria
	Weight loss
	Dry mouth
	Tingling of extremities

Because most of these data are from long-term studies (up to 40 weeks of treatment), it is probable that many of the adverse experiences reported are due to causes other than the drug. Approximately 10% of patients given indapamide discontinued treatment in long-term trials because of reactions either related or unrelated to the drug.

Clinical hypokalemia (i.e., lowered serum potassium concentration with concomitant clinical signs or symptoms) occurred in 3% and 7% of patients given indapamide 2.5 mg and 5.0 mg, respectively. In a long-term study of both doses (157 patients given indapamide), potassium supplementation was given to 12% of patients on indapamide 2.5 mg and 27% of patients on indapamide 5.0 mg.

As expected in long-term clinical trials, many patients experienced single instances of abnormal clinical laboratory test results. However, over time, the mean changes in selected values are slight, as shown in the table below:
[See table below].

Other adverse reactions reported with antihypertensive/diuretics are jaundice (intrahepatic cholestatic jaundice), sialadenitis, xanthopsia, photosensitivity, purpura, necrotizing angiitis, fever, respiratory distress (including pneumonitis), and anaphylactic reactions; also, agranulocytosis, leukopenia, thrombocytopenia, and aplastic anemia. These reactions should be considered as possible occurrences with clinical usage of LOZOL.

OVERDOSAGE

Symptoms of overdosage include nausea, vomiting, weakness, gastrointestinal disorders and disturbances of electrolyte balance. In severe instances, hypotension and depressed respiration may be observed. If this occurs, support of respiration and cardiac circulation should be instituted. There is no specific antidote. An evacuation of the stomach is recommended by emesis and gastric lavage after which the electrolyte and fluid balance should be evaluated carefully.

DOSAGE AND ADMINISTRATION

Hypertension and edema of congestive heart failure: The adult starting dose for hypertension or edema of congestive heart failure is 2.5 mg as a *single daily dose* taken in the morning. If the response to 2.5 mg is not satisfactory after one (edema) to four (hypertension) weeks, the daily dose may be increased to 5.0 mg taken once daily.

If the antihypertensive response to indapamide is insufficient, LOZOL may be combined with other antihypertensive drugs, with careful monitoring of blood pressure. It is recommended that the usual dose of other agents be reduced by 50% during initial combination therapy. As the blood pressure response becomes evident, further dosage adjustments may be necessary.

In general, doses of 5.0 mg and larger have not appeared to provide additional effects on blood pressure or heart failure, but are associated with a greater degree of hypokalemia. There is little clinical trial experience in patients with doses greater than 5.0 mg once a day.

HOW SUPPLIED

LOZOL (indapamide). White, round film-coated tablets of 2.5 mg in bottles of 100 (NDC 0075-0082-00), 1,000 (NDC 0075-0082-99), and in unit-dose blister packs, boxes of 100 (10 × 10 strips) (NDC 0075-0082-62).

Keep tightly closed. Store at room temperature; avoid excessive heat. Dispense in tight containers as defined in USP.

CAUTION

Federal (U.S.A.) law prohibits dispensing without prescription.

Revised: 5/88
RORER PHARMACEUTICALS
a division of
RORER PHARMACEUTICAL CORPORATION
Fort Washington, PA, U.S.A. 19034
Shown in Product Identification Section, page 426

PRODUCT OVERVIEW

KEY FACTS

M.V.I.®–12 makes available a combination of important oil-soluble and water-soluble vitamins in an aqueous solution for intravenous infusion after dilution.

MAJOR USES

M.V.I.®–12 is indicated as daily multivitamin maintenance dosage for adults and children age 11 years and above receiving parenteral nutrition.

SAFETY INFORMATION

M.V.I.®–12 is contraindicated in patients with known hypersensitivity to any of the vitamins or pre-existing hypervitaminosis. The vitamin preparation is for intravenous infusion only after dilution in not less than 500 mL of infusion fluid.

PRESCRIBING INFORMATION

For dilution in intravenous infusions only
M.V.I.®–12 ℞
[ĕm-vē-ī-twĕlv]
Multi-Vitamin Infusion
M.V.I.®–12 Multi-Dose
Multi-Vitamin Infusion
M.V.I.®–12 UNIT VIAL
Multi-Vitamin Infusion

DESCRIPTION

M.V.I.–12 and M.V.I.–12 Multi-Dose are sterile products consisting of two vials labeled Vial 1 and Vial 2 in 5 mL single-dose vials and 50 mL multiple-dose vials respectively.
Each 5 mL in Vial 1† provides:

ascorbic acid (vitamin C)	100 mg
vitamin A* (retinol)	1 mg (a)
ergocalciferol* (vitamin D)	5 mcg (b)
thiamine (vitamin B₁)	
(as the hydrochloride)	3 mg
riboflavin (vitamin B₂) (as riboflavin-5 phosphate sodium)	3.6 mg
pyridoxine HCl (vitamin B₆)	4 mg
niacinamide	40 mg
dexpanthenol (d-pantothenyl alcohol)	15 mg
vitamin E* (dl-alpha tocopheryl acetate)	10 mg (c)

† with propylene glycol 30% and gentisic acid ethanolamide 2% as stabilizers and preservatives, sodium hydroxide for pH adjustment, polysorbate 80 1.6%, polysorbate 20 0.028%, butylated hydroxytoluene 0.002%, butylated hydroxyanisole 0.0005%.
* Oil-soluble vitamins A, D, and E water solubilized with polysorbate 80.
(a) 1 mg vitamin A equals 3,300 USP units.
(b) 5 mcg ergocalciferol equals 200 USP units.
(c) 10 mg vitamin E equals 10 USP units.
Each 5 mL in Vial 2 provides:

biotin	60 mcg
folic acid	400 mcg
cyanocobalamin (vitamin B₁₂)	5 mcg

with propylene glycol 30%; and citric acid, sodium citrate, and sodium hydroxide for pH adjustment.
M.V.I.–12 UNIT VIAL is a sterile product in a two-chambered single-dose vial which must be mixed just prior to use.
Each 10 mL of the mixed solution provides:

ascorbic acid (vitamin C)	100 mg
vitamin A‡ (retinol)	1 mg (a)
ergocalciferol‡ (vitamin D)	5 mcg (b)
thiamine (vitamin B₁)	
(as the hydrochloride)	3 mg
riboflavin (vitamin B₂) (as riboflavin-5 phosphate sodium)	3.6 mg
pyridoxine HCl (vitamin B₆)	4 mg
niacinamide	40 mg
dexpanthenol (d-pantothenyl alcohol)	15 mg
vitamin E‡ (dl-alpha tocopheryl acetate)	10 mg (c)
biotin	60 mcg
folic acid	400 mcg
cyanocobalamin (vitamin B₁₂)	5 mcg

with propylene glycol 30% and gentisic acid ethanolamide 1% as stabilizers and preservatives and citric acid, sodium citrate and sodium hydroxide for pH adjustment, polysorbate 80 0.8%, polysorbate 20 0.014%, butylated hydroxytoluene 0.001%, butylated hydroxyanisole 0.0003%.

	Serum Electrolytes (mEq/L)			Serum Uric Acid (mg/dL)	BUN (mg/dL)
	Potassium	Sodium	Chloride		
Indapamide 2.5 mg (n=76)	−0.4	−0.6	−3.6	0.7	−0.1
Indapamide 5.0 mg (n=81)	−0.6	−0.7	−5.1	1.1	1.4

Mean Changes from Baseline after 40 Weeks of Treatment

‡Oil-soluble vitamins A, D, and E water solubilized with polysorbate 80.

(a) 1 mg vitamin A equals 3,300 USP units.

(b) 5 mcg ergocalciferol equals 200 USP units.

(c) 10 mg vitamin E equals 10 USP units.

"Aqueous" multivitamin formula for intravenous infusion: M.V.I.–12 (Multi-Vitamin Infusion) makes available a combination of important oil-soluble and water-soluble vitamins in an aqueous solution, formulated specially for incorporation into intravenous infusions. Through special processing techniques, the liposoluble vitamins A, D, and E have been solubilized in an aqueous medium with polysorbate 80, permitting intravenous administration of these vitamins.

INDICATIONS AND USAGE

This formulation is indicated as daily multivitamin maintenance dosage for adults and children aged 11 years and above receiving parenteral nutrition.

It is also indicated in other situations where administration by the intravenous route is required. Such situations include surgery, extensive burns, fractures and other trauma, severe infectious diseases, and comatose states, which may provoke a "stress" situation with profound alterations in the body's metabolic demands and consequent tissue depletion of nutrients.

The physician should not await the development of clinical signs of vitamin deficiency before initiating vitamin therapy. The use of a multivitamin product obviates the need to speculate on the status of individual vitamin nutriture.

M.V.I.–12 (administered in intravenous fluids under proper dilution) contributes intake of these necessary vitamins, except vitamin K, toward maintaining the body's normal resistance and repair processes.

Patients with multiple vitamin deficiencies or with markedly increased requirements may be given multiples of the daily dosage for two or more days as indicated by the clinical status.

M.V.I.–12 does not contain vitamin K, which may have to be administered separately.

Clinical testing indicates that some patients do not maintain adequate levels of certain vitamins when this formulation in recommended amounts is the sole source of vitamins. No vitamin deficiencies were clinically evident, but blood levels of vitamins A, C, D, and folic acid declined in a number of subjects who received this formulation as the only vitamin source for 4 to 6 months. Therefore, in patients for whom total parenteral nutrition will be continued for long periods of time, these vitamins should be monitored. If deficiencies appear to be developing, multiples of the formulation (1.5 to 3 times) may be needed for a period of time. When multiples of the formulation are used for more than a few weeks, vitamins A and D should be monitored occasionally to be certain that an excess accumulation of these vitamins is not occurring.

CONTRAINDICATIONS

Known hypersensitivity to any of the vitamins in this product or a pre-existing hypervitaminosis.

PRECAUTIONS

Drug Interactions: M.V.I.–12 (Multi-Vitamin Infusion) is not physically compatible with DIAMOX® (acetazolamide) 500 mg, DIURIL® Intravenous Sodium (chlorothiazide sodium) 500 mg, or moderately alkaline solutions. ACHROMYCIN® (tetracycline HCl) 500 mg may not be physically compatible with M.V.I.–12. It has been reported that folic acid is unstable in the presence of calcium salts such as calcium gluconate. Some of the vitamins in M.V.I.–12 may react with vitamin K bisulfite. Direct addition of M.V.I.–12 to intravenous fat emulsions is not recommended.

Carcinogenicity: Carcinogenicity studies have not been performed.

Pregnancy: Pregnant women should follow the U.S. Recommended Daily Allowances for their condition, because their vitamin requirements may exceed those of nonpregnant women.

Nursing Mothers: Lactating women should follow the U.S. Recommended Daily Allowances for their condition, because their vitamin requirements may exceed those of nonlactating women.

Pediatric Use: Safety and effectiveness in children below the age of 11 years have not been established.

ADVERSE REACTIONS

There have been rare reports of anaphylactoid reactions following large intravenous doses of thiamine. The risk, however, is negligible if thiamine is coadministered with other vitamins in the B group. There have been no reports of fatal anaphylactoid reactions associated with M.V.I.–12.

There have been rare reports of the following types of reactions:

Dermatologic—rash, erythema, pruritis

CNS—headache, dizziness, agitation, anxiety

Ophthalmic—diplopia

Allergic—urticaria, periorbital and digital edema

OVERDOSAGE

The possibility of hypervitaminosis A or D should be borne in mind.

DOSAGE AND ADMINISTRATION

M.V.I.–12 is ready for immediate use in adults and children aged 11 years and above when added to intravenous infusion fluids.

For multiple doses, the Pharmacy Bulk Package is prepared by aseptically transferring the contents of Vial 1 to Vial 2. Mix the solution gently. The mixed solution can be stored in a refrigerator and used within 24 hours. The mixed solution will provide 10 10-mL doses.

Directions for using UNIT VIAL: Remove the protective plastic cap, turn the plunger-stopper 90° and press down firmly to force liquid in the upper chamber and the center seal into the lower compartment. Gently agitate to mix solution. Sterilize the rubber stopper in the usual manner and insert needle squarely through the center of plunger-stopper until tip is just visible. Invert vial and withdraw dose in the usual manner. Vial should be mixed just prior to use. Mixed solution may be stored refrigerated at 2°–8°C for up to 24 hours.

M.V.I.–12 should not be given as a direct, undiluted intravenous injection as it may give rise to dizziness, faintness, and possible tissue irritation.

For intravenous feeding, one daily dose of M.V.I.–12 (5 mL of Vial 1 plus 5 mL of Vial 2, or 10 mL of mixed UNIT VIAL) added directly to not less than 500 mL, preferably 1,000 mL, of intravenous dextrose, saline or similar infusion solutions. Parenteral drug products should be inspected visually for particulate matter and discoloration prior to administration, whenever solution and container permit.

After M.V.I.–12 is diluted in an intravenous infusion, the resulting solution should be refrigerated unless it is to be administered immediately and, in any event, should be administered within 48 hours. Some of the vitamins in this product, particularly A and D and riboflavin, are light sensitive, and exposure to light should be minimized.

STORE AT 2°–8°C (36°–46°F).

HOW SUPPLIED

M.V.I.®–12—Boxes of 25 (NDC 0053-1199-31) and cartons of 100. Each box contains two vials—Vial 1 (5 mL) and Vial 2 (5 mL), both vials to be used for a single dose.

M.V.I.®–12 Multi-Dose—Boxes of 20 vials, 50 mL each (10 Vial 1 and Vial 2) (NDC 0053-1199-10). Both solutions to be used for a single dose.

M.V.I.®–12 UNIT VIAL—Boxes of 25 two-chambered 10 mL vials (NDC 0053-1199-35).

CAUTION

Federal (U.S.A.) law prohibits dispensing without prescription.

Revised: August 1988

ARMOUR PHARMACEUTICAL COMPANY

Kankakee, Illinois 60901, U.S.A.

For dilution in intravenous infusions only

M.V.I.® Pediatric   ℞

[ĕm-vē-i pē″dē-ăt′rĭk]

Multi-Vitamins for Infusion

PRODUCT OVERVIEW

KEY FACTS

M.V.I.® Pediatric provides a combination of important oil-soluble vitamins for reconstitution and incorporation into intravenous infusions.

MAJOR USES

M.V.I.® Pediatric is indicated as daily multivitamin maintenance dosage for infants and children up to 11 years of age receiving parenteral nutrition.

SAFETY INFORMATION

M.V.I.® Pediatric is contraindicated in patients with known hypersensitivity to any of the vitamins or pre-existing hypervitaminosis. The vitamin preparation is for intravenous infusion only after reconstitution and incorporation in not less than 100 mL of infusion fluid.

PRESCRIBING INFORMATION

For dilution in intravenous infusions only

M.V.I.® Pediatric   ℞

[ĕm-vē-i pē″dē-ăt′rĭk]

Multi-Vitamins for Infusion

DESCRIPTION

M.V.I.® Pediatric is a lyophilized, sterile powder intended for reconstitution and dilution in intravenous infusions. Each 5 mL of reconstituted product provides:

ascorbic acid (vitamin C).............................. 80 mg

vitamin A† (retinol).. 0.7 mg (a)

ergocalciferol† (vitamin D)........................... 10 mcg (b)

thiamine (vitamin B₁)

(as the hydrochloride) .... 1.2 mg

riboflavin (vitamin B₂) (as ribo-

flavin-5-phosphate sodium) .... 1.4 mg

pyridoxine (vitamin B₆)

(as the hydrochloride) .... 1 mg

niacinamide.. 17 mg

dexpanthenol (d-pantothenyl

alcohol) .... 5 mg

vitamin E† (dl-alpha

tocopheryl acetate)..................................... 7 mg (c)

biotin .... 20 mcg

folic acid .... 140 mcg

cyanocobalamin (vitamin B₁₂)...................... 1 mcg

phytonadione (vitamin K₁)............................ 200 mcg

with mannitol 375 mg, sodium hydroxide for pH adjustment, polysorbate 80 50 mg, polysorbate 20 0.8 mg, butylated hydroxytoluene 58 mcg, butylated hydroxyanisole 14 mcg.

† Oil-soluble vitamins A, D and E water-solubilized with polysorbate 80.

(a) 0.7 mg vitamin A equals 2,300 USP units.

(b) 10 mcg ergocalciferol equals 400 USP units.

(c) 7 mg vitamin E equals 7 USP units.

Multivitamin formula for intravenous infusion:

M.V.I.® Pediatric (Multi-Vitamins for Infusion) provides a combination of important oil-soluble and water-soluble vitamins, formulated especially for incorporation into intravenous infusions after reconstitution. Through special processing techniques, the liposoluble vitamins A, D and E have been water solubilized with polysorbate 80, permitting intravenous administration of these vitamins.

INDICATIONS AND USAGE

This formulation is indicated as daily multivitamin maintenance dosage for infants and children up to 11 years of age receiving parenteral nutrition.

It is also indicated in other situations where administration by the intravenous route is required. Such situations include surgery, extensive burns, fractures and other trauma, severe infectious diseases, and comatose states, which may provoke a "stress" situation with profound alterations in the body's metabolic demands and consequent tissue depletion of nutrients.

The physician should not await the development of clinical signs of vitamin deficiency before initiating vitamin therapy. The use of a multivitamin product obviates the need to speculate on the status of individual vitamin nutriture.

M.V.I.® Pediatric (reconstituted and administered in intravenous fluids under proper dilution) contributes intake of these necessary vitamins toward maintaining the body's normal resistance and repair processes.

Patients with multiple vitamin deficiencies or with markedly increased requirements may be given multiples of the daily dosage for two or more days as indicated by the clinical status.

CONTRAINDICATIONS

Known hypersensitivity to any of the vitamins in this product or a pre-existing hypervitaminosis.

PRECAUTIONS

General: Unlike the adult formulation, M.V.I.®–12, this product contains phytonadione (vitamin K₁).

Adequate blood levels of vitamin E are achieved when M.V.I.® Pediatric is given to infants at the recommended dosage. Larger doses or supplementation with oral or parenteral vitamin E are not recommended because elevated blood levels of vitamin E may result.

Studies have shown that vitamin A may adhere to plastic resulting in inadequate vitamin A administration in the doses recommended with M.V.I.® Pediatric. Additional vitamin A supplementation may be required.

Drug Interactions: M.V.I.® Pediatric is not physically compatible with DIAMOX® (acetazolamide) 500 mg, DIURIL® Intravenous Sodium (chlorothiazide sodium) 500 mg, aminophylline 125 mg, ampicillin 500 mg, or moderately alkaline solutions. ACHROMYCIN® (tetracycline HCl) 500 mg may not be physically compatible with M.V.I.® Pediatric. It has been reported that folic acid is unstable in the presence of calcium salts such as calcium gluconate. Direct addition of M.V.I.® Pediatric to intravenous fat emulsions is not recommended.

Carcinogenicity: Carcinogenicity studies have not been performed.

ADVERSE REACTIONS

There have been rare reports of anaphylactoid reactions following large intravenous doses of thiamine. The risk, however, is negligible if the thiamine is coadministered with other vitamins in the B group. There have been no reports of

Continued on next page

This product information was prepared in September, 1989. Information concerning these products may be obtained by addressing Rorer Pharmaceutical Corporation, 500 Virginia Drive, Fort Washington, PA 19034.

Rorer Pharm.—Cont.

fatal anaphylactoid reactions associated with M.V.I. Pediatric.

There have been rare reports of the following types of reactions:

Dermatologic—rash, erythema, pruritis
CNS—headache, dizziness, agitation, anxiety
Ophthalmic—diplopia
Allergic—urticaria, periorbital and digital edema

OVERDOSAGE

The possibility of hypervitaminosis A or D should be borne in mind.

DOSAGE AND ADMINISTRATION

The single-dose vial of M.V.I.® Pediatric is reconstituted by adding 5 mL of Sterile Water for Injection USP, Dextrose Injection USP 5%, or Sodium Chloride Injection to the 10-mL vial. The Pharmacy Bulk Package is reconstituted by adding 24 mL of Sterile Water for Injection USP, Dextrose Injection USP 5%, or Sodium Chloride Injection to the 50-mL vial. This bulk package provides five 5 mL doses. Since the solution contains no preservative, all five doses should be withdrawn for dispensing with one vial entry. The vial may be swirled gently after the addition of the water to hasten reconstitution. The reconstituted solution is ready within three minutes for immediate use. The amount to be administered should be added to appropriate intravenous infusion fluids (see below).

The reconstituted M.V.I.® Pediatric should not be given as a direct, undiluted intravenous injection as it may give rise to dizziness, faintness and possible tissue irritation.

For a single dose, 5 mL of reconstituted M.V.I.® Pediatric should be added directly to not less than 100 mL of intravenous dextrose, saline or similar infusion solutions.

<u>Infants weighing less than 1 kg:</u> The daily dose is 30% (1.5 mL) of a single full dose (5 mL). Do not exceed this daily dose.

<u>Infants weighing 1 to 3 kg:</u> The daily dose is 65% (3.25 mL) of a single full dose (5 mL). Multiples of this recommended dose should not be given to infants weighing less than 3 kg.

<u>Infants and children weighing 3 kg or more up to 11 years of age:</u> The daily dose is 5 mL unless there is clinical or laboratory evidence for increasing or decreasing the dosage. Discard any unused portion.

Parenteral drug products should be inspected visually for particulate matter and discoloration prior to administration, whenever solution and container permit.

After M.V.I.® Pediatric is reconstituted and diluted in an intravenous infusion, the resulting solution should be refrigerated unless it is to be administered immediately and, in any event, should be administered within 24 hours. Some of the vitamins in this product, particularly vitamins A and D and riboflavin, are light sensitive and exposure to light should be minimized.

HOW SUPPLIED

Boxes of 25 single dose vials (NDC 0053-0815-35) and boxes of 5 single use multiple dose vials (NDC 0053-0815-25).

Store at controlled room temperature between 15°–30°C (59°–86°F).

CAUTION

Federal (U.S.A.) law prohibits dispensing without prescription.

Revised: August 1988

ARMOUR PHARMACEUTICAL COMPANY
Kankakee, Illinois 60901, U.S.A.

NICOBID® Tempules®
(niacin)
TIMED–RELEASE NICOTINIC ACID SUPPLEMENT

DESCRIPTION

Each black-and-clear Tempule (timed-release capsule) contains 125 mg niacin (nicotinic acid); each green-and-clear Tempule (timed-release capsule) contains 250 mg niacin (nicotinic acid); and each opaque blue and white Tempule (timed-release capsule) contains 500 mg niacin (nicotinic acid). Nicobid Tempules® provide the full actions of niacin (nicotinic acid). Portions of the pellets contained in the Tempule are released immediately. The remainder is released over several hours.

USES

Nicobid (niacin) is used in all those conditions in which niacin (nicotinic acid) supplementation is indicated. It has the advantage of a slower release of niacin (nicotinic acid) than conventional tablet dosage forms. This may permit its use by those who do not tolerate the tablets.

CAUTIONS

Nicobid should not be used by persons with a known sensitivity to niacin (nicotinic acid) and by persons with heart or gallbladder disease, gout, arterial bleeding, glaucoma, diabetes, impaired liver function, peptic ulcer, or by pregnant women. Patients taking hypertensive drugs should consult a physician before taking Nicobid.

SIDE EFFECTS

Temporary flushing and feeling of warmth may be expected. These seldom reach levels so as to necessitate discontinuance. If these symptoms persist, discontinue use and consult a physician. Temporary headache, itching and tingling, gastric disturbances, skin rash and allergies may occur.

DOSAGE

Usual adult dose—one Tempule 125 mg, 250 mg or 500 mg morning and evening. Before exceeding usual adult dose consult a physician.

KEEP OUT OF THE REACH OF CHILDREN
Revised: 2/88
RORER PHARMACEUTICALS
a division of
RORER PHARMACEUTICAL CORPORATION
Fort Washington, PA, U.S.A. 19034
Shown in Product Identification Section, page 426

NICOLAR®
[nic′ō-lär″]
(niacin tablets)

℞

DESCRIPTION

Nicolar® (niacin tablets) is a scored yellow-colored tablet containing 500 mg of niacin (nicotinic acid).

The tablets also contain microcrystalline cellulose, FD&C yellow No. 5 (tartrazine) (see PRECAUTIONS), magnesium stearate, povidone, and colloidal silica.

ACTIONS

Niacin functions in the body as a component of two hydrogen transporting coenzymes: Coenzyme I (Nicotinamide Adenine Dinucleotide [NAD], sometimes called Diphosphopyridine Nucleotide [DPN]) and Coenzyme II (Nicotinamide Adenine Dinucleotide Phosphate [NADP], sometimes called Triphosphopyridine Nucleotide [TPN]). Niacin, in addition to its functions as a vitamin, exerts several distinctive pharmacologic effects which vary according to the dosage level employed.

Niacin, in large doses, causes a reduction in serum lipids. The exact mechanism of this action is unknown.

INDICATIONS

Since no drug is innocuous, strict attention should be paid to the indications and contraindications, particularly when selecting drugs for long-term use.

Nicolar® (niacin tablets) is indicated as adjunctive therapy in patients with significant hyperlipidemia (elevated cholesterol and/or triglycerides) who do not respond adequately to diet and weight loss.

Notice: It has not been established whether the drug-induced lowering of serum cholesterol or triglyceride levels has a beneficial effect, no effect, or a detrimental effect on the morbidity or mortality due to atherosclerosis including coronary heart disease. Investigations now in progress may yield an answer to this question.

CONTRAINDICATIONS

Niacin is contraindicated in patients with a known idiosyncrasy to niacin, with hepatic dysfunction, with active peptic ulcer or with arterial bleeding.

WARNINGS

Use of this drug in pregnancy, lactation or in women of child-bearing age requires that the potential benefits of the drug be weighed against its possible hazards to the mother and child. Although fetal abnormalities have not been reported with this drug, its use as an antilipidemic agent requires high dosages, and animal reproduction or teratology studies have not been done. There are insufficient studies done for usage in children.

Keep out of reach of children.

PRECAUTIONS

Great caution must be exercised when niacin is used in patients with coronary disease or gallbladder disease. Patients with a past history of jaundice, liver disease or peptic ulcer should be observed closely while taking the medication.

Frequent monitoring of liver function tests and blood glucose should be performed during therapy to ascertain that the drug has no adverse effects on these organ systems.

Antihypertensive drugs of the adrenergic-blocking type may have an additive vasodilating effect and produce postural hypotension.

Elevated uric acid levels have occurred, therefore use with caution in patients predisposed to gout.

Drug Interactions: Antihypertensive drugs may have an additive vasodilating effect and produce postural hypotension.

Diabetic or potential diabetic patients should be observed closely in the event of decreased glucose tolerance. Adjustment of diet and/or hypoglycemic therapy may be necessary. This product contains FD&C Yellow No. 5 (tartrazine) which may cause allergic-type reactions (including bronchial asthma) in certain susceptible persons. Although the overall incidence of FD&C Yellow No. 5 (tartrazine) sensitivity in the general population is low, it is frequently seen in patients who also have aspirin hypersensitivity.

ADVERSE REACTIONS

Atrial fibrillation and other cardiac arrhythmias
Severe generalized flushing
Decreased glucose tolerance
Activation of peptic ulcers
Abnormalities of hepatic functional tests
Jaundice
Gastrointestinal disorders
Dryness of the skin
Acanthosis Nigricans
Pruritus
Hyperuricemia
Toxic amblyopia
Hypotension
Transient headache

OVERDOSAGE

High doses of nicotinic acid may produce temporary flushing, pruritus, and gastrointestinal distress.

DOSAGE AND ADMINISTRATION

Usually Recommended Adult Dosage—1 to 2 grams three times a day. The dosage must be adjusted to the response of the patient.

Start with two tablets (1 g) three times a day with food or after meals, taken with cold liquids, if necessary, to facilitate swallowing. Since low doses may control hyperlipidemia in some patients, the dosage should be individualized according to the effect on serum lipid levels. If the plasma cholesterol and/or triglyceride level does not show a decrease after a reasonable time at this dosage, an increase in dosage may be considered but requires careful titration and observation of the patient for unwanted effects. The dosage may be increased every 2 to 4 weeks, but in no case should the dosage exceed 6 grams/day.

Since flushing, pruritus and gastrointestinal distress appear frequently and tend to be dose-related, increase the dosage gradually in increments of 500 mg (1 tablet) while carefully observing the patient and monitoring the plasma cholesterol and/or triglyceride level for therapeutic response and for adverse effects.

Where the observed adverse reactions or potential hazards exceed the benefits of use, dosage should be reduced to the minimum recommended dosage and, where necessary, discontinued entirely.

HOW SUPPLIED

Nicolar® (niacin tablets) is available in bottles of 100 scored tablets, (NDC 0075-2850-01). Each tablet contains 500 mg of nicotinic acid (identified by the code NE).

Dispense in a tight container as defined in the USP. Store at controlled room temperature, 59°–86°F (15°–30°C).

Caution: Federal (U.S.A.) law prohibits dispensing without prescription.

Rev. 5/88
RORER PHARMACEUTICALS
a division of
RORER PHARMACEUTICAL CORPORATION
Fort Washington, PA, U.S.A. 19034
Shown in Product Identification Section, page 426

NITROLINGUAL® SPRAY
(nitroglycerin lingual aerosol)
0.4 mg/metered dose

℞

PRODUCT OVERVIEW

KEY FACTS

Nitrolingual® Spray is a metered-dose aerosol containing 200 doses of nitroglycerin. Each metered dose of Nitrolingual Spray delivers 0.4 mg of nitroglycerin per spray emission. Nitrolingual Spray offers guaranteed potency for 3 years from date of manufacture.

MAJOR USES

Nitrolingual® Spray is indicated for acute relief or prophylaxis of angina pectoris due to coronary artery insufficiency.

SAFETY INFORMATION

Nitrolingual® Spray is contraindicated in patients who have shown purported hypersensitivity or idiosyncrasy to it or to other nitrates or nitrites. Tolerance to this drug and cross-tolerance to other nitrates and nitrites may occur. Severe hypotension may occur even with small doses of nitroglycerin. Adverse reaction, particularly headache and hypotension, is generally dose-related. Epinephrine is ineffective in reversing the severe hypotensive events associated with overdosage. It and related compounds are contraindicated in this situation.

NOTE: THE SPRAY SHOULD NOT BE INHALED.

PRESCRIBING INFORMATION

NITROLINGUAL® SPRAY   ℞
(nitroglycerin lingual aerosol)
0.4 mg/metered dose

DESCRIPTION

Nitroglycerin, an organic nitrate, is a vasodilator which has effects on both arteries and veins. The chemical name for nitroglycerin is 1,2,3-propanetriol trinitrate ($C_3H_5N_3O_9$). The compound has a molecular weight of 227.09. The chemical structure is:

$$CH_2-ONO_2$$
$$CH\ -ONO_2$$
$$CH_2-ONO_2$$

Nitrolingual Spray (nitroglycerin lingual aerosol 0.4 mg) is a metered dose aerosol containing nitroglycerin in propellants (dichlorodifluoromethane and dichlorotetrafluoroethane). Each metered dose of Nitrolingual Spray delivers 0.4 mg of nitroglycerin per spray emission. This product delivers nitroglycerin in the form of spray droplets onto or under the tongue. Inactive ingredients: caprylic/capric/diglyceryl succinate, ether, flavors.

CLINICAL PHARMACOLOGY

The principal pharmacological action of nitroglycerin is relaxation of vascular smooth muscle, producing a vasodilator effect on both peripheral arteries and veins with more prominent effects on the latter. Dilation of the post-capillary vessels, including large veins, promotes peripheral pooling of blood and decreases venous return to the heart, thereby reducing left ventricular end-diastolic pressure (preload). Arteriolar relaxation reduces systemic vascular resistance and arterial pressure (afterload).

The mechanism by which nitroglycerin relieves angina pectoris is not fully understood. Myocardial oxygen consumption or demand (as measured by the pressure-rate product, tension-time index, and stroke-work index) is decreased by both the arterial and venous effects of nitroglycerin and presumably, a more favorable supply-demand ratio is achieved. While the large epicardial coronary arteries are also dilated by nitroglycerin, the extent to which this action contributes to relief of exertional angina is unclear.

Nitroglycerin is rapidly metabolized *in vivo*, with a liver reductase enzyme having primary importance in the formation of glycerol nitrate metabolites and inorganic nitrate. Two active major metabolites, 1, 2- and 1,3-dinitroglycerols, the products of hydrolysis, although less potent as vasodilators, have longer plasma half-lives than the parent compound. The dinitrates are further metabolized to mononitrates (considered biologically inactive with respect to cardiovascular effects) and ultimately glycerol and carbon dioxide.

Therapeutic doses of nitroglycerin may reduce systolic, diastolic, and mean arterial blood pressure. Effective coronary perfusion pressure is usually maintained, but can be compromised if blood pressure falls excessively or increased heart rate decreases diastolic filling time.

Elevated central venous and pulmonary capillary wedge pressures, pulmonary vascular resistance, and systemic vascular resistance are also reduced by nitroglycerin therapy. Heart rate is usually slightly increased, presumably a reflex response to the fall in blood pressure. Cardiac index may be increased, decreased, or unchanged. Patients with elevated left ventricular filling pressure and systemic vascular resistance values in conjunction with a depressed cardiac index are likely to experience an improvement in cardiac index. On the other hand, when filling pressures and cardiac index are normal, cardiac index may be slightly reduced.

A pharmacokinetic study in 13 healthy men showed no statistically significant differences between the mean values for maximum plasma concentration and time to achieve maximum plasma level with equal doses (0.8 mg) of Nitrolingual Spray and sublingual nitroglycerin tablets. Peak plasma concentration after 0.8 mg of Nitrolingual occurred within 4 minutes and the apparent plasma half-life was approximately 5 minutes. In a randomized, double-blind study in patients with exertional angina pectoris dose-related increases in exercise tolerance and time to achieve angina were seen following doses of 0.2, 0.4, and 0.8 mg delivered by metered spray.

INDICATIONS AND USAGE

Nitrolingual Spray is indicated for acute relief of an attack or prophylaxis of angina pectoris due to coronary artery disease.

CONTRAINDICATIONS

Nitrolingual Spray is contraindicated in patients who have shown purported hypersensitivity or idiosyncrasy to it or other nitrates or nitrites.

WARNINGS

The use of any form of nitroglycerin during the early days of acute myocardial infarction requires particular attention to hemodynamic monitoring and clinical status.

PRECAUTIONS

General—Severe hypotension, particularly with upright posture, may occur even with small doses of nitroglycerin. The drug, therefore, should be used with caution in subjects who may have volume depletion from diuretic therapy or in patients who have low systolic blood pressure (e.g. below 90 mm Hg). Paradoxical bradycardia and increased angina pectoris may accompany nitroglycerin-induced hypotension. Nitrate therapy may aggravate the angina caused by hypertrophic cardiomyopathy.

Tolerance to this drug and cross-tolerance to other nitrates and nitrites may occur. Tolerance to the vascular and antianginal effects of nitrates has been demonstrated in clinical trials, experience through occupational exposure, and in isolated tissue experiments in the laboratory.

In industrial workers continuously exposed to nitroglycerin, tolerance clearly occurs. Moreover, physical dependence also occurs since chest pain, acute myocardial infarction, and even sudden death have occurred during temporary withdrawal of nitroglycerin from the workers. In various clinical trials in angina patients, there are reports of anginal attacks being more easily provoked and of rebound in the hemodynamic effects soon after nitrate withdrawal. The relative importance of these observations to the routine, clinical use of nitroglycerin is not known.

Drug Interactions: Alcohol may enhance sensitivity to the hypotensive effects of nitrates. Nitroglycerin acts directly on vascular muscle. Therefore, any other agents that depend on vascular smooth muscle as the final common path can be expected to have decreased or increased effect depending upon the agent.

Marked symptomatic orthostatic hypotension has been reported when calcium channel blockers and oral controlled-release nitroglycerin were used in combination. Dose adjustments of either class of agents may be necessary.

Carcinogenesis, Mutagenesis, Impairment of Fertility: No long-term studies in animals have been performed to evaluate carcinogenic potential of Nitrolingual Spray.

Pregnancy: Pregnancy Category C—Animal reproduction studies have not been conducted with Nitrolingual Spray. It is not known whether nitroglycerin can cause fetal harm when administered to a pregnant woman or can affect reproduction capacity. Nitroglycerin should be given to a pregnant woman only if clearly needed.

Nursing Mothers: It is not known whether nitroglycerin is excreted in human milk. Because many drugs are excreted in human milk, caution should be exercised when Nitrolingual Spray is administered to a nursing woman.

Pediatric Use: The safety and effectiveness of nitroglycerin in children have not been established.

ADVERSE REACTIONS

Adverse reaction to Nitrolingual Spray, particularly headache and hypotension, is generally dose-related. In clinical trials at various doses of nitroglycerin, the following adverse have been observed:

Headache, which may be severe and persistent, is the most commonly reported side effect of nitroglycerin with an incidence on the order of about 50% in some studies. Cutaneous vasodilation with flushing may occur. Transient episodes of dizziness and weakness, as well as other signs of cerebral ischemia associated with postural hypotension, may occasionally develop. An occasional individual may exhibit marked sensitivity to the hypotensive effects of nitrates and severe responses (nausea, vomiting, weakness, restlessness, pallor, perspiration, and collapse) may occur even with therapeutic doses. Drug rash and/or exfoliative dermatitis have been reported in patients receiving nitrate therapy. Nausea and vomiting appear to be uncommon.

OVERDOSAGE

Signs and Symptoms:

Nitrate overdosage may result in: severe hypotension; persistent throbbing headache; vertigo; palpitation; visual disturbance; flushing and perspiring skin (later becoming cold and cyanotic); nausea and vomiting (possibly with colic and even bloody diarrhea); syncope (especially in the upright posture); methemoglobinemia with cyanosis and anorexia; initial hypernea, dyspnea, and slow breathing; slow pulse (dicrotic and intermittent); heart block; increased intracranial pressure with cerebral symptoms of confusion and moderate fever; paralysis and coma followed by clonic convulsions, and possibly death due to circulatory collapse.

Treatment of Overdosage:

Keep the patient recumbent in a shock position and comfortably warm. Gastric lavage may be of use if the medication has only recently been swallowed. Passive movement of the extremities may aid venous return. Administer oxygen and artificial ventilation, if necessary. If methemoglobinemia is present, administration of methylene blue (1% solution), 1–2 mg per kilogram of body weight intravenously, may be required.

Methemoglobinemia:

Case reports of clinically significant methemoglobinemia are rare at conventional doses of organic nitrates. The formation of methemoglobin is dose-related and in the case of genetic abnormalities of hemoglobin that favor methemoglobin formation, even conventional doses of organic nitrates could produce harmful concentrations of methemoglobin.

WARNING

Epinephrine is ineffective in reversing the severe hypotensive events associated with overdosage. It and related compounds are contraindicated in this situation.

DOSAGE AND ADMINISTRATION

At the onset of an attack, one or two metered doses should be sprayed onto or under the tongue. No more than three metered doses are recommended within a 15-minute period. If the chest pain persists, prompt medical attention is recommended. Nitrolingual Spray may be used prophylactically five to ten minutes prior to engaging in activities which might precipitate an acute attack.

During application the patient should rest, ideally in the sitting position. The canister should be held vertically with the valve head uppermost and the spray orifice as close to the mouth as possible. The dose should preferably be sprayed onto the tongue by pressing the button firmly and the mouth should be closed immediately after each dose. THE SPRAY SHOULD NOT BE INHALED. Patients should be instructed to familiarize themselves with the position of the spray orifice, which can be identified by the finger rest on top of the valve, in order to facilitate orientation for administration at night.

HOW SUPPLIED

Nitrolingual Spray, 13.8 g (Net Contents) containing 200 metered doses, box of one. (NDC 0075-0820-80)

Do not expose to heat or store at temperatures above 120°F (49°C).

CAUTION

Federal (U.S.A.) law prohibits dispensing without prescription.

Rev. 4/88

Manufactured by:
G. Pohl-Boskamp GmbH & Co., D-2214
Hohenlockstedt, West Germany

Distributed by:
RORER PHARMACEUTICALS
a division of
RORER PHARMACEUTICAL CORPORATION
Fort Washington, PA, U.S.A. 19034
Shown in Product Identification Section, page 426

NITROSPAN®   ℞
[nī'trō-span"]
(nitroglycerin)
sustained-release capsules
2.5 mg capsules
6.5 mg capsules

DESCRIPTION

Nitroglycerin, an organic nitrate, is a vasodilator which has effects on both arteries and veins. The chemical name for nitroglycerin is 1,2,3 propanetriol trinitrate ($C_3H_5N_3O_9$). The compound has a molecular weight of 227.09. The chemical structure is:

$$CH_2-ONO_2$$
$$CH\ -ONO_2$$
$$CH_2-ONO_2$$

Nitrospan® is provided in two strengths. Each Nitrospan sustained-release capsule contains 2.5 mg or 6.5 mg nitroglycerin in a sustained-released vehicle.

The inactive ingredients contained in both the 2.5 mg and the 6.5 mg capsules are: cornstarch, ethylcellulose, lactose, pharmaceutical glaze, sucrose, and talc. Nitrospan 6.5 mg also contains Yellow 6.

CLINICAL PHARMACOLOGY

The principal pharmacological action of nitroglycerin is relaxation of vascular smooth muscle, producing a vasodilator effect on both peripheral arteries and veins with more predominant effects on the latter. Dilation of the postcapillary vessels, including large veins, promotes peripheral pooling of blood and decreases venous return to the heart, thereby reducing left ventricular end-diastolic pressure (preload). Arteriolar relaxation reduces systemic vascular resistance and arterial pressure (afterload).

The mechanism by which nitroglycerin relieves angina pectoris is not fully understood. Myocardial oxygen consumption or demand (as measured by the pressure-rate product,

Continued on next page

This product information was prepared in September, 1989. Information concerning these products may be obtained by addressing Rorer Pharmaceutical Corporation, 500 Virginia Drive, Fort Washington, PA 19034.

Rorer Pharm.—Cont.

tension-time index, and stroke work index) is decreased by both the arterial and venous effects of nitroglycerin and, presumably, a more favorable supply-demand ratio is achieved. While the large epicardial coronary arteries are also dilated by nitroglycerin, the extent to which this action contributes to relief of exertional angina is unclear.

Nitroglycerin is rapidly metabolized *in vivo*, with a liver reductase enzyme having primary importance in the formation of glycerol nitrate metabolites and inorganic nitrate. Two active major metabolites, 1–2 and 1–3 dinitroglycerols, the products of hydrolysis, although less potent as vasodilators, have longer plasma half-lives than the parent compound, and appear in substantial concentration. The dinitrates are further metabolized to mononitrates (considered biologically inactive with respect to cardiovascular effects) and ultimately glycerol and carbon dioxide. There is extensive first-pass deactivation by the liver of nitroglycerin following gastrointestinal absorption, but the hepatic reductase activity may be saturated by some doses of oral nitroglycerin, resulting in prolonged pharmacologic effects. Hemodynamic studies employing plethysmographic methods in human volunteers have demonstrated that oral nitroglycerin (single dose 6.5 mg) has biologic effects significantly different from placebo for up to 8 hours.

Adequate studies defining the pharmacokinetics of Nitrospan have not been reported. The clinical relevance of nitroglycerin blood levels has not been established, since therapeutic levels of the drug and metabolites have not been defined. Therapeutic doses of nitroglycerin reduce systolic and mean arterial blood pressures, especially when the patient assumes upright posture. Systolic blood pressure is decreased for up to 4 hours after a single dose of 6.5 mg of swallowed controlled-release nitroglycerin.

Clinical studies indicate that oral controlled-release nitroglycerin may reduce abnormally elevated left ventricular end-diastolic pressure (LVEDP), a hemodynamic occurrence during acute episodes of angina pectoris. Although there have been no reported, invasively measured, hemodynamic studies of Nitrospan in patients with angina pectoris, controlled clinical trials in patients with congestive heart failure have shown significant decreases in mean LVEDP for as long as 4 hours after a single dose (6.5–19.5 mg) of oral nitroglycerin. The onset of hemodynamic effect from the swallowed form of nitroglycerin is not sufficiently rapid to be of use in aborting an acute episode of angina pectoris.

INDICATIONS AND USAGE

Nitrospan is indicated for the prevention of angina pectoris due to coronary artery disease. Controlled clinical trials have demonstrated that this form of nitroglycerin is effective in improving exercise tolerance in patients with exertional angina pectoris. Controlled clinical studies of 2.6 mg and larger (6.5–26 mg) doses in patients with angina pectoris have shown improvement in treadmill exercise time for at least 4 hours after dosing.

CONTRAINDICATIONS

Nitroglycerin is contraindicated in patients who have shown acute or recent myocardial infarction, severe anemia, closed-angle glaucoma, postural hypotension, increased intracranial pressure, hypersensitivity to nitroglycerin or other nitrates or nitrites.

WARNINGS

This form of nitroglycerin is not intended for immediate relief of anginal attacks. The use of any form of nitroglycerin during the early days of acute myocardial infarction requires particular attention to hemodynamic monitoring and clinical status. In general, a long-acting dosage form such as Nitrospan should not be used because its effects are difficult to terminate rapidly should excessive hypotension or tachycardia develop.

PRECAUTIONS

General: Intraocular pressure may be increased; therefore, caution is required in administering to patients with glaucoma. Severe hypotension, particularly with upright posture, may occur even with small doses of nitroglycerin. The drug therefore should be used with caution in subjects who may have volume depletion from diuretic therapy or in patients who have low systolic blood pressure (e.g., below 90 mm Hg). Paradoxical bradycardia and increased angina pectoris may accompany nitroglycerin-induced hypotension.

Nitrate therapy may aggravate the angina caused by hypertrophic cardiomyopathy.

If blurring of vision, dryness of mouth or lack of benefit occurs, the drug should be discontinued.

Tolerance to this drug and cross-tolerance to other nitrates and nitrites may occur. Tolerance to the vascular and antianginal effects of nitrates has been demonstrated in clinical trials, experience through occupational exposure, and in isolated tissue experiments in the laboratory.

The importance of tolerance to the use of nitroglycerin in the management of patients with angina pectoris has not been

determined. In controlled clinical trials in patients with angina pectoris, sustained therapy with some nitrate preparations resulted in significantly less and shorter duration of improvement in exercise time on stress testing than did acute therapy. However, a controlled study of repetitive doses of oral nitroglycerin showed treadmill performance to be significantly better with drug than with placebo in 18 patients with angina pectoris after 2 weeks of therapy.

In industrial workers continuously exposed to nitroglycerin, tolerance clearly occurs. Moreover, physical dependence also occurs since chest pain, acute myocardial infarction, and even sudden death have occurred during temporary withdrawal of nitroglycerin from the workers. In various clinical trials of angina patients, there are reports of anginal attacks being more easily provoked and of rebound in the hemodynamic effects soon after nitrate withdrawal. The relative importance of these observations to the routine, clinical use of nitroglycerin are not known. However, it seems prudent to gradually withdraw patients from nitroglycerin when the therapy is being terminated, rather than stopping the drug abruptly.

Drug Interactions: Alcohol may enhance sensitivity to the hypotensive effects of nitrates.

Adverse reactions (see below) are enhanced by ingestion of alcohol, which appears to increase absorption from the gastrointestinal tract.

Nitroglycerin acts directly on vascular muscle. Therefore, any other agents that depend on vascular smooth muscle as the final common path can be expected to have decreased or increased effect, depending on the agent.

Marked symptomatic orthostatic hypotension has been reported when calcium channel blockers and oral controlled-release nitroglycerin were used in combination. Dose adjustments of either class of agents may be necessary.

Carcinogenesis, Mutagenesis, Impairment of Fertility: No long-term studies in animals have been performed to evaluate carcinogenic potential of Nitrospan.

Pregnancy: Pregnancy Category C. Animal reproduction studies have not been conducted with Nitrospan. It is also not known whether nitroglycerin can cause fetal harm when administered to a pregnant woman or can affect reproduction capacity. Nitroglycerin should be given to a pregnant woman only if clearly needed.

Nursing Mothers: It is not known whether nitroglycerin is excreted in human milk. Because many drugs are excreted in human milk, caution should be exercised when Nitrospan is administered to a nursing woman.

Pediatric Use: Safety and effectiveness in children have not been established.

ADVERSE REACTIONS

Adverse reactions to Nitrospan, particularly headache and hypotension, are generally dose-related and may disappear with a reduction in dosage. In clinical trials at various doses of nitroglycerin, the following adverse effects have been observed:

Headache, which may be severe and persistent, is the most commonly reported side effect of nitroglycerin, with an incidence in the order of about 50% in some studies. Cutaneous vasodilation with flushing may occur. Transient episodes of dizziness and weakness, as well as other signs of cerebral ischemia associated with postural hypotension, may occasionally develop. An occasional individual may exhibit marked sensitivity to the hypotensive effects of nitrates and severe responses (nausea, vomiting, weakness, restlessness, pallor, perspiration, and collapse) may occur even with therapeutic doses of nitrates. Drug rash and/or exfoliative dermatitis have been reported in patients receiving nitrate therapy. Nausea and vomiting appear to be uncommon.

OVERDOSAGE

Signs and Symptoms: Nitrate overdosage may result in: Severe hypotension, persistent throbbing headache, vertigo, palpitation, visual disturbance, flushing and perspiring skin (later becoming cold and cyanotic), nausea and vomiting (possibly with colic and even bloody diarrhea), syncope (especially in the upright posture), methemoglobinemia with cyanosis and anorexia, initial hyperpnea, dyspnea and slow breathing, slow pulse (dicrotic and intermittent), heart block, increased intracranial pressure with cerebral symptoms of confusion and moderate fever, paralysis and coma followed by clonic convulsions, and possibly death due to circulatory collapse.

Treatment of Overdosage: Keep the patient recumbent in a shock position and comfortably warm. Gastric lavage may be of use if the medication has only recently been swallowed. Passive movement of the extremities may aid venous return. Administer oxygen and artificial ventilation if necessary. If methemoglobinemia is present, administration of methylene blue (1% solution), 1–2 mg/kg intravenously, may be required.

Methemoglobin: Case reports of clinically significant methemoglobinemia are rare at conventional doses of organic nitrates. The formation of methemoglobin is dose-related and in the case of genetic abnormalities of hemoglobin that favor methemoglobin formation, even conventional doses of

organic nitrates could produce harmful concentrations of methemoglobin.

WARNING: Epinephrine is ineffective in reversing the severe hypotensive events associated with overdose. It and related compounds are contraindicated in this situation.

DOSAGE AND ADMINISTRATION

The usual starting dose for Nitrospan (nitroglycerin) is 2.5 mg taken 3 to 4 times daily. Controlled trials have been carried out to 5 hours after dosing; therefore, it is not known whether the drug is effective in prevention of exertional angina beyond 5 hours after dosing.

Nitrospan should be TITRATED upward until a dose effective in controlling angina is determined or until side effects limit the dose. The dose generally may be increased by 2.5-mg increments 2 to 4 times daily over a period of days or weeks. Doses as high as 26 mg given 4 times daily have been reported effective in angina pectoris patients.

Administer the smallest effective dose 3 to 4 times daily unless clinical response suggests a different regimen. Discontinue if not effective. At initiation of therapy or change in dosage, the blood pressure (patient standing) should be monitored.

Nitrospan Capsules must be swallowed. They are NOT FOR CHEWING OR FOR SUBLINGUAL USE. Nitrospan Capsules are not intended for immediate relief of anginal attacks.

HOW SUPPLIED

Nitrospan (nitroglycerin) 2.5 mg Capsules are available in bottles of 100 (NDC 0075-0150-00), and 6.5 mg Capsules are available in bottles of 60 (NDC 0075-0151-60).

Store capsules at controlled room temperature, 59°–86°F (15°–30°C). Dispense only in original unopened container.

CAUTION

Federal (U.S.A.) law prohibits dispensing without prescription.

Revised: July 1988

RORER PHARMACEUTICALS

a division of

RORER PHARMACEUTICAL CORPORATION

Fort Washington, PA, U.S.A. 19034

PARATHAR™　　　　　　　　　　　　　　　　　　　℞

[par'əthär]

(teriparatide acetate)

for Injection, Synthetic

(human parathyroid hormone 1-34)

10 mL Vial with Diluent

DESCRIPTION

Parathar™ (teriparatide acetate) for Injection, Synthetic contains teriparatide acetate (hPTH 1-34), a synthetic polypeptide hormone consisting of the 1-34 fragment of human parathyroid hormone, the biologically active N-terminal region of the 84 amino acid native hormone.

The structure of teriparatide acetate is represented by the following amino acid sequence:

H_2N-Ser-Val-Ser-Glu-Ile-Gln-Leu-Met-His-
Asn-Leu-Gly-Lys-His-Leu-Asn-Ser-Met-
Glu-Arg-Val-Glu-Trp-Leu-Arg-Lys-Lys-Leu-
Gln-Asp-Val-His-Asn-Phe-OH XCH_3COOH, X=6-9

Parathar is a sterile, lyophilized white powder providing 200 units hPTH activity per vial with 20 mg gelatin, and hydrochloric acid to adjust pH. It may contain up to 35% extraneous peptides, the chemical structures of which have not been determined. The product is for I.V. infusion after reconstitution with accompanying diluent.

CLINICAL PHARMACOLOGY

Parathyroid hormone is secreted by the four parathyroid glands found on or embedded in the two lateral lobes of the thyroid gland. hPTH 1-34 acts on bone to mobilize calcium and on the kidney to reduce calcium clearance, increase phosphate excretion, stimulate the release of cyclic AMP in the urine, and stimulate the conversion of 25-hydroxy-vitamin D_3 (25-OH-D_3) to the active form 1, 25-dihydroxyvitamin D_3 [1, 25 (OH)$_2$$D_3$].

The initial effect of teriparatide acetate on bone is to promote an increased rate of release of calcium from bone mineral into blood. The action may be mediated by an effect on osteocytes or osteoclasts.

The kidney effects, which may be due to a direct action of the hormone on its receptors, include a reduction of calcium clearance and an inhibition of tubular phosphate reabsorption as well as an increased excretion of sodium and potassium. Parathyroid hormone stimulates the conversion of 25-OH-D to 1,25(OH)$_2$D by the kidney.

Intestinal transport of calcium is increased by the PTH indirectly by increasing renal 1,25(OH)$_2$D production.

The primary mode of action is the stimulation of adenylate cyclase in the involved organ.

INDICATIONS AND USAGE

Parathar (teriparatide acetate) for Injection, Synthetic is indicated as a diagnostic agent to assist in establishing the diagnosis in patients presenting with clinical and laboratory evidence of hypocalcemia due to either hypoparathyroidism or pseudohypoparathyroidism. The test will distinguish between hypoparathyroidism and pseudohypoparathyroidism, but not between these conditions and normal. The discriminant power of Parathar's effect on urinary cAMP is much greater than that of the effect on urinary phosphate.

CONTRAINDICATIONS

Known hypersensitivity to teriparatide acetate or to any components of the preparation.

WARNINGS

Allergic Reactions: Because teriparatide acetate is a peptide, the possibility of a systemic allergic reaction cannot be overlooked. The usual provisions should be made for the emergency treatment of such a reaction should it occur.

PRECAUTIONS

1. General: The administration of Parathar could lead to hypercalcemia. Parathar is not intended for recurrent or chronic use.
2. Carcinogenesis, Mutagenesis, Impairment of Fertility: No studies have been performed to evaluate the carcinogenic or mutagenic potential of Parathar or its effect on fertility.
3. Pregnancy/Teratogenic Effects: Pregnancy—Category C: Animal reproduction studies have not been conducted with Parathar. It is also not known whether Parathar can cause fetal harm when administered to a pregnant woman or can affect reproduction capacity. Parathar should be given to a pregnant woman only if clearly needed.
4. Nursing Mother: It is not known to what degree Parathar is excreted in human milk, but the peptide would not be expected to be absorbed in an active form from the infant's gastrointestinal tract. However, caution should be exercised when Parathar is administered to a nursing woman.
5. Pediatric Use: There is limited data on safety in children. The use of Parathar in children 3 years of age and older was uneventful and the response to the drug followed expected patterns.

ADVERSE REACTIONS

Cardiovascular
A hypertensive crisis occurred in one patient 8 hours after a study. This patient had had previous hypertensive episodes not related to teriparatide acetate injection.
Metabolic/Nutritional
Hypocalcemia was not reversed in one patient, and a hypocalcemic convulsion occurred $4\frac{1}{2}$ hours following injection; this was corrected by calcium administration.
Gastrointestinal
Nausea, abdominal cramps, urge to defecate, and diarrhea were reported. The incidence of each of these adverse reactions was less then 2.0%.
Other
Tingling of the extremities, metallic taste, and pain at the injection site have been reported during or shortly following the infusion. The incidence of each of these adverse reactions was less than 2.0%.

OVERDOSAGE

Parathar given repeatedly in doses in excess of 500 units may produce hypercalcemia. In those who are borderline hypercalcemic (10.5 mg/dl), a dose of 200 units could produce mild hypercalcemia for a brief period. If hypercalcemia develops, the drug should be discontinued and steps should be taken to ensure adequate hydration.

DOSAGE AND ADMINISTRATION

Diagnostic use in patients with hypocalcemia: The recommended dose for adults is 200 units of Parathar. Reconstitute by adding the 10 mL diluent to the 10 mL Parathar vial. The 10 mL of solution is infused intravenously over a 10-minute period. In children 3 years of age or older, the recommended dose is 3 units per kg of body weight, up to a maximum of 200 units. Reconstituted solution should be used within 4 hours. Discard any unused portion.
Parenteral drug products should be inspected visually for particulate matter and discoloration prior to administration, whenever solution and container permit.
Modified Ellsworth Howard Test: Test subjects should be in a fasting state when starting the test period. An active urine output should be initiated and maintained by the ingestion of 200 mL of water per hour for 2 hours prior to study and continuing through the study. A baseline urine collection should be made in the 60-minute period preceding the Parathar infusion. Following the hPTH (1-34) infusion (time 0), urine should be collected as separate collections in the 0–30 minute, 30–60 minute and 60–120 minute postinfusion time periods. Confidence in the test will be influenced by adequate hydration and urine flow and complete collection of urine specimens.

INTERPRETATION OF TEST

The measurement of urinary cAMP and phosphate must be corrected for creatinine excretion.
In the clinical trials, patients with hypoparathyroidism showed a tenfold or greater increase over baseline of urinary cAMP at the 0–30 minute postinfusion period, and 92 per-

cent of these patients showed a threefold or greater urinary phosphate excretion in the 0–60 minute collection.
Patients with end-organ resistance pseudohypoparathyroidism showed a blunted response of less than sixfold increase of urinary cAMP excretion over baseline in the 0–30 minute period, and 88 percent showed a less than threefold increase in urinary phosphate excretion in the 0–60 minute collection period.
Although this test does not discriminate between normal and abnormal in most cases, it does discriminate between hypoparathyroidism and pseudohypoparathyroidism. The change in the urinary cAMP excretion in the 0–30 minute period is the most sensitive indicator for separation of hypoparathyroidisms.

HOW SUPPLIED

Parathar (teriparatide acetate) for Injection, Synthetic is supplied in a 10 mL vial as a sterile, lyophilized powder containing 200 units hPTH activity with a 10 mL vial of diluent (NDC 0075-2050-53).
Store at controlled room temperature, 59°–86°F (15°–30°C).
Caution: Federal (U.S.A.) law prohibits dispensing without prescription.
23785/11-87
RORER PHARMACEUTICALS
a division of
RORER PHARMACEUTICAL CORPORATION
Fort Washington, PA, U.S.A. 19034

PAREPECTOLIN®   Ⓒ
Antidiarrheal

FORMULA

Paregoric (equivalent) ....(1 fl dram) 3.7 mL
Contains opium (¼ grain) ....15 mg/fl oz
(Warning: May be habit forming.)
Pectin ....(2½ grains) 162 mg
Kaolin ....(85 grains) 5.5 g

INACTIVE INGREDIENTS

Alcohol 0.69%, benzoic acid, carboxymethylcellulose sodium, ethylparaben, flavors, glycerin, propylparaben, saccharin sodium, purified water.

INDICATIONS

For symptomatic relief of diarrhea.

CONTRAINDICATIONS

Paregoric should not be used to treat diarrhea caused by poisons, toxins, or infectious agents until the gastrointestinal tract has been cleared of the causative agent.

ACTIONS

The kaolin adsorbs irritants and forms a protective coating on intestinal mucosa. Kaolin enhances stool formation; however, total water loss may be unchanged. Pectin acts to consolidate the stool. Paregoric is very useful in diarrhea because it has a soothing action and allays discomfort of intestinal grippe.

ADVANTAGES

Parepectolin contains paregoric (equivalent) and effectively controls both diarrhea and colicky cramps. It is prepared as a stable suspension with a pleasant taste for oral administration.

DIRECTIONS FOR USE

Adults and Children over 12 years of age: One or two tablespoonfuls after each loose bowel movement not to exceed 8 tablespoonfuls in 12 hours.
Children 6 to 12 years of age: One or two teaspoonfuls after each loose bowel movement not to exceed 8 teaspoonfuls in 12 hours.
Children 3 to 6 years of age: 1½ teaspoonfuls after each loose bowel movement not to exceed 6 teaspoonfuls in 12 hours.
Children under 3 years of age: Not to be administered unless directed by a doctor.

WARNING

As with any drug, if you are pregnant or nursing a baby, seek the advice of a health professional before using this product. In case of accidental overdose, seek professional assistance or contact a poison control center immediately.
Diarrhea may be serious. Do not use for more than 2 days or in the presence of high fever or in infants or children under 3 years of age unless directed by physician.
KEEP OUT OF THE REACH OF CHILDREN/STORE AT ROOM TEMPERATURE
How Supplied: Bottles of 4 oz. (118 mL) (NDC 0075-0660-60) and 8 oz. (237 mL) (NDC 0075-0660-66) fluid ounces.
RORER PHARMACEUTICALS
a division of
RORER PHARMACEUTICAL CORPORATION
Fort Washington, PA, U.S.A. 19034

PERTOFRANE®   ℞
[pert 'ō-frān "]
(desipramine hydrochloride, USP)
25 mg capsules
50 mg capsules

COMPOSITION

Each capsule provides 25 mg or 50 mg desipramine hydrochloride. The capsules also contain lactose, magnesium stearate, and talc.

DESCRIPTION

PERTOFRANE (desipramine hydrochloride) is a metabolite of imipramine hydrochloride. It is a dibenzazepine derivative, representing the desmethyl analog of imipramine hydrochloride. Chemically it is 10,11-dihydro-5-[3-(methylamino) propyl]-5H-dibenz [b.f] azepine monohydrochloride, and differs from the parent substance by having only one methyl group on the side chain nitrogen. It has the following structure:

Desipramine hydrochloride is a white, crystalline substance with a molecular weight of 302.8. It is soluble to the extent of about 10% w/v in water, and melts within a range of 5° between 208-218°C.

ACTIONS

PERTOFRANE has been found in some studies to have a more rapid onset of action than imipramine; antidepressant efficacy is similar though potency on a weight basis may be less. The earliest manifestations consist mainly of an increase in psychomotor activity. Full treatment benefit is seldom attained before the end of the second week.
PERTOFRANE is not a monoamine oxidase inhibitor and does not act primarily as a central nervous system stimulant. Like all tricyclic antidepressants, PERTOFRANE blocks the re-uptake of norepinephrine by adrenergic nerve terminals. Demethylated analogs such as desipramine are more potent in increasing norepinephrine turnover rate than the methylated compounds. However, the exact mechanism of action of tricyclics in depression is still unknown.
A mechanism of action proposed for antidepressant drugs, the biogenic amine theory postulates that some, if not all, depression is associated with a deficiency or depletion of catecholamines and that some antidepressant drugs increase the amount of amine available at the synaptic receptor.
Desipramine is metabolized in the liver and approximately 70% is excreted in the urine.

INDICATIONS

PERTOFRANE is indicated for the relief of mental depression (see Note before How Supplied section for additional information on depressive symptomatologies often responsive to this drug).

CONTRAINDICATIONS

The use of PERTOFRANE concomitantly or within two weeks of the administration of MAO inhibitors is contraindicated. Hyperpyretic crises or severe convulsive seizures may occur in patients receiving such combinations. The potentiation of adverse reactions can be serious or even fatal. When it is desired to substitute PERTOFRANE in patients receiving a monoamine oxidase inhibitor, as long an interval should elapse as the clinical situation allows with a minimum of 14 days. Initial dosage should be low and increases should be gradual and cautiously prescribed.
The drug is contraindicated following recent myocardial infarction.
Patients with a known hypersensitivity to tricyclic antidepressants should not be given PERTOFRANE.

WARNINGS

As with other potent antidepressants, an activation of the psychosis may occasionally be observed in schizophrenic patients.
Due to the drug's atropine-like effects and its sympathomimetic potentiation, PERTOFRANE should be used only with the greatest care in patients with narrow-angle glaucoma and with urethral or ureteral spasm.
Likewise only when patient need outweighs the risk of serious adverse reactions should the drug be used in the pres-

Continued on next page

This product information was prepared in September, 1989. Information concerning these products may be obtained by addressing Rorer Pharmaceutical Corporation, 500 Virginia Drive, Fort Washington, PA 19034.

Rorer Pharm.—Cont.

ence of any of the following conditions: severe coronary heart disease with ECG abnormalities, progressive heart failure, angina pectoris, paroxysmal tachycardia and active seizure disorder (this agent has been shown to lower the seizure threshold).

In some instances, desipramine and the parent compound, imipramine, have been shown to block the pharmacologic action of the antihypertensive, guanethidine, and related adrenergic neuron-blocking agents.

Hypertensive episodes have been observed during surgery in patients on desipramine hydrochloride therapy.

The concurrent use of other central nervous system drugs or alcohol may potentiate the adverse effects of desipramine hydrochloride. Since many such drugs may be used during surgery, it is recommended that desipramine hydrochloride be discontinued for as long as the clinical situation will allow prior to elective surgery.

In patients who may use alcohol excessively, it should be borne in mind that the potentiation may increase the danger inherent in any suicide attempt or overdosage.

Patients should be cautioned about the possibility of impaired ability to operate a motor vehicle or other dangerous machinery.

Usage in Pregnancy: Although teratogenic studies in mice, rats and rabbits have revealed no adverse effects, safe use of this drug in women who are or may become pregnant has not been definitely established. Therefore, PERTOFRANE should be withheld from these women unless the clinical situation warrants the potential risk.

In view of the lack of experience in children, the drug is not recommended for use in patients under twelve years of age. Elderly and adolescent patients can usually be managed on lower dosage than that recommended for other patients and may not tolerate higher doses as well because of an increased incidence of adverse reactions.

PRECAUTIONS

It should be kept in mind that the possibility of suicide in seriously depressed patients is inherent in the illness and may persist until remission occurs. These patients require careful supervision and protective measures during therapy. Anxiety and increased agitation have been reported, particularly where depression is not the primary disorder. A shift to hypomanic or manic excitement may occur during therapy. Such reactions may necessitate discontinuation of the drug. Although the anticholinergic activity of the drug is weak, in susceptible patients and in those receiving anticholinergic drugs (including antiparkinsonism agents), atropine-like effects may be more pronounced (e.g., paralytic ileus). Caution should be observed in prescribing the drug in hyperthyroid patients and in those receiving thyroid medications. Transient cardiac arrhythmias have occurred in rare instances.

Steady-state serum concentrations of tricyclic antidepressants are reported to fluctuate significantly as cimetidine is either added or deleted from the drug regimen. Serious anticholinergic symptoms (severe dry mouth, urinary retention, blurred vision) have been associated with elevations in serum levels of the tricyclic antidepressants when cimetidine is added to the drug regimen. Additionally, higher than expected steady-state serum concentrations of tricyclic antidepressant have been observed when therapy is initiated in patients already taking cimetidine. Alternatively, decreases in steady-state serum concentrations of tricyclic antidepressant have been reported in well-controlled patients on concurrent therapy, upon discontinuance of cimetidine. Therapeutic efficacy of the tricyclic antidepressant may be compromised in these patients.

In all patients undergoing extended courses of therapy, periodic blood and liver studies for signs of toxicity should supplement careful clinical observations.

ADVERSE REACTIONS

PERTOFRANE is well tolerated by most patients and severe complications or adverse reactions are infrequent. Those most often reported cause little discomfort and seldom require discontinuation of the drug.

Nervous System: Dizziness, drowsiness, insomnia, headache and disturbed visual accommodation have been reported with the drug. In addition, tremor, unsteadiness, tinnitus and paresthesias have been reported. Occasionally, mild extrapyramidal activity, falling, and neuromuscular incoordination have been seen. A confusional state (with such symptoms as hallucinations and disorientation) may be produced, particularly in older patients and at higher dosage, and may require discontinuation of the drug. Changes in EEG patterns have been observed. Epileptiform seizures may occur. The syndrome of inappropriate ADH (antidiuretic hormone) secretion may occur. A reduction in dosage may help control some of these adverse reactions.

Gastrointestinal Tract: Anorexia, dryness of the mouth, nausea, epigastric distress, constipation and diarrhea have been reported in patients receiving PERTOFRANE.

Skin: Skin rashes (including photosensitization), perspiration and flushing sensations have been reported during therapy.

Liver: Transient jaundice, apparently of an obstructive nature, and liver damage have been observed in rare cases. Elevation in transaminase and changes in alkaline phosphatase have occurred and should indicate repeated liver-function profiles. If progressive elevation occurs, the drug should be discontinued.

Blood Elements: Bone-marrow depression, agranulocytosis, thrombocytopenia and purpura have been reported. If these occur, the drug should be discontinued. Transient eosinophilia has been observed in some instances.

Cardiovascular System: Orthostatic hypotension and tachycardia have been observed but seldom require discontinuation of treatment. Patients who require concomitant vasodilating therapy should be carefully supervised, particularly during the initial phases.

Genitourinary System: Urinary frequency or retention and impotence have been reported.

Endocrine System: Occasional hormonal effects, including gynecomastia, galactorrhea and breast enlargement have been reported with PERTOFRANE (desipramine hydrochloride). In addition, decreased libido and estrogenic effect have been noted. The exact relationship of these adverse effects to the administration of the drug has not been established.

Sensitivity: Urticaria and rare instances of drug fever and cross-sensitivity with imipramine have been observed.

WITHDRAWAL SYMPTOMS

Abrupt cessation of treatment after prolonged administration may produce nausea, headache and malaise. These are not indicative of addiction. Rare instances have been reported of mania or hypomania occurring within 2–7 days following cessation of chronic therapy with tricyclic antidepressants.

DOSAGE AND ADMINISTRATION

All Patients Except Geriatric and Adolescent: The usual dosage range is from 75 to 150 mg/day in divided doses or as a single daily dose. Titration to a maintenance dose should be based on clinical response and tolerance by starting in the low dose range and increasing dosage when required. When necessary, dosage may be increased, after initiation of therapy, up to 200 mg daily in divided doses. Continued therapy at the optimal dosage level should be maintained during the active phase of the depression.

It is recommended that a lower maintenance dosage be continued for at least two months after a satisfactory response has been achieved. This, too, may be given on a once-daily schedule for convenience and compliance.

In cases of relapse due to premature withdrawal of the drug, a prompt response may be obtained by immediate resumption of treatment.

Geriatric and Adolescent Patients: Elderly and adolescent patients can usually be managed on lower dosage and may not tolerate higher doses as well as other patients. Therapy in these age groups may be initiated with 25 to 50 mg daily. Dosage may be increased according to response and tolerance to a maximum of 100 mg daily. It is recommended that a lower maintenance dosage be continued for at least two months after a satisfactory response has been achieved. Therapy may be given in divided doses or as a single daily dose.

OVERDOSAGE

Signs and Symptoms: These may vary in severity depending on several factors, including the amount absorbed, age, interval between ingestion and start of treatment, etc. In infants and young children, especially, acute overdosage in any amount must be considered serious and potentially fatal. CNS abnormalities may include drowsiness, stupor, coma, ataxia, restlessness, agitation, hyperactive reflexes, muscle rigidity, athetoid and choreiform movements, and convulsions.

Cardiac abnormalities may include arrhythmia, tachycardia, ECG evidence of impaired conduction, and signs of congestive failure.

Respiratory depression, cyanosis, hypotension, shock, vomiting, hyperpyrexia, mydriasis, and diaphoresis may also be present.

Treatment: Because CNS involvement, respiratory depression and cardiac arrhythmia can occur suddenly, hospitalization and close observation are necessary, even when the amount ingested is thought to be small or the initial degree of intoxication appears slight or moderate. All patients with ECG abnormalities should have continuous cardiac monitoring for at least 72 hours and be closely observed until well after cardiac status has returned to normal; relapses may occur after apparent recovery.

The *slow* intravenous administration of physostigmine salicylate has been reported to reverse most of the cardiovascular and CNS effects of overdosage with tricyclic antidepressants. In adults, 1 to 3 mg has been reported to be effective. In children, start with 0.5 mg and repeat at 5-minute intervals to determine the minimum effective dose; do not exceed 2 mg. Because of the short duration of action of physostigmine, repeat the effective dose at 30- to 50-minute intervals, as necessary. Avoid rapid injection to reduce the possibility of physostigmine-induced convulsions.

In the alert patient, empty the stomach promptly by induced emesis followed by lavage. In the obtunded patient, secure the airway with a cuffed endotracheal tube before beginning lavage (do not induce emesis). Continue lavage for 24 hours or longer, depending on the apparent severity of intoxication. Use normal or half-normal saline to avoid water intoxication, especially in children. Instillation of activated charcoal slurry may help reduce absorption of desipramine.

Minimize external stimulation to reduce the tendency to convulsions. If anticonvulsants are necessary, diazepam, short-acting barbiturates, paraldehyde or methocarbamol may be useful. Do not use barbiturates if MAO inhibitors have been taken recently.

Maintain adequate respiratory exchange. Do not use respiratory stimulants.

Shock should be treated with supportive measures, such as intravenous fluids, oxygen and corticosteroids. Digitalis may increase conduction abnormalities and further irritate an already sensitized myocardium. If congestive heart failure necessitates rapid digitalization, particular care must be exercised.

Hyperpyrexia should be controlled by whatever external means are available, including ice packs and cooling sponge baths, if necessary.

Hemodialysis, peritoneal dialysis, exchange transfusions and forced diuresis have been generally reported as ineffective because of the rapid fixation of desipramine in tissues. Blood desipramine levels may not correlate with the degree of intoxication, and are unreliable indicators in the clinical management of the patient.

NOTE

Depressions which are most responsive to PERTOFRANE may be described in terms of "target symptoms." These include:

Despondency, sadness and depressed mood

Fatigue

Lack of interest and emotional response

Helplessness, hopelessness, pessimism and despair

Feelings of incapacity and inferiority

Psychomotor retardation and inhibition

Delusions of guilt and unworthiness

Psychosomatic complaints

Insomnia

Anorexia and weight loss

Depression-related anxiety and agitation

Suicidal drive

It should be borne in mind that these "target symptoms" of depression assume their proper significance only after careful history, physical and mental evaluations and other investigative procedures have confirmed a diagnosis of one of the several types of depression.

HOW SUPPLIED

25 mg Capsules (pink), bottles of 100 (NDC 0075-0160-00). 50 mg Capsules (maroon and pink), bottles of 100 (NDC 0075-0161-00).

Store at room temperature; avoid excessive heat.

CAUTION

Federal (U.S.A.) law prohibits dispensing without prescription.

Revised: May 1988

RORER PHARMACEUTICALS

a division of

RORER PHARMACEUTICAL CORPORATION

Fort Washington, PA, U.S.A. 19034

REGROTON®   ℞

[rĕ-grō-tŏn]

Each tablet provides:
chlorthalidone USP 50 mg
reserpine USP 0.25 mg

DEMI-REGROTON®   ℞

Each tablet provides:
chlorthalidone USP 25 mg
reserpine USP 0.125 mg
Oral antihypertensives

DESCRIPTION

REGROTON and DEMI-REGROTON are drug combinations of two well-known antihypertensive agents, chlorthalidone and reserpine. DEMI-REGROTON provides one-half the amount of both agents as REGROTON, for flexibility of dosage in patient management.

Chemistry: A monosulfamyl diuretic, chlorthalidone differs from thiazide diuretics in that a double-ring system is incorporated in its structure. Chemically, it is 2-Chloro-5-(1-hydroxy-3-oxo-1-isoindolinyl) benzenesulfonamide, with the following structural formula:

[See Chemical Formula at top of next column].

Chlorthalidone is practically insoluble in water, in ether, and in chloroform; soluble in methanol; slightly soluble in alcohol.

Reserpine is a pure crystalline alkaloid from the root of Rauwolfia serpentina. It has the following structural formula:

Reserpine is insoluble in water; freely soluble in acetic acid and in chloroform; slightly soluble in benzene; very slightly soluble in alcohol and in ether.

REGROTON and DEMI-REGROTON contain the following inactive ingredients: cornstarch, gelatin, glycerin, lactose, magnesium stearate, silica, talc, and other ingredients. REGROTON also contains FD&C Red No. 40 and FD&C Blue No. 1.

ACTIONS

The pharmacologic effects are those of the constituent drugs. Chlorthalidone produces a saluretic effect in humans, beginning within two hours after an oral dose and continuing for as long as 72 hours. Copious diuresis is produced, with greatly increased excretion of sodium and chloride.

Reserpine, because it reduces arterial blood pressure and exerts a sedative effect, is particularly useful in the therapy of hypertension with related emotional disturbance. Reserpine is characterized by slow onset of action and sustained effect. Both its cardiovascular and central nervous system effects may persist following withdrawal of the drug. (See Precautions.)

Both chlorthalidone and reserpine have prolonged action, and the combination is thus able to exert a smooth and concerted effect over a long period. The two drugs appear to enhance each other, and this gives the combination a high degree of effectiveness. When considered necessary, the combination may be prescribed together with other antihypertensive agents, which may then be given in lower dosage with lessened chance of side reactions.

ANIMAL PHARMACOLOGY

In animal biochemical studies, chlorthalidone is absorbed slowly from the gastrointestinal tract, due to low solubility. After passage to the liver, some of the drug enters the general circulation, while some is excreted in the bile, to be reabsorbed later. In the general circulation, the drug is distributed widely to the tissues, but is taken up in the highest concentrations in the kidneys, where amounts have been found 72 hours after ingestion, long after it has disappeared from other tissues. The drug is excreted unchanged in the urine. The high renal concentration of chlorthalidone may be casually associated with the prolonged saluretic effect of the drug. Chlorthalidone appears to inhibit sodium and chloride reabsorption in the cortical diluting segment of ascending limb of Henle's loop. The reduction of plasma volume following diuresis is a probable mechanism in the initial antihypertensive action of the drug.

Reserpine probably produces its sedative and hypotensive effects through a depletion in tissue stores of catecholamines. The antihypertensive action of reserpine is probably due to loss of epinephrine and norepinephrine from peripheral sites. By contrast, its sedative and tranquilizing properties are thought to be related to depletion of 5-hydroxytryptamine from the brain.

INDICATION

Treatment of hypertension. (See box warning.)

CONTRAINDICATIONS

Patients with a history of mental depression, demonstrated hypersensitivity, and most cases of severe renal or hepatic diseases are the only contraindications.

WARNINGS

These fixed combination drugs are not indicated for initial therapy of hypertension. Hypertension requires therapy titrated to the individual patient. If the fixed combination represents the dosage so determined, its use may be more convenient in patient management. The treatment of hypertension is not static, but must be reevaluated as conditions in each patient warrant.

These drugs should be used with caution in severe renal disease, since products containing chlorthalidone or similar drugs may precipitate azotemia. Cumulative effects of the drug may develop in patients with impaired renal function. They should be used with caution in patients with impaired hepatic function or progressive liver disease, since minor alterations of fluid and electrolyte balance may precipitate hepatic coma.

REGROTON or DEMI-REGROTON may add to or potentiate the action of other antihypertensive drugs. Potentiation occurs with ganglionic or peripheral adrenergic-blocking drugs.

Sensitivity reactions may occur in patients with a history of allergy or bronchial asthma.

Reserpine may cause mental depression. Recognition of depression may be difficult because this condition may often be disguised by somatic complaints (Masked Depression). The drug should be discontinued at first signs of depression such as despondency, early morning insomnia, loss of appetite, impotence, or self-deprecation. Drug induced depression may persist for several months after drug withdrawal and may be severe enough to result in suicide. In patients who have had depression, the drug should not be started. Electroshock therapy should not be given to patients taking reserpine, since severe and even fatal reactions have occurred. The drug should be stopped at least seven days before giving electroshock therapy.

In susceptible patients, peptic ulcer may be precipitated or activated, in which case the drug should be discontinued.

Usage in Pregnancy: Reproduction studies with chlorthalidone in various animal species at multiples of the human dose showed no significant level of teratogenicity; no fetal or congenital abnormalities were observed. Animal data should not be extrapolated for clinical application.

Thiazides cross the placental barrier and appear in cord blood. The use of chlorthalidone and related drugs in pregnant women requires that the anticipated benefits of the drug be weighed against possible hazards to the fetus. These hazards include fetal or neonatal jaundice, thrombocytopenia, and possibly other adverse reactions which have occurred in the adult.

Nursing Mothers: Thiazides and reserpine cross the placental barrier and appear in cord blood and breast milk. Increased respiratory secretions, nasal congestion, cyanosis and anorexia may occur in infants born to reserpine-treated mothers. If use of the drug is deemed essential, the patient should stop nursing.

PRECAUTIONS

Antihypertensive therapy with chlorthalidone/reserpine combinations should always be initiated cautiously in postsympathectomy patients and in those receiving ganglionic-blocking agents, other potent antihypertensive drugs, or curare. At least a one-half reduction in the usual dosage of such agents may be advisable. Careful and continuous supervision of patients on such multiple-drug regimens is necessary.

Since some patients receiving Rauwolfia preparations have experienced hypotension when undergoing surgery, it may be advisable to discontinue chlorthalidone/reserpine combination drugs about two weeks prior to elective surgical procedures. Emergency surgery may be carried out by using, if necessary, anticholinergic or adrenergic drugs to prevent vagocirculatory responses; other supportive measures may be used as indicated.

Because of the possibility of progression of renal damage, periodic kidney function tests are indicated. In case of a rising BUN, the drug should be stopped.

The drug should be discontinued in cases of aggravated liver dysfunction (hepatic coma may be precipitated).

Periodic determination of serum electrolytes to detect possible electrolyte imbalance should be performed at appropriate intervals.

All patients receiving chlorthalidone should be observed for clinical signs of fluid or electrolyte imbalance; namely, hyponatremia, hypochloremic alkalosis, and hypokalemia. Serum and urine electrolyte determinations are particularly important when the patient is vomiting excessively or receiving parenteral fluids. Medication such as digitalis may also influence serum electrolytes. Warning signs, irrespective of cause, are: Dryness of mouth, thirst, weakness, lethargy, drowsiness, restlessness, muscle pains or cramps, muscular fatigue, hypotension, oliguria, tachycardia, and gastrointestinal disturbances such as nausea and vomiting.

Hypokalemia may develop with chlorthalidone as with any other potent diuretic, especially with brisk diuresis, when severe cirrhosis is present, or during concomitant use of corticosteroids or ACTH.

Interference with adequate oral electrolyte intake will also contribute to hypokalemia. Digitalis therapy may exagger-

ate metabolic effects of hypokalemia especially with reference to myocardial activity.

Any chloride deficit is generally mild and usually does not require specific treatment except under extraordinary circumstances (as in liver disease or renal disease). Dilutional hyponatremia may occur in edematous patients in hot weather; appropriate therapy is water restriction, rather than administration of salt except in rare instances when the hyponatremia is life threatening. In actual salt depletion, appropriate replacement is the therapy of choice.

Hyperuricemia may occur or frank gout may be precipitated in certain patients receiving chlorthalidone.

Insulin requirements in diabetic patients may be increased, decreased, or unchanged. Latent diabetes mellitus may become manifest during chlorthalidone administration.

Chlorthalidone and related drugs may decrease arterial responsiveness to norepinephrine. This diminution is not sufficient to preclude effectiveness of the pressor agent for therapeutic use.

Chlorthalidone and related drugs may decrease serum PBI levels without signs of thyroid disturbance.

Because reserpine increases gastrointestinal motility and secretion, REGROTON or DEMI-REGROTON should be used cautiously in patients with ulcerative colitis or gallstones, where biliary colic may be precipitated. In susceptible patients, bronchial asthma may occur.

Animal tumorigenicity: Rodent studies have shown that reserpine is an animal tumorigen, causing an increased incidence of mammary fibroadenomas in female mice, malignant tumors of the seminal vesicles in male mice, and malignant adrenal medullary tumors in male rats. These findings arose in two-year studies in which the drug was administered in the feed at concentrations of 5 and 10 ppm—about 100 to 300 times the usual human dose. The breast neoplasms are thought to be related to reserpine's prolactin-elevating effect. Several other prolactin-elevating drugs have also been associated with an increased incidence of mammary neoplasia in rodents.

The extent to which these findings indicate a risk to humans is uncertain. Tissue culture experiments show that about one third of human breast tumors are prolactin-dependent in vitro, a factor of considerable importance if the use of the drug is contemplated in a patient with previously detected breast cancer. The possibility of an increased risk of breast cancer in reserpine users has been studied extensively; however, no firm conclusion has emerged. Although a few epidemiologic studies have suggested a slightly increased risk (less than twofold in all studies except one) in women who have used reserpine, other studies of generally similar design have not confirmed this. Epidemiologic studies conducted using other drugs (neuroleptic agents) that, like reserpine, increase prolactin levels and, therefore, would be considered rodent mammary carcinogens, have not shown an association between chronic administration of the drug and human mammary tumorigenesis. While long-term clinical observation has not suggested such an association, the available evidence is considered too limited to be conclusive at this time. An association of reserpine intake with pheochromocytoma or tumors of the seminal vesicles has not been explored.

ADVERSE REACTIONS

Clinical trials indicate that the combination of chlorthalidone with reserpine is generally well tolerated. The adverse reactions most frequently seen include anorexia, gastric irritation, nausea, vomiting, diarrhea, constipation, nasal congestion, muscle cramps, dizziness, weakness, headache, drowsiness, and mental depression. Skin rashes, urticaria, and a case of ecchymosis have been reported. (Other dermatologic manifestations may occur—see below.)

A decreased glucose tolerance evidenced by hyperglycemia and glycosuria may develop inconsistently. This condition, usually reversible on discontinuation of therapy, responds to control with antidiabetic treatment. Diabetics and those predisposed should be checked regularly.

Hyperuricemia may be observed on occasion and acute attacks of gout have been precipitated. In cases where prolonged and significant elevation of blood uric acid concentration is considered potentially deleterious, concomitant use of a uricosuric agent is effective in reversing hyperuricemia without loss of diuretic and/or antihypertensive activity.

In addition to the reactions listed above, certain adverse reactions attributable to the drugs' components are shown below. Since REGROTON and DEMI-REGROTON combine chlorthalidone and reserpine in relatively small doses, such reactions may be less than when those drugs are used in full dosage.

Chlorthalidone: Idiosyncratic drug reactions such as aplastic anemia, purpura, thrombocytopenia, leukopenia, agranu-

Continued on next page

This product information was prepared in September, 1989. Information concerning these products may be obtained by addressing Rorer Pharmaceutical Corporation, 500 Virginia Drive, Fort Washington, PA 19034.

Rorer Pharm.—Cont.

locytosis, necrotizing angiitis and Lyell's syndrome (toxic epidermal necrolysis) have occurred, but are rare.

The remote possibility of pancreatitis should be considered when epigastric pain or unexplained gastrointestinal symptoms develop after prolonged administration.

Other reported reactions include restlessness, transient myopia, impotence or dysuria, and orthostatic hypotension, which may be potentiated when chlorthalidone is combined with alcohol, barbiturates, or narcotics. Since jaundice, xanthopsia, paresthesia, and photosensitization have been documented in related compounds, the possibility of these reactions should be kept in mind.

Reserpine: The sedative effect of reserpine may lead to drowsiness or lassitude in some patients. Frequently, this effect disappears with continued administration. Nasal stuffiness sometimes occurs. Gastrointestinal reactions include increased gastric secretions, loose stools, or increased bowel frequency.

Symptoms of mental depression may occur in a small percentage of patients, although the recommended dosage of REGROTON contains substantially less reserpine than that usually implicated in such reactions. The same is true of other rare side effects recorded for reserpine, which include bradycardia and ectopic cardiac rhythms (especially when used with digitalis), pruritus, eruptions and/or flushing of skin, angina pectoris, headache, dizziness, paradoxical anxiety, nightmare, dull sensorium, muscular aches, a reversible paralysis agitans-like syndrome, blurred vision, conjunctival infection, uveitis, optic atrophy and glaucoma, increased susceptibility to colds, dyspnea, weight gain, decreased libido or impotence, dryness of the mouth, deafness, and anorexia.

DOSAGE AND ADMINISTRATION

Selection of drug and dosage should be determined by individual titration. (See box warning.) According to the requirement, the recommended dose of either REGROTON or DEMI-REGROTON is usually *one tablet once a day.* Some patients may require two tablets once a day. Divided doses are unnecessary, and a single dose given in the morning with food is recommended.

Maintenance: Maintenance dosage must be individually adjusted. Mild cases may be adequately controlled with one DEMI-REGROTON tablet daily. Optimal lowering of elevated blood pressure may require two weeks or more in some cases because of the slow onset of action of reserpine.

Combination With Other Drugs: In more severe cases, if the response to a chlorthalidone/reserpine combination alone is inadequate, potent antihypertensives may be added gradually in dosages at least 50% lower than those usually employed. Such patients should be supervised carefully and continuously. As soon as desired blood pressure levels have been attained, the lowest effective maintenance dosage should be followed.

OVERDOSAGE

Adverse reactions resulting from accidental acute overdosage may include nausea, weakness, dizziness, syncope, and disturbances of electrolyte balance. There is no specific antidote. However, the following is recommended: Gastric lavage followed by supportive treatment, including intravenous dextrose-saline with potassium chloride if necessary, to be given with the usual caution. If marked hypotension results from overdosage, it can be treated with vasopressor drugs.

HOW SUPPLIED

REGROTON is available as pink, uniquely-shaped* tablets, bottles of 100 (NDC 0070-0031-00); DEMI-REGROTON as white, uniquely-shaped* tablets, bottles of 100 (NDC 0070-0032-00). Store at controlled room temperature between 15°–30°C (59°–86°F). Dispense in tight, light-resistant containers as defined in USP.

*The distinctive design of REGROTON and DEMI-REGROTON tablets is patented by Rorer Pharmaceutical Corporation. U.S. Pat. No. Des. 286,919.

CAUTION

Federal (U.S.A.) law prohibits dispensing without prescription.

Revised May 1988

RORER PHARMACEUTICALS

a division of

RORER PHARMACEUTICAL CORPORATION

Fort Washington, PA, U.S.A. 19034

Shown in Product Identification Section, page 426

SLO–BID™   ℞

[slō'bid"]
(theophylline, anhydrous)
50 mg, 75 mg, 100 mg, 125 mg, 200 mg, and 300 mg
Gyrocaps®
Timed-Release Capsules

PRODUCT OVERVIEW

KEY FACTS

Slo-bid™ Gyrocaps® contain theophylline, anhydrous in the form of long-acting beads within a dye-free hard gelatin capsule for oral administration (intact or sprinkled). Theophylline is a bronchodilator and is a member of the xanthine class of chemical compounds.

MAJOR USES

Slo-bid™ is indicated for relief and/or prevention of symptoms of asthma and reversible bronchospasm associated with chronic bronchitis and emphysema.

SAFETY INFORMATION

Slo-bid™ is contraindicated in persons who have shown hypersensitivity to any of the components of this product. It is not intended for patients experiencing an acute episode of bronchospasm. Such patients require *rapid* relief of symptoms and should be treated with an immediate-release or intravenous theophylline preparation. Status asthmaticus should be considered a medical emergency. Adverse reactions are usually due to overdose.

PRESCRIBING INFORMATION

SLO–BID™   ℞

[slō'bid"]
(theophylline, anhydrous)
50 mg, 75 mg, 100 mg, 125 mg, 200 mg and 300 mg
Gyrocaps®
Timed-Release Capsules

DESCRIPTION

Slo-bid™ Gyrocaps® contain 50 mg, 100 mg, 200 mg, or 300 mg theophylline, anhydrous in the form of long-acting beads within a dye-free hard gelatin capsule and are intended for oral administration. Theophylline is a bronchodilator structurally classified as a xanthine derivative.

Slo-bid Gyrocaps can be administered with a 12-hour dosing interval for a majority of patients and a 24-hour dosing interval for selected patients (see DOSAGE and ADMINISTRATION section for description of appropriate patient population).

Theophylline is $1H$ -Purine-2,6-dione,3,7-dihydro-1,3-dimethyl represented by the following structural formula:

Theophylline is a white, odorless, crystalline powder having a bitter taste.

CLINICAL PHARMACOLOGY

Theophylline directly relaxes the smooth muscle of the bronchial airways and pulmonary blood vessels, thus acting as a bronchodilator and smooth muscle relaxant. It has also been demonstrated that aminophylline has a potent effect on diaphragmatic contractility in normal persons and may then be capable of reducing fatigability and thereby improve contractility in patients with chronic obstructive airways disease. The exact mode of action remains unsettled. Although theophylline does cause inhibition of phosphodiesterase with a resultant increase in intracellular cyclic AMP, other agents similarly inhibit the enzyme producing a rise of cyclic AMP but are unassociated with any demonstrable bronchodilation. Other mechanisms proposed include an effect on translocation of intracellular calcium; prostaglandin antagonism; stimulation of catecholamines endogenously; inhibition of cyclic guanosine monophosphate metabolism and adenosine receptor antagonism. None of these mechanisms has been proved, however.

In vitro, theophylline has been shown to act synergistically with beta agonists, and there are now available data that do demonstrate an additive effect *in vivo* with combined use.

Pharmacokinetics:

The half-life of theophylline is influenced by a number of known variables. It may be prolonged in chronic alcoholics, particularly those with liver disease (cirrhosis or alcoholic liver disease), in patients with congestive heart failure and in those patients taking certain other drugs (See PRECAUTIONS, Drug Interactions).

Newborns and neonates have extremely slow clearance rates compared to older infants and children, i.e., those over one year. Older children have rapid clearance rates while most nonsmoking adults have clearance rates between these two extremes. In premature neonates the decreased clearance is

related to oxidative pathways that have yet to be established.

Theophylline Elimination Characteristics
Half-life (in hours)

	Range	Mean
Children	1–9	3.7
Adults	3–15	7.7

In cigarette smokers (1–2 packs/day) the mean half-life is 4–5 hours, much shorter than in nonsmokers. The increase in clearance associated with smoking is presumably due to stimulation of the hepatic metabolic pathway by components of cigarette smoke. The duration of this effect after cessation of smoking is unknown but may require 6 months to 2 years before the rate approaches that of the nonsmoker.

In a single-dose bioavailability study in 18 normal subjects, 300 mg sustained-release Slo-bid Gyrocaps produced mean peak serum concentrations of 3.5 ± 0.7 µg/mL at a mean time of 7.8 ± 1.8 hours after dosing. Subjects fasted overnight before dosing and four hours after the dose. When compared to a syrup dosage form, relative bioavailability of Slo-bid Gyrocaps was about 91%. At steady state in a multiple-dose bioavailability study in 18 normal subjects with q12h dosing (600–1000 mg/day), the mean peak-trough variation was 3.5 ± 0.9 µg/mL. The mean C_{max} and C_{min} were 12.9 ± 3.0 and 9.4 ± 2.5 µg/mL, respectively. The mean percent fluctuation $[(C_{max}-C_{min}/C_{min}) \times 100]$ was $40 \pm 15\%$. Subjects fasted 12 hours before the dose and 4 hours after the dose was administered on the days that the blood samples were drawn. A multiple-dose bioequivalence study with 15 asthmatic children, ages 9–16, comparing Slo-bid Gyrocaps administered as intact capsules and as the beaded contents sprinkled on applesauce with b.i.d. dosing (150–600 mg/dose) indicated no significant differences in maximum and minimum theophylline concentrations, time to achieve peak concentration, and peak-trough differences. The bioavailability as measured by comparing area under the curves (AUC $_{0-12}$ hours granules/AUC $_{0-12\ hours}$ capsules) was 0.990 ± 0.214. Taking Slo-bid immediately after a high-fat content meal may result in a decrease in the rate of absorption (lower C_{max} and later T_{max}) but with no significant difference in the extent of absorption (see PRECAUTIONS, Drug-Food Interactions). In a single-dose bioavailability study, 24 normal adult nonsmoking subjects were given 900 mg sustained-release Slo-bid Gyrocaps with food and under fasting conditions. Results (mean $\pm$ S.D.) showed:

	Food	Fasting
AUC O → ∞	260.5 ± 60.6	280.5 ± 68.7
(mcg-hr/mL)		
C_{max} (mcg/mL)	10.57 ± 2.00	12.49 ± 2.15
T_{max} (hr)	9.8 ± 2.1	7.0 ± 1.4

Steady-state pharmacokinetics were determined in 26 normal male volunteers (with theophylline clearance rates less than or equal to 5.0 L/hr and/or a theophylline elimination half-life of 6 to 12 hours) who received 900 mg of theophylline per day for five days. Twenty-six were dosed with three 300 mg sustained-release Slo-bid Gyrocaps administered 24 hours apart immediately after the consumption of breakfast, and seventeen were dosed with one 300 mg, one 100 mg, and one 50 mg Slo-bid Gyrocap administered 12 hours apart (immediately after consuming breakfast and two hours after the consumption of dinner).

The pharmacokinetic parameters obtained for the sustained-release Slo-bid Gyrocaps given as 900 mg once daily in the morning after a high-fat content breakfast were essentially the same as those parameters obtained after Slo-bid Gyrocaps administered in the widely-acceptable, approved manner of twice-daily. In particular, the area-under-the-curve values were 238 ± 27 (S.D.) and 251 ± 29 µg-hr/mL for the products administered q24h and q12h, respectively. Mean C_{max} values of 13.2 ± 2.0 µg/mL and 12.2 ± 2.2 µg/mL and C_{min} values of 5.9 ± 1.0 µg/mL and 8.6 ± 1.1 µg/mL were obtained after q24h and q12h administration, respectively. The mean percent fluctuation $[(C_{max}-C_{min}/C_{min} \times 100)]$ was $140 \pm 66\%$ (S.D.) and $40 \pm 15\%$ (S.D.) when Slo-bid was given once- or twice-daily, respectively.

INDICATIONS AND USAGE

For relief and/or prevention of symptoms from asthma and reversible bronchospasm associated with chronic bronchitis and emphysema.

CONTRAINDICATIONS

Slo-bid is contraindicated in individuals who have shown hypersenitivity to any of the components of this product. It is also contraindicated in patients with active peptic ulcer disease and in individuals with underlying seizure disorders (unless receiving appropriate anticonvulsant medication).

WARNINGS

Serum levels above 20 µg/mL are rarely found after appropriate administration of the recommended doses. However, in individuals in whom theophylline plasma clearance is reduced *for any reason,* even conventional doses may result in increased serum levels and potential toxicity. Reduced theophylline clearance has been documented in the following readily identifiable groups: 1) patients with impaired renal or liver function; 2) patients over 55 years of age, particularly males and those with chronic lung disease; 3) those with cardiac failure from any cause; 4) patients with sustained high fever; 5) neonates and infants under 1 year of age; and 6) those patients taking certain drugs (see PRECAUTIONS, Drug Interactions). Frequently, such patients have markedly prolonged theophylline serum levels following discontinuation of the drug.

Reduction of dosage and laboratory monitoring is especially appropriate in the above individuals.

Serious side effects such as ventricular arrhythmias, convulsions or even death may appear as the first sign of toxicity without any previous warning. Less serious signs of theophylline toxicity (i.e., nausea and restlessness) may occur frequently when initiating therapy but are usually transient; when such signs are persistent during maintenance therapy, they are often associated with serum concentrations above 20 μg/mL. Stated differently, *serious toxicity is not reliably preceded by less severe side effects.* A serum concentration measurement is the only reliable method of identifying a potential for life-threatening toxicity.

Many patients who require theophylline exhibit tachycardia due to their underlying disease process, so the cause/effect relationship to elevated serum theophylline concentrations may not be appreciated.

Theophylline products may cause dysrhythmia and/or worsen preexisting arrhythmias and any significant change in rate and/or rhythm warrants monitoring and further investigation.

Studies in laboratory animals (minipigs, rodents and dogs) recorded the occurrence of cardiac arrhythmias and sudden death (with histologic evidence of myocardial necrosis) when beta agonists and methylxanthines were administered concurrently. The significance of these findings when applied to humans is currently unknown.

PRECAUTIONS

General: On the average, theophylline half-life is shorter in cigarette and marijuana smokers than in nonsmokers, but smokers can have half-lives as long as nonsmokers. Theophylline should not be administered concurrently with other xanthine preparations. Use with caution in patients with hypoxemia, hypertension or with a history of peptic ulcer. Theophylline may occasionally act as a local irritant to the GI tract, although GI symptoms are more commonly centrally mediated and associated with serum drug concentrations over 20 μg/mL.

Information for Patients:
The physician should reinforce the importance of taking only the prescribed dose at the prescribed time intervals. The patient should alert the physician if symptoms occur repeatedly, especially near the end of a dosing interval. When prescribing administration by the sprinkle method, details of the proper technique should be explained to the patient.

Laboratory Test: Serum levels should be monitored periodically to determine the theophylline levels associated with observed clinical response and to identify the potential for toxicity. For such measurements, the serum sample should be obtained at the time of peak concentration, approximately 5-9 hours after the morning dose. It is important that the patient has not missed or taken additional doses during the previous 48 hours and that dosing intervals have been reasonably equally spaced.

DOSE ADJUSTMENT BASED ON SERUM THEOPHYLLINE MEASUREMENTS WHEN THESE INSTRUCTIONS HAVE NOT BEEN FOLLOWED MAY RESULT IN RECOMMENDATIONS THAT PRESENT RISK OF TOXICITY TO THE PATIENT.

Drug Interactions:
Drug-Drug: Toxic synergism with ephedrine has been documented and may occur with some other sympathomimetic bronchodilators. In addition, the following drug interactions have been demonstrated:
Theophylline with:

Allopurinol (high dose)	Increased serum theophylline levels
Cimetidine	Increased serum theophylline levels
Erythromycin, Troleandomycin	Increased serum theophylline levels
Lithium carbonate	Increased renal excretion of lithium
Oral contraceptives	Increased serum theophylline levels
Phenytoin	Decreased theophylline and phenytoin serum levels
Rifampin	Decreased serum theophylline levels

Drug-Food: Taking Slo-bid immediately after a high-fat content meal such as 8 ounces whole milk, 2 fried eggs, 2 strips bacon, one bran muffin with butter, 2 ounces hash brown potatoes (about 789 calories, including approximately 49 gm of fat) may result in a decrease in the rate of absorption, but with no significant difference in the extent of absorption (see CLINICAL PHARMACOLOGY, Pharmacokinetics). The influence of the type and amount of other foods,

as well as the time interval between drug and food, has not been studied.

Drug/Laboratory Test Interactions: Currently available analytic methods, including high-pressure liquid chromatography and immunoassay techniques, for measuring serum theophylline levels are specific. Metabolites and other drugs generally do not affect the results. Other new analytic methods are also now in use. The physician should be aware of the laboratory method used and whether other drugs will interfere with the assay for theophylline.

Carcinogenesis, Mutagenesis, Impairment of Fertility: Long-term carcinogenicity studies have not been performed with theophylline.

Chromosome-breaking activity was detected in human cell cultures at concentrations of theophylline up to 50 times the therapeutic serum concentrations in humans. Theophylline was not mutagenic in the dominant lethal assay in male mice given theophylline intraperitoneally in doses up to 30 times the maximum daily human oral dose.

Studies to determine the effect on fertility have not been performed with theophylline.

Pregnancy: Pregnancy Category C—Animal reproduction studies have not been conducted with theophylline. It is also not known whether theophylline can cause fetal harm when administered to a pregnant woman or can affect reproduction capacity. Theophylline should be given to a pregnant woman only if clearly needed.

Nursing Mothers: Theophylline is distributed into breast milk and may cause irritability or other signs of toxicity in nursing infants. Because of the potential for serious adverse reactions in nursing infants from theophylline, a decision should be made whether to discontinue nursing or to discontinue the drug, taking into account the importance of the drug to the mother.

Pediatric Use: Safety and effectiveness of Slo-bid Gyrocaps administered:
1. Every 24 hours in children under 12 years of age, have not been established.
2. Every 12 hours in children under 6 years of age, have not been established.

ADVERSE REACTIONS

The following adverse reactions have been observed, but there has not been enough systematic collection of data to support an estimate of their frequency. The most consistent adverse reactions are usually due to overdosage.

Gastrointestinal: nausea, vomiting, epigastric pain, hematemesis, diarrhea.

Central Nervous System: headaches, irritability, restlessness, insomnia, reflex hyperexcitability, muscle twitching, clonic and tonic generalized convulsions.

Cardiovascular: palpitation, tachycardia, extrasystoles, flushing, hypotension, circulatory failure, ventricular arrhythmias.

Respiratory: tachypnea

Renal: potentiation of diuresis.

Other: alopecia, hyperglycemia, inappropriate ADH syndrome, rash.

OVERDOSAGE:

Management: It is suggested that the management principles (consistent with the clinical status of the patient when first seen) outlined below be instituted and that simultaneous contact with a Regional Poison Control Center be established. In this way both updated information and individualization regarding therapy may be provided.

1. When potential oral overdose is established and seizure has not occurred:
   a) If patient is alert and seen soon after ingestion, induction of emesis may be of value. Gastric lavage has been demonstrated to be of no value in influencing outcome in patients who present more than 1 hour after ingestion.
   b) Administer a cathartic. Sorbitol solution is reported to be of value.
   c) Administer repeated doses of activated charcoal and monitor theophylline serum levels.
   d) Prophylactic administration of phenobarbital has been shown to increase the seizure threshold in laboratory animals, and administration of this drug may be of value.
2. If patient presents with a seizure:
   a) Establish an airway
   b) Administer oxygen
   c) Treat the seizure with intravenous diazepam 0.1 to 0.3 mg/kg up to 10 mg. If seizures cannot be controlled, the use of general anesthesia should be considered.
   d) Monitor vital signs, maintain blood pressure and provide adequate hydration.
3. Postseizure Coma
   a) Maintain airway and oxygenation
   b) If a result of oral medication, follow above recommendations to prevent absorption of drug, but intubation and lavage will have to be performed instead of inducing emesis and the cathartic and charcoal will need to be introduced via a large-bore gastric lavage tube

c) Continue to provide full supportive care and adequate hydration until the drug is metabolized. In general, drug metabolism is sufficiently rapid so as not to warrant dialysis. If repeated oral activated charcoal is ineffective (as noted by stable or rising serum levels), charcoal hemoperfusion may be indicated.

DOSAGE AND ADMINISTRATION

Taking Slo-bid immediately after a high-fat-content meal may alter its rate of absorption (see CLINICAL PHARMACOLOGY and PRECAUTIONS, Drug-Food Interactions). However, the differences are usually small and Slo-bid may normally be administered without regard to meals.

Effective use of theophylline (i.e., the concentration of drug in the serum associated with optimal benefit and minimal risk of toxicity) is considered to occur when the theophylline concentration is maintained from 10 to 20 μg/mL. The early studies from which these levels were derived were carried out in patients immediately or shortly after recovery from acute exacerbations of their disease (some hospitalized with status asthmaticus).

Although the 20 μg/mL level remains appropriate as a critical value (above which toxicity is more likely to occur) for safety purposes, additional data are now available that indicate that the serum theophylline concentrations required to produce maximum physiologic benefit may, in fact, fluctuate with the degree of bronchospasm present and are variable. Therefore, the physician should individualize the range appropriate to the patient's requirements, based on both symptomatic response and improvement in pulmonary function. It should be stressed that serum theophylline concentrations maintained at the upper level of the 10 to 20 mcg/mL range may be associated with potential toxicity when factors known to reduce theophylline clearance are operative. (See WARNINGS).

If it is not possible to obtain serum level determinations, restriction of the daily dose (in otherwise healthy adults) to not greater than 13 mg/kg/day, to a maximum of 900 mg, in divided doses will result in relatively few patients exceeding serum levels of 20 μg/mL and the resultant greater risk of toxicity.

Caution should be exercised for younger children who cannot complain of minor side effects. Older adults, those with cor pulmonale, congestive heart failure, and/or liver disease may have unusually low dosage requirements and thus may experience toxicity at the maximal dosage recommended below.

Theophylline does not distribute into fatty tissue. Dosage should be calculated on the basis of lean (ideal) body weight where mg/kg doses are presented.

Frequency of Dosing: When immediate-release products with rapid absorption are used, dosing to maintain serum levels generally requires administration every 6 hours. This is particularly true in children, but dosing intervals up to 8 hours may be satisfactory in adults since they eliminate the drug at a slower rate. Some children, and adults requiring higher than average doses (those having rapid rates of clearance, e.g., half-lives of under 6 hours) may benefit and be more effectively controlled during chronic therapy when given products with sustained-release characteristics since these provide longer dosing intervals and/or less fluctuation in serum concentration between dosing. Those sustained-release products which provide flexibility in dosage through formulations of varying strengths are also helpful in controlling serum levels. Dosage guidelines are approximations only and the wide range of theophylline clearance between individuals (particularly those with concomitant disease) make indiscriminate usage hazardous.

Dosage Guidelines:
I. Acute Symptoms
NOTE: Status asthmaticus should be considered a medical emergency and is defined as that degree of bronchospasm that is not rapidly responsive to usual doses of conventional bronchodilators. Optimal therapy for such patients frequently requires both *additional medication* parenterally administered, and *close monitoring*, preferably in an intensive care setting.

Slo-bid is not intended for patients experiencing an acute episode of bronchospasm (associated with asthma, chronic bronchitis, or emphysema). Such patients require *rapid* relief of symptoms and should be treated with an immediate-release or intravenous theophylline preparation (or other bronchodilators) and not with controlled-release products.

II. Chronic Therapy
A. Initiating Therapy with an Immediate-Release Product

Continued on next page

This product information was prepared in September, 1989. Information concerning these products may be obtained by addressing Rorer Pharmaceutical Corporation, 500 Virginia Drive, Fort Washington, PA 19034.

Rorer Pharm.—Cont.

It is recommended that the appropriate dosage be established using an immediate-release preparation. A dosage form that allows small incremental doses is desirable for initiation therapy. A liquid preparation should be considered for children to permit easier and more accurate dosage adjustment. Slow clinical titration is generally preferred to help assure acceptance and safety of the medication and to allow the patient to develop tolerance to transient caffeine-like side effects. Then, if the total 24-hour dose can be given by one of the available strengths of this product, the patient can usually be switched to Slo-bid, giving one third of the daily dose at 8-hour intervals or one half the daily dose at 12-hour intervals. Patients who metabolize theophylline rapidly, such as the young, smokers, and some nonsmoking adults are the most likely candidates for dosing at 8-hour intervals. Such patients can generally be identified as having trough serum concentrations lower than desired or repeatedly exhibiting symptoms near the end of a dosing interval.

B. Initiating Therapy with Slo-bid Gyrocaps

Alternatively, therapy can be initiated with Slo-bid Gyrocaps since they are available in dosage strengths that permit titration and adjustments of dosage (in adults and older children). Children weighing less than 25 kg should have their daily dosage requirements established with Slo-Phyllin 80 mg Syrup to permit small dosage increments.

Initial Dose: 16 mg/kg 24 hours or 400 mg/24 hours (whichever is less) of anhydrous theophylline in 2 or 3 divided doses at 8- or 12-hour intervals.

Increasing Dose: The above dosage may be increased in approximately 25-percent increments at 3-day intervals so long as the drug is tolerated. Following each adjustment, if the clinical response is satisfactory and serum levels can be measured, then such measurements should be obtained as directed under section IV (below). If serum levels cannot be obtained, then that dosage level should be maintained. Dosage increases may be made in this manner until the maximum dose indicated in section III (below) is reached.

It is important that no patient be maintained on any dosage that is not tolerated. When instructing patients to increase dosage according to the schedule above, they should be told not to take a subsequent dose if apparent side effects occur and to resume therapy at a lower dose once adverse effects have disappeared.

C. Sprinkling Contents on Food

Slo-bid Gyrocaps may be administered by carefully opening the capsule and sprinkling the beaded contents on a spoonful of soft food such as applesauce or pudding; the soft food should be swallowed immediately without chewing and followed with a glass of cool water or juice to ensure complete swallowing of the beads. It is recommended that the food used should not be hot and should be soft enough to be swallowed without chewing. Any bead/food mixture should be used immediately and not stored for future use. SUBDIVIDING THE CONTENTS OF A CAPSULE IS NOT RECOMMENDED.

D. Once-Daily Dosing

The slow absorption rate of this preparation may allow once-daily administration in adult non-smokers with appropriate total body clearance and other patients with low dosage requirements. Once-daily dosing should be considered only after the patient has been gradually and satisfactorily titrated to therapeutic levels with q12h dosing. Once-daily dosing should be based on twice the q12h dose and should be initiated at the end of the last q12h dosing interval. The trough concentration (C_{min}) obtained following conversion to once-daily dosing may be lower (especially in high clearance patients) and the peak concentration (C_{max}) may be higher (especially in low clearance patients) than that obtained with q12h dosing. If symptoms recur, or signs of toxicity appear during the once-daily dosing interval, dosing on the q12h basis should be reinstituted.

It is essential that serum theophylline concentrations be monitored before and after transfer to once-daily dosing. Food and posture, along with changes associated with circadian rhythm, may influence the rate of absorption and/or clearance rates of theophylline from controlled-release dosage forms administered at night. The exact relationship of these and other factors to nighttime serum concentrations and the clinical significance of such findings require additional study. Therefore, it is

not recommended that Slo-bid, when used as a once-a-day product, be administered at night.

III. Maximum Dose of Theophylline Where the Serum Concentration is Not Measured: *WARNING: DO NOT ATTEMPT TO MAINTAIN ANY DOSE THAT IS NOT TOLERATED. Not to exceed the following:*
[See table below].

IV. Measurement of Serum Theophylline Concentrations During Chronic Therapy: If the above maximum doses are to be maintained or exceeded, serum theophylline measurement is essential (See PRECAUTIONS, Laboratory Tests for guidance).

V. Final adjustment of Dosage:
Dosage adjustment after serum theophylline measurement

If serum theophylline is:		Directions:
Within desired range		Maintain dosage if tolerated.
Too high	20 to 25 µg/mL	Decrease doses by about 10% and recheck serum level after 3 days.
	25 to 30 µg/mL	Skip next dose and decrease subsequent doses by about 25%. Recheck serum level after 3 days.
	Over 30 µg/mL	Skip next 2 doses and decrease subsequent doses by 50%. Recheck serum level after 3 days.
Too low		Increase dosage by 25% at 3-day intervals until either the desired serum concentration and/or clinical response is achieved. The total daily dose may need to be administered at more frequent intervals if symptoms occur repeatedly at the end of a dosing interval.

The serum concentration may be rechecked at appropriate intervals, but at least at the end of any adjustment period. When the patient's condition is otherwise clinically stable and none of the recognized factors which alter elimination are present, measurement of serum levels need be repeated only every 6 to 12 months.

STORAGE CONDITIONS

Store at room temperature. Protect from excessive heat, light and moisture.

CAUTION

Federal (U.S.A.) law prohibits dispensing without prescription. Keep this and all medications out of the reach of children.

HOW SUPPLIED

Slo-bid Gyrocaps are identified as follows:
50 mg—Clear (cap) and opaque white (body) capsule with WHR 50 printed in red on cap and body
75 mg—Opaque white (cap) and clear (body) capsule with 75 printed in red
100 mg—Clear capsule with WHR 100 printed in red
125 mg—Opaque white (cap) and opaque white (body) capsule with 125 printed in red
200 mg—Opaque white (cap) and clear (body) capsule with WHR 200 printed in red
300 mg—Opaque white capsule with WHR 300 printed in red
Slo-bid Gyrocaps 50 mg are available in bottles of 100 (NDC 0075-0057-00), bottles of 1000 (NDC 0075-0057-99) and in unit dose 10 x 10 (NDC 0075-0057-62), Slo-bid Gyrocaps 75 mg are available in bottles of 100 (NDC 0075-1075-00) and in unit dose 10 x 10 (NDC 0075-1075-62), Slo-bid Gyrocaps 100 mg are available in bottles of 100 (NDC 0075-0100-00), bottles of 1000 (NDC 0075-0100-99) and in unit dose 10 x 10 (NDC 0075-0100-62), Slo-bid Gyrocaps 125 mg are available in bottles of 100 (NDC 0075-1125-00) and in unit dose 10 x 10 (NDC 0075-1125-62), Slo-bid Gyrocaps 200 mg are available in bottles of 100 (NDC 0075-0200-00), bottles of 1000 (NDC 0075-0200-99) and in unit dose 10 x 10 (NDC 0075-0200-62), and Slo-bid Gyrocaps 300 mg are available in bottles of 100 (NDC 0075-0300-00), bottles of 1000 (NDC 0075-0300-99) and in unit dose 10 x 10 (NDC 0075-0300-62), and are manufactured by:

RORER PHARMACEUTICALS
a division of
Rorer Pharmaceutical Corporation
Fort Washington, PA, U.S.A. 19034
Rev. 12/88

Shown in Product Identification Section, page 426

SLO-PHYLLIN®   ℞
[*slō″fil′in*]
(theophylline, anhydrous)
60 mg, 125 mg, 250 mg Gyrocaps®, Timed-Release Capsules

DESCRIPTION

Slo-Phyllin® Gyrocaps® contain 60 mg, 125 mg, or 250 mg theophylline, anhydrous, in the form of long-acting dye-free beads within a hard gelatin capsule and are intended for oral administration. Theophylline is a bronchodilator and is a member of the xanthine class of chemical compounds related to both theobromine and caffeine. Theophylline is a white, odorless, crystalline powder having a bitter taste. Theophylline is 1 *H*-Purine-2,6-dione, 3,7-dihydro-1,3-dimethyl, represented by the following structural formula:

Inactive ingredients in all strengths of Slo-Phyllin Gyrocaps are: FD&C Blue No. 1, gelatin, pharmaceutical glaze, silicon dioxide, sodium bisulfite, sodium lauryl sulfate, starch, sucrose, talc, titanium dioxide. The 60 mg gyrocaps also contain D&C Yellow No. 10, FD&C Red No. 40, FD&C Blue No. 2, iron oxide, propylene glycol. The 125 mg gyrocaps also contain D&C Yellow No. 10, D&C Red No. 28, FD&C Red No. 40, dimethylpolysiloxane, methylparaben, propylparaben, may contain soya lecithin. The 250 mg gyrocaps also contain D&C Red No. 28, dimethylpolysiloxane, may contain soya lecithin.

CLINICAL PHARMACOLOGY

Theophylline directly relaxes the smooth muscle of the bronchial airways and pulmonary blood vessels, thus acting mainly as a brochodilator and smooth muscle relaxant. The drug also produces other actions typical of the xanthine derivatives: cardiac stimulation, coronary vasodilatation, stimulation of skeletal muscle, cerebral stimulation, and diuresis. The action of theophylline may be mediated through inhibition of phosphodiesterase and a resultant increase in intracellular cyclic AMP.

In vitro, theophylline has been shown to act synergistically with beta agonists that increase intracellular cyclic AMP through the stimulation of adenyl cyclase but synergism has not been demonstrated in patient studies. More data are needed to determine if theophylline and beta agonists have a clinically important additive effect *in vivo.* Apparently, no development of tolerance occurs with chronic use of theophylline.

Pharmacokinetics: The half-life of theophylline is influenced by a number of known variables. It is prolonged in patients suffering from chronic alcoholism, impaired hepatic or renal function, congestive heart failure, and in patients receiving macrolide antibiotics and cimetidine. Older adults (over age 55) and patients with chronic obstructive pulmonary disease, with or without cor pulmonale, may also have much slower clearance rates. For such patients, the theophylline half-life may exceed 24 hours.

Newborns and neonates have extremely slow clearance rates compared to older infants (over 6 months) and children, and may also have a theophylline half-life of over 24 hours. High fever for prolonged periods may also reduce the rate of theophylline elimination.

Representative Theophylline

Serum Half-Lives	Half-Life (hours)
Adults	
nonsmokers	7-9
smokers	4-5
congestive heart failure	24
Children (6-16 years)	3-5

The half-life of theophylline in smokers (1 to 2 packs/day) averages 4-5 hours, much shorter than the half-life in non-smokers, which averages 7-9 hours. The increase in theophylline clearance caused by smoking is probably the result of induction of drug-metabolizing enzymes that do not readily normalize after cessation of smoking. It appears that between 3 months and 2 years may be necessary for normalization of the effect of smoking on theophylline pharmacokinetics.

In a single-dose bioavailability study in 20 normal subjects, sustained-release Slo-Phyllin Gyrocaps were compared to the immediate-release Slo-Phyllin 80 mg Syrup. The mean bioavailability of the three strengths of Slo-Phyllin Gyrocaps ranged between 90% and 95%. A dose of 250 mg Slo-Phyllin Gyrocaps produced a mean peak serum concentration of 4.0 ± 0.8 µg/mL at a mean time of 4.8 hours after a single dose. At steady state in a multiple-dose bioavailability study, Slo-

			Dose per 8 hours	Dose per 12 hours
Age	6–9 years	24 mg/kg/day	8.0 mg/kg	12.0 mg/kg
Age	9–12 years	20 mg/kg/day	6.7 mg/kg	10.0 mg/kg
Age	12–16 years	18 mg/kg/day	6.0 mg/kg	9.0 mg/kg
Age	over 16 years	13 mg/kg/day	4.3 mg/kg	6.5 mg/kg
		OR 900 mg		
		(WHICHEVER IS LESS)		

Phyllin Gyrocaps were compared to Slo-Phyllin 80 mg Syrup. Doses of 2.6 to 5.6 mg/kg (mean dose of 4.2 mg/kg) of Slo-Phyllin Gyrocaps were administered q8h in 17 normal subjects. The mean peak serum concentration was 17.4 ± 0.9 μg/mL and the mean trough was 10.4 ± 0.7 μg/mL. In both of these studies, subjects fasted overnight before dosing and four hours after the first dose.

A multiple-dose bioequivalence study with 14 asthmatic children, ages 10–12, comparing Slo-Phyllin Gyrocaps administered as intact capsules and as the beaded contents sprinkled on applesauce with q8h dosing (125–250 mg/day) indicated no significant differences in maximum and minimum theophylline concentrations, time to achieve peak concentration, and peak-trough differences. The bioavailability as measured by comparing areas under the curves (AUC_{0-8} hours granules/$AUC_{0-8 \ hours}$ capsules) was 0.999 ± 0.324.

INDICATIONS AND USE
For relief and/or prevention of symptoms of asthma and reversible bronchospasm associated with chronic bronchitis and emphysema.

CONTRAINDICATIONS
Slo-Phyllin Gyrocaps are contraindicated in individuals who have shown hypersensitivity to any of their components.

WARNINGS
Status asthmaticus should be considered a medical emergency and is defined as that degree of bronchospasm which is not rapidly responsive to usual doses of conventional bronchodilators. Optimal therapy for such patients frequently requires both *additional medication*, parenterally administered, and *close monitoring*, preferably in an intensive care setting. Although increasing the dose of theophylline may bring about relief, such treatment may be associated with toxicity. The likelihood of such toxicity developing increases significantly when the serum theophylline concentration exceeds 20 μg/mL. Therefore, determination of serum theophylline levels is recommended to assure maximal benefit without excessive risk.

Serum levels above 20 μg/mL are rarely found after appropriate administration of the recommended doses. However, in individuals in whom theophylline plasma clearance is reduced *for any reason*, even conventional doses may result in increased serum levels and potential toxicity. Reduced theophylline clearance has been documented in the following readily identifiable groups: (1) patients with impaired renal or liver function, (2) patients over 55 years of age, particularly males and those with chronic lung disease, (3) those with cardiac failure from any cause, (4) neonates, and (5) those patients taking certain drugs (macrolide antibiotics and cimetidine). Decreased clearance of theophylline may be associated with either influenza immunization or active infection with influenza.

Reduction of dosage and laboratory monitoring is especially appropriate in the above individuals.

Less serious signs of theophylline toxicity, i.e., nausea and restlessness, may appear in up to 50% of patients. Unfortunately, however, serious side effects such as ventricular arrhythmias, convulsions, or even death may appear as the first sign of toxicity without any previous warning. Stated differently, *serious toxicity is not reliably preceded by less severe side effects.*

Many patients who require theophylline may exhibit tachycardia due to their underlying disease process so that the cause/effect relationship to elevated serum theophylline concentrations may not be appreciated.

Theophylline products may cause dysrhythmia and/or worsen preexisting arrhythmias and any significant change in rate and/or rhythm warrants monitoring and further investigation.

The occurrence of arrhythmias and sudden death (with histological evidence of necrosis of the myocardium) has been recorded in laboratory animals (minipigs, rodents, and dogs) when theophylline and beta agonists were administered concomitantly, although not when either was administered alone. The significance of these findings when applied to human usage is currently unknown.

PRECAUTIONS
General: Mean half-life in smokers is shorter than nonsmokers. Therefore, smokers may require larger or more frequent doses of theophylline. Morphine and curare should be used with caution in patients with airway obstruction as they may suppress respiration and stimulate histamine release. Alternative drugs should be used when possible. Theophylline should not be administered concurrently with other xanthine preparations. Use with caution in patients with severe cardiac disease, severe hypoxemia, hypertension, hyperthyroidism, acute myocardial injury, cor pulmonale, congestive heart failure, alcoholism, liver disease, and in the elderly, especially males, and neonates. Great caution should be used in giving theophylline to patients with congestive heart failure. Frequently such patients have shown markedly prolonged theophylline blood levels with theophylline persisting in serum for long periods following discontinuation of the drug. Use theophylline cautiously in pa-

tients with a history of peptic ulcer. Theophylline may occasionally act as a local gastrointestinal irritant, although GI symptoms are more commonly centrally mediated and associated with serum drug concentrations over 20 μg/mL.

Information for Patients: The physician should reinforce the importance of taking only the prescribed dose at the prescribed time intervals. The patient should alert the physician if symptoms occur repeatedly, especially near the end of a dosing interval.

Drug Interactions:

Drug-Drug: Toxic synergism with ephedrine has been documented and may occur with some other sympathomimetic bronchodilators. In addition, the following drug interactions have been demonstrated:

DRUG	EFFECT
Aminophylline with lithium carbonate	Increased excretion of lithium carbonate
Aminophylline with propranolol	Increased theophylline serum concentrations. Antagonism of propranolol effects
Theophylline with troleandomycin or erythromycin	Increased theophylline serum concentrations
Theophylline with cimetidine	Increased theophylline serum concentrations

Drug-Food: Slo-Phyllin Gyrocaps have not been adequately studied to determine whether its bioavailability is altered when it is given with food.

Available data suggest that drug administration at the time of food ingestion may influence the absorption characteristics of some or all theophylline controlled-release products resulting in serum values different from those found after administration in the fasting state.

A drug-food effect, if any, would likely have its greatest clinical significance when high theophylline serum levels are being maintained and/or when large single doses (greater than 13 mg/kg or 900 mg) of a controlled-release product are given. The influence of the type and amount of food on performance of controlled-release theophylline products is under study at this time.

Drug/Laboratory Test Interactions: When plasma levels of theophylline are measured by spectrophotometric methods, coffee, tea, cola beverages, chocolate, and acetaminophen contribute falsely high values.

Carcinogenesis, Mutagenesis, Impairment of Fertility
Long-term animal studies have not been performed to evaluate the carcinogenic potential, mutagenic potential, or the effect on fertility by xanthine compounds.

Pregnancy: Pregnancy Category C
Animal reproduction studies have not been conducted with theophylline. It is not known whether theophylline can cause fetal harm when administered to a pregnant woman or can affect reproduction capacity. Theophylline should be given to a pregnant woman only if clearly needed.

Nursing Mothers: It has been reported that theophylline distributes readily into breast milk and may cause adverse effects in the infant. Caution must be used if prescribing xanthines to a mother who is nursing, taking into account the risk-benefit of this therapy.

Pediatric Use: Safety and effectiveness in children under 6 years of age have not been established with this product.

ADVERSE REACTIONS
The most consistent adverse reactions are usually due to overdose and are:

Gastrointestinal: nausea, vomiting, epigastric pain, hematemesis, and diarrhea.

Central Nervous System: headaches, irritability, restlessness, insomnia, reflex hyperexcitability, muscle twitching, and clonic and tonic generalized convulsions.

Cardiovascular: palpitation, tachycardia, extrasystoles, flushing, hypotension, circulatory failure, and ventricular arrhythmias.

Respiratory: tachypnea.

Renal: albuminuria, increased excretion of renal tubular cells and red blood cells, potentiation of diuresis.

Other: hyperglycemia and inappropriate ADH syndrome and rash.

OVERDOSAGE
Management:
A. If potential oral overdose is established and seizure has not occurred
  1. Induce vomiting
  2. Administer a cathartic (this is particularly important if sustained-release preparations have been taken)
  3. Administer activated charcoal
  4. Monitor vital signs, maintain blood pressure and provide adequate hydration

B. If patient is having a seizure
  1. Establish an airway
  2. Administer oxygen
  3. Treat the seizure with intravenous diazepam 0.1 to 0.3 mg/kg up to a total dose of 10 mg
  4. Monitor vital signs, maintain blood pressure and provide adequate hydration
C. Postseizure Coma
  1. Maintain airway and oxygenation
  2. If a result of oral medication, follow above recommendations to prevent absorption of drug, but intubation and lavage will have to be performed instead of inducing emesis and the cathartic and charcoal will need to be introduced via a large-bore gastric lavage tube.
  3. Continue to provide full supportive care and adequate hydration while waiting for drug to be metabolized. In general, the drug is metabolized sufficiently rapidly so as to not warrant consideration of dialysis. However, if serum levels exceed 50 μg/mL, charcoal hemoperfusion may be indicated.

DOSAGE AND ADMINISTRATION
Studies to determine the bioavailability of Slo-Phyllin Gyrocaps when administered with food are being initiated. (See PRECAUTIONS, Drug-Food Interactions.)

For most patients, *effective use* of theophylline, i.e., associated with optimal likelihood of benefit combined with minimal risk of toxicity, is considered to occur when serum levels are maintained between 10 and 20 μg/mL. Levels above 20 μg/mL may produce toxicity, and in a small number of patients, toxicity may even be seen with serum levels between 15–20 μg/mL, particularly during initiation of therapy.

There is considerable variation from patient to patient in the dosage required to achieve and maintain therapeutic and safe levels, primarily due to variable rates of elimination. Therefore, it is essential that not only must dosage be individualized, but titration and monitoring of serum levels be utilized where available. When serum concentration cannot be obtained, restriction of dosage to the amounts and intervals recommended in the guidelines listed below becomes essential. Dosage should be calculated on the basis of lean (ideal) body weight where mg/kg doses are presented. Theophylline does not distribute into fatty tissue.

Frequency of Dosing: When immediate-release products with rapid absorption (such as tablets or liquid) are used, dosing to maintain serum levels generally requires administration every 6 hours. This is particularly true in children, but dosing intervals up to 8 hours may be satisfactory in adults since they eliminate the drug at a slower rate. Some children, and adults requiring higher-than-average doses (those having rapid rates of clearance, e.g., half-lives of under 6 hours) may benefit and be more effectively controlled during chronic therapy when given products with sustained-release characteristics since these provide longer dosing intervals and/or less fluctuation in serum concentration between dosing. Those sustained-release products which provide flexibility in dosage through formulations of varying strengths are also helpful in controlling serum levels. Dosage guidelines are approximations only and the wide range of theophylline clearance between individuals (particularly those with concomitant disease) make indiscriminate usage hazardous.

As a practical consideration, it is not always possible to obtain serum level determinations. Under such conditions, restriction of the daily dose (*in otherwise healthy adults*) to not greater than 13 mg/kg/day (or up to 900 mg) of anhydrous theophylline in divided doses will result in relatively few patients exceeding serum levels of 20 μg/mL and the resultant risk of toxicity.

Dosage Guidelines:
I. Acute Symptoms
Slo-Phyllin Gyrocaps are not intended for patients experiencing an acute episode of bronchospasm (associated with asthma, chronic bronchitis, or emphysema). Such patients require *rapid* relief of symptoms and should be treated with an immediate-release or intravenous theophylline preparation (or other bronchodilators) and not with controlled-release products.

II. Chronic Therapy
A. Initiating Therapy with an Immediate-Release Product
It is recommended that the appropriate dosage be established using an immediate-release preparation. Children weighing less than 25 kg should have their daily dosage requirements established with Slo-Phyllin 80 mg Syrup to permit small dosage increments. Slow clinical titration is generally preferred to help ensure acceptance and safety of the medication. Then, if the total 24-hour dose

Continued on next page

This product information was prepared in September, 1989. Information concerning these products may be obtained by addressing Rorer Pharmaceutical Corporation, 500 Virginia Drive, Fort Washington, PA 19034.

Rorer Pharm.—Cont.

can be given by use of the sustained-release product, the patient can usually be switched to Slo-Phyllin Gyrocaps, giving one third of the daily dose at 8-hour intervals or one half the daily dose at 12-hour intervals. Patients who metabolize theophylline rapidly, such as the young, smokers, and some nonsmoking adults are the most likely candidates for dosing at 8-hour intervals. Such patients can generally be identified as having trough serum concentrations lower than desired, or repeatedly exhibiting symptoms near the end of a dosing interval.

B. Initiating Therapy with Slo-Phyllin Gyrocaps

Alternatively, therapy can be initiated with Slo-Phyllin Gyrocaps since they are available in dosage strengths which permit titration and adjustments of dosage (in adults and older children).

Initial Dose:

16 mg/kg/24 hours or 400 mg/24 hours (whichever is less) of anhydrous theophylline in 2 or 3 divided doses at 8- or 12-hour intervals.

Increasing Dose:

The above dosage may be increased in approximately 25-percent increments at 3-day intervals so long as the drug is tolerated, until the maximum dose indicated in section III below is reached.

C. Sprinkling Contents on Food

Slo-Phyllin Gyrocaps may be administered by carefully opening the capsule and sprinkling the beaded contents on a spoonful of soft food such as applesauce or pudding; the soft food should be swallowed immediately without chewing and followed with a glass of cool water or juice to ensure complete swallowing of the beads. It is recommended that the food used should not be hot and should be soft enough to be swallowed without chewing. Any bead/food mixture should be used immediately and not stored for future use. Until additional bioavailability data are available, it is recommended that dosing not take place at mealtime until a study is completed to show the effect of taking Slo-Phyllin Gyrocaps with food as compared to the fasting state.

III. Maximum Dose of Theophylline Where the Serum Concentration Is Not Measured

[See table below].

IV. Measurement of Serum Theophylline Concentrations During Chronic Therapy

If the above maximum doses are to be maintained or exceeded, serum theophylline measurement is recommended. The serum sample should be obtained at the time of peak absorption, 1 to 2 hours after administration for immediate-release products and 4 hours after dosing for Slo-Phyllin Gyrocaps. It is important that the patient will have missed *no* doses during the previous 48 hours and that dosing intervals will have been reasonably typical with no added doses during that period of time. DOSAGE ADJUSTMENT BASED ON SERUM THEOPHYLLINE MEASUREMENTS WHEN THESE INSTRUCTIONS HAVE NOT BEEN FOLLOWED MAY RESULT IN RECOMMENDATIONS THAT PRESENT RISK OF TOXICITY TO THE PATIENT.

V. Final Adjustment of Dosage: (see Table 1)

Table 1—Dosage adjustment after serum theophylline measurement

If serum theophylline is:		Directions:
With normal limits	10 to 20 µg/mL	Maintain dosage if tolerated. Recheck serum theophylline concentration at 6- to 12-month intervals.*
Too high	20 to 25 µg/mL	Decrease doses by about 10%. Recheck serum theophylline concentration at 6- to 12-month intervals.*
	25 to 30 µg/mL	Skip next dose and decrease subsequent doses by about 25%.
	Over 30 µg/mL	Skip next 2 doses and decrease subsequent doses by 50%. Recheck serum theophylline.
Too low	7.5 to 10 µg/mL	Increase dose by about 25%.** Recheck serum theophylline concentration at 6- to 12-month intervals.*
	5 to 7.5 µg/mL	Increase dose by about 25% to the nearest dose increment and recheck serum theophylline for guidance and further dosage adjustment (another increase will probably be needed, but this provides a safety check).

*Finer adjustments in dosage may be needed for some patients.

**The total daily dose may need to be administered at more frequent intervals if symptoms occur repeatedly at the end of a dosing interval.

From the *Journal of Respiratory Diseases* 2 (7):16, 1981

Caution should be exercised for younger children who cannot complain of minor side effects. Older adults, those with cor pulmonale, congestive heart failure, and/or liver disease may have unusually low dosage requirements and thus may experience toxicity at the maximal dosage recommended above. It is important that no patient be maintained on any dosage that is not tolerated. In instructing the patients to increase dosage according to the schedule above, they should be instructed not to take a subsequent dose if apparent side effects occur and to resume therapy at a lower dose once adverse effects have disappeared.

HOW SUPPLIED

Slo-Phyllin® Gyrocaps® 60 mg are available in bottles of 100 (NDC-0075-1354-00).

Slo-Phyllin® Gyrocaps® 125 mg are available in bottles of 100 (NDC-0075-1355-00), 1000 (NDC-0075-1355-99) and unit dose strip packages (NDC-0075-1355-62).

Slo-Phyllin® Gyrocaps® 250 mg are available in bottles of 100 (NDC-0075-1356-00), 1000 (NDC-0075-1356-99) and unit dose strip packages (NDC-0075-1356-62).

Slo-Phyllin® Gyrocaps® are identified as follows:

60-mg—white capsule with WHR 1354 printed in black on body and cap, containing dye-free beads

125-mg—brown capsule with WHR 1355 printed in white on body and cap, containing dye-free beads

250-mg—purple capsule with WHR 1356 printed in white on body and cap, containing dye-free beads

STORAGE CONDITIONS

Store at room temperature. Protect from excessive heat, light, and moisture.

CAUTION

Federal (U.S.A.) law prohibits dispensing without prescription.

Keep this and all medications out of the reach of children.

Rev. 6/88

Manufactured by
CORD LABORATORIES, INC.
Broomfield, CO 80020
for
RORER PHARMACEUTICALS
a division of
Rorer Pharmaceutical Corporation
Fort Washington, PA, U.S.A. 19034
Shown in Product Identification Section, page 426

SLO-PHYLLIN®

[slō "fil 'in]
100 mg and 200 mg Tablets
(theophylline tablets USP)
80 mg Syrup 80 mg/15mL
(theophylline, anhydrous)

℞

DESCRIPTION

Slo-Phyllin® Tablets (theophylline tablets, USP) are scored, dye-free tablets providing 100 mg or 200 mg of theophylline anhydrous, USP.

Slo-Phyllin® 80 mg Syrup (theophylline, anhydrous) is a nonalcoholic, sugar-free solution containing per 15 mL theophylline, anhydrous, USP 80 mg with sodium benzoate, NF, 18 mg and methylparaben, NF, 3 mg added as preservatives.

Both tablets and syrup are intended for oral administration. Theophylline is a bronchodilator structurally classified as a xanthine derivative.

Theophylline is a 1*H*-Purine-2,6-dione, 3,7-dihydro, 1,3-dimethyl, represented by the following structural formula:

Theophylline is a white odorless crystalline powder having a bitter taste.

Syrup inactive ingredients are citric acid, FD&C Red No. 3, FD&C Yellow No. 6, flavors, glycerin, methylparaben, propylene glycol, saccharin sodium, sodium benzoate, sorbitol, purified water.

Tablets: 100 mg inactive ingredients are lactose, magnesium stearate, microcrystalline cellulose, sodium starch glycolate; 200 mg inactive ingredients are magnesium stearate, microcrystalline cellulose, sodium starch glycolate.

CLINICAL PHARMACOLOGY

Theophylline directly relaxes the smooth muscle of the bronchial airways and pulmonary blood vessels, thus acting mainly as a bronchodilator and smooth muscle relaxant. It has also been demonstrated that aminophylline has a potent effect on diaphragmatic contractility in normal persons and may then be capable of reducing fatigability and thereby improve contractility in patients with chronic obstructive airways disease. The exact mode of action remains unsettled. Although theophylline does cause inhibition of phosphodiesterase with a resultant increase in intracellular cyclic AMP, other agents similarly inhibit the enzyme producing a rise of cyclic AMP but are unassociated with any demonstrable bronchodilation. Other mechanisms proposed include an effect on translocation of intracellular calcium; prostaglandin antagonism; stimulation of catecholamines endogenously; inhibition of cyclic guanosine monophosphate metabolism and adenosine receptor antagonism. None of these mechanisms has been proved, however.

In vitro, theophylline has been shown to act synergistically with beta-agonists and there are now available data that do demonstrate an additive effect *in vivo* with combined use.

Pharmacokinetics: The half-life of theophylline is influenced by a number of known variables. It may be prolonged in chronic alcoholics, particularly those with liver disease (cirrhosis or alcoholic liver disease), in patients with congestive heart failure and in those patients taking certain other drugs (see PRECAUTIONS, Drug Interactions).

Newborns and neonates have extremely slow clearance rates compared to older infants and children, i.e., those over one year. Older children have rapid clearance rates while most nonsmoking adults have clearance rates between these two extremes. In premature neonates the decreased clearance is related to oxidative pathways that have yet to be established.

Theophylline Elimination Characteristics
Half-Life (in hours)

	Range	Mean
Children	1– 9	3.7
Adults	3–15	7.7

In cigarette smokers (1–2 packs/day) the mean half-life is 4–5 hours, much shorter than in nonsmokers. The increase in clearance associated with smoking is presumably due to stimulation of the hepatic metabolic pathway by components of cigarette smoke. The duration of this effect after smoking is unknown but may require 6 months to 2 years before the rate approaches that of the nonsmoker.

In single-dose bioavailability studies in normal volunteers, 300 mg Slo-Phyllin Syrup produced mean peak serum concentrations of 7.90 ± 1.67 µg/mL at a mean time of 1.43 ± 0.87 hours after dosing. At steady state in multiple-dose bioavailability studies with four times a day dosing (600–1000 mg/day), the mean peak-trough variation was 4.39 ± 0.77 µg/mL.

In a single-dose three-way cross-over bioavailability study, 400 mg each of the 100 mg Slo-Phyllin tablet, the 200 mg tablet and Slo-Phyllin Syrup were given to 19 volunteers. The respective means ± standard error for the bioequivalence parameters were: peak concentration (C_{max}) 11.18 ± 0.38, 10.91 ± 0.39 and 11.17 ± 0.40 µg/mL; time of peak concentration (T_{max}) 1.67 ± 0.17, 1.84 ± 0.17 and 2.18 ± 0.21 hours; area under the curve, 0 to infinity ($AUC_{0-\infty}$) 120.53 ± 9.80, 121.29 ± 9.61 and 127.37 ± 9.40. There were no statistical differences between the formulations with regard to C_{max}, T_{max} or $AUC_{0-\infty}$. Bioavailability relative to the Syrup was 95% for the 100 mg tablet and 96% for the 200 mg tablet.

WARNING: DO NOT ATTEMPT TO MAINTAIN ANY DOSE THAT IS NOT TOLERATED.

Not to exceed the following:

				Dose per 8 hours	Dose per 12 hours
Age	6–9	years	24 mg/kg /day	8.0 mg/kg	12.0 mg/kg
Age	9–12	years	20 mg/kg/day	6.7 mg/kg	10.0 mg/kg
Age	12–16	years	18 mg/kg/day	6.0 mg/kg	9.0 mg/kg
Age	over 16	years	13 mg/kg/day	4.3 mg/kg	6.5 mg/kg

OR 900 mg
(WHICHEVER IS LESS)

INDICATIONS AND USE

For relief and/or prevention of symptoms of asthma and reversible bronchospasm associated with chronic bronchitis and emphysema.

CONTRAINDICATIONS

Slo-Phyllin Tablets and Syrup are contraindicated in individuals who have shown hypersensitivity to any of the components. It is also contraindicated in patients with active peptic ulcer disease, and in individuals with underlying seizure disorders (unless receiving appropriate anticonvulsant medication).

WARNINGS

Serum levels above 20 μg/mL are rarely found after appropriate administration of the recommended doses. However, in individuals in whom theophylline plasma clearance is reduced *for any reason*, even conventional doses may result in increased serum levels and potential toxicity. Reduced theophylline clearance has been documented in the following readily identifiable groups: 1) patients with impaired liver function; 2) patients over 55 years of age, particularly males and those with chronic lung disease; 3) those with cardiac failure from any cause; 4) patients with sustained high fever; 5) neonates and infants under 1 year of age; and 6) those patients taking certain drugs (see PRECAUTIONS, Drug Interactions). Frequently, such patients have markedly prolonged theophylline serum levels following discontinuation of the drug.

Reduction of dosage and laboratory monitoring is especially appropriate in the above individuals.

Serious side effects such as ventricular arrhythmias, convulsions, or even death may appear as the first sign of toxicity without any previous warning. Less serious signs of theophylline toxicity (i.e., nausea and restlessness) may occur frequently when initiating therapy, but are usually transient; when such signs are persistent during maintenance therapy, they are often associated with serum concentrations above 20 μg/mL. Stated differently, *serious toxicity is not reliably preceded by less severe side effects.* A serum concentration measurement is the only reliable method of identifying a potential for life-threatening toxicity.

Many patients who require theophylline exhibit tachycardia due to their underlying disease process, so the cause/effect relationship to elevated serum theophylline concentrations may not be appreciated.

Theophylline products may cause dysrhythmia and/or worsen preexisting arrhythmias and any significant change in rate and/or rhythm warrants monitoring and further investigation.

Studies in laboratory animals (minipigs, rodents, and dogs) recorded the occurrence of cardiac arrhythmias and sudden death (with histologic evidence of myocardial necrosis) when beta-agonists and methylxanthines were administered concurrently. The significance of these findings when applied to humans is currently unknown.

PRECAUTIONS

General: On the average, theophylline half-life is shorter in cigarette and marijuana smokers than in nonsmokers, but smokers can have half lives as long as nonsmokers.

Theophylline should not be administered concurrently with other xanthine preparations. Use with caution in patients with hypoxemia, hypertension, or with a history of peptic ulcer. Theophylline may occasionally act as a local irritant to the GI tract, although GI symptoms are more commonly centrally mediated and associated with serum drug concentrations over 20 μg/mL.

Information for Patients: The physician should reinforce the importance of taking only the prescribed dose at the prescribed time intervals.

Laboratory Tests: Serum levels should be monitored periodically to determine the theophylline level associated with observed clinical response and to identify the potential for toxicity. For such measurements, the serum sample should be obtained at the time of peak concentration, 1 to 2 hours after administration for immediate-release products. It is important that the patient has not missed or taken additional doses during the previous 48 hours and that dosing intervals have been reasonably equally spaced. DOSAGE ADJUSTMENT BASED ON SERUM THEOPHYLLINE MEASUREMENTS WHEN THESE INSTRUCTIONS HAVE NOT BEEN FOLLOWED MAY RESULT IN RECOMMENDATIONS THAT PRESENT RISK OF TOXICITY TO THE PATIENT.

Drug Interactions: Toxic synergism with ephedrine has been documented and may occur with other sympathomimetic bronchodilators. In addition, the following drug interactions have been demonstrated:

Theophylline with:

Allopurinol (high-dose)	Increased serum theophylline levels
Cimetidine	Increased serum theophylline levels
Erythromycin, Troleandomycin	Increased serum theophylline levels
Lithium Carbonate	Increased renal excretion of lithium
Oral Contraceptives	Increased serum theophylline levels
Phenytoin	Decreased theophylline and phenytoin serum levels
Rifampin	Decreased serum theophylline levels

Drug/Laboratory Test Interactions: Currently available analytical methods, including high pressure liquid chromatography and immunoassay techniques, for measuring serum theophylline levels are specific. Metabolites and other drugs generally do not affect the results. Other new analytic methods are also now in use. The physician should be aware of the laboratory method used and whether other drugs will interfere with the assay for theophylline.

Carcinogenesis, Mutagenesis, and Impairment of Fertility: Long-term carcinogenicity studies have not been performed with theophylline.

Chromosome-breaking activity was detected in human cell cultures at concentrations of theophylline up to 50 times the therapeutic serum concentration in humans. Theophylline was not mutagenic in the dominant lethal assay in male mice given theophylline intraperitoneally in doses up to 30 times the maximum daily human oral dose.

Studies to determine the effect on fertility have not been performed with theophylline.

Pregnancy: Category C—Animal reproduction studies have not been conducted with theophylline. It is also not known whether theophylline can cause fetal harm when administered to a pregnant woman or can affect reproduction capacity. Theophylline should be given to a pregnant woman only if clearly needed.

Nursing Mothers: Theophylline is distributed into breast milk and may cause irritability or other signs of toxicity in nursing infants. Because of the potential for serious adverse reactions in nursing infants from theophylline, a decision should be made whether to discontinue nursing or to discontinue the drug, taking into account the importance of the drug to the mother.

Pediatric Use: Sufficient numbers of infants under the age of 1 year have not been studied in clinical trials to support use in this age group; however, there is evidence recorded that the use of dosage recommendations for older infants and young children (16 mg/kg/24 hours) may result in the development of toxic serum levels. Such findings very probably reflect differences in the metabolic handling of the drug related to absent or undeveloped enzyme systems. Consequently, prescribers of the drug for this age group should carefully consider the associated benefits and risks. If used, the maintenance dose must be conservative and in accord with the following guidelines:

Initial Maintenance Dosage

Premature infants:
Up to 24 days postnatal age—1.0 mg/kg q12h
Beyond 24 days postnatal age—1.5 mg/kg q12h
Infants 6 to 52 weeks:
[(0.2 × age in weeks) + 5.0] × kg body wt = 24 hour dose in mg.
Up to 26 weeks, divide into q8h dosing intervals.
From 26–52 weeks, divide into q6h dosing intervals.
Final Dosage should be guided by serum concentration after a steady state (no further accumulation of drug) has been achieved.

ADVERSE REACTIONS

The following adverse reactions have been observed, but there has not been enough systematic collection of data to support an estimate of their frequency. The most consistent adverse reactions are usually due to overdosage.

Gastrointestinal: nausea, vomiting, epigastric pain, hematemesis, diarrhea.

Central Nervous System: headaches, irritability, restlessness, insomnia, reflex hyperexcitability, muscle twitching, clonic and tonic generalized convulsions.

Cardiovascular: palpitation, tachycardia, extrasystoles, flushing, hypotension, circulatory failure, ventricular arrhythmias.

Respiratory: tachypnea.

Renal: potentiation of diuresis.

Other: alopecia, hyperglycemia, inappropriate ADH syndrome, rash.

OVERDOSAGE

Management: It is suggested that the management principles (consistent with the clinical status of the patient when first seen) outlined below be instituted and that simultaneous contact with a Regional Poison Control Center be established. In this way both updated information and individualization regarding required therapy may be provided.

1. When potential oral overdose is established and seizure has not occurred:
   a) If patient is alert and seen soon after ingestion, induction of emesis may be of value. Gastric lavage has been demonstrated to be of no value in influencing outcome in patients who present more than 1 hour after ingestion.
   b) Administer a cathartic. Sorbitol solution is reported to be of value.
   c) Administer repeated doses of activated charcoal and monitor theophylline serum levels.
   d) Prophylactic administration of phenobarbitol has been shown to increase the seizure threshold in laboratory animals, and administration of this drug may be of value.
2. If patient presents with a seizure:
   a) Establish an airway.
   b) Administer oxygen.
   c) Treat the seizure with intravenous diazepam 0.1 to 0.3 mg/kg up to 10 mg. If seizures cannot be controlled, the use of general anesthesia should be considered.
   d) Monitor vital signs, maintain blood pressure and provide adequate hydration.
3. If postseizure coma is present:
   a) Maintain airway and oxygenation.
   b) Follow above recommendations to prevent absorption of drug, but intubation and lavage will have to be performed instead of inducing emesis and the cathartic and charcoal will need to be introduced via a large-bore gastric lavage tube.
   c) Continue to provide full supportive care and adequate hydration until the drug is metabolized. In general, drug metabolism is sufficiently rapid so as not to warrant dialysis. If repeated oral activated charcoal is ineffective (as noted by stable or rising serum levels), charcoal hemoperfusion may be indicated.

DOSAGE AND ADMINISTRATION

Effective use of theophylline (i.e., the concentration of drug in the serum associated with optimal benefit and minimal risk of toxicity) is considered to occur when the theophylline concentration is maintained from 10 to 20 μg/mL. The early studies from which these levels were derived were carried out in patients immediately or shortly after recovery from acute exacerbations of their disease (some hospitalized with status asthmaticus).

Although the 20 μg/mL level remains appropriate as a critical value (above which toxicity is more likely to occur) for safety purposes, additional data are now available which indicate that the serum theophylline concentrations required to produce maximum physiologic benefit may, in fact, fluctuate with the degree of bronchospasm present and are variable. Therefore, the physician should individualize the range appropriate to the patient's requirements, based on both symptomatic response and improvement in pulmonary function. It should be stressed that serum theophylline concentrations maintained at the upper level of the 10 to 20 μg/mL range may be associated with potential toxicity when factors known to reduce theophylline clearance are operative. (See WARNINGS.)

If it is not possible to obtain serum level determinations, restriction of the daily dose (*in otherwise healthy adults*) to not greater than 13 mg/kg/day to a maximum of 900 mg of anhydrous theophylline in divided doses will result in relatively few patients exceeding serum levels of 20 μg/mL and the resultant greater risk of toxicity.

Caution should be exercised for younger children who cannot complain of minor side effects. Older adults, those with cor pulmonale, congestive heart failure, and/or liver disease may have unusually low dosage requirements and thus may experience toxicity at the maximal dosage recommended below.

Theophylline does not distribute into fatty tissue. Dosage should be calculated on the basis of lean (ideal) body weight where mg/kg doses are presented.

Frequency of Dosing: When immediate-release products with rapid absorption are used, dosing to maintain serum levels generally requires administration every 6 hours. This is particularly true in children, but dosing intervals up to 8 hours may be satisfactory in adults since they eliminate the drug at a slower rate. Some children, and adults requiring higher than average doses (those having rapid rates of clearance, e.g., half-lives of under 6 hours) may benefit and be more effectively controlled during chronic therapy when given products with sustained-release characteristics, since these provide longer dosing intervals and/or less fluctuation in serum concentration between dosing.

Dosage guidelines are approximations only and the wide range of theophylline clearance between individuals (particularly those with concomitant disease) make indiscriminate usage hazardous.

Continued on next page

This product information was prepared in September, 1989. Information concerning these products may be obtained by addressing Rorer Pharmaceutical Corporation, 500 Virginia Drive, Fort Washington, PA 19034.

Rorer Pharm.—Cont.

Dosage Guidelines:

I.   Acute symptoms of asthma or bronchospasm requiring rapid attainment of theophylline serum levels:

NOTE: Status asthmaticus should be considered a medical emergency and is defined as that degree of bronchospasm which is not rapidly responsive to usual doses of conventional bronchodilators. Optimal therapy for such patients frequently requires both *additional medication*, parenterally administered, and *close monitoring*, preferably in an intensive care setting.

A.   Patients not currently receiving theophylline products:

	Theophylline Dosage Oral	
	Loading	Maintenance
Children age: 1 to 9 years	5 mg/kg	4 mg/kg q 6 hours
Children age: 9 to 16 years and smokers	5 mg/kg	3 mg/kg q 6 hours
Otherwise healthy nonsmoking adults	5 mg/kg	3 mg/kg q 8 hours
Older patients and patients with cor pulmonale	5 mg/kg	2 mg/kg q 8 hours
Patients with congestive heart failure	5 mg/kg	1–2 mg/kg q 12 hours

B.   Patients currently receiving theophylline products:

Determine, where possible, the time, amount, dosage form, and route of administration of the last dose the patient received.

The loading dose for theophylline is based on the principle that each 0.5 mg/kg of theophylline administered as a loading dose will result in a 1.0 µg/mL increase in serum theophylline concentration. Ideally, the loading dose should be deferred if a serum theophylline concentration can be obtained rapidly.

If this is not possible, the clinician must exercise judgment in selecting a dose based on the potential for benefit and risk. When there is sufficient respiratory distress to warrant a small risk, then 2.5 mg/kg of theophylline administered in rapidly absorbed form is likely to increase serum concentration by approximately 5 µg/mL. If the patient is not experiencing theophylline toxicity, this is unlikely to result in dangerous adverse effects.

Subsequent to the decision regarding use of a loading dose for this group of patients, the maintenance dosage recommendations are the same as those described above.

II.   Chronic Therapy:

Theophylline is a treatment for relief and/or prevention of symptoms from asthma and reversible bronchospasm associated with chronic bronchitis and emphysema. A dosage form that allows small incremental doses is desirable for initiating therapy. A liquid preparation should be considered for children to permit easier and more accurate dosage adjustment. Slow clinical titration is generally preferred to assure acceptance and safety of the medication, and to allow the patient to develop tolerance to transient caffeine-like side effects.

Initial Dose: 16 mg/kg/24 hours or 400 mg/24 hours (whichever is less) of anhydrous theophylline in divided doses at 6- or 8-hour intervals.

Increasing Dose: The above dosage may be increased in approximately 25 percent increments at 3-day intervals so long as the drug is tolerated, until clinical response is satisfactory or the maximum dose indicated in section III (below) is reached. The serum concentration may be checked at these intervals, but at a minimum should be determined at the end of this adjustment period.

It is important that no patient be maintained on any dosage that is not tolerated. When instructing patients to increase dosage according to the schedule above, they should be told not to take a subsequent dose if apparent side effects occur and to resume therapy at a lower dose once adverse effects have disappeared.

III.   Maximum Dose of Theophylline Where the Serum Concentration Is Not Measured:

WARNING: DO NOT ATTEMPT TO MAINTAIN ANY DOSE THAT IS NOT TOLERATED.

Not to exceed the following (or 900 mg, whichever is less):

Age 1–9 years	24 mg/kg day
Age 9–12 years	20 mg/kg day
Age 12–16 years	18 mg/kg day
Age 16 years or older	13 mg/kg day

IV.   Measurement of Serum Theophylline Concentrations During Chronic Therapy:

If the above maximum doses are to be maintained or exceeded, serum theophylline measurement is essential (see PRECAUTIONS, Laboratory Tests for guidance).

V.   Final Adjustment of Dosage:

Dosage adjustment after serum theophylline measurement

If serum theophylline is:		Directions:
Within desired range		Maintain dosage if tolerated.
Too high	20 to 25 µg/mL	Decrease doses by about 10% and recheck serum level after 3 days.
	25 to 30 µg/mL	Skip the next dose and decrease subsequent doses by about 25%. Recheck serum level after 3 days.
	Over 30 µg/mL	Skip next 2 doses and decrease subsequent doses by 50%. Recheck serum level after 3 days.
Too low		Increase dosage by 25% at 3-day intervals until either the desired serum concentration and/or clinical response is achieved. The total daily dose may need to be administered at more frequent intervals if symptoms occur repeatedly at the end of a dosing interval.

The serum concentration may be rechecked at appropriate intervals, but at least at the end of any adjustment period. When the patient's condition is otherwise clinically stable and none of the recognized factors that alter elimination are present, measurement of serum levels need to be repeated only every 6 to 12 months.

HOW SUPPLIED

Slo-Phyllin 100 mg Tablets (theophylline, tablets, USP), scored, dye-free, white, round, convex tablet, imprinted "WHR 351" in bottles of 100 (NDC 0075-0351-68) and in unit dose packages of 100 tablets (NDC 0075-0351-01).

Slo-Phyllin 200 mg Tablets (theophylline, tablets, USP), scored, dye-free, white, flat-faced tablet, imprinted "WHR 352" in bottles of 100 (NDC 0075-0352-68) and in unit dose packages of 100 tablets (NDC 0075-0352-01).

Slo-Phyllin 80 mg Syrup (theophylline anhydrous, 80 mg per 15 mL) nonalcoholic, orange color in 16 fl oz (NDC 0075-3650-16).

STORAGE CONDITIONS

Store at room temperature. Protect from excessive heat, light, and moisture.

CAUTION

Federal (U.S.A.) law prohibits dispensing without prescription.

Keep this and all medications out of the reach of children.
Rev. 7/87
RORER PHARMACEUTICALS
a division of
RORER PHARMACEUTICAL CORPORATION
Fort Washington, PA, U.S.A. 19034

CAPSULES, SYRUP
[slō "fil 'in]
(theophylline—guaifenesin)

DESCRIPTION

Each Slo-Phyllin® GG gelatin capsule or tablespoonful (15 mL) of liquid contains 150 mg of theophylline (anhydrous) and 90 mg of guaifenesin, as an oral bronchodilator-expectorant.

Theophylline (1H-Purine-2,6-dione, 3,7-dihydro-1, 3-dimethyl-), a xanthine compound, is a white, odorless crystalline powder having a bitter taste.

Guaifenesin (1,2-Propanediol, 3-[2-methoxyphenoxy]-), a guaiacol compound, is a white to slightly yellow crystalline powder with a bitter, aromatic taste.

Slo-Phyllin® GG capsules inactive ingredients: black iron oxide, dimethylpolysiloxane, FD&C Blue No. 1, gelatin, glycerin, lecithin, methylparaben, pharmaceutical glaze, polyethylene glycol, propylparaben, sorbitol, titanium dioxide.

Slo-Phyllin® GG syrup inactive ingredients: citric acid, flavors, glycerin, methylparaben, propylene glycol, sodium benzoate, saccharin sodium, sorbitol, sucrose, purified water.

Theophylline   Guaifenesin

CLINICAL PHARMACOLOGY

Theophylline: Theophylline directly relaxes the smooth muscle of the bronchial airways and pulmonary blood vessels, thus acting mainly as a bronchodilator, pulmonary vasodilator and smooth muscle relaxant. The drug also possesses other actions typical of the xanthine derivatives: coronary vasodilator, diuretic, cardiac stimulant, cerebral stimulant, and skeletal muscle stimulant. The actions of theophylline may be mediated through inhibition of phosphodiesterase and a resultant increase in intracellular cyclic AMP, which could mediate smooth muscle relaxation. At concentrations higher than attained *in vivo*, theophylline also inhibits the release of histamine by mast cells.

In vitro, theophylline has been shown to react synergistically with beta agonists that increase intracellular cyclic AMP through the stimulation of adenyl cyclase (isoproterenol), but synergism has not been demonstrated in patient studies and more data are needed to determine if theophylline and beta agonists have clinically important additive effects *in vivo*.

Apparently, no development of tolerance occurs with chronic use of theophylline. The half-life is shortened with cigarette smoking. The half-life is prolonged in alcoholism, reduced hepatic or renal function, congestive heart failure, and in patients receiving antibiotics such as TAO (troleandomycin), erthromycin and clindamycin. High fever for prolonged periods may decrease theophylline elimination.
[See table below].

Newborn infants have extremely slow clearances and half-lives exceeding 24 hours which approach those seen for older children after about 3–6 months.

Older adults with chronic obstructive pulmonary disease, any patients with cor pulmonale or other causes of heart failure, and patients with liver pathology may have much lower clearances with half-lives that may exceed 24 hours. The half-life of theophylline in smokers (1 to 2 packs/day) averaged 4 to 5 hours among various studies, much shorter than the half-life in nonsmokers, who averaged about 7 to 9 hours. The increase in theophylline clearance caused by smoking is probably the result of induction of drug-metabolizing enzymes that do not readily normalize after cessation of smoking. It appears that between 3 months and 2 years may be necessary for normalization of the effect of smoking on theophylline pharmacokinetics.

Guaifenesin:

Guaifenesin increases respiratory tract secretions, possibly by stimulating the Goblet cells.

Guaifenesin appears to be well absorbed, but its pharmacokinetics have not been thoroughly studied.

INDICATIONS AND USAGE

For relief and/or prevention of symptoms of asthma and reversible bronchospasm associated with chronic bronchitis and emphysema.

CONTRAINDICATIONS

In individuals who have shown hypersensitivity to any of the components.

WARNINGS

Status asthmaticus is a medical emergency. Optimal therapy frequently requires additional medication including corticosteroids when the patient is not rapidly responsive to bronchodilators. Excessive theophylline doses may be associated

Theophylline Elimination Characteristics

	Theophylline Clearance Rates (mean±S.D.)	Half-life Average (mean±S.D.)
Children (over 6 months of age)	1.45±.58 mL/kg/min	3.7±1.1 hours
Adult nonsmokers with uncomplicated asthma	.65±.19 mL/kg/min	8.7±2.2 hours

with toxicity. Therefore, monitoring of serum theophylline levels is recommended to ensure maximal benefit without excessive risk. Incidence of toxicity increases at levels greater than 20 μg/mL. Morphine, curare, and stilbamidine should be used with caution in patients with airflow obstruction since they stimulate histamine release and can induce asthmatic attacks. They may also suppress respiration leading to respiratory failure. Alternative drugs should be chosen whenever possible.

There is an excellent correlation between high blood levels of theophylline resulting from conventional doses and associated clinical manifestations of toxicity in (1) patients with lowered body plasma clearances (due to transient cardiac decompensation), (2) patients with liver dysfunction or chronic obstructive pulmonary disease, (3) patients who are older than 55 years of age, particularly males. There are often no early signs of less serious theophylline toxicity such as nausea and restlessness, which may appear in up to 50 percent of patients prior to onset of convulsions. Ventricular arrhythmias or seizures may be the first signs of toxicity. Many patients who have higher theophylline serum levels exhibit tachycardia.

Theophylline products may worsen pre-existing arrhythmias.

PRECAUTIONS

General: Theophylline.

Mean half-life in smokers is shorter than nonsmokers; therefore, smokers may require larger doses of theophylline. Theophylline should not be administered concurrently with other xanthine medications. Use with caution in patients with severe cardiac disease, severe hypoxemia, hypertension, hyperthyroidism, acute myocardial injury, cor pulmonale, congestive heart failure, liver disease, and in the elderly (especially males) and in neonates. Great caution should especially be used in giving theophylline to patients in congestive heart failure. Such patients have shown markedly prolonged theophylline blood level curves with theophylline persisting in serum for long periods following discontinuation of the drug.

Use theophylline cautiously in patients with a history of peptic ulcer. Theophylline may occasionally act as a local irritant to G.I. tract although gastrointestinal symptoms are more commonly central and associated with serum concentrations over 20 μg/mL.

DRUG INTERACTIONS

Toxic synergism with ephedrine has been documented and may occur with some other sympathomimetic bronchodilators.

DRUG	EFFECT
Aminophylline with Lithium Carbonate	Increased excretion of Lithium Carbonate
Aminophylline with Propranolol	Antagonism of Propranolol effect
Theophylline with Furosemide	Increased Diuresis of Furosemide
Theophylline with Hexamethonium	Decreased Hexamethonium-induced chronotropic effect
Theophylline with Reserpine	Reserpine-induced Tachycardia
Theophylline with Chlordiazepoxide	Chlordiazepoxide-induced fatty acid mobilization
Theophylline with Cyclamycin (TAO= troleandomycin): erythromycin, clindamycin, lincomycin	Increased Theophylline plasma levels

DRUG/LABORATORY TEST INTERACTIONS

Theophylline may increase uric acid levels and urinary catecholamines. Metabolites of guaifenesin may contribute to increased urinary 5-hydroxy-indoleacetic acid readings, when determined with nitrosonaphthol reagent.

Carcinogenesis, Mutagenesis, Impairment of Fertility

Long-term animal studies have not been performed to evaluate the carcinogenic potential, mutagenic potential, or the effect on fertility by xanthine compounds.

USAGE IN PREGNANCY

Teratogenic effects:

Pregnancy Category C—Animal reproduction studies have not been conducted with **Slo-Phyllin® GG**. It is also not known whether **Slo-Phyllin® GG** can cause fetal harm when administered to a pregnant woman or can affect reproduc-

Group	Oral Loading Dose (Theophylline)	Maintenance Dose For Next 12 hours (Theophylline)	Maintenance Dose Beyond 12 hours (Theophylline)
1. Children 6 months to 9 years	6 mg/kg	4 mg/kg q4hrs	4 mg/kg q6hrs
2. Children age 9–16 and young adult smokers	6 mg/kg	3 mg/kg q4hrs	3 mg/kg q6hrs
3. Otherwise healthy nonsmoking adults	6 mg/kg	3 mg/kg q6hrs	3 mg/kg q8hrs
4. Older patients and patients with cor pulmonale	6 mg/kg	2 mg/kg q6hrs	2 mg/kg q8hrs
5. Patients with congestive heart failure, liver failure	6 mg/kg	2 mg/kg q8hrs	1–2 mg/kg q12hrs

tion capacity. Therefore, it should be given to a pregnant woman only if clearly needed.

Nonteratogenic effects:

Theophylline may be excreted in the milk and cause irritability in the nursing infant. Therefore, caution should be exercised when **Slo-Phyllin® GG** is administered to a nursing mother.

ADVERSE REACTIONS

The frequency of adverse reactions is related to serum theophylline levels and is usually not a problem at levels below 20 μg/mL. The most consistent adverse reactions are usually due to overdosage and, while all have not been reported with **Slo-Phyllin® GG**, the following reactions may be considered when theophylline is administered. Central nervous system: clonic and tonic generalized convulsions, muscle twitching, reflex hyperexcitability, headaches, insomnia, restlessness, and irritability. Cardiovascular: circulatory failure, life-threatening ventricular arrhythmias, hypotension, extrasystoles, tachycardia, palpitation, and flushing. Gastrointestinal: hematemesis, vomiting, diarrhea, epigastric pain, and nausea. Renal: increased excretion of renal tubular cells and red blood cells, albuminuria, and potentiation of diuresis. Respiratory: tachypnea. Other: hyperglycemia and inappropriate ADH syndrome.

OVERDOSAGE

Symptoms:

Nervousness, agitation, headache, insomnia, vomiting, tachycardia, extrasystoles, hyperreflexia, fasciculations and clonic and tonic convulsions. Children may be particularly prone to restlessness and hyperactivity that can proceed to convulsions.

Management:

A. If potential oral overdose is established and seizure has not occurred:
1) Induce vomiting.
2) Administer a cathartic (this is particularly important if sustained-release preparations have been taken).
3) Administer activated charcoal.
4) Monitor vital signs, maintain blood pressure and provide adequate hydration.

B. If patient is having a seizure:
1) Establish an airway.
2) Administer oxygen.
3) Treat the seizure with intravenous diazepam, 0.1 to 0.3 mg/kg up to 10 mg.
4) Monitor vital signs, maintain blood pressure and provide adequate hydration.

C. Postseizure coma:
1) Maintain airway and oxygenation.
2) If a result of oral medication, follow above recommendations to prevent absorption of drug, but intubation and lavage will have to be performed instead of inducing emesis, and the cathartic and charcoal will need to be introduced via a large-bore gastric lavage tube.
3) Continue to provide full supportive care and adequate hydration while waiting for drug to be metabolized. In general, the drug is metabolized sufficiently rapidly enough so as not to warrant consideration of dialysis.

D. Animal studies suggest that phenobarbital may decrease theophylline toxicity. There are as yet, however, insufficient data to recommend pretreatment of an overdosage with phenobarbital.

GENERAL

The oral LD$_{50}$ of theophylline in mice is 350 mg/kg. The oral LD$_{50}$ of guaifenesin in mice is 1725 mg/kg. In humans, adverse reactions often occur when serum theophylline levels exceed 20 μg/mL. Information on physiological variables which influence excretion of theophylline can be found under the heading "Clinical Pharmacology."

DOSAGE AND ADMINISTRATION

General

Therapeutic serum levels associated with optimal likelihood for benefit and minimal risk of toxicity are considered to be between 10 μg/mL and 20 μg/mL. Levels above 20 μg/mL may produce toxic effects. There is great variation from patient to patient in dosage needed in order to achieve a therapeutic blood level because of variable rates of elimination. Because of this wide variation from patient to patient, and

the relatively narrow therapeutic blood level range, dosage must be individualized and monitoring of serum theophylline levels is highly recommended.

Dosage should be calculated on the basis of lean (ideal) body weight where mg/kg doses are stated. Theophylline does not distribute into fatty tissue.

Giving theophylline with food may prevent the rare case of stomach irritation, and although absorption may be slower, it is still complete.

When rapidly absorbed products such as solutions and soft gelatin capsules with rapid dissolution are used, dosing to maintain "around the clock" blood levels generally requires administration every 6 hours to obtain the greatest efficacy for clinical use in children; dosing intervals up to 8 hours may be satisfactory for adults because of their slower elimination. Children and adults requiring higher-than-average doses may benefit from products with slower absorption which may allow longer dosing intervals and/or less fluctuation in serum concentration over a dosing interval during chronic therapy.

Acute Symptoms of Asthma Requiring Rapid Theophyllinization

Note: Due to their slower rate of absorption, sustained-release theophylline products are not designed for use in conditions requiring rapid theophyllinization.

I. Not currently receiving theophylline products.

II. Those currently receiving theophylline products: Determine, where possible, the time, amount, route of administration and form of the patient's last dose.

The loading dose for theophylline will be based on the principle that each 0.5 mg/kg of theophylline administered as a loading dose will result in a 1 μg/mL increase in serum theophylline concentration. Ideally, then, the loading dose should be deferred if a serum theophylline concentration can be rapidly obtained. If this is not possible, the clinician must exercise his judgment in selecting a dose based on the potential for benefit and risk. When there is sufficient respiratory distress to warrant a small risk, 2.5 mg/kg of theophylline is likely to increase the serum concentration when administered as a loading dose in rapidly absorbed form by only about 5 μg/mL. If the patient is not already experiencing theophylline toxicity, this is unlikely to result in dangerous adverse effects.

Subsequent to the modified decision regarding loading dose in this group of patients, the subsequent maintenance dosage recommendations are the same as those described above. [See table above].

COMMENTS

To achieve optimal therapeutic theophylline dosage, it is recommended to monitor serum theophylline concentration. However, it is not always possible or practical to obtain a serum theophylline level.

Patients should be closely monitored for signs of toxicity. The present data suggest that the above dosage recommendations will achieve therapeutic serum concentrations with minimal risk of toxicity for most patients. However, some risk of toxic serum concentrations is still present. Adverse reactions to theophylline often occur when serum theophylline levels exceed 20 μg/mL.

CHRONIC ASTHMA

Theophyllinization is a treatment of first choice for the management of chronic asthma (to prevent symptoms and maintain patent airways). Slow clinical titration is generally preferred to ensure acceptance and safety of the medication.

Initial Dose: 16 mg/kg/day or 400 mg/day (whichever is lower) in 3 to 4 divided doses at 6- to 8-hour intervals for the Syrup and Capsules.

Increased Dose: The above dosage may be increased in approximately 25 percent increments at 2- to 3-day intervals so long as no intolerance is observed, until the maximum indicated below is reached.

Continued on next page

This product information was prepared in September, 1989. Information concerning these products may be obtained by addressing Rorer Pharmaceutical Corporation, 500 Virginia Drive, Fort Washington, PA 19034.

Rorer Pharm.—Cont.

Maximum Dose Without Measurement of Serum Concentration: Not to exceed the following: (WARNING: DO NOT ATTEMPT TO MAINTAIN ANY DOSE THAT IS NOT TOLERATED.)

Age 6 months to 9 years—24 mg/kg/day
Age 9 to 12 years—20 mg/kg/day
Age 12 to 16 years—18 mg/kg/day
Age > 16 years—13 mg/kg/day or 900 mg/day (WHICHEVER IS LESS)

Note: Use ideal body weight for obese patients.

Measurement of Serum Theophylline Concentration During Chronic Therapy:
If the above maximum doses are to be maintained or exceeded, serum theophylline measurement is recommended. This should be obtained at the approximate time of peak absorption during chronic therapy for the product used (1 to 2 hours for liquids, soft gelatin capsules, and plain uncoated tablets that undergo rapid dissolution, 3 to 5 hours for sustained-release preparations). It is important that the patient will have missed *no* doses during the previous 48 hours and that dosing intervals will have been reasonably typical with no added doses during that period of time. DOSAGE ADJUSTMENT BASED ON SERUM THEOPHYLLINE MEASUREMENTS WHEN THESE INSTRUCTIONS HAVE NOT BEEN FOLLOWED MAY RESULT IN RECOMMENDATIONS THAT PRESENT RISK OF TOXICITY TO THE PATIENT.

Final Dosage Adjustment: Caution should be exercised for younger children who cannot complain of minor side effects. Older adults, those with cor pulmonale, congestive heart failure, and/or liver disease may have unusually low dosage requirements and thus may experience toxicity at the maximal dosage recommended above.

It is important that no patient be maintained on any dosage that he is not tolerating. In instructing patients to increase dosage according to the schedule above, they should be instructed not to take a subsequent dose if apparent side effects occur and to resume therapy at a lower dose once adverse effects have disappeared.

Caution: Federal (U.S.A.) law prohibits dispensing without prescription.

KEEP THIS AND ALL MEDICATION OUT OF THE REACH OF CHILDREN.

HOW SUPPLIED

Slo-Phyllin® GG Syrup is lemon-vanilla flavored, nonalcoholic, dye-free, and each 15 mL tablespoonful contains theophylline, anhydrous, 150 mg and guaifenesin 90 mg. Available in 16 oz. bottles (NDC 0075–0357-16).

Slo-Phyllin® GG Capsules are white, liquid filled, soft gelatin capsules each containing theophylline, anhydrous, 150 mg and guaifenesin 90 mg. Available in bottles of 100 capsules (NDC 0075–0358-00).

[See table below.]

Rev 3/88

Slo-Phyllin® GG Syrup
Manufactured by
RORER PHARMACEUTICALS
a division of
Rorer Pharmaceutical Corporation
Fort Washington, PA, U.S.A. 19034
Slo-Phyllin® GG Capsules
Manufactured by
R. P. SCHERER CORPORATION
Troy, MI 48084
For
RORER PHARMACEUTICALS
a division of
RORER PHARMACEUTICAL CORPORATION
Fort Washington, PA, U.S.A. 19034
Shown in Product Identification Section, page 426

ARMOUR® THYROID Tablets   ℞
[thī´roid]
(THYROID TABLETS, U.S.P.)

DESCRIPTION

Armour® Thyroid Tablets (Thyroid Tablets, USP) for oral use are natural preparations derived from porcine thyroid glands. (T_3 liothyronine is approximately four times as potent as T_4 levothyroxine on a microgram for microgram basis.) They provide 38 mcg levothyroxine (T_4) and 9 mcg liothyronine (T_3) per grain of thyroid. The inactive ingredients are calcium stearate, dextrose and mineral oil.

STRUCTURAL FORMULAS

Liothyronine (T_3)

Levothyroxine (T_4)

CLINICAL PHARMACOLOGY

The steps in the synthesis of the thyroid hormones are controlled by thyrotropin (Thyroid Stimulating Hormone, TSH) secreted by the anterior pituitary. This hormone's secretion is in turn controlled by a feedback mechanism effected by the thyroid hormones themselves and by thyrotropin releasing hormone (TRH), a tripeptide of hypothalamic origin. Endogenous thyroid hormone secretion is suppressed when exogenous thyroid hormones are administered to euthyroid individuals in excess of the normal gland's secretion.

The mechanisms by which thyroid hormones exert their physiologic action are not well understood. These hormones enhance oxygen consumption by most tissues of the body, increase the basal metabolic rate, and the metabolism of carbohydrates, lipids, and proteins. Thus, they exert a profound influence on every organ system in the body and are of particular importance in the development of the central nervous system.

The normal thyroid gland contains approximately 200 mcg of levothyroxine (T_4) per gram of gland, and 15 mcg of liothyronine (T_3) per gram. The ratio of these two hormones in the circulation does not represent the ratio in the thyroid gland, since about 80 percent of peripheral liothyronine (T_3) comes from monodeiodination of levothyroxine (T_4). Peripheral monodeiodination of levothyroxine (T_4) at the 5 position (inner ring) also results in the formation of reverse liothyronine (T_3), which is calorigenically inactive.

Liothyronine (T_3) levels are low in the fetus and newborn, in old age, in chronic caloric deprivation, hepatic cirrhosis, renal failure, surgical stress, and chronic illnesses representing what has been called the "T_3 thyronine syndrome."

Pharmacokinetics—Animal studies have shown that levothyroxine (T_4) is only partially absorbed from the gastrointestinal tract. The degree of absorption is dependent on the vehicle used for its administration and by the character of the intestinal contents, the intestinal flora, including plasma protein, and soluble dietary factors, all of which bind thyroid and thereby make it unavailable for diffusion. Only 41 percent is absorbed when given in a gelatin capsule as opposed to a 74 percent absorption when given with an albumin carrier.

Depending on other factors, absorption has varied from 48 to 79 percent of the administered dose. Fasting increases absorption. Malabsorption syndromes, as well as dietary factors, (children's soybean formula, concomitant use of anionic exchange resins such as cholestyramine) cause excessive fecal loss. Liothyronine (T_3) is almost totally absorbed, 95 percent in 4 hours. The hormones contained in the natural preparations are absorbed in a manner similar to the synthetic hormones.

More than 99 percent of circulating hormones are bound to serum proteins, including thyroid-binding globulin (TBg), thyroid-binding prealbumin (TBPA), and albumin (TBa), whose capacities and affinities vary for the hormones. The higher affinity of levothyroxine (T_4) for both TBg and TBPA as compared to liothyronine (T_3) partially explains the higher serum levels and longer half-life of the former hormone. Both protein-bound hormones exist in reverse equilibrium with minute amounts of free hormone, the latter accounting for the metabolic activity.

Deiodination of levothyroxine (T_4) occurs at a number of sites, including liver, kidney, and other tissues. The conjugated hormone, in the form of glucuronide or sulfate, is found in the bile and gut where it may complete an enterohepatic circulation. Eighty-five percent of levothyroxine (T_4) metabolized daily is deiodinated.

INDICATIONS AND USAGE

Armour Thyroid Tablets are indicated:
1. As replacement or supplemental therapy in patients with hypothyroidism of any etiology, except transient hypothyroidism during the recovery phase of subacute thyroiditis. This category includes cretinism, myxedema, and ordinary hypothyroidism in patients of any age (children, adults, the elderly), or state (including pregnancy); primary hypothyroidism resulting from functional deficiency, primary atrophy, partial or total absence of thyroid gland, or the effects of surgery, radiation, or drugs, with or without the presence of goiter; and secondary (pituitary), or tertiary (hypothalamic) hypothyroidism (See WARNINGS).
2. As pituitary TSH suppressants, in the treatment or prevention of various types of euthyroid goiters, including thyroid nodules, subacute or chronic lymphocytic thyroiditis (Hashimoto's), multinodular goiter, and in the management of thyroid cancer.
3. As diagnostic agents in suppression tests to differentiate suspected mild hyperthyroidism or thyroid gland autonomy.

CONTRAINDICATIONS

Thyroid hormone preparations are generally contraindicated in patients with diagnosed but as yet uncorrected adrenal cortical insufficiency, untreated thyrotoxicosis, and apparent hypersensitivity to any of their active or extraneous constituents. There is no well-documented evidence from the literature, however, of true allergic or idiosyncratic reactions to thyroid hormone.

WARNINGS

> Drugs with thyroid hormone activity, alone or together with other therapeutic agents, have been used for the treatment of obesity. In euthyroid patients, doses within the range of daily hormonal requirements are ineffective for weight reduction. Larger doses may produce serious or even life-threatening manifestations of toxicity, particularly when given in association with sympathomimetic amines such as those used for their anorectic effects.

The use of thyroid hormones in the therapy of obesity, alone or combined with other drugs, is unjustified and has been shown to be ineffective. Neither is their use justified for the treatment of male or female infertility unless this condition is accompanied by hypothyroidism.

PRECAUTIONS

General—Thyroid hormones should be used with great caution in a number of circumstances where the integrity of the cardiovascular system, particularly the coronary arteries, is suspected. These include patients with angina pectoris or the elderly, in whom there is a greater likelihood of occult cardiac disease. In these patients therapy should be initiated with low doses, i.e. 15–30 mg Armour Thyroid. When, in such patients, a euthyroid state can only be reached at the expense of an aggravation of the cardiovascular disease, thyroid hormone dosage should be reduced.

Thyroid hormone therapy in patients with concomitant diabetes mellitus or diabetes insipidus or adrenal cortical insufficiency aggravates the intensity of their symptoms. Appropriate adjustments of the various therapeutic measures directed at these concomitant endocrine diseases are required. The therapy of myxedema coma requires simultaneous administration of glucocorticoids (See DOSAGE AND ADMINISTRATION).

Hypothyroidism decreases and hyperthyroidism increases the sensitivity to oral anticoagulants. Prothrombin time should be closely monitored in thyroid-treated patients on oral anticoagulants and dosage of the latter agents adjusted on the basis of frequent prothrombin time determinations. In infants, excessive doses of thyroid hormone preparations may produce craniosynostosis.

Body Weight		Dosage of *Slo-Phyllin® GG* Syrup Calculated at Approximately:		
Expressed in		3mg	4mg	5mg
Kilos	Lbs	Per Kilo	Per Kilo	Per Kilo
9	20	½ tsp.	¾ tsp.	1 tsp.
18	40	1 tsp.	1½ tsp.	2 tsp.
27	60	1½ tsp.	2 tsp.	2¾ tsp.
36	79	2 tsp.	3 tsp.	3½ tsp.
45	99	2¾ tsp.	3½ tsp.	4½ tsp.
54	118	3¼ tsp.	4½ tsp.	5½ tsp.

Administered every six (6) hours.

Information for the Patient—Patients on thyroid hormone preparations and parents of children on thyroid therapy should be informed that:

1. Replacement therapy is to be taken essentially for life, with the exception of cases of transient hypothyroidism, usually associated with thyroiditis, and in those patients receiving a therapeutic trial of the drug.
2. They should immediately report during the course of therapy any signs or symptoms of thyroid hormone toxicity, e.g., chest pain, increased pulse rate, palpitations, excessive sweating, heat intolerance, nervousness, or any other unusual event.
3. In case of concomitant diabetes mellitus, the daily dosage of antidiabetic medication may need readjustment as thyroid hormone replacement is achieved. If thyroid medication is stopped, a downward readjustment of the dosage of insulin or oral hypoglycemic agent may be necessary to avoid hypoglycemia. At all times, close monitoring of urinary glucose levels is mandatory in such patients.
4. In case of concomitant oral anticoagulant therapy, the prothrombin time should be measured frequently to determine if the dosage of oral anticoagulants is to be readjusted.
5. Partial loss of hair may be experienced by children in the first few months of thyroid therapy, but this is usually a transient phenomenon and later recovery is usually the rule.

Laboratory Tests—Treatment of patients with thyroid hormones requires the periodic assessment of thyroid status by means of appropriate laboratory tests besides the full clinical evaluation. The TSH suppression test can be used to test the effectiveness of any thyroid preparation bearing in mind the relative insensitivity of the infant pituitary to the negative feedback effect of thyroid hormones. Serum T_4 levels can be used to test the effectiveness of all thyroid medications except T_3. When the total serum T_4 is low but TSH is normal, a test specific to assess unbound (free) T_4 levels is warranted. Specific measurements of T_4 and T_3 by competitive protein binding or radioimmunoassay are not influenced by blood levels of organic or inorganic iodine.

Drug Interactions—Oral Anticoagulants—Thyroid hormones appear to increase catabolism of vitamin K-dependent clotting factors. If oral anticoagulants are also being given, compensatory increases in clotting factor synthesis are impaired. Patients stabilized on oral anticoagulants who are found to require thyroid replacement therapy should be watched very closely when thyroid is started. If a patient is truly hypothyroid, it is likely that a reduction in anticoagulant dosage will be required. No special precautions appear to be necessary when oral anticoagulant therapy is begun in a patient already stabilized on maintenance thyroid replacement therapy.

Insulin or Oral Hypoglycemics—Initiating thyroid replacement therapy may cause increases in insulin or oral hypoglycemic requirements. The effects seen are poorly understood and depend upon a variety of factors such as dose and type of thyroid preparations and endocrine status of the patient. Patients receiving insulin or oral hypoglycemics should be closely watched during initiation of thyroid replacement therapy.

Cholestyramine or Colestipol—Cholestyramine or colestipol binds both levothyroxine (T_4) and liothyronine (T_3) in the intestine, thus impairing absorption of these thyroid hormones. In vitro studies indicate that the binding is not easily removed. Therefore, four to five hours should elapse between administration of cholestyramine or colestipol and thyroid hormones.

Estrogen, Oral Contraceptives—Estrogens tend to increase serum thyroxine-binding globulin (TBg). In a patient with a nonfunctioning thyroid gland who is receiving thyroid replacement therapy, free levothyroxine (T_4) may be decreased when estrogens are started thus increasing thyroid requirements. However, if the patient's thyroid gland has sufficient function, the decreased free levothyroxine (T_4) will result in a compensatory increase in levothyroxine (T_4) output by the thyroid. Therefore, patients without a functioning thyroid gland who are on thyroid replacement therapy may need to increase their thyroid dose if estrogens or estrogen-containing oral contraceptives are given.

Drug/Laboratory Test Interactions—The following drugs or moieties are known to interfere with laboratory tests performed in patients on thyroid hormone therapy: androgens, corticosteroids, estrogens, oral contraceptives containing estrogens, iodine-containing preparations, and the numerous preparations containing salicylates.

1. Changes in TBg concentration should be taken into consideration in the interpretation of levothyroxine (T_4) and liothyronine (T_3) values. In such cases, the unbound (free) hormone should be measured. Pregnancy, estrogens, and estrogen-containing oral contraceptives increase TBg concentrations. TBg may also be increased during infectious hepatitis. Decreases in TBg concentrations are observed in nephrosis, acromegaly, and after androgen or corticosteroid therapy. Familial hyper- or hypothyroxine-binding-globulinemias have been described. The incidence of TBg

deficiency approximates 1 in 9,000. The binding of thyroxine by TBPA is inhibited by salicylates.
2. Medicinal or dietary iodine interferes with all in vivo tests of radio-iodine uptake, producing low uptakes which may not be relative of a true decrease in hormone synthesis.
3. The persistence of clinical and laboratory evidence of hypothyroidism in spite of adequate dosage replacement indicates either poor patient compliance, poor absorption, excessive fecal loss, or inactivity of the preparation. Intracellular resistance to thyroid hormone is quite rare.

Carcinogenesis, Mutagenesis, and Impairment of Fertility—A reportedly apparent association between prolonged thyroid therapy and breast cancer has not been confirmed and patients on thyroid for established indications should not discontinue therapy. No confirmatory long-term studies in animals have been performed to evaluate carcinogenic potential, mutagenicity, or impairment of fertility in either males or females.

Pregnancy-Category A—Thyroid hormones do not readily cross the placental barrier. The clinical experience to date does not indicate any adverse effect on fetuses when thyroid hormones are administered to pregnant women. On the basis of current knowledge, thyroid replacement therapy to hypothyroid women should not be discontinued during pregnancy.

Nursing Mothers—Minimal amounts of thyroid hormones are excreted in human milk. Thyroid is not associated with serious adverse reactions and does not have a known tumorigenic potential. However, caution should be exercised when thyroid is administered to a nursing woman.

Pediatric Use—Pregnant mothers provide little or no thyroid hormone to the fetus. The incidence of congenital hypothyroidism is relatively high (1:4,000) and the hypothyroid fetus would not derive any benefit from the small amounts of hormone crossing the placental barrier. Routine determinations of serum T_4 and/or TSH is strongly advised in neonates in view of the deleterious effects of thyroid deficiency on growth and development.

Treatment should be initiated immediately upon diagnosis, and maintained for life, unless transient hypothyroidism is suspected; in which case, therapy may be interrupted for 2 to 8 weeks after the age of 3 years to reassess the condition. Cessation of therapy is justified in patients who have maintained a normal TSH during those 2 to 8 weeks.

ADVERSE REACTIONS

Adverse reactions other than those indicative of hyperthyroidism because of therapeutic overdosage, either initially or during the maintenance period, are rare (See OVERDOSAGE).

OVERDOSAGE

Signs and Symptoms—Excessive doses of thyroid result in a hypermetabolic state resembling in every respect the condition of endogenous origin. The condition may be self-induced.

Treatment of Overdosage—Dosage should be reduced or therapy temporarily discontinued if signs and symptoms of overdosage appear.

Treatment may be reinstituted at a lower dosage. In normal individuals, normal hypothalamic-pituitary-thyroid axis function is restored in 6 to 8 weeks after thyroid suppression. Treatment of acute massive thyroid hormone overdosage is aimed at reducing gastrointestinal absorption of the drugs and counteracting central and peripheral effects, mainly those of increased sympathetic activity. Vomiting may be induced initially if further gastrointestinal absorption can reasonably be prevented and barring contraindications such as coma, convulsions, or loss of the gagging reflex. Treatment is symptomatic and supportive. Oxygen may be administered and ventilation maintained. Cardiac glycosides may be indicated if congestive heart failure develops. Measures to control fever, hypoglycemia, or fluid loss should be instituted if needed. Antiadrenergic agents, particularly propranolol, have been used advantageously in the treatment of increased sympathetic activity. Propranolol may be administered intravenously at a dosage of 1 to 3 mg over a 10-minute period or orally, 80 to 160 mg/day, initially, especially when no contraindications exist for its use.

DOSAGE AND ADMINISTRATION

The dosage of thyroid hormones is determined by the indication and must in every case be individualized according to patient response and laboratory findings.

Thyroid hormones are given orally. In acute, emergency conditions, injectable levothyroxine sodium (T_4) may be given intravenously when oral administration is not feasible or desirable, as in the treatment of myxedema coma, or during total parenteral nutrition. Intramuscular administration is not advisable because of reported poor absorption.

Hypothyroidism—Therapy is usually instituted using low doses, with increments which depend on the cardiovascular status of the patient. The usual starting dose is 30 mg Armour Thyroid, with increments of 15 mg every 2 to 3 weeks. A lower starting dosage, 15 mg/day, is recommended in patients with long standing myxedema, particularly if cardiovascular impairment is suspected, in which case extreme caution is recommended. The appearance of angina is

an indication for a reduction in dosage. Most patients require 60–120 mg/day. Failure to respond to doses of 180 mg suggests lack of compliance or malabsorption. Maintenance dosages of 60–120 mg/day usually result in normal serum T_4 and T_3 levels. Adequate therapy usually results in normal TSH and T_4 levels after 2 to 3 weeks of therapy. Readjustment of thyroid hormone dosage should be made within the first four weeks of therapy, after proper clinical and laboratory evaluations, including serum levels of T_4, bound and free, and TSH.

Liothyronine (T_3) may be used in preference to levothyroxine (T_4) during radio-isotope scanning procedures, since induction of hypothyroidism in those cases is more abrupt and can be of shorter duration. It may also be preferred when impairment of peripheral conversion of levothyroxine (T_4) and liothyronine (T_3) is suspected.

Myxedema Coma—Myxedema coma is usually precipitated in the hypothyroid patient of long-standing by intercurrent illness or drugs such as sedatives and anesthetics and should be considered a medical emergency. Therapy should be directed at the correction of electrolyte disturbances and possible infection besides the administration of thyroid hormones. Corticosteroids should be administered routinely. Levothyroxine (T_4) and liothyronine (T_3) may be administered via a nasogastric tube but the preferred route of administration of both hormones is intravenous. Levothyroxine sodium (T_4) is given at a starting dose of 400 mcg (100 mcg/mL) given rapidly, and is usually well tolerated, even in the elderly. This initial dose is followed by daily supplements of 100 to 200 mcg given IV. Normal T_4 levels are achieved in 24 hours followed in 3 days by threefold elevation of T_3. Oral therapy with thyroid hormone would be resumed as soon as the clinical situation has been stabilized and the patient is able to take oral medication.

Thyroid Cancer—Exogenous thyroid hormone may produce regression of metastases from follicular and papillary carcinoma of the thyroid and is used as ancillary therapy of these conditions with radioactive iodine. TSH should be suppressed to low or undetectable levels. Therefore, larger amounts of thyroid hormone than those used for replacement therapy are required. Medullary carcinoma of the thyroid is usually unresponsive to this therapy.

Thyroid Suppression Therapy—Administration of thyroid hormone in doses higher than those produced physiologically by the gland results in suppression of the production of endogenous hormone. This is the basis for the thyroid suppression test and is used as an aid in the diagnosis of patients with signs of mild hyperthyroidism in whom base line laboratory tests appear normal, or to demonstrate thyroid gland autonomy in patients with Grave's ophthalmopathy. ^{131}I uptake is determined before and after the administration of the exogenous hormone. A 50 percent or greater suppression of uptake indicates a normal thyroid-pituitary axis and thus rules out thyroid gland autonomy.

For adults, the usual suppressive dose of levothyroxine (T_4) is 1.56 mg/kg of body weight per day given for 7 to 10 days. These doses usually yield normal serum T_4 and T_3 levels and lack of response to TSH.

Thyroid hormones should be administered cautiously to patients in whom there is strong suspicion of thyroid gland autonomy, in view of the fact that the exogenous hormone effects will be additive to the endogenous source.

Pediatric Dosage—Pediatric dosage should follow the recommendations summarized in Table 1. In infants with congenital hypothyroidism, therapy with full doses should be instituted as soon as the diagnosis has been made.

Recommended Pediatric Dosage for Congenital Hypothyroidism

	Armour Thyroid Tablets	
Age	Dose per day	Daily dose per kg of body weight
0–6 mos	15–30 mg	4.8–6 mg
6–12 mos	30–45 mg	3.6–4.8 mg
1–5 yrs	45–60 mg	3–3.6 mg
6–12 yrs	60–90 mg	2.4–3 mg
Over 12 yrs	Over 90 mg	1.2–1.8 mg

Table 1

HOW SUPPLIED

Armour Thyroid tablets (thyroid tablets, USP) are supplied as follows: 15 mg (¼ gr) are available in bottles of 100 (NDC 0075-3510-06). 30 mg (½ gr) are available in bottles of 100

Continued on next page

This product information was prepared in September, 1989. Information concerning these products may be obtained by addressing Rorer Pharmaceutical Corporation, 500 Virginia Drive, Fort Washington, PA 19034.

Rorer Pharm.—Cont.

(NDC 0075-3520-06), 1000 (NDC 0075-3520-02), drums of 50,000 (NDC 0075-3520-50), and unit dose cartons of 100 (NDC 0075-3520-04). 60 mg (1 gr) are available in bottles of 100 (NDC 0075-3532-06), 1000 (NDC 0075-3532-02), 5000 (NDC 0075-3532-03), drums of 50,000 (NDC 0075-3532-50) and unit dose cartons of 100 (NDC 0075-3532-04). 90 mg (1½ gr) are available in bottles of 100 (NDC 0075-3540-06). 120 mg (2 gr) are available in bottles of 100 (NDC 0075-3550-06), 1000 (NDC 0075-3550-02), drums of 50,000 (NDC 0075-3550-50) and unit dose cartons of 100 (NDC 0075-3550-05). 180 mg (3 gr) are available in bottles of 100 (NDC 0075-3555-06), and 1000 (NDC 0075-3555-02). 240 mg (4 gr) are available in bottles of 100 (NDC 0075-3556-06). 300 mg (5 gr) are available in bottles of 100 (NDC 0075-3560-06). The bottles of 100 are special dispensing bottles with child-resistant closures.

NOTE: (T_3 liothyronine is approximately four times as potent as T_4 levothyroxine on a microgram for microgram basis.)

Tablets should be stored at controlled room temperature, 59°–86°F (15°–30°C), in capped bottles or unbroken plastic strip packing.

CAUTION

Federal (U.S.A.) law prohibits dispensing without prescription.
Revised: December 1988
RORER PHARMACEUTICALS
a division of
RORER PHARMACEUTICAL CORPORATION
Fort Washington, PA, U.S.A. 19034
Shown in Product Identification Section, page 426

THYROLAR® Tablets   ℞

[thī-rō-lär]
(Liotrix Tablets, USP)

DESCRIPTION

Thyrolar® Tablets (Liotrix Tablets, USP) contain triiodothyronine (T_3 liothyronine) sodium and tetraiodothyronine (T_4 levothyroxine) sodium in the amounts listed in the "How Supplied" section. (T_3 liothyronine sodium is approximately four times as potent at T_4 thyroxine on a microgram for microgram basis.)

The inactive ingredients are calcium phosphate, microcrystalline cellulose, corn starch, lactose, and magnesium stearate. The tablets also contain the following dyes: Thyrolar® ¼-FD&C Blue #1 and FD&C Red #40; Thyrolar® ½-FD&C Red #40 and D&C Yellow #10; Thyrolar® 1-FD&C Red #40; Thyrolar® 2-FD&C Blue #1, FD&C Red #40, and D&C Yellow #10; Thyrolar® 3-FD&C Red #40 and D&C Yellow #10.

STRUCTURAL FORMULAS

Liothyronine (T_3) Sodium

$$HO-\bigcirc-O-\bigcirc-CH_2-\underset{H}{\overset{NH_2}{C}}-COONa$$

Levothyroxine (T_4) Sodium

$$HO-\bigcirc-O-\bigcirc-CH_2-\underset{H}{\overset{NH_2}{C}}-COONa \cdot xH_2O$$

CLINICAL PHARMACOLOGY

The steps in the synthesis of the thyroid hormones are controlled by thyrotropin (Thyroid Stimulating Hormone, TSH) secreted by the anterior pituitary. This hormone's secretion is in turn controlled by a feedback mechanism effected by the thyroid hormones themselves and by thyrotropin releasing hormone (TRH), a tripeptide of hypothalamic origin. Endogenous thyroid hormone secretion is suppressed when exogenous thyroid hormones are administered to euthyroid individuals in excess of the normal gland's secretion.

The mechanisms by which thyroid hormones exert their physiologic action are not well understood. These hormones enhance oxygen consumption by most tissues of the body, increase the basal metabolic rate, and the metabolism of carbohydrates, lipids, and proteins. Thus, they exert a profound influence on every organ system in the body and are of particular importance in the development of the central nervous system.

The normal thyroid gland contains approximately 200 mcg of levothyroxine (T_4) per gram of gland, and 15 mcg of triio-

dothyronine (T_3) per gram. The ratio of these two hormones in the circulation does not represent the ratio in the thyroid gland, since about 80 percent of peripheral triiodothyronine comes from monodeiodination of levothyroxine. Peripheral monodeiodination of levothyroxine at the 5 position (inner ring) also results in the formation of reverse triiodothyronine (T_3), which is calorigenically inactive.

Triiodothyronine (T_3) levels are low in the fetus and newborn, in old age, in chronic caloric deprivation, hepatic cirrhosis, renal failure, surgical stress, and chronic illnesses representing what has been called the "low triiodothyronine syndrome."

Pharmacokinetics—Animal studies have shown that T_4 is only partially absorbed from the gastrointestinal tract. The degree of absorption is dependent on the vehicle used for its administration and by the character of the intestinal contents, the intestinal flora, including plasma protein, soluble dietary factors, all of which bind thyroid and thereby make it unavailable for diffusion. Only 41 percent is absorbed when given in a gelatin capsule as opposed to a 74 percent absorption when given with an albumin carrier.

Depending on other factors, absorption has varied from 48 to 79 percent of the administered dose. Fasting increases absorption. Malabsorption syndromes, as well as dietary factors (children's soybean formula, concomitant use of anionic exchange resins such as cholestyramine) cause excessive fecal loss. T_3 is almost totally absorbed, 95 percent in 4 hours. The hormones contained in the natural preparations are absorbed in a manner similar to the synthetic hormones.

More than 99 percent of circulating hormones are bound to serum proteins, including thyroid-binding globulin (TBg), thyroid-binding prealbumin (TBPA), and albumin (TBa), whose capacities and affinities vary for the hormones. The higher affinity of levothyroxine (T_4) for both TBg and TBPA as compared to triiodothyronine (T_3) partially explains the higher serum levels and longer half-life of the former hormone. Both protein-bound hormones exist in reverse equilibrium with minute amounts of free hormone, the latter accounting for the metabolic activity.

Deiodination of levothyroxine (T_4) occurs at a number of sites, including liver, kidney, and other tissues. The conjugated hormone, in the form of glucuronide or sulfate, is found in the bile and gut where it may complete an enterohepatic circulation. Eighty-five percent of levothyroxine (T_4) metabolized daily is deiodinated.

INDICATIONS AND USAGE

Thyrolar® Tablets are indicated:
1. As replacement or supplemental therapy in patients with hypothyroidism of any etiology, except transient hypothyroidism during the recovery phase of subacute thyroiditis. This category includes cretinism, myxedema, and ordinary hypothyroidism in patients of any age (children, adults, the elderly), or state (including pregnancy); primary hypothyroidism resulting from functional deficiency, primary atrophy, partial or total absence of thyroid gland, or the effects of surgery, radiation, or drugs, with or without the presence of goiter; and secondary (pituitary), or tertiary (hypothalamic) hypothyroidism (See WARNINGS).
2. As pituitary TSH suppressants, in the treatment or prevention of various types of euthyroid goiters, including thyroid nodules, sub-acute or chronic lymphocytic thyroiditis (Hashimoto's), multinodular goiter, and in the management of thyroid cancer.
3. As diagnostic agents in suppression tests to differentiate suspected mild hyperthyroidism or thyroid gland autonomy.

CONTRAINDICATIONS

Thyroid hormone preparations are generally contraindicated in patients with diagnosed but as yet uncorrected adrenal cortical insufficiency, untreated thyrotoxicosis, and apparent hypersensitivity to any of their active or extraneous constituents. There is no well documented evidence from the literature, however, of true allergic or idiosyncratic reactions to thyroid hormone.

WARNINGS

> Drugs with thyroid hormone activity, alone or together with other therapeutic agents, have been used for the treatment of obesity. In euthyroid patients, doses within the range of daily hormonal requirements are ineffective for weight reduction. Larger doses may produce serious or even life-threatening manifestations of toxicity, particularly when given in association with sympathomimetic amines such as those used for their anorectic effects.

The use of thyroid hormones in the therapy of obesity, alone or combined with other drugs, is unjustified and has been shown to be ineffective. Neither is their use justified for the treatment of male or female infertility unless this condition is accompanied by hypothyroidism.

PRECAUTIONS

General—Thyroid hormones should be used with great caution in a number of circumstances where the integrity of the cardiovascular system, particularly the coronary arteries, is suspected. These include patients with angina pectoris or the elderly, in whom there is a greater likelihood of occult cardiac disease. In these patients therapy should be initiated with low doses, i.e., one tablet of Thyrolar® ¼ or Thyrolar® ½. When, in such patients, a euthyroid state can only be reached at the expense of an aggravation of the cardiovascular disease, thyroid hormone dosage should be reduced. Thyroid hormone therapy in patients with concomitant diabetes mellitus or diabetes insipidus or adrenal cortical insufficiency aggravates the intensity of their symptoms. Appropriate adjustments of the various therapeutic measures directed at these concomitant endocrine diseases are required. The therapy of myxedema coma requires simultaneous administration of glucocorticoids (See DOSAGE AND ADMINISTRATION).

Hypothyroidism decreases and hyperthyroidism increases the sensitivity to oral anticoagulants. Prothrombin time should be closely monitored in thyroid treated patients on oral anticoagulants and dosage of the latter agents adjusted on the basis of frequent prothrombin time determinations. In infants, excessive doses of thyroid hormone preparations may produce craniosynostosis.

Information for the Patient—Patients on thyroid hormone preparations and parents of children on thyroid therapy should be informed that:
1. Replacement therapy is to be taken essentially for life, with the exception of cases of transient hypothyroidism, usually associated with thyroiditis, and in those patients receiving a therapeutic trial of the drug.
2. They should immediately report during the course of therapy any signs or symptoms of thyroid hormone toxicity, e.g., chest pain, increased pulse rate, palpitations, excessive sweating, heat intolerance, nervousness, or any other unusual event.
3. In case of concomitant diabetes mellitus, the daily dosage of antidiabetic medication may need readjustment as thyroid hormone replacement is achieved. If thyroid medication is stopped, a downward readjustment of the dosage of insulin or oral hypoglycemic agent may be necessary to avoid hypoglycemia. At all times, close monitoring of urinary glucose levels is mandatory in such patients.
4. In case of concomitant oral anticoagulant therapy, the prothrombin time should be measured frequently to determine if the dosage of oral anticoagulants is to be readjusted.
5. Partial loss of hair may be experienced by children in the first few months of thyroid therapy, but this is usually a transient phenomenon and later recovery is usually the rule.

Laboratory Tests—Treatment of patients with thyroid hormones requires the periodic assessment of thyroid status by means of appropriate laboratory tests besides the full clinical evaluation. The TSH suppression test can be used to test the effectiveness of any thyroid preparation bearing in mind the relative insensitivity of the infant pituitary to the negative feedback effect of thyroid hormones. Serum T_4 levels can be used to test the effectiveness of all thyroid medications except T_3. When the total serum T_4 is low but TSH is normal, a test specific to assess unbound (free) T_4 levels is warranted. Specific measurements of T_4 and T_3 by competitive protein binding or radioimmunoassay are not influenced by blood levels of organic or inorganic iodine.

Drug Interactions—Oral Anticoagulants—Thyroid hormones appear to increase catabolism of vitamin K-dependent clotting factors. If oral anticoagulants are also being given, compensatory increases in clotting factor synthesis are impaired. Patients stabilized on oral anticoagulants who are found to require thyroid replacement therapy should be watched very closely when thyroid is started. If a patient is truly hypothyroid, it is likely that a reduction in anticoagulant dosage will be required. No special precautions appear to be necessary when oral anticoagulant therapy is begun in a patient already stabilized on maintenance thyroid replacement therapy.

Insulin or Oral Hypoglycemics—Initiating thyroid replacement therapy may cause increases in insulin or oral hypoglycemic requirements. The effects seen are poorly understood and depend upon a variety of factors such as dose and type of thyroid preparations and endocrine status of the patient. Patients receiving insulin or oral hypoglycemics should be closely watched during initiation of thyroid replacement therapy.

Cholestyramine or Colestipol—Cholestyramine or colestipol binds both T_4 and T_3 in the intestine, thus impairing absorption of these thyroid hormones. In vitro studies indicate that the binding is not readily removed. Therefore, four to five hours should elapse between administration of cholestyramine or colestipol and thyroid hormones.

Estrogen, Oral Contraceptives—Estrogens tend to increase serum thyroxine-binding globulin (TBg). In a patient with a nonfunctioning thyroid gland who is receiving thyroid replacement therapy, free levothyroxine may be decreased when estrogens are started, thus increasing thyroid requirements. However, if the patient's thyroid gland has sufficient function, the decreased free thyroxine will result in a compensatory increase in thyroxine output by the thyroid. Therefore, patients without a functioning thyroid gland who are on thyroid replacement therapy may need to increase their thyroid dose if estrogens or estrogen-containing oral contraceptives are given.

Drug/Laboratory Test Interactions—The following drugs or moieties are known to interfere with laboratory tests performed in patients on thyroid hormone therapy: androgens, corticosteroids, estrogens, oral contraceptives containing estrogens, iodine-containing preparations, and the numerous preparations containing salicylates.

1. Changes in TBg concentration should be taken into consideration in the interpretation of T_4 and T_3 values. In such cases, the unbound (free) hormone should be measured. Pregnancy, estrogens, and estrogen-containing oral contraceptives increase TBg concentrations. TBg may also be increased during infectious hepatitis. Decreases in TBg concentrations are observed in nephrosis, acromegaly, and after androgen or corticosteroid therapy. Familial hyper- or hypothyroxine-binding-globulinemias have been described. The incidence of TBg deficiency approximates 1 in 9,000. The binding of thyroxine by TBPA is inhibited by salicylates.

2. Medicinal or dietary iodine interferes with all *in vivo* tests of radio-iodine uptake, producing low uptakes which may not be relative of a true decrease in hormone synthesis.

3. The persistence of clinical and laboratory evidence of hypothyroidism in spite of adequate dosage replacement indicates either poor patient compliance, poor absorption, excessive fecal loss, or inactivity of the preparation. Intracellular resistance to thyroid hormone is quite rare.

Carcinogenesis, Mutagenesis, and Impairment of Fertility—A reportedly apparent association between prolonged thyroid therapy and breast cancer has not been confirmed and patients on thyroid for established indications should not discontinue therapy. No confirmatory long-term studies in animals have been performed to evaluate carcinogenic potential, mutagenicity, or impairment of fertility in either males or females.

Pregnancy-Category A—Thyroid hormones do not readily cross the placental barrier. The clinical experience to date does not indicate any adverse effect on fetuses when thyroid hormones are administered to pregnant women. On the basis of current knowledge, thyroid replacement therapy to hypothyroid women should not be discontinued during pregnancy.

Nursing Mothers—Minimal amounts of thyroid hormones are excreted in human milk. Thyroid is not associated with serious adverse reactions and does not have a known tumorigenic potential. However, caution should be exercised when thyroid is administered to a nursing woman.

Pediatric Use—Pregnant mothers provide little or no thyroid hormone to the fetus. The incidence of congenital hypothyroidism is relatively high (1:4000) and the hypothyroid fetus would not derive any benefit from the small amounts of hormone crossing the placental barrier. Routine determinations of serum (T_4) and/or TSH is strongly advised in neonates in view of the deleterious effects of thyroid deficiency on growth and development.

Treatment should be initiated immediately upon diagnosis, and maintained for life, unless transient hypothyroidism is suspected; in which case, therapy may be interrupted for 2 to 8 weeks after the age of 3 years to reassess the condition. Cessation of therapy is justified in patients who have maintained a normal TSH during those 2 to 8 weeks.

ADVERSE REACTIONS

Adverse reactions other than those indicative of hyperthyroidism because of therapeutic overdosage, either initially or during the maintenance period, are rare (See OVERDOSAGE).

OVERDOSAGE

Signs and Symptoms—Excessive doses of thyroid result in a hypermetabolic state resembling in every respect the condition of endogenous origin. The condition may be self-induced.

Treatment of Overdosage—Dosage should be reduced or therapy temporarily discontinued if signs and symptoms of overdosage appear.

Treatment may be reinstituted at a lower dosage. In normal individuals, normal hypothalamic-pituitary-thyroid axis function is restored in 6 to 8 weeks after thyroid suppression. Treatment of acute massive thyroid hormone overdosage is aimed at reducing gastrointestinal absorption of the drugs and counteracting central and peripheral effects, mainly those of increased sympathetic activity. Vomiting may be induced initially if further gastrointestinal absorption can reasonably be prevented and barring contraindications such as coma, convulsions, or loss of the gagging reflex. Treatment is symptomatic and supportive. Oxygen may be administered and ventilation maintained. Cardiac glycosides may be indicated if congestive heart failure develops. Measures to control fever, hypoglycemia, or fluid loss should be instituted if

needed. Antiadrenergic agents, particularly propranolol, have been used advantageously in the treatment of increased sympathetic activity. Propranolol may be administered intravenously at a dosage of 1 to 3 mg over a 10 minute period or orally, 80 to 160 mg/day, initially, especially when no contraindications exist for its use.

DOSAGE AND ADMINISTRATION

The dosage of Thyrolar® Tablets (Liotrix Tablets, USP) is determined by the indication and must in every case be individualized according to patient response and laboratory findings.

Thyroid hormones are given orally. In acute, emergency conditions, injectable sodium levothyroxine may be given intravenously when oral administration is not feasible or desirable, as in the treatment of myxedema coma, or during total parenteral nutrition. Intramuscular administration is not advisable because of reported poor absorption.

Hypothyroidism—Therapy is usually instituted using low doses with increments which depend on the cardiovascular status of the patient. The usual starting dose is one tablet of Thyrolar® ½ with increments of one tablet of Thyrolar® ¼ every 2 to 3 weeks. A lower starting dosage, one tablet of Thyrolar® ¼/day, is recommended in patients with long-standing myxedema, particularly if cardiovascular impairment is suspected, in which case extreme caution is recommended. The appearance of angina is an indication for a reduction in dosage. Most patients require one tablet of Thyrolar® 1 to one tablet of Thyrolar® 2 per day. Failure to respond to doses of one tablet of Thyrolar® 3 suggests lack of compliance or malabsorption. Maintenance dosages of one tablet of Thyrolar® 1 to one tablet of Thyrolar® 2 per day usually result in normal serum levothyroxine (T_4) and triiodothyronine (T_3) levels. Adequate therapy usually results in normal TSH and T_4 levels after 2 to 3 weeks of therapy. Readjustment of thyroid hormone dosage should be made within the first four weeks of therapy, after proper clinical and laboratory evaluations, including serum levels of T_4, bound and free, and TSH.

T_3 may be used in preference to levothyroxine (T_4) during radio-isotope scanning procedures, since induction of hypothyroidism in those cases is more abrupt and can be of shorter duration. It may also be preferred when impairment of peripheral conversion of T_4 and T_3 is suspected.

Myxedema Coma—Myxedema coma is usually precipitated in the hypothyroid patient of long-standing by intercurrent illness or drugs such as sedatives and anesthetics and should be considered a medical emergency. Therapy should be directed at the correction of electrolyte disturbances and possible infection besides the administration of thyroid hormones. Corticosteroids should be administered routinely. T_4 and T_3 may be administered via a nasogastric tube but the preferred route of administration of both hormones is intravenous. Sodium levothyroxine (T_4) is given at a starting dose of 400 mcg (100 mcg/ml) given rapidly, and is usually well tolerated, even in the elderly. This initial dose is followed by daily supplements of 100 to 200 mcg given IV. Normal T_4 levels are achieved in 24 hours followed in 3 days by threefold elevation of T_3. Oral therapy with thyroid hormone would be resumed as soon as the clinical situation has been stabilized and the patient is able to take oral medication.

Thyroid Cancer—Exogenous thyroid hormone may produce regression of metastases from follicular and papillary carcinoma of the thyroid and is used as ancillary therapy of these conditions with radioactive iodine. TSH should be suppressed to low or undetectable levels. Therefore, larger amounts of thyroid hormone than those used for replacement therapy are required. Medullary carcinoma of the thyroid is usually unresponsive to this therapy.

Thyroid Suppression Therapy—Administration of thyroid hormone in doses higher than those produced physiologically by the gland results in suppression of the production of endogenous hormone. This is the basis for the thyroid suppression test and is used as an aid in the diagnosis of patients with signs of mild hyperthyroidism in whom base line laboratory tests appear normal, or to demonstrate thyroid gland autonomy in patients with Grave's ophthalmopathy. [131]I uptake is determined before and after the administration of the exogenous hormone. A fifty percent or greater suppression of uptake indicates a normal thyroid-pituitary axis and thus rules out thyroid gland autonomy.

For adults, the usual suppressive dose of levothyroxine (T_4) is 1.56 mcg/kg of body weight per day given for 7 to 10 days. These doses usually yield normal serum T_4 and T_3 levels and lack of response to TSH.

Thyroid hormones should be administered cautiously to patients in whom there is strong suspicion of thyroid gland

autonomy, in view of the fact that the exogenous hormone effects will be additive to the endogenous source.

Pediatric Dosage—Pediatric dosage should follow the recommendations summarized in Table 1. In infants with congenital hypothyroidism, therapy with full doses should be instituted as soon as the diagnosis has been made.

Recommended Pediatric Dosage for
Congenital Hypothyroidism

Age	Dose per day in mcg		
	T_3/T_4	to	T_3/T_4
0–6 mos	3.1/12.5	to	6.25/25
6–12 mos	6.25/25	to	9.35/37.5
1–5 yrs	9.35/37.5	to	12.5/50
6–12 yrs	12.5/50	to	18.75/75
Over 12 yrs		over	18.75/75

Table 1

HOW SUPPLIED

Thyrolar® Tablets (Liotrix Tablets, USP) are available in five potencies, coded as follows:

[See table above.]

Name	Composition (T_3/T_4 per tablet)	Color	Armacode®
Thyrolar®—¼(0075–3900–06)	3.1 mcg/12.5 mcg	Violet/White	YC
Thyrolar®—½(0075–3905–06)	6.25 mcg/25 mcg	Peach/White	YD
Thyrolar®—1 (0075–3910–06)	12.5 mcg/50 mcg	Pink/White	YE
Thyrolar®—2 (0075–3915–06)	25 mcg/100 mcg	Green/White	YF
Thyrolar®—3 (0075–3920–06)	37.5 mcg/150 mcg	Yellow/White	YH

Supplied in bottles of 100, two-layered compressed tablets. Tablets should be stored at controlled room temperature, 59°–86°F (15°–30°C) in tight, light-resistant containers.

Note: (T_3) liothyronine sodium is approximately four times as potent as T_4 thyroxine on a microgram for microgram basis.)

CAUTION

Federal (U.S.A.) law prohibits dispensing without prescription.

Rev. 12/87

RORER PHARMACEUTICALS
a division of
RORER PHARMACEUTICAL CORPORATION
Fort Washington, PA, U.S.A. 19034

Shown in Product Identification Section, page 426

TUSSAR® DM   OTC

[tŭs 'är]

Cold/Cough Syrup
Non-narcotic, Alcohol Free
Antitussive/Nasal Decongestant/Antihistaminic

Each 5 mL (one teaspoonful) contains:
Dextromethorphan
  Hydrobromide, U.S.P. ....15 mg
Chlorpheniramine Maleate, U.S.P. ....2 mg
Pseudoephedrine Hydrochloride, U.S.P. ....30 mg
Inactive ingredients: artificial flavor, citric acid, F.D.&C. Red No. 40, glucose, glycerin, methylparaben, sodium citrate, sucrose and water.

INDICATIONS

For the temporary relief of cough due to common cold and minor throat and bronchial irritation. TUSSAR DM provides relief of nasal congestion, runny nose, and watery eyes as may occur in allergic rhinitis (such as hay fever).

DIRECTIONS FOR USE

ADULTS AND CHILDREN OVER 12 YEARS OF AGE—One or two teaspoonfuls (5 or 10 mL) every 6 to 8 hours, not to exceed eight teaspoonfuls in any 24-hour period.
CHILDREN 6–12 YEARS OF AGE—One teaspoonful (5 mL) every 6 to 8 hours, not to exceed four teaspoonfuls in any 24-hour period.
CHILDREN UNDER 6 YEARS OF AGE—Not to be administered unless directed by a doctor.

WARNINGS

A persistent cough may be a sign of a serious condition. If cough persists for more than one week, tends to recur, or is accompanied by fever, rash, or persistent headache, consult a doctor. Do not take this product for persistent and chronic cough such as occurs with smoking, asthma, or emphysema, unless directed by a doctor. If drowsiness, sleeplessness, nervousness, or dizziness occurs, do not drive a car or operate

Continued on next page

This product information was prepared in September, 1989. Information concerning these products may be obtained by addressing Rorer Pharmaceutical Corporation, 500 Virginia Drive, Fort Washington, PA 19034.

Rorer Pharm.—Cont.

machinery. May cause excitability, especially in children. Do not exceed recommended dosage. Do not take this product if you have heart disease, high blood pressure, thyroid disease, diabetes, or difficulty in urination. As with any drug, if you are pregnant or nursing a baby, seek the advice of a health professional before using this product.

Store at controlled room temperature between 15°–30°C (59°–86°F).

KEEP OUT OF THE REACH OF CHILDREN.

8/88

RORER PHARMACEUTICALS
a division of
RORER PHARMACEUTICAL CORPORATION
Fort Washington, PA, U.S.A. 19034

TUSSAR®-2　　　　　　　　　　　　　　　Ⓒ
[tŭs-är]
**(exempt narcotic cough
suppressant/antihistaminic/expectorant)**

Each 5 mL (one teaspoonful) contains:
Codeine Phosphate, U.S.P. ....10 mg
WARNING—MAY BE HABIT-FORMING.
Chlorpheniramine Maleate, U.S.P. ....2 mg
Guaifenesin, U.S.P. ....100 mg
Alcohol 6%
Inactive ingredients: artificial flavors, citric acid, D&C Yellow No. 10, FD&C Blue No. 1, glucose, methylparaben, methyl salicylate, propylene glycol, saccharin, sodium citrate, sucrose, water.

INDICATIONS

Tussar-2 temporarily relieves cough due to common cold and minor throat and bronchial irritation; provides temporary relief of nasal congestion, runny nose and watery eyes as may occur in allergic rhinitis (such as hay fever). The antitussive, codeine, calms the cough control center and relieves coughing. The expectorant, guaifenesin, increases the flow of natural secretions making a dry cough more productive.

WARNINGS

A persistent cough may be a sign of a serious condition. If cough persists for more than one week, tends to recur, or is accompanied by fever, rash, or persistent headache, consult a doctor. May cause or aggravate constipation. Do not take this product if you have a chronic pulmonary disease, shortness of breath, or excessive secretions, unless directed by a doctor. If drowsiness occurs, do not drive a car or operate machinery. Do not exceed recommended dosage. As with any drug, if you are pregnant or nursing a baby, seek the advice of a health professional before using this product.

DIRECTIONS FOR USE

Adults and children 12 years of age and over—One teaspoonful (5 mL) every 4 to 6 hours, not to exceed 6 teaspoonfuls in any 24-hour period. Not to be administered to infants or children under 12 unless directed by a doctor.

Store at controlled room temperature between 59°–86°F [15°–30°C].

1/89

RORER PHARMACEUTICALS
a division of
RORER PHARMACEUTICAL CORPORATION
Fort Washington, PA, U.S.A. 19034

TUSSAR® SF (Sugar Free)　　　　　　　　　Ⓒ
[tŭs-är]
**(exempt narcotic cough
suppressant/antihistaminic/expectorant)**

Formulation identical to Tussar®-2, except Tussar SF contains saccharin-sorbitol base and F.D.&C. Red No. 40 for patients who must limit sugar intake. Alcohol content 12 percent instead of 6 percent.

RORER PHARMACEUTICALS
a division of
RORER PHARMACEUTICAL CORPORATION
Fort Washington, PA, U.S.A. 19034

Products are cross-indexed by
generic and chemical names
in the
YELLOW SECTION

Ross Laboratories
COLUMBUS, OH 43216

ADVANCE®
[ad-vans ']
Nutritional Beverage With Iron
● **Concentrated Liquid**
● **Ready To Feed**

(See PDR For Nonprescription Drugs)

ALIMENTUM®
[al "ah-men 'tum]
**Protein Hydrolysate Formula
With Iron**
● **Ready To Feed**

(See PDR For Nonprescription Drugs)

CLEAR EYES®　　　　　　　　　　　　　OTC
[klēr īz]
Lubricating Eye Redness Reliever

DESCRIPTION

Clear Eyes is a sterile, isotonic buffered solution containing the active ingredients naphazoline hydrochloride (0.012%) and glycerin (0.2%) as well as boric acid, purified water and sodium borate. Edetate disodium 0.1% and benzalkonium chloride 0.01% are added as preservatives. (Contains vasoconstrictor.)

INDICATIONS

Clear Eyes is a decongestant ophthalmic solution specially designed for temporary relief of redness and drying due to minor eye irritation caused by dust, smoke, smog, sun glare, wearing contact lenses, colds, allergies, swimming, reading, driving, TV or close work. Clear Eyes contains laboratory tested and scientifically blended ingredients, including an effective vasoconstrictor which narrows swollen blood vessels and rapidly whitens reddened eyes in a formulation which produces a refreshing, soothing effect. Clear Eyes is a sterile, isotonic solution compatible with the natural fluids of the eye.

WARNINGS

To avoid contamination of this product, do not touch tip of container to any surface. Replace cap after using. If you experience eye pain, changes in vision, continued redness or irritation of the eye, or if the condition worsens or persists for more than 72 hours, discontinue use and consult a doctor. If you have glaucoma, do not use this product except under the advice and supervision of a doctor. Overuse of this product may produce increased redness of the eye. If solution changes color or becomes cloudy, do not use. REMOVE CONTACT LENSES BEFORE USING. KEEP THIS AND ALL DRUGS OUT OF THE REACH OF CHILDREN.

DOSAGE AND ADMINISTRATION

Instill 1 or 2 drops in the affected eye(s) up to four times daily.

HOW SUPPLIED

In 0.2-fl-oz, 0.5-fl-oz and 1.0-fl-oz plastic dropper bottles.
(FAN 2222-03)

EAR DROPS BY MURINE　　　　　　　　　OTC
See Murine Ear Wax Removal
System/Murine Ear Drops

ENRICH®
[en-rich ']
Liquid Nutrition with Fiber

USAGE

As a high-fiber liquid food providing complete, balanced nutrition, Enrich helps patients maintain normal bowel function. Enrich may be useful for patients with intolerance (ie, diarrhea or constipation) to low-residue feedings. Enrich can be used as a full liquid diet or liquid supplement. Enrich may be fed orally or by tube. Two cans daily provide at least one third of recommended daily fiber, vitamin, and protein intake for most patients.

DOSAGE AND ADMINISTRATION

Shake well. Enrich is ready to use and does not require dilution. Enrich may be stored unopened at room temperature. Once opened, any unused Enrich should be covered and refrigerated; discard if not used within 48 hours.
Oral Feeding: May be used for total nutrition, or with and between meals for added nutritional support. Enrich may be fed at room temperature or chilled.

Tube Feeding: Follow physician's instructions. Adjust flow rate, volume and dilution according to patient's condition and tolerance. Gavage feed at room temperature with a 10Fr or larger tube. Use a pump with smaller tubes. Additional fluid requirements should be met by giving water with or after feedings. Avoid contamination during preparation and use.

Enrich is not recommended for situations requiring a low-residue feeding.

Not for parenteral use.

AVAILABILITY

Ready To Use:
8-fl-oz cans; 4 six-packs per case; Vanilla, No. 759; Chocolate, No. 756.
32-fl-oz cans; 6 per case; Vanilla, No. 706.

COMPOSITION

Ready To Use Vanilla (Chocolate flavor has similar composition. For specific information, see product label.)

INGREDIENTS

Ⓓ-D Water, hydrolyzed cornstarch, sucrose, corn oil, sodium and calcium caseinates, soy fiber (a source of dietary fiber), soy protein isolate, natural and artificial flavor, potassium citrate, magnesium chloride, soy lecithin, calcium phosphate tribasic, sodium citrate, potassium chloride, choline chloride, ascorbic acid, zinc sulfate, ferrous sulfate, alpha-tocopheryl acetate, niacinamide, calcium pantothenate, manganese sulfate, thiamine chloride hydrochloride, pyridoxine hydrochloride, cupric sulfate, riboflavin, vitamin A palmitate, folic acid, biotin, potassium iodide, phylloquinone, cyanocobalamin and vitamin D_3.

Nutrients (Grams/8 fl oz): Protein, 9.4; Fat, 8.8; Carbohydrate, 38.3†; Water, 196. Calories per fl oz, 32.5; Calories per mL, 1.1.

† Includes 5 g soy fiber (a source of dietary fiber that provides 10 Calories and 3.4 g total dietary fiber).
(FAN 574-03)

ENSURE®
[en-shur ']
Liquid Nutrition

USAGE

For complete, balanced nutrition. Ensure can be used as a full liquid diet or liquid supplement. Ensure may be fed orally or by tube (nasogastric, nasoduodenal, jejunal). Ensure is useful whenever the patient's medical, surgical or psychological state precludes normal food intake and/or leads to inadequate nutrition. Two quarts (2000 Calories) of Ensure meets or surpasses 100% of the U.S. RDA for vitamins and minerals for adults and children 4 or more years of age.

DOSAGE AND ADMINISTRATION

Ready To Use
Shake well. May be stored unopened at room temperature. Once opened, Ensure should be covered and refrigerated; discard if not used within 48 hours. Ensure may be fed at room temperature or chilled.
Powder: To prepare an 8-fl-oz glassful; put ¾ cup of cold water in a glass. Gradually stir in ½ cup Ensure Powder and mix until dissolved. Reconstituted Ensure should be used promptly or be covered, refrigerated and used within 24 hours. Opened can should be covered with overcap and stored in a cool, dry place, but not refrigerated. Once opened, use contents within 3 weeks.
Oral Feeding: May be used for total nutrition, or with and between meals.
Tube Feeding: Follow physician's instructions. Adjust flow rate, volume and dilution according to patient's condition and tolerance. Additional fluid requirements should be met by giving water with or after feedings. Avoid contamination during preparation and use.
Not for parenteral use.

AVAILABILITY

Ready To Use:
8-fl-oz bottles; 24 per case; Vanilla, No. 708.
8-fl-oz cans; 4 six-packs per case; Chocolate, No. 701; Black Walnut, No. 703; Coffee, No. 704; Strawberry, No. 705; Eggnog, No. 710; Vanilla, No. 711.
32-fl-oz cans; 6 per case; Vanilla, No. 733; Chocolate, No. 799.
Powder:
14-oz (400 g) cans; 6 per case; Vanilla, No. 750.

COMPOSITION

Ready To Use Vanilla (Other flavors and Vanilla Powder at standard dilution have similar composition and nutrient values. For specific information, see product labels.)

INGREDIENTS

Ⓓ-D Water, corn syrup, sucrose, corn oil, sodium and calcium caseinates, soy protein isolate, potassium citrate, magnesium chloride, soy lecithin, calcium phosphate tribasic, sodium citrate, natural and artificial flavor, potassium chloride, ascorbic acid, choline chloride, carrageenan, zinc sul-

fate, ferrous sulfate, alpha-tocopheryl acetate, niacinamide, calcium pantothenate, manganese sulfate, thiamine chloride hydrochloride, pyridoxine hydrochloride, riboflavin, cupric sulfate, vitamin A palmitate, folic acid, biotin, potassium iodide, phylloquinone and vitamin D_3.
Nutrients (Grams/8 fl oz): Protein, 8.8; Fat, 8.8; Carbohydrate, 34.3; Water, 200. Calories per mL, 1.06; Calories per fl oz, 31.3.
(FAN 574-03)

ENSURE® HN
[en-shur´]
High Nitrogen Liquid Nutrition

USAGE
As an all-purpose, high-nitrogen, low-residue liquid food, Ensure HN provides complete, balanced nutritional support for patients with decreased energy requirements or for those with increased protein needs. Ensure HN can be used as a full liquid diet or liquid supplement. Ensure HN may be fed orally or by tube.

DOSAGE AND ADMINISTRATION
Shake well. May be stored unopened at room temperature. Once opened, Ensure HN should be covered and refrigerated; discard if not used within 48 hours. Ensure HN may be fed at room temperature or chilled.
Oral Feeding: May be used for total nutrition, or with and between meals.
Tube Feeding: Follow physician's instructions. Adjust flow rate, volume and dilution according to patient's condition and tolerance. Additional fluid requirements should be met by giving water with or after feedings. Avoid contamination during preparation and use.
Not for parenteral use.

AVAILABILITY
Ready To Use:
8-fl-oz cans; 4 six-packs per case; Chocolate, No. 712; Vanilla, No. 719.
32-fl-oz cans; 6 per case; Vanilla, No. 732.

COMPOSITION
Ready To Use Vanilla (Chocolate flavor has similar composition. For specific information, see product label.)

INGREDIENTS
Ⓤ-D Water, corn syrup, sodium and calcium caseinates, sucrose, corn oil, soy protein isolate, potassium citrate, magnesium chloride, calcium phosphate tribasic, soy lecithin, natural and artificial flavor, sodium citrate, choline chloride, ascorbic acid, potassium phosphate dibasic, potassium chloride, carrageenan, zinc sulfate, ferrous sulfate, alpha-tocopheryl acetate, niacinamide, calcium pantothenate, manganese sulfate, thiamine chloride hydrochloride, pyridoxine hydrochloride, cupric sulfate, riboflavin, vitamin A palmitate, folic acid, biotin, potassium iodide, phylloquinone, cyanocobalamin and vitamin D_3.
Nutrients (Grams/8 fl oz): Protein, 10.5; Fat, 8.4; Carbohydrate, 33.4; Water, 199. Calories per mL, 1.06; Calories per fl oz, 31.3.
(FAN 574-03)

ENSURE PLUS®
[en-shur´]
High Calorie Liquid Nutrition

USAGE
As a high-calorie liquid food providing complete, balanced nutrition. Caloric density is 1500 Calories per liter, 50% more than that of most other liquid feedings. Ensure Plus is intended for use when extra calories and correspondingly higher concentrations of protein and most other nutrients are needed to achieve a required calorie intake in a limited volume. When used to provide total nutrition, Ensure Plus can deliver the high-calorie intakes required by patients who are nutritionally depleted, and who may not be able to tolerate large-volume intakes. As a dietary supplement, Ensure Plus can supply extra calories and protein for those patients unable to consume adequate nutrition.

DOSAGE AND ADMINISTRATION
Shake well. May be stored unopened at room temperature. Once opened, Ensure Plus should be covered and refrigerated; discard if not used within 48 hours. Ensure Plus may be fed at room temperature or chilled.
Oral Feeding: May be used for total nutrition, or with and between meals.
Tube Feeding: Follow physician's instructions. Adjust flow rate, volume and dilution according to patient's condition and tolerance. Additional fluid requirements should be met by giving water with or after feedings. Avoid contamination during preparation and use.

Not for parenteral use.

AVAILABILITY
8-fl-oz bottles; 24 per case; Vanilla, No. 741.
8-fl-oz cans; 4 six-packs per case; Chocolate, No. 702; Vanilla, No. 707; Eggnog, No. 716; Coffee, No. 717; Strawberry, No. 718.
32-fl-oz cans; 6 per case; Vanilla, No.688; Chocolate, No. 698.

COMPOSITION
Ready To Use Vanilla (Other flavors have similar composition. For specific information, see product labels.)

INGREDIENTS
Ⓤ-D Water, corn syrup, corn oil, sodium and calcium caseinates, sucrose, soy protein isolate, magnesium chloride, potassium citrate, calcium phosphate tribasic, soy lecithin, natural and artificial flavor, sodium citrate, potassium chloride, choline chloride, ascorbic acid, zinc sulfate, ferrous sulfate, alpha-tocopheryl acetate, carrageenan, niacinamide, calcium pantothenate, manganese sulfate, thiamine chloride hydrochloride, pyridoxine hydrochloride, riboflavin, cupric sulfate, vitamin A palmitate, folic acid, biotin, potassium iodide, phylloquinone, cyanocobalamin and vitamin D_3.
Nutrients (Grams/8 fl oz): Protein, 13.0; Fat, 12.6; Carbohydrate, 47.3; Water, 182. Calories per mL, 1.5; Calories per fl oz, 44.4.
(FAN 574-03)

ENSURE PLUS® HN
[en-shur´]
High Calorie, High Nitrogen Liquid Nutrition

USAGE
As a high-calorie, high-nitrogen liquid food, Ensure Plus HN provides complete, balanced nutrition. It is most appropriate for patients with increased calorie and protein needs, or for those patients whose volume intake is limited. Ensure Plus HN can be used as a full liquid diet or liquid supplement. Ensure Plus HN may be fed orally or by tube (nasogastric or nasoduodenal).

DOSAGE AND ADMINISTRATION
Ready To Use: Shake well. May be stored unopened at room temperature. Once opened, Ensure Plus HN should be covered and refrigerated; discard if not used within 48 hours. Ensure Plus HN may be fed at room temperature or chilled.
Ready-To-Hang Enteral Feeding Container: ENTIRE FEEDING MUST BE USED WITHIN 24 HOURS AFTER FOIL IS BROKEN. DO NOT remove protective cap until ready to attach feeding set. THOROUGHLY wash hands with soap and water before handling container or feeding set. Turn container upside down and SHAKE VIGOROUSLY, using a twisting motion. DO NOT touch any part of container or feeding set that comes in contact with the formula. Remove protective cap from container and discard, taking special care NOT to touch foil cover. Swab foil cover with alcohol prior to use. Attach feeding set as instructed on package insert.
Oral Feeding: May be used for total nutrition, or with and between meals.
Tube Feeding: Follow physician's instructions. Adjust flow rate, volume and dilution according to patient's condition and tolerance. Additional fluid requirements should be met by giving water with or after feedings. Avoid contamination during preparation and use.
Not for parenteral use.

AVAILABILITY
Ready To Use:
8-fl-oz cans; 4 six-packs per case; Vanilla, No. 721; Chocolate, No. 631.
1-liter Ross Ready-To-Hang® Enteral Feeding Containers; 8 per case; No. 681.

COMPOSITION
Ready To Use Vanilla (Chocolate flavor has similar composition. For specific information, see product label.)

INGREDIENTS
Ⓤ-D Water, hydrolyzed cornstarch, sodium and calcium caseinates, corn oil, sucrose, minerals (magnesium chloride, potassium citrate, calcium phosphate tribasic, sodium citrate, zinc sulfate, ferrous sulfate, manganese sulfate, cupric sulfate, potassium iodide), soy protein isolate, soy lecithin, vitamins (choline chloride, ascorbic acid, alpha-tocopheryl acetate, niacinamide, calcium pantothenate, thiamine chloride hydrochloride, pyridoxine hydrochloride, riboflavin, vitamin A palmitate, folic acid, biotin, phylloquinone, cyanocobalamin, vitamin D_3), natural and artificial flavor, and carrageenan.
Nutrients (Grams/8 fl oz): Protein, 14.8; Fat, 11.8; Carbohydrate, 47.3; Water, 182. Calories per mL, 1.5; Calories per fl oz, 44.4.
(FAN 446-03)

ENSURE® PUDDING
[en-shur´]

USAGE
To provide balanced nutrition in a delicious, easy-to-eat form. Ensure Pudding is appropriate for any patient who is able to eat semisolid or solid food. It may be particularly useful for patients with impaired swallowing. Each 5-oz serving provides at least 17% of the U.S. RDA for vitamins and minerals for adults and children 4 or more years of age. Suitable for puréed, mechanical soft and soft diets.

AVAILABILITY
Ready To Eat: 5-oz cans; 12 four-packs per case; Chocolate, No. 790; Vanilla, No. 792; Tapioca, No. 794; Butterscotch, No. 798.

COMPOSITION
Vanilla (Other flavors have similar composition. For specific information, see product packaging.)

INGREDIENTS
K DAIRY Nonfat milk, water, sucrose, partially hydrogenated soybean oil, modified food starch, magnesium sulfate, sodium stearoyl lactylate, sodium phosphate dibasic, artificial flavor, ascorbic acid, zinc sulfate, alpha-tocopheryl acetate, choline chloride, ferrous sulfate, calcium pantothenate, artificial colors (including FD&C yellow no. 5 and FD&C yellow no. 6), manganese sulfate, cupric sulfate, vitamin A palmitate, thiamine chloride hydrochloride, pyridoxine hydrochloride, riboflavin, folic acid, biotin, phylloquinone, vitamin D_3 and cyanocobalamin.
Nutrients Per 5-oz Serving: Protein, 6.8 g; Fat, 9.7 g; Carbohydrate, 34.0 g; Minerals (Ash), 0.6 g; Water, 91 g. Calories per serving, 250.
(FAN 574-02)

GLUCERNA®
[glu-ser´nah]
Specialized Nutrition with Fiber
for Patients with Abnormal Glucose
Tolerance

USAGE
As a high-fiber, low-carbohydrate, enteral formula providing complete nutrition for patients with abnormal glucose tolerance. Glucerna has a unique formulation designed to maintain or improve nutritional status, yet enhance blood glucose control. Glucerna can be used as a tube feeding or oral supplement in persons with type I or type II diabetes mellitus or stress-induced hyperglycemia.

DOSAGE AND ADMINISTRATION
Shake well. May be stored unopened at room temperature. Once opened, Glucerna should be covered and refrigerated; discard if not used within 48 hours.
Oral Feeding: Glucerna may be fed at room temperature or chilled.
Tube Feeding: Follow physician's instructions. Adjust flow rate, volume and dilution according to patient's condition and tolerance. Gavage feed at room temperature with a 10Fr or larger tube. Use a pump with smaller tubes. Additional fluid requirements should be met by giving water with or after feedings. Avoid contamination during preparation and use.
Not for parenteral use.

AVAILABILITY
Ready To Use:
8-fl-oz cans; 4 six-packs per case; Vanilla, No. 50240.

INGREDIENTS
Ⓤ-D Water, hydrolyzed cornstarch, hi-oleic safflower oil, sodium caseinate, soy fiber, fructose, sodium calcium caseinate, soy oil, soy lecithin, magnesium chloride, calcium phosphate tribasic, sodium citrate, natural and artificial flavors, potassium chloride, m-inositol, potassium citrate, choline chloride, potassium phosphate dibasic, ascorbic acid, L-carnitine, taurine, zinc sulfate, ferrous sulfate, alpha-tocopheryl acetate, niacinamide, calcium pantothenate, manganese sulfate, thiamine chloride hydrochloride, pyridoxine hydrochloride, cupric sulfate, riboflavin, vitamin A palmitate, folic acid, sodium molybdate, biotin, chromium chloride, sodium selenite, potassium iodide, phylloquinone, cyanocobalamin and vitamin D_3.
Nutrients (Grams/8 fl oz): Protein, 9.9; Fat, 13.2; Carbohydrate, 22.2*; L-carnitine, 0.034; Taurine, 0.025; m-Inositol, 0.20; Water, 207. Calories per mL, 1.0; Calories per fl oz, 29.6.
*Includes soy fiber (a source of dietary fiber that provides 10 Calories and 3.4 g total dietary fiber).
(FAN 562-01)

Continued on next page

Ross—Cont.

INTROLITE™
[in 'trah-līt]
Transitional Liquid Nutrition

USAGE
As a fortified, half-calorie liquid food for introductory tube feeding. Introlite may also be used as a source of hydration when used as an adjunct to a full-strength enteral formula. 1000-mL container is prefilled for one-step preparation of tube feeding.

DOSAGE AND ADMINISTRATION
Ready-To-Hang Enteral Feeding Container:
ENTIRE FEEDING MUST BE USED WITHIN 24 HOURS AFTER FOIL IS BROKEN. DO NOT remove protective cap until ready to attach feeding set. THOROUGHLY wash hands with soap and water before handling container or feeding set. Turn container upside down and SHAKE VIGOROUSLY, using a twisting motion. DO NOT touch any part of container or feeding set that comes in contact with the formula. Remove protective cap from container and discard, taking special care NOT to touch foil cover. Swab foil cover with alcohol prior to use. Attach feeding set as instructed on package insert.
Tube Feeding: Follow physician's instructions. Adjust flow rate and volume according to patient's condition and tolerance. Additional fluid requirements should be met by giving water between or after feedings. Avoid contamination during preparation and use.
Not for parenteral use.

AVAILABILITY
Ready To Use:
1-liter Ross Ready-To-Hang® Enteral Feeding Containers; 8 per case; No. 669.

INGREDIENTS
Ⓤ-D Water, hydrolyzed cornstarch, sodium and calcium caseinates, minerals (sodium citrate, calcium phosphate tribasic, magnesium chloride, potassium phosphate dibasic, potassium citrate, magnesium sulfate, potassium chloride, zinc sulfate, ferrous sulfate, manganese sulfate, cupric sulfate, potassium iodide), medium-chain triglycerides (fractionated coconut oil), corn oil, soy protein isolate, soy oil, vitamins (ascorbic acid, choline chloride, alpha-tocopheryl acetate, niacinamide, calcium pantothenate, thiamine chloride hydrochloride, pyridoxine hydrochloride, riboflavin, vitamin A palmitate, folic acid, biotin, phylloquinone, cyanocobalamin, and vitamin D₃), carrageenan and soy lecithin.
Nutrients (Grams/liter): Protein, 22.2; Fat, 18.4; Carbohydrate, 70.5; Water, 920. Calories per mL, 0.53.
(FAN 551-01)

ISOMIL®
[ī'sō-mil]
Soy Protein Formula With Iron
- **Powder**
- **Concentrated Liquid**
- **Ready To Feed**

(See PDR For Nonprescription Drugs)

ISOMIL® SF
[ī'sō-mil]
Sucrose-Free Soy Protein Formula With Iron
- **Concentrated Liquid**
- **Ready To Feed**

(See PDR For Nonprescription Drugs)

JEVITY®
[jev 'ə-tē "]
Isotonic Liquid Nutrition with Fiber

USAGE
As a fiber-containing, isotonic, high-nitrogen, nutritionally complete liquid food for tube feeding. The fiber source and fiber level in Jevity help patients maintain normal bowel function and may be useful in the dietary management of tube-feeding bowel patterns such as diarrhea and constipation. The high-nitrogen and concentrated vitamin/mineral content of Jevity makes it ideal for tube feeders whose caloric intake is not high.
The ultra-trace minerals chromium, selenium and molybdenum and the conditionally essential nutrients carnitine and taurine have been added in amounts comparable to those in a typical diet.

DOSAGE AND ADMINISTRATION
Ready To Use:
Shake well. May be stored unopened at room temperature. Once opened, Jevity should be covered and refrigerated; discard if not used within 48 hours.
Ready-To-Hang Enteral Feeding Container:
ENTIRE FEEDING MUST BE USED WITHIN 24 HOURS AFTER FOIL IS BROKEN. DO NOT remove protective cap until ready to attach feeding set. THOROUGHLY wash hands with soap and water before handling container or feeding set. Turn container upside down and SHAKE VIGOROUSLY, using a twisting motion. DO NOT touch any part of container or feeding set that comes in contact with the formula. Remove protective cap from container and discard, taking special care NOT to touch foil cover. Swab foil cover with alcohol prior to use. Attach feeding set as instructed on package insert.
Oral Feeding: May be used for total or supplemental nutrition. It may be fed at room temperature or chilled.
Tube Feeding: Follow physician's instructions. Adjust flow rate, volume and dilution according to patient's condition and tolerance. Gavage feed at room temperature with a 10 Fr or larger tube; use a pump with smaller tubes. Do not chill Jevity prior to feeding by tube, since chilling increases viscosity. Additional fluid requirements should be met by giving water with or after feedings or when flushing the tube. Avoid contamination during preparation and use.
Not for parenteral use.

AVAILABILITY
Ready To Use:
8-fl-oz cans; 4 six-packs per case; No. 143.
32-fl-oz cans; 6 per case; No. 50330.
1-liter Ross Ready-To-Hang® Enteral Feeding Containers; 8 per case; No. 682.

COMPOSITION
INGREDIENTS
Ⓤ-D Water, hydrolyzed cornstarch, sodium and calcium caseinates, soy fiber (a source of dietary fiber), medium-chain triglycerides (fractionated coconut oil), corn oil, soy oil, calcium phosphate tribasic, potassium citrate, magnesium chloride, soy lecithin, sodium citrate, potassium chloride, magnesium sulfate, choline chloride, ascorbic acid, taurine, L-carnitine, zinc sulfate, ferrous sulfate, alpha-tocopheryl acetate, niacinamide, calcium pantothenate, manganese sulfate, thiamine chloride hydrochloride, pyridoxine hydrochloride, cupric sulfate, riboflavin, vitamin A palmitate, folic acid, sodium molybdate, chromium chloride, biotin, potassium iodide, sodium selenite, phylloquinone, cyanocobalamin and vitamin D₃.
Nutrients (Grams/8 fl oz): Protein, 10.5; Fat, 8.7; Carbohydrate, 35.9*; L-carnitine, 0.027; Taurine, 0.027; Water, 197. Calories per mL, 1.06; Calories per fl oz, 31.3.
*Includes soy fiber (a source of dietary fiber that provides 10 Calories and 3.4 g total dietary fiber).
(FAN 574-02)

MURINE®   OTC
[mur 'ēn]
Eye Lubricant

DESCRIPTION
Murine Eye Lubricant is a sterile buffered solution containing the active ingredients 1.4% polyvinyl alcohol and 0.6% povidone. Also contains benzalkonium chloride, dextrose, disodium edetate, potassium chloride, purified water, sodium bicarbonate, sodium chloride, sodium citrate and sodium phosphate (mono- and dibasic).

INDICATIONS
Murine is a clear, buffered, sterile solution formulated to more closely match the natural fluid of the eye for gentle, soothing relief from minor eye irritation while moisturizing and preventing dryness. Use as desired to temporarily relieve minor eye irritation, dryness and burning due to dust, smoke, smog, sun glare, wearing contact lenses, colds, allergies, swimming, reading, driving, TV or close work.

WARNING
To avoid contamination of this product, do not touch tip of container to any other surface. Replace cap after using. If you experience eye pain, changes in vision, continued redness or irritation of the eye, or if the condition worsens or persists for more than 72 hours, discontinue use and consult a doctor. If solution changes color or becomes cloudy, do not use. REMOVE CONTACT LENSES BEFORE USING. KEEP THIS AND ALL DRUGS OUT OF THE REACH OF CHILDREN.

DOSAGE AND ADMINISTRATION
Instill 1 or 2 drops in the affected eye(s) as needed.

HOW SUPPLIED
In 0.2-fl-oz, 0.5-fl-oz and 1.0-fl-oz plastic dropper bottles.
(FAN 2202-04)

MURINE® PLUS   OTC
[mur 'ēn]
Lubricating Eye Redness Reliever

DESCRIPTION
Murine Plus is a sterile, non-staining buffered solution containing the active ingredients 1.4% polyvinyl alcohol, 0.6% povidone and 0.05% tetrahydrozoline hydrochloride. Also contains benzalkonium chloride, dextrose, disodium edetate, potassium chloride, purified water, sodium bicarbonate, sodium chloride, sodium citrate and sodium phosphate (mono- and dibasic).

INDICATIONS
Murine Plus is an isotonic, sterile, ophthalmic solution, formulated to more closely match the natural fluid of the eye. It contains demulcents for gentle, soothing relief from minor eye irritation as well as the sympathomimetic agent, tetrahydrozoline hydrochloride, which produces local vasoconstriction in the eye. Thus, the drug effectively narrows swollen blood vessels locally and provides symptomatic relief of edema and hyperemia of conjunctival tissues due to eye allergies, minor local irritations and conjunctivitis. Use up to 4 times daily, to remove redness due to minor eye irritation caused by dust, smoke, smog, sun glare, wearing contact lenses, colds, allergies, swimming, reading, driving, TV or close work. The effect of Murine Plus is prompt (apparent within minutes) and sustained.

WARNING
To avoid contamination of this product, do not touch tip of container to any surface. Replace cap after using. If you experience eye pain, changes in vision, continued redness or irritation of the eye, or if the condition worsens or persists for more than 72 hours, discontinue use and consult a doctor. If you have glaucoma, do not use this product except under the advice and supervision of a doctor. Overuse of this product may produce increased redness of the eye. If solution changes color or becomes cloudy, do not use. REMOVE CONTACT LENSES BEFORE USING. KEEP THIS AND ALL DRUGS OUT OF THE REACH OF CHILDREN.

DOSAGE AND ADMINISTRATION
Instill 1 or 2 drops in the affected eye(s) up to four times daily.

HOW SUPPLIED
In 0.5-fl-oz and 1.0-fl-oz plastic dropper bottles.
(FAN 2202-04)

MURINE® EAR WAX REMOVAL   OTC
SYSTEM/MURINE® EAR DROPS
[mur 'ēn]
Carbamide Peroxide Ear Wax Removal Aid

DESCRIPTION
Active Ingredient: Carbamide Peroxide 6.5%. Also Contains: Alcohol (6.3%), Glycerin, Polysorbate 20 and other ingredients. A 1.0 fl oz soft bulb ear washer is also included. The Murine Ear Wax Removal System is the only complete self-treatment system on the market for ear wax removal. Application of carbamide peroxide drops followed by warm water irrigation is an effective, medically recommended way to help loosen hardened ear wax.

ACTIONS
The carbamide peroxide formula in Murine Ear Drops is an aid in the removal of hardened cerumen from the ear canal. Anhydrous glycerin penetrates and softens wax while the release of oxygen from carbamide peroxide provides a mechanical action resulting in the loosening of the softened wax accumulation. It is usually necessary to remove the loosened wax by gently flushing the ear with warm water using the soft bulb ear syringe provided.

INDICATIONS
The Murine Ear Wax Removal System is indicated for occasional use as an aid to soften, loosen and remove excessive ear wax.

CAUTION
Do not use if you have ear drainage or discharge, ear pain, irritation, or rash in the ear or are dizzy; consult a doctor. Do not use if you have an injury or perforation (hole) of the eardrum or after ear surgery, unless directed by a doctor.
Do not use for more than 4 days; if excessive ear wax remains after use of this product, consult a doctor. Avoid contact with the eyes. Keep this and all medicines out of the reach of children.

DOSAGE AND ADMINISTRATION
FOR USE IN THE EAR ONLY. Adults and children over 12 years: Tilt head sideways and place 5 to 10 drops into ear. Tip of applicator should not enter ear canal. Keep drops in ear for several minutes by keeping head tilted or placing cotton in ear.

Use twice daily for up to 4 days if needed, or as directed by a doctor. Any wax remaining after treatment may be removed by gently flushing the ear with warm water, using a soft bulb ear syringe. Children under 12 years: Consult a doctor.

Used regularly, the Murine Ear Wax Removal System helps keep the ear canal free from blockage due to accumulated ear wax.

HOW SUPPLIED

The Murine Ear Wax Removal System contains 0.5-fl-oz drops and a 1.0-fl-oz soft bulb ear syringe.

Also available in 0.5-fl-oz drops only, Murine Ear Drops.
(FAN 2223)

OSMOLITE®

[oz 'mō-līt]
Isotonic Liquid Nutrition

USAGE

As an isotonic liquid food providing complete, balanced nutrition. Osmolite has been designed for patients particularly sensitive to hyperosmotic feedings. Osmolite may be used as a tube feeding (nasogastric, nasoduodenal or jejunal) or as an oral feeding. Two quarts (2000 Calories) of Osmolite meet or surpass 100% of the U.S. RDA for vitamins and minerals for adults and children 4 or more years of age.

DOSAGE AND ADMINISTRATION

Ready To Use in bottles and cans:
Shake well. May be stored unopened at room temperature. Once opened, Osmolite should be covered and refrigerated; discard if not used within 48 hours. Osmolite may be fed at room temperature or chilled.

Ready-To-Hang Enteral Feeding Container:
ENTIRE FEEDING MUST BE USED WITHIN 24 HOURS AFTER FOIL IS BROKEN. DO NOT remove protective cap until ready to attach feeding set. THOROUGHLY wash hands with soap and water before handling container or feeding set. Turn container upside down and SHAKE VIGOROUSLY, using a twisting motion. DO NOT touch any part of container or feeding set that comes in contact with the formula. Remove protective cap from container and discard, taking special care NOT to touch foil cover. Swab foil cover with alcohol prior to use. Attach feeding set as instructed on package insert.

Oral Feeding: May be used for total nutrition, or with and between meals.

Tube Feeding: Follow physician's instructions. Adjust flow rate, volume and dilution according to patient's condition and tolerance. Additional fluid requirements should be met by giving water with or after feedings. Avoid contamination during preparation and use.

Not for parenteral use.

AVAILABILITY

Ready To Use:
8-fl-oz bottles; 24 per case; No. 715.
8-fl-oz cans; 4 six-packs per case; No. 709.
32-fl-oz cans; 6 per case; No. 738.
1-liter Ross Ready-To-Hang® Enteral Feeding Containers; 8 per case; No. 50350.

COMPOSITION

INGREDIENTS

Ⓓ-D Water, hydrolyzed cornstarch, casein, medium-chain triglycerides (fractionated coconut oil), corn oil, soy protein isolate, soy oil, potassium citrate, soy lecithin, calcium phosphate tribasic, magnesium chloride, choline chloride, ascorbic acid, magnesium sulfate, carrageenan, sodium citrate, zinc sulfate, ferrous sulfate, alpha-tocopheryl acetate, niacinamide, calcium pantothenate, manganese sulfate, thiamine chloride hydrochloride, pyridoxine hydrochloride, riboflavin, cupric sulfate, vitamin A palmitate, folic acid, biotin, potassium iodide, phylloquinone, cyanocobalamin and vitamin D_3.

Nutrients (Grams/8 fl oz): Protein, 8.8; Fat, 9.1; Carbohydrate, 34.3; Water, 199. Calories per mL, 1.06; Calories per fl oz, 31.3.
(FAN 574-05)

OSMOLITE® HN

[oz 'mō-līt]
High Nitrogen Isotonic Liquid Nutrition

USAGE

As a high-nitrogen, isotonic liquid food providing complete, balanced nutrition. Osmolite HN was designed to meet the needs of tube-fed patients with decreased energy requirements, increased protein needs, with intolerance to hyperosmolar feedings or with fat maldigestion/malabsorption. Osmolite HN helps tube-fed patients get the vitamins, minerals and protein they need when their volume intake is low.

DOSAGE AND ADMINISTRATION

Ready To Use in bottles and cans:
Shake well. May be stored unopened at room temperature. Once opened, Osmolite HN should be covered and refrigerated; discard if not used within 48 hours. Osmolite HN may be fed at room temperature or chilled.

Ready-To-Hang Enteral Feeding Container:
ENTIRE FEEDING MUST BE USED WITHIN 24 HOURS AFTER FOIL IS BROKEN. DO NOT remove protective cap until ready to attach feeding set. THOROUGHLY wash hands with soap and water before handling container or feeding set. Turn container upside down and SHAKE VIGOROUSLY, using a twisting motion. DO NOT touch any part of container or feeding set that comes in contact with the formula. Remove protective cap from container and discard, taking special care NOT to touch foil cover. Swab foil cover with alcohol prior to use. Attach feeding set as instructed on package insert.

Oral Feeding: May be used for total nutrition, or with and between meals.

Tube Feeding: Follow physician's instructions. Adjust flow rate, volume and dilution according to patient's condition and tolerance. Additional fluid requirements should be met by giving water with or after feedings. Avoid contamination during preparation and use.

Not for parenteral use.

AVAILABILITY

Ready To Use:
8-fl-oz bottles; 24 per case; No. 736.
8-fl-oz cans; 4 six-packs per case; No. 735.
32-fl-oz cans; 6 per case; No. 739.
1-liter Ross Ready-To-Hang® Enteral Feeding Containers; 8 per case; No. 668.

COMPOSITION

INGREDIENTS

Ⓓ-D Water, hydrolyzed cornstarch, sodium and calcium caseinates, medium-chain triglycerides (fractionated coconut oil), corn oil, soy protein isolate, soy oil, potassium citrate, magnesium chloride, calcium phosphate tribasic, soy lecithin, sodium citrate, choline chloride, ascorbic acid, potassium chloride, potassium phosphate dibasic, carrageenan, zinc sulfate, ferrous sulfate, alpha-tocopheryl acetate, niacinamide, calcium pantothenate, manganese sulfate, thiamine chloride hydrochloride, pyridoxine hydrochloride, cupric sulfate, riboflavin, vitamin A palmitate, folic acid, biotin, potassium iodide, phylloquinone, cyanocobalamin and vitamin D_3.

Nutrients (Grams/8 fl oz): Protein, 10.5; Fat, 8.7; Carbohydrate, 33.4; Water, 199. Calories per mL, 1.06; Calories per fl oz, 31.3.
(FAN 574-05)

PEDIAFLOR® Drops   ℞

[pē 'dē-a-flor "]
Sodium Fluoride Oral Solution, USP

DESCRIPTION

One dropperful (1.0 mL) provides:
Fluoride ....0.5 mg
  (as sodium fluoride ....1.1mg)

Inactive Ingredients: Alcohol less than 0.5%, citric acid, methylparaben, propylparaben, sorbitol, water, artificial flavoring and other ingredients.

INDICATIONS AND USAGE

As an aid in the prevention of dental caries in infants and children.

CONTRAINDICATIONS

Should be used only where the fluoride content of the drinking water supply is known to be 0.7 parts per million or less.

PRECAUTIONS

The recommended dosage should not be exceeded since chronic overdosage of fluoride may result in mottling of tooth enamel and osseous changes.

OVERDOSAGE

In children, acute ingestion of 10 to 20 mg of sodium fluoride may cause excessive salivation and gastrointestinal disturbances; 500 mg may be fatal. Oral and/or intravenous fluids containing calcium may be indicated.

DOSAGE AND ADMINISTRATION

Daily dosage—under 2 years of age, one-half dropperful or less daily; 2 years of age, one dropperful daily; 3 years of age or older, two dropperfuls or less daily; or as directed by physician or dentist.

AVAILABILITY

50-mL bottles, calibrated dropper enclosed; ℞;NDC 0074-0101-50.

PEDIALYTE®

[pē 'dē-ah-līt "]
Oral Electrolyte Maintenance Solution

USAGE

For maintenance of water and electrolytes during mild or moderate diarrhea in infants and children; for maintenance of water and electrolytes following corrective parenteral therapy for severe diarrhea.

Features:

- Ready To Use—no mixing or dilution necessary.
- Balanced electrolytes to replace stool losses and provide maintenance requirements.
- Provides glucose to promote sodium and water absorption.
- Fruit-flavored form available to enhance compliance in older infants and children.
- Plastic quart bottles are resealable, easy to pour and easy to measure.
- No coloring added.
- Widely available in grocery, drug and convenience stores.

AVAILABILITY

32-fl-oz plastic bottles; 8 per case; Unflavored, No. 336—NDC 0074-6470-32; Fruit-flavored, No. 365—NDC 0074-6471-32. 8-fl-oz bottles; 4 six-packs per case; Unflavored, No. 160—NDC 0074-6470-08. For hospital use, Pedialyte is available in the Ross Hospital Formula System.

DOSAGE

See Administration Guide for maintenance of body water and electrolytes in mild or moderate diarrhea (Pedialyte Unflavored or Fruit-Flavored) and management of mild to moderate dehydration secondary to moderate to severe diarrhea (Rehydralyte® Oral Electrolyte Rehydration Solution).

Pedialyte (Unflavored or Fruit-Flavored) or Rehydralyte should be offered frequently in amounts tolerated. Total daily intake should be adjusted to meet individual needs, based on thirst and response to therapy. The suggested intakes for maintenance are based on water requirements for ordinary energy expenditure.[1] The suggested intakes for replacement are based on fluid losses of 5% or 10% of body weight, including maintenance requirement.
[See table on next page].

COMPOSITION

Unflavored Pedialyte (Fruit-Flavored Pedialyte has similar composition and nutrient value. For specific information, see product label.)

INGREDIENTS

(Pareve, Ⓓ) Water, dextrose, potassium citrate, sodium chloride and sodium citrate.

Provides:	Per 8 Fl Oz	Per Liter	Per 32 Fl Oz
Sodium (mEq)	10.6	45	42.4
Potassium (mEq)	4.7	20	18.8
Chloride (mEq)	8.3	35	33.2
Citrate (mEq)	7.1	30	28.4
Dextrose (g)	5.9	25	23.6
Calories	24	100	96

(FAN 387-01)

PEDIASURE®

[pē 'dē-ah-shur "]
Liquid Nutrition for Children

USAGE

As a nutritionally complete, balanced, isotonic liquid food especially designed for tube or oral feeding of children 1 to 6 years of age. May be used as the sole source of nutrition or as a supplement. PediaSure meets or exceeds 100% of the NAS-NRC RDAs for protein, vitamins and minerals for children 1 to 6 years of age in 1100 mL. Calcium/phosphorus ratio of 1.2:1 meets recommendations by the American Academy of Pediatrics Committee on Nutrition (AAP-CON) for growing children. Fortified with biotin, choline, inositol, taurine and L-carnitine.

DOSAGE AND ADMINISTRATION

Shake well. Do not add water for a 1 Cal/mL (30 Cal/fl oz) feeding. May be stored (unopened) and fed at room temperature. Once opened, unused PediaSure should be covered and refrigerated; discard if not used within 48 hours.

Oral Feeding: May be used for total nutritional support or as a supplemental feeding with and between meals. PediaSure is delicious when chilled.

Tube Feeding: Follow physician's instructions. When initiating feeding, adjust flow rate, volume and dilution according to patient's condition and tolerance. Avoid contamination during preparation and use. Additional fluid requirement should be met by giving water orally with or between feedings, or when flushing the feeding tube.

Continued

Ross—Cont.

Not for parenteral use.
Not intended for infants under 1 year of age unless specified by a physician.

AVAILABILITY
Ready To Use:
8-fl-oz cans; 4 six-packs per case; Vanilla, No. 373.

INGREDIENTS
Ⓤ-D Water, hydrolyzed cornstarch, sucrose, sodium caseinate, high oleic safflower oil, soy oil, fractionated coconut oil (medium-chain triglycerides), minerals (calcium phosphate tribasic, potassium citrate, magnesium chloride, potassium phosphate dibasic, potassium chloride, ferrous sulfate, zinc sulfate, manganese sulfate, cupric sulfate, potassium iodide), whey protein concentrate, natural and artifical flavor, vitamins (choline chloride, ascorbic acid, m-inositol, alpha-tocopheryl acetate, niacinamide, calcium pantothenate, thiamine chloride hydrochloride, pyridoxine hydrochloride, riboflavin, vitamin A palmitate, folic acid, biotin, phylloquinone, vitamin D₃, cyanocobalamin), mono- and diglycerides, soy lecithin, carrageenan, taurine and L-carnitine.

Nutrients (Grams/8 fl oz): Protein, 7.1; Fat, 11.8; Carbohydrate, 26; Water, 200. Calories per mL, 1.0; Calories per fl oz, 29.6.

(FAN 508-01)

PEDIAZOLE® ℞
[pē'dē-e-zōl″]
erythromycin ethylsuccinate
and sulfisoxazole acetyl for oral suspension

PRODUCT OVERVIEW
KEY FACTS
Pediazole Suspension provides a combination of erythromycin ethylsuccinate and sulfisoxazole acetyl in a convenient single prescription. This strawberry-banana flavored suspension provides 200 mg erythromycin activity and the equivalent of 600 mg of sulfisoxazole per teaspoonful (5 mL). Keep suspension refrigerated. Pediazole is available in 100 mL, 150 mL, 200 mL and 250 mL bottles.

MAJOR USES
Pediazole is indicated for the treatment of acute otitis media in children that is caused by susceptible strains of *Hemophilus influenzae* (including ampicillin-resistant strains).

SAFETY INFORMATION
Pediazole Suspension is contraindicated for patients with known hypersensitivity to erythromycin or sulfonamides. It is also contraindicated for use in infants less than 2 months of age and for women who are pregnant or nursing. Fatalities associated with the administration of sulfonamides have occurred due to severe reactions. Pediazole should be discontinued at the first appearance of skin rash or any sign of adverse reaction. Complete blood counts should be done frequently in patients receiving sulfonamide therapy.
Erythromycin therapy in patients receiving high doses of theophylline may be associated with an increase of serum theophylline levels and potential theophylline toxicity. Caution should be exercised in use of sulfonamide therapy in those patients with impaired renal or hepatic function, history of severe allergy or bronchial asthma, or a deficiency in the glucose-6-phosphate dehydrogenase. Adequate fluid intake must be maintained during Pediazole therapy.

PRESCRIBING INFORMATION

PEDIAZOLE® ℞
[pē'dē-e-zōl″]
erythromycin ethylsuccinate
and sulfisoxazole acetyl for oral suspension

DESCRIPTION
Pediazole is a combination of erythromycin ethylsuccinate, USP and sulfisoxazole acetyl, USP. When reconstituted with water as directed on the label, the granules form a white, strawberry-banana flavor suspension which provides 200 mg erythromycin activity and the equivalent of 600 mg of sulfisoxazole per teaspoonful (5 mL).
Erythromycin is produced by a strain of *Streptomyces erythraeus* and belongs to the macrolide group of antibiotics. It is basic and readily forms salts and esters. Erythromycin ethylsuccinate is an ester of erythromycin.
Sulfisoxazole acetyl or N¹-acetyl sulfisoxazole is an ester of sulfisoxazole. Chemically, sulfisoxazole is N¹-(3,4-dimethyl-5-isoxazolyl) sulfanilamide.
Inactive Ingredients: Citric acid, magnesium aluminum silicate, poloxamer, sodium carboxymethylcellulose, sodium citrate, sucrose, artificial flavoring and other ingredients.

ACTIONS
Clinical Pharmacology: Orally administered erythromycin ethylsuccinate suspension is reliably and readily absorbed and serum levels are comparable when administered to patients in either the fasting or non-fasting state. After absorption, erythromycin diffuses readily into most body fluids. In the presence of normal hepatic function, erythromycin is concentrated in the liver and excreted in the bile; the effect of hepatic dysfunction on excretion of erythromycin by the liver into the bile is not known. After oral administration, less than 5 percent of the activity of the administered dose can be recovered in the urine.
Erythromycin crosses the placental barrier but fetal plasma levels are generally low.
Sulfisoxazole acetyl is deacetylated by enzymatic hydrolysis in the gastrointestinal tract from which it is readily absorbed as sulfisoxazole. Sulfisoxazole exists in the blood primarily bound to serum proteins as well as conjugated and in the active or free form. Metabolic pathways include N⁴-acetylation and oxidation with approximately 80 percent of an administered dose being excreted by the kidney within 24 hours.
Serum half-life for total erythromycin and free sulfisoxazole is about 1.5 and 6 hours, respectively.
Microbiology: Pediazole has been formulated to contain sulfisoxazole for concomitant use with erythromycin. The mode of action of erythromycin is by inhibition of protein synthesis without affecting nucleic acid synthesis. Sulfonamides, including sulfisoxazole, possess bacteriostatic activity. This bacteriostatic agent acts by means of competitively inhibiting bacterial synthesis of folic acid (pteroylglutamic acid) from para-aminobenzoic acid. Resistance to erythromycin blood levels ordinarily achieved has been demonstrated by some strains of *Hemophilus influenzae*. Pediazole is usually active against *Hemophilus influenzae in vitro*, including ampicillin-resistant strains.
Quantitative methods that require measurements of zone diameters give the most precise estimates of antibiotic susceptibility. One such standardized procedure, the ASM-2 method published by the National Committee for Clinical Laboratory Standards (NCCLS), has been recommended for use with discs to test susceptibility to erythromycin and sulfisoxazole. Interpretation involves correlation of the diameters obtained in the disc test with Minimal Inhibitory Concentrations (MIC) values for erythromycin and sulfisoxazole. If the standardized ASM-2 procedure of disc susceptibility is used, a 15 mcg erythromycin disc should give a zone diameter of at least 18 mm when tested against an erythromycin-susceptible bacterial strain and a 250-300 mcg sulfisoxazole disc should give a zone diameter of at least 17 mm when tested against a sulfisoxazole-susceptible bacterial strain.
In vitro sulfonamide sensitivity tests are not always reliable because media containing excessive amounts of thymidine are capable of reversing the inhibitory effect of sulfonamides which may result in false resistant reports. The tests must be carefully coordinated with bacteriological and clinical responses. When the patient is already taking sulfonamides follow-up cultures should have aminobenzoic acid added to the isolation media but not to subsequent susceptibility test media.

INDICATION
For treatment of ACUTE OTITIS MEDIA in children that is caused by susceptible strains of *Hemophilus influenzae*.

CONTRAINDICATIONS
Known hypersensitivity to either erythromycin or sulfonamides.
Infants less than 2 months of age.
Pregnancy at term and during the nursing period, because sulfonamides pass into the placental circulation and are excreted in human breast milk and may cause kernicterus in the infant.

WARNINGS
FATALITIES ASSOCIATED WITH THE ADMINISTRATION OF SULFONAMIDES, ALTHOUGH RARE, HAVE OCCURRED DUE TO SEVERE REACTIONS INCLUDING STEVENS-JOHNSON SYNDROME, TOXIC EPIDERMAL NECROLYSIS, FULMINANT HEPATIC NECROSIS, AGRANULOCYTOSIS, APLASTIC ANEMIA, AND OTHER BLOOD DYSCRASIAS.
Clinical signs such as sore throat, fever, pallor, rash, purpura, or jaundice may be early indications of serious reactions.
PEDIAZOLE SHOULD BE DISCONTINUED AT THE FIRST APPEARANCE OF SKIN RASH OR ANY SIGN OF ADVERSE REACTION. In some instances a skin rash may be followed by a more severe reaction, such as Stevens-Johnson syndrome, toxic epidermal necrolysis, hepatic necrosis and serious blood disorders.
COMPLETE BLOOD COUNT SHOULD BE DONE FREQUENTLY IN PATIENTS RECEIVING SULFONAMIDES.
Usage in Pregnancy (SEE ALSO: CONTRAINDICATIONS): The safe use of erythromycin or sulfonamides in pregnancy has not been established. The teratogenic potential of most sulfonamides has not been thoroughly investigated in either animals or humans. However, a significant increase in the incidence of cleft palate and other bony abnormalities of offspring has been observed when certain sulfonamides of the short, intermediate and long-acting types were given to pregnant rats and mice at high oral doses (7 to 25 times the human therapeutic dose).
The frequency of renal complications is considerably lower in patients receiving the most soluble sulfonamides such as sulfisoxazole. Urinalysis with careful microscopic examina-

Pedialyte, Rehydralyte Administration Guide

For Infants and Young Children

Age	2 Weeks	3 Months	6 Months	9 Months	1	1½	2	2½ Years	3	3½	4
Approximate Weight²											
(lb)	7	13	17	20	23	25	28	30	32	35	38
(kg)	3.2	6.0	7.8	9.2	10.2	11.4	12.6	13.6	14.6	16.0	17.0
PEDIALYTE UNFLAVORED or FRUIT-FLAVORED fl oz/day for maintenance*	13 to 16	28 to 32	34 to 40	38 to 44	41 to 46	45 to 50	48 to 53	51 to 56	54 to 58	56 to 60	57 to 62
REHYDRALYTE fl oz/day for Replacement for 5% Dehydration (including maintenance)*	18 to 21	38 to 42	47 to 53	53 to 59	58 to 63	64 to 69	69 to 74	74 to 79	78 to 82	83 to 87	85 to 90
REHYDRALYTE fl oz/day for Replacement for 10% Dehydration (including maintenance)*	23 to 26	48 to 52	60 to 66	68 to 74	75 to 80	83 to 88	90 to 95	97 to 102	102 to 106	110 to 114	113 to 118

Administration Guide does not apply to infants less than 1 week of age. For children over 4 years, maintenance intakes may exceed 2 qt daily.

1. Extrapolated from Barness L: Nutrition and nutritional disorders, in Behrman RE, Vaughan VC III: *Nelson Textbook of Pediatrics*, ed 12. Philadelphia, WB Saunders Co, 1983, pp 136-138.
2. Weight based on the 50th percentile of weight for age of the National Center for Health Statistics (NCHS) reference data. Hamill PVV, Drizd TA, Johnson CL, et al: Physical growth: National Center for Health Statistics percentiles. *Am J Clin Nutr* 1979; 32:607-629.
   Fluid intakes do not take into account ongoing stool losses. Fluid loss in the stool should be replaced by consumption of an ⸱xtra amount of Pedialyte or Rehydralyte equal to stool losses in addition to the amounts given in this Administration ⸱uide.

tion should be obtained frequently in patients receiving sulfonamides.

PRECAUTIONS

Erythromycin is principally excreted by the liver. Caution should be exercised in administering the antibiotic to patients with impaired hepatic function. There have been reports of hepatic dysfunction, with or without jaundice occurring in patients receiving oral erythromycin products.

Recent data from studies of erythromycin reveal that its use in patients who are receiving high doses of theophylline may be associated with an increase of serum theophylline levels and potential theophylline toxicity. In case of theophylline toxicity and/or elevated serum theophylline levels, the dose of theophylline should be reduced while the patient is receiving concomitant erythromycin therapy.

Surgical procedures should be performed when indicated.

Sulfonamide therapy should be given with caution to patients with impaired renal or hepatic function and in those patients with a history of severe allergy or bronchial asthma. In the presence of a deficiency in the enzyme glucose-6-phosphate dehydrogenase, hemolysis may occur. This reaction is frequently dose-related. Adequate fluid intake must be maintained in order to prevent crystalluria and renal stone formation.

ADVERSE REACTIONS

The most frequent side effects of oral erythromycin preparations are gastrointestinal, such as abdominal cramping and discomfort, and are dose-related. Nausea, vomiting and diarrhea occur infrequently with usual oral doses. During prolonged or repeated therapy, there is a possibility of overgrowth of nonsusceptible bacteria or fungi. If such infections occur, the drug should be discontinued and appropriate therapy instituted. The overall incidence of these latter side effects reported for the combined administration of erythromycin and a sulfonamide is comparable to those observed in patients given erythromycin alone. Mild allergic reactions such as urticaria and other skin rashes have occurred. Serious allergic reactions, including anaphylaxis, have been reported with erythromycin.

There have been isolated reports of reversible hearing loss occurring chiefly in patients with renal insufficiency and in patients receiving high doses of erythromycin.

The following untoward effects have been associated with the use of sulfonamides:

Blood Dyscrasias: Agranulocytosis, aplastic anemia, thrombocytopenia, leukopenia, hemolytic anemia, purpura, hypoprothrombinemia and methemoglobinemia.

Allergic Reactions: Erythema multiforme (Stevens-Johnson syndrome), generalized skin eruptions, epidermal necrolysis, urticaria, serum sickness, pruritus, exfoliative dermatitis, anaphylactoid reactions, periorbital edema, conjunctival and scleral injection, photosensitization, arthralgia and allergic myocarditis.

Gastrointestinal Reactions: Nausea, emesis, abdominal pains, hepatitis, diarrhea, anorexia, pancreatitis and stomatitis.

CNS Reactions: Headache, peripheral neuritis, mental depression, convulsions, ataxia, hallucinations, tinnitus, vertigo and insomnia.

Miscellaneous Reactions: Drug fever, chills and toxic nephrosis with oliguria or anuria. Periarteritis nodosa and LE phenomenon have occurred.

The sulfonamides bear certain chemical similarities to some goitrogens, diuretics (acetazolamide and the thiazides) and oral hypoglycemic agents. Goiter production, diuresis and hypoglycemia have occurred rarely in patients receiving sulfonamides. Cross-sensitivity may exist with these agents. Rats appear to be especially susceptible to the goitrogenic effects of sulfonamides, and long-term administration has produced thyroid malignancies in the species.

DOSAGE AND ADMINISTRATION

PEDIAZOLE SHOULD NOT BE ADMINISTERED TO INFANTS UNDER 2 MONTHS OF AGE BECAUSE OF CONTRAINDICATIONS OF SYSTEMIC SULFONAMIDES IN THIS AGE GROUP.

For Acute Otitis Media in Children: The dose of Pediazole can be calculated based on the erythromycin component (50 mg/kg/day) or the sulfisoxazole component (150 mg/kg/day to a maximum of 6 g/day). Pediazole should be administered in equally divided doses four times a day for 10 days. Pediazole may be administered without regard to meals.

The following approximate dosage schedule is recommended for using Pediazole:

Children: Two months of age or older

Weight	Dose—every 6 hours
Less than 8 kg (18 lb)	Adjust dosage by body weight
8 kg (18 lb)	½ teaspoonful (2.5 mL)
16 kg (35 lb)	1 teaspoonful (5 mL)
24 kg (53 lb)	1½ teaspoonfuls (7.5 mL)
Over 45 kg (over 100 lb)	2 teaspoonfuls (10 mL)

HOW SUPPLIED

Pediazole Suspension is available for teaspoon dosage in 100-mL (**NDC** 0074-8030-13), 150-mL (**NDC** 0074-8030-43), 200-mL (**NDC** 0074-8030-53) and 250 mL (**NDC** 0074-8030-73) bottles, in the form of granules to be reconstituted with water. The suspension provides erythromycin ethylsuccinate equivalent to 200 mg erythromycin activity and sulfisoxazole acetyl equivalent to 600 mg sulfisoxazole per teaspoonful (5 mL).

(.9830)

POLYCOSE®

[*pol 'ē-kōs*]
Glucose Polymers

USAGE

As a source of calories (derived solely from carbohydrate) for persons with increased caloric needs or those unable to meet their caloric needs with their normal diet. Polycose is particularly useful in supplying carbohydrate calories for protein-, electrolyte- and fat-restricted diets.

DOSAGE AND ADMINISTRATION

Polycose may be added to tube-feeding formulas and most foods and beverages, or mixed in water, in amounts determined by taste, caloric requirement and tolerance. Small, frequent feedings are more desirable than large amounts given infrequently. Polycose may be used for extended periods with diets containing all other essential nutrients, or as an oral adjunct to intravenous administration of nutrients. Polycose is not a balanced diet and should not be used as a sole source of nutrition. Undiluted Polycose should not be fed without physician supervision.

Refrigerate dissolved Polycose Powder and opened Polycose Liquid and discard unused portion after 24 hours. Concentrated solutions become more viscous when cold; thus serving Polycose at room temperature is advised.

NOT FOR PARENTERAL USE.

Precaution (For Infant Use): Not to be fed undiluted. Use only as specifically directed by a physician.

AVAILABILITY

Powder: 12.3 oz (350g) cans; 6 per case; No. 746.
Liquid: (43% solution): 4.2-fl-oz bottles; 48 per case; No. 431.

COMPOSITION

Powder: (Pareve, Ⓤ) Glucose polymers derived from controlled hydrolysis of cornstarch.

Nutrients (per 100 grams):

Carbohydrate		94 g
Water		6 g
Calcium	Does not exceed	30 mg (1.5 mEq)
Sodium	Does not exceed	110 mg (4.8 mEq)
Potassium	Does not exceed	10 mg (0.3 mEq)
Chloride	Does not exceed	223 mg (6.3 mEq)
Phosphorus	Does not exceed	5 mg

Approximate Caloric Equivalents:

1 level teaspoonful (2 g) = 8 Calories; 1 level tablespoonful (6 g) = 23 Calories; ¼ cup (25 g) = 95 Calories; ⅓ cup (33 g) = 125 Calories; ½ cup (50 g) = 190 Calories; 1 cup (100 g) = 380 Calories.

(FAN 366-01)

COMPOSITION

Liquid: (Pareve, Ⓤ) Water and glucose polymers derived from controlled hydrolysis of cornstarch.

Nutrients (per 100 mL):

Carbohydrate		50 g
Water		70 g
Calcium	Does not exceed	20 mg (1.0 mEq)
Sodium	Does not exceed	70 mg (3.0 mEq)
Potassium	Does not exceed	6 mg (0.15 mEq)
Chloride	Does not exceed	140 mg (3.9 mEq)
Phosphorus	Does not exceed	3 mg

Approximate Caloric Equivalents:

1 mL = 2 Calories; 1 fl oz = 60 Calories; 100 mL = 200 Calories.

(FAN 366-01)

PRAMET® FA   ℞

[*pram 'et*]
**Vitamin/Mineral Prescription
for Expectant and
New Mothers**

DESCRIPTION

Each Pramet FA Filmtab® Film-Sealed oral tablet provides:

Vitamins

Vitamin A (as acetate, may contain palmitate) 1.2 mg	4000	I.U.
Vitamin D (cholecalciferol, 10 mcg)	400	I.U.
Vitamin C (ascorbic acid)	100	mg
Folic Acid	1	mg
Vitamin B₁ (thiamine mononitrate)	3	mg
Vitamin B₂ (riboflavin)	2	mg
Niacinamide	10	mg
Vitamin B₆ (pyridoxine hydrochloride)	5	mg
Vitamin B₁₂ (cyanocobalamin)	3	mcg
Pantothenic Acid (as calcium pantothenate)	0.92	mg
Minerals		
Calcium (as calcium carbonate)	250	mg
Iodine (as calcium iodate)	100	mcg
Elemental Iron* (300 mg ferrous sulfate USP)	60	mg
Copper (as cupric chloride)	0.15	mg

* In controlled-release form—Gradumet®

Inactive Ingredients: Cellulosic polymers, corn starch, DC Yellow No. 10, FDC Blue No. 1, magnesium stearate, methyl acrylate-methyl methacrylate copolymer, microcrystalline cellulose, polyethylene glycols, povidone, propylene glycol, talc, titanium dioxide and vanillin.

INDICATIONS AND USAGE

To help prevent vitamin and mineral deficiencies during and after pregnancy and for treatment of megaloblastic anemias. 1 mg of folic acid has been found to be effective therapy for megaloblastic anemias of pregnancy and lactation.

WARNING

Folic acid alone is improper therapy in the treatment of pernicious anemia and other megaloblastic anemias where vitamin B₁₂ is deficient.

PRECAUTION

Folic acid may mask the presence of pernicious anemia in that hematologic remission may occur while neurologic manifestations remain progressive.

ADVERSE REACTION

Allergic sensitization has been reported following both oral and parenteral administration of folic acid.

OVERDOSAGE

Acute overdosage of iron may cause nausea and vomiting and, in severe cases, cardiovascular collapse and death. The estimated lethal dose of orally ingested elemental iron is 300 mg per kg body weight. Serum iron and total iron-binding capacity may be used as guides for use of chelating agents such as deferoxamine.

DOSAGE AND ADMINISTRATION

One tablet daily, or as directed by physician.

HOW SUPPLIED

100-tablet bottles; ℞; **NDC** 0074-0147-01.

(.9830)

PRAMILET® FA   ℞

[*pram 'e-let*]
**Prenatal Vitamin/Mineral Preparation
With Folic Acid**

DESCRIPTION

Each Pramilet FA Filmtab® Film-Sealed oral tablet provides:

Vitamins

Vitamin A (as acetate, may contain palmitate) 1.2 mg	4000	I.U.
Vitamin D (cholecalciferol, 10 mcg)	400	I.U.
Vitamin C (as sodium ascorbate)	60	mg
Folic Acid	1	mg
Vitamin B₁ (thiamine mononitrate)	3	mg
Vitamin B₂ (riboflavin)	2	mg
Niacinamide	10	mg
Vitamin B₆ (pyridoxine hydrochloride)	3	mg
Vitamin B₁₂ (cyanocobalamin)	3	mcg
Calcium Pantothenate	1	mg
Minerals		
Calcium (as calcium carbonate)	250	mg
Iodine (as calcium iodate)	100	mcg
Elemental Iron (as ferrous fumarate)	40	mg
Magnesium (as magnesium oxide)	10	mg
Copper (as cupric chloride)	0.15	mg
Zinc (as zinc oxide)	0.085	mg

Inactive Ingredients: Carmine No. 40, cellulosic polymers, corn starch, crospovidone, FDC Blue No. 1, propylene glycol, magnesium stearate, povidone, sorbic acid, sorbitan monooleate, titanium dioxide, vanillin and other ingredients.

INDICATIONS AND USAGE

To help prevent vitamin and mineral deficiencies during and after pregnancy and for treatment of megaloblastic anemias.

Continued on next page

Ross—Cont.

1 mg of folic acid has been found to be effective therapy for megaloblastic anemias of pregnancy and lactation.

WARNING
Folic acid alone is improper therapy in the treatment of pernicious anemia and other megaloblastic anemias where vitamin B_{12} is deficient.

PRECAUTION
Folic acid may mask the presence of pernicious anemia in that hematologic remission may occur while neurologic manifestations remain progressive.

ADVERSE REACTION
Allergic sensitization has been reported following both oral and parenteral administration of folic acid.

OVERDOSAGE
Acute overdosage of iron may cause nausea and vomiting and, in severe cases, cardiovascular collapse and death. The estimated lethal dose of orally ingested elemental iron is 300 mg per kg body weight. Serum iron and total iron-binding capacity may be used as guides for use of chelating agents such as deferoxamine.

DOSAGE AND ADMINISTRATION
One tablet daily, or as directed by physician.

HOW SUPPLIED
100-tablet bottles; ℞ NDC 0074-0121-01.
(.6821)

PROMOD®
[prō'mod]
Protein Supplement

USAGE
For providing extra protein to individuals who have increased protein needs and those who are unable to meet their protein needs with a normal diet. ProMod may be added to an oral supplement, an enteral tube feeding or table foods. It may also be useful in controlling protein intake in protein-restricted diets when the protein level of regular food or enteral products is inappropriate.

DOSAGE AND ADMINISTRATION
Instructions for Use: Designed to be added to an enteral formula, food or beverage. Use the enclosed scoop or standard household measures to add the recommended amount of protein (see table). Opened can should be covered with overcap and stored in a cool, dry place but not refrigerated. Once opened, use contents within 1 month. After mixing, enteral nutritional products should be used promptly, or covered, refrigerated and used within 24 hours. When mixed with prepared foods, use promptly or store appropriately.
Mixing with Liquids: For best results, mix ProMod with a small amount of the liquid or water to make a smooth paste, then gradually add the remaining liquid to the mixture while stirring. For blender mixing, combine ProMod with the desired amount of liquid and briefly blend at the lowest speed to minimize foaming.
Mixing with Foods: ProMod may be mixed directly into prepared foods such as mashed potatoes, oatmeal, gravy or soup.
ProMod is not a balanced diet and should not be used as a sole source of nutrition. ProMod is for enteral use only and should be used as directed by a physician or other health care professional.
Not for parenteral use.

PRECAUTION (For Infant Use)
Use only as directed by a physician.
Availability:
Powder: 9.7 oz (275 g) cans; 6 per case; No. 775.
Composition:
Ingredients: Ⓤ-D Whey protein concentrate and soy lecithin.

Nutrients:		Per 5 g Protein (one scoop)	
Protein		5.0	g
Fat	Does not exceed	0.60	g
Carbohydrate	Does not exceed	0.67	g
Water		0.60	g
Calcium	Does not exceed	44	mg (2.20 mEq)
Sodium	Does not exceed	15	mg (0.65 mEq)
Potassium	Does not exceed	65	mg (1.66 mEq)
Phosphorus	Does not exceed	33	mg
Calories		28	

Approximate Protein Equivalents:

Amount of ProMod Protein Supplement	Amount of Protein
1 scoop (6.6 g)	5 g
1 level teaspoonful (1.3 g)	1 g
1 level tablespoonful (4.0 g)	3 g
¼ cup (16 g)	12 g
⅓ cup (22 g)	16 g
½ cup (32 g)	24 g
1 cup (64 g)	48 g

Typical Amino Acid Composition Per 100 g Protein*—
Essential Amino Acids: Histidine, 1.9 g; Isoleucine, 6.2 g; Leucine, 10.8 g; Lysine, 9.3 g; Methionine, 2.2 g; Phenylalanine, 3.6 g; Threonine, 7.3 g; Tryptophan, 1.9 g; Valine, 6.0 g.
Non-Essential Amino Acids:
Alanine, 5.3 g; Arginine, 2.6 g; Aspartic Acid, 11.2 g; Cystine, 2.6 g; Glutamic Acid, 18.2 g; Glycine, 2.1 g; Proline, 6.5 g; Serine, 5.6 g; Tyrosine, 3.4 g.
* 100 grams of ProMod protein yields approximately 105 grams of individual amino acids.
(FAN 534-02)

PULMOCARE®
[pul'mō-kār]
Specialized Nutrition for Pulmonary Patients

USAGE
For the dietary management of respiratory insufficiency, the high-fat and low-carbohydrate content of Pulmocare is designed to reduce carbon dioxide production. Pulmocare can be used for enteral tube feeding or for oral supplementation and is appropriate for ambulatory or ventilator-dependent patients.

DOSAGE AND ADMINISTRATION
Shake well. May be stored unopened at room temperature. Once opened, Pulmocare should be covered and refrigerated; discard if not used within 48 hours. Pulmocare may be fed at room temperature or chilled.
Oral Feeding: May be used as total or supplemental nutrition for patients on a low-carbohydrate diet.
Tube Feeding: Follow physician's instructions. Adjust flow rate, volume and dilution according to patient's condition and tolerance. Additional fluid requirements should be met by giving water with or after feedings. Avoid contamination during preparation and use.
Not for parenteral use.

AVAILABILITY
8-fl-oz cans; 4 six-packs per case; Vanilla, No. 699; Strawberry, No. 50180.

COMPOSITION
Ready To Use Vanilla.

INGREDIENTS
Ⓤ-D Water, corn oil, sodium and calcium caseinates, sucrose, hydrolyzed cornstarch, magnesium chloride, soy lecithin, calcium phosphate tribasic, potassium citrate, sodium citrate, natural and artificial flavor, potassium phosphate dibasic, choline chloride, ascorbic acid, sodium chloride, zinc sulfate, ferrous sulfate, alpha-tocopheryl acetate, niacinamide, carrageenan, calcium pantothenate, cupric sulfate, thiamine chloride hydrochloride, pyridoxine hydrochloride, riboflavin, manganese sulfate, vitamin A palmitate, folic acid, biotin, potassium iodide, phylloquinone, cyanocobalamin and vitamin D_3.
Nutrients (Grams/8 fl oz): Protein, 14.8; Fat, 21.8; Carbohydrate, 25.0; Water, 186. Calories per mL, 1.5; Calories per fl oz, 44.4.
(FAN 574-03)

REHYDRALYTE®
[rē-hī'drə-līt]
Oral Electrolyte Rehydration Solution

USAGE
For replacement of water and electrolytes lost during moderate to severe diarrhea.
Features:
- Ready To Use—no mixing or dilution necessary.
- Safe, economical alternative to IV therapy.
- 75 mEq of sodium per liter for effective replacement of fluid deficits.
- 2½% glucose solution to promote sodium and water absorption and provide energy.
- Widely available in pharmacies.

AVAILABILITY
8-fl-oz bottles; 4 six-packs per case; No. 162; NDC 0074-0162-01.

DOSAGE
(See Administration Guide under Pedialyte)

INGREDIENTS
(Pareve, Ⓤ) Water, dextrose, sodium chloride, potassium citrate and sodium citrate.

Provides:	Per 8 Fl Oz	Per Liter
Sodium (mEq)	17.7	75
Potassium (mEq)	4.7	20
Chloride (mEq)	15.4	65
Citrate (mEq)	7.1	30
Dextrose (g)	5.9	25
Calories	24	100

(FAN 437-01)

RONDEC® Oral Drops   ℞
[ron'dek]
RONDEC® Syrup   ℞
RONDEC® Tablet   ℞
RONDEC–TR® Tablet   ℞

PRODUCT OVERVIEW
KEY FACTS
Rondec products contain the antihistamine carbinoxamine maleate and the decongestant pseudoephedrine hydrochloride. Rondec Oral Drops, Rondec Syrup, Rondec Tablets are immediate release dosage forms. Rondec-TR Tablet uses a gradual release mechanism allowing twice daily dosing.

MAJOR USES
Rondec products provide symptomatic relief of seasonal and perennial allergic rhinitis and vasomotor rhinitis.

SAFETY INFORMATION
Use with caution in patients with hypertension or ischemic heart disease, persons over age 60, and nursing mothers. Safety for use in pregnancy has not been established.

PRESCRIBING INFORMATION
RONDEC® Oral Drops   ℞
[ron'dek]
RONDEC® Syrup   ℞
RONDEC® Tablet   ℞
RONDEC-TR® Tablet   ℞

DESCRIPTION
Antihistamine/Decongestant for oral use

For infants
RONDEC® Oral Drops
Each dropperful (1 mL) contains carbinoxamine maleate, 2 mg; pseudoephedrine hydrochloride, 25 mg.
Inactive Ingredients: Citric acid, DC Red No. 33, FDC Yellow No. 6, glycerin, methylparaben, propylparaben, purified water, sodium benzoate, sodium citrate, sorbitol and artificial flavoring.

For young children
RONDEC® Syrup
Each teaspoonful (5 mL) contains carbinoxamine maleate, 4 mg; pseudoephedrine hydrochloride, 60 mg.
Inactive Ingredients: Citric acid, DC Red No. 33, FDC Yellow No. 6, glycerin, methylparaben, propylparaben, purified water, sodium benzoate, sodium citrate, sorbitol and artificial flavoring.

For adults and children 6 years and over
RONDEC® Tablet
Each Filmtab® tablet contains carbinoxamine maleate, 4 mg; pseudoephedrine hydrochloride, 60 mg.
Inactive Ingredients: Castor oil, cellulosic polymers, FDC Yellow No. 6, lactose, polacrilin potassium, povidone, stearic acid, titanium dioxide and vanillin.

For adults and children 12 years and over
RONDEC-TR® Tablet
Each timed-release Filmtab tablet contains carbinoxamine maleate, 8 mg; pseudoephedrine hydrochloride, 120 mg.
Inactive Ingredients: Castor oil, cellulosic polymers, confectioner's sugar, corn starch, FDC Blue No. 1, lactose, magnesium stearate, methyl acrylate-methyl methacrylate copolymer, microcrystalline cellulose, povidone, propylene glycol, sorbitan monooleate and titanium dioxide.

Carbinoxamine maleate (2-[p-Chloro-α-[2-(dimethylamino) ethoxy] benzyl] pyridine maleate) is one of the ethanolamine class of H_1 antihistamines.

Pseudoephedrine hydrochloride (Benzenemethanol, α-[1-(methylamino)ethyl]-, [S-(R*, R*)]-, hydrochloride) is the hydrochloride of pseudoephedrine, a naturally occurring dextrorotatory stereoisomer of ephedrine.

CLINICAL PHARMACOLOGY
Antihistaminic and decongestant actions.
Carbinoxamine maleate possesses H_1 antihistaminic activity and mild anticholinergic and sedative effects. Serum half-life for carbinoxamine is estimated to be 10 to 20 hours. Virtually no intact drug is excreted in the urine.

Pseudoephedrine hydrochloride is an oral sympathomimetic amine that acts as a decongestant to respiratory tract mucous membranes. While its vasoconstrictor action is similar to that of ephedrine, pseudoephedrine has less pressor effect in normotensive adults. Serum half-life for pseudoephedrine is 6 to 8 hours. Acidic urine is associated with faster elimination of the drug. About one half of the administered dose is excreted in the urine.

INDICATIONS AND USAGE
For symptomatic relief of seasonal and perennial allergic rhinitis and vasomotor rhinitis.
Rondec Oral Drops, Rondec Syrup and Rondec Tablet are immediate-release dosage forms allowing titration of dose up to four times a day.

Rondec-TR Tablet utilizes a gradual-release mechanism providing approximately a 12-hour therapeutic effect, thus allowing twice-daily dosage.

CONTRAINDICATIONS

Patients with hypersensitivity or idiosyncrasy to any ingredients, patients taking monoamine oxidase (MAO) inhibitors, patients with narrow-angle glaucoma, urinary retention, peptic ulcer, severe hypertension or coronary artery disease, or patients undergoing an asthmatic attack.

WARNINGS

Use in Pregnancy: Safety for use during pregnancy has not been established.
Nursing Mothers: Use with caution in nursing mothers.
Special Risk Patients: Use with caution in patients with hypertension or ischemic heart disease, and persons older than 60 years.

PRECAUTIONS

Use with caution in patients with hypertension, heart disease, asthma, hyperthyroidism, increased intraocular pressure, diabetes mellitus and prostatic hypertrophy.
Information for Patients: Avoid alcohol and other CNS depressants while taking these products. Patients sensitive to antihistamines may experience moderate to severe drowsiness. Patients sensitive to sympathomimetic amines may note mild CNS stimulation. While taking these products, exercise care in driving or operating appliances, machinery, etc.
Drug Interactions: Antihistamines may enhance the effects of tricyclic antidepressants, barbiturates, alcohol, and other CNS depressants. MAO inhibitors prolong and intensify the anticholinergic effects of antihistamines. Sympathomimetic amines may reduce the antihypertensive effects of reserpine, veratrum alkaloids, methyldopa and mecamylamine. Effects of sympathomimetics are increased with MAO inhibitors and beta-adrenergic blockers.
Pregnancy Category C.: Animal reproduction studies have not been conducted with these products. It is also not known whether these products can cause fetal harm when administered to a pregnant woman or affect reproduction capacity. Give to pregnant women only if clearly needed.

ADVERSE REACTIONS

Antihistamines: Sedation, dizziness, diplopia, vomiting, diarrhea, dry mouth, headache, nervousness, nausea, anorexia, heartburn, weakness, polyuria and dysuria and, rarely, excitability in children.
Sympathomimetic Amines: Convulsions, CNS stimulation, cardiac arrhythmias, respiratory difficulty, increased heart rate or blood pressure, hallucinations, tremors, nervousness, insomnia, weakness, pallor and dysuria.

OVERDOSAGE

No information is available as to specific results of an overdose of these products. The signs, symptoms and treatment described below are those of H_1 antihistamine and ephedrine overdose.
Symptoms: Should antihistamine effects predominate, central action constitutes the greatest danger. In the small child, symptoms include excitation, hallucination, ataxia, incoordination, tremors, flushed face and fever. Convulsions, fixed and dilated pupils, coma and death may occur in severe cases. In the adult, fever and flushing are uncommon; excitement leading to convulsions and postictal depression is often preceded by drowsiness and coma. Respiration is usually not seriously depressed; blood pressure is usually stable.
Should sympathomimetic symptoms predominate, central effects include restlessness, dizziness, tremor, hyperactive reflexes, talkativeness, irritability and insomnia. Cardiovascular and renal effects include difficulty in micturition, headache, flushing, palpitation, cardiac arrhythmias, hypertension with subsequent hypotension and circulatory collapse. Gastrointestinal effects include dry mouth, metallic taste, anorexia, nausea, vomiting, diarrhea and abdominal cramps.
Treatment: *a*) Evacuate stomach as condition warrants. Activated charcoal may be useful. *b*) Maintain a nonstimulating environment. *c*) Monitor cardiovascular status. *d*) Do not give stimulants. *e*) Reduce fever with cool sponging. *f*) Support respiration. *g*) Use sedatives or anticonvulsants to control CNS excitation and convulsions. *h*) Physostigmine may reverse anticholinergic symptoms. *i*) Ammonium chloride may acidify the urine to increase excretion of pseudoephedrine. *j*) Further care is symptomatic and supportive.

DOSAGE AND ADMINISTRATION

Age	Dose*	Frequency*
Rondec Oral Drops		
for oral use only		
1–3 months	¼ dropperful (¼ mL)	q.i.d.
3–6 months	½ dropperful (½ mL)	q.i.d.
6–9 months	¾ dropperful (¾ mL)	q.i.d.
9–18 months	1 dropperful (1 mL)	q.i.d.

Rondec Syrup and
Rondec Tablet

18 months–		
6 years	½ teaspoonful (2.5 mL)	q.i.d.
adults and		
children	1 teaspoonful (5 mL)	q.i.d.
6 years and	or	
over	1 tablet	

Rondec-TR Tablet

adults and children		
12 years and over	1 tablet	b.i.d.

*In mild cases or in particularly sensitive patients, less frequent or reduced doses may be adequate.

HOW SUPPLIED

Rondec Oral Drops, berry-flavored, in 30-mL bottles for dropper dosage, NDC 0074-5783-30. Calibrated shatterproof dropper enclosed in each carton. Container meets safety closure requirements. Avoid exposure to excessive heat.
Rondec Syrup, berry-flavored, in 16-fl-oz (1-pint) bottles, NDC 0074-5782-16; and 4-fl-oz bottles, NDC 0074-5782-04. Dispense in USP tight glass container. Avoid exposure to excessive heat.
Rondec Tablet, Filmtab tablets, in bottles of 100, NDC 0074-5726-13; and bottles of 500, NDC 0074-5726-53. Each orange-colored tablet marked with Ross "R" and the number 5726 for professional identification. Dispense in USP tight container.
Rondec-TR Tablet, Filmtab tablets, in bottles of 100, NDC 0074-6240-13. Each blue-colored tablet marked with Ross "R" and the number 6240 for professional identification. Dispense in USP tight container.
(.9820)

RONDEC®–DM Syrup ℞
[ron 'dek]
RONDEC®–DM Oral Drops ℞

PRODUCT OVERVIEW

KEY FACTS

Rondec-DM products contain the antihistamine carbinoxamine maleate, the decongestant pseudoephedrine hydrochloride, and the nonnarcotic antitussive dextromethorphan hydrobromide.

MAJOR USES

Rondec-DM products are indicated for relief of cough and upper respiratory symptoms, including nasal congestion, associated with allergy or the common cold.

SAFETY INFORMATION

Use with caution in patients with hypertension or ischemic heart disease, persons over 60, and nursing mothers. Safety for use during pregnancy has not been established.

PRESCRIBING INFORMATION

RONDEC®–DM Syrup ℞
[ron 'dek]
RONDEC®–DM Oral Drops ℞

DESCRIPTION

Antihistamine/Decongestant/Antitussive for oral use.
For adults and children
Rondec®-DM Syrup
Each teaspoonful (5 mL) contains carbinoxamine maleate, 4 mg; pseudoephedrine hydrochloride, 60 mg; dextromethorphan hydrobromide, 15 mg.
Inactive Ingredients: Citric acid, DC Red No. 33, FDC Blue No. 1, glycerin, menthol, purified water, sodium benzoate, sodium citrate, sorbitol, natural and artificial flavoring and other ingredients.
For infants
Rondec®-DM Oral Drops
Each dropperful (1 mL) contains carbinoxamine maleate, 2 mg; pseudoephedrine hydrochloride, 25 mg; dextromethorphan hydrobromide, 4 mg.
Inactive Ingredients: Citric acid, DC Red No. 33, FDC Blue No. 1, glycerin, menthol, purified water, sodium benzoate, sodium citrate, sorbitol, natural and artificial flavoring and other ingredients.
Carbinoxamine maleate (2-[p-Chloro-α-[2-(dimethylamino) ethoxy]benzyl]pyridine maleate) is one of the ethanolamine class of H_1 antihistamines.
Pseudoephedrine hydrochloride (Benzenemethanol, α-[1-(methylamino) ethyl]-, [S-(R*, R*)]-, hydrochloride) is the hydrochloride of pseudoephedrine, a naturally occurring dextrorotatory stereoisomer of ephedrine.
Dextromethorphan hydrobromide (Morphinan, 3-methoxy-17-methyl-, (9α, 13α, 14α)-, hydrobromide, monohydrate) is the hydrobromide of d-form racemethorphan.

CLINICAL PHARMACOLOGY

Antihistaminic, decongestant and antitussive actions.
Carbinoxamine maleate possesses H_1 antihistaminic activity and mild anticholinergic and sedative effects. Serum half-

---

life for carbinoxamine is estimated to be 10 to 20 hours. Virtually no intact drug is excreted in the urine.
Pseudoephedrine hydrochloride is an oral sympathomimetic amine that acts as a decongestant to respiratory tract mucous membranes. While its vasoconstrictor action is similar to that of ephedrine, pseudoephedrine has less pressor effect in normotensive adults. Serum half-life for pseudoephedrine is 6 to 8 hours. Acidic urine is associated with faster elimination of the drug. About one half of the administered dose is excreted in the urine.
Dextromethorphan hydrobromide is a nonnarcotic antitussive with effectiveness equal to codeine. It acts in the medulla oblongata to elevate the cough threshold. Dextromethorphan does not produce analgesia or induce tolerance, and has no potential for addiction. At usual doses, it will not depress respiration or inhibit ciliary activity. Dextromethorphan is rapidly metabolized, with trace amounts of the parent compound in blood and urine. About one half of the administered dose is excreted in the urine as conjugated metabolites.

INDICATIONS AND USAGE

For relief of coughs and upper respiratory symptoms, including nasal congestion, associated with allergy or the common cold.

CONTRAINDICATIONS

Patients with hypersensitivity or idiosyncrasy to any ingredients, patients taking monoamine oxidase (MAO) inhibitors, patients with narrow-angle glaucoma, urinary retention, peptic ulcer, severe hypertension or coronary artery disease, or patients undergoing an asthmatic attack.

WARNINGS

Use in Pregnancy: Safety for use during pregnancy has not been established.
Nursing Mothers: Use with caution in nursing mothers.
Special Risk Patients: Use with caution in patients with hypertension or ischemic heart disease, and persons older than 60 years.

PRECAUTIONS

Before prescribing medication to suppress or modify cough, identify and provide therapy for the underlying cause of cough.
Use with caution in patients with hypertension, heart disease, asthma, hyperthyroidism, increased intraocular pressure, diabetes mellitus and prostatic hypertrophy.
Information for Patients: Avoid alcohol and other CNS depressants while taking these products. Patients sensitive to antihistamines may experience moderate to severe drowsiness. Patients sensitive to sympathomimetic amines may note mild CNS stimulation. While taking these products, exercise care in driving or operating appliances, machinery, etc.
Drug Interactions: Antihistamines may enhance the effects of tricyclic antidepressants, barbiturates, alcohol, and other CNS depressants. MAO inhibitors prolong and intensify the anticholinergic effects of antihistamines. Sympathomimetic amines may reduce the antihypertensive effects of reserpine, veratrum alkaloids, methyldopa and mecamylamine. Effects of sympathomimetics are increased with MAO inhibitors and beta-adrenergic blockers. The cough-suppressant action of dextromethorphan and narcotic antitussives are additive.
Pregnancy Category C.: Animal reproduction studies have not been conducted with Rondec-DM. It is also not known whether these products can cause fetal harm when administered to a pregnant woman or affect reproduction capacity. Give to pregnant women only if clearly needed.

ADVERSE REACTIONS

Antihistamines: Sedation, dizziness, diplopia, vomiting, diarrhea, dry mouth, headache, nervousness, nausea, anorexia, heartburn, weakness, polyuria and dysuria and, rarely, excitability in children.
Sympathomimetic Amines: Convulsions, CNS stimulation, cardiac arrhythmias, respiratory difficulty, increased heart rate or blood pressure, hallucinations, tremors, nervousness, insomnia, weakness, pallor and dysuria.
Dextromethorphan: Drowsiness and GI disturbance.

OVERDOSAGE

No information is available as to specific results of an overdose of these products. The signs, symptoms and treatment described below are those of H_1 antihistamine, ephedrine and dextromethorphan overdose.
Symptoms: Should antihistamine effects predominate, central action constitutes the greatest danger. In the small child, predominant symptoms are excitation, hallucination, ataxia, incoordination, tremors, flushed face and fever. Convulsions, fixed and dilated pupils, coma and death may occur in severe cases. In the adult, fever and flushing are uncommon; excitement leading to convulsions and postictal depression is often preceded by drowsiness and coma. Respiration is usually not seriously depressed; blood pressure is usually stable.

Continued on next page

Ross—Cont.

Should sympathomimetic symptoms predominate, central effects include restlessness, dizziness, tremor, hyperactive reflexes, talkativeness, irritability and insomnia. Cardiovascular and renal effects include difficulty in micturition, headache, flushing, palpitation, cardiac arrhythmias, hypertension with subsequent hypotension and circulatory collapse. Gastrointestinal effects include dry mouth, metallic taste, anorexia, nausea, vomiting, diarrhea and abdominal cramps.

Dextromethorphan may cause respiratory depression with a large overdose.

Treatment: *a*) Evacuate stomach as condition warrants. Activated charcoal may be useful. *b*) Maintain a nonstimulating environment. *c*) Monitor cardiovascular status. *d*) Do not give stimulants. *e*) Reduce fever with cool sponging. *f*) Treat respiratory depression with naloxone if dextromethorphan toxicity is suspected. *g*) Use sedatives or anticonvulsants to control CNS excitation and convulsions. *h*) Physostigmine may reverse anticholinergic symptoms. *i*) Ammonium chloride may acidify the urine to increase urinary excretion of pseudoephedrine. *j*) Further care is symptomatic and supportive.

DOSAGE AND ADMINISTRATION

Age	Dose*	Frequency*
Rondec-DM Syrup		
18 months–	½ teaspoonful	
6 years	(2.5 mL)	q.i.d.
adults and	1 teaspoonful	
children 6	(5 mL)	q.i.d.
years and over		

Rondec-DM Oral Drops
for oral use only

1–3 months	¼ dropperful (¼ mL)	q.i.d.
3–6 months	½ dropperful (½ mL)	q.i.d.
6–9 months	¾ dropperful (¾ mL)	q.i.d.
9–18 months	1 dropperful (1 mL)	q.i.d.

*In mild cases or in particularly sensitive patients, less frequent or reduced doses may be adequate.

HOW SUPPLIED

Rondec-DM Syrup, grape-flavored, in 16-fl-oz (1-pint) bottles, **NDC 0074-5640-16**; and 4-fl-oz bottles, **NDC 0074-5640-04**. Dispense in USP tight, light-resistant, glass container. Avoid exposure to excessive heat.

Rondec-DM Oral Drops, grape-flavored, in 30-mL bottles for dropper dosage. Calibrated, shatterproof dropper enclosed in each carton. Container meets safety closure requirements. **NDC 0074-5639-30**. Avoid exposure to excessive heat.
(.7890)

ROSS HOSPITAL FORMULA SYSTEM
Products for hospital nursery use

ADVANCE®
Nutritional Beverage With Iron
    Availability: Ready To Feed
    8-fl-oz nursing bottles; 24 per case; No. 804.

ALIMENTUM®
Protein Hydrolysate Formula With Iron
    Availability: Ready To Feed
    8-fl-oz nursing bottles; 24 per case; No. 862.

ISOMIL® 20 (20 Cal/fl oz)
Soy Protein Formula With Iron
    Availability: Ready To Feed
    4-fl-oz nursing bottles; 48 per case; No. 406.
    8-fl-oz nursing bottles; 24 per case; No. 871.

ISOMIL® SF 20
Sucrose-Free Soy Protein Formula With Iron
    Availability: Ready To Feed
    8-fl-oz nursing bottles; 24 per case; No. 801.

PEDIALYTE®
Oral Electrolyte Maintenance Solution
    Availability: Ready To Use
    8-fl-oz nursing bottles; 24 per case; No. 806.

SIMILAC® 13 (13 Cal/fl oz)
Low-Iron Infant Formula
    Availability: Ready To Feed
    4-fl-oz nursing bottles; 48 per case; No. 408.

SIMILAC® WITH IRON 13
Infant Formula
    Availability: Ready To Feed
    4-fl-oz nursing bottles; 48 per case; No. 413.

SIMILAC® 20 (20 Cal/fl oz)
Low-Iron Infant Formula
    Availability: Ready To Feed
    4-fl-oz nursing bottles; 48 per case; No. 415.
    8-fl-oz nursing bottles; 24 per case; No. 841.

SIMILAC® WITH IRON 20
Infant Formula
    Availability: Ready To Feed
    4-fl-oz nursing bottles; 48 per case; No. 426.
    8-fl-oz nursing bottles; 24 per case; No. 858.

SIMILAC® 24 (24 Cal/fl oz)
Low-Iron Infant Formula
    Availability: Ready To Feed
    4-fl-oz nursing bottles; 48 per case; No. 404.

SIMILAC® WITH IRON 24
Infant Formula
    Availability: Ready To Feed
    4-fl-oz nursing bottles; 48 per case; No. 403.

SIMILAC® 27 (27 Cal/fl oz)
Low-Iron Infant Formula
    Availability: Ready To Feed
    4-fl-oz nursing bottles; 48 per case; No. 427.

SIMILAC NATURAL CARE®
Low-Iron Human Milk Fortifier
    Availability: Ready To Use
    4-fl-oz nursing bottles; 48 per case; No. 443.

SIMILAC® PM 60/40
Low-Iron Infant Formula
    Availability: Ready To Feed
    4-fl-oz nursing bottles; 48 per case; No. 424.

SIMILAC® SPECIAL CARE® 20 (20 Cal/fl oz)
Low-Iron Premature Infant Formula
    Availability: Ready To Feed
    4-fl-oz nursing bottles; 48 per case; No. 439.

SIMILAC® SPECIAL CARE® 24 (24 Cal/fl oz)
Low-Iron Premature Infant Formula
    Availability: Ready To Feed
    4-fl-oz nursing bottles; 48 per case; No. 433.

SIMILAC® SPECIAL CARE® WITH IRON 24
Premature Infant Formula
    Availability: Ready To Feed
    4-fl-oz nursing bottles; 48 per case; No. 478.

STERILIZED WATER
    Availability: Ready To Feed
    4-fl-oz nursing bottles; 48 per case; No. 432.
    8-fl-oz nursing bottles; 24 per case; No. 879.

5% GLUCOSE WATER
    Availability: Ready To Feed
    4-fl-oz nursing bottles; 48 per case; No. 405.

10% GLUCOSE WATER
    Availability: Ready To Feed
    4-fl-oz nursing bottles; 48 per case; No. 410.

ROSS SLD®
Surgical Liquid Diet

USAGE
A low-residue formula for patients requiring a clear liquid diet (ie, pre- and post-surgery, prior to diagnostic testing), and as a low-fat diet. Provides calories, high-quality protein, vitamins and minerals in a delicious-tasting fruit-punch flavor. Ross SLD may also be useful as a high-protein, vitamin and mineral supplement for patients receiving enteral nutritional support.

DOSAGE AND ADMINISTRATION
Instructions for Use: For one serving: pour 6 fl oz (³⁄₄ cup) water into a container. Add ⅓ level measuring cup or one packet of SLD and stir until powder dissolves. (If using a blender, low speed is recommended to reduce foaming.) The contents of one can will make approximately 10 servings. To prepare, mix entire contents of can with 7½ cups water. Use within 6 hours or store covered in refrigerator and use within 48 hours. Stir before use. STORAGE: Opened can should be covered with overcap and stored in a cool, dry place but not refrigerated. Once the can is opened, use contents within 1 month. Store unopened powder in a cool, dry place.
CAUTION: Ross SLD is a low-fat product that should be used only under medical supervision. This product and other clear liquid diets should not be used as the sole source of nutrition for extended periods of time. Not intended for infants.
NOT FOR PARENTERAL USE.
Availability: 13.5 oz (383 g) cans; 6 per case; Fruit punch flavor, No. 674.
1.35 oz (38.3 g) packets; 6 packets per carton; 4 cartons per case; Fruit punch flavor, No. 673.

COMPOSITION
Powder

INGREDIENTS
Ⓤ Sugar (sucrose), egg white solids, hydrolyzed cornstarch, calcium glycerophosphate, citric acid, magnesium carbonate, natural and artificial flavor, ammonium phosphate dibasic, choline bitartrate, potassium citrate, sodium citrate, ascorbic acid, potassium chloride, artificial color, zinc sulfate, ferrous sulfate, alpha-tocopheryl acetate, vitamin A palmitate, niacinamide, manganese glycerophosphate, calcium pantothenate, copper gluconate, vitamin D_3, pyridoxine hydrochloride, thiamine mononitrate, riboflavin, folic acid, biotin, potassium iodide, phylloquinone and cyanocobalamin.

Nutrients:	Per 140 Calories (1 Serving)	Per 840 Calories (6 Servings)
Protein, g	7.5	45
Fat, g	0.1	0.6
Carbohydrate, g	27.3	163.8
Water, g... does not exceed	1.9	11.4

(FAN 574-01)

ROSS METABOLIC FORMULA SYSTEM

A line of products designed to meet the special nutrient needs of infants, children and adults with inherited metabolic disorders requiring specific nutrition support tailored to their condition.

Available from Ross Laboratories are formulas for the following conditions:

    Glutaric Aciduria Type I
    Homocystinuria
    Hypermethioninemia
    Maple syrup urine disease
       (branched-chain ketoaciduria)
    Methylmalonic acidemia
    Phenylketonuria
    Propionic acidemia
    Tyrosinemias

ANALOG® MSUD
Amino Acid-Modified Infant Formula With Iron
Isoleucine-, Leucine-, and Valine-Free

USAGE
When an isoleucine-, leucine- and valine-free formula is needed for the nutrition support of infants with branched-chain ketoaciduria (maple syrup urine disease).

AVAILABILITY
Powder: 3.5-oz (100 g) containers; 10 per case; No. 355.

ANALOG® XMET
Amino Acid-Modified Infant Formula With Iron
Methionine-Free

USAGE
When a methionine-free formula is needed for the nutrition support of infants with vitamin B_6 non-responsive homocystinuria or hypermethioninemia.

AVAILABILITY
Powder: 3.5-oz (100 g) containers; 10 per case; No. 356.

ANALOG® XMET, THRE, VAL, ISOLEU
Amino Acid-Modified Infant Formula With Iron
Methionine-, Threonine- and Valine-Free; Low-Isoleucine

USAGE
When a methionine-, threonine- and valine-free; low-isoleucine formula is needed for the nutrition support of infants with methylmalonic or propionic acidemia.

AVAILABILITY
Powder: 3.5-oz (100 g) containers; 10 per case; No. 359.

ANALOG® XP
Amino Acid-Modified Infant Formula With Iron
Phenylalanine-Free

USAGE
When a phenylalanine-free formula is needed for the nutrition support of infants with phenylketonuria (PKU).

AVAILABILITY
Powder: 3.5-oz (100 g) containers; 10 per case; No. 350.

ANALOG® XPHEN, TYR
Amino Acid-Modified Infant Formula With Iron
Phenylalanine- and Tyrosine-Free

USAGE
When a phenylalanine- and tyrosine-free formula is needed for the nutrition support of infants with tyrosinemia.

AVAILABILITY
Powder: 3.5-oz (100 g) containers; 10 per case; No. 354.

ANALOG® XPHEN, TYR, MET
Amino Acid-Modified Infant Formula With Iron
Phenylalanine-, Tyrosine- and Methionine-Free

USAGE
When a phenylalanine-, tyrosine- and methionine-free formula is needed for the nutrition support of infants with tyrosinemia type 1.

AVAILABILITY

Powder: 3.5-oz (100 g) containers; 10 per case; No. 357.

CALCILO XD®
**Low-Calcium/Vitamin D-Free
Low-Iron Infant Formula**

USAGE

For use in the nutrition support of infants with hypercalcemia when a low-calcium/vitamin D-free formula is needed.

AVAILABILITY

Powder: 14.1 oz cans, measuring scoop enclosed; 6 per case; No. 378.

PROVIMIN®
**Protein-Vitamin-Mineral
Formula Component**

USAGE

For use as the protein base in the preparation of liquid diets for feeding infants and children with chronic diarrhea and other malabsorptive disorders that require restriction of fat and carbohydrate intake.

AVAILABILITY

Powder: 5.3-oz (150 g) cans, measuring scoop enclosed; 6 per case; No. 50260.

RCF®
**Ross Carbohydrate Free
Low-Iron Soy Protein Formula Base**

USAGE

For use in the dietary management of persons unable to tolerate the type or amount of carbohydrate in milk or conventional infant formulas: many of these patients have intractable diarrhea and are not able to tolerate other formulas. This product has been formulated to contain no carbohydrate, which must be added before feeding.

AVAILABILITY

Concentrated Liquid: 13-fl-oz cans; 12 per case; No. 108.

SIMILAC® PM 60/40
[*sim 'e-lak*]
Low-Iron Infant Formula

USAGE

For infants in the lower range of homeostatic capacity; those who are predisposed to hypocalcemia; and those whose renal, digestive or cardiovascular functions would benefit from lowered mineral levels.

AVAILABILITY

Powder: 1-lb cans, measuring scoop enclosed; 6 per case; No. 00850.
For hospital use, Ready To Feed Similac PM 60/40 in disposable nursing bottles is available in the Ross Hospital Formula System. (Ready To Feed has similar composition and nutrient values as Powder. For specific information see bottle tray.)

MAXAMAID® MSUD
**Dietary Supplement for Maple Syrup
Urine Disease (MSUD)**

USAGE

An artificially orange-flavored powder containing no isoleucine, leucine or valine. For the dietary management of Maple Syrup Urine Disease (MSUD) in children 1 to 8 years of age.

AVAILABILITY

Powder: 7-oz (200 g) containers; 10 per case; Orange, No. 345.

MAXAMAID® XLYS, TRY
**Dietary Supplement for
Glutaric Aciduria Type 1**

USAGE

An artificially orange-flavored powder containing no lysine or tryptophan. For the dietary management of glutaric aciduria type 1 in children 1 to 19 years of age.

AVAILABILITY

Powder: 7-oz (200 g) containers; 10 per case; Orange, No. 371.

MAXAMAID® XMET
**Dietary Supplement for Vitamin B₆
Nonresponsive Homocystinuria due
to Cystathionine-β-synthase
Deficiency or Hypermethioninemia**

USAGE

An artificially orange-flavored powder containing no methionine. For the dietary management of vitamin B₆ nonre-

sponsive homocystinuria due to cystathionine-β-synthase deficiency or hypermethioninemia.

AVAILABILITY

Powder: 7-oz (200 g) containers; 10 per case; Orange, No. 366.

MAXAMAID® XMET, THRE, VAL, ISOLEU
**Dietary Supplement for Methylmalonic
Acidemia or Propionic Acidemia**

USAGE

An artificially orange-flavored powder containing no methionine, threonine or valine and low in isoleucine. For the dietary management of methylmalonic acidemia or propionic acidemia.

AVAILABILITY

Powder: 7-oz (200 g) containers; 10 per case; Orange, No. 376.

MAXAMAID® XP
Dietary Supplement for Phenylketonuria

USAGE

An artificially orange-flavored powder containing no phenylalanine. For the dietary management of phenylketonuria (PKU) in children 1 to 8 years of age.

AVAILABILITY

Powder: 7-oz (200 g) containers; 10 per case; Orange, No. 344; Unflavored, No. 363.

MAXAMAID® XPHEN, TYR
Dietary Supplement for Tyrosinemia

USAGE

An artificially orange-flavored powder containing no phenylalanine or tyrosine. For the dietary management of tyrosinemia in children 1 to 8 years of age.

AVAILABILITY

Powder: 7-oz (200 g) containers; 10 per case; Orange, No. 362.

MAXAMUM® MSUD
**Dietary Supplement for Maple Syrup
Urine Disease (MSUD)**

USAGE

An artificially orange-flavored powder containing no isoleucine, leucine or valine. For the dietary management of maple syrup urine disease (MSUD) in individuals over 8 years of age and women in the childbearing years.

AVAILABILITY

Powder: 7-oz (200 g) containers; 10 per case; Orange, No. 375.

MAXAMUM® XP
Dietary Supplement for Phenylketonuria

USAGE

An artificially orange-flavored powder containing no phenylalanine. For the dietary management of phenylketonuria (PKU) in pregnant women, women in the childbearing years and individuals over 8 years of age.

AVAILABILITY

Powder: 7-oz (200 g) containers; 10 per case; Orange, No. 346; Unflavored, No. 369.

SELSUN BLUE®   OTC
[*sel 'sen blü*]
**Dandruff Shampoo
(selenium sulfide lotion, 1%)**

Selsun Blue is a non-prescription anti-dandruff shampoo containing the active ingredient selenium sulfide, 1%, in a freshly scented, pH balanced formula to leave hair clean and manageable. Available in Dry, Oily, Normal, Extra Conditioning and Extra Medicated formulas (contains 0.5% menthol).

INACTIVE INGREDIENTS

Dry formula—Acetylated lanolin alcohol, ammonium laureth sulfate, ammonium lauryl sulfate, cetyl acetate, citric acid, cocamide DEA, cocamidopropyl betaine, DMDM hydantoin, FD&C blue No. 1, fragrance, hydroxypropyl methylcellulose, magnesium aluminum silicate, polysorbate 80, sodium chloride, titanium dioxide, water and other ingredients.
Normal formula—Ammonium laureth sulfate, ammonium lauryl sulfate, citric acid, cocamide DEA, cocamidopropyl betaine, DMDM hydantoin, FD&C blue No. 1, fragrance, hydroxypropyl methylcellulose, magnesium aluminum silicate, sodium chloride, titanium dioxide, water and other ingredients.
Oily formula—Ammonium laureth sulfate, ammonium lauryl sulfate, citric acid, cocamide DEA, cocamidopropyl betaine, DMDM hydantoin, FD&C blue No. 1, fragrance, hydrox-

ypropyl methylcellulose, magnesium aluminum silicate, sodium chloride, titanium dioxide, water and other ingredients.
Extra Conditioning formula—Acetylated lanolin alcohol, aloe, ammonium laureth sulfate, ammonium lauryl sulfate, cetyl acetate, citric acid, cocamide DEA, cocamidopropyl betaine, DMDM hydantoin, FD&C blue No. 1, fragrance, glycol distearate, hydroxypropyl methylcellulose, magnesium aluminum silicate, polysorbate 80, propylene glycol, sodium chloride, TEA-lauryl sulfate, titanium dioxide, water and other ingredients.
Extra Medicated formula—Ammonium laureth sulfate, ammonium lauryl sulfate, citric acid, cocamide DEA, cocamidopropyl betaine, DMDM hydantoin, D&C red No. 33, FD&C blue No. 1, fragrance, hydroxypropyl methylcellulose, magnesium aluminum silicate, sodium chloride, TEA-lauryl sulfate, water and other ingredients.

Clinical testing has shown Selsun Blue to be as safe and effective as other leading shampoos in helping control dandruff symptoms with regular use.

DIRECTIONS

Shake well before using. Lather, rinse thoroughly and repeat. For best results, use at least twice a week for effective dandruff control.

PRECAUTIONS

For external use only. Keep out of eyes—if this happens, rinse thoroughly with water. If used just before or after bleaching, tinting or permanent waving, rinse hair for at least five minutes in cool running water. If irritation occurs, discontinue use. Keep out of the reach of children.

HOW SUPPLIED

4-, 7- and 11-fl-oz plastic bottles.
(FAN 2137-02)

SIMILAC®
[*sim 'e-lak*]
Low-Iron Infant Formula
- Powder
- Concentrated Liquid
- Ready To Feed

(See PDR For Nonprescription Drugs)

SIMILAC® SPECIAL CARE® WITH IRON 24
Premature Infant Formula
- Ready To Feed

(See PDR For Nonprescription Drugs)

SIMILAC® WITH IRON
[*sim 'e-lak*]
Infant Formula
- Powder
- Concentrated Liquid
- Ready To Feed

(See PDR For Nonprescription Drugs)

TRONOLANE®   OTC
[*tron 'e-lān*]
**Anesthetic Cream for Hemorrhoids
Anesthetic Suppositories for Hemorrhoids**

DESCRIPTION

The active ingredient in Tronolane is a topical anesthetic agent (Cream: pramoxine hydrochloride 1%; Suppositories: pramoxine 1% as pramoxine and pramoxine HCl), chemically unrelated to the benzoate esters of the "caine" type, which is chemically designated as a 4-n-butoxyphenyl gammamorpholinopropylether hydrochloride. The cream contains the following inactive ingredients: A non-greasy zinc oxide cream base containing beeswax, cetyl alcohol, cetyl esters wax, glycerin, methylparaben, propylparaben, sodium lauryl sulfate, water and zinc oxide. The suppository contains the following inactive ingredients: A base containing hydrogenated cocoa glycerides and zinc oxide.

INDICATIONS

Tronolane is a topical anesthetic indicated for the temporary relief of the pain, burning, itching and discomfort that accompany hemorrhoids. It has a soothing, lubricant action on mucous membranes.
Tronolane contains a rapidly acting topical anesthetic producing analgesia that lasts up to 5 hours. Because the drug is chemically unrelated to other anesthetics, cross-sensitization is unlikely. Patients who are already sensitized to the "caine" anesthetics can generally use Tronolane.
The emollient/emulsion base of Tronolane cream provides soothing lubrication making bowel movements more com-

Continued on next page

Ross—Cont.

fortable. Tronolane cream is in a nondrying base that is nongreasy and nonstaining to undergarments.

WARNINGS

If bleeding is present, consult physician. Certain persons can develop allergic reactions to ingredients in this product. During treatment, if condition worsens or persists 7 days, consult physician. For children under 12 years, use only as directed by physician. Keep out of the reach of children. As with any drug, if you are pregnant or nursing a baby, we recommend that you seek the advice of a health professional before using this product.

DOSAGE AND ADMINISTRATION

CREAM: Apply up to five times daily, especially morning, night, and after bowel movements, or as directed by physician.

External—Apply liberally to affected area. *Intrarectal*—Remove cap from tube and attach clean applicator. Remove protective cover from clean applicator. Squeeze tube to fill applicator and lubricate tip with cream. Gently insert applicator into rectum and squeeze tube again. Thoroughly cleanse applicator after use.

SUPPOSITORIES: Use up to five times daily, especially morning, night, and after bowel movements, or as directed by physician. Detach one suppository from pack. Separate foil at rounded end and peel apart until the suppository is exposed. Insert suppository into the rectum, rounded end first.

HOW SUPPLIED

Tronolane is available in 1-oz and 2-oz cream tubes and 10 and 20 count suppository boxes.
(FAN 2093)

TWOCAL® HN
[tü´kal]
High Nitrogen Liquid Nutrition

USAGE

As a high-calorie, high-nitrogen liquid food, TwoCal HN delivers 100% of the U.S. RDA for vitamins and minerals in only 950 mL (1 quart). TwoCal HN is most appropriate for use in severely hypermetabolic and fluid-restricted patients. As a concentrated source of nutrition, TwoCal HN is an excellent dietary supplement when voluntary food intake is inadequate to meet nutrient needs.

DOSAGE AND ADMINISTRATION

Shake well. May be stored unopened at room temperature. Once opened, TwoCal HN should be covered and refrigerated; discard if not used within 48 hours. TwoCal HN may be fed at room temperature or chilled.

Oral Feeding: May be used for total nutrition, or with and between meals.

Tube Feeding: Follow physician's instructions. Adjust flow rate, volume and dilution according to patient's condition and tolerance. When used as the sole source of nutrition, products containing 2 Cal/mL may provide inadequate water for most patients.

Monitor hydration status; additional fluid requirements should be met by giving water with or after feedings or by parenteral routes. Avoid contamination during preparation and use.

NOT FOR PARENTERAL USE.

AVAILABILITY

Ready To Use:
8-fl-oz cans; 4 six-packs per case; Vanilla, No. 729.

COMPOSITION

Ready To Use Vanilla

INGREDIENTS

Ⓓ-D Water, hydrolyzed cornstarch, corn oil, sodium calcium caseinate, sucrose, medium-chain triglycerides (fractionated coconut oil), potassium citrate, soy lecithin, magnesium chloride, calcium phosphate tribasic, natural and artificial flavors, ascorbic acid, sodium citrate, choline chloride, zinc sulfate, ferrous sulfate, alpha-tocopheryl acetate, niacinamide, calcium pantothenate, manganese sulfate, cupric sulfate, thiamine chloride hydrochloride, pyridoxine hydrochloride, vitamin A palmitate, riboflavin, folic acid, biotin, potassium iodide, phylloquinone, cyanocobalamin and vitamin D₃.

Nutrients (grams/8 fl oz): Protein, 19.8; Fat, 21.5; Carbohydrate, 51.4; Water, 169. Calories per mL, 2.0; Calories per fl oz, 59.4.
(FAN 574-05)

VARI-FLAVORS® Flavor Pacs
[var´ē-flā´´verz]

USAGE

To provide flavor variety for patients receiving full liquid diets and liquid supplements.

AVAILABILITY

One-gram packets; 24 per dispenser carton; Pecan, No. 720; Cherry, No. 722; Lemon, No. 724; Orange, No. 726; Strawberry, No. 728; Assorted flavors, No. 730.

INSTRUCTIONS FOR USE

Tap Pac lightly to shake contents to bottom. Tear off corner of packet. Pour contents into suitable dry serving container. Add 8 ounces of one of the Ross Medical Nutritional products. Allow flavor to dissolve for a few seconds. Stir until flavor is mixed and serve.

COMPOSITION

(Pareve, Ⓤ) Dextrose, artificial flavor and color (Strawberry and Cherry); Dextrose, artificial flavor and artificial color [including FD&C Yellow No. 6]. (Orange); Dextrose and artificial flavor (Pecan); Dextrose, artificial flavor and FD & C Yellow #5 (Lemon).

When used as directed, Vari-Flavors contribute trace amounts of minerals and less than 1 gram of dextrose. The addition of a single Vari-Flavors Pac (1 gram) to one serving of a Ross Medical Nutritional product or Ross New Direction® Nutritional Beverage increases total calories per 8-oz serving by approximately 4 Calories.
(FAN 242)

VI-DAYLIN® ADC VITAMINS Drops
[vī´´dā´lin]
Dietary Supplement of Vitamins A, D and C

DESCRIPTION

One dropperful (1.0 mL) provides:

Vitamins			% U.S. RDA*	% U.S. RDA**
Vitamin A	1500	I.U.	100	60
Vitamin D	400	I.U.	100	100
Vitamin C	35	mg	100	87

INGREDIENTS

Propylene glycol, polysorbate 80, ascorbic acid, methylparaben (preservative), vitamin A palmitate, propylparaben (preservative), and ergocalciferol in corn oil, in a glycerin-water vehicle with added artificial pineapple-fruit flavoring and caramel coloring. Contains only a trace (less than ½%) of alcohol.

Contains no sugar.

*% U.S. Recommended Daily Allowance for infants.
**% U.S. Recommended Daily Allowance for children under 4 years of age.

INDICATIONS AND USAGE

Dietary supplement of vitamins A, D and C for infants and children under 4 years of age.

DOSAGE AND ADMINISTRATION

One dropperful daily, or as directed by physician.

HOW SUPPLIED

50-mL Spil-gard® bottles, calibrated dropper enclosed; OTC; List No. 0105-04.

VI-DAYLIN® ADC VITAMINS + IRON Drops
[vī´´dā´lin]
Dietary Supplement of Vitamins A, D and C with Iron

DESCRIPTION

One dropperful (1.0 mL) provides:

Vitamins			% U.S. RDA*	% U.S. RDA**
Vitamin A	1500	I.U.	100	60
Vitamin D	400	I.U.	100	100
Vitamin C	35	mg	100	87
Minerals				
Iron	10	mg	66	100

INGREDIENTS

Polysorbate 80, ferrous sulfate, ascorbic acid, vitamin A palmitate, benzoic acid (preservative), methylparaben (preservative), and ergocalciferol in a glycerin-water vehicle with added artificial flavoring and coloring.

Contains no sugar.

*% U.S. Recommended Daily Allowance for infants.
**% U.S. Recommended Daily Allowance for children under 4 years of age.

INDICATIONS AND USAGE

Dietary supplement of vitamins A, D and C with iron for infants and children under 4 years of age.

DOSAGE AND ADMINISTRATION

One dropperful daily, or as directed by physician.

HOW SUPPLIED

50-mL Spil-gard® bottles; calibrated dropper enclosed; OTC; List No. 0117-01.

VI-DAYLIN® MULTIVITAMIN Drops
[vī´´dā´lin]
Multivitamin Supplement

DESCRIPTION

One dropperful (1.0 mL) provides:

Vitamins			% U.S. RDA*	% U.S. RDA**
Vitamin A	1500	I.U.	100	60
Vitamin D	400	I.U.	100	100
Vitamin E	5	I.U.	100	50
Vitamin C	35	mg	100	87
Thiamine (Vitamin B₁)	0.5	mg	100	71
Riboflavin (Vitamin B₂)	0.6	mg	100	75
Niacin	8	mg	100	88
Vitamin B₆	0.4	mg	100	57
Vitamin B₁₂	1.5	mcg	75	50

INGREDIENTS

Ascorbic acid, d-alpha-tocopheryl acid succinate, niacinamide, benzoic acid (preservative), ferric ammonium citrate (stabilizer), vitamin A palmitate, riboflavin-5'-phosphate sodium, methylparaben (preservative), thiamine hydrochloride, pyridoxine hydrochloride, ergocalciferol in corn oil, disodium edetate (stabilizer) and cyanocobalamin in a glycerin-water vehicle with added artificial flavoring. Contains only a trace (less than ½%) of alcohol.

Contains no sugar.

*% U.S. Recommended Daily Allowance for infants.
**% U.S. Recommended Daily Allowance for children under 4 years of age.

INDICATIONS AND USAGE

Multivitamin supplement for infants and children under 4 years of age.

DOSAGE AND ADMINISTRATION

One dropperful daily, or as directed by physician.

HOW SUPPLIED

50-mL Spil-gard® bottles, calibrated dropper enclosed; OTC; List No. 0103-04.

VI-DAYLIN® MULTIVITAMIN + IRON Drops
[vī´´dā´lin]
Multivitamin/Iron Supplement

DESCRIPTION

One dropperful (1.0 mL) provides:

Vitamins			% U.S. RDA*	% U.S. RDA**
Vitamin A	1500	I.U.	100	60
Vitamin D	400	I.U.	100	100
Vitamin E	5	I.U.	100	50
Vitamin C	35	mg	100	87
Thiamine (Vitamin B₁)	0.5	mg	100	71
Riboflavin (Vitamin B₂)	0.6	mg	100	75
Niacin	8	mg	100	88
Vitamin B₆	0.4	mg	100	57
Minerals				
Iron	10	mg	66	100

INGREDIENTS

Ferrous sulfate, ascorbic acid, d-alpha-tocopheryl acid succinate, niacinamide, vitamin A palmitate, benzoic acid (preservative), riboflavin-5'-phosphate sodium, thiamine hydrochloride, methylparaben (preservative), pyridoxine hydrochloride, and ergocalciferol in corn oil, in a glycerin-water vehicle with added artificial coloring and flavoring. Contains only a trace (less than ½%) of alcohol.

Contains no sugar.

*% U.S. Recommended Daily Allowance for infants.
**% U.S. Recommended Daily Allowance for children under 4 years of age.

INDICATIONS AND USAGE

Multivitamin supplement with iron for infants and children under 4 years of age.

ADMINISTRATION AND DOSAGE

One dropperful daily, or as directed by physician.

HOW SUPPLIED

50-mL Spil-gard® bottles, calibrated dropper enclosed; OTC; List No. 0116-01.

VI-DAYLIN®/F ADC VITAMINS Drops With Fluoride℞
[vī″dā′lin]
ADC Vitamins/Fluoride

DESCRIPTION

One dropperful (1.0 mL) provides:
Fluoride   0.25 mg

Vitamins			% U.S. RDA*	% U.S. RDA**
Vitamin A	1500	I.U.	100	60
Vitamin D	400	I.U.	100	100
Vitamin C	35	mg	100	87

Active Ingredients: Ascorbic acid, vitamin A palmitate, sodium fluoride and ergocalciferol.
Inactive Ingredients: Alcohol approximately 0.3%, caramel coloring, corn oil, glycerin, methylparaben, polysorbate 80, propylene glycol, propylparaben, water, artificial and natural flavoring, and other ingredients.
Contains no sugar.
 *%U.S. Recommended Daily Allowance for infants.
**% U.S. Recommended Daily Allowance for children under 4 years of age.

INDICATIONS AND USAGE

As an aid in the prevention of dental caries in infants and children, and in the prophylaxis of vitamin A, D and C deficiencies.

CONTRAINDICATIONS

Should be used only where the fluoride content of the drinking water supply is known to be 0.7 parts per million or less.

PRECAUTIONS

The recommended dosage should not be exceeded since chronic overdosage of fluoride may result in mottling of tooth enamel and osseous changes.

OVERDOSAGE

In children, acute ingestion of 10 to 20 mg of sodium fluoride may cause excessive salivation and gastrointestinal disturbances; 500 mg may be fatal. Oral and/or intravenous fluids containing calcium may be indicated.

DOSAGE AND ADMINISTRATION

One dropperful daily, or as directed by physician or dentist.

HOW SUPPLIED

50-mL Spil-gard® bottles, calibrated dropper enclosed; ℞; NDC 0074-1106-50.

VI-DAYLIN®/F ADC VITAMINS + IRON℞ Drops With Fluoride
[vī″dā′lin]
ADC Vitamins/Fluoride/Iron Supplement

DESCRIPTION

One dropperful (1.0 mL) provides:
Fluoride   0.25 mg

Vitamins			% U.S. RDA*	% U.S. RDA**
Vitamin A	1500 I.U.		100	60
Vitamin D	400 I.U.		100	100
Vitamin C	35 mg		100	87
Minerals				
Iron	10 mg		66	100

Active Ingredients: Ascorbic acid, ferrous sulfate, vitamin A palmitate, sodium fluoride and ergocalciferol.
Inactive Ingredients: Benzoic acid, caramel coloring, glycerin, methylparaben, polysorbate 80, water, artificial flavoring and other ingredients.
Contains no sugar.
 *%U.S. Recommended Daily Allowance for infants.
**%U.S. Recommended Daily Allowance for children under 4 years of age.

INDICATIONS AND USAGE

As an aid in the prevention of dental caries in infants and children, and in the prophylaxis of iron and vitamin A, D and C deficiencies.

CONTRAINDICATIONS

Should be used only where the fluoride content of the drinking water supply is known to be 0.7 parts per million or less.

PRECAUTIONS

The recommended dosage should not be exceeded since chronic overdosage of fluoride may result in mottling of tooth enamel and osseous changes. In infants, oral iron-containing preparations may cause temporary darkening of the membrane covering the teeth.

OVERDOSAGE

In children, acute ingestion of 10 to 20 mg of sodium fluoride may cause excessive salivation and gastrointestinal disturbances; 500 mg may be fatal. Oral and/or intravenous fluids containing calcium may be indicated.
Acute overdosage of iron may cause nausea and vomiting and, in severe cases, cardiovascular collapse and death. The estimated lethal dose of orally ingested elemental iron is 300 mg per kg body weight. Serum iron and total iron-binding capacity may be used as guides for use of chelating agents such as deferoxamine.

DOSAGE AND ADMINISTRATION

One dropperful daily, or as directed by physician or dentist.

HOW SUPPLIED

50-mL Spil-gard® bottles, calibrated dropper enclosed; ℞; NDC 0074-8929-50.

VI-DAYLIN®/F MULTIVITAMIN Drops With Fluoride℞
[vī″dā′lin]
Multivitamins/Fluoride

DESCRIPTION

One dropperful (1.0 mL) provides:
Fluoride   0.25 mg

Vitamins			% U.S. RDA*	% U.S. RDA**
Vitamin A	1500	I.U.	100	60
Vitamin D	400	I.U.	100	100
Vitamin E	5	I.U.	100	50
Vitamin C	35	mg	100	87
Thiamine (Vitamin B₁)	0.5	mg	100	71
Riboflavin (Vitamin B₂)	0.6	mg	100	75
Niacin	8	mg	100	88
Vitamin B₆	0.4	mg	100	57

Active Ingredients: Ascorbic acid, niacinamide, d-alpha tocopheryl acid succinate, riboflavin-5′-phosphate sodium, sodium fluoride, vitamin A palmitate, thiamine hydrochloride, pyridoxine hydrochloride and ergocalciferol.
Inactive Ingredients: Alcohol less than 0.1%, benzoic acid, caramel coloring, corn oil, glycerin, methylparaben, water, natural flavoring and other ingredients. No artificial sweeteners.
Contains no sugar.
 *%U.S. Recommended Daily Allowance for infants.
**%U.S. Recommended Daily Allowance for children under 4 years of age.

INDICATIONS AND USAGE

As an aid in the prevention of dental caries in infants and children, and in the prophylaxis of appropriate vitamin deficiencies.

CONTRAINDICATIONS

Should be used only where the fluoride content of the drinking water supply is known to be 0.7 parts per million or less.

PRECAUTIONS

The recommended dosage should not be exceeded since chronic overdosage of fluoride may result in mottling of tooth enamel and osseous changes.

OVERDOSAGE

In children, acute ingestion of 10 to 20 mg of sodium fluoride may cause excessive salivation and gastrointestinal disturbances; 500 mg may be fatal. Oral and/or intravenous fluids containing calcium may be indicated.

DOSAGE AND ADMINISTRATION

One dropperful daily, or as directed by physician or dentist.

HOW SUPPLIED

50-mL Spil-gard® bottles, calibrated dropper enclosed; ℞; NDC 0074-1104-50.

VI-DAYLIN®/F MULTIVITAMIN + IRON Drops With Fluoride℞
[vī″dā′lin]
Multivitamins/Fluoride/Iron Supplement

DESCRIPTION

One dropperful (1.0 mL) provides:
Fluoride   0.25 mg

Vitamins			% U.S. RDA*	% U.S. RDA**
Vitamin A	1500	I.U.	100	60
Vitamin D	400	I.U.	100	100
Vitamin E	5	I.U.	100	50
Vitamin C	35	mg	100	87
Thiamine (Vitamin B₁)	0.5	mg	100	71
Riboflavin (Vitamin B₂)	0.6	mg	100	75
Niacin	8	mg	100	88
Vitamin B₆	0.4	mg	100	57
Minerals				
Iron	10	mg	66	100

Active Ingredients: Ascorbic acid, ferrous sulfate, niacinamide, d-alpha tocopheryl acid succinate, vitamin A palmitate, riboflavin-5′-phosphate sodium, thiamine hydrochloride, sodium fluoride, pyridoxine hydrochloride and ergocalciferol.
Inactive Ingredients: Alcohol less than 0.1%, benzoic acid, caramel coloring, corn oil, glycerin, methylparaben, water, natural flavoring and other ingredients.
Contains no sugar.
 *%U.S. Recommended Daily Allowance for infants.
**%U.S. Recommended Daily Allowance for children under 4 years of age.

INDICATIONS AND USAGE

As an aid in the prevention of dental caries in infants and children and in the prophylaxis of iron and appropriate vitamin deficiencies.

CONTRAINDICATIONS

Should be used only where the fluoride content of the drinking water supply is known to be 0.7 parts per million or less.

PRECAUTIONS

The recommended dosage should not be exceeded since chronic overdosage of fluoride may result in mottling of tooth enamel and osseous changes. In infants, oral iron-containing preparations may cause temporary darkening of the membrane covering the teeth.

OVERDOSAGE

In children, acute ingestion of 10 to 20 mg of sodium fluoride may cause excessive salivation and gastrointestinal disturbances; 500 mg may be fatal. Oral and/or intravenous fluids containing calcium may be indicated.
Acute overdosage of iron may cause nausea and vomiting and, in severe cases, cardiovascular collapse and death. The estimated lethal dose of orally ingested elemental iron is 300 mg per kg body weight. Serum iron and total iron-binding capacity may be used as guides for use of chelating agents such as deferoxamine.

DOSAGE AND ADMINISTRATION

One dropperful daily, or as directed by physician or dentist.

HOW SUPPLIED

50-mL Spil-gard® bottles, calibrated dropper enclosed; ℞; NDC 0074-8928-50.

VI-DAYLIN® MULTIVITAMIN Chewable Tablets
[vī″dā′lin]
Multivitamin Supplement

DESCRIPTION

Each chewable tablet provides:

Vitamins			%U.S. RDA*	%U.S. RDA**
Vitamin A	2500	I.U.	100	50
Vitamin D	400	I.U.	100	100
Vitamin E	15	I.U.	150	50
Vitamin C	60	mg	150	100
Folic Acid	0.3	mg	150	75
Thiamine (Vitamin B₁)	1.05	mg	150	70
Riboflavin (Vitamin B₂)	1.2	mg	150	70
Niacin	13.5	mg	150	67
Vitamin B₆	1.05	mg	150	52
Vitamin B₁₂	4.5	mcg	150	75

INGREDIENTS

Sucrose and dextrins, sodium ascorbate, niacinamide, dl-alpha tocopheryl acetate, ascorbic acid, vitamin A palmitate, riboflavin, pyridoxine hydrochloride, thiamine mononitrate, cholecalciferol, folic acid and cyanocobalamin. Made with natural sweeteners, artificial flavoring and artificially colored with natural ingredients.
 *% U.S. Recommended Daily Allowance for children under 4 years of age.
**% U.S. Recommended Daily Allowance for adults and children 4 or more years of age.

INDICATIONS AND USAGE

Multivitamin supplement for children and adults.

DOSAGE AND ADMINISTRATION

One chewable tablet daily, or as directed by physician.

HOW SUPPLIED

100-tablet bottles; OTC; List No. 4519-13.

Continued on next page

Ross—Cont.

VI-DAYLIN® MULTIVITAMIN + IRON
Chewable Tablets
[vī"dā'lin]
Multivitamin/Iron Supplement

DESCRIPTION
Each chewable tablet provides:

Vitamins			% U.S. RDA*	% U.S. RDA**
Vitamin A	2500	I.U.	100	50
Vitamin D	400	I.U.	100	100
Vitamin E	15	I.U.	150	50
Vitamin C	60	mg	150	100
Folic Acid	0.3	mg	150	75
Thiamine (Vitamin B$_1$)	1.05	mg	150	70
Riboflavin (Vitamin B$_2$)	1.2	mg	150	70
Niacin	13.5	mg	150	67
Vitamin B$_6$	1.05	mg	150	52
Vitamin B$_{12}$	4.5	mcg	150	75
Minerals				
Iron	12	mg	120	66

INGREDIENTS
Sucrose and dextrins, mannitol, sodium ascorbate, niacinamide, ferrous fumarate, dl-alpha tocopheryl acetate, ascorbic acid, vitamin A palmitate, riboflavin, pyridoxine hydrochloride, thiamine mononitrate, cholecalciferol, folic acid and cyanocobalamin. Made with natural sweeteners, artificial flavoring and FD&C Yellow No. 6.
  *%U.S. Recommended Daily Allowance for children under 4 years of age.
  **%U.S. Recommended Daily Allowance for adults and children 4 or more years of age.

INDICATIONS AND USAGE
Multivitamin supplement with iron for children and adults.

DOSAGE AND ADMINISTRATION
One tablet daily, or as directed by physician.

HOW SUPPLIED
100-tablet bottles; OTC; List No. 4520-13.

VI-DAYLIN®/F MULTIVITAMIN ℞
Chewable Tablets With Fluoride
[vī"dā'lin]
Multivitamins/Fluoride

DESCRIPTION
Each chewable tablet provides:
Fluoride (as sodium fluoride) 1 mg

Vitamins			%U.S. RDA*	%U.S. RDA**
Vitamin A (as palmitate, 0.75 mg)	2500	I.U.	100	50
Vitamin D (as cholecalciferol, 10 mcg)	400	I.U.	100	100
Vitamin E (as dl-alpha tocopheryl acetate)	15	I.U.	150	50
Vitamin C (as sodium ascorbate, 40 mg; ascorbic acid, 20 mg)	60	mg	150	100
Folic Acid	0.3	mg	150	75
Vitamin B$_1$ (as thiamine mononitrate)	1.05	mg	150	70
Vitamin B$_2$ (as riboflavin)	1.2	mg	150	70
Niacin (as niacinamide)	13.5	mg	150	67
Vitamin B$_6$ (as pyridoxine hydrochloride)	1.05	mg	150	52
Vitamin B$_{12}$ (as cyanocobalamin)	4.5	mcg	150	75

  *%U.S. Recommended Daily Allowance for children under 4 years of age.
  **%U.S. Recommended Daily Allowance for adults and children 4 or more years of age.

INACTIVE INGREDIENTS
Cellulosic polymers, citric acid, corn starch, DC Yellow No. 10, dextrin, FDC Yellow No. 6, magnesium stearate, sucrose, artificial flavoring and other ingredients.

INDICATIONS AND USAGE
As an aid in the prevention of dental caries in children, and in the prophylaxis of appropriate vitamin deficiencies.

CONTRAINDICATIONS
Should be used only where the fluoride content of the drinking water supply is known to be 0.7 parts per million or less.

PRECAUTIONS
The recommended dosage should not be exceeded since chronic overdosage of fluoride may result in mottling of tooth enamel and osseous changes.

OVERDOSAGE
In children, acute ingestion of 10 to 20 mg of sodium fluoride may cause excessive salivation and gastrointestinal disturbances: 500 mg may be fatal. Oral and/or intravenous fluids containing calcium may be indicated.

DOSAGE AND ADMINISTRATION
Children 3 years of age or older, 1 chewable tablet daily; age 2 to 3 years, ½ chewable tablet daily; or as directed by physician or dentist.

HOW SUPPLIED
100-tablet bottles; ℞; NDC 0074-7626-13.

VI-DAYLIN®/F MULTIVITAMIN + IRON ℞
Chewable Tablets With Fluoride
[vī"dā'lin]
Multivitamins/Fluoride/Iron

DESCRIPTION
Each chewable tablet provides:
Fluoride (as sodium fluoride) 1 mg

Vitamins			% U.S. RDA*	% U.S. RDA**
Vitamin A (as palmitate, 0.75 mg)	2500	I.U.	100	50
Vitamin D (as cholecalciferol, 10 mcg)	400	I.U.	100	100
Vitamin E (as dl-alpha tocopheryl acetate)	15	I.U.	150	50
Vitamin C (as sodium ascorbate, 40 mg; ascorbic acid, 20 mg)	60	mg	150	100
Folic Acid	0.3	mg	150	75
Vitamin B$_1$ (as thiamine mononitrate)	1.05	mg	150	70
Vitamin B$_2$ (as riboflavin)	1.2	mg	150	70
Niacin (as niacinamide)	13.5	mg	150	67
Vitamin B$_6$ (as pyridoxine hydrochloride)	1.05	mg	150	52
Vitamin B$_{12}$ (as cyanocobalamin)	4.5	mcg	150	75
Minerals				
Iron (as ferrous fumarate)	12	mg	120	66

  *%U.S. Recommended Daily Allowance for children under 4 years of age.
  **%U.S. Recommended Daily Allowance for adults and children 4 or more years of age.

INACTIVE INGREDIENTS
Carmine No. 40, cellulosic polymers, citric acid, corn starch, dextrin, FDC Yellow No. 6, magnesium stearate, mannitol, sodium chloride, sucrose, tricalcium phosphate, artificial flavoring and other ingredients.

INDICATIONS AND USAGE
As an aid in the prevention of dental caries in children, and in the prophylaxis of iron and appropriate vitamin deficiencies.

CONTRAINDICATIONS
Should be used only where the fluoride content of the drinking water supply is known to be 0.7 parts per million or less.

PRECAUTIONS
The recommended dosage should not be exceeded since chronic overdosage of fluoride may result in mottling of tooth enamel and osseous changes.

OVERDOSAGE
In children, acute ingestion of 10 to 20 mg of sodium fluoride may cause excessive salivation and gastrointestinal disturbances; 500 mg may be fatal. Oral and/or intravenous fluids containing calcium may be indicated.
Acute overdosage of iron may cause nausea and vomiting and, in severe cases, cardiovascular collapse and death. The estimated lethal dose of orally ingested elemental iron is 300 mg per kg body weight. Serum iron and total iron-binding capacity may be used as guides for use of chelating agents such as deferoxamine.

DOSAGE AND ADMINISTRATION
Children 3 years of age or older, one chewable tablet daily; age 2-3 years, ½ chewable tablet daily; or as directed by physician or dentist.

HOW SUPPLIED
100-tablet bottles; ℞; NDC 0074-7621-13.

VI-DAYLIN® MULTIVITAMIN Liquid
[vī"dā'lin]
Multivitamin Supplement

DESCRIPTION
One teaspoonful (5.0 mL) provides:

Vitamins			% U.S. RDA*	% U.S. RDA**
Vitamin A	2500	I.U.	100	50
Vitamin D	400	I.U.	100	100
Vitamin E	15	I.U.	150	50
Vitamin C	60	mg	150	100
Thiamine (Vitamin B$_1$)	1.05	mg	150	70
Riboflavin (Vitamin B$_2$)	1.2	mg	150	70
Niacin	13.5	mg	150	67
Vitamin B$_6$	1.05	mg	150	52
Vitamin B$_{12}$	4.5	mcg	150	75

  *% U.S. Recommended Daily Allowance for children under 4 years of age.
  **% U.S. Recommended Daily Allowance for adults and children 4 or more years of age.

INGREDIENTS
Glucose, sucrose, ascorbic acid, polysorbate 80, d-alpha tocopheryl acetate, niacinamide, acacia, cysteine hydrochloride (stabilizer), benzoic acid (preservative), vitamin A palmitate, methylparaben (preservative), pyridoxine hydrochloride, riboflavin, thiamine hydrochloride, ergocalciferol in corn oil, and cyanocobalamin in an aqueous vehicle with added natural citrus flavor and artificial color. Contains only a trace of alcohol (not more than ½%).

INDICATIONS AND USAGE
Multivitamin supplement for children and adults.

DOSAGE AND ADMINISTRATION
One teaspoonful daily, or as directed by physician.

HOW SUPPLIED
16-fl-oz (pint) bottles; OTC; List No. 3606-03.
8-fl-oz bottles; OTC; List No. 3606-02.

VI-DAYLIN® MULTIVITAMIN + IRON Liquid
[vī"dā'lin]
Multivitamin/Iron Supplement

DESCRIPTION
One teaspoonful (5.0 mL) provides:

Vitamins			% U.S. RDA*	% U.S. RDA**
Vitamin A	2500	I.U.	100	50
Vitamin D	400	I.U.	100	100
Vitamin E	15	I.U.	150	50
Vitamin C	60	mg	150	100
Thiamine (Vitamin B$_1$)	1.05	mg	150	70
Riboflavin (Vitamin B$_2$)	1.2	mg	150	70
Niacin	13.5	mg	150	67
Vitamin B$_6$	1.05	mg	150	52
Vitamin B$_{12}$	4.5	mcg	150	75
Minerals				
Iron	10	mg	100	55

  *% U.S. Recommended Daily Allowance for children under 4 years of age.
  **% U.S. Recommended Daily Allowance for adults and children 4 or more years of age.

INGREDIENTS
Glucose, sucrose, ascorbic acid, ferrous gluconate, polysorbate 80, d-alpha tocopheryl acetate, citric acid, niacinamide, acacia, cysteine hydrochloride (stabilizer), benzoic acid (preservative), methylparaben (preservative), vitamin A palmitate, riboflavin-5'-phosphate sodium, pyridoxine hydrochloride, thiamine hydrochloride, propylparaben (preservative), ergocalciferol in corn oil, and cyanocobalamin in an aqueous vehicle with added natural citrus flavor and artificial color. Contains only a trace of alcohol (not more than ½%).

INDICATIONS AND USAGE
Multivitamin supplement with iron for children and adults.

DOSAGE AND ADMINISTRATION
One teaspoonful daily, or as directed by physician.

HOW SUPPLIED
16-fl-oz (pint) bottles; OTC; List No. 6992-03.
8-fl-oz bottles; OTC; List No. 6992-02.

VITAL® HIGH NITROGEN
[vī'tel]
Nutritionally Complete
Partially Hydrolyzed Diet

USAGE

As a source of total or supplemental nutrition for patients with impaired gastrointestinal function (limited digestion/absorption). VITAL HIGH NITROGEN may be used as a tube feeding (nasogastric, nasoduodenal or jejunal) or as an oral feeding. Five servings (1500 Calories) meet or surpass 100% of the daily U.S. RDA for vitamins and minerals for adults and children 4 or more years of age.

DOSAGE AND ADMINISTRATION

Instructions for Use: [Standard Dilution—One packet of powder (79 g) mixed in 255 mL (8.5 fl oz) of water yields approximately 300 mL.] Pour 255 mL (8.5 fl oz) of cold water into a container. Empty contents of one packet into container and mix until powder dissolves. Prepare only the amount intended for a single day's feeding. Refrigerate after preparation. Store unopened powder in a cool, dry place.
Oral Feeding: Serving Vital High Nitrogen chilled enhances its flavor and increases palatability. May be used for total nutrition, or with and between meals.
Tube Feeding: Follow physician's instructions. Adjust flow rate, volume and dilution according to patient's condition and tolerance. Additional fluid requirements should be met by giving water orally with or after feedings. Avoid contamination during preparation and use.
Not for parenteral use.

AVAILABILITY

Powder: 2.79 oz (79 g) packets; 24 packets per case; Vanilla, No. 766.

COMPOSITION

Ingredients: Hydrolyzed cornstarch, protein components (partially hydrolyzed whey, meat and soy), sucrose, safflower oil, medium-chain triglycerides (fractionated coconut oil), artificial and natural flavor, magnesium sulfate, calcium phosphate tribasic, potassium phosphate dibasic, L-tyrosine, magnesium chloride, L-leucine, L-valine, L-isoleucine, L-phenylalanine, L-histidine, ascorbic acid, choline chloride, L-methionine, sodium chloride, L-threonine, mono- and di-glycerides, soy lecithin, L-tryptophan, zinc sulfate, ferrous sulfate, niacinamide, alpha-tocopheryl acetate, calcium pantothenate, manganese sulfate, thiamine chloride hydrochloride, pyridoxine hydrochloride, riboflavin, cupric sulfate, vitamin A palmitate, potassium citrate, folic acid, biotin, potassium iodide, phylloquinone, cyanocobalamin and vitamin D_3.

Nutrients: (grams)	Per 300 Calories* (1 packet)	Per 1500 Calories* (5 packets)
Protein	12.5	62.5
Fat	3.25	16.25
Carbohydrate	55.4	277
Water (Max)	5.2	26.0

*In standard dilution (79 g of Vital High Nitrogen Powder mixed in 255 mL of water).
(FAN 574-03)

EDUCATIONAL MATERIAL

A complete program of educational services for health professionals and patients is available.
Contact your local Ross representative.

Roxane Laboratories, Inc.
P.O. 16532
COLUMBUS, OH 43216-6532

HOSPITAL UNIT DOSE

Hospital Unit Dose—Roxane, was developed to aid in improved drug distribution and administration. With Hospital Unit Dose, each single unit of medication moves from our quality controlled production lines to the patient's bedside in tamper resistant containers, labeled for positive identification, thus protecting dosage integrity to the point of administration.
The following products are currently available in Hospital Unit Dose:

Acetaminophen Elixir (lime) 325mg/10.15mL, 650mg/20.3mL
Acetaminophen Elixir (cherry) 160mg/5mL, 325mg/10.15mL, 650mg/20.3mL

Acetaminophen Suppositories 120mg, 650mg
Acetaminophen Tablets USP 325mg, 500mg, 650mg
Acetaminophen 120mg and Codeine Phosphate 12mg Elixir USP
Acetaminophen 300mg and Codeine Phosphate 30mg Tablets USP
Acetaminophen 300mg and Codeine Phosphate 60mg Tablets USP
Aluminum Hydroxide Gel USP (Flavored) 2700mg/30mL
Aluminum Hydroxide, Concentrate, 2700mg/20mL, 4050mg/30mL
Aluminum Hydroxide Tablets 500mg
Aluminum and Magnesium Hydroxides with Simethicone I 15mL, 30mL
Aluminum and Magnesium Hydroxides with Simethicone II 15mL, 30mL
Aminophylline Tablets USP 100mg, 200mg
Aminophylline Oral Solution USP 210mg/10mL, 315mg/15mL
Amitriptyline Hydrochloride Tablets USP 10mg, 25mg, 50mg, 75mg, 100mg, 150mg
Aromatic Cascara Fluidextract USP 5mL
Aromatic Castor Oil USP 30mL, 60mL
Ascorbic Acid Tablets USP 250mg, 500mg
Bisacodyl Suppositories USP 10mg
Bisacodyl Tablets USP 5mg
Calcium Carbonate Tablets USP 1250mg
Calcium Carbonate Oral Suspension 1250mg/5mL
Calcium Gluconate Tablets USP 500mg
Castor Oil USP 30mL, 60mL
Chloral Hydrate Syrup USP 500mg/10mL, 1g/10mL
Chloral Hydrate Capsules USP 500mg
Chlorpheniramine Maleate Tablets USP 4mg
Cocaine Hydrochloride Topical Solution 4%/4mL, 10%/4mL
Codeine Sulfate Tablets USP 15mg, 30mg, 60mg
Dexamethasone Oral Solution 0.5mg/5mL, 2mg/20mL
Dexamethasone Tablets USP 0.5mg, 0.75mg, 1mg, 1.5mg, 2mg, 4mg, 6mg
Diazepam Oral Solution 5 mg/5 mL, 10 mg/10 mL
Diazepam Tablets USP 2mg, 5mg, 10mg
Digoxin Elixir USP
DHT (Dihydrotachysterol) Tablets USP 0.125mg, 0.2mg
Diluent (Flavored) for Oral Use 15mL
Diphenhydramine Hydrochloride Elixir USP 25mg/10mL
Diphenhydramine Hydrochloride Capsules USP 50mg
Diphenoxylate Hydrochloride 2.5mg and Atropine Sulfate 0.025mg Tablets USP
Diphenoxylate Hydrochloride and Atropine Sulfate Oral Solution USP 4mL, 10mL
Docusate Sodium Capsules USP 50mg, 100mg, 250mg
Docusate Sodium Syrup USP 50mg/15mL, 100mg/30mL
Docusate Sodium 100mg with Casanthranol 30mg Capsules
Ferrous Sulfate Oral Solution 300mg/5mL
Ferrous Sulfate Tablets USP 300mg
Furosemide Oral Solution 40mg/5mL, 80mg/10mL
Furosemide Tablets USP 20mg, 40mg, 80mg
Guaifenesin Syrup USP 100mg/5mL, 200mg/10mL, 300mg/15mL
Haloperidol Tablets USP 0.5 mg, 1 mg, 2 mg, 5 mg, 10 mg and 20 mg
Hydromorphone Hydrochloride Tablets USP 2mg, 4mg
Imipramine Hydrochloride Tablets USP 10mg, 25mg, 50mg
Indomethacin Capsules USP 25mg, 50mg
Ipecac Syrup USP 15mL, 30mL
Isoetharine Inhalation Solution USP 0.1%, 2.5mL
Isoetharine Inhalation Solution USP 0.125%, 4mL
Isoetharine Inhalation Solution USP 0.167%, 3mL
Isoetharine Inhalation Solution USP 0.2%, 2.5mL
Isoetharine Inhalation Solution USP 0.25%, 2mL
Kaolin-Pectin Suspension 30mL
Levorphanol Tartrate Tablets USP 2 mg
Lidocaine Viscous 2% 20mL
Lithium Carbonate Capsules USP 150mg, 300mg, 600mg
Lithium Carbonate Tablets USP 300mg
Lithium Citrate Syrup 8 mEq per 5mL, 16 mEq per 10mL
Magaldrate Oral Suspension USP 30mL
Magnesia and Alumina Oral Suspension USP 30mL
Metaproterenol Sulfate Syrup USP 5mg/2.5 mL, 10mg/5mL, 20mg/10mL
Methadone Hydrochloride Oral Solution USP 5mg/5mL, 10mg/10mL
Methadone Hydrochloride Tablets USP 5mg, 10mg
Methyldopa Tablets USP 125mg, 250mg, 500mg
Milk of Magnesia USP 15mL, 30mL
Milk of Magnesia Concentrated Flavored 10mL, 15mL, 20mL
Milk of Magnesia—Cascara Suspension Concentrated 15mL
Milk of Magnesia—Mineral Oil Emulsion 30mL
Milk of Magnesia—Mineral Oil Emulsion (Flavored) 30mL
Mineral Oil-Light Sterile 10mL, 30mL
Mineral Oil USP 30mL
Morphine Sulfate Tablets 15mg, 30mg
Morphine Sulfate Oral Solution 10mg/5mL, 20mg/10mL
Neomycin Sulfate Tablets USP 500mg
Paregoric USP 5mL

Phenobarbital Elixir USP 20mg/5mL, 30mg/7.5mL
Phenobarbital Tablets USP 15mg, 30mg, 60mg, 100mg
Potassium Chloride Oral Solution USP 10% (15mEq/11.25mL), (20mEq/15mL), (30mEq/22.5mL), (40mEq/30mL)
Prednisolone Tablets USP 5mg
Prednisone Oral Solution 5mg/5mL, 10mg/10mL
Prednisone Tablets USP 1mg, 2.5mg, 5mg, 10mg, 20mg, 50mg
Propantheline Bromide Tablets USP 15mg
Propoxyphene Hydrochloride Capsules USP 65mg
Propranolol Hydrochloride Tablets USP 10mg, 20mg, 40mg, 60mg, 80mg, 90mg
Propranolol Hydrochloride Oral Solution 20 mg/5 mL and 40 mg/5 mL
Pseudoephedrine Hydrochloride Tablets USP 30mg, 60mg
Quinidine Gluconate Sustained Release Tablets 324mg
Quinidine Sulfate Tablets USP 200mg, 300mg
Roxanol UD (morphine sulfate concentrated oral solution)
Roxanol SR Tablets (morphine sulfate sustained release tablets) 30mg
Roxicet Oral Solution (oxycodone hydrochloride 5mg and acetaminophen 325mg/5mL)
Roxicet Tablets (oxycodone hydrochloride 5mg and acetaminophen 325mg)
Roxicet 5/500 Caplets (oxycodone and acetaminophen tablets USP)
Roxicodone Oral Solution (oxycodone hydrochloride oral solution USP 5mg/5mL)
Roxicodone Tablets (oxycodone hydrochloride tablets USP 5mg)
Roxiprin Tablets (oxycodone hydrochloride 4.5mg, oxycodone terephalate 0.38mg, and aspirin 325mg tablets USP)
Sodium Chloride Inhalation Solution USP (Normal Saline) Sterile 0.9% 3mL, 5mL
Sodium Phosphates Oral Solution USP 30mL
Sodium Polystyrene Sulfonate Suspension 60mL, and 120mL Enema Package
Terpin Hydrate and Codeine Elixir USP 5mL
Theophylline Oral Solution 80mg/15mL, 100mg/18.75mL, 160mg/30mL
Thioridazine Hydrochloride Tablets USP 10mg, 25mg, 50mg, 100mg
Torecan Tablets (thiethylperazine tablets USP)
As research continues, new Roxane Laboratories' products will be available in Hospital Unit Dose packages.

DHT™
Dihydrotachysterol
Tablets USP and Intensol

℞

DESCRIPTION

Each tablet contains:
Dihydrotachysterol .... 0.125 mg, 0.2 mg, or 0.4 mg
Each mL of Intensol contains:
Dihydrotachysterol .... 0.2 mg
Dihydrotachysterol is a synthetic reduction product of tachysterol, a close isomer of vitamin D. Chemically Dihydrotachysterol is 9, 10- Secoergosta-5,7,22-tri-en-3β- ol. Dihydrotachysterol acts as a blood calcium regulator.

CLINICAL PHARMACOLOGY

Dyhydrotachysterol is hydroxylated in the liver to 25-hydroxydihydrotachysterol, which is the major circulating active form of the drug. It does not undergo further hydroxylation by the kidney and therefore is the analogue of 1,25-dihydroxyvitamin D. Dihydrotachysterol is effective in the elevation of serum calcium by stimulating intestinal calcium absorption and mobilizing bone calcium in the absence of parathyroid hormone and of functioning renal tissue. Dihydrotachysterol also increases renal phosphate excretion. In contrast to parathyroid extract, Dihydrotachysterol is active when taken orally, exerts a slow but persistent effect, and may be used for long periods without increasing the dosage or causing tolerance. Dihydrotachysterol is faster-acting than pharmacologic doses of vitamin D and is less persistent after cessation of treatment, thus decreasing the risk of accumulation and of hypercalcemia.

INDICATIONS AND USAGE

Dihydrotachysterol is indicated for the treatment of acute, chronic, and latent forms of postoperative tetany, idiopathic tetany, and hypoparathyroidism.

CONTRAINDICATIONS

Contraindicated in patients with hypercalcemia, abnormal sensitivity to the effects of vitamin D, and hypervitaminosis D.

PRECAUTIONS

General: The difference between therapeutic dose and intoxicating dose may be small in any patient and therefore dosage must be individualized and periodically reevaluated.

Continued on next page

Roxane—Cont.

In patients with renal osteodystrophy accompanied by hyperphosphatemia, maintenance of a normal serum phosphorus level by dietary phosphate restriction and/or administration of aluminum gels as intestinal phosphate binders is essential to prevent metastatic calcification.

Because of its effect on serum calcium, Dihydrotachysterol should be administered to pregnant patients or to patients with renal stones only when, in the judgment of the physician, the potential benefits outweigh the possible hazards.

Laboratory tests: To prevent hypercalcemia, treatment should always be controlled by regular determinations of blood calcium level, which should be maintained within the normal range.

Drug interactions: Administration of thiazide diuretics to hypoparathyroid patients who are concurrently being treated with Dihydrotachysterol may cause hypercalcemia.

Pregnancy: Teratogenic effects —Pregnancy Category C: Animal reproduction studies have shown fetal abnormalities in several species associated with hypervitaminosis D. These are similar to the supravalvular aortic stenosis syndrome described in infants by Black in England (1963). This syndrome was characterized by supravalvular aortic stenosis, elfin facies, and mental retardation.

There are no adequate and well-controlled studies in pregnant women. Dihydrotachysterol should be used during pregnancy only if the potential benefit justifies the potential risk to the fetus.

Nursing mothers: It is not known whether this drug is excreted in human milk. Because many drugs are excreted in human milk, caution should be exercised when Dihydrotachysterol is administered to a nursing woman.

OVERDOSAGE

The effects of Dihydrotachysterol can persist for up to one month after cessation of treatment.

Manifestations: Toxicity associated with Dihydrotachysterol is similar to that seen with large doses of vitamin D. Overdosage is manifested by symptoms of hypercalcemia, i.e., weakness, headache, anorexia, nausea, vomiting, abdominal cramps, diarrhea, constipation, vertigo, tinnitus, ataxia, hypotonia, lethargy, depression, amnesia, disorientation, hallucinations, syncope, and coma. Impairment of renal function may result in polyuria, polydipsia, and albuminuria. Widespread calcification of soft tissues, including heart, blood vessels, kidneys, and lungs, can occur. Death can result from cardiovascular or renal failure.

Treatment: Treatment of overdosage consists of withdrawal of Dihydrotachysterol, bed rest, liberal intake of fluids, a low-calcium diet, and administration of a laxative. Hypercalcemic crisis with dehydration, stupor, coma, and azotemia requires more vigorous treatment. The first step should be hydration of the patient. Intravenous saline may quickly and significantly increast urinary calcium excretion. A loop diuretic (furosemide or ethacrynic acid) may be given with the saline infusion to further increase renal calcium excretion. Other reported therapeutic measures include dialysis or the administration of citrates, sulfates, phosphates, corticosteroids, EDTA (ethylenediaminetetraacetic acids), and mithramycin via appropriate regimens.

DOSAGE AND ADMINISTRATION

The dosage depends on the nature and seriousness of the disorder and should be adapted to each individual patient. Serum calcium levels should be maintained between 9 to 10 mg per 100 mL.

The following dosage schedule will serve as a guide:

Initial dose: 0.8 mg to 2.4 mg daily for several days.

Maintenance dose: 0.2 mg to 1.0 mg daily as required for normal serum calcium levels. The average maintenance dose is 0.6 mg daily. This dose may be supplemented with 10 to 15 grams of calcium lactate or gluconate by mouth daily.

HOW SUPPLIED

0.125 mg white tablets.
NDC 0054-8172-25: Unit dose, 10 tablets per strip, 10 strips per shelf pack, 10 shelf packs per shipper.
NDC 0054-4190-19: Bottles of 50 tablets.

0.2 mg pink tablets.
NDC 0054-8182-25: Unit dose, 10 tablets per strip, 10 strips per shelf pack, 10 shelf packs per shipper.
NDC 0054-4189-25: Bottles of 100 tablets.

0.4 mg white tablets.
NDC 0054-4191-19: Bottles of 50 tablets.

Intensol 0.2 mg/mL
NDC 0054-3170-44: Bottles of 30 mL with calibrated dropper (graduated 0.25 mL to 1.0 mL)

LITHIUM CARBONATE   ℞
CAPSULES USP 150 mg, 300 mg, and 600 mg
TABLETS USP 300 mg

WARNING
Lithium toxicity is closely related to serum lithium levels, and can occur at doses close to therapeutic levels. Facilities for prompt and accurate serum lithium determinations should be available before initiating therapy.

DESCRIPTION

Each tablet for oral administration contains:
  Lithium Carbonate .... 300 mg
Each capsule for oral administration contains:
  Lithium Carbonate .... 150 mg, 300 mg, or 600 mg

Inactive Ingredients:
The capsules contain talc, gelatin, FD&C Red No. 40, titanium dioxide, and the imprinting ink contains FD&C Blue No. 2, FD&C Yellow No. 6, FD&C Red No. 40, synthetic black iron oxide, and pharmaceutical glaze. The tablets contain calcium stearate, microcrystalline cellulose, povidone, sodium lauryl sulfate, and sodium starch glycolate.

Lithium Carbonate is a white, light alkaline powder with molecular formula Li_2CO_3 and molecular weight 73.89. Lithium is an element of the alkali-metal group with atomic number 3, atomic weight 6.94 and an emission line at 671 nm on the flame photometer. Lithium acts as an antimanic.

CLINICAL PHARMACOLOGY

Preclinical studies have shown that lithium alters sodium transport in nerve and muscle cells and effects a shift toward intraneuronal metabolism of catecholamines, but the specific biochemical mechanism of lithium action in mania is unknown.

INDICATIONS AND USAGE

Lithium carbonate is indicated in the treatment of manic episodes of Bipolar Disorder. Bipolar Disorder, Manic (DSM-III) is equivalent to Manic Depressive illness, Manic, in the older DSM-II terminology.

Lithium is also indicated as a maintenance treatment for individuals with a diagnosis of Bipolar Disorder. Maintenance therapy reduces the frequency of manic episodes and diminishes the intensity of those episodes which may occur. Typical symptoms of mania include pressure of speech, motor hyperactivity, reduced need for sleep, flight of ideas, grandiosity, or poor judgment, aggressiveness, and possibly hostility. When given to a patient experiencing a manic episode, lithium may produce a normalization of symptomatology within 1 to 3 weeks.

CONTRAINDICATIONS

Lithium should generally not be given to patients with significant renal or cardiovascular disease, severe debilitation or dehydration, or sodium depletion, and to patients receiving diuretics, since the risk of lithium toxicity is very high in such patients. If the psychiatric indication is life-threatening, and if such a patient fails to respond to other measures, lithium treatment may be undertaken with extreme caution, including daily serum lithium determinations and adjustment to the usualy low doses ordinarily tolerated by these individuals. In such instances, hospitlization is a necessity.

WARNINGS

Lithium may cause fetal harm when administered to a pregnant woman. There have been reports of lithium having adverse effects on nidation in rats, embryo viability in mice, and metabolism in-vitro of rat testis and human spermatozoa have been attributed to lithium, as have teratogenicity in submammalian species and cleft palates in mice. Studies in rats, rabbits and monkeys have shown no evidence of lithium-induced teratology. Data from lithium birth registries suggest an increase in cardiac and other anomalies, especially Ebstein's anomaly. If the patient becomes pregnant while taking lithium, she should be apprised of the potential risk to the fetus. If possible, lithium should be withdrawn for at least the first trimester unless it is determined that this would seriously endanger the mother.

Chronic lithium therapy may be associated with diminution of renal concentrating ability, occasionally presenting as nephrogenic diabetes insipidus, with polyuria and polydipsia. Such patients should be carefully managed to avoid dehydration with resulting lithium retention and toxicity. This condition is usually reversible when lithium is discontinued. Morphologic changes with glomerular and interstitial fibrosis and nephron-atrophy have been reported in patients on chronic lithium therapy. Morphologic changes have been seen in bipolar patients never exposed to lithium. The relationship between renal functional and morphologic changes and their association with lithium therapy has not been established. To date, lithium in therapeutic doses has not been reported to cause end-stage renal disease.

When kidney function is assessed, for baseline data prior to starting lithium therapy or thereafter, routine urinalysis and other tests may be used to evaluate tubular function

(e.g., urine specific gravity or osmolality following a period of water deprivation, or 24-hour urine volume) and glomerular function (e.g., serum creatinine or creatinine clearance). During lithium therapy, progressive or sudden changes in renal function, even within the normal range, indicate the need for reevaluation of treatment.

Lithium toxicity is closely related to serum lithium levels, and can occur at doses close to therapeutic levels (see DOSAGE AND ADMINISTRATION).

PRECAUTIONS

General: The ability to tolerate lithium is greater during the acute manic phase and decreases when manic symptoms subside (See DOSAGE AND ADMINISTRATION).

The distribution space of lithium approximates that of total body water. Lithium is primarily excreted in urine with insignificant excretion in feces. Renal excretion of lithium is proportional to its plasma concentration. The half-life of elimination of lithium is approximately 24 hours. Lithium decreases sodium reabsorption by the renal tubules which could lead to sodium depletion. Therefore, it is essential for the patient to maintain a normal diet, including salt, and an adequate fluid intake (2500-3000 mL) at least during the initial stabilization period. Decreased tolerance to lithium has been reported to ensue from protracted sweating or diarrhea and, if such occur, supplemental fluid and salt should be administered.

In addition to sweating and diarrhea, concomitant infection with elevated temperatures may also necessitate a temporary reduction or cessation of medication.

Previously existing underlying thyroid disorders do not necessarily constitute a contraindication to lithium treatment; where hypothyroidism exists, careful monitoring of thyroid function during lithium stabilization and maintenance allows for correction of changing thyroid parameters, if any. Where hypothyroidism occurs during lithium stabilization and maintenance, supplemental thyroid treatment may be used.

Information for the patients: Outpatients and their families should be warned that the patient must discontinue lithium therapy and contact his physician if such clinical signs of lithium toxicity as diarrhea, vomiting, tremor, mild ataxia, drowsiness, or muscular weakness occur.

Lithium may impair mental and/or physical abilities. Caution patients about activities requiring alertness (e.g., operating vehicles or machinery).

Drug interactions: *Combined use of haloperidol and lithium:* An encephalopathic syndrome (characterized by weakness, lethargy, fever, tremulousness and confusion, extrapyramidal symptoms, leucocytosis, elevated serum enzymes, BUN and FBS) followed by irreversible brain damage has occurred in a few patients treated with lithium plus haloperidol. A causal relationship between these events and the concomitant administration of lithium and haloperidol has not been established; however, patients receiving such combined therapy should be monitored closely for early evidence of neurological toxicity and treatment discontinued promptly if such signs appear.

The possibility of similar adverse interactions with other antipsychotic medication exists.

Lithium may prolong the effects of neuromuscular blocking agents. Therefore, neuromuscular blocking agents should be given with caution to patients receiving lithium.

Indomethacin and piroxicam have been reported to increase significantly steady state plasma lithium levels. In some cases lithium toxicity has resulted from such interactions. There is also evidence that other non-steroidal, anti-inflammatory agents may have a similar effect. When such combinations are used, increased plasma lithium level monitoring is recommended.

There is evidence that the angiotensin converting enzyme inhibitors, enalapril and captopril, may substantially increase steady state plasma lithium levels, sometimes resulting in lithium toxicity. When such combinations are used, the lithium dose may need to be decreased, and increased plasma lithium level monitoring is recommended.

Pregnancy: Teratogenic effects—Pregnancy Category D, See "Warnings" section.

Nursing mothers: Lithium is excreted in human milk. Nursing should not be undertaken during lithium therapy except in rare and unusual circumstances where, in the view of the physician, the potential benefits to the mother outweigh possible hazards to the child.

Usage in Children: Since information regarding the safety and effectiveness of lithium in children under 12 years of age is not available, its use in such patients is not recommended at this time. There has been a report of a transient syndrome of acute dystonia and hyperreflexia occurring in a 15 kg child who ingested 300 mg lithium carbonate.

ADVERSE REACTIONS

Lithium toxicity: The likelihood of toxicity increases with increasing serum lithium levels. Serum lithium levels greater than 1.5 mEq/l carry a greater risk than lower levels. However, patients sensitive to lithium may exhibit toxic signs at serum levels below 1.5 mEq/l.

Diarrhea, vomiting, drowsiness, muscular weakness and lack of coordination may be early signs of lithium toxicity, and can occur at lithium levels below 2.0 mEq/l. At higher levels, giddiness, ataxia, blurred vision, tinnitus and a large output of dilute urine may be seen. Serum lithium levels above 3.0 mEq/l may produce a complex clinical picture involving multiple organs and organ systems. Serum lithium levels should not be permitted to exceed 2.0 mEq/l during the acute treatment phase.

Fine hand tremor, polyuria and mild thirst may occur during initial therapy for the acute manic phase, and may persist throughout treatment. Transient and mild nausea and general discomfort may also appear during the first few days of lithium administration.

These side effects are an inconvenience rather than a disabling condition, and usually subside with continued treatment or a temporary reduction or cessation of dosage. If persistent, a cessation of dosage is indicated.

The following adverse reactions have been reported and do not appear to be directly related to serum lithium levels.

Neuromuscular: tremor, muscle hyperirritability (fasciculations, twitching, clonic movements of whole limbs), ataxia, choreo-athetotic movements, hyperactive deep tendon reflexes.

Central Nervous System: Blackout spells, epileptiform seizures, slurred speech, dizziness, vertigo, incontinence of urine or feces, somnolence, psychomotor retardation, restlessness, confusion, stupor, coma, acute dystonia, downbeat nystagmus.

Cardiovascular: cardiac arrhythmia, hypotension, peripheral circulatory collapse.

Neurological: Cases of pseudotumor cerebri (increased intracranial pressure and papilledema) have been reported with lithium use. If undetected, this condition may result in enlargement of the blind spot, constriction of visual fields and eventual blindness due to optic atrophy. Lithium should be discontinued, if clinically possible, if this syndrome occurs.

Gastrointestinal: anorexia, nausea, vomiting, diarrhea.

Genitourinary: albuminuria, oliguria, polyuria, glycosuria.

Dermatologic: drying and thinning of hair, anesthesia of skin, chronic folliculitis, xerosis cutis, alopecia and exacerbation of psoriasis.

Autonomic Nervous System: blurred vision, dry mouth.

Miscellaneous: fatigue, lethargy, tendency to sleep, dehydration, weight loss, transient scotomata.

Thyroid Abnormalities: euthyroid goiter and/or hypothyroidism (including myxedema) accompanied by lower T_3 and T_4. Iodine 131 uptake may be elevated. (See PRECAUTIONS). Paradoxically, rare cases of hyperthyroidism have been reported.

EEG Changes: diffuse slowing, widening of frequency spectrum, potentiation and disorganization of background rhythm.

EKG Changes: reversible flattening, isoelectricity or inversion of T-waves.

Miscellaneous: fatigue, lethargy, transient scotomata, dehydration, weight loss, tendency to sleep.

Miscellaneous reactions unrelated to dosage are: transient electroencephalographic and electrocardiographic changes, leucocytosis, headache, diffuse nontoxic goiter with or without hypothyroidism, transient hyperglycemia, generalized pruritis with or without rash, cutaneous ulcers, albuminuria, worsening of organic brain syndromes, excessive weight gain, edematous swelling of ankles or wrists, and thirst or polyuria, sometimes resembling diabetes insipidus, and metallic taste.

A single report has been received of the development of painful discoloration of fingers and toes and coldness of the extremities within one day of the starting of treatment of lithium. The mechanism through which these symptoms (resembling Raynaud's Syndrome) developed is not known. Recovery followed discontinuance.

OVERDOSAGE

The toxic levels for lithium are close to the therapeutic levels. It is therefore important that patients and their families be cautioned to watch for early symptoms and to discontinue the drug and inform the physician should they occur. Toxic symptoms are listed in detail under ADVERSE REACTIONS.

Treatment: No specific antidote for lithium poisoning is known. Early symptoms of lithium toxicity can usually be treated by reduction or cessation of dosage of the drug and resumption of the treatment at a lower dose after 24 to 48 hours. In severe cases of lithium poisoning, the first and foremost goal of treatment consists of elimination of this ion from the patient.

Treatment is essentially the same as that used in barbiturate poisoning: 1) gastric lavage, 2) correction of fluid and electrolyte imbalance and 3) regulation of kidney functioning. Urea, mannitol, and aminophylline all produce significant increases in lithium excretion. Hemodialysis is an effective and rapid means of removing the ion from the severely toxic patient. Infection prophylaxis, regular chest X-rays, and preservation of adequate respiration are essential.

DOSAGE AND ADMINISTRATION

Acute Mania: Optimal patient response to Lithium Carbonate usually can be established and maintained with 600 mg t.i.d. Such doses will normally produce an effective serum lithium level ranging between 1.0 and 1.5 mEq/l. Dosage must be individualized according to serum levels and clinical response. Regular monitoring of the patient's clinical state and of serum lithium levels is necessary. Serum levels should be determined twice per week during the acute phase, and until the serum level and clinical condition of the patient have been stabilized.

Long-term Control: The desirable serum lithium levels are 0.6 to 1.2 mEq/l. Dosage will vary from one individual to another, but usually 300 mg t.i.d. or q.i.d. will maintain this level. Serum lithium levels in uncomplicated cases receiving maintenance therapy during remission should be monitored at least every two months.

Patients abnormally sensitive to lithium may exhibit toxic signs at serum levels of 1.0 to 1.5 mEq/l. Elderly patients often respond to reduced dosage, and may exhibit signs of toxicity at serum levels ordinarily tolerated by other patients.

N.B.: Blood samples for serum lithium determination should be drawn immediately prior to the next dose when lithium concentrations are relatively stable (i.e., 8–12 hours after the previous dose.) Total reliance must not be placed on serum levels alone. Accurate patient evaluation requires both clinical and laboratory analysis.

HOW SUPPLIED

Lithium Carbonate Tablets USP

300 mg white, scored tablets (Identified 54 452)

NDC 0054-8528-25: Unit dose, 10 tablets per strip, 10 strips per shelf pack, 10 shelf packs per shipper.

(For Institutional Use Only).

NDC 0054-4527-25: Bottles of 100 tablets.

NDC 0054-4527-31: Bottles of 1000 tablets.

Lithium Carbonate Capsules USP

150 mg white opaque colored capsules (size 4) (Identified 54 213).

NDC 0054-8526-25: Unit dose, 10 capsules per strip, 10 strips per shelf pack, 10 shelf packs per shipper.

(For Institutional Use Only).

NDC 0054-2526-25: Bottles of 100 capsules.

NDC 0054-2526-31: Bottles of 1000 capsules.

300 mg flesh-colored capsules (size 2) (Identified 54 463).

NDC 0054-8527-25: Unit dose, 10 capsules per strip, 10 strips per shelf pack, 10 shelf packs per shipper.

(For Institutional Use Only).

NDC 0054-2527-25: Bottles of 100 capsules.

NDC 0054-2527-31: Bottles of 1000 capsules.

600 mg white opaque/flesh colored capsules (size 0) (Identified 54 702).

NDC 0054-8531-25: Unit dose, 10 capsules per strip, 10 strips per shelf pack, 10 shelf packs per shipper.

(For Institutional Use Only.)

NDC 0054-2531-25: Bottles of 100 capsules.

NDC 0054-2531-31: Bottles of 1000 capsules.

LITHIUM CITRATE SYRUP USP   ℞

8 mEq of Lithium per 5 mL, 16mEq of Lithium per 10 mL

SUGAR FREE

FOR ORAL ADMINISTRATION ONLY

DESCRIPTION

Lithium Citrate Syrup is a palatable oral dosage form of lithium ion. Lithium citrate is prepared in solution from lithium hydroxide and citric acid in a ratio approximating di-lithium citrate:

Each 5 mL of Lithium Citrate Syrup contains 8 mEq of lithium ion (Li+), equivalent to the amount of lithium in 300 mg of lithium carbonate and alcohol 0.3% v/v.

Inactive ingredients:

The syrup contains alcohol, sorbitol, flavoring, water, and other ingredients.

Lithium is an element of the alkali-metal group with atomic number 3, atomic weight 6.94, and an emission line at 671 nm on the flame photometer.

HOW SUPPLIED

Lithium Citrate Syrup, 8 mEq per 5 mL

NDC 0054-8529-04: Unit dose Patient Cup™ filled to deliver 5 mL, ten 5 mL Patient Cups™ per shelf pack, ten shelf packs per shipper. (For Institutional Use Only.)

NDC 0054-3527-63: Bottles of 500 mL.

Lithium Citrate Syrup, 16 mEq per 10 mL

NDC 0054-8530-04: Unit dose Patient Cup™ filled to deliver 10 mL, ten 10 mL Patient Cups™ per shelf pack, ten shelf packs per shipper. (For Institutional Use Only.)

Refer to Lithium Carbonate Capsules and Tablets heading for complete text.

MARINOL®   ℃ ℞
(Dronabinol)

(WARNING: May be habit forming)

DESCRIPTION

Each capsule for oral administration contains:

Dronabinol .... 2.5 mg, 5 mg, or 10 mg

(Warning: May be habit forming)

MARINOL brand of dronabinol (delta-9-tetrahydrocannabinol, THC), [(6aR-trans)-6a,7,8,10a-tetrahydro-6,6,9-trimethyl-3-pentyl-6H-dibenzo[b,d]pyran-1-ol] is the principal psychoactive substance present in *Cannabis sativa L.* (marijuana). It has the empirical formula $C_{21}H_{30}O_2$ with the molecular weight of 314.45. It has the following structural formula:

MARINOL is chemically synthesized and formulated in sesame oil and encapsulated in round soft gelatin capsules for oral administration.

CLINICAL PHARMACOLOGY

Non-therapeutic Effects

Dronabinol, commonly known as delta-9-THC, is one of the major active substances in marijuana. For practical purposes, the non-therapeutic effects of dronabinol may be considered essentially identical to those of marijuana and other centrally active cannabinoids. MARINOL is highly abusable and can produce both physical and psychological dependence.

Dronabinol has complex effects upon the central nervous system. Subjects using cannabis may experience changes in mood (euphoria, detachment, depression, anxiety, panic, paranoia, etc.), decrements in cognitive performance and memory, a decreased ability to control drives and impulses, and alterations in the experience of reality (e.g., distortions in the perception of objects and the sense of time, hallucinations, etc.). These latter phenomena appear to be more common when larger doses of dronabinol are administered; however, a full blown picture of psychosis (psychotic organic brain syndrome) may occur in patients receiving doses within the lower portion of the therapeutic range.

Reliable information on the behavioral effects of chronic dronabinol use is not available; however, it has been reported that chronic use of cannabis may be associated with decrements in motivation, cognition, judgment, etc. (Whether these impairments reflect the underlying character of individuals chronically abusing cannabis or are a result of the use of cannabis is not known.)

Dronabinol, used within or slightly above the recommended dose range, has several systemic effects of interest. It characteristically causes an increase in heart rate and conjunctival injection. Its effects on blood pressure are inconsistent, but occasional subjects have experienced orthostatic hypotension and/or fainting upon standing. In one study, a slight, but consistent, decrease in oral temperature was recorded. The potential of dronabinol to cause tolerance and physical dependence was examined in a 30 day rising dose tolerance study. Following thirty days of use, tolerance developed to the cardiovascular and subjective effects of dronabinol administered at doses up to 210 mg/day. An initial tachycardia induced by dronabinol was replaced successively by normal sinus rhythm and then bradycardia. A fall in supine blood pressure, made worse by standing, was also observed initially. Within days, however, these effects disappeared, indicating the development of tolerance.

A withdrawal syndrome, consisting of irritability, insomnia, and restlessness, was observed in some subjects within 12 hours following abrupt withdrawal of dronabinol. The syndrome reached its peak intensity at 24 hours when subjects exhibited "hot flashes", sweating, rhinorrhea, loose stools, hiccoughs and anorexia. The syndrome was essentially complete within 96 hours. Electroencephalographic changes recorded following dronabinol discontinuation were consistent with a withdrawal syndrome. While on drug, dronabinol produced a decrease in REM sleep. Following discontinuation, a marked rebound of REM sleep occurred. Several subjects reported impressions of disturbed sleep for several weeks after discontinuing high dose dronabinol. Dronabinol is not an opioid, and does not cause opioid-like effects upon respiration or pupil size.

Continued on next page

Roxane—Cont.

Metabolism and Pharmacokinetics

Reliable information on the pharmacokinetics of MARINOL is not yet available. The following summary highlights important aspects of the literature concerning the absorption, distribution, metabolism and elimination of dronabinol; however, differences in the preparation, formulation and method of administration make it difficult to extrapolate this information directly to the drug product, MARINOL. Following oral administration, dronabinol has a systemic availability of 10 to 20% relative to an I.V. dose, indicating that the drug undergoes extensive first pass metabolism. Numerous metabolites have been identified, including 11-hydroxy-tetrahydrocannabinol, which is psychoactive. Dronabinol has a volume of distribution about 100 times as large as the plasma volume.

The maximum plasma concentrations of dronabinol, the 11-hydroxy metabolite, and several other metabolites occur approximately 2 to 3 hours after oral dosing. Biliary excretion is the major route of elimination. Within 72 hours following oral administration, approximately 50% of the dose is recovered in feces; another ten to fifteen percent appears in the urine either unchanged or as a metabolite. Renal clearance in normals is approximately one-tenth of the glomerular filtration rate.

The elimination phase of dronabinol exhibits biphasic kinetics with an alpha half-life of about 4 hours and a terminal half-life of 25 to 36 hours. The principal active metabolite, 11-OH-delta-9-THC, appears in the plasma in roughly the same mg quantities as its parent. The terminal plasma half-life for the 11-OH-delta-9-THC is approximately 15–18 hours. Thus, extended use of MARINOL at the doses recommended in this labeling may cause the accumulation of toxic amounts of dronabinol and its metabolites.

INDICATIONS AND USAGE

MARINOL is indicated for the treatment of the nausea and vomiting associated with cancer chemotherapy in patients who have failed to respond adequately to conventional antiemetic treatments. This restriction is required because a substantial proportion of patients treated with MARINOL can be expected to experience disturbing psychotomimetic reactions not observed with other antiemetic agents.

Because of its potential to alter the mental state, MARINOL is intended for use under circumstances that permit close supervision of the patient by a responsible individual. MARINOL is highly abusable and controlled under Schedule II of the Controlled Substances Act. Prescriptions of MARINOL should be limited to the amount necessary for a single cycle of chemotherapy (i.e., a few days).

Evidence supporting the efficacy of MARINOL in the treatment of nausea and vomiting induced by cancer chemotherapy was obtained from a variety of sources. The most persuasive evidence was obtained in subjects being treated with MOPP for Hodgkin's and non-Hodgkin's lymphomas. Other evidence supports the conclusion that MARINOL is effective against nausea and vomiting induced by other cancer chemotherapy regimens employed in the treatment of a wide variety of tumor types.

CONTRAINDICATIONS

MARINOL is contraindicated in patients whose nausea and vomiting arises from any cause other than cancer chemotherapy.

MARINOL is contraindicated in any patient known to be hypersensitive to either dronabinol or sesame oil.

WARNINGS

Because of its profound effects on the mental status, patients should be warned not to drive, operate complex machinery, or engage in any activity requiring sound judgment and unimpaired coordination while receiving treatment with MARINOL. The effects of MARINOL may persist for a variable and unpredictable period of time following its oral administration. Dronabinol is highly lipid soluble and its metabolites may persist in tissues, including plasma, for days. Because of individual variation in response and tolerance to the effects of MARINOL, the physician should determine on clinical grounds the period of patient supervision required. Patients receiving MARINOL should be closely observed, if possible within an inpatient setting. This is especially important during the treatment of naive patients. However, even patients experienced with MARINOL (or cannabis) may have serious untoward responses not predicted by prior uneventful exposures. Because a psychotic patient is a potential danger to him/herself and/or others, any patient who has a psychotic experience with MARINOL should be closely observed in an appropriate setting until his/her mental state returns to normal. The patient should not be given additional doses of MARINOL until he/she has been examined, and the circumstances evaluated, by a physician. If the clinical situation warrants it, a lower dose of MARINOL may be administered under very close supervision. The patient should be counseled about the experience and should share in the decision about further use of MARINOL.

MARINOL should not be taken with alcohol, sedatives, hypnotics, or other psychotomimetic substances.

PRECAUTIONS

General: Because it may cause a general increase in central sympathomimetic activity, MARINOL should be used with caution in persons with hypertension or heart disease. MARINOL should be used cautiously in manic, depressive, or schizophrenic patients as the symptoms of these disease states may be unmasked by the use of cannabinoids.

MARINOL should be used with caution in individuals receiving other psychoactive drugs.

Information for Patients: Persons taking MARINOL should be alerted to the additive central nervous system depression resulting from simultaneous use of MARINOL and alcohol or barbiturates. This combination should be avoided. Operation of machinery or a motor vehicle should be avoided during MARINOL therapy. Patients using MARINOL should be made aware of possible changes in mood and other adverse behavioral effects of the drug so as to avoid panic in the event of such manifestations. Patients should remain under supervision of a responsible adult while using MARINOL.

Drug Interactions: The effects of MARINOL on blood ethanol levels are complex. During sub-chronic MARINOL administration (60 mg/day) for ten days, absorption of ethanol was delayed, resulting in lower and delayed peak blood alcohol levels. Metabolism of ethanol was increased in some subjects and decreased in others. The overall rate of ethanol disappearance was decreased by about ten percent.

Carcinogenesis, Mutagenesis, and Impairment of Fertility: Carcinogenicity studies have not been performed with MARINOL. Reproductive studies in mice (approximately 32–400 times the human dose) and rats (approximately 8–32 times the human dose) demonstrate that MARINOL causes a decrease in pregnancy rate. In a long-term rat study (77 days), oral administration of MARINOL at doses 3–17 times the human dose reduced ventral prostate, seminal vesicle and epididymal weights and caused a decrease in seminal fluid volume. Decreases in spermatogenesis, number of developing germ cells, and number of Leydig cells in the testis were also observed. However, sperm count, mating success and testosterone levels were not affected. The significance of these animal findings in humans is not known.

Pregnancy: Pregnancy Category B. Reproduction studies have been performed in mice, rats and rabbits at doses up to 400 times, 32 times, and 10 times the human dose, respectively, and have revealed no evidence of teratogenicity due to MARINOL. At these dose levels in mice and rats, which produced substantial reductions in maternal weight gain, MARINOL caused a decrease in the number of viable pups, an increase in fetal mortality and an increase in early resorptions. Such effects were dose dependent and less apparent at lower doses which produced less maternal toxicity. There are, however, no adequate and well-controlled studies in pregnant women. Because animal reproduction studies are not always predictive of human response, this drug should be used during pregnancy only if clearly needed.

Nursing Mothers: MARINOL is concentrated and secreted in human milk and is absorbed by the nursing baby. Because the effects on the infant of chronic exposure to MARINOL and its metabolites are unknown, nursing mothers should not use MARINOL.

ADVERSE REACTIONS

In controlled clinical trials, the most frequently reported adverse reactions involved the central nervous system. In decreasing order of frequency these events were drowsiness, dizziness, muddled thinking and brief impairment of coordination, sensory and perceptual functions. Easy laughing, elation and heightened awareness, often termed a "high", was observed in 24% of MARINOL patients.

The incidences listed in the following table are derived from comparative double-blind, crossover or parallel design trials in which patients received MARINOL, an active control drug (usually prochlorperazine) or placebo.

The figures cited cannot be used to predict precisely the incidence of untoward events in the course of usual medical practice where patient characteristics and other factors often differ from those obtained in the clinical trials. Furthermore, these figures should not be compared with those obtained in other clinical studies involving related drug products and placebo, as each group of drug trials are conducted under a different set of conditions.

FREQUENCY OF ADVERSE EFFECTS FROM CONTROLLED STUDIES

Body System/ Adverse Reaction	MARINOL (n=317) %	Control (n=263) %	Placebo (n=68) %
CENTRAL NERVOUS SYSTEM:			
Drowsiness	48	33	49
Dizziness	21	5	1
Anxiety	16	3	24
Muddled Thinking	12	1	1
Perceptual Difficulties	11	1	0
Coordination Impairment	9	2	10
Irritability/Weird Feeling	7	3	0
Depression	7	3	15
Weak, Sluggish	6	3	1
Headache	6	4	4
Hallucinations	5	0	0
Memory Lapse	5	1	0
Unsteadiness, Ataxia	4	1	0
Paranoia	2	1	0
Depersonalization	2	0	0
Disorientation, Confusion	1	0	2
AUTONOMIC NERVOUS SYSTEM:			
Dry Mouth	3	1	1
Paresthesia	3	0	1
Visual Distortions	3	0	0
CARDIOVASCULAR:			
Tachycardia	1	1	0
Postural Hypotension	1	0	0

In addition to the events enumerated above, the following have been reported at a frequency below one percent: CENTRAL NERVOUS SYSTEM: tinnitus, nightmares; AUTONOMIC NERVOUS SYSTEM: speech difficulty, facial flushing, perspiring; CARDIOVASCULAR: syncope; GASTROINTESTINAL: diarrhea, fecal incontinence; MUSCULOSKELETAL: muscular pains.

DRUG ABUSE AND DEPENDENCE

MARINOL is highly abusable and controlled as delta-9-tetrahydrocannabinol under Schedule II of the Controlled Substances Act. Prescriptions of MARINOL should be limited to the amount necessary for a single cycle of chemotherapy (i.e., a few days).

It is not known what proportion of individuals exposed chronically to MARINOL or other cannabinoids will develop either psychological or physical dependence. Long-term use of these compounds has been associated with disorders of motivation, judgment, and cognition. It is not clear, though, if this is a manifestation of the underlying personalities of chronic users of this class of drugs, or if cannabinoids are directly responsible for these effects. An abstinence syndrome has been reported following discontinuation of high doses of delta-9-THC (210 mg per day). The acute phase was characterized by psychic distress, insomnia, and signs of autonomic hyperactivity (sweating, rhinorrhea, loose stools, hiccoughs). A protracted abstinence phase may have occurred as subjects reported sleep disturbances for several weeks after delta-9-THC discontinuation.

OVERDOSAGE

Signs and symptoms of overdosage are an extension of the psychotomimetic and physiologic effects of MARINOL, and, therefore, the clinical picture of overdosage may vary widely from patient to patient. Overdosages may be considered to be of two types: those at therapeutic doses, and those at higher, non-therapeutic doses.

Overdosage at Prescribed Dosages

Overdosage may be considered to have occurred even at prescribed dosages if disturbing psychiatric symptoms have occurred. In these cases, the patient should be observed in a quiet environment and supportive measures, including reassurance, should be used. Subsequent doses should be held until the patient has returned to baseline; routine dosing may then be resumed if clinically indicated, though this should be at a lower dosage. In controlled clinical trials, all such disturbing reactions spontaneously disappeared within 24 hours without specific medical therapy.

Particular attention should be paid to the vital signs in these patients, as tachycardia and both hyper- and hypotension are common adverse reactions. These signs should be monitored and treated, if necessary, in the usual manner according to the judgment of the physician.

Overdosage at Multiples of Prescribed Dosages

No cases of overdosage in multiples of prescribed dosages were reported in the controlled clinical studies. Few deaths have been reported from the use of dronabinol in any of its many forms (e.g., hashish, marijuana, etc.). Two incidents of death following the ingestion of large overdoses of Indian Hemp have been reported, while one death resulting from smoking cannabis herb and/or resin has appeared. No estimate of actual dosages was provided in either case. However, from a case of severe coma due to cannabis in a young French soldier, who recovered with conventional supportive therapy (intubation, I.V. fluids), it has been estimated that the acute lethal intravenous dose of dronabinol would be on the order of 1000–2000 mg total dose. Although this is a crude extrapolation at best, it represents a five to ten-fold multiple of the maximum oral dose recommended for MARINOL in a twenty-four hour period.

DOSAGE AND ADMINISTRATION

MARINOL is best administered at an initial dose of 5 mg/M², given 1–3 hours prior to the administration of chemotherapy, then every 2–4 hours after chemotherapy is given, for a total of 4–6 doses/day. Should the 5 mg/M² dose prove to be ineffective, and in the absence of significant side effects, the dose may be escalated by 2.5 mg/M² increments to a maximum of 15 mg/M² per dose. Caution should be exercised, however, as the incidence of disturbing psychiatric symptoms increases significantly at this maximum dose.

HOW SUPPLIED

MARINOL CAPSULES (Dronabinol solution in soft gelatin capsules).

2.5 mg white capsules (Identified RL).
NDC 0054-8541-11: Unit dose, 25 capsules per card (reverse numbered), 1 card per shipper.
NDC 0054-2601-11: Bottles of 25 capsules.
5 mg dark brown capsules (Identifed RL)
NDC 0054-8542-11: Unit dose, 25 capsules per card (reverse numbered), 1 card per shipper.
NDC 0054-2602-11: Bottles of 25 capsules.
10 mg orange capsules (Identifed RL)
NDC 0054-8543-11: Unit dose, 25 capsules per card (reverse numbered), 1 card per shipper.
NDC 0054-2603-11: Bottles of 25 capsules.
MARINOL capsules should be preserved in a well sealed container, and stored in a cool place
MARINOL® is a registered trademark of and is marketed under license from Unimed, Inc.

DEA ORDER FORM REQUIRED.
Shown in Product Identification Section, page 426

METHADONE HYDROCHLORIDE   ©℞
ORAL SOLUTION USP
TABLETS USP

(WARNING: May be habit forming)

CONDITIONS FOR DISTRIBUTION AND
USE OF METHADONE PRODUCTS:
Code of Federal Regulations,
Title 21, Sec. 291.505

METHADONE PRODUCTS, WHEN USED FOR TREATMENT OF NARCOTIC ADDICTION IN DETOXIFICATION OR MAINTENANCE PROGRAMS, SHALL BE DISPENSED ONLY BY APPROVED HOSPITAL PHARMACIES, APPROVED COMMUNITY PHARMACIES, AND MAINTENANCE PROGRAMS APPROVED BY THE FOOD AND DRUG ADMINISTRATION AND THE DESIGNATED STATE AUTHORITY.
APPROVED MAINTENANCE PROGRAMS SHALL DISPENSE AND USE METHADONE IN ORAL FORM ONLY AND ACCORDING TO THE TREATMENT REQUIREMENTS STIPULATED IN THE FEDERAL METHADONE REGULATIONS (21 CFR 291.505). FAILURE TO ABIDE BY THE REQUIREMENTS IN THESE REGULATIONS MAY RESULT IN CRIMINAL PROSECUTION, SEIZURE OF THE DRUG SUPPLY, REVOCATION OF THE PROGRAM APPROVAL, AND INJUNCTION PRECLUDING OPERATION OF THE PROGRAM.
A METHADONE PRODUCT, WHEN USED AS AN ANALGESIC, MAY BE DISPENSED IN ANY LICENSED PHARMACY.

DESCRIPTION

Each 5 mL of Methadone Hydrochloride Oral Solution contains:
Methadone Hydrochloride .... 5 mg or 10 mg
    (Warning: May be habit forming)
Alcohol 8%
Each tablet for oral administration contains:
Methadone Hydrochloride .... 5 mg or 10 mg
    (Warning: May be habit forming)
Inactive Ingredients:
The oral solution contains alcohol, FD&C Red No. 40, FD&C Yellow No. 6, flavoring, glycol, sorbitol, water, and other ingredients.
The tablets contain magnesium stearate, microcrystalline cellulose, and starch (corn).
Chemically, Methadone Hydrochloride is 3-Heptanone, 6-(dimethylamino)-4,4-diphenyl-, hydrochloride.
Methadone Hydrochloride acts as a narcotic analgesic.

CLINICAL PHARMACOLOGY

Methadone Hydrochloride is a synthetic narcotic analgesic with multiple actions quantitatively similar to those of morphine, the most prominent of which involve the central nervous system and organs composed of smooth muscle. The principal actions of therapeutic value are analgesia and sedation and detoxification or temporary maintenance in narcotic addiction. The methadone abstinence syndrome, although qualitatively similar to that of morphine, differs in that the onset is slower, the course is more prolonged, and the symptoms are less severe.
When administered orally, methadone is approximately one-half as potent as when given parenterally. Oral administration results in a delay of the onset, a lowering of the peak, and an increase in the duration of analgesic effect.

INDICATIONS AND USAGE

Methadone Hydrochloride is indicated for relief of severe pain, for detoxification treatment of narcotic addiction, and for temporary maintenance treatment of narcotic addiction.

Note

If methadone is administered for treatment of heroin dependence for more than three weeks, the procedure passes from treatment of the acute withdrawal syndrome (detoxification) to maintenance therapy. Maintenance treatment is permitted to be undertaken only by approved methadone programs. This does not preclude the maintenance treatment of an addict who is hospitalized for medical conditions other than addiction and who requires temporary maintenance during the critical period of his stay or whose enrollment has been verified in a program which has approval for maintenance treatment with methadone.

CONTRAINDICATIONS

Hypersensitivity to methadone.

WARNINGS

Methadone Hydrochloride Tablets are for oral administration only and *must not* be used for injection. It is recommended that Methadone Hydrochloride Tablets, if dispensed, be packaged in child-resistant containers and kept out of the reach of children to prevent accidental ingestion.

Methadone Hydrochloride, a narcotic, is a Schedule II controlled substance under the Federal Controlled Substances Act. Appropriate security measures should be taken to safeguard stocks of methadone against diversion.
DRUG DEPENDENCE — METHADONE CAN PRODUCE DRUG DEPENDENCE OF THE MORPHINE TYPE AND, THEREFORE, HAS THE POTENTIAL FOR BEING ABUSED. PSYCHIC DEPENDENCE, PHYSICAL DEPENDENCE, AND TOLERANCE MAY DEVELOP UPON REPEATED ADMINISTRATION OF METHADONE, AND IT SHOULD BE PRESCRIBED AND ADMINISTERED WITH THE SAME DEGREE OF CAUTION APPROPRIATE TO THE USE OF MORPHINE.
Interaction with Other Central-Nervous-System Depressants —Methadone should be used with caution and in reduced dosage in patients who are concurrently receiving other narcotic analgesics, general anesthetics, phenothiazines, other tranquilizers, sedative-hypnotics, tricyclic antidepressants, and other C.N.S. depressants (including alcohol). Respiratory depression, hypotension, and profound sedation or coma may result.
Anxiety —Since methadone, as used by tolerant subjects at a constant maintenance dosage, is not a tranquilizer, patients who are maintained on this drug will react to life problems and stresses with the same symptoms of anxiety as do other individuals. The physician should not confuse such symptoms with those of narcotic abstinence and should not attempt to treat anxiety by increasing the dosage of methadone. The action of methadone in maintenance treatment is limited to the control of narcotic symptoms and is ineffective for relief of general anxiety.
Head Injury and Increased Intracranial Pressure —The respiratory depressant effects of methadone and its capacity to elevate cerebrospinal-fluid pressure may be markedly exaggerated in the presence of increased intracranial pressure. Furthermore, narcotics produce side effects that may obscure the clinical course of patients with head injuries. In such patients, methadone must be used with caution and only if it is deemed essential.
Asthma and Other Respiratory Conditions — Methadone should be used with caution in patients having an acute asthmatic attack, in those with chronic obstructive pulmonary disease or cor pulmonale, and in individuals with a substantially decreased respiratory reserve, preexisting respiratory depression, hypoxia, or hypercapnia. In such patients, even usual therapeutic doses of narcotics may decrease respiratory drive while simultaneously increasing airway resistance to the point of apnea.
Hypotensive Effect —The administration of methadone may result in severe hypotension in an individual whose ability to maintain his blood pressure has already been compromised by a depleted blood volume or concurrent administration of such drugs as the phenothiazines or certain anesthetics.
Use in Ambulatory Patients —Methadone may impair the mental and/or physical abilities required for the performance of potentially hazardous tasks, such as driving a car or operating machinery. The patient should be cautioned accordingly.
Methadone, like other narcotics, may produce orthostatic hypotension in ambulatory patients.
Use in Pregnancy —Safe use in pregnancy has not been established in relation to possible adverse effects on fetal development. Therefore, methadone should not be used in pregnant

women unless, in the judgment of the physician, the potential benefits outweigh the possible hazards.
Methadone is not recommended for obstetric analgesia because its long duration of action increases the probability of respiratory depression in the newborn.
Use in Children —Methadone is not recommended for use as an analgesic in children, since documented clinical experience has been insufficient to establish a suitable dosage regimen for the pediatric age group.

PRECAUTIONS

Interaction with Pentazocine —**Patients who are addicted to heroin or who are on the methadone maintenance program may experience withdrawal symptoms when given pentazocine.**
Interaction with Rifampin —The concurrent administration of rifampin may possibly reduce the blood concentration of methadone. The mechanism by which rifampin may decrease blood concentrations of methadone is not fully understood, although enhanced microsomal drug-metabolized enzymes may influence drug disposition.
Acute Abdominal Conditions —The administration of methadone or other narcotics may obscure the diagnosis or clinical course in patients with acute abdominal conditions.
Interaction with Monoamine Oxidase (MAO) Inhibitors —Therapeutic doses of meperidine have precipitated severe reactions in patients concurrently receiving monoamine oxidase inhibitors or those who have received such agents within 14 days. Similar reactions thus far have not been reported with methadone; but if the use of methadone is necessary in such patients, a sensitivity test should be performed in which repeated small incremental doses are administered over the course of several hours while the patient's condition and vital signs are under careful observation.
Special-Risk Patients —Methadone should be given with caution and the initial dose should be reduced in certain patients, such as the elderly or debilitated and those with severe impairment of hepatic or renal function, hypothyroidism, Addison's disease, prostatic hypertrophy, or urethral stricture.

ADVERSE REACTIONS

THE MAJOR HAZARDS OF METHADONE, AS OF OTHER NARCOTIC ANALGESICS, ARE RESPIRATORY DEPRESSION AND, TO A LESSER DEGREE, CIRCULATORY DEPRESSION. RESPIRATORY ARREST, SHOCK, AND CARDIAC ARREST HAVE OCCURRED.
The most frequently observed adverse reactions include lightheadedness, dizziness, sedation, nausea, vomiting, and sweating. These effects seem to be more prominent in ambulatory patients and in those who are not suffering severe chronic pain. In such individuals, lower doses are advisable. Some adverse reactions may be alleviated in the ambulatory patient if he lies down.
Other adverse reactions include the following:
Central Nervous System —Euphoria, dysphoria, weakness, headache, insomnia, agitation, disorientation, and visual disturbances.
Gastrointestinal —Dry mouth, anorexia, constipation, and biliary tract spasm.
Cardiovascular —Flushing of the face, bradycardia, palpitation, faintness, and syncope.
Genitourinary —Urinary retention or hesitancy, antidiuretic effect, and reduced libido and/or potency.
Allergic —Pruritus, urticaria, other skin rashes, edema, and, rarely, hemorrhagic urticaria.

ADMINISTRATION AND DOSAGE

For relief of Severe Pain —Dosage should be adjusted according to the severity of the pain and the response of the patient. Occasionally it may be necessary to exceed the usual dosage recommended in cases of exceptionally severe chronic pain or in those patients who have become tolerant to the analgesic effect of narcotics.
For severe acute pain, the usual adult dose is 2.5 mg to 10 mg every three to four hours as necessary.
For Detoxification Treatment —THE DRUG SHALL BE ADMINISTERED DAILY UNDER CLOSE SUPERVISION AS FOLLOWS:
A detoxification treatment course shall not exceed 21 days and may not be repeated earlier than four weeks after completion of the preceding course.
The oral form of administration is preferred. However, if the patient is unable to ingest oral medication, he may be started on the parenteral form initially.
In detoxification, the patient may receive methadone when there are significant symptoms of withdrawal. The dosage schedules indicated below are recommended but could be varied in accordance with clinical judgment. Initially, a single dose of 15 to 20 mg of methadone will often be sufficient to suppress withdrawal symptoms. Additional methadone may be provided if withdrawal symptoms are not suppressed or if symptoms reappear. When patients are physically dependent on high doses, it may be necessary to exceed these levels. Forty mg per day in single or divided doses will usu-

Continued on next page

Roxane—Cont.

ally constitute an adequate stabilizing dosage level. Stabilization can be continued for two to three days, and then the amount of methadone normally will be gradually decreased. The rate at which methadone is decreased will be determined separately for each patient. The dose of methadone can be decreased on a daily basis or at two-day intervals, but the amount of intake shall always be sufficient to keep withdrawal symptoms at a tolerable level. In hospitalized patients, a daily reduction of 20 percent of the total dose may be tolerated and may cause little discomfort. In ambulatory patients, a somewhat slower schedule may be needed. If methadone is administered for more than three weeks, the procedure is considered to have progressed from detoxification or treatment of the acute withdrawal syndrome to maintenance treatment, even though the goal and intent may be eventual total withdrawal.

OVERDOSAGE

Symptoms—Serious overdosage of methadone is characterized by respiratory depression (a decrease in respiratory rate and/or tidal volume, Cheyne-Stokes respiration, cyanosis), extreme somnolence progressing to stupor or coma, maximally constricted pupils, skeletal-muscle flaccidity, cold and clammy skin, and sometimes, bradycardia and hypotension. In severe overdosage, particularly by the intravenous route, apnea, circulatory collapse, cardiac arrest, and death may occur.

Treatment—Primary attention should be given to the reestablishment of adequate respiratory exchange through provision of a patent airway and institution of assisted or controlled ventilation. If a nontolerant person, especially a child, takes a large dose of methadone, effective narcotic antagonists are available to counteract the potentially lethal respiratory depression. **The physician must remember, however, that methadone is a long-acting depressant (36 to 48 hours), whereas the antagonists act for much shorter periods (one to three hours).** The patient must, therefore, be monitored continuously for recurrence of respiratory depression and treated repeatedly with the narcotic antagonist as needed. If the diagnosis is correct and respiratory depression is due only to overdosage of methadone, the use of other respiratory stimulants is not indicated.

An antagonist should not be administered in the absence of clinically significant respiratory or cardiovascular depression. Intravenously administered narcotic antagonists (naloxone and nalorphine) are the drugs of choice to reverse signs of intoxication. These agents should be given repeatedly until the patient's status remains satisfactory. The hazard that the narcotic agent will further depress respiration is less likely with the use of naloxone.

Oxygen, intravenous fluids, vasopressors, and other supportive measures should be employed as indicated.

Note

IN AN INDIVIDUAL PHYSICALLY DEPENDENT ON NARCOTICS, THE ADMINISTRATION OF THE USUAL DOSE OF A NARCOTIC ANTAGONIST WILL PRECIPITATE AN ACUTE WITHDRAWAL SYNDROME. THE SEVERITY OF THIS SYNDROME WILL DEPEND ON THE DEGREE OF PHYSICAL DEPENDENCE AND THE DOSE OF THE ANTAGONIST ADMINISTERED. THE USE OF A NARCOTIC ANTAGONIST IN SUCH A PERSON SHOULD BE AVOIDED IF POSSIBLE. IF IT MUST BE USED TO TREAT SERIOUS RESPIRATORY DEPRESSION IN THE PHYSICALLY DEPENDENT PATIENT, THE ANTAGONIST SHOULD BE ADMINISTERED WITH EXTREME CARE AND BY TITRATION WITH SMALLER THAN USUAL DOSES OF THE ANTAGONIST.

HOW SUPPLIED

Methadone Hydrochloride Oral Solution USP
5 mg per 5 mL
NDC 0054-8548-16: Unit dose Patient Cup™ filled to deliver 5 mL (Methadone Hydrochloride 5 mg), ten 5 mL Patient Cups™ per shelf pack, 4 shelf packs per shipper.
NDC 0054-8549-16: Unit dose Patient Cup™ filled to deliver 10 mL (Methadone Hyrdochloride 10 mg), ten 10 mL Patient Cups™ per shelf pack, 4 shelf packs per shipper.
NDC 0054-3555-63: Bottles of 500 mL
10 mg per 5 mL
NDC 0054-3556-63: Bottles of 500 mL
Methadone Hydrochloride Tablets USP
5 mg white, scored identified (54210) tablets.
NDC 0054-4570-25: Bottle of 100 tablets.
NDC 0054-8553-24: Unit dose, 25 tablets per card (reverse numbered), 4 cards per shipper.
10 mg white, scored identified (54142) tablets.
NDC 0054-4571-25: Bottle of 100 tablets.
NDC 0054-8554-24: Unit dose, 25 tablets per card (reverse numbered), 4 cards per shipper.

MORPHINE SULFATE IMMEDIATE RELEASE   Ⓒ ℞
ORAL SOLUTION
(WARNING: May be habit forming.)
MORPHINE SULFATE IMMEDIATE RELEASE   Ⓒ ℞
TABLETS
(WARNING: May be habit forming.)

DESCRIPTION

Each 5 mL of Morphine Sulfate Oral Solution contains:
Morphine Sulfate .... 10 or 20 mg
(WARNING: May be habit forming.)
Each tablet for oral administration contains:
Morphine Sulfate .... 15 or 30 mg
(WARNING: May be habit forming.)

HOW SUPPLIED

Morphine Sulfate Oral Solution
(Unflavored).
10 mg per 5 mL.
NDC 0054-8585-16: Unit dose Patient Cup™ filled to deliver 5 mL (10 mg Morphine Sulfate), ten 5 mL Patient Cups™ per shelf pack, four shelf packs per shipper.
NDC 0054-8586-16: Unit dose Patient Cup™ filled to deliver 10 mL (20 mg Morphine Sulfate), ten 10 mL Patient Cups™ per shelf pack, four shelf packs per shipper.
NDC 0054-3785-49: 100 mL "Unit of use" calibrated bottle.
NDC 0054-3785-63: Bottles of 500 mL.
20 mg per 5 mL.
NDC 0054-3786-49: 100 mL "Unit of Use" calibrated bottle.
NDC 0054-3786-63: Bottles of 500 mL.
Tablets
15 mg white scored, identified (54/733) tablets.
NDC 0054-8582-24: Unit dose, 25 tablets per card (reverse numbered), 4 cards per shipper.
NDC 0054-4582-25: Bottles of 100 tablets.
30 mg white scored, identified (54/262) tablets.
NDC 0054-8583-24: Unit dose, 25 tablets per card (reverse numbered), 4 cards per shipper.
NDC 0054-4583-25: Bottles of 100 Tablets.
DEA Order Form Required

POTASSIUM CHLORIDE   ℞
ORAL SOLUTION USP

DESCRIPTION

Potassium Chloride Oral Solution USP: 10 or 20%:
Each 30 mL 10% solution contains potassium 40 mEq and chloride 40 mEq
Each 30 mL 20% solution contains potassium 80 mEq and chloride 80 mEq
The 10% solution is cocoanut flavored, and the 20% solution is grapefruit flavored. Alcohol 5%.
Potassium Chloride is chemically KCl. Potassium Chloride is an electrolyte replenisher.

HOW SUPPLIED

POTASSIUM CHLORIDE ORAL SOLUTION USP, 10%
15 mEq of potassium per 11.25 mL
NDC 0054-8711-04: Unit dose Patient Cups™ filled to deliver 11.25 mL, ten 11.25 mL Patient Cups™ per shelf pack, ten shelf packs per shipper.
20 mEq of potassium per 15 mL
NDC 0054-8714-04: Unit dose Patient Cups™ filled to deliver 15mL, ten 15mL patient Cups™ per shelf pack, ten shelf packs per shipper.
30 mEq of potassium per 22.5 mL
NDC 0054-8712-04: Unit dose Patient Cups™ filled to deliver 22.5 mL, ten 22.5 mL Patient Cups™ per shelf pack, ten shelf packs per shipper.
40 mEq of potassium per 30 mL
NDC 0054-8713-04: Unit dose Patient Cups™ filled to deliver 30mL, ten 30mL Patient Cups™ per shelf pack, ten shelf packs per shipper.
NDC 0054-3716-63: Bottles of 500 mL.
NDC 0054-3716-68: Bottles of 1 liter.
POTASSIUM CHLORIDE ORAL SOLUTION USP, 20%
80 mEq of potassium per 30 mL
NDC 0054-3714-63: Bottles of 500 mL.
NDC 0054-3714-68: Bottles of 1 liter.

PREDNISONE TABLETS USP   ℞
1 mg, 2.5 mg, 5 mg, 10 mg, 20 mg, or 50 mg

HOW SUPPLIED

1 mg white, scored tablets, gluten-free (Identified 54 092).
NDC 0054-8739-25: Unit dose, 10 tablets per strip, 10 strips per shelf pack, 10 shelf packs per shipper.
NDC 0054-4741-25: Bottles of 100 tablets.
2.5 mg white, scored tablets, gluten-free (Identified 54 339).
NDC 0054-8740-25: Unit dose, 10 tablets per strip, 10 strips per shelf pack, 10 shelf packs per shipper.
NDC 0054-4742-25: Bottles of 100 tablets.
5 mg white, scored tablets, gluten-free (Identified 54 612).
NDC 0054-8724-25: Unit dose, 10 tablets per strip, 10 strips per shelf pack, 10 shelf packs per shipper.
NDC 0054-4728-25: Bottles of 100 tablets.
NDC 0054-4728-31: Bottles of 1000 tablets.
10 mg white, scored tablets, gluten-free (Identified 54 899).
NDC 0054-8725-25: Unit dose, 10 tablets per strip, 10 strips per shelf pack, 10 shelf packs per shipper.
NDC 0054-4730-25: Bottles of 100 tablets.
NDC 0054-4730-29: Bottles of 500 tablets.
20 mg white, scored tablets, gluten-free (Identified 54 760).
NDC 0054-8726-25: Unit dose, 10 tablets per strip, 10 strips per shelf pack, 10 shelf packs per shipper.
NDC 0054-4729-25: Bottles of 100 tablets.
NDC 0054-4729-29: Bottles of 500 tablets.
50 mg white, scored tablets, gluten-free (Identified 54 343).
NDC 0054-8729-25: Unit dose, 10 tablets per strip, 10 strips per shelf pack, 10 shelf packs per shipper.
NDC 0054-4733-25: Bottles of 100 tablets.

ROXANOL™   Ⓒ ℞
[rox'-ĕ-nŭl]
Morphine Sulfate Immediate Release, Concentrated Oral Solution
20 mg per mL

(WARNING: May be habit forming.)

ROXANOL 100™
Morphine Sulfate Immediate Release, Concentrated Oral Solution
100 mg per 5 mL

(WARNING: May be be habit forming.)

DESCRIPTION

Each mL of Roxanol™ contains:
Morphine Sulfate .... 20 mg
(Warning: May be habit forming.)
Each 5 mL of Roxanol 100™ contains:
Morphine Sulfate .... 100 mg
(Warning: May be habit forming.)
Chemically, Morphine Sulfate is, Morphinan-3,6-diol, 7,8-didehydro-4,5-epoxy-17-methyl-, $(5\alpha,6\alpha)$-, sulfate (2:1) (salt), pentahydrate.
Morphine Sulfate acts as a narcotic analgesic.

CLINICAL PHARMACOLOGY

The major effects of morphine are on the central nervous system and the bowel. Opioids act as agonists, interacting with stereospecific and saturable binding sites or receptors in the brain and other tissues.
Morphine is about two-thirds absorbed from the gastrointestinal tract with the maximum analgesic effect occurring 60 minutes post administration.

INDICATIONS AND USAGE

Morphine is indicated for the relief of severe acute and severe chronic pain.

CONTRAINDICATIONS

Hypersensitivity to morphine; respiratory insufficiency or depression; severe CNS depression; attack of bronchial asthma; heart failure secondary to chronic lung disease; cardiac arrhythmias; increased intracranial or cerebrospinal pressure; head injuries; brain tumor; acute alcoholism; delirium tremens; convulsive disorders; after biliary tract surgery; suspected surgical abdomen; surgical anastomosis; concomitantly with MAO inhibitors or within 14 days of such treatment.

WARNINGS

Morphine can cause tolerance, psychological and physical dependence. Withdrawal will occur on abrupt discontinuation or administration of a narcotic antagonist.
Interaction with Other Central-Nervous-System Depressants—Morphine should be used with caution and in reduced dosage in patients who are concurrently receiving other narcotic analgesics, general anesthetics, phenothiazines, other tranquilizers, sedative-hypnotics, tricyclic antidepressants, and other CNS depressants (including alcohol). Respiratory depression, hypotension, and profound sedation or coma may result.

PRECAUTIONS

General:
Head Injury and Increased Intracranial Pressure—The respiratory depressant effects of morphine and its capacity to elevate cerebrospinal-fluid pressure may be markedly exaggerated in the presence of increased intracranial pressure. Furthermore, narcotics produce side effects that may obscure the clinical course of patients with head injuries. In such patients, morphine must be used with caution and only if it is deemed essential.
Asthma and Other Respiratory Conditions—Morphine should be used with caution in patients having an acute asthmatic attack, in those with chronic obstructive pulmonary disease or cor pulmonale, and in individuals with a substan-

tially decreased respiratory reserve, preexisting respiratory depression, hypoxia, or hypercapnia. In such patients, even usual therapeutic doses of narcotics may decrease respiratory drive while simultaneously increasing airway resistance to the point of apnea.

Hypotensive Effect—The administration of morphine may result in severe hypotension in an individual whose ability to maintain his blood pressure has already been compromised by a depleted blood volume or concurrent administration of such drugs as the phenothiazines or certain anesthetics.

Special-Risk Patients—Morphine should be given with caution and the initial dose should be reduced in certain patients, such as the elderly or debilitated and those with severe impairment of hepatic or renal function, hypothyroidism, Addison's disease, prostatic hypertrophy, or urethral stricture.

Acute Abdominal Conditions—The administration of morphine or other narcotics may obscure the diagnosis or clinical course in patients with acute abdominal conditions.

Information for patients:

Use in Ambulatory Patients—Morphine may impair the mental and/or physical abilities required for the performance of potentially hazardous tasks, such as driving a car or operating machinery. The patient should be cautioned accordingly.

Morphine, like other narcotics, may produce orthostatic hypotension in ambulatory patients.

Patients should be cautioned about the combined effects of alcohol or other central nervous system depressants with morphine.

Drug interactions:

Generally, effects of morphine may be potentiated by alkalizing agents and antagonized by acidifying agents. Analgesic effect of morphine is potentiated by chlorpromazine and methocarbamol. CNS depressants such as anaesthetics, hypnotics, barbiturates, phenothiazines, chloral hydrate, glutethimide, sedatives, MAO inhibitors (including procarbazine hydrochloride), antihistamines, β-blockers (propranolol), alcohol, furazolidone and other narcotics may enhance the depressant effects of morphine.

Morphine may increase anticoagulant activity of coumarin and other anticoagulants.

Carcinogenicity/Mutagenicity:

Long-term studies to determine the carcinogenic and mutagenic potential of morphine are not available.

Pregnancy:

Teratogenic Effects—Pregnancy Category C: Animal production studies have not been conducted with morphine. It is also not known whether morphine can cause fetal harm when administered to a pregnant woman or can affect reproduction capacity. Morphine should be given to a pregnant woman only if clearly needed.

Labor and Delivery:

Morphine readily crosses the placental barrier and, if administered during labor, may lead to respiratory depression in the neonate.

Nursing Mothers:

Morphine has been detected in human milk. For this reason, caution should be exercised when morphine is administered to a nursing woman.

Pediatric Usage:

Safety and effectiveness in children have not been established.

ADVERSE REACTIONS

THE MAJOR HAZARDS OF MORPHINE AS OF OTHER NARCOTIC ANALGESICS, ARE RESPIRATORY DEPRESSION AND, TO A LESSER DEGREE, CIRCULATORY DEPRESSION, RESPIRATORY ARREST, SHOCK, AND CARDIAC ARREST HAVE OCCURRED.

The most frequently observed adverse reactions include lightheadedness, dizziness, sedation, nausea, vomiting, and sweating. These effects seem to be more prominent in ambulatory patients and in those who are not suffering severe pain. In such individuals, lower doses are advisable. Some adverse reactions may be alleviated in the ambulatory patient if he lies down.

Other adverse reactions include the following:

Central Nervous System—Euphoria, dysphoria, weakness, headache, insomnia, agitation, disorientation, and visual disturbances.

Gastrointestinal—Dry mouth, anorexia, constipation, and biliary tract spasm.

Cardiovascular—Flushing of the face, bradycardia, palpitation, faintness, and syncope.

Genitourinary—Urinary retention or hesitancy, anti-diuretic effect, and reduced libido and/or potency.

Allergic—Pruritus, urticaria, other skin rashes, edema, and, rarely hemorrhagic urticaria.

Treatment of the most frequent adverse reactions:

Constipation—Ample intake of water or other liquids should be encouraged. Concomitant administration of a stool softener and a peristaltic stimulant with the narcotic analgesic can be an effective preventive measure for those patients in need of therapeutics. If elimination does not occur for two

days, an enema should be administered to prevent impaction.

In the event diarrhea occurs, see page around a fecal impaction is a possible cause to consider before antidiarrheal measures are employed.

Nausea and Vomiting—Phenothiazines and antihistamines can be effective treatments for nausea of the medullary and vestibular sources respectively. However, these drugs may potentiate the side effects of the narcotics or the antinauseant.

Drowsiness (sedation)—Once pain control is achieved, undesirable sedation can be minimized by titrating the dosage to a level that just maintains a tolerable pain or pain free state.

DRUG ABUSE AND DEPENDENCE

Morphine Sulfate, narcotic, is a Schedule II controlled substance under the Federal Controlled Substance Act. As with other narcotics, some patients may develop a physical and psychological dependence on morphine. They may increase dosage without consulting a physician and subsequently may develop a physical dependence on the drug. In such cases, abrupt discontinuance may precipitate typical withdrawal symptoms, including convulsions. Therefore the drug should be withdrawn gradually from any patient known to be taking excessive dosages over a long period of time.

In treating the terminally ill patient the benefit of pain relief may outweigh the possibility of drug dependence. *The chance of drug dependence is substantially reduced when the patient is placed on scheduled narcotic programs instead of a "pain to relief-of-pain" cycle typical of a PRN regimen.*

OVERDOSAGE

Signs and Symptoms: Serious overdose with morphine is characterized by respiratory depression (a decrease in respiratory rate and/or tidal volume, Cheyne-Stokes respiration, cyanosis), extreme somnolence progressing to stupor or coma, skeletal muscle flaccidity, cold or clammy skin, and sometimes bradycardia and hypotension. In severe overdosage, apnea, circulatory collapse, cardiac arrest and death may occur.

Treatment: Primary attention should be given to the reestablishment of adequate respiratory exchange through provision of a patent airway and the institution of assisted or controlled ventilation. The narcotic antagonist naloxone is a specific antidote against respiratory depression which may result from overdosage or unusual sensitivity to narcotics, including morphine. Therefore, an appropriate dose of naloxone (usual initial adult dose: 0.4 mg) should be administered, preferably by the intravenous route and simultaneously with efforts at respiratory resuscitation. Since the duration of action of morphine may exceed that of the antagonist, the patient should be kept under continued surveillance and repeated doses of the antagonist should be administered as needed to maintain adequate respiration.

An antagonist should not be administered in the absence of clinically significant respiratory or cardiovascular depression.

Oxygen, intravenous fluids, vasopressors and other supportive measures should be employed as indicated.

Gastric emptying may be useful in removing unabsorbed drug.

DOSAGE AND ADMINISTRATION

ROXANOL™ and ROXANOL 100™—Usual Adult Oral Dose: 10 to 30 mg every 4 hours or as directed by physician. Dosage is a patient dependent variable, therefore increased dosage may be required to achieve adequate analgesia.

For control of chronic, agonizing pain in patients with certain terminal disease, this drug should be administered on a regularly scheduled basis, every 4 hours, at the lowest dosage level that will achieve adequate analgesia.

Note: Medication may suppress respiration in the elderly, the very ill, and those patients with respiratory problems, therefore lower doses may be required.

Morphine Dosage Reduction: During the first two to three days of effective pain relief, the patient may sleep for many hours. This can be misinterpreted as the effect of excessive analgesic dosing rather than the first sign of relief in a pain exhausted patient. The dose, therefore, should be maintained for at least three days before reduction, if respiratory activity and other vital signs are adequate.

Following successful relief of severe pain, periodic attempts to reduce the narcotic dose should be made. Smaller doses or complete discontinuation of the narcotic analgesic may become feasible due to a physiologic change or the improved mental state of the patient.

HOW SUPPLIED

Roxanol™

(Morphine Sulfate Immediate Release, Concentrated Oral Solution)

20 mg per mL

NDC 0054-3751-44: Bottle of 30 mL with calibrated dropper.

NDC 0054-3751-50: Bottle of 120 mL with calibrated dropper.

Roxanol 100™

(Morphine Sulfate Immediate Release, Concentrated Oral Solution)

100 mg per 5 mL

NDC 0054-3751-58: Bottle of 240 mL with calibrated patient spoon.

DEA Order Form Required

Shown in Product Identification Section, page 426

ROXANOL SR™   Ⓒ ℞

[*rox '-ĕ-nŭl SR*]

(MORPHINE SULFATE)

Sustained Release Tablets

(WARNING: May be habit forming.)

NOTE

THIS IS A SUSTAINED RELEASE DOSAGE FORM. TABLET MUST BE SWALLOWED WHOLE. DO NOT BREAK THE TABLET IN HALF. DO NOT CRUSH OR CHEW.

THE SUSTAINED RELEASE OF DRUG FROM THE DOSAGE FORM SHOULD BE TAKEN INTO CONSIDERATION IN EVENT OF ADVERSE REACTIONS OR OVERDOSAGE.

DESCRIPTION

Each tablet for oral administration contains:

Morphine Sulfate .... 30 mg

(WARNING: May be habit forming.)

In a tablet that provides for sustained release of the medication.

Refer to Roxanol™ (morphine sulfate concentrated oral solution) 20 mg/mL for the complete text.

INDICATIONS AND USAGE

Morphine is indicated for the relief of severe chronic pain.

ADVERSE REACTIONS

NOTE: THE SUSTAINED RELEASE OF THE DRUG FROM THE DOSAGE FORM SHOULD BE TAKEN INTO CONSIDERATION IN THE EVENT OF OCCURRING ADVERSE REACTIONS.

DOSAGE AND ADMINISTRATION

ROXANOL SR™ Tablets—The usual starting dose for patients with severe chronic pain is 30 mg every 8 hours. Patients with terminal cancer may require higher doses for adequate relief. The dose and/or dosage interval should be adjusted according to the severity of pain, as well as the patient's underlying disease, age, and size.

Note: Medication may suppress respiration in the elderly, the very ill, and those patients with respiratory problems, therefore lower doses or longer dosing intervals may be required.

NOTE: TABLET MUST BE SWALLOWED WHOLE. DO NOT BREAK THE TABLET IN HALF. DO NOT CRUSH OR CHEW.

HOW SUPPLIED

ROXANOL SR™ (Morphine Sulfate)

Sustained Release Tablets

30 mg white tablets (Identified 54 090).

NDC 0054-8780-24: Unit dose, 25 tablets per card (reverse numbered), 4 cards per shipper.

NDC 0054-4780-19: Bottles of 50 tablets.

NDC 0054-4780-25: Bottles of 100 tablets.

NDC 0054-4780-27: Bottles of 250 tablets.

Shown in Product Identification Section, page 426

ROXICET™ Tablets   Ⓒ ℞

[*rox-ĕ-cĕt*]

Oxycodone and Acetaminophen Tablets USP

(Oxycodone Hydrochloride 5 mg and Acetaminophen 325 mg)

(WARNING: May be habit forming)

ROXICET™ Oral Solution   Ⓒ ℞

Oxycodone and Acetaminophen Oral Solution

(Oxycodone Hydrochloride 5 mg and Acetaminophen 325 mg Oral Solution per 5 mL)

(WARNING: May be habit forming)

DESCRIPTION

Each tablet contains:

Oxycodone Hydrochloride+ .... 5 mg

(**Warning:** May Be Habit Forming)

Acetaminophen .... 325 mg

Each 5 mL contains:

Oxycodone Hydrochloride+ .... 5 mg

(**Warning:** May Be Habit Forming)

Acetaminophen .... 325 mg

Alcohol 0.4%

(+5 mg Oxycodone HCl is equivalent to 4.4815 mg Oxycodone)

Continued on next page

Roxane—Cont.

Acetaminophen, 4'-hydroxyacetanilide, is a non-opiate, non-salicylate analgesic and antipyretic which occurs as a white, odorless, crystalline powder, possessing a slightly bitter taste.

The oxycodone component is 14-hydroxydihydrocodeinone, a white, odorless crystalline powder which is derived from the opium alkaloid, thebaine.

CLINICAL PHARMACOLOGY

The principal analgesic ingredient, oxycodone, is a semisynthetic narcotic with multiple actions qualitatively similar to those of morphine; the most prominent of these involve the central nervous system and organs composed of smooth muscle. The princpal actions of therapeutic value of oxycodone are analgesia and sedation.

Oxycodone is similar to codeine and methadone in that it retains at least one half of its analgesic activity when administered orally.

Acetaminophen is distributed throughout most fluids of the body, and is metabolized primarily in the liver. Little unchanged drug is excreted in the urine, but most metabolic products appear in the urine within 24 hours.

INDICATIONS AND USAGE

For the relief of moderate to moderately severe pain.

CONTRAINDICATIONS

Hypersensitivity to oxycodone or acetaminophen.

WARNINGS

Drug Dependence: Oxycodone can produce drug dependence of the morphine type and, therefore, has the potential for being abused. Psychic dependence, physical dependence and tolerance may develop upon repeated administration of this drug, and it should be prescribed and administered with the same degree of caution appropriate to the use of other oral narcotic-containing medications. Like other narcotic-containing medications, this drug is subject to the Federal Controlled Substances Act.

PRECAUTIONS

1. *General*
   Head injury and increased intracranial pressure: The respiratory depressant effects of narcotics and their capacity to elevate cerebrospinal fluid pressure may be markedly exaggerated in the presence of head injury, other intracranial lesions or a pre-existing increase in intracranial pressure. Furthermore, narcotics produce adverse reactions which may obscure the clinical course of patients with head injuries.
   Acute abdominal conditions: The administration of products containing oxycodone or other narcotics may obscure the diagnosis or clinical course in patients with acute abdominal conditions.
   Special risk patients: Oxycodone and Acetaminophen should be given with caution to certain patients such as the elderly or debilitated, and those with severe impairment of hepatic or renal function, hypothyroidism, Addison's disease and prostatic hypertrophy or urethral stricture.

2. *Information for Patients:* Oxycodone may impair the mental and/or physical abilities required for the performance of potentially hazardous tasks such as driving a car or operating machinery. The patient taking this drug should be cautioned accordingly.

3. *Drug Interactions:* Patients receiving other narcotic analgesics, general anesthetics, phenothiazines, other tranquilizers, sedative-hypnotics, or other CNS depressants (including alcohol) concomitantly with oxycodone and acetaminonphen may exhibit an additive CNS depression. When such therapy is contemplated, the dose of one or both agents should be reduced.
   The use of MAO inhibitors or tricyclic antidepressants with oxycodone preparations may increase the effect of either the antidepressant or oxycodone. The concurrent use of anticholinergics with oxycodone may produce paralytic ileus.

4. *Usage In Pregnancy:* Pregnancy Category C. Animal reproductive studies have not been conducted with oxycodone and acetaminophen. It is also not known whether oxycodone and acetaminophen can cause fetal harm when administered to a pregnant woman or can affect reproductive capacity. Oxycodone and acetaminophen should not be given to a pregnant woman unless in the judgment of the physician the potential benefits outweigh the possible hazards.
   Nonteratogenic Effects: Use of narcotics during pregnancy may produce physical dependence in the neonate.
   Labor and Delivery: As with all narcotics, administration of oxycodone and acetaminophen to the mother shortly before delivery may result in some degree of respiratory depression in the newborn and the mother, especially if higher doses are used.

5. *Nursing Mothers:* It is not known whether the components of this drug are excreted in human milk. Because

many drugs are excreted in human milk, caution should be exercised when oxycodone and acetaminophen is administered to a nursing mother.

6. *Pediatric Use:* Safety and effectiveness in children have not been established.

ADVERSE REACTIONS

The most frequently observed adverse reactions include light headedness, dizziness, sedation, nausea and vomiting. These effects seem to be more prominent in ambulatory than in non-ambulatory patients, and some of these adverse reactions may be alleviated if the patient lies down.

Other adverse reactions include euphoria, dysphoria, constipation, skin rash and pruritus. At higher doses, oxycodone has most of the disadvantages of morphine including respiratory depression.

DRUG ABUSE AND DEPENDENCE

Oxycodone and Acetaminophen tablets and oral solution are a Schedule II controlled substance.

Oxycodone can produce drug dependence and has the potential for being abused. (see WARNINGS.)

OVERDOSAGE

Acetaminophen:
Signs and Symptoms: In acute acetaminophen overdosage, dose-dependent, potentially fatal hepatic necrosis is the most serious adverse effect. Renal tubular necrosis, hypoglycemic coma and thrombocytopenia may also occur.

In adults, hepatic toxicity has rarely been reported with acute overdoses of less than 10 grams and fatalities with less than 15 grams. Importantly, young children seem to be more resistant than adults to the hepatotoxic effect of an acetaminophen overdose. Despite this, the measures outlined below should be initiated in any adult or child suspected of having ingested an acetaminophen overdose.

Early symptoms following a potentially hepatotoxic overdose may include: nausea, vomiting, diaphoresis and general malaise. Clinical and laboratory evidence of hepatic toxicity may not be apparent until 48 to 72 hours post-ingestion.

Treatment: The stomach should be emptied promptly by lavage or by induction of emesis with syrup of ipecac. Patients' estimates of the quantity of a drug ingested are notoriously unreliable. Therefore, if an acetaminophen overdose is suspected, a serum acetaminophen assay should be obtained as early as possible, but no sooner than four hours following ingestion. Liver function studies should be obtained initially and repeated at 24-hour intervals.

The antidote, N-acetylcysteine, should be administered as early as possible, preferably within 16 hours of the overdose ingestion for optimal results, but in any case, within 24 hours. Following recovery, there are no residual, structural or functional hepatic abnormalities.

Oxycodone:
Signs and Symptoms: Serious overdose with oxycodone is characterized by respiratory depression (a decrease in respiratory rate and/or tidal volume, Cheyne-Stokes respiration, cyanosis), extreme somnolence progressing to stupor or coma, skeletal muscle flaccidity, cold and clammy skin, and sometimes bradycardia and hypotension. In severe overdosage, apnea, circulatory collapse, cardiac arrest and death may occur.

Treatment: Primary attention should be given to the reestablishment of adequate respiratory exchange through provision of a patent airway and the institution of assisted or controlled ventilation. The narcotic antagonist naloxone is a specific antidote against respiratory depression which may result from overdosage or unusual sensitivity to narcotics, including oxycodone. Therefore, an appropriate dose of naloxone hydrochloride (usual initial adult dose 0.4 mg to 2 mg) should be administered, preferably by the intravenous route, and simultaneously with efforts at respiratory resuscitation (see package insert). Since the duration of action of oxycodone may exceed that of the antagonist, the patient should be kept under continued surveillance and repeated doses of the antagonist should be administered as needed to maintain adequate respiration.

An antagonist should not be administered in the absence of clinically significant respiratory or cardiovascular depression. Oxygen, intravenous fluids, vasopressors and other supportive measures should be employed as indicated.

Gastric emptying may be useful in removing unabsorbed drug.

DOSAGE AND ADMINISTRATION

Dosage should be adjusted according to the severity of the pain and response of the patient. However, it should be kept in mind that tolerance to oxycodone can develop with continued use and that the incidence of untoward effects is dose related. This product is inappropriate even in high doses for severe or intractable pain.

Tablets:
The usual adult dose is one tablet every six hours as needed for pain.

Oral Solution:
The usual adult dose is 5 mL (one teaspoonful) every six hours as needed for pain.

HOW SUPPLIED

ROXICET™ Tablets, Oxycodone and Acetaminophen Tablets USP (Oxycodone Hydrochloride 5 mg and Acetaminophen 325 mg) white scored tablets (Identified 54 543).
NDC 0054-8650-24: Unit dose, 25 tablets per card (reverse numbered), 4 cards per shipper.
NDC 0054-4650-25: Bottles of 100 tablets.
NDC 0054-4650-29: Bottles of 500 tablets.
ROXICET™ Oral Solution,
Oxycodone and Acetaminophen Oral Solution (Oxycodone Hydrochloride 5 mg amd Acetaminophen 325 mg Oral Solution per 5 mL)
NDC 0054-8648-16: Unit dose Patient Cups™ filled to deliver 5 mL (Oxycodone Hydrochloride 5 mg, Acetaminophen 325 mg), ten 5 mL Patient Cups™ per shelf pack, 4 shelf packs per shipper.
NDC 0054-3686-63: Bottles of 500 mL.
Store at Controlled Room Temperature (15°–30°C (59°–86°F).
DEA Order Form Required.
Caution: Federal law prohibits dispensing without prescription.

ROXICODONE™   Ⓒ ℞
[rox-ē-cō-dōne]
(oxycodone hydrochloride)
Tablets USP and Oral Solution USP

DESCRIPTION

Each tablet contains:
Oxycodone Hydrochloride .... 5 mg
    (WARNING: May be habit forming)
Each 5 mL Oral Solution contains:
Oxycodone Hydrochloride .... 5 mg
    (WARNING: May be habit forming)
Inactive Ingredients:
The tablets contain microcrystalline cellulose and stearic acid.

The oral solution contains alcohol, FD&C Red No. 40, flavoring, glycol, sorbitol, water, and other ingredients.
Oxycodone is 14-hydroxydihydrocodeinone, a white odorless crystalline powder which is derived from the opium alkaloid, thebaine.

ACTIONS

The analgesic ingredient, oxycodone, is a semisynthetic narcotic with multiple actions qualitatively similar to those of morphine; the most prominent of these involve the central nervous system and organs composed of smooth muscle. The principal actions of therapeutic value of oxycodone are analgesia and sedation.

Oxycodone is similar to codeine and methadone in that it retains at least one half of its analgesic activity when administered orally.

INDICATIONS

For the relief of moderate to moderately severe pain.

CONTRAINDICATIONS

Hypersensitivity to oxycodone.

WARNINGS

Drug Dependence: Oxycodone can produce drug dependence of the morphine type, and therefore, has the potential for being abused. Psychic dependence, physical dependence and tolerance may develop upon repeated administration of this drug, and it should be prescribed and administered with the same degree of caution appropriate to the use of other oral narcotic-containing medications. Like other narcotic-containing medications, this drug is subject to the Federal Controlled Substances Act.

Usage in ambulatory patients: Oxycodone may impair the mental and/or physical abilities required for the performance of potentially hazardous tasks such as driving a car or operating machinery. The patient using this drug should be cautioned accordingly.

Interaction with other central nervous system depressants: Patients receiving other narcotic analgesics, general anesthetics, phenothiazines, other tranquilizers, sedative-hypnotics or other CNS depressants (including alcohol) concomitantly with oxycodone hydrochloride may exhibit an additive CNS depression. When such combined therapy is contemplated, the dose of one or both agents should be reduced.

Usage in pregnancy: Safe use in pregnancy has not been established relative to possible adverse effects on fetal development. Therefore, this drug should not be used in pregnant women unless, in the judgment of the physician, the potential benefits outweigh the possible hazards.

Usage in children: This drug should not be administered to children.

PRECAUTIONS

Head injury and increased intracranial pressure: The respiratory depressant effects of narcotics and their capacity to elevate cerebrospinal fluid pressure may be markedly exaggerated in the presence of head injury, other intracranial lesions or a pre-existing increase in intracranial pressure. Furthermore, narcotics produce adverse reactions which may obscure the clinical course of patients with head injuries.

Acute abdominal conditions: The administration of this drug or other narcotics may obscure the diagnosis or clinical course in patients with acute abdominal conditions.

Special risk patients: This drug should be given with caution to certain patients such as the elderly, or debilitated, and those with severe impairment of hepatic or renal function, hypothyroidism, Addison's disease and prostatic hypertrophy or urethral stricture.

ADVERSE REACTIONS

The most frequently observed adverse reactions include light headedness, dizziness, sedation, nausea and vomiting. These effects seem to be more prominent in ambulatory than in nonambulatory patients, and some of these adverse reactions may be alleviated if the patient lies down.

Other adverse reactions include euphoria, dysphoria, constipation, skin rash and pruritus.

DOSAGE AND ADMINISTRATION

Dosage should be adjusted to the severity of the pain and the response of the patient. It may occasionally be necessary to exceed the usual dosage recommended below in cases of more severe pain or in those patients who have become tolerant to the analgesic effects of narcotics. This drug is given orally. The usual adult dose is one 5 mg tablet or 5 mL every 6 hours as needed for pain.

DRUG INTERACTIONS

The CNS depressant effects of oxycodone hydrochloride may be additive with that of other CNS depressants. See WARNINGS.

MANAGEMENT OF OVERDOSAGE

Signs and Symptoms: Serious overdose of oxycodone hydrochloride is characterized by respiratory depression (a decrease in respiratory rate and/or tidal volume, Cheyne-Stokes respiration, cyanosis), extreme somnolence progressing to stupor or coma, skeletal muscle flaccidity, cold and clammy skin, and sometimes bradycardia and hypotension. In severe overdosage, apnea, circulatory collapse, cardiac arrest and death may occur.

Treatment: Primary attention should be given to the reestablishment of adequate respiratory exchange through provision of a patent airway and the institution of assisted or controlled ventilation. The narcotic antagonist naloxone is a specific antidote against respiratory depression which may result from overdosage or unusual sensitivity to narcotics, including oxycodone. Therefore, an appropriate dose of naloxone (usual initial adult dose: 0.4 mg) should be administered, preferably by the intravenous route, simultaneously with efforts at respiratory resuscitation. Since the duration of action of oxycodone may exceed that of the antagonist, the patient should be kept under continued surveillance and repeated doses of the antagonist should be administered as needed to maintain adequate respiration.

An antagonist should not be administered in the absence of clinically significant respiratory or cardiovascular depression.

Oxygen, intravenous fluids, vasopressors and other supportive measures should be employed as indicated.

Gastric emptying may be useful in removing unabsorbed drug.

HOW SUPPLIED

5 mg white scored tablets. (Identified 54 582).
NDC 0054-8657-24: Unit dose, 25 tablets per card (reverse numbered), 4 cards per shipper.
NDC 0054-4657-25: Bottles of 100 tablets.

5 mg per 5 mL oral solution.
NDC 0054-8545-16: Unit dose Patient Cups™ filled to deliver 5 mL (oxycodone hydrochloride 5 mg), ten 5 mL Patient Cups™ per shelf pack, 4 shelf packs per shipper.
NDC 0054-3682-63: Bottles of 500 mL.

DEA Order Form Required

SODIUM POLYSTYRENE SULFONATE SUSPENSION USP   ℞

DESCRIPTION

Each 60 mL contains:
Sodium Polystyrene Sulfonate USP .... 15 g
Sorbitol USP.. 14.1 g
Alcohol 0.1%
The suspension is caramel-cherry-flavored and also contains Propylene Glycol USP, Microcrystalline Cellulose and Carboxymethylcellulose Sodium, Methylparaben, NF, Propylparaben NF, Saccharin Sodium USP, Flavors, and Purified Water USP.

The sodium content of the suspension is 1500 mg (65 mEq) per 60 mL. It is a brown, slightly viscous suspension with an *in-vitro* exchange capacity of approximately 3.1 mEqu (*in-vivo* approximately 1 mEq) of potassium per 4 mL (1 gram) of suspension. This product may be administered either orally or rectally.

ACTION

The action of this product is to partially release sodium ions from the resin, and replace them by potassium ions as the resin passes along the intestine or is retained in the colon after administration by enema. For the most part, this action occurs in the large intestine, which excretes potassium ions to a greater degree than does the small intestine. The efficiency of this process is limited and unpredictably variable. It commonly approximates the order of 33%, but the range is so large that definitive indices of electrolyte balance must be clearly monitored. Frequent serum potassium determinations, at least once every 24 hours, should be done in order to adjust the individual dosage. The action of this product can be accomplished by either oral administration or by retention enema.

INDICATION

Sodium Polystyrene Sulfonate suspension is indicated for treatment of hyperkalemia.

WARNINGS

Since the effective lowering of serum potassium with this product may take hours to days, treatment with this drug alone may be insufficient to rapidly correct severe hyperkalemia associated with states of rapid tissue breakdown (e.g., burns and renal failure) or hyperkalemia so marked as to constitute a medical emergency. Therefore, other definitive measures, including dialysis, should always be considered and may be imperative. Serious potassium deficiency can occur from Sodium Polystyrene Sulfonate therapy. The effect must be carefully controlled by frequent serum potassium determinations within each 24 hour period. Since intracellular potassium deficiency is not always reflected by serum potassium levels, the level at which treatment with this product should be discontinued must be determined individually for each patient. Important aids in making this determination are the patient's clinical condition and electrocardiogram. Early clinical signs of severe hypokalemia include a pattern of irritable confusion and delayed thought processes. Electrocardiographically, severe hypokalemia is often associated with a lengthened Q-T interval, widening, flattening, or inversion of the T wave, and prominant U waves. Also, cardiac arrhythmias may occur, such as premature atrial, nodal, and ventricular contractions, and supraventricular and ventricular tachycardias. The toxic effects of digitalis are likely to be exaggerated. Marked hypokalemia can also be manifested by severe muscle weakness, at times extending into frank paralysis.

Like all cation-exchange resins, Sodium Polystyrene Sulfonate is not totally selective (for potassium) in its actions, and small amounts of other cations such as magnesium and calcium can also be lost during treatment. Accordingly, patients receiving the product should be monitored for all applicable electrolyte disturbances. Systemic alkalosis has been reported after cation-exchange resins were administered orally in combination with nonabsorbable cation-donating antacids and laxatives such as magnesium hydroxide and aluminum carbonate. Magnesium hydroxide should not be administered with the product. One case of grand mal seizure has been reported in a patient with chronic hypocalemia of renal failure who was given Sodium Polystyrene Sulfonate with magnesium hydroxide as a laxative. Also, the simultaneous oral administration of the product with nonabsorbable cation-donating antacids and laxatives may reduce the resin's potassium exchange capacity.

PRECAUTIONS

Caution is advised when the product is administered to patients who cannot tolerate even a small increase in sodium loads (i.e., severe congestive heart failure, severe hypertension, or marked edema). In such instances compensatory restriction of sodium intake from other sources may be indicated.

If constipation occurs, patients should be treated with sorbital (from 10 to 20 mL of 70% syrup every 2 hours or as needed to produce 1 or 2 watery stools daily), a measure which also reduces any tendency to fecal impaction.

ADVERSE REACTIONS

The product may cause some degree of gastric irritation. Anorexia, nausea, vomiting, and constipation may occur especially if high doses are given. Also, hypokalemia, hypocalcemia, and significant sodium retention may occur. Occasionally diarrhea develops. Large doses in elderly individuals may cause fecal impaction (see Precautions). This effect may be obviated through usage of the resin in enemas as described under Dosage and Administration. Intestinal obstruction due to concretions of aluminum hydroxide, when used in combination with the product, has been reported.

DOSAGE AND ADMINISTRATION

Oral Administration
The average daily adult dose is 15 g (60 mL) to 60 g (240 mL) of suspension. This is best provided by administering 15 g (60 mL) of Sodium Polystyrene Sulfonate suspension one to four times daily. Each 60 mL of Sodium Polystyrene Sulfonate suspension contains 1500 mg (65 mEq) of sodium. Since the

in-vivo efficiency of sodium-potassium exchange resins is approximately 33%, about one-third of the resin's actual sodium content is being delivered to the body.

In smaller children and infants, lower doses should be employed by using as a guide a rate of 1 mEq of potassium per gram of resin as the basis for calculation.

The suspension may be introduced into the stomach through a plastic tube and, if desired, mixed with a diet appropriate for a patient in renal failure.

The suspension may also be given, although with less effective results, as a retention enema for adults of 30 g (120 mL) to 50 g (200 mL) every six hours. The enema should be retained as long as possible and **followed by a clensing enema.** After an **initial cleansing enema,** Sodium Polystyrene Sulfonate suspension is administered at body temperature by using a soft, large size (French 28) rubber tube and is inserted into the rectum for a distance of about 20 cm, with the tip well into the sigmoid colon and taped in place. The suspension is flushed with 50 or 100 mL of fluid, following which the tube is clamped and left in place. If back leakage occurs, the hips are elevated on pillows or a knee-chest position is taken temporarily. The suspension is kept in the sigmoid colon for several hours, if possible. **Then the colon is irrigated with a nonsodium containing solution at body temperature in order to remove the resin.** Two quarts of flushing solution may be necessary. The returns are drained constantly through a Y tube connection.

The intensity and duration of therapy depend upon the severity and resistance of hyperkalemia.

Sodium Polystyrene Sulfonate suspension should not be heated for to do so may alter the exchange properties of the resin.

HOW SUPPLIED

NDC 0054-8816-11: Unit dose bottle filled to deliver 60 mL, 10 bottles per shipper.
NDC 0054-8815-01: Unit dose enema bottle filled to contain 120 mL (for use in delivering the suspension rectally through appropriate tubing).
NDC 0054-8817-55: Unit dose enema bottle filled to contain 200 mL (for use in delivering the suspension rectally through appropriate tubing).
NDC 0054-3805-63: Bottle of 500 mL.

TORECAN®   ℞
(thiethylperazine maleate tablets USP)
(thiethylperazine malate injection USP)
(for intramuscular use only)
(thiethylperazine maleate suppositories USP)

Caution: Federal law prohibits dispensing without prescription.

DESCRIPTION

Torecan® (thiethylperazine) is a phenothiazine. Thiethylperazine is characterized by a substituted thioethyl group at position 2 in the phenothiazine nucleus, and a piperazine moiety in the side chain. The chemical designation is: 2-ethyl-mercapto-10-[3'(1''-methyl-piperazinyl-4'')-propyl-1']-phenothiazine. Thiethylperazine has the following structural formula:

Tablet, 10 mg, for oral administration
ACTIVE INGREDIENT: thiethylperazine maleate USP, 10 mg. *INACTIVE INGREDIENTS:* acacia, carnauba wax, FD&C Yellow No. 5 aluminum lake (tartrazine), FD&C Yellow No. 6 aluminum lake, gelatin, lactose, magnesium stearate, povidone, sodium benzoate, sorbitol, starch, stearic acid, sucrose, talc, titanium dioxide.

Ampul, 2 ml, for intramuscular administration
ACTIVE INGREDIENT: thiethylperazine malate USP, 10 mg per 2 ml. *INACTIVE INGREDIENTS:* sodium metabisulfite NF, 0.5 mg; ascorbic acid USP, 2.0 mg; sorbitol NF, 40 mg; carbon dioxide gas q.s.; water for injection USP, q.s. to 2 ml.

Suppository, 10 mg, for rectal administration
ACTIVE INGREDIENT: thiethylperazine maleate USP, 10 mg. *INACTIVE INGREDIENT:* cocoa butter NF.

Continued on next page

Roxane—Cont.

ACTIONS

The pharmacodynamic action of Torecan® (thiethylperazine) in humans is unknown. However, a direct action of Torecan on both the CTZ and the vomiting center may be concluded from induced vomiting experiments in animals.

INDICATIONS

Torecan® (thiethylperazine) is indicated for the relief of nausea and vomiting.

CONTRAINDICATIONS

Severe central nervous system (CNS) depression and comatose states.

In patients who have demonstrated a hypersensitivity reaction (e.g., blood dyscrasias, jaundice) to phenothiazines.

Because severe hypotension has been reported after the intravenous administration of phenothiazines, this route of administration is contraindicated.

Usage in Pregnancy: Torecan® (thiethylperazine) is contraindicated in pregnancy.

WARNINGS

Torecan® (thiethylperazine) injection contains sodium metabisulfite, a sulfite that may cause allergic-type reactions including anaphylactic symptoms and life-threatening or less severe asthmatic episodes in certain susceptible people. The overall prevalence of sulfite sensitivity in the general population is unknown and probably low. Sulfite sensitivity is seen more frequently in asthmatic than in nonasthmatic people.

Phenothiazines are capable of potentiating CNS depressants (e.g., anesthetics, opiates, alcohol, etc.) as well as atropine and phosphorus insecticides.

Since Torecan® (thiethylperazine) may impair mental and/or physical ability required in the performance of potentially hazardous tasks such as driving a car or operating machinery, it is recommended that patients be warned accordingly.

Postoperative Nausea and Vomiting: With the use of this drug to control postoperative nausea and vomiting occurring in patients undergoing elective surgical procedures, restlessness and postoperative CNS depression during anesthesia recovery may occur. Possible postoperative complications of a severe degree of any of the known reactions of this class of drug must be considered. Postural hypotension may occur after an initial injection, rarely with the tablet or suppository.

The administration of epinephrine should be avoided in the treatment of drug-induced hypotension in view of the fact that phenothiazines may induce a reversed epinephrine effect on occasion.

Should a vasoconstrictive agent be required, the most suitable are norepinephrine bitartrate and phenylephrine.

The use of this drug has not been studied following intracardiac and intracranial surgery.

Usage in Pediatrics: The safety and efficacy of Torecan in children under 12 years of age has not been established.

Nursing Mothers: Information is not available concerning the secretion of Torecan in the milk of nursing mothers. As a general rule, nursing should not be undertaken while a patient is on a drug, since many drugs are secreted in human milk.

PRECAUTIONS

Abnormal movements such as extrapyramidal symptoms (E.P.S.) (e.g., dystonia, torticollis, dysphasia, oculogyric crises, akathisia) have occurred. Convulsions have also been reported. The varied symptom complex is more likely to occur in young adults and children. Extrapyramidal effects must be treated by reduction of dosage or cessation of medication.

Torecan® (thiethylperazine) tablets contain FD&C Yellow No. 5 (tartrazine) which may cause allergic-type reactions (including bronchial asthma) in certain susceptible individuals. Although the overall incidence of FD&C Yellow No. 5 (tartrazine) sensitivity in the general population is low, it is frequently seen in patients who also have aspirin hypersensitivity.

Postoperative Nausea and Vomiting: When used in the treatment of the nausea and/or vomiting associated with anesthesia and surgery, it is recommended that Torecan® (thiethylperazine) should be administered by deep intramuscular injection at or shortly before the termination of anesthesia.

ADVERSE REACTIONS

Central Nervous System: Serious: Convulsions have been reported. Extrapyramidal symptoms (E.P.S.) may occur, such as dystonia, torticollis, oculogyric crises, akathisia and gait disturbances. Others: Occasional cases of dizziness, headache, fever and restlessness have been reported. Drowsiness may occur on occasion, following an initial injection. Generally this effect tends to subside with continued therapy or is usually alleviated by a reduction in dosage.

Autonomic Nervous System: Dryness of the mouth and nose, blurred vision, tinnitus. An occasional case of sialorrhea together with altered gustatory sensation has been observed.

Endocrine System: Peripheral edema of the arms, hands and face.

Hepatotoxicity: An occasional case of cholestatic jaundice has been observed.

Other: An occasional case of cerebral vascular spasm and trigeminal neuralgia has been reported.

Phenothiazine Derivatives: The physician should be aware that the following have occurred with one or more phenothiazines and should be considered whenever one of these drugs is used:

Blood Dyscrasias Serious—Agranulocytosis, leukopenia, thrombocytopenia, aplastic anemia, pancytopenia. Other —Eosinophilia, leukocytosis.

Autonomic Reactions Miosis, obstipation, anorexia, paralytic ileus.

Cutaneous Reactions Serious—Erythema, exfoliative dermatitis, contact dermatitis.

Hepatotoxicity Serious—Jaundice, biliary stasis.

Cardiovascular Effects Serious—Hypotension, rarely leading to cardiac arrest; electrocardiographic (ECG) changes.

Extrapyramidal Symptoms Serious—Akathisia, agitation, motor restlessness, dystonic reactions, trismus, torticollis, opisthotonos, oculogyric crises, tremor, muscular rigidity, akinesia—some of which have persisted for several months or years especially in patients of advanced age with brain damage.

Endocrine Disturbances Menstrual irregularities, altered libido, gynecomastia, weight gain. False positive pregnancy tests have been reported.

Urinary Disturbances Retention, incontinence.

Allergic Reactions Serious—Fever, laryngeal edema, angioneurotic edema, asthma.

Others: Hyperpyrexia, Behavioral effects suggestive of a paradoxical reaction have been reported. These include excitement, bizarre dreams, aggravation of psychoses and toxic confusional states. While there is no evidence at present that ECG changes observed in patients receiving phenothiazines are in any way precursors of any significant disturbance of cardiac rhythm, it should be noted that sudden and unexpected deaths apparently due to cardiac arrest have been reported in a few instances in hospitalized psychotic patients previously showing characteristic ECG changes. A peculiar skin-eye syndrome has also been recognized as a side effect following long-term treatment with certain phenothiazines. This reaction is marked by progressive pigmentation of areas of the skin or conjunctiva and/or accompanied by discoloration of the exposed sclera and cornea. Opacities of the anterior lens and cornea described as irregular or stellate in shape have also been reported.

Drug Interactions: Phenothiazines are capable of potentiating CNS depressants (e.g., anesthetics, opiates, alcohol, etc.) as well as atropine and phosphorus insecticides.

Phenothiazines may induce a reversed epinephrine effect on occasion.

DOSAGE AND ADMINISTRATION

Adult: Usual daily dose range is 10 mg to 30 mg. *ORAL:* One tablet one to three times daily. *INTRAMUSCULAR:* 2 ml IM, one to three times daily. (See PRECAUTIONS.) *SUPPOSITORY:* Insert one suppository, one to three times daily.

Children: Appropriate dosage of Torecan® (thiethylperazine) has not been determined in children.

HOW SUPPLIED

Tablets Each tablet contains 10 mg thiethylperazine maleate, USP. Bottles of 100.

Ampuls: Each 2 ml ampul contains in aqueous solution 10 mg thiethylperazine malate, USP. Boxes of 20 and 100.

Storage: Below 86°F; protect from light.
Administer only if clear and colorless.

Suppositories: Each containing 10 mg thiethylperazine maleate, USP. Packages of 12.

Storage: Below 77°F; tight container (sealed foil).

Manufactured by
Sandoz Pharmaceuticals Corporation
East Hanover, NJ 07936
Distributed by
Roxane Laboratories Inc.
Columbus OH 43216

EDUCATIONAL MATERIAL

Booklets
"Oral Morphine in Advanced Cancer," Robert G. Twycross and Sylvia A. Lack, Practical guidelines on the considerations which must be taken into account when initiating oral morphine therapy, free to physicians and pharmacists

"Oral Morphine—Information for Patients, Families, and Friends," Robert G. Twycross and Sylvia A. Lack, free to physicians, pharmacists, and patients.

Software Diskette
"A Decision Model for the Treatment of Cancer Pain," Charles S. Cleeland and Armando Rotondi. Continuing education for physicians, pharmacists, and nurses. Information for ordering available.

Audiocassette
"Current Concepts in Pain Management and Supportive Care in Patients with Cancer." Continuing education program free to physicians and pharmacists.

Rugby Laboratories, Inc.
100 BANKS AVENUE
ROCKVILLE CENTRE, NY 11570

PARTIAL PRODUCT LISTING:

NDC # 0536-	PRODUCT	
3007	ACETAZOLAMIDE Tablets 250 mg	℞
2110	ACETIC ACID Otic Solution w/HYDROCORTISONE	℞
3027	ALLOPURINOL Tablets 100 mg	℞
3028	ALLOPURINOL Tablets 300 mg	℞
3085	AMANTADINE HCl SG Capsules 100 mg	℞
3044	AMILORIDE w/HYDROCHLORTHIAZIDE Tablets 5 mg/50 mg	℞
3072	AMITRIPTYLINE HCl Tablets 25 mg	℞
3073	AMITRIPTYLINE HCl Tablets 50 mg	℞
3075	AMITRIPTYLINE HCl Tablets 100 mg	℞
0070	AMOXICILLIN Capsules 250 mg	℞
0080	AMOXICILLIN Capsules 500 mg	℞
0016	AMPICILLIN Capsules 500 mg	℞
4050	ANTIBIOTIC EAR Solution	℞
4071	ANTIBIOTIC EAR Suspension	℞
0082	APAP w/CODEINE Elixir	ⓒⱽ/℞
3227	APAP w/CODEINE Tablets 30 mg	ⓒⁱⁱⁱ/℞
3215	APAP w/CODEINE Tablets 60 mg	ⓒⁱⁱⁱ/℞
3219	APAP w/OXYCODONE Capsules 500 mg/5 mg	ⓒⁱⁱ/℞
4959	BACLOFEN USP Tablets 10 mg	℞
4960	BACLOFEN USP Tablets 20 mg	℞
4310	BETAMETHASONE Cream NF 0.1%	℞
3415	CARBAMAZEPINE Tablets 200 mg	℞
3435	CARISOPRODOL Tablets 350 mg	℞
3429	CARISOPRODOL/ASPIRIN Tablets 200 mg/325 mg	℞
3491	CHLORDIAZEPOXIDE/AMITRIPTYLINE HCl Tablets 5/12.5 mg	ⓒⁱⱽ/℞
3492	CHLORDIAZEPOXIDE/AMITRIPTYLINE HCl Tablets 10/25 mg	ⓒⁱⱽ/℞
0120	CEPHALEXIN Capsules 250 mg	℞
0130	CEPHALEXIN Capsules 500 mg	℞
0118	CEPHALEXIN Powder 250 mg/5 cc	℞
0180	CEPHRADINE Capsules 250 mg	℞
0185	CEPHRADINE Capsules 500 mg	℞
3488	CHLORDIAZEPOXIDE HCl Caps 10 mg	ⓒⁱⱽ/℞
3461	CHLOROTHIAZIDE Tablets 0.5 gm	℞
3465	CHLORPROPAMIDE Tablets 250 mg	℞
3444	CHLORZOXAZONE Tablets 500 mg	℞
3490	CLINDEX Capsules	℞
3466	CLOFIBRATE SG Capsules 500 mg	℞
3523	CLONIDINE HCl Tablets 0.1 mg	℞
3524	CLONIDINE HCl Tablets 0.2 mg	℞
3526	CLONIDINE HCl Tablets 0.3 mg	℞
4940	CLORAZEPATE DIPOTASSIUM Tablets 3.75 mg	ⓒⁱⱽ/℞
4941	CLORAZEPATE DIPOTASSIUM Tablets 7.5 mg	ⓒⁱⱽ/℞
4942	CLORAZEPATE DIPOTASSIUM Tablets 15 mg	ⓒⁱⱽ/℞
3516	CONJUGATED ESTROGEN Tabs 0.625 mg	℞
3522	CONJUGATED ESTROGEN Tabs 1.25 mg	℞
5658	CYCLOBENZAPRINE HCl Tablets 10 mg	℞
4963	DANAZOL Capsules 200 mg	℞
4957	DESIPRAMINE FC Tablets 75 mg	℞
4958	DESIPRAMINE FC Tablets 100 mg	℞
4163	DEXAMETHASONE ACETATE LA Suspension 8 mg/cc	℞
3580	DEXAMETHASONE CT Tablets 4 mg	℞
3592	DIAZEPAM Tablets 5 mg	ⓒⁱⱽ/℞
3593	DIAZEPAM Tablets 10 mg	ⓒⁱⱽ/℞
1180	DICLOXACILLIN Capsules 250 mg	℞
1190	DICLOXACILLIN Capsules 500 mg	℞
3367	DICYCLOMINE Capsules 10 mg	℞
3377	DICYCLOMINE Tablets 20 mg	℞
3701	DIETHYLPROPION HCl TD Tabs 75 mg	ⓒⁱⱽ/℞
3763	DIPHENOXYLATE HCl and ATROPINE SULFATE Tablets 2.5 mg	ⓒⱽ/℞
3758	DIPHENHYDRAMINE HCl Capsules 25 mg	℞
3762	DIPHENHYDRAMINE HCl Capsules 50 mg	℞

3570	DIPYRIDAMOLE FC Tablets 25 mg	℞
3571	DIPYRIDAMOLE FC Tablets 50 mg	℞
3572	DIPYRIDAMOLE FC Tablets 75 mg	℞
3596	DISOPYRAMIDE PHOSPHATE Caps 150 mg	℞
3728	DOXEPIN HCl Capsules 25 mg	℞
3729	DOXEPIN HCl Capsules 50 mg	℞
3737	DOXEPIN HCl Capsules 75 mg	℞
3730	DOXEPIN HCl Capsules 100 mg	℞
3738	DOXEPIN HCl Capsules 150 mg	℞
0230	DOXYCYCLINE HYCLATE Caps 100 mg	℞
0340	DOXYCYCLINE HYCLATE Tablets 100 mg	℞
3798	EQUAZINE-M Tablets	ℂⱽ/℞
0354	ERYTHYROMYCIN ER Capsules 250 mg	℞
0335	ERYTHROMYCIN ESTOLATE Suspension 125 mg/5 mL	℞
0337	ERYTHROMYCIN ESTOLATE Suspension 250 mg/5 mL	℞
0360	ERYTHROMYCIN ETHYLSUCCINATE Suspension 200 mg/5 mL	℞
0351	ERYTHROMYCIN ETHYLSUCCINATE Tablets 400 mg	℞
0371	ERYTHROMYCIN ETHYLSUCCINATE Suspension 400 mg/5 mL	℞
0250	ERYTHROMYCIN STEARATE Tabs 250 mg	℞
0265	ERYTHROMYCIN STEARATE Tabs 500 mg	℞
3813	FENOPROFEN CALCIUM Tablets 600 mg	℞
0720	FLUOCINOLONE ACETATE Topical Solution 0.01%	℞
4350	FLUOCINONIDE Cream	℞
3818	FLUPHENAZINE HCl Tablets 5 mg	℞
3819	FLUPHENAZINE HCl Tablets 10 mg	℞
3795	FLURAZEPAM HCl Capsules 15 mg	ℂⱽ/℞
3796	FLURAZEPAM HCl Capsules 30 mg	ℂⱽ/℞
3840	FUROSEMIDE Tablets 20 mg	℞
3841	FUROSEMIDE Tablets 40 mg	℞
3835	FUROSEMIDE Tablets 80 mg	℞
4055	GENORA® ORAL CONTRACEPTIVE Tablets 1/35 6x28	℞
4058	GENORA® ORAL CONTRACEPTIVE Tablets 1/35 3x21	℞
4056	GENORA® ORAL CONTRACEPTIVE Tablets 1/50 6x21	℞
4059	GENORA® ORAL CONTRACEPTIVE Tablets 1/50 3x21	℞
4480	GENTAMICIN Ointment 0.1%	℞
0925	GENTAMICIN Ophthalmic Solution Sterile	℞
3856	GERIMAL Oral Tablets 1 mg	℞
1371	GRANUMED Aerosol Spray	℞
3871	GUIATEX LA Tablets	℞
0840	GUIATUSSIN w/CODEINE Syrup	ℂⱽ/℞
1011	HALOPERIDOL CONCENTRATE 2 mg/mL	℞
3889	HALOPERIDOL Tablets 1 mg	℞
3899	HALOPERIDOL Tablets 2 mg	℞
3879	HALOPERIDOL Tablets 5 mg	℞
3880	HALOPERIDOL Tablets 10 mg	℞
3881	HALOPERIDOL Tablets 20 mg	℞
1245	HEMORRHOIDAL HC Suppositories	℞
3862	HYDRALAZINE HCl CT Tablets 25 mg	℞
3885	HYDRALAZINE PLUS Capsules 25/25	℞
3922	HYDROCHLORTHIAZIDE Tablets 25 mg	℞
3921	HYDROCHLORTHIAZIDE Tablets 50 mg	℞
3923	HYDROCHLORTHIAZIDE Tablets 100 mg	℞
3914	HYDROCODONE w/APAP Tablets	ℂ/℞
0611	HYDROCORTISONE Cream Plain 2.5%	℞
0501	HYDROCORTISONE Cream USP 1%	℞
4286	HYDROCORTISONE Lotion 1%	℞
3884	HYDROPINE H.P. Tablets	℞
3874	HYDROXYZINE HCl FC Tablets 10 mg	℞
3875	HYDROXYZINE HCl FC Tablets 25 mg	℞
1002	HYDROXYZINE HCl Syrup	℞
3893	HYDROXYZINE PAMOATE Capsules 25 mg	℞
3894	HYDROXYZINE PAMOATE Capsules 50 mg	℞
3977	IBUPROFEN Tablets 400 mg	℞
3978	IBUPROFEN Tablets 600 mg	℞
3979	IBUPROFEN Tablets 800 mg	℞
3930	IMIPRAMINE HCl Tablets 25 mg	℞
3931	IMIPRAMINE HCl Tablets 50 mg	℞
3981	INDOMETHACIN Capsules 25 mg	℞
3982	INDOMETHACIN Capsules 50 mg	℞
3980	INDOMETHACIN ER Capsules 75 mg	℞
1390	IOPHEN DM Liquid	℞
1012	IOPHEN-C Liquid	℞
4856	ISOCET Tablets	℞
3937	ISOLLYL Improved Tablets	℞
3942	ISOLLYL w/CODEINE Capsules ½ gr	ℂⁱⁱⁱ/℞
3943	ISOSORBIDE DINITRATE Oral Tabs 10 mg	℞
3927	ISOSORBIDE DINITRATE Oral Tabs 20 mg	℞
4296	ISOSORBIDE DINITRATE TD Tabs 40 mg	℞
3952	LEVOTHYROXINE SODIUM Tablets 0.1 mg	℞
1262	LINDANE Lotion USP	℞
1270	LINDANE Shampoo	℞
3959	LORAZEPAM Tablets 0.5 mg	ℂⱽ/℞
3960	LORAZEPAM Tablets 1 mg	ℂⱽ/℞
3961	LORAZEPAM Tablets 2 mg	ℂⱽ/℞
4827	MAPROTILINE HCl Tablets 50 mg	℞

4002	MECLOFENAMATE Capsules 50 mg	℞
4003	MECLOFENAMATE Capsules 100 mg	℞
3995	MEDROXYPROGESTERONE ACETATE Tablets 10 mg	℞
4822	MEGESTROL ACETATE Tablets 40 mg	℞
4006	MEPROBAMATE Tablets 400 mg	ℂⱽ/℞
1462	METAPROTERENOL Syrup	℞
4027	METHOCARBAMOL Tablets 750 mg	℞
4041	METHYCLOTHIAZIDE Tablets 5 mg	℞
4021	METHYLDOPA FC Tablets 250 mg	℞
4023	METHYLDOPA FC Tablets 500 mg	℞
3996	METHYLDOPA/HYDROCHLORTHIAZIDE Tablets 250 mg/15 mg	℞
3997	METHYLDOPA/HYDROCHLORTHIAZIDE Tablets 250 mg/25 mg	℞
4029	METHYLPHENIDATE HCl Tabs 5 mg	ℂⁱⁱ/℞
4035	METHYLPHENIDATE HCl Tabs 10 mg	ℂⁱⁱ/℞
4030	METHYLPHENIDATE HCl Tabs 20 mg	ℂⁱⁱ/℞
4036	METHYLPREDNISOLONE Tablets 4 mg	℞
4036	METHYLPREDNISOLONE Tablets 4 mg 21 pack	℞
4042	METOCLOPRAMIDE HCl Tablets 10 mg	℞
4018	METRONIDAZOLE FC Tablets 250 mg	℞
4019	METRONIDAZOLE FC Tablets 500 mg	℞
4043	MINOXIDIL Tablets 10 mg	℞
5411	NANDROLONE DECANOATE Injection 100 mg/mL	℞
4831	NITROFURANTOIN Macro-Crystal Capsules 50 mg	℞
4832	NITROFURANTOIN Macro-Crystal Capsules 100 mg	℞
4083	NITROGLYCERIN TD Capsules 2.5 mg	℞
4084	NITROGLYCERIN TD Capsules 6.5 mg	℞
4090	NITROGLYCERIN TD Capsules 9 mg	℞
4098	NITROGLYCERIN TRANSDERMAL SYSTEM 5 mg/24 hrs	℞
4111	NITROGLYCERIN TRANSDERMAL SYSTEM 10 mg/24 hrs	℞
4830	NYSTATIN Cream	℞
1220	NYSTATIN Oral Suspension USP	℞
4094	NYSTATIN Oral Tablets	℞
4091	NYSTATIN VAGINAL Tabs w/Applicator	℞
4097	ORPHENADRINE CITRATE Tablets 100 mg	℞
4115	OXAZEPAM Capsules 15 mg	ℂⱽ/℞
4116	OXAZEPAM Capsules 30 mg	ℂⱽ/℞
4124	PAVAGEN TD Capsules 150 mg	℞
2520	PENICILLIN V Tablets 250 mg	℞
2537	PENICILLIN V Tablets 500 mg	℞
4131	PERPHENAZINE Tablets 2 mg	℞
4132	PERPHENAZINE Tablets 4 mg	℞
4147	PERPHENAZINE Tablets 8 mg	℞
4134	PERPHENAZINE Tablets 16 mg	℞
3077	PERPHENAZINE/AMITRIPTYLINE Tablets 2/10	℞
3082	PERPHENAZINE/AMITRIPTYLINE Tablets 2/25	℞
3083	PERPHENAZINE/AMITRIPTYLINE Tablets 4/25	℞
3084	PERPHENAZINE/AMITRIPTYLINE Tablets 4/50	℞
4234	PHENERBEL-S Tablets	℞
4299	PHENYLBUTAZONE FC Tablets 100 mg	℞
3764	PHENYTOIN SODIUM Capsules 1½ gr	℞
4300	PHENYTOIN SODIUM Extended Action Capsules 100 mg	℞
4312	POLY-VITAMIN FLUORIDE Tabs 0.5 mg	℞
4307	POLY-VITAMIN FLUORIDE Tabs 1.0 mg	℞
4322	POTASSIUM CHLORIDE Extended Release Tablets 8 mEq	℞
4323	POTASSIUM CHLORIDE Extended Release Tablets 10 mEq	℞
3773	POTASSIUM CHLORIDE USP Powder 20 mEq	℞
3777	POTASSIUM Effervescent Tablets 25 mEq	℞
1825	POVIDINE Solution	℞
4336	PRAZEPAM Capsules 5 mg	ℂⱽ/℞
4337	PRAZEPAM Capsules 10 mg	ℂⱽ/℞
4845	PRAZOSIN HCl Capsules 1 mg	℞
4846	PRAZOSIN HCl Capsules 2 mg	℞
4847	PRAZOSIN HCl Capsules 5 mg	℞
4325	PREDNISONE CT Tablets 10 mg	℞
4324	PREDNISONE Tablets 5 mg White	℞
4326	PREDNISONE Tablets 20 mg	℞
4339	PRENATAL PLUS Improved FC Tablets	℞
4366	PROBENECID Tablets 0.5 gm	℞
4365	PROBEN-C Tablets	℞
4357	PROCAINAMIDE SR Tablets 500 mg	℞
4358	PROCAINAMIDE SR Tablets 750 mg	℞
4359	PROCAINAMIDE SR Tablets 1000 mg	℞
4414	PROCHLORPERAZINE Tablets 10 mg	℞
1872	PROMETHAZINE VC w/CODEINE Syrup	ℂⱽ/℞
1805	PROMETHAZINE w/CODEINE Syrup	ℂⱽ/℞
4361	PROPOXYPHENE NAPSYLATE w/APAP Tablets 100 mg/650 mg	ℂⱽ/℞

4387	PROPOXYPHENE w/APAP Tablets 65 mg/650 mg	ℂⱽ/℞
4374	PROPOXYPHENE w/ASPIRIN & CAFFEINE Capsules	ℂⱽ/℞
4309	PROPRANOLOL HCl Tablets 10 mg	℞
4313	PROPRANOLOL HCl Tablets 20 mg	℞
4314	PROPRANOLOL HCl Tablets 40 mg	℞
4316	PROPRANOLOL HCl Tablets 80 mg	℞
4911	PROPRANOLOL E.R. Capsules 60 mg	℞
4912	PROPRANOLOL E.R. Capsules 80 mg	℞
4913	PROPRANOLOL E.R. Capsules 120 mg	℞
4914	PROPRANOLOL E.R. Capsules 160 mg	℞
4402	PROPRANOLOL/HYDROCHLORTHIAZIDE Tablets 40 mg/25 mg	℞
4403	PROPRANOLOL/HYDROCHLORTHIAZIDE Tablets 80 mg/25 mg	℞
4434	QUINIDINE GLUCONATE TD Tablets 324 mg	℞
4432	QUINIDINE SULFATE Tablets 200 mg	℞
4429	QUINIDINE SULFATE Tablets 300 mg	℞
4427	QUININE SULFATE Captabs 325 mg	℞
4426	QUININE SULFATE Tablets 260 mg	℞
1980	SELENIUM SULFIDE Lotion 2½%	℞
4547	SODIUM FLUORIDE Chewable Tabs 2.2 mg	℞
4575	SPIRONOLACTONE Tablets 25 mg	℞
4576	SPIROZIDE Tablets	℞
4617	SULFASALAZINE Tablets 500 mg	℞
0050	SULFIMYCIN Oral Suspension	℞
4628	TEMAZEPAM Capsules 15 mg	ℂⱽ/℞
4629	TEMAZEPAM Capsules 30 mg	ℂⱽ/℞
2040	TERPIN HYDRATE w/CODEINE Elixir	ℂⱽ/℞
9490	TESTOSTERONE CYPIONATE Solution 200 mg/cc	℞
1820	TETRACYCLINE Capsules 250 mg	℞
1870	TETRACYCLINE Capsules 500 mg	℞
4651	THEOPHYLLINE TD Tablets 200 mg	℞
4652	THEOPHYLLINE TD Tablets 300 mg	℞
4642	THIORIDAZINE FC Tablets 25 mg	℞
4643	THIORIDAZINE FC Tablets 50 mg	℞
4644	THIORIDAZINE FC Tablets 100 mg	℞
4646	THIORIDAZINE FC Tablets 200 mg	℞
4515	THIOTHIXENE Capsules 2 mg	℞
4516	THIOTHIXENE Capsules 5 mg	℞
4517	THIOTHIXENE Capsules 10 mg	℞
4518	THIOTHIXENE Capsules 20 mg	℞
4739	TOLAZAMIDE Tablets 250 mg	℞
4744	TOLAZAMIDE Tablets 500 mg	℞
4687	TRAZODONE HCl Tablets 50 mg	℞
4688	TRAZODONE HCl Tablets 100 mg	℞
4689	TRAZODONE HCl Tablets 150 mg	℞
9810	TRIAMCINOLONE ACETONIDE Injection 40 mg/mL	℞
5225	TRIAMCINOLONE Cream 0.1%	℞
5180	TRIAMCINOLONE Ointment 0.1%	℞
4926	TRIAMTERENE HYDROCHLORTHIAZIDE Capsules 50 mg/25 mg	℞
4956	TRIAMTERENE HYDROCHLORTHIAZIDE Tablets 75 mg/50 mg	℞
4734	TRIFLUOPERAZINE SC Tablets 2 mg	℞
4735	TRIFLUOPERAZINE SC Tablets 5 mg	℞
4733	TRIFLUOPERAZINE SC Tablets 10 mg	℞
4686	TRIMETHOPRIM Tablets 100 mg	℞
4692	TRIMETH/SULFA Tablets	℞
4693	TRIMETH/SULFA D/S Tablets	℞
1725	TRIMETH/SULFA Pediatric Suspension	℞
5280	TRIPLE SULFA VAGINAL Cream 2.75 oz	℞
4721	TRI-HYDROSERPINE Tablets	℞
4910	TRI-STATIN II Cream	℞
8520	TRI-VITAMINS w/FLUORIDE Drops 0.25 mg	℞
4779	VALPROIC ACID SG Capsules 250 mg	℞
2390	VALPROIC ACID Syrup 250 mg	℞
4812	VERAPAMIL HCl Tablets 80 mg	℞
4813	VERAPAMIL HCl Tablets 120 mg	℞

GENORA® 0.5/35–21 Tablets   ℞
(norethindrone and ethinyl estradiol)
GENORA® 1/35–21 Tablets   ℞
(norethindrone and ethinyl estradiol)
GENORA® 1/50–21 Tablets   ℞
(norethindrone and mestranol)
GENORA® 0.5/35–28 Tablets   ℞
(norethindrone and ethinyl estradiol)
GENORA® 1/35–28 Tablets   ℞
(norethindrone and ethinyl estradiol)
GENORA® 1/50–28 Tablets   ℞
(norethindrone and mestranol)

PRODUCT OVERVIEW

KEY FACTS

The Rugby distributed line of oral contraceptives includes
Genora® 0.5/35, Genora® 1/35, and Genora® 1/50 containing norethindrone (0.5 mg., 1.0 mg.) and either ethinyl

Continued on next page

Rugby—Cont.

estradiol (0.035 mg.) or mestranol (0.05 mg.), each of the oral contraceptive products is available in both 28-day (including 7 days of inert tablets) and 21-day dosage regimens.

MAJOR USES
Each of the Rugby distributed oral contraceptive products is highly effective in the prevention of pregnancy.

SAFETY INFORMATION
See complete safety information set forth below.

PRESCRIBING INFORMATION

GENORA® 0.5/35–21 Tablets   ℞
(norethindrone and ethinyl estradiol)
GENORA® 1/35–21 Tablets   ℞
(norethindrone and ethinyl estradiol)
GENORA® 1/50–21 Tablets   ℞
(norethindrone and mestranol)
GENORA® 0.5/35–28 Tablets   ℞
(norethindrone and ethinyl estradiol)
GENORA® 1/35–28 Tablets   ℞
(norethindrone and ethinyl estradiol)
GENORA® 1/50–28 Tablets   ℞
(norethindrone and mestranol)

DESCRIPTION
GENORA® 0.5/35-21 Tablets provide an oral contraceptive regimen consisting of 21 white tablets containing norethindrone 0.5 mg and ethinyl estradiol 0.035 mg.
GENORA® 1/35-21 Tablets provide an oral contraceptive regimen consisting of 21 pale blue tablets containing norethindrone 1 mg and ethinyl estradiol 0.035 mg.
GENORA® 1/50-21 Tablets provide an oral contraceptive regimen consisting of 21 white tablets containing norethindrone 1 mg and mestranol 0.05 mg.
GENORA® 0.5/35-28 Tablets provide a continuous oral contraceptive regimen consisting of 21 white tablets containing norethindrone 0.5 mg and ethinyl estradiol 0.035 mg followed by 7 peach tablets containing inert ingredients.
GENORA® 1/35-28 Tablets provide a continuous oral contraceptive regimen consisting of 21 pale blue tablets containing norethindrone 1 mg and ethinyl estradiol 0.035 mg followed by 7 peach tablets containing inert ingredients.
Genora® 1/50-28 Tablets provide a continuous oral contraceptive regimen consisting of 21 white tablets containing norethindrone 1 mg and mestranol 0.05 mg followed by 7 peach tablets containing inert ingredients.

Norethindrone is a potent progestational agent with the chemical name 17-hydroxy-19-nor-17α-pregn-4-en-20-yn-3-one. Ethinyl estradiol is an estrogen with the chemical name 19-nor-17α-pregna-1, 3, 5(10) trien-20-yne-3, 17-diol. Mestranol is an estrogen with the chemical name 3-methoxy-19-nor-17α-pregna-1,3,5(10) -trien-20-yn-17-ol.

Inactive ingredients: Each tablet contains the following inactive ingredients: lactose, magnesium stearate, povidone, starch, and one or more of the following FDA certified dyes: FD&C Blue No. 1, FD&C Yellow No. 6.

CLINICAL PHARMACOLOGY
Combination oral contraceptives act by suppression of gonadotrophins. Although the primary mechanism of this action is inhibition of ovulation, other alterations include changes in the cervical mucus (which increase the difficulty of sperm entry into the uterus) and the endometrium (which may reduce the likelihood of implantation).
The primary mechanism through which Genora® prevents conception is not known, but progestogen-only contraceptives are known to alter the cervical mucus, exert a progestational effect on the endometrium, interfering with implantation, and, in some patients, suppress ovulation.

INDICATIONS AND USAGE
Oral contraceptives are indicated for the prevention of pregnancy in women who elect to use these products as a method of contraception.
Oral contraceptives are highly effective. Table I lists the typical accidental pregnancy rates for users of combination oral contraceptives and other methods of contraception.[1] The efficacy of these contraceptives methods, except sterilization, depends upon the reliability with which they are used. Correct and consistent use of methods can result in lower failure rates.

TABLE I: LOWEST EXPECTED AND TYPICAL FAILURE RATES DURING THE FIRST YEAR OF CONTINUOUS USE OF A METHOD
% of Women Experiencing an Accidental Pregnancy in the First Year of Continuous Use

Method	Lowest Expected[a]	Typical[b]
(No Contraception)	(89)	(89)
Oral Contraceptives		3
combined	0.1	N/A[c]
progestogen only	0.5	N/A[c]
Diaphragm with spermicidal cream or jelly	3	18
Spermicides alone (foam, creams, jellies, and vaginal suppositories)	3	21
Vaginal Sponge		
Nulliparous	5	18
Multiparous	>8	>28
IUD (medicated)	1	6[d]
Condom without spermicides	2	12
Periodic abstinence (all methods)	2–10	20
Female sterilization	0.2	0.4
Male sterilization	0.1	0.15

Adapted from J. Trussell and K. Kost, Table 11[1]

[a] The authors' best guess of the percentage of women expected to experience an accidental pregnancy among couples who initiate a method (not necessarily for the first time) and who use it consistently and correctly during the first year if they do not stop for any other reason.
[b] This term represents "typical" couples who initiate use of a method (not necessarily for the first time), who experience an accidental pregnancy during the first year if they do not stop use for any other reason. The authors derive these data largely from the National Surveys of Family Growth (NSFG), 1976 and 1982.
[c] N/A—Data not available from the NSFG, 1976 and 1982.
[d] Combined typical rate for both medicated and non-medicated IUD. The rate for the medicated IUD alone is not available.

CONTRAINDICATIONS
Oral contraceptives should not be used in women who have the following conditions:
- Thrombophlebitis or thromboembolic disorders
- A past history of deep vein thrombophlebitis or thromboembolic disorders
- Cerebral vascular or coronary artery disease
- Known or suspected carcinoma of the breast
- Carcinoma of the endometrium, and known or suspected estrogen-dependent neoplasia
- Undiagnosed abnormal genital bleeding
- Cholestatic jaundice of pregnancy or jaundice with prior pill use
- Hepatic adenomas, carcinomas or benign liver tumors
- Known or suspected pregnancy

WARNINGS

> **Cigarette smoking increases the risk of serious cardiovascular side effects from oral contraceptive use. This risk increases with age and with heavy smoking (15 or more cigarettes per day) and is quite marked in women over 35 years of age. Women who use oral contraceptives should be strongly advised not to smoke.**

The use of oral contraceptives is associated with increased risks of several serious conditions including myocardial infarction, thromboembolism, stroke, hepatic neoplasia and gallbladder disease, although the risk of serious morbidity and mortality increases significantly in the presence of other underlying risk factors such as hypertension, hyperlipidemias, hypercholesterolemia, obesity and diabetes.[2–5] Practitioners prescribing oral contraceptives should be familiar with the following information to these risks:
The information contained in this package insert is principally based on studies carried out in patients who used oral contraceptives with formulations containing 0.05 mg or higher of estrogen[6–11] The effects of long-term use with lower dose formulations of both estrogens and progestogens remain to be determined.
Throughout this labeling, epidemiological studies reported are of two types: retrospective or case control studies and prospective or cohort studies. Case control studies provide a measure of the relative risk of a disease. Relative risk, the *ratio* of the incidence of a disease among oral contraceptives users to that among non-users, cannot be assessed directly from case control studies, but the odds ratio obtained is a measure of relative risk. The relative risk does not provide information on the actual clinical occurrence of a disease. Cohort studies provide not only a measure of the relative risk but a measure of attributable risk, which is the *difference* in the incidence of disease between oral contraceptive users and non-users. The attributable risk does provide information about the actual occurrence of a disease in the population.[12–13]

1. THROMBOEMBOLIC DISORDERS AND OTHER VASCULAR PROBLEMS
a. Myocardial Infarction
An increased risk of myocardial infarction has been attributed to oral contraceptive use. This risk is primarily in smokers or women with other underlying risk factors for coronary artery disease such as hypertension, hypercholesterolemia, morbid obesity and diabetes.[2–5,13] The relative risk of heart attack for current oral contraceptive users has been estimated to be 2 to 6.[2,14–19] The risk is very low under the age of 30. However, there is the possibility of a risk of cardiovascular disease even in very young women who take oral contraceptives.
Smoking in combination with oral contraceptive use has been shown to contribute substantially to the incidence of myocardial infarctions in women 35 or older, with smoking accounting for the majority of excess cases.[20]
Mortality rates associated with circulatory disease have been shown to increase substantially in smokers over the age of 35 and non-smokers over the age of 40 among women who use oral contraceptives (see Table II).[16]

TABLE II: CIRCULATORY DISEASE MORTALITY RATES PER 100,000 WOMAN YEARS BY AGE, SMOKING STATUS AND ORAL CONTRACEPTIVE USE

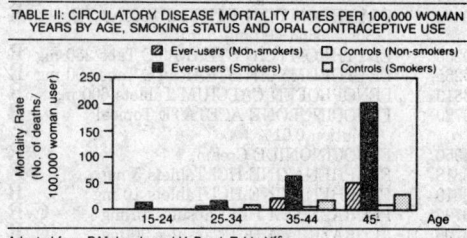

Adapted from P.M. Layde and V. Beral, Table V[16]

Oral contraceptives may compound the effects of well-known risk factors for coronary artery disease, such as hypertension, diabetes, hyperlipidemias, hypercholesterolemia, age and obesity.[3,13,21] In particular, some progestogens are known to decrease HDL cholesterol and impair oral glucose tolerance, while estrogens may create a state of hyperinsulinism.[21–25] Oral contraceptives have been shown to increase blood pressure among users (see WARNINGS, section 9). Similar effects on risk factors have been associated with an increased risk of heart disease. Oral contraceptives must be used with caution in women with cardiovascular disease risk factors.

b. Thromboembolism
An increased risk of thromboembolic and thrombotic disease associated with the use of oral contraceptives is well established. Case control studies have found the relative risk of users compared to non-users to be 3 for the first episode of superficial venous thrombosis, 4 to 11 for deep vein thrombosis or pulmonary embolism, and 1.5 to 6 for women with predisposing conditions for venous thromboembolic disease.[12,13,26–31] One cohort study has shown the relative risk to be somewhat lower, about 3 for new cases (subjects with no past history of venous thrombosis or varicose veins) and about 4.5 for new cases requiring hospitalization.[32] The risk of thromboembolic disease due to oral contraceptives is not related to length of use and disappears after pill use is stopped.[12]
A 2- to 6-fold increase in relative risk of post-operative thromboembolic complications has been reported with the use of oral contraceptives.[18] If feasible, oral contraceptives should be discontinued at least 4 weeks prior to and for 2 weeks after elective surgery and during and following prolonged immobilization. Since the immediate postpartum period also is associated with an increased risk of thromboembolism, oral contraceptives should be started no earlier than 4 to 6 weeks after delivery in women who elect not to breast feed.[33]

c. Cerebrovascular diseases
An increase in both the relative and attributable risks of cerebrovascular events (thrombotic and hemorrhagic strokes) has been shown in users of oral contraceptives. In general, the risk is greatest among older (>35 years), hypertensive women who also smoke. Hypertension was found to be a risk factor for both users and non-users for both types of strokes while smoking interacted to increase the risk for hemorrhagic strokes.[34]
In a large study, the relative risk of thrombotic strokes has been shown to range from 3 for normotensive users to 14 for users with severe hypertension.[35] The relative risk of hemorrhagic stroke is reported to be 1.2 for non-smokers who used oral contraceptives, 2.6 for smokers who did not use oral contraceptives, 7.6 for smokers who used oral contraceptives, 1.8 for normotensive users and 25.7 for users with severe hypertension.[35] The attributable risk also is greater in women 35 or older and among smokers.[13]

d. Dose-related risk of vascular disease from oral contraceptives.
A positive association has been observed between the amount of estrogen and progestogen in oral contraceptives and the risk of vascular disease.[36–38] A decline in serum high density lipoproteins (HDL) has been reported with some progestational agents.[22–24] A decline in serum high density lipo-

proteins has been associated with an increased incidence of ischemic heart disease.[39] Because estrogens increase HDL cholesterol, the net effect of an oral contraceptive depends on a balance achieved between doses of estrogen and progestogen and the nature and absolute amount of progestogens used in the contraceptives. The amount of both hormones should be considered in the choice of oral contraceptives.[37] Minimizing exposure to estrogen and progestogen is in keeping with good principles of therapeutics. For any particular estrogen/progestogen combination, the dosage regimen prescribed should be one which contains the least amount of estrogen and progestogen that is compatible with a low failure rate and the needs of the individual patient. New acceptors of oral contraceptive agents should be started on preparations containing the lowest estrogen content that produces satisfactory results for the individual.

e. Persistence of risk of vascular disease

There are three studies which have shown persistence of risk of vascular disease for ever-users of oral contraceptives.[17,34,40] In a study in the United States, the risk of developing myocardial infarction after discontinuing oral contraceptives persists for at least 9 years for women 40–49 years who had used oral contraceptives for 5 or more years, but this increased risk was not demonstrated in other age groups.[17] In another study in Great Britain, the risk of developing cerebrovascular disease persisted for at least 6 years after discontinuation of oral contraceptives, although excess risk was very small.[40] Subarachnoid hemorrhage also has a significantly increased relative risk after termination of use of oral contraceptives.[34] However, these studies were performed with oral contraceptives formulations containing 0.05 mg or higher of estrogen.

2. ESTIMATES OF MORTALITY FROM CONTRACEPTIVES USE

One study gathered data from a variety of sources which have estimated the mortality rates associated with different methods of contraception at different ages (see Table III).[41] These estimates include the combined risk of death associated with contraceptive methods plus the risk attributable to pregnancy in the event of method failure. Each method of contraception has its specific benefits and risks. The study concluded that with the exception of oral contraceptive users 35 and older who smoke and 40 and older who do not smoke, mortality associated with all methods of birth control is low and below that associated with childbirth. However, smokers 35 and older and non-smokers 40 and older who use oral contraceptives have an increase in morality greater than those using other methods of birth control. These facts must be weighed in conjunction with failure rates for other methods and the risk associated with subsequent pregnancy (see Table I).

[See table above].

3. CARCINOMA OF THE BREAST AND REPRODUCTIVE ORGANS

Numerous epidemiological studies have been performed on the incidence of breast, endometrial, ovarian and cervical cancer in women using oral contraceptives. The evidence in the literature suggests that use of oral contraceptives is not associated with an increase in the risk of developing breast cancer, regardless of the age and parity of first use or with most of the marketed brands and doses.[42,43] The Cancer and Steroid Hormone study also showed no latent effect on the risk of breast cancer for at least a decade following long-term use.[43] A few studies have shown a slightly increased relative risk of developing breast cancer,[44–47] although the methodology of these studies, which included differences in examination of users and non-users and differences in age at start of use, has been questioned.[47–49]

Some studies suggest that oral contraceptive use has been associated with an increase in the risk of cervical intraepithelial neoplasia in some populations of women.[50–53] However, there continues to be controversy about the extent to which such findings may be due to differences in sexual behavior and other factors.

In spite of many studies of the relationship between oral contraceptive use and breast or cervical cancers, a cause and effect relationship has not been established.

4. HEPATIC NEOPLASIA

Benign hepatic adenomas are associated with oral contraceptives use although the incidence of benign tumors is rare in the United States. Indirect calculations have estimated the attributable risk to be in the range of 3.3 cases per 100,000 for users, a risk that increases after 4 or more years of use.[54] Rupture of rare, benign, hepatic adenomas may cause death through intra-abdominal hermorrhage.[55–56] Studies in the United States and Britain have shown an increased risk of developing hepatocellular carcinoma in long-term (>8 years) oral contraceptive users.[57–59] However, these cancers are extremely rare in the United States and the attributable risk (the excess incidence) of liver cancers in oral contraceptive users is less than 1 per 1,000,000 users.

5. OCULAR LESIONS

There have been clinical case reports of retinal thrombosis associated with the use of oral contraceptives. Oral contraceptives should be discontinued if there is unexplained partial or complete loss of vision; onset of proptosis or diplopia; papilledema; or retinal vascular lesions. Appropriate diagnostic and therapeutic measures should be undertaken immediately.

6. ORAL CONTRACEPTIVE USE BEFORE OR DURING EARLY PREGNANCY

Extensive epidemiological studies have revealed no increased risk of birth defects in women who have used oral contraceptives prior to pregnancy.[60–62] More recent studies do not suggest a teratogenic effect, particularly insofar as cardiac anomalies and limb reduction defects are concerned, when taken inadvertently during early pregnancy.[60,61,63,64] The administration of oral contraceptives to induce withdrawal bleeding should not be used as a test for pregnancy. Oral contraceptives should not be used during pregnancy to treat threatened or habitual abortion.

It is recommended that for any patient who has missed 2 consecutive periods, pregnancy should be ruled out before continuing oral contraceptive use. If the patient has not adhered to the prescribed schedule, the possibility of pregnancy should be considered at the time of the first missed period. Oral contraceptive use should be discontinued if pregnancy is confirmed.

7. GALLBLADDER DISEASE

Earlier studies have reported an increased lifetime relative risk of gallbladder surgery in users of oral contraceptives and estrogens.[65–66] More recent studies, however, have shown that the relative risk of developing gallbladder disease among oral contraceptive users may be minimal.[67] The recent findings of minimal risk may be related to the use of oral contraceptive formulations containing lower hormonal doses of estrogens and progestogens.[68]

8. CARBOHYDRATE AND LIPID METABOLIC EFFECTS

Oral contraceptives have been shown to impair oral glucose tolerance.[69] Oral contraceptives containing greater than 0.075 mg of estrogen cause glucose intolerance with impaired insulin secretion, while lower doses of estrogen may produce less glucose intolerance.[70] Progestogens increase insulin secretion and create insulin resistance, this effect varying with different progestational agents.[25,71] However, in the non-diabetic woman, oral contraceptives appear to have no effect on fasting blood glucose.[69] Because of these demonstrated effects, prediabetic and diabetic women should be carefully observed while taking oral contraceptives.

Some women may develop persistent hypertriglyceridemia while on the pill.[72] As discussed earlier (see WARNINGS, sections 1a. and 1d.), changes in serum triglycerides and lipoprotein levels have been reported in oral contraceptives users.[23]

9. ELEVATED BLOOD PRESSURE

An increase in blood pressure has been reported in women taking oral contraceptives. The incidence of risk also was reported to increase with continued use and among older women.[66] Data from the Royal College of General Practitioners and subsequent randomized trials have shown that the incidence of hypertension increases with increasing concentrations of progestogens.

Women with a history of hypertension or hypertension-related diseases or renal disease should be encouraged to use another method of contraception. If women elect to use oral contraceptives, they should be monitored closely and if significant elevation of blood pressure occurs oral contraceptives should be discontinued. For most women, elevated blood pressure will return to normal after stopping oral contraceptives and there is no difference in the occurrence of hypertension among ever- and never-users.[73–75]

10. HEADACHE

The onset or exacerbation of migraine or development of headache with a new pattern which is recurrent, persistent or severe requires discontinuation of oral contraceptives and evaluation of the cause.

11. BLEEDING IRREGULARITIES

Breakthrough bleeding and spotting are sometimes encountered in patients on oral contraceptives, especially during the first 3 months of use. Non-hormonal causes should be considered and adequate diagnostic measures taken to rule out malignancy or pregnancy in the event of breakthrough bleeding, as in the case of any abnormal vaginal bleeding. If pathology has been excluded, time or a change to another formulation may solve the problem. In the event of amenorrhea, pregnancy should be ruled out.

Some women may encounter post-pill amenorrhea or oligomenorrhea, especially when such a condition was pre-existent.

PRECAUTIONS

1. PHYSICAL EXAMINATION AND FOLLOW-UP

A complete medical history and physical examination should be taken prior to the initiation or reinstitution of oral contraceptives and at least annually during use of oral contraceptives. These physical examinations should include special reference to blood pressure, breasts, abdomen and pelvic organs, including cervical cytology and relevant laboratory tests. In case of undiagnosed, persistent or recurrent abnormal vaginal bleeding, appropriate diagnostic measures, should be conducted to rule out malignancy. Women with a strong family history of breast cancer or who have breast nodules should be monitored with particular care.

2. LIPID DISORDERS

Women who are being treated for hyperlipidemias should be followed closely if they elect to use oral contraceptives. Some progestogens may elevate LDL levels and may render the control of hyperlipidemias more difficult.

3. LIVER FUNCTION

If jaundice develops in any woman receiving oral contraceptives the medication should be discontinued. Steroid hormones may be poorly metabolized in patients with impaired liver function.

4. FLUID RETENTION

Oral contraceptives may cause some degree of fluid retention. They should be prescribed with caution, and only with careful monitoring, in patients with conditions which might be aggravated by fluid retention.

5. EMOTIONAL DISORDERS

Women with a history of depression should be carefully observed and the drug discontinued if depression recurs to a serious degree.

6. CONTACT LENSES

Contact lens wearers who develop visual changes or changes in lens tolerance should be assessed by an ophthalmologist.

7. DRUG INTERACTIONS

Reduced efficacy and increased incidence of breakthrough bleeding and menstrual irregularities have been associated with concomitant use of rifampin. A similar association though less marked, has been suggested with barbiturates, phenylbutazone, phenytoin sodium, and possibly with griseofulvin, ampicillin and tetracyclines.[76]

8. INTERACTIONS WITH LABORATORY TESTS

Certain endocrine and liver function tests and blood components may be affected by oral contraceptives:

a. Increased prothrombin and factors VII, VIII, IX, and X; decreased antithrombin 3; increased norepinephrine-induced platelet aggregability.

b. Increased thyroid binding globulin (TBG) leading to increased circulating total thyroid hormone, as measured by protein-bound iodine (PBI), T4 by column or by radioimmunoassay. Free T3 resin uptake is decreased, reflecting the elevated TBG. Free T4 concentration is unaltered.

c. Other binding proteins may be elevated in serum.

d. Sex steroid binding globulins are increased and result in elevated levels of total circulating sex steroids and corticords; however, free or biologically active levels remain unchanged.

TABLE III: ESTIMATED ANNUAL NUMBER OF BIRTH-RELATED OR METHOD-RELATED DEATHS ASSOCIATED WITH CONTROL OF FERTILITY PER 100,000 NONSTERILE WOMEN, BY FERTILITY CONTROL METHOD ACCORDING TO AGE

Method of control and outcome	15–19	20–24	25–29	30–34	35–39	40–44
No fertility control methods*	7.0	7.4	9.1	14.8	25.7	28.2
Oral contraceptives non-smoker**	0.3	0.5	0.9	1.9	13.8	31.6
Oral contraceptives smoker**	2.2	3.4	6.6	13.5	51.1	117.2
IUD**	0.8	0.8	1.0	1.0	1.4	1.4
Condom*	1.1	1.6	0.7	0.2	0.3	0.4
Diaphragm/Spermicide*	1.9	1.2	1.2	1.3	2.2	2.8
Periodic abstinence*	2.5	1.6	1.6	1.7	2.9	3.6

*Deaths are birth-related
**Deaths are method-related

Estimates adapted from H.W. Ory, Table 3[41]

Continued on next page

Rugby—Cont.

e. Triglycerides may be increased.

f. Glucose tolerance may be decreased.

g. Serum folate levels may be depressed by oral contraceptives therapy. This may be of clinical significance if a woman becomes pregnant shortly after discontinuing oral contraceptives.

9. CARCINOGENESIS

See WARNINGS section.

10. PREGNANCY

Pregnancy Category X. See CONTRAINDICATIONS and WARNINGS sections.

11. NURSING MOTHERS

Small amounts of oral contraceptives steroids have been identified in the milk of nursing mothers and a few adverse effects on the child have been reported, including jaundice and breast enlargement. In addition, oral contraceptives given in the postpartum period may interfere with lactation by decreasing the quantity and quality of breast milk. If possible, the nursing mother should be advised not to use oral contraceptives but to use other forms of contraception until she has completely weaned her child.

INFORMATION FOR THE PATIENT
See PATIENT LABELING printed below.

ADVERSE REACTIONS
An increased risk of the following serious adverse reactions has been associated with the use of oral contraceptives (see WARNINGS section):

- Thrombophlebitis
- Arterial thromboembolsim
- Pulmonary embolism
- Myocardial infarction
- Cerebral hemorrhage
- Cerebral thrombosis
- Hypertension
- Gallbladder disease
- Hepatic adenomas, carcinomas or benign liver tumors

There is evidence of an association between the following conditions and the use of oral contraceptives, although additional confirmatory studies are needed:

- Mesenteric thrombosis
- Retinal thrombosis

The following adverse reactions have been reported in patients receiving oral contraceptives and are believed to be drug related:

- Nausea
- Vomiting
- Gastrointestinal symptoms (such as abdominal cramps and bloating)
- Breakthrough bleeding
- Spotting
- Change in menstrual flow
- Amenorrhea
- Temporary infertility after discontinuation of treatment
- Edema
- Melasma which may persist
- Breast changes: tenderness, enlargement, secretion
- Change in weight (increase or decrease)
- Change in cervical erosion and secretion
- Diminution in lactation when given immediately postpartum
- Cholestatic jaundice
- Migraine
- Rash (allergic)
- Mental depression
- Reduced tolerance to carbohydrates
- Vaginal candidiasis
- Change in corneal curvature (steepening)
- Intolerance to contact lenses

The following adverse reactions have been reported in users of oral contraceptives and the association has been neither confirmed nor refuted:

- Pre-menstrual syndrome
- Cataracts
- Changes in appetite
- Cystitis-like syndrome
- Headache
- Nervousness
- Dizziness
- Hirsutism
- Loss of scalp hair
- Erythema multiforme
- Erythema nodosum
- Hemorrhagic eruption
- Vaginitis
- Porphyria
- Impaired renal function
- Hemolytic uremic syndrome
- Budd-Chiari syndrome
- Acne
- Changes in libido

- Colitis

OVERDOSAGE
Serious ill effects have not been reported following acute ingestion of large doses of oral contraceptives by young children. Overdosage may cause nausea, and withdrawal bleeding may occur in females.

NON-CONTRACEPTIVE HEALTH BENEFITS
The following non-contraceptive health benefits related to the use of oral contraceptives are supported by epidemiological studies which largely utilized oral contraceptive formulations containing estrogen doses exceeding 0.035 mg of ethinyl estradiol or 0.05 mg of mestranol.[6-11]

Effects on menses:
- Increased menstrual cycle regularity
- Decreased blood loss and decreased incidence of iron deficiency anemia
- Decreased incidence of dysmenorrhea

Effects related to inhibition of ovulation:
- Decreased incidence of functional ovarian cysts
- Decreased incidence of ectopic pregnancies

Effects from long-term use:
- Decreased incidence of fibroadenomas and fibrocystic disease of the breast
- Decreased incidence of acute pelvic inflammatory disease
- Decreased incidence of endometrial cancer
- Decreased incidence of ovarian cancer

DOSAGE AND ADMINISTRATION
To achieve maximum contraceptive effectiveness, oral contraceptives must be taken exactly as described and at intervals not exceeding 24 hours.

21-Day Regimen Dosage Schedule: For the initial cycle of therapy the first tablet may be taken on Day 5 of the menstrual cycle, counting the first day of menstrual flow as Day 1 (DAY 5 START). One tablet is taken each evening at bedtime for 21 days. No tablets are taken for 7 days, then, whether bleeding has stopped or not, a new course is started of one tablet a day for 21 days. This institutes a three weeks on, one week off dosage regimen.

28-Day Regimen Dosage Schedule: For the initial cycle of therapy the first tablet may be taken on the first Sunday after menstrual flow begins (SUNDAY START). When menstrual flow begins on Sunday, the first tablet is taken on that day. One white or pale blue tablet is taken each evening at bedtime for 21 days. Then the peach tablets are taken, one each evening at bedtime for 7 days. After all 28 tablets have been taken, whether bleeding has stopped or not, repeat the same dosage schedule beginning on the following day.

INSTRUCTIONS TO PATIENTS
- To achieve maximum contraceptive effectiveness, the oral contraceptive pill must be taken exactly as directed and at intervals not exceeding 24 hours.
- Important: Women should be instructed to use an additional method of protection until after the first 7 days of administration *in the initial cycle.*
- Due to the normally increased risk of thromboembolism occurring in postpartum, women should be instructed not to initiate treatment with oral contraceptives earlier than 4 weeks after a full-term delivery. If pregnancy is terminated in the first 12 weeks, the patient should be instructed to start oral contraceptives immediately or within 7 days. If pregnancy is terminated after 12 weeks, the patient should be instructed to start oral contraceptives after 2 weeks.[33,77]
- If spotting or breakthrough bleeding should occur, the patient should continue the medication according to the schedule. Should spotting or breakthrough bleeding persist, the patient should notify her physician.
- If the patient misses 1 pill, she should be instructed to take it as soon as she remembers and then take the next pill at the regular time. If the patient has missed 2 pills, she should take 1 of the missed pills as soon as she remembers and discard the other missed pill. She should then take her next pill at the regular time. Furthermore, she should use an additional method of contraception in addition to taking her pills for the remainder of the cycle.
- If the patient has missed more than 2 pills, she should be instructed to discontinue taking the remaining pills and to use an alternative method of contraception until pregnancy has been ruled out.
- Use of oral contraceptives in the event of a missed menstrual period:
  1. If the patient has not adhered to the prescribed dosage regimen, the possibility of pregnancy should be considered after the first missed period and oral contraceptives should be withheld until pregnancy has been ruled out.
  2. If the patient has adhered to the prescribed regimen and misses 2 consecutive periods, pregnancy should be ruled out before continuing the contraceptive regimen.

HOW SUPPLIED
Genora® 0.5/35-21 and Genora® 0.5/35-28 (norethindrone and ethinyl estradiol tablets), Genora® 1/50-21 and Genora® 1/50-28 (norethindrone and mestranol tablets) and Genora® 1/35-21 and Genora® 1/35-28 (norethindrone and ethinyl estradiol tablets) are available in 21-tablet or 28-tablet blisters.

Each 28-tablet blister contains 7 inert tablets. Tablet dispensers are provided with the blisters.

CAUTION: Federal law prohibits dispensing without prescription.

REFERENCES
1. Trussell, J., et al.: *Stud Fam Plann* 18(5):237–283, 1987. 2. Mann, J., et al.: *Br Med J* 2(5956):241–245, 1975. 3. Knopp, R.H.: *J Reprod Med* 31(9):913–921, 1986. 4. Mann, J.I., et al.: *Br Med J* 2:445–447, 1976. 5. Ory, H.: *JAMA* 237:2619–2622, 1977. 6. The Cancer and Steroid Hormone Study of the Centers for Disease Control: *JAMA* 249(2):1596–1599, 1983. 7. The Cancer and Steroid Hormone Study of the Centers for Disease Control: *JAMA* 257(6):796–800, 1987. 8. Ory, H.W.: *JAMA* 228(1):68–69, 1974. 9. Ory, H.W., et al.: *N Engl J Med* 294:419–422, 1976. 10. Ory, H.W.: *Fam Plann Perspect* 14:182–184, 1982. 11. Ory, H.W., et al.: *Making Choices*, New York, The Alan Guttmacher Institute, 1983. 12. Stadel, B.: *N Engl J Med* 305(11):612–618, 1981. 13. Stadel, B: *N Engl J Med* 305(12):672–677, 1981. 14. Adam, S., et al.: *Br J Obstet Gynecol* 88:838–845, 1981. 15. Mann, J., et al.: *Br Med J* 2(5965):245–248, 1975. 16. Royal College of General Practitioners' Oral Contraceptive Study: *Lancet* 1:541–546, 1981. 17. Slone, D., et al.: *N Engl J Med* 305(8):420–424, 1981. 18. Vessey, M.P.: *Br J Fam Plann* 6 (supplement:1–12, 1980. 19. Russell-Briefel, R., et al.: *Prev Med* 15:352–362, 1986. 20. Goldbaum, G., et al.: *JAMA* 258(10):1339–1342, 1987. 21. LaRosa, J.C.: *J Reprod Med* 31(9):906–912, 1986. 22. Krauss, R.M., et al.: *Am J Obstet Gynecol* 145:446–452, 1983. 23. Wahl, P., et al.: *N Engl J Med* 308(15):862–867, 1983. 24. Wynn, V., et al.: *Am J Obstet Gynecol* 142(6):766–771, 1982. 25. Wynn V., et al.: *J Reprod Med* 31(9):892–897, 1986. 26. Inman, W.H., et al.: *Br Med J* 2(5599):193–199, 1968. 27. Maguire, M.G., et al.: *Am J Epidemiol* 110(2):188–195, 1979. 28. Petitti, D., et al.: *JAMA* 242(11):1150–1154, 1979. 29. Vessey, M.P., et al.: *Br Med J* 2(5599):199–205, 1968. 30. Vessey, M.P., et al.: *Br Med J* 2(5658):651–657, 1969. 31. Porter, J.B., et al.: *Obstet Gynecol* 59(3):299–302, 1982. 32. Vessey, M.P., et al.: *J Biosoc Sci* 8:373–427, 1976. 33. Mishell, D.R., et al.: *Reproductive Endocrinology*, Philadelphia, F.A. Davis Co., 1979. 34. Petitti, D.B., et al.: *Lancet* 2:234–236, 1978. 35. Collaborative Group for the Study of Stroke in Young Women: *JAMA* 231(7):718–722, 1975. 36. Inman, W.H., et al.: *Br Med J* 2:203–209, 1970. 37. Meade, T.W., et al.: *Br Med J* 280 (6224): 1157–1161, 1980. 38. Kay, C.R.: *Am J Obstet Gynecol* 142(6):762–765, 1982. 39. Gordon, T., et al.: *Am J Med* 62:707–714, 1977. 40. Royal College of General Practitioners' Oral Contraception Study: *J Coll Gen Pract* 33:75–82, 1983. 41. Ory, H.W.: *Fam Plann Perspect* 15(2):57–63, 1983. 42. Paul, C., et al.: *Br Med J* 293:723–725, 1986. 43. The Cancer and Steroid Hormone Study of the Centers for Disease Control: *N Engl J Med* 315(7):405–411, 1986. 44. Pike, M.C., et al.: *Lancet* 2:926–929, 1983. 45. Miller, D.R., et al.: *Obstet Gynecol* 68:863–868, 1986. 46. Olsson, H., et al.: *Lancet* 2:748–749, 1985. 47. McPherson, K., et al.: *Br J Cancer* 56:653–660, 1987. 48. Huggins, G.R., et al.: *Fertil Steril* 47(5):733–761, 1987. 49. McPherson, K., et al.: *Br Med J* 293:709–710, 1986. 50. Ory, H., et al.: *Am J Obstet Gynecol* 124(6):573–577, 1976. 51. Vessey, M.P., et al.: *Lancet*, 2:930, 1983. 52. Brinton, L.A., et al.: *Int J Cancer* 38:339–344, 1986. 53. WHO Collaborative Study of Neoplasia and Steroid Contraceptives: *Br Med J* 290:961–965, 1985. 54. Rooks, J.B., et al.: *JAMA* 242(7):644–648, 1979. 55. Bein, N.N., et al.: *Br J Surg* 64:433–435, 1977. 56. Klatskin, G.: *Gastroenterology* 73:386–394, 1977. 57. Henderson, B.E., et al.: *Br J Cancer* 48:437–440, 1983. 58. Neuberger, J., et al.: *Br Med J* 292:1355–1357, 1986. 59. Forman, D., et al.: *Br Med J* 292:1357–1361, 1986. 60. Harlap, S., et al.: *Obstet Gynecol* 55(4):447–452, 1980. 61. Savolainen, E., et al.: *Am J Obstet Gynecol* 140(5):521–524, 1981. 62. Janerich, D.T., et al.: *Am J Epidemiol* 112(1):73–79, 1980. 63. Ferencz, C., et al.: *Teratology* 21:225–239, 1980. 64. Rothman, K.J., et al.: *Am J Epidemiol* 109(4):433–439, 1979. 65. Boston Collaborative Drug Surveillance Program: *Lancet* 1:1399–1404, 1973. 66. Royal College of General Practitioners: *Oral contraceptives and health*. New York, Pittman, 1974. 67. Rome Group for the Epidemiology and Prevention of Cholelithiasis: *Am J Epidemiol* 119(5):796–805, 1984. 68. Strom, B.L., et al.: *Clin Pharmacol Ther* 39(3):335–341, 1986. 69. Perlman, J.A., et al.: *J Chornic Dis* 38(10):857–864, 1985. 70. Wynn, V., et al.: *Lancet* 1:1045–1049, 1979. 71. Wynn, V.: *Progesterone and Progestin*, New York, Raven Press, 1983. 72. Wynn, V., et al.: *Lancet* 2:720–723, 1966. 73. Fisch, I.R., et al.: *JAMA* 237(23):2499–2503, 1977. 74. Laragh, J.H.: *Am J Obstet Gynecol* 126(1):141–147, 1976. 75. Ramcharan, S., et al.: *Pharmacology of Steroid Contraceptive Drugs*, New York, Raven Press, 1977. 76. Stockley, I.: *Pharm J* 216:140–143, 1976. 77. Dickey, R.P.: *Managing Contraceptive Pill Patients*, Oklahoma, Creative Informatics Inc., 1984.

DETAILED PATIENT LABELING

INTRODUCTION

Any woman who considers using oral contraceptives ("birth control pills" or "the pill") should understand the benefits and risks of using this form of birth control. This leaflet will give you much of the information you will need to make this decision and will also help you determine if you are at risk of developing any of the serious side effects of the pill. It will tell you how to use the pill properly so that it will be as effective as possible. However, this leaflet is not a replacement for a careful discussion between you and your health care provider. You should discuss the information provided in this leaflet with him or her, both when you first start taking the pill and during your regular visits. You also should follow the advice of your health care provider with regard to regular check-ups while you are on the pill.

EFFECTIVENESS OF ORAL CONTRACEPTIVES

Oral contraceptives are used to prevent pregnancy and are more effective than other non-surgical methods of birth control. When they are taken correctly, without missing any pills, the chance of becoming pregnant is less than 1% (1 pregnancy per 100 women per year of use). Typical failure rates are actually 3% per year. The chance of becoming pregnant increases with each missed pill during a menstrual cycle.

In comparison, typical failure rates for other non-surgical methods of birth control during the first year are as follows:
IUD: 6%
Diaphragm with spermicides: 18%
Spermicides alone: 21%
Vaginal sponge: 18 to 30%
Condom alone: 12%
Periodic abstinence: 20%
No methods: 89%

WHO SHOULD NOT TAKE ORAL CONTRACEPTIVES

> Cigarette smoking increases the risk of serious cardio-vascular side effects from oral contraceptive use. This risk increases with age and with heavy smoking (15 or more cigarettes per day) and is quite marked in women over 35 years of age. Women who use oral contraceptives are strongly advised not to smoke.

Some women should not use the pill. For example, you should not take the pill if you are pregnant or think you may be pregnant. You also should not use the pill if you have any of the following conditions:
- A history of heart attack or stroke
- Blood clots in the legs (thrombophlebitis), brain (stroke), lungs (pulmonary embolism), or eyes
- A history of blood clots in the deep veins of your legs
- Chest pain (angina pectoris)
- Known or suspected breast cancer or cancer of the lining of the uterus, cervix or vagina
- Unexplained vaginal bleeding (until a diagnosis is reached by your doctor)
- Yellowing of the whites of the eyes or of the skin (jaundice) during pregnancy or during previous use of the pill
- Liver tumor (benign or cancerous)
- Known or suspected pregnancy

Tell your health care provider if you have ever had any of these conditions. Your health care provider can recommend a safer method of birth control.

OTHER CONSIDERATIONS BEFORE TAKING ORAL CONTRACEPTIVES

Tell your health care provider if you have or have had:
- Breast nodules, fibrocystic disease of the breast, an abnormal breast x-ray or mammogram
- Diabetes
- Elevated cholesterol or triglycerides
- High blood pressure
- Migraine or other headaches or epilepsy
- Mental depression
- Gallbladder, heart or kidney disease
- History of scanty or irregular menstrual periods

Women with any of these conditions should be checked often by their health care provider if they choose to use oral contraceptives.

Also, be sure to inform your doctor or health care provider if you smoke or are on any medications.

RISKS OF TAKING ORAL CONTRACEPTIVES

1. Risk of developing blood clots

Blood clots and blockage of blood vessels are the most serious side effects of taking oral contraceptives. In particular, a clot in the legs can cause thrombophlebitis and a clot that travels to the lungs can cause a sudden blocking of the vessel carrying blood to the lungs. Rarely, clots occur in the blood vessels of the eye and may cause blindness, double vision, or impaired vision.

If you take oral contraceptives and need elective surgery, need to stay in bed for a prolonged illness or have recently delivered a baby, you may be at risk of developing blood clots.

ESTIMATED ANNUAL NUMBER OF BIRTH-RELATED OR METHOD-RELATED DEATHS ASSOCIATED WITH CONTROL OF FERTILITY PER 100,000 NONSTERILE WOMEN, BY FERTILITY CONTROL METHOD ACCORDING TO AGE

Method of control and outcome	15–19	20–24	25–29	30–34	35–39	40–44
No fertility control methods*	7.0	7.4	9.1	14.8	25.7	28.2
Oral contraceptives non-smoker**	0.3	0.5	0.9	1.9	13.8	31.6
Oral contraceptives smoker**	2.2	3.4	6.6	13.5	51.1	117.2
IUD**	0.8	0.8	1.0	1.0	1.4	1.4
Condom*	1.1	1.6	0.7	0.2	0.3	0.4
Diaphragm/Spermicide*	1.9	1.2	1.2	1.3	2.2	2.8
Periodic abstinence*	2.5	1.6	1.6	1.7	2.9	3.6

*Deaths are birth-related
**Deaths are method-related

You should consult your doctor about stopping oral contraceptives three to four weeks before surgery and not taking oral contraceptives for two weeks after surgery or during bed rest. You should also not take oral contraceptives soon after delivery of a baby. It is advisable to wait for at least four weeks after delivery if you are not breast feeding. If you are breast feeding, you should wait until you have weaned your child before using the pill (see GENERAL PRECAUTIONS, While Breast Feeding).

2. Heart attacks and strokes

Oral contraceptives may increase the tendency to develop strokes (stoppage or rupture of blood vessels in the brain) and angina pectoris and heart attacks (blockage of blood vessels in the heart). Any of these conditions can cause death or temporary or permanent disability.

Smoking greatly increases the possibility of suffering heart attacks and strokes. Furthermore, smoking and the use of oral contraceptives greatly increase the chances of developing and dying of heart disease.

3. Gallbladder disease

Oral contraceptive users may have a greater risk than non-users of having gallbladder disease, although this risk may be related to pills containing high doses of estrogen.

4. Liver tumors

In rare cases, oral contraceptives can cause benign but dangerous liver tumors. These benign liver tumors can rupture and cause fatal internal bleeding. In addition, a possible but not definite association has been found with the pill and liver cancers in 2 studies, in which a few women who developed these very rare cancers were found to have used oral contraceptives for long periods. However, liver cancers are extremely rare.

5. Cancer of the breast and reproductive organs

There is, at present, no confirmed evidence that oral contraceptives increase the risk of cancer of the reproductive organs in human studies. Several studies have found no overall increase in the risk of developing breast cancer. However, women who use oral contraceptives and have a strong family history of breast cancer or who have breast nodules or abnormal mammograms should be followed closely by their doctors.

Some studies have found an increase in the incidence of cancer of the cervix in women who use oral contraceptives. However, this finding may be related to factors other than the use of oral contraceptives.

ESTIMATED RISK OF DEATH FROM A BIRTH CONTROL METHOD OR PREGNANCY

All methods of birth control and pregnancy are associated with a risk of developing certain diseases which may lead to disability or death. An estimate of the number of deaths associated with different methods of birth control and pregnancy has been calculated and is shown in the following table: [See table above].

In the above table, the risk of death from any birth control method is less than the risk of childbirth except for oral contraceptive users over the age of 35 who smoke and pill users over the age of 40 even if they do not smoke. It can be seen from the table that for women aged 15 to 39 the risk of death is highest with pregnancy (7–26 deaths per 100,000 women, depending on age). Among pill users who do not smoke the risk of death is always lower than that associated with pregnancy for any age group, although over the age of 40 the risk increases to 32 deaths per 100,000 women compared to 28 associated with pregnancy at that age. However, for pill users who smoke and are over the age of 35 the estimated number of deaths exceeds those for other methods of birth control. If a woman is over the age of 40 and smokes, her estimated risk of death is 4 times higher (117/100,000 women) than the estimated risk associated with pregnancy (28/100,000 women) in that age group.

According to this table, for women who do not smoke and are under the age of 35, the possible risk of death from oral contraceptive use is low compared to the pregnancy-related risk of death associated with no fertility control method or the failure of other methods of contraception.

WARNING SIGNALS

If any of these adverse effects occur while you are taking oral contraceptives, call your doctor immediately:
- Sharp chest pain, coughing of blood or sudden shortness of breath (indicating a possible clot in the lung)
- Pain in the calf (indicating a possible clot in the leg)
- Crushing chest pain or heaviness in the chest (indicating a possible heart attack)
- Sudden severe headache or vomiting, dizziness or fainting, disturbances of vision or speech, weakness, or numbness in an arm or leg (indicating a possible stroke)
- Sudden partial or complete loss of vision (indicating a possible clot in the eye)
- Breast lumps (indicating possible breast cancer or fibrocystic disease of the breast: ask your doctor or health care provider to show you how to examine your breasts)
- Severe pain or tenderness in the stomach area (indicating a possible ruptured liver tumor)
- Difficulty in sleeping, weakness, lack of energy, fatigue or change in mood (possibly indicating severe depression)
- Jaundice or a yellowing of the skin or eyeballs, accompanied frequently by fever, fatigue, loss of appetite, dark colored urine or light colored bowel movements (indicating possible liver problems)

SIDE EFFECTS OF ORAL CONTRACEPTIVES

1. Vaginal bleeding

Irregular vaginal bleeding or spotting may occur while you are taking the pill. Irregular bleeding may vary from slight staining between menstrual periods to breakthrough bleeding which is a flow much like a regular period. Irregular bleeding occurs most often during the first few months of oral contraceptive use but may also occur after you have been taking the pill for some time. Such bleeding may be temporary and usually does not indicate any serious problem. It is important to continue taking your pills on schedule. If the bleeding occurs in more than 1 cycle or lasts for more than a few days, talk to your doctor or health care provider.

2. Contact lenses

If you wear contact lenses and notice a change in vision or an inability to wear your lenses, contact your doctor or health care provider.

3. Fluid retention

Oral contraceptives may cause edema (fluid retention) with swelling of the fingers or ankles and may raise your blood pressure. If you experience fluid retention, contact your doctor or health care provider.

4. Melasma (Mask of Pregnancy)

A spotty darkening of the skin is possible, particularly of the face.

5. Other side effects

Other side effects may include change in appetite, headache, nervousness, depression, dizziness, loss of scalp hair, rash, and vaginal infections.

If any of these side effects occur, contact your doctor or health care provider.

GENERAL PRECAUTIONS

1. Missed periods and use of oral contraceptives before or during early pregnancy

At times you may not menstruate regularly after you have completed taking a cycle of pills. If you have taken your pills regularly and miss 1 menstrual period, continue taking your pills for the next cycle but be sure to inform your health care provider before doing so. If you have not taken the pills daily as instructed and miss 1 menstrual period, or if you miss 2 consecutive menstrual periods, you may be pregnant. You should stop taking oral contraceptives until you are sure you are not pregnant and continue to use another method of contraception.

There is no conclusive evidence that oral contraceptive use is associated with an increase in birth defects when taken inadvertently during early pregnancy. Previously, a few studies had reported that oral contraceptives might be associated

Continued on next page

Rugby—Cont.

with birth defects but these studies have not been confirmed. Nevertheless, oral contraceptives or any other drugs should not be used during pregnancy unless clearly necessary and prescribed by your doctor. You should check with your doctor about risks to your unborn child from any medication taken during pregnancy.

2. While breast feeding

If you are breast feeding, consult your doctor before starting oral contraceptives. Some of the drug will be passed on to the child in the milk. A few adverse effects on the child have been reported, including yellowing of the skin (jaundice) and breast enlargement. In addition, oral contraceptives may decrease the amount and quality of your milk. If possible, use another method of contraception while breast feeding. You should consider starting oral contraceptives only after you have weaned your child completely.

3. Laboratory tests

If you are scheduled for any laboratory tests, tell your doctor you are taking birth control pills. Certain blood tests may be affected by birth control pills.

4. Drug interactions

Certain drugs may interact with birth control pills to make them less effective in preventing pregnancy or cause an increase in breakthrough bleeding. Such drugs include rifampin, drugs used for epilepsy such as barbiturates (for example, phenobarbital), and phenytoin (Dilantin is one brand of this drug), phenylbutazone (Butazolidin is one brand of this drug) and possibly certain antibiotics. You may need to use additional contraception when you take drugs which can make oral contraceptives less effective.

HOW TO TAKE ORAL CONTRACEPTIVES

1. General instructions

- You must take your pill every day according to the instructions. Oral contraceptives are most effective if taken no more than 24 hours apart. Take your pill at the same time every day so that you are less likely to forget to take it. You will then maintain the proper amount of drug in your body.
- If you are scheduled for surgery or you need prolonged bed rest you should advise your doctor that you are on the pill and stop taking the pill 4 weeks before surgery to avoid an increased risk of blood clots. It is also advisable not to start oral contraceptives sooner than 4 weeks after delivery of a baby.
- When you first begin to use the pill, you should use an additional method of protection until you have taken your first 7 pills.

Your physician has prescribed one of the following dosage schedules. Please follow the instructions appropriate for your schedule.

21-Day Schedule: Consider the first day of menstrual flow as Day 1 of the menstrual cycle and take the first white or pale blue tablet on Day 5 of the menstrual cycle, whether or not the flow has stopped. Take another tablet at the same time each day, preferably at bedtime, for 21 days. Then wait 7 days, during which time a menstrual period usually occurs, and begin taking one tablet every day on the 8th day after you took your last tablet, whether or not the menstrual flow has stopped. This cycle is repeated 21 days on tablets and 7 days off tablets until time for the physician's examination and tablet refill.

28-Day Schedule: Take the first white or pale blue tablet on the first Sunday after your menstrual flow begins. If it begins on Sunday, take the first white or pale blue tablet that day. Follow the sequence around the card and continue taking another tablet at the same time each day, preferably at bedtime, for 21 days. Then take a peach tablet each day for 7 days and expect a menstrual period during this week. The peach tablets contain no active drug and are included simply for your convenience—to eliminate the need for counting days. After all 28 pills have been taken, whether menstrual flow has stopped or not, take the first white or pale blue tablet of the next cycle without any interruption. With the 28-day package, tablets are taken every day of the year with no gap between cycles.

2. Missed periods/breakthrough bleeding

At times, there may be no menstrual period after you complete a cycle of pills. If you miss 1 menstrual period but have taken the pills *exactly as you were supposed to,* continue as usual into the next cycle. If you have not taken the pills correctly, and have missed a menstrual period, *you may be pregnant* and you should stop taking oral contraceptives until your doctor determines whether or not you are pregnant. Until you can get to your doctor, use another form of contraception. If you miss 2 consecutive menstrual periods, you should stop taking the pills until it is determined that you are not pregnant.

Even if spotting or breakthrough bleeding should occur, continue the medication according to the schedule. Should spotting or breakthrough bleeding persist, you should notify your physician.

3. If you forget to take your pill

If you miss only 1 pill in a cycle, the chance of becoming pregnant is small. Take the missed pill as soon as you realize that you have forgotten it. Since the risk of pregnancy increases with each additional pill you skip, it is very important that you take each pill according to schedule.

If you miss 2 pills in a row, you should take 1 of the missed pills as soon as you remember, discard the other missed pill and take your regular pill for that day at the proper time. Furthermore, you should use an additional method of contraception in addition to taking your pills for the remainder of the cycle. If more than 2 pills in a row have been missed, discontinue taking your pills immediately and use an additional method of contraception until you have a period or your doctor determines that you are not pregnant. Missing peach pills in the 28-day schedule does not increase your chances of becoming pregnant.

4. Pregnancy due to pill failure

When taken correctly, the incidence of pill failure resulting in pregnancy is approximately 1% (i.e., 1 pregnancy per 100 women per year). If failure occurs, the risk to the fetus is minimal. The typical failure rate of large numbers of pill users is less than 3% when women who miss pills are included. If you become pregnant, you should discuss your pregnancy with your doctor.

5. Pregnancy after stopping the pill

There may be some delay in becoming pregnant after you stop using oral contraceptives, especially if you had irregular menstrual cycles before you used oral contraceptives. It may be advisable to postpone conception until you begin menstruating regularly once you have stopped taking the pill and desire pregnancy.

There does not appear to be any increase in birth defects in newborn babies when pregnancy occurs soon after stopping the pill.

6. Overdosage

Serious ill effects have not been reported following ingestion of large doses of oral contraceptives by young children. Overdosage may cause nausea and withdrawal bleeding in females. In case of overdosage, contact your health care provider or pharmacist.

7. Other information

Your health care provider will take a medical and family history and will examine you before prescribing oral contraceptives. You should be reexamined at least once a year. Be sure to inform your health care provider if there is a family history of any of the conditions listed previously in this leaflet. Be sure to keep all appointments with your health care provider because this is a time to determine if there are early signs of side effects of oral contraceptive use.

Do not use the drug for any condition other than the one for which it was prescribed. This drug has been prescribed specifically for you; do not give it to others who may want birth control pills.

If you want more information about birth control pills, ask your doctor or health care provider. They have a more technical leaflet called **PHYSICIAN LABELING** which you may wish to read.

NON-CONTRACEPTIVE HEALTH BENEFITS

In addition to preventing pregnancy, use of oral contraceptives may provide certain non-contraceptive health benefits:

- Menstrual cycles may become more regular
- Blood flow during menstruation may be lighter and less iron may be lost. Therefore, anemia due to iron deficiency is less likely to occur.
- Pain or other symptoms during menstruation may be encountered less frequently
- Ectopic (tubal) pregnancy may occur less frequently
- Non-cancerous cysts or lumps in the breast may occur less frequently
- Acute pelvic inflammatory disease may occur less frequently
- Oral contraceptive use may provide some protection against developing two forms of cancer: cancer of the ovaries and cancer of the lining of the uterus.

BRIEF SUMMARY

PATIENT PACKAGE INSERT

Oral contraceptives, also known as "birth control pills" or "the pill," are taken to prevent pregnancy and, when used correctly, have a failure rate of about 1% per year when used without missing any pills. The typical failure rate of large numbers of pill users is less than 3% per year when women who miss pills are included. For most women, oral contraceptives are also free of serious or unpleasant side effects. However, forgetting to take oral contraceptives considerably increases the chances of pregnancy.

For the majority of women, oral contraceptives can be taken safely, but there are some women who are at high risk of developing certain serious diseases that can be life-threatening or may cause temporary or permanent disability. The risks associated with taking oral contraceptives increase significantly if you:

- Smoke
- Are over the age of 40
- Have high blood pressure, diabetes or high cholesterol
- Have or have had clotting disorders, heart attack, stroke, angina pectoris, cancer of the breast or sex organs, jaundice or malignant or benign liver tumors

You should not take the pill if you suspect you are pregnant or have unexplained vaginal bleeding.

> **Cigarette smoking increases the risk of serious cardiovascular side effects from oral contraceptive use. This risk increases with age and with heavy smoking (15 or more cigarettes per day) and is quite marked in women over 35 years of age. Women who use oral contraceptives are strongly advised not to smoke.**

Most side effects of the pill are not serious. The most common such effects are nausea, vomiting, bleeding between menstrual periods, weight gain, breast tenderness and difficulty wearing contact lenses. These side effects, especially nausea and vomiting, may subside within the first 3 months of use. The serious side effects of the pill occur very infrequently, especially if you are in good health and are young. However, you should know that the following medical conditions have been associated with or made worse by the pill:

1. Blood clots in the legs (thrombophlebitis) or lungs (pulmonary embolism), stoppage or rupture of a blood vessel in the brain (stroke), blockage of blood vessels in the heart (heart attack or angina pectoris), eye or other organs of the body. As mentioned above, smoking increases the risk of heart attacks and strokes and subsequent serious medical consequences.
2. Liver tumors, which may rupture and cause severe bleeding. A possible but not definite association has been found with the pill and liver cancer. However, liver cancers are extremely rare.
3. High blood pressure, although blood pressure usually returns to normal when the pill is stopped.

The symptoms associated with these serious side effects are discussed in the detailed leaflet given to you with your supply of pills. Notify your doctor or health care provider if you notice any unusual physical disturbances while taking the pill. In addition, drugs such as rifampin, as well as some anticonvulsants and some antibiotics, may decrease oral contraceptive effectiveness.

Studies to date of women taking the pill have not shown an increase in the incidence of cancer of the breast or cervix. There is, however, insufficient evidence to rule out the possibility that the pill may cause such cancers.

Taking the pill may provide some important non-contraceptive health benefits. These include less painful menstruation, less menstrual blood loss and anemia, fewer acute pelvic infections, and fewer cancers of the ovary and the lining of the uterus.

Be sure to discuss any medical condition you may have with your health care provider. Your health care provider will take a medical and family history before prescribing oral contraceptives and will examine you. You should be reexamined at least once a year while taking oral contraceptives. The detailed patient information leaflet gives you further information which you should read and discuss with your health care provider.

Manufactured for
RUGBY LABORATORIES, INC.
ROCKVILLE CENTRE, N.Y. 11570
Manufactured by
SYNTEX GENERAL PRODUCTS, INC.
HUMACAO, PUERTO RICO 00661
02-121-25-02   © SGPI MAY 1989
Shown in Product Identification Section, page 427

Russ Pharmaceuticals, Inc.
**22 INVERNESS CENTER PARKWAY
SUITE 400
BIRMINGHAM, AL 35242**

FEMCET®   ℞

DESCRIPTION

Each FEMCET® capsule for oral administration contains:
Butalbital* .... 50 mg
*WARNING: May be habit forming.
Acetaminophen .... 325 mg
Caffeine .... 40 mg
Butalbital, 5-allyl-5-isobutylbarbituric acid, a white, odorless, crystalline powder having a slightly bitter taste, is a short to intermediate-acting barbiturate. Its structure is as follows:
[See Chemical Formula at top of next page].
Acetaminophen, 4'-hydroxyacetanilide, is a non-opiate, non-salicylate analgesic and antipyretic which occurs as a white,

$C_{11}H_{16}N_2O_3$ M.W. 224.26

odorless, crystalline powder possessing a slightly bitter taste. Its structure is as follows:

$C_8H_9NO_2$ M.W. 151.16

Caffeine, 1,3,7-trimethylxanthine, is a central nervous system stimulant which occurs as a white powder or white glistening needles. It also has a bitter taste. Its structure is as follows:

$C_8H_{10}N_4O_2$ M.W. 194.19

CLINICAL PHARMACOLOGY

Pharmacologically, FEMCET® combines the analgesic properties of acetaminophen-caffeine with the anxiolytic and muscle relaxant properties of butalbital.

INDICATIONS AND USAGE

FEMCET® is indicated for the relief of the symptom complex of tension (or muscle contraction) headache.

CONTRAINDICATIONS

Hypersensitivity to acetaminophen, caffeine or barbiturates. Patients with porphyria.

PRECAUTIONS

General: Barbiturates should be administered with caution, if at all, to patients who are mentally depressed, have suicidal tendencies, or a history of drug abuse.

Elderly or debilitated patients may react to barbiturates with marked excitement, depression, and confusion. In some persons, barbiturates repeatedly produce excitement rather than depression.

Information for Patients: Practitioners should give the following information and instructions to patients receiving barbiturates:

A. The use of barbiturates carries with it an associated risk of psychological and/or physical dependence. The patient should be warned against increasing the dose of the drug without consulting a physician.

B. Barbiturates may impair mental and/or physical abilities required for the performance of potentially hazardous tasks (e.g., driving, operating machinery, etc.).

C. Alcohol should not be consumed while taking barbiturates. Concurrent use of barbiturates with other CNS depressants (e.g., alcohol, narcotics, tranquilizers, and antihistamines) may result in additional CNS depressant effects.

Drug Interactions: Patients receiving narcotic analgesics, antipsychotics, antianxiety agents, or other CNS depressants (including alcohol) concomitantly with FEMCET® may exhibit additive CNS depressant effects.

  Drugs: Butalbital w/coumarin anticoagulants.

  Effect: Decreased effect of anticoagulant because of increased metabolism resulting from enzyme induction.

  Drugs: Butalbital w/tricyclic antidepressants.

  Effect: Decreased blood levels of the antidepressant.

Usage in Pregnancy: Adequate studies have not been performed in animals to determine whether this drug affects fertility in males or females, has teratogenic potential or has other adverse effects on the fetus. There are no well-controlled studies in pregnant women. Although there is no clearly defined risk, one cannot exclude the possibility of infrequent or subtle damage to the human fetus. FEMCET® should be used in pregnant women only when clearly needed.

Nursing Mothers: The effects of FEMCET® on infants of nursing mothers are not known. Barbiturates are excreted in the breast milk of nursing mothers. The serum levels in infants are believed to be insignificant with therapeutic doses.

Pediatric Use: Safety and effectiveness in children below the age of 12 have not been established.

ADVERSE REACTIONS

The most frequent adverse reactions are drowsiness and dizziness. Less frequent adverse reactions are lightheadedness and gastrointestinal disturbances including nausea, vomiting, and flatulence. Mental confusion or depression can occur due to intolerance or overdosage of butalbital.

DRUG ABUSE AND DEPENDENCE

Prolonged use of barbiturates can produce drug dependence, characterized by psychic dependence, and tolerance. The abuse liability of FEMCET® is similar to that of other barbiturate-containing drug combinations. Caution should be exercised when prescribing medication for patients with a known propensity for taking excessive quantities of drugs, which is not uncommon in patients with chronic tension headache.

OVERDOSAGE

The toxic effects of acute overdosage of FEMCET® (Butalbital, Acetaminophen and Caffeine capsules) are attributable mainly to its barbiturate component, and, to a lesser extent, acetaminophen. Because toxic effects of caffeine occur in very high dosages only, the possibility of significant caffeine toxicity from FEMCET® overdosage is unlikely.

Barbiturate:

Signs and Symptoms: Drowsiness; confusion; coma; respiratory depression; hypotension; shock.

Treatment: 1) Maintenance of an adequate airway, with assisted respiration and oxygen administration as necessary. 2) Monitoring of vital signs and fluid balance. 3) If the patient is conscious and has not lost the gag reflex, emesis may be induced with ipecac. Care should be taken to prevent pulmonary aspiration of vomitus. After completion of vomiting, 30 grams of activated charcoal in a glass of water may be administered. 4) If emesis is contraindicated, gastric lavage may be performed with a cuffed endotracheal tube in place with the patient in the facedown position. Activated charcoal may be left in the emptied stomach and a saline cathartic administered. 5) Fluid therapy and other standard treatment for shock, if needed. 6) If renal function is normal, forced diuresis may aid in the elimination of the barbiturate. Alkalinization of the urine increases renal excretion of some barbiturates, especially phenobarbital. 7) Although not recommended as a routine procedure, hemodialysis may be used in severe barbiturate intoxications or if the patient is anuric or in shock.

Acetaminophen:

Signs and Symptoms: In acute acetaminophen overdosage, dose-dependent, potentially fatal hepatic necrosis is the most serious adverse effect. Renal tubular necrosis, hypoglycemic coma, and thrombocytopenia may also occur.

In adults, hepatic toxicity has rarely been reported with acute overdoses of less than 10 grams and fatalities with less than 15 grams. Importantly, young children seem to be more resistant than adults to the hepatotoxic effect of an acetaminophen overdose.

Early symptoms following a potentially hepatotoxic overdose may include: nausea, vomiting, diaphoresis, and general malaise. Clinical and laboratory evidence of hepatic toxicity may not be apparent until 48 to 72 hours post-ingestion.

Treatment: The stomach should be emptied promptly by lavage or by induction of emesis with syrup of ipecac. Patients' estimates of the quantity of a drug ingested are notoriously unreliable. Therefore, if an acetaminophen overdose is suspected, a serum acetaminophen assay should be obtained as early as possible, but no sooner than four hours following ingestion. Liver function studies should be obtained initially and repeated at 24-hour intervals.

The antidote, N-acetylcysteine, should be administered as early as possible, preferably within 16 hours of the overdose ingestion for optimal results, but in any case, within 24 hours. Following recovery, there are no residual, structural or functional hepatic abnormalities.

DOSAGE AND ADMINISTRATION

One or two capsules every four hours as needed. Do not exceed 6 capsules per day.

HOW SUPPLIED

FEMCET® is supplied in bottles of 100 (NDC 50474-703-01), opaque lavender capsules, imprinted "RUSS 702."

Storage: Store at controlled room temperature, 15°–30°C (59°–86°F).

Dispense in a tight, light-resistant container as defined in the USP/NF.

CAUTION

Federal law prohibits dispensing without prescription.

Manufactured for:
RUSS PHARMACEUTICALS, INC.
Birmingham, AL 35242
Manufactured by:
D. M. GRAHAM LABORATORIES, INC.
Hobart, NY 13788

Rev. 9/88

LORTAB® Tablets
LORTAB® Liquid
[lŏr′tab]

DESCRIPTION

Each LORTAB® 2.5 mg tablet contains:

Hydrocodone Bitartrate* .... 2.5 mg

  *WARNING: May be habit forming.

Acetaminophen.................................500 mg

Also contains colloidal silicon dioxide, croscarmellose sodium, microcrystalline cellulose, polyvinylpyrrolidone, starch (derived from corn), stearic acid and sugar spheres which are composed of starch (derived from corn), sucrose and FD&C Red #3.

Each LORTAB® 5 mg tablet contains:

Hydrocodone Bitartrate* .... 5 mg

  *WARNING: May be habit forming.

Acetaminophen.................................500 mg

Also contains cornstarch, FD&C Blue #1, gelatin, magnesium stearate, microcrystalline cellulose, sugar spheres, povidone, pregelatinized starch, sodium starch glycolate.

Each LORTAB® 7.5 mg tablet contains:

Hydrocodone Bitartrate* .... 7.5 mg

  *WARNING: May be habit forming.

Acetaminophen.................................500 mg

Also contains colloidal silicon dioxide, croscarmellose sodium, microcrystalline cellulose, povidone, starch (derived from corn), stearic acid and sugar spheres which are composed of starch (derived from corn), sucrose, FD&C Blue #1 and D&C Yellow #10.

Each 5cc (1 teaspoonful) LORTAB® LIQUID contains:

Hydrocodone Bitartrate* .... 2.5 mg

  *WARNING: May be habit forming.

Acetaminophen.................................120 mg

Alcohol 7%

Also contains citric acid, glycerin, methylparaben, propylene glycol, propylparaben, purified water, saccharin sodium, sorbitol solution, and sucrose with natural and artificial flavor, and the following coloring agents: FD&C Yellow #10 and FD&C Blue #1.

Hydrocodone bitartrate is an opioid analgesic and antitussive and occurs as fine, white crystals or as a crystalline powder. It is affected by light. The chemical name is: 4,5α-epoxy-3-methoxy-17-methylmorphinan-6-one tartrate (1:1) hydrate (2:5). Its structure is as follows:

$C_{18}H_{21}NO_3 \cdot C_4H_6O_6 \cdot 2\frac{1}{2}H_2O$ M.W. 494.50

Acetaminophen, 4'-hydroxyacetanilide is a non-opiate, non-salicylate analgesic, and antipyretic which occurs as a white, odorless crystalline powder, possessing a slightly bitter taste. Its structure is as follows:

$C_8H_9NO_2$ M.W. 151.16

CLINICAL PHARMACOLOGY

Hydrocodone: Hydrocodone is a semisynthetic narcotic analgesic and antitussive with multiple actions qualitatively similar to those of codeine. Most of these involve the central nervous system and smooth muscle. The precise mechanism of action of hydrocodone and other opiates is not known, although it is believed to relate to the existence of opiate receptors in the central nervous system. In addition to analgesia, narcotics may produce drowsiness, changes in mood and mental clouding.

Radioimmunoassay techniques have recently been developed for the analysis of hydrocodone in human plasma. After a 10 mg oral dose of hydrocodone bitartrate, a mean peak serum drug level of 23.6 ng/mL and an elimination half-life of 3.8 hours were found.

Acetaminophen: The analgesic action of acetaminophen involves peripheral and central influences, but the specific mechanism is as yet undetermined. Antipyretic activity is mediated through hypothalamic heat regulating centers. Acetaminophen inhibits prostaglandin synthetase. Therapeutic doses of acetaminophen have negligible effects on the cardiovascular or respiratory systems; however, toxic doses may cause circulatory failure and rapid, shallow breathing. Acetaminophen is rapidly and almost completely absorbed from the gastrointestinal tract, producing maximum serum concentrations within 30 minutes to one hour. The plasma half-life in adults and children ranges from 0.90 hours to 3.25

Continued on next page

Russ—Cont.

hours with an average of approximately 2 hours. The drug distributes uniformly in most body fluids and is approximately 25% protein bound. Acetaminophen is conjugated in the liver, with less than 3% of the dose excreted unchanged in 24 hours. The primary metabolic pathway is conjugation to sulfate and glucuronide by-products. A minor oxidative pathway forms cysteine and mercapturic acid. These compounds are subsequently excreted by the kidneys into the urine.

INDICATIONS AND USAGE
For the relief of moderate to moderately severe pain.

CONTRAINDICATIONS
Hydrocodone Bitartrate and Acetaminophen Tablets and Liquid: Hypersensitivity or intolerance to hydrocodone or acetaminophen.

WARNINGS
Hydrocodone: Respiratory Depression: At high doses or in sensitive patients, hydrocodone may produce dose-related respiratory depression by acting directly on the brain stem respiratory center. Hydrocodone also affects the center that controls respiratory rhythm, and may produce irregular and periodic breathing.

Head Injury and Increased Intracranial Pressure: The respiratory depressant effects of narcotics and their capacity to elevate cerebrospinal fluid pressure may be markedly exaggerated in the presence of head injury, other intracranial lesions or a pre-existing increase in intracranial pressure. Furthermore, narcotics produce adverse reactions which may obscure the clinical course of patients with head injuries.

Acute Abdominal Conditions: The administration of narcotics may obscure the diagnosis or clinical course of patients with acute abdominal conditions.

PRECAUTIONS
Special Risk Patients (Acetaminophen): As with any narcotic analgesic agent, Hydrocodone Bitartrate and Acetaminophen Tablets and Liquid should be used with caution in elderly or debilitated patients and those with severe impairment of hepatic or renal function, hypothyroidism, Addison's disease, prostatic hypertrophy or urethral stricture. The usual precautions should be observed and the possibility of respiratory depression should be kept in mind.

Information for Patients: Hydrocodone Bitartrate and Acetaminophen Tablets and Liquid like all narcotics, may impair the mental and/or physical abilities required for the performance of potentially hazardous tasks such as driving a car or operating machinery; patients should be cautioned accordingly.

Cough Reflex: Hydrocodone suppresses the cough reflex; as with all narcotics, caution should be exercised when Hydrocodone Bitartrate and Acetaminophen Tablets and Liquid are used postoperatively and in patients with pulmonary disease.

Drug Interactions
Hydrocodone: Patients receiving other narcotic analgesics, antipsychotics, antianxiety agents, or other CNS depressants (including alcohol) concomitantly with Hydrocodone Bitartrate and Acetaminophen Tablets and Liquid may exhibit additive CNS depression. When combined therapy is contemplated, the dose of one or both agents should be reduced.

The use of MAO inhibitors or tricyclic antidepressants with hydrocodone preparations may increase the effect of either the antidepressant or hydrocodone.

The concurrent use of anticholinergics with hydrocodone, as with all narcotics, may produce paralytic ileus.

Pregnancy:
Teratogenic Effects: Pregnancy Category C.
Hydrocodone: Hydrocodone has been shown to be teratogenic in hamsters when given in doses 700 times the human dose. There are no adequate and well-controlled studies in pregnant women. Hydrocodone Bitartrate and Acetaminophen Tablets and Liquid should be used during pregnancy only if the potential benefit justifies the potential risk to the fetus.

Nonteratogenic Effects:
Hydrocodone: Babies born to mothers who have been taking opioids regularly prior to delivery will be physically dependent. The withdrawal signs include irritability and excessive crying, tremors, hyperactive reflexes, increased respiratory rate, increased stools, sneezing, yawning, vomiting, and fever. The intensity of the syndrome does not always correlate with the duration of maternal opioid use or dose. There is no consensus on the best method of managing withdrawal. Chlorpromazine 0.7 to 1 mg/kg q6h, and paregoric 2 to 4 drops/kg q4h, have been used to treat withdrawal symptoms in infants. The duration of therapy is 4 to 28 days, with the dosage decreased as tolerated.

Labor and Delivery: As with all narcotics, administration of Hydrocodone Bitartrate and Acetaminophen Tablets and Liquid to the mother shortly before delivery may result in

some degree of respiratory depression in the newborn, especially if higher doses are used.

Nursing Mothers: It is not known whether hydrocodone is excreted in human milk. Because many drugs are excreted in human milk and because of the potential for serious adverse reactions in nursing infants from Hydrocodone Bitartrate and Acetaminophen Tablets and Liquid, a decision should be made whether to discontinue nursing or to discontinue the drug, taking into account the importance of the drug to the mother.

Pediatric Use: Safety and effectiveness in children have not been established.

ADVERSE REACTIONS
The most frequently observed adverse reactions include lightheadedness, dizziness, sedation, nausea and vomiting. These effects seem to be more prominent in ambulatory than in nonambulatory patients and some of these adverse reactions may be alleviated if the patient lies down.
Other adverse reactions include:

Central Nervous System:
Hydrocodone: Drowsiness, mental clouding, lethargy, impairment of mental and physical performance, anxiety, fear, dysphoria, dizziness, psychic dependence, mood changes.

Gastrointestinal System:
Hydrocodone: The antiemetic phenothiazines are useful in suppressing the nausea and vomiting which may occur (see above); however, some phenothiazine derivatives seem to be antianalgesic and to increase the amount of narcotic required to produce pain relief, while other phenothiazines reduce the amount of narcotic required to produce a given level of analgesia. Prolonged administration of Hydrocodone Bitartrate and Acetaminophen Tablets and Liquid may produce constipation.

Genitourinary System:
Ureteral spasm, spasm of vesical sphincters and urinary retention have been reported.

Respiratory Depression:
Hydrocodone: Hydrocodone bitartrate may produce dose-related respiratory depression by acting directly on the brain stem respiratory center. Hydrocodone also affects the center that controls respiratory rhythm, and may produce irregular and periodic breathing.

If significant respiratory depression occurs, it may be antagonized by the use of naloxone hydrochloride. Apply other supportive measures when indicated.

DRUG ABUSE AND DEPENDENCE
Hydrocodone Bitartrate and Acetaminophen Tablets and Liquid are subject to the Federal Controlled Substance Act [Schedule CIII].

Psychic dependence, physical dependence, and tolerance may develop upon repeated administration of narcotics; therefore, Hydrocodone Bitartrate and Acetaminophen Tablets and Liquid should be prescribed and administered with caution. However, psychic dependence is unlikely to develop when Hydrocodone Bitartrate and Acetaminophen Tablets and Liquid are used for a short time for the treatment of pain.

Physical dependence, the condition in which continued administration of the drug is required to prevent the appearance of a withdrawal syndrome, assumes clinically significant proportions only after several weeks of continued narcotic use, although some mild degree of physical dependence may develop after a few days of narcotic therapy. Tolerance, in which increasingly large doses are required in order to produce the same degree of analgesia, is manifested initially by shortened duration of analgesic effect, and subsequently by decreases in the intensity of analgesia. The rate of development of tolerance varies among patients.

OVERDOSAGE
Acetaminophen:
Signs and Symptoms: In acute acetaminophen overdosage, dose-dependent, potentially fatal hepatic necrosis is the most serious adverse effect. Renal tubular necrosis, hypoglycemic coma, and thrombocytopenia may also occur.

In adults, hepatic toxicity has rarely been reported with acute overdoses of less than 10 grams and fatalities with less than 15 grams. Importantly, young children seem to be more resistant than adults to the hepatotoxic effect of an acetaminophen overdose. Despite this, the measures outlined below should be initiated in any adult or child suspected of having ingested an acetaminophen overdosage.

Early symptoms following a potentially hepatotoxic overdose may include: nausea, vomiting, diaphoresis and general malaise. Clinical and laboratory evidence of hepatic toxicity may not be apparent until 48 to 72 hours post-ingestion.

Treatment: The stomach should be emptied promptly by lavage or by induction of emesis with syrup of ipecac. Patients' estimates of the quantity of a drug ingested are notoriously unreliable. Therefore, if an acetaminophen overdose is suspected, a serum acetaminophen assay should be obtained as early as possible, but no sooner than four hours following ingestion. Liver function studies should be obtained initially and repeated at 24-hour intervals. The antidote, N-acetylcysteine, should be administered as early as possible, preferably

within 16 hours of the overdose ingestion for optimal results, but in any case, within 24 hours. Following recovery, there are no residual, structural or functional hepatic abnormalities.

Hydrocodone:
Signs and Symptoms: Serious overdose with hydrocodone is characterized by respiratory depression (a decrease in respiratory rate and/or tidal volume, Cheyne-Stokes respiration, cyanosis), extreme somnolence progressing to stupor or coma, skeletal muscle flaccidity, cold and clammy skin, and sometimes bradycardia and hypotension. In severe overdosage, apnea, circulatory collapse, cardiac arrest and death may occur.

Treatment: Primary attention should be given to the reestablishment of adequate respiratory exchange through provision of a patent airway and the institution of assisted or controlled ventilation. The narcotic antagonist naloxone is a specific antidote against respiratory depression which may result from overdosage or unusual sensitivity to narcotics, including hydrocodone. Therefore, an appropriate dose of naloxone hydrochloride (see package insert) should be administered, preferably by the intravenous route, and simultaneously with efforts at respiratory resuscitation. Since the duration of action of hydrocodone may exceed that of the antagonist, the patient should be kept under continued surveillance and repeated doses of the antagonist should be administered as needed to maintain adequate respiration.

A narcotic antagonist should not be administered in the absence of clinically significant respiratory or cardiovascular depression. Oxygen, intravenous fluids, vasopressors and other supportive measures should be employed as indicated. Gastric emptying may be useful in removing unabsorbed drug.

DOSAGE AND ADMINISTRATION
Dosage should be adjusted according to the severity of the pain and the response of the patient. However, tolerance to hydrocodone can develop with continued use and the incidence of untoward effects is dose related.

The usual adult dosage for LORTAB® 2.5 mg tablets is one or two tablets every four to six hours as needed for pain. The total 24 hour dose should not exceed 8 tablets.

The usual adult dosage for LORTAB® 5 mg tablets is one or two tablets every four to six hours as needed for pain. The total 24 hour dose should not exceed 8 tablets.

The usual adult dosage for LORTAB® 7.5 mg tablets is one tablet every four to six hours as needed for pain. The total 24 hour dose should not exceed 6 tablets.

The usual adult dosage for LORTAB® Liquid is for adults: 1 tablespoonful (15 cc) every 4 hours as needed (up to 6 tablespoonfuls in 24 hours).

HOW SUPPLIED
LORTAB® 2.5 mg tablets (hydrocodone bitartrate and acetaminophen tablets) contain hydrocodone bitartrate 2.5 mg and acetaminophen 500 mg. They are supplied as white with pink specks, capsule-shaped, bisected tablets, debossed "RUSS 901" in containers of 24 tablets (NDC 50474-925-24) and in containers of 100 tablets (NDC 50474-925-01).

LORTAB® 5 mg tablets (hydrocodone bitartrate and acetaminophen tablets) contain hydrocodone bitartrate 5 mg and acetaminophen 500 mg. They are supplied as white with blue specks, capsule-shaped, bisected tablets, debossed "RUSS 902" in bottles of 100 (NDC 50474-902-01), 500 (NDC 50474-902-50) and in hospital unit-dose packages of 100 (NDC 50474-902-60).

LORTAB® 7.5 mg tablets (hydrocodone bitartrate and acetaminophen tablets) contain hydrocodone bitartrate 7.5 mg and acetaminophen 500 mg. They are supplied as white with green specks, capsule-shaped, bisected tablets, debossed "RUSS 903" in containers of 24 tablets (NDC 50474-907-24), in containers of 100 tablets (NDC 50474-907-01), in containers of 500 tablets (NDC 50474-907-50) and in hospital unit-dose packages of 100 (NDC 50474-907-60).

LORTAB® Liquid, (colored green, tropical punch flavored), is supplied in bottles of 1 pint (NDC 50474-905-16) and 4 oz. (NDC 50474-905-04).

STORAGE
Store at controlled room temperature, 15°–30°C (59°–86°F). Protect from moisture.
DISPENSE IN A TIGHT, LIGHT-RESISTANT CONTAINER AS DEFINED IN THE USP/NF WITH A CHILD-RESISTANT CLOSURE.

CAUTION
Federal law prohibits dispensing without prescription.

Schedule CIII Controlled Substances (Narcotic).

Manufactured For:
RUSS PHARMACEUTICALS, INC.
Birmingham, Alabama 35242
Lortab 2.5 mg, Lortab 7.5 mg and Lortab Liquid Manufactured By:
MIKART, INC.
Atlanta, GA 30318

Lortab 5 mg Manufactured By:
D. M. GRAHAM LABORATORIES, INC.
Hobart, NY 13788

Revised 12/88
Shown in Product Identification Section, page 427

LORTAB® ASA   ⓒ R̶
[lŏr'tab]
Hydrocodone Bitartrate and Aspirin Tablets
5 mg/500 mg

DESCRIPTION

Each tablet contains:
Hydrocodone Bitartrate* .... 5 mg
*WARNING: May be habit forming.
Aspirin ....500 mg
Hydrocodone bitartrate is an opioid analgesic and antitussive and occurs as fine, white crystals or as a crystalline powder. It is affected by light. The chemical name is: 4,5α-epoxy-3-methoxy-17-methylmorphinan-6-one tartrate (1:1) hydrate (2:5). Its structure is as follows:

$C_{18}H_{21}NO_3 \cdot C_4H_6O_6 \cdot 2\frac{1}{2}H_2O$ M.W. 494.50

Aspirin, salicylic acid acetate, is a nonopiate, salicylate analgesic, anti-inflammatory, and antipyretic which occurs as a white, crystalline tabular or needle like powder and is odorless or has a faint odor. Its structure is as follows:

$C_9H_8O_4$ M.W. 180.16

Inactive Ingredients: D&C Red #7 Lake, Pregelatinized Starch and Stearic Acid.

CLINICAL PHARMACOLOGY

Hydrocodone: Hydrocodone is a semisynthetic narcotic analgesic and antitussive with multiple actions qualitatively similar to those of codeine. Most of these involve the central nervous system and smooth muscle. The precise mechanism of action of hydrocodone and other opiates is not known, although it is believed to relate to the existence of opiate receptors in the central nervous system. In addition to analgesia, narcotics may produce drowsiness, changes in mood and mental clouding.

Radioimmunoassay techniques have recently been developed for the analysis of hydrocodone in human plasma. After a 10 mg oral dose of hydrocodone bitartrate, a mean peak serum drug level of 23.6 ng/ml and an elimination half-life of 3.8 hours were found.

Aspirin: The analgesic, anti-inflammatory and antipyretic effects of aspirin are believed to result from inhibition of the synthesis of certain prostaglandins. Aspirin interferes with clotting mechanisms primarily by diminishing platelet aggregation; at high doses prothrombin synthesis can be inhibited.

Aspirin in solution is rapidly absorbed from the stomach and from the upper small intestine. About 50 percent of an oral dose is absorbed in 30 minutes and peak plasma concentrations are reached in about 40 minutes. Higher than normal stomach pH or the presence of food slightly delays absorption.

Once absorbed, aspirin is mainly hydrolyzed to salicylic acid and distributed to all body tissues and fluids, including fetal tissue, breast milk and the central nervous system (CNS). Highest concentrations are found in plasma, liver, renal cortex, heart and lung.

From 50 to 80 percent of salicylic acid and it metabolites in plasma are loosely bound to protein. The plasma half-life of total salicylate is about 3.0 hours, with a 650 mg dose. Higher doses of aspirin cause increases in plasma salicylate half-life. Almost all of a therapeutic dose of aspirin is excreted through the kidneys, either as salicylic acid or it metabolites. Renal clearance of salicylate is greatly augmented by an alkaline urine, as is produced by concurrent administration of sodium bicarbonate or potassium citrate.

Toxic salicylate blood levels are usually above 30 mg/100 ml. The single lethal dose of aspirin in normal adults is approximatey 25–30 g, but patients have recovered from much larger doses with appropriate treatment.

INDICATIONS AND USAGE

For the relief of moderate to moderately severe pain.

CONTRAINDICATIONS

Hydrocodone Bitartrate 5mg and Aspirin 500mg Tablets are contraindicated under the following conditions:

(1) hypersensitivity or intolerance to hydrocodone or aspirin.
(2) severe bleeding, disorders of coagulation or primary hemostasis, including hemophilia, hypoprothrombinemia, von Willebrand's disease, thrombocytopenias, thrombasthenia and other ill-defined hereditary platelet dysfunctions, severe vitamin K deficiency and severe liver damage.
(3) anticoagulant therapy.
(4) peptic ulcer, or other serious gasrointestinal lesions.

WARNINGS

Drugs of this class, salicylates, have been reported to be associated with the development of Reyes Syndrome in children or teenagers with chicken pox, influenza, and influenza-like infections.

Hydrocodone: Respiratory Depression: At high doses or in sensitive patients, hydrocodone may produce dose-related respiratory depression by acting directly on the brain stem respiratory center. Hydrocodone also affects the center that controls respiratory rhythm, and may produce irregular and periodic breathing.

Head Injury and Increased Intracranial Pressure: The respiratory depressant effects of narcotics and their capacity to elevate cerebrospinal fluid pressure may be markedly exaggerated in the presence of head injury, other intracranial lesions or a pre-existing increase in intracranial pressure. Furthermore, narcotics produce adverse reactions which may obscure the clinical course of patients with head injuries.

Acute Abdominal Conditions: The administration of narcotics may obscure the diagnosis or clinical course of patients with acute abdominal conditions.

Aspirin: Allergic Reactions: Therapeutic doses of aspirin can cause anaphylactic shock and other severe allergic reactions. A history of allergy is often lacking.

Bleeding: Significant bleeding can result from aspirin therapy in patients with peptic ulcer or other gastrointestinal lesions, and in patients with bleeding disorders. Aspirin administered preoperatively may prolong bleeding time.

PRECAUTIONS

Special Risk Patients: As with any narcotic analgesic agent, Hydrocodone Bitartrate 5mg and Aspirin 500mg Tablets should be used with caution in elderly or debilitated patients and those with severe impairment of hepatic or renal function, gallbladder disease or gallstones, respiratory impairment, cardiac arrhythmias, inflammatory disorders of the gastrointestinal tract, hypothyroidism, Addison's disease, prostatic hypertrophy or urethral stricture, coagulation disorders, head injuries or acute abdominal conditions. The usual precautions should be observed and the possibility of respiratory depression should not be overlooked.

Precautions should be taken when administering salicylates to persons with known allergies. Hypersensitivity to aspirin is particularly likely in patients with nasal polyps, and relatively common with asthma.

Information for Patients: Hydrocodone Bitartrate 5mg and Aspirin 500mg Tablets, like all narcotics, may impair the mental and/or physical abilities required for the performance of potentially hazardous tasks such as driving a car or operating machinery; patients should be cautioned accordingly.

Cough Reflex: Hydrocodone suppresses the cough reflex; as with all narcotics, caution should be exercised when Hydrocodone Bitartrate 5mg and Aspirin 500mg Tablets are used postoperatively and in patients with pulmonary disease.

Laboratory Tests: Hypersensitivity to aspirin cannot be detected by skin testing or radioimmunoassay procedures.

Drug Interactions
Hydrocodone: Patients receiving other narcotic analgesics, antipsychotics, antianxiety agents, or other CNS depressants (including alcohol) concomitantly with Hydrocodone Bitartrate 5mg and Aspirin 500mg Tablets may exhibit additive CNS depression. When combined therapy is contemplated, the dose of one or both agents should be reduced.
The use of MAO inhibitors or tricyclic antidepressants with hydrocodone preparations may increase the effect of either the antidepressant or hydrocodone.
The concurrent use of anticholinergics with hydrocodone, as with all narcotics, may produce paralytic ileus.
Aspirin: Aspirin may *enhance* the effects of:
(1) oral anticoagulants, causing bleeding by inhibiting prothrombin formation in the liver and displacing anticoagulants from plasma protein binding sites.
(2) oral antidiabetic agents and insulin, causing hypoglycemia by contributing an additive effect, and by displacing the oral antidiabetic agents from secondary binding sites.

(3) 6-mercaptopurine and methotrexate, causing bone marrow toxicity and blood dyscrasias by displacing these drugs from secondary binding sites.
(4) non-steroidal anti-inflammatory agents increasing the risk of peptic ulceration and bleeding by contributing additive effects.
(5) corticosteroids, potentiating anti-inflammatory effects by displacing steroids from protein binding sites. Aspirin intoxication may occur with corticosteroid withdrawal because steroids promote renal clearance of salicylates.
Aspirin may *diminish* the effects of uricosuric agents, such as probenecid and sulfinpyrazone, in the treatment of gout by competing for protein binding sites.
Drug/Laboratory Test Interactions:
Aspirin: Aspirin may interfere with the following laboratory determinations.
In blood: serum amylase, fasting blood glucose, carbon dioxide, cholesterol, protein, protein bound iodine, uric acid, prothrombin time, bleeding time and spectrophotometric detection of barbiturates.
In urine: glucose, 5-hydroxyindoleacetic acid, Gerhardt ketone, vanillylmandelic acid (VMA), protein, uric acid, and diacetic acid.
Pregnancy:
Teratogenic Effects: Pregnancy Category C.
Hydrocodone: Hydrocodone has been shown to be teratogenic in hamsters when given in doses 700 times the human dose. There are no adequate and well-controlled studies in pregnant women. Hydrocodone Bitartrate 5mg and Aspirin 500mg Tablets should be used during pregnancy only if the potential benefit justifies the potential risk to the fetus.
Aspirin: Reproductive studies in rats and mice have shown aspirin to be teratogenic and embryocidal at four to six times the human therapeutic dose. Studies in pregnant women, however, have not shown that aspirin increases the risk of abnormalities when administered during the first trimester of pregnancy. In controlled studies involving 41,337 pregnant women and their offspring, there was no evidence that aspirin taken during pregnancy caused stillbirth, neonatal death or reduced birthweight. In controlled studies of 50,282 pregnant women and their offspring, aspirin administration in moderate and heavy doses during the first four months of pregnancy showed no teratogenic effect.
Nonteratogenic Effects:
Hydrocodone: Babies born to mothers who have been taking opioids regularly prior to delivery will be physically dependent. The withdrawal signs include irritability and excessive crying, tremors, hyperactive reflexes, increased respiratory rate, increased stools, sneezing, yawning, vomiting, and fever. The intensity of the syndrome does not always correlate with the duration of maternal opioid use or dose. There is no consensus on the best method of managing withdrawal. Chlorpromazine 0.7 to 1 mg/kg q6h, and paregoric 2 to 4 drops/kg q4h, have been used to treat withdrawal symptoms in infants. The duration of therapy is 4 to 28 days, with the dosage decreased as tolerated.
Aspirin: Therapeutic doses of aspirin in pregnant women close to term may cause bleeding in the mother, fetus, or neonate. During the last six months of pregnancy, regular use of aspirin in high doses may prolong pregnancy and delivery.
Labor and Delivery: As with all narcotics, administration of Hydrocodone Bitartrate 5mg and Aspirin 500mg Tablets to the mother shortly before delivery may result in some degree of respiratory depression in the newborn, especially if higher doses are used. Ingestion of aspirin prior to delivery may prolong delivery or lead to bleeding in the mother or neonate.
Nursing Mothers: Aspirin is excreted in human milk in a small amount; the significance of its effect on nursing infants is not known. It is not known whether hydrocodone is excreted in human milk. Because many drugs are excreted in human milk and because of the potential for serious adverse reactions in nursing infants, a decision should be made whether to discontinue nursing or to discontinue the drug, taking into account the importance of the drug to the mother.
Pediatric Use: Safety and effectiveness in children have not been established.

ADVERSE REACTIONS

The most frequently observed adverse reactions include lightheadedness, sedation, nausea and vomiting. These effects seem to be more prominent in ambulatory than in nonambulatory patients and some of these adverse reactions may be alleviated if the patient lies down.
Other adverse reactions include:
Central Nervous System:
Hydrocodone: Drowsiness, mental clouding, lethargy, impairment of mental and physical performance, anxiety, fear, dysphoria, dizziness, psychic dependence, mood changes.
Aspirin: Headache, drowsiness and mental confusion can occur in response to chronic use of large doses.

Continued on next page

Russ—Cont.

Gastrointestinal System:
Hydrocodone: The antiemetic phenothiazines are useful in suppressing the nausea and vomiting which may occur (see above); however, some phenothiazine derivatives seem to be antianalgesic and to increase the amount of narcotic required to produce pain relief, while other phenothiazines reduce the amount of narcotic required to produce a given level of analgesia. Prolonged administration of Hydrocodone Bitartrate 5mg and Aspirin 500mg Tablets may produce constipation.
Aspirin: Some patients are unable to take aspirin or other salicylates without developing nausea or vomiting. Occasional patients respond to aspirin (usually large doses) with dyspepsia or heartburn, which may be accompanied by occult bleeding. Excessive bruising or bleeding is sometimes seen in patients with mild disorders or primary hemostasis who regularly use low doses of aspirin.
Prolonged use of aspirin can cause painless erosion of gastric mucosa, occult bleeding and infrequently, iron-deficiency anemia. High doses of aspirin can exacerbate symptoms of peptic ulcer and, occasionally, cause extensive bleeding. Excessive bleeding can follow injury or surgery in patients with or without known bleeding disorders who have taken therapeutic doses of aspirin within the preceding 10 days. Hepatotoxicity has been reported in association with prolonged use of large doses of aspirin in patients with lupus erythematosus, rheumatoid arthritis and rheumatic disease.
Hematologic:
Aspirin: Bone marrow depression, manifested by weakness, fatigue or abnormal bruising or bleeding, has occasionally been reported with aspirin.
In patients with glucose-6-phosphate dehydrogenase deficiency, aspirin can cause a mild degree of hemolytic anemia.
Respiratory:
Hydrocodone: Hydrocodone bitartrate may produce dose-related respiratory depression by acting directly on the brain stem respiratory center. Hydrocodone also affects centers that control repiratory rhythm, and may produce irregular and periodic breathing.
If significant respiratory depression occurs, it may be antagonized by the use of naloxone hydrochloride. Apply other supportive measures when indicated.
Aspirin: Hyperpnea and hyperventilation can occur in response to chronic use of large doses.
Cardiovascular:
Aspirin: Tachycardia can occur in response to chronic use of large doses of aspirin.
Genitourinary:
Hydrocodone: Ureteral spasm, spasm of vesical sphincters and urinary retention have been reported.
Metabolic:
Aspirin: In hyperuricemic persons, low doses of aspirin may reduce the effectiveness of uricosuric therapy or precipitate an attack of gout.
Allergic:
Aspirin: Therapeutic doses of aspirin can induce mild or severe allergic reactions manifested by skin rashes, urticaria, angioedema, rhinorrhea, asthma, abdominal pain, nausea, vomiting, or anaphylactic shock. A history of allergy is often lacking, and allergic reactions may occur even in patients who have previously taken aspirin without any ill effects. Allergic reactions to aspirin are most likely to occur in patients with a history of allergic disease, especially in patients with nasal polyps or asthma.
Other:
Aspirin: Sweating and thirst can occur in response to chronic use of large doses of aspirin.

DRUG ABUSE AND DEPENDENCE

Hydrocodone Bitartrate 5mg and Aspirin 500mg Tablets are subject to the Federal Controlled Substance Act [Schedule CIII].
Psychic dependence, physical dependence, and tolerance may develop upon repeated administration of narcotics; therefore, Hydrocodone Bitartrate 5mg and Aspirin 500mg Tablets should be prescribed and administered with caution. However, psychic dependence is unlikely to develop when Hydrocodone Bitartrate 5mg and Aspirin 500mg Tablets are used for a short time for the treatment of pain.
Physical dependence, the condition in which continued administration of the drug is required to prevent the appearance of a withdrawal syndrome, assumes clinically significant proportions only after several weeks of continued narcotic use, although some mild degree of physical dependence may develop after a few days of narcotic therapy. Tolerance, in which increasingly large doses are required in order to produce the same degree of analgesia, is manifested initially by shortened duration of analgesic effect, and subsequently by decreases in the intensity of analgesia. The rate of development of tolerance varies among patients.

OVERDOSAGE

Hydrocodone:
Signs and Symptoms: Serious overdose with hydrocodone is characterized by respiratory depression (a decrease in respiratory rate and/or tidal volume, Cheyne-Stokes respiration, cyanosis), extreme somnolence progressing to stupor or coma, skeletal muscle flaccidity, cold and clammy skin, and sometimes bradycardia and hypotension. In severe overdosage, apnea, circulatory collapse, cardiac arrest and death may occur.
Treatment: Primary attention should be given to the reestablishment of adequate respiratory exchange through provision of a patent airway and institution of assisted or controlled ventilation. If significant respiratory depression occurs, it may be antagonized by the use of naloxone hydrochloride intravenously (see package insert for dosage and full information). Naloxone promptly reverses the effects of morphine-like opioid antagonists such as hydrocodone. In patients who are physically dependent, small doses of naloxone may be sufficient not only to antagonize respiratory depression, but also to precipitate withdrawal phenomena. The dose of naloxone should therefore be adjusted accordingly in such patients. Since the duration of action of hydrocodone may exceed that of the antagonist, the patient should be kept under continued surveillance and repeated doses of the antagonist should be administered as needed to maintain adequate respiration.
A narcotic antagonist should not be administered in the absence of clinically significant respiratory or cardiovascular depression. Oxygen, intravenous fluids, vasopressors and other supportive measures should be employed as indicated. Gastric emptying may be useful in removing unabsorbed drug.
Aspirin:
Signs and Symptoms: The most severe manifestations from aspirin results from cardiovascular and respiratory insufficiency secondary to acid-base and electrolyte disturbances, complicated by hyperthermia and dehydration.
Respiratory alkalosis is characteristic of the early phase of intoxication with aspirin while hyperventilation is occurring, but is quickly followed by metabolic acidosis in most people with severe intoxication.
Concentrations of aspirin in plasma above 30 mg/100 ml are associated with toxicity (See Clinical Pharmacology Section for information on factors influencing aspirin blood levels.) The single lethal dose of aspirin in adults is probably about 25–30 g. but is not known with certainty.
Hemodialysis and peritoneal dialysis can be performed to reduce the body aspirin content.
Treatment: Treatment consists primarily of supporting vital functions, increasing salicylate elimination, and correcting the acid-base imbalance due primarily to salicylism. Gastric emptying (Syrup of Ipecac) and/or lavage is recommended as soon as possible after ingestion, even if the patient has vomited spontaneously. Administration of activated charcoal as a slurry is beneficial after lavage and/or emesis, if less than three hours have passed since ingestion. Charcoal adsorption should *not* be employed prior to emesis or lavage.
Severity of aspirin intoxication is determined by measuring the blood salicylate level. Acid-base status should be closely followed with serial blood gas and serum pH measurements. Fluid and electrolyte balance should also be regularly monitored.
In severe cases, hyperthermia and hypovolemia are the major immediate threats to life. Children should be sponged with tepid water. Replacement fluid should be administered intravenously and augmented with sufficient bicarbonate to correct acidosis, with monitoring of plasma electrolytes and pH, to promote alkaline diuresis of salicylate if renal function is normal. Complete control may also require infusion of glucose to control hypoglycemia.
In patients with renal insufficiency or in cases of life-threatening intoxication, dialysis is usually required. Peritoneal dialysis or exchange transfusion is indicated in infants and young children and hemodialysis in older patients.

DOSAGE AND ADMINISTRATION

Dosage should be adjusted according to the severity of the pain and the response of the patient. However, tolerance to hydrocodone can develop with continued use and the incidence of untoward effects is dose related.
The usual adult dosage is one or two tablets every four to six hours as needed for pain.
Hydrocodone Bitartrate 5mg and Aspirin 500mg Tablets should be taken with food or a full glass of milk or water to lessen gastric irritation.

HOW SUPPLIED

Dark pink capsule shaped tablet containing 5mg of Hydrocodone Bitartrate (WARNING: may be habit forming) and 500mg Aspirin. Each tablet is debossed with the Russ logo on one side and the number 500 on the other side.

Supplied in bottles of 100 tablets (NDC 50474-500-01).

STORAGE

Store at controlled room temperature, 15°–30°C (59°–86°F). Protect from moisture.
DISPENSE IN A TIGHT, LIGHT-RESISTANT CONTAINER AS DEFINED IN THE USP/NF WITH A CHILD-RESISTANT CLOSURE.

CAUTION

Federal law prohibits dispensing without prescription.
A Schedule CIII Controlled Substance (Narcotic).
Manufactured For:
RUSS PHARMACEUTICALS, INC.
Birmingham, Alabama 35242
Manufactured By:
CENTRAL PHARMACEUTICALS, INC.
Seymour, IN 47274
Revised March 1988
Shown in Product Identification Section, page 427

Rystan Company, Inc.
47 CENTER AVENUE
P.O. BOX 214
LITTLE FALLS, NJ 07424-0214

CHLORESIUM®
[klor-eez'ium]
Ointment and Solution
Healing and Deodorizing Agent

COMPOSITION
Ointment: 0.5% Chlorophyllin Copper Complex in a hydrophilic base. Solution: 0.2% Chlorophyllin Copper Complex in isotonic saline solution.

ACTIONS AND USES
To promote normal healing, relieve pain and inflammation and reduce malodors in wounds, burns, surface ulcers, cuts, abrasions and skin irritations.

ADMINISTRATION AND DOSAGE
Ointment: Apply generously and cover with gauze, linen or other appropriate dressing. Dressings preferably changed no more often than every 48 to 72 hours. Solution: Apply full strength as continuous wet dressing, or instill directly into sinus tracts, fistulae, deep ulcers or cavities. As a mouthwash, use half strength.

SIDE EFFECTS
CHLORESIUM Ointment and Solution are soothing and nontoxic. Sensitivity reactions are extremely rare, and only a few instances of slight itching or irritation have been reported.

HOW SUPPLIED
Ointment: 1 oz. and 4 oz. tubes, 1 lb. jars (NDC 0263-5155-01 and -04, -16). Solution: 8 oz. and 32 oz. bottles. (NDC 0263-5158-08 and -32)

DERIFIL® Tablets
[der'ah-fil]
Internal Deodorant

COMPOSITION
100 mg chlorophyllin copper complex per tablet.

ACTIONS AND USES
Oral deodorant for internal use: 1. an aid to reduce fecal or urinary odor due to incontinence, 2: an aid to reduce odor from colostomies or ileostomies.

ADMINISTRATION AND DOSAGE
Adults and children 12 years of age and over: Oral dosage is one to two tablets daily. Children under 12 years of age: Consult a doctor. In ostomies, tablets may be either taken by mouth or placed in the appliance.

SIDE EFFECTS
No toxic effects have been reported from use of DERIFIL Tablets at the recommended dosage over long periods. A temporary mild laxative effect may be noted, and the fecal discharge is commonly stained dark green.

HOW SUPPLIED
Bottles of 30 (NDC 0263-5001-03), 100 (NDC 0263-5001-10), and 1000 tablets (NDC 0263-5001-11).

PANAFIL® Ointment   ℞
[pan 'ah-fil]
PANAFIL®—WHITE Ointment   ℞

CAUTION
Federal law prohibits dispensing without prescription.

DESCRIPTION
PANAFIL® Ointment is an enzymatic debriding-healing ointment which contains standardized papain 10%, urea USP 10% and chlorophyllin copper complex 0.5% in a hydrophilic base. Inactive ingredients are: White Petrolatum, USP; Propylene Glycol, USP; Stearyl Alcohol, NF; Sorbitan Monostearate, NF; Polyoxyl 40 Stearate, NF; Boric Acid, NF; Sodium Borate, NF; Chlorobutanol (Anhydrous), NF as a preservative. PANAFIL-WHITE is identical except that the chlorophyllin copper complex is omitted.

CLINICAL PHARMACOLOGY
Papain, the proteolytic enzyme derived from the fruit of carica papaya, is a potent digestant of nonviable protein matter, but is harmless to viable tissue. It has the unique advantage of being active over a wide pH range, 3 to 12. Despite its recognized value as a digestive agent, papain is relatively ineffective when used alone as a debriding agent, primarily because it requires the presence of activators to exert its digestive function.

Urea is combined with papain to provide two supplementary chemical actions: 1) to expose by solvent action the activators of papain (sulfhydryl groups) which are always present, but not necessarily accessible, in the nonviable tissue or debris of lesions, and 2) to denature the nonviable protein matter in lesions and thereby render it more susceptible to enzymatic digestion. In pharmacologic studies involving digestion of beef powder, Miller[1] showed that the combination of papain and urea produced twice as much digestion as papain alone. Chlorophyllin copper complex adds healing action to the cleansing action of the proteolytic papain-urea combination. The basic wound-healing properties of chlorophyllin copper complex are promotion of healthy granulations, control of local inflammation and reduction of wound odors.[2] Specifically, chlorophyllin copper complex inhibit the hemagglutinating and inflammatory properties of protein degradation products in the wound, including the products of enzymatic digestion, thus providing an additional protective factor.[1,3] The incorporation of chlorophyllin copper complex in PANAFIL® Ointment permits its continuous use for as long as desired to help produce and then maintain a clean wound base and to promote healing.

INDICATIONS AND USES
Ointment is suggested for treatment of acute and chronic lesions such as varicose, diabetic and decubitus ulcers, burns, postoperative wounds, pilonidal cyst wounds, carbuncles and miscellaneous traumatic or infected wounds.

Ointment is applied continuously throughout treatment of these conditions (1) for enzymatic debridement of necrotic tissue and liquefaction of fibrinous, purulent debris, (2) to keep the wound clean, and simultaneously (3) to promote normal healing.

CONTRAINDICATIONS
None known.

PRECAUTIONS
See Dosage and Administration.
Not to be used in eyes.

ADVERSE REACTIONS
Ointment is generally well tolerated and nonirritating. A small percentage of patients may experience a transient "burning" sensation on application of the ointment. Occasionally, the profuse exudate resulting from enzymatic digestion may cause irritation. In such cases, more frequent changes of dressings until exudate diminishes will alleviate discomfort.

DOSAGE AND ADMINISTRATION
Apply Ointment directly to lesion and cover with gauze or linen dressing. When practicable, daily or twice daily changes of dressings are preferred. Longer intervals between redressings (two or three days) have proved satisfactory, and Ointment may be applied under pressure dressings. At each redressing, the lesion should be irrigated with isotonic saline solution or other mild cleansing solution (except hydrogen peroxide solution, which may inactivate the papain) to remove any accumulation of liquefied necrotic material.

NOTE
Papain may also be inactivated by the salts of heavy metals (lead, silver, mercury, etc.) Contact with medications containing these metals should be avoided.

HOW SUPPLIED
PANAFIL—1 oz. tubes, (NDC 0263-5145-01).
1 lb. jars, (NDC 0263-5145-16).
PANAFIL-WHITE—1 oz. tubes, (NDC-0263-5148-01)

REFERENCES
1. Miller, J.M.: The Interaction of Papain, Urea and Water-Soluble Chlorophyll in a Proteolytic Ointment for Infected Wounds, Surgery 43:939, 1958.
2. Smith, L.W.: The Present Status of Topical Chlorophyll Therapy, New York J. Med. 55:2041, 1955.
3. Barnard, R.D.: Elucidation of Chemically Defined Haptenes For Competitive Inhibition of Aggression Activity, Immunol 8:78, 1954.

PROPHYLLIN®
[pro-fil'in]
Wet Dressing Powder and Ointment

COMPOSITION
Each 2.3 gm. powder packet (or teaspoonful of bulk powder) in 8 ounces of water makes a solution containing 1% Sodium Propionate and 0.0025% Chlorophyllin Copper Complex. Ointment: 5% Sodium Propionate and 0.0125% Chlorophyllin Copper Complex in an emollient base.

ACTION AND USES
Antifungal, antibacterial, antipruritic, antiinflammatory. Solution is nonastringent and nonirritating. Useful in dermatophytosis, contact dermatoses, eczemas, minor burns.

ADMINISTRATION AND DOSAGE
Use solution as wet dressing, soak or mouthwash. Half-strength solution (one packet in 16 oz. water) may be preferred for footbath or in severe inflammation. Ointment: Apply liberally several times daily and on retiring.

HOW SUPPLIED
Powder: Cartons of 12 packets and in 4 oz. jars (NDC 0263-5182-12 and 04). Ointment: 1 oz. tubes (NDC 0263-5185-01).

Sandoz Pharmaceuticals/
Consumer Division
Division of Sandoz, Inc.
EAST HANOVER, NJ 07936

ACID MANTLE® CREME   OTC
[ă'sĭd-mănt'l]

DESCRIPTION
A greaseless, water-miscible preparation containing buffered aluminum acetate. Other ingredients: aluminum sulfate, calcium acetate, cetearyl alcohol, glycerin, light mineral oil, methylparaben, purified water, sodium lauryl sulfate, synthetic beeswax, white petrolatum, white potato dextrin. May also contain: ammonium hydroxide, citric acid.

INDICATIONS
A vehicle for compatible topical drugs. Restores and maintains protective acidity of the skin. Provides relief from mild skin irritation due to exposure to soaps, detergents, chemicals, alkalis. Aids in the treatment of diaper rash, acne, eczema and dry, rough, scaly skin from varied causes.

APPLICATION
Apply several times daily, especially after wet work.

CAUTION
Limited compatibility and stability with Vitamin A, neomycin and water-soluble antibiotics. For external use only. Not for ophthalmic use.

HOW SUPPLIED
1 oz tubes; 4 oz and 1 lb jars.

CAMA® ARTHRITIS PAIN RELIEVER   OTC
[kă'măh]

(See PDR For Nonprescription Drugs)

DORCOL® CHILDREN'S COUGH   OTC
SYRUP
[door'call]

DESCRIPTION
Each teaspoonful (5 ml) of DORCOL Children's Cough Syrup contains: pseudoephedrine hydrochloride 15 mg, guaifenesin 50 mg and dextromethorphan hydrobromide 5 mg. Other ingredients: benzoic acid, Blue 1, edetate disodium, flavors, glycerin, propylene glycol, purified water, Red 40, sodium hydroxide, sucrose, tartaric acid.

INDICATIONS
Temporarily relieves your child's cough due to minor throat and bronchial irritation as may occur with the common cold. Helps loosen phlegm (mucus) and bronchial secretions to rid the bronchial passageways of bothersome mucus. Relieves irritated membranes in the respiratory passageways by preventing dryness through increased mucus flow. Temporarily relieves nasal stuffiness due to the common cold, hay fever or other upper respiratory allergies. Promotes nasal and/or sinus drainage.

CONTRAINDICATIONS
Hypersensitivity to any of the ingredients. The use of sympathomimetic agents such as pseudoephedrine hydrochloride is contraindicated in patients with severe hypertension, severe coronary artery disease or in those taking monoamine oxidase inhibitors.

PRECAUTIONS
Exercise prescribing caution in patients with persistent or chronic cough such as occurs with chronic bronchitis or bronchial asthma or with cough that is accompanied by excessive secretions. Use with caution in patients with hypertension, hyperthyroidism, cardiovascular disease, diabetes mellitus, elevated intraocular pressure, prostatic hypertrophy or impaired hepatic function.

ADVERSE REACTIONS
Mild CNS stimulation, gastrointestinal upsets, headache, drowsiness or dizziness may occur.

DOSAGE AND ADMINISTRATION
Bottle label dosage reads:
By age: Children 2 to under 6 years:
                     1 teaspoonful every 4 hours
Children 6 to under 12 years: 2 teaspoonfuls every 4 hours
By weight: Children 25 to 45 pounds:
                     1 teaspoonful every 4 hours
Children 46 to 85 pounds: 2 teaspoonfuls every 4 hours
Children under 2 years—consult physician.
Unless directed by a physician, do not exceed 4 doses in 24 hours.
The suggested dosage for pediatric patients 3 months to under 12 months of age is 3 drops per kilogram of body weight administered every 4 hours. The suggested dosage for patients 12 months to under 24 months of age is 7 drops (0.2 ml) per kilogram of body weight administered every 4 hours. A maximum of 4 doses per 24 hours is recommended.

HOW SUPPLIED
DORCOL Children's Cough Syrup (grape colored), in 4 fl oz and 8 fl oz plastic bottles with tamper-evident band around child-resistant cap.

DORCOL® CHILDREN'S DECONGESTANT   OTC
LIQUID
[door'call]

DESCRIPTION
Each teaspoonful (5 ml) of DORCOL Children's Decongestant Liquid contains pseudoephedrine hydrochloride 15 mg. Other ingredients: benzoic acid, edetate disodium, flavors, purified water, sodium hydroxide, sorbitol, sucrose, Yellow 10. Contains FD&C Yellow No. 6 as a color additive.

INDICATIONS
Provides temporary relief of nasal congestion due to the common cold, hay fever or other upper respiratory allergies, or associated with sinusitis. Reduces swelling of nasal passages to restore freer breathing through the nose. Promotes nasal and sinus drainage; relieves sinus pressure.

CONTRAINDICATIONS
Hypersensitivity to any of the components. The use of sympathomimetic agents such as pseudoephedrine hydrochloride is contraindicated in patients with severe hypertension, severe coronary artery disease or in those taking monoamine oxidase inhibitors.

PRECAUTIONS
Exercise prescribing caution in patients with hypertension, cardiovascular disease, diabetes mellitus, hyperthyroidism, elevated intraocular pressure or prostatic hypertrophy.

ADVERSE REACTIONS
Mild CNS stimulation or dizziness may occur. Headache and drowsiness have been reported. Large doses may cause lightheadedness, nausea and/or vomiting.

DOSAGE AND ADMINISTRATION
Bottle label dosage reads:
By age:
   Children 2 to under 6 years:
                     1 teaspoonful every 4 to 6 hours
   Children 6 years: 2 teaspoonfuls every 4 to 6 hours
By weight:
   Children 25 to 45 pounds
                     1 teaspoonful every 4 to 6 hours
   Children 46 to 85 pounds
                     2 teaspoonfuls every 4 to 6 hours

Continued on next page

Sandoz Consumer—Cont.

Children under 2 years—consult physician.
Unless directed by a physician, do not exceed 4 doses in 24 hours.
The suggested dosage for pediatric patients 3 months to under 12 months of age is 3 drops per kilogram of body weight every 4 to 6 hours. The suggested dosage for patients 12 months to under 24 months of age is 7 drops (0.2 ml) per kilogram of body weight every 4 to 6 hours. A maximum of 4 doses per 24 hours is recommended.

HOW SUPPLIED
DORCOL Children's Decongestant Liquid (pale orange), in 4 fl oz bottles with tamper-evident band around child-resistant cap.

DORCOL® CHILDREN'S FEVER & PAIN   OTC
REDUCER
[door'call]

DESCRIPTION
Each teaspoonful (5 ml) of DORCOL Children's Fever & Pain Reducer contains acetaminophen 160 mg. Other ingredients: benzoic acid, edetate disodium, flavors, glycerin, polyethylene glycol, purified water, Red 40, sodium chloride, sucrose.

INDICATIONS
Provides analgesic/antipyretic action for infants and children with conditions requiring relief of pain or reduction of fever.

CONTRAINDICATIONS
Hypersensitivity to any of the ingredients. Repeated administration of acetaminophen is contraindicated in patients with anemia or renal or hepatic disease.

PRECAUTIONS
Acetaminophen is relatively nontoxic in therapeutic doses. However, it should be used with caution in patients with preexisting anemia, since cyanosis may not be apparent despite very high levels of methemoglobin.

ADVERSE REACTIONS
Acetaminophen has rarely been found to produce any side effects. Sensitivity reactions have been reported.

DOSAGE AND ADMINISTRATION
Bottle label dosage reads:
Children under 2 years—consult physician.
By age:

Children 2 to under 4 years:	1 teaspoonful
Children 4 to under 6 years:	1½ teaspoonfuls
Children 6 years of age:	2 teaspoonfuls

By weight:

Children 25 to 35 pounds:	1 teaspoonful
Children 36 to 45 pounds:	1½ teaspoonfuls
Children 46 to 60 pounds:	2 teaspoonfuls

Give every 4 hours while symptoms persist or as directed by a physician. Unless directed by a physician, do not exceed 5 doses in 24 hours.
The suggested dosage for pediatric patients 3 months to under 12 months of age is 3 drops per kilogram of body weight. The suggested dosage for patients 12 months to under 24 months of age is 7 drops (0.2 ml) per kilogram of body weight. Give dose every 4 hours while symptoms persist. A maximum of 5 doses per 24 hours is recommended.

HOW SUPPLIED
DORCOL Children's Fever & Pain Reducer (red), in 4 fl oz bottles with tamper-evident band around child-resistant cap.

DORCOL® CHILDREN'S LIQUID COLD   OTC
FORMULA
[door'call]

DESCRIPTION
Each teaspoonful (5 ml) of DORCOL Children's Liquid Cold Formula contains pseudoephedrine hydrochloride 15 mg and chlorpheniramine maleate 1 mg. Other ingredients: benzoic acid, Blue 1, flavors, purified water, Red 40, sorbitol, sucrose, Yellow 10. May also contain sodium hydroxide.

INDICATIONS
Provides temporary relief of nasal congestion, sneezing and rhinorrhea due to the common cold, hay fever or other upper respiratory allergies, or associated with sinusitis. Reduces swelling of nasal passages and restores freer breathing through the nose. Promotes nasal and sinus drainage; relieves sinus pressure.

CONTRAINDICATIONS
Hypersensitivity to any of the ingredients. The use of sympathomimetic agents such as pseudoephedrine hydrochloride is contraindicated in patients with severe hypertension, severe coronary artery disease or in those taking monoamine oxi-

dase inhibitors. Antihistamines such as chlorpheniramine maleate should not be administered to premature or newborn infants or be used to treat lower respiratory tract symptoms.

PRECAUTIONS
Exercise prescribing caution in patients with hypertension, cardiovascular disease, diabetes mellitus, hyperthyroidism, elevated intraocular pressure, prostatic hypertrophy, bladder neck obstruction or chronic pulmonary disease.

ADVERSE REACTIONS
Mild CNS stimulation, drowsiness, blurred vision, dry mouth, tachycardia, dizziness, gastrointestinal upset may occur occasionally. May produce thickening of bronchial secretions.

DOSAGE AND ADMINISTRATION
Bottle label dosage reads:
Children under 6 years—consult physician.
By age:

    Children 6 to under 12 years:
        2 teaspoonfuls every 4 to 6 hours
By weight:
    Children 45 to 85 pounds:
        2 teaspoonfuls every 4 to 6 hours
Unless directed by a physician, do not exceed 4 doses in 24 hours.
The suggested dosage for pediatric patients 3 months to under 12 months of age is 2 drops per kilogram of body weight every 4 to 6 hours. The suggested dosage for patients 12 months to under 24 months of age is 5 drops (0.2 ml) per kilogram of body weight every 4 to 6 hours. The suggested dosage for patients 2 years to under 6 years is 1 teaspoonful every 4 to 6 hours. A maximum of 4 doses per 24 hours is recommended.

HOW SUPPLIED
DORCOL Children's Liquid Cold Formula (light brown), in 4 fl oz bottles with tamper-evident band around child-resistant cap.

TRIAMINIC® ALLERGY TABLETS   OTC
[trī"ah-mĭn'ĭc]

(See PDR For Nonprescription Drugs)

TRIAMINIC® CHEWABLE TABLETS   OTC
For Children
[trī"ah-mĭn'ĭc]

(See PDR For Nonprescription Drugs)

TRIAMINIC® COLD TABLETS   OTC
[trī"ah-mĭn'ĭc]

DESCRIPTION
Each TRIAMINIC Cold Tablet contains phenylpropanolamine hydrochloride 12.5 mg and chlorpheniramine maleate 2 mg. Other ingredients: calcium stearate, colloidal silicon dioxide, flavor, lactose, methylcellulose, methylparaben, microcrystalline cellulose, polyethylene glycol, povidone, pregelatinized starch, Red 40, saccharin sodium, titanium dioxide. Contains FD&C Yellow No. 6 as a color additive.

INDICATIONS
For the temporary relief of nasal congestion, runny nose and sneezing that may occur with the common cold or with hay fever or other upper respiratory allergies. Promotes nasal and sinus drainage.

CONTRAINDICATIONS
Hypersensitivity to any of the ingredients. The use of sympathomimetic agents such as phenylpropanolamine hydrochloride is contraindicated in patients with severe hypertension, severe coronary artery disease or in those taking monoamine oxidase inhibitors. Antihistamines such as chlorpheniramine maleate should not be used to treat lower respiratory tract symptoms.

PRECAUTIONS
Exercise prescribing caution in patients with hypertension, cardiovascular disease, diabetes mellitus, hyperthyroidism, elevated intraocular pressure, prostatic hypertrophy, bladder neck obstruction or chronic pulmonary disease. Alcoholic beverages and other CNS depressants may potentiate the sedative effects of antihistamines. Use with caution in pregnant and nursing women.

ADVERSE REACTIONS
Mild CNS stimulation, drowsiness, blurred vision, dry mouth, tachycardia, dizziness or gastrointestinal upset may occur. May produce thickening of bronchial secretions.

DOSAGE AND ADMINISTRATION
Adults — 2 tablets every 4 hours. Children 6-12 years — 1 tablet every 4 hours.

HOW SUPPLIED
TRIAMINIC Cold Tablets (orange), imprinted "DORSEY" on one side, "TRIAMINIC" on the other, in blister packs of 24.

TRIAMINIC® EXPECTORANT   OTC
[trī"ah-mĭn'ĭc]

DESCRIPTION
Each teaspoonful (5 ml) of TRIAMINIC Expectorant contains phenylpropanolamine hydrochloride 12.5 mg and guaifenesin 100 mg. Other ingredients: alcohol (5%), benzoic acid, edetate disodium, flavors, purified water, saccharin, saccharin sodium, sodium hydroxide, sorbitol, sucrose, Yellow 10. Contains FD&C Yellow No. 6 as a color additive.

INDICATIONS
Provides prompt relief of cough and nasal congestion due to the common cold. The expectorant component helps loosen bronchial secretions and rid the bronchial passageways of bothersome mucus. The decongestant and expectorant are provided in an antihistamine-free formula.

CONTRAINDICATIONS
Hypersensitivity to any of the ingredients. The use of sympathomimetic agents such as phenylpropanolamine hydrochloride is contraindicated in patients with severe hypertension, severe coronary artery disease or in those taking monoamine oxidase inhibitors.

PRECAUTIONS
Exercise prescribing caution in patients with persistent or chronic cough such as occurs with chronic bronchitis or bronchial asthma. Use with caution in patients with hypertension, hyperthyroidism, cardiovascular disease or diabetes mellitus. Use with caution in pregnant and nursing women.

ADVERSE REACTIONS
Mild CNS stimulation, drowsiness, headache or gastrointestinal upsets may occur.

DOSAGE AND ADMINISTRATION
Bottle label dosage reads: Adults—2 teaspoonfuls every 4 hours. Children 6–12 years—1 teaspoonful every 4 hours. Children 2–6 years—½ teaspoonful every 4 hours. Children under 2 years—consult physician.
The suggested dosage for pediatric patients 3 months to under 12 months of age is 2 drops per kg of body weight administered every 4 hours. The suggested dosage for patients 12 months to under 24 months of age is 3 drops per kg of body weight administered every 4 hours.

HOW SUPPLIED
TRIAMINIC Expectorant (yellow), in 4 fl oz and 8 fl oz plastic bottles with tamper-evident band around child-resistant cap.

TRIAMINIC® EXPECTORANT DH   ⑪
[trī"ah-mĭn'ĭc]

DESCRIPTION
Each teaspoonful (5 ml) of TRIAMINIC Expectorant DH contains: hydrocodone bitartrate 1.67 mg (Warning: May be habit forming), phenylpropanolamine hydrochloride 12.5 mg, pheniramine maleate 6.25 mg, pyrilamine maleate 6.25 mg, and guaifenesin 100 mg. Other ingredients: alcohol (5%), benzoic acid, Blue 1, flavors, purified water, saccharin sodium, sorbitol, sucrose, Yellow 10. Contains FD&C Yellow No. 6 as a color additive.
Phenylpropanolamine hydrochloride, a sympathomimetic drug, is structurally related to ephedrine and amphetamine. Pheniramine maleate is an antihistamine of the alkylamine class while pyrilamine maleate belongs to the ethylenediamine class.
The expectorant component is guaifenesin (3-(o-methoxyphenoxy)-1,2- propanediol) which helps loosen and thus clear the bronchial passageways of bothersome, thickened mucus. The antitussive component, hydrocodone, is 7,8 dihydrocodeinone, a derivative of codeine.

CLINICAL PHARMACOLOGY
Phenylpropanolamine presumably acts on α-adrenergic receptors in the mucosa of the respiratory tract producing vasoconstriction which results in shrinkage of swollen mucous membranes, reduction of tissue hyperemia, edema and nasal congestion, and an increase in nasal airway patency. Antihistamines competitively act as H_1 receptor antagonists of histamine. They exhibit anticholinergic (drying) and sedative side effects. There are several classes of antihistamines which vary with respect to potency, dosage and the relative incidence of side effects. Antihistamines inhibit the effects of histamine on capillary permeability and on vascular, bronchial and many other types of smooth muscle.
By increasing respiratory tract fluid, guaifenesin reduces the viscosity of tenacious secretions and acts as an expectorant. The drug is effective in productive as well as nonproductive cough, but is of particular value in dry, nonproduc-

tive cough which tends to injure the mucous membranes of the air passages.
Hydrocodone is a centrally acting narcotic antitussive providing cough relief for up to 6 hours.

INDICATIONS
For relief of troublesome cough, nasal congestion and postnasal drip associated with colds, nasal allergies, sinusitis, and rhinitis. Also effective for relief of severe, prolonged or refractory cough associated with other respiratory disorders. For the relief of symptoms associated with allergic rhinitis such as sneezing, rhinorrhea, pruritus and lacrimation.

CONTRAINDICATIONS
TRIAMINIC Expectorant DH is contraindicated in patients exhibiting hypersensitivity to any of the ingredients. Antihistamines are contraindicated in patients receiving monoamine oxidase inhibitors since these agents may prolong and intensify the anticholinergic effects of antihistamines (see Drug Interactions). Antihistamines *should not* be used to treat lower respiratory tract symptoms or be given to premature or newborn infants. Sympathomimetic agents such as phenylpropanolamine are contraindicated in patients with severe hypertension, severe coronary artery disease and in those taking monoamine oxidase inhibitors. Narcotic analgesics are contraindicated in patients with acute respiratory depression. Continuous dosage over an extended period is generally contraindicated since hydrocodone can cause addiction.
Nursing Mothers: Because of the higher risk of antihistamines for premature and newborn infants, antihistamine therapy is contraindicated in nursing mothers.

WARNINGS
TRIAMINIC Expectorant DH can produce drug dependence, and therefore has the potential for abuse.
Sympathomimetic agents should be used with caution in patients with hypertension, hyperthyroidism, diabetes mellitus and cardiovascular disease. Antihistamines should be used with caution in patients with narrow angle glaucoma, stenosing peptic ulcer, pyloroduodenal obstruction, symptomatic prostatic hypertrophy, bladder neck obstruction or chronic pulmonary disease. Narcotic analgesics should be used with caution in patients with chronic respiratory impairment, cardiac arrhythmias, history of convulsions, history of drug dependence, gallbladder disease or impaired renal or hepatic function.
Use in the Elderly (Approximately 60 Years or Older): Antihistamines are more likely to cause dizziness, sedation and hypotension in elderly patients. Overdosage of sympathomimetic agents in this age group may cause hallucinations, convulsions, CNS depression or death. Geriatric patients may be more susceptible to the effects of hydrocodone, especially the respiratory depressant effects.

PRECAUTIONS
General: Use with caution in patients with hypertension, hyperthyroidism, diabetes mellitus, cardiovascular disease, bronchial asthma, increased intraocular pressure (see WARNINGS). Before prescribing medication to suppress or modify cough, it is important to ascertain that the underlying cause of cough is identified, that modification of cough does not increase the risk of clinical complications, and that appropriate therapy for the primary disease is provided.
Information for Patients: Patients should be informed of the potential for sedation or drowsiness and cautioned about engaging in activities requiring mental alertness such as driving or operating machinery. The concomitant consumption of alcoholic beverages or other sedative drugs should be avoided.
Drug Interactions:
(1) Monoamine oxidase inhibitors: MAO inhibitors may prolong and intensify the anticholinergic effects of antihistamines and potentiate the pressor effects of sympathomimetics.
(2) Alcohol and CNS depressants: These agents potentiate the sedative effects of antihistamines and hydrocodone. The CNS and respiratory depressant effects of some opioids may be exaggerated and prolonged by phenothiazines, alcohol, CNS depressants, MAO inhibitors, and tricyclic antidepressants; the mechanism of this supraadditive effect is not fully understood, but may involve alterations in the rate of metabolic transformation of the opioid or alterations in neurotransmitters involved in opioid actions.
(3) Certain antihypertensives: Sympathomimetics may reduce the antihypertensive effects of methyldopa, mecamylamine, reserpine and veratrum alkaloids.
Drug/Laboratory Test Interactions: Guaifenesin or its metabolites may cause color interference with the VMA test for catechols. It may also falsely elevate the level of urinary 5HIAA in certain serotonin metabolite chemical tests because of color interference.
Carcinogenesis, Mutagenesis, Impairment of Fertility: No data are available on the long-term potential for carcinogenicity, mutagenicity or impairment of fertility in animals or humans.

Pregnancy: *Pregnancy Category C* — Animal reproduction studies have not been conducted. Safe use in pregnancy has not been established relative to possible adverse effects on fetal development. Therefore, this product should not be used in pregnant patients unless, in the judgement of the physician, the potential benefits outweigh possible hazards.
Nursing Mothers: See CONTRAINDICATIONS.
Pediatric Use: TRIAMINIC Expectorant DH is intended for administration to children 1 to 12 years of age (see DOSAGE AND ADMINISTRATION). It is important to note the variability of response infants and small children exhibit to antihistamines and sympathomimetics. As in adults, the combination of an antihistamine and sympathomimetic can elicit either mild stimulation or mild sedation in children. In the young child, mild stimulation is the response most frequently seen. In infants and children, overdosage of antihistamines may cause hallucinations, convulsions or death. Pediatric patients may be more susceptible to the effects of hydrocodone, especially the respiratory depressant effects.

ADVERSE REACTIONS
The most frequent adverse reactions are underlined.
(1) General: urticaria, drug rash, anaphylactic shock, photosensitivity, excessive perspiration, chills, dryness of mouth, nose and throat.
(2) Cardiovascular System: hypotension, headache, palpitations, tachycardia, extrasystoles.
(3) Hematologic System: hemolytic anemia, thrombocytopenia, agranulocytosis.
(4) Nervous System: sedation, sleepiness, dizziness, disturbed coordination, fatigue, confusion, restlessness, excitation, nervousness, tremor, irritability, insomnia, euphoria, paresthesias, blurred vision, diplopia, vertigo, tinnitus, acute labyrinthitis, hysteria, neuritis, convulsions, CNS depression, hallucinations.
(5) GI System: epigastric distress, anorexia, nausea, vomiting, diarrhea, constipation.
(6) GU System: urinary frequency, difficult urination, urinary retention, early menses.
(7) Respiratory System: thickening of bronchial secretions, tightness of chest and wheezing, nasal stuffiness.
DRUG ABUSE AND DEPENDENCE: Tolerance and physical dependence may occur following prolonged administration of hydrocodone.

OVERDOSAGE
Symptoms: The triad of coma, pinpoint pupils, and depressed respiration strongly suggest hydrocodone poisoning. Serious overdose with TRIAMINIC Expectorant DH may be characterized by respiratory depression, extreme somnolence progressing to stupor or coma, convulsions, skeletal muscle flaccidity, cold and clammy skin, and sometimes bradycardia and hypotension. In severe overdosage, apnea, circulatory collapse, cardiac arrest and death may occur. In the presence of fever and dehydration excitation may occur in children.
Treatment of Overdosage: Primary attention should be given to the reestablishment of adequate respiratory exchange through provision of patent airway and the institution of assisted or controlled ventilation. The narcotic antagonists naloxone and levallorphan are specific antidotes against respiratory depression which may result from overdosage or unusual sensitivity to narcotics, including hydrocodone. An appropriate dose of one of these antagonists should be administered, preferably by the intravenous route, simultaneously with efforts at respiratory resuscitation. The fact that an opioid antagonist may precipitate withdrawal symptoms in patients who are physically dependent on hydrocodone must be kept in mind and dosage titrated accordingly. Since the duration of action of hydrocodone may exceed that of the antagonist, the patient should be kept under continued surveillance and repeated doses of the antagonist should be administered as needed to maintain adequate respiration. Oxygen, intravenous fluids, vasopressors and other supportive measures should be employed as indicated, including treatment for anticholinergic drug intoxication. Gastric emptying may be useful in removing unabsorbed drug. Activated charcoal may be of benefit.

DOSAGE AND ADMINISTRATION
Adults—2 teaspoonfuls every 4 hours; children 6 to 12—1 teaspoonful every 4 hours; children 1 to 6—1/2 teaspoonful every 4 hours.

HOW SUPPLIED
TRIAMINIC Expectorant DH (green), in pint bottles. Store at room temperature. TRIAMINIC Expectorant DH is a Schedule III controlled substance.

TRIAMINIC® EXPECTORANT WITH CODEINE   Ⓥ
[trĭ″ah-mĭn′ĭc]

DESCRIPTION
Each teaspoonful (5 ml) of TRIAMINIC Expectorant with Codeine contains: codeine phosphate 10 mg (Warning: May

be habit forming), phenylpropanolamine hydrochloride 12.5 mg, and guaifenesin 100 mg. Other ingredients: alcohol (5%), benzoic acid, Blue 1, flavors, purified water, saccharin sodium, sorbitol, sucrose. Yellow 10.

INDICATIONS
For use in providing temporary relief of coughs and nasal congestion due to the common cold, when the antitussive properties of codeine are desired. The expectorant component helps loosen bronchial secretions. The ingredients are provided in an antihistamine-free formula.

CONTRAINDICATIONS
Hypersensitivity to any of the ingredients. The use of sympathomimetic agents such as phenylpropanolamine hydrochloride is contraindicated in those patients with severe hypertension, severe coronary artery disease or in those taking monoamine oxidase inhibitors. Continuous dosage over an extended period is generally contraindicated since codeine phosphate may cause addiction.

PRECAUTIONS
Exercise prescribing caution in patients with persistent or chronic cough such as occurs with chronic bronchitis, bronchial asthma, or emphysema. Use with caution in patients with hypertension, hyperthyroidism, cardiovascular disease, diabetes mellitus, chronic pulmonary disease or shortness of breath. Exercise caution in prescribing this product to children taking other drugs. Pediatric and geriatric patients may be more susceptible to the effects of codeine, especially the respiratory depressant effects. Tolerance and physical dependence may occur following prolonged administration. Use with caution in pregnant and nursing women.

ADVERSE REACTIONS
Nausea, vomiting, constipation, dizziness, sedation or mild CNS stimulation may occur.

DOSAGE AND ADMINISTRATION
Bottle label dosage reads: Adults—2 teaspoonfuls every 4 hours. Children 6 to 12 years—1 teaspoonful every 4 hours. Children 2 to 6 years—1/2 teaspoonful every 4 hours. Children under 2 years—consult physician.
The suggested dosage in pediatric patients 3 months to 2 years of age is 2 drops per kilogram of body weight administered every 4 hours.

HOW SUPPLIED
TRIAMINIC Expectorant with Codeine (green), in pint bottles. TRIAMINIC Expectorant with Codeine is a Schedule V controlled substance.

TRIAMINIC® NITE LIGHT™   OTC
Nighttime Cough and Cold Medicine for Children
[trĭ″ah-mĭn′ĭc]

DESCRIPTION
Each teaspoonful (5 ml) of Triaminic® Nite Light™ contains: Pseudoephedrine hydrochloride 15 mg, chlorpheniramine maleate 1 mg, dextromethorphan hydrobromide 7.5 mg in a palatable non-alcoholic vehicle. Other ingredients: benzoic acid, Blue 1, citric acid, flavors, propylene glycol, purified water, Red 33, dibasic sodium phosphate, sorbitol, sucrose.

INDICATIONS
Temporarily quiets your child's cough associated with the common cold. Also, provides temporary relief of nasal stuffiness, sneezing, runny nose, and itchy watery eyes caused by the common cold, hay fever or other upper respiratory allergies.

WARNINGS
Do not exceed recommended dosage or take for more than 7 days. A persistent cough may be a sign of a serious condition. If symptoms persist for more than one week, tend to recur, or are accompanied by fever, rash, or persistent headache, consult a physician. May cause excitability especially in children. Unless directed by a physician, do not take this product: 1) if cough is accompanied by excessive phlegm (mucus), 2) for persistent or chronic cough such as occurs with smoking, asthma or emphysema, or 3) if you have heart disease, high blood pressure, thyroid disease, diabetes, asthma, glaucoma, difficulty in breathing, enlargement of the prostate gland. May cause marked drowsiness. Alcohol, sedatives, and tranquilizers may increase the drowsiness effect. Avoid alcoholic beverages while taking this product. Use caution when driving a motor vehicle or operating machinery. As with any drug, if you are pregnant or nursing a baby, seek the advice of a health professional before using this product. Keep this and all drugs out of the reach of children. In case of accidental overdose, seek professional assistance, or call a Poison Control Center immediately.

Continued on next page

Sandoz Consumer—Cont.

DRUG INTERACTION PRECAUTION.
Do not take this product if you are taking a prescription drug for high blood pressure or depression, or if you are taking sedatives or tranquilizers, without first consulting your physician.

DOSAGE AND ADMINISTRATION
Children 12 and over (96+ lbs.)—4 teaspoonfuls every 6–8 hours. Children 6 to under 12 years (48–95 lbs.)—2 teaspoonfuls every 6–8 hours. Unless directed by physician, do not exceed 4 doses in 24 hours. For convenience, a True-Dose™ dosage cup is provided with each 4 fl. oz. and 8 fl. oz. bottle.

PROFESSIONAL LABELING
The suggested dosage for pediatric patients is:

3 to under 12 months ... ¼ teaspoon or 1.25 ml
  (12–17 lbs.)
12 months to under 2 years ... ½ teaspoon or 2.5 ml
  (18–23 lbs.)
2 to under 6 years ... 1 teaspoonful or 5 ml

HOW SUPPLIED
Triaminic® Nite Light™ Nighttime Cough and Cold Medicine for Children, in 4 fl. oz. and 8 fl. oz. plastic bottles packaged in cartons with tamper-evident band around child-resistant cap.

TRIAMINIC® ORAL INFANT DROPS ℞
[trī″ah-mĭn′ĭc]

DESCRIPTION
Each ml of TRIAMINIC Oral Infant Drops contains: phenylpropanolamine hydrochloride 20 mg, pheniramine maleate 10 mg, and pyrilamine maleate 10 mg. Other ingredients: benzoic acid, flavor, glycerin, purified water, Red 33, saccharin sodium, sorbitol, sucrose. Contains FD&C Yellow No. 6 as a color additive.

This product combines the nasal decongestant properties of phenylpropanolamine hydrochloride with the antihistaminic activities of pheniramine maleate and pyrilamine maleate.

Phenylpropanolamine hydrochloride, a sympathomimetic drug, is structurally related to ephedrine and amphetamine. Pheniramine maleate is an antihistamine of the alkylamine class while pyrilamine maleate belongs to the ethylenediamine class.

CLINICAL PHARMACOLOGY
Phenylpropanolamine presumably acts on α-adrenergic receptors in the mucosa of the respiratory tract producing vasoconstriction which results in shrinkage of swollen mucous membranes, reduction of tissue hyperemia, edema and nasal congestion, and an increase in nasal airway patency. Antihistamines competitively act as H_1 receptor antagonists of histamine. They exhibit anticholinergic (drying) and sedative side effects. There are several classes of antihistamines which vary with respect to potency, dosage and the relative incidence of side effects. Antihistamines inhibit the effects of histamine on capillary permeability and on vascular, bronchial and many other types of smooth muscle.

INDICATIONS AND USAGE
For relief from such symptoms as nasal congestion and postnasal drip associated with colds, allergies, sinusitis and rhinitis. Also for relief of symptoms associated with allergic rhinitis such as sneezing, rhinorrhea, pruritus and lacrimation.

CONTRAINDICATIONS
TRIAMINIC Oral Infant Drops are contraindicated in patients exhibiting hypersensitivity to any of the ingredients. Antihistamines are contraindicated in patients receiving monoamine oxidase inhibitors since these agents may prolong and intensify the anticholinergic and CNS depressant effects of antihistamines (see Drug Interactions). Antihistamines should not be used to treat lower respiratory tract symptoms or be given to premature or newborn infants. Sympathomimetic agents such as phenylpropanolamine are contraindicated in patients with severe hypertension, severe coronary artery disease and in those taking monoamine oxidase inhibitors.

WARNINGS
Sympathomimetic agents should be used with caution in patients with hypertension, hyperthyroidism, diabetes mellitus and cardiovascular disease. Antihistamines should be used with caution in patients with narrow angle glaucoma, stenosing peptic ulcer, pyloroduodenal obstruction, symptomatic prostatic hypertrophy, bladder neck obstruction or chronic pulmonary disease.

PRECAUTIONS
General: see WARNINGS.
Information For Patients: Mothers should be informed of the potential for sedation or drowsiness. When prescribing antihistamine preparations, patients should be cautioned against mechanical activity requiring alertness.
Drug Interactions:
(1) Monoamine oxidase inhibitors: MAO inhibitors prolong and intensify the anticholinergic effects of antihistamines and potentiate the pressor effects of sympathomimetics.
(2) Alcohol and CNS depressants: These agents potentiate the sedative effects of antihistamines.
(3) Certain antihypertensives: Sympathomimetics may reduce the antihypertensive effects of methyldopa, mecamylamine, reserpine and veratrum alkaloids.
Carcinogenesis, Mutagenesis, Impairment Of Fertility: No data are available on the long-term potential for carcinogenicity, mutagenicity or impairment of fertility in animals or humans.
Pediatric Use: TRIAMINIC Oral Infant Drops have been formulated to provide safe and effective symptomatic relief for infants and small children. Precise dosage (on a body weight basis) is facilitated through the use of the plastic squeeze bottle with attached dropper tip (see DOSAGE AND ADMINISTRATION). It is important to note the variability of response infants and small children exhibit to antihistamines and sympathomimetics. As in adults, the combination of an antihistamine and sympathomimetic can elicit either mild stimulation or mild sedation in children. In the young child, mild stimulation is the response most frequently seen. In infants and children, overdosage of antihistamines may cause hallucinations, convulsions or death.

ADVERSE REACTIONS
The most frequent adverse reactions are underlined.
(1) *General:* urticaria, drug rash, anaphylactic shock, photosensitivity, excessive perspiration, chills, dryness of mouth, nose, and throat.
(2) *Cardiovascular System:* hypotension, headache, palpitations, tachycardia, extrasystoles.
(3) *Hematologic System:* hemolytic anemia, thrombocytopenia, agranulocytosis.
(4) *Nervous System:* sedation, sleepiness, dizziness, disturbed coordination, fatigue, confusion, restlessness, excitation, nervousness, tremor, irritability, insomnia, euphoria, paresthesias, blurred vision, diplopia, vertigo, tinnitus, acute labyrinthitis, hysteria, neuritis, convulsions, CNS depression, hallucinations.
(5) *GI System:* epigastric distress, anorexia, nausea, vomiting, diarrhea, constipation.
(6) *GU System:* urinary frequency, difficult urination, urinary retention.
(7) *Respiratory System:* thickening of bronchial secretions, tightness of chest and wheezing, nasal stuffiness.

OVERDOSAGE
TRIAMINIC product overdosage reactions may vary from central nervous system depression to stimulation. Stimulation is particularly likely in children. Atropine-like signs and symptoms—dry mouth; fixed, dilated pupils; flushing—and gastrointestinal symptoms may also occur.
If vomiting has not occurred spontaneously, the conscious patient should be induced to vomit. This is best done by having the patient drink a glass of water or milk after which they should be made to gag. Precautions against aspiration must be taken, especially in infants and children.
If vomiting is unsuccessful, gastric lavage is indicated within 3 hours after ingestion, and even later if large amounts of milk or cream were given beforehand. Isotonic and ½ isotonic saline is the lavage solution of choice.
Saline cathartics, such as milk of magnesia, draw water by osmosis into the bowel and therefore are valuable for their action in rapid dilution of bowel content.
Stimulants should *not* be used. Vasopressors may be used to treat hypotension.

DOSAGE AND ADMINISTRATION
1 drop per 2 pounds of body weight administered orally 4 times daily. The prescribed number of drops may be put directly into child's mouth or on a spoon for administration.

HOW SUPPLIED
TRIAMINIC Oral Infant Drops, in 15 ml plastic squeeze bottles which deliver approximately 24 drops per ml. Store TRIAMINIC Oral Infant Drops at room temperature.

TRIAMINIC® SYRUP OTC
[trī″ah-mĭn′ĭc]

DESCRIPTION
Each teaspoonful (5 ml) of TRIAMINIC Syrup contains phenylpropanolamine hydrochloride 12.5 mg and chlorpheniramine maleate 2 mg in a nonalcoholic vehicle. Other ingredients: benzoic acid, edetate disodium, flavors, purified water, sodium hydroxide, sorbitol, sucrose. Contains FD&C Yellow No. 6 as a color additive.

INDICATIONS
Provides temporary relief of nasal congestion, runny nose and sneezing that may occur with the common cold or with hay fever or other upper respiratory allergies. Relieves itching of the nose or throat and itchy, watery eyes.

CONTRAINDICATIONS
Hypersensitivity to any of the ingredients. The use of sympathomimetic agents such as phenylpropanolamine hydrochloride is contraindicated in patients with severe hypertension, severe coronary artery disease or in those taking monoamine oxidase inhibitors. Antihistamines such as chlorpheniramine maleate should not be administered to premature or newborn infants or be used to treat lower respiratory tract symptoms.

PRECAUTIONS
Exercise prescribing caution in patients with hypertension, cardiovascular disease, diabetes mellitus, hyperthyroidism, elevated intraocular pressure, prostatic hypertrophy, bladder neck obstruction or chronic pulmonary disease. Alcoholic beverages and other CNS depressants may potentiate the sedative effects of antihistamines. Use with caution in pregnant and nursing women.

ADVERSE REACTIONS
Mild CNS stimulation, drowsiness, blurred vision, dry mouth, tachycardia, dizziness, gastrointestinal upset may occur occasionally. May produce thickening of bronchial secretions.

DOSAGE AND ADMINISTRATION
Bottle label dosage reads: Adults—2 teaspoonfuls every 4 hours. Children 6–12 years—1 teaspoonful every 4 hours. Children under 6 years—consult physician.
The suggested dosage for pediatric patients 3 months to under 12 months of age is 1 drop per kg of body weight administered every 4 hours. The suggested dosage for patients 12 months to under 24 months of age is 3 drops per kg of body weight administered every 4 hours. The suggested dosage for patients 2 to under 6 years is ½ teaspoonful every 4 hours.

HOW SUPPLIED
TRIAMINIC Syrup (orange), in 4 fl oz and 8 fl oz plastic bottles with tamper-evident band around child-resistant cap.

TRIAMINIC® TR TABLETS ℞
[trī″ah mĭn′ĭc]
(Timed Release)

DESCRIPTION
Each TRIAMINIC TR Tablet (Timed Release) contains: phenylpropanolamine hydrochloride 50 mg, pheniramine maleate 25 mg, and pyrilamine maleate 25 mg. Other ingredients: acacia, colloidal silicon dioxide, lactose, magnesium stearate, methylcellulose, methylparaben, pharmaceutical glaze, polyethylene glycol, povidone, starch, stearic acid, sucrose, talc, titanium dioxide, Yellow 10. Contains FD&C Yellow No. 6 as a color additive.

This product combines the nasal decongestant properties of phenylpropanolamine hydrochloride with the antihistaminic activities of pheniramine maleate and pyrilamine maleate.

Phenylpropanolamine hydrochloride, a sympathomimetic drug, is structurally related to ephedrine and amphetamine. Pheniramine maleate is an antihistamine of the alkylamine class while pyrilamine maleate belongs to the ethylenediamine class.

CLINICAL PHARMACOLOGY
Phenylpropanolamine presumably acts on α-adrenergic receptors in the mucosa of the respiratory tract producing vasoconstriction which results in shrinkage of swollen mucous membranes, reduction of tissue hyperemia, edema and nasal congestion, and an increase in nasal airway patency. Antihistamines competitively act as H_1 receptor antagonists of histamine. They exhibit anticholinergic (drying) and sedative side effects. There are several classes of antihistamines which vary with respect to potency, dosage and the relative incidence of side effects. Antihistamines inhibit the effects of histamine on capillary permeability and on vascular, bronchial and many other types of smooth muscle.

INDICATIONS AND USAGE
For relief from such symptoms as nasal congestion and postnasal drip associated with colds, allergies, sinusitis and rhinitis. Also for the relief of symptoms associated with allergic rhinitis such as sneezing, rhinorrhea, pruritus and lacrimation.

CONTRAINDICATIONS
TRIAMINIC TR Tablets are contraindicated in patients exhibiting hypersensitivity to any of the ingredients. Antihistamines are contraindicated in patients receiving monoamine oxidase inhibitors since these agents may prolong and intensify the anticholinergic effects of antihistamines (see Drug Interactions). Antihistamines should not be used to treat lower respiratory tract symptoms. Sympathomimetic agents such as phenylpropanolamine are contraindicated in patients with severe hypertension, severe coronary artery disease and in those taking monoamine oxidase inhibitors.

Nursing Mothers: Because of the higher risk of antihistamines for premature or newborn infants, antihistamine therapy is contraindicated in nursing mothers.

WARNINGS

Sympathomimetic agents should be used with caution in patients with hypertension, hyperthyroidism, diabetes mellitus and cardiovascular disease. Antihistamines should be used with caution in patients with narrow angle glaucoma, stenosing peptic ulcer, pyloroduodenal obstruction, symptomatic prostatic hypertrophy, bladder neck obstruction or chronic pulmonary disease.

Use In The Elderly (approximately 60 years or older): Antihistamines are more likely to cause dizziness, sedation and hypertension in elderly patients. Overdosage of sympathomimetic agents in this age group may cause hallucinations, convulsions, CNS depression or death.

PRECAUTIONS

General: See WARNINGS.

Information For Patients: Patients should be informed of the potential for sedation or drowsiness and cautioned about driving or operating machinery. The concomitant consumption of alcoholic beverages or other sedative drugs should be avoided.

Drug Interactions:

(1) Monoamine oxidase inhibitors: MAO inhibitors may prolong and intensify the anticholinergic effects of antihistamines and potentiate the pressor effects of sympathomimetics.

(2) Alcohol and CNS depressants: These agents potentiate the sedative effects of antihistamines.

(3) Certain antihypertensives: Sympathomimetics may reduce the antihypertensive effects of methyldopa, mecamylamine, reserpine and veratrum alkaloids.

Carcinogenesis, Mutagenesis, Impairment of Fertility: No data are available on the long-term potential for carcinogenicity, mutagenicity or impairment of fertility in animals or humans.

Pregnancy: *Pregnancy Category C* —Animal reproduction studies have not been conducted. Safe use in pregnancy has not been established relative to possible adverse effects on fetal development. Therefore, TRIAMINIC TR Tablets should not be used in pregnant patients unless, in the judgment of the physician, the potential benefits outweigh possible hazards.

Nursing Mothers: See CONTRAINDICATIONS.

ADVERSE REACTIONS

The most frequent adverse reactions are underlined.

(1) *General:* urticaria, drug rash, anaphylactic shock, photosensitivity, excessive perspiration, chills, dryness of mouth, nose and throat.

(2) *Cardiovascular System:* hypotension, headache, palpitations, tachycardia, extrasystoles.

(3) *Hematologic System:* hemolytic anemia, thrombocytopenia, agranulocytosis.

(4) *Nervous System:* sedation, sleepiness, dizziness, disturbed coordination, fatigue, confusion, restlessness, excitation, nervousness, tremor, irritability, insomia, euphoria, paresthesias, blurred vision, diplopia, vertigo, tinnitus, acute labyrinthitis, hysteria, neuritis, convulsions, CNS depression, hallucinations.

(5) *GI System:* epigastic distress, anorexia, nausea, vomiting, diarrhea, constipation.

(6) *GU System:* urinary frequency, difficult urination, urinary retention, early menses.

(7) *Respiratory System:* thickening of bronchial secretions, tightness of chest and wheezing, nasal stuffiness.

OVERDOSAGE

TRIAMINIC TR Tablets overdosage reactions may vary from central nervous system depression to stimulation. Stimulation is particularly likely in children. Atropine-like signs and symptoms—dry mouth; fixed, dilated pupils; flushing —and gastrointestinal symptoms may also occur.

If vomiting has not occurred spontaneously, the conscious patient should be induced to vomit. This is best done by having the patient drink a glass of water or milk after which they should be made to gag. Precautions against aspiration must be taken, especially in infants and children.

If vomiting is unsuccessful, gastric lavage is indicated within 3 hours after ingestion, and even later if large amounts of milk or cream were given beforehand. Isotonic and ½ isotonic saline is the lavage solution of choice.

Saline cathartics, such as milk of magnesia, by osmosis draw water into the bowel and therefore are valuable for their action in rapid dilution of bowel content.

Stimulants should *not* be used. Vasopressors may be used to treat hypotension.

DOSAGE AND ADMINISTRATION

TRIAMINIC TR Tablets (Timed Release): Adults and children over 12 years—1 tablet swallowed whole, in the morning, midafternoon and before retiring.

HOW SUPPLIED

TRIAMINIC TR Tablets (Timed Release) (yellow, round, film-coated, imprinted "DORSEY" on one side and "TRIAMINIC TR" on the other), in bottles of 100 and 250.

TRIAMINIC–DM® SYRUP   OTC
[trī"ah-mĭn'ĭc]

DESCRIPTION

Each teaspoonful (5 ml) of TRIAMINIC-DM Syrup contains phenylpropanolamine hydrochloride 12.5 mg and dextromethorphan hydrobromide 10 mg in a nonalcoholic vehicle. Other ingredients: benzoic acid, Blue 1, flavors, propylene glycol, purified water, Red 40, sodium chloride, sorbitol, sucrose.

INDICATIONS

Provides relief of cough due to minor throat and bronchial irritation as may occur with the common cold or inhaled irritants. Promotes nasal and sinus drainage. The decongestant and antitussive are provided in an alcohol-free and antihistamine-free formula.

CONTRAINDICATIONS

Hypersensitivity to any of the ingredients. The use of sympathomimetic agents such as phenylpropanolamine hydrochloride is contraindicated in patients with severe hypertension, severe coronary artery disease or in those taking monoamine oxidase inhibitors.

PRECAUTIONS

Exercise prescribing caution in patients with persistent or chronic cough such as occurs with chronic bronchitis, bronchial asthma or emphysema. Use with caution in patients with hypertension, hyperthyroidism, cardiovascular disease or diabetes mellitus. Use with caution in pregnant and nursing women.

ADVERSE REACTIONS

Mild CNS stimulation, dizziness, headache or gastrointestinal upsets may occur.

DOSAGE AND ADMINISTRATION

Bottle label dosage reads: Adults—2 teaspoonfuls every 4 hours. Children 6–12 years—1 teaspoonful every 4 hours. Children 2–6 years—½ teaspoonful every 4 hours. Children under 2 years—consult physician.

The suggested dosage for pediatric patients 3 months to under 12 months of age is 1 drop per kg of body weight administered every 4 hours. The suggested dosage for patients 12 months to under 24 months of age is 3 drops per kg of body weight administered every 4 hours.

HOW SUPPLIED

TRIAMINIC-DM Syrup (dark red), in 4 fl oz and 8 fl oz plastic bottles with tamper-evident band around child-resistant cap.

TRIAMINIC-12® TABLETS   OTC
[trī"ah-mĭn'ĭc]

DESCRIPTION

Each TRIAMINIC-12 Tablet contains phenylpropanolamine hydrochloride 75 mg and chlorpheniramine maleate 12 mg. Other ingredients: acetylated monoglycerides, carnauba wax, colloidal silicon dioxide, ethylcellulose, lactose, hydroxypropyl methylcellulose, Red 30, stearic acid, titanium dioxide. Contains FD&C Yellow No. 6 as a color additive. TRIAMINIC-12 Tablets contain the nasal decongestant, phenylpropanolamine, and the antihistamine, chlorpheniramine, in a formulation providing 12 hours of symptomatic relief.

INDICATIONS

For the temporary relief of nasal congestion due to the common cold, hay fever or other upper respiratory allergies and associated with sinusitis. Helps decongest sinus openings, sinus passages; promotes nasal and/or sinus drainage; temporarily restores freer breathing through the nose.

For temporary relief of running nose, sneezing, itching of the nose or throat and itchy and watery eyes as may occur in allergic rhinitis (such as hay fever).

DOSAGE

Adults and children over 12 years of age—1 tablet swallowed whole every 12 hours.

NOTE: The nonactive portion of the tablet that supplies the active ingredients may occasionally appear in the stool as a soft mass.

WARNINGS

This product is not recommended for use in children under 12 years of age. Use with caution in patients with high blood pressure, heart disease, diabetes, thyroid disease, asthma, glaucoma or difficulty in urination due to enlargement of the prostate gland. Do not exceed the recommended dosage because at higher doses nervousness, dizziness, or sleeplessness

may occur. This preparation may cause drowsiness; this preparation may cause excitability, especially in children.

CAUTION

Patients should be advised to avoid driving a motor vehicle or operating heavy machinery. Patients should also be advised to avoid alcoholic beverages while taking this product. Use with caution in pregnant and nursing women.

DRUG INTERACTION PRECAUTION

Use with caution in patients presently taking a prescription antihypertensive or antidepressant drug containing a monoamine oxidase inhibitor.

HOW SUPPLIED

TRIAMINIC-12 Tablets (orange), imprinted "DORSEY" on one side, "TRIAMINIC 12" on the other, in blister packs of 10 and 20.

TRIAMINICIN® TABLETS   OTC
[trī"ah-mĭn'ĭ-sĭn]

(See PDR For Nonprescription Drugs)

TRIAMINICOL® MULTI-SYMPTOM   OTC
COLD TABLETS
[trī"ah-mĭn'ĭ-call]

DESCRIPTION

Each TRIAMINICOL Multi-Symptom Cold Tablet contains: phenylpropanolamine hydrochloride 12.5 mg, chlorpheniramine maleate 2 mg, and dextromethorphan hydrobromide 10 mg. Other ingredients: calcium stearate, colloidal silicon dioxide, lactose, methylcellulose, methylparaben, microcrystalline cellulose, polyethylene glycol, povidone, pregelatinized starch, Red 40, titanium dioxide.

INDICATIONS

Provides relief of runny nose, nasal congestion and sneezing that may occur with the common cold. Suppresses cough due to minor throat and bronchial irritation. Promotes nasal and sinus drainage.

CONTRAINDICATIONS

Hypersensitivity to any of the ingredients. The use of sympathomimetic agents such as phenylpropanolamine hydrochloride is contraindicated in patients with severe hypertension, severe coronary artery disease and in those taking monoamine oxidase inhibitors. Antihistamines should not be administered to premature or newborn infants or be used to treat lower respiratory tract symptoms.

PRECAUTIONS

Exercise prescribing caution in patients with hypertension, cardiovascular disease, diabetes mellitus, hyperthyroidism, elevated intraocular pressure, prostatic hypertrophy, bladder neck obstruction or chronic pulmonary disease. Use with caution in patients with persistent or chronic cough such as occurs with chronic bronchitis, bronchial asthma or emphysema. Alcoholic beverages and other CNS depressants may potentiate the sedative effects of antihistamines. Use with caution in pregnant and nursing women.

ADVERSE REACTIONS

Mild CNS stimulation, drowsiness, blurred vision, dry mouth, tachycardia, dizziness or gastrointestinal upset may occur. May produce thickening of bronchial secretions.

DOSAGE AND ADMINISTRATION

Adults—2 tablets every 4 hours. Children 6–12 years—1 tablet every 4 hours.

HOW SUPPLIED

TRIAMINICOL Multi-Symptom Cold Tablets (cherry pink), imprinted "DORSEY" on one side, "TRIAMINICOL" on the other, in blister packs of 24.

TRIAMINICOL® MULTI-SYMPTOM RELIEF   OTC
[trī"ah-mĭn'ĭ-call]

DESCRIPTION

Each teaspoonful (5 ml) of TRIAMINICOL Multi-Symptom Relief contains: phenylpropanolamine hydrochloride 12.5 mg, chlorpheniramine maleate 2 mg, and dextromethorphan hydrobromide 10 mg, in a palatable nonalcoholic vehicle. Other ingredients: benzoic acid, flavors, propylene glycol, purified water, Red 40, saccharin sodium, sodium chloride, sorbitol, sucrose.

INDICATIONS

Provides relief of runny nose, nasal congestion and sneezing that may occur with the common cold. Suppresses cough due to minor throat and bronchial irritation. Promotes nasal and sinus drainage.

Continued on next page

Sandoz Consumer—Cont.

CONTRAINDICATIONS

Hypersensitivity to any of the ingredients. The use of sympathomimetic agents such as phenylpropanolamine hydrochloride is contraindicated in patients with severe hypertension, severe coronary artery disease and in those taking monoamine oxidase inhibitors. Antihistamines should not be administered to premature or newborn infants or be used to treat lower respiratory tract symptoms.

PRECAUTIONS

Exercise prescribing caution in patients with hypertension, cardiovascular disease, diabetes mellitus, hyperthyroidism, elevated intraocular pressure, prostatic hypertrophy, bladder neck obstruction or chronic pulmonary disease. Use caution in patients with persistent or chronic cough such as occurs with chronic bronchitis, bronchial asthma or emphysema. Alcoholic beverages and other CNS depressants may potentiate the sedative effects of antihistamines. Use with caution in pregnant and nursing women.

ADVERSE REACTIONS

Mild CNS stimulation, drowsiness, blurred vision, dry mouth, tachycardia, dizziness or gastrointestinal upset may occur. May produce thickening of bronchial secretions. May cause excitability, especially in children.

DOSAGE AND ADMINISTRATION

Bottle label dosage reads: Adults—2 teaspoonfuls every 4 hours. Children 6–12 years—1 teaspoonful every 4 hours. Children under 6 years—consult physician.

The suggested dosage for pediatric patients 3 months to under 12 months of age is 1 drop per kg of body weight administered every 4 hours. The suggested dosage for patients 12 months to under 24 months of age is 3 drops per kg of body weight administered every 4 hours. The suggested dosage for children 2 to under 6 years is ½ teaspoonful every 4 hours.

HOW SUPPLIED

TRIAMINICOL Multi-Symptom Relief (red), in 4 fl oz and 8 fl oz plastic bottles with tamper-evident band around child-resistant cap.

Sandoz Pharmaceuticals Corp.
Dorsey Division
Sandoz Division
ROUTE 10
EAST HANOVER, NJ 07936

ASBRON G® Elixir and   ℞
[az'bron]
ASBRON G® Inlay-Tabs®

The following prescribing information is based on official labeling in effect on August 1, 1989.

DESCRIPTION

Each ASBRON G® Inlay-Tab® and tablespoonful (15 ml) of Asbron G® Elixir contains: theophylline sodium glycinate 300 mg (equivalent to 150 mg theophylline), guaifenesin 100 mg. The elixir supplies the active ingredients in a solution containing 15% alcohol by volume. Asbron G® contains a bronchodilator and an expectorant.

Theophylline sodium glycinate, a methylxanthine, is a white crystalline powder that is freely soluble in water, has a slight ammoniacal odor and a bitter taste. It is an equimolar mixture of theophylline sodium and glycine buffered by an additional mole of the essential amino acid, glycine.

The expectorant component is guaifenesin (formerly called glyceryl guaiacolate) which helps loosen and thus clear the bronchial passageways of bothersome, thickened mucus. Guaifenesin, 3-(o-methoxyphenoxy)-1,2-propanediol, occurs as a fine, white powder having a bitter, aromatic taste and a slight odor of guaiacol. The powder tends to become lumpy on storage. It is freely soluble in alcohol and soluble in water.

Asbron G® Elixir
Active Ingredients: Guaifenesin USP and Theophylline Sodium Glycinate USP

Inactive Ingredients: Alcohol, Benzoic Acid, Blue 1, Citric Acid, Natural and Artificial Flavorings, Purified Water, Saccharin, Saccharin Sodium, Sodium Chloride, Sorbitol, Sucrose and Yellow 10.

Asbron G® Inlay-Tabs®
Active Ingredients: Guaifenesin USP and Theophylline Sodium Glycinate USP
Inactive Ingredients: Blue 1, Calcium Stearate, Calcium Sulfate, Colloidal Silicon Dioxide, Sodium Starch Glycolate, Starch, Stearic Acid, Sucrose and Yellow 10.

CLINICAL PHARMACOLOGY

Theophylline sodium glycinate is more stable in the presence of hydrochloric acid due to the buffering action of glycine with subsequent reduction of the chance of theophylline precipitation in the stomach. This and the high solubility of the product are suggested as the reasons why this product has better gastric tolerance than aminophylline.

Theophylline, the active ingredient of theophylline sodium glycinate, accounts for 50% of the weight of this compound. Theophylline sodium glycinate is highly effective in relaxing the smooth muscle of the bronchioles and the pulmonary blood vessels, thus acting primarily as a bronchodilator, pulmonary vasodilator and smooth muscle relaxant. Like other xanthines, theophylline sodium glycinate is a coronary vasodilator, a diuretic, a cerebral, cardiac and skeletal muscle stimulant.

Theophylline acts by inhibiting phosphodiesterase which causes an increase in intracellular cyclic AMP. This action produces smooth muscle relaxation and inhibits the release of histamine and other bronchoconstricting mediators from mast cells.

In vitro, using human white blood cells, theophylline has been shown to react synergistically with beta agonists to increase intracellular cyclic AMP. More data is required to clearly establish if theophylline and the beta agonists are synergistic or additive in vivo.

Even after prolonged therapy, it has not been possible to demonstrate the development of tolerance to theophylline sodium glycinate.

The half-life of theophylline varies from individual to individual. Since effective bronchodilatation depends upon maintaining serum theophylline levels between 10-20 mg/dl (10-20 mcg/ml), the determination of serum theophylline can be of value.

The half-life of theophylline is prolonged in alcoholism, in patients with reduced hepatic or renal function, congestive heart failure and in patients receiving antibiotics such as triacetyloleandomycin, erythromycin, clindamycin and lincomycin. Fever can also prolong theophylline half-life.

Cigarette smoking (1-2 packs per day) enhances theophylline elimination. The half-life of theophylline is shortened with cigarette smoking. This effect is probably related to the induction of enzymes and requires between three months and two years to normalize after stopping tobacco usage.

By increasing respiratory tract fluid, guaifenesin reduces the viscosity of tenacious secretions and acts as an expectorant. The drug is effective in productive as well as nonproductive cough, but is of particular value in dry, nonproductive cough which tends to injure the mucous membranes of the air passages.

[See table below].

INDICATIONS AND USAGE

For relief of acute bronchial asthma and for reversible bronchospasm associated with chronic bronchitis and emphysema.

CONTRAINDICATIONS

Asbron G® Inlay-Tabs® and Asbron G® Elixir are contraindicated in individuals who have shown hypersensitivity to any of the components.

Drug	Effect
Aminophylline with Lithium Carbonate	Increased excretion of Lithium Carbonate
Aminophylline with Propranolol	Antagonism of Propranolol effect
Theophylline with Furosemide	Increased Diuresis
Theophylline with Hexamethonium	Decreased Hexamethonium-induced chronotropic effect
Theophylline with Reserpine	Reserpine-induced Tachycardia
Theophylline with Cimetidine	Increased theophylline blood levels
Theophylline with clindamycin, troleandomycin, erythromycin, lincomycin	Increased theophylline blood levels

WARNINGS

There is an excellent correlation between high theophylline blood levels and the clinical manifestations of toxicity in (1) patients with lowered body plasma clearances (due to transient cardiac decomposition), (2) chronic obstructive lung disease or patients with liver dysfunction, (3) patients who are older than 55 years of age, particularly males.

There are often no early signs of theophylline toxicity such as nausea and restlessness which may appear in up to 50% of patients. Convulsions or ventricular arrhythmias may be the first signs of toxicity.

Excessive doses of theophylline sodium glycinate may be expected to be toxic and serum theophylline levels are recommended to monitor therapy. The incidence of toxicity increases significantly at levels greater than 20 mcg/ml. Many patients who have higher theophylline serum levels exhibit tachycardia. Theophylline products often worsen preexisting arrhythmias.

Asbron G® Inlay-Tabs®, Asbron G® Elixir and other oral theophylline compounds should never be used to treat status asthma.

PRECAUTIONS

General: Theophylline should be used with caution in patients with severe cardiovascular disease, severe hypoxemia, hypertension, hyperthyroidism, acute myocardial injury, obstructive lung disease, liver disease, in the elderly and in neonates.

Great caution should be used in giving theophylline to patients in congestive heart failure. Such patients have markedly prolonged theophylline blood levels which have persisted for long periods after discontinuation of the drug.

Smokers have a shorter mean half-life of theophylline than nonsmokers and may require larger doses of theophylline.

Theophylline sodium glycinate should not be administered concurrently with other theophylline containing products.

Theophylline should be given with caution to patients with a history of peptic ulcer. Theophylline may act as a local irritant in the gastrointestinal tract.

Information for Patients: The importance of adherence to the prescribed dosage regimen should be stressed. Patients should be informed of symptoms associated with theophylline toxicity such as nausea and restlessness.

Laboratory Tests: There is great patient-to-patient variation in the serum half-life of theophylline. Therefore, when possible, serum theophylline levels should be measured to assist in titration of dosage.

Drug Interactions: The use of theophylline sodium glycinate with ephedrine and other sympathomimetic bronchodilators may result in a significant increase in side effects. [See table above].

Drug/Laboratory Test Interactions
Theophylline has been shown to increase the urinary excretion of catecholamines. The VMA test for catechols may be falsely elevated by guaifenesin. Theophylline may increase the apparent serum uric acid in certain manual or automated chemical procedures by being treated as if it were uric acid. Guaifenesin may increase renal clearance for urate and thereby lower the serum uric acid. It may also falsely elevate the level of urinary 5HIAA in certain serotonin metabolite chemical tests.

Carcinogenesis, Mutagenesis, Impairment of Fertility: No data are available on the long-term potential for carcinogenicity, mutagenicity or impairment of fertility in animals or humans.

Pregnancy: *Pregnancy Category C*—Animal reproduction studies have not been conducted with Asbron G®. Safe use in pregnancy has not been established relative to possible adverse effects on fetal development. Therefore, theophylline should not be used in pregnant patients unless, in the judgment of the physician, the potential benefits outweigh possible hazards.

Nursing Mothers: It is not known whether this drug is excreted in human milk. Because many drugs are excreted in human milk, caution should be observed when Asbron G® Inlay-Tabs® or Asbron G® Elixir is administered to a nursing mother.

Pediatric Use: See Dosage and Administration Section for mg/kg dosage in pediatric patients.

ADVERSE REACTIONS

Included in this listing which follows are adverse reactions, some of which may have been reported with theophylline sodium glycinate. However, pharmacological similarities

THEOPHYLLINE ELIMINATION CHARACTERISTICS

Group	Theophylline Renal Clearance Rates	Half-Life Average
1. Children	1.4 ml/kg/min	3.5 hours
2. Adults with uncomplicated asthma	1.2 ml/kg/min	7 hours
3. Older adults with chronic obstructive pulmonary disease	0.6 ml/kg/min	up to 24 hours
4. Adults with chronic obstructive pulmonary disease and cor pulmonale or other causes of heart failure and liver pathology	0.6 ml/kg/min and less	may exceed 24 hours
5. Young smokers	Not available	4.3 hours

among the xanthine drugs require that each of the reactions be considered when theophylline is administered. The most consistent adverse reactions are usually due to overdosage of theophylline sodium glycinate and are:

1. Gastrointestinal: nausea, vomiting, epigastric pain, hematemesis, diarrhea.
2. Central Nervous System: headaches, irritability, restlessness, insomnia, reflex hyperexcitability, muscle twitching, clonic and tonic generalized convulsions.
3. Cardiovascular: palpitation, tachycardia, extrasystoles, flushing hypotension, circulatory failure, life-threatening ventricular arrhythmias.
4. Respiratory: tachypnea.
5. Renal: albuminuria, increased excretion of renal tubular cells and red blood cells; potentiation of diuresis.
6. Others: hyperglycemia and inappropriate ADH syndrome.

OVERDOSAGE (Management):

A. If potential oral overdose is established and seizure has not occurred: (1) induce vomiting and resort to gastric lavage if the patient fails to vomit within 20-30 minutes; (2) administer a cathartic (this is particularly important if sustained-release preparations have been taken) and activated charcoal after successful vomiting has been induced or adequate gastric lavage performed.

B. If patient is having a seizure: (1) establish an airway; (2) administer O$_2$; (3) treat the seizure with intravenous diazepam 0.1 to 0.3 mg/kg up to 10 mg; (4) monitor vital signs, maintain blood pressure and provide adequate hydration.

C. Post-Seizure Coma: (1) maintain airway and oxygenation; (2) if a result of oral medication, follow above recommendations to prevent absorption of drug, but tracheal intubation and lavage will have to be performed instead of inducing emesis, and the cathartic and charcoal will need to be introduced via a large bore gastric lavage tube; (3) continue to provide full supportive care and adequate hydration while waiting for drug to be metabolized. In general, the drug is metabolized sufficiently rapidly so as to not warrant consideration of dialysis.

DOSAGE AND ADMINISTRATION

Therapeutic serum levels associated with optimal likelihood for benefit and minimal risk of toxicity are between 10-20 mcg/ml. There is great variation from patient to patient in the dosage of theophylline needed to achieve a therapeutic blood level because of variable rates of elimination. Because of this and because of the relatively narrow therapeutic blood level range associated with optimal results, the monitoring of serum theophylline levels is highly recommended. (See Laboratory Tests)

Usual Dosage: Adults—1 or 2 tablets or tablespoonfuls (15-30 ml), 3 or 4 times daily. Children 6 to 12—2 or 3 teaspoonfuls (10-15 ml), 3 or 4 times daily. Children 3 to 6—1 to 1½ teaspoonfuls (5-7.5 ml), 3 or 4 times daily. Children 1 to 3—½ to 1 teaspoonful (2.5-5 ml), 3 or 4 times daily.

Dosage Titration:

A. FOR PATIENTS NOT CURRENTLY RECEIVING THEOPHYLLINE PRODUCTS:

[See table above].

B. FOR PATIENTS CURRENTLY RECEIVING THEOPHYLLINE PRODUCTS: Determine, where possible, the time, amount, route of administration and form of the patient's last dose of theophylline.

The loading dose of theophylline will be based on the principle that each 0.5 mg/kg of theophylline administered as a loading dose will result in a 1 mcg/ml increase in serum theophylline concentration. Ideally, then, the loading dose should be deferred if a serum theophylline concentration can be rapidly obtained. If this is not possible, the clinician must exercise his judgment in selecting a dose based on the potential for benefit and risk. When there is sufficient respiratory distress to warrant a small risk, 2.5 mg/kg of theophylline is likely to increase the serum concentration when administered as a loading dose in rapidly absorbed form by only about 5 mcg/ml. If the patient is not already experiencing theophylline toxicity, this is unlikely to result in dangerous adverse effects.

Measurement of serum theophylline concentration during chronic therapy:

Blood for peak theophylline determinations should be obtained 1-2 hours after a dose of theophylline sodium glycinate. When determining theophylline serum concentrations in patients who have received chronic therapy, it is essential to establish that no doses were omitted in the 48 hours prior

	Oral Loading Dose (Theophylline Sodium Glycinate)	Maintenance Dose For Next 12 Hours (Theophylline Sodium Glycinate)	Maintenance Dose Beyond 12 Hours (Theophylline Sodium Glycinate)
1. Infants	8 mg/kg *(4 mg/kg)	3-8 mg/kg q6h *(1.5-4.0 mg/kg q6h)	4-6 mg/kg q6h *(2-3 mg/kg q6h)**
2. Children 6 months to 9 years	12 mg/kg *(6 mg/kg)	8 mg/kg q4h *(4 mg/kg q4h)	8 mg/kg q6h *(4 mg/kg q6h)
3. Children age 9-16 and young adult smokers	12 mg/kg *(6 mg/kg)	6 mg/kg q4h *(3 mg/kg q4h)	6 mg/kg q6h *(3 mg/kg q6h)
4. Otherwise healthy nonsmoking adults	12 mg/kg *(6 mg/kg)	6 mg/kg q6h *(3 mg/kg q6h)	6 mg/kg q8h *(3 mg/kg q8h)
5. Older patients and patients with Cor pulmonale	12 mg/kg *(6 mg/kg)	4 mg/kg q6h *(2 mg/kg q6h)	4 mg/kg q8h *(2 mg/kg q8h)
6. Patients with congestive heart failure, liver failure	12 mg/kg *(6 mg/kg)	4 mg/kg q8h *(2 mg/kg q8h)	2-4 mg/kg q12h *(1-2 mg/kg q12h)

Equivalent theophylline dosage indicated in parenthesis and marked with an asterisk (*).
** PEDIATRICS, Vol. 55, No. 5, May 1975.

to the determination. Missed doses could result in recommendations of future doses that would cause serious toxicity due to overdosage.

DOSAGE ADJUSTMENT BASED ON SERUM THEOPHYLLINE MEASUREMENTS WHEN THESE INSTRUCTIONS HAVE NOT BEEN FOLLOWED MAY RESULT IN RECOMMENDATIONS THAT PRESENT RISK OF TOXICITY TO THE PATIENT.

PATIENTS SHOULD NEVER BE MAINTAINED ON A DOSAGE OF THEOPHYLLINE THAT IS NOT WELL TOLERATED. Patients experiencing toxic side effects should be instructed to skip the next regular dose and to resume theophylline therapy at a lower dosage when all side effects have disappeared.

Maximum Dose Without Measurement of Serum Concentration: Not to exceed the following: (WARNING: DO NOT ATTEMPT TO MAINTAIN ANY DOSAGE THAT IS NOT WELL TOLERATED.)

[See table below].

Use ideal (lean) body weight for obese patients in computing dosage.

Dosage should always be calculated on the basis of ideal (lean) body weight when mg/kg doses are stated. Theophylline does not distribute into fatty tissues. NEVER ATTEMPT TO MAINTAIN A DOSAGE THAT IS NOT WELL TOLERATED BY THE PATIENT.

HOW SUPPLIED

Asbron G® Inlay-Tabs® (green, round, compressed tablet with white inlay) in bottles of 100. Asbron G® Elixir (green) in pint bottles.

Company's Product Identification Mark(s): Tablets imprinted "Asbron G" on one side, "78-202" on the other.

[ASB-Z3 Issued June 22, 1987]

BELLADENAL® Tablets   ℞
[bel-ad 'in-ol]
BELLADENAL-S® Tablets

The following prescribing information is based on official labeling in effect on August 1, 1989.

DESCRIPTION

Each Belladenal® Tablet and Belladenal-S® Tablet contains 0.25 mg Bellafoline® (levorotatory alkaloids of belladonna) and 50 mg phenobarbital, USP. (Warning: May be habit forming.)

Belladenal Tablets

Active Ingredients: Bellafoline (levorotatory alkaloids of belladonna) and phenobarbital, USP.

Inactive Ingredients: gelatin, lactose, malic acid, starch, stearic acid, and sucrose.

Belladenal-S Tablets

Active Ingredients: Bellafoline (levorotatory alkaloids of belladonna) and phenobarbital, USP.

Inactive Ingredients: colloidal silicon dioxide, color additives including FD&C Blue #1, FD&C Red #4, FD&C Yellow #5 (tartrazine), FD&C Yellow #6 (Sunset Yellow), gelatin, lac-

tose, magnesium stearate, malic acid, polyvinyl acetate resins, stearic acid, and sucrose.

CLINICAL PHARMACOLOGY

The antispasmodic-anticholinergic action of Belladenal is due to the presence of the natural levorotatory alkaloids of belladonna (Bellafoline). One Belladenal or Belladenal-S tablet provides the antispasmodic-anticholinergic activity equivalent to 0.83 ml of tincture of belladonna. Phenobarbital is a central nervous system sedative.

INDICATIONS AND USAGE

Based on a review of this drug by the National Academy of Sciences—National Research Council and/or other information, FDA has classified the indications as follows:

"Possibly" effective: As adjunctive therapy in the treatment of peptic ulcer and in the treatment of the irritable bowel syndrome (irritable colon, spastic colon, mucous colitis) and acute enterocolitis.

Final classification of the less-than-effective indications requires further investigation.

CONTRAINDICATIONS

Glaucoma, elevated intraocular pressure, advanced hepatic or renal disease, or pulmonary insufficiency. Phenobarbital is contraindicated in patients with a history of manifest or latent porphyria. Phenobarbital is contraindicated in those patients in whom the drug produces restlessness and/or excitement. Belladenal is contraindicated in patients with a demonstrated hypersensitivity to any of the components.

PRECAUTIONS

General

Due to the presence of a barbiturate, may be habit forming. Caution is advised in the elderly.

Information for Patients

Do not operate a motor vehicle or other hazardous equipment after taking Belladenal. Alcohol increases the sedative effects of this medication.

Laboratory Tests

Progress of patients with gastric ulcer may be followed radiologically or by gastroscopy. Problems related to lower bowel function may be checked by X-ray, stool examination or sigmoidoscopy.

Drug Interactions

1. Oral Anticoagulants: Phenobarbital may lower the plasma levels of dicumarol (name previously used: bishydroxycoumarin) and may cause a decrease in anticoagulant activity as measured by the prothrombin time. More frequent monitoring of prothrombin time responses is indicated whenever phenobarbital is initiated or discontinued, and the dosage of anticoagulants should be adjusted accordingly.

2. CNS Depressants: Combined administration of phenobarbital and CNS depressants such as alcohol, tricyclic antidepressants, phenothiazines and narcotic analgesics may result in a potentiation of the depressant action.

3. Hepatic Metabolism: Through the mechanism of enzyme induction caused by phenobarbital, a number of substances have been shown to be metabolized at an increased rate. In these cases, clinical responses should be closely monitored and appropriate dosage adjustments made. Included are such substances as griseofulvin, quinidine, doxycycline and estrogen. Although the meaning of published reports regarding the effects of phenobarbital on estrogen metabolism are unclear at this time, if avoidance

Age	Theophylline Sodium Glycinate	Equivalent Theophylline
Under 9 years	48 mg/kg/day	24 mg/kg/day
9-12 years	40 mg/kg/day	20 mg/kg/day
12-16 years	36 mg/kg/day	18 mg/kg/day
Over 16 years	26 mg/kg/day or 1800 mg/day (WHICHEVER IS LESS)	13 mg/kg/day or 900 mg/day (WHICHEVER IS LESS)

Continued on next page

Sandoz Pharm.—Cont.

of pregnancy is critical, consideration should be given to alternative methods of contraception.

4. *Phenytoin, Sodium Valproate, Valproic Acid:* The effect of barbiturates on the metabolism of phenytoin appears to be variable. Some investigators report an accelerating effect, while others report no effect. Because the effect of barbiturates on the metabolism of phenytoin is not predictable, phenytoin and barbiturate blood levels should be monitored more frequently if these drugs are given concurrently. Sodium valproate and valproic acid appear to decrease barbiturate metabolism; therefore, barbiturate blood levels should be monitored and appropriate dosage adjustments made as indicated.

5. *Tricylic Antidepressants:* Due to the presence of levorotatory alkaloids of belladonna, concomitant administration of tricyclic antidepressants may result in additive anticholinergic effects.

Drug/Laboratory Test Interactions

Belladonna does not appear to alter laboratory tests. Barbiturates may lower serum bilirubin and icterus index, increase or give false + values for BSP and PBI, and either raise or lower prothrombin time.

Carcinogenesis, Mutagenesis, Impairment of Fertility

Animal studies have not been conducted with Belladenal to assess its carcinogenicity, or potential for mutagenesis or fertility impairment. However, in more than 50 years of clinical use, there has been no indication of such effects.

Pregnancy

Teratogenic effects—Pregnancy Category C. Animal reproduction studies have not been conducted with Belladenal. It is also not known whether Belladenal can cause fetal harm when administered to a pregnant woman or can affect reproduction capacity. Belladenal should be given to a pregnant woman only if clearly needed. In more than 50 years of clinical use, however, there have been no reports of teratogenicity or congenital abnormality attributed to ingestion of Belladenal.

Chronic overuse of the phenobarbital contained in Belladenal during late pregnancy can result in respiratory depression and undue sedation in the newborn infant.

Labor and Delivery

Belladenal, a smooth muscle antispasmodic agent, is not intended for use during labor or delivery.

Nursing Mothers

Repetitive use of phenobarbital by the mother may permit drug transfer to the infant via breast milk, causing undue sedation. Belladonna alkaloids may also be transmitted to the nursing infant via breast milk, possibly resulting in depressed gastrointestinal motility and other anticholinergic effects. Therefore, it is recommended that nursing mothers avoid use of Belladenal.

Pediatric Use

(See DOSAGE AND ADMINISTRATION).

Tartrazine Reaction

Belladenal-S tablets contain FD&C Yellow #5 (tartrazine) which may cause allergic-type reactions (including bronchial asthma) in certain susceptible individuals. Although the overall incidence of FD&C Yellow #5 (tartrazine) sensitivity in the general population is low, it is frequently seen in patients who also have aspirin hypersensitivity.

ADVERSE REACTIONS

The most frequently reported adverse reactions are dry mouth, drowsiness, and blurred vision. Dizziness, skin rash, headache, pruritus, flushing and urinary retention have been reported.

DRUG ABUSE AND DEPENDENCE

During 50 years of clinical use of Belladenal there have been no reports of physical or psychological dependence, drug tolerance, habituation, chronic abuse, or symptoms of withdrawal involving Belladenal. Nevertheless, the propensity for barbiturate abuse among susceptible drug users is common knowledge.

OVERDOSAGE

Signs, Symptoms and Laboratory Findings of Acute Overdosage

The adverse effects of an overdose of Belladenal are due primarily to its barbiturate component. These may include:

Drowsiness, confusion, incoordination and coma.

Respiratory depression, which is early in onset, pronounced and persistent.

Hypotension, followed by a typical shock-like state in more severe cases.

Renal failure.

Signs and symptoms of belladonna overdosage may include:

Dilated pupils, blurring of vision and photophobia.

Hot, dry skin and dry mouth.

Hyperpyrexia, which may be alarming in infants.

Rapid pulse and respiration.

Urinary retention.

Restlessness, weakness, incoordination, memory lapses, disorientation, hallucinations, delirium and coma.

Circulatory and respiratory depression, with death usually due to respiratory failure.

Because reports of acute Belladenal® overdosage are not available, the lethal dose of this drug has not been established.

Phenobarbital drug blood concentrations of 40–60 mg/liter are considered toxic; levels of 80–150 mg/liter have been cited as lethal (C.L. Winek).

The minimum lethal dose of phenobarbital is estimated to be approxiamtely 2 Gm. Blood levels of about 8–10 mg per 100 ml, representing an ingested dose of about 5 Gm, have been found in fatal cases. However, recovery has followed considerably higher doses and blood levels. An oral dose of 1 Gm of most barbiturates produces significant toxic effects in adults. The fatal dose of Bellafoline® (levorotatory alkaloids of belladonna) has not been established. However, it is about one-half as toxic as atropine, the fatal dose of which is likewise unknown. Although doses of 1000 mg atropine have been survived by adults, 10 mg may be lethal in a child.

While the minimum lethal dose of the combined ingredients of Belladenal has not been established, data on the constituents of Belladenal administered orally to rats are available as follows:

Component	MLD mg/Kg	LD$_{50}$mg/Kg
Bellafoline	2.5	—
Phenobarbital	—	660

Treatment

Treatment is directed mainly toward the toxic effects of the barbiturate overdosage. However, the added toxic effects of the belladonna alkaloids must also be considered.

The therapeutic procedures most commonly employed are as follows:

ELIMINATION OF THE OFFENDING DRUG:

1. *Emesis*—If the patient is conscious, vomiting should be induced mechanically or with emetics.

2. *Gastric lavage*—This should be performed if the pharyngeal and laryngeal reflexes are present and if less than four hours have elapsed since ingestion. Gastric lavage on an unconscious patient should not be attempted unless cuffed endotracheal intubation has been performed to prevent aspiration and pulmonary implications.

3. *Catharsis*—Following gastric lavage, a saline cathartic [sodium or magnesium sulfate 30 Gm (1 oz.) in 250 ml (1 cup) of water] may be introduced and left in the stomach.

4. *Diuresis*—This should be encouraged with the administration of intravenous fluids, assisted, if necessary, by 100–150 mg 25% mannitol solution given slowly intravenously. NOTE: Mannitol should not be mixed with blood in a transfusion set as red cell crenation and agglutination may occur.

5. *Alkalinization of the urine (see CAUTION)*—Intravenous isotonic sodium bicarbonate solution accelerates urinary excretion of barbiturates. Maximum alkalinization may be more successful if the sodium bicarbonate infusion is accompanied by acetazolamide (Diamox®) 250 mg in a single I.V. injection every six hours.

CAUTION: Urinary alkalinization should be performed with care in children.

6. *Peritoneal dialysis and hemodialysis*—These have been used with success in acute barbiturate intoxication and may be life-saving. However, before embarking on either method, the risks inherent to these procedures must be carefully weighed against the risk of not using them at all.

MAINTENANCE OF ADEQUATE PULMONARY VENTILATION

Respiratory depression is an early and often profound manifestation of acute barbiturate poisoning. Meticulous attention to this aspect of treatment is essential.

Diligent pharyngeal and tracheal suction should be performed to remove excess mucous secretions. Judicious administration of oxygen is also indicated. However, oxygen without assisted respiration must be used with caution, as its use in hypoventilation hypoxia may result in further respiratory depression and hypercapnia. In more critical cases, endotracheal intubation and tracheotomy, with or without assisted respiration, may be necessary.

CORRECTION OF HYPOTENSION

Vigorous treatment is essential, as circulatory collapse and renal failure are not infrequent causes of death.

1. *Mild cases*—The usual head-down position and other supportive measures may be adequate.

2. *Severe cases*—Levarterenol barbiturate (Levophed®) 0.2% solution, 4 ml in 1000 ml 5% dextrose water solution given intravenously with the usual precautions and serial blood pressure monitoring; or phenylephrine hydrochloride (Neo-Synephrine®) 10 mg in 500 ml 5% dextrose water solution given intravenously with serial blood pressure monitoring may be used.

CNS STIMULATION

Considerable controversy exists over the use of an analeptic drug in acute barbiturate poisoning. Many investigators feel that analeptics are of benefit in coma involving severe cardiovascular or respiratory depression. However, there are no studies which have proved the merit of these drugs, and at best they are ancillary to general supportive therapy. Further, because severe belladonna alkaloid poisoning has a tendency to induce convulsions, the use of analeptic drugs in Belladenal poisoning must be approached with caution.

SPECIAL FEATURES DUE TO BELLADONNA OVERDOSAGE

If the peripheral effects of belladonna overdosage become prominent, they may be neutralized with the administration of neostigmine methylsulfate (Prostigmin®) 0.5–2.5 mg intramuscularly or by slow intravenous injection repeated every 3–4 hours if necessary.

GENERAL SUPPORTIVE MEASURES

1. *Good nursing care* is of primary importance, particularly in the comatose patient, and should include regular observation and accurate recording of the vital signs and depth of coma, maintenance of a free airway, frequent turning and other routine measures usually adopted with unconscious patients.

2. *Careful supervision and recording* of fluid intake and output is essential.

3. *Normal body temperature* must be maintained. This is particularly important in infants who are especially liable to hyperpyrexia.

4. *Prophylactic antibiotic therapy* in the comatose patient is a matter of individual physician preference. Because the incidence of pulmonary complications is high, the consensus of published opinion favors the use of prophylactic penicillin.

DOSAGE AND ADMINISTRATION

Belladenal Tablets

Adults:	2 to 4 tablets per day, in divided doses of ¼ to ½ tablet.*
Children:	¼ to ½ tablet* one to four times daily, according to age.

Belladenal-S® Tablets

Adults:	One tablet in the morning and one at night.

*Tablets are scored so that they can be divided easily.

HOW SUPPLIED

Belladenal Tablets (compressed, white, scored) in bottles of 100. Belladenal-S Tablets (compressed, scored tablets of tricolored pattern: salmon pink, emerald green and white) in bottles of 100.

Company's Product Identification Mark(s): Belladenal Tablets embossed 78-28 on one side and scored on reverse side. Belladenal-S Tablets embossed 78-27 on one side and scored on reverse side.

[BED-Z17 Issued May 1, 1987]

BELLERGAL–S® Tablets   ℞
[*bel 'er-gal*]

The following prescribing information is based on official labeling in effect on August 1, 1989.

Autonomic Stabilizer

DESCRIPTION

Each Bellergal-S Tablet contains: phenobarbital, USP, (Warning: may be habit forming), 40 mg; ergotamine tartrate, USP, 0.6 mg; Bellafoline® (levorotatory alkaloids of belladonna) 0.2 mg.

Inactive Ingredients: colloidal silicon dioxide, color additives including FD&C Blue #1, FD&C Red #40, FD&C Yellow #5, FD&C Yellow #6 (Sunset Yellow); gelatin, lactose, magnesium stearate, malic acid, polyvinyl acetate resins, stearic acid, sucrose and tartaric acid.

CLINICAL PHARMACOLOGY

Based on the concept that functional disorders frequently involve hyperactivity of both the sympathetic and parasympathetic nervous systems, the ingredients in Bellergal-S are combined to provide a balanced preparation designed to correct imbalance of the autonomic nervous system. The integrated action of Bellergal-S is effected through the combined administration of ergotamine and the levorotatory alkaloids of belladonna, specific inhibitors of the sympathetic and parasympathetic respectively, reinforced by the synergistic action of phenobarbital in dampening the cortical centers. It should be noted that on a weight basis the levorotatory alkaloids of belladonna have approximately twice the pharmacological effect as do the usual racemic mixtures.

INDICATIONS AND USAGE

Bellergal-S is employed in the management of disorders characterized by nervous tension and exaggerated autonomic response: *Menopausal disorders* with hot flushes, sweats, restlessness and insomnia; *cardiovascular disorders* with palpitation, tachycardia, chest oppression and vasomotor disturbances; *gastrointestinal disorders* with hypermotility, hypersecretion, "nervous stomach," and alternately diarrhea and constipation; interval treatment of *recurrent, throbbing headache.*

CONTRAINDICATIONS

Peripheral vascular disease, coronary heart disease, hypertension, impaired hepatic or renal function, sepsis, pregnancy, nursing mothers and glaucoma. The concomitant administration of ergotamine and dopamine should be avoided, due to the increased potential for ischemic vasoconstriction. Phenobarbital is contraindicated in patients with a history of manifest or latent porphyria. Phenobarbital is contraindicated in those patients in whom the drug produces restlessness and/or excitement. Bellergal-S is contraindicated in patients with a demonstrated hypersensitivity to any of the components.

WARNINGS

Total weekly dosage of ergotamine tartrate should not exceed 10 mg. (This dosage corresponds to 16 Bellergal-S tablets). Due to presence of a barbiturate, may be habit forming.

PRECAUTIONS

Even though the ergotamine tartrate content of this product is low and untoward effects have been rare and of minor significance, caution should be exercised if large or prolonged dosage is contemplated, and physicians should be alert to possible peripheral vascular complications in patients sensitive to ergot. Due to the presence of the anticholinergic agent, special caution should be exercised in the use of this drug in patients with bronchial asthma or obstructive uropathy.

Bellergal-S contains FD&C Yellow No. 5 (tartrazine) which may cause allergic-type reactions (including bronchial asthma) in certain susceptible individuals. Although the overall incidence of FD&C Yellow No. 5 (tartrazine) sensitivity in the general population is low, it is frequently seen in patients who also have aspirin hypersensitivity.

Information for Patients: Patients on large or prolonged dosage should be asked to report numbness or tingling of extremities, claudication or other symptoms of peripheral vasoconstriction.

Drug Interactions:
1. *Oral Anticoagulants:* Phenobarbital may lower the plasma levels of dicumarol (name previously used: bishydroxycoumarin) and may cause a decrease in anticoagulant activity as measured by the prothrombin time. More frequent monitoring of prothrombin time responses is indicated whenever phenobarbital is initiated or discontinued, and the dosage of anticoagulants should be adjusted accordingly.
2. *CNS Depressants:* Combined administration of phenobarbital and CNS depressants such as alcohol, tricyclic antidepressants, phenothiazines and narcotic analgesics may result in a potentiation of the depressant action.
3. *Beta Adrenergic Blocking Agents:* Although proof is lacking, several reports in the literature suggest a possible interaction between ergot alkaloids and beta adrenergic blocking agents. This interaction may result in excessive vasoconstriction. Although many patients can apparently take propranolol and ergot alkaloids without ill effects, there is enough evidence of an interaction to dictate closer surveillance of patients so treated.
4. *Hepatic Metabolism:* Through the mechanism of enzyme induction caused by phenobarbital, a number of substances have been shown to be metabolized at an increased rate. In these cases, clinical responses should be closely monitored and appropriate dosage adjustments made. Included are such substances as griseofulvin, quinidine, doxycycline and estrogen. Although the meaning of published reports regarding the effects of phenobarbital on estrogen metabolism are unclear at this time, if avoidance of pregnancy is critical, consideration should be given to alternative methods of contraception.
5. *Phenytoin, Sodium Valproate, Valproic Acid:* The effect of barbiturates on the metabolism of phenytoin appears to be variable. Some investigators report an accelerating effect, while others report no effect. Because the effect of barbiturates on the metabolism of phenytoin is not predictable, phenytoin and barbiturate blood levels should be monitored more frequently if these drugs are given concurrently. Sodium valproate and valproic acid appear to decrease barbiturate metabolism; therefore, barbiturate blood levels should be monitored and appropriate dosage adjustments made as indicated.
6. *Tricyclic Antidepressants:* Due to the presence of levoratatory alkaloids of belladonna, concomitant administra-

tion of tricyclic antidepressants may result in additive anticholinergic effects.

Carcinogenesis: No data are available on the long-term potential for carcinogenicity in animals or humans.

Pregnancy: *Pregnancy Category X*—due to the potential uterotonic effects of the ergot alkaloids, the use of Bellergal-S® during pregnancy is contraindicated. See "Contraindications" section.

Nursing Mothers: A number of ergot alkaloids inhibit the secretion of prolactin. Therefore, Bellergal-S is contraindicated in nursing mothers. See "Contraindications" section.

Pediatric Use: Safety and effectiveness in children have not been established.

ADVERSE REACTIONS

Tingling and other paresthesias of the extremities, blurred vision, palpitations, dry mouth, decreased sweating, decreased gastrointestinal motility, urinary retention, tachycardia, flushing, and drowsiness occur rarely.

DRUG ABUSE AND DEPENDENCE

Barbiturates may be habit-forming. Tolerance, psychological dependence, and physical dependence may occur especially following prolonged use of high doses. Daily administration in excess of 400 mg of pentobarbital or secobarbital for approximately 90 days is likely to produce some degree of physical dependence. By way of comparison, the phenobarbital component of Bellergal-S at the highest recommended daily dosage amounts to 80 mg.

OVERDOSAGE

Management of Overdosage: While severe symptoms of overdosage with Bellergal-S have not been reported, theoretically they could occur. It is imperative to note that overdosage symptoms with Bellergal-S may be attributable to any one or more of the three active ingredients. Which toxic manifestation might predominate in any individual case would be impossible to predict but one should be alert to the various possibilities. When anticholinergic/antispasmodic drugs are taken in sufficient overdose to produce such severe symptoms, prompt treatment should be instituted. Gastric lavage and other measures to limit intestinal absorption should be initiated without delay.

Cholinesterase inhibitors administered parenterally may be necessary for treatment of the serious manifestation of anticholinergic overdosage. Additionally, symptomatic therapy, including oxygen, sedatives and control of hyperthermia may be necessary.

Acute barbiturate overdosage symptoms with Bellergal-S, while possible, have not been reported. While the usual procedures for handling barbiturate poisoning should be employed, keep in mind the possibility of anticholinergic overdosing effects.

Acute ergot overdosage symptoms with Bellergal-S, while possible, have not been reported. The usual procedures for handling ergot overdosage include the administration of a peripheral vasodilator to counteract the vasospasm.

DOSAGE AND ADMINISTRATION

One in the morning and one in the evening.

HOW SUPPLIED

Compressed tablets of tri-colored pattern: dark green, orange and light lemon yellow, in bottles of 100. (NDC 0078-0031-05)

Company's Product Identification Mark(s):
BELLERGAL-S Tablets scored on one side, embossed "78-31" other side.

[BEG-Z15 Issued May 1, 1987]
Shown in Product Identification Section, page 427

CAFERGOT®   ℞
[kaf'er-got]
(ergotamine tartrate and caffeine) tablets, USP
(ergotamine tartrate and caffeine) suppositories, USP
CAFERGOT® P-B
Tablets and Suppositories

The following prescribing information is based on official labeling in effect on August 1, 1989.

DESCRIPTION

CAFERGOT®—
Tablet:
ergotamine tartrate, USP .... 1 mg
caffeine, USP .... 100 mg
Inactive Ingredients: acacia, carnauba wax, lactose, methylparaben, povidone, propylparaben, sodium benzoate, sorbitol, starch, stearic acid, sucrose, synthetic black ferric oxide, synthetic red ferric oxide, synthetic yellow ferric oxide, talc, tartaric acid and titanium dioxide.
Suppository:
ergotamine tartrate, USP .... 2 mg
caffeine, USP .... 100 mg
Inactive Ingredients: tartaric acid, NF, and cocoa butter, NF

CAFERGOT® P-B—
Tablet:
ergotamine tartrate, USP .... 1 mg
caffeine, USP .... 100 mg
Bellafoline® (levoratatory alkaloids
    of belladonna) .... 0.125 mg
pentobarbital sodium, USP .... 30 mg
    Warning: May be habit forming.
Inactive Ingredients: acacia, carnauba wax, color additives including D&C Yellow #10, FD&C Blue #1, FD&C Yellow #6 (Sunset Yellow), lactose, malic acid, mixed parabens, povidone, sodium benzoate, starch, stearic acid, sucrose, talc, tartaric acid and titanium dioxide
Suppository:
ergotamine tartrate, USP .... 2 mg
caffeine, USP .... 100 mg
Bellafoline® (levoratatory alkaloids
    of belladonna) .... 0.25 mg
pentobarbital, USP .... 60 mg
    Warning: May be habit forming.
Inactive Ingredients: tartaric acid, NF, malic acid, NF, and cocoa butter, NF

Cafergot Suppositories and Cafergot P-B Suppositories are *sealed* in foil to afford protection from cocoa butter leakage. If an unavoidable period of exposure to heat softens the suppository, it should be chilled in ice-cold water to solidify it before removing the foil.

ACTIONS

Ergotamine is an alpha adrenergic blocking agent with a direct stimulating effect on the smooth muscle of peripheral and cranial blood vessels and produces depression of central vasomotor centers. The compound also has the properties of serotonin antagonism. In comparison to hydrogenated ergotamine, the adrenergic blocking actions are less pronounced and vasoconstrictive actions are greater.

Caffeine, also a cranial vasoconstrictor, is added to further enhance the vasoconstrictive effect without the necessity of increasing ergotamine dosage.

For individuals experiencing excessive nausea and vomiting during migraine attacks the further addition of the anticholinergic and antiemetic alkaloids of belladonna and pentobarbital for reduction of nervous tension has been provided. Many migraine patients experience excessive nausea and vomiting during attacks, making it impossible for them to retain any oral medication. In such cases, therefore, the only practical means of medication is through the rectal route where medication may reach the cranial vessels directly, evading the splanchnic vasculature and the liver.

INDICATIONS

Cafergot
Indicated as therapy to abort or prevent vascular headache, e.g., migraine, migraine variants, or so-called "histaminic cephalalgia".

Cafergot P-B
Indicated as therapy to abort or prevent vascular headache complicated by tension and gastrointestinal disturbances.

CONTRAINDICATIONS

Peripheral vascular disease, coronary heart disease, hypertension, impaired hepatic or renal function, sepsis and pregnancy. Hypersensitivity to any of the components.

PRECAUTIONS

Although signs and symptoms of ergotism rarely develop even after long term intermittent use of the orally or rectally administered drugs, care should be exercised to remain within the limits of recommended dosage.

Ergotism is manifested by intense arterial vasoconstriction, producing signs and symptoms of peripheral vascular ischemia. Ergotamine induces vasoconstriction by a direct action on vascular smooth muscle. In chronic intoxication with ergot derivatives, headache, intermittent claudication, muscle pains, numbness, coldness and pallor of the digits may occur. If the condition is allowed to progress untreated, gangrene can result.

While most cases of ergotism associated with ergotamine treatment result from frank overdosage, some cases have involved apparent hypersensitivity. There are few reports of ergotism among patients taking doses within the recommended limits or for brief periods of time. In rare instances, patients, particularly those who have used the medication indiscriminately over long periods of time, may display withdrawal symptoms consisting of rebound headache upon discontinuation of the drug.

There have been reports of drug abuse and psychological dependence in patients on Cafergot® (ergotamine tartrate and caffeine) therapy. Due to the chronicity of vascular headaches, it is imperative that patients be advised not to exceed recommended dosages with long-term use to avoid ergotism.

ADVERSE REACTIONS

Vasoconstrictive complications, at times of a serious nature, may occur. These include pulselessness, weakness, muscle pains and paresthesias of the extremities and precordial distress and pain. Although these effects occur most com-

Continued on next page

Sandoz Pharm.—Cont.

monly with long-term therapy at relatively high doses, they have also been reported with short-term or normal doses. Other adverse effects include transient tachycardia or bradycardia, nausea, vomiting, localized edema and itching. Drowsiness may occur with Cafergot P-B.

DOSAGE AND ADMINISTRATION

Procedure: For the best results, dosage should start at the first sign of an attack. Adults: *Orally*—2 tablets at start of attack; 1 additional tablet every ½ hour, if needed for full relief (maximum 6 tablets per attack, 10 per week). *Rectally* —1 suppository at start of attack; second suppository after 1 hour, if needed for full relief (maximum 2 suppositories per attack, 5 per week).

MAXIMUM ADULT DOSAGE

Orally: Total dose for any one attack should not exceed 6 tablets.
Rectally: Two suppositories is the maximum dose for an individual attack.
Total weekly dosage should not exceed 10 tablets or 5 suppositories.
In carefully selected patients, with due consideration of maximum dosage recommendations, administration of the drug at bedtime may be an appropriate short-term preventive measure.

OVERDOSAGE

The toxic effects of an acute overdosage of Cafergot® (ergotamine tartrate and caffeine) are due primarily to the ergotamine component. The amount of caffeine is such that its toxic effects will be overshadowed by those of ergotamine. Symptoms include vomiting, numbness, tingling, pain and cyanosis of the extremities associated with diminished or absent peripheral pulses; hypertension or hypotension; drowsiness, stupor, coma, convulsions and shock. A case has been reported of reversible bilateral papillitis with ring scotomata in a patient who received five times the recommended daily adult dose over a period of 14 days.
Treatment consists of removal of the offending drug by induction of emesis, gastric lavage, and catharsis. Maintenance of adequate pulmonary ventilation, correction of hypotension, and control of convulsions are important considerations. Treatment of peripheral vasospasm should consist of warmth, but not heat, and protection of the ischemic limbs. Vasodilators may be used with benefit but caution must be exercised to avoid aggravating an already existent hypotension.

HOW SUPPLIED

Cafergot Tablets: shell pink colored, sugar coated. Bottles of 250 and cartons of three SigPak® (dispensing unit) packages, each containing 30 tablets in individual blisters. Cafergot Suppositories: sealed in fuchsia-colored aluminum foil in boxes of 12. Cafergot P-B Tablets: bright green, sugar coated. Bottles of 250 and cartons of three SigPak® (dispensing unit) packages, each containing 30 tablets in individual blisters. Cafergot P-B Suppositories: sealed in blue aluminum foil in boxes of 12.
Company's Product Identification Mark(s): Cafergot Tablets imprinted "CAFERGOT" on one side, triangle (S) other side.
Cafergot P-B Tablets imprinted "78-36" on one side, triangle (S) other side.
Cafergot Suppositories imprinted "triangle (S) CAFERGOT® SUPPOSITORY 78-33 SANDOZ".
Cafergot P-B Suppositories imprinted "triangle (S) CAFERGOT® P-B SUPPOSITORY 78-35 SANDOZ".
[CAF-Z24 Issued May 15, 1987]
Shown in Product Identification Section, page 427

CEDILANID®-D   ℞
[sē-de-lan'id]
(deslanoside) injection, USP

The following prescribing information is based on official labeling in effect on August 1, 1989.

DESCRIPTION

The cardiac (or digitalis) glycosides are a closely related group of drugs having in common specific and powerful effects on the myocardium. These drugs are found in a number of plants. Typically, the glycosides are composed of three portions, a steroid nucleus, a lactone ring, and a sugar (hence "glycosides").
Cedilanid-D (deslanoside) is provided as ampul solution containing the cardioactive glycoside, desacetyl lanatoside C. This agent is prepared by controlled alkaline hydrolysis of lanatoside C, a glycoside obtained from digitalis lanata.
Supplied in ampuls of 2 ml. Each 2 ml contains:
deslanoside, USP .... 0.4 mg
citric acid, USP, qs to .... pH 6.2±0.3
sodium phosphate, USP .... 10.7 mg
alcohol, USP .... 9.8% by vol.

glycerin, USP .... 15% by wt.
water for injection, USP, qs to 2 ml

ACTION

The digitalis glycosides have qualitatively the same therapeutic effect on the heart. They (1) increase the force of myocardial contraction, (2) increase the refractory period of the atrioventricular (A-V) node, and (3) to a lesser degree, affect the sinoatrial (S-A) node and conduction system via the parasympathetic and sympathetic nervous systems.
Cedilanid-D (deslanoside) has its onset of action in about 5 minutes after intravenous administration and reaches peak effect in 2-4 hours. Therapeutic action persists for 2 to 5 days.

INDICATIONS

1. "Congestive heart failure," all degrees, is the primary indication. The increased cardiac output results in diuresis and general amelioration of the disturbances characteristic of right (venous congestion, edema) and left (dyspnea, orthopnea, cardiac asthma) heart failure.
   Digitalis, generally, is most effective in "low output" failure and less effective in "high output" (bronchopulmonary insufficiency, infection, hyperthyroidism) heart failure.
   Digitalis should be continued after failure is abolished unless some known precipitating factor is corrected.
2. "Atrial fibrillation"— especially when the ventricular rate is elevated. Digitalis rapidly reduces ventricular rates and eliminates the pulse deficit. Palpitation, precordial distress or weakness are relieved and any concomitant congestive failure ameliorated.
   Digitalis is continued in doses necessary to maintain the desired ventricular rate and other clinical effects.
3. "Atrial flutter" digitalis slows the heart and regular sinus rhythm may appear. Frequently the flutter is converted to atrial fibrillation with a slow ventricular rate. Stopping digitalis at this point may be followed by restoration of sinus rhythm, especially if the flutter was of the paroxysmal type. It is preferable, however, to continue digitalis if failure ensues or if atrial flutter is a frequent occurrence.
4. "Paroxysmal atrial tachycardia" digitalis may be used, especially if it is resistant to lesser measures. Depending on the urgency, a more rapid acting parenteral preparation may be preferable to initiate digitalization, although if failure has ensued or paroxysms recur frequently, digitalis is maintained by oral administration.
   Digitalis is not indicated in sinus tachycardia or premature systoles in the absence of heart failure.
   "Cardiogenic shock"—the value of digitalis is not established, but the drug is often employed, especially when the condition is accompanied by pulmonary edema. Digitalis seems to adversely affect shock due to infections.

CONTRAINDICATIONS

The presence of toxic effects (See "Overdosage") induced by any digitalis preparation is an absolute contraindication to all of the glycosides.
"Allergy," though rare, does occur. It may not extend to all preparations and another may be tried.
"Ventricular Fibrillation"
"Ventricular tachycardia," unless congestive failure supervenes after a protracted episode not itself due to digitalis.

WARNINGS

Many of the arrhythmias for which digitalis is advised are identical with those reflecting digitalis intoxication. If the possibility of digitalis intoxication cannot be excluded, cardiac glycosides should be temporarily withheld if permitted by the clinical situation.
The patient with congestive heart failure may complain of nausea and vomiting. These symptoms may also be indications of digitalis intoxication. A clinical determination of the cause of these symptoms must be attempted before further drug administration.

PRECAUTIONS

"Potassium depletion" sensitizes the myocardium to digitalis and toxicity is apt to develop even with usual dosage. Hypokalemia also tends to reduce the positive inotropic effect of digitalis.
Potassium wastage may result from diuretic, corticosteroid, hemodialysis and other therapy. It is apt to accompany malnutrition, old age and long-standing congestive heart failure.
"Acute myocardial infarction," severe pulmonary disease, or far advanced heart failure are apt to be more sensitive to digitalis and more prone to disturbances of rhythm.
"Calcium" affects contractility and excitability of the heart in a manner similar to that of digitalis. Calcium may produce serious arrhythmias in digitalized patients.
"Myxedema"—Digitalis requirements are less because excretion rate is decreased and blood levels are significantly higher.
"Incomplete AV block," especially patients subject to Stokes Adams attacks, may develop advanced or complete heart

block. Heart failure in these patients can usually be controlled by other measures and by increasing the heart rate.
"Chronic constrictive pericarditis," is apt to respond unfavorably.
"Idiopathic hypertrophic subaortic stenosis" must be managed extremely carefully. Unless cardiac failure is severe it is doubtful whether digitalis should be employed.
"Renal insufficiency" delays the excretion of digitalis and dosage must be adjusted accordingly in patients with renal disease.
NOTE: This applies also to potassium administration should it become necessary.
Electrical conversion of arrhythmias may require adjustment of digitalis dosage.

ADVERSE REACTIONS

Gynecomastia, uncommon.

OVERDOSAGE, TOXIC EFFECTS

"Gastrointestinal" anorexia, nausea, vomiting, diarrhea—are the most common early symptoms of overdosages in the adult.
Uncontrolled heart failure may also produce such symptoms.
"Central Nervous System"—headache, weakness, apathy, visual disturbances.
"Cardiac Disturbances"———
Arrhythmias —"ventricular premature beats" is the most common.
Paroxysmal and nonparoxysmal nodal rhythms, atrioventricular (inference) dissociation and paroxysmal atrial tachycardia (PAT) with block are also common arrhythmias due to digitalis overdosage.
Conduction Disturbances—excessive slowing of the pulse is a clinical sign of digitalis overdosage. Atrioventricular block of increasing degree, may proceed to complete heart block.
NOTE: The electrocardiogram is fundamental in determining the presence and nature of these toxic disturbances. Digitalis may also induce other changes (as of the ST segment), but these provide no measure of the degree of digitalization.

TREATMENT OF TOXIC ARRHYTHMIAS

Digitalis is discontinued until after all signs of toxicity are abolished. This may be all that is necessary if toxic manifestations are not severe and appear after the time for peak effect of the drug.
Potassium salts are commonly used. Potassium chloride in divided doses totaling 4 to 6 gm for adults provided renal function is adequate.
When correction of the arrhythmia is urgent, potassium is administered intravenously in a solution of 5 percent dextrose in water, a total of 40-100 mEq. (40 mEq per 500 ml) at the rate of 40 mEq per hour unless limited by pain due to local irritation.
Additional amounts may be given if the arrhythmia is uncontrolled and the potassium well tolerated.
Electrocardiographic monitoring is indicated to avoid potassium toxicity, e.g. peaking of T waves.

CAUTION

Potassium should not be used and may be dangerous for severe or complete heart block due to digitalis and not related to any tachycardia.
Chelating agents to bind calcium may also be used to counteract the arrhythmia effect of digitalis toxicity, hypokalemia and of elevated serum calcium which may also precipitate digitalis toxicity.
Four grams (0.8 percent solution) of the disodium salt of EDTA is dissolved in 500 ml of 5 percent dextrose in water (50 mg per ml) and administered over a period of 2 hours unless the arrhythmia is controlled before the infusion is completed.
A continuous electrocardiogram should be observed so that the infusion may be promptly stopped when the desired effect is achieved.
Other counteracting agents are: Quinidine, procainamide, and beta adrenergic blocking agents.

DOSAGE AND ADMINISTRATION

"Parenteral" administration should be used only when the drug cannot be taken orally, or rapid digitalization is very urgent.
Parenteral digitalization can be obtained within 12 hours by giving 8 ml (1.6 mg) *either intramuscularly* or *intravenously*. By the I.V. route the dose may be given as one injection or in portions of 4 ml each. By I.M. route, 4 ml portions are injected at each of 2 sites.
After parenteral digitalization with Cedilanid®-D (deslanoside) maintenance therapy may be accomplished by starting administration of an oral preparation, within 12 hours.

HOW SUPPLIED

Ampuls, 2 ml size (2 ml contains 0.4 mg deslanoside, USP) Boxes of 20 ampuls.
Being chemically pure and of constant potency, deslanoside, USP is standardized by weight; the ampul solution of

Cedilanid-D (deslanoside) contains in each 2 ml:
deslanoside, USP .... 0.4 mg
citric acid, USP qs to .... pH 6.2±0.3
sodium phosphate, USP .... 10.7 mg
alcohol, USP .... 9.8% by vol.
glycerin, USP .... 15% by wt.
water for injection, USP, qs to 2 ml
[CED-Z19 Issued February 16, 1987]

D.H.E. 45® Injection   ℞

(dihydroergotamine mesylate) injection, USP

The following prescribing information is based on official labeling in effect on August 1, 1989.

DESCRIPTION

D.H.E. 45® is hydrogenated ergotamine as the mesylate. It is a clear, colorless, stable ampul solution containing per ml:
dihydroergotamine
   mesylate, USP .... 1 mg
methanesulfonic acid/sodium
   hydroxide .... qs to pH 3.6±0.4
alcohol, USP .... 6.1% by vol.
glycerin, USP .... 15% by wt.
water for injection, USP, qs to .... 1 ml

ACTIONS

Dihydroergotamine is an alpha adrenergic blocking agent with a direct stimulating effect on the smooth muscle of peripheral and cranial blood vessels, and produces depression of central vasomotor centers. The compound also has the properties of serotonin antagonism. In comparison to ergotamine, the adrenergic blocking actions are more pronounced, the vasoconstrictive actions somewhat less pronounced, and there is reduced incidence and degree of nausea and vomiting.
Onset of action occurs in 15 to 30 minutes following intramuscular administration and persists for 3-4 hours.
Repeated dosage at 1 hour intervals up to 3 hours may be required to obtain maximal effect.

INDICATIONS

As therapy to abort or prevent vascular headache, e.g., migraine, migraine variants, or so-called "histaminic cephalalgia" when rapid control is desired or when other routes of administration are not feasible.

CONTRAINDICATIONS

Peripheral vascular disease, coronary heart disease, hypertension, impaired hepatic or renal function, sepsis and pregnancy. Hypersensitivity.

ADVERSE REACTIONS

Numbness and tingling of fingers and toes, muscle pains in the extremities, weakness in the legs, precordial distress and pain, transient tachycardia or bradycardia, nausea, vomiting, localized edema and itching.

DOSAGE AND ADMINISTRATION

For vascular headache, 1 ml intramuscularly at first warning sign of headache, repeated at 1 hour intervals to a total of 3 ml. Optimal results are obtained by titrating the dose for several headaches to find the minimal effective dose for each patient and this dose should then be employed at onset of subsequent attacks. Where more rapid effect is desired, the intravenous route may be employed to a maximum of 2 ml. Total weekly dosage should not exceed 6 ml.

OVERDOSAGE

Failure to observe the upper limits of repeated parenteral dosage may result in eventual onset of the peripheral toxic signs and symptoms of ergotism. Treatment includes discontinuance of the drug, warmth, vasodilators, and good nursing care to prevent tissue damage.

HOW SUPPLIED

As a clear, colorless and stable solution in ampuls containing:
dihydroergotamine
   mesylate, USP .... 1 mg
methanesulfonic acid/sodium
   hydroxide .... qs to pH 3.6±0.4
alcohol, USP .... 6.1% by vol.
glycerin, USP .... 15% by wt.
water for injection, USP, qs to .... 1 ml
Ampuls, 1 ml size—boxes of 20.
To assure constant potency, protect the ampuls from light and heat. In the event the ampul solution becomes discolored, it should not be used.
[D.H.E.-Z19 Issued February 15, 1988]

DIAPID® Nasal Spray   ℞

[dī'a-pid "]

(lypressin nasal solution, USP)

The following prescribing information is based on official labeling in effect on August 1, 1989.

DESCRIPTION

Diapid® (lypressin nasal solution, USP) Nasal Spray contains synthetic lysine-8-vasopressin with an activity of 50 USP Posterior Pituitary (Pressor) Units per ml (0.185 mg/ml).
The molecular formula of lysine-8-vasopressin is $C_{46}H_{65}N_{13}O_{12}S_2$; its structural formula may be represented as follows:

Phe		Gln
Tyr		Asn
Cys		Cys
		Pro
		Lys
		GlyNH$_2$

It is an antidiuretic with vasoconstrictor activity.
Diapid (lypressin nasal solution, USP) Nasal Spray is provided for intra-nasal administration as a solution containing per 1 ml, 50 USP Posterior Pituitary (Pressor) Units of synthetic lysine-8-vasopressin and the following inactive ingredients: acetic acid, NF, chlorobutanol, NF, (max. 0.1%), citric acid, USP, disodium phosphate, USP, glycerin, USP, methylparaben, NF, propylparaben, NF, purified water, USP, sodium acetate, USP, sodium chloride, USP, sorbitol solution, USP.

CLINICAL PHARMACOLOGY

Lysine-8-vasopressin is a polypeptide and is one of the two known naturally occurring molecular forms of mammalian posterior pituitary antidiuretic hormone. It is identical to the vasopressin produced naturally in swine pituitaries. This synthetic vasopressin differs from that produced in humans in that it contains lysine instead of arginine in its structure. It is present as a protein-free substance in Diapid® (lypressin nasal solution, USP) Nasal Spray. Unlike preparations of posterior pituitary antidiuretic hormone of animal origin, Diapid (lypressin nasal solution, USP) Nasal Spray is completely free of oxytocin and foreign proteins.
The principal pharmacologic action of lysine-8-vasopressin, the active ingredient of Diapid (lypressin nasal solution, USP) Nasal Spray, is similar to that of arginine-8-vasopressin, the posterior pituitary antidiuretic hormone occurring in man. Diapid (lypressin nasal solutin, USP) Nasal Spray increases the rate of reabsorption of solute free water from the distal renal tubules, without significantly modifying the rate of glomerular filtration, producing a fall in free water clearance and an increase in urinary osmolality. The rates of solute and creatinine excretion noted with therapeutic doses of Diapid® (lypressin nasal solution, USP) Nasal Spray suggest that sodium clearance and glomerular filtration rates are essentially unaltered by this hormone. Diapid (lypressin nasal solution, USP) Nasal Spray is relatively free of oxytocin activity when used within the recommended therapeutic dose levels.
It possesses little pressor activity, the ratio of pressor to antidiuretic activity being in the range of 1:1000.
The antidiuretic effect produced by Diapid (lypressin nasal solution, USP) Nasal Spray begins rapidly and usually reaches a peak within 30 to 120 minutes. Its usual duration of action is 3 to 8 hours.

INDICATIONS

Diapid (lypressin nasal solution, USP) Nasal Spray is indicated for the control or prevention of the symptoms and complications of diabetes insipidus due to deficiency of endogenous posterior pituitary antidiuretic hormone in both children and adults. These symptoms and complications include polydipsia, polyuria, and dehydration. It is particularly useful in patients with diabetes insipidus who have become unresponsive to other forms of therapy or who experience various types of local and/or systemic reactions, allergic reactions, or other undesirable effects (e.g., excessive fluid retention) from preparations of posterior pituitary antidiuretic hormone of animal origin.

CONTRAINDICATIONS

Hypersensitivity. (See Precautions)

WARNINGS

Cardiovascular pressor effects with Diapid® (lypressin nasal solution, USP) Nasal Spray are minimal or absent when it is administered as a nasal spray in therapeutic doses. Nevertheless, it should be used with caution in patients for whom such effects would not be desirable because mild blood pressure elevation has been noted in unanesthetized subjects who received lypressin intravenously. Large doses intranasally may cause coronary artery constriction and caution should be observed in treating patients with coronary artery disease. There have been reports of acute myocardial infarction in patients taking Diapid (lypressin nasal solution, USP) Nasal Spray.[1]

[1] Adverse reaction file, Sandoz Pharmaceuticals

PRECAUTIONS

General
The effectiveness of Diapid (lypressin nasal solution, USP) Nasal Spray may be lessened in patients with nasal congestion, allergic rhinitis, and upper respiratory infections because these conditions may interfere with absorption of the drug by the nasal mucosa. In this event, larger doses of Diapid® (lypressin nasal solution, USP) Nasal Spray, or adjunctive therapy, may be needed.
Patients with a known sensitivity to antidiuretic hormone should be tested for sensitivity to Diapid (lypressin nasal solution, USP) Nasal Spray. (See Contraindications)
Information For Patients
Diapid (lypressin nasal solution, USP) Nasal Spray is indicated for the treatment of diabetes insipidus, a disorder in which the lack of a specific hormone, vasopressin, prevents the kidneys from conserving water. As a result, excess urine is produced which can lead to dehydration. The symptoms of this disorder are mainly excessive urination and thirst. Diapid (lypressin nasal solution, USP) Nasal Spray provides the body with a synthetic form of vasopressin and thus prevents these symptoms.
Patients should be instructed on how to regulate their daily dosage according to their degree of excessive urination and thirst. Once established, daily requirements should remain stable for a long period of time. In case of nasal congestion due to allergic conditions or upper respiratory tract infections which interferes with the absorption of the drug by the nasal mucosa, patients may require larger doses of Diapid (lypressin nasal solution, USP) Nasal Spray or an alternate form of therapy. Patients should be advised to consult their physician if this circumstance arises.
To assure a uniform delivery of spray with Diapid® (lypressin nasal solution, USP) Nasal Spray, the bottle should be held upright and the patient should be sitting or standing with the head upright.
Diapid (lypressin nasal solution, USP) Nasal Spray is indicated for use in the treatment of diabetes insipidus *only*. It should not be used in the therapy of other disorders or conditions.
Carcinogenesis, Mutagenesis, Impairment of Fertility
No long-term studies in animals have been performed to evaluate carcinogenic potential. Reproductive studies have not been conducted in animals or humans to test whether lypressin constitutes a potential problem in relation to mutagenesis or impairment of fertility in either females or males. However, as a posterior pituitary antidiuretic hormone it is unlikely to evoke detrimental reproductive effects. Commercially available since September, 1970, lypressin has not been reported to have been related to any instance of fetal abnormality, infertility or impotence.
Pregnancy Category C
Animal reproduction studies have not been conducted with Diapid (lypressin nasal solution, USP) Nasal Spray. It is not known whether Diapid (lypressin nasal solution, USP) Nasal Spray can cause fetal harm when administered to a pregnant woman or can affect reproduction capacity. Diapid® (lypressin nasal solution, USP) Nasal Spray should be given to a pregnant woman only if clearly needed.
Nursing Mothers
It is not known whether this drug is excreted in human milk. Because many drugs are excreted in human milk, a decision should be made whether to discontinue nursing or to discontinue the drug, taking into account the importance of the drug to the mother.
Pediatric Use
The usual dosage in children is the same as for adults (See Dosage and Administration). Safety and efficacy have not been demonstrated in children less than six weeks of age.

ADVERSE REACTIONS

Cardiovascular pressor effects with Diapid® (lypressin nasal solution, USP) Nasal Spray are minimal when it is administered as a nasal spray in therapeutic doses. (See Warnings)
With clinical use of Diapid (lypressin nasal solution, USP) Nasal Spray adverse reactions, in general, have been infrequent and mild. Such reactions have included rhinorrhea, nasal congestion, irritation and pruritus of the nasal passages, nasal ulceration, headache, conjunctivitis, heartburn secondary to excessive nasal administration with drippage into the pharynx, abdominal and muscle cramps and increased bowel movements. Periorbital edema, with itching, has been reported. Inadvertent inhalation of Diapid (lypres-

Continued on next page

Sandoz Pharm.—Cont.

sin nasal solution, USP) Nasal Spray has resulted in substernal tightness, coughing, and transient dyspnea. Tolerance or tachyphylaxis to Diapid (lypressin nasal solution, USP) Nasal Spray has not been reported to date.

Hypersensitivity manifested by positive skin test has been reported.

DRUG ABUSE AND DEPENDENCE
There have been no reports of drug abuse or dependence with Diapid® (lypressin nasal solution, USP) Nasal Spray.

OVERDOSAGE
The lethal dose of Diapid (lypressin nasal solution, USP) Nasal Spray has not been established. The I.V. LD$_{50}$ of Diapid (lypressin nasal solution, USP) in rats is 7266 mg/kg. The oral or intraperitoneal administration of Diapid (lypressin nasal solution, USP) Nasal Spray to rats in doses up to 20ml (1000 I.U.)/100 gm resulted in no deaths.

Diapid (lypressin nasal solution, USP) Nasal Spray is a polypeptide and is therefore subject to inactivation by the proteolytic enzymes of the alimentary tract. Hence, Diapid (lypressin nasal solution, USP) Nasal Spray is NOT ABSORBED from the gastrointestinal tract, and, for this reason, ingestion of this drug is not likely to have toxic effects. The only reasonable route of significant acute overdosage with Diapid (lypressin nasal solution, USP) Nasal Spray is by excessive use of the nasal spray.

Inadvertent or intentional excessive use of Diapid (lypressin nasal solution, USP) Nasal Spray may result in significant water retention, and if the overdosage is high enough and associated with a very high fluid intake, the possibility of water intoxication does arise. The symptoms of water intoxication include headache, anorexia, nausea, vomiting, abdominal pain, lethargy, drowsiness, unconsciousness and grand mal-type seizures. The dilution factor associated with marked water retention lowers the electrolyte concentration in the blood.

A patient being treated with Diapid® (lypressin nasal solution, USP) Nasal Spray for diabetes insipidus misunderstood the therapeutic recommendations and used the spray vigorously according to thirst. As a result, marked water retention with related hyponatremia developed. These conditions were relieved by decreasing the frequency of use of the nasal spray.

The treatment of Diapid (lypressin nasal solution, USP) Nasal Spray overdose should include the following:

1) Discontinue the drug and restrict fluid intake. As the duration of action of Diapid (lypressin nasal solution, USP) Nasal Spray is from 3 to 8 hours, these measures alone usually suffice for simple water retention.
2) Correction of electrolyte imbalance as indicated in water intoxication with the I.V. administration of 200–300 ml of 5% saline solution over several hours sufficient to raise the serum sodium to a level at which the symptoms will improve.
3) When there is the possibility of congestive heart failure due to the fluid overload, the simultaneous administration of furosemide with the hypertonic saline usually causes a diuresis sufficient to reduce cardiac overload. Potassium and other electrolyte levels must be monitored with the use of furosemide.
4) If I.V. fluid administration is considered necessary when the serum sodium has been raised to normal, the slow infusion of isotonic saline is advised to maintain normal serum sodium levels.

DOSAGE AND ADMINISTRATION
Patients should be instructed to administer 1 or 2 sprays of Diapid® (lypressin nasal solution, USP) Nasal Spray to one or both nostrils whenever frequency of urination becomes increased or significant thirst develops. (One spray provides approximately 2 USP Posterior Pituitary [Pressor] Units.) The usual dosage for adults and children 6 weeks and older is 1 or 2 sprays in each nostril 4 times daily. An additional dose at bedtime is often helpful to eliminate nocturia, if it is not controlled with the regular daily dosage. For patients requiring more than 2 sprays per nostril every 4 to 6 hours, it is recommended that the time interval between doses be reduced rather than increasing the number of sprays at each dose. (More than 2 or 3 sprays in each nostril usually results in wastage because the unabsorbed excess will drain posteriorly, by way of the nasopharynx, into the digestive tract where it will be inactivated.)

Diapid (lypressin nasal solution, USP) Nasal Spray permits individualization of dosage necessary to control the symptoms of diabetes insipidus. Patients quickly learn to regulate their dosage in accordance with their degree of polyuria and thirst, and once determined, daily requirements remain fairly stable for months or years. Although most patients require 1 or 2 sprays of Diapid (lypressin nasal solution, USP) Nasal Spray in each nostril 4 times daily, dosage has ranged from 1 spray per day at bedtime to 10 sprays in each nostril every 3-4 hours. Requirements of the larger doses may represent greater severity of disease or other phenom-

ena, such as poor nasal absorption. A seeming requirement for large doses of lypressin may be due to the presence of mixed hypothalamic-hypophyseal and nephrogenic diabetes insipidus, the latter condition being unresponsive to administration of antidiuretic hormone.

Diapid (lypressin nasal solution, USP) Nasal Spray is conveniently administered, from a compact and portable, plastic squeeze bottle, by inserting the nozzle of the bottle into the nostril and squeezing once firmly to deliver each short spray. *NOTE: To assure that a uniform, well-diffused spray is delivered, the bottle of Diapid (lypressin nasal solution, USP) Nasal Spray should be held upright and the patient should be in a vertical position with head upright.*

SUPPLIED
Diapid (lypressin nasal solution, USP) Nasal Spray is supplied in a plastic bottle that contains 8 ml of solution. Each ml of solution contains lypressin (0.185 mg) equivalent to 50 USP Posterior Pituitary (Pressor) Units. Store and dispense below 72°F.

[DIA-Z15 Issued June 1, 1988]

FIOGESIC® Tablets
[fē-ō-je zik]

The following prescribing information is based on official labeling in effect on August 1, 1989.

COMPOSITION
Each tablet contains pseudoephedrine HCl, USP, 30 mg and aspirin, USP, 325 mg. Other ingredients: calcium stearate, lactose, microcrystalline cellulose, pregelatinized starch, sodium starch glycolate, starch, color additives including FD&C Yellow No. 6 (Sunset Yellow) and FD&C Yellow No. 10.

INDICATIONS
For the temporary relief of nasal congestion due to the common cold, hay fever or associated with sinusitis. For the temporary relief of occasional minor aches, pains and headache.

CONTRAINDICATIONS
Sensitivity to any of the ingredients.

WARNINGS
Children and teenagers should not use this medicine for chicken pox or flu symptoms before a doctor is consulted about Reye syndrome, a rare but serious illness reported to be associated with aspirin. Unless directed by a doctor: 1) do not take this product if you are allergic to aspirin or if you have asthma; 2) do not take this product if you have heart disease, high blood pressure, thyroid disease, diabetes, or difficulty in urination due to enlargement of the prostate gland, and 3) do not take this product during the last three months of pregnancy. Do not exceed recommended dosage because at higher doses nervousness, dizziness, or sleeplessness may occur. Do not take this product for more than 7 days. If symptoms do not improve, are accompanied by fever, or new symptoms occur, consult a doctor. Stop taking this product if ringing in the ears or other symptoms occur. Drink a full glass of water with each dose. Caution: Do not take this product if you are presently taking a prescription drug for anticoagulation (thinning the blood), diabetes, gout or arthritis or if you have stomach distress, ulcers or bleeding problems except under the advice and supervision of a physician. Drug Interaction Precaution: Do not take this product if you are presently taking a prescription drug for high blood pressure or depression, without first consulting your doctor. As with any drug, if you are pregnant or nursing a baby, seek the advice of a health professional before using this product.

SIDE EFFECTS
Drowsiness, blurred vision, cardiac palpitations, flushing, dizziness, nervousness, or gastrointestinal upsets may occur occasionally.

DOSAGE
Adult and children 12 years and older; 2 tablets every 4 hours while symptoms persist or as directed by a physician. Do not take more than 4 doses in 24 hours.

SUPPLIED
FIOGESIC Oblong Inlay Tablets (white with yellow inlay) in bottles of 100.

Company's Product Identification Mark(s)
Tablets embossed FIOGESIC on one side, SANDOZ other side.

FIORICET®   ℞
[fē "or 'i-set]
TABLETS

The following prescribing information is based on offical labeling in effect on August 1, 1989.

DESCRIPTION
Each Fioricet® tablet for oral administration contains:
Butalbital*, USP .... 50 mg
  *WARNING: May be habit forming

Acetaminophen, USP .... 325 mg
Caffeine, USP .... 40 mg
Active Ingredients: butalbital, USP, acetaminophen, USP and caffeine, USP.
Inactive Ingredients: crospovidone, FD&C Blue #1, magnesium stearate, microcrystalline cellulose, povidone, pregelatinized starch and stearic acid.

Butalbital, 5-allyl-5-isobutylbarbituric acid, a white, odorless crystalline powder having a slightly bitter taste, is a short to intermediate-acting barbiturate. Its structure is as follows:

$C_{11}H_{16}N_2O_3$ M.W. 224.26

Acetaminophen, 4'-hydroxyacetanilide, is a non-opiate, non-salicylate analgesic, and antipyretic which occurs as a white, odorless crystalline powder possessing a slightly bitter taste. Its structure is as follows:

$C_8H_9NO_2$ M.W. 151.16

Caffeine, 1,3,7-trimethylxanthine, is a central nervous system stimulant which occurs as a white powder or white glistening needles. It also has a bitter taste. Its structure is as follows:

$C_8H_{10}N_4O_2$ M.W. 194.19

CLINICAL PHARMACOLOGY
Pharmacologically, Fioricet® combines the analgesic properties of acetaminophen-caffeine with the anxiolytic and muscle relaxant properties of butalbital.

INDICATIONS AND USAGE
Fioricet® is indicated for the relief of the symptom complex of tension (or muscle contraction) headache.

CONTRAINDICATIONS
Hypersensitivity to acetaminophen, caffeine or barbiturates. Patients with porphyria.

PRECAUTIONS
General: Barbiturates should be administered with caution, if at all, to patients who are mentally depressed, have suicidal tendencies, or a history of drug abuse.

Elderly or debilitated patients may react to barbiturates with marked excitement, depression, and confusion. In some persons, barbiturates repeatedly produce excitement rather than depression.

Information for Patients: Practitioners should give the following information and instructions to patients receiving barbiturates.

1. The use of barbiturates carries with it an associated risk of psychological and/or physical dependence. The patient should be warned against increasing the dose of the drug without consulting a physician.
2. Barbiturates may impair mental and/or physical abilities required for the performance of potentially hazardous tasks (e.g., driving, operating machinery, etc.).
3. Alcohol should not be consumed while taking barbiturates. Concurrent use of the barbiturates with other CNS depressants (e.g., alcohol, narcotics, tranquilizers, and antihistamines) may result in additional CNS depressant effects.

Drug Interactions: Patients receiving narcotic analgesics, antipsychotics, antianxiety agents, or other CNS depressants (including alcohol) concomitantly with Fioricet® may exhibit additive CNS depressant effects.

DRUGS	EFFECT
Butalbital w/coumarin anticoagulants	Decreased effect of anticoagulant because of increased metabolism resulting from enzyme induction.
Butalbital w/tricycle antidepressants	Decreased blood levels of the depressant.

Usage in Pregnancy: Adequate studies have not been performed in animals to determine whether this drug affects fertility in males or females, has teratogenic potential or has other adverse effects on the fetus. There are no well-controlled studies in pregnant women. Although there is no clearly defined risk, one cannot exclude the possibility of infrequent or subtle damage to the human fetus. Fioricet® should be used in pregnant women only when clearly needed.

Nursing Mothers: The effects of Fioricet® on infants of nursing mothers are not known. Barbiturates are excreted in the breast milk of nursing mothers. The serum levels in infants are believed to be insignificant with therapeutic doses.

Pediatric Use: Safety and effectiveness in children below the age of 12 have not been established.

ADVERSE REACTIONS

The most frequent adverse reactions are drowsiness and dizziness. Less frequent adverse reactions are light-headedness and gastrointestinal disturbances including nausea, vomiting, and flatulence. Mental confusion or depression can occur due to intolerance or overdosage of butalbital.

DRUG ABUSE AND DEPENDENCE

Prolonged use of barbiturates can produce drug dependence, characterized by psychic dependence and tolerance. The abuse liability of Fioricet® is similar to that of other barbiturate-containing drug combinations. Caution should be exercised when prescribing medication for patients with a known propensity for taking excessive quantities of drugs, which is not uncommon in patients with chronic tension headache.

OVERDOSAGE

The toxic effects of acute overdosage of Fioricet® are attributable mainly to its barbiturate component, and, to a lesser extent, acetaminophen. Because toxic effects of caffeine occur in very high dosages only, the possibility of significant caffeine toxicity from Fioricet® overdosage is unlikely.

Barbiturate

Signs and Symptoms: Drowsiness, confusion, coma; respiratory depression; hypotension; shock.

Treatment:

1. Maintenance of an adequate airway, with assisted respiration and oxygen administration as necessary.
2. Monitoring of vital signs and fluid balance.
3. If the patient is conscious and has not lost the gag reflex, emesis may be induced with ipecac. Care should be taken to prevent pulmonary aspiration of vomitus. After completion of vomiting, 30 grams activated charcoal in a glass of water may be administered.
4. If emesis is contraindicated, gastric lavage may be performed with a cuffed endotracheal tube in place with the patient in the face-down position. Activated charcoal may be left in the emptied stomach and a saline cathartic administered.
5. Fluid therapy and other standard treatment for shock, if needed.
6. If renal function is normal, forced diuresis may aid in the elimination of the barbiturate. Alkalinization of the urine increases renal excretion of some barbiturates, especially phenobarbital.
7. Although not recommended as a routine procedure, hemodialysis may be used in severe barbiturate intoxication or if the patient is anuric or in shock.

Acetaminophen

Signs and Symptoms: In acute acetaminophen overdosage, dose-dependent, potentially fatal hepatic necrosis is the most serious adverse effect. Renal tubular necrosis, hypoglycemic coma, and thrombocytopenia may also occur.

In adults, hepatic toxicity has rarely been reported with acute overdoses of less than 10 grams and fatalities with less than 15 grams. Importantly, young children seem to be more resistant than adults to the hepatotoxic effect of an acetaminophen overdose.

Early symptoms following a potentially hepatotoxic overdose may include: nausea, vomiting, diaphoresis and general malaise. Clinical and laboratory evidence of hepatic toxicity may not be apparent until 48 to 72 hours post-ingestion.

Treatment: The stomach should be emptied promptly by lavage or by induction of emesis with syrup of ipecac. Patients' estimates of the quantity of a drug ingested are notoriously unreliable. Therefore, if an acetaminophen overdose is suspected, a serum acetaminophen assay should be obtained as early as possible, but no sooner than four hours following ingestion. Liver function studies should be obtained initially and repeated at 24-hour intervals.

The antidote, N-acetylcysteine, should be administered as early as possible, preferably within 16 hours of the overdose ingestion for optimal results, but in any case, within 24 hours. Following recovery, there are no residual, structural or functional hepatic abnormalities.

DOSAGE AND ADMINISTRATION

One or 2 tablets every 4 hours as needed. Do not exceed 6 tablets per day.

HOW SUPPLIED

Fioricet® (butalbital 50 mg, acetaminophen 325 mg and caffeine 40 mg) is available as a light-blue, round compressed tablet, embossed "FIORICET" and triangle "S" on one side, three-head profile on other side. Bottles of 100 (NDC 0078-0084-05) and 500 (NDC 0078-0084-08). SandoPak® (unit-dose) packages of 100, 10 blisters strips of 10 tablets (NDC 0078-0084-06).

Store and dispense: Store below 86°F; dispense in a tight container.

[FCT-Z10 Issued August 1, 1989]

Shown in Product Identification Section, page 427

FIORINAL®   ⓒ
[fē-ōr'i-nol]
Tablets and Capsules

The following prescribing information is based on official labeling in effect on August 1, 1989.

DESCRIPTION

Each Fiorinal® Tablet or Capsule for oral administration contains: butalbital, USP, 50 mg (Warning: May be habit forming); aspirin, USP, 325 mg; caffeine, USP, 40 mg. Butalbital, 5-allyl-5-isobutyl-barbituric acid, a white odorless crystalline powder; is a short- to intermediate-acting barbiturate.

$$CH_2=CHCH_2 \quad (CH_3)_2CHCH_2$$

Tablets

Active Ingredients: aspirin, USP, butalbital, USP, and caffeine, USP.

Inactive Ingredients: alginic acid, lactose, microcrystalline cellulose, povidone, stearic acid, and another ingredient.

Capsules

Active Ingredients: aspirin, USP, butalbital, USP, and caffeine, USP.

Inactive Ingredients: D&C Yellow #10, gelatin, microcrystalline cellulose, sodium lauryl sulfate, starch, and talc.

May Also Include: benzyl alcohol, butylparaben, color additives including FD&C Blue #1, FD&C Green #3, FD&C Yellow #6, edetate calcium disodium, methylparaben, propylparaben, silicon dioxide, and sodium propionate.

ACTIONS

Pharmacologically, Fiorinal® combines the analgesic properties of aspirin with the anxiolytic and muscle relaxant properties of butalbital.

The clinical effectiveness of Fiorinal® in tension headache has been established in double-blind, placebo-controlled, multi-clinic trials. A factorial design study compared Fiorinal® with each of its major components. This study demonstrated that each component contributes to the efficacy of Fiorinal® in the treatment of the target symptoms of tension headache (headache pain, psychic tension, and muscle contraction in the head, neck and shoulder region). For each symptom and the symptom complex as a whole, Fiorinal® was shown to have significantly superior clinical effects to either component alone.

INDICATIONS

Fiorinal® is indicated for the relief of the symptom complex of tension (or muscle contraction) headache.

CONTRAINDICATIONS

Hypersensitivity to aspirin, caffeine, or barbiturates. Patients with porphyria.

WARNINGS

Drug Dependency: Prolonged use of barbiturates can produce drug dependence, characterized by psychic dependence, and less frequently, physical dependence and tolerance. The abuse liability of Fiorinal® is similar to that of other barbiturate-containing drug combinations. Caution should be exercised when prescribing medication for patients with a known propensity for taking excessive quantities of drugs, which is not uncommon in patients with chronic tension headache.

Use in Ambulatory Patients: Fiorinal® may impair the mental and/or physical abilities required for the performance of potentially hazardous tasks, such as driving a car or operating machinery. The patient should be cautioned accordingly. Central Nervous System depressant effects of butalbital may be additive with those of other CNS depressants. Concurrent use with other sedative-hypnotics or alcohol should be avoided. When such combined therapy is necessary, the dose of one or more agents may need to be reduced.

Use in Pregnancy: Adequate studies have not been performed in animals to determine whether this drug affects fertility in males or females, has teratogenic potential, or has other adverse effects on the fetus. While there are no well-controlled studies in pregnant women, over twenty years of marketing and clinical experience does not include any positive evidence of adverse effects on the fetus. Although there is no clearly defined risk, such experience cannot exclude the possibility of infrequent or subtle damage to the human fetus. Fiorinal® should be used in pregnant women only when clearly needed.

Nursing Mothers: The effects of Fiorinal® on infants of nursing mothers are not known. Salicylates and barbiturates are excreted in the breast milk of nursing mothers. The serum levels in infants are believed to be insignificant with therapeutic doses.

PRECAUTIONS

Salicylates should be used with extreme caution in the presence of peptic ulcer or coagulation abnormalities.

Pediatric Use: Safety and effectiveness in children below the age of 12 have not been established.

ADVERSE REACTIONS

The most frequent adverse reactions are drowsiness and dizziness. Less frequent adverse reactions are lightheadedness and gastrointestinal disturbances including nausea, vomiting, and flatulence. A single incidence of bone marrow suppression has been reported with the use of Fiorinal®. Several cases of dermatological reactions including toxic epidermal necrolysis and erythema multiforme have been reported.

OVERDOSAGE

The toxic effects of acute overdosage of Fiorinal® are attributable mainly to its barbiturate component, and, to a lesser extent, aspirin. Because toxic effects of caffeine occur in very high dosages only, the possibility of significant caffeine toxicity from Fiorinal® overdosage is unlikely. Symptoms attributable to *acute barbiturate poisoning* include drowsiness, confusion, and coma; respiratory depression; hypotension; shock. Symptoms attributable to *acute aspirin poisoning* include hyperpnea; acid-base disturbances with development of metabolic acidosis; vomiting and abdominal pain; tinnitus; hyperthermia; hypoprothrombinemia; restlessness; delirium; convulsions. *Acute caffeine poisoning* may cause insomnia, restlessness, tremor, and delirium; tachycardia and extrasystoles. *Treatment* consists primarily of management of barbiturate intoxication and the correction of the acid-base imbalance due to salicylism. Vomiting should be induced mechanically or with emetics in the conscious patient. Gastric lavage may be used if the pharyngeal and laryngeal reflexes are present and if less than 4 hours have elapsed since ingestion. A cuffed endotracheal tube should be inserted before gastric lavage of the unconscious patient and when necessary to provide assisted respiration. Diuresis, alkalinization of the urine, and correction of electrolyte disturbances should be accomplished through administration of intravenous fluids such as 1% sodium bicarbonate in 5% dextrose in water. Meticulous attention should be given to maintaining adequate pulmonary ventilation. Correction of hypotension may require the administration of levarterenol bitartrate or phenylephrine hydrochloride by intravenous infusion. In severe cases of intoxication, peritoneal dialysis, hemodialysis, or exchange transfusion may be lifesaving. Hypoprothrombinemia should be treated with Vitamin K, intravenously.

DOSAGE AND ADMINISTRATION

One or 2 tablets or capsules every 4 hours. Total daily dose should not exceed 6 tablets or capsules.

HOW SUPPLIED

Fiorinal® Capsules: Color is bright Kelly green and lime green, in packages of 100 (NDC 0078-0103-05) and 500 (NDC 0078-0103-08). Also available in ControlPak® package, 25 capsules (continuous reverse numbered roll of sealed blisters) (NDC 0078-0103-13). Fiorinal® Tablets: White, compressed tablet in packages of 100 (NDC 0078-0104-05) and 1000 (NDC 0078-0104-09).

Company's Product Identification Mark(s): Tablets embossed "FIORINAL" on one side, "SANDOZ" on other side, and Capsules imprinted "FIORINAL 78–103" on each half of capsule.

[FIO-ZZ29 Issued July 1, 1989]

Shown in Product Identification Section, page 427

FIORINAL® with CODEINE   ⓒ
[fē-ōr'i-nol]
Capsules

The following prescribing information is based on official labeling in effect on August 1, 1989.

DESCRIPTION

Contents per Fiorinal® with Codeine No. 3 Capsule:

codeine phosphate, USP .... 30 mg (½ gr)
    Warning: May be habit forming.
butalbital, USP .... 50 mg
    Warning: May be habit forming.
caffeine, USP .... 40 mg
aspirin, USP .... 325 mg

Butalbital, 5-allyl-5-isobutyl-barbituric acid, a white odorless crystalline powder, is a short to intermediate-acting barbiturate. Its molecular weight is 224.26 and its empirical formula is $C_{11}H_{16}N_2O_3$. The structural formula is as follows: [See Chemical Formula at top of next page].

Continued on next page

Sandoz Pharm.—Cont.

Inactive Ingredients: D&C Yellow #10, FD&C Blue #1, FD&C Red #3, FD&C Yellow #6, gelatin, microcrystalline cellulose, sodium lauryl sulfate, starch, talc, titanium dioxide.

May Also Include: benzyl alcohol, butylparaben, edetate calcium disodium, glycerin, methylparaben, propylparaben, silicon dioxide, sodium propionate.

CLINICAL PHARMACOLOGY

Fiorinal® with Codeine combines the analgesic properties of aspirin and codeine with the anxiolytic and muscle relaxant properties of butalbital.

Pharmacokinetics

Aspirin

The systemic availability of aspirin after an oral dose is highly dependent on the dosage form, the presence of food, the gastric emptying time, gastric pH, antacids, buffering agents and particle size. These factors affect not necessarily the extent of absorption of total salicylates but more the stability of aspirin prior to absorption.

During the absorption process and after absorption, aspirin is mainly hydrolyzed to salicylic acid and distributed to all body tissues and fluids, including fetal tissues, breast milk and the central nervous system (CNS). Highest concentrations are found in plasma, liver, renal cortex, heart and lung. In plasma, about 50%–80% of the salicylic acid and its metabolites are loosely bound to plasma proteins.

The clearance of total salicylates is subject to saturable kinetics; however, first-order elimination kinetics are still a good approximation for doses up to 650 mg. The plasma half-life for aspirin is about 12 minutes and for salicylic acid and/or total salicylates is about 3.0 hours.

The elimination of therapeutic doses is through the kidneys either as salicylic acid or other biotransformation products. The renal clearance is greatly augmented by an alkaline urine as is produced by concurrent administration of sodium bicarbonate or potassium citrate.

The biotransformation of aspirin occurs primarily in the hepatocytes. The major metabolites are salicyluric acid (75%), the phenolic and acyl glucuronides of salicylate (15%), and gentisic and gentisuric acid (<1%).

The bioavailability of the aspirin component for Fiorinal® with Codeine capsules is equivalent to that of a solution showing only a slightly slower rate of absorption. Peak concentrations are achieved about 30 minutes after a dose. See *Overdosage Section* for toxic information.

Codeine

Codeine is readily absorbed from the gastrointestinal tract, and is rapidly distributed from blood to body tissues. During distribution it is taken up preferentially by parenchymatous organs such as liver, spleen and kidney. It passes the blood-brain barrier and is found in fetal tissue and breast milk. The drug is not bound to plasma proteins nor does it accumulate in body tissues.

The elimination of codeine is primarily through the kidney. The plasma half-life is about 2.9 hours. The urinary excretion products represent about 90% of the dose within 24 hours and consist of free and glucuronide-conjugated codeine (about 70%), free and conjugated norcodeine (about 10%), free and conjugated morphine (about 10%), normorphine (under 4%) and hydrocodone (<1%). The remainder of the dose appears in the feces.

At therapeutic doses, the analgesic effect reaches peak within 2 hours and persists for 4–6 hours. Blood concentrations causing CNS depression begin at 500–1900 ng/mL. The bioavailability of the codeine component for Fiorinal® with Codeine capsules is equivalent to that of a solution. Peak concentrations of 198 ng/mL were obtained at 1 hour after a 60 mg dose.

See *OVERDOSAGE* for toxic information.

Butalbital

Butalbital is well absorbed from the gastrointestinal tract and is expected to distribute to most of the tissues in the body. Barbiturates, in general, may appear in milk and readily cross the placental barrier. They are bound to plasma and tissue proteins to a varying degree and binding increases directly as a function of lipid solubility.

Elimination of butalbital is primarily via the kidney (59–88% of the dose) as unchanged drug or metabolites. The plasma half-life is about 35 hours. Urinary excretion products included parent drug (about 3.6% of the dose), 5-isobutyl-5-(2,3-dihydroxypropyl)barbituric acid (about 24% of the dose), 5-allyl-5(3-hydroxy-2-methyl-1-propyl)barbituric acid (about 4.8% of dose), products with the barbituric acid ring hydrolyzed with excretion of urea (about 14% of the dose) as well as unidentified materials. Of the material excreted in the urine, 32% was conjugated.

The bioavailability of the butalbital component for Fiorinal® with Codeine capsules is equivalent to that of a solution except for a decrease in the rate of absorption. A peak concentration of 2020 ng/mL is obtained at about 1.5 hours after a 100 mg dose.

See *OVERDOSAGE* for toxic information.

Caffeine

Like most xanthines, caffeine is rapidly absorbed and distributed in all body tissues and fluids, including the CNS, fetal tissues and breast milk.

Caffeine is cleared rapidly through metabolism and excretion in the urine. The plasma half-life is about 3 hours. Hepatic biotransformation prior to excretion results in about equal amounts of 1-methyl-xanthine and 1-methyluric acid. Of the 70% of the dose that has been recovered in the urine, only 3% was unchanged drug.

The bioavailability of the caffeine component for Fiorinal® with Codeine capsules is equivalent to that of a solution except for a slightly longer time to peak. A peak concentration of 1660 ng/mL was obtained in less than an hour for an 80 mg dose.

See *OVERDOSAGE* for toxic information.

INDICATIONS

Fiorinal® with Codeine raises the threshold of pain and discomfort and can be used in a great variety of painful conditions short of those which require morphine.

Fiorinal® with Codeine is indicated for all types of pain associated with medical and surgical aftercare, postpartum pain, dysmenorrhea, neuritis, pleurisy, sciatica, neuralgia, sinusitis, pharyngitis, tonsillitis, otitis, febrile diseases, dental pain following extractions, headache, bursitis, arthritis, rheumatism, low back pain, dislocations, strains, sprains, fractures, etc.

CONTRAINDICATIONS

Fiorinal® with Codeine is contraindicated under the following conditions:

1) hypersensitivity or intolerance to aspirin, caffeine, butalbital or codeine
2) peptic ulcer or other serious gastrointestinal lesions, and
3) patients with porphyria.

WARNINGS

Care should be taken when administering salicylates to persons with known allergies. Hypersensitivity to aspirin is particularly likely in patients with nasal polyps, and relatively common in those with asthma.

PRECAUTIONS

Information for Patients

Take medication with food or full glass of water or milk to minimize gastrointestinal irritation.

Fiorinal® with Codeine may impair the mental and/or physical abilities required for performance of potentially dangerous tasks such as driving a car or operating machinery. The patient should be cautioned accordingly.

Central Nervous System depressant effects of butalbital and codeine may be additive with those of other CNS depressants. Concurrent use with sedative-hypnotics or alcohol should be avoided. When such combined therapy is necessary, the dose of one or more agents may need to be reduced. Codeine and butalbital may be habit-forming when used over long periods or in high doses. Patients should take Fiorinal® with Codeine only for as long as prescribed, in the amounts prescribed, and no more frequently than prescribed.

Keep medication out of reach of children; overdose is especially dangerous in young children.

Usage in Pregnancy

Category C. Adequate studies have not been performed in animals to determine whether this drug affects fertility in males or females, has teratogenic potential, or has other adverse effects on the fetus. While there are no well-controlled studies in pregnant women, over twenty years of marketing and clinical experience does not include any positive evidence of adverse effects on the fetus. Although there is no clearly defined risk, such experience cannot exclude the possibility of infrequent or subtle damage to the human fetus. Fiorinal® with Codeine capsules should be used in pregnant women only when clearly needed.

Nursing Mothers

The effects of Fiorinal® with Codeine capsules on infants or nursing mothers are not known. Salicylates, codeine, caffeine, and barbiturates are excreted in the breast milk of nursing mothers. Caution should be exercised when Fiorinal® with Codeine is administered to a nursing woman.

Pediatric Use

Safety and effectiveness in children below the age of 12 have not been established.

ADVERSE REACTIONS

Nausea, vomiting, constipation, dizziness, weakness, drowsiness, and lethargy are the most common side effects. A single incidence of bone marrow suppression has been reported with the use of Fiorinal®. Several cases of dermatological reactions including toxic epidermal necrolysis and erthema multiforme have been reported. Overdosage is primarily manifested by drowsiness.

DRUG ABUSE AND DEPENDENCE

Fiorinal® with Codeine is controlled by the Drug Enforcement Administration and is classified under Schedule III.

Codeine

Codeine can produce drug dependence of the morphine type and, therefore, has the potential for being abused. Psychological dependence, physical dependence and tolerance may develop upon repeated administration and it should be prescribed and administered with the same degree of caution appropriate to the use of other oral narcotic medications.

Butalbital

Barbiturates may be habit forming: Tolerance, psychological dependence, and physical dependence may occur especially following prolonged use of high doses of barbiturates. The average daily dose for the barbiturate addict is usually about 1,500 mg. As tolerance to barbiturates develops, the amount needed to maintain the same level of intoxication increases; tolerance to a fatal dosage, however, does not increase more than two-fold. As this occurs, the margin between an intoxication dosage and fatal dosage becomes smaller. The lethal dose of a barbiturate is far less if alcohol is also ingested. Major withdrawal symptoms (convulsions and delirium) may occur within 16 hours and last up to 5 days after abrupt cessation of these drugs. Intensity of withdrawal symptoms gradually declines over a period of approximately 15 days.

Treatment of barbiturate dependence consists of cautious and gradual withdrawal of the drug. Barbiturate-dependent patients can be withdrawn by using a number of different withdrawal regimens. One method involves initiating treatment at the patient's regular dosage level and gradually decreasing the daily dosage as tolerated by the patient.

OVERDOSAGE

The toxic effects of acute overdosage of Fiorinal® with Codeine capsules are attributable mainly to its barbiturate component, and, to a lesser extent, codeine and aspirin. Because toxic effects of caffeine occur in very high dosages only, the possibility of significant caffeine toxicity from Fiorinal® with Codeine overdosage is unlikely.

Signs and Symptoms

Symptoms attributable to *acute barbiturate poisoning* include drowsiness, confusion, and coma; respiratory depression; hypotension; shock. Symptoms attributable to *acute aspirin poisoning* include hyperpnea; acid-base disturbances with development of metabolic acidosis; vomiting and abdominal pain; tinnitus, hyperthermia; hypoprothrombinemia; restlessness; delirium; convulsions. Symptoms of *acute codeine poisoning* include the triad of: pinpoint pupils, marked depression of respiration, and loss of consciousness. Convulsions may occur.

Treatment

Treatment consists primarily of management of barbiturate intoxication, reversal of the effects of codeine, and the correction of the acid-base imbalance due to salicylism. Vomiting should be induced mechanically or with emetics in the conscious patient. Gastric lavage may be used if the pharyngeal and laryngeal reflexes are present and if less than four hours have elapsed since ingestion. A cuffed endotracheal tube should be inserted before gastric lavage of the unconscious patient and when necessary to provide assisted respiration. Diuresis, alkalinization of the urine, and correction of electrolyte disturbances should be accomplished through administration of intravenous fluids such as 1% sodium bicarbonate in 5% dextrose in water.

Meticulous attention should be given to maintaining adequate pulmonary ventilation. The narcotic antagonist naloxone is a specific antidote for respiratory depression which may result from overdosage or unusual sensitivity to narcotics. A narcotic antagonist should not be administered in the absence of clinically significant respiratory or cardiovascular depression. NOTE: Respiratory depression caused by barbiturates will *not* respond to narcotic antagonists. Unwitting overdosage with narcotic antagonists may occur in an attempt to reverse respiratory depression caused by mixed barbiturate-codeine intoxication.

Correction of hypotension may require the administration of levarterenol bitartrate or phenylephrine hydrochloride by intravenous infusion. In severe cases of intoxication, peritoneal dialysis, hemodialysis, or exchange transfusion may be lifesaving. Hypoprothrombinemia should be treated with vitamin K, intravenously. Methemoglobinemia over 30% should be treated with methylene blue administered slowly intravenously.

Toxic and Lethal Doses

Butalbital: toxic dose 1.0 g (adult); lethal dose 2.0–5.0 g
Aspirin: toxic blood level > 30 mg/100 ml; lethal dose 10–30g (adult)

Caffeine: toxic dose > 1.0 g; lethal dose unknown
Codeine: lethal dose 0.5–1.0 g (adult)

DOSAGE AND ADMINISTRATION

One or two capsules every four hours. Total daily dose should not exceed six capsules.

HOW SUPPLIED

Fiorinal with Codeine Capsules

30 mg (½ gr) imprinted "Sandoz triangle F-C#3" on one half, "SANDOZ 78-107" other half, color is blue and yellow.

Packaging

Fiorinal with Codeine No. 3 (½ gr) in bottles of 100 capsules and in ControlPak® package, 25 capsules (continuous reverse-numbered roll of sealed blisters).

[FWC-Z25 Issued April 15, 1989]

Shown in Product Identification Section, page 427

HYDERGINE®   ℞

[hī'der-jēn]
(ergoloid mesylates) tablets, USP (ORAL)
(ergoloid mesylates) tablets, USP
  (SUBLINGUAL)
(ergoloid mesylates) liquid
HYDERGINE® LC
(ergoloid mesylates) liquid capsules

The following prescribing information is based on official labeling in effect on August 1, 1989.

DESCRIPTION AND TYPE

Hydergine tablet 1 mg, Hydergine sublingual tablet 1 mg and Hydergine LC (liquid capsule) 1 mg, each contains ergoloid mesylates USP as follows: dihydroergocornine mesylate 0.333 mg, dihydroergocristine mesylate 0.333 mg, and dihydroergocryptine (dihydro-alpha-ergocryptine and dihydro-beta-ergocryptine in the proportion of 2:1) mesylate 0.333 mg, representing a total of 1 mg.
Inactive Ingredients:
1 mg, Oral Tablets: lactose, povidone, starch, stearic acid, and talc
1 mg, Sublingual Tablets: gelatin, mannitol, starch, stearic acid, and sucrose
Liquid Capsules: ascorbic acid, gelatin, glycerin, methyl paraben, polyethylene glycol, propyl paraben, propylene glycol, sorbitol, and titanium dioxide
Hydergine sublingual tablet 0.5 mg, each contains ergoloid mesylates USP as follows: dihydroergocornine mesylate 0.167 mg, dihydroergocristine mesylate 0.167 mg, and dihydroergocryptine (dihydro-alpha-ergocryptine and dihydro-beta-ergocryptine in the proportion of 2:1) mesylate 0.167 mg, representing a total of 0.5 mg.
Inactive Ingredients: gelatin, mannitol, starch, stearic acid, and sucrose.
Hydergine liquid 1 mg/ml, each ml contains ergoloid mesylates USP as follows: dihydroergocornine mesylate 0.333 mg, dihydroergocristine mesylate 0.333 mg, and dihydroergocryptine (dihydro-alpha-ergocryptine and dihydro-beta-ergocryptine in the proportion of 2:1) mesylate 0.333 mg, representing a total of 1 mg; alcohol, USP, 30% by volume.
Inactive Ingredients: alcohol, glycerin, propylene glycol, and purified water

Pharmacokinetic Properties

Pharmacokinetic studies have been performed in normal volunteers with the help of radiolabelled drug as well as employing a specific radioimmunoassay technique. From the urinary excretion quotient of orally and intravenously administered tritium-labelled Hydergine® (ergoloid mesylates) the absorption of ergoloid was calculated to be 25%. Following oral administration, peak levels of 0.5 ng Eq/ml/mg were achieved within 1.5-3 hr. Bioavailability studies with the specific radioimmunoassay confirm that ergoloid is rapidly absorbed from the gastrointestinal tract, with mean peak levels of 0.05-0.13 ng/ml/mg (with extremes of 0.03 and 0.18 ng/ml/mg) achieved within 0.6-1.3 hr. (with extremes of 0.4 and 2.8 hrs.). The finding of lower peak levels of ergoloid compared to the total drug-metabolite composite is consistent with a considerable first pass liver metabolism, with less than 50% of the therapeutic moiety reaching the systemic circulation. The elimination of radioactivity, representing ergoloid plus metabolites bearing the radiolabel, was biphasic with half-lives of 4 and 13 hr. The mean half-life of unchanged ergoloid in plasma is about 2.6-5.1 hr; after 3 half-lives ergoloid plasma levels are less than 10% of radioactivity levels, and by 24 hr no ergoloid is detectable.
Bioequivalence studies were performed comparing Hydergine® oral tablets (administered orally) with Hydergine sublingual tablets (administered sublingually), Hydergine oral tablets with Hydergine liquid and Hydergine oral tablets with Hydergine LC (liquid capsules). The oral tablet, sublingual tablet and liquid capsule oral forms were shown to be bioequivalent. Within the bioequivalence limits, the liquid capsule showed a statistically significant (12%) greater bioavailability than the oral tablet. In the study comparing the oral tablet and liquid forms, both forms tested showed an equivalent rate of absorption and an equivalent peak plasma concentration (C_{max}).

ACTIONS

There is no specific evidence which clearly establishes the mechanism by which Hydergine® (ergoloid mesylates) preparations produce mental effects, nor is there conclusive evidence that the drug particularly affects cerebral arteriosclerosis or cerebrovascular insufficiency.

INDICATIONS

A proportion of individuals over sixty who manifest signs and symptoms of an idiopathic decline in mental capacity (i.e., cognitive and interpersonal skills, mood, self-care, apparent motivation) can experience some symptomatic relief upon treatment with Hydergine (ergoloid mesylates) preparations. The identity of the specific trait(s) or condition(s), if any, which would usefully predict a response to Hydergine (ergoloid mesylates) therapy is not known. It appears, however, that those individuals who do respond come from groups of patients who would be considered clinically to suffer from some ill-defined process related to aging or to have some underlying dementing condition (i.e., primary progressive dementia, Alzheimer's dementia, senile onset, multi-infarct dementia).
Before prescribing Hydergine (ergoloid mesylates), the physician should exclude the possibility that the patient's signs and symptoms arise from a potentially reversible and treatable condition. Particular care should be taken to exclude delirium and dementiform illness secondary to systemic disease, and dementiform illness secondary to systemic disease, primary neurological disease, or primary disturbance of mood. Hydergine (ergoloid mesylates) preparations are not indicated in the treatment of acute or chronic psychosis, regardless of etiology (see CONTRAINDICATIONS section).
The decision to use Hydergine (ergoloid mesylates) in the treatment of an individual with a symptomatic decline in mental capacity of unknown etiology should be continually reviewed since the presenting clinical picture may subsequently evolve sufficiently to allow a specific diagnosis and a specific alternative treatment. In addition, continued clinical evaluation is required to determine whether any initial benefit conferred by Hydergine (ergoloid mesylates) therapy persists with time.
The efficacy of Hydergine (ergoloid mesylates) was evaluated using a special rating scale known as the SCAG (Sandoz Clinical Assessment-Geriatric). The specific items on this scale on which modest but statistically significant changes were observed at the end of twelve weeks include: mental alertness, confusion, recent memory, orientation, emotional lability, self-care, depression, anxiety/fears, cooperation, sociability, appetite, dizziness, fatigue, bothersome(ness), and an overall impression of clinical status.

CONTRAINDICATIONS

Hydergine (ergoloid mesylates) preparations are contraindicated in individuals who have previously shown hypersensitivity to the drug. Hydergine (ergoloid mesylates) preparations are also contraindicated in patients who have psychosis, acute or chronic, regardless of etiology.

PRECAUTIONS

Practitioners are advised that because the target symptoms are of unknown etiology, careful diagnosis should be attempted before prescribing Hydergine (ergoloid mesylates) preparations.

ADVERSE REACTIONS

Hydergine (ergoloid mesylates) preparations have not been found to produce serious side effects. Some sublingual irritation with the sublingual tablets, transient nausea, and gastric disturbances have been reported. Hydergine (ergoloid mesylates) preparations do not possess the vasoconstrictor properties of the natural ergot alkaloids.

DOSAGE AND ADMINISTRATION

1 mg three times daily.
Alleviation of symptoms is usually gradual and results may not be observed for 3-4 weeks.

HOW SUPPLIED

Hydergine tablets (for oral use):
1 mg, round, white, embossed. Packages of 100 and 500.
Hydergine sublingual tablets:
1 mg, oval, white, packages of 100 and 1000.
0.5 mg, round, white, packages of 100 and 1000.
Hydergine liquid:
1 mg/ml. Bottles of 100 ml with an accompanying dropper graduated to deliver 1 mg.
Hydergine LC (liquid capsule):
1 mg, oblong, off-white, packages of 100 and 500. (Encapsulated by R. P. Scherer, N.A., Clearwater, Florida 33518)
Company's Product Identification Mark(s): Hydergine Tablets (for oral use): embossed "HYDERGINE 1" on one side, triangle (S) other side.
Hydergine Sublingual Tablets: 1 mg, embossed "HYDERGINE" on one side, "78-77" other side. 0.5 mg., embossed "HYDERGINE 0.5" on one side, triangle (S) other side.
Hydergine LC (liquid capsules): branded "HYDERGINE LC 1 mg" on one side, triangle (S) other side.

[HYD-ZZ25 Issued October 1, 1985]

Shown in Product Identification Section, page 427

KLORVESS® EFFERVESCENT   ℞
GRANULES, and
[klor'ves"]
KLORVESS® (potassium chloride)
10% LIQUID

The following prescribing information is based on official labeling in effect on August 1, 1989.

DESCRIPTION

KLORVESS® EFFERVESCENT GRANULES: Each packet (2.8 g) contains 20 mEq each of potassium and chloride supplied by potassium chloride 1.125 g, potassium bicarbonate 0.5 g, lysine hydrochloride 0.913 g in a sodium-, sugar- and carbohydrate-free effervescent formulation. Dissolution of the packet contents in water provides the potassium and chloride available for oral ingestion as potassium chloride, potassium bicarbonate, potassium citrate and lysine hydrochloride.
Active Ingredients: lysine hydrochloride USP, potassium bicarbonate USP and potassium chloride USP
Inactive Ingredients: citric acid, flavorings, polyethylene glycol and saccharin
KLORVESS® (potassium chloride) 10% LIQUID: Each tablespoonful (15 ml) contains 20 mEq of potassium chloride (provided by potassium chloride 1.5 g), in a palatable, cherry and pit flavored vehicle, alcohol 0.75%.
Active Ingredient: potassium chloride USP
Inactive Ingredients: alcohol, malic acid, natural flavor, purified water, saccharin sodium, sodium benzoate and sucrose

INDICATIONS

For the prevention and treatment of potassium depletion and hypokalemic-hypochloremic alkalosis. Deficits of body potassium and chloride can occur as a consequence of therapy with potent diuretic agents and adrenal corticosteroids.

CONTRAINDICATIONS

Severe renal impairment characterized by azotemia or oliguria, untreated Addison's disease, Familial Periodic Paralysis, acute dehydration, heat cramps, patients receiving aldosterone-inhibiting or potassium-sparing diuretic agents, or hyperkalemia from any cause.

PRECAUTIONS

In response to a rise in the concentration of body potassium, renal excretion of the ion is increased. In the presence of normal renal function and hydration, it is difficult to produce potassium intoxication by oral potassium salt supplements.
Since the extent of potassium deficiency cannot be accurately determined, it is prudent to proceed cautiously in undertaking potassium replacement. Periodic evaluations of the patient's clinical status, serum electrolytes and the EKG should be carried out when replacement therapy is undertaken. This is particularly important in patients with cardiac disease and those patients receiving digitalis.
High serum concentrations of potassium may cause death through cardiac depression, arrhythmia or cardiac arrest. To minimize gastrointestinal irritation associated with potassium chloride preparations, patients should dissolve the packet contents of KLORVESS® EFFERVESCENT GRANULES in 3 to 4 ounces of cold water, fruit juice, or other liquid, or dilute each tablespoonful of KLORVESS® (potassium chloride) 10% LIQUID in 3 to 4 ounces of cold water. Both of these solutions should be ingested slowly with or immediately after meals.

ADVERSE REACTIONS

Abdominal discomfort, diarrhea, nausea and vomiting may occur with the use of potassium salts.
The symptoms and signs of potassium intoxication include paresthesias, heaviness, muscle weakness and flaccid paralysis of the extremities. Potassium intoxication can produce listlessness, mental confusion, a fall in blood pressure, shock, cardiac arrhythmias, heart block and cardiac arrest.
The EKG picture of hyperkalemia is characterized by the early appearance of tall, peaked T waves. The R wave is decreased in amplitude and the S wave deepens; the QRS complex widens progressively. The P wave widens and decreases in amplitude until it disappears. Occasionally, an apparent elevation of the RS-T junction and a cove plane RS-T segment and T wave will be noted in AVL.

DOSAGE AND ADMINISTRATION

KLORVESS® EFFERVESCENT GRANULES: Adults—One packet (20 mEq each of potassium and chloride) completely dissolved in 3 to 4 ounces of cold water, fruit juice or other liquid 2 to 4 times daily depending upon the requirements of the patient.
KLORVESS® (potassium chloride) 10% LIQUID: Adults—One tablespoonful (15 ml) of KLORVESS LIQUID (20 mEq

Continued on next page

Sandoz Pharm.—Cont.

of potassium chloride) completely diluted in 3 to 4 ounces of cold water 2 to 4 times daily depending upon the requirements of the patient.

Both of these solutions should be ingested slowly with meals or immediately after eating. Deviations from these recommended dosages may be indicated in certain cases of hypokalemia based upon the patient's status. The average total daily dosage must be governed by the patient's response as determined by frequent evaluation of serum electrolytes, EKG and clinical status.

OVERDOSAGE

Potassium intoxication may result from overdosage of potassium or from therapeutic dosage in conditions stated under "Contraindications." Hyperkalemia, when detected, must be treated immediately because lethal levels can be reached in a few hours.

Treatment of Hyperkalemia:

1. Dextrose solution, 10 or 25% containing 10 units of crystalline insulin per 20 g dextrose, given IV in a dose of 300 to 500 ml in an hour.
2. Adsorption and exchange of potassium using sodium or ammonium cycle cation exchange resins, orally and as retention enema. (Caution: Ammonium compounds should not be used in patients with hepatic cirrhosis.)
3. Hemodialysis and peritoneal dialysis.
4. The use of potassium-containing foods or medicaments must be eliminated.

In digitalized patients too rapid a lowering of plasma potassium concentration can cause digitalis toxicity.

HOW SUPPLIED

KLORVESS® EFFERVESCENT GRANULES—packages of 30 packets (2.8 g each). KLORVESS® (potassium chloride) 10% LIQUID (dark red) – as a cherry and pit flavored liquid in pint bottles.

NOTE: Occasionally, KLORVESS® GRANULES packets may appear to be slightly swollen due to a small amount of moisture that may have been included during packaging. The quality of the product is not affected.

[KLO-Z4 Issued February 20, 1986]

KLORVESS®   ℞
[klor'ves ″]
EFFERVESCENT TABLETS

The following prescribing information is based on official labeling in effect on August 1, 1989.

DESCRIPTION

Each dry, sodium- and sugar-free effervescent tablet contains 20 mEq each of potassium and chloride supplied by potassium chloride 1.125 g, potassium bicarbonate 0.5 g, lysine hydrochloride 0.913 g. Dissolution of the tablet in water provides the potassium and chloride available for oral ingestion as potassium chloride, potassium bicarbonate, potassium citrate and lysine hydrochloride

Active Ingredients: lysine hydrochloride USP, potassium bicarbonate USP and potassium chloride USP

Inactive Ingredients: citric acid, flavorings, polyethylene glycol and saccharin

INDICATIONS

For the prevention and treatment of potassium depletion and hypokalemic-hypochloremic alkalosis. Deficits of body potassium and chloride can occur as a consequence of therapy with potent diuretic agents and adrenal corticosteroids.

CONTRAINDICATIONS

Severe renal impairment characterized by azotemia or oliguria, untreated Addison's disease, Familial Periodic Paralysis, acute dehydration, heat cramps, patients receiving aldosterone-inhibiting or potassium-sparing diuretic agents, or hyperkalemia from any cause.

PRECAUTIONS

In response to a rise in the concentration of body potassium, renal excretion of the ion is increased. In the presence of normal renal function and hydration, it is difficult to produce potassium intoxication by oral potassium salt supplements.

Since the extent of potassium deficiency cannot be accurately determined, it is prudent to proceed cautiously in undertaking potassium replacement. Periodic evaluations of the patient's clinical status, serum electrolytes and the EKG should be carried out when replacement therapy is undertaken. This is particularly important in patients with cardiac disease and those patients receiving digitalis.

High serum concentrations of potassium may cause death through cardiac depression, arrhythmia or cardiac arrest. To minimize gastrointestinal irritation associated with potassium chloride preparations, patients should dissolve each Klorvess® Effervescent Tablet in 3 or 4 ounces of cold water or fruit juice. This solution should be ingested slowly with or immediately after meals.

ADVERSE REACTIONS

Abdominal discomfort, diarrhea, nausea and vomiting may occur with the use of potassium salts.

The symptoms and signs of potassium intoxication include paresthesias, heaviness, muscle weakness and flaccid paralysis of the extremities. Potassium intoxication can produce listlessness, mental confusion, a fall in blood pressure, shock, cardiac arrhythmias, heart block and cardiac arrest.

The EKG picture of hyperkalemia is characterized by the early appearance of tall, peaked T waves. The R wave is decreased in amplitude and the S wave deepens; the QRS complex widens progressively. The P wave widens and decreases in amplitude until it disappears. Occasionally, an apparent elevation of the RS-T junction and a cove-plane RS-T segment and T wave will be noted in AVL.

DOSAGE AND ADMINISTRATION

Adults—One Klorvess® Effervescent Tablet (20 mEq each of potassium and chloride) completely dissolved in 3 to 4 ounces of cold water or fruit juice 2 to 4 times daily depending upon the requirements of the patient.

The solution should be ingested slowly with meals or immediately after eating. Deviations from these recommended dosages may be indicated in certain cases of hypokalemia based upon the patient's status. The average total daily dosage must be governed by the patient's response as determined by frequent evaluation of serum electrolytes, EKG and clinical status.

OVERDOSAGE

Potassium intoxication may result from overdosage of potassium or from therapeutic dosage in conditions stated under "Contraindications." Hyperkalemia, when detected, must be treated immediately because lethal levels can be reached in a few hours.

Treatment of Hyperkalemia:

1. Dextrose solution, 10 or 25% containing 10 units of crystalline insulin per 20 g dextrose, given IV in a dose of 300 to 500 ml in an hour.
2. Adsorption and exchange of potassium using sodium or ammonium cycle cation exchange resins, orally and as retention enema. (Caution: Ammonium compounds should not be used in patients with hepatic cirrhosis.)
3. Hemodialysis and peritoneal dialysis.
4. The use of potassium-containing foods or medicaments must be eliminated.

In digitalized patients too rapid a lowering of plasma potassium concentration can cause digitalis toxicity.

HOW SUPPLIED

Klorvess® Effervescent Tablets (white)—60 and 1000 tablets. Each tablet is individually foil wrapped.

[KLO-ZZ3 Issued February 20, 1986]

MELLARIL®   ℞
[mel'ah-ril ″]
(thioridazine) HCl tablets, USP
(thioridazine) HCl oral solution, USP
MELLARIL-S®
(thioridazine) oral suspension, USP

The following prescribing information is based on official labeling in effect on August 1, 1989.

DESCRIPTION

Mellaril® (thioridazine) is 2- methylmercapto -10- [2 - (N-methyl -2- piperidyl) ethyl] phenothiazine.

The presence of a thiomethyl radical (S-CH$_3$) in position 2, conventionally occupied by a halogen, is unique and could account for the greater toleration obtained with recommended doses of thioridazine as well as a greater specificity of psychotherapeutic action.

10 mg, 15 mg, 25 mg, 50 mg, 100 mg, 150 mg, 200 mg Tablets
Active Ingredient: thioridazine HCl, USP
10 mg Tablets
Inactive Ingredients: acacia, calcium sulfate dihydrate, carnauba wax, D&C Yellow #10, FD&C Blue #1, FD&C Yellow #6, gelatin, lactose, methylparaben, povidone, propylparaben, sodium benzoate, starch, stearic acid, sucrose, talc, titanium dioxide, and other ingredients
15 mg Tablets
Inactive Ingredients: acacia, calcium sulfate dihydrate, carnauba wax, D&C Red #7, gelatin, lactose, methylparaben, povidone, propylparaben, starch, stearic acid, sucrose, talc, titanium dioxide, and other ingredients

25 mg Tablets
Inactive Ingredients: acacia, calcium sulfate dihydrate, carnauba wax, gelatin, lactose, methylparaben, povidone, propylparaben, sodium benzoate, starch, stearic acid, sucrose, synthetic iron oxide, talc, titanium dioxide, and other ingredients
50 mg Tablets
Inactive Ingredients: acacia, calcium sulfate dihydrate, carnauba wax, gelatin, lactose, sodium benzoate, starch, stearic acid, sucrose, talc, titanium dioxide, and other ingredients
100 mg Tablets
Inactive Ingredients: acacia, calcium sulfate dihydrate, carnauba wax, D&C Yellow #10, FD&C Blue #1, FD&C Blue #2, FD&C Yellow #6, lactose, povidone, sodium benzoate, sorbitol, starch, stearic acid, sucrose, talc, titanium dioxide, and other ingredients
150 mg Tablets
Inactive Ingredients: acacia, calcium sulfate dihydrate, carnauba wax, D&C Yellow #10, FD&C Green #3, FD&C Yellow #6, lactose, methylparaben, povidone, propylparaben, sodium benzoate, starch, stearic acid, sucrose, talc, titanium dioxide, and other ingredients
200 mg Tablets
Inactive Ingredients: acacia, calcium sulfate dihydrate, carnauba wax, D&C Red #7, gelatin, lactose, magnesium stearate, methylparaben, povidone, propylparaben, starch, stearic acid, sucrose, talc, titanium dioxide, and other ingredients
30 mg, and 100 mg Concentrate
Active Ingredient: thioridazine HCl, USP
30 mg Concentrate
Inactive Ingredients: alcohol 3.0%, flavor, methylparaben, propylparaben, purified water, and sorbitol solution. May contain sodium hydroxide or hydrochloric acid to adjust the pH.
100 mg Concentrate
Inactive Ingredients: alcohol 4.2%, flavor, glycerin, methylparaben, propylparaben, purified water, sorbitol solution, and sucrose. May contain sodium hydroxide or hydrochloric acid to adjust pH.
25 mg, and 100 mg Suspension
Active Ingredient: thioridazine base
25 mg Suspension
Inactive Ingredients: carbomer 934, flavor, polysorbate 80, purified water, sodium hydroxide, and sucrose
100 mg Suspension
Inactive Ingredients: carbomer 934, D&C Yellow #10, FD&C Yellow #6, flavor, polysorbate 80, purified water, sodium hydroxide, and sucrose

CLINICAL PHARMACOLOGY

Mellaril® (thioridazine) is effective in reducing excitement, hypermotility, abnormal initiative, affective tension and agitation through its inhibitory effect on psychomotor functions. Successful modification of such symptoms is the prerequisite for, and often the beginning of, the process of recovery in patients exhibiting mental and emotional disturbances.

Thioridazine's basic pharmacological activity is similar to that of other phenothiazines, but certain specific qualities have come to light which support the observation that the clinical spectrum of this drug shows significant differences from those of the other agents of this class. Minimal antiemetic activity and minimal extrapyramidal stimulation, notably pseudoparkinsonism, are distinctive features of this drug.

INDICATIONS

For the management of manifestations of psychotic disorders.

For the short-term treatment of moderate to marked depression with variable degrees of anxiety in adult patients and for the treatment of multiple symptoms such as agitation, anxiety, depressed mood, tension, sleep disturbances, and fears in geriatric patients.

For the treatment of severe behavioral problems in children marked by combativeness and/or explosive hyperexcitable behavior (out of proportion to immediate provocations), and in the short-term treatment of hyperactive children who show excessive motor activity with accompanying conduct disorders consisting of some or all of the following symptoms: impulsivity, difficulty sustaining attention, aggressivity, mood lability, and poor frustration tolerance.

CONTRAINDICATIONS

In common with other phenothiazines, Mellaril® (thioridazine) is contraindicated in severe central nervous system depression or comatose states from any cause. It should also be noted that hypertensive or hypotensive heart disease of extreme degree is a contraindication of phenothiazine administration.

WARNINGS

Tardive Dyskinesia: Tardive dyskinesia, a syndrome consisting of potentially irreversible, involuntary, dyskinetic movements may develop in patients treated with neuroleptic (antipsychotic) drugs. Although the prevalence of the syndrome appears to be highest among the elderly, especially elderly women, it is impossible to rely upon prevalence estimates to predict, at the inception of neuroleptic treatment, which patients are likely to develop the syndrome. Whether neuroleptic drug products differ in their potential to cause tardive dyskinesia is unknown.

Both the risk of developing the syndrome and the likelihood that it will become irreversible are believed to increase as the duration of treatment and the total cumulative dose of neuroleptic drugs administered to the patient increase. However, the syndrome can develop, although much less commonly, after relatively brief treatment periods at low doses. There is no known treatment for established cases of tardive dyskinesia, although the syndrome may remit, partially or completely, if neuroleptic treatment is withdrawn. Neuroleptic treatment, itself, however, may suppress (or partially suppress) the signs and symptoms of the syndrome and thereby may possibly mask the underlying disease process. The effect that symptomatic suppression has upon the long-term course of the syndrome is unknown.

Given these considerations, neuroleptics should be prescribed in a manner that is most likely to minimize the occurrence of tardive dyskinesia. Chronic neuroleptic treatment should generally be reserved for patients who suffer from a chronic illness that, 1) is known to respond to neuroleptic drugs, and, 2) for whom alternative, equally effective, but potentially less harmful treatments are *not* available or appropriate. In patients who do require chronic treatment, the smallest dose and the shortest duration of treatment producing a satisfactory clinical response should be sought. The need for continued treatment should be reassessed periodically.

If signs and symptoms of tardive dyskinesia appear in a patient on neuroleptics, drug discontinuation should be considered. However, some patients may require treatment despite the presence of the syndrome.

(For further information about the description of tardive dyskinesia and its clinical detection, please refer to the sections on *Information for Patients* and ADVERSE REACTIONS.)

It has been suggested in regard to phenothiazines in general, that people who have demonstrated a hypersensitivity reaction (e.g. blood dyscrasias, jaundice) to one may be more prone to demonstrate a reaction to others. Attention should be paid to the fact that phenothiazines are capable of potentiating central nervous system depressants (e.g. anesthetics, opiates, alcohol, etc.) as well as atropine and phosphorus insecticides. Physicians should carefully consider benefit versus risk when treating less severe disorders.

Reproductive studies in animals and clinical experience to date have failed to show a teratogenic effect with Mellaril® (thioridazine). However, in view of the desirability of keeping the administration of all drugs to a minimum during pregnancy. Mellaril® (thioridazine) should be given only when the benefits derived from treatment exceed the possible risks to mother and fetus.

Neuroleptic Malignant Syndrome (NMS)

A potentially fatal symptom complex sometimes referred to as Neuroleptic Malignant Syndrome (NMS) has been reported in association with antipsychotic drugs. Clinical manifestations of NMS are hyperpyrexia, muscle rigidity, altered mental status and evidence of autonomic instability (irregular pulse or blood pressure, tachycardia, diaphoresis, and cardiac dysrhythmias).

The diagnostic evaluation of patients with this syndrome is complicated. In arriving at a diagnosis, it is important to identify cases where the clinical presentation includes both serious medical illness (e.g., pneumonia, systemic infection, etc.) and untreated or inadequately treated extrapyramidal signs and symptoms (EPS). Other important considerations in the differential diagnosis include central anticholinergic toxicity, heat stroke, drug fever and primary central nervous system (CNS) pathology.

The management of NMS should include 1) immediate discontinuation of antipsychotic drugs and other drugs not essential to concurrent therapy, 2) intensive symptomatic treatment and medical monitoring, and 3) treatment of any concomitant serious medical problems for which specific treatments are available. There is no general agreement about specific pharmacological treatment regimens for uncomplicated NMS.

If a patient requires antipsychotic drug treatment after recovery from NMS, the potential reintroduction of drug therapy should be carefully considered. The patient should be carefully monitored, since recurrences of NMS have been reported.

PRECAUTIONS

Leukopenia and/or agranulocytosis and convulsive seizures have been reported but are infrequent. Mellaril® (thioridazine) has been shown to be helpful in the treatment of behavioral disorders in epileptic patients, but anticonvulsant medication should also be maintained. Pigmentary retinopathy, which has been observed primarily in patients taking larger than recommended doses, is characterized by diminution of

visual acuity, brownish coloring of vision, and impairment of night vision; examination of the fundus discloses deposits of pigment. The possibility of this complication may be reduced by remaining within the recommended limits of dosage. Where patients are participating in activities requiring complete mental alertness (e.g., driving) it is advisable to administer the phenothiazines cautiously and to increase the dosage gradually. Female patients appear to have a greater tendency to orthostatic hypotension than male patients. The administration of epinephrine should be avoided in the treatment of drug-induced hypotension in view of the fact that phenothiazines may induce a reversed epinephrine effect on occasion. Should a vasoconstrictor be required, the most suitable are levarterenol and phenylephrine.

Neuroleptic drugs elevate prolactin levels; the elevation persists during chronic administration. Tissue culture experiments indicate that approximately one-third of human breast cancers are prolactin dependent in vitro, a factor of potential importance if the prescription of these drugs is contemplated in a patient with a previously detected breast cancer. Although disturbances such as galactorrhea, amenorrhea, gynecomastia, and impotence have been reported, the clinical significance of elevated serum prolactin levels is unknown for most patients. An increase in mammary neoplasms has been found in rodents after chronic administration of neuroleptic drugs. Neither clinical studies nor epidemiologic studies conducted to date, however, have shown an association between chronic administration of these drugs and mammary tumorigenesis; the available evidence is considered too limited to be conclusive at this time.

Concurrent administration of propranolol (100 mg to 800 mg daily) has been reported to produce increases in plasma levels of thioridazine (approximately 50 to 400 percent) and its metabolites (approximately 80 to 300 percent).

Pindolol: Concurrent administration of pindolol and thioridazine have resulted in moderate dose related increases in the serum levels of thioridazine and two of its metabolites, as well as higher than expected serum pindolol levels.

It is recommended that a daily dose in excess of 300 mg. be reserved for use only in severe neuropsychiatric conditions.

Information for Patients: Given the likelihood that some patients exposed chronically to neuroleptics will develop tardive dyskinesia, it is advised that all patients in whom chronic use is contemplated be given, if possible, full information about this risk. The decision to inform patients and /or their guardians must obviously take into account the clinical circumstances and the competency of the patient to understand the information provided.

ADVERSE REACTIONS

In the recommended dosage ranges with Mellaril® (thioridazine), most side effects are mild and transient.

Central Nervous System: Drowsiness may be encountered on occasion, especially where large doses are given early in treatment. Generally, this effect tends to subside with continued therapy or a reduction in dosage. Pseudoparkinsonism and other extrapyramidal symptoms may occur but are infrequent. Nocturnal confusion, hyperactivity, lethargy, psychotic reactions, restlessness and headache have been reported but are extremely rare.

Autonomic Nervous System: Dryness of mouth, blurred vision, constipation, nausea, vomiting, diarrhea, nasal stuffiness, and pallor have been seen.

Endocrine System: Galactorrhea, breast engorgement, amenorrhea, inhibition of ejaculation and peripheral edema have been described.

Skin: Dermatitis and skin eruptions of the urticarial type have been observed infrequently. Photosensitivity is extremely rare.

Cardiovascular System: ECG changes have been reported (see *Phenothiazine Derivatives: Cardiovascular Effects*).

Other: Rare cases described as parotid swelling have been reported following administration of Mellaril® (thioridazine).

Phenothiazine Derivatives:

It should be noted that efficacy, indications and untoward effects have varied with the different phenothiazines. It has been reported that old age lowers the tolerance for phenothiazines. The most common neurological side effects in these patients are parkinsonism and akathisia. There appears to be an increased risk of agranulocytosis and leukopenia in the geriatric population. The physician should be aware that the following have occurred with one or more phenothiazines and should be considered whenever one of these drugs is used:

Autonomic Reactions: Miosis, obstipation, anorexia, paralytic ileus.

Cutaneous Reactions: Erythema, exfoliative dermatitis, contact dermatitis.

Blood Dyscrasias: Agranulocytosis, leukopenia, eosinophilia, thrombocytopenia, anemia, aplastic anemia, pancytopenia.

Allergic Reactions: Fever, laryngeal edema, angioneurotic edema, asthma.

Hepatotoxicity: Jaundice, biliary stasis.

Cardiovascular Effects: Changes in the terminal portion of the electrocardiogram, including prolongation of the Q-T interval, lowering and inversion of the T-wave and appearance of a wave tentatively identified as a bifid T or a U wave have been observed in some patients receiving the phenothiazine tranquilizers, including Mellaril® (thioridazine). To date, these appear to be due to altered repolarization and not related to myocardial damage. They appear to be reversible. While there is no evidence at present that these changes are in any way precursors of any significant disturbance of cardiac rhythm, it should be noted that several sudden and unexpected deaths apparently due to cardiac arrest have occurred in patients previously showing characteristic electrocardiographic changes while taking the drug. The use of periodic electrocardiograms has been proposed but would appear to be of questionable value as a predictive device. Hypotension, rarely resulting in cardiac arrest.

Extrapyramidal Symptoms: Akathisia, agitation, motor restlessness, dystonic reactions, trismus, torticollis, opisthotonus, oculogyric crises, tremor, muscular rigidity, akinesia.

Tardive Dyskinesia: Chronic use of neuroleptics may be associated with the development of tardive dyskinesia. The salient features of this syndrome are described in the *WARNINGS* section and below.

The syndrome is characterized by involuntary choreoathetoid movements which variously involve the tongue, face, mouth, lips, or jaw (e.g. protrusion of the tongue, puffing of cheeks, puckering of the mouth, chewing movements), trunk and extremities. The severity of the syndrome and the degree of impairment produced vary widely.

The syndrome may become clinically recognizable either during treatment, upon dosage reduction, or upon withdrawal of treatment. Movements may decrease in intensity and may disappear altogether if further treatment with neuroleptics is withheld. It is generally believed that reversibility is more likely after short rather than long-term neuroleptic exposure. Consequently, early detection of tardive dyskinesia is important. To increase the likelihood of detecting the syndrome at the earliest possible time, the dosage of neuroleptic drug should be reduced periodically (if clinically possible) and the patient observed for signs of the disorder. This maneuver is critical, for neuroleptic drugs may mask the signs of the syndrome.

Neuroleptic Malignant Syndrome: Chronic use of neuroleptics may be associated with the development of Neuroleptic Malignant Syndrome (NMS). The salient features of this syndrome are described in the *WARNINGS* section and below. Clinical manifestations of NMS are hyperpyrexia, muscle rigidity, altered mental status and evidence of autonomic instability (irregular pulse or blood pressure, tachycardia, diaphoresis, and cardiac dysrhythmias).

Endocrine Disturbances: Menstrual irregularities, altered libido, gynecomastia, lactation, weight gain, edema. False positive pregnancy tests have been reported.

Urinary Disturbances: Retention, incontinence.

Others: Hyperpyrexia. Behavioral effects suggestive of a paradoxical reaction have been reported. These include excitement, bizarre dreams, aggravation of psychoses, and toxic confusional states. More recently, a peculiar skin-eye syndrome has been recognized as a side effect following long-term treatment with phenothiazines. This reaction is marked by progressive pigmentation of areas of the skin or conjunctiva and/or accompanied by discoloration of the exposed sclera and cornea. Opacities of the anterior lens and cornea described as irregular or stellate in shape have also been reported. Systemic lupus erythematosus-like syndrome.

DOSAGE

Dosage must be individualized according to the degree of mental and emotional disturbance. In all cases, the smallest effective dosage should be determined for each patient.

Adults: *Psychotic manifestations:* The usual starting dose is 50 to 100 mg three times a day, with a gradual increment to a maximum of 800 mg daily if necessary. Once effective control of symptoms has been achieved, the dosage may be reduced gradually to determine the minimum maintenance dose. The total daily dosage ranges from 200 to 800 mg, divided into two to four doses.

For the short-term treatment of moderate to marked depression with variable degrees of anxiety in adult patients and for the treatment of multiple symptoms such as agitation, anxiety, depressed mood, tension, sleep disturbances, and fears in geriatric patients: The usual starting dose is 25 mg three times a day. Dosage ranges from 10 mg two to four times a day in milder cases to 50 mg three or four times a day for more severely disturbed patients. The total daily dosage range is from 20 mg to a maximum of 200 mg.

Children: Mellaril® (thioridazine) is not intended for children under 2 years of age. For children aged 2 to 12 the dosage of thioridazine hydrochloride ranges from 0.5 mg to a maximum of 3.0 mg/Kg per day. For children with moderate disorders 10 mg two or three times a day is the usual starting

Continued on next page

Sandoz Pharm.—Cont.

dose. For hospitalized, severely disturbed, or psychotic children, 25 mg two or three times daily is the usual starting dose. Dosage may be increased gradually until optimum therapeutic effect is obtained or the maximum has been reached.

HOW SUPPLIED

MELLARIL® (thioridazine) HCl
Tablets: 10 mg, 15 mg, 25 mg, 50 mg, 100 mg, 150 mg and 200 mg thioridazine hydrochloride, USP. Packages of 100, 500 and 1000 tablets. Also, for wholly tax-supported institutions only, packages of 4800 (48 × 100) and 5000 tablets. Store and dispense: Below 86°F; tight container.
Concentrate—30 mg/ml: Each ml contains 30 mg thioridazine hydrochloride, USP, alcohol, USP, 3.0% by volume. Immediate containers: Amber glass bottles of 4 fl. oz (118 ml) as follows:
4 fl. oz bottles, in cartons of 12 bottles, with an accompanying dropper graduated to deliver 10 mg, 25 mg and 50 mg of thioridazine hydrochloride, USP. Also, for wholly tax-supported institutions only, gallon cartons of 32 x 4 oz. bottles, each with the same dropper.
Concentrate—100 mg/ml: Each ml contains 100 mg thioridazine hydrochloride, USP, alcohol, 4.2% by volume, *4 fl. oz bottles,* in cartons of 12 bottles, with an accompanying dropper graduated to deliver 100 mg, 150 mg and 200 mg of thioridazine hydrochloride.
Store & dispense: Below 86°F; tight, amber glass bottle.
The concentrate may be diluted with distilled water, acidified tap water, or suitable juices. Each dose should be so diluted just prior to administration—preparation and storage of bulk dilutions is not recommended.
MELLARIL-S® (thioridazine)
Suspension—25 mg/5 ml: Each 5 ml contains thioridazine, USP, equivalent to 25 mg thioridazine hydrochloride, USP. Buttermint-flavored in pint bottles.
Suspension—100 mg/5 ml: Each 5 ml contains thioridazine, USP, equivalent to 100 mg thioridazine hydrochloride, USP. Buttermint-flavored in pint bottles.
Store and dispense: Below 77°F; tight, amber glass bottle.
Additional information available to physicians.
Company's Product Identification Mark(s): 10 mg and 15 mg tablets branded with NDC number on one side, triangle (S) other side. All other tablet strengths branded MELLARIL & strength on one side, triangle (S) other side.
Shown in Product Identification Section, page 427
[MEL-Z44 Issued June 1, 1988]

MESANTOIN® Tablets ℞
[*meh-san'toyn*]
(mephenytoin) tablets, USP

The following prescribing information is based on official labeling in effect on August 1, 1989.

DESCRIPTION

Mesantoin® (mephenytoin) is 3- methyl 5,5-phenyl-ethyl-hydantoin. It may be considered to be the hydantoin homolog of the barbiturate mephobarbital. Mesantoin (mephenytoin) has the following structure:

Active Ingredient: mephenytoin, USP
Inactive Ingredients: D&C Red #3, gelatin, lactose, starch, stearic acid and sucrose

ACTIONS

Mephenytoin exhibits pharmacologic effects similar to both diphenylhydantoin and the barbiturates in antagonizing experimental seizures in laboratory animals. Mephenytoin produces behavioral and electroencephalographic effects in man which are similar to those produced by barbiturates.

INDICATIONS

For the control of grand mal, focal, Jacksonian, and psychomotor seizures in those patients who have been refractory to less toxic anticonvulsants.

CONTRAINDICATIONS

Hypersensitivity to hydantoin products.

WARNINGS

Mephenytoin should be used only after safer anticonvulsants have been given an adequate trial and have failed.
As with all anticonvulsants, dose reduction must be gradual so as to minimize the risk of precipitating seizures.
Patients should be cautioned about possible additive effects of alcohol and other CNS depressants. Acute alcohol intoxication may increase the anticonvulsant effect due to decreased metabolic breakdown. Chronic alcohol abuse may

result in decreased anticonvulsant effect due to enzyme induction.

Usage in Pregnancy
The effects of mephenytoin in human pregnancy and nursing infants are unknown.
Recent reports suggest an association between the use of anticonvulsant drugs by women with epilepsy and an elevated incidence of birth defects in children born to these women. Data are more extensive with respect to diphenylhydantoin and phenobarbital, but these are also the most commonly prescribed anticonvulsants; less systematic or anecdotal reports suggest a possible similar association with the use of all known anticonvulsant drugs.
The reports suggesting an elevated incidence of birth defects in children of drug-treated epileptic women cannot be regarded as adequate to prove a definite cause and effect relationship. There are intrinsic methodologic problems in obtaining adequate data on drug teratogenicity in humans; the possibility also exists that other factors, e.g., genetic factors or the epileptic condition itself, may be more important than drug therapy in leading to birth defects. The great majority of mothers on anticonvulsant medication deliver normal infants. It is important to note that anticonvulsant drugs should not be discontinued in patients in whom the drug is administered to prevent major seizures because of the strong possibility of precipitating status epilepticus with attendant hypoxia and threat to life. In individual cases where the severity and frequency of the seizure disorder are such that the removal of medication does not pose a serious threat to the patient, discontinuation of the drug may be considered prior to and during pregnancy, although it cannot be said with any confidence that even minor seizures do not pose some hazards to the developing embryo or fetus.
The prescribing physician will wish to weigh these considerations in treating or counseling epileptic women of child-bearing potential.

PRECAUTIONS

The patient taking Mesantoin® (mephenytoin) must be kept under close medical supervision at all times since serious adverse reactions may emerge.
Because the primary site of degradation is the liver, it is recommended that screening tests of liver function precede introduction of the drug.
Some patients may show side reactions as the result of individual sensitivity. These reactions can be broken down into three types respectively according to severity: 1) blood dyscrasias; 2) skin and mucous membrane manifestations; and 3) central effects. The blood, skin and mucous membrane manifestations are the more important since they can be more serious in nature. Since mephenytoin has been reported to produce blood dyscrasia in certain instances, the patient must be instructed that in the event any unusual symptoms develop (e.g. sore throat, fever, mucous membrane bleeding, glandular swelling, cutaneous reaction), he must discontinue the drug and report for examination immediately. It is recommended that blood examinations be made (total white cell count and differential count) during the initial phase of administration. Such tests are best made: a) before starting medication; b) after 2 weeks on a low dosage; c) again after 2 weeks when full dosage is reached; d) thereafter, monthly for a year; e) from then on, every 3 months. If the neutrophils drop to between 2500 and 1600/cu.mm., counts are made every 2 weeks. Stop medication if the count drops to 1600.

ADVERSE REACTIONS

A number of side effects and toxic reactions have been reported with Mesantoin (mephenytoin) as well as with other hydantoin compounds. Many of these appear to be dose related while others seem to be a manifestation of a hypersensitivity reaction to these drugs.
Blood Dyscrasias
Leukopenia, neutropenia, agranulocytosis, thrombocytopenia and pancytopenia have occurred. Eosinophilia, monocytosis, and leukocytosis have been described. Simple anemia, hemolytic anemia, megaloblastic anemia and aplastic anemia have occurred but are uncommon.
Skin and Mucous Membrane Manifestations
Maculopapular, morbilliform, scarlatiniform, urticarial, purpuric (associated with thrombocytopenia) and non-specific skin rashes have been reported. Exfoliative dermatitis, erythema multiforme (Stevens-Johnson Syndrome), toxic epidermal necrolysis and fatal dermatitides have been described on rare occasions. Skin pigmentation and rashes associated with a lupus erythematosus syndrome have also been reported.
Central Effects
Drowsiness is dose-related and may be reduced by a reduction in dose. Ataxia, diplopia, nystagmus, dysarthria, fatigue, irritability, choreiform movements, depression and tremor have been encountered.
Nervousness, nausea, vomiting, sleeplessness and dizziness may occur during the initial stages of therapy. Generally, these symptoms are transient, often disappearing with continued treatment.

Mental confusion and psychotic disturbances and increased seizures have been reported, but a definite causal relationship with the drug is uncertain.
Miscellaneous
Hepatitis, jaundice and nephrosis have been reported but a definite cause and effect relationship between the drug and these effects has not been established.
Alopecia, weight gain, edema, photophobia, conjunctivitis and gum hyperplasia have been encountered.
Polyarthropathy, pulmonary fibrosis, lupus erythematosus syndrome, and lymphadenopathy which simulates Hodgkin's Disease have also been observed.

DOSAGE AND ADMINISTRATION

Dosage of antiepileptic therapy should be adjusted to the needs of the individual patient. Maintenance dosage is that smallest amount of antiepileptic necessary to suppress seizures completely or reduce their frequency. Optimum dosage is attained by starting with ½ or 1 tablet of Mesantoin (mephenytoin) per day during the first week and thereafter increasing the daily dose by ½ or 1 tablet at weekly intervals. No dose should be increased until it has been taken for at least one week.
The average dose of Mesantoin for adults ranges from 2 to 6 tablets (0.2 to 0.6 Gm.) daily. In some instances it may be necessary to administer as much as 8 tablets or more daily in order to obtain full seizure control. Children usually require from 1 to 4 tablets (0.1 Gm. to 0.4 Gm.) according to nature of seizures and age.
When the physician wishes to replace the anticonvulsant now being employed with Mesantoin (mephenytoin), he should give ½ or 1 tablet of Mesantoin (mephenytoin) daily during the first week and gradually increase the daily dose at weekly intervals while gradually reducing that of the drug being discontinued. The transition can be made smoothly over a period of three to six weeks. If seizures are not completely controlled with the dose so attained, the daily dose should then be increased by a one-tablet increment at weekly intervals to the point of maximum effect. If the patient had also been receiving phenobarbital, it is well to continue it until the transition is completed, at which time gradual withdrawal of the phenobarbital may be tried.

HOW SUPPLIED

Each tablet contains 100 mg mephenytoin and is scored to permit half-tablet dosage. Packages of 100 tablets. (Pale pink, compressed, scored).
Company's Product Identification Mark(s): Tablets embossed 78/52 and scored on one side, triangle S SANDOZ other side.
[MES—Z16 Issued July 27, 1987]

METAPREL® ℞
(metaproterenol sulfate USP)
INHALATION AEROSOL BRONCHODILATOR

CAUTION: Federal law prohibits dispensing without prescription.
The following prescribing information is based on official labeling in effect on August 1, 1989.

PRESCRIBING INFORMATION

DESCRIPTION

Metaprel® (metaproterenol sulfate USP) Inhalation Aerosol is a bronchodilator administered by oral inhalation. Each Metaprel® (metaproterenol sulfate USP) Inhalation Aerosol contains 150 mg of metaproterenol sulfate as a micronized powder. This is sufficient medication for 200 inhalations. Each metered dose delivers through the mouthpiece 0.65 mg of metaproterenol sulfate (each mL contains 15 mg). The inert ingredients are dichlorodifluoromethane, dichlorotetrafluoroethane, and trichloromonofluoromethane as propellants, and soya lecithin.
Metaprel® (metaproterenol sulfate USP), 1-(3,5-dihydroxyphenyl)-2-isopropylaminoethanol sulfate, is a white, crystalline, racemic mixture of 2 optically active isomers. It has the following chemical structure:

metaproterenol sulfate
(Metaprel)®

isoproterenol hydrochloride
$(C_{11}H_{17}NO_3)_2 \cdot H_2SO_4$ Mol. wt. 520.59

CLINICAL PHARMACOLOGY

In vitro studies and *in vivo* pharmacologic studies have demonstrated that Metaprel® (metaproterenol sulfate USP) has a preferential effect on beta-2 adrenergic receptors compared with isoproterenol. While it is recognized that beta-2 adrenergic receptors are the predominant receptors in bronchial smooth muscle, recent data indicate that there is a population of beta-2 receptors in the human heart existing in a concentration between 10%–50%. The precise function of these, however, is not yet established. *(See WARNINGS)*
The pharmacologic effects of beta adrenergic agonist drugs, including Metaprel® (metaproterenol sulfate USP), are at least in part attributable to stimulation through beta adrenergic receptors of intracellular adenyl cyclase, the enzyme which catalyzes the conversion of adenosine triphosphate (ATP) to cyclic-3′, 5′-adenosine monophosphate (c-AMP). Increased c-AMP levels are associated with relaxation of bronchial smooth muscle and inhibition of release of mediators of immediate hypersensitivity from cells, especially from mast cells.

Pharmacokinetics

Absorption, biotransformation, and excretion studies in humans following administration by inhalation have shown that approximately 3% of the actuated dose is absorbed intact through the lungs. The major metabolite, metaproterenol-3-O-sulfate, is produced in the gastrointestinal tract. Metaprel® (metaproterenol sulfate USP) is not metabolized by catechol-O-methyltransferase nor have glucuronide conjugates been isolated to date.
Pulmonary function tests performed concomitantly usually show improvement following aerosol Metaprel® (metaproterenol sulfate USP) administration, e.g., an increase in the 1-second forced expiratory volume (FEV_1), maximum expiratory flow rate, forced vital capacity, and/or a decrease in airway resistance. The resultant decrease in airway obstruction may relieve the dyspnea associated with bronchospasm.
Controlled single- and multiple-dose studies have been performed with pulmonary function monitoring. The duration of effect of a *single dose* of 2–3 inhalations of Metaprel® (metaproterenol sulfate USP) (that is, the period of time during which there is a 20% or greater increase in FEV_1) has varied from 1–5 hours.
In repetitive-dosing studies (up to q.i.d.), the duration of effect for a similar dose of Metaprel® (metaproterenol sulfate USP) has ranged from about 1–2.5 hours. Present studies are inadequate to explain the divergence in duration of the FEV_1 effect between single- and repetitive-dosing studies, respectively.
Recent studies in laboratory animals (minipigs, rodents, and dogs) recorded the occurrence of cardiac arrhythmias and sudden death (with histologic evidence of myocardial necrosis) when beta agonists and methylxanthines were administered concurrently. The significance of these findings when applied to humans is currently unknown.

INDICATIONS AND USAGE

Metaprel® (metaproterenol sulfate USP) is indicated as a bronchodilator for bronchial asthma and for reversible bronchospasm which may occur in association with bronchitis and emphysema.

CONTRAINDICATIONS

Use in patients with cardiac arrhythmias associated with tachycardia is contraindicated.
Although rare, immediate hypersensitivity reactions can occur. Therefore, Metaprel® (metaproterenol sulfate USP) Inhalation Aerosol is contraindicated in patients with a history of hypersensitivity to any of its components.

WARNINGS

Fatalities have been reported following excessive use of Metaprel® (metaproterenol sulfate USP) as with other sympathomimetic inhalation preparations, and the exact cause is unknown. Cardiac arrest was noted in several cases.
Metaprel® (metaproterenol sulfate USP), like other beta adrenergic agonists, can produce a significant cardiovascular effect in some patients, as measured by pulse rate, blood pressure, symptoms, and/or ECG changes. As with other beta adrenergic agonists, Metaprel® (metaproterenol sulfate USP) can produce paradoxical bronchospasm (which can be life threatening). If it occurs, the preparation should be discontinued immediately and alternative therapy instituted.
Metaprel® (metaproterenol sulfate USP) should not be used more often than prescribed. Patients should be advised to contact their physician in the event that they do not respond to their usual dose of a sympathomimetic amine aerosol.

PRECAUTIONS

General: Extreme care must be exercised with respect to the administration of additional sympathomimetic agents.

Since metaproterenol is a sympathomimetic amine, it should be used with caution in patients with cardiovascular disorders, including ischemic heart disease, hypertension or cardiac arrhythmias, in patients with hyperthyroidism or diabetes mellitus, and in patients who are unusually responsive to sympathomimetic amines or who have convulsive disorders. Significant changes in systolic and diastolic blood pressure could be expected to occur in some patients after use of any beta adrenergic bronchodilator.

Information for Patients

Appropriate care should be exercised when considering the administration of additional sympathomimetic agents. A sufficient interval of time should elapse prior to administration of another sympathomimetic agent.

Drug Interactions

Other beta adrenergic aerosol bronchodilators should not be used concomitantly with Metaprel® (metaproterenol sulfate USP) because they may have additive effects. Beta adrenergic agonists should be administered with caution to patients being treated with monoamine oxidase inhibitors or tricyclic antidepressants, since the action of beta adrenergic agonists on the vascular system may be potentiated.

Carcinogenesis/Mutagenesis/Impairment of Fertility

In an 18-month study in mice, Metaprel® (metaproterenol sulfate USP) produced an increase in benign ovarian tumors in females at doses corresponding to 320 and 640 times the maximum recommended dose (based on a 50 kg individual). In a 2-year study in rats, a non-significant incidence of benign leiomyomata of the mesovarium was noted at 640 times the maximum recommended dose. The relevance of these findings to man is not known. Mutagenic studies with Metaprel® (metaproterenol sulfate USP) have not been conducted. Reproduction studies in rats revealed no evidence of impaired fertility.

Pregnancy: Teratogenic Effects

Pregnancy Category C. Metaprel® (metaproterenol sulfate USP) has been shown to be teratogenic and embryotoxic in rabbits when given in doses corresponding to 640 times the maximum recommended dose. These effects included skeletal abnormalities, hydrocephalus, and skull bone separation. Results of other studies in rabbits, rats, or mice have not revealed any teratogenic, embryocidal, or fetotoxic effects. There are no adequate and well-controlled studies in pregnant women. Metaprel® (metaproterenol sulfate USP) should be used during pregnancy only if the potential benefit justifies the potential risk to the fetus.

Nursing Mothers

It is not known whether Metaprel® (metaproterenol sulfate USP) is excreted in human milk; therefore, Metaprel® (metaproterenol sulfate USP) should be used during nursing only if the potential benefit justifies the possible risk to the newborn.

Pediatric Use

Safety and effectiveness in children below the age of 12 have not been established. Studies are currently under way in this age group.

ADVERSE REACTIONS

Adverse reactions are similar to those noted with other sympathomimetic agents.
The most frequent adverse reaction to Metaprel® (metaproterenol sulfate USP) administered by metered-dose inhaler among 251 patients in 90-day controlled clinical trials was nervousness. This was reported in 6.8% of patients. Less frequent adverse experiences, occurring in 1%–4% of patients were headache, dizziness, palpitations, gastrointestinal distress, tremor, throat irritation, nausea, vomiting, cough, and asthma exacerbation. Tachycardia occurred in less than 1% of patients.

OVERDOSAGE

The expected symptoms with overdosage are those of excessive beta-stimulation and/or any of the symptoms listed under adverse reactions, e.g. angina, hypertension or hypotension, arrhythmias, nervousness, headache, tremor, dry mouth, palpitation, nausea, dizziness, fatigue, malaise, and insomnia.
Treatment consists of discontinuation of metaproterenol together with appropriate symptomatic therapy.

DOSAGE AND ADMINISTRATION

The usual single dose is 2–3 inhalations. With repetitive dosing, inhalation should usually not be repeated more often than about every 3–4 hours. Total dosage per day should not exceed 12 inhalations.
Metaprel® (metaproterenol sulfate USP) Inhalation Aerosol is not recommended for children under 12 years of age. It is recommended that the physician titrate dosage according to each individual patient's response to therapy.

HOW SUPPLIED

Each Metaprel® (metaproterenol sulfate USP) Inhalation Aerosol contains 150 mg of metaproterenol sulfate as a micronized powder in inert propellants. This is sufficient medication for 200 inhalations. Each metered dose delivers through the mouthpiece 0.65 mg metaproterenol sulfate (each mL contains 15 mg). Metaprel® (metaproterenol sul-

fate USP) Inhalation Aerosol with Mouthpiece (NDC 0078-0209-57), net contents 14 g (10 mL), equipped with a purple protective cap. Metaprel® (metaproterenol sulfate USP) Inhalation Aerosol Refill (NDC 0078-0209-53), net contents 14 g (10 mL).

Storage

Store between 59°F (15°C) and 77°F (25°C). Avoid excessive humidity.

INSTRUCTIONS FOR USE

1. Insert metal canister into clear end of mouthpiece.
2. Remove protective cap, invert canister and shake thoroughly.

3. Enclose mouthpiece with the lips. The base of the canister should be held vertically.

4. Exhale deeply, then inhale slowly through the mouth and at the same time firmly press once on the upended canister base; continue to inhale deeply. Hold your breath for a few seconds and then remove the mouthpiece from the mouth and exhale slowly.
5. One inhalation is often enough to obtain relief. The inhalation can be repeated once or twice if necessary, or as your physician directs. Wait at least 2 minutes before repeating the inhalation. In most cases, the dose should not be repeated more often than every 3–4 hours. No more than 12 inhalations should be taken in 1 day.
6. Replace protective cap after use.

WARNING: Do not exceed the dose prescribed by your physician. If difficulty in breathing persists, contact your physician immediately.
Note: When full, the container holds enough medication for at least 200 inhalations. Check regularly, by shaking the cylinder or container, to determine whether it contains any medication. When it first seems empty, there are still about 10 doses left. Refill containers for the plastic mouthpiece are available when prescribed by your physician.
Keep the mouthpiece clean. Wash with hot water. If soap is used, rinse thoroughly with plain water.
Never open the container holding the medication. Opening it is dangerous and renders the contents useless.
Caution: Contents under pressure. Do not puncture or incinerate container. Do not expose to heat or store at temperatures above 120°F. Keep out of reach of small children.
Manufactured by:
3M Health Care Specialties Division
Bldg. 225-1N, 3M Center
St. Paul, MN 55144-1000
Distributed by:
SANDOZ
PHARMACEUTICALS
CORPORATION
EAST HANOVER, N.J. 07936
Licensed from Boehringer Ingelheim Pharmaceuticals, Inc.
(MTP-ZZ(200)1   Issued June 1, 1989

METAPREL®   ℞
(metaproterenol sulfate USP)
Syrup—10 mg/5 mL
Tablets 10 mg; 20 mg
Oral Bronchodilator

The following prescribing information is based on official labeling in effect on August 1, 1989.

DESCRIPTION

Syrup: Each 5 mL of Metaprel® (metaproterenol sulfate) syrup contains metaproterenol sulfate USP 10 mg. Inactive Ingredients: edetate disodium, flavor, hydroxyethyl cellulose, methylparaben, propylparaben, purified water, Red 40, saccharin, sorbitol.

Continued on next page

Sandoz Pharm.—Cont.

Tablets: Each Metaprel® (metaproterenol sulfate) tablet, 10 mg and 20 mg, contains metaproterenol sulfate USP 10 mg and 20 mg respectively.

Other Ingredients: colloidal silicon dioxide, dibasic calcium phosphate, lactose, magnesium stearate, starch.

Chemically, Metaprel® (metaproterenol sulfate) is 1-(3, 5-dihydroxyphenyl)-2-isopropyl-aminoethanol sulfate, a white, crystalline, racemic mixture of two optically active isomers.

Metaproterenol Sulfate USP:

Isoproterenol Hydrochloride:

It differs from isoproterenol hydrochloride by having two hydroxyl groups attached at the meta positions on the benzene ring rather than one at the meta and one at the para position.

ACTIONS

Metaprel® (metaproterenol sulfate) is a potent beta-adrenergic stimulator. It is postulated that beta-adrenergic stimulants produce many of their pharmacological effects by activation of adenyl cyclase, the enzyme which catalyzes the conversion of adenosine triphosphate to cyclic adenosine monophosphate.

Absorption, biotransformation and excretion studies in humans following oral administration, have indicated that an average of 40 percent of the drug is absorbed; it is not metabolized by catechol-O-methyltransferase or sulfatase enzymes in the gut but is excreted primarily as glucuronic acid conjugates.

Syrup: When administered orally, Metaprel® (metaproterenol sulfate) decreases reversible bronchospasm. Pulmonary function tests performed after the administration of Metaprel® (metaproterenol sulfate) usually show improvement, e.g., an increase in the one-second forced expiratory volume (FEV_1), an increase in maximum expiratory flow rate, an increase in peak expiratory flow rate, an increase in forced vital capacity, and/or a decrease in airway resistance. The decrease in airway obstruction may relieve the dyspnea associated with bronchospasm. Pulmonary function has been monitored in controlled single-and multiple-dose studies. The duration of effect of a single dose of Metaprel® (metaproterenol sulfate) Syrup (that is, the period of time during which there is a 15 percent or greater increase in mean FEV_1) was up to four hours.

Tablets: When administered orally, Metaprel® (metaproterenol sulfate) decreases reversible bronchospasm. Pulmonary function tests performed concomitantly usually show improvement following Metaprel® (metaproterenol sulfate) administration, e.g., an increase in the one-second forced expiratory volume (FEV_1), an increase in maximum expiratory flow rate, an increase in forced vital capacity, and/or a decrease in airway resistance. The resultant decrease in airway obstruction may relieve the dyspnea associated with bronchospasm.

Controlled single- and multiple-dose studies have been performed with pulmonary function monitoring. The mean duration of effect of a single dose of 20 mg of Metaprel® (metaproterenol sulfate) (that is, the period of time during which there is a 15 percent or greater increase in FEV_1) was up to four hours. Four controlled multiple-dose 60-day studies, comparing the effectiveness of metaproterenol sulfate tablets with ephedrine tablets, have been performed. Because of difficulties in study design, only one study was available which could be analyzed in depth. This study showed a loss of efficacy with time for both metaproterenol sulfate and ephedrine. Therefore, the physician should take this phenomenon into account in evaluating the individual patient's overall management. Further studies are in progress to adequately explain these results.

Recent studies in laboratory animals (minipigs, rodents and dogs), recorded the occurrence of cardiac arrhythmias and sudden death (with histologic evidence of myocardial necrosis) when beta agonists and methylxanthines were adminis-

tered concurrently. The significance of these findings when applied to humans is currently unknown.

INDICATIONS

Metaprel® (metaproterenol sulfate) is indicated as a bronchodilator for bronchial asthma, and for reversible bronchospasm which may occur in association with bronchitis and emphysema.

CONTRAINDICATIONS

Use in patients with cardiac arrhythmias associated with tachycardia is contraindicated.

Although rare, immediate hypersensitivity reactions can occur. Therefore, Metaprel® (metaproterenol sulfate) is contraindicated in patients with a history of hypersensitivity to any of its components.

PRECAUTIONS

Extreme care must be exercised with respect to the administration of additional sympathomimetic agents. A sufficient interval of time should elapse prior to administration of another sympathomimetic agent.

Because metaproterenol sulfate is a sympathomimetic drug, it should be used with great caution in patients with hypertension, coronary artery disease, congestive heart failure, hyperthyroidism and diabetes, or when there is sensitivity to sympathomimetic amines.

Usage in Pregnancy: Safety in pregnancy has not been established. Metaproterenol should not be used except with caution during pregnancy, weighing the drug's benefit to the patient against potential risk to the fetus. Studies of metaproterenol in mice, rats and rabbits have revealed no significant teratogenic effects at oral doses up to 50 mg/kg (31 times the recommended daily human oral dose). In rabbits, fetal loss and teratogenic effects have been observed at and above oral doses of 50 and 100 mg/kg, respectively.

ADVERSE REACTIONS

Adverse reactions such as tachycardia, hypertension, palpitations, nervousness, tremor, nausea and vomiting have been reported. These reactions are similar to those noted with other sympathomimetic agents.

DOSAGE AND ADMINISTRATION

Syrup: Children aged 6–9 years or weight under 60 lbs—one teaspoonful three or four times a day. Children over 9 years or weight over 60 lbs—two teaspoonfuls three or four times a day. Experience in children under the age of six is limited to seventy-eight children. Of this number, forty were treated with metaproterenol sulfate for at least one month. In this group, daily doses of approximately 1.3 to 2.6 mg/kg were well tolerated. Adults—two teaspoonfuls three or four times a day.

Tablets: The usual adult dose is 20 mg three or four times a day. Children aged 6–9 years or weight under 60 lbs—10 mg three or four times a day. Over 9 years or weight over 60 lbs—20 mg three or four times a day. Metaprel® tablets are not recommended for use in children under 6 years at this time. (Please refer to the Actions section for further information on clinical experience with this product.)

If Metaprel® (metaproterenol sulfate) is administered before or after other sympathomimetic bronchodilators, caution should be exercised with respect to possible potentiation of adrenergic effects.

SYMPTOMS OF OVERDOSAGE

The symptoms of overdosage are those of excessive beta-adrenergic stimulation listed under Adverse Reactions.

HOW SUPPLIED

Syrup: Metaprel® (metaproterenol sulfate) is available as a cherry-flavored syrup, 10 mg per teaspoonful (5 mL), in pint bottles.

Tablets: Metaprel® (metaproterenol sulfate) Tablets, 10 mg, white, scored, round, imprinted "78-212" on one side, "10" on the other. Metaprel® (metaproterenol sulfate) Tablets, 20 mg, white, scored, round, imprinted "78-213" on one side, "20" on the other. Both strengths are available in bottles of 100.

Metaprel® (metaproterenol sulfate) is also available as a micronized powder in 15 cc metered dose inhalers and as a 5% inhalant solution in bottles of 10 mL. For details on Metaprel® (metaproterenol sulfate) Metered Dose Inhalers and Metaprel® (metaproterenol sulfate) Inhalant Solution 5% please refer to separate Product Information.

CAUTION

Federal law prohibits dispensing without prescription.
Under license from
Boehringer Ingelheim Pharmaceuticals, Inc.
[MTP-Z2 Issued August 1, 1986]

METHERGINE®   ℞

[meth 'er-gin]
(methylergonovine maleate) injection, USP
(methylergonovine maleate) tablets, USP

The following prescribing information is based on official labeling in effect on August 1, 1989.

DESCRIPTION

Methergine® (methylergonovine maleate) is a semi-synthetic ergot alkaloid used for the prevention and control of postpartum hemorrhage.

Methergine® (methylergonovine maleate) is available in sterile ampuls of 1 mL, containing 0.2 mg methylergonovine maleate for intramuscular or intravenous injection and in tablets for oral ingestion containing 0.2 mg methylergonovine maleate.

Tablet
Active Ingredient: methylergonovine maleate USP, 0.2 mg
Inactive Ingredients: acacia, carnauba wax, D&C Red #7, FD&C Blue #1, lactose, mixed parabens, povidone, sodium benzoate, starch, stearic acid, sucrose, talc, tartaric acid, and titanium dioxide

Ampul, 1 mL, clear, colorless solution
Active Ingredient: methylergonovine maleate USP, 0.2 mg
Inactive Ingredients: tartaric acid NF 0.25 mg, sodium chloride USP 3 mg, water for injection USP qs to 1 mL
Chemically, methylergonovine maleate is designated as 9, 10-didehydro-N-[(S)-1-(hydroxymethyl) propyl]-6-methylergoline-8β-carboxamide maleate (1:1) (salt)
Its structural formula is:

CLINICAL PHARMACOLOGY

Methergine® (methylergonovine maleate) acts directly on the smooth muscle of the uterus and increases the tone, rate, and amplitude of rhythmic contractions. Thus, it induces a rapid and sustained tetanic uterotonic effect which shortens the third stage of labor and reduces blood loss. The onset of action after i.v. administration is immediate; after i.m. administration, 2 to 5 minutes, and after oral administration, 5 to 10 minutes.

Pharmacokinetic studies have utilized radioimmunoassay techniques. After i.v. injection of 0.2 mg., Methergine (methylergonovine maleate) is rapidly distributed from plasma to peripheral tissues within an alpha-phase half-life of 2 to 3 minutes or less. The beta-phase elimination half-life is 20 to 30 minutes or more, but clinical effects continue for about 3 hours.[1,2]

Intramuscular injection of 0.2 mg afforded peak plasma concentrations of over 3 mg/mL at t_{max} of 0.5 hours. After 2 hours, total plasma clearance was 120 to 240 mL/minute. After oral administration, bioavailability was reported as 60% with no cumulation after repeated doses. During delivery, with parenteral injection, bioavailability increased to 78%.

Excretion is rapid and appears to be partially renal and partially hepatic. Whether the drug is able to penetrate the blood/brain barrier has not been determined.

INDICATIONS AND USAGE

For routine management after delivery of the placenta; postpartum atony and hemorrhage; subinvolution. Under full obstetric supervision, it may be given in the second stage of labor following delivery of the anterior shoulder.

CONTRAINDICATIONS

Hypertension; toxemia; pregnancy; and hypersensitivity.

WARNINGS

This drug should not be administered i.v. routinely because of the possibility of inducing sudden hypertensive and cerebrovascular accidents. If i.v. administration is considered essential as a lifesaving measure, Methergine® (methylergonovine maleate) should be given slowly over a period of no less than 60 seconds with careful monitoring of blood pressure.

PRECAUTIONS

General
Caution should be exercised in the presence of sepsis, obliterative vascular disease, hepatic or renal involvement. Also use with caution during the second stage of labor. The necessity for manual removal of a retained placenta should occur only rarely with proper technique and adequate allowance of time for its spontaneous separation.

Drug Interactions
Caution should be exercised when Methergine® (methylergonovine maleate) is used concurrently with other vasoconstrictors or ergot alkaloids.

Carcinogenesis, mutagenesis, impairment of fertility
No long-term studies have been performed in animals to evaluate carcinogenic potential. The effect of the drug on fertility has not been determined.

Pregnancy

Category C. Animal reproductive studies have not been conducted with Methergine® (methylergonovine maleate). It is also not known whether methylergonovine maleate can cause fetal harm or can affect reproductive capacity. Use of Methergine® (methylergonovine maleate) is contraindicated during pregnancy (See Indications).

Labor and Delivery

The uterotonic effect of Methergine® (methylergonovine maleate) is utilized after delivery to assist involution and decrease hemorrhage, shortening the third stage of labor.

Nursing Mothers

Methergine® (methylergonovine maleate) may be administered orally for a maximum of one week postpartum to control uterine bleeding. Recommended dosage is one tablet (0.2 mg) three or four times daily. At this dosage level a small quantity of drug appears in mothers' milk. Adverse effects have not been described, but caution should be exercised when Methergine® (methylergonovine maleate) is administered to a nursing woman.

ADVERSE REACTIONS

The most common adverse reaction is hypertension associated in several cases with seizure and/or headache. Hypotension has also been reported. Nausea and vomiting have occurred occasionally. Rarely observed reactions have included, in order of severity: transient chest pains, dyspnea, hematuria, thrombophlebitis, water intoxication, hallucinations, leg cramps, dizziness, tinnitus, nasal congestion, diarrhea, diaphoresis, palpitation and foul taste.[3]

DRUG ABUSE AND DEPENDENCE

Methergine® (methylergonovine maleate) has not been associated with drug abuse or dependence of either a physical or psychological nature.

OVERDOSE

Symptoms of acute overdose may include: nausea, vomiting, abdominal pain, numbness, tingling of the extremities, rise in blood pressure, in severe cases followed by hypotension, respiratory depression, hypothermia, convulsions and coma. Because reports of overdosage with Methergine® (methylergonovine maleate) are infrequent, the lethal dose in humans has not been established. The oral LD_{50} (in mg/kg) for the mouse is 187, the rat 93, and the rabbit 4.5.[4] Several cases of accidental Methergine® (methylergonovine maleate) injection in newborn infants have been reported, and in such cases 0.2 mg represents an overdose of great magnitude. However, recovery occurred in all but one case following a period of respiratory depression, hypothermia, hypertonicity with jerking movements, and, in one case, a single convulsion.

Also, several children one to three years of age have accidentally ingested up to 10 tablets (2 mg) with no apparent ill effects. A postpartum patient took 4 tablets at one time in error and reported paresthesias and clamminess as her only symptoms.

Treatment of acute overdosage is symptomatic and includes the usual procedures of:

1. removal of offending drug by inducing emesis, gastric lavage, catharsis, and supportive diuresis.
2. maintenance of adequate pulmonary ventilation, especially if convulsions or coma develop.
3. correction of hypotension with pressor drugs as needed.
4. control of convulsions with standard anticonvulsant agents.
5. control of peripheral vasospasm with warmth to the extremities if needed.[5]

DOSAGE AND ADMINISTRATION

Parenteral drug products should be inspected visually for particulate matter and discoloration prior to administration.

Intramuscularly

One mL, 0.2 mg, after delivery of the anterior shoulder, after delivery of the placenta, or during the puerperium. May be repeated as required, at intervals of 2–4 hours.

Intravenously

Dosage same as intramuscular. (See "Warning" section.)

Orally

One tablet, 0.2 mg, 3 or 4 times daily in the puerperium for a maximum of 1 week.

HOW SUPPLIED

Tablets

0.2 mg round, coated, orchid, branded "78-54" one side, "SANDOZ" other side. Bottles of 100 (NDC 0078-0054-05) and 1000 (NDC 0078-0054-09). SandoPak® (unit dose) packages of 100, 10 blister strips of 10 tablets (NDC 0078-0054-06).

Ampuls

1 mL size, boxes of 20 (NDC 0078-0053-03), and 50 (NDC 0078-0053-04).

Store and dispense

Tablets—

Below 77°F; tight, light-resistant container

Ampuls—

Below 77°F; protect from light — administer only if solution is clear and colorless.

References

1. Mantyla, R. and Kants, J: Clinical Pharmacokinetics of Methylergometrine (Methylergonovine). Int. J. Clin. Pharmacol. Ther. Toxicol. 19(9):386–391, 1981.
2. Iwamura, S. and Kambegawa, A: Determination of Methylergometrine and Dihydroergotoxine in Biological Fluids. J. Pharm. Dyn. 4:275–281, 1981.
3. Information on Adverse Reactions supplied by Medical Services Dept., Sandoz Pharmaceuticals, E. Hanover, N.J., based on computerized clinical reports.
4. Berde, B. and Schild, H.O.: *Ergot Alkaloids and Related Compounds*, Springer-Verlag, New York, 1978, p. 810
5. Treatment of Acute Overdosage. Sandoz Dorsey Rx Products. Sandoz Inc., Medical Services Department.

Company's Product Identification Mark(s): Tablets imprinted "78-54" on on side, "SANDOZ" other side.

[Met-Z20 Issued June 30, 1989]

NEO-CALGLUCON® (CALCIUM GLUBIONATE) Syrup, USP

[nē 'ō cal "glū 'kon]

(calcium glubionate)

Palatable and Readily Absorbable Calcium Supplement.

The following prescribing information is based on official labeling in effect on August 1, 1989

DESCRIPTION

Each teaspoonful (5 ml) of NEO-CALGLUCON® (calcium glubionate) Syrup, USP contains: glubionate calcium 1.8 g, (calcium content 115 mg—providing the same amount as 1.2 g calcium gluconate). Other ingredients: benzoic acid, caramel, citric acid, flavors, purified water, saccharin sodium, sorbitol, sucrose.

Adequate calcium intake is particularly important during periods of bone growth in childhood and adolescence, during pregnancy and lactation. An adequate supply of calcium is considered necessary in adults, especially those over 40, to prevent a negative calcium balance which may contribute to the development of osteoporosis. The following are the US Government Recommended Daily Allowances (US RDA) of calcium.

Age Period	Calcium Requirements
Infants	0.6 g
Children under 4 years	0.8 g
Adults and children over 4	1.0 g
Pregnant and lactating women	1.3 g

Eight ounces of whole milk provide approximately 267 mg of calcium. One tablespoonful (15 ml) of NEO-CALGLUCON® (calcium glubionate) Syrup, USP contains 345 mg of calcium.

NEO-CALGLUCON® (calcium glubionate) Syrup, USP

	Grams of Supplemental Calcium Provided Daily	Percentage of US Recommended Daily Allowance (US RDA)
I. As a Dietary Supplement: Adults and children 4 or more years of age—1 tablespoonful 3 times daily.	1.0 g	104
Pregnant or lactating women— 1 tablespoonful 4 times daily.	1.4 g	106
Children under 4 years of age— 2 teaspoonfuls 3 times daily.	0.7 g	86
Infants—1 teaspoonful 5 times daily (may be taken undiluted, mixed with infant's formula or fruit juice).	0.6 g	96
(Part of need is supplied by diet)		

NEO-CALGLUCON® (calcium glubionate) Syrup, USP

	Grams of Supplemental Ca Provided Daily
II. In the treatment of Calcium Deficiency States: *Tetany of the Newborn* (Tetany of the newborn appears to be a transient physiologic hypoparathyroidism related to the maturation of the parathyroid glands. Adequate parathyroid gland function usually occurs within one week after birth.) Serum calcium should be determined before therapy is instituted. Hypocalcemia is defined as a serum calcium below 8 mg/100 ml or 4 mEq/liter. It is advisable to lower the calcium and phosphorus loads in the feeding as well as to provide extra calcium. Intravenous administration of calcium solutions may be necessary for prompt relief of symptoms. Dose: Infants with confirmed hypocalcemia may be benefited by the oral administration of calcium salts so as to provide ELEMENTAL CALCIUM in a dosage of 50 to 150 mg/kg/day divided into three or more doses. (NEO-CALGLUCON® (calcium glubionate) Syrup, USP contains 115 mg ELEMENTAL CALCIUM per 5 ml teaspoon.) The lower dosage range should be employed if calcium is also being provided by the parenteral route. Whole milk formulas which are high in phosphorus should be eliminated in order to increase the calcium/phosphorus ratio. Supplemental oral calcium should be gradually reduced over a period of two or three weeks after the condition has completely stabilized.	See left-hand column
Hypoparathyroidism Acute Intravenous administration of calcium solutions may be necessary for prompt correction of hypocalcemia. Supplementary calcium should be given orally as soon as possible. Dose: 1–3 tablespoonfuls 3 times daily	1.0–3.1
Chronic Dose: 1–3 tablespoonfuls daily	0.3–1.0
Pseudohypoparathyroidism Dose: 1–3 tablespoonfuls daily	0.3–1.0
Osteoporosis, postmenopausal and senile Dose: 1–2 tablespoonfuls 3 times daily	1.0–2.1

Rickets and Osteomalacia

Treatment of these disorders consists of the administration of Vitamin D orally. The addition of calcium to the therapeutic regimen may be desirable to provide calcium needed for remineralization and to avoid hypocalcemia which occurs not infrequently in the early days of treatment. Dosages should be those recommended above under Dietary Supplement.

Continued on next page

Sandoz Pharm.—Cont.

INDICATIONS

1. As a *dietary supplement* where calcium intake may be inadequate:
   a. childhood and adolescence
   b. pregnancy
   c. lactation
   d. postmenopausal females and in the aged
2. In the *treatment* of calcium deficiency states which may occur in diseases such as:
   a. tetany of the newborn*
   b. hypoparathyroidism, acute* and chronic
   c. pseudohypoparathyroidism
   d. postmenopausal and senile osteoporosis
   e. rickets and osteomalacia
   *As a supplement to parenterally administered calcium.

CONTRAINDICATIONS

Patients with renal calculi.

WARNINGS

Certain dietary substances interfere with the absorption of calcium. These include oxalic acid (found in large quantities in rhubarb and spinach), phytic acid (bran and whole cereals) and phosphorus (milk and other dairy products). Administration of corticosteroids may interfere with calcium absorption.

PRECAUTIONS

When calcium is administered in therapeutic amounts for prolonged periods, hypercalcemia and hypercalciuria may result. This is most likely to occur in patients with hypoparathyroidism who are receiving high doses of Vitamin D. It can be avoided by frequent checks of plasma and urine calcium levels. Urine calcium levels may rise before plasma calcium levels. The former may be checked by determining 24-hour calcium excretion or by the Sulkowitch test.

ADVERSE REACTIONS

NEO-CALGLUCON® (calcium glubionate) Syrup, USP is exceptionally well tolerated. Gastrointestinal disturbances are exceedingly rare. A fatal case of hypercalcemia associated with an overdose of NEO-CALGLUCON® (calcium glubionate) Syrup, USP has been reported in a two pound neonate. Symptoms of hypercalcemia include anorexia, nausea, vomiting, constipation, abdominal pain, dryness of the mouth, thirst and polyuria.

DOSAGE AND ADMINISTRATION

NEO-CALGLUCON® (calcium glubionate) Syrup, USP should be administered before meals to enhance absorption. [See table on preceding page].

HOW SUPPLIED

NEO-CALGLUCON® (calcium glubionate) Syrup, USP (straw yellow) in pint bottles.

PAMELOR®   ℞
[*pam'ah-lar"*]
(nortriptyline HCl), capsules, USP
(nortriptyline HCl) oral solution, USP

The following prescribing information is based on official labeling in effect on August 1, 1989.

DESCRIPTION

Pamelor® (nortriptyline HCl) is 5-(3-methylamino propylidene)-10, 11-dihydro-5H-dibenzo [a,d] cycloheptene hydrochloride. Its molecular weight is 299.8, and its empirical formula is $C_{19}H_{21}N \cdot HCl$.
The structural formula is as follows:

$$=CH-CH_2-CH_2-NH-CH_3 \cdot HCl$$

10 mg, 25 mg, 50 mg and 75 mg, Capsules
Active Ingredient: nortriptyline HCl, USP
10 mg, 25 mg, and 75 mg, Capsules
Inactive Ingredients: D&C Yellow #10, FD&C Yellow #6, gelatin, silicon fluid, sodium lauryl sulfate, starch, and titanium dioxide
May Also Include: benzyl alcohol, butylparaben, edetate calcium disodium, methylparaben, propylparaben, silicon dioxide, and sodium propionate
50 mg, Capsules

Inactive Ingredients: gelatin, silicon fluid, sodium lauryl sulfate, starch, and titanium dioxide
May Also Include: benzyl alcohol, butylparaben, edetate calcium disodium, methylparaben, propylparaben, silicon dioxide, sodium bisulfite (capsule shell only), and sodium propionate
Solution
Active Ingredient: nortriptyline HCl, USP
Inactive Ingredients: alcohol, benzoic acid, flavoring, purified water, and sorbitol

ACTIONS

The mechanism of mood elevation by tricyclic antidepressants is at present unknown. Pamelor® (nortriptyline HCl) is not a monoamine oxidase inhibitor. It inhibits the activity of such diverse agents as histamine, 5-hydroxytryptamine, and acetylcholine. It increases the pressor effect of norepinephrine but blocks the pressor response of phenethylamine. Studies suggest that Pamelor® (nortriptyline HCl) interferes with the transport, release, and storage of catecholamines. Operant conditioning techniques in rats and pigeons suggest that Pamelor® (nortriptyline HCl) has a combination of stimulant and depressant properties.

INDICATIONS

Pamelor® (nortriptyline HCl) is indicated for the relief of symptoms of depression. Endogenous depressions are more likely to be alleviated than are other depressive states.

CONTRAINDICATIONS

The use of Pamelor® (nortriptyline HCl) or other tricyclic antidepressants concurrently with a monoamine oxidase (MAO) inhibitor is contraindicated. Hyperpyretic crises, severe convulsions, and fatalities have occurred when similar tricyclic antidepressants were used in such combinations. It is advisable to have discontinued the MAO inhibitor for at least two weeks before treatment with Pamelor® (nortriptyline HCl) is started. Patients hypersensitive to Pamelor® (nortriptyline HCl) should not be given the drug.
Cross-sensitivity between Pamelor® (nortriptyline HCl) and other dibenzazepines is a possibility.
Pamelor® (nortriptyline HCl) is contraindicated during the acute recovery period after myocardial infarction.

WARNINGS

Patients with cardiovascular disease should be given Pamelor® (nortriptyline HCl) only under close supervision because of the tendency of the drug to produce sinus tachycardia and to prolong the conduction time. Myocardial infarction, arrhythmia, and strokes have occurred. The antihypertensive action of guanethidine and similar agents may be blocked. Because of its anticholinergic activity, Pamelor® (nortriptyline HCl) should be used with great caution in patients who have glaucoma or a history of urinary retention.
Patients with a history of seizures should be followed closely when Pamelor® (nortriptyline HCl) is administered, inasmuch as this drug is known to lower the convulsive threshold. Great care is required if Pamelor® (nortriptyline HCl) is given to hyperthyroid patients or to those receiving thyroid medication, since cardiac arrhythmias may develop.
Pamelor® (nortriptyline HCl) may impair the mental and/or physical abilities required for the performance of hazardous tasks, such as operating machinery or driving a car; therefore, the patient should be warned accordingly.
Excessive consumption of alcohol in combination with nortriptyline therapy may have a potentiating effect, which may lead to the danger of increased suicidal attempts or overdosage, especially in patients with histories of emotional disturbances or suicidal ideation.
The concomitant administration of quinidine and nortriptyline may result in a significantly longer plasma half-life, higher A.U.C. and lower clearance of nortriptyline.
Use in Pregnancy—Safe use of Pamelor® (nortriptyline HCl) during pregnancy and lactation has not been established; therefore, when the drug is administered to pregnant patients, nursing mothers, or women of childbearing potential, the potential benefits must be weighed against the possible hazards. Animal reproduction studies have yielded inconclusive results.
Use in Children—This drug is not recommended for use in children, since safety and effectiveness in the pediatric age group have not been established.

PRECAUTIONS

The use of Pamelor® (nortriptyline HCl) in schizophrenic patients may result in an exacerbation of the psychosis or may activate latent schizophrenic symptoms. If the drug is given to overactive or agitated patients, increased anxiety and agitation may occur. In manic-depressive patients, Pamelor® (nortriptyline HCl) may cause symptoms of the manic phase to emerge.
Administration of reserpine during therapy with a tricyclic antidepressant has been shown to produce a "stimulating" effect in some depressed patients.

Troublesome patient hostility may be aroused by the use of Pamelor® (nortriptyline HCl). Epileptiform seizures may accompany its administration, as is true of other drugs of its class.
Close supervision and careful adjustment of the dosage are required when Pamelor® (nortriptyline HCl) is used with other anticholinergic drugs and sympathomimetic drugs. Concurrent administration of cimetidine and tricyclic antidepressants can produce clinically significant increases in the plasma concentrations of the tricyclic antidepressant. The patient should be informed that the response to alcohol may be exaggerated.
When it is essential, the drug may be administered with electroconvulsive therapy, although the hazards may be increased. Discontinue the drug for several days, if possible, prior to elective surgery.
The possibility of a suicidal attempt by a depressed patient remains after the initiation of treatment; in this regard, it is important that the least possible quantity of drug be dispensed at any given time.
Both elevation and lowering of blood sugar levels have been reported.
A case of significant hypoglycemia has been reported in a type II diabetic patient maintained on chlorpropamide (250 mg/day), after the addition of nortriptyline (125 mg/day).

ADVERSE REACTIONS

Note: Included in the following list are a few adverse reactions that have not been reported with this specific drug. However, the pharmacologic similarities among the tricyclic antidepressant drugs require that each of the reactions be considered when nortriptyline is administered.
Cardiovascular—Hypotension, hypertension, tachycardia, palpitation, myocardial infarction, arrhythmias, heart block, stroke.
Psychiatric—Confusional states (especially in the elderly) with hallucinations, disorientation, delusions; anxiety, restlessness, agitation; insomnia, panic, nightmares; hypomania; exacerbation of psychosis.
Neurologic—Numbness, tingling, paresthesias of extremities; incoordination, ataxia, tremors; peripheral neuropathy; extrapyramidal symptoms; seizures, alteration in EEG patterns; tinnitus.
Anticholinergic—Dry mouth and, rarely, associated sublingual adenitis; blurred vision, disturbance of accommodation, mydriasis; constipation, paralytic ileus; urinary retention, delayed micturition, dilation of the urinary tract.
Allergic—Skin rash, petechiae, urticaria, itching, photosensitization (avoid excessive exposure to sunlight); edema (general or of face and tongue), drug fever, cross-sensitivity with other tricyclic drugs.
Hematologic—Bone-marrow depression, including agranulocytosis; eosinophilia; purpura; thrombocytopenia.
Gastrointestinal—Nausea and vomiting, anorexia, epigastric distress, diarrhea, peculiar taste, stomatitis, abdominal cramps, black-tongue.
Endocrine—Gynecomastia in the male, breast enlargement and galactorrhea in the female; increased or decreased libido, impotence; testicular swelling; elevation or depression of blood sugar levels; syndrome of inappropriate ADH (antidiuretic hormone) secretion.
Other—Jaundice (simulating obstructive); altered liver function; weight gain or loss; perspiration; flushing; urinary frequency, nocturia; drowsiness, dizziness, weakness, fatigue; headache; parotid swelling; alopecia.
Withdrawal Symptoms—Though these are not indicative of addiction, abrupt cessation of treatment after prolonged therapy may produce nausea, headache, and malaise.

DOSAGE AND ADMINISTRATION

Pamelor® (nortriptyline HCl) is not recommended for children.
Pamelor® (nortriptyline HCl) is administered orally in the form of capsules or liquid. Lower than usual dosages are recommended for elderly patients and adolescents. Lower dosages are also recommended for outpatients than for hospitalized patients who will be under close supervision. The physician should initiate dosage at a low level and increase it gradually, noting carefully the clinical response and any evidence of intolerance. Following remission, maintenance medication may be required for a longer period of time at the lowest dose that will maintain remission.
If a patient develops minor side effects, the dosage should be reduced. The drug should be discontinued promptly if adverse effects of a serious nature or allergic manifestations occur.
Usual Adult Dose—25 mg three or four times daily; dosage should begin at a low level and be increased as required. As an alternate regimen, the total daily dosage may be given once-a-day. When doses above 100 mg daily are administered, plasma levels of nortriptyline should be monitored and maintained in the optimum range of 50-150 ng/mL. Doses above 150 mg per day are not recommended.
Elderly and Adolescent Patients—30 to 50 mg per day, in divided doses, or the total daily dosage may be given once-a-day.

OVERDOSAGE

Toxic overdosage may result in confusion, restlessness, agitation, vomiting, hyperpyrexia, muscle rigidity, hyperactive reflexes, tachycardia, ECG evidence of impaired conduction, shock, congestive heart failure, stupor, coma, and C.N.S. stimulation with convulsions followed by respiratory depression. Deaths have occurred following overdosage with drugs of this class.

No specific antidote is known. General supportive measures are indicated, with gastric lavage. Respiratory assistance is apparently the most effective measure when indicated. The use of CNS depressants may worsen the prognosis.

The administration of barbiturates for control of convulsions alleviates an increase in the cardiac work load but should be undertaken with caution to avoid potentiation of respiratory depression.

Intramuscular paraldehyde or diazepam provides anticonvulsant activity with less respiratory depression than do the barbiturates; diazepam seems to be preferred.

The use of digitalis and/or physostigmine may be considered in case of serious cardiovascular abnormalities or cardiac failure.

The value of dialysis has not been established.

HOW SUPPLIED

Capsules: Pamelor® (nortriptyline HCl) USP, equivalent to 10 mg, 25 mg, 50 mg and 75 mg base, are supplied in bottles of 100 and 500 and in boxes of 100 individually labeled blisters, each containing one capsule.

10 mg capsules branded "SANDOZ 78–86" on one half, "PAMELOR 10 mg" other half; 25 mg capsules branded "SANDOZ 78–87" on one half, "PAMELOR 25 mg" other half; 50 mg capsules branded "SANDOZ 78–78" on one half, "PAMELOR 50 mg" other half; and 75 mg capsules branded "SANDOZ 78–79" on one half, "PAMELOR 75 mg" other half.

Store and Dispense: Below 86°F; tight container.
Solution: Pamelor® (nortriptyline HCl) USP, equivalent to 10 mg base per 5 mL is supplied in 16-fluid-ounce bottles. Alcohol content 4%.
Store and Dispense: Below 86°F; tight, light-resistant container.

[PAM-Z17]
Shown in Product Identification Section, page 427

PARLODEL®   ℞

[*par'lō-del"*]
SnapTabs™
(bromocriptine mesylate) TABLETS, USP
(bromocriptine mesylate) CAPSULES

The following prescribing information is based on official labeling in effect August 1, 1989.

DESCRIPTION

Parlodel® (bromocriptine mesylate) is an ergot derivative with potent dopamine receptor agonist activity. Each Parlodel® (bromocriptine mesylate) SnapTab™ for oral administration contains 2½ mg and each capsule contains 5 mg bromocriptine (as the mesylate). Parlodel® (bromocriptine mesylate) is chemically designated as (1) Ergotaman-3′,6′,18-trione,2-bromo-12′-hydroxy-2′-(1-methylethyl) -5′- (2-methylpropyl)-,(5′α) monomethanesulfonate (salt); (2) 2-bromoergocryptine monomethanesulfonate (salt).*
Structural Formula

2.5 mg SnapTabs™
Active Ingredient: bromocriptine mesylate, USP
Inactive Ingredients: colloidal silicon dioxide, lactose, magnesium stearate, povidone, starch, and another ingredient
5 mg Capsules
Active Ingredient: bromocriptine mesylate, USP
Inactive Ingredients: colloidal silicon dioxide, gelatin, lactose, magnesium stearate, red iron oxide, silicon dioxide, sodium bisulfite, sodium lauryl sulfate, starch, titanium dioxide, yellow iron oxide, and another ingredient

CLINICAL PHARMACOLOGY

Parlodel® (bromocriptine mesylate) is a dopamine receptor agonist, which activates post-synaptic dopamine receptors. The dopaminergic neurons in the tuberoinfundibular process modulate the secretion of prolactin from the anterior pituitary by secreting a prolactin inhibitory factor (thought to be dopamine); in the corpus striatum the dopaminergic neurons are involved in the control of motor function. Clinically, Parlodel® (bromocriptine mesylate) significantly reduces plasma levels of prolactin in patients with physiologically elevated prolactin as well as in patients with hyperprolactinemia. The inhibition of physiological lactation as well as galactorrhea in pathological hyperprolactinemic states is obtained at dose levels that do not affect secretion of other tropic hormones from the anterior pituitary. Experiments have demonstrated that bromocriptine induces long lasting stereotyped behavior in rodents and turning behavior in rats having unilateral lesions in the substantia nigra. These actions, characteristic of those produced by dopamine, are inhibited by dopamine antagonists and suggest a direct action of bromocriptine on striatal dopamine receptors.

Parlodel® (bromocriptine mesylate) is a nonhormonal, nonestrogenic agent that inhibits the secretion of prolactin in humans, with little or no effect on other pituitary hormones, except in patients with acromegaly, where it lowers elevated blood levels of growth hormone in the majority of patients.

In about 75% of cases of amenorrhea and galactorrhea, Parlodel® (bromocriptine mesylate) therapy suppresses the galactorrhea completely, or almost completely, and reinitiates normal ovulatory menstrual cycles.

Menses are usually reinitiated prior to complete suppression of galactorrhea; the time for this on average is 6–8 weeks. However, some patients respond within a few days, and others may take up to 8 months.

Galactorrhea may take longer to control depending on the degree of stimulation of the mammary tissue prior to therapy. At least a 75% reduction in secretion is usually observed after 8–12 weeks. Some patients may fail to respond even after 12 months of therapy.

Parlodel® (bromocriptine mesylate), by virtue of its ability to inhibit prolactin secretion, acts to prevent physiological lactation in women when therapy is started after delivery and continued for two to three weeks. There is no evidence that Parlodel® (bromocriptine mesylate) acts on the mammary tissues to prevent lactation, as is the case with estrogen containing preparations.

In many acromegalic patients, Parlodel® (bromocriptine mesylate) produces a prompt and sustained reduction in circulating levels of serum growth hormone.

Parlodel® (bromocriptine mesylate) produces its therapeutic effect in the treatment of Parkinson's disease, a clinical condition characterized by a progressive deficiency in dopamine synthesis in the substantia nigra, by directly stimulating the dopamine receptors in the corpus striatum. In contrast, levodopa exerts its therapeutic effect only after conversion to dopamine by the neurons of the substantia nigra, which are known to be numerically diminished in this patient population.

PHARMACOKINETICS

The pharmacokinetics and metabolism of bromocriptine in human subjects were studied with the help of radioactively labeled drug. Twenty-eight percent of an oral dose was absorbed from the gastrointestinal tract. The blood levels following a 2½ mg dose were in the range of 2–3 ng equivalents/mL. Plasma levels were in the range of 4–6 ng equivalents/mL indicating that the red blood cells did not contain appreciable amounts of drug and/or metabolites. *In vitro* experiments showed that the drug was 90–96% bound to serum albumin.

Bromocriptine was completely metabolized prior to excretion. The major route of excretion of absorbed drug was via the bile. Only 2.5–5.5% of the dose was excreted in the urine. Almost all (84.6%) of the administered dose was excreted in the feces in 120 hours.

INDICATIONS AND USAGE

Hyperprolactinemia-associated Dysfunctions
Parlodel® (bromocriptine mesylate) is indicated for the treatment of dysfunctions associated with **hyperprolactinemia** including **amenorrhea** with or without **galactorrhea, infertility or hypogonadism.** Parlodel® (bromocriptine mesylate) treatment is indicated in patients with **prolactin-secreting adenomas,** which may be the basic underlying endocrinopathy contributing to the above clinical presentations. **Reduction** in **tumor size** has been demonstrated in both male and female patients with macroadenomas. In cases where adenectomy is elected, a course of Parlodel® (bromocriptine mesylate) therapy may be used to reduce the tumor mass prior to surgery.
Prevention of Physiological Lactation
Parlodel® (bromocriptine mesylate) SnapTabs™ are indicated for the prevention of physiological lactation (secretion, congestion, and engorgement) occurring:
1. After parturition when the mother elects not to breast feed the infant, or when breast feeding is contraindicated.
2. After stillbirth or abortion.
The physician should keep in mind that the incidence of significant painful engorgement is low and usually responsive to appropriate supportive therapy. In contrast with supportive therapy, Parlodel® (bromocriptine mesylate) prevents the secretion of prolactin, thus inhibiting lactogenesis and the subsequent development of secretion, congestion and engorgement.

Once Parlodel® (bromocriptine mesylate) therapy is stopped, 18% to 40% of patients experience rebound of breast secretion, congestion or engorgement, which is usually mild to moderate in severity.
Acromegaly
Parlodel® (bromocriptine mesylate) therapy is indicated in the treatment of acromegaly. Parlodel® (bromocriptine mesylate) therapy, alone or as adjunctive therapy with pituitary irradiation or surgery, reduces serum growth hormone by 50% or more in approximately one-half of patients treated, although not usually to normal levels.

Since the effects of external pituitary radiation may not become maximal for several years, adjunctive therapy with Parlodel® (bromocriptine mesylate) offers potential benefit before the effects of irradiation are manifested.
Parkinson's Disease
Parlodel® (bromocriptine mesylate) SnapTabs™ or capsules are indicated in the treatment of the signs and symptoms of idiopathic or postencephalitic Parkinson's disease. As adjunctive treatment to levodopa (alone or with a peripheral decarboxylase inhibitor), Parlodel® (bromocriptine mesylate) therapy may provide additional therapeutic benefits in those patients who are currently maintained on optimal dosages of levodopa, those who are beginning to deteriorate (develop tolerance) to levodopa therapy, and those who are experiencing "end of dose failure" on levodopa therapy. Parlodel® (bromocriptine mesylate) therapy may permit a reduction of the maintenance dose of levodopa and, thus may ameliorate the occurence and/or severity of adverse reactions associated with long-term levodopa therapy such as abnormal involuntary movements (e.g., dyskinesias) and the marked swings in motor function ("on-off" phenomenon). Continued efficacy of Parlodel® (bromocriptine mesylate) therapy during treatment of more than two years has not been established.

Data are insufficient to evaluate potential benefit from treating newly diagnosed Parkinson's disease with Parlodel® (bromocriptine mesylate). Studies have shown, however, significantly more adverse reactions (notably nausea, hallucinations, confusion and hypotension) in Parlodel® (bromocriptine mesylate) treated patients than in levodopa/carbidopa treated patients. Patients unresponsive to levodopa are poor candidates for Parlodel® (bromocriptine mesylate) therapy.

CONTRAINDICATIONS

Uncontrolled hypertension, toxemia of pregnancy, sensitivity to any ergot alkaloids.

WARNINGS

Since hyperprolactinemia with amenorrhea/galactorrhea and infertility has been found in patients with pituitary tumors, a complete evaluation of the pituitary is indicated before treatment with Parlodel® (bromocriptine mesylate).

If pregnancy occurs during Parlodel® (bromocriptine mesylate) administration, careful observation of these patients is mandatory. Prolactin-secreting adenomas may expand and compression of the optic or other cranial nerves may occur, emergency pituitary surgery becoming necessary. In most cases, the compression resolves following delivery. Reinitiation of Parlodel® (bromocriptine mesylate) treatment has been reported to produce improvement in the visual fields of patients in whom nerve compression has occurred during pregnancy. The safety of Parlodel® (bromocriptine mesylate) treatment during pregnancy to the mother and fetus has not been established.

Symptomatic hypotension can occur in patients treated with Parlodel® (bromocriptine mesylate) for any indication.

In postpartum studies with Parlodel® (bromocriptine mesylate), decreases in supine systolic and diastolic pressures of greater than 20 mm and 10 mm Hg, respectively, have been observed in almost 30% of patients receiving Parlodel® (bromocriptine mesylate). On occasion, the drop in supine systolic pressure was as much as 50–59 mm of Hg. Since decreases in blood pressure are frequently noted during the puerperium independent of drug therapy, it is likely that many of these decreases in blood pressure observed with Parlodel® (bromocriptine mesylate) therapy were not drug induced. **While hypotension during the start of therapy with Parlodel® (bromocriptine mesylate) occurs in some patients, 50 cases of hypertension have been reported, sometimes at the initiation of therapy, but often developing in the second week of therapy. Seizures have been reported in 38 cases (including 4 cases of status epilepticus), both with and without the prior development of hypertension occurring mostly in postpartum patients up to 14 days after initiation of treatment. Fifteen cases of stroke during Parlodel® (bromocriptine mesylate) therapy have been reported mostly in postpartum patients whose prenatal and obstetric courses had been**

Continued on next page

Sandoz Pharm.—Cont.

uncomplicated. Many of these patients experiencing seizures and/or strokes reported developing a constant and often progressively severe headache hours to days prior to the acute event. Some cases of strokes and seizures during therapy with Parlodel® (bromocriptine mesylate) were also preceded by visual disturbances (blurred vision, and transient cortical blindness). Four cases of acute myocardial infarction have been reported, including 3 cases receiving Parlodel® (bromocriptine mesylate) for the prevention of physiological lactation. The relationship of these adverse reactions to Parlodel® (bromocriptine mesylate) administration is not certain. The use of Parlodel® (bromocriptine mesylate) is not recommended for patients with uncontrolled hypertension or toxemia of pregnancy. Although there is no conclusive evidence which demonstrates the interaction between Parlodel® (bromocriptine mesylate) and other ergot alkaloids, the concomitant use of these medications is not recommended. Particular attention should be paid to patients who have recently received other drugs that can alter the blood pressure. Parlodel® (bromocriptine mesylate) therapy for the prevention of postpartum lactation should not be initiated until the vital signs have been stabilized and no sooner than four hours after delivery. Periodic monitoring of the blood pressure, particularly during the first weeks of therapy and especially during the postpartum period, is prudent. If hypertension, severe, progressive, or unremitting headache (with or without visual disturbance), or evidence of CNS toxicity develops, drug therapy should be discontinued and the patient should be evaluated promptly.

Long-term treatment (6–36 months) with Parlodel® (bromocriptine mesylate) in doses ranging from 20–100 mg/day has been associated with pulmonary infiltrates, pleural effusion and thickening of the pleura in a few patients. In those instances in which Parlodel® (bromocriptine mesylate) treatment was terminated, the changes slowly reverted towards normal.

PRECAUTIONS

General

Safety and efficacy of Parlodel® (bromocriptine mesylate) have not been established in patients with renal or hepatic disease. Care should be exercised when administering Parlodel® (bromocriptine mesylate) therapy concomitantly with other medications known to lower blood pressure.

Hyperprolactinemic States

The relative efficacy of Parlodel® (bromocriptine mesylate) versus surgery in preserving visual fields is not known. Patients with rapidly progressive visual field loss should be evaluated by a neurosurgeon to help decide on the most appropriate therapy. Since pregnancy is often the therapeutic objective in many hyperprolactinemic patients presenting with amenorrhea/galactorrhea and hypogonadism (infertility) a careful assessment of the pituitary is essential to detect the presence of a prolactin secreting adenoma. Patients not seeking pregnancy, or those harboring large adenomas, should be advised to use contraceptive measures, other than the oral contraceptives, during treatment with Parlodel® (bromocriptine mesylate). Since pregnancy may occur prior to reinitiation of menses, a pregnancy test is recommended at least every four weeks during the amenorrheic period, and, once menses are reinitiated, every time a patient misses a menstrual period. Treatment with Parlodel® (bromocriptine mesylate) SnapTabs™ or capsules should be discontinued as soon as pregnancy has been established. Patients must be monitored closely throughout pregnancy for signs and symptoms that may signal the enlargement of a previously undetected or existing prolactin-secreting tumor. Discontinuation of Parlodel® (bromocriptine mesylate) treatment in patients with known macroadenomas has been associated with rapid regrowth of tumor and increase in serum prolactin in most cases.

Use in Pregnancy

In human studies with Parlodel® (bromocriptine mesylate) there have been 1276 reported pregnancies, which have yielded 1109 live and 4 stillborn infants from women who took Parlodel® (bromocriptine mesylate) during pregnancy. The majority of these patients received Parlodel® (bromocriptine mesylate) therapy during the first two to three weeks of pregnancy and several received the drug for up to three months and 5 were treated for the entire period of gestation. Several studies in the literature reported on the use of Parlodel® (bromocriptine mesylate) during the final weeks of pregnancy to reduce plasma levels of prolactin in cases where possible pituitary tumor expansion occurred. Among the 1113 infants, 37 cases of congenital anomalies have been reported. There were 9 major malformations which included 3 limb reduction defects and 28 minor malformations which include 8 hip dislocations. The total incidence of malformations (3.3%) and the incidence of spontaneous abortions (11%) in this group of pregnancies does not exceed that generally reported for the population at large. There were three hydatidiform moles, two of which occurred in the same patient.

Physiological Lactation

Decreases in the blood pressure are common during the puerperium and, since Parlodel® (bromocriptine mesylate) therapy is known to produce hypotension and, rarely, hypertension in some patients, the drug should not be administered until the vital signs have been stabilized. Because the development of hypertension may be delayed, it is prudent to monitor the blood pressure periodically during the first weeks of therapy. If hypertension, severe, progressive, or unremitting headache (with or without visual disturbance), or evidence of CNS toxicity develops, drug therapy should be discontinued and the patient should be evaluated promptly.

Acromegaly

Cold sensitive digital vasospasm has been observed in some acromegalic patients treated with Parlodel® (bromocriptine mesylate). The response, should it occur, can be reversed by reducing the dose of Parlodel® (bromocriptine mesylate) and may be prevented by keeping the fingers warm. Cases of severe gastrointestinal bleeding from peptic ulcers have been reported, some fatal. Although there is no evidence that Parlodel® (bromocriptine mesylate) increases the incidence of peptic ulcers in acromegalic patients, symptoms suggestive of peptic ulcer should be investigated thoroughly and treated appropriately.

Possible tumor expansion while receiving Parlodel® (bromocriptine mesylate) therapy has been reported in a few patients. Since the natural history of growth hormone secreting tumors is unknown, all patients should be carefully monitored and, if evidence of tumor expansion develops, discontinuation of treatment and alternative procedures considered.

Parkinson's Disease

Safety during long-term use for more than two years at the doses required for parkinsonism has not been established. As with any chronic therapy, periodic evaluation of hepatic, hematopoietic, cardiovascular, and renal function is recommended. Symptomatic hypotension can occur and, therefore, caution should be exercised when treating patients receiving antihypertensive drugs.

High doses of Parlodel® (bromocriptine mesylate) may be associated with confusion and mental disturbances. Since parkinsonian patients may manifest mild degrees of dementia, caution should be used when treating such patients. Parlodel® (bromocriptine mesylate) administered alone or concomitantly with levodopa may cause hallucinations (visual or auditory). Hallucinations usually resolve with dosage reduction; occasionally, discontinuation of Parlodel® (bromocriptine mesylate) is required. Rarely, after high doses, hallucinations have persisted for several weeks following discontinuation of Parlodel® (bromocriptine mesylate). As with levodopa, caution should be exercised when administering Parlodel® (bromocriptine mesylate) to patients with a history of myocardial infarction who have a residual atrial, nodal, or ventricular arrhythmia.

Retroperitoneal fibrosis has been reported in a few patients receiving long-term therapy (2–10 years) with Parlodel® (bromocriptine mesylate) in doses ranging from 30 to 140 mg daily.

Nursing Mothers

Since it prevents lactation, Parlodel® (bromocriptine mesylate) should not be administered to mothers who elect to breast feed infants.

Pediatric Use

Safety and efficacy of Parlodel® (bromocriptine mesylate) have not been established in children under the age of 15.

INFORMATION FOR PATIENTS

When initiating therapy, all patients receiving Parlodel® (bromocriptine mesylate) should be cautioned with regard to engaging in activities requiring rapid and precise responses, such as driving an automobile or operating machinery since dizziness (8–16%), drowsiness (8%), faintness, fainting (8%), and syncope (less than 1%) have been reported early in the course of therapy. Patients receiving Parlodel® (bromocriptine mesylate) for hyperprolactinemic states associated with macroadenoma or those who have had previous transsphenoidal surgery, should be told to report any persistent watery nasal discharge to their physician. Patients receiving Parlodel® (bromocriptine mesylate) for treatment of a macroadenoma should be told that discontinuation of drug may be associated with rapid regrowth of the tumor and recurrence of their original symptoms. Patients receiving Parlodel® (bromocriptine mesylate) for the prevention of physiological lactation should be advised to stop the drug and seek prompt medical attention including blood pressure evaluation should severe, progressive, or unremitting headache develop during therapy.

DRUG INTERACTIONS

Lack or decrease in efficacy may occur in patients receiving Parlodel® (bromocriptine mesylate) when they are treated concurrently with drugs which have dopamine antagonist activity, e.g. phenothiazines, butyrophenones. This may be a problem particularly for patients treated with Parlodel® (bromocriptine mesylate) for macroadenomas. Although there is no conclusive evidence demonstrating interactions between Parlodel® (bromocriptine mesylate) and other ergot derivatives, the concomitant use of these medications is not recommended.

ADVERSE REACTIONS

Hyperprolactinemic Indications

The incidence of adverse effects is quite high (69%) but these are generally mild to moderate in degree. Therapy was discontinued in approximately 5% of patients because of adverse effects. These in decreasing order of frequency are: nausea (49%), headache (19%), dizziness (17%), fatigue (7%), lightheadedness (5%), vomiting (5%), abdominal cramps (4%), nasal congestion (3%), constipation (3%), diarrhea (3%) and drowsiness (3%).

A slight hypotensive effect may accompany Parlodel® (bromocriptine mesylate) treatment. The occurence of adverse reactions may be lessened by temporarily reducing dosage to one-half SnapTab™ two or three times daily. A few cases of cerebrospinal fluid rhinorrhea have been reported in patients receiving Parlodel® (bromocriptine mesylate) for treatment of large prolactinomas. This has occurred rarely, usually only in patients who have received previous transsphenoidal surgery, pituitary radiation, or both, and who were receiving Parlodel® (bromocriptine mesylate) for tumor recurrence. It may also occur in previously untreated patients whose tumor extends into the sphenoid sinus.

Physiological Lactation

Twenty-three percent of patients treated within the recommended dosage range for the prevention of physiological lactation had at least one side effect, but they were generally mild to moderate in degree. Therapy was discontinued in approximately 3% of patients. The most frequently occurring adverse reactions were: headache (10%), dizziness (8%), nausea (7%), vomiting (3%), fatigue (1.0%), syncope (0.7%), diarrhea (0.4%) and cramps (0.4%). Decreases in blood pressure (≥ 20 mm Hg systolic and ≥ 10 mm Hg diastolic) occurred in 28% of patients at least once during the first three postpartum days; these were usually of a transient nature. Reports of fainting in the puerperium may possibly be related to this effect. Serious adverse reactions reported include 38 cases of seizures (including 4 cases of status epilepticus), 15 cases of stroke, and 3 cases of myocardial infarction among postpartum patients. Seizure cases were not necessarily accompanied by the development of hypertension. An unremitting and often progressively severe headache, sometimes accompanied by visual disturbance, often preceded by hours to days many cases of seizure and/or stroke. Most patients had shown no evidence of toxemia during the pregnancy. One stroke case was associated with sagittal sinus thrombosis, and another was associated with cerebral and cerebellar vasculitis. One case of myocardial infarction was associated with unexplained disseminated intravascular coagulation and a second occurred in conjunction with use of another ergot alkaloid. The relationship of these adverse reactions to Parlodel® (bromocriptine mesylate) administration has not been established.

Acromegaly

The most frequent adverse reactions encountered in acromegalic patients treated with Parlodel® (bromocriptine mesylate) were: nausea (18%), constipation (14%), postural/orthostatic hypotension (6%), anorexia (4%), dry mouth/nasal stuffiness (4%), indigestion/dyspepsia (4%), digital vasospasm (3%), drowsiness/tiredness (3%) and vomiting (2%). Less frequent adverse reactions (less than 2%) were: gastrointestinal bleeding, dizziness, exacerbation of Raynaud's Syndrome, headache and syncope. Rarely (less than 1%) hair loss, alcohol potentiation, faintness, lightheadedness, arrhythmia, ventricular tachycardia, decreased sleep requirement, visual hallucinations, lassitude, shortness of breath, bradycardia, vertigo, paresthesia, sluggishness, vasovagal attack, delusional psychosis, paranoia, insomnia, heavy headedness, reduced tolerance to cold, tingling of ears, facial pallor and muscle cramps have been reported.

Parkinson's Disease

In clinical trials in which bromocriptine was administered with concomitant reduction in the dose of levodopa/carbidopa, the most common newly appearing adverse reactions were: nausea, abnormal involuntary movements, hallucinations, confusion, "on-off" phenomenon, dizziness, drowsiness, faintness/fainting, vomiting, asthenia, abdominal discomfort, visual disturbance, ataxia, insomnia, depression, hypotension, shortness of breath, constipation, and vertigo. Less common adverse reactions which may be encountered include: anorexia, anxiety, blepharospasm, dry mouth, dysphagia, edema of the feet and ankles, erythromelalgia, epileptiform seizure, fatigue, headache, lethargy, mottling of skin, nasal stuffiness, nervousness, nightmares, paresthesia, skin rash, urinary frequency, urinary incontinence, urinary retention, and rarely, signs and symptoms of ergotism such as tingling of fingers, cold feet, numbness, muscle cramps of feet and legs or exacerbation of Raynaud's syndrome.

Abnormalities in laboratory tests may include elevations in blood urea nitrogen, SGOT, SGPT, GGPT, CPK, alkaline phosphatase and uric acid, which are usually transient and not of clinical significance.

DOSAGE AND ADMINISTRATION

General

It is recommended that Parlodel® (bromocriptine mesylate) be taken with food. Patients should be evaluated frequently during dose escalation to determine the lowest dosage that produces a therapeutic response.

Hyperprolactinemic Indications

The initial dosage of Parlodel® (bromocriptine mesylate) is one-half to one $2\frac{1}{2}$ mg SnapTab™ daily. An additional $2\frac{1}{2}$ mg SnapTab™ may be added to the treatment regimen as tolerated every 3–7 days until an optimal therapeutic response is achieved. The therapeutic dosage usually is 5–7.5 mg and ranges from 2.5–15 mg/day.

In order to reduce the likelihood of prolonged exposure to Parlodel® (bromocriptine mesylate) should an unsuspected pregnancy occur, a mechanical contraceptive should be used in conjunction with Parlodel® (bromocriptine mesylate) therapy until normal ovulatory menstrual cycles have been restored. Contraception may then be discontinued in patients desiring pregnancy.

Thereafter, if menstruation does not occur within 3 days of the expected date, Parlodel® (bromocriptine mesylate) therapy should be discontinued and a pregnancy test performed.

Prevention of Physiological Lactation

Therapy should be started only after the patient's vital signs have been stabilized and no sooner than four hours after delivery. The recommended therapeutic dosage is one $2\frac{1}{2}$ mg SnapTab™ of Parlodel® (bromocriptine mesylate) twice daily. The usual dosage range is 2.5–7.5 mg daily. Parlodel® (bromocriptine mesylate) therapy should be continued for 14 days; however, therapy may be given for up to 21 days if necessary.

Acromegaly

Virtually all acromegalic patients receiving therapeutic benefit from Parlodel® (bromocriptine mesylate) also have reductions in circulating levels of growth hormone. Therefore periodic assessment of circulating levels of growth hormone will, in most cases, serve as a guide in determining the therapeutic potential of Parlodel® (bromocriptine mesylate). If, after a brief trial with Parlodel® (bromocriptine mesylate) therapy, no significant reduction in growth hormone levels has taken place, careful assessment of the clinical features of the disease should be made, and if no change has occurred, dosage adjustment or discontinuation of therapy should be considered.

The initial recommended dosage is $\frac{1}{2}$ to one $2\frac{1}{2}$ mg Parlodel® (bromocriptine mesylate) SnapTab™ on retiring (with food) for 3 days. An additional $\frac{1}{2}$ to 1 SnapTab™ should be added to the treatment regimen as tolerated every 3–7 days until the patient obtains optimal therapeutic benefit. Patients should be reevaluated monthly and the dosage adjusted based on reductions of growth hormone or clinical response. The usual optimal therapeutic dosage range of Parlodel® (bromocriptine mesylate) varies from 20 to 30 mg per day in most patients. The maximal dosage should not exceed 100 mg per day.

Patients treated with pituitary irradiation should be withdrawn from Parlodel® (bromocriptine mesylate) therapy on a yearly basis to assess both the clinical effects of radiation on the disease process as well as the effects of Parlodel® (bromocriptine mesylate) therapy. Usually a four to eight week withdrawal period is adequate for this purpose. Recurrence of the signs/symptoms or increases in growth hormone indicate the disease process is still active and further courses of Parlodel® (bromocriptine mesylate) should be considered.

Parkinson's Disease

The basic principle of Parlodel® (bromocriptine mesylate) therapy is to initiate treatment at a low dosage and, on an individual basis, increase the daily dosage slowly until a maximum therapeutic response is achieved. The dosage of levodopa during this introductory period should be maintained, if possible. The initial dose of Parlodel® (bromocriptine mesylate) is $\frac{1}{2}$ of a $2\frac{1}{2}$ mg SnapTab™ twice daily with meals. Assessments are advised at two week intervals during dosage titration to ensure that the lowest dosage producing an optimal therapeutic response is not exceeded. If necessary, the dosage may be increased every 14 to 28 days by $2\frac{1}{2}$ mg per day with meals. Should it be advisable to reduce the dosage of levodopa because of adverse reactions, the daily dosage of Parlodel® (bromocriptine mesylate), if increased, should be accomplished gradually in small ($2\frac{1}{2}$ mg) increments.

The safety of Parlodel® (bromocriptine mesylate) has not been demonstrated in dosages exceeding 100 mg per day.

HOW SUPPLIED

SnapTabs™, $2\frac{1}{2}$ mg

Round, white, scored SnapTabs™, each containing $2\frac{1}{2}$ mg bromocriptine (as the mesylate) in packages of 30 (NDC 0078-0017-15) and 100 (NDC 0078-0017-05). Embossed "PARLODEL $2\frac{1}{2}$" on one side and scored on reverse side.

Capsules, 5 mg

Caramel and white capsules, each containing 5 mg bromocriptine (as the mesylate) in packages of 30 (NDC 0078-0102-

15) and 100 (NDC 0078-0102-05). Imprinted "PARLODEL 5 mg" on one half and triangle (S) on other half.

Store and Dispense

Below 77°F; tight, light-resistant container.
[PAR-Z20 ISSUED JULY 15, 1988]
*U.S. Pat. Nos. 3.752.814 and 3.752.888
Shown in Product Identification Section, page 427

RESTORIL®   ℞
[res 'tah-ril "]
(temazepam) capsules

The following prescribing information is based on official labeling in effect on August 1, 1989.

DESCRIPTION

Restoril® (temazepam) is a benzodiazepine hypnotic agent. The chemical name is 7-chloro-1,3-dihydro-3-hydroxy-1-methyl-5-phenyl- $2H$ -1,4-benzodiazepin-2-one, and the structural formula is:

$C_{16}H_{13}ClN_2O_2$ Mo. wt. 300.74

Temazepam is a white, crystalline substance, very slightly soluble in water and sparingly soluble in alcohol USP. It has a molecular weight of 300.7.

Restoril® (temazepam) capsules, 15 mg and 30 mg, are for oral administration.

15 mg, and 30 mg Capsules
Active Ingredient: temazepam
15 mg. Capsules
Inactive Ingredients: FD&C Blue #1, FD&C Red #3, gelatin, lactose, magnesium stearate, sodium lauryl sulfate, synthetic red ferric oxide, and titanium dioxide.
May also include: benzyl alcohol, butylparaben, edetate calcium disodium, methylparaben, propylparaben, silicon dioxide, sodium propionate, and another ingredient.
30 mg, Capsules
Inactive Ingredients: FD&C Blue #1, FD&C Red #3, gelatin, lactose, magnesium stearate, sodium lauryl sulfate and titanium dioxide.
May also include: benzyl alcohol, butylparaben, edetate, calcium disodium, methylparaben, propylparaben, silicon dioxide, sodium propionate, and another ingredient.

CLINICAL PHARMACOLOGY

Restoril® (temazepam) improved sleep parameters in clinical studies. Residual medication effects ("hangover") were essentially absent. Early morning awakening, a particular problem in the geriatric patient, was significantly reduced. In sleep laboratory studies, Restoril® (temazepam) significantly improved sleep maintenance parameters [e.g., wake time after sleep onset, total sleep time, and the number of nocturnal awakenings]. There was no significant reduction in sleep latency. REM sleep was essentially unchanged, slow wave sleep was decreased, and no rebound effects occurred in these sleep stages. Transient sleep disturbance, mainly during the first night, occurred after withdrawal of the drug. In these studies, there was no evidence of tolerance when patients were given Restoril® (temazepam) nightly for approximately one month.

A single and a multiple dose absorption, distribution, metabolism, and excretion (ADME) study using ³H-labeled drug, as well as a bioavailability study, were carried out in normal volunteers. Absorption was complete and detectable blood levels were achieved at 20-40 minutes; peak concentration was reached at 2-3 hours. There was minimal (approximately 8%) first pass metabolism.

The only significant metabolite present in blood was the O-conjugate. The unchanged drug was 96% bound to plasma proteins. The blood level decline of the parent drug was biphasic with the short half-life ranging from 0.4-0.6 hours and the terminal half-life from 9.5-12.4 hours (mean: 10 hours), depending on the study population and method of determination. Metabolites were formed with a half-life of 10 hours and excreted with a half-life of approximately 2 hours. Thus, formation of the major metabolite is the rate limiting step in the biodisposition of temazepam. There is no accumulation of metabolites. The area under the blood concentration/time curve was directly proportional to the dose in the 0-45 mg range.

Temazepam was completely metabolized prior to excretion; 80%–90% of the dose appeared in the urine. The major metabolite was the O-conjugate of temazepam (90%); the O-conjugate of N-demethyl temazepam was a minor metabolite (7%). There were no active metabolites.

At a dose of 30 mg once a day for 8 weeks, no evidence of enzyme induction was found in man.

The steady state plasma concentration measured under therapeutic sleep laboratory conditions was 382 $\pm$ 192 ng/mL, 2.5 hours after a 30 mg dose, and 26 ng/mL at 24 hours. On a once-a-day regimen, steady state was attained on the third day.

INDICATIONS AND USAGE

Restoril® (temazepam) is indicated for the relief of insomnia associated with the complaints of difficulty in falling asleep, frequent nocturnal awakenings, and/or early morning awakenings. In clinical trials there is a perception by patients that Restoril® (temazepam) decreases sleep latency, but sleep laboratory studies have not confirmed such an effect when the drug was administered within 30 minutes of retiring.

Since insomnia is often transient and intermittent, the prolonged administration of Restoril® (temazepam) is generally not necessary or recommended. Restoril® (temazepam) has been employed for sleep maintenance for up to 35 consecutive nights of drug administration in sleep laboratory studies.

Since insomnia may be a symptom of several other disorders, the possibility that the complaint may be related to a condition for which there is more specific treatment should be considered.

CONTRAINDICATIONS

Benzodiazepines may cause fetal damage when administered during pregnancy. An increased risk of congenital malformations associated with the use of diazepam and chlordiazepoxide during the first trimester of pregnancy has been suggested in several studies. Transplacental distribution has resulted in neonatal CNS depression following the ingestion of therapeutic doses of a benzodiazepine hypnotic during the last weeks of pregnancy.

Reproduction studies in animals with temazepam were performed in rats and rabbits. In a perinatal-postnatal study in rats, oral doses of 60 mg/kg/day resulted in increasing nursling mortality. Teratology studies in rats demonstrated increased fetal resorptions at doses of 30 and 120 mg/kg in one study and increased occurrence of rudimentary ribs, which are considered skeletal variants, in a second study at doses of 240 mg/kg or higher. In rabbits, occasional abnormalities such as exencephaly and fusion or asymmetry of ribs were reported without dose relationship. Although these abnormalities were not found in the concurrent control group, they have been reported to occur randomly in historical controls. At doses of 40 mg/kg or higher, there was an increased incidence of the 13th rib variant when compared to the incidence in concurrent and historical controls.

Restoril® (temazepam) is contraindicated in pregnant women. If there is a likelihood of the patient becoming pregnant while receiving temazepam, she should be warned of the potential risk to the fetus. Patients should be instructed to discontinue the drug prior to becoming pregnant. The possibility that a woman of childbearing potential may be pregnant at the time of institution of therapy should be considered.

WARNINGS

Patients receiving Restoril® (temazepam) should be cautioned about possible combined effects with alcohol and other CNS depressants.

Withdrawal symptoms (of the barbiturate type) have occurred after the abrupt discontinuation of benzodiazepines (see *DRUG ABUSE AND DEPENDENCE*).

PRECAUTIONS

General

Since the risk of the development of oversedation, dizziness, confusion, and/or ataxia increases, substantially with larger doses of benzodiazepines in elderly and debilitated patients, 15 mg of Restoril® (temazepam) is recommended as the initial dosage for such patients.

Restoril® (temazepam) should be administered with caution in severely depressed patients or those in whom there is any evidence of latent depression; it should be recognized that suicidal tendencies may be present and protective measures may be necessary.

The usual precautions should be observed in patients with impaired renal or hepatic function and in patients with chronic pulmonary insufficiency.

If Restoril® (temazepam) is to be combined with other drugs having known hypnotic properties or CNS-depressant effects, consideration should be given to potential additive effects.

The possibility of a synergistic effect exists with the co-administration of Restoril® (temazepam) and diphenhydramine. One case of stillbirth at term has been reported 8 hours after a pregnant patient received Restoril® (temazepam) and diphenhydramine. A cause and effect relationship has not yet been determined (see *CONTRAINDICATIONS*).

Continued on next page

Sandoz Pharm.—Cont.

Information for Patients

Patients receiving Restoril® (temazepam) should be cautioned about possible combined effects with alcohol and other CNS depressants. Patients should be cautioned not to operate machinery or drive a motor vehicle after ingesting the drug.

Patients should also be advised that, because benzodiazepines may produce psychological and physical dependence, they should consult with their physician before increasing the dose. In addition, they should be cautioned that a temporary disturbance of nocturnal sleep and other symptoms may result from discontinuation of the drug. Patients taking 30 mg or more for more than a few nights should be advised not to abruptly discontinue this drug without first consulting with their physician.

Laboratory Tests

The usual precautions should be observed in patients with impaired renal or hepatic function and in patients with chronic pulmonary insufficiency. Abnormal liver function tests as well as blood dyscrasias have been reported with benzodiazepines.

Carcinogenesis, Impairment of Fertility

No carcinogenic potential was demonstrated in long-term studies in mice and rats. Fertility in male and female rats was not adversely affected by Restoril® (temazepam).

Pregnancy

Pregnancy Category X. See *CONTRAINDICATIONS*.

Nursing Mothers

It is not known whether this drug is excreted in human milk. Because many drugs are excreted in human milk, caution should be exercised when Restoril® (temazepam) is administered to a nursing woman.

Pediatric Use

Safety and effectiveness in children below the age of 18 years have not been established.

ADVERSE REACTIONS

During clinical studies in which 795 patients received Restoril® (temazepam), the drug was well tolerated. Side effects were usually mild and transient. These 795 patients included 175 subjects who received Restoril® (temazepam) during daytime waking hours, sometimes in excess of recommended therapeutic dosage, in studies to evaluate dosage levels for safety and pharmacokinetic profiles.

The most common adverse reactions were drowsiness (17%), dizziness (7%), and lethargy (5%).

Other side effects include confusion, euphoria, and relaxed feeling (2%–3%). Less commonly reported were weakness, anorexia and diarrhea (1%–2%). Rarely reported were tremor, ataxia, lack of concentration, loss of equilibrium, falling, and palpitations (less than 1%).

Hallucinations, horizontal nystagmus, and paradoxical reactions, including excitement, stimulation, and hyperactivity were rare (less than 0.5%).

DRUG ABUSE AND DEPENDENCE

Controlled Substance

Restoril® (temazepam) is a controlled substance in Schedule IV.

Abuse and Dependence

Withdrawal symptoms, similar in character to those noted with barbiturates and alcohol (convulsions, tremor, abdominal, and muscle cramps, vomiting, and sweating), have occurred following abrupt discontinuance of benzodiazepines. The more severe withdrawal symptoms have usually been limited to those patients who received excessive doses over an extended period of time. Generally milder withdrawal symptoms (e.g., dysphoria and insomnia) have been reported following abrupt discontinuance of benzodiazepines taken continuously at therapeutic levels for several months. Consequently, after extended therapy at doses higher than 15 mg, abrupt discontinuation should generally be avoided and a gradual dosage tapering schedule followed. As with any hypnotic, caution must be exercised in administering Restoril® (temazepam) to individuals known to be addiction-prone or to those whose history suggests they may increase the dosage on their own initiative. It is desirable to limit repeated prescriptions without adequate medical supervision.

OVERDOSAGE

Manifestations of acute overdosage of Restoril® (temazepam) can be expected to reflect the CNS effects of the drug and include somnolence, confusion, and coma, with reduced or absent reflexes, respiratory depression, and hypotension. If the patient is conscious, vomiting should be induced mechanically or with emetics. Gastric lavage should be employed utilizing concurrently a cuffed endotracheal tube if the patient is unconscious to prevent aspiration and pulmonary complications. Maintenance of adequate pulmonary ventilation is essential. The use of pressor agents intravenously may be necessary to combat hypotension. Fluids should be administered intravenously to encourage diuresis. The value of dialysis has not been determined. If excitation occurs, barbiturates should not be used. It should be borne in mind that multiple agents may have been ingested.

The oral LD_{50} was 1963 mg/kg in mice, 1833 mg/kg in rats, and > 2400 mg/kg in rabbits.

DOSAGE AND ADMINISTRATION

The recommended usual adult dose is 30 mg before retiring. In some patients, 15 mg may be sufficient. As with all medications, dosage should be individualized for maximal beneficial effects. In elderly and/or debilitated patients it is recommended that therapy be initiated with 15 mg until individual responses are determined.

HOW SUPPLIED

Restoril® (temazepam) Capsules

15 mg, maroon and pink, imprinted "RESTORIL 15 mg" and "FOR SLEEP" twice on each capsule; 30 mg, maroon and blue, imprinted "RESTORIL 30 mg" and "FOR SLEEP" twice on each capsule. Supplied in bottles of 100, 15 mg (NDC 0078-0098-05), and 30 mg (NDC 0078-0099-05) and bottles of 500, 15 mg (NDC 0078-0098-08) and 30 mg (NDC 0078-0099-08). ControlPak® (continuous reverse-numbered roll of sealed blisters) packages of 25 capsules, 15 mg (NDC 0078-0098-13) and 30 mg (NDC 0078-0099-13). SandoPak® (unit-dose) packages of 100 individually labeled blisters, each containing one capsule, 15 mg (NDC 0078-0098-06) and 30 mg (NDC 0078-0099-06).

[RES-Z12 Issued July 10, 1989]
Shown in Product Identification Section, page 427

SANDIMMUNE® Oral Solution ℞
[san'di-mewn]
(cyclosporine)
SANDIMMUNE® I.V. ℞
(cyclosporine)

The following prescribing information is based on official labeling in effect on August 1, 1989.

> **WARNING**
>
> Only physicians experienced in immunosuppressive therapy and management of organ transplant patients should prescribe Sandimmune® (cyclosporine) Oral Solution and I.V. Patients receiving the drug should be managed in facilities equipped and staffed with adequate laboratory and supportive medical resources. The physician responsible for maintenance therapy should have complete information requisite for the follow-up of the patient.
> Sandimmune® (cyclosporine) Oral Solution and I.V. should be administered with adrenal corticosteroids but not with other immunosuppressive agents. Increased susceptibility to infection and the possible development of lymphoma may result from immunosuppression.

> The absorption of cyclosporine during chronic administration of Sandimmune® (cyclosporine) Oral Solution was found to be erratic. It is recommended that patients taking the oral solution over a period of time be monitored at repeated intervals for cyclosporine blood levels and subsequent dose adjustments be made in order to avoid toxicity due to high levels and possible organ rejection due to low absorption of cyclosporine. This is of special importance in liver transplants. (See Dosage and Administration section.)

DESCRIPTION

Cyclosporine, the active principle in Sandimmune® (cyclosporine) is a cyclic polypeptide immunosuppressant agent consisting of 11 amino acids. It is produced as a metabolite by the fungus species Tolypocladium inflatum Gams. Chemically, cyclosporine is designated as [R-[R*,R*-(E)]]-cyclic-(L-alanyl-D-alanyl-N-methyl-L-leucyl-N-methyl-L-leucyl-N-methyl-L-valyl-3-hydroxy-N,4-dimethyl-L-2-amino-6-octenoyl-L-α-amino-butyryl-N-methylglycyl-N-methyl-L-leucyl-L-valyl-N-methyl-L-leucyl).

Sandimmune® (cyclosporine) Oral Solution is available in 50 mL bottles.

Each mL contains:

cyclosporine .... 100 mg
alcohol, Ph. Helv. .... 12.5% by volume
dissolved in an olive oil, Ph. Helv./Labrafil® M 1944CS (polyoxyethylated oleic glycerides) vehicle which must be further diluted with milk, chocolate milk or orange juice before oral administration.

Sandimmune® (cyclosporine) I.V. is available in a 5 mL sterile ampul for I.V. administration.

Each mL contains:

cyclosporine .... 50 mg
*Cremophor® EL .... 650 mg
  (polyoxyethylated castor oil)
alcohol, Ph. Helv. .... 32.9% by volume
nitrogen .... qs
which must be diluted further with 0.9% Sodium Chloride Injection or 5% Dextrose Injection before use.
The chemical structure of cyclosporine (also known as cyclosporin A) is:

* Cremophor is the registered trademark of BASF Aktiengesellschaft.

CLINICAL PHARMACOLOGY

Sandimmune® (cyclosporine) is a potent immunosuppressive agent which in animals prolongs survival of allogeneic transplants involving skin, heart, kidney, pancreas, bone marrow, small intestine and lung. Sandimmune® (cyclosporine) has been demonstrated to suppress some humoral immunity and to a greater extent, cell-mediated reactions such as allograft rejection, delayed hypersensitivity, experimental allergic encephalomyelitis, Freund's adjuvant arthritis and graft vs. host disease in many animal species for a variety of organs.

Successful kidney, liver and heart allogeneic transplants have been performed in man using Sandimmune® (cyclosporine).

The exact mechanism of action of Sandimmune® (cyclosporine) is not known. Experimental evidence suggests that the effectiveness of cyclosporine is due to specific and reversible inhibition of immunocompetent lymphocytes in the G_0 or G_1-phase of the cell cycle. T-lymphocytes are preferentially inhibited. The T-helper cell is the main target, although the T-suppressor cell may also be suppressed. Sandimmune® (cyclosporine) also inhibits lymphokine production and release including interleukin-2 or T-cell growth factor (TCGF). No functional effects on phagocytic (changes in enzyme secretions not altered, chemotactic migration of granulocytes, macrophage migration, clearance *in vivo*) or tumor cells (growth rate, metastasis) can be detected in animals. Sandimmune® (cyclosporine) does not cause bone marrow suppression in animal models or man.

The absorption of cyclosporine from the gastrointestinal tract is incomplete and variable. Peak concentrations (C_{max}) in blood and plasma are achieved at about 3.5 hours. C_{max} and area under the plasma or blood concentration/time curve (AUC) increase with the administered dose; for blood the relationship is curvilinear (parabolic) between 0 and 1400 mg. As determined by a specific assay, C_{max} is approximately 1.0 ng/mL/mg of dose for plasma and 2.7 to 1.4 ng/mL/mg of dose for blood (for low to high doses). Compared to an intravenous infusion, the absolute bioavailability of the oral solution is approximately 30% based upon the results in two patients.

Cyclosporine is distributed largely outside the blood volume. In blood the distribution is concentration dependent. Approximately 33–47% is in plasma, 4–9% in lymphocytes, 5–12% in granulocytes and 41–58% in erythrocytes. At high concentrations, the uptake by leukocytes and erythrocytes becomes saturated. In plasma, approximately 90% is bound to proteins, primarily lipoproteins.

The disposition of cyclosporine from blood is biphasic with a terminal half-life of approximately 19 hours (range: 10–27 hours). Elimination is primarily biliary with only 6% of the dose excreted in the urine.

Cyclosporine is extensively metabolized but there is no major metabolic pathway. Only 0.1% of the dose is excreted in the urine as unchanged drug. Of 15 metabolites characterized in human urine, 7 have been assigned structures. The major pathways consist of hydroxylation of the Cγ-carbon of two of the leucine residues, Cη-carbon hydroxylation and cyclic ether formation (with oxidation of the double bond) in the side chain of the amino acid 3-hydroxyl-N,4-dimethyl-L-2-amino-6-octenoic acid and N-demethylation of N-methyl leucine residues. Hydrolysis of the cyclic peptide chain or conjugation of the above metabolites do not appear to be important biotransformation pathways.

INDICATIONS AND USAGE

Sandimmune® (cyclosporine) Oral Solution and I.V. are indicated for the prophylaxis of organ rejection in kidney, liver and heart allogeneic transplants. They are always to be used with adrenal corticosteroids. The drug may also be used in the treatment of chronic rejection in patients previously treated with other immunosuppressive agents.

Because of the risk of anaphylaxis, Sandimmune® (cyclosporine) I.V. should be reserved for patients who are unable to take the oral solution.

CONTRAINDICATIONS

Sandimmune® (cyclosporine) I.V. is contraindicated in patients with a hypersensitivity to Sandimmune® (cyclosporine) and/or Cremophor® EL (polyoxyethylated castor oil).

WARNINGS

SEE BOXED WARNINGS

Sandimmune® (cyclosporine), when used in high doses, can cause hepatotoxicity and nephrotoxicity.

It is not unusual for serum creatinine and BUN levels to be elevated during Sandimmune® (cyclosporine) therapy. These elevations in renal transplant patients do not necessarily indicate rejection, and each patient must be fully evaluated before dosage adjustment is initiated.

Nephrotoxicity has been noted in 25% of cases of renal transplantation, 38% of cases of cardiac transplantation and 37% of cases of liver transplantation. Mild nephrotoxicity was generally noted two to three months after transplant and consisted of an arrest in the fall of the pre-operative elevations of BUN and creatinine at a range of 35–45 mg/dl and 2.0–2.5 mg/dl respectively. These elevations were often responsive to dosage reduction.

More overt nephrotoxicity was seen early after transplantation and was characterized by a rapidly rising BUN and creatinine. Since these events are similar to rejection episodes care must be taken to differentiate between them. This form of nephrotoxicity is usually responsive to Sandimmune® (cyclosporine) dosage reduction.

Impaired renal function at any time requires close monitoring, and frequent dosage adjustment may be indicated. In patients with persistent high elevations of BUN and creatinine who are unresponsive to dosage adjustments, consideration should be given to switching to other immunosuppressive therapy. In the event of severe and unremitting rejection, it is preferable to allow the kidney transplant to be rejected and removed rather than increase the Sandimmune® (cyclosporine) dosage to a very high level in an attempt to reverse the rejection. Occasionally patients have developed a syndrome of thrombocytopenia and microangiopathic hemolytic anemia which may result in graft failure. Neither the pathogenesis nor the management of this syndrome is clear. Significant hyperkalemia and hyperuricemia have been seen occasionally in individual patients.

Hepatotoxicity has been noted in 4% of cases of renal transplantation, 7% of cases of cardiac transplantation and 4% of cases of liver transplantation. This was usually noted during the first month of therapy when high doses of Sandimmune® (cyclosporine) were used and consisted of elevations of hepatic enzymes and bilirubin. The chemistry elevations usually decreased with a reduction in dosage.

Lymphomas have developed in patients receiving Sandimmune® (cyclosporine) and other forms of immunosuppressive therapy after transplantation though no causal relationship has been established. With Sandimmune® (cyclosporine), some patients have developed a lymphoproliferative disorder which regresses when the drug is discontinued.

There have been reports of convulsions in adult and pediatric patients receiving cyclosporine, particularly in combination with high dose methylprednisolone.

Rarely (approximately 1 in 1000), patients receiving Sandimmune® (cyclosporine) I.V. have experienced anaphylactic reactions. Although the exact cause of these reactions is unknown, it is believed to be due to the Cremophor® EL (polyoxyethylated castor oil) used as the vehicle for the I.V. formulation. These reactions have consisted of flushing of the face and upper thorax, acute respiratory distress with dyspnea and wheezing, blood pressure changes and tachycardia. One patient died after respiratory arrest and aspiration pneumonia. In some cases, the reaction subsided after the infusion was stopped.

Patients receiving Sandimmune® (cyclosporine) I.V. should be under continuous observation for at least the first 30 minutes following start of the infusion and at frequent intervals thereafter. If anaphylaxis occurs, the infusion should be stopped. An aqueous solution of epinephrine 1:1000 should be available at the bedside as well as a source of oxygen.

Anaphylactic reactions have not been reported with the Oral Solution which lacks Cremophor® EL. In fact, patients experiencing anaphylactic reactions have been treated subsequently with the Oral Solution without incident.

Sandimmune® (cyclosporine) Oral Solution and I.V. should not be used concomitantly with other immunosuppressive agents except adrenal corticosteroids. Immunosuppression can lead to increased susceptibility to infection and the possible development of lymphoma. [See Boxed Warning.]

Care should be taken in using Sandimmune® (cyclosporine) with nephrotoxic drugs. [See Precautions.]

PRECAUTIONS

General: Patients with malabsorption may have difficulty in achieving therapeutic levels with Sandimmune® (cyclosporine) Oral Solution.

Given its hyperkalemic effect, cyclosporine should not be used concomitantly with potassium-sparing diuretics.

Hypertension is a fairly common side effect of Sandimmune® (cyclosporine) therapy (see Adverse Reactions). In

Body System/ Adverse Reaction	Randomized Kidney Patients		All Sandimmune® Patients		
	Sandimmune® (N=227) %	Azathioprine (N=228) %	Kidney (N=705) %	Heart (N=112) %	Liver (N=75) %
Genitourinary					
Renal Dysfunction	32	6	25	38	37
Cardiovascular					
Hypertension	26	18	13	53	27
Cramps	4	<1	2	<1	0
Skin					
Hirsutism	21	<1	21	28	45
Acne	6	8	2	2	1
Central Nervous System					
Tremor	12	0	21	31	55
Convulsions	3	1	1	4	5
Headache	2	<1	2	15	4
Gastrointestinal					
Gum Hyperplasia	4	0	9	5	16
Diarrhea	3	<1	3	4	8
Nausea/Vomiting	2	<1	4	10	4
Hepatotoxicity	<1	<1	4	7	4
Abdominal Discomfort	<1	0	<1	7	0
Autonomic Nervous System					
Paresthesia	3	0	1	2	1
Flushing	<1	0	4	0	4
Hematopoietic					
Leukopenia	2	19	<1	6	0
Lymphoma	<1	0	1	6	1
Respiratory					
Sinusitis	<1	0	4	3	7
Miscellaneous					
Gynecomastia	<1	0	<1	4	3

some patients with cardiac transplants antihypertensive therapy was required.

Information for Patients: Patients should be informed of the necessity of repeated laboratory tests while they are receiving the drug. They should be given careful dosage instructions, advised of the potential risks during pregnancy and informed of the increased risk of neoplasia.

Laboratory Tests: Renal and liver functions should be assessed repeatedly by measurement of BUN, serum creatinine, serum bilirubin and liver enzymes.

Drug Interactions: Care should be taken using Sandimmune® (cyclosporine) with nephrotoxic drugs since potential synergies of nephrotoxicity may occur. Drugs which have been reported to increase the hepatic metabolism of cyclosporine and *decrease* its plasma levels include rifampin, phenytoin, phenobarbital and I.V. sulfatrimethoprim; drugs which have been reported to *increase* the plasma concentration of cyclosporine by decreasing its metabolism include high dose methylprednisolone, erythromycin and the antifungal agents, ketoconazole and amphotericin B. Monitoring of plasma or blood levels of cyclosporine and appropriate dosage adjustment are essential when these drugs are used concomitantly.

Carcinogenesis, Mutagenesis and Impairment of Fertility: Cyclosporine gave no evidence of mutagenic or teratogenic effects in appropriate test systems. Only at dose levels toxic to dams, were adverse effects seen in reproduction studies in rats. (See Pregnancy.)

Carcinogenicity studies were carried out in male and female rats and mice. In the 78 week mouse study, at doses of 1, 4 and 16 mg/kg/day, evidence of a statistically significant trend was found for lymphocytic lymphomas in females, and the incidence of hepatocellular carcinomas in mid-dose males significantly exceeded the control value. In the 24 month rat study, conducted at 0.5, 2 and 8 mg/kg/day, pancreatic islet cell adenomas significantly exceeded the control rate in the low dose level. The hepatocellular carcinomas and pancreatic islet cell adenomas were not dose related.

No impairment in fertility was demonstrated in studies in male and female rats.

Pregnancy: Pregnancy Category C. Sandimmune® (cyclosporine) Oral Solution has been shown to be embryo- and fetotoxic in rats and rabbits when given in doses 2–5 times the human dose. At toxic doses (rats at 30 mg/kg/day and rabbits at 100 mg/kg/day), Sandimmune® (cyclosporine) Oral Solution was embryo- and fetotoxic as indicated by increased pre- and postnatal mortality and reduced fetal weight together with related skeletal retardations. In the well-tolerated dose range (rats at up to 17 mg/kg/day and rabbits at up to 30 mg/kg/day), Sandimmune® (cyclosporine) Oral Solution proved to be without any embryolethal or teratogenic effects.

There are no adequate and well-controlled studies in pregnant women. Sandimmune® (cyclosporine) should be used during pregnancy only if the potential benefit justifies the potential risk to the fetus.

Nursing Mothers: Since Sandimmune® (cyclosporine) is excreted in human milk, nursing should be avoided.

Pediatric Use: Although no adequate and well-controlled studies have been conducted in children, patients as young as 6 months of age have received the drug with no unusual adverse effects.

ADVERSE REACTIONS

The principal adverse reactions of Sandimmune® (cyclosporine) therapy are renal dysfunction, tremor, hirsutism, hypertension and gum hyperplasia.

The following reactions occurred in 3% or greater of 892 patients involved in clinical trials of kidney, heart and liver transplants:

[See table above].

The following reactions occurred in 2% or less of patients: allergic reactions, anemia, anorexia, confusion, conjunctivitis, edema, fever, brittle fingernails, gastritis, hearing loss, hiccups, hyperglycemia, muscle pain, peptic ulcer, thrombocytopenia, tinnitus.

The following reactions occurred rarely: anxiety, chest pain, constipation, depression, hair breaking, hematuria, joint pain, lethargy, mouth sores, myocardial infarction, night sweats, pancreatitis, pruritus, swallowing difficulty, tingling, upper GI bleeding, visual disturbance, weakness, weight loss.

[See table on top next page].

Cremophor® EL is known to cause hyperlipemia and electrophoretic abnormalities of lipoproteins. These effects are reversible upon discontinuation of treatment but are usually not a reason to stop treatment.

OVERDOSAGE

There is a minimal experience with overdosage. Because of the slow absorption of Sandimmune® (cyclosporine) Oral Solution, forced emesis would be of value up to 2 hours after administration. Transient hepatotoxicity and nephrotoxicity may occur which should resolve following drug withdrawal. General supportive measures and symptomatic treatment should be followed in all cases of overdosage. Sandimmune® (cyclosporine) is not dialyzable to any great extent, nor is it cleared well by charcoal hemoperfusion. The oral LD_{50} is 2329 mg/kg in mice, 1480 mg/kg in rats, and >1000 mg/kg in rabbits. The I.V. LD_{50} is 148 mg/kg in mice, 104 mg/kg in rats, and 46 mg/kg in rabbits.

DOSAGE AND ADMINISTRATION

Sandimmune® (cyclosporine) Oral Solution

The initial dose of Sandimmune® (cyclosporine) Oral Solution should be given 4–12 hours prior to transplantation as a single dose of 15 mg/kg per day (14–18 mg/kg per day were used in most clinical trials). This daily single dose is continued postoperatively for one to two weeks and then tapered by 5% per week to a maintenance level of 5–10 mg/kg per day. In several studies pediatric patients tolerated and required higher doses of cyclosporine. Some centers have successfully tapered the cyclosporine dose to as low as 3 mg/kg in selected renal transplant patients without an apparent rise in rejection rate.

In one large controlled study in renal transplantation, a lower initial dose of 10 mg/kg/day was used after a preoperative oral dose of 20 mg/kg. In this study, however, dosage was adjusted to achieve specific *plasma* levels as determined by

Continued on next page

Sandoz Pharm.—Cont.

RENAL TRANSPLANT PATIENTS IN WHOM THERAPY WAS DISCONTINUED

Reason for Discontinuation	Randomized Patients Sandimmune® (N=227) %	Azathioprine (N=228) %	All Sandimmune® Patients (N=705) %
Renal Toxicity	5.7	0	5.4
Infection	0	0.4	0.9
Lack of Efficacy	2.6	0.9	1.4
Acute Tubular Necrosis	2.6	0	1.0
Lymphoma/ Lymphoproliferative Disease	0.4	0	0.3
Hypertension	0	0	0.3
Hematological Abnormalities	0	0.4	0
Other	0	0	0.7

Sandimmune® (cyclosporine) was discontinued on a temporary basis and then restarted in 18 additional patients.

INFECTIOUS COMPLICATIONS IN THE RANDOMIZED RENAL TRANSPLANT PATIENTS

Complication	Cyclosporine Treatment (N=227) % of Complications	Standard Treatment* (N=228) % of Complications
Septicemia	5.3	4.8
Abcesses	4.4	5.3
Systemic Fungal Infection	2.2	3.9
Local Fungal Infection	7.5	9.6
Cytomegalovirus	4.8	12.3
Other Viral Infections	15.9	18.4
Urinary Tract Infections	21.1	20.2
Wound and Skin Infections	7.0	10.1
Pneumonia	6.2	9.2

* Some patients also received ALG.

radioimmunoassay (RIA). During the first few weeks after transplant, trough *plasma* levels of 150–250 ng/mL were sought. By three months post-transplant, trough *plasma* levels of 50–150 ng/mL were sought. These values correspond to trough *whole blood* levels of 450–750 ng/mL and 150–450 ng/mL. Overt nephrotoxicity was uncommon in that trial (although BUN and creatinine were somewhat increased on the average), perhaps because of the lower dose. Such a dose should not be considered, however, unless cyclosporine level monitoring can be obtained.

Adjunct steroid therapy is to be used. Study centers used prednisone in different tapering schedules with seemingly similar results. One center started with 2.0 mg/kg/day for days 0–4, tapered to 1.0 mg/kg/day by 1 week, 0.6 mg/kg/day by 2 weeks, 0.3 mg/kg/day by 1 month and reached a maintenance dose of 0.15 mg/kg/day by 2 months. Another center started with a 200 mg dose initially, tapered by 40 mg/day until reaching 20 mg/day and continued at this level for 60 days. A further reduction to 10 mg/day was made during the following months. In all centers adjustments in dosage were made according to the clinical situation.

To make Sandimmune® (cyclosporine) Oral Solution more palatable, the oral solution may be diluted with milk, chocolate milk, or orange juice preferably at room temperature. Take the prescribed amount of Sandimmune® (cyclosporine) from the container using the pipette supplied, after removal from the protective cover, and transfer the solution to a glass of milk, chocolate milk, or orange juice. Stir well and drink at once. Do not allow to stand before drinking. It is best to use a glass container and rinse it with more diluent to ensure that the total dose is taken. After use, dry the outside of the pipette with a clean towel and replace it in the protective cover. To avoid turbidity, do not rinse the pipette with water or other cleaning agents.

Sandimmune® (cyclosporine) I.V. Note: Anaphylactic reactions have occurred with Sandimmune® (cyclosporine) I.V. (See WARNINGS).

Patients unable to take Sandimmune® (cyclosporine) Oral Solution pre- or postoperatively may be treated with the I.V. concentrate. **Sandimmune® (cyclosporine) I.V. concentrate is administered at one third the oral dose.** The initial dose of Sandimmune® (cyclosporine) I.V. should be given 4–12 hours prior to transplantation as a single I.V. dose of 5–6 mg/kg per day. This daily single dose is continued postoperatively until the patient can tolerate the oral solution. Patients should be switched to Sandimmune® (cyclosporine) Oral Solution as soon as possible after surgery. In pediatric usage, the same dose and dosing regimen may be used. Adjunct steroid therapy is to be used. (See above.)

Immediately before use, the I.V. concentrate should be diluted 1 mL Sandimmune® (cyclosporine) I.V. in 20 mL to 100 mL 0.9% Sodium Chloride Injection or 5% Dextrose Injection and given in a slow intravenous infusion over approximately 2 to 6 hours.

The Cremophor® EL contained in the concentrate for intravenous infusion can cause phthalate stripping from PVC.

Parenteral drug products should be inspected visually for particulate matter and discoloration prior to administration, whenever solution and container permit.

Blood Level Monitoring: Several study centers have found blood level monitoring of cyclosporine useful in patient management. While no fixed relationships have yet been established, 24 hour trough values of 250–800 ng/mL (whole blood, RIA) or 50–300 ng/mL (plasma, RIA) appear to minimize side effects and rejection events. Blood level monitoring is not a replacement for renal function monitoring with serum creatinines, creatinine clearance or tissue biopsies.

HOW SUPPLIED

Sandimmune® (cyclosporine) Oral Solution is supplied in 50 mL bottles containing 100 mg of cyclosporine per mL (NDC 0078-0110-22). A graduated pipette for dispensing is provided. Sandimmune® (cyclosporine) Oral Solution should be stored and dispensed in the original container at temperatures below 86°F (30°C). Do not store in the refrigerator. Once opened, the contents must be used within 2 months.
Sandimmune® (cyclosporine) I.V. for intravenous infusion is supplied as a 5 mL sterile ampul containing 50 mg of cyclosporine per mL, in boxes of 10 ampuls (NDC 0078-0109-01). Sandimmune® (cyclosporine) I.V. should be stored at temperatures below 86°F (30°C) and protected from light. Protect from freezing.
Manufactured by SANDOZ Ltd.
Basle, Switzerland for
SANDOZ Pharmaceuticals Corporation
East Hanover, N.J. 07936
     [SDI-Z7 Issued April 1, 1988]
Shown in Product Identification Section, page 427

**IMMUNE GLOBULIN   ℞
INTRAVENOUS (HUMAN)
SANDOGLOBULIN®**
[san 'dō-glob "ü-lin]
Lyophilized Preparation

The following prescribing information is based on official labeling in effect on August 1, 1989.

DESCRIPTION

Immune Globulin Intravenous (Human)* Sandoglobulin® is a polyvalent antibody product containing in concentrated form all the IgG antibodies which regularly occur in the donor population. This immunoglobulin preparation is produced by cold alcohol precipitation from the plasma of over 8,000 volunteer U.S. donors. Part of the fractionation may be performed by another US-licensed manufacturer. Before pooling, the single donor units of plasma have been found non-reactive for hepatitis B surface antigen (HBsAg) using an FDA approved test. Sandoglobulin® (IGIV) is made suitable for intravenous use by treatment at acid pH in the presence of trace amounts of pepsin (1, 2). The preparation contains at least 96% of IgG and upon reconstitution has a pH of 6.6 ± 0.2. Most of the immunoglobulins are monomeric (7 S) IgG; the remainder consists of dimeric IgG and a small amount of polymeric IgG, traces of IgA and IgM and immunoglobulin fragments (3). The distribution of the IgG subclasses corresponds to that of normal serum (4, 5, 6). Final container lyophilized units are prepared so as to contain 1, 3 or 6 g protein and 1.67, 5 or 10 g sucrose, respectively, as well as small quantities of NaCl. The lyophilized powder is devoid of any preservatives and reconstitutes with 0.9% saline to a sterile 3% or 6% protein solution containing 5% or 10% sucrose, respectively.

*Hereinafter referred to as IGIV.

CLINICAL PHARMACOLOGY

This product contains a broad spectrum of antibody specificities against bacterial and viral antigens, that are capable of both opsonization and neutralization of microbes and toxins. The 3 week half-life of Immune Globulin Intravenous, (Human) Sandoglobulin® corresponds to that of Immune Globulin (Human) for intramuscular use, although individual variations in half-time have been observed (7, 8). Appropriate doses of Sandoglobulin® (IGIV) restore abnormally low immunoglobulin G levels to the normal range. 100% of the infused dose is available in the recipient's circulation immediately after infusion. After approximately 6 days an equilibrium is reached between the intra- and extravascular compartments. This is distributed approximately 50% intravascular and 50% extravascular. In comparison, after the intramuscular injection of an intramuscular immune globulin, the IgG requires 2–5 days to reach its maximum concentration in the intravascular compartment. This concentration corresponds to about 40% of the injected dose (8).
While Sandoglobulin® (IGIV) has been shown to be effective in some cases of idiopathic thrombocytopenic purpura (ITP) (see INDICATIONS AND USAGE), the mechanism of action in ITP has not been fully elucidated.
Toxicity from overdose has not been observed on regimens of 0.4 g per kg body weight each day for 5 days (9, 10, 11). Sucrose is added to Sandoglobulin® (IGIV) for reasons of stability, solubility and safety.
The intravenous administration of the sucrose used for stabilizing Immune Globulin Intravenous (Human) Sandoglobulin® is considered to be innocuous (12). Because sucrose is excreted unchanged in the urine when given intravenously, Sandoglobulin® (IGIV) may be given to diabetics, without compensatory changes in insulin dosage regimen.

INDICATIONS AND USAGE

Immunodeficiency
Sandoglobulin® (IGIV) is indicated for the maintenance treatment of patients with primary immunodeficiencies, e.g., in common variable immunodeficiency, severe combined immunodeficiency and primary immunoglobulin deficiency syndromes such as X-linked agammaglobulinemia (10, 13, 14, 15). Sandoglobulin® (IGIV) is preferable to intramuscular Immune Globulin (Human) preparations in treating patients who require an immediate and high increase in the intravascular immunoglobulin level (8), in patients with limited muscle mass, and in patients with bleeding tendencies for whom intramuscular injections are contraindicated. The infusions must be repeated at regular intervals.

Idiopathic Thrombocytopenic Purpura
ACUTE
A controlled study was performed in children in which Sandoglobulin® (IGIV) was compared with steroids for the treatment of acute (defined as less than 6 months duration) ITP. In this study sequential platelet levels of 30,000, 100,000 and 150,000/µl were all achieved faster with Sandoglobulin® (IGIV) than steroids and without any of the side effects associated with steroids (9, 16). However, it should be noted that many cases of acute ITP in childhood resolve spontaneously within weeks to months. Immune Globulin Intravenous (Human) Sandoglobulin® has been used with good results in the treatment of acute ITP in adult patients (18, 20, 21). In a study involving ten adults with ITP of less than 16 weeks duration, Sandoglobulin® (IGIV) therapy raised the platelet count to the normal range after a five day course. This effect lasted a mean of over 173 days (22).
CHRONIC
Children and adults with chronic (defined as greater than 6 months duration) ITP have also shown an increase (albeit temporary) in platelet counts upon administration of Sandoglobulin® (IGIV) (16, 17, 19, 22, 24). Therefore, in situations that require a rapid rise in platelet count, for example prior to surgery or in control of excessive bleeding, use of Sandoglobulin® (IGIV) should be considered. In children with chronic ITP, Sandoglobulin® (IGIV) therapy resulted in a mean rise in platelet count of 312,000/µl and an average duration of increase lasting 63 days (17). Sandoglobulin® (IGIV) therapy may be considered as a means to defer splenectomy (24). In adults, Sandoglobulin® (IGIV) therapy has been shown to be effective in maintaining the platelet count in an acceptable range with or without periodic booster therapy. The mean rise in platelet count was 93,000/µl and the average duration of the increase was 20-24 days (17, 22). However, it should be noted that not all patients will respond. Even in those patients who do respond, this treatment should not be considered to be curative.

CONTRAINDICATIONS

As with all blood products containing IgA, Sandoglobulin® (IGIV) is contraindicated in patients with selective IgA deficiency, who possess antibody to IgA. It may also be contraindicated in patients who have had severe systemic reactions to the intravenous or intramuscular administration of human immune globulin.

WARNINGS

Patients with agamma- or extreme hypogammaglobulinemia who have never before received immunoglobulin substitution treatment or whose time from last treatment is greater than 8 weeks, may be at risk of developing inflammatory reactions on rapid infusion of Immune Globulin Intravenous (Human) Sandoglobulin® (over 20 drops [1 mL] per minute). These reactions are manifested by a rise in temperature, chills, nausea and vomiting. The patient's vital signs should be monitored continuously and he should be carefully observed throughout the infusion, since these reactions on rare occasions may lead to shock. Epinephrine should be available for treatment of an acute anaphylactic reaction. Particular care should be exercised when Sandoglobulin® (IGIV) is administered to patients with paraproteins (15).

PRECAUTIONS

It is generally advisable not to dilute plasma derivatives with other infusable drugs. Sandoglobulin® (IGIV) should be given by a separate infusion line. No other medications or fluids should be mixed with the Sandoglobulin® (IGIV) preparation.

Pregnancy

Pregnancy Category C. Animal reproduction studies have not been conducted with Sandoglobulin® (IGIV). It is also not known whether Sandoglobulin® (IGIV) can cause fetal harm when administered to a pregnant woman or can affect reproduction capacity. Sandoglobulin® (IGIV) should be given to a pregnant woman only if clearly needed (21).

Pediatric Use

High dose administration of Immune Globulin Intravenous (Human) Sandoglobulin® in children with acute or chronic idiopathic thrombocytopenic purpura did not reveal any pediatric-specific hazard (9).

ADVERSE REACTIONS

Adverse reactions to Sandoglobulin® (IGIV) are rare and occur in less than 1% of patients who are not immunodeficient. Agammaglobulinemic and hypogammaglobulinemic patients who have never received immunoglobulin substitution therapy whose time from last treatment is greater than 8 weeks may show adverse reactions if the initial infusion flow rate exceeds 20 drops (1 mL) per minute. This occurs in approximately 10% of such cases.

These reactions, which generally become apparent only 30 minutes to one hour after the beginning of the infusion, are as follows: flushing of the face, feelings of tightness in the chest, chills, fever, dizziness, nausea, diaphoresis and hypotension. In such cases the infusion should be temporarily stopped until the symptoms have subsided. Immediate anaphylactoid and hypersensitivity reactions due to previous sensitization of the recipient to certain antigens, most commonly IgA, may be observed in exceptional cases, described under CONTRAINDICATIONS (10, 11, 23).

In patients with ITP, who received higher doses (0.4 g/kg/day or greater) 2.9% of infusions many result in adverse reactions (16). Headache generally mild, is the most common symptom noted, occurring during or following 2% of infusions.

DOSAGE AND ADMINISTRATION

Adult and child substitution therapy

The usual dose of Sandoglobulin® (IGIV) in immunodeficiency syndromes is 0.2 g per kg of body weight administered once a month by intravenous infusion. If the clinical response is inadequate, the dose may be increased to 0.3 g per kg of body weight or the infusion may be repeated more frequently than once a month (10, 13, 14, 15).

The first infusion of Immune Globulin Intravenous (Human) Sandoglobulin® in previously untreated agammaglobulinemic or hypogammaglobulinemic patients must be given as a 3% immunoglobulin solution (use the total volume of fluid provided to reconstitute the lyophilized product). Start with a flow rate of 10 to 20 drops (0.5 to 1.0 mL) per minute. After 15–30 minutes the rate of infusion may be further increased to 30 to 50 drops (1.5 to 2.5 mL) per minute. Subsequent infusions may be administered at a rate of 40 to 50 drops (2.0 to 2.5 mL) per minute.

After the first bottle of 3% solution is infused and the patient shows good tolerance, subsequent bottles may be infused as a 6% solution (Use half the volume of fluid provided to reconstitute the lyophilized product). In this case the initial rate of infusion should be 20 to 30 drops (1.0 to 1.5 mL) per minute, increased after 15–30 minutes to a maximum of 50 drops (2.5 mL) per minute.

Recent investigations confirm that Sandoglobulin® (IGIV) is well tolerated and not likely to produce side effects when infused at these rates (11). However, the first infusion of Sandoglobulin® (IGIV) in previously untreated agamma-

globulinemic and hypogammaglobulinemic patients may lead to systemic side effects. Some of the effects may occur as a result of the reaction between the antibodies administered and free antigens in the blood and tissues of the immunodeficient recipient (11, 23). When free antigen is no longer present, further administration of Sandoglobulin® (IGIV) to immunodeficient patients as well as to normal individuals usually does not cause further untoward side effects.

Therapy of idiopathic thrombocytopenic purpura (ITP)

INDUCTION

0.4 g per kg of body weight on 2 to 5 consecutive days.

ACUTE ITP-CHILDHOOD

In acute ITP of childhood, if an initial platelet count response to the first two doses is adequate (30-50,000/μl), therapy may be discontinued after the second day of the five day course (16).

MAINTENANCE-Chronic ITP

In adults and children, if after induction therapy the platelet count falls to less than 30,000/μl and/or the patient manifests clinically significant bleeding, 0.4 g/kg of body weight may be given as a single infusion. If an adequate response does not result, the dose can be increased to 0.8-1.0 g/kg of body weight given as a single infusion (18, 26).

Reconstitution: Preparation of a 3% or 6% solution

For a 3% solution:

1. Tear off the protective caps from the bottles containing the solvent and the Immune Globulin Intravenous (Human) Sandoglobulin®. Disinfect both rubber stoppers with alcohol.
2. Remove the protective cover from one end of the transfer set and insert the needle through the rubber stopper into the bottle containing the solvent.
3. Remove the cover from the other needle and plunge the inverted Sandoglobulin® (IGIV) bottle onto it, as shown in 3.
4. Invert the two bottles, so that the solvent flows into the Sandoglobulin® (IGIV) bottle.
5. Discard the empty solvent bottle and the transfer set.

For a 6% solution*:
1. Follow steps 1–3 aforementioned.
2. Invert the two bottles, so that the solvent flows into the Immune Globulin Intravenous (Human) (Sandoglobulin)® bottle. Use half the solvent by removing the solvent bottle with transfer needle as soon as the fluid reaches the 6% mark printed on the Sandoglobulin® (IGIV) label.
   Note: The 6% mark is printed on the label only to provide general guidance in preparing a solution containing approximately 6 g protein per 100 mL. If an exact dosage of a 6% solution is required, reconstitute with diluent by using a hypodermic needle and syringe; e.g.,

    for 1 g vial use 16.5 mL diluent,
    for 3 g vial use 50 mL diluent,
    for 6 g vial use 100 mL diluent.

3. Discard any unused solvent and the transfer set.
   To reconstitute Sandoglobulin® (IGIV) from the multivial bulk packs use sterile saline (0.9% NaCl injection, USP) solution drawn up with a sterile hypodermic syringe and needle. Observing aseptic precautions, add the saline to the Sandoglobulin® (IGIV) vials in the following quantities. For a 3% solution add 100 mL saliine to a 3 g vial or 200 mL saline to a 6 g vial. For a 6% solution add 50 mL saline to a 3 g vial or 100 mL to a 6 g vial.
   Sandoglobulin® (IGIV) normally dissolves within a few minutes, though in exceptional cases it may take up to 20 minutes.

DO NOT SHAKE! Excessive shaking will cause foaming.

Any undissolved particles should respond to careful rotation of the bottle. Avoid foaming.

Parenteral drug products should be inspected visually for particulate matter and discoloration prior to administration, whenever solution and container permit. Begin administration promptly after reconstitution. Partially used vials should be discarded.

PROCEED WITH INFUSION ONLY IF SOLUTION IS CLEAR AND AT APPROXIMATELY ROOM TEMPERATURE!

HOW SUPPLIED

Immune Globulin Intravenous (Human) Sandoglobulin® is supplied as a kit containing the lyophilized preparation, sterile Sodium Chloride Injection USP, one double-ended spike for reconstitution and complete directions for use. Sandoglobulin® (IGIV) kits are available in three package sizes:

- 1 g Sandoglobulin® (IGIV) and 33 mL reconstitution fluid
- 3 g Sandoglobulin® (IGIV) and 100 mL reconstitution fluid
- 6 g Sandoglobulin® (IGIV) and 200 mL reconstitution fluid

Alternatively, Sandoglobulin® (IGIV) bulk packs contain ten 3 g or ten 6 g vials without diluent or double-ended spikes.

STORAGE

Sandoglobulin® (IGIV) should be stored at room temperature not exceeding 25°C (77°F). The preparation should not be used after the expiration date printed on the label.

CAUTION

U.S. Federal law prohibits dispensing without prescription.

REFERENCES

1. Römer J, Morgenthaler JJ, Scherz, R, et al: Characterization of various immunoglobulin-preparations for intravenous application. I. Protein composition and antibody content. *Vox. Sang.* 42:62–73 1982.
2. Römer J, Späth, PJ, Skvaril F, et al: Characterization of various immunoglobulin preparations for intravenous application. II. Complement activation and binding to Staphylococcus protein A. *Vox. Sang.* 42:74–80 1982.
3. Römer J, Späth PJ: Molecular composition of immunoglobulin preparations and its relation to complement activation, in Nydegger, UE (ed): *Immunohemotherapy: A Guide to Immunoglobulin Prophylaxis and Therapy.* London, Academic Press, 1981, p 123.
4. Skvaril F, Roth-Wicky B, and Barandun S: IgG subclasses in human-γ-globulin preparations for intravenous use and their reactivity with Staphylococcus protein A. *Vox. Sang.* 38:147 1980.
5. Skvaril F: Qualitative and quantitative aspects of IgG subclasses in i.v. immunoglobulin preparations, in Nydegger, UE (ed): *Immunohemotherapy: A Guide to Immunoglobulin Prophylaxis and Therapy.* London, Academic Press, 1981, p 113.
6. Skvaril F, and Barandun S: In vitro characterization of immunoglobulins for intravenous use, in Alving BM, Finlayson JS (eds): *Immunoglobulins: Characteristics and Uses of Intravenous Preparations,* DHHS Publication No. (FDA)-80-9005. US Government Printing Office, 1980, pp. 201–206.
7. Morell A, and Skvaril F: Struktur und biologische Eigenschaften von Immunoglobulinen und γ-Globulin-Präparaten. II. Eigenschaften von γ-Globulin-Präparaten. *Schweiz Med Wochenschr* 110:80, 1980.
8. Morell A, Schürch B, Ryser D, et al: In vivo behavior of gamma globulin preparations. *Vox. Sang.* 38:272 1980.
9. Imbach P, Barandun S, d'Apuzzo V, et al: High-dose intravenous gamma globulin for idiopathic thrombocytopenic purpura in childhood. *Lancet* 1:1228, 1981.
10. Barandun S, Morell A, Skvaril F: Clinical experiences with immunoglobulin for intravenous use, in Alving BM, Finlayson JS (eds): *Immunoglobulins: Characteristics and Uses of Intravenous Preparations.* DHHS Publication No. (FDA)-80-9005. US Government Printing Office, 1980, pp. 31–35.
11. Barandun S, Morell A: Adverse reactions to immunoglobulin preparations, in Nydegger UE (ed): *Immunohemotherapy: A Guide to Immunoglobulin Prophylaxis and Therapy.* London, Academic Press, 1981, p223.

Continued on next page

Sandoz Pharm.—Cont.

12. Wade A (ed): *Martindale: The Extra Pharmacopoeia*, ed 27. London, The Pharmaceutical Press, 1979, p 65.

13. Joller PW, Barandun S, Hitzig WH: Neue Möglichkeiten der Immunoglobulin-Ersatztherapie bei Antikörpermangel. Syndrom. *Schweiz Med. Wochaenschr* 110:1451, 1980.

14. Barandun S, Imbach P, Morell A, et al: Clinical indications for immunoglobulin infusion, in Nydegger, UE (ed): *Immunohemotherapy: A Guide to Immunoglobulin Prophylaxis and Therapy*. London, Academic Press, 1981, p 275.

15. Cunningham-Rundles C, Smithwick EM, Siegal FP, et al: Treatment of primary humoral immunodeficiency disease with intravenous (pH 4.0 treated) gamma globulin, in Nydegger UE (ed): *Immunohemotherapy: A Guide to Immunoglobulin Prophylaxis and Therapy*. London, Academic Press, 1981, p 283.

16. Imbach P. Wagner HP, Berchtold W, et al: Intravenous immunoglobulin versus oral corticosteroids in acute immune thrombocytopenic purpura in childhood. *Lancet* 2:464, 1985.

17. Bussel JB, Kimberly RP, Inman RD, et al: Intravenous gammaglobulin for chronic idiopathic thrombocytopenic purpura. *Blood* 62:480–486, 1983.

18. Fehr J, Hofmann V, Kappeler U: Transient reversal of thrombocytopenia in idiopathic thrombocytopenic purpura by high-dose intravenous gamma globulin. *N Engl J Med* 306:1254, 1982.

19. Abe T, Matsuda J, Kawasugi K, et al: Clinical effect of intravenous immunoglobulin in chronic idiopathic thrombocytopenic purpura. *Blut* 47:69–75, 1983.

20. Mueller-Eckhardt C, Küenzlen E, Thilo-Körner D, et al: High-dose intravenous immunoglobulin for posttransfusion purpura. *N Engl J Med* 308:287, 1983.

21. Wenske G, Gaedicke G, Küenzlen E, et al: Treatment of idiopathic thrombocytopenic purpura in pregnancy by high-dose intravenous immunoglobulin. *Blut* 46:347–353, 1983.

22. Newland AC, Treleaven JG, Minchinton B, et al: High-dose intravenous IgG in adults with autoimmune thrombocytopenia. *Lancet* 1:84–87, 1983.

23. Cunningham-Rundles C, Day NK, Wahn V, et al: Reactions to intravenous gamma globulin infusions and immune complex formation, in Nydegger UE (ed): *Immunohemotherapy: A Guide to Immunoglobulin Prophylaxis and Therapy*. London, Academic Press, 1981, p 447.

24. Bussel JB, Schulman I, Hilgartner MW, et al: Intravenous use of gamma globulin in the treatment of chronic immune thrombocytopenic purpura as a means to defer splenectomy. *J Pediatr* 103:651–654, 1983.

25. Gardi A: Quality control in the production of an immunoglobulin for intravenous use. *Blut* 48:337–344, 1984.

26. Bussel JB, Pham LC, Hilgartner MW, et al: Long-term maintenance of adults with ITP using intravenous gamma globulin. Abstract, *American Society of Hemotology*, New Orleans, December, 1985.

Manufactured by:
CENTRAL LABORATORY
BLOOD TRANSFUSION SERVICE
SWISS RED CROSS
Wankdorfstrasse 10
3000 Berne 22
Switzerland
U.S. License No. 647
Distributed by:
SANDOZ Pharmaceuticals Corporation
East Hanover, N.J. 07936
[SGL-Z10 Issued March 17, 1989]
Shown in Product Identification Section, page 427

SANDOSTATIN® ℞

[san'dō-stat-in]
(octreotide acetate)
Injection
The following prescribing information is based on official labeling in effect on August 1, 1989.

DESCRIPTION

Sandostatin® (octreotide acetate) Injection, a cyclic octapeptide prepared as a clear sterile solution of octreotide, acetate salt, in buffered sodium chloride for administration by deep subcutaneous (intrafat) injection. Octreotide acetate, known chemically as L-Cysteinamide, D-phenylalanyl-L-cysteinyl-L- phenylalanyl-D-tryptophyl-L-lysyl-L-threonyl-N[2-hydroxy-1- (hydroxymethyl)propyl] cyclic (2->7)-disulfide, [R-(R*, R*)] acetate salt, is a long-acting octapeptide with pharmacologic actions mimicking those of the natural hormone somatostatin.

Sandostatin® (octreotide acetate) Injection is available as sterile 1 mL ampuls in three strengths, containing 0.05, 0.1 or 0.5 mg. octreotide (as acetate).

Each ampul also contains:
acetic acid, glacial, USP .... 2.0 mg
sodium acetate trihydrate, USP .... 2.0 mg
sodium chloride, USP .... 7.0 mg
water for injection, USP .... qs to 1 mL
Acetic acid and sodium acetate trihydrate are added to provide a buffered solution, pH 4.2 ± 0.3.
The molecular weight of octreotide acetate is 1019.3 (free peptide, $C_{49}H_{66}N_{10}O_{10}S_2$) and its amino acid sequence is:

H-D-Phe-Cys-Phe-D-Trp-Lys-Thr-Cys-Thr-ol,
x CH$_3$COOH   where x = 1.4 to 2.5

CLINICAL PHARMACOLOGY

Sandostatin® (octreotide acetate) exerts pharmacological actions similar to the natural hormone somatostatin. In normal subjects, it has the ability to suppress secretion of serotonin and the gastroenteropancreatic peptides: gastrin, vasoactive intestinal peptide, insulin, glucagon, secretin, motilin, and pancreatic polypeptide. In addition, Sandostatin® (octreotide acetate) suppresses growth hormone. In animals, Sandostatin® (octreotide acetate) is a more potent inhibitor of growth hormone, glucagon, and insulin release than natural somatostatin with greater selectivity for growth hormone and glucagon suppression. Sandostatin® (octreotide acetate), like somatostatin, decreases splanchnic blood flow.

By virtue of these pharmacological actions, Sandostatin® (octreotide acetate) has been used to treat the symptoms associated with metastatic carcinoid tumors (flushing and diarrhea), and Vasoactive Intestinal Peptide (VIP) secreting adenomas (watery diarrhea).

Pharmacokinetics

After subcutaneous injection, octreotide is absorbed rapidly and completely from the injection site. Peak concentrations of 5.5 ng/mL (100 mcg dose) were reached 0.4 hours after dosing. Relative to an equivalent intravenous dose, the bioavailability of a subcutaneous dose was estimated to be 80–135%. This was established based on the respective plasma concentrations determined by a radioimmunoassay, the specificity of which remains to be completely defined. Peak concentrations and area under the curve values were dose proportional both after s.c. or i.v. single doses up to 400 mcg and with multiple doses of 200 mcg t.i.d. (600 mcg/day). Clearance was reduced by about 66% suggesting non-linear kinetics of the drug at daily doses of 600 mcg/day as compared to 150 mcg/day. The relative decrease in clearance with doses above 600 mcg/day is not defined.

The distribution of octreotide from plasma was rapid (tα½ = 0.2 h) and the volume of distribution was estimated to be 13.6 L. In blood, the distribution into the erythrocytes was found to be negligible and about 65% was bound in the plasma in a concentration-independent manner. Binding was mainly to lipoprotein and, to a lesser extent, to albumin. The elimination of octreotide from plasma had an apparent half-life of 1.5 hours compared with 1 to 3 minutes with the natural hormone. The duration of action of Sandostatin® (octreotide acetate) is variable but extends up to 12 hours depending upon the type of tumor. About 32% of the dose is excreted unchanged into the urine.

In patients with severe renal failure requiring dialysis, clearance was reduced to about half that found in normal subjects (from approximately 10 L/h to 4.5 L/h). The effect of hepatic diseases on the disposition of octreotide is unknown.

INDICATIONS AND USAGE

General

Sandostatin® (octreotide acetate) therapy is indicated for control of symptoms in patients with metastatic carcinoid and vasoactive intestinal peptide-secreting tumors (VIPomas).

Data are insufficient to determine whether Sandostatin® (octreotide acetate) decreases the size, rate of growth, or development of metastases in patients with these tumors. Sandostatin® (octreotide acetate) has been used in patients ranging in age from 1 month to 83 years without any drug limiting toxicity.

Carcinoid Tumors

Sandostatin® (octreotide acetate) is indicated for the symptomatic treatment of patients with metastatic carcinoid tumors where it suppresses or inhibits the severe diarrhea and flushing episodes associated with the disease.

Vasoactive Intestinal Peptide Tumors (VIPomas)

Sandostatin® (octreotide acetate) is indicated for the treatment of the profuse watery diarrhea associated with VIP-secreting tumors. Significant improvement has been noted in the overall condition of these otherwise therapeutically unresponsive patients. Therapy with Sandostatin® (octreotide acetate) results in improvement in electrolyte abnormalities, e.g., hypokalemia, often enabling reduction of fluid and electrolyte support.

CONTRAINDICATIONS

Sensitivity to this drug or any of its components.

WARNINGS

Sandostatin® (octreotide acetate) therapy, like the natural hormone, somatostatin, may be associated with cholelithia-sis, presumably by altering fat absorption and possibly by decreasing the motility of the gallbladder. Because patients with somatostatinomas have been reported to be at risk for these dysfunctions, patients being treated with Sandostatin® (octreotide acetate) should be monitored periodically for gallbladder disease. Surgical intervention has been required in a few patients who developed severe abdominal pain associated with cholelithiasis while on Sandostatin® (octreotide acetate) therapy.

It is recommended that patients on extended therapy be evaluated periodically using ultrasound evaluations of the gallbladder and bile ducts.

PRECAUTIONS

General

In the treatment of patients with carcinoid syndrome or VIPomas, dosage adjustment may be required to maintain symptomatic control.

Sandostatin® (octreotide acetate) therapy is occasionally associated with mild transient hypo- or hyperglycemia due to alterations in the balance between the counterregulatory hormones; insulin, glucagon, and growth hormone. Patients should be closely observed on introduction of Sandostatin® (octreotide acetate) therapy and at each change of dosage for symptomatic evidence of hyper- or hypoglycemia.

Data on the effect of chronic therapy with Sandostatin® (octreotide acetate) on hypothalamic/pituitary function has not been obtained. A progressive drop in T$_4$ levels has been reported, culminating in clinical and biochemical hypothyroidism after 19 months of therapy in one clinical trial patient (carcinoid) receiving 1500 mcg of Sandostatin® (octreotide acetate) daily. Therefore, baseline and periodic thyroid function tests using total and free T$_4$ are advised to monitor patients.

In insulin-dependent diabetics, reduction of insulin requirements may result following initiation of Sandostatin® (octreotide acetate) therapy.

There is evidence that Sandostatin® (octreotide acetate) therapy may alter absorption of dietary fats in some patients. It is suggested that periodic quantitative 72-hour fecal fat and serum carotene determinations be performed to aid in the assessment of possible drug-induced aggravation of fat malabsorption.

In patients with severe renal failure requiring dialysis, the half-life of the drug may be increased, necessitating adjustment of the maintenance dosage.

Because decreased gallbladder contractility and bile stasis may result from treatment with Sandostatin® (octreotide acetate), baseline and periodic ultrasonography may be useful to assess the presence of gallstones (See WARNINGS).

Information for Patients

Careful instruction in sterile subcutaneous injection technique should be given to the patients and to other persons who may administer Sandostatin® (octreotide acetate) Injection.

Laboratory Tests

Laboratory tests that may be helpful as biochemical markers in determining and following patient response depend on the specific tumor. Based on diagnosis, measurement of the following substances may be useful in monitoring the progress of therapy:

Carcinoid: 5-HIAA (urinary 5-hydroxyindole acetic acid), plasma serotonin, plasma Substance P

VIPoma: VIP (plasma vasoactive intestinal peptide)

Baseline and periodic total and/or free T$_4$ measurements should be performed during chronic therapy (See PRECAUTIONS—General).

Drug Interactions

Many patients with carcinoid syndrome or VIPomas being treated with Sandostatin® (octreotide acetate) have also been, or are being, treated with many other drugs to control the symptomatology or progression of the disease, generally without serious drug interaction. Included are chemotherapeutic agents, H$_2$ antagonists, antimotility agents, drugs affecting glycemic states, solutions for electrolyte and fluid support or hyperalimentation, antihypertensive diuretics, and antidiarrheal agents.

Where symptoms are severe and Sandostatin® (octreotide acetate) therapy is added to other therapies used to control glycemic states such as sulfonylureas, insulin, diazoxide and to beta blockers or agents for the control of fluid and electrolyte balance, patients must be monitored closely and adjustment made in the other therapies as the symptoms of the disease are controlled. Evidence currently available suggests these imbalances in fluid and electrolytes or glycemic states are secondary to correction of pre-existing abnormalities and not to a direct metabolic action of Sandostatin® (octreotide acetate). Adjustment of the dosage of drugs, such as insulin, affecting glucose metabolism may be required following initiation of Sandostatin® (octreotide acetate) therapy in patients with diabetes.

Since Sandostatin® (octreotide acetate) has been associated with alterations in nutrient absorption, its effect on absorption of any orally administered drugs should be carefully considered. A single case of transplant rejection episode (renal/whole pancreas) in a patient immunosuppressed with cyclosporine has been reported. Sandostatin® (octreotide acetate) treatment to reduce exocrine secretion and close a fistula in this patient resulted in decreases in blood levels of cyclosporine and may have contributed to the rejection episode.

Drug Laboratory Test Interactions
No known interference exists with clinical laboratory tests, including amine or peptide determinations.

Carcinogenesis/Mutagenesis/Impairment of Fertility
Studies in laboratory animals have demonstrated no mutagenic potential of Sandostatin® (octreotide acetate). No long-term studies in animals to assess carcinogenicity have been completed. Sandostatin® (octreotide acetate) did not impair fertility in rats at doses up to 1 mg/kg/day.

Pregnancy Category B
Reproduction studies have been performed in rats and rabbits at doses up to 30 times the highest human dose and have revealed no evidence of impaired fertility or harm to the fetus due to Sandostatin® (octreotide acetate). There are, however, no adequate and well-controlled studies in pregnant women. Because animal reproduction studies are not always predictive of human response, this drug should be used during pregnancy only if clearly needed.

Nursing Mothers
It is not known whether this drug is excreted in human milk. Because many drugs are excreted in milk, caution should be exercised when Sandostatin® (octreotide acetate) is administered to a nursing woman.

Pediatric Use
Experience with Sandostatin® (octreotide acetate) in the pediatric population is limited. The youngest patient to receive the drug was 1 month old. Doses of 1–10 mcg/kg body weight were well tolerated in the young patients. A single case of an infant (nesidio-blastosis) was complicated by a seizure thought to be independent of Sandostatin® (octreotide acetate) therapy.

ADVERSE REACTIONS
The incidence of adverse reactions by patient group and in the total cohort (N = 491) of patients follows. These adverse reactions were largely of mild to moderate severity and of short duration.
[See table right].
In addition, the following infrequent reactions were reported (fewer than 1% of patients):

Gastrointestinal
Constipation, flatulence, hepatitis, jaundice, slight increase in liver enzymes, rectal disorder (spasm), GI bleeding, stomach swollen, heartburn, fluttering sensation, abnormal stools, and cholelithiasis.

Integumentary
Hair loss, thinning of skin, skin flaking, bruising, bleeding from a superficial wound, pruritus, and rash.

Musculoskeletal
Backache pain, muscle pain, muscle cramping, joint pain, shoulder and leg pain, leg cramps, and chest pain.

Cardiovascular
Shortness of breath, hypertensive reaction, thrombophlebitis, ischemia, congestive heart failure, hypertension, palpitations, orthostatic BP decrease, and chest pain.

CNS
Anxiety, anorexia, convulsions, depression, drowsiness, vertigo, hyperesthesia, pounding in head, insomnia, irritability, libido decrease/frigidity, forgetfulness, malasie, nervousness, shakiness, syncope, tremor, and Bells' Palsy.

Respiratory
Rhinorrhea

Endocrine
Galactorrhea
Clinical hypothyroidism requiring thyroid hormone replacement was observed after 19 months of therapy with 1500 mcg daily of Sandostatin® (octreotide acetate) in a clinical trial patient. A progressive fall to low total and free T_4 values was observed, without an elevated TSH, indicative of hypothalamic-pituitary dysfunction, probably related to Sandostatin® (octreotide acetate) therapy.

Urogenital
Oliguria, pollakiuria, prostatitis, and urine hyperosmolarity.

Autonomic
Burning sensation, dry mouth, numbness, hyperhidrosis, hyperdipsia, warm feeling, and visual disturbance.

Miscellaneous
Chills, fever, throat discomfort, increased CPK, arm pain, and eyes burning.
Evaluation of 20 patients treated for at least 6 months has failed to demonstrate titers of antibodies exceeding background levels.

OVERDOSAGE
Specific information on Sandostatin® (octreotide acetate) overdosage is not available as no frank overdosage has occurred in any patient to date. Bolus i.v. injections of 1000 mcg given to healthy volunteers have been tolerated without serious complication.

Adverse Reactions Occurring in 3 to 10% of Patients

| | Number Reporting | | |
Reaction	Carcinoid and VIPoma Patients N = 211 (%)	Other Patients N = 280 (%)	Total N = 491 (%)
Nausea	16 (7.6)	31 (11.1)	47 (9.6)
Injection Site Pain	16 (7.6)	21 (7.5)	37 (7.5)
Diarrhea	10 (4.7)	24 (8.6)	34 (6.9)
Abdominal Pain/ Discomfort	6 (2.8)	27 (9.6)	33 (6.7)
Loose Stools	3 (1.4)	18 (6.4)	21 (4.3)
Vomiting	4 (1.9)	15 (5.4)	19 (3.9)

Adverse Reactions Occurring in 1 to 3% of Patients

| | Number Reporting | | |
Reaction	Carcinoid and VIPoma Patients N = 211(%)	Other Patients N = 280(%)	Total N = 491(%)
Headache	3 (1.4)	7 (2.5)	10 (2.0)
Fat Malabsorption	5 (2.4)	3 (1.1)	8 (1.6)
Dizziness/ Light-headedness	3 (1.4)	5 (1.8)	8 (1.6)
Hyperglycemia	3 (1.4)	5 (1.8)	8 (1.6)
Fatigue	2 (0.9)	5 (1.8)	7 (1.4)
Flushing	3 (1.4)	4 (1.4)	7 (1.4)
Hypoglycemia	1 (0.5)	5 (1.8)	6 (1.2)
Edema	2 (0.9)	3 (1.1)	5 (1.0)
Asthenia/Weakness	4 (1.9)	1 (0.4)	5 (1.0)
Injection Site/ Wheal/Erythema	4 (1.9)	1 (0.4)	5 (1.0)

Based on the pharmacological properties of Sandostatin® (octreotide acetate), acute overdosage may be expected to produce hyper- or hypoglycemia, depending on the endocrine status of the patient and type of peptide-secreting tumor involved. Hyper- and hypoglycemia may be manifested by neurologic and mental disturbances such as loss of sensory or motor function, incoordination, visual blurring, dizziness, drowsiness, and disturbed consciousness. These conditions should resolve with temporary withdrawal of the drug and symptomatic treatment.
The i.v. LD_{50} is 72 mg/kg in mice and 18 mg/kg in rats.

DOSAGE AND ADMINISTRATION
Parenteral drug products should be inspected visually for particulate matter and discoloration prior to administration. **Do not use if particulates and/or discoloration are observed.** Subcutaneous injection is the recommended route of administration of Sandostatin® (octreotide acetate) for control of symptoms in most instances. Intravenous bolus injections have been used under emergency conditions. Multiple injections at the same site within short periods of time should be avoided. The initial dosage is 50 mcg, administered subcutaneously, once or twice daily. Thereafter, the number of injections and dosage may be increased gradually based on patient tolerability and response. Dosage information for patients with specific tumors follows. The drug is usually given in a b.i.d. or t.i.d. schedule.

Carcinoid Tumors
The suggested daily dosage of Sandostatin® (octreotide acetate) during the first two weeks of therapy ranges from 100 to 600 mcg per day in two to four divided doses (mean daily dosage is 300 mcg). In the clinical studies, the **median** daily maintenance dosage was approximately 450 mcg, but clinical and biochemical benefits were obtained in some patients with as little as 50 mcg, while others required doses up to 1500 mcg per day. However, experience with doses above 750 mcg per day is limited.

VIPomas
Daily dosages of 200 to 300 mcg in two to four divided doses are recommended during the initial 2 weeks of therapy (range 150 to 750 mcg) to control symptoms of the disease. On an individual basis, dosage may be adjusted to achieve a therapeutic response, but usually doses above 450 mcg per day are not required.

HOW SUPPLIED
Sandostatin® (octreotide acetate) Injection is available as a one mL ampul in packages of 20 and 50 as follows:
0.05 mg octreotide (as acetate)
Package of 20 ampuls (NDC 0078-0180-03)
Package of 50 ampuls (NDC 0078-0180-04)
0.1 mg octreotide (as acetate)
Package of 20 ampuls (NDC 0078-0181-03)
Package of 50 ampuls (NDC 0078-0181-04)
0.5 mg octreotide (as acetate)
Package of 20 ampuls (NDC 0078-0182-03)
Package of 50 ampuls (NDC 0078-0182-04)
Sandostatin® (octreotide acetate) is also available as a patient home administration starter kit containing an ampul

opener, alcohol swabs and the following one mL drug ampuls:
0.05 mg octreotide (as acetate)
Package of 30 ampuls (NDC 0078-0180-15)
0.1 mg octreotide (as acetate)
Package of 30 ampuls (NDC 0078-0181-15)
0.5 mg octreotide (as acetate)
Package of 18 ampuls (NDC 0078-0182-17)

Storage
For prolonged storage, Sandostatin® (octreotide acetate) ampuls should be stored in the refrigerator at 2°–8°C (36°–46°F). Ampuls can be stored at room temperature (20°–30°C or 70°–86°F) for the day they will be used.
Manufactured by
Sandoz, Ltd., Basle, Switerland
for
SANDOZ
PHARMACEUTICALS
CORPORATION
EAST HANOVER, NJ 07936
© 1989 Sandoz Pharmaceuticals Corporation
SDS-Z1 Issued January 1, 1989
Shown in Product Identification Section, page 427

SANOREX®
[san 'ŏ-rex ″]
(mazindol) tablets, USP

The following prescribing information is based on official labeling in effect on August 1, 1989.

DESCRIPTION
Sanorex® (mazindol) is an imidazoiso-indole anorectic agent. It is chemically designated as 5-p-chloro-phenyl-5-hydroxy-2, 3- dihydro-5H-imidazo (2,1-a) isoindole, a tautomeric form of 2-[2'-(p-chlorobenzoyl) phenyl]-2-imidazoline, and has the following structure:

Mazindol
1 mg. and 2 mg, Tablets
Active Ingredient: mazindol, USP
Inactive Ingredients: calcium sulfate dihydrate, lactose, magnesium stearate, povidone, starch and talc

Continued on next page

Sandoz Pharm.—Cont.

ACTIONS

Sanorex®, (mazindol), although an isoindole, has pharmacologic activity similar in many ways to the prototype drugs used in obesity, the amphetamines. Actions include central nervous system stimulation in humans and animals, as well as such amphetamine-like effects in animals as the production of stereotyped behavior. Animal experiments also suggest certain differences from phenethylamine anorectic drugs, e.g., amphetamine, with respect to site and mechanism of action; for example, mazindol appears to exert its primary effects on the limbic system. The significance of these differences for humans is uncertain. It does not cause brain norepinephrine depletion in animals; on the other hand, it does appear to inhibit storage site uptake of norepinephrine as is suggested by its marked potentiation of the effect of exogenous norepinephrine on blood pressure in dogs (see WARNINGS) and on smooth muscle contraction *in vitro.* Tolerance has been demonstrated with all drugs of this class in which this phenomenon has been studied.

Drugs used in obesity are commonly known as "anorectics" or "anorexigenics." It has not been established, however, that the action of such drugs in treating obesity is exclusively one of appetite suppression. Other central nervous system actions, or metabolic effects may be involved as well. Adult obese subjects instructed in dietary management and treated with anorectic drugs, lose more weight on the average than those treated with placebo and diet, as determined in relatively short-term clinical trials.

The average magnitude of increased weight loss of drug-treated patients over placebo-treated patients in studies of anorectics in general is ordinarily only a fraction of a pound a week. The rate of weight loss is greatest in the first weeks of therapy for both drug and placebo subjects and tends to decrease in succeeding weeks.

The amount of weight loss associated with the use of Sanorex® (mazindol), as with other anorectic drugs, varies from trial to trial, and the increased weight loss appears to be related in part to variables other than the drugs prescribed, such as the interaction between physician-investigator and the patient, the population treated, and the diet prescribed. The importance of non-drug factors in such weight loss has not been elucidated.

The natural history of obesity is measured in years, whereas, most studies cited are restricted to a few weeks' duration; thus, the total impact of drug-induced weight loss over that of diet alone must be considered clinically limited.

INDICATION

Sanorex® (mazindol) is indicated in the management of exogenous obesity as a short-term (a few weeks) adjunct in a regimen of weight reduction based on caloric restriction. The limited usefulness of agents of this class (see ACTIONS) should be measured against possible risk factors inherent in their use, such as those described below.

CONTRAINDICATIONS

Glaucoma; hypersensitivity or idiosyncrasy to Sanorex (mazindol).

Agitated states.

Patients with a history of drug abuse.

During or within 14 days following the administration of monoamine oxidase inhibitors, (hypertensive crises may result).

WARNINGS

Tolerance to the effect of many anorectic drugs may develop within a few weeks; if this occurs, the recommended dose should not be exceeded in an attempt to increase the effect; rather, the drug should be discontinued.

Sanorex® (mazindol) may impair the ability of the patient to engage in potentially hazardous activities such as operating machinery or driving a motor vehicle; the patient should therefore be cautioned accordingly.

Drug Interactions: Sanorex® (mazindol) may decrease the hypotensive effect of guanethidine; patients should be monitored accordingly.

Sanorex® (mazindol) may markedly potentiate the pressor effect of exogenous catecholamines. If it should be necessary to give a pressor amine agent (e.g., levarterenol or isoproterenol) to a patient in shock (e.g., from a myocardial infarction) who has recently been taking Sanorex® (mazindol) extreme care should be taken in monitoring blood pressure at frequent intervals and initiating pressor therapy with a low initial dose and careful titration.

Drug Dependence: Sanorex® (mazindol) shares important pharmacological properties with amphetamines. Amphetamines and related stimulant drugs have been extensively abused and can produce tolerance and severe psychologic dependence. In this regard, the manifestations of chronic overdosage or withdrawal of Sanorex® (mazindol) have not been determined in humans. Abstinence effects have been observed in dogs after abrupt cessation for prolonged periods. There was some self-administration of the drug in monkeys. EEG studies and "liking" scores in human subjects yielded equivocal results. While the abuse potential of Sanorex® (mazindol) has not been further defined, the possibility of dependence should be kept in mind when evaluating the desirability of including Sanorex® (mazindol) as part of a weight reduction program.

Usage in Pregnancy: Sanorex® (mazindol) was studied in reproduction experiments in rats and rabbits and an increase in neonatal mortality and a possible increased incidence of rib anomalies in rats were observed at relatively high doses.

Although these studies have not indicated important adverse effects, use of mazindol by women who are or may become pregnant requires that the potential benefit be weighed against the possible hazard to mother and infant.

Usage in Children: Sanorex® (mazindol) is not recommended for use in children under 12 years of age.

PRECAUTIONS

Insulin requirements in diabetes mellitus may be altered in association with the use of mazindol and the concomitant dietary regimen.

The least amount feasible should be prescribed or dispensed at one time in order to minimize the possibility of overdosage.

Use only with caution in hypertension with monitoring of blood pressure, since evidence is insufficient to rule out a possible adverse effect on blood pressure in some hypertensive patients. The drug is not recommended in severely hypertensive patients. The drug is not recommended for patients with symptomatic cardiovascular disease including arrhythmias.

ADVERSE REACTIONS

The most common adverse effects of Sanorex® (mazindol) are dry mouth, tachycardia, constipation, nervousness and insomnia.

Cardiovascular: Palpitation, tachycardia.

Central Nervous System: Overstimulation, restlessness, dizziness, insomnia, dysphoria, tremor, headache, depression, drowsiness, weakness.

Gastrointestinal: Dryness of the mouth, unpleasant taste, diarrhea, constipation, nausea, other gastrointestinal disturbances.

Skin: Rash, excessive sweating, clamminess.

Endocrine: Impotence, changes in libido have rarely been observed with Sanorex® (mazindol).

Eye: Treatment of dogs with high doses of Sanorex® (mazindol) for long periods resulted in some corneal opacities, reversible on cessation of medication. No such effect has been observed in humans.

DOSAGE AND ADMINISTRATION

Usual dosage is 1 mg three times daily, one hour before meals, or 2 mg once daily, one hour before lunch. The lowest effective dose should be used. To determine the lowest effective dose, therapy with Sanorex® (mazindol) may be initiated at 1 mg once a day, and adjusted to the need and response of the patient. Should G.I. discomfort occur, Sanorex® (mazindol) may be taken with meals.

OVERDOSAGE

There are no data as yet on acute overdosage with Sanorex® (mazindol) in humans.

Manifestations of acute overdosage with amphetamines and related substances include restlessness, tremor, rapid respiration, dizziness. Fatigue and depression may follow the stimulatory phase of overdosage. Cardiovascular effects include tachycardia, hypertension and circulatory collapse. Gastrointestinal symptoms include nausea, vomiting and abdominal cramps. While similar manifestations of overdosage may be seen with Sanorex® (mazindol), their exact nature has yet to be determined. The management of acute intoxication is largely symptomatic. Data are not available on the treatment of acute intoxication with Sanorex® (mazindol) by hemodialysis or peritoneal dialysis, but the substance is poorly soluble except at very acid pH.

HOW SUPPLIED

Sanorex® (mazindol) is available in 1 mg elliptical, white tablets, embossed "SANOREX" one side, "78–71" other side; and in 2 mg round, white scored tablets, embossed "78/66" one side, "SANDOZ" other side, in packages of 100.

[SNX-Z13 Issued February 2, 1987]

SANSERT®   ℞

[san 'surt]

(methysergide maleate) tablets, USP

The following prescribing information is based on official labeling in effect on August 1, 1989.

> **WARNING**
> Retroperitoneal Fibrosis, Pleuropulmonary Fibrosis and Fibrotic Thickening of Cardiac Valves May Occur in Patients Receiving Long-term Methysergide Maleate Therapy. Therefore, This Preparation Must be Reserved for Prophylaxis in Patients Whose Vascular Headaches Are Frequent and/or Severe and Uncontrollable and Who Are Under Close Medical Supervision.
>
> (See Also "Warnings" Section.)

DESCRIPTION

Sansert® (methysergide maleate) is a partially synthetic compound structurally related to lysergic acid butanolamide, well-known as methylergonovine in obstetrical practice as an oxytocic agent.

SANSERT
(methysergide maleate)

Methylation in the number 1 position of the ring structure enormously enhances the antagonism to serotonin which is present to a much lesser degree in the partially methylated compound (methylergonovine maleate) as well as profoundly altering other pharmacologic properties.

Active Ingredient: methysergide maleate, USP

Inactive Ingredients: acacia, carnauba wax, colloidal silicon dioxide, FD&C Blue #1, FD&C Yellow #5, gelatin, lactose, malic acid, povidone, sodium benzoate, starch, stearic acid, sucrose, talc, and titanium dioxide

ACTIONS

Sansert® (methysergide maleate) has been shown, *in vitro* and *in vivo,* to inhibit or block the effects of serotonin, a substance which may be involved in the mechanism of vascular headaches. Serotonin has been variously described as a central neurohumoral agent or chemical mediator, as a "headache substance" acting directly or indirectly to lower pain threshold (others in this category include tyramine; polypeptides, such as bradykinin; histamine; and acetylcholine), as an intrinsic "motor hormone" of the gastrointestinal tract, and as a "hormone" involved in connective tissue reparative processes. Suggestions have been made by investigators as to the mechanism whereby methysergide produces its clinical effects, but this has not been finally established.

INDICATIONS

For the prevention or reduction of intensity and frequency of vascular headaches in the following kinds of patients:

1. Patients suffering from one or more severe vascular headaches per week.

2. Patients suffering from vascular headaches that are uncontrollable or so severe that preventive therapy is indicated regardless of the frequency of the attack.

CONTRAINDICATIONS

Pregnancy, peripheral vascular disease, severe arteriosclerosis, severe hypertension, coronary artery disease, phlebitis or cellulitis of the lower limbs, pulmonary disease, collagen diseases or fibrotic processes, impaired liver or renal function, valvular heart disease, debilitated states and serious infections.

WARNINGS

With long-term, uninterrupted administration, retroperitoneal fibrosis or related conditions—pleuropulmonary fibrosis and cardiovascular disorders with murmurs or vascular bruits have been reported. Patients must be warned to report immediately the following symptoms: cold, numb, and painful hands and feet; leg cramps on walking; any type of girdle, flank, or chest pain, or any associated symptomatology. Should any of these symptoms develop, methysergide should be discontinued. Continuous administration should not exceed 6 months. There must be a drug-free interval of 3-4 weeks after each 6-month course of treatment. The dosage should be reduced gradually during the last 2-3 weeks of each treatment course to avoid "headache rebound."

The drug is not recommended for use in children.

PRECAUTIONS

All patients receiving Sansert® (methysergide maleate) should remain under constant supervision of the physician and be examined regularly for the development of fibrotic or vascular complications. (See Adverse Reactions.)

The manifestations of retroperitoneal fibrosis, pleuropulmonary fibrosis, and vascular shutdown have shown a high incidence of regression once Sansert (methysergide maleate) is withdrawn. These facts should be borne in mind to avoid unnecessary surgical intervention. Cardiac murmurs, which may indicate endocardial fibrosis, have shown varying degrees of regression, with complete disappearance in some and persistence in others.

Sansert® (methysergide maleate) has been specifically designed for the prophylaxis of vascular headache and has no place in the management of the acute attack.

Sansert® (methysergide maleate) tablets contain FD&C Yellow No. 5 (tartrazine) which may cause allergic-type reactions (including bronchial asthma) in certain susceptible individuals. Although the overall incidence of FD&C Yellow No. 5 (tartrazine) sensitivity in the general population is low, it is frequently seen in patients who also have aspirin hypersensitivity.

ADVERSE REACTIONS

Within the recommended dose levels, the following side effects have been reported:

1) Fibrotic Complications

Fibrotic changes have been observed in the retroperitoneal, pleuropulmonary, cardiac, and other tissues, either singly or, very rarely, in combination.

Retroperitoneal Fibrosis: This non-specific fibrotic process is usually confined to the retroperitoneal connective tissue above the pelvic brim and may present clinically with one or more symptoms such as general malaise, fatigue, weight loss, backache, low grade fever (elevated sedimentation rate), urinary obstruction (girdle or flank pain, dysuria, polyuria, oliguria, elevated BUN), vascular insufficiency of the lower limbs (leg pain, Leriche syndrome, edema of legs, thrombophlebitis). The single most useful diagnostic procedure in suspected cases of retroperitoneal fibrosis is intravenous pyelography. Typical deviation and obstruction of one or both ureters may be observed.

Pleuropulmonary Complications: A similar nonspecific fibrotic process, limited to the pleural and immediately subjacent pulmonary tissues, usually presents clinically with dyspnea, tightness and pain in the chest, pleural friction rubs, and pleural effusion. These findings may be confirmed by chest X-ray.

Cardiac Complications: Nonrheumatic fibrotic thickenings of the aortic root and of the aortic and mitral valves usually present clinically with cardiac murmurs and dyspnea.

Other Fibrotic Complications: Several cases of fibrotic plaques, simulating Peyronie's disease have been described.

2) Cardiovascular Complications

Encroachment of retroperitoneal fibrosis on the aorta, inferior vena cava and their common major iliac branches may result in vascular insufficiency of the lower limbs, the presenting features of which are mentioned under retroperitoneal fibrosis.

Intrinsic vasoconstriction of large and small arteries, involving one or more vessels or merely a segment of a vessel, may occur at any stage of therapy. Depending on the vessel involved, this complication may present with chest pain, abdominal pain, or cold, numb, painful extremities with or without paresthesias and diminished or absent pulses. Progression to ischemic tissue damage has rarely been reported. Prompt withdrawal of the drug at the first signs of impaired circulation is recommended (See Warnings) to obviate such effects.

Postural hypotension and tachycardia have also been observed.

3) Gastrointestinal Symptoms

Nausea, vomiting, diarrhea, heartburn, abdominal pain. These effects tend to appear early and can frequently be obviated by gradual introduction of the medication and by administration of the drug with meals.

Constipation and elevation of gastric HCl have also been reported.

4) CNS Symptoms

Insomnia, drowsiness, mild euphoria, dizziness, ataxia, lightheadedness, hyperesthesia, unworldly feelings (described variously as "dissociation," "hallucinatory experiences," etc.). Some of these symptoms may be associated with vascular headaches, per se, and may, therefore, be unrelated to the drug.

5) Dermatological Manifestations

Facial flush, telangiectasia, and nonspecific rashes have rarely been reported. Increased hair loss may occur, but in many instances the tendency has abated despite continued therapy.

6) Edema

Peripheral edema, and more rarely, localized brawny edema may occur.

Dependent edema has responded to lowered doses, salt restriction, or diuretics.

7) Weight Gain

Weight gain may be a reason to caution patients regarding their caloric intake.

8) Hematological Manifestations

Neutropenia, eosinophilia.

9) Miscellaneous

Weakness, arthralgia, myalgia.

DOSAGE AND ADMINISTRATION

Usual adult dose 4 to 8 mg daily. Tablets to be given with meals.

Note: There must be a medication-free interval of 3-4 weeks after every 6-month course of treatment (see WARNINGS).

No pediatric dosage has been established.

If, after a 3-week trial period, efficacy has not been demonstrated, longer administration of Sansert® (methysergide maleate) is unlikely to be of benefit.

HOW SUPPLIED

Bottles of 100 tablets, each tablet containing 2 mg of methysergide maleate, USP.

Company's Product Identification Mark(s): Imprinted 78-58 on one side, SANDOZ other side.

[SAN-Z21 Issued July 15, 1986]

SYNTOCINON® INJECTION   ℞

[sin "tō 'si-non]
(oxytocin injection, USP)

The following prescribing information is based on official labeling in effect on August 1, 1989.

DESCRIPTION

Syntocinon® (oxytocin) injection is a synthetic nonapeptide. For intravenous or intramuscular administration.

Each 1 mL of Syntocinon solution contains 10 USP or International Units of oxytocin and the following inactive ingredients:

sodium acetate, USP	1 mg
sodium chloride, USP	0.017 mg
chlorobutanol, NF	0.5%
alcohol, USP	0.61% by vol.
acetic acid, NF, qs to	pH 4 ± .3
water for injection, USP, qs to	1 ml

The Syntocinon® solution in each ampul is sterile.

Syntocinon® (oxytocin) is a cyclic (1–6) nonapeptide with the following chemical name:

Glycinamide,   L-cysteinyl-L-tyrosyl-L-isoleucyl-L-glutaminyl-L-asparaginyl-L-cysteinyl-L-prolyl-L-leucyl-, cyclic (1–6)-disulfide

Its Chemical Abstract Registry number is: 50-56-6; and its chemical formula is shown below:

$$\underset{\substack{|\\ \underset{3}{Ileu} - \underset{2}{Tyr} - \underset{1}{Cys}}}{\overset{4\quad\;\;5\qquad\quad 6\;\;\;7\;\;\;8\;\;\;9}{Glu(NH_2)-Asp(NH_2)-Cys-Pro-Leu-Gly(NH_2)}}$$

oxytocin

CLINICAL PHARMACOLOGY

The pharmacologic and clinical properties of Syntocinon® (oxytocin) are identical with the naturally occurring oxytocic principle of the posterior lobe of the pituitary. Syntocinon® (oxytocin) injection does not contain the amino acids characteristic of vasopressin, and therefore has fewer and less severe cardiovascular effects. Syntocinon® (oxytocin) exerts a selective action on the smooth musculature of the uterus, particularly toward the end of pregnancy, during labor and immediately following delivery. Oxytocin stimulates rhythmic contractions of the uterus, increases the frequency of existing contractions, and raises the tone of the uterine musculature.

Syntocinon® (oxytocin), when given in appropriate doses during pregnancy, is capable of eliciting graded increases in uterine motility from a moderate increase in the rate and force of spontaneous motor activity to sustained tetanic contraction.

Syntocinon® (oxytocin) is promptly effective after parenteral administration. Following intramuscular injection, the myotonic effect on the uterus appears in 3–7 minutes, and persists for 30–60 minutes. With intravenous injection, the uterine effect appears within one minute and is of more brief duration.

INDICATIONS AND USAGE

> **IMPORTANT NOTICE**
>
> Syntocinon® (oxytocin) injection is indicated for the medical rather than the elective induction of labor. Available data and information are inadequate to define the benefits to risks considerations in the use of the drug product for elective induction. Elective induction of labor is defined as the initiation of labor for convenience in an individual with a term pregnancy who is free of medical indications.

Antepartum: Syntocinon® (oxytocin) is indicated for the initiation or improvement of uterine contractions, where this is desirable and considered suitable, in order to achieve early vaginal delivery for fetal or maternal reasons. It is indicated for (1) induction of labor in patients with a medical indication for the initiation of labor, such as Rh problems, maternal diabetes, pre-eclampsia at or near term, when delivery is in the best interest of mother and fetus or when membranes are prematurely ruptured and delivery is indicated; (2) stimulation or reinforcement of labor, as in selected cases of uterine inertia; (3) as adjunctive therapy in the management of incomplete or inevitable abortion. In the first trimester currettage is generally considered primary ther-

---

apy. In the second trimester abortion, oxytocin infusion will often be successful in emptying the uterus. Other means of therapy, however, may be required in such cases.

Postpartum: Syntocinon® (oxytocin) injection is indicated to produce uterine contractions during the third stage of labor and to control postpartum bleeding or hemorrhage.

CONTRAINDICATIONS

Syntocinon® (oxytocin) injection is contraindicated in any of the following conditions: Significant cephalopelvic disproportion; unfavorable fetal positions or presentations which are undeliverable without conversion prior to delivery, (transverse lies); i.e., in obstetrical emergencies where the benefit-to-risk ratio for either the fetus or the mother favors surgical intervention; in cases of fetal distress where delivery is not imminent; prolonged use in uterine inertia or severe toxemia; hypertonic uterine patterns; patients with hypersensitivity to the drug; induction or augmentation of labor in those cases where vaginal delivery is contraindicated, such as cord presentation or prolapse, total placenta previa, and vasa previa.

WARNINGS

Syntocinon® (oxytocin) when given for induction or stimulation of labor, must be administered only by the intravenous route and with adequate medical supervision in a hospital.

PRECAUTIONS

General: All patients receiving intravenous oxytocin must be under continuous observation by trained personnel with a thorough knowledge of the drug and qualified to identify complications. A physician qualified to manage any complications should be immediately available.

When properly administered, oxytocin should stimulate uterine contractions similar to those seen in normal labor. Overstimulation of the uterus by improper administration can be hazardous to both mother and fetus. Even with proper administration and adequate supervision, hypertonic contractions can occur in patients whose uteri are hypersensitive to oxytocin.

Except in unusual circumstances, oxytocin should not be administered in the following conditions: prematurity, borderline cephalopelvic disproportion, previous major surgery on the cervix or uterus including cesarean section, over-distention of the uterus, grand multiparity, or invasive cervical carcinoma. Because of the variability of the combinations of factors which may be present in the conditions listed above, the definition of "unusual circumstances" must be left to the judgment of the physician. The decision can only be made by carefully weighing the potential benefits which oxytocin can provide in a given case against rare but definite potential for the drug to produce hypertonicity or tetanic spasm.

Maternal deaths due to hypertensive episodes, subarachnoid hemorrhage, rupture of the uterus, and fetal deaths due to various causes have been reported associated with the use of parental oxytocic drugs for induction of labor or for augmentation in the first and second stages of labor.

Oxytocin has been shown to have an intrinsic antidiuretic effect, acting to increase water reabsorption from the glomerular filtrate. Consideration should, therefore, be given to the possibility of water intoxication, particularly when oxytocin is administered continuously by infusion and the patient is receiving fluids by mouth.

Drug Interactions: Severe hypertension has been reported when oxytocin was given three to four hours following prophylactic administration of a vasoconstrictor in conjunction with caudal block anesthesia. Cyclopropane anesthesia may modify oxytocin's cardiovascular effects, so as to produce unexpected results such as hypotension. Maternal sinus bradycardia with abnormal atrioventricular rhythms has also been noted when oxytocin was used concomitantly with cyclopropane anesthesia.

Carcinogenesis, Mutagenesis, Impairment of Fertility: There are no animal or human studies on the carcinogenicity and mutagenicity of this drug, nor is there any information on its effect on fertility.

Pregnancy: Teratogenic Effects. Animal reproduction studies have not been conducted with oxytocin. There are no known indications for use in the first trimester of pregnancy other than in relation to spontaneous or induced abortion. Based on the wide experience with this drug and its chemical structure and pharmacological properties, it would not be expected to present a risk of fetal abnormalities when used as indicated.

Nonteratogenic Effects. See **ADVERSE REACTIONS** in the fetus or infant.

Labor and Delivery: see **INDICATIONS AND USAGE.**

Nursing Mothers: Syntocinon® (oyxtocin) may be found in small quantities in mother's milk. If a patient requires the drug postpartum to control severe bleeding, she should not commence nursing until the day after Syntocinon has been discontinued.

Pediatric Use: Syntocinon® (oxytocin) is not intended for use in children.

Continued on next page

Sandoz Pharm.—Cont.

ADVERSE REACTIONS

The following adverse reactions have been reported in the mother.

Anaphylactic reaction
Postpartum hemorrhage
Cardiac arrhythmia
Fatal afibrinogenemia
Nausea
Vomiting
Premature ventricular contractions
Pelvic hematoma
Excessive dosage or hypersensitivity to the drug may result in uterine hypertonicity, spasm, tetanic contraction, or rupture of the uterus.

The possibility of increased blood loss and afibrinogenemia should be kept in mind when administering the drug.

Severe water intoxication with convulsions and coma has occurred, associated with a slow oxytocin infusion over a 24-hour period. Maternal death due to oxytocin-induced water intoxication has been reported.

The following adverse reactions have been reported in the fetus or infant:

Due to induced uterine motility:
Bradycardia
Premature ventricular contractions and other arrhythmias
Permanent CNS or brain damage
Fetal death

Due to use of oxytocin in the mother:
Low Apgar scores at 5 minutes
Neonatal jaundice
Neonatal retinal hemorrhage

DRUG ABUSE AND DEPENDENCE

There is no evidence that Syntocinon® (oxytocin) has been abused or has provoked drug dependence.

OVERDOSAGE

Overdosage with oxytocin depends essentially on uterine hyperactivity, whether or not due to hypersensitivity to this agent. Hyperstimulation with strong (hypertonic) or prolonged (tetanic) contractions, or a resting tone of 15 to 20 mm H_2O or more between contractions can lead to tumultuous labor, uterine rupture, cervical and vaginal lacerations, postpartum hemorrhage, uteroplacental hypoperfusion, and variable deceleration of fetal heart, fetal hypoxia, hypercapnia or death. Water intoxication with convulsions, which is caused by the inherent antidiuretic effect of oxytocin, is a serious complication that may occur if large doses (40 to 50 mL/minute) are infused for long periods. Treatment of water intoxication consists of discontinuation of oxytocin, restriction of fluid intake, diuresis, IV hypertonic saline solution, correction of electrolyte imbalance, control of convulsions with judicious use of a barbiturate, and special nursing care for the comatose patient.

DOSAGE AND ADMINISTRATION

Dosage of oxytocin is determined by uterine response. The following dosage information is based upon the various regimens and indications in general use. Parenteral drug products should be inspected visually for particulate matter and discoloration prior to administration, wherever solution and container permit.

A. Induction or Stimulation of Labor
Intravenous infusion (drip method) is the only acceptable method of administration for the induction or stimulation of labor.

Accurate control of the rate of infusion flow is essential. An infusion pump or other such device and frequent monitoring of strength of contractions and fetal heart rate are necessary for the safe administration of oxytocin for the induction or stimulation of labor. If uterine contractions become too powerful, the infusion can be abruptly stopped, and oxytocic stimulation of the uterine musculature will soon wane.
1. An intravenous infusion of non-oxytocin containing solution should be started. Physiologic electrolyte solution should be used except under unusual circumstances.
2. To prepare the usual solution for infusion, the contents of one 1-mL ampul are combined aseptically with 1,000 mL of nonhydrating diluent. The combined solution, rotated in the infusion bottle to insure thorough mixing contains 10 mU/mL. Add the container with dilute oxytocic solution to the system through use of a constant infusion pump or other such device, to control accurately the rate of infusion.
3. The initial dose should be no more than 1–2 mU/minute. The dose may be gradually increased in increments of no more than 1 to 2 mU/minute until a contraction pattern has been established, which is similar to normal labor.
4. The fetal heart rate, resting uterine tone, and the frequency, duration, and force of contractions should be monitored.
5. The oxytocin infusion should be discontinued immediately in the event of uterine hyperactivity or fetal distress. Oxygen should be administered to the mother. The mother

and the fetus must be evaluated by the responsible physician.
B. Control of Postpartum Uterine Bleeding
1. *Intravenous Infusion (Drip Method):* To control postpartum bleeding, 10–40 units of oxytocin may be added to 1,000 mL of a nonhydrating diluent and run at a rate necessary to control uterine atony.
2. *Intramuscular Administration:* 1 mL (10 units) of oxytocin can be given after delivery of the placenta.
C. Treatment of Incomplete or Inevitable Abortion
Intravenous infusion with physiologic saline solution, 500 mL, or 5% dextrose in physiologic saline solution to which 10 units of Syntocinon® (oxytocin) have been added should be infused at a rate of 20–40 drops/per minute.

HOW SUPPLIED

Ampuls: 1 mL (10 USP units) size, boxes of 20 (NDC 0078-0060-03), 50 (NDC 0078-0060-04) and 100 (NDC 0078-0060-05).

Store and dispense: Below 77°F; DO NOT FREEZE
[SYT-Z20 Issued July 15, 1986]

SYNTOCINON® NASAL SPRAY   ℞

[*sin "tō 'si-non*]
(oxytocin nasal solution, USP)

The following prescribing information is based on official labeling in effect on August 1, 1989.

DESCRIPTION

Each mL contains 40 USP Units (International Units) Syntocinon® (oxytocin) and the following: dried sodium phosphate, USP; citric acid, USP; sodium chloride, USP; glycerin, USP; sorbitol solution, USP; methylparaben, NF; propylparaben, NF; chlorobutanol, NF max. 0.05%, purified water, USP.

Oxytocin is one of the polypeptide hormones of the posterior lobe of the pituitary gland. The pharmacologic and clinical properties of Syntocinon® (oxytocin nasal solution, USP), Nasal Spray are identified with *the oxytocic and the galactokinetic* principle of the natural hormone.

Synthetic oxytocin has the formula $C_{43}H_{66}N_{12}O_{12}S_2$, with a molecular weight of 1007.19. It is represented structurally[1] as:

$$\begin{array}{ccccccc}
4 & 5 & 6 & 7 & 8 & 9 \\
Glu(NH_2)-Asp(NH_2)-Cys-Pro-Leu-Gly(NH_2) \\
| & & & & & | \\
Ile & Tyr & & & & H-Cys \\
3 & 2 & & & & 1
\end{array}$$

Oxytocin

Since oxytocin, a polypeptide, is subject to inactivation by the proteolytic enzymes of the alimentary tract, it is *not absorbed from the gastrointestinal tract.*

CLINICAL PHARMACOLOGY

Syntocinon® (oxytocin nasal solution, USP) Nasal Spray acts specifically on the myoepithelial elements surrounding the alveoli of the breast, and making up the walls of the lactiferous ducts, causing their smooth muscle fibers to contract and thus force milk into the large ducts or sinuses where it is more readily available to the baby. Oxytocin does not possess galactopoietic properties and its use is intended only for the purpose of milk ejection.
Pharmacokinetics: Syntocinon® (oxytocin nasal solution, USP) Nasal Spray is promptly absorbed by the nasal mucosa to enter the systemic circulation. Intranasal application of the spray preparation, however, is a practical and effective method of administration. Half-life is extremely short—less than 10 minutes—and oxytocin is then rapidly removed from plasma by the kidney, liver, and lactating mammary gland. The enzyme oxytocinase is believed to be elaborated by placental and uterine tissues. This enzyme inactivates the hormone by cleavage of the cysteine-tyrosine peptide bond. Excretion is mainly urinary following inactivation of metabolites.[2]

INDICATIONS AND USAGE

Syntocinon® (oxytocin nasal solution, USP) Nasal Spray is indicated to assist initial postpartum milk ejection from the breasts once milk formation has commenced.

CONTRAINDICATIONS

Pregnancy and hypersensitivity are the only known contraindications.

PRECAUTIONS

General: No particular information regarding any special care to be exercised by the practitioner for safe and effective use of the drug is known at this time.
Information for Patients: The squeeze bottle should be held in upright position when administering drug to the nose and patient should be in a sitting position rather than lying down. If preferred, the solution can be instilled in drop form by inverting the squeeze bottle and exerting very gentle pressure on its walls.
Carcinogenesis, Mutagenesis, Impairment of Fertility: There are no animal or human studies on the carcinogenicity and

mutagenicity of this drug, nor is there any information on its effect on fertility.
Pregnancy: Category X. (See Contraindications.) Syntocinon® (oxytocin nasal solution, USP) Nasal Spray is contraindicated during pregnancy since it may provoke a uterotonic effect to precipitate contractions and abortion. Its proper use is during the first week postpartum, as needed.
Nursing Mothers: While harmful effects on the newborn have not been reported, it should be noted that Syntocinon® (oxytocin nasal solution, USP) Nasal Spray is intended to be used only for **initial** milk propulsion and ejection during the first week postpartum, and not for continued use. Caution shall be exercised when Syntocinon® (oxytocin nasal solution, USP) Nasal Spray is administered to a nursing mother since oxytocin is known to be excreted in human milk.

ADVERSE REACTIONS

Lack of efficacy has been the most frequent adverse effect (seven cases), followed by nasal irritation and/or rhinorrhea, uterine bleeding, excessive uterine contractions, and lacrimation.
One case each of seizure and "psychotic state" are the most severe reactions reported. No other reactions have been described.[3]

DRUG ABUSE AND DEPENDENCE

These problems have not been encountered with Syntocinon® (oxytocin nasal solution, USP) Nasal Spray. This may be due to the fact that synthetic oxytocin acts like the natural posterior pituitary hormone. Also, its clinical use is limited to the first week following delivery, to assist in initial milk letdown.

OVERDOSAGE

No case of overdosage with Syntocinon® (oxytocin nasal solution, USP) Nasal Spray has been reported since the preparation became commercially available in 1961. It is theoretically possible for very large doses to be self-administered depending on the topical tolerance of the nasal mucosa. With such massive use, painful uterine contractions could be induced, although these effects persist for only about 15 minutes.[4] Also, an antidiuretic effect could occur resulting in water intoxification. Should this ensue, diuresis should be forced with appropriate agents such as furosemide.[5]

DOSAGE AND ADMINISTRATION

One spray into one or both nostrils two to three minutes before nursing or pumping of breasts.

HOW SUPPLIED

Syntocinon® (oxytocin nasal solution, USP) Nasal Spray in squeeze bottles containing 2 mL oxytocin solution, NDC 0078-0061-23 or 5 mL oxytocin solution, NDC 0078-0061-25.
Store and dispense: Below 77°F; DO NOT FREEZE

REFERENCES

1. U.S.P. XXI, p. 777.
2. Goodman and Gilman: The Pharmacological Basis of Therapeutics. Sixth Ed., 937–8.
3. Data collected by the Medical Services Department. Sandoz Pharmaceuticals Corporation.
4. Borglin, N.E.: The use of intranasal oxytocin for the induction of labor. Zbl. Gynak. **85**: 193–199 (Feb. 9) 1963.
5. Sandoz Overdosage Manual, 1984, Syntocinon Injection.
[SYT-ZZ13 ISSUED JULY 15, 1988]

TAVIST® (clemastine)
Syrup 0.5 mg-5 mL
(present as clemastine
fumarate 0.67 mg/5 mL)

The following prescribing information is based on official labeling in effect on August 1, 1989.

DESCRIPTION

Each teaspoonful (5 mL) of Tavist® (clemastine fumarate) Syrup for oral administration contains clemastine 0.5 mg (present as clemastine fumarate 0.67 mg). Other ingredients: alcohol 5.5%, flavors, methylparaben, propylene glycol, propylparaben, purified water, saccharin sodium, sorbitol in a buffered solution. Tavist® (clemastine fumarate) belongs to the benzhydryl ether group of antihistaminic compounds. The chemical name is (+)-(2R)-2-[2-[[(R)-p-Chloro-α-methyl-α-phenylbenzyl]-oxy] ethyl]-1-methylpyrrolidine fumarate and has the following structural formula:

*U.S. Patent No. 3,097,212.
AHFS Classification 4:00
CAS Registration Number 14976-57-9

Clemastine fumarate occurs as a colorless to faintly yellow, practically odorless, crystalline powder. Tavist® (clemastine fumarate) Syrup has an approximate pH of 6.2.

CLINICAL PHARMACOLOGY

Tavist® (clemastine fumarate) is an antihistamine with anticholinergic (drying) and sedative side effects. Antihistamines competitively antagonize various physiological effects of histamine including increased capillary permeability and dilatation, the formation of edema, the "flare" and "itch" response, and gastrointestinal and respiratory smooth muscle constriction. Within the vascular tree, H_1-receptor antagonists inhibit both the vasoconstrictor and vasodilator effects of histamine. Depending on the dose, H_1- receptor antagonists can produce CNS stimulation or depression. Most antihistamines exhibit central and/or peripheral anticholinergic activity. Antihistamines act by competitively blocking H_1-receptor sites. Antihistamines do not pharmacologically antagonize or chemically inactivate histamine, nor do they prevent the release of histamine.

PHARMACOKINETICS

Antihistamines are well-absorbed following oral administration. Chlorpheniramine maleate, clemastine fumarate, and diphenhydramine hydrochloride achieve peak blood levels within 2–5 hours following oral administration. The absorption of antihistamines is often partially delayed by the use of controlled release dosage forms. In these instances, plasma concentrations from identical doses of the immediate and controlled release dosage forms will not be similar.

Tissue distribution of the antihistamines in humans has not been established.

Antihistamines appear to be metabolized in the liver chiefly via mono- and didemethylation and glucuronide conjugation. Antihistamine metabolites and small amounts of unchanged drug are excreted in the urine. Small amounts of the drugs may also be excreted in breast milk.

In normal human subjects who received histamine injections over a 24-hour period, the antihistaminic activity of Tavist® (clemastine fumarate) reached a peak at 5–7 hours, persisted for 10–12 hours and, in some cases, for as long as 24 hours. Pharmacokinetic studies in man utilizing ^{3}H and ^{14}C labeled compound demonstrates that: Tavist® (clemastine fumarate) is rapidly absorbed from the gastrointestinal tract, peak plasma concentrations are attained in 2–4 hours, and urinary excretion is the major mode of elimination.

INDICATIONS AND USAGE

Tavist® (clemastine fumarate) Syrup is indicated for the relief of symptoms associated with allergic rhinitis such as sneezing, rhinorrhea, pruritus and lacrimation. Tavist (clemastine fumarate) Syrup is indicated for use in pediatric populations (age 6 years through 12) and adults (see *DOSAGE AND ADMINISTRATION*).

It should be noted that Tavist® (clemastine fumarate) is indicated for the relief of mild uncomplicated allergic skin manifestations of urticaria and angioedema at the 2 mg dosage level only.

CONTRAINDICATIONS

Antihistamines are contraindicated in patients hypersensitive to the drug or to other antihistamines of similar chemical structure (see *PRECAUTIONS —Drug Interactions*).

Antihistamines *should not* be used *in newborn or premature infants*. Because of the higher risk of antihistamines for infants generally and for newborns and prematures in particular, antihistamine therapy is contraindicated in *nursing mothers* (See *PRECAUTIONS —Nursing Mothers*).

WARNINGS

Antihistamines should be used with considerable caution in patients with: narrow angle glaucoma, stenosing peptic ulcer, pyloroduodenal obstruction, symptomatic prostatic hypertrophy, and bladder neck obstruction.

Use with CNS Depressants: Tavist® (clemastine fumarate) has additive effects with alcohol and other CNS depressants (hypnotics, sedatives, tranquilizers, etc.)

Use in Activities Requiring Mental Alertness: Patients should be warned about engaging in activities requiring mental alertness such as driving a car or operating appliances, machinery, etc.

Use in the Elderly (approximately 60 years or older): Antihistamines are more likely to cause dizziness, sedation, and hypotension in elderly patients.

PRECAUTIONS

General: Tavist® (clemastine fumarate) should be used with caution in patients with: history of bronchial asthma, increased intraocular pressure, hyperthyroidism, cardiovascular disease, and hypertension.

Information for Patients:
Patients taking antihistamines should receive the following information and instructions:
1. Antihistamines are prescribed to reduce allergic symptoms.

2. Patients should be questioned regarding a history of glaucoma, peptic ulcer, urinary retention, or pregnancy before starting antihistamine therapy.
3. Patients should be told not to take alcohol, sleeping pills, sedatives, or tranquilizers while taking antihistamines.
4. Antihistamines may cause drowsiness, dizziness, dry mouth, blurred vision, weakness, nausea, headache, or nervousness in some patients.
5. Patients should avoid driving a car or working with hazardous machinery until they assess the effects of this medicine.
6. Patients should be told to store this medicine in a tightly closed container in a dry, cool place away from heat or direct sunlight and out of the reach of children.

Drug Interactions:
Additive CNS depression may occur when antihistamines are administered concomitantly with other CNS depressants including barbiturates, tranquilizers, and alcohol. Patients receiving antihistamines should be advised against the concurrent use of other CNS depressant drugs.

Monoamine oxidase (MAO) inhibitors prolong and intensify the anticholinergic effects of antihistamines.

Carcinogenesis, Mutagenesis, Impairment of Fertility:
Carcinogenesis and Mutagenesis: In a 2-year oral study in the rat at a dose of 84 mg/kg (about 500 times the adult human dose) and an 85-week oral study in the mouse at 206 mg/kg (about 1300 times the adult human dose), clemastine fumarate showed no evidence of carcinogenesis. No mutagenic studies have been conducted with clemastine fumarate.

Impairment of Fertility: Oral doses of clemastine fumarate in the rat produced a decrease in mating ability of the male at 312 times the adult human dose. This effect was not found at 156 times the adult human dose.

Pregnancy —*Pregnancy Category B:* Oral reproduction studies performed with clemastine fumarate in rats and rabbits at doses up to 312 and 188 times the adult human doses respectively, have revealed no evidence of teratogenic effects.

There are no adequate and well-controlled studies of Tavist® (clemastine fumarate) Syrup in pregnant women. Because animal reproduction studies are not always predictive of human response, this drug should be used in pregnancy only if clearly needed.

Nursing Mothers:
Although quantitative determinations of antihistaminic drugs in breast milk have not been reported, qualitative tests have documented the excretion of diphenhydramine, pyrilamine, and tripelennamine in human milk.

Because of the potential for adverse reactions in nursing infants from antihistamines, a decision should be made whether to discontinue nursing or to discontinue the drug.

Pediatric Use: The safety and efficacy of Tavist® (clemastine fumarate) Syrup has been confirmed in the pediatric population (age 6 years through 12). Safety and dose tolerance studies have confirmed children 6 through 11 years tolerated dosage ranges of 0.75 to 2.25 mg clemastine. In infants and children particularly, antihistamines in overdosage may produce hallucinations, convulsions, and death. Symptoms of antihistamine toxicity in children may include fixed dilated pupils, flushed face, dry mouth, fever, excitation, hallucinations, ataxia, incoordination, athetosis, tonic-clonic convulsions, and postictal depression (see *OVERDOSAGE*).

ADVERSE REACTIONS

The most frequent adverse reactions are underlined:

Nervous System: Sedation, sleepiness, dizziness, disturbed coordination, fatigue, confusion, restlessness, excitation, nervousness, tremor, irritability, insomnia, euphoria, paresthesia, blurred vision, diplopia, vertigo, tinnitus, acute labyrinthitis, hysteria, neuritis, convulsions.

Gastrointestinal System: Epigastric distress, anorexia, nausea, vomiting, diarrhea, constipation.

Respiratory System: Thickening of bronchial secretions, tightness of chest and wheezing, nasal stuffiness.

Cardiovascular System: Hypotension, headache, palpitations, tachycardia, extrasystoles.

Hematologic System: Hemolytic anemia, thrombocytopenia, agranulocytosis.

Genitourinary System: Urinary frequency, difficult urination, urinary retention, early menses.

General: Urticaria, drug rash, anaphylactic shock, photosensitivity, excessive perspiration, chills, dryness of mouth, nose, and throat.

OVERDOSAGE

Antihistamine overdosage reactions may vary from central nervous system depression to stimulation. In children, stimulation predominates initially in a syndrome which may include excitement, hallucinations, ataxia, incoordination, muscle twitching, athetosis, hyperthermia, cyanosis convulsions, tremors, and hyperreflexia followed by postictal depression and cardio-respiratory arrest. Convulsions in children may be preceded by mild depression. Dry mouth, fixed, dilated pupils, flushing of the face, and fever are common. In adults, CNS depression, ranging from drowsiness to coma, is

more common. The convulsant dose of antihistamines lies near the lethal dose. Convulsions indicate a poor prognosis. In both children and adults, coma and cardiovascular collapse may occur. Deaths are reported especially in infants and children.

There is no specific therapy for acute overdosage with antihistamines. The latent period from ingestion to appearance of toxic effects is characteristically short ($\frac{1}{2}$–2 hours). General symptomatic and supportive measures should be instituted promptly and maintained for as long as necessary.

Since overdoses of other classes of drugs (i.e., tricyclic antidepressants)may also present anticholinergic symptomatology, appropriate toxicological analysis should be performed as soon as possible to identify the causative agent.

In the conscious patient, vomiting should be induced even though it may have occured spontaneously. If vomiting cannot be induced, gastric lavage is indicated. Adequate precautions must be taken to protect against aspiration, especially in infants and children. Charcoal slurry or other suitable agents should be instilled into the stomach after vomiting or lavage. Saline cathartics or milk of magnesia may be of additional benefit.

In the unconscious patient, the airway should be secured with a cuffed endotracheal tube before attempting to evacuate the gastric contents. Intensivesupportive and nursing care is indicated, as for any comatose patient.

If breathing is significantly impaired, maintenance of an adequate airway and mechanical support of respiration is the most effective means of providing adequate oxygenation.

Hypotension is an early sign of impending cardiovascular collapse and should be treated vigorously. Although general supportive measuresare important, specific treatment with intravenous infusion of a vasopressor titrated to maintain adequate blood pressure may be necessary.

Do not use with CNS stimulants.

Convulsions should be controlled by careful administration of diazepam or a short-acting barbiturate, repeated as necessary. Physostigmine may also be considered for use in controlling centrally mediated convulsions.

Ice packs and cooling sponge baths, not alcohol, can aid in reducing the fever commonly seen in children.

A more detailed review of antihistamine toxicology and overdose management is available in Gosselin, R.E., et al., "Clinical Toxicology of Commercial Products."

DOSAGE AND ADMINISTRATION

DOSAGE SHOULD BE INDIVIDUALIZED ACCORDING TO THE NEEDS AND RESPONSE OF THE PATIENT.

Pediatric: Children aged 6 to 12 years:
For Symptoms of Allergic Rhinitis—The starting dose is 1 teaspoonful (0.5 mg clemastine) twice daily. Since single doses of up to 2.25 mg clemastine were well tolerated by this age group, dosage may be increased as required, but not to exceed 6 teaspoonful daily (3 mg clemastine).

For Urticaria and Angioedema—The starting dose is 2 teaspoonful (1 mg clemastine) twice daily, not to exceed 6 teaspoonful daily (3 mg clemastine).

Adults and Children 12 Years and Over:
For Symptoms of Allergic Rhinitis—The starting dose is 2 teaspoonsful (1.0 mg clemastine) twice daily. Dosage may be increased as required, but not to exceed 12 teaspoonsful daily (6 mg clemastine).

For Urticaria and Angioedema—The starting dose is 4 teaspoonsful (2 mg clemastine) twice daily, not to exceed 12 teaspoonsful daily (6 mg clemastine).

HOW SUPPLIED

Tavist® (clemastine fumarate) Syrup: clemastine 0.5 mg/5 mL (present as clemastine fumarate 0.67 mg/5 mL). A clear, colorless liquid with a citrus flavor, in 4 fl. oz. bottle (NDC 0078-0222-31).

STORE AND DISPENSE

Below 77°F (25°C) tight, amber glass bottle. Store in an upright position.

[TAS-Z3 Issued April 1, 1986]

TAVIST-1® **(clemastine fumarate)**   ℞
[*tav ′ist*]
Tablets, USP 1.34 mg
TAVIST® **(clemastine fumarate)**
Tablets, USP 2.68 mg

The following prescribing information is based on official labeling in effect on August 1, 1989.

DESCRIPTION

TAVIST® (clemastine fumarate) belongs to the benzhydryl ether group of antihistaminic compounds. The chemical name is (+)-2-[2-[(p- chloro-α-methyl-α-phenylbenzyl) oxy] ethyl]-1-methylpyrrolidine hydrogen fumarate.
[See Chemical Formula at top of next page].

Continued on next page

Sandoz Pharm.—Cont.

*U.S. Patent No. 3,097,212

1.34 mg and 2.68 mg, Tablets
Active Ingredient: clemastine fumarate, USP
Inactive Ingredients: lactose, povidone, starch, stearic acid, and talc

ACTIONS

TAVIST® (clemastine fumarate) is an antihistamine with anticholinergic (drying) and sedative side effects. Antihistamines appear to compete with histamine for cell receptor sites on effector cells. The inherently long duration of antihistaminic effects of TAVIST® (clemastine fumarate) has been demonstrated in wheal and flare studies. In normal human subjects who received histamine injections over a 24-hour period, the antihistaminic activity of TAVIST® (clemastine fumarate) reached a peak at 5–7 hours, persisted for 10–12 hours and, in some cases, for as long as 24 hours. Pharmacokinetic studies in man utilizing ^3H and ^{14}C labeled compound demonstrates that: TAVIST® (clemastine fumarate) is rapidly and nearly completely absorbed from the gastrointestinal tract, peak plasma concentrations are attained in 2–4 hours, and urinary excretion is the major mode of elimination.

INDICATIONS

TAVIST-1® (clemastine fumarate) Tablets 1.34 mg are indicated for the relief of symptoms associated with allergic rhinitis such as sneezing, rhinorrhea, pruritus and lacrimation. TAVIST® (clemastine fumarate) Tablets 2.68 mg are indicated for the relief of symptoms associated with allergic rhinitis such as sneezing, rhinorrhea, pruritus, and lacrimation. TAVIST® (clemastine fumarate) Tablets 2.68 mg are also indicated for the relief of mild, uncomplicated allergic skin manifestations of urticaria and angioedema.
It should be noted that TAVIST® (clemastine fumarate) is indicated for the dermatologic indications at the 2.68 mg dosage level only.

CONTRAINDICATIONS

Use in Nursing Mothers: Because of the higher risk of antihistamines for infants generally and for newborns and prematures in particular, antihistamine therapy is contraindicated in nursing mothers.
Use in Lower Respiratory Disease: Antihistamines *should not* be used to treat lower respiratory tract symptoms including asthma.
Antihistamines are also contraindicated in the following conditions:
Hypersensitivity to TAVIST® (clemastine fumarate) or other antihistamines of similar chemical structure.
Monamine oxidase inhibitor therapy (see Drug Interaction Section).

WARNINGS

Antihistamines should be used with considerable caution in patients with: narrow angle glaucoma, stenosing peptic ulcer, pyloroduodenal obstruction, symptomatic prostatic hypertrophy, and bladder neck obstruction.
Use in Children: Safety and efficacy of TAVIST® (clemastine fumarate) have not been established in children under the age of 12.
Use in Pregnancy: Experience with this drug in pregnant women is inadequate to determine whether there exists a potential for harm to the developing fetus.
Use with CNS Depressants: TAVIST® (clemastine fumarate) has additive effects with alcohol and other CNS depressants (hypnotics, sedatives, tranquilizers, etc.).
Use in Activities Requiring Mental Alertness: Patients should be warned about engaging in activities requiring mental alertness such as driving a car or operating appliances, machinery, etc.
Use in the Elderly (approximately 60 years or older): Antihistamines are more likely to cause dizziness, sedation, and hypotension in elderly patients.

PRECAUTIONS

TAVIST® (clemastine fumarate) should be used with caution in patients with: history of bronchial asthma, increased intraocular pressure, hyperthyroidism, cardiovascular disease, and hypertension.
Drug Interactions: MAO inhibitors prolong and intensify the anticholinergic (drying) effects of antihistamines.

ADVERSE REACTIONS

Transient drowsiness, the most common adverse reaction associated with TAVIST® (clemastine fumarate), occurs relatively frequently and may require discontinuation of therapy in some instances.
Antihistaminic Compounds: It should been noted that the following reactions have occurred with one or more antihistamines and, therefore, should be kept in mind when prescribing drugs belonging to this class, including TAVIST. The most frequent adverse reactions are underlined.

1. *General:* Urticaria, drug rash, anaphylactic shock, photosensitivity, excessive perspiration, chills, dryness of mouth, nose, and throat.
2. *Cardiovascular System:* Hypotension, headache, palpitations, tachycardia, extrasystoles.
3. *Hematologic System:* Hemolytic anemia, thrombocytopenia, agranulocytosis.
4. *Nervous System:* Sedation, sleepiness, dizziness, disturbed coordination, fatigue, confusion, restlessness, excitation, nervousness, tremor, irritability, insomnia, euphoria, paresthesias, blurred vision, diplopia, vertigo, tinnitus, acute labyrinthitis, hysteria, neuritis, convulsions.
5. *GI System:* Epigastric distress, anorexia, nausea, vomiting, diarrhea, constipation.
6. *GU System:* Urinary frequency, difficult urination, urinary retention, early menses.
7. *Respiratory System:* Thickening of bronchial secretions, tightness of chest and wheezing, nasal stuffiness.

OVERDOSAGE

Antihistamine overdosage reactions may vary from central nervous system depression to stimulation. Stimulation is particularly likely in children. Atropine-like signs and symptoms: dry mouth; fixed, dilated pupils; flushing; and gastrointestinal symptoms may also occur.
If vomiting has not occurred spontaneously the conscious patient should be induced to vomit. This is best done by having him drink a glass of water or milk after which he should be made to gag. Precautions against aspiration must be taken, especially in infants and children.
If vomiting is unsuccessful gastric lavage is indicated within 3 hours after ingestion and even later if large amounts of milk or cream were given beforehand. Isotonic and $\frac{1}{2}$ isotonic saline is the lavage solution of choice.
Saline cathartics, such as milk of magnesia, by osmosis draw water into the bowel and therefore, are valuable for their action in rapid dilution of bowel content.
Stimulants should *not* be used.
Vasopressors may be used to treat hypotension.

DOSAGE AND ADMINISTRATION

DOSAGE SHOULD BE INDIVIDUALIZED ACCORDING TO THE NEEDS AND RESPONSE OF THE PATIENT.
TAVIST-1® (clemastine fumarate) Tablets 1.34 mg: The recommended starting dose is one tablet twice daily. Dosage may be increased as required, but not to exceed six tablets daily.
TAVIST® (clemastine fumarate) Tablets 2.68 mg: The maximum recommended dosage is one tablet three times daily. Many patients respond favorably to a single dose which may be repeated as required, but not to exceed three tablets daily.

HOW SUPPLIED

TAVIST-1® (clemastine fumarate) Tablets: 1.34 mg clemastine fumarate. White, oval compressed, scored tablet, packages of 100.
TAVIST® (clemastine fumarate) Tablets: 2.68 mg clemastine fumarate. White, round compressed tablet, packages of 100.
Company's Product Identification Mark(s): Tavist-1® (clemastine fumarate) Tablets: 1.34 mg, embossed "78-75" on one side, "TAVIST 1" on the other.
Tavist Tablets: 2.68 mg, embossed "78/72" and scored on one side, "TAVIST" on the other.
[TAV-Z3 Issued July 15, 1986]
Shown in Product Identification Section, page 427

TAVIST-D® ℞

[tav 'ist]
(clemastine fumarate USP
phenylpropanolamine HCl USP)
Tablets

The following prescribing information is based on official labeling in effect on August 1, 1989.

DESCRIPTION

Each TAVIST-D® (clemastine fumarate/phenylpropanolamine HCl) Tablet contains 1.34 mg clemastine fumarate (equivalent to 1 mg of the free base) and 75 mg phenylpropanolamine hydrochloride. The clemastine fumarate is in the outer shell of the tablet and is immediately released upon dissolution. The tablet's core is a sustained-release matrix which releases the phenylpropanolamine hydrochloride over a 12-hour period at a rate that produces blood levels bio-equivalent to those obtained by the administration of 25 mg standard release tablets of phenylpropanolamine hydrochloride every four hours for three doses. Clemastine fumarate belongs to the benzhydryl ether group of antihistaminic compounds. The chemical name is (+)-2-[2-[(p-chloro-α-methyl-α-phenyl benzyl) oxy] ethyl]-1-methylpyrrolidine hydrogen fumarate and the structural formula is:

Phenylpropanolamine hydrochloride is a sympathomimetic, orally effective nasal decongestant. Sympathomimetic compounds, whether catecholamines or noncatecholamines, can be regarded as compounds produced by substitution on the phenylethylamine nucleus common to all these sympathomimetic products, whether their action is on the Alpha receptors of the sympathetic nervous system or on Beta-1 or Beta-2 receptors. The chemical name for phenylpropanolamine hydrochloride is α-(1-Aminoethyl)benzenemethanol hydrochloride, and the structural formula is:

Active Ingredient: clemastine fumarate, USP phenylpropanolamine HCl, USP
Inactive Ingredients: colloidal silicon dioxide, D&C Yellow #10, dibasic calcium phosphate dihydrate, lactose, magnesium stearate, methylcellulose, polyethylene glycol, povidone, starch, synthetic polymers, and titanium dioxide

CLINICAL PHARMACOLOGY

Clemastine fumarate is an antihistamine with anticholinergic (drying) and sedative side effects. Antihistamines appear to compete with histamine for cell receptor sites on effector cells. The inherently long duration of antihistaminic effects of clemastine fumarate has been demonstrated in wheal and flare studies. In normal human subjects who received intradermal histamine injections over a 24-hour period, the antihistaminic activity of clemastine fumarate, as demonstrated by inhibition of the wheal and flare reaction, reached a peak at 5–7 hours, persisted for 10–12 hours and, in some cases, for as long as 24 hours. Pharmacokinetic studies in man utilizing ^3H and ^{14}C labeled compound demonstrate that clemastine fumarate is rapidly and nearly completely absorbed from the gastrointestinal tract, peak plasma concentrations are attained in 2–4 hours, and urinary excretion is the major mode of elimination.
Phenylpropanolamine hydrochloride is an Alpha adrenergic stimulator producing nasal decongestion by constriction of arterioles and precapillary arterioles in the nasal mucosa. Phenylpropanolamine hydrochloride is one of the most widely used oral nasal decongestants; it is similar in action to ephedrine, but produces less central nervous system stimulation.
In adult subjects who were given one TAVIST-D® (clemastine fumarate/phenylpropanolamine HCl) Tablet, the average peak plasma concentration of phenylpropanolamine was 85.4 ng/ml ± 13.1 (S.D.) which occurred at about 4.3 hours. In this crossover study these same subjects were given a 25 mg phenylpropanolamine hydrochloride tablet every 4 hours for 3 consecutive doses plus a single dose of a TAVIST-1 Tablet (clemastine fumarate 1.34 mg). The average peak concentration of phenylpropanolamine was found to be 67.6 ng/ml ± 11.6 (S.D.) which occurred at about 8.2 hours.
In another study, adult subjects received TAVIST-D® Tablets every 12 hours for 4 consecutive days. The average peak concentration of phenylpropanolamine was found to be 117.29 ng/ml ± 14.52 (S.D.) which occurred at about 6.2 hours after the morning dose. In this crossover study these same subjects received a 25 mg phenylpropanolamine hydrochloride tablet every 4 hours for 4 consecutive days. In addition they received a TAVIST-1 Tablet (clemastine fumarate 1.34 mg) every 12 hours for 4 consecutive days. The average peak concentration of phenylpropanolamine was found to be 107.92 ng/ml ± 15.97 (S.D.) which occurred at about 4.8 hours after the first dose in the morning.

INDICATIONS AND USAGE

TAVIST-D® (clemastine fumarate/phenylpropanolamine HCl) Tablets are indicated for the relief of symptoms associated with allergic rhinitis such as sneezing, rhinorrhea, pruritus of the eyes, nose or throat, lacrimation and nasal congestion.

CONTRAINDICATION

Tavist-D® Tablets are contraindicated in patients hypersensitive to any of the components. Antihistamines should not be used in newborn or premature infants or in nursing mothers. Antihistamines should not be used to treat lower respiratory tract symptoms including asthma. Tavist-D® Tablets are contraindicated in patients receiving monoamine oxidase inhibitors (see PRECAUTIONS—Drug Interactions) and in patients with severe hypertension or severe coronary artery disease.

WARNINGS

Antihistamines such as clemastine fumarate should be used with considerable caution in patients with narrow angle glaucoma, stenosing peptic ulcer, pyloroduodenal obstruction, symptomatic prostatic hypertrophy, and bladder neck obstruction. Sympathomimetic drugs such as phenylpropanolamine hydrochloride should be used with caution in hypertension, cardiovascular disease, diabetes mellitus, and uncontrolled hyperthyroidism.

Use with CNS Depressants: Antihistamines have additive effects with alcohol and other CNS depressants (hypnotics, sedatives, tranquilizers, etc.).

Use in Activities Requiring Mental Alertness: Patients should be warned about engaging in activities requiring mental alertness such as driving a car or operating appliances, machinery, etc.

Use in the Elderly (approximately 60 years or older): Antihistamines are more likely to cause dizziness, sedation and hypotension in elderly patients. Overdosages of sympathomimetics in this age group may cause hallucinations, convulsions, CNS depression and death in elderly patients.

Use in Children: Safety and effectiveness of TAVIST-D® (clemastine fumarate/phenylpropanolamine HCl) have not been established in children under the age of 12. In infants and children, especially, antihistamines in *overdosage* may cause hallucinations, convulsions or death. As in adults antihistamines may diminish mental alertness, but they may also produce excitation, particularly in young children.

PRECAUTIONS

General: TAVIST-D® (clemastine fumarate/phenylpropanolamine HCl) Tablets should be used with caution in patients with: History of bronchial asthma, increased intraocular pressure, hyperthyroidism, cardiovascular disease, hypertension, diabetes mellitus, and prostate disease. (See WARNINGS.)

Information for Patients: Patients should be informed of the potential for sedation or drowsiness and warned about driving or operating machinery. The concomitant consumption of alcoholic beverages or other sedative drugs should be avoided.

Due to the inherently long-acting nature of clemastine fumarate and due to the sustained-release of phenylpropanolamine hydrochloride from the tablet's core, TAVIST-D® Tablets provide prolonged symptomatic relief (10–14 hours).

Drug Interactions:
(1) Monoamine oxidase inhibitors; MAO inhibitors prolong and intensify the anticholinergic effects of antihistamines and potentiate the pressor effects of sympathomimetics.
(2) Alcohol and CNS depressants: These agents potentiate the sedative effects of antihistamines.
(3) Certain antihypertensives: Sympathomimetics may reduce the antihypertensive effects of methyldopa, mecamylamine, reserpine and veratrum alkaloids.

Carcinogenesis and Mutagenesis: Carcinogenic studies have not been conducted on the drug combination of clemastine fumarate/phenylpropanolamine hydrochloride. In a two-year oral study in the rat at a dose of 84 mg/Kg (about 1500 times the human dose) and an 85-week oral study in the mouse at 206 mg/Kg (about 3800 times the human dose), clemastine fumarate showed no evidence of carcinogenesis. No mutagenic studies have been conducted with clemastine fumarate, phenylpropanolamine hydrochloride or the drug combination.

Impairment of Fertility: Oral doses of clemastine fumarate alone in the rat produced a decrease in mating ability of the male at 933 times the human dose. This effect was not found at 466 times the human dose.

Pregnancy—*Pregnancy Category B:* Oral reproduction studies performed with clemastine fumarate alone in rats and rabbits at doses up to 933 and 560 times the human dose, respectively, have revealed no evidence of teratogenic effects. Reproduction studies have not been conducted with phenylpropanolamine hydrochloride.

Oral reproduction studies on the drug combination in a ratio of 1 part of clemastine fumarate to 49 parts of phenylpropanolamine hydrochloride in rats and rabbits at doses up to 100 and 67 times the human dose, respectively, have revealed no evidence of teratogenic effects. Adverse reactions attributed to the pharmacological effects of phenylpropanolamine were as follows: Rats—Impaired weight gain and deaths in dams at 33 times the human dose and a slight increase in pre-implantation loss and prenatal deaths, and reduced fetal weights at 100 times the human dose. Rabbits—Increased maternal deaths at 20 times the human dose, and increased maternal deaths and weight loss plus a slight increase in

prenatal deaths (within normal limits) at 67 times the human dose.

There are no adequate and well controlled studies of TAVIST-D® (clemastine fumarate/phenylpropanolamine HCl) Tablets in pregnant women. Because animal reproductive studies are not always predictive of human response, this drug should be used in pregnancy only if clearly needed.

Nursing Mothers: See CONTRAINDICATIONS:

ADVERSE REACTIONS

Antihistaminic Compounds: It should be noted that the following reactions have occurred with one or more antihistamines and, therefore, should be kept in mind when prescribing drugs belonging to this class, including clemastine fumarate. The most frequent adverse reactions reported with clemastine fumarate are underlined.

1. *General:* Urticaria, drug rash, anaphylactic shock, photosensitivity, excessive perspiration, chills, dryness of mouth, nose and throat.
2. *Cardiovascular System:* Hypotension, headache, palpitations, tachycardia, extrasystoles.
3. *Hematologic System:* Hemolytic anemia, thrombocytopenia, agranulocytosis.
4. *Nervous System:* <u>Sedation</u>, <u>sleepiness</u>, <u>dizziness</u>, <u>disturbed coordination</u>, fatigue, confusion, restlessness, excitation, nervousness, tremor, irritability, insomnia, euphoria, paresthesias, blurred vision, diplopia, vertigo, tinnitus, acute labyrinthitis, hysteria, neuritis, convulsions.
5. *GI System:* <u>Epigastric distress</u>, anorexia, nausea, vomiting, diarrhea, constipation.
6. *GU System:* Urinary frequency, difficult urination, urinary retention, early menses.
7. *Respiratory System:* <u>Thickening of bronchial secretions</u>, tightness of chest and wheezing, nasal stuffiness.

Sympathomimetic Compounds:

Nervous System: At higher doses may cause drowsiness, dizziness, nervousness, or sleeplessness, and especially in children may cause excitability. Phenylpropanolamine hydrochloride may cause elevated blood pressure and tachyarrhythmias, especially in hyperthyroid patients.

OVERDOSAGE

Antihistamine overdosage reactions may vary from central nervous system depression to stimulation. Stimulation is particularly likely in children. Atropine-like signs and symptoms: dry mouth; fixed, dilated pupils; flushing; and gastrointestinal symptoms may also occur.

Overdosage of the phenylpropanolamine hydrochloride may produce tachycardia, pupillary dilatation, excitation and arrhythmias.

If vomiting has not occurred spontaneously the conscious patient should be induced to vomit. This is best done by having the patient drink a glass of water or milk along with an appropriate amount of Syrup of Ipecac. Precautions against aspiration must be taken, especially in infants and children.

If vomiting is unsuccessful in 20 minutes, gastric lavage is indicated within 3 hours after ingestion and even later if large amounts of milk or cream were given beforehand. Isotonic and ½ isotonic saline is the lavage solution of choice.

Saline cathartics, such as milk of magnesia, by osmosis draw water into the bowel and therefore are valuable for their action in rapid dilution of bowel content.

Stimulants should *not* be used.

Activated charcoal has been demonstrated to interfere with phenylpropanolamine absorption.

The value of dialysis has not been established.

The concentration of phenylpropanolamine hydrochloride or clemastine fumarate in biological fluids associated with toxicity is not known.

The amount of TAVIST-D® in single doses associated with significant signs of overdose or death is not known.

The oral LD_{50} for a mixture containing 50 mg phenylpropanolamine hydrochloride and 1.34 mg clemastine fumarate is 1277 mg/Kg in mice, 602 mg/Kg in rats and 634 mg/Kg in rabbits.

DOSAGE AND ADMINISTRATION

Adults and children twelve years and over: One tablet swallowed whole every twelve hours.

HOW SUPPLIED

TAVIST-D® (clemastine fumarate/phenylpropanolamine HCl) Tablets: containing 1.34 mg clemastine fumarate (equivalent to 1 mg of the free base) and 75 mg phenylpropanolamine hydrochloride. White, round, film-coated multiple compressed tablet, packages of 100 (NDC 0078-0221-05). TAVIST-D® Tablets should be stored and dispensed below 86°F in a tight, light-resistant container.

Company's Product Identification Mark(s): Tavist-D® Tablets embossed "TAVIST-D" on one side and "78-221" on the other.

[TAD-Z4 Issued April 15, 1986]

Shown in Product Identification Section, page 427

VISKEN®   ℞

[*vis'kin*]

(pindolol) tablets, USP

The following prescribing information is based on official labeling in effect on August 1, 1989.

DESCRIPTION

Visken® (pindolol), a synthetic beta-adrenergic receptor blocking agent with intrinsic sympathomimetic activity is 4-(2-hydroxy-3-isopropylaminopropoxy)-indole.

Molecular Weight—248.3

Pindolol is a white to off-white odorless powder soluble in organic solvents and aqueous acids.

5 mg. and 10 mg. Tablets

Active Ingredient: pindolol

Inactive Ingredients: colloidal silicon dioxide, magnesium stearate, microcrystalline cellulose, and pregelatinized starch

CLINICAL PHARMACOLOGY

Visken® (pindolol) is a non-selective beta-adrenergic antagonist (beta-blocker) which possesses intrinsic sympathomimetic activity (ISA) in therapeutic dosage ranges but does not possess quinidine-like membrane stabilizing activity.

PHARMACODYNAMICS

In standard pharmacologic tests in man and animals, Visken® (pindolol) attenuates increases in heart rate, systolic blood pressure, and cardiac output resulting from exercise and isoproterenol administration, thus confirming its beta-blocking properties. The ISA or partial agonist activity of Visken® (pindolol) is mediated directly at the adrenergic receptor sites and may be blocked by other beta-blockers. In catecholamine depleted animal experiments, ISA is manifested as an increase in the inotropic and chronotropic activity of the myocardium. In man, ISA is manifested by a smaller reduction in the resting heart rate (4–8 beats/min) than is seen with drugs lacking ISA. There is also a smaller reduction in resting cardiac output. The clinical significance of this observation has not been evaluated and there is no evidence, or reason to believe, that exercise cardiac output is less affected by Visken® (pindolol).

Visken® (pindolol) has been shown in controlled, double-blind clinical studies to be an effective antihypertensive agent when used as monotherapy, or when added to therapy with thiazide-type diuretics. Divided dosages in the range of 10 mg—60 mg daily have been shown to be effective. As monotherapy, Visken® (pindolol) is as effective as propranolol, α-methyldopa, hydrochlorothiazide and chlorthalidone in reducing systolic and diastolic blood pressure. The effect on blood pressure is not orthostatic, i.e. Visken® (pindolol) was equally effective in reducing the supine and standing blood pressure.

In open, long-term studies up to four (4) years, no evidence of diminution of the blood pressure lowering response was observed.

An average 3 pound increase in body weight has been noted in patients treated with Visken® (pindolol) alone, a larger increase than was observed with propranolol or placebo. The weight gain appeared unrelated to blood pressure response and was not associated with an increased risk of heart failure, although edema was more common than in control patients. Visken® (pindolol) does not have a consistent effect on plasma renin activity.

The mechanism of the antihypertensive effects of beta-blocking agents has not been established, but several mechanisms have been postulated: 1) an effect on the central nervous system resulting in a reduced sympathetic outflow to the periphery, 2) competitive antagonism of catecholamines at peripheral (especially cardiac) adrenergic receptor sites, leading to decreased cardiac output, 3) an inhibition of renin release. These mechanisms appear less likely for pindolol than other beta-blockers in view of the modest effect on resting cardiac output and renin.

Beta-blockade therapy is useful when it is necessary to suppress the effects of beta-adrenergic agonists in order to achieve therapeutic goals. However, in certain clinical situations, (e.g., cardiac failure, heart block, bronchospasm) the preservation of an adequate sympathetic tone may be necessary to maintain vital functions. Although a beta-antagonist with ISA such as Visken® (pindolol) does not eliminate sympathetic tone entirely, there is no controlled evidence that it is safer than other beta-blockers in such conditions as heart failure, heart block, or bronchospasm or is less likely to cause

Continued on next page

Sandoz Pharm.—Cont.

those conditions. In single dose studies of the effects of beta-blockers on FEV_1, Visken® (pindolol) was indistinguishable from other non-cardioselective agents in its reduction of FEV_1, and its reduction in the effectiveness of an exogenous beta agonist.

Exacerbation of angina and, in some cases, myocardial infarction and ventricular dysrhythmias have been reported after abrupt discontinuation of therapy with beta-adrenergic blocking agents in patients with coronary artery disease. Abrupt withdrawal of these agents in patients without coronary artery disease has resulted in transient symptoms, including tremulousness, sweating, palpitation, headache, and malaise. Several mechanisms have been proposed to explain these phenomena, among them increased sensitivity to catecholamines because of increased numbers of beta receptors.

Pharmacokinetics and Metabolism: Visken® (pindolol) is rapidly and reproducibly absorbed (greater than 95%), achieving peak plasma concentrations within one hour of drug administration. Visken® (pindolol) has no significant first-pass effect. The blood concentrations are proportional in a linear manner to the administered dose in the range of 5–20 mg. Upon repeated administration to the same subject, variation is minimal. After a single dose, intersubject variation for peak plasma concentrations was about 4 fold (e.g. 45–167 ng/ml for a 20 mg dose). Upon multiple dosing, intersubject variation decreased to 2–2.5 fold. Visken® (pindolol) is only 40% bound to plasma proteins and is evenly distributed between plasma and red cells. The volume of distribution in healthy subjects is about 2 L/kg.

Visken® (pindolol) undergoes extensive metabolism in animals and man. In man, 35–40% is excreted unchanged in the urine and 60–65% is metabolized primarily to hydroxy-metabolites which are excreted as glucuronides and ethereal sulfates. The polar metabolites are excreted with a half-life of approximately 8 hours and thus multiple dosing therapy (q.8H) results in a less than 50% accumulation in plasma. About 6–9% of an administered intravenous dose is excreted by the bile into the feces.

The disposition of Visken® (pindolol) after oral administration is monophasic with a half-life in healthy subjects or hypertensive patients with normal renal function of approximately 3–4 hours. Following t.i.d. administration (q.8H), no significant accumulation of Visken® (pindolol) is observed. In elderly hypertensive patients with normal renal function, the half-life of Visken® (pindolol) is more variable, averaging about 7 hours, but with values as high as 15 hours.

In hypertensive patients with renal diseases, the half-life is within the range expected for healthy subjects. However, a significant decrease (50%) in volume of distribution (V_D) is observed in uremic patients and V_D appears to be directly correlated to creatinine clearance. Therefore, renal drug clearance is significantly reduced in uremic patients, resulting in a significant decrease in urinary excretion of unchanged drug. Uremic patients with a creatinine clearance of less than 20 mL/min generally excreted less than 15% of the administered dose unchanged in the urine.

In patients with histologically diagnosed cirrhosis of the liver, the elimination of Visken® (pindolol) was more variable in rate and generally significantly slower than in healthy subjects. The total body clearance of Visken® (pindolol) in cirrhotic patients ranged from about 50 ml/min to 300 ml/min and was directly correlated to antipyrine clearance. The half-life ranges from 2.5 hours to greater than 30 hours. These findings strongly suggest that caution should be exercised in dosage adjustments of Visken® (pindolol) in such patients.

The bioavailability of Visken® (pindolol) is not significantly affected by co-administration of food, hydralazine, hydrochlorothiazide or aspirin. Visken® (pindolol) has no effect on warfarin activity or the clinical effectiveness of digoxin, although small transient decreases in plasma digoxin concentrations were noted.

INDICATIONS AND USAGES

Visken® (pindolol) is indicated in the management of hypertension. It may be used alone or concomitantly with other antihypertensive agents, particularly with a thiazide type diuretic.

CONTRAINDICATIONS

Visken® (pindolol) is contraindicated in: 1) bronchial asthma; 2) overt cardiac failure; 3) cardiogenic shock; 4) second and third degree heart block; 5) severe bradycardia; (see Warnings).

WARNINGS

Cardiac Failure: Sympathetic stimulation may be a vital component supporting circulatory function in patients with congestive heart failure, and its inhibition by beta-blockade may precipitate more severe failure. Although beta-blockers should be avoided in overt congestive heart failure, if necessary, Visken® (pindolol) can be used with caution in patients with a history of failure who are well-compensated, usually with digitalis and diuretics. Beta-adrenergic block-

ing agents do not abolish the inotropic action of digitalis on heart muscle.

In Patients Without A History of Cardiac Failure: In patients with latent cardiac insufficiency, continued depression of the myocardium with beta-blocking agents over a period of time can in some cases lead to cardiac failure. At the first sign or symptom of impending cardiac failure, patients should be fully digitalized and/or be given a diuretic, and the response observed closely. If cardiac failure continues, despite adequate digitalization and diuretic, Visken® (pindolol) therapy should be withdrawn (gradually if possible).

Exacerbation of Ischemic Heart Disease Following Abrupt Withdrawal: Hypersensitivity to catecholamines has been observed in patients withdrawn from beta-blocker therapy; exacerbation of angina and, in some cases, myocardial infarction have occurred after *abrupt* discontinuation of such therapy. When discontinuing chronically administered Visken® (pindolol), particularly in patients with ischemic heart disease, the dosage should be gradually reduced over a period of one to two weeks and the patient should be carefully monitored. If angina markedly worsens or acute coronary insufficiency develops, Visken® (pindolol) administration should be reinstituted promptly, at least temporarily, and other measures appropriate for the management of unstable angina should be taken. Patients should be warned against interruption or discontinuation of therapy without the physician's advice. Because coronary artery disease is common and may be unrecognized, it may be prudent not to discontinue Visken® (pindolol) therapy abruptly even in patients treated only for hypertension.

Nonallergic Bronchospasm (e.g., chronic bronchitis, emphysema)—Patients with Bronchospastic Diseases Should in General Not Receive Beta-Blockers: Visken® (pindolol) should be administered with caution since it may block bronchodilation produced by endogenous or exogenous catecholamine stimulation of $beta_2$ receptors.

Major Surgery: Because beta blockade impairs the ability of the heart to respond to reflex stimuli and may increase the risks of general anesthesia and surgical procedures, resulting in protracted hypotension or low cardiac output, it has generally been suggested that such therapy should be withdrawn several days prior to surgery. Recognition of the increased sensitivity to catecholamines of patients recently withdrawn from beta-blocker therapy, however, has made this recommendation controversial. If possible, beta-blockers should be withdrawn well before surgery takes place. In the event of emergency surgery, the anesthesiologist should be informed that the patient is on beta-blocker therapy.

The effects of Visken® (pindolol) can be reversed by administration of beta-receptor agonists such as isoproterenol, dopamine, dobutamine, or levarterenol. Difficulty in restarting and maintaining the heart beat has also been reported with beta-adrenergic receptor blocking agents.

Diabetes and Hypoglycemia: Beta-adrenergic blockade may prevent the appearance of premonitory signs and symptoms (e.g., tachycardia and blood pressure changes) of acute hypoglycemia. This is especially important with labile diabetics. Beta-blockade also reduces the release of insulin in response to hyperglycemia; therefore, it may be necessary to

adjust the dose of antidiabetic drugs.

Thyrotoxicosis: Beta-adrenergic blockade may mask certain clinical signs (e.g., tachycardia) of hyperthyroidism. Patients suspected of developing thyrotoxicosis should be managed carefully to avoid abrupt withdrawal of beta-blockade which might precipitate a thyroid crisis.

PRECAUTIONS

Impaired Renal or Hepatic Function: Beta-blocking agents should be used with caution in patients with impaired hepatic or renal function. Poor renal function has only minor effects on Visken® (pindolol) clearance, but poor hepatic function may cause blood levels of Visken® (pindolol) to increase substantially.

Information for Patients: Patients, especially those with evidence of coronary artery insufficiency, should be warned against interruption or discontinuation of Visken® (pindolol) therapy without the physician's advice. Although cardiac failure rarely occurs in properly selected patients, patients being treated with beta-adrenergic blocking agents should be advised to consult the physician at the first sign or symptom of impending failure.

Drug Interactions: Catecholamine-depleting drugs (e.g., reserpine) may have an additive effect when given with beta-blocking agents. Patients receiving Visken® (pindolol) plus a catecholamine depleting agent should, therefore, be closely observed for evidence of hypotension and/or marked bradycardia which may produce vertigo, syncope, or postural hypotension.

Visken® (pindolol) has been used with a variety of antihypertensive agents, including hydrochlorothiazide, hydralazine, and guanethidine without unexpected adverse interactions.

Visken® (pindolol) has been shown to increase serum thioridazine levels when both drugs are co-administered. Visken® (pindolol) levels may also be increased with this combination.

Carcinogenesis, Mutagenesis, Impairment of Fertility: In chronic oral toxicologic studies (one to two years) in mice, rats, and dogs, Visken® (pindolol) did not produce any significant toxic effects. In two-year oral carcinogenicity studies in rats and mice in doses as high as 59 mg/kg/day and 124 mg/kg/day (50 and 100 times the maximum recommended human dose), respectively, Visken® (pindolol) did not produce any neoplastic, preneoplastic, or nonneoplastic pathologic lesions. In fertility and general reproductive performance studies in rats, Visken® (pindolol) caused no adverse effects at a dose of 10 mg/kg.

In the male fertility and general reproductive performance test in rats, definite toxicity characterized by mortality and decreased weight gain was observed in the group given 100 mg/kg/day. At 30 mg/kg/day, decreased mating was associated with testicular atrophy and/or decreased spermatogenesis. This response is not clearly drug related, however, as there was no dose response relationship within this experiment and no similar effect on testes of rats administered Visken® (pindolol) as a dietary admixture for 104 weeks. There appeared to be an increase in prenatal mortality in

	Adverse Reactions which were Volunteered or Elicited (and at least possibly drug related)		
Body System/Adverse Reactions	Visken® (pindolol) (N = 322) %	Active Controls* (N = 188) %	Placebo (N = 78) %
Central Nervous System			
Bizarre or Many Dreams	5	0	6
Dizziness	9	11	1
Fatigue	8	4	4
Hallucinations	<1	0	0
Insomnia	10	3	10
Nervousness	7	3	5
Weakness	4	2	1
Autonomic Nervous System			
Paresthesia	3	1	6
Cardiovascular			
Dyspnea	5	4	6
Edema	6	3	1
Heart Failure	<1	<1	0
Palpitations	<1	1	0
Musculoskeletal			
Chest Pain	3	1	3
Joint Pain	7	4	4
Muscle Cramps	3	1	0
Muscle Pain	10	9	8
Gastrointestinal			
Abdominal Discomfort	4	4	5
Nausea	5	2	1
Skin			
Pruritus	1	<1	0
Rash	<1	<1	1

*Active Controls: Patients received either propranolol, α-methyldopa or a diuretic (hydrochlorothiazide or chlorthalidone).

males given 100 mg/kg but development of offspring was not impaired.

In females administered Visken® (pindolol) prior to mating through day 21 of lactation, mating behavior was decreased at 100 mg/kg and 30 mg/kg. At these dosages there also was increased mortality of offspring. Prenatal mortality was increased at 10 mg/kg but there was not a clear dose response relationship in this experiment. There was an increased resorption rate at 100 mg/kg observed in females necropsied on the 15th day of gestation.

Pregnancy—Category B: Studies in rats and rabbits exceeding 100 times the maximum recommended human doses, revealed no embryotoxicity or teratogenicity. Since there are no adequate and well-controlled studies in pregnant women, and since animal reproduction studies are not always predictive of human response, Visken® (pindolol), as with any drug, should be employed during pregnancy only if the potential benefit justifies the potential risk to the fetus. **Nursing Mothers:** Since Visken® (pindolol) is secreted in human milk, nursing should not be undertaken by mothers receiving the drug. **Pediatric Use:** Safety and effectiveness in children have not been established.

CLINICAL LABORATORY

Minor persistent elevations in serum transaminases (SGOT, SGPT) have been noted in 7% of patients during Visken® (pindolol) administration, but progressive elevations were not observed and liver injury has not been reported in the medical literature over a ten (10) year period of marketing. Alkaline phosphatase, lactic acid dehydrogenase (LDH) and uric acid are also elevated on rare occasions. The significance of these findings is unknown.

ADVERSE REACTIONS

Most adverse reactions have been mild. The incidences listed in the following table are derived from 12 week comparative double-blind, parallel design trials in hypertensive patients given Visken® (pindolol) as monotherapy, given various active control drugs as monotherapy, or given placebo. Data for Visken® (pindolol) and the positive controls were pooled from several trials because no striking differences were seen in the individual studies, with one exception. When considering all adverse reactions reported, the frequency of edema was noticeably higher in positive control trials (16% Visken® (pindolol) vs 9% positive control) than in placebo controlled trials (6% Visken® (pindolol) vs 3% placebo). The table includes adverse reactions either volunteered or elicited, and at least possibly drug related, which were reported in greater than 2% of Visken® (pindolol) patients and other selected important reactions.

[See table on bottom preceding page].

The following selected (potentially important) adverse reactions were seen in 2% or fewer patients and their relationship to Visken® (pindolol) is uncertain. CENTRAL NERVOUS SYSTEM: anxiety, lethargy; AUTONOMIC NERVOUS SYSTEM: visual disturbances, hyperhidrosis; CARDIOVASCULAR: bradycardia, claudication, cold extremities, heart block, hypotension, syncope, tachycardia, weight gain; GASTROINTESTINAL: diarrhea, vomiting; RESPIRATORY: wheezing; UROGENITAL: impotence, pollakiuria; MISCELLANEOUS: eye discomfort or burning eyes.

POTENTIAL ADVERSE EFFECTS

In addition, other adverse effects not listed above have been reported with other beta-adrenergic blocking agents and should be considered potential adverse effects of Visken® (pindolol).

Central Nervous System: Reversible mental depression progressing to catatonia; an acute reversible syndrome characterized by disorientation for time and place, short-term memory loss, emotional lability, slightly clouded sensorium, and decreased performance on neuropsychometrics.
Cardiovascular: Intensification of AV block. (See CONTRAINDICATIONS).
Allergic: Erythematous rash; fever combined with aching and sore throat; laryngospasm; respiratory distress.
Hematologic: Agranulocytosis; thrombocytopenic and nonthrombocytopenic purpura.
Gastrointestinal: Mesenteric arterial thrombosis; ischemic colitis.
Miscellaneous: Reversible alopecia; Peyronie's disease.
The oculomucocutaneous syndrome associated with the beta-blocker practolol has not been reported with Visken® (pindolol) during investigational use and extensive foreign experience amounting to over 4 million patient-years.

OVERDOSAGE

No specific information on emergency treatment of overdosage is available. Therefore, on the basis of the pharmacologic actions of Visken® (pindolol), the following general measures should be employed as appropriate in addition to gastric lavage:

Excessive Bradycardia: administer atropine; if there is no response to vagal blockade, administer isoproterenol cautiously.
Cardiac Failure: digitalize the patient and/or administer

diuretic. It has been reported that glucagon may be useful in this situation.
Hypotension: administer vasopressors, e.g., epinephrine or levarterenol, with serial monitoring of blood pressure. (There is evidence that epinephrine may be the drug of choice.)
Bronchospasm: administer a beta$_2$ stimulating agent such as isoproterenol and/or a theophylline derivative.
A case of an acute overdosage has been reported with an intake of 500 mg of Visken® (pindolol) by a hypertensive patient. Blood pressure increased and heart rate was ≥ 80 beat/min. Recovery was uneventful. In another case 250 mg of Visken® (pindolol) was taken with 150 mg diazepam and 50 mg nitrazepam, producing coma and hypotension. The patient recovered in 24 hours.

DOSAGE AND ADMINISTRATION

The dosage of Visken® (pindolol) should be individualized. The recommended initial dose of Visken® (pindolol) is 5 mg b.i.d. alone or in combination with other antihypertensive agents. An antihypertensive response usually occurs within the first week of treatment. Maximal response, however, may take as long as or occasionally longer than two weeks. If a satisfactory reduction in blood pressure does not occur within 3–4 weeks, the dose may be adjusted in increments of 10 mg per day at these intervals up to a maximum of 60 mg per day.

HOW SUPPLIED

White, round, scored tablets: 5 mg (NDC 0078-0111-05) and 10 mg (NDC 0078-0073-05), packages of 100.
Company's Product Identification Mark(s): 5 mg tablets embossed "VISKEN 5" on one side, and "78-111" and scored on other side.
10 mg tablets embossed "VISKEN 10" on one side, and "78-73" and scored on other side.
[VIS-Z8 Issued July 15, 1988]
Shown in Product Identification Section, page 427

Savage Laboratories
a division of Altana Inc.
60 BAYLIS ROAD
MELVILLE, NY 11747

ALPHATREX®   R
[al "fah-trex ']
(betamethasone dipropionate)
Cream, USP 0.05%
Ointment, USP 0.05%
Lotion, USP 0.05%
For Dermatologic Use Only–Not for Ophthalmic Use

DESCRIPTION

Alphatrex® Cream, Ointment and Lotion contain Betamethasone Dipropionate USP (Pregna-1, 4-diene-3, 20-dione, 9-fluoro-11-hydroxy-16-methyl-17, 21-bis (1-oxopropoxy)-(11β, 16β)-); it has a molecular formula of $C_{28}H_{37}FO_7$, and a molecular weight of 504.59 (CAS Registry Number 5593-20-4).
Each gram of the 0.05% Cream contains 0.64 mg betamethasone dipropionate (equivalent to 0.5 mg betamethasone) in a soft, white, hydrophilic cream of purified water, mineral oil, white petrolatum, polyethylene glycol 1000 monocetyl ether, cetostearyl alcohol, monobasic sodium phosphate and phosphoric acid or sodium hydroxide; chlorocresol is present as a preservative. Betamethasone Dipropionate Cream contains no parabens.
Each gram of the 0.05% Ointment contains 0.64 mg betamethasone dipropionate (equivalent to 0.5 mg betamethasone) in an ointment base of mineral oil and white petrolatum. Betamethasone Dipropionate Ointment contains no parabens.
Each gram of the 0.05% Lotion contains 0.64 mg of betamethasone dipropionate (equivalent to 0.5 mg betamethasone) in a vehicle of isopropyl alcohol and purified water slightly thickened with carbomer 934P. Phosphoric acid or sodium hydroxide is used to adjust pH.

CLINICAL PHARMACOLOGY

Topical corticosteroids share anti-inflammatory, anti-pruritic and vasoconstrictive actions. The mechanism of anti-inflammatory activity of the topical corticosteroids is unclear. Various laboratory methods, including vasoconstrictor assays, are used to compare and predict potencies and/or clinical efficacies of the topical corticosteroids. There is some evidence to suggest that a recognizable correlation exists between vasoconstrictor potency and therapeutic efficacy in man.
Pharmacokinetics: The extent of percutaneous absorption of topical corticosteroids is determined by many factors including the vehicle, the integrity of the epidermal barrier, and the use of occlusive dressings. Topical corticosteroids can be absorbed from normal intact skin. Inflammation and/or other disease processes in the skin increase percutaneous absorption. Occlusive dressings substantially increase the

percutaneous absorption of topical corticosteroids. (See DOSAGE AND ADMINISTRATION) Once absorbed through the skin, topical corticosteroids are handled through pharmacokinetic pathways similar to systemically administered corticosteroids. Corticosteroids are bound to plasma proteins in varying degrees. Corticosteroids are metabolized primarily in the liver and are then excreted by the kidneys. Some of the topical corticosteroids and their metabolites are also excreted into the bile.

INDICATIONS AND USAGE

Topical corticosteroids are indicated for the relief of the inflammatory and pruritic manifestations of corticosteroid-responsive dermatoses.

CONTRAINDICATIONS

Topical corticosteroids are contraindicated in those patients with a history of hypersensitivity to any of the components of the preparation.

PRECAUTIONS

General: Systemic absorption of topical corticosteroids has produced reversible hypothalamic-pituitary-adrenal (HPA) axis suppression, manifestations of Cushing's syndrome, hyperglycemia, and glucosuria in some patients. Conditions which augment systemic absorption include the application of the more potent steroids, use over large surface areas, prolonged use, and the addition of occlusive dressings. (See DOSAGE AND ADMINISTRATION) Therefore, patients receiving a large dose of a potent topical steroid applied to a large surface area should be evaluated periodically for evidence of HPA axis suppression by using the urinary free cortisol and ACTH stimulation tests. If HPA axis suppression is noted, an attempt should be made to withdraw the drug, to reduce the frequency of application, or to substitute a less potent steroid. Recovery of HPA axis function is generally prompt and complete upon discontinuation of the drug. Infrequently, signs and symptoms of steroid withdrawal may occur, requiring supplemental systemic corticosteroids. Children may absorb proportionally larger amounts of topical corticosteroids and thus be more susceptible to systemic toxicity (See PRECAUTIONS-Pediatric Use). If irritation develops topical corticosteroids should be discontinued and appropriate therapy instituted. In the presence of dermatological infections, the use of an appropriate antifungal or antibacterial agent should be instituted. If a favorable response does not occur promptly, the corticosteroid should be discontinued until the infection has been adequately controlled.
Information for the Patient: Patients using topical corticosteroids should receive the following information and instructions:
1. This medication is to be used as directed by the physician. It is for external use only. Avoid contact with the eyes.
2. Patients should be advised not to use this medication for any disorder other than for which it was prescribed.
3. The treated skin area should not be bandaged or otherwise covered or wrapped as to be occlusive. (See DOSAGE AND ADMINISTRATION)
4. Patients should report any signs of local adverse reactions.
5. Parents of pediatric patients should be advised not to use tight fitting diapers or plastic pants on a child being treated in the diaper area, as these garments may constitute occlusive dressings. (See DOSAGE AND ADMINISTRATION)
Laboratory Tests: The following tests may be helpful in evaluating the HPA axis suppression: Urinary free cortisol test; ACTH stimulation test.
Carcinogenesis, Mutagenesis, and Impairment of Fertility: Long-term animal studies have not been performed to evaluate the carcinogenic potential or the effect on fertility of topical corticosteroids. Studies to determine mutagenicity with prednisolone and hydrocortisone have revealed negative results.
Pregnancy Category C: Corticosteroids are generally teratogenic in laboratory animals when administered systemically at relatively low dosage levels. The more potent corticosteroids have been shown to be teratogenic after dermal application in laboratory animals. There are no adequate and well-controlled studies in pregnant women on teratogenic effects from topically applied corticosteroids. Therefore, topical corticosteroids should be used during pregnancy only if the potential benefit justifies the potential risk to the fetus. Drugs of this class should not be used extensively on pregnant patients, in large amounts, or for prolonged periods of time.
Nursing Mothers: It is not known whether topical administration of corticosteroids could result in sufficient systemic absorption to produce detectable quantities in breast milk. Systemically administered corticosteroids are secreted into breast milk in quantities *not* likely to have a deleterious effect on the infant. Nevertheless, caution should be exercised when topical corticosteroids are administered to a nursing woman.
Pediatric Use: *Pediatric patients may demonstrate greater susceptibility to topical corticosteroid-induced HPA axis sup-*

Continued on next page

Savage—Cont.

pression and Cushing's syndrome than mature patients because of a larger skin surface area to body weight ratio. Hypothalamic-pituitary-adrenal (HPA) axis suppression, Cushing's syndrome, and intracranial hypertension have been reported in children receiving topical corticosteroids. Manifestations of adrenal suppression in children include linear growth retardation, delayed weight gain, low plasma cortisol levels, and absence of response to ACTH stimulation. Manifestations of intracranial hypertension include bulging fontanelles, headaches, and bilateral papilledema. Administration of topical corticosteroids to children should be limited to the least amount compatible with an effective therapeutic regimen. Chronic corticosteroid therapy may interfere with the growth and development of children.

ADVERSE REACTIONS

The following local adverse reactions are reported infrequently when Alphatrex products are used as recommended in the DOSAGE AND ADMINISTRATION section. These reactions are listed in an approximate decreasing order of occurrence: burning, itching, irritation, dryness, folliculitis, hypertrichosis, acneiform eruptions, hypopigmentation, perioral dermatitis, allergic contact dermatitis, maceration of the skin, secondary infection, skin atrophy, striae and miliaria.

Systemic absorption of topical corticosteroids has produced reversible hypothalamic-pituitary-adrenal (HPA) axis suppression, manifestations of Cushing's syndrome, hyperglycemia and glucosuria in some patients.

OVERDOSAGE

Topically applied corticosteroids can be absorbed in sufficient amounts to produce systemic effects (See PRECAUTIONS).

DOSAGE AND ADMINISTRATION

Alphatrex® Cream and Ointment are applied to the affected skin areas as a thin film once daily. In some cases, twice daily dosage may be necessary.

Apply a few drops of Alphatrex® Lotion to the affected skin areas and massage lightly until it disappears. Apply twice daily, in the morning and night. If an infection develops, appropriate antimicrobial therapy should be instituted.

Alphatrex® products should not be used with occlusive dressings.

HOW SUPPLIED

Alphatrex® Cream, USP 0.05%
  NDC 0281-0055-15, 15 gram tube
  NDC 0281-0055-46, 45 gram tube
Alphatrex® Ointment, USP 0.05%
  NDC 0281-0056-15, 15 gram tube
  NDC 0281-0056-46, 45 gram tube
Alphatrex® Lotion, USP 0.05%
  NDC 0281-0057-60, 60 ml bottle
Shake well before using.

Caution: Federal law prohibits dispensing without prescription.

BETATREX®   ℞
[ba"tah-trex']
(betamethasone valerate)
Cream, USP 0.1%
Ointment, USP 0.1%
Lotion, USP 0.1%
For Dermatologic Use Only—Not for Ophthalmic Use

DESCRIPTION

Betatrex® Cream, Ointment and Lotion contain Betamethasone Valerate USP (Pregna-1, 4-diene-3, 20-dione, 9-fluoro-11, 21-dihydroxy-16-methyl-17-[(1-oxopentyl)oxy]-, $(11\beta, 16\beta)$-); it has a molecular formula of $C_{27}H_{37}FO_6$ and a molecular weight of 476.58 (CAS Registry Number 2152-44-5).

Each gram of the 0.1% cream contains 1.2 mg Betamethasone Valerate (equivalent to 1.0 mg Betamethasone) in a soft, white hydrophilic cream of Water, Mineral Oil, White Petrolatum, Polyethylene Glycol 1000 Monocetyl Ether, Cetostearyl Alcohol, Monobasic Sodium Phosphate and Phosphoric Acid or Sodium Hydroxide; Chlorocresol is present as a preservative. Betamethasone Valerate Cream contains no parabens.

Each gram of the 0.1% ointment contains 1.2 mg Betamethasone Valerate (equivalent to 1.0 mg Betamethasone) in an ointment base of White Petrolatum and Mineral Oil. Betamethasone Valerate Ointment contains no parabens.

Each gram of the 0.1% lotion contains 1.2 mg Betamethasone Valerate (equivalent to 1.0 mg Betamethasone) in a vehicle of Isopropyl Alcohol and Water slightly thickened with Carbomer 934P. Phosphoric Acid or Sodium Hydroxide are used to adjust the pH.

CLINICAL PHARMACOLOGY

Topical corticosteroids share anti-inflammatory, anti-pruritic and vasoconstrictive actions. The mechanism of anti-inflammatory activity of the topical corticosteroids is unclear. Various laboratory methods, including vasoconstrictor assays, are used to compare and predict potencies and/or clinical efficacies of the topical corticosteroids. There is some evidence to suggest that a recognizable correlation exists between vasoconstrictor potency and therapeutic efficacy in man.

Pharmacokinetics: The extent of percutaneous absorption of topical corticosteroids is determined by many factors including the vehicle, the integrity of the epidermal barrier, and the use of occlusive dressings. Topical corticosteroids can be absorbed from normal intact skin. Inflammation and/or other disease processes in the skin increase percutaneous absorption. Occlusive dressings substantially increase the percutaneous absorption of topical corticosteroids. Thus occlusive dressings may be a valuable therapeutic adjunct for treatment of resistant dermatoses (See DOSAGE AND ADMINISTRATION). Once absorbed through the skin, topical corticosteroids are handled through pharmacokinetic pathways similar to systemically administered corticosteroids. Corticosteroids are bound to plasma proteins in varying degrees. Corticosteroids are metabolized primarily in the liver and are then excreted by the kidneys. Some of the topical corticosteroids and their metabolites are also excreted into the bile.

INDICATIONS AND USAGE

Topical corticosteroids are indicated for the relief of the inflammatory and pruritic manifestations of corticosteroid-responsive dermatoses.

CONTRAINDICATIONS

Topical corticosteroids are contraindicated in those patients with a history of hypersensitivity to any of the components of the preparation.

PRECAUTIONS

General: Systemic absorption of topical corticosteroids has produced reversible hypothalamic-pituitary-adrenal (HPA) axis suppression, manifestations of Cushing's syndrome, hyperglycemia, and glucosuria in some patients. Conditions which augment systemic absorption include the application of the more potent steroids, use over large surface areas, prolonged use, and the addition of occlusive dressings. Therefore, patients receiving a large dose of a potent topical steroid applied to a large surface area or under an occlusive dressing should be evaluated periodically for evidence of HPA axis suppression by using the urinary free cortisol and ACTH stimulation tests. If HPA axis suppression is noted, an attempt should be made to withdraw the drug, to reduce the frequency of application, or to substitute a less potent steroid. Recovery of HPA axis function is generally prompt and complete upon discontinuation of the drug. Infrequently, signs and symptoms of steroid withdrawal may occur, requiring supplemental systemic corticosteroids. Children may absorb proportionally larger amounts of topical corticosteroids and thus be more susceptible to systemic toxicity (See PRECAUTIONS-Pediatric Use). If irritation develops, topical corticosteroids should be discontinued and appropriate therapy instituted. In the presence of dermatological infections, the use of an appropriate antifungal or antibacterial agent should be instituted. If a favorable response does not occur promptly, the corticosteroid should be discontinued until the infection has been adequately controlled.

Information for the Patient: Patients using topical corticosteroids should receive the following information and instructions:
1. This medication is to be used as directed by the physician. It is for external use only. Avoid contact with the eyes.
2. Patients should be advised not to use this medication for any disorder other than for which it was prescribed.
3. The treated skin area should not be bandaged or otherwise covered or wrapped as to be occlusive unless directed by the physician.
4. Patients should report any signs of local adverse reactions especially under occlusive dressing.
5. Parents of pediatric patients should be advised not to use tight fitting diapers or plastic pants on a child being treated in the diaper area, as these garments may constitute occlusive dressings.

Laboratory Tests: The following tests may be helpful in evaluating the HPA axis suppression: Urinary free cortisol test. ACTH stimulation test.

Carcinogenesis, Mutagenesis, and Impairment of Fertility: Long-term animal studies have not been performed to evaluate the carcinogenic potential or the effect on fertility of topical corticosteroids. Studies to determine mutagenicity with prednisolone and hydrocortisone have revealed negative results.

Pregnancy Category C: Corticosteroids are generally teratogenic in laboratory animals when administered systemically at relatively low dosage levels. The more potent corticosteroids have been shown to be teratogenic after dermal ap-

plication in laboratory animals. There are no adequate and well-controlled studies in pregnant women on teratogenic effects from topically applied corticosteroids. Therefore, topical corticosteroids should be used during pregnancy only if the potential benefit justifies the potential risk to the fetus. Drugs of this class should not be used extensively on pregnant patients, in large amounts, or for prolonged periods of time.

Nursing Mothers: It is not known whether topical administration of corticosteroids could result in sufficient systemic absorption to produce detectable quantities in breast milk. Systemically administered corticosteroids are secreted into breast milk in quantities *not* likely to have a deleterious effect on the infant. Nevertheless, caution should be exercised when topical corticosteroids are administered to a nursing woman.

Pediatric Use: *Pediatric patients may demonstrate greater susceptibility to topical corticosteroid-induced HPA axis suppression and Cushing's syndrome than mature patients because of a larger skin surface area to body weight ratio.* Hypothalamic-pituitary-adrenal (HPA) axis suppression, Cushing's syndrome, and intracranial hypertension have been reported in children receiving topical corticosteroids. Manifestations of adrenal suppression in children include linear growth retardation, delayed weight gain, low plasma cortisol levels, and absence of response to ACTH stimulation. Manifestations of intracranial hypertension include bulging fontanelles, headaches, and bilateral papilledema. Administration of topical corticosteroids to children should be limited to the least amount compatible with an effective therapeutic regimen. Chronic corticosteroid therapy may interfere with the growth and development of children.

ADVERSE REACTIONS

The following local adverse reactions are reported infrequently with topical corticosteroids, but may occur more frequently with the use of occlusive dressings. These reactions are listed in an approximate decreasing order of occurrence: burning, itching, irritation, dryness, folliculitis, hypertrichosis, acneiform eruptions, hypopigmentation, perioral dermatitis, allergic contact dermatitis, maceration of the skin, secondary infection, skin atrophy, striae and miliaria.

OVERDOSAGE

Topically applied corticosteroids can be absorbed in sufficient amounts to produce systemic effects (See PRECAUTIONS)

DOSAGE AND ADMINISTRATION

Betatrex® Cream: Apply a thin film to the affected skin areas one to three times a day. Dosage once or twice a day is often effective.

Betatrex® Ointment: Apply a thin film to the affected skin areas one to three times a day. Dosage once or twice a day is often effective.

Betatrex® Lotion: Apply a few drops of Betatrex Lotion to the affected area and massage lightly until it disappears. Apply twice daily, in the morning and at night. Dosage may be increased in stubborn cases. Following improvement, apply once daily. For the most effective and economical use, apply nozzle very close to affected area and gently squeeze bottle. Shake well before using. Store at controlled room temperature 15–30°C (59°–86°F).

HOW SUPPLIED

Betatrex® Cream USP, 0.1%
  NDC 0281-3510-44, 15 gram tube
  NDC 0281-3510-50, 45 gram tube
Betratrex® Ointment USP, 0.1%
  NDC 0281-3516-44, 15 gram tube
  NDC 0281-3516-50, 45 gram tube
Betatrex® Lotion USP, 0.1%
  NDC 0281-3519-46, 60 ml bottle

CAUTION

Federal law prohibits dispensing without prescription.

BREXIN® L.A. Capsules   ℞
[brex'in]
(chlorpheniramine maleate, pseudoephedrine hydrochloride)

DESCRIPTION

Each red and clear colored capsule contains chlorpheniramine maleate USP 8 mg. and pseudoephedrine hydrochloride USP 120 mg. in a specially prepared base containing benzyl alcohol, butyl paraben, carboxymethylcellulose sodium, edetate calcium disodium, FD&C blue #1, FD&C red #3, FD&C red #40, gelatin, methylparaben, pharmaceutical glaze, propylparaben, sodium lauryl sulfate, sodium propionate, starch, sucrose and other ingredients.

HOW SUPPLIED

NDC 0281-1934-53, Brexin® L.A. bottle of 100 capsules.
Distributed by Savage Laboratories
Shown in Product Identification Section, page 427

CHROMAGEN®   ℞
[kro"mah-jen]
Soft Gelatin Capsules

DESCRIPTION
CONTENTS: Each maroon soft gelatin capsule contains: ferrous fumarate USP 200 mg, ascorbic acid USP 250 mg, cyanocobalamin USP 10 mcg, desiccated stomach substance 100 mg.

DISCUSSION: The amount of elemental iron and the absorption of the iron components of commercial iron preparations vary widely. It is further established that certain "accessory components" may be included to enhance abosorption and utilization of iron. Chromagen® Capsules are formulated to provide the essential factors for a complete, versatile hematinic.

ACTIONS
HIGH ELEMENTAL IRON CONTENT: Ferrous fumarate, used in Chromagen® Capsules, is an organic iron complex which has a higher elemental iron content than any other hematinic salt—33%. This compares with 20% for ferrous sulfate and 12% for ferrous gluconate.[1,2]

MORE COMPLETE ABSORPTION: It has been repeatedly shown that ascorbic acid, when given in sufficient amounts, can increase the absorption of ferrous iron from the gastrointestinal tract. [3,4,5,6,7,8,9] The absorption-promoting effect is mainly due to the reducing action of ascorbic acid within the gastrointestinal lumen, which helps to prevent or delay the information of insoluble or less dissociated ferric compounds.[3]

Iron absorption has been shown to increase sharply with increasing amounts of ascorbic acid, showing a gain in absorption of approximately 40% at 250 mg. Above 250 mg, the gain becomes insignificant, with an additional gain of only approximately 8% at 500 mg.[3] Each Chromagen® Capsule contains 250 mg of ascorbic acid, believed to be the optimal amount.

PROMOTES MOVEMENT OF PLASMA IRON: Ascorbic acid also plays an important role in the movement of plasma iron to storage depots in the tissues.[10] The action, which leads to the transport of plasma iron to ferritin, presumably involves its reducing effect, converting transferrin iron from the ferric to the ferrous state.[5] There is also evidence that ascorbic acid improves iron utilization, presumably as a further result of its reducing action,[6,9] and some evidence that it may have a direct effect upon erythropoiesis. Ascorbic acid is further alleged to enhance the conversion of folic acid to a more physiologically active form, folinic acid, which would make it even more important in the treatment of anemia since it would aid in the utilization of dietary folic acid.[11]

EXCELLENT ORAL TOLERATION: Ferrous fumarate is used in Chromagen® Capsules because it is less likely to cause the gastric disturbances so often associated with oral iron therapy. Ferrous fumarate has a low ionization constant and high solubility in the entire pH range of the gastrointestinal tract. It does not precipitate proteins or have the astringency of more ionizable forms or iron, and does not interfere with proteolytic or diastatic activities of the digestive system. Because of excellent oral toleration, Chromagen® Capsules can usually be administered between meals when iron absorption is maximal.

FACILITATES ABSORPTION OF VITAMIN B₁₂: It is now known that "Intrinsic Factor" is essential for the adequate alimentary absorption of vitamin B₁₂[12,13,14,15] The chemical structure of intrinsic factor is still undetermined and it has not yet been isolated in pure form;[16] however, the inclusion of desiccated stomach substance and vitamin B₁₂ will furnish sufficient intrinsic factor to assure absorption of the vitamin.

TOXICITY: Ferrous fumarate was found to be the least toxic of three popular oral iron salts, with an oral LD_{50} of 630 mg/kg. In the same report, the LD_{50} of ferrous gluconate was reported to be 320 mg/kg and ferrous sulfate 230 mg/kg.[1,17]

INDICATIONS
For the treatment of all anemias responsive to oral iron therapy, such as hypochromic anemia associated with pregnancy, chronic or acute blood loss, dietary restriction, metabolic disease and post-surgical convalescence.

CONTRAINDICATIONS
Hemochromatosis and hemosiderosis are contraindications to iron therapy.

SIDE EFFECTS
Average capsule doses in sensitive individuals or excessive dosage may cause nausea, skin rash, vomiting, diarrhea, precordial pain, or flushing of the face and extremities.

DOSAGE AND ADMINISTRATION
Usual adult dose is 1 soft gelatin capsule daily.

HOW SUPPLIED
Chromagen® Capsules:

NDC 0281-4285-53, bottle of 100
NDC 0281-4285-56, bottle of 500
CAUTION: Federal law prohibits dispensing without prescription.

BIBLIOGRAPHY
[1]Berk, M.S. and Novich, M.A.: "Treatment of Iron Deficiency Anemia With Ferrous Fumarate," Am. J. Obst. & Gynec., 203–206, 1962. [2]Shapleigh, J.B., and Montgomery, A.; Am. Pract & Dig. Treat 10–461, 1959. [3]Brise, H. and Hallberg. L.: "Effect of Ascorbic Acid on Iron Absorption," Acta. Med. Scand. 171:376, 51–58, 1962. [4]New Drugs, p.309, AMA, Chicago, 1966. [5]Mazur, A., Green, S. and Carleton, A.: "Mechanism of Plasma Iron Incorporation into Hepatic Ferritin," j. of Bio. Chem. 3:595–603, 1960. [6]Greenberg, S.M., Tucker, A.E., Mathues, H. and J.D.: "Iron Absorption and Metabolism, I. Interrelationship of Ascorbic Acid and Vitamin E", J. Nutrition 63:19–31, 1957. [7]Moore, C.V., and Dubach, R.: "Observations on the Absorption of Iron From Foods Tagged with Radioiron," Trans. Assoc. Amer. Physic. 64:245, 1951. [8]Steinkamp, R., Dubach, R. and Moore, C.V.: "Studies in Iron Transportation and Metabolism," Arch. Int. Med. 95:181, 1955. [9]Gorten, M.K. and Bradley, J.E.: "The Treatment of Nutritional Anemia in Infancy and Childhood with Oral Iron and Ascorbic Acid," J. Pediatrics, 45:1, 1954. [10]Mazur, A.: "Role of Ascorbic Acid in the Incorportion of Plasma Iron into Ferritin," An. N.Y. Acad. Sci. 92:223–229, 1961. [11]Cox, E.V. et al.: "The Anemia of Scurvy," Amer. J. Med. 42:220–227, 1967. [12]Berk, L. et al.: "Observations on the Etiologic Relationship of Achylia Gastrica to Pernicious Anemia, X," N. Eng. J. Med. 239:911–913, 1948. [13]Hall, B.E.: "Studies on the Nature of the Intrinsic Factor of Castle," Brit. Med. J. 2:585–589, 1950. [14]Wallerstein, R.O. et al.: "Observations on the Etiologic Relationship of Achylia Gastrica to Pericious Anemia, XV," J. Lab & Clin. Med. 41:363–375, 1953. [15]Castle, W.B.: "Observations on the Etiologic Relationship of Achylia Gastrica to Pernicious Anemia, 1," Am. J. Med. Sc. 178:748–764, 1929. [16]Goodman, L.S. and Gilman, A.: The Pharmacological Basis of Therapeutics, 2 ed., P. 1482, N.Y., 1958. [17]Berenbaum, M.C. et al.: Blood, 15:540, 1960.

Manufactured by R.P. Scherer Corporation, St. Petersburg, Florida 33702
Distributed by
SAVAGE LABORATORIES
a division of Altana Inc.
MELVILLE, NEW YORK 11747   R9/87
Shown in Product Identification Section, page 427

DILOR® Tablets   ℞
[dī'lor]
(dyphylline)

COMPOSITION
Each blue, scored tablet contains dyphylline (dihydroxypropyl theophylline) 200 mg. and the following inactive ingredients: colloidal silicon dioxide, corn starch, food starch, povidone, sodium lauryl sulfate, stearic acid and artificial coloring.

Each white scored tablet contains dyphylline (dihydroxypropyl theophylline) 400 mg and the following inactive ingredients: colloidal silicon dioxide, corn starch, food starch, povidone, sodium lauryl sulfate and stearic acid.

DESCRIPTION
Dyphylline [7-(2,3-Dihydroxypropyl) theophylline] $[C_{10}H_{14}N_4O_4]$ is a white, extremely bitter, amorphous solid, freely soluble in water and soluble to the extent of 2 gm in 100 ml alcohol.

ACTIONS
As a xanthine derivative, dyphylline possesses the peripheral vasodilator and bronchodilator actions characteristic of theophylline. It has diuretic and myocardial stimulant effects, and is effective orally. Dyphylline may show fewer side effects than aminophylline, but its blood levels and possibly its activity are also lower.

INDICATIONS
For relief of acute bronchial asthma and for reversible bronchospasm associated with chronic bronchitis and emphysema.

CONTRAINDICATIONS
In individuals who have shown hypersensitivity to any of its components. Dyphylline should not be administered concurrently with other xanthine preparations.

WARNINGS
Status asthmaticus is a medical emergency. Excessive doses may be expected to be toxic. In children treated with dyphylline elixir, the alcoholic vehicle of the drug product poses a truly significant factor of drug dependence including all three components of tolerance, physical dependence and compulsive abuse.

Usage in Pregnancy: Safe use in pregnancy has not been established relative to possible adverse effects on fetal development. Therefore, dyphylline should not be used in pregnant women unless, in the judgment of the physician, the potential benefits outweigh the possible hazards.

PRECAUTIONS
Use with caution in patients with severe cardiac disease, hypertension, hyperthyroidism, or acute myocardial injury. Particular caution in dose administration must be exercised in patients with peptic ulcers, since the condition may be exacerbated. Chronic oral administration in high doses (500 to 1,000 mg.) is usually associated with gastrointestinal irritation. Great caution should be used in giving dyphylline to patients in congestive heart failure. Such patients have shown markedly prolonged blood level curves which have persisted for long periods following discontinuation of the drug.

ADVERSE REACTIONS
Note: Included in this listing which follows are a few adverse reactions which may not have been reported with this specific drug. However, pharmacological similarities among the xanthine drugs require that each of the reactions be considered when dyphylline is administered. The most consistent adverse reactions are: 1. Gastrointestinal irritation: nausea, vomiting, and epigastric pain, generally preceded by headache, hematemesis, diarrhea. 2. Central nervous system stimulation: irritability, restlessness, insomnia, reflex hyperexcitability, muscle twitching, clonic and tonic generalized convulsions, agitation. 3. Cardiovascular: palpitation, tachycardia, extra systoles, flushing, marked hypotension, and circulatory failure. 4. Respiratory: tachypnea, respiratory arrest. 5. Renal: albuminuria, increased excretion of renal tubule and red blood cells. 6. Others: fever, dehydration.

OVERDOSAGE
Symptoms:
In infants and small children: agitation, headache, hyperreflexia, fasciculations, and clonic and tonic convulsions. In adults: nervousness, insomnia, nausea, vomiting, tachycardia and extra systoles.
Therapy:
Discontinue drug immediately.
No specific treatment.
Ipecac syrup for oral ingestion.
Avoid sympathomimetics.
Supportive treatment for hypotension, seizure, arrhythmias and dehydration.
Sedatives such as short acting barbiturates will help control central nervous system stimulation.
Restore the acid-base balance with lactate or bicarbonate.
Oxygen and antibiotics provide supportive treatment as indicated.

DRUG INTERACTIONS
Toxic synergism with ephedrine and other sympathomimetic bronchodilator drugs may occur.
Recent controlled studies suggest that the addition of ephedrine to adequate dosage regimens of dyphylline produces no increase in effectiveness over that of dyphylline alone, but does produce an increase in toxic effects.

DOSAGE AND ADMINISTRATION
When administered orally it produces less nausea than aminophylline and other alkaline theophylline compounds. Absorption orally appears to be faster on an empty stomach; preferably the drug is to be given at six hour intervals. Adults: Usual Adult Dose: 15 mg/kg every 6 hours up to 4 times a day. The dosage should be individualized by titration to the condition and response of the patient.
Pulmonary functional measurements before and after a period of treatment allow an objective assessment of whether or not therapy should be continued in patients with chronic bronchitis and emphysema.

HOW SUPPLIED
Dilor® Tablets

200 mg–	NDC 0281-1115-53, Bottle of 100.
	NDC 0281-1115-57, Bottle of 1000.
	NDC 0281-1115-63, Unit dose, Box of 100
400 mg–	NDC 0281-1116-53, Bottle of 100.
	NDC 0281-1116-57, Bottle of 1000.
	NDC 0281-1116-63, Unit dose, Box of 100

ALSO AVAILABLE
Dilor® Elixir, dyphylline 160 mg/15 ml; and Dilor® Injectable, dyphylline 250 mg/ml.
Shown in Product Identification Section, page 427

DILOR-G®   ℞
[dī'lor]
(dyphylline, guaifenesin USP)

COMPOSITION
Each pink, scored tablet contains dyphylline 200 mg, guaifenesin USP 200 mg and the following inactive ingredients:

Continued on next page

Savage—Cont.

colloidal silicon dioxide, corn starch, food starch, povidone, stearic acid and artificial coloring.

Each teaspoonful (5 ml) of the liquid contains dyphylline 100 mg, guaifenesin USP 100 mg, in a mint flavored base of citric acid, glycerin, saccharin sodium, sorbitol, sucrose, artificial coloring and flavoring, purified water, veltol and sodium hydroxide to adjust pH. Methylparaben and propylparaben are added as preservatives. Contains no alcohol.

HOW SUPPLIED
Dilor-G® Tablets
  NDC 0281-1124-53, bottle of 100.
  NDC 0281-1124-57, bottle of 1000.
  NDC 0281-1124-63, unit dose, box of 100.
Dilor-G® Liquid
  NDC 0281-1127-74, pint.
  NDC 0281-1127-76, gallon.
   Shown in Product Identification Section, page 427

ETHIODOL®   ℞
[ĕ-thī'ŏ'dŏl]
(brand of ethiodized oil injection)

DESCRIPTION
Ethiodol, brand of ethiodized oil, is a sterile injectable radioopaque diagnostic agent for use in hysterosalpingography and lymphography. It contains 37% iodine (475 mg/ml) organically combined with ethyl esters of fatty acids (primarily as ethyl monoiodostearate and ethyl diiodostearate) of poppyseed oil. Stabilized with poppyseed oil, 1%. The precise structure of Ethiodol is unknown at this time. Ethiodol is a straw to amber colored, oil fluid, which because of simplified molecular structure, possesses a greatly reduced viscosity (1.280 specific gravity at 15°C yields viscosity of 0.5 to 1.0 poise). This high fluidity provides a new flexibility for radiographic exploration.

HOW SUPPLIED
Ethiodol® (brand of ethiodized oil for injection) is supplied in a box of two 10 ml ampules, NDC 0281-7062-37.

MYTREX®   ℞
[my"trex']
(nystatin-triamcinolone acetonide)
Cream USP and Ointment USP

For Dermatologic Use Only
Not for Ophthalmic Use

DESCRIPTION
MYTREX® (nystatin-triamcinolone acetonide) Cream and Ointment contain the antifungal agent Nystatin and the synthetic corticosteroid Triamcinolone Acetonide.

Nystatin is a polyene antimycotic obtained from *Streptomyces noursei*. It is a yellow to light tan powder with a cereal-like odor, very slightly soluble in water, and slightly to sparingly soluble in alcohol. It has an empirical formula of $C_{47}H_{75}NO_{17}$ and a molecular weight of 926.13 (CAS Registry Number 1400-61-9).

Triamcinolone Acetonide is designated chemically as Pregna-1, 4-diene-3, 20-dione, 9-fluoro-11, 21-dihydroxy-16,17-[(1-methylethylidene)bis(oxy)]-, (11β, 16α)-; The white to cream crystalline powder has a slight odor, is practically insoluble in water, and very soluble in alcohol. It has an empirical formula of $C_{24}H_{31}FO_6$ and a molecular weight of 434.50 (CAS Registry Number 76-25-5).

Each gram of MYTREX® (nystatin-triamcinolone acetonide) Cream contains 100,000 units of nystatin and 1.0 mg of triamcinolone acetonide in a cream base containing polyoxyethylene fatty alcohol ether, white petrolatum, glyceryl monostearate, polyethylene glycol 400 monostearate, sorbitol solution, simethicone emulsion, propylene glycol, aluminum hydroxide gel, polysorbate 60, titanium dioxide, and purified water with benzyl alcohol as a preservative. Hydrochloric acid or sodium hydroxide to adjust pH.

Each gram of MYTREX® (nystatin-triamcinolone acetonide) Ointment contains 100,000 units of nystatin and 1.0 mg of triamcinolone acetonide in a base of polyethylene and mineral oil.

CLINICAL PHARMACOLOGY
NYSTATIN
Nystatin exerts its antifungal activity against a variety of pathogenic and nonpathogenic yeasts and fungi by binding to sterols in the cell membrane. The binding process renders the cell membrane incapable of functioning as a selective barrier. Nystatin provides specific anticandidal activity to *Candida* (Monilia) *albicans* and other *Candida* species, but it is not active against bacteria, protozoa, trichomonads, or viruses. Nystatin is not absorbed from intact skin or mucous membranes.

TRIAMCINOLONE ACETONIDE
Triamcinolone Acetonide is primarily effective because of its anti-inflammatory, anti-pruritic and vasoconstrictive actions, characteristic of the topical corticosteroid class of drugs. The pharmacological effects of the topical corticosteroids are well known; however, mechanism of their dermatologic actions are unclear. Various laboratory methods, including vasoconstrictor assays, are used to compare and predict potencies and/or clinical efficacies of the topical corticosteroids. There is some evidence to suggest that a recognizable correlation exists between vasoconstrictor potency and therapeutic efficacy in man.

Pharmacokinetics: The extent of percutaneous absorption of topical corticosteroids is determined by many factors including the vehicle, the integrity of the epidermal barrier and the use of occlusive dressings (see DOSAGE AND ADMINISTRATION). Topical corticosteroids can be absorbed from normal intact skin. Inflammation and/or other disease processes in the skin increase percutaneous absorption. Occlusive dressings substantially increase the percutaneous absorption of topical corticosteroids (see DOSAGE AND ADMINISTRATION). Once absorbed through the skin, topical corticosteroids are handled through pharmacokinetic pathways similar to systemically administered corticosteroids. Corticosteroids are bound to plasma proteins in varying degrees. Corticosteroids are metabolized primarily in the liver and then excreted by the kidneys. Some of the topical corticosteroids and their metabolites are also excreted into the bile.

NYSTATIN and TRIAMCINOLONE ACETONIDE
Patients having mild to severe manifestations of cutaneous candidiasis, treated with combined nystatin and triamcinolone acetonide show a faster and more pronounced clearing of erythema and pruritis than patients treated with nystatin or triamcinolone acetonide alone.

INDICATIONS AND USAGE
MYTREX® (nystatin-triamcinolone acetonide) Cream and Ointment is indicated for the treatment of cutaneous candidiasis; it has been demonstrated that the nystatin-steroid combination provides greater benefit than the nystatin component alone during the first few days of treatment.

CONTRAINDICATIONS
This preparation is contraindicated in those patients with a history of hypersensitivity to any of its components.

PRECAUTIONS
General: Systemic absorption of topical corticosteroids has produced reversible hypothalamic-pituitary-adrenal (HPA) axis suppression, manifestations of Cushing's syndrome, hyperglycemia, and glucosuria in some patients. Conditions which augment systemic absorption include the application of the more potent steroids, use over large surface areas, prolonged use, and the addition of occlusive dressings (see DOSAGE AND ADMINISTRATION). Therefore, patients receiving a large dose of any potent topical steroid applied to a large surface area should be evaluated periodically for evidence of HPA axis suppression by using the urinary free cortisol and ACTH stimulation tests, and for impairment of thermal homeostasis. If HPA axis suppression or elevation of the body temperature occurs, an attempt should be made to withdraw the drug, to reduce the frequency of application, or to substitute a less potent steroid. Recovery of HPA axis function and thermal homeostasis are generally prompt and complete upon discontinuation of the drug. Infrequently, signs and symptoms of steroid withdrawal may occur, requiring supplemental systemic corticosteroids. Children may absorb proportionally larger amounts of topical corticosteroids and thus be more susceptible to systemic toxicity (See PRECAUTIONS, Pediatric Use). If irritation or hypersensitivity develops with the combination nystatin and triamcinolone acetonide, treatment should be discontinued and appropriate therapy instituted.

Information for the Patient: Patients using this medication should receive the following information and instructions:
1. This medication is to be used as directed by the physician. It is for external use only. Avoid contact with the eyes.
2. Patients should be advised not to use this medication for any disorder other than for which it was prescribed.
3. The treated skin area should not be bandaged or otherwise covered or wrapped as to be occluded (see DOSAGE AND ADMINISTRATION).
4. Patients should report any signs of local adverse reactions.
5. When using this medication in the inguinal area, patients should be advised to apply cream or ointment sparingly and to wear loose fitting clothing.
6. Parents of pediatric patients should be advised not to use tight-fitting diapers or plastic pants on a child being treated in the diaper area, as these garments may constitute occlusive dressings.
7. Patients should be advised on preventive measures to avoid reinfection.

Laboratory Tests: If there is a lack of therapeutic response, appropriate microbiological studies (e.g., KOH smears and/or cultures) should be repeated to confirm the diagnosis and rule out other pathogens, before instituting another course of therapy. The following tests may be helpful in evaluating

hypothalamic-pituitary-adrenal (HPA) axis suppression due to the corticosteroid: Urinary free cortisol test; ACTH stimulation test.

Carcinogenesis, Mutagenesis, and Impairment of Fertility: Long-term animal studies have not been performed to evaluate the carcinogenic or mutagenic potential or possible impairment of fertility in males or females.

Pregnancy Category C: There are no teratogenic studies with combined nystatin and triamcinolone acetonide. Corticosteroids are generally teratogenic in laboratory animals when administered systemically at relatively low dosage levels. The more potent corticosteroids have been shown to be teratogenic after dermal application in laboratory animals. Therefore, any topical corticosteroid preparation should be used during pregnancy only if the potential benefit justifies the potential risk to the fetus. Topical preparations containing corticosteroids should not be used extensively on pregnant patients, in large amounts, or for prolonged periods of time.

Nursing Mothers: It is not known whether any component of this preparation is excreted in human milk. Because many drugs are excreted in human milk, caution should be exercised during use of this preparation by a nursing woman.

Pediatric Use: In clinical studies of a limited number of pediatric patients ranging in age from 2 months through twelve years, Nystatin-Triamcinolone Acetonide Cream cleared or significantly ameliorated the disease state in most patients. *Pediatric patients may demonstrate greater susceptibility to topical corticosteroid-induced hypothalamic-pituitary-adrenal (HPA) axis suppression and Cushing's syndrome than mature patients because of a larger skin surface area to body weight ratio.* HPA axis suppression, Cushing's syndrome, and intracranial hypertension have been reported in children receiving topical corticosteroids. Manifestations of adrenal suppression in children include linear growth retardation, delayed weight gain, low plasma cortisol levels, and absence of response to ACTH stimulation. Manifestations of intracranial hypertension include bulging fontanelles, headaches and bilateral papilledema. Administration of topical corticosteroids to children should be limited to the least amount compatible with an effective therapeutic regimen. Chronic corticosteroid therapy may interfere with the growth and development of children.

ADVERSE REACTIONS
A single case (approximately one percent of patients studied) of acneiform eruption occurred with the use of combined nystatin and triamcinolone acetonide in clinical studies. Nystatin is virtually nontoxic and nonsensitizing and is well tolerated by all age groups, even during prolonged use. Rarely, irritation may occur.

The following local adverse reactions are reported infrequently with topical corticosteroids. These reactions are listed in an approximate decreasing order of occurrence: burning, itching, irritation, dryness, folliculitis, hypertrichosis, acneiform eruptions, hypopigmentation, perioral dermatitis, allergic contact dermatitis, maceration of the skin, secondary infection, skin atrophy, striae and miliaria.

OVERDOSAGE
Topically applied corticosteroids can be absorbed in sufficient amounts to produce systemic effects (see PRECAUTIONS, General). However, acute overdosage and serious adverse effects with dermatologic use are unlikely.

DOSAGE AND ADMINISTRATION
Apply MYTREX® (nystatin-triamcinolone acetonide) Cream to the affected area twice daily in the morning and the evening by gently and thoroughly massaging the preparation into the skin. A thin film of MYTREX® Ointment is usually applied to the affected areas twice daily in the morning and evening. The cream or ointment should be discontinued if symptoms persist after 25 days of therapy. (See PRECAUTIONS, Laboratory Tests). MYTREX® (nystatin-triamcinolone acetonide) Cream and Ointment should not be used with occlusive dressings.

HOW SUPPLIED
MYTREX® Cream
12 × 1.5 Gram Foilpac—NDC 0281-0081-08
15 Gram Tube—NDC 0281-0081-15
30 Gram Tube—NDC 0281-0081-30
60 Gram Tube—NDC 0281-0081-60
   Shown in Product Identification Section, page 427
MYTREX® Ointment
15 gram tube—NDC 0281-0089-15
30 gram tube—NDC 0281-0089-30
60 gram tube—NDC 0281-0089-60
Store at room temperature. Avoid freezing.

CAUTION
Federal law prohibits dispensing without prescription.

NYSTEX™ ℞
[nī'stex]
(nystatin cream USP and ointment USP)

DESCRIPTION
NYSTEX™ (nystatin USP) Cream contains the antifungal antibiotic nystatin at a concentration of 100,000 units per gram in an aqueous, vanishing cream base containing polysorbate 60, aluminum hydroxide compressed gel, titanium dioxide, glyceryl monostearate, polyethylene glycol monostearate 400, simethicone, sorbic acid, propylene glycol, ethylenediamine, polyoxyethylene fatty alcohol ether, sorbitol solution, methyl paraben, propyl paraben, hydrochloric acid, white petrolatum, and purified water.
NYSTEX™ (nystatin USP) Ointment contains 100,000 units nystatin per gram in a polyethylene and mineral oil base.

HOW SUPPLIED
NYSTEX™ Cream
  NDC 0281-3208-44, 15 gram tube
  NDC 0281-3208-45, 30 gram tube
NYSTEX™ Ointment
  NDC 0281-3212-44, 15 gram tube

NYSTEX™ ℞
[nī'stex]
(nystatin oral suspension USP)

DESCRIPTION
Nystatin is an antifungal antibiotic that is both fungistatic and fungicidal in vitro against a wide variety of yeasts and yeastlike fungi. It is a polyene antibiotic of undetermined structural formula that is obtained from *Streptomyces noursei*. Nystex™ Oral Suspension contains 100,000 units nystatin per ml in a vehicle containing alcohol USP (not more than 1% by volume), mint blend flavoring, dibasic sodium phosphate USP, glycerin USP, purified water USP, silicon dioxide, sucrose NF (50%) and methylparaben NF (0.12%) and propylparaben NF (0.03%) as preservatives.

HOW SUPPLIED
Nystex™ Oral Suspension (NDC 0281-0037-60) is available as a pleasant-tasting, ready-to-use suspension containing 100,000 units nystatin per ml in 60 ml bottles (each supplied with a calibrated dropper).

STORAGE
Store at room temperaure; avoid freezing.

TRYSUL® ℞
[trī'sul]
(triple sulfa vaginal cream)

DESCRIPTION
Active Ingredients: sulfathiazole 3.42%, sulfacetamide 2.86%, sulfabenzamide 3.70% and urea 0.64%.
In a Base Containing: Glyceryl monostearate, cetyl alcohol, stearic acid, lecithin, peanut oil, diethylaminoethyl steramide, phosphoric acid, propylene glycol, ethoxylated cholesterol, methyl paraben 0.15% and propyl paraben 0.05% as preservatives, and purified water.

HOW SUPPLIED
NDC 0281-3790-47, Trysul® 78 g tube with measured dose applicator.

IDENTIFICATION PROBLEM?
Consult PDR's
Product Identification Section
where you'll find over 1700
products pictured actual size
and in full color.

Schering Corporation
a wholly-owned subsidiary of Schering-Plough Corporation
GALLOPING HILL ROAD
KENILWORTH, NJ 07033

Product Identification Codes
To provide quick and positive identification of Schering Products, we have imprinted the product identification number of the National Drug Code on most tablets and capsules. In some cases, identification letters also appear.
Additionally, the following telephone numbers are provided for inquires:

  Professional Services Department
  9:00 AM to 5:00 PM EST
  1-800-526-4099

After regular hours and on weekends: (201) 298-4000
For convenience, a complete list of all Schering products and their identification codes, where appropriate, follow:

Product Listing

Product	Code	
A&D™ Ointment*		OTC
AFRIN®*		OTC
oxymetazoline HCl		
Nasal Spray 0.05%		
Menthol Nasal Spray 0.05%		
Nose Drops 0.05%		
Pediatric Nose Drops 0.025%		
AFRINOL®*		OTC
pseudoephedrine sulfate		
Repetabs Tablets Long-Acting		
Nasal Decongestant	AFRINOL	
CELESTONE®		℞
betamethasone, USP		
Phosphate Injection†		
Soluspan® Suspension		
Syrup†		
Tablets 0.6 mg†	011/BDA	
CHLOR-TRIMETON®*		OTC
chlorpheniramine maleate		
Allergy Syrup		
Allergy Tablets 4 mg	080	
Long-Acting Allergy		
Repetabs® Tablets 8 mg	374	
Maximum Strength		
Allergy Repetabs® Tablets 12 mg	009	
CHLOR-TRIMETON®*		OTC
chlorpheniramine maleate/		
pseudoephedrine sulfate		
Decongestant Tablets	901	
Long-Acting Decongestant		
Repetabs® Tablets		
CHLOR-TRIMETON® †		℞
chlorpheniramine maleate, USP		
Injection 10 mg/ml		
COD LIVER OIL CONCENTRATE*		OTC
Capsules		
Tablets		
Tablets with Vitamin C		
COMPLEX 15®*		OTC
Face Cream		
Hand and Body Cream		
Hand and Body Lotion		
CORICIDIN®*		OTC
D® Decongestant Tablets	307	
DEMILETS® Tablets		
Nasal Mist		
Sinus Caplets		
(Maximum Strength)		
Tablets	522	
DEMAZIN®*		OTC
Timed-Release Tablets	751	
Syrup		
DERMOLATE®*		OTC
hydrocortisone 0.5%		
Anti-Itch Cream		
DIPROLENE®		℞
augmented betamethasone dipropionate		
AF Cream 0.05%		
Cream 0.05%		
Lotion 0.05%		
Ointment 0.05%		
DIPROSONE®		℞
betamethasone dipropionate, USP		
Aerosol 0.1%		
Cream 0.05%		
Lotion 0.05%		
Ointment 0.05%		
DISOPHROL®*		OTC
CHRONOTAB® Tablets	555	
DISOPHROL® †	WBS	OTC
Tablets		

Product	Code	
DRIXORAL®* Sustained-Action		OTC
Tablets		
DRIXORAL®PLUS		OTC
Sustained-Action Tablets		
DRIXORAL® Syrup		OTC
ELOCON®		℞
Mometasone furoate		
Cream 0.1%		
Lotion 0.1%		
Ointment 0.1%		
EMKO®*		OTC
BECAUSE® Contraceptor®*		
PRE-FIL® Vaginal Contraceptive Foam		
Vaginal Contraceptive Foam		
ESTINYL® Tablets		℞
estinyl estradiol, USP		
0.02 mg	298	
0.05 mg	070	
0.5 mg	150	
Eulexin® Capsules		℞
flutamide	525	
125 mg		
ETRAFON® Tablets		℞
perphenazine, USP-amitriptyline		
hydrochloride, USP		
Tablets (2–10)	ANA/287	
Tablets (2–25)	ANC/598	
A Tablets (4–10)	ANB/119	
Forte Tablets (4–25)	ANE/720	
FULVICIN® P/G Tablets		℞
ultramicrosize griseofulvin, USP		
125 mg	228	
165 mg	654	
250 mg	507	
330 mg	352	
FULVICIN U/F® Tablets		℞
griseofulvin, (microsize), USP		
250 mg	AUF/948	
500 mg	AUG/496	
GARAMYCIN® Injectables		℞
gentamicin sulfate, USP		
Disposable Syringes 1.5 ml (60 mg)		
Disposable Syringes 2.0 ml (80 mg)		
Injectable 2 ml vial (80 mg)		
Injectable 20 ml vial (800 mg)		
Intrathecal 2 ml (4 mg) ampul		
Pediatric Injectable 2 ml vial (20 mg)		
I.V. Piggyback Injection–		
60 ml (60 mg), 80 ml (80 mg)		
GARAMYCIN® Topicals		℞
gentamicin sulfate, USP		
Cream		
Ointment		
Ophthalmic Ointment		
Ophthalmic Solution		
GYNE-LOTRIMIN®		℞
clotrimazole, USP		
Vaginal Cream 1%		
Vaginal Tablets 100 mg	734	
Vaginal Tablets 500 mg	396	
HYPERSTAT® I.V. Injection		℞
diazoxide, USP		
INHAL-AID®		℞
Drug Delivery System for Metered		
Dose Inhalers		
INSPIREASE®		℞
Drug Delivery System for use with		
Metered Dose Inhalers		
INTRON® A		℞
Interferon alfa-2b, recombinant		
Injection		
LOTRIMIN®		℞
clotrimazole, USP		
Cream 1%		
Lotion 1%		
Solution 1%		
LOTRISONE® Cream		℞
clotrimazole, USP, betamethasone		
dipropionate, USP		
METICORTEN® Tablets†		℞
prednisone, USP		
1 mg	843	
METIMYD®†		℞
prednisolone acetate, USP/		
sulfacetamide sodium, USP		
Ophthalmic Ointment		
Ophthalmic Suspension		
MIRADON® Tablets		℞
anisindione, USP		

Continued on next page

Information on Schering products appearing on these pages is effective as of September 30, 1989.

Schering—Cont.

MOL-IRON®*			OTC
Tablets			
Tablets with Vitamin C			
NAQUA® Tablets†			℞
trichlormethiazide, USP			
	2 mg	AHG/822	
	4 mg	AHH/547	
NAQUIVAL® Tablets†			℞
trichlormethiazide,			
USP/reserpine, USP		AHT/394	
NETROMYCIN®			℞
netilmicin sulfate			
Injection		100 mg/ml	
NORMODYNE®			℞
labetalol HCl			
Tablets	100 mg	244	
	200 mg	752	
	300 mg	438	
Injection		5 mg/ml	
NORMOZIDE®			℞
labetalol/hydrochlorothiazide, USP			
Tablets	100 mg/25 mg	235	
	200 mg/25 mg	227	
	300 mg/25 mg	391	
OCUCLEAR Eye Drops			OTC
oxymetazoline 0.025%			
OPTIMINE® Tablets			℞
azatadine maleate, USP		282	
OPTIMYD® Ophthalmic Solution†			℞
prednisolone sodium phosphate, USP/			
sulfacetamide sodium, USP			
ORETON®†			℞
methyltestosterone, USP			
Methyl Tablets	10 mg	311	
Methyl Buccal Tablets		970	
OTOBIOTIC® Otic Solution†			℞
polymyxin B sulfate, USP and			
hydrocortisone, USP			
PAXIPAM® Tablets ℂ†			℞
halazepam, USP			
	20 mg	251	
	40 mg	538	
PERMITIL®			℞
fluphenazine hydrochloride, USP			
Oral Concentrate			
Tablets	2.5 mg	WDR/442	
	5 mg	WFF/550	
	10 mg	WFG/316	
POLARAMINE®			℞
dexchlorpheniramine maleate, USP			
Expectorant†			
Repetabs® Tablets	4 mg	095	
	6 mg	148	
Syrup			
Tablets	2 mg	AGT/820	
PROVENTIL®			℞
albuterol			
Inhaler			
PROVENTIL®			℞
albuterol sulfate			
Solution for Inhalation 0.083%/0.5%			
Syrup			
Repetabs® Tablets	4 mg	431	
Tablets	02 mg	252	
	4 mg	573	
RELA® Tablets†			℞
carisoprodol, USP		AHR/160	
SEBIZON® Lotion†			℞
sulfacetamide sodium, USP 10%			
SODIUM SULAMYD®			℞
sulfacetamide sodium, USP			
Ophthalmic Ointment 10%			
Ophthalmic Solution 10%			
Ophthalmic Solution 30% w/v			
SOLGANAL® Suspension			℞
aurothioglucose, USP			
THEOVENT® Long-Acting Capsules†			℞
theophylline anhydrous, USP			
	125 mg	402	
	250 mg	753	
TINACTIN®*			OTC
tolnaftate, USP			
Cream 1%			
Jock Itch Cream			
Jock Itch Spray Powder			
Liquid 1% Aerosol			
Powder 1%			
Powder 1% Aerosol			
Solution 1%			
TINDAL® Tablets†		BBA/968	℞
acetophenazine maleate, USP			

TRILAFON®			℞
perphenazine, USP			
Concentrate			
Injection			
Tablets	2 mg	ADH/705	
	4 mg	ADK/940	
	8 mg	ADJ/313	
	16 mg	ADM/077	
TRINALIN® Long-Acting			℞
Antihistamine/Decongestant			
Repetabs® Tablets		703	
VALISONE®†			℞
betamethasone valerate, USP			
Cream 0.1%			
Lotion 0.1%			
Ointment 0.1%			
Reduced Strength Cream 0.01%			
VANCENASE®			℞
beclomethasone dipropionate, USP			
Nasal Inhaler			
AQ Nasal Spray 0.042%			
VANCERIL® Oral Inhaler			℞
beclomethasone dipropionate, USP			

* For complete prescribing information see PDR For Non-prescription Drugs.

† For complete prescribing information contact the Schering Professional Services Department.

CELESTONE® SOLUSPAN® *   ℞

[se-les 'tōn]

Suspension

brand of sterile betamethasone sodium phosphate

and betamethasone acetate suspension,

USP

6 mg per ml

DESCRIPTION

Each ml of CELESTONE SOLUSPAN* Suspension contains: 3.0 mg betamethasone as betamethasone sodium phosphate; 3.0 mg betamethasone acetate; 7.1 mg dibasic sodium phosphate; 3.4 mg monobasic sodium phosphate; 0.1 mg edetate disodium; and 0.2 mg benzalkonium chloride. It is a sterile, aqueous suspension with a pH between 6.8 and 7.2.

The formula for betamethasone sodium phosphate is $C_{22}H_{28}FNa_2O_8P$ with a molecular weight of 516.41. Chemically it is 9-Fluoro-11β, 17,21-trihydroxy-16β-methylpregna-1,4-diene-3,20-dione 21-(disodium phosphate).

The formula for betamethasone acetate is $C_{24}H_{31}FO_6$ with a molecular weight of 434.50. Chemically it is 9-Fluoro-11β,17,21-trihydroxy-16β-methylpregna-1, 4-diene-3, 20-dione 21-acetate.

Betamethasone sodium phosphate is a white to practically white, odorless powder, and is hygroscopic. It is freely soluble in water and in methanol, but is practically insoluble in acetone and in chloroform.

Betamethasone acetate is a white to creamy white, odorless powder that sinters and resolidifies at about 165°C, and remelts at about 200°C–220°C with decomposition. It is practically insoluble in water, but freely soluble in acetone, and is soluble in alcohol and in chloroform.

*brand of rapid and repository injectable.

ACTIONS

Naturally occurring glucocorticoids (hydrocortisone), which also have salt-retaining properties, are used as replacement therapy in adrenocortical deficiency states. Their synthetic analogs are primarily used for their potent anti-inflammatory effects in disorders of many organ systems.

Betamethasone sodium phosphate, a soluble ester, provides prompt activity, while betamethasone acetate is only slightly soluble and affords sustained activity.

Glucocorticoids cause profound and varied metabolic effects. In addition, they modify the body's immune responses to diverse stimuli.

INDICATIONS

When oral therapy is not feasible and the strength, dosage form, and route of administration of the drug reasonably lend the preparation to the treatment of the condition, CELESTONE SOLUSPAN Suspension for **intramuscular use** is indicated as follows:

Endocrine disorders: Primary or secondary adrenocortical insufficiency (hydrocortisone or cortisone is the drug of choice; synthetic analogs may be used in conjunction with mineralocorticoids where applicable; in infancy, mineralocorticoid supplementation is of particular importance). Acute adrenocortical insufficiency (hydrocortisone or cortisone is the drug of choice; mineralocorticoid supplementation may be necessary, particularly when synthetic analogs are used). Preoperatively and in the event of serious trauma or illness, in patients with known adrenal insufficiency or when adrenocortical reserve is doubtful. Shock unresponsive to conventional therapy if adrenocortical insufficiency exists or is suspected. Congenital adrenal hyperplasia. Nonsuppurative thyroiditis. Hypercalcemia associated with cancer.

Rheumatic disorders: As adjunctive therapy for short-term administration (to tide the patient over an acute episode or exacerbation) in: post-traumatic osteoarthritis; synovitis of osteoarthritis; rheumatoid arthritis; acute and subacute bursitis; epicondylitis; acute nonspecific tenosynovitis; acute gouty arthritis; psoriatic arthritis; ankylosing spondylitis; juvenile rheumatoid arthritis (selected cases may require low-dose maintenance therapy).

Collagen disease: During an exacerbation or as maintenance therapy in selected cases of: systemic lupus erythematosus; acute rheumatic carditis.

Dermatologic diseases: Pemphigus: severe erythema multiforme (Stevens-Johnson syndrome); exfoliative dermatitis; bullous dermatitis herpetiformis; severe seborrheic dermatitis; severe psoriasis; mycosis fungoides.

Allergic states: Control of severe or incapacitating allergic conditions intractable to adequate trials of conventional treatment in: bronchial asthma; contact dermatitis; atopic dermatitis; serum sickness; seasonal or perennial allergic rhinitis; drug hypersensitivity reactions; urticarial transfusion reactions; acute noninfectious laryngeal edema (epinephrine is the drug of first choice).

Ophthalmic diseases: Severe, acute and chronic allergic and inflammatory processes involving the eye, such as: herpes zoster ophthalmicus; iritis, iridocyclitis; chorioretinitis; diffuse posterior uveitis and choroiditis; optic neuritis; sympathetic ophthalmia; anterior segment inflammation; allergic conjunctivitis; allergic corneal marginal ulcer; keratitis.

Gastrointestinal diseases: To tide the patient over a critical period of disease in: ulcerative colitis—(systemic therapy); regional enteritis—(systemic therapy).

Respiratory diseases: Symptomatic sarcoidosis; berylliosis; fulminating or disseminated pulmonary tuberculosis, when concurrently with appropriate antituberculous chemotherapy; aspiration pneumonitis; Loffler's syndrome not manageable by other means.

Hematologic disorders: Acquired (autoimmune) hemolytic anemia. Secondary thrombocytopenia in adults. Erythroblastopenia (RBC anemia). Congenital (erythroid) hypoplastic anemia.

Neoplastic diseases: For palliative management of: leukemias and lymphomas in adults; acute leukemia of childhood.

Edematous state: To induce diuresis or remission of proteinuria in the nephrotic syndrome, without uremia, of the idiopathic type or that due to lupus erythematosus.

Miscellaneous: Tuberculous meningitis with subarachnoid block or impending block when used concurrently with appropriate antituberculous chemotherapy. Trichinosis with neurologic or myocardial involvement.

When the strength and dosage form of the drug lend the preparation to the treatment of the condition, the **intra-articular or soft tissue administration** of CELESTONE SOLU-SPAN Suspension is indicated as adjunctive therapy for short-term administration (to tide the patient over an acute episode or exacerbation) in: synovitis of osteoarthritis; rheumatoid arthritis; acute and subacute bursitis; acute gouty arthritis; epicondylitis; acute nonspecific tenosynovitis; post-traumatic osteoarthritis.

When the strength and dosage form of the drug lend the preparation to the treatment of the condition, the **intralesional administration** of CELESTONE SOLUSPAN Suspension is indicated for: keloids; localized hypertrophic, infiltrated, inflammatory lesions of lichen planus, psoriatic plaques, granuloma annulare, and lichen simplex chronicus (neurodermatitis); discoid lupus erythematosus; necrobiosis lipoidica diabeticorum; alopecia areata.

CELESTONE SOLUSPAN Suspension may also be useful in cystic tumors of an aponeurosis or tendon (ganglia).

CONTRAINDICATIONS

CELESTONE SOLUSPAN Suspension is contraindicated in systemic fungal infections.

WARNINGS

CELESTONE SOLUSPAN should not be administered intravenously.

In patients on corticosteroid therapy subjected to any unusual stress, increased dosage of rapidly acting corticosteroids before, during, and after the stressful situation is indicated.

Corticosteroids may mask some signs of infection, and new infections may appear during their use. There may be decreased resistance and inability to localize infection when corticosteroids are used.

Prolonged use of corticosteroids may produce posterior subcapsular cataracts, glaucoma with possible damage to the optic nerves, and may enhance the establishment of secondary ocular infections due to fungi or viruses.

CELESTONE SOLUSPAN contains two betamethasone esters one of which, betamethasone sodium phosphate, disappears rapidly from the injection site. The potential for systemic effect produced by the soluble portion of CELESTONE SOLUSPAN should therefore be taken into account by the physician when using the drug.

Average and large doses of cortisone or hydrocortisone can cause elevation of blood pressure, salt and water retention, and increased excretion of potassium. These effects are less likely to occur with the synthetic derivatives except when used in large doses. Dietary salt restriction and potassium supplementation may be necessary. All corticosteroids increase calcium excretion.

While on Corticosteroid Therapy Patients Should Not Be Vaccinated Against Smallpox. Other Immunization Procedures Should Not Be Undertaken in Patients Who Are on Corticosteroids, Especially in High Doses, Because of Possible Hazards of Neurological Complications and Lack of Antibody Response.

The use of CELESTONE SOLUSPAN Suspension in active tuberculosis should be restricted to those cases of fulminating or disseminated tuberculosis in which the corticosteroid is used for the management of the disease in conjunction with appropriate antituberculous regimen.

If corticosteroids are indicated in patients with latent tuberculosis or tuberculin reactivity, close observation is necessary as reactivation of the disease may occur. During prolonged corticosteroid therapy, these patients should receive chemoprophylaxis.

Because rare instances of anaphylactoid reactions have occurred in patients receiving parenteral corticosteroid therapy, appropriate precautionary measures should be taken prior to administration, especially when the patient has a history of allergy to any drug.

Usage in pregnancy: Since adequate human reproduction studies have not been done with corticosteroids, the use of these drugs in pregnancy, nursing mothers, or women of childbearing potential requires that the possible benefits of the drug be weighed against the potential hazards to the mother and embryo or fetus. Infants born of mothers who have received substantial doses of corticosteroids during pregnancy should be carefully observed for signs of hypoadrenalism.

PRECAUTIONS

Drug-induced secondary adrenocortical insufficiency may be minimized by gradual reduction of dosage. This type of relative insufficiency may persist for months after discontinuation of therapy; therefore, in any situation of stress occurring during that period, hormone therapy should be reinstituted. Since mineralocorticoid secretion may be impaired, salt and/or a mineralocorticoid should be administered concurrently.

There is an enhanced effect of corticosteroids in patients with hypothyroidism and in those with cirrhosis.

Corticosteroids should be used cautiously in patients with ocular herpes simplex for fear of corneal perforation.

The lowest possible dose of corticosteroid should be used to control the condition under treatment, and when reduction in dosage is possible, the reduction must be gradual.

Psychic derangements may appear when corticosteroids are used, ranging from euphoria, insomnia, mood swings, personality changes, and severe depression to frank psychotic manifestations. Also, existing emotional instability or psychotic tendencies may be aggravated by corticosteroids.

Aspirin should be used cautiously in conjunction with corticosteroids in hypoprothrombinemia.

Steroids should be used with caution in nonspecific ulcerative colitis, if there is a probability of impending perforation, abscess or other pyogenic infection, also in diverticulitis, fresh intestinal anastomoses, active or latent peptic ulcer, renal insufficiency, hypertension, osteoporosis, and myasthenia gravis.

Growth and development of infants and children on prolonged corticosteroid therapy should be carefully followed.

The following additional precautions also apply for parenteral corticosteroids. **Intra-articular injection of a corticosteroid may produce systemic as well as local effects.**

Appropriate examination of any joint fluid present is necessary to exclude a septic process.

A marked increase in pain accompanied by local swelling, further restriction of joint motion, fever, and malaise are suggestive of septic arthritis. If this complication occurs and the diagnosis of sepsis is confirmed, appropriate antimicrobial therapy should be instituted.

Local injection of a steroid into a previously infected joint is to be avoided.

Corticosteroids should not be injected into unstable joints. The slower rate of absorption by intramuscular administration should be recognized.

ADVERSE REACTIONS

Fluid and electrolyte disturbances: sodium retention; fluid retention; congestive heart failure in susceptible patients; potassium loss; hypokalemic alkalosis; hypertension.

Musculoskeletal: muscle weakness; steroid myopathy; loss of muscle mass; osteoporosis; vertebral compression fractures; aseptic necrosis of femoral and humeral heads; pathologic fracture of long bones.

Gastrointestinal: peptic ulcer with possible subsequent perforation and hemorrhage; pancreatitis; abdominal distension; ulcerative esophagitis.

Dermatologic: impaired wound healing; thin fragile skin; petechiae and ecchymoses; facial erythema; increased sweating; may suppress reactions to skin tests.

Neurological: convulsions; increased intracranial pressure with papilledema (pseudotumor cerebri) usually after treatment; vertigo; headache.

Endocrine: menstrual irregularities; development of Cushingoid state; suppression of growth in children; secondary adrenocortical and pituitary unresponsiveness, particularly in times of stress, as in trauma, surgery, or illness; decreased carbohydrate tolerance; manifestations of latent diabetes mellitus; increased requirements for insulin or oral hypoglycemic agents in diabetics.

Ophthalmic: posterior subcapsular cataracts; increased intraocular pressure; glaucoma; exophthalmos.

Metabolic: negative nitrogen balance due to protein catabolism.

The following *additional* adverse reactions are related to parenteral corticosteroid therapy: rare instances of blindness associated with intralesional therapy around the face and head; hyperpigmentation or hypopigmentation; subcutaneous and cutaneous atrophy; sterile abscess; post-injection flare (following intra-articular use); charcot-like arthropathy.

DOSAGE AND ADMINISTRATION

The initial dosage of CELESTONE SOLUSPAN Suspension may vary from 0.5 to 9.0 mg per day depending on the specific disease entity being treated. In situations of less severity, lower doses will generally suffice while in selected patients higher initial doses may be required. Usually the parenteral dosage ranges are one-third to one-half the oral dose given every 12 hours. However, in certain overwhelming, acute, life-threatening situations, administration in dosages exceeding the usual dosages may be justified and may be in multiples of the oral dosages.

The initial dosage should be maintained or adjusted until a satisfactory response is noted. If after a reasonable period of time there is a lack of satisfactory clinical response, CELESTONE SOLUSPAN Suspension should be discontinued and the patient transferred to other appropriate therapy. *It Should Be Emphasized That Dosage Requirements Are Variable and Must Be Individualized on the Basis of the Disease Under Treatment and the Response of the Patient.* After a favorable response is noted, the proper maintenance dosage should be determined by decreasing the initial drug dosage in small decrements at appropriate time intervals until the lowest dosage which will maintain an adequate clinical response is reached. It should be kept in mind that constant monitoring is needed in regard to drug dosage. Included in the situations which may make dosage adjustments necessary are changes in clinical status secondary to remissions or exacerbations in the disease process, the patient's individual drug responsiveness, and the effect of patient exposure to stressful situations not directly related to the disease entity under treatment; in this latter situation it may be necessary to increase the dosage of CELESTONE SOLUSPAN Suspension for a period of time consistent with the patient's condition. If after long-term therapy the drug is to be stopped, it is recommended that it be withdrawn gradually rather than abruptly.

If coadministration of a local anesthetic is desired, CELESTONE SOLUSPAN Suspension may be mixed with 1% or 2% lidocaine hydrochloride, using the formulations which do not contain parabens. Similar local anesthetics may also be used. Diluents containing methylparaben, propylparaben, phenol, etc., should be avoided since these compounds may cause flocculation of the steroid. The required dose of CELESTONE SOLUSPAN Suspension is first withdrawn from the vial into the syringe. The local anesthetic is then drawn in, and the syringe shaken briefly. **Do not inject local anesthetics into the vial of CELESTONE SOLUSPAN Suspension.**

Bursitis, tenosynovitis, peritendinitis. In acute subdeltoid, subacromial, olecranon, and prepatellar bursitis, one intrabursal injection of 1.0 ml CELESTONE SOLUSPAN Suspension can relieve pain and restore full range of movement. Several intrabursal injections of corticosteroids are usually required in recurrent acute bursitis and in acute exacerbations of chronic bursitis. Partial relief of pain and some increase in mobility can be expected in both conditions after one or two injections. Chronic bursitis may be treated with reduced dosage once the acute condition is controlled. In tenosynovitis and tendinitis, three or four local injections at intervals of one to two weeks between injections are given in most cases. Injections should be made into the affected tendon sheaths rather than into the tendons themselves. In ganglions of joint capsules and tendon sheaths, injection of 0.5 ml directly into the ganglion cysts has produced marked reduction in the size of the lesions. *Rheumatoid arthritis and osteoarthritis.* Following intra-articular administration of 0.5 to 2.0 ml of CELESTONE SOLUSPAN Suspension, relief of pain, soreness, and stiffness may be experienced. Duration of relief varies widely in both diseases. Intra-articular Injection—CELESTONE SOLUSPAN Suspension is well tolerated in joints and periarticular tissues. There is virtually no

pain on injection, and the "secondary flare" that sometimes occurs a few hours after intra-articular injection of corticosteroids has not been reported with CELESTONE SOLUSPAN Suspension. Using sterile technique, a 20- to 24-gauge needle on an empty syringe is inserted into the synovial cavity, and a few drops of synovial fluid are withdrawn to confirm that the needle is in the joint. The aspirating syringe is replaced by a syringe containing CELESTONE SOLUSPAN Suspension and injection is then made into the joint.

Recommended Doses for Intra-articular Injection

Size of joint	Location	Dose (ml)
Very Large	Hip	1.0-2.0
Large	Knee, Ankle, Shoulder	1.0
Medium	Elbow, Wrist	0.5-1.0
Small (Metacarpophalangeal, interphalangeal)	Hand	0.25-0.5
(Sternoclavicular)	Chest	

A portion of the administered dose of CELESTONE SOLUSPAN Suspension is absorbed systemically following intra-articular injection. In patients being treated concomitantly with oral or parenteral corticosteroids, especially those receiving large doses, the systemic absorption of the drug should be considered in determining intra-articular dosage. *Dermatologic conditions.* In intralesional treatment, 0.2 ml/sq. cm. of CELESTONE SOLUSPAN Suspension is injected intradermally (not subcutaneously) using a tuberculin syringe with a 25-gauge, ½-inch needle. Care should be taken to deposit a uniform depot of medication intradermally. A total of no more than 1.0 ml. at weekly intervals is recommended. *Disorders of the foot.* A tuberculin syringe with a 25-gauge, ¾-inch needle is suitable for most injections into the foot. The following doses are recommended at intervals of three days to a week.

Diagnosis	CELESTONE SOLUSPAN Suspension Dose (ml)
Bursitis	
under heloma durum or heloma molle	0.25-0.5
under calcaneal spur	0.5
over hallux rigidus or digiti quinti varus	0.5
Tenosynovitis, periostitis of cuboid	0.5
Acute gouty arthritis	0.5-1.0

HOW SUPPLIED

CELESTONE SOLUSPAN Suspension, 5 ml multiple-dose vial, box of one (NDC-0085-0566-05). **Shake well before using. Store between 2° and 25°C (36° and 77°F). Protect from light.** Revised 7/83

Copyright © 1969, 1983, Schering Corporation, USA. All rights reserved.

COMPLEX 15®
Phospholipid Moisturizer

(See PDR For Nonprescription Drugs)

DIPROLENE®   ℞
brand of augmented betamethasone dipropionate*
AF CREAM, 0.05 %
CREAM, 0.05%
OINTMENT, 0.05%
LOTION, 0.05%
(Potency expressed as betamethasone)
***Vehicle augments the penetration of the steroid**
For Dermatologic Use Only—Not for Ophthalmic Use

DESCRIPTION

DIPROLENE® products contain betamethasone dipropionate, USP, a synthetic adrenocorticosteroid for dermatologic use. Betamethasone, an analog of prednisolone, has a high degree of corticosteroid activity and a slight degree of miner-

Continued on next page

Information on Schering products appearing on these pages is effective as of September 30, 1989.

Schering—Cont.

alocorticoid activity. Betamethasone dipropionate is the 17,21-dipropionate ester of betamethasone.

Chemically, betamethasone dipropionate is 9-fluoro-11β, 17,21-trihydroxy-16β-methylpregna-1, 4-diene-3; 20-dione 17, 21-dipropionate, with the empirical formula $C_{28}H_{37}FO_7$, and a molecular weight of 504.6.

Betamethasone dipropionate is a white to creamy white, odorless crystalline powder, insoluble in water.

Each gram of DIPROLENE **AF Cream** 0.05% contains: 0.64 mg betamethasone dipropionate, USP (equivalent to 0.5 mg betamethasone), in an emollient cream base of purified water, chlorocresol, propylene glycol, white petrolatum, white wax, cyclomethicone, sorbitol solution, glyceryl monooleate, ceteareth-30, carbomer 940 and sodium hydroxide.

Each gram of DIPROLENE **Cream** 0.05% contains: 0.64 mg betamethasone dipropionate, USP (equivalent to 0.5 mg betamethasone), in an improved cream base of purified water, propylene glycol, carbomer 940, sodium hydroxide and titanium dioxide.

Each gram of DIPROLENE **Lotion** 0.05% contains: 0.64 mg betamethasone dipropionate, USP (equivalent to 0.5 mg betamethasone), in a lotion base of purified water, isopropyl alcohol (30%), hydroxypropylcellulose, propylene glycol, sodium phosphate, phosphoric acid and sodium hydroxide used to adjust the pH to 4.5.

Each gram of DIPROLENE **Ointment** 0.05% contains: 0.64 mg betamethasone dipropionate, USP (equivalent to 0.5 mg betamethasone), in ACTIBASE™, an optimized vehicle of propylene glycol, propylene glycol stearate, white wax and white petrolatum.

CLINICAL PHARMACOLOGY

The corticosteroids are a class of compounds comprising steroid hormones secreted by the adrenal cortex and their synthetic analogs. In pharmacologic doses, corticosteroids are used primarily for their anti-inflammatory and/or immunosuppressive effects.

Topical corticosteroids, such as betamethasone dipropionate, are effective in the treatment of corticosteroid-responsive dermatoses primarily because of their anti-inflammatory, anti-pruritic, and vasoconstrictive actions. However, while the physiologic, pharmacologic, and clinical effects of the corticosteroids are well-known, the exact mechanisms of their actions in each disease are uncertain. Betamethasone dipropionate, a corticosteroid, has been shown to have topical (dermatologic) and systemic pharmacologic and metabolic effects characteristic of this class of drugs.

Pharmacokinetics: The extent of percutaneous absorption of topical corticosteroids is determined by many factors including the vehicle, the integrity of the epidermal barrier, and the use of occlusive dressings. (See **DOSAGE AND ADMINISTRATION** section.)

Topical corticosteroids can be absorbed through normal intact skin. Inflammation and/or other disease processes in the skin may increase percutaneous absorption. Occlusive dressings substantially increase the percutaneous absorption of topical corticosteroids. (See **DOSAGE AND ADMINISTRATION** section.)

Once absorbed through the skin, topical corticosteroids enter pharmacokinetic pathways similar to systemically administered corticosteroids. Corticosteroids are bound to plasma proteins in varying degrees, are metabolized primarily in the liver and excreted by the kidneys. Some of the topical corticosteroids and their metabolites are also excreted into the bile. DIPROLENE **AF Cream** was applied once daily at 7 grams per day for one week to diseased skin, in patients with psoriasis or atopic dermatitis, to study its effects on the hypothalamic-pituitary-adrenal (HPA) axis. The results suggested that the drug caused a slight lowering of adrenal corticosteroid secretion, although in no case did plasma cortisol levels go below the lower limit of the normal range.

At 14 g per day (applied as 7 g twice daily), DIPROLENE **Cream** depressed the plasma levels of adrenal cortical hormones following application for 8 days to diseased skin in patients with psoriasis. Adrenal output in these patients returned to normal shortly after treatment cessation. At 7 g per day (applied once daily or as 3.5 g twice daily), DIPROLENE **Cream** was shown to cause inhibition of the hypothalamic-pituitary-adrenal (HPA) axis following application for one, two, or three weeks to diseased skin, in patients with psoriasis or atopic dermatitis. HPA axis inhibition in these patients was transient, and returned to normal during treatment, or shortly after treatment cessation.

DIPROLENE **Lotion** was applied once daily at 7 mL per day for 21 days to diseased skin (in patients with scalp psoriasis), to study its effects on the hypothalamic-pituitary-adrenal (HPA) axis. In 2 out of 11 patients, the drug lowered plasma cortisol levels below normal limits. Adrenal depression in these patients was transient, and returned to normal within a week. In one of these patients, plasma cortisol levels returned to normal while treatment continued.

At 14 g per day, DIPROLENE **Ointment** was shown to depress the plasma levels of adrenal cortical hormones following repeated application to diseased skin in patients with psoriasis. Adrenal depression in these patients was transient, and rapidly returned to normal upon cessation of treatment. At 7 g per day (3.5 g bid), DIPROLENE **Ointment** was shown to cause minimal inhibition of the hypothalamic-pituitary-adrenal (HPA) axis when applied two times daily for two to three weeks, in normal patients and in patients with psoriasis and eczematous disorders.

With 6 to 7 g of DIPROLENE **Ointment** applied once daily for 3 weeks, no significant inhibition of the HPA axis was observed in patients with psoriasis and atopic dermatitis, as measured by plasma cortisol and 24 hour urinary 17-hydroxycorticosteroid levels.

INDICATIONS AND USAGE

DIPROLENE **AF Cream** and **Ointment** are indicated for relief of the inflammatory and pruritic manifestations of corticosteroid-responsive dermatoses.

DIPROLENE **Cream** and **Lotion** are intended for short-term treatment of the inflammatory and pruritic manifestations of moderate to severe corticosteroid-responsive dermatoses. Treatment beyond two weeks is not recommended for DIPROLENE **Cream** and DIPROLENE **Lotion**. The total dosage should not exceed 45 g per week for DIPROLENE **Cream** and 50 mL per week for DIPROLENE **Lotion** because of potential for the drug to suppress the hypothalamic-pituitary-adrenal axis. DIPROLENE **Cream** is not recommended for use in children under 12 years of age.

CONTRAINDICATIONS

DIPROLENE products are contraindicated in patients who are hypersensitive to betamethasone dipropionate, to other corticosteroids, or to any ingredient in these preparations.

PRECAUTIONS

General: DIPROLENE **Cream** is a highly potent topical corticosteroid that has been shown to suppress the HPA axis at doses as low as 7 g per day. DIPROLENE **Lotion** is a highly potent topical corticosteroid that has been shown to suppress the HPA axis at 7 mL per day.

Systemic absorption of topical corticosteroids has produced reversible HPA axis suppression, manifestations of Cushing's syndrome, hyperglycemia, and glucosuria in some patients.

Conditions which augment systemic absorption include the application of the more potent corticosteroids, use over large surface areas, prolonged use, and the addition of occlusive dressings. (See **DOSAGE AND ADMINISTRATION** section.)

Therefore, patients receiving a large dose of a potent topical steroid applied to a large surface area should be evaluated periodically for evidence of HPA axis suppression by using the urinary free cortisol and ACTH stimulation tests. If HPA axis suppression is noted, an attempt should be made to withdraw the drug, to reduce the frequency of application, or to substitute a less potent steroid.

Recovery of HPA axis function is generally prompt and complete upon discontinuation of the drug. Infrequently, signs and symptoms of steroid withdrawal may occur, requiring supplemental systemic corticosteroids.

Children may absorb proportionally larger amounts of topical corticosteroids and thus be more susceptible to systemic toxicity. (See **PRECAUTIONS—Pediatric Use**.)

If irritation develops, topical corticosteroids should be discontinued and appropriate therapy instituted.

In the presence of dermatological infections, the use of an appropriate antifungal or antibacterial agent should be instituted. If a favorable response does not occur promptly, the corticosteroid should be discontinued until the infection has been adequately controlled.

Information for Patients: Patients using topical corticosteroids should receive the following information and instructions. This information is intended to aid in the safe and effective use of this medication. It is not a disclosure of all possible adverse or intended effects.

1. This medication is to be used as directed by the physician and should not be used longer than the prescribed time period. It is for external use only. Avoid contact with the eyes.
2. Patients should be advised not to use this medication for any disorder other than that for which it was prescribed.
3. The treated skin areas should not be bandaged or otherwise covered or wrapped so as to be occlusive. (See **DOSAGE AND ADMINISTRATION** section.)
4. Patients should report any sign of local adverse reactions.

Laboratory Tests: The following tests may be helpful in evaluating HPA axis suppression:
Urinary free cortisol test
ACTH stimulation test

Carcinogenesis, Mutagenesis, and Impairment of Fertility: Long-term animal studies have not been performed to evaluate the carcinogenic potential or the effect on fertility of topically applied corticosteroids.

Studies to determine mutagenicity with prednisolone and hydrocortisone have revealed negative results.

Pregnancy Category C: Corticosteroids are generally teratogenic in laboratory animals when administered systemically at relatively low dosage levels. The more potent corticosteroids have been shown to be teratogenic after dermal application in laboratory animals. Betamethasone dipropionate has not been tested for teratogenicity by this route, however, it appears to be fairly well-absorbed percutaneously. There are no adequate and well-controlled studies of the teratogenic effects of topically applied corticosteroids in pregnant women. Therefore, topical corticosteroids should be used during pregnancy only if the potential benefit justifies the potential risk to the fetus. Drugs of this class should not be used extensively on pregnant patients, in large amounts, or for prolonged periods of time.

Nursing Mothers: It is not known whether topical administration of corticosteroids can result in sufficient systemic absorption to produce detectable quantities in breast milk. Systemically administered corticosteroids are secreted into breast milk in quantities not likely to have a deleterious effect on the infant. Nevertheless, a decision should be made whether to discontinue nursing or to discontinue the drug, taking into account the importance of the drug to the mother.

Pediatric Use: Use of DIPROLENE **AF Cream**, DIPROLENE **Cream** and DIPROLENE **Ointment** in children under 12 years is not recommended. The safety and efficacy of DIPROLENE **Lotion** when used in children under 12 years of age have not been established.

Pediatric patients may demonstrate greater susceptibility to topical corticosteroid-induced HPA axis suppression and Cushing's syndrome than mature patients because of a larger skin surface area to body weight ratio.

Hypothalamic-pituitary-adrenal (HPA) axis suppression Cushing's syndrome, and intracranial hypertension have been reported in children receiving topical corticosteroids. Manifestations of adrenal suppression in children include linear growth retardation, delayed weight gain, low plasma cortisol levels, and absence of response to ACTH stimulation. Manifestations of intracranial hypertension include bulging fontanelles, headaches, and bilateral papilledema. Chronic corticosteroid therapy may interfere with the growth and development of children.

ADVERSE REACTIONS

The only local adverse reaction reported to be possibly or probably related to treatment with DIPROLENE **AF Cream** during controlled clinical studies was stinging. It occurred in 0.4% of the 242 patients or subjects involved in the studies. The overall incidence of drug-related adverse reactions in the DIPROLENE **Cream** clinical studies was 10%. The local adverse reactions that were reported to be possibly or probably related to treatment with DIPROLENE **Cream** during controlled clinical studies involving 815 patients were as follows: burning/stinging 6%, dry skin 4%, pruritus 2%, irritation 1%, telangiectasia, erythema, cracking/tightening of the skin, follicular rash, and skin atrophy each occurred in less than 1% of patients.

The overall incidence of drug-related adverse reactions in the DIPROLENE **Lotion** clinical studies was 5%. The adverse reactions that were reported to be possibly or probably related to treatment with DIPROLENE **Lotion** during controlled clinical studies involving 327 patients or normal volunteers were as follows: folliculitis occurred in 2%, burning and acneiform papules each occurred in 1%, and hyperesthesia and irritation each occurred in less than 1% of patients. The local adverse reactions that were reported with DIPROLENE **Ointment** applied either once or twice a day during clinical studies are as follows: erythema, 3 per 767 patients; folliculitis, 2 per 767 patients; pruritus, 2 per 767 patients; vesiculation, 1 per 767 patients.

The following local adverse reactions are reported infrequently when topical corticosteroids are used as recommended. These reactions are listed in approximate decreasing order of occurrence: burning, itching, irritation, dryness, folliculitis, hypertrichosis, acneiform eruptions, hypopigmentation, perioral dermatitis, allergic contact dermatitis, maceration of the skin, secondary infection, skin atrophy, striae, miliaria.

OVERDOSAGE

Topically applied corticosteroids can be absorbed in sufficient amounts to produce systemic effects. (See **PRECAUTIONS.**)

DOSAGE AND ADMINSTRATION

Apply a thin film of DIPROLENE **AF Cream** or DIPROLENE **Ointment** to the affected skin areas once or twice daily. Treatment with either DIPROLENE **AF Cream** or **Ointment** should be limited to 45 g per week.

Apply a thin film of DIPROLENE **Cream** to the affected skin areas once or twice daily. DIPROLENE **Cream** is potent; therefore, treatment must be limited to 14 days, and amounts greater than 45 g per week should not be used.

Apply a few drops of DIPROLENE **Lotion** to the affected area once or twice daily and massage lightly until the lotion disappears. Treatment must be limited to 14 days, and amounts greater than 50 mL per week should not be used.

DIPROLENE products are not to be used with occlusive dressings.

HOW SUPPLIED

DIPROLENE **AF Cream** 0.05% is supplied in 15-(NDC 0085-0517- 01), and 45-gram (NDC 0085-0517-02) tubes; boxes of one.
Store between 2° and 30°C (36° and 86°F).
DIPROLENE **Cream** 0.05% is supplied in 15-(NDC 0085-0728-01), and 45-gram (NDC 0085-0728-02) tubes; boxes of one.
Store between 2° and 30°C (36 ° and 86°F).
DIPROLENE **Lotion** 0.05% is supplied in 30 mL (29 g) (NDC 0085- 0962-01), and 60 mL (58 g) (NDC 0085-0962-02), plastic squeeze bottles; boxes of one.
Store between 2° and 30°C (36° and 86°F).
DIPROLENE **Ointment** 0.05% is supplied in 15- (NDC 0085-0575- 02), and 45-gram (NDC 0085-0575-03) tubes; boxes of one.
Store between 2° and 30°C (36° and 86°F).
Revised 6/89
Copyright © 1983, 1984, 1986, 1987, 1988, 1989, Schering Corporation. All rights reserved.

DRIXORAL PLUS
Sustained-Action Tablets

(See PDR For Nonprescription Drugs)
Shown in Product Identification Section, page 428

ELOCON®   ℞

[el 'ŏ-con]
brand of mometasone furoate
Cream 0.1%
For Dermatologic Use Only
Not for Ophthalmic Use

DESCRIPTION

ELOCON® Cream contains mometasone furoate for dermatologic use. Mometasone furoate is a synthetic corticosteroid with anti-inflammatory activity.
Chemically, mometasone furoate is 9α,21-Dichloro-11β,17-dihydroxy-16α-methylpregna-1,4 diene-3,20 dione 17-(2-furoate), with the empirical formula $C_{27}H_{30}Cl_2O_6$, and a molecular weight of 521.4.
Mometasone furoate is a white to off-white powder practically insoluble in water, slightly soluble in octanol, and moderately soluble in ethyl alcohol.
Each gram of ELOCON Cream 0.1% contains: 1 mg mometasone furoate in a cream base of hexylene glycol, phosphoric acid, propylene glycol stearate, stearyl alcohol and ceteareth-20, titanium dioxide, aluminum starch octenylsuccinate, white wax, white petrolatum and purified water.

CLINICAL PHARMACOLOGY

The corticosteroids are a class of compounds comprising steroid hormones secreted by the adrenal cortex and their synthetic analogs. In pharmacologic doses corticosteroids are used primarily for their anti-inflammatory and/or immunosuppressive effects.
Topical corticosteroids, such as mometasone furoate, are effective in the treatment of corticosteroid-response dermatoses primarily because of their anti-inflammatory, antipruritic, and vasoconstrictive actions. However, while the physiologic, pharmacologic, and clinical effects of the corticosteroids are well known, the exact mechanisms of their actions in each disease are uncertain. Mometasone furoate has been shown to have topical (dermatologic) and systemic pharmacologic and metabolic effects characteristic of this class of drugs.
Pharmacokinetics: The extent of percutaneous absorption of topical corticosteroids is determined by many factors including the vehicle, the integrity of the epidermal barrier, and the use of occlusive dressings. (See **DOSAGE AND ADMINISTRATION**.) Topical corticosteroids can be absorbed from normal intact skin.
The percutaneous absorption of ^{3}H-mometasone furoate was evaluated in rabbits following topical application of both cream (0.1%) and ointment (0.1%) formulations. Approximately 5% of the topically applied dose was systemically absorbed following topical application of the cream and 6% following application of the ointment formulation. Based upon these results, it was concluded that mometasone furoate is absorbed to a similar extent following application of either cream or ointment formulations. Percutaneous absorption studies of ^{3}H-mometasone furoate ointment in rats and dogs have shown that approximately 2.5% of a topically applied dose was absorbed by rats and 2% by dogs.
The percutaneous absorption of ^{3}H-mometasone furoate was also studied in man following topical application of an ointment (0.1%) formulation. Results showed that only about 0.7% of the steroid was systemically absorbed following 8 hours of contact without occlusion. Minimal absorption would be anticipated with the cream formulation.
Inflammation and/or other disease processes in the skin increase percutaneous absorption. Occlusive dressings substantially increase the percutaneous absorption of topical corticosteroids. (See **DOSAGE AND ADMINISTRATION.**)
In a study of the effects of mometasone furoate cream on the hypothalamic-pituitary-adrenal (HPA) axis, fifteen grams were applied twice daily for seven days to six patients with psoriasis or atopic dermatitis. The cream was applied without occlusion to at least 30% of the body surface. The results suggest that the drug caused a slight lowering of adrenal corticosteroid secretion, although in no case did plasma cortisol levels go below the lower limit of the normal range.
Once absorbed through the skin, topical corticosteroids are handled through pharmacokinetic pathways similar to systemically administered corticosteroids. Corticosteroids are bound to plasma proteins in varying degrees. Corticosteroids are metabolized primarily in the liver and are then excreted by the kidneys. Some of the topical corticosteroids and their metabolites are also excreted into the bile.

INDICATIONS AND USAGE

ELOCON Cream is indicated for the relief of the inflammatory and pruritic manifestations of corticosteroid-responsive dermatoses.

CONTRAINDICATIONS

ELOCON Cream is contraindicated in patients who are hypersensitive to mometasone furoate, to other corticosteroids, or to any ingredient in this preparation.

PRECAUTIONS

General: Systemic absorption of potent topical corticosteroids has produced reversible hypothalamic-pituitary-adrenal (HPA) axis suppression, manifestations of Cushing's syndrome, hyperglycemia, and glucosuria in some patients. Conditions which augment systemic absorption include application of steroids in optimized vehicles, use over large surface areas, prolonged use, use in areas where the epidermal barrier is disrupted, and the use of occlusive dressings. (See **DOSAGE AND ADMINISTRATION**.)
Patients receiving a large dose of a potent topical steroid applied to a large surface area or under an occlusive dressing should be evaluated periodically for evidence of HPA axis suppression by using the urinary free cortisol and ACTH stimulation tests. If HPA axis suppression is noted, an attempt should be made to withdraw the drug, to reduce the frequency of application, or to substitute a less potent steroid.
Recovery of HPA axis function is generally prompt and complete upon discontinuation of the drug. Infrequently, signs and symptoms of steroid withdrawal may occur, requiring supplemental systemic corticosteroids.
Children may absorb proportionally larger amounts of topical corticosteroids and thus be more susceptible to systemic toxicity. (See **PRECAUTIONS—Pediatric Use.**)
If irritation develops, topical corticosteroids should be discontinued and appropriate therapy instituted.
In the presence of dermatological infections, use of an appropriate antifungal or antibacterial agent should be instituted. If a favorable response does not occur promptly, the corticosteroid should be discontinued until the infection has been adequately controlled.
Information for Patients: Patients using topical corticosteroids should receive the following information and instructions. This information is intended to aid in the safe and effective use of this medication. It is not a disclosure of all possible adverse or intended effects.
1. This medication is to be used as directed by the physician. It is for external use only. Avoid contact with the eyes.
2. Patients should be advised not to use this medication for any disorder other than that for which it was prescribed.
3. The treated skin area should not be bandaged or otherwise covered or wrapped so as to be occlusive unless directed by the physician. (See **DOSAGE AND ADMINISTRATION.**)
4. Patients should report any signs of local adverse reactions.
5. Parents of pediatric patients should be advised not to use tight-fitting diapers or plastic pants on a child being treated in the diaper area, as these garments may constitute occlusive dressing. (See **DOSAGE AND ADMINISTRATION.**)
Laboratory Tests: The following tests may be helpful in evaluating HPA axis suppression:
  Urinary free cortisol test
  ACTH stimulation test
Carcinogenesis, Mutagenesis, and Impairment of Fertility: Long-term animal studies have not been performed to evaluate the carcinogenic potential or the effect on fertility of topical corticosteroids.
Genetic toxicity studies with mometasone furoate, which included the Ames test, mouse lymphoma assay, and a micronucleus test, did not reveal any mutagenic potential.
Pregnancy Category C: Corticosteroids are generally teratogenic in laboratory animals when administered systemically at relatively low dosage levels. Corticosteroids have been shown to be teratogenic after dermal application in laboratory animals. There are no adequate and well-controlled studies of teratogenic effects from topically applied corticosteroids in pregnant women. Therefore, topical corticosteroids should be used during pregnancy only if the potential benefit justifies the potential risk to the fetus. Drugs of this class should not be used extensively on pregnant patients, in large amounts, or for prolonged periods.
Nursing Mothers: It is not known whether topical administration of corticosteroids could result in sufficient systemic absorption to produce detectable quantities in breast milk. Systemically administered corticosteroids are secreted into breast milk in quantities not likely to have a deleterious effect on the infant. Nevertheless, a decision should be made whether to discontinue nursing or to discontinue the drug taking into account the importance of the drug to the mother.
Pediatric Use: *Pediatric patients may demonstrate greater susceptibility to topical corticosteroid-induced HPA axis suppression and Cushing's syndrome than mature patients because of a larger skin surface area to body weight ratio.*
Hypothalamic-pituitary-adrenal (HPA) axis suppression, Cushing's syndrome, and intracranial hypertension have been reported in children receiving topical corticosteroids. Manifestations of adrenal suppression in children include linear growth retardation, delayed weight gain, low plasma cortisol levels, and absence of response to ACTH stimulation. Manifestations of intracranial hypertension include bulging fontanelles, headaches, and bilateral papilledema.
Administration of topical corticosteroids to children should be limited to the least amount compatible with an effective therapeutic regimen. Chronic corticosteroid therapy may interfere with the growth and development of children.

ADVERSE REACTIONS

The following local adverse reactions were reported with ELOCON Cream during clinical studies with 319 patients: burning, 1; pruritus, 1; and signs of skin atrophy, 3.
The following local adverse reactions have been reported infrequently when other topical dermatologic corticosteroids have been used as recommended. These reactions are listed in an approximate decreasing order of occurrence: burning, itching, irritation, dryness, folliculitis, hypertrichosis, acneiform eruptions, hypopigmentation, perioral dermatitis, allergic contact dermatitis, maceration of the skin, secondary infection, skin atrophy, striae, miliaria.

OVERDOSAGE

Topically applied corticosteroids can be absorbed in sufficient amounts to produce systemic effects. (See **PRECAUTIONS.**)

DOSAGE AND ADMINISTRATION

Apply a thin film of ELOCON Cream to the affected skin areas once daily. Do not use occlusive dressings.

HOW SUPPLIED

ELOCON Cream 0.1% is supplied in 15 g (NDC 0085-0567-01) and 45 g (NDC 0085-0567-02) tubes; boxes of one.
Store ELOCON Cream between 2° and 30°C (36° and 86°F).
Copyright © 1987, Schering Corporation. All rights reserved.

ELOCON®   ℞

[el 'ŏ-con]
brand of mometasone furoate
Lotion 0.1%
For Dermatologic Use Only
Not for Ophthalmic Use

DESCRIPTION

ELOCON Lotion 0.1% contains mometasone furoate for dermatologic use. Mometasone furoate is a synthetic corticosteroid with anti-inflammatory activity.
Chemically, mometasone furoate is 9α, 21-Dichloro-11β, 17-dihydroxy-16α-methylpregna-1, 4-diene-3, 20 dione 17-(2-furoate), with the empirical formula $C_{27}H_{30}Cl_2O_6$, and a molecular weight of 521.4.
Mometasone furoate is a white to off-white powder practically insoluble in water, slightly soluble in octanol, and moderately soluble in ethyl alcohol.
Each gram of ELOCON Lotion 0.1% contains: 1 mg of mometasone furoate in a lotion base of isopropyl alcohol (40%), propylene glycol, hydroxypropylcellulose, sodium phosphate and water. May also contain phosphoric acid and sodium hydroxide used to adjust the pH to approximately 4.5.

CLINICAL PHARMACOLOGY

The corticosteroids are a class of compounds comprising steroid hormones secreted by the adrenal cortex and their synthetic analogs. In pharmacologic doses corticosteroids are used primarily for their anti-inflammatory and/or immunosuppressive effects.

Continued on next page

Information on Schering products appearing on these pages is effective as of September 30, 1989.

Schering—Cont.

Topical corticosteroids, such as mometasone furoate, are effective in the treatment of corticosteroid-responsive dermatoses primarily because of their anti-inflammatory, antipruritic, and vasoconstrictive actions. However, while the physiologic, pharmacologic, and clinical effects of the corticosteroids are well known, the exact mechanisms of their actions in each disease are uncertain. Mometasone furoate has been shown to have topical (dermatologic) and systemic pharmacologic and metabolic effects characteristic of this class of drugs.

Pharmacokinetics: The extent of percutaneous absorption of topical corticosteroids is determined by many factors including the vehicle, the integrity of the epidermal barrier, and the use of occlusive dressings. (See **DOSAGE AND ADMINISTRATION.**) Topical corticosteroids can be absorbed from normal intact skin.

A study using a radio-labelled ^{3}H mometasone furoate ointment (0.1%) formulation was performed in man to measure systemic absorption and excretion. Results showed that approximately 0.7% of the steroid was absorbed during 8 hours of contact, without occlusion, with intact skin of normal volunteers. A similar minimal degree of absorption of the corticosteroid from the lotion formulation would be anticipated. Inflammation and/or disease processes in the skin increase percutaneous absorption. Occlusive dressings substantially increase the percutaneous absorption of topical corticosteroids. (See **DOSAGE AND ADMINSTRATION.**)

Mometasone furoate lotion was applied at 15 mL twice daily (30 mL per day) to diseased skin (patients with scalp and body psoriasis) of four patients for seven days, to study its effects on the hypothalamic-pituitary-adrenal (HPA) axis. Plasma cortisol levels for each of the four patients remained well within the normal range and changed little from baseline.

Once absorbed through the skin, topical corticosteroids are handled through pharmacokinetic pathways similar to systemically administered corticosteroids. Corticosteroids are bound to plasma proteins in varying degrees. Corticosteroids are metabolized primarily in the liver and are then excreted by the kidneys. Some of the topical corticosteroids and their metabolites are also excreted into the bile.

INDICATIONS AND USAGE

ELOCON Lotion is indicated for the relief of the inflammatory and pruritic manifestations of corticosteroid-responsive dermatoses.

CONTRAINDICATIONS

ELOCON Lotion is contraindicated in patients who are hypersensitive to mometasone furoate, to other corticosteroids, or to any ingredient in this preparation.

PRECAUTIONS

General: Systemic absorption of potent topical corticosteroids has produced reversible hypothalamic-pituitary-adrenal (HPA) axis suppression, manifestations of Cushing's syndrome, hyperglycemia, and glucosuria in some patients. Conditions which augment systemic absorption include application of more potent steroids, use over large surface areas, prolonged use, use in areas where the epidermal barrier is disrupted, and the use of occlusive dressings. (See **DOSAGE AND ADMINISTRATION.**)

Patients receiving a large dose of a potent topical steroid applied to a large surface area or under an occlusive dressing should be evaluated periodically for evidence of HPA axis suppression by using the urinary free cortisol and ACTH stimulation tests. If HPA axis suppression is noted, an attempt should be made to withdraw the drug, to reduce the frequency of application, or to substitute a less potent steroid.

Recovery of HPA axis function is generally prompt and complete upon discontinuation of the drug. Infrequently, signs and symptoms of steroid withdrawal may occur, requiring supplemental systemic corticosteroids.

Children may absorb proportionally larger amounts of topical corticosteroids and thus be more susceptible to systemic toxicity. (See **PRECAUTIONS—Pediatric Use.**)

If irritation develops, topical corticosteroids should be discontinued and appropriate therapy instituted.

In the presence of dermatological infections, use of an appropriate antifungal or antibacterial agent should be instituted. If a favorable response does not occur promptly, the corticosteroid should be discontinued until the infection has been adequately controlled.

Information for Patients: Patients using topical corticosteroids should receive the following information and instructions. This information is intended to aid in the safe and effective use of this medication. It is not a disclosure of all possible adverse or intended effects.

1. This medication is to be used by the physician. It is for external use only. Avoid contact with the eyes.
2. Patients should be advised not to use this medication for any disorder other than that for which it was prescribed.

3. The treated skin area should not be bandaged or otherwise covered or wrapped as to be occlusive unless directed by the physician. (See **DOSAGE AND ADMINISTRATION**).
4. Patients should report any signs of local adverse reactions.
5. Parents of pediatric patients should be advised not to use tight-fitting diapers or plastic pants on a child being treated in the diaper area, as these garments may constitute occlusive dressing. (See **DOSAGE AND ADMINISTRATION.**)

Laboratory Tests: The following tests may be helpful in evaluating HPA axis suppression:

Urinary free cortisol test

ACTH stimulation test

Carcinogenesis, Mutagenesis, and Impairment of Fertility: Long-term animal studies have not been performed to evaluate the carcinogenic potential or the effect on fertility of topical corticosteroids.

Genetic toxicity studies with mometasone furoate, which included the Ames test, mouse lymphoma assay, and a micronucleus test, did not reveal any mutagenic potential.

Pregnancy Category C: Corticosteroids are generally teratogenic in laboratory animals when administered systemically at relatively low dosage levels. Corticosteroids have been shown to be teratogenic after dermal application in laboratory animals. There are no adequate and well-controlled studies of teratogenic effects from topically applied corticosteroids in pregnant women. Therefore, topical corticosteroids should be used during pregnancy only if the potential benefit justifies the potential risk to the fetus. Drugs of this class should not be used extensively on pregnant patients, in large amounts, or for prolonged periods.

Nursing Mothers: It is not known whether topical administration of corticosteroids could result in sufficient systemic absorption to produce detectable quantities in breast milk. Systemically administered corticosteroids are secreted into breast milk in quantities not likely to have a deleterious effect on the infant. Nevertheless, a decision should be made whether to discontinue nursing or to discontinue the drug, taking into account the importance of the drug to the mother.

Pediatric Use: Pediatric patients may demonstrate greater susceptibility to topical corticosteroid-induced HPA axis suppression and Cushing's Syndrome than mature patients because of a larger skin surface area to body weight ratio. Hypothalamic-pituitary-adrenal (HPA) axis suppression, Cushing's syndrome, and intracranial hypertension have been reported in children receiving topical corticosteroids. Manifestations of adrenal suppression in children include linear growth retardation, delayed weight gain, low plasma cortisol levels, and absence of response to ACTH stimulation. Manifestations of intracranial hypertension include bulging fontanelles, headaches, and bilateral papilledema. Administration of topical corticosteroids to children should be limited to the least amount compatible with an effective therapeutic regimen. Chronic corticosteroid therapy may interfere with the growth and development of children.

ADVERSE REACTIONS

The following local adverse reactions were reported with ELOCON Lotion during clinical studies with 209 patients; acneiform reaction, 2; burning, 4; and itching, 1. In an irritation/sensitization study with 156 normal subjects, folliculitis was reported in 4.

The following local adverse reactions have been reported infrequently when other topical dermatologic corticosteroids have been used as recommended. These reactions are listed in an approximate decreasing order of occurrence; burning, itching, irritation, dryness, folliculitis, hypertrichosis, acneiform eruptions, hypopigmentation, perioral dermatitis, allergic contact dermatitis, maceration of the skin, secondary infection, skin atrophy, striae, miliaria.

OVERDOSAGE

Topically applied corticosteroids can be absorbed in sufficient amounts to produce systemic effects. (See **PRECAUTIONS.**)

DOSAGE AND ADMINISTRATION

Apply a few drops of ELOCON Lotion to the affected areas once daily and massage lightly until it disappears. For the most effective and economical use, hold the nozzle of the bottle very close to the affected areas and gently squeeze.

HOW SUPPLIED

ELOCON Lotion 0.1% is supplied in 30 mL (27.5 g) (NDC-0085-0854-01) and 60 mL (55 g) (NDC-0085-0854-02) bottles; boxes of one.

Store ELOCON Lotion between 2° and 30°C (36° and 86°F).
Revised 3/89

ELOCON®   R

[el 'ō-con]
brand of mometasone furoate
Ointment 0.1%
For Dermatologic Use Only
Not for Ophthalmic Use

DESCRIPTION

ELOCON® Ointment contains mometasone furoate for dermatologic use. Mometasone furoate is a synthetic corticosteroid with anti-inflammatory activity.

Chemically, mometasone furoate is $9\alpha,21$-Dichloro-$11\beta,17$-dihydroxy-16α-methylpregna-1,4-diene-3,20 dione 17-(2-furoate), with the empirical formula $C_{27}H_{30}Cl_2O_6$, and a molecular weight of 521.4.

Mometasone furoate is a white to off-white powder practically insoluble in water, slightly soluble in octanol, and moderately soluble in ethyl alcohol.

Each gram of ELOCON Ointment 0.1% contains: 1 mg mometasone furoate in an ointment base of hexylene glycol, propylene glycol stearate, white wax, white petrolatum and purified water. May also contain phosphoric acid.

CLINICAL PHARMACOLOGY

The corticosteroids are a class of compounds comprising steroid hormones secreted by the adrenal cortex and their synthetic analogs. In pharmacologic doses corticosteroids are used primarily for their anti-inflammatory and/or immunosuppressive effects.

Topical corticosteroids, such as mometasone furoate, are effective in the treatment of corticosteroid-responsive dermatoses primarily because of their anti-inflammatory, antipruritic, and vasoconstrictive actions. However, while the physiologic, pharmacologic, and clinical effects of the corticosteroids are well known, the exact mechanisms of their actions in each disease are uncertain. Mometasone furoate has been shown to have topical (dermatologic) and systemic pharmacologic and metabolic effects characteristic of this class of drugs.

Pharmacokinetics: The extent of percutaneous absorption of topical corticosteroids is determined by many factors including the vehicle, the integrity of the epidermal barrier, and the use of occlusive dressings. (See **DOSAGE AND ADMINISTRATION.**) Topical corticosteroids can be absorbed from normal intact skin.

A study utilizing a radio-labelled ^{3}H mometasone furoate ointment formulation was performed to measure systemic absorption and excretion. Results showed that approximately 0.7% of the steroid was absorbed during 8 hours of contact, without occlusion, with intact skin of normal volunteers.

Inflammation and/or other disease processes in the skin increase percutaneous absorption. Occlusive dressings substantially increase the percutaneous absorption of topical corticosteroids. (See **DOSAGE AND ADMINISTRATION.**)

In a study of the effects of mometasone furoate ointment on the hypothalamic-pituitary-adrenal axis, 15 grams were applied twice daily for seven days to six patients with psoriasis or atopic dermatitis. The ointment was applied without occlusion to at least 30% of the body surface. The results suggest that the drug caused a slight lowering of adrenal corticosteroid secretion, although in no case did plasma cortisol levels go below the lower limit of the normal range.

Once absorbed through the skin, topical corticosteroids are handled through pharmacokinetic pathways similar to systemically administered corticosteroids. Corticosteroids are bound to plasma proteins in varying degrees. Corticosteroids are metabolized primarily in the liver and are then excreted by the kidneys. Some of the topical corticosteroids and their metabolites are also excreted into the bile.

INDICATIONS AND USAGE

ELOCON Ointment is indicated for the relief of the inflammatory and pruritic manifestations of corticosteroid-responsive dermatoses.

CONTRAINDICATIONS

ELOCON Ointment is contraindicated in patients who are hypersensitive to mometasone furoate, to other corticosteroids, or to any ingredient in this preparation.

PRECAUTIONS

General: Systemic absorption of potent topical corticosteroids has produced reversible hypothalamic-pituitary-adrenal (HPA) axis suppression, manifestations of Cushing's syndrome, hyperglycemia, and glucosuria in some patients. Conditions which augment systemic absorption include application of more potent steroids, use over large surface areas, prolonged use, use in areas where the epidermal barrier is disrupted, and the use of occlusive dressings. (See **DOSAGE AND ADMINISTRATION.**)

Patients receiving a large dose of a potent topical steroid applied to a large surface area or under an occlusive dressing should be evaluated periodically for evidence of HPA axis suppression by using the urinary free cortisol and ACTH stimulation tests. If HPA axis suppression is noted, an attempt should be made to withdraw the drug, to reduce the frequency of application, or to substitute a less potent steroid.

Recovery of HPA axis function is generally prompt and complete upon discontinuation of the drug. Infrequently, signs and symptoms of steroid withdrawal may occur, requiring supplemental systemic corticosteroids.

Children may absorb proportionally larger amounts of topical corticosteroids and thus be more susceptible to systemic toxicity. (See PRECAUTIONS—Pediatric Use.)

If irritation develops, topical corticosteroids should be discontinued and appropriate therapy instituted.

In the presence of dermatological infections, use of an appropriate antifungal or antibacterial agent should be instituted. If a favorable response does not occur promptly, the corticosteroid should be discontinued until the infection has been adequately controlled.

Information for Patients: Patients using topical corticosteroids should receive the following information and instructions. This information is intended to aid in the safe and effective use of this medication. It is not a disclosure of all possible adverse or intended effects.

1. This medication is to be used as directed by the physician. It is for external use only. Avoid contact with the eyes.
2. Patients should be advised not to use this medication for any disorder other than that for which it was prescribed.
3. The treated skin area should not be bandaged or otherwise covered or wrapped so as to be occlusive unless directed by the physician. (See DOSAGE AND ADMINISTRATION.)
4. Patients should report any signs of local adverse reactions.
5. Parents of pediatric patients should be advised not to use tight-fitting diapers or plastic pants on a child being treated in the diaper area, as these garments may constitute occlusive dressing. (See DOSAGE AND ADMINISTRATION.)

Laboratory Tests: The following tests may be helpful in evaluating HPA axis suppression:

Urinary free cortisol test
ACTH stimulation test

Carcinogenesis, Mutagenesis, and Impairment of Fertility: Long-term animal studies have not been performed to evaluate the carcinogenic potential or the effect on fertility of topical corticosteroids.

Genetic toxicity studies with mometasone furoate, which included the Ames test, mouse lymphoma assay, and a micronucleus test, did not reveal any mutagenic potential.

Pregnancy Category C: Corticosteroids are generally teratogenic in laboratory animals when administered systemically at relatively low dosage levels. Corticosteroids have been shown to be teratogenic after dermal application in laboratory animals. There are no adequate and well-controlled studies of teratogenic effects from topically applied corticosteroids in pregnant women. Therefore, topical corticosteroids should be used during pregnancy only if the potential benefit justifies the potential risk to the fetus. Drugs of this class should not be used extensively on pregnant patients, in large amounts, or for prolonged periods.

Nursing Mothers: It is not known whether topical administration of corticosteroids could result in sufficient systemic absorption to produce detectable quantities in breast milk. Systemically administered corticosteroids are secreted into breast milk in quantities not likely to have a deleterious effect on the infant. Nevertheless, a decision should be made whether to discontinue nursing or to discontinue the drug, taking into account the importance of the drug to the mother.

Pediatric Use: *Pediatric patients may demonstrate greater susceptibility to topical corticosteroid-induced HPA axis suppression and Cushing's syndrome than mature patients because of a larger skin surface area to body weight ratio.*

Hypothalamic-pituitary-adrenal (HPA) axis suppression, Cushing's syndrome, and intracranial hypertension have been reported in children receiving topical corticosteroids. Manifestations of adrenal suppression in children include linear growth retardation, delayed weight gain, low plasma cortisol levels, and absence of response to ACTH stimulation. Manifestations of intracranial hypertension include bulging fontanelles, headaches, and bilateral papilledema.

Administration of topical corticosteroids to children should be limited to the least amount compatible with an effective therapeutic regimen. Chronic corticosteroid therapy may interfere with the growth and development of children.

ADVERSE REACTIONS

The following local adverse reactions were reported with ELOCON Ointment during clinical studies with 812 patients: burning, 13; pruritus, 8; skin atrophy, 8; tingling/stinging, 7; and furunculosis, 3.

The following local adverse reactions have been reported infrequently when other topical dermatologic corticosteroids have been used as recommended. These reactions are listed in an approximate decreasing order of occurrence: burning, itching, irritation, dryness, folliculitis, hypertrichosis, acneiform eruptions, hypopigmentation, perioral dermatitis, al-

lergic contact dermatitis, maceration of the skin, secondary infection, skin atrophy, striae, miliaria.

OVERDOSAGE

Topically applied corticosteroids can be absorbed in sufficient amounts to produce systemic effects. (See PRECAUTIONS.)

DOSAGE AND ADMINISTRATION

Apply a thin film of ELOCON Ointment to the affected skin areas once daily. Do not use occlusive dressings.

HOW SUPPLIED

ELOCON Ointment 0.1% is supplied in 15 g (NDC 0085-0370-01) and 45 g (NDC 0085-0370-02) tubes; boxes of one.

Store ELOCON Ointment between 2° and 30°C (36° and 86°F).

Copyright © 1987, Schering Corporation. All rights reserved.

ESTINYL® ℞

[es'ti-nil]
**brand of ethinyl estradiol,
Tablets, USP**

WARNINGS

1. ESTROGENS HAVE BEEN REPORTED TO INCREASE THE RISK RATIO OF ENDOMETRIAL CARCINOMA.

Three independent case control studies have reported an increased risk ratio of endometrial cancer in postmenopausal women exposed to exogenous estrogens for prolonged periods.[1-3] This risk ratio was independent of the other risk factors for endometrial cancer. These studies are further supported by the report that incidence rates of endometrial cancer have increased sharply since 1969 in eight different areas of the United States with population-based cancer reporting systems, an increase which may be related to the rapidly expanding use of estrogens during the last decade.[4]

The three case control studies reported that the risk ratio of endometrial cancer in estrogen users was about 4.5 to 13.9 times greater than in nonusers. The risk ratio appears to depend on both duration of treatment[1] and on estrogen dose.[3] In view of these reports, when estrogens are used for the treatment of menopausal symptoms, the lowest dose that will control symptoms should be utilized and medication should be discontinued as soon as possible. When prolonged treatment is medically indicated, the patient should be reassessed on at least a semiannual basis to determine the need for continued therapy. Although the evidence must be considered preliminary, one study suggests that cyclic administration of low doses of estrogen may carry less risk than continuous administration[3]; it therefore appears prudent to utilize such a regimen.

Close clinical surveillance of all women taking estrogens is important. In all cases of undiagnosed persistent or recurring abnormal vaginal bleeding, adequate diagnostic measures should be undertaken to rule out malignancy.

There is no evidence at present that "natural" estrogens are more or less hazardous than "synthetic" estrogens at equiestrogenic doses.

2. ESTROGENS SHOULD NOT BE USED DURING PREGNANCY.

The use of estrogens during early pregnancy may seriously damage the offspring. It has been reported that females exposed in utero to diethylstilbestrol, a nonsteroidal estrogen, may have an increased risk of developing in later life a form of vaginal or cervical cancer that is ordinarily extremely rare.[5,6] This risk has been estimated statistically as not greater than 4 per 1000 exposures.[7] In certain studies, a high percentage of such exposed women (from 30 to 90 percent) have been found to have vaginal adenosis,[8-11] epithelial changes of the vagina and cervix. Although these changes are histologically benign, it is not known whether they are precursors of malignancy. Although similar data are not available with the use of other estrogens, it cannot be presumed they would not induce similar changes. Exposure to diethylstilbestrol has also been associated with adverse effects on reproductive performance, including increased rates of spontaneous abortion, ectopic pregnancy, premature deliveries, and perinatal deaths. Several reports suggest an association between intrauterine fetal exposure to female sex hormones and congenital anomalies, including congenital heart defects and limb reduction defects.[12-15] One case control study[15] estimated a 4.7 fold increased risk of limb reduction defects in infants exposed in utero to sex hormones (oral contraceptives, hormone withdrawal tests for pregnancy, or attempted treatment for threatened abortion). Some of these exposures were very short and involved only a few days of treatment. The data suggest

that the risk of limb reduction defects in exposed fetuses is somewhat less than 1 per 1000.

In the past, estrogens have been used during pregnancy in an attempt to treat threatened or habitual abortion. There is considerable evidence that estrogens are ineffective for these indications.

If ESTINYL Tablets are used during pregnancy, or if the patient becomes pregnant while taking this drug, she should be apprised of the potential risks to the fetus, and the advisability of pregnancy continuation.

DESCRIPTION

ESTINYL Tablets contain ethinyl estradiol, USP, a potent synthetic estrogen having the chemical name, 19-Nor-17α-pregna-1,3,5(10)-trien-20-yne-3,17-diol; the chemical formula $C_{20}H_{24}O_2$; and a molecular weight of 296.41.

Ethinyl estradiol is a white to creamy white, odorless, crystalline powder. It is insoluble in water, soluble in alcohol, chloroform, ether and vegetable oils.

Biologically, estrogens may be defined as compounds capable of stimulating female secondary sex characteristics. Chemically, there are different groups of estrogens, depending on whether they are natural or synthetic, steroidal or nonsteroidal. Natural human estrogens are ultimately formed from either androstenedione or testosterone as immediate precursors. Ethinyl estradiol is a synthetic, steroidal estrogen.

ESTINYL, for oral administration, is available in tablets containing 0.02, 0.05, or 0.5 mg ethinyl estradiol, USP.

The inactive ingredients for ESTINYL Tablets 0.02 mg include: acacia, butylparaben, calcium phosphate, calcium sulfate, carnauba wax, corn starch, gelatin, FD&C Blue No. 2 Al Lake, FD&C Yellow No. 5, FD&C Yellow No. 5 Al Lake, FD&C Yellow No. 6 Al Lake, lactose, magnesium stearate, potato starch, sodium phosphate, sugar, and white wax. May also contain talc.

The inactive ingredients for ESTINYL Tablets 0.05 mg include: acacia, butylparaben, calcium phosphate, calcium sulfate, carnauba wax, corn starch, FD&C Blue No. 1, FD&C Red No. 3, gelatin, lactose, magnesium stearate, potato starch, sodium phosphate, and white wax. May also contain talc.

The inactive ingredients for ESTINYL Tablets 0.5 mg include: corn starch, FD&C Yellow No. 6, lactose, magnesium stearate, and sodium phosphate.

CLINICAL PHARMACOLOGY

Ethinyl estradiol is a synthetic derivative of the natural estrogen, estradiol.

Ethinyl estradiol, like estradiol, promotes growth of the endometrium and thickening, stratification and cornification of the vagina. It causes growth of the ducts of the mammary glands, but inhibits lactation. It also inhibits the anterior pituitary and causes capillary dilatation, fluid retention and protein anabolism.

Estradiol is the major estrogen in premenopausal women, with up to 100 to 600 mcg being secreted daily by the ovary. Natural estrogens are poorly effective when given by mouth. Apparently this is due to rapid clearance of the endogenous hormone from blood, along with a "first-pass-effect" after oral administration. The addition of a 17-alpha-ethinyl group to estradiol increases potency and enhances oral activity by impeding hepatic degradation. The oral efficacy of ethinyl estradiol is related to slower elimination than estradiol from the circulation. A part of ingested ethinyl estradiol is excreted in glucuronide form via urine in animals and in man, but also extensive metabolism of the steroid nucleus occurs. The major metabolism takes place mainly in the liver. Large amounts of ethinyl estradiol metabolites are excreted via human bile, much similar to what has been reported for estradiol. However, unlike estradiol, ethinyl estradiol metabolites do not exclusively leave via urine. Urinary recovery is much less than that of estradiol and substantial amounts of ethinyl estradiol metabolites appear in human feces. Quantitatively, the major metabolic pathway for ethinyl estradiol, both in rats and in humans, is aromatic hydroxylation, as it is for the natural estrogens.

Rapid and complete absorption follows oral intake of ethinyl estradiol. Elimination of ethinyl estradiol from plasma proceeds slower than that of estradiol. After oral administration, an initial peak occurs in plasma at 2 to 3 hours, with a secondary peak at about 12 hours after dosing; the second peak is interpreted as evidence for extensive enterohepatic circulation of ethinyl estradiol.

INDICATIONS AND USAGE

ESTINYL Tablets are indicated in the treatment of: 1) Moderate to severe *vasomotor* symptoms associated with the menopause. (There is no evidence that estrogens are effective for nervous symptoms or depression which might occur

Continued on next page

Schering—Cont.

during menopause, and they should not be used to treat these conditions.) 2) Female hypogonadism. 3) Prostatic carcinoma—palliative therapy of advanced disease. 4) Breast cancer (for palliation only) in appropriately selected women, such as those who are more than 5 years postmenopausal with progressing inoperable or radiation-resistant disease. ETHINYL ESTRADIOL HAS NOT BEEN SHOWN TO BE EFFECTIVE FOR ANY PURPOSE DURING PREGNANCY AND ITS USE MAY CAUSE SEVERE HARM TO THE FETUS (SEE BOXED **WARNINGS**).

The lowest effective dose appropriate for the specific indication should be utilized. Studies of the addition of a progestin for seven or more days of a cycle of estrogen administration have reported a lowered incidence of endometrial hyperplasia. Morphological and biochemical studies of endometrium suggest that 10 to 13 days of progestin are needed to provide maximal maturation of the endometrium and to eliminate any hyperplastic changes. Whether this will provide protection from endometrial carcinoma has not been clearly established. There are possible additional risks which may be associated with the inclusion of progestin in estrogen replacement regimens. The potential risks include adverse effects on carbohydrate and lipid metabolism. The choice of progestin and dosage may be important to minimizing these adverse effects.

CONTRAINDICATIONS

Estrogens should not be used in women (or men) with any of the following conditions:
1. Known or suspected cancer of the breast except in appropriately selected patients being treated for metastatic disease.
2. Known or suspected estrogen-dependent neoplasia.
3. Known or suspected pregnancy (see boxed **WARNINGS**).
4. Undiagnosed abnormal genital bleeding.
5. Active thrombophlebitis or thromboembolic disorders.
6. A past history of thrombophlebitis, thrombosis or thromboembolic disorders associated with previous estrogen use (except when used in treatment of breast or prostatic malignancy).

WARNINGS

1. *Induction of malignant neoplasms.* Long-term continuous administration of natural and synthetic estrogens in certain animal species increases the frequency of carcinomas of the breast, cervix, vagina, and liver. There is now evidence that estrogens increase the risk of carcinoma of the endometrium in humans. (See boxed **WARNINGS**.)

At the present time there is no satisfactory evidence that estrogens given to postmenopausal women increase the risk of cancer of the breast,[16] although a recent long-term follow-up of a single physician's practice has raised this possibility.[17] Because of the animal data, there is a need for caution in prescribing estrogens for women with a strong family history of breast cancer or who have breast nodules, fibrocystic disease, or abnormal mammograms.

Estrogens have been reported to be associated with carcinoma of the male breast and suspicious lesions in males receiving estrogen therapy should be investigated accordingly.

2. *Gallbladder disease.* A recent study has reported a 2- to 3-fold increase in the risk of surgically confirmed gallbladder disease in women receiving postmenopausal estrogens,[16] similar to the 2-fold increase previously noted in users of oral contraceptives.[18,22] In the case of oral contraceptives, the increased risk appeared after two years of use.[22]

3. *Effects similar to those caused by estrogen-progestagen oral contraceptives.* There are several serious adverse effects of oral contraceptives, most of which have not, up to now, been documented as consequences of postmenopausal estrogen therapy. This may reflect the comparatively low doses of estrogen used in postmenopausal women. It would be expected that the larger doses of estrogen used to treat prostatic or breast cancer are more likely to result in these adverse effects, and, in fact, it has been shown that there is an increased risk of thrombosis in men receiving estrogens for prostatic cancer.[19-22]

a. *Thromboembolic disease* It is now well established that users of oral contraceptives have an increased risk of various thromboembolic and thrombotic vascular diseases, such as thrombophlebitis, pulmonary embolism, stroke and myocardial infarction.[22-29] Cases of retinal thrombosis, mesenteric thrombosis, and optic neuritis have been reported in oral contraceptive users. There is evidence that the risk of several of these adverse reactions is related to the dose of the drug.[30,31] An increased risk of postsurgery thromboembolic complications has also been reported in users of oral contraceptives.[32,33] If feasible, estrogen should be discontinued at least 4 weeks before surgery of the type associated with an increased risk of thromboembolism, or during periods of immobilization.

While an increased rate of thromboembolic and thrombotic disease in postmenopausal users of estrogen has not been found,[16,34] this does not rule out the possibility that such an increase may be present or that subgroups of women who have underlying risk factors or who are receiving relatively large doses of estrogens may have increased risk. Therefore, estrogens should not be used in persons with active thrombophlebitis or thromboembolic disorders, and they should not be used (except in treatment of malignancy) in persons with a history of such disorders in association with estrogen use. They should be used with caution in patients with cerebral vascular or coronary artery disease and only for those in whom estrogens are clearly needed.

Large doses of estrogen (5 mg conjugated estrogens per day), comparable to those used to treat cancer of the prostate and breast, have been shown in a large prospective clinical trial in men[35] to increase the risk of nonfatal myocardial infarction, pulmonary embolism and thrombophlebitis. When estrogen doses of this size are used, any of the thromboembolic and thrombotic adverse effects associated with oral contraceptive use should be considered a clear risk.

b. *Hepatic adenoma* Benign hepatic adenomas appear to be associated with the use of oral contraceptives.[36-38] Although benign, and rare, these may rupture and may cause death through intra-abdominal hemorrhage. Such lesions have not yet been reported in association with other estrogen or progestagen preparations but should be considered in estrogen users having abdominal pain and tenderness, abdominal mass, or hypovolemic shock. Hepatocellular carcinoma has also been reported in women taking estrogen-containing oral contraceptives.[37] The relationship of this malignancy to these drugs is not known at this time.

c. *Elevated blood pressure* Increased blood pressure is not uncommon in women using oral contraceptives. There is now a report that this may occur with use of estrogens in the menopause[39] and blood pressure should be monitored with estrogen use, especially if high doses are used.

d. *Glucose tolerance* A worsening of glucose tolerance has been observed in a significant percentage of patients on estrogen-containing oral contraceptives. For this reason, diabetic patients should be carefully observed while receiving estrogen.

4. *Hypercalcemia.* Administration of estrogens may lead to severe hypercalcemia in patients with breast cancer and bone metastases. If this occurs, the drug should be stopped and appropriate measures taken to reduce the serum calcium level.

PRECAUTIONS

General Precautions:

1. A complete medical and family history should be taken prior to the initiation of any estrogen therapy. The pretreatment and periodic physical examinations should include special reference to blood pressure, breasts, abdomen, and pelvic organs, and should include a Papanicolaou smear. As a general rule, estrogen should not be prescribed for longer than one year without another physical examination being performed.

2. Fluid retention—Because estrogens may cause some degree of fluid retention, conditions which might be influenced by this factor, such as epilepsy, migraine, and cardiac or renal dysfunction, require careful observation.

3. Certain patients may develop undesirable manifestations of excessive estrogenic stimulation, such as abnormal or excessive uterine bleeding, mastodynia, etc.

4. Oral contraceptives appear to be associated with an increased incidence of mental depression.[22] Although it is not clear whether this is due to the estrogenic or progestagenic component of the contraceptive, patients with a history of depression should be carefully observed.

5. Preexisting uterine leiomyomata may increase in size during estrogen use.

6. The pathologist should be advised of estrogen therapy when relevant specimens are submitted.

7. Patients with a past history of jaundice during pregnancy have an increased risk of recurrence of jaundice while receiving estrogen-containing oral contraceptive therapy. If jaundice develops in any patient receiving estrogen, the medication should be discontinued while the cause is investigated.

8. Estrogens may be poorly metabolized in patients with impaired liver function and they should be administered with caution in such patients.

9. Because estrogens influence the metabolism of calcium and phosphorus, they should be used with caution in patients with metabolic bone diseases that are associated with hypercalcemia or in patients with renal insufficiency.

10. Because of the effects of estrogens on epiphyseal closure, they should be used judiciously in young patients in whom bone growth is not complete.

11. ESTINYL Tablets, .02 mg contain FD&C Yellow No. 5 (tartrazine) which may cause allergic-type reactions (including bronchial asthma) in certain susceptible individuals. Although the overall incidence of FD&C Yellow No. 5 (tartrazine) sensitivity in the general population is low, it is frequently seen in patients who also have aspirin hypersensitivity.

Information for the Patient: See text of Patient Package Insert.

Drug/Laboratory Test Interactions: Certain endocrine and liver function tests may be affected by estrogen-containing oral contraceptives. The following similar changes may be expected with larger doses of estrogen:

Increased sulfobromophthalein retention; increased prothrombin and factors VII, VIII, IX, and X; decreased antithrombin 3; increased norepinephrine-induced platelet aggregation; increased thyroid binding globulin (TBG) leading to increased circulating total thyroid hormone, as measured by PBI, T4 by column, or T4 by radioimmunoassay. Free T3 resin uptake is decreased, reflecting the elevated TBG; free T4 concentration is unaltered; impaired glucose tolerance; decreased pregnanediol excretion; reduced response to metyrapone test; reduced serum folate concentration; increased serum triglyceride and phospholipid concentration.

Carcinogenesis, Mutagenesis, Impairment of Fertility: See boxed **WARNINGS**.

Pregnancy Category X. See **CONTRAINDICATIONS** and boxed **WARNINGS**.

Nursing Mothers: Because of the potential for tumorigenicity shown for ethinyl estradiol in animal and human studies, a decision should be made whether to discontinue nursing or to discontinue the drug, taking into account the importance of the drug to the mother.

Pediatric Use: Safety and effectiveness in children have not been established.

ADVERSE REACTIONS

(See **WARNINGS** regarding induction of neoplasia, adverse effects on the fetus, increased incidence of gallbladder disease, and adverse effects similar to those of oral contraceptives, including thromboembolism.) The following additional adverse reactions have been reported with estrogenic therapy, including oral contraceptives:

Genitourinary system: Breakthrough bleeding, spotting, change in menstrual flow; dysmenorrhea; premenstrual-like syndrome; amenorrhea during and after treatment; increase in size of uterine fibromyomata; vaginal candidiasis; change in cervical eversion and in degree of cervical secretion; cystitis-like syndrome.

Breasts: Tenderness, enlargement, secretion.

Gastrointestinal: Nausea, vomiting; abdominal cramps, bloating; cholestatic jaundice.

Skin: Chloasma or melasma which may persist when drug is discontinued; erythema multiforme; erythema nodosum; hemorrhagic eruption; loss of scalp hair; hirsutism.

Eyes: Steepening of corneal curvature; intolerance to contact lenses.

CNS: Headache, migraine, dizziness; mental depression; chorea.

Miscellaneous: Increase or decrease in weight; reduced carbohydrate tolerance; aggravation of porphyria; edema; changes in libido.

ACUTE OVERDOSAGE

Numerous reports of ingestion of large doses of estrogen-containing oral contraceptives by young children indicate that serious ill effects do not occur. Overdosage of estrogen may cause nausea, and withdrawal bleeding may occur in females.

DOSAGE AND ADMINISTRATION

1. *Given cyclically for short-term use only.*

For treatment of moderate to severe *vasomotor* symptoms associated with the menopause: The lowest dose that will control symptoms should be chosen and medication should be discontinued as promptly as possible. Administration should be cyclic (e.g., 3 weeks on and 1 week off). Attempts to discontinue or taper medication should be made at 3- to 6-month intervals. The usual dosage range is one 0.02 mg or 0.05 mg tablet daily. In some instances, the effective dose may be as low as one 0.02 mg tablet every other day. A useful dosage schedule for early menopause, while spontaneous menstruation continues, is 0.05 mg once a day for twenty-one days and then a rest period for seven days. For the initial treatment of the late menopause, the same regimen is indicated with the 0.02 mg ESTINYL Tablet for the first few cycles, after which the 0.05 mg dosage may be substituted. In more severe cases, such as those due to surgical and roentgenologic castration, one 0.05 mg tablet may be administered three times daily at the start of treatment. With adequate clinical improvement, usually obtainable in a few weeks, the dosage may be reduced to one 0.05 mg tablet daily and the patient continued thereafter on a maintenance dosage as in the average case.

2. *Given cyclically.*

Female hypogonadism: One 0.05 mg tablet is given one to three times daily during the first two weeks of a theoretical menstrual cycle. This is followed by progesterone during the last half of the arbitrary cycle. This regimen is continued for three to six months. The patient is then allowed to go untreated for two months to determine whether or not she can maintain the cycle without hormonal therapy. If not, additional courses of therapy may be prescribed.

3. *Given chronically.*

Inoperable progressing prostatic cancer: From three 0.05 mg to four 0.5 mg tablets may be administered daily for palliation.

Inoperable progressing breast cancer in appropriately selected postmenopausal women (See **INDICATIONS AND USAGE**): Two 0.5 mg tablets three times daily for palliation. Treated patients with an intact uterus should be monitored closely for signs of endometrial cancer and appropriate diagnostic measures should be taken to rule out malignancy in the event of persistent or recurring abnormal vaginal bleeding.

HOW SUPPLIED

ESTINYL Tablets 0.02 mg, beige, sugar-coated tablets branded in black with the Schering trademark and product identification number, 298; bottles of 100 (NDC 0085-0298-03) and 250 (NDC 0085-0298-06).

ESTINYL Tablets 0.05 mg, pink, sugar-coated tablets branded in black with the Schering trademark and product identification number, 070; bottles of 100 (NDC 0085-0070-03) and 250 (NDC 0085-0070-06).

ESTINYL Tablets 0.5 mg, peach-colored, compressed, scored tablets impressed with the Schering trademark and product identification number, 150; bottle of 100 (NDC 0085-0150-03).

Store between 2° and 30° C (36° and 86° F).

Patient package inserts are being dispensed with this product. They are available to physicians upon request. Physician references available on request.

Copyright © 1968, 1983, 1986, Schering Corporation, USA. All rights reserved.

Shown in Product Identification Section, page 428
Rev. 1/86

ETRAFON®   ℞

[ĕ'trah-fon]

brand of perphenazine, USP—amitriptyline hydrochloride, USP

  ETRAFON 2–10 TABLETS (2–10)
  ETRAFON TABLETS (2–25)
  ETRAFON-A TABLETS (4–10)
  ETRAFON-FORTE TABLETS (4–25)

DESCRIPTION

ETRAFON Tablets contain perphenazine, USP and amitriptyline hydrochloride, USP. Perphenazine is a piperazinyl phenothiazine having the chemical formula, $C_{21}H_{26}ClN_3OS$. Amitriptyline hydrochloride is a dibenzocycloheptadiene derivative having the chemical formula, $C_{20}H_{23}N.HCl$.

ETRAFON Tablets are available in multiple strengths to afford dosage flexibility for optimum management. They are available as ETRAFON 2-10 Tablets, 2 mg perphenazine and 10 mg amitriptyline hydrochloride; ETRAFON Tablets, 2 mg perphenazine and 25 mg amitriptyline hydrochloride; ETRAFON-A Tablets, 4 mg perphenazine and 10 mg amitriptyline hydrochloride; and ETRAFON-FORTE Tablets, 4 mg perphenazine and 25 mg amitriptyline hydrochloride.

The inactive ingredients for ETRAFON 2-10 Tablets (2-10) include: acacia, butylparaben, calcium phosphate, calcium sulfate, carnauba wax, corn starch, D&C Yellow No. 10 Al Lake, FD&C Yellow No. 6 Al Lake, gelatin, lactose, magnesium stearate, potato starch, sugar, and white wax. May also contain talc.

The inactive ingredients for ETRAFON Tablets (2-25) include: acacia, butylparaben, calcium phosphate, calcium sulfate, carnauba wax, corn starch, D&C Red No. 30 Al Lake, FD&C Yellow No. 6 Al Lake, gelatin, lactose, magnesium stearate, potato starch, sugar, and white wax. May also contain talc.

The inactive ingredients for ETRAFON-A Tablets (4-10) include: acacia, butylparaben, calcium phosphate, calcium sulfate, carnauba wax, corn starch, FD&C Yellow No. 6, gelatin, lactose, magnesium stearate, potato starch, sugar, and white wax. May also contain talc.

The inactive ingredients for ETRAFON-FORTE Tablets (4-25) include: acacia, butylparaben, calcium phosphate, calcium sulfate, carnauba wax, corn starch, FD&C Red No. 40 Al Lake, FD&C Yellow No. 6 Al Lake, gelatin, lactose, magnesium stearate, potato starch, sugar, and white wax. May also contain talc.

ACTIONS

ETRAFON combines the tranquilizing action of perphenazine with the antidepressant properties of amitriptyline hydrochloride. Perphenazine acts on the central nervous system and has a greater behavioral potency than other phenothiazine derivatives whose side chains do not contain a piperazine moiety. Amitriptyline hydrochloride is a tricyclic antidepressant. It is not a monoamine oxidase inhibitor, but its mechanism of action in man is not known, it does not act primarily by stimulation of the central nervous system.

INDICATIONS

ETRAFON Tablets are indicated for the treatment of patients with moderate to severe anxiety and/or agitation and depressed mood; patients with depression in whom anxiety and/or agitation are moderate or severe; patients with anxiety and depression associated with chronic physical disease; patients in whom depression and anxiety cannot be clearly differentiated.

Schizophrenic patients who have associated symptoms of depression should be considered for therapy with ETRAFON.

CONTRAINDICATIONS

ETRAFON Tablets are contraindicated in comatose or greatly obtunded patients and in patients receiving large doses of central nervous system depressants (barbiturates, alcohol, narcotics, analgesics, or antihistamines); in the presence of existing blood dyscrasias, bone marrow depression, or liver damage; and in patients who have shown hypersensitivity to ETRAFON Tablets, its components, or related compounds.

ETRAFON Tablets are also contraindicated in patients with suspected or established subcortical brain damage, with or without hypothalamic damage, since a hyperthermic reaction with temperatures in excess of 104°F may occur in such patients, sometimes not until 14 to 16 hours after drug administration. Total body ice-packing is recommended for such a reaction; antipyretics may also be useful.

ETRAFON should not be given concomitantly with a monoamine oxidase inhibiting compound. Hyperpyretic crises, severe convulsions and deaths have occurred in patients receiving tricyclic antidepressant and monoamine oxidase inhibiting drugs simultaneously. In patients who have been receiving a monoamine oxidase inhibitor, it is recommended that two weeks or longer elapse before the start of treatment with ETRAFON Tablets to permit recovery from the effects of the MAO inhibitor and to avoid possible potentiation. Treatment with ETRAFON Tablets should be initiated cautiously in such patients, with gradual increase in dosage until a satisfactory response is obtained.

Amitriptyline hydrochloride is not recommended for use during the acute recovery phase following myocardial infarction.

WARNINGS

Tardive dyskinesia, a syndrome consisting of potentially irreversible, involuntary, dyskinetic movements, may develop in patients treated with neuroleptic (antipsychotic) drugs. Although the prevalence of the syndrome appears to be highest among the elderly, especially elderly women, it is impossible to rely upon prevalence estimates to predict, at the inception of neuroleptic treatment, which patients are likely to develop the syndrome. Whether neuroleptic drug products differ in their potential to cause tardive dyskinesia is unknown.

Both the risk of developing the syndrome and the likelihood that it will become irreversible are believed to increase as the duration of treatment and the total cumulative dose of neuroleptic drugs administered to the patient increase. However, the syndrome can develop, although much less commonly, after relatively brief treatment periods at low doses.

There is no known treatment for established cases of tardive dyskinesia, although the syndrome may remit, partially or completely, if neuroleptic treatment is withdrawn. Neuroleptic treatment itself, however, may suppress (or partially suppress) the signs and symptoms of the syndrome, and thereby may possibly mask the underlying disease process. The effect that symptomatic suppression has upon the long-term course of the syndrome is unknown.

Given these considerations, neuroleptics should be prescribed in a manner that is most likely to minimize the occurrence of tardive dyskinesia. Chronic neuroleptic treatment should generally be reserved for patients who suffer from a chronic illness that, 1) is known to respond to neuroleptic drugs, and, 2) for whom alternative, equally effective, but potentially less harmful treatments are not available or appropriate. In patients who do require chronic treatment, the smallest dose and the shortest duration of treatment producing a satisfactory clinical response should be sought. The need for continued treatment should be reassessed periodically.

If signs and symptoms of tardive dyskinesia appear in a patient on neuroleptics, drug discontinuation should be considered. However, some patients may require treatment despite the presence of the syndrome.

(For further information about the description of tardive dyskinesia and its clinical detection, please refer to **Information for Patients** and **Adverse Reactions**.)

NEUROLEPTIC MALIGNANT SYNDROME (NMS)

A potentially fatal symptom complex sometimes referred to as Neuroleptic Malignant Syndrome (NMS) has been reported in association with antipsychotic drugs. Clinical manifestations of NMS are hyperpyrexia, muscle rigidity, altered mental status and evidence of autonomic instability (irregular pulse or blood pressure, tachycardia, diaphoresis, and cardiac dysrhythmias).

The diagnostic evaluation of patients with this syndrome is complicated. In arriving at a diagnosis, it is important to identify cases where the clinical presentation includes both serious medical illness (e.g., pneumonia, systemic infection, etc.) and untreated or inadequately treated extrapyramidal signs and symptoms (EPS). Other important considerations in the differential diagnosis include central anticholinergic toxicity, heat stroke, drug fever and primary central nervous system (CNS) pathology.

The management of NMS should include 1) immediate discontinuation of antipsychotic drugs and other drugs not essential to concurrent therapy, 2) intensive symptomatic treatment and medical monitoring, and 3) treatment of any concomitant serious medical problems for which specific treatments are available. There is no general agreement about specific pharmacological treatment regimens for uncomplicated NMS.

If a patient requires antipsychotic drug treatment after recovery from NMS, the potential reintroduction of drug therapy should be carefully considered. The patient should be carefully monitored, since recurrences of NMS have been reported.

Patients with cardiovascular disorders should be watched closely. Tricyclic antidepressant drugs, including amitriptyline hydrochloride, particularly when given in high doses, have been reported to produce arrhythmias, sinus tachycardia, and prolongation of the conduction time. Myocardial infarction and stroke have been reported with drugs of this class.

ETRAFON should not be given concomitantly with guanethidine or similarly acting compounds, since amitriptyline, like other tricyclic antidepressants, may block the antihypertensive effect of these compounds.

If hypotension develops, epinephrine should not be administered, since its action is blocked and partially reversed by perphenazine. If a vasopressor is needed, norepinephrine may be used. Severe, acute hypotension has occurred with the use of phenothiazines and is particularly likely to occur in patients with mitral insufficiency or pheochromocytoma. Rebound hypertension may occur in pheochromocytoma patients.

Perphenazine can lower the convulsive threshold in susceptible individuals; it should be used with caution in alcohol withdrawal and in patients with convulsive disorders. If the patient is being treated with an anticonvulsant agent, increased dosage of that agent may be required when ETRAFON Tablets are used concomitantly.

Because of the anticholinergic activity of amitriptyline hydrochloride, ETRAFON should be used with caution in patients with glaucoma, increased intraocular pressure, and those in whom urinary retention is present or anticipated. In patients with angle-closure glaucoma, even average doses may precipitate an attack.

Close supervision is required when amitriptyline hydrochloride is given to hyperthyroid patients or those receiving thyroid medication.

ETRAFON Tablets may impair the mental and/or physical abilities required for the performance of potentially hazardous tasks, such as driving a car or operating machinery, the patient should be warned accordingly.

Usage in Children: Since a dosage for children has not been established, ETRAFON is not recommended for use in children.

Usage in Pregnancy: Safe use of ETRAFON Tablets during pregnancy and lactation has not been established; therefore, in administering the drug to pregnant patients, nursing mothers, or women who may become pregnant, the possible benefits must be weighed against the possible hazards to mother and child.

PRECAUTIONS

The possibility of suicide in depressed patients remains during treatment and until significant remission occurs. This type of patient should not have access to large quantities of this drug.

Perphenazine

As with all phenothiazine compounds, perphenazine should not be used indiscriminately. Caution should be observed in giving it to patients who have previously exhibited severe adverse reactions to other phenothiazines. Some of the untoward actions of perphenazine tend to appear more frequently when high doses are used. However, as with other phenothiazine compounds, patients receiving perphenazine in any dosage should be kept under close supervision.

Neuroleptic drugs elevate prolactin levels; the elevation persists during chronic administration. Tissue culture experiments indicate that approximately one-third of human breast cancers are prolactin dependent *in vitro*, a factor of potential importance if the prescription of these drugs is contemplated in a patient with a previously detected breast cancer. Although disturbances such as galactorrhea, amenorrhea, gynecomastia, and impotence have been reported, the clinical significance of elevated serum prolactin levels is unknown for most patients. An increase in mammary neo-

Continued on next page

Schering—Cont.

plasms has been found in rodents after chronic administration of neuroleptic drugs. Neither clinical studies nor epidemiologic studies conducted to date, however, have shown an association between chronic administration of these drugs and mammary tumorigenesis; the available evidence is considered too limited to be conclusive at this time.

The antiemetic effect of perphenazine may obscure signs of toxicity due to overdosage of other drugs, or render more difficult the diagnosis of disorders such as brain tumors or intestinal obstruction.

A significant, not otherwise explained, rise in body temperature may suggest individual intolerance to perphenazine, in which case ETRAFON should be discontinued.

Patients on large doses of a phenothiazine drug who are undergoing surgery should be watched carefully for possible hypotensive phenomena. Moreover, reduced amounts of anesthetics or central nervous system depressants may be necessary.

Since phenothiazines and central nervous system depressants (opiates, analgesics, antihistamines, barbiturates) can potentiate each other, less than the usual dosage of the added drug is recommended, and caution is advised, when they are administered concomitantly.

Use with caution in patients who are receiving atropine or related drugs because of additive anticholinergic effects and also in patients who will be exposed to extreme heat or organic phosphate insecticides.

The use of alcohol should be avoided, since additive effects and hypotension may occur. Patients should be cautioned that their response to alcohol may be increased while they are being treated with ETRAFON Tablets. The risk of suicide and the danger of overdose may be increased in patients who use alcohol excessively due to its potentiation of the drug's effect.

Blood counts and hepatic and renal functions should be checked periodically. The appearance of signs of blood dyscrasias requires the discontinuance of the drug and institution of appropriate therapy. If abnormalities in hepatic tests occur, phenothiazine treatment should be discontinued. Renal function in patients on long-term therapy should be monitored; if blood urea nitrogen (BUN) becomes abnormal, treatment with the drug should be discontinued.

The use of phenothiazine derivatives in patients with diminished renal function should be undertaken with caution.

Use with caution in patients suffering from respiratory impairment due to acute pulmonary infections, or in chronic respiratory disorders such as severe asthma or emphysema. In general, phenothiazines do not produce psychic dependence. Gastritis, nausea and vomiting, dizziness, and tremulousness have been reported following abrupt cessation of high-dose therapy. Reports suggest that these symptoms can be reduced by continuing concomitant antiparkinson agents for several weeks after the phenothiazine is withdrawn.

The possibility of liver damage, corneal and lenticular deposits, and irreversible dyskinesias should be kept in mind when patients are on long-term therapy.

Because photosensitivity has been reported, undue exposure to the sun should be avoided during phenothiazine treatment.

Information for Patients: This information is intended to aid in the safe and effective use of this medication. It is not a disclosure of all possible adverse or intended effects.

Given the likelihood that a substantial proportion of patients exposed chronically to neuroleptics will develop tardive dyskinesia, it is advised that all patients in whom chronic use is contemplated be given, if possible, full information about this risk. The decision to inform patients and/or their guardians must obviously take into account the clinical circumstances and the competency of the patients to understand the information provided.

Amitriptyline Hydrochloride

In manic-depressive psychosis, depressed patients may experience a shift toward the manic phase if they are treated with an antidepressant drug. Patients with paranoid symptomatology may have an exaggeration of such symptoms. The tranquilizing effect of ETRAFON has seemed to reduce the likelihood of this effect.

When amitriptyline hydrochloride is given with anticholinergic agents or sympathomimetic drugs, including epinephrine combined with local anesthetics, close supervision and careful adjustment of dosages are required.

Paralytic ileus may occur in patients taking tricyclic antidepressants in combination with anticholinergic-type drugs. Concurrent use of large doses of ethchlorvynol should be used with caution, since transient delirium has been reported in patients receiving this drug in combination with amitriptyline hydrochloride.

This drug may enhance the response to alcohol and the effects of barbiturates and other CNS depressants.

Concurrent administration of amitriptyline hydrochloride and electroshock therapy may increase the hazards of ther-

apy. Such treatment should be limited to patients for whom it is essential.

Discontinue the drug several days before elective surgery, if possible.

Both elevation and lowering of blood sugar levels have been reported.

The usefulness of amitriptyline in the treatment of depression has been amply demonstrated; however, it should be realized that abuse of amitriptyline among a narcotic-dependent population is not uncommon.

Concurrent administration of cimetidine and tricyclic antidepressants can produce clinically significant increases in the plasma concentrations of the tricyclic antidepressant. Serious anticholinergic symptoms (severe dry mouth, urinary retention, blurred vision) have been associated with elevations in the serum levels of the tricyclic antidepressant when cimetidine is added to the drug regimen. Additionally, higher than expected steady-state serum concentrations of the tricyclic antidepressant have been observed when therapy is initiated in patients taking cimetidine.

Alternatively, decreases in the steady-state serum concentration of the tricyclic antidepressant have been reported in well-controlled patients on concurrent therapy upon discontinuance of cimetidine. The therapeutic efficacy of the tricyclic antidepressant may be compromised in these patients as the cimetidine is discontinued.

ADVERSE REACTIONS

Adverse reactions to ETRAFON Tablets are the same as those to its components, perphenazine and amitriptyline hydrochloride. There have been no reports of effects peculiar to the combination of these components in ETRAFON Tablets.

Perphenazine

Not all of the following adverse reactions have been reported with perphenazine; however, pharmacological similarities among various phenothiazine derivatives require that each be considered. With the piperazine group (of which perphenazine is an example), the extrapyramidal symptoms are more common, and others (e.g., sedative effects, jaundice, and blood dyscrasias) are less frequently seen.

CNS Effects: *Extrapyramidal reactions:* opisthotonus, trismus, torticollis, retrocollis, aching and numbness of the limbs, motor restlessness, oculogyric crisis, hyperreflexia, dystonia, including protrusion, discoloration, aching and rounding of the tongue, tonic spasm of the masticatory muscles, tight feeling in the throat, slurred speech, dysphagia, akathisia, dyskinesia, parkinsonism, and ataxia. Their incidence and severity usually increase with an increase in dosage, but there is considerable individual variation in the tendency to develop such symptoms. Extrapyramidal symptoms can usually be controlled by the concomitant use of effective antiparkinsonian drugs, such as benztropine mesylate, and/or by reduction in dosage.

In some instances, however, these extrapyramidal reactions may persist after discontinuation of treatment with perphenazine.

Persistent tardive dyskinesia: As with all antipsychotic agents, tardive dyskinesia may appear in some patients on long-term therapy or may appear after drug therapy has been discontinued. Although the risk appears to be greater in elderly patients on high-dose therapy, especially females it may occur in either sex and in children. The symptoms are persistent and in some patients appear to be irreversible. The syndrome is characterized by rhythmical, involuntary movements of the tongue, face, mouth or jaw (eg, protrusion of tongue, puffing of cheeks, puckering of mouth, chewing movements). Sometimes these may be accompanied by involuntary movements of the extremities. There is no known effective treatment for tardive dyskinesia; antiparkinsonism agents usually do not alleviate the symptoms of this syndrome. It is suggested that all antipsychotic agents be discontinued if these symptoms appear. Should it be necessary to reinstitute treatment, or increase the dosage of the agent, or switch to a different antipsychotic agent, the syndrome may be masked. It has been reported that fine, vermicular movements of the tongue may be an early sign of the syndrome, and if the medication is stopped at that time the syndrome may not develop.

Other CNS effects include cerebral edema; abnormality of cerebrospinal fluid proteins; convulsive seizures, particularly in patients with EEG abnormalities or a history of such disorders; and headaches.

Neuroleptic malignant syndrome has been reported in patients treated with neuroleptic drugs (see WARNINGS for further information).

Drowsiness may occur, particularly during the first or second week, after which it generally disappears. If troublesome, lower the dosage. Hypnotic effects appear to be minimal, especially in patients who are permitted to remain active.

Adverse behavioral effects include paradoxical exacerbation of psychotic symptoms, catatonic-like states, paranoid reactions, lethargy, paradoxical excitement, restlessness, hyperactivity, nocturnal confusion, bizarre dreams, and insomnia.

Hyperreflexia has been reported in the newborn when a phenothiazine was used during pregnancy.

Autonomic Effects: dry mouth or salivation, nausea, vomiting, diarrhea, anorexia, constipation, obstipation, fecal impaction, urinary retention, frequency or incontinence, polyuria, bladder paralysis, nasal congestion, pallor, myosis, mydriasis, blurred vision, glaucoma, perspiration, hypertension, hypotension, and a change in pulse rate occasionally may occur. Significant autonomic effects have been infrequent in patients receiving less than 24 mg perphenazine daily.

Adynamic ileus occasionally occurs with phenothiazine therapy and if severe can result in complications and death. It is of particular concern in psychiatric patients, who may fail to seek treatment of the condition.

Allergic Effects: urticaria, erythema, eczema, exfoliative dermatitis, pruritus, photosensitivity, asthma, fever, anaphylactoid reactions, laryngeal edema, and angioneurotic edema; contact dermatitis in nursing personnel administering the drug; and in extremely rare instances, individual idiosyncrasy or hypersensitivity to phenothiazines has resulted in cerebral edema, circulatory collapse, and death.

Endocrine Effects: lactation, galactorrhea, moderate breast enlargement in females and gynecomastia in males on large doses, disturbances in the menstrual cycle, amenorrhea, changes in libido, inhibition of ejaculation, false positive pregnancy tests, hyperglycemia, hypoglycemia, glycosuria, syndrome of inappropriate ADH (antidiuretic hormone) secretion.

Cardiovascular Effects: Postural hypotension, tachycardia (especially with sudden marked increase in dosage), bradycardia, cardiac arrest, faintness, and dizziness. Occasionally the hypotensive effect may produce a shock-like condition. ECG changes, nonspecific, (quinidine-like effect) usually reversible, have been observed in some patients receiving phenothiazine tranquilizers.

Sudden death has occasionally been reported in patients who have received phenothiazines. In some cases the death was apparently due to cardiac arrest; in others the cause appeared to be asphyxia due to failure of the cough reflex. In some patients, the cause could not be determined nor could it be established that the death was due to the phenothiazine.

Hematological Effects: agranulocytosis, eosinophilia, leukopenia, hemolytic anemia, thrombocytopenic purpura, and pancytopenia. Most cases of agranulocytosis have occurred between the fourth and tenth weeks of therapy. Patients should be watched closely especially during that period for the sudden appearance of sore throat or signs of infection. If white blood cell and differential cell counts show significant cellular depression, discontinue the drug and start appropriate therapy. However, a slightly lowered white count is not in itself an indication to discontinue the drug.

Other Effects: Special considerations in long-term therapy include pigmentation of the skin, occurring chiefly in the exposed areas; ocular changes consisting of deposition of fine particulate matter in the cornea and lens, progressing in more severe cases to star-shaped lenticular opacities; epithelial keratopathies; and pigmentary retinopathy. Also noted: peripheral edema, reversed epinephrine effect, increase in PBI not attributable to an increase in thyroxine, parotid swelling (rare), hyperpyrexia, systemic lupus erythematosus-like syndrome, increases in appetite and weight, polyphagia, photophobia, and muscle weakness.

Liver damage (biliary stasis) may occur. Jaundice may occur, usually between the second and fourth weeks of treatment, and is regarded as a hypersensitivity reaction. Incidence is low. The clinical picture resembles infectious hepatitis but with laboratory features of obstructive jaundice. It is usually reversible; however, chronic jaundice has been reported.

Amitriptyline Hydrochloride

Although activation of latent schizophrenia has been reported with antidepressant drugs, including amitriptyline hydrochloride, it may be prevented with ETRAFON Tablets in some cases because of the antipsychotic effect of perphenazine. A few instances of epileptiform seizures have been reported in chronic schizophrenic patients during treatment with amitriptyline hydrochloride.

Note: Included in the listing which follows are a few adverse reactions which have not been reported with this specific drug. However, pharmacological similarities among the tricyclic antidepressant drugs require that each of the reactions be considered when amitriptyline hydrochloride is administered.

Allergic: Rash, pruritus, urticaria, photosensitization, edema of face and tongue.

Anticholinergic: Dry mouth, blurred vision, disturbance of accommodation, constipation, paralytic ileus, urinary retention, dilatation of urinary tract.

Cardiovascular: Hypotension, hypertension, tachycardia, palpitations, myocardial infarction, arrhythmias, heart block, stroke.

CNS and Neuromuscular: Confusional states, disturbed concentration, disorientation, delusions, hallucinations, excitement, jitteriness, anxiety, restlessness, insomnia, nightmares, numbness, tingling, and paresthesias of the extremities, peripheral neuropathy, incoordination, ataxia, tremors, seizures, alteration in EEG patterns, extrapyramidal symptoms, tinnitus.

Endocrine: Testicular swelling and gynecomastia in the male, breast enlargement and galactorrhea in the female, increased or decreased libido, elevation and lowering of blood sugar levels, syndrome of inappropriate ADH (antidiuretic hormone secretion).

Gastrointestinal: Nausea, epigastric distress, heartburn, vomiting, anorexia, stomatitis, peculiar taste, diarrhea, jaundice, parotid swelling, black tongue. Rarely hepatitis has occurred (including altered liver function and jaundice).

Hematologic: Bone marrow depression including agranulocytosis, leukopenia, eosinophilia, purpura, thrombocytopenia.

Other: Dizziness, weakness, fatigue, headache, weight gain or loss, increased perspiration, urinary frequency, mydriasis, drowsiness, alopecia.

Withdrawal Symptoms: Abrupt cessation of treatment after prolonged administration may produce nausea, headache, and malaise. These are not indicative of addiction.

DOSAGE AND ADMINISTRATION

Initial Dosage

In psychoneurotic patients whose anxiety and depression warrant combined therapy, one ETRAFON Tablet (2–25) or one ETRAFON-FORTE Tablet (4–25) three or four times a day is recommended.

In elderly patients, adolescents and other patients as indicated, one ETRAFON-A Tablet (4–10) may be administered three or four times a day as initial dosage. This dosage may be adjusted as required to produce an adequate response.

In more severely ill patients with schizophrenia, two ETRAFON-FORTE Tablets (4–25) three times a day are recommended as the initial dosage. If necessary, a fourth dose may be given at bedtime. The total daily dosage should not exceed eight tablets of any strength.

Maintenance Dosage

Depending on the condition being treated, the onset of therapeutic response may vary from a few days to a few weeks or even longer. After a satisfactory response is noted, dosage should be reduced to the smallest dose which is effective for relief of the symptoms for which ETRAFON Tablets are being administered. A useful maintenance dosage is one ETRAFON Tablet (2–25) or one ETRAFON-FORTE Tablet (4–25) two to four times a day. In some patients, maintenance dosage is required for many months.

ETRAFON 2–10 Tablets (2–10) and ETRAFON-A Tablets (4–10) can be used to increase flexibility in adjusting maintenance dosage to the lowest amount consistent with relief of symptoms.

OVERDOSAGE

In the event of overdosage, emergency treatment should be started immediately. All patients suspected of having taken an overdose should be hospitalized as soon as possible.

Manifestations: Overdosage of perphenazine primarily involves the extrapyramidal mechanism and produces the same side effects described under ADVERSE REACTIONS, but to a more marked degree. It is usually evidenced by stupor or coma; children may have convulsive seizures.

High doses of ETRAFON Tablets may cause temporary confusion, disturbed concentration, or transient visual hallucinations. Overdosage may cause drowsiness; hypothermia; tachycardia and other arrhythmic abnormalities—for example, bundle branch block; ECG evidence of impaired conduction; congestive heart failure; dilated pupils; convulsions; severe hypotension; stupor; and coma. Other symptoms may be agitation, hyperactive reflexes, muscle rigidity, vomiting, hyperpyrexia, or any of the adverse reactions listed for perphenazine or amitriptyline hydrochloride.

Overdosage with tricyclic antidepressants (TCAs), such as imipramine, doxepin, or amitriptyline may result in plasma TCA levels of 1,000 ng/ml or higher. Such levels more accurately define patients who are at risk for major medical complications of overdosage than does the amount of drug ingested based on patient history. In one study, all patients with TCA levels of this magnitude had a QRS duration of 100 msec or more on a routine ECG within the first 24 hours following overdose.

In the absence of TCA blood level determinations, a QRS of 100 msec or more suggests a greater likelihood of serious complications.

Oculomotor paresis (loss of conjugate movement in the so-called doll's eyes maneuver) as a manifestation of amitriptyline overdosage has been reported as being significant in the differential diagnosis of a patient in light coma.

Treatment: Treatment is symptomatic and supportive. There is no specific antidote. The patient should be induced to vomit even if emesis has occurred spontaneously. Pharmacologic vomiting by the administration of ipecac syrup is a preferred method. It should be noted that ipecac has a central mode of action in addition to its local gastric irritant properties, and the central mode of action may be blocked by the antiemetic effect of ETRAFON Tablets. Vomiting should not be induced in patients with impaired consciousness. The action of ipecac is facilitated by physical activity and by the administration of 8 to 12 fluid ounces of water. If emesis does not occur within 15 minutes, the dose of ipecac should be repeated. Precautions against aspiration must be taken, especially in infants and children. Following emesis, any drug remaining in the stomach may be adsorbed by activated charcoal administered as a slurry with water. If vomiting is unsuccessful or contraindicated, gastric lavage should be performed. Isotonic and one-half isotonic saline are the lavage solutions of choice. Saline cathartics, such as milk of magnesia, draw water into the bowel by osmosis and therefore may be valuable for their action in rapid dilution of bowel content.

Standard measures (oxygen, intravenous fluids, corticosteroids) should be used to manage circulatory shock or metabolic acidosis. An open airway and adequate fluid intake should be maintained. Body temperature should be regulated. Hypothermia is expected, but severe hyperthermia may occur and must be treated vigorously. (See CONTRAINDICATIONS.)

An electrocardiogram should be taken and close monitoring of cardiac function instituted if there is any sign of abnormality. Cardiac arrhythmias may be treated with neostigmine, pyridostigmine, or propranolol. Digitalis should be considered for cardiac failure. Close monitoring of cardiac function is advisable for not less than five days.

Vasopressors such as norepinephrine may be used to treat hypotension, but epinephrine should NOT be used.

The intravenous administration of 1 to 3 mg physostigmine salicylate has been reported to reverse the symptoms of tricyclic antidepressant poisoning and therefore, should be considered in the symptomatic treatment of the central anticholinergic effects due to overdosage with ETRAFON Tablets. Because physostigmine is rapidly metabolized, it should be re-administered as required, especially if life-threatening signs, such as arrhythmias, convulsions, or deep coma recur or persist.

Anticonvulsants (an inhalation anesthetic, diazepam, or paraldehyde) are recommended for control of convulsions, since perphenazine increases the central nervous system depressant action, but not the anticonvulsant action of barbiturates.

If acute parkinson-like symptoms result from perphenazine intoxication, benztropine mesylate or diphenhydramine may be administered.

Central nervous system depression may be treated with non-convulsant doses of CNS stimulants. Avoid stimulants that may cause convulsions (e.g., picrotoxin and pentylenetetrazol).

Signs of arousal may not occur for 48 hours.

Dialysis is of no value because of low plasma concentrations of the drug.

Since overdosage is often deliberate, patients may attempt suicide by other means during the recovery phase. Deaths by deliberate or accidental overdosage have occurred with this class of drugs.

HOW SUPPLIED

ETRAFON 2–10 Tablets (perphenazine 2 mg and amitriptyline hydrochloride 10 mg): deep yellow, sugar-coated tablets branded in blue-black with the Schering trademark and either product identification letters, ANA, or number, 287; bottles of 100 (NDC 0085-0287-04) and 500 (NDC 0085-0287-07) and box of 100 for unit-dose dispensing (10 strips of 10 tablets each) (NDC 0085-0287-08).

ETRAFON Tablets (perphenazine 2 mg and amitriptyline hydrochloride 25 mg): pink, sugar-coated tablets branded in red with the Schering trademark and either product identification letters, ANC or number, 598; bottles of 100 (NDC 0085-0598-04) and 500 (NDC 0085-0598-07) and box of 100 for unit-dose dispensing (10 strips of 10 tablets each) (NDC 0085-0598-08).

ETRAFON-A Tablets (perphenazine 4 mg and amitriptyline hydrochloride 10 mg): orange, sugar-coated tablets branded in blue-black with the Schering trademark and either product identification letters, ANB, or number, 119; bottles of 100 (NDC 0085-0119-04) and box of 100 for unit-dose dispensing (10 strips of 10 tablets each) (NDC 0085-0119-08).

ETRAFON-FORTE Tablets (perphenazine 4 mg and amitriptyline hydrochloride 25 mg): red, sugar-coated tablets branded in blue with the Schering trademark and either product identification letters, ANE, or number, 720; bottles of 100 (NDC 0085-0720-04) and 500 (NDC 0085-0720-07) and box of 100 for unit-dose dispensing (10 strips of 10 tablets each) (NDC 0085-0720-08).

Store ETRAFON 2-10, 4-10, 2-25 and 4-25 Tablets between 2° and 30°C (36° and 86°F). In addition, protect unit-dose packages from excessive moisture.

Revised 6/87

Shown in Product Identification Section, page 428

EULEXIN® ℞
brand of flutamide
Capsules

DESCRIPTION

EULEXIN Capsules contain flutamide, a nonsteroid, orally active antiandrogen having the chemical name, 2-methyl-N-[4-nitro-3-(trifluoromethyl)phenyl] propanamide.

Each capsule contains 125 mg flutamide. The compound is a buff to yellow powder with a molecular weight of 276.2.

The inactive ingredients for EULEXIN Capsules include: corn starch, lactose, magnesium stearate, povidone, and sodium lauryl sulfate. Gelatin capsule shells may contain methylparaben, propylparaben, butylparaben and the following dye systems: FD&C Blue 1, FD&C Yellow 6 and either FD&C Red 3 or FD&C Red 40 plus D&C Yellow 10, with titanium dioxide and other inactive ingredients.

CLINICAL PHARMACOLOGY

General: In animal studies. flutamide demonstrates potent antiandrogenic effects. It exerts its antiandrogenic action by inhibiting androgen uptake and/or by inhibiting nuclear binding of androgen in target tissues or both. Prostatic carcinoma is known to be androgen-sensitive and responds to treatment that counteracts the effect of androgen and/or removes the source of androgen, e.g., castration.

Pharmacokinetics: Analysis of plasma, urine, and feces following a single oral 200 mg dose of tritium-labeled flutamide to human volunteers showed that the drug is rapidly and completely absorbed. It is excreted mainly in the urine with only 4.2% of the dose excreted in the feces over 72 hours. The composition of plasma radioactivity showed that flutamide is rapidly and extensively metabolized, with flutamide comprising only 2.5% of plasma radioactivity one hour after administration. At least six metabolites have been identified in plasma. The major plasma metabolite is a biologically active alpha-hydroxylated derivative which accounts for 23% of the plasma tritium one hour after drug administration.

The major urinary metabolite is 2-amino-5-nitro-4-(trifluoromethyl)phenol.

Following a single 250 mg oral dose to normal adult volunteers, low plasma levels of varying amounts of flutamide were detected. The biologically active alpha-hydroxylated metabolite reaches maximum plasma levels in about two hours, indicating that it is rapidly formed from flutamide. The plasma half-life for this metabolite is about 6 hours.

Following multiple oral dosing of 250 mg t.i.d. in normal geriatric volunteers, flutamide and its active metabolite approached steady-state plasma levels (based on pharmacokinetic stimulations) after the fourth flutamide dose. The half-life of the active metabolite in geriatric volunteers after a single flutamide dose is about 8 hours and at steady-state is 9.6 hours.

Flutamide, *in vivo*, at steady-state plasma concentrations of 24 to 78 ng/mL is 94% to 96% bound to plasma proteins. The active metabolite of flutamide, *in vivo*, at steady-state plasma concentrations of 1556 to 2284 ng/mL, is 92% to 94% bound to plasma proteins.

In male rats neither flutamide nor any of its metabolites are preferentially accumulated in any tissue except the prostate after an oral 5 mg/kg dose of ¹⁴C-flutamide. Total drug levels were highest 6 hours after drug administration in all tissues. Levels declined at roughly similar rates to low levels at 18 hours. The major metabolite was present at higher concentrations than flutamide in all tissues studied.

Elevations of plasma testosterone and estradiol levels have been noted following flutamide administration.

Clinical Studies: Flutamide has been demonstrated to interfere with testosterone at the cellular level. This can complement medical castration achieved with leuprolide, which suppresses testicular androgen production by inhibiting luteinizing horome secretion.

To study the effects of combination therapy, 617 patients (311 leuprolide + flutamide, 306 leuprolide + placebo) with previously untreated advanced prostatic carcinoma were enrolled in a large multi-centered, controlled clinical trial. Three and one-half years after the study was initiated, median survival had been reached. The median actuarial survival time is 34.9 months for patients treated with leuprolide and flutamide versus 27.9 months for patients treated with leuprolide alone. This seven month increment represents 25% improvement in overall survival with the flutamide therapy. Analysis of progression free survival showed a 2.6 month improvement in patients who received leuprolide plus flutamide, a 19% increment over leuprolide and placebo.

Continued on next page

Schering—Cont.

INDICATIONS AND USAGE

EULEXIN Capsules are indicated for use in combination with LHRH agonistic analogues (such as leuprolide acetate) for the treatment of metastatic prostatic carcinoma (stage D_2). To achieve the benefit of the adjunctive therapy with EULEXIN, treatment must be started simultaneously using both drugs.

CONTRAINDICATIONS

EULEXIN Capsules are contraindicated in patients who are hypersensitive to flutamide or any component of this preparation.

WARNINGS

Gynecomastia occurred in 9% of patients receiving flutamide together with medical castration.

Flutamide may cause fetal harm when administered to a pregnant woman. There was decreased 24-hour survival in the offspring of rats treated with flutamide at doses of 30, 100, or 200 mg/kg/day (approximately 3, 9, and 19 times the human dose) during pregnancy. A slight increase in minor variations in the development of the sternebra and vertebra was seen in fetuses of rats at the two higher doses. Feminization of the males also occurred at the two higher dose levels. There was a decreased survival rate in the offspring of rabbits receiving the highest dose (15 mg/kg/day; equal to 1.4 times the human dose).

PRECAUTIONS

Information for Patients: Patients should be informed that EULEXIN and the drug used for medical castration should be administered concomitantly, and that they should not interrupt their dosing or stop taking these medications without consulting their physician.

Laboratory Tests: Periodic liver function tests may be considered in patients on long-term treatment with EULEXIN Capsules since transient abnormalities of transaminases have been reported; however, fewer than 1% of the patients treated with the combination had transaminases greater than five to greater than ten times the normal values.

Drug Interactions: Interactions between EULEXIN Capsules and leuprolide have not occurred. Interactions between EULEXIN Capsules and other drugs have not been reported.

Carcinogenesis, Mutagenesis, Impairment of Fertility: No carcinogenicity studies were performed with flutamide. However, daily administration of flutamide to rats for 52 weeks at doses of 30, 90, or 180 mg/kg/day (approximately 3, 8, or 17 times the human dose) produced testicular interstitial cell adenomas at all doses.

Flutamide did not demonstrate DNA modifying activity in the Ames *Salmonella*/microsome Mutagenesis Assay. Dominant lethal tests in rats were negative.

Reduced sperm counts were observed during a six-week study of flutamide monotherapy in normal voluneers. Flutamide did not affect estrous cycles or interfere with the mating behavior of male and female rats when the drug was administered at 25 and 75 mg/kg/day prior to mating. Males treated with 160 mg/kg/day (30 times the minimum effective antiandrogenic dose) failed to mate; mating behavior returned to normal after dosing was stopped. Conception rates were decreased in all dosing groups. Suppression of spermatogenesis was observed in rats dosed for 52 weeks at approximately 3, 8, or 17 times the human dose and in dogs dosed for 78 weeks at 1.4, 2.3, and 3.7 times the human dose.

Pregnancy: Pregnancy Category D. See **WARNINGS** section.

ADVERSE REACTIONS

The following adverse experiences were reported during treatment with EULEXIN Capsules in combination with LHRH-agonist.

The most frequently reported (greater than 5%) adverse experiences during treatment with EULEXIN Capsules in combination with a LHRH agonist are listed in the table below. For comparison, adverse experiences seen with a LHRH agonist and placebo are also listed in the following table.

	(n=294) Flutamide + LHRH-agonist % All	(n=285) Placebo + LHRH-agonist % All
Hot Flashes	61	57
Loss of Libido	36	31
Impotence	33	29
Diarrhea	12	4
Nausea/Vomiting	11	10
Gynecomastia	9	11
Other	7	9
Other GI	6	4

As shown in the table, for both treatment groups, the most frequently occurring adverse experiences (hot flashes, impotence, loss of libido) were those known to be associated with low serum androgen levels and known to occur with LHRH-agonists alone.

The only notable difference was the higher incidence of diarrhea in the flutamide + LHRH-agonist group (12%), which was severe in five percent as opposed to the placebo + LHRH-agonist (4%), which was severe in less than one percent.

In addition, the following adverse reactions were reported during treatment with flutamide + LHRH-agonist. No causal relatedness of these reactions to drug treatment has been made, and some of the adverse experiences reported are those that commonly occur in elderly patients.

Cardiovascular System: hypertension in 1% of patients.

Central Nervous System: CNS (drowsiness/confusion/depression/anxiety/nervousness) reactions occurred in 1% of patients.

Endocrine System: gynecomastia in 9% of patients.

Gastrointestinal System: nausea/vomiting occurred in 11%; diarrhea 12% and other GI disorders occurred in 6% of patients. Liver: elevation of serum enzymes, as well as clinically evident hepatitis, that appears to be causally related, has been reported with flutamide monotherapy.

Respiratory System: pulmonary symptoms in less than 1% of patients.

Skin: irritation at the injection site and rash occurred in 3% of patients. Photosensitivity reactions have been reported in five patients.

Other: edema, hematopoietic (hemoglobin/WBC/platelets) symptoms and anorexia occurred in 4% of patients; neuromuscular, hepatic, genital-urinary symptoms occurred in 2% of patients.

Laboratory Values: Laboratory abnormalities included elevated SGOT and SGPT and bilirubin values, which occurred in 7 patients. In addition, there were 11 patients who had elevated creatinine values (these values changed from WHO grades 0 to 2 at baseline, to grades 3 or 4 some time during treatment).

OVERDOSAGE

In animal studies with flutamide alone, signs of overdose included hypoactivity, piloerection, slow respiration, ataxia, and/or lacrimation, anorexia, tranquilization, and emesis. Clinical trials have been conducted with flutamide in doses up to 1500 mg per day for periods up to 36 weeks with no serious adverse effects reported. Those adverse reactions reported included gynecomastia, breast tenderness and some increases in SGOT. The single dose of flutamide ordinarily associated with symptoms of overdose or considered to be life-threatening has not been established.

Since EULEXIN is highly protein bound, dialysis may not be of any use as treatment for overdose. As in the management of overdosage with any drug, it should be borne in mind that multiple agents may have been taken. If vomiting does not occur spontaneously, it should be induced if the patient is alert. General supportive care, including frequent monitoring of the vital signs and close observation of the patient, is indicated.

DOSAGE AND ADMINISTRATION

The recommended dosage is two capsules three times a day at eight hour intervals for a total daily dosage of 750 mg.

HOW SUPPLIED

EULEXIN Capsules, 125 mg, are available as opaque, two-toned brown capsules, imprinted with "Schering 525". They are supplied as follows:

NDC 0085-0525-04—Bottles of 100
NDC 0085-0525-05—Bottles of 500
NDC 0085-0525-03—Unit Dose packages of 100 (10 × 10's)

Store between 2° and 30°C (36° and 86°F).

1/89

Copyright © 1989, Schering Corporation. All rights reserved.

Shown in Product Identification Section, page 428

FULVICIN® P/G ℞
[*ful 'vĭ-sin*]
brand of ultramicrosize griseofulvin,
  Tablets, USP

DESCRIPTION

FULVICIN P/G Tablets contain ultramicrosize crystals of griseofulvin, an antibiotic derived from a species of *Penicillium*. Griseofulvin crystals are partly dissolved in polyethylene glycol 6000 and partly dispersed throughout the tablet matrix.

Each FULVICIN P/G Tablet contains 125 mg or 250 mg griseofulvin ultramicrosize.

The inactive ingredients for FULVICIN P/G Tablets, 125 or 250 mg, include: corn starch, lactose, magnesium stearate, PEG, and sodium lauryl sulfate.

ACTIONS

Microbiology Griseofulvin is fungistatic with *in vitro* activity against various species of *Microsporum*, *Epidermophyton*, and *Trichophyton*. It has no effect on bacteria or on other genera of fungi.

Human Pharmacology: Following oral administration, griseofulvin is deposited in the keratin precursor cells and has a greater affinity for diseased tissue. The drug is tightly bound to the new keratin which becomes highly resistant to fungal invasions.

The efficiency of gastrointestinal absorption of ultramicrocrystalline griseofulvin is approximately one and one-half times that of the conventional microsized griseofulvin. This factor permits the oral intake of two-thirds as much ultramicrocrystalline griseofulvin as the microsize form. However, there is currently no evidence that this lower dose confers any significant clinical differences with regard to safety and/or efficacy.

INDICATIONS

FULVICIN P/G Tablets are indicated for the treatment of ringworm infections of the skin, hair, and nails, namely: tinea corporis, tinea pedis, tinea cruris, tinea barbae, tinea capitis, tinea unguium (onychomycosis) when caused by one or more of the following genera of fungi: *Trichophyton rubrum*, *Trichophyton tonsurans*, *Trichophyton mentagrophytes*, *Trichophyton interdigitale*, *Trichophyton verrucosum*, *Trichophyton megninii*, *Trichophyton gallinae*, *Trichophyton crateriforme*, *Trichophyton sulphureum*, *Trichophyton schoenleinii*, *Microsporum audouini*, *Microsporum canis*, *Microsporum gypseum*, and *Epidermophyton floccosum*.

Note: Prior to therapy, the type of fungi responsible for the infection should be identified.

The use of this drug is not justified in minor or trivial infections which will respond to topical agents alone.

Griseofulvin is not effective in the following: bacterial infections, candidiasis (moniliasis), histoplasmosis, actinomycosis, sporotrichosis, chromoblastomycosis, coccidioidomycosis, North American blastomycosis, cryptococcosis (torulosis), tinea versicolor, and nocardiosis.

CONTRAINDICATIONS

This drug is contraindicated in patients with porphyria, hepatocellular failure, and in individuals with a history of hypersensitivity to griseofulvin.

Rare cases of conjoined twins have been reported in patients taking griseofulvin during the first trimester of pregnancy. Griseofulvin should not be prescribed to pregnant patients or to women contemplating pregnancy.

WARNINGS

Prophylactic Usage: Safety and efficacy of griseofulvin for prophylaxis of fungal infections have not been established.

Animal Toxicology: Chronic feeding of griseofulvin, at levels ranging from 0.5–2.5% of the diet, resulted in the development of liver tumors in several strains of mice, particularly in males. Smaller particle sizes result in an enhanced effect. Lower oral dosage levels have not been tested. Subcutaneous administration of relatively small doses of griseofulvin once a week during the first three weeks of life has also been reported to induce hepatomata in mice. Thyroid tumors, mostly adenomas but some carcinomas, have been reported in male rats receiving griseofulvin at levels of 2.0%, 1.0%, and 0.2% of the diet, and in female rats receiving the two higher dose levels. Although studies in other animal species have not yielded evidence of tumorigenicity, these studies were not of adequate design to form a basis for conclusions in this regard.

In subacute toxicity studies, orally administered griseofulvin produced hepatocellular necrosis in mice, but this has not been seen in other species. Disturbances in porphyrin metabolism have been reported in griseofulvin-treated laboratory animals. Griseofulvin has been reported to have a colchicine-like effect on mitosis and cocarcinogenicity with methylcholanthrene in cutaneous tumor induction in laboratory animals.

Usage in Pregnancy: Griseofulvin should not be prescribed to pregnant patients or to women contemplating pregnancy (see **CONTRAINDICATIONS**).

Animal Reproduction Studies: It has been reported in the literature that griseofulvin was found to be embryotoxic and teratogenic on oral administration to pregnant rats. Pups with abnormalities have been reported in the litters of a few bitches treated with griseofulvin.

Suppression of spermatogenesis has been reported to occur in rats, but investigation in man failed to confirm this.

PRECAUTIONS

Patients on prolonged therapy with any potent medication should be under close observation. Periodic monitoring of organ system function, including renal, hepatic, and hematopoietic, should be done.

Since griseofulvin is derived from species of *Penicillium*, the possibility of cross-sensitivity with penicillin exists; however, known penicillin-sensitive patients have been treated without difficulty.

Since a photosensitivity reaction is occasionally associated with griseofulvin therapy, patients should be warned to avoid exposure to intense natural or artificial sunlight.

Lupus erythematosus or lupus-like syndromes, or exacerbation of existing lupus, have been reported in patients receiving griseofulvin.

Drug Interactions

Griseofulvin decreases the activity of warfarin-type anticoagulants so that patients receiving these drugs concomitantly may require dosage adjustment of the anticoagulant during and after griseofulvin therapy.

Barbiturates usually depress griseofulvin activity, and concomitant administration may require a dosage adjustment of the antifungal agent.

The effects of alcohol may be potentiated by griseofulvin, producing such effects as tachycardia and flush.

Griseofulvin may potentiate an increase in hepatic enzymes that metabolize estrogens at an increased rate, including the estrogen component of oral contraceptives, thereby causing possible decreased contraceptive effects and menstrual irregularities.

ADVERSE REACTIONS

When adverse reactions occur, they are most commonly of the hypersensitivity type, such as skin rashes, urticaria, and rarely, angioneurotic edema, and may necessitate withdrawal of therapy and appropriate countermeasures. Paresthesias of the hands and feet have been reported rarely after extended therapy. Other side effects reported occasionally are oral thrush, nausea, vomiting, epigastric distress, diarrhea, headache, fatigue, dizziness, insomnia, mental confusion, and impairment of performance of routine activities. Proteinuria, nephrosis, leukopenia, hepatic toxicity, GI bleeding and menstrual irregularities have been reported rarely. Administration of the drug should be discontinued if granulocytopenia occurs.

When rare, serious reactions occur with griseofulvin, they are usually associated with high dosages, long periods of therapy, or both.

DOSAGE AND ADMINISTRATION

Accurate diagnosis of the infecting organism is essential. Identification should be made either by direct microscopic examination of a mounting of infected tissue in a solution of potassium hydroxide or by culture on an appropriate medium.

Medication must be continued until the infecting organism is completely eradicated as indicated by appropriate clinical or laboratory examination. Representative treatment periods are tinea capitis, 4 to 6 weeks; tinea corporis, 2 to 4 weeks; tinea pedis, 4 to 8 weeks; tinea unguium—depending on rate of growth—fingernails, at least 4 months; toenails, at least 6 months.

General measures in regard to hygiene should be observed to control sources of infection or reinfection. Concomitant use of appropriate topical agents is usually required particularly in treatment of tinea pedis. In some forms of athlete's foot, yeasts and bacteria may be involved as well as fungi. Griseofulvin will not eradicate the bacterial or monilial infection.

Adults: Daily administration of 375 mg (as a single dose or in divided amounts) will give a satisfactory response in most patients with tinea corporis, tinea cruris, and tinea capitis. For those fungus infections more difficult to eradicate, such as tinea pedis and tinea unguium, a divided dose of 750 mg is recommended.

Children: Approximately 3.3 mg per pound of body weight per day of ultramicrosize griseofulvin is an effective dose for most children. On this basis, the following dosage schedule is suggested: Children weighing 35 to 60 pounds—125 mg to 187.5 mg daily. Children weighing over 60 pounds—187.5 mg to 375 mg daily.

Children 2 years of age and younger—dosage has not been established.

Clinical experience with griseofulvin in children with tinea capitis indicates that a single daily dose is effective. Clinical relapse will occur if the medication is not continued until the infecting organism is eradicated.

HOW SUPPLIED

FULVICIN P/G Tablets, 125 mg, white, compressed, scored tablets impressed with the Schering trademark and product identification numbers, 228; bottle of 100 (NDC 0085-0228-03).

FULVICIN P/G Tablets, 250 mg, white, compressed, scored tablets impressed with the Schering trademark and product identification numbers, 507; bottle of 100 (NDC 0085-0507-03).

Store at controlled room temperature 59°F to 86°F (15°C to 30°C).

Revised 4/87

Shown in Product Identification Section, page 428

FULVICIN® P/G 165 and 330   ℞

[ful′vĭ-sin]

brand of ultramicrosize griseofulvin
  Tablets, USP

DESCRIPTION

FULVICIN P/G Tablets contain ultramicrosize crystals of griseofulvin, an antibiotic derived from a species of *Penicillium*. Griseofulvin crystals are partly dissolved in polyethylene glycol 8000 and partly dispersed throughout the tablet matrix.

Each FULVICIN P/G Tablet contains 165 mg or 330 mg ultramicrosize griseofulvin, USP.

The inactive ingredients for FULVICIN P/G 165 and 330 Tablets include: corn starch, lactose, magnesium stearate, PEG, and sodium lauryl sulfate.

ACTIONS

Microbiology: Griseofulvin is fungistatic with *in vitro* activity against various species of *Microsporum, Epidermophyton,* and *Trichophyton*. It has no effect on bacteria or on other genera of fungi.

Human Pharmacology: Following oral administration, griseofulvin is deposited in the keratin precursor cells and has a greater affinity for diseased tissue. The drug is tightly bound to the new keratin which becomes highly resistant to fungal invasions.

The efficiency of gastrointestinal absorption of ultramicrocrystalline griseofulvin is approximately one and one-half times that of the conventional microsize griseofulvin. This factor permits the oral intake of two-thirds as much ultramicrocrystalline griseofulvin as the microsize form. However, there is currently no evidence that this lower dose confers any significant clinical differences with regard to safety and/or efficacy.

INDICATIONS

FULVICIN P/G Tablets are indicated for the treatment of ringworm infections of the skin, hair, and nails, namely: tinea corporis, tinea pedis, tinea cruris, tinea barbae, tinea capitis, tinea unguium (onychomycosis) when caused by one or more of the following genera of fungi: *Trichophyton rubrum, Trichophyton tonsurans, Trichophyton mentagrophytes, Trichophyton interdigitale, Trichophyton verrucosum, Trichophyton megninii, Trichophyton gallinae, Trichophyton crateriforme, Trichophyton sulphureum, Trichophyton schoenleinii, Microsporum audouini, Microsporum canis, Microsporum gypseum,* and *Epidermophyton floccosum.*

Note: Prior to therapy, the type of fungi responsible for the infection should be identified.

The use of this drug is not justified in minor or trivial infections which will respond to topical agents alone.

Griseofulvin is not effective in the following: bacterial infections, candidiasis (moniliasis), histoplasmosis, actinomycosis, sporotrichosis, chromoblastomycosis, coccidioidomycosis, North American blastomycosis, cryptococcosis (torulosis), tinea versicolor, and nocardiosis.

CONTRAINDICATIONS

This drug is contraindicated in patients with porphyria, hepatocellular failure, and in individuals with a history of hypersensitivity to griseofulvin.

Rare cases of conjoined twins have been reported in patients taking griseofulvin during the first trimester of pregnancy. Griseofulvin should not be prescribed to pregnant patients or to women contemplating pregnancy.

WARNINGS

Prophylactic Usage: Safety and efficacy of griseofulvin for prophylaxis of fungal infections have not been established.

Animal Toxicology: Chronic feeding of griseofulvin, at levels ranging from 0.5–2.5% of the diet, resulted in the development of liver tumors in several strains of mice, particularly in males. Smaller particle sizes result in an enhanced effect. Lower oral dosage levels have not been tested. Subcutaneous administration of relatively small doses of griseofulvin once a week during the first three weeks of life has also been reported to induce hepatomata in mice. Thyroid tumors, mostly adenomas but some carcinomas, have been reported in male rats receiving griseofulvin at levels of 2.0%, 1.0%, and 0.2% of the diet, and in female rats receiving the two higher dose levels. Although studies in other animal species have not yielded evidence of tumorigenicity, these studies were not of adequate design to form a basis for conclusions in this regard.

In subacute toxicity studies, orally administered griseofulvin produced hepatocellular necrosis in mice, but this has not been seen in other species. Disturbances in porphyrin metabolism have been reported in griseofulvin-treated laboratory animals. Griseofulvin has been reported to have a colchicine-like effect on mitosis and cocarcinogenicity with methylcholanthrene in cutaneous tumor induction in laboratory animals.

Usage in Pregnancy: Griseofulvin should not be prescribed to pregnant patients or to women contemplating pregnancy (see *CONTRAINDICATIONS).*

Animal Reproduction Studies: It has been reported in the literature that griseofulvin was found to be embryotoxic and teratogenic on oral administration to pregnant rats. Pups with abnormalities have been reported in the litters of a few bitches treated with griseofulvin.

Suppression of spermatogenesis has been reported to occur in rats, but investigation in man failed to confirm this.

PRECAUTIONS

Patients on prolonged therapy with any potent medication should be under close observation. Periodic monitoring of organ system function, including renal, hepatic, and hematopoietic, should be done.

Since griseofulvin is derived from species of *Penicillium,* the possibility of cross-sensitivity with penicillin exists; however, known penicillin-sensitive patients have been treated without difficulty.

Since a photosensitivity reaction is occasionally associated with griseofulvin therapy, patients should be warned to avoid exposure to intense natural or artificial sunlight.

Lupus erythematosus or lupus-like syndromes, or exacerbation of existing lupus, have been reported in patients receiving griseofulvin.

Drug Interactions: Griseofulvin decreases the activity of warfarin-type anticoagulants so that patients receiving these drugs concomitantly may require dosage adjustment of the anticoagulant during and after griseofulvin therapy.

Barbiturates usually depress griseofulvin activity, and concomitant administration may require a dosage adjustment of the antifungal agent.

The effects of alcohol may be potentiated by griseofulvin, producing such effects as tachycardia and flush.

Griseofulvin may potentiate an increase in hepatic enzymes that metabolize estrogens at an increased rate, including the estrogen component of oral contraceptives, thereby causing possible decreased contraceptive effects and menstrual irregularities.

ADVERSE REACTIONS

When adverse reactions occur, they are most commonly of the hypersensitivity type, such as skin rashes, urticaria, and rarely, angioneurotic edema, and may necessitate withdrawal of therapy and appropriate countermeasures. Paresthesias of the hands and feet have been reported rarely after extended therapy. Other side effects reported occasionally are oral thrush, nausea, vomiting, epigastric distress, diarrhea, headache, fatigue, dizziness, insomnia, mental confusion, and impairment of performance of routine activities. Proteinuria, nephrosis, leukopenia, hepatic toxicity, GI bleeding and menstrual toxicity have been reported rarely. Administration of the drug should be discontinued if granulocytopenia occurs.

When rare, serious reactions occur with griseofulvin, they are usually associated with high dosages, long periods of therapy, or both.

DOSAGE AND ADMINISTRATION

Accurate diagnosis of the infecting organism is essential. Identification should be made either by direct microscopic examination of a mounting of infected tissue in a solution of potassium hydroxide or by culture on an appropriate medium.

Medication must be continued until the infecting organism is completely eradicated as indicated by appropriate clinical or laboratory examination. Representative treatment periods are tinea capitis, 4 to 6 weeks, tinea corporis, 2 to 4 weeks, tinea pedis, 4 to 8 weeks, tinea unguium—depending on rate of growth—fingernails, at least 4 months; toenails, at least 6 months.

General measures in regard to hygiene should be observed to control sources of infection or reinfection. Concomitant use of appropriate topical agents is usually required particularly in treatment of tinea pedis. In some forms of athlete's foot, yeasts and bacteria may be involved as well as fungi. Griseofulvin will not eradicate the bacterial or monilial infection.

Adults: Daily administration of 330 mg (as a single dose or in divided amounts) will give a satisfactory response in most patients with tinea corporis, tinea cruris, and tinea capitis. For those fungus infections more difficult to eradicate, such as tinea pedis and tinea unguium, a divided daily dosage of 660 mg is recommended.

Children: Approximately 3.3 mg per pound of body weight per day is an effective dose for most children. On this basis, the following dosage schedule is suggested: Children weighing 30 to 50 pounds—82.5 mg to 165 mg daily. Children weighing over 50 pounds—165 mg to 330 mg daily.

Children 2 years of age and younger—dosage has not been established.

Clinical experience with griseofulvin in children with tinea capitis indicates that a single daily dose is effective. Clinical relapse will occur if the medication is not continued until the infecting organism is eradicated.

HOW SUPPLIED

FULVICIN P/G 165 Tablets, 165 mg, off-white, oval, compressed, scored tablets impressed with the product name (FULVICIN P/G) and product identification numbers, 654; bottle of 100 (NDC 0085-0654-03).

Continued on next page

Schering—Cont.

FULVICIN P/G 330 Tablets, 330 mg, off-white, oval, compressed, scored tablets impressed with the product name (FULVICIN P/G) and product identification numbers, 352; bottle of 100 (NDC 0085-0352-03).

Store between 2° and 30°C (36° and 86°F).
Revised 4/87
Copyright © 1976, 1987, Schering Corporation, USA. All rights reserved.

Shown in Product Identification Section, page 428

FULVICIN-U/F®   ℞
[ful′vĭ-sin]
brand of griseofulvin,
    Tablets, USP

DESCRIPTION
FULVICIN-U/F Tablets contain microsize crystals of griseofulvin, an antibiotic derived from a species of *Penicillium*. Each FULVICIN-U/F Tablet contains 250 or 500 mg of microsized griseofulvin.
The inactive ingredients for FULVICIN-U/F Tablets, 250 or 500 mg, include: magnesium stearate, pluronic F-68 (poloxamer 188), potato starch, and silica.

ACTIONS
Microbiology: Griseofulvin is fungistatic with *in vitro* activity against various species of *Microsporum, Epidermophyton,* and *Trichophyton.* It has no effect on bacteria or on other genera of fungi.
Human Pharmacology: Griseofulvin absorption from the gastrointestinal tract varies considerably among individuals mainly because of insolubility of the drug in aqueous media of the upper G.I. tract. The peak serum level found in fasting adults given 0.5 g occurs at about four hours and ranges between 0.5 to 1.5 mcg/ml. The serum level may be increased by giving the drug with a meal with a high fat content.
Griseofulvin is deposited in the keratin precursor cells and has a greater affinity for diseased tissue. The drug is tightly bound to the new keratin which becomes highly resistant to fungal invasions.

INDICATIONS
FULVICIN-U/F Tablets are indicated for the treatment of ringworm infections of the skin, hair, and nails, namely: tinea corporis, tinea pedis, tinea cruris, tinea barbae, tinea capitis, tinea unguium (onychomycosis) when caused by one or more of the following genera of fungi: *Trichophyton rubrum, Trichophyton tonsurans, Trichophyton mentagrophytes, Trichophyton interdigitale, Trichophyton verrucosum, Trichophyton megninii, Trichophyton gallinae, Trichophyton crateriforme, Trichophyton sulphureum, Trichophyton schoenleinii, Microsporum audouini, Microsporum canis, Microsporum gypseum,* and *Epidermophyton floccosum.*
Note: Prior to therapy, the type of fungi responsible for the infection should be identified.
The use of this drug is not justified in minor or trivial infections which will respond to topical agents alone.
Griseofulvin is not effective in the following: bacterial infections, candidiasis (moniliasis), histoplasmosis, actinomycosis, sporotrichosis, chromoblastomycosis, coccidioidomycosis, North American blastomycosis, cryptococcosis (torulosis), tinea versicolor, and nocardiosis.

CONTRAINDICATIONS
This drug is contraindicated in patients with porphyria, hepatocellular failure, and in individuals with a history of hypersensitivity to griseofulvin.
Rare cases of conjoined twins have been reported in patients taking griseofulvin during the first trimester of pregnancy. Griseofulvin should not be prescribed to pregnant patients or to women contemplating pregnancy.

WARNINGS
Prophylactic usage: Safety and efficacy of griseofulvin for prophylaxis of fungal infections have not been established.
Animal toxicology: Chronic feeding of griseofulvin, at levels ranging from 0.5-2.5% of the diet, resulted in the development of liver tumors in several strains of mice, particularly in males. Smaller particle sizes result in an enhanced effect. Lower oral dosage levels have not been tested. Subcutaneous administration of relatively small doses of griseofulvin, once a week, during the first three weeks of life has also been reported to induce hepatomata in mice. Thyroid tumors, mostly adenomas but some carcinomas, have been reported in male rats receiving griseofulvin at levels of 2.0%, 1.0%, and 0.2% of the diet, and in female rats receiving the two higher dose levels. Although studies in other animal species have not yielded evidence of tumorigenicity, these studies were not of adequate design to form a basis for conclusions in this regard.
In subacute toxicity studies, orally administered griseofulvin produced hepatocellular necrosis in mice, but this has not been seen in other species. Disturbances in porphyrin metab-

olism have been reported in griseofulvin-treated laboratory animals. Griseofulvin has been reported to have a colchicine-like effect on mitosis and cocarcinogenicity with methylcholanthrene in cutaneous tumor induction in laboratory animals.
Usage in pregnancy: Griseofulvin should not be prescribed to pregnant patients or to women contemplating pregnancy (see **CONTRAINDICATIONS**).
Animal reproduction studies: It has been reported in the literature that griseofulvin was found to be embryotoxic and teratogenic on oral administration to pregnant rats. Pups with abnormalities have been reported in the litters of a few bitches treated with griseofulvin.
Suppression of spermatogenesis has been reported to occur in rats, but investigation in man failed to confirm this.

PRECAUTIONS
Patients on prolonged therapy with any potent medication should be under close observation. Periodic monitoring of organ system functions, including renal, hepatic, and hematopoietic, should be done.
Since griseofulvin is derived from species of *Penicillium,* the possibility of cross sensitivity with penicillin exists; however, known penicillin-sensitive patients have been treated without difficulty.
Since a photosensitivity reaction is occasionally associated with griseofulvin therapy, patients should be warned to avoid exposure to intense natural or artificial sunlight.
Lupus erythematosus or lupus-like syndromes, or exacerbation of existing lupus, have been reported in patients receiving griseofulvin.
Drug Interactions: Griseofulvin decreases the activity of warfarin-type anticoagulants so that patients receiving these drugs concomitantly may require dosage adjustment of the anticoagulant during and after griseofulvin therapy.
Barbiturates usually depress griseofulvin activity and concomitant administration may require a dosage adjustment of the antifungal agent.
The effects of alcohol may be potentiated by griseofulvin, producing such effects as tachycardia and flush.
Griseofulvin may potentiate an increase in hepatic enzymes that metabolize estrogens at an increased rate, including the estrogen component of oral contraceptives, thereby causing possible decreased contraceptive effects and menstrual irregularities.

ADVERSE REACTIONS
When adverse reactions occur, they are most commonly of the hypersensitivity type, such as skin rashes, urticaria, and rarely, angioneurotic edema, and may necessitate withdrawal of therapy and appropriate countermeasures. Paresthesias of the hands and feet have been reported rarely after extended therapy. Other side effects reported occasionally are oral thrush, nausea, vomiting, epigastric distress, diarrhea, headache, fatigue, dizziness, insomnia, mental confusion, and impairment of performance of routine activities. Proteinuria, nephrosis, leukopenia, hepatic toxicity, GI bleeding and menstrual irregularities have been reported rarely. Administration of the drug should be discontinued if granulocytopenia occurs.
When rare, serious reactions occur with griseofulvin, they are usually associated with high dosages, long periods of therapy, or both.

DOSAGE AND ADMINISTRATION
Accurate diagnosis of the infecting organism is essential. Identification should be made either by direct microscopic examination of a mounting of infected tissue in a solution of potassium hydroxide or by culture on an appropriate medium.
Medication must be continued until the infecting organism is completely eradicated as indicated by appropriate clinical or laboratory examination. Representative treatment periods are for tinea capitis, four to six weeks; tinea corporis, two to four weeks; tinea pedis, four to eight weeks; tinea unguium, depending on the rate of growth, fingernails, at least four months; toenails, at least six months.
General measures in regard to hygiene should be observed to control sources of infection or reinfection. Concomitant use of appropriate topical agents is usually required, particularly in treatment of tinea pedis. In some forms of athlete's foot, yeasts and bacteria may be involved as well as fungi. Griseofulvin will not eradicate the bacterial or monilial infection.
Adults: Daily administration of 500 mg (as a single dose or in divided amounts), will give a satisfactory response in most patients with tinea corporis, tinea cruris, and tinea capitis. For those fungus infections more difficult to eradicate, such as tinea pedis and tinea unguium, daily dosage of 1.0 g is recommended.
Children: Approximately 5 mg per pound of body weight per day is an effective dose for most children. On this basis the following dosage schedule for children is suggested:
Children weighing 30 to 50 pounds—125 mg to 250 mg daily.
Children weighing over 50 pounds—250 mg to 500 mg daily.
Clinical experience with griseofulvin in children with tinea capitis indicates that a single daily dose is effective. Clinical

relapse will occur if the medication is not continued until the infecting organism is eradicated.

HOW SUPPLIED
FULVICIN-U/F Tablets, 250 mg: white, compressed, scored tablets impressed with the Schering trademark and product identification letters, AUF, or numbers, 948; bottles of 60 (NDC 0085-0948-03) and 250 (NDC 0085-0948-06).
FULVICIN-U/F Tablets, 500 mg: white, compressed, scored tablets impressed with the Schering trademark and product identification letters, AUG, or numbers, 496; bottles of 60 (NDC 0085-0496-03) and 250 (NDC 0085-0496-06).
Store between 2° and 30° C (36° and 86° F).
Revised 4/87
Copyright © 1968, 1987, Schering Corporation, USA. All rights reserved.

Shown in Product Identification Section, page 428

GARAMYCIN®   ℞
[gar-ah-mī′sin]
brand of gentamicin sulfate
    Cream, USP 0.1%
    Ointment, USP 0.1%
For Dermatologic Use only
Not For Ophthalmic Use

DESCRIPTION
Each gram of GARAMYCIN **Cream** 0.1% contains 1.7 mg gentamicin sulfate, USP equivalent to 1.0 mg gentamicin base, with 1.0 mg methylparaben and 4.0 mg butylparaben as preservatives, in a bland emulsion-type vehicle composed of stearic acid, propylene glycol stearate, isopropyl myristate, propylene glycol, polysorbate 40, sorbitol solution and purified water.
Each gram of GARAMYCIN **Ointment** 0.1% contains 1.7 mg gentamicin sulfate, USP equivalent to 1.0 mg gentamicin base, with 0.5 mg methylparaben and 0.1 mg propylparaben as preservatives in a bland, unctuous petrolatum base.

ACTIONS
GARAMYCIN, a wide-spectrum antibiotic, provides highly effective topical treatment in primary and secondary bacterial infections of the skin. GARAMYCIN may clear infections that have not responded to other topical antibiotic agents. In impetigo contagiosa and other primary skin infections, treatment three or four times daily with GARAMYCIN usually clears the lesions promptly. In secondary skin infections, GARAMYCIN facilitates the treatment of the underlying dermatosis by controlling the infection. Bacteria susceptible to the action of GARAMYCIN include sensitive strains of streptococci (group A beta-hemolytic, alpha-hemolytic), *Staphylococcus aureus* (coagulase-positive, coagulase-negative, and some penicillinase-producing strains), and the gram-negative bacteria, *Pseudomonas aeruginosa, Aerobacter aerogenes, Escherichia coli, Proteus vulgaris,* and *Klebsiella pneumoniae.*

INDICATIONS
Primary skin infections: Impetigo contagiosa, superficial folliculitis, ecthyma, furunculosis, sycosis barbae, and pyoderma gangrenosum. *Secondary skin infections:* Infectious eczematoid dermatitis, pustular acne, pustular psoriasis, infected seborrheic dermatitis, infected contact dermatitis (including poison ivy), infected excoriations, and bacterial superinfections of fungal or viral infections. Note: GARAMYCIN is a bactericidal agent that is not effective against viruses or fungi in skin infections. GARAMYCIN is useful in the treatment of infected skin cysts and certain other skin abscesses when preceded by incision and drainage to permit adequate contact between the antibiotic and the infecting bacteria. Good results have been obtained in the treatment of infected stasis and other skin ulcers, infected superficial burns, paronychia, infected insect bites and stings, infected lacerations and abrasions, and wounds from minor surgery. Patients sensitive to neomycin can be treated with gentamicin, although regular observation of patients sensitive to topical antibiotics is advisable when such patients are treated with any topical antibiotic. GARAMYCIN **Ointment** helps retain moisture and has been useful in infection on dry eczematous or psoriatic skin. GARAMYCIN **Cream** is recommended for wet, oozing primary infections, and greasy, secondary infections, such as pustular acne or infected seborrheic dermatitis. If a water-washable preparation is desired, GARAMYCIN **Cream** is preferable. GARAMYCIN **Ointment** and **Cream** have been used successfully in infants over one year of age as well as in adults and children.

CONTRAINDICATIONS
This drug is contraindicated in individuals with a history of sensitivity reactions to any of its components.

PRECAUTIONS
Use of topical antibiotics occasionally allows overgrowth of nonsusceptible organisms, including fungi. If this occurs, or if irritation, sensitization, or superinfection develops, treatment with gentamicin should be discontinued and appropriate therapy instituted.

ADVERSE REACTIONS

In patients with dermatoses treated with gentamicin, irritation (erythema and pruritus) that did not usually require discontinuance of treatment has been reported in a small percentage of cases. There was no evidence of irritation or sensitization, however, in any of these patients patch-tested subsequently with gentamicin on normal skin. Possible photosensitization has been reported in several patients but could not be elicited in these patients by reapplication of gentamicin followed by exposure to ultraviolet radiation.

DOSAGE AND ADMINISTRATION

A small amount of GARAMYCIN **Cream** or **Ointment** should be applied gently to the lesions three or four times daily. The area treated may be covered with a gauze dressing if desired. In impetigo contagiosa, the crusts should be removed before application of GARAMYCIN to permit maximum contact between the antibiotic and the infection. Care should be exercised to avoid further contamination of the infected skin. Infected stasis ulcers have responded well to GARAMYCIN under gelatin packing.

HOW SUPPLIED

GARAMYCIN **Cream** 0.1% (NDC-0085-0008-05) and GARAMYCIN **Ointment** 0.1% (NDC-0085-0343-05), 15 g tubes. **Store between 2° and 30° C (36° and 86° F).**
Rev. 8/85
Copyright © 1966, 1981 Schering Corporation, USA. All rights reserved.

GARAMYCIN®   ℞

[gar-ah-mī'sin]
brand of gentamicin sulfate
  Ophthalmic Solution, USP—Sterile
  Ophthalmic Ointment, USP—Sterile
Each ml or gram contains gentamicin sulfate, USP equivalent to 3.0 mg gentamicin

DESCRIPTION

Gentamicin sulfate is a water-soluble antibiotic of the aminoglycoside group active against a wide variety of pathogenic gram-negative and gram-positive bacteria.
GARAMYCIN **Ophthalmic Solution** is a sterile, aqueous solution buffered to approximately pH 7 for use in the eye. Each ml. contains gentamicin sulfate, USP (equivalent to 3.0 mg gentamicin), disodium phosphate, monosodium phosphate, sodium chloride, and benzalkonium chloride as a preservative.
GARAMYCIN **Ophthalmic Ointment** is a sterile ointment, each gram containing gentamicin sulfate, USP (equivalent to 3.0 mg gentamicin) in a bland base of white petrolatum, with methylparaben and propylparaben as preservatives.

ACTIONS

The gram-positive bacteria against which gentamicin sulfate is active include coagulase-positive and coagulase-negative staphylococci, including certain strains that are resistant to penicillin; Group A beta-hemolytic and nonhemolytic streptococci; and *Diplococcus pneumoniae*. The gram-negative bacteria against which gentamicin sulfate is active include certain strains of *Pseudomonas aeruginosa*, indole-positive and indole-negative *Proteus* species, *Escherichia coli, Klebsiella pneumoniae* (Friedlander's bacillus), *Haemophilus influenza* and *Haemophilus aegyptius* (Koch-Weeks bacillus), *Aerobacter aerogenes, Moraxella lacunata* (diplobacillus of Morax-Axenfeld), and *Neisseria* species, including *Neisseria gonorrhoeae*. Although significant resistant organisms have not been isolated from patients treated with gentamicin at the present time, this may occur in the future as resistance has been produced with difficulty *in vitro* by repeated exposures.

INDICATIONS

GARAMYCIN **Ophthalmic Solution** and **Ointment** are indicated in the topical treatment of infections of the external eye and its adnexa caused by susceptible bacteria. Such infections embrace conjunctivitis, keratitis and keratoconjunctivitis, corneal ulcers, blepharitis and blepharoconjunctivitis, acute meibomianitis, and dacryocystitis.

CONTRAINDICATIONS

GARAMYCIN **Ophthalmic Solution** and **Ointment** are contraindicated in patients with known hypersensitivity to any of the components.

WARNINGS

GARAMYCIN **Ophthalmic Solution** is not for injection. It should never be injected subconjunctivally, nor should it be directly introduced into the anterior chamber of the eye.

PRECAUTIONS

Prolonged use of topical antibiotics may give rise to overgrowth of nonsusceptible organisms, such as fungi. Should this occur, or if irritation or hypersensitivity to any component of the drug develops, discontinue use of the preparation and institute appropriate therapy.

Ophthalmic ointments may retard corneal healing.

ADVERSE REACTIONS

Transient irritation has been reported with the use of GARAMYCIN **Ophthalmic Solution.**
Occasional burning or stinging may occur with the use of GARAMYCIN **Ophthalmic Ointment.**

DOSAGE AND ADMINISTRATION

GARAMYCIN **Ophthalmic Solution:** instill one or two drops into the affected eye every four hours. In severe infections, dosage may be increased to as much as two drops once every hour.
GARAMYCIN **Ophthalmic Ointment:** apply a small amount to the affected eye two to three times a day.

HOW SUPPLIED

GARAMYCIN **Ophthalmic Solution**—Sterile, 5 ml. plastic dropper bottle, box of one (NDC 0085-0899-05).
GARAMYCIN **Ophthalmic Ointment**—Sterile, 3.5 g, box of one (NDC 0085-0151-05).
Store GARAMYCIN Ophthalmic Ointment and Solution between 2° and 30°C (36° and 86°F).
Revised 8/85
Copyright © 1969, 1981, Schering Corporation, USA. All rights reserved.

GARAMYCIN® Injectable   ℞

[gar-ah-mī'sin]
brand of gentamicin sulfate injection, USP
  40 mg per ml
Each ml contains gentamicin sulfate, USP equivalent to 40 mg gentamicin.
For Parenteral Administration

WARNINGS

Patients treated with aminoglycosides should be under close clinical observation because of the potential toxicity associated with their use.
As with other aminoglycosides, GARAMYCIN Injectable is potentially nephrotoxic. The risk of nephrotoxicity is greater in patients with impaired renal function and in those who receive high dosage or prolonged therapy.
Neurotoxicity manifested by ototoxicity, both vestibular and auditory, can occur in patients treated with GARAMYCIN Injectable primarily in those with preexisting renal damage and in patients with normal renal function treated with higher doses and/or for longer periods than recommended. Aminoglycoside-induced ototoxicity is usually irreversible. Other manifestations of neurotoxicity may include numbness, skin tingling, muscle twitching and convulsions.
Renal and eighth cranial nerve function should be closely monitored, especially in patients with known or suspected reduced renal function at onset of therapy, and also in those whose renal function is initially normal but who develop signs of renal dysfunction during therapy. Urine should be examined for decreased specific gravity, increased excretion of protein, and the presence of cells or casts. Blood urea nitrogen, serum creatinine, or creatinine clearance should be determined periodically. When feasible, it is recommended that serial audiograms be obtained in patients old enough to be tested, particularly high-risk patients. Evidence of ototoxicity (dizziness, vertigo, tinnitus, roaring in the ears or hearing loss) or nephrotoxicity requires dosage adjustment or discontinuance of the drug.
As with the other aminoglycosides, on rare occasions changes in renal and eighth cranial nerve function may not become manifest until soon after completion of therapy.
Serum concentrations of aminoglycosides should be monitored when feasible to assure adequate levels and to avoid potentially toxic levels. When monitoring gentamicin peak concentrations, dosage should be adjusted so that prolonged levels above 12 mcg/ml are avoided. When monitoring gentamicin trough concentrations, dosage should be adjusted so that levels above 2 mcg/ml are avoided. Excessive peak and/ or trough serum concentrations of aminoglycosides may increase the risk of renal and eighth cranial nerve toxicity. In the event of overdose or toxic reactions, hemodialysis may aid in the removal of gentamicin from the blood, especially if renal function is, or becomes, compromised. The rate of removal of gentamicin is considerably less by peritoneal dialysis than by hemodialysis.
Concurrent and/or sequential systemic or topical use of other potentially neurotoxic and/or nephrotoxic drugs, such as cisplatin, cephaloridine, kanamycin, amikacin, neomycin, polymyxin B, colistin, paromomycin, streptomycin, tobramycin, vancomycin, and viomycin, should be avoided. Other factors which may increase patient risk of toxicity are advanced age and dehydration.

The concurrent use of gentamicin with potent diuretics, such as ethacrynic acid or furosemide, should be avoided, since certain diuretics by themselves may cause ototoxicity. In addition, when administered intravenously, diuretics may enhance aminoglycoside toxicity by altering the antibiotic concentration in serum and tissue.

DESCRIPTION

Gentamicin sulfate, USP, a water-soluble antibiotic of the aminoglycoside group, is derived from *Micromonospora purpurea*, an actinomycete. GARAMYCIN Injectable is a sterile, aqueous solution for parenteral administration. Each ml contains gentamicin sulfate, USP equivalent to 40 mg gentamicin base, 1.8 mg methylparaben and 0.2 mg propylparaben as preservatives, 3.2 mg sodium bisulfite, and 0.1 mg edetate disodium.

CLINICAL PHARMACOLOGY

After intramuscular administration of GARAMYCIN Injectable, peak serum concentrations usually occur between 30 and 60 minutes and serum levels are measurable for six to eight hours. When gentamicin is administered by intravenous infusion over a two-hour period, the serum concentrations are similar to those obtained by intramuscular administration.
In patients with normal renal function, peak serum concentrations of gentamicin (mcg/ml) are usually up to four times the single intramuscular dose (mg/kg); for example, a 1.0 mg/kg injection in adults may be expected to result in a peak serum concentration up to 4 mcg/ml; a 1.5 mg/kg dose may produce levels up to 6 mcg/ml. While some variation is to be expected due to a number of variables such as age, body temperature surface area and physiologic differences, the individual patient given the same dose tends to have similar levels in repeated determinations. Gentamicin administered at 1.0 mg/kg every eight hours for the usual 7- to 10-day treatment period to patients with normal renal function does not accumulate in serum.
Gentamicin, like all aminoglycosides, may accumulate in the serum and tissues of patients treated with higher doses and/or for prolonged periods, particularly in the presence of impaired renal function. In adult patients, treatment with gentamicin dosages of 4 mg/kg/day or higher for seven to ten days may result in a slight, progressive rise in both peak and trough concentrations. In patients with impaired renal function, gentamicin is cleared from the body more slowly than in patients with normal renal function. The more severe the impairment, the slower the clearance. (Dosage must be adjusted.)
Since gentamicin is distributed in extracellular fluid, peak serum concentrations may be lower than usual in adult patients who have a large volume of this fluid. Serum concentrations of gentamicin in febrile patients may be lower than those in afebrile patients given the same dose. When body temperature returns to normal, serum concentrations of the drug may rise. Febrile and anemic states may be associated with a shorter than usual serum half-life. (Dosage adjustment is usually not necessary.) In severely burned patients, the half-life may be significantly decreased and resulting serum concentrations may be lower than anticipated from the mg/kg dose.
Protein-binding studies have indicated that the degree of gentamicin binding is low; depending upon the methods used for testing, this may be between 0 and 30%.
After initial administration to patients with normal renal function, generally 70% or more of the gentamicin dose is recoverable in the urine in 24 hours; concentrations in urine above 100 mcg/ml may be achieved. Little, if any, metabolic transformation occurs; the drug is excreted principally by glomerular filtration. After several days of treatment, the amount of gentamicin excreted in the urine approaches the daily dose administered. As with other aminoglycosides, a small amount of the gentamicin dose may be retained in the tissues, especially in the kidneys. Minute quantities of aminoglycosides have been detected in the urine weeks after drug administration was discontinued. Renal clearance of gentamicin is similar to that of endogenous creatinine.
In patients with marked impairment of renal function, there is a decrease in the concentration of aminoglycosides in urine and in their penetration into defective renal parenchyma. This decreased drug excretion, together with the potential nephrotoxicity of aminoglycosides, should be considered when treating such patients who have urinary tract infections.
Probenecid does not affect renal tubular transport of gentamicin.
The endogenous creatinine clearance rate and the serum creatinine level have a high correlation with the half-life of

Continued on next page

Schering—Cont.

gentamicin in serum. Results of these tests may serve as guides for adjusting dosage in patients with renal impairment (see DOSAGE AND ADMINISTRATION).

Following parenteral administration, gentamicin can be detected in serum, lymph, tissues, sputum, and in pleural, synovial, and peritoneal fluids. Concentrations in renal cortex sometimes may be eight times higher than the usual serum levels. Concentrations in bile, in general, have been low and have suggested minimal biliary excretion. Gentamicin crosses the peritoneal as well as the placental membranes. Since aminoglycosides diffuse poorly into the subarachnoid space after parenteral administration, concentrations of gentamicin in cerebrospinal fluid are often low and dependent upon dose, rate of penetration, and degree of meningeal inflammation. There is minimal penetration of gentamicin into ocular tissues following intramuscular or intravenous administration.

Microbiology: *In vitro* tests have demonstrated that gentamicin is a bactericidal antibiotic which acts by inhibiting normal protein synthesis in susceptible microorganisms. It is active against a wide variety of pathogenic bacteria including *Escherichia coli*, *Proteus* species, (indole-positive and indole-negative), *Pseudomonas aeruginosa*, species of the *Klebsiella-Enterobacter-Serratia* group. *Citrobacter* species and *Staphylococcus* species (including penicillin- and methicillin-resistant strains). Gentamicin is also active *in vitro* against species of *Salmonella* and *Shigella*. The following bacteria are usually resistant to aminoglycoside: *Streptococcus pneumoniae*, most species of streptococci, particularly group D and anaerobic organisms, such as *Bacteroides* species or *Clostridium* species.

In vitro studies have shown that an aminoglycoside combined with an antibiotic that interferes with cell wall synthesis may act synergistically against some group D streptococcal strains. The combination of gentamicin and penicillin G has a synergistic bactericidal effect against virtually all strains of *Streptococcus faecalis* and its varieties (S. faecalis var. *liquifaciens, S. faecalis* var. *zymogenes), S. faecium* and *S. durans*. An enhanced killing effect against many of these strains has also been shown *in vitro* with combinations of gentamicin and ampicillin, carbenicillin, nafcillin, or oxacillin.

The combined effect of gentamicin and carbenicillin is synergistic for many strains of *Pseudomonas aeruginosa*. *In vitro* synergism against other gram-negative organisms has been shown with combinations of gentamicin and cephalosporins. Gentamicin may be active against clinical isolates of bacteria resistant to other aminoglycosides. Bacteria resistant to one aminoglycoside may be resistant to one or more other aminoglycosides. Bacterial resistance to gentamicin is generally developed slowly.

Susceptibility Testing: If the disc method of susceptibility testing used is that described by Bauer *et al*. (*Am J Clin Path* 45:493, 1966; *Federal Register* 37:20525-20529, 1972), a disc containing 10 mcg of gentamicin should give a zone of inhibition of 15mm or more to indicate susceptibility of the infecting organism. A zone of 12mm or less indicates that the infecting organism is likely to be resistant. Zones greater than 12mm and less than 15mm indicate intermediate susceptibility. In certain conditions it may be desirable to do additional susceptibility testing by the tube or agar dilution method; gentamicin substance is available for this purpose.

INDICATIONS AND USAGE

GARAMYCIN Injectable is indicated in the treatment of serious infections caused by susceptible strains of the following microorganisms: *Pseudomonas aeruginosa, Proteus* species (indole-positive and indole-negative), *Escherichia coli, Klebsiella-Enterobacter-Serratia* species, *Citrobacter* species and *Staphylococcus* species (coagulase-positive and coagulase-negative).

Clinical studies have shown GARAMYCIN Injectable to be effective in bacterial neonatal sepsis; bacterial septicemia; and serious bacterial infections of the central nervous system (meningitis), urinary tract, respiratory tract, gastrointestinal tract (including peritonitis), skin, bone and soft tissue (including burns). Aminoglycosides, including gentamicin, are not indicated in uncomplicated initial episodes of urinary tract infections unless the causative organisms are susceptible to these antibiotics and are not susceptible to antibiotics having less potential for toxicity.

Specimens for bacterial culture should be obtained to isolate and identify causative organisms and to determine their susceptibility to gentamicin.

GARAMYCIN may be considered as initial therapy in suspected or confirmed gram-negative infections, and therapy may be instituted before obtaining results of susceptibility testing. The decision to continue therapy with this drug should be based on the results of susceptibility tests, the severity of the infection, and the important additional concepts contained in the "WARNINGS Box" above. If the causative organisms are resistant to gentamicin, other appropriate therapy should be instituted.

In serious infections when the causative organisms are unknown, GARAMYCIN may be administered as initial therapy in conjunction with a penicillin-type or cephalosporin-type drug before obtaining results of susceptibility testing. If anaerobic organisms are suspected as etiologic agents, consideration should be given to using other suitable antimicrobial therapy in conjunction with gentamicin. Following identification of the organism and its susceptibility, appropriate antibiotic therapy should then be continued.

GARAMYCIN has been used effectively in combination with carbenicillin for the treatment of life-threatening infections caused by *Pseudomonas aeruginosa*. It has also been found effective when used in conjunction with a penicillin-type drug for the treatment of endocarditis caused by group D streptococci.

GARAMYCIN Injectable has also been shown to be effective in the treatment of serious staphylococcal infections. While not the antibiotic of first choice, GARAMYCIN Injectable may be considered when penicillins or other less potentially toxic drugs are contraindicated and bacterial susceptibility tests and clinical judgment indicate its use. It may also be considered in mixed infections caused by susceptible strains of staphylococci and gram-negative organisms.

In the neonate with suspected bacterial sepsis or staphylococcal pneumonia, a penicillin-type drug is also usually indicated as concomitant therapy with gentamicin.

CONTRAINDICATIONS

Hypersensitivity to gentamicin is a contraindication to its use. A history of hypersensitivity or serious toxic reactions to other aminoglycosides may contraindicate use of gentamicin because of the known cross-sensitivity of patients to drugs in this class.

WARNINGS

(See boxed **WARNINGS**.) Aminoglycosides can cause fetal harm when administered to a pregnant woman. Aminoglycoside antibiotics cross the placenta, and there have been several reports of total irreversible bilateral congenital deafness in children whose mothers received streptomycin during pregnancy. Serious side effects to mother, fetus, or newborn have not been reported in the treatment of pregnant women with other aminoglycosides. Animal reproduction studies conducted on rats and rabbits did not reveal evidence of impaired fertility or harm to the fetus due to gentamicin sulfate.

It is not known whether gentamicin sulfate can cause fetal harm when administered to a pregnant woman or can affect reproduction capacity. If gentamicin is used during pregnancy or if the patient becomes pregnant while taking gentamicin, she should be apprised of the potential hazard to the fetus.

GARAMYCIN Injectable contains sodium bisulfite, a sulfite that may cause allergic-type reactions including anaphylactic symptoms and life-threatening or less severe asthmatic episodes in certain susceptible people. The overall prevalence of sulfite sensitivity in the general population is unknown and probably low. Sulfite sensitivity is seen more frequently in asthmatic than in nonasthmatic people.

PRECAUTIONS

Neurotoxic and nephrotoxic antibiotics may be absorbed in significant quantities from body surfaces after local irrigation or application. The potential toxic effect of antibiotics administered in this fashion should be considered.

Increased nephrotoxicity has been reported following concomitant administration of aminoglycoside antibiotics and cephalosporins.

Neuromuscular blockade and respiratory paralysis have been reported in the cat receiving high doses (40 mg/kg) of gentamicin. The possibility of these phenomena occurring in man should be considered if aminoglycosides are administered by any route to patients receiving anesthetics, or to patients receiving neuromuscular blocking agents, such as succinylcholine, tubocurarine, or decamethonium, or in patients receiving massive transfusions of citrate-anticoagulated blood. If neuromuscular blockade occurs, calcium salts may reverse it.

Aminoglycosides should be used with caution in patients with neuromuscular disorders, such as myasthenia gravis, since these drugs may aggravate muscle weakness because of their potential curare-like effects on the neuromuscular junction. During or following gentamicin therapy, paresthesias, tetany, positive Chvostek and Trousseau signs, and mental confusion have been described in patients with hypomagnesemia, hypocalcemia, and hypokalemia. When this has occurred in infants, tetany and muscle weakness have been described. Both adults and infants required appropriate corrective electrolyte therapy.

Elderly patients may have reduced renal function which may not be evident in the results of routine screening tests, such as BUN or serum creatinine. A creatinine clearance determination may be more useful. Monitoring of renal function during treatment with gentamicin, as with other aminoglycosides, is particularly important in such patients. A Fanconi-like syndrome, with aminoaciduria and metabolic acido-

sis, has been reported in some adults and infants being given gentamicin injections.

Cross-allergenicity among aminoglycosides has been demonstrated.

Patients should be well hydrated during treatment.

Although the *in vitro* mixing of gentamicin and carbenicillin results in a rapid and significant inactivation of gentamicin, this interaction has not been demonstrated in patients with normal renal function who received both drugs by different routes of administration. A reduction in gentamicin serum half-life has been reported in patients with severe renal impairment receiving carbenicillin concomitantly with gentamicin.

Treatment with gentamicin may result in overgrowth of nonsusceptible organisms. If this occurs, appropriate therapy is indicated.

See "WARNINGS Box" regarding concurrent use of potent diuretics and regarding concurrent and/or sequential use of other neurotoxic and/or nephrotoxic antibiotics and for other essential information.

Usage in Pregnancy—Safety for use in pregnancy has not been established.

ADVERSE REACTIONS

Nephrotoxicity Adverse renal effects, as demonstrated by the presence of casts, cells, or protein in the urine or by rising BUN, NPN, serum creatinine or oliguria, have been reported. They occur more frequently in patients with a history of renal impairment and in patients treated for longer periods or with larger dosage than recommended.

Neurotoxicity Serious adverse effects on both vestibular and auditory branches of the eighth cranial nerves have been reported, primarily in patients with renal impairment (especially if dialysis is required), and in patients on high doses and/or prolonged therapy. Symptoms include dizziness, vertigo, tinnitus, roaring in the ears and hearing loss, which, as with the other aminoglycosides, may be irreversible. Hearing loss is usually manifested initially by diminution of high-tone acuity. Other factors which may increase the risk of toxicity include excessive dosage, dehydration and previous exposure to other ototoxic drugs.

Peripheral neuropathy or encephalopathy, including numbness, skin tingling, muscle twitching, convulsions, and a myasthenia gravis-like syndrome, have been reported.

Note: The risk of toxic reactions is low in patients with normal renal function who do not receive GARAMYCIN Injectable at higher doses or for longer periods of time than recommended.

Other reported adverse reactions possibly related to gentamicin include: respiratory depression, lethargy, confusion, depression, visual disturbances, decreased appetite, weight loss, and hypotension and hypertension; rash, itching, urticaria, generalized burning, laryngeal edema, anaphylactoid reactions, fever, and headache, nausea, vomiting, increased salivation, and stomatitis; purpura, pseudotumor cerebri, acute organic brain syndrome, pulmonary fibrosis, alopecia, joint pain, transient hepatomegaly, and splenomegaly.

Laboratory abnormalities possibly related to gentamicin include: increased levels of serum transaminase (SGOT, SGPT), serum LDH and bilirubin; decreased serum calcium, magnesium, sodium and potassium; anemia, leukopenia, granulocytopenia, transient agranulocytosis, eosinophilia, increased and decreased reticulocyte counts, and thrombocytopenia. While clinical laboratory test abnormalities may be isolated findings, they may also be associated with clinically related signs and symptoms. For example, tetany and muscle weakness may be associated with hypomagnesemia, hypocalcemia, and hypokalemia.

While local tolerance of GARAMYCIN Injectable is generally excellent, there has been an occasional report of pain at the injection site. Subcutaneous atrophy or fat necrosis suggesting local irritation has been reported rarely.

OVERDOSAGE

In the event of overdose or toxic reactions, hemodialysis may aid in the removal of gentamicin from the blood, and is especially important if renal function is, or becomes, compromised. The rate of removal of gentamicin is considerably less by peritoneal dialysis than it is by hemodialysis.

DOSAGE AND ADMINISTRATION

GARAMYCIN Injectable may be given intramuscularly or intravenously. The patient's pretreatment body weight should be obtained for calculation of correct dosage. The dosage of aminoglycosides in obese patients should be based on an estimate of the lean body mass. It is desirable to limit the duration of treatment with aminoglycosides to short term.

DOSAGE FOR PATIENTS WITH NORMAL RENAL FUNCTION

Adults: The recommended dosage of GARAMYCIN Injectable for patients with serious infections and normal renal function is 3 mg/kg/day, administered in three equal doses every eight hours (Table I).

For patients with life-threatening infections, dosages up to 5 mg/kg/day may be administered in three or four equal doses. This dosage should be reduced to 3 mg/kg/day as soon as clinically indicated (Table I).

It is desirable to measure periodically both peak and trough serum concentrations of gentamicin when feasible during therapy to assure adequate but not excessive drug levels. For example, the peak concentration (at 30 to 60 minutes after intramuscular injection) is expected to be in the range of 4 to 6 mcg/ml. When monitoring peak concentrations after intramuscular or intravenous administration, dosage should be adjusted so that prolonged levels above 12 mcg/ml are avoided. When monitoring trough concentrations (just prior to the next dose), dosage should be adjusted so that levels above 2 mcg/ml are avoided. Determination of the adequacy of a serum level for a particular patient must take into consideration the susceptibility of the causative organism, the severity of the infection, and the status of the patient's host-defense mechanisms.

In patients with extensive burns, altered pharmacokinetics may result in reduced serum concentrations of aminoglycosides. In such patients treated with gentamicin, measurement of serum concentrations is recommended as a basis for dosage adjustment.

TABLE I
DOSAGE SCHEDULE GUIDE FOR ADULTS WITH NORMAL RENAL FUNCTION
(Dosage at Eight-Hour Intervals)
40 mg per ml

Patient's Weight*		Usual Dose For Serious Infections 1 mg/kg q8h (3 mg/kg/day)		Dose for Life-Threatening Infections (Reduce as Soon as Clinically Indicated) 1.7 mg/kg q8h** (5 mg/kg/day)	
kg	(lb)	$\frac{mg}{dose}$ q8h	$\frac{ml}{dose}$	$\frac{mg}{dose}$ q8h	$\frac{ml}{dose}$
40	(88)	40	1.0	66	1.6
45	(99)	45	1.1	75	1.9
50	(110)	50	1.25	83	2.1
55	(121)	55	1.4	91	2.25
60	(132)	60	1.5	100	2.5
65	(143)	65	1.6	108	2.7
70	(154)	70	1.75	116	2.9
75	(165)	75	1.9	125	3.1
80	(176)	80	2.0	133	3.3
85	(187)	85	2.1	141	3.5
90	(198)	90	2.25	150	3.75
95	(209)	95	2.4	158	4.0
100	(220)	100	2.5	166	4.2

* The dosage of aminoglycosides in obese patients should be based on an estimate of the lean body mass.
** For q6h schedules, dosage should be recalculated.

Children: 6 to 7.5 mg/kg/day. (2.0 to 2.5 mg/kg administered every 8 hours.)
Infants and Neonates: 7.5 mg/kg/day. (2.5 mg/kg administered every 8 hours.)
Premature or Full-Term Neonates One Week of Age or Less: 5 mg/kg/day. (2.5 mg/kg administered every 12 hours.)
For further information concerning the use of gentamicin in infants and children, see GARAMYCIN Pediatric Injectable Product Information.

The usual duration of treatment for all patients is seven to ten days. In difficult and complicated infections, a longer course of therapy may be necessary. In such cases, monitoring of renal, auditory, and vestibular functions is recommended, since toxicity is more apt to occur with treatment extended for more than ten days. Dosage should be reduced if clinically indicated.

For Intravenous Administration
The intravenous administration of gentamicin may be particularly useful for treating patients with bacterial septicemia or those in shock. It may also be the preferred route of administration for some patients with congestive heart failure, hematologic disorders, severe burns, or those with reduced muscle mass. For intermittent intravenous administration in adults, a single dose of GARAMYCIN Injectable may be diluted in 50 to 200 ml of sterile isotonic saline solution or in a sterile solution of dextrose 5% in water; in infants and children, the volume of diluent should be less. The solution may be infused over a period of one-half to two hours.

The recommended dosage for intravenous and intramuscular administration is identical.

GARAMYCIN Injectable should not be physically premixed with other drugs, but should be administered separately in accordance with the recommended route of administration and dosage schedule.

DOSAGE FOR PATIENTS WITH IMPAIRED RENAL FUNCTION
Dosage must be adjusted in patients with impaired renal function to assure therapeutically adequate, but not excessive, blood levels. Whenever possible, serum concentrations of gentamicin should be monitored. One method of dosage adjustment is to increase the interval between administration of the usual doses. Since the serum creatinine concentration has a high correlation with the serum half-life of gentamicin, this laboratory test may provide guidance for adjustment of the interval between doses. The interval between doses (in hours) may be approximated by multiplying the serum creatinine level (mg/100 ml) by 8. For example, a patient weighing 60 kg with a serum creatinine level of 2.0 mg/100 ml could be given 60 mg (1 mg/kg) every 16 hours (2×8).

In patients with serious systemic infections and renal impairment, it may be desirable to administer the antibiotic more frequently but in reduced dosage. In such patients, serum concentrations of gentamicin should be measured so that adequate but not excessive levels result. A peak and trough concentration measured intermittently during therapy will provide optimal guidance for adjusting dosage. After the usual initial dose, a rough guide for determining reduced dosage at eight-hour intervals is to divide the normally recommended dose by the serum creatinine level (Table II). For example, after an initial dose of 60 mg (1 mg/kg), a patient weighing 60 kg with a serum creatinine level of 2.0 mg/100 ml could be given 30 mg every eight hours $(60 \div 2)$. It should be noted that the status of renal function may be changing over the course of the infectious process. It is important to recognize that deteriorating renal function may require a greater reduction in dosage than that specified in the above guidelines for patients with stable renal impairment.

TABLE II
DOSAGE ADJUSTMENT GUIDE FOR PATIENTS WITH RENAL IMPAIRMENT
(Dosage at Eight-Hour Intervals After the Usual Initial Dose)

Serum Creatinine (mg %)	Approximate Creatinine Clearance Rate (ml/min/1.73M^2)	Percent of Usual Doses Shown in Table I
≤ 1.0	> 100	100
1.1–1.3	70–100	80
1.4–1.6	55–70	65
1.7–1.9	45–55	55
2.0–2.2	40–45	50
2.3–2.5	35–40	40
2.6–3.0	30–35	35
3.1–3.5	25–30	30
3.6–4.0	20–25	25
4.1–5.1	15–20	20
5.2–6.6	10–15	15
6.7–8.0	< 10	10

In adults with renal failure undergoing hemodialysis, the amount of gentamicin removed from the blood may vary depending upon several factors including the dialysis method used. An eight-hour hemodialysis may reduce serum concentrations of gentamicin by approximately 50%. The recommended dosage at the end of each dialysis period is 1 to 1.7 mg/kg depending upon the severity of infection. In children, a dose of 2 mg/kg may be administered.

The above dosage schedules are not intended as rigid recommendations but are provided as guides to dosage when the measurement of gentamicin serum levels is not feasible.

A variety of methods are available to measure gentamicin concentrations in body fluids; these include microbiologic, enzymatic and radioimmunoassay techniques.

HOW SUPPLIED
GARAMYCIN Injectable, 40 mg per ml, for parenteral administration, is supplied in 2 ml (80 mg) vials, boxes of 25 (NDC 0085-0069-04); 20 ml vials, box of 5 (NDC 0085-0069-08); and in 1.5 ml (60 mg) (NDC 0085-0069-05) and 2 ml (80 mg) (NDC 0085-0069-06) disposable syringes, each in boxes of 1 and 10.

Also available, GARAMYCIN Pediatric Injectable, 10 mg per ml, for parenteral administration, supplied in 2 ml (20 mg) vials, box of one (NDC 0085-0013-05).

GARAMYCIN Injectable is a clear, stable solution that requires no refrigeration.

Store between 2° and 30°C (36° and 86°F).
Schering Pharmaceutical Corporation (PR)
Manati, Puerto Rico 00701
An Affiliate of Schering Corporation
Kenilworth, NJ 07033
Copyright © 1968, 1983, 1986, 1987, Schering Corporation, USA. All rights reserved.
Revised 1/87

GARAMYCIN® PEDIATRIC
[gar-ah-mī'sin]
Injectable
brand of gentamicin sulfate injection, USP
10 mg per ml
Each ml contains gentamicin sulfate, USP equivalent to 10 mg gentamicin.
For Parenteral Administration

WARNINGS
Patients treated with aminoglycosides should be under close clinical observation because of the potential toxicity associated with their use.

As with other aminoglycosides, GARAMYCIN Pediatric Injectable is potentially nephrotoxic. The risk of nephrotoxicity is greater in patients with impaired renal function and in those who receive high dosage or prolonged therapy.

Neurotoxicity manifested by ototoxicity, both vestibular and auditory, can occur in patients treated with GARAMYCIN Pediatric Injectable, primarily in those with pre-existing renal damage and in patients with normal renal function treated with higher doses and/or for longer periods than recommended. Aminoglycoside-induced ototoxicity is usually irreversible. Other manifestations of neurotoxicity may include numbness, skin tingling, muscle twitching, and convulsions.

Renal and eighth cranial nerve function should be closely monitored, especially in patients with known or suspected reduced renal function at onset of therapy, and also in those whose renal function is initially normal but who develop signs of renal dysfunction during therapy. Urine should be examined for decreased specific gravity, increased excretion of protein, and the presence of cells or casts. Blood urea nitrogen, serum creatinine, or creatinine clearance should be determined periodically. When feasible, it is recommended that serial audiograms be obtained in patients old enough to be tested, particularly high-risk patients. Evidence of ototoxicity (dizziness, vertigo, tinnitus, roaring in the ears or hearing loss) or nephrotoxicity requires dosage adjustment or discontinuance of the drug. As with the other aminoglycosides, on rare occasions changes in renal and eighth cranial nerve function may not become manifest until soon after completion of therapy.

Serum concentrations of aminoglycosides should be monitored when feasible to assure adequate levels and to avoid potentially toxic levels. When monitoring gentamicin peak concentrations, dosage should be adjusted so that prolonged levels above 12 mcg/ml are avoided. When monitoring gentamicin trough concentrations, dosage should be adjusted so that levels above 2 mcg/ml are avoided. Excessive peak and/or trough serum concentrations of aminoglycosides may increase the risk of renal and eighth cranial nerve toxicity. In the event of overdose or toxic reactions, hemodialysis may aid in the removal of gentamicin from the blood, especially if renal function is, or becomes, compromised. The rate of removal of gentamicin is considerably less by peritoneal dialysis than by hemodialysis.

In the newborn infant, exchange transfusions may also be considered.

Concurrent and/or sequential systemic or topical use of other potentially neurotoxic and/or nephrotoxic drugs, such as cisplatin, cephaloridine, kanamycin, amikacin, neomycin, polymyxin B, colistin, paromomycin, streptomycin, tobramycin, vancomycin, and viomycin, should be avoided. Another factor which may increase patient risk of toxicity is dehydration.

The concurrent use of gentamicin with potent diuretics, such as ethacrynic acid or furosemide, should be avoided, since certain diuretics by themselves may cause ototoxicity. In addition, when administered intravenously, diuretics may enhance aminoglycoside toxicity by altering the antibiotic concentration in serum and tissue.

DESCRIPTION
Gentamicin sulfate, USP, a water-soluble antibiotic of the aminoglycoside group, is derived from *Micromonospora purpurea*, an actinomycete. GARAMYCIN Pediatric Injectable is a sterile, aqueous solution for parenteral administration. Each ml contains gentamicin sulfate, USP equivalent to 10 mg gentamicin base, 1.3 mg methylparaben and 0.2 mg propylparaben as preservatives, 3.2 mg sodium bisulfite and 0.1 mg edetate disodium.

Continued on next page

Information on Schering products appearing on these pages is effective as of September 30, 1989.

Schering—Cont.

CLINICAL PHARMACOLOGY

After intramuscular administration of GARAMYCIN Pediatric Injectable, peak serum concentrations usually occur between 30 and 60 minutes and serum levels are measurable for 6 to 12 hours. In infants, a single dose of 2.5 mg/kg usually provides a peak serum level in the range of 3 to 5 mcg/ml. When gentamicin is administered by intravenous infusion over a two-hour period, the serum concentrations are similar to those obtained by intramuscular administration. Age markedly affects the peak concentrations: in one report, a 1 mg/kg dose produced mean peak concentrations of 1.58, 2.03, and 2.81 mcg/ml in patients 6 months to 5 years old, 5 to 10 years old, and over 10 years old, respectively. In infants one week to six months of age, the half-life is 3 to 3½ hours. In full-term and large premature infants less than one week old, the approximate serum half-life of gentamicin is 5½ hours. In small premature infants, the half-life is inversely related to birth weight. In premature infants weighing less than 1500 grams, the half-life is 11½ hours; in those weighing 1500 to 2000 grams, the half-life is 8 hours; in those weighing over 2000 grams, the half-life is approximately 5 hours. While some variation is to be expected due to a number of variables such as age, body temperature, surface area and physiologic differences, the individual patient given the same dose tends to have similar levels in repeated determinations.

Gentamicin, like all aminoglycosides, may accumulate in the serum and tissues of patients treated with higher doses and/or for prolonged periods, particularly in the presence of impaired or immature renal function. In patients with immature or impaired renal function, gentamicin is cleared from the body more slowly than in patients with normal renal function. The more severe the impairment, the slower the clearance. (Dosage must be adjusted.)

Since gentamicin is distributed in extracellular fluid, peak serum concentrations may be lower than usual in patients who have a large volume of this fluid. Serum concentrations of gentamicin in febrile patients may be lower than those in afebrile patients given the same dose. When body temperature returns to normal, serum concentrations of the drug may rise. Febrile and anemic states may be associated with a shorter than usual serum half-life. (Dosage adjustment is usually not necessary.) In severely burned patients, the half-life may be significantly decreased and resulting serum concentrations may be lower than anticipated from the mg/kg/dose.

Protein-binding studies have indicated that the degree of gentamicin binding is low, depending upon the methods used for testing, this may be between 0 and 30%.

In neonates less than 3 days old, approximately 10% of the administered dose is excreted in 12 hours; in infants 5 to 40 days old, approximately 40% is excreted over the same period. Excretion of gentamicin correlates with postnatal age and creatinine clearance. Thus, with increasing postnatal age and concomitant increase in renal maturity, gentamicin is excreted more rapidly. Little, if any metabolic transformation occurs; the drug is excreted principally by glomerular filtration. After several days of treatment, the amount of gentamicin excreted in the urine approaches, but does not equal, the daily dose administered. As with other aminoglycosides, a small amount of the gentamicin dose may be retained in the tissues, especially in the kidneys. Minute quantities of aminoglycosides have been detected in the urine of some patients weeks after drug administration was discontinued. Renal clearance of gentamicin is similar to that of endogenous creatinine.

In patients with marked impairment of renal function, there is a decrease in the concentration of aminoglycosides in urine and in their penetration into defective renal parenchyma. This decreased drug excretion, together with the potential nephrotoxicity of aminoglycosides, should be considered when treating such patients who have urinary tract infections.

Probenecid does not affect renal tubular transport of gentamicin.

The endogenous creatinine clearance rate and the serum creatinine level have a high correlation with the half-life of gentamicin in serum. Results of these tests may serve as guides for adjusting dosage in patients with renal impairment (see DOSAGE AND ADMINISTRATION).

Following parenteral administration, gentamicin can be detected in serum, lymph, tissues, sputum and in pleural, synovial, peritoneal fluids. Concentrations in renal cortex sometimes may be eight times higher than the usual serum levels. Concentrations in bile, in general, have been low and have suggested minimal biliary excretion. Gentamicin crosses the peritoneal as well as the placental membranes. Since aminoglycosides diffuse poorly into the subarachnoid space after parenteral administration, concentrations of gentamicin in cerebrospinal fluid are often low and dependent upon dose, rate of penetration, and degree of meningeal inflammation. There is minimal penetration of gentamicin into ocular tissues following intramuscular or intravenous administration.

Microbiology: *In vitro* tests have demonstrated that gentamicin is a bactericidal antibiotic which acts by inhibiting normal protein synthesis in susceptible microorganisms. It is active against a wide variety of pathogenic bacteria including *Escherichia coli*, *Proteus* species (indole-positive and indole-negative), *Pseudomonas aeruginosa*, species of *Klebsiella-Enterobacter-Serratia* group, *Citrobacter* species, and *Staphylococcus* species (including penicillin- and methicillin-resistant strains). Gentamicin is also active *in vitro* against species of *Salmonella* and *Shigella*. The following bacteria are usually resistant to aminoglycosides: *Streptococcus pneumoniae*, most species of streptococci, particularly group D and anaerobic organisms, such as *Bacteroides* species or *Clostridium* species.

In vitro studies have shown that an aminoglycoside combined with an antibiotic that interferes with cell wall synthesis may act synergistically against some group D streptococcal strains. The combination of gentamicin and penicillin G has a synergistic bactericidal effect against virtually all strains of *Streptococcus faecalis* and its varieties (*S. faecalis* var. *liquifaciens, S. faecalis* var. *zymogenes), S. faecium* and *S. durans*. An enhanced killing effect against many of these strains has also been shown *in vitro* with combinations of gentamicin and ampicillin, carbenicillin, nafcillin, or oxacillin.

The combined effect of gentamicin and carbenicillin is synergistic for many strains of *Pseudomonas aeruginosa*. *In vitro* synergism against other gram-negative organisms has been shown with combinations of gentamicin and cephalosporins. Gentamicin may be active against clinical isolates of bacteria resistant to other aminoglycosides. Bacteria resistant to one aminoglycoside may be resistant to one or more other aminoglycosides. Bacterial resistance to gentamicin is generally developed slowly.

Susceptibility Testing: If the disc method of susceptibility testing used is that described by Bauer *et al* (*Am J Clin Path* 45:493, 1966; *Federal Register* 37:20525–20529, 1972), a disc containing 10 mcg of gentamicin should give a zone of inhibition of 15 mm or more to indicate susceptibility of the infecting organism. A zone of 12 mm or less indicates that the infecting organism is likely to be resistant. Zones greater than 12mm and less than 15mm indicate intermediate susceptibility. In certain conditions it may be desirable to do additional susceptibility testing by the tube or agar dilution method; gentamicin substance is available for this purpose.

INDICATIONS AND USAGE

GARAMYCIN Pediatric Injectable is indicated in the treatment of serious infections caused by susceptible strains of the following microorganisms: *Pseudomonas aeruginosa*, *Proteus* species (indole-positive and indole-negative), *Escherichia coli*, *Klebsiella-Enterobacter-Serratia* species, *Citrobacter* species, and *Staphyloccous* species (coagulase-positive and coagulase-negative).

Clinical studies have shown GARAMYCIN Pediatric Injectable to be effective in bacterial neonatal sepsis; bacterial septicemia; and serious bacterial infections of the central nervous system (meningitis), urinary tract, respiratory tract, gastrointestinal tract (including peritonitis), skin, bone and soft tissue (including burns).

Aminoglycosides, including gentamicin, are not indicated in uncomplicated initial episodes of urinary tract infections unless the causative organisms are susceptible to these antibiotics and are not susceptible to antibiotics having less potential for toxicity.

Specimens for bacterial culture should be obtained to isolate and identify causative organisms and to determine their susceptibility to gentamicin.

GARAMYCIN may be considered as initial therapy in suspected or confirmed gram-negative infections, and therapy may be instituted before obtaining results of susceptibility testing. The decision to continue therapy with this drug should be based on the results of susceptibility tests, the severity of the infection, and the important additional concepts contained in the "WARNINGS Box" above. If the causative organisms are resistant to gentamicin, other appropriate therapy should be instituted.

In serious infections when the causative organisms are unknown, GARAMYCIN may be administered as initial therapy in conjunction with a penicillin-type or cephalosporin-type drug before obtaining results of susceptibility testing. If anaerobic organisms are suspected as etiologic agents, consideration should be given to using other suitable antimicrobial therapy in conjunction with gentamicin. Following identification of the organism and its susceptibility, appropriate antibiotic therapy should then be continued.

GARAMYCIN has been used effectively in combination with carbenicillin for the treatment of life-threatening infections caused by *Pseudomonas aeruginosa*. It has also been found effective when used in conjunction with a penicillin-type drug for the treatment of endocarditis caused by group D streptococci.

GARAMYCIN Pediatric Injectable has also been shown to be effective in the treatment of serious staphylococcal infections. While not the antibiotic of first choice, GARAMYCIN Pediatric Injectable may be considered when penicillins or other less potentially toxic drugs are contraindicated and bacterial susceptibility tests and clinical judgment indicate its use. It may also be considered in mixed infections caused by susceptible strains of staphylococci and gram-negative organisms.

In the neonate with suspected bacterial sepsis or staphylococcal pneumonia, a penicillin-type drug is also usually indicated as concomitant therapy with gentamicin.

CONTRAINDICATIONS

Hypersensitivity to gentamicin is a contraindication to its use. A history of hypersensitivity or serious toxic reactions to other aminoglycosides may contraindicate use of gentamicin because of the known cross-sensitivity of patients to drugs in this class.

WARNINGS

(See boxed **WARNINGS**.) Aminoglycosides can cause fetal harm when administered to a pregnant woman. Aminoglycoside antibiotics cross the placenta, and there have been several reports of total irreversible bilateral congenital deafness in children whose mothers received streptomycin during pregnancy. Serious side effects to mother, fetus, or newborn have not been reported in the treatment of pregnant women with other aminoglycosides. Animal reproduction studies conducted on rats and rabbits did not reveal evidence of impaired fertility or harm to the fetus due to gentamicin sulfate.

It is not known whether gentamicin sulfate can cause fetal harm when administered to a pregnant woman or can affect reproduction capacity. If gentamicin is used during pregnancy or if the patient becomes pregnant while taking gentamicin, she should be apprised of the potential hazard to the fetus.

GARAMYCIN Pediatric Injectable contains sodium bisulfite, a sulfite that may cause allergic-type reactions including anaphylactic symptoms and life-threatening or less severe asthmatic episodes in certain susceptible people. The overall prevalence of sulfite sensitivity in the general population is unknown and probably low. Sulfite sensitivity is seen more frequently in asthmatic than in nonasthmatic people.

PRECAUTIONS

Neurotoxic and nephrotoxic antibiotics may be absorbed in significant quantities from body surfaces after local irrigation or application. The potential toxic effect of antibiotics administered in this fashion should be considered.

Increased nephrotoxicity has been reported following concomitant administration of aminoglycoside antibiotics and cephalosporins.

Neuromuscular blockade and respiratory paralysis have been reported in the cat receiving high doses (40 mg/kg) of gentamicin. The possibility of these phenomena occurring in man should be considered if aminoglycosides are administered by any route to patients receiving anesthetics, or to patients receiving neuromuscular blocking agents, such as succinylcholine, tubocurarine, or decamethonium, or in patients receiving massive transfusions of citrate-anticoagulated blood. If neuromuscular blockade occurs, calcium salts may reverse it.

Aminoglycosides should be used with caution in patients with neuromuscular disorders, such as myasthenia gravis, since these drugs may aggravate muscle weakness because of their potential curare-like effects on the neuromuscular junction. During or following gentamicin therapy, paresthesias, tetany, positive Chvostek and Trousseau signs, and mental confusion have been described in patients with hypomagnesemia, hypocalcemia, and hypokalemia. When this has occurred in infants, tetany and muscle weakness have been described. Both adults and infants required appropriate corrective electrolyte therapy.

A Fanconi-like syndrome, with aminoaciduria and metabolic acidosis, has been reported in some adults and infants being given gentamicin injections.

Cross-allergenicity among aminoglycosides has been demonstrated.

Patients should be well hydrated during treatment.

Although the *in vitro* mixing of gentamicin and carbenicillin results in a rapid and significant inactivation of gentamicin, this interaction has not been demonstrated in patients with normal renal function who received both drugs by different routes of administration. A reduction in gentamicin serum half-life has been reported in patients with severe renal impairment receiving carbenicillin concomitantly with gentamicin.

Treatment with gentamicin may result in overgrowth of nonsusceptible organisms. If this occurs, appropriate therapy is indicated.

See "WARNINGS Box" regarding concurrent use of potent diuretics and regarding concurrent and/or sequential use of other neurotoxic and/or nephrotoxic antibiotics and for other essential information.

Usage in Pregnancy—Safety for use in pregnancy has not been established.

ADVERSE REACTIONS

Nephrotoxicity Adverse renal effects, as demonstrated by the presence of casts, cells or protein in the urine or by rising BUN, NPN, serum creatinine or oliguria, have been reported. They occur more frequently in patients treated for longer periods or with larger dosages than recommended.

Neurotoxicity Serious adverse effects on both vestibular and auditory branches of the eighth cranial nerves have been reported, primarily in patients with renal impairment (especially if dialysis is required), and in patients on high doses and/or prolonged therapy. Symptoms include dizziness, vertigo, tinnitus, roaring in the ears and hearing loss, which, as with the other aminoglycosides, may be irreversible. Hearing loss is usually manifested initially by diminution of high-tone acuity. Other factors which may increase the risk of toxicity include excessive dosage, dehydration and previous exposure to other ototoxic drugs.

Peripheral neuropathy or encephalopathy, including numbness, skin tingling, muscle twitching, convulsions, and a myasthenia gravis-like syndrome, have been reported.

Note: The risk of toxic reactions is low in neonates, infants and children with normal renal function who do not receive GARAMYCIN Pediatric Injectable at higher doses or for longer periods of time than recommended.

Other reported adverse reactions possibly related to gentamicin include: respiratory depression, lethargy, confusion, depression, visual disturbances, decreased appetite, weight loss and hypotension and hypertension; rash, itching, urticaria, generalized burning, laryngeal edema, anaphylactoid reactions, fever, and headache; nausea, vomiting, increased salivation, and stomatitis; purpura, pseudotumor cerebri, acute organic brain syndrome, pulmonary fibrosis, alopecia, joint pain, transient hepatomegaly, and splenomegaly.

Laboratory abnormalities possibly related to gentamicin include: increased levels of serum transaminase (SGOT, SGPT), serum LDH and bilirubin; decreased serum calcium, magnesium, sodium, and potassium; anemia, leukopenia, granulocytopenia, transient agranulocytosis, eosinophilia, increased and decreased reticulocyte counts, and thrombocytopenia.

While clinical laboratory test abnormalities may be isolated findings, they may also be associated with clinically related signs and symptoms. For example, tetany and muscle weakness may be associated with hypomagnesemia, hypocalcemia, and hypokalemia.

While local tolerance of GARAMYCIN Pediatric Injectable is generally excellent, there has been an occasional report of pain at the injection site. Subcutaneous atrophy or fat necrosis suggesting local irritation has been reported rarely.

OVERDOSAGE

In the event of overdose or toxic reactions, hemodialysis may aid in the removal of gentamicin from the blood, and is especially important if renal function is, or becomes, compromised. The rate of removal of gentamicin is considerably less by peritoneal dialysis than it is by hemodialysis. In the newborn infant, exchange transfusions may also be considered.

DOSAGE AND ADMINISTRATION

GARAMYCIN Pediatric Injectable may be given intramuscularly or intravenously. The patient's pretreatment body weight should be obtained for calculation of correct dosage. The dosage of aminoglycosides in obese patients should be based on an estimate of the lean body mass. It is desirable to limit the duration of treatment with aminoglycosides to short term.

DOSAGE FOR PATIENTS WITH NORMAL RENAL FUNCTION

Children: 6 to 7.5 mg/kg/day. (2.0 to 2.5 mg/kg administered every 8 hours.)

Infants and Neonates: 7.5 mg/kg/day. (2.5 mg/kg administered every 8 hours.)

Premature or Full-Term Neonates One Week of Age or Less: 5 mg/kg/day. (2.5 mg/kg administered every 12 hours.)

It is desirable to measure periodically both peak and trough serum concentrations of gentamicin when feasible during therapy to assure adequate but not excessive drug levels. For example, the peak concentration (at 30 to 60 minutes after intramuscular injection) is expected to be in the range of 3 to 5 mcg/ml. When monitoring peak concentrations after intramuscular or intravenous administration, dosage should be adjusted so that prolonged levels above 12 mcg/ml are avoided. When monitoring trough concentrations (just prior to the next dose), dosage should be adjusted so that levels above 2 mcg/ml are avoided. Determination of the adequacy of a serum level for a particular patient must take into consideration the susceptibility of the causative organism, the severity of the infection, and the status of the patient's host-defense mechanisms.

In patients with extensive burns, altered pharmacokinetics may result in reduced serum concentrations of aminoglycosides. In such patients treated with gentamicin, measurement of serum concentrations is recommended as a basis for dosage adjustment.

The usual duration of treatment is seven to ten days. In difficult and complicated infections, a longer course of therapy may be necessary. In such cases monitoring of renal, auditory, and vestibular functions is recommended, since toxicity is more apt to occur with treatment extended for more than ten days. Dosage should be reduced if clinically indicated.

For Intravenous Administration

The intravenous administration of gentamicin may be particularly useful for treating patients with bacterial septicemia or those in shock. It may also be the preferred route of administration for some patients with congestive heart failure, hematologic disorders, severe burns, or those with reduced muscle mass.

For intermittent intravenous administration, a single dose of GARAMYCIN Pediatric Injectable may be diluted in sterile isotonic saline solution or in a sterile solution of dextrose 5% in water. The solution may be infused over a period of one-half to two hours.

The recommended dosage of intravenous and intramuscular administration is identical.

GARAMYCIN Pediatric Injectable should not be physically premixed with other drugs, but should be administered separately in accordance with the recommended route of administration and dosage schedule.

DOSAGE FOR PATIENTS WITH IMPAIRED RENAL FUNCTION

Dosage must be adjusted in patients with impaired renal function to assure therapeutically adequate, but not excessive, blood levels. Whenever possible, serum concentrations of gentamicin should be monitored. One method of dosage adjustment is to increase the interval between administration of the usual doses. Since the serum creatinine concentration has a high correlation with the serum half-life of gentamicin, this laboratory test may provide guidance for adjustment of the interval between doses. In adults, the interval between doses (in hours) may be approximated by multiplying the serum creatinine level (mg/100 ml) by 8. For example, a patient weighing 60 kg with a serum creatinine level of 2.0 mg/100 ml could be given 60 mg (1 mg/kg) every 16 hours (2 × 8). These guidelines may be considered when treating infants and children with serious renal impairment. In patients with serious systemic infections and renal impairment, it may be desirable to administer the antibiotic more frequently but in reduced dosage. In such patients, serum concentrations of gentamicin should be measured so that adequate but not excessive levels result.

A peak and trough concentration measured intermittently during therapy will provide optimal guidance for adjusting dosage. After the usual initial dose, a rough guide for determining reduced dosage at eight-hour intervals is to divide the normally recommended dose by the serum creatinine level (Table 1). For example, after an initial dose of 20 mg (2.0 mg/kg), a child weighing 10 kg with a serum creatinine level of 2.0 mg/100 ml could be given 10 mg every eight hours (20 ÷ 2). It should be noted that the status of renal function may be changing over the course of the infectious process. It is important to recognize that deteriorating renal function may require a greater reduction in dosage than that specified in the above guidelines for patients with stable renal impairment.

TABLE 1
DOSAGE ADJUSTMENT GUIDE FOR PATIENTS WITH RENAL IMPAIRMENT
(Dosage at Eight-Hour Intervals
After the Usual Initial Dose)

Serum Creatinine (mg %)	Approximate Creatinine Clearance Rate (ml/min/1.73M^2)	Percent of Usual Doses Shown Above
≤ 1.0	> 100	100
1.1–1.3	70–100	80
1.4–1.6	55–70	65
1.7–1.9	45–55	55
2.0–2.2	40–45	50
2.3–2.5	35–40	40
2.6–3.0	30–35	35
3.1–3.5	25–30	30
3.6–4.0	20–25	25
4.1–5.1	15–20	20
5.2–6.6	10–15	15
6.7–8.0	< 10	10

In patients with renal failure undergoing hemodialysis, the amount of gentamicin removed from the blood may vary depending upon several factors including the dialysis method used. An eight-hour hemodialysis may reduce serum concentrations of gentamicin by approximately 50%. In children, the recommended dose at the end of each dialysis period is 2.0 to 2.5 mg/kg depending upon the severity of infection.

The above dosage schedules are not intended as rigid recommendations but are provided as guides to dosage when the measurement of gentamicin serum levels is not feasible.

A variety of methods are available to measure gentamicin concentrations in body fluids; these include microbiologic, enzymatic and radioimmunoassay techniques.

HOW SUPPLIED

GARAMYCIN Pediatric Injectable, 10 mg per ml, for parenteral administration, supplied in 2 ml (20 mg) vials; box of one (NDC 0085-0013-05).

Also available, GARAMYCIN Injectable, 40 mg per ml, for parenteral administration, supplied in 2 ml (80 mg) vials, boxes of 25 (NDC 0085-0069-04); 20 ml vials, box of 5 (NDC 0085-0069-08); and in 1.5 ml (60 mg) (NDC 0085-0069-05) and 2 ml (80 mg) (NDC 0085-0069-06) disposable syringes, boxes of 1.

GARAMYCIN Pediatric Injectable is a clear, stable solution that requires no refrigeration.

Store between 2° and 30°C (36° and 86°F).

Schering Pharmaceutical Corporation (PR)
Manati, Puerto Rico 00701
An Affiliate of Schering Corporation
Kenilworth, NJ 07033

Copyright © 1968, 1983, 1986, 1987, Schering Corporation, USA.
All rights reserved.
Revised 1/87

GARAMYCIN® I.V.   ℞
[*gar-ah-mī'sin*]
Piggyback Injection   **Sterile**
brand of gentamicin sulfate, USP
1 mg per ml
Each ml contains gentamicin sulfate, USP
equivalent to 1 mg gentamicin.
For Intermittent Intravenous Infusion

WARNINGS

Patients treated with aminoglycosides should be under close clinical observation because of the potential toxicity associated with their use.

As with other aminoglycosides, gentamicin sulfate is potentially nephrotoxic. The risk of nephrotoxicity is greater in patients with impaired renal function and in those who receive high dosage or prolonged therapy.

Neurotoxicity manifested by ototoxicity, both vestibular and auditory, can occur in patients treated with gentamicin sulfate, primarily in those with preexisting renal damage and in patients with normal renal function treated with higher doses and/or for longer periods than recommended. Aminoglycoside-induced ototoxicity is usually irreversible. Other manifestations of neurotoxicity may include numbness, skin tingling, muscle twitching and convulsions.

Renal and eighth cranial nerve function should be closely monitored, especially in patients with known or suspected reduced renal function at onset of therapy, and also in those whose renal function is initially normal but who develop signs of renal dysfunction during therapy. Urine should be examined for decreased specific gravity, increased excretion of protein, and the presence of cells or casts. Blood urea nitrogen, serum creatinine, or creatinine clearance should be determined periodically. When feasible, it is recommended that serial audiograms be obtained in patients old enough to be tested, particularly high-risk patients. Evidence of ototoxicity (dizziness, vertigo, tinnitus, roaring in the ears or hearing loss) or nephrotoxicity requires dosage adjustment or discontinuance of the drug. As with the other aminoglycosides, on rare occasions changes in renal and eighth cranial nerve function may not become manifest until soon after completion of therapy.

Serum concentrations of aminoglycosides should be monitored when feasible to assure adequate levels and to avoid potentially toxic levels. When monitoring gentamicin peak concentrations, dosage should be adjusted so that prolonged levels above 12 mcg/ml are avoided. When monitoring gentamicin trough concentrations, dosage should be adjusted so that levels above 2 mcg/ml are avoided. Excessive peak and/or trough serum concentrations of aminoglycosides may increase the risk of renal and eighth cranial nerve toxicity. In the event of overdose or toxic reactions, hemodialysis may aid in the removal of gentamicin from the blood, especially if renal function is, or becomes, compromised. The rate of removal of gentamicin is considerably less by peritoneal dialysis than by hemodialysis.

Continued on next page

Schering—Cont.

Concurrent and/or sequential systemic or topical use of other potentially neurotoxic and/or nephrotoxic drugs, such as cisplatin, cephaloridine, kanamycin, amikacin, neomycin, polymyxin B, colistin, paromomycin, tobramycin, vancomycin, and viomycin, should be avoided. Other factors which may increase patient risk of toxicity are advanced age and dehydration.

The concurrent use of gentamicin with potent diuretics, such as ethacrynic acid or furosemide, should be avoided, since certain diuretics by themselves may cause ototoxicity. In addition, when administered intravenously, diuretics may enhance aminoglycoside toxicity by altering the antibiotic concentration in serum and tissue.

DESCRIPTION

Gentamicin sulfate, USP, a water-soluble antibiotic of the aminoglycoside group, is derived from *Micromonospora purpurea*, an actinomycete. GARAMYCIN I.V. Piggyback Injection is a sterile, aqueous solution for intravenous infusion. Each ml contains gentamicin sulfate, USP, equivalent to 1 mg gentamicin base; and 8.9 mg sodium chloride. It does not contain preservatives.

CLINICAL PHARMACOLOGY

When gentamicin sulfate is administered by intravenous infusion over a two-hour period, the serum concentrations are similar to those obtained by intramuscular administration. Peak serum concentrations following intravenous administration occur 30 to 60 minutes following cessation of infusion. Serum levels are measurable for 6 to 8 hours.

In patients with normal renal function, peak serum concentrations of gentamicin (mcg/ml) are usually up to four times the single intramuscular dose (mg/kg); for example, a 1.0 mg/kg injection in adults may be expected to result in a peak serum concentration up to 4 mcg/ml; a 1.5 mg/kg dose may produce levels up to 6 mcg/ml. While some variation is to be expected due to a number of variables such as age, body temperature, surface area, and physiologic differences, the individual patient given the same dose tends to have similar levels in repeated determinations. Gentamicin administered at 1.0 mg/kg every eight hours for the usual 7- to 10-day treatment period to patients with normal renal function does not accumulate in the serum.

Gentamicin, like all aminoglycosides, may accumulate in the serum and tissues of patients treated with higher doses and/or for prolonged periods, particularly in the presence of impaired renal function. In adult patients, treatment with gentamicin dosages of 4 mg/kg/day or higher for seven to ten days may result in a slight, progressive rise in both peak and trough concentrations. In patients with impaired renal function, gentamicin is cleared from the body more slowly than in patients with normal renal function. The more severe the impairment, the slower the clearance. (Dosage must be adjusted.)

Since gentamicin is distributed in extracellular fluid, peak serum concentrations may be lower than usual in adult patients who have a large volume of this fluid. Serum concentrations of gentamicin in febrile patients may be lower than those in afebrile patients given the same dose. When body temperature returns to normal, serum concentrations of the drug may rise. Febrile and anemic states may be associated with a shorter than usual serum half-life. (Dosage adjustment is usually not necessary.) In severely burned patients, the half-life may be significantly decreased and resulting serum concentrations may be lower than anticipated from the mg/kg dose.

Protein-binding studies have indicated that the degree of gentamicin binding is low; depending upon the methods used for testing, this may be between 0 and 30%.

After initial administration to patients with normal renal function, generally 70% or more of the gentamicin dose is recoverable in the urine in 24 hours; concentrations in urine above 100 mcg/ml may be achieved. Little, if any, metabolic transformation occurs; the drug is excreted principally by glomerular filtration. After several days of treatment, the amount of gentamicin excreted in the urine approaches the daily dose administered. As with other aminoglycosides, a small amount of the gentamicin dose may be retained in the tissues, especially in the kidneys. Minute quantities of aminoglycosides have been detected in the urine weeks after drug administration was discontinued. Renal clearance of gentamicin is similar to that of endogenous creatinine.

In patients with marked impairment of renal function, there is a decrease in the concentration of aminoglycosides in urine and in their penetration into defective renal parenchyma. This decreased drug excretion, together with the potential nephrotoxicity of aminoglycosides, should be considered when treating such patients who have urinary tract infections.

Probenecid does not affect renal tubular transport of gentamicin.

The endogenous creatinine clearance rate and the serum creatinine level have a high correlation with the half-life of gentamicin in serum. Results of these tests may serve as guides for adjusting dosage in patients with renal impairment (see DOSAGE AND ADMINISTRATION).

Following parenteral administration, gentamicin can be detected in serum, lymph, tissues, sputum, and in pleural, synovial, and peritoneal fluids. Concentrations in renal cortex sometimes may be eight times higher than the usual serum levels. Concentrations in bile, in general, have been low and have suggested minimal biliary excretion. Gentamicin crosses the peritoneal as well as the placental membranes. Since aminoglycosides diffuse poorly into the subarachnoid space after parenteral administration, concentrations of gentamicin in cerebrospinal fluid are often low and dependent upon dose, rate of penetration, and degree of meningeal inflammation. There is minimal penetration of gentamicin into ocular tissues following intramuscular or intravenous administration.

Microbiology: *In vitro* tests have demonstrated that gentamicin is a bactericidal antibiotic which acts by inhibiting normal protein synthesis in susceptible microorganisms. It is active against a wide variety of pathogenic bacteria including *Escherichia coli*, *Proteus* species (indole-positive and indole-negative), *Pseudomonas aeruginosa*, species of the *Klebsiella-Enterobacter-Serratia* group, *Citrobacter* species and *Staphylococcus* species (including penicillin- and methicillin-resistant strains). Gentamicin is also active *in vitro* against species of *Salmonella* and *Shigella*. The following bacteria are usually resistant to aminoglycosides: *Streptococcus pneumoniae*, most species of streptococci, particularly group D and anaerobic organisms, such as *Bacteroides* species or *Clostridium* species.

In vitro studies have shown that an aminoglycoside combined with an antibiotic that interferes with cell wall synthesis may act synergistically against some group D streptococcal strains. The combination of gentamicin and penicillin G has a synergistic bactericidal effect against virtually all strains of *Streptococcus faecalis* and its varieties *(S. faecalis* var. *liquifaciens*, *S. faecalis* var. *zymogenes), S. faecium* and *S. durans*. An enhanced killing effect against many of these strains has also been shown *in vitro* with combinations of gentamicin and ampicillin, carbenicillin, nafcillin, or oxacillin.

The combined effect of gentamicin and carbenicillin is synergistic for many strains of *Pseudomonas aeruginosa*. *In vitro* synergism against other gram-negative organisms has been shown with combinations of gentamicin and cephalosporins. Gentamicin may be active against clinical isolates of bacteria resistant to other aminoglycosides.

Bacteria resistant to one aminoglycoside may be resistant to one or more other aminoglycosides. Bacterial resistance to gentamicin is generally developed slowly.

Susceptibility Testing: If the disc method of susceptibility testing used is that described by Bauer *et al (Am J Clin Path* 45:493, 1966; *Federal Register* 37:20525-20529, 1972), a disc containing 10 mcg of gentamicin should give a zone of inhibition of 15mm or more to indicate susceptibility of the infecting organism. A zone of 12mm or less indicates that the infecting organism is likely to be resistant. Zones greater than 12mm and less than 15mm indicate intermediate susceptibility. In certain conditions it may be desirable to do additional susceptibility testing by the tube or agar dilution method; gentamicin substance is available for this purpose.

INDICATIONS AND USAGE

GARAMYCIN I.V. Piggyback Injection is indicated in the treatment of serious infections caused by susceptible strains of the following microorganisms: *Pseudomonas aeruginosa*, *Proteus* species (indole-positive and indole-negative), *Escherichia coli*, *Klebsiella-Enterobacter-Serratia* species, *Citrobacter* species and *Staphylococcus* species (coagulase-postive and coagulase-negative).

Clinical studies have shown GARAMYCIN to be effective in bacterial neonatal sepsis; bacterial septicemia; and serious bacterial infections of the central nervous system (meningitis), urinary tract, respiratory tract, gastrointestinal tract (including peritonitis), skin, bone and soft tissue (including burns). Aminoglycosides, including gentamicin, are not indicated in uncomplicated initial episodes of urinary tract infections unless the causative organisms are susceptible to these antibiotics and are not susceptible to antibiotics having less potential for toxicity.

Specimens for bacterial culture should be obtained to isolate and identify causative organisms and to determine their susceptibility to gentamicin.

GARAMYCIN may be considered as initial therapy in suspected or confirmed gram-negative infections, and therapy may be instituted before obtaining results of susceptibility testing. The decision to continue therapy with this drug should be based on the results of susceptibility tests, the severity of the infection, and the important additional concepts contained in the "WARNINGS Box" above. If the causative organisms are resistant to gentamicin, other appropriate therapy should be instituted.

In serious infections when the causative organisms are unknown, GARAMYCIN may be administered as initial therapy in conjunction with a penicillin-type or cephalosporin-type drug before obtaining results of susceptibility testing. If anaerobic organisms are suspected as etiologic agents, consideration should be given to using other suitable antimicrobial therapy in conjunction with gentamicin. Following identification of the organism and its susceptibility, appropriate antibiotic therapy should then be continued.

GARAMYCIN has been used effectively in combination with carbenicillin for the treatment of life-threatening infections caused by *Pseudomonas aeruginosa*. It has also been found effective when used in conjunction with a penicillin-type drug for the treatment of endocarditis caused by group D streptococci.

GARAMYCIN has also been shown to be effective in the treatment of serious staphylococcal infections. While not the antibiotic of first choice, GARAMYCIN may be considered when penicillins or other less potentially toxic drugs are contraindicated and bacterial susceptibility tests and clinical judgment indicate its use. It may also be considered in mixed infections caused by susceptible strains of staphylococci and gram-negative organisms.

In the neonate with suspected bacterial sepsis or staphylococcal pneumonia, a penicillin-type drug is also usually indicated as concomitant therapy with gentamicin.

CONTRAINDICATIONS

Hypersensitivity to gentamicin is a contraindication to its use. A history of hypersensitivity or serious toxic reactions to other aminoglycosides may contraindicate use of gentamicin because of the known cross-sensitivity of patients to drugs in this class.

WARNINGS

(See boxed **WARNINGS**.) Aminoglycosides can cause fetal harm when administered to a pregnant woman. Aminoglycoside antibiotics cross the placenta, and there have been several reports of total irreversible bilateral congenital deafness in children whose mother received streptomycin during pregnancy. Serious side effects to mother, fetus, or newborn have not been reported in the treatment of pregnant women with other aminoglycosides. Animal reproduction studies conducted on rats and rabbits did not reveal evidence of impaired fertility or harm to the fetus due to gentamicin sulfate.

It is not known whether gentamicin sulfate can cause fetal harm when administered to a pregnant woman or can affect reproduction capacity. If gentamicin is used during pregnancy or if the patient becomes pregnant while taking gentamicin, she should be apprised of the potential hazard to the fetus.

PRECAUTIONS

Neurotoxic and nephrotoxic antibiotics may be absorbed in significant quantities from body surfaces after local irrigation or application. The potential toxic effect of antibiotics administered in this fashion should be considered.

Increased nephrotoxicity has been reported following concomitant administration of aminoglycoside antibiotics and cephalosporins. Neuromuscular blockade and respiratory paralysis have been reported in the cat receiving high doses (40 mg/kg) of gentamicin. The possibility of these phenomena occurring in man should be considered if aminoglycosides are administered by any route to patients receiving anesthetics, or to patients receiving neuromuscular blocking agents, such as succinylcholine, tubocurarine, or decamethonium, or in patients receiving massive transfusions of citrate-anticoagulated blood. If neuromuscular blockade occurs, calcium salts may reverse it.

Aminoglycosides should be used with caution in patients with neuromuscular disorders, such as myasthenia gravis, since these drugs may aggravate muscle weakness because of their potential curare-like effects on the neuromuscular junction. During or following gentamicin therapy, paresthesias, tetany, positive Chvostek and Trousseau signs, and mental confusion have been described in patients with hypomagnesemia, hypocalcemia, and hypokalemia. When this has occurred in infants, tetany and muscle weakness have been described. Both adults and infants required appropriate corrective electrolyte therapy.

Elderly patients may have reduced renal function which may not be evident in the results of routine screening tests, such as BUN or serum creatinine. A creatinine clearance determination may be more useful. Monitoring of renal function during treatment with gentamicin, as with other aminoglycosides, is particularly important in such patients. A Fanconi-like syndrome, with aminoaciduria and metabolic acidosis, has been reported in some adults and infants being given gentamicin injections.

Cross-allergenicity among aminoglycosides has been demonstrated.

Patients should be well hydrated during treatment.

Although the *in vitro* mixing of gentamicin and carbenicillin results in a rapid and significant inactivation of gentamicin, this interaction has not been demonstrated in patients with normal renal function who received both drugs by different routes of administration. A reduction in gentamicin serum half-life has been reported in patients with severe renal impairment receiving carbenicillin concomitantly with gentamicin.

Treatment with gentamicin may result in overgrowth of nonsusceptible organisms. If this occurs, appropriate therapy is indicated.

See "WARNINGS Box" regarding concurrent use of potent diuretics and regarding concurrent and/or sequential use of other neurotoxic and/or nephrotoxic antibiotics and for other essential information.

Usage in Pregnancy—Safety for use in pregnancy has not been established.

ADVERSE REACTIONS

Nephrotoxicity Adverse renal effects, as demonstrated by the presence of casts, cells, or protein in the urine or by rising BUN, NPN, serum creatinine or oliguria, have been reported. They occur more frequently in patients with a history of renal impairment and in patients treated for longer periods or with larger dosage than recommended.

Neurotoxicity Serious adverse effects on both vestibular and auditory branches of the eighth nerve have been reported, primarily in patients with renal impairment (especially if dialysis is required), and in patients on high doses and/or prolonged therapy. Symptoms include dizziness, vertigo, tinnitus, roaring in the ears and hearing loss, which, as with the other aminoglycosides, may be irreversible. Hearing loss is usually manifested initially by diminution of high-tone acuity. Other factors which may increase the risk of toxicity include excessive dosage, dehydration and previous exposure to other ototoxic drugs.

Peripheral neuropathy or encephalopathy, including numbness, skin tingling, muscle twitching, convulsions, and a myasthenia gravis-like syndrome, have been reported.

Note: The risk of toxic reactions is low in patients with normal renal function who do not receive GARAMYCIN at higher doses or for longer periods of time than recommended.

Other reported adverse reactions possibly related to gentamicin include: respiratory depression, lethargy, confusion, depression, visual disturbances, decreased appetite, weight loss, and hypotension and hypertension; rash, itching, urticaria, generalized burning, laryngeal edema, anaphylactoid reactions, fever, and headache; nausea, vomiting, increased salivation, and stomatitis; purpura, pseudotumor cerebri, acute organic brain syndrome, pulmonary fibrosis, alopecia, joint pain, transient hepatomegaly, and splenomegaly.

Laboratory abnormalities possibly related to gentamicin include: increased levels of serum transaminase (SGOT, SGPT), serum LDH and bilirubin; decreased serum calcium, magnesium, sodium and potassium; anemia, leukopenia, granulocytopenia, transient agranulocytosis, eosinophilia, increased and decreased reticulocyte counts, and thrombocytopenia. While clinical laboratory test abnormalities may be isolated findings, they may also be associated with clinically related signs and symptoms. For example, tetany and muscle weakness may be associated with hypomagnesemia, hypocalcemia, and hypokalemia.

While local tolerance of GARAMYCIN is generally excellent, there has been an occasional report of pain at the injection site. Subcutaneous atrophy or fat necrosis suggesting local irritation has been reported rarely.

OVERDOSAGE

In the event of overdose or toxic reactions, hemodialysis may aid in the removal of gentamicin from the blood, and is especially important if renal function is, or becomes, compromised. The rate of removal of gentamicin is considerably less by peritoneal dialysis than it is by hemodialysis.

DOSAGE AND ADMINISTRATION

GARAMYCIN I.V. Piggyback Injection should only be administered intravenously. This product does not contain a preservative system; the contents must be used promptly after the seal is broken. Any unused portion must be discarded. DO NOT RETAIN FOR LATER USE.

It is desirable to limit the duration of treatment with aminoglycosides to short-term.

The usual duration of treatment for all patients is seven to ten days. In difficult and complicated infections, a longer course of therapy may be necessary. In such cases monitoring of renal, auditory, and vestibular functions is recommended, since toxicity is more apt to occur with treatment extended for more than ten days. Dosage should be reduced if clinically indicated.

The patient's pretreatment body weight should be obtained for calculation of correct dosage. The dosage of aminoglycosides in obese patients should be based on an estimate of the lean body mass.

In patients with extensive burns, altered pharmacokinetics may result in reduced serum concentrations of aminoglycosides. In such patients treated with gentamicin, measurement of serum concentrations is recommended as a basis for dosage adjustment.

It is desirable to measure periodically both peak and trough serum concentrations of gentamicin when feasible during

Garamycin I.V.

TABLE I
DOSAGE SCHEDULE GUIDE FOR ADULTS WITH NORMAL RENAL FUNCTION
(Dosage at Eight-Hour Intervals)
1 mg/ml

Patient's Weight* kg (lb)	Usual Dose for Serious Infections 1 mg/kg q8h (3 mg/kg/day)	Dose for Life-Threatening Infections (Reduce As Soon As Clinically Indicated) 1.7 mg/kg q8h** (5 mg/kg/day)
	mg/dose	mg/dose
40 (88)	40	66
45 (99)	45	75
50 (110)	50	83
55 (121)	55	91
60 (132)	60	100
65 (143)	65	108
70 (154)	70	116
75 (165)	75	125
80 (176)	80	133
85 (187)	85	141
90 (198)	90	150
95 (209)	95	158
100 (220)	100	166

* The dosage of aminoglycosides in obese patients should be based on an estimate of the lean body mass.
** For q6h schedules, dosage should be recalculated.

therapy to assure adequate but not excessive drug levels. For example, the peak concentrations (at 30 to 60 minutes following cessation of infusion) is expected to be in the range of 4 to 6 mcg/ml. When monitoring peak concentrations, dosage should be adjusted so that prolonged levels above 12 mcg/ml are avoided. When monitoring trough concentrations (just prior to the next dose), dosage should be adjusted so that levels above 2 mcg/ml are avoided. Determination of the adequacy of a serum level for a particular patient must take into consideration the susceptibility of the causative organism, the severity of the infection, and the status of the patient's host-defense mechanisms.

The intravenous administration of gentamicin may be particularly useful for treating patients with bacterial septicemia or those in shock. It may also be the preferred route of administration for some patients with congestive heart failure, hematologic disorders, severe burns, or those with reduced muscle mass. The solution may be infused over a period of one-half to two hours.

GARAMYCIN I.V. Piggyback Injection should not be physically premixed with other drugs but should be administered separately in accordance with the recommended route of administration and dosage schedule.

The dosage recommendations which follow are not intended as rigid schedules, but are provided as guides for initial therapy or when the measurement of gentamicin serum levels during therapy is not feasible.

DOSAGE FOR PATIENTS WITH NORMAL RENAL FUNCTION

Adults: The recommended dosage of GARAMYCIN I.V. Piggyback Injection for patients with serious infections and normal renal function is 3 mg/kg/day, administered in three equal doses every eight hours (Table I).

For patients with life-threatening infections, dosages up to 5 mg/kg/day may be administered in three or four equal doses. This dosage should be reduced to 3 mg/kg/day as soon as clinically indicated (Table I).

[See table above].

Children: 6 to 7.5 mg/kg/day (2.0 to 2.5 mg/kg administered every 8 hours.)

Infants and Neonates: 7.5 mg/kg/day (2.5 mg/kg administered every 8 hours).

Premature or Full-Term Neonates one week of age or less: 5 mg/kg/day (2.5 mg/kg administered every 12 hours).

Note: For further information concerning the use of gentamicin in infants and children, see GARAMYCIN Pediatric Injectable Product Information.

DOSAGE FOR PATIENTS WITH IMPAIRED RENAL FUNCTION

Dosage must be adjusted in patients with impaired renal function to assure therapeutically adequate, but not excessive, blood levels. Whenever possible, serum concentrations of gentamicin should be monitored. One method of dosage adjustment is to increase the interval between administration of the usual doses. Since the serum creatinine concentration has a high correlation with the serum half-life of gentamicin, this laboratory test may provide guidance for adjustment of the interval between doses. The interval between doses (in hours) may be approximated by multiplying the serum creatinine level (mg/100 ml) by 8. For example, a patient weighing 60 kg with a serum creatinine level of 2.0 mg/100 ml could be given 60 mg (1 mg/kg every 16 hours (2 × 8).

In patients with serious systemic infections and renal impairment, it may be desirable to administer the antibiotic more frequently but in reduced dosage. In such patients, serum concentrations of gentamicin should be measured so that adequate but not excessive levels result. A peak and trough concentration measured intermittently during therapy will provide optimal guidance for adjusting dosage. After the usual initial dose, a rough guide for determining reduced dosage at eight-hour intervals is to divide the normally recommended dose by the serum creatinine level (Table II). For example, after an initial dose of 60 mg (1 mg/kg), a patient weighing 60 kg with a serum creatinine level of 2.0 mg/100 ml could be given 30 mg every eight hours (60 ÷ 2). It should be noted that the status of renal function may be changing over the course of the infectious process.

It is important to recognize that deteriorating renal function may require a greater reduction in dosage than that specified in the above guidelines for patients with stable renal impairment.

[See table on next page].

In adults with renal failure undergoing hemodialysis, the amount of gentamicin removed from the blood may vary depending upon several factors including the dialysis method used. An eight-hour hemodialysis may reduce serum concentrations of gentamicin by approximately 50%. The recommended dosage at the end of each dialysis period is 1 mg/kg to 1.7 mg/kg depending upon the severity of infection. In children, a dose of 2 mg/kg may be administered.

A variety of methods are available to measure gentamicin concentrations in body fluids; these include microbiologic, enzymatic and radio-immunoassay techniques.

INSTRUCTIONS FOR THE ADMINISTRATION OF GARAMYCIN I.V. PIGGYBACK INJECTION (For proper apparatus setup see Instruction Sheet).

THIS PRODUCT IS IN A READY-TO-USE FORM AND IS INTENDED FOR USE ONLY AS AN I.V. PIGGYBACK.

If the prescribed dose is exactly 60 or 80 mg, use the appropriate unit; if the prescribed dose is higher or lower than that of the supplied unit, adjustments can be made in either piggyback unit. If the dose is higher that the contents of the 80 mg unit, the additional amount should be removed from a vial of GARAMYCIN Injectable (40 mg/ml) and added to the 80 mg piggyback unit. If the prescribed dose is less, decrements can be made by removing and discarding the appropriate amount from either unit. It should be kept in mind that **each ml of the piggyback unit contains 1 mg of gentamicin.**

The following are specific examples of dosage adjustment:

- to prepare a 90 mg dose, remove ¼ ml from a vial of GARAMYCIN Injectable (40 mg/ml) and add to the 80 mg piggyback unit.
- to prepare a 70 mg dose, either remove and discard 10 ml from the 80 mg piggyback unit or add the 10 ml from the 80 mg piggyback unit to the 60 mg piggyback unit.
- to prepare a 40 mg dose, remove and discard 20 ml from the 60 mg piggyback unit.

Observe all precautions for sterile technique when adding or removing contents of these units.

Continued on next page

Information on Schering products appearing on these pages is effective as of September 30, 1989.

Schering—Cont.

HOW SUPPLIED

GARAMYCIN I.V. Piggyback Injection, 1 mg per ml, for intravenous infusion, is supplied in 60 ml (60 mg) (NDC 0085-0527-03) and 80 ml (80 mg) (NDC 0085-0527-04) units; boxes of one.

Store between 2° and 30°C (36° and 86°F).

Also available, GARAMYCIN Injectable, 40 mg per ml, for parenteral administration, is supplied in 2 ml (80 mg) vials, boxes of 25 (NDC 0085-0069-04); and 20 ml vials, box of 5 (NDC 0085-0069-08); and in 1.5 ml (60 mg) NDC 0085-0069-05) and 2 ml (80 mg) (NDC 0085-0069-06) disposable syringes, each in boxes of 1 and 10.
GARAMYCIN Pediatric Injectable, 10 mg per ml, for parenteral administration, supplied in 2 ml (20 mg) vials; box of one (NDC 0085-0013-05).
GARAMYCIN Products are clear, stable solutions that require no refrigeration.

> Schering Pharmaceutical
> Corporation (P.R.),
> Manati, Puerto Rico 00701
> An Affiliate of Schering
> Corporation, Kenilworth,
> N.J. 07033 USA

Revised 2/86
Copyright © 1968, 1983, 1986, Schering Corporation, USA. All rights reserved.

GARAMYCIN® Intrathecal   ℞
[gar-ah-mī'sin]
brand of gentamicin sulfate, USP
Injection 2.0 mg/ml
FOR DIRECT ADMINISTRATION INTO
THE CEREBROSPINAL FLUID SPACES
OF THE CENTRAL NERVOUS SYSTEM

WARNINGS

GARAMYCIN Intrathecal Injection is intended as adjunctive therapy in patients with central nervous system infections.
Since patients considered for treatment with GARAMYCIN Intrathecal Injection will usually be receiving concomitant treatment with intramuscular or intravenous gentamicin sulfate, all warnings and precautions for this or other concomitantly administered agents must be observed. Moreover, when the drug is administered by more than one route, additive effects must be considered. (See GARAMYCIN Injectable or GARAMYCIN Pediatric Injectable Product Information.) Laboratory studies in animals have shown that gentamicin sulfate, when administered directly into the central nervous system, has caused neurologic disturbances, including adverse effects on the eighth cranial nerve. The risk of direct administration of a potentially neurotoxic drug into the cerebrospinal fluid spaces of the central nervous system must be weighed against the potential benefit to be derived from this route of administration.

DESCRIPTION

Gentamicin sulfate, USP, a water-soluble antibiotic of the aminoglycoside group, is derived from *Micromonospora purpurea,* an actinomycete. GARAMYCIN Intrathecal Injection is a sterile, aqueous solution for direct administration into the cerebrospinal fluid spaces of the central nervous system.

Each ml contains: gentamicin sulfate, USP equivalent to 2.0 mg gentamicin base; and 8.5 mg sodium chloride.

CLINICAL PHARMACOLOGY

Since gentamicin sulfate and other aminoglycosides diffuse poorly into the subarachnoid space after systemic administration, concentrations of these antibiotics in the lumbar or ventricular cerebrospinal fluid (CSF) are often low. Following intramuscular or intravenous administration of the usual doses, gentamicin concentrations in CSF in the absence of infection are usually less than 1 mcg/ml. In acute meningitis, slightly higher concentrations are obtained but these vary and are usually well below the peak serum concentration. CSF concentrations which are attained following intravenous or intramuscular administration of gentamicin sulfate tend to become lower as meningeal inflammation subsides. GARAMYCIN Intrathecal Injections are intended to increase the concentration of gentamicin in the CSF when used as part of the management of patients with central nervous system infections.
When GARAMYCIN Intrathecal Injection is given concomitantly with systemically administered gentamicin sulfate, the CSF levels are substantially increased depending upon the location of the injection. Peak CSF concentrations which follow intralumbar administration generally occur at 1 to 6 hours after injection.
Factors which affect the concentration of gentamicin in the CSF following injection into cerebrospinal fluid spaces are the dose administered, the site of the injection (intralumbar, intraventricular), the volume in which the dose is diluted, and the presence or absence of obstruction to the CSF flow. There appears to be considerable inter-patient variation.
The half-life of gentamicin in the CSF of adults who received intralumbar injections is approximately 5.5 hours; this is somewhat longer than that in serum.
In one pharmacokinetic study in adults, a 3 to 4 mg intralumbar injection resulted in a mean CSF concentration of 6.2 mcg/ml 24 hours after injection. The mean CSF concentration was noted to decrease with time; during days 1 through 6 of treatment with GARAMYCIN Intrathecal Injection by the intralumbar route, the mean 24-hour concentration was 9.9 mcg/ml, while during days 7 through 13, the mean concentration was 3.7 mcg/ml.
In another study in adults, CSF levels were measured at varying intervals after intralumbar administration of gentamicin sulfate. During days 1 through 6 of treatment, a 4 mg dose produced a mean CSF level of 2.4 mcg/ml 24 hours after injection, while during days 7 through 13, the same dose produced a mean 24-hour level of 0.5 mcg/ml.
Following intralumbar administration there may be limited upward diffusion of the drug, presumably because of the direction of the CSF flow. Intraventricular administration produces high concentrations in the ventricles and throughout the central nervous system. Adequate levels will usually result from dosing every 24 hours, but it is desirable to manage each patient's infection with serial monitoring of gentamicin serum and CSF concentrations.
Microbiology: *In vitro* tests have demonstrated that gentamicin is a bactericidal antibiotic which acts by inhibiting normal protein synthesis in susceptible microorganisms. It is active against a wide variety of pathogenic bacteria including *Escherichia coli, Proteus* species (indole-positive and indole-negative), *Pseudomonas aeruginosa,* species of the *Klebsiella-Enterobacter-Serratia* group, *Citrobacter* species, and *Staphylococcus* species (including penicillin- and methicillin-resistant strains). Gentamicin is also active *in vitro* against species of *Salmonella* and *Shigella.* The following bacteria are usually resistant to aminoglycosides: *Streptococcus pneumoniae,* most species of streptococci, particularly group D and anaerobic organisms, such as *Bacteroides* species or *Clostridium* species.

In vitro studies have shown that an aminoglycoside combined with an antibiotic that interferes with cell wall synthesis may act synergistically against some group D streptococcal strains. The combination of gentamicin sulfate and penicillin G has a synergistic bactericidal effect against virtually all strains of *Streptococcus faecalis* and its varieties (*S. faecalis* var. *liquifaciens, S. faecalis* var. *zymogenes), S. faecium* and *S. durans.* An enhanced killing effect against many of these strains has also been shown *in vitro* with combinations of gentamicin and ampicillin, carbenicillin, nafcillin, or oxacillin.
The combined effect of gentamicin and carbenicillin is synergistic for many strains of *Pseudomonas aeruginosa.*
Gentamicin may be active against clinical isolates of bacteria resistant to other aminoglycosides. However, bacteria resistant to one aminoglycoside may be resistant to one or more other aminoglycosides.
Susceptibility Testing: If the disc method of susceptibility testing used is that described by Bauer *et al* (*Am J Clin Path* **45**:493, 1966; *Federal Register* **37**:20525–20529, 1972), a disc containing 10 mcg of gentamicin, when tested against a bacterial strain susceptible to gentamicin, should give a zone of inhibition of $\geq$ 15mm. A zone of $\leq$ 12 mm indicates that the infecting organism is likely to be resistant. Zones greater than 12mm and less than 15mm indicate intermediate susceptibility. In certain conditions it may be desirable to do additional susceptibility testing by the broth or agar dilution method; gentamicin substance is available for this purpose.

INDICATIONS AND USAGE

GARAMYCIN Intrathecal Injection is indicated as adjunctive therapy to systemically administered gentamicin sulfate in the treatment of serious central nervous system infections (meningitis, ventriculitis) caused by susceptible *Pseudomonas* species.
Bacteriologic tests should be performed to determine that the causative organisms are *Pseudomonas* species susceptible to gentamicin.

CONTRAINDICATIONS

Hypersensitivity to gentamicin sulfate is a contraindication to its use. A history of hypersensitivity or serious toxic reactions to aminoglycosides may also contraindicate use of gentamicin sulfate because of the known cross-sensitivity of patients to drugs in this class.

WARNINGS

(See "WARNINGS Box" above and the WARNINGS listed in the Product Information for GARAMYCIN Injectable and GARAMYCIN Pediatric Injectable.)

PRECAUTIONS

(See PRECAUTIONS listed in the Product Information for GARAMYCIN Injectable and GARAMYCIN Pediatric Injectable.)
In a patient with a seven-year history of multiple sclerosis who was treated with gentamicin sulfate by intralumbar injection, disseminated microscopic lesions of the brain stem were reported at autopsy. Lesions observed were: tissue rarefaction with loss and marked swelling of axis cylinders with occasional calcification, loss of oligodendroglia and astroglia, and a poor inflammatory response.
Safety and efficacy in children below the age of three months have not been established.

ADVERSE REACTIONS

Local tolerance to GARAMYCIN Intrathecal Injection has been good. Local reactions of arachnoiditis or burning at the injection site have been reported rarely.
Because the recommended dosage of GARAMYCIN Intrathecal Injection is low, the potential for systemic adverse effects is minimal. However, GARAMYCIN Intrathecal Injection is recommended as adjunctive therapy with other antibiotics, such as parenteral gentamicin sulfate, which should be administered in full therapeutic dosages. Evidence of eighth nerve dysfunction, changes in renal function, leg cramps, rash, fever, convulsions, and an increase in cerebrospinal fluid protein have been reported in patients who were treated concomitantly with GARAMYCIN Intrathecal Injection and the parenteral preparation of gentamicin.
Administration of excessive (40 to 160 mg) doses of the parenteral formulation of gentamicin sulfate (which contains a preservative system) by the various intrathecal routes has been reported to produce neuromuscular disturbances, e.g., ataxia, paresis, and incontinence.

DOSAGE AND ADMINISTRATION

GARAMYCIN Intrathecal Injection is intended for administration directly into the cerebrospinal fluid spaces of the central nervous system.
The dosage will vary depending upon factors, such as age and weight of the patient, site of injection, degree of obstruction to cerebrospinal fluid flow and the amount of cerebrospinal fluid estimated to be present. In general, the recommended dose for infants 3 months of age and older (see PRECAUTIONS) and children is 1 to 2 mg once a day. For adults, 4 to 8 mg may be administered once a day.

Garamycin I.V.

TABLE II
DOSAGE ADJUSTMENT GUIDE FOR PATIENTS WITH RENAL IMPAIRMENT
(Dosage at Eight-Hour Intervals After the Usual Initial Dose)

Serum Creatinine (mg %)	Approximate Creatinine Clearance Rate (ml/min/1.73M²)	Percent of Usual Doses Shown in Table I
≤1.0	>100	100
1.1-1.3	70-100	80
1.4-1.6	55-70	65
1.7-1.9	45-55	55
2.0-2.2	40-45	50
2.3-2.5	35-40	40
2.6-3.0	30-35	35
3.1-3.5	25-30	30
3.6-4.0	20-25	25
4.1-5.1	15-20	20
5.2-6.6	10-15	15
6.7-8.0	<10	10

Administration of GARAMYCIN Intrathecal Injection should be continued as long as sensitive organisms are demonstrated in the cerebrospinal fluid. Since the intralumbar or intraventricular dose is administered immediately after specimens are taken for laboratory study, treatment should usually be continued for at least one day after negative results have been obtained from CSF cultures and/or stained smears.

The suggested method for administering GARAMYCIN Intrathecal Injection into the lumbar area is as follows: the desired quantity of GARAMYCIN Intrathecal Injection is drawn up carefully from the ampule into a 5- or 10-ml sterile syringe. After the lumbar puncture is performed and a specimen of the spinal fluid is removed for laboratory tests, the syringe containing GARAMYCIN Intrathecal Injection is inserted into the hub of the spinal needle. A quantity of cerebrospinal fluid (approximately 10% of the estimated total CSF volume) is allowed to flow into the syringe and mix with the GARAMYCIN Intrathecal Injection. The resultant solution is then injected over a period of 3 to 5 minutes with the bevel of the needle directed upward.

If the cerebrospinal fluid is grossly purulent, or if it is unobtainable, GARAMYCIN Intrathecal Injection may be diluted with sterile normal saline before injection.

GARAMYCIN Intrathecal Injection may also be administered directly into the subdural space or directly into the ventricles, including administration by use of an implanted reservoir.

HOW SUPPLIED

GARAMYCIN Intrathecal Injection, 2.0 mg per ml, is supplied in 2 ml ampules; box of 25.

Store below 30°C (86°F).

NOTE: This preparation does not contain any preservative. Once opened, contents should be used immediately and unused portions should be discarded.

ANIMAL PHARMACOLOGY AND TOXICOLOGY

In dogs, an 8-hour perfusion of the ventriculosubarachnoid system with a solution containing 40 mcg/ml (~5 mg or ~0.3 mg/kg) gentamicin produced no seizure activity or change in vital signs during administration. No morphological changes were observed when the dogs were sacrificed at 10 and 90 days following infusion.

The effects of repeated intrathecal injections of gentamicin at 0.1 and 0.3 mg/kg were evaluated in tranquilized beagle puppies. Transient flaccid paralysis was observed on the first day when the drug was administered rapidly (i.e., in less than 5 seconds), but no adverse effects were observed thereafter when the drug was administered less rapidly (i.e., over a period of approximately 30 seconds). No drug-related changes were found on histological examination of the cerebellum, brain stem or cephalic cord. In cats, gentamicin administered intracisternally at one-hour intervals in doses of up to 50 mg/kg did not produce any abnormalities in the electroencephalogram. In another study in cats, gentamicin sulfate given daily by the intracisternal route for up to 7 days caused neurologic disturbances, including adverse effects on the eighth cranial nerve.

In rabbits intracisternal injection of gentamicin at doses 50 and 100 times the therapeutic dose produced peak CSF concentrations of 160 and 180 mcg/ml, respectively. These doses were associated with changes in the myelin sheath predominantly of the lateral columns of the upper cervical cord, and some changes in glial cells and lesions in the medulla oblongata. In addition to a high incidence of mortality, the animals demonstrated weakness, ataxia and paralysis. At doses of one and ten times the therapeutic dose (providing peak levels of 16.5 and 40 mcg/ml CSF), no morphologic changes occurred and there were no drug-related symptoms identified.

Schering Pharmaceutical Corporation (PR)
Manati, Puerto Rico 00701
An Affiliate of Schering Corporation
Kenilworth, New Jersey 07033
Copyright © 1979, 1983, Schering Corporation, USA. All rights reserved.
Revised 7/83

GYNE–LOTRIMIN®   ℞
[gī"ne-lo'trim-in]
brand of clotrimazole
Vaginal Tablets, USP
Vaginal Cream, USP 1%

DESCRIPTION

GYNE-LOTRIMIN is clotrimazole [1-(o-Chloro-α, α-diphenylbenzyl) imidazole], a synthetic antifungal agent having the chemical formula $C_{22}H_{17}ClN_2$.

Each GYNE-LOTRIMIN **Vaginal Tablet** contains 100 mg clotrimazole, USP dispersed in lactose, povidone, corn starch, and magnesium stearate.

Each applicatorful of GYNE-LOTRIMIN **Vaginal Cream** contains approximately 50 mg clotrimazole, USP dispersed in sorbitan monostearate, polysorbate 60, cetyl esters wax, cetearyl alcohol, 2-octyldodecanol, purified water, and as preservative, benzyl alcohol (1%).

ACTIONS

Clotrimazole is a broad-spectrum antifungal agent that inhibits the growth of pathogenic yeasts. Clotrimazole exhibits fungicidal activity *in vitro* against *Candida albicans* and other species of the genus *Candida*.

No single-step or multiple-step resistance to clotrimazole has developed during successive passages of *Candida albicans*.

INDICATIONS

GYNE-LOTRIMIN **Vaginal Cream** and **Tablets** are indicated for the local treatment of patients with vulvovaginal candidiasis (moniliasis). The diagnosis should be confirmed by KOH smears and/or cultures. Other pathogens commonly associated with vulvovaginitis (*Trichomonas* and *Hemophilus vaginalis*) should be ruled out by appropriate laboratory methods.

The 3-day regimen of GYNE-LOTRIMIN **Vaginal Tablets** did not prove to be effective in pregnant patients.

Studies with clotrimazole cream have shown that women taking oral contraceptives had a cure rate similar to those not taking oral contraceptives.

CONTRAINDICATIONS

GYNE-LOTRIMIN **Vaginal Tablets** and **Vaginal Cream** are contraindicated in women who have shown hypersensitivity to any of the components of the preparation.

PRECAUTIONS

Laboratory Tests: If there is a lack of response to GYNE-LOTRIMIN, appropriate microbiological studies should be repeated to confirm the diagnosis and rule out other pathogens before instituting another course of antimycotic therapy.

Application of ^{14}C-labeled clotrimazole has shown negligible absorption (peak of 0.03 mcg/ml of serum 24 hours after insertion of a 100 mg tablet; peak serum level of 0.01 mcg/ml 24 hours after insertion of vaginal cream containing 50 mg of active drug) from both normal and inflamed human vaginal mucosa.

Usage in Pregnancy: While GYNE-LOTRIMIN **Vaginal Tablets** and **Vaginal Cream** have not been studied in the first trimester of pregnancy, use in the second and third trimesters has not been associated with ill effects. Follow-up reports now available on 71 neonates of 177 pregnant patients treated with GYNE-LOTRIMIN **Vaginal Tablets** reveal no adverse effects or complications attributable to GYNE-LOTRIMIN therapy.

ADVERSE REACTIONS

Eighteen (1.6%) of the 1116 patients treated with GYNE-LOTRIMIN **Vaginal Tablets** in double-blind studies reported complaints during therapy that were possibly drug-related. Mild burning occurred in six patients while other complaints, such as skin rash, itching, vulval irritation, lower abdominal cramps and bloating, slight cramping, slight urinary frequency, and burning or irritation in the sexual partner, occurred rarely.

Three (0.5%) of the 653 patients treated with GYNE-LOTRIMIN **Vaginal Cream** reported complaints during therapy that were possibly drug-related. Vaginal burning occurred in one patient; erythema, irritation and burning in another; intercurrent cystitis was reported in the third.

DOSAGE AND ADMINISTRATION

GYNE-LOTRIMIN **Vaginal Cream** has been found to be effective when used from seven to fourteen days; studies have shown that patients treated for fourteen days had a significantly higher cure rate. The recommended dose is one applicatorful of cream (approximately 5 grams) inserted intravaginally for seven to fourteen consecutive days, preferably at bedtime.

GYNE-LOTRIMIN **Vaginal Tablets:** Two tablets inserted intravaginally at bedtime for three nights or one tablet inserted intravaginally at bedtime for seven nights.

In the event of treatment failure, other pathogens commonly responsible for vaginitis should be ruled out before instituting another course of antimycotic therapy.

HOW SUPPLIED

GYNE-LOTRIMIN **Vaginal Tablets,** 100 mg, white, uncoated tablets impressed with the trademark GYNE-LOTRIMIN and/or the Schering trademark and product identification number, 734; carton of six tablets for three-day treatment regimen and carton of seven tablets for seven-day treatment regimen; with plastic applicator and patient instructions.
Store between 2° and 30°C (36° and 86°F).

GYNE-LOTRIMIN **Vaginal Cream 1%** is supplied in 45-gram tubes with a measured-dose applicator; box of one for seven-day treatment; box of two for fourteen-day treatment.
Store between 2° and 30°C (36° and 86°F).

Copyright © 1976, 1982, Schering Corporation, USA. Rev. 8/82

Shown in Product Identification Section, page 428

GYNE-LOTRIMIN® 500 mg   ℞
[gī"ne-lo'trim-in]
brand of clotrimazole
Vaginal Tablets

DESCRIPTION

Each GYNE-LOTRIMIN 500 mg Vaginal Tablet contains 500 mg clotrimazole (the active ingredient) dispersed in lactose, microcrystalline cellulose, lactic acid, corn starch, crospovidone, calcium lactate, magnesium stearate, silicon dioxide and hydroxypropyl methylcellulose. Chemically, clotrimazole is [1-(o-Chloro-α, α-diphenylbenzyl) imidazole], a synthetic antifungal agent having the chemical formula $C_{22}H_{17}ClN_2$, and a molecular weight of 344.84.

Clotrimazole is an odorless, white crystalline substance, practically insoluble in water, sparingly soluble in ether, soluble in carbon tetrachloride, and very soluble in ethanol and chloroform.

CLINICAL PHARMACOLOGY

Serum levels and levels in vaginal secretions of clotrimazole were measured in six healthy volunteers who had one 500 mg vaginal tablet inserted. Although serum levels of clotrimazole were higher than those in other volunteers given 100 mg and 200 mg vaginal tablets, these levels did not exceed 10 nanograms/ml. It has been estimated that three to ten percent of a vaginal dose of clotrimazole may be absorbed, but the drug rapidly and efficiently degrades to microbiologically inactive metabolites. The clotrimazole concentrations remaining in vaginal secretions were still in the mg/ml range for 48 hours and in two of the six subjects at 72 hours.

The findings of high clotrimazole concentrations in vaginal secretions for up to 72 hours and low concentrations in the serum suggest that nearly all the clotrimazole given in the 500 mg vaginal tablet remains in the vagina for 48 hours, and in some cases 72 hours, in fungicidal concentrations.

Clotrimazole is a broad-spectrum antifungal agent. It has been postulated that the compound affects the permeability characteristics of the membrane allowing the leakage of essential intracellular components with a consequent inhibition of the synthesis of such macromolecules as protein, lipid, DNA, and polysaccharides.

At concentrations as low as 2–5 µg/ml, clotrimazole exhibits fungicidal activity *in vitro* against *Candida albicans* and other species of the genus *Candida*.

No single-step or multiple-step resistance to clotrimazole has developed during successive passages of *Candida albicans*.

INDICATIONS

GYNE-LOTRIMIN 500 mg Vaginal Tablets are indicated for the local treatment of vulvovaginal candidiasis when one day therapy is felt warranted. In the case of severe vulvovaginitis due to candidiasis, longer antimycotic therapy is recommended. The diagnosis should be confirmed by KOH smears and/or cultures. Other pathogens commonly associated with vulvovaginitis, *Trichomonas* and *Gardnerella (Haemophilus) vaginalis*, should be ruled out by appropriate laboratory methods.

CONTRAINDICATIONS

GYNE-LOTRIMIN 500 mg Vaginal Tablets are contraindicated in women who have shown hypersensitivity to any components of the preparation.

WARNINGS

None

PRECAUTIONS

If there is a lack of response to GYNE-LOTRIMIN 500 mg Vaginal Tablets, appropriate microbiological studies should be repeated to confirm the diagnosis and rule out other pathogens before instituting another course of antimycotic therapy.

Carcinogenesis: No long term studies in animals have been performed to evaluate the carcinogenic potential of GYNE-LOTRIMIN 500 mg Vaginal Tablets intravaginally. A long term study in rats (Wistar strains) where clotrimazole was administered orally provided no indication of carcinogenicity.

Usage in Pregnancy: Pregnancy Category B: The disposition of ^{14}C-clotrimazole has been studied in humans and animals. Clotrimazole is poorly absorbed following intravaginal administration to humans whereas it is rather well absorbed after oral administration.

In clinical trials, use of vaginally applied clotrimazole in pregnant women in their second and third trimesters has not been associated with ill effects. There are, however, no adequate and well-controlled studies in pregnant women during the first trimester of pregnancy.

Continued on next page

Information on Schering products appearing on these pages is effective as of September 30, 1989.

Schering—Cont.

Studies in pregnant rats given repeated intravaginal doses up to 100 mg/kg/day have revealed no evidence of harm to the fetus due to clotrimazole.

Repeated high oral doses of clotrimazole in rats and mice ranging from 50 to 120 mg/kg resulted in embryotoxicity (possibly secondary to maternal toxicity), impairment of mating, decreased litter size and number of viable young and decreased pup survival to weaning. However, clotrimazole was not teratogenic in mice, rabbits and rats at oral doses up to 200, 180 and 100 mg/kg, respectively. Oral absorption in the rat amounts to approximately 90% of the administered dose.

Because animal reproduction studies are not always predictive of human response, this drug should be used only if clearly indicated during the first trimester of pregnancy.

ADVERSE REACTIONS

Of 297 patients in double-blind studies with the 500 mg vaginal tablet, 3 of 149 patients treated with active drug and 3 of 148 patients treated with placebo reported complaints during therapy that were possibly drug related. In the active drug group, vomiting occurred in one patient, vaginal soreness with coitus in another, and complaints of vaginal irritation, itching, burning and dyspareunia in the third patient. In the placebo group, clitoral irritation occurred in one patient and dysuria, described as remotely related to drug, in the other. A third patient in the placebo group developed bacterial vaginitis which the investigator classed as possibly related to drug.

Eighteen (1.6%) of the 1116 patients treated with GYNE-LOTRIMIN in other formulations in double-blind studies reported complaints during therapy that were possibly drug-related. Mild burning occurred in six patients while other complaints such as skin rash, itching, vulval irritation, lower abdominal cramps and bloating, slight cramping, slight urinary frequency, and burning or irritation in the sexual partner, occurred rarely.

OVERDOSAGE

No data available.

DRUG ABUSE AND DEPENDENCE

Drug abuse and dependence with GYNE-LOTRIMIN 500 mg Vaginal Tablets has not been reported.

DOSAGE AND ADMINISTRATION

The recommended dose is one tablet inserted intravaginally one time only, preferably at bedtime. In the event of treatment failure, that is, persistence of signs and symptoms of vaginitis after five days, other pathogens commonly responsible for vaginitis should be ruled out before instituting another course of antimycotic therapy.

HOW SUPPLIED

GYNE-LOTRIMIN 500 mg Vaginal Tablets are white, bullet shaped, uncoated tablets, coded with Schering on one side and 396 on the other, supplied as a single 500 mg tablet with plastic applicator and patient instructions (NDC 0085-0396-01).

Store below 30°C (86°F).

Revised 6/86

Copyright ©1986. Schering Corporation, USA. All rights reserved.

Shown in Product Identification Section, page 428.

HYPERSTAT® I.V.   ℞

[hi'per-stat]
brand of diazoxide, USP
Injection
For Intravenous Use In
Hospitalized Patients Only

DESCRIPTION

HYPERSTAT I.V. Injection is a nondiuretic benzothiadiazine antihypertensive agent. Each ampule (20 ml) contains 300 mg diazoxide, USP, in a clear, sterile, colorless aqueous solution; the pH is adjusted to approximately 11.6 with sodium hydroxide.

Diazoxide is 7-chloro-3-methyl-$2H$-1,2,4-benzothiadiazine 1,1-dioxide, with the empirical formula $C_8H_7ClN_2O_2S$, and the molecular weight 230.7. It is a white crystalline powder practically insoluble to sparingly soluble in water.

CLINICAL PHARMACOLOGY

HYPERSTAT I.V. Injection produces a prompt reduction of blood pressure in man by relaxing smooth muscle in the peripheral arterioles. Cardiac output is increased as blood pressure is reduced. Studies in animals demonstrate that coronary blood flow is maintained, while renal blood flow is increased after an initial decrease.

Transient hyperglycemia occurs in the majority of patients treated with HYPERSTAT, but usually requires treatment only in patients with diabetes mellitus. It will respond to the usual management measures, including insulin.

Blood glucose levels should be monitored especially in patients with diabetes and in those requiring multiple injections of diazoxide. Cataracts have been observed in a few animals receiving repeated daily doses of intravenous diazoxide.

Since diazoxide causes sodium retention, repeated injections may precipitate edema and congestive heart failure. Increased volume of extracellular fluid may be a cause of treatment failure in nonresponsive patients. The increase in fluid volume characteristically responds to diuretic agents if adequate renal function exists. Concurrently administered thiazide diuretics may be expected to potentiate the antihypertensive and hyperuricemic actions of diazoxide. (See **Drug Interactions**.)

Diazoxide is extensively bound to serum protein (>90%). The plasma half-life is 28 ± 8.3 hours; however, the duration of its antihypertensive effect is variable, generally lasting less than 12 hours.

INDICATIONS AND USAGE

HYPERSTAT I.V. Injection is indicated for short-term use in the emergency reduction of blood pressure in severe, nonmalignant and malignant hypertension in hospitalized adults; and in acute severe hypertension in hospitalized children, when prompt and urgent decrease of diastolic pressure is required. Treatment with orally effective antihypertensive agents should not be instituted until blood pressure has stabilized. The use of HYPERSTAT I.V. Injection for longer than 10 days is not recommended.

HYPERSTAT I.V. Injection is ineffective against hypertension due to pheochromocytoma.

CONTRAINDICATIONS

HYPERSTAT I.V. Injection should not be used in the treatment of compensatory hypertension, such as that associated with aortic coarctation or arteriovenous shunt, and should not be used in patients hypersensitive to diazoxide, other thiazides, or other sulfonamide-derived drugs.

WARNINGS

Rapid decrease of blood pressure Caution must be observed when reducing severely elevated blood pressure. Diazoxide should only be administered utilizing the new 150 mg minibolus dosage. The use of a 300 mg intravenous dose of diazoxide has been associated with angina and with myocardial and cerebral infarction. One instance of optic nerve infarction was reported when a 100 mmHg reduction in diastolic pressure occurred over ten minutes following a single 300 mg bolus. In one prospective trial conducted in patients with severe hypertension and coexistent coronary artery disease, a 50% incidence of ischemic changes in the electrocardiogram was observed following single 300 mg bolus injections of diazoxide. The desired blood pressure lowering should therefore be achieved over as long a period of time as is compatible with the patient's status. At least several hours and preferably one or two days is tentatively recommended. Improved safety with equal efficacy can be achieved by administering HYPERSTAT I.V. Injection as a mini-bolus dose (1 to 3 mg/kg every 5 to 15 minutes up to a maximum of 150 mg in a single injection) until a diastolic blood pressure below 100 mmHg is achieved. HYPERSTAT I.V. Injection should not be administered in a bolus dose of 300 mg since this mode of administration is less predictable and less controllable than the minibolus dosage. If hypotension severe enough to require therapy results from the reduction in blood pressure, it will usually respond to the Trendelenberg maneuver. If necessary, sympathomimetic agents such as dopamine or norepinephrine may be administered.

Special attention is required for patients with diabetes mellitus and those in whom retention of salt and water may present serious problems.

Myocardial Lesions in Animals Intravenous administration of diazoxide in dogs has induced subendocardial necrosis and necrosis of papillary muscles. These lesions, which are also produced by other vasodilator drugs (i.e., hydralazine, minoxidil) and by catecholamines, are presumed to be related to anoxia resulting from a combination of reflex tachycardia and decreased perfusion.

PRECAUTIONS

General: HYPERSTAT (diazoxide) I.V. Injection is an effective antihypertensive agent requiring close monitoring of the patient's blood pressure at frequent intervals. Its administration may occasionally cause hypotension requiring treatment with sympathomimetic drugs. Therefore, HYPERSTAT, I.V. Injection should be used primarily in the hospital or where adequate facilities exist to treat such untoward responses.

HYPERSTAT I.V. Injection should be administered only into a peripheral vein. Because the alkalinity of the solution is irritating to tissue, avoid extravascular injection or leakage. Subcutaneous administration has produced inflammation and pain without subsequent necrosis. If leakage into subcutaneous tissue occurs, the area should be treated with warm compresses and rest.

HYPERSTAT I.V. Injection should be used with care in patients who have impaired cerebral or cardiac circulation,

that is, patients in whom abrupt reduction in blood pressure might be detrimental or those in whom mild tachycardia or decreased blood perfusion may be deleterious (see **Warnings**). Prolonged hypotension should be avoided so as not to aggravate preexisting renal failure.

Information for Patients: During and immediately following intravenous injection of HYPERSTAT I.V. Injection, the patient should remain supine.

Laboratory Tests: Diagnostic laboratory tests necessary to establish the patient's condition and status should be carried out prior to treatment with HYPERSTAT I.V. Injection. During and following treatment with HYPERSTAT I.V. Injection, laboratory tests to monitor the effects of treatment with this drug and the patient's condition should be done. Among the tests (not necessarily inclusive) are: hematologic (hematocrit, hemoglobin, white blood cell and platelet counts); metabolic (glucose, uric acid, total protein, albumin); electrolyte (sodium, potassium) and osmolality; renal function (creatinine, urine-protein); electrocardiogram.

Drug Interactions: Diazoxide is highly bound to serum protein. It can be expected to displace other substances which are also bound to protein, such as bilirubin or coumarin and its derivatives, resulting in higher blood levels of these substances.

An undesirable hypotension may result when diazoxide is administered to patients who have received other antihypertensive medication within six hours.

One patient in a clinical study exhibited excessive hypotension after concomitant administration of HYPERSTAT with hydralazine and methyldopa. An episode of maternal hypotension and fetal bradycardia occurred in a patient in labor who received both reserpine and hydralazine prior to administration of diazoxide. Neonatal hyperglycemia following intrapartum administration of HYPERSTAT I.V. Injection has also been reported.

HYPERSTAT I.V. Injection should not be administered within six hours of the administration of: hydralazine, reserpine, alphaprodine, methyldopa, beta-blockers, prazosin, minoxidil, the nitrites and other papaverine-like compounds. Concomitant administration with thiazides or other commonly used diuretics may be expected to potentiate the hyperuricemic and antihypertensive effects of diazoxide.

Drug/Laboratory Test Interactions: The hyperglycemic and hyperuricemic effects of diazoxide preclude proper assessment of these metabolic states. Increased renin secretion, IgG concentrations and decreased cortisol secretion have also been noted. Diazoxide inhibits glucagon-stimulated insulin release and will cause a false-negative insulin response to glucagon. In the rat, dog and monkey, diazoxide increased serum free fatty acids and decreased plasma insulin levels.

Carcinogenesis, Mutagenesis, Impairment of Fertility: No long-term animal dosing study has been done to evaluate the carcinogenic potential of diazoxide. No laboratory studies of mutagenic potential or animal studies of effects on fertility have been done.

Pregnancy Category C: Diazoxide has been shown to reduce fetal and/or pup survival; and to reduce fetal growth in rats, rabbits, and dogs at daily doses of 30, 21, or 10 mg/kg, respectively. In rats treated at term, diazoxide, at doses of 10 mg/kg and above, prolonged parturition.

The safety of HYPERSTAT I.V. Injection in pregnancy has not been established.

Non-teratogenic Effects: Diazoxide crosses the placental barrier and appears in cord blood. When given to the mother prior to delivery the drug may produce fetal or neonatal hyperbilirubinemia, thrombocytopenia, altered carbohydrate metabolism, and possibly other side effects that have occurred in adults.

Labor and Delivery: HYPERSTAT I.V. Injection is not indicated for use in pregnancy. Intravenous administration of the drug during labor may cause cessation of uterine contractions, requiring administration of an oxytocic agent.

Nursing Mothers: Information is not available concerning the passage of HYPERSTAT in breast milk. Because many drugs are excreted in human milk and because of the potential for adverse reactions in nursing infants from diazoxide, a decision should be made whether to discontinue nursing or to discontinue the drug, taking into account the importance of the drug to the mother.

Pediatric Use: See **Indications and Usage**.

ADVERSE REACTIONS

It is reasonable to speculate that the currently recommended mini-bolus dosing regimen, which has replaced the 300 mg bolus dose in clinical practice, will result in adverse effects which are of similar character but of lesser frequency and severity.

In clinical experience with the rapid bolus administration of 300 mg, the most common adverse reactions reported were: hypotension (7%); nausea and vomiting (4%); dizziness and weakness (2%). Additional adverse reactions reported with bolus administration of 300 mg were as follows:

Cardiovascular: sodium and water retention after repeated injections, especially important in patients with impaired cardiac reserve; hypotension to shock levels; myocardial ischemia, usually transient and manifested by angina, atrial and ventricular arrhythmias, and marked electrocardiographic changes, but occasionally leading to myocardial infarction; optic nerve infarction following too rapid decrease in severely elevated blood pressure; supraventricular tachycardia and palpitation; bradycardia; chest discomfort or nonanginal "tightness in the chest."

Central Nervous System: cerebral ischemia, usually transient but occasionally leading to infarction and manifested by unconsciousness, convulsions, paralysis, confusion, or focal neurological deficit such as numbness of the hands; vasodilative phenomena, such as orthostatic hypotension, sweating, flushing, and generalized or localized sensations of warmth; various transient neurological findings secondary to alteration in regional blood flow to brain, such as headache (sometimes throbbing), dizziness, lightheadedness, sleepiness (also reported as lethargy, somnolence or drowsiness), euphoria or "funny feeling," ringing in the ears and momentary hearing loss, and weakness of short duration; apprehension or anxiety.

Gastrointestinal: rarely, acute pancreatitis; nausea, vomiting and/or abdominal discomfort, anorexia; alteration in taste, parotid swelling; salivation; dry mouth; lacrimation; ileus; constipation and diarrhea.

Other: hyperglycemia in diabetic patients, especially after repeated injections; hyperosmolar coma in an infant; transient hyperglycemia in nondiabetic patients; transient retention of nitrogenous wastes; various respiratory findings secondary to the relaxation of smooth muscle, such as dyspnea, cough and choking sensation; warmth or pain along the injected vein; cellulitis without sloughing and/or phlebitis at the injection site of extravasation; back pain and increased nocturia; hypersensitivity reactions, such as rash, leukopenia and fever; papilledema induced by plasma volume expansion secondary to the administration of diazoxide reported in a patient who had received eleven injections (300 mg/dose) over a 22-day period; malaise and blurred vision; transient cataract in an infant; hirsutism and decreased libido.

OVERDOSAGE

Overdosage of HYPERSTAT I.V. Injection may cause an undesirable hypotension. Usually, this can be controlled with the Trendelenberg maneuver. If necessary, sympathomimetic agents, such as dopamine or norepinephrine, may be administered. Failure of blood pressure to rise in response to such agents suggests that the hypotension may have been caused by something other than diazoxide. Excessive hyperglycemia resulting from overdosage will respond to conventional therapy of hyperglycemia.

DOSAGE AND ADMINISTRATION

HYPERSTAT I.V. Injection was originally recommended for use by bolus administration of 300 mg. Recent studies have shown that minibolus administration of HYPERSTAT I.V. Injection i.e., doses of 1 to 3 mg/kg repeated at intervals of 5 to 15 minutes is as effective in reducing blood pressure. Minibolus administration usually provides a more gradual reduction in blood pressure and thus may be expected to reduce the circulatory and neurological risks associated with acute hypotension.

HYPERSTAT I.V. Injection is administered undiluted and rapidly by intravenous injections of 1 to 3 mg/kg up to a maximum of 150 mg in a single injection. This dose may be repeated at intervals of 5 to 15 minutes until a satisfactory reduction in blood pressure (diastolic pressure below 100 mmHg) has been achieved.

With the patient recumbent, the calculated dose of HYPERSTAT I.V. Injection is administered intravenously in 30 seconds or less.

HYPERSTAT I.V. Injection should only be given into a peripheral vein. Do no administer it intramuscularly, subcutaneously, or into body cavities. Avoid extravasation of the drug into subcutaneous tissues.

Following the use of HYPERSTAT I.V. Injection, the blood pressure should be monitored closely until it has stabilized. Thereafter, measurements made hourly during the balance of the effect should indicate any unusual response. A further decrease in blood pressure 30 minutes or more after injection should be investigated for causes other than the action of HYPERSTAT I.V. Injection. It is preferable that the patient remain supine for at least one hour after injection. In ambulatory patients, the blood pressure should also be measured with the patient standing before surveillance is ended. Repeated administration of HYPERSTAT I.V. Injection at intervals of 4 to 24 hours usually will maintain the blood pressure below pretreatment levels until a regimen of oral antihypertensive medication can be instituted. The interval between injections may be adjusted by the duration of the response to each injection. It is usually unnecessary to continue treatment with HYPERSTAT I.V. Injection for more than four to five days.

Since repeated administration of HYPERSTAT I.V. Injection can lead to sodium and water retention, administration of a diuretic may be necessary both for maximal blood pres-

sure reduction and to avoid congestive heart failure. (See **Clinical Pharmacology**.)

Parenteral drug products should be inspected visually for particulate matter and discoloration prior to administration whenever solution & container permit.

HOW SUPPLIED

HYPERSTAT I.V. Injection is supplied in a 20 ml. ampule, containing 300 mg diazoxide, in a clear, sterile, colorless aqueous solution; box of one ampule. (NDC 0085-0201-05).

Protect from light and freezing. Store between 36° and 86°F (2° and 30°C).

Revised 2/85

INHAL-AID®
Drug Delivery System for Metered Dose Inhalers.

PRESCRIBING INFORMATION:

Inhal-Aid is a drug delivery system that helps deliver oral aerosolized medication from metered dose inhalers (MDIs) to the lungs. It can improve the delivery of these medications by making it simpler for patients to use them. Studies document that almost half of the patients who use MDIs use them incorrectly because they have difficulty coordinating inhalation with the fast release of medication from the MDI. This is a major factor limiting aerosol delivery to the airways. Inhal-Aid's collecting chamber holds the medication and allows patients to breathe medication through the mouthpiece without having to carefully time inhalation with activation of the MDI.

The incentive flow indicator provides a visual means of identifying inspiratory effort and sustained breathing via a sensitive float mechanism activated by the patient's negative inspiratory effort. The design is such that children can adequately perform the maneuver.

CAUTION

The usual caution should be exercised in dosing medications and evaluating patient response. The prescribing information for the marketed MDIs varies with respect to dosing, administration, etc. We recommend that these be followed when using Inhal-Aid.

INHAL-AID contains a clear plastic **collecting chamber** and can be utilized with any of the currently marketed metered-dose inhalers via a **universal adapter.** Connected at the end opposite the universal adapter is a T-tube with a **mouthpiece** on one end, a one-way valve on the other and a vertical **incentive indicator** (incentive spirometer device). The junction between the collecting chamber and the mouthpiece-containing T-tube also contains a **one-way valve.** Inhaling through the mouthpiece draws air through four small holes in the collecting chamber. The contents of the 700-mL collecting chamber are thus progressively inhaled with each successive inspiration by passing through the one-way valve in the collecting chamber through the mouthpiece and into the lungs. Exhaled air passes straight through the T-tube and out the one-way valve opposite the mouthpiece. The aerosol in the collecting chamber therefore leaves only during inhalation and cannot be blown out through the venting holes during exhalation.

NOTE: INHAL-AID should be replaced every 9–12 months or as needed. A prescription will be needed to obtain a new one.

Assembly Instructions

1. Mouthpiece and incentive indicator assembled. The incentive indicator has 4 parts:
   A. Orange cap
   B. Outer flow-tube
   C. Inner flow-tube
   D. Orange float
2. Small rubber valve.
3. Large rubber valve.
4. Collecting chamber (700 mL reservoir); the 2 parts are held together by prongs fitting into the 4 small openings.
5. Blue rubber "spray inhaler" adapter.
6. Typical "spray inhaler" and mouthpiece (not included).

7. Extra set of rubber valves.
8. Nose clips.

INHAL-AID is supplied partly assembled. The parts include:
— collecting chamber (4) with blue rubber "spray inhaler" (metered dose inhaler-MDI) adapter (5) attached
— mouthpiece with incentive indicator attached (1)
— package of extra rubber valves (7)
— nose clips (8)

Your patient should:

1. Remove the parts. Place the collecting chamber on a flat surface. Check to see that the small rubber valve (2) is firmly in place.

2. Connect the mouthpiece (with incentive indicator attached) to the opening that has the small rubber valve. Check to see that the large rubber valve (3) at the back of the mouthpiece is firmly in place.
3. Check the INHAL-AID. If it is assembled correctly, patients should be able to breathe freely and see the orange float go up to the top of the incentive indicator as they breathe in.
4. To administer the medication, connect the MDI with mouthpiece to the blue rubber adapter. The incentive indicator and MDI container must point upward. This is necessary for INHAL-AID to work properly.
5. INHAL-AID comes with nose clips for patients who may have trouble breathing **only** through their mouth.
6. The small and large rubber valves are needed for INHAL-AID to function properly. A package of extra valves is included in case the original set is damaged or lost.

DIRECTIONS FOR USE:

Your patient should:

1. Shake MDI and its mouthpiece before placing it straight into the blue rubber adapter as far as it will go. The incentive indicator and "spray inhaler" container should both point upward. The blue adapter has one side with a smaller opening and one side with a larger opening. The mouthpiece of the MDI should fit snugly.

2. Place mouthpiece in mouth and close lips tightly around it.
3. Push the top of the MDI down with a finger while supporting the bottom with the thumb to release medication into the collecting chamber.

NOTE: Patients should be reminded of the correct dosage schedule.

4. **Breathe in slowly** through the mouthpiece. By teaching patients to **slowly raise** the orange float to the top of the incentive indicator and to keep it at the top as long as possible, they can improve the delivery of medication to their lungs.
5. **Once a breath is taken, hold while slowly counting to five,** when possible. This can help to increse the amount of medication that stays in the lungs.
6. **Breathe out slowly through** the mouthpiece. Do not remove the mouthpiece from the mouth.

Continued on next page

Schering—Cont.

7. Repeat the breathing in and out steps (numbers 4, 5, 6) four more times keeping the lips closed tightly around the mouthpiece. This will help to get the medication from the collecting chamber.

IMPORTANT CLEANING INSTRUCTIONS

Your patient should:

1. Remove the incentive indicator unit from the mouthpiece. The incentive indicator should not be taken apart or washed.
2. Remove mouthpiece (with incentive indicator attached) from the collecting chamber.
3. Take the collecting chamber apart by holding each of the two halves and twisting to release the prongs while pulling apart. (To put the chamber back together, place the prongs into the small openings and snap closed.)
4. Rinse the INHAL-AID parts with **warm, not hot, water.** After rinsing, shake parts to remove most of the water and let air-dry in a clean dust-free area before reassembling. **Do not dry** near artificial heat source such as a dishwasher or oven.

NOTE: Inhal-Aid is designed for single-patient use and single-drug use. Even if the patient cannot exactly follow each step, the rising orange float (slowly moving it off the bottom of the incentive indicator) shows that medication is being delivered. Replace the Inhal-Aid every 9–12 months or as needed.

Children and other first time users should practice the breathing in and out steps before using the medication.

CAUTION: Federal law restricts this device to sale by or on the order of a physician.

References

1. Sackner MA, Brown LK, Kim CS: *Chest 80* (suppl): 915–918, 1981. 2. Tobin MJ, Jenouri G, Danta I, et al; *Am Rev Respir Dis* 126:670–675, 1982. 3. Saunders KB: *Br. Med J* 1:1037–1038, 1965. 4. Gayrard P, Orehek J: *Respiration* 40:47–52, 1980. 5. Shim C, Williams MH Jr: *Am. J. Med* 69:891–894, 1980

Rev. 2/89

Distributed By: Schering Corporation, Kenilworth, NJ 07033 USA

Copyright © 1988, 1989 Schering Corporation, USA
All rights reserved

INSPIREASE®
Drug Delivery System for use with metered dose inhalers

Prescribing Information

DESCRIPTION

InspirEase® is an effective and easy-to-use portable drug delivery system for metered dose inhalers (MDIs). Its components are a replaceable reservoir bag and two mouthpieces adaptable to most of the MDIs currently available.

A carrying case is supplied for transporting and storing InspirEase and the MDI container.

Typical "Spray Inhaler" (Metered Dose Inhaler)*

INDICATIONS

InspirEase improves the distribution and deposition in the lungs of aerosolized medication from MDIs.

1. Minimal patient skill is required for use.
   A significant number of patients fail to derive full benefit from their MDIs. This is sometimes due to inadequate instruction or to misuse of the device by anxious, breathless patients. The correct use of an MDI requires greater skill than is immediately apparent.[1–5]
   Studies have demonstrated that nearly 50% of patients had difficulty coordinating MDI activation with inspiration.[3–5] This is a major factor limiting aerosol delivery to the airways.[2] With MDIs alone, the patient has to carefully time each inspiraton with activation of the inhaler.
   InspirEase eliminates the need for the patient to coordinate inspiration with activation of the MDI.

---

2. Medication is more effectively delivered to the airways. With InspirEase, medication is more effectively delivered to the airways—less is deposited on the oropharynx, because the aerosol particles are inhaled slowly and evenly. The reservoir bag acts as a collecting chamber for the medication emitted from MDIs. This permits the patient to calmly inhale medication and rebreathe with a second breath.
3. Proper breathing technique is encouraged.
   InspirEase has visual and auditory signals to help patients assess the rate and depth of each inhalation. Slow, deep inspiration results in deflation of the reservoir bag and *no* whistling sound. Rapid inspiration (greater than 0.3 L/s) produces a whistling sound from the flow rate monitor. This signals the patients to inhale more slowly. Patients can see and feel the bag collapsing.
   The volume of the fully extended reservoir bag is approximately 700 ml, which is approximately 1½ to 2 times the average adult tidal volume.

CAUTION

The usual caution should be exercised in dosing medications and evaluating patient response. The prescribing information for the marketed MDIs varies with respect to dosing, administration, etc. We recommend that these be followed when using InspirEase.

DIRECTIONS FOR USE

Your patient should:

1. Connect the mouthpiece to the reservoir bag by lining up the *locking tabs* with the opening in the reservoir bags. Push in and twist to lock.

2. Untwist the reservoir bag gently to open it to its full size. Shake "spray inhaler" well before placing its stem into the *mouthpiece*. Make sure it fits snugly.

3. Place mouthpiece in mouth and close lips tightly around it.
4. Press down on the "spray inhaler" to release one dose of medication into the bag.
   IMPORTANT NOTE: Follow your doctor's instructions regarding the number of doses you should take and when to take them.

5. Breathe in *slowly* through the mouthpiece. If you hear a whistling sound, breathe slower until no sound can be heard.

6. Breathe in the entire contents of the bag. You will know to stop when the bag collapses and you cannot breathe in anymore.

---

7. *Hold his or her breath while slowly counting to five.*
8. Breathe out slowly into the bag.

9. Repeat the inhale/exhale cycle (steps 5 through 8) a second time, keeping lips tightly closed around the mouthpiece.

IMPORTANT NOTE: Repeat steps 2 through 9 for each dose of medication prescribed by your doctor.

10. Remove the mouthpiece from mouth. Take drug canister off the reservoir bag. Unlock mouthpiece from the bag and store all components in carrying case.

IMPORTANT CLEANING INSTRUCTIONS

Your patients should:

1. Clean only the mouthpiece thoroughly with warm (not hot) running water *at least* once a day. *InspirEase® is not dishwasher safe. Always clean by hand.*
2. The clear plastic reed section of the mouthpiece should not be touched due to potential breakage. We recommend a visual inspection of the reed section for signs of breakage prior to each use. If reed breakage occurs, replace mouthpiece immediately; otherwise replace mouthpiece as needed every six months.
3. After cleaning, wait until mouthpiece is *completely dry* before storing in carrying case. Do not place near artificial heat such as dishwasher or oven.
4. We recommend that the reservoir bag be replaced every two to three weeks or as needed. *However, if there is a hole or tear in it, replace immediately.*

NOTE: You will need a doctor's prescription for replacement bags or a new starter kit.

InspirEase is designed for use with most "spray inhaler" (metered dose inhaler) containers currently available; for single-patient use and single-dose use.

The usual caution should be exercised in dosing medications and evaluating patient response.

The prescribing information for the marketed MDIs varies with respect to dosing, administration, etc. We recommend that these be followed when using InspirEase.

CAUTION: Federal law restricts this device to sale by or on the order of a physician.

Rev. 3/89

REFERENCES

1. Sackner MA, Brown LK, Kim CS: *Chest* 80 (suppl): 915–918, 1981. **2.** Tobin MJ, Jenouri G, Danta I, et al: *Am Rev Respir Dis* 126:670–675, 1982. **3.** Saunders KB:*Br Med J* 1:1037–1038, 1965. **4.** Gayrard P, Orehek J: *Respiration* 40:47–52, 1980. **5.** Shim C, Williams MH Jr: *Am J Med* 69:891–894, 1980.

Distributed by: Schering Corporation, Kenilworth, NJ 07033 USA

Copyright© 1987, 1989 Schering Corporation, USA
All rights reserved.

INTRON® A   ℞
Interferon alfa-2b
recombinant
   For Injection

DESCRIPTION

INTRON A Interferon alfa-2b, recombinant for intramuscular, subcutaneous or intralesional Injection is a purified sterile, lyophilized recombinant interferon formulation. The 3 million, 5 million, 25 million and 50 million IU packages are for use by intramuscular or subcutaneous injection. The 10 million IU package is for intramuscular, subcutaneous, or intralesional injection. (See **WARNINGS** and **PRECAUTIONS**.)

Interferon alfa-2b, recombinant is a water soluble protein with a molecular weight of 19,271 daltons produced by recombinant DNA techniques. It is obtained from the bacterial fermentation of a strain of *Escherichia coli* bearing a genetically engineered plasmid containing an interferon alfa-2b gene from human leukocytes. The fermentation is carried out in a defined nutrient medium containing the antibiotic tetracycline hydrochloride at a concentration of 5 to 10 mg/L; the presence of this antibiotic is not detectable in the final product. The specific activity of Interferon alfa-2b, recombinant is approximately 2×10^8 IU/mg protein.

The content of Interferon alfa-2b, recombinant is expressed in terms of International Units (IU). International Units are determined by comparison of the antiviral activity of the interferon alfa-2b, recombinant with the activity of the international reference preparation of human leukocyte interferon established by the World Health Organization (WHO). Each vial of INTRON A contains either 3 million, 5 million, 10 million, 25 million or 50 million IU of interferon alfa-2b, recombinant, 20 mg glycine, 2.3 mg sodium phosphate dibasic, 0.55 mg sodium phosphate monobasic, and 1.0 mg human albumin are also present. Based on the specific activity of INTRON A as approximately 2×10^8 IU/mg protein, the corresponding mg quantities of interferon alfa-2b, recombinant in the vials described above are approximately 0.015 mg, 0.025 mg, 0.05 mg, 0.125 mg, and 0.25 mg protein, respectively. Prior to administration, the lyophilized powder is to be reconstituted with Diluent for INTRON A Interferon alfa-2b, recombinant (bacteriostatic water for injection) provided (see diluent label for preservative). (See **DOSAGE AND ADMINISTRATION**.)

Lyophilized INTRON A is a white to cream colored powder.

CLINICAL PHARMACOLOGY

General: The interferons are a family of naturally occurring, small protein molecules with molecular weights of approximately 15,000 to 21,000 daltons. They are produced and secreted by cells in response to viral infections or to various synthetic and biological inducers. Three major classes of interferons have been identified: alpha, beta, and gamma. These three classes are not homogenous, and each may contain several different molecular species of interferon. As an example, at least 14 genetically distinct human alpha interferons have been identified thus far. INTRON A has been classified as an alpha interferon.

Interferons exert their cellular activities by binding to specific membrane receptors on the cell surface. Preliminary studies to characterize these membrane receptors and to determine the subsequent fate of the human interferon-receptor complex have been carried out using ^{125}I-labeled interferon alfa-2b, recombinant. Human interferon receptors, as isolated from human lymphoblastoid (Daudi) cells, appear to be highly asymmetric membrane proteins. They exhibit selectivity for human but not murine interferons, suggesting species-specificity. Studies with other interferons have demonstrated varying degrees of species-specificity.

The results of several studies suggest that once bound to the cell membrane, interferon initiates a complex sequence of intracellular events that include the induction of certain enzymes. It is thought that this process, at least in part, is responsible for the various cellular responses to interferon, including inhibition of virus replication in virus-infected cells, suppression of cell proliferation, and such immunomodulating activities as enhancement of the phagocytic activity of macrophages and augmentation of the specific cytotoxicity of lymphocytes for target cells. Any of these activities might contribute to interferon's therapeutic effects.

Preclinical Pharmacology INTRON A Interferon alfa-2b, recombinant for Injection has exhibited antiproliferative effects in preclinical studies employing both cell culture systems and human tumor xenografts in animals, and has demonstrated significant immunomodulatory activity *in vitro*. The clinical significance of these findings is unknown.

The antiproliferative activity of INTRON A was evaluated *in vitro* using mouse and human leukemia cell lines, and human osteosarcoma, melanoma, and normal amnion cells. No activity was seen in mouse leukemia cells, which again suggests species-specificity.

The immunomodulating activity of INTRON A was demonstrated *in vitro* by its augmentation of the spontaneous "natural killer" activity of human lymphocytes, its enhancement of the tumoricidal activity of human monocytes against human tumor cells, and its induction of Class I histocompatibility antigens on the surface of a number of cell types. These effects appear to be dose-dependent.

In vivo studies of INTRON A showed inhibition of tumor growth. INTRON A injected *intralesionally* (0.2 million or 0.8 million IU once daily for 7 days) delayed the development and reduced the volume of human osteosarcoma implants in athymic mice. The effect was dose-related. Additionally, *subcutaneous* administration of INTRON A at a dose of 0.2 million IU/day inhibited the growth of implanted human breast tumor xenografts in athymic mice by about 50% after 23 days. INTRON A has not been shown to be effective in the treatment of osteosarcoma or carcinoma of the breast in humans.

Pharmacokinetics The pharmacokinetics of INTRON A were studied in 12 healthy male volunteers following single doses of 5 million IU/m^2 administered intramuscularly, subcutaneously and as a 30-minute intravenous infusion in a cross-over design. INTRON A concentrations were determined using a radioimmunoassay (RIA) with a detection limit equal to 10 IU/mL.

The mean serum concentration of INTRON A following intramuscular and subcutaneous injections were comparable. The maximum serum concentrations obtained via these routes were approximately 18 to 116 IU/mL and occurred 3 to 12 hours after administration. The elimination half-lives of INTRON A following both intramuscular and subcutaneous injections were approximately two to three hours. Serum concentrations were below the detection limit by 16 hours after the injections.

After intravenous administration, serum concentrations of INTRON A peaked (135 to 273 IU/mL) by the end of the infusion, then declined at a slightly more rapid rate than after intramuscular or subcutaneous drug administration, becoming undetectable four hours after the infusion. The elimination half-life was approximately two hours.

Urine concentrations of INTRON A following a single dose (5 million IU/m^2) were not detectable after any of the parenteral routes of administration. This result was expected since preliminary studies with isolated and perfused rabbit kidneys have shown that the kidney may be the main site of interferon catabolism.

There is no pharmacokinetic data available for the intralesional route of administration.

Hairy Cell Leukemia: In clinical trials in patients with hairy cell leukemia, there was depression of circulating red blood cells, white blood cells and platelets during the first one to two months of treatment with INTRON A Interferon alfa-2b, recombinant for Injection. Subsequently, both splenectomized and non-splenectomized patients with hairy cell leukemia, treated with INTRON A achieved substantial and sustained improvements in granulocytes, platelets, and hemoglobin levels in 75% of treated patients and at least some improvement (minor responses) occurred in 90%. For the entire study group median platelet counts were within the normal range after 2 months, median hemoglobin levels were in the normal range after 4 months and median granulocyte counts were in the normal range after 5 months of treatment. Responses of blood cell elements were similar in splenectomized and non-splenectomized patients except that median platelet counts after maximum response was to a level of 100,000/mm^3 in the latter group.

Treatment with INTRON A resulted in a decrease in bone marrow hypercellularity and hairy cell infiltrates. The hairy cell index (HCI), which represents the percent of bone marrow cellularity times the percent of hairy cell infiltrate, was greater than or equal to 50% at the beginning of the study in 87% of patients. The percentage of patients with such an HCI decreased to 25% after six months and to 14% after one year. These results indicate that even though hematologic improvement had occurred earlier, prolonged treatment with INTRON A may be required to obtain maximal reduction in tumor cell infiltrates in the bone marrow.

The percentage of patients with hairy cell leukemia who required red blood cell or platelet transfusions decreased significantly during treatment with INTRON A. Additionally, the percentage of patients with confirmed and serious infections declined during treatment with INTRON A as granulocyte counts improved.

The responses observed in non-splenectomized patients included reversal of splenomegaly and of abnormalities in blood cell counts attributable to hypersplenism. In some cases there was reversal of clinically significant hypersplenism that may have resulted in need for splenectomy.

Reduced risk of major complications of hairy cell leukemia (serious infections, bleeding diatheses, transfusion requirements) were apparent within 3 months of initiation of treatment in comparisons of INTRON A treated patients to a control group. No deaths occurred in patients treated with INTRON A during the subsequent 9 months of treatment and follow up, while the mortality rate in the control group was 20% in the same time interval based on probability of survival analysis.

Subsequent follow-up with a median time of approximately 40 months demonstrated an overall survival of 87.8%. In a comparable historical control group, followed for 24 months, overall median survival was approximately 40%.

During the initial 3 months of treatment, there may be interferon-mediated suppression of hematopoiesis.

Serum Neutralizing Antibodies In a multicenter controlled clinical trial involving 145 hairy cell leukemia patients, no serum neutralizing antibodies were detected in the 90 patients evaluated.

In AIDS-Related Kaposi's Sarcoma patients treated with INTRON A, one out of 24 patients have developed detectable serum neutralizing antibodies.

Serum neutralizing antibodies have been detected in less than 3% of patients treated with higher doses of INTRON A in malignancies other than hairy cell leukemia or AIDS-

Related Kaposi's Sarcoma. The clinical significance of these findings is unknown.

Condylomata Acuminata: Condylomata acuminata (venereal or genital warts) are associated with infections of the human papilloma virus (HPV), especially HPV type-6 and possibly type-11. Given the antiviral and antiproliferative activities of interferons and the viral etiology of condylomata, placebo-controlled clinical trials were conducted to evaluate the efficacy and safety of intralesional injections of INTRON A Interferon alfa-2b, recombinant for Injection in the treatment of condylomata acuminata.

In the three controlled double-blind clinical trials conducted to determine the efficacy of INTRON A in condyloma, a total of 192 patients were evaluable for efficacy (a total of 224 were evaluable for safety). These patients were injected intralesionally with 1 million IU of INTRON A per lesion. Up to five lesions per patient were treated three times a week for three weeks, and the patients were then observed for up to 16 weeks after the full treatment course. These studies showed that INTRON A was significantly more effective than placebo in the treatment of condylomata, as measured by disappearance of lesions, decreases in lesion size, and by an overall change in disease status. In the 192 patients evaluated, 42% experienced clearing of all treated lesions, while 24% experienced marked ($\geq 75\%$ to $<100\%$) and 18% experienced moderate ($\geq 50\%$ to $<75\%$) reduction in lesion size, and 10% of patients had a slight reduction ($<50\%$) in lesion size. Therefore, in these studies, 84% of patients experienced either lesion clearing or marked to moderate reduction in lesion size. INTRON A was effective in treating lesions of all sizes.

In one of these studies involving 125 patients in whom multiple (up to three) lesions were treated, a significant number of patients whose lesions were treated with INTRON A (54 patients out of 125 or 43%) experienced complete clearing of all treated lesions at one time or another during the course of the study. Of these 54 patients, 81% remained cleared of all treated lesions 16 weeks after treatment was initiated.

In this study, the percentage of patients who had one, two or three lesions treated and had all respective treated lesions cleared after one course of therapy ranged from 31 to 56%. Those patients who did not achieve total clearing of all their treated lesions had these same lesions treated with a second course of therapy. During this second course of treatment, 38 to 67% of patients had clearing of all treated lesions. Overall percentage of patients who had all their treated lesions clear after two courses of treatment ranged from 57 to 85%.

Also from the above study, the INTRON A treated lesions showed improvement within two to four weeks after the start of treatment. In 64% (68 patients out of 107) of those patients who experienced lesion clearing, or marked ($\geq 75\%$ to $<100\%$) or moderate ($\geq 50\%$ to $<75\%$) reduction in lesion size, the maximal response to INTRON A therapy was noted four to eight weeks after initiation of treatment. Additionally, a greater number of placebo-treated patients experienced exacerbations of their lesions during the post-treatment period, than did patients treated with INTRON A.

There was no significant difference in the clearing of lesions between those patients who had received other prior therapies for condylomata and those who had not. However, patients having condylomata for a shorter duration had better responses to treatment with INTRON A than those with lesions of a longer duration. There was no difference in response to treatment of penile, vulvar or perianal condylomata or of condylomata appearing in heavily or lightly keratinized areas.

Serum neutralizing activity was detected in 0.8% of patients (2 out of 260) evaluate who received INTRON A intralesionally. The significance of the appearance of serum neutralizing activity is not known.

AIDS-Related Kaposi's Sarcoma: Kaposi's Sarcoma (KS) is a common manifestation of the Acquired Immune Deficiency Syndrome (AIDS). Kaposi's Sarcoma lesions are usually cutaneous but may also occur throughout the gastrointestinal tract and occasionally affect visceral organs. They frequently are very numerous and may be painful and disfiguring.

INTRON A Interferon alfa-2b, recombinant for Injection was administered to AIDS-Related Kaposi's Sarcoma patients in three separate clinical trials to evaluate efficacy and safety. A total of 144 patients were treated in these studies.

The first clinical trial was a randomized study comparing the efficacy and safety of subcutaneous low dose (1 million IU/m^2 INTRON A) versus intravenous high dose (50 million IU/m^2 INTRON A) therapy. Both treatments were administered daily for 5 days every other week. Preliminary results showed objective responses in both regimens, but a shorter time to response and a higher response rate occurred with

Continued on next page

Information on Schering products appearing on these pages is effective as of September 30, 1989.

Schering—Cont.

the 50 million IU/m^2 regimen. This study showed significantly greater activity in patients who were asymptomatic (afebrile and without weight loss) than in those with systemic symptoms (57% vs. 23%).

In the second clinical study patients with AIDS-Related KS received 30 million IU/m^2 of INTRON A, subcutaneously three times per week (TIW). Doses were adjusted for patient tolerance. In this study the average weekly dose delivered in the first four weeks was 150 million IU; at the end of twelve weeks this averaged 110 million IU/week; and by twenty-four weeks averaged 75 million IU/week. A response rate of 44% was obtained in asymptomatic patients versus 7% in symptomatic patients. The median time to response was approximately 2 months and the median duration of response was approximately three months for the asymptomatic patients. For the symptomatic patients, the median time to response was one month and median duration of response was also one month. Baseline T4/T8 ratios were 0.46 for responders vs. 0.33 for nonresponders.

In a third study INTRON A was administered daily as a subcutaneous injection of 35 million IU/d for 12 weeks. Maintenance treatment, with every other day dosing, was continued for up to one year in patients achieving antitumor and antiviral responses. The median time to response was 2 months and median duration of response 5 months in the asymptomatic patients.

In all studies, the likelihood of response has been greatest in patients with relatively intact immune systems as assessed by baseline T4 counts (interchangeable with CD4) or T4/T8 ratios. Results at doses of 30 million IU/m^2 TIW and 35 million IU/daily, subcutaneously were similar and are provided together in Tables 1 and 2 below. These tables demonstrate the relationship of response to baseline T4 count or T4/T8 ratio in both asymptomatic (subtype A) and symptomatic (subtype B) patients in the 30 million IU/m^2 TIW dose and the 35 million IU/d dose.

TABLE 1
*RESPONSE BY BASELINE T4 COUNT**
30 million IU/m^2
TIW, SC and 35 million IU Daily, SC

	Asymptomatic	Symptomatic
T4 ≤ 200	4/14(29%)	0/19(0%)
200 ≤ T4 ≤ 400	6/12(50%)	0/5(0%)
	58%	
T4 > 400	5/7(71%)	0/0(0%)

TABLE 2
*RESPONSE BY T4/T8 RATIOS**
30 million IU/m^2
TIW, SC and 35 million IU Daily, SC

	Asymptomatic	Symptomatic
T4/T8 ≤ 0.25	1/13(8%)	0/21(0%)
0.25 ≤ T4/T8 ≤ 0.50	13/21(62%)	3/14(21%)
	60%	
0.50 ≤ T4/T8	11/19(58%)	0/3(0%)

*Data for T4, T4/T8, and asymptomatic and symptomatic classification was not available for all patients.

In the 30 million IU study group, there were 7% (5/72) of patients who were complete responders and 22% (16/72) of the patients were partial responders. The 35 million IU study had 13% (3/23 patients) complete responders and 17% (4/23) of the patients were partial responders.

For patients who received 30 million IU, TIW, the median survival time is longer in patients with T4 greater than 200 (30.7 months) than in patients with T4 less than or equal to 200 (8.9 months). Among responders, the median survival time was 22.6 months versus 9.7 months in non-responders.

INDICATIONS AND USAGE

General: INTRON A Interferon alfa-2b, recombinant for Injection is indicated for the treatment of hairy cell leukemia, selected cases of condylomata acuminata involving external surfaces of the genital and perianal areas, and AIDS-Related Kaposi's Sarcoma in select patients 18 years or older.

Hairy Cell Leukemia: INTRON A for Injection is indicated for the treatment of patients 18 years of age or older with hairy cell leukemia. Studies have shown that INTRON A can produce clinically meaningful regression or stabilization of this disease, both in previously splenectomized and non-splenectomized patients.

Prior to initiation of therapy, tests should be performed to quantitate peripheral blood hemoglobin, platelets, granulocytes and hairy cells and bony marrow hairy cells. These parameters should be monitored periodically during treatment to determine whether response to treatment has occurred. If a patient does not respond within 6 months, treatment should be discontinued. If a response to treatment does occur, treatment usually should be continued until no further improvement is observed and these laboratory parameters have been stable for about 3 months (see **DOSAGE AND ADMINISTRATION**). It is not known whether continued treatment after that time point is beneficial. Studies are in progress to evaluate this question.

The 50 million IU strength is not to be used for the treatment of hairy cell leukemia.

Condylomata Acuminata: INTRON A is indicated also for intralesional treatment of selected cases of condylomata acuminata involving external surfaces of the genital and perianal areas (see **DOSAGE AND ADMINISTRATION**). The 3 million, 5 million, and 25 million IU strengths are not to be used for the intralesional treatment of condylomata since the dilution required for intralesional use would result in a hypertonic solution. The 50 million IU strength is not to be used for the treatment of condylomata.

In selecting patients for treatment with INTRON A, the physician should consider the nature of the patient's lesion and the patient's past treatment history, in addition to the patient's ability to comply with the treatment regimen. INTRON A offers an additional approach to treatment in condyloma and is particularly useful for those patients who do not respond satisfactorily to other treatment modalities (e.g., podophyllin resin, surgery, cryotherapy, chemotherapy, and laser therapy), or whose lesions are more readily treatable by INTRON A Interferon alfa-2b, recombinant for Injection than by other treatments.

The use of this product in adolescents has not been studied. Interferon alpha has been shown to affect the menstrual cycle and decrease serum estradiol and progesterone levels in females. Consideration should be given as to whether the adolescent patient should be treated.

AIDS-Related Kaposi's Sarcoma: INTRON A is also indicated for the treatment of select patients, above 18 years of age with AIDS-Related Kaposi's Sarcoma. Studies have demonstrated a greater likelihood of response to INTRON A therapy in patients who are without systemic symptoms, who have limited lymphadenopathy and who have a relatively intact immune system.

Lesion measurements and blood counts should be performed prior to initiation of therapy and should be monitored periodically during treatment to determine whether response to treatment or disease stabilization has occurred.

When disease stabilization or a response to treatment occurs, treatment should continue until there is no further evidence of tumor or until discontinuation is required by evidence of a severe opportunistic infection or adverse effect.

CONTRAINDICATIONS

INTRON A is contraindicated in patients with a history of hypersensitivity to interferon alfa or any component of the injection.

WARNINGS

Moderate to severe adverse experiences may require modification of the patient's dosage regimen, or in some cases, termination of therapy with INTRON A.

Because of the fever and other "flu-like" symptoms associated with INTRON A administration, it should be used cautiously in patients with debilitating medical conditions, such as those with a history of cardiovascular disease (e.g., unstable angina, uncontrolled congestive heart failure), pulmonary disease (e.g., chronic obstructive pulmonary disease), or diabetes mellitus prone to ketoacidosis. Caution should also be observed in patients with coagulation disorders (e.g., thrombophlebitis, pulmonary embolism) or severe myelosuppression.

Hairy Cell Leukemia: Patients with platelet counts of less than 50,000/mm^3 should not be administered INTRON A intramuscularly, but instead by subcutaneous administration. The 50 million IU strength is not to be used for the treatment of hairy cell leukemia.

Cardiovascular adverse experiences, which include significant hypotension, arrhythmia, or tachycardia of 150 beats per minute or greater, were observed in approximately 3% of the patients studied who had various malignancies and were treated at doses higher than those for hairy cell leukemia. Transient reversible cardiomyopathy was reported in approximately 2% of the AIDS-Related Kaposi's Sarcoma patients treated with INTRON A Injection. Cardiomyopathy has also been reported in AIDS patients not receiving INTRON A therapy. The incidence of these complications in patients with preexisting heart disease is unknown. Hypotension may occur during administration, or up to two days post therapy, and may require supportive therapy including fluid replacement to maintain intravascular volume. Supraventricular arrhythmias occurred rarely and appeared to be correlated with preexisting conditions, and prior therapy with cardiotoxic agents. These adverse experiences were controlled by modifying the dose or discontinuing treatment, but may require specific additional therapy.

Those patients with a recent history of myocardial infarction and/or previous or current arrhythmic disorder, who require INTRON A Interferon alfa-2b, recombinant for Injection therapy, should be closely monitored (see **Laboratory Tests**). Central nervous system effects manifested by depression, confusion and other alterations of mental status were observed in about 2% of hairy cell leukemia patients treated with INTRON A. The overall incidence in a larger patient population with other malignancies treated with higher doses of INTRON A was 10%. More significant obtundation

and coma have been observed in some patients, usually elderly, treated at higher doses for other malignant diseases. These effects are usually rapidly reversible. In a few severe episodes, full resolution of symptoms has taken up to three weeks. Patients should be closely monitored until resolution of these effects. Discontinuation of INTRON A therapy may be required. Narcotics, hypnotics, or sedatives may be used concurrently with caution.

Laboratory abnormalities which occurred in hairy cell leukemia patients included elevated SGOT and SGPT, which occurred in 4% and 13% of patients, respectively. The overall incidences of laboratory abnormalities in a larger patient population with other malignancies, and treated at higher doses were somewhat higher. These included elevated liver function tests (SGOT, SGPT in 10% of patients) and reductions in granulocyte (20% of patients) and platelet counts (18% of patients) (see **Laboratory Tests**). These abnormalities are usually mild to moderate and transient. Severe abnormalities of these laboratory parameters are usually rapidly reversible upon cessation or reduction of INTRON A therapy.

Condylomata Acuminata: The 3 million, 5 million, and 25 million IU strengths are not to be used for the intralesional treatment of condylomata since the dilution required for the intralesional use would result in a hypertonic solution. The 50 million IU strength is not to be used for the treatment of condylomata.

AIDS-Related Kaposi's Sarcoma: INTRON A should not be used for patients with rapidly progressive visceral disease (see **CLINICAL PHARMACOLOGY**). Also, of note, there may be synergistic adverse effects between INTRON A and zidovudine (AZT). Patients receiving concomitant zidovudine have had a higher incidence of neutropenia than that expected with zidovudine alone. Careful monitoring of the WBC count is indicated in all patients who are myelosuppressed and in all patients receiving other myelosuppressive medications. The effects of INTRON A when combined with other drugs used in the treatment of AIDS-Related disease are unknown.

PRECAUTIONS

General: Acute serious hypersensitivity reactions (e.g., urticaria, angioedema, bronchoconstriction, anaphylaxis) have not been observed, but might occur, in patients receiving INTRON A; however, if such an acute reaction develops, the drug should be discontinued immediately and appropriate medical therapy instituted. Transient rashes have occurred in some patients following injection, but have not necessitated treatment interruption.

Variations in dosage, routes of administration, and adverse reactions exist among different brands of Interferon. Therefore, do not use different brands of Interferon in any single treatment regimen.

Information for Patients: Patients being treated with INTRON A Injection should be directed in its appropriate use, informed of benefits and risks associated with treatment and referred to the PATIENT INFORMATION SHEET. This information is intended to aid in the safe and effective use of this medication. It is not a disclosure of all possible adverse or intended effects.

If home use is prescribed, a puncture resistant container for the disposal of used syringes and needles should be supplied to the patient. Patients should be thoroughly instructed in the importance of proper disposal and cautioned against any reuse of needles and syringes. The full container should be disposed of according to the directions provided by the physician (see **PATIENT INFORMATION SHEET**).

Patients should be cautioned not to change brands of Interferon without medical consultation as a change in dosage may result.

Patients receiving treatment for AIDS-Related KS should be cautioned against performing tasks that would require complete mental alertness, such as operating machinery or driving a motor vehicle.

The most common adverse experiences occurring with INTRON A Interferon alfa-2b, recombinant for Injection therapy are "flu-like" symptoms, such as fever, headache, fatigue, anorexia, nausea, or vomiting (see **ADVERSE REACTIONS** section) and appear to decrease in severity as treatment continues. Some of these "flu-like" symptoms may be minimized by bedtime administration. Acetaminophen may be used to prevent or partially alleviate the fever and headache.

It is advised that patients be well hydrated especially during the initial stages of treatment.

Laboratory Tests: In addition to those tests normally required for monitoring patients, the following laboratory tests are recommended for all patients on INTRON A therapy, prior to beginning treatment and then periodically thereafter.

● Standard hematologic tests—including complete blood counts and differential as well as platelet counts.
● Blood chemistries—electrolytes and liver function tests. Those patients who have preexisting cardiac abnormalities and/or are in advanced stages of cancer, should have electro-

cardiograms taken prior to and during the course of treatment.

Mild to moderate leukopenia and elevated serum liver enzyme (SGOT) levels have been reported with intralesional administration of INTRON A (see **ADVERSE REACTIONS** section); therefore, the monitoring of these laboratory parameters should be considered.

Transient reversible cardiomyopathy was reported in approximately 2% of the AIDS-Related Kaposi's Sarcoma patients treated with INTRON A Injection. Cardiomyopathy has also been reported in AIDS patients not receiving INTRON A therapy.[2] Baseline chest X-rays are suggested and should be repeated if clinically indicated.

Carcinogenesis, Mutagenesis, Impairment of Fertility: Studies with INTRON A have not been performed to determine carcinogenicity, or the effect on fertility.

Interferon may impair fertility. In studies of interferon use in non-human primates, abnormalities of the menstrual cycle have been observed. Decreases in serum estradiol and progesterone concentrations have been reported in women treated with human leukocyte interferon.[1] Therefore, fertile women should not receive INTRON A unless they are using effective contraception during the therapy period. INTRON A should be used with caution in fertile men.

Mutagenicity studies with INTRON A revealed no adverse effects.

Studies in mice, rats, and monkeys injected with INTRON A Injection for up to one month have revealed no evidence of toxicity. However, due to the known species-specificity of interferon, the effects in animals are unlikely to be predictive of those in man.

Pregnancy Category C: INTRON A has been shown to have abortifacient effects in *Macaca mulatta* (rhesus monkeys) at 90 and 180 times the intramuscular or subcutaneous dose of 2 million IU/m^2. Although abortion was observed in all dose groups (7.5 million, 15 million, and 30 million IU/kg), it was only statistically significant versus control at the mid and high dose groups (corresponding to 90 and 180 times the intramuscular or subcutaneous dose of 2 million IU/m^2). There are no adequate and well controlled studies in pregnant women. INTRON A should be used during pregnancy only if the potential benefit justifies the potential risk to the fetus.

Nursing Mothers: It is not known whether this drug is excreted in human milk. However, studies in mice have shown that mouse interferons are excreted into the milk. Because of the potential for serious adverse reactions from INTRON A Interferon alfa-2b, recombinant for Injection in nursing infants, a decision should be made whether to discontinue nursing or to discontinue the drug, taking into account the importance of the drug to the mother.

Pediatric Use: Safety and effectiveness have not been established in patients below the age of 18 years.

ADVERSE REACTIONS

Hairy Cell Leukemia: The following adverse reactions were reported to be possibly or probably related to INTRON A therapy during clinical trials in 145 patients with hairy cell leukemia. Most of the adverse reactions reported were mild to moderate and diminished in severity and number with continued therapy. The most frequently reported adverse reactions were flu-like symptoms, particularly fever (68%), fatigue (61%), and chills (46%). Other adverse reactions which were reported in 5% or more patients included:

Application Site Disorders (20%).

Central and Peripheral Nervous System—Paresthesia and depression, each occurred in 6%, anxiety in 5%.

Flu-like Symptoms (other)—Myalgia and headache (39% in each), unspecified flu-like symptoms (37%), anorexia, back pain, dry mouth (19% in each), pain (unspecified) (18%), taste alteration (13%), dizziness (12%), arthralgia and increased sweating (8% in each) and asthenia (7%).

Gastrointestinal System—Nausea (21%), diarrhea (18%), and vomiting (6%).

Skin and Appendages—Rashes (25%), pruritus (11%), dry skin (9%), and dermatitis and alopecia (8% in each).

Other—Vision disorders (7%).

The following adverse reactions were reported in less than 5% of patients: amnesia, confusion, decreased libido, hypertonia, hypoesthesia, migraine, somnolence, flushing, leg cramps, rhinitis, abdominal pain, eructation, gynecomastia, arthrosis, bone disorder, stye, hearing disorders, urticaria, pharyngitis, stomatitis.

Miscellaneous adverse events, such as palpitation, postural hypotension, impaired consciousness, tremor, constipation, thirst, chest pain, coughing, dyspnea, impotence, acne, erythema, nail disorder, micturition disorder, nocturia, and weight decrease, were also rarely observed (less than 1%).

All of the previously described adverse reactions which occurred in patients with hairy cell leukemia were also observed in patients receiving higher doses for other malignancies. The incidence of most adverse reactions were similar between the two groups, with some being higher in patients who received higher doses of INTRON A. In studies of patients with malignancies other than hairy cell leukemia, hematologic and hepatic toxicities were more common in patients receiving individual injections greater than 10 mil-

lion IU, than in patients receiving less than this amount. Hematologic, hepatic, cardiovascular and neurologic toxicities were more common in patients receiving more than 30 million IU per injection than in patients receiving less than that amount. Some additional adverse effects which occurred in patients treated for malignancies other than hairy cell leukemia included malaise (11%), hypotension (8%), herpes simplex (3%), epistaxis (2%), hypertension (2%), tachycardia (3%), and eye pain (3%).

Adverse experiences occurring in less than 1% of these patients and observed only in patients with malignancies other than hairy cell leukemia are as follows: hot flashes, purpura, bradycardia, cardiac failure, arrhythmia, atrial fibrillation, peripheral ischemia, agitation, coma, impaired concentration, emotional lability, extrapyramidal disorder, paresis, parosmia, speech disorder, abnormal thinking, dehydration, nasal congestion, bilirubinemia, dyspepsia, loose stools, melena, increased saliva, abscess, conjunctivitis, furunculosis, viral and fungal infection, moniliasis, pneumonia, sepsis, sinusitis, hypercalcemia, virilism, bronchospasm, cyanosis, wheezing, respiratory disorder, nonherpetic cold sores, epidermal necrolysis, syncope, hematuria, polyuria, cachexia, edema, earache, impotence, lacrimal gland disorder, lymphadenopathy, muscle weakness, tinnitus, and vertigo.

Abnormal Laboratory Test Values The percentage of patients with hairy cell leukemia or with other types of malignancies who experienced a significant abnormal laboratory test value (values that changed from WHO Grades 0, 1 or 2 at baseline to WHO Grades 3 or 4 during treatment) at least once during their treatment is shown in the following table:

ABNORMAL LABORATORY TEST VALUES

	Hairy Cell Leukemia (N=145)	Overall Safety Summary* (N=867)
SGOT	4%	11%
SGPT	13%	10%
Alkaline Phosphatase	4%	6%
Lactate Dehydrogenase	0%	3%
BUN	0%	<1%
Creatinine	0%	0%
White Blood Cell Count	NA	22%
Granulocyte Count	NA	26%
Hemoglobin Level	NA	5%
Platelet Count	NA	8%

*Patients with hairy cell are included in the overall summary.

NA—Not Applicable—Patients' initial hematologic laboratory test values were abnormal due to their condition.

Condylomata Acuminata: The adverse experiences listed below were reported to be possibly or probably related to intralesional treatment with INTRON A Interferon alfa-2b, recombinant for Injection during clinical trials involving 352 condyloma patients. These patients were injected intralesionally with 1 million IU per lesion. Up to 5 lesions were treated for a total of up to 5 million IU of INTRON A per treatment.

Each patient was treated up to three times a week for three weeks, and then observed for up to 16 weeks after treatment. Eighty-eight percent (311 of 352) of those patients treated with INTRON A for condyloma who were evaluable for safety, reported an adverse reaction some time during treatment. All 40 patients who had five warts treated, reported some type of adverse reaction during treatment. Most of the following reported adverse reactions were mild to moderate and were transient and rapidly reversible, and did not interfere with therapy. The frequency of these reactions decreased markedly over the course of treatment, with most reactions occurring during the first week of treatment. Few patients reported treatment-related adverse experiences after treatment with INTRON A ended. The incidence of these adverse experiences includes all experiences reported throughout the course of the study (overall incidence). The incidence at any weekly interval was lower than the overall incidences cited below. The incidence of the adverse reactions reported increased when the number of treated lesions increased from one to five.

The most frequently reported adverse reactions were flu-like symptoms, primarily fever (56%), headache (47%), myalgia (44%) and chills (45%). These reactions were mostly mild and transient and were considered to be alleviated by administration of acetaminophen.

In addition, the following adverse reactions were reported:
Autonomic Nervous System—Increased sweating (2%).
Body as a Whole—Fatigue (18%), malaise (14%), back pain (6%), weakness (4%), pain (3%), and leg cramps (2%).
Central and Peripheral Nervous Systems—Dizziness (9%), and confusion (4%).
Gastrointestinal System—Nausea (17%), diarrhea, dyspepsia, and vomiting (2% in each).
Musculoskeletal System—Arthralgia (9%).
Psychiatric Disorders—Depression and somnolence (3% in each).

Those adverse reactions which were reported by 1% of patients treated with INTRON A Interferon alfa-2b, recombinant for Injection include: hot flushes, hypoesthesia, paresthesia, tremor, vertigo, abdominal pain, anorexia, thirst,

arthrosis, emotional lability, epistaxis, agitation, nervousness, herpes simplex, nasal congestion, pharyngitis, pruritus, urticaria, eye pain and lymphadenopathy.

The adverse reactions which were reported rarely (less than 1% of patients) include: flushing, syncope, chest pain, weight decrease, edema (peripheral and swollen lips), abnormal coordination, hypertonia, esophagitis, loose stools, palpitations, rectal bleeding after stool, tachycardia, arthritis, purpura, anxiety, impaired concentration, insomnia, leukorrhea, menorrhagia, fungal infection, moniliasis, photosensitivity reaction, skin discoloration, taste alteration, abnormal vision, conjunctivitis, and photophobia.

Application Site Disorders The frequency of reporting application site disorders (such as burning, itching and pain) for patients treated with INTRON A or placebo were similar (20%); therefore, these adverse reactions were probably due to the manipulation of the lesions rather than to INTRON A therapy.

Abnormal Laboratory Test Values An assessment of laboratory values obtained before, during, and after treatment indicated that abnormalities occurred primarily as lowering of WBC counts (17%) and elevated SGOT levels (12%). Elevations in SGOT levels also occurred in placebo-treated patients (8%). The majority of these laboratory abnormalities in INTRON A treated patients involved increases of one WHO grade, and were generally mild to moderate and were transient.

Adverse Reactions After Retreatment with INTRON A Adverse reactions, application site disorders, and abnormal laboratory test values, reported by patients who were retreated with INTRON A, were qualitatively and quantitatively similar to those reported above.

AIDS-Related Kaposi's Sarcoma: The incidence and severity of adverse experiences in AIDS-Related Kaposi's Sarcoma patients is similar to those reported in other clinical trials of patients with malignancies who were treated with INTRON A. More severe toxicities are observed at higher doses and may be difficult for patients to tolerate. Adverse experiences in AIDS-Related Kaposi's Sarcoma patients are usually mild or moderate in severity and consist primarily of flu-like symptoms. Adverse reactions of any type occurred in 100% of the 74 patients treated subcutaneously with 30 million IU/m^2 three times a week and in 97% of patients who received 35 million IU of INTRON A subcutaneously per day.

The most frequently reported adverse experiences were flu-like symptoms which occurred in 45% (33/74) of patients receiving 30 million IU/m^2 TIW and in 79% (23/29) of the patients receiving 35 million IU/day.

Other treatment-related adverse experiences which occurred most frequently are shown in the following table: [See table on next page].

In the 30 million IU/m^2 TIW study, severe adverse experiences included: fatigue (20%), flu-like symptoms (15%), anorexia (12%), dry mouth (4%), headache (4%), confusion (3%), fever (3%), myalgia (3%), and nausea and vomiting (1% each). The severe adverse reactions reported for patients who received the 35 million IU per day included: fever (24%), fatigue (17%), flu-like symptoms (14%), dyspnea (14%), headache (10%), pharyngitis (7%), and ataxia, confusion, dysphagia, GI hemorrhage, abnormal hepatic function, increased SGOT, myalgia, cardiomyopathy, face edema, depression, emotional lability, suicide attempt, chest pain, and coughing (1 patient each). Overall, the incidence of severe toxicity was higher among patients who received the 35 million IU per day dose.

Other infrequent treatment-related adverse reactions for the 30 million IU TIW study included: pruritus (7%); and abdominal pain, malaise, taste perversion and weight loss (5% each); and dyspepsia, malaise, and maculopapular rash (4% each); and pain, insomnia, and somnolence (3% each). Those adverse experiences reported as occurring in only 1 patient each included: back pain, flushing, impaired consciousness, eructation, thirst, epistaxis, gingival bleeding, agitation, anxiety, anemia, taste loss, hematuria and abnormal vision.

In the patient group receiving 35 million IU INTRON A Interferon alfa-2b, recombinant for Injection per day, less common adverse reactions were reported as: face edema (10%); and aphasia, ataxia, CNS dysfunction, tremor, dysphagia, stomatitis, abnormal hepatic function, gingival bleeding, purpura, paroniria, pleural pain, rhinitis, skin disorder, taste perversion, micturition frequency, granulocytopenia and leukopenia, photophobia (2 patients each); and back pain, pain, weight decrease, edema, peripheral edema, hypotension, neuropathy, gastric ulcer, gum hyperplasia, rectal hemorrhage, oral leukoplakia, GI mucosal discoloration, earache, tinnitus, increased BUN, periorbital edema, arthralgia, epistaxis, thrombocytopenia, amnesia, anxiety,

Continued on next page

Information on Schering products appearing on these pages is effective as of September 30, 1989.

Schering—Cont.

apathy, aggravated depression, insomnia, nervousness, neurosis, impotence, herpes simplex, viral infection, pneumonia, respiratory disorder, abnormal hair texture, skin depigmentation, urticaria, hematuria, micturition disorder, polyuria, eye pain (1 patient each).

Abnormal Laboratory Test Values Laboratory test abnormalities occurred mostly in total white blood cell count, granulocyte count, and liver enzyme levels. Treatment-related changes in laboratory test values from WHO grade 0, 1, or 2 to WHO grades 3 or 4 for the 30 million IU/m^2 and the 35 million IU/d dosing regimens are shown in the following table:

ABNORMAL LABORATORY TEST VALUES

	Number of Patients (%)	
Laboratory Tests	30 million IU/m^2 TIW	35 million IU/d
Hemoglobin	1/73 (1%)	4/26 (15%)
White Blood Cell Count	7/73 (10%)	6/27 (22%)
Granulocyte Count	22/71 (31%)	11/28 (39%)
Platelet Count	none	2/26 (8%)
SGOT	8/72 (11%)	11/27 (41%)
SGPT	7/69 (10%)	4/27 (15%)

DOSAGE AND ADMINISTRATION

IMPORTANT: INTRON A dosing regimens are different for each of the following indications described in this section of the product information sheet.

Hairy Cell Leukemia: The recommended dosage of INTRON A for Injection for the treatment of hairy cell leukemia is 2 million IU/m^2 administered intramuscularly (see **WARNINGS**) or subcutaneously 3 times a week. The 50 million IU strength is not to be used for the treatment of hairy cell leukemia. Higher doses are not recommended. The normalization of one or more hematologic variables usually begins within 2 months of initiation of therapy. Improvement in all three hematologic variables may require 6 months or more of therapy.

This dosage regimen should be maintained unless the disease progresses rapidly, or severe intolerance is manifested. If severe adverse reactions develop, the dosage should be modified (50% reduction) or therapy should be temporarily discontinued until the adverse reactions abate. If persistent or recurrent intolerance develops following adequate dosage adjustment, or disease progresses, treatment with INTRON A Interferon alfa-2b, recombinant for Injection should be discontinued. The minimum effective dose of INTRON A has not been established.

At the discretion of the physician, the patient may self-administer the dose. (See illustrated PATIENT INFORMATION SHEET for instructions.) The medication may be administered at bedtime.

Condylomata Acuminata: The 10 million IU vial of INTRON A must be reconstituted with 1 mL of Diluent for INTRON A Interferon alfa-2b, recombinant (bacteriostatic water for injection), to provide the proper concentration of INTRON A for the treatment of condylomata. Do not use the 3, 5, or 25 million IU vials for treatment of condylomata acuminata since the dilution required for intralesional treatment would result in a hypertonic solution. The 50 million IU vial is not to be used for the treatment of condylomata. Additionally, do not reconstitute the 10 million IU vial with more than 1 mL of diluent, since the injection would be subpotent.

Inject 1.0 million IU of INTRON A (0.1 mL of reconstituted INTRON A) into each lesion three times per week on alternate days, for three weeks. The injection should be administered intralesionally using a Tuberculin or similar syringe and a 25–30 gauge needle. The needle should be directed at the center of the base of the wart and at an angle almost parallel to the plane of the skin (approximating that in the commonly used PPD test). This will deliver the interferon to the dermal core of the lesion, infiltrating the lesion and causing a small wheal. Care should be taken not to go beneath the lesion too deeply; subcutaneous injection should be avoided, since this area is below the base of the lesion. Do not inject too superficially since this will result in possible leakage, infiltrating only the keratinized layer, and not the dermal core. As many as 5 lesions can be treated at one time. To re-

Treatment-Related Adverse Experiences in AIDS-Related KS Patients
Dosing Regimens

ADVERSE EXPERIENCE	30 million IU/m^2, TIW/SC N=74	35 million IU/d/SC N=29
		Percentage (%) of patients
Flu-like symptoms	45	79
Other Flu-like Symptoms		
fatigue	84	48
fever	47	55
anorexia	38	41
headache	36	21
myalgia	34	28
rigors	30	14
dry mouth	22	28
dizziness	7	24
increased sweating	4	21
chest pain	1	28
asthenia	11	0
Central and Peripheral Nervous System Disorders		
confusion	12	10
hypoesthesia	0	10
paresthesia	3	21
Gastrointestinal System Disorders		
abdominal pain	5	21
constipation	1	10
diarrhea	18	45
nausea	28	21
vomiting	11	14
gingivitis	0	14
loose stools	0	10
Psychiatric Disorders		
depression	9	28
concentration impaired	3	14
amnesia	0	14
Resistance Mechanism Disorders		
moniliasis	0	17
Respiratory System Disorders		
dyspnea	1	34
coughing	0	31
pharyngitis	1	31
sinusitis	0	21
nonproductive coughing	0	14
nasal congestion	0	10
Skin and Appendages Disorders		
alopecia	12	31
rash	9	10
dry skin	9	10

duce side effects, INTRON A may be administered in the evening, when possible. Additionally, acetaminophen may be administered at the time of injection to alleviate some of the potential side effects.

The maximum response usually occurs four to eight weeks after initiation of the first treatment course. If results at 12 to 16 weeks after the initial treatment course has concluded are not satisfactory, a second course of treatment using the above dosage schedule may be instituted providing that clinical symptoms and signs, or changes in laboratory parameters (liver function tests, WBC and platelets) do not preclude such a course of action.

Patients with six to ten condylomata may receive a second (sequential) course of treatment at the above dosage schedule, to treat up to five additional condylomata per course of treatment. Patients with greater than ten condylomata may receive additional sequences depending on how large a number of condylomata are present.

AIDS-Related Kaposi's Sarcoma: The recommended dosage of INTRON A is 30 million IU/m^2 three times a week administered subcutaneously or intramuscularly.

The selected dosage regimen should be maintained unless the disease progresses rapidly or severe intolerance is manifested. If severe adverse reactions develop, the dosage should be modified (50% reduction) or therapy should be temporarily discontinued until the adverse reactions abate. When patients initiate therapy at 30 million IU/m^2 TIW, the average dose tolerated at the end of 12 weeks of therapy is 110 million IU/week and 75 million IU/week at the end of 24 weeks of therapy.

When disease stabilization or a response to treatment occurs, treatment should continue until there is no further evidence of tumor until discontinuation is required by evidence of a severe opportunistic infection or adverse effect.

Preparation and Administration of INTRON A Interferon alfa-2b, recombinant for Injection

Reconstitution of lyophilized INTRON A Interferon alfa-2b, recombinant for Injection Inject the amount of Diluent for INTRON A (bacteriostatic water for injection) stated in the appropriate chart below (diluent is supplied in either a vial or syringe, see **HOW SUPPLIED** below), into the vial of INTRON A. Agitate gently to hasten complete dissolution of the powder. The appropriate dose of INTRON A should then be withdrawn and injected intramuscularly, subcutaneously, or intralesionally. (See **PATIENT INFORMATION SHEET** for detailed instructions.)

After preparation and administration of INTRON A, it is essential to follow the procedure for proper disposal of syringes and needles. (See **PATIENT INFORMATION SHEET** for detailed instructions.)

HAIRY CELL LEUKEMIA

Vial Strength	mL Diluent	Final Concentration
3 million IU	1	3 million IU/mL
5 million IU	1	5 million IU/mL
10 million IU	2	5 million IU/mL
25 million IU	5	5 million IU/mL

CONDYLOMATA ACUMINATA

Vial Strength	mL Diluent	Final Concentration
*10 million IU	1	10 million IU/mL

* *IMPORTANT:* For patients with condylomata acuminata, reconstitute the 10 million IU vial with only 1 mL of the diluent provided to reach a final concentration of 10 million IU/mL to be administered intralesionally. (See **DOSAGE AND ADMINISTRATION, Condylomata Acuminata**.)

AIDS-RELATED KAPOSI'S SARCOMA

Vial Strength	mL Diluent	Final Concentration
50 million IU	1	50 million IU/mL

IMPORTANT: This vial size is to be used only for treatment of patients with AIDS-Related Kaposi's Sarcoma (see **DOSAGE AND ADMINISTRATION, AIDS-Related Kaposi's Sarcoma**).

Stability After reconstitution with Diluent for INTRON A (bacteriostatic water for injection) the solution is stable for one month at 2° to 8°C (36° to 46°F). The reconstituted solution is clear and colorless to light yellow.

Parenteral drug products should be inspected visually for particulate matter and discoloration prior to administration, whenever solution and container permit.

INTRON A may be administered using either sterilized glass or plastic disposable syringes.

HOW SUPPLIED

INTRON A Interferon alfa-2b, recombinant for Injection, 3 million IU per vial and Diluent for INTRON A Interferon alfa-b, recombinant (bacteriostatic water for injection) 1 mL per vial or syringe; boxes containing 1 vial of INTRON A for Injection and 1 vial of Diluent for INTRON A Interferon alfa-2b, recombinant (bacteriostatic water for injection) (NDC 0085-0647-03), and boxes containing 1 vial of INTRON A for Injection and 1 syringe of Diluent for INTRON A Interferon alfa-2b, recombinant (bacteriostatic water for injection) (NDC 0085-0647-04).

INTRON A Interferon alfa-2b, recombinant for Injection, 5 million IU per vial and Diluent for INTRON A Interferon alfa-2b, recombinant (bacteriostatic water for injection) 1 mL per vial; boxes containing 1 vial of INTRON A for Injection and 1 vial of Diluent for INTRON A Interferon alfa-2b, recombinant (bacteriostatic water for injection) (NDC 0085-0120-02).

INTRON A Interferon alfa-2b, recombinant for Injection, 10 million IU per vial and Diluent for INTRON A Interferon alfa-2b, recombinant (bacteriostatic water for injection) 2 mL per vial; boxes containing 1 vial of INTRON A for Injection and 1 vial of Diluent for INTRON A Interferon alfa-2b, recombinant (bacteriostatic water for injection) (NDC 0085-0571-02).

INTRON A Interferon alfa-2b, recombinant for Injection, 25 million IU per vial and Diluent for INTRON A Interferon alfa-2b, recombinant (bacteriostatic water for injection) 5 mL per vial; boxes containing 1 vial of INTRON A for Injection and 1 vial of Diluent for INTRON A Interferon alfa-2b, recombinant (bacteriostatic water for injection) (NDC 0085-0285-02).

INTRON A Interferon alfa-2b, recombinant for Injection, 50 million IU per vial and Diluent for INTRON A Interferon alfa-2b, recombinant (bacteriostatic water for injection) 1 mL per vial; boxes containing 1 vial of INTRON A for Injection and 1 vial of Diluent for INTRON A Interferon alfa-2b, recombinant (bacteriostatic water for injection) (NDC 0085-0539-01).

Store INTRON A for Injection both before and after reconstitution between 2° and 8°C (36° and 46°F).

Revised 11/88   B-16147605

REFERENCES

1. Kauppila A, et al; *Int J Cancer*, 29:291–294, 1982.
2. Cohen I, et al; *N Engl J Med*, 315:628–630, 1986.
U.S. Patents 4,530,901 & 4,496,537

LOTRIMIN®   ℞

[lo'trim-in]
brand of clotrimazole
   Cream, USP 1%
   Lotion, USP 1%
   Solution, USP 1%
For Dermatologic Use Only—
Not For Ophthalmic Use

DESCRIPTION

LOTRIMIN products contain clotrimazole, USP, a synthetic antifungal agent having the chemical name [1-(o-Chloro-α,α-diphenylbenzyl)imidazole]; the empirical formula, $C_{22}H_{17}ClN_2$; and a molecular weight of 344.84.

Clotrimazole is an odorless, white crystalline substance. It is practically insoluble in water, sparingly soluble in ether and very soluble in polyethylene glycol 400, ethanol and chloroform.

Each gram of LOTRIMIN **Cream** contains 10 mg clotrimazole, USP in a vanishing cream base of sorbitan monostearate, polysorbate 60, cetyl esters wax, cetearyl alcohol, 2-octyldodecanol, purified water and, as preservative, benzyl alcohol (1%).

Each gram of LOTRIMIN **Lotion** contains 10 mg clotrimazole, USP dispersed in an emulsion vehicle composed of sorbitan monostearate, polysorbate 60, cetyl esters wax, cetearyl alcohol, 2-octyldodecanol, purified water; benzyl alcohol (1%) as preservative; sodium phosphate dibasic and sodium biphosphate to adjust pH.

Each ml of LOTRIMIN **Solution** contains 10 mg clotrimazole, USP in a nonaqueous vehicle of polyethylene glycol 400.

CLINICAL PHARMACOLOGY

Clotrimazole is a broad-spectrum antifungal agent that is used for the treatment of dermal infections caused by various species of pathogenic dermatophytes, yeasts, and *Malassezia furfur.* The primary action of clotrimazole is against dividing and growing organisms.

In vitro, clotrimazole exhibits fungistatic and fungicidal activity against isolates of *Trichophyton rubrum, Trichophyton mentagrophytes, Epidermophyton floccosum, Microsporum canis,* and *Candida* species, including *Candida albicans*. In general, the *in vitro* activity of clotrimazole corresponds to that of tolnaftate and griseofulvin against the mycelia of dermatophytes (*Trichophyton, Microsporum,* and *Epidermophyton*), and to that of the polyenes (amphotericin B and nystatin) against budding fungi (*Candida*). Using an *in vivo* (mouse) and an *in vitro* (mouse kidney homogenate) testing system, clotrimazole and miconazole were equally effective in preventing the growth of the pseudomycelia and mycelia of *Candida albicans.*

Strains of fungi having a natural resistance to clotrimazole are rare. Only a single isolate of *Candida guilliermondi* has been reported to have primary resistance to clotrimazole.

No single-step or multiple-step resistance to clotrimazole has developed during successive passages of *Candida albicans* and *Trichophyton mentagrophytes*. No appreciable change in sensitivity was detected after successive passages of isolates of *C. albicans, C. krusei,* or *C. pseudotropicalis* in liquid or solid media containing clotrimazole. Also, resistance could

not be developed in chemically induced mutant strains of polyene-resistant isolates of *C. albicans*. Slight, reversible resistance was noted in three isolates of *C. albicans* tested by one investigator. There is a single report that records the clinical emergence of a *C. albicans* strain with considerable resistance to flucytosine and miconazole, and with cross-resistance to clotrimazole; the strain remained sensitive to nystatin and amphotericin B.

In studies of the mechanism of action, the minimum fungicidal concentration of clotrimazole caused leakage of intracellular phosphorus compounds into the ambient medium with concomitant breakdown of cellular nucleic acids and accelerated potassium efflux. Both these events began rapidly and extensively after addition of the drug.

Clotrimazole appears to be well absorbed in humans following oral administration and is eliminated mainly as inactive metabolites. Following topical and vaginal administration, however, clotrimazole appears to be minimally absorbed.

Six hours after the application of radioactive clotrimazole 1% cream and 1% solution onto intact and acutely inflamed skin, the concentration of clotrimazole varied from 100 mcg/cm³ in the stratum corneum to 0.5 to 1 mcg/cm³ in the stratum reticulare, and 0.1 mcg/cm³ in the subcutis. No measurable amount of radioactivity (≤0.001 mcg/ml) was found in the serum within 48 hours after application under occlusive dressing of 0.5 ml of the solution or 0.8 g of the cream. Only 0.5% or less of the applied radioactivity was excreted in the urine.

Following intravaginal administration of 100 mg ^{14}C-clotrimazole vaginal tablets to nine adult females, an average peak serum level, corresponding to only 0.03 µg equivalents/ml of clotrimazole, was reached one to two days after application. After intravaginal administration of 5 g of 1% ^{14}C-clotrimazole vaginal cream, containing 50 mg active drug, to five subjects (one with candidal colpitis), serum levels corresponding to approximately 0.01 µg equivalents/ml were reached between 8 and 24 hours after application.

INDICATIONS AND USAGE

LOTRIMIN products are indicated for the topical treatment of the following dermal infections: tinea pedis, tinea cruris, and tinea corporis due to *Trichophyton rubrum, trichophyton mentagrophytes, Epidermophyton floccosum,* and *Microsporum canis;* candidiasis due to *Candida albicans;* and tinea versicolor due to *Malassezia furfur.*

CONTRAINDICATIONS

LOTRIMIN products are contraindicated in individuals who have shown hypersensitivity to any of their components.

WARNINGS

LOTRIMIN products are not for ophthalmic use.

PRECAUTIONS

General: If irritation or sensitivity develops with the use of clotrimazole, treatment should be discontinued and appropriate therapy instituted.

Information For Patients:
This information is intended to aid in the safe and effective use of this medication. It is not a disclosure of all possible adverse or intended effects.
The patient should be advised to:
1. Use the medication for the full treatment time even though the symptoms may have improved. Notify the physician if there is no improvement after four weeks of treatment.
2. Inform the physician if the area of application shows signs of increased irritation (redness, itching, burning, blistering, swelling, oozing) indicative of possible sensitization.
3. Avoid sources of infection or reinfection.

Laboratory Tests: If there is lack of response to clotrimazole, appropriate microbiological studies should be repeated to confirm the diagnosis and rule out other pathogens before instituting another course of antimycotic therapy.

Drug Interactions: Synergism or antagonism between clotrimazole and nystatin, or amphotericin B, or flucytosine against strains of *C. albicans* has not been reported.

Carcinogenesis, Mutagenesis, Impairment of Fertility: An 18-month oral dosing study with clotrimazole in rats has not revealed any carcinogenic effect.

In tests for mutagenesis, chromosomes of the spermatophores of Chinese hamsters which had been exposed to clotrimazole were examined for structural changes during the metaphase. Prior to testing, the hamsters had received five oral clotrimazole doses of 100 mg/kg body weight. The results of this study showed that clotrimazole had no mutagenic effect.

Usage in Pregnancy: Pregnancy Category B: The disposition of ^{14}C-clotrimazole has been studied in humans and animals. Clotrimazole is very poorly absorbed following dermal application or intravaginal administration to humans. (See **Clinical Pharmacology.**)

In clinical trials, use of vaginally applied clotrimazole in pregnant women in their second and third trimesters has not been associated with ill effects. There are, however, no adequate and well-controlled studies in pregnant women during the first trimester of pregnancy.

Studies in pregnant rats with intravaginal doses up to 100 mg/kg have revealed no evidence of harm to the fetus due to clotrimazole.

High oral doses of clotrimazole in rats and mice ranging from 50 to 120 mg/kg resulted in embryotoxicity (possibly secondary to maternal toxicity), impairment of mating, decreased litter size and number of viable young and decreased pup survival to weaning. However, clotrimazole was not teratogenic in mice, rabbits and rats at oral doses up to 200, 180 and 100 mg/kg, respectively. Oral absorption in the rat amounts to approximately 90% of the administered dose. Because animal reproduction studies are not always predictive of human response, this drug should be used only if clearly indicated during the first trimester of pregnancy.

Nursing Mothers: It is not known whether this drug is excreted in human milk. Because many drugs are excreted in human milk, caution should be exercised when clotrimazole is used by a nursing woman.

Pediatric Use: Safety and effectiveness in children have been established for clotrimazole when used as indicated and in the recommended dosage.

ADVERSE REACTIONS

The following adverse reactions have been reported in connection with the use of clotrimazole: erythema, stinging, blistering, peeling, edema, pruritus, urticaria, burning, and general irritation of the skin.

OVERDOSAGE

Acute overdosage with topical application of clotrimazole is unlikely and would not be expected to lead to a life-threatening situation.

DOSAGE AND ADMINISTRATION

Gently massage sufficient LOTRIMIN into the affected and surrounding skin areas twice a day, in the morning and evening.

Clinical improvement, with relief of pruritus, usually occurs within the first week of treatment with LOTRIMIN. If the patient shows no clinical improvement after four weeks of treatment with LOTRIMIN, the diagnosis should be reviewed.

HOW SUPPLIED

LOTRIMIN **Cream** 1% is supplied in 15, 30, 45 and 90-g tubes (NDC 0085-0613-02, 05, 04, 03, respectively); boxes of one.
LOTRIMIN **Lotion** 1% is supplied in 30 ml bottles (NDC 0085-0707-02); boxes of one.
Shake well before using.
LOTRIMIN **Solution** 1% is supplied in 10 ml and 30 ml plastic bottles (NDC 0085-0182-02, 04, respectively); boxes of one.
Store LOTRIMIN products between 2° and 30°C (36° and 86°F).

Rev. 1/87

LOTRISONE®   ℞

[lō'trĭ-sōn]
brand of clotrimazole
and betamethasone
dipropionate
Cream, USP

For Dermatologic Use Only—
Not for Ophthalmic Use

DESCRIPTION

LOTRISONE Cream contains a combination of clotrimazole, USP, a synthetic antifungal agent, and betamethasone dipropionate, USP, a synthetic corticosteroid, for dermatologic use.

Chemically, clotrimazole is 1-(o -Chloro-α,α-diphenyl benzyl) imidazole, with the empirical formula $C_{22}H_{17}ClN_2$ and a molecular weight of 344.8.

Clotrimazole is an odorless, white crystalline powder, insoluble in water and soluble in ethanol.

Betamethasone dipropionate has the chemical name 9-Fluoro-11β, 17,21-trihydroxy-16β-methylpregna-1,4-diene-3,20-dione 17,21-dipropionate, with the empirical formula $C_{28}H_{37}FO_7$ and a molecular weight of 504.6.

Betamethasone dipropionate is a white to creamy white, odorless crystalline powder, insoluble in water.

Each gram of LOTRISONE Cream contains 10.0 mg clotrimazole, USP, and 0.64 mg betamethasone dipropionate, USP (equivalent to 0.5 mg betamethasone), in a hydrophilic emollient cream consisting of purified water, mineral oil, white petrolatum, cetearyl alcohol, ceteareth-30, propylene glycol, sodium phosphate monobasic, and phosphoric acid; benzyl alcohol as preservative.

Continued on next page

Information on Schering products appearing on these pages is effective as of September 30, 1989.

Schering—Cont.

LOTRISONE is a smooth, uniform, white to off-white cream.

CLINICAL PHARMACOLOGY

Clotrimazole

Clotrimazole is a broad-spectrum, antifungal agent that is used for the treatment of dermal infections caused by various species of pathogenic dermatophytes, yeasts, and *Malassezia furfur*. The primary action of clotrimazole is against dividing and growing organisms.

In vitro, clotrimazole exhibits fungistatic and fungicidal activity against isolates of *Trichophyton rubrum, Trichophyton mentagrophytes, Epidermophyton floccosum* and *Microsporum canis*. In general, the *in vitro* activity of clotrimazole corresponds to that of tolnaftate and griseofulvin against the mycelia of dermatophytes (*Trichophyton, Microsporum,* and *Epidermophyton*).

In vivo studies in guinea pigs infected with *Trichophyton mentagrophytes* have shown no measurable loss of clotrimazole activity due to combination with betamethasone dipropionate.

Strains of fungi having a natural resistance to clotrimazole have not been reported.

No single-step or multiple-step resistance to clotrimazole has developed during successive passages of *Trichophyton mentagrophytes*.

In studies of the mechanism of action in fungal cultures, the minimum fungicidal concentration of clotrimazole caused leakage of intracellular phosphorous compounds into the ambient medium with concomitant breakdown of cellular nucleic acids, and accelerated potassium efflux. Both of these events began rapidly and extensively after addition of the drug to the cultures.

Clotrimazole appears to be minimally absorbed following topical application to the skin. Six hours after the application of radioactive clotrimazole 1% cream and 1% solution onto intact and acutely inflamed skin, the concentration of clotrimazole varied from 100 mcg/cm^3 in the stratum corneum, to 0.5 to 1 mcg/cm^3 in the stratum reticulare, and 0.1 mcg/cm^3 in the subcutis. No measureable amount of radioactivity (<0.001 mcg/ml) was found in the serum within 48 hours after application under occlusive dressing of 0.5 ml of the solution or 0.8 g of the cream.

Betamethasone dipropionate

Betamethasone dipropionate, a corticosteroid, is effective in the treatment of corticosteroid-responsive dermatoses primarily because of its anti-inflammatory, antipruritic, and vasoconstrictive actions. However, while the physiologic, pharmacologic, and clinical effects of corticosteroids are well-known, the exact mechanisms of their actions in each disease are uncertain. Betamethasone dipropionate, a corticosteroid, has been shown to have topical (dermatologic) and systemic pharmacologic and metabolic effects characteristic of this class of drugs.

Pharmacokinetics: The extent of percutaneous absorption of topical corticosteroids is determined by many factors including the vehicle, the integrity of the epidermal barrier, and the use of occlusive dressings. (See **Dosage and Administration** section.)

Topical corticosteroids can be absorbed from normal intact skin. Inflammation and/or other disease processes in the skin increase percutaneous absorption. Occlusive dressings substantially increase the percutaneous absorption of topical corticosteroids. (See **Dosage and Administration** section.)

Once absorbed through the skin, topical corticosteroids are handled through pharmacokinetic pathways similar to systemically administered corticosteroids. Corticosteroids are bound to plasma proteins in varying degrees. Corticosteroids are metabolized primarily in the liver and are then excreted by the kidneys. Some of the topical corticosteroids and their metabolities are also excreted into the bile.

Clotrimazole and betamethasone dipropionate

In clinical studies of tinea corporis, tinea cruris and tinea pedis, patients treated with LOTRISONE Cream showed a better clinical response at the first return visit, than patients treated with clotrimazole cream. In tinea corporis and tinea cruris, the patient returned three days after starting treatment, and in tinea pedis, after one week. Mycological cure rates observed in patients treated with LOTRISONE Cream were as good as or better than in those patients treated with clotrimazole cream.

In these same clinical studies, patients treated with LOTRISONE Cream showed statistically significantly better clinical responses and mycological cure rates when compared with patients treated with betamethasone dipropionate cream.

INDICATIONS AND USAGE

LOTRISONE Cream is indicated for the topical treatment of the following dermal infections: tinea pedis, tinea cruris, and tinea corporis due to *Trichophyton rubrum, Trichophyton mentagrophytes, Epidermophyton floccosum,* and *Microsporum canis*.

CONTRAINDICATIONS

LOTRISONE Cream is contraindicated in patients who are sensitive to clotrimazole, betamethasone dipropionate, other corticosteroids or imidazoles, or to any ingredient in this preparation.

PRECAUTIONS

General: Systemic absorption of topical corticosteroids has produced reversible hypothalamic-pituitary-adrenal (HPA) axis suppression, manifestations of Cushing's syndrome, hyperglycemia, and glucosuria in some patients.

Conditions which augment systemic absorption include the application of the more potent steroids, use over large surface areas, prolonged use, and the addition of occlusive dressings. (See **Dosage and Administration** section.)

Therefore, patients receiving a large dose of a potent topical steroid applied to a large surface area should be evaluated periodically for evidence of HPA axis suppression by using the urinary free cortisol and ACTH stimulation tests. If HPA axis suppression is noted, an attempt should be made to withdraw the drug, to reduce the frequency of application, or to substitute a less potent steroid.

Recovery of HPA axis function is generally prompt and complete upon discontinuation of the drug. Infrequently, signs and symptoms of steroid withdrawal may occur, requiring supplemental systemic corticosteroids.

Children may absorb proportionally larger amounts of topical corticosteroids and thus be more susceptible to systemic toxicity. (See **Precautions-Pediatric Use.**)

If irritation or hypersensitivity develops with the use of LOTRISONE Cream, treatment should be discontinued and appropriate therapy instituted.

Information for Patients Patients using LOTRISONE Cream should receive the following information and instructions:

1. This medication is to be used as directed by the physician. It is for external use only. Avoid contact with the eyes.
2. The medication is to be used for the full prescribed treatment time, even though the symptoms may have improved. Notify the physician if there is no improvement after one week of treatment for tinea cruris or tinea corporis, or after two weeks for tinea pedis.
3. Patients should be advised not to use this medication for any disorder other than for which it was prescribed.
4. The treated skin areas should not be bandaged or otherwise covered or wrapped as to be occluded. (See **Dosage and Administration** section.)
5. When using this medication in the groin area, patients should be advised to use the medication for two weeks only, and to apply the cream sparingly. The physician should be notified if the condition persists after two weeks. Patients should also be advised to wear loose fitting clothing. (See **Dosage and Administration** section.)
6. Patients should report any signs of local adverse reactions.
7. Parents of pediatric patients should be advised not to use tight-fitting diapers or plastic pants on a child being treated in the diaper area, as these garments may constitute occlusive dressing. (See **Dosage and Administration** section.)
8. Patients should avoid sources of infection or reinfection.

Laboratory Tests: If there is a lack of response to LOTRISONE Cream, appropriate microbiological studies should be repeated to confirm the diagnosis and rule out other pathogens before instituting another course of antimycotic therapy.

The following tests may be helpful in evaluating HPA axis suppression due to the corticosteroid component:

   Urinary free cortisol test

   ACTH stimulation test

Carcinogenesis, Mutagenesis, Impairment of Fertility: There are no animal or laboratory studies with the combination clotrimazole and betamethasone dipropionate to evaluate carcinogenesis, mutagenesis or impairment of fertility.

An 18-month oral dosing study with clotrimazole in rats has not revealed any carcinogenic effect.

In tests for mutagenesis, chromosomes of the spermatophores of Chinese hamsters which have been exposed to clotrimazole were examined for structural changes during the metaphase. Prior to testing, the hamsters had received five oral clotrimazole doses of 100 mg/kg body weight. The results of this study showed that clotrimazole had no mutagenic effect.

Pregnancy Category C: There have been no teratogenic studies performed with the combination clotrimazole and betamethasone dipropionate.

Studies in pregnant rats with intravaginal doses up to 100 mg/kg have revealed no evidence of harm to the fetus due to clotrimazole.

High oral doses of clotrimazole in rats and mice ranging from 50 to 120 mg/kg resulted in embryotoxicity (possibly secondary to maternal toxicity), impairment of mating, decreased litter size and number of viable young and decreased pup survival to weaning. However, clotrimazole was not teratogenic in mice, rabbits and rats at oral doses up to 200, 180

and 100 mg/kg, respectively. Oral absorption in the rat amounts to approximately 90% of the administered dose. Corticosteroids are generally teratogenic in laboratory animals when administered systemically at relatively low dosage levels. The more potent corticosteroids have been shown to be teratogenic after dermal application in laboratory animals.

There are no adequate and well-controlled studies in pregnant women on teratogenic effects from a topically applied combination of clotrimazole and betamethasone dipropionate. Therefore, LOTRISONE Cream should be used during pregnancy only if the potential benefit justifies the potential risk to the fetus.

Drugs containing corticosteroids should not be used extensively on pregnant patients, in large amounts, or for prolonged periods of time.

Nursing Mothers: It is not known whether this drug is excreted in human milk. Because many drugs are excreted in human milk, caution should be exercised when LOTRISONE Cream is used by a nursing woman.

Pediatric Use: Safety and effectiveness in children below the age of 12 have not been established with LOTRISONE Cream. However, dosage forms containing concentrations of clotrimazole and of betamethasone dipropionate found in LOTRISONE Cream have been demonstrated to be safe and effective when used as indicated and in the recommended dosages.

Pediatric patients may demonstrate greater susceptibility to topical corticosteroid-induced HPA axis suppression and Cushing's syndrome than mature patients because of a larger skin surface area to body weight ratio.

Hypothalamic-pituitary-adrenal (HPA) axis suppression, Cushing's syndrome, and intracranial hypertension have been reported in children receiving topical corticosteroids. Manifestations of adrenal suppression in children include linear growth retardation, delayed weight gain, low plasma cortisol levels, and absence of response to ACTH stimulation. Manifestations of intracranial hypertension include bulging fontanelles, headaches, and bilateral papilledema.

Administration of topical dermatologics containing a corticosteroid to children should be limited to the least amount compatible with an effective therapeutic regimen. Chronic corticosteroid therapy may interfere with the growth and development of children.

ADVERSE REACTIONS

The following adverse reactions have been reported in connection with the use of LOTRISONE Cream: paresthesia in 5 of 270 patients, maculopapular rash, edema, and secondary infection, each in 1 of 270 patients.

Adverse reactions reported with the use of clotrimazole are as follows: erythema, stinging, blistering, peeling, edema, pruritus, urticaria, and general irritation of the skin.

The following local adverse reactions are reported infrequently when topical corticosteroids are used as recommended. These reactions are listed in an approximate decreasing order of occurrence: burning, itching, irritation, dryness, folliculitis, hypertrichosis, acneiform eruptions, hypopigmentation, perioral dermatitis, allergic contact dermatitis, maceration of the skin, secondary infection, skin atrophy, striae, and miliaria.

OVERDOSAGE

Acute overdosage with topical application of LOTRISONE Cream is unlikely and would not be expected to lead to a life-threatening situation.

Topically applied corticosteroids can be absorbed in sufficient amounts to produce systemic effects. (See **Precautions.**)

DOSAGE AND ADMINISTRATION

Gently massage sufficient LOTRISONE Cream into the affected and surrounding skin areas twice a day, in the morning and evening for two weeks in tinea cruris and tinea corporis, and for four weeks in tinea pedis. The use of LOTRISONE Cream for longer than four weeks is not recommended.

Clinical improvement, with relief of erythema and pruritus, usually occurs within three to five days of treatment. If a patient with tinea cruris and tinea corporis shows no clinical improvement after one week of treatment with LOTRISONE Cream, the diagnosis should be reviewed. In tinea pedis, the treatment should be applied for two weeks prior to making that decision.

Treatment with LOTRISONE Cream should be discontinued if the condition persists after two weeks in tinea cruris and tinea corporis, and after four weeks in tinea pedis. Alternate therapy may then be instituted with LOTRIMIN Cream, a product containing an antifungal only.

LOTRISONE Cream should not be used with occlusive dressings.

HOW SUPPLIED

LOTRISONE Cream is supplied in 15-gram (NDC 0085-0924-01), and 45-gram tubes (NDC 0085-0924-02); boxes of one.

NETROMYCIN® ℞
brand of netilmicin sulfate
Injection, USP 100 mg/ml

WARNINGS

Patients treated with aminoglycosides should be under close clinical observation because of the potential toxicity associated with the use of these drugs.

Netilmicin has potent neuromuscular blocking potential. Neuromuscular blockade and respiratory paralysis have been reported in animals receiving netilmicin. The possibility of these phenomena occurring in man should be considered if aminoglycosides are administered by any route to patients receiving neuromuscular blocking agents, such as succinylcholine, tubocurarine, or decamethonium, or to patients receiving massive transfusions of citrate-anticoagulated blood. If neuromuscular blockade occurs, calcium salts may lessen it, but mechanical respiratory assistance may also be necessary.

As with other aminoglycosides, netilmicin sulfate injection is potentially nephrotoxic. The risk is greater in patients with impaired renal function, in those who receive high dosage or prolonged therapy, and in the elderly.

Neurotoxicity manifested by ototoxicity, both vestibular and auditory, can occur in patients treated with netilmicin, primarily in those with preexisting renal damage and in patients treated with higher doses and/or for longer periods than recommended. Aminoglycoside-induced ototoxicity is usually irreversible. Other manifestations of aminoglycoside-induced neurotoxicity include numbness, skin tingling, muscle twitching, and convulsions.

Renal and eighth cranial nerve functions should be closely monitored, especially in patients with known or suspected impairment of renal function either at onset of therapy or during therapy. Urine should be examined for increased excretion of protein, the presence of cells or casts, and decreased specific gravity. Serum creatinine concentration or blood urea nitrogen should be determined periodically. A more precise measure of glomerular filtration rate is a carefully conducted determination of creatinine clearance rate or, often more practically, an estimate of creatinine clearance based on published nomograms or equations. (See **DOSAGE AND ADMINISTRATION.**) When feasible it is recommended that serial audiograms be obtained in patients old enough to be tested, particularly in high-risk patients. The dosage of netilmicin should be reduced or administration discontinued if evidence of drug-induced auditory or vestibular toxicity (dizziness, vertigo, tinnitus, nystagmus, or hearing loss) develops during therapy. If evidence of nephrotoxicity occurs, dosage should be adjusted. (See **DOSAGE AND ADMINISTRATION, DOSAGE FOR IMPAIRED RENAL FUNCTION.**) As with other aminoglycosides, on rare occasions changes in renal and eighth cranial nerve functions may not become manifest until soon after completion of therapy.

Serum concentrations of aminoglycosides should be monitored when feasible to assure adequate levels and to avoid potentially toxic levels. After administration of an appropriate dose of netilmicin, peak serum concentrations occur approximately 30 to 60 minutes after an intramuscular injection or at the end of a one hour intravenous infusion. Dosage should be adjusted so that prolonged peak serum concentrations above 16 mcg/ml are avoided.

When monitoring trough concentrations, dosage should be adjusted so that levels above 4 mcg/ml are avoided.

Excessive peak and/or trough serum concentrations of aminoglycosides may increase the risk of renal and eighth cranial nerve toxicity. In the event of overdose or toxic reactions, hemodialysis may aid in removal of netilmicin from the blood, especially if renal function is, or becomes, compromised. Removal of netilmicin by peritoneal dialysis is at a rate considerably less than by hemodialysis.

Concurrent and/or sequential systemic or topical use of other potentially neurotoxic and/or nephrotoxic drugs, such as: cephaloridine, amphotericin B, streptomycin, kanamycin, acyclovir, gentamicin, tobramycin, amikacin, neomycin, vancomycin, bacitracin, polymyxin B, colistin, paromomycin, viomycin, or cisplatin should be avoided. The concurrent use of aminoglycosides with potent diuretics, such as ethacrynic acid or furosemide, should be avoided since certain diuretics by themselves may cause ototoxicity. In addition, when administered intravenously, diuretics may enhance aminoglycoside

---

toxicity by altering the antibiotic concentration in the serum and tissues. Other factors which may increase patient risk of toxicity are advanced age and dehydration.

DESCRIPTION

NETROMYCIN Injection contains netilmicin sulfate, USP in clear, sterile aqueous solution with a pH range of 3.5 to 6.0 for intramuscular or intravenous administration. Netilmicin is a semisynthetic, water-soluble antibiotic of the aminoglycoside group, derived from sisomicin. Its chemical name is: O-3-Deoxy-4-C-methyl-3-(methylamino)-β-L-arabinopyranosyl (1→4)-O-[2,6-diamino-2,3,4,6-tetradeoxy-α-D-$glycero$-hex-4-enopyranosyl-(1→6)]-2-deoxy-N^3-ethyl-L-streptamine sulfate (2:5) (salt).

Each ml of NETROMYCIN Injection contains netilmicin sulfate, USP equivalent to 100 mg netilmicin; 10 mg benzyl alcohol as a preservative; 0.1 mg edetate disodium; 2.4 mg sodium metabisulfite; 0.8 mg sodium sulfite; and water for injection, q.s.

CLINICAL PHARMACOLOGY

Netilmicin is rapidly and completely absorbed after intramuscular injection. Peak serum levels, after intramuscular injection, usually occur within 30 to 60 minutes and levels are measurable for 12 hours. In adult volunteers with normal renal function, peak serum concentrations of netilmicin in mcg/ml are usually about 3 to 3.5 times the single intramuscular dose in mg/kg. For example, a dose of 2.0 mg/kg may be expected to result in a peak serum concentration of approximately 7 mcg/ml. At eight or more hours after administration of a dose in the recommended range, serum levels are usually less than 3 mcg/ml. When a single dose of netilmicin is administered by 60-minute intravenous infusion, the peak serum concentrations are similar to those obtained by intramuscular administration. Following a rapid intravenous injection of netilmicin, levels in serum may be transiently 2 to 3 times higher than those of the 60-minute infusion. Netilmicin rapidly distributes to tissues.

The half-life of netilmicin after single doses is usually 2 to 2.5 hours, a half-life which is very similar to that of gentamicin, and is independent of the route of administration. The half-life increases as the dose increases (e.g., 2.2 hours after a 1 mg/kg dose to 3 hours after a 3 mg/kg dose). Approximately 80% of the administered dose is excreted in the urine within 24 hours; the urine netilmicin concentration after a dose often exceeds 100 mcg/ml. There is no evidence of metabolic transformation of netilmicin. The drug is excreted principally by glomerular filtration. Probenecid does not affect renal tubular transport of aminoglycosides. The volume of distribution of netilmicin is approximately 20% of body weight; total body clearance is about 80 ml/min and renal clearance is about 60 ml/min. In multiple-dose studies in volunteers when the drug was administered every 12 hours at doses ranging from 1.0 to 4.0 mg/kg, steady-state levels were obtained by the second day.

The serum levels at steady-state were less than 20% higher than those of the first dose. As with other aminoglycosides, the half-life of netilmicin increases, and its renal clearance decreases with decreasing renal function.

The endogenous creatinine clearance rate and the serum creatinine level have a high correlation with the half-life of netilmicin. Results of these tests can serve as a guide for adjusting dosage in patients with renal impairment.

In patients with marked impairment of renal function, there is a decrease in the concentration of aminoglycosides in urine and in their penetration into defective renal parenchyma. This should be considered when treating patients with urinary tract infections. In one study of adults with renal failure undergoing hemodialysis, netilmicin serum levels were reduced by approximately 63% over an 8-hour dialysis session. Shorter dialysis sessions will remove less drug. No hemodialysis information is available for children. Aminoglycosides are also removed by peritoneal dialysis but at a rate considerably less than by hemodialysis.

Since netilmicin is distributed in extracellular fluid, peak serum concentrations may be lower than usual in patients whose extracellular fluid volume is expanded (e.g., patients with edema or ascites). Serum concentrations of aminoglycosides in febrile patients may be lower than those in afebrile patients given the same dose. When body temperature returns to normal, serum concentrations of the drug may rise. Both febrile and anemic states may be associated with a shorter than usual half-life. (Dosage adjustment is usually not necessary.)

In severely burned patients, the half-life of aminoglycosides may be significantly decreased, and serum concentrations resulting from a particular dose may be lower than anticipated.

The elimination half-life of netilmicin in neonates during the first week of life is inversely correlated with body weight, ranging from approximately 8 hours for neonates weighing 1.5 to 2.0 kg to approximately 4.5 hours for 3.0 to 4.0 kg neonates. The elimination half-life of infants and children 6 weeks of age and older is 1.5 to 2.0 hours.

Following parenteral administration, aminoglycosides can be detected in serum, tissues, and sputum and in pericardial, pleural, synovial, and peritoneal fluids. A variety of methods are available to measure netilmicin concentrations in body fluids; these include microbiologic, enzymatic, and radioimmunoassay techniques. Concentrations in renal cortex may be markedly higher than the usual serum levels.

Minute quantities of aminoglycosides have been detected in the urine for up to 30 days after discontinuing administration. Hepatic secretion is minimal. As with all aminoglycosides, netilmicin diffuses poorly into the subarachnoid space after parenteral administration. Concentrations of netilmicin in cerebrospinal fluid are often low and dependent upon dose and the degree of meningeal inflammation. Netilmicin crosses the placenta and has been detected in cord blood and in the fetus. Studies in nursing mothers indicate that small amounts of the drug is excreted in breast milk. Netilmicin is poorly absorbed from the intact gastrointestinal tract after oral administration. As with other aminoglycosides, the binding of netilmicin to serum proteins is low (0–30%).

Microbiology: Netilmicin is a rapidly acting, broad-spectrum bactericidal antibiotic which appears to act by inhibiting normal protein synthesis in susceptible microorganisms. Netilmicin is active *in vitro* against a wide variety of pathogenic bacteria, primarily gram-negative bacilli and also a few gram-positive organisms including *Citrobacter, Enterobacter, Escherichia coli, Klebsiella* species, *Proteus mirabilis, Pseudomonas aeruginosa, Salmonella* species, *Shigella* species, and *Staphylococcus* species (penicillin- and methicillin-resistant strains).

Netilmicin is also active *in vitro* against some isolates of *Acinetobacter* and *Neisseria* species, indole-positive *Proteus* species, *Pseudomonas* and *Serratia* species. In addition, netilmicin is active *in vitro* against many strains which have acquired resistance to other aminoglycosides. Such resistance is usually caused by aminoglycoside modifying (inactivating) enzymes. In general, netilmicin is active against organisms which inactivate aminoglycosides by either phosphorylation or adenylylation; it has variable activity against acetylating strains, depending on the specific type. For example, the susceptibility of *Serratia* species producing a combination of adenylylating and acetylating enzymes varies according to the level of acetylating enzyme present. Netilmicin is active *in vitro* against certain strains of gram-negative bacteria resistant to gentamicin and tobramycin: *Citrobacter, Enterobacter* species, *Escherichia coli, Klebsiella, Proteus* (indole-positive), *Pseudomonas, Salmonella,* and *Shigella* species. Netilmicin is active *in vitro* against certain staphylococci resistant to amikacin and tobramycin. Like other aminoglycosides, netilmicin is not active against bacteria with reduced permeability to this class of antibiotics.

Most species of streptococci and anaerobic organisms, such as *Bacteroides* and *Clostridium* species, are resistant to aminoglycosides.

The *in vitro* activity of netilmicin and of other aminoglycosides is affected by media pH, protein content, divalent cation concentration, and inoculum size.

Netilmicin acts synergistically *in vitro* with members of the penicillin class of antibiotics against *Streptococcus faecalis*. It also acts synergistically with those penicillins which are active alone against many strains of *Pseudomonas*. In addition, many, but not all isolates of *Serratia* which are resistant to multiple antibiotics, are inhibited by synergistic combinations of netilmicin with carbenicillin, azlocillin, mezlocillin, cefamandole, cefotaxime, or moxalactam. Tests for antibiotic synergy are necessary.

Susceptibility Testing: Quantitative methods that require measurements of zone diameters give the most precise estimates of antibiotic susceptibility. One such procedure has been recommended for use with discs to test susceptibility to netilmicin. Interpretation involves correlation of the diameters obtained in the disc test with minimal inhibitory concentration (MIC) values for netilmicin.

Reports from the laboratory giving results of the standardized single disc susceptibility test (Bauer, et al. Am J Clin Path 1966; 45:493 and Federal Register 37:20525–20529, 1972), using a 30 mcg netilmicin disc should be interpreted according to the following criteria:

Organisms producing zones of 15 mm or greater, or MIC's of 8.0 mcg or less are considered susceptible, indicating that the tested organism is likely to respond to therapy.

Resistant organisms produce zones of 12 mm or less or MIC's of 16 mcg or greater. A report of "resistant" from the laboratory indicates that the infecting organism is not likely to respond to therapy.

Zones greater than 12 mm and less than 15 mm, or MIC's of greater than 8.0 mcg and less than 16 mcg, indicate intermediate susceptibility. A report of "intermediate" susceptibility suggests that the organism would be susceptible if the

Continued on next page

Schering—Cont.

infection is confined to tissues and fluids (e.g., urine), in which high antibiotic levels are attained.

Control organisms are recommended for susceptibility testing. Each time the test is performed one or more of the following organisms should be included: *Escherichia coli* ATCC 25922, *Staphylococcus aureus* ATCC 25923, and *Pseudomonas aeruginosa* ATCC 27853. The control organisms should produce zones of inhibition within the following ranges:

Escherichia coli (ATCC 25922) 22–30 mm
Staphylococcus aureus (ATCC 25923) 22–31 mm
Pseudomonas aeruginosa (ATCC 27853) 17–23 mm

In certain circumstances, particularly with strains of *Pseudomonas aeruginosa*, it may be desirable to do additional susceptibility testing by the tube or agar dilution method. Netilmicin sulfate powder, a diagnostic reagent, is available for this purpose.

The MIC values of netilmicin for the control strains are the following:

Escherichia coli (ATCC 25922) 0.25–0.5 mcg/ml
Staphylococcus aureus (ATCC 25923) 0.125–0.25 mcg/ml
Pseudomonas aeruginosa (ATCC 27853) 4–8 mcg/ml in media supplemented with calcium and magnesium.

INDICATIONS AND USAGE

Netilmicin sulfate injection is indicated for the short-term treatment of patients of all ages, including neonates, infants, and children with serious or life-threatening bacterial infections caused by susceptible strains of the designated microorganisms in the diseases listed below:

COMPLICATED URINARY TRACT infections caused by *Escherichia coli, Klebsiella pneumoniae, Pseudomonas aeruginosa, Enterobacter* species, *Proteus mirabilis, Proteus* species (indole-positive), *Serratia** and *Citrobacter* species, and *Staphylococcus aureus.***

SEPTICEMIA caused by *Escherichia coli, Klebsiella pneumoniae, Pseudomonas aeruginosa, Enterobacter* and *Serratia** species, and *Proteus mirabilis.*

SKIN AND SKIN STRUCTURE infections caused by *Escherichia coli, Klebsiella pneumoniae, Pseudomonas aeruginosa, Enterobacter* and *Serratia** species. *Proteus mirabilis, Proteus* species (indole-positive), and *Staphylococcus aureus*** (pencillinase- and non-penicillinase-producing strains).

INTRA-ABDOMINAL infections including peritonitis and intra-abdominal abscess caused by *Escherichia coli, Klebsiella pneumoniae, Pseudomonas aeruginosa, Enterobacter* species, *Proteus mirabilis, Proteus* species (indole-positive), and *Staphylococcus aureus*** (penicillinase- and non-penicillinase-producing strains).

LOWER RESPIRATORY TRACT infections caused by *Escherichia coli, Klebsiella pneumoniae, Pseudomonas aeruginosa, Enterobacter* and *Serratia** species, *Proteus mirabilis, Proteus* species (indole-positive), and *Staphylococcus aureus*** (penicillinase- and non-penicillinase-producing strains).

* (See **Microbiology** Section.)

** While not the antibiotic class of first choice, aminoglycosides, including netilmicin, may be considered for the treatment of serious staphylococcal infections when penicillins or other less potentially toxic drugs are contraindicated and bacterial susceptibility tests and clinical judgment indicate their use. They may also be considered in mixed infections caused by susceptible strains of staphylococci and gram-negative organisms.

Aminoglycosides are indicated for those infections for which less potentially toxic antimicrobial agents are ineffective or contraindicated. They are not indicated in the treatment of uncomplicated initial episodes of urinary tract infection unless the causative organisms are resistant to antimicrobial agents having less potential toxicity.

Netilmicin sulfate injection may be considered as initial therapy in suspected or confirmed gram-negative infections, and therapy may be instituted before obtaining results of susceptibility testing. The decision to continue therapy with netilmicin should be based on the results of susceptibility tests, the severity of the infection, and the important additional concepts contained in the "**WARNINGS** Box" above. If the causative organisms are resistant to netilmicin, other appropriate therapy should be instituted.

In serious infections when the causative organisms are unknown, netilmicin may be administered as initial therapy in conjunction with a penicillin-type or cephalosporin-type drug before obtaining results of susceptibility testing. In neonates with suspected sepsis, a penicillin-type drug is also usually indicated as concomitant therapy with netilmicin. If anaerobic organisms are suspected as etiologic agents, other suitable antimicrobial therapy should also be given. Following identification of the organism and its susceptibility, appropriate antibiotic therapy should then be continued. Netilmicin sulfate injection has been used effectively in combination with carbenicillin or ticarcillin for the treatment of life-threatening infections caused by *Pseudomonas aeruginosa.*

Clinical studies have shown that netilmicin has been effective in the treatment of serious infections caused by some organisms resistant to other aminoglycosides, *i.e.,* gentamicin, tobramycin, and/or amikacin.

Specimens for bacterial culture should be obtained to isolate and identify causative organisms and to determine their susceptibility to netilmicin.

CONTRAINDICATION

Hypersensitivity to netilmicin or to any of the ingredients of the preparation is a contraindication to its use. See **WARNINGS** if patient is hypersensitive to another aminoglycoside.

WARNINGS

(See "**WARNINGS** Box" above.) If the patient has a history of hypersensitivity or serious toxic reaction to another aminoglycoside, netilmicin should be used very cautiously, if at all, because cross-sensitivity to drugs in this class has been reported.

Aminoglycosides can cause fetal harm when administered to a pregnant woman. Aminoglycoside antibiotics cross the placenta and there have been several reports of total irreversible bilateral congenital deafness in children whose mothers received streptomycin during pregnancy. Although serious side effects to fetus or newborn have not been reported in the treatment of pregnant women with other aminoglycosides, the potential for harm exists. Reproduction studies in netilmicin have been performed in rats and rabbits using intramuscular and subcutaneous doses approximately 13–15 times the highest adult human dose and have revealed no evidence of impairment of fertility or harm to the fetus. Moreover, there was no evidence of ototoxicity in the offspring of rats treated subcutaneously with netilmicin throughout pregnancy and during the subsequent lactation period. It is not known whether netilmicin sulfate can cause fetal harm when administered to a pregnant women or can affect reproduction capacity. However, if this drug is used during pregnancy, or if the patient becomes pregnant while taking this drug, the patient should be apprised of the potential hazard to the fetus.

NETROMYCIN Injection contains sodium metabisulfite and sodium sulfite, which may cause allergic-type reactions including anaphylactic symptoms and life-threatening or less severe asthmatic episodes in certain susceptible people. The overall prevalence of sulfite sensitivity in the general population is unknown and probably low. Sulfite sensitivity is seen more frequently in asthmatic than in nonasthmatic people.

PRECAUTIONS

General: Neurotoxic and nephrotoxic antibiotics may be almost completely absorbed from body surfaces (except the urinary bladder) after local irrigation and after topical application during surgical procedures. The potential toxic effects of antibiotics administered in this fashion (neuromuscular blockade, respiratory paralysis, oto- and nephrotoxicity) should be considered. (See "**WARNINGS** Box.")

Increased nephrotoxicity has been reported following concomitant administration of aminoglycoside antibiotics with some cephalosporins.

Aminoglycosides should be used with caution in patients with neuromuscular disorders, such as myasthenia gravis, or infant botulism, since these drugs may aggravate muscle weakness because of their potential curare-like effect on the neuromuscular junction.

During or following netilmicin therapy, parasthesias, tetany, positive Chvostek and Trousseau signs, and mental confusion have been described in patients with hypomagnesemia, hypocalcemia, and hypokalemia. When this has occurred in infants, tetany and muscle weakness has been described. Both adults and infants required appropriate corrective electrolyte therapy.

Elderly patients may have reduced renal function which may not be evident in the results of routine screening tests, such as BUN or serum creatinine levels. Determination of creatinine clearance or an estimate based on published nomograms or equations may be more useful. Monitoring of renal function during treatment with netilmicin, as with other aminoglycosides, is particularly important in such patients. A Fanconi-like syndrome, with aminoaciduria and metabolic acidosis, has been reported in some adults and infants being given netilmicin injections.

Patients should be well hydrated during treatment.

Treatment with netilmicin may result in overgrowth of nonsusceptible organisms. If this occurs, appropriate therapy is indicated.

Laboratory Tests: *Tests of renal function:* Urine should be examined periodically for increased excretion of protein and the presence of cells and casts, keeping in mind the effects of the primary illness on these tests. One or more of the following laboratory measurements should be obtained at the onset of therapy, periodically during therapy, and at, or shortly after, the end of therapy:

- creatinine clearance rate (either carefully measured or estimated from published nomograms or equations based on the patient's age, sex, body weight, and serum creatinine concentration) (preferred over BUN);

- serum creatinine concentration (preferred over BUN);
- blood urea nitrogen (BUN).

More frequent testing is desirable if renal function is changing.

See also "**PRECAUTIONS, General**" above regarding elderly patients.

Test of eighth cranial nerve functions: Serial audiometric tests are suggested, particularly when renal function is impaired and/or prolonged aminoglycoside therapy is required; such tests should also be repeated periodically after treatment if there is evidence of a hearing deficit or vestibular abnormality before or during therapy, or when consecutive or concomitant use of other potentially ototoxic drugs is unavoidable.

Drug Interactions: *In vitro* mixing of an aminoglycoside with beta-lactam-type antibiotics (penicillins or cephalosporins) may result in a significant mutual inactivation. Even when an aminoglycoside and a penicillin-type drug are administered separately by different routes, a reduction in aminoglycoside serum half-life or serum levels has been reported in patients with impaired renal function and in some patients with normal renal function. Usually, such inactivation of the aminoglycoside is clinically significant only in patients with severely impaired renal function. (See also "Drug/Laboratory Test Interactions.") See "**WARNINGS** Box" regarding concurrent use of potent diuretics, concurrent and/or sequential use of other neurotoxic and/or nephrotoxic antibiotics, and for other essential information. See also "**PRECAUTIONS, General**."

Drug/Laboratory Test Interactions: Concomitant cephalosporin therapy may spuriously elevate creatinine determinations.

The inactivation between aminoglycosides and beta-lactam antibiotics described in "**Drug Interactions**" may continue in specimens of body fluids collected for assay, resulting in inaccurate, false low aminoglycoside readings. Such specimens should be properly handled, *i.e.,* assayed promptly, frozen, or treated with beta-lactamase.

Carcinogenesis, Mutagenesis, Impairment of Fertility: Lifetime carcinogenicity tests have been undertaken in the mouse and rat and no drug-related tumors were observed. Similarly, mutagenesis tests with netilmicin have proven negative, and no impairment in fertility has been observed in the rat.

Pregnancy Category D: (See **WARNINGS** Section.)

Nursing Mothers: Clinical studies in nursing mothers indicate that small amounts of netilmicin are excreted in breast milk. Because of the potential for serious adverse reactions from aminoglycosides in nursing infants, a decision should be made whether to discontinue nursing or to discontinue the drug, taking into account the importance of the drug to the mother.

Pediatric Use: Aminoglycosides should be used with caution in prematures and neonates because of the renal immaturity of these patients and the resulting prolongation of serum half-life of these drugs (also see **DOSAGE AND ADMINISTRATION** for use in Neonates and Children.)

ADVERSE REACTIONS

Nephrotoxicity—Adverse renal effects due to netilmicin were reported in 7 per 100 patients.

They were demonstrated by a rise in serum creatinine and may have been accompanied by oliguria; the presence of casts, cells or protein in the urine; by rising levels of BUN; or by decreasing creatinine clearance rates. These effects occurred more frequently in the elderly, in patients with a history of renal impairment, and in patients treated for longer periods or with larger doses than recommended. While permanent impairment of renal function may occur following aminoglycoside therapy, observed renal impairment associated with netilmicin was usually mild and reversible after treatment ended while the drug was being excreted.

Neurotoxicity—Adverse effects on both the auditory and vestibular branches of the eighth cranial nerves have been reported.

Audiometric changes associated with netilmicin occurred in approximately 4 per 100 patients. Subjective netilmicin-related hearing loss occurred in about 1 per 250 patients. Vestibular abnormalities related to netilmicin were seen in 1 per 150 patients. Factors which may increase the risk of aminoglycoside-induced ototoxicity include renal impairment (especially if dialysis is required), excessive dosage, dehydration, concomitant administration of ethacrynic acid or furosemide, or previous exposure to other ototoxic drugs. Peripheral neuropathy or encephalopathy including numbness, skin tingling, muscle twitching, convulsions, and myasthenia gravis-like syndrome have been reported.

Symptoms include dizziness, vertigo, tinnitus, nystagmus, and hearing loss. Aminoglycoside-induced ototoxicity is usually irreversible. Cochlear damage is usually manifested initially by small changes in audiometric test results at the higher frequencies and may not be associated with subjective hearing loss. Vestibular dysfunction is usually manifested by nystagmus, vertigo, nausea, vomiting, or acute Meniere's syndrome.

The risk of toxic reactions is low in patients with normal renal function who do not receive netilmicin injection at higher doses or for longer periods of time than recommended. Some patients who have had previous neurotoxic reactions to other aminoglycosides have been treated with netilmicin without further neurotoxicity.

Neuromuscular blockade manifested as acute muscular paralysis and apnea can occur following treatment with aminoglycosides. (See "WARNINGS Box.")

The approximate incidence of other reported adverse reactions to netilmicin injection follows: increased levels of serum transaminase (SGOT or SGPT), alkaline phosphatase, or bilirubin in 15 patients per 1000; rash or itching in 4 or 5 patients per 1000; eosinophilia in 4 patients per 1000; thrombocytosis in 2 patients per 1000; prolonged prothrombin time in 1 patient per 1000; fever in 1 patient per 1000.

Fewer than one patient per 1000 was reported to have netilmicin-related anemia, leukopenia, thrombocytopenia, leukemoid reaction, immature circulating white blood cells, hyperkalemia, vomiting, diarrhea, palpitations, hypotension, headache, disorientation, blurred vision, or paresthesias. Local tolerance to intramuscular injection and intravenous infusion of netilmicin is generally excellent, but approximately four patients per 1000 have had severe pain, and similar numbers had induration or hematomas.

OVERDOSAGE

In the event of overdosage or toxic reaction, netilmicin can be removed from the blood by hemodialysis, and is especially important if renal function is, or becomes, compromised. Although there is no specific information concerning removal of netilmicin by peritoneal dialysis, other aminoglycosides are known to be removed by this method but at a rate considerably less than by hemodialysis.

DOSAGE AND ADMINISTRATION

Netilmicin injection may be given intramuscularly or intravenously. (See **CLINICAL PHARMACOLOGY.**) The recommended dosage for both methods of administration is identical.

The patient's pretreatment body weight should be obtained for calculation of correct dosage. The dosage of aminoglycosides in obese patients should be based on an estimate of the lean body mass.

The status of renal function should be estimated by measurement of the serum creatinine concentration or calculation of the endogenous creatinine clearance rate. The blood urea nitrogen (BUN) level is much less reliable for this purpose. Reassessment of renal function should be made periodically during therapy.

In patients with extensive body surface burns, altered pharmacokinetics may result in reduced serum concentrations of aminoglycosides. Measurement of netilmicin serum concentrations is particularly important as a basis for dosage adjustment in such patients.

Duration of Treatment: It is desirable to limit the duration of treatment with aminoglycosides to short-term whenever feasible. The usual duration of treatment for all patients is seven to fourteen days. In complicated infections, a longer course of therapy may be necessary. Although prolonged courses of netilmicin injection have been well tolerated, it is particularly important that patients treated for longer than the usual period be carefully monitored for changes in renal, auditory, and vestibular functions. Dosage should be adjusted if clinically indicated.

Measurement of Serum Concentrations: It is desirable to measure both peak and trough serum concentrations of netilmicin to determine the adequacy and safety of the administered dosage.

When such measurements are feasible, they should be carried out periodically during therapy. Peak serum concentrations are expected to range from 4 to 12 mcg/ml. Dosage should be adjusted to attain the desired peak and trough concentrations and to avoid prolonged peak serum concentrations above 16 mcg/ml. When monitoring trough concentrations (just prior to the next dose), dosage should be adjusted so that levels above 4 mcg/ml are avoided. Inter-patient variation of aminoglycoside serum concentrations occurs in patients with normal or abnormal renal function. Generally, desirable peak and trough concentrations will be in the range of 6–10 and 0.5–2 mcg/ml, respectively.

Determination of the adequacy of a serum level for a particular patient must take into consideration the susceptibility of the causative organism, the severity of the infection, and the status of the patient's host-defense mechanisms.

The dosage recommendations which follow are not intended as rigid schedules, but are provided as guides for initial therapy, or for when the measurement of netilmicin serum levels during therapy is not feasible.

DOSAGE FOR PATIENTS WITH NORMAL RENAL FUNCTION

Table I shows the recommended dosage of netilmicin injection for patients of various ages with normal renal function. [See table above.]

Although a causal relationship has not been established, administration of injections preserved with benzyl alcohol

has been associated with toxicity in neonates. Caution should be used with NETROMYCIN Injection (100 mg/ml) is administered to neonates and children.

    Neonates (less than 6 weeks): 4.0 to 6.5 mg/kg/day given as 2.0 to 3.25 mg/kg every 12 hours.

    Infants and Children (6 weeks through 12 years): 5.5 to 8.0 mg/kg/day given either as 1.8 to 2.7 mg/kg every 8 hours, or as 2.7 to 4.0 mg/kg every 12 hours.

DOSAGE FOR PATIENTS WITH IMPAIRED RENAL FUNCTION

Dosage must be individualized in patients with impaired renal function to ensure therapeutic levels are attained. There are several methods of doing this; however, dosage adjustment based upon the measurement of serum drug concentrations during treatment is the most accurate.

If netilmicin serum concentrations are not available and renal function is stable, serum creatinine and creatinine clearance values are the most reliable, readily available indicators of the degree of renal impairment for use as a guide for dosage adjustment.

It is also important to recognize that deteriorating renal function may require a greater reduction in dosage than that specified in the guidelines given below for patients with stable renal impairment.

The initial or loading dose is the same as that for a patient with normal renal function. A number of methods are available to adjust the total daily dosage for the degree of renal impairment. Three suggested methods are:

1) Divide the suggested dosage value for patients with normal renal function from Table I above by the serum creatinine level to obtain the adjusted size of each dose.

2) If the creatinine clearance rate is known or can be estimated from the serum creatinine levels using the formula given below, the adjusted daily dose of netilmicin may be determined by multiplying the dose given in Table I by:

$$\frac{\text{Patient's Creatinine Clearance Rate}}{\text{Normal Creatinine Clearance Rate}}$$

3) Alternatively, the following graph may be used to obtain the percentage of the dose selected from Table I, which should be administered at 8-hour intervals:

REDUCED DOSAGE GRAPH

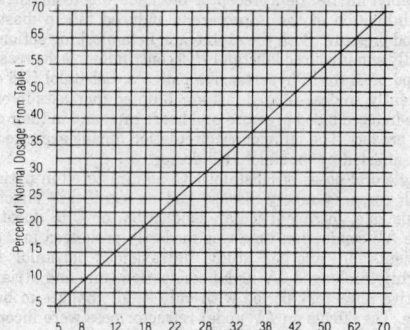

Creatinine Clearance Rate
ml/min/1.73 m²

Creatinine clearance can be estimated from serum creatinine levels by the following formula for adult males; multiply by 0.85 for adult females (Nephron, 1976; 16:31–41):

$$C_{cr} = \frac{(140 - \text{Age})(\text{Wt. Kg})}{72 \times S_{cr}(\text{mg}/100 \text{ ml})}$$

The adjusted total daily dose may be administered as one dose at 24-hour intervals, or as 2 or 3 equally divided doses at 12-hour or 8-hour intervals, respectively. Generally, each individual dose should not exceed 3.25 mg/kg. In adults with renal failure who are undergoing hemodialysis, the amount of netilmicin removed from the blood may vary depending upon the dialysis equipment and methods used. (See **CLINICAL PHARMACOLOGY.**) In adults, a dose of 2.0 mg/kg at the end of each dialysis period is recommended until the results of tests measuring netilmicin serum levels become available. Dosage should then be appropriately adjusted based on these tests.

ALTERNATE DOSING METHOD FOR PATIENTS WITH NORMAL OR IMPAIRED RENAL FUNCTION

An alternate method of determining a dosage regimen (dose and dosing interval) applicable to all ages and all states of renal function (both normal and abnormal) is to employ pharmacokinetic parameters derived from measurements of serum concentrations.

Following the administration of an initial dose of netilmicin and the determination of drug serum concentrations in post-infusion blood samples, the drug's half-life and the patient's elimination rate constant and volume of distribution can be calculated. Desired peak and trough serum levels for a particular patient are then selected by taking into consideration the susceptibility of the causative organism, the severity of infection, and the status of the patient's host-defense mechanisms. The dosage regimen (dose and dosing interval) is then determined using standardized formulae and the appropriate computer program, and the dosage regimen can be adjusted to the nearest practical interval and amount.

ADDITION OF NETILMICIN SULFATE TO VARIOUS INTRAVENOUS PREPARATIONS

In adults, a single dose of netilmicin injection may be diluted to 50 to 200 ml of one of the parenteral solutions listed below. In infants and children, the volume of diluent should be less according to the fluid requirements of the patient. The solution may be infused over a period of one-half to two hours. Tested at concentrations of 2.1 to 3.0 mg/ml, netilmicin sulfate has been shown to be stable in the following large volume parenteral solutions for up to 72 hours when stored in glass containers, both when refrigerated and at room temperature. Use after this time period is not recommended. [See table on next page].

Parenteral drug products should be inspected visually for particulate matter and discoloration prior to administration, whenever solution and container permit.

HOW SUPPLIED

NETROMYCIN Injection 100 mg/ml is supplied in 1.5 ml vials, box of 10 (NDC 0085-0264-02). **Store between 2° and 30°C (36°and 86°F).**

Continued on next page

Information on Schering products appearing on these pages is effective as of September 30, 1989.

Table I
DOSAGE GUIDE FOR ADULTS WITH NORMAL RENAL FUNCTION

Patient's Weight*		For Complicated Urinary Tract Infections, Give 3.0–4.0 mg/kg/day as 1.5–2.0 mg/kg EVERY 12 HOURS	For Serious Systemic Infections Give 4.0–6.5 mg/kg/day as 1.3–2.2 mg/kg EVERY 8 HOURS	2.0–3.25 mg/kg EVERY 12 HOURS
kg	(lb)	mg/dose	mg/dose	mg/dose
40	(88)	60– 80	52– 88	80–130
45	(99)	68– 90	59– 99	90–146
50	(110)	75–100	65–110	100–163
55	(121)	83–110	72–121	110–179
60	(132)	90–120	78–132	120–195
65	(143)	98–130	85–143	130–211
70	(154)	105–140	91–154	140–228
75	(165)	113–150	98–165	150–244
80	(176)	120–160	104–176	160–260
85	(187)	128–170	111–187	170–276
90	(198)	135–180	117–198	180–293
95	(209)	143–190	124–209	190–309
100	(220)	150–200	130–220	200–325

* The dosage of aminoglycosides in obese patients should be based on an estimate of the lean body mass.

Schering—Cont.

TABLE II
LARGE VOLUME PARENTERAL SOLUTIONS IN WHICH
NETILMICIN SULFATE IS STABLE

Products/Compositions Tested	Other Trade Names and Manufacturers
	(Solutions of Same Composition)
Sterile Water for Injection 0.9% Sodium Chloride Injection alone or with 5% Dextrose 5% or 10% Dextrose Injection in Water, or 5% Dextrose in Polysal Injection, or 5% Dextrose with Electrolyte #48 or #75 Ringer's and Lactated Ringer's, and Lactated Ringer's with 5% Dextrose Injection	
10% Travert with Electrolyte #2 or #3 Injection (Travenol)	Electrolyte #3 (Cooke & Crowley's Solution) with 10% Inverted Sugar Injection (Cutter)
Isolyte E, M, or P with 5% Dextrose Injection 10% Dextran 40 or 6% Dextran 75 in 5% Dextrose Injection	
Plasma-Lyte 56 or 148 Injection with 5% Dextrose (Travenol)	Normosol-M or R in D5-W (Abbott), Isolyte H or S with 5% Dextrose (McGaw), Polyonic R-148 or M-56 with 5% Dextrose (Cutter)
Plasma-Lyte M Injection 5% Dextrose (Travenol)	Polysal M with 5% Dextrose (Cutter)
Ionosol B in D5-W 5% Amigen Injection alone or with 5% Dextrose Normosol-R	Polyonic R-148 (Cutter), Isolyte S (McGaw) Plasma-Lyte 148 Injection in Water (Travenol)
Polysal (Plain) Aminosol 5% Injection Fre-Amine II 8.5% Injection Plasma-Lyte 148 Injection (approx. pH 7.4) (Travenol) 10% Fructose Injection	Normosol-R pH 7.4 (Abbott)

ANIMAL PHARMACOLOGY AND/OR ANIMAL TOXICOLOGY

Netilmicin sulfate, administered by the intravenous and intramuscular routes, has been compared to kanamycin, sisomicin, gentamicin, amikacin, and tobramycin in studies ranging in duration from two weeks to three months. Among the aminoglycosides, netilmicin is one of the more potent neuromuscular-blocking agents; however, in six different species, netilmicin sulfate has proven to be the least nephrotoxic and ototoxic of these aminoglycosides, using morphological as well as functional end points. In the clinical trials nephrotoxicity and ototoxicity occurred at about the same frequency in netilmicin-treated patients as in those treated with other aminoglycosides.

Schering Biochem Corporation,
Manati, Puerto Rico 00701
An Affiliate of Schering Corporation,
Kenilworth, NJ 07033

Revised 1/87
Copyright © 1980, 1983, 1984, 1987, Schering Corporation,
USA. All rights reserved.

NORMODYNE®   ℞
[nŏr-mŏ- dĭn]
brand of labetalol hydrochloride
Injection

DESCRIPTION

NORMODYNE (labetalol HCl) is an adrenergic receptor blocking agent that has both selective alpha$_1$- and nonselective beta-adrenergic receptor blocking actions in a single substance.

Labetalol HCl is 5-[1-hydroxy-2-1[(1-methyl-3- phenylpropyl) amino]ethyl]salicylamide monohydrochloride.

Labetalol HCl has the empirical formula $C_{19}H_{24}N_2O_3HCl$ and a molecular weight of 364.9. It has two asymmetric centers and therefore exists as a molecular complex of two diastereoisomeric pairs.

Labetalol HCl is a white or off-white crystalline powder, soluble in water.

NORMODYNE (labetalol HCl) Injection is a clear, colorless to light yellow aqueous sterile isotonic solution for intravenous injection. It has a pH range of 3.0 to 4.0. Each mL contains 5 mg labetalol HCl, 45 mg anhydrous dextrose, 0.10 mg edetate disodium; 0.80 mg methylparaben and 0.10 mg propylparaben as preservatives; citric acid monohydrate and sodium hydroxide, as necessary, to bring the solution into the pH range.

CLINICAL PHARMACOLOGY

NORMODYNE (labetalol HCl) combines both selective, competitive alpha$_1$- adrenergic blocking and nonselective, competitive beta-adrenergic blocking activity in a single substance. In man, the ratios of alpha- to beta-blockade have been estimated to be approximately 1:3 and 1:7 following oral and intravenous administration, respectively. Beta$_2$-agonist activity has been demonstrated in animals with minimal beta$_1$- agonist (ISA) activity detected. In animals, at doses greater than those required for alpha or beta-adrenergic blockade, a membrane stabilizing effect has been demonstrated.

Pharmacodynamics: The capacity of labetalol HCl to block alpha receptors in man has been demonstrated by attenuation of the pressor effect of phen-ylephrine and by a significant reduction of the pressor response caused by immersing the hand in ice-cold water ("cold-pressor test"). Labetalol HCl's beta$_1$-receptor blockade in man was demonstrated by a small decrease in the resting heart rate, attenuation of tachycardia produced by isoproterenol or exercise, and by attenuation of the reflex tachycardia to the hypotension produced by amyl nitrite. Beta$_2$-receptor blockade was demonstrated by inhibition of the isoproterenol-induced fall in diastolic blood pressure. Both the alpha- and beta-blocking actions of orally administered labetalol HCl contribute to a decrease in blood pressure in hypertensive patients. Labetalol HCl consistently, in dose-related fashion, blunted increases in exercise-induced blood pressure and heart rate, and in their double product. The pulmonary circulation during exercise was not affected by labetalol HCl dosing.

Single oral doses of labetalol HCl administered in patients with coronary artery disease had no significant effect on sinus rate, intraventricular conduction, or QRS duration. The AV conduction time was modestly prolonged in 2 of 7 patients. In another study, intravenous labetalol HCl slightly prolonged AV nodal conduction time and atrial effective refractory period with only small changes in heart rate. The effects on AV nodal refractoriness were inconsistent.

Labetalol HCl produces dose-related falls in blood pressure without reflex tachycardia and without significant reduction in heart rate, presumably through a mixture of its alpha-blocking and beta-blocking effects. Hemodynamic effects are variable with small nonsignificant changes in cardiac output seen in some studies but not others, and small decreases in total peripheral resistance. Elevated plasma renins are reduced.

Doses of labetalol HCl that controlled hypertension did not affect renal function in mild to severe hypertensive patients with normal renal function.

Due to the alpha$_1$-receptor blocking activity of labetalol HCl, blood pressure is lowered more in the standing than in the supine position, and symptoms of postural hypotension can occur. During dosing with intravenous labetalol HCl, the contribution of the postural component should be considered when positioning patients for treatment, and patients should not be allowed to move to an erect position unmonitored until their ability to do so is established.

In a clinical pharmacologic study in severe hypertensives, an initial 0.25 mg/kg injection of labetalol HCl, administered to patients in the supine postition, decreased blood pressure by an average of 11/7 mmHg. Additional injections of 0.5 mg/kg at 15-minute intervals up to a total cumulative dose of 1.75 mg/kg. of labetalol HCl caused further dose-related decreases in blood pressure. Some patients required cumulative doses of up to 3.25 mg/kg. The maximal effect of each dose level occurred within 5 minutes. Following discontinuation of intravenous treatment with labetalol HCl, the blood pressure rose gradually and progressively, approaching pretreatment baseline values within an average of 16–18 hours in the majority of patients.

Similar results were obtained in the treatment of patients with severe hypertension requiring urgent blood pressure reduction with an initial dose of 20 mg (which corresponds to 0.25 mg/kg for an 80 kg patient) followed by additional doses of either 40 or 80 mg at 10-minute intervals to achieve the desired effect or up to a cumulative dose of 300 mg. Labetalol HCl administered as a continuous intravenous infusion, with a mean dose of 136 mg (27 to 300 mg) over a period of 2 to 3 hours (mean of 2 hours and 39 minutes) lowered the blood pressure by an average of 60/35 mmHg.

Exacerbation of angina and, in some cases, myocardial infarction and ventricular dysrhythmias have been reported after abrupt discontinuation of therapy with beta-adrenergic blocking agents in patients with coronary artery disease. Abrupt withdrawal of these agents in patients without coronary artery disease has resulted in transient symptoms, including tremulousness, sweating, palpitation, headache, and malaise. Several mechanisms have been proposed to explain these phenomena, among them increased sensitivity to catecholamines because of increased numbers of beta receptors. Although beta-adrenergic receptor blockade is useful in the treatment of angina and hypertension, there are also situations in which sympathetic stimulation is vital. For example, in patients with severely damaged hearts, adequate ventricular function may depend on sympathetic drive. Beta-adrenergic blockade may worsen AV block by preventing the necessary facilitating effects of sympathetic activity on conduction. Beta$_2$- adrenergic blockade results in passive bronchial constriction by interfering with endogenous adrenergic bronchodilator activity in patients subject to bronchospasm and may also interfere with exogenous bronchodilators in such patients.

Pharmacokinetics and Metabolism Following intravenous infusion, the elimination half-life is about 5.5 hours and the total body clearance is approximately 33 mL/min/kg. The plasma half-life of labetalol following oral administration is about six to eight hours. In patients with decreased hepatic or renal function, the elimination half-life of labetalol is not altered, however, the relative bioavailability in hepatically impaired patients is increased due to decreased "first-pass" metabolism.

The metabolism of labetalol is mainly through conjugation to glucuronide metabolites. These metabolites are present in plasma and are excreted in the urine and, via the bile, into the feces. Approximately 55 to 60% of a dose appears in the urine as conjugates or unchanged labetalol within the first 24 hours of dosing.

Labetalol has been shown to cross the placental barrier in humans. Only negligible amounts of the drug crossed the blood- brain barrier in animal studies. Labetalol is approximately 50% protein bound. Neither hemodialysis nor peritoneal dialysis removes a significant amount of labetalol HCl from the general circulation (<1%).

INDICATIONS AND USAGE

NORMODYNE (labetalol HCl) Injection is indicated for control of blood pressure in severe hypertension.

CONTRAINDICATIONS

NORMODYNE (labetalol HCl) Injection is contraindicated in bronchial asthma, overt cardiac failure, greater than first degree heart block, cardiogenic shock, and severe bradycardia. (See **WARNINGS**.)

WARNINGS

Hepatic Injury Severe hepatocellular injury, confirmed by rechallenge in at least one case, occurs rarely with labetalol therapy. The hepatic injury is usually reversible, but hepatic necrosis and death have been reported. Injury has occurred after both short- and long-term treatment and may be slowly progressive despite minimal symptomatology. Appropriate laboratory testing should be done at the first symptom/sign of liver dysfunction (e.g., pruritus, dark urine, persistent anorexia, jaundice, right upper quadrant tenderness, or unexplained "flu-like" symptoms). If the patient has laboratory evidence of liver injury or jaundice, labetalol should be stopped and not restarted.

Cardiac Failure Sympathetic stimulation is a vital component supporting circulatory function in congestive heart failure. Beta blockade carries a potential hazard of further depressing myocardial contractility and precipitating more severe failure. Although beta-blockers should be avoided in overt congestive heart failure, if necessary, labetalol HCl can be used with caution in patients with a history of heart failure who are well-compensated. Congestive heart failure has been observed in patients receiving labetalol HCl. Labetalol HCl does not abolish the inotropic action of digitalis on heart muscle.

In Patients Without a History of Cardiac Failure In patients with latent cardiac insufficiency, continued depression of the myocardium with beta-blocking agents over a period of time can in some cases lead to cardiac failure. At the first sign or symptom of impending cardiac failure, patients should be fully digitalized and/or be given a diuretic, and the response observed closely. If cardiac failure continues, despite adequate digitalization and diuretic, NORMODYNE (labetalol HCl) therapy should be withdrawn (gradually if possible).

Ischemic Heart Disease Angina pectoris has not been reported upon labetalol HCl discontinuation. However, following abrupt cessation of therapy with some beta-blocking agents in patients with coronary artery disease, exacerbations of angina pectoris and, in some cases, myocardial infarction have been reported. Therefore, such patients should be cautioned against interruption of therapy without the physician's advice. Even in the absence of overt angina pectoris, when discontinuation of NORMODYNE (labetalol HCl) is planned, the patient should be carefully observed and should be advised to limit physical activity. If angina markedly worsens or acute coronary insufficiency develops, NORMODYNE (labetalol HCl) administration should be reinstituted promptly, at least temporarily, and other measures appropriate for the management of unstable angina should be taken.

Nonallergic Bronchospasm (e.g., chronic bronchitis and emphysema). Since NORMODYNE (labetalol HCl) Injection at the usual intravenous therapeutic doses has not been studied in patients with nonallergic bronchospastic disease, it should not be used in such patients.

Pheochromocytoma Intravenous labetalol HCl has been shown to be effective in lowering the blood pressure and relieving symptoms in patients with pheochromocytoma; higher than usual doses may be required. However, paradoxical hypertensive responses have been reported in a few patients with this tumor; therefore, use caution when administering labetalol HCl to patients with pheochromocytoma.

Diabetes Mellitus and Hypoglycemia Beta-adrenergic blockade may prevent the appearance of premonitory signs and symptoms (e.g., tachycardia) of acute hypoglycemia. This is especially important with labile diabetics. Beta-blockade also reduces the release of insulin in response to hyperglycemia; it may therefore be necessary to adjust the dose of anti-diabetic drugs.

Major Surgery The necessity or desirability of withdrawing beta-blocking therapy prior to major surgery is controversial. Protracted severe hypotension and difficulty in restarting or maintaining a heart beat have been reported with beta-blockers. The effect of labetalol HCl's alpha-adrenergic activity has not been evaluated in this setting. A synergism between labetalol HCl and halothane anesthesia has been shown (see **Drug Interactions**).

Rapid Decreases of Blood Pressure Caution must be observed when reducing severely elevated blood pressure. Although such findings have not been reported with intravenous labetalol HCl, a number of adverse reactions, including cerebral infarction, optic nerve infarction, angina and ischemic changes in the electrocardiogram, have been reported with other agents when severely elevated blood pressure was reduced over time courses of several hours to as long as one or two days. The desired blood pressure lowering should therefore be achieved over as long a period of time as is compatible with the patient's status.

PRECAUTIONS

General: *Impaired Hepatic Function* may diminish metabolism of NORMODYNE (labetalol HCl) Injection.

Hypotension Symtomatic postural hypotension (incidence 58%) is likely to occur if patients are tilted or allowed to assume the upright position within 3 hours of receiving NORMODYNE (labetalol HCl) Injection. Therefore, the patient's ability to tolerate an upright position should be established before permitting any ambulation.

Jaundice or Hepatic Dysfunction (see **WARNINGS**.)

Information for Patients: The following information is intended to aid in the safe and effective use of this medica-

Labetalol HCl									
Daily Dose (mg)	200	300	400	600	800	900	1200	1600	2400
Number of Patients	522	181	606	608	503	117	411	242	175
Dizziness (%)	2	3	3	3	5	1	9	13	16
Fatigue	2	1	4	4	5	3	7	6	10
Nausea	<1	0	1	2	4	0	7	11	19
Vomiting	0	0	<1	<1	<1	0	1	2	3
Dyspepsia	1	0	2	1	1	0	2	2	4
Paresthesias	2	0	2	2	1	1	2	5	5
Nasal Stuffiness	1	1	2	2	2	2	4	5	6
Ejaculation Failure	0	2	1	2	3	0	4	3	5
Impotence	1	1	1	1	2	4	3	4	3
Edema	1	0	1	1	1	0	1	2	2

tion. It is not a disclosure of all possible adverse or intended effects. During and immediately following (for up to 3 hours) NORMODYNE Injection, the patient should remain supine. Subsequently, the patient should be advised on how to proceed gradually to become ambulatory, and should be observed at the time of first ambulation.

When the patient is started on NORMODYNE Tablets, following adequate control of blood pressure with NORMODYNE Injection, appropriate directions for titration of dosage should be provided. (See **DOSAGE AND ADMINISTRATION**.)

As with all drugs with beta-blocking activity, certain advice to patients being treated with labetalol HCl is warranted. While no incident of the abrupt withdrawal phenomenon (exacerbation of angina pectoris) has been reported with labetalol HCl, dosing with NORMODYNE Tablets should not be interrupted or discontinued without a physician's advice. Patients being treated with NORMODYNE Tablets should consult a physician at any signs or symptoms of impending cardiac failure or hepatic dysfunction (see **WARNINGS**.) Also transient scalp tingling may occur, usually when treatment with NORMODYNE Tablets is initiated (see **ADVERSE REACTIONS**).

Laboratory Tests: Routine laboratory tests are ordinarily not required before or after intravenous labetalol HCl. In patients with concomitant illnesses, such as impaired renal function, appropriate tests should be done to monitor these conditions.

Drug Interactions: Since NORMODYNE (labetalol HCl) Injection may be administered to patients already being treated with other medications, including other antihypertensive agents, careful monitoring of these patients is necessary to detect and treat promptly any undesired effect from concomitant administration.

In one survey, 2.3% of patients taking labetalol HCl orally in combination with tricyclic antidepressants experienced tremor as compared to 0.7% reported to occur with labetalol HCl alone. The contribution of each of the treatments to this adverse reaction is unknown but the possibility of a drug interaction cannot be excluded.

Drugs possessing beta-blocking properties can blunt the bronchodilator effect of beta-receptor agonist drugs in patients with bronchospasm; therefore, doses greater than the normal anti- asthmatic dose of beta-agonist bronchodilator drugs may be required.

Cimetidine has been shown to increase the bioavailability of labetalol HCl administered orally. Since this could be explained either by enhanced absorption or by an alteration of hepatic metabolism of labetalol HCl, special care should be used in establishing the dose required for blood pressure control in such patients.

Synergism has been shown between halothane anesthesia and intravenously administered labetalol HCl. During controlled hypotensive anesthesia using labetalol HCl in association with halothane, high concentrations (3% or above) of halothane should not be used because the degree of hypotension will be increased and because of the possibility of a large reduction in cardiac output and an increase in central venous pressure. The anesthesiologist should be informed when a patient is receiving labetalol HCl.

Labetalol HCl blunts the reflex tachycardia produced by nitroglycerin without preventing its hypotensive effect. If labetalol HCl is used with nitroglycerin in patients with angina pectoris, additional antihypertensive effects may occur.

Drug/Laboratory Test Interactions: The presence of labetalol metabolites in the urine may result in falsely elevated levels of urinary catecholamines, metanephrine, normetanephrine, and vanillylmandelic acid (VMA) when measured by fluorimetric or photometric methods. In screening patients suspected of having a pheochromocytoma and being treated with labetalol HCl, a specific method, such as high performance liquid chromatographic assay with solid phase extraction (e.g., *J Chromatogr* 385:241, 1987) should be employed in determining levels of catecholamines.

Labetalol HCl has also been reported to produce a false-positive test for amphetamine when screening urine for the presence of drugs using the commercially available assay methods Toxi-Lab A® (thin-layer chromatographic assay) and Emit-d.a.u.® (radioenzymatic assay). When patients being treated with labetalol have a positive urine test for amphetamine using these techniques, confirmation should be made

by using more specific methods, such as a gas chromatographic-mass spectrometer technique.

Carcinogenesis, Mutagenesis, Impairment of Fertility: Long-term oral dosing studies with labetalol HCl for 18 months in mice and for 2 years in rats showed no evidence of carcinogenesis. Studies with labetalol HCl, using dominant lethal assays in rats and mice, and exposing microorganisms according to modified Ames tests, showed no evidence of mutagenesis.

Pregnancy Category C: Teratogenic studies have been performed with labetalol in rats and rabbits at oral doses up to approximately 6 and 4 times the maximum recommended human dose (MRHD), respectively. No reproducible evidence of fetal malformations was observed. Increased fetal resorptions were seen in both species at doses approximating the MRHD. A teratology study performed with labetalol in rabbits at intravenous doses up to 1.7 times the MRHD revealed no evidence of drug related harm to the fetus. There are no adequate and well-controlled studies in pregnant women. Labetalol should be used during pregnancy only if the potential benefit justifies the potential risk to the fetus.

Nonteratogenic Effects: Transient hypotension, bradycardia, and hypoglycemia have been rarely observed in infants of mothers who were treated with labetalol HCl for hypertension during pregnancy. Oral administration of labetalol to rats during late gestation through weaning at doses of 2 to 4 times the MRHD caused a decrease in neonatal survival.

Labor and Delivery: Labetalol HCl given to pregnant women with hypertension did not appear to affect the usual course of labor and delivery.

Nursing Mothers: Small amounts of labetalol (approximately 0.004% of the maternal dose) are excreted in human milk. Caution should be exercised when NORMODYNE (labetalol HCl) Injection is administered to a nursing woman.

Pediatric Use: Safety and effectiveness in children have not been established.

ADVERSE REACTIONS

NORMODYNE (labetalol HCl) Injection is usually well tolerated. Most adverse effects have been mild and transient and in controlled trials involving 92 patients did not require labetalol HCl withdrawal. Symptomatic postural hypotension (incidence 58%) is likely to occur if patients are tilted or allowed to assume the upright position within 3 hours of receiving NORMODYNE (labetalol HCl) Injection. Moderate hypotension occurred in 1 of 100 patients while supine. Increased sweating was noted in 4 of 100 patients, and flushing occurred in 1 of 100 patients.

The following also were reported with NORMODYNE Injection with the incidence per 100 patients as noted:

Cardiovascular System Ventricular arrhythmia in 1.

Central and Peripheral Nervous Systems Dizziness in 9; tingling of the scalp/ skin 7; hypoesthesia (numbness), and vertigo 1 each.

Gastrointestinal System Nausea in 13; vomiting 4; dyspepsia and taste distortion, 1 each.

Metabolic Disorders Transient increases in blood urea nitrogen and serum creatinine levels occurred in 8 of 100 patients; these were associated with drops in blood pressure, generally in patients with prior renal insufficiency.

Psychiatric Disorders Somnolence/yawning in 3.

Respiratory System Wheezing in 1.

Skin Pruritus in 1.

The incidence of adverse reactions depends upon the dose of labetalol HCl. The largest experience is with oral labetalol HCl (see NORMODYNE Tablet Product Information for details). Certain of the side effects increased with increasing oral dose as shown in the table below which depicts the entire U.S. therapeutic trials data base for adverse reactions that are clearly or possibly dose related.

[See table above].

The oculomucocutaneous syndrome assoicated with the beta-blocker practolol has not been reported with labetalol HCl during investigational use and extensive foreign marketing experience.

Continued on next page

Information on Schering products appearing on these pages is effective as of September 30, 1989.

Schering—Cont.

Clinical Laboratory Tests: Among patients dosed with NORMODYNE (labetalol HCl) Tablets, there have been reversible increases of serum transaminases in 4% of patients tested, and more rarely, reversible increases in blood urea.

OVERDOSAGE

Overdosage with NORMODYNE (labetalol HCl) Injection causes excessive hypotension that is posture sensitive, and sometimes, excessive bradycardia. Patients should be placed supine and their legs raised if necessary to improve the blood supply to the brain. If overdosage with labetalol HCl follows oral ingestion, gastric lavage or pharmacologically induced emesis (using syrup of ipecac) may be useful for removal of the drug shortly after ingestion. The following additional measures should be employed if necessary: *Excessive bradycardia*-administer atropine or epinephrine. *Cardiac failure*-administer a digitalis glycoside and a diuretic. Dopamine or dobutamine may also be useful. *Hypotension*-administer vasopressors, eg. norepinephrine. There is pharmacological evidence that norepinephrine may be the drug of choice. *Bronchospasm*- administer epinephrine and/or an aerosolized beta$_2$- agonist. *Seizures*-administer diazepam.

In severe beta-blocker overdose resulting in hypotension and/or bradycardia, glucagon has been shown to be effective when administered in large doses (5 to 10 mg rapidly over 30 seconds, followed by continuous infusion of 5 mg/hr that can be reduced as the patient improves).

Neither hemodialysis nor peritoneal dialysis removes a significant amount of labetalol HCl from the general circulation ($<$1%).

The oral LD_{50} value of labetalol HCl in the mouse is approximately 600 mg/kg and in the rat is greater than 2 g/kg. The intravenous LD_{50} in these species is 50 to 60 mg/kg.

DOSAGE AND ADMINISTRATION

NORMODYNE (labetalol HCl) Injection is intended for intravenous use in hospitalized patients. DOSAGE MUST BE INDIVIDUALIZED depending upon the severity of hypertension and the repsonse of the patient during dosing.

Patients should always be kept in a supine position during the period of intravenous drug administration. A substantial fall in blood pressure on standing should be expected in these patients. The patient's ability to tolerate an upright position should be established before permitting any ambulation, such as using toilet facilities.

Either of two methods of administration of NORMODYNE Injection may be used: a) repeated intravenous injections, b) slow continuous infusion.

Repeated Intravenous Injection: Initially, NORMODYNE (labetalol HCl) Injection should be given in a dose of 20 mg labetalol HCl (which corresponds to 0.25 mg/kg for an 80 kg patient) by slow intravenous injection over a two-minute period.

Immediately before the injection and at five and ten minutes after injection, supine blood pressure should be measured to evaluate response. Additional injections of 40 mg or 80 mg can be given at ten minute intervals until a desired supine blood pressure is achieved or a total of 300 mg labetalol HCl has been injected. The maximum effect usually occurs within 5 minutes of each injection.

Slow Continuous Infusion: NORMODYNE (labetalol HCl) Injection is prepared for intravenous continuous infusion by diluting the contents with commonly used intravenous fluids (see below). Examples of methods of preparing the infusion solution are:

The contents of either two 20 mL vials (40 mL), or one 40 mL vial, are added to 160 mL of a commonly used intravenous fluid such that the resultant 200 mL of solution contains 200 mg of labetalol HCl, 1 mg/mL. The diluted solution should be administered at a rate of 2 mL/min to deliver 2 mg/min.

Alternatively the contents of either two 20 mL vials (40 mL), or one 40 mL vial, of NORMODYNE (labetalol HCl) Injection are added to 250 mL of a commonly used intravenous fluid. The resultant solution will contain 200 mg of labetalol HCl, approximately 2 mg/3 mL. The diluted solution should be administered at a rate of 3 mL/min to deliver approximately 2 mg/min.

The rate of infusion of the diluted solution may be adjusted according to the blood pressure response, at the discretion of the physician. To facilitate a desired rate of infusion, the diluted solution can be infused using a controlled administration mechanism, e.g., graduated burette or mechanically driven infusion pump.

Since the half life of labetalol is 5 to 8 hours, steady- state blood levels (in the face of a constant rate of infusion) would not be reached during the usual infusion time period. The infusion should be continued until a satisfactory response is obtained and should then be stopped and oral labetalol HCl started (see below). The effective intravenous dose is usually in the range of 50 to 200 mg. A total dose of up to 300 mg may be required in some patients.

Blood Pressure Monitoring: The blood pressure should be monitored during and after completion of the infusion or intravenous injections. Rapid or excessive falls in either systolic or diastolic blood pressure during intravenous treatment should be avoided. In patients with excessive systolic hypertension, the decrease in systolic pressure should be used as indicator of effectiveness in addition to the response of the diastolic pressure.

Initiation of Dosing with NORMODYNE (labetalol HCl) Tablets: Subsequent oral dosing with NORMODYNE (labetalol HCl) Tablets should begin when it has been established that the supine diastolic blood pressure has begun to rise. The recommended initial dose is 200 mg, followed in 6–12 hours by an additional dose of 200 or 400 mg, depending on the blood pressure response. Thereafter, *inpatient titration with NORMODYNE (labetalol HCl) Tablets* may proceed as follows:

Inpatient Titration Instructions

Regimen	Daily Dose*
200 mg bid	400 mg
400 mg bid	800 mg
800 mg bid	1600 mg
1200 mg bid	2400 mg

* If needed, the total daily dose may be given in three divided doses.

While in the hospital, the dosage of NORMODYNE Tablets may be increased at one day intervals to achieve the desired blood pressure reduction.

For subsequent outpatient titration or maintenance dosing see NORMODYNE Tablets Product Information **DOSAGE AND ADMINISTRATION** for additional recommendations.

Compatibility with commonly used intravenous fluids. Parenteral drug products should be inspected visually for particulate matter and discoloration prior to administration, whenever solution and container permit.

NORMODYNE (labetalol HCl) Injection was tested for compatibility with commonly used intravenous fluids at final concentrations of 1.25 mg to 3.75 mg labetalol HCl per mL of the mixture. NORMODYNE Injection was found to be compatible with and stable (for 24 hours refrigerated or at room temperature) in mixtures with the following solutions:

Ringers Injection, USP
Lactated Ringers Injection, USP
5% Dextrose and Ringers Injection
5% Lactated Ringers and 5% Dextrose Injection
5% Dextrose Injection, USP
0.9% Sodium Chloride Injection, USP
5% Dextrose and 0.2% Sodium Chloride Injection, USP
2.5% Dextrose and 0.45% Sodium Chloride Injection, USP
5% Dextrose and 0.9% Sodium Chloride Injection, USP
5% Dextrose and 0.33% Sodium Chloride Injection, USP
NORMODYNE (labetalol HCl) Injection was NOT compatible with 5% Sodium Bicarbonate Injection, USP.

HOW SUPPLIED

NORMODYNE (labetalol HCl) Injection, 5 mg/mL, is supplied in 20 mL (100 mg) (NDC-0085-0362-07) and 40 mL (200 mg) (NDC- 0085- 0362-06) multi-dose vials, boxes of 1; 4 mL (20 mg) (NDC-0085- 0362-08) and 4 mL (40 mg) (NDC-0085-0362-09) single-dose, prefilled, disposable syringes, boxes of 1.

Store between 2° and 30°C (36° and 86°F). Do not freeze. Protect syringe from light.

Note: To insure patient safety, the needle and the prefilled syringes should be handled with care and should be destroyed and discarded if damaged in any manner. If the cannula is bent, no attempt should be made to straighten it. To prevent needle-stick injuries, needles should not be recapped, purposely bent, or broken by hand.

Schering Corporation
Kenilworth, NJ 07033 USA

Revised 4/89   B-14525629
Copyright © 1984, 1985, 1986, 1988, 1989, Schering Corporation. All rights reserved.

NORMODYNE®   ℞
brand of
labetalol hydrochloride
Tablets

DESCRIPTION

NORMODYNE (labetalol HCl) is an adrenergic receptor blocking agent that has both selective alpha$_1$-and non-selective beta-adrenergic receptor blocking actions in a single substance.

Labetalol HCl is 5-[1-hydroxy-2[(1-methyl-3-phenylpropyl) amino] ethyl]salicylamide monohydrochloride.

Labetalol HCl has the empirical formula $C_{19}H_{24}N_2O_3 \cdot HCl$ and a molecular weight of 364.9. It has two asymmetric centers and therefore exists as a molecular complex of two diastereoisomeric pairs.

Labetalol HCl is a white or off-white crystalline powder, soluble in water.

NORMODYNE Tablets contain 100 mg, 200 mg or 300 mg labetalol HCl and are taken orally.

The inactive ingredients for NORMODYNE Tablets, 100 mg, include: corn starch, FD&C Blue No. 2 Al Lake, FD&C Yellow No. 6 Al Lake, hydroxypropyl methylcellulose, lactose, magnesium stearate, methylparaben, PEG and propylparaben. May also contain: potato starch and wheat starch.

The inactive ingredients for NORMODYNE Tablets, 200 mg, include: corn starch, hydroxypropyl methylcellulose, lactose, magnesium stearate, methylparaben, PEG, propylparaben and titanium dioxide. May also contain: potato starch and wheat starch.

The inactive ingredients for NORMODYNE Tablets, 300 mg, include: corn starch, FD&C Blue No. 2 Al Lake, hydroxypropyl methylcellulose, lactose, magnesium stearate, methylparaben, PEG and propylparaben. May also contain: potato starch and wheat starch.

CLINICAL PHARMACOLOGY

NORMODYNE (labetalol HCl) combines both selective, competitive alpha$_1$-adrenergic blocking and nonselective, competitive beta-adrenergic blocking activity in a single substance. In man, the ratios of alpha- to beta-blockade have been estimated to be approximately 1:3 and 1:7 following oral and intravenous administration, respectively. Beta$_2$-agonist activity has been demonstrated in animals with minimal beta$_1$-agonist (ISA) activity detected. In animals, at doses greater than those required for alpha or beta-adrenergic blockade, a membrane-stabilizing effect has been demonstrated.

Pharmacodynamics The capacity of labetalol HCl to block alpha receptors in man has been demonstrated by attenuation of the pressor effect of phenylephrine and by a significant reduction of the pressor response caused by immersing the hand in ice-cold water ("cold-pressor test"). Labetalol HCl's beta$_1$-receptor blockade in man was demonstrated by a small decrease in the resting heart rate, attenuation of tachycardia produced by isoproterenol or exercise, and by attenuation of the reflex tachycardia to the hypotension produced by amyl nitrite. Beta$_2$-receptor blockade was demonstrated by inhibition of the isoproterenol-induced fall in diastolic blood pressure. Both the alpha- and beta-blocking actions of orally administered labetalol HCl contribute to a decrease in blood pressure in hypertensive patients. Labetalol HCl consistently, in dose-related fashion, blunted increases in exercise-induced blood pressure and heart rate, and in their double product. The pulmonary circulation during exercise was not affected by labetalol HCl dosing.

Single oral doses of labetalol HCl administered in patients with coronary artery disease had no significant effect on sinus rate, intraventricular conduction, or QRS duration. The AV conduction time was modestly prolonged in 2 of 7 patients. In another study, intravenous labetalol HCl slightly prolonged AV nodal conduction time and atrial effective refractory period with only small changes in heart rate. The effects on AV nodal refractoriness were inconsistent.

Labetalol HCl produces dose-related falls in blood pressure without reflex tachycardia and without significant reduction in heart rate, presumably through a mixture of its alpha-blocking and beta-blocking effects. Hemodynamic effects are variable with small nonsignificant changes in cardiac output seen in some studies but not others, and small decreases in total peripheral resistance. Elevated plasma renins are reduced.

Doses of labetalol HCl that controlled hypertension did not affect renal function in mild to severe hypertensive patients with normal renal function.

Due to the alpha$_1$-receptor blocking activity of labetalol HCl, blood pressure is lowered more in the standing than in the supine position, and symptoms of postural hypotension (2%), including rare instances of syncope, can occur. Following oral administration, when postural hypotension has occurred, it has been transient and is uncommon when the recommended starting dose and titration increments are closely followed (see **DOSAGE AND ADMINISTRATION**). Symptomatic postural hypotension is most likely to occur 2 to 4 hours after a dose, especially following the use of large initial doses or upon large changes in dose.

The peak effects of single oral doses of labetalol HCl occur within 2 to 4 hours. The duration of effect depends upon dose, lasting at least 8 hours following single oral doses of 100 mg and more than 12 hours following single oral doses of 300 mg. The maximum, steady-state blood pressure response upon oral, twice-a-day dosing occurs within 24 to 72 hours.

The antihypertensive effect of labetalol HCl has a linear correlation with the logarithm of labetalol plasma concentration, and there is also a linear correlation between the reduction in exercise-induced tachycardia occurring at two hours after oral administration of labetalol HCl and the logarithm of the plasma concentration.

About 70% of the maximum beta-blocking effect is present for five hours after the administration of a single oral dose of 400 mg, with suggestion that about 40% remains at eight hours.

The anti-anginal efficacy of labetalol HCl has not been studied. In 37 patients with hypertension and coronary artery disease, labetalol HCl did not increase the incidence or severity of angina attacks.

Exacerbation of angina and, in some cases, myocardial infarction and ventricular dysrhythmias have been reported after abrupt discontinuation of therapy with beta-adrenergic blocking agents in patients with coronary artery disease. Abrupt withdrawal of these agents in patients without coronary artery disease has resulted in transient symptoms, including tremulousness, sweating, palpitation, headache, and malaise. Several mechanisms have been proposed to explain these phenomena, among them increased sensitivity to catecholamines because of increased numbers of beta receptors. Although beta-adrenergic receptor blockade is useful in the treatment of angina and hypertension, there are also situations in which sympathetic stimulation is vital. For example, in patients with severely damaged hearts, adequate ventricular function may depend on sympathetic drive. Beta-adrenergic blockade may worsen AV block by preventing the necessary facilitating effects of sympathetic activity on conduction. Beta$_2$-adrenergic blockade results in passive bronchial constriction by interfering with endogenous adrenergic bronchodilator activity in patients subject to bronchospasm and may also interfere with exogenous bronchodilators in such patients.

Pharmacokinetics and Metabolism Labetalol HCl is completely absorbed from the gastrointestinal tract with peak plasma levels occurring one to two hours after oral administration. The relative bioavailability of labetalol HCl tablets compared to an oral solution is 100%. The absolute bioavailability (fraction of drug reaching systemic circulation) of labetalol when compared to an intravenous infusion is 25%; this is due to extensive "first-pass" metabolism. Despite "first-pass" metabolism there is a linear relationship between oral doses of 100 to 3000 mg and peak plasma levels. The absolute bioavailability of labetalol is increased when administered with food.

The plasma half-life of labetalol following oral administration is about six to eight hours. Steady-state plasma levels of labetalol during repetitive dosing are reached by about the third day of dosing. In patients with decreased hepatic or renal function, the elimination half-life of labetalol is not altered; however, the relative bioavailability in hepatically impaired patients is increased due to decreased "first-pass" metabolism.

The metabolism of labetalol is mainly through conjugation to glucuronide metabolites. These metabolites are present in plasma and are excreted in the urine and, via the bile, into the feces. Approximately 55 to 60% of a dose appears in the urine as conjugates or unchanged labetalol within the first 24 hours of dosing.

Labetalol has been shown to cross the placental barrier in humans. Only negligible amounts of the drug crossed the blood-brain barrier in animal studies. Labetalol is approximately 50% protein bound. Neither hemodialysis nor peritoneal dialysis removes a significant amount of labetalol HCl from the general circulation (<1%).

INDICATIONS AND USAGE

NORMODYNE (labetalol HCl) Tablets are indicated in the management of hypertension. NORMODYNE Tablets may be used alone or in combination with other antihypertensive agents, especially thiazide and loop diuretics.

CONTRAINDICATIONS

NORMODYNE (labetalol HCl) Tablets are contraindicated in bronchial asthma, overt cardiac failure, greater than first degree heart block, cardiogenic shock, and severe bradycardia (see **WARNINGS**).

WARNINGS

Hepatic Injury Severe hepatocellular injury, confirmed by rechallenge in at least one case, occurs rarely with labetalol therapy. The hepatic injury is usually reversible, but hepatic necrosis and death have been reported. Injury has occurred after both short- and long-term treatment and may be slowly progressive despite minimal symptomatology. Appropriate laboratory testing should be done at the first symptom/sign of liver dysfunction (e.g., pruritis, dark urine, persistent anorexia, jaundice, right upper quadrant tenderness, or unexplained "flu-like" symptoms). If the patient has laboratory evidence of liver injury or jaundice, labetalol should be stopped and not restarted.

Cardiac Failure Sympathetic stimulation is a vital component supporting circulatory function in congestive heart failure. Beta blockade carries a potential hazard of further depressing myocardial contractility and precipitating more severe failure. Although beta-blockers should be avoided in overt congestive heart failure, if necessary, labetalol HCl can be used with caution in patients with a history of heart failure who are well-compensated. Congestive heart failure has been observed in patients receiving labetalol HCl. Labetalol HCl does not abolish the inotropic action of digitalis on heart muscle.

In Patients Without a History of Cardiac Failure In patients with latent cardiac insufficiency, continued depression of the myocardium with beta-blocking agents over a period of time can, in some cases, lead to cardiac failure. At the first sign or symptom of impending cardiac failure, patients should be fully digitalized and/or be given a diuretic, and the response observed closely. If cardiac failure continues, despite adequate digitalization and diuretic, NORMODYNE (labetalol HCl) therapy should be withdrawn (gradually if possible).

Exacerbation of Ischemic Heart Disease Following Abrupt Withdrawal Angina pectoris has not been reported upon labetalol HCl discontinuation. However, hypersensitivity to catecholamines has been observed in patients withdrawn from beta-blocker therapy; exacerbation of angina and, in some cases, myocardial infarction have occurred after *abrupt* discontinuation of such therapy. When discontinuing chronically administered NORMODYNE (labetalol HCl), particularly in patients with ischemic heart disease, the dosage should be gradually reduced over a period of one to two weeks and the patient should be carefully monitored. If angina markedly worsens or acute coronary insufficiency develops, NORMODYNE (labetalol HCl) administration should be reinstituted promptly, at least temporarily, and other measures appropriate for the management of unstable angina should be taken. Patients should be warned against interruption or discontinuation of therapy without the physician's advice. Because coronary artery disease is common and may be unrecognized, it may be prudent not to discontinue NORMODYNE (labetalol HCl) therapy abruptly even in patients treated only for hypertension.

Nonallergic Bronchospasm (e.g., chronic bronchitis and emphysema) Patients with bronchospastic disease should, in general, not receive beta-blockers. NORMODYNE may be used with caution, however, in patients who do not respond to, or cannot tolerate, other antihypertensive agents. It is prudent, if NORMODYNE is used, to use the smallest effective dose, so that inhibition of endogenous or exogenous beta-agonists is minimized.

Pheochromocytoma Labetalol HCl has been shown to be effective in lowering the blood pressure and relieving symptoms in patients with pheochromocytoma. However, paradoxical hypertensive responses have been reported in a few patients with this tumor; therefore, use caution when administering labetalol HCl to patients with pheochromocytoma.

Diabetes Mellitus and Hypoglycemia Beta-adrenergic blockade may prevent the appearance of premonitory signs and symptoms (e.g., tachycardia) of acute hypoglycemia. This is especially important with labile diabetics. Beta-blockade also reduces the release of insulin in response to hyperglycemia; it may therefore be necessary to adjust the dose of antidiabetic drugs.

Major Surgery The necessity or desirability of withdrawing beta-blocking therapy prior to major surgery is controversial. Protracted severe hypotension and difficulty in restarting or maintaining a heart beat have been reported with beta-blockers. The effect of labetalol HCl's alpha-adrenergic activity has not been evaluated in this setting.

A synergism between labetalol HCl and halothane anesthesia has been shown (see **Drug Interactions**).

PRECAUTIONS

General: *Impaired Hepatic Function* NORMODYNE (labetalol HCl) Tablets should be used with caution in patients with impaired hepatic function since metabolism of the drug may be diminished.

Jaundice or Hepatic Dysfunction (see **WARNINGS**).

Information for Patients
As with all drugs with beta-blocking activity, certain advice to patients being treated with labetalol HCl is warranted. This information is intended to aid in the safe and effective use of this medication. It is not a disclosure of all possible adverse or intended effects. While no incident of the abrupt withdrawal phenomenon (exacerbation of angina pectoris) has been reported with labetalol HCl, dosing with NORMODYNE Tablets should not be interrupted or discontinued without a physician's advice. Patients being treated with NORMODYNE Tablets should consult a physician at any signs or symptoms of impending cardiac failure or hepatic dysfunction (see **WARNINGS**). Also, transient scalp tingling may occur, usually when treatment with NORMODYNE Tablets is initiated (see **ADVERSE REACTIONS**).

Laboratory Tests
As with any new drug given over prolonged periods, laboratory parameters should be observed over regular intervals. In patients with concomitant illnesses, such as impaired renal function, appropriate tests should be done to monitor these conditions.

Drug Interactions
In one survey, 2.3% of patients taking labetalol HCl in combination with tricyclic antidepressants experienced tremor as compared to 0.7% reported to occur with labetalol HCl alone. The contribution of each of the treatments to this adverse reaction is unknown but the possibility of a drug interaction cannot be excluded.

Drugs possessing beta-blocking properties can blunt the bronchodilator effect of beta-receptor agonist drugs in patients with bronchospasm; therefore, doses greater than the normal anti-asthmatic dose of beta-agonist bronchodilator drugs may be required.

Cimetidine has been shown to increase the bioavailability of labetalol HCl. Since this could be explained either by enhanced absorption or by an alteration of hepatic metabolism of labetalol HCl, special care should be used in establishing the dose required for blood pressure control in such patients. Synergism has been shown between halothane anesthesia and intravenously administered labetalol HCl. During controlled hypotensive anesthesia using labetalol HCl in association with halothane, high concentrations (3% or above) of halothane should not be used because the degree of hypotension will be increased and because of the possibility of a large reduction in cardiac output and an increase in central venous pressure. The anesthesiologist should be informed when a patient is receiving labetalol HCl.

Labetalol HCl blunts the reflex tachycardia produced by nitroglycerin without preventing its hypotensive effect. If labetalol HCl is used with nitroglycerin in patients with angina pectoris, additional antihypertensive effects may occur.

Drug/Laboratory Test Interactions
The presence of labetalol metabolites in the urine may result in falsely elevated levels of urinary catecholamines, metanephrine, normetanephrine, and vanillylmandelic acid (VMA) when measured by fluorimetric or photometric methods. In screening patients suspected of having a pheochromocytoma and being treated with labetalol HCl, a specific method, such as a high performance liquid chromatographic assay with solid phase extraction (e.g. *J Chromatogr* 385:241,1987) should be employed in determining levels of catecholamines.

Labetalol HCl has also been reported to produce a false-positive test for amphetamine when screening urine for the presence of drugs using the commercially available assay methods Toxi-Lab A® (thin-layer chromatographic assay) and Emit-d.a.u.® (radioenzymatic assay). When patients being treated with labetalol have a positive urine test for amphetamine using these techniques, confirmation should be made by using more specific methods, such as a gas chromatographic-mass spectrometer technique.

Carcinogenesis, Mutagenesis, Impairment of Fertility
Long-term oral dosing studies with labetalol HCl for 18 months in mice and for 2 years in rats showed no evidence of carcinogenesis. Studies with labetalol HCl, using dominant lethal assays in rats and mice, and exposing microorganisms according to modified Ames tests, showed no evidence of mutagenesis.

Pregnancy Category C
Teratogenic studies have been performed with labetalol in rats and rabbits at oral doses up to approximately 6 and 4 times the maximum recommended human dose (MRHD), respectively. No reproducible evidence of fetal malformations was observed. Increased fetal resorptions were seen in both species at doses approximating the MRHD. A teratology study performed with labetalol in rabbits at intravenous doses up to 1.7 times the MRHD revealed no evidence of drug related harm to the fetus. There are no adequate and well-controlled studies in pregnant women. Labetalol should be used during pregnancy only if the potential benefit justifies the potential risk to the fetus.

Nonteratogenic Effects
Transient hypotension, bradycardia, and hypoglycemia have been rarely observed in infants of mothers who were treated with labetalol HCl for hypertension during pregnancy. Oral administration of labetalol to rats during late gestation through weaning at doses of 2 to 4 times the MRHD caused a decrease in neonatal survival.

Labor and Delivery
Labetalol HCl given to pregnant women with hypertension did not appear to affect the usual course of labor and delivery.

Nursing Mothers
Small amounts of labetalol (approximately 0.004% of the maternal dose) are excreted in human milk. Caution should be exercised when NORMODYNE Tablets are administered to a nursing woman.

Pediatric Use
Safety and effectiveness in children have not been established.

ADVERSE REACTIONS

Most adverse effects are mild, transient and occur early in the course of treatment. In controlled clinical trials of 3 to 4 months duration, discontinuation of NORMODYNE (labetalol HCl) Tablets due to one or more adverse effects was required in 7% of all patients. In these same trials, beta-blocker control agents led to discontinuation in 8 to 10% of patients, and a centrally acting alpha-agonist in 30% of patients.

Continued on next page

Information on Schering products appearing on these pages is effective as of September 30, 1989.

Schering—Cont.

The incidence rates of adverse reactions listed in the following table were derived from multicenter controlled clinical trials, comparing labetalol HCl, placebo, metoprolol and propranolol, over treatment periods of 3 and 4 months. Where the frequency of adverse effects for labetalol HCl and placebo is similar, causal relationship is uncertain. The rates are based on adverse reactions considered probably drug-related by the investigator. If all reports are considered, the rates are somewhat higher (e.g., dizziness 20%, nausea 14%, fatigue 11%), but the overall conclusions are unchanged. [See table below].

The adverse effects were reported spontaneously and are representative of the incidence of adverse effects that may be observed in a properly selected hypertensive patient population, (i.e., a group excluding patients with bronchospastic disease, overt congestive heart failure, or other contraindications to beta-blocker therapy.

Clinical trials also included studies utilizing daily doses up to 2400 mg in more severely hypertensive patients. Certain of the side effects increased with increasing dose as shown in the table below which depicts the entire U.S. therapeutic trials data base for adverse reactions that are clearly or possibly drug related.
[See table above].

In addition, a number of other less common adverse events have been reported:

Body as a Whole Fever
Cardiovascular Postural hypotension, including rarely, syncope.
Central and Peripheral Nervous Systems Paresthesias, most frequently described as scalp tingling. In most cases, it was mild, transient and usually occurred at the beginning of treatment.
Collagen Disorders Systemic lupus erythematosus; positive antinuclear factor (ANF).
Eyes Dry eyes.
Immunological System Antimitochondrial antibodies.
Liver and Biliary System Hepatic necrosis; hepatitis; cholestatic jaundice, elevated liver function tests.
Musculo-Skeletal System Muscle cramps; toxic myopathy.
Respiratory System Bronchospasm.
Skin and Appendages Rashes of various types, such as generalized maculo-papular; lichenoid; urticarial; bullous lichen planus; psoriaform; facial erythema; Peyronie's disease; reversible alopecia.
Urinary System Difficulty in micturition, including acute urinary bladder retention.

Following approval for marketing in the United Kingdom, a monitored release survey involving approximately 6,800 patients was conducted for further safety and efficacy evaluation of this product. Results of this survey indicate that the type, severity, and incidence of adverse effects were comparable to those cited above.

Potential Adverse Effects
In addition, other adverse effects not listed above have been reported with other beta-adrenergic blocking agents.

Labetalol HCl

Daily Dose (mg)	200	300	400	600	800	900	1200	1600	2400
Number of Patients	522	181	606	608	503	117	411	242	175
Dizziness (%)	2	3	3	3	5	1	9	13	16
Fatigue	2	1	4	4	5	3	7	6	10
Nausea	<1	0	1	2	4	0	7	11	19
Vomting	0	0	<1	<1	<1	0	1	2	3
Dyspepsia	1	0	2	1	1	0	2	2	4
Paresthesias	2	0	2	2	1	1	2	5	5
Nasal Stuffiness	1	1	2	2	2	2	4	5	6
Ejaculation Failure	0	2	1	2	3	0	4	3	5
Impotence	1	1	1	1	2	4	3	4	3
Edema	1	0	1	1	1	0	1	2	2

Central Nervous System Reversible mental depression progressing to catatonia; an acute reversible syndrome characterized by disorientation for time and place, short-term memory loss, emotional lability, slightly clouded sensorium, and decreased performance on neuropsychometrics.
Cardiovascular Intensification of AV block. See **CONTRAINDICATIONS**.
Allergic Fever combined with aching and sore throat; laryngospasm; respiratory distress.
Hematologic Agranulocytosis; thrombocytopenic or nonthrombocytopenic purpura.
Gastrointestinal Mesenteric artery thrombosis; ischemic colitis.

The oculomucocutaneous syndrome associated with the beta-blocker practolol has not been reported with labetalol HCl.

Clinical Laboratory Tests
There have been reversible increases of serum transaminases in 4% of patients treated with labetalol HCl and tested, and more rarely, reversible increases in blood urea.

OVERDOSAGE

Overdosage with NORMODYNE (labetalol HCl) Tablets causes excessive hypotension that is posture sensitive, and sometimes, excessive bradycardia. Patients should be placed supine and their legs raised if necessary to improve the blood supply to the brain. If overdosage with labetalol HCl follows oral ingestion, gastric lavage or pharmacologically induced emesis (using syrup of ipecac) may be useful for removal of the drug shortly after ingestion. The following additional measures should be employed if necessary: *Excessive bradycardia*—administer atropine or epinephrine. *Cardic failure*—administer a digitalis glycoside and a diuretic. Dopamine or dobutamine may also be useful. *Hypotension*—administer vasopressors, e.g., norepinephrine. There is pharmacological evidence that norepinephrine may be the drug of choice. *Bronchospasm*—administer epinephrine and/or an aerosolized beta$_2$-agonist. *Seizures*—administer diazepam.

In severe beta-blocker overdose resulting in hypotension and/or bradycardia, glucagon has been shown to be effective when administered in large doses (5 to 10 mg rapidly over 30 seconds, followed by continuous infusion of 5 mg/hr that can be reduced as the patient improves).

Neither hemodialysis nor peritoneal dialysis removes a significant amount of labetalol HCl from the general circulation (<1%).

The oral LD$_{50}$ value of labetalol HCl in the mouse is approximately 600 mg/kg and in the rat is greater than 2 g/kg. The intravenous LD$_{50}$ in these species is 50 to 60 mg/kg.

DOSAGE AND ADMINISTRATION

DOSAGE MUST BE INDIVIDUALIZED. The recommended initial dose is 100 mg twice daily whether used alone or added to a diuretic regimen. After 2 or 3 days, using standing blood pressure as an indicator, dosage may be titrated in increments of 100 mg bid every 2 or 3 days. The usual maintenance dosage of labetalol HCl is between 200 and 400 mg twice daily.

Since the full antihypertensive effect of labetalol HCl is usually seen within the first one to three hours of the initial dose or dose increment, the assurance of a lack of an exaggerated hypotensive response can be clinically established in the office setting. The antihypertensive effects of continued dosing can be measured at subsequent visits, approximately 12 hours after a dose, to determine whether further titration is necessary.

Patients with severe hypertension may require from 1200 mg to 2400 mg per day, with or without thiazide diuretics. Should side effects (principally nausea or dizziness) occur with these doses administered bid, the same total daily dose administered bid may improve tolerability and facilitate further titration. Titration increments should not exceed 200 mg bid.

When a diuretic is added, an additive antihypertensive effect can be expected. In some cases this may necessitate a labetalol HCl dosage adjustment. As with most antihypertensive drugs, optimal dosages of NORMODYNE Tablets are usually lower in patients also receiving a diuretic.

When transferring patients from other antihypertensive drugs, NORMODYNE Tablets should be introduced as recommended and the dosage of the existing therapy progressively decreased.

HOW SUPPLIED

NORMODYNE (labetalol HCl) Tablets, 100 mg, light-brown, round, scored, film-coated tablets engraved on one side with Schering and product identification numbers 244, and on the other side the number 100 for the strength and "NORMODYNE"; bottles of 100 (NDC-0085-0244-04), 500 (NDC-0085-0244-05), bottles of 1000 (NDC-0085-0244-07), and box of 100 for unit-dose dispensing (NDC-0085-0244-08).

NORMODYNE (labetalol HCl) Tablets, 200 mg, white, round, scored, film-coated tablets engraved on one side with Schering and product identification numbers 752, and on the other side the number 200 for the strength and "NORMODYNE"; bottles of 100 (NDC-0085-0752-04), 500 (NDC-0085-0752-05), bottles of 1000 (NDC-0085-0752-07), box of 100 for unit-dose dispensing (NDC-0085-0752-08).

NORMODYNE (labetalol HCl) Tablets, 300 mg, blue, round, film-coated tablets engraved on one side with Schering and product identification numbers 438, and on the other side the number 300 for the strength and "NORMODYNE"; bottles of 100 (NDC-0085-0438-03), 500 (NDC-0085-0438-05), box of 100 for unit-dose dispensing (NDC-0085-0438-06).

NORMODYNE (labetalol HCl) Tablets should be stored between 2° and 30°C (36° and 86°F).

NORMODYNE (labetalol HCl) Tablets in the unit-dose boxes should be protected from excessive moisture.

Schering Corporation
Kenilworth, NJ 07033 USA

Rev. 4/89   B-16098914
Copyright© 1984, 1985, 1986, 1987, 1988, 1989, Schering Corporation. All rights reserved.

Shown in Product Identification Section, page 428

	Labetalol HCl (N=227) %	Placebo (N=98) %	Propranolol (N=84) %	Metoprolol (N=49) %
Body as a whole				
fatigue	5	0	12	12
asthemia	1	1	1	0
headache	2	1	1	2
Gastrointestinal				
nausea	6	1	1	2
vomiting	<1	0	0	0
dyspepsia	3	1	1	0
abdominal pain	0	0	1	2
diarrhea	<1	0	2	0
taste distortion	1	0	0	0
Central and Peripheral Nervous Systems				
dizziness	11	3	4	4
paresthesias	<1	0	0	0
drowsiness	<1	2	2	2
Autonomic Nervous System				
nasal stuffiness	3	0	0	0
ejaculation failure	2	0	0	0
impotence	<1	0	1	3
increased sweating	<1	0	0	0
Cardiovascular				
edema	1	0	0	0
postural hypotension	1	0	0	0
bradycardia	0	0	5	12
Respiratory				
dyspnea	2	0	1	2
Skin				
rash	1	0	0	0
Special Senses				
vision abnormality	1	0	0	0
vertigo	2	1	0	0

NORMOZIDE®   ℞
brand of labetalol hydrochloride and
hydrochlorothiazide, USP
Tablets

DESCRIPTION

NORMOZIDE® Tablets combine three modes of antihypertensive action: the vasodilating and beta-adrenergic blocking activity of NORMODYNE® (labetalol hydrochloride), plus the known antihypertensive effect of a thiazide diuretic, hydrochlorothiazide.

Labetalol HCl is Benzamide, 2-hydroxy-5-[1-hydroxy-2-[(1-methyl-3-phenylpropyl)amino]ethyl]-, monohydrochloride.
Labetalol HCl is a white or off-white crystalline powder, soluble in water, having the empirical formula $C_{19}H_{24}N_2O_3 \cdot HCl$, a molecular weight of 364.9, and two asymmetric centers; therefore, it exists as a molecular complex of two diastereoisomeric pairs.

Hydrochlorothiazide is 6-Chloro-3,4-dihydro-2H-1,2, 4-benzothiadizine-7-sulfonamide 1,1-dioxide.

Hydrochlorothiazide is a white or practically white crystalline compound, practically insoluble in water but soluble in sodium hydroxide. It has the empirical formula $C_7H_8ClN_3O_4S_2$ and a molecular weight of 297.73.

NORMOZIDE Tablets are available in several strengths and are taken orally. They are available as: 100 mg labetalol HCl/25 mg hydrochlorothiazide; 200 mg labetalol HCl/25 mg hydrochlorothiazide; and 300 mg labetalol HCl/25 mg hydrochlorothiazide.

The inactive ingredients for NORMOZIDE Tablets, 100/25 mg, include: corn starch, FD&C Blue No. 2 Al Lake, FD&C Yellow No. 6 Al Lake, hydroxypropyl methylcellulose, lactose, magnesium stearate, methylparaben, PEG, and propylparaben.

The inactive ingredients for NORMOZIDE Tablets, 200/25 mg. include: corn starch, hydroxypropyl methylcellulose, lactose, magnesium stearate, methylparaben, PEG, propylparaben, and titanium dioxide.

The inactive ingredients for NORMOZIDE Tablets, 300/25 mg, include: corn starch, FD&C Blue No. 2 Al Lake, hydroxypropyl methylcellulose, lactose, magnesium stearate, methylparaben, PEG, and propylparaben.

CLINICAL PHARMACOLOGY

NORMOZIDE Tablets: The antihypertensive effects of labetalol and hydrochlorothiazide are additive. Studies have shown that there is no interference with bioavailability when these agents are given together in the single combination tablet. Therefore, this combination provides a convenient formulation for the concomitant administration of these two entites.

Labetalol HCl: Labetalol HCl combines both selective, competitive alpha$_1$-adrenergic blocking and nonselective, competitive beta-adrenergic blocking activity in a single substance. In man, the ratios of alpha- to beta-blockade have been estimated to be approximately 1:3 and 1:7 following oral and intravenous administration, respectively. Beta$_2$-agonist activity has been demonstrated in animals with minimal beta$_1$-agonist (ISA) activity detected. In animals, at doses greater than those required for alpha- or beta-adrenergic blockade, a membrane-stabilizing effect has been demonstrated.

Pharmacodynamics The capacity of labetalol HCl to block alpha receptors in man has been demonstrated by attenuation of the pressor effect of phenylephrine and by a significant reduction of the pressor response caused by immersing the hand in ice-cold water ("cold-pressor test"). Labetalol HCL's beta$_1$-receptor blockade in man was demonstrated by a small decrease in the resting heart rate, attenuation of tachycardia produced by isoproterenol or exercise, and by attenuation of the reflex tachycardia to the hypotension produced by amyl nitrite. Beta$_2$-receptor blockade was demonstrated by inhibition of the isoproterenol-induced fall in diastolic blood pressure. Both the alpha- and beta-blocking actions of orally administered labetalol HCl contribute to a decrease in blood pressure in hypertensive patients. Labetalol HCl consistently, in dose-related fashion, blunted increases in exercise-induced blood pressure and heart rate, and in their double product. The pulmonary circulation during exercise was not affected by labetalol HCl dosing.

Single oral doses of labetalol HCl administered to patients with coronary artery disease had no significant effect on sinus rate, intraventricular conduction, or QRS duration. The AV conduction time was modestly prolonged in 2 of 7 patients. In another study, intravenous labetalol HCl slightly prolonged AV nodal conduction time and atrial effective refractory period with only small changes in heart rate. The effects on AV nodal refractoriness were inconsistent.

Labetalol HCl produces dose-related falls in blood pressure without reflex tachycardia and without significant reduction in heart rate, presumably through a mixture of its alpha-blocking and beta-blocking effects. Hemodynamic effects are variable with small nonsignificant changes in cardiac output seen in some studies but not others, and small decreases in total peripheral resistance. Elevated plasma renins are reduced.

Doses of labetalol HCl that controlled hypertension did not affect renal function in mild to severe hypertensive patients with normal renal function.

Due to the alpha$_1$-receptor blocking activity of labetalol HCl, blood pressure is lowered more in the standing than in the supine position, and symptoms of postural hypotension (2%), including rare instances of syncope, can occur. Following oral administration, when postural hypotension has occurred, it has been transient and is uncommon when the recommended starting dose and titration increments are closely followed (see **DOSAGE AND ADMINISTRATION** section of the NORMODYNE® Tablets package insert).

Symptomatic postural hypotension is most likely to occur 2 to 4 hours after a dose, especially following the use of large initial doses or upon large changes in dose.

The peak effects of single oral doses of labetalol HCl occur within 2 to 4 hours. The duration of effect depends upon dose, lasting at least 8 hours following single oral doses of 100 mg and more than 12 hours following single oral doses of 300 mg. The maximum, steady-state blood pressure response upon oral, twice-a-day dosing occurs within 24 to 72 hours.

The antihypertensive effect of labetalol has a linear correlation with the logarithm of labetalol plasma concentration, and there is also a linear correlation between the reduction in exercise-induced tachycardia at two hours after oral administration of labetalol HCl and the logarithm of the plasma concentration.

About 70% of the maximum beta-blocking effect is present for five hours after the administration of a single oral dose of 400 mg with suggestion that about 40% remains at eight hours.

The anti-anginal efficacy of labetalol HCl has not been studied. In 37 patients with hypertension and coronary artery disease, labetalol HCl did not increase the incidence or severity of angina attacks.

Exacerbation of angina and, in some cases, myocardial infarction and ventricular dysrhythmias have been reported after abrupt discontinuation of therapy with beta-adrenergic blocking agents in patients with coronary artery disease. Abrupt withdrawal of these agents in patients without coronary artery disease has resulted in transient symptoms, including tremulousness, sweating, palpitation, headache, and malaise. Several mechanisms have been proposed to explain these phenomena, among them increased sensitivity to catecholamines because of increased numbers of beta receptors. Although beta-adrenergic receptor blockade is useful in the treatment of hypertension, there are also situations in which sympathetic stimulation is vital. For example, in patients with severely damaged hearts, adequate ventricular function may depend on sympathetic drive. Beta-adrenergic blockade may worsen AV block by preventing the necessary facilitating effects of sympathetic activity on conduction. Beta$_2$-adrenergic blockade results in passive bronchial constriction by interfering with endogenous adrenergic bronchodilator activity in patients subject to bronchospasm and may also interfere with exogenous bronchodilators in such patients.

Pharmacokinetics and Metabolism Labetalol HCl is completely absorbed from the gastrointestinal tract with peak plasma levels occurring one to two hours after oral administration. The relative bioavailability of labetalol HCl tablets compared to an oral solution is 100%. The absolute bioavailability (fraction of drug reaching systemic circulation) of labetalol when compared to an intravenous infusion is 25%; this is due to extensive "first-pass" metabolism. Despite "first-pass" metabolism there is a linear relationship between oral doses of 100 to 3000 mg and peak plasma levels. The absolute bioavailability of labetalol is increased when administered with food.

The plasma half-life of labetalol following oral administration is about six to eight hours. Steady-state plasma levels of labetalol during repetitive dosing are reached by about the third day of dosing. In patients with decreased hepatic or renal function, the elimination half-life of labetalol is not altered; however, the relative bioavailability in hepatically impaired patients is increased due to decreased "first-pass" metabolism.

The metabolism of labetalol is mainly through conjugation to glucuronide metabolites. These metabolites are present in plasma and are excreted in the urine and, via the bile, into the feces. Approximately 55 to 60% of a dose appears in the urine as conjugates or unchanged labetalol within the first 24 hours of dosing.

Labetalol has been shown to cross the placental barrier in humans. Only negligible amounts of the drug crossed the blood-brain barrier in animal studies. Labetalol is approximately 50% protein bound. Neither hemodialysis nor peritoneal dialysis removes a significant amount of labetalol HCl from the general circulation ($< 1\%$).

Hydrochlorothiazide: Hydrochlorothiazide is a diuretic/antihypertensive.

Thiazides affect the renal tubular mechanism of electrolyte reabsorption. At maximal therapeutic dosage, all thiazides are approximately equal in their diuretic potency.

Thiazides increase excretion of sodium and chloride in approximately equivalent amounts. Natriuresis may be accompanied by some loss of potassium and bicarbonate. Following oral administration, the diuretic action of hydrochlorothiazide occurs within two hours with the peak effect occurring in about four hours. Its action persists for approximately 6 to 12 hours. Thiazides are eliminated rapidly by the kidney.

Thiazide diuretics have antihypertensive activity *per se* in hypertensive patients and also may augment the actions of other antihypertensive drugs. The full mechanism of antihypertensive action is not known.

Therapy for hypertension is often initiated with a thiazide diuretic which induces diuresis, natriuresis, depletion of extracellular fluid, and reduction of cardiac output. Direct arteriolar dilatation may play a role. Thiazides do not affect normal blood pressure.

Plasma renin activity is elevated during thiazide therapy. The aldosterone secretion rate is increased slightly but significantly; this contributes to the hypokalemia caused by thiazides.

INDICATIONS AND USAGE

NORMOZIDE (labetalol HCl/hydrochlorothiazide) Tablets are indicated in the management of hypertension.

THIS FIXED COMBINATION DRUG IS NOT INDICATED FOR INITIAL THERAPY OF HYPERTENSION. IF THE FIXED COMBINATION REPRESENTS THE DOSE TITRATED TO AN INDIVIDUAL PATIENT'S NEEDS, IT MAY BE MORE CONVENIENT THAN THE SEPARATE COMPONENTS.

CONTRAINDICATIONS

Labetalol HCl is contraindicated in bronchial asthma, overt cardiac failure, greater than first degree heart block, cardiogenic shock, and severe bradycardia. (See **WARNINGS**.) Hydrochlorothiazide is contraindicated in patients with anuria or hypersensitivity to this or other sulfonamide-derived drugs.

WARNINGS

Labetalol HCL: *Hepatic Injury* Severe hepatocellular injury, confirmed by rechallenge in at least one case, occurs rarely with labetalol therapy. The hepatic injury is usually reversible, but hepatic necrosis and death have been reported. Injury has occurred after both short- and long-term treatment and may be slowly progressive despite minimal symptomatology. Appropriate laboratory testing should be done at the first symptom/sign of liver dysfunction (e.g. pruritus, dark urine, persistent anorexia, jaundice, right upper quadrant tenderness, or unexplained "flu-like" symptoms). If the patient has laboratory evidence of liver injury or jaundice, labetalol should be stopped and not restarted.

Cardiac Failure Sympathetic stimulation is a vital component supporting circulatory function in congestive heart failure. Beta blockade carries a potential hazard of further depressing myocardial contractility and precipitating more severe failure. Although beta-blockers should be avoided in overt congestive heart failure, if necessary, labetalol HCl can be used with caution in patients with a history of heart failure who are well-compensated. Congestive heart failure has been observed in patients receiving labetalol HCl. Labetalol HCl does not abolish the inotropic action of digitalis on heart muscle.

In Patients Without a History of Cardiac Failure In patients with latent cardiac insufficiency, continued depression of the myocardium with beta-blocking agents over a period of time can in some cases lead to cardiac failiure. At the first sign or symptom of impending cardiac failure, patients should be fully digitalized and/or be given additional diuretic and the response observed closely. If cardiac failure continues despite adequate digitalization and diuretic, NORMOZIDE therapy should be withdrawn (gradually if possible).

Exacerbation of Ischemic Heart Disease Following Abrupt Withdrawal Angina pectoris has not been reported upon labetalol HCl discontinuation. However, hypersensitivity to catecholamines has been observed in patients withdrawn from beta-blocker therapy; exacerbation of angina and, in some cases, myocardial infarction have occurred after *abrupt* discontinuation of such therapy. When discontinuing chronically administered NORMOZIDE Tablets, particularly in patients with ischemic heart disease, the dosage should be gradually reduced over a period of one to two weeks and the patient should be carefully monitored. If angina markedly worsens or acute coronary insufficiency develops, labetalol HCl therapy should be reinstituted promptly, at least temporarily, and other measures appropriate for the management of unstable angina should be taken. Patients should be warned against interruption or discontinuation of therapy without the physician's advice. Because coronary artery disease is common and may be unrecognized, it may be prudent not to discontinue NORMODIZE therapy abruptly in patients treated for hypertension.

Bronchospastic Disease Patients with bronchospastic disease should, in general, not receive antihypertensive drugs possessing beta-blocking properties. Because of labetalol's alpha$_1$-blockade and beta$_2$-agonist actions on airway smooth muscle, however, it may be used with caution in patients who cannot tolerate other antihypertensive treatment. It is nevertheless prudent, if labetalol is used, to use the smallest effective dose, so that inhibition of endogenous or exogenous beta-agonists is minimized.

Continued on next page

Information on Schering products appearing on these pages is effective as of September 30, 1989.

Schering—Cont.

Pheochromocytoma: Labetalol HCl has been shown to be effective in lowering the blood pressure and relieving symptoms in patients with pheochromocytoma. However, paradoxical hypertensive responses have been reported in a few patients with this tumor; therefore, use caution when administering labetalol HCl to patients with pheochromocytoma.

Diabetes Mellitus and Hypoglycemia Beta-adrenergic blockade may prevent the appearance of premonitory signs and symptoms (e.g., tachycardia) of acute hypoglycemia. This is especially important with labile diabetics. Beta-blockade also reduces the release of insulin in response to hyperglycemia; it may therefore be necessary to adjust the dose of antidiabetic drugs.

Major Surgery The necessity or desirability of withdrawing beta-blocking therapy prior to major surgery is controversial. Protracted severe hypotension and difficulty in restarting or maintaining a heart beat have been reported with beta-blockers. The effect of labetalol HCl's alpha-adrenergic activity has not been evaluated in this setting.

A synergism between labetalol HCl and halothane anesthesia has been shown (see **Drug Interactions**).

Hydrochlorothiazide: Thiazides should be used with caution in severe renal disease. In patients with renal disease, thiazides may precipitate azotemia. Cumulative effects of the drug may develop in patients with impaired renal function.

Thiazides should also be used with caution in patients with impaired hepatic function or progressive liver disease, since minor alterations of fluid and electrolyte balance may precipitate hepatic coma.

Thiazides may add to or potentiate the action of other antihypertensive drugs. Potentiation occurs with ganglionic or peripheral adrenergic-blocking drugs.

Sensitivity reactions may occur in patients with a history of allergy or bronchial asthma. The possibility of exacerbation or activation of systemic lupus erythematosus has been reported.

Diabetes mellitus, which has been latent, may become manifest during thiazide therapy.

PRECAUTIONS

General—*Labetalol HCl:* *Impaired Hepatic Function* Labetalol HCl should be used with caution in patients with impaired hepatic function since metabolism of the drug may be diminished.

Jaundice or Hepatic Dysfunction (see **WARNINGS**).

General—*Hydrochlorothiazide:* Serum and urine electrolyte determinations are particularly important when the patient is vomiting excessively, having diarrhea, or receiving parenteral fluids. Thiazides may cause hyponatremia, hypochloremic alkalosis, hypokalemia, hypmagnesemia, and changes in serum and urine calcium. All patients receiving thiazide therapy should be observed for the following clinical warning signs of fluid or electrolyte imbalance, irrespective of cause: dryness of mouth, thirst, weakness, lethargy, drowsiness, restlessness, muscular pains, cramps, or fatigue, hypotension, oliguria, tachycardia, and gastrointestinal disturbances such as nausea and vomiting.

Hypokalemia may develop, especially with brisk diuresis, when severe cirrhosis is present, during concomitant use of corticosteroids or ACTH, or after prolonged therapy. Interference with adequate oral electrolyte intake will also contribute to hypokalemia. Hypokalemia can sensitize or exaggerate the response of the heart to the toxic effects of digitalis (e.g., increased ventricular irritability). Hypokalemia may be avoided or treated by use of potassium supplements such as foods with a high potassium content.

Any chloride deficit is generally mild and usually does not require specific treatment except under extraordinary circumstances (as in liver or renal disease). Dilutional hyponatremia may occur in edematous patients in hot weather; appropriate therapy is water restriction rather than administration of salt, except in rare instances when the hyponatremia is life-threatening. In actual salt depletion, appropriate replacement is the therapy of choice.

Hyperuricemia may occur or acute gout may be precipitated in certain patients receiving thiazides.

The antihypertensive effects of the drug may be enhanced in the postsympathectomy patient.

If progressive renal impairment becomes evident, consider withholding or discontinuing diuretic therapy.

Thiazides may decrease urinary calcium excretion. Thiazides may cause intermittent and slight elevation of serum calcium in the absence of known disorders of calcium metabolism. Marked hypercalcemia may be evidence of hidden hyperparathyroidism.

Information for Patients: As with all drugs with beta-blocking activity, certain advice to patients being treated with labetalol HCl is warranted. This information is intended to aid in the safe and effective use of this medication. It is not a disclosure of all possible adverse or intended effects. While no incident of the abrupt withdrawal phenomenon (exacerbation of angina pectoris) has been reported with labetalol

HCl, dosing with NORMOZIDE Tablets should not be interrupted or discontinued without a physician's advice. Patients being treated with NORMOZIDE Tablets should consult a physician at any signs or symptoms of impending cardiac failure or hepatic dysfunction (see **WARNINGS**). Also, transient scalp tingling may occur, usually when treatment with labetalol is initiated (see **ADVERSE REACTIONS**).

Laboratory Tests: As with any new drug given over prolonged periods, laboratory parameters should be observed over regular intervals. In patients with concomitant illnesses, such as impaired renal function, appropriate tests should be done to monitor these conditions.

Periodic determination of serum electrolytes to detect possible electrolyte imbalance from the thiazide should be performed at appropriate intervals.

Drug Interactions—*Labetalol HCl:* In one survey, 2.3% of patients taking labetalol HCl in combination with tricyclic antidepressants experienced tremor as compared to 0.7% reported to occur with labetalol HCl alone. The contribution of each of the treatments to this adverse reaction is unknown but the possibility of a drug interaction cannot be excluded. Drugs possessing beta-blocking properties can blunt the bronchodilator effect of beta-receptor agonist drugs in patients with bronchospasm; therefore, doses greater than the normal anti-asthmatic dose of beta-agonist bronchodilator drugs may be required.

Cimetidine has been shown to increase the bioavailability of labetalol HCl. Since this could be explained either by enhanced absorption or by an alteration of hepatic metabolism of labetalol HCl, special care should be used in establishing the dose required for blood pressure control in such patients. Synergism has been shown between halothane anesthesia and intravenously administered labetalol HCl. During controlled hypotensive anesthesia using labetalol HCl in association with halothane, high concentrations (3% or above) of halothane should not be used because the degree of hypotension will be increased and because of the possibility of a large reduction in cardiac output and an increase in central venous pressure. The anesthesiologist should be informed when a patient is receiving labetalol HCl.

Labetalol HCl blunts the reflex tachycardia produced by nitroglycerin without preventing its hypotensive effect. If labetalol HCl is used with nitroglycerin in patients with angina pectoris, additional antihypertensive effects may occur.

Hydrochlorothiazide: Insulin requirements in diabetic patients may be increased, decreased, or unchanged.

Thiazide drugs may increase the responsiveness to tubocurarine.

Thiazides may decrease arterial responsiveness to norepinephrine. This diminution is not sufficient to preclude effectiveness of the pressor agent for therapeutic use.

Lithium generally should not be given with diuretics because they reduce its renal clearance and add a high risk of lithium toxicity.

In some patients, the administration of a non-steroidal anti-inflammatory agent can reduce the diuretic, natriuretic, and antihypertensive effects of loop, potassium-sparing and thiazide diuretics. Therefore, when NORMOZIDE and nonsteroidal anti-inflammatory agents are used concomitantly, the patient should be observed closely to determine if the desired effect of the diuretic is obtained.

Drug/Laboratory Test Interactions—*Labetalol HCl:* The presence of labetalol metabolites in the urine may result in falsely elevated levels of urinary catecholamines, metanephrine, normetanephrine, and vanillylmandelic acid (VMA) when measured by fluorimetric or photometric methods. In screening patients suspected of having a pheochromocytoma and being treated with labetalol HCl, a specific method, such as a high performance liquid chromatographic assay with solid phase extraction (e.g. *J Chromotogr* 385:241,1987) should be employed in determining levels of catecholamines. Labetalol HCl has also been reported to produce a false-positive test for amphetamine when screening urine for the presence of drugs using the commercially available assay methods Toxi-Lab A® (thin-layer chromatographic assay) and Emit-d.a.u.® (radioenzymatic assay). When patients being treated with labetalol have a positive urine test for amphetamine using these techniques, confirmation should be made by using more specific methods, such as a gas chromatographic-mass spectrometer technique.

Hydrochlorothiazide: Thiazides should be discontinued before carrying out tests for parathyroid function.

Thiazides may decrease serum protein-bound iodine (PBI) levels without signs of thyroid disturbances.

Carcinogenesis, Mutagenesis, Impairment of Fertility—*Labetalol HCl:* Long-term oral dosing studies with labetalol HCl for 18 months in mice and for 2 years in rats showed no evidence of carcinogenesis. Studies with labetalol HCl, using dominant lethal assays in rats and mice, and exposing microorganisms according to modified Ames test, showed no evidence of mutagenesis.

Hydrochlorothiazide: Hydrochlorothiazide is presently under study for carcinogenesis in rats and mice in the National Toxicology Research and Testing Program.

Hydrochlorothiazide was not mutagenic in *in vitro* Ames Mutagenicity assay of *Salmonella typhimurium* strains TA

98, TA 100, TA 1535, TA 1537 and TA 1538 or in *in vivo* mutagenicity assays of mouse germinal cell chromosomes and chinese hamster bone marrow cell chromosomes. It was, however, mutagenic in inducing non-disjunction (96% frequency) in diploid strains of *Aspergillus nidulans*. Hydrochlorothiazide had no adverse effects on fertility in rats at a dose equivalent to the recommended maximum human dose and in mice at dose equivalent of 25 times the recommended maximum human dose (4 mg/kg, assumed body weight of 50 kg).

Pregnancy Category C: Reproduction studies performed in rats and rabbits dosed orally with labetalol HCl at doses up to ten times and 8 times the human dose, respectively, revealed no evidence of impaired fertility or harm to the fetus. The combination of labetalol HCl and hydrochlorothiazide was not teratogenic in rats and rabbits at oral doses up to approximately 15 and 80 times the maximum recommended human dose (MRHD) of labetalol (1200 mg) and hydrochlorothiazide (50 mg), respectively. In rabbits, maternal toxicity was observed with consequent fetotoxicity at the lowest dose tested (3.5 and 20 times the MRHD of labetalol and hydrochlorothiazide, respectively). Consequently, the combination of labetalol and hydrochlorothiazide appeared to be more toxic only in maternal rabbits than was either of the drugs given alone. No such effects were seen in rats.

Teratogenic studies have been performed with labetalol in rats and rabbits at oral doses up to approximately 6 and 4 times the MRHD, respectively. No reproducible evidence of fetal malformations was observed. Increased fetal resorptions were seen in both species at doses approximating the MRHD. A teratology study performed with labetalol in rabbits at intravenous doses up to 1.7 times the MRHD revealed no evidence of drug related harm to the fetus.

Available information indicates that hydrochlorothiazide at doses as high as 330 times the recommended maximum human dose was not teratogenic in pregnant rats.

There are no adequate and well-controlled studies in pregnant women. NORMOZIDE Tablets should be used during pregnancy only if the potential benefit justifies the potential risk to the fetus.

Nonteratogenic Effects—*HCl:* Transient hypotension, bradycardia, and hypoglycemia have been rarely observed in infants of mothers who were treated with labetalol HCl for hypertension during pregnancy. Oral administration of labetalol to rats during late gestation through weaning at doses of 2 to 4 times the MRHD caused a decrease in neonatal survival.

Hydrochlorothiazide: Thiazides cross the placental barrier and appear in cord blood. The use of thiazides in pregnant women requires that the anticipated benefit be weighed against possible hazards to the fetus. These hazards include fetal or neonatal jaundice, thrombocytopenia, and possible other adverse reactions that have occurred in the adult.

Labor and Delivery: Labetalol HCl given to pregnant women with hypertension did not appear to affect the usual course of labor and delivery.

Nursing Mothers: Small amounts of labetalol (approximately 0.004% of the maternal dose) are excreted in human milk.

However, thiazides appear in greater amounts in breast milk. Because of the potential for serious adverse reactions in nursing infants from hydrochlorothiazide, a decision should be made whether to discontinue nursing or to discontinue the drug, taking into account the importance of the drug to the mother.

Caution should be exercised when NORMOZIDE Tablets are administered to a nursing woman.

Pediatric Use: Safety and effectiveness in children have not been established.

ADVERSE REACTIONS

In general, the adverse effects of the combination are the sum of the adverse effects of the two components.

Labetalol HCl: Most adverse effects are mild, transient and occur early in the course of treatment. In controlled clinical trials of 3 to 4 months duration, discontinuation of NORMODYNE® (labetalol HCl) Tablets due to one or more adverse effects was required in 7% of all patients. In these same trials, other agents with solely beta-blocking activity used in the control groups led to discontinuation in 8 to 10% of patients, and a centrally acting alpha-agonist in 30% of patients.

The incidence rates of adverse reactions listed in the following table were derived from multicenter controlled clinical trials, comparing labetalol HCl, placebo, metoprolol and propranolol as monotherapy, over treatment periods of 3 and 4 months. Where the frequency of adverse effects for labetalol HCl and placebo is similar, causal relationship is uncertain. The rates are based on adverse reactions considered probably drug-related by the investigator. If all reports are considered, the rates are somewhat higher (e.g., dizziness 20%, nausea 14%, fatigue 11%), but the overall conclusions are unchanged.

[See table on top next page].

The adverse effects were reported spontaneously and are representative of the incidence of adverse effects that may be observed in a properly selected hypertensive patient population, i.e., a group excluding patients with bronchospastic disease, overt congestive heart failure, or other contraindications to beta-blocker therapy.

In other studies with labetalol HCl utilizing daily doses up to 2400 mg, certain of the side effects increased with increasing labetalol dose, including dizziness, fatigue, nausea, paresthesias, nasal stuffiness, ejaculation failure and impotence.

Labetalol HCl/Hydrochlorothiazide: The incidence rates of adverse reactions noted in the following table were derived from multicenter controlled clinical trials of three months duration comparing labetalol HCl plus hydrochlorothiazide (HCTZ) to labetalol HCl or hydrochlorothiazide alone. The rates are based on adverse reactions considered probably drug-related by the investigators. If all reports are considered, the rates are somewhat higher (e.g., dizziness 16%, headache 11%, fatigue 9%), but the overall conclusions are unchanged.

[See table below].

In addition, a number of other less common adverse events in patients who were taking labetalol HCl have been reported.
Body as A whole   Fever.
Cardiovascular   Postural hypotension, including rarely, syncope.
Central and Peripheral Nervous Systems   Paresthesias, most frequently described as scalp tingling. In most cases, it was mild, transient and usually occurred at the beginning of treatment.
Collagen Disorders   Systemic lupus erythematosus; positive antinuclear factor (ANF).
Eyes   Dry eyes.
Immunological System   Antimitochondrial antibodies.
Liver and Biliary System   Hepatic necrosis, hepatitis, cholestatic jaundice, elevated liver function tests.
Musculo-Skeletal System   Muscle cramps, toxic myopathy.
Respiratory System   Bronchospasm.
Skin and Appendages   Rashes of various types, such as generalized maculo-papular; lichenoid; urticarial; bullous lichen planus; psoriaform; facial erythema; Peyronie's disease; reversible alopecia.
Urinary System   Difficulty in micturition, including acute urinary bladder retention.

Following approval for marketing in the United Kingdom, a monitored release survey involving approximately 6,800

	Labetalol HCl (N=227) %	Placebo (N=98) %	Propranolol (N=84) %	Metoprolol (N=49) %
Body as a whole				
fatigue	5	0	12	12
asthenia	1	1	1	0
headache	2	1	1	2
Gastrointestinal				
nausea	6	1	1	2
vomiting	<1	0	0	0
dyspepsia	3	1	1	0
abdominal pain	0	0	1	2
diarrhea	<1	0	2	0
taste distortion	1	0	0	0
Central and Peripheral Nervous System				
dizziness	11	3	4	4
paresthesia (usually scalp tingling)	<1	0	0	0
drowsiness	<1	2	2	2
Autonomic Nervous System				
nasal stuffiness	3	0	0	0
ejaculation failure	2	0	0	0
impotence	1	0	1	3
increased sweating	<1	0	0	0
Cardiovascular				
edema	1	0	0	0
postural hypotension	1	0	0	0
bradycardia	0	0	5	12
Respiratory				
dyspnea	2	0	1	2
Skin				
rash	1	0	0	0
Special Senses				
vision abnormality	1	0	0	0
vertigo	2	1	0	0

patients was conducted for further safety and efficacy evaluation of this product. Results of this survey indicate that the type, severity, and incidence of adverse effects were comparable to those cited above.

Potential Adverse Effects: In addition, other adverse effects not listed above have been reported with other beta-adrenergic blocking agents.

	Labetalol/HCTZ (N=208) %	HCTZ (N=95) %	Labetalol (N=106) %
Body as a whole			
asthenia	1	2	0
leg cramps	1	0	0
fatigue	1	1	2
headache	<1	0	0
malaise	<1	0	0
pain	<1	0	0
rigors	0	0	1
gout	<1	0	0
increased appetite	<1	0	0
creatine phosphokinase	<1	0	0
hypokalemia	1	0	0
Gastrointestinal			
abdominal pain	0	1	0
constipation	<1	0	1
dyspepsia	<1	0	0
flatulence	<1	0	0
gastritis	1	0	0
nausea	2	0	0
Central and Peripheral Nervous System			
dizziness	6	2	3
decreased libido	<1	0	0
paresthesia (usually scalp tingling)	<1	0	0
insomnia	0	1	1
paroniria	0	0	1
somnolence	<1	1	0
Cardiovascular			
postural hypotension	<1	0	0
Autonomic Nervous System			
ejaculation failure	<1*	0**	0***
impotence	1*	1**	0***
Respiratory System			
bronchospasm	<1	0	0
rhinitis	<1	0	0
Skin and Appendages			
rash	<1	0	0
Urinary System			
micturition frequency	<1	0	0
nocturia	<1	1	0
polyuria	<1	0	0
urinary retention	<1	0	0
Vision			
abnormal vision	<1	0	0

* Based on a male population of 108
** Based on a male population of 39
*** Based on a male population of 65

Central Nervous System   Reversible mental depression progressing to catatonia; an acute reversible syndrome characterized by disorientation for time and place, short-term memory loss, emotional lability, slightly clouded sensorium, and decreased performance on neuropsychometrics.
Cardiovascular   Intensification of AV block. See **CONTRAINDICATIONS.**
Allergic   Fever combined with aching and sore throat; laryngospasm; respiratory distress.
Hematologic   Agranulocytosis; thrombocytopenic or nonthrombocytopenic purpura.
Gastrointestinal   Mesenteric artery thrombosis; ischemic colitis.

The oculomucocutaneous syndrome associated with the beta-blocker practolol has not been reported with labetalol HCl.

Hydrochlorothiazide: Adverse reactions reported include:
Gastrointestinal System   Anorexia, gastric irritation, nausea, vomiting, cramping, diarrhea, constipation, jaundice (intrahepatic cholestatic jaundice), pancreatitis, sialadenitis.
Central Nervous System   Dizziness, vertigo, paresthesias, headache, xanthopsia.
Hematologic   Leukopenia, agranulocytosis, thrombocytopenia, aplastic anemia, hemolytic anemia.
Cardiovascular   Orthostatic hypotension may occur and may be aggravated by alcohol, barbiturates, or narcotics.
Hypersensitivity   Purpura, photosensitivity, rash, urticaria, necrotizing angiitis (vasculitis, cutaneous vasculitis), fever, respiratory distress including pneumonitis and pulmonary edema, anaphylactic reactions.
Other   Hyperglycemia, glycosuria, hyperuricemia, muscle spasm, weakness, restlessness, transient blurred vision, severe fluid and electrolyte derangements (rarely).

Whenever adverse reactions are moderate or severe, thiazide dosage should be reduced or therapy withdrawn.

Clinical Laboratory Tests *Labetalol HCl:* There have been reversible increases of serum transaminases in 4% of patients treated with labetalol HCl and tested, and more rarely, reversible increases in blood urea.

OVERDOSAGE

Labetalol HCl: Overdosage with labetalol HCl causes excessive hypotension which is posture sensitive, and sometimes, excessive bradycardia. Patients should be placed supine and their legs raised if necessary to improve the blood supply to the brain. If overdosage with labetalol HCl follows oral ingestion, gastric lavage or pharmacologically induced emesis (using syrup of ipecac) may be useful for removal of the drug shortly after ingestion. The following additional measures should be employed if necessary: *Excessive bradycardia* —administer atropine or epinephrine. *Cardiac failure* —administer a digitalis glycoside and a diuretic. Dopamine or dobutamine may also be useful. *Hypotension* —administer vasopres-

Continued on next page

Information on Schering products appearing on these pages is effective as of September 30, 1989.

Schering—Cont.

sors, eg, norepinephrine. There is pharmacological evidence that norepinephrine may be the drug of choice. *Bronchospasm*—administer epinephrine and/or an aerosolized beta$_2$-agonist. *Seizures*—administer diazepam.

In severe beta-blocker overdose resulting in hypotension and/or bradycardia, glucagon has been shown to be effective when administered in large doses (5 to 10 mg rapidly over 30 seconds, followed by continuous infusion of 5 mg/hr that can be reduced as the patient improves).

Neither hemodialysis nor peritoneal dialysis removes a significant amount of labetalol HCl from the general circulation (< 1%).

The oral LD_{50} value of labetalol HCl in the mouse is approximatey 600 mg/kg and in the rat is greater than 2 g/kg. The intravenous LD_{50} in these species is 50 to 60 mg/kg.

Hydrochlorothiazide: Overdosage symptoms include: electrolyte imbalance and signs of potassium deficiency such as confusion, dizziness, muscular weakness and gastrointestinal disturbances. General supportive measures include replacement of fluids and electrolytes.

DOSAGE AND ADMINISTRATION

DOSAGE MUST BE INDIVIDUALIZED. The fixed combination is indicated for patients who, after titration, need the dose of each component present in the combination. (See **INDICATIONS AND USAGE.**)

The recommended initial dose of labetalol is 100 mg twice daily whether used alone or added to a diuretic regimen. After 2 or 3 days using standing blood pressure as an indicator, dosage may be titrated in increments of 100 mg b.i.d. every 2 or 3 days. The usual maintenance dose of labetalol is between 200 and 400 mg twice daily, although doses up to 1200–2400 mg have been used.

Hydrochlorothiazide is generally started at 25 mg twice daily although lower doses may be effective in some patients. Most patients do not need doses greater than 25 mg b.i.d. although doses of 50 mg b.i.d. have been used, and the larger doses caused increased hypokalemia, hyperuricemia and hyperglycemia.

The usual dose of NORMOZIDE Tablets is 200/25 mg to 400/25 mg twice daily. If larger doses than 800 mg of labetalol are needed, it should be added as the single entity, unless there is a specific need and intent to increase the hydrochlorothiazide.

HOW SUPPLIED

NORMOZIDE (100 mg labetalol HCl/25 mg hydrochlorothiazide) Tablets: light brown, capsule-shaped, film-coated tablets engraved on one side with NORMOZIDE and the other side engraved with the number 235; bottles of 100 (NDC 0085-0235-02).

NORMOZIDE (200 mg labetalol HCl/25 mg hydrochlorothiazide) Tablets: white, capsule-shaped, film-coated tablets engraved on one side with NORMOZIDE and the other side engraved with the number 227; bottles of 100 (NDC 0085-0227-02).

NORMOZIDE (300 mg labetalol HCl/25 mg hydrochlorothiazide) Tablets: blue, capsule-shaped, film-coated tablets engraved on one side with NORMOZIDE and the other side engraved with the number 391; bottles of 100 (NDC 0085-0391-02).

Store NORMOZIDE (labetalol HCl/hydrochlorothiazide) Tablets between 2° and 30° C (36° and 86° F); protect unit-dose boxes from excessive moisture.

Schering Corporation
Kenilworth, NJ 07033 USA

Rev 4/89   B-16100315
Copyright © 1987, 1988, 1989. Schering Corporation. All rights reserved.

Shown in Product Identification Section, page 428

OCUCLEAR Eye Drops

(See PDR For Nonprescription Drugs)

OPTIMINE®   ℞
[*op ʹtĭ-mēn*]
brand of azatadine maleate, USP
Tablets

DESCRIPTION

OPTIMINE Tablets contain azatadine maleate, an antihistamine having the empirical formula, $C_{20}H_{22}N_2 \cdot 2C_4H_4O_4$, the chemical name, 6,11-Dihydro-11-(1-methyl-4- piperidylidene)-5H-benzo[5,6]cyclohepta [1,2-β] pyridine maleate (1:2). The molecular weight of azatadine maleate is 522.54. It is a white to off-white powder and is very soluble in water and soluble in alcohol.

Each OPTIMINE Tablet contains 1 mg azatadine maleate, USP. They also contain: corn starch, lactose, magnesium stearate and povidone.

CLINICAL PHARMACOLOGY

Azatadine maleate is an antihistamine related to cyproheptadine, with antiserotonin, anticholinergic (drying), and sedative effects.

Antihistamines competitively antagonize those pharmacological effects of histamine which are mediated through activation of histamine H_1-receptor sites on effector cells. Histamine-related allergic reactions and tissue injury are blocked or diminished in intensity. Antihistamines antagonize the vasodilator effect of endogenously released histamine, especially in small vessels, and mitigate the effect of histamine which results in increased capillary permeability and edema formation. As consequences of these actions, antihistamines antagonize the physiological manifestations of histamine release in the nose following antigen-antibody interactions, such as congestion related to vascular engorgement, mucosal edema, and profuse, watery secretion, and irritation and sneezing resulting from histamine action on afferent nerve terminals.

Pharmacokinetic studies in normal volunteers dosed orally with radio-labeled azatadine maleate show that the drug is readily absorbed with peak plasma levels at about four hours after dosing. Approximately 50% of the drug is excreted in the urine within five days after administration of a single dose, and no evidence of drug accumulation was seen after daily dosing for 30 days. The elimination half-life of azatadine maleate, based on plasma radioactivity, was approximately 9 hours. Approximately 20% of the drug is excreted unchanged and extensive conjugation of the drug and its metabolites occurs. Azatadine maleate is minimally bound to plasma protein.

While the antihistamines have not been studied for passage through the blood-brain and placental barriers, the occurrence of pharmacologic effects in the central nervous system and in the newborn indicate presence of the drug.

INDICATIONS AND USAGE

OPTIMINE Tablets are indicated for the treatment of perennial and seasonal allergic rhinitis and chronic urticaria.

CONTRAINDICATIONS

Antihistamines *should NOT* be used to treat lower respiratory tract symptoms, including asthma.

Antihistamines, including azatadine maleate, are also contraindicated in patients hypersensitive to this medication and to other antihistamines of similar chemical structure, and in patients receiving monoamine oxidase inhibitor therapy. (See Drug Interactions.)

WARNINGS

Antihistamines should be used with caution in patients with narrow angle glaucoma, stenosing peptic ulcer; pyloroduodenal obstruction; and urinary bladder obstruction due to symptomatic prostatic hypertrophy and narrowing of the bladder neck.

Use with CNS Depressants: Antihistamines have additive effects with alcohol and other CNS depressants (hypnotics, sedatives, tranquilizers, etc.).

Use in Activities Requiring Mental Alertness: Patients should be warned about engaging in activities requiring mental alertness, such as driving a car or operating certain appliances, machinery, etc., until their response to this medication has been determined.

Use in Patients approximately 60 years or older: Antihistamines are more likely to cause dizziness, sedation, and hypotension in patients over 60 years of age.

PRECAUTIONS

General: Azatadine maleate has an atropine-like action and therefore should be used with caution in patients with: a history of bronchial asthma; increased intraocular pressure; hyperthyroidism; cardiovascular disease; hypertension.

Information for Patients: This information is intended to aid in the safe and effective use of this medication. It is not a disclosure of all possible adverse or intended effects.

1. Antihistamines may cause drowsiness.

2. Patients taking antihistamines should not engage in activities requiring mental alertness, such as driving a car or operating machinery, certain appliances, etc., until their response to this medication has been determined.

3. Alcohol or other sedative drugs may enhance the drowsiness caused by antihistamines.

4. Patients should not take this medication if they are receiving a monoamine oxidase (MAO) inhibitor, or if they are receiving oral anticoagulants.

5. This medication should not be given to children less than 12 years of age.

Drug Interactions: MAO inhibitors prolong and intensify the anticholinergic and sedative effects of antihistamines. Additive effects may occur from the concomitant use of antihistamines with tricyclic antidepressants. (See also WARNINGS.) The action of oral anticoagulants may be diminished by antihistamines.

Drug/Laboratory Test Interaction: Antihistamines should be discontinued about four days prior to skin testing procedures since these drugs may prevent or diminish otherwise positive reactions to dermal reactivity indicators.

Carcinogenesis, Mutagenesis, and Impairment of Fertility: Long-term oral dosing studies with azatadine maleate in rats and mice showed no evidence of carcinogenesis. No mutagenic effect was seen in a dominant lethal assay study in mice dosed with azatadine maleate orally and intraperitoneally. There was no impairment of fertility in rats fed azatadine maleate at doses greater than 150 times the recommended human daily dose.

Pregnancy Category B: Reproduction studies have been performed in rats and rabbits at doses up to 188 times and 38 times, respectively, the human dose and have revealed no evidence of impaired fertility or harm to the fetus due to azatadine maleate. There are, however, no adequate and well-controlled studies in pregnant women. Because animal reproduction studies are not always predictive of human response, this drug should be used during pregnancy only if clearly needed. (See **Non-Teratogenic Effects.**)

Non-Teratogenic Effects: Antihistamines should not be used in the third trimester of pregnancy because newborns and premature infants may have severe reactions, such as convulsions, to them.

Nursing Mothers: It is not known whether this drug is excreted in human milk. However, certain antihistamines are known to be excreted in human milk in low concentration. Because of the higher risk of antihistamines for infants generally and for newborns and prematures in particular, a decision should be made whether to discontinue nursing or to discontinue the drug, taking into account the importance of the drug to the mother.

Pediatric Use: Safety and effectiveness in children below the age of 12 years have not been established.

ADVERSE REACTIONS

Slight to moderate drowsiness may occur with azatadine maleate. Other possible side effects common to antihistamines in general include: (the most frequent are underlined).

General: urticaria, drug rash, anaphylactic shock, photosensitivity, excessive perspiration, chills, dryness of mouth, nose, and throat.

Cardiovascular: hypotension, headache, palpitations, tachycardia, extrasystoles.

Hematologic: hemolytic anemia, hypoplastic anemia, thrombocytopenia, agranulocytosis.

Nervous: <u>sedation, sleepiness, dizziness</u>, vertigo, tinnitus, acute labyrinthitis, <u>disturbed coordination</u>, fatigue, confusion, restlessness, excitation, nervousness, tremor, irritability, insomnia, euphoria, paresthesias, blurred vision diplopia, hysteria, neuritis, convulsions.

Gastrointestinal: <u>epigastric distress</u>, anorexia, nausea, vomiting, diarrhea, constipation.

Genitourinary: urinary frequency, difficult urination, urinary retention, early menses.

Respiratory: <u>thickening of bronchial secretions</u>, tightness of chest and wheezing, nasal stuffiness.

DRUG ABUSE AND DEPENDENCE

There is no information to indicate that abuse or dependency occurs with azatadine maleate.

Overdosage: In the event of overdosage, emergency treatment should be started immediately.

Manifestations: Antihistamine overdosage effects may vary from central nervous system depression (sedation, apnea, diminished mental alertness, cardiovascular collapse) to stimulation (insomnia, hallucinations, tremors or convulsions) to death. Other signs and symptoms may be dizziness, tinnitus, ataxia, blurred vision, and hypotension. Stimulation is particularly likely in children, as are atropine-like signs and symptoms (dry mouth; fixed, dilated pupils; flushing; hyperthermia; and gastrointestinal symptoms).

Treatment: The patient should be induced to vomit, even if emesis has occurred spontaneously. Pharmacologic vomiting by the administration of ipecac syrup is a preferred method. However, vomiting should not be induced in patients with impaired consciousness. The action of ipecac is facilitated by physical activity and by the administration of 8 to 12 fluid ounces of water. If emesis does not occur within fifteen minutes, the dose of ipecac should be repeated. Precautions against aspiration must be taken, especially in infants and children. Following emesis, any drug remaining in the stomach may be adsorbed by activated charcoal administered as a slurry with water. If vomiting is unsuccessful or contraindicated, gastric lavage should be performed. Physiologic saline solution is the lavage solution of choice, particularly in children. In adults, tap water can be used; however, as much as possible of the amount administered should be removed before the next instillation. Saline cathartics, such as milk of magnesia, draw water into the bowel by osmosis and, therefore, may be valuable for their action in rapid dilution of bowel content. Dialysis is of little value in antihistamine poisoning. After emergency treatment, the patient should continue to be medically monitored.

Treatment of the signs and symptoms of overdosage is symptomatic and supportive. <u>Stimulants</u> (analeptic agents) should <u>not</u> be used. Vasopressors may be used to treat hypotension. Short acting barbiturates, diazepam, or paraldehyde may be administered to control seizures. Hyperpyrexia, especially in children, may require treatment with tepid water sponge baths or a hypothermic blanket. Apnea is treated with ventilatory support.

DOSAGE AND ADMINISTRATION

DOSAGE SHOULD BE INDIVIDUALIZED ACCORDING TO THE NEEDS AND THE RESPONSE OF THE PATIENT. **OPTIMINE Tablets are not recommended for use in children under 12 years of age.**
The usual adult dosage is 1 or 2 mg, twice a day.

HOW SUPPLIED

OPTIMINE Tablets, 1 mg. white, compressed, scored tablets impressed with the Schering trademark and product identification numbers, 282; bottle of 100 (NDC 0085-0282-03).
Store between 2°and 30°C (36°and 86°F).
Revised 12/85
Copyright © 1973, 1981, 1985, Schering Corporation, USA. All rights reserved.
Shown in Product Identification Section, page 428

PERMITIL®

[per′mĭ-til]
brand of fluphenazine hydrochloride
Tablets, USP
Oral Concentrate

℞

DESCRIPTION

PERMITIL products are formulations of fluphenazine hydrochloride, USP, a phenothiazine of the piperazine group. It is available as **Tablets**, 2.5, 5, and 10 mg fluphenazine hydrochloride and as an **Oral Concentrate**, 5 mg fluphenazine hydrochloride per mL and alcohol 1%.
The inactive ingredients for PERMITIL **Tablets** 2.5 mg include: calcium phosphate, FD&C Yellow No. 6, lactose, magnesium stearate, pregelatinized starch and starch.
The inactive ingredients for PERMITIL **Tablets** 5 mg include: calcium phosphate, D&C Red No. 33, FD&C Red No. 40, FD&C Yellow No. 6, lactose, magnesium stearate, pregelatinized starch and starch.
The inactive ingredients for PERMITIL **Tablets** 10 mg include: calcium phosphate, D&C Red No. 27 Lake, D&C Red No. 30 Lake, FD&C Yellow No. 6 Lake, lactose, magnesium stearate, pregelatinized starch and starch.
The inactive ingredients for PERMITIL **Oral Concentrate** include: alcohol, methylparaben, propylparaben, sodium phosphate, and water. Sodium hydroxide is used for adjusting the pH.

ACTIONS

Fluphenazine hydrochloride has actions at all levels of the central nervous system, as well as on other organ systems. However, the site and mechanism of action of therapeutic effect are not known.

INDICATIONS

PERMITIL **Tablets** and **Oral Concentrate** are indicated for the management of manifestations of psychotic disorders. PERMITIL has not been shown effective in the management of behavioral complications in patients with mental retardation.

CONTRAINDICATIONS

PERMITIL is contraindicated in comatose or greatly obtunded patients and in patients receiving large doses of central nervous system depressants (barbiturates, alcohol, narcotics, analgesics, or antihistamines); in the presence of existing blood dyscrasias, bone marrow depression, or liver damage; and in patients who have shown hypersensitivity to PERMITIL products, their components, or related compounds.
PERMITIL is also contraindicated in patients with suspected or established subcortical brain damage, with or without hypothalamic damage, since a hyperthermic reaction with temperatures in excess of 104° F may occur in such patients, sometimes not until 14 to 16 hours after drug administration. Total body ice-packing is recommended for such a reaction; antipyretics may also be useful.

WARNINGS

Tardive dyskinesia, a syndrome consisting of potentially irreversible, involuntary, dyskinetic movements, may develop in patients treated with neuroleptic (antipsychotic) drugs. Although the prevalence of the syndrome appears to be highest among the elderly, especially elderly women, it is impossible to rely upon prevalence estimates to predict, at the inception of neuroleptic treatment, which patients are likely to develop the syndrome. Whether neuroleptic drug products differ in their potential to cause tardive dyskinesia is unknown.
Both the risk of developing the syndrome and the likelihood that it will become irreversible are believed to increase as the duration of treatment and the total cumulative dose of neuroleptic drugs administered to the patient increase. However, the syndrome can develop, although much less commonly, after relatively brief treatment periods at low doses.

There is no known treatment for established cases of tardive dyskinesia, although the syndrome may remit, partially or completely, if neuroleptic treatment is withdrawn. Neuroleptic treatment itself, however, may suppress (or partially suppress) the signs and symptoms of the syndrome, and thereby may possibly mask the underlying disease process. The effect that symptomatic suppression has upon the long-term course of the syndrome is unknown.
Given these considerations, neuroleptics should be prescribed in a manner that is most likely to minimize the occurrence of tardive dyskinesia. Chronic neuroleptic treatment should generally be reserved for patients who suffer from a chronic illness that, 1) is known to respond to neuroleptic drugs, and, 2) for whom alternative, equally effective, but potentially less harmful treatments are *not* available or appropriate. In patients who do require chronic treatment, the smallest dose and the shortest duration of treatment producing a satisfactory clinical response should be sought. The need for continued treatment should be reassessed periodically.
If signs and symptoms of tardive dyskinesia appear in a patient on neuroleptics, drug discontinuation should be considered. However, some patients may require treatment despite the presence of the syndrome.
(For further information about the description of tardive dyskinesia and its clinical detection, please refer to **Information for Patients** and **ADVERSE REACTIONS**.)
NEUROLEPTIC MALIGNANT SYNDROME (NMS)
A potentially fatal symptom complex sometimes referred to as Neuroleptic Malignant Syndrome (NMS) has been reported in association with antipsychotic drugs. Clinical manifestations of NMS are hyperpyrexia, muscle rigidity, altered mental status and evidence of autonomic instability (irregular pulse or blood pressure, tachycardia, diaphoresis, and cardiac dysrhythmias).
The diagnostic evaluation of patients with this syndrome is complicated. In arriving at a diagnosis, it is important to identify cases where the clinical presentation includes both serious medical illness (e.g., pneumonia, systemic infection, etc.) and untreated or inadequately treated extrapyramidal signs and symptoms (EPS). Other important considerations in the differential diagnosis include central anticholinergic toxicity, heat stroke, drug fever and primary central nervous system (CNS) pathology.
The management of NMS should include 1) immediate discontinuation of antipsychotic drugs and other drugs not essential to concurrent therapy, 2) intensive symptomatic treatment and medical monitoring, and 3) treatment of any concomitant serious medical problems for which specific treatments are available. There is no general agreement about specific pharmacological treatment regimens for uncomplicated NMS.
If a patient requires antipsychotic drug treatment after recovery from NMS, the potential reintroduction of drug therapy should be carefully considered. The patient should be carefully monitored, since recurrences of NMS have been reported.
If hypotension develops, epinephrine should not be administered since its action is blocked and partially reversed by fluphenazine hydrochloride. If a vasopressor is needed, norepinephrine may be used. Severe, acute hypotension has occurred with the use of phenothiazines and is particularly likely to occur in patients with mitral insufficiency or pheochromocytoma. Rebound hypertension may occur in pheochromocytoma patients.
PERMITIL can lower the convulsive threshold in susceptible individuals; it should be used with caution in alcohol withdrawal and in patients with convulsive disorders. If the patient is being treated with an anticonvulsant agent, increased dosage of that agent may be required when PERMITIL is used concomitantly.
PERMITIL should be used with caution in patients with psychic depression.
Fluphenazine hydrochloride may impair the mental and/or physical abilities required for the performance of hazardous tasks such as driving a car or operating machinery; therefore, the patient should be warned accordingly.
Usage in Children Safety and effectiveness in children have not been established; therefore, PERMITIL is not recommended for use in children.
Usage in Pregnancy Safe use of fluphenazine hydrochloride during pregnancy and lactation has not been established; therefore, in administering the drug to pregnant patients, nursing mothers, or women who may become pregnant, the possible benefits must be weighed against the possible hazards to mother and child.

PRECAUTIONS

The possibility of suicide in depressed patients remains during treatment and until significant remission occurs. This type of patient should not have access to large quantities of this drug.
As with all phenothiazine compounds, fluphenazine hydrochloride should not be used indiscriminately. Caution should be observed in giving it to patients who have previously exhibited severe adverse reactions to other phenothiazines.

Some of the untoward actions of fluphenazine hydrochloride tend to appear more frequently when high doses are used. However, as with other phenothiazine compounds, patients receiving PERMITIL in any dosage should be kept under close supervision.
Neuroleptic drugs elevate prolactin levels; the elevation persists during chronic administration. Tissue culture experiments indicate that approximately one-third of human breast cancers are prolactin dependent *in vitro*, a factor of potential importance if the prescription of these drugs is contemplated in a patient with a previously detected breast cancer. Although disturbances such as galactorrhea, amenorrhea, gynecomastia, and impotence have been reported, the clinical significance of elevated serum prolactin levels is unknown for most patients. An increase in mammary neoplasms has been found in rodents after chronic administration of neuroleptic drugs. Neither clinical studies nor epidemiologic studies conducted to date, however, have shown an association between chronic administration of these drugs and mammary tumorigenesis; the available evidence is considered too limited to be conclusive at this time.
The antiemetic effect of fluphenazine hydrochloride may obscure signs of toxicity due to overdosage of other drugs, or render more difficult the diagnosis of disorders such as brain tumors or intestinal obstruction.
A significant, not otherwise explained, rise in body temperature may suggest individual intolerance to fluphenazine hydrochloride; in which case it should be discontinued.
Patients on large doses of a phenothiazine drug who are undergoing surgery should be watched carefully for possible hypotensive phenomena. Moreover, reduced amounts of anesthetics or central nervous system depressants may be necessary.
Since phenothiazines and central nervous system depressants (opiates, analgesics, antihistamines, barbiturates) can potentiate each other, less than the usual dosage of the added drug is recommended; caution is advised when they are administered concomitantly.
Use with caution in patients who are receiving atropine or related drugs because of additive anticholinergic effects and also in patients who will be exposed to extreme heat or phosphorus insecticides.
The use of alcohol should be avoided since additive effects and hypotension may occur. Patients should be cautioned that their response to alcohol may be increased while they are being treated with PERMITIL. The risk of suicide and the danger of overdose may be increased in patients who use alcohol excessively due to its potentiation of the drug's effect.
Blood counts and hepatic and renal functions should be checked periodically. The appearance of signs of blood dyscrasias requires the discontinuance of the drug and institution of appropriate therapy. If abnormalities in hepatic tests occur, phenothiazine treatment should be discontinued. Renal function in patients on long-term therapy should be monitored: if blood urea nitrogen (BUN) becomes abnormal, treatment with the drug should be discontinued.
The use of phenothiazine derivatives in patients with diminished renal function should be undertaken with caution.
Use with caution in patients suffering from respiratory impairment due to acute pulmonary infections, or in chronic respiratory disorders such as severe asthma or emphysema.
In general, phenothiazines, including fluphenazine hydrochloride, do not produce psychic dependence. Gastritis, nausea and vomiting, dizziness, and tremulousness have been reported following abrupt cessation of high-dose therapy. Reports suggest that these symptoms can be reduced by continuing concomitant antiparkinson agents for several weeks after the phenothiazine is withdrawn.
The possibility of liver damage, corneal and lenticular deposits, and irreversible dyskinesias should be kept in mind when patients are on long-term therapy.
Because photosensitivity has been reported, undue exposure to the sun should be avoided during phenothiazine treatment.
Information for Patients: This information is intended to aid in the safe and effective use of this medication. It is not a disclosure of all possible adverse or intended effects.
Given the likelihood that a substantial proportion of patients exposed chronically to neuroleptics will develop tardive dyskinesia, it is advised that all patients in whom chronic use is contemplated be given, if possible, full information about this risk. The decision to inform patients and/or their guardians must obviously take into account the clinical circumstances and the competency of the patient to understand the information provided.

ADVERSE REACTIONS

Not all of the following adverse reactions have been reported with this specific drug; however, pharmacological similarities among various phenothiazine derivatives require that

Continued on next page

Schering—Cont.

each be considered. With the piperazine group (of which fluphenazine hydrochloride is an example), the extrapyramidal symptoms are more common, and others (e.g., sedative effects, jaundice, and blood dyscrasias) are less frequently seen.

CNS Effects: *Extrapyramidal reactions:* opisthotonus, trismus, torticollis, retrocollis, aching and numbness of the limbs, motor restlessness, oculogyric crisis, hyperreflexia, dystonia, including protrusion, discoloration, aching and rounding of the tongue, tonic spasm of the masticatory muscles, tight feeling in the throat, slurred speech, dysphagia, akathisia, dyskinesia, parkinsonism, and ataxia. Their incidence and severity usually increase with an increase in dosage, but there is considerable individual variation in the tendency to develop such symptoms. Extrapyramidal symptoms can usually be controlled by the concomitant use of effective antiparkinsonian drugs, such as benztropine mesylate, and/or by reduction in dosage. In some instances, however, these extrapyramidal reactions may persist after discontinuation of treatment with fluphenazine.

Persistent tardive dyskinesia: As with all antipsychotic agents, tardive dyskinesia may appear in some patients on long-term therapy or may appear after drug therapy has been discontinued. Although the risk appears to be greater in elderly patients on high-dose therapy, especially females, it may occur in either sex and in children. The symptoms are persistent and in some patients appear to be irreversible. The syndrome is characterized by rhythmical, involuntary movements of the tongue, face, mouth or jaw (e.g., protrusion of tongue, puffing of cheeks, puckering of mouth, chewing movements). Sometimes these may be accompanied by involuntary movements of the extremities. There is no known effective treatment for tardive dyskinesia; antiparkinsonism agents usually do not alleviate the symptoms of this syndrome. It is suggested that all antipsychotic agents be discontinued if these symptoms appear. Should it be necessary to reinstitute treatment, or increase the dosage of the agent, or switch to a different antipsychotic agent the syndrome may be masked. It has been reported that fine, vermicular movements of the tongue may be an early sign of the syndrome, and if the medication is stopped at that time the syndrome *may not* develop.

Other CNS effects: include cerebral edema; abnormality of cerebrospinal fluid proteins; convulsive seizures, particularly in patients with EEG abnormalities or a history of such disorders; and headaches.

Neuroleptic malignant syndrome has been reported in patients treated with neuroleptic drugs. (see **WARNINGS** for additional information). There is no specific treatment; the neuroleptic drug should be stopped immediately.

Drowsiness may occur, particularly during the first or second week, after which it generally disappears. If troublesome, lower the dosage. Hypnotic effects appear to be minimal, especially in patients who are permitted to remain active.

Adverse behavioral effects include paradoxical exacerbation of psychotic symptoms, catatonic-like states, paranoid reactions, lethargy, paradoxical excitement, restlessness, hyperactivity, nocturnal confusion, bizarre dreams, and insomnia. Hyperreflexia has been reported in the newborn when a phenothiazine was used during pregnancy.

Autonomic Effects: dry mouth or salivation, nausea, vomiting, diarrhea, anorexia, constipation, obstipation, fecal impaction, urinary retention, frequency or incontinence, bladder paralysis, polyuria, nasal congestion, pallor, myosis, mydriasis, blurred vision, glaucoma, perspiration, hypertension, hypotension, and change in pulse rate occasionally may occur. Significant autonomic effects have been infrequent in patients receiving less than 6 mg fluphenazine hydrochloride daily.

Adynamic ileus occasionally occurs with phenothiazine therapy and if severe, can result in complications and death. It is of particular concern in psychiatric patients who may fail to seek treatment of the condition.

Allergic Effects: urticaria, erythema, eczema, exfoliative dermatitis, pruritus, photosensitivity, asthma, fever, anaphylactoid reactions, laryngeal edema, and angioneurotic edema; contact dermatitis in nursing personnel administering the drug; and in extremely rare instances, individual idiosyncrasy or hypersensitivity to phenothiazines has resulted in cerebral edema, circulatory collapse, and death.

Endocrine Effects: lactation, galactorrhea, moderate breast enlargement in females and gynecomastia in males on large doses, disturbances in the menstrual cycle, amenorrhea, changes in libido, inhibition of ejaculation, syndrome of inappropriate ADH (antidiuretic hormone) secretion, false positive pregnancy tests, hyperglycemia, hypoglycemia, glycosuria.

Cardiovascular Effects: postural hypotension, tachycardia (especially with sudden marked increase in dosage), bradycardia, cardiac arrest, faintness, and dizziness. Occasionally the hypotensive effect may produce a shock-like condition.

ECG changes, nonspecific, (quinidine-like effect) usually reversible, have been observed in some patients receiving phenothiazine tranquilizers.

Sudden death has occasionally been reported in patients who have received phenothiazines. In some cases the death was apparently due to cardiac arrest; in others, the cause appeared to be asphyxia due to failure of the cough reflex. In some patients, the cause could not be determined nor could it be established that the death was due to the phenothiazine.

Hematological Effects: agranulocytosis, eosinophilia, leukopenia, hemolytic anemia, thrombocytopenic purpura, and pancytopenia. Most cases of agranulocytosis have occurred between the fourth and tenth weeks of therapy. Patients should be watched closely especially during that period for the sudden appearance of sore throat or signs of infection. If white blood cell and differential cell counts show significant cellular depression, discontinue the drug and start appropriate therapy. However, a slightly lowered white count is not in itself an indication to discontinue the drug.

Other Effects: Special considerations in long-term therapy include pigmentation of the skin, occurring chiefly in the exposed areas; ocular changes consisting of deposition of fine particulate matter in the cornea and lens, progressing in more severe cases to star-shaped lenticular opacities; epithelial keratopathies; and pigmentary retinopathy. Also noted: peripheral edema, reversed epinephrine effect, increase in PBI not attributable to an increase in thyroxine, parotid swelling (rare), hyperpyrexia, systemic lupus erythematosus-like syndrome, increases in appetite and weight, polyphagia, photophobia, and muscle weakness.

Liver damage (biliary stasis) may occur. Jaundice may occur usually between the second and fourth weeks of treatment and is regarded as a hypersensitivity reaction. Incidence is low. The clinical picture resembles infectious hepatitis but with laboratory features of obstructive jaundice. It is usually reversible; however, chronic jaundice has been reported.

DOSAGE AND ADMINISTRATION

In all cases the smallest effective dose should be used. Doses should be initiated at a low level and increased gradually to determine clinical response. Patients who are acutely ill may respond to lower doses than those who are chronically ill. Acutely ill patients may require a rapid increase of dosage. Elderly and debilitated patients and adolescents may respond to low dosages. Outpatients should receive smaller dosages than are given to hospitalized patients who are under close supervision.

Adults: The total daily dose ranges from 0.5 mg to 10 mg and is usually administered in divided doses. In general, a daily dose in excess of 3 mg is rarely necessary. A dose in excess of 20 mg should be used with caution.

Administration of an adequate dose should be continued for sufficiently long periods in order to obtain maximum benefits. After maximum therapeutic response is obtained, dosage may be decreased gradually to the minimal effective maintenance dose.

Geriatric patients: Reduced dosage is usually recommended.

PERMITIL **Oral Concentrate** is a palatable liquid preparation, suitable for administration only with the following diluents: water, saline, Seven-Up, homogenized milk, carbonated orange beverage, and pineapple, apricot, prune, orange, V-8, tomato, and grapefruit juices.

PERMITIL **Oral Concentrate** should not be mixed with beverages containing caffeine (coffee, cola), tannics (tea), or pectinates (apple juice) since physical incompatability may result.

OVERDOSAGE

In the event of overdosage, emergency treatment should be started immediately. All patients suspected of having taken an overdose should be hospitalized as soon as possible.

Manifestations: Overdosage of fluphenazine hydrochloride primarily involves the extrapyramidal mechanism and produces the same side effects described under ADVERSE REACTIONS, but to a more marked degree. It is usually evidenced by stupor or coma; children may have convulsive seizures.

Treatment: Treatment is symptomatic and supportive. There is no specific antidote. The patient should be induced to vomit even if emesis has occurred spontaneously. Pharmacologic vomiting by the administration of ipecac syrup is a preferred method. It should be noted that ipecac has a central mode of action in addition to its local gastric irritant properties, and the central mode of action may be blocked by the antiemetic effect of PERMITIL.

Vomiting should not be induced in patients with impaired consciousness. The action of ipecac is facilitated by physical activity and by the administration of 8 to 12 fluid ounces of water. If emesis does not occur within 15 minutes, the dose of ipecac should be repeated. Precautions against aspiration must be taken, especially in infants and children. Following emesis, any drug remaining in the stomach may be adsorbed by activated charcoal administered as a slurry with water. If vomiting is unsuccessful or contraindicated, gastric lavage should be performed. Isotonic and one-half isotonic saline are the lavage solutions of choice. Saline cathartics, such as

milk of magnesia, draw water into the bowel by osmosis and therefore may be valuable for their action in rapid dilution of bowel content.

Standard measures (oxygen, intravenous fluids, corticosteroids) should be used to manage circulatory shock or metabolic acidosis. An open airway and adequate fluid intake should be maintained. Body temperature should be regulated. Hypothermia is expected, but severe hyperthermia may occur and must be treated vigorously. (See CONTRAINDICATIONS.)

An electrocardiogram should be taken and close monitoring of cardiac function instituted if there is any sign of abnormality. Cardiac arthythmias may be treated with neostigmine, pyridostigmine, or propranolol. Digitalis should be considered for cardiac failure. Close monitoring of cardiac function is advisable for not less than five days. Vasopressors such as norepinephrine may be used to treat hypotension, but epinephrine should NOT be used.

Anticonvulsants (an inhalation anesthetic, diazepam or paraldehyde) are recommended for control of convulsions, since fluphenazine hydrochloride increases the central nervous system depressant action, but not the anticonvulsant action of barbiturates.

If acute parkinson-like symptoms result from fluphenazine hydrochloride intoxication, benztropine mesylate or diphenhydramine may be administered.

Central nervous system depression may be treated with nonconvulsant doses of CNS stimulants. Avoid stimulants that may cause convulsions (e.g., picrotoxin and pentylenetetrazol).

Signs of arousal may not occur for 48 hours.

Dialysis is of no value because of low plasma concentrations of the drug.

Since overdosage is often deliberate, patients may attempt suicide by other means during the recovery phase. Deaths by deliberate or accidental overdosage have occurred with this class of drugs.

HOW SUPPLIED

PERMITIL **Tablets**, 2.5 mg, compressed, scored, light orange, oval tablets impressed with the Schering trademark and product identification letters, WDR, or number, 442; bottle of 100 (NDC 0085-0442-04).

PERMITIL **Tablets**, 5 mg, compressed, scored, purple-pink, oval tablets impressed with the Schering trademark and product identification letters WFF, or number, 550; bottle of 100 (NDC 0085-0550-04).

PERMITIL **Tablets**, 10 mg, compressed, scored, light red, oval tablets impressed with the Schering trademark and product identification letters, WFG, or number, 316; bottle of 1000 (NDC 0085-0316-05).

PERMITIL **Oral Concentrate**, 5 mg per mL, a straw-colored, unflavored syrup containing alcohol 1%; bottle of 4 fluid ounces (118 mL), with dropper calibrated both in mg of fluphenazine hydrochloride and in mL of concentrate (NDC 0085-0296-05). **Protect from light and dispense only in amber bottles.**

Store PERMITIL Tablets and Oral Concentrate between 2° and 30°C (36° and 86°F).

Rev. 3/88

Shown in Product Identification Section, page 428

POLARAMINE®   ℞

[po-lar'ah-mēn]
brand of dexchlorpheniramine maleate
REPETABS® Tablets
Tablets, USP
Syrup, USP

DESCRIPTION

POLARAMINE products contain dexchlorpheniramine maleate, USP, an antihistamine having the formula, $C_{16}H_{19}ClN_2 \cdot C_4H_4O_4$, and a molecular weight of 390.87. Chemically, it is (+)-2-[p - Chloro - α - [2 - (dimethylamino)ethyl]benzyl] pyridine maleate (1:1).

POLARAMINE REPETABS (brand of repeat-action tablets) **Tablets** (4 mg and 6 mg) contain, respectively, 2 or 3 mg dexchlorpheniramine maleate, USP in an outer layer for prompt effect and 2 or 3 mg, respectively, in an inner core for release three to six hours after ingestion.

The inactive ingredients for POLARAMINE REPETABS 4 mg include: acacia, butylparaben, calcium phosphate, calcium sulfate, carnauba wax, corn starch, diatomaceous earth, FD&C Red No. 40 Al Lake, FD&C Yellow No. 6 Al Lake, kaolin, lactose, magnesium stearate, neutral soap, oleic acid, potato starch, rosin, stearic acid, sugar, talc, white wax, and zein.

The inactive ingredients for POLARAMINE REPETABS 6 mg include: acacia, butylparaben, calcium phosphate, calcium sulfate, carnauba wax, corn starch, diatomaceous earth, FD&C Red No. 40 Al Lake, FD&C Yellow No. 6 Al Lake, kaolin, lactose, magnesium stearate, neutral soap, oleic acid, potato starch, rosin, stearic acid, sugar, talc, white wax, and zein.

POLARAMINE **Tablets** contain 2 mg dexchlorpheniramine maleate, USP. The inactive ingredients include: corn starch, D&C Red No. 27 Al Lake, D&C Red No. 30 Al Lake, FD&C Yellow No. 6 Al Lake, lactose, magnesium stearate, and potato starch.

POLARAMINE **Syrup** contains 2 mg dexchlorpheniramine maleate, USP per 5 ml. The inactive ingredients include: alcohol (6%), FD&C Red No. 40, FD&C Yellow No. 6, flavors, menthol, methylparaben, propylene glycol, propylparaben, sodium chloride, sodium citrate, sorbitol, sugar, and water. Dexchlorpheniramine maleate is a white, odorless, crystalline powder which in aqueous solution has a pH of between 4 and 5. It is freely soluble in water, soluble in alcohol and in chloroform, but only slightly soluble in benzene or ether.

CLINICAL PHARMACOLOGY

POLARAMINE (dexchlorpheniramine maleate) is an antihistamine with anticholinergic properties. It is capable of producing a slight to moderate sedative effect. Antihistamines appear to compete with histamine for receptor sites on effector cells and are of value clinically in the prevention and relief of many allergic manifestations.

In vitro and *in vivo* assays of the antihistamine potencies of the optically active isomers of chlorpheniramine demonstrate that the predominant activity is in the dextro-isomer. The dextro-isomer is approximately two times more active than the racemic compound. Since dexchlorpheniramine is the dextro-isomer and active moiety of chlorpheniramine, it can be assumed that experience with chlorpheniramine also applies to dexchlorpheniramine.

Chlorpheniramine maleate 4 mg given to fasting human volunteers produced prompt blood levels after oral administration. Peak blood levels were approximately 7 ng/ml at an average time of 3 hours after administration. The half-life of chlorpheniramine maleate ranged from 20 to 24 hours. Following a single dose of tritium-labeled chlorpheniramine maleate to humans, the drug was found to be extensively metabolized whether given orally or by intravenous administration. The drug and metabolites were primarily excreted in the urine, with 19% of the dose appearing in 24 hours and a total of 34% in 48 hours.

Another study in volunteers has demonstrated that a **REPETABS Tablet** containing 12 mg chlorpheniramine maleate gives essentially identical plasma levels of drug as 12 mg of chlorpheniramine given in divided doses.

In a study in normal volunteers, a high flow rate of acidic urine resulted in a high excretion rate of chlorpheniramine maleate. Over a concentration range of 0.28 to 1.24 mcg/ml of plasma, chlorpheniramine maleate was 72 to 69% bound to plasma protein, respectively.

INDICATIONS AND USAGE

POLARAMINE is indicated for the treatment of perennial and seasonal allergic rhinitis; vasomotor rhinitis; allergic conjunctivitis; mild, uncomplicated allergic skin manifestations of urticaria and angioedema; amelioration of allergic reactions to blood or plasma; and dermographism. They are also indicated as therapy for anaphylactic reactions adjunctive to epinephrine and other standard measures after the acute manifestations have been controlled.

CONTRAINDICATIONS

Hypersensitivity to dexchlorpheniramine maleate or other antihistamines of similar chemical structure contraindicates the use of POLARAMINE.

Drug products containing dexchlorpheniramine maleate should not be used in newborn or premature infants because of the possibility of severe reactions such as convulsions.

Antihistamines *should not* be used to treat lower respiratory tract symptoms. Antihistamines are also contraindicated for use in conjunction with monoamine oxidase inhibitor therapy.

WARNINGS

Dexchlorpheniramine, as with all antihistamines, should be used with caution in patients with narrow angle glaucoma, stenosing peptic ulcer, pyloroduodenal obstruction, symptomatic prostatic hypertrophy, and bladder neck obstruction.

Overdoses of antihistamines may cause hallucinations, convulsions, or death, especially in infants and children.

Products containing dexchlorpheniramine maleate have additive effects with alcohol and other CNS depressants (hypnotics, sedatives, tranquilizers, etc.). Patients should not engage in activities requiring mental alertness, such as driving a car or operating machinery.

Antihistamines are more likely to cause dizziness, sedation, and hypotension in elderly patients (approximately 60 years or older).

PRECAUTIONS

General: Dexchlorpheniramine maleate has an atropine-like action and therefore products containing it should be used with caution in patients with: a history of bronchial asthma; increased intraocular pressure; hyperthyroidism; cardiovascular disease; hypertension.

Information for Patients:

1. Dexchlorpheniramine may cause slight to moderate drowsiness.
2. Patients should not engage in activities requiring mental alertness, such as driving or operating machinery.
3. Alcohol or other sedative drugs may enhance the drowsiness caused by antihistamines.
4. Patients should not take POLARAMINE in conjunction with a monoamine oxidase inhibitor or oral anticoagulant.

Drug Interactions: Dexchlorpheniramine maleate may cause severe hypotension when given in conjunction with a monoamine oxidase inhibitor.

Alcohol and other sedative drugs will potentiate the sedative effects of dexchlorpheniramine. (See WARNINGS.)

Carcinogenesis, Mutagenesis, Impairment of Fertility: Although there have been no oncogenic or mutagenic studies on dexchlorpheniramine, a 103-week oncogenic study in rats on the racemic mixture, chlorpheniramine, did not produce an increase in the incidence of tumors in the drug-treated groups, as compared with the controls.

An Ames mutagenicity test performed on chlorpheniramine and its nitrosation product was negative. An early study in rats with chlorpheniramine maleate revealed a reduction in fertility in female rats at doses approximately 67 times the human dose. More recent studies in rabbits and rats, using more appropriate methodology and doses up to approximately 50 and 85 times the human dose, showed no reduction in fertility in the animals.

Pregnancy Category B: Reproduction studies have been performed in rabbits and rats at doses up to 50 times and 85 times the human dose, respectively, and have revealed no evidence of harm to the fetus due to chlorpheniramine maleate. (See above, "Impairment of Fertility.") There are, however, no adequate and well-controlled studies in pregnant women. Because animal reproduction studies are not always predictive of human response, this drug should be used during the first two trimesters of pregnancy only if clearly needed. Dexchlorpheniramine maleate should not be used in the third trimester of pregnancy because newborn and premature infants may have severe reactions to antihistamines. (See CONTRAINDICATIONS.)

Nonteratogenic Effects: Studies of chlorpheniramine maleate done in rats revealed a decrease in the postnatal survival rate of pups of animals dosed with 33 and 67 times the human dose.

Nursing Mothers: It is not known whether this drug is excreted in human milk. Because certain other antihistamines are known to be excreted in human milk, and because dexchlorpheniramine maleate is contraindicated in newborn and premature infants, caution should be exercised when it is administered to a nursing woman.

Pediatric Use: Safety and effectiveness of the 4 and 6 mg **REPETABS Tablets** in children below the ages of 6 and 12 years, respectively, have not been established. Safety and effectiveness of the **Tablets** and **Syrup** in children below the age of 2 years have not been established.

ADVERSE REACTIONS

Slight to moderate drowsiness is the most frequent side effect of dexchlorpheniramine maleate. Other possible side effects of antihistamines include:

General: urticaria, drug rash, anaphylactic shock, photosensitivity, excessive perspiration, chills, dryness of mouth, nose, and throat.

Cardiovascular System: headache, palpitations, tachycardia, extrasystoles, hypotension.

Hematologic System: hemolytic anemia, hypoplastic anemia, thrombocytopenia, agranulocytosis.

Nervous System: sedation, dizziness, vertigo, tinnitus, acute labyrinthitis, disturbed coordination, fatigue, confusion, restlessness, excitation, nervousness, tremor, irritability, insomnia, euphoria, paresthesias, blurred vision, hysteria, neuritis, convulsions.

Gastrointestinal System: epigastric distress, anorexia, nausea, vomiting, diarrhea, constipation.

Genitourinary System: urinary frequency, difficult urination, urinary retention, early menses.

Respiratory System: thickening of bronchial secretions, tightness of chest, wheezing, nasal stuffiness.

OVERDOSAGE

In the event of overdosage, emergency treatment should be started immediately.

Manifestations of antihistamine overdosage may vary from central nervous system depression (sedation, apnea, diminished mental alertness, cardiovascular collapse) to stimulation (insomnia, hallucinations, tremors, or convulsions) to death. Other signs and symptoms may be dizziness, tinnitus, ataxia, blurred vision, and hypotension. Stimulation is particularly likely in children, as are atropine-like signs and symptoms (dry mouth; fixed, dilated pupils; flushing; hyperthermia; and gastrointestinal symptoms).

Treatment—The patient should be induced to vomit, even if emesis has occurred spontaneously. Pharmacologic vomiting by the administration of ipecac syrup is a preferred method.

However, vomiting should not be induced in patients with impaired consciousness. The action of ipecac is facilitated by physical activity and by the administration of eight to twelve fluid ounces of water. If emesis does not occur within fifteen minutes, the dose of ipecac should be repeated. Precautions against aspiration must be taken, especially in infants and children. Following emesis, any drug remaining in the stomach may be adsorbed by activated charcoal administered as a slurry with water. If vomiting is unsuccessful or contraindicated, gastric lavage should be performed. Isotonic and one-half isotonic saline are the lavage solutions of choice. Saline cathartics, such as milk of magnesia, draw water into the bowel by osmosis and therefore may be valuable for their action in rapid dilution of bowel content. Dialysis is of little value in antihistamine poisoning. After emergency treatment, the patient should continue to be medically monitored. Treatment of the signs and symptoms of overdosage is symptomatic and supportive. Stimulants (analeptic agents) should *not* be used. Vasopressors may be used to treat hypotension. Short-acting barbiturates, diazepam, or paraldehyde may be administered to control seizures. Hyperpyrexia, especially in children, may require treatment with tepid water sponge baths or a hypothermic blanket. Apnea is treated with ventilatory support.

In mice, the oral LD_{50} of dexchlorpheniramine is 258 mg/kg. In humans, the estimated lethal dose of racemic chlorpheniramine is 5 to 10 mg/kg. Thus a dose of 2.5 to 5 mg/kg of dexchlorpheniramine should be similarly regarded.

DOSAGE AND ADMINISTRATION

DOSAGE SHOULD BE INDIVIDUALIZED ACCORDING TO THE NEEDS AND RESPONSE OF THE PATIENT.

POLARAMINE **REPETABS Tablets**—*Adults and children 12 years or older:* one 4 or 6 mg POLARAMINE REPETABS Tablet at bedtime or every 8 to 10 hours during the day.

Children 6 to 12 years: one 4 mg REPETABS Tablet daily, taken preferably at bedtime.

POLARAMINE **Tablets**—*Adults and children 12 years of age and over:* one tablet every 4 to 6 hours. *Children 6 through 11 years:* one-half tablet every 4 to 6 hours. *Children 2 through 5 years:* one-quarter tablet every 4 to 6 hours.

POLARAMINE **Syrup**—*Adults and children 12 years of age and over:* 1 teaspoonful (2 mg) every 4 to 6 hours. *Children 6 through 11 years:* one-half teaspoonful (1 mg) every 4 to 6 hours. *Children 2 through 5 years:* one-quarter teaspoonful ($\frac{1}{2}$ mg) every 4 to 6 hours.

HOW SUPPLIED

POLARAMINE **REPETABS Tablets,** 4 mg, light red, sugar-coated, oval tablets branded in blue-black with the Schering trademark and product identification number, 095; bottle of 100.

POLARAMINE **REPETABS Tablets,** 6 mg, bright red, sugar-coated, oval tablets branded in white with the Schering trademark and product identification number, 148; bottle of 100.

POLARAMANE **Tablets,** 2 mg, red, compressed, oval tablets impressed with the Schering trademark and either product identification letters, AGT, or number, 820; bottle of 100.

POLARAMINE **Syrup,** 2 mg per 5 ml, red-orange-colored, orange-like flavored liquid; 16-fluid ounce (473 ml) bottle.

Store POLARAMINE between 2° and 30°C (36° and 86°F).

Rev. 1/89

Shown in Product Identification Section, page 428

PROVENTIL® Inhaler   ℞
[pro-ven 'til]
brand of albuterol
Bronchodilator Aerosol
FOR ORAL INHALATION ONLY

DESCRIPTION

The active component of PROVENTIL Inhaler is albuterol (α^1-[(tert -butylamino)methyl] -4- hydroxy-m -xylene-α,α'-diol), a relatively selective beta$_2$-adrenergic bronchodilator. Albuterol is the official generic name in the United States. The international generic name for the drug is salbutamol. The molecular weight of albuterol is 239.3, and the empirical formula is $C_{13}H_{21}NO_3$. Albuterol is a white to off-white crystalline solid. It is soluble in ethanol, sparingly soluble in water, and very soluble in chloroform.

PROVENTIL Inhaler is a metered-dose aerosol unit for oral inhalation. It contains a microcrystalline suspension of albuterol in propellants (trichloromonofluoromethane and dichlorodifluoromethane) with oleic acid. Each actuation

Continued on next page

Information on Schering products appearing on these pages is effective as of September 30, 1989.

Schering—Cont.

delivers from the mouthpiece 90 mcg of albuterol. Each canister provides at least 200 inhalations.

CLINICAL PHARMACOLOGY

The prime action of beta-adrenergic drugs is to stimulate adenyl cyclase, the enzyme which catalyzes the formation of cyclic-3',5'-adenosine monophosphate (cyclic AMP) from adenosine triphosphate (ATP). The cyclic AMP thus formed mediates the cellular responses. By virtue of its relatively selective action on beta$_2$- adrenoceptors, albuterol relaxes smooth muscle of the bronchi, uterus, and vascular supply to skeletal muscle, but may have less cardiac stimulant effects than does isoproterenol.

Albuterol is longer acting than isoproterenol by any route of administration in most patients because it is not a substrate for the cellular uptake processes for catecholamines nor for catechol-O-methyl transferase.

Because of its gradual absorption from the bronchi, systemic levels of albuterol are low after inhalation of recommended doses. Studies undertaken with four subjects administered tritiated albuterol, resulted in maximum plasma concentrations occurring within two to four hours. Due to the sensitivity of the assay method, the metabolic rate and half-life of elimination of albuterol in plasma could not be determined. However, urinary excretion provided data indicating that albuterol has an elimination half-life of 3.8 hours. Approximately 72 percent of the inhaled dose is excreted within 24 hours in the urine, and consists of 28 percent of unchanged drug and 44 percent as metabolite.

Results of animal studies show that albuterol does not pass the blood-brain barrier.

The effects of rising doses of albuterol and isoproterenol aerosols were studied in volunteers and asthmatic patients. Results in normal volunteers indicated that albuterol is $\frac{1}{2}$ to $\frac{1}{4}$ as active as isoproterenol in producing increases in heart rate. In asthmatic patients similar cardiovascular differentiation between the two drugs was also seen.

INDICATIONS AND USAGE

PROVENTIL Inhaler is indicated for the prevention and relief of bronchospasm in patients with reversible obstructive airway disease, and for the prevention of exercise-induced bronchospasm.

In controlled clinical trials the onset of improvement in pulmonary function was within 15 minutes, as determined by both maximal midexpiratory flow rate (MMEF) and FEV$_1$. MMEF measurements also showed that near maximum improvement in pulmonary function generally occurs within 60 to 90 minutes following 2 inhalations of albuterol and that clinically significant improvement generally continues for 3 to 4 hours in most patients. In clinical trials, some patients with asthma showed a therapeutic response (defined by maintaining FEV$_1$ values 15 percent or more above baseline) which was still apparent at 6 hours. Continued effectiveness of albuterol was demonstrated over a 13-week period in these same trials.

In clinical studies, 2 inhalations of albuterol taken approximately 15 minutes prior to exercise, prevented exercise-induced bronchospasm, as demonstrated by the maintenance of FEV$_1$ within 80 percent of baseline values in the majority of patients. One of these studies also evaluated the duration of the prophylactic effect to repeated exercise challenges, which was evident at 4 hours in the majority of patients, and at 6 hours in approximately one third of the patients.

CONTRAINDICATIONS

PROVENTIL Inhaler is contraindicated in patients with a history of hypersensitivity to any of its components.

WARNINGS

As with other adrenergic aerosols, the potential for paradoxical bronchospasm should be kept in mind. If it occurs, the preparation should be discontinued immediately and alternative therapy instituted.

Fatalities have been reported in association with excessive use of inhaled sympathomimetic drugs. The exact cause of death is unknown, but cardiac arrest following the unexpected development of a severe acute asthmatic crisis and subsequent hypoxia is suspected.

The contents of PROVENTIL Inhaler are under pressure. Do not puncture. Do not use or store near heat or open flame. Exposure to temperatures above 120°F may cause bursting. Never throw container into fire or incinerator. Keep out of reach of children.

PRECAUTIONS

Although it has less effect on the cardiovascular system than isoproterenol at recommended dosages, albuterol is a sympathomimetic amine and as such should be used with caution in patients with cardiovascular disorders, including coronary insufficiency and hypertension, in patients with hyperthyroidism or diabetes mellitus, and in patients who are unusually responsive to sympathomimetic amines.

Large doses of intravenous albuterol have been reported to aggravate preexisting diabetes and ketoacidosis. The rele-

vance of this observation to the use of PROVENTIL Inhaler is unknown, since the aerosol dose is much lower than the doses given intravenously.

Although there have been no reports concerning the use of PROVENTIL Inhaler during labor and delivery, it has been reported that high doses of albuterol administered intravenously inhibit uterine contractions. Although this effect is extremely unlikely as a consequence of aerosol use, it should be kept in mind.

Information For Patients: The action of PROVENTIL Inhaler may last up to six hours and therefore it should not be used more frequently than recommended. Increasing the number or frequency of doses without consulting your physician can be dangerous. If recommended dosage does not provide relief of symptoms or symptoms become worse, seek immediate medical attention. While taking PROVENTIL Inhaler, other inhaled medicines should not be used unless prescribed.

See Illustrated Patient Instructions For Use.

Drug Interactions: Other sympathomimetic aerosol bronchodilators should not be used concomitantly with albuterol. If additional adrenergic drugs are to be administered by any route, they should be used with caution to avoid deleterious cardiovascular effects.

Albuterol should be administered with caution to patients being treated with monoamine oxidase inhibitors or tricyclic antidepressants, since the action of albuterol on the vascular system may be potentiated.

Beta-receptor blocking agents and albuterol inhibit the effect of each other.

Carcinogenesis, Mutagenesis, and Impairment of Fertility: In a 2 year study in the rat, albuterol sulfate caused a significant dose-related increase in the incidence of benign leiomyomas of the mesovarium at doses corresponding to 111, 555, and 2,800 times the maximum human inhalational dose. In another study this effect was blocked by the coadministration of propranolol. The relevance of these findings to humans is not known. An 18-month study in mice revealed no evidence of tumorigenicity. Studies with albuterol revealed no evidence of mutagenesis. Reproduction studies in rats revealed no evidence of impaired fertility.

Teratogenic Effects — Pregnancy Category C: Albuterol has been shown to be teratogenic in mice when given in doses corresponding to 14 times the human dose. There are no adequate and well-controlled studies in pregnant women. Albuterol should be used during pregnancy only if the potential benefit justifies the potential risk to the fetus. A reproduction study in CD-1 mice with albuterol (0.025, 0.25, and 2.5 mg/kg, corresponding to 1.4, 14, and 140 times the maximum human inhalational dose) showed cleft palate formation in 5 of 111 (4.5 percent) fetuses at 0.25 mg/kg and in 10 of 108 (9.3 percent) fetuses at 2.5 mg/kg. None were observed at 0.025 mg/kg. Cleft palate also occurred in 22 of 72 (30.5 percent) fetuses treated with 2.5 mg/kg isoproterenol (positive control). A reproduction study in Stride Dutch rabbits revealed cranioschisis in 7 of 19 (37 percent) fetuses at 50 mg/kg, corresponding to 2,800 times the maximum human inhalational dose.

Nursing Mothers: It is not known whether this drug is excreted in human milk. Because of the potential for tumorigenicity shown for albuterol in animal studies, a decision should be made whether to discontinue nursing or to discontinue the drug, taking into account the importance of the drug to the mother.

Pediatric Use: Safety and effectiveness in children below the age of 12 years have not been established.

ADVERSE REACTIONS

The adverse reactions of albuterol are similar in nature to those of other sympathomimetic agents, although the incidence of certain cardiovascular effects is less with albuterol. A 13-week double-blind study compared albuterol and isoproterenol aerosols in 147 asthmatic patients. The results of this study showed that the incidence of cardiovascular effects was: palpitations, less than 10 per 100 with albuterol and less than 15 per 100 with isoproterenol; tachycardia, 10 per 100 with both albuterol and isoproterenol; and increased blood pressure, less than 5 per 100 with both albuterol and isoproterenol. In the same study, both drugs caused tremor or nausea in less than 15 patients per 100; dizziness or heartburn in less than 5 per 100 patients. Nervousness occurred in less than 10 per 100 patients receiving albuterol and in less than 15 per 100 patients receiving isoproterenol. Rare cases of urticaria, angioedema, rash, bronchospasm and oropharyngeal edema have been reported after the use of inhaled albuterol.

In addition, albuterol, like other sympathomimetic agents, can cause adverse reactions such as hypertension, angina, vomiting, vertigo, central nervous system stimulation, insomnia, headache, unusual taste, and drying or irritation of the oropharynx.

OVERDOSAGE

Exaggeration of the effects listed in ADVERSE REACTIONS can occur. Anginal pain and hypertension may result.

As with all sympathomimetic aerosol medications, cardiac arrest and even death may be associated with abuse.

The oral LD$_{50}$ in male and female rats and mice was greater than 2,000 mg/kg. The aerosol LD$_{50}$ could not be determined. Dialysis is not appropriate treatment for overdosage of PROVENTIL Inhaler. The judicious use of a cardioselective beta-receptor blocker, such as metoprolol tartrate, is suggested, bearing in mind the danger of inducing an asthmatic attack.

DOSAGE AND ADMINISTRATION

For treatment of acute episodes of bronchospasm or prevention of asthmatic symptoms, the usual dosage for adults and children 12 years and older is 2 inhalations repeated every 4 to 6 hours; in some patients, 1 inhalation every 4 hours may be sufficient. More frequent administration or a larger number of inhalations is not recommended. For maintenance therapy or prevention of exacerbation of bronchospasm, 2 inhalations, 4 times a day should be sufficient. The use of PROVENTIL Inhaler can be continued as medically indicated to control recurring bouts of bronchospasm. During this time most patients gain optimal benefit from regular use of the inhaler. Safe usage for periods extending over several years has been documented.

If a previously effective dosage regimen fails to provide the usual relief, medical advice should be sought immediately as this is often a sign of seriously worsening asthma which would require reassessment of therapy.

Exercise-Induced Bronchospasm Prevention: The usual dosage for adults and children 12 years and older is 2 inhalations, 15 minutes prior to exercise.

For treatment, see above.

HOW SUPPLIED

PROVENTIL Inhaler, 17.0 g canister; box of one. Each actuation delivers 90 mcg of albuterol from the mouthpiece. It is supplied with an oral adapter and patient's instructions (NDC-0085-0614-02). PROVENTIL Inhaler REFILL canister, 17.0g, with patient's instructions; box of one (NDC-0085-0614-03).

Store between 15° and 30°C (59° and 86°F). Failure to use product within this temperature range may result in improper dosing. Shake well before using.

Copyright© 1981, 1985, 1986, Schering Corporation, USA. All rights reserved.

Revised 2/86

Shown in Product Identification Section, page 428

PROVENTIL®
brand of albuterol sulfate
    Solution for Inhalation 0.5%*
    Solution for Inhalation 0.083%*
    (*Potency expressed as albuterol)

℞

DESCRIPTION

PROVENTIL, brand of albuterol sulfate, Solution for Inhalation, is a relatively selective beta$_2$-adrenergic bronchodilator (see **CLINICAL PHARMACOLOGY** section below). Albuterol sulfate has the chemical name α^1-[(*tert*-Butylamino) methyl]-4-hydroxy-*m*-xylene-α,α'diol sulfate (2:1) (salt).

Albuterol sulfate has a molecular weight of 576.7 and the empirical formula $(C_{13}H_{21}NO_3)_2 \cdot H_2SO_4$. Albuterol sulfate is a white crystalline powder, soluble in water and slightly soluble in ethanol.

The international generic name for albuterol base is salbutamol.

PROVENTIL Solution for Inhalation is available in two concentrations. The 0.5% solution is in concentrated form. Dilute 0.5 ml of the solution to 3 ml with normal saline solution prior to administration. The 0.083% solution requires no dilution prior to administration.

Each ml of PROVENTIL Solution for Inhalation (0.5%) contains 5 mg of albuterol (as 6.0 mg of albuterol sulfate) in an aqueous solution containing benzalkonium chloride; sulfuric acid is used to adjust the pH between 3 and 5. PROVENTIL Solution for Inhalation (0.5%) contains no sulfiting agents. It is supplied in 20 ml bottles.

Each ml of PROVENTIL Solution for Inhalation (0.083%) contains 0.83 mg of albuterol (as 1.0 mg of albuterol sulfate) in an isotonic aqueous solution containing sodium chloride and benzalkonium chloride; sulfuric acid is used to adjust the pH between 3 and 5. PROVENTIL Solution for Inhalation (0.083%) contains no sulfiting agents. It is supplied in 3 ml bottles for unit-dose dispensing.

PROVENTIL Solution for Inhalation is a clear, colorless to light yellow solution.

CLINICAL PHARMACOLOGY

The prime action of beta-adrenergic drugs is to stimulate adenyl cyclase, the enzyme which catalyzes the formation of cyclic-3', 5'-adenosine monophosphate (cyclic AMP) from adenosine triphosphate (ATP). The cyclic AMP thus formed mediates the cellular responses. *In vitro* studies and *in vivo* pharmacologic studies have demonstrated that albuterol has a preferential effect on beta$_2$-adrenergic receptors compared with isoproterenol. While it is recognized that beta$_2$-adrenergic receptors are the predominant receptors in bronchial smooth muscle, recent data indicate that 10 to 50% of the beta receptors in the human heart may be $beta_2$ receptors. The precise function of these receptors, however, is not yet established. Albuterol has been shown in most controlled clinical trials to have more effect on the respiratory tract, in the form of bronchial smooth muscle relaxation, than isoproterenol at comparable doses while producing fewer cardiovascular effects. Controlled clinical studies and other clinical experience have shown that inhaled albuterol, like other beta-adrenergic agonist drugs, can produce a significant cardiovascular effect in some patients, as measured by pulse rate, blood pressure, symptoms, and/or ECG changes.

Albuterol is longer acting than isoproterenol in most patients by any route of administration because it is not a substrate for the cellular uptake processes for catecholamines nor for catechol-O-methyl transferase.

Studies in asthmatic patients have shown that less than 20% of a single albuterol dose was absorbed following either IPPB or nebulizer administration; the remaining amount was recovered from the nebulizer and apparatus and expired air. Most of the absorbed dose was recovered in the urine 24 hours after drug administration. Following a 3.0 mg dose of nebulized albuterol, the maximum albuterol plasma level at 0.5 hours was 2.1 ng/ml (range 1.4 to 3.2ng/ml). There was a significant dose-related response in FEV_1 and peak flow rate (PFR). It has been demonstrated that following oral administration of 4 mg albuterol, the elimination half-life was five to six hours.

Animal studies show that albuterol does not pass the blood-brain barrier. Recent studies in laboratory animals (minipigs, rodents, and dogs) recorded the occurrence of cardiac arrhythmias and sudden death (with histologic evidence of myocardial necrosis) when beta-agonists and methylxanthines were administered concurrently. The significance of these findings when applied to humans is currently unknown.

In controlled clinical trials, most patients exhibited an onset of improvement in pulmonary function within 5 minutes as determined by FEV_1. FEV_1 measurements also showed that the maximum average improvement in pulmonary function usually occurred at approximately 1 hour following inhalation of 2.5 mg of albuterol by compressor-nebulizer, and remained close to peak for 2 hours. Clinically significant improvement in pulmonary function (defined as maintenance of a 15% or more increase in FEV_1 over baseline values) continued for 3 to 4 hours in most patients and in some patients continued up to 6 hours.

In repetitive dose studies, continued effectiveness was demonstrated throughout the three-month period of treatment in some patients.

INDICATIONS AND USAGE
PROVENTIL Solution for Inhalation is indicated for the relief of bronchospasm in patients with reversible obstructive airway disease and acute attacks of bronchospasm.

CONTRAINDICATIONS
PROVENTIL Solution for Inhalation is contraindicated in patients with a history of hypersensitivity to any of its components.

WARNINGS
As with other inhaled beta-adrenergic agonists, PROVENTIL Solution for Inhalation can produce paradoxical bronchospasm, which can be life threatening. If it occurs, the preparation should be discontinued immediately and alternative therapy instituted.

Fatalities have been reported in association with excessive use of inhaled sympathomimetic drugs and with the home use of sympathomimetic nebulizers. It is, therefore, essential that the physician instruct the patient in the need for further evaluation if his/her asthma becomes worse. In individual patients, any $beta_2$-adrenergic agonist, including albuterol solution for inhalation, may have a clinically significant cardiac effect.

Immediate hypersensitivity reactions may occur after administration of albuterol as demonstrated by rare cases of urticaria, angioedema, rash, bronchospasm, and oropharyngeal edema.

PRECAUTIONS
General: Albuterol, as with all sympathomimetic amines, should be used with caution in patients with cardiovascular disorders, especially coronary insufficiency, cardiac arrhythmias and hypertension, in patients with convulsive disorders, hyperthyroidism or diabetes mellitus, and in patients who are unusually responsive to sympathomimetic amines. Large doses of intravenous albuterol have been reported to aggravate preexisting diabetes mellitus and ketoacidosis. Additionally, beta-agonists, including albuterol, when given intravenously may cause a decrease in serum potassium, possibly through intracellular shunting. The decrease is usually transient, not requiring supplementation. The relevance of these observations to the use of PROVENTIL Solution for Inhalation is unknown.

Information For Patients: The action of PROVENTIL Solution for Inhalation may last up to six hours and therefore it should not be used more frequently than recommended. Do

not increase the dose or frequency of medication without medical consultation. If symptoms get worse, medical consultation should be sought promptly. While taking PROVENTIL Solution for Inhalation, other anti-asthma medicines should not be used unless prescribed.

See illustrated "Patient's Instructions for Use."

Drug Interactions: Other sympathomimetic aerosol bronchodilators or epinephrine should not be used concomitantly with albuterol.

Albuterol should be administered with extreme caution to patients being treated with monoamine oxidase inhibitors or tricyclic antidepressants, since the action of albuterol on the vascular system may be potentiated.

Beta-receptor blocking agents and albuterol inhibit the effect of each other.

Carcinogenesis, Mutagenesis, and Impairment of Fertility: Albuterol sulfate, like other agents in its class, caused a significant dose-related increase in the incidence of benign leiomyomas of the mesovarium in a 2-year study in the rat, at oral doses corresponding to 10, 50 and 250 times the maximum human nebulizer dose. In another study, this effect was blocked by the coadministration of propranolol. The relevance of these findings to humans is not known. An 18-month study in mice and a lifetime study in hamsters revealed no evidence of tumorigenicity. Studies with albuterol revealed no evidence of mutagenesis. Reproduction studies in rats revealed no evidence of impaired fertility.

Teratogenic Effects—Pregnancy Category C: Albuterol has been shown to be teratogenic in mice when given subcutaneously in doses corresponding to the human nebulization dose. There are no adequate and well-controlled studies in pregnant women. Albuterol should be used during pregnancy only if the potential benefit justifies the potential risk to the fetus. A reproduction study in CD-1 mice with albuterol (0.025, 0.25 and 2.5 mg/kg subcutaneously, corresponding to 0.1, 1, and 12.5 times the maximum human nebulization dose, respectively) showed cleft palate formation in 5 of 111 (4.5%) of fetuses at 0.25 mg/kg and in 10 of 108 (9.3%) of fetuses at 2.5 mg/kg. None were observed at 0.025 mg/kg. Cleft palate also occurred in 22 of 72 (30.5%) of fetuses treated with 2.5 mg/kg isoproterenol (positive control). A reproduction study in Stride Dutch rabbits revealed cranioschisis in 7 of 19 (37%) of fetuses at 50 mg/kg, corresponding to 250 times the maximum human nebulization dose,.

Labor and Delivery: Oral albuterol has been shown to delay preterm labor in some reports. There are presently no well controlled studies which demonstrate that it will stop preterm labor or prevent labor at term. Therefore, cautious use of PROVENTIL Solution for Inhalation is required in pregnant patients when given for relief of bronchospasm so as to avoid interference with uterine contractibility.

Nursing Mothers: It is not known whether this drug is excreted in human milk. Because of the potential for tumorigenicity shown for albuterol in some animal studies, a decision should be made whether to discontinue nursing or to discontinue the drug, taking into account the importance of the drug to the mother.

Pediatric Use: Safety and effectiveness of albuterol solution for inhalation in children below the age of 12 years have not been established.

ADVERSE REACTIONS
The results of clinical trials with PROVENTIL Solution for Inhalation in 135 patients showed the following side effects which were considered probably or possibly drug related: *Central Nervous System:* tremors (20%), dizziness (7%), nervousness (4%), headache (3%), insomnia (1%). *Gastrointestinal:* nausea (4%), dyspepsia (1%). *Ear, Nose and Throat:* pharyngitis (<1%), nasal congestion (1%). *Cardiovascular:* tachycardia (1%), hypertension (1%). *Respiratory:* bronchospasm (8%), cough (4%), bronchitis (4%), wheezing (1%).

No clinically relevant laboratory abnormalities related to PROVENTIL Solution for Inhalation administration were determined in these studies.

In comparing the adverse reactions reported for patients treated with PROVENTIL Solution for Inhalation with those of patients treated with isoproterenol during clinical trials of three months, the following moderate to severe reactions, as judged by the investigators, were reported. This table does no include mild reactions.

Percent Incidence of Moderate To Severe Reactions

Reaction	Albuterol N=65	Isoproterenol N=65
Central Nervous System		
Tremors	10.7%	13.8%
Headache	3.1%	1.5%
Insomnia	3.1%	1.5%
Cardiovascular		
Hypertension	3.1%	3.1%
Arrhythmias	0%	3.0%
**Palpitation	0%	22.0%
Respiratory		
*Bronchospasm	15.4%	18%
Cough	3.1%	5%
Bronchitis	1.5%	5%
Wheeze	1.5%	1.5%
Sputum Increase	1.5%	1.5%
Dyspnea	1.5%	1.5%
Gastrointestinal		
Nausea	3.1%	0
Dyspepsia	1.5%	0
Systemic		
Malaise	1.5%	0

* In most cases of bronchospasm, this item was generally used to describe exacerbations in the underlying pulmonary disease.

** The finding of no arrhythmias and no palpitations after albuterol administration in this clinical study should not be interpreted as indicating that these adverse effects can not occur after the administration of inhaled albuterol.

Rare cases of urticaria, angioedema, rash, bronchospasm and oropharyngeal edema have been reported after the use of inhaled albuterol.

OVERDOSAGE
Manifestations of overdosage may include anginal pain, hypertension, hypokalemia, and exaggeration of the pharmacological effects listed in **ADVERSE REACTIONS**.

The oral LD_{50} in rats and mice was greater than 2,000 mg/kg. The inhalational LD_{50} could not be determined. There is insufficient evidence to determine if dialysis is beneficial for overdosage of PROVENTIL Solution for Inhalation.

DOSAGE AND ADMINISTRATION
The usual dosage for adults and children 12 years and older is 2.5 mg of albuterol administered 3 to 4 times daily by nebulization. More frequent administration or higher doses is not recommended. To administer 2.5 mg of albuterol, either dilute 0.5 ml of the 0.5% solution for inhalation to a total volume of 3 ml with normal saline solution, or administer the contents of one unit-dose bottle (3 ml of 0.083% nebulizer solution) by nebulization. The flow rate is regulated to suit the particular nebulizer so that the PROVENTIL Solution for Inhalation will be delivered over approximately 5 to 15 minutes.

The use of PROVENTIL Solution for Inhalation can be continued as medically indicated to control recurring bouts of bronchospasm. During treatment, most patients gain optimum benefit from regular use of the nebulizer solution.

If a previously effective dosage regimen fails to provide the usual relief, medical advice should be sought immediately, as this is often a sign of seriously worsening asthma which would require reassessment of therapy.

HOW SUPPLIED
PROVENTIL Solution for Inhalation, 0.5%, is a clear, colorless to light yellow solution, and is supplied in bottles of 20 ml (NDC-0085-0208-02) with accompanying calibrated dropper; boxes of one. **Store between 2° and 30°C (36° and 86°F).** PROVENTIL Solution for Inhalation, 0.083%, is a clear, colorless to light yellow solution, and is supplied in unit-dose bottles of 3 ml each, boxes of 25 (NDC-0085-0209-01). **Store between 2° and 25°C (36° and 77°F).**

Revised

Copyright © 1986, 1987 Schering Corporation, Kenilworth, NJ 07033. All rights reserved.

PROVENTIL®   ℞
brand of albuterol sulfate
Syrup

DESCRIPTION
PROVENTIL Syrup contains albuterol sulfate, a relatively selective $beta_2$-adrenergic bronchodilator. Albuterol sulfate has the chemical name α^1-[($tert$-Butylamino)methyl]-4-hydroxy-m-xylene-α,α'-diol sulfate (2:1) (salt).

Albuterol sulfate has a molecular weight of 576.7 and the empirical formula $(C_{13}H_{21}NO_3)_2 \cdot H_2SO_4$. Albuterol sulfate is a white crystalline powder, soluble in water and slightly soluble in ethanol.

The international generic name for albuterol base is salbutamol.

PROVENTIL Syrup contains 2 mg of albuterol as 2.4 mg of albuterol sulfate in each teaspoonful (5 ml).

The inactive ingredients for Proventil Syrup include: citric acid, FD&C Yellow No. 6, flavor, hydroxypropyl methylcellulose, saccharin, sodium benzoate, sodium citrate and water.

CLINICAL PHARMACOLOGY
The prime action of beta-adrenergic drugs is to stimulate adenyl cyclase, the enzyme which catalyzes the formation of cyclic-3′,5′-adenosine monophosphate (cyclic AMP) from

Continued on next page

Information on Schering products appearing on these pages is effective as of September 30, 1989.

Schering—Cont.

adenosine triphosphate (ATP). The cyclic AMP thus formed mediates the cellular responses. Based on pharmacologic studies in animals, albuterol appears to exert direct and preferential action on beta$_2$-adrenoceptors including those of the bronchial tree and uterus, and may have less cardiac stimulant effect than isoproterenol, when given in the usual recommended dose.

Albuterol is longer acting than isoproterenol in most patients by any route of administration because it is not a substrate for the cellular uptake processes for catecholamines nor for catechol-O-methyl transferase.

After oral administration of 10 ml PROVENTIL Syrup (4 mg albuterol) in normal volunteers, albuterol is rapidly absorbed. Maximum plasma albuterol concentrations of about 18 ng/ml are achieved within 2 hours and the drug is eliminated with a half-life of about 5 hours. In other studies, the analysis of urine samples of patients given 8 mg tritiated albuterol orally showed that 76% of the dose was excreted over 3 days, with the majority of the dose being excreted within the first 24 hours. Sixty percent of this radioactivity was shown to be the metabolite. Feces collected over this period contained 4% of the administered dose.

Animal studies show that albuterol does not pass the blood-brain barrier.

INDICATIONS AND USAGE

PROVENTIL Syrup is indicated for the relief of bronchospasm in adults and in children 2 years of age and older with reversible obstructive airway disease.

In controlled clinical trials in patients with asthma, the onset of improvement in pulmonary function, as measured by maximal midexpiratory flow rate (MMEF) and forced expiratory volume in one second (FEV$_1$), was within 30 minutes after a dose of PROVENTIL Syrup. Peak improvement of pulmonary function occurred between 2 to 3 hours. In a controlled clinical trial involving 55 children, clinically significant improvement (defined as maintenance of mean values over baseline of 15% or 20% or more in the FEV$_1$ and MMEF respectively) continued to be recorded up to 6 hours. No decrease in the effectiveness was reported in one uncontrolled study of 32 children who took PROVENTIL Syrup for a 3 month period.

CONTRAINDICATIONS

PROVENTIL Syrup is contraindicated in patients with a history of hypersensitivity to any of its components.

PRECAUTIONS

General: Although albuterol usually has minimal effects on the beta$_1$-adrenoceptors of the cardiovascular system at the recommended dosage, occasionally the usual cardiovascular and CNS stimulatory effects common to all sympathomimetic agents have been seen with patients treated with albuterol necessitating discontinuation. Therefore, albuterol should be used with caution in patients with cardiovascular disorders, including coronary insufficiency and hypertension, in patients with hyperthyroidism or diabetes mellitus, and in patients who are unusually responsive to sympathomimetic amines.

Large doses of intravenous albuterol have been reported to aggravate preexisting diabetes mellitus and ketoacidosis. Additionally, albuterol and other beta-agonists, when given intravenously, may cause a decrease in serum potassium, possibly through intracellular shunting. The decrease is usually transient, not requiring supplementation. The relevance of these observations to the use of PROVENTIL Syrup is unknown.

Information for Patients: The action of PROVENTIL Syrup may last up to six hours and therefore it should not be taken more frequently than recommended. Do not increase the dose or frequency of medication without medical consultation. If symptoms get worse, medical consultation should be sought promptly.

Drug Interactions: The concomitant use of PROVENTIL Syrup and other oral sympathomimetic agents is not recommended since such combined use may lead to deleterious cardiovascular effects. This recommendation does not preclude the judicious use of an aerosol bronchodilator of the adrenergic stimulant type in patients receiving PROVENTIL Syrup. Such concomitant use, however, should be individualized and not given on a routine basis. If regular coadministration is required, then alternative therapy should be considered.

Albuterol should be administered with extreme caution to patients being treated with monoamine oxidase inhibitors or tricyclic antidepressants since the action of albuterol on the vascular system may be potentiated.

Beta-receptor blocking agents and albuterol inhibit the effect of each other.

Carcinogenesis, Mutagenesis, and Impairment of Fertility: Albuterol sulfate, like other agents in its class, caused a significant dose-related increase in the incidence of benign leiomyomas of the mesovarium in a 2-year study in the rat, at doses corresponding to 2, 9, and 46 times the maximum hu-

man (child weighing 21 kg) oral dose. In another study this effect was blocked by the coadministration of propranolol. The relevance of these findings to humans is not known. An 18-month study in mice and a lifetime study in hamsters revealed no evidence of tumorigenicity. Studies with albuterol revealed no evidence of mutagenesis. Reproduction studies in rats revealed no evidence of impaired fertility.

Teratogenic Effects—Pregnancy Category C: Albuterol has been shown to be teratogenic in mice when given subcutaneously in doses corresponding to 0.2 times the maximum human (child weighing 21 kg) oral dose. There are no adequate and well-controlled studies in pregnant women. Albuterol should be used during pregnancy only if the potential benefit justifies the potential risk to the fetus. A reproduction study in CD-1 mice with albuterol showed cleft palate formation in 5 of 111 (4.5%) fetuses at 0.25 mg/kg and in 10 of 108 (9.3%) fetuses at 2.5 mg/kg; none was observed at 0.025 mg/kg. Cleft palate also occurred in 22 of 72 (30.5%) fetuses treated with 2.5 mg/kg isoproterenol (positive control). A reproduction study in Stride Dutch rabbits revealed cranioschisis in 7 of 19 (37%) fetuses at 50 mg/kg, corresponding to 46 times the maximum human (child weighing 21 kg) oral dose of albuterol sulfate.

Labor and Delivery: Oral albuterol has been shown to delay preterm labor in some reports. There are presently no well-controlled studies which demonstrate that it will stop preterm labor or prevent labor at term. Therefore, cautious use of PROVENTIL Syrup is required in pregnant patients when given for relief of bronchospasm so as to avoid interference with uterine contractility. Use in such patients should be restricted to those patients in whom the benefits clearly outweigh the risks.

Nursing Mothers: It is not know whether this drug is excreted in human milk. Because of the potential for tumorigenicity shown for albuterol in animal studies, a decision should be made whether to discontinue nursing or to discontinue the drug, taking into account the importance of the drug to the mother.

Pediatric Use: Safety and effectiveness in children below the age of 2 years have not yet been adequately demonstrated.

ADVERSE REACTIONS

The adverse reactions to albuterol are similar in nature to those of other sympathomimetic agents. The most frequent adverse reactions to PROVENTIL Syrup in adults and older children were tremor, 10 of 100 patients; nervousness and shakiness, each 9 of 100 patients. Other reported adverse reactions were headache, 4 of 100 patients; dizziness and increased appetite, each 3 of 100 patients; hyperactivity and excitement, each 2 of 100 patients; tachycardia, epistaxis, irritable behavior, and sleeplessness, each 1 of 100 patients. The following adverse effects occurred in less than 1 of 100 patients each: muscle spasm; disturbed sleep, epigastric pain; cough; palpitations; stomach ache; irritable behavior; dilated pupils; sweating; chest pain; weakness.

In young children 2 to 6 years of age, some adverse reactions were noted more frequently than in adults and older children. Excitement was noted in approximately 20% of patients and nervousness in 15%. Hyperkinesia occurred in 4% of patients; insomnia, tachycardia, and gastrointestinal symptoms in 2% each. Anorexia, emotional lability, pallor, fatigue, and conjunctivitis were seen in 1%.

In addition, albuterol, like other sympathomimetic agents, can cause adverse reactions such as hypertension, angina, vomiting, vertigo, central nervous system stimulation, unusual taste, and drying or irritation of the oropharynx.

The reactions are generally transient in nature, and it is usually not necessary to discontinue treatment with PROVENTIL Syrup. In selected cases, however, dosage may be reduced temporarily; after the reaction has subsided, dosage should be increased in small increments to the optimal dosage.

OVERDOSAGE

Manifestations of overdosage include anginal pain, hypertension, hypokalemia, and exaggeration of the effects listed in Adverse Reactions.

The oral LD$_{50}$ in rats and mice was greater than 2,000 mg/kg. Dialysis is not appropriate treatment for overdosage of PROVENTIL Syrup. The judicious use of a cardioselective beta-receptor blocker, such as metoprolol tartrate, is suggested, bearing in mind the danger of inducing an asthmatic attack.

DOSAGE AND ADMINISTRATION

The following dosages of PROVENTIL Syrup are expressed in terms of albuterol base.

Usual Dose: The usual starting dosage for adults and children over age 14 is 2 mg (1 teaspoonful) or 4 mg (2 teaspoonfuls) three or four times a day.

The usual starting dosage for children 6 to 14 years of age is 2 mg (1 teaspoonful) three or four times a day.

For children 2 to 6 years of age, dosing should be initiated at 0.1 mg/kg of body weight three times a day. This starting dose should not exceed 2 mg (1 teaspoonful) three times a day.

Dosage Adjustment: For adults and children above age 14, dosage above 4 mg four times a day should be used *only* when the patient fails to respond. If a favorable response does not occur, the dosage may be cautiously increased stepwise, but not to exceed 8 mg four times a day.

For children from 6 to 14 years of age who fail to respond to the initial starting dosage of 2 mg four times a day, the dosage may be cautiously increased stepwise, but not to exceed 24 mg per day (given in divided doses).

For children 2 to 6 years of age who do not respond satisfactorily to the initial dosage, the dose may be increased stepwise to 0.2 mg/kg of body weight three times a day, but not to exceed a maximum of 4 mg (2 teaspoonfuls) given three times a day.

For elderly patients and those sensitive to beta-adrenergic stimulation, the initial dose should be restricted to 2 mg three or four times a day and individually adjusted thereafter.

HOW SUPPLIED

PROVENTIL Syrup, a clear orange-yellow liquid with a strawberry flavor, contains 2 mg albuterol as the sulfate per 5 ml, bottles of 16 fluid ounces (NDC 0085-0315-02).

Store between 2° and 30°C (36° and 86°F).

Revised 5/86

Copyright © 1982, 1985, 1986. Schering Corporation, USA. All rights reserved.

PROVENTIL®   ℞

[pro-ven'til]

brand of albuterol sulfate
  REPETABS® brand of
  extended-release Tablets
PROVENTIL®
brand of albuterol sulfate
  Tablets

DESCRIPTION

PROVENTIL REPETABS Tablets and PROVENTIL Tablets contain albuterol sulfate, a relatively selective beta$_2$-adrenergic bronchodilator. Albuterol sulfate has the chemical name α^1-[($tert$-Butylamino)methyl]-4-hydroxy-m-xylene-α-α'-diol sulfate (2:1) (salt).

Albuterol sulfate has a molecular weight of 576.7 and the empirical formula $(C_{13}H_{21}NO_3)_2 \cdot H_2SO_4$. Albuterol sulfate is a white crystalline powder, soluble in water and slightly soluble in ethanol.

The World Health Organization recommended name for albuterol base is salbutamol.

Each PROVENTIL REPETABS Tablet contains a total of 4 mg (2 mg in the coating for immediate release and 2 mg in the core for release after several hours) of albuterol as 4.8 mg of albuterol sulfate.

Each PROVENTIL Tablet contains 2 or 4 mg of albuterol as 2.4 and 4.8 mg of albuterol sulfate, respectively.

The inactive ingredients for PROVENTIL REPETABS Tablets include: acacia, butylparaben, calcium sulfate, carnauba wax, corn starch, gum rosin, lactose, magnesium stearate, oleic acid, sugar, talc, titanium dioxide, tribasic calcium phosphate, white neutral sodium soap, white wax, and zein. The inactive ingredients for PROVENTIL Tablets, 2 and 4 mg include: lactose, corn starch, and magnesium stearate.

CLINICAL PHARMACOLOGY

In vitro studies and *in vivo* pharmacologic studies have demonstrated that PROVENTIL has a preferential effect on beta$_2$-adrenergic receptors compared with isoproterenol. While it is recognized that beta$_2$-adrenergic receptors are the predominant receptors in bronchial smooth muscle, recent data indicate that there is a population of beta$_2$-receptors in the human heart, existing in a concentration between 10–50%. The precise function of these receptors, however, is not yet established.

Albuterol is longer acting than isoproterenol in most patients by any route of administration because it is not a substrate for the cellular uptake processes for catecholamines nor for catechol-O-methyl transferase.

Albuterol is rapidly and well absorbed following oral administration. In studies involving normal volunteers, the mean steady state peak and trough plasma levels of albuterol were 6.7 and 3.8 ng/ml, respectively, following dosing with a 2 mg PROVENTIL Tablet every 6 hours and 14.8 and 8.6 ng/ml, respectively, following dosing with a 4 mg PROVENTIL Tablet every 6 hours. Maximum albuterol plasma levels are usually obtained between 2 and 3 hours after dosing and the elimination half-life is 5 to 6 hours. These data indicate that albuterol administered orally, is dose proportional and exhibits dose independent pharmacokinetics.

In other studies, the analysis of urine samples of subjects given tritiated albuterol (4–10 mg) orally showed that 65% to 90% of the dose was excreted over 3 days, with the majority of the dose being excreted within the first 24 hours. Sixty percent of this radioactivity was shown to be the metabolite of albuterol. Feces collected over this period contained 4% of the administered dose.

PROVENTIL REPETABS Tablets have been formulated to provide a duration of action of up to 12 hours. In studies conducted in normal volunteers, the mean steady state peak and trough plasma levels of albuterol were 6.5 and 3.0 ng/ml, respectively, following dosing with a 4 mg PROVENTIL REPETABS Tablet every 12 hours. In addition, it has been shown that administration of a 4 mg PROVENTIL REPETABS Tablet every 12 hours is bioequivalent to administration of a 2 mg PROVENTIL Tablet every 6 hours.

Animal studies show that albuterol does not pass the blood-brain barrier. Recent studies in laboratory animals (minipigs, rodents, and dogs) recorded the occurrence of cardiac arrhythmias and sudden death (with histologic evidence of myocardial necrosis) when beta-agonists and methylxanthines were administered concurrently. The significance of these findings when applied to humans is currently unknown.

In controlled clinical trials in patients with asthma, the onset of improvement in pulmonary function, as measured by maximal midexpiratory flow rate, MMEF, was noted within 30 minutes after a dose of PROVENTIL Tablets with peak improvement occurring between 2 to 3 hours. In controlled clinical trials, in which measurements were conducted for 6 hours, significant clinical improvement in pulmonary function (defined as maintaining a 15% or more increase in FEV_1 and a 20% or more increase in MMEF over baseline values) was observed in 60% of patients at 4 hours and in 40% at 6 hours. In other single dose, controlled clinical trials, clinically significant improvement was observed in at least 40% of the patients at 8 hours with the 4 mg PROVENTIL Tablet. No decrease in the effectiveness of PROVENTIL Tablets has been reported in patients who received long-term treatment with the drug in uncontrolled studies for periods up to 6 months.

In another controlled clinical study in asthmatic patients, it has been demonstrated that the initiation of therapy with either the 4 mg PROVENTIL REPETABS Tablet dosed every 12 hours, or the 2 mg PROVENTIL Tablet dosed every 6 hours, achieve therapeutically equivalent effects.

INDICATIONS AND USAGE
PROVENTIL REPETABS Tablets and PROVENTIL Tablets are indicated for the relief of bronchospasm in patients with reversible obstructive airway disease.

CONTRAINDICATIONS
PROVENTIL REPETABS Tablets and PROVENTIL Tablets are contraindicated in patients with a history of hypersensitivity to any of their components.

PRECAUTIONS
General: Since albuterol is a sympathomimetic amine, it should be used with caution in patients with cardiovascular disorders, including ischemic heart disease, hypertension or cardiac arrhythmias, in patients with hyperthyroidism or diabetes mellitus, and in patients who are unusually responsive to sympathomimetic amines or who have convulsive disorders. Significant changes in systolic and diastolic blood pressure could be expected to occur in some patients after use of any beta adrenergic bronchodilator.

Large doses of intravenous albuterol have been reported to aggravate preexisting diabetes mellitus and ketoacidosis. Additionally, albuterol and other beta agonists, when given intravenously, may cause a decrease in serum potassium, possibly through intracellular shunting. The decrease is usually transient, not requiring supplementation. The relevance of these observations to the use of PROVENTIL REPETABS Tablets and PROVENTIL Tablets is unknown.

Information for Patients: Patients being treated with PROVENTIL REPETABS Tablets or PROVENTIL Tablets should receive the following information and instructions. This information is intended to aid in the safe and effective use of this medication. It is not a disclosure of all possible adverse or intended effects.

PROVENTIL REPETABS Tablets and PROVENTIL Tablets should not be taken more frequently than recommended. Do not increase the dose or frequency of medication, or add other medications to your therapy without medical consultation. If symptoms get worse, medical consultation should be sought promptly. If pregnant or nursing, consult with your physician.

Drug Interactions: The concomitant use of PROVENTIL REPETABS Tablets or PROVENTIL Tablets and other oral sympathomimetic agents is not recommended since such combined use may lead to deleterious cardiovascular effects. This recommendation does not preclude the judicious use of an aerosol bronchodilator of the adrenergic stimulant type in patients receiving PROVENTIL REPETABS Tablets or PROVENTIL Tablets. Such concomitant use, however, should be individualized and not given on a routine basis. If regular coadministration is required, then alternative therapy should be considered.

Albuterol should be administered with extreme caution to patients being treated with monoamine oxidase inhibitors or tricyclic antidepressants, since the action of albuterol on the vascular system may be potentiated.

Beta-receptor blocking agents and albuterol inhibit the effect of each other.

Carcinogenesis, Mutagenesis, and Impairment of Fertility: Albuterol sulfate, like other agents in its class, caused a significant dose-related increase in the incidence of benign leiomyomas of the mesovarium in a 2-year study in the rat, at doses corresponding to 3, 16, and 78 times the maximum human oral dose. In another study, this effect was blocked by the coadministration of propranolol. The relevance of these findings to humans is not known. An 18-month study in mice and a lifetime study in hamsters revealed no evidence of tumorigenicity.

Studies with albuterol revealed no evidence of mutagenesis. Reproduction studies in rats revealed no evidence of impaired fertility.

Teratogenic Effects—Pregnancy Category C: Albuterol has been shown to be teratogenic in mice when given subcutaneously in doses corresponding to 0.4 times the maximum human oral dose. There are no adequate and well-controlled studies in pregnant women. Albuterol should be used during pregnancy only if the potential benefit justifies the potential risk to the fetus. A reproduction study in CD-1 mice with albuterol showed cleft palate formation in 5 of 111 (4.5%) fetuses at 0.25 mg/kg and in 10 of 108 (9.3%) fetuses at 2.5 mg/kg; none were observed at 0.025 mg/kg. Cleft palate also occurred in 22 of 72 (30.5%) fetuses treated with 2.5 mg/kg isoproterenol (positive control). A reproduction study in Stride Dutch rabbits revealed cranioschisis in 7 of 19 (37%) fetuses at 50 mg/kg, corresponding to 78 times the maximum human oral dose of albuterol.

Labor and Delivery: Oral albuterol has been shown to delay preterm labor in some reports. There are presently no well-controlled studies which demonstrate that it will stop preterm labor or prevent labor at term. Therefore, cautious use of PROVENTIL REPETABS Tablets and PROVENTIL Tablets is required in pregnant patients when given for relief of bronchospasm so as to avoid interference with uterine contractibility.

Nursing Mothers: It is not known whether this drug is excreted in human milk. Because of the potential for tumorigenicity shown for albuterol in some animal studies, a decision should be made whether to discontinue nursing or to discontinue the drug, taking into account the importance of the drug to the mother.

Pediatric Use: Safety and effectiveness in children below the age of 6 years for PROVENTIL Tablets, and below the age of 12 years for PROVENTIL REPETABS Tablets have not been established.

ADVERSE REACTIONS
The adverse reactions to albuterol are similar in nature to those of other sympathomimetic agents. The most frequent adverse reactions to PROVENTIL Tablets were nervousness and tremor, with each occurring in approximately 20 of 100 patients (20%). Other reported reactions were headache, 7 of 100 patients (7%); tachycardia and palpitations, 5 of 100 patients (5%); muscle cramps, 3 of 100 patients (3%); insomnia, nausea, weakness, and dizziness, each occurred in 2 of 100 patients (2%). Drowsiness, flushing, restlessness, irritability, chest discomfort, and difficulty in micturition each occurred in less than 1 of 100 patients (less than 1%).

In a clinical study of one week duration comparing a 4 mg PROVENTIL REPETABS Tablet administered every 12 hours, to a 2 mg PROVENTIL Tablet administered every 6 hours, the following adverse reactions considered to be possibly or probably treatment related were reported: nervousness in 1 of 50 (2%) and 3 of 50 patients (6%) for PROVENTIL REPETABS and PROVENTIL Tablets, respectively; nausea in 2 of 50 (4%) for both; vomiting in 1 of 50 (2%) and 2 of 50 (4%) for PROVENTIL REPETABS and PROVENTIL Tablets, respectively; somnolence in 1 of 50 (2%) for both. The following adverse reactions were reported for PROVENTIL Tablets only, tremor in 3 of 50 patients (6%), tinnitus, dyspepsia, and rash each occurred in 1 of 50 patients (2%). Although not reported for PROVENTIL REPETABS Tablets in the above study, there have been reports of tremor in other trials. When all clinical experience is considered, the incidence of tremor is approximately the same as that seen with PROVENTIL Tablets.

In addition to those adverse reactions reported above, albuterol, like other sympathomimetic agents, can cause adverse reactions such as hypertension, angina, vomiting, vertigo, central nervous system stimulation, unusual taste, and drying or irritation of the oropharynx.

The reactions are generally transient in nature, and it is usually not necessary to discontinue treatment with PROVENTIL REPETABS Tablets or PROVENTIL Tablets. In selected cases, however, dosage may be reduced temporarily; after the reaction has subsided, dosage should be increased in small increments to the optimal dosage.

OVERDOSAGE
Manifestations of overdosage include anginal pain, hypertension, hypokalemia and exaggeration of the pharmacological effects listed in ADVERSE REACTIONS.

The oral LD_{50} in rats and mice was greater than 2,000 mg/kg.

There is insufficient evidence to determine if dialysis is beneficial for overdosage of PROVENTIL REPETABS Tablets or PROVENTIL Tablets.

DOSAGE AND ADMINISTRATION
The following dosages of PROVENTIL REPETABS Tablets and PROVENTIL Tablets are expressed in terms of albuterol base.

PROVENTIL REPETABS Tablets
Usual Dose The usual starting dosage of PROVENTIL REPETABS Tablets for adults and children 12 years and over is 4 or 8 mg (one or two tablets) every 12 hours.

Dosage Adjustment Doses above 8 mg twice a day of PROVENTIL REPETABS Tablets should be used only when the patient fails to respond. If a favorable response does not occur with the 4 mg initial dosage, it should be cautiously increased stepwise up to a maximum of 16 mg twice a day. The total daily dose should not exceed 32 mg in adults and children 12 years and over.

Switching to PROVENTIL REPETABS Tablets Patients currently maintained on PROVENTIL Tablets can be switched to PROVENTIL REPETABS Tablets. For example, the administration of a 4 mg PROVENTIL REPETABS Tablet every 12 hours is equivalent to one 2 mg PROVENTIL Tablet every 6 hours. Multiples of this regimen up to the maximum recommended daily dose also apply.

PROVENTIL Tablets
Usual Dose The usual starting dosage for children 6 to 12 years of age is 2 mg three or four times a day.

The usual starting dosage for adults and children 12 years and over is 2 mg or 4 mg three or four times a day.

Dosage Adjustment For children from 6 to 12 years of age who fail to respond to the initial starting dosage of 2 mg four times a day, the dosage may be cautiously increased stepwise, but not to exceed 24 mg per day (given in divided doses). For adults and children 12 years and over, a dosage above 4 mg four times a day should be used only when the patient fails to respond. If a favorable response does not occur with the 4 mg initial dosage, it should be cautiously increased stepwise up to a maximum of 8 mg four times a day as tolerated.

Elderly Patients and Those Sensitive to Beta-Adrenergic Stimulators An initial dose of 2 mg three or four times a day is recommended for elderly patients and for those with a history of unusual sensitivity to beta-adrenergic stimulators. If adequate bronchodilation is not obtained, dosage may be increased gradually to as much as 8 mg three or four times a day.

The total daily dose should not exceed 32 mg in adults and children 12 years and over.

HOW SUPPLIED
PROVENTIL REPETABS Tablets, 4 mg albuterol as the sulfate (2 mg in the coating for immediate release and 2 mg in the core for release after several hours), white, round, coated tablets, branded in red on one side with the Schering trademark, and product identifications numbers, 431, bottles of 100 (NDC 0085-0431-02) and boxes of 100 for unit dose dispensing (NDC 0085-0431-04).

PROVENTIL Tablets, 2 mg albuterol as the sulfate, white, round, compressed tablets, impressed with the product name (PROVENTIL) and the number 2 on one side, and product identification numbers, 252, and scored on the other, bottles of 100 (NDC 0085-0252-02) and 500 (NDC 0085-0252-03).

PROVENTIL Tablets, 4 mg albuterol as the sulfate, white, round, compressed tablets, impressed with the product name (PROVENTIL) and the number 4 on one side, and product identification numbers, 573, and scored on the other, bottles of 100 (NDC 0085-0573-02) and 500 (NDC 0085-0573-03).

Store PROVENTIL REPETABS Tablets and PROVENTIL Tablets between 2° and 30°C (36° and 86°F). Protect PROVENTIL REPETABS Tablets in the unit dose box from excessive moisture.

Shown in Product Identification Section, page 428

Sodium SULAMYD®   ℞

[*so'dē-um soo'lah-mĭd*]

brand of sulfacetamide sodium

   Ophthalmic Solution, USP 30%—Sterile
   Ophthalmic Solution, USP 10%—Sterile
   Ophthalmic Ointment, USP 10%—Sterile

DESCRIPTION
Sodium SULAMYD is available in three ophthalmic forms: **Ophthalmic Solution 30%** contains in each ml of sterile aqueous solution 300 mg sulfacetamide sodium, USP, 1.5 mg sodium thiosulfate, with 0.5 mg methylparaben and 0.1 mg

Continued on next page

Information on Schering products appearing on these pages is effective as of September 30, 1989.

Schering—Cont.

propylparaben added as preservatives, and monobasic sodium phosphate as buffer.

Ophthalmic Solution 10% contains in each ml of sterile aqueous solution 100 mg sulfacetamide sodium, USP, 3.1 mg sodium thiosulfate, and 5 mg methylcellulose, with 0.5 mg methylparaben and 0.1 mg propylparaben added as preservatives and monobasic sodium phosphate as buffer.

Ophthalmic Ointment 10% is a sterile ointment, each gram containing 100 mg sulfacetamide sodium, USP, with 0.5 mg methylparaben, 0.1 mg propylparaben and 0.25 mg benzalkonium chloride added as preservatives, and sorbitan monolaurate and water in a bland, unctuous, petrolatum base.

ACTIONS

Sodium SULAMYD exerts a bacteriostatic effect against a wide range of gram-positive and gram-negative microorganisms by restricting, through competition with para-aminobenzoic acid, the synthesis of folic acid which bacteria require for growth.

INDICATIONS

Sodium SULAMYD is indicated for the treatment of conjunctivitis, corneal ulcer, and other superficial ocular infections due to susceptible microorganisms, and as adjunctive treatment in systemic sulfonamide therapy of trachoma.

CONTRAINDICATIONS

Sodium SULAMYD is contraindicated in individuals with known or suspected sensitivity to sulfonamides or to any of the ingredients of the preparations.

PRECAUTIONS

Sodium SULAMYD products are incompatible with silver preparations. Ophthalmic ointments may retard corneal healing. Non-susceptible organisms, including fungi, may proliferate with the use of these preparations. Sulfonamides are inactivated by the para-aminobenzoic acid present in purulent exudates.

Sensitization may recur when a sulfonamide is re-administered irrespective of the route of administration, and cross sensitivity between different sulfonamides may occur. If signs of sensitivity or other untoward reactions occur, discontinue use of the preparation.

ADVERSE REACTIONS

Sulfacetamide sodium may cause local irritation, stinging and burning. While the irritation may be transient, occasionally, use of the medication has to be discontinued.

Although sensitivity reactions to sulfacetamide sodium are rare, an isolated incident of Stevens-Johnson syndrome was reported in a patient who had experienced a previous bullous drug reaction to an orally administered sulfonamide and a single instance of local hypersensitivity was reported which progressed to a fatal syndrome resembling systemic lupus erythematosus.

DOSAGE AND ADMINISTRATION

Sodium SULAMYD Ophthalmic Solution 30%. *For conjunctivitis or corneal ulcer:* instill one drop into lower conjunctival sac every two hours or less frequently according to severity of infection. *For trachoma:* Two drops every two hours; concomitant systemic sulfonamide therapy is indicated.

Sodium SULAMYD Ophthalmic Solution 10%. One or two drops into the lower conjunctival sac every two or three hours during the day and less often at night.

Sodium SULAMYD Ophthalmic Ointment 10%. Apply a small amount four times daily and at bedtime. The ointment may be used adjunctively with either of the solution forms.

HOW SUPPLIED

Sodium SULAMYD Ophthalmic Ointment 10%, 3.5 g tube (NDC 0085-0066-03), box of one. **Store away from heat.**

Sodium SULAMYD Ophthalmic Solution 30%, 15 ml dropper bottle (NDC 0085-0717-06), box of one. **Store between 2° and 30°C (36° and 86°F).**

Sodium SULAMYD Ophthalmic Solution 10%, 5 ml dropper bottle (NDC 0085-0946-03), box of 25; 15 ml dropper bottle (NDC 0085-0946-06), box of one. **Store between 2° and 30°C (36° and 86°F).**

On long standing, sulfonamide solutions will darken in color and should be discarded.

Revised 10/84

SOLGANAL®   ℞

[sol'gah-nal]
brand of sterile aurothioglucose
Suspension, USP
FOR INTRAMUSCULAR
INJECTION ONLY—
NOT FOR INTRAVENOUS USE

WARNINGS

> Physicians planning to use SOLGANAL Suspension should thoroughly familiarize themselves with its toxicity and its benefits. The possibility of toxic reactions should always be explained to the patient before starting therapy. Patients should be warned to report promptly any symptom suggesting toxicity. Before **each** injection of SOLGANAL Suspension, the physician should review the results of laboratory work and see the patient to determine the presence or absence of adverse reactions, since some of these can be severe or even fatal.

DESCRIPTION

SOLGANAL is a sterile suspension, for **intramuscular injection only.** SOLGANAL Suspension is an antiarthritic agent which is absorbed gradually following intramuscular injection, producing a therapeutically desired prolonged effect. Each ml contains 50 mg of aurothioglucose, USP in sterile sesame oil with 2% aluminum monostearate; 1 mg propylparaben is added as preservative. Aurothioglucose contains approximately 50% gold by weight.

The empirical formula for aurothioglucose is $C_6H_{11}AuO_5S$; the molecular weight is 392.18. Chemically it is (1-Thio-D-glucopyranosato) gold.

Aurothioglucose is a nearly odorless, yellow powder which is stable in air. An aqueous solution is unstable on long standing. Aurothioglucose is freely soluble in water but practically insoluble in acetone, in alcohol, in chloroform, and in ether.

CLINICAL PHARMACOLOGY

Although the mechanism of action is not well understood, gold compounds have been reported to decrease synovial inflammation and retard cartilage and bone destruction.

Gold is absorbed from injection sites, reaching peak concentration in blood in four to six hours. Following a single intramuscular injection of 50 mg SOLGANAL Suspension in each of two patients, peak serum levels were about 235 mcg/dl in one patient and 450 mcg/dl in the other. In plasma, 95% is bound to the albumin fraction. Approximately 70% of the gold is eliminated in the urine and approximately 30% in the feces. When a standard weekly treatment schedule is followed, approximately 40% of the administered dose is excreted each week, and the remainder is excreted over a longer period. The biological half-life of gold salts following a single 50 mg dose has been reported to range from 3 to 27 days. Following successive weekly doses, the half-life increases and may be 14 to 40 days after the third dose and up to 168 days after the eleventh weekly dose.

After the initial injection, the serum level of gold rises sharply and declines over the next week. Peak levels with aqueous preparations are higher and decline faster than those with oily preparations. Weekly administration produces a continuous rise in the basal value for several months, after which the serum level becomes relatively stable. After a standard weekly dose, considerable individual variation in the levels of gold has been found. A steady decline in gold levels occurs when the interval between injections is lengthened, and small amounts may be found in the serum for months after discontinuance of therapy. The incidence of toxic reactions is apparently unrelated to the plasma level of gold, but it may be related to the cumulative body content of gold.

Storage of gold in human tissues is dependent upon organ mass as well as upon the concentration of gold. Therefore, tissues having the highest gold levels (weight/weight) do not necessarily contain the greatest total amounts of gold. The major depots, in decreasing order of total gold content, are the bone marrow, liver, skin, and bone, accounting for approximately 85% of body gold. The highest concentrations of gold are found in the lymph nodes, adrenal glands, liver, kidneys, bone marrow, and spleen. Relatively small concentrations are found in articular structures.

Gold passes the blood-brain barrier in hamsters.

Transfer of gold across the human placenta at the twentieth week of pregnancy has been documented. The placenta showed numerous gold deposits and smaller amounts were detected in the fetal liver and kidneys; other tissues provided no evidence of gold deposition.

Gold is excreted into human milk in significant amounts and trace amounts can be demonstrated in the blood of nursing infants. (See PRECAUTIONS, "Nursing Mothers.")

INDICATIONS AND USAGE

SOLGANAL Suspension is indicated for the adjunctive treatment of early active rheumatoid arthritis (both of the adult and juvenile types) not adequately controlled by other anti-inflammatory agents and conservative measures. In chronic, advanced cases of rheumatoid arthritis, gold therapy is less valuable.

Antirheumatic measures such as salicylates and other anti-inflammatory drugs (both steroidal and non-steroidal) may be continued after initiation of gold therapy. After improvement commences, these measures may be discontinued slowly as symptoms permit.

See Precautions, "*Laboratory Tests*" and **Dosage and Administration.**

CONTRAINDICATIONS

A history of known hypersensitivity to any component of SOLGANAL Suspension contraindicates its use. Gold therapy is contraindicated in patients with uncontrolled diabetes mellitus, severe debilitation, systemic lupus erythematosus, renal disease, hepatic dysfunction, uncontrolled congestive heart failure, marked hypertension, agranulocytosis, other blood dyscrasias, or hemorrhagic diathesis; or if there is a history of infectious hepatitis. Patients who recently have had radiation, and those who have developed severe toxicity from previous exposure to gold or other heavy metals should not receive SOLGANAL Suspension.

Urticaria, eczema, and colitis are also contraindications.

Gold therapy is usually contraindicated in pregnancy. (See PRECAUTIONS, "*Usage in Pregnancy*".)

Gold salts should not be used with penicillamine (See MANAGEMENT OF ADVERSE REACTIONS) or antimalarials. The safety of coadministration with immunosuppressive agents other than corticosteroids has not been established.

WARNINGS

The following signs should be considered danger signals of gold toxicity, and no additional injection should be given unless further studies reveal some other cause for their presence: rapid reduction of hemoglobin, leukopenia (WBC below 4000/cu mm), eosinophilia above 5%, platelet count below 100,000/cu mm, albuminuria, hematuria, pruritus, dermatitis, stomatitis, jaundice, and petechiae.

Effects that may occur immediately following an injection, or at any time during gold therapy, include: anaphylactic shock, syncope, bradycardia, thickening of the tongue, difficulty in swallowing and breathing, and angioneurotic edema. If such effects are observed, treatment with SOLGANAL Suspension should be discontinued.

Tolerance to gold usually decreases with advancing age. Diabetes mellitus or congestive heart failure should be under control before gold therapy is instituted.

SOLGANAL Suspension should be used with extreme caution in patients with: skin rash, hypersensitivity to other medications, or a history of renal or liver disease.

PRECAUTIONS

General: Before **each** injection, the physician should personally check the patient for adverse reactions and inquiry should be made regarding pruritus, rash, sore mouth, indigestion, and metallic taste. The patient should be observed for at least 15 minutes following each injection. (See also "*Laboratory Tests*".)

Patients with HLA-D locus histocompatibility antigens DRw2 and DRw3 may have a genetic predisposition to develop certain toxic reactions, such as proteinuria, during treatment with gold or D-penicillamine.

SOLGANAL Suspension should be used with caution in patients with compromised cardiovascular or cerebral circulation.

Information for Patients:

1. Promptly report to the physician any unusual symptoms such as pruritus (itching), rash, sore mouth, indigestion, or metallic taste.
2. Increased joint pain may occur for one or two days after an injection and usually subsides after the first few injections.
3. Exposure to sunlight or artificial ultraviolet light should be minimized.
4. Careful oral hygiene is recommended in conjunction with therapy.
5. Patients should be aware of potential hazards if they become pregnant while receiving gold therapy. (See "*Usage in Pregnancy*".)

Laboratory Tests: Before treatment is started, a complete blood count, platelet count, and urinalysis should be done to serve as reference points. Since gold therapy is usually contraindicated in pregnant patients, pregnancy should be ruled out before treatment is started. Throughout the treatment period, urinalysis should be repeated prior to each injection, and complete blood cell and platelet counts should be performed every two weeks. A platelet count is indicated any time that purpura or ecchymosis occurs.

Drug Interactions: Drug interactions have not been reported. (See **Contraindications**.)

Carcinogenesis, Mutagenesis, and Impairment of Fertility: Renal adenomas developed in rats receiving an injectable gold product similar to SOLGANAL Suspension at doses of 2 mg/kg weekly for 46 weeks, followed by 6 mg/kg daily for 47 weeks. These doses were higher and administered more frequently than the recommended human doses. The adenomas were similar histologically to those produced by chronic administration of other gold compounds and heavy metals, such as lead or nickel.

Renal tubular cell neoplasia consisting of renal adenoma and adenocarcinoma were noted in a dose-response relationship in another study in rats using daily intramuscular doses of 3 mg/kg and 6 mg/kg for up to 2 years. These doses were higher and were administered more frequently than the recommended human doses. In this same study, sarcomas at the injection site occurred in some rats but their numbers were not sufficient to demonstrate a dose-response relationship.

No report of renal adenoma or sarcoma at the injection site in man in association with the use of SOLGANAL Suspension has been received.

Gold compounds have not been studied for evaluation of mutagenesis.

Gold sodium thiomalate given subcutaneously did not adversely affect fertility or reproductive performance.

Usage in Pregnancy: Gold therapy is usually contraindicated in pregnant patients. The patient should be warned about the hazards of becoming pregnant while on gold therapy. Rheumatoid arthritis frequently improves when the patient becomes pregnant, thereby eliminating the need for gold therapy. The potential nephrotoxicity of gold should not be superimposed on the increased renal burden which normally occurs in pregnancy and hence, gold therapy should be discontinued upon recognition of pregnancy unless continued use is required in an individual case. The slow excretion of gold and its persistence in body tissues after discontinuation of treatment should be kept in mind when a woman of child-bearing potential being treated with gold plans to become pregnant.

Pregnancy Category C: Gold sodium thiomalate administered subcutaneously, a route not used clinically, has been shown to be teratogenic during the organogenic period in rats and rabbits when given in doses 140 and 175 times, respectively, the usual human dose. Hydrocephalus and microphthalmia were the malformations observed in rats when gold sodium thiomalate was administered at a dose of 25 mg/kg/day from day 6 through day 15 of gestation. In rabbits, limb defects and gastroschisis were the malformations observed when gold sodium thiomalate was administered at doses of 20 to 45 mg/kg/day from day 6 through day 18 of gestation.

Gold compounds administered orally to rabbits from days 6 through 18 of pregnancy resulted in the occurrence of abdominal defects, such as gastroschisis and umbilical hernia; anomalies of the brain, heart, lung, and skeleton; and microphthalmia.

The administration of excessive doses of gold-containing compounds during pregnancy in the above studies was toxic to the mothers and their embryos; the embryotoxic effects probably were secondary to maternal toxicity. Therefore, the significance of these findings in relation to human use is unknown.

There are no adequate and well-controlled studies with SOLGANAL Suspension in pregnant women. Extensive clinical experience with SOLGANAL Suspension has not demonstrated human teratogenicity.

Nursing Mothers: Gold has been demonstated in the milk of lactating mothers. In one patient, a total dose of 135 mg of gold thioglucose was given during the postpartum period. Samples of the maternal milk and urine, and samples of red blood cells and serum of the mother and child were evaluated by atomic absorption spectrophotometry. Trace amounts of gold appeared in the serum and red blood cells of the nursing offspring. It has been postulated that this may be the cause of unexplained rashes, nephritis, hepatitis, and hematologic aberrations in the nursing infants of mothers treated with gold. Because of the potential for serious adverse reactions in nursing infants, a decision should be made whether to discontinue nursing or to discontinue the gold therapy, taking into account the importance of the drug to the mother. The slow excretion of gold and its persistence in the mother after discontinuation of treatment should be kept in mind.

Pediatric Use: Safety and effectiveness in children below the age of six years have not been established.

ADVERSE REACTIONS

Adverse reactions to gold therapy may occur at any time during treatment or many months after therapy has been discontinued. The incidence of toxic reactions is apparently unrelated to the plasma level of gold, but it may be related to the cumulative body content of gold. Higher than conventional dosage schedules may increase the occurrence and severity of toxicity. Severe effects are most common after 300 to 500 mg have been administered.

Cutaneous Reactions: Dermatitis is the most common reaction. Pruritus should be considered a warning signal of an impending cutaneous reaction. Erythema and occasionally the more severe reactions such as papular, vesicular, and exfoliative dermatitis leading to alopecia and shedding of the nails may occur. Chrysiasis (gray-to-blue pigmentation) has been reported, especially on photoexposed areas. Gold dermatitis may be aggravated by exposure to sunlight, or an actinic rash may develop.

Mucous Membrane Reactions: Stomatitis is the second most common adverse reaction. Shallow ulcers on the buccal membranes, on the borders of the tongue and on the palate, diffuse glossitis, or gingivitis may be preceded by the sensation of metallic taste. Careful oral hygiene is recommended. Inflammation of the upper respiratory tract, pharyngitis, gastritis, colitis, tracheitis, and vaginitis have also been reported. Conjunctivitis is rare.

Renal Reactions: Nephrotic syndrome or glomerulitis with hematuria, which is usually relatively mild, subsides completely if recognized early and treatment is discontinued. These reactions become severe and chronic if gold therapy is continued after their onset. Therefore, it is important to perform a urinalysis before each injection and to discontinue treatment promptly if proteinuria or hematuria develops.

Hematologic Reactions: Although rare, blood dyscrasias, including granulocytopenia, agranulocytosis, thrombocytopenia with or without purpura, leukopenia, eosinophilia, panmyelopathy, hemorrhagic diathesis, and hypoplastic and aplastic anemia, have been reported. These reactions may occur separately or in combination.

Nitritoid and Allergic Reactions: These reactions, which may rarely occur with SOLGANAL Suspension and which resemble anaphylactoid effects, include flushing, fainting, dizziness, sweating, malaise, weakness, nausea, and vomiting.

Miscellaneous Reactions: On rare occasions, gastrointestinal symptoms, i.e., nausea, vomiting, colic, anorexia, abdominal cramps, diarrhea, ulcerative enterocolitis, and headache have been reported.

There have been rare reports of iritis and corneal ulcers. Transient, asymptomatic gold deposits in the cornea or conjunctiva may occur.

Other reported reactions include encephalitis, immunological destruction of the synovia, EEG abnormalities, intrahepatic cholestasis, hepatitis with jaundice, toxic hepatitis, acute yellow atrophy, peripheral neuritis, gold bronchitis, pulmonary injury manifested by interstitial pneumonitis or fibrosis, fever, and partial or complete hair loss.

Less common but more severe effects that may occur shortly after an injection or at any time during gold therapy include: anaphylactic shock, syncope, bradycardia, thickening of the tongue, difficulty in swallowing and breathing, and angioneurotic edema. If they are observed, treatment with SOLGANAL Suspension should be discontinued.

Arthralgia may occur for one or two days after an injection and usually subsides after the first few injections. The mechanism of the transient increase in rheumatic symptoms after injection of gold (the so-called nonvasomotor postinjection reaction) is unknown. These reactions are usually mild but occasionally may be so severe that treatment is stopped prematurely.

MANAGEMENT OF ADVERSE REACTIONS

In the event of toxic reactions, gold therapy should be discontinued immediately.

In the presence of mild reactions, it may be sufficient to discontinue the administration of SOLGANAL Suspension for a short period and then to resume treatment with smaller doses.

Dermatitis and pruritus may respond to soothing lotions, other appropriate antipruritic treatment, or topical glucocorticoids.

If dermatitis or stomatitis becomes severe or spreads, systemic glucocorticoid treatment may be indicated. For renal, hematologic, and most other adverse reactions, glucocorticoids may be required in larger doses and for a longer time than for dermatologic reactions. Often this treatment may be required for many months because of the slow elimination of gold from the body.

If severe adverse reactions do not improve with steroid treatment in patients who receive large doses of gold, a chelating agent, such as dimercaprol (BAL), may be used. In one case, it was reported that penicillamine was beneficial in the treatment of gold-induced thrombocytopenia. Adjunctive use of an anabolic steroid with other drugs (i.e., BAL, penicillamine, and corticosteroids) may contribute to recovery of bone marrow deficiency.

In the presence of severe or idiosyncratic reactions, treatment with SOLGANAL Suspension should not be reinstituted.

OVERDOSAGE

Overdosage resulting from too rapid increases in dosing with SOLGANAL Suspension will be manifested by rapid appearance of toxic reactions, particularly those relating to renal damage, such as hematuria, proteinuria, and to hematologic effects, such as thrombocytopenia and granulocytopenia. Other toxic effects, including fever, nausea, vomiting, diarrhea, and various skin disorders such as papulovesicular lesions, urticaria, and exfoliative dermatitis, all attended with severe pruritus, may develop. Treatment consists of prompt discontinuation of the medication, and early administration of dimercaprol. Specific supportive therapy should be given for the renal and hematologic complications. (See also MANAGEMENT OF ADVERSE REACTIONS above).

DOSAGE AND ADMINISTRATION

Adults—The usual dosage schedule for the intramuscular administration of SOLGANAL is as follows: first dose, 10 mg; second and third doses, 25 mg; fourth and subsequent doses, 50 mg. The interval between doses is one week. The 50 mg dose is continued at weekly intervals until 0.8 to 1.0 g SOLGANAL has been given. If the patient has improved and has exhibited no sign of toxicity, the 50 mg dose may be continued many months longer, at three- to four-week intervals. A weekly dose above 50 mg is usually unnecessary and contraindicated; the tendency in gold therapy is toward lower dosage. With this in mind, it may eventually be established that a 25 mg dose is the one of choice. If no improvement has been demonstrated after a total administration of 1.0 g of SOLGANAL Suspension, the necessity for gold therapy should be reevaluated.

Children 6 to 12 years—one-fourth of the adult dose, governed chiefly by body weight, not to exceed 25 mg per dose. SOLGANAL Suspension should be injected **intramuscularly,** (preferably intragluteally), **never intravenously.** The patient should be lying down and should remain recumbent for approximately 10 minutes after the injection. The vial should be thoroughly shaken in order to suspend all of the active material. Heating the vial to body temperature (by immersion in warm water) will facilitate drawing the suspension into the syringe. An 18-gauge, 1½-inch needle is recommended for depositing the preparation deep into the muscular tissue. For obese patients, an 18-gauge, 2-inch needle may be used. The site usually selected for injection is the upper outer quadrant of the gluteal region.

NOTE: Shake the vial in horizontal position before the dose is withdrawn. Needle and syringe must be dry. The patient should be observed for at least 15 minutes following each injection.

HOW SUPPLIED

SOLGANAL Suspension is available in 10 ml multiple-dose vials containing 5% (50 mg/ml) aurothioglucose; box of one. **Shake well before using. Store between 0° and 30°C (32° and 86°F). Protect from light. Store in carton until contents are used.**

Copyright © 1963, 1984, Schering Corporation, USA. All rights reserved.

TRILAFON®   ℞

[*tri'lah-fon*]
brand of perphenazine, USP
   Tablets
   Concentrate
   Injection

DESCRIPTION

TRILAFON products contain perphenazine, USP (4-[3-(2-chlorophenothiazin-10-yl)propyl]-1-piperazineethanol), a piperazinyl phenothiazine having the chemical formula, $C_{21}H_{26}ClN_3OS$. It is available as **Tablets,** 2, 4, 8 and 16 mg; **Concentrate,** 16 mg perphenazine per 5 mL and alcohol less than 0.1%; and **Injection,** perphenazine 5 mg per 1 mL.

The inactive ingredients for TRILAFON **Tablets,** 2, 4, 8 and 16 mg. include: acacia, black iron oxide, butylparaben, calcium phosphate, calcium sulfate, carnauba wax, corn starch, gelatin, lactose, magnesium stearate, potato starch, sugar, titanium dioxide, white wax and other ingredients. May also contain talc.

The inactive ingredients for TRILAFON **Concentrate** include: alcohol, citric acid, flavors, menthol, sodium phosphate, sorbitol, sugar, and water.

The inactive ingredients for TRILAFON **Injection** include: citric acid, sodium bisulfite, sodium hydroxide, and water.

ACTIONS

Perphenazine has actions at all levels of the central nervous system, particularly the hypothalamus. However, the site and mechanism of action of therapeutic effect are not known.

INDICATIONS

Perphenazine is indicated for use in the management of the manifestations of psychotic disorders; and for the control of severe nausea and vomiting in adults.

Continued on next page

Information on Schering products appearing on these pages is effective as of September 30, 1989.

Schering—Cont.

TRILAFON has not been shown effective in the management of behavioral complications in patients with mental retardation.

CONTRAINDICATIONS

TRILAFON products are contraindicated in comatose or greatly obtunded patients and in patients receiving large doses of central nervous system depressants (barbiturates, alcohol, narcotics, analgesics, or antihistamines); in the presence of existing blood dyscrasias, bone marrow depression, or liver damage; and in patients who have shown hypersensitivity to TRILAFON products, their components, or related compounds.

TRILAFON products are also contraindicated in patients with suspected or established subcortical brain damage, with or without hypothalamic damage, since a hyperthermic reaction with temperatures in excess of 104°F may occur in such patients, sometimes not until 14 to 16 hours after drug administration. Total body ice-packing is recommended for such a reaction; antipyretics may also be useful.

WARNINGS

Tardive dyskinesia, a syndrome consisting of potentially irreversible, involuntary, dyskinetic movements, may develop in patients treated with neuroleptic (antipsychotic) drugs. Although the prevalence of the syndrome appears to be highest among the elderly, especially elderly women, it is impossible to rely upon prevalence estimates to predict, at the inception of neuroleptic treatment, which patients are likely to develop the syndrome. Whether neuroleptic drug products differ in their potential to cause tardive dyskinesia is unknown.

Both the risk of developing the syndrome and the likelihood that it will become irreversible are believed to increase as the duration of treatment and the total cumulative dose of neuroleptic drugs administered to the patient increase. However, the syndrome can develop, although much less commonly, after relatively brief treatment periods at low doses.

There is no known treatment for established cases of tardive dyskinesia, although the syndrome may remit, partially or completely, if neuroleptic treatment is withdrawn. Neuroleptic treatment itself, however, may suppress (or partially suppress) the signs and symptoms of the syndrome, and thereby may possibly mask the underlying disease process. The effect that symptomatic suppression has upon the long-term course of the syndrome is unknown.

Given these considerations, neuroleptics should be prescribed in a manner that is most likely to minimize the occurrence of tardive dyskinesia. Chronic neuroleptic treatment should generally be reserved for patients who suffer from a chronic illness that, 1) is known to respond to neuroleptic drugs, and 2) for whom alternative, equally effective, but potentially less harmful treatments are not available or appropriate. In patients who do require chronic treatment, the smallest dose and the shortest duration of treatment producing a satisfactory clinical response should be sought. The need for continued treatment should be reassessed periodically.

If signs and symptoms of tardive dyskinesia appear in a patient on neuroleptics, drug discontinuation should be considered. However, some patients may require treatment despite the presence of the syndrome.

(For further information about the description of tardive dyskinesia and its clinical detection, please refer to **Information for Patients** and **Adverse Reactions**.)

TRILAFON **Injection** contains sodium bisulfite, a sulfite that may cause allergic-type reactions including anaphylactic symptoms and life-threatening or less severe asthmatic episodes in certain susceptible people. The overall prevalence of sulfite sensitivity is seen more frequently in asthmatic than in non-asthmatic people.

NEUROLEPTIC MALIGNANT SYNDROME (NMS)

A potentially fatal symptom complex sometimes referred to as Neuroleptic Malignant Syndrome (NMS) has been reported in association with antipsychotic drugs. Clinical manifestations of NMS are hyperpyrexia, muscle rigidity, altered mental status and evidence of autonomic instability (irregular pulse or blood pressure, tachycardia, diaphoresis, and cardiac dysrhythmias).

The diagnostic evaluation of patients with this syndrome is complicated. In arriving at a diagnosis, it is important to identify cases where the clinical presentation includes both serious medical illness (e.g., pneumonia, systemic infection, etc.) and untreated or inadequately treated extrapyramidal signs and symptoms (EPS). Other important considerations in the differential diagnosis include central anticholinergic toxicity, heat stroke, drug fever and primary central nervous system (CNS) pathology.

The management of NMS should include 1) immediate discontinuation of antipsychotic drugs and other drugs not essential to concurrent therapy, 2) intensive symptomatic treatment and medical monitoring, and 3) treatment of any concomitant serious medical problems for which specific treatments are available. There is no general agreement about specific pharmacological treatment regimens for uncomplicated NMS.

If a patient requires antipsychotic drug treatment after recovery from NMS, the potential reintroduction of drug therapy should be carefully considered. The patient should be carefully monitored, since recurrences of NMS have been reported.

If hypotension develops, epinephrine should not be administered since its action is blocked and partially reversed by perphenazine. If a vasopressor is needed, norepinephrine may be used. Severe, acute hypotension has occurred with the use of phenothiazines and is particularly likely to occur in patients with mitral insufficiency or pheochromocytoma. Rebound hypertension may occur in pheochromocytoma patients.

TRILAFON products can lower the convulsive threshold in susceptible individuals; they should be used with caution in alcohol withdrawal and in patients with convulsive disorders. If the patient is being treated with an anticonvulsant agent, increased dosage of that agent may be required when TRILAFON products are used concomitantly.

TRILAFON products should be used with caution in patients with psychic depression.

Perphenazine may impair the mental and/or physical abilities required for the performance of hazardous tasks such as driving a car or operating machinery; therefore, the patient should be warned accordingly.

TRILAFON products are not recommended for children under 12 years of age.

Usage in Pregnancy: Safe use of TRILAFON during pregnancy and lactation has not been established; therefore, in administering the drug to pregnant patients, nursing mothers, or women who may become pregnant, the possible benefits must be weighed against the possible hazards to mother and child.

PRECAUTIONS

The possibility of suicide in depressed patients remains during treatment and until significant remission occurs. This type of patient should not have access to large quantities of this drug.

As with all phenothiazine compounds, perphenazine should not be used indiscriminately. Caution should be observed in giving it to patients who have previously exhibited severe adverse reactions to other phenothiazines. Some of the untoward actions of perphenazine tend to appear more frequently when high doses are used. However, as with other phenothiazine compounds, patients receiving TRILAFON products in any dosage should be kept under close supervision.

Neuroleptic drugs elevate prolactin levels; the elevation persists during chronic administration. Tissue culture experiments indicate that approximately one-third of human breast cancers are prolactin dependent *in vitro*, a factor of potential importance if the prescription of these drugs is contemplated in a patient with a previously detected breast cancer. Although disturbances such as galactorrhea, amenorrhea, gynecomastia, and impotence have been reported, the clinical significance of elevated serum prolactin levels is unknown for most patients. An increase in mammary neoplasms has been found in rodents after chronic administration of neuroleptic drugs. Neither clinical studies nor epidemiologic studies conducted to date, however, have shown an association between chronic administration of these drugs and mammary tumorigenesis; the available evidence is considered too limited to be conclusive at this time.

The antiemetic effect of perphenazine may obscure signs of toxicity due to overdosage of other drugs, or render more difficult the diagnosis of disorders such as brain tumors or intestinal obstruction.

A significant, not otherwise explained, rise in body temperature may suggest individual intolerance to perphenazine, in which case it should be discontinued.

Patients on large doses of a phenothiazine drug who are undergoing surgery should be watched carefully for possible hypotensive phenomena. Moreover, reduced amounts of anesthetics or central nervous system depressants may be necessary.

Since phenothiazines and central nervous system depressants (opiates, analgesics, antihistamines, barbiturates) can potentiate each other, less than the usual dosage of the added drug is recommended, and caution is advised, when they are administered concomitantly.

Use with caution in patients who are receiving atropine or related drugs because of additive anticholinergic effects and also in patients who will be exposed to extreme heat or phosphorus insecticides.

The use of alcohol should be avoided, since additive effects and hypotension may occur. Patients should be cautioned that their response to alcohol may be increased while they are being treated with TRILAFON products. The risk of suicide and the danger of overdose may be increased in patients who use alcohol excessively due to its potentiation of the drug's effect.

Blood counts and hepatic and renal functions should be checked periodically. The appearance of signs of blood dyscrasias requires the discontinuance of the drug and institution of appropriate therapy. If abnormalities in hepatic tests occur, phenothiazine treatment should be discontinued. Renal function in patients on long-term therapy should be monitored; if blood urea nitrogen (BUN) becomes abnormal, treatment with the drug should be discontinued.

The use of phenothiazine derivatives in patients with diminished renal function should be undertaken with caution.

Use with caution in patients suffering from respiratory impairment due to acute pulmonary infections, or in chronic respiratory disorders such as severe asthma or emphysema.

In general, phenothiazines, including perphenazine, do not produce psychic dependence. Gastritis, nausea and vomiting, dizziness, and tremulousness have been reported following abrupt cessation of high-dose therapy. Reports suggest that these symptoms can be reduced by continuing concomitant antiparkinson agents for several weeks after the phenothiazine is withdrawn.

The possibility of liver damage, corneal and lenticular deposits, and irreversible dyskinesias should be kept in mind when patients are on long-term therapy.

Because photosensitivity has been reported, undue exposure to the sun should be avoided during phenothiazine treatment.

Information for Patients: This information is intended to aid in the safe and effective use of this medication. It is not a disclosure of all possible adverse or intended effects.

Given the likelihood that a substantial proportion of patients exposed chronically to neuroleptics will develop tardive dyskinesia, it is advised that all patients in whom chronic use is contemplated be given, if possible, full information about this risk. The decision to inform patients and/or their guardians must obviously take into account the clinical circumstances and the competency of the patient to understand the information provided.

ADVERSE REACTIONS

Not all of the following adverse reactions have been reported with this specific drug; however, pharmacological similarities among various phenothiazine derivatives require that each be considered. In the case of the piperazine group (of which perphenazine is an example) the extrapyramidal symptoms are more common, and others (e.g., sedative effects, jaundice, and blood dyscrasias) are less frequently seen.

CNS Effects: *Extrapyramidal reactions:* opisthotonus, trismus, torticollis, retrocollis, aching and numbness of the limbs, motor restlessness, oculogyric crisis, hyperreflexia, dystonia, including protrusion, discoloration, aching and rounding of the tongue, tonic spasm of the masticatory muscles, tight feeling in the throat, slurred speech, dysphagia, akathisia, dyskinesia, parkinsonism, and ataxia. Their incidence and severity usually increase with an increase in dosage, but there is considerable individual variation in the tendency to develop such symptoms. Extrapyramidal symptoms can usually be controlled by the concomitant use of effective antiparkinsonian drugs, such as benztropine mesylate, and/or by reduction in dosage. In some instances, however, these extrapyramidal reactions may persist after discontinuation of treatment with perphenazine.

Persistent tardive dyskinesia: As with all antipsychotic agents, tardive dyskinesia may appear in some patients on long-term therapy or may appear after drug therapy has been discontinued. Although the risk appears to be greater in elderly patients on high-dose therapy, especially females, it may occur in either sex and in children. The symptoms are persistent and in some patients appear to be irreversible. The syndrome is characterized by rhythmical, involuntary movements of the tongue, face, mouth, or jaw (e.g. protrusion of tongue, puffing of cheeks, puckering of mouth, chewing movements). Sometimes these may be accompanied by involuntary movements of the extremities. There is no known effective treatment for tardive dyskinesia; antiparkinsonism agents usually do not alleviate the symptoms of this syndrome. It is suggested that all antipsychotic agents be discontinued if these symptoms appear. Should it be necessary to reinstitute treatment, or increase the dosage of the agent, or switch to a different antipsychotic agent, the syndrome may be masked. It has been reported that fine, vermicular movements of the tongue may be an early sign of the syndrome, and if the medication is stopped at that time the syndrome may not develop.

Other CNS effects include cerebral edema; abnormality of cerebrospinal fluid proteins; convulsive seizures, particularly in patients with EEG abnormalities or a history of such disorders, and headaches.

Neuroleptic malignant syndrome has been reported in patients treated with neuroleptic drugs (see WARNINGS for further information).

Drowsiness may occur, particularly during the first or second week, after which it generally disappears. If troublesome, lower the dosage. Hypnotic effects appear to be minimal, especially in patients who are permitted to remain active.

Adverse behavioral effects include paradoxical exacerbation of psychotic symptoms, catatonic-like states, paranoid reactions, lethargy, paradoxical excitement, restlessness, hyperactivity, nocturnal confusion, bizarre dreams, and insomnia. Hyperreflexia has been reported in the newborn when a phenothiazine was used during pregnancy.

Autonomic Effects: dry mouth or salivation, nausea, vomiting, diarrhea, anorexia, constipation, obstipation, fecal impaction, urinary retention, frequency or incontinence, bladder paralysis, polyuria, nasal congestion, pallor, myosis, mydriasis, blurred vision, glaucoma, perspiration, hypertension, hypotension, and change in pulse rate occasionally may occur. Significant autonomic effects have been infrequent in patients receiving less than 24 mg perphenazine daily.

Adynamic ileus occasionally occurs with phenothiazine therapy and if severe can result in complications and death. It is of particular concern in psychiatric patients, who may fail to seek treatment of this condition.

Allergic Effects: urticaria, erythema, eczema, exfoliative dermatitis, pruritus, photosensitivity, asthma, fever, anaphylactoid reactions, laryngeal edema, and angioneurotic edema; contact dermatitis in nursing personnel administering the drug, and in extremely rare instances, individual idiosyncrasy or hypersensitivity to phenothiazines has resulted in cerebral edema, circulatory collapse, and death.

Endocrine Effects: lactation, galactorrhea, moderate breast enlargement in females and gynecomastia in males on large doses, disturbances in the menstrual cycle, amenorrhea, changes in libido, inhibition of ejaculation, syndrome of inappropriate ADH (antidiuretic hormone) secretion, false positive pregnancy tests, hyperglycemia, hypoglycemia, glycosuria.

Cardiovascular Effects: postural hypotension, tachycardia (especially with sudden marked increase in dosage), bradycardia, cardiac arrest, faintness, and dizziness. Occasionally the hypotensive effect may produce a shock-like condition. ECG changes, nonspecific, (quinidine-like effect) usually reversible, have been observed in some patients receiving phenothiazine tranquilizers.

Sudden death has occasionally been reported in patients who have received phenothiazines. In some cases the death was apparently due to cardiac arrest; in others, the cause appeared to be asphyxia due to failure of the cough reflex. In some patients, the cause could not be determined nor could it be established that the death was due to the phenothiazine.

Hematological Effects: agranulocytosis, eosinophilia, leukopenia, hemolytic anemia, thrombocytopenic purpura, and pancytopenia. Most cases of agranulocytosis have occurred between the fourth and tenth weeks of therapy. Patients should be watched closely especially during that period for the sudden appearance of sore throat or signs of infection. If white blood cell and differential cell counts show significant cellular depression, discontinue the drug and start appropriate therapy. However, a slightly lowered white count is not in itself an indication to discontinue the drug.

Other Effects: Special considerations in long-term therapy include pigmentation of the skin, occurring chiefly in the exposed areas, ocular changes consisting of deposition of fine particulate matter in the cornea and lens, progressing in more severe cases to star-shaped lenticular opacities; epithelial keratopathies; and pigmentary retinopathy. Also noted: peripheral edema, reversed epinephrine effect, increase in PBI not attributable to an increase in thyroxine, parotid swelling (rare), hyperpyrexia, systemic lupus erythematosus-like syndrome, increases in appetite and weight, polyphagia, photophobia, and muscle weakness.

Liver damage (biliary stasis) may occur. Jaundice may occur, usually between the second and fourth weeks of treatment and is regarded as a hypersensitivity reaction. Incidence is low. The clinical picture resembles infectious hepatitis but with laboratory features of obstructive jaundice. It is usually reversible; however, chronic jaundice has been reported.

Side effects with intramuscular TRILAFON Injection have been infrequent and transient. Dizziness or significant hypotension after treatment with TRILAFON Injection is a rare occurrence.

DOSAGE AND ADMINISTRATION

Dosage must be individualized and adjusted according to the severity of the condition and the response obtained. As with all potent drugs, the best dose is the lowest dose that will produce the desired clinical effect. Since extrapyramidal symptoms increase in frequency and severity with increased dosage, it is important to employ the lowest effective dose. These symptoms have disappeared upon reduction of dosage, withdrawal of the drug or administration of an anti-parkinsonian agent.

Prolonged administration of doses exceeding 24 mg daily should be reserved for hospitalized patients or patients under continued observation for early detection and management of adverse reactions. An antiparkinsonian agent, such as trihexyphenidyl hydrochloride or benztropine mesylate, is valuable in controlling drug-induced, extrapyramidal symptoms.

TRILAFON Tablets

Suggested dosages for **Tablets** for various conditions follow:
Moderately disturbed non-hospitalized psychotic patients:
Tablets 4 to 8 mg t.i.d., initially; reduce as soon as possible to minimum effective dosage.
Hospitalized psychotic patients: **Tablets** 8 to 16 mg b.i.d. to q.i.d.; avoid dosages in excess of 64 mg daily.
Severe nausea and vomiting in adults: **Tablets** 8 to 16 mg daily in divided doses; 24 mg occasionally may be necessary; early dosage reduction is desirable.

TRILAFON INJECTION—Intramuscular Administration

The injection is used when rapid effect and prompt control of acute or intractable conditions is required or when oral administration is not feasible. TRILAFON Injection, administered by deep intramuscular injection, is well tolerated. The injection should be given with the patient seated or recumbent, and the patient should be observed for a short period after administration.

Therapeutic effect is usually evidenced in 10 minutes and is maximal in 1 to 2 hours. The average duration of effective action is 6 hours, occasionally 12 to 24 hours.

Pediatric dosage has not yet been established. Children over 12 years may receive the lowest limit of adult dosage.

The usual initial dose is 5 mg (1 mL). This may be repeated every 6 hours. Ordinarily, the total daily dosage should not exceed 15 mg in ambulatory patients or 30 mg in hospitalized patients. When required for satisfactory control of symptoms in severe conditions, an initial 10 mg intramuscular dose may be given. Patients should be placed on oral therapy as soon as practicable. Generally, this may be achieved within 24 hours. In some instances, however, patients have been maintained on injectable therapy for several months. It has been established that TRILAFON Injection is more potent than TRILAFON Tablets. Therefore, equal or higher dosage should be used when the patient is transferred to oral therapy after receiving the injection.

Psychotic conditions: While 5 mg of the Injection has a definite tranquilizing effect, it may be necessary to use 10 mg doses to initiate therapy in severely agitated states. Most patients will be controlled and amendable to oral therapy within a maximum of 24 to 48 hours. Acute conditions (hysteria, panic reaction) often respond well to a single dose whereas in chronic conditions, several injections may be required. When transferring patients to oral therapy, it is suggested that increased dosage be employed to maintain adequate clinical control. This should be followed by gradual reduction to the minimal maintenance dose which is effective.

Severe nausea and vomiting in adults: To obtain rapid control of vomiting, administer 5 mg (1 mL); in rare instances it may be necessary to increase the dose to 10 mg, in general, higher doses should be given only to hospitalized patients.

TRILAFON Injection—Intravenous Administration

The intravenous administration of TRILAFON Injection is seldom required. This route of administration should be used with particular caution and care and only when absolutely necessary to control severe vomiting, intractable hiccoughs, or acute conditions, such as violent retching during surgery. Its use should be limited to recumbent, hospitalized adults in doses not exceeding 5 mg. When employed in this manner, intravenous injection ordinarily should be given as a diluted solution by either fractional injection or a slow drip infusion. In the surgical patient, slow infusion of no more than 5 mg is preferred. When administered in divided doses, TRILAFON Injection should be diluted to 0.5 mg/mL (1 mL mixed with 9 mL of physiologic saline solution), and not more than 1 mg per injection given at not less than one-to two-minute intervals. Intravenous injection should be discontinued as soon as symptoms are controlled and should not exceed 5 mg. The possibility of hypotensive and extrapyramidal side effects should be considered and appropriate means for management kept available. Blood pressure and pulse should be monitored continuously during intravenous administration. Pharmacologic and clinical studies indicate that intravenous administration of norepinephrine should be useful in alleviating the hypotensive effect.

TRILAFON Concentrate

In hospitalized psychotic patients, the usual dosage range is 8 to 16 mg b.i.d. to q.i.d., depending on the severity of symptoms and individual response. Although a number of investigators have employed higher dosages, a total daily dose of more than 64 mg ordinarily is not required. The **Concentrate** should be diluted only with water, saline, Seven-Up, homogenized milk, carbonated orange drink and pineapple, apricot, prune, orange. V-8, tomato, and grapefruit juices. Trilafon **Concentrate** should not be mixed with beverages containing caffeine (coffee, cola) tannics (tea), or pectinates (apple juice) since physical incompatibility may result. Suggested dilution is approximately two fluid ounces of diluent for each 5 mL (16 mg) teaspoonful of TRILAFON **Concentrate**. For convenience in measuring smaller doses, a graduated dropper marked to measure 8 mg or 4 mg is supplied with each bottle.

OVERDOSAGE

In the event of overdosage, emergency treatment should be started immediately. All patients suspected of having taken an overdose should be hospitalized as soon as possible.

Manifestations: Overdosage of perphenazine primarily involves the extrapyramidal mechanism and produces the same side effects described under ADVERSE REACTIONS, but to a more marked degree. It is usually evidenced by stupor or coma; children may have convulsive seizures.

Treatment: Treatment is symptomatic and supportive. There is no specific antidote. The patient should be induced to vomit even if emesis has occurred spontaneously. Pharmacologic vomiting by the administration of ipecac syrup is a preferred method. It should be noted that ipecac has a central mode of action in addition to its local gastric irritant properties, and the central mode of action may be blocked by the antiemetic effect of TRILAFON products. Vomiting should not be induced in patients with impaired consciousness. The action of ipecac is facilitated by physical activity and by the administration of 8 to 12 fluid ounces of water. If emesis does not occur within 15 minutes, the dose of ipecac should be repeated. Precautions against aspiration must be taken, especially in infants and children. Following emesis, any drug remaining in the stomach may be adsorbed by activated charcoal administered as a slurry with water. If vomiting is unsuccessful or contraindicated, gastric lavage should be performed. Isotonic and one-half isotonic saline are the lavage solutions of choice. Saline cathartics, such as milk of magnesia, draw water into the bowel by osmosis and therefore may be valuable for their action in rapid dilution of bowel content.

Standard measures (oxygen, intravenous fluids, corticosteroids) should be used to manage circulatory shock or metabolic acidosis. An open airway and adequate fluid intake should be maintained. Body temperature should be regulated. Hypothermia is expected, but severe hyperthermia may occur and must be treated vigorously. (See CONTRAINDICATIONS.)

An electrocardiogram should be taken and close monitoring of cardiac function instituted if there is any sign of abnormality. Cardiac arrhythmias may be treated with neostigmine, pyridostigmine, or propranolol. Digitalis should be considered for cadiac failure. Close monitoring of cardiac function is advisable for not less than five days. Vasopressors such as norepinephrine may be used to treat hypotension, but epinephrine should NOT be used.

Anticonvulsants (an inhalation anesthetic, diazepam, or paraldehyde) are recommended for control of convulsions, since perphenazine increases the central nervous system depressant action, but not the anticonvulsant action of barbiturates.

If acute parkinson-like symptoms result from perphenazine intoxication, benztropine mesylate or diphenhydramine may be administered.

Central nervous system depression may be treated with non-convulsant doses of CNS stimulants. Avoid stimulants that may cause convulsions (e.g., picrotoxin and pentylenetetrazol).

Signs of arousal may not occur for 48 hours.

Dialysis is of no value because of low plasma concentrations of the drug.

Since overdosage is often deliberate, patients may attempt suicide by other means during the recovery phase. Deaths by deliberate or accidental overdosage have occurred with this class of drugs.

HOW SUPPLIED

TRILAFON **Tablets** (2 mg): gray, sugar-coated tablets branded in black with the Schering trademark and either product identification letters, ADH, or numbers 705; bottles of 100 (NDC 0085-0705-04) and 500 (NDC 0085-0705-06).

TRILAFON **Tablets** (4 mg): gray, sugar-coated tablets branded in green with the Schering trademark and either product identification letters, ADK, or numbers, 940; bottles of 100 (NDC 0085-0940-05) and 500 (NDC 0085-0940-04).

TRILAFON **Tablets** (8 mg): gray, sugar-coated tablets branded in blue with the Schering trademark and either product identification letters, ADJ, or numbers 313; bottles of 100 (NDC 0085-0313-05) and 500 (NDC 0085-0313-04).

TRILAFON **Tablets** (16 mg): gray, sugar-coated tablets branded in red with the Schering trademark and either product identification letters, ADM, or numbers, 077; bottles of 100 (NDC 0085-0077-05) and 500 (NDC 0085-0077-04).

TRILAFON **Concentrate**, 16 mg per 5 mL, 4 fluid ounce (118 mL) bottle with graduated dropper (NDC 0085-0363-02). The **Concentrate** is light-sensitive and should be dispensed in amber bottles. **Protect from light. Store in carton until contents are used. Shake well.**

Continued on next page

Information on Schering products appearing on these pages is effective as of September 30, 1989.

Schering—Cont.

TRILAFON Injection, 5 mg per mL, 1-mL ampul for intramuscular or intravenous use, box of 100 (NDC 0085-0012-04). Keep package closed to protect from light. Exposure may cause discoloration. Slight yellowish discoloration will not alter potency or therapeutic efficacy; if markedly discolored, ampul should be discarded. **Protect from light. Store in carton until contents are used.**

Store all TRILAFON Tablets and TRILAFON Concentrate between 2° and 30°C (36° and 86°F).

Revised 1/88

Copyright©1969, 1988, Schering Corporation, USA. All rights reserved.

Shown in Product Identification Section, page 428

TRINALIN®   ℞

[*trĭn 'a-lin*]

brand of azatadine maleate, USP and pseudoephedrine sulfate, USP

Long-Acting Antihistamine/Decongestant
REPETABS® **Tablets**

DESCRIPTION

TRINALIN Long-Acting Antihistamine/Decongestant REPETABS (brand of repeat-action tablets) Tablets) contain 1 mg azatadine maleate, USP in the tablet coating and 120 mg pseudoephedrine sulfate, USP, equally distributed between the tablet coating and the barrier-coated core. Following ingestion, the two active components in the coating are quickly liberated; release of the decongestant in the core is delayed for several hours.

Azatadine maleate is an antihistamine having the empirical formula, $C_{20}H_{22}N_2 \cdot 2C_4H_4O_4$, the chemical name, 6,11-Dihydro-11-(1-methyl-4-piperidylidene)-5*H*-benzo-[5,6]cyclohepta[1,2-*b*] pyridine maleate (1:2).

The molecular weight of azatadine maleate is 522.54. Azatadine maleate is a white to off-white powder and is very soluble in water and soluble in alcohol.

Pseudoephedrine sulfate, a sympathomimetic amine, is a salt of pseudoephedrine, one of the naturally occurring alkaloids obtained from various species of the plant *Ephedra*. The empirical formula for pseudoephedrine sulfate is $(C_{10}H_{15}NO)_2 \cdot H_2SO_4$; the chemical name is Benzenemethanol, α-[1-(methylamino)ethyl]-, [*S*-(*R**, *R**)]-, sulfate (2:1) (salt).

The molecular weight of pseudoephedrine sulfate is 428.56. It is a white to off-white crystal or powder, very soluble in water, freely soluble in alcohol, and sparingly soluble in chloroform.

The inactive ingredients for TRINALIN REPETABS Tablets are: Acacia, Butylparaben, Calcium Sulfate, Carnauba Wax, Corn Starch, D&C Red No. 30 Al Lake, FD&C Yellow No. 6 Al Lake, Gelatin, Lactose, Magnesium Stearate, Neutral Soap, Oleic Acid, Povidone, Rosin, Sugar, Talc, White Wax, and Zein.

CLINICAL PHARMACOLOGY

Azatadine maleate is an antihistamine, related to cyproheptadine, with antiserotonin, anticholinergic (drying), and sedative effects. Antihistamines appear to compete with histamine for histamine H_1-receptor sites on effector cells. The antihistamines antagonize those pharmacological effects of histamine which are mediated through activation of H_1-receptor sites and thereby reduce the intensity of allergic reactions and tissue injury response involving histamine release. Antihistamines antagonize the vasodilator effect of endogenously released histamine, especially in small vessels, and mitigate the effect of histamine which results in increased capillary permeability and edema formation. As consequences of these actions, antihistamines antagonize the physiological manifestations of histamine release in the nose following antigen-antibody interaction, such as congestion related to vascular engorgement, mucosal edema, and profuse, watery secretion, and irritation and sneezing resulting from histamine action on afferent nerve terminals.

Pseudoephedrine sulfate (d-isoephedrine sulfate) is an orally effective nasal decongestant which appears to exert its sympathomimetic effect indirectly, predominantly through release of adrenergic mediators from post-ganglionic nerve terminals. In effective recommended oral dosage, pseudoephedrine sulfate produces minimal other sympathomimetic effects, such as pressor activity and CNS stimulation. Use of an orally administered vasoconstrictor for shrinkage of congested nasal mucosa has several advantages: a) it produces a gradual but sustained decongestant effect, causing little, if any "rebound" congestion; b) it facilitates shrinkage of swollen mucosa in upper respiratory areas that are relatively inaccessible to topically applied sprays or drops; c) it relieves nasal obstruction without the additional irritation that may result from local medication.

Pseudoephedrine passes through the blood-brain and placental barriers. While the antihistamines have not been studied systematically for passage through these barriers, the occurrence of pharmacologic effects in the central nervous system and in newborns indicate presence of the drug.

Following administration of the two drugs to normal volunteers in either a single TRINALIN REPETABS Tablet or similar doses in two conventional pseudoephedrine sulfate tablets and a conventional tablet of azatadine maleate, the blood levels of pseudoephedrine and the urinary excretion of azatadine showed that the TRINALIN REPETABS Tablets are bioequivalent to the conventional dosage forms. The apparent elimination half-life of pseudoephedrine in TRINALIN REPETABS Tablets was approximately $6\frac{1}{2}$ hours. The apparent elimination of half-life of azatadine maleate (available from the outer layer of the TRINALIN REPETABS Tablets or from the conventional azatadine maleate tablet) was approximately 12 hours.

INDICATIONS AND USAGE

TRINALIN Long-Acting Antihistamine/Decongestant REPETABS Tablets are indicated for the relief of the symptoms of upper respiratory mucosal congestion in perennial and allergic rhinitis, and for the relief of nasal congestion and eustachian tube congestion. Analgesics, antibiotics, or both may be administered concurrently, when indicated.

CONTRAINDICATIONS

Antihistamines should not be used to treat lower respiratory tract symptoms, including asthma.

This product is contraindicated in patients with narrow-angle glaucoma or urinary retention, and in patients receiving monoamine oxidase (MAO) inhibitor therapy or within ten days of stopping such treatment. (See Drug Interactions section.) It is also contraindicated in patients with severe hypertension, severe coronary artery disease, hyperthyroidism, and in those who have shown hypersensitivity or idiosyncrasy to its components, to adrenergic agents, or to other drugs of similar chemical structures. Manifestations of patient idiosyncrasy to adrenergic agents include: insomnia, dizziness, weakness, tremor, or arrhythmias.

WARNINGS

TRINALIN REPETABS Tablets should be used with considerable caution in patients with: stenosing peptic ulcer, pyloroduodenal obstruction, urinary bladder obstruction due to symptomatic prostatic hypertrophy, or narrowing of the bladder neck. It should also be administered with caution to patients with cardiovascular disease, including hypertension or ischemic heart disease; increased intraocular pressure (See CONTRAINDICATIONS); diabetes mellitus, or in patients receiving digitalis or oral anticoagulants.

Central nervous system stimulation and convulsions or cardiovascular collapse with accompanying hypotension may be produced by sympathomimetics.

Do not exceed recommended dosage.

Use in Activities Requiring Mental Alertness: Patients should be warned about engaging in activities requiring mental alertness, such as driving a car or operating appliances, machinery, etc.

Use in Patients Approximately 60 Years and Older: Antihistamines are more likely to cause dizziness, sedation, and hypotension in patients over 60 years of age. In these patients, sympathomimetics are also more likely to cause adverse reactions, such as confusion, hallucinations, convulsions, CNS depression, and death. For this reason, before considering the use of a repeat-action formulation, the safe use of a short-acting sympathomimetic in that particular patient should be demonstrated.

PRECAUTIONS

General: Because of the atropine-like action of antihistamines, this product should be used with caution in patients with a history of bronchial asthma.

Information for Patients:

1. Products containing antihistamines may cause drowsiness.
2. Patients should not engage in activities requiring mental alertness, such as driving or operating machinery or appliances.
3. Alcohol or other sedative drugs may enhance the drowsiness caused by antihistamines.
4. Patients should not take TRINALIN REPETABS Tablets if they are receiving a monoamine oxidase inhibitor or within 10 days of stopping such treatment, or if they are receiving oral anticoagulants.
5. This medication should not be given to children less than 12 years of age.

Drug Interactions: MAO inhibitors prolong and intensify the effects of antihistamines. Concomitant use of antihistamines with alcohol, tricyclic antidepressants, barbiturates, or other central nervous system depressants may have an additive effect.

When sympathomimetic drugs are given to patients receiving monoamine oxidase inhibitors, hypertensive reactions, including hypertensive crises, may occur. The antihypertensive effects of methyldopa, mecamylamine, reserpine, and veratrum alkaloids may be reduced by sympathomimetics. Beta-adrenergic blocking agents may also interact with sympathomimetics. Increased ectopic pacemaker activity can occur when pseudoephedrine is used concomitantly with digitalis. Antacids increase the rate of absorption of pseudoephedrine, while kaolin decreases it.

Drug/Laboratory Test Interactions: The *in vitro* addition of pseudoephedrine to sera containing the cardiac isoenzyme MB of serum creatine phosphokinase progressively inhibits the activity of the enzyme. The inhibition becomes complete over six hours.

Carcinogenesis, Mutagenesis, and Impairment of Fertility: There is no animal or laboratory study of the mixture of azatadine maleate and pseudoephedrine sulfate to evaluate carcinogenesis or mutagenesis. Reproduction studies of this mixture in rats showed no evidence of impaired fertility.

Pregnancy Category C: Retarded fetal development and the presence of angulated hyoid wings were seen in the offspring of pregnant rabbits administered TRINALIN at about 12.5 times and 5 times the recommended human dosage, respectively; increased resorption was noted at about 25 times the human dosage. A decreased survival rate at day 21 was seen in rat pups born of mothers given TRINALIN during pregnancy at a dose about 12.5 times the human dosage. There are no adequate and well-controlled studies in pregnant women. TRINALIN REPETABS Tablets should be used during pregnancy only if the potential benefits to the mother justify the potential risks to the infant. (See Nonteratogenic Effects.)

Nonteratogenic Effects: Antihistamines should not be used in the third trimester of pregnancy, because newborns and premature infants may have severe reactions to them such as convulsions.

Nursing Mothers: It is not known whether these drugs are excreted in human milk. However, certain antihistamines and sympathomimetics are known to be excreted in human milk. Because of the higher risks of antihistamines for infants generally and for newborns and prematures in particular, a decision should be made whether to discontinue nursing or to discontinue the drug, taking into account the importance of the drug to the mother.

There is a report of irritability, excessive crying and disturbed sleeping patterns in a nursing infant whose mother had taken a product containing an antihistamine and pseudoephedrine.

Pediatric use: Safety and effectiveness in children below the age of 12 years have not been established.

ADVERSE REACTIONS

The following adverse reactions are associated with antihistamine and sympathomimetic drugs. (Those adverse reactions which occur most frequently with the antihistamines are underlined.)

General: Urticaria, drug rash, anaphylactic shock, photosensitivity, excessive perspiration, chills, dryness of mouth, nose, and throat.

Cardiovascular: Hypertension (see CONTRAINDICATIONS and WARNINGS), hypotension, arrhythmias and cardiovascular collapse, headache, palpitations, extrasystoles, tachycardia, angina.

Hematologic: Hemolytic anemia, hypoplastic anemia, thrombocytopenia, agranulocytosis.

Central Nervous System: Sedation, sleepiness, dizziness, vertigo, tinnitus, acute labyrinthitis, disturbed coordination, fatigue, mydriasis, confusion, restlessness, excitation, nervousness, tension, tremor, irritability, insomnia, euphoria, paresthesias, blurred vision, hysteria, neuritis, convulsions, fear, anxiety, hallucinations, CNS depression, weakness, pallor.

Gastrointestinal: Epigastric distress, anorexia, nausea, vomiting, diarrhea, constipation, abdominal cramps.

Genitourinary: Urinary frequency, urinary retention, dysuria, early menses.

Respiratory: Thickening of bronchial secretions, tightness of chest and wheezing, nasal stuffiness, respiratory difficulty.

DRUG ABUSE AND DEPENDENCE

There is no information to indicate that abuse or dependency occurs with azatadine maleate.

Pseudoephedrine, like other central nervous system stimulants, has been abused. At high doses, subjects commonly experience an elevation of mood, a sense of increased energy and alertness, and decreased appetite. Some individuals become anxious, irritable, and loquacious. In addition to the marked euphoria, the user experiences a sense of markedly enhanced physical strength and mental capacity. With continued use, tolerance develops, the user increases the dose, and toxic signs and symptoms appear. Depression may follow rapid withdrawal.

OVERDOSAGE

In the event of overdosage, emergency treatment should be started immediately.

Manifestations of overdosage may vary from central nervous system depression (sedation, apnea, diminished mental alertness, cyanosis, coma, cardiovascular collapse) to stimulation (insomnia, hallucinations, tremors, or convulsions) to death. Other signs and symptoms may be euphoria, excitement, tachycardia, palpitations, thirst, perspiration, nausea, dizziness, tinnitus, ataxia, blurred vision, and hypertension or hypotension. Stimulation is particularly likely in children, as are atropine-like signs and symptoms (dry mouth; fixed, dilated pupils, flushing; hyperthermia; and gastrointestinal symptoms).

In large doses sympathomimetics may give rise to giddiness, headache, nausea, vomiting, sweating, thirst, tachycardia, precordial pain, palpitations, difficulty in micturition, muscular weakness and tenseness, anxiety, restlessness, and insomnia. Many patients can present a toxic psychosis with delusions and hallucinations. Some may develop cardiac arrhythmias, circulatory collapse, convulsions, coma, and respiratory failure.

The oral LD_{50} of the mixture of the two drugs in mature rats and mice was greater than 1700 mg/kg and 600 mg/kg, respectively.

Treatment —The patient should be induced to vomit, even if emesis has occurred spontaneously. Pharmacologically induced vomiting by the administration of ipecac syrup is a preferred method. However, vomiting should not be induced in patients with impaired consciousness. The action of ipecac is facilitated by physical activity and by the administration of eight to twelve fluid ounces of water. If emesis does not occur within fifteen minutes, the dose of ipecac should be repeated. Precautions against aspiration must be taken, especially in infants and children. Following emesis, any drug remaining in the stomach may be adsorbed by activated charcoal administered as a slurry with water. If vomiting is unsuccessful or contraindicated, gastric lavage should be performed. Isotonic and one-half isotonic saline are the lavage solutions of choice. Saline cathartics, such as milk of magnesia, draw water into the bowel by osmosis and therefore may be valuable for their action in rapid dilution of bowel content. Dialysis is of little value in antihistamine poisoning. After emergency treatment the patient should continue to be medically monitored.

Treatment of the signs and symptoms of overdosage is symptomatic and supportive. Stimulants (analeptic agents) should <u>not</u> be used. Vasopressors may be used to treat hypotension. Short-acting barbiturates, diazepam, or paraldehyde may be administered to control seizures. Hyperpyrexia, especially in children, may require treatment with tepid water sponge baths or a hypothermic blanket. Apnea is treated with ventilatory support.

DOSAGE AND ADMINISTRATION

TRINALIN REPETABS Tablets ARE NOT INTENDED FOR USE IN CHILDREN UNDER 12 YEARS OF AGE. The usual adult dosage is one tablet twice a day.

HOW SUPPLIED

TRINALIN REPETABS Tablets contain 1 mg azatadine maleate and 120 mg pseudoephedrine sulfate. TRINALIN REPETABS Tablets are coral-colored, sugar-coated tablets branded in black with the Schering trademark, or the product name and product identification numbers, 703; bottle of 100 (NDC-0085-0703-04).

Store between 2° and 30°C (36° and 86°F).

Copyright © 1981, 1985, 1987, 1988 Schering Corporation, USA. All rights reserved.
Revised 8/88

Shown in Product Identification Section, page 428

VANCENASE® Nasal Inhaler ℞

[van 'sen-ās]
brand of beclomethasone dipropionate, USP
For Nasal Inhalation Only

DESCRIPTION

Beclomethasone dipropionate, USP, the active component of VANCENASE Nasal Inhaler, is an anti-inflammatory steroid having the chemical name, 9-Chloro-11β,17,21-trihydroxy-16β-methylpregna-1,4-diene-3,20-dione 17, 21-dipropionate.

Beclomethasone dipropionate is a white to creamy-white odorless powder with a molecular weight of 521.25. It is very slightly soluble in water; very soluble in chloroform; and freely soluble in acetone and in alcohol.

VANCENASE Nasal Inhaler is a metered-dose aerosol unit containing a microcrystalline suspension of beclomethasone dipropionate-trichloromonofluoromethane clathrate in a mixture of propellants (trichloromonofluoromethane and dichlorodifluoromethane) with oleic acid. Each canister contains beclomethasone dipropionate-trichloromonofluoromethane clathrate having a molecular proportion of beclomethasone dipropionate to trichloromonofluoromethane between 3:1 and 3:2. Each actuation delivers from the nasal adapter a quantity of clathrate equivalent to 42 mcg of beclomethasone dipropionate, USP. The contents of one canister provide at least 200 metered doses.

CLINICAL PHARMACOLOGY

Beclomethasone 17,21-dipropionate is a diester of beclomethasone, a synthetic halogenated corticosteroid. Animal studies showed that beclomethasone dipropionate has potent glucocorticoid and weak mineralocorticoid activity. The mechanisms for the anti-inflammatory action of beclomethasone dipropionate are unknown. The precise mechanism of the aerosolized drug's action in the nose is also unknown. Biopsies of nasal mucosa obtained during clinical studies showed no histopathologic changes when beclomethasone dipropionate was administered intranasally.

The effects of beclomethasone dipropionate on hypothalamic-pituitary-adrenal (HPA) function have been evaluated in adult volunteers, by other routes of administration. Studies are currently being undertaken with beclomethasone dipropionate by the intranasal route, which may demonstrate that there is more or that there is less absorption by this route of administration. There was no suppression of early morning plasma cortisol concentrations when beclomethasone dipropionate was administered in a dose of 1000 mcg/day for one month as an oral aerosol or for three days by intramuscular injection. However, partial suppression of plasma cortisol concentration was observed when beclomethasone dipropionate was administered in doses of 2000 mcg/day either by oral aerosol or intramuscularly. Immediate suppression of plasma cortisol concentrations was observed after single doses of 4000 mcg of beclomethasone dipropionate. Suppression of HPA function (reduction of early morning plasma cortisol levels) has been reported in adult patients who received 1600 mcg daily doses of oral beclomethasone dipropionate for one month. In clinical studies using beclomethasone dipropionate intranasally, there was no evidence of adrenal insufficiency.

Beclomethasone dipropionate is sparingly soluble. When given by nasal inhalation in the form of an aqueous or aerosolized suspension, the drug is deposited primarily in the nasal passages. A portion of the drug is swallowed. Absorption occurs rapidly from all respiratory and gastrointestinal tissues. There is no evidence of tissue storage of beclomethasone dipropionate or its metabolites. *In vitro* studies, have shown that tissue other than the liver (lung slices) can rapidly metabolize beclomethasone dipropionate to beclomethasone 17-monopropionate and more slowly to free beclomethasone (which has very weak anti-inflammatory activity). However, irrespective of the route of entry, the principal route of excretion of the drug and its metabolites is the feces. In humans, 12% to 15% of an orally administered dose of beclomethasone dipropionate is excreted in the urine as both conjugated and free metabolites of the drug.

Studies have shown that the degree of binding to plasma proteins is 87%.

INDICATIONS AND USAGE

VANCENASE Nasal Inhaler is indicated for the relief of the symptoms of seasonal or perennial rhinitis, in those cases poorly responsive to conventional treatment.

VANCENASE is also indicated for the prevention of recurrence of nasal polyps following surgical removal.

Clinical studies in seasonal and perennial rhinitis have shown that improvement is usually apparent within a few days. However, symptomatic relief may not occur in some patients for as long as two weeks. Although systemic effects are minimal at recommended doses, VANCENASE should not be continued beyond three weeks in the absence of significant symptomatic improvement. VANCENASE should not be used in the presence of untreated localized infection involving the nasal mucosa.

Clinical studies have shown that treatment of the symptoms associated with nasal polyps may have to be continued for several weeks or more before a therapeutic result can be fully assessed. Recurrence of symptoms due to polyps can occur after stopping treatment, depending on the severity of the disease.

CONTRAINDICATIONS

Hypersensitivity to any of the ingredients of this preparation contraindicates its use.

WARNINGS

The replacement of a systemic corticosteroid with VANCENASE Nasal Inhaler can be accompanied by signs of adrenal insufficiency.

Careful attention must be given when patients previously treated for prolonged periods with systemic corticosteroids are transferred to VANCENASE Nasal Inhaler. This is particularly important in those patients who have associated asthma or other clinical conditions, where too rapid a decrease in systemic corticosteroids may cause a severe exacerbation of their symptoms.

Studies have shown that the combined administration of alternate day prednisone systemic treatment and orally inhaled beclomethasone increased the likelihood of HPA suppression compared to a therapeutic dose of either one alone. Therefore, VANCENASE treatment should be used with caution in patients already on alternate day prednisone regimens for any disease.

If recommended doses of intranasal beclomethasone are exceeded or if individuals are particularly sensitive or predisposed by virtue of recent systemic steroid therapy, symptoms of hypercorticism may occur, including very rare cases of menstrual irregularities, acneiform lesions, and cushingoid features. If such changes occur, VANCENASE Nasal Inhaler should be discontinued slowly, consistent with accepted procedures for discontinuing oral steroid therapy.

PRECAUTIONS

General: During withdrawal from oral steroids, some patients may experience symptoms of withdrawal, e.g., joint and/or muscular pain, lassitude, and depression.

Extremely rare instances of nasal septum perforation and increased intraocular pressure have been reported following the intranasal application of aerosolized corticosteroids.

In clinical studies with beclomethasone dipropionate administered intranasally, the development of localized infections of the nose and pharynx with *Candida albicans* has occurred only rarely. When such an infection develops, it may require treatment with appropriate local therapy or discontinuance of treatment with VANCENASE Nasal Inhaler.

Beclomethasone dipropionate is absorbed into the circulation. Use of excessive doses of VANCENASE Nasal Inhaler may suppress HPA function.

VANCENASE should be used with caution, if at all, in patients with active or quiescent tuberculous infections of the respiratory tract, or in untreated fungal, bacterial, systemic viral infections, or ocular herpes simplex.

For VANCENASE to be effective in the treatment of nasal polyps, the aerosol must be able to enter the nose. Therefore, treatment of nasal polyps with VANCENASE should be considered adjunctive therapy to surgical removal and/or the use of other medications which will permit effective penetration of VANCENASE into the nose. Nasal polyps may recur after any form of treatment.

As with any long-term treatment, patients using VANCENASE over several months or longer should be examined periodically for possible changes in the nasal mucosa.

Because of the inhibitory effect of corticosteroids on wound healing, patients who have experienced recent nasal septal ulcers, nasal surgery, or trauma should not use a nasal corticosteroid until healing has occurred.

Although systemic effects have been minimal with recommended doses, this potential increases with excessive doses. Therefore, larger than recommended doses should be avoided.

Information for Patients: Patients should use VANCENASE Nasal Inhaler at regular intervals since its effectiveness depends on its regular use. The patient should take the medication as directed. It is not acutely effective and the prescribed dosage should not be increased. Instead, nasal vasoconstrictors or oral antihistamines may be needed until the effects of VANCENASE Nasal Inhaler are fully manifested. One to two weeks may pass before full relief is obtained. The patient should contact the doctor if symptoms do not improve, or if the condition worsens, or if sneezing or nasal irritation occurs. For the proper use of this unit and to attain maximum improvement, the patient should read and follow the accompanying PATIENT'S INSTRUCTIONS carefully.

Carcinogenesis, Mutagenesis, Impairment of Fertility: Treatment of rats for a total of 95-weeks, 13 weeks by inhalation and 82 weeks by the oral route, resulted in no evidence of carcinogenic activity. Mutagenic studies have not been performed.

Impairment of fertility, as evidenced by inhibition of the estrus cycle in dogs, was observed following treatment by the oral route. No inhibition of the estrus cycle in dogs was seen following treatment with beclomethasone dipropionate by the inhalation route.

Pregnancy Category C: Like other corticoids, parenteral (subcutaneous) beclomethasone dipropionate has been shown to be teratogenic and embryocidal in the mouse and rabbit when given in doses approximately ten times the human dose. In these studies beclomethasone was found to produce fetal resorption, cleft palate, agnathia, microstomia, absence of tongue, delayed ossification, and agenesis of the thymus. No teratogenic or embryocidal effects have been seen in the rat when beclomethasone dipropionate was administered by inhalation at ten times the human dose or orally at 1000 times the human dose. There are no adequate and well-controlled studies in pregnant women. Beclomethasone dipropionate should be used during pregnancy only if the potential benefit justifies the potential risk to the fetus.

Nonteratogenic Effects: Hypoadrenalism may occur in infants born of mothers receiving corticosteroids during pregnancy. Such infants should be carefully observed.

Nursing Mothers: It is not known whether beclomethasone dipropionate is excreted in human milk. Because other corticosteroids are excreted in human milk, caution should be exercised when VANCENASE Nasal Inhaler is administered to nursing women.

Pediatric Use: Safety and effectiveness in children below the age of 6 years have not been established.

Continued on next page

Information on Schering products appearing on these pages is effective as of September 30, 1989.

Schering—Cont.

ADVERSE REACTIONS

In general, side effects in clinical studies have been primarily associated with the nasal mucous membranes. Adverse reactions reported in controlled clinical trials and long-term open studies in patients treated with VANCENASE are described below.

Sensations of irritation and burning in the nose (11 per 100 patients) following the use of VANCENASE Nasal Inhaler have been reported. Also, occasional sneezing attacks (10 per 100 patients) have occurred immediately following the use of the intranasal inhaler. This symptom may be more common in children.

Rhinorrhea may occur occasionally (1 per 100 patients). Localized infections of the nose and pharynx with *Candida albicans* have occurred rarely. (See PRECAUTIONS.) Transient episodes of epistaxis or bloody discharge from the nose have been reported in 2 per 100 patients. Ulceration of the nasal mucosa has been reported rarely.

Extremely rare instances of nasal septum perforation and increased intraocular pressure have been reported following the intranasal administration of aerosolized corticosteroids (see **PRECAUTIONS**). Rare cases of immediate and delayed hypersensitivity reactions, including urticaria, angioedema, rash, and bronchospasm have been reported following the oral and intranasal inhalation of beclomethasone.

Systemic corticosteroid side effects were not reported during the controlled clinical trials. If recommended doses are exceeded, however, or if individuals are particularly sensitive, symptoms of hypercorticism, i.e., Cushing's syndrome could occur.

DOSAGE AND ADMINISTRATION

Adults and Children 12 years of age and over: the usual dosage is one inhalation (42 mcg) in each nostril two to four times a day (total dose 168–336 mcg/day). Patients can often be maintained on a maximum dose of one inhalation in each nostril three times a day (252 mcg/day).

Children 6 to 12 years of age: the usual dosage is one inhalation in each nostril three times a day (252 mcg/day). VANCENASE Nasal Inhaler is not recommended for children below 6 years of age since safety and efficacy studies have not been conducted in this age group.

In patients who respond to VANCENASE Nasal Inhaler, an improvement of the symptoms of seasonal or perennial rhinitis usually becomes apparent within a few days after the start of VANCENASE Nasal Inhaler therapy. However, symptomatic relief may not occur in some patients for as long as two weeks. VANCENASE Nasal Inhaler should not be continued beyond three weeks in the absence of significant symptomatic improvement.

The therapeutic effects of corticosteroids, unlike those of decongestants, on seasonal or perennial rhinitis or on nasal polyps are not immediate. This should be explained to the patient in advance in order to ensure cooperation and continuation of treatment with the prescribed dosage regimen.

VANCENASE Nasal Inhaler is not recommended for children below 6 years of age.

In the presence of excessive nasal mucus secretion or edema of the nasal mucosa, the drug may fail to reach the site of intended action. In such cases it is advisable to use a nasal vasoconstrictor during the first two to three days of VANCENASE Nasal Inhaler therapy.

Directions for Use: Illustrated PATIENT INSTRUCTIONS for proper use accompany each package of VANCENASE Nasal Inhaler.

CONTENTS UNDER PRESSURE. Do not puncture. Do not use or store near heat or open flame. Exposure to temperatures above 120°F may cause bursting. Never throw container into fire or incinerator. Keep out of reach of children.

OVERDOSAGE

When used at excessive doses, systemic corticosteroid effects such as hypercorticism and adrenal suppression may appear. If such changes occur, VANCENASE Nasal Inhaler should be discontinued slowly consistent with accepted procedures for discontinuing oral steroid therapy.

The oral LD_{50} of beclomethasone dipropionate is greater than 1 g/kg in rodents. One canister of VANCENASE Nasal Inhaler contains 8.4 mg of beclomethasone dipropionate, therefore acute overdosage is unlikely.

HOW SUPPLIED

VANCENASE Nasal Inhaler, 16.8 g canister; box of one. Supplied with nasal adapter and PATIENT'S INSTRUCTIONS; (NDC 0085-0041-06).

Store between 15° and 30°C (36° and 86°F). Failure to use the product within this temperature range may result in improper dosing. Shake well before using. Revised 5/88

Shown in Product Identification Section, page 428

VANCENASE® AQ

[*van-sen-ase AQ*]
brand of beclomethasone dipropionate, monohydrate
Nasal Spray 0.042%*
FOR INTRANASAL USE ONLY
*calculated on the dried basis

DESCRIPTION

Beclomethasone dipropionate, monohydrate, the active component of VANCENASE AQ Nasal Spray, is an anti-inflammatory steroid having the chemical name, 9-Chloro-11β, 17, 21-trihydroxy-16β-methylpregna-1, 4-diene-3, 20-dione 17,21-dipropionate, monohydrate.

Beclomethasone dipropionate, monohydrate is a white to creamy-white, odorless powder with a molecular weight of 539.06. It is very slightly soluble in water; very soluble in chloroform; and freely soluble in acetone and in alcohol.

VANCENASE AQ Nasal Spray is a metered-dose, manual pump spray unit containing a microcrystalline suspension of beclomethasone dipropionate, monohydrate equivalent to 0.042% w/w beclomethasone dipropionate calculated on the dried basis in an aqueous medium containing microcrystalline cellulose and carboxymethylcellulose sodium, dextrose, benzalkonium chloride, polysorbate 80 and 0.25% v/w phenylethyl alcohol; hydrochloric acid may be added to adjust pH. The pH is between 4.5 and 7.0.

After initial priming (3 to 4 actuations), each actuation of the pump delivers from the nasal adapter 100 mg of suspension containing beclomethasone dipropionate, monohydrate equivalent to 42 mcg beclomethasone dipropionate. Each bottle of VANCENASE AQ Nasal Spray will provide at least 200 metered doses.

CLINICAL PHARMACOLOGY

Beclomethasone 17,21-dipropionate is a diester of beclomethasone, a synthetic halogenated corticosteroid. Animal studies show that beclomethasone dipropionate has potent glucocorticosteroid and weak mineralocorticosteroid activity. The mechanisms for the anti-inflammatory action of beclomethasone dipropionate are unknown. The precise mechanism of the aerosolized drug's action in the nose is also unknown. Biopsies of nasal mucosa obtained during clinical studies showed no histopathologic changes when beclomethasone dipropionate was administered intranasally.

The effects of beclomethasone dipropionate on hypothalamic-pituitary-adrenal (HPA) function have been evaluated in adult volunteers by other routes of administration. Studies with beclomethasone dipropionate by the intranasal route may demonstrate that there is more or that there is less absorption by this route of administration. There was no suppression of early morning plasma cortisol concentrations when beclomethasone dipropionate was administered in a dose of 1000 mcg/day for one month as an oral aerosol or for three days by intramuscular injection. However, partial suppression of plasma cortisol concentration was observed when beclomethasone dipropionate was administered in doses of 2000 mcg/day either by oral aerosol or intramuscular injection. Immediate suppression of plasma cortisol concentrations was observed after single doses of 4000 mcg of beclomethasone dipropionate. Suppression of HPA function (reduction of early morning plasma cortisol levels) has been reported in adult patients who received 1600 mcg daily doses of oral beclomethasone dipropionate for one month. In clinical studies using beclomethasone dipropionate aerosol intranasally, there was no evidence of adrenal insufficiency. The effect of VANCENASE AQ Nasal Spray on HPA function was not evaluated but would not be expected to differ from intranasal beclomethasone dipropionate aerosol.

In one study in asthmatic children, the administration of inhaled beclomethasone at recommended daily doses for at least one year was associated with a reduction in nocturnal cortisol secretion. The clinical significance of this finding is not clear. It reinforces other evidence, however, that topical beclomethasone may be absorbed in amounts that can have systemic effects and that physicians should be alert for evidence of systemic effects, especially in chronically treated patients (see **PRECAUTIONS**).

Beclomethasone dipropionate is sparingly soluble. When given by nasal inhalation in the form of an aqueous or aerosolized suspension, the drug is deposited primarily in the nasal passages. A portion of the drug is swallowed. Absorption occurs rapidly from all respiratory and gastrointestinal tissues. There is no evidence of tissue storage of beclomethasone dipropionate or its metabolites. *In vitro* studies have shown that tissue other than the liver (lung slices) can rapidly metabolize beclomethasone dipropionate to beclomethasone 17-monopropionate and more slowly to free beclomethasone (which has very weak anti-inflammatory activity). However, irrespective of the route of entry the principal route of excretion of the drug and its metabolites is the feces. In humans, 12% to 15% of an orally administered dose of beclomethasone dipropionate is excreted in the urine as both conjugated and free metabolites of the drug.

Studies have shown that the degree of binding to plasma proteins is 87%.

INDICATIONS AND USAGE

VANCENASE AQ (beclomethasone dipropionate, monohydrate) Nasal Spray is indicated for the relief of the symptoms of seasonal or perennial allergic and non-allergic (vasomotor) rhinitis. Results from two clinical trials have shown that significant symptomatic relief was obtained within three days. However, symptomatic relief may not occur in some patients for as long as two weeks. VANCENASE AQ Nasal Spray should not be continued beyond three weeks in the absence of significant symptomatic improvement. VANCENASE AQ Nasal Spray should not be used in the presence of untreated localized infection involving the nasal mucosa.

VANCENASE AQ Nasal Spray is also indicated for the prevention of recurrence of nasal polyps following surgical removal.

Clinical studies have shown that treatment of the symptoms associated with nasal polyps may have to be continued for several weeks or more before a therapeutic result can be fully assessed. Recurrence of symptoms due to polyps can occur after stopping treatment, depending on the severity of the disease.

CONTRAINDICATIONS

Hypersensitivity to any of the ingredients of this preparation contraindicates its use.

WARNINGS

The replacement of a systemic corticosteroid with VANCENASE AQ Nasal Spray can be accompanied by signs of adrenal insufficiency.

Careful attention must be given when patients previously treated for prolonged periods with systemic corticosterioids are transferred to VANCENASE AQ Nasal Spray. This is particularly important in those patients who have associated asthma or other clinical conditions, where too rapid a decrease in systemic corticosteroids may cause a severe exacerbation of their symptoms.

Studies have shown that the combined administration of alternate day prednisone systemic treatment and orally inhaled beclomethasone increased the likelihood of HPA suppression compared to a therapeutic dose of either one alone. Therefore, VANCENASE AQ Nasal Spray treatment should be used with caution in patients already on alternate day prednisone regimens for any disease.

If recommended doses of intranasal beclomethasone are exceeded or if individuals are particularly sensitive or predisposed by virtue of recent systemic steroid therapy, symptoms of hypercorticism may occur, including very rare cases of menstrual irregularities, acneiform lesions, and cushingoid features. If such changes occur, VANCENASE AQ Nasal Spray should be discontinued slowly, consistent with accepted procedures for discontinuing oral steroid therapy.

PRECAUTIONS

General: During withdrawal from oral steroids, some patients may experience symptoms of withdrawal, e.g., joint and/or muscular pain, lassitude and depression. Rarely, immediate hypersensitivity reactions may occur after the intranasal administration of beclomethasone.

Extremely rare instances of wheezing, nasal septum perforation and increased intraocular pressure have been reported following the intranasal application of aerosolized corticosteroids. Although these have not been observed in clinical trials with VANCENASE AQ Nasal Spray, vigilance should be maintained.

In clinical studies with beclomethasone dipropionate administered intranasally, the development of localized infections of the nose and pharynx with *Candida albicans* has occurred only rarely. When such an infection develops, it may require treatment with appropriate local therapy or discontinuance of treatment with VANCENASE AQ Nasal Spray.

If persistent nasopharyngeal irritation occurs, it may be an indication for stopping VANCENASE AQ Nasal Spray.

Beclomethasone dipropionate is absorbed into the circulation. Use of excessive doses of VANCENASE AQ Nasal Spray may suppress HPA function.

VANCENASE AQ Nasal Spray should be used with caution, if at all, in patients with active or quiescent tuberculous infections of the respiratory tract; in untreated fungal, bacterial, or systemic viral infections; or ocular herpes simplex.

For VANCENASE AQ Nasal Spray to be effective in the treatment of nasal polyps, the spray must be able to enter the nose. Therefore, treatment of nasal polyps with VANCENASE AQ Nasal Spray should be considered adjunctive therapy to surgical removal and/or the use of other medications that will permit effective penetration of VANCENASE

AQ Nasal Spray into the nose. Nasal polyps may recur after any form of treatment.

As with any long-term treatment, patients using VANCENASE AQ Nasal Spray over several months or longer should be examined periodically for possible changes in the nasal mucosa.

Because of the inhibitory effect of cortiocosteroids on wound healing, patients who have experienced recent nasal septal ulcers, nasal surgery, or trauma should not use a nasal corticosteroid until healing has occurred.

Although systemic effects have been minimal with recommended doses, this potential increases with excessive doses. Therefore, larger than recommended doses should be avoided.

Information for Patients: Patients being treated with VANCENASE AQ Nasal Spray should receive the following information and instructions. This information is intended to aid in the safe and effective use of medication. It is not a disclosure of all possible adverse or intended effects. Patients should use VANCENASE AQ Nasal Spray at regular intervals since its effectiveness depends on its regular use. The patient should take the medication as directed. It is not acutely effective and the prescribed dosage should not be increased. Instead, nasal vasoconstrictors or oral antihistamines may be needed until the effects of VANCENASE AQ Nasal Spray are fully manifested. One or two weeks may pass before full relief is obtained. The patient should contact the doctor if symptoms do not improve, or if the condition worsens, or if sneezing or nasal irritation occurs. For the proper use of this unit and to attain maximum improvement, the patient should read and follow the accompanying Patient's Instructions carefully.

Carcinogenesis, Mutagenesis, Impairment or Fertility: Treatment of rats for a total of 95 weeks, 13 weeks by inhalation and 82 weeks by the oral route, resulted in no evidence of carcinogenic activity. Mutagenic studies have not been performed.

Impairment of fertility, as evidenced by inhibition of the estrous cycle in dogs, was observed following treatment by the oral route. No inhibition of the estrous cycle in dogs was seen following treatment with beclomethasone dipropionate by the inhalation route.

Pregnancy: Teratogenic Effects: Pregnancy Category C: Like other corticoids, parenteral (subcutaneous) beclomethasone dipropionate has been shown to be teratogenic and embryocidal in the mouse and rabbit when given in doses approximately ten times the human dose. In these studies beclomethasone was found to produce fetal resorption, cleft palate, agnathia, microstomia, absence of tongue, delayed ossification, and agenesis of the thymus. No teratogenic or embryocidal effects have been seen in the rat when beclomethasone dipropionate was administered by inhalation at ten times the human dose or orally at 1000 times the human dose. There are no adequate and well-controlled studies in pregnant women. Beclomethasone dipropionate should be used during pregnancy only if the potential benefit justifies the potential risk to the fetus.

Nonteratogenic Effects: Hypoadrenalism may occur in infants born of mothers receiving corticosteroids during pregnancy. Such infants should be carefully observed.

Nursing Mothers: It is not known whether beclomethasone dipropionate is excreted in human milk. Because other corticosteroids are excreted in human milk, caution should be exercised when VANCENASE AQ Nasal Spray is administered to nursing women.

Pediatric Use: Safety and effectiveness in children below 6 years of age have not been established.

ADVERSE REACTIONS

In general, side effects in clinical studies have been primarily associated with irritation of the nasal mucous membranes. Rarely, immediate hypersensitivity reactions may occur after the intranasal administration of beclomethasone.

Adverse reactions reported in controlled clinical trials and open studies in patients treated with VANCENASE AQ Nasal Spray are described below.

Mild nasopharyngeal irritation following the use of beclomethasone aqueous nasal spray has been reported in up to 24% of patients treated, including occasional sneezing attacks (about 4%) occurring immediately following use of the inhaler. In patients experiencing these symptoms, none had to discontinue treatment. The incidence of transient irritation and sneezing was approximately the same in the group of patients who received placebo in these studies, implying that these complaints may be related to vehicle components of the formulation.

Fewer than 5 per 100 patients reported headache, nausea, or lightheadedness following the use of VANCENASE AQ (beclomethasone dipropionate, monohydrate) Nasal Spray. Fewer than 3 per 100 patients reported nasal stuffiness, nosebleeds, rhinorrhea, or tearing eyes.

Extremely rare instances of wheezing, nasal septum perforation and increased intraocular pressure have been reported following the intranasal administration of aerosolized corticosteroids (see **PRECAUTIONS**).

OVERDOSAGE

When used at excessive doses, systemic corticosteroid effects such as hypercorticism and adrenal suppression may appear. If such changes occur, VANCENASE AQ Nasal Spray should be discontinued slowly consistent with accepted procedures for discontinuing oral steroid therapy. The oral LD_{50} of beclomethasone dipropionate is greater than 1 g/kg in rodents. One bottle of VANCENASE AQ Nasal Spray contains beclomethasone dipropionate, monohydrate equivalent to 10.5 mg of beclomethasone dipropionate; therefore, acute overdosage is unlikely.

DOSAGE AND ADMINISTRATION

Adults and Children 6 Years of Age and Older: The usual dosage is 1 or 2 inhalations (42 to 84 mcg) in each nostril twice a day (total dose 168 to 336 mcg/day).

In patients who respond to VANCENASE AQ Nasal Spray, an improvement of the symptoms of seasonal or perennial rhinitis usually becomes apparent within a few days after the start of VANCENASE AQ Nasal Spray therapy. However, symptomatic relief may not occur in some patients for as long as two weeks. VANCENASE AQ Nasal Spray should not be continued beyond three weeks in the absence of significant symptomatic improvement.

The therapeutic effects of corticosteroids, unlike those of decongestants, are not immediate. This should be explained to the patient in advance in order to ensure cooperation and continuation of treatment with the prescribed dosage regimen.

VANCENASE AQ Nasal Spray is not recommended for children below 6 years of age.

In the presence of excessive nasal mucus secretion or edema of the nasal mucosa, the drug may fail to reach the site of intended action. In such cases, it is advisable to use a nasal vasoconstrictor during the first 2 to 3 days of VANCENASE AQ Nasal Spray therapy.

Directions for Use: Illustrated Patient's Instructions for proper use accompany each package of VANCENASE AQ Nasal Spray.

HOW SUPPLIED

VANCENASE AQ (beclomethasone dipropionate, monohydrate) Nasal Spray, 0.042%* is supplied in an amber glass bottle fitted with a metering atomizing pump and nasal adapter in a box of one (NDC 0085-0259-02) with patient's instructions for use. Each bottle contains 25 g of suspension.
*Calculated on the dried basis.

Store between 15° and 30°C (59° and 86°F).
SHAKE WELL BEFORE EACH USE.
Revised 9/88

Shown in Product Identification Section, page 428

VANCERIL® Inhaler ℞
[van 'ser-il]
brand of beclomethasone dipropionate, USP
FOR ORAL INHALATION ONLY

DESCRIPTION

Beclomethasone dipropionate, USP, the active component of VANCERIL Inhaler, is an anti-inflammatory steroid having the chemical name 9-Chloro-11β,17-21-trihydroxy-16 β-methylpregna-1,4-diene-3, 20-dione 17,21-dipropionate.

VANCERIL Inhaler is a metered-dose aerosol unit containing a microcrystalline suspension of beclomethasone dipropionate-trichloromonofluoromethane clathrate in a mixture of propellants (trichloromonofluoromethane and dichlorodifluoromethane) with oleic acid. Each canister contains beclomethasone dipropionate-trichloromonofluoromethane clathrate having a molecular proportion of beclomethasone dipropionate, USP, to trichloromonofluoromethane between 3:1 and 3:2. Each actuation delivers from the mouthpiece a quantity of clathrate equivalent to 42 mcg of beclomethasone dipropionate, USP. The contents of one canister provide at least 200 oral inhalations.

CLINICAL PHARMACOLOGY

Beclomethasone 17,21-dipropionate is a diester of beclomethasone, a synthetic corticosteroid which is chemically related to dexamethasone. Beclomethasone differs from dexamethasone only in having a chlorine at the 9-alpha in place of a fluorine and in having a 16β-methyl group instead of a 16 alpha-methyl group. Animal studies showed that beclomethasone dipropionate has potent anti-inflammatory activity. When administered systemically to mice, the anti-inflammatory activity was accompanied by other typical features of glucocorticoid action including thymic involution, liver glycogen deposition, and pituitary-adrenal suppression. However, after systemic administration to rats, the anti-inflammatory action was associated with little or no effect on other tests of glucocorticoid activity.

Beclomethasone dipropionate is sparingly soluble and is poorly mobilized from subcutaneous or intramuscular injection sites. However, systemic absorption occurs after all routes of administration. When given to animals in the form of an aerosolized suspension of the trichloromonofluoromethane clathrate, the drug is deposited in the mouth and nasal passages, the trachea and principal bronchi, and in the lung; a considerable portion of the drug is also swallowed. Absorption occurs rapidly from all respiratory and gastrointestinal tissues, as indicated by the rapid clearance of radioactively labeled drug from local tissues and appearance of tracer in the circulation. There is no evidence of tissue storage of beclomethasone dipropionate or its metabolites. Lung slices can metabolize beclomethasone dipropionate rapidly to beclomethasone 17-monopropionate and more slowly to free beclomethasone (which has very weak anti-inflammatory activity). However, irrespective of the route of administration (injection, oral, or aerosol), the principal route of excretion of the drug and its metabolites is the feces. Less than 10% of the drug and its metabolites is excreted in the urine. In humans, 12% to 15% of an orally administered dose of beclomethasone dipropionate was excreted in the urine as both conjugated and free metabolites of the drug.

The mechanisms responsible for the anti-inflammatory action of beclomethasone dipropionate are unknown. The precise mechanism of the aerosolized drug's action in the lung is also unknown.

INDICATIONS

VANCERIL Inhaler is indicated only for patients who require chronic treatment with corticosteroids for control of the symptoms of bronchial asthma. Such patients would include those already receiving systemic corticosteroids, and selected patients who are inadequately controlled on a nonsteroid regimen and in whom steroid therapy has been withheld because of concern over potential adverse effects.

VANCERIL Inhaler is NOT indicated:
1. For relief of asthma which can be controlled by bronchodilators and other non-steroid medications.
2. In patients who require systemic corticosteroid treatment infrequently.
3. In the treatment of non-asthmatic bronchitis.

CONTRAINDICATIONS

VANCERIL Inhaler is contraindicated in the primary treatment of status asthmaticus or other acute episodes of asthma where intensive measures are required.

Hypersensitivity to any of the ingredients of this preparation contraindicates its use.

WARNINGS

Particular care is needed in patients who are transferred from systemically active corticosteroids to VANCERIL Inhaler because deaths due to adrenal insufficiency have occurred in asthmatic patients during and after transfer from systemic corticosteroids to aerosol beclomethasone dipropionate. After withdrawal from systemic corticosteroids, a number of months are required for recovery of hypothalamic-pituitary-adrenal (HPA) function. During this period of HPA suppression, patients may exhibit signs and symptoms of adrenal insufficiency when exposed to trauma, surgery or infections, particularly gastroenteritis. Although VANCERIL Inhaler may provide control of asthmatic symptoms during these episodes, it does NOT provide the systemic steroid which is necessary for coping with these emergencies.

During periods of stress or a severe asthmatic attack, patients who have been withdrawn from systemic corticosteroids should be instructed to resume systemic steroids (in large doses) immediately and to contact their physician for further instruction. These patients should also be instructed to carry a warning card indicating that they may need supplementary systemic steroids during periods of stress or a severe asthma attack. To assess the risk of adrenal insuffficiency in emergency situations, routine tests of adrenal cortical function, including measurement of early morning resting cortisol levels, should be performed periodically in all patients. An early morning resting cortisol level may be accepted as normal only if it falls at or near the normal mean level.

Localized infections with *Candida albicans* or *Aspergillus niger* have occurred frequently in the mouth and pharynx and occasionally in the larynx. Positive cultures for oral *Candida* may be present in up to 75% of patients. Although the frequency of clinically apparent infection is considerably lower, these infections may require treatment with appropriate antifungal therapy or discontinuance of treatment with VANCERIL Inhaler.

Continued on next page

Information on Schering products appearing on these pages is effective as of September 30, 1989.

Schering—Cont.

VANCERIL Inhaler is not to be regarded as a bronchodilator and is not indicated for rapid relief of bronchospasm.

Patients should be instructed to contact their physician immediately when episodes of asthma which are not responsive to bronchodilators occur during the course of treatment with VANCERIL. During such episodes, patients may require therapy with systemic corticosteroids.

There is no evidence that control of asthma can be achieved by the administration of VANCERIL in amounts greater than the recommended doses.

Transfer of patients from systemic steroid therapy to VANCERIL Inhaler may unmask allergic conditions previously suppressed by the systemic steroid therapy, e.g., rhinitis, conjunctivitis, and eczema.

PRECAUTIONS

During withdrawal from oral steroids, some patients may experience symptoms of systemically active steroid withdrawal, e.g., joint and/or muscular pain, lassitude and depression, despite maintenance or even improvement of respiratory function (See DOSAGE AND ADMINISTRATION for details).

In responsive patients, beclomethasone dipropionate may permit control of asthmatic symptoms without suppression of HPA function, as discussed below (See CLINICAL STUDIES). Since beclomethasone dipropionate is absorbed into the circulation and can be systemically active, the beneficial effects of VANCERIL Inhaler in minimizing or preventing HPA dysfunction may be expected only when recommended dosages are not exceeded.

The long-term effects of beclomethasone dipropionate in human subjects are still unknown. In particular, the local effects of the agent on developmental or immunologic processes in the mouth, pharynx, trachea, and lung are unknown. There is also no information about the possible long-term systemic effects of the agent.

The potential effects of VANCERIL on acute, recurrent, or chronic pulmonary infections, including active or quiescent tuberculosis, are not known. Similarly, the potential effects of long-term administration of the drug on lung or other tissues are unknown.

Pulmonary infiltrates with eosinophilia may occur in patients on VANCERIL Inhaler therapy. Although it is possible that in some patients this state may become manifest because of systemic steroid withdrawal when inhalational steroids are administered, a causative role for beclomethasone dipropionate and/or its vehicle cannot be ruled out.

Use in Pregnancy: Glucocorticoids are known teratogens in rodent species and beclomethasone dipropionate is no exception.

Teratology studies were done in rats, mice, and rabbits treated with subcutaneous beclomethasone dipropionate. Beclomethasone dipropionate was found to produce fetal resorptions, cleft palate, agnathia, microstomia, absence of tongue, delayed ossification and partial agenesis of the thymus. Well-controlled trials relating to fetal risk in humans are not available. Glucocorticoids are secreted in human milk. It is not known whether beclomethasone dipropionate would be secreted in human milk but it is safe to assume that it is likely. The use of beclomethasone dipropionate in pregnancy, nursing mothers, or women of childbearing potential requires that the possible benefits of the drug be weighed against the potential hazards to the mother, embryo, or fetus. Infants born of mothers who have received substantial doses of corticosteroids during pregnancy should be carefully observed for hypoadrenalism.

ADVERSE REACTIONS

Deaths due to adrenal insufficiency have occurred in asthmatic patients during and after transfer from systemic corticosteroids to aerosol beclomethasone dipropionate (See WARNINGS).

Suppression of HPA function (reduction of early morning plasma cortisol levels) has been reported in adult patients who received 1600 mcg daily doses of VANCERIL for one month. A few patients on VANCERIL have complained of hoarseness or dry mouth.

Rare cases of immediate and delayed hypersensitivity reactions, including urticaria, angioedema, rash and bronchospasm have been reported following the oral and intranasal inhalation of beclomethasone.

DOSAGE AND ADMINISTRATION

Adults: The usual recommended dosage is two inhalations (84 mcg) given three or four times a day. Alternatively, four inhalations (168 mcg) given twice daily has been shown to be effective in some patients. In patients with severe asthma, it is advisable to start with 12 to 16 inhalations a day and adjust the dosage downward according to the response of the patient. The maximal daily intake should not exceed 20 inhalations, 840 mcg (0.84 mg), in adults.

Children 6 to 12 years of age: The usual recommended dosage is one or two inhalations (42 to 84 mcg) given three or four times a day according to the response of the patient.

Alternatively, four inhalations (168 mcg) given twice daily has been shown to be effective in some patients. The maximal daily intake should not exceed ten inhalations, 420 mcg (0.42 mg), in children 6 to 12 years of age. Insufficient clinical data exist with respect to the administration of VANCERIL Inhaler in children below the age of 6.

Rinsing the mouth after inhalation is advised.

Patients receiving bronchodilators by inhalation should be advised to use the bronchodilator before VANCERIL Inhaler in order to enhance penetration of beclomethasone dipropionate into the bronchial tree. After use of an aerosol bronchodilator, several minutes should elapse before use of the VANCERIL Inhaler to reduce the potential toxicity from the inhaled fluorocarbon propellants in the two aerosols.

Different considerations must be given to the following groups of patients in order to obtain the full therapeutic benefit of VANCERIL Inhaler.

Patients not receiving systemic steroids: The use of VANCERIL Inhaler is straightforward in patients who are inadequately controlled with non-steroid medications but in whom systemic steroid therapy has been withheld because of concern over potential adverse reactions. In patients who respond to VANCERIL, an improvement in pulmonary function is usually apparent within one to four weeks after the start of VANCERIL Inhaler.

Patients receiving systemic steroids: In those patients dependent on systemic steroids, transfer to VANCERIL and subsequent management may be more difficult because recovery from impaired adrenal function is usually slow. Such suppression has been known to last for up to 12 months. Clinical studies, however, have demonstrated that VANCERIL may be effective in the management of these asthmatic patients and may permit replacement or significant reduction in the dosage of systemic corticosteroids.

The patient's asthma should be reasonably stable before treatment with VANCERIL Inhaler is started. Initially, the aerosol should be used concurrently with the patient's usual maintenance dose of systemic steroid. After approximately one week, gradual withdrawal of the systemic steroid is started by reducing the daily or alternate daily dose. The next reduction is made after an interval of one or two weeks, depending on the response of the patient. Generally, these decrements should not exceed 2.5 mg of prednisone or its equivalent. A slow rate of withdrawal cannot be overemphasized. During withdrawal, some patients may experience symptoms of systemically active steroid withdrawal, e.g., joint and/or muscular pain, lassitude and depression, despite maintenance or even improvement of respiratory function. Such patients should be encouraged to continue with the Inhaler but should be watched carefully for objective signs of adrenal insufficiency, such as hypotension and weight loss. If evidence of adrenal insufficiency occurs, the systemic steroid dose should be boosted temporarily and thereafter further withdrawal should continue more slowly. During periods of stress or a severe asthma attack, transfer patients will require supplementary treatment with systemic steroids. Exacerbations of asthma which occur during the course of treatment with VANCERIL Inhaler should be treated with a short course of systemic steroid which is gradually tapered as these symptoms subside. There is no evidence that control of asthma can be achieved by administration of VANCERIL in amounts greater than the recommended doses.

Directions for Use: Illustrated patient instructions for proper use accompany each package of VANCERIL Inhaler. CONTENTS UNDER PRESSURE. Do not puncture. Do not use or store near heat or open flame. Exposure to temperatures above 120°F. may cause bursting. Never throw container into fire or incinerator. Keep out of reach of children.

HOW SUPPLIED

VANCERIL Inhaler 16.8 g canister supplied with an oral adapter and patient's instructions; box of one. (NDC-0085-0736-04).

Store between 15° and 30°C (59° and 86°F). Failure to use the product within this temperature range may result in improper dosing.

ANIMAL PHARMACOLOGY AND TOXICOLOGY

Studies in a number of animal species including rats, rabbits, and dogs have shown no unusual toxicity during acute experiments. However, the effects of beclomethasone dipropionate in producing signs of glucocorticoid excess during chronic administration by various routes were dose related.

CLINICAL STUDIES

The effects of beclomethasone dipropionate on hypothalamic-pituitary-adrenal (HPA) function have been evaluated in adult volunteers. There was no suppression of early morning plasma cortisol concentrations when beclomethasone dipropionate was administered in a dose of 1000 mcg/day for one month as an aerosol or for three days by intramuscular injection. However, partial suppression of plasma cortisol concentration was observed when beclomethasone dipropionate was administered in doses of 2000 mcg/day either intramuscularly or by aerosol. Immediate suppression of plasma corti-

sol concentrations was observed after single doses of 4000 mcg of beclomethasone dipropionate.

In one study, the effects of beclomethasone dipropionate on HPA function were examined in patients with asthma. There was no change in basal early morning plasma cortisol concentrations or in the cortisol responses to tetracosactrin (ACTH 1:24) stimulation after daily administration of 400, 800 or 1200 mcg of beclomethasone dipropionate for 28 days. After daily administration of 1600 mcg each day for 28 days, there was a slight reduction in basal cortisol concentrations and a statistically significant (p < .01) reduction in plasma cortisol responses to tetracosactrin stimulation. The effects of a more prolonged period of beclomethasone dipropionate administration on HPA function have not been evaluated. However, a number of investigators have noted that when systemic corticosteroid therapy in asthmatic subjects can be replaced with recommended doses of beclomethasone dipropionate, there is gradual recovery of endogenous cortisol concentrations to the normal range. There is still no documented evidence of recovery from other adverse systemic corticosteroid-induced reactions during prolonged therapy of patients with beclomethasone dipropionate.

Clinical experience has shown that some patients with bronchial asthma who require corticosteroid therapy for control of symptoms can be partially or completely withdrawn from systemic corticosteroid if therapy with beclomethasone dipropionate aerosol is substituted. Beclomethasone dipropionate aerosol is not effective for all patients with bronchial asthma or at all stages of the disease in a given patient.

The early clinical experience has revealed several new problems which may be associated with the use of beclomethasone dipropionate by inhalation for treatment of patients with bronchial asthma:

1. There is a risk of adrenal insufficiency when patients are transferred from systemic corticosteroids to aerosol beclomethasone dipropionate. Although the aerosol may provide adequate control of asthma during the transfer period, it does not provide the systemic steroid which is needed during acute stress situations. Deaths due to adrenal insufficiency have occurred in asthmatic patients during and after transfer from systemic corticosteroids to aerosol beclomethasone dipropionate. (See WARNINGS.)

2. Transfer of patients from systemic steroid therapy to beclomethasone dipropionate aerosol may unmask allergic conditions which were previously controlled by the systemic steroid therapy, e.g., rhinitis, conjunctivitis, and eczema.

3. Localized infections with Candida albicans or Aspergillus niger have occurred frequently in the mouth and pharynx and occasionally in the larynx. It has been reported that up to 75% of the patients who receive prolonged treatment with beclomethasone dipropionate have positive oral cultures for Candida albicans. The incidence of clinically apparent infection is considerably lower but may require therapy with appropriate antifungal agents or discontinuation of treatment with beclomethasone dipropionate aerosol.

The long-term effects of beclomethasone dipropionate in human subjects are still unknown. In particular, the local effects of the agent on developmental or immunologic processes in the mouth, pharynx, trachea and lung are unknown. There is also no information about the possible long-term systemic effects of the agent. The possible relevance of the data in animal studies to results in human subjects cannot be evaluated.

Revised 1/89

Shown in Product Identification Section, page 428

Schiapparelli Searle
BOX 5110
CHICAGO, IL 60680

Alphabetic Product Listing

Lactulose, 3036, Syrup USP, 10 g/15 ml
Lactulose, 3056, Syrup USP, 10 g/15 ml
Norethin 1/35E-21, Dispenser, 221, Tablet, 1 mg/35 mcg
Norethin 1/35E-28, Dispenser, 221 (231), Tablet, 1 mg/ 35 mcg
Norethin 1/50M-21, Dispenser, 431, Tablet, 1 mg/50 mcg
Norethin 1/50M-28, Dispenser, 431 (441), Tablet, 1 mg/ 50 mcg
Pro-Banthine, 601, Tablet, 15 mg
Pro-Banthine, Unit Dose, 601, Tablet, 15 mg
Pro-Banthine, 611, Tablet, 7½ mg

* When the product ID # is not the same as the NDC #, the NDC # appears in parentheses.

DIULO®   ℞
[dĭ'ū-lō]
(metolazone)

DO NOT INTERCHANGE

DO NOT INTERCHANGE DIULO TABLETS AND OTHER FORMULATIONS OF METOLAZONE THAT SHARE ITS SLOW AND INCOMPLETE BIOAVAILABILITY AND ARE NOT THERAPEUTICALLY EQUIVALENT AT THE SAME DOSES TO MYKROX™ TABLETS, A MORE RAPIDLY AVAILABLE AND COMPLETELY BIOAVAILABLE METOLAZONE PRODUCT. FORMULATIONS BIOEQUIVALENT TO DIULO AND FORMULATIONS BIOEQUIVALENT TO MYKROX SHOULD NOT BE INTERCHANGED FOR ONE ANOTHER.

DESCRIPTION

Diulo tablets for oral administration contain 2½, 5, or 10 mg of metolazone, a diuretic/saluretic/antihypertensive drug of the quinazoline class.
Metolazone has the molecular formula $C_{16}H_{16}ClN_3O_3S$, the chemical name 7-chloro-1,2,3,4-tetrahydro-2-methyl-3- (2-methylphenyl) -4-oxo-6-quinazolinesulfonamide, and a molecular weight of 365.83. The structural formula is:

Metolazone is only sparingly soluble in water, but more soluble in plasma, blood, alkali, and organic solvents.
Diulo tablets also contain magnesium stearate, microcrystalline cellulose, and dye: 2½ mg—D&C Red No. 33: 5 mg—FD&C Blue No. 2; 10 mg—D&C Yellow No. 10 and FD&C Yellow No. 6.

CLINICAL PHARMACOLOGY

Diulo is a quinazoline diuretic, with properties generally similar to the thiazide diuretics. The actions of Diulo (metolazone) result from interference with the renal tubular mechanism of electrolyte reabsorption. Diulo acts primarily to inhibit sodium reabsorption at the cortical diluting site and to a lesser extent in the proximal convoluted tubule. Sodium and chloride ions are excreted in approximately equivalent amounts. The increased delivery of sodium to the distal-tubular exchange site results in increased potassium excretion. Diulo does not inhibit carbonic anhydrase. A proximal action has been shown in humans by increased excretion of phosphate and magnesium ions and by a markedly increased fractional excretion of sodium in patients with severely compromised glomerular filtration. This action has been demonstrated in animals by micropuncture studies.
When Diulo tablets are given, diuresis and saluresis usually begin within one hour and may persist for 24 hours or more. For most patients, the duration of effect can be varied by adjusting the daily dose. High doses may prolong the effect. A single daily dose is recommended. When a desired therapeutic effect has been obtained, it may be possible to reduce dosage to a lower maintenance level.
The diuretic potency of Diulo at maximum therapeutic dosage is approximately equal to thiazide diuretics. However, unlike thiazides, Diulo may produce diuresis in patients with glomerular filtration rates below 20 ml/min.
Diulo (metolazone) and furosemide administered concurrently have produced marked diuresis in some patients where edema or ascites was refractory to treatment with maximum recommended doses of these or other diuretics administered alone. The mechanism of this interaction is unknown (see *Drug interactions* and *Warnings*).
Maximum blood levels of metolazone are found approximately eight hours after dosing. A small fraction of metolazone is metabolized. Most of the drug is excreted in the unconverted form in the urine.

INDICATIONS AND USAGE

Diulo is indicated for the treatment of salt and water retention including:
—edema accompanying congestive heart failure;
—edema accompanying renal diseases, including the nephrotic syndrome and states of diminished renal function.
Diulo is also indicated for the treatment of hypertension, alone or in combination with other antihypertensive drugs of a different class. Mykrox (metolazone) tablets, a more rapidly available form of metolazone, are intended for the treatment of new patients with mild to moderate hypertension. A dose titration is necessary if Mykrox tablets are to be substituted for Diulo in the treatment of hypertension. See package circular for Mykrox tablets (Fisons Pharmaceuticals).
Usage in pregnancy: The routine use of diuretics in an otherwise healthy woman is inappropriate and exposes mother and fetus to unnecessary hazard. Diuretics do not prevent development of toxemia of pregnancy, and there is no evidence that they are useful in the treatment of developed toxemia.
Edema during pregnancy may arise from pathologic causes or from the physiologic and mechanical consequences of pregnancy. Diulo is indicated in pregnancy when edema is due to pathologic causes, just as it is in the absence of pregnancy (see *Precautions*). Dependent edema in pregnancy resulting from restriction of venous return by the expanded uterus is properly treated through elevation of the lower extremities and use of support hose; use of diuretics to lower intravascular volume in this case is illogical and unnecessary. There is hypervolemia during normal pregnancy which is harmful to neither the fetus nor the mother (in the absence of cardiovascular disease), but which is associated with edema, including generalized edema, in the majority of pregnant women. If this edema produces discomfort, increased recumbency will often provide relief. In rare instances, this edema may cause extreme discomfort which is not relieved by rest. In these cases, a short course of diuretics may be appropriate.

CONTRAINDICATIONS

Anuria, hepatic coma or pre-coma, known allergy, or hypersensitivity to metolazone.

WARNINGS

Rapid onset hyponatremia: Rarely, the rapid onset of severe hyponatremia and/or hypokalemia has been reported following initial doses of thiazide and non-thiazide diuretics. When symptoms consistent with severe electrolyte imbalance appear rapidly, drug should be discontinued and supportive measures should be initiated immediately. Parenteral electrolytes may be required. Appropriateness of therapy with this class of drugs should be carefully reevaluated.
Hypokalemia: Hypokalemia may occur with consequent weakness, cramps, and cardiac dysrhythmias. Serum potassium should be determined at regular intervals, and dose reduction, potassium supplementation, or addition of a potassium-sparing diuretic instituted whenever indicated. Hypokalemia is a particular hazard in patients who are digitalized or who have or have had a ventricular arrhythmia; dangerous or fatal arrhythmias may be precipitated. Hypokalemia is dose related.
Lithium: In general, diuretics should not be given concomitantly with lithium because they reduce its renal clearance and add a high risk of lithium toxicity. Read prescribing information for lithium preparations before use of such concomitant therapy.
Concomitant therapy
Furosemide: Unusually large or prolonged losses of fluids and electrolytes may result when Diulo is administered concomitantly to patients receiving furosemide (see *Drug interactions*).
Other antihypertensive drugs: When Diulo is used with other antihypertensive drugs, particular care must be taken to avoid excessive reduction of blood pressure, especially during initial therapy.
Cross-allergy: Cross-allergy, while not reported to date, theoretically may occur when Diulo is given to patients known to be allergic to sulfonamide-derived drugs, thiazides, or quinethazone.

PRECAUTIONS

DO NOT INTERCHANGE

DO NOT INTERCHANGE DIULO TABLETS AND OTHER FORMULATIONS OF METOLAZONE THAT SHARE ITS SLOW AND INCOMPLETE BIOAVAILABILITY AND ARE NOT THERAPEUTICALLY EQUIVALENT AT THE SAME DOSES TO MYKROX TABLETS, A MORE RAPIDLY AVAILABLE AND COMPLETELY BIOAVAILABLE METOLAZONE PRODUCT. FORMULATIONS BIOEQUIVALENT TO DIULO AND FORMULATIONS BIOEQUIVALENT TO MYKROX SHOULD NOT BE INTERCHANGED FOR ONE ANOTHER.

General

Fluid and electrolytes: All patients receiving therapy with Diulo tablets should have serum electrolyte measurements done at appropriate intervals and be observed for clinical signs of fluid and/or electrolyte imbalance: namely, hyponatremia, hypochloremic alkalosis, and hypokalemia. In patients with severe edema accompanying cardiac failure or renal disease, a low-salt syndrome may be produced, especially with hot weather and a low-salt diet. Serum and urine electrolyte determinations are particularly important when the patient has protracted vomiting, severe diarrhea, or is receiving parenteral fluids. Warning signs of imbalance are: dryness of mouth, thirst, weakness, lethargy, drowsiness, restlessness, muscle pains or cramps, muscle fatigue, hypotension, oliguria, tachycardia, and gastrointestinal disturbances such as nausea and vomiting. Hyponatremia may occur at any time during long-term therapy and, on rare occasions, may be life threatening.
The risk of hypokalemia is increased when larger doses are used, when diuresis is rapid, when severe liver disease is present, when corticosteroids are given concomitantly, when oral intake is inadequate, or when excess potassium is being lost extrarenally, such as with vomiting or diarrhea.
Glucose tolerance: Metolazone may raise blood glucose concentrations possibly causing hyperglycemia and glycosuria in patients with diabetes or latent diabetes.
Hyperuricemia: Diulo regularly causes an increase in serum uric acid and can occasionally precipitate gouty attacks even in patients without a prior history of them.
Azotemia: Azotemia, presumably prerenal azotemia, may be precipitated during the administration of Diulo. If azotemia and oliguria worsen during treatment of patients with severe renal disease, Diulo should be discontinued.
Renal impairment: Use caution when administering Diulo tablets to patients with severely impaired renal function. As most of the drug is excreted by the renal route, accumulation may occur.
Orthostatic hypotension: Orthostatic hypotension may occur; this may be potentiated by alcohol, barbiturates, narcotics, or concurrent therapy with other antihypertensive drugs.
Hypercalcemia: Use of other diuretics has been associated on rare occasions with pathological changes in the parathyroid glands. This possibility should be considered with clinical use of Diulo tablets. Hypercalcemia has been noted in a few patients treated with metolazone.
Systemic lupus erythematosus: Thiazide diuretics have exacerbated or activated systemic lupus erythematosus and this possibility should be considered with Diulo (metolazone) tablets.
Information for patients: Patients should be informed of possible adverse effects, advised to take the medication as directed, and promptly report any possible adverse reactions to the treating physician.
Drug interactions
Diuretics: Furosemide and probably other loop diuretics given concomitantly with metolazone can cause unusually large or prolonged losses of fluid and electrolytes (see *Warnings*).
Other antihypertensives: When Diulo tablets are used with other antihypertensive drugs, care must be taken, especially during initial therapy. Dosage adjustments of other antihypertensives may be necessary.
Alcohol, barbiturates, and narcotics: The hypotensive effects of these drugs may be potentiated by the volume contraction that may be associated with metolazone therapy.
Digitalis glycosides: Diuretic-induced hypokalemia can increase the sensitivity of the myocardium to digitalis. Serious arrhythmias can result.
Corticosteroids or ACTH: May increase the risk of hypokalemia and increase salt and water retention.
Lithium: Serum lithium levels may increase (see *Warnings*).
Curariform drugs: Diuretic-induced hypokalemia may enhance neuromuscular blocking effects of curariform drugs (eg, tubocurarine)—the most serious effect would be respiratory depression which could proceed to apnea. Accordingly, it may be advisable to discontinue Diulo tablets three days before elective surgery.
Salicylates and other nonsteroidal anti-inflammatory drugs: May decrease the antihypertensive effects of Diulo tablets.
Sympathomimetics: Metolazone may decrease arterial responsiveness to norepinephrine, but this diminution is not sufficient to preclude effectiveness of the pressor agent for therapeutic use.
Insulin and oral antidiabetic agents: See *Glucose tolerance* under *Precautions: General.*
Methenamine: Efficacy may be decreased due to urinary alkalizing effect of metolazone.
Drug/Laboratory test interactions: None reported.
Carcinogenesis, mutagenesis, impairment of fertility: Mice and rats given metolazone for 1½ to 2 years at daily doses of 2, 10, and 50 mg/kg (approximately 13, 67, and 333 times the average human dose of 0.15 mg/kg) showed no evidence that metolazone caused an increased number of tumors. The small number of animals examined histologically and poor survival in the mice limit the conclusions that can be reached from these studies.

Continued on next page

Schiapparelli Searle—Cont.

Reproductive performance has been evaluated in mice and rats. There is no evidence that metolazone possesses the potential for altering reproductive capacity in mice. In a rat study, in which males were treated orally with metolazone at doses of 2, 10, and 50 mg/kg for 127 days prior to mating with untreated females, an increased number of resorption sites was observed in dams mated with males from the 50 mg/kg group. In addition, the fetal weight of offspring was decreased and the pregnancy rate was reduced in dams mated with males from the 10 and 50 mg/kg groups.

Pregnancy

Teratogenic effects: Pregnancy Category B. Reproduction studies performed in mice, rabbits, and rats treated during the appropriate period of gestation at doses up to 50 mg/kg/day (333 times an average human dose of Diulo) have revealed no evidence of harm to the fetus due to metolazone. There are, however, no adequate and well-controlled studies in pregnant women. Because animal reproduction studies are not always predictive of human response, Diulo tablets should be used during pregnancy only if clearly needed. Metolazone crosses the placental barrier and appears in cord blood.

Nonteratogenic effects: The use of Diulo tablets in pregnant women requires that the anticipated benefit be weighed against possible hazards to the fetus. These hazards include fetal or neonatal jaundice, thrombocytopenia, and possibly other adverse reactions which have occurred in the adult. It is not known what effect the use of the drug during pregnancy has on the later growth, development, and functional maturation of the child. No such effects have been reported with metolazone.

Labor and delivery: Based on clinical studies in which women received metolazone in late pregnancy until the time of delivery, there is no evidence that the drug has any adverse effects on the normal course of labor or delivery.

Nursing mothers: Metolazone appears in breast milk. Because of the potential for serious adverse reactions in nursing infants from metolazone, a decision should be made whether to discontinue nursing or to discontinue the drug, taking into account the importance of the drug to the mother.

Pediatric use: Safety and effectiveness in children have not been established and such use is not recommended.

ADVERSE REACTIONS

Diulo is usually well tolerated, and most reported adverse reactions have been mild and transient. Many Diulo-related adverse reactions represent extensions of its expected pharmacologic activity and can be attributed to either its antihypertensive action or its renal/metabolic actions. The following adverse reactions have been reported. Several are single or comparably rare occurrences. Adverse reactions are listed in decreasing order of severity within body systems.

Cardiovascular: Chest pain/discomfort, orthostatic hypotension, excessive volume depletion, hemoconcentration, venous thrombosis, palpitations.

Central and peripheral nervous system: Syncope, neuropathy, vertigo, paresthesias, psychotic depression, impotence, dizziness/light-headedness, drowsiness, fatigue, weakness, restlessness (sometimes resulting in insomnia), headache.

Dermatologic/Hypersensitivity: Necrotizing angiitis (cutaneous vasculitis), purpura, dermatitis (photosensitivity), urticaria, and skin rashes.

Gastrointestinal: Hepatitis, intrahepatic cholestatic jaundice, pancreatitis, vomiting, nausea, epigastric distress, diarrhea, constipation, anorexia, abdominal bloating.

Hematologic: Aplastic/hypoplastic anemia, agranulocytosis, leukopenia.

Metabolic: Hypokalemia, hyponatremia, hyperuricemia, hypochloremia, hypochloremic alkalosis, hyperglycemia, glycosuria, increase in serum urea nitrogen (BUN) or creatinine, hypophosphatemia.

Musculoskeletal: Joint pain, acute gouty attacks, muscle cramps or spasm.

Other: Transient blurred vision, chills.

In addition, adverse reactions reported with similar antihypertensive-diuretics, but which have not been reported to date for Diulo, include: bitter taste, dry mouth, sialadenitis, xanthopsia, respiratory distress (including pneumonitis), thyrombocytopenia, and anaphylactic reactions. These reactions should be considered as possible occurrences with clinical usage of Diulo.

Whenever adverse reactions are moderate or severe, Diulo dosage should be reduced or therapy withdrawn.

OVERDOSAGE

Intentional overdosage has been reported rarely with metolazone and similar diuretic drugs.

Signs and symptoms: Orthostatic hypotension, dizziness, drowsiness, syncope, electrolyte abnormalities, hemoconcentration, and hemodynamic changes due to plasma volume depletion may occur. In some instances depressed respiration may be observed. At high doses, lethargy of varying de-

gree may progress to coma within a few hours. The mechanism of CNS depression with thiazide overdosage is unknown. Also, GI irritation and hypermotility may occur. Temporary elevation of BUN has been reported, especially in patients with impairment of renal function. Serum electrolyte changes and cardiovascular and renal function should be closely monitored.

Treatment: There is no specific antidote available but immediate evacuation of stomach contents is advised. Dialysis is not likely to be effective. Care should be taken when evacuating the gastric contents to prevent aspiration, especially in the stuporous or comatose patient. Supportiye measures should be initiated as required to maintain hydration, electrolyte balance, respiration, and cardiovascular and renal function.

DOSAGE AND ADMINISTRATION

Effective dosage of Diulo (metolazone) should be individualized according to indication and patient response. A single daily dose is recommended. Therapy with Diulo should be titrated to gain an initial therapeutic response and to determine the minimal dose possible to maintain the desired therapeutic response.

Usual single daily dosage schedules

Suitable initial dosages will usually fall in the ranges given. Edema of cardiac failure:

    Diulo 5 to 20 mg once daily.

Edema of renal disease:

    Diulo 5 to 20 mg once daily.

Mild to moderate essential hypertension:

    Diulo 2½ to 5 mg once daily.

    New patients—Mykrox (metolazone) tablets (see Mykrox package circular). If considered desirable to switch patients currently on Diulo to Mykrox, the dose should be determined by titration starting at one tablet (½ mg) once daily and increasing to two tablets (1 mg) once daily if needed.

Treatment of edematous states

The time interval required for the initial dosage to produce an effect may vary. Diuresis and saluresis usually begin within one hour and persist for 24 hours or longer. When a desired therapeutic effect has been obtained, it may be advisable to reduce the dose if possible. The daily dose depends on the severity of the patient's condition, sodium intake, and responsiveness. A decision to change the daily dose should be based on the results of thorough clinical and laboratory evaluations. If antihypertensive drugs or diuretics are given concurrently with Diulo, more careful dose adjustment may be necessary. For patients who tend to experience paroxysmal nocturnal dyspnea, it may be advisable to employ a larger dose to ensure prolongation of diuresis and saluresis for a full 24-hour period.

Treatment of hypertension

The time interval required for the initial dosage regimen to show effect may vary from three or four days to three to six weeks in the treatment of elevated blood pressure. Doses should be adjusted at appropriate intervals to achieve maximum therapeutic effect.

HOW SUPPLIED

Diulo (metolazone) is supplied as tablets containing 2½, 5, and 10 mg of metolazone.

Diulo 2½-mg tablets are round, pink tablets with 2.5 debossed on one side and 501 on the other side.

Diulo 5-mg tablets are round, blue tablets with 5 debossed on one side and 511 on the other side.

Diulo 10-mg tablets are round, yellow tablets with 10 debossed on one side and 521 on the other side.

Diulo 2½ mg, 5 mg, and 10 mg are available in bottles of 100 tablets.

Store at room temperature. Dispense in a tight, light-resistant container.

Caution: Federal law prohibits dispensing without prescription.

Diulo is manufactured for G.D. Searle & Co.

RF138

FLAGYL® I.V.   ℞
[flaj 'yl]
(metronidazole hydrochloride)
Single-Dose, 500 mg, glass
  vials (lyophilized powder)
    NSN 6505-01-153-4364 (VA)

FLAGYL® I.V. RTU®   ℞
(metronidazole injection USP) Ready-to-Use
Single-Dose, 500 mg/100 ml,
  RTU plastic containers
    NSN 6505-01-139-4931 (VA)
Sterile
For Intravenous Infusion Only

WARNING

Metronidazole has been shown to be carcinogenic in mice and rats (see *Warnings*). Its use, therefore, should be reserved for the conditions described in the *Indications and Usage* section below.

DESCRIPTION

Flagyl I.V., sterile (metronidazole hydrochloride), and Flagyl I.V. RTU, sterile (metronidazole), are parenteral dosage forms of the synthetic antibacterial agents 1-(β-hydroxyethyl)-2-methyl-5-nitroimidazole hydrochloride and 1-(β-hydroxyethyl)-2-methyl-5-nitroimidazole, respectively.

metronidazole hydrochloride   metronidazole

Each single-dose vial of lyophilized Flagyl I.V. contains sterile, nonpyrogenic metronidazole hydrochloride, equivalent to 500 mg metronidazole, and 415 mg mannitol.

Each Flagyl I.V. RTU 100-ml single-dose plastic container contains a sterile, nonpyrogenic, isotonic, buffered solution of 500 mg metronidazole, 47.6 mg sodium phosphate, 22.9 mg citric acid, and 790 mg sodium chloride in Water for Injection USP. Flagyl I.V. RTU has a tonicity of 310 mOsm/L and a pH of 5 to 7. Each container contains 14 mEq of sodium. The plastic container is fabricated from a specially formulated polyvinyl chloride plastic. Water can permeate from inside the container into the overwrap in amounts insufficient to affect the solution significantly. Solutions in contact with the plastic container can leach out certain of its chemical components in very small amounts within the expiration period, eg, di 2-ethylhexyl phthalate (DEHP), up to 5 parts per million. However, the safety of the plastic has been confirmed in tests in animals according to USP biological tests for plastic containers as well as by tissue culture toxicity studies.

CLINICAL PHARMACOLOGY

Metronidazole is a synthetic antibacterial compound. Disposition of metronidazole in the body is similar for both oral and intravenous dosage forms, with an average elimination half-life in healthy humans of eight hours.

The major route of elimination of metronidazole and its metabolites is via the urine (60–80% of the dose), with fecal excretion accounting for 6–15% of the dose. The metabolites that appear in the urine result primarily from side-chain oxidation [1-(β-hydroxyethyl) -2- hydroxymethyl-5-nitroimidazole and 2-methyl-5-nitroimidazole-1-yl-acetic acid] and glucuronide conjugation, with unchanged metronidazole accounting for approximately 20% of the total. Renal clearance of metronidazole is approximately 10 ml/min/1.73 m^2.

Metronidazole is the major component appearing in the plasma, with lesser quantities of the 2-hydroxymethyl metabolite also being present. Less than 20% of the circulating metronidazole is bound to plasma proteins. Both the parent compound and the metabolite possess *in vitro* bactericidal activity against most strains of anaerobic bacteria.

Metronidazole appears in cerebrospinal fluid, saliva, and breast milk in concentrations similar to those found in plasma. Bactericidal concentrations of metronidazole have also been detected in pus from hepatic abscesses.

Plasma concentrations of metronidazole are proportional to the administered dose. An eight-hour intravenous infusion of 100–4,000 mg of metronidazole in normal subjects showed a linear relationship between dose and peak plasma concentration.

In patients treated with Flagyl I.V., using a dosage regimen of 15 mg/kg loading dose followed six hours later by 7.5 mg/kg every six hours, peak steady-state plasma concentrations of metronidazole averaged 25 mcg/ml with trough (minimum) concentrations averaging 18 mcg/ml.

Decreased renal function does not alter the single-dose pharmacokinetics of metronidazole. However, plasma clearance of metronidazole is decreased in patients with decreased liver function.

In one study newborn infants appeared to demonstrate diminished capacity to eliminate metronidazole. The elimination half-life, measured during the first three days of life, was inversely related to gestational age. In infants whose gestational ages were between 28 and 40 weeks, the corresponding elimination half-lives ranged from 109 to 22.5 hours.

Microbiology: Metronidazole is active *in vitro* against most obligate anaerobes, but does not appear to possess any clinically relevant activity against facultative anaerobes or obligate aerobes. Against susceptible organisms, metronidazole is generally bactericidal at concentrations equal to or slightly higher than the minimal inhibitory concentrations. Metronidazole has been shown to have *in vitro* and clinical activity against the following organisms:

Anaerobic gram-negative bacilli, including:
Bacteroides species, including the *Bacteroides fragilis* group (*B. fragilis, B. distasonis, B. ovatus, B. thetaiotaomicron, B. vulgatus*)
Fusobacterium species.
Anaerobic gram-positive bacilli, including:
Clostridium species and susceptible strains of *Eubacterium*
Anaerobic gram-positive cocci, including:
Peptococcus species
Peptostreptococcus species

Susceptibility Tests: Bacteriologic studies should be performed to determine the causative organisms and their susceptibility to metronidazole; however, the rapid, routine susceptibility testing of individual isolates of anaerobic bacteria is not always practical, and therapy may be started while awaiting these results.

Quantitative methods give the most accurate estimates of susceptibility to antibacterial drugs. A standardized agar dilution method and a broth microdilution method are recommended.[1]

Control strains are recommended for standardized susceptibility testing. Each time the test is performed, one or more of the following strains should be included: *Clostridium perfringens* ATCC 13124, *Bacteroides fragilis* ATCC 25285, and *Bacteroides thetaiotaomicron* ATCC 29741. The mode metronidazole MICs for those three strains are reported to be 0.25, 0.25, and 0.5 mcg/ml, respectively.

A clinical laboratory test is considered under acceptable control if the results of the control strains are within one doubling dilution of the mode MICs reported for metronidazole.

A bacterial isolate may be considered susceptible if the MIC value for metronidazole is not more than 16 mcg/ml. An organism is considered resistant if the MIC is greater than 16 mcg/ml. A report of "resistant" from the laboratory indicates that the infecting organism is not likely to respond to therapy.

INDICATIONS AND USAGE

Treatment of Anaerobic Infections

Flagyl I.V. (metronidazole hydrochloride) and Flagyl I.V. RTU (metronidazole) are indicated in the treatment of serious infections caused by susceptible anaerobic bacteria. Indicated surgical procedures should be performed in conjunction with Flagyl I.V. or Flagyl I.V. RTU therapy. In a mixed aerobic and anaerobic infection, antibiotics appropriate for the treatment of the aerobic infection should be used in addition to Flagyl I.V. or Flagyl I.V. RTU.

Flagyl I.V. and Flagyl I.V. RTU are effective in *Bacteroides fragilis* infections resistant to clindamycin, chloramphenicol, and penicillin.

INTRA-ABDOMINAL INFECTIONS, including peritonitis, intra-abdominal abscess, and liver abscess, caused by *Bacteroides* species including the *B. fragilis* group (*B. fragilis, B. distasonis, B. ovatus, B. thetaiotaomicron, B. vulgatus), Clostridium* species, *Eubacterium* species, *Peptococcus* species, and *Peptostreptococcus* species.

SKIN AND SKIN STRUCTURE INFECTIONS caused by *Bacteroides* species including the *B. fragilis* group, *Clostridium* species, *Peptococcus* species, *Peptostreptococcus* species, and *Fusobacterium* species.

GYNECOLOGIC INFECTIONS, including endometritis, endomyometritis, tubo-ovarian abscess, and postsurgical vaginal cuff infection, caused by *Bacteroides* species including the *B. fragilis* group, *Clostridium* species, *Peptococcus* species, and *Peptostreptococcus* species.

BACTERIAL SEPTICEMIA caused by *Bacteroides* species including the *B. fragilis* group, and *Clostridium* species.

BONE AND JOINT INFECTIONS, as adjunctive therapy, caused by *Bacteroides* species including the *B. fragilis* group.

CENTRAL NERVOUS SYSTEM (CNS) INFECTIONS, including meningitis and brain abscess, caused by *Bacteroides* species including the *B. fragilis* group.

LOWER RESPIRATORY TRACT INFECTIONS, including pneumonia, empyema, and lung abscess, caused by *Bacteroides* species including the *B. fragilis* group.

ENDOCARDITIS caused by *Bacteroides* species including the *B. fragilis* group.

Prophylaxis

The prophylactic administration of Flagyl I.V. or Flagyl I.V. RTU preoperatively, intraoperatively, and postoperatively may reduce the incidence of postoperative infection in patients undergoing elective colorectal surgery which is classified as contaminated or potentially contaminated.

Prophylactic use of Flagyl I.V. or Flagyl I.V. RTU should be discontinued within 12 hours after surgery. If there are signs of infection, specimens for cultures should be obtained for the identification of the causative organism(s) so that appropriate therapy may be given (see *Dosage and Administration*).

CONTRAINDICATIONS

Flagyl I.V. and Flagyl I.V. RTU are contraindicated in patients with a prior history of hypersensitivity to metronidazole or other nitroimidazole derivatives.

WARNINGS

Convulsive Seizures and Peripheral Neuropathy: Convulsive seizures and peripheral neuropathy, the latter characterized mainly by numbness or paresthesia of an extremity, have been reported in patients treated with metronidazole. The appearance of abnormal neurologic signs demands the prompt evaluation of the benefit/risk ratio of the continuation of therapy.

PRECAUTIONS

General: Patients with severe hepatic disease metabolize metronidazole slowly, with resultant accumulation of metronidazole and its metabolites in the plasma. Accordingly, for such patients, doses below those usually recommended should be administered cautiously.

Administration of solutions containing sodium ions may result in sodium retention. Care should be taken when administering Flagyl I.V. RTU to patients receiving corticosteroids or to patients predisposed to edema.

Known or previously unrecognized candidiasis may present more prominent symptoms during therapy with Flagyl I.V. or Flagyl I.V. RTU and requires treatment with a candicidal agent.

Laboratory Tests: Metronidazole is a nitroimidazole, and Flagyl I.V. or Flagyl I.V. RTU should be used with care in patients with evidence of or history of blood dyscrasia. A mild leukopenia has been observed during its administration; however, no persistent hematologic abnormalities attributable to metronidazole have been observed in clinical studies. Total and differential leukocyte counts are recommended before and after therapy.

Drug Interactions: Metronidazole has been reported to potentiate the anticoagulant effect of warfarin and other oral coumarin anticoagulants, resulting in a prolongation of prothrombin time. This possible drug interaction should be considered when Flagyl I.V. or Flagyl I.V. RTU is prescribed for patients on this type of anticoagulant therapy.

The simultaneous administration of drugs that induce microsomal liver enzymes, such as phenytoin or phenobarbital, may accelerate the elimination of metronidazole, resulting in reduced plasma levels; impaired clearance of phenytoin has also been reported.

The simultaneous administration of drugs that decrease microsomal liver enzyme activity, such as cimetidine, may prolong the half-life and decrease plasma clearance of metronidazole.

Alcoholic beverages should not be consumed during metronidazole therapy because abdominal cramps, nausea, vomiting, headaches, and flushing may occur.

Psychotic reactions have been reported in alcoholic patients who are using metronidazole and disulfiram concurrently. Metronidazole should not be given to patients who have taken disulfiram within the last two weeks.

Drug/Laboratory Test Interactions: Metronidazole may interfere with certain types of determinations of serum chemistry values, such as aspartate aminotransferase (AST, SGOT), alanine aminotransferase (ALT, SGPT), lactate dehydrogenase (LDH), triglycerides, and hexokinase glucose. Values of zero may be observed. All of the assays in which interference has been reported involve enzymatic coupling of the assay to oxidation-reduction of nicotine adenine dinucleotide $(NAD^+ \rightleftarrows NADH)$. Interference is due to the similarity in absorbance peaks of NADH (340 nm) and metronidazole (322 nm) at pH 7.

Carcinogenesis, Mutagenesis, Impairment of Fertility: Tumorigenicity in Rodents—Metronidazole has shown evidence of carcinogenic activity in studies involving chronic, oral administration in mice and rats, but similar studies in the hamster gave negative results. Also, metronidazole has shown mutagenic activity in a number of *in vitro* assay systems, but studies in mammals (*in vivo*) failed to demonstrate a potential for genetic damage.

Pregnancy: Teratogenic Effects—Pregnancy Category B. Metronidazole crosses the placental barrier and enters the fetal circulation rapidly. Reproduction studies have been performed in rats at doses up to five times the human dose and have revealed no evidence of impaired fertility or harm to the fetus due to metronidazole. Metronidazole administered intraperitoneally to pregnant mice at approximately the human dose caused fetotoxicity; administered orally to pregnant mice, no fetotoxicity was observed. There are, however, no adequate and well-controlled studies in pregnant women. Because animal reproduction studies are not always predictive of human response, and because metronidazole is a carcinogen in rodents, these drugs should be used during pregnancy only if clearly needed.

Nursing Mothers: Because of the potential for tumorigenicity shown for metronidazole in mouse and rat studies, a decision should be made whether to discontinue nursing or to discontinue the drug, taking into account the importance of the drug to the mother. Metronidazole is secreted in breast milk in concentrations similar to those found in plasma.

Pediatric Use: Safety and effectiveness in children have not been established.

ADVERSE REACTIONS

Two serious adverse reactions reported in patients treated with Flagyl I.V. or Flagyl I.V. RTU have been convulsive seizures and peripheral neuropathy, the latter characterized mainly by numbness or paresthesia of an extremity. Since persistent peripheral neuropathy has been reported in some patients receiving prolonged oral administration of Flagyl® (metronidazole), patients should be observed carefully if neurologic symptoms occur and a prompt evaluation made of the benefit/risk ratio of the continuation of therapy.

The following reactions have also been reported during treatment with Flagyl I.V. (metronidazole hydrochloride) or Flagyl I.V. RTU (metronidazole):

Gastrointestinal: Nausea, vomiting, abdominal discomfort, diarrhea, and an unpleasant metallic taste.

Hematopoietic: Reversible neutropenia (leukopenia).

Dermatologic: Erythematous rash and pruritus.

Central Nervous System: Headache, dizziness, syncope, ataxia, and confusion.

Local Reactions: Thrombophlebitis after intravenous infusion. This reaction can be minimized or avoided by avoiding prolonged use of indwelling intravenous catheters.

Other: Fever. Instances of a darkened urine have also been reported, and this manifestation has been the subject of a special investigation. Although the pigment which is probably responsible for this phenomenon has not been positively identified, it is almost certainly a metabolite of metronidazole and seems to have no clinical significance.

The following adverse reactions have been reported during treatment with oral Flagyl (metronidazole):

Gastrointestinal: Nausea, sometimes accompanied by headache, anorexia, and occasionally vomiting; diarrhea, epigastric distress, abdominal cramping, and constipation.

Mouth: A sharp, unpleasant metallic taste is not unusual. Furry tongue, glossitis, and stomatitis have occurred; these may be associated with a sudden overgrowth of *Candida* which may occur during effective therapy.

Hematopoietic: Reversible neutropenia (leukopenia); rarely, reversible thrombocytopenia.

Cardiovascular: Flattening of the T-wave may be seen in electrocardiographic tracings.

Central Nervous System: Convulsive seizures, peripheral neuropathy, dizziness, vertigo, incoordination, ataxia, confusion, irritability, depression, weakness, and insomnia.

Hypersensitivity: Urticaria, erythematous rash, flushing, nasal congestion, dryness of mouth (or vagina or vulva), and fever.

Renal: Dysuria, cystitis, polyuria, incontinence, a sense of pelvic pressure, and darkened urine.

Other: Proliferation of *Candida* in the vagina, dyspareunia, decrease of libido, proctitis, and fleeting joint pains sometimes resembling "serum sickness." If patients receiving metronidazole drink alcoholic beverages, they may experience abdominal distress, nausea, vomiting, flushing, or headache. A modification of the taste of alcoholic beverages has also been reported.

Crohn's disease patients are known to have an increased incidence of gastrointestinal and certain extraintestinal cancers. There have been some reports in the medical literature of breast and colon cancer in Crohn's disease patients who have been treated with metronidazole at high doses for extended periods of time. A cause and effect relationship has not been established. Crohn's disease is not an approved indication for Flagyl I.V. or Flagyl I.V. RTU.

OVERDOSAGE

Use of dosages of Flagyl I.V. (metronidazole hydrochloride) higher than those recommended has been reported. These include the use of 27 mg/kg three times a day for 20 days, and the use of 75 mg/kg as a single loading dose followed by 7.5 mg/kg maintenance doses. No adverse reactions were reported in either of the two cases.

Single oral doses of metronidazole, up to 15 g, have been reported in suicide attempts and accidental overdoses. Symptoms reported include nausea, vomiting, and ataxia.

Oral metronidazole has been studied as a radiation sensitizer in the treatment of malignant tumors. Neurotoxic effects, including seizures and peripheral neuropathy, have been reported after 5 to 7 days of doses of 6 to 10.4 g every other day.

Treatment: There is no specific antidote for overdose; therefore, management of the patient should consist of symptomatic and supportive therapy.

DOSAGE AND ADMINISTRATION

In elderly patients the pharmacokinetics of metronidazole may be altered and therefore monitoring of serum levels may be necessary to adjust the metronidazole dosage accordingly.

Continued on next page

Schiapparelli Searle—Cont.

Treatment of Anaerobic Infections

The recommended dosage schedule for *adults* is:

Loading dose:
15 mg/kg infused over one hour (approximately 1 g for a 70-kg adult).

Maintenance Dose:
7.5 mg/kg infused over one hour every six hours (approximately 500 mg for a 70-kg adult). The first maintenance dose should be instituted six hours following the initiation of the loading dose.

Parenteral therapy may be changed to oral Flagyl (metronidazole) when conditions warrant, based upon the severity of the disease and the response of the patient to Flagyl I.V. or Flagyl I.V. RTU (metronidazole) treatment. The usual adult oral dosage is 7.5 mg/kg every six hours.

A maximum of 4 g should not be exceeded during a 24-hour period.

Patients with severe hepatic disease metabolize metronidazole slowly, with resultant accumulation of metronidazole and its metabolites in the plasma. Accordingly, for such patients, doses below those usually recommended should be administered cautiously. Close monitoring of plasma metronidazole levels[2] and toxicity is recommended.

In patients receiving Flagyl I.V. or Flagyl I.V. RTU in whom gastric secretions are continuously removed by nasogastric aspiration, sufficient metronidazole may be removed in the aspirate to cause a reduction in serum levels.

The dose of Flagyl I.V. or Flagyl I.V. RTU should not be specifically reduced in anuric patients since accumulated metabolites may be rapidly removed by dialysis.

The usual duration of therapy is 7 to 10 days; however, infections of the bone and joint, lower respiratory tract, and endocardium may require longer treatment.

Prophylaxis

For surgical prophylactic use, to prevent postoperative infection in contaminated or potentially contaminated colorectal surgery, the recommended dosage schedule for adults is:

a. 15 mg/kg infused over 30 to 60 minutes and completed approximately one hour before surgery; followed by

b. 7.5 mg/kg infused over 30 to 60 minutes at 6 and 12 hours after the initial dose.

It is important that (1) administration of the initial preoperative dose be completed approximately one hour before surgery so that adequate drug levels are present in the serum and tissues at the time of initial incision, and (2) Flagyl I.V. or Flagyl I.V. RTU be administered, if necessary, at 6-hour intervals to maintain effective drug levels. Prophylactic use of Flagyl I.V. or Flagyl I.V. RTU should be limited to the day of surgery only, following the above guidelines.

CAUTION: Flagyl I.V. (metronidazole hydrochloride) or Flagyl I.V. RTU (metronidazole) is to be administered by slow intravenous drip infusion only, either as a continuous or intermittent infusion. I.V. admixtures containing metronidazole and other drugs should be avoided. Additives should not be introduced into the Flagyl I.V. RTU solution. If used with a primary intravenous fluid system, the primary solution should be discontinued during metronidazole infusion. DO NOT USE EQUIPMENT CONTAINING ALUMINUM (EG, NEEDLES, CANNULAE) THAT WOULD COME IN CONTACT WITH THE DRUG SOLUTION.

FLAGYL I.V.

Flagyl I.V. **cannot** be given by direct intravenous injection (I.V. bolus) because of the low pH (0.5 to 2.0) of the reconstituted product. **FLAGYL I.V. MUST BE FURTHER DILUTED AND NEUTRALIZED FOR I.V. INFUSION.**

Flagyl I.V. is prepared for use in two steps:

NOTE: ORDER OF MIXING IS IMPORTANT

A. Reconstitution

B. Dilution in intravenous solution followed by pH neutralization with sodium bicarbonate injection into the dilution.

Reconstitution: To prepare the solution, add 4.4 ml of one of the following diluents and mix thoroughly: Sterile Water for Injection, USP; Bacteriostatic Water for Injection, USP; 0.9% Sodium Chloride Injection, USP; or Bacteriostatic 0.9% Sodium Chloride Injection, USP. The resultant approximate withdrawal volume is 5.0 ml with an approximate concentration of 100 mg/ml.

The pH of the reconstituted product will be in the range of 0.5 to 2.0. Reconstituted Flagyl I.V. is clear, and pale yellow to yellow-green in color.

Dilution in Intravenous Solutions: Properly reconstituted Flagyl I.V. (metronidazole hydrochloride) may be added to a glass or plastic I.V. container not to exceed a concentration of 8 mg/ml. Any of the following intravenous solutions may be used: 0.9% Sodium Chloride Injection, USP; 5% Dextrose Injection, USP; or Lactated Ringer's Injection, USP.

NEUTRALIZATION IS REQUIRED PRIOR TO ADMINISTRATION.

The final product should be mixed thoroughly and used within 24 hours.

Neutralization For Intravenous Infusion: Neutralize the intravenous solution containing Flagyl I.V. with approximately 5 mEq of sodium bicarbonate injection for each 500 mg of Flagyl I.V. used. Mix thoroughly. The pH of the neutralized intravenous solution will be approximately 6.0 to 7.0. Carbon dioxide gas will be generated with neutralization. It may be necessary to relieve gas pressure within the container.

Note: When the contents of one vial (500 mg) are diluted and neutralized to 100 ml, the resultant concentration is 5 mg/ml. Do not exceed an 8 mg/ml concentration of Flagyl I.V. in the neutralized intravenous solution, since neutralization will decrease the aqueous solubility and precipitation may occur. DO NOT REFRIGERATE NEUTRALIZED SOLUTIONS; otherwise, precipitation may occur.

Storage and Stability: Reconstituted vials of Flagyl I.V. are chemically stable for 96 hours when stored below 86°F (30°C) in room light.

Use diluted and neutralized intravenous solutions containing Flagyl I.V. within 24 hours of mixing.

FLAGYL I.V. RTU

Flagyl I.V. RTU is a ready-to-use isotonic solution. **NO DILUTION OR BUFFERING IS REQUIRED.** Do not refrigerate. Each container of Flagyl I.V. RTU contains 14 mEq of sodium.

Directions for use of plastic container:

CAUTION: Do not use plastic containers in series connections. Such use could result in air embolism due to residual air (approximately 15 ml) being drawn from the primary container before administration of the fluid from the secondary container is complete.

To open. Tear overwrap down side at slit and remove solution container. Some opacity of the plastic due to moisture absorption during the sterilization process may be observed. This is normal and does not affect the solution quality or safety. The opacity will diminish gradually. Check for minute leaks by squeezing inner bag firmly. If leaks are found discard solution as sterility may be impaired.

Preparation for administration:

1. Suspend container from eyelet support.
2. Remove plastic protector from outlet port at bottom of container.
3. Attach administration set. Refer to complete directions accompanying set.

Parenteral drug products should be inspected visually for particulate matter and discoloration prior to administration, whenever solution and container permit. Do not use if cloudy or precipitated or if the seal is not intact.

Use sterile equipment. It is recommended that the intravenous administration apparatus be replaced at least once every 24 hours.

HOW SUPPLIED

FLAGYL I.V.

Flagyl I.V., sterile (metronidazole hydrochloride), is supplied in single-dose lyophilized vials each containing 500 mg metronidazole equivalent, individually packaged in cartons of 10 vials.

Flagyl I.V., prior to reconstitution, should be stored below 86°F (30°C) and protected from light.

FLAGYL I.V. RTU

Flagyl I.V. RTU, sterile (metronidazole), is supplied in 100-ml single-dose plastic containers, each containing an isotonic, buffered solution of 500 mg metronidazole, individually packaged in boxes of 24.

Flagyl I.V. RTU should be stored at controlled room temperature, 59° to 86° F (15° to 30°C), and protected from light during storage.

1. Proposed standard: PSM-11—Proposed Reference Dilution Procedure for Antimicrobic Susceptibility Testing of Anaerobic Bacteria, National Committee for Clinical Laboratory Standards; and Sutter, et al.: Collaborative Evaluation of a Proposed Reference Dilution Method of Susceptibility Testing of Anaerobic Bacteria, Antimicrob. Agents Chemother. *16:* 495–502 (Oct.) 1979; and Tally, et al.: *In Vitro* Activity of Thienamycin, Antimicrob. Agents Chemother. *14:* 436–438 (Sept.) 1978.

2. Ralph, E.D., and Kirby, W.M.M.: Bioassay of Metronidazole With Either Anaerobic or Aerobic Incubation, J. Infect. Dis. *132:* 587–591 (Nov.) 1975; or Gulaid, et al.: Determination of Metronidazole and Its Major Metabolites in Biological Fluids by High Pressure Liquid Chromatography, Br. J. Clin. Pharmacol. *6:* 430–432, 1978.　　A05034-4

Shown in Product Identification Section, page 428

NORETHIN 1/35E™–21　　℞
NORETHIN 1/35E™–28　　℞

[*nor'ĕ-thin*]

(norethindrone and ethinyl estradiol tablets USP)

NORETHIN 1/50M™–21　　℞
NORETHIN 1/50M™–28　　℞

[*nor'ĕ-thin*]

(norethindrone and mestranol tablets USP)

DESCRIPTION

Norethin 1/35E™-21 and Norethin 1/35E™-28. Each white tablet contains 1 mg of norethindrone and 35 mcg of ethinyl estradiol. Each blue tablet in the Norethin 1/35E™-28 package is a placebo containing inert ingredients.

Norethin 1/50M™-21 and Norethin 1/50M™-28. Each white tablet contains 1 mg of norethindrone and 50 mcg of mestranol. Each blue tablet in the Norethin 1/50M™-28 package is a placebo containing inert ingredients.

In addition to the active ingredients listed with each tablet, all active tablets contain the following inert ingredients: calcium acetate (hydrous), corn starch, dibasic calcium phosphate (anhydrous), hydrogenated castor oil, and povidone. All placebo tablets are composed of calcium sulfate (dihydrate), corn starch, FD&C Blue No. 1 Lake, magnesium stearate, and sucrose.

The chemical name for norethindrone is 17-hydroxy-19-nor-17α-pregn-4-en-20-yn-3-one. The chemical name for ethinyl estradiol is 19-nor-17α-pregna-1,3,5(10)-trien-20-yne-3,17-diol. The chemical name for mestranol is 3-methoxy-19-nor-17α-pregna-1,3,5(10)-trien-20-yn-17-ol. Their structural formulas are as follows:

norethindrone

mestranol

ethinyl estradiol

Therapeutic Class:　　Oral contraceptive.

CLINICAL PHARMACOLOGY

Combination oral contraceptives act primarily through the mechanism of gonadotropin suppression due to the estrogenic and progestational activity of their components. Although the primary mechanism of action is inhibition of ovulation, alterations in the genital tract, including changes in the cervical mucus (which reduce sperm penetration) and the endometrium (which reduce the likelihood of implantation) may also contribute to contraceptive effectiveness.

INDICATIONS AND USAGE

Oral contraceptives are indicated for the prevention of pregnancy in women who elect to use oral contraceptives as a method of contraception.

Oral contraceptives are highly effective.[176] The pregnancy rate in women using conventional combination oral contraceptives (containing 35 mcg or more of ethinyl estradiol or 50 mcg or more of mestranol) is generally reported to be less than 1 pregnancy per 100 woman-years of use. Slightly higher rates (somewhat more than 1 pregnancy per 100 woman-years of use) are reported for some combination products containing 35 mcg or less of ethinyl estradiol, and rates on the order of 3 pregnancies per 100 woman-years are reported for the progestogen-only oral contraceptives.

These rates are derived from separate studies conducted by different investigators in several population groups; therefore, a precise comparison cannot be made. Furthermore, pregnancy rates tend to be lower as clinical studies are continued, possibly due to selective retention in the longer studies of those patients who accept the treatment regimen and do not discontinue as a result of adverse reactions, pregnancy, or other reasons. In Table 1 ranges of pregnancy rates as reported in the literature[1] are shown for other means of contraception. The efficacy of these means of contraception, except for the IUD, depends upon the degree of adherence to the method.

Table 1
Pregnancies per 100 Woman-Years

Method	Range
IUD	<1 to 6
Diaphragm with spermicidal cream or gel	2 to 20
Condom	3 to 36
Spermicidal aerosol foams	2 to 29
Spermicidal gels and creams	4 to 36
Periodic abstinence (rhythm), all types	<1 to 47
1. Calendar method	14 to 47
2. Temperature method	1 to 20
3. Temperature method (intercourse only in postovulatory phase)	<1 to 7
4. Mucus method	1 to 25
No contraception	60 to 80

Dose-Related Risk of Thromboembolism from Oral Contraceptives: Studies have shown a positive association between the dose of estrogens in oral contraceptives and the risk of thromboembolism[2,96,97] (see *Warning* No. 1). For this reason, it is prudent and in keeping with good principles of therapeutics to minimize exposure to estrogen. The oral contraceptive product prescribed for any given patient should be that product which contains the least amount of estrogen that is compatible with an acceptable pregnancy rate and patient acceptance. It is recommended that new users of oral contraceptives be started on preparations containing 50 mcg or less of estrogen.

CONTRAINDICATIONS

Oral contraceptives should not be used in women with any of the following conditions:

1. Thrombophlebitis or thromboembolic disorders.
2. A past history of deep vein thrombophlebitis or thromboembolic disorders.
3. Cerebral vascular disease, myocardial infarction or coronary artery disease, or a past history of these conditions.
4. Known or suspected carcinoma of the breast.
5. Known or suspected estrogen-dependent neoplasia.
6. Undiagnosed abnormal genital bleeding.
7. Known or suspected pregnancy (see *Warning* No. 5).
8. Past or present, benign or malignant liver tumors among women who developed these tumors during the use of oral contraceptives or other estrogen-containing products (see *Warning* No. 4).

WARNINGS

Cigarette-smoking increases the risk of serious cardiovascular side effects from oral contraceptive use. This risk increases with age and with heavy smoking (15 or more cigarettes per day) and is quite marked in women over 35 years of age. Women who use oral contraceptives should be strongly advised not to smoke.

The use of oral contraceptives is associated with increased risk of several serious conditions including venous and arterial thromboembolism, thrombotic and hemorrhagic stroke, myocardial infarction, visual disorders, liver tumors or other liver lesions, gallbladder disease, hypertension, and fetal abnormalities. Practitioners prescribing oral contraceptives should be familiar with the following information relating to these and other risks.

1. Thromboembolic Disorders and Other Vascular Problems. An increased risk of thromboembolic and thrombotic disease associated with the use of oral contraceptives is well established. One study in Great Britain[3] demonstrated an increased relative risk for fatal venous thromboembolism; several British[4,5,14,22,92,156] and U.S.[6-8,93,98-101,126] studies demonstrated an increased relative risk for nonfatal venous thromboembolism. U.S. studies[6,9,10,99,101-103] demonstrated an increased relative risk for stroke, which had not been shown in prior British studies.[3-5] In these studies it was estimated that users of oral contraceptives were 1.9 to 11 times more likely than nonusers to manifest these diseases without evident cause (Table 2). In a British study of idiopathic deep vein thrombosis and pulmonary embolism, the projected annual hospitalization rates for women aged 16–40 were 47 per 100,000 users and 5 for nonusers.[77] In one British mortality study,[3] overall excess mortality due to pulmonary embolism or stroke was on the order of 1.3 to 3.4 deaths annually per 100,000 users and increased with age.

Cerebrovascular Disorders: In a collaborative U.S. study[9,10] of cerebrovascular disorders in women with and without predisposing causes, it was estimated that the risk of hemorrhagic stroke was 2.0 times greater in users than in

nonusers, and the risk of thrombotic stroke was 4.0[10] to 9.5[9] times greater in users than in nonusers (Table 2). Analysis of mortality trends in 21 countries indicates that, since oral contraceptives first became available, changes in mortality from nonrheumatic heart disease and hypertension, cerebrovascular disease, and all nonrheumatic cardiovascular disease among women aged 15 to 44 years have been associated with changes in the prevalence of oral contraceptive use in each country.[11]

Table 2. *Summary of Relative Risks of Thromboembolic Disorders and Other Vascular Problems in Oral Contraceptive Users Compared with Nonusers.*

Disorders	Relative Risk
Idiopathic thrombo-embolic disease	2 to 11 times greater
Postsurgery thromboem-bolic complications	4 to 7 times greater
Thrombotic stroke	4 to 9.5 times greater
Hemorrhagic stroke	2.0 to 2.3 times greater
Myocardial infarction	2 to 12 times greater

In May 1974 the Royal College of General Practitioners[12] issued an interim report of its continuing large-scale prospective study comparing a user group with a nonuser group. It stated: "A statistically significant higher rate of reporting of cerebrovascular accidents in Takers is evident, but the numbers are too small to justify an estimation of the degree of risk." A 1981 analysis of data from this study was reported[13] to show a 4-fold increased mortality from circulatory diseases, mainly from myocardial infarction and hemorrhagic stroke, in users. The excess mortality was associated with age and smoking in users. A 1983 analysis[138] of arterial diseases reported a significantly increased incidence of cerebrovascular disease among current oral contraceptive users. Risk appeared to increase with duration of use up to 8 years. Categories with a significantly increased incidence included cerebral thrombosis or embolism, and transient ischemic attacks, but not hemorrhagic strokes. Incidence of peripheral arterial thromboembolism, Raynaud's disease, and acute myocardial infarction was increased in current users. Women aged 30 years and older had appreciably higher rates of arterial disease than did younger women. Smoking increased the risk for older women in each usage group, the greatest risk being in current users aged 35 years and older who smoked. Expressed as the percentage of women diagnosed as having an arterial disease who died of that disease, the case-fatality rates were 2 to 3 times greater for users who smoked than for women in the other groups.

In October 1976 an interim report was issued on the long-term follow-up study of the British Family Planning Association.[14] There was a highly significant association between oral contraceptive use and stroke, although total numbers were small in this study also. The increase in risk of venous thrombosis and pulmonary embolism among users was about 4-fold and was statistically highly significant. In later reports[15] it was noted that mortality from nonrheumatic heart disease was greater in women who had ever used oral contraceptives. A 1984 report[147] on stroke found pill use to be a significant risk factor for nonhemorrhagic stroke, but not for subarachnoid hemorrhage. Smoking and hypertension were significant risk factors only for the latter.

In the Walnut Creek prospective study,[99,101,102] the risk of subarachnoid hemorrhage was associated with heavy smoking, age, and use of the pill.

Myocardial Infarction: An increased risk of myocardial infarction associated with the use of oral contraceptives has been reported in Great Britain,[16-19,136,138,180] confirming a previously suspected association.[3] The morbidity study[16,17] found that the greater the number of underlying risk factors for coronary artery disease (cigarette-smoking, hypertension, hypercholesterolemia, obesity, diabetes, history of preeclamptic toxemia), the higher the risk of developing myocardial infarction, regardless of whether the patient was an oral contraceptive user or not. Oral contraceptives were considered an additional risk factor.

The annual excess rate of fatal myocardial infarction in British oral contraceptive users was estimated to be approximately 3.5 cases per 100,000 women users in the 30- to 39-year age group and 20 per 100,000 women users in the 40- to 44-year age group.[19] (These estimates are based on British vital statistics, which show acute myocardial infarction death rates 2 to 3 times less than in the U.S. for women in these age groups. In an attempt to extrapolate these figures to U.S. women, it was estimated that the annual excess rates in users were 25.7 cases per 100,000 for women aged 30–39 with predisposing conditions versus 1.5 cases without; corresponding estimates for women aged 40–44 were 86.2 versus 5.1.[78]) The annual excess rate of hospitalization for nonfatal myocardial infarction in married British oral contraceptive users was estimated to be approximately 3.5 per 100,000 women users in the 30- to 39-year age group and 47 per 100,000 women users in the 40- to 44-year age group.[16]

Smoking is considered a major predisposing condition to myocardial infarction. In terms of relative risk, it has been estimated[20] that oral contraceptive users who do not smoke are about twice as likely to have a fatal myocardial infarc-

tion as nonusers who do not smoke. Oral contraceptive users who are also smokers have about a 5-fold increased risk of fatal infarction compared to users who do not smoke, but about a 10- to 12-fold increased risk compared to nonusers who do not smoke. Furthermore, the amount of smoking is also an important factor. In determining the importance of these relative risks, however, the baseline rates for various age groups, as shown in Table 3, must be given serious consideration. The importance of other predisposing conditions mentioned above in determining relative and absolute risks has not been quantified; it is likely that the same synergistic action exists, but perhaps to a lesser extent.

Similar findings relating nonfatal and fatal myocardial infarction, oral contraceptives, smoking, and age were subsequently published in the U.S.[91,99,104-108,152] and by the Royal College of General Practitioners in Great Britain.[13,138,190]

Table 3. *Estimated Annual Mortality Rate per 100,000 Women from Myocardial Infarction by Use of Oral Contraceptives, Smoking Habits, and Age in Years[20]*

	Myocardial infarction			
	Women aged 30–39		Women aged 40–44	
Smoking habits	Users	Non-users	Users	Non-users
All smokers	10.2	2.6	62.0	15.9
Heavy*	13.0	5.1	78.7	31.3
Light	4.7	0.9	28.6	5.7
Nonsmokers	1.8	1.2	10.7	7.4
Smokers and nonsmokers	5.4	1.9	32.8	11.7

*15 or more cigarettes per day

Risk of Dose: Reports of thromboembolism following the use of oral contraceptives containing 50 mcg or more of estrogen received by drug safety committees in Great Britain, Sweden, and Denmark were compared with the distribution expected from market research estimates of sales.[2] A positive correlation was found between the dose of estrogen and the reporting of thromboembolism, including coronary thrombosis, in excess of that predicted by sales estimates. Preparations containing 100 mcg or more of estrogen were associated with a higher risk of thromboembolism than those containing 50 to 80 mcg of estrogen. The authors' analysis did suggest, however, that the quantity of estrogen may not be the sole factor involved. Any influence on the part of the progestogens was not considered, which may have been responsible for certain discrepancies in the data. No significant differences were detected between preparations containing the same dose of estrogen nor between the two estrogens ethinyl estradiol and mestranol. A subsequent study of a similar nature in Great Britain found a positive association between the dose of progestogen or estrogen and certain thromboembolic conditions,[96] which is consistent with findings of the Royal College study.[12,92,135] Swedish authorities noted decreased reporting of thromboembolic episodes when higher estrogen preparations were no longer prescribed.[97] Careful epidemiologic studies to determine the degree of thromboembolic risk associated with progestogen-only oral contraceptives have not been performed. Cases of thromboembolic disease have been reported in women using these products, and they should not be presumed to be free of excess risk.

The relative risk of oral contraceptive use one month prior to hospitalization for various types of thromboembolism was calculated in a U.S. retrospective case-control study.[8] If no account is taken of the relative estrogenic potency of different estrogens and if any possible influence of the different progestogenic components is ignored, the products employed may be divided into those containing less than 100 mcg and those containing 100 mcg or more of estrogen. For all cases combined, the larger-dose category was associated with only a slightly higher relative risk; for the idiopathic subgroup, the relative risk was approximately doubled with the larger estrogen content, but the confidence limits overlapped considerably and the differences, therefore, were not statistically significant. Apparently there was less of an increased relative risk for the subgroup with predispositions to thromboembolism.[98]

In the British Family Planning Association study, no nonhemorrhagic strokes occurred during 9,100 woman-years of current use of pills containing less than 50 mcg of estrogen, in contrast to 13 observed during 39,400 woman-years of current use of pills with higher doses.[147] The incidence of venous thromboembolism was greater for those women using pills containing 50 mcg or more of estrogen than for those using pills with less than 50 mcg estrogen.[173]

A decline of serum high density lipoproteins (HDL) has been reported with increasing progestational activity,[165,167,168,182] and decreased HDL has been associated with an increased incidence of ischemic heart disease.[169] The amount of both

Continued on next page

Schiapparelli Searle—Cont.

steroids should be another consideration in the choice of an oral contraceptive.

The risk of thromboembolic and thrombotic disorders, both in users and in nonusers of oral contraceptives, increases with age. Oral contraceptives have been considered an independent risk factor for these events.

Persistence of Risk: A 1977 analysis[13a] of the mortality data from the prospective study of the Royal College of General Practitioners (RCGP) suggested that the risk of circulatory disease increases with the duration of oral contraceptive use and may persist after discontinuation. The ratio of the mortality rate from circulatory disease in former users to that in controls was 4.3 to 1 (P < 0.01), and was still 3.7 to 1 even after excluding the two deaths from malignant hypertension, where use was stopped because of the onset of hypertension. For the category of fatal subarachnoid hemorrhage, the rate ratio comparing former users to controls was also statistically significant.

In 1981, a new analysis of the RCGP mortality data[13] showed significantly increased risk ratios in former users for the categories of all nonrheumatic heart disease plus hypertension (4.6 to 1), cerebrovascular disease (3.6 to 1), as well as the subcategory of subarachnoid hemorrhage (4.5 to 1). Overall, the incidence of fatal circulatory disease for former users was 4.3 times that of the controls.

A 1983 analysis of the incidence of arterial disease in the RCGP study[138] showed that the incidence of all cerebrovascular disease, fatal and nonfatal, was significantly greater in former users than in controls (risk ratio = 2.6) and remained elevated for at least 6 years after discontinuation of oral contraceptives. Former users had significantly increased rates for cerebral thrombosis (4 vs 0), transient ischemic attacks (8.7 to 1), and "other" cerebrovascular disease (3.8 to 1).

In the Walnut Creek prospective study,[102] former use of oral contraceptives was significantly associated with increased risk of subarachnoid hemorrhage, the relative risk being 5.3. In a U.S. hospital-based, case-control study,[137] when the duration of oral contraceptive use was considered, the data suggested that the rate of myocardial infarction is increased approximately 2- to 3-fold in older women who had used oral contraceptives for more than 10 years before discontinuation. The excess risk associated with long-term use was evident in subjects who had stopped less than 5 years previously, as well as in those who had stopped 5 to 9 years previously. Whether the excess risk persisted for more than 10 years after discontinuation could not be assessed because of a paucity of data.

In summary, persistence of risk after discontinuation of oral contraceptives has been reported for circulatory disease in general,[13,13a] for nonrheumatic heart disease,[13,137] and for cerebrovascular disease,[13,138] including subarachnoid hemorrhage,[13,13a,102] cerebral thrombosis,[138] and transient ischemic attacks.[138]

Estimate of Excess Mortality from Circulatory Diseases: A large prospective study[13] carried out in the U.K. provided estimates of the mortality rate per 100,000 women per year from diseases of the circulatory system for users and nonusers of oral contraceptives according to age, smoking habits, and duration of use. The overall annual excess death rate from circulatory diseases for oral contraceptive users was estimated at 23 per 100,000 for women of all ages. The rates for nonsmokers and smokers, respectively, were: ages 25–34, 2 and 10 per 100,000; ages 35–44, 15 and 48 per 100,000; and ages 45 and older, 41 and 179 per 100,000. The risk was statistically significant only in cigarette-smokers over age 34. The majority of deaths were due to subarachnoid hemorrhage or ischemic heart disease. Relative risk for women who had ever used oral contraceptives rose with increasing parity, a new observation that needs confirmation.

The available data from a variety of sources have been analyzed[21,163] to estimate the risk of death associated with various methods of contraception. The estimates of risk of death for each method included the combined risk of the contraceptive method (eg, thromboembolic and thrombotic disease in the case of oral contraceptives) plus the risk attributable to pregnancy or abortion in the event of method failure. This latter risk varies with the effectiveness of the contraceptive method. The findings of this analysis are shown in Figure 1.[21] The study concluded that the mortality associated with all methods of birth control is low and below that associated with childbirth, except for that associated with oral contraceptives in women over 40 who smoke. (The rates given for pill only/smokers for each age group are for smokers as a class. For "heavy" smokers [more than 15 cigarettes a day], the rates given would be about double; for "light" smokers [less than 15 cigarettes a day], about 50 percent.[20]) The mortality associated with oral contraceptive use in nonsmokers over 40 is higher than with any other method of contraception in that age group. The lowest mortality is associated with the condom or diaphragm backed up by early legal abortion.

Figure 1. Estimated annual number of deaths associated with control of fertility and no control per 100,000 nonsterile women by regimen of control and age of woman.

The risk of thromboembolic and thrombotic disease associated with oral contraceptives increases with age after approximately age 30 and, for myocardial infarction, is further increased by hypertension, hypercholesterolemia, obesity, diabetes, or history of preeclamptic toxemia, and especially by cigarette-smoking.[20,78,79]

Based on the data currently available, the following table gives a gross estimate of the risk of death from circulatory disorders associated with the use of oral contraceptives:

Table 4. *Smoking Habits and Other Predisposing Conditions—Risk Associated with Use of Oral Contraceptives*

Age	Below 30	30–39	40+
Heavy smokers	C	B	A
Light smokers	D	C	B
Nonsmokers (no predisposing conditions)	D	C,D	C
Nonsmokers (other predisposing conditions)	C	C,B	B,A

A—Use associated with very high risk.
B—Use associated with high risk.
C—Use associated with moderate risk.
D—Use associated with low risk.

The physician and patient should be alert to the earliest manifestations of thromboembolic and thrombotic disorders (eg, thrombophlebitis, pulmonary embolism, cerebrovascular insufficiency, coronary artery disease or myocardial infarction, retinal thrombosis, and mesenteric thrombosis). Should any of these occur or be suspected, the drug should be discontinued immediately.

A 4- to 7-fold increased risk of postsurgery thromboembolic complications has also been reported in oral contraceptive users.[22,23] If feasible, oral contraceptives should be discontinued at least 4 weeks before elective surgery or during periods of prolonged immobilization. The decision as to when to resume oral contraception following major surgery or bed rest should balance the recognized risks of postsurgery thromboembolic complications with the need to reinstate contraceptive practices.

The Royal College of General Practitioners in a large prospective study reported a higher incidence of superficial and deep vein thrombosis in users, the former being correlated with the progestogen dose. The RCGP data suggest that the presence of varicose veins substantially increases the risk of superficial venous thrombosis of the leg, the risk depending upon the severity of the varicosities. The evidence suggests that the presence of varicose veins has little effect on the development of deep vein thrombosis in the leg.[92] Other prospective studies have also reported a higher incidence of venous thrombosis in users.[14,99–101,109]

2. *Ocular Lesions.* There have been reports of neuro-ocular lesions such as optic neuritis or retinal thrombosis associated with the use of oral contraceptives. Discontinue medication if there is unexplained, gradual or sudden, partial or complete loss of vision; proptosis or diplopia; papilledema; or any evidence of retinal vascular lesions. Appropriate diagnostic and therapeutic measures should be instituted.

3. *Carcinoma.* Long-term continuous administration of either natural or synthetic estrogens in certain animal species increases the frequency of certain carcinomas, and/or nonmalignant neoplasms, such as those of the breast, uterus, cervix, vagina, ovary, liver, and pituitary. Certain synthetic progestogens, none currently contained in oral contraceptives, have been noted to increase the incidence of mammary nodules, benign and malignant, in dogs.

There is now evidence that estrogens increase the risk of carcinoma of the endometrium in humans. In several independent, retrospective case-control studies,[24–28,80,93] an increased relative risk (2.2 to 13.9 times) was reported, associating endometrial carcinoma with the prolonged use of estrogens in postmenopausal women who took estrogen replacement medication to relieve menopausal symptoms. This risk was independent of the other known risk factors for endometrial cancer and appeared to depend both on duration of treatment[24,27,28] and on estrogen dose.[26–28] These findings are supported by the observation that incidence rates of endometrial cancer have increased sharply since 1969 in 8 different areas of the U.S. with population-based cancer-reporting systems, an increase which may be related to the rapidly expanding use of estrogens during the past decade.[29] There is no evidence at present that "natural" estrogens are more or less hazardous than "synthetic" estrogens at equiestrogenic doses.

One publication[30] reported on the first 30 cases submitted by physicians to a registry of cases of adenocarcinoma of the endometrium in women under 40 on oral contraceptives. Of the adenocarcinomas found in women without predisposing risk factors for adenocarcinoma of the endometrium (eg, irregular bleeding at the time oral contraceptives were first given, polycystic ovaries), nearly all occurred in women who had used a sequential oral contraceptive. These products are no longer marketed. No statistical association has been reported suggesting an increased risk of endometrial cancer in users of conventional combination or progestogen-only oral contraceptives, although individual cases have been reported.

Several studies[7,31–35,39,99,121,122] have reported no increased risk of breast cancer in women taking oral contraceptives or estrogens; however, several other studies have provided inconsistent data reflecting increased risk in various subgroups. In one study,[36,37] while no overall increased risk of breast cancer was noted in women treated with oral contraceptives, a greater risk was suggested for the subgroups of oral contraceptive users with documented benign breast disease and for long-term (2–4 years) users. Other studies[123,142,175] reported increased risk of breast cancer in women who had used the pill for more than 4 years before their first full-term pregnancy. One other study[38] indicated an increasing risk of breast cancer in women taking menopausal estrogens, which increased with duration of follow-up. Several other studies have also shown oral contraceptives[127–129,133,140,141,144,146,148] or estrogens[130,145] to be associated with breast cancer, particularly in connection with other risk factors[127–129] (eg, family history, previous breast biopsy, late age of first delivery) and long duration of use.[127,128,130,146,161] Several recent studies report increased risk in: nulliparous women aged 20–44 with menarche before age 13 who took the pill for 8 or more years[185]; a two-fold overall increased risk for ever-users, with significant risk for subroups aged 30–39 at interview, for long-term (>5 years) users, and for parous women taking the pill for 1–4 years before the first term pregnancy or for < 1 years or >4 years after[186]; age 30–34 at time of diagnosis, and when standardized for age, those who were para 1, and among the latter, those with 2 or more years of use.[187] A reduced occurrence of benign breast tumors in users of oral contraceptives has been well documented.[7,12,14,31,36,39,40,86,99] Some epidemiologic studies[41,81–84,99,109,120,143,149,150,162,170,189] have suggested an increased risk of cervical dysplasia, intraepithelial neoplasia, erosion, and carcinoma in long-term pill users; however, cause and effect has not been established. There have been other reports of microglandular dysplasia of the cervix in users.

In summary, there is at present no consistent evidence from human studies of an increased risk of cancer associated with oral contraceptives.[42] Close clinical surveillance of all women taking oral contraceptives is, nevertheless, essential. In all cases of undiagnosed persistent or recurrent abnormal vaginal bleeding, nonfunctional causes should be borne in mind and appropriate diagnostic measures should be taken to rule out malignancy. Women who have a strong family history of breast cancer or who have breast nodules, fibrocystic disease, recurrent cystic mastitis, abnormal mammograms, or cervical dysplasia should be monitored with particular care if they elect to use oral contraceptives.

4. *Hepatic Lesions (adenomas, hepatomas, hamartomas, regenerating nodules, focal nodular hyperplasia, hemangiomas, peliosis hepatis, sinusoidal dilatation, hepatocellular carcinoma, etc).* Benign hepatic adenomas and other hepatic lesions have been associated with the use of oral contraceptives.[43,45,46,85] One study[46] reported that oral contraceptive formulations with high "hormonal potency" were associated with a higher risk than lower-potency formulations, as was age over 30 years. Although benign, these hepatic lesions may rupture and may cause death through intra-abdominal hemorrhage. This has been reported in short-term as well as long-term users of oral contraceptives. Two studies related risk with duration of use of the contraceptive, the risk being much greater after 4 or more years of oral contraceptive use.[45,46] Long-term users of oral contraceptives have an estimated annual incidence of hepatocellular adenoma of 3 to 4 per 100,000.[46] While such hepatic lesions are rare, they should be considered in women presenting with abdominal pain and tenderness, abdominal mass, or shock. Patients with liver tumors have demonstrated variable clinical features, which may make preoperative diagnosis difficult. About one quarter of the cases presented because of abdominal masses; up to one half had signs and symptoms of acute intraperitoneal hemorrhage. Routine radiologic and laboratory studies may not be helpful. Liver scans may clearly show a focal defect. Hepatic arteriography or computed tomography may be useful procedures in diagnosing primary liver neoplasms.

Cases of hepatocellular carcinoma have been reported in women taking oral contraceptives. The relationship of these drugs to this type of malignancy is not known at this time, although epidemiologic studies[157-159] have estimated a relative risk as high as 7 to 20 for users for 8 or more years as compared to nonusers.[158,159] There is also evidence that oral contraceptives are associated with cancer of the bile duct.[172,177-179]

Oral contraceptives are contraindicated if there are past or present, benign or malignant liver tumors among women who developed these tumors during the use of oral contraceptives or other estrogen-containing products.

5. *Use In or Immediately Preceding Pregnancy, Birth Defects in Offspring, and Malignancy in Offspring.* The use of female sex hormones, both estrogens and progestogens, during early pregnancy may seriously damage the offspring. It has been reported that females exposed in utero to diethylstilbestrol and other nonsteroidal estrogens have an increased risk of developing in later life a form of vaginal or cervical cancer that is ordinarily extremely rare.[47,48] This risk has been estimated to be on the order of 1 in 1,000 exposures or less.[49,50,171] The excess incidence for dysplasia and carcinoma in situ has been estimated at 7.8 cases per 1,000 woman-years.[154] Although there is no evidence at the present time that oral contraceptives further enhance the risk of developing this type of malignancy, such patients should be monitored with particular care if they elect to use oral contraceptives instead of other methods of contraception. Furthermore, a high percentage of such exposed women (from 30% to 90%) have been found to have adenosis (epithelial changes) of the vagina and cervix.[51-55] Although these changes are histologically benign, it is not known whether this condition is a precursor of malignancy. DES-exposed daughters appear to have an increased risk of unfavorable outcome of pregnancy.[110-112] DES-exposed male children may develop abnormalities of the urogenital tract[56-58,131] and sperm.[131] Although similar data are not available for the use of other estrogens, it cannot be presumed that they would not induce similar changes.

Several reports suggest an association between fetal exposure to female sex hormones, including oral contraceptives, and congenital anomalies,[59-64,94,113-116, 174] including multiple congenital anomalies described by the acronym VACTERL, for vertebral, anal, cardiac, tracheoesophageal, renal, and limb defects.[61,62,113] There appears to be a preferential expression of these defects by exposed male offspring.[63,65,115,124] In one case-control study[63] it was estimated that there was a 4.7-fold increased risk of limb-reduction defects in infants exposed in utero to sex hormones (oral contraceptives, hormonal withdrawal tests for pregnancy, or attempted treatment for threatened abortion). Some of these exposures were very short and involved only a few days of treatment. It is reported that the risk of cardiac anomalies and of limb-reduction defects in exposed fetuses is about 1 in 1,000 live births. In a large prospective study,[64] cardiovascular defects in children born to women who received female hormones, including oral contraceptives, during early pregnancy occurred at a rate of 18.2 per 1,000 births, compared to 7.8 per 1,000 for children not so exposed in utero. These results are statistically significant. Female hormone exposure in utero during the first trimester has been reported to be associated with an increased risk of testicular[183] and ovarian[184] cancer. The incidence of twin births may be increased for women who conceive shortly after discontinuing use of the pill.[14,63,117,118,124]

In the past, female sex hormones have been used during pregnancy in an attempt to treat threatened or habitual abortion. There is considerable evidence that estrogens are ineffective for these indications, and there is no evidence from well-controlled studies that progestogens are effective for these uses. An increased incidence of spontaneous abortion associated with lethal chromosome abnormalities (trisomy, triploidy) was reported with high-dose oral contraceptives.[66] However, a recent study including low-dose oral contraceptives did not confirm this effect.[164] Whether there is an overall increase in spontaneous abortion of pregnancies conceived soon after stopping the oral contraceptives is unknown. A highly significant (P < 0.001) increase of lymphocytic chromosome aberrations in oral contraceptive users has been reported.[160]

The safety of this product in pregnancy has not been demonstrated. Pregnancy should be ruled out before initiating or continuing the contraceptive regimen. Pregnancy should always be considered if withdrawal bleeding does not occur. It is recommended that for any patient who has missed 2 consecutive periods, pregnancy should be ruled out before continuing the contraceptive regimen. If the patient has not adhered to the prescribed schedule, the possibility of pregnancy should be considered at the time of the first missed period, and further use of oral contraceptives should be withheld until pregnancy has been ruled out. If pregnancy is confirmed, oral contraceptive use should not be resumed and the patient should be apprised of the potential risks to the fetus, and the advisability of continuation of the pregnancy should be discussed in the light of these risks.

It is recommended that women who discontinue oral contraceptives with the intent of becoming pregnant use an alternative form of contraception for a period of time before attempting to conceive. Many clinicians recommend 3 months, although no precise information is available on which to base this recommendation.

The administration of progestogen-only or progestogen-estrogen combinations to induce withdrawal bleeding should not be used as a test of pregnancy.

6. *Gallbladder Disease.* Reports of studies[7,8,12,14,33] indicate an increased risk for surgically confirmed gallbladder disease in users of oral contraceptives or estrogens. In one study,[12] an increased risk appeared after 2 years of use and doubled after 4 or 5 years of use. In one of the other studies[7] an increased risk was apparent between 6 and 12 months of use. Bile duct carcinoma has been reported.[172,177-179]

7. *Carbohydrate and Lipid Metabolism.* A decrease in glucose tolerance has been observed in a significant percentage of patients on oral contraceptives. For this reason, prediabetic and diabetic patients should be carefully observed while receiving oral contraceptives. An increase in triglycerides, total phospholipids, and lipoproteins has been observed in patients receiving oral contraceptives.[67,165] The clinical significance of this finding remains to be defined.

8. *Elevated Blood Pressure.* An increase in blood pressure has been reported in patients receiving oral contraceptives.[12,69,109] There is evidence that the degree of hypertension may correlate directly with increasing dosage of progestogen.[86] In some women, hypertension may occur within a few months of beginning oral contraceptive use. The prevalence of hypertension in users is low in the first year of use, and may be no higher than that in a comparable group of nonusers. The prevalence in users increases, however, with longer exposure and, in the fifth year of use, is 2½ to 3 times the reported prevalence in the first year. Age is also strongly correlated with the development of hypertension in oral contraceptive users.

Women with a history of elevated blood pressure (hypertension), preexisting renal disease, a history of toxemia or elevated blood pressure during pregnancy, a familial tendency to hypertension or its consequences, or a history of excessive weight gain or fluid retention during the menstrual cycle may be more likely to develop elevation of blood pressure when given oral contraceptives and, therefore, should be monitored closely.[68] Even though elevated blood pressure may remain within the "normal" range, the clinical implications of elevations should not be ignored and close surveillance is indicated, particularly for women with other risk factors for cardiovascular disease or stroke.[69] High blood pressure may or may not persist after discontinuation of the oral contraceptive.

9. *Headache.* The onset or exacerbation of migraine or development of headache of a new pattern which is recurrent, persistent, or severe, requires discontinuation of oral contraceptives and evaluation of the cause.

10. *Bleeding Irregularities.* Breakthrough bleeding, spotting, and amenorrhea are frequent reasons for discontinuance of oral contraceptives. In breakthrough bleeding, as in all cases of irregular or abnormal vaginal bleeding, nonfunctional causes should be borne in mind. In patients with undiagnosed persistent or recurrent abnormal vaginal bleeding, adequate diagnostic measures are indicated to rule out pregnancy or malignancy. If a pathologic basis has been excluded, passage of time or a change to another formulation may correct the bleeding problem. A change to an oral contraceptive with a higher estrogen content, while potentially useful in minimizing menstrual irregularity, should be made only when considered necessary since this may increase the risk of thromboembolic disease.

Women with a past history of oligomenorrhea or secondary amenorrhea or young women who have not established regular cycles may have a tendency to remain anovulatory or to become amenorrheic after discontinuation of oral contraceptives. Women with these preexisting problems should be informed of these possibilities and encouraged to use other contraceptive methods. Post-use anovulation, possibly prolonged, may also occur in women without previous irregularities. A higher incidence of galactorrhea and of pituitary tumors (eg, adenomas) has been associated with amenorrhea in former users compared with nonusers.[87] One study[70] reported a 16-fold increased prevalence of pituitary prolactin-secreting tumors among patients with postpill amenorrhea when galactorrhea was present. A case-control study[44] reported an increased risk of galactorrhea following discontinuation of oral contraceptives by women who did not have pituitary tumors.

11. *Ectopic Pregnancy.* Contraceptive failure may result in either ectopic or intrauterine pregnancy. In failures with combination-type oral contraceptives, the ratio of ectopic to intrauterine pregnancies is no higher than in women who are not receiving oral contraceptives.

12. *Breast Feeding.* Oral contraceptives given in the postpartum period may interfere with lactation. There may be a decrease in the quantity and quality of the breast milk. Furthermore, a small fraction of the hormonal agents in oral contraceptives has been identified in the milk of mothers receiving these drugs.[71,88,89] The effects, if any, on the breast-fed child have not been determined. If feasible, the use of oral contraceptives should be deferred until the infant has been weaned.

13. *Infertility.* There is evidence of fertility impairment in women discontinuing oral contraceptives in comparison with those discontinuing other methods.[14,90,132,155] While the impairment diminishes with time, there is still an appreciable difference in the results in nulliparous women aged 25 to 29 at 30 months after discontinuation of birth control; the difference is negligible after 48 months. However, among nulliparas aged 30–34, the impairment persists up to 72 months and appears more severe for users for 2 or more years. For parous women aged 25 to 34 the difference is no longer apparent 30 months after cessation of contraception.

PRECAUTIONS

General. 1. A complete medical and family history should be taken and a thorough physical examination should be performed prior to the initiation of oral contraceptives. The pretreatment and periodic physical examinations should include special reference to blood pressure, breasts, abdomen, and pelvic organs, including a Pap smear and relevant laboratory tests. As a general rule, oral contraceptives should not be prescribed for longer than one year without the performance of another physical examination (see *Warnings*).

2. Preexisting uterine leiomyomata may increase in size during oral contraceptive use. While unconfirmed, an increased risk of fibroids with oral contraceptives containing ethynodiol diacetate has been reported.[166]

3. Oral contraceptives appear to be associated with an increased incidence of mental depression. Therefore, patients with a history of depression should be carefully observed and the drug discontinued if depression recurs to a serious degree. Patients becoming significantly depressed while taking oral contraceptives should stop the medication and use an alternative method of contraception in an attempt to determine whether the symptom is drug related.

4. Oral contraceptives may cause some degree of fluid retention. They should be prescribed with caution, and only with careful monitoring, in patients with conditions which might be aggravated by fluid retention, such as convulsive disorders, migraine syndrome, asthma, or cardiac, hepatic, or renal dysfunction.

5. Patients with a past history of jaundice during pregnancy have an increased risk of recurrence of jaundice and should be carefully observed while receiving oral contraceptives. If jaundice develops in any patient receiving such drugs, the medication should be discontinued while the cause is investigated. Cholestatic jaundice has been reported after combined treatment with oral contraceptives and troleandomycin. Hepatotoxicity following a combination of oral contraceptives and cyclosporine has also been reported.

6. Steroid hormones may be poorly metabolized in patients with impaired liver function and should be administered with caution in such patients.

7. Oral contraceptive users may have disturbances in normal tryptophan metabolism, which may result in a relative pyridoxine deficiency. The clinical significance of this is unknown, although megaloblastic anemia has been reported.

8. Serum folate levels may be depressed by oral contraceptive therapy. Since the pregnant woman is predisposed to folate deficiency and the incidence of folate deficiency increases with lengthening gestation, it is possible that if a woman becomes pregnant shortly after stopping oral contraceptives, she may have a greater chance of developing

Continued on next page

Schiapparelli Searle—Cont.

folate deficiency and complications attributable to this deficiency.

9. The pathologist should be advised of oral contraceptive therapy when relevant specimens are submitted.

10. Certain endocrine and liver function tests may be affected by estrogen-containing oral contraceptives. Therefore, it is recommended that any abnormal tests be repeated after the drug has been withdrawn for two months. The following alterations in laboratory results have been observed with the use of oral contraceptives:

a. Hepatic function: Increased sulfobromophthalein retention and other abnormalities in tests of liver function.

b. Coagulation tests: Increased prothrombin and coagulation factors VII, VIII, IX, and X; decreased antithrombin III; increased platelet aggregability.

c. Thyroid function: Increased thyroid-binding globulin (TBG) leading to increased circulating total thyroid hormone, as measured by protein-bound iodine (PBI) or T^4 by column or radioimmunoassay. Free T^3 resin uptake is decreased, reflecting the elevated TBG; free T^4 concentration is unaltered.

d. Decreased pregnanediol excretion.

e. Reduced response to metyrapone test.

f. Increased blood transcortin and corticosteroid levels.

g. Increased blood triglyceride and phospholipid concentrations.

h. Reduced serum folate concentration.

i. Impaired glucose tolerance.

j. Altered plasma levels of trace minerals (eg, increased ceruloplasmin).

11. The influence of prolonged oral contraceptive therapy on pituitary, ovarian, adrenal, hepatic, or uterine function, or on the immune response, has not been established.

12. Treatment with oral contraceptives may mask the onset of the climacteric. (See *Warnings* section regarding risks in this age group.)

13. The prevalence of cervical *Chlamydia trachomatis* and *Neisseria gonorrhoeae* in oral contraceptive users is increased several-fold.[151,191] It should not be assumed that oral contraceptives afford protection against pelvic inflammatory disease from *Chlamydia*.[151] HIV seropositivity in female African prostitutes was significantly associated with a history of taking oral medications for the prevention of pregnancy and/or of sexually transmitted diseases.[181,188]

Information for the Patient. See patient labeling printed at end.

Drug Interactions. Oral contraceptives may be rendered less effective and increased incidence of breakthrough bleeding may occur by virtue of drug interaction with rifampin, isoniazid, ampicillin, neomycin, penicillin V, tetracycline, chloramphenicol, sulfonamides, nitrofurantoin, griseofulvin, barbiturates, phenytoin, carbamazepine, primidone, phenylbutazone, analgesics, tranquilizers, and antimigraine preparations.[72–74,95,125,153] Oral contraceptives may alter the effectiveness of other types of drugs, such as oral anticoagulants, anticonvulsants, tranquilizers (eg, diazepam), tricyclic antidepressants, antihypertensive agents (eg, guanethidine), theophylline, caffeine, vitamins, hypoglycemic agents, clofibrate, glucocorticoids, and acetaminophen.[72,119,134,139,153] (See *Precaution* No. 5.)

Carcinogenesis. See *Warnings* No. 3 and 4 for information on the carcinogenic potential of oral contraceptives.

Pregnancy. Pregnancy category X. See *Contraindication* No. 7 and *Warning* No. 5.

Nursing Mothers. See *Warning* No. 12.

ADVERSE REACTIONS

An increased risk of the following serious adverse reactions has been associated with the use of oral contraceptives (see *Warnings*):

Thrombophlebitis and thrombosis
Pulmonary embolism
Arterial thromboembolism
Raynaud's disease
Myocardial infarction and coronary thrombosis
Cerebral thrombosis
Cerebral hemorrhage
Hypertension
Gallbladder disease
Budd-Chiari syndrome
Benign adenomas and other hepatic lesions, with or without intra-abdominal bleeding
Hepatocellular carcinoma
Congenital anomalies

There is evidence of an association between the following conditions and the use of oral contraceptives, although confirmatory studies have not been done:

Mesenteric thrombosis
Neuro-ocular lesions (eg, retinal thrombosis and optic neuritis)

The following adverse reactions have been reported in patients receiving oral contraceptives and are believed to be drug related:

Nausea and vomiting
(Usually the most common adverse reactions, occurring in approximately 10% or fewer patients during the first cycle. Other reactions, as a general rule, are seen much less frequently or only occasionally.)
Gastrointestinal symptoms (eg, abdominal cramps and bloating)
Breakthrough bleeding
Spotting
Change in menstrual flow
Dysmenorrhea
Amenorrhea during and after use
Infertility after discontinuation
Edema
Chloasma or melasma, which may persist when the drug is discontinued
Breast changes: tenderness, enlargement, and secretion
Change in weight (increase or decrease)
Change in cervical erosion and secretion
Endocervical hyperplasia
Possible diminution in lactation when given immediately post partum
Cholestatic jaundice
Migraine
Increase in size of uterine leiomyomata
Rash (allergic)
Mental depression
Reduced tolerance to carbohydrates
Vaginal candidiasis
Change in corneal curvature (steepening)
Intolerance to contact lenses

The following adverse reactions or conditions have been reported in users of oral contraceptives, and the association has been neither confirmed nor refuted:

Premenstrual-like syndrome
Cataracts
Changes in libido
Chorea
Changes in appetite
Cystitis-like syndrome
Headache
Paresthesia
Nervousness
Dizziness
Auditory disturbances
Rhinitis
Fatigue
Backache
Hirsutism
Loss of scalp hair
Erythema multiforme
Erythema nodosum
Hemorrhagic eruption
Herpes gestationis
Hidradenitis suppurativa
Hemolytic uremic syndrome
Malignant hypertension
Impaired renal function
Acute renal failure, sometimes irreversible
Itching
Vaginitis
Porphyria
Premature ventricular contractions
Electrocardiogram abnormalities
Pulmonary hypertension
Thrombotic thrombocytopenic purpura
Anemia
Pancreatitis
Hepatitis
Colitis
Crohn's disease
Gingivitis
Dry socket
Lupus erythematosus
Rheumatoid arthritis
Pituitary tumors (eg, adenoma) with amenorrhea and/or galactorrhea after OC use
Malignant melanoma
Endometrial, cervical, breast, and bile duct carcinoma (see *Warning* No. 3)

ACUTE OVERDOSAGE

Serious ill effects have not been reported following the acute ingestion of large doses of oral contraceptives by young children.[75,76] Overdosage may cause nausea, and withdrawal bleeding might occur in females.

DOSAGE AND ADMINISTRATION

Each package contains 21 or 28 tablets in numbered rows of 7 tablets each. The days of the week are printed above the columns.

To achieve maximum contraceptive effectiveness, oral contraceptives must be taken exactly as directed and at intervals of 24 hours.

IMPORTANT: During the first week of *initial* use of oral contraceptives, the patient should be instructed to use an additional method of contraception. The possibility of ovulation and conception prior to initiation of oral contraceptives should be considered.

Dosage Schedules
21-Day Schedules

For use with Norethin 1/35E™-21 and Norethin 1/50M™-21.

Sunday Schedule: The patient starts taking tablets on the first Sunday after the menstrual period begins. If the menstrual period begins on a Sunday, the first tablet is taken that same day. The three rows of tablets are completed, in order, followed by 7 days with no tablets. The next cycle is begun, as before, on a Sunday.

Day-5 Schedule: The patient starts taking tablets on day 5 of the menstrual cycle, counting day 1 as the first day of menstrual flow. The initial tablet is in row #1, the day of the week corresponding to day 5 of the cycle. When row #3 has been completed, any tablets remaining in row #1 should be taken. After 7 days of no tablets, the next cycle is begun on the same day of the week as the first cycle.

Postpartum Administration. Norethin 1/35E™-21 and Norethin 1/50M™-21 oral contraceptives may be prescribed at the first postpartum examination regardless of whether or not the patient has experienced spontaneous menstruation. In non-nursing mothers, administration may be initiated immediately after delivery if desired or on the first Sunday after delivery. If preferred the tablets may be started on the day the patient leaves the hospital. (For nursing mothers, see *Warning* No. 12.) Increased risk of thromboembolism during the postpartum period must be considered. (See *Contraindications, Warnings, and Precautions.*)

28-Day Schedules

For use with Norethin 1/35E™-28 and Norethin 1/50M™-28.

Sunday Schedule: The patient starts taking tablets on the first Sunday after the menstrual period begins. If the menstrual period begins on a Sunday, the first tablet is taken that same day. The four rows of tablets are completed in order, and the next cycle is started the next day, Sunday.

If one or more placebo tablets are missed, the next cycle should be started as scheduled on the next Sunday. Risk of pregnancy is not increased by missing placebo tablets, if the schedule of active tablets is followed.

Day-5 Schedule: The patient starts taking white tablets on day 5 of the menstrual cycle, counting day 1 as the first day of menstrual flow. The initial white tablet is in row #1, the day of the week corresponding to day 5 of the cycle. When row #3 has been completed, any white tablets remaining in row #1 should be taken. **The patient must take all of the white tablets before taking any blue placebo tablets in row #4.** After all of the white tablets are used, the patient takes the blue placebo tablets in row #4 for one week (7 days). The patient begins the next cycle on the same day of the week as she began the first cycle.

If one or more placebo tablets are missed, the next cycle should be started as scheduled on the same day of the week as the previous cycle. Risk of pregnancy is not increased by missing placebo tablets, if the schedule of active tablets is followed.

Postpartum Administration. Norethin 1/35E™-28 and Norethin 1/50M™-28 oral contraceptives may be prescribed at the first postpartum examination regardless of whether or not the patient has experienced spontaneous menstruation. In non-nursing mothers, administration may be initiated immediately after delivery if desired or on the first Sunday after delivery. If preferred the tablets may be started on the day the patient leaves the hospital. (For nursing mothers, see *Warning* No. 12.) Increased risk of thromboembolism during the postpartum period must be considered. (See *Contraindications, Warnings, and Precautions.*)

Special Notes

Spotting or Breakthrough Bleeding. If spotting (bleeding insufficient to require a pad) or breakthrough bleeding (heavier bleeding similar to a menstrual flow) occurs when these products are used for contraception the patient should continue taking her tablets as directed. The incidence of spotting or breakthrough bleeding is minimal, most frequently occurring in the first cycle. Ordinarily spotting or breakthrough bleeding will stop within a week. Usually the patient will begin to cycle regularly within two or three courses of tablet-taking. In the event of spotting or breakthrough bleeding organic causes should be borne in mind. (See *Warning* No. 10.)

Missed Menstrual Periods. Withdrawal flow will normally occur two or three days after the last active tablet is taken. Failure of withdrawal bleeding ordinarily does not mean that the patient is pregnant, providing the dosage schedule has been correctly followed. (See *Warning* No. 5.)

If the patient has *not* adhered to the prescribed dosage regimen, the possibility of pregnancy should be considered after the first missed period, and oral contraceptives should be withheld until pregnancy has been ruled out.

If the patient has adhered to the prescribed regimen and misses two consecutive periods, pregnancy should be ruled out before continuing the contraceptive regimen.

The first intermenstrual interval after discontinuing the tablets is usually prolonged; consequently, a patient for whom a 28-day cycle is usual might not begin to menstruate for 35 days or longer. Ovulation in such prolonged cycles will occur correspondingly later in the cycle. Posttreatment cycles after the first one, however, are usually typical for the individual woman prior to taking tablets. (See *Warnings* No. 10 and 11.)

Missed Tablets (Contraception). If a woman misses taking one active tablet the missed tablet should be taken as soon as it is remembered. In addition, the next tablet should be taken at the usual time. If two consecutive active tablets are missed the dosage should be doubled for the next two days. The regular schedule should then be resumed, but an additional method of protection is recommended for the remainder of the cycle.

While there is little likelihood of ovulation if only one active tablet is missed, the possibility of spotting or breakthrough bleeding is increased and should be expected if two or more successive active tablets are missed. However, the possibility of ovulation increases with each successive day that scheduled active tablets are missed.

HOW SUPPLIED

Norethin 1/35E:

Each white Norethin 1/35E tablet is round in shape, with a debossed SEARLE on one side and 221 on the other side, and contains 1 mg of norethindrone and 35 mcg of ethinyl estradiol.

Norethin 1/35E^{TM}*-21* (NDC 0014-0221-06) is packaged in cartons of six tablet dispensers of 21 tablets each.

Norethin 1/35E^{TM}*-28* (NDC 0014-0231-06) is packaged in cartons of six tablet dispensers. Each dispenser contains 21 white tablets and 7 blue placebo tablets. (Placebo tablets have a debossed SEARLE on one side and a "P" on the other side.)

Norethin 1/50M:

Each white Norethin 1/50M tablet is round in shape, with a debossed SEARLE on one side and 431 on the other side, and contains 1 mg of norethindrone and 50 mcg of mestranol.

Norethin 1/50M^{TM}*-21* (NDC 0014-0431-06) is packaged in cartons of six tablet dispensers of 21 tablets each.

Norethin 1/50M^{TM}*-28* (NDC 0014-0441-06) is packaged in cartons of six tablet dispensers. Each dispenser contains 21 white tablets and 7 blue placebo tablets. (Placebo tablets have a debossed SEARLE on one side and a "P" on the other side.)

Caution: Federal law prohibits dispensing without prescription.

REFERENCES

1. Population Reports, Series H, No. 2 (May) 1974; Series I, No. 1 (June) 1974; Series B, No. 3 (May) 1979; Series H, No. 3 (Jan.) 1975; Series H, No. 4 (Jan.) 1976; Population Information Program, Geo. Washington U. Medical Center, Washington, D.C. **2.** Inman, W. H. W., et al.: Br. Med. J. *2*:203 (April 25) 1970. **3.** Inman, W. H. W., et al.: Br. Med. J. *2*:193 (April 27) 1968. **4.** Royal College of General Practitioners: J. Coll. Gen. Pract. *13*:267 (May) 1967. **5.** Vessey, M. P., et al.: Br. Med. J. *2*:651 (June 14) 1969. **6.** Sartwell, P. E., et al.: Am. J. Epidemiol. *90*:365 (Nov.) 1969.**7.** Boston Collaborative Drug Surveillance Programme: Lancet *1*:1399 (June 23) 1973. **8.** Stolley, P.D., et al.: Am. J. Epidemiol. *102*:197 (Sept.) 1975. **9.** Collaborative Group for the Study of Stroke in Young Women: N. Engl. J. Med. *288*:871 (April 26) 1973. **10.** Collaborative Group for the Study of Stroke in Young Women: J.A.M.A. *231*:718 (Feb. 17) 1975. **11.** Beral, V.: Lancet *2*:1047 (Nov. 13) 1976. **12.** Royal College of General Practitioners: Oral Contraceptives and Health, New York, Pitman Publ. Corp., May 1974. **13.** Layde, P., et al.: Lancet *1*:541 (March 7) 1981. **13a.** Beral, V., et al.: Lancet *2*:727 (Oct. 8) 1977. **14.** Vessey, M., et al.: J. Biosoc. Sci. *8*:373 (Oct.) 1976. **15.** Vessey, M., et al.: Lancet *2*:731 (Oct. 8) 1977; *1*:549 (March 7) 1981. **16.** Mann, J. I., et al.: Br. Med. J. *2*:241 (May 3) 1975. **17.** Mann, J. I., et al.: Br. Med. J. *3*:631 (Sept. 13) 1975. **18.** Mann, J. I., et al.: Br. Med. J. *2*:245 (May 3) 1975. **19.** Mann, J. I., et al.: Br. Med. J. *2*:445 (Aug. 21) 1976. **20.** Jain, A. K.: Stud. Fam. Plann. *8*:50 (March) 1977. **21.** Tietze, C.: Fam. Plann. Perspect. *9*:74 (March-April) 1977. **22.** Vessey, M. P., et al.: Br. Med. J. *3*:123 (July 18) 1970. **23.** Greene, G. R., et al.: Am. J. Public Health *62*:680 (May) 1972. **24.** Ziel, H. K., et al.: N. Engl. J. Med. *293*:1167 (Dec. 4) 1975. **25.** Smith, D. C., et al.: N. Engl. J. Med. *293*:1164 (Dec. 4) 1975. **26.** Mack, T. M., et al.: N. Engl. J. Med. *294*:1262 (June 3) 1976. **27.** Gray, L. A., et al.: Obstet. Gynecol. *49*:385 (April) 1977. **28.** McDonald, T. W., et al.: Am. J. Obstet. Gynecol. *127*:572 (March 15) 1977. **29.** Weiss, N. S., et al.: N. Engl. J. Med. *294*:1259 (June 3) 1976. **30.** Silverberg, S. G., et al.: Cancer *39*:592 (Feb.) 1977. **31.** Vessey, M. P., et al.: Br. Med. J. *3*:719 (Sept. 23) 1972. **32.** Vessey, M. P., et al.: Lancet *1*:941 (April 26) 1975. **33.** Boston Collaborative Drug Surveillance Program: N. Engl. J. Med. *290*:15 (Jan. 3) 1974. **34.** Arthes, F. G., et al.: Cancer *28*:1391 (Dec.) 1971. **35.** Casagrande, J., et al.: J. Natl. Cancer Inst. *56*:839 (April) 1976. **36.** Fasal, E., et al.: J. Natl. Cancer Inst. *55*:767 (Oct.) 1975. **37.** Paffenbarger, R. S., et al.: Cancer *39*:1887 (April Suppl.) 1977. **38.** Hoover, R., et al.: N. Engl. J. Med. *295*:401 (Aug. 19) 1976. **39.** Kelsey, J. L., et al.: Am. J. Epidemiol. *107*:236 (March) 1978. **40.** Ory, H., et al.: N. Engl. J. Med. *294*:419 (Feb. 19) 1976. **41.** Stern, E., et al.: Science *196*:1460 (June 24) 1977. **42.** Population Reports, Series A, No. 4 (May) 1977: Population Information Program, Geo. Washington U. Medical Center, Washington, D.C. **43.** Baum, J. K., et al.: Lancet *2*:926 (Oct. 27) 1973. **44.** Taler, S.J., et al.: Obstet. Gynecol. *65*:665 (May) 1985. **45.** Edmondson, H. A., et al.: N. Engl. J. Med. *294*:470 (Feb. 26) 1976. **46.** Rooks, J. B., et al.: J.A.M.A. *242*:644 (Aug. 17) 1979. **47.** Herbst, A. L., et al.: N. Engl. J. Med. *284*:878 (April 22) 1971. **48.** Greenwald, P., et al.: N. Engl. J. Med. *285*:390 (Aug. 12) 1971. **49.** Lanier, A. P., et al.: Mayo Clin. Proc. *48*:793 (Nov.) 1973. **50.** Herbst, A. L., et al.: Am. J. Obstet. Gynecol. *128*:43 (May 1) 1977. **51.** Herbst, A. L., et al.: Obstet. Gynecol. *40*:287 (Sept.) 1972. **52.** Herbst, A. L., et al.: Am. J. Obstet. Gynecol. *118*:607 (March 1) 1974. **53.** Herbst, A. L., et al.: N. Engl. J. Med. *292*:334 (Feb. 13) 1975. **54.** Stafl, A., et al.: Obstet. Gynecol. *43*:118 (Jan.) 1974. **55.** Sherman, A. I., et al.: Obstet. Gynecol. *44*:531 (Oct.) 1974. **56.** Bibbo, M., et al.: J. Reprod. Med. *15*:29 (July) 1975. **57.** Gill, W., et al.: J. Reprod. Med. *16*:147 (April) 1976. **58.** Henderson, B., et al.: Pediatrics *58*:505 (Oct.) 1976. **59.** Gal, I., et al.: Nature *240*:241 (Nov. 24) 1972. **60.** Levy, E. P., et al.: Lancet *1*:611 (March 17) 1973. **61.** Nora, J. J., et al.: Lancet *1*:941 (April 28) 1973. **62.** Nora, A. H., et al.: Arch. Environ. Health *30*:17 (Jan.) 1975; Adv. Plann. Parent. *12*:156, 1978. **63.** Janerich, D. T., et al.: N. Engl. J. Med. *291*:697 (Oct. 3) 1974. **64.** Heinonen, O. P., et al.: N. Engl. J. Med. *296*:67 (Jan. 13) 1977. **65.** Nora, J. J., et al.: N. Engl. J. Med. *291*:731 (Oct. 3) 1974. **66.** Carr, D. H.: Can. Med. Assoc. J. *103*:343 (Aug. 15 & 29) 1970. **67.** Wynn, V., et al.: Lancet *2*:720 (Oct. 1) 1966. **68.** Laragh, J. H.: Am. J. Obstet. Gynecol. *126*:141 (Sept.) 1976. **69.** Fisch, I. R., et al.: J.A.M.A. *237*:2499 (June 6) 1977. **70.** Van Campenhout, J., et al.: Fertil. Steril. *28*:728 (July) 1977. **71.** Laumas, K. R., et al.: Am. J. Obstet. Gynecol. *98*:411 (June 1) 1967. **72.** Stockley, I.: Pharmaceut. J. *216*:140 (Feb. 14) 1976. **73.** Hempel, E., et al.: Drugs *12*:442 (Dec.) 1976. **74.** Bessot, J.-C., et al.: Nouv. Presse Med. *6*:1568 (April 30) 1977. **75.** Francis, W. G., et al.: Can. Med. Assoc. J. *92*:191 (Jan. 23) 1965. **76.** Verhulst, H. L., et al.: J. Clin. Pharmacol. *7*:9 (Jan.-Feb.) 1967. **77.** Vessey, M. P., et al.: Br. Med. J. *2*:199 (April 27) 1968. **78.** Ory, H. W.: J.A.M.A. *237*:2619 (June 13) 1977. **79.** Jain, A. K.: Am. J. Obstet. Gynecol. *126*:301 (Oct. 1) 1976. **80.** Ziel, H. K., et al.: Am. J. Obstet. Gynecol. *124*:735 (April 1) 1976. **81.** Peritz, E., et al.: Am. J. Epidemiol. *106*:462 (Dec.) 1977. **82.** Ory, H. W., et al.: in Garattini, S., and Berendes, H. (eds.): Pharmacology of Steroid Contraceptive Drugs, Raven Press, N.Y., 1977. **83.** Goldacre, M. J., et al.: Br. Med. J. *1*:748 (March 25) 1978. **84.** Meisels, A., et al.: Cancer *40*:3076 (Dec.) 1977. **85.** Klatskin, G.: Gastroenterology *73*:386 (Aug.) 1977. **86.** Kay, C. R.: Lancet *1*:624 (March 19) 1977. **87.** March, C. M., et al.: Fertil. Steril. *28*:346 (March) 1977. **88.** Saxena, B. N., et al.: Contraception *16*:605 (Dec.) 1977. **89.** Nilsson, S., et al.: Contraception *17*:131 (Feb.) 1978. **90.** Vessey, M. P., et al.: Br. Med. J. *1*:265 (Feb. 4) 1978. **91.** Jick, H., et al.: J.A.M.A. *239*:1403, 1407 (April 3) 1978. **92.** Kay, C. R.: J. R. Coll. Gen. Pract. *28*:393 (July) 1978. **93.** Hoogerland, D. L., et al.: Gynecol. Oncol. *6*:451 (Oct.) 1978. **94.** Lorber, C. A., et al.: Fertil. Steril. *31*:21 (Jan.) 1979. **95.** Bacon, J. F., et al.: Br. Med. J. *280*:293 (Feb. 2) 1980. **96.** Meade, T. W., et al.: Br. Med. J. *280*:1157 (May 10) 1980. **97.** Böttiger, L. E., et al.: Lancet *1*:1097 (May 24) 1980. **98.** Maguire, M. G., et al.: Am. J. Epidemiol. *110*:188 (Aug.) 1979. **99.** Ramcharan, S., et al.: The Walnut Creek Contraceptive Drug Study, Vol. 3, U.S. Govt. Ptg. Off., 1981; J. Reprod. Med. *25*:346 (Dec.) 1980. **100.** Petitti, D. B., et al.: Am. J. Epidemiol. *108*:480 (Dec.) 1978. **101.** Petitti, D. B., et al.: J.A.M.A. *242*:1150 (Sept. 14) 1979. **102.** Petitti, D. B., et al.: Lancet *2*:234 (July 29) 1978. **103.** Jick, H., et al.: Ann. Int. Med. *88*:58 (July) 1978. **104.** Jick, H., et al.: J.A.M.A. *240*:2548 (Dec. 1) 1978. **105.** Shapiro, S., et al.: Lancet *1*:743 (April 7) 1979. **106.** Rosenberg, L., et al.: Am. J. Epidemiol. *111*:59 (Jan.) 1980. **107.** Kreuger, D. E., et al.: Am. J. Epidemiol. *111*:655 (June) 1980. **108.** Arthes, F. G., et al.: Chest *70*:574 (Nov.) 1976. **109.** Hoover, R., et al.: Am. J. Public Health *68*:335 (April) 1978. **110.** Herbst, A. L., et al.: J. Reprod. Med. *24*:62 (Feb.) 1980. **111.** Barnes, A. B., et al.: N. Engl. J. Med. *302*:609 (March 13) 1980. **112.** Cousins, L., et al.: Obstet. Gynecol. *56*:70 (July) 1980. **113.** Nora, J. J., et al.: J.A.M.A. *240*:837 (Sept. 1) 1978. **114.** Aarskog, D.: N. Engl. J. Med. *300*:75 (Jan. 11) 1979. **115.** Janerich, D. T., et al.: Am. J. Epidemiol. *112*:73 (July) 1980. **116.** Kasan, P. N., et al.: Br. J. Obstet. Gynaecol. *87*:545 (July) 1980. **117.** Rothman, K. J.: N. Engl. J. Med. *297*:468 (Sept. 1) 1977. **118.** Bracken, M. B.: Am. J. Obstet. Gynecol. *133*:432 (Feb. 15) 1979. **119.** De Teresa, E., et al.: Br. Med. J. *2*:1260 (Nov. 17) 1979. **120.** Swan, S., et al.: Am. J. Obstet. Gynecol. *139*:52 (Jan. 1) 1981. **121.** Kay, C. R.: Br. Med. J. *282*:2089 (June 27) 1981. **122.** Vessey, M. P., et al.: Br. Med. J. *282*:2093 (June 27) 1981. **123.** Pike, M. C., et al.: Br. J. Cancer *43*:72 (Jan.) 1981. **124.** Harlap, S., et al.: Obstet. Gynecol. *55*:447 (April) 1980. **125.** Back, D. J., et al.: Drugs *21*:46 (Jan.) 1981. **126.** Porter, J. B., et al.: Obstet. Gynecol. *66*:1 (July) 1985. **127.** Lees, A.W., et al.: Int. J. Cancer *22*:700, 1978. **128.** Brinton, L. A., et al.: J. Natl. Cancer Inst. (JNCI) *62*:37 (Jan.) 1979. **129.** Black, M. M.: Pathol. Res. Pract. *166*:491, 1980; Cancer *46*:2747 (Dec.) 1980; Cancer *51* : 2147 (June 1) 1983. **130.** Hoover, R., et al.: JNCI *67*:815 (Oct.) 1981. **131.** Gill, W. B., et al.: J. Urol. *122*:36 (July) 1979. **132.** Linn, S., et al.: J.A.M.A. *247*:629 (Feb. 5) 1982. **133.** Clavel, F., et al.: Bull. Cancer (Paris) *68*:449 (Dec.) 1981. **134.** Abernethy, D. R., et al.: N. Engl. J. Med. *306*:791 (April 1) 1982. **135.** Kay, C. R.: Am. J. Obstet. Gynecol. *142*:762 (March 15) 1982. **136.** Adam, S. A., et al.: Br. J. Obstet. Gynaecol. *88*:838 (Aug.) 1981. **137.** Slone, D., et al.: N. Engl. J. Med. *305*:420 (Aug. 20) 1981. **138.** Layde, P.M., et al.: J.R. Coll. Gen. Pract. *33*:75 (Feb.) 1983. **139.** Abernethy, D. R., et al.: Obstet. Gynecol. *60*:338 (Sept.) 1982. **140.** Brinton, L.A., et al.: Int. J. Epidemiol. *11*:316, 1982. **141.** Harris, N.V., et al.: Am. J. Epidemiol. *116*: 643 (Oct.) 1982. **142.** Pike, M.C., et al.: Lancet *2*:926 (Oct. 22) 1983. **143.** Vessey, M.P., et al.: Lancet *2*:930 (Oct. 22) 1983. **144.** Jick, H., et al.: Am. J. Epidemiol. *112*:577 (Nov.) 1980. **145.** Jick, H., et al.: Am. J. Epidemiol. *112*:586 (Nov.) 1980. **146.** McPherson, K., et al.: Lancet *2*:1414 (Dec. 17) 1983. **147.** Vessey, M.P., et al.: Br. Med. J. *289*:530 (Sept. 1) 1984. **148.** Olsson, H., et al.: Lancet *1*:748 (March 30) 1985. **149.** Thomas, D.B., et al.: Br. Med. J. *290*:961 (March 30) 1985. **150.** Dallenbach-Hellweg, G.: Path. Res. Pract. *179*:38, 1984. **151.** Washington, A.E., et al.: J.A.M.A. *253*:2246 (April 19) 1985. **152.** Rosenberg, L., et al.: J.A.M.A. *253*:2965 (May 24/31) 1985. **153.** Baciewicz, A.M.: Therap. Drug Monitor. *7*:26 (March) 1985. **154.** Robboy, S.J., et al.: J.A.M.A. *252*:2979 (Dec. 7) 1984. **155.** Vessey, M.P., et al.: Br. J. Fam. Plann. *11*:120 (Jan.) 1986. **156.** Vessey, M.P., et al.: Br. Med. J. *292*:526 (Feb. 22) 1986. **157.** Henderson, B.E., et al.: Br. J. Cancer *48*:437 (July) 1983. **158.** Neuberger, J., et al.: Br. Med. J. *292*:1355 (May 24) 1986. **159.** Forman, D., et al.: Br. Med. J. *292*:1357 (May 24) 1986. **160.** Pinto, M.R.: Mutat. Res. *169*:149 (March) 1986. **161.** Meirik, O., et al.: Lancet *2*:650 (Sept. 20) 1986. **162.** Brinton, L.A., et al.: Int. J. Cancer *38*:339 (Sept.) 1986.**163.** Ory, H.: Fam. Plann. Perspect. *15*:57 (March-April) 1983. **164.** Harlap, S., et al.: Teratology *31*:381 (June) 1985. **165.** Tikkanen, M.J.: J. Reprod. Med. *31*:898 (Sept.) 1986. **166.** Ross, R.K.: Br. Med. J. *293*:359 (Aug. 9) 1986. **167.** Lipson, A., et al.: Contraception *34*:121 (Aug.) 1986. **168.** Bradley, D. D., et al.: N. Engl. J. Med. *299*:17 (July 6) 1978. **169.** Gordon, T., et al.: Am. J. Med. *62*:707 (May) 1977. **170.** Ebeling, K., et al.: Int. J. Cancer *39*:427 (April) 1987. **171.** Melnick, S., et al.: N. Engl. J. Med. *316*:514 (Feb. 26) 1987. **172.** Ellis, E.F., et al.: Lancet *1*:207 (Jan. 28) 1978. **173.** Vessey, M., et al.: Br. Med. J. *292*:526 (Feb. 22) 1986. **174.** Sainz, M.P., et al.: Med. Clin. (Barcelona) *89*:272, 1987. **175.** McPherson, K., et al.: Br. J. Cancer *56*:653 (Nov.) 1987. **176.** Trussell, J., et al.: Stud. Fam. Plann. *18*:227 (Sept./Oct.) 1987. **177.** Littlewood, E.R., et al.: Lancet *1*:310 (Feb. 4) 1980. **178.** Caggiano, V., et al.: Lancet *2*:365 (Aug. 16) 1980. **179.** Yen, S., et al.: Cancer *59*:2112 (June) 1987. **180.** Mant, D., et al.: J Epidemiol. Commun. Hlth. *41*:215 (Sept.) 1987. **181.** Plummer, F.A., et al.: Second Internat. Symp. AIDS and Assoc. Cancers in Africa, abst. S.9.3, 1987. **182.** Burkman, R.T., et al.: Obstet. Gynecol. *71*:33 (Jan.) 1987. **183.** Depue, R.H., et al.: JNCI *71*:1151 (Dec.) 1983. **184.** Walker, A.H., et al.: Br. J. Cancer *57*:418 (April) 1988. **185.** Stadel, B.V., et al.: Contraception *38*:287 (Sept.) 1988. **186.** Miller, D.R., et al.: Am. J. Epidemiol. *129*:269 (Feb.) 1989. **187.** Kay, C.R., et al.: Br. J. Cancer *58*:675 (Nov.) 1988. **188.** Mann, J.M., et al.: AIDS *2*:249, 1988. **189.** Beral, V., et al.: Lancet *2*:1331 (Dec. 10) 1988. **190.** Croft, P., et al.: Br. Med. J. *298*:165 (Jan. 21) 1989. **191.** Louv, W.C., et al.: Am. J. Obstet. Gynecol. *160*:396 (Feb.) 1989.

BRIEF SUMMARY OF PATIENT LABELING

Cigarette-smoking increases the risk of serious adverse effects on the heart and blood vessels from oral contraceptive use. This risk increases with age and with heavy smoking (15 or more cigarettes per day) and is quite marked in women over 35 years of age. Women who use oral contraceptives should not smoke.

In the detailed leaflet, "What You Should Know About Oral Contraceptives," which you have received, the risks and bene-

Continued on next page

Schiapparelli Searle—Cont.

fits of oral contraceptives are discussed in much more detail. This leaflet also provides information on other forms of contraception. Please take time to read it carefully for it may have been recently revised.

If you have any questions or problems regarding this information, contact your doctor.

Oral contraceptives taken as directed are about 99% effective in preventing pregnancy. (The mini-pill, however, is somewhat less effective.) Forgetting to take your pills increases the chance of pregnancy.

Women who have or have had clotting disorders, cancer of the breast or sex organs, unexplained vaginal bleeding, stroke, heart attack, chest pains on exertion (angina pectoris), liver tumors associated with the use of the pill or with other estrogen-containing products, or who suspect they may be pregnant should not use oral contraceptives.

Most side effects of the pill are not serious. The most common side effects are nausea, vomiting, bleeding between menstrual periods, weight gain, and breast tenderness. However, proper use of oral contraceptives requires that they be taken under your doctor's continuing supervision, because they can be associated with serious side effects which may be fatal. Fortunately, these are very uncommon, but the risks may persist after use of the pill is discontinued. The serious side effects are:

1. Blood clots in the legs, arms, lungs, brain, heart, eyes, abdomen, or elsewhere in the body.
2. Bleeding in the brain (hemorrhage) as a result of bursting of a blood vessel.
3. Disorders of vision.
4. Liver tumors, which may rupture and cause severe bleeding.
5. Birth defects if the pill is taken during pregnancy.
6. High blood pressure.
7. Gallbladder disease.

The symptoms associated with these serious side effects are discussed in the detailed leaflet given you with your supply of pills. Notify your doctor if you notice any unusual physical disturbance while taking the pill.

Breast cancer and other cancers have developed in certain animals when given the estrogens in oral contraceptives for long periods. These findings suggest that oral contraceptives may also cause cancer in humans. However, studies to date in women taking currently marketed oral contraceptives have not confirmed that oral contraceptives cause cancer in humans.

Caution: Oral contraceptives are of no value in the prevention or treatment of venereal disease.

Various drugs, such as antibiotics, may also decrease the effectiveness of oral contraceptives.

DETAILED PATIENT LABELING: WHAT YOU SHOULD KNOW ABOUT ORAL CONTRACEPTIVES

Oral contraceptives (the pill) are the most effective way (except for sterilization) to prevent pregnancy if you follow the directions for their use and are careful not to skip doses or take them irregularly. They are also convenient and, for most women, free of serious or unpleasant side effects. Oral contraceptives must always be taken under the continuing supervision of a doctor.

It is important that any woman who considers using an oral contraceptive understands the risks involved. Although the oral contraceptives have important advantages over other methods of contraception, they have certain risks that no other method has. Only you can decide whether the advantages are worth these risks. This leaflet will tell you about the most important risks. It will explain how you can help your doctor prescribe the pill as safely as possible by telling him/her about yourself and being alert for the earliest signs of trouble. And it will tell you how to use the pill properly, so that it will be as effective as possible. THERE IS MORE DETAILED INFORMATION AVAILABLE IN THE LEAFLET PREPARED FOR DOCTORS. Your pharmacist can show you a copy; you may need your doctor's help in understanding parts of it.

Caution: Oral contraceptives are of no value in the prevention or treatment of venereal disease.

> **Cigarette-smoking increases the risk of serious adverse effects on the heart and blood vessels from oral contraceptive use. This risk increases with age and with heavy smoking (15 or more cigarettes per day) and is quite marked in women over 35 years of age. Women who use oral contraceptives should not smoke.**

WHO SHOULD NOT USE ORAL CONTRACEPTIVES

You should not use oral contraceptives:

A. If you have any of the following conditions:
1. Blood clots in the legs, lungs, eyes, or elsewhere in the body.
2. Chest pains on exertion (angina pectoris).
3. Known or suspected cancer of the breast or sex organs, such as the womb (uterus), vagina, or cervix.
4. Unusual vaginal bleeding that has not been diagnosed by your doctor.
5. Known or suspected pregnancy (one or more menstrual periods missed).

B. If you have had any of the following conditions:
1. Heart attack or stroke (clots or bleeding in the brain).
2. Blood clots in the legs, lungs, eyes, or elsewhere in the body.
3. Liver tumor associated with use of the pill or other estrogen-containing products.

C. If you have scanty or irregular periods or are a young woman without a regular cycle, you should use another method of contraception because, if you use the pill, you may have difficulty becoming pregnant or may fail to have menstrual periods after discontinuing the pill.

DECIDING TO USE ORAL CONTRACEPTIVES

If you do not have any of the conditions listed above and are thinking about using oral contraceptives, to help you decide, you need information about the advantages and risks of oral contraceptives and of other contraceptive methods as well. This leaflet describes the advantages and risks of oral contraceptives. Except for sterilization, the intrauterine device (IUD), and abortion, which have their own specific risks, the only risks of other methods of contraception are those due to pregnancy should the method fail. Your doctor can answer questions you may have with respect to other methods of contraception, and further questions you may have on oral contraceptives after reading this leaflet.

1. *What Oral Contraceptives Are and How They Work.* Oral contraceptives are of two types. The most common, often simply called "the pill," is a *combination* of an estrogen and a progestogen, the two kinds of female hormones. The amount of estrogen and progestogen can vary, but the amount of estrogen is more important because both the effectiveness and some of the dangers of oral contraceptives have been related to the amount of estrogen. This combination oral contraceptive works principally by preventing release of an egg from the ovary during the cycle in which the pills are taken. When the amount of estrogen is 50 micrograms or more, and the pill is taken as directed, oral contraceptives are more than 99% effective (that is, there would be less than 1 pregnancy in 100 women using the pill for one year). Pills that contain 20 to 35 micrograms of estrogen vary slightly in effectiveness, ranging from 98% to more than 99% effective.

The second type of oral contraceptive, often called the mini-pill, contains only a progestogen. It works in part by preventing release of an egg from the ovary, but also by keeping sperm from reaching the egg and by making the womb (uterus) less receptive to any fertilized egg that reaches it. The mini-pill is less effective than the combination oral contraceptive, about 97% effective. In addition, the mini-pill has a tendency to cause irregular bleeding, which may be quite inconvenient, or cessation of bleeding entirely. The mini-pill is used despite its lower effectiveness in the hope that it will prove not to have some of the serious side effects of the estrogen-containing pill, but it is not yet certain that the mini-pill does in fact have fewer serious side effects. The following discussion, while based mainly on information about the combination pills, should be considered to apply as well to the mini-pill.

2. *Other Nonsurgical Ways to Prevent Pregnancy.* As this leaflet will explain, oral contraceptives have several serious risks. Other methods of contraception have lesser risks or none at all. They are also less effective than oral contraceptives, but, used properly, may be effective enough for many women. The following table gives reported pregnancy rates (the number of women out of 100 who would become pregnant in one year) for these methods:

Pregnancies per 100 Women per Year

Method	Range
Intrauterine device (IUD)	less than 1 to 6
Diaphragm with spermicidal cream or jelly	2 to 20
Condom (rubber)	3 to 36
Spermicidal aerosol foams	2 to 29
Spermicidal jellies or creams	4 to 36
Periodic abstinence (rhythm), all types	less than 1 to 47
1. Calendar method	14 to 47
2. Temperature method	1 to 20
3. Temperature method (intercourse only in postovulatory phase)	less than 1 to 7
4. Mucus method	1 to 25
No contraception	60 to 80

These figures (except for the IUD) vary widely because people differ in how well they use each method. Very faithful users of the various methods obtain the best results, except for users of the periodic abstinence (rhythm) calendar method. Effective use of these methods, except for the IUD, requires somewhat more effort than simply taking a single pill every day, but it is an effort that many couples undertake successfully. Your doctor can tell you a great deal more about these methods of contraception and their effectiveness.

3. *The Dangers of Oral Contraceptives.*

a. *Circulatory disorders (blood clots, strokes, and heart attacks).* Blood clots occasionally form in the blood vessels of the body and, though rare, are the most common of the serious side effects of oral contraceptives. Clotting can result in a stroke (a clot in the brain), a heart attack (a clot in a blood vessel of the heart), or a pulmonary embolus (a clot that forms in the legs or abdominal region, then breaks off and travels to the lungs), or loss of a limb (a clot in a blood vessel in, or leading to, an arm or leg). Clots can also form in the blood vessels of the intestines or liver. Any of these events can be fatal (lead to death). Clots also occur rarely in the blood vessels of the eye, resulting in blindness or impairment of vision in that eye. There is some evidence that the risk of clotting may increase with higher estrogen doses. It is therefore important for your doctor to keep the dose of estrogen as low as possible, so long as the oral contraceptive used has an acceptable pregnancy rate and doesn't cause unacceptable changes in the menstrual pattern. Higher doses of progestogen have also been suggested as increasing the risk of clotting. Furthermore, cigarette-smoking by oral contraceptive users increases the risk of serious adverse effects on the heart and blood vessels. This risk increases with age and with heavy smoking (15 or more cigarettes per day) and begins to become quite marked in women over 35 years of age. For this reason, women who use oral contraceptives should not smoke.

The risk of abnormal clotting increases with age both in users and in nonusers of oral contraceptives, but the increased risk with the oral contraceptives appears to be present at all ages.

The risks of circulatory disorders may persist or continue after the pill is stopped. This has been reported for circulatory disorders in general, for heart disease or heart attacks, and for strokes caused either by a bursting blood vessel in the brain or by blood clots in the brain.

For oral contraceptive users in general, it has been estimated that in women between the ages of 25 and 34 the risk of death due to circulatory disorders in nonsmokers is about 1 in 23,000 per year. In contrast, for nonusers of the pill the risk is about 1 in 37,000 per year. Estimates of the risk of death due to circulatory disorders can be made, depending upon the woman's age, whether or not she uses oral contraceptives, and whether or not she smokes cigarettes. In the age group 25–34 years, women who use the pill have a risk of 1 in 7,000 (for smokers) to 1 in 23,000 (for nonsmokers) per year. This may be compared to the corresponding risk in women who have not used the pill: 1 in 24,000 (for smokers) to 1 in 37,000 (for nonsmokers) per year. The risks are greater in older women; thus, in the age group 35–44 years, women who use the pill have a risk of 1 in 1,600 (for smokers) to 1 in 4,700 (for nonsmokers) per year. The corresponding risk for women who have not used the pill is 1 in 6,600 (for smokers) to 1 in 16,000 (for nonsmokers) per year.

For women aged 16 to 40 it is estimated that about 1 in 2,000 using oral contraceptives will be hospitalized each year because of abnormal clotting in the veins or lungs. Among nonusers of the same age, about 1 in 20,000 would be hospitalized each year for these disorders.

Disease of the arteries characterized by paleness, numbness, or tingling in the fingers or toes has been reported to be more common in pill users.

Strokes are caused by a bursting blood vessel in the brain (hemorrhage) or a loss of blood circulation to the brain due to blood clots. When they occur, paralysis of all or part of the body may result; death can result. The risk of strokes due to clots or hemorrhages in the brain has been reported to be increased in pill users when compared with nonusers.

It has been estimated that pill users are twice as likely as nonusers to have a stroke due to a bursting blood vessel in the brain. It has further been estimated that pill users are 4 to 10 times as likely as nonusers to have a stroke due to clotting in a blood vessel in or leading to the brain.

It has been reported that women using the pill may have a greater risk of heart attack than nonusers. Even without the pill the risk of having a heart attack increases with age and is also increased by additional risk factors such as high blood pressure, high blood cholesterol, obesity, diabetes, cigarette-smoking, or the occurrence during pregnancy of high blood pressure, swelling of the legs, or protein in the urine. Without any risk factors present, the use of oral contraceptives alone may double the risk of heart attack. However, the combination of cigarette-smoking, especially heavy smoking, and oral contraceptive use greatly increases the risk of heart attack. Oral contraceptive users who smoke are about five times more likely to have a heart attack than users who do not smoke, and about ten times more likely to have a heart attack than nonusers who do not smoke. It has been estimated that among women between the ages of 30 and 39 who smoke have about a 1 in 10,000 chance each year of having a fatal heart attack compared to about a 1 in 50,000 chance in users who do not smoke, and about a 1 in 100,000 chance in nonusers who do not smoke. In the age group 40 to 44, the risk is about 1 in 1,700 per year for users who smoke compared to about 1 in 10,000 for users who do not smoke, and to about 1 in 14,000 per year for nonusers who do not smoke. Heavy smoking (about 15 cigarettes or more a day) further increases the risk. If you do not smoke and have none of the other heart attack risk factors described above, you will have a smaller risk than listed. If you have several heart attack risk factors, the risk may be considerably greater than listed. The above are average figures for Great Britain; comparable estimates for the U.S. have been higher.

Oral contraceptives should never be used at any age by women who have had a stroke, a heart attack, or chest pains on exertion (angina pectoris), or who have had blood clots in the legs, lungs, or elsewhere.

Anyone using the pill who has severe leg or chest pains, coughs up blood, has difficulty in breathing, severe headache or vomiting, dizziness or fainting, disturbances of vision or speech, weakness, numbness, or pain in an arm or leg should call her doctor immediately and stop taking the pill, and use another method of contraception.

b. *Formation of tumors.* When certain animals are given the female sex hormone estrogen (which is an ingredient in oral contraceptives) continuously for long periods, cancers may develop in organs such as the breast, cervix, vagina, liver, womb, ovary, and pituitary.

These findings suggest that oral contraceptives may cause cancer in humans. However, studies to date in women taking currently marketed oral contraceptives have not confirmed that oral contraceptives cause cancer in humans, but it remains possible they will be discovered in the future to do so. Although several studies have reported no overall increase in breast cancer in oral contraceptive users, other studies have reported increases in certain groups of women who have used oral contraceptives. Such groups reported to be at increased risk have differed from one study to another. Examples of such subgroups are: (a) women aged 20–44 without children who had their first menstrual period before age 13 and who took the pill for 8 or more years; (b) women aged 30–39, users for more than 5 years, and women with children who took the pill for 1–4 years before their first term pregnancy or for less than one year or more than 4 years after delivery; (c) women aged 30–34, and women with one child who took the pill for 2 or more years; (d) women already having benign (noncanceorus) breast disease (for example, cysts); (e) long-term (2–4 years) users; and (f) women having other risk factors (such as family history of breast cancer, a previous breast biopsy, or delay in having a first child). Women with a family history of breast cancer or who have breast nodules (lumps), fibrocystic disease (breast cysts), or abnormal mammograms (x-ray pictures of the breasts), or who were exposed to the estrogen diethylstilbestrol (DES) during their mother's pregnancy, or who have abnormal Pap smears should be followed very closely by their doctors if they choose to use oral contraceptives instead of another method of contraception. Many studies have shown that women taking oral contraceptives have less risk of getting benign (noncancerous) breast disease than those who have not used oral contraceptives. There is strong evidence that estrogens (one component of combination-type oral contraceptives), when given for periods of more than one year to women after the menopause (change-of-life), increase the risk of cancer of the womb (uterus). There is also some evidence that the sequential oral contraceptive, a kind of oral contraceptive that is no longer sold, may increase the risk of cancer of the womb. There is no evidence, however, that the oral contraceptives now available increase the risk of this type of cancer, although some individual cases have been reported. Cancer of the cervix may develop more readily in long-term users of the pill, particularly if they have had preexisting abnormal Pap smears. Cervical erosion and cell abnormalities, as well as chlamydial and gonococcal infections, have been reported to be more frequent in pill users. Unconfirmed observations have reported a greater use of oral contraceptives among African prostitutes testing positive for the AIDS virus.

Very rarely, oral contraceptive users may have a noncancerous tumor of the liver. These tumors do not spread, but they may rupture and cause internal bleeding, which may be fatal. This has been reported in short-term as well as long-term users, although increasing duration of use increases the risk. Long-term users have an estimated annual incidence of 3 to 4 per 100,000. One study reported that oral contraceptive products with a high "hormonal potency" were associated with a higher risk than lower-potency products, as was age over 30 years. Cases of cancer of the liver have been reported in women using oral contraceptives also. Users for 8 or more years were estimated to be 7 to 20 times more likely to develop this cancer than were nonusers. An increased risk of cancer of the bile ducts also has been reported.

A type of skin cancer that has been linked to exposure to sunlight (malignant melanoma) has been reported to be more frequent among pill users. It was not possible to determine what the effect was of greater exposure to sunlight in users.

c. *Dangers to a developing baby if oral contraceptives are used in or immediately preceding pregnancy.* Oral contraceptives should not be taken by pregnant women because they may damage the developing baby. There is an increased risk to the baby of abnormalities of such parts of the body as the backbone, anus, heart, windpipe, esophagus, kidneys, arms, and legs. In addition, the developing female child whose mother has received DES, a synthetic estrogen, during pregnancy has a risk of getting cancer of the vagina or cervix in her teens or young adulthood. This risk is estimated to be about 1 in 1,000 exposures or less. DES-exposed daughters appear to have an increased risk of unfavorable outcome of pregnancy. Abnormalities of the urinary and sex organs and sperm have been reported in DES-exposed male babies as well. It is possible that other estrogens, such as the estrogens in oral contraceptives, could have the same effect in the baby if the mother takes them during pregnancy. It has been reported that there is an increased risk of a type of cancer of the testes and ovaries in people whose mothers received female hormones (including oral contraceptives) during early pregnancy.

Occasionally women who are taking the pill miss periods. It has been reported to occur as frequently as several times each year in some women, depending on various factors such as age and prior history. (Your doctor is the best source of information about this.) The pill should not be used when you are pregnant or suspect you may be pregnant. Very rarely, women who are using the pill as directed become pregnant. The likelihood of becoming pregnant is higher if you occasionally miss one or two pills. Therefore, if you miss a period you should consult your physician before continuing to take the pill. If you miss a period, especially if you have not taken the pill regularly, you should use an alternative method of contraception until pregnancy has been ruled out; if you have missed more than one pill at any time, you should immediately start using an additional method of contraception and complete your pill cycle.

You should not attempt to become pregnant for at least three months after discontinuing oral contraceptives. Use another method of contraception during this period of time. The reason for this is that during this period there may be an increased risk of miscarriage and deformity to the baby, or an increased chance of having twins. Whether there is an overall increase in miscarriage in women who become pregnant soon after stopping the pill as compared with women who did not use the pill is not known, but it is possible that there may be.

If, however, you do become pregnant soon after stopping oral contraceptives, and do not have a miscarriage, there is no evidence that the baby has an increased risk of being abnormal.

d. *Gallbladder disease.* Women who use oral contraceptives have a greater risk than nonusers of having gallbladder disease requiring surgery. The increased risk may first appear within one year of use and may double after 4 or 5 years of use. Cancer of the ducts that collect bile may be more frequent in pill users.

e. *Other side effects of oral contraceptives.* Some women using oral contraceptives experience unpleasant side effects from the pill which are not dangerous and are not likely to damage their health. Some of these side effects are similar to symptoms women experience in early pregnancy and may be temporary. Your breasts may feel tender, be enlarged, or have a discharge; nausea and vomiting or other stomach or intestinal problems may occur; you may gain or lose weight, and your ankles may swell. A spotty darkening of the skin, particularly of the face, is possible and may persist after the drug is discontinued. An allergic or other type of rash or vaginal yeast infection may occur. You may notice unexpected vaginal bleeding, change in discharge, or changes in your menstrual period. Irregular bleeding is frequently seen when the mini-pill or the combination oral contraceptives containing less than 50 micrograms of estrogen are used. These should all be reported to your doctor.

Other side effects include worsening of migraine, asthma, convulsive disorders (such as epilepsy), and kidney, liver, or heart disease because of a tendency for water to be retained in the body when oral contraceptives are used. Other side effects are painful periods; growth of preexisting fibroid tumors of the womb; mental depression; and liver problems with jaundice (yellowing of the whites of the eyes or of the skin). Your doctor may find that levels of sugar and fatty substances in your blood are elevated; the long-term effects of these changes are not known. Some women develop high blood pressure while taking oral contraceptives, which ordinarily, but not always, returns to the original levels when the oral contraceptive is stopped. The degree of blood pressure rise may be related to the amount of progestogen in the pill. Women with a history of increased blood pressure, kidney disease, or toxemia during pregnancy (increased blood pressure, swelling of the legs, protein in the urine, or convulsions), or a family tendency to high blood pressure or its consequences (stroke, heart disease, kidney disease, blood vessel problems), or a history of excessive weight gain or swelling of the legs during their menstrual cycle, may be more likely to develop increased blood pressure when given

oral contraceptives; therefore, they should have their blood pressure taken frequently. High blood pressure predisposes one to stroke, heart attacks, kidney disease, and other diseases of the blood vessels. The effect of prolonged use of oral contraceptives on several of your organs (pituitary, liver, ovaries, womb, and adrenals) or immune system is not known at this time.

Increased damage to the chromosomes of white blood cells has been reported in pill users. The significance for cancer or birth defects is unknown.

Other conditions, although not proved to be caused by oral contraceptives, are occasionally reported. These include more frequent urination and some discomfort when urinating, kidney disease, nervousness, dizziness, hearing problems, inflammation of the nasal passages, loss of scalp hair, an increase in body hair, an increase or decrease in sex drive, appetite changes, gum disease, dry socket, cataracts, a need for a change in contact lens prescription or inability to use contact lenses, tiredness, backache, vaginal infections, itching, anemia, blood cell breakdown with kidney failure, headache, symptoms similar to those you get before a period; breast, womb, cervical, and liver cancer; inflammation of the pancreas, liver, or large or small intestine; chorea (spasmodic movements), burning or prickly sensation, rheumatoid arthritis, pulmonary hypertension, abnormal heart rhythm or electrocardiogram, and a bruising disease caused by decreased blood platelets (TTP).

After you stop using oral contraceptives, there may be a delay before you are able to become pregnant or before you resume having menstrual periods. This is especially true of women who had irregular menstrual cycles prior to the use of oral contraceptives.

One study showed that this delay in becoming pregnant can persist up to 72 months after stopping the pill if you have never had children and are over 30 years old. The delay appears to be more severe if the pill has been used for 2 years or more by such women. For women who have had children, the delay can persist to 30 months, regardless of age. For women who have not had children and who are less than 30, the delay may persist to 48 months. Very rarely there may be secretions from the breast associated with the absence of periods, which might be due to a noncancerous tumor of the pituitary gland requiring surgery. This may occur more frequently in former users of the pill than in nonusers. As discussed previously, you should wait at least three months after stopping the pill before you try to become pregnant. During the first three months after stopping oral contraceptives, use another form of contraception. You should consult your doctor before resuming use of oral contraceptives after childbirth, especially if you plan to nurse your baby. Drugs in oral contraceptives are known to appear in the milk, and the long-range effect on babies is not known at this time. Furthermore, oral contraceptives may cause a decrease in your milk supply as well as in the quality of the milk.

4. *Comparison of the Risks of Oral Contraceptives and Other Contraceptive Methods.*

The many studies on the risks and effectiveness of oral contraceptives and other methods of contraception have been

Figure 1. Estimated annual number of deaths associated with control of fertility and no control per 100,000 nonsterile women by regimen of control and age of woman.

Annual deaths

Regimen of control:　No method　Abortion only
Pill only/nonsmokers　Pill only/smokers　IUDs only
Traditional contraception only (diaphragm or condom)　Traditional contraception and abortion

Continued on next page

Schiapparelli Searle—Cont.

analyzed to estimate the risk of death associated with various methods of contraception. This risk has two parts: (a) the risk of the method itself (for example, the risk that oral contraceptives might cause death due to abnormal blood clotting), and (b) the risk of death due to pregnancy or abortion in the event the method should fail. The results of this analysis are shown in the following bar graph. The height of the bars indicates the number of deaths per 100,000 women each year. There are six sets of bars, each set referring to a specific age group of women. Within each set of bars, there is a single bar for each of the different contraceptive methods.

For oral contraceptives, there are two bars—one for smokers and the other for nonsmokers. The analysis is based on present knowledge and new information could, of course, alter it. The analysis shows that the risk of death from all methods of birth control is low and below that associated with the risks of childbirth, *except for oral contraceptives in women over 40 who smoke.* The risk of death associated with pill use in nonsmokers over 40 is higher than with any other method of contraception in that age group. It shows that the lowest risk of death is associated with the condom or diaphragm (traditional contraception) backed up by early legal abortion in case of failure of the condom or diaphragm to prevent pregnancy. Also, at any age, the risk of death (due to unexpected pregnancy) from use of traditional contraception, even without a backup of abortion, is generally the same as, or less than, that from use of oral contraceptives.

HOW TO USE ORAL CONTRACEPTIVES AS SAFELY AND EFFECTIVELY AS POSSIBLE, ONCE YOU HAVE DECIDED TO USE THEM

1. *What to Tell Your Doctor.* You can make use of the pill as safe as possible, by telling your doctor if you have any of the following:

a. Conditions that mean you should not use oral contraceptives:

If you *now* have any of the following:
1. Blood clots in the legs, lungs, eyes, or elsewhere in the body.
2. Chest pains on exertion (angina pectoris).
3. Known or suspected cancer of the breast or sex organs, such as the womb (uterus), vagina, or cervix.
4. Unusual vaginal bleeding that has not been diagnosed by your doctor.
5. Known or suspected pregnancy (one or more menstrual periods missed).

If you have *ever* had any of the following:
1. Heart attack or stroke (clots or bleeding in the brain).
2. Blood clots in the legs, lungs, eyes, or elsewhere in the body.
3. Liver tumor associated with use of the pill or other estrogen-containing products.

b. Inform your doctor of the following conditions since s/he will want to watch them closely or they might cause him/her to suggest another method of contraception:
A family history of breast cancer
Breast nodules (lumps), fibrocystic disease (breast cysts), abnormal mammograms (x-ray pictures of the breasts), or abnormal Pap smears
Diabetes
High blood pressure
High blood cholesterol
Cigarette-smoking
Migraine
Heart or kidney disease
Asthma
Problems during a prior pregnancy
Epilepsy
Mental depression
Fibroid tumors of the womb
History of jaundice (yellowing of the whites of the eyes or of the skin)
Gallbladder disease
Varicose veins
Tuberculosis
Plans for elective surgery
Previous problems with your periods (irregularities)
Use of any of the following kinds of drugs, which might interact with the pill: antibiotics (such as rifampin, ampicillin, and tetracycline), sulfa drugs, drugs for epilepsy or migraine, painkillers, tranquilizers, sedatives or sleeping pills, blood-thinning drugs, cortisone-like drugs, vitamins, drugs being used for the treatment of depression, high blood pressure, high blood sugar (diabetes), elevated blood lipids, or asthma.

c. Once you are using oral contraceptives, you should be alert for signs of a serious adverse effect and call your doctor immediately if any of these occur:

Sharp pain in the chest, coughing up of blood, or sudden shortness of breath (indicating possible clots in the lungs).

Pain in the calf (possible clot in the leg).
Crushing chest pain or heaviness (indicating possible heart attack).
Sudden severe headache or vomiting, dizziness or fainting, disturbance of vision or speech, or weakness or numbness in an arm or leg (indicating a possible stroke).
Sudden partial or complete loss of vision (indicating a possible clot in the blood vessels of the eye).
Abnormal vaginal bleeding.
Breast discharge or lumps (you should ask your doctor to show you how to examine your own breasts).
Severe and/or persistent pain or a mass in the abdomen (indicating a possible tumor of the liver which might have ruptured).
Severe depression.
Yellowing of the whites of the eyes or of the skin (jaundice).
Unusual swelling.
Other unusual conditions.

2. *How to Take the Pill So That It Is Most Effective. Dosage Schedules.* See later sections in this leaflet concerning spotting, breakthrough bleeding, forgotten pills, and missed menstruation.

Each tablet dispenser contains 21 or 28 tablets in numbered rows of 7 tablets each. The days of the week are printed above the columns. To remove a pill, press down on it. The pill will be released through the back of the dispenser.
Read the information below carefully because maximum contraceptive effectiveness of oral contraceptives depends on your taking the pills exactly as directed, every day, and at time intervals of 24 hours. It is recommended that you take your pill at the same time every day.

The first time you take the pill, use another method of contraception in addition, until you have taken the first 7 pills.

21-Day Schedules

For use with Norethin 1/35E™-21 and Norethin 1/50M™-21.

Sunday Schedule: Start taking the pills on the first Sunday after the menstrual period begins. If it begins on a Sunday, start taking the pills that same day. Begin with row #1, Sunday, and take one pill every day, at the same time, in order, for 21 days. Then stop taking the pills for one week (7 days). Begin the next cycle, as before, on Sunday.

Day-5 Schedule: Start taking the pills on day 5 of the menstrual cycle, counting day 1 as the first day of menstrual flow. Begin with row #1 on the day of the week corresponding to day 5. Take a pill every day, at the same time, for 21 days. Complete row #3, then take any pills remaining in row #1. Then stop taking the pill for one week (7 days). Begin the next cycle on the same day of the week as you began the first cycle.

28-Day Schedules

For use with Norethin 1/35E™-28 and Norethin 1/50M™-28.

Sunday Schedule: The first pill in row #1 must be taken on the first Sunday after menstrual flow begins, or on that same day if it begins on Sunday. Take one pill every day, at the same time, and in order. When you finish row #1, begin with Sunday in row #2, and so on. After you have taken 28 pills, begin a new cycle, on Sunday, just as described. Take a pill faithfully every day, even if menstrual flow stops while you are still taking the blue pills in row #4. If you miss one or more of the blue pills (row #4), your chances of becoming pregnant will not increase providing the white pill schedule has been followed.

Day-5 Schedule: Start taking the white pills on day 5 of the menstrual cycle, counting day 1 as the first day of menstrual flow. Begin with row #1 on the day of the week corresponding to day 5. Take a pill every day, at the same time, for 21 days. Complete row #3, then take any white pills remaining in row #1. **Take all of the white pills before taking any blue placebo pills in row #4.** After all of the white pills are used, take the blue placebo pills in row #4 for one week (7 days). Begin the next cycle on the same day of the week as you began the first cycle. Take a pill faithfully every day, even if menstrual flow stops while you are still taking the blue pills in row #4. If you miss one or more of the blue pills (row #4), your chances of becoming pregnant will not increase providing the white pill schedule has been followed.

Take your pill faithfully every "pill day"!
It is important that you take a pill without fail every pill day, at intervals of 24 hours, for two reasons. First, your ovaries may release an egg and therefore you may become pregnant if you do not take your pills regularly. Second, you may spot or start to flow between your periods. This may be inconvenient.

Take your pill at the same time every day!
You are probably wondering why the same time of day is important. By taking your pill at the same time every day it becomes a good habit, and you are much less likely to forget. You may wish to keep your pills in the medicine cabinet near your toothbrush as a reminder to take them when you brush

your teeth at night. The best time to take your daily pill may be either with your evening meal or at bedtime. You may find it helpful to associate your pill-taking with something else you do every day at a particular time.
Another very important reason for you to take your pills as "regular as clockwork" is that you are protected best when you take one every 24 hours; they are made to work that way. Just remember that once every day is not the same as once every 24 hours. Here is why: Suppose you were to take your Monday pill in the morning when you get up, and then not take your Tuesday pill till the evening before you go to bed. True, you will have taken a pill each day, on Monday and on Tuesday—but the time between pill-taking will probably have been more than 36 hours, or more than $1\frac{1}{2}$ days! You might spot. Chances are you would still be protected and would not get pregnant, but why risk it when it is so easy to guarantee yourself maximal protection by taking your pill faithfully every pill day and at the same time every pill day? In summary, you should take the pills exactly as directed and at intervals of 24 hours in order to achieve maximum contraceptive effectiveness.
Spotting. This is a slight staining between your menstrual periods which may not even require a pad. Some women spot even though they take their pills exactly as directed. Many women spot although they have never taken the pills. Spotting does not mean that your ovaries are releasing an egg. Spotting may be the result of irregular pill-taking. Getting back on schedule will usually stop it.
If you should spot while taking the pills you should not be alarmed because spotting usually stops by itself within a few days. It seldom occurs after the first pill cycle. Consult your doctor if spotting persists for more than a few days or if it occurs after the second cycle.
Unexpected (Breakthrough) Bleeding. Unexpected (breakthrough) bleeding does not mean your ovaries have released an egg. It seldom occurs, but when it does happen it is most common in the first pill cycle. It is a flow much like a regular period, requiring the use of a pad or tampon.
If you experience breakthrough bleeding use a pad or tampon and continue with your schedule. Usually your periods will become regular within a few cycles. Breakthrough bleeding will seldom bother you again.
Consult your doctor if breakthrough bleeding does not stop within a week or if it occurs after the second cycle.
Forgotten Pills. There is little likelihood of your getting pregnant if only one active pill is missed; however, the possibility increases with each successive day that the scheduled active pills are missed. If you forget to take a pill one day, take two the next day—the one you forgot as soon as you remember and your regular pill at your usual time.
If you forget your pills (except the inactive blue pills in Norethin 1/35E™-28 and Norethin 1/50M™-28) on two consecutive days, do not be surprised if you spot or start to flow. You should take two pills each day for the next two days, and use an additional method of protection for the remainder of the cycle.
If you are using Norethin 1/35E™-28 or Norethin 1/50M™-28 and forget to take one or more blue pills, begin a new cycle on the same day of the week as you began the previous cycle; use a new package and start taking the white pills. Missing the blue pills does not increase your chances of getting pregnant providing the white pill schedule has been followed.
Missed Menstruation. At times there may be no menstrual period after a cycle of pills. Therefore, if you miss one menstrual period but have taken the pills *exactly as you were supposed to,* continue as usual into the next cycle. You may wish to call your doctor. If you have not taken the pills correctly and miss a menstrual period, *you may be pregnant* and should stop taking oral contraceptives until your doctor determines whether or not you are pregnant. Until you can get to your doctor, use another form of contraception. If two consecutive menstrual periods are missed, you should stop taking the pills until it is determined whether you are pregnant. If you do become pregnant while using oral contraceptives, you should discuss the risks to the developing baby with your doctor.

3. *Periodic Examinations.* Your doctor will take a complete medical and family history before prescribing oral contraceptives. At that time and about once a year thereafter, s/he will generally examine your blood pressure, breasts, abdomen, and internal female organs (including a Pap smear test for cancer of the cervix) and perform certain laboratory tests. Certain health problems or conditions in your medical or family history may require that your doctor see you more frequently while you are taking the pill.

SUMMARY

Oral contraceptives are the most effective method, except sterilization, for preventing pregnancy. Other methods, when used conscientiously, are also very effective and have fewer risks. The serious side effects of oral contraceptives are uncommon, but the risk of experiencing them may persist after discontinuing the pill. The pill is a very convenient method for preventing pregnancy.

Women who use oral contraceptives should not smoke.
If you have certain conditions or have had these conditions in the past, you should not use oral contraceptives because of increased risk. These conditions are listed in this leaflet. If you do not have these conditions, and decide to use the pill, please read this leaflet carefully so that you can use the pill safely and effectively.

Based on your doctor's assessment of your medical needs, this drug has been prescribed for you. Do not give it to anyone else.

See your doctor regularly, ask any questions you may have about the use of the pill, and report any special problems that may arise.

Be certain to read new revisions of this leaflet. You may check the date of the most recent revision by phoning the manufacturer toll free at 1-800-323-4204 or by writing to the address below.

Address medical inquiries to:
G.D. Searle & Co.
Medical & Scientific Information Department
4901 Searle Parkway
Skokie, IL 60077   AO5604-2

PRO-BANTHĪNE® Tablets   ℞
[prō-ban′thīne]
(propantheline bromide USP)

DESCRIPTION
Pro-Banthine oral tablets contain 15 mg or 7½ mg of the anticholinergic propantheline bromide, (2-hydroxyethyl)-diisopropylmethylammonium bromide xanthene-9-carboxylate.
The structural formula of Pro-Banthine is

Propantheline bromide is very soluble in water, alcohol, and chloroform, but it is practically insoluble in ether and in benzene. Its molecular weight is 448.40.
Inactive ingredients include calcium carbonate, corn starch, edible ink, flavor, lactose, magnesium carbonate, magnesium stearate, sucrose, talc, titanium dioxide, and waxes. The 15-mg tablet also contains red oxide and yellow oxide as coloring agents.

CLINICAL PHARMACOLOGY
Pro-Banthine inhibits gastrointestinal motility and diminishes gastric acid secretion. The drug also inhibits the action of acetylcholine at the postganglionic nerve endings of the parasympathetic nervous system.
Propantheline bromide is extensively metabolized in man primarily by hydrolysis to the inactive materials xanthene-9-carboxylic acid and (2-hydroxyethyl) diisopropylmethylammonium bromide. After a single 30-mg oral dose given as two 15-mg tablets the mean peak plasma concentration of propantheline was 21 ng/ml at one hour in six healthy subjects.
The plasma elimination half-life of propantheline is about 1.6 hours. Approximately 70% of the dose is excreted in the urine, mostly as metabolites. The urinary excretion of propantheline is about 3% after oral tablet administration.

INDICATIONS AND USAGE
Pro-Banthine is effective as adjunctive therapy in the treatment of peptic ulcer.

CONTRAINDICATIONS
Pro-Banthine (propantheline bromide) is contraindicated in patients with:
1. Glaucoma, since mydriasis is to be avoided.
2. Obstructive disease of the gastrointestinal tract (pyloroduodenal stenosis, achalasia, paralytic ileus, etc).
3. Obstructive uropathy (eg, bladder-neck obstruction due to prostatic hypertrophy).
4. Intestinal atony of elderly or debilitated patients.
5. Severe ulcerative colitis or toxic megacolon complicating ulcerative colitis.
6. Unstable cardiovascular adjustment in acute hemorrhage.
7. Myasthenia gravis.

WARNINGS
In the presence of a high environmental temperature, heat prostration (fever and heat stroke due to decreased sweating) can occur with the use of Pro-Banthine.
Diarrhea may be an early symptom of incomplete intestinal obstruction, especially in patients with ileostomy or colostomy. In this instance treatment with Pro-Banthine would be inappropriate and possibly harmful.

With overdosage, a curare-like action may occur (ie, neuromuscular blockade leading to muscular weakness and possible paralysis).
Pro-Banthine may cause increased heart rate and, therefore, should be used with caution in patients with heart disease.

PRECAUTIONS
General: Pro-Banthine (propantheline bromide) should be used with caution in the elderly and in all patients with autonomic neuropathy, hepatic or renal disease, hyperthyroidism, coronary heart disease, congestive heart failure, cardiac tachyarrhythmias, hypertension, or hiatal hernia associated with reflux esophagitis, since anticholinergics may aggravate this condition.
In patients with ulcerative colitis, large doses of Pro-Banthine may suppress intestinal motility to the point of producing paralytic ileus and, for this reason, may precipitate or aggravate toxic megacolon, a serious complication of the disease.
Information for patients: Pro-Banthine may produce drowsiness or blurred vision. The patient should be cautioned regarding activities requiring mental alertness, such as operating a motor vehicle or other machinery or performing hazardous work, while taking this drug.
Drug interactions: Anticholinergics may delay absorption of other medication given concomitantly.
Excessive cholinergic blockade may occur if Pro-Banthine is given concomitantly with belladonna alkaloids, synthetic or semisynthetic anticholinergic agents, narcotic analgesics such as meperidine, Type 1 antiarrhythmic drugs (eg, disopyramide, procainamide, or quinidine), antihistamines, phenothiazines, tricyclic antidepressants, or other psychoactive drugs. Pro-Banthine may also potentiate the sedative effect of phenothiazines. Increased intraocular pressure may result from concurrent administration of anticholinergics and corticosteroids.
Concurrent use of Pro-Banthine with slow-dissolving tablets of digoxin may cause increased serum digoxin levels. This interaction can be avoided by using only those digoxin tablets that rapidly dissolve by USP standards.
Carcinogenesis, mutagenesis, impairment of fertility: No long-term fertility, carcinogenicity, or mutagenicity studies have been done with Pro-Banthine.
Pregnancy: Pregnancy Category C. Animal reproduction studies have not been conducted with Pro-Banthine. It is also not known whether Pro-Banthine can cause fetal harm when administered to a pregnant woman or can affect reproductive capacity. Pro-Banthine should be given to a pregnant woman only if clearly needed.
Nursing mothers: It is not known whether this drug is excreted in human milk. Because many drugs are excreted in human milk, caution should be exercised when Pro-Banthine is administered to a nursing woman. Suppression of lactation may occur with anticholinergic drugs.
Pediatric use: Safety and effectiveness in children have not been established.

ADVERSE REACTIONS
Varying degrees of drying of salivary secretions may occur as well as decreased sweating. Ophthalmic side effects include blurred vision, mydriasis, cycloplegia, and increased ocular tension. Other reported adverse reactions include urinary hesitancy and retention, tachycardia, palpitations, loss of the sense of taste, headache, nervousness, mental confusion, drowsiness, weakness, dizziness, insomnia, nausea, vomiting, constipation, bloated feeling, impotence, suppression of lactation, and allergic reactions or drug idiosyncrasies, including anaphylaxis, urticaria, and other dermal manifestations.

OVERDOSAGE
The symptoms of overdosage with Pro-Banthine progress from an intensification of the usual side effects to CNS disturbances (from restlessness and excitement to psychotic behavior), circulatory changes (flushing, fall in blood pressure, circulatory failure), respiratory failure, paralysis, and coma.
Measures to be taken are (1) immediate induction of emesis or lavage of the stomach, (2) injection of physostigmine 0.5 to 2 mg intravenously, repeated as necessary up to a total of 5 mg, and (3) monitoring of vital signs and managing as necessary.
Fever may be treated symptomatically (cooling blanket or alcohol sponging). Excitement of a degree which demands attention may be managed with thiopental sodium 2% solution given slowly intravenously, or diazepam, 5 to 10 mg intravenously or 10 mg intramuscularly. In the event of progression of the curare-like effect to paralysis of the respiratory muscles, mechanical respiration should be instituted and maintained until effective respiratory action returns.
The oral LD$_{50}$ of propantheline bromide is 780 mg/kg in the mouse and 370 mg/kg in the rat.

DOSAGE AND ADMINISTRATION
The usual initial adult dosage of Pro-Banthine tablets is 15 mg taken 30 minutes before each meal and 30 mg at bedtime (a total of 75 mg daily). Subsequent dosage adjustment

should be made according to the patient's individual response and tolerance. The administration of one 7½-mg tablet three times a day is convenient for patients with mild manifestations, for geriatric patients, and for those of small stature.

HOW SUPPLIED
Pro-Banthine 15-mg tablets are round, peach colored, sugar coated, with SEARLE imprinted on one side and 601 on the other side; bottles of 100 and 500, and cartons containing 100 unit-dose, individually blister-sealed tablets.
Pro-Banthine 7½-mg tablets are round, white, sugar coated, with SEARLE imprinted on one side and 611 on the other side; bottles of 100.
Store below 86°F (30°C).
Caution: Federal law prohibits dispensing without prescription.

A05876

The preceding prescribing information for Schiapparelli Searle products was current on September 1, 1989.

Schmid Laboratories, Inc.
ROUTE 46 WEST
LITTLE FALLS, NJ 07424-0415

KORO-FLEX®   ℞
ARCING SPRING DIAPHRAGM

DESCRIPTION
The KORO-FLEX (R) ARCING SPRING DIAPHRAGM is made of natural, dipped, latex rubber. The contouring spring is actually 5 (five) springs in one.

ACTION
When compressed, it assumes a half moon shape which facilitates introduction beyond the cervix for simple, correct placement. When properly fitted, it will help to prevent sperm from entering the cervical canal. It also holds the spermicide in place.

INDICATIONS
KORO-FLEX Diaphragms, when used in conjunction with an appropriate spermicide such as KOROMEX (R) CONTRACEPTIVE CRYSTAL CLEAR GEL, KOROMEX (R) CONTRACEPTIVE JELLY or KOROMEX (R) CONTRACEPTIVE CREAM, are indicated for the prevention of pregnancy in women who choose diaphragms as their method of contraception.

PRECAUTIONS
While there has been no established link between the use of a diaphragm and Toxic Shock Syndrome (TSS), a few women wearing diaphragms have developed symptoms of the condition. In many of these situations, the women wore the diaphragm for more than 24 hours. It should be recommended, therefore, that the diaphragm not be worn continuously for more than 24 hours.
Symptoms of TSS include sudden high fever (generally 102°F or over), vomiting, diarrhea, dizziness, fainting, or near fainting when standing up and a rash that resembles sunburn. Other signs of TSS may include sore throat, weakness, aching of muscles and joints, and redness of the eyes. If the woman experiences a high fever and one or more other TSS symtoms, she should be instructed to remove the diaphragm and contact her physician immediately.
An increased risk of developing Urinary Tract infections among some users of diaphragms has been suggested. Physicians may wish to reevaluate the diaphragm size being used or consider alternate methods of contraception for those diaphragm-using patients experiencing an unacceptable number of Urinary Tract Infections.

INSTRUCTIONS
To be effective, the diaphragm should always be used with a contraceptive gel, jelly or cream. This must be spread around the inner surface of the diaphragm as well as on the rim. Proper placement of the diaphragm is essential.
The diaphragm may be inserted up to 6 (six) hours before intercourse. If more than 6 (six) hours has elapsed after insertion of the diaphragm or for each repeated intercourse, an additional applicatorful of contraceptive gel, jelly, or cream must be used. The diaphragm SHOULD NOT be removed for this additional application.
The diaphragm must be left in place for at least 6 (six) hours after the last intercourse. If the diaphragm is removed before the six (6) hour time period, the chances of becoming pregnant could be greatly increased. However, the diaphragm should be removed as soon after six (6) hours as practicable, but in no event should the diaphragm be left in place more than 24 hours.

Continued on next page

Schmid—Cont.

Douching is not necessary. However, if recommended, the woman must wait for a full 6 (six) hours after the last intercourse.

The woman should wash her hands thoroughly before inserting or removing the diaphragm. When the diaphragm is in use, the woman should avoid applying body lubricants, vaginal lubricants, cold cream soaps, or powders that contain petroleum. These products can weaken rubber. The diaphragm should be checked every year. The woman may need a replacement or the size required may have changed. The diaphragm must be rechecked after a weight change (up or down) of more than ten pounds, after an abortion, after giving birth, or after any vaginal or pelvic surgery. The diaphragm may become dislodged when the woman is on top during intercourse. The diaphragm is an effective method of birth control if it is used properly and used every time intercourse occurs. Although no contraceptive provides 100% protection, the Koromex Diaphragm when properly used, effectively aids in the prevention of pregnancy.

HOW SUPPLIED
KORO-FLEX ARCING SPRING DIAPHRAGMS are available in two convenient packages: KORO-FLEX ARCING SPRING DIAPHRAGM KIT (stock #136), contains trial sizes of KOROMEX CONTRACEPTIVE CRYSTAL CLEAR GEL, KOROMEX CONTRACEPTIVE JELLY, KOROMEX CONTRACEPTIVE CREAM, and a white plastic case. Available in sizes 60 mm–95 mm in 5 mm gradations.
KORO-FLEX ARCING SPRING DIAPHRAGM COMPACT SET (stock #536), contains a regular tube of KOROMEX CONTRACEPTIVE CRYSTAL CLEAR GEL, trial sizes of KOROMEX CONTRACEPTIVE JELLY and KOROMEX CONTRACEPTIVE CREAM, a gel/jelly/cream applicator, white plastic case, and a convenient zippered pouch. Available in sizes 60 mm–95 mm in 5 mm gradations.

KOROMEX®
COIL SPRING DIAPHRAGM　　　　　　　　　℞

DESCRIPTION
The KOROMEX COIL SPRING DIAPHRAGM is made of natural, dipped, latex rubber. The plated spring is tension-controlled.

ACTION
When properly fitted, it will help to prevent sperm from entering the cervical canal. It also holds the spermicide in place.

INDICATIONS
KOROMEX Diaphragms, when used in conjunction with an appropriate spermicide such as KOROMEX (R) CONTRACEPTIVE CRYSTAL CLEAR GEL, KOROMEX (R) CONTRACEPTIVE JELLY or KOROMEX (R) CONTRACEPTIVE CREAM, are indicated for the prevention of pregnancy in women who choose diaphragms as their method of contraception.

PRECAUTIONS
While there has been no established link between use of a diaphragm and Toxic Shock Syndrome (TSS), a few women wearing diaphragms have developed symptoms of the condition. In many of these situations, the women wore the diaphragm for more than 24 hours. It should be recommended therefore, that the diaphragm not be worn continuously for more than 24 hours.
Symptoms of TSS include sudden high fever (generally 102°F or over), vomiting, diarrhea, dizziness, fainting, or near fainting when standing up, and a rash that resembles sunburn. Other signs of TSS may include: sore throat, weakness, aching of muscles and joints, and redness of the eyes. If the women experiences a high fever and one or more other TSS symptoms, she should be instructed to remove the diaphragm and contact her physician immediately.
An increased risk of developing Urinary Tract infections among some users of diaphragms has been suggested. Physicians may wish to reevaluate the diaphragm size being used or consider alternate methods of contraception for those diaphragm-using patients experiencing an unacceptable number of Urinary Tract Infections.

INSTRUCTIONS
To be effective, the diaphragm should always be used with a contraceptive gel, jelly, or cream. This must be spread around the inner surface of the diaphragm as well as on the rim. Proper placement of the diaphragm is essential.
The diaphragm may be inserted up to 6 (six) hours before intercourse. If more than 6 (six) hours has elapsed after insertion of the diaphragm or for each repeated intercourse, an additional applicatorful of contraceptive gel, jelly, or cream must be used. The diaphragm SHOULD NOT be removed for this additional application.
The diaphragm must be left in place for at least 6 (six) hours after the last intercourse. If the diaphragm is removed before

the six (6) hour time period, the chances of becoming pregnant could be greatly increased. However, the diaphragm should be removed as soon after six (6) hours as practicable, but in no event should the diaphragm be left in place more than 24 hours.
Douching is not necessary. However, if recommended, the woman must wait a full 6 (six) hours after the last intercourse.
The woman should wash her hands thoroughly before inserting or removing the diaphragm. When the diaphragm is in use, the woman should avoid applying body lubricants, vaginal lubricants, cold cream soaps, or powders that contain petroleum. These products can weaken rubber. The diaphragm should be checked every year. The woman may need a replacement or the size required may have changed. The diaphragm must be rechecked after a weight change (up or down) of more than ten pounds, after an abortion, after giving birth, or after any vaginal or pelvic surgery. The diaphragm may become dislodged when the woman is on top during intercourse. The diaphragm is an effective method of birth control if it is used properly and used every time intercourse occurs. Although no contraceptive provides 100% protection, the Koromex Diaphragm when properly used, effectively aids in the prevention of pregnancy.

HOW SUPPLIED
KOROMEX COIL SPRING DIAPHRAGMS are available in two convenient packages: KOROMEX COIL SPRING DIAPHRAGM KIT (stock #131), contains trial sizes of KOROMEX CONTRACEPTIVE CRYSTAL CLEAR GEL, KOROMEX CONTRACEPTIVE JELLY, KOROMEX CONTRACEPTIVE CREAM, and a white plastic case. Available in sizes 50 mm–95 mm in 5 mm gradations.
KOROMEX COIL SPRING DIAPHRAGM COMPACT SET (Stock #541), contains a regular tube of KOROMEX CONTRACEPTIVE CRYSTAL CLEAR GEL, trial sizes of KOROMEX CONTRACEPTIVE JELLY and KOROMEX CONTRACEPTIVE CREAM, a diaphragm introducer, a gel/jelly/cream applicator, white plastic case, and a convenient zippered pouch. Available in sizes 60 mm–95 mm in 5 mm gradations.

VAGISEC PLUS® SUPPOSITORIES　　　　℞
[vaj 'ĕ-sĕk "]
VAGISEC® MEDICATED DOUCHE LIQUID CONCENTRATE

DESCRIPTION
VAGISEC PLUS SUPPOSITORIES contain a combination of trichomonacidal and bactericidal agents and provide continued medication by gradual liquefaction. Each vaginal suppository contains the following ingredients:

9-aminoacridine HCl	6.00 mg.
Polyoxyethylene nonyl phenol	5.25 mg.
Sodium edetate	0.66 mg.
Sodium dioctyl sulfosuccinate	0.07 mg.

in a polyethylene glycol base containing glycerin and citric acid.
VAGISEC MEDICATED DOUCHE LIQUID CONCENTRATE contains a combination of polyoxyethylene nonyl phenol, sodium edetate, and sodium dioctyl sulfosuccinate, a complex proven to be effective trichomonacide when used as a vaginal douche (Vagisec Liquid).

CLINICAL PHARMACOLOGY
9-aminoacridine is a broad-spectrum anti-infective of extensive medical acceptance for the topical treatment of bacterial infections. The combination of polyoxyethylene nonyl phenol, sodium edetate, and sodium dioctyl sulfosuccinate is a trichomonacide which when in solution and diluted disintegrates the flagellates through marked changes in surface tension.

INDICATIONS AND USAGE
The Vagisec Liquid/Suppository regimen is indicated for the specific treatment, in adults, of vaginitis, as evidenced by pruritus, malodorous leukorrhea, erythema of the vaginal mucosa, dyspareunia, caused by Trichomonas vaginalis and mixed vaginal infections complicated by a bacterial moiety. The presence of trichomonads can be established by a hanging drop mount preparation of the discharge from the posterior fornix and confirmed by cultures grown on STS medium; the atypical bacterial moiety can be identified by examination of gram-stained preparations of smeared vaginal secretions.

CONTRAINDICATIONS
Douching is not recommended during pregnancy. VAGISEC Medicated Douche and VAGISEC PLUS Suppositories are spermicidal and should not be used when the patient is trying to conceive.

PRECAUTIONS
General: The full course of therapy must be completed to eliminate the infecting micro-organisms from the vagina. It is generally desirable to continue treatment through the menses in order to guard against potential flare-ups since

the presence of blood favors the rapid growth of Trichomonas. Recurrence of vaginitis often indicates extravaginal foci or infection in cervical, vestibular and urethral glands, etc. or reinfection by the sexual partner.
Information for Patients: During treatment, patient should refrain from intercourse, or the partner should wear a prophylactic. To prevent flare-ups after completion of therapy and for continued vaginal cleanliness, the patient is advised to continue with VAGISEC Liquid as a regular douche, but no more than twice weekly unless otherwise directed by physician.
Laboratory Tests: No patient should be considered cured until cultures on STS medium and gram-stained preparations of smeared vaginal secretions, taken at monthly intervals for 3 months following treatment, show absence of trichomonads and a return to the normal vaginal bacterial flora.

ADVERSE REACTIONS
No significant adverse reactions have been reported to date for Vagisec Plus Suppositories or Vagisec Liquid. Any minor irritation is generally relieved by discontinuance of douche for 24 hours.

OVERDOSAGE
Antidote: Copious use of water. The dilute Vagisec solution is non-toxic.

DOSAGE & ADMINISTRATION
Office Treatment (Adult): For the treatment of vaginal trichomoniasis and mixed vaginal infections, best results are obtained by scrubbing the vagina with VAGISEC Liquid, diluted 1:100 by the physician in the office: 3 scrubs the first week, 2 the second. A suppository is inserted after each office scrub in the Liquid/Suppository regimen. Patient should be instructed to continue treatment at home. *Home Treatment:* The combination douche and suppositories (Liquid/Suppository regimen) is recommended for home use. The usual daily home treatment is VAGISEC Medicated Douche in the morning, followed by a VAGISEC PLUS Suppository inserted deep in the vagina, using tip of finger, and a second suppository inserted in like manner at bedtime for a period of 14 days. Treatment should be omitted the night and morning preceding an office visit. In chronic or stubborn cases, therapy may be repeated with no interval between courses. The Liquid/Suppository regimen may be continued throughout the menstrual cycle. It is advisable to continue treatment through two menstrual periods. Patients should be reexamined 3 days after home treatment has been discontinued. The full course of therapy must be completed to eliminate the infecting micro-organisms from the vagina. No patient should be considered cured until vaginal smears or cultures, taken at monthly intervals for 3 months following treatment, show absence of trichomonads and a return to the normal vaginal flora.

HOW SUPPLIED
VAGISEC PLUS® SUPPOSITORIES—box of 28 plastic-wrapped 3 gram suppositories. VAGISEC® MEDICATED DOUCHE LIQUID CONCENTRATE—4 oz. plastic bottle with instructions for dilution and douching.

CAUTION
Federal law prohibits dispensing VAGISEC PLUS Suppositories without prescription.

Scholl, Inc.
3030 JACKSON AVENUE
MEMPHIS, TN 38151

DR. SCHOLL'S® ATHLETE'S FOOT　　　OTC
SPRAY LIQUID
(Tolnaftate 1%)

DESCRIPTION
Contains a clinically proven ingredient to <u>cure</u> Athlete's Foot. Kills Athlete's Foot fungi, even in most stubborn cases. Soothes and cools burning, itching feet. Promotes healing and prevents recurrence. To prevent reinfection, continue daily bathing of feet and application of Dr. Scholl's Athlete's Foot Spray Liquid, Powder or Shaker Powder.

DIRECTIONS
Thoroughly wash and dry infected areas twice daily. Shake can well. Hold can 4 to 6 inches away. Spray liberally on entire infected area. Continue treatment for 2 weeks after symptoms disappear.

CAUTION
For external use only. Avoid getting into eyes. Do not use on nail or scalp infections. If symptoms do not improve in 10 days, or irritation occurs, discontinue use and consult your doctor.

WARNING — FLAMMABLE

DO NOT SPRAY WHILE SMOKING OR NEAR FIRE. DO NOT PUNCTURE OR INCINERATE CONTAINER OR PLACE WHERE TEMPERATURE EXCEEDS 120°F. USE ONLY AS DIRECTED. INTENTIONAL MISUSE BY DELIBERATELY CONCENTRATING AND INHALING THE CONTENTS CAN BE HARMFUL OR FATAL. KEEP OUT OF REACH OF CHILDREN. IN CASE OF ACCIDENTAL INGESTION, SEEK PROFESSIONAL ASSISTANCE OR CONTACT A POISON CONTROL CENTER IMMEDIATELY.

ACTIVE INGREDIENT

TOLNAFTATE 1%
Also contains Alcohol 36%
w/w (from SD alcohol 40),
BHT, isobutane, PPG-12-
buteth-16.
A FOOT COMFORT® PRODUCT
Distributed by
© Scholl, Inc.
Memphis, TN 38151
Shown in Product Identification Section, page 429

DR. SCHOLL'S® ATHLETE'S FOOT SPRAY POWDER   OTC

Tolnaftate 1%
Advanced Formula—Super Moisture Absorption

DESCRIPTION

Dr. Scholl's® Athlete's Foot Spray Powder with a super moisture-absorbing formula aids in the drying of naturally moist areas on the feet and between the toes and contains a clinically proven ingredient that kills athlete's foot fungi on contact. Also soothes and cools burning, itching feet.
To prevent infection, follow a regular daily hygiene program for feet. After bathing and drying feet carefully, apply Dr. Scholl's Athlete's Foot Spray Powder or Shaker Powder as directed.

DIRECTIONS

Thoroughly wash and dry infected areas twice daily. Shake can well. Hold can 4 to 6 inches away. Spray liberally between toes, on feet, in shoes and socks. Continue treatment for 2 weeks after symptoms disappear.

CAUTION

For external use only. Avoid getting into eyes. If symptoms do not improve in 10 days, or irritation occurs, discontinue use and consult your doctor. Do not use on nail or scalp infections.

WARNING — FLAMMABLE

DO NOT SPRAY WHILE SMOKING OR NEAR FIRE. DO NOT PUNCTURE OR INCINERATE CONTAINER OR PLACE WHERE TEMPERATURE EXCEEDS 120°F. USE ONLY AS DIRECTED. INTENTIONAL MISUSE BY DELIBERATELY CONCENTRATING AND INHALING THE CONTENTS CAN BE HARMFUL OR FATAL. KEEP OUT OF REACH OF CHILDREN. IN CASE OF ACCIDENTAL INGESTION, SEEK PROFESSIONAL ASSISTANCE OR CONTACT A POISON CONTROL CENTER IMMEDIATELY.

ACTIVE INGREDIENT

TOLNAFTATE 1%
Also contains: Alcohol 14% w/w (from SD alcohol 40), BHT, Isobutane, PPG-12-Buteth-16, Silica, Talc.
A FOOT COMFORT® PRODUCT
Distributed by
© Scholl, Inc.
Memphis, TN 38151
Shown in Product Identification Section, page 429

DR. SCHOLL'S® SMOOTH TOUCH DEEP MOISTURIZING CREAM   OTC

(Urea 5%)

DESCRIPTION

Unlike some general purpose lotions, Smooth Touch® Deep Moisturizing Cream's unique formula:
- Penetrates deeper to soften and smooth extra-dry and calloused skin on your feet
- Enhances skin's natural ability to absorb moisture
- Contains rich, non-greasy emollients that absorb quickly.

DIRECTIONS

Massage into skin once or twice daily or as often as needed to keep feet feeling soft and smooth. Regular use helps prevent the buildup of hard, dry skin.
Use also to soften and smooth extra dry skin on hands and elbows.
For additional ways to treat your feet to softness, Dr. Scholl's® Smooth Touch™ makes a complete line of foot and leg toiletries.

INGREDIENTS

Water, Petrolatum, Urea, Glyceryl Stearate Se, Methyl Hydroxystearate, Cocoa Butter, Stearic Acid, Triethanolamine Carbomer 934, Lanolin, Methylparaben, Fragrance, Imidazolidinyl Urea, Dimethicone, Propylparaben, Disodium EDTA.
Distribted by
© 1987 Scholl, Inc.
Memphis, TN 38151
Shown in Product Identification Section, page 429

DR. SCHOLL'S® SOAP'N SOAK®   OTC INSTANT FOOT BATH

DESCRIPTION

Just add a packet of this special formula to warm water and start soaking away foot discomfort. Your feet will feel refreshed, relaxed, revitalized. Dr. Scholl's SOAP'N SOAK is the perfect "pick-up" at the end of a busy day.

DIRECTIONS

Mix 1 packet in basin for every 2 quarts of warm water. Soak feet for up to fifteen minutes. For additional stimulation, massage feet briskly during soaking. To soften corns and callouses, soak feet daily.
FOR EXTERNAL USE ONLY—KEEP OUT OF REACH OF CHILDREN

INGREDIENTS

Soap, sodium, bicarbonate, sodium borate, sodium sesquicaronate, bran, fragrance, FD&C blue No. 1.
WARNING
If you have diabetes or poor circulation, consult your physician or podiatrist before using.
©Scholl, Inc.
Memphis, TN 38151
Shown in Product Identification Section, page 429

DR. SCHOLL'S® SUPER DEODORANT FOOT POWDER   OTC

(Aluminum Chlorhydrate 15%)

DESCRIPTION

Specially formulated to help eliminate offensive foot odors and absorb excessive perspiration associated with Bromidrosis, a functional disorder of the sweat glands.

DIRECTIONS

Bathe feet and dry thoroughly. Shake powder between toes, on tops and soles of feet. Also use daily inside shoes and in stockings to reduce excessive moisture. May also be used under arms.

CAUTION

Keep out of children's reach. In case of accidental ingestion, seek professional assistance, or contact a poison control center immediately.
AVOID CONTACT WITH EYES

INGREDIENTS

Talc, Aluminum Chlorhydrate, Salicylic Acid, Boric Acid, Fragrance.
A FOOT COMFORT® PRODUCT
© 1984 Scholl, Inc
Memphis, TN 38151
Shown in Product Identification Section, page 429

DR. SCHOLL'S® TRITIN™ ANTIFUNGAL POWDER   OTC

(Tolnaftate 1%)

DESCRIPTION

Triple Protection for maximum confidence... This advanced formula provides protection against athlete's foot, foot odor and wetness, in just one product...
1 Cures and prevents athlete's foot. Highly effective antifungal kills fungi on contact; prevents reinfection.
2 Fights odor all day. Leaves clean, fresh scent.
3 Controls wetness. Developed to absorb up to 50% more moisture than other leading antifungal brands.
Nothing works harder or longer than Tritin powder's 3-way protection... so you feel confident all day.

DIRECTIONS

Thoroughly wash and dry feet twice daily. Sprinkle powder on top and bottom of feet, as well as between toes, in shoes and socks. For athlete's foot, pay special attention to infected areas. Use daily to prevent reinfection.

CAUTION

For external use only. Keep out of eyes. Do not use on nail or scalp infections. If symptoms do not improve in 2 weeks, or irritation occurs, discontinue use and consult your doctor. Keep out of reach of children.

ACTIVE INGREDIENT

TOLNAFTATE 1%.
Other Ingredients: Talc, Cellulose, Fragrance, Starch/Acrylates/Acrylamide Copolymer.
© 1987 Scholl, Inc.
Memphis, TN 38151
Shown in Product Identification Section, page 429

DR. SCHOLL'S® TRITIN™ ANTIFUNGAL SPRAY POWDER   OTC

(Tolnaftate 1%)

DESCRIPTION

Triple Protection for maximum confidence. This advanced formula provides protection against athlete's foot, foot odor and wetness, in just one product.
1 Cures and prevents athlete's foot. Highly effective antifungal kills fungi on contact; prevents reinfection.
2 Fights odor all day. Leaves clean, fresh scent.
3 Controls wetness. Developed to absorb up to 50% more moisture than other leading antifungal brands.
Nothing works harder or longer than Tritin powder's 3-way protection... so you feel confident all day.

DIRECTIONS

Thoroughly wash and dry feet twice daily. Shake can well. Hold can 4–6 inches away. Spray top and bottom of feet, as well as between toes, in shoes and socks. For athlete's foot, pay special attention to infected areas. Use daily to prevent reinfection.

CAUTION

For external use only. Keep out of eyes. Do not use on nail or scalp infections. If symptoms do not improve in 2 weeks, or irritation occurs, discontinue use and consult your doctor.

WARNING — FLAMMABLE

Do not spray while smoking or near fire. Do not puncture or incinerate container or place where temperature exceeds 120°F. Use only as directed. Intentional misuse by deliberately concentrating and inhaling the contents can be harmful or fatal. Keep out of reach of children.

ACTIVE INGREDIENT

TOLNAFTATE 1%.
Other Ingredients: Isobutane, SD Alcohol 40 (14% w/w), Talc, Silica, PPG-12-Buteth-16, Fragrance, BHT.
© 1987 Scholl, Inc.
Memphis, TN 38151
Shown in Product Identification Section, page 429

DR. SCHOLL'S WORK DAY®   OTC

Super Comfort Insoles

DESCRIPTION

Work Day Insoles are made from a technologically advanced material that's so durable, they're guaranteed to cushion your feet day after day for a full six months. This fabric-covered breathable foam helps keep your feet cool and dry.

DIRECTIONS

Insert insole with cloth side up.

GUARANTEE

Dr. Scholl's Work Day Insoles are guaranteed for six months. If you are dissatisfied with this product, return the used insoles to Scholl, Inc., P.O. Box 377, Dept. AB, Memphis, TN 38151 for refund or replacement.

ALSO AVAILABE

- AIR-PILLO® DOUBLE COMFORT INSOLES
- FRESH STEP® SCENTED COMFORT INSOLES
- ODOR ATTACKERS® ODOR PREVENTING INSOLES, REGULAR & HEAVY DUTY
- WARM-EZE® SHEEP WOOL FLEECE INSOLES
- THERMA-CUSHION® INSULATING INSOLES
- HIDDEN COMFORT® HALF INSOLES

©1985 Scholl, Inc.
Memphis, TN 38151
Shown in Product Identification Section, page 429

Products are
listed alphabetically
in the
PINK SECTION.

Schwarz Pharma

Kremers Urban Company
P.O. BOX 2038
5600 W. COUNTY LINE ROAD
MILWAUKEE, WI 53201

CALCIFEROL™ Products
[kal-si 'fur-ol]
CALCIFEROL™ Drops   OTC
(ergocalciferol oral solution USP)
8,000 USP Units/mL
CALCIFEROL™ Tablets   ℞
(ergocalciferol tablets USP)
50,000 USP Units
CALCIFEROL™ in Oil Injection   ℞
(ergocalciferol)
500,000 Units/mL

DEPONIT®   ℞
[dĕp 'ō-nĭt]
(nitroglycerin transdermal delivery system)
5 mg/24 hours, 10 mg/24 hours

DESCRIPTION

Deponit is a unique nitroglycerin-containing transdermal delivery system. A multilayered self-adhesive film, the system contains nitroglycerin in a matrix composed of lactose, plasticizer, medical adhesive, polyisobutylene, and aluminized plastic for controlled release of the active agent through the skin into the systemic circulation. For the 24 hours during which the system is applied to the intact skin, its technology is intended to deliver an accurate dosage with no premature release of the nitroglycerin or undesired accumulation on the skin. Nitroglycerin (glyceryl trinitrate) is a vasodilator for the relief and prevention of anginal attacks. Deponit is available in two strengths which release either 5 mg or 10 mg of nitroglycerin during a 24-hour period. The 5 mg/24 hr system has a 16 cm^2 releasing surface and contains 16 mg nitroglycerin. The 10 mg/24 hr system has a 32 cm^2 releasing surface and contains 32 mg nitroglycerin. The Deponit system is approximately 0.3 mm thick, insoluble in water, and, as illustrated below, consists of two main elements:
1. A flexible, flesh-colored waterproof covering foil.
2. A multilayered adhesive film that constitutes simultaneously the drug reservoir and the release-control system.

- Covering foil
- Adhesive multilayered drug reservoir with the release-control system
- Protective foil with the special peel-off aid

The system is protected by an aluminum foil which has a patented S-shaped opening to facilitate its removal prior to use of the system.

CLINICAL PHARMACOLOGY

When the Deponit system is applied to the skin, nitroglycerin is continuously released for absorption directly into the systemic circulation. Thus, active drug reaches the target organs (heart, extremities) before deactivation by the liver. Nitroglycerin is a smooth-muscle relaxant with vascular effects manifested predominantly by venous dilatation and pooling. The major beneficial effect of nitroglycerin in angina pectoris is a reduction in myocardial oxygen consumption, secondary to vascular smooth-muscle relaxation with resultant reduction in cardiac preload and afterload. In recent years there has been increasing recognition of a direct vasodilator effect of nitroglycerin on the coronary vessels. In a bioavailability study using healthy volunteers,[1] transdermal absorption of nitroglycerin from the Deponit system achieved steady-state venous plasma levels and maintained these levels for 24 hours. Detectable plasma levels were attained within 30 minutes after application of the system and were still detectable 30 minutes after removal of the system. The amount of nitroglycerin released (5 mg/24 hr or 10 mg/24 hr) represents the mean release rate of nitroglycerin from the system as determined from healthy volunteers, and hence, the amount potentially available through the skin.

Absorption will vary among individuals. Precise definition of "therapeutic plasma level" is not known at this time.

INDICATIONS AND USAGE
This drug product has been conditionally approved by the FDA for the prevention and treatment of angina pectoris due to coronary artery disease. The conditional approval reflects a determination that the drug may be marketed while further investigation of its effectiveness is undertaken. A final evaluation of the effectiveness of the product will be announced by the FDA.

CONTRAINDICATIONS

Nitroglycerin is contraindicated in patients known to be intolerant of organic nitrate drugs and in patients with marked anemia.

WARNINGS

In patients with acute myocardial infarction or congestive heart failure, nitroglycerin should be used under careful clinical and/or hemodynamic monitoring.
In terminating treatment of patients with angina, both the dosage and frequency of application must be gradually reduced over a period of 4 to 6 weeks to prevent the sudden withdrawal reactions which are characteristic of vasodilators in the nitroglycerin class.
Transdermal nitroglycerin systems should be removed before attempting defibrillation or cardioversion because of the potential for altered electrical conductivity which may enhance the possibility of arcing, a phenomenon associated with the use of defibrillators.

PRECAUTIONS

Symptoms of hypotension, such as faintness, weakness, or dizziness, particularly orthostatic hypotension, may be due to overdosage. When these symptoms occur, the dosage should be reduced or use of the product discontinued.
Deponit is not intended for use in treatment of acute anginal attacks. For this purpose, occasional use of sublingual nitrates may be necessary.
Pregnancy—Pregnancy Category C:
Animal reproduction studies have not been conducted with nitroglycerin. It is not known whether nitroglycerin can cause fetal harm when administered to a pregnant woman or can affect reproduction capacity. Nitroglycerin should be given to a pregnant woman only if clearly needed.
Nursing Mothers:
It is not known whether nitroglycerin is excreted in human milk. Because many drugs are excreted in human milk, caution should be exercised when the preparation is administered to a nursing woman.

ADVERSE REACTIONS

Transient headache is the most common side effect, especially when higher doses of the drug are used. These headaches should be treated with mild analgesics while Deponit therapy is continued. When such headaches are unresponsive to treatment, the dosage should be reduced or use of the product discontinued.
Adverse reactions reported less frequently include hypotension, increased heart rate, faintness, flushing, dizziness, nausea, vomiting, and dermatitis. Except for dermatitis these symptoms are attributable to the known pharmacologic effects of nitroglycerin, but may be symptoms of overdosage. When they persist, the Deponit dose should be reduced or use of the product discontinued.

DOSAGE AND ADMINISTRATION

Deponit can be applied as a single system or as multiples, depending upon the clinical requirements. Dosage should be titrated to achieve the optimal therapeutic effect by monitoring clinical response, side effects, heart rate, and the effect of therapy upon blood pressure.
Deponit should be removed from the single-unit package just prior to use. The protective aluminum precut S-shaped foil is removed according to the "Patient Instructions," and the system is applied with a firm pressure on a convenient skin site, preferably on the chest, innerside of the upper arm, or shoulders. Deponit should not be applied to the distal parts of extremities.
Each system is designed to remain in place for 24 hours; however, the treatment site should be changed daily to minimize skin irritation and should be intact, clean, and dry. If necessary, hair may be removed by clipping.
Therapy should be initiated with application of a single Deponit system, delivering 5 mg every 24 hours. Response in terms of satisfactory control of anginal symptoms without

adverse effects should be evaluated to determine the optimal dose. Some patients may require adjustment of dosage to provide a better clinical response. This can be achieved by removing the system delivering 5 mg/24 hours, and applying a larger system delivering 10 mg/24 hours or a multiple of either system, depending on the dose required to achieve the desired effect.
After 24 hours, the system should be removed and discarded. Because no adhesive residue remains on the skin, there is no need to use a solvent.

STORAGE CONDITIONS

Store at controlled room temperature below 25°C (77°F). Do not refrigerate.
Patient Instructions for Application
A leaflet describing use of Deponit is provided with each package.

HOW SUPPLIED

Deponit® (nitroglycerin transdermal delivery system) is packaged in cartons containing unit doses of 30 flesh-colored systems on aluminum backings.
[See table below].
Caution: Federal law prohibits dispensing without prescription.

REFERENCE

1. Data on file.
U S Pat No. 4,524,095 and 4,769,028
Manufactured for
SCHWARZ
PHARMA
Kremers Urban Company
Milwaukee, WI 53201
by Lohmann, Neuwied, West Germany
Shown in Product Identification Section, page 429

FEDAHIST® Decongestant Syrup

(See PDR For Nonprescription Drugs)

FEDAHIST® Tablets

(See PDR For Nonprescription Drugs)

FEDAHIST® Expectorant Syrup

(See PDR For Nonprescription Drugs)

FEDAHIST® Expectorant Pediatric Drops

(See PDR For Nonprescription Drugs)

FEDAHIST® TIMECAPS™   ℞
FEDAHIST® GYROCAPS®   ℞
[fed 'a-hist ']

DESCRIPTION

FEDAHIST® TIMECAPS™ contain 120 mg pseudoephedrine hydrochloride USP and 8 mg chlorpheniramine maleate USP in a timed-release formulation designed for oral b.i.d. dosage.
FEDAHIST® GYROCAPS® contain 65 mg pseudoephedrine hydrochloride USP and 10 mg chlorpheniramine maleate USP in a timed-release formulation designed for oral b.i.d. dosage.
Pseudoephedrine hydrochloride is a nasal decongestant. The empirical formula is $C_{10}H_{15}NO \cdot HCl$ and the molecular weight is 201.70. Chemically, it is benzenemethanol,α-[1-(methylamino) ethyl]-, [S-(R*,R*)]-, hydrochloride. Chlorpheniramine maleate is an antihistamine. The empirical formula is $C_{16}H_{19}ClN_2 \cdot C_4H_4O_4$ and the molecular weight is 390.87. Chemically, it is 2-[p-chloro-α-[2-(dimethylamino)ethyl]benzyl] pyridine maleate (1:1).
FEDAHIST TIMECAPS also contain as inactive ingredients: FD&C Blue #1, gelatin, pharmaceutical glaze, starch, sucrose, and other ingredients.
FEDAHIST GYROCAPS also contain as inactive ingredients: D&C Yellow #10, FD&C Blue #1, FD&C Blue #2, FD&C Yellow #6, gelatin, pharmaceutical glaze, silicon dioxide, sodium lauryl sulfate, starch, sucrose, titanium dioxide, and other ingredients.

CLINICAL PHARMACOLOGY

Pseudoephedrine is an orally active sympathomimetic amine and exerts a decongestant action on the nasal mucosa. Pseudoephedrine produces peripheral effects similar to those of ephedrine and central effects similar to, but less intense than amphetamines. It has the potential for excitatory side effects. At the recommended oral dosages it has little or no pressor effect in normotensive adults. The serum half-life of pseudoephedrine is approximately 4 to 6 hours. The serum half-life is decreased with increased excretion of drug at urine pH lower than 6 and may be increased with decreased excretion at urine pH higher than 8.

Nitroglycerin released *in vivo*	Total drug content/system	System size	Carton size
5 mg/24 hr	16 mg	16 cm^2	30 Systems (**NDC** 0091-4195-01)
10 mg/24 hr	32 mg	32 cm^2	30 Systems (**NDC** 0091-4196-01)

Chlorpheniramine is an antihistamine that possesses anticholinergic and sedative effects. It is considered one of the most effective and least toxic of the histamine antagonists. Chlorpheniramine is a H_1 receptor antagonist. It antagonizes many of the pharmacologic actions of histamine. It prevents released histamine from dilating capillaries and causing edema of the respiratory mucosa. Chlorpheniramine is well absorbed and has a duration of action of 4 to 6 hours (the TIMECAPS and GYROCAPS formulation provide a continuous therapeutic effect for up to 12 hours). Its half-life in serum is 12 to 16 hours. Degradation products of chlorpheniramine's metabolic transformation by the liver are almost completely excreted in 24 hours.

FEDAHIST TIMECAPS release 120 mg pseudoephedrine and 8 mg chlorpheniramine at a controlled and predictable rate for 12 hours. FEDAHIST GYROCAPS release 65 mg pseudoephedrine and 10 mg chlorpheniramine at a controlled and predictable rate for 12 hours. Peak blood levels occur in 4 hours for pseudoephedrine and 6 hours for chlorpheniramine. The apparent plasma half-life is approximately 6 hours for pseudoephedrine and 16 hours for chlorpheniramine. The relative bioavailability of the timed-release dosage form is approximately 85% and 100% for the immediate-release dosage forms for pseudoephedrine and chlorpheniramine, respectively.

INDICATIONS AND USAGE

FEDAHIST is indicated for the relief of nasal congestion and eustachian tube congestion associated with the common cold, sinusitis, and acute upper respiratory infections. FEDAHIST is also indicated for symptomatic relief of perennial and seasonal allergic rhinitis and vasomotor rhinitis. Decongestants in combination with antihistamines have been used to relieve eustachian tube congestion associated with acute eustachian salpingitis, aerotitis, and serous otitis media.

CONTRAINDICATIONS

Sympathomimetic amines are contraindicated in patients with severe hypertension, severe coronary artery disease and in patients on MAO inhibitor therapy. Antihistamines are contraindicated in patients with narrow-angle glaucoma, urinary retention, peptic ulcer, during an asthmatic attack and in patients receiving MAO inhibitors.

Hypersensitivity: Contraindicated in patients with hypersensitivity or idiosyncrasy to sympathomimetic amines. FEDAHIST is also contraindicated in patients hypersensitive to chlorpheniramine and other antihistamines of similar chemical structure.

Nursing Mothers: Contraindicated because of the higher than usual risk for infants from sympathomimetic amines.

Newborn or Premature Infants: FEDAHIST should not be administered to premature or full-term infants.

WARNINGS

Sympathomimetic amines should be used judiciously and sparingly in patients with hypertension, diabetes mellitus, ischemic heart disease, increased intraocular pressure, hyperthyroidism or prostatic hypertrophy (see **CONTRAINDICATIONS**). Sympathomimetics may produce CNS stimulation and convulsions or cardiovascular collapse with accompanying hypotension. Chlorpheniramine maleate has an atropine-like action and should be used with caution in patients with increased intraocular pressure, cardiovascular disease, hypertension or in patients with a history of bronchial asthma (see **CONTRAINDICATIONS**). Antihistamines may cause excitability, especially in children. Do not exceed recommended dosage because at higher doses nervousness, dizziness, or sleeplessness may occur.

Use in the Elderly: The elderly (60 years and older) are more likely to have adverse reactions to sympathomimetics. Overdosage of sympathomimetics in this age group may cause hallucinations, convulsions, CNS depression and death.

PRECAUTIONS

General:
Should be used with caution in patients with diabetes, hypertension, cardiovascular disease and hyperreactivity to ephedrine. The antihistamine may cause drowsiness, therefore ambulatory patients who operate machinery or motor vehicles should be cautioned accordingly.

Information for Patients:
Antihistamines may impair mental and physical abilities required for the performance of potentially hazardous tasks, such as driving a vehicle or operating machinery, and may impair mental alertness in children.

Drug Interactions:
MAO inhibitors and beta adrenergic blockers increase the effect of sympathomimetics. Sympathomimetics may reduce the antihypertensive effects of methyldopa, mecamylamine, reserpine and veratrum alkaloids. Concomitant use of antihistamines with alcohol, tricyclic antidepressants, barbiturates and other CNS depressants may have an additive effect.

Laboratory Test Interactions:
Antihistamines may suppress the wheal and flare reactions to antigen skin testing. Considerable interindividual variation in the extent and duration of suppression have been reported, depending on the antigen and test technique, antihistamine and dosage regimen, time since the last dose and individual response to testing. In one study, usual oral dosages of chlorpheniramine suppressed the wheal response for about 2 days after the last dose. Whenever possible, antihistamines should be discontinued about 4 days prior to skin testing procedures since they may prevent otherwise positive reactions to dermal reactivity indicators.

Carcinogenesis, Mutagenesis, Impairment of Fertility:
No long-term or reproduction studies in animals have been performed with FEDAHIST to evaluate its carcinogenic, mutagenic, and impairment of fertility potential.

Pregnancy —Pregnancy Category C:
Animal reproduction studies have not been conducted with FEDAHIST. It is not known whether FEDAHIST can cause fetal harm when administered to a pregnant woman or can affect reproduction capacity. FEDAHIST may be given to a pregnant woman only if clearly needed.

Nursing Mothers:
Pseudoephedrine is contraindicated in nursing mothers because of the higher than usual risk for infants from sympathomimetic amines.

ADVERSE REACTIONS

Hyperreactive individuals may display ephedrine-like reactions such as tachycardia, palpitations, headache, dizziness or nausea. Patients sensitive to antihistamines may experience mild sedation.

Sympathomimetic drugs have been associated with certain untoward reactions including fear, anxiety, tenseness, restlessness, tremor, weakness, pallor, respiratory difficulty, dysuria, insomnia, hallucinations, convulsions, CNS depression, arrhythmias, and cardiovascular collapse with hypotension.

Possible side effects of antihistamines are drowsiness, restlessness, dizziness, weakness, dry mouth, anorexia, nausea, headache, nervousness, blurring of vision, heartburn, dysuria, and very rarely, dermatitis. Patient idiosyncrasy to adrenergic agents may be manifested by insomnia, dizziness, weakness, tremor or arrhythmias.

OVERDOSAGE

Symptoms: Manifestations of antihistamine overdosage may vary from central nervous system depression (sedation, apnea, cardiovascular collapse) to stimulation (insomnia, hallucinations, tremors or convulsions). Other signs and symptoms may be dizziness, tinnitus, ataxia, blurred vision and hypotension. Stimulation is particularly likely in children, as are atropine-like signs and symptoms (dry mouth, dilated pupils, flushing, hyperthermia, and gastrointestinal symptoms).

Treatment Recommendations: The patient should be induced to vomit even if emesis has occurred spontaneously; however, vomiting should not be induced in patients with impaired consciousness. Precautions against aspiration should be taken, especially in infants and children.

Ipecac Syrup is the preferred method for inducing vomiting. The action of ipecac is facilitated by physical activity and the administration of eight to twelve fluid ounces of water. If emesis does not occur in fifteen minutes, the dose of ipecac should be repeated. Following emesis, any drug remaining in the stomach may be absorbed by activated charcoal administered as a slurry with water.

If vomiting is unsuccessful or contraindicated, gastric lavage should be performed. Isotonic and one-half isotonic saline are the lavage solutions of choice. Saline cathartics, such as milk of magnesia, draw water into the bowel by osmosis and, therefore, may be valuable for their action of rapid dilution of bowel content.

Treatment of the signs and symptoms of overdosage is symptomatic and supportive. Vasopressors may be used to treat hypotension. Short-acting barbiturates, diazepam or paraldehyde may be administered to control seizures. Hyperpyrexia, especially in children, may require treatment with tepid water sponge baths or a hypothermic blanket. Apnea is treated with ventilatory support. Stimulants (analeptic agents) should not be used.

The LD_{50} for pseudoephedrine is 202 mg/kg delivered intraperitoneally to rats. When given orally to mice, the LD_{50} for chlorpheniramine is 162 mg/kg.

DOSAGE AND ADMINISTRATION

FEDAHIST TIMECAPS: *Adults and children 12 years of age and older:* One TIMECAP every 12 hours not to exceed 2 TIMECAPS in 24 hours. Not recommended for children under 12 years of age.

FEDAHIST GYROCAPS: *Adults and children 12 years of age and older:* One GYROCAP every 12 hours not to exceed 2 GYROCAPS in 24 hours. Not recommended for children under 12 years of age.

HOW SUPPLIED

FEDAHIST TIMECAPS are clear capsules containing white and blue beadlets and imprinted with "KREMERS URBAN" and "055".

　Bottles of 100 capsules　　　　NDC 0091-0055-01
FEDAHIST GYROCAPS are white and yellow capsules containing white and green beadlets and imprinted with "KREMERS URBAN" AND "053".

　Bottles of 100 capsules　　　　NDC 0091-1053-01
Store at controlled room temperature 15°–30°C (59°–86°F).

CAUTION

Federal law prohibits dispensing without prescription.
　Mfd. by:
　Central Pharmaceuticals, Inc.
　Seymour, Indiana 47274
　For:
　SCHWARZ
　PHARMA
　Kremers Urban Company
　Milwaukee, Wisconsin 53201
　Shown in Product Identification Section, page 429

KUTRASE® Capsules　　　　℞
[*qū 'trās*]

DESCRIPTION

KUTRASE® Capsules contain four standardized digestive enzymes: lipase, amylase, protease, cellulase, and hyoscyamine sulfate USP and phenyltoloxamine citrate. Lipase, amylase, protease and cellulase are derived from fungal, plant and animal sources and are oral digestive enzyme supplements. Hyoscyamine sulfate USP is one of the principal anticholinergic/antispasmodic components of belladonna alkaloids. Phenyltoloxamine citrate is a non-barbiturate sedative. Each capsule contains:

lipase	75 mg
amylase	30 mg
protease	6 mg
cellulase	2 mg
hyoscyamine sulfate USP	0.0625 mg
phenyltoloxamine citrate	15 mg

Each capsule also contains as inactive ingredients: D&C Yellow #10, ethylcellulose, FD&C Green #3, FD&C Yellow #6, gelatin, lactose, magnesium stearate, titanium dioxide, vanillin and other ingredients.

CLINICAL PHARMACOLOGY

Diminution of secretions from exocrine glands is often a result of the normal aging process. KUTRASE provides a balanced combination of natural proteolytic, amylolytic, cellulolytic and lipolytic enzymes to enhance digestion of proteins, starch and fat in the gastrointestinal tract. These enzymes do not exert any systemic pharmacologic effects. KUTRASE should be considered an enzyme supplement and not an enzyme replacement therapy. Enzymes in KUTRASE are basically derived from fungal and plant sources and possess a broad spectrum of pH activity. Enzymes are promptly released from the capsule and are bioavailable for digestion of food in the stomach and intestines. Hyoscyamine sulfate provides a potent spasmolytic effect in reducing gastrointestinal hypermotility and intestinal spasm. A mild sedative effect is provided by phenyltoloxamine citrate.

INDICATIONS AND USAGE

KUTRASE is indicated for the relief of the symptoms of functional indigestion devoid of organic pathology commonly referred to as nervous indigestion and colloquially as "butterflies". The symptoms are bloating, gas, and fullness.

CONTRAINDICATIONS

Glaucoma, obstructive uropathy, obstructive disease of the gastrointestinal tract (as in achalasia, pyloroduodenal stenosis); paralytic ileus, intestinal atony of the elderly or debilitated patients; unstable cardiovascular status in acute hemorrhage; severe ulcerative colitis; toxic megacolon complicating ulcerative colitis; myasthenia gravis, or a hypersensitivity to any of the ingredients.

WARNINGS

Do not administer to patients who are allergic to pork products. In the presence of high environmental temperature, heat prostration can occur with drug use (fever and heat stroke due to decreased sweating). Diarrhea may be an early symptom of incomplete intestinal obstruction, especially in patients with ileostomy or colostomy. In this instance, treatment with this drug would be inappropriate. KUTRASE may produce drowsiness or blurred vision. In this event, the patient should be warned not to engage in activities requiring mental alertness such as operating a motor vehicle or other machinery or to perform hazardous work while taking this drug.

Continued on next page

Schwarz Pharma—Cont.

PRECAUTIONS

General:
Use with caution in patients with autonomic neuropathy, hyperthyroidism, coronary heart disease, congestive heart failure, cardiac arrhythmias, and hypertension. Investigate any tachycardia before giving any anticholinergic drug since they may increase the heart rate. Use with caution in patients with hiatal hernia associated with reflux esophagitis.

Information for Patients:
If capsules are opened, avoid inhalation of the powder. Sensitive individuals may experience allergic reactions.

Carcinogenesis, Mutagenesis, Impairment of Fertility:
Long-term studies in animals have not been performed to evaluate the carcinogenic, mutagenic or impairment of fertility potential of KUTRASE.

Pregnancy-Pregnancy Category C:
Animal reproduction studies have not been conducted with KUTRASE. It is also not known whether KUTRASE can cause fetal harm when administered to a pregnant woman or can affect reproduction capacity. KUTRASE should be given to a pregnant woman only if clearly needed.

Nursing Mothers:
Hyoscyamine sulfate is excreted in human milk. It is not known whether the enzymes or phenyltoloxamine citrate are excreted in human milk. Caution should be exercised when KUTRASE is administered to a nursing woman.

ADVERSE REACTIONS

Occasionally a slight looseness of the stools may be noticed. If so, dosage should be reduced. Finely powdered pancreatic enzyme may be irritating to the mucous membranes and respiratory tract. Inhalation of the airborne powder may precipitate an asthma attack in sensitive individuals. Other adverse reactions may include dryness of the mouth; urinary hesitancy and retention; blurred vision; tachycardia; palpitations; mydriasis; cycloplegia; increased ocular tension; headache; nervousness; drowsiness; weakness; suppression of lactation; allergic reactions or drug idiosyncrasies; urticaria and other dermal manifestations and decreased sweating.

OVERDOSAGE

The signs and symptoms of overdose are headache, nausea, vomiting, blurred vision, dilated pupils, hot dry skin, dizziness, dryness of the mouth, difficulty in swallowing. Measures to be taken are immediate lavage of the stomach and injection of physostigmine 0.5 to 2 mg intravenously and repeated as necessary up to a total of 5 mg. Fever may be treated symptomatically. Excitement to a degree which demands attention may be managed with sodium thiopental 2% solution given slowly intravenously. In the event of paralysis of the respiratory muscles, artificial respiration should be instituted.

DOSAGE AND ADMINISTRATION

1 or 2 capsules taken with each meal or snack. Dosage may be adjusted according to the conditions and severity of symptoms to assure symptomatic control with a minimum of adverse effects.

HOW SUPPLIED

KUTRASE Capsules are green and white capsules and are imprinted "KREMERS URBAN" and "475."

Bottles of 100 capsules	NDC 0091-3475-01
Bottles of 500 capsules	NDC 0091-3475-05

Store at controlled room temperature 15°–30°C (59°–86°F).

CAUTION

Federal law prohibits dispensing without prescription.
Shown in Product Identification Section, page 429

KU-ZYME® Capsules   ℞
[qū' zīm]

DESCRIPTION

KU-ZYME® Capsules contain four standardized enzymes: lipase, amylase, protease and cellulase. They are derived from fungal, plant and animal sources and are designed for oral digestive enzyme supplement therapy.
Each capsule contains:

lipase	75 mg
amylase	30 mg
protease	6 mg
cellulase	2 mg

Each capsule also contains as inactive ingredients: D&C Yellow #10, FD&C Yellow #6, gelatin, lactose, magnesium stearate, titanium dioxide, vanillin and other ingredients.

CLINICAL PHARMACOLOGY

Diminution of secretions from exocrine glands is often a result of the normal aging process. KU-ZYME provides a balanced combination of natural proteolytic, amylolytic, cellulolytic and lipolytic enzymes to enhance digestion of proteins, starch and fat in the gastrointestinal tract. These en-

zymes do not exert any systemic pharmacologic effects. KU-ZYME should be considered an enzyme supplement and not an enzyme replacement therapy. Enzymes in KU-ZYME are basically derived from fungal and plant sources and possess a broad spectrum of pH activity. Enzymes are promptly released from the capsule and are bioavailable for digestion of food in the stomach and intestines.

INDICATIONS AND USAGE

For the relief of functional indigestion when due to enzyme deficiency or imbalance. KU-ZYME relieves symptoms due to faulty digestion including the sensation of fullness after meals, dyspepsia, flatulence, abdominal distention and intolerance to certain foods.

CONTRAINDICATIONS

There are no known contraindications to the administration of digestive enzymes. These enzymes do not attack living tissues and do not present any danger to the patient with ulceration or inflammation in the digestive tract.

WARNINGS

Do not administer to patients who are allergic to pork products.

PRECAUTIONS

Information for Patients:
If capsules are opened, avoid inhalation of the powder. Sensitive individuals may experience allergic reactions.

Carcinogenesis, Mutagenesis, Impairment of Fertility:
Long-term studies in animals have not been performed to evaluate carcinogenic, mutagenic or impairment of fertility potential of KU-ZYME.

Pregnancy-Pregnancy Category C:
Animal reproduction studies have not been conducted with KU-ZYME. It is also not known whether KU-ZYME can cause fetal harm when administered to a pregnant woman or can affect reproduction capacity. KU-ZYME should be given to a pregnant woman only if clearly needed.

Nursing Mothers:
It is not known whether KU-ZYME is excreted in human milk. Because many drugs are excreted in human milk, caution should be exercised when KU-ZYME is administered to a nursing woman.

ADVERSE REACTIONS

Virtually unknown. Occasionally, a slight looseness of the stool may be noticed. If so, dosage should be reduced. Finely powdered pancreatic enzyme may be irritating to the mucous membranes and respiratory tract. Inhalation of the airborne powder may precipitate an asthma attack in sensitive individuals.

OVERDOSAGE

No systemic toxicity occurs. Excessive dosage may, however, produce a laxative effect.

DOSAGE AND ADMINISTRATION

1 or 2 capsules taken with each meal or snack. Dosage may be adjusted depending on individual requirements for relief of symptoms due to digestive enzyme deficiency. In patients who experience difficulty in swallowing the capsule, it may be opened and the contents sprinkled on the food. When opening the capsules, avoid inhalation of the powder (see PRECAUTIONS and ADVERSE REACTIONS).

HOW SUPPLIED

KU-ZYME Capsules are yellow and white capsules and are imprinted "KREMERS URBAN" and "522".

Bottles of 100 capsules	NDC 0091-3522-01
Bottles of 500 capsules	NDC 0091-3522-05

Store at controlled room temperature 15°–30°C (59°–86°F).

CAUTION

Federal law prohibits dispensing without prescription.
Shown in Product Identification Section, page 429

KU-ZYME® HP Capsules   ℞
[qū' zīm]
(pancrelipase capsules USP)

DESCRIPTION

KU-ZYME® HP Capsules (pancrelipase capsules USP) contain standardized lipase, amylase and protease obtained from hog pancreas and are designed for oral digestive enzyme replacement therapy. Each capsule contains:

lipase	8,000 USP units
protease	30,000 USP units
amylase	30,000 USP units

Each capsule also contains as inactive ingredients: gelatin, lactose, magnesium stearate, titanium dioxide and other ingredients.

CLINICAL PHARMACOLOGY

Pancrelipase USP is a pancreatic enzyme concentrate which hydrolyzes fats to glycerol and fatty acids, changes protein into proteoses and derived substances, and converts starch into dextrins and sugars. The administration of pancrelipase

reduces the fat and nitrogen content in the stool. Pancreatic enzymes are normally secreted in great excess. Generally, steatorrhea and malabsorption occur only after a 90 percent or greater reduction in secretion of lipase and proteolytic enzymes. It has been estimated that approximately 8,000 units of lipase per hour should be delivered into the duodenum postprandially. Even if all the enzymes taken orally reached the proximal intestine in active form, ingestion of 24,000 units of lipase (8,000 units per hour) for 3 postprandial hours would be required. If one could deliver sufficient pancreatic enzymes to the small intestine, malabsorption could be corrected. It is rarely possible to achieve complete relief of steatorrhea although major improvement in fat absorption can be achieved in most patients.

INDICATIONS

KU-ZYME HP is effective in patients with deficient exocrine pancreatic secretions. Thus, KU-ZYME HP may be used as enzyme replacement therapy in cystic fibrosis, chronic pancreatitis, post pancreatectomy, in ductal obstructions caused by cancer of the pancreas, pancreatic insufficiency and for steatorrhea of malabsorption syndrome and post gastrectomy (Billroth II and Total). May also be used as a presumptive test for pancreatic function, especially in pancreatic insufficiency due to chronic pancreatitis.

CONTRAINDICATIONS

There are no known contraindications for the use of pancrelipase although sensitivity to pork protein may preclude its use.

WARNINGS

Pancreatic exocrine replacement therapy should not delay or supplant treatment of the primary disorder. Use with caution in patients known to be hypersensitive to pork or enzymes.

PRECAUTIONS

Information for Patients:
If capsules are opened, avoid inhalation of the powder. Sensitive individuals may experience allergic reactions.

Drug Interactions:
The serum iron response to oral iron may be decreased by concomitant administration of pancreatic extracts.

Carcinogenesis, Mutagenesis, and Impairment of Fertility:
Long-term studies in animals have not been performed to evaluate the carcinogenic, mutagenic or impairment of fertility potential of KU-ZYME HP.

Pregnancy-Pregnancy Category C:
Animal reproduction studies have not been conducted with KU-ZYME HP. It is also not known whether KU-ZYME HP can cause fetal harm when administered to a pregnant woman or can affect reproduction capacity. KU-ZYME HP should be given to a pregnant woman only if clearly needed.

Nursing Mothers:
It is not known whether KU-ZYME HP is excreted in human milk. Because many drugs are excreted in human milk, caution should be exercised when KU-ZYME HP is administered to a nursing woman.

ADVERSE REACTIONS

High doses may cause nausea, abdominal cramps and/or diarrhea in certain patients. Finely powdered pancreatic enzyme concentrate may be irritating to the mucous membranes and respiratory tract. Inhalation of the airborne powder may precipitate an asthma attack in sensitive individuals. Extremely high doses of exogenous pancreatic enzymes have been associated with hyperuricemia and hyperuricosuria.

DOSAGE AND ADMINISTRATION

1 to 3 capsules taken with each meal or snack. Dosage may be adjusted depending on individual requirements for control of steatorrhea. In severe deficiencies the dose may be increased to 8 capsules with meals or the frequency of administration may increase to hourly intervals if nausea, cramps and/or diarrhea do not occur.

HOW SUPPLIED

KU-ZYME® HP Capsules (pancrelipase capsules USP) are white opaque capsules and are imprinted "KREMERS URBAN" and "525."

Bottles of 100 capsules	NDC 0091-3525-01

Store at a temperature not exceeding 25°C (77°F).

CAUTION

Federal law prohibits dispensing without prescription.
Shown in Product Identification Section, page 429

LACTRASE® Capsules   OTC
[lăk 'trās]
(lactase)

DESCRIPTION

LACTRASE® Capsules contain 250 mg of standardized lactase. Lactase is a natural enzyme used in the treatment of lactose intolerance. Lactase is produced by a unique fermentation process. The chemical name of lactase is beta-D-galactosidase. Each capsule also contains as inactive ingredients: gelatin, magnesium stearate, maltodextrin, red iron oxide, titanium dioxide, yellow iron oxide and other ingredients.

ACTION

Though lactase is normally present in adequate quantities in infants, in many populations its concentration naturally declines starting at about 4–5 years of age and is low in a substantial number of individuals by their teens or early 20's. Within certain geographic and ethnic groups, especially in adult Blacks, Orientals, American Indians, and Eastern European Jews, the lactase activity may be low even earlier. Although many of them can easily digest smaller quantities of lactose in milk, after consumption of an excessive volume of milk or dairy products, they may exhibit symptoms of lactose intolerance.

Lactose is a non-absorbable disaccharide found as a common constituent in most dairy products. Under normal conditions, dietary lactose is hydrolyzed in the jejunum and proximal ileum by beta-D-galactosidase or lactase. Lactase is produced in the brush border of the columnar epithelial cells of the intestinal villi. Lactase hydrolyzes lactose into two monosaccharides, glucose and galactose, that are readily absorbed by the intestine.

When available lactase is insufficient to split the lactose, the unabsorbable sugar remains in the small intestine for an extended period, presenting an osmotic load that increases and retains intraluminal fluid and intensifies intestinal motility; thus the individual reports a bloated feeling and cramps. The undigested lactose is decomposed by the intestinal flora in the lower intestine and excessive carbon dioxide and hydrogen is produced. These gases contribute to flatulence and increased abdominal discomfort. The lactic acid and other short chain acids raise the osmolality, hinder fluid reabsorption and decrease transit time of the contents of the colon, leading to diarrhea. Often hydrogen is noticed in the expired breath of a lactase deficient patient.

INDICATIONS

LACTRASE is indicated for individuals exhibiting symptoms of lactose intolerance or lactase insufficiency as identified by a lactose tolerance test or by exhibiting gastrointestinal disturbances after consumption of milk or dairy products.

PRECAUTIONS

It should be noted that in diabetic persons who use LACTRASE, the milk sugar will be metabolically available and may result in increased blood glucose levels. Individuals with galactosemia may not have milk in any form, lactase enzyme modified or not.

DIRECTIONS

Generally, one or two LACTRASE Capsules swallowed with milk or dairy products is all that is necessary to digest the milk sugar contained in a normal serving. If the individual is severely intolerant to lactose, additional capsules may be taken until a satisfactory response is achieved as recognized by resolution of the symptoms. LACTRASE Capsules are safe to take and higher quantities in severe cases will be well-tolerated.

If the individual cannot swallow capsules, the contents of the capsules may be sprinkled onto dairy products before consuming. LACTRASE will not alter the taste of the dairy product when used in this manner.

Milk may also be pre-treated with LACTRASE; simply add the contents from one or two capsules to each quart of milk, shake gently, and store the milk in the refrigerator for 24 hours. LACTRASE will break down milk sugars to digestible simple sugars. LACTRASE powder will not alter the appearance of milk, however the taste may be slightly sweeter than untreated milk.

HOW SUPPLIED

LACTRASE Capsules are opaque orange and opaque white and are imprinted, "KREMERS URBAN" and "505". They are supplied in blister packs containing 10 capsules (NDC 0091-3505-10) or 30 capsules (NDC 0091-3505-03) and in bottles containing 100 capsules (NDC 0091-3505-01).

Store at controlled room temperature 15°–30°C (59°–86°F).

Shown in Product Identification Section, page 429

LEVSIN® PRODUCTS ℞
[lev'sin]
(hyoscyamine sulfate USP)
LEVSIN®/SL Tablets
LEVSIN® Tablets
LEVSIN® Elixir
LEVSIN® Drops (Oral Solution)
LEVSIN® Injection
LEVSINEX™ TIMECAPS™

DESCRIPTION

LEVSIN® (hyoscyamine sulfate USP) is one of the principal anticholinergic/antispasmodic components of belladonna alkaloids. The empirical formula is $(C_{17}H_{23}NO_3)_2 \cdot H_2SO_4 \cdot 2H_2O$ and the molecular weight is 712.85. Chemically, it is benzeneacetic acid, α-(hydroxymethyl)-,8-methyl-8-azabicyclo [3.2.1.] oct-3-yl ester, [3(S)-endo]-,sulfate (2:1), dihydrate.

LEVSIN/SL Tablets contain 0.125 mg hyoscyamine sulfate formulated for sublingual administration. However, the tablets may also be chewed or taken orally. Each tablet also contains as inactive ingredients: colloidal silicon dioxide, dextrates, FD&C Green #3, flavor, mannitol, and stearic acid.

LEVSIN Tablets contain 0.125 mg hyoscyamine sulfate formulated for oral administration. Each tablet also contains as inactive ingredients: acacia, confectioner's sugar, corn starch, lactose, powdered cellulose and stearic acid.

LEVSIN Elixir contains 0.125 mg hyoscyamine sulfate per 5 mL (teaspoonful) with 20% alcohol for oral use. LEVSIN Elixir also contains as inactive ingredients: FD&C Red #40, FD&C Yellow #6, flavor, glycerin, purified water, sorbitol solution and sucrose.

LEVSIN Drops, oral solution, contain 0.125 mg hyoscyamine sulfate per mL with 5% alcohol. LEVSIN Drops also contain as inactive ingredients: FD&C Red #40, FD&C Yellow #6, flavor, glycerin, purified water, sodium citrate, sorbitol solution, and sucrose.

LEVSIN Injection is a sterile solution containing 0.5 mg hyoscyamine sulfate per mL. The 1 mL ampuls contain as inactive ingredients: water for injection, pH is adjusted with hydrochloric acid when necessary. The 10 mL multiple-dose vials contain as inactive ingredients: benzyl alcohol 1.5%, sodium metabisulfite 0.1%, isotonic sodium chloride, and water for injection.

LEVSINEX TIMECAPS contain 0.375 mg hyoscyamine sulfate in a timed-release formulation designed for oral b.i.d. dosage. Each TIMECAP also contains as inactive ingredients: corn starch, D&C Red #28, FD&C Blue #1, FD&C Blue #2, FD&C Red #3, FD&C Red #40, FD&C Yellow #6, gelatin, sucrose, titanium dioxide and other ingredients.

CLINICAL PHARMACOLOGY

LEVSIN inhibits specifically the actions of acetylcholine on structures innervated by postganglionic cholinergic nerves and on smooth muscles that respond to acetylcholine but lack cholinergic innervation. These peripheral cholinergic receptors are present in the autonomic effector cells of the smooth muscle, cardiac muscle, the sinoatrial node, the atrioventricular node, and the exocrine glands. It is completely devoid of any action in the autonomic ganglia. LEVSIN inhibits gastrointestinal propulsive motility and decreases gastric acid secretion. LEVSIN also controls excessive pharyngeal, tracheal and bronchial secretions.

LEVSIN is absorbed totally and completely by sublingual administration as well as oral administration. Once absorbed, LEVSIN disappears rapidly from the blood and is distributed throughout the entire body. The half-life of LEVSIN is 3 ½ hours. LEVSIN is partly hydrolyzed to tropic acid and tropine but the majority of the drug is excreted in the urine unchanged within the first 12 hours. Only traces of this drug are found in breast milk. LEVSIN passes the blood brain barrier and the placental barrier.

LEVSINEX TIMECAPS release 0.375 mg hyoscyamine sulfate at a controlled and predictable rate for 12 hours. Peak blood levels occur in 2 ½ hours and the apparent plasma half-life is approximately 7 hours. The relative bioavailability of the timed-release dosage form is approximately 81% that of the immediate-release dosage form. The urinary excretion from both the immediate-release dosage form and the timed-release dosage form is equal and uniform over a 24 hour period.

INDICATIONS AND USAGE

LEVSIN is effective as adjunctive therapy in the treatment of peptic ulcer. It can also be used to control gastric secretion, visceral spasm, and hypermotility in spastic colitis, spastic bladder, cystitis, pylorospasm, and associated abdominal cramps. May be used in functional intestinal disorders to reduce symptoms such as those seen in mild dysenteries, diverticulitis, and acute enterocolitis. For use as adjunctive therapy in the treatment of irritable bowel syndrome (irritable colon, spastic colon, mucous colitis) and functional gastrointestinal disorders. Also as adjunctive therapy in the treatment of neurogenic bowel disturbances including the splenic flexure syndrome and neurogenic colon. Also used in the treatment of infant colic (elixir and drops). LEVSIN is indicated along with morphine or other narcotics in symptomatic relief of biliary and renal colic; as a "drying agent" in the relief of symptoms of acute rhinitis; in the therapy of parkinsonism to reduce rigidity and tremors and to control associated sialorrhea and hyperhidrosis. May be used in the therapy of poisoning by anticholinesterase agents.

Parenterally administered LEVSIN is also effective in reducing duodenal motility to facilitate the diagnostic radiologic procedure, hypotonic duodenography. LEVSIN may be used to reduce pain and hypersecretion in pancreatitis. LEVSIN may also be used in certain cases of partial heart block associated with vagal activity.

IN ANESTHESIA:

LEVSIN Injection is indicated as a pre-operative antimuscarinic to reduce salivary, tracheobronchial, and pharyngeal secretions; to reduce the volume and acidity of gastric secretions, and to block cardiac vagal inhibitory reflexes during induction of anesthesia and intubation. LEVSIN protects against the peripheral muscarinic effects such as bradycardia and excessive secretions produced by halogenated hydrocarbons and cholinergic agents such as physostigmine, neostigmine, and pyridostigmine given to reverse the actions of curariform agents.

IN UROLOGY:

LEVSIN Injection may also be used intravenously to improve radiologic visibility of the kidneys.

CONTRAINDICATIONS

Glaucoma; obstructive uropathy (for example, bladder neck obstruction due to prostatic hypertrophy); obstructive disease of the gastrointestinal tract (as in achalasia, pyloroduodenal stenosis); paralytic ileus, intestinal atony of elderly or debilitated patients; unstable cardiovascular status in acute hemorrhage; severe ulcerative colitis; toxic megacolon complicating ulcerative colitis; myasthenia gravis.

WARNINGS

In the presence of high environmental temperature, heat prostration can occur with drug use (fever and heat stroke due to decreased sweating). Diarrhea may be an early symptom of incomplete intestinal obstruction, especially in patients with ileostomy or colostomy. In this instance, treatment with this drug would be inappropriate and possibly harmful. Like other anticholinergic agents, LEVSIN may produce drowsiness or blurred vision. In this event, the patient would be warned not to engage in activities requiring mental alertness such as operating a motor vehicle or other machinery or to perform hazardous work while taking this drug.

The 10 mL multiple-dose vial of LEVSIN Injection contains sodium metabisulfite, a sulfite that may cause allergic-type reactions including anaphylactic symptoms and life-threatening or less severe asthmatic episodes in certain susceptible people. The overall prevalence of sulfite sensitivity in the general population is unknown and probably low. Sulfite sensitivity is seen more frequently in asthmatic than in nonasthmatic people.

PRECAUTIONS

General:
Use with caution in patients with: autonomic neuropathy, hyperthyroidism, coronary heart disease, congestive heart failure, cardiac arrhythmias, and hypertension. Investigate any tachycardia before giving any anticholinergic drug since they may increase the heart rate. Use with caution in patients with hiatal hernia associated with reflux esophagitis.

Information for Patients:
LEVSIN may cause drowsiness, dizziness or blurred vision; patients should observe caution before driving, using machinery or performing other tasks requiring mental alertness.

Use of LEVSIN may decrease sweating resulting in heat prostration, fever or heat stroke; febrile patients or those who may be exposed to elevated environmental temperatures should use caution.

Drug Interactions:
Additive adverse effects resulting from cholinergic blockade may occur when LEVSIN is administered concomitantly with other antimuscarinics, amantadine, haloperidol, phenothiazines, monoamine oxidase (MAO) inhibitors, tricyclic antidepressants or some antihistamines.

Antacids may interfere with the absorption of LEVSIN; take LEVSIN before meals and antacids after meals.

Carcinogenesis, Mutagenesis, Impairment of Fertility:
No long term studies in animals have been performed to determine the carcinogenic, mutagenic or impairment of fertility potential of LEVSIN; however, over 30 years of marketing experience shows no demonstrable evidence of a problem.

Pregnancy—Pregnancy Category C:
Animal reproduction studies have not been conducted with LEVSIN. It is also not known whether LEVSIN can cause fetal harm when administered to a pregnant woman or can affect reproduction capacity. LEVSIN should be given to a pregnant woman only if clearly needed.

Nursing Mothers:
LEVSIN is excreted in human milk. Caution should be exercised when LEVSIN is administered to a nursing woman.

ADVERSE REACTIONS

Adverse reactions may include dryness of the mouth; urinary hesitancy and retention; blurred vision; tachycardia; palpitations; mydriasis; cycloplegia; increased ocular tension; headache; nervousness; drowsiness; weakness; suppression of lactation; allergic reactions or drug idiosyncrasies; urticaria and other dermal manifestations; and decreased sweating.

Continued on next page

Schwarz Pharma—Cont.

DRUG ABUSE AND DEPENDENCE

The information on drug abuse and dependence is limited to uncontrolled data derived from marketing experience. Such experience has revealed no evidence of drug abuse and dependence associated with LEVSIN.

OVERDOSAGE

The signs and symptoms of overdose are headache, nausea, vomiting, blurred vision, dilated pupils, hot dry skin, dizziness, dryness of the mouth, difficulty in swallowing. Measures to be taken are immediate lavage of the stomach and injection of physostigmine 0.5 to 2 mg intravenously and repeated as necessary up to a total of 5 mg. Fever may be treated symptomatically (tepid water sponge baths, hypothermic blanket). Excitement to a degree which demands attention may be managed with sodium thiopental 2% solution given slowly intravenously or chloral hydrate (100–200 mL of a 2% solution) by rectal infusion. In the event of progression of the curare-like effect to paralysis of the respiratory muscles, artificial respiration should be instituted and maintained until effective respiratory action returns. In rats, the LD_{50} for LEVSIN is 375 mg/kg. LEVSIN is dialyzable.

DOSAGE AND ADMINISTRATION

Dosage may be adjusted according to the conditions and severity of symptoms.

LEVSIN/SL Tablets: The tablets may be taken sublingually or orally. *Adults and children 12 years of age and older:* 1 to 2 tablets every four hours or as needed. Do not exceed 12 tablets in 24 hours. *Children 2 to under 12 years of age:* ½ to 1 tablet every four hours or as needed. Do not exceed 6 tablets in 24 hours.

LEVSIN Tablets: The tablets may be taken orally or sublingually. *Adults and children 12 years of age and older:* 1 to 2 tablets every four hours or as needed. Do not exceed 12 tablets in 24 hours.

Children 2 to under 12 years of age: ½ to 1 tablet every four hours or as needed. Do not exceed 6 tablets in 24 hours.

LEVSIN Elixir: *Adults and children 12 years of age and older:* 1 to 2 teaspoonfuls every four hours or as needed. Do not exceed 12 teaspoonfuls in 24 hours.

Children 2 to under 12 years of age: ¼ to 1 teaspoonful every four hours or as needed. Do not exceed 6 teaspoonfuls in 24 hours.

The following dosage guide is based upon body weight. The doses may be repeated every four hours or as needed.

Body Weight	Usual Dose
10 kg (22 lb)	¼ tsp
20 kg (44 lb)	½ tsp
40 kg (88 lb)	¾ tsp
50 kg (110 lb)	1 tsp

LEVSIN Drops: *Adults and children 12 years of age and older:* 1 to 2 mL every four hours or as needed. Do not exceed 12 mL in 24 hours.

Children 2 to under 12 years of age: ¼ to 1 mL every four hours or as needed. Do not exceed 6 mL in 24 hours.

Children under 2 years of age: The following dosage guide is based upon body weight. The doses may be repeated every four hours or as needed.

Body Weight	Usual Dose	Do Not Exceed in 24 Hours
2.3 kg (5 lb)	3 drops	18 drops
3.4 kg (7.5 lb)	4 drops	24 drops
5 kg (11 lb)	5 drops	30 drops
7 kg (15 lb)	6 drops	36 drops
10 kg (22 lb)	8 drops	48 drops
15 kg (33 lb)	11 drops	66 drops

LEVSIN Injection: The dose may be administered subcutaneously, intramuscularly, or intravenously without dilution.

Gastrointestinal Disorders: The usual adult recommended dose is 0.5 to 1.0 mL (0.25 to 0.5 mg). Some patients may need only a single dose; others may require administration two, three, or four times a day at four hour intervals.

Hypotonic Duodenography: The usual adult recommended dose is 0.5 to 1.0 mL (0.25 to 0.5 mg) administered 5 to 10 minutes prior to the diagnostic procedure.

Anesthesia: Adults and children over 2 years of age: As a pre-anesthetic medication, the recommended dose is 5 µg (0.005 mg) per kg of body weight. This dose is usually given 30 to 60 minutes prior to the anticipated time of induction of anesthesia or at the time the pre-anesthetic narcotic or sedative is administered.

LEVSIN Injection may be used during surgery to reduce drug-induced bradycardia. It should be administered intravenously in increments of 0.25 mL and repeated as needed. To achieve reversal of neuromuscular blockade, the recommended dose is 0.2 mg (0.4 mL) LEVSIN Injection for every 1 mg neostigmine or the equivalent dose of physostigmine or pyridostigmine.

Parenteral drug products should be inspected visually for particulate matter and discoloration prior to administration, whenever solution and container permit.

LEVSINEX TIMECAPS: *Adults and children 12 years of age and older:* 1 to 2 TIMECAPS every 12 hours. Dosage may be adjusted to 1 TIMECAP every 8 hours if needed. Do not exceed 4 TIMECAPS in 24 hours.

Children 2 to under 12 years of age: 1 TIMECAP every 12 hours. Do not exceed 2 TIMECAPS in 24 hours.

HOW SUPPLIED

LEVSIN/SL Tablets (hyoscyamine sulfate tablets USP, 0.125 mg) are pale blue-green, peppermint-flavored, octagonal shaped, scored, and embossed with "SCHWARZ" on one side and "532" on the other.

Bottles of 100 tablets	NDC 0091-3532-01
Bottles of 500 tablets	NDC 0091-3532-05

LEVSIN Tablets (hyoscyamine sulfate tablets USP, 0.125 mg) are white and scored with "K-U" on one side and "531" imprinted on the other.

Bottles of 100 tablets	NDC 0091-3531-01
Bottles of 500 tablets	NDC 0091-3531-05

LEVSIN Elixir (hyoscyamine sulfate elixir USP, 0.125 mg/5mL) is orange colored and orange flavored with 20% alcohol. Pint (473 mL) bottles (NDC 0091-4532-16).

LEVSIN Drops (hyoscyamine sulfate oral solution USP, 0.125 mg/mL) are orange colored, orange flavored and contain 5% alcohol. 15 mL bottle with dropper (NDC 0091-4538-15).

LEVSIN Injection (hyoscyamine sulfate injection USP, 0.5 mg/mL) is a clear, colorless and sterile solution. Box of 5-1mL ampuls (NDC 0091-1536-05), 10 mL vial (NDC 0091-1536-10).

LEVSINEX TIMECAPS (hyoscyamine sulfate USP, 0.375 mg, timed release) are brown and clear capsules containing brown and white beadlets and imprinted with "KREMERS URBAN" and "537." Bottles of 100 capsules (NDC 0091-3537-01).

LEVSIN with Phenobarbital Products, call K-U (1-800-558-5114) for complete prescribing information.

LEVSIN with Phenobarbital Tablets [0.125 mg hyoscyamine sulfate/15 mg phenobarbital (Warning: May be habit forming)] are pink and scored with "K-U" on one side and "534" on the other.

Bottles of 100 tablets	NDC 0091-3534-01
Bottles of 500 tablets	NDC 0091-3534-05

LEVSIN with Phenobarbital Elixir [0.125 mg hyoscyamine sulfate/15 mg phenobarbital (Warning: May be habit forming)] per 5 mL, is red colored and raspberry flavored and contains 20% alcohol. Pint (473 mL) bottles (NDC 0091-4530-16).

LEVSIN-PB Drops [0.125 mg hyoscyamine sulfate/15 mg phenobarbital (Warning: May be habit forming)] per mL oral solution, is red colored and cherry flavored and contain 5% alcohol. 15 mL bottle with dropper (NDC 0091-4536-15).

LEVSINEX with Phenobarbital TIMECAPS [0.375 mg hyoscyamine sulfate/45 mg phenobarbital (Warning: May be habit forming)] are pink and clear capsules containing pink and white beadlets and imprinted with "KREMERS URBAN" and "539." Bottles of 100 capsules (NDC 0091-3539-01).

Store at controlled room temperatue 15°–30°C (59°–86°F).

CAUTION

Federal law prohibits dispensing without prescription.

Shown in Product Identification Section, page 429

PRE-PEN®   ℞

[prē'pen]

(benzylpenicilloyl polylysine injection USP)

Skin Test Antigen

DESCRIPTION

PRE-PEN® (benzylpenicilloyl polylysine injection USP) is a skin test antigen used in assessing a patient's allergy status to penicillin.

PRE-PEN is a sterile solution of benzylpenicilloyl polylysine in a concentration of 6.0×10^{-5}M (benzylpenicilloyl) in 0.01 M phosphate buffer and 0.15 M sodium chloride and water for injection. The benzylpenicilloyl polylysine in PRE-PEN is a derivative of poly-l-lysine, where the epsilon amino groups are substituted with benzylpenicilloyl groups (50-70%) forming benzylpenicilloyl alpha amide. Each single dose ampul contains 0.25 mL of PRE-PEN.

CLINICAL PHARMACOLOGY

PRE-PEN reacts specifically with benzylpenicilloyl skin sensitizing antibodies (reagins: IgE class) to initiate release of chemical mediators which produce an immediate wheal and flare reaction at a skin test site. All individuals exhibiting a positive skin test to PRE-PEN possess reagins against the benzylpenicilloyl group which is a haptene. A haptene is a low molecular weight chemical which, when conjugated to a carrier, e.g., poly-l-lysine, has the properties under appropriate conditions of an antigen with the haptene's specificity. It is to be noted that individuals who have previously received therapeutic penicillin may have positive skin test reactions to PRE-PEN as well as to a number of other non-benzylpenicilloyl haptenes. The latter are designated as minor determinants, in that they are present in lesser amounts than the major determinant, benzylpenicilloyl. The minor

determinants may nevertheless be associated with examples of significant clinical hypersensitivity.

Virtually everyone who receives penicillin develops specific antibodies to the drug as measured by hemagglutination studies, but (a) positive skin tests to various penicillin and penicillin-derived reagents become positive in less than 10% of patients who have tolerated penicillin in the past and (b) allergic responses are infrequent (less than 1%).

Many individuals reacting positively to PRE-PEN will not develop a systemic allergic reaction on subsequent exposure to therapeutic penicillin. Thus, the PRE-PEN skin test facilitates assessing the local allergic skin reactivity of a patient to benzylpenicilloyl.

INDICATIONS AND USAGE

PRE-PEN is useful as an adjunct in assessing the risk of administering penicillin (benzylpenicillin or penicillin G) when it is the preferred drug of choice in adult patients who have previously received penicillin and have a history of clinical penicillin hypersensitivity. In this situation, a negative skin test to PRE-PEN is associated with an incidence of allergic reactions of less than 5% after the administration of therapeutic penicillin, whereas the incidence may be more than 20% in the presence of a positive skin test to PRE-PEN. These allergic reactions are predominantly dermatologic. Because of the extremely low incidence of anaphylactic reactions, there are insufficient data at present to document that a decreased incidence of anaphylactic reactions following the administration of penicillin will occur in patients with a negative skin test to PRE-PEN. Similarly, when deciding the risk of proposed penicillin treatment, there are not enough data at present to permit relative weighing in individual cases of a history of clinical penicillin hypersensitivity as compared to positive skin tests to PRE-PEN and/or minor penicillin determinants.

It should be borne in mind that no reagent, test, or combination of tests will completely assure that a reaction to penicillin therapy will not occur.

CONTRAINDICATIONS

PRE-PEN is contraindicated in those patients who have exhibited either a systemic or marked local reaction to its previous administration. Patients known to be extremely hypersensitive to penicillin should not be skin tested.

WARNINGS

There are insufficient data to assess the potential danger of sensitization to repeated skin testing with PRE-PEN.

Rarely, a systemic allergic reaction (see below) may follow a skin test with PRE-PEN. This can be avoided by making the first application by scratch test and very carefully following the instructions below in administering the intradermal test, using the intradermal route only if the scratch test has been entirely negative.

Skin testing with penicillin and/or other penicillin-derived reagents should not be performed simultaneously.

PRECAUTIONS

General:

There are insufficient data derived from well-controlled studies to determine the value of the PRE-PEN skin test as a means of assessing the risk of administering therapeutic penicillin (when penicillin is the preferred drug of choice) in the following situations:

(1)   Adult patients who give no history of clinical penicillin hypersensitivity.

(2)   Pediatric patients.

In addition, there are no data at present to assess the clinical value of PRE-PEN where exposure to penicillin is suspected as a cause of a drug reaction and in patients who are undergoing routine allergy evaluation.

Furthermore, there are no data relating the clinical value of PRE-PEN skin tests to the risk of administering semi-synthetic penicillins (phenoxymethyl penicillin, ampicillin, carbenicillin, dicloxacillin, methicillin, nafcillin, oxacillin, phenethicillin) and cephalosporin-derived antibiotics.

Recognition that the following clinical outcomes are possible makes it imperative for the physician to weigh risk to benefit in every instance where the decision to administer or not to administer penicillin is based in part on a PRE-PEN skin test.

(1)   An allergic reaction to therapeutic penicillin may occur in a patient with a negative skin test to PRE-PEN.

(2)   It is possible for a patient to have an anaphylactic reaction to therapeutic penicillin in the presence of a negative PRE-PEN skin test and a negative history of clinical penicillin hypersensitivity.

(3)   If penicillin is the absolute drug of choice in a life-threatening situation, successful desensitization with therapeutic penicillin may be possible irrespective of a positive skin test and/or a positive history of clinical penicillin hypersensitivity.

Pregnancy-Pregnancy Category C:

Animal reproduction studies have not been conducted with PRE-PEN. It is not known whether PRE-PEN can cause fetal harm when administered to a pregnant woman or can affect reproduction capacity. The hazards of skin testing in such patients should be weighed against the hazard of penicillin therapy without skin testing.

ADVERSE REACTIONS

Occasionally, patients may develop an intense local inflammatory response at the skin test site. Rarely, patients will develop a systemic allergic reaction, manifested by generalized erythema, pruritus, angioneurotic edema, urticaria, dyspnea, and/or hypotension. The usual methods of treating a skin test antigen-induced reaction—the application of a venous occlusion tourniquet proximal to the skin test site and administration of epinephrine (and, at times, an injection of an antihistamine) — are recommended and will usually control the reaction. As a rule, systemic allergic reactions following skin test procedures are of short duration and controllable, but the patient should be kept under observation for several hours.

DOSAGE AND ADMINISTRATION

SKIN TESTING DOSAGE AND TECHNIQUE

Scratch Testing:

Skin testing is usually performed on the inner volar aspect of the forearm. The skin test material should always be applied first by the scratch technique. After preparing the skin surface, a sterile 20 gauge needle should be used to make a 3–5 mm scratch of the epidermis. Very little pressure is required to break the epidermal continuity. If bleeding occurs, prepare a second site and scratch more lightly with the needle—sufficient to produce a non-bleeding scratched surface. Apply a small drop of PRE-PEN solution to the scratch and rub gently with an applicator, toothpick, or the side of the needle. Observe for the appearance of a wheal, erythema, and the occurrence of itching at the test site during the succeeding 15 minutes at which time the solution over the scratch is wiped off. A positive reaction is unmistakable and consists of the development within 10 minutes of a pale wheal, usually with pseudopods, surrounding the scratch site and varying in diameter from 5 to 15 mm (or more). This wheal may be surrounded by a variable diameter of erythema, and accompanied by a variable degree of itching. The most sensitive individuals develop itching almost instantly, and the wheal and erythema are prompt in their appearance. As soon as a positive response as defined above is clearly evident, the solution over the scratch should be immediately wiped off. If the scratch test is either negative or equivocally positive (less than 5 mm wheal and little or no erythema, and no itching), an intradermal test may be performed.

The Intradermal Test:

Using a tuberculin syringe with a ⅜″ to ⅝″ long, 26 to 30 gauge, short bevel needle, withdraw the contents of the ampul. Prepare a sterile skin test area on the upper, outer arm, sufficiently below the deltoid muscle to permit proximal application of a tourniquet later, if necessary. Be sure to eject all air from the syringe through the needle, then insert the needle, bevel up, immediately below the skin surface. Inject an amount of PRE-PEN sufficient to raise the smallest possible perceptible bleb. This volume will be between 0.01 and 0.02 mL. Using a separate syringe and needle, inject a like amount of saline as a control at least 1½ inches removed from the test site. Most skin reactions will develop within 5–15 minutes and response to the skin test is read as follows:

(—) Negative response—no increase in size of original bleb and/or no greater reaction than the control site.

(±) Ambiguous response—wheal being only slightly larger than initial injection bleb, with or without accompanying erythematous flare and larger than the control site.

(+) Positive response—itching and marked increase in size of original bleb. Wheal may exceed 20 mm in diameter and exhibit pseudopods.

The control site should be completely reactionless. If it exhibits a wheal greater than 2–3 mm, repeat the test, and if the same reaction is observed, a physician experienced with allergy skin testing should be consulted.

Parenteral drug products should be inspected visually for particulate matter and discoloration prior to administration, whenever solution and container permit.

HOW SUPPLIED

PRE-PEN (benzylpenicilloyl polylysine injection USP) is a clear, colorless, sterile solution supplied in ampuls containing 0.25 mL.

Boxes of five—single dose ampuls........NDC 0091-1640-05
PRE-PEN is stable only when kept under refrigeration. It is, therefore, recommended that test materials subjected to ambient temperatures for over a day be discarded.

CAUTION

Federal law prohibits dispensing without prescription.
Mfd. by:
Ben Venue Laboratories
Bedford, Ohio 44146

For:
SCHWARZ PHARMA
Kremers Urban Company
Milwaukee, Wisconsin 53201

EDUCATIONAL MATERIAL

Booklet
"Good news for people who can't digest milk . . . Cheers! " For people who cannot digest dairy products because they lack the enzymes necessary for the digestion of milk sugar, this pamphlet explains how the problem comes about, its symptoms and how it can be treated with LACTRASE®, an enzyme supplement. A table addressing the lactose content of food is included.
FREE TO HEALTH PROFESSIONALS AND CONSUMERS

Sclavo Inc.
5 MANSARD COURT
WAYNE, NJ 07470

COMPLETE INFORMATION FOR THE BELOW LISTED PRODUCTS IS FURNISHED IN THE PACKAGING.

DIPHTHERIA ANTITOXIN (equine) USP ℞
DIPHTHERIA AND TETANUS ℞
   TOXOIDS ADSORBED, USP
   (For Pediatric Use)
Sclavo-PPD Solution (Mantoux) ℞
   Tuberculin Purified Protein
   Derivative (PPD)
   Tween Stabilized Solution
** SclavoTest®-PPD** ℞
   Tuberculin Purified Protein
   Derivative (PPD)
   Multiple Puncture Device
For product information, consult Diagnostic Product Information Section.
TETANUS ANTITOXIN (equine) USP ℞
TETANUS TOXOID, ADSORBED, USP ℞
TETANUS AND DIPHTHERIA ℞
   TOXOIDS ADSORBED, USP
   For Adult Use

EDUCATIONAL MATERIAL

SclavoTest Brochure Free on Request to Physicians
"Tuberculin Skin Testing: Mantoux or Multiple Puncture Device" Paper by J. J. Piecoro, Jr., Pharm D, H. David Wilson, M.D. and Irene G. Melvin, M.S. Available on request to physicians free.

Scot-Tussin Pharmacal Co., Inc.
50 CLEMENCE STREET
P.O. BOX 8217
CRANSTON, RI 02920-0217

S-T FORTE™ SUGAR-FREE ©
S-T FORTE™ Syrup

Complete prescribing information is furnished in the packaging.

COMPOSITION

Each 5 ml (1 teaspoonful) contains:
Hydrocodone Bitartrate, USP ....2.5 mg
   (**Warning:** May be habit forming)
Phenylephrine HCl, USP ....5 mg
Phenylpropanolamine HCl, USP ....5 mg
Pheniramine Maleate, USP ....13.33 mg
Guaifenesin, USP ....80 mg
Alcohol 5 per cent by vol.

HOW SUPPLIED

Syrup: Pints (NDC 0372-0004-16); Gallons (NDC 0372-0004-28).
Sugar-Free: Pints (NDC 0372-0005-16); Gallons (NDC 0372-0005-28).

SCOT-TUSSIN® SUGAR-FREE; DM OTC
ALCOHOL & CHOLESTEROL-FREE
SORBITOL & SODIUM SACCHARIN
& DECONGESTANT-FREE
COUGH & COLD MEDICINE

COMPOSITION

Each 5 ml (1 teaspoonful) contains:
Dextromethorphan HBr., USP .... 15 mg.
Chlorpheniramine Maleate, USP .... 2 mg.
Recommended for use by diabetics and others on sugar restricted diets.

HOW SUPPLIED

Bottles of 4 fl. oz. (NDC 0372-0036-04)

SCOT-TUSSIN® Sugar-Free Expectorant OTC
Decongestant, Sodium, Cholesterol, Dye-Free, Cough Formula

COMPOSITION

Each 5 ml (1 teaspoonful) contains:
Guaifenesin, USP ....100 mg
Alcohol 3.5 per cent
Recommended for use by diabetics and others on sugar restricted diets.

HOW SUPPLIED

Bottles of 4 fl. oz. (NDC 0372-0006-04).

TUSSIREX™ SUGAR-FREE; ALCOHOL-FREE, ©
CHOLESTEROL & DYE-FREE
TUSSIREX™ ALCOHOL, CHOLESTEROL & DYE-FREE
Syrup (with sugar)

Complete prescribing information is furnished in the packaging.

COMPOSITION

Each 5 ml (1 teaspoonful) contains:
Codeine Phosphate, USP ....10 mg
   (**Warning:** May be habit forming)
Pheniramine Maleate, USP ....13.33 mg
Phenylephrine HCl., USP ....4.17 mg
Sodium Citrate, USP ....83.33 mg
Sodium Salicylate, USP ....83.33 mg
Caffeine Citrate, USP ....25 mg

HOW SUPPLIED

Both Tussirex™ Sugar-Free (lemon flavor), and Tussirex™ Syrup "Dye-Free" are available: Sugar-Free (NDC 0372-0018 4 ozs & pints; Syrup NDC 0372-0017 4ozs & pints.

G. D. Searle & Co.
BOX 5110
CHICAGO, IL 60680

Alphabetic Product Listing*
Product, ID# (NDC†), Form, Strength
*Aldactazide, 1011, Tablet, 25 mg/25 mg
*Aldactazide, 1021, Tablet, 50 mg/50 mg
*Aldactone, 1001, Tablet, 25 mg
*Aldactone, 1041, Tablet, 50 mg
*Aldactone, 1031, Tablet, 100 mg
*Aminophyllin, 1231, Tablet, 100 mg
*Aminophyllin, 1251, Tablet, 200 mg
*Calan, 40(1771), Tablet, 40 mg
*Calan, 80(1851), Tablet, 80 mg
*Calan, 120(1861), Tablet, 120 mg
*Calan SR, 240, (1891), Caplet, 240 mg
Cytotec, 1461, Tablet, 200 mcg
Cytotec, 1461, Unit Dose, Tablet, 200 mcg
*Demulen 1/35-21, Compack, 151, Tablet, 1 mg/35 mcg
*Demulen 1/35-21, Refill, 151, Tablet, 1 mg/35 mcg
*Demulen 1/35-28, Compack, 151 (0161), Tablet, 1 mg/35 mcg
*Demulen 1/35-28, Refill, 151 (0161), Tablet, 1 mg/35 mcg
*Demulen 1/50-21, Compack, 71, Tablet, 1 mg/50 mcg
*Demulen 1/50-21, Refill, 71, Tablet, 1 mg/50 mcg
*Demulen 1/50-28, Compack, 71 (0081), Tablet, 1 mg/50 mcg
*Demulen 1/50-28, Refill, 71 (0081), Tablet, 1 mg/50 mcg
Dramamine Injection, 1703, Ampul, 50 mg/1 ml
Dramamine Injection, 1724, Vial, 250 mg/5 ml
*Dramamine, 1736, Liquid, 12.5 mg/4 ml, 16 oz
*Dramamine, 1701, Unit Dose, Tablet, 50 mg, 100s
*Enovid, 51, Tablet, 5 mg/75 mcg
*Enovid, 101, Tablet, 10 mg (9.85 mg/0.15 mg)
*Flagyl, 1831, Tablet, 250 mg
*Flagyl, 500 (1821), Tablet, 500 mg

Continued on next page

G.D. Searle & Co.—Cont.

*Lomotil Ⓒ, 61, Tablet, 2.5 mg/0.025 mg
*Lomotil Ⓒ, Liquid, 66, 2.5 mg/0.025 mg per 5 ml
 Nitrodisc, 2058, 5 mg/24 hr
 Nitrodisc, 2078, 7.5 mg/24 hr
 Nitrodisc, 2068, 10 mg/24 hr
*Norpace, 2752, Capsule, 100 mg
*Norpace, 2762, Capsule, 150 mg
*Norpace CR, 2732, Capsule, 100 mg
*Norpace CR, 2742, Capsule, 150 mg
*Theo-24, 2832, Capsule, 100 mg
*Theo-24, 2842, Capsule, 200 mg
*Theo-24, 2852, Capsule, 300 mg

---

* Products of Searle & Co., San Juan, PR 00936.

† When the product ID # is not the same as the NDC #, the NDC # appears in parentheses.

Various educational materials are available for physicians, pharmacists, nurses, physicians' assistants, and patients (through the physician). Please ask your Searle representative for information about these materials.

ALDACTAZIDE®   ℞
[al-dac 'tuh "zīde]
(spironolactone with hydrochlorothiazide)

Warning

Spironolactone, an ingredient of Aldactazide, has been shown to be a tumorigen in chronic toxicity studies in rats (see *Warnings*). Aldactazide should be used only in those conditions described under *Indications and Usage*. Unnecessary use of this drug should be avoided.
Fixed-dose combination drugs are not indicated for initial therapy of edema or hypertension. Edema or hypertension requires therapy titrated to the individual patient. If the fixed combination represents the dosage so determined, its use may be more convenient in patient management. The treatment of hypertension and edema is not static but must be reevaluated as conditions in each patient warrant.

DESCRIPTION

Aldactazide oral tablets contain:
spironolactone .... 25 mg
hydrochlorothiazide .... 25 mg
                    or
spironolactone .... 50 mg
hydrochlorothiazide .... 50 mg

Spironolactone (Aldactone®), an aldosterone antagonist, is 17- hydroxy-7α-mercapto-3-oxo-17α-pregn-4-ene- 21- carboxylic acid γ-lactone acetate and has the following structural formula:

Spironolactone is practically insoluble in water, soluble in alcohol, and freely soluble in benzene and in chloroform.
Hydrochlorothiazide, a diuretic and antihypertensive, is 6-chloro-3, 4-dihydro-2H-1,2,4-benzothiadiazine-7-sulfonamide 1,1-dioxide and has the following structural formula:

Hydrochlorothiazide is slightly soluble in water and freely soluble in sodium hydroxide solution.
Inactive ingredients include calcium sulfate, corn starch, flavor, hydroxypropyl cellulose, hydroxypropyl methylcellulose, iron oxide, magnesium stearate, polyethylene glycol, povidone, and titanium dioxide.

CLINICAL PHARMACOLOGY

Mechanism of action: Aldactazide is a combination of two diuretic agents with different but complementary mechanisms and sites of action, thereby providing additive diuretic and antihypertensive effects. Additionally, the spironolac-

tone component helps to minimize the potassium loss characteristically induced by the thiazide component.
The diuretic effect of spironolactone is mediated through its action as a specific pharmacologic antagonist of aldosterone, primarily by competitive binding of receptors at the aldosterone-dependent sodium-potassium exchange site in the distal convoluted renal tubule. Hydrochlorothiazide promotes the excretion of sodium and water primarily by inhibiting their reabsorption in the cortical diluting segment of the distal renal tubule.
Aldactazide is effective in significantly lowering the systolic and diastolic blood pressure in many patients with essential hypertension, even when aldosterone secretion is within normal limits.
Both spironolactone and hydrochlorothiazide reduce exchangeable sodium, plasma volume, body weight, and blood pressure. The diuretic and antihypertensive effects of the individual components are potentiated when spironolactone and hydrochlorothiazide are given concurrently.
Pharmacokinetics: In the human, the bioavailability of both spironolactone and hydrochlorothiazide from orally administered Aldactazide 25 mg/25 mg uncoated tablets and Aldactazide film-coated tablets has been evaluated in hypertensive subjects. Equivalent doses of the film-coated tablets, which contain microcrystalline spironolactone, showed 20% to 25% higher bioavailability of spironolactone compared to the uncoated Aldactazide tablets. Hydrochlorothiazide bioavailability was similar in the film-coated and uncoated tablets.
Spironolactone is rapidly and extensively metabolized. The primary metabolite is canrenone, which attains peak serum levels at two to four hours following single oral administration. Canrenone plasma concentrations decline in two distinct phases, being rapid in the first 12 hours and slower from 12 to 96 hours. The log-linear phase half-life of canrenone, following multiple doses of Aldactone (spironolactone), is between 13 and 24 hours. Both spironolactone and canrenone are more than 90% bound to plasma proteins. The metabolites of spironolactone are excreted primarily in urine, but also in bile.
Hydrochlorothiazide is rapidly absorbed following oral administration. Onset of action of hydrochlorothiazide is observed within one hour and persists for 6 to 12 hours. Hydrochlorothiazide plasma concentrations attain peak levels at one to two hours and decline with a half-life of four to five hours. Hydrochlorothiazide undergoes only slight metabolic alteration and is excreted in urine. It is distributed throughout the extracellular space, with essentially no tissue accumulation except in the kidney.

INDICATIONS AND USAGE

Spironolactone, an ingredient of Aldactazide, has been shown to be a tumorigen in chronic toxicity studies in rats (see *Warnings* section). Aldactazide should be used only in those conditions described below. Unnecessary use of this drug should be avoided.
Aldactazide is indicated for:
Edematous conditions for patients with:
   Congestive heart failure: For the management of edema and sodium retention when the patient is only partially responsive to, or is intolerant of, other therapeutic measures. The treatment of diuretic-induced hypokalemia in patients with congestive heart failure when other measures are considered inappropriate. The treatment of patients with congestive heart failure taking digitalis when other therapies are considered inadequate or inappropriate.
   Cirrhosis of the liver accompanied by edema and/or ascites: Aldosterone levels may be exceptionally high in this condition. Aldactazide is indicated for maintenance therapy together with bed rest and the restriction of fluid and sodium.
   The nephrotic syndrome: For nephrotic patients when treatment of the underlying disease, restriction of fluid and sodium intake, and the use of other diuretics do not provide an adequate response.
Essential hypertension
   For patients with essential hypertension in whom other measures are considered inadequate or inappropriate. In hypertensive patients for the treatment of a diuretic-induced hypokalemia when other measures are considered inappropriate.
Usage in Pregnancy. The routine use of diuretics in an otherwise healthy woman is inappropriate and exposes mother and fetus to unnecessary hazard. Diuretics do not prevent development of toxemia of pregnancy, and there is no satisfactory evidence that they are useful in the treatment of developing toxemia.
Edema during pregnancy may arise from pathologic causes or from the physiologic and mechanical consequences of pregnancy. Aldactazide is indicated in pregnancy when edema is due to pathologic causes just as it is in the absence of pregnancy (however, see *Warnings* section). Dependent edema in pregnancy, resulting from restriction of venous return by the expanded uterus, is properly treated through elevation of the lower extremities and use of support hose;

use of diuretics to lower intravascular volume in this case is unsupported and unnecessary. There is hypervolemia during normal pregnancy which is harmful to neither the fetus nor the mother (in the absence of cardiovascular disease), but which is associated with edema, including generalized edema, in the majority of pregnant women. If this edema produces discomfort, increased recumbency will often provide relief. In rare instances, this edema may cause extreme discomfort which is not relieved by rest. In these cases, a short course of diuretics may provide relief and may be appropriate.

CONTRAINDICATIONS

Aldactazide is contraindicated in patients with anuria, acute renal insufficiency, significant impairment of renal excretory function, or hyperkalemia, and in patients who are allergic to thiazide diuretics or to other sulfonamide-derived drugs. Aldactazide may also be contraindicated in acute or severe hepatic failure.

WARNINGS

Potassium supplementation, either in the form of medication or as a diet rich in potassium, should not ordinarily be given in association with Aldactazide therapy. Excessive potassium intake may cause hyperkalemia in patients receiving Aldactazide (see *Precautions* section). Aldactazide should not be administered concurrently with other potassium-sparing diuretics. Spironolactone, when used with ACE inhibitors, even in the presence of a diuretic, has been associated with severe hyperkalemia. Extreme caution should be exercised when Aldactazide is given concomitantly with ACE inhibitors (see *Precautions*).
Sulfonamide derivatives, including thiazides, have been reported to exacerbate or activate systemic lupus erythematosus.
Spironolactone has been shown to be a tumorigen in chronic toxicity studies performed in rats, with its proliferative effects manifested on endocrine organs and the liver. In one study using 25, 75, and 250 times the usual daily human dose (2 mg/kg) there was a statistically significant dose-related increase in benign adenomas of the thyroid and testes. In female rats there was a statistically significant increase in malignant mammary tumors at the mid-dose only. In male rats there was a dose-related increase in proliferative changes in the liver. At the highest dosage level (500 mg/kg), the range of effects included hepatocytomegaly, hyperplastic nodules, and hepatocellular carcinoma; the last was not statistically significant at a value of p = 0.05. A dose-related (above 20 mg/kg/day) incidence of myelocytic leukemia was observed in rats fed daily doses of potassium canrenoate for a period of one year. In long-term (two-year) oral carcinogenicity studies of potassium canrenoate in the rat, myelocytic leukemia and hepatic, thyroid, testicular, and mammary tumors were observed. Potassium canrenoate did not produce a mutagenic effect in tests using bacteria or yeast. It did produce a positive mutagenic effect in several *in vitro* tests in mammalian cells following metabolic activation. In an *in vivo* mammalian system potassium canrenoate was not mutagenic. Canrenone and canrenoic acid are the major metabolites of potassium canrenoate. Spironolactone is also metabolized to canrenone. An increased incidence of leukemia was not observed in chronic rat toxicity studies conducted with spironolactone at doses up to 500 mg/kg/day.

PRECAUTIONS

Patients receiving Aldactazide therapy should be carefully evaluated for possible disturbances of fluid and electrolyte balance. Hyperkalemia may occur in patients with impaired renal function or excessive potassium intake and can cause cardiac irregularities, which may be fatal. Consequently, no potassium supplement should ordinarily be given with Aldactazide. Hyperkalemia can be treated promptly by the rapid intravenous administration of glucose (20% to 50%) and regular insulin, using 0.25 to 0.5 units of insulin per gram of glucose. This is a temporary measure to be repeated as required. Aldactazide use should be discontinued and potassium intake (including dietary potassium) restricted.
Hypokalemia may develop as a result of profound diuresis, particularly when Aldactazide is used concomitantly with loop diuretics, glucocorticoids, or ACTH. Hypokalemia may exaggerate the effects of digitalis therapy. Potassium depletion may induce signs of digitalis intoxication at previously tolerated dosage levels.
Concomitant administration of potassium-sparing diuretics and ACE inhibitors or indomethacin has been associated with severe hyperkalemia.
Warning signs of possible fluid and electrolyte imbalance include dryness of the mouth, thirst, weakness, lethargy, drowsiness, restlessness, muscle pains or cramps, muscular fatigue, hypotension, oliguria, tachycardia, and gastrointestinal symptoms.
Aldactazide therapy may cause a transient elevation of BUN. This appears to represent a concentration phenomenon rather than renal toxicity, since the BUN level returns to normal after use of Aldactazide is discontinued. Progressive elevation of BUN is suggestive of the presence of preexisting renal impairment.

Reversible hyperchloremic metabolic acidosis, usually in association with hyperkalemia, has been reported to occur in some patients with decompensated hepatic cirrhosis, even in the presence of normal renal function.

Dilutional hyponatremia, manifested by dryness of the mouth, thirst, lethargy, and drowsiness, and confirmed by a low serum sodium level, may be induced, especially when Aldactazide is administered in combination with other diuretics. A true low-salt syndrome may rarely develop with Aldactazide therapy and may be manifested by increasing mental confusion similar to that observed with hepatic coma. This syndrome is differentiated from dilutional hyponatremia in that it does not occur with obvious fluid retention. Its treatment requires that diuretic therapy be discontinued and sodium administered.

Gynecomastia may develop in association with the use of spironolactone; physicians should be alert to its possible onset. The development of gynecomastia appears to be related to both dosage level and duration of therapy and is normally reversible when Aldactazide is discontinued. In rare instances some breast enlargement may persist when Aldactazide is discontinued.

Thiazides have been demonstrated to alter the metabolism of uric acid and carbohydrates, with possible development of hyperuricemia, gout, and decreased glucose tolerance. Thiazides may temporarily exaggerate abnormalities of glucose metabolism in diabetic patients or cause abnormalities to appear in patients with latent diabetes.

The antihypertensive effects of hydrochlorothiazide may be enhanced in patients who have undergone sympathectomy. Pathologic changes in the parathyroid gland with hypercalcemia and hypophosphatemia have been observed in patients on prolonged thiazide therapy. Thiazides may also decrease serum PBI levels without evidence of alteration of thyroid function.

A determination of serum electrolytes to detect possible electrolyte imbalance should be performed at periodic intervals. Both spironolactone and hydrochlorothiazide reduce the vascular responsiveness to norepinephrine. Therefore, caution should be exercised in the management of patients subjected to regional or general anesthesia while they are being treated with Aldactazide. Thiazides may also increase the responsiveness to tubocurarine.

Spironolactone has been shown to increase the half-life of digoxin. This may result in increased serum digoxin levels and subsequent digitalis toxicity. It may be necessary to reduce the maintenance and digitalization doses when spironolactone is administered, and the patient should be carefully monitored to avoid over- or underdigitalization.

Hydrochlorothiazide may raise the concentration of blood uric acid. Dosage adjustment of antigout medications may be necessary. Hydrochlorothiazide may also raise blood glucose concentrations. Dosage adjustments of insulin or hypoglycemic medications may be necessary. Concurrent use of diuretics with lithium is not recommended as it may produce lithium toxicity.

Several reports of possible interference with digoxin radioimmunoassays by spironolactone, or its metabolites, have appeared in the literature. Neither the extent nor the potential clinical significance of its interference (which may be assay-specific) has been fully established.

Usage in Pregnancy. Spironolactone or its metabolites may, and hydrochlorothiazide does, cross the placental barrier. Therefore, the use of Aldactazide in pregnant women requires that the anticipated benefit be weighed against possible hazards to the fetus. These hazards include fetal or neonatal jaundice, thrombocytopenia, and possible other adverse reactions which have been reported in the adult.

Nursing Mothers. Canrenone, a metabolite of spironolactone, and hydrochlorothiazide appear in breast milk. If use of these drugs is deemed essential, an alternative method of infant feeding should be instituted.

ADVERSE REACTIONS

Gynecomastia is observed not infrequently. A few cases of agranulocytosis have been reported in patients taking spironolactone. Other adverse reactions that have been reported in association with the use of spironolactone are: gastrointestinal symptoms including cramping and diarrhea, drowsiness, lethargy, headache, maculopapular or erythematous cutaneous eruptions, urticaria, mental confusion, drug fever, ataxia, inability to achieve or maintain erection, irregular menses or amenorrhea, postmenopausal bleeding, hirsutism, deepening of the voice, gastric bleeding, ulceration, gastritis, and vomiting. Carcinoma of the breast has been reported in patients taking spironolactone, but a cause and effect relationship has not been established.

Adverse reactions reported in association with the use of thiazides include: gastrointestinal symptoms (anorexia, nausea, vomiting, diarrhea, abdominal cramps), purpura, thrombocytopenia, leukopenia, agranulocytosis, dermatologic symptoms (cutaneous eruptions, pruritus, erythema multiforme), paresthesia, acute pancreatitis, jaundice, dizziness, vertigo, headache, xanthopsia, photosensitivity, necrotizing angiitis, aplastic anemia, orthostatic hypotension, muscle spasm, weakness, restlessness, and hypokalemia.

Adverse reactions are usually reversible upon discontinuation of Aldactazide.

DOSAGE AND ADMINISTRATION

Optimal dosage should be established by individual titration of the components (see Box Warning).

Edema in adults (*congestive heart failure, hepatic cirrhosis, or nephrotic syndrome*). The usual maintenance dose of Aldactazide is 100 mg each of spironolactone and hydrochlorothiazide daily, administered in a single dose or in divided doses, but may range from 25 mg to 200 mg of each component daily depending on the response to the initial titration. In some instances it may be desirable to administer separate tablets of either Aldactone (spironolactone) or hydrochlorothiazide in addition to Aldactazide in order to provide optimal individual therapy.

The onset of diuresis with Aldactazide occurs promptly and, due to prolonged effect of the spironolactone component, persists for two to three days after Aldactazide is discontinued.

Edema in children. The usual daily maintenance dose of Aldactazide should be that which provides 0.75 to 1.5 mg of spironolactone per pound of body weight (1.65 to 3.3 mg/kg).

Essential hypertension. Although the dosage will vary depending on the results of titration of the individual ingredients, many patients will be found to have an optimal response to 50 mg to 100 mg each of spironolactone and hydrochlorothiazide daily, given in a single dose or in divided doses.

Concurrent potassium supplementation is not recommended when Aldactazide is used in the long-term management of hypertension or in the treatment of most edematous conditions, since the spironolactone content of Aldactazide is usually sufficient to minimize loss induced by the hydrochlorothiazide component.

HOW SUPPLIED

Aldactazide tablets containing 25 mg of spironolactone (Aldactone) and 25 mg of hydrochlorothiazide are round, tan, film coated, with SEARLE and 1011 debossed on one side and ALDACTAZIDE and 25 on the other side, supplied as:

NDC Number	Size
0014-1011-31	bottle of 100
0014-1011-51	bottle of 500
0014-1011-52	bottle of 1000
0014-1011-55	bottle of 2500
0014-1011-34	carton of 100 unit dose

Aidactazide tablets containing 50 mg of spironolactone (Aldactone) and 50 mg of hydrochlorothiazide are oblong, tan, scored, film coated, with SEARLE and 1021 debossed on the scored side and ALDACTAZIDE and 50 on the other side, supplied as:

NDC Number	Size
0014-1021-31	bottle of 100
0014-1021-34	carton of 100 unit dose

Store below 86°F (30°C).

Caution: Federal law prohibits dispensing without prescription.

AO5388-1

Shown in Product Identification Section, page 429

ALDACTONE® ℞
[*al-dac'tone*]
(spironolactone)

Warning

Spironolactone has been shown to be a tumorigen in chronic toxicity studies in rats (see *Warnings*). Aldactone should be used only in those conditions described under *Indications and Usage*. Unnecessary use of this drug should be avoided.

DESCRIPTION

Aldactone oral tablets contain 25 mg, 50 mg, or 100 mg of the aldosterone antagonist spironolactone, 17-hydroxy-7α-mercapto-3-oxo-17α-pregn-4-ene-21-carboxylic acid γ-lactone acetate, which has the following structural formula:

Spironolactone is practically insoluble in water, soluble in alcohol, and freely soluble in benzene and in chloroform.

Inactive ingredients include calcium sulfate, corn starch, flavor, hydroxypropyl methylcellulose, iron oxide, magnesium stearate, polyethylene glycol, povidone, and titanium dioxide.

CLINICAL PHARMACOLOGY

Mechanism of action: Aldactone (spironolactone) is a specific pharmacologic antagonist of aldosterone, acting primarily through competitive binding of receptors at the aldosterone-dependent sodium-potassium exchange site in the distal convoluted renal tubule. Aldactone causes increased amounts of sodium and water to be excreted, while potassium is retained. Aldactone acts both as a diuretic and as an antihypertensive drug by this mechanism. It may be given alone or with other diuretic agents which act more proximally in the renal tubule.

Aldosterone antagonist activity: Increased levels of the mineralocorticoid, aldosterone, are present in primary and secondary hyperaldosteronism. Edematous states in which secondary aldosteronism is usually involved include congestive heart failure, hepatic cirrhosis, and the nephrotic syndrome. By competing with aldosterone for receptor sites, Aldactone provides effective therapy for the edema and ascites in those conditions. Aldactone counteracts secondary aldosteronism induced by the volume depletion and associated sodium loss caused by active diuretic therapy.

Aldactone is effective in lowering the systolic and diastolic blood pressure in patients with primary hyperaldosteronism. It is also effective in most cases of essential hypertension, despite the fact that aldosterone secretion may be within normal limits in benign essential hypertension.

Through its action in antagonizing the effect of aldosterone, Aldactone inhibits the exchange of sodium for potassium in the distal renal tubule and helps to prevent potassium loss. Aldactone has not been demonstrated to elevate serum uric acid, to precipitate gout, or to alter carbohydrate metabolism.

Pharmacokinetics: In the human, the bioavailability of spironolactone from orally administered Aldactone 25-mg and 100-mg film-coated tablets, which contain microcrystalline spironolactone, has been evaluated in hypertensive subjects. Equivalent doses showed 35% and 20% higher bioavailability of spironolactone from the 25-mg and 100-mg film-coated tablets, respectively, compared to the 25-mg uncoated Aldactone tablets.

Spironolactone is rapidly and extensively metabolized. The primary metabolite is canrenone, which attains peak serum levels at two to four hours following single oral administration. In the dose range of 25 mg to 200 mg, an approximately linear relationship exists between a single dose of spironolactone and plasma levels of canrenone. Plasma concentrations of canrenone decline in two distinct phases, the first phase lasting from 3 to 12 hours, being more rapid than the second phase lasting from 12 to 96 hours. Canrenone clearance data, following multiple doses of spironolactone, indicate that accumulation of canrenone in the body with 100 mg once a day would be lower than with 25 mg four times a day. Both spironolactone and canrenone are more than 90% bound to plasma proteins. The metabolites of spironolactone are excreted primarily in urine, but also in bile.

INDICATIONS AND USAGE

Aldactone (spironolactone) is indicated in the management of:

Primary hyperaldosteronism for:
Establishing the diagnosis of primary hyperaldosteronism by therapeutic trial.
Short-term preoperative treatment of patients with primary hyperaldosteronism.
Long-term maintenance therapy for patients with discrete aldosterone-producing adrenal adenomas who are judged to be poor operative risks or who decline surgery.
Long-term maintenance therapy for patients with bilateral micro- or macronodular adrenal hyperplasia (idiopathic hyperaldosteronism).

Edematous conditions for patients with:
Congestive heart failure: For the management of edema and sodium retention when the patient is only partially responsive to, or is intolerant of, other therapeutic measures. Aldactone is also indicated for patients with congestive heart failure taking digitalis when other therapies are considered inappropriate.

Cirrhosis of the liver accompanied by edema and/or ascites: Aldosterone levels may be exceptionally high in this condition. Aldactone is indicated for maintenance therapy together with bed rest and the restriction of fluid and sodium.

The nephrotic syndrome: For nephrotic patients when treatment of the underlying disease, restriction of fluid and sodium intake, and the use of other diuretics do not provide an adequate response.

Essential hypertension
Usually in combination with other drugs, Aldactone is indicated for patients who cannot be treated adequately

Continued on next page

G.D. Searle & Co.—Cont.

with other agents or for whom other agents are considered inappropriate.

Hypokalemia

For the treatment of patients with hypokalemia when other measures are considered inappropriate or inadequate. Aldactone is also indicated for the prophylaxis of hypokalemia in patients taking digitalis when other measures are considered inadequate or inappropriate.

Usage in Pregnancy. The routine use of diuretics in an otherwise healthy woman is inappropriate and exposes mother and fetus to unnecessary hazard. Diuretics do not prevent development of toxemia of pregnancy, and there is no satisfactory evidence that they are useful in the treatment of developing toxemia.

Edema during pregnancy may arise from pathologic causes or from the physiologic and mechanical consequences of pregnancy.

Aldactone is indicated in pregnancy when edema is due to pathologic causes just as it is in the absence of pregnancy (however, see *Warnings* section). Dependent edema in pregnancy, resulting from restriction of venous return by the expanded uterus, is properly treated through elevation of the lower extremities and use of support hose; use of diuretics to lower intravascular volume in this case is unsupported and unnecessary. There is hypervolemia during normal pregnancy which is harmful to neither the fetus nor the mother (in the absence of cardiovascular disease), but which is associated with edema, including generalized edema, in the majority of pregnant women. If this edema produces discomfort, increased recumbency will often provide relief. In rare instances, this edema may cause extreme discomfort which is not relieved by rest. In these cases, a short course of diuretics may provide relief and may be appropriate.

CONTRAINDICATIONS

Aldactone is contraindicated for patients with anuria, acute renal insufficiency, significant impairment of renal excretory function, or hyperkalemia.

WARNINGS

Potassium supplementation, either in the form of medication or as a diet rich in potassium, should not ordinarily be given in association with Aldactone therapy. Excessive potassium intake may cause hyperkalemia in patients receiving Aldactone (see *Precautions* section). Aldactone should not be administered concurrently with other potassium-sparing diuretics. Aldactone, when used with ACE inhibitors, even in the presence of a diuretic, has been associated with severe hyperkalemia. Extreme caution should be exercised when Aldactone is given concomitantly with ACE inhibitors (see *Precautions: Drug interactions*).

Spironolactone has been shown to be a tumorigen in chronic toxicity studies performed in rats, with its proliferative effects manifested on endocrine organs and the liver. In one study using 25, 75, and 250 times the usual daily human dose (2 mg/kg) there was a statistically significant dose-related increase in benign adenomas of the thyroid and testes. In female rats there was a statistically significant increase in malignant mammary tumors at the mid-dose only. In male rats there was a dose-related increase in proliferative changes in the liver. At the highest dosage level (500 mg/kg) the range of effects included hepatocytomegaly, hyperplastic nodules, and hepatocellular carcinoma; the last was not statistically significant at a value of p = 0.05. A dose-related (above 20 mg/kg/day) incidence of myelocytic leukemia was observed in rats fed daily doses of potassium canrenoate for a period of one year. In long-term (two-year) oral carcinogenicity studies of potassium canrenoate in the rat, myelocytic leukemia and hepatic, thyroid, testicular, and mammary tumors were observed. Potassium canrenoate did not produce a mutagenic effect in tests using bacteria or yeast. It did produce a positive mutagenic effect in several *in vitro* tests in mammalian cells following metabolic activation. In an *in vivo* mammalian system potassium canrenoate was not mutagenic. Canrenone and canrenoic acid are the major metabolites of potassium canrenoate. Spironolactone is also metabolized to canrenone. An increased incidence of leukemia was not observed in chronic rat toxicity studies conducted with spironolactone at doses up to 500 mg/kg/day.

PRECAUTIONS

General: Because of the diuretic action of Aldactone (spironolactone), patients should be carefully evaluated for possible disturbances of fluid and electrolyte balance. Hyperkalemia may occur in patients with impaired renal function or excessive potassium intake and can cause cardiac irregularities, which may be fatal. Consequently, no potassium supplement should ordinarily be given with Aldactone. Hyperkalemia can be treated promptly by the rapid intravenous administration of glucose (20% to 50%) and regular insulin, using 0.25 to 0.5 units of insulin per gram of glucose. This is a temporary measure to be repeated as required. Aldactone use should be discontinued and potassium intake (including dietary potassium) restricted.

Reversible hyperchloremic metabolic acidosis, usually in association with hyperkalemia, has been reported to occur in some patients with decompensated hepatic cirrhosis, even in the presence of normal renal function.

Hyponatremia, manifested by dryness of the mouth, thirst, lethargy, and drowsiness, and confirmed by a low serum sodium level, may be caused or aggravated, especially when Aldactone is administered in combination with other diuretics.

Gynecomastia may develop in association with the use of spironolactone; physicians should be alert to its possible onset. The development of gynecomastia appears to be related to both dosage level and duration of therapy and is normally reversible when Aldactone is discontinued. In rare instances some breast enlargement may persist when Aldactone is discontinued.

Aldactone therapy may cause a transient elevation of BUN, especially in patients with preexisting renal impairment. Aldactone may cause mild acidosis.

A determination of serum electrolytes to detect possible electrolyte imbalance should be performed at periodic intervals.

Drug interactions: When used in combination with other diuretics or antihypertensive agents, Aldactone potentiates their effects. Therefore, the dosage of such drugs, particularly the ganglionic blocking agents, should be reduced by at least 50% when Aldactone is added to the regimen.

Concomitant administration of potassium-sparing diuretics with ACE inhibitors or indomethacin has been associated with severe hyperkalemia.

Spironolactone reduces the vascular responsiveness to norepinephrine. Therefore, caution should be exercised in the management of patients subjected to regional or general anesthesia while they are being treated with Aldactone.

Spironolactone has been shown to increase the half-life of digoxin. This may result in increased serum digoxin levels and subsequent digitalis toxicity. It may be necessary to reduce the maintenance and digitalization doses when spironolactone is administered, and the patient should be carefully monitored to avoid over- or underdigitalization.

Drug/Laboratory test interactions: Several reports of possible interference with digoxin radioimmunoassays by spironolactone, or its metabolites, have appeared in the literature. Neither the extent nor the potential clinical significance of its interference (which may be assay-specific) has been fully established.

Usage in pregnancy: Spironolactone or its metabolites may cross the placental barrier. Therefore, the use of Aldactone in pregnant women requires that the anticipated benefit be weighed against possible hazard to the fetus.

Nursing mothers: Canrenone, a metabolite of spironolactone, appears in breast milk. If use of the drug is deemed essential, an alternative method of infant feeding should be instituted.

ADVERSE REACTIONS

Gynecomastia is observed not infrequently. A few cases of agranulocytosis have been reported in patients taking spironolactone. Other adverse reactions that have been reported in association with Aldactone are: gastrointestinal symptoms including cramping and diarrhea, drowsiness, lethargy, headache, maculopapular or erythematous cutaneous eruptions, urticaria, mental confusion, drug fever, ataxia, inability to achieve or maintain erection, irregular menses or amenorrhea, postmenopausal bleeding, hirsutism, deepening of the voice, gastric bleeding, ulceration, gastritis, and vomiting. Carcinoma of the breast has been reported in patients taking spironolactone, but a cause and effect relationship has not been established.

Adverse reactions are usually reversible upon discontinuation of the drug.

DOSAGE AND ADMINISTRATION

Primary hyperaldosteronism. Aldactone may be employed as an initial diagnostic measure to provide presumptive evidence of primary hyperaldosteronism while patients are on normal diets.

    Long test: Aldactone (spironolactone) is administered at a daily dosage of 400 mg for three to four weeks. Correction of hypokalemia and of hypertension provides presumptive evidence for the diagnosis of primary hyperaldosteronism.

    Short test: Aldactone is administered at a daily dosage of 400 mg for four days. If serum potassium increases during Aldactone administration but drops when Aldactone is discontinued, a presumptive diagnosis of primary hyperaldosteronism should be considered.

After the diagnosis of hyperaldosteronism has been established by more definitive testing procedures, Aldactone may be administered in doses of 100 to 400 mg daily in preparation for surgery. For patients who are considered unsuitable for surgery, Aldactone may be employed for long-term maintenance therapy at the lowest effective dosage determined for the individual patient.

Edema in adults (*congestive heart failure, hepatic cirrhosis, or nephrotic syndrome*). An initial daily dosage of 100 mg of Aldactone administered in either single or divided doses is

recommended, but may range from 25 to 200 mg daily. When given as the sole agent for diuresis, Aldactone should be continued for at least five days at the initial dosage level, after which it may be adjusted to the optimal therapeutic or maintenance level administered in either single or divided daily doses. If, after five days, an adequate diuretic response to Aldactone has not occurred, a second diuretic which acts more proximally in the renal tubule may be added to the regimen. Because of the additive effect of Aldactone when administered concurrently with such diuretics, an enhanced diuresis usually begins on the first day of combined treatment; combined therapy is indicated when more rapid diuresis is desired. The dosage of Aldactone should remain unchanged when other diuretic therapy is added.

Edema in children. The initial daily dosage should provide approximately 1.5 mg of Aldactone per pound of body weight (3.3 mg/kg) administered in either single or divided doses.

Essential hypertension. For adults, an initial daily dosage of 50 to 100 mg of Aldactone administered in either single or divided doses is recommended. Aldactone may also be given with diuretics which act more proximally in the renal tubule or with other antihypertensive agents. Treatment with Aldactone should be continued for at least two weeks, since the maximum response may not occur before this time. Subsequently, dosage should be adjusted according to the response of the patient.

Hypokalemia. Aldactone in a dosage ranging from 25 mg to 100 mg daily is useful in treating a diuretic-induced hypokalemia, when oral potassium supplements or other potassium-sparing regimens are considered inappropriate.

HOW SUPPLIED

Aldactone 25-mg tablets are round, light yellow, film coated, with SEARLE and 1001 debossed on one side and ALDACTONE and 25 on the other side, supplied as:

NDC Number	Size
0014-1001-31	bottle of 100
0014-1001-51	bottle of 500
0014-1001-52	bottle of 1000
0014-1001-55	bottle of 2500
0014-1001-34	carton of 100 unit dose

Aldactone 50-mg tablets are oval, light orange, scored, film coated, with SEARLE and 1041 debossed on the scored side and ALDACTONE and 50 on the other side, supplied as:

NDC Number	Size
0014-1041-31	bottle of 100
0014-1041-34	carton of 100 unit dose

Aldactone 100-mg tablets are round, peach colored, scored, film coated, with SEARLE and 1031 debossed on the scored side and ALDACTONE and 100 on the other side, supplied as:

NDC Number	Size
0014-1031-31	bottle of 100
0014-1031-34	carton of 100 unit dose

Store below 86°F (30°C).

Caution: Federal law prohibits dispensing without prescription.

AO5449-1

Shown in Product Identification Section, page 429

AMINOPHYLLIN™ Tablets   ℞

[ă-mĭ-nŏph ′yl-lĭn]
(aminophylline)

DESCRIPTION

Each oral tablet contains 100 mg or 200 mg of aminophylline USP calculated as the dihydrate, which is equivalent to 79 mg and 158 mg of anhydrous theophylline, respectively. Aminophylline USP (anhydrous) is a soluble complex containing approximately 85% anhydrous theophylline and 15% ethylenediamine. Aminophylline is white or slightly yellowish granules or powder, having a slight ammoniacal odor and a bitter taste.

The structural formula of aminophylline (3,7-dihydro-1,3-dimethyl-1*H*-purine-2,6-dione; 1,2-ethanediamine) is:

Inactive ingredients of Aminophyllin 100-mg tablets include acacia, corn starch, magnesium stearate, potassium phosphate, sodium sulfate, and sodium sulfite. Inactive ingredients of Aminophyllin 200-mg tablets include corn starch, magnesium stearate, potassium phosphate, sodium sulfite, and talc.

ACTIONS

Aminophylline directly relaxes the smooth muscle of the bronchial airways and pulmonary blood vessels, thus acting mainly as a bronchodilator, pulmonary vasodilator, and smooth muscle relaxant. The drug also possesses other actions typical of the xanthine derivatives: coronary vasodilator, diuretic, cardiac stimulant, cerebral stimulant, and skeletal muscle stimulant.

INDICATIONS AND USAGE

Aminophyllin Tablets are indicated for the relief and/or prevention of symptoms from asthma and reversible bronchospasm associated with chronic bronchitis and emphysema.

CONTRAINDICATIONS

Aminophylline should not be administered to patients with active peptic ulcer disease, since it may increase the volume and acidity of gastric secretions.

Patients with a history of hypersensitivity to aminophylline or theophylline should not be treated with the drug.

Aminophylline should not be administered with other xanthine preparations.

WARNINGS

Excessive doses may be expected to be toxic. Some children may be unusually sensitive to aminophylline. Toxic synergism with ephedrine and other sympathomimetic bronchodilator drugs may occur. Halothane anesthesia in the presence of aminophylline may produce sinus tachycardia or ventricular arrhythmias.

Contains sodium sulfite, a sulfite that may cause allergic-type reactions including anaphylactic symptoms and life-threatening or less severe asthmatic episodes in certain susceptible people. The overall prevalence of sulfite sensitivity in the general population is unknown and probably low. Sulfite sensitivity is seen more frequently in asthmatic than in nonasthmatic people.

Usage in Pregnancy. Safe use in pregnancy has not been established relative to possible adverse effects on fetal development. Therefore, aminophylline should not be used in pregnant women unless, in the judgment of the physician, the potential benefits outweigh the possible hazards.

PRECAUTIONS

Use with caution in patients with severe cardiac disease, hypertension, hyperthyroidism, acute myocardial injury, cor pulmonale, severe hypoxemia, hepatic impairment, or alcoholism, and in the elderly (especially males) and in neonates. Particular caution in dose administration must be exercised in patients with a history of peptic ulcer since the condition may be exacerbated. Chronic oral administration in high doses may be associated with gastrointestinal irritation.

Caution should be used in giving aminophylline to patients in congestive heart failure. Serum levels in such patients have persisted for long periods following discontinuation of the drug.

Theophylline half-life is shorter in smokers than nonsmokers; therefore, smokers may require larger or more frequent doses.

Aminophylline may lower the seizure threshold.

Elevated serum levels of theophylline may occur in patients treated concomitantly with aminophylline and cimetidine, troleandomycin, erythromycin, allopurinol, or oral contraceptive steroids. The addition of ephedrine or other sympathomimetic drugs to regimens of aminophylline increases the toxicity potential and may result in symptoms of overdosage, due to the additive pharmacological effects of these compounds. Co-medication with phenobarbital, phenytoin, or rifampin may increase theophylline clearance and an increase of the aminophylline dose may be required. The excretion of lithium carbonate is increased in patients receiving aminophylline. Aminophylline may antagonize the effects of propranolol.

Consumption of coffee, tea, cola beverages, chocolate, or acetaminophen contributes to falsely high serum theophylline levels when theophylline is measured spectrophotometrically without previous isolation by chromatography.

Mutagenesis: Theophylline has been shown to be mutagenic in *Escherichia coli* and other lower organisms (*Euglena gracilis* and *Ophiostoma multiannulatum*) and to produce chromosome breaks in cultured mouse cells and cultured human lymphocytes. The drug had no mutagenic activity *in vivo* in a dominant lethal test using mice.

Limited animal studies have shown teratogenic activity of theophylline in mice and rats.

Theophylline is excreted in breast milk and may cause adverse effects in the infant. Caution must be used when prescribing aminophylline to a nursing mother, taking into account the risk/benefit of this therapy.

Due to the marked variation in theophylline metabolism in infants under 6 months of age, aminophylline is not recommended for this age group.

ADVERSE REACTIONS

The most consistent adverse reactions observed with *therapeutic* amounts of aminophylline are:

1. Gastrointestinal: Nausea, vomiting, anorexia, bitter aftertaste, dyspepsia, heavy feeling in the stomach, and gastrointestinal distress.

2. Central nervous system: Dizziness, vertigo, lightheadedness, headache, nervousness, insomnia, and agitation.
3. Cardiovascular: Palpitation, tachycardia, flushing, and extrasystoles.
4. Respiratory: Increase in respiratory rate.
5. Dermatologic: Urticaria.

OVERDOSAGE

The most consistent reactions observed with *toxic* overdoses of aminophylline are:

1. Gastrointestinal: Nausea, vomiting, epigastric pain, hematemesis, and diarrhea.
2. Central nervous system: In addition to those cited above, the patient may exhibit hyperreflexia, fasciculations, and clonic and tonic convulsions. These are especially prone to occur in cases of overdosage in infants and small children.
3. Cardiovascular: In addition to those outlined above, marked hypotension and circulatory failure may be manifest.
4. Respiratory: Tachypnea and respiratory arrest may occur.
5. Renal: Albuminuria and microhematuria may occur. Increased excretion of renal tubular cells has been observed.
6. General systemic effects: Syncope, collapse, fever, and dehydration.

Management of Toxic Symptoms:

1. Discontinue drug immediately.
2. There is no known specific antidote.
3. Gastric lavage.
4. Emetic medication may be of value.
5. Avoid administration of sympathomimetic drugs.
6. Intravenous fluids, oxygen, and other supportive measures to prevent hypotension and overcome dehydration.
7. Central nervous system stimulation and seizures may respond to short-acting barbiturates.
8. Monitor serum levels until below 20 mcg/ml.

DOSAGE AND ADMINISTRATION

The oral dose for adults should be adjusted according to the need and response of the patient. Usually a daily dose in the range of 600 to 1600 mg, administered in 3 or 4 divided doses, will provide the desired therapeutic effect. Similarly, the dose for children should be adjusted according to the response. An oral dose of 12 mg/kg/24 hours, administered in four divided doses, will usually provide the desired therapeutic effect in children.

Therapeutic serum levels are considered to be between 10 mcg/ml and 20 mcg/ml. Levels above 20 mcg/ml may produce toxic effects. There is great variation from patient to patient in dosage needed to achieve a therapeutic serum level and in the duration of action of oral aminophylline. Because of these wide variations and the relatively narrow therapeutic serum level range, dosage must be individualized with monitoring of theophylline serum levels, particularly when prolonged use is planned.

HOW SUPPLIED

Aminophyllin Tablets are supplied as:

Round, white, scored tablets with 1231 debossed on the scored side and SEARLE on the other side, each tablet containing 100 mg of aminophylline.

NDC Number	Size
0014-1231-31	bottle of 100
0014-1231-52	bottle of 1,000
0014-1231-34	carton of 100 unit dose

Oval, white, scored tablets with 1251 debossed on the scored side and SEARLE on the other side, each tablet containing 200 mg of aminophylline.

NDC Number	Size
0014-1251-31	bottle of 100
0014-1251-52	bottle of 1,000
0014-1251-34	carton of 100 unit dose

Dispense in a tight, non-PVC container.

Caution: Federal law prohibits dispensing without prescription.

AO5232

CALAN® Tablets ℞
[cal 'an]
(verapamil hydrochloride)

PRODUCT OVERVIEW

KEY FACTS

Calan, a calcium ion antagonist, exerts its pharmacologic effects by modulating the influx of ionic calcium across the cell membrane of the arterial smooth muscle as well as in conductile and contractile myocardial cells. Calan increases myocardial oxygen supply, reduces myocardial oxygen consumption, and is a potent inhibitor of coronary artery spasm, making it an effective antianginal agent. By decreasing the influx of calcium, Calan prolongs the effective refractory

period within the AV node and slows AV conduction in a rate-related manner, thereby slowing the ventricular rate in patients with chronic atrial flutter or fibrillation. Calan exerts antihypertensive effects by decreasing systemic vascular resistance, usually without orthostatic decreases in blood pressure or reflex tachycardia.

MAJOR USES

Calan Tablets are indicated for: angina at rest, including vasospastic and unstable angina; chronic stable angina; control (in association with digitalis) of ventricular rate at rest and during stress in patients with chronic atrial flutter and/or atrial fibrillation; prophylaxis of repetitive paroxysmal supraventricular tachycardia; management of essential hypertension.

SAFETY INFORMATION

See complete safety information set forth below.

PRESCRIBING INFORMATION

CALAN® Tablets ℞
[cal 'an]
(verapamil hydrochloride)

DESCRIPTION

Calan (verapamil HCl) is a calcium ion influx inhibitor (slow-channel blocker or calcium ion antagonist) available for oral administration in film-coated tablets containing 40 mg, 80 mg, or 120 mg of verapamil hydrochloride.

The structural formula of verapamil HCl is

$$CH_3O-\text{---}-C(CH_3)_2NCH_2CH_2-\text{---}-OCH_3 \cdot HCl$$

$$C_{27}H_{38}N_2O_4 \cdot HCl \qquad M.W.= 491.08$$

Benzeneacetonitrile, α-[3-[[2-(3, 4-dimethoxyphenyl) ethyl] methylamino]propyl]-3,4-dimethoxy-α- (1-methylethyl) hydrochloride.

Verapamil HCl is an almost white, crystalline powder, practically free of odor, with a bitter taste. It is soluble in water, chloroform, and methanol. Verapamil HCl is not chemically related to other cardioactive drugs.

Inactive ingredients include microcrystalline cellulose, corn starch, gelatin, hydroxypropyl cellulose, hydroxypropyl methylcellulose, iron oxide colorant, lactose, magnesium stearate, polyethylene glycol, talc, and titanium dioxide.

CLINICAL PHARMACOLOGY

Calan is a calcium ion influx inhibitor (slow-channel blocker or calcium ion antagonist) that exerts its pharmacologic effects by modulating the influx of ionic calcium across the cell membrane of the arterial smooth muscle as well as in conductile and contractile myocardial cells.

Mechanism of action

Angina: The precise mechanism of action of Calan as an antianginal agent remains to be fully determined, but includes the following two mechanisms:

1. *Relaxation and prevention of coronary artery spasm:* Calan dilates the main coronary arteries and coronary arterioles, both in normal and ischemic regions, and is a potent inhibitor of coronary artery spasm, whether spontaneous or ergonovine-induced. This property increases myocardial oxygen delivery in patients with coronary artery spasm and is responsible for the effectiveness of Calan in vasospastic (Prinzmetal's or variant) as well as unstable angina at rest. Whether this effect plays any role in classical effort angina is not clear, but studies of exercise tolerance have not shown an increase in the maximum exercise rate–pressure product, a widely accepted measure of oxygen utilization. This suggests that, in general, relief of spasm or dilation of coronary arteries is not an important factor in classical angina.

2. *Reduction of oxygen utilization:* Calan regularly reduces the total peripheral resistance (afterload) against which the heart works both at rest and at a given level of exercise by dilating peripheral arterioles. This unloading of the heart reduces myocardial energy consumption and oxygen requirements and probably accounts for the effectiveness of Calan in chronic stable effort angina.

Arrhythmia: Electrical activity through the AV node depends, to a significant degree, upon calcium influx through the slow channel. By decreasing the influx of calcium, Calan prolongs the effective refractory period within the AV node and slows AV conduction in a rate-related manner. This property accounts for the ability of Calan to slow the ventricular rate in patients with chronic atrial flutter or atrial fibrillation.

Normal sinus rhythm is usually not affected, but in patients with sick sinus syndrome, Calan may interfere with sinusnode impulse generation and may induce sinus arrest or sinoatrial block. Atrioventricular block can occur in patients without preexisting conduction defects (see *Warnings*).

Continued on next page

G.D. Searle & Co.—Cont.

Calan decreases the frequency of episodes of paroxysmal supraventricular tachycardia.

Calan does not alter the normal atrial action potential or intraventricular conduction time, but in depressed atrial fibers it decreases amplitude, velocity of depolarization, and conduction velocity. Calan may shorten the antegrade effective refractory period of the accessory bypass tract. Acceleration of ventricular rate and/or ventricular fibrillation has been reported in patients with atrial flutter or atrial fibrillation and a coexisting accessory AV pathway following administration of verapamil (see *Warnings*).

Calan has a local anesthetic action that is 1.6 times that of procaine on an equimolar basis. It is not known whether this action is important at the doses used in man.

Essential hypertension: Calan exerts antihypertensive effects by decreasing systemic vascular resistance, usually without orthostatic decreases in blood pressure or reflex tachycardia; bradycardia (rate less than 50 beats/min) is uncommon (1.4%). During isometric or dynamic exercise Calan does not alter systolic cardiac function in patients with normal ventricular function.

Calan does not alter total serum calcium levels. However, one report suggested that calcium levels above the normal range may alter the therapeutic effect of Calan.

Pharmacokinetics and metabolism: More than 90% of the orally administered dose of Calan is absorbed. Because of rapid biotransformation of verapamil during its first pass through the portal circulation, bioavailability ranges from 20% to 35%. Peak plasma concentrations are reached between 1 and 2 hours after oral administration. Chronic oral administration of 120 mg of verapamil HCl every 6 hours resulted in plasma levels of verapamil ranging from 125 to 400 ng/ml, with higher values reported occasionally. A non-linear correlation between the verapamil dose administered and verapamil plasma levels does exist. In early dose titration with verapamil a relationship exists between verapamil plasma concentration and prolongation of the PR interval. However, during chronic administration this relationship may disappear. The mean elimination half-life in single-dose studies ranged from 2.8 to 7.4 hours. In these same studies, after repetitive dosing, the half-life increased to a range from 4.5 to 12.0 hours (after less than 10 consecutive doses given 6 hours apart). Half-life of verapamil may increase during titration. Aging may affect the pharmacokinetics of verapamil. Elimination half-life may be prolonged in the elderly. In healthy men, orally administered Calan undergoes extensive metabolism in the liver. Twelve metabolites have been identified in plasma; all except norverapamil are present in trace amounts only. Norverapamil can reach steady-state plasma concentrations approximately equal to those of verapamil itself. The cardiovascular activity of norverapamil appears to be approximately 20% that of verapamil. Approximately 70% of an administered dose is excreted as metabolites in the urine and 16% or more in the feces within 5 days. About 3% to 4% is excreted in the urine as unchanged drug. Approximately 90% is bound to plasma proteins. In patients with hepatic insufficiency, metabolism is delayed and elimination half-life prolonged up to 14 to 16 hours (see *Precautions*); the volume of distribution is increased and plasma clearance reduced to about 30% of normal. Verapamil clearance values suggest that patients with liver dysfunction may attain therapeutic verapamil plasma concentrations with one third of the oral daily dose required for patients with normal liver function.

After four weeks of oral dosing (120 mg q.i.d.), verapamil and norverapamil levels were noted in the cerebrospinal fluid with estimated partition coefficient of 0.06 for verapamil and 0.04 for norverapamil.

Hemodynamics and myocardial metabolism: Calan reduces afterload and myocardial contractility. Improved left ventricular diastolic function in patients with IHSS and those with coronary heart disease has also been observed with Calan therapy. In most patients, including those with organic cardiac disease, the negative inotropic action of Calan is countered by reduction of afterload, and cardiac index is usually not reduced. However, in patients with severe left ventricular dysfunction (eg, pulmonary wedge pressure above 20 mm Hg or ejection fraction less than 30%), or in patients taking beta-adrenergic blocking agents or other cardiodepressant drugs, deterioration of ventricular function may occur (see *Drug interactions*).

Pulmonary function: Calan does not induce bronchoconstriction and, hence, does not impair ventilatory function.

INDICATIONS AND USAGE

Calan tablets are indicated for the treatment of the following:

Angina

1. Angina at rest, including:
   —Vasospastic (Prinzmetal's variant) angina
   —Unstable (crescendo, pre-infarction) angina
2. Chronic stable angina (classic effort-associated angina)

Arrhythmias

1. In association with digitalis for the control of ventricular rate at rest and during stress in patients with chronic atrial flutter and/or atrial fibrillation (see *Warnings: Accessory bypass tract*)
2. Prophylaxis of repetitive paroxysmal supraventricular tachycardia

Essential hypertension

CONTRAINDICATIONS

Verapamil HCl tablets are contraindicated in:
1. Severe left ventricular dysfunction (see *Warnings*)
2. Hypotension (systolic pressure less than 90 mm Hg) or cardiogenic shock
3. Sick sinus syndrome (except in patients with a functioning artificial ventricular pacemaker)
4. Second- or third-degree AV block (except in patients with a functioning artificial ventricular pacemaker)
5. Patients with atrial flutter or atrial fibrillation and an accessory bypass tract (eg, Wolff-Parkinson-White, Lown-Ganong-Levine syndromes). (See *Warnings*.)
6. Patients with known hypersensitivity to verapamil hydrochloride.

WARNINGS

Heart failure: Verapamil has a negative inotropic effect, which in most patients is compensated by its afterload reduction (decreased systemic vascular resistance) properties without a net impairment of ventricular performance. In clinical experience with 4,954 patients, 87 (1.8%) developed congestive heart failure or pulmonary edema. Verapamil should be avoided in patients with severe left ventricular dysfunction (eg, ejection fraction less than 30%) or moderate to severe symptoms of cardiac failure and in patients with any degree of ventricular dysfunction if they are receiving a beta-adrenergic blocker (see *Drug interactions*). Patients with milder ventricular dysfunction should, if possible, be controlled with optimum doses of digitalis and/or diuretics before verapamil treatment. **(Note interactions with digoxin under *Precautions*.)**

Hypotension: Occasionally, the pharmacologic action of verapamil may produce a decrease in blood pressure below normal levels, which may result in dizziness or symptomatic hypotension. The incidence of hypotension observed in 4,954 patients enrolled in clinical trials was 2.5%. In hypertensive patients, decreases in blood pressure below normal are unusual. Tilt-table testing (60 degrees) was not able to induce orthostatic hypotension.

Elevated liver enzymes: Elevations of transaminases with and without concomitant elevations in alkaline phosphatase and bilirubin have been reported. Such elevations have sometimes been transient and may disappear even with continued verapamil treatment. Several cases of hepatocellular injury related to verapamil have been proven by rechallenge; half of these had clinical symptoms (malaise, fever, and/or right upper quadrant pain), in addition to elevation of SGOT, SGPT, and alkaline phosphatase. Periodic monitoring of liver function in patients receiving verapamil is therefore prudent.

Accessory bypass tract (Wolff-Parkinson-White or Lown-Ganong-Levine): Some patients with paroxysmal and/or chronic atrial fibrillation or atrial flutter and a coexisting accessory AV pathway have developed increased antegrade conduction across the accessory pathway bypassing the AV node, producing a very rapid ventricular response or ventricular fibrillation after receiving intravenous verapamil (or digitalis). Although a risk of this occurring with oral verapamil has not been established, such patients receiving oral verapamil may be at risk and its use in these patients is contraindicated (see *Contraindications*). Treatment is usually DC-cardioversion. Cardioversion has been used safely and effectively after oral Calan.

Atrioventricular block: The effect of verapamil on AV conduction and the SA node may cause asymptomatic first-degree AV block and transient bradycardia, sometimes accompanied by nodal escape rhythms. PR-interval prolongation is correlated with verapamil plasma concentrations especially during the early titration phase of therapy. Higher degrees of AV block, however, were infrequently (0.8%) observed. Marked first-degree block or progressive development to second- or third-degree AV block requires a reduction in dosage or, in rare instances, discontinuation of verapamil HCl and institution of appropriate therapy, depending on the clinical situation.

Patients with hypertrophic cardiomyopathy (IHSS): In 120 patients with hypertrophic cardiomyopathy (most of them refractory or intolerant to propranolol) who received therapy with verapamil at doses up to 720 mg/day, a variety of serious adverse effects was seen. Three patients died in pulmonary edema; all had severe left ventricular outflow obstruction and a past history of left ventricular dysfunction. Eight other patients had pulmonary edema and/or severe hypotension; abnormally high (greater than 20 mm Hg) pulmonary wedge pressure and a marked left ventricular outflow obstruction were present in most of these patients. Concomitant administration of quinidine (see *Drug interactions*)

preceded the severe hypotension in 3 of the 8 patients (2 of whom developed pulmonary edema). Sinus bradycardia occurred in 11% of the patients, second-degree AV block in 4%, and sinus arrest in 2%. It must be appreciated that this group of patients had a serious disease with a high mortality rate. Most adverse effects responded well to dose reduction, and only rarely did verapamil use have to be discontinued.

PRECAUTIONS

General

Use in patients with impaired hepatic function: Since verapamil is highly metabolized by the liver, it should be administered cautiously to patients with impaired hepatic function. Severe liver dysfunction prolongs the elimination half-life of verapamil to about 14 to 16 hours; hence, approximately 30% of the dose given to patients with normal liver function should be administered to these patients. Careful monitoring for abnormal prolongation of the PR interval or other signs of excessive pharmacologic effects (see *Overdosage*) should be carried out.

Use in patients with attenuated (decreased) neuromuscular transmission: It has been reported that verapamil decreases neuromuscular transmission in patients with Duchenne's muscular dystrophy, and that verapamil prolongs recovery from the neuromuscular blocking agent vecuronium. It may be necessary to decrease the dosage of verapamil when it is administered to patients with attenuated neuromuscular transmission.

Use in patients with impaired renal function: About 70% of an administered dose of verapamil is excreted as metabolites in the urine. Verapamil is not removed by hemodialysis. Until further data are available, verapamil should be administered cautiously to patients with impaired renal function. These patients should be carefully monitored for abnormal prolongation of the PR interval or other signs of overdosage (see *Overdosage*).

Drug interactions

Beta-blockers: Controlled studies in small numbers of patients suggest that the concomitant use of Calan and oral beta-adrenergic blocking agents may be beneficial in certain patients with chronic stable angina or hypertension, but available information is not sufficient to predict with confidence the effects of concurrent treatment in patients with left ventricular dysfunction or cardiac conduction abnormalities. Concomitant therapy with beta-adrenergic blockers and verapamil may result in additive negative effects on heart rate, atrioventricular conduction and/or cardiac contractility.

In one study involving 15 patients treated with high doses of propranolol (median dose, 480 mg/day; range, 160 to 1,280 mg/day) for severe angina, with preserved left ventricular function (ejection fraction greater than 35%), the hemodynamic effects of additional therapy with verapamil HCl were assessed using invasive methods. The addition of verapamil to high-dose beta-blockers induced modest negative inotropic and chronotropic effects that were not severe enough to limit short-term (48 hours) combination therapy in this study. These modest cardiodepressant effects persisted for greater than 6 but less than 30 hours after abrupt withdrawal of beta-blockers and were closely related to plasma levels of propranolol. The primary verapamil/beta-blocker interaction in this study appeared to be hemodynamic rather than electrophysiologic.

In other studies verapamil did not generally induce significant negative inotropic, chronotropic, or dromotropic effects in patients with preserved left ventricular function receiving low or moderate doses of propranolol (less than or equal to 320 mg/day); in some patients, however, combined therapy did produce such effects. Therefore, if combined therapy is used, close surveillance of clinical status should be carried out. Combined therapy should usually be avoided in patients with atrioventricular conduction abnormalities and those with depressed left ventricular function.

Asymptomatic bradycardia (36 beats/min) with a wandering atrial pacemaker has been observed in a patient receiving concomitant timolol (a beta-adrenergic blocker) eyedrops and oral verapamil.

A decrease in metoprolol clearance has been observed when verapamil and metoprolol were administered together. A similar effect has not been seen when verapamil and atenolol were given together.

Digitalis: Clinical use of verapamil in digitalized patients has shown the combination to be well tolerated if digoxin doses are properly adjusted. However, chronic verapamil treatment can increase serum digoxin levels by 50% to 75% during the first week of therapy, and this can result in digitalis toxicity. In patients with hepatic cirrhosis the influence of verapamil on digoxin kinetics is magnified. Verapamil may reduce total body clearance and extrarenal clearance of digitoxin by 27% and 29%, respectively. Maintenance and digitalization doses should be reduced when verapamil is administered, and the patient should be reassessed to avoid over- or underdigitalization. Whenever overdigitalization is suspected, the daily dose of digitalis should be reduced or temporarily discontinued. On discontinuation of Calan use, the patient should be reassessed to avoid under-digitalization.

Antihypertensive agents: Verapamil administered concomitantly with oral antihypertensive agents (eg, vasodilators, angiotensin-converting enzyme inhibitors, diuretics, beta-blockers) will usually have an additive effect on lowering blood pressure. Patients receiving these combinations should be appropriately monitored. Concomitant use of agents that attenuate alpha-adrenergic function with verapamil may result in a reduction in blood pressure that is excessive in some patients. Such an effect was observed in one study following the concomitant administration of verapamil and prazosin.

Antiarrhythmic agents:
Disopyramide: Until data on possible interactions between verapamil and disopyramide are obtained, disopyramide should not be administered within 48 hours before or 24 hours after verapamil administration.
Flecainide: A study in healthy volunteers showed that the concomitant administration of flecainide and verapamil may have additive effects on myocardial contractility, AV conduction, and repolarization. Concomitant therapy with flecainide and verapamil may result in additive negative inotropic effect and prolongation of atrioventricular conduction.
Quinidine: In a small number of patients with hypertrophic cardiomyopathy (IHSS), concomitant use of verapamil and quinidine resulted in significant hypotension. Until further data are obtained, combined therapy of verapamil and quinidine in patients with hypertrophic cardiomyopathy should probably be avoided.
The electrophysiologic effects of quinidine and verapamil on AV conduction were studied in 8 patients. Verapamil significantly counteracted the effects of quinidine on AV conduction. There has been a report of increased quinidine levels during verapamil therapy.
Other:
Nitrates: Verapamil has been given concomitantly with short- and long-acting nitrates without any undesirable drug interactions. The pharmacologic profile of both drugs and the clinical experience suggest beneficial interactions.
Cimetidine: The interaction between cimetidine and chronically administered verapamil has not been studied. Variable results on clearance have been obtained in acute studies of healthy volunteers; clearance of verapamil was either reduced or unchanged.
Lithium: Pharmacokinetic and pharmacodynamic interactions between oral verapamil and lithium have been reported. The former may result in a lowering of serum lithium levels in patients receiving chronic stable oral lithium therapy. The latter may result in an increased sensitivity to the effects of lithium. Patients receiving both drugs must be monitored carefully.
Carbamazepine: Verapamil therapy may increase carbamazepine concentrations during combined therapy. This may produce carbamazepine side effects such as diplopia, headache, ataxia, or dizziness.
Rifampin: Therapy with rifampin may markedly reduce oral verapamil bioavailability.
Phenobarbital: Phenobarbital therapy may increase verapamil clearance.
Cyclosporin: Verapamil therapy may increase serum levels of cyclosporin.
Inhalation anesthetics: Animal experiments have shown that inhalation anesthetics depress cardiovascular activity by decreasing the inward movement of calcium ions. When used concomitantly, inhalation anesthetics and calcium antagonists, such as verapamil, should each be titrated carefully to avoid excessive cardiovascular depression.
Neuromuscular blocking agents: Clinical data and animal studies suggest that verapamil may potentiate the activity of neuromuscular blocking agents (curare-like and depolarizing). It may be necessary to decrease the dose of verapamil and/or the dose of the neuromuscular blocking agent when the drugs are used concomitantly.
Carcinogenesis, mutagenesis, impairment of fertility: An 18-month toxicity study in rats, at a low multiple (6-fold) of the maximum recommended human dose, and not the maximum tolerated dose, did not suggest a tumorigenic potential. There was no evidence of a carcinogenic potential of verapamil administered in the diet of rats for two years at doses of 10, 35, and 120 mg/kg/day or approximately 1, 3.5, and 12 times, respectively, the maximum recommended human daily dose (480 mg/day or 9.6 mg/kg/day).
Verapamil was not mutagenic in the Ames test in 5 test strains at 3 mg per plate with or without metabolic activation.
Studies in female rats at daily dietary doses up to 5.5 times (55 mg/kg/day) the maximum recommended human dose did not show impaired fertility. Effects on male fertility have not been determined.
Pregnancy: Pregnancy Category C. Reproduction studies have been performed in rabbits and rats at oral doses up to 1.5 (15 mg/kg/day) and 6 (60 mg/kg/day) times the human oral daily dose, respectively, and have revealed no evidence of teratogenicity. In the rat, however, this multiple of the human dose was embryocidal and retarded fetal growth and development, probably because of adverse maternal effects reflected in reduced weight gains of the dams. This oral dose has also been shown to cause hypotension in rats. There are no adequate and well-controlled studies in pregnant women. Because animal reproduction studies are not always predictive of human response, this drug should be used during pregnancy only if clearly needed. Verapamil crosses the placental barrier and can be detected in umbilical vein blood at delivery.

Labor and delivery: It is not known whether the use of verapamil during labor or delivery has immediate or delayed adverse effects on the fetus, or whether it prolongs the duration of labor or increases the need for forceps delivery or other obstetric intervention. Such adverse experiences have not been reported in the literature, despite a long history of use of verapamil in Europe in the treatment of cardiac side effects of beta-adrenergic agonist agents used to treat premature labor.

Nursing mothers: Verapamil is excreted in human milk. Because of the potential for adverse reactions in nursing infants from verapamil, nursing should be discontinued while verapamil is administered.

Pediatric use: Safety and efficacy of Calan in children below the age of 18 years have not been established.

Animal pharmacology and/or animal toxicology: In chronic animal toxicology studies verapamil caused lenticular and/or suture line changes at 30 mg/kg/day or greater, and frank cataracts at 62.5 mg/kg/day or greater in the beagle dog but not in the rat. Development of cataracts due to verapamil has not been reported in man.

ADVERSE REACTIONS

Serious adverse reactions are uncommon when Calan therapy is initiated with upward dose titration within the recommended single and total daily dose. See *Warnings* for discussion of heart failure, hypotension, elevated liver enzymes, AV block, and rapid ventricular response. The following reactions to orally administered verapamil occurred at rates greater than 1.0% or occurred at lower rates but appeared clearly drug-related in clinical trials in 4,954 patients:

Constipation	7.3%	Dyspnea	1.4%
Dizziness	3.3%	Bradycardia	
Nausea	2.7%	(HR < 50/min)	1.4%
Hypotension	2.5%	AV block	
Headache	2.2%	total (1°, 2°, 3°)	1.2%
Edema	1.9%	2° and 3°	0.8%
CHF/Pulmonary		Rash	1.2%
edema	1.8%	Flushing	0.6%
Fatigue	1.7%		

Elevated liver enzymes (see *Warnings*)

In clinical trials related to the control of ventricular response in digitalized patients who had atrial fibrillation or flutter, ventricular rates below 50 at rest occurred in 15% of patients and asymptomatic hypotension occurred in 5% of patients.
The following reactions, reported in 1.0% or less of patients, occurred under conditions (open trials, marketing experience) where a causal relationship is uncertain; they are listed to alert the physician to a possible relationship:
Cardiovascular: angina pectoris, atrioventricular dissociation, chest pain, claudication, myocardial infarction, palpitations, purpura (vasculitis), syncope.
Digestive system: diarrhea, dry mouth, gastrointestinal distress, gingival hyperplasia.
Hemic and lymphatic: ecchymosis or bruising.
Nervous system: cerebrovascular accident, confusion, equilibrium disorders, insomnia, muscle cramps, paresthesia, psychotic symptoms, shakiness, somnolence.
Skin: arthralgia and rash, exanthema, hair loss, hyperkeratosis, macules, sweating, urticaria, Stevens-Johnson syndrome, erythema multiforme.
Special senses: blurred vision.
Urogenital: gynecomastia, increased urination, spotty menstruation, impotence.
Treatment of acute cardiovascular adverse reactions: The frequency of cardiovascular adverse reactions that require therapy is rare; hence, experience with their treatment is limited. Whenever severe hypotension or complete AV block occurs following oral administration of verapamil, the appropriate emergency measures should be applied immediately; eg, intravenously administered norepinephrine bitartrate, atropine sulfate, isoproterenol HCl (all in the usual doses), or calcium gluconate (10% solution). In patients with hypertrophic cardiomyopathy (IHSS), alpha-adrenergic agents (phenylephrine HCl, metaraminol bitartrate, or methoxamine HCl) should be used to maintain blood pressure, and isoproterenol and norepinephrine should be avoided. If further support is necessary, dopamine HCl or dobutamine HCl may be administered. Actual treatment and dosage should depend on the severity of the clinical situation and the judgment and experience of the treating physician.

OVERDOSAGE

Treatment of overdosage should be supportive. Beta-adrenergic stimulation or parenteral administration of calcium solutions may increase calcium ion flux across the slow channel, and have been used effectively in treatment of deliberate overdosage with verapamil. Verapamil cannot be removed by hemodialysis. Clinically significant hypotensive reactions or fixed high-degree AV block should be treated with vasopressor agents or cardiac pacing, respectively. Asystole should be handled by the usual measures, including cardiopulmonary resuscitation.

DOSAGE AND ADMINISTRATION

The dose of verapamil must be individualized by titration. The usefulness and safety of dosages exceeding 480 mg/day have not been established; therefore, this daily dosage should not be exceeded. Since the half-life of verapamil increases during chronic dosing, maximum response may be delayed.
Angina: Clinical trials show that the usual dose is 80 mg to 120 mg three times a day. However, 40 mg three times a day may be warranted in patients who may have an increased response to verapamil (eg, decreased hepatic function, elderly, etc). Upward titration should be based on therapeutic efficacy and safety evaluated approximately eight hours after dosing. Dosage may be increased at daily (eg, patients with unstable angina) or weekly intervals until optimum clinical response is obtained.
Arrhythmias: The dosage in digitalized patients with chronic atrial fibrillation (see *Precautions*) ranges from 240 to 320 mg/day in divided (t.i.d. or q.i.d.) doses. The dosage for prophylaxis of PSVT (non-digitalized patients) ranges from 240 to 480 mg/day in divided (t.i.d or q.i.d.) doses. In general, maximum effects for any given dosage will be apparent during the first 48 hours of therapy.
Essential hypertension: Dose should be individualized by titration. The usual initial monotherapy dose in clinical trials was 80 mg three times a day (240 mg/day). Daily dosages of 360 and 480 mg have been used but there is no evidence that dosages beyond 360 mg provided added effect. Consideration should be given to beginning titration at 40 mg three times per day in patients who might respond to lower doses, such as the elderly or people of small stature. The antihypertensive effects of Calan are evident within the first week of therapy. Upward titration should be based on therapeutic efficacy, assessed at the end of the dosing interval.

HOW SUPPLIED

Calan 40-mg tablets are round, pink, film coated, with CALAN debossed on one side and 40 on the other, supplied as:

NDC Number	Size
0014-1771-31	bottle of 100

Calan 80-mg tablets are oval, peach colored, scored, film coated, with CALAN debossed on one side and 80 on the other, supplied as:

NDC Number	Size
0014-1851-31	bottle of 100
0014-1851-51	bottle of 500
0014-1851-52	bottle of 1,000
0014-1851-34	carton of 100 unit dose

Calan 120-mg tablets are oval, brown, scored, film coated, with CALAN 120 debossed on one side, supplied as:

NDC Number	Size
0014-1861-31	bottle of 100
0014-1861-51	bottle of 500
0014-1861-52	bottle of 1,000
0014-1861-34	carton of 100 unit dose

Store at 59° to 86°F (15° to 30°C) and protect from light. Dispense in tight, light-resistant containers.
Caution: Federal law prohibits dispensing without prescription.

A05295-2

Shown in Product Identification Section, page 429

CALAN® SR   ℞
[cal'an ess ar]
(verapamil hydrochloride)
Sustained-Release Oral Caplets

PRODUCT OVERVIEW

KEY FACTS
Calan SR, a calcium ion antagonist designed for sustained-release in the gastrointestinal tract, exerts an antihypertensive effect by decreasing systemic vascular resistance, usually without orthostatic decreases in blood pressure or reflex tachycardia.

Continued on next page

G.D. Searle & Co.—Cont.

MAJOR USE
Calan SR is indicated for the management of essential hypertension.

SAFETY INFORMATION
See complete safety information set forth below.

<u>PRESCRIBING INFORMATION</u>

CALAN® SR   ℞
[cal'an ess ar]
(verapamil hydrochloride)
Sustained-Release Oral Caplets

DESCRIPTION
Calan SR (verapamil hydrochloride) is a calcium ion influx inhibitor (slow-channel blocker or calcium ion antagonist). Calan SR is available for oral administration as light green, capsule-shaped, scored, film-coated tablets (caplets) containing 240 mg of verapamil hydrochloride. The caplets are designed for sustained release of the drug in the gastrointestinal tract; sustained-release characteristics are not altered when the caplet is divided in half.
The structural formula of verapamil HCl is

$C_{27}H_{38}N_2O_4 \cdot HCl$ M.W.= 491.08

Benzeneacetonitrile, α-[3-[[2-(3, 4-dimethoxyphenyl)
ethyl] methylamino]propyl]-3,4-dimethoxy-α-
(1-methylethyl) hydrochloride

Verapamil HCl is an almost white, crystalline powder, practically free of odor, with a bitter taste. It is soluble in water, chloroform, and methanol. Verapamil HCl is not chemically related to other cardioactive drugs.
Inactive ingredients include alginate, carnauba wax, D&C Yellow No. 10 Lake, FD&C Blue No. 2 Lake, hydroxypropyl methylcellulose, magnesium stearate, microcrystalline cellulose, polyethylene glycol, talc, and titanium dioxide.

CLINICAL PHARMACOLOGY
Calan (verapamil HCl) is a calcium ion influx inhibitor (slow-channel blocker or calcium ion antagonist) that exerts its pharmacologic effects by modulating the influx of ionic calcium across the cell membrane of the arterial smooth muscle as well as in conductile and contractile myocardial cells.
Mechanism of action
Essential hypertension: Verapamil exerts antihypertensive effects by decreasing systemic vascular resistance, usually without orthostatic decreases in blood pressure or reflex tachycardia; bradycardia (rate less than 50 beats/min) is uncommon (1.4%). During isometric or dynamic exercise Calan does not alter systolic cardiac function in patients with normal ventricular function.
Calan does not alter total serum calcium levels. However, one report suggested that calcium levels above the normal range may alter the therapeutic effect of Calan.
Other pharmacologic actions of Calan include the following:
Calan dilates the main coronary arteries and coronary arterioles, both in normal and ischemic regions, and is a potent inhibitor of coronary artery spasm, whether spontaneous or ergonovine-induced. This property increases myocardial oxygen delivery in patients with coronary artery spasm and is responsible for the effectiveness of Calan in vasospastic (Prinzmetal's or variant) as well as unstable angina at rest. Whether this effect plays any role in classical effort angina is not clear, but studies of exercise tolerance have not shown an increase in the maximum exercise rate–pressure product, a widely accepted measure of oxygen utilization. This suggests that, in general, relief of spasm or dilation of coronary arteries is not an important factor in classical angina.
Calan regularly reduces the total systemic resistance (afterload) against which the heart works both at rest and at a given level of exercise by dilating peripheral arterioles. Electrical activity through the AV node depends, to a significant degree, upon calcium influx through the slow channel. By decreasing the influx of calcium, Calan prolongs the effective refractory period within the AV node and slows AV conduction in a rate-related manner.
Normal sinus rhythm is usually not affected, but in patients with sick sinus syndrome, Calan may interfere with sinus-node impulse generation and may induce sinus arrest or sinoatrial block. Atrioventricular block can occur in patients without preexisting conduction defects (see *Warnings*).
Calan does not alter the normal atrial action potential or intraventricular conduction time, but depresses amplitude, velocity of depolarization, and conduction in depressed atrial fibers. Calan may shorten the antegrade effective refractory period of the accessory bypass tract.

Acceleration of ventricular rate and/or ventricular fibrillation has been reported in patients with atrial flutter or atrial fibrillation and a coexisting accessory AV pathway following administration of verapamil (see *Warnings*).
Calan has a local anesthetic action that is 1.6 times that of procaine on an equimolar basis. It is not known whether this action is important at the doses used in man.
Pharmacokinetics and metabolism: With the immediate-release formulation, more than 90% of the orally administered dose of Calan is absorbed. Because of rapid biotransformation of verapamil during its first pass through the portal circulation, bioavailability ranges from 20% to 35%. Peak plasma concentrations are reached between 1 and 2 hours after oral administration. Chronic oral administration of 120 mg of verapamil HCl every 6 hours resulted in plasma levels of verapamil ranging from 125 to 400 ng/ml, with higher values reported occasionally. A nonlinear correlation between the verapamil dose administered and verapamil plasma level does exist. In early dose titration with verapamil a relationship exists between verapamil plasma concentration and prolongation of the PR interval. However, during chronic administration this relationship may disappear. The mean elimination half-life in single-dose studies ranged from 2.8 to 7.4 hours. In these same studies, after repetitive dosing, the half-life increased to a range from 4.5 to 12.0 hours (after less than 10 consecutive doses given 6 hours apart). Half-life of verapamil may increase during titration. Aging may affect the pharmacokinetics of verapamil. Elimination half-life may be prolonged in the elderly. In multiple-dose studies under fasting conditions, the bioavailability, measured by AUC, of Calan SR was similar to Calan (immediate release); rates of absorption were of course different.
In a randomized, single-dose, crossover study using healthy volunteers, administration of 240 mg Calan SR with food produced peak plasma verapamil concentrations of 79 ng/ml; time to peak plasma verapamil concentration of 7.71 hours; and AUC (0–24 hr) of 841 ng·hr/ml). When Calan SR was administered to fasting subjects, peak plasma verapamil concentration was 164 ng/ml; time to peak plasma verapamil concentration was 5.21 hours; and AUC (0–24 hr) was 1,478 ng·hr/ml. Similar results were demonstrated for plasma norverapamil. Food thus produces decreased bioavailability (AUC) but a narrower peak-to-trough ratio. Good correlation of dose and response is not available, but controlled studies of Calan SR have shown effectiveness of doses similar to the effective doses of Calan (immediate release).
In hypertensive patients, plasma verapamil levels are not related to antihypertensive efficacy at the dosages usually administered (240 to 480 mg/day).
In healthy men, orally administered Calan undergoes extensive metabolism in the liver. Twelve metabolites have been identified in plasma; all except norverapamil are present in trace amounts only. Norverapamil can reach steady-state plasma concentrations approximately equal to those of verapamil itself. The cardiovascular activity of norverapamil appears to be approximately 20% that of verapamil. Approximately 70% of an administered dose is excreted as metabolites in the urine and 16% or more in the feces within 5 days. About 3% to 4% is excreted in the urine as unchanged drug. Approximately 90% is bound to plasma proteins. In patients with hepatic insufficiency, metabolism of immediate-release verapamil is delayed and elimination half-life prolonged up to 14 to 16 hours (see *Precautions*); the volume of distribution is increased and plasma clearance reduced to about 30% of normal. Verapamil clearance values suggest that patients with liver dysfunction may attain therapeutic verapamil plasma concentrations with one third of the oral daily dose required for patients with normal liver function.
After four weeks of oral dosing (120 mg q.i.d.), verapamil and norverapamil levels were noted in the cerebrospinal fluid with estimated partition coefficient of 0.06 for verapamil and 0.04 for norverapamil.
Hemodynamics and myocardial metabolism: Calan reduces afterload and myocardial contractility. Improved left ventricular diastolic function in patients with IHSS and those with coronary heart disease has also been observed with Calan. In most patients, including those with organic cardiac disease, the negative inotropic action of Calan is countered by reduction of afterload, and cardiac index is usually not reduced. However, in patients with severe left ventricular dysfunction (eg, pulmonary wedge pressure above 20 mm Hg or ejection fraction less than 30%), or in patients taking beta-adrenergic blocking agents or other cardiodepressant drugs, deterioration of ventricular function may occur (see *Drug interactions*).
Pulmonary function: Calan does not induce bronchoconstriction and, hence, does not impair ventilatory function.

INDICATIONS AND USAGE
Calan SR is indicated for the management of essential hypertension.

CONTRAINDICATIONS
Verapamil HCl caplets are contraindicated in:
1. Severe left ventricular dysfunction (see *Warnings*)
2. Hypotension (systolic pressure less than 90 mm Hg) or cardiogenic shock
3. Sick sinus syndrome (except in patients with a functioning artificial ventricular pacemaker)
4. Second- or third-degree AV block (except in patients with a functioning artificial ventricular pacemaker)
5. Patients with atrial flutter or atrial fibrillation and an accessory bypass tract (eg, Wolff-Parkinson-White, Lown-Ganong-Levine syndromes). (See *Warnings*.)
6. Patients with known hypersensitivity to verapamil hydrochloride.

WARNINGS
Heart failure: Verapamil has a negative inotropic effect, which in most patients is compensated by its afterload reduction (decreased systemic vascular resistance) properties without a net impairment of ventricular performance. In clinical experience with 4,954 patients, 87 (1.8%) developed congestive heart failure or pulmonary edema. Verapamil should be avoided in patients with severe left ventricular dysfunction (eg, ejection fraction less than 30%) or moderate to severe symptoms of cardiac failure and in patients with any degree of ventricular dysfunction if they are receiving a beta-adrenergic blocker (see *Drug interactions*). Patients with milder ventricular dysfunction should, if possible, be controlled with optimum doses of digitalis and/or diuretics before verapamil treatment. **(Note interactions with digoxin under** *Precautions.***)**
Hypotension: Occasionally, the pharmacologic action of verapamil may produce a decrease in blood pressure below normal levels, which may result in dizziness or symptomatic hypotension. The incidence of hypotension observed in 4,954 patients enrolled in clinical trials was 2.5%. In hypertensive patients, decreases in blood pressure below normal are unusual. Tilt-table testing (60 degrees) was not able to induce orthostatic hypotension.
Elevated liver enzymes: Elevations of transaminases with and without concomitant elevations in alkaline phosphatase and bilirubin have been reported. Such elevations have sometimes been transient and may disappear even in the face of continued verapamil treatment. Several cases of hepatocellular injury related to verapamil have been proven by rechallenge; half of these had clinical symptoms (malaise, fever, and/or right upper quadrant pain) in addition to elevation of SGOT, SGPT, and alkaline phosphatase. Periodic monitoring of liver function in patients receiving verapamil is therefore prudent.
Accessory bypass tract (Wolff-Parkinson-White or Lown-Ganong-Levine): Some patients with paroxysmal and/or chronic atrial fibrillation or atrial flutter and a coexisting accessory AV pathway have developed increased antegrade conduction across the accessory pathway bypassing the AV node, producing a very rapid ventricular response or ventricular fibrillation after receiving intravenous verapamil (or digitalis). Although a risk of this occurring with oral verapamil has not been established, such patients receiving oral verapamil may be at risk and its use in these patients is contraindicated (see *Contraindications*). Treatment is usually DC-cardioversion. Cardioversion has been used safely and effectively after oral Calan.
Atrioventricular block: The effect of verapamil on AV conduction and the SA node may cause asymptomatic first-degree AV block and transient bradycardia, sometimes accompanied by nodal escape rhythms. PR-interval prolongation is correlated with verapamil plasma concentrations, especially during the early titration phase of therapy. Higher degrees of AV block, however, were infrequently (0.8%) observed. Marked first-degree block or progressive development to second- or third-degree AV block requires a reduction in dosage or, in rare instances, discontinuation of verapamil HCl and institution of appropriate therapy, depending upon the clinical situation.
Patients with hypertrophic cardiomyopathy (IHSS): In 120 patients with hypertrophic cardiomyopathy (most of them refractory or intolerant to propranolol) who received therapy with verapamil at doses up to 720 mg/day, a variety of serious adverse effects was seen. Three patients died in pulmonary edema; all had severe left ventricular outflow obstruction and a past history of left ventricular dysfunction. Eight other patients had pulmonary edema and/or severe hypotension; abnormally high (greater than 20 mm Hg) pulmonary wedge pressure and a marked left ventricular outflow obstruction were present in most of these patients. Concomitant administration of quinidine (see *Drug interactions*) preceded the severe hypotension in 3 of the 8 patients (2 of whom developed pulmonary edema). Sinus bradycardia occurred in 11% of the patients, second-degree AV block in 4%, and sinus arrest in 2%. It must be appreciated that this group of patients had a serious disease with a high mortality rate. Most adverse effects responded well to dose reduction, and only rarely did verapamil use have to be discontinued.

PRECAUTIONS

General

Use in patients with impaired hepatic function: Since verapamil is highly metabolized by the liver, it should be administered cautiously to patients with impaired hepatic function. Severe liver dysfunction prolongs the elimination half-life of immediate-release verapamil to about 14 to 16 hours; hence, approximately 30% of the dose given to patients with normal liver function should be administered to these patients. Careful monitoring for abnormal prolongation of the PR interval or other signs of excessive pharmacologic effects (see *Overdosage*) should be carried out.

Use in patients with attenuated (decreased) neuromuscular transmission: It has been reported that verapamil decreases neuromuscular transmission in patients with Duchenne's muscular dystrophy, and that verapamil prolongs recovery from the neuromuscular blocking agent vecuronium. It may be necessary to decrease the dosage of verapamil when it is administered to patients with attenuated neuromuscular transmission.

Use in patients with impaired renal function: About 70% of an administered dose of verapamil is excreted as metabolites in the urine. Verapamil is not removed by hemodialysis. Until further data are available, verapamil should be administered cautiously to patients with impaired renal function. These patients should be carefully monitored for abnormal prolongation of the PR interval or other signs of overdosage (see *Overdosage*).

Drug interactions

Beta-blockers: Concomitant therapy with beta-adrenergic blockers and verapamil may result in additive negative effects on heart rate, atrioventricular conduction and/or cardiac contractility. The combination of sustained-release verapamil and beta-adrenergic blocking agents has not been studied. However, there have been reports of excessive bradycardia and AV block, including complete heart block, when the combination has been used for the treatment of hypertension. For hypertensive patients, the risks of combined therapy may outweigh the potential benefits. The combination should be used only with caution and close monitoring.

Asymptomatic bradycardia (36 beats/min) with a wandering atrial pacemaker has been observed in a patient receiving concomitant timolol (a beta-adrenergic blocker) eyedrops and oral verapamil.

A decrease in metoprolol clearance has been observed when verapamil and metoprolol were administered together. A similar effect has not been seen when verapamil and atenolol were given together.

Digitalis: Clinical use of verapamil in digitalized patients has shown the combination to be well tolerated if digoxin doses are properly adjusted. However, chronic verapamil treatment can increase serum digoxin levels by 50% to 75% during the first week of therapy, and this can result in digitalis toxicity. In patients with hepatic cirrhosis the influence of verapamil on digoxin kinetics is magnified. Verapamil may reduce total body clearance and extrarenal clearance of digitoxin by 27% and 29%, respectively. Maintenance digitalis doses should be reduced when verapamil is administered, and the patient should be carefully monitored to avoid over- or underdigitalization. Whenever overdigitalization is suspected, the daily dose of digitalis should be reduced or temporarily discontinued. On discontinuation of Calan use, the patient should be reassessed to avoid underdigitalization.

Antihypertensive agents: Verapamil administered concomitantly with oral antihypertensive agents (eg, vasodilators, angiotensin-converting enzyme inhibitors, diuretics, beta-blockers) will usually have an additive effect on lowering blood pressure. Patients receiving these combinations should be appropriately monitored. Concomitant use of agents that attenuate alpha-adrenergic function with verapamil may result in a reduction in blood pressure that is excessive in some patients. Such an effect was observed in one study following the concomitant administration of verapamil and prazosin.

Antiarrhythmic agents:

Disopyramide: Until data on possible interactions between verapamil and disopyramide phosphate are obtained, disopyramide should not be administered within 48 hours before or 24 hours after verapamil administration.

Flecainide: A study in healthy volunteers showed that the concomitant administration of flecainide and verapamil may have additive effects on myocardial contractility, AV conduction, and repolarization. Concomitant therapy with flecainide and verapamil may result in additive negative inotropic effect and prolongation of atrioventricular conduction.

Quinidine: In a small number of patients with hypertrophic cardiomyopathy (IHSS), concomitant use of verapamil and quinidine resulted in significant hypotension. Until further data are obtained, combined therapy of verapamil and quinidine in patients with hypertrophic cardiomyopathy should probably be avoided.

The electrophysiologic effects of quinidine and verapamil on AV conduction were studied in 8 patients. Verapamil significantly counteracted the effects of quinidine on AV conduction. There has been a report of increased quinidine levels during verapamil therapy.

Other:

Nitrates: Verapamil has been given concomitantly with short- and long-acting nitrates without any undesirable drug interactions. The pharmacologic profile of both drugs and the clinical experience suggest beneficial interactions.

Cimetidine: The interaction between cimetidine and chronically administered verapamil has not been studied. Variable results on clearance have been obtained in acute studies of healthy volunteers; clearance of verapamil was either reduced or unchanged.

Lithium: Pharmacokinetic and pharmacodynamic interactions between oral verapamil and lithium have been reported. The former may result in a lowering of serum lithium levels in patients receiving chronic stable oral lithium therapy. The latter may result in an increased sensitivity to the effects of lithium. Patients receiving both drugs must be monitored carefully.

Carbamazepine: Verapamil therapy may increase carbamazepine concentrations during combined therapy. This may produce carbamazepine side effects such as diplopia, headache, ataxia, or dizziness.

Rifampin: Therapy with rifampin may markedly reduce oral verapamil bioavailability.

Phenobarbital: Phenobarbital therapy may increase verapamil clearance.

Cyclosporin: Verapamil therapy may increase serum levels of cyclosporin.

Inhalation anesthetics: Animal experiments have shown that inhalation anesthetics depress cardiovascular activity by decreasing the inward movement of calcium ions. When used concomitantly, inhalation anesthetics and calcium antagonists, such as verapamil, should each be titrated carefully to avoid excessive cardiovascular depression.

Neuromuscular blocking agents: Clinical data and animal studies suggest that verapamil may potentiate the activity of neuromuscular blocking agents (curare-like and depolarizing). It may be necessary to decrease the dose of verapamil and/or the dose of the neuromuscular blocking agent when the drugs are used concomitantly.

Carcinogenesis, mutagenesis, impairment of fertility: An 18-month toxicity study in rats, at a low multiple (6-fold) of the maximum recommended human dose, and not the maximum tolerated dose, did not suggest a tumorigenic potential. There was no evidence of a carcinogenic potential of verapamil administered in the diet of rats for two years at doses of 10, 35, and 120 mg/kg/day or approximately 1, 3.5, and 12 times, respectively, the maximum recommended human daily dose (480 mg/day or 9.6 mg/kg/day).

Verapamil was not mutagenic in the Ames test in 5 test strains at 3 mg per plate with or without metabolic activation.

Studies in female rats at daily dietary doses up to 5.5 times (55 mg/kg/day) the maximum recommended human dose did not show impaired fertility. Effects on male fertility have not been determined.

Pregnancy: Pregnancy Category C. Reproduction studies have been performed in rabbits and rats at oral doses up to 1.5 (15 mg/kg/day) and 6 (60 mg/kg/day) times the human oral daily dose, respectively, and have revealed no evidence of teratogenicity. In the rat, however, this multiple of the human dose was embryocidal and retarded fetal growth and development, probably because of adverse maternal effects reflected in reduced weight gains of the dams. This oral dose has also been shown to cause hypotension in rats. There are no adequate and well-controlled studies in pregnant women. Because animal reproduction studies are not always predictive of human response, this drug should be used during pregnancy only if clearly needed. Verapamil crosses the placental barrier and can be detected in umbilical vein blood at delivery.

Labor and delivery: It is not known whether the use of verapamil during labor or delivery has immediate or delayed adverse effects on the fetus, or whether it prolongs the duration of labor or increases the need for forceps delivery or other obstetric intervention. Such adverse experiences have not been reported in the literature, despite a long history of use of verapamil in Europe in the treatment of cardiac side effects of beta-adrenergic agonist agents used to treat premature labor.

Nursing mothers: Verapamil is excreted in human milk. Because of the potential for adverse reactions in nursing infants from verapamil, nursing should be discontinued while verapamil is administered.

Pediatric use: Safety and efficacy of Calan SR in children below the age of 18 years have not been established.

Animal pharmacology and/or animal toxicology: In chronic animal toxicology studies verapamil caused lenticular and/or suture line changes at 30 mg/kg/day or greater, and frank cataracts at 62.5 mg/kg/day or greater in the beagle dog but not in the rat. Development of cataracts due to verapamil has not been reported in man.

ADVERSE REACTIONS

Serious adverse reactions are uncommon when verapamil therapy is initiated with upward dose titration within the recommended single and total daily dose. See *Warnings* for discussion of heart failure, hypotension, elevated liver enzymes, AV block, and rapid ventricular response. The following reactions to orally administered verapamil occurred at rates greater than 1.0% or occurred at lower rates but appeared clearly drug-related in clinical trials in 4,954 patients:

Constipation	7.3%	Dyspnea	1.4%
Dizziness	3.3%	Bradycardia	
Nausea	2.7%	(HR < 50/min)	1.4%
Hypotension	2.5%	AV block	
Headache	2.2%	total 1°, 2°, 3°	1.2%
Edema	1.9%	2° and 3°	0.8%
CHF, Pulmonary		Rash	1.2%
edema	1.8%	Flushing	0.6%
Fatigue	1.7%		

Elevated liver enzymes (see *Warnings*)

In clinical trials related to the control of ventricular response in digitalized patients who had atrial fibrillation or flutter, ventricular rates below 50/min at rest occurred in 15% of patients and asymptomatic hypotension occurred in 5% of patients.

The following reactions, reported in 1% or less of patients, occurred under conditions (open trials, marketing experience) where a causal relationship is uncertain; they are listed to alert the physician to a possible relationship:

Cardiovascular: angina pectoris, atrioventricular dissociation, chest pain, claudication, myocardial infarction, palpitations, purpura (vasculitis), syncope.

Digestive system: diarrhea, dry mouth, gastrointestinal distress, gingival hyperplasia.

Hemic and lymphatic: ecchymosis or bruising.

Nervous system: cerebrovascular accident, confusion, equilibrium disorders, insomnia, muscle cramps, paresthesia, psychotic symptoms, shakiness, somnolence.

Skin: arthralgia and rash, exanthema, hair loss, hyperkeratosis, macules, sweating, urticaria, Stevens-Johnson syndrome, erythema multiforme.

Special senses: blurred vision.

Urogenital: gynecomastia, increased urination, spotty menstruation, impotence.

Treatment of acute cardiovascular adverse reactions: The frequency of cardiovascular adverse reactions that require therapy is rare; hence, experience with their treatment is limited. Whenever severe hypotension or complete AV block occurs following oral administration of verapamil, the appropriate emergency measures should be applied immediately; eg, intravenously administered norepinephrine bitartrate, atropine sulfate, isoproterenol HCl (all in the usual doses), or calcium gluconate (10% solution). In patients with hypertrophic cardiomyopathy (IHSS), alpha-adrenergic agents (phenylephrine HCl, metaraminol bitartrate, or methoxamine HCl) should be used to maintain blood pressure, and isoproterenol and norepinephrine should be avoided. If further support is necessary, dopamine HCl or dobutamine HCl may be administered. Actual treatment and dosage should depend on the severity of the clinical situation and the judgment and experience of the treating physician.

OVERDOSAGE

Treatment of overdosage should be supportive. Beta-adrenergic stimulation or parenteral administration of calcium solutions may increase calcium ion flux across the slow channel, and have been used effectively in treatment of deliberate overdosage with verapamil. Verapamil cannot be removed by hemodialysis. Clinically significant hypotensive reactions or fixed high-degree AV block should be treated with vasopressor agents or cardiac pacing, respectively. Asystole should be handled by the usual measures, including cardiopulmonary resuscitation.

DOSAGE AND ADMINISTRATION

Essential hypertension: The dose of Calan SR should be individualized by titration and the drug should be administered with food. The usual daily dose of sustained-release verapamil HCl in clinical trials has been 240 mg given by mouth once daily in the morning. However, 120 mg (½ caplet) a day may be warranted in patients who may have an increased response to verapamil (eg, the elderly or small people). Upward titration should be based on therapeutic efficacy and safety evaluated approximately 24 hours after dosing. The antihypertensive effects of verapamil are evident within the first week of therapy.

If adequate response is not obtained, the dose may be titrated upward in the following manner:

  a) 240 mg (1 caplet) each morning,

  b) 240 mg (1 caplet) each morning plus 120 mg (½ caplet) each evening,

  c) 240 mg (1 caplet) every twelve hours.

Continued on next page

G.D. Searle & Co.—Cont.

When switching from immediate-release Calan to Calan SR the total daily dose in milligrams may remain the same.

HOW SUPPLIED

Calan SR 240-mg caplets are light green, capsule shaped, scored, film coated, with CALAN debossed on one side and SR 240 on the other, supplied as:

NDC Number	Size
0014-1891-31	bottle of 100
0014-1891-34	carton of 100 unit dose

Store at 59° to 86°F (15° to 30°C) and protect from light and moisture. Dispense in tight, light-resistant containers.

Caution: Federal law prohibits dispensing without prescription.

Manufactured for Searle & Co.

A05290-3

Shown in Product Identification Section, page 429

CYTOTEC® ℞
[sī-tō-tĕc]
(misoprostol)

CONTRAINDICATIONS AND WARNINGS

Cytotec (misoprostol) is contraindicated, because of its abortifacient property, in women who are pregnant. (See *Precautions.*) Patients must be advised of the abortifacient property and warned not to give the drug to others. Cytotec should not be used in women of childbearing potential unless the patient requires nonsteroidal anti-inflammatory drug (NSAID) therapy and is at high risk of complications from gastric ulcers associated with use of the NSAID, or is at high risk of developing gastric ulceration. In such patients, Cytotec may be prescribed if the patient

- is capable of complying with effective contraceptive measures.
- has received both oral and written warnings of the hazards of misoprostol, the risk of possible contraception failure, and the danger to other women of childbearing potential should the drug be taken by mistake.
- has had a negative *serum* pregnancy test within two weeks prior to beginning therapy.
- will begin Cytotec only on the second or third day of the next normal menstrual period.

DESCRIPTION

Cytotec oral tablets contain 200 mcg of misoprostol, a synthetic prostaglandin E_1 analog.

Misoprostol contains approximately equal amounts of the two diastereomers presented below with their enantiomers indicated by (±):

$C_{22}H_{38}O_5$ M.W. = 382.5
(±)methyl 11α, 16-dihydroxy-16-methyl-9-oxoprost-13E-en-1-oate

Misoprostol is a water-soluble, viscous liquid.

Inactive ingredients of tablets are hydrogenated castor oil, hydroxypropyl methylcellulose, microcrystalline cellulose, and sodium starch glycolate.

CLINICAL PHARMACOLOGY

Pharmacokinetics: Misoprostol is extensively absorbed, and undergoes rapid de-esterification to its free acid, which is responsible for its clinical activity and, unlike the parent compound, is detectable in plasma. The alpha side chain undergoes beta oxidation and the beta side chain undergoes omega oxidation followed by reduction of the ketone to give prostaglandin F analogs.

In normal volunteers, Cytotec (misoprostol) is rapidly absorbed after oral administration with a T_{max} of misoprostol

---

acid of 12 ± 3 minutes and a terminal half-life of 20–40 minutes.

There is high variability of plasma levels of misoprostol acid between and within studies but mean values after single doses show a linear relationship with dose over the range of 200–400 mcg. No accumulation of misoprostol acid was noted in multiple dose studies; plasma steady state was achieved within two days.

Maximum plasma concentrations of misoprostol acid are diminished when the dose is taken with food and total availability of misoprostol acid is reduced by use of concomitant antacid. Clinical trials were conducted with concomitant antacid, however, so this effect does not appear to be clinically important.

Mean ± SD	C_{max}(pg/ml)	AUC (0-4) (pg·hr/ml)	T_{max}(min)
Fasting	811 ± 317	417 ± 135	14 ± 8
With Antacid	689 ± 315	349 ± 108*	20 ± 14
With High Fat Breakfast	303 ± 176*	373 ± 111	64 ± 79*

*Comparisons with fasting results statistically significant, $p < 0.05$.

After oral administration of radiolabeled misoprostol, about 80% of detected radioactivity appears in urine. Pharmacokinetic studies in patients with varying degrees of renal impairment showed an approximate doubling of $T_{1/2}$, C_{max}, and AUC compared to normals, but no clear correlation between the degree of impairment and AUC. In subjects over 64 years of age, the AUC for misoprostol acid is increased. No routine dosage adjustment is recommended in older patients or patients with renal impairment, but dosage may need to be reduced if the usual dose is not tolerated.

Cytotec does not affect the hepatic mixed function oxidase (cytochrome P-450) enzyme systems in animals.

Drug interaction studies between misoprostol and several nonsteroidal anti-inflammatory drugs showed no effect on the kinetics of ibuprofen or diclofenac, and a 20% decrease in aspirin AUC, not thought to be clinically significant.

Pharmacokinetic studies also showed a lack of drug interaction with antipyrine and propranolol when these drugs were given with misoprostol. Misoprostol given for one week had no effect on the steady state pharmacokinetics of diazepam when the two drugs were administered two hours apart.

The serum protein binding of misoprostol acid is less than 90% and is concentration-independent in the therapeutic range.

Pharmacodynamics: Misoprostol has both antisecretory (inhibiting gastric acid secretion) and (in animals) mucosal protective properties. NSAIDs inhibit prostaglandin synthesis, and a deficiency of prostaglandins within the gastric mucosa may lead to diminishing bicarbonate and mucus secretion and may contribute to the mucosal damage caused by these agents. Misoprostol can increase bicarbonate and mucus production, but in man this has been shown at doses 200 mcg and above that are also antisecretory. It is therefore not possible to tell whether the ability of misoprostol to prevent gastric ulcer is the result of its antisecretory effect, its mucosal protective effect, or both.

In vitro studies on canine parietal cells using tritiated misoprostol acid as the ligand have led to the identification and characterization of specific prostaglandin receptors. Receptor binding is saturable, reversible, and stereospecific. The sites have a high affinity for misoprostol, for its acid metabolite, and for other E type prostaglandins, but not for F or I prostaglandins and other unrelated compounds, such as histamine or cimetidine. Receptor-site affinity for misoprostol correlates well with an indirect index of antisecretory activity. It is likely that these specific receptors allow misoprostol taken with food to be effective topically, despite the lower serum concentrations attained.

Misoprostol produces a moderate decrease in pepsin concentration during basal conditions, but not during histamine stimulation. It has no significant effect on fasting or postprandial gastrin nor on intrinsic factor output.

Effects on gastric acid secretion: Misoprostol, over the range of 50–200 mcg, inhibits basal and nocturnal gastric acid secretion, and acid secretion in response to a variety of stimuli, including meals, histamine, pentagastrin, and coffee. Activity is apparent 30 minutes after oral administration and persists for at least 3 hours. In general, the effects of 50 mcg were modest and shorter lived, and only the 200-mcg dose had substantial effects on nocturnal secretion or on histamine and meal-stimulated secretion.

Uterine effects: Cytotec has been shown to produce uterine contractions that may endanger pregnancy. (See *Contraindications* and *Warnings.*) In studies in women undergoing elective termination of pregnancy during the first trimester, Cytotec caused partial or complete expulsion of the uterine contents in 11% of the subjects and increased uterine bleeding in 41%.

Other pharmacologic effects: Cytotec does not produce clinically significant effects on serum levels of prolactin, gonadotropins, thyroid-stimulating hormone, growth hor-

---

mone, thyroxine, cortisol, gastrointestinal hormones (somatostatin, gastrin, vasoactive intestinal polypeptide, and motilin), creatinine, or uric acid. Gastric emptying, immunologic competence, platelet aggregation, pulmonary function, or the cardiovascular system are not modified by recommended doses of Cytotec.

Clinical studies: In a series of small short-term (about one week) placebo-controlled studies in healthy human volunteers, doses of misoprostol were evaluated for their ability to prevent NSAID-induced mucosal injury. Studies of 200 mcg q.i.d. of misoprostol with tolmetin and naproxen, and of 100 and 200 mcg q.i.d. with ibuprofen, all showed reduction of the rate of significant endoscopic injury from about 70–75% on placebo to 10–30% on misoprostol. Doses of 25–200 mcg q.i.d. reduced aspirin-induced mucosal injury and bleeding.

Preventing gastric ulcers caused by nonsteroidal anti-inflammatory drugs (NSAIDs): Two 12-week, randomized, double-blind trials in osteoarthritic patients who had gastrointestinal symptoms but no ulcer on endoscopy while taking an NSAID compared the ability of 200 mcg of Cytotec, 100 mcg of Cytotec, and placebo to prevent gastric ulcer (GU) formation. Patients were approximately equally divided between ibuprofen, piroxicam, and naproxen, and continued this treatment throughout the 12 weeks. The 200-mcg dose caused a marked, statistically significant reduction in gastric ulcers in both studies. The lower dose was somewhat less effective, with a significant result in only one of the studies. [See table on next page].

In these trials there were no significant differences between Cytotec and placebo in relief of day or night abdominal pain. No effects of Cytotec in preventing duodenal ulcers was demonstrated, but relatively few duodenal lesions were seen.

In another clinical trial, 239 patients receiving aspirin 650–1300 mg q.i.d. for rheumatoid arthritis and who had endoscopic evidence of duodenal and/or gastric inflammation were randomized to misoprostol 200 mcg q.i.d. or placebo for eight weeks while continuing to receive aspirin. The study evaluated the possible interference of Cytotec on the efficacy of aspirin in these patients with rheumatoid arthritis by analyzing joint tenderness, joint swelling, physician's clinical assessment, patient's assessment, change in ARA classification, change in handgrip strength, change in duration of morning stiffness, patient's assessment of pain at rest, movement, interference with daily activity, and ESR. Cytotec did not interfere with the efficacy of aspirin in these patients with rheumatoid arthritis.

INDICATIONS AND USAGE

Cytotec (misoprostol) is indicated for the prevention of NSAID (nonsteroidal anti-inflammatory drugs, including aspirin)-induced gastric ulcers in patients at high risk of complications from a gastric ulcer, eg, the elderly and patients with concomitant debilitating disease, as well as patients at high risk of developing gastric ulceration, such as patients with a history of ulcer. Cytotec has not been shown to prevent duodenal ulcers in patients taking NSAIDs. Cytotec should be taken for the duration of NSAID therapy. Cytotec has been shown to prevent gastric ulcers in controlled studies of three months' duration. It had no effect, compared to placebo, on gastrointestinal pain or discomfort associated with NSAID use.

CONTRAINDICATIONS

See boxed *CONTRAINDICATIONS AND WARNINGS*.

Cytotec should not be taken by anyone with a history of allergy to prostaglandins.

WARNINGS

See boxed *CONTRAINDICATIONS AND WARNINGS*.

PRECAUTIONS

Information for patients: Women of childbearing potential should be told that they must not be pregnant when Cytotec therapy is initiated, and that they must use an effective contraception method while taking Cytotec.

See boxed *CONTRAINDICATIONS AND WARNINGS*.

Patients should be advised of the following:

Cytotec is intended for administration along with nonsteroidal anti-inflammatory drugs (NSAIDs), including aspirin, to decrease the chance of developing an NSAID-induced gastric ulcer.

Cytotec should be taken only according to the directions given by a physician.

If the patient has questions about or problems with Cytotec, the physician should be contacted promptly.

THE PATIENT SHOULD NOT GIVE CYTOTEC TO ANYONE ELSE. Cytotec has been prescribed for the patient's specific condition, may not be the correct treatment for another person, and may be dangerous to the other person if she were to become pregnant.

Keep Cytotec out of reach of children.

SPECIAL NOTE FOR WOMEN: Cytotec must not be used by pregnant women. Cytotec may cause miscarriage. Miscarriages caused by Cytotec may be incomplete which could lead to potentially dangerous bleeding.

Cytotec is available only as a unit-of-use package that contains a leaflet containing patient information. See *Patient Information* at the end of this labeling.

Drug interactions: See *Clinical Pharmacology.* Cytotec has not been shown to interfere with the beneficial effects of aspirin on signs and symptoms of rheumatoid arthritis. Cytotec does not exert clinically significant effects on the absorption, blood levels, and antiplatelet effects of therapeutic doses of aspirin. Cytotec has no clinically significant effect on the kinetics of diclofenac or ibuprofen.

Animal toxicology: A reversible increase in the number of normal surface gastric epithelial cells occurred in the dog, rat, and mouse. No such increase has been observed in humans administered Cytotec for up to one year.

An apparent response of the female mouse to Cytotec in long-term studies at 100 to 1000 times the human dose was hyperostosis, mainly of the medulla of sternebrae. Hyperostosis did not occur in long-term studies in the dog and rat and has not been seen in humans treated with Cytotec.

Carcinogenesis, mutagenesis, impairment of fertility: There was no evidence of an effect of Cytotec on tumor occurrence or incidence in rats receiving daily doses up to 150 times the human dose for 24 months. Similarly, there was no effect of Cytotec on tumor occurrence or incidence in mice receiving daily doses up to 1000 times the human dose for 21 months. The mutagenic potential of Cytotec was tested in several *in vitro* assays, all of which were negative.

Misoprostol, when administered to breeding male and female rats at doses 6.25 times to 625 times the maximum recommended human therapeutic dose, produced dose-related pre- and post-implantation losses and a significant decrease in the number of live pups born at the highest dose. These findings suggest the possibility of a general adverse effect on fertility in males and females.

Pregnancy: Pregnancy Category X. See boxed *CONTRAINDICATIONS AND WARNINGS.*

Nonteratogenic effects: Cytotec may endanger pregnancy (may cause miscarriage) and thereby cause harm to the fetus when administered to a pregnant woman. Cytotec produces uterine contractions, uterine bleeding, and expulsion of the products of conception. Miscarriages caused by Cytotec may be incomplete. In studies in women undergoing elective termination of pregnancy during the first trimester, Cytotec caused partial or complete expulsion of the products of conception in 11% of the subjects and increased uterine bleeding in 41% of cases. If a woman is or becomes pregnant while taking this drug, the drug should be discontinued and the patient apprised of the potential hazard to the fetus.

Teratogenic effects: Cytotec is not fetotoxic or teratogenic in rats and rabbits at doses 625 and 63 times the human dose, respectively.

Nursing mothers: See *Contraindications.* It is unlikely that Cytotec is excreted in human milk since it is rapidly metabolized throughout the body. However, it is not known if the active metabolite (misoprostol acid) is excreted in human milk. Therefore, Cytotec should not be administered to nursing mothers because the potential excretion of misoprostol acid could cause significant diarrhea in nursing infants.

Pediatric use: Safety and effectiveness in children below the age of 18 years have not been established.

ADVERSE REACTIONS

The following have been reported as adverse events in subjects receiving Cytotec:

Gastrointestinal: In subjects receiving Cytotec 400 or 800 mcg daily in clinical trials, the most frequent gastrointestinal adverse events were diarrhea and abdominal pain. The incidence of diarrhea at 800 mcg in controlled trials in patients on NSAIDs ranged from 14–40% and in all studies (over 5,000 patients) averaged 13%. Abdominal pain occurred in 13–20% of patients in NSAID trials and about 7% in all studies, but there was no consistent difference from placebo.

Diarrhea was dose related and usually developed early in the course of therapy (after 13 days), usually was self-limiting (often resolving after 8 days), but sometimes required discontinuation of Cytotec (2% of the patients). The incidence of diarrhea can be minimized by administering after meals and at bedtime, and by avoiding coadministration of Cytotec with magnesium-containing antacids.

Gynecological: Women who received Cytotec during clinical trials reported the following gynecological disorders: spotting (0.7%), cramps (0.6%), hypermenorrhea (0.5%), menstrual disorder (0.3%) and dysmenorrhea (0.1%). Postmenopausal vaginal bleeding may be related to Cytotec administration. If it occurs, diagnostic workup should be undertaken to rule out gynecological pathology.

Elderly: There were no significant differences in the safety profile of Cytotec in approximately 500 ulcer patients who were 65 years of age or older compared with younger patients.

Additional adverse events which were reported are categorized as follows:

Incidence greater than 1%: In clinical trials, the following adverse reactions were reported by more than 1% of the subjects receiving Cytotec and may be causally related to the

drug: nausea (3.2%), flatulence (2.9%), headache (2.4%), dyspepsia (2.0%), vomiting (1.3%), and constipation (1.1%). However, there were no significant differences between the incidences of these events for Cytotec and placebo.

Causal relationship unknown: The following adverse events were infrequently reported. Causal relationships between Cytotec and these events have not been established but cannot be excluded.

Body as a whole: aches/pains, asthenia, fatigue, fever, rigors, weight changes.

Skin: rash, dermatitis, alopecia, pallor, breast pain.

Special senses: abnormal taste, abnormal vision, conjunctivitis, deafness, tinnitus, earache.

Respiratory: upper respiratory tract infection, bronchitis, bronchospasm, dyspnea, pneumonia, epistaxis.

Cardiovascular: chest pain, edema, diaphoresis, hypotension, hypertension, arrhythmia, phlebitis, increased cardiac enzymes, syncope.

Gastrointestinal: GI bleeding, GI inflammation/infection, rectal disorder, abnormal hepatobiliary function, gingivitis, reflux, dysphagia, amylase increase.

Metabolic: glycosuria, gout, increased nitrogen, increased alkaline phosphatase.

Genitourinary: polyuria, dysuria, hematuria, urinary tract infection.

Nervous system/Psychiatric: anxiety, change in appetite, depression, drowsiness, dizziness, thirst, impotence, loss of libido, sweating increase, neuropathy, neurosis.

Musculoskeletal: arthralgia, myalgia, muscle cramps, stiffness, back pain.

Blood/Coagulation: anemia, abnormal differential, thrombocytopenia, purpura, ESR increased.

OVERDOSAGE

The toxic dose of Cytotec in humans has not been determined. Cumulative total daily doses of 1600 mcg have been tolerated, with only symptoms of gastrointestinal discomfort being reported. In animals, the acute toxic effects are diarrhea, gastrointestinal lesions, focal cardiac necrosis, hepatic necrosis, renal tubular necrosis, testicular atrophy, respiratory difficulties, and depression of the central nervous system. Clinical signs that may indicate an overdose are sedation, tremor, convulsions, dyspnea, abdominal pain, diarrhea, fever, palpitations, hypotension, or bradycardia. Symptoms should be treated with supportive therapy.

It is not known if misoprostol acid is dialyzable. However, because misoprostol is metabolized like a fatty acid, it is unlikely that dialysis would be appropriate treatment for overdosage.

DOSAGE AND ADMINISTRATION

The recommended adult oral dose of Cytotec for the prevention of NSAID-induced gastric ulcers is 200 mcg four times daily with food. If this dose cannot be tolerated, a dose of 100 mcg can be used. (See *Clinical Pharmacology: Clinical studies.*) Cytotec should be taken for the duration of NSAID therapy as prescribed by the physician. Cytotec should be taken with a meal, and the last dose of the day should be at bedtime.

Renal impairment: Adjustment of the dosing schedule in renally impaired patients is not routinely needed, but dosage can be reduced if the 200-mcg dose is not tolerated. (See *Clinical Pharmacology.*)

Prevention of Gastric Ulcers Induced by Ibuprofen, Piroxicam, or Naproxen
[No. of patients with ulcer(s) (%)]

Therapy	Therapy Duration			
	4 weeks	8 weeks	12 weeks	
Study No 1				
Cytotec 200 mcg q.i.d. (n=74)	1 (1.4)	0	0	1 (1.4)*
Cytotec 100 mcg q.i.d. (n=77)	3 (3.9)	1 (1.3)	1 (1.3)	5 (6.5)*
Placebo (n=76)	11 (14.5)	4 (5.3)	4 (5.3)	19 (25.0)
Study No. 2				
Cytotec 200 mcg q.i.d. (n=65)	1 (1.5)	1 (1.5)	0	2 (3.1)*
Cytotec 100 mcg q.i.d. (n=66)	2 (3.0)	2 (3.0)	1 (1.5)	5 (7.6)
Placebo (n=62)	6 (9.7)	2 (3.2)	3 (4.8)	11 (17.7)
*Studies No. 1 & No. 2***				
Cytotec 200 mcg q.i.d. (n=139)	2 (1.4)	1 (0.7)	0	3 (2.2)*
Cytotec 100 mcg q.i.d. (n=143)	5 (3.5)	3 (2.1)	2 (1.4)	10 (7.0)*
Placebo (n=138)	17 (12.3)	6 (4.3)	7 (5.1)	30 (21.7)

*Statistically significantly different from placebo at the 5% level.
**Combined data from Study No. 1 and Study No. 2.

HOW SUPPLIED

Cytotec 200-mcg tablets are white, hexagonal, with SEARLE debossed above and 1461 debossed below the line on one side and a double stomach debossed on the other side; supplied as:

NDC Number	Size
0025-1461-31	unit-of-use bottle of 100
0025-1461-34	carton of 100 unit dose

Store below 86°F (30°C) in a dry area.

Caution: Federal law prohibits dispensing without prescription.

PATIENT INFORMATION

Cytotec (misoprostol) is being prescribed by your doctor to decrease the chance of getting stomach ulcers related to the arthritis/pain medication that you need.

Cytotec can cause miscarriage, often associated with potentially dangerous bleeding. This may result in hospitalization, surgery, infertility, or death. **Do not take it if you are pregnant and do not become pregnant while taking this medicine.**

If you become pregnant during Cytotec therapy, stop taking Cytotec and contact your physician immediately.

Take Cytotec only according to the directions given by your physician.

Do not give Cytotec to anyone else. It has been prescribed for your specific condition, may not be the correct treatment for another person, and would be dangerous if the other person were pregnant.

Keep out of the reach of children.

A05418

Shown in Product Identification Section, page 429

DEMULEN® 1/35–21 ℞
DEMULEN® 1/35–28 ℞
DEMULEN® 1/50–21 ℞
DEMULEN® 1/50–28 ℞
[dem ′ū-len]
(ethynodiol diacetate with ethinyl estradiol)

ENOVID® 5 mg ℞
ENOVID® 10 mg ℞
[ē-nov ′id]
(norethynodrel with mestranol)

PRODUCT OVERVIEW

KEY FACTS

The Searle line of oral contraceptives contains two fixed-dose combination oral contraceptives (DEMULEN 1/35-21 and DEMULEN 1/35-28) containing ethynodiol diacetate (1 mg) with ethinyl estradiol (35 mcg) and two fixed-dose combination oral contraceptives (DEMULEN 1/50-21 and DEMULEN 1/50-28) containing ethynodiol diacetate (1 mg) with ethinyl estradiol (50 mcg). DEMULEN 1/35-21 and DEMULEN 1/50-21 are 21-day dosage regimens. DEMULEN 1/35-28 and DEMULEN 1/50-28 are 28-day dosage regimens (including 7 days of inert tablets). These forms are packaged in Compack® tablet dispensers. ENOVID 5 mg (not an oral contraceptive) contains 5 mg of norethynodrel and 75 mcg of mestranol. ENOVID 10 mg (not an oral

Continued on next page

G.D. Searle & Co.—Cont.

contraceptive) contains 9.85 mg of norethynodrel and 0.15 mg of mestranol.

MAJOR USES
DEMULEN 1/35 and DEMULEN 1/50 are highly effective in preventing pregnancy. ENOVID 5 mg and ENOVID 10 mg are indicated for treatment of endometriosis and hypermenorrhea, and for the production of cyclic withdrawal bleeding.

SAFETY INFORMATION
See complete safety information set forth below.

PRESCRIBING INFORMATION

DEMULEN® 1/35–21   ℞
DEMULEN® 1/35–28   ℞
DEMULEN® 1/50–21   ℞
DEMULEN® 1/50–28   ℞
[dem 'ū-len]
(ethynodiol diacetate with ethinyl estradiol)

ENOVID® 5 mg   ℞
ENOVID® 10 mg   ℞
[ē-nov 'id]
(norethynodrel with mestranol)

DESCRIPTION
Demulen 1/35-21 and Demulen 1/35-28. Each white tablet contains 1 mg of ethynodiol diacetate and 35 mcg of ethinyl estradiol, and the inactive ingredients include calcium acetate, calcium phosphate, corn starch, hydrogenated castor oil, and povidone. Each blue tablet in the Demulen 1/35-28 package is a placebo containing no active ingredients, and the inactive ingredients include calcium sulfate, corn starch, FD&C Blue No. 1 Lake, magnesium stearate, and sucrose.
Demulen 1/50-21 and Demulen 1/50-28. Each white tablet contains 1 mg of ethynodiol diacetate and 50 mcg of ethinyl estradiol, and the inactive ingredients include calcium acetate, calcium phosphate, corn starch, hydrogenated castor oil, and povidone. Each pink tablet in the Demulen 1/50-28 package is a placebo containing no active ingredients, and the inactive ingredients include calcium sulfate, corn starch, FD&C Red No. 3, FD&C Yellow No. 6, magnesium stearate, and sucrose.
Enovid 5 mg. Each tablet contains 5 mg of norethynodrel and 75 mcg of mestranol. Inactive ingredients include acacia, corn starch, FD&C Red No. 3, FD&C Yellow No. 6, magnesium stearate, sodium phosphate, sodium sulfate, and sucrose.
Enovid 10 mg. Each tablet contains 9.85 mg of norethynodrel and 0.15 mg of mestranol. Inactive ingredients include acacia, corn starch, FD&C Red No. 40, FD&C Yellow No. 6, magnesium stearate, and sodium sulfate.
The chemical name for norethynodrel is 17α-ethynyl-17-hydroxy-5(10)-estren-3-one, for mestranol it is 3-methoxy-19-nor-17α-pregna-1,3,5(10)-trien-20-yn-17-ol, for ethynodiol diacetate it is 19-nor-17α-pregn-4-en-20-yne-3β,17-diol diacetate, and for ethinyl estradiol it is 19-nor-17α-pregna-1,3,5(10)-trien-20-yne-3,17-diol. Their structural formulas are as follows:

ethynodiol
diacetate

mestranol

ethinyl
estradiol

norethynodrel

Therapeutic Class: Oral contraceptive (except for Enovid 5 mg and 10 mg). Estrogen-progestogen combination (Enovid 5 mg and 10 mg only).

CLINICAL PHARMACOLOGY
Combination oral contraceptives act primarily through the mechanism of gonadotropin suppression due to the estrogenic and progestational activity of their components. Although the primary mechanism of action is inhibition of ovulation, alterations in the genital tract, including changes in the cervical mucus (which reduce sperm penetration) and the endometrium (which reduce the likelihood of implantation) may also contribute to contraceptive effectiveness.
Enovid 5 mg or Enovid 10 mg, when used for the treatment of endometriosis, may be administered to induce changes in areas of endometriosis similar to those that occur during pregnancy. In many instances when Enovid 5 mg or Enovid 10 mg is taken continuously the areas of endometriosis develop a decidua-like response followed by necrosis, which may result in destruction of the abnormally located tissue and resolution of the lesions.

INDICATIONS AND USAGE
Demulen 1/35 and Demulen 1/50 are indicated for the prevention of pregnancy in women who elect to use oral contraceptives as a method of contraception.
Enovid 5 mg and Enovid 10 mg are indicated for the treatment of endometriosis, for the treatment of hypermenorrhea, and for the production of cyclic withdrawal bleeding.
NOTE: The contraindication, warning, precaution, and adverse reaction information in this leaflet also applies when Enovid 5 mg or when Enovid 10 mg is prescribed.
Oral contraceptives are highly effective.[176] The pregnancy rate in women using conventional combination oral contraceptives (containing 35 mcg or more of ethinyl estradiol or 50 mcg or more of mestranol) is generally reported to be less than 1 pregnancy per 100 woman-years of use. Slightly higher rates (somewhat more than 1 pregnancy per 100 woman-years of use) are reported for some combination products containing 35 mcg or less of ethinyl estradiol, and rates on the order of 3 pregnancies per 100 woman-years are reported for the progestogen-only oral contraceptives.
These rates are derived from separate studies conducted by different investigators in several population groups; therefore, a precise comparison cannot be made. Furthermore, pregnancy rates tend to be lower as clinical studies are continued, possibly due to selective retention in the longer studies of those patients who accept the treatment regimen and do not discontinue as a result of adverse reactions, pregnancy, or other reasons. In Table 1 ranges of pregnancy rates as reported in the literature[1] are shown for other means of contraception. The efficacy of these means of contraception, except for the IUD, depends upon the degree of adherence to the method.
In clinical trials with Demulen 1/50, 2,256 patients completed 30,409 cycles, and a total of 30 pregnancies were reported. This represents a pregnancy rate of 1.18 per 100 woman-years.
In clinical trials with Demulen 1/35, 1,231 patients completed 14,641 cycles, and a total of 15 pregnancies were reported. This represents a pregnancy rate of 1.23 per 100 woman-years.
In clinical trials with Demulen 1/35, the incidence of delayed or breakthrough bleeding was 44% at cycle 6. However, only 9.9% of the patients dropped out of the study due to bleeding.

Table 1
Pregnancies per 100 Woman-Years

Method	Range
IUD	<1 to 6
Diaphragm with spermicidal cream or gel	2 to 20
Condom	3 to 36
Spermicidal aerosol foams	2 to 29
Spermicidal gels and creams	4 to 36
Periodic abstinence (rhythm), all types	<1 to 47
1. Calendar method	14 to 47
2. Temperature method	1 to 20
3. Temperature method (intercourse only in postovulatory phase)	<1 to 7
4. Mucus method	1 to 25
No contraception	60 to 80

Dose-related Risk of Thromboembolism from Oral Contraceptives: Studies have shown a positive association be-

tween the dose of estrogens in oral contraceptives and the risk of thromboembolism[2,96,97] (see *Warning* No. 1). For this reason, it is prudent and in keeping with good principles of therapeutics to minimize exposure to estrogen. The oral contraceptive product prescribed for any given patient should be that product which contains the least amount of estrogen that is compatible with an acceptable pregnancy rate and patient acceptance. It is recommended that new users of oral contraceptives be started on preparations containing 50 mcg or less of estrogen.

CONTRAINDICATIONS
Oral contraceptives should not be used in women with any of the following conditions:
1. Thrombophlebitis or thromboembolic disorders.
2. A past history of deep vein thrombophlebitis or thromboembolic disorders.
3. Cerebral vascular disease, myocardial infarction or coronary artery disease, or a past history of these conditions.
4. Known or suspected carcinoma of the breast.
5. Known or suspected estrogen-dependent neoplasia.
6. Undiagnosed abnormal genital bleeding.
7. Known or suspected pregnancy (see *Warning* No. 5).
8. Past or present, benign or malignant liver tumors among women who developed these tumors during the use of oral contraceptives or other estrogen-containing products (see *Warning* No. 4).

WARNINGS

> **Cigarette-smoking increases the risk of serious cardiovascular side effects from oral contraceptive use. This risk increases with age and with heavy smoking (15 or more cigarettes per day) and is quite marked in women over 35 years of age. Women who use oral contraceptives should be strongly advised not to smoke.**
>
> The use of oral contraceptives is associated with increased risk of several serious conditions including venous and arterial thromboembolism, thrombotic and hemorrhagic stroke, myocardial infarction, visual disorders, liver tumors or other liver lesions, gallbladder disease, hypertension, and fetal abnormalities. Practitioners prescribing oral contraceptives should be familiar with the following information relating to these and other risks.

1. Thromboembolic Disorders and Other Vascular Problems. An increased risk of thromboembolic and thrombotic disease associated with the use of oral contraceptives is well established. One study in Great Britain[3] demonstrated an increased relative risk for fatal venous thromboembolism; several British[4,5,14,22,92,156] and U.S. [6–8,23,98–101,126] studies demonstrated an increased relative risk for nonfatal venous thromboembolism. U.S. studies[6,9,10,99,101–103] demonstrated an increased relative risk for stroke, which had not been shown in prior British studies.[3–5] In these studies it was estimated that users of oral contraceptives were 1.9 to 11 times more likely than nonusers to manifest these diseases without evident cause (Table 2). In a British study of idiopathic deep vein thrombosis and pulmonary embolism, the projected annual hospitalization rates for women aged 16–40 were 47 per 100,000 users and 5 for nonusers.[77] In one British mortality study,[3] overall excess mortality due to pulmonary embolism or stroke was on the order of 1.3 to 3.4 deaths annually per 100,000 users and increased with age.
Cerebrovascular Disorders: In a collaborative U.S. study[9,10] of cerebrovascular disorders in women with and without predisposing causes, it was estimated that the risk of hemorrhagic stroke was 2.0 times greater in users than in nonusers, and the risk of thrombotic stroke was 4.0[10] to 9.5[9] times greater in users than in nonusers (Table 2). Analysis of mortality trends in 21 countries indicates that, since oral contraceptives first became available, changes in mortality from nonrheumatic heart disease and hypertension, cerebrovascular disease, and all nonrheumatic cardiovascular disease among women aged 15 to 44 years have been associated with changes in the prevalence of oral contraceptive use in each country.[11]

Table 2. *Summary of Relative Risks of Thromboembolic Disorders and Other Vascular Problems in Oral Contraceptive Users Compared with Nonusers.*

Disorders	Relative Risk
Idiopathic thromboembolic disease	2 to 11 times greater
Postsurgery thromboembolic complications	4 to 7 times greater
Thrombotic stroke	4 to 9.5 times greater
Hemorrhagic stroke	2.0 to 2.3 times greater
Myocardial infarction	2 to 12 times greater

In May 1974 the Royal College of General Practitioners[12] issued an interim report of its continuing large-scale prospective study comparing a user group with a nonuser group. It stated: "A statistically significant higher rate of reporting of cerebrovascular accidents in Takers is evident, but the numbers are too small to justify an estimation of the degree of risk." A 1981 analysis of data from this study was reported[13] to show a 4-fold increased mortality from circulatory diseases, mainly from myocardial infarction and hemorrhagic stroke, in users. The excess mortality was associated with age and smoking in users. A 1983 analysis[138] of arterial diseases reported a significantly increased incidence of cerebrovascular disease among current oral contraceptive users. Risk appeared to increase with duration of use up to 8 years. Categories with a significantly increased incidence included cerebral thrombosis or embolism, and transient ischemic attacks, but not hemorrhagic strokes. Incidence of peripheral arterial thromboembolism, Raynaud's disease, and acute myocardial infarction was increased in current users. Women aged 30 years and older had appreciably higher rates of arterial disease than did younger women. Smoking increased the risk for older women in each usage group, the greatest risk being in current users aged 35 years and older who smoked. Expressed as the percentage of women diagnosed as having an arterial disease who died of that disease, the case-fatality rates were 2 to 3 times greater for users who smoked than for women in the other groups.

In October 1976 an interim report was issued on the long-term follow-up study of the British Family Planning Association.[14] There was a highly significant association between oral contraceptive use and stroke, although total numbers were small in this study also. The increase in risk of venous thrombosis and pulmonary embolism among users was about 4-fold and was statistically highly significant. In later reports[15] it was noted that mortality from nonrheumatic heart disease was greater in women who had ever used oral contraceptives. A 1984 report[147] on stroke found pill use to be a significant risk factor for nonhemorrhagic stroke, but not for subarachnoid hemorrhage. Smoking and hypertension were significant risk factors only for the latter.

In the Walnut Creek prospective study,[99,101,102] the risk of subarachnoid hemorrhage was associated with heavy smoking, age, and use of the pill.

Myocardial Infarction: An increased risk of myocardial infarction associated with the use of oral contraceptives has been reported in Great Britain,[16-19,136,138,180] confirming a previously suspected association.[3] The morbidity study[16,17] found that the greater the number of underlying risk factors for coronary artery disease (cigarette-smoking, hypertension, hypercholesterolemia, obesity, diabetes, history of preeclamptic toxemia), the higher the risk of developing myocardial infarction, regardless of whether the patient was an oral contraceptive user or not. Oral contraceptives were considered an additional risk factor.

The annual excess rate of fatal myocardial infarction in British oral contraceptive users was estimated to be approximately 3.5 cases per 100,000 women users in the 30- to 39-year age group and 20 per 100,000 women users in the 40- to 44-year age group.[19] (These estimates are based on British vital statistics, which show acute myocardial infarction death rates 2 to 3 times less than in the U.S. for women in these age groups. In an attempt to extrapolate these figures to U.S. women, it was estimated that the annual excess rates in users are 25.7 cases per 100,000 for women aged 30–39 with predisposing conditions versus 1.5 cases without; corresponding estimates for women aged 40–44 were 86.2 versus 5.1.[78]) The annual excess rate of hospitalization for nonfatal myocardial infarction in married British oral contraceptive users was estimated to be approximately 3.5 per 100,000 women users in the 30- to 39-year age group and 47 per 100,000 women users in the 40- to 44-year age group.[16] Smoking is considered a major predisposing condition to myocardial infarction. In terms of relative risk, it has been estimated[20] that oral contraceptive users who do not smoke are about twice as likely to have a fatal myocardial infarction as nonusers who do not smoke. Oral contraceptive users who are also smokers have about a 5-fold increased risk of fatal infarction compared to users who do not smoke, but about a 10- to 12-fold increased risk compared to nonusers who do not smoke. Furthermore, the amount of smoking is also an important factor. In determining the importance of these relative risks, however, the baseline rates for various age groups, as shown in Table 3, must be given serious consideration. The importance of other predisposing conditions mentioned above in determining relative and absolute risks has not been quantified; it is likely that the same synergistic action exists, but perhaps to a lesser extent.

Similar findings relating nonfatal and fatal myocardial infarction, oral contraceptives, smoking, and age were subsequently published in the British literature[91,99,104-108,152] and by the Royal College of General Practitioners in Great Britain.[13,138,190]

Table 3. *Estimated Annual Mortality Rate per 100,000 Women from Myocardial Infarction by Use of Oral Contraceptives, Smoking Habits, and Age in Years.*[20]

| | Myocardial infarction | | | |
| | Women aged 30–39 | | Women aged 40–44 | |
Smoking habits	Users	Non-users	Users	Non-users
All smokers	10.2	2.6	62.0	15.9
Heavy*	13.0	5.1	78.7	31.3
Light	4.7	0.9	28.6	5.7
Nonsmokers	1.8	1.2	10.7	7.4
Smokers and nonsmokers	5.4	1.9	32.8	11.7

*15 or more cigarettes per day

Risk of Dose: Reports of thromboembolism following the use of oral contraceptives containing 50 mcg or more of estrogen received by drug safety committees in Great Britain, Sweden, and Denmark were compared with the distribution expected from market research estimates of sales.[2] A positive correlation was found between the dose of estrogen and the reporting of thromboembolism, including coronary thrombosis, in excess of that predicted by sales estimates. Preparations containing 100 mcg or more of estrogen were associated with a higher risk of thromboembolism than those containing 50 to 80 mcg of estrogen. The authors' analysis did suggest, however, that the quantity of estrogen may not be the sole factor involved. Any influence on the part of the progestogens was not considered, which may have been responsible for certain discrepancies in the data. No significant differences were detected between preparations containing the same dose of estrogen nor between the two estrogens ethinyl estradiol and mestranol. A subsequent study of a similar nature in Great Britain found a positive association between the dose of progestogen or estrogen and certain thromboembolic conditions,[96] which is consistent with findings of the Royal College study.[12,92,135] Swedish authorities noted decreased reporting of thromboembolic episodes when higher estrogen preparations were no longer prescribed.[97] Careful epidemiologic studies to determine the degree of thromboembolic risk associated with progestogen-only oral contraceptives have not been performed. Cases of thromboembolic disease have been reported in women using these products, and they should not be presumed to be free of excess risk.

The relative risk of oral contraceptive use one month prior to hospitalization for various types of thromboembolism was calculated in a U.S. retrospective case-control study.[8] If no account is taken of the relative estrogenic potency of different estrogens and if any possible influence of the different progestogenic components is ignored, the products employed may be divided into those containing less than 100 mcg and those containing 100 mcg or more of estrogen. For all cases combined, the larger-dose category was associated with only a slightly higher relative risk; for the idiopathic subgroup, the relative risk was approximately doubled with the larger estrogen content, but the confidence limits overlapped considerably and the differences, therefore, were not statistically significant. Apparently there was less of an increased relative risk for the subgroup with predispositions to thromboembolism.[98]

In the British Family Planning Association study, no nonhemorrhagic strokes occurred during 9,100 woman-years of current use of pills containing less than 50 mcg of estrogen, in contrast to 13 observed during 39,400 woman-years of current use of pills with higher doses.[147] The incidence of venous thromboembolism was greater for those women using pills containing 50 mcg or more of estrogen than for those using pills with less than 50 mcg estrogen.[173]

A decline of serum high density lipoproteins (HDL) has been reported with increasing progestational activity,[165,167,168,182] and decreased HDL has been associated with an increased incidence of ischemic heart disease.[169] The amount of both steroids should be another consideration in the choice of an oral contraceptive.

The risk of thromboembolic and thrombotic disorders, both in users and in nonusers of oral contraceptives, increases with age. Oral contraceptives have been considered an independent risk factor for these events.

Persistence of Risk: A 1977 analysis[13a] of the mortality data from the prospective study of the Royal College of General Practitioners (RCGP) suggested that the risk of circulatory disease increases with the duration of oral contraceptive use and may persist after discontinuation. The ratio of the mortality rate from circulatory disease in former users to that in controls was 4.3 to 1 (P < 0.01), and was still 3.7 to 1 even after excluding the two deaths from malignant hypertension, where use was stopped because of the onset of hypertension. For the category of fatal subarachnoid hemorrhage, the rate ratio comparing former users to controls was also statistically significant.

In 1981, a new analysis of the RCGP mortality data[13] showed significantly increased risk ratios in former users for the categories of all nonrheumatic heart disease plus hypertension (4.6 to 1), cerebrovascular disease (3.6 to 1), as well as the subcategory of subarachnoid hemorrhage (4.5 to 1). Overall, the incidence of fatal circulatory disease for former users was 4.3 times that of the controls.

A 1983 analysis of the incidence of arterial disease in the RCGP study[138] showed that the incidence of all cerebrovascular disease, fatal and nonfatal, was significantly greater in former users than in controls (risk ratio = 2.6) and remained elevated for at least 6 years after discontinuation of oral contraceptives. Former users had significantly increased rates for cerebral thrombosis (4 vs 0), transient ischemic attacks (8.7 to 1), and "other" cerebrovascular disease (3.8 to 1). In the Walnut Creek prospective study,[102] former use of oral contraceptives was significantly associated with increased risk of subarachnoid hemorrhage, the relative risk being 5.3. In a U.S. hospital-based, case-control study,[137] when the duration of oral contraceptive use was considered, the data suggested that the rate of myocardial infarction is increased approximately 2- to 3-fold in older women who had used oral contraceptives for more than 10 years before discontinuation. The excess risk associated with long-term use was evident in subjects who had stopped less than 5 years previously, as well as in those who had stopped 5 to 9 years previously. Whether the excess risk persisted for more than 10 years after discontinuation could not be assessed because of a paucity of data.

In summary, persistence of risk after discontinuation of oral contraceptives has been reported for circulatory disease in general,[13,13a] for nonrheumatic heart disease,[13,137] and for cerebrovascular disease,[13,138] including subarachnoid hemorrhage,[13,13a,102] cerebral thrombosis,[138] and transient ischemic attacks.[138]

Estimate of Excess Mortality from Circulatory Diseases: A large prospective study[13] carried out in the U.K. provided estimates of the mortality rate per 100,000 women per year from diseases of the circulatory system for users and nonusers of oral contraceptives according to age, smoking habits, and duration of use. The overall annual excess death rate from circulatory diseases for oral contraceptive users was estimated at 23 per 100,000 for women of all ages. The rates for nonsmokers and smokers, respectively, were: ages 25–34, 2 and 10 per 100,000; ages 35–44, 15 and 48 per 100,000; and ages 45 and older, 41 and 179 per 100,000. The risk was statistically significant only in cigarette-smokers over age 34. The majority of deaths were due to subarachnoid hemorrhage or ischemic heart disease. Relative risk for women who had ever used oral contraceptives rose with increasing parity, a new observation that needs confirmation.

The available data from a variety of sources have been analyzed[21,163] to estimate the risk of death associated with various methods of contraception. The estimates of risk of death for each method included the combined risk of the contraceptive method (eg, thromboembolic and thrombotic disease in the case of oral contraceptives) plus the risk attributable to pregnancy or abortion in the event of method failure. This latter risk varies with the effectiveness of the contraceptive method. The findings of this analysis are shown in Figure 1.[21] The study concluded that the mortality associated with

Figure 1. Estimated annual number of deaths associated with control of fertility and no control per 100,000 nonsterile women by regimen of control and age of woman.

Annual deaths

Age: 15-19, 20-24, 25-29, 30-34, 35-39, 40-44

Regimen of control:
- No method
- Abortion only
- Pill only/nonsmokers
- Pill only/smokers
- IUDs only
- Traditional contraception only (diaphragm or condom)
- Traditional contraception and abortion

Continued on next page

G.D. Searle & Co.—Cont.

all methods of birth control is low and below that associated with childbirth, except for that associated with oral contraceptives in women over 40 who smoke. (The rates given for pill only/smokers for each age group are for smokers as a class. For "heavy" smokers [more than 15 cigarettes a day], the rates given would be about double; for "light" smokers [less than 15 cigarettes a day], about 50 percent.[20]) The mortality associated with oral contraceptive use in nonsmokers over 40 is higher than with any other method of contraception in that age group. The lowest mortality is associated with the condom or diaphragm backed up by early legal abortion.

The risk of thromboembolic and thrombotic disease associated with oral contraceptives increases with age after approximately age 30 and, for myocardial infarction, is further increased by hypertension, hypercholesterolemia, obesity, diabetes, or history of preeclamptic toxemia, and especially by cigarette-smoking.[20,78,79]

Based on the data currently available, the following table gives a gross estimate of the risk of death from circulatory disorders associated with the use of oral contraceptives:

Table 4. *Smoking Habits and Other Predisposing Conditions—Risk Associated with Use of Oral Contraceptives.*

Age	Below 30	30–39	40+
Heavy smokers	C	B	A
Light smokers	D	C	B
Nonsmokers (no predisposing conditions)	D	C,D	C
Nonsmokers (other predisposing conditions)	C	C,B	B,A

A—Use associated with very high risk.
B—Use associated with high risk.
C—Use associated with moderate risk.
D—Use associated with low risk.

The physician and patient should be alert to the earliest manifestations of thromboembolic and thrombotic disorders (eg, thrombophlebitis, pulmonary embolism, cerebrovascular insufficiency, coronary artery disease or myocardial infarction, retinal thrombosis, and mesenteric thrombosis). Should any of these occur or be suspected, the drug should be discontinued immediately.

A 4- to 7-fold increased risk of postsurgery thromboembolic complications has also been reported in oral contraceptive users.[22,23] If feasible, oral contraceptives should be discontinued at least 4 weeks before elective surgery or during periods of prolonged immobilization. The decision as to when to resume oral contraception following major surgery or bed rest should balance the recognized risks of postsurgery thromboembolic complications with the need to reinstate contraceptive practices.

The Royal College of General Practitioners in a large prospective study reported a higher incidence of superficial and deep vein thrombosis in users, the former being correlated with the progestogen dose. The RCGP data suggest that the presence of varicose veins substantially increases the risk of superficial venous thrombosis of the leg, the risk depending upon the severity of the varicosities. The evidence suggests that the presence of varicose veins has little effect on the development of deep vein thrombosis in the leg.[92] Other prospective studies have also reported a higher incidence of venous thrombosis in users.[14,99-101,109]

2. *Ocular Lesions.* There have been reports of neuro-ocular lesions such as optic neuritis or retinal thrombosis associated with the use of oral contraceptives. Discontinue medication if there is unexplained, gradual or sudden, partial or complete loss of vision; proptosis or diplopia; papilledema; or any evidence of retinal vascular lesions. Appropriate diagnostic and therapeutic measures should be instituted.

3. *Carcinoma.* Long-term continuous administration of either natural or synthetic estrogens in certain animal species increases the frequency of certain carcinomas, and/or nonmalignant neoplasms, such as those of the breast, uterus, cervix, vagina, ovary, liver, and pituitary. Certain synthetic progestogens, none currently contained in oral contraceptives, have been noted to increase the incidence of mammary nodules, benign and malignant, in dogs.

There is now evidence that estrogens increase the risk of carcinoma of the endometrium in humans. In several independent, retrospective case-control studies,[24-28,80,93] an increased relative risk (2.2 to 13.9 times) was reported, associating endometrial carcinoma with the prolonged use of estrogens in postmenopausal women who took estrogen replacement medication to relieve menopausal symptoms. This risk was independent of the other known risk factors for endometrial cancer and appeared to depend both on duration of treatment[24,27,28] and on estrogen dose.[26-28] These findings are supported by the observation that incidence rates of endometrial cancer have increased sharply since 1969 in 8 different areas of the U.S. with population-based cancer-reporting systems, an increase which may be related to the rapidly expanding use of estrogens during the past decade.[29] There is no evidence at present that "natural" estrogens are more or less hazardous than "synthetic" estrogens at equiestrogenic doses.

One publication[30] reported on the first 30 cases submitted by physicians to a registry of cases of adenocarcinoma of the endometrium in women under 40 on oral contraceptives. Of the adenocarcinomas found in women without predisposing risk factors for adenocarcinoma of the endometrium (eg, irregular bleeding at the time oral contraceptives were first given, polycystic ovaries), nearly all occurred in women who had used a sequential oral contraceptive. These products are no longer marketed. No statistical association has been reported suggesting an increased risk of endometrial cancer in users of conventional combination or progestogen-only oral contraceptives, although individual cases have been reported.

Several studies[7,31-35,39,99,121,122] have reported no increased risk of breast cancer in women taking oral contraceptives or estrogens; however, several other studies have provided inconsistent data reflecting increased risk in various subgroups. In one study,[36,37] while no overall increased risk of breast cancer was noted in women treated with oral contraceptives, a greater risk was suggested for the subgroups of oral contraceptive users with documented benign breast disease and for long-term (2–4 years) users. Other studies[123,142,175] reported increased risk of breast cancer in women who had used the pill for more than 4 years before their first full-term pregnancy. One other study[38] indicated an increasing risk of breast cancer in women taking menopausal estrogens, which increased with duration of follow-up. Several other studies have shown oral contraceptives[127-129,133,140,141,144,146,148] or estrogens[130,145] to be associated with breast cancer, particularly in connection with other risk factors[127-129] (eg, family history, previous breast biopsy, late age of first delivery) and long duration of use.[127,128,130,146,161] Several recent studies report increased risk in: nulliparous women aged 20–44 with menarche before age 13 who took the pill for 8 or more years[185]; a twofold overall increased risk for ever-users, with significant risk for subgroups aged 30–39 at interview, for long-term (>5 years) users, and for parous women taking the pill for 1–4 years before the first term pregnancy or for <1 year or >4 years after[186]; age 30–34 at time of diagnosis, and when standardized for age, those who were para 1, and among the latter, those with 2 or more years of use.[187] A reduced occurrence of benign breast tumors in users of oral contraceptives has been well documented.[7,12,14,31,36,39,40,86,99] Some epidemiologic studies[41,81-84,99,109,120,143,149,150,162,170,189] have suggested an increased risk of cervical dysplasia, intraepithelial neoplasia, erosion, and carcinoma in long-term pill users; however, cause and effect has not been established. There have been other reports of microglandular dysplasia of the cervix in users.

In summary, there is at present no consistent evidence from human studies of an increased risk of cancer associated with oral contraceptives.[42] Close clinical surveillance of all women taking oral contraceptives is, nevertheless, essential. In all cases of undiagnosed persistent or recurrent abnormal vaginal bleeding, nonfunctional causes should be borne in mind and appropriate diagnostic measures should be taken to rule out malignancy. Women who have a strong family history of breast cancer or who have breast nodules, fibrocystic disease, recurrent cystic mastitis, abnormal mammograms, or cervical dysplasia should be monitored with particular care if they elect to use oral contraceptives.

4. *Hepatic Lesions (adenomas, hepatomas, hamartomas, regenerating nodules, focal nodular hyperplasia, hemangiomas, peliosis hepatis, sinusoidal dilatation, hepatocellular carcinoma, etc).* Benign hepatic adenomas and other hepatic lesions have been associated with the use of oral contraceptives.[43,45,46,85] One study[46] reported that oral contraceptive formulations with high "hormonal potency" were associated with a higher risk than lower-potency formulations, as was age over 30 years. Although benign, these hepatic lesions may rupture and may cause death through intra-abdominal hemorrhage. This has been reported in short-term as well as long-term users of oral contraceptives. Two studies related risk with duration of use of the contraceptive, the risk being much greater after 4 or more years of oral contraceptive use.[45,46] Long-term users of oral contraceptives have an estimated annual incidence of hepatocellular adenoma of 3 to 4 per 100,000.[46] While such hepatic lesions are rare, they should be considered in women presenting with abdominal pain and tenderness, abdominal mass, or shock. Patients with liver tumors have demonstrated variable clinical features, which may make preoperative diagnosis difficult. About one quarter of the cases presented because of abdominal masses; up to one half had signs and symptoms of acute intraperitoneal hemorrhage. Routine radiologic and laboratory studies may not be helpful. Liver scans may clearly show a focal defect. Hepatic arteriography or computed tomography may be useful procedures in diagnosing primary liver neoplasms.

Cases of hepatocellular carcinoma have been reported in women taking oral contraceptives. The relationship of these drugs to this type of malignancy is not known at this time, although epidemiologic studies[157-159] have estimated a relative risk as high as 7 to 20 for users for 8 or more years as compared to nonusers.[158,159] There is also evidence that oral contraceptives are associated with cancer of the bile duct.[172,177-179]

Oral contraceptives are contraindicated if there are past or present, benign or malignant liver tumors among women who developed these tumors during the use of oral contraceptives or other estrogen-containing products.

5. *Use In or Immediately Preceding Pregnancy, Birth Defects in Offspring, and Malignancy in Offspring.* The use of female sex hormones, both estrogens and progestogens, during early pregnancy may seriously damage the offspring. It has been reported that females exposed in utero to diethylstilbestrol and other nonsteroidal estrogens have an increased risk of developing in later life a form of vaginal or cervical cancer that is ordinarily extremely rare.[47,48] This risk has been estimated to be on the order of 1 in 1,000 exposures or less.[49,50,171] The excess incidence for dysplasia and carcinoma in situ has been estimated at 7.8 cases per 1,000 woman-years.[154] Although there is no evidence at the present time that oral contraceptives further enhance the risk of developing this type of malignancy, such patients should be monitored with particular care if they elect to use oral contraceptives instead of other methods of contraception. Furthermore, a high percentage of such exposed women (from 30% to 90%) have been found to have adenosis (epithelial changes) of the vagina and cervix.[51-55] Although these changes are histologically benign, it is not known whether this condition is a precursor of malignancy. DES-exposed daughters appear to have an increased risk of unfavorable outcome of pregnancy.[110-112] DES-exposed male children may develop abnormalities of the urogenital tract[56-58,131] and sperm.[131] Although similar data are not available for the use of other estrogens, it cannot be presumed that they would not induce similar changes.

Several reports suggest an association between fetal exposure to female sex hormones, including oral contraceptives, and congenital anomalies,[59-64,94,113-116,174] including multiple congenital anomalies described by the acronym VACTERL, for vertebral, anal, cardiac, tracheoesophageal, renal, and limb defects.[61,62,113] There appears to be a preferential expression of these defects by exposed male offspring.[63,65,115,124] In one case-control study[63] it was estimated that there was a 4.7-fold increased risk of limb-reduction defects in infants exposed in utero to sex hormones (oral contraceptives, hormonal withdrawal tests for pregnancy, or attempted treatment for threatened abortion). Some of these exposures were very short and involved only a few days of treatment. It is reported that the risk of cardiac anomalies and of limb reduction defects in exposed fetuses is about 1 in 1,000 live births. In a large prospective study,[64] cardiovascular defects in children born to women who received female hormones, including oral contraceptives, during early pregnancy occurred at a rate of 18.2 per 1,000 births, compared to 7.8 per 1,000 for children not so exposed in utero. These results are statistically significant. Female hormone exposure in utero during the first trimester has been reported to be associated with an increased risk of testicular[183] and ovarian[184] cancer. The incidence of twin births may be increased for women who conceive shortly after discontinuing use of the pill.[14,63,117,118,124]

In the past, female sex hormones have been used during pregnancy in an attempt to treat threatened or habitual abortion. There is considerable evidence that estrogens are ineffective for these indications, and there is no evidence from well-controlled studies that progestogens are effective for these uses. An increased incidence of spontaneous abortion associated with lethal chromosome abnormalities (trisomy, triploidy) was reported with high-dose oral contraceptives.[66] However, a recent study including low-dose oral contraceptives did not confirm this effect.[164] Whether there is an overall increase in spontaneous abortion of pregnancies conceived soon after stopping the oral contraceptives is unknown. A highly significant (P < 0.001) increase of lymphocytic chromosome aberrations in oral contraceptive users has been reported.[160]

The safety of this product in pregnancy has not been demonstrated. Pregnancy should be ruled out before initiating or continuing the contraceptive regimen. Pregnancy should always be considered if withdrawal bleeding does not occur. It is recommended that for any patient who has missed 2 consecutive periods, pregnancy should be ruled out before continuing the contraceptive regimen. If the patient has not adhered to the prescribed schedule, the possibility of pregnancy should be considered at the time of the first missed period, and further use of oral contraceptives should be withheld until pregnancy has been ruled out. If pregnancy is confirmed, oral contraceptive use should not be resumed and the patient should be apprised of the potential risks to the fetus, and the advisability of continuation of the pregnancy should be discussed in the light of these risks.

It is recommended that women who discontinue oral contraceptives with the intent of becoming pregnant use an alternative form of contraception for a period of time before attempting to conceive. Many clinicians recommend 3 months, although no precise information is available on which to base this recommendation.

The administration of progestogen-only or progestogen-estrogen combinations to induce withdrawal bleeding should not be used as a test of pregnancy.

6. *Gallbladder Disease.* Reports of studies[7,8,12,14,33] indicate an increased risk for surgically confirmed gallbladder disease in users of oral contraceptives or estrogens. In one study,[12] an increased risk appeared after 2 years of use and doubled after 4 or 5 years of use. In one of the other studies[7] an increased risk was apparent between 6 and 12 months of use. Bile duct carcinoma has been reported.[172,177–179]

7. *Carbohydrate and Lipid Metabolism.* A decrease in glucose tolerance has been observed in a significant percentage of patients on oral contraceptives. For this reason, prediabetic and diabetic patients should be carefully observed while receiving oral contraceptives. An increase in triglycerides, total phospholipids, and lipoproteins has been observed in patients receiving oral contraceptives.[67,165] The clinical significance of this finding remains to be defined.

8. *Elevated Blood Pressure.* An increase in blood pressure has been reported in patients receiving oral contraceptives.[12,69,109] There is evidence that the degree of hypertension may correlate directly with increasing dosage of progestogen.[86] In some women, hypertension may occur within a few months of beginning oral contraceptive use. The prevalence of hypertension in users is low in the first year of use, and may be no higher than that in a comparable group of nonusers. The prevalence in users increases, however, with longer exposure and, in the fifth year of use, is 2½ to 3 times the reported prevalence in the first year. Age is also strongly correlated with the development of hypertension in oral contraceptive users.

Women with a history of elevated blood pressure (hypertension), preexisting renal disease, a history of toxemia or elevated blood pressure during pregnancy, a familial tendency to hypertension or its consequences, or a history of excessive weight gain or fluid retention during the menstrual cycle may be more likely to develop elevation of blood pressure when given oral contraceptives and, therefore, should be monitored closely.[68] Even though elevated blood pressure may remain within the "normal" range, the clinical implications of elevations should not be ignored and close surveillance is indicated, particularly for women with other risk factors for cardiovascular disease or stroke.[69] High blood pressure may or may not persist after discontinuation of the oral contraceptive.

9. *Headache.* The onset or exacerbation of migraine or development of headache of a new pattern which is recurrent, persistent, or severe, requires discontinuation of oral contraceptives and evaluation of the cause.

10. *Bleeding Irregularities.* Breakthrough bleeding, spotting, and amenorrhea are frequent reasons for discontinuance of oral contraceptives. In breakthrough bleeding, as in all cases of irregular or abnormal vaginal bleeding, nonfunctional causes should be borne in mind. In patients with undiagnosed persistent or recurrent abnormal vaginal bleeding, adequate diagnostic measures are indicated to rule out pregnancy or malignancy. If a pathologic basis has been excluded, passage of time or a change to another formulation may correct the bleeding problem. A change to an oral contraceptive with a higher estrogen content, while potentially useful in minimizing menstrual irregularity, should be made only when considered necessary since this may increase the risk of thromboembolic disease.

Women with a past history of oligomenorrhea or secondary amenorrhea or young women who have not established regular cycles may have a tendency to remain anovulatory or to become amenorrheic after discontinuation of oral contraceptives. Women with these preexisting problems should be informed of these possibilities and encouraged to use other contraceptive methods. Post-use anovulation, possibly prolonged, may also occur in women without previous irregularities. A higher incidence of galactorrhea and of pituitary tumors (eg, adenomas) has been associated with amenorrhea in former users compared with nonusers.[87] One study[70] reported a 16-fold increased prevalence of pituitary prolactin-secreting tumors among patients with postpill amenorrhea when galactorrhea was present. A case-control study[44] reported an increased risk of galactorrhea following discontinuation of oral contraceptives by women who did not have pituitary tumors.

11. *Ectopic Pregnancy.* Contraceptive failure may result in either ectopic or intrauterine pregnancy. In failures with combination-type oral contraceptives, the ratio of ectopic to intrauterine pregnancies is no higher than in women who are not receiving oral contraceptives.

12. *Breast Feeding.* Oral contraceptives given in the postpartum period may interfere with lactation. There may be a decrease in the quantity and quality of the breast milk. Furthermore, a small fraction of the hormonal agents in oral contraceptives has been identified in the milk of mothers receiving these drugs.[71,88,89] The effects, if any, on the breast-fed child have not been determined. If feasible, the use of oral contraceptives should be deferred until the infant has been weaned.

13. *Infertility.* There is evidence of fertility impairment in women discontinuing oral contraceptives in comparison with those discontinuing other methods.[14,90,132,155] While the impairment diminishes with time, there is still an appreciable difference in the results in nulliparous women aged 25 to 29 at 30 months after discontinuation of birth control; the difference is negligible after 48 months. However, among nulliparas aged 30–34, the impairment persists up to 72 months and appears more severe for users for 2 or more years. For parous women aged 25 to 34 the difference is no longer apparent 30 months after cessation of contraception.

PRECAUTIONS

General. 1. A complete medical and family history should be taken and a thorough physical examination should be performed prior to the initiation of oral contraceptives. The pretreatment and periodic physical examinations should include special reference to blood pressure, breasts, abdomen, and pelvic organs, including a Pap smear and relevant laboratory tests. As a general rule, oral contraceptives should not be prescribed for longer than one year without the performance of another physical examination (see *Warnings*).

2. Preexisting uterine leiomyomata may increase in size during oral contraceptive use. While unconfirmed, an increased risk of fibroids with oral contraceptives containing ethynodiol diacetate has been reported.[166]

3. Oral contraceptives appear to be associated with an increased incidence of mental depression. Therefore, patients with a history of depression should be carefully observed and the drug discontinued if depression recurs to a serious degree. Patients becoming significantly depressed while taking oral contraceptives should stop the medication and use an alternative method of contraception in an attempt to determine whether the symptom is drug related.

4. Oral contraceptives may cause some degree of fluid retention. They should be prescribed with caution, and only with careful monitoring, in patients with conditions which might be aggravated by fluid retention, such as convulsive disorders, migraine syndrome, asthma, or cardiac, hepatic, or renal dysfunction.

5. Patients with a past history of jaundice during pregnancy have an increased risk of recurrence of jaundice and should be carefully observed while receiving oral contraceptives. If jaundice develops in any patient receiving such drugs, the medication should be discontinued while the cause is investigated. Cholestatic jaundice has been reported after combined treatment with oral contraceptives and troleandomycin. Hepatotoxicity following a combination of oral contraceptives and cyclosporine has also been reported.

6. Steroid hormones may be poorly metabolized in patients with impaired liver function and should be administered with caution in such patients.

7. Oral contraceptive users may have disturbances in normal tryptophan metabolism, which may result in a relative pyridoxine deficiency. The clinical significance of this is unknown, although megaloblastic anemia has been reported.

8. Serum folate levels may be depressed by oral contraceptive therapy. Since the pregnant woman is predisposed to folate deficiency and the incidence of folate deficiency increases with lengthening gestation, it is possible that if a woman becomes pregnant shortly after stopping oral contraceptives, she may have a greater chance of developing folate deficiency and complications attributable to this deficiency.

9. The pathologist should be advised of oral contraceptive therapy when relevant specimens are submitted.

10. Certain endocrine and liver function tests may be affected by estrogen-containing oral contraceptives. Therefore, it is recommended that any abnormal tests be repeated after the drug has been withdrawn for two months. The following alterations in laboratory results have been observed with the use of oral contraceptives:

a. Hepatic function: Increased sulfobromophthalein retention and other abnormalities in tests of liver function.

b. Coagulation tests: Increased prothrombin and coagulation factors VII, VIII, IX, and X; decreased antithrombin III; increased platelet aggregability.

c. Thyroid function: Increased thyroid-binding globulin (TBG) leading to increased circulating total thyroid hormone, as measured by protein-bound iodine (PBI) or T^4 by column or radioimmunoassay. Free T^3 resin uptake is decreased, reflecting the elevated TBG; free T^4 concentration is unaltered.

d. Decreased pregnanediol excretion.

e. Reduced response to metyrapone test.

f. Increased blood transcortin and corticosteroid levels.

g. Increased blood triglyceride and phospholipid concentrations.

h. Reduced serum folate concentration.

i. Impaired glucose tolerance.

j. Altered plasma levels of trace minerals (eg, increased ceruloplasmin).

11. The influence of prolonged oral contraceptive therapy on pituitary, ovarian, adrenal, hepatic, or uterine function, or on the immune response, has not been established.

12. Treatment with oral contraceptives may mask the onset of the climacteric. (See *Warnings* section regarding risks in this age group.)

13. The prevalence of cervical *Chlamydia trachomatis* and *Neisseria gonorrhoeae* in oral contraceptive users is increased several-fold.[151,191] It should not be assumed that oral contraceptives afford protection against pelvic inflammatory disease from *Chlamydia*.[151] HIV seropositivity in female African prostitutes was significantly associated with a history of taking oral medications for the prevention of pregnancy and/or of sexually transmitted diseases.[181,188]

Information for the Patient. See patient labeling printed at end.

Drug Interactions. Oral contraceptives may be rendered less effective and increased incidence of breakthrough bleeding may occur by virtue of drug interaction with rifampin, isoniazid, ampicillin, neomycin, penicillin V, tetracycline, chloramphenicol, sulfonamides, nitrofurantoin, griseofulvin, barbiturates, phenytoin, carbamazepine, primidone, phenylbutazone, analgesics, tranquilizers, and antimigraine preparations.[72–74,95,125,153] Oral contraceptives may alter the effectiveness of other types of drugs, such as oral anticoagulants, anticonvulsants, tranquilizers (eg, diazepam), tricyclic antidepressants, antihypertensive agents (eg, guanethidine), theophylline, caffeine, vitamins, hypoglycemic agents, clofibrate, glucocorticoids, and acetaminophen.[72,119,134,139,153] (See *Precaution* No. 5).

Carcinogenesis. See *Warnings* No. 3 and 4 for information on the carcinogenic potential of oral contraceptives.

Pregnancy. Pregnancy category X. See *Contraindication* No. 7 and *Warning* No. 5.

Nursing Mothers. See *Warning* No. 12.

ADVERSE REACTIONS

An increased risk of the following serious adverse reactions has been associated with the use of oral contraceptives (see *Warnings*):

    Thrombophlebitis and thrombosis
    Pulmonary embolism
    Arterial thromboembolism
    Raynaud's disease
    Myocardial infarction and coronary thrombosis
    Cerebral thrombosis
    Cerebral hemorrhage
    Hypertension
    Gallbladder disease
    Budd-Chiari syndrome
    Benign adenomas and other hepatic lesions, with or without intra-abdominal bleeding
    Hepatocellular carcinoma
    Congenital anomalies

There is evidence of an association between the following conditions and the use of oral contraceptives, although confirmatory studies have not been done:

    Mesenteric thrombosis
    Neuro-ocular lesions (eg, retinal thrombosis and optic neuritis)

The following adverse reactions have been reported in patients receiving oral contraceptives and are believed to be drug related:

    Nausea and vomiting
        (Usually the most common adverse reactions, occurring in approximately 10% or fewer patients during the first cycle. Other reactions, as a general rule, are seen much less frequently or only occasionally.)
    Gastrointestinal symptoms (eg, abdominal cramps and bloating)
    Breakthrough bleeding
    Spotting
    Change in menstrual flow
    Dysmenorrhea
    Amenorrhea during and after use
    Infertility after discontinuation
    Edema
    Chloasma or melasma, which may persist when the drug is discontinued
    Breast changes: tenderness, enlargement, and secretion
    Change in weight (increase or decrease)
    Change in cervical erosion and secretion
    Endocervical hyperplasia
    Possible diminution in lactation when given immediately post partum

Continued on next page

G.D. Searle & Co.—Cont.

Cholestatic jaundice
Migraine
Increase in size of uterine leiomyomata
Rash (allergic)
Mental depression
Reduced tolerance to carbohydrates
Vaginal candidiasis
Change in corneal curvature (steepening)
Intolerance to contact lenses

The following adverse reactions or conditions have been reported in users of oral contraceptives, and the association has been neither confirmed nor refuted:

Premenstrual-like syndrome
Cataracts
Changes in libido
Chorea
Changes in appetite
Cystitis-like syndrome
Headache
Paresthesia
Nervousness
Dizziness
Auditory disturbances
Rhinitis
Fatigue
Backache
Hirsutism
Loss of scalp hair
Erythema multiforme
Erythema nodosum
Hemorrhagic eruption
Herpes gestationis
Hidradenitis suppurativa
Hemolytic uremic syndrome
Malignant hypertension
Impaired renal function
Acute renal failure, sometimes irreversible
Itching
Vaginitis
Porphyria
Premature ventricular contractions
Electrocardiogram abnormalities
Pulmonary hypertension
Thrombotic thrombocytopenic purpura
Anemia
Pancreatitis
Hepatitis
Colitis
Crohn's disease
Gingivitis
Dry socket
Lupus erythematosus
Rheumatoid arthritis
Pituitary tumors (eg, adenoma) with amenorrhea and/or galactorrhea after OC use
Malignant melanoma
Endometrial, cervical, breast, and bile duct carcinoma (see *Warning* No. 3)

ACUTE OVERDOSAGE

Serious ill effects have not been reported following the acute ingestion of large doses of oral contraceptives by young children.[75,76] Overdosage may cause nausea, and withdrawal bleeding might occur in females.

DOSAGE AND ADMINISTRATION

Contraception: Demulen 1/35-21, Demulen 1/35-28, Demulen 1/50-21, and Demulen 1/50-28.
To achieve maximum contraceptive effectiveness, oral contraceptives must be taken exactly as directed and at intervals of 24 hours.
IMPORTANT: The patient should be instructed to use an additional method of protection until after the first week of administration *in the initial cycle*. The possibility of ovulation and conception prior to initiation of use should be considered.
Demulen 1/35-21, Demulen 1/35-28, Demulen 1/50-21, and Demulen 1/50-28. Dosage Schedules: The Demulen 1/35-21 and Demulen 1/50-21 Compack® tablet dispensers contain 21 tablets arranged in three numbered rows of 7 tablets each. The Demulen 1/35-28 and Demulen 1/50-28 tablet dispensers contain 21 white active tablets arranged in three numbered rows of 7 tablets each, followed by a fourth row of 7 pink (blue for Demulen 1/35-28) placebo tablets.
Days of the week are printed above the tablets, starting with Sunday on the left.
Two dosage schedules are described, one of which may be more convenient or suitable than the other for an individual patient.
Schedule #1: Sunday Start: The patient begins taking Demulen 1/35-21, Demulen 1/35-28, Demulen 1/50-21, or Demulen 1/50-28 from the first row of her package, one tablet daily, starting on the first Sunday after the onset of men-

struation. If the patient's period begins on a Sunday she takes her first tablet that very same day. The 21st tablet or the 28th tablet, depending on whether the patient is taking the 21- or 28-tablet course, will then be taken on a Saturday.
Subsequent Cycles:
21-tablet course—The patient begins a new 21-tablet course on the eighth day, Sunday, after taking her last tablet. All subsequent cycles will also begin on Sunday, one tablet being taken each day for three weeks followed by a week of no pill-taking.
28-tablet course—The patient begins a new 28-tablet course on the next day, Sunday, and all subsequent cycles will also begin on Sunday, one tablet being taken each and every day.
With a Sunday-start schedule, a woman whose period begins on the day of or one to four days before taking the first tablet should expect a diminution of flow and fewer menstrual days. The initial cycle will likely be shortened by from one to five days. Thereafter, cycles should be about 28 days in length.
Schedule #2: Day 5 Start: The patient begins taking Demulen 1/35-21 or Demulen 1/50-21 from the first row of her package, one tablet daily, starting with the pill day which corresponds to day 5 of her menstrual cycle; the first day of menstruation is counted as day 1. After the last (Saturday) tablet in row #3 has been taken, if any remain in the first row, the patient completes her 21-tablet schedule starting with Sunday in row #1.
Subsequent Cycles: The patient begins a new 21-tablet course on the eighth day after taking her last tablet, again starting the same day of the week on which she began her first course. All subsequent cycles will also begin on that same day, one tablet being taken each day for three weeks followed by a week of no pill-taking.
Hypermenorrhea; Production of Cyclic Withdrawal Bleeding: Enovid 5 mg or 10 mg only. Most patients with hypermenorrhea may be expected to respond to Enovid 5-mg or 10-mg therapy within 24 to 48 hours. Regular withdrawal bleeding may then be induced by cyclic administration. Vaginal bleeding at times other than the regular menstrual period requires that a diagnosis be established prior to beginning therapy.
For emergency control of severe bleeding in patients with hypermenorrhea give 20 to 30 mg of Enovid daily until the bleeding is controlled, then reduce the daily dose to 10 mg and continue through day 24 of the cycle. Then discontinue Enovid and withdrawal flow usually will begin approximately two to three days later.
Cyclic withdrawal bleeding may be produced after treatment in this initial cycle by giving the patient 5 to 10 mg of Enovid 5 mg or 10 mg daily from day 5 through day 24 of the next two or three cycles. A new course of Enovid therapy should be started on day 5 of her menstrual cycle or eight days after the last pill from the previous cycle, whichever occurs first. The first day of menstruation is counted as day 1.
Endometriosis: Enovid 5 mg or 10 mg only. A daily dose of Enovid should be given for six to nine months or longer on the following schedule: 5 or 10 mg should be given for two weeks beginning on day 5 of a menstrual cycle. This daily dose should be given continuously (without cyclic interruption) and increased 5 or 10 mg at two-week intervals until the patient is receiving 20 mg daily. This dose of 20 mg should be continued for six to nine months and further increased (up to 40 mg daily) if breakthrough bleeding occurs.
Therapy may be discontinued after six months if the disease is mild and the lesions are no longer palpable. If the disorder is more severe continue treatment for nine months or longer. When surgery is contemplated, prior administration of Enovid may facilitate the surgical procedure. (See *Warning* No. 1 concerning discontinuation prior to elective surgery.)
Special Notes: *Spotting or Breakthrough Bleeding.* If spotting (bleeding insufficient to require a pad) or breakthrough bleeding (heavier bleeding similar to a menstrual flow) occurs when these products are used for contraception the patient should continue taking her tablets as directed. The incidence of spotting or breakthrough bleeding is minimal, most frequently occurring in the first cycle. Ordinarily spotting or breakthrough bleeding will stop within a week. Usually the patient will begin to cycle regularly within two or three courses of tablet-taking. If breakthrough bleeding occurs while the patient is taking Enovid for hypermenorrhea she should immediately increase the daily dosage by 5 or 10 mg until bleeding has been controlled for three days, after which the original dosage usually may be resumed. In the event of spotting or breakthrough bleeding organic causes should be borne in mind. (See *Warning* No. 10.)
Missed Menstrual Periods. Withdrawal flow will normally occur two or three days after the last active tablet is taken. Failure of withdrawal bleeding ordinarily does not mean that the patient is pregnant, providing the dosage schedule has been correctly followed. (See *Warning* No. 5.)
If the patient has *not* adhered to the prescribed dosage regimen, the possibility of pregnancy should be considered after the first missed period, and oral contraceptives should be withheld until pregnancy has been ruled out.

If the patient has adhered to the prescribed regimen and misses two consecutive periods, pregnancy should be ruled out before continuing the contraceptive regimen.
The first intermenstrual interval after discontinuing the tablets is usually prolonged; consequently, a patient for whom a 28-day cycle is usual might not begin to menstruate for 35 days or longer. Ovulation in such prolonged cycles will occur correspondingly later in the cycle. Posttreatment cycles after the first one, however, are usually typical for the individual woman prior to taking tablets. (See *Warnings* No. 10 and 11.)
Missed Tablets (Contraception). If a woman misses taking one active tablet the missed tablet should be taken as soon as it is remembered. In addition, the next tablet should be taken at the usual time. If two consecutive active tablets are missed the dosage should be doubled for the next two days. The regular schedule should then be resumed, but an additional method of protection is recommended for the remainder of the cycle.
While there is little likelihood of ovulation if only one active tablet is missed, the possibility of spotting or breakthrough bleeding is increased and should be expected if two or more successive active tablets are missed. However, the possibility of ovulation increases with each successive day that scheduled active tablets are missed.
If one or more placebo tablets of Demulen 1/35-28 or Demulen 1/50-28 are missed, the Demulen 1/35-28 or Demulen 1/50-28 schedule should be resumed on the following Sunday (the eighth day after the last white tablet was taken). Omission of placebo tablets in the 28-tablet courses does not increase the possibility of conception provided that this schedule is followed.

HOW SUPPLIED

Demulen 1/35: Each white Demulen 1/35 tablet is round in shape, with a debossed SEARLE on one side and 151 design on the other side, and contains 1 mg of ethynodiol diacetate and 35 mcg of ethinyl estradiol.
Demulen 1/35-21 is packaged in cartons of 6 and 24 Compack tablet dispensers of 21 tablets each, and in cartons of 12 Compack refills of 21 tablets each.
Demulen 1/35-28 is packaged in cartons of 6 and 24 Compack tablet dispensers and in cartons of 12 Compack refills. Each Compack and refill contains 21 white Demulen 1/35 tablets and 7 blue placebo tablets. (Placebo tablets have a debossed SEARLE on one side and a "P" on the other side.)
Demulen: 1/50: Each white Demulen 1/50 tablet is round in shape, with a debossed SEARLE on one side and 71 on the other side, and contains 1 mg of ethynodiol diacetate and 50 mcg of ethinyl estradiol.
Demulen 1/50-21 is packaged in cartons of 6 and 24 Compack tablet dispensers of 21 tablets each, and in cartons of 12 Compack refills of 21 tablets each.
Demulen 1/50-28 is packaged in cartons of 6 and 24 Compack tablet dispensers and in cartons of 12 Compack refills. Each Compack and refill contains 21 white Demulen 1/50 tablets and 7 pink placebo tablets. (Placebo tablets have a debossed SEARLE on one side and a "P" on the other side.)
Enovid 5 mg: Each Enovid 5 mg tablet is pink, round in shape, with a debossed SEARLE on one side and 51 on the other side, and contains 5 mg of norethynodrel and 75 mcg of mestranol. Enovid 5 mg is packaged in bottles of 100 tablets each.
Enovid 10 mg: Each Enovid 10 mg tablet is coral colored, round in shape, with a debossed SEARLE 10 on one side and 101 on the other side, and contains 9.85 mg of norethynodrel and 0.15 mg of mestranol. Enovid 10 mg is packaged in bottles of 50 tablets each.

Caution: Federal law prohibits dispensing without prescription.

REFERENCES

1. Population Reports, Series H, No. 2 (May) 1974; Series I, No. 1 (June) 1974; Series B, No. 3 (May) 1979; Series H, No. 3 (Jan.) 1975; Series H, No. 4 (Jan.) 1976; Population Information Program, Geo. Washington U. Medical Center, Washington, D.C. **2.** Inman, W. H. W., et al.: Br. Med. J. *2*:203 (April 25) 1970. **3.** Inman, W. H. W., et al.: Br. Med. J. *2*:193 (April 27) 1968. **4.** Royal College of General Practitioners: J. Coll. Gen. Pract. *13*:267 (May) 1967. **5.** Vessey, M. P., et al.: Br. Med. J. *2*:651 (June 14) 1969. **6.** Sartwell, P. E.: Am. J. Epidemiol. *90*:365 (Nov.) 1969. **7.** Boston Collaborative Drug Surveillance Programme: Lancet *1*:1399 (June 23) 1973. **8.** Stolley, P.D., et al.: Am. J. Epidemiol. *102*:197 (Sept.) 1975. **9.** Collaborative Group for the Study of Stroke in Young Women: N. Engl. J. Med. *288*:871 (April 26) 1973. **10.** Collaborative Group for the Study of Stroke in Young Women: J.A.M.A. *231*:718 (Feb. 17) 1975. **11.** Beral, V.: Lancet *2*:1047 (Nov. 13) 1976. **12.** Royal College of General Practitioners: Oral Contraceptives and Health, New York, Pitman Publ. Corp., May 1974. **13.** Layde, P., et al.: Lancet *1*:541 (March 7) 1981. **13a.** Beral, V., et al.: Lancet *2*:727 (Oct. 8) 1977. **14.** Vessey, M., et al.: J. Biosoc. Sci. *8*:373 (Oct.) 1976. **15.** Vessey, M., et al.: Lancet *2*:731 (Oct. 8) 1977; *1*:549 (March 7) 1981. **16.** Mann, J. I., et al.: Br. Med. J. *2*:241 (May 3) 1975. **17.** Mann, J. I., et al.: Br. Med. J. *3*:631 (Sept. 13)

1975. **18.** Mann, J. I., et al.: Br. Med. J. *2* :245 (May 3) 1975. **19.** Mann, J. I., et al.: Br. Med. J. *2* :445 (Aug. 21) 1976. **20.** Jain, A. K.: Stud. Fam. Plann. *8* :50 (March) 1977. **21.** Tietze, C.: Fam. Plann. Perspect. *9* :74 (March-April) 1977. **22.** Vessey, M. P., et al.: Br. Med. J. *3* :123 (July 18) 1970. **23.** Greene, G. R., et al.: Am. J. Public Health *62* :680 (May) 1972. **24.** Ziel, H. K., et al.: N. Engl. J. Med. *293* :1167 (Dec. 4) 1975. **25.** Smith, D. C., et al.: N. Engl. J. Med. *293* :1164 (Dec. 4) 1975. **26.** Mack, T. M., et al.: N. Engl. J. Med. *294* :1262 (June 3) 1976. **27.** Gray, L. A., et al.: Obstet. Gynecol. *49* :385 (April) 1977. **28.** McDonald, T. W., et al.: Am. J. Obstet. Gynecol. *127* :572 (March 15) 1977. **29.** Weiss, N. S., et al.: N. Engl. J. Med. *294* :1259 (June 3) 1976.

30. Silverberg, S. G., et al.: Cancer *39* :592 (Feb.) 1977. **31.** Vessey, M. P., et al.: Br. Med. J. *3* :719 (Sept. 23) 1972. **32.** Vessey, M. P., et al.: Lancet *1* :941 (April 26) 1975. **33.** Boston Collaborative Drug Surveillance Program: N. Engl. J. Med. *290* :15 (Jan. 3) 1974. **34.** Arthes, F. G., et al.: Cancer *28* :1391 (Dec.) 1971. **35.** Casagrande, J., et al.: J. Natl. Cancer Inst. *56* :839 (April) 1976. **36.** Fasal, E., et al.: J. Natl. Cancer Inst. *55* :767 (Oct.) 1975. **37.** Paffenbarger, R. S., et al.: Cancer *39* :1887 (April Suppl.) 1977. **38.** Hoover, R., et al.: N. Engl. J. Med. *295* :401 (Aug. 19) 1976. **39.** Kelsey, J. L., et al.: Am. J. Epidemiol. *107* :236 (March) 1978.

40. Ory, H., et al.: N. Engl. J. Med. *294* :419 (Feb. 19) 1976. **41.** Stern, E., et al.: Science *196* :1460 (June 24) 1977. **42.** Population Reports, Series A, No. 4 (May) 1977: Population Information Program, Geo. Washington U. Medical Center, Washington, D.C. **43.** Baum, J. K., et al.: Lancet *2* :926 (Oct. 27) 1973. **44.** Taler, S.J., et al.: Obstet. Gynecol. *65* :665 (May) 1985. **45.** Edmondson, H. A., et al.: N. Engl. J. Med. *294* :470 (Feb. 26) 1976. **46.** Rooks, J. B., et al.: J.A.M.A. *242* :644 (Aug. 17) 1979. **47.** Herbst, A. L., et al.: N. Engl. J. Med. *284* :878 (April 22) 1971. **48.** Greenwald, P., et al.: N. Engl. J. Med. *285* :390 (Aug. 12) 1971. **49.** Lanier, A. P., et al.: Mayo Clin. Proc. *48* :793 (Nov.) 1973.

50. Herbst, A. L., et al.: Am. J. Obstet. Gynecol. *128* :43 (May 1) 1977. **51.** Herbst, A. L., et al.: Obstet. Gynecol. *40* :287 (Sept.) 1972. **52.** Herbst, A. L., et al.: Am. J. Obstet. Gynecol. *118* :607 (March 1) 1974. **53.** Herbst, A. L., et al.: N. Engl. J. Med. *292* :334 (Feb. 13) 1975. **54.** Stafl, A., et al.: Obstet. Gynecol. *43* :118 (Jan.) 1974. **55.** Sherman, A. I., et al.: Obstet. Gynecol. *44* :531 (Oct.) 1974. **56.** Bibbo, M., et al.: J. Reprod. Med. *15* :29 (July) 1975. **57.** Gill, W., et al.: J. Reprod. Med. *16* :147 (April) 1976. **58.** Henderson, B., et al.: Pediatrics *58* :505 (Oct.) 1976. **59.** Gal, I., et al.: Nature *240* :241 (Nov. 24) 1972.

60. Levy, E. P., et al.: Lancet *1* :611 (March 17) 1973. **61.** Nora, J. J., et al.: Lancet *1* :941 (April 28) 1973. **62.** Nora, A. H., et al.: Arch. Environ. Health *30* :17 (Jan.) 1975; Adv. Plann. Parent. *12* :156, 1978. **63.** Janerich, D. T., et al.: N. Engl. J. Med. *291* :697 (Oct. 3) 1974. **64.** Heinonen, O. P., et al.: N. Engl. J. Med. *296* :67 (Jan. 13) 1977. **65.** Nora, J. J., et al.: N. Engl. J. Med. *291* :731 (Oct. 3) 1974. **66.** Carr, D. H.: Can. Med. Assoc. J. *103* :343 (Aug. 15 & 29) 1970. **67.** Wynn, V., et al.: Lancet *2* :720 (Oct. 1) 1966. **68.** Laragh, J. H.: Am. J. Obstet. Gynecol. *126* :141 (Sept.) 1976. **69.** Fisch, I. R., et al.: J.A.M.A. *237* :2499 (June 6) 1977.

70. Van Campenhout, et al.: Fertil. Steril. *28* :728 (July) 1977. **71.** Laumas, K. R., et al.: Am. J. Obstet. Gynecol. *98* :411 (June 1) 1967. **72.** Stockley, I.: Pharmaceut. J. *216* :140 (Feb. 14) 1976. **73.** Hempel, E., et al.: Zentralbl. Gynaekol. *95* :1451 (Nov. 2) 1973; cited in Int. Plann. Parent. Fed. Med. Bull. *10* : (Dec.) 1976. **74.** Bessot, J.-C., et al.: Nouv. Presse Med. *6* :1568 (April 30) 1977. **75.** Francis, W. G., et al.: Can. Med. Assoc. J. *92* :191 (Jan. 23) 1965. **76.** Verhulst, H., et al.: J. Clin. Pharmacol. *7* :9 (Jan.-Feb.) 1967. **77.** Vessey, M. P., et al.: Br. Med. J. *2* :199 (April 27) 1968. **78.** Ory, H. W.: J.A.M.A. *237* :2619 (June 13) 1977. **79.** Jain, A. K.: Am. J. Obstet. Gynecol. *126* :301 (Oct. 1) 1976.

80. Ziel, H. K., et al.: Am. J. Obstet. Gynecol. *124* :735 (April 1) 1976. **81.** Peritz, E., et al.: Am. J. Epidemiol. *106* :462 (Dec.) 1977. **82.** Ory, H. W., et al.: in Garattini, S., and Berendes, H. (eds.): Pharmacology of Steroid Contraceptive Drugs, Raven Press, N.Y., 1977. **83.** Goldacre, M. J., et al.: Br. Med. J. *1* :748 (March 25) 1978. **84.** Meisels, A., et al.: Cancer *40* :3076 (Dec.) 1977. **85.** Klatskin, G.: Gastroenterology *73* :386 (Aug.) 1977. **86.** Kay, C. R.: Lancet *1* :624 (March 19) 1977. **87.** March, C. M., et al.: Fertil. Steril. *28* :346 (March) 1977. **88.** Saxena, B. N., et al.: Contraception *16* :605 (Dec.) 1977. **89.** Nilsson, S., et al.: Contraception *17* :131 (Feb.) 1978.

90. Vessey, M. P., et al.: Br. Med. J. *1* :265 (Feb. 4) 1978. **91.** Jick, H., et al.: J.A.M.A. *239* :1403, 1407 (April 3) 1978. **92.** Kay, C. R.: J. R. Coll. Gen. Pract. *28* :393 (July) 1978. **93.** Hoogerland, D. L., et al.: Gynecol. Oncol. *6* :451 (Oct.) 1978. **94.** Lorber, C. A., et al.: Fertil. Steril. *31* :21 (Jan.) 1979. **95.** Bacon, J. F., et al.: Br. Med. J. *280* :293 (Feb. 2) 1980. **96.** Meade, T. W., et al.: Br. Med. J. *280* :1157 (May 10) 1980. **97.** Böttiger, L. E., et al.: Lancet *1* :1097 (May 24) 1980. **98.** Maguire, M. G., et al.: Am. J. Epidemiol. *110* :188 (Aug.) 1979. **99.** Ramcharan, S., et al.: The Walnut Creek Contraceptive Drug Study, Vol. 3, U.S. Govt. Ptg. Off., 1981; J. Reprod. Med. *25* :346 (Dec.) 1980.

100. Petitti, D. B., et al.: Am. J. Epidemiol. *108* :480 (Dec.) 1978. **101.** Petitti, D. B., et al.: J.A.M.A. *242* :1150 (Sept. 14) 1979. **102.** Petitti, D. B., et al.: Lancet *2* :234 (July 29) 1978. **103.** Jick, H., et al.: Ann. Int. Med. *88* :58 (July) 1978. **104.** Jick, H., et al.: J.A.M.A. *240* :2548 (Dec. 1) 1978. **105.** Shapiro, S., et al.: Lancet *1* :743 (April 7) 1979. **106.** Rosenberg, L., et al.: Am. J. Epidemiol. *111* :59 (Jan.) 1980. **107.** Kreuger, D. E., et al.: Am. J. Epidemiol. *111* :655 (June) 1980. **108.** Arthes, F. G., et al.: Chest *70* :574 (Nov.) 1976. **109.** Hoover, R., et al.: Am. J. Public Health *68* :335 (April) 1978.

110. Herbst, A. L., et al.: J. Reprod. Med. *24* :62 (Feb.) 1980. **111.** Barnes, A. B., et al.: N. Engl. J. Med. *302* :609 (March 13) 1980. **112.** Cousins, L., et al.: Obstet. Gynecol. *56* :70 (July) 1980. **113.** Nora, J. J., et al.: J.A.M.A. *240* :837 (Sept. 1) 1978. **114.** Aarskog, D.: N. Engl. J. Med. *300* :75 (Jan. 11) 1979. **115.** Janerich, D. T., et al.: Am. J. Epidemiol. *112* :73 (July) 1980. **116.** Kasan, P. N., et al.: Br. J. Obstet. Gynaecol. *87* :545 (July) 1980. **117.** Rothman, K. J.: N. Engl. J. Med. *297* :468 (Sept. 1) 1977. **118.** Bracken, M. B.: Am. J. Obstet. Gynecol. *133* :432 (Feb. 15) 1979. **119.** De Teresa, E., et al.: Br. Med. J. *2* :1260 (Nov. 17) 1979.

120. Swan, S., et al.: Am. J. Obstet. Gynecol. *139* :52 (Jan. 1) 1981. **121.** Kay, C. R.: Br. Med. J. *282* :2089 (June 27) 1981. **122.** Vessey, M. P., et al.: Br. Med. J. *282* :2093 (June 27) 1981. **123.** Pike, M. C., et al.: Br. J. Cancer *43* :72 (Jan.) 1981. **124.** Harlap, S., et al.: Obstet. Gynecol. *55* :447 (April) 1980. **125.** Back, D. J., et al.: Drugs *21* :46 (Jan.) 1981. **126.** Porter, J. B., et al.: Obstet. Gynecol. *66* :1 (July) 1985. **127.** Lees, A.W., et al.: Int. J. Cancer *22* :700, 1978. **128.** Brinton, L. A., et al.: J. Natl. Cancer Inst. (JNCI) *62* :37 (Jan.) 1979. **129.** Black, M. M.: Pathol. Res. Pract. *166* :491, 1980; Cancer *46* :2747 (Dec.) 1980; Cancer *51* : 2147 (June 1) 1983. **130.** Hoover, R., et al.: JNCI *67* :815 (Oct.) 1981. **131.** Gill, W. B., et al.: J. Urol. *122* :36 (July) 1979. **132.** Linn, S., et al.: J.A.M.A. *247* :629 (Feb. 5) 1982. **133.** Clavel, F., et al.: Bull. Cancer (Paris) *68* :449 (Dec.) 1981. **134.** Abernethy, D. R., et al.: N. Engl. J. Med. *306* :791 (April 1) 1982. **135.** Kay, C. R.: Am. J. Obstet. Gynecol. *142* :762 (March 15) 1982. **136.** Adam, S. A., et al.: Br. J. Obstet. Gynaecol. *88* :838 (Aug.) 1981. **137.** Slone, D., et al.: N. Engl. J. Med. *305* :420 (Aug. 20) 1981. **138.** Layde, P.M., et al.: J.R. Coll. Gen. Pract. *33* :75 (Feb.) 1983. **139.** Abernethy, D. R., et al.: Obstet. Gynecol. *60* :338 (Sept.) 1982.

140. Brinton, L.A., et al.: Int. J. Epidemiol. *11* :316, 1982. **141.** Harris, N.V., et al.: Am. J. Epidemiol. *116:* 643 (Oct.) 1982. **142.** Pike, M.C., et al.: Lancet *2* :926 (Oct. 22) 1983. **143.** Vessey, M.P., et al.: Lancet *2* :930 (Oct. 22) 1983. **144.** Jick, H., et al.: Am. J. Epidemiol. *112* :577 (Nov.) 1980. **145.** Jick, H., et al.: Am. J. Epidemiol. *112* :586 (Nov.) 1980. **146.** McPherson, K., et al.: Lancet *2* :1414 (Dec. 17) 1983. **147.** Vessey, M.P., et al.: Br. Med. J. *289* :530 (Sept. 1) 1984. **148.** Olsson, H., et al.: Lancet *1* :748 (March 30) 1985. **149.** Thomas, D.B., et al.: Br. Med. J. *290* :961 (March 30) 1985.

150. Dallenbach-Hellweg, G.: Path. Res. Pract. *179* :38, 1984. **151.** Washington, A.E., et al.: J.A.M.A. *253* :2246 (April 19) 1985. **152.** Rosenberg, L., et al.: J.A.M.A. *253* :2965 (May 24/31) 1985. **153.** Baciewicz, A.M.: Therap. Drug Monitor. *7* :26 (March) 1985. **154.** Robboy, S.J., et al.: J.A.M.A. *252* :2979 (Dec. 7) 1984. **155.** Vessey, M.P., et al.: Br. J. Fam. Plann. *11* :120 (Jan.) 1986. **156.** Vessey, M.P., et al.: Br. Med. J. *292* :526 (Feb. 22) 1986. **157.** Henderson, B.E., et al.: Br. J. Cancer *48* :437 (July) 1983. **158.** Neuberger, J., et al.: Br. Med. J. *292* :1355 (May 24) 1986. **159.** Forman, D., et al.: Br. Med. J. *292* :1357 (May 24) 1986.

160. Pinto, M.R.: Mutat. Res. *169* :149 (March) 1986. **161.** Meirik, O., et al.: Lancet *2* :650 (Sept. 20) 1986. **162.** Brinton, L.A., et al.: Int. J. Cancer *38* :339 (Sept.) 1986. **163.** Ory, H.: Fam. Plann. Perspect. *15* :57 (March-April) 1983. **164.** Harlap, S., et al.: Teratology *31* :381 (June) 1985. **165.** Tikkanen, M.J.: J. Reprod. Med. *31* :898 (Sept.) 1986. **166.** Ross, R.K.: Br. Med. J. *293* :359 (Aug. 9) 1986. **167.** Lipson, A.: Contraception *34* :121 (Aug.) 1986. **168.** Bradley, D. D., et al.: N. Engl. J. Med. *299* :17 (July 6) 1978. **169.** Gordon, T., et al.: Am. J. Med. *62* :707 (May) 1977.

170. Ebeling, K., et al.: Int. J. Cancer *39* :427 (April) 1987. **171.** Melnick, S., et al.: N. Engl. J. Med. *316* :514 (Feb. 26) 1987. **172.** Ellis, E.F., et al.: Lancet *1* :207 (Jan. 28) 1978. **173.** Vessey, M., et al.: Br. Med. J. *292* :526 (Feb. 22) 1986. **174.** Sainz, M.P., et al.: Med. Clin. (Barcelona) *89* :272, 1987. **175.** McPherson, K., et al.: Br. J. Cancer *56* :653 (Nov.) 1987. **176.** Trussell, J., et al.: Stud. Fam. Plann. *18* :227 (Sept./Oct.) 1987. **177.** Littlewood, E.R., et al.: Lancet *1* :310 (Feb. 4) 1980. **178.** Caggiano, V., et al.: Lancet *2* :365 (Aug. 16) 1980. **179.** Yen, S., et al.: Cancer *59* :2112 (June) 1987.

180. Mant, D., et al.: J Epidemiol. Commun. Hlth. *41* :215 (Sept.) 1987. **181.** Plummer, F.A., et al.: Second Internat. Symp. AIDS and Assoc. Cancers in Africa, abst. S.9.3, 1987. **182.** Burkman, R.T., et al.: Obstet. Gynecol. *71* :33 (Jan.) 1987. **183.** Depue, R.H., et al.: JNCI *71* :1151 (Dec.) 1983. **184.** Walker, A.H., et al.: Br. J. Cancer *57* :418 (April) 1988. **185.** Stadel, B.V., et al.: Contraception *38* :287 (Sept.) 1988. **186.** Miller, D.R., et al.: Am. J. Epidemiol. *129* :269 (Feb.) 1989. **187.** Kay, C.R., et al.: Br. J. Cancer *58* :675 (Nov.) 1988. **188.** Mann, J.M., et al.: AIDS *2* :249, 1988. **189.** Beral, V., et al.: Lancet *2* :1331 (Dec. 10) 1988.

190. Croft, P., et al.: Br. Med. J. *298* :165 (Jan. 21) 1989. **191.** Louv, W.C., et al.: Am. J. Obstet. Gynecol. *160* :396 (Feb.) 1989.

BRIEF SUMMARY OF PATIENT LABELING

Cigarette-smoking increases the risk of serious adverse effects on the heart and blood vessels from oral contraceptive use. This risk increases with age and with heavy smoking (15 or more cigarettes per day) and is quite marked in women over 35 years of age. Women who use oral contraceptives should not smoke.

In the detailed leaflet, "What You Should Know About Oral Contraceptives," which you have received, the risks and benefits of oral contraceptives are discussed in much more detail. This leaflet also provides information on other forms of contraception. Please take time to read it carefully for it may have been recently revised.

If you have any questions or problems regarding this information, contact your doctor.

Oral contraceptives taken as directed are about 99% effective in preventing pregnancy. (The mini-pill, however, is somewhat less effective.) Forgetting to take your pills increases the chance of pregnancy.

Women who have or have had clotting disorders, cancer of the breast or sex organs, unexplained vaginal bleeding, stroke, heart attack, chest pains on exertion (angina pectoris), liver tumors associated with the use of the pill or with other estrogen-containing products, or who suspect they may be pregnant should not use oral contraceptives.

Most side effects of the pill are not serious. The most common side effects are nausea, vomiting, bleeding between menstrual periods, weight gain, and breast tenderness. However, proper use of oral contraceptives requires that they be taken under your doctor's continuing supervision, because they can be associated with serious side effects which may be fatal. Fortunately, these are very uncommon, but the risks may persist after use of the pill is discontinued. The serious side effects are:

1. Blood clots in the legs, arms, lungs, brain, heart, eyes, abdomen, or elsewhere in the body.
2. Bleeding in the brain (hemorrhage) as a result of bursting of a blood vessel.
3. Disorders of vision.
4. Liver tumors, which may rupture and cause severe bleeding.
5. Birth defects if the pill is taken during pregnancy.
6. High blood pressure.
7. Gallbladder disease.

The symptoms associated with these serious side effects are discussed in the detailed leaflet given you with your supply of pills. Notify your doctor if you notice any unusual physical disturbance while taking the pill.

Breast cancer and other cancers have developed in certain animals when given the estrogens in oral contraceptives for long periods. These findings suggest that oral contraceptives may also cause cancer in humans. However, studies to date in women taking currently marketed oral contraceptives have not confirmed that oral contraceptives cause cancer in humans.

Caution: Oral contraceptives are of no value in the prevention or treatment of venereal disease.

Various drugs, such as antibiotics, may also decrease the effectiveness of oral contraceptives.

DETAILED PATIENT LABELING:
WHAT YOU SHOULD KNOW
ABOUT ORAL CONTRACEPTIVES

Please take the time to read this booklet carefully for it may have been recently revised.

Oral contraceptives (the pill) are the most effective way (except for sterilization) to prevent pregnancy if you follow the directions for their use and are careful not to skip doses or take them irregularly. They are also convenient and, for most women, free of serious or unpleasant side effects. Oral contraceptives must always be taken under the continuing supervision of a doctor.

It is important that any woman who considers using an oral contraceptive understands the risks involved. Although the oral contraceptives have important advantages over other methods of contraception, they have certain risks that no other method has. Only you can decide whether the advantages are worth these risks. This leaflet will tell you about the most important risks. It will explain how you can help your doctor prescribe the pill as safely as possible by telling him/her about yourself and being alert for the earliest signs of trouble. And it will tell you how to use the pill properly, so that it will be as effective as possible. THERE IS MORE DETAILED INFORMATION AVAILABLE IN THE LEAFLET PREPARED FOR DOCTORS. Your pharmacist can show you a copy; you may need your doctor's help in understanding parts of it.

Enovid 5 mg or 10 mg can be prescribed as a treatment for endometriosis and as a treatment for hypermenorrhea and regulating periods. If you are taking Enovid 5 mg or 10 mg

Continued on next page

G.D. Searle & Co.—Cont.

for one of these conditions, the warning information in this detailed leaflet also applies, so please read this leaflet.
Caution: Oral contraceptives are of no value in the prevention or treatment of venereal disease.

> Cigarette-smoking increases the risk of serious adverse effects on the heart and blood vessels from oral contraceptive use. This risk increases with age and with heavy smoking (15 or more cigarettes per day) and is quite marked in women over 35 years of age. Women who use oral contraceptives should not smoke.

WHO SHOULD NOT USE ORAL CONTRACEPTIVES
You should not use oral contraceptives:
A. If you have any of the following conditions:
   1. Blood clots in the legs, lungs, eyes, or elsewhere in the body.
   2. Chest pains on exertion (angina pectoris).
   3. Known or suspected cancer of the breast or sex organs, such as the womb (uterus), vagina, or cervix.
   4. Unusual vaginal bleeding that has not been diagnosed by your doctor.
   5. Known or suspected pregnancy (one or more menstrual periods missed).
B. If you have had any of the following conditions:
   1. Heart attack or stroke (clots or bleeding in the brain).
   2. Blood clots in the legs, lungs, eyes, or elsewhere in the body.
   3. Liver tumor associated with use of the pill or other estrogen-containing products.
C. If you have scanty or irregular periods or are a young woman without a regular cycle, you should use another method of contraception because, if you use the pill, you may have difficulty becoming pregnant or may fail to have menstrual periods after discontinuing the pill.

DECIDING TO USE ORAL CONTRACEPTIVES.
If you do not have any of the conditions listed above and are thinking about using oral contraceptives, to help you decide, you need information about the advantages and risks of oral contraceptives and of other contraceptive methods as well. This leaflet describes the advantages and risks of oral contraceptives. Except for sterilization, the intrauterine device (IUD), and abortion, which have their own specific risks, the only risks of other methods of contraception are those due to pregnancy should the method fail. Your doctor can answer questions you may have with respect to other methods of contraception, and further questions you may have on oral contraceptives after reading this leaflet.

1. *What Oral Contraceptives Are and How They Work.*
Oral contraceptives are of two types. The most common, often simply called "the pill," is a *combination* of an estrogen and a progestogen, the two kinds of female hormones. The amount of estrogen and progestogen can vary, but the amount of estrogen is more important because both the effectiveness and some of the dangers of oral contraceptives have been related to the amount of estrogen. This combination oral contraceptive works principally by preventing release of an egg from the ovary during the cycle in which the pills are taken. When the amount of estrogen is 50 micrograms or more, and the pill is taken as directed, oral contraceptives are more than 99% effective (that is, there would be less than 1 pregnancy in 100 women using the pill for one year). Pills that contain 20 to 35 micrograms of estrogen vary slightly in effectiveness, ranging from 98% to more than 99% effective. The second type of oral contraceptive, often called the mini-pill, contains only a progestogen. It works in part by preventing release of an egg from the ovary, but also by keeping sperm from reaching the egg and by making the womb (uterus) less receptive to any fertilized egg that reaches it. The mini-pill is less effective than the combination oral contraceptive, about 97% effective. In addition, the mini-pill has a tendency to cause irregular bleeding, which may be quite inconvenient, or cessation of bleeding entirely. The mini-pill is used despite its lower effectiveness in the hope that it will prove not to have some of the serious side effects of the estrogen-containing pill, but it is not yet certain that the mini-pill does in fact have fewer serious side effects. The following discussion, while based mainly on information about the combination pills, should be considered to apply as well to the mini-pill.

2. *Other Nonsurgical Ways to Prevent Pregnancy.*
As this leaflet will explain, oral contraceptives have several serious risks. Other methods of contraception have lesser risks or none at all. They are also less effective than oral contraceptives, but, used properly, may be effective enough for many women. The following table gives reported pregnancy rates (the number of women out of 100 who would become pregnant in one year) for these methods:

Pregnancies per 100 Women per Year	
Method	*Range*
Intrauterine device (IUD)	less than 1 to 6
Diaphragm with spermicidal cream or jelly	2 to 20
Condom (rubber)	3 to 36
Spermicidal aerosol foams	2 to 29
Spermicidal jellies or creams	4 to 36
Periodic abstinence (rhythm), all types	less than 1 to 47
1. Calendar method	14 to 47
2. Temperature method	1 to 20
3. Temperature method (intercourse only in postovulatory phase)	less than 1 to 7
4. Mucus method	1 to 25
No contraception	60 to 80

These figures (except for the IUD) vary widely because people differ in how well they use each method. Very faithful users of the various methods obtain the best results, except for users of the periodic abstinence (rhythm) calendar method. Effective use of these methods, except for the IUD, requires somewhat more effort than simply taking a single pill every day, but it is an effort that many couples undertake successfully. Your doctor can tell you a great deal more about these methods of contraception and their effectiveness.

3. *The Dangers of Oral Contraceptives.*
a. *Circulatory disorders (blood clots, strokes, and heart attacks).* Blood clots occasionally form in the blood vessels of the body and, though rare, are the most common of the serious side effects of oral contraceptives. Clotting can result in a stroke (a clot in the brain), a heart attack (a clot in a blood vessel of the heart), or a pulmonary embolus (a clot that forms in the legs or abdominal region, then breaks off and travels to the lungs), or loss of a limb (a clot in a blood vessel in, or leading to, an arm or leg). Clots can also form in the blood vessels of the intestines or liver. Any of these events can be fatal (lead to death). Clots also occur rarely in the blood vessels of the eye, resulting in blindness or impairment of vision in that eye. There is some evidence that the risk of clotting may increase with higher estrogen doses. It is therefore important for your doctor to keep the dose of estrogen as low as possible, so long as the oral contraceptive used has an acceptable pregnancy rate and doesn't cause unacceptable changes in the menstrual pattern. Higher doses of progestogen have also been suggested as increasing the risk of clotting. Furthermore, cigarette-smoking by oral contraceptive users increases the risk of serious adverse effects on the heart and blood vessels. This risk increases with age and with heavy smoking (15 or more cigarettes per day) and begins to become quite marked in women over 35 years of age. For this reason, women who use oral contraceptives should not smoke.
The risk of abnormal clotting increases with age both in users and in nonusers of oral contraceptives, but the increased risk with the oral contraceptives appears to be present at all ages.
The risks of circulatory disorders may persist or continue after the pill is stopped. This has been reported for circulatory disorders in general, for heart disease or heart attacks, and for strokes caused either by a bursting blood vessel in the brain or by blood clots in the brain.
For oral contraceptive users in general, it has been estimated that in women between the ages of 25 and 34 the risk of death due to circulatory disorders in nonsmokers is about 1 in 23,000 per year. In contrast, for nonusers of the pill the risk is about 1 in 37,000 per year. Estimates of the risk of death due to circulatory disorders can be made, depending upon the woman's age, whether or not she uses oral contraceptives, and whether or not she smokes cigarettes. In the age group 25–34 years, women who use the pill have a risk of 1 in 7,000 (for smokers) to 1 in 23,000 (for nonsmokers) per year. This may be compared to the corresponding risk in women who have not used the pill: 1 in 24,000 (for smokers) to 1 in 37,000 (for nonsmokers) per year. The risks are greater in older women; thus, in the age group 35–44 years, women who use the pill have a risk of 1 in 1,600 (for smokers) to 1 in 4,700 (for nonsmokers) per year. The corresponding risk for women who have not used the pill is 1 in 6,600 (for smokers) to 1 in 16,000 (for nonsmokers) per year.
For women aged 16 to 40 it is estimated that about 1 in 2,000 using oral contraceptives will be hospitalized each year because of abnormal clotting in the veins or lungs. Among nonusers of the same age, about 1 in 20,000 would be hospitalized each year for these disorders.
Disease of the arteries characterized by paleness, numbness, or tingling in the fingers or toes has been reported to be more common in pill users.
Strokes are caused by a bursting blood vessel in the brain (hemorrhage) or a loss of blood circulation to the brain due to blood clots. When they occur, paralysis of all or part of the body may result; death can result. The risk of strokes due to clots or hemorrhages in the brain has been reported to be increased in pill users when compared with nonusers.

It has been estimated that pill users are twice as likely as nonusers to have a stroke due to a bursting blood vessel in the brain. It has further been estimated that pill users are 4 to 10 times as likely as nonusers to have a stroke due to clotting in a blood vessel in or leading to the brain.
It has been reported that women using the pill may have a greater risk of heart attack than nonusers. Even without the pill the risk of having a heart attack increases with age and is also increased by additional risk factors such as high blood pressure, high blood cholesterol, obesity, diabetes, cigarette-smoking, or the occurrence during pregnancy of high blood pressure, swelling of the legs, or protein in the urine. Without any risk factors present, the use of oral contraceptives alone may double the risk of heart attack. However, the combination of cigarette-smoking, especially heavy smoking, and oral contraceptive use greatly increases the risk of heart attack. Oral contraceptive users who smoke are about five times more likely to have a heart attack than users who do not smoke, and about ten times more likely to have a heart attack than nonusers who do not smoke. It has been estimated that users between the ages of 30 and 39 who smoke have about a 1 in 10,000 chance each year of having a fatal heart attack compared to about a 1 in 50,000 chance in users who do not smoke, and about a 1 in 100,000 chance in nonusers who do not smoke. In the age group 40 to 44, the risk is about 1 in 1,700 per year for users who smoke compared to about 1 in 10,000 for users who do not smoke, and to about 1 in 14,000 per year for nonusers who do not smoke. Heavy smoking (about 15 cigarettes or more a day) further increases the risk. If you do not smoke and have none of the other heart attack risk factors described above, you will have a smaller risk than listed. If you have several heart attack risk factors, the risk may be considerably greater than listed. The above are average figures for Great Britain; comparable estimates for the U.S. have been higher.
Oral contraceptives should never be used at any age by women who have had a stroke, a heart attack, or chest pains on exertion (angina pectoris), or who have had blood clots in the legs, lungs, or elsewhere.
Anyone using the pill who has severe leg or chest pains, coughs up blood, has difficulty in breathing, severe headache or vomiting, dizziness or fainting, disturbances of vision or speech, weakness, numbness, or pain in an arm or leg should call her doctor immediately and stop taking the pill, and use another method of contraception.
b. *Formation of tumors.* When certain animals are given the female sex hormone estrogen (which is an ingredient in oral contraceptives) continuously for long periods, cancers may develop in organs such as the breast, cervix, vagina, liver, womb, ovary, and pituitary.
These findings suggest that oral contraceptives may cause cancer in humans. However, studies to date in women taking currently marketed oral contraceptives have not confirmed that oral contraceptives cause cancer in humans, but it remains possible they will be discovered in the future to do so. Although several studies have reported no overall increase in breast cancer in oral contraceptive users, other studies have reported increases in certain groups of women who have used oral contraceptives. Such groups reported to be at increased risk have differed from one study to another. Examples of such subgroups are: (a) women aged 20–44 without children who had their first menstrual period before age 13 and who took the pill for 8 or more years; (b) women aged 30–39, users for more than 5 years, and women with children who took the pill for 1–4 years before their first term pregnancy or for less than one year or more than 4 years after delivery; (c) women aged 30–34, and women with one child who took the pill for 2 or more years; (d) women already having benign (noncancerous) breast disease (for example, cysts); (e) long-term (2–4 years) users; and (f) women having other risk factors (such as family history of breast cancer, a previous breast biopsy, or delay in having a first child). Women with a family history of breast cancer or who have breast nodules (lumps), fibrocystic disease (breast cysts), or abnormal mammograms (x-ray pictures of the breasts), or who were exposed to the estrogen diethylstilbestrol (DES) during their mother's pregnancy, or who have abnormal Pap smears should be followed very closely by their doctors if they choose to use oral contraceptives instead of another method of contraception. Many studies have shown that women taking oral contraceptives have less risk of getting benign (noncancerous) breast disease than those who have not used oral contraceptives. There is strong evidence that estrogens (one component of combination-type oral contraceptives), when given for periods of more than one year to women after the menopause (change-of-life), increase the risk of cancer of the womb (uterus). There is also some evidence that the sequential oral contraceptive, a kind of oral contraceptive that is no longer sold, may increase the risk of cancer of the womb. There is no evidence, however, that the oral contraceptives now available increase the risk of this type of cancer, although some individual cases have been reported. Cancer of the cervix may develop more readily in long-term users of the pill, particularly if they have had preexisting abnormal Pap smears. Cervical erosion and cell

abnormalities, as well as chlamydial and gonococcal infections, have been reported to be more frequent in pill users. Unconfirmed observations have reported a greater use of oral contraceptives among African prostitutes testing positive for the AIDS virus.

Very rarely, oral contraceptive users may have a noncancerous tumor of the liver. These tumors do not spread, but they may rupture and cause internal bleeding, which may be fatal. This has been reported in short-term as well as long-term users, although increasing duration of use increases the risk. Long-term users have an estimated annual incidence of 3 to 4 per 100,000. One study reported that oral contraceptive products with a high "hormonal potency" were associated with a higher risk than lower-potency products, as was age over 30 years. Cases of cancer of the liver have been reported in women using oral contraceptives also. Users for 8 or more years were estimated to be 7 to 20 times more likely to develop this cancer than were nonusers. An increased risk of cancer of the bile ducts also has been reported.

A type of skin cancer that has been linked to exposure to sunlight (malignant melanoma) has been reported to be more frequent among pill users. It was not possible to determine what the effect was of greater exposure to sunlight in users.

c. *Dangers to a developing baby if oral contraceptives are used in or immediately preceding pregnancy.* Oral contraceptives should not be taken by pregnant women because they may damage the developing baby. There is an increased risk to the baby of abnormalities of such parts of the body as the backbone, anus, heart, windpipe, esophagus, kidneys, arms, and legs. In addition, the developing female child whose mother has received DES, a synthetic estrogen, during pregnancy has a risk of getting cancer of the vagina or cervix in her teens or young adulthood. This risk is estimated to be about 1 in 1,000 exposures or less. DES-exposed daughters appear to have an increased risk of unfavorable outcome of pregnancy. Abnormalities of the urinary and sex organs and sperm have been reported in DES-exposed male babies as well. It is possible that other estrogens, such as the estrogens in oral contraceptives, could have the same effect in the baby if the mother takes them during pregnancy. It has been reported that there is an increased risk of a type of cancer of the testes and ovaries in people whose mothers received female hormones (including oral contraceptives) during early pregnancy.

Occasionally women who are taking the pill miss periods. It has been reported to occur as frequently as several times each year in some women, depending on various factors such as age and prior history. (Your doctor is the best source of information about this.) The pill should not be used when you are pregnant or suspect you may be pregnant. Very rarely, women who are using the pill as directed become pregnant. The likelihood of becoming pregnant is higher if you occasionally miss one or two pills. Therefore, if you miss a period you should consult your physician before continuing to take the pill. If you miss a period, especially if you have not taken the pill regularly, you should use an alternative method of contraception until pregnancy has been ruled out; if you have missed more than one pill at any time, you should immediately start using an additional method of contraception and complete your pill cycle.

You should not attempt to become pregnant for at least three months after discontinuing oral contraceptives. Use another method of contraception during this period of time. The reason for this is that during this period there may be an increased risk of miscarriage and deformity to the baby, or an increased chance of having twins. Whether there is an overall increase in miscarriage in women who become pregnant soon after stopping the pill as compared with women who did not use the pill is not known, but it is possible that there may be.

If, however, you do become pregnant soon after stopping oral contraceptives, and do not have a miscarriage, there is no evidence that the baby has an increased risk of being abnormal.

d. *Gallbladder disease.* Women who use oral contraceptives have a greater risk than nonusers of having gallbladder disease requiring surgery. The increased risk may first appear within one year of use and may double after 4 or 5 years of use. Cancer of the ducts that collect bile may be more frequent in pill users.

e. *Other side effects of oral contraceptives.* Some women using oral contraceptives experience unpleasant side effects from the pill which are not dangerous and are not likely to damage their health. Some of these side effects are similar to symptoms women experience in early pregnancy and may be temporary. Your breasts may feel tender, be enlarged, or have a discharge; nausea and vomiting or other stomach or intestinal problems may occur; you may gain or lose weight, and your ankles may swell. A spotty darkening of the skin, particularly of the face, is possible and may persist after the drug is discontinued. An allergic or other type of rash or vaginal yeast infection might occur. You may notice unexpected vaginal bleeding, change in discharge, or changes in your menstrual period. Irregular bleeding is frequently seen when the mini-pill or the combination oral contraceptives containing less than 50 micrograms of estrogen are used. These should all be reported to your doctor.

Other side effects include worsening of migraine, asthma, convulsive disorders (such as epilepsy), and kidney, liver, or heart disease because of a tendency for water to be retained in the body when oral contraceptives are used. Other side effects are painful periods; growth of preexisting fibroid tumors of the womb; mental depression; and liver problems with jaundice (yellowing of the whites of the eyes or of the skin). Your doctor may find that levels of sugar and fatty substances in your blood are elevated; the long-term effects of these changes are not known. Some women develop high blood pressure while taking oral contraceptives, which ordinarily, but not always, returns to the original levels when the oral contraceptive is stopped. The degree of blood pressure rise may be related to the amount of progestogen in the pill. Women with a history of increased blood pressure, kidney disease, or toxemia during pregnancy (increased blood pressure, swelling of the legs, protein in the urine, or convulsions), or a family tendency to high blood pressure or its consequences (stroke, heart disease, kidney disease, blood vessel problems), or a history of excessive weight gain or swelling of the legs during their menstrual cycle, may be more likely to develop increased blood pressure when given oral contraceptives; therefore, they should have their blood pressure taken frequently. High blood pressure predisposes one to stroke, heart attacks, kidney disease, and other diseases of the blood vessels. The effect of prolonged use of oral contraceptives on several of your organs (pituitary, liver, ovaries, womb, and adrenals) or immune system is not known at this time.

Increased damage to the chromosomes of white blood cells has been reported in pill users. The significance for cancer or birth defects is unknown.

Other conditions, although not proved to be caused by oral contraceptives, are occasionally reported. These include more frequent urination and some discomfort when urinating, kidney disease, nervousness, dizziness, hearing problems, inflammation of the nasal passages, loss of scalp hair, an increase in body hair, an increase or decrease in sex drive, appetite changes, gum disease, dry socket, cataracts, a need for a change in contact lens prescription or inability to use contact lenses, tiredness, backache, vaginal infections, itching, anemia, blood cell breakdown with kidney failure, headache, symptoms similar to those you get before a period; breast, womb, cervical, and liver cancer; inflammation of the pancreas, liver, or large or small intestine; chorea (spasmodic movements), burning or prickly sensation, rheumatoid arthritis, pulmonary hypertension, abnormal heart rhythm or electrocardiogram, and a bruising disease caused by decreased blood platelets (TTP).

After you stop using oral contraceptives, there may be a delay before you are able to become pregnant or before you resume having menstrual periods. This is especially true of women who had irregular menstrual cycles prior to the use of oral contraceptives.

One study showed that this delay in becoming pregnant can persist up to 72 months after stopping the pill if you have never had children and are over 30 years old. The delay appears to be more severe if the pill has been used for 2 years or more by such women. For women who have had children, the delay can persist to 30 months, regardless of age. For women who have not had children and who are less than 30, the delay may persist to 48 months. Very rarely there may be secretions from the breast associated with the absence of periods, which might be due to a noncancerous tumor of the pituitary gland requiring surgery. This may occur more frequently in former users of the pill than in nonusers. As discussed previously, you should wait at least three months after stopping the pill before you try to become pregnant. During the first three months after stopping oral contraceptives, use another form of contraception. You should consult your doctor before resuming use of oral contraceptives after childbirth, especially if you plan to nurse your baby. Drugs in oral contraceptives are known to appear in the milk, and the long-range effect on babies is not known at this time. Furthermore, oral contraceptives may cause a decrease in your milk supply as well as in the quality of the milk.

4. *Comparison of the Risks of Oral Contraceptives and Other Contraceptive Methods.*

The many studies on the risks and effectiveness of oral contraceptives and other methods of contraception have been analyzed to estimate the risk of death associated with various methods of contraception. This risk has two parts: (a) the risk of the method itself (for example, the risk that oral contraceptives might cause death due to abnormal blood clotting), and (b) the risk of death due to pregnancy or abortion in the event the method should fail. The results of this analysis are shown in the following bar graph. The height of the bars indicates the number of deaths per 100,000 women each year. There are six sets of bars, each set referring to a specific age group of women. Within each set of bars, there is a single bar for each of the different contraceptive methods.

For oral contraceptives, there are two bars—one for smokers and the other for nonsmokers. The analysis is based on present knowledge and new information could, of course, alter it. The analysis shows that the risk of death from all methods of birth control is low and below that associated with the risks of childbirth, *except for oral contraceptives in women over 40 who smoke.* The risk of death associated with pill use in nonsmokers over 40 is higher than with any other method of contraception in that age group. It shows that the lowest risk of death is associated with the condom or diaphragm (traditional contraception) backed up by early legal abortion in case of failure of the condom or diaphragm to prevent pregnancy. Also, at any age, the risk of death (due to unexpected pregnancy) from use of traditional contraception, even without a backup of abortion, is generally the same as, or less than, that from use of oral contraceptives.

Figure 1. Estimated annual number of deaths associated with control of fertility and no control per 100,000 nonsterile women by regimen of control and age of woman.

HOW TO USE ORAL CONTRACEPTIVES AS SAFELY AND EFFECTIVELY AS POSSIBLE, ONCE YOU HAVE DECIDED TO USE THEM

1. *What to Tell Your Doctor.* You can make use of the pill as safe as possible, by telling your doctor if you have any of the following:

a. Conditions that mean you should not use oral contraceptives:

If you *now* have any of the following:

1. Blood clots in the legs, lungs, eyes, or elsewhere in the body.
2. Chest pains on exertion (angina pectoris).
3. Known or suspected cancer of the breast or sex organs, such as the womb (uterus), vagina, or cervix.
4. Unusual vaginal bleeding that has not been diagnosed by your doctor.
5. Known or suspected pregnancy (one or more menstrual periods missed).

If you have *ever* had any of the following:

1. Heart attack or stroke (clots or bleeding in the brain).
2. Blood clots in the legs, lungs, eyes, or elsewhere in the body.
3. Liver tumor associated with use of the pill or other estrogen-containing products.

b. Inform your doctor of the following conditions since s/he will want to watch them closely or they might cause him/her to suggest another method of contraception:

A family history of breast cancer
Breast nodules (lumps), fibrocystic disease (breast cysts), abnormal mammograms (x-ray pictures of the breasts), or abnormal Pap smears
Diabetes
High blood pressure
High blood cholesterol
Cigarette-smoking
Migraine
Heart or kidney disease
Asthma
Problems during a prior pregnancy
Epilepsy

Continued on next page

G.D. Searle & Co.—Cont.

Mental depression

Fibroid tumors of the womb

History of jaundice (yellowing of the whites of the eyes or of the skin)

Gallbladder disease

Varicose veins

Tuberculosis

Plans for elective surgery

Previous problems with your periods (irregularities)

Use of any of the following kinds of drugs, which might interact with the pill: antibiotics (such as rifampin, ampicillin, and tetracycline), sulfa drugs, drugs for epilepsy or migraine, painkillers, tranquilizers, sedatives or sleeping pills, blood-thinning drugs, cortisone-like drugs, vitamins, drugs being used for the treatment of depression, high blood pressure, high blood sugar (diabetes), elevated blood lipids, or asthma.

c. Once you are using oral contraceptives, you should be alert for signs of a serious adverse effect and call your doctor immediately if any of these occur:

Sharp pain in the chest, coughing up of blood, or sudden shortness of breath (indicating possible clots in the lungs).

Pain in the calf (possible clot in the leg).

Crushing chest pain or heaviness (indicating possible heart attack).

Sudden severe headache or vomiting, dizziness or fainting, disturbance of vision or speech, or weakness or numbness in an arm or leg (indicating a possible stroke).

Sudden partial or complete loss of vision (indicating a possible clot in the blood vessels of the eye).

Abnormal vaginal bleeding.

Breast discharge or lumps (you should ask your doctor to show you how to examine your own breasts).

Severe and/or persistent pain or a mass in the abdomen (indicating a possible tumor of the liver, which might have ruptured).

Severe depression.

Yellowing of the whites of the eyes or of the skin (jaundice).

Unusual swelling.

Other unusual conditions.

2. *How to Take the Pill So That It Is Most Effective. Dosage Schedules.* See later sections in this leaflet concerning spotting, breakthrough bleeding, forgotten pills, and missed menstruation.

When you first begin to use the pill, you should use an additional method of protection until you have taken your first seven pills.

To remove a pill, press down on it. The pill will drop through a hole in the bottom of the Compack®.

The Two "three weeks on—one week off" Schedules. Your Demulen 1/35-21 or Demulen 1/50-21 Compack contains 21 tablets arranged in three numbered rows with the days of the week printed above them.

Day-5 Schedule. If you are to begin on day 5, count the day you start to menstruate as day 1 and determine which day to start. Start in row #1 with the pill under the day which corresponds to day 5 after your flow began. Continue to take one pill each day on consecutive days of the week.

After the last (Saturday) pill in row #3 has been taken, if any remain in the first row, complete your 21-pill schedule by taking one pill daily starting with Sunday in row #1. Then stop for one week before starting to take the pills again. Begin your next pill cycle on the same day of the week that you began the first cycle.

Sunday Schedule. Start taking the pills on the first Sunday after your period begins unless your period begins on Sunday. If your period begins on Sunday start taking the pill that very same day.

Begin in row #1 and take your pills, one each day on consecutive days, for three weeks (21 days), then stop taking them for one week (7 days) before starting to take the pills again on Sunday.

Whether you begin on "day 5" or on Sunday, continue taking your pills as directed, month after month, regardless of whether your flow has or has not ceased or whether you may have experienced spotting or unexpected (breakthrough) bleeding during your pill cycle. You will probably have your period about every 28 days.

The "Pill-a-day" Schedule. Your Demulen 1/35-28 or Demulen 1/50-28 Compack contains 28 pills arranged in four numbered rows of seven pills each with the days of the week printed above them.

You must take your pills in order, one each day. Begin with the Sunday pill in row #1.

1—Start taking the pills on the first Sunday after your period begins unless your period begins on Sunday. *If your period begins on Sunday start taking the pills that very same day.*

2—Continue to take one pill each day on consecutive days of the week.

3—After the Saturday pill in row #1 has been taken begin taking pills in row #2, and so on, until the Saturday pill in row #4 has been taken.

4—Replace the Refill in your Compack at once, and begin a new pill cycle the next day, starting with the Sunday pill in row #1.

You will probably have your period about every 28 days, while you are taking the pink (blue for Demulen 1/35-28) pills.

Continue your pill-a-day schedule, month after month, regardless of whether your flow ceases while you are taking the colored pills, or whether you experience spotting or unexpected (breakthrough) bleeding during a cycle.

Take your pill faithfully every "pill day"!

It is important that you take a pill without fail every pill day, at intervals of 24 hours, for two reasons: First, your ovaries may release an egg and therefore you may become pregnant if you do not take your pills regularly. Second, you may spot or start to flow between your periods. This may be inconvenient.

Take your pill at the same time every day!

You are probably wondering why the same time of day is important. By taking your pill at the same time every day it becomes a good habit, and you are much less likely to forget. You may wish to keep your pills in the medicine cabinet near your toothbrush as a reminder to take them when you brush your teeth at night. The best time to take your daily pill may be either with your evening meal or at bedtime. You may find it helpful to associate your pill-taking with something else you do every day at a particular time.

Another very important reason for you to take your pills as "regular as clockwork" is that you are protected best when you take one every 24 hours; they are made to work that way. Just remember that once every day is not the same as once every 24 hours. Here is why: Suppose you were to take your Monday pill in the morning when you get up, and then not take your Tuesday pill till the evening before you go to bed. True, you will have taken a pill each day, on Monday and on Tuesday—but the time between pill-taking will probably have been more than 36 hours, or more than 1½ days! You might spot. Chances are you would still be protected and would not get pregnant, but why risk it when it is so easy to guarantee yourself maximal protection by taking your pill faithfully every pill day and at the same time every pill day? In summary, you should take the pills exactly as directed and at intervals of 24 hours in order to achieve maximum contraceptive effectiveness.

Spotting. This is a slight staining between your menstrual periods which may not even require a pad. Some women spot even though they take their pills exactly as directed. Many women spot although they have never taken the pills. Spotting does not mean that your ovaries are releasing an egg. Spotting may be the result of irregular pill-taking. Getting back on schedule will usually stop it.

If you should spot while taking the pills you should not be alarmed because spotting usually stops by itself within a few days. It seldom occurs after the first pill cycle. Consult your doctor if spotting persists for more than a few days or if it occurs after the second cycle.

Unexpected (Breakthrough) Bleeding. Unexpected (breakthrough) bleeding does not mean your ovaries have released an egg. It seldom occurs, but when it does happen it is most common in the first pill cycle. It is a flow much like a regular period, requiring the use of a pad or tampon.

If you experience breakthrough bleeding use a pad or tampon and continue with your schedule. Usually your periods will become regular within a few cycles. Breakthrough bleeding will seldom bother you again.

Consult your doctor if breakthrough bleeding does not stop within a week or if it occurs after the second cycle.

Forgotten Pills. There is little likelihood of your getting pregnant if only one active pill is missed; however, the possibility increases with each successive day that the scheduled active pills are missed. If you forget to take a pill one day, take two the next day—the one you forgot as soon as you remember and your regular pill at your usual time.

If you forget your pills (except the inactive colored pills in Demulen 1/35-28 or Demulen 1/50-28) on two consecutive days, do not be surprised if you spot or start to flow. You should take two pills each day for the next two days, and use an additional method of protection for the remainder of the cycle.

If you are using Demulen 1/35-28 or Demulen 1/50-28 and forget to take one or more colored pills, begin a new cycle on the next Sunday; use a new package and start taking the white pills. Missing the colored pills does not increase your chances of getting pregnant providing the white pill schedule has been followed.

Missed Menstruation. At times there may be no menstrual period after a cycle of pills. Therefore, if you miss one menstrual period but have taken the pills *exactly as you were supposed to,* continue as usual into the next cycle. You may wish to call your doctor. If you have not taken the pills correctly and miss a menstrual period, *you may be pregnant* and should stop taking oral contraceptives until your doctor determines

whether or not you are pregnant. Until you can get to your doctor, use another form of contraception. If two consecutive menstrual periods are missed, you should stop taking the pills until it is determined whether you are pregnant. If you do become pregnant while using oral contraceptives, you should discuss the risks to the developing baby with your doctor.

3. *Periodic Examinations.* Your doctor will take a complete medical and family history before prescribing oral contraceptives. At that time and about once a year thereafter, s/he will generally examine your blood pressure, breasts, abdomen, and internal female organs (including a Pap smear test for cancer of the cervix) and perform certain laboratory tests. Certain health problems or conditions in your medical or family history may require that your doctor see you more frequently while you are taking the pill.

4. *Using Enovid.* Dosage schedules for Enovid must be individualized for each patient; please follow the directions of your doctor.

SUMMARY

Oral contraceptives are the most effective method, except sterilization, for preventing pregnancy. Other methods, when used conscientiously, are also very effective and have fewer risks. The serious side effects of oral contraceptives are uncommon, but the risk of experiencing them may persist after discontinuing the pill. The pill is a very convenient method for preventing pregnancy.

Women who use oral contraceptives should not smoke.

If you have certain conditions or have had these conditions in the past, you should not use oral contraceptives because of increased risk. These conditions are listed in this leaflet. If you do not have these conditions, and decide to use the pill, please read this leaflet carefully so that you can use the pill safely and effectively.

Based on your doctor's assessment of your medical needs, this drug has been prescribed for you. Do not give it to anyone else.

See your doctor regularly, ask any questions you may have about the use of the pill, and report any special problems that may arise.

Be certain to read new revisions of this leaflet. You may check the date of the most recent revision by phoning the manufacturer toll free at 1-800-323-4204 or by writing to the address below.

Address medical inquiries to:

G.D. Searle & Co.

Medical and Scientific Information Department

4901 Searle Parkway

Skokie, IL 60077   AO5479-1

These products are shown in the Product Identification Section, page 429

DRAMAMINE® Liquid   **OTC**

[*dram¹uh-meen*]

(dimenhydrinate syrup USP)

DRAMAMINE® Tablets   **OTC**

(dimenhydrinate tablets USP)

DRAMAMINE INJECTION™   ℞

(dimenhydrinate injection USP)

DESCRIPTION

Dimenhydrinate, an antinauseant/antiemetic, is the 8-chlorotheophylline (8-chloro-3,7-dihydro-1,3-dimethyl-1H-purine-2,6-dione) salt of diphenhydramine (2-diphenylmethoxy-N,N-dimethylethanamine). The structural formula of dimenhydrinate is

Dimenhydrinate contains not less than 53% and not more than 56% of diphenhydramine, and not less than 44% and not more than 47% of 8-chlorotheophylline, calculated on the dried basis.

Dramamine Injection ampuls and vials contain a sterile solution of dimenhydrinate 50 mg/ml in benzyl alcohol 5%, propylene glycol 50%, and water for injection.

Inactive ingredients of Dramamine tablets include acacia, carboxymethylcellulose sodium, corn starch, magnesium stearate, and sodium sulfate. Inactive ingredients of Dramamine liquid include cherry flavor, coloring, ethyl alcohol 5%, glycerin, methylparaben, sucrose, and water.

CLINICAL PHARMACOLOGY

While the precise mode of action of dimenhydrinate is not known, it has a depressant action on hyperstimulated labyrinthine function.

INDICATIONS AND USAGE

Dramamine is indicated for the prevention and treatment of the nausea, vomiting, or vertigo/dizziness of motion sickness.

CONTRAINDICATIONS

Neonates and patients with a history of hypersensitivity to dimenhydrinate or its components (diphenhydramine or 8-chlorotheophylline) should not be treated with Dramamine Injection.

WARNINGS

Injection:

Caution should be used when Dramamine is taken in conjunction with certain antibiotics that may cause ototoxicity, since Dramamine is capable of masking ototoxic symptoms and an irreversible state may be reached. As with any drug, pregnant or nursing women should seek the advice of a health professional before using this product.

This drug may impair the mental and/or physical abilities required for the performance of potentially hazardous tasks, such as driving a vehicle or operating machinery. The concomitant use of alcohol or other central nervous system depressants may have an additive effect. Therefore, patients should be warned accordingly.

Dimenhydrinate should be used with caution in patients having conditions which might be aggravated by anticholinergic therapy (ie, prostatic hypertrophy, stenosing peptic ulcer, pyloroduodenal obstruction, bladder neck obstruction, narrow-angle glaucoma, bronchial asthma, or cardiac arrhythmias).

This preparation should not be injected intra-arterially.

Usage in Children: For infants and children especially, antihistamines in overdosage may cause hallucinations, convulsions, or death.

As in adults, antihistamines may diminish mental alertness in children. In the young child, particularly, they may produce excitation.

Oral: Do not take this product if you have asthma, glaucoma, emphysema, chronic pulmonary disease, shortness of breath, difficulty in breathing, or difficulty in urination due to enlargement of the prostate gland unless directed by a doctor. Do not give to children under 2 years of age unless directed by a doctor. May cause marked drowsiness; alcohol, sedatives, and tranquilizers may increase the drowsiness effect. Avoid alcoholic beverages while taking this product. Do not take this product if you are taking sedatives or tranquilizers, without first consulting your doctor. Use caution when driving a motor vehicle or operating machinery. As with any drug, if you are pregnant or nursing a baby, seek the advice of a health professional before using this product.

PRECAUTIONS

General: Drowsiness may be experienced by some patients, especially with high dosage. This condition frequently is not undesirable in conditions for which the drug is used.

Information for Patients: Because of the potential for drowsiness, patients taking Dramamine should be cautioned against operating automobiles or dangerous machinery. See *Warnings.*

Carcinogenesis, mutagenesis, impairment of fertility: Mutagenicity screening tests performed with dimenhydrinate, diphenhydramine, and 8-chlorotheophylline produced positive results in the bacterial systems and negative results in the mammalian systems. There are no human data that indicate Dramamine is a carcinogen or mutagen or that it impairs fertility.

Pregnancy: Pregnancy Category B. Reproduction studies have been performed in rats at doses up to 20 times the human dose, and in rabbits at doses up to 25 times the human dose (on an mg/kg basis), and have revealed no evidence of impaired fertility or harm to the fetus due to Dramamine. There are no adequate and well-controlled studies in pregnant women. However, clinical studies in pregnant women have not indicated that Dramamine increases the risk of abnormalities when administered in any trimester of pregnancy. It would appear that the possibility of fetal harm is remote when the drug is used during pregnancy. Nevertheless, because the studies in humans cannot rule out the possibility of harm, Dramamine should be used during pregnancy only if clearly needed.

Nursing mothers: Small amounts of dimenhydrinate are excreted in breast milk. Because of the potential for adverse reactions in nursing infants from dimenhydrinate, a decision should be made whether to discontinue nursing or to discontinue the drug, taking into account the importance of the drug to the mother.

ADVERSE REACTIONS

The most frequent adverse reaction to Dramamine (dimenhydrinate) is drowsiness. Dizziness may also occur. Symptoms of dry mouth, nose and throat, blurred vision, difficult or painful urination, headache, anorexia, nervousness, restlessness or insomnia (especially in children), skin rash, thickening of bronchial secretions, tachycardia, epigastric distress, lassitude, excitation, and nausea have been reported.

OVERDOSAGE

Drowsiness is the usual clinical side effect. Convulsions, coma, and respiratory depression may occur with massive overdosage. No specific antidote is known. If respiratory depression occurs, mechanically assisted respiration should be initiated and oxygen administered. Convulsions should be treated with appropriate doses of diazepam. Phenobarbital (5 to 6 mg/kg) may be given to control convulsions in children.

The oral LD_{50} in mice and rats is 203 mg/kg and 1320 mg/kg, respectively. The intraperitoneal LD_{50} in mice is 149 mg/kg.

DOSAGE AND ADMINISTRATION

Dramamine Tablets: To prevent motion sickness, the first dose should be taken ½ to 1 hour before starting your activity. Additional medication depends on travel conditions. *Adult and children 12 years of age and over:* 1 to 2 tablets every 4 to 6 hours, not to exceed 8 tablets in 24 hours or as directed by a doctor. *Children 6 to under 12 years:* ½ to 1 tablet every 6 to 8 hours, not to exceed 3 tablets in 24 hours or as directed by a doctor. *Children 2 to under 6 years:* Up to ½ tablet every 6 to 8 hours, not to exceed 1½ tablets in 24 hours or as directed by a doctor. Not for frequent or prolonged use except on advice of a doctor. Do not exceed recommended dosage.

Dramamine Liquid: To prevent motion sickness, the first dose should be taken ½ to 1 hour before starting your activity. Additional medication depends on travel conditions. *Adult and children 12 years of age and over:* 4 to 7 teaspoonfuls every 4 to 6 hours, not to exceed 26 teaspoonfuls in 24 hours or as directed by a doctor. *Children 6 to under 12 years:* 2 to 4 teaspoonfuls every 6 to 8 hours, not to exceed 10 teaspoonfuls in 24 hours or as directed by a doctor. *Children 2 to under 6 years:* 1 to 2 teaspoonfuls every 6 to 8 hours, not to exceed 5 teaspoonfuls in 24 hours or as directed by a doctor. Not for frequent or prolonged use except on advice of a doctor. Do not exceed recommended dosage.

Dramamine Injection (dimenhydrinate injection) is indicated when the oral form is impractical.

Adults: Nausea or vomiting may be expected to be controlled for approximately 4 hours with 50 mg, and prevented by a similar dose every 4 hours. Its administration may be attended by some degree of drowsiness in some patients, and 100 mg every 4 hours may be given in conditions in which drowsiness is not objectionable or is even desirable.

For *intramuscular* administration, each milliliter (50 mg) of solution is injected as needed, but for *intravenous* administration, each milliliter (50 mg) of solution must be diluted in 10 ml of 0.9% Sodium Chloride Injection USP and injected over a period of 2 minutes.

Pediatric: For intramuscular administration, 1.25 mg/kg of body weight or 37.5 mg/m² of body surface area is administered four times daily. The maximum dose should not exceed 300 mg daily.

Parenteral drug products should be inspected visually for particulate matter and discoloration prior to administration, whenever solution and container permit. Use only if solution is clear and vial seal is intact.

HOW SUPPLIED

Dramamine (dimenhydrinate) is supplied in the following dosage forms and package sizes:

For oral use—**tablets,** scored, white, 50 mg, with SEARLE debossed on one side and 1701 on the other side; cartons of 100 single-dose individually blister-sealed tablets; **liquid,** 15.62 mg/5 ml ethyl alcohol 5%, bottles of 16 fl oz.

Dramamine Injection (dimenhydrinate) is supplied in 1-ml ampuls, each containing 50 mg of dimenhydrinate, in cartons of 25, and in 5-ml (50 mg/ml, 250 mg total) vials in cartons of 25.

Dramamine Liquid and Tablets are manufactured by Searle & Co. Dramamine ampuls and vials are manufactured for G. D. Searle & Co.

[*Please note: Other sizes of Dramamine Tablets and Liquid are also shown in the PDR For Nonprescription Drugs.*]

A05100-1

ENOVID® 5 mg ℞
ENOVID® 10 mg ℞
[*ē-nov'id*]
(norethynodrel with mestranol)

See Demulen products under this manufacturer for Enovid 5 mg and Enovid 10 mg prescribing information.

FLAGYL® Tablets ℞
[*flaj'yl*]
(metronidazole)

WARNING

Metronidazole has been shown to be carcinogenic in mice and rats (see *Warnings*). Unnecessary use of the drug should be avoided. Its use should be reserved for the conditions described in the *Indications and Usage* section below.

DESCRIPTION

Flagyl (metronidazole) is an oral synthetic antiprotozoal and antibacterial agent, 1-(β-hydroxyethyl)-2-methyl-5-nitroimidazole, which has the following structural formula:

Flagyl tablets contain 250 mg or 500 mg of metronidazole. Inactive ingredients include cellulose, FD&C Blue No. 2 Lake, hydroxypropyl cellulose, hydroxypropyl methylcellulose, polyethylene glycol, stearic acid, and titanium dioxide.

CLINICAL PHARMACOLOGY

Disposition of metronidazole in the body is similar for both oral and intravenous dosage forms, with an average elimination half-life in healthy humans of eight hours.

The major route of elimination of metronidazole and its metabolites is via the urine (60–80% of the dose), with fecal excretion accounting for 6–15% of the dose. The metabolites that appear in the urine result primarily from side-chain oxidation [1-(β-hydroxyethyl)- 2-hydroxymethyl-5-nitroimidazole and 2-methyl-5-nitroimidazole-1-yl-acetic acid] and glucuronide conjugation, with unchanged metronidazole accounting for approximately 20% of the total. Renal clearance of metronidazole is approximately 10 ml/min/1.73 m². Metronidazole is the major component appearing in the plasma, with lesser quantities of the 2-hydroxymethyl metabolite also being present. Less than 20% of the circulating metronidazole is bound to plasma proteins. Both the parent compound and the metabolite possess *in vitro* bactericidal activity against most strains of anaerobic bacteria and *in vitro* trichomonacidal activity.

Metronidazole appears in cerebrospinal fluid, saliva, and breast milk in concentrations similar to those found in plasma. Bactericidal concentrations of metronidazole have also been detected in pus from hepatic abscesses.

Following oral administration metronidazole is well absorbed, with peak plasma concentrations occurring between one and two hours after administration. Plasma concentrations of metronidazole are proportional to the administered dose. Oral administration of 250 mg, 500 mg, or 2,000 mg produced peak plasma concentrations of 6 mcg/ml, 12 mcg/ml, and 40 mcg/ml, respectively. Studies reveal no significant bioavailability differences between males and females; however, because of weight differences, the resulting plasma levels in males are generally lower.

Decreased renal function does not alter the single-dose pharmacokinetics of metronidazole. However, plasma clearance of metronidazole is decreased in patients with decreased liver function.

Microbiology:

Trichomonas vaginalis, Entamoeba histolytica. Flagyl (metronidazole) possesses direct trichomonacidal and amebacidal activity against *T. vaginalis* and *E. histolytica.* The *in vitro* minimal inhibitory concentration (MIC) for most strains of these organisms is 1 mcg/ml or less.

Anaerobic Bacteria. Metronidazole is active *in vitro* against most obligate anaerobes, but does not appear to possess any clinically relevant activity against facultative anaerobes or obligate aerobes. Against susceptible organisms, metronidazole is generally bactericidal at concentrations equal to or slightly higher than the minimal inhibitory concentrations.

Metronidazole has been shown to have *in vitro* and clinical activity against the following organisms:

Anaerobic gram-negative bacilli, including:
   Bacteroides species including the *Bacteroides fragilis* group (*B. fragilis, B. distasonis, B. ovatus, B. thetaiotaomicron, B. vulgatus*)
   Fusobacterium species
Anaerobic gram-positive bacilli, including:
   Clostridium species and susceptible strains of *Eubacterium*
Anaerobic gram-positive cocci, including:
   Peptococcus species
   Peptostreptococcus species

Susceptibility Tests: Bacteriologic studies should be performed to determine the causative organisms and their susceptibility to metronidazole; however, the rapid, routine susceptibility testing of individual isolates of anaerobic bacteria is not always practical, and therapy may be started while awaiting these results.

Quantitative methods give the most precise estimates of susceptibility to antibacterial drugs. A standardized agar dilution method and a broth microdilution method are recommended.[1]

Control strains are recommended for standardized susceptibility testing. Each time the test is performed, one or more of the following strains should be included: *Clostridium perfringens* ATCC 13124, *Bacteroides fragilis* ATCC 25285, and *Bacteroides thetaiotaomicron* ATCC 29741. The mode metronida-

Continued on next page

G.D. Searle & Co.—Cont.

zole MICs for those three strains are reported to be 0.25, 0.25, and 0.5 mcg/ml, respectively.

A clinical laboratory is considered under acceptable control if the results of the control strains are within one doubling dilution of the mode MICs reported for metronidazole.

A bacterial isolate may be considered susceptible if the MIC value for metronidazole is not more than 16 mcg/ml. An organism is considered resistant if the MIC is greater than 16 mcg/ml. A report of "resistant" from the laboratory indicates that the infecting organism is not likely to respond to therapy.

INDICATIONS AND USAGE

Symptomatic Trichomoniasis. Flagyl is indicated for the treatment of symptomatic trichomoniasis in females and males when the presence of the trichomonad has been confirmed by appropriate laboratory procedures (wet smears and/or cultures).

Asymptomatic Trichomoniasis. Flagyl is indicated in the treatment of asymptomatic females when the organism is associated with endocervicitis, cervicitis, or cervical erosion. Since there is evidence that presence of the trichomonad can interfere with accurate assessment of abnormal cytological smears, additional smears should be performed after eradication of the parasite.

Treatment of Asymptomatic Consorts. *T. vaginalis* infection is a venereal disease. Therefore, asymptomatic sexual partners of treated patients should be treated simultaneously if the organism has been found to be present, in order to prevent reinfection of the partner. The decision as to whether to treat an asymptomatic male partner who has a negative culture or one for whom no culture has been attempted is an individual one. In making this decision, it should be noted that there is evidence that a woman may become reinfected if her consort is not treated. Also, since there can be considerable difficulty in isolating the organism from the asymptomatic male carrier, negative smears and cultures cannot be relied upon in this regard. In any event, the consort should be treated with Flagyl in cases of reinfection.

Amebiasis. Flagyl is indicated in the treatment of acute intestinal amebiasis (amebic dysentery) and amebic liver abscess.

In amebic liver abscess, Flagyl therapy does not obviate the need for aspiration or drainage of pus.

Anaerobic Bacterial Infections. Flagyl is indicated in the treatment of serious infections caused by susceptible anaerobic bacteria. Indicated surgical procedures should be performed in conjunction with Flagyl therapy. In a mixed aerobic and anaerobic infection, antibiotics appropriate for the treatment of the aerobic infection should be used in addition to Flagyl.

In the treatment of most serious anaerobic infections, Flagyl I.V.™ (metronidazole hydrochloride) or Flagyl I.V.™ RTU® (metronidazole) is usually administered initially. This may be followed by oral therapy with Flagyl (metronidazole) at the discretion of the physician.

INTRA-ABDOMINAL INFECTIONS, including peritonitis, intra-abdominal abscess, and liver abscess, caused by *Bacteroides* species including the *B. fragilis* group (*B. fragilis, B. distasonis, B. ovatus, B. thetaiotaomicron, B. vulgatus*), *Clostridium* species, *Eubacterium* species, *Peptococcus* species, and *Peptostreptococcus* species.

SKIN AND SKIN STRUCTURE INFECTIONS caused by *Bacteroides* species including the *B. fragilis* group, *Clostridium* species, *Peptococcus* species, *Peptostreptococcus* species, and *Fusobacterium* species.

GYNECOLOGIC INFECTIONS, including endometritis, endomyometritis, tubo-ovarian abscess, and postsurgical vaginal cuff infection, caused by *Bacteroides* species including the *B. fragilis* group, *Clostridium* species, *Peptococcus* species, and *Peptostreptococcus* species.

BACTERIAL SEPTICEMIA caused by *Bacteroides* species including the *B. fragilis* group, and *Clostridium* species.

BONE AND JOINT INFECTIONS, as adjunctive therapy, caused by *Bacteroides* species including the *B. fragilis* group.

CENTRAL NERVOUS SYSTEM (CNS) INFECTIONS, including meningitis and brain abscess, caused by *Bacteroides* species including the *B. fragilis* group.

LOWER RESPIRATORY TRACT INFECTIONS, including pneumonia, empyema, and lung abscess, caused by *Bacteroides* species including the *B. fragilis* group.

ENDOCARDITIS caused by *Bacteroides* species including the *B. fragilis* group.

CONTRAINDICATIONS

Flagyl is contraindicated in patients with a prior history of hypersensitivity to metronidazole or other nitroimidazole derivatives.

In patients with trichomoniasis, Flagyl is contraindicated during the first trimester of pregnancy. (See *Warnings.*)

WARNINGS

Convulsive Seizures and Peripheral Neuropathy: Convulsive seizures and peripheral neuropathy, the latter characterized

mainly by numbness or paresthesia of an extremity, have been reported in patients treated with metronidazole. The appearance of abnormal neurologic signs demands the prompt discontinuation of Flagyl therapy. Flagyl should be administered with caution to patients with central nervous system diseases.

PRECAUTIONS

General: Patients with severe hepatic disease metabolize metronidazole slowly, with resultant accumulation of metronidazole and its metabolites in the plasma. Accordingly, for such patients, doses below those usually recommended should be administered cautiously.

Known or previously unrecognized candidiasis may present more prominent symptoms during therapy with Flagyl and requires treatment with a candicidal agent.

Information for patients: Alcoholic beverages should be avoided while taking Flagyl and for at least one day afterward. See *Drug interactions.*

Laboratory tests: Flagyl (metronidazole) is a nitroimidazole and should be used with care in patients with evidence of or history of blood dyscrasia. A mild leukopenia has been observed during its administration; however, no persistent hematologic abnormalities attributable to metronidazole have been observed in clinical studies. Total and differential leukocyte counts are recommended before and after therapy for trichomoniasis and amebiasis, especially if a second course of therapy is necessary, and before and after therapy for anaerobic infection.

Drug interactions: Metronidazole has been reported to potentiate the anticoagulant effect of warfarin and other oral coumarin anticoagulants, resulting in a prolongation of prothrombin time. This possible drug interaction should be considered when Flagyl is prescribed for patients on this type of anticoagulant therapy.

The simultaneous administration of drugs that induce microsomal liver enzymes, such as phenytoin or phenobarbital, may accelerate the elimination of metronidazole, resulting in reduced plasma levels; impaired clearance of phenytoin has also been reported.

The simultaneous administration of drugs that decrease microsomal liver enzyme activity, such as cimetidine, may prolong the half-life and decrease plasma clearance of metronidazole. In patients stabilized on relatively high doses of lithium, short-term Flagyl therapy has been associated with elevation of serum lithium and, in a few cases, signs of lithium toxicity. Serum lithium and serum creatinine levels should be obtained several days after beginning metronidazole to detect any increase that may precede clinical symptoms of lithium intoxication.

Alcoholic beverages should not be consumed during Flagyl therapy and for at least one day afterward because abdominal cramps, nausea, vomiting, headaches, and flushing may occur.

Psychotic reactions have been reported in alcoholic patients who are using metronidazole and disulfiram concurrently. Metronidazole should not be given to patients who have taken disulfiram within the last two weeks.

Drug/Laboratory test interactions: Metronidazole may interfere with certain types of determinations of serum chemistry values, such as aspartate aminotransferase (AST, SGOT), alanine aminotransferase (ALT, SGPT), lactate dehydrogenase (LDH), triglycerides, and hexokinase glucose. Values of zero may be observed. All of the assays in which interference has been reported involve enzymatic coupling of the assay to oxidation-reduction of nicotine adenine dinucleotide ($NAD^+ \rightleftharpoons NADH$). Interference is due to the similarity in absorbance peaks of NADH (340 nm) and metronidazole (322 nm) at pH 7.

Carcinogenesis, mutagenesis, impairment of fertility:

Tumorigenicity studies in rodents: Metronidazole has shown evidence of carcinogenic activity in a number of studies involving chronic, oral administration in mice and rats. Prominent among the effects in the mouse was the promotion of pulmonary tumorigenesis. This has been observed in all six reported studies in that species, including one study in which the animals were dosed on an intermittent schedule (administration during every fourth week only). At very high dose levels (approx. 500 mg/kg/day) there was a statistically significant increase in the incidence of malignant liver tumors in males. Also, the published results of one of the mouse studies indicate an increase in the incidence of malignant lymphomas as well as pulmonary neoplasms associated with lifetime feeding of the drug. All these effects are statistically significant.

Several long-term, oral-dosing studies in the rat have been completed. There were statistically significant increases in the incidence of various neoplasms, particularly in mammary and hepatic tumors, among female rats administered metronidazole over those noted in the concurrent female control groups.

Two lifetime tumorigenicity studies in hamsters have been performed and reported to be negative.

Mutagenicity studies: Although metronidazole has shown mutagenic activity in a number of *in vitro* assay systems,

studies in mammals (*in vivo*) have failed to demonstrate a potential for genetic damage.

Pregnancy: Teratogenic Effects—Pregnancy Category B. Metronidazole crosses the placental barrier and enters the fetal circulation rapidly. Reproduction studies have been performed in rats at doses up to five times the human dose and have revealed no evidence of impaired fertility or harm to the fetus due to metronidazole. Metronidazole administered intraperitoneally to pregnant mice at approximately the human dose caused fetotoxicity; administered orally to pregnant mice, no fetotoxicity was observed. There are, however, no adequate and well-controlled studies in pregnant women. Because animal reproduction studies are not always predictive of human response, and because metronidazole is a carcinogen in rodents, this drug should be used during pregnancy only if clearly needed (see *Contraindications*). Use of Flagyl for trichomoniasis in the second and third trimesters should be restricted to those in whom local palliative treatment has been inadequate to control symptoms.

Nursing mothers: Because of the potential for tumorigenicity shown for metronidazole in mouse and rat studies, a decision should be made whether to discontinue nursing or to discontinue the drug, taking into account the importance of the drug to the mother. Metronidazole is secreted in breast milk in concentrations similar to those found in plasma.

Pediatric use: Safety and effectiveness in children have not been established, except for the treatment of amebiasis.

ADVERSE REACTIONS

Two serious adverse reactions reported in patients treated with Flagyl (metronidazole) have been convulsive seizures and peripheral neuropathy, the latter characterized mainly by numbness or paresthesia of an extremity. Since persistent peripheral neuropathy has been reported in some patients receiving prolonged administration of Flagyl, patients should be specifically warned about these reactions and should be told to stop the drug and report immediately to their physicians if any neurologic symptoms occur.

The most common adverse reactions reported have been referable to the gastrointestinal tract, particularly nausea reported by about 12% of patients, sometimes accompanied by headache, anorexia, and occasionally vomiting; diarrhea; epigastric distress; and abdominal cramping. Constipation has also been reported.

The following reactions have also been reported during treatment with Flagyl (metronidazole):

Mouth: A sharp, unpleasant metallic taste is not unusual. Furry tongue, glossitis, and stomatitis have occurred; these may be associated with a sudden overgrowth of *Candida* which may occur during effective therapy.

Hematopoietic: Reversible neutropenia (leukopenia); rarely, reversible thrombocytopenia.

Cardiovascular: Flattening of the T-wave may be seen in electrocardiographic tracings.

Central Nervous System: Convulsive seizures, peripheral neuropathy, dizziness, vertigo, incoordination, ataxia, confusion, irritability, depression, weakness, and insomnia.

Hypersensitivity: Urticaria, erythematous rash, flushing, nasal congestion, dryness of the mouth (or vagina or vulva), and fever.

Renal: Dysuria, cystitis, polyuria, incontinence, and a sense of pelvic pressure. Instances of darkened urine have been reported by approximately one patient in 100,000. Although the pigment which is probably responsible for this phenomenon has not been positively identified, it is almost certainly a metabolite of metronidazole and seems to have no clinical significance.

Other: Proliferation of *Candida* in the vagina, dyspareunia, decrease of libido, proctitis, and fleeting joint pains sometimes resembling "serum sickness." If patients receiving Flagyl drink alcoholic beverages, they may experience abdominal distress, nausea, vomiting, flushing, or headache. A modification of the taste of alcoholic beverages has also been reported.

Crohn's disease patients are known to have an increased incidence of gastrointestinal and certain extraintestinal cancers. There have been some reports in the medical literature of breast and colon cancer in Crohn's disease patients who have been treated with metronidazole at high doses for extended periods of time. A cause and effect relationship has not been established. Crohn's disease is not an approved indication for Flagyl.

OVERDOSAGE

Single oral doses of metronidazole, up to 15 g, have been reported in suicide attempts and accidental overdoses. Symptoms reported include nausea, vomiting, and ataxia.

Oral metronidazole has been studied as a radiation sensitizer in the treatment of malignant tumors. Neurotoxic effects, including seizures and peripheral neuropathy, have been reported after 5 to 7 days of doses of 6 to 10.4 g every other day.

Treatment: There is no specific antidote for Flagyl overdose; therefore, management of the patient should consist of symptomatic and supportive therapy.

DOSAGE AND ADMINISTRATION

In elderly patients the pharmacokinetics of metronidazole may be altered and therefore monitoring of serum levels may be necessary to adjust the metronidazole dosage accordingly.

Trichomoniasis:

In the Female:

One-day treatment—two grams of Flagyl, given either as a single dose or in two divided doses of one gram each given in the same day.

Seven-day course of treatment—250 mg three times daily for seven consecutive days. There is some indication from controlled comparative studies that cure rates as determined by vaginal smears, signs and symptoms, may be higher after a seven-day course of treatment than after a one-day treatment regimen.

The dosage regimen should be individualized. Single-dose treatment can assure compliance, especially if administered under supervision, in those patients who cannot be relied on to continue the seven-day regimen. A seven-day course of treatment may minimize reinfection of the female long enough to treat sexual contacts. Further, some patients may tolerate one course of therapy better than the other.

Pregnant patients should not be treated during the first trimester with either regimen. If treated during the second or third trimester, the one-day course of therapy should not be used, as it results in higher serum levels which reach the fetal circulation. (See *Contraindications* and *Precautions.*)

When repeat courses of the drug are required, it is recommended that an interval of four to six weeks elapse between courses and that the presence of the trichomonad be reconfirmed by appropriate laboratory measures. Total and differential leukocyte counts should be made before and after re-treatment.

In the Male: Treatment should be individualized as for the female.

Amebiasis:

Adults:

For acute intestinal amebiasis (acute amebic dysentery): 750 mg orally three times daily for 5 to 10 days.

For amebic liver abscess: 500 mg or 750 mg orally three times daily for 5 to 10 days.

Children: 35 to 50 mg/kg/24 hours, divided into three doses, orally for 10 days.

Anaerobic Bacterial Infections: In the treatment of most serious anaerobic infections, Flagyl I.V.™ (metronidazole hydrochloride) or Flagyl I.V.™RTU® (metronidazole) is usually administered initially.

The usual adult *oral* dosage is 7.5 mg/kg every six hours (approx. 500 mg for a 70-kg adult). A maximum of 4 g should not be exceeded during a 24-hour period.

The usual duration of therapy is 7 to 10 days; however, infections of the bone and joint, lower respiratory tract, and endocardium may require longer treatment.

Patients with severe hepatic disease metabolize metronidazole slowly, with resultant accumulation of metronidazole and its metabolites in the plasma. Accordingly, for such patients, doses below those usually recommended should be administered cautiously. Close monitoring of plasma metronidazole levels[2] and toxicity is recommended.

The dose of Flagyl should not be specifically reduced in anuric patients since accumulated metabolites may be rapidly removed by dialysis.

HOW SUPPLIED

Flagyl 250-mg tablets are round, blue, film coated, with SEARLE and 1831 debossed on one side and FLAGYL and 250 on the other side; bottles of 50, 100, 250, 1,000, and 2,500, and cartons of 100 unit-dose individually blister-sealed tablets.

Flagyl 500-mg tablets are oblong, blue, film coated, with FLAGYL debossed on one side and 500 on the other side; bottles of 50, 100, and 500, and cartons of 100 unit-dose individually blister-sealed tablets.

Storage and Stability: Store below 86°F (30°C) and protect from light.

---

1. Proposed standard: PSM-11—Proposed Reference Dilution Procedure for Antimicrobic Susceptibility Testing of Anaerobic Bacteria, National Committee for Clinical Laboratory Standards; and Sutter, et al.: Collaborative Evaluation of a Proposed Reference Dilution Method of Susceptibility Testing of Anaerobic Bacteria, Antimicrob. Agents Chemother. 16: 495–502 (Oct.) 1979; and Tally, et al.: *In Vitro* Activity of Thienamycin, Antimicrob. Agents Chemother. 14: 436–438 (Sept.) 1978.
2. Ralph, E.D., and Kirby, W.M.M.: Bioassay of Metronidazole With Either Anaerobic or Aerobic Incubation, J. Infect. Dis. 132: 587–591 (Nov.) 1975; or Gulaid, et al.: Determination of Metronidazole and Its Major Metabolites in Biological Fluids by High Pressure Liquid Chromatography, Br. J. Clin. Pharmacol. 6: 430–432, 1978.   A05709-3

Shown in Product Identification Section, page 429

LOMOTIL® Liquid   ©

LOMOTIL® Tablets   ©

[lō-mō'til]

(diphenoxylate hydrochloride with atropine sulfate)

DESCRIPTION

Each Lomotil tablet and each 5 ml of Lomotil liquid for oral use contains:

diphenoxylate hydrochloride .... 2.5 mg

(Warning—May be habit forming.)

atropine sulfate .... 0.025 mg

Diphenoxylate hydrochloride, an antidiarrheal, is ethyl 1-(3-cyano-3,3-diphenylpropyl)-4-phenylisonipecotate monohydrochloride and has the following structural formula:

Atropine sulfate, an anticholinergic, is endo-(±)-α-(hydroxymethyl) benzeneacetic acid 8-methyl-8-azabicyclo[3.2.1] oct-3-yl ester sulfate (2:1) (salt) monohydrate and has the following structural formula:

Inactive ingredients of Lomotil tablets include acacia, corn starch, magnesium stearate, sorbitol, sucrose, and talc. Inactive ingredients of Lomotil liquid include cherry flavor, citric acid, ethyl alcohol 15%, FD&C Yellow No. 6, glycerin, sodium phosphate, sorbitol, and water.

IMPORTANT INFORMATION

Lomotil is classified as a Schedule V controlled substance by federal law. Diphenoxylate hydrochloride is chemically related to the narcotic meperidine. Therefore, in case of overdosage, treatment is similar to that for meperidine or morphine intoxication, in which prolonged and careful monitoring is essential. Respiratory depression may be evidenced as late as 30 hours after ingestion and may recur in spite of an initial response to narcotic antagonists. A subtherapeutic amount of atropine sulfate is present to discourage deliberate overdosage. LOMOTIL IS *NOT* AN INNOCUOUS DRUG AND DOSAGE RECOMMENDATIONS SHOULD BE STRICTLY ADHERED TO, ESPECIALLY IN CHILDREN. KEEP THIS AND ALL MEDICATIONS OUT OF REACH OF CHILDREN.

CLINICAL PHARMACOLOGY

Diphenoxylate is rapidly and extensively metabolized in man by ester hydrolysis to diphenoxylic acid (difenoxine), which is biologically active and the major metabolite in the blood. After a 5-mg oral dose of carbon-14 labeled diphenoxylate hydrochloride in ethanolic solution was given to three healthy volunteers, an average of 14% of the drug plus its metabolites was excreted in the urine and 49% in the feces over a four-day period. Urinary excretion of the unmetabolized drug constituted less than 1% of the dose, and diphenoxylic acid plus its glucuronide conjugate constituted about 6% of the dose. In a 16-subject crossover bioavailability study, a linear relationship in the dose range of 2.5 to 10 mg was found between the dose of diphenoxylate hydrochloride (given as Lomotil liquid) and the peak plasma concentration, the area under the plasma concentration-time curve, and the amount of diphenoxylic acid excreted in the urine. In the same study the bioavailability of the tablet compared with an equal dose of the liquid was approximately 90%. The average peak plasma concentration of diphenoxylic acid following ingestion of four 2.5-mg tablets was 163 ng/ml at about 2 hours, and the elimination half-life of diphenoxylic acid was approximately 12 to 14 hours.

In dogs, diphenoxylate hydrochloride has a direct effect on circular smooth muscle of the bowel that conceivably results in segmentation and prolongation of gastrointestinal transit time. The clinical antidiarrheal action of diphenoxylate hydrochloride may thus be a consequence of enhanced segmentation that allows increased contact of the intraluminal contents with the intestinal mucosa.

INDICATIONS AND USAGE

Lomotil is effective as adjunctive therapy in the management of diarrhea.

CONTRAINDICATIONS

Lomotil is contraindicated in patients with

1. Known hypersensitivity to diphenoxylate or atropine.
2. Obstructive jaundice.
3. Diarrhea associated with pseudomembranous enterocolitis or enterotoxin-producing bacteria.

WARNINGS

LOMOTIL IS *NOT* AN INNOCUOUS DRUG AND DOSAGE RECOMMENDATIONS MUST BE STRICTLY ADHERED TO, ESPECIALLY IN CHILDREN. LOMOTIL IS NOT RECOMMENDED FOR CHILDREN UNDER 2 YEARS OF AGE. OVERDOSAGE MAY RESULT IN SEVERE RESPIRATORY DEPRESSION AND COMA, POSSIBLY LEADING TO PERMANENT BRAIN DAMAGE OR DEATH (SEE *OVERDOSAGE*). THEREFORE, KEEP THIS MEDICATION OUT OF THE REACH OF CHILDREN.

THE USE OF LOMOTIL SHOULD BE ACCOMPANIED BY APPROPRIATE FLUID AND ELECTROLYTE THERAPY, WHEN INDICATED. IF SEVERE DEHYDRATION OR ELECTROLYTE IMBALANCE IS PRESENT, LOMOTIL SHOULD BE WITHHELD UNTIL APPROPRIATE CORRECTIVE THERAPY HAS BEEN INITIATED. DRUG-INDUCED INHIBITION OF PERISTALSIS MAY RESULT IN FLUID RETENTION IN THE INTESTINE, WHICH MAY FURTHER AGGRAVATE DEHYDRATION AND ELECTROLYTE IMBALANCE.

LOMOTIL SHOULD BE USED WITH SPECIAL CAUTION IN YOUNG CHILDREN BECAUSE THIS AGE GROUP MAY BE PREDISPOSED TO DELAYED DIPHENOXYLATE TOXICITY AND BECAUSE OF THE GREATER VARIABILITY OF RESPONSE IN THIS AGE GROUP.

Antiperistaltic agents may prolong and/or worsen diarrhea associated with organisms that penetrate the intestinal mucosa (toxigenic *E. coli, Salmonella, Shigella*), and pseudomembranous enterocolitis associated with broad-spectrum antibiotics. Antiperistaltic agents should not be used in these conditions.

In some patients with acute ulcerative colitis, agents that inhibit intestinal motility or prolong intestinal transit time have been reported to induce toxic megacolon. Consequently, patients with acute ulcerative colitis should be carefully observed and Lomotil therapy should be discontinued promptly if abdominal distention occurs or if other untoward symptoms develop.

Since the chemical structure of diphenoxylate hydrochloride is similar to that of meperidine hydrochloride, the concurrent use of Lomotil with monoamine oxidase (MAO) inhibitors may, in theory, precipitate hypertensive crisis.

Lomotil should be used with extreme caution in patients with advanced hepatorenal disease and in all patients with abnormal liver function since hepatic coma may be precipitated.

Diphenoxylate hydrochloride may potentiate the action of barbiturates, tranquilizers, and alcohol. Therefore, the patient should be closely observed when any of these are used concomitantly.

PRECAUTIONS

General: Since a subtherapeutic dose of atropine has been added to the diphenoxylate hydrochloride, consideration should be given to the precautions relating to the use of atropine. In children, Lomotil should be used with caution since signs of atropinism may occur even with recommended doses, particularly in patients with Down's syndrome.

Information for patients: INFORM THE PATIENT (PARENT OR GUARDIAN) NOT TO EXCEED THE RECOMMENDED DOSAGE AND TO KEEP LOMOTIL OUT OF THE REACH OF CHILDREN AND IN A CHILD-RESISTANT CONTAINER. INFORM THE PATIENT OF THE CONSEQUENCES OF OVERDOSAGE, INCLUDING SEVERE RESPIRATORY DEPRESSION AND COMA, POSSIBLY LEADING TO PERMANENT BRAIN DAMAGE OR DEATH. Lomotil may produce drowsiness or dizziness. The patient should be cautioned regarding activities requiring mental alertness, such as driving or operating dangerous machinery. Potentiation of the action of alcohol, barbiturates, and tranquilizers with concomitant use of Lomotil should be explained to the patient. The physician should also provide the patient with other information in this labeling, as appropriate.

Drug interactions: Known drug interactions include barbiturates, tranquilizers, and alcohol. Lomotil may interact with MAO inhibitors (see *Warnings*).

In studies with male rats, diphenoxylate hydrochloride was found to inhibit the hepatic microsomal enzyme system at a dose of 2 mg/kg/day. Therefore, diphenoxylate has the potential to prolong the biological half-lives of drugs for which the rate of elimination is dependent on the microsomal drug metabolizing enzyme system.

Carcinogenesis, mutagenesis, impairment of fertility: No long-term study in animals has been performed to evaluate carcinogenic potential. Diphenoxylate hydrochloride was

Continued on next page

G.D. Searle & Co.—Cont.

administered to male and female rats in their diets to provide dose levels of 4 and 20 mg/kg/day throughout a three-litter reproduction study. At 50 times the human dose (20 mg/kg/day), female weight gain was reduced and there was a marked effect on fertility as only 4 of 27 females became pregnant in three test breedings. The relevance of this finding to usage of Lomotil in humans is unknown.

Pregnancy: Pregnancy Category C. Diphenoxylate hydrochloride has been shown to have an effect on fertility in rats when given in doses 50 times the human dose (see above discussion). Other findings in this study include a decrease in maternal weight gain of 30% at 20 mg/kg/day and of 10% at 4 mg/kg/day. At 10 times the human dose (4 mg/kg/day), average litter size was slightly reduced.

Teratology studies were conducted in rats, rabbits, and mice with diphenoxylate hydrochloride at oral doses of 0.4 to 20 mg/kg/day. Due to experimental design and small numbers of litters, embryotoxic, fetotoxic, or teratogenic effects cannot be adequately assessed. However, examination of the available fetuses did not reveal any indication of teratogenicity.

There are no adequate and well-controlled studies in pregnant women. Lomotil should be used during pregnancy only if the anticipated benefit justifies the potential risk to the fetus.

Nursing mothers: Caution should be exercised when Lomotil is administered to a nursing woman, since the physicochemical characteristics of the major metabolite, diphenoxylic acid, are such that it may be excreted in breast milk and since it is known that atropine is excreted in breast milk.

Pediatric use: Lomotil may be used as an adjunct to the treatment of diarrhea but should be accompanied by appropriate fluid and electrolyte therapy, if needed. LOMOTIL IS NOT RECOMMENDED FOR CHILDREN UNDER 2 YEARS OF AGE. Lomotil should be used with special caution in young children because of the greater variability of response in this age group. See *Warnings* and *Dosage and Administration*. In case of accidental ingestion by children, see *Overdosage* for recommended treatment.

ADVERSE REACTIONS

At *therapeutic* doses, the following have been reported; they are listed in decreasing order of severity, but not of frequency:

Nervous system: numbness of extremities, euphoria, depression, malaise/lethargy, confusion, sedation/drowsiness, dizziness, restlessness, headache.

Allergic: anaphylaxis, angioneurotic edema, urticaria, swelling of the gums, pruritus.

Gastrointestinal system: toxic megacolon, paralytic ileus, pancreatitis, vomiting, nausea, anorexia, abdominal discomfort.

The following atropine sulfate effects are listed in decreasing order of severity, but not of frequency: hyperthermia, tachycardia, urinary retention, flushing, dryness of the skin and mucous membranes. These effects may occur especially in children.

THIS MEDICATION SHOULD BE KEPT IN A CHILD-RESISTANT CONTAINER AND OUT OF THE REACH OF CHILDREN SINCE AN OVERDOSAGE MAY RESULT IN SEVERE RESPIRATORY DEPRESSION AND COMA, POSSIBLY LEADING TO PERMANENT BRAIN DAMAGE OR DEATH.

DRUG ABUSE AND DEPENDENCE

Controlled substance: Lomotil is classified as a Schedule V controlled substance by federal regulation. Diphenoxylate hydrochloride is chemically related to the narcotic analgesic meperidine.

Drug abuse and dependence: In doses used for the treatment of diarrhea, whether acute or chronic, diphenoxylate has not produced addiction.

Diphenoxylate hydrochloride is devoid of morphine-like subjective effects at therapeutic doses. At high doses it exhibits codeine-like subjective effects. The dose which produces antidiarrheal action is widely separated from the dose which causes central nervous system effects. The insolubility of diphenoxylate hydrochloride in commonly available aqueous media precludes intravenous self-administration. A dose of 100 to 300 mg/day, which is equivalent to 40 to 120 tablets, administered to humans for 40 to 70 days, produced opiate withdrawal symptoms. Since addiction to diphenoxylate hydrochloride is possible at high doses, the recommended dosage should not be exceeded.

OVERDOSAGE

RECOMMENDED DOSAGE SCHEDULES SHOULD BE STRICTLY FOLLOWED. THIS MEDICATION SHOULD BE KEPT IN A CHILD-RESISTANT CONTAINER AND OUT OF THE REACH OF CHILDREN, SINCE AN OVERDOSAGE MAY RESULT IN SEVERE, EVEN FATAL, RESPIRATORY DEPRESSION.

Diagnosis: Initial signs of overdosage may include dryness of the skin and mucous membranes, mydriasis, restlessness, flushing, hyperthermia, and tachycardia followed by lethargy or coma, hypotonic reflexes, nystagmus, pinpoint pupils, and respiratory depression. Respiratory depression may be evidenced as late as 30 hours after ingestion and may recur in spite of an initial response to narcotic antagonists. TREAT ALL POSSIBLE LOMOTIL OVERDOSAGES AS SERIOUS AND MAINTAIN MEDICAL OBSERVATION FOR AT LEAST 48 HOURS, PREFERABLY UNDER CONTINUOUS HOSPITAL CARE.

Treatment: In the event of overdose, induction of vomiting, gastric lavage, establishment of a patent airway, and possibly mechanically assisted respiration are advised. *In vitro* and animal studies indicate that activated charcoal may significantly decrease the bioavailability of diphenoxylate. In non-comatose patients, a slurry of 100 g of activated charcoal can be administered immediately after the induction of vomiting or gastric lavage.

A pure narcotic antagonist (eg, naloxone) should be used in the treatment of respiratory depression caused by Lomotil. When a narcotic antagonist is administered intravenously, the onset of action is generally apparent within two minutes. It may also be administered subcutaneously or intramuscularly, providing a slightly less rapid onset of action but a more prolonged effect.

To counteract respiratory depression caused by Lomotil overdosage, the following dosage schedule for the narcotic antagonist naloxone hydrochloride should be followed:

Adult dosage: The usual initial adult dose of naloxone hydrochloride is 0.4 mg (1 ml) administered intravenously. If respiratory function does not adequately improve after the initial dose, the same I.V. dose may be repeated at two- to three-minute intervals.

Children: The usual initial dose of naloxone hydrochloride for children is 0.01 mg/kg of body weight administered intravenously and repeated at two- to three-minute intervals if necessary.

Following initial improvement of respiratory function, repeated doses of naloxone hydrochloride may be required to counteract recurrent respiratory depression. Supplemental intramuscular doses of naloxone hydrochloride may be utilized to produce a longer-lasting effect.

Since the duration of action of diphenoxylate hydrochloride is longer than that of naloxone hydrochloride, improvement of respiration following administration may be followed by recurrent respiratory depression. Consequently, continuous observation is necessary until the effect of diphenoxylate hydrochloride on respiration has passed. This effect may persist for many hours. The period of observation should extend over at least 48 hours, preferably under continuous hospital care. Although signs of overdosage and respiratory depression may not be evident soon after ingestion of diphenoxylate hydrochloride, respiratory depression may occur from 12 to 30 hours later.

DOSAGE AND ADMINISTRATION

DO NOT EXCEED RECOMMENDED DOSAGE.

Adults: The recommended initial dosage is two Lomotil tablets four times daily or 10 ml (two regular teaspoonfuls) of Lomotil liquid four times daily (20 mg per day). Most patients will require this dosage until initial control has been achieved, after which the dosage may be reduced to meet individual requirements. Control may often be maintained with as little as 5 mg (two tablets or 10 ml of liquid) daily. Clinical improvement of acute diarrhea is usually observed within 48 hours. If clinical improvement of chronic diarrhea after treatment with a maximum daily dose of 20 mg of diphenoxylate hydrochloride is not observed within 10 days, symptoms are unlikely to be controlled by further administration.

Children: Lomotil is not recommended in children under 2 years of age and should be used with special caution in young children (see Warnings and Precautions). The nutritional status and degree of dehydration must be considered. In children under 13 years of age, use Lomotil liquid. Do not use Lomotil tablets for this age group.

Only the plastic dropper should be used when measuring Lomotil liquid for administration to children.

Dosage schedule for children: The recommended initial total daily dosage of Lomotil liquid for children is 0.3 to 0.4 mg/kg, administered in four divided doses. The following table provides an *approximate* initial daily dosage recommendation for children.

Age (years)	Approximate weight (kg)	Approximate weight (lb)	Dosage in ml (four times daily)
2	11–14	24–31	1.5–3.0
3	12–16	26–35	2.0–3.0
4	14–20	31–44	2.0–4.0
5	16–23	35–51	2.5–4.5
6–8	17–32	38–71	2.5–5.0
9–12	23–55	51–121	3.5–5.0

These pediatric schedules are the best approximation of an average dose recommendation which may be adjusted downward according to the overall nutritional status and degree of dehydration encountered in the sick child. Reduction of dosage may be made as soon as initial control of symptoms has been achieved. Maintenance dosage may be as low as one-fourth of the initial daily dosage. If no response occurs within 48 hours, Lomotil is unlikely to be effective.

KEEP THIS AND ALL MEDICATIONS OUT OF THE REACH OF CHILDREN.

HOW SUPPLIED

Tablets—round, white, with SEARLE debossed on one side and 61 on the other side and containing 2.5 mg of diphenoxylate hydrochloride and 0.025 mg of atropine sulfate, supplied as:

NDC Number	Size
0014-0061-31	bottle of 100
0014-0061-51	bottle of 500
0014-0061-52	bottle of 1,000
0014-0061-55	bottle of 2,500
0014-0061-34	carton of 100 unit dose

Liquid—containing 2.5 mg of diphenoxylate hydrochloride and 0.025 mg of atropine sulfate per 5 ml; bottles of 2 fl oz (NDC Number 0014-0066-02). Dispense only in original container.

A plastic dropper calibrated in increments of ½ ml (¼ mg) with a capacity of 2 ml (1 mg) accompanies each 2-oz bottle of Lomotil liquid. Only this plastic dropper should be used when measuring Lomotil liquid for administration to children.

A05758-1

Shown in Product Identification Section, page 429

NITRODISC®   ℞
[nī′trō′disc]
(nitroglycerin transdermal system)
5 mg/24 hr; 7.5 mg/24 hr; 10 mg/24 hr

DESCRIPTION

Nitrodisc incorporates a patented Microseal Drug Delivery™ system consisting of a solid, nitroglycerin-impregnated polymer bonded to a flexible, nonsensitizing adhesive bandage. It is designed to be applied topically. Nitrodisc provides constant and controlled drug delivery over a uniform skin surface area for 24 hours.

Nitrodisc is available in three strengths which release 5 mg, 7.5 mg, or 10 mg of nitroglycerin during a 24-hour period. The 5 mg/24 hr system contains 16 mg of nitroglycerin over an 8 cm² releasing surface. The 7.5 mg/24 hr system contains 24 mg of nitroglycerin over a 12 cm² releasing surface. The 10 mg/24 hr system contains 32 mg of nitroglycerin over a 16 cm² releasing surface (see HOW SUPPLIED section).

Inactive ingredients are lactose, isopropyl palmitate, mineral oil, polyethylene glycol, water, silicone rubber, plasticizers, aluminum foil laminate, polyethylene foam, and acrylic adhesive.

CLINICAL PHARMACOLOGY

When Nitrodisc is applied to the skin, nitroglycerin is absorbed continuously through the skin into the systemic circulation. This results in active drug reaching the target organs (heart and peripheral vasculature) before being inactivated by the liver. Nitroglycerin is a smooth muscle relaxant with vascular effects manifested predominantly by venous dilation and pooling. The major beneficial effect of nitroglycerin in angina pectoris is due to a reduction in myocardial oxygen consumption secondary to vascular smooth muscle relaxation and consequent reduced cardiac preload and afterload. In addition, a direct effect of nitroglycerin on the coronary vessels is recognized as well.

In normal volunteers, transdermal absorption of nitroglycerin from Nitrodisc occurred in a continuous and well-controlled manner for a minimum of 24 hours. Detectable plasma levels were attained within 1 hour after the application of the disc and remained at a similar level for 24 hours. Precise definition of "therapeutic plasma level" is not known at this time. Plasma levels of nitroglycerin were still detectable 30 minutes after removal of the system.

The amount of nitroglycerin released (5 mg/24 hr, 7.5 mg/24 hr, or 10 mg/24 hr) represents the mean release rate of nitroglycerin from the disc as determined from healthy volunteers and, hence, the amount potentially available for absorption through the skin. Absorption will vary among individuals.

INDICATIONS AND USAGE

Nitrodisc has been conditionally approved by the FDA for the prevention and treatment of angina pectoris due to coronary artery disease. The conditional approval reflects a determination that the drug may be marketed while further investigation of its effectiveness is undertaken. A final evaluation of the effectiveness of the product will be announced by the FDA.

CONTRAINDICATIONS

Nitrodisc (nitroglycerin) is contraindicated in patients known to be intolerant of organic nitrate drugs and in patients with marked anemia.

WARNINGS

In patients with acute myocardial infarction or congestive heart failure, Nitrodisc should be used under careful clinical and/or hemodynamic monitoring.

In terminating treatment of patients with angina, both the dosage and frequency of application must be gradually reduced over a period of 4 to 6 weeks to prevent potential withdrawal reactions, which are characteristic of all vasodilators in the nitrate class.

PRECAUTIONS

Symptoms of hypotension, such as faintness, weakness, or dizziness, particularly orthostatic hypotension, may be due to overdosage. When these symptoms occur, the dosage should be reduced or use of the product discontinued. Nitrodisc is not intended for immediate relief of anginal attacks. For this purpose, occasional use of sublingual preparations may be necessary.

Pregnancy: Pregnancy Category C. Animal reproduction studies have not been conducted with Nitrodisc. It is also not known whether nitroglycerin can cause fetal harm when administered to a pregnant woman or can affect reproduction capacity. Nitroglycerin should be given to a pregnant woman only if clearly needed.

Nursing mothers: It is not known whether nitroglycerin is excreted in human milk. Because many drugs are excreted in human milk, caution should be exercised when Nitrodisc is administered to a nursing woman.

ADVERSE REACTIONS

Transient headache is the most common side effect, especially when higher doses of the drug are used. These headaches should be treated with mild analgesics while Nitrodisc therapy is continued. When such headaches are unresponsive to treatment, the nitroglycerin dosage should be reduced or use of the product discontinued.

Adverse reactions reported less frequently include hypotension, increased heart rate, faintness, flushing, dizziness, nausea, vomiting, and dermatitis. With the exception of dermatitis, these symptoms are attributable to the known pharmacologic effects of nitroglycerin, but may be symptoms of overdosage. When they persist, Nitrodisc (nitroglycerin) dose should be reduced or use of the product discontinued.

DOSAGE AND ADMINISTRATION

Nitrodisc should be applied once each day. To use Nitrodisc, follow the instructions accompanying the package. Nitrodisc should be applied to an intact skin site free of hair and not subject to excessive movement. It should not be applied to the distal parts of the extremities. A suitable area should be shaved free of hair, if necessary. The application site should be changed slightly each time to avoid undue skin irritation. A new Nitrodisc should be applied if the product loosens. The optimal dosage regimen should be selected based upon the clinical response, the side effects, and the effects of therapy upon blood pressure and heart rate. It is recommended that therapy be initiated with Nitrodisc 5 mg/24 hr and that Nitrodisc 7.5 mg/24 hr or Nitrodisc 10 mg/24 hr be utilized when a greater response is desired. In the event that higher doses are necessary, multiple discs may be applied.

PATIENT INSTRUCTIONS FOR APPLICATION

These are provided with the product.

HOW SUPPLIED

Nitrodisc	5 mg/ 24 hr	7.5 mg/ 24 hr	10 mg/ 24 hr
Drug released per 24 hours	5 mg	7.5 mg	10 mg
Total drug content	16 mg	24 mg	32 mg
Drug releasing surface	8 cm²	12 cm²	16 cm²

Nitrodisc (nitroglycerin transdermal system) is supplied in cartons of 30 discs and in cartons of 30 and 100 discs (labeled for institutional use). Store at a controlled room temperature of 59°–86°F (15°–30°C). **Do not refrigerate.** Extremes of temperature and/or humidity should be avoided.

Caution: Federal law prohibits dispensing without prescription.

A05582-1

Shown in Product Identification Section, page 429

NORPACE® Capsules   ℞

[*nor'pāce*]

(disopyramide phosphate)

100 mg-NSN 6505-01-220-6314 (VA)

150 mg-NSN 6505-01-220-6313 (VA)

(bottles of 120 capsules)

NORPACE® CR Capsules   ℞

(disopyramide phosphate extended-release)

100 mg-NSN 6505-01-158-2170 (VA)

150 mg-NSN 6505-01-158-6361 (VA)

(bottles of 100 capsules)

PRODUCT OVERVIEW

KEY FACTS

Norpace and Norpace CR are Type 1 antiarrhythmics. Norpace is an immediate-release capsule. Norpace CR is a controlled-release capsule, designed to afford a gradual and consistent release of disopyramide with the benefit of less frequent dosing. At therapeutic levels, Norpace shortens the sinus node recovery time, lengthens the effective refractory period of the atrium, and has a minimal effect on the effective refractory period of the AV node.

MAJOR USES

Norpace and Norpace CR are indicated for the suppression and prevention of recurrence of unifocal and multifocal premature (ectopic) ventricular contractions, paired premature ventricular contractions (couplets), and episodes of ventricular tachycardia.

SAFETY INFORMATION

See complete prescribing information set forth below.

PRESCRIBING INFORMATION

NORPACE® Capsules   ℞

[*nor'pāce*]

(disopyramide phosphate)

100 mg-NSN 6505-01-220-6314 (VA)

150 mg-NSN 6505-01-220-6313 (VA)

(bottles of 120 capsules)

NORPACE® CR Capsules   ℞

(disopyramide phosphate extended-release)

100 mg-NSN 6505-01-158-2170 (VA)

150 mg-NSN 6505-01-158-6361 (VA)

(bottles of 100 capsules)

DESCRIPTION

Norpace (disopyramide phosphate) is an antiarrhythmic drug available for oral administration in immediate-release and controlled-release capsules containing 100 mg or 150 mg of disopyramide base, present as the phosphate. The base content of the phosphate salt is 77.6%. The structural formula of Norpace is:

α-[2-(diisopropylamino) ethyl]-α-phenyl-2-pyridine-acetamide phosphate

Norpace is freely soluble in water, and the free base (pKa 10.4) has an aqueous solubility of 1 mg/ml. The chloroform:water partition coefficient of the base is 3.1 at pH 7.2.

Norpace is a racemic mixture of *d* - and *l* -isomers. This drug is not chemically related to other antiarrhythmic drugs.

Norpace CR (controlled-release) capsules are designed to afford a gradual and consistent release of disopyramide. Thus, for maintenance therapy, Norpace CR provides the benefit of less frequent dosing (every 12 hours) as compared with the every-6-hour dosage schedule of immediate-release Norpace capsules.

Inactive ingredients of Norpace include corn starch, edible ink, FD&C Red No. 3, FD&C Yellow No. 6, gelatin, lactose, talc, and titanium dioxide; the 150-mg capsule also contains FD&C Blue No. 1.

Inactive ingredients of Norpace CR include corn starch, D&C Yellow No. 10, edible ink, ethylcellulose, FD&C Blue No. 1, gelatin, shellac, sucrose, talc, and titanium dioxide; the 150-mg capsule also contains FD&C Red No. 3 and FD&C Yellow No. 6.

CLINICAL PHARMACOLOGY

Mechanisms of Action

Norpace (disopyramide phosphate) is a Type 1 antiarrhythmic drug (ie, similar to procainamide and quinidine). *In animal studies* Norpace decreases the rate of diastolic depolarization (phase 4) in cells with augmented automaticity, decreases the upstroke velocity (phase 0) and increases the action potential duration of normal cardiac cells, decreases the disparity in refractoriness between infarcted and adjacent normally perfused myocardium, and has no effect on alpha- or beta-adrenergic receptors.

Electrophysiology

In man, Norpace at therapeutic plasma levels shortens the sinus node recovery time, lengthens the effective refractory period of the atrium, and has a minimal effect on the effective refractory period of the AV node. Little effect has been shown on AV-nodal and His-Purkinje conduction times or QRS duration. However, prolongation of conduction in accessory pathways occurs.

Hemodynamics

At recommended oral doses, Norpace rarely produces significant alterations of blood pressure in patients without congestive heart failure (see *Warnings*). With intravenous Norpace, either increases in systolic/diastolic or decreases in systolic blood pressure have been reported, depending on the infusion rate and the patient population. Intravenous Norpace may cause cardiac depression with an approximate mean 10% reduction of cardiac output, which is more pronounced in patients with cardiac dysfunction.

Anticholinergic Activity

The *in vitro* anticholinergic activity of Norpace is approximately 0.06% that of atropine; however, the usual dose for Norpace is 150 mg every 6 hours and for Norpace CR 300 mg every 12 hours, compared to 0.4–0.6 mg for atropine (see *Warnings* and *Adverse Reactions* for anticholinergic side effects).

Pharmacokinetics

Following oral administration of immediate-release Norpace, disopyramide phosphate is rapidly and almost completely absorbed, and peak plasma levels are usually attained within 2 hours. The usual therapeutic plasma levels of disopyramide base are 2–4 mcg/ml, and at these concentrations protein binding varies from 50–65%. Because of concentration-dependent protein binding, it is difficult to predict the concentration of the free drug when total drug is measured.

The mean plasma half-life of disopyramide in healthy humans is 6.7 hours (range of 4 to 10 hours). In six patients with impaired renal function (creatinine clearance less than 40 ml/min), disopyramide half-life values were 8 to 18 hours.

After the oral administration of 200 mg of disopyramide to 10 cardiac patients with borderline to moderate heart failure, the time to peak serum concentration of 2.3 ± 1.5 hours (mean $\pm$ SD) was increased, and the mean peak serum concentration of 4.8 ± 1.6 mcg/ml was higher than in healthy volunteers. After intravenous administration in these same patients, the mean elimination half-life was 9.7 ± 4.2 hours (range in healthy volunteers of 4.4 to 7.8 hours). In a second study of the oral administration of disopyramide to 7 patients with heart disease, including left ventricular dysfunction, the mean plasma half-life was slightly prolonged to 7.8 $\pm$ 1.9 hours (range of 5 to 9.5 hours).

In healthy men about 50% of a given dose of disopyramide is excreted in the urine as the unchanged drug, about 20% as the mono-N-dealkylated metabolite, and 10% as the other metabolites. The plasma concentration of the major metabolite is approximately one tenth that of disopyramide. Altering the urinary pH in man does not affect the plasma half-life of disopyramide.

In a crossover study in healthy subjects, the bioavailability of disopyramide from Norpace CR capsules was similar to that from the immediate-release capsules. With a single 300-mg oral dose peak disopyramide plasma concentrations of 3.23 ± 0.75 mcg/ml (mean $\pm$ SD) at 2.5 ± 2.3 hours were obtained with two 150-mg immediate-release capsules and 2.22 ± 0.47 mcg/ml at 4.9 ± 1.4 hours with two 150-mg Norpace CR capsules. The elimination half-life of disopyramide was 8.31 ± 1.83 hours with the immediate-release capsules and 11.65 ± 4.72 hours with Norpace CR capsules. The amount of disopyramide and mono-N-dealkylated metabolite excreted in the urine in 48 hours was 128 and 48 mg, respectively, with the immediate-release capsules, and 112 and 33 mg, respectively, with Norpace CR capsules. The differences in the urinary excretion of either constituent were not statistically significant.

Following multiple doses, steady-state plasma levels of between 2 and 4 mcg/ml were attained following either 150 mg every-6-hour dosing with immediate-release capsules or 300 mg every-12-hour dosing with Norpace CR capsules.

INDICATIONS AND USAGE

Norpace or Norpace CR should be prescribed only after appropriate electrocardiographic assessment.

Norpace and Norpace CR are indicated for suppression and prevention of recurrence of the following cardiac arrhythmias when they occur singly or in combination:

1. Unifocal premature (ectopic) ventricular contractions.
2. Premature (ectopic) ventricular contractions of multifocal origin.

Continued on next page

G.D. Searle & Co.—Cont.

3. Paired premature ventricular contractions (couplets).
4. Episodes of ventricular tachycardia (persistent ventricular tachycardia is ordinarily treated with DC-cardioversion).

In controlled trials of ambulatory patients, 150 mg of Norpace every 6 hours was as effective as 325 mg of quinidine every 6 hours in reducing the frequency of ventricular ectopic activity. Norpace was equally effective in digitalized and nondigitalized patients. Norpace is also equally effective in the treatment of primary cardiac arrhythmias and those which occur in association with organic heart disease, including coronary artery disease.

Oral disopyramide phosphate has not been adequately studied in patients with acute myocardial infarction or in patients with persistent ventricular tachycardia or atrial arrhythmias.

Norpace CR should not be used initially if rapid establishment of disopyramide plasma levels is desired.

Type 1 antiarrhythmic drugs are usually not effective in treating arrhythmias secondary to digitalis intoxication and, therefore, Norpace or Norpace CR is not indicated for such cases.

The value of antiarrhythmic drugs in preventing sudden death in patients with serious ventricular ectopic activity has not been established.

CONTRAINDICATIONS

Norpace and Norpace CR are contraindicated in the presence of cardiogenic shock, preexisting second- or third-degree AV block (if no pacemaker is present), congenital Q-T prolongation, or known hypersensitivity to the drug.

WARNINGS

Negative Inotropic Properties:
Heart Failure/Hypotension
Norpace or Norpace CR may cause or worsen congestive heart failure or produce severe hypotension as a consequence of its negative inotropic properties. Hypotension has been observed primarily in patients with primary cardiomyopathy or inadequately compensated congestive heart failure. Norpace or Norpace CR should not be used in patients with uncompensated or marginally compensated congestive heart failure or hypotension unless the congestive heart failure or hypotension is secondary to cardiac arrhythmia. Patients with a history of heart failure may be treated with Norpace or Norpace CR, but careful attention must be given to the maintenance of cardiac function, including optimal digitalization. If hypotension occurs or congestive heart failure worsens, Norpace or Norpace CR should be discontinued and, if necessary, restarted at a lower dosage only after adequate cardiac compensation has been established.

QRS Widening
Although it is unusual, significant widening (greater than 25%) of the QRS complex may occur during Norpace or Norpace CR administration; in such cases Norpace or Norpace CR should be discontinued.

Q-T Prolongation
As with other Type 1 antiarrhythmic drugs, prolongation of the Q-T interval (corrected) and worsening of the arrhythmia, including ventricular tachycardia and ventricular fibrillation, may occur. Patients who have evidenced prolongation of the Q-T interval in response to quinidine may be at particular risk. In general, Type 1A antiarrhythmic drugs have been associated with torsade de pointes. If a Q-T prolongation of greater than 25% is observed and if ectopy continues, the patient should be monitored closely, and consideration be given to discontinuing Norpace or Norpace CR.

Hypoglycemia
In rare instances significant lowering of blood glucose values has been reported during Norpace administration. The physician should be alert to this possibility, especially in patients with congestive heart failure, chronic malnutrition, hepatic, renal, or other diseases, or drugs (eg, beta adrenoceptor blockers, alcohol) which could compromise preservation of the normal glucoregulatory mechanisms in the absence of food. In these patients the blood glucose levels should be carefully followed.

Concomitant Antiarrhythmic Therapy
The concomitant use of Norpace or Norpace CR with other Type 1 antiarrhythmic agents (such as quinidine or procainamide) and/or propranolol should be reserved for patients with life-threatening arrhythmias who are demonstrably unresponsive to single-agent antiarrhythmic therapy. Such use may produce serious negative inotropic effects, or may excessively prolong conduction. This should be considered particularly in patients with any degree of cardiac decompensation or those with a prior history thereof. Patients receiving more than one antiarrhythmic drug must be carefully monitored.

Heart Block
If first-degree heart block develops in a patient receiving Norpace or Norpace CR, the dosage should be reduced. If the block persists despite reduction of dosage, continuation of the drug must depend upon weighing the benefit being obtained against the risk of higher degrees of heart block. Development of second- or third-degree AV block or unifascicular, bifascicular, or trifascicular block requires discontinuation of Norpace or Norpace CR therapy, unless the ventricular rate is adequately controlled by a temporary or implanted ventricular pacemaker.

Anticholinergic Activity
Because of its anticholinergic activity, disopyramide phosphate should not be used in patients with glaucoma, myasthenia gravis, or urinary retention unless adequate overriding measures are taken; these consist of the topical application of potent miotics (eg, pilocarpine) for patients with glaucoma, and catheter drainage or operative relief for patients with urinary retention. Urinary retention may occur in patients of either sex as a consequence of Norpace or Norpace CR administration, but males with benign prostatic hypertrophy are at particular risk. In patients with a family history of glaucoma, intraocular pressure should be measured before initiating Norpace or Norpace CR therapy. Disopyramide phosphate should be used with special care in patients with myasthenia gravis since its anticholinergic properties could precipitate a myasthenic crisis in such patients.

PRECAUTIONS

General
Atrial Tachyarrhythmias
Patients with atrial flutter or fibrillation should be digitalized prior to Norpace or Norpace CR administration to ensure that drug-induced enhancement of AV conduction does not result in an increase of ventricular rate beyond physiologically acceptable limits.

Conduction Abnormalities
Care should be taken when prescribing Norpace or Norpace CR for patients with sick sinus syndrome (bradycardia-tachycardia syndrome), Wolff-Parkinson-White syndrome (WPW), or bundle branch block. The effect of disopyramide phosphate in these conditions is uncertain at present.

Cardiomyopathy
Patients with myocarditis or other cardiomyopathy may develop significant hypotension in response to the usual dosage of disopyramide phosphate, probably due to cardiodepressant mechanisms. Therefore, a loading dose of Norpace should not be given to such patients, and initial dosage and subsequent dosage adjustments should be made under close supervision (see *Dosage and Administration*).

Renal Impairment
More than 50% of disopyramide is excreted in the urine unchanged. Therefore Norpace dosage should be reduced in patients with impaired renal function (see *Dosage and Administration*). The electrocardiogram should be carefully monitored for prolongation of PR interval, evidence of QRS widening, or other signs of overdosage (see *Overdosage*). Norpace CR is not recommended for patients with severe renal insufficiency (creatinine clearance 40 ml/min or less).

Hepatic Impairment
Hepatic impairment also causes an increase in the plasma half-life of disopyramide. Dosage should be reduced for patients with such impairment. The electrocardiogram should be carefully monitored for signs of overdosage (see *Overdosage*).

Patients with cardiac dysfunction have a higher potential for hepatic impairment; this should be considered when administering Norpace or Norpace CR.

Potassium Imbalance
Antiarrhythmic drugs may be ineffective in patients with hypokalemia, and their toxic effects may be enhanced in patients with hyperkalemia. Therefore, potassium abnormalities should be corrected before starting Norpace or Norpace CR therapy.

Drug Interactions
If phenytoin or other hepatic enzyme inducers are taken concurrently with Norpace or Norpace CR, lower plasma levels of disopyramide may occur. Monitoring of disopyramide plasma levels is recommended in such concurrent use to avoid ineffective therapy. Other antiarrhythmic drugs (eg, quinidine, procainamide, lidocaine, propranolol) have occasionally been used concurrently with Norpace. Excessive widening of the QRS complex and/or prolongation of the Q-T interval may occur in these situations (see *Warnings*). In healthy subjects, no significant drug-drug interaction was observed when Norpace was coadministered with either propranolol or diazepam. Concomitant administration of Norpace and quinidine resulted in slight increases in plasma disopyramide levels and slight decreases in plasma quinidine levels. Norpace does not increase serum digoxin levels.

Carcinogenesis, Mutagenesis, Impairment of Fertility
Eighteen months of Norpace administration to rats, at oral doses up to 400 mg/kg/day (about 30 times the usual daily human dose of 600 mg/day, assuming a patient weight of at least 50 kg), revealed no evidence of carcinogenic potential.

An evaluation of mutagenic potential by Ames test was negative. Norpace, at doses up to 250 mg/kg/day, did not adversely affect fertility of rats.

Pregnancy
Teratogenic Effects: Pregnancy Category C. Norpace was associated with decreased numbers of implantation sites and decreased growth and survival of pups when administered to pregnant rats at 250 mg/kg/day (20 or more times the usual daily human dose of 12 mg/kg, assuming a patient weight of at least 50 kg), a level at which weight gain and food consumption of dams were also reduced. Increased resorption rates were reported in rabbits at 60 mg/kg/day (5 or more times the usual daily human dose). Effects on implantation, pup growth and survival were not evaluated in rabbits. There are no adequate and well-controlled studies in pregnant women. Norpace or Norpace CR should be used during pregnancy only if the potential benefit justifies the potential risk to the fetus.

Nonteratogenic Effects: Norpace has been reported to stimulate contractions of the pregnant uterus. Disopyramide has been found in human fetal blood.

Labor and Delivery
It is not known whether the use of Norpace or Norpace CR during labor or delivery has immediate or delayed adverse effects on the fetus, or whether it prolongs the duration of labor or increases the need for forceps delivery or other obstetric intervention.

Nursing Mothers
Studies in rats have shown that the concentration of disopyramide and its metabolites is between one and three times greater in milk than it is in plasma. Following oral administration, disopyramide has been detected in human milk at a concentration not exceeding that in plasma. Because of the potential for serious adverse reactions in nursing infants from Norpace or Norpace CR, a decision should be made whether to discontinue nursing or to discontinue the drug, taking into account the importance of the drug to the mother.

ADVERSE REACTIONS

The adverse reactions which were reported in Norpace clinical trials encompass observations in 1,500 patients, including 90 patients studied for at least 4 years. The most serious adverse reactions are hypotension and congestive heart failure. The most common adverse reactions, which are dose dependent, are associated with the anticholinergic properties of the drug. These may be transitory, but may be persistent or can be severe. Urinary retention is the most serious anticholinergic effect.

The following reactions were reported in 10–40% of patients:
Anticholinergic: dry mouth (32%), urinary hesitancy (14%), constipation (11%)

The following reactions were reported in 3–9% of patients:
Anticholinergic: blurred vision, dry nose/eyes/ throat
Genitourinary: urinary retention, urinary frequency and urgency
Gastrointestinal: nausea, pain/bloating/gas
General: dizziness, general fatigue/muscle weakness, headache, malaise, aches/pains

The following reactions were reported in 1–3% of patients:
Genitourinary: impotence
Cardiovascular: hypotension with or without congestive heart failure, increased congestive heart failure (see *Warnings*), cardiac conduction disturbances (see *Warnings*), edema/weight gain, shortness of breath, syncope, chest pain
Gastrointestinal: anorexia, diarrhea, vomiting
Dermatologic: generalized rash/dermatoses, itching
Central nervous system: nervousness
Other: hypokalemia, elevated cholesterol/triglycerides

The following reactions were reported in less than 1%:
Depression, insomnia, dysuria, numbness/tingling, elevated liver enzymes, AV block, elevated BUN, elevated creatinine, decreased hemoglobin/hematocrit

Hypoglycemia has been reported in association with Norpace administration (see *Warnings*).

Infrequent occurrences of reversible cholestatic jaundice, fever, and respiratory difficulty have been reported in association with disopyramide therapy, as have rare instances of thrombocytopenia, reversible agranulocytosis, and gynecomastia. Some cases of LE (lupus erythematosus) symptoms have been reported; most cases occurred in patients who had been switched to disopyramide from procainamide following the development of LE symptoms. Rarely, acute psychosis has been reported following Norpace therapy, with prompt return to normal mental status when therapy was stopped. The physician should be aware of these possible reactions and should discontinue Norpace or Norpace CR therapy promptly if they occur.

OVERDOSAGE

Symptoms
Deliberate or accidental overdose of oral disopyramide may be followed by apnea, loss of consciousness, cardiac arrhythmias, and loss of spontaneous respiration. Death has occurred following overdose.

Toxic plasma levels of disopyramide produce excessive widening of the QRS complex and Q-T interval, worsening of congestive heart failure, hypotension, varying kinds and degrees of conduction disturbance, bradycardia, and finally asystole. Obvious anticholinergic effects are also observed.

The approximate oral LD_{50} of disopyramide phosphate is 580 and 700 mg/kg for rats and mice, respectively.

Treatment

Experience indicates that prompt and vigorous treatment of overdosage is necessary even in the absence of symptoms. Such treatment may be lifesaving. No specific antidote for disopyramide phosphate has been identified. Treatment should be symptomatic and may include induction of emesis or gastric lavage, administration of a cathartic followed by activated charcoal by mouth or stomach tube, intravenous administration of isoproterenol and dopamine, insertion of an intra-aortic balloon for counterpulsation, and mechanically assisted ventilation. Hemodialysis or, preferably, hemoperfusion with charcoal may be employed to lower serum concentration of the drug.

The electrocardiogram should be monitored, and supportive therapy with cardiac glycosides and diuretics should be given as required.

If progressive AV block should develop, endocardial pacing should be implemented. In case of any impaired renal function, measures to increase the glomerular filtration rate may reduce the toxicity (disopyramide is excreted primarily by the kidney).

The anticholinergic effects can be reversed with neostigmine at the discretion of the physician.

Altering the urinary pH in humans does not affect the plasma half-life or the amount of disopyramide excreted in the urine.

DOSAGE AND ADMINISTRATION

The dosage of Norpace or Norpace CR must be individualized for each patient on the basis of response and tolerance. The usual adult dosage of Norpace or Norpace CR is 400 to 800 mg per day given in divided doses. The recommended dosage for most adults is 600 mg/day given in divided doses (either 150 mg every 6 hours for immediate-release Norpace or 300 mg every 12 hours for Norpace CR). For patients whose body weight is less than 110 pounds (50 kg), the recommended dosage is 400 mg/day given in divided doses (either 100 mg every 6 hours for immediate-release Norpace or 200 mg every 12 hours for Norpace CR).

For patients with cardiomyopathy or possible cardiac decompensation, a loading dose, as discussed below, should not be given and initial dosage should be limited to 100 mg of immediate-release Norpace every 6 to 8 hours. Subsequent dosage adjustments should be made gradually, with close monitoring for the possible development of hypotension and/or congestive heart failure (see *Warnings*).

For patients with moderate renal insufficiency (creatinine clearance greater than 40 ml/min) or hepatic insufficiency, the recommended dosage is 400 mg/day given in divided doses (either 100 mg every 6 hours for immediate-release Norpace or 200 mg every 12 hours for Norpace CR).

For patients with severe renal insufficiency (C_{cr} 40 ml/min or less) the recommended dosage regimen of immediate-release Norpace is 100 mg at intervals shown in the table below, with or without an initial loading dose of 150 mg.

IMMEDIATE-RELEASE NORPACE
DOSAGE INTERVAL FOR PATIENTS
WITH RENAL INSUFFICIENCY

Creatinine clearance (ml/min)	40–30	30–15	less than 15
Approximate maintenance-dosing interval	q 8 hr	q 12 hr	q 24 hr

The above dosing schedules are for Norpace immediate-release capsules; Norpace CR is not recommended for patients with severe renal insufficiency.

For patients in whom rapid control of ventricular arrhythmia is essential, an initial loading dose of 300 mg of immediate-release Norpace (200 mg for patients whose body weight is less than 110 pounds) is recommended, followed by the appropriate maintenance dosage. Therapeutic effects are usually attained 30 minutes to 3 hours after administration of a 300-mg loading dose. If there is no response or evidence of toxicity within 6 hours of the loading dose, 200 mg of immediate-release Norpace every 6 hours may be prescribed instead of the usual 150 mg. If there is no response to this dosage within 48 hours, either Norpace should then be discontinued or the physician should consider hospitalizing the patient for careful monitoring while subsequent immediate-release Norpace doses of 250 mg or 300 mg every 6 hours are given. A limited number of patients with severe refractory ventricular tachycardia have tolerated daily doses of Norpace up to 1600 mg per day (400 mg every 6 hours) resulting

in disopyramide plasma levels up to 9 mcg/ml. If such treatment is warranted, it is essential that patients be hospitalized for close evaluation and continuous monitoring.

Norpace CR should not be used initially if rapid establishment of disopyramide plasma levels is desired.

Transferring to Norpace or Norpace CR

The following dosage schedule based on theoretical considerations rather than experimental data is suggested for transferring patients with normal renal function from either quinidine sulfate or procainamide therapy (Type 1 antiarrhythmic agents) to Norpace or Norpace CR therapy:

Norpace or Norpace CR should be started using the regular maintenance schedule **without a loading dose** 6–12 hours after the last dose of quinidine sulfate or 3–6 hours after the last dose of procainamide.

In patients in whom withdrawal of quinidine sulfate or procainamide is likely to produce life-threatening arrhythmias, the physician should consider hospitalization of the patient. When transferring a patient from immediate-release Norpace to Norpace CR, the maintenance schedule of Norpace CR may be started 6 hours after the last dose of immediate-release Norpace.

Pediatric Dosage

Controlled clinical studies have not been conducted in pediatric patients; however, the following suggested dosage table is based on published clinical experience.

Total daily dosage should be divided and equal doses administered orally every 6 hours or at intervals according to individual patient needs. Disopyramide plasma levels and therapeutic response must be monitored closely. Patients should be hospitalized during the initial treatment period, and dose titration should start at the lower end of the ranges provided below.

SUGGESTED TOTAL DAILY DOSAGE*

Age (years)	Disopyramide (mg/kg body weight/day)
Under 1	10 to 30
1 to 4	10 to 20
4 to 12	10 to 15
12 to 18	6 to 15

* Dosage is expressed in milligrams of disopyramide base. Since Norpace (disopyramide phosphate) 100-mg capsules contain 100 mg of disopyramide base, the pharmacist can readily prepare a 1-mg/ml to 10-mg/ml liquid suspension by adding the entire contents of Norpace capsules to cherry syrup, NF. The resulting suspension, when refrigerated, is stable for one month and should be thoroughly shaken before the measurement of each dose. The suspension should be dispensed in an amber glass bottle with a child-resistant closure.

Norpace CR capsules should not be used to prepare the above suspension.

HOW SUPPLIED

Norpace (disopyramide phosphate) is supplied in hard gelatin capsules containing either 100 mg or 150 mg of disopyramide base, present as the phosphate.

Norpace 100-mg capsules are white and orange, with markings SEARLE, 2752, NORPACE, and 100 MG.

NDC Number	Size
0014-2752-31	bottle of 100
0014-2752-51	bottle of 500
0014-2752-52	bottle of 1,000
0014-2752-34	carton of 100 unit dose

Norpace 150-mg capsules are brown and orange, with markings SEARLE, 2762, NORPACE, and 150 MG.

NDC Number	Size
0014-2762-31	bottle of 100
0014-2762-51	bottle of 500
0014-2762-52	bottle of 1,000
0014-2762-34	carton of 100 unit dose

Norpace CR (disopyramide phosphate) Controlled-Release is supplied as specially prepared controlled-release beads in hard gelatin capsules containing either 100 mg or 150 mg of disopyramide base, present as the phosphate.

Norpace CR 100-mg capsules are white and light green, with markings SEARLE, 2732, NORPACE CR, and 100 mg.

NDC Number	Size
0014-2732-31	bottle of 100
0014-2732-51	bottle of 500
0014-2732-34	carton of 100 unit dose

Norpace CR 150-mg capsules are brown and light green, with markings SEARLE, 2742, NORPACE CR, and 150 mg.

NDC Number	Size
0014-2742-31	bottle of 100
0014-2742-51	bottle of 500
0014-2742-34	carton of 100 unit dose

Store below 86°F (30°C).

Caution: Federal law prohibits dispensing without prescription.

AO5851-2

Shown in Product Identification Section, page 429

THEO-24®   Ŗ

[thē′ō-24]
(theophylline anhydrous)

DESCRIPTION

Theo-24 oral capsules contain 100 mg, 200 mg, or 300 mg of anhydrous theophylline, a bronchodilator, in a controlled-release formulation which allows a 24-hour dosing interval for appropriate patients.

The structural formula of theophylline, 3,7-dihydro-1,3-dimethyl-1H -purine-2,6-dione, is:

Theophylline is a white, odorless, crystalline powder having a bitter taste.

Inactive ingredients are edible ink, ethylcellulose, gelatin, shellac, silicon dioxide, starch, sucrose, talc, titanium dioxide, and coloring agents: 100-mg—includes FD&C Yellow No. 6; 200-mg—FD&C Red No. 3 and other colors; 300-mg—FD&C Blue No. 1 and other colors.

CLINICAL PHARMACOLOGY

Theophylline directly relaxes the smooth muscle of the bronchial airways and pulmonary blood vessels, thus acting mainly as a bronchodilator and smooth muscle relaxant. The drug also possesses other actions typical of the xanthine derivatives: coronary vasodilation, cardiac stimulation, diuresis, cerebral stimulation, and skeletal muscle stimulation. The actions of theophylline may be mediated through inhibition of phosphodiesterase and a resultant increase in intracellular cyclic AMP. *In vitro*, theophylline also has been shown to act synergistically with beta agonists that increase intracellular cyclic AMP through the stimulation of adenyl cyclase. More data are needed to determine if theophylline and beta agonists have a clinically important additive effect *in vivo*.

Pharmacokinetics:

Theophylline Elimination Characteristics

	Theophylline Clearance Rates (mean ± S.D.)	Half-Life Average (mean ± S.D.)
Children (over 6 months of age)	1.45 ± 0.58 ml/kg/min	3.7 ± 1.1 hr
Adult nonsmokers with uncomplicated asthma	0.65 ± 0.19 ml/kg/min	8.7 ± 2.2 hr

The half-life of theophylline is prolonged in patients with alcoholism, reduced hepatic or renal function, or congestive heart failure, and in patients receiving cimetidine or macrolide antibiotics such as troleandomycin and erythromycin. High fever for prolonged periods may reduce the rate of theophylline elimination.

Newborn infants have extremely slow theophylline clearance rates. The theophylline half-life in newborn infants may exceed 24 hours. Not until the age of 6 months do clearance rates approach those seen in older children.

Patients over age 55 and patients with chronic obstructive pulmonary disease, cardiac failure, or liver insufficiency may have much slower clearance rates with half-lives that exceed 24 hours.

The average half-life of theophylline in smokers (1 to 2 packs/day) is 4 to 5 hours; the average half-life in nonsmokers is 7 to 10 hours. The increase in theophylline clearance caused by smoking is probably the result of induction of drug-metabolizing enzymes. The effect of smoking on theophylline pharmacokinetics may persist for 3 months to 2 years after smoking is discontinued.

Tolerance does not appear to develop during long-term use of theophylline.

Theo-24 capsules contain hundreds of coated beads of theophylline. Each bead is an individual controlled-release delivery system. After dissolution of the capsules these beads are released and distributed in the gastrointestinal tract, thus minimizing the probability of high local concentrations of theophylline at any particular site.

Following the single-dose administration (8 mg/kg) of Theo-24 to 20 normal subjects who had fasted overnight and 2 hours after morning dosing, peak serum theophylline concentrations of 4.8 ± 1.5 (S.D.) mcg/ml were obtained at 13.3 ±4.7 (S.D.) hours. The fraction of the amount of the dose

Continued on next page

G.D. Searle & Co.—Cont.

absorbed was approximately 13% at 3 hours, 31% at 6 hours, 55% at 12 hours, 70% at 16 hours, and 88% at 24 hours. The extent of theophylline bioavailability from Theo-24 was comparable to the most widely used 12-hour controlled-release product when both products were administered every 12 hours.

In a 6-day multiple-dose study involving 18 subjects (with theophylline clearance rates between 0.57 and 1.02 ml/kg/min) who had fasted overnight and 2 hours after morning dosing, Theo-24 given once daily in a dose of 1500 mg produced serum theophylline levels that ranged between 5.7 mcg/ml and 22 mcg/ml. The mean minimum and maximum values were 11.6 mcg/ml and 18.1 mcg/ml, respectively, with an average peak-trough difference of 6.5 mcg/ml. A 24-hour single-dose study demonstrated an approximately proportional increase in serum levels as the dose was increased from 600 to 1500 mg.

Taking Theo-24 with a high-fat-content meal may result in a significant increase in peak serum level and in the extent of absorption of theophylline as compared to administration in the fasted state (see *Precautions: Drug/Food interactions*).

INDICATIONS AND USAGE

Theo-24 is indicated for the relief and/or prevention of symptoms of asthma and for reversible bronchospasm associated with chronic bronchitis and emphysema.

CONTRAINDICATIONS

Theo-24 (theophylline anhydrous) is contraindicated in patients who have shown hypersensitivity to theophylline.

WARNINGS

Status asthmaticus is a medical emergency and is defined as that degree of bronchospasm not rapidly responsive to recommended doses of usual bronchodilators. Oral theophylline alone is not appropriate treatment for status asthmaticus. Patients with status asthmaticus require *medication administered parenterally* and *close monitoring*, preferably in an intensive-care setting.

Optimum therapeutic response occurs in many patients when the serum theophylline concentration is 10 to 20 mcg/ml. In other patients satisfactory results (as determined by both relief of symptoms and improvement in pulmonary function) may be obtained at lower levels. In still others, adequate response may require higher levels. The physician should adjust the desired serum concentration range to the patients' requirements, keeping in mind that *an increased probability of toxicity exists when levels exceed 20 mcg/ml.* Therefore, in order to assure maximum benefit without excessive risk, measurement of serum levels is highly recommended.

Serum levels above 20 mcg/ml are rarely found after appropriate administration of the recommended doses. However, in individuals in whom theophylline plasma clearance is reduced *for any reason*, even conventional doses may result in increased serum levels with subsequent toxicity. Reduced theophylline clearance has been documented in the following readily identifiable groups:

1. Patients with impaired renal or liver function.
2. Patients over 55 years of age, particularly males and those with chronic lung disease.
3. Patients with cardiac failure from any cause.
4. Neonates.
5. Patients taking certain drugs (eg, macrolide antibiotics, cimetidine, or oral contraceptive steroids). See *Precautions.*

Decreased clearance of theophylline may be associated with either influenza immunization or active influenza, and with other viral infections. Reduction of dosage and measurement of serum theophylline levels are especially appropriate in the above individuals.

Although the effects of theophylline are dose related, *serious toxicity is not reliably preceded by less severe side effects.* Ventricular arrhythmias, convulsions, or even death may appear as the first sign of toxicity without previous warning. Less serious signs of theophylline toxicity (ie, nausea and restlessness) may occur frequently when initiating therapy, but are usually transient; when such signs are persistent during maintenance therapy, they are often associated with serum concentrations above 20 mcg/ml.

Patients who require theophylline may exhibit tachycardia due to the underlying disease process so that the cause/effect relationship to elevated serum theophylline concentrations will not be recognized.

Theophylline products may cause arrhythmias or worsen preexisting arrhythmias. Any significant change in cardiac rate and/or rhythm warrants monitoring and further investigation. Halothane anesthesia in the presence of theophylline may produce sinus tachycardia or ventricular arrhythmias.

In minipigs, rodents, and dogs, arrhythmia and sudden death (with histological evidence of myocardial necrosis) have been observed when theophylline and beta agonists were administered concomitantly but not when either was administered alone. The significance of these findings for human use is unknown.

PRECAUTIONS

General: Use with caution in patients with severe cardiac disease, hypertension, acute myocardial injury, congestive heart failure, cor pulmonale, severe hypoxemia, hyperthyroidism, hepatic impairment, or alcoholism, and in the elderly (especially males) and in neonates. Particular caution should be used in administering theophylline to patients with congestive heart failure. Reduced theophylline clearance in these patients may cause serum theophylline levels to persist long after the drug is discontinued.

Individuals who are rapid metabolizers of theophylline (such as the young, smokers, and some nonsmoking adults) may not be suitable candidates for once-a-day dosing. Dividing the daily dose into two doses may be indicated if symptoms of bronchospasm occur repeatedly, especially near the end of a 24-hour dosing interval, or if the patient exhibits wider peak-trough differences than desired.

Convulsions may occur in patients with theophylline overdosage when serum theophylline concentrations exceed 30 mcg/ml. Theophylline may lower the seizure threshold. Theophylline should not be administered concomitantly with other xanthine medications.

Methylxanthines are known to increase gastric acidity. Therefore, theophylline should be used cautiously in patients with a history of peptic ulcer since the disease may be exacerbated. Theophylline may occasionally act as a local irritant to the gastrointestinal tract, although gastrointestinal symptoms are more commonly mediated through the central nervous system and are usually associated with serum drug concentrations over 20 mcg/ml.

Information for patients: Patients should be instructed to take this medication in the morning, at approximately the same time each day, and to not exceed the prescribed dose.

Patients who require a relatively high dose of theophylline (ie, a dose equal to or greater than 900 mg or 13 mg/kg, whichever is less) should be informed of important considerations relating to time of drug administration and meal content (see *Precautions: Drug/Food interactions; and Dosage and Administration*).

As with any controlled-release theophylline product the patient should alert the physician if symptoms occur repeatedly, especially near the end of a dosing interval.

Laboratory tests: The determination of serum theophylline levels is highly recommended.

Drug interactions

Drug/Drug interactions: Elevated serum levels of theophylline may occur in patients treated concomitantly with theophylline and cimetidine, ranitidine, troleandomycin, erythromycin, allopurinol, or oral contraceptive steroids. Therefore, such patients should be watched carefully for signs of theophylline toxicity and the dose of theophylline decreased if necessary. Increased toxicity may occur when ephedrine or other sympathomimetic drugs are given concomitantly with theophylline. Co-medication with phenobarbital, phenytoin, or rifampin may increase theophylline clearance and an increase of the theophylline dose may be required. The excretion of lithium carbonate is increased in patients receiving aminophylline (theophylline with ethylenediamine). Aminophylline may antagonize the effects of propranolol.

Drug/Food interactions: Taking Theo-24 less than one hour before a high-fat-content meal, such as 8 oz whole milk, 2 fried eggs, 2 bacon strips, 2 oz hashed brown potatoes, and 2 slices of buttered toast (about 985 calories, including approximately 71 g of fat) may result in a significant increase in peak serum level and in the extent of absorption of theophylline as compared to administration in the fasted state. In some cases (especially with doses of 900 mg or more taken less than one hour before a high-fat-content meal) serum theophylline levels may exceed the 20 mcg/ml level, above which theophylline toxicity is more likely to occur.

Drug/Laboratory test interactions: Consumption of coffee, tea, cola beverages, chocolate, or acetaminophen contributes to falsely high serum theophylline levels when theophylline is measured spectrophotometrically without previous isolation by chromatography.

Carcinogenesis, mutagenesis, and impairment of fertility: Theophylline has been shown to be mutagenic in *Escherichia coli* and other lower organisms (*Euglena gracilis* and *Ophiostoma multiannulatum*) and to produce chromosome breaks in cultured mouse cells and cultured human lymphocytes. The drug had no mutagenic activity *in vivo* in a dominant lethal test using mice. Long-term animal studies have not been performed with theophylline to evaluate carcinogenic potential, mutagenic potential, or effect on fertility.

Pregnancy: Pregnancy Category C. Limited animal studies have shown teratogenic activity of theophylline in mice and rats. It is not known whether theophylline can cause fetal harm when administered to a pregnant woman or can affect reproductive capacity. Xanthines should be given to a pregnant woman only if clearly needed.

Nursing mothers: Theophylline is excreted in breast milk and may cause adverse effects in the infant. Caution must be used when prescribing theophylline to a nursing mother, taking into account the risk/benefit of this therapy.

Pediatric use: Safety and effectiveness in children under 12 years of age have not been established with this product.

ADVERSE REACTIONS

The most consistent adverse reactions are usually due to overdose and are:

1. Gastrointestinal: nausea, vomiting, epigastric pain, hematemesis, diarrhea.
2. Central nervous system: headaches, irritability, restlessness, insomnia, reflex hyperexcitability, muscle twitching, clonic and tonic generalized convulsions, coma.
3. Cardiovascular: palpitation, tachycardia, extrasystoles, flushing, hypotension, circulatory failure, ventricular arrhythmias.
4. Respiratory: tachypnea.
5. Renal: albuminuria, microhematuria, potentiation of diuresis.
6. Other: hyperglycemia and inappropriate ADH (antidiuretic hormone) syndrome, rash.

OVERDOSAGE

Management

If overdose following oral administration is suspected and a seizure has not occurred:

A. Induce vomiting or perform gastric lavage.
B. Administer activated charcoal.
C. Administer a cathartic, particularly if a controlled-release preparation has been taken.

If patient is having a seizure:

A. Establish an airway.
B. Administer oxygen.
C. Treat the seizure with intravenous diazepam, 0.1 to 0.3 mg/kg up to a total dose of 10 mg.
D. Monitor vital signs, maintain blood pressure, and provide adequate hydration.

If patient is in post-seizure coma:

A. Maintain airway and oxygenation.
B. Gastric lavage must be performed and a cathartic and activated charcoal introduced via a large-bore tube.
C. Continue to provide full supportive care and adequate hydration while waiting for drug to be metabolized. The drug is metabolized rapidly enough by most patients so that dialysis is usually not needed. If serum levels exceed 50 mcg/ml, charcoal hemoperfusion may be indicated.

DOSAGE AND ADMINISTRATION

Patients who require a relatively high dose of theophylline (ie, a dose equal to or greater than 900 mg or 13 mg/kg, whichever is less) should not take Theo-24 less than one hour before a high-fat-content meal since this may result in a significant increase in peak serum level and in the extent of absorption of theophylline as compared to administration in the fasted state (see *Precautions: Drug/Food interactions*).

Effective use of theophylline (ie, the concentration of drug in the serum associated with optimal benefit and minimal risk of toxicity) is considered to occur when the theophylline concentration is maintained from 10 to 20 mcg/ml. The early studies from which these levels were derived were carried out in patients immediately or shortly after recovery from acute exacerbations of their disease (some hospitalized with status asthmaticus).

Although the 20 mcg/ml level remains appropriate as a critical value (above which toxicity is more likely to occur) for safety purposes, additional data are now available which indicate that the serum theophylline concentrations required to produce maximum physiologic benefit may, in fact, fluctuate with the degree of bronchospasm present and are variable. Therefore, the physician should individualize the range appropriate to the patient's requirements, based on both symptomatic response and improvement in pulmonary function. It should be stressed that serum theophylline concentrations maintained at the upper level of the 10 to 20 mcg/ml range may be associated with potential toxicity when factors known to reduce theophylline clearance are operative. (See *Precautions*, including *Drug interactions*.)

Theo-24, like other controlled-release theophylline products, is intended for patients with relatively continuous or recurring symptoms who have a need to maintain therapeutic serum levels of theophylline. It is not intended for patients experiencing an acute episode of bronchospasm (associated with asthma, chronic bronchitis, or emphysema). Such patients require *rapid* relief of symptoms and should be treated with an immediate-release or intravenous theophylline preparation (or other bronchodilators) and not with controlled-release products.

Patients who metabolize theophylline at a normal or slow rate are reasonable candidates for once-daily dosing with Theo-24. Patients who metabolize theophylline rapidly (eg, the young, smokers, and some nonsmoking adults) who have symptoms repeatedly at the end of a dosing interval, will require either increased doses given once a day, or preferably, are likely to be better controlled by a schedule of twice-daily dosing. Those patients who require increased daily doses are more likely to experience relatively wide peak-trough differences and may be candidates for twice-a-day dosing with Theo-24.

Patients should be instructed to take this medication each morning at approximately the same time and not to exceed the prescribed dose.

Recent studies suggest that dosing of controlled-release theophylline products at night (after the evening meal) results in serum concentrations of theophylline which are not identical to those recorded during waking hours and may be characterized by early trough and delayed peak levels. This appears to occur whether the drug is given as an immediate-release, controlled-release, *or* intravenous product. To avoid this phenomenon when two doses per day are prescribed, it is recommended that the second dose be given 10 to 12 hours after the morning dose and before the evening meal.

Food and posture, along with changes associated with circadian rhythm, may influence the rate of absorption and/or clearance rates of theophylline from controlled-release dosage forms administered at night. The exact relationship of these and other factors to nighttime serum concentrations and the clinical significance of such findings require additional study. Therefore, it is not recommended that Theo-24 (when used as a once-a-day product) be administered at night.

Since there is a wide variation from patient to patient in the total dose of theophylline required to attain the desired level in the serum, it is essential that the dose be titrated and that serum levels be monitored before and after *transfer* to any sustained-release product.

When serum levels are not measured, the initial dosage should be restricted to the amount recommended below (see *Initiation of Therapy*).

As a practical consideration, it is not always possible to obtain serum level determinations. Under such conditions, restriction of the daily dose (in otherwise healthy adults) to not greater than 13 mg/kg/day (or 900 mg, whichever is lower) will result in relatively few patients exceeding serum levels of 20 mcg/ml, thereby reducing the risk of developing toxicity.

Dosage Guidelines

WARNING: DO NOT ATTEMPT TO MAINTAIN ANY DOSE THAT IS NOT TOLERATED. Dosage guidelines are approximations only, and the wide range of clearance of theophylline among individuals (particularly those with concomitant disease) makes indiscriminate usage hazardous. Because a high-fat-content meal may significantly increase the peak level and extent of absorption of theophylline from Theo-24, patients receiving large single doses (ie, equal to or greater than 900 mg or 13 mg/kg, whichever is less) should be instructed to avoid eating a high-fat-content morning meal or to take their medication at least one hour before eating. If the physician cannot be assured that the patient will follow this regimen, then the patient should be placed on a twice-daily dosing regimen.

For patients receiving lower once-daily single doses (less than 900 mg), very high peak levels are less likely to occur when Theo-24 (theophylline anhydrous) is taken with food. With close monitoring, patients less certain to observe the fasting requirements could be treated with once-daily dosing.

It is recommended that dosing be considered in three stages: (I) initiation of therapy with Theo-24, (II) titration and adjustment, and (III) chronic maintenance:

I. Initiation of Therapy with Theo-24:

A. *Transfer of patients* already on established daily doses of theophylline (whether stabilized on immediate- or controlled-release products) can be accomplished by administering the total daily dosage as a single dose given in the morning (eg, 300 mg of an immediate-release product given t.i.d. should be given as 900 mg of Theo-24. The initial transfer should not be made at doses exceeding 900 mg/day or 13 mg/kg/day, whichever is less. Subsequent dose titration should be done on the basis of serum levels and with appropriate attention to the time of drug administration and meal content as noted above.

It must be recognized that the peak and trough serum theophylline levels produced by once-daily dosing may vary (usually wider peak-trough differences) from those produced by the previous product and/or dosage regimen.

B. *For initiation of therapy with Theo-24* in patients who are not currently taking a theophylline product, the total daily dose, administered in the morning, must be established in accordance with the following guidelines:

Body Weight	Daily Dose
Children	
30 to 35 kg	300 mg
35 kg and above	400 mg
Adults	400 mg

Theophylline does not distribute into fatty tissue. Therefore, dosage should be calculated on the basis of lean (ideal) body weight where mg/kg doses are presented.

If appropriate serum theophylline concentrations or adequate improvement in pulmonary function is not obtained after 3 days, the instructions in Part II (below) should be followed.

II. Titration and Adjustment of Dose:

This phase of adjustment should be implemented either by the use of serum concentration measurements or by empirical principles when serum level determinations are not available.

A. *If serum levels can be measured:*

After 3 days' therapy with Theo-24, serum levels should be determined for peak concentration (sample obtained 12 hours after the morning dose) and trough concentration (24 hours after the morning dose). It is important that the patient has not missed or added any dose during the 72-hour period and that dosing intervals have been reasonably consistent. DOSE ADJUSTMENT BASED ON MEASUREMENTS WHEN THESE INSTRUCTIONS HAVE NOT BEEN FOLLOWED MAY RESULT IN TOXICITY.

Based on the results of the peak-trough values obtained, *three possibilities* exist:

1. The values of serum theophylline concentration fall within the desired range. If this result is obtained, the dosage should be maintained if it is tolerated.
2. If the serum theophylline concentration is too high, the dosage should be reduced as follows:
   a. If the values are between 20 and 25 mcg/ml, the daily dose may be reduced by about 10% and serum theophylline levels should be rechecked after 3 days.
   b. If the values are between 25 and 30 mcg/ml, the next dose should be skipped and the daily dose reduced by about 25%. The serum concentration should be rechecked after 3 days.
   c. If the values are over 30 mcg/ml, the next dose should be skipped and the daily dose reduced by 50%. The serum concentration should be rechecked after 3 days.
3. If the serum theophylline concentration is too low, the dosage should be increased at 3-day intervals by 100 mg or 200 mg (or 25% of the current dose), depending upon the desired goal. The serum concentration may be rechecked at appropriate intervals, but at least at the end of this adjustment period.

B. *If serum levels cannot be measured:*

1. If the clinical response is satisfactory then the total daily dose should be maintained.
2. If the response is unsatisfactory (due to persistence of symptoms or minimal improvement in measured function) after 3 days, then the dose may be increased by 100-mg increments. Reevaluation should be undertaken every 3 days.
3. If the response is still unsatisfactory and there are no adverse reactions, the dose may be cautiously adjusted upward in increments of 100 mg/day at 3- to 5-day intervals up to 900 mg (or 13 mg/kg/day, whichever is less).
4. If a response is accompanied by adverse reactions, then the next dose should be withheld or reduced by 25% depending on the severity of the reactions.

III. Chronic Maintenance:

After the dose is established theophylline serum concentrations usually remain stable. However, as noted elsewhere (see *Precautions* and *Warnings*), certain exogenous and endogenous factors alter theophylline elimination (including concomitant disease and drug interactions) which require drug monitoring and adjustments in total daily dose requirements while such factors are operative.

Older adults, those with cor pulmonale, congestive heart failure, and/or liver disease may have unusually low dosage requirements and thus may experience toxicity at the minimal dosage recommended above.

If the patient's condition is otherwise clinically stable and none of the recognized factors which alter elimination are present, measurement of serum levels need be repeated only every 6 to 12 months.

HOW SUPPLIED

Theo-24 (theophylline anhydrous) is supplied in controlled-release capsules containing 100, 200, or 300 mg of anhydrous theophylline.

Theo-24 100-mg capsules are gold and clear, with markings Theo-24, 100 mg, SEARLE, and 2832.

Theo-24 200-mg capsules are orange and clear, with markings Theo-24, 200 mg, SEARLE, and 2842.

Theo-24 300-mg capsules are red and clear, with markings Theo-24, 300 mg, SEARLE, and 2852.

Available in bottles of 100, 500 (except 100 mg), and cartons of 100 unit-dose individually blister-sealed capsules.

Caution: Federal law prohibits dispensing without prescription.

A05325

Shown in Product Identification Section, page 430

The preceding prescribing information for G.D. Searle & Co. products was current on September 1, 1989.

SERES Laboratories, Inc.
**3331 INDUSTRIAL DRIVE
BOX 470
SANTA ROSA, CA 95402**

CANTHARONE®   ℞
[kan'tha-rone]
**(cantharidin collodion)
For External Use Only
For Doctor's Use Only**

DESCRIPTION

CANTHARONE, cantharidin collodion, is a topical liquid containing 0.7% cantharidin, acetone, pyroxylin, castor oil and camphor.

HOW SUPPLIED

7.5 mL bottles (NDC 50694-096-01). Close tightly immediately after use. Keep away from heat.
Revised July, 1989
Direct inquiries to Kathryn MacLeod, Ph.D.

CANTHARONE® PLUS   ℞
[kan'tha rone PLUS]
**For External Use Only
For Doctor's Use Only**

DESCRIPTION

CANTHARONE PLUS is a topical liquid containing 30% salicylic acid, 2% podophyllin B.P., 1% cantharidin, octylphenylpolyethylene glycol, cellosolve, ethocel, pyroxylin, castor oil and acetone.

HOW SUPPLIED

7.5 mL bottles (NDC 50694-097-01). Close tightly immediately after use. Keep away from heat. Do not refrigerate.

SPECIAL WARNING

Do not dispense under any circumstances.
Revised July, 1989
Direct inquiries to Kathryn MacLeod, Ph.D.

NIGHT CAST™ Regular Formula
(Medicated Acne Mask-lotion)

DESCRIPTION

Contains 4% sulfur, 1.5% salicylic acid and 33% alcohol in a non-comedogenic vehicle.

HOW SUPPLIED

4 fl. oz. in a plastic dispenser bottle.
(NDC 50694-201-04)   Revised May 1987
Direct inquiries to Kathryn MacLeod, Ph.D.

NIGHT CAST™ Special Formula
(Medicated Acne Mask-lotion)

DESCRIPTION

Contains 8% sulfur, 2% resorcinol and 31% alcohol in a non-comedogenic vehicle.

HOW SUPPLIED

4 fl. oz. in a plastic dispenser bottle.
(NDC 50694-202-04)   Revised May 1987
Direct inquiries to Kathryn MacLeod, Ph.D.

Products are cross-indexed
by product classifications
in the
BLUE SECTION

Serono Laboratories, Inc.
100 LONGWATER CIRCLE
NORWELL, MA 02061

Serono Laboratories, Inc. will be pleased to answer inquiries about the following products:

METRODIN® ℞
[me 'trō-dēn]
(urofollitropin for injection)
FOR INTRAMUSCULAR USE ONLY

PRODUCT OVERVIEW

KEY FACTS
Metrodin® is a purified, lyophilized preparation of urofollitropin for injection containing 75 IU follicle stimulating hormone activity and less than 1 IU luteinizing hormone activity per ampule. It is administered by intramuscular injection immediately after reconstitution with Sodium Chloride for Injection, USP.

MAJOR USES
Metrodin® is indicated for the induction of ovulation in patients with polycystic ovarian disease, who have an elevated LH/FSH ratio and who have failed to respond adequately to clomiphene citrate therapy. Treatment with Metrodin® alone, in most cases, results only in follicular growth and maturation. Ovulation is induced with human chorionic gonadotropin (hCG: Profasi®).
Metrodin® and hCG may also be used to stimulate the development of multiple oocytes in ovulatory patients participating in an in vitro fertilization program.

SAFETY INFORMATION
Metrodin® should not be administered to patients who have previously demonstrated hypersensitivity to gonadotropins. In rare instances, women may experience the Ovarian Hyperstimulation Syndrome, which may require hospitalization. This risk can be minimized through careful patient monitoring. The patient should be advised of the possibility of multiple gestation occurring with Metrodin® therapy.

PRESCRIBING INFORMATION

METRODIN® ℞
[me 'trō-dēn]
(urofollitropin for injection)
FOR INTRAMUSCULAR USE ONLY

DESCRIPTION
Metrodin® (urofollitropin for injection) is a preparation of gonadotropin extracted from the urine of postmenopausal women. Each ampule of Metrodin® contains 75 IU of follicle-stimulating hormone (FSH) activity in not more than 0.83 mg of extract, plus 10 mg lactose in a sterile, lyophilized form. Metrodin® is administered by intramuscular injection.
Metrodin® contains an acidic, water soluble glycoprotein biologically standardized for FSH gonadotropin activity in terms of the Second International Reference Preparation for Human Menopausal Gonadotropins established in September, 1964 by the Expert Committee on Biological Standards of the World Health Organization. Negligible amounts of LH (less than 1 IU per 75 IU FSH) activity are contained in Metrodin®.
Therapeutic Class: Infertility.

CLINICAL PHARMACOLOGY
Metrodin® stimulates ovarian follicular growth in women who do not have primary ovarian failure. Treatment with Metrodin® in most instances results only in follicular growth and maturation. In order to effect ovulation in the absence of an endogenous LH surge, human chorionic gonadotropin (hCG) must be given following the administration of Metrodin® when clinical and laboratory assessment of the patient indicates that sufficient follicular maturation has occurred.

INDICATIONS AND USAGE
Metrodin® and hCG given in a sequential manner are indicated for the induction of ovulation in patients with polycystic ovarian disease who have an elevated LH/FSH ratio and who have failed to respond to adequate clomiphene citrate therapy.
Metrodin® and hCG may also be used to stimulate the development of multiple oocytes in ovulatory patients participating in an in vitro fertilization program.
Selection of Patients:
1. Before treatment with Metrodin® is instituted, a thorough gynecologic and endocrinologic evaluation must be performed. This should include a hysterosalpingogram (to rule out uterine and tubal pathology) and documentation of anovulation by means of basal body temperature, serial vaginal smears, examination of cervical mucus, determination of serum (or urine) progesterone, urinary preg-

nanediol and endometrial biopsy. Patients with tubal pathology should receive Metrodin® only if enrolled in an in vitro fertilization program.
2. Primary ovarian failure should be excluded by the determination of gonadotropin levels.
3. Careful examination should be made to rule out the presence of early pregnancy.
4. Patients in late reproductive life have a greater predilection to endometrial carcinoma as well as a higher incidence of anovulatory disorders. Cervical dilation and curettage should always be done for diagnosis before starting Metrodin® therapy in such patients who demonstrate abnormal uterine bleeding or other signs of endometrial abnormalities.
5. Evaluation of the husband's fertility potential should be included in the workup.

CONTRAINDICATIONS
Metrodin is contraindicated in women who exhibit:
1. High levels of **both** LH and FSH indicating primary ovarian failure.
2. Uncontrolled thyroid or adrenal dysfunction.
3. An organic intracranial lesion such as a pituitary tumor.
4. The presence of any cause of infertility other than anovulation, as stated in the indications unless they are candidates for in vitro fertilization.
5. Abnormal bleeding of undetermined origin.
6. Ovarian cysts or enlargement not due to polycystic ovary syndrome.
7. Prior hypersensitivity to urofollitropin.
8. Metrodin® is contraindicated in women who are pregnant and may cause fetal harm when administered to a pregnant woman. There are limited human data on the effects of Metrodin® when administered during pregnancy.

WARNINGS
Metrodin® is a drug that should only be used by physicians who are thoroughly familiar with infertility problems. It is a potent gonadotropic substance capable of causing mild to severe adverse reactions. Gonadotropin therapy requires a certain time commitment by physicians and supportive health professionals, and its use requires the availability of appropriate monitoring facilities. (See Precautions/Laboratory Tests). It must be used with a great deal of care.
Overstimulation of the Ovary During Metrodin® Therapy: Ovarian Enlargement: Mild to moderate uncomplicated ovarian enlargement which may be accompanied by abdominal distension and/or abdominal pain occurs in approximately 20% of those treated with Metrodin® and hCG and generally regresses without treatment within two or three weeks.
In order to minimize the hazard associated with the occasional abnormal ovarian enlargement which may occur with Metrodin®-hCG therapy, the lowest dose consistent with expectation of good results should be used. Careful monitoring of ovarian response can further minimize the risk of overstimulation.
If the ovaries are abnormally enlarged on the last day of Metrodin® therapy, hCG should not be administered in this course of therapy; this will reduce the chances of development of the Ovarian Hyperstimulation Syndrome.
The Ovarian Hyperstimulation Syndrome (OHSS): OHSS is a medical event distinct from uncomplicated ovarian enlargement. OHSS may progress rapidly to become a serious medical event. It is characterized by an apparent dramatic increase in vascular permeability which can result in a rapid accumulation of fluid in the peritoneal cavity, thorax, and potentially, the pericardium. The early warning signs of development of OHSS are severe pelvic pain, nausea, vomiting and weight gain. The following symptomatology has been seen with cases of OHSS: abdominal pain, abdominal distension, gastrointestinal symptoms including nausea, vomiting and diarrhea, severe ovarian enlargement, weight gain, dyspnea, and oliguria. Clinical evaluation may reveal hypovolemia, hemoconcentration, electrolyte imbalances, ascites, hemoperitoneum, pleural effusions, hydrothorax, acute pulmonary distress, and thromboembolic events (see "Pulmonary and Vascular Complications" below).
OHSS occurred in approximately 6.0% of patients treated with Metrodin® therapy in the initial clinical trials, in patients treated for anovulation due to polycystic ovarian disease. During studies for in vitro fertilization, four cases of the Ovarian Hyperstimulation Syndrome were reported following 1,586 treatment cycles (0.25%). Cases of OHSS are more common, more severe, and more protracted if pregnancy occurs. OHSS develops rapidly; therefore, patients should be followed for at least two weeks after hCG administration. Most often, OHSS occurs after treatment has been discontinued and reaches its maximum at about seven to ten days following treatment. Usually, OHSS resolves spontaneously with the onset of menses. If there is evidence that OHSS may be developing prior to hCG administration (see Precautions/Laboratory Tests), the hCG should be withheld.
If OHSS occurs, treatment should be stopped and the patient should be hospitalized. Treatment is primarily symptomatic

and should consist of bed rest, fluid and electrolyte management, and analgesics if needed. The phenomenon of hemoconcentration associated with fluid loss into the peritoneal cavity, pleural cavity, and the pericardial cavity has been seen to occur and should be thoroughly assessed in the following manner: 1) fluid intake and output, 2) weight, 3) hematocrit, 4) serum and urinary electrolytes, 5) urine specific gravity, 6) BUN and creatinine, and 7) abdominal girth. These determinations are to be performed daily or more often if the need arises.
With OHSS there is an increased risk of injury to the ovary. The ascitic, pleural, and pericardial fluid should not be removed unless absolutely necessary to relieve symptoms such as pulmonary distress or cardiac tamponade. Pelvic examination may cause rupture of an ovarian cyst, which may result in hemoperitoneum, and should therefore be avoided. If this does occur, and if bleeding becomes such that surgery is required, the surgical treatment should be designed to control bleeding and to retain as much ovarian tissue as possible. Intercourse should be prohibited in those patients in whom significant ovarian enlargement occurs after ovulation because of the danger of hemoperitoneum resulting from ruptured ovarian cysts.
The management of OHSS may be divided into three phases: the acute, the chronic, and the resolution phases. Because the use of diuretics can accentuate the diminished intravascular volume, diuretics should be avoided except in the late phase of resolution as described below.
Acute Phase: Management during the acute phase should be designed to prevent hemoconcentration due to loss of intravascular volume to the third space and to minimize the risk of thromboembolic phenomena and kidney damage. Treatment is designed to normalize electrolytes while maintaining an acceptable but somewhat reduced intravascular volume. Full correction of the intravascular volume deficit may lead to an unacceptable increase in the amount of third space fluid accumulation. Management includes administration of limited intravenous fluids, electrolytes, and human serum albumin. Monitoring for the development of hyperkalemia is recommended.
Chronic Phase: After stabilizing the patient during the acute phase, excessive fluid accumulation in the third space should be limited by instituting severe potassium, sodium, and fluid restriction.
Resolution Phase: A fall in hematocrit and an increasing urinary output without an increased intake are observed due to the return of third space fluid to the intravascular compartment. Peripheral and/or pulmonary edema may result if the kidneys are unable to excrete third space fluid as rapidly as it is mobilized. Diuretics may be indicated during the resolution phase if necessary to combat pulmonary edema.
Pulmonary and Vascular Complications: The following paragraph describes serious medical events reported following menotropins therapy. Although these events have not been reported following Metrodin® therapy, the physician must be aware that these events may occur.
Serious pulmonary conditions (e.g., atelectasis, acute respiratory distress syndrome) have been reported. In addition, thromboembolic events both in association with, and separate from the Ovarian Hyperstimulation Syndrome have been reported. Intravascular thrombosis and embolism, which may originate in venous or arterial vessels, can result in reduced blood flow to critical organs or the extremities. Sequelae of such events have included venous thrombophlebitis, pulmonary embolism, pulmonary infarction, cerebral vascular occlusion (stroke), and arterial occlusion resulting in loss of limb. In rare cases, pulmonary complications and/or thromboembolic events have resulted in death.
Multiple Births: Reports of multiple births have been associated with Metrodin®-hCG treatment, including triplet and quintuplet gestations. In clinical studies with Metrodin®, 83% of the pregnancies following therapy resulted in single births and 17% in multiple births. The patient and her husband should be advised of the potential risk of multiple births before starting treatment.

PRECAUTIONS
General: Careful attention should be given to diagnosis in candidates for Metrodin® therapy (see "Indications and Usage—Selection of Patients").
Information for Patients: Prior to therapy with Metrodin®, patients should be informed of the duration of treatment and monitoring of their condition that will be required. Possible adverse reactions (see "Adverse Reactions" section) and the risk of multiple births should also be discussed.
Laboratory Tests: In most instances treatment with Metrodin® results only in follicular growth and maturation. In order to effect ovulation, hCG must be given following the administration of Metrodin® when clinical assessment of the patient indicates that sufficient follicular maturation has occurred. This may be directly estimated by measuring serum (or urinary) estrogen levels and sonographic visualization of the ovaries. The combination of both estradiol levels and ultrasonography are useful for monitoring the growth and development of follicles, timing hCG administration, as

well as minimizing the risk of the Ovarian Hyperstimulation Syndrome and multiple gestation.

Other clinical parameters which may have potential use for monitoring menotropins therapy include:

a) Changes in the vaginal cytology,
b) Appearance and volume of the cervical mucus,
c) Spinnbarkeit, and
d) Ferning of the cervical mucus.

The above clinical indices provide an indirect estimate of the estrogenic effect upon the target organs, and therefore should only be used adjunctively with more direct estimates of follicular development, i.e., serum estradiol and ultrasonography.

The clinical confirmation of ovulation, with the exception of pregnancy, is obtained by direct and indirect indices of progesterone production. The indices most generally used are as follows:

a) A rise in basal body temperature,
b) Increase in serum progesterone, and
c) Menstruation following the shift in basal body temperature.

When used in conjunction with indices of progesterone production, sonographic visualization of the ovaries will assist in determining if ovulation has occurred. Sonographic evidence of ovulation may include the following:

a) Fluid in the cul-de-sac,
b) Ovarian stigmata, and
c) Collapsed follicle.

Because of the subjectivity of the various tests for the determination of follicular maturation and ovulation, it cannot be overemphasized that the physician should choose tests with which he/she is thoroughly familiar.

Drug Interactions: No clinically significant drug/drug or drug/food interactions have been reported during Metrodin® therapy.

Carcinogenesis and Mutagenesis: Long-term toxicity studies in animals have not been performed to evaluate the carcinogenic potential of Metrodin®.

Pregnancy Category X: See "Contraindications" section.

Nursing Mothers: It is not known whether this drug is excreted in human milk. Because many drugs are excreted in human milk, caution should be exercised if Metrodin® is administered to a nursing woman.

ADVERSE REACTIONS

The following adverse reactions, reported during Metrodin® therapy, are listed in decreasing order of potential severity:

1. Ovarian Hyperstimulation Syndrome (See "Warnings" above.),
2. Mild to moderate ovarian enlargement,
3. Ovarian cysts,
4. Abdominal pain,
5. Sensitivity to Metrodin®,
   (Febrile reactions which may be accompanied by chills, musculoskeletal aches or pain, malaise and fatigue have occurred after the administration of Metrodin®. It is not clear whether or not these were pyrogenic responses or possible allergic reactions.)
6. Gastrointestinal symptoms (nausea, vomiting, diarrhea, abdominal cramps, bloating),
7. Pain, rash, swelling and/or irritation at the site of injection,
8. Breast tenderness,
9. Headache, and
10. Dermatological symptoms (dry skin, body rash, hair loss, hives).

The following medical events have been reported subsequent to pregnancies resulting from Metrodin® therapy:

1. Ectopic pregnancy
2. Congenital abnormalities.
   (Three incidents of chromosomal abnormalities and four birth defects have been reported following Metrodin®-hCG or Metrodin®, Pergonal®-hCG therapy in clinical trials for stimulation prior to in vitro fertilization. The aborted pregnancies included one Trisomy 13, one Trisomy 18, and one fetus with multiple congenital anomalies (hydrocephaly, omphalocele, and meningocele). One meningocele, one external ear defect, one dislocated hip and ankle, and one dilated cardiomyopathy in the presence of maternal Systemic Lupus Erythematosis were reported. None of these events were thought to be drug-related. The incidence does not exceed that found in the general population.)

In addition, the following adverse reactions have been reported during menotropins therapy and, therefore, may also occur during Metrodin® therapy:

1. Pulmonary and vascular complications (See "Warnings" above.)
2. Hemoperitoneum.

DRUG ABUSE AND DEPENDENCE

There have been no reports of abuse or dependence with Metrodin®.

OVERDOSAGE

Aside from possible ovarian hyperstimulation and multiple gestations (see "Warnings"), little is known concerning the consequences of acute overdosage with Metrodin®.

DOSAGE AND ADMINISTRATION

Dosage: The dose of Metrodin® to produce maturation of the follicle must be individualized for each patient. It is recommended that the initial dose to any patient should be 75 IU of Metrodin® per day, **ADMINISTERED INTRAMUSCULARLY,** for seven to twelve days followed by hCG, 5,000 U to 10,000 U, one day after the last dose of Metrodin®. Administration of Metrodin® may exceed 12 days if inadequate follicle development is indicated by estrogen and/or ultrasound measurement. The patient should be treated until indices of estrogenic activity, as indicated under "Precautions" above, are equivalent to or greater than those of the normal individual. If serum or urinary estradiol determinations or ultrasonographic visualizations are available, they may be useful as a guide to therapy. If the ovaries are abnormally enlarged on the last day of Metrodin® therapy, hCG should not be administered in this course of therapy; this will reduce the chances of development of the Ovarian Hyperstimulation Syndrome. If there is evidence of ovulation but no pregnancy, repeat this dosage regimen for at least two more courses before increasing the dose of Metrodin® to 150 IU of FSH per day for seven to twelve days. As before, this dose should be followed by 5,000 U to 10,000 U of hCG one day after the last dose of Metrodin®. If evidence of ovulation is present, but pregnancy does not ensue, repeat the same dose for two more courses. Doses larger than this are not routinely recommended.

During treatment with both Metrodin® and hCG and during a two week post-treatment period, patients should be examined at least every other day for signs of excessive ovarian stimulation. It is recommended that Metrodin® administration be stopped if the ovaries become abnormally enlarged or abdominal pain occurs. Most of the Ovarian Hyperstimulation Syndrome occurs after treatment has been discontinued and reaches its maximum at about seven to ten days post-ovulation. Patients should be followed for at least two weeks after hCG administration.

The couple should be encouraged to have intercourse daily, beginning on the day prior to the administration of hCG until ovulation becomes apparent from the indices employed for the determination of progestational activity. Care should be taken to insure insemination. In the light of the foregoing indices and parameters mentioned, it should become obvious that, unless a physician is willing to devote considerable time to these patients and be familiar with and conduct the necessary laboratory studies, he/she should not use Metrodin®.

In Vitro Fertilization

For in vitro fertilization, therapy with Metrodin® should be initiated in the early follicular phase (cycle day 2 or 3) at a dose of 150 IU per day, until sufficient follicular development is attained. In most cases, therapy should not exceed ten days.

Administration: Dissolve the contents of one ampule of Metrodin® in one to two mL of sterile saline and **ADMINISTER INTRAMUSCULARLY** immediately. Any unused reconstituted material should be discarded.

Parenteral drug products should be inspected visually, for particulate matter and discoloration prior to administration, whenever solution and container permit.

HOW SUPPLIED

Metrodin® is supplied in a sterile, lyophilized form as a white to off-white powder or pellet in snap-top ampules containing 75 IU FSH activity. The following package combinations are available:

—1 ampule 75 IU Metrodin® and 1 ampule 2 mL Sodium Chloride Injection (USP), NDC 44087-6075-1
—10 ampules 75 IU Metrodin® and 10 ampules 2 mL Sodium Chloride Injection (USP), NDC 44087-6075-3

Lyophilized powder may be stored refrigerated or at room temperature (3°–25°C/37°–77°F). Protect from light. Use immediately after reconstitution. Discard unused material.

CLINICAL STUDIES

The results of the clinical experience and effectiveness of the administration of Metrodin® to 80 PCO patients in 189 courses of therapy are summarized below. All patients had received extensive prior therapy with clomiphene citrate, without success, and many had failed to conceive or hyperstimulated following treatment with Pergonal®.

	%
Patients ovulating	88
Patients pregnant	30
Patients aborting	25*
Multiple pregnancies	17*
Hyperstimulation syndrome (% patients)	6

* Based on total pregnancies.

CAUTION

Federal law prohibits dispensing without prescription.

Manufactured for:
SERONO LABORATORIES, INC.
Randolph, MA 02368 U.S.A.
by Laboratoires Serono SA
Aubonne, Switzerland
©SERONO LABORATORIES, INC. 1986, 1989
Revised: January, 1989

PERGONAL®   ℞
[per'go-nal]
(menotropins for injection, USP)
FOR INTRAMUSCULAR USE ONLY

PRODUCT OVERVIEW

KEY FACTS

Pergonal® is a purified, lyophilized preparation of gonadotropins and contains equal amounts of follicle stimulating hormone and luteinizing hormone. Pergonal® is administered by intramuscular injection immediately after reconstitution with Sodium Chloride for Injection, USP.

MAJOR USES

Women: Pergonal® is used to stimulate follicular development in hypogonadotropic anovulatory women who do not have primary ovarian failure.

Men: Pergonal® is used concomitantly with Profasi® (hCG) to stimulate spermatogenesis in men with infertility due to primary or secondary hypogonadotropic hypogonadism.

SAFETY INFORMATION

Pergonal® is contraindicated in individuals who have previously demonstrated hypersensitivity to the drug. In rare instances, women may experience excessive ovarian enlargement, ascites, and pleural effusion requiring hospitalization. The risk can be minimized through careful patient monitoring. Multiple births, 75% of which are twins, have been reported in 20% of pregnancies resulting from Pergonal® therapy.

PRESCRIBING INFORMATION

DESCRIPTION

Pergonal® (menotropins for injection, USP) is a purified preparation of gonadotropins extracted from the urine of postmenopausal women. Each ampule of Pergonal® contains 75 IU or 150 IU of follicle-stimulating hormone (FSH) activity and 75 IU or 150 IU of luteinizing hormone (LH) activity, respectively, plus 10 mg lactose in a sterile, lyophilized form. Pergonal® is administered by intramuscular injection.

Pergonal® is biologically standardized for FSH and LH (ICSH) gonadotropin activities in terms of the Second International Reference Preparation for Human Menopausal Gonadotropins established in September, 1964 by the Expert Committee on Biological Standards of the World Health Organization.

Both FSH and LH are glycoproteins that are acidic and water soluble. Therapeutic class: Infertility.

CLINICAL PHARMACOLOGY

Women:

Pergonal® administered for seven to twelve days produces ovarian follicular growth in women who do not have primary ovarian failure. Treatment with Pergonal® in most instances results only in follicular growth and maturation. In order to effect ovulation, human chorionic gonadotropin (hCG) must be given following the administration of Pergonal® when clinical assessment of the patient indicates that sufficient follicular maturation has occurred.

Men:

Pergonal® administered concomitantly with human chorionic gonadotropin (hCG) for at least three months induces spermatogenesis in men with primary or secondary pituitary hypofunction who have achieved adequate masculinization with prior hCG therapy.

INDICATIONS AND USAGE

Women:

Pergonal® and hCG given in a sequential manner are indicated for the induction of ovulation and pregnancy in the anovulatory infertile patient, in whom the cause of anovulation is functional and is not due to primary ovarian failure.

Men:

Pergonal® with concomitant hCG is indicated for the stimulation of spermatogenesis in men who have primary or secondary hypogonadotropic hypogonadism.

Pergonal® with concomitant hCG has proven effective in inducing spermatogenesis in men with primary hypogonadotropic hypogonadism due to a congenital factor or prepubertal hypophysectomy and in men with secondary hypogonadotropic hypogonadism due to hypophysectomy, craniopharyngioma, cerebral aneurysm or chromophobe adenoma.

Continued on next page

Serono—Cont.

SELECTION OF PATIENTS

Women:

1. Before treatment with Pergonal® is instituted, a thorough gynecologic and endocrinologic evaluation must be performed. This should include a hysterosalpingogram (to rule out uterine and tubal pathology) and documentation of anovulation by means of basal body temperature, serial vaginal smears, examination of cervical mucus, determination of serum (or urine) progesterone, urinary pregnanediol and endometrial biopsy.
2. Primary ovarian failure should be excluded by the determination of gonadotropin levels.
3. Careful examination should be made to rule out the presence of an early pregnancy.
4. Patients in late reproductive life have a greater predilection to endometrial carcinoma as well as a higher incidence of anovulatory disorders. Cervical dilation and curettage should always be done for diagnosis before starting Pergonal® therapy in such patients who demonstrate abnormal uterine bleeding or other signs of endometrial abnormalities.
5. Evaluation of the husband's fertility potential should be included in the workup.

Men:

Patient selection should be made based on a documented lack of pituitary function. Prior to hormonal therapy, these patients will have low testosterone levels and low or absent gonadotropin levels. Patients with primary hypogonadotropic hypogonadism will have a subnormal development of masculinization, and those with secondary hypogonadotropic hypogonadism will have decreased masculinization.

CONTRAINDICATIONS

Women:

Pergonal® is contraindicated in women who have:

1. A high FSH level indicating primary ovarian failure.
2. Uncontrolled thyroid and adrenal dysfunction.
3. An organic intracranial lesion such as a pituitary tumor.
4. The presence of any cause of infertility other than anovulation.
5. Abnormal bleeding of undetermined origin.
6. Ovarian cysts or enlargement not due to polycystic ovary syndrome.
7. Prior hypersensitivity to menotropins.
8. Pergonal® is contraindicated in women who are pregnant and may cause fetal harm when administered to a pregnant woman. There are limited human data on the effects of Pergonal® when administered during pregnancy.

Men:

Pergonal® is contraindicated in men who have:

1. Normal gonadotropin levels indicating normal pituitary function.
2. Elevated gonadotropin levels indicating primary testicular failure.
3. Infertility disorders other than hypogonadotropic hypogonadism.

WARNINGS

Pergonal® is a drug that should only be used by physicians who are thoroughly familiar with infertility problems. It is a potent gonadotropic substance capable of causing mild to severe adverse reactions in women. Gonadotropin therapy requires a certain time commitment by physicians and supportive health professionals, and its use requires the availability of appropriate monitoring facilities (see "Precautions—Laboratory Tests"). In female patients it must be used with a great deal of care.

Overstimulation of the Ovary During Pergonal® Therapy:
Ovarian Enlargement: Mild to moderate uncomplicated ovarian enlargement which may be accompanied by abdominal distension and/or abdominal pain occurs in approximately 20% of those treated with Pergonal® and hCG, and generally regresses without treatment within two or three weeks.

In order to minimize the hazard associated with the occasional abnormal ovarian enlargement which may occur with Pergonal®-hCG therapy, the lowest dose consistent with expectation of good results should be used. Careful monitoring of ovarian response can further minimize the risk of overstimulation.

If the ovaries are abnormally enlarged on the last day of Pergonal® therapy, hCG should not be administered in this course of therapy; this will reduce the chances of development of the Ovarian Hyperstimulation Syndrome.

The Ovarian Hyperstimulation Syndrome (OHSS): OHSS is a medical event distinct from uncomplicated ovarian enlargement. OHSS may progress rapidly to become a serious medical event. It is characterized by an apparent dramatic increase in vascular permeability which can result in a rapid accumulation of fluid in the peritoneal cavity, thorax, and potentially, the pericardium. The early warning signs of development of OHSS are severe pelvic pain, nausea, vomiting, and weight gain. The following symptomatology has

been seen with cases of OHSS: abdominal pain, abdominal distension, gastrointestinal symptoms including nausea, vomiting and diarrhea, severe ovarian enlargement, weight gain, dyspnea, and oliguria. Clinical evaluation may reveal hypovolemia, hemoconcentration, electrolyte imbalances, ascites, hemoperitoneum, pleural effusions, hydrothorax, acute pulmonary distress, and thromboembolic events (see "Pulmonary and Vascular Complications" below).

OHSS occurs in approximately 0.4% of patients when the recommended dose is administered and in 1.3% of patients when higher than recommended doses are administered. Cases of OHSS are more common, more severe and more protracted if pregnancy occurs. OHSS develops rapidly; therefore patients should be followed for at least two weeks after hCG administration. Most often, OHSS occurs after treatment has been discontinued and reaches its maximum at about seven to ten days following treatment. Usually, OHSS resolves spontaneously with the onset of menses. If there is evidence that OHSS may be developing prior to hCG administration (see "Precautions—Laboratory Tests"), the hCG should be withheld.

If OHSS occurs, treatment should be stopped and the patient hospitalized. Treatment is primarily symptomatic, consisting of bed rest, fluid and electrolyte management, and analgesics if needed. The phenomenon of hemoconcentration associated with fluid loss into the peritoneal cavity, pleural cavity, and the pericardial cavity has been seen to occur and should be thoroughly assessed in the following manner: 1) fluid intake and output, 2) weight, 3) hematocrit, 4) serum and urinary electrolytes, 5) urine specific gravity, 6) BUN and creatinine, and 7) abdominal girth. These determinations are to be performed daily or more often if the need arises.

With OHSS there is an increased risk of injury to the ovary. The ascitic, pleural, and pericardial fluid should not be removed unless absolutely necessary to relieve symptoms such as pulmonary distress or cardiac tamponade. Pelvic examination may cause rupture of an ovarian cyst, which may result in hemoperitoneum, and should therefore be avoided. If this does occur, and if bleeding becomes such that surgery is required, the surgical treatment should be designed to control bleeding and to retain as much ovarian tissue as possible. Intercourse should be prohibited in those patients in whom significant ovarian enlargement occurs after ovulation because of the danger of hemoperitoneum resulting from ruptured ovarian cysts.

The management of OHSS may be divided into three phases: the acute, the chronic, and the resolution phases. Because the use of diuretics can accentuate the diminished intravascular volume, diuretics should be avoided except in the late phase of resolution as described below.

Acute Phase: Management during the acute phase should be designed to prevent hemoconcentration due to loss of intravascular volume to the third space and to minimize the risk of thromboembolic phenomena and kidney damage. Treatment is designed to normalize electrolytes while maintaining an acceptable but somewhat reduced intravascular volume. Full correction of the intravascular volume deficit may lead to an unacceptable increase in the amount of third space fluid accumulation. Management includes administration of limited intravenous fluids, electrolytes, and human serum albumin. Monitoring for the development of hyperkalemia is recommended.

Chronic Phase: After stabilizing the patient during the acute phase, excessive fluid accumulation in the third space should be limited by instituting severe potassium, sodium, and fluid restriction.

Resolution Phase: A fall in hematocrit and an increasing urinary output without an increased intake are observed due to the return of third space fluid to the intravascular compartment. Peripheral and/or pulmonary edema may result if the kidneys are unable to excrete third space fluid as rapidly as it is mobilized. Diuretics may be indicated during the resolution phase if necessary to combat pulmonary edema.

Pulmonary and Vascular Complications: Serious pulmonary conditions (e.g., atelectasis, acute respiratory distress syndrome) have been reported. In addition, thromboembolic events both in association with, and separate from, the Ovarian Hyperstimulation Syndrome have been reported following Pergonal® therapy. Intravascular thrombosis and embolism, which may originate in venous or arterial vessels, can result in reduced blood flow to critical organs or the extremities. Sequelae of such events have included venous thrombophlebitis, pulmonary embolism, pulmonary infarction, cerebral vascular occlusion (stroke), and arterial occlusion resulting in loss of limb. In rare cases, pulmonary complications and/or thromboembolic events have resulted in death.

Multiple Births: Data from a clinical trial revealed the following results regarding multiple births: Of the pregnancies following therapy with Pergonal® and hCG, 80% resulted in single births, 15% in twins, and 5% of the total pregnancies resulted in three or more concepti. The patient and her husband should be advised of the frequency and potential hazards of multiple gestation before starting treatment.

PRECAUTIONS

General: Careful attention should be given to diagnosis in the selection of candidates for Pergonal® therapy (see "Indications and Usage—Selection of Patients").

Information for Patients: Prior to therapy with Pergonal®, patients should be informed of the duration of treatment and the monitoring of their condition that will be required. Possible adverse reactions (see "Adverse Reactions" section) and the risk of multiple births should also be discussed.

Laboratory Tests:

Women:

Treatment for Induction of Ovulation

In most instances, treatment with Pergonal® results only in follicular growth and maturation. In order to effect ovulation, hCG must be given following the administration of Pergonal® when clinical assessment of the patient indicates that sufficient follicular maturation has occurred. This may be directly estimated by measuring serum (or urinary) estrogen levels and sonographic visualization of the ovaries. The combination of both estradiol levels and ultrasonography are useful for monitoring the growth and development of follicles, timing hCG administration, as well as minimizing the risk of the Ovarian Hyperstimulation Syndrome and multiple gestation.

Other clinical parameters which may have potential use for monitoring menotropins therapy include:

a) Changes in the vaginal cytology;
b) Appearance and volume of the cervical mucus;
c) Spinnbarkeit; and
d) Ferning of the cervical mucus.

The above clinical indices provide an indirect estimate of the estrogenic effect upon the target organs, and therefore should only be used adjunctively with more direct estimates of follicular development, i.e., serum estradiol and ultrasonography.

The clinical confirmation of ovulation, with the exception of pregnancy, is obtained by direct and indirect indices of progesterone production. The indices most generally used are as follows:

a) A rise in basal body temperature;
b) Increase in serum progesterone, and
c) Menstruation following the shift in basal body temperature.

When used in conjunction with indices of progesterone production, sonographic visualization of the ovaries will assist in determining if ovulation has occurred. Sonographic evidence of ovulation may include the following:

a) Fluid in the cul-de-sac;
b) Ovarian stigmata; and
c) Collapsed follicle.

Because of the subjectivity of the various tests for the determination of follicular maturation and ovulation, it cannot be overemphasized that the physician should choose tests with which he/she is thoroughly familiar.

Drug Interactions: No clinically significant drug/drug or drug/food adverse interactions have been reported during Pergonal® therapy.

Carcinogenesis and Mutagenesis: Long-term toxicity studies in animals have not been performed to evaluate the carcinogenic potential of Pergonal®.

Pregnancy: Pregnancy Category X. See "Contraindications" section.

Nursing Mothers: It is not known whether this drug is excreted in human milk. Because many drugs are excreted in human milk, caution should be exercised if Pergonal® is administered to a nursing woman.

ADVERSE REACTIONS

Women:

The following adverse reactions, reported during Pergonal® therapy, are listed in decreasing order of potential severity:

1. Pulmonary and vascular complications (see "Warnings")
2. Ovarian Hyperstimulation Syndrome (see "Warnings")
3. Hemoperitoneum
4. Mild to moderate ovarian enlargement
5. Ovarian cysts
6. Abdominal pain
7. Sensitivity to Pergonal®
   Febrile reactions after the administration of Pergonal® have occurred. It is not clear whether or not these were pyrogenic responses or possible allergic reactions. In addition, reports of "flu-like symptoms" including fever, chills, musculoskeletal aches, joint pains, nausea, headache and malaise have been received.
8. Gastrointestinal symptoms (nausea, vomiting, diarrhea, abdominal cramps, bloating)
9. Pain, rash, swelling and/or irritation at the site of injection
10. Body rashes
11. Dizziness, tachycardia, dyspnea, tachypnea

The following medical events have been reported subsequent to pregnancies resulting from Pergonal® therapy:

1. Ectopic pregnancy
2. Congenital abnormalities

From a study of 287 completed pregnancies following Pergonal®-hCG therapy five incidents of birth defects were reported (1.7%). One infant had multiple congenital anomalies consisting of imperforate anus, aplasia of the sigmoid colon, third degree hypospadias, cecovesicle fistula, bifid scrotum, meningocele, bilateral internal tibial torsion, and right metatarsus adductus. Another infant was born with an imperforate anus and possible congenital heart lesions; another had a supernumerary digit; another was born with hypospadias and exstrophy of the bladder; and the fifth child had Down's syndrome. None of the investigators felt that these defects were drug-related. Subsequently one report of an infant death due to hydrocephalus and cardiac anomalies has been received.

Men:
1. Gynecomastia may occur occasionally during Pergonal®-hCG therapy. This is a known effect of hCG treatment.
2. Erythrocytosis (hct 50%, hgb 17.8 g%) was recorded in one patient.

DRUG ABUSE AND DEPENDENCE
There have been no reports of abuse or dependence with Pergonal®.

OVERDOSAGE
Aside from possible ovarian hyperstimulation (see "Warnings"), little is known concerning the consequences of acute overdosage with Pergonal®.

DOSAGE AND ADMINISTRATION
Women:
1. Dosage:
The dose of Pergonal® to produce maturation of the follicle must be individualized for each patient. It is recommended that the initial dose to any patient should be 75 IU of FSH/LH per day, **ADMINISTERED INTRAMUSCULARLY,** for seven to twelve days followed by hCG, 5,000 U to 10,000 U, one day after the last dose of Pergonal®. Administration of Pergonal® should not exceed 12 days in a single course of therapy. The patient should be treated until indices of estrogenic activity, as indicated under "Precautions" above, are equivalent to or greater than those of the normal individual. If serum or urinary estradiol determinations or ultrasonographic visualizations are available, they may be useful as a guide to therapy. If the ovaries are abnormally enlarged on the last day of Pergonal® therapy, hCG should not be administered in this course of therapy; this will reduce the chances of development of the Ovarian Hyperstimulation Syndrome. If there is evidence of ovulation but no pregnancy, repeat this dosage regime for at least two more courses before increasing the dose of Pergonal® to 150 IU of FSH/LH per day for seven to twelve days. As before, this dose should be followed by 5,000 U to 10,000 U of hCG one day after the last dose of Pergonal®. A Pergonal® dose of 150 IU of FSH/LH per day has proven to be the most effective dose. If evidence of ovulation is present, but pregnancy does not ensue, repeat the same dose for two more courses. Doses larger than this are not routinely recommended.

During treatment with both Pergonal® and hCG and during a two-week post-treatment period, patients should be examined at least every other day for signs of excessive ovarian stimulation. It is recommended that Pergonal® administration be stopped if the ovaries become abnormally enlarged or abdominal pain occurs. Most of the Ovarian Hyperstimulation Syndrome occurs after treatment has been discontinued and reaches its maximum at about seven to ten days post-ovulation. Patients should be followed for at least two weeks after hCG administration. The couple should be encouraged to have intercourse daily, beginning on the day prior to the administration of hCG until ovulation becomes apparent from the indices employed for the determination of progestational activity. Care should be taken to insure insemination. In the light of the foregoing indices and parameters mentioned, it should become obvious that, unless a physician is willing to devote considerable time to these patients and be familiar with and conduct the necessary laboratory studies, he/she should not use Pergonal®.

2. Administration:
Dissolve the contents of one ampule of Pergonal® in one to two ml of sterile saline and **ADMINISTER INTRAMUSCULARLY** immediately. Any unused reconstituted material should be discarded. Parenteral drug products should be inspected visually for particulate matter and discoloration prior to administration, whenever solution and container permit.

Men:
1. Dosage:
Prior to concomitant therapy with Pergonal® and hCG, pretreatment with hCG alone (5,000 U three times a week) is required. Treatment should continue for a period sufficient to achieve serum testosterone levels within the normal range and masculinization as judged by the appearance of secondary sex characteristics. Such pretreatment

	% Pts. Ovul.	% Pts. Preg.	% Abort.	% Multi Preg.	% Twins	% 3 or More Concepti	% Hyperstim. Syndr.
Primary Amenorrhea	62	22	14	25	25	0	0
Secondary Amenorrhea	61	28	24	28	18	10	1.9
Secondary Amen. with Galactorrhea	77	42	21	41	31	10	1.2
Polycystic Ovaries	76	26	39	17	17	0	1.1
Anovulatory Cycles	77	24	15	14	9	5	2.0
Miscellaneous	83	20	36	2	2	0	0.1

may require four to six months, then the recommended dose of Pergonal® is 75 IU FSH/LH **ADMINISTERED INTRAMUSCULARLY,** three times a week and the recommended dose of hCG is 2,000 U twice a week. Therapy should be carried on for a minimum of four more months to insure detecting spermatozoa in the ejaculate, as it takes 74± 4 days in the human male for germ cells to reach the spermatozoa stage.

If the patient has not responded with evidence of increased spermatogenesis at the end of four months of therapy, treatment may continue with 75 IU FSH/LH three times a week, or the dose can be increased to 150 IU FSH/LH three times a week, with the hCG dose unchanged.

2. Administration:
Dissolve the contents of one ampule of Pergonal® in one to two ml of sterile saline and **ADMINISTER INTRAMUSCULARLY** immediately. Any unused reconstituted material should be discarded. Parenteral drug products should be inspected visually for particulate matter and discoloration prior to administration, whenever solution and container permit.

HOW SUPPLIED
Pergonal® is supplied in a sterile lyophilized form as a white to off-white powder or pellet in snap-top ampules containing 75 IU or 150 IU FSH/LH activity. The following package combinations are available:
—1 ampule 75 IU Pergonal® and 1 ampule 2 ml Sodium Chloride Injection (USP), NDC 44087-0571-7.
—10 ampules 75 IU Pergonal® and 10 ampules 2 ml Sodium Chloride Injection (USP), NDC 44087-5075-3.
—1 ampule 150 IU Pergonal® and 1 ampule 2 ml Sodium Chloride Injection (USP), NDC 44087-5150-1.
By biological assay, one IU of LH for the Second International Reference Preparation (2nd-IRP) for hMG is biologically equivalent to approximately ½ U of hCG.
Lyophilized powder may be stored refrigerated or at room temperature (3–25°C/37–77°F). Protect from light. Use immediately after reconstitution. Discard unused material.

CLINICAL STUDIES
Women:
The results of the clinical experience and effectiveness of the administration of Pergonal® to 1,286 patients in 3,002 courses of therapy are summarized below. The values include patients who were treated with other than the recommended dosage regime. The values for the presently recommended dosage regime are essentially the same.

	%
Patients ovulating	75
Patients pregnant	25
Patients aborting	25*
Multiple pregnancies	20†
Twins	15†
Three or more concepti	5†
Fetal abnormalities	1.7†
Hyperstimulation syndrome	1.3

* Based on total pregnancies
† Based on total deliveries
Results by diagnosis group are summarized below. (These values include patients who were treated with other than the present recommended dosage regime):
[See table above].

Men:
Clinical results of the treatment of men with primary or secondary hypogonadotropic hypogonadism are as follows:
In the Serono Cooperative study, with an adequate treatment period of 3 to 8 months, 60 of 70 men with primary hypogonadotropic hypogonadism and 8 of 11 men with secondary hypogonadotropic hypogonadism responded with mean increases in their sperm counts from less than 5 to 24 million spermatozoa per milliliter of ejaculate. Forty-one wives of 54 men with primary hypogonadotropic hypogonadism desiring offspring and 7 wives of men with secondary hypogonadotropic hypogonadism conceived. Patients treated with Pergonal® and hCG for less than 3 months or with Pergonal® alone did not respond to therapy.
A world-wide data search revealed that of 160 recorded pregnancies as the result of use of Pergonal®-hCG in men, there were 7 spontaneous abortions, one ectopic pregnancy and 3 congenital anomalies at birth (esophageal atresia in a female

infant which was later corrected by surgery, unilateral cryptorchidism, inguinal hernia).

Caution: Federal law prohibits dispensing without prescription.

Manufactured for:
© SERONO LABORATORIES, INC.
Randolph, MA 02368 USA
by: Laboratoires Serono, SA
Aubonne, Switzerland
© SERONO LABORATORIES, INC. 1988
Revised: June, 1988

PROFASI®   ℞
[pro'fah-se]
(human chorionic gonadotropin, USP)
FOR INTRAMUSCULAR USE ONLY

PRODUCT OVERVIEW

KEY FACTS
Profasi® is a lyophilized preparation of human chorionic gonadotropin. It is administered by intramuscular injection after reconstitution with Bacteriostatic Water for Injection, USP.

MAJOR USES
Women: Profasi® is used to induce ovulation in women who have been appropriately treated with Pergonal®.
Men: Profasi® is used to treat hypogonadotropic males, or to treat prepubertal cryptorchidism not due to anatomical obstruction.

SAFETY INFORMATION
Profasi® should not be administered to patients who have previously demonstrated hypersensitivity to human chorionic gonadotropin. Women who have experienced excessive ovarian enlargement and overstimulation while undergoing Pergonal® treatment should not be given HCG. When treating prepubertal cryptorchidism, therapy should be discontinued if signs of precocious puberty occur.

PRESCRIBING INFORMATION

PROFASI®   ℞
[pro'fah-se]
(human chorionic gonadotropin, USP)
FOR INTRAMUSCULAR USE ONLY

DESCRIPTION
Human chorionic gonadotropin (HCG), a polypeptide hormone produced by the human placenta, is composed of an alpha and a beta sub-unit. The alpha sub-unit is essentially identical to the alpha sub-units of the human pituitary gonadotropins, luteinizing hormone (LH) and follicle-stimulating hormone (FSH), as well as to the alpha sub-unit of human thyroid-stimulating hormone (TSH). The beta sub-units of these hormones differ in amino acid sequence.
Chorionic Gonadotropin is a water soluble glycoprotein derived from human pregnancy urine. The sterile lyophilized powder is stable. When reconstituted the solution should be refrigerated and should be used within 60 days.
Each vial when reconstituted will contain:
Chorionic Gonadotropin: 5,000 USP Units or 10,000 USP Units, Mannitol: 100 mg with Dibasic Sodium Phosphate and Monobasic Sodium Phosphate to adjust pH.
In addition, when reconstituted with the diluent provided (Bacteriostatic Water for Injection, USP containing 0.9% v/v Benzyl Alcohol) each serum vial will contain Benzyl Alcohol 0.9%.

CLINICAL PHARMACOLOGY
The action of HCG is virtually identical to that of pituitary LH, although HCG appears to have a small degree of FSH activity as well. It stimulates production of gonadal steroid hormones by stimulating the interstitial cells (Leydig cells) of the testis to produce androgens and the corpus luteum of the ovary to produce progesterone. Androgen stimulation in the male leads to the development of secondary sex characteristics and may stimulate testicular descent when no anatomical impediment to descent is present. This descent is

Continued on next page

Serono—Cont.

usually reversible when HCG is discontinued. During the normal menstrual cycle, LH participates with FSH in the development and maturation of the normal ovarian follicle, and the mid-cycle LH surge triggers ovulation. HCG can substitute for LH in this function.

During a normal pregnancy, HCG secreted by the placenta maintains the corpus luteum after LH secretion decreases, supporting continued secretion of estrogen and progesterone and preventing menstruation. HCG HAS NO KNOWN EFFECT ON FAT MOBILIZATION, APPETITE OR SENSE OF HUNGER, OR BODY FAT DISTRIBUTION.

INDICATIONS AND USAGE

HCG HAS NOT BEEN DEMONSTRATED TO BE EFFECTIVE ADJUNCTIVE THERAPY IN THE TREATMENT OF OBESITY. THERE IS NO SUBSTANTIAL EVIDENCE THAT IT INCREASES WEIGHT LOSS BEYOND THAT RESULTING FROM CALORIC RESTRICTION, THAT IT CAUSES A MORE ATTRACTIVE OR "NORMAL" DISTRIBUTION OF FAT, OR THAT IT DECREASES THE HUNGER AND DISCOMFORT ASSOCIATED WITH CALORIE-RESTRICTED DIETS.

1. Prepubertal cryptorchidism not due to anatomical obstruction. In general, HCG is thought to induce testicular descent in situations when descent would have occurred at puberty. HCG thus may help predict whether or not orchiopexy will be needed in the future. Although, in some cases, descent following HCG administration is permanent, in most cases, the response is temporary. Therapy is usually instituted between the ages of 4 and 9.
2. Selected cases of hypogonadotropic hypogonadism (hypogonadism secondary to a pituitary deficiency) in males.
3. Induction of ovulation and pregnancy in the anovulatory, infertile woman in whom the cause of anovulation is secondary and not due to primary ovarian failure, and who has been appropriately pre-treated with human menotropins.

CONTRAINDICATIONS

Precocious puberty, prostatic carcinoma or other androgen-dependent neoplasm, prior allergic reaction to HCG.

WARNINGS

HCG should be used in conjunction with human menopausal gonadotropins only by physicians experienced with infertility problems who are familiar with the criteria for patient selection, contraindications, warnings, precautions, and adverse reactions described in the package insert for menotropins. The principal serious adverse reactions during this use are: (1) Ovarian hyperstimulation, a syndrome of sudden ovarian enlargement, ascites with or without pain, and/or pleural effusion, (2) Rupture of ovarian cysts with resultant hemoperitoneum, (3) Multiple births, and (4) Arterial thromboembolism.

PRECAUTIONS

1. Induction of androgen secretion by HCG may induce precocious puberty in patients treated for cryptorchidism. Therapy should be discontinued if signs of precocious puberty occur.
2. Since androgens may cause fluid retention, HCG should be used with caution in patients with cardiac or renal disease, epilepsy, migraine, or asthma.

ADVERSE REACTIONS

Headache, irritability, restlessness, depression, fatigue, edema, precocious puberty, gynecomastia, pain at the site of injection.

DOSAGE AND ADMINISTRATION

(Intramuscular Use Only): The dosage regimen employed in any particular case will depend upon the indication for use, the age and weight of the patient, and the physician's preference. The following regimens have been advocated by various authorities.

Prepubertal cryptorchidism not due to anatomical obstruction:

1. 4,000 USP Units three times weekly for three weeks.
2. 5,000 USP Units every second day for four injections.
3. 15 injections of 500 to 1,000 USP Units over a period of six weeks.
4. 500 USP Units three times weekly for four to six weeks. If this course of treatment is not successful, another is begun one month later, giving 1,000 USP Units per injection.

Selected cases of hypogonadotropic hypogonadism in males:

1. 500 to 1,000 USP Units three times a week for three weeks, followed by the same dose twice a week for three weeks.
2. 4,000 USP Units three times weekly for six to nine months, following which the dosage may be reduced to 2,000 USP Units three times weekly for an additional three months.

Induction of ovulation and pregnancy in the anovulatory, unfertile woman in whom the cause of anovulation is secondary and not due to primary ovarian failure and who has been appropriately pre-treated with human menotropins (see prescribing information for menotropins for dosage and administration for that drug product):

5,000 to 10,000 USP Units one day following the last dose of menotropins (a dosage of 10,000 USP Units is recommended in the labeling for menotropins).

HOW SUPPLIED

Regular 10 ml lyophilized multiple dose vial
5,000 USP Units per Vial—NDC 44087-8005-3
10,000 USP Units per Vial—NDC 44087-8010-3
with 10 ml vial Bacteriostatic Water for Injection, USP (containing Benzyl Alcohol 0.9% v/v).

CAUTION

Federal law prohibits dispensing without prescription.

DIRECTIONS FOR RECONSTITUTION

TWO-VIAL PACKAGE: Withdraw sterile air from lyophilized vial and inject into diluent vial. Remove up to 10 ml from the diluent and add to the lyophilized vial; agitate gently until solution is complete.

© Serono Laboratories, Inc. 1984
Revised: September 1988

SEROPHENE®   ℞

[se'ro-fēn]
(clomiphene citrate tablets, USP)

PRODUCT OVERVIEW

KEY FACTS

Serophene® is an orally administered, non-steroidal compound with some estrogenic activity. The exact mechanism of action is unknown, although it appears to involve the pituitary by stimulating release of pituitary gonadotropins to mediate ovulation.

MAJOR USES

Serophene® is effective in inducing ovulation in infertile women with physiological indications of normal estrogen production. Reduced estrogen levels, while less favorable, do not prevent successful therapy.

SAFETY INFORMATION

Serophene® is contraindicated in patients who have previously experienced hypersensitivity to clomiphene citrate. Visual disturbances, vasomotor flushes, and ovarian enlargement occasionally occur. Because the teratogenic potential of clomiphene citrate is unknown, it should not be administered during pregnancy. Multiple births occur in approximately 10% of pregnancies resulting from clomiphene citrate therapy; the vast majority of these are twins.

PRESCRIBING INFORMATION

SEROPHENE®   ℞

[se'ro-fēn]
(clomiphene citrate tablets, USP)

DESCRIPTION

Each scored white tablet contains:
Clomiphene Citrate USP 50 mg. Clomiphene citrate is designated chemically as 2-[p-(2-chloro-1,2-diphenylvinyl) phenoxy] triethylamine dihydrogen citrate and is represented structurally as:

$$(C_2H_5)_2NCH_2CH_2O-C_6H_4-C=C-C_6H_4-C_6H_8O_7$$ (Cl)

clomiphene citrate, USP (Serophene®)

As shown, one molecule of citric acid is chemically bound with one molecule of the organic base, clomiphene. Clomiphene citrate is a chemical analog of other triarylethylene compounds such as chlorotrianisene and the cholesterol inhibitor, triparanol.

ACTIONS

Clomiphene citrate, an orally-administered, non-steroidal agent, may induce ovulation in selected anovulatory women. It is a drug of considerable pharmacologic potency. Careful evaluation and selection of the patient and close attention to the timing of the dose is mandatory prior to treatment with clomiphene citrate. Conservative selection and management of the patient contribute to successful therapy of anovulation. Clomiphene citrate induces ovulation in most selected anovulatory patients. The various criteria for ovulation include: an ovulation peak of estrogen excretion followed by a biphasic basal body temperature curve, urinary excretion of pregnanediol at post-ovulatory levels, and endometrial histologic findings characteristic of the luteal phase.

A review of eleven publications appearing between 1964 and 1978 showed that pregnancy occurred in 35% of 5154 patients with ovulatory dysfunction who received clomiphene citrate.

[See table below].

Clomiphene citrate therapy appears to mediate ovulation through increased output of pituitary gonadotropins. These stimulate the maturation and endocrine activity of the ovarian follicle which is followed by the development and function of the corpus luteum. Increased urinary excretion of gonadotropins and estrogen suggest involvement of the pituitary.

Studies with ^{14}C labeled clomiphene citrate have shown that it is readily absorbed orally in humans, and is excreted principally in the feces. An average of 51% of the administered dose was excreted after 5 days. After intravenous administration 37% was excreted in 5 days. The appearance of ^{14}C in the feces six weeks after administration suggests that the remaining drug and/or metabolites are slowly excreted from a sequestered enterohepatic recirculation pool.

INDICATIONS

Clomiphene citrate is indicated for the treatment of ovulatory failure in patients desiring pregnancy, and whose husbands are fertile and potent. Impediments to this goal must be excluded or adequately treated before beginning therapy. Administration of clomiphene citrate is indicated only in patients with demonstrated ovulatory dysfunction and in whom the following conditions apply:

1. Normal liver function.
2. Physiologic indications of normal endogenous estrogen (as estimated from vaginal smears, endometrial biopsy, assay of urinary estrogen, or from bleeding in response to progesterone). Reduced estrogen levels, while less favorable, do not prevent successful therapy.
3. Clomiphene citrate therapy is not effective for those patients with primary pituitary or ovarian failure. It cannot substitute for appropriate therapy of other disturbances leading to ovulatory dysfunction, e.g., diseases of the thyroid or adrenals.
4. Particularly careful evaluation prior to clomiphene citrate therapy should be done in patients with abnormal uterine bleeding. It is most important that neoplastic lesions are detected.

CONTRAINDICATIONS

Pregnancy

Although no direct effect of clomiphene citrate therapy on the human fetus has been seen, clomiphene citrate should not be administered in cases of suspected pregnancy as such effects have been reported in animals. To prevent inadvertent clomiphene citrate administration during early pregnancy, the basal body temperature should be recorded throughout all treatment cycles, and therapy should be discontinued if pregnancy is suspected. If the basal body temperature following clomiphene citrate is biphasic and is not followed by menses, the possibility of an ovarian cyst and/or pregnancy should be excluded. Until the correct diagnosis has been determined, the next course of therapy should be delayed.

Liver Disease

Patients with liver disease or a history of liver dysfunction should not receive clomiphene citrate therapy.

Abnormal Uterine Bleeding

Clomiphene citrate is contraindicated in patients with abnormal uterine bleeding.

PREGNANCIES FOLLOWING CLOMIPHENE CITRATE USP[a]		(Range)
Number of Patients	= 5154	
Percent of Patients Ovulating[b]	= 75	(50-94)%
Percent of Ovulatory Cycles	= 53	(33-69)%
Percent of Patients Pregnant	= 35	(11-52)%
Percent Patients Pregnant	= 46	(22-61)%
Percent Patients Ovulating		
Percent Live Births	= 86	(74-99.8)%
Percent Abortions	= 14	(0.2-26)%
Percent of Single Births	= 90	(67-100)%
Percent Surviving	= 99	(98.2-100)%
Percent of Multiple Births	= 10	(0-33)%
Percent Surviving	= 96	(82-100)%

a) includes patients receiving other than recommended dosage regimen.
b) average from studies.

WARNINGS

Visual Symptoms

Patients should be warned that blurring and/or other visual symptoms may occur occasionally with clomiphene citrate therapy. These may make activities such as driving or operating machinery more hazardous than usual, particularly under conditions of variable lighting. While their significance is not yet understood (see ADVERSE REACTIONS), patients having any visual symptoms, should discontinue treatment and have a complete ophthalmologic evaluation.

PRECAUTIONS

Diagnosis Prior to Clomiphene Citrate Therapy

Careful evaluation should be given to candidates for clomiphene citrate therapy. A complete pelvic examination should be performed prior to treatment and repeated before each subsequent course. Clomiphene citrate should not be given to patients with an ovarian cyst, as further ovarian enlargement may result.

Since the incidence of endometrial carcinoma and of ovulatory disorders increases with age, endometrial biopsy should always exclude the former as causative in such patients. If abnormal uterine bleeding is present, full diagnostic measures are necessary.

Ovarian Overstimulation During Treatment with Clomiphene Citrate

To minimize the hazard associated with the occasional abnormal ovarian enlargement during clomiphene citrate therapy (see ADVERSE REACTIONS), the lowest dose producing good results should be chosen. Some patients with polycystic ovary syndrome are unusually sensitive to gonadotropin and may have an exaggerated response to usual doses of clomiphene citrate. Maximal enlargement of the ovary, whether abnormal or physiologic, does not occur until several days after discontinuation of clomiphene citrate. The patient complaining of pelvic pains after receiving clomiphene citrate should be examined carefully. If enlargement of the ovary occurs, clomiphene citrate therapy should be withheld until the ovaries have returned to pretreatment size, and the dosage or duration of the next course should be reduced. The ovarian enlargement and cyst formation following clomiphene citrate therapy regress spontaneously within a few days or weeks after discontinuing treatment. Therefore, unless a strong indication for laparotomy exists, such cystic enlargement always should be managed conservatively.

Multiple Pregnancy

In the reviewed publications, the incidence of multiple pregnancies was increased during those cycles in which clomiphene citrate was given. Among the 1803 pregnancies on which the outcome was reported, 90% were single and 10% twins. Less than 1% of the reported deliveries resulted in triplets or more.

Of these multiple pregnancies, 96-99% resulted in the births of live infants. The patient and her husband should be advised of the frequency and potential hazards of multiple pregnancy before starting treatment.

ADVERSE REACTIONS

Symptoms

Side effects are not prominent at the recommended dosage of clomiphene citrate, and infrequently interfere with treatment. Side effects tend to occur more frequently at higher doses and in the longer treatment courses used in some early studies. The more common side effects and the percent of patients experiencing them include vasomotor flushes (11%), abdominal discomfort (7.4%), abnormal uterine bleeding (0.5%), ovarian enlargement (14%), breast tenderness (2.1%), and visual symptoms (1.6%). The vasomotor symptoms resemble menopausal "hot flushes", and are not usually severe. They promptly disappear after treatment is discontinued. Abdominal discomfort may resemble ovulatory (mittelschmerz) or premenstrual phenomena, or that due to ovarian enlargement. In addition, nausea and vomiting (2.1%), nervousness and insomnia (1.9%), headache (1%), dizziness and lightheadedness (1%), increased urination (0.9%), depression and fatigue (0.8%), urticaria and allergic dermatitis (0.6%), weight gain (0.4%), and reversible hair loss (0.3%) have been reported.

When clomiphene citrate is administered at the recommended dose, abnormal ovarian enlargement (see PRECAUTIONS) is infrequent, although the usual cyclic variation in ovarian size may be exaggerated. Similarly, mid-cycle ovarian pain (mittelschmerz) may be accentuated. With prolonged or higher dosage, ovarian enlargement and cyst formation (usually luteal) may occur more often and the luteal phase of the cycle may be prolonged. Patients with polycystic ovary disease may be unusually sensitive to clomiphene therapy. Rare occurrences of massive ovarian enlargement have been reported, for example, in a patient with polycystic ovary syndrome whose clomiphene citrate therapy consisted of 100 mg daily for 14 days. Since abnormal ovarian enlargement usually regresses spontaneously, most of these patients should be treated conservatively.

The incidence of visual symptoms (see WARNINGS for further recommendations), usually described as "blurring" or

spots or flashes (scintillating scotomata), correlates with increasing total dose. The symptoms disappear within a few days or weeks after clomiphene citrate is discontinued. This may be due to intensification and/or prolongation of after-images. Symptoms often appear first, or are accentuated, upon exposure to a more brightly lit environment. While measured visual acuity has not generally been affected, in one patient taking 200 mg daily, visual blurring developed on the seventh day of treatment, and progressed to severe diminution of visual acuity by the tenth day. No other abnormality was coincident, and the visual acuity was normal by the third day after treatment was stopped. Ophthalmologically definable scotomata and electroretinographic retinal function changes have also been reported.

BSP Laboratory Studies

Greater than 5% retention of sulfobromophthalein (BSP) has been reported in approximately 10 to 20% of patients in whom it was measured. Retention was usually minimal but was elevated during prolonged clomiphene citrate administration or with apparently unrelated liver disease. In some patients, pre-existing BSP retention decreased even though clomiphene citrate therapy was continued. Other liver function tests were usually normal.

Other Laboratory Studies

Clomiphene citrate has not been reported to cause a significant abnormality in hematologic or renal tests, in protein bound iodine, or in serum cholesterol levels.

Birth Defects

Of 1803 births following clomiphene citrate administration, 45 infants with birth defects were reported for a cumulative rate of 2.5%.

Six cases of Down's Syndrome, one neonatal death with multiple malformations and one case each of the following were reported: extropia, club foot, tibial torsion, blocked tear duct and hemangioma. The other congenital abnormalities were not described. The investigators did not report that these were presumed to be due to therapy. The cumulative rate of congenital abnormalities does not exceed that reported in the general population.

DOSAGE AND ADMINISTRATION

General Considerations

Physicians experienced in managing gynecologic or endocrine disorders should supervise the work-up and treatment of candidate patients for clomiphene citrate therapy. Patients should be chosen for clomiphene citrate therapy only after careful diagnostic evaluation (see INDICATIONS). The plan of therapy should be outlined in advance. Impediments to achieving the goal of therapy must be excluded or adequately treated before beginning clomiphene citrate.

In determining a starting dose schedule, efficacy must be balanced against potential side effects. For example, the available data so far suggests that ovulation and pregnancy are slightly more attainable with 100 mg/day for 5 days than with 50 mg/day for 5 days. As the dosage is increased, however, ovarian overstimulation and other side effects may be expected to increase. Although the data do not yet establish a relationship between dose level and multiple births, it is reasonable that such a correlation exists on pharmacologic grounds.

For these reasons, treatment of the usual patient should initiate with a 50 mg daily dose for 5 days. The dose may be increased only in those patients who do not respond to the first course (see RECOMMENDED DOSAGE). Special treatment with lower dosage over shorter duration is particularly recommended if unusual sensitivity to pituitary gonadotropin is suspected, including patients with polycystic ovary syndrome (see PRECAUTIONS).

Recommended Dosage

The recommended dosage for the first course of clomiphene citrate is 50 mg (1 tablet) daily for 5 days. Therapy may be started at any time if the patient has had no recent uterine bleeding. If progestin-induced bleeding is intended, or if spontaneous uterine bleeding occurs prior to therapy, the regimen of 50 mg daily for 5 days should be started on or about the fifth day of the cycle. When ovulation occurs at this dosage, there is no advantage to increasing the dose in subsequent cycles of treatment.

If ovulation does not appear to have occurred after the first course of therapy, a second course of 100 mg daily (two 50 mg tablets given as a single daily dose) for 5 days may be started. This course may begin as early as 30 days after the previous one. Increasing the dosage or duration of therapy beyond 100 mg/day for 5 days should not be undertaken.

The majority of patients who respond do so during the first course of therapy, and 3 courses constitute an adequate therapeutic trial. If ovulatory menses do not occur, the diagnosis should be re-evaluated. Treatment beyond this is not recommended in the patient who does not exhibit evidence of ovulation.

Pregnancy

Properly timed coitus is very important for good results. For regularity of cyclic ovulatory response it is also important that each course of clomiphene citrate be started on or about the fifth day of the cycle, once ovulation has been established. As with other therapeutic modalities, Serophene®

therapy follows the rule of diminishing returns, such that likelihood of conception diminishes with each succeeding course of therapy. If pregnancy has not been achieved after 3 ovulatory responses to Serophene, further treatment is not generally recommended. Before starting treatment, patients should be advised of the possibility and potential hazards of multiple pregnancy if conception occurs following clomiphene citrate therapy.

Long-Term Cyclic Therapy —Not Recommended

Since the relative safety of long-term cyclic therapy has not yet been conclusively demonstrated, and since the majority of patients will ovulate following 3 courses, long-term cyclic therapy is not recommended.

HOW SUPPLIED

Serophene is available as 50 mg scored white tablets in the following package combinations:
● 1 carton 10 tablets, NDC 44087-8090-6
Each carton contains 2 strips of 5 tablets each.
● 1 carton 30 tablets, NDC 44087-8090-1
Each carton contains 3 strips of 10 tablets, each in a 2 × 5 arrangement.

Protect from light, moisture, and excessive heat. Dispense in well-closed, light resistant container as defined in the USP, with child resistant closure.

PRODUCT INFORMATION

AVAILABLE ONLY ON PRESCRIPTION.

© Serono Laboratories, Inc. 1982
Revised: 2/88

For additional information, please contact:
Serono Laboratories, Inc.
Medical Information Services
100 Longwater Circle
Norwell, MA 02061
800-283-8088 (Toll free)
617-982-9000

Sigma-Tau Pharmaceuticals, Inc.
200 ORCHARD RIDGE DRIVE
GAITHERSBURG, MARYLAND 20878

CARNITOR® ℞
(Levocarnitine) Tablets (330 mg.)
[kar'nĭ-tor]

CARNITOR® ℞
(Levocarnitine) Oral Solution
(1.0 gm per 10 ml multidose)
For oral use only. Not for parenteral use.

DESCRIPTION

CARNITOR (Levocarnitine) is L-beta-hydroxy-gamma-trimethylamino butyric acid (inner salt). As a bulk drug substance it is a white powder with a melting point of 196–197°C and is readily soluble in water. The L-isomer of carnitine is the biologically active form. Its chemical structure is:

$$CH_3-N^+-CH_2-CH-CH_2-COO^-$$

with CH_3 groups and OH.

Each CARNITOR (Levocarnitine) Tablet contains 330 mg of levocarnitine and the inactive ingredients magnesium stearate, microcrystalline cellulose and povidone.

Each 118 ml container of the CARNITOR (Levocarnitine) Oral Solution contains 1 gm of levocarnitine/10 ml., sucrose syrup, D, L-malic acid, red colors and artificial cherry flavor. Methyl paraben NF and Propylparaben NF are added as preservatives. The pH is approximately 5.

CLINICAL PHARMACOLOGY

CARNITOR (Levocarnitine) is a naturally occurring substance required in mammalian energy metabolism. It has been shown to facilitate long-chain fatty acid entry into cellular mitochondria, therefore delivering substrate for oxidation and subsequent energy production. Fatty acids are utilized as an energy substrate in all tissues except the brain. In skeletal and cardiac muscle they serve as major fuel. Primary systemic carnitine deficiency is characterized by low plasma, RBC, and tissue levels. The resulting impairment in fatty acid metabolism manifests itself as elevated triglycerides and free fatty acids, diminished ketogenesis, and lipid infiltration of liver and muscle.

Severe chronic carnitine deficiency may be associated with hypoglycemia, progressive myasthenia, hypotonia, lethargy, hepatomegaly, encephalopathy, hepatic coma, cardiomegaly, congestive heart failure, cardiac arrest, neurologic dis-

Continued on next page

Sigma-Tau—Cont.

turbances, and impaired growth and development in infants. Published reports and clinical studies with CARNITOR (Levocarnitine) have shown that administration of CARNITOR (Levocarnitine) to patients with plasma deficiency of carnitine results in increased levels and, in some patients, reversal of complications associated with impaired fat utilization.

BIOAVAILABILITY

The bioavailability/pharmacokinetics of CARNITOR (Levocarnitine) Tablets and the Oral Solution preparation have not been determined in well controlled studies.

METABOLISM AND EXCRETION

The majority of body carnitine is excreted in the urine and feces. In renal failure, carnitine levels may rise.

INDICATIONS AND USAGE

CARNITOR (Levocarnitine) is indicated in the treatment of primary systemic carnitine deficiency.

CONTRAINDICATIONS

None known.

WARNINGS

None.

PRECAUTIONS

General

CARNITOR (Levocarnitine) Oral Solution is for oral/internal use only.

Not for parenteral use.

Gastrointestinal reactions may result from too rapid consumption of carnitine. CARNITOR (Levocarnitine) Oral Solution may be consumed alone, or dissolved in drinks or other liquid foods to reduce taste fatigue. It should be consumed slowly and doses should be spaced evenly throughout the day to maximize tolerance.

Carcinogenesis, Mutagenesis, impairment of fertility

Mutagenicity tests have been performed in Salmonella typhimurium, Saccharomyces cerevisiae, and Schizosaccharomyces pombe that do not indicate that CARNITOR (Levocarnitine) is mutagenic. Long-term animal studies have not been conducted to evaluate the carcinogenicity of the compound.

Usage in pregnancy

Pregnancy Category B Reproductive studies have been performed in rats and rabbits using parenteral administration at doses equivalent on a mg/kg basis to the suggested oral adult dosage and have revealed no harm to the fetus due to CARNITOR (Levocarnitine). There are, however, no adequate and well controlled studies in pregnant women. Because animal reproduction studies are not always predictive of human response, this drug should be used during pregnancy only if clearly needed.

Nursing mothers

Levocarnitine is a normal component of human milk. Levocarnitine supplementation in nursing mothers has not been studied.

Pediatric use

See Dosage and Administration.

ADVERSE REACTIONS

Various mild gastrointestinal complaints have been reported during the long-term administration of oral L- or D, L-carnitine; these include transient nausea and vomiting, abdominal cramps, and diarrhea. Mild myasthenia has been described only in uremic patients receiving D,L-carnitine. Gastrointestinal adverse reactions with CARNITOR (Levocarnitine) Oral Solution dissolved in liquids might be avoided by a slow consumption of the solution or by a greater dilution. Decreasing the dosage often diminishes or eliminates drug-related patient body odor or gastrointestinal symptoms when present. Tolerance should be monitored very closely during the first week of administration, and after any dosage increases.

OVERDOSAGE

There have been no reports of toxicity from carnitine overdosage. The oral LD_{50} of levocarnitine in mice is 19.2 g/kg. Carnitine may cause diarrhea. Overdosage should be treated with supportive care.

DOSAGE AND ADMINISTRATION

CARNITOR (Levocarnitine) Tablets.

Adults: The recommended oral dosage for adults is 990 mg. two or three times a day using the 330 mg. tablets, depending on clinical response.

Infants and children: The recommended oral dosage for infants and children is between 50 and 100 mg/kg/day in divided doses, with a maximum of 3 grams/day. Dosage should begin at 50 mg/kg/day. The exact dosage will depend on clinical response. Monitoring should include periodic blood chemistries, vital signs, plasma carnitine concentrations and overall clinical condition.

CARNITOR (Levocarnitine) Oral Solution.
For oral use only. **Not for parenteral use.**

Adults: The recommended dosage of levocarnitine is one to three 1–3 g/day for a 50 kg subject which is equivalent to 10–30 ml/day of Carnitor (Levocarnitine) Oral Solution. Higher doses should be administered only with caution and only where clinical and biochemical considerations make it seem likely that higher doses will be of benefit. Dosage should start at 1 g/day, (10 ml/day), and be increased slowly while assessing tolerance and therapeutic response. Monitoring should include periodic blood chemistries, vital signs, plasma carnitine concentrations, and overall clinical condition.

Infants and children: The recommended dosage of levocarnitine is 50–100 mg/kg/day which is equivalent to 0.5 ml/kg/day CARNITOR (Levocarnitine) Oral Solution. Higher doses should be administered only with caution and only where clinical and biochemical considerations make it seem likely that higher doses will be of benefit. Dosage should start at 50 mg/kg/day, and be increased slowly to a maximum of 3 g/day (30 ml/day) while assessing tolerance and therapeutic response. Monitoring should include periodic blood chemistries, vital signs, plasma carnitine concentrations, and overall clinical condition.

CARNITOR (Levocarnitine) Oral Solution may be consumed alone or dissolved in drink or other liquid food. Doses should be spaced evenly throughout the day (every three or four hours), preferably during or following meals and should be consumed slowly in order to maximize tolerance.

HOW SUPPLIED

CARNITOR (Levocarnitine) Tablets are supplied as 330 mg., individually foil wrapped tablets in boxes of 90 (NDC 54482-144-07). Store at room temperature (25° C).

CARNITOR (Levocarnitine) Oral Solution is supplied in 118 ml (4 fl. oz.) multiple-unit plastic containers. The multiple-unit containers are packaged 24 per case. (NDC 54482-145-08). Store at room temperature (25° C).

CAUTION

Federal (U.S.A.) law prohibits dispensing without prescription.

CARNITOR (Levocarnitine) Oral Solution manufactured for: Sigma-Tau, Inc.

By: Barre-National, Inc. Baltimore, MD 21207-2642

REFERENCES

1. Bohmer T. Rynding A, Solberg HE: Carnitine levels in human serum in health and disease. **Clin Chim Acta 57**:55–61, 1974.
2. Brooks H, Goldberg L, Holland R et al: Carnitine-induced effects on cardiac and peripheral hemodynamics. **J Clin Pharmacol 17**:561–578, 1977.
3. Christiansen R, Bremer J: Active transport of butyrobetaine and carnitine into isolated liver cells. **Biochem Biophys Acta 448**:562–577, 1977.
4. Lindstedt S, Lindstedt G: Distribution and excretion of carnitine $^{14}CO_2$ in the rat. **Acta Chim Scand 15**:701–702, 1961.
5. Rebouche CJ, Engel Ag: Carnitine metabolism and deficiency syndromes. **Mayo Clin Proc 58**:533–540, 1983.
6. Rebouche CJ, Paulson DJ: Carnitine metabolism and function in humans. **Ann Rev Nutr 6**:41–68, 1986.

SmithKline Consumer Products
A SmithKline Beckman Company
P.O. BOX 8082
PHILADELPHIA, PA 19101

ECOTRIN®
Enteric-Coated Aspirin
Antiarthritic, Antiplatelet

DESCRIPTION

'Ecotrin' is enteric-coated aspirin (acetylsalicylic acid, ASA) available in tablet and caplet forms in 325 mg. and 500 mg. dosage units.

The enteric coating covers a core of aspirin and is designed to resist disintegration in the stomach, dissolving in the more neutral-to-alkaline environment of the duodenum. Such action helps to protect the stomach from injury that may result from ingestion of plain, buffered or highly buffered aspirin (see SAFETY).

INDICATIONS

'Ecotrin' is indicated for:

- conditions requiring chronic or long-term aspirin therapy for pain and/or inflammation, e.g., rheumatoid arthritis, juvenile rheumatoid arthritis, systemic lupus erythematosus, osteoarthritis (degenerative joint disease), ankylosing spondylitis, psoriatic arthritis, Reiter's syndrome and fibrositis,
- antiplatelet indications of aspirin (see the ANTIPLATELET EFFECT section) and

- situations in which compliance with aspirin therapy may be affected because of the gastrointestinal side effects of plain, i.e., non-enteric-coated, or buffered aspirin.

DOSAGE

For analgesic or anti-inflammatory indications, the OTC maximum dosage for aspirin is 4000 mg. per day in divided doses, i.e., 2-325 mg. tablets or caplets q4h or 3-325 mg. tablets or caplets or 2-500 mg. tablets or caplets q6h.

For antiplatelet effect dosage: see the ANTIPLATELET EFFECT section.

Under a physician's direction, the dosage can be increased or otherwise modified as appropriate to the clinical situation. When 'Ecotrin' is used for anti-inflammatory effect, the physician should be attentive to plasma salicylate levels, and may also caution the patient to be alert to the development of tinnitus as an indicator of elevated salicylate levels. It should be noted that patients with a high frequency hearing loss (such as may occur in older individuals) may have difficulty perceiving the tinnitus. Tinnitus would then not be a reliable indicator in such individuals.

INACTIVE INGREDIENTS

Inactive ingredients (listed for individuals with specific allergies): Cellulose, Cellulose Acetate Phthalate, D&C Yellow 10, Diethyl Phthalate, FD&C Yellow 6 (Sunset Yellow) as a color additive, Silicon Dioxide, Sodium Starch Glycolate, Starch, Stearic Acid, Titanium Dioxide, and trace amounts of other inactive ingredients.

BIOAVAILABILITY

The bioavailability of aspirin from 'Ecotrin' has been demonstrated in a number of salicylate excretion studies. The studies show levels of salicylate (and metabolites) in urine excreted over 48 hours for 'Ecotrin' do not differ statistically from plain, i.e., non-enteric-coated, aspirin.

Plasma studies, in which 'Ecotrin' has been compared with plain aspirin in steady-state studies over eight days, also demonstrate that 'Ecotrin' provides plasma salicylate levels not statistically different from plain aspirin.

Information regarding salicylate levels over a range of doses was generated in a study in which 24 healthy volunteers (12 male and 12 female) took daily (divided) doses of either 2600 mg., 3900 mg., or 5200 mg. of 'Ecotrin'. Plasma salicylate levels generally acknowledged to be anti-inflammatory (15 mg./dL.) were attained at daily doses of 5200 mg., on Day 2 by females and Day 3 by males. At 3900 mg., anti-inflammatory levels were attained at Day 3 by females and Day 4 by males.

Dissolution of the enteric coating occurs at a neutral-to-basic pH and is therefore dependent on gastric emptying into the duodenum. With continued dosing, appropriate plasma levels are maintained.

SAFETY

The safety of 'Ecotrin' has been demonstrated in a number of endoscopic studies comparing 'Ecotrin', plain aspirin, as well as plain buffered and "arthritis-strength" buffered preparations. In these studies, all forms of aspirin were dosed to the OTC maximum (3900–4000 mg. per day) for up to 14 days. The normal healthy volunteers participating in these studies were gastroscoped before and after the courses of treatment, and 14-day drug-free periods followed active drug. Compared to all the other preparations, there was statistically significantly less gastric damage during the 'Ecotrin' courses. There was also statistically less duodenal damage when compared with the plain, i.e., non-enteric-coated, aspirin.

Details of studies demonstrating the safety and bioavailability of 'Ecotrin' are available to health care professionals. Write: Medical Affairs Department, SmithKline Consumer Products, P.O. Box 8082, Philadelphia, PA 19101.

WARNING

Consumer Warning: Children and teenagers should not use this medicine for chicken pox or flu symptoms before a doctor is consulted about Reye syndrome, a rare but serious illness reported to be associated with aspirin. If pain persists for more than 10 days, or if redness is present, or in arthritic or rheumatic conditions affecting children under 12, consult a physician immediately. Discontinue use if dizziness, ringing in ears, or impaired hearing occurs. If you experience persistent or unexplained stomach upset, consult a physician. Keep this and all drugs out of children's reach. In case of accidental overdose, seek professional assistance or contact a poison control center immediately. As with any medicine, if you are pregnant or nursing a baby, seek the advice of a health professional before using this product. Store at controlled room temperature (59°–86°F.).

Professional Warning: There have been occasional reports in the literature concerning individuals with impaired gastric emptying in whom there may be retention of one or more 'Ecotrin' tablets over time. This unusual phenomenon may occur as a result of outlet obstruction from ulcer disease alone or combined with hypotonic gastric peristalsis. Because of the integrity of the enteric coating in an acidic environment, these tablets may accumulate and form a bezoar in the stomach. Individuals with this condition may present with complaints of early satiety or of vague upper abdominal distress. Diagnosis may be made by endoscopy or by abdominal films which show opacities suggestive of a mass of small tablets (*Ref.: Bogacz, K. and Caldron, P.: Enteric-coated Aspirin Bezoar: Elevation of Serum Salicylate Level by Barium Study. Amer. J. Med. 1987:83, 783-6.*). Management may vary according to the condition of the patient. Options include: gastrotomy and alternating slightly basic and neutral lavage (*Ref.: Baum, J.: Enteric-Coated Aspirin and the Problem of Gastric Retention. J. Rheum., 1984:11, 250-1.*). While there have been no clinical reports, it has been suggested that such individuals may also be treated with parenteral cimetidine (to reduce acid secretion) and then given sips of slightly basic liquids to effect gradual dissolution of the enteric coating. Progress may be followed with plasma salicylate levels or via recognition of tinnitus by the patient.

It should be kept in mind that individuals with a history of partial or complete gastrectomy may produce reduced amounts of acid and therefore have less acidic gastric pH. Under these circumstances, the benefits offered by the acid-resistant enteric coating may not exist.

ANTIPLATELET EFFECT

FDA has approved the professional labeling of aspirin to reduce the risk of death and/or nonfatal myocardial infarction (MI) in patients with a previous infarction or unstable angina pectoris. Previously, wording was added to the professional labeling of aspirin approving its use in reducing the risk of transient ischemic attacks in men.
Labeling for both indications follows:

Aspirin for Myocardial Infarction
Indication: Aspirin is indicated to reduce the risk of death and/or nonfatal myocardial infarction in patients with a previous infarction or unstable angina pectoris.
Clinical Trials: The indication is supported by the results of six, large, randomized multicenter, placebo-controlled studies involving 10,816 predominantly male, post-myocardial infarction (MI) patients and one randomized placebo-controlled study of 1,266 men with unstable angina.[1-7] Therapy with aspirin was begun at intervals after the onset of acute MI varying from less than three days to more than five years and continued for periods of from less than one year to four years. In the unstable angina study, treatment was started within one month after the onset of unstable angina and continued for 12 weeks, and patients with complicating conditions such as congestive heart failure were not included in the study.
Aspirin therapy in MI patients was associated with about a 20 percent reduction in the risk of subsequent death and/or nonfatal reinfarction, a median absolute decrease of 3 percent from the 12 to 22 percent event rates in the placebo groups. In aspirin-treated unstable angina patients, the reduction in risk was about 50 percent, a reduction in event rate in the placebo group over the 12 weeks of the study. Daily dosage of aspirin in the post-myocardial infarction studies was 300 mg. in one study and 900 to 1500 mg. in five studies. A dose of 325 mg. was used in the study of unstable angina.

Adverse Reactions
Gastrointestinal Reactions: Doses of 1000 mg. per day of aspirin caused gastrointestinal symptoms and bleeding that in some cases were clinically significant. In the largest post-infarction study (the Aspirin Myocardial Infarction Study [AMIS] with 4,500 people), the percentage incidences of gastrointestinal symptoms of a standard, solid-tablet formulation and placebo-treated subjects, respectively, were: stomach pain (14.5%; 4.4%); heartburn (11.9%; 4.8%); nausea and/or vomiting (7.6%; 2.1%); hospitalization for gastrointestinal disorder (4.9%; 3.5%). In the AMIS and other trials, aspirin-treated patients had increased rates of gross gastrointestinal bleeding. Symptoms and signs of gastrointestinal irritation were not significantly increased in subjects treated for unstable angina with buffered aspirin in solution.
Cardiovascular and Biochemical: In the AMIS trial, the dosage of 1000 mg. per day of aspirin was associated with small increases in systolic blood pressure (BP) (average 1.5 to 2.1 mmHg) and diastolic BP (0.5 to 0.6 mmHg), depending upon whether maximal or last available readings were used. Blood urea nitrogen and uric acid levels were also increased, but by less than 1.0 mg.%. Subjects with marked hypertension or renal insufficiency had been excluded from the trial so that the clinical importance of these observations for such subjects or for any subjects treated over more prolonged periods is not known. It is recommended that patients placed on long-term aspirin treatment, even at doses of 300 mg. per day, be seen at regular intervals to assess changes in these measurements.
Sodium in Buffered Aspirin for Solution Formulations: One tablet daily of buffered aspirin in solution adds 553 mg. of sodium to that in the diet and may not be tolerated by patients with active sodium-retaining states such as congestive heart or renal failure. This amount of sodium adds about 30 percent to the 70 to 90 meq. intake suggested as appropriate for dietary hypertension in the 1984 Report of the Joint National Committee on Detection, Evaluation, and Treatment of High Blood Pressure.[8]

Dosage and Administration: Although most of the studies used dosages exceeding 300 mg. daily, two trials used only 300 mg. and pharmacologic data indicate that this dose inhibits platelet function fully. Therefore, 300 mg. or a conventional 325 mg. aspirin dose daily is a reasonable, routine dose that would minimize gastrointestinal adverse reactions for both solid, oral dosage forms (buffered and plain aspirin) and buffered aspirin in solution.

References:
1. Elwood, P.C., et al.: A Randomized Controlled Trial of Acetylsalicylic Acid in the Secondary Prevention of Mortality from Myocardial Infarction, *Br. Med. J.* 1:436–440, 1974.
2. The Coronary Drug Project Research Group: Aspirin in Coronary Heart Disease, *J. Chronic Dis.* 29:625–642, 1976.
3. Breddin, K., et al.: Secondary Prevention of Myocardial Infarction: A Comparison of Acetylsalicylic Acid, Phenprocoumon or Placebo, *Homeostasis* 470:263–268, 1979.
4. Aspirin Myocardial Infarction Study Research Group: A Randomized Controlled Trial of Aspirin in Persons Recovered from Myocardial Infarction, *J.A.M.A.* 243:661–669, 1980.
5. Elwood, P.C., and Sweetnam, P.M.: Aspirin and Secondary Mortality After Myocardial Infarction, *Lancet* pp. 1313–1315, Dec. 22–29, 1979.
6. The Persantine-Aspirin Reinfarction Study Research Group, Persantine and Aspirin in Coronary Heart Disease, *Circulation* 62:449–469, 1980.
7. Lewis, H.D., et al.: Protective Effects of Aspirin Against Acute Myocardial Infarction and Death in Men with Unstable Angina, Results of a Veterans Administration Cooperative Study, *N. Engl. J. Med.* 309:396–403, 1983.
8. 1984 Report of the Joint National Committee on Detection, Evaluation, and Treatment of High Blood Pressure, U.S. Department of Health and Human Services and U.S. Public Health Service, National Institutes of Health. NIH Pub. No. 84-1088.

"ASPIRIN FOR TRANSIENT ISCHEMIC ATTACKS"

Indication
For reducing the risk of recurrent Transient Ischemic Attacks (TIA's) or stroke in men who have had transient ischemia of the brain due to fibrin platelet emboli. There is inadequate evidence that aspirin or buffered aspirin is effective in reducing TIA's in women at the recommended dosage. There is no evidence that aspirin or buffered aspirin is of benefit in the treatment of completed strokes in men or women.
Clinical Trials
The indication is supported by the results of a Canadian study (1) in which 585 patients with threatened stroke were followed in a randomized clinical trial for an average of 26 months to determine whether aspirin or sulfinpyrazone, singly or in combination, was superior to placebo in preventing transient ischemic attacks, stroke or death. The study showed that, although sulfinpyrazone had no statistically significant effect, aspirin reduced the risk of continuing transient ischemic attacks, stroke or death by 19 percent and reduced the risk of stroke or death by 31 percent. Another aspirin study carried out in the United States with 178 patients, showed a statistically significant number of "favorable outcomes," including reduced transient ischemic attacks, stroke and death (2).
Precautions
Patients presenting with signs and symptoms of TIA's should have a complete medical and neurologic evaluation. Consideration should be given to other disorders that resemble TIA's. Attention should be given to risk factors: it is important to evaluate and treat, if appropriate, other diseases associated with TIA's and stroke, such as hypertension and diabetes.
Concurrent administration of absorbable antacids at therapeutic doses may increase the clearance of salicylates in some individuals. The concurrent administration of nonabsorbable antacids may alter the rate of absorption of aspirin, thereby resulting in a decreased acetylsalicylic acid/salicylate ratio in plasma. The clinical significance of these decreases in available aspirin is unknown.
Aspirin at dosages of 1,000 milligrams per day has been associated with small increases in blood pressure, blood urea nitrogen, and serum uric acid levels. It is recommended that patients placed on long-term aspirin treatment be seen at regular intervals to assess changes in these measurements.
Adverse Reactions:
At dosages of 1,000 milligrams or higher of aspirin per day, gastrointestinal side effects include stomach pain, heartburn, nausea and/or vomiting, as well as increased rates of gross gastrointestinal bleeding.
Dosage and Administration
Adult dosage for men is 1,300 milligrams a day, in divided doses of 650 milligrams twice a day or 325 milligrams four times a day.
REFERENCES
(1) The Canadian Cooperative Study Group, "Randomized Trial of Aspirin and Sulfinpyrazone in Threatened Stroke," *New England Journal of Medicine,* 299:53, 1978.
(2) Fields, W. S., et al., "Controlled Trial of Aspirin in Cerebral Ischemia," *Stroke* 8:301-316, 1977."

SUPPLIED

'Ecotrin' Tablets
325 mg. in bottles of 100, 250 and 1000.
500 mg. in bottles of 60 and 150.
'Ecotrin' Caplets
325 mg. in bottles of 75.
500 mg. in bottles of 50.
TAMPER-RESISTANT PACKAGE FEATURES:
● The carton has been sealed at the factory with a clear overwrap printed with "safety sealed."
● Bottle has imprinted "SKCP" seal under cap.
● The words ECOTRIN REG or ECOTRIN MAX appear on each tablet or caplet (see product illustration printed on carton).
● DO NOT USE THIS PRODUCT IF ANY OF THESE TAMPER-RESISTANT FEATURES ARE MISSING OR BROKEN. IF YOU HAVE ANY QUESTIONS, PLEASE CALL 1-800-543-3434 TOLL FREE.

FEOSOL® CAPSULES
Hematinic

DESCRIPTION
'Feosol' Capsules provide the body with ferrous sulfate—iron in its most efficient form—for simple iron deficiency and iron-deficiency anemia. The special targeted-release capsule formulation—ferrous sulfate in pellets—reduces stomach upset, a common problem with iron.

FORMULA
Each capsule contains 159 mg. of dried ferrous sulfate USP (50 mg. of elemental iron), equivalent to 250 mg. of ferrous sulfate USP. Inactive Ingredients (listed for individuals with specific allergies): Benzyl Alcohol, Cetylpyridinium Chloride, D&C Red 33, Yellow 10, FD&C Blue 1, Red 3, Red 40, Gelatin, Glyceryl Stearates, Iron Oxide, Polyethylene Glycol, Povidone, Sodium Lauryl Sulfate, Starch, Sucrose, White Wax, and trace amounts of other inactive ingredients.

DOSAGE
Adults: 1 or 2 capsules daily or as directed by a physician. Children: As directed by a physician.
TAMPER-RESISTANT PACKAGE FEATURES:
● The carton is protected by a clear overwrap printed with "safety sealed"; do not use if overwrap is missing or broken.
● Each capsule is encased in a plastic cell with a foil back; do not use if cell or foil is broken.
● Each FEOSOL capsule is protected by a red Perma-Seal™ band which bonds the two capsule halves together; do not use if capsule is broken or band is missing or broken.
● A package insert is provided for information on tamper-resistant packaging.

WARNING
Do not exceed recommended dosage. The treatment of any anemic condition should be under the advice and supervision of a physician. Iron-containing medication may occasionally cause constipation or diarrhea. Since oral iron products interfere with absorption of oral tetracycline antibiotics, these products should not be taken within two hours of each other. Keep this and all drugs out of the reach of children. In case of accidental overdose, seek professional assistance or contact a poison control center immediately. As with any drug, if you are pregnant or nursing a baby, seek the advice of a health professional before using this product.
Store at controlled room temperature (59°–86°F.).

HOW SUPPLIED
Packages of 30 and 60 capsules, bottle of 500's; in Single Unit Packages of 100 capsules (intended for institutional use only).
Also available in Tablets and Elixir.

FEOSOL® ELIXIR
Hematinic

DESCRIPTION
'Feosol' Elixir, an unusually palatable iron elixir, provides the body with ferrous sulfate—iron in its most efficient form. The standard elixir for simple iron deficiency and iron-deficiency anemia when the need for such therapy has been determined by a physician. Each 5 ml. (1 teaspoonful) contains ferrous sulfate, USP, 220 mg. (44 mg. of elemental iron); alcohol, 5%.
Inactive Ingredients (listed for individuals with specific allergies): Citric Acid, FD&C Yellow 6 (Sunset Yellow) as a color additive, Flavors, Glucose, Saccharin Sodium, Sucrose, Purified Water.

USUAL DOSAGE
Adults—1 to 2 teaspoonsful three times daily preferably between meals. Children—½ to 1 teaspoonful three times

Continued on next page

SmithKline Consumer—Cont.

daily preferably between meals. Infants—as directed by physician. Mix with water or fruit juice to avoid temporary staining of teeth; do not mix with milk or wine-based vehicles.

TAMPER-RESISTANT PACKAGE FEATURE: IMPRINTED SEAL AROUND BOTTLE CAP; DO NOT USE IF BROKEN.

WARNING

The treatment of any anemic condition should be under the advice and supervision of a physician. Since oral iron products interfere with absorption of oral tetracycline antibiotics, these products should not be taken within two hours of each other. Occasional gastrointestinal discomfort (such as nausea) may be minimized by taking with meals and by beginning with one teaspoonful the first day, two the second, etc. until the recommended dosage is reached. Iron-containing medication may occasionally cause constipation or diarrhea, and liquids may cause temporary staining of the teeth (this is less likely when diluted). Keep this and all drugs out of reach of children. In case of accidental overdose, seek professional assistance or contact a poison control center immediately. As with any drug, if you are pregnant or nursing a baby, seek the advice of a health professional before using this product.
Store at controlled room temperature (59°–86°F.).

HOW SUPPLIED

A clear orange liquid in 16 fl. oz. bottles.

ALSO AVAILABLE

'Feosol' Tablets, 'Feosol' Capsules.

FEOSOL® TABLETS
Hematinic

PRODUCT INFORMATION

'Feosol' Tablets provide the body with ferrous sulfate, iron in its most efficient form, for iron deficiency and iron-deficiency anemia when the need for such therapy has been determined by a physician. The distinctive triangular-shaped tablet has a coating to prevent oxidation and improve palatability.

FORMULA

Active Ingredient: Each tablet contains 200 mg. of dried ferrous sulfate USP (65 mg. of elemental iron), equivalent to 325 mg. (5 grains) of ferrous sulfate USP. Inactive Ingredients (listed for individuals with specific allergies): Calcium Sulfate, D&C Yellow 10, FD&C Blue 2, Glucose, Hydroxypropyl Methylcellulose, Mineral Oil, Polyethylene Glycol, Sodium Lauryl Sulfate, Starch, Stearic Acid, Talc, Titanium Dioxide and trace amounts of other inactive ingredients.

USUAL DOSAGE

Adults—one tablet 3 to 4 times daily, after meals and upon retiring. Children 6 to 12 years—one tablet three times a day after meals. Children under 6 years and infants—use 'Feosol' Elixir.

TAMPER-RESISTANT PACKAGE FEATURES:

○ The carton has been sealed at the factory with a clear overwrap printed with "safety sealed."
○ Bottle has imprinted "SKCP" seal under cap.
○ FEOSOL Tablets are triangular shaped (see product illustration printed on carton).

CAUTION: DO NOT USE THIS PRODUCT IF ANY OF THESE TAMPER-RESISTANT FEATURES ARE MISSING OR BROKEN. IF YOU HAVE ANY QUESTIONS, PLEASE CALL 1-800-543-3434 TOLL FREE.

WARNINGS

Do not exceed recommended dosage. The treatment of any anemic condition should be under the advice and supervision of a physician. Since oral iron products interfere with absorption of oral tetracycline antibiotics, these products should not be taken within two hours of each other. Occasional gastrointestinal discomfort (such as nausea) may be minimized by taking with meals and by beginning with one tablet the first day, two the second, etc. until the recommended dosage is reached. Iron-containing medication may occasionally cause constipation or diarrhea. Keep this and all drugs out of reach of children. In case of accidental overdose, seek professional assistance or contact a poison control center immediately. As with any drug, if you are pregnant or nursing a baby, seek the advice of a health professional before using this product.
Store at controlled room temperature (59°–86°F.).

HOW SUPPLIED

Bottles of 100 or 1000 tablets; in Single Unit Packages of 100 tablets (intended for institutional use only).
Also available in Capsules and Elixir.

TELDRIN®
Chlorpheniramine maleate
Timed-Release Allergy Capsules

Antihistamine

FORMULA

Active Ingredient: Each capsule contains Chlorpheniramine Maleate, 12 mg. Inactive Ingredients (listed for individuals with specific allergies): Benzyl Alcohol, Cetylpyridinium Chloride, D&C Red 33, Ethylcellulose, FD&C Green 3, Red 3, Red 40, Yellow 6 (Sunset Yellow) as a color additive, Gelatin, Hydrogenated Castor Oil, Silicon Dioxide, Sodium Lauryl Sulfate, Starch, Sucrose, and trace amounts of other inactive ingredients.

DESCRIPTION

Each 'Teldrin' Timed-Release capsule contains chlorpheniramine maleate, Maximum Strength 12 mg., so formulated that a portion of the antihistamine dose is released initially, and the remaining medication is released gradually over a prolonged period.

INDICATIONS FOR USE

Hay fever and allergies are caused by grass and tree pollen, dust and pollution. 'Teldrin' provides up to 12 hours of relief from hay fever/upper respiratory allergy symptoms; sneezing; runny nose; itchy, watery eyes.

DOSAGE

Adults and children over 12 years of age: Just one capsule in the morning, and one in the evening. Do not give to children under 12 without the advice and consent of a physician. Not to exceed 24 mg. (2 capsules of 12 mg.) in 24 hours.

TAMPER-RESISTANT PACKAGE FEATURES

⊙ The carton is protected by a clear overwrap printed with "safety sealed"; do not use if overwrap is missing or broken.
⊙ Each capsule is encased in a plastic cell with a foil back; do not use if the cell or foil is broken.
⊙ Each 'TELDRIN' capsule is protected by a green PERMA-SEAL™ band which bonds the two capsule halves together; do not use if capsule or band is broken.
⊙ A package insert is provided for information on tamper-resistant packaging.

WARNING

Do not take this product if you have asthma, glaucoma, or difficulty in urination due to enlargement of the prostate gland, except under the advice and supervision of a physician. Do not drive or operate heavy machinery as this preparation may cause drowsiness. Avoid alcoholic beverages while taking this product. May cause excitability, especially in children. Keep this and all drugs out of the reach of children. In case of accidental overdose, seek professional assistance or contact a poison control center immediately. As with any drug, if you are pregnant or nursing a baby, seek the advice of a health professional before using this product. Store at controlled room temperature (59°–86°F.).

HOW SUPPLIED

Packages of 12, 24 and 48 capsules.

Smith Kline & French
Laboratories
Division of SmithKline Beckman Corporation
1500 SPRING GARDEN ST.
P.O. BOX 7929
PHILADELPHIA, PA 19101

SK&F Lab Co.
Cidra, P.R. 00639
Subsidiary of SmithKline Beckman Corporation

SK&F PRODUCT CODE INDEX

Code	Product, Form and Strength
C44	'Compazine' *Spansule* capsules 10 mg
C46	'Compazine' *Spansule* capsules 15 mg
C47	'Compazine' *Spansule* capsules 30 mg
C60	'Compazine' Suppositories 2 ½ mg
C61	'Compazine' Suppositories 5 mg
C62	'Compazine' Suppositories 25 mg
C66	'Compazine' Tablets 5 mg
C67	'Compazine' Tablets 10 mg
C69	'Compazine' Tablets 25 mg
D14	'Cytomel' Tablets 5 mcg
D16	'Cytomel' Tablets 25 mcg
D17	'Cytomel' Tablets 50 mcg
D62	'Darbid' Tablets 5 mg
E12	'Dexedrine' *Spansule* capsules 5 mg
E13	'Dexedrine' *Spansule* capsules 10 mg
E14	'Dexedrine' *Spansule* capsules 15 mg
E19	'Dexedrine' Tablets 5 mg
E33	'Dibenzyline' Capsules 10 mg
J09	'Eskalith' Tablets 300 mg
J10	'Eskalith' Controlled Release Tablets 450 mg
S03	*'Stelazine' Tablets 1 mg
S04	*'Stelazine' Tablets 2 mg
S06	*'Stelazine' Tablets 5 mg
S07	*'Stelazine' Tablets 10 mg
T63	'Thorazine' *Spansule* capsules 30 mg
T64	'Thorazine' *Spansule* capsules 75 mg
T66	'Thorazine' *Spansule* capsules 150 mg
T67	'Thorazine' *Spansule* capsules 200 mg
T69	'Thorazine' *Spansule* capsules 300 mg
T70	'Thorazine' Suppositories 25 mg
T71	'Thorazine' Suppositories 100 mg
T73	'Thorazine' Tablets 10 mg
T74	'Thorazine' Tablets 25 mg
T76	'Thorazine' Tablets 50 mg
T77	'Thorazine' Tablets 100 mg
T79	'Thorazine' Tablets 200 mg

* A product of SK&F Lab Co., Cidra, P.R. 00639, Subsidiary of SmithKline Beckman Corporation, Philadelphia, Pa.

ANCEF®   ℞
[an-sef']
(brand of sterile cefazolin sodium and cefazolin sodium injection)

PRODUCT OVERVIEW

KEY FACTS

'Ancef' is a semi-synthetic cephalosporin for parenteral administration. 'Ancef' has proven to be active against a number of gram-positive and gram-negative organisms *in vitro* and in clinical infections.

MAJOR USES

'Ancef' is indicated in the treatment of serious infections due to susceptible organisms listed below in the full prescribing information. These include infections of the urinary tract, respiratory tract, skin and skin structure, biliary tract, bone and joint and genital infections, as well as septicemia and endocarditis. 'Ancef' is also indicated for perioperative prophylaxis in patients undergoing surgical procedures classified as contaminated or potentially contaminated.

SAFETY INFORMATION

'Ancef' is contraindicated in patients with known allergy to cephalosporins. Careful inquiry should be made concerning previous hypersensitivity to cephalosporins and penicillin. 'Ancef' should be administered cautiously to penicillin-sensitive patients. Serious acute hypersensitivity reactions may require epinephrine and other emergency measures. Because pseudomembranous colitis has been reported with the use of cephalosporins, it is important to consider its diagnosis in patients who develop diarrhea in association with antibiotic use.

PRESCRIBING INFORMATION

ANCEF®   ℞
[an-sef']
(brand of sterile cefazolin sodium and cefazolin sodium injection)

DESCRIPTION

Ancef (sterile cefazolin sodium, SK&F) is a semi-synthetic cephalosporin for parenteral administration. It is the sodium salt of 3- {[(5-methyl-1, 3, 4-thiadiazol-2-yl) thio]-methyl}-8-oxo-7- [2-(1H-tetrazol -1- yl) acetamido] -5- thia-1-azabicyclo [4.2.0] oct-2-ene-2-carboxylic acid.
The sodium content is 46 mg. per gram of cefazolin.
'Ancef' in lyophilized form is supplied in vials equivalent to 250 mg., 500 mg. or 1 gram of cefazolin, in "Piggyback" Vials for intravenous admixture equivalent to 500 mg. or 1 gram of cefazolin; and in Pharmacy Bulk Vials equivalent to 5 grams or 10 grams of cefazolin.
'Ancef' is also supplied as a frozen, sterile, nonpyrogenic solution of cefazolin sodium in an iso-osmotic diluent in plastic containers. After thawing, the solution is intended for intravenous use.
The plastic container is fabricated from specially formulated polyvinyl chloride. Solutions in contact with the plastic container can leach out certain of its chemical components in very small amounts within the expiration period, e.g., di 2-ethylhexyl phthalate (DEHP), up to 5 parts per million. However, the safety of the plastic has been confirmed in tests in animals according to the USP biological tests for plastic containers as well as by tissue culture toxicity studies.

CLINICAL PHARMACOLOGY

Human Pharmacology: After intramuscular administration of 'Ancef' to normal volunteers, the mean serum concentrations were 37 mcg./ml. at one hour and 3 mcg./ml. at eight hours following a 500 mg. dose, and 64 mcg./ml. at one hour and 7 mcg./ml. at eight hours following a 1 gram dose. Studies have shown that following intravenous administration of 'Ancef' to normal volunteers, mean serum concentrations peaked at approximately 185 mcg./ml. and were approximately 4 mcg./ml. at eight hours for a 1 gram dose.

The serum half-life for 'Ancef' is approximately 1.8 hours following I.V. administration and approximately 2.0 hours following I.M. administration.

In a study (using normal volunteers) of constant intravenous infusion with dosages of 3.5 mg./kg. for one hour (approximately 250 mg.) and 1.5 mg./kg. the next two hours (approximately 100 mg.), 'Ancef' produced a steady serum level at the third hour of approximately 28 μg./ml.

Studies in patients hospitalized with infections indicate that Ancef (sterile cefazolin sodium, SK&F) produces mean peak serum levels approximately equivalent to those seen in normal volunteers.

Bile levels in patients without obstructive biliary disease can reach or exceed serum levels by up to five times; however, in patients with obstructive biliary disease, bile levels of 'Ancef' are considerably lower than serum levels (< 1.0 μg./ml.).

In synovial fluid, the 'Ancef' level becomes comparable to that reached in serum at about four hours after drug administration.

Studies of cord blood show prompt transfer of 'Ancef' across the placenta. 'Ancef' is present in very low concentrations in the milk of nursing mothers.

'Ancef' is excreted unchanged in the urine. In the first six hours approximately 60% of the drug is excreted in the urine and this increases to 70%–80% within 24 hours. 'Ancef' achieves peak urine concentrations of approximately 2400 μg./ml. and 4000 μg./ml. respectively following 500 mg. and 1 gram intramuscular doses.

In patients undergoing peritoneal dialysis (2 l./hr.), 'Ancef' produced mean serum levels of approximately 10 and 30 μg./ml. after 24 hours' instillation of a dialyzing solution containing 50 mg./l. and 150 mg./l., respectively. Mean peak levels were 29 μg./ml. (range 13–44 μg./ml.) with 50 mg./l. (three patients), and 72 μg./ml. (range 26–142 μg./ml.) with 150 mg./l. (six patients). Intraperitoneal administration of 'Ancef' is usually well tolerated.

Controlled studies on adult normal volunteers, receiving 1 gram 4 times a day for 10 days, monitoring CBC, SGOT, SGPT, bilirubin, alkaline phosphatase, BUN, creatinine, and urinalysis, indicated no clinically significant changes attributed to 'Ancef'.

Microbiology: *In vitro* tests demonstrate that the bactericidal action of cephalosporins results from inhibition of cell wall synthesis. Ancef (sterile cefazolin sodium, SK&F) is active against the following organisms *in vitro* and in clinical infections:

Staphylococcus aureus (including penicillinase-producing strains)

Staphylococcus epidermidis

Methicillin-resistant staphylococci are uniformly resistant to cefazolin

Group A beta-hemolytic streptococci and other strains of streptococci (many strains of enterococci are resistant)

Streptococcus pneumoniae (formerly *D. pneumoniae*)

Escherichia coli

Proteus mirabilis

Klebsiella species

Enterobacter aerogenes

Hemophilus influenzae

Most strains of indole positive Proteus (*Proteus vulgaris*), *Enterobacter cloacae, Morganella morganii,* and *Providencia rettgeri* are resistant. *Serratia, Pseudomonas, Mima, Herellea* species are almost uniformly resistant to cefazolin.

Disk Susceptibility Tests

Disk diffusion technique—Quantitative methods that require measurement of zone diameters give the most precise estimates of antibiotic susceptibility. One such procedure[1] has been recommended for use with disks to test susceptibility to cefazolin.

Reports from a laboratory using the standardized single-disk susceptibility test[1] with a 30 mcg. cefazolin disk should be interpreted according to the following criteria:

Susceptible organisms produce zones of 18 mm. or greater, indicating that the tested organism is likely to respond to therapy.

Organisms of intermediate susceptibility produce zones 15 to 17 mm., indicating that the tested organism would be susceptible if high dosage is used or if the infection is confined to tissues and fluids (e.g., urine), in which high antibiotic levels are attained.

Resistant organisms produce zones of 14 mm. or less, indicating that other therapy should be selected.

For gram-positive isolates, a zone of 18 mm. is indicative of a cefazolin-susceptible organism when tested with either the cephalosporin-class disk (30 mcg. cephalothin) or the cefazolin disk (30 mcg. cefazolin).

Gram-negative organisms should be tested with the cefazolin disk (using the above criteria), since cefazolin has been shown by *in vitro* tests to have activity against certain strains of *Enterobacteriaceae* found resistant when tested with the cephalothin disk. Gram-negative organisms having zones of less than 18 mm. around the cephalothin disk may be susceptible to cefazolin.

Standardized procedures require use of control organisms. The 30 mcg. cefazolin disk should give zone diameter between 23 and 29 mm. for *E. coli* ATCC 25922 and between 29 and 35 mm. for *S. aureus* ATCC 25923.

The cefazolin disk should not be used for testing susceptibility to other cephalosporins.

Dilution techniques—A bacterial isolate may be considered susceptible if the minimal inhibitory concentration (MIC) for cefazolin is not more than 16 mcg. per ml. Organisms are considered resistant if the MIC is equal to or greater than 64 mcg. per ml.

The range of MIC's for the control strains are as follows:

S. aureus ATCC 25923, 0.25-1.0 mcg./ml.

E. coli ATCC 25922, 1.0-4.0 mcg./ml.

INDICATIONS AND USAGE

Ancef (sterile cefazolin sodium, SK&F) is indicated in the treatment of the following serious infections due to susceptible organisms:

RESPIRATORY TRACT INFECTIONS due to *Streptococcus pneumoniae* (formerly *D. pneumoniae*), *Klebsiella* species, *Hemophilus influenzae, Staphylococcus aureus* (penicillin-sensitive and penicillin-resistant), and group A beta-hemolytic streptococci.

Injectable benzathine penicillin is considered to be the drug of choice in treatment and prevention of streptococcal infections, including the prophylaxis of rheumatic fever.

'Ancef' is effective in the eradication of streptococci from the nasopharynx; however, data establishing the efficacy of 'Ancef' in the subsequent prevention of rheumatic fever are not available at present.

URINARY TRACT INFECTIONS due to *Escherichia coli, Proteus mirabilis, Klebsiella* species, and some strains of enterobacter and enterococci.

SKIN AND SKIN STRUCTURE INFECTIONS due to *Staphylococcus aureus* (penicillin-sensitive and penicillin-resistant), group A beta-hemolytic streptococci and other strains of streptococci.

BILIARY TRACT INFECTIONS due to *Escherichia coli*, various strains of streptococci, *Proteus mirabilis, Klebsiella* species and *Staphylococcus aureus*.

BONE AND JOINT INFECTIONS due to *Staphylococcus aureus*.

GENITAL INFECTIONS (i.e., prostatitis, epididymitis) due to *Escherichia coli, Proteus mirabilis, Klebsiella* species, and some strains of enterococcus.

SEPTICEMIA due to *Streptococcus pneumoniae* (formerly *D. pneumoniae*), *Staphylococcus aureus* (penicillin-sensitive and penicillin-resistant), *Proteus mirabilis, Escherichia coli,* and *Klebsiella* species.

ENDOCARDITIS due to *Staphylococcus aureus* (penicillin-sensitive and penicillin-resistant) and group A beta-hemolytic streptococci.

Appropriate culture and susceptibility studies should be performed to determine susceptibility of the causative organism to 'Ancef'.

PERIOPERATIVE PROPHYLAXIS: The prophylactic administration of 'Ancef' preoperatively, intraoperatively, and postoperatively may reduce the incidence of certain postoperative infections in patients undergoing surgical procedures which are classified as contaminated or potentially contaminated (e.g., vaginal hysterectomy, and cholecystectomy in high-risk patients such as those over 70 years of age, with acute cholecystitis, obstructive jaundice, or common duct bile stones).

The perioperative use of 'Ancef' may also be effective in surgical patients in whom infection at the operative site would present a serious risk (e.g., during open-heart surgery and prosthetic arthroplasty).

The prophylactic administration of 'Ancef' should usually be discontinued within a 24-hour period after the surgical procedure. In surgery where the occurrence of infection may be particularly devastating (e.g., open-heart surgery and prosthetic arthroplasty), the prophylactic administration of 'Ancef' may be continued for 3 to 5 days following the completion of surgery.

If there are signs of infection, specimens for cultures should be obtained for the identification of the causative organism so that appropriate therapy may be instituted. (See DOSAGE AND ADMINISTRATION.)

CONTRAINDICATIONS

ANCEF (STERILE CEFAZOLIN SODIUM, SK&F) IS CONTRAINDICATED IN PATIENTS WITH KNOWN ALLERGY TO THE CEPHALOSPORIN GROUP OF ANTIBIOTICS.

WARNINGS

BEFORE CEFAZOLIN THERAPY IS INSTITUTED, CAREFUL INQUIRY SHOULD BE MADE CONCERNING PREVIOUS HYPERSENSITIVITY REACTIONS TO CEPHALOSPORINS AND PENICILLIN. CEPHALOSPORIN C DERIVATIVES SHOULD BE GIVEN CAUTIOUSLY IN PENICILLIN-SENSITIVE PATIENTS.

SERIOUS ACUTE HYPERSENSITIVITY REACTIONS MAY REQUIRE EPINEPHRINE AND OTHER EMERGENCY MEASURES.

There is some clinical and laboratory evidence of partial cross-allergenicity of the penicillins and the cephalosporins. Patients have been reported to have had severe reactions (including anaphylaxis) to both drugs.

Any patient who has demonstrated some form of allergy, particularly to drugs, should receive antibiotics cautiously. No exception should be made with regard to 'Ancef'.

Pseudomembranous colitis has been reported with the use of cephalosporins (and other broad-spectrum antibiotics); therefore, it is important to consider its diagnosis in patients who develop diarrhea in association with antibiotic use.

Treatment with broad-spectrum antibiotics alters normal flora of the colon and may permit overgrowth of clostridia. Studies indicate a toxin produced by *Clostridium difficile* is one primary cause of antibiotic-associated colitis. Cholestyramine and colestipol resins have been shown to bind the toxin *in vitro*.

Mild cases of colitis may respond to drug discontinuance alone.

Moderate to severe cases should be managed with fluid, electrolyte and protein supplementation as indicated.

When the colitis is not relieved by drug discontinuance or when it is severe, oral vancomycin is the treatment of choice for antibiotic-associated pseudomembranous colitis produced by *C. difficile*. Other causes of colitis should also be considered.

PRECAUTIONS

General—Prolonged use of Ancef (sterile cefazolin sodium, SK&F) may result in the overgrowth of nonsusceptible organisms. Careful clinical observation of the patient is essential.

When 'Ancef' is administered to patients with low urinary output because of impaired renal function, lower daily dosage is required (see DOSAGE AND ADMINISTRATION).

As with other beta-lactam antibiotics, seizures may occur if inappropriately high doses are administered to patients with impaired renal function (see DOSAGE AND ADMINISTRATION).

'Ancef', as with all cephalosporins, should be prescribed with caution in individuals with a history of gastrointestinal disease, particularly colitis.

Drug Interactions—Probenecid may decrease renal tubular secretion of cephalosporins when used concurrently, resulting in increased and more prolonged cephalosporin blood levels.

Drug/Laboratory Test Interactions—A false positive reaction for glucose in the urine may occur with Benedict's solution, Fehling's solution, or with Clinitest® tablets, but not with enzyme-based tests such as Clinistix® and Tes-Tape®. Positive direct and indirect antiglobulin (Coombs) tests have occurred; these may also occur in neonates whose mothers received cephalosporins before delivery.

Carcinogenesis/Mutagenesis — Mutagenicity studies and long-term studies in animals to determine the carcinogenic potential of Ancef (sterile cefazolin sodium, SK&F) have not been performed.

Pregnancy — Teratogenic Effects — Pregnancy Category B. Reproduction studies have been performed in rats, mice and rabbits at doses up to 25 times the human dose and have revealed no evidence of impaired fertility or harm to the fetus due to 'Ancef'. There are, however, no adequate and well-controlled studies in pregnant women. Because animal reproduction studies are not always predictive of human response, this drug should be used during pregnancy only if clearly needed.

Labor and Delivery—When cefazolin has been administered prior to caesarean section, drug levels in cord blood have been approximately one quarter to one third of maternal drug levels. The drug appears to have no adverse effect on the fetus.

Nursing Mothers—'Ancef' is present in very low concentrations in the milk of nursing mothers. Caution should be exercised when 'Ancef' is administered to a nursing woman.

Pediatric Use—Safety and effectiveness for use in prematures and infants under one month of age have not been established. See DOSAGE AND ADMINISTRATION for recommended dosage in children over one month.

ADVERSE REACTIONS

The following reactions have been reported:

Gastrointestinal: Diarrhea, oral candidiasis (oral thrush), vomiting, nausea, stomach cramps, anorexia. Symptoms of pseudomembranous colitis can appear during antibiotic treatment. Nausea and vomiting have been reported rarely.

Allergic: Anaphylaxis, eosinophilia, itching, drug fever, skin rash.

Continued on next page

Smith Kline &French—Cont.

Hematologic: Neutropenia, leukopenia, thrombocythemia.

Hepatic and Renal: Transient rise in SGOT, SGPT, BUN and alkaline phosphatase levels has been observed without clinical evidence of renal or hepatic impairment.

Local Reactions: Rare instances of phlebitis have been reported at site of injection. Pain at the site of injection after intramuscular administration has occurred infrequently. Some induration has occurred.

Other Reactions: Genital and anal pruritus (including vulvar pruritus, genital moniliasis, and vaginitis).

DOSAGE AND ADMINISTRATION
Usual Adult Dosage

Type of Infection	Dose	Frequency
Moderate to severe infections	500 mg. to 1 gram	every 6 to 8 hrs.
Mild infections caused by susceptible gram + cocci	250 mg. to 500 mg.	every 8 hours
Acute, uncomplicated urinary tract infections	1 gram	every 12 hours
Pneumococcal pneumonia	500 mg.	every 12 hours
Severe, life-threatening infections (e.g., endocarditis, septicemia)*	1 gram to 1.5 grams	every 6 hours

* In rare instances, doses of up to 12 grams of 'Ancef' per day have been used.

Perioperative Prophylactic Use

To prevent postoperative infection in contaminated or potentially contaminated surgery, recommended doses are:

a. 1 gram I.V. or I.M. administered ½ hour to 1 hour prior to the start of surgery.

b. For lengthy operative procedures (e.g., 2 hours or more), 500 mg. to 1 gram I.V. or I.M. during surgery (administration modified depending on the duration of the operative procedure).

c. 500 mg. to 1 gram I.V. or I.M. every 6 to 8 hours for 24 hours postoperatively.

It is important that (1) the preoperative dose be given just (½ to 1 hour) prior to the start of surgery so that adequate antibiotic levels are present in the serum and tissues at the time of initial surgical incision; and (2) 'Ancef' be administered, if necessary, at appropriate intervals during surgery to provide sufficient levels of the antibiotic at the anticipated moments of greatest exposure to infective organisms.

In surgery where the occurrence of infection may be particularly devastating (e.g., open-heart surgery and prosthetic arthroplasty), the prophylactic administration of Ancef (sterile cefazolin sodium, SK&F) may be continued for 3 to 5 days following the completion of surgery.

Dosage Adjustment for Patients with Reduced Renal Function

'Ancef' may be used in patients with reduced renal function with the following dosage adjustments: Patients with a creatinine clearance of 55 ml./min. or greater or a serum creatinine of 1.5 mg. % or less can be given full doses. Patients with creatinine clearance rates of 35 to 54 ml./min. or serum creatinine of 1.6 to 3.0 mg. % can also be given full doses but dosage should be restricted to at least 8 hour intervals. Patients with creatinine clearance rates of 11 to 34 ml./min. or serum creatinine of 3.1 to 4.5 mg. % should be given ½ the usual dose every 12 hours. Patients with creatinine clearance rates of 10 ml./min. or less or serum creatinine of 4.6 mg. % or greater should be given ½ the usual dose every 18 to 24 hours. All reduced dosage recommendations apply after an initial loading dose appropriate to the severity of the infection. Patients undergoing peritoneal dialysis: See Human Pharmacology.

Pediatric Dosage

In children, a total daily dosage of 25 to 50 mg. per kg. (approximately 10 to 20 mg. per pound) of body weight, divided into three or four equal doses, is effective for most mild to moderately severe infections. Total daily dosage may be increased to 100 mg. per kg. (45 mg. per pound) of body weight for severe infections. Since safety for use in premature infants and in infants under one month has not been established, the use of Ancef (sterile cefazolin sodium, SK&F) in these patients is not recommended.

Pediatric Dosage Guide

Weight		25 mg./kg./Day Divided into 3 Doses		25 mg./kg./Day Divided into 4 Doses	
Lbs.	Kg.	Approximate Single Dose mg./q8h	Vol. (ml.) needed with dilution of 125 mg./ml.	Approximate Single Dose mg./q6h	Vol. (ml.) needed with dilution of 125 mg./ml.
10	4.5	40 mg.	0.35 ml.	30 mg.	0.25 ml.
20	9.0	75 mg.	0.60 ml.	55 mg.	0.45 ml.
30	13.6	115 mg.	0.90 ml.	85 mg.	0.70 ml.
40	18.1	150 mg.	1.20 ml.	115 mg.	0.90 ml.
50	22.7	190 mg.	1.50 ml.	140 mg.	1.10 ml.

Weight		50 mg./kg./Day Divided into 3 Doses		50 mg./kg./Day Divided into 4 Doses	
Lbs.	Kg.	Approximate Single Dose mg./q8h	Vol. (ml.) needed with dilution of 225 mg./ml.	Approximate Single Dose mg./q6h	Vol. (ml.) needed with dilution of 225 mg./ml.
10	4.5	75 mg.	0.35 ml.	55 mg.	0.25 ml.
20	9.0	150 mg.	0.70 ml.	110 mg.	0.50 ml.
30	13.6	225 mg.	1.00 ml.	170 mg.	0.75 ml.
40	18.1	300 mg.	1.35 ml.	225 mg.	1.00 ml.
50	22.7	375 mg.	1.70 ml.	285 mg.	1.25 ml.

In children with mild to moderate renal impairment (creatinine clearance of 70 to 40 ml./min.), 60 percent of the normal daily dose given in equally divided doses every 12 hours should be sufficient. In patients with moderate impairment (creatinine clearance of 40 to 20 ml./min.), 25 percent of the normal daily dose given in equally divided doses every 12 hours should be adequate. Children with severe renal impairment (creatinine clearance of 20 to 5 ml./min.) may be given 10 percent of the normal daily dose every 24 hours. All dosage recommendations apply after an initial loading dose.

RECONSTITUTION

Preparation of Parenteral Solution

Parenteral drug products should be SHAKEN WELL when reconstituted, and inspected visually for particulate matter prior to administration. If particulate matter is evident in reconstituted fluids, the drug solutions should be discarded. When reconstituted or diluted according to the instructions below, Ancef (sterile cefazolin sodium, SK&F) is stable for 24 hours at room temperature or for 96 hours if stored under refrigeration. Reconstituted solutions may range in color from pale yellow to yellow without a change in potency.

Single-Dose Vials

For I.M. injection, I.V. direct (bolus) injection, or I.V. infusion, reconstitute with Sterile Water for Injection according to the following table. SHAKE WELL.

Vial Size	Amount of Diluent	Approximate Concentration	Approximate Available Volume
250 mg.	2.0 ml.	125 mg./ml.	2.0 ml.
500 mg.	2.0 ml.	225 mg./ml.	2.2 ml.
1 gram	2.5 ml.	330 mg./ml.	3.0 ml.

Pharmacy Bulk Vials

Add Sterile Water for Injection, Bacteriostatic Water for Injection, or Sodium Chloride Injection according to the table below. SHAKE WELL.

Vial Size	Amount of Diluent	Approximate Concentration	Approximate Available Volume
5 grams	23 ml.	1 gram/5 ml.	26 ml.
	48 ml.	1 gram/10 ml.	51 ml.
10 grams	45 ml.	1 gram/5 ml.	51 ml.
	96 ml.	1 gram/10 ml.	102 ml.

"Piggyback" Vials

Reconstitute with 50 to 100 ml. of Sodium Chloride Injection or other I.V. solution listed under ADMINISTRATION. When adding diluent to vial, allow air to escape by using a small vent needle or by pumping the syringe. SHAKE WELL. Administer with primary I.V. fluids, as a single dose.

ADMINISTRATION

Intramuscular Administration—Reconstitute vials with Sterile Water for Injection according to the dilution table above. Shake well until dissolved. 'Ancef' should be injected into a large muscle mass. Pain on injection is infrequent with 'Ancef'.

Intravenous Administration—Direct (bolus) injection: Following reconstitution according to the above table, further dilute vials with approximately 5 ml. Sterile Water for Injection. Inject the solution slowly over 3 to 5 minutes, directly or through tubing for patients receiving parenteral fluids (see list below).

Intermittent or continuous infusion: Dilute reconstituted 'Ancef' in 50 to 100 ml. of one of the following solutions:

  Sodium Chloride Injection, USP
  5% or 10% Dextrose Injection, USP
  5% Dextrose in Lactated Ringer's Injection, USP
  5% Dextrose and 0.9% Sodium Chloride Injection, USP
  5% Dextrose and 0.45% Sodium Chloride Injection, USP
  5% Dextrose and 0.2% Sodium Chloride Injection, USP
  Lactated Ringer's Injection, USP
  Invert Sugar 5% or 10% in Sterile Water for Injection
  Ringer's Injection, USP
  5% Sodium Bicarbonate Injection, USP

DIRECTIONS FOR USE OF ANCEF (CEFAZOLIN SODIUM INJECTION, SK&F) PLASTIC CONTAINERS

'Ancef' supplied as a frozen, sterile, nonpyrogenic solution in plastic containers is to be administered either as a continuous or intermittent infusion.

Thaw container at room temperature. After thawing, check for minute leaks by squeezing bag firmly. If leaks are found, discard solution as sterility may be impaired. Additives should not be introduced into this solution. Do not use if the solution is cloudy or precipitated or if the seal is not intact. After thawing, the solution is stable for 48 hours at room temperature and 10 days if stored under refrigeration (5℃). DO NOT REFREEZE.

Use sterile equipment. It is recommended that the intravenous administration apparatus be replaced at least once every 48 hours.

CAUTION: Do not use plastic containers in series connections. Such use could result in air embolism due to residual air being drawn from the primary container before administration of the fluid from the secondary container is complete.

Preparation for administration:

1. Suspend container from eyelet support.
2. Remove plastic protector from outlet port at bottom of container.
3. Attach administration set. Refer to complete directions accompanying set.

HOW SUPPLIED

Ancef (sterile cefazolin sodium, SK&F)—supplied in vials equivalent to 250 mg., 500 mg. or 1 gram of cefazolin; in "Piggyback" Vials for intravenous admixture equivalent to 500 mg. or 1 gram of cefazolin; and in Pharmacy Bulk Vials equivalent to 5 grams or 10 grams of cefazolin.

Ancef (cefazolin sodium injection, SK&F) as a frozen, sterile, nonpyrogenic solution in plastic containers—supplied in 50 ml. single-dose containers equivalent to 500 mg. or 1 gram of cefazolin in 5% Dextrose (D5W). Do not store above −20℃. 'Ancef' supplied as a frozen, sterile, nonpyrogenic solution in plastic containers is manufactured for Smith Kline &French Laboratories by Travenol Laboratories, Inc., Deerfield, IL 60015.

Military—Vial, 5 gram, 100 ml., 10's, 6505-01-058-2046; 10 gram, 100 ml., 6505-01-184-1574.

1 Bauer, A.W.; Kirby, W.M.M.; Sherris, J.C., and Turck, M.: Antibiotic Testing by a Standardized Single Disc Method, Am. J. Clin. Path. 45:493, 1966. Standardized Disc Susceptibility Test, Federal Register 39:19182-19184, 1974.

                       AF:L40

Shown in Product Identification Section, page 430

ANSPOR®   ℞

[*an-spore*']
(brand of cephradine)
Capsules, 250 mg. and 500 mg.
and
for Oral Suspension, 125 mg./5 ml. and
250 mg./5 ml.

('Anspor' is manufactured for Smith Kline &French Laboratories, Division of SmithKline Beckman Corporation, Philadelphia, Pa., by Squibb Manufacturing, Inc., Humacao, P.R., Subsidiary of E.R. Squibb & Sons, Inc.)

DESCRIPTION

Cephradine is a semisynthetic cephalosporin antibiotic chemically designated as (6R, 7R)-7-[(R)-2-amino-2-(1, 4-cyclohexadien-1-yl)acetamido]-3-methyl-8-oxo-5-thia-1-azabicyclo[4.2.0]oct-2-ene-2-carboxylic acid.

Capsules—Each Anspor (cephradine, SK&F) capsule contains cephradine as follows: 250 mg.—opaque orange cap and opaque white body imprinted with the product name ANSPOR, SKF and 250; 500 mg.—opaque orange cap and body imprinted with the product name ANSPOR, SKF and 500. Inactive ingredients consist of FD&C Red No. 3, FD&C Yellow No. 6, gelatin, lactose, magnesium stearate, talc, titanium dioxide and trace amounts of other inactive ingredients.

For Oral Suspension—When reconstituted as directed, the fruit-flavored suspension contains cephradine as follows: 125 mg./5 ml. (yellow-orange) or 250 mg./5 ml. (red). Inactive ingredients consist of citric acid, FD&C Red No. 40 (250 mg./5 ml. strength), FD&C Yellow No. 6 (125 mg./5 ml. strength), flavors, guar gum, methylcellulose, sodium citrate and sucrose.

CLINICAL PHARMACOLOGY

Human Pharmacology: Anspor (cephradine, SK&F) is acid stable. It is rapidly absorbed after oral administration in the fasting state. Following doses of 250 mg. and 500 mg. in normal adult volunteers, average peak serum levels within one hour were approximately 9 and 16.5 mcg. per ml. respectively. The presence of food in the gastrointestinal tract delays the absorption but does not affect the total amount of cephradine absorbed. Over 90 percent of the drug is excreted unchanged in the urine within 6 hours. Peak urine concentrations are approximately 1600 mcg. per ml. following a 250 mg. dose and 3200 mcg. per ml. following a 500 mg. dose.

Microbiology: In vitro tests demonstrate that the cephalosporins are bactericidal because of their inhibition of cell-wall synthesis. Cephradine is active against the following organisms in vitro and in clinical infections:

Beta-hemolytic streptococci
Staphylococci, including coagulase-positive, coagulase-negative, and penicillinase-producing strains
Streptococcus pneumoniae (formerly D. pneumoniae)
Escherichia coli
Proteus mirabilis
Klebsiella sp.
Hemophilus influenzae

Note—Some strains of enterococci (Streptococcus faecalis) are resistant to cephradine. It is not active against most strains of Enterobacter sp., Pr. morganii, and Pr. vulgaris. It has no activity against Pseudomonas or Herellea species. When tested by in vitro methods, staphylococci exhibit cross-resistance between cephradine and methicillin-type antibiotics.

Disc Susceptibility Tests: Quantitative methods that require measurement of zone diameters give the most precise estimates of antibiotic susceptibility. One recommended procedure (21 CFR § 460.1) uses cephalosporin class discs for testing susceptibility; interpretations correlate zone diameters of this disc test with MIC values for cephradine. With this procedure, a report from the laboratory of "resistant" indicates that the infecting organism is not likely to respond to therapy. A report of "intermediate susceptibility" suggests that the organism would be susceptible if the infection is confined to the urinary tract, as high antibiotic levels can be obtained in the urine, or if high dosage is used in other types of infection.

INDICATIONS AND USAGE

Anspor (cephradine, SK&F) Capsules and 'Anspor' for Oral Suspension are indicated in the treatment of the following infections when caused by susceptible strains of designated microorganisms:

Infections of the respiratory tract (e.g., tonsillitis, pharyngitis, and lobar pneumonia) caused by group A beta-hemolytic streptococci and Streptococcus pneumoniae (formerly D. pneumoniae).

(Penicillin is the usual drug of choice in the treatment and prevention of streptococcal infections, including the prophylaxis of rheumatic fever. 'Anspor' is generally effective in the eradication of streptococci from the nasopharynx; substantial data establishing the efficacy of 'Anspor' in the subsequent prevention of rheumatic fever are not available at present.)

Otitis media caused by group A beta-hemolytic streptococci, Streptococcus pneumoniae (formerly D. pneumoniae), Hemophilus influenzae and staphylococci.

Skin and skin structure infections caused by staphylococci (penicillin-susceptible and penicillin-resistant) and beta-hemolytic streptococci.

Infections of the urinary tract, including prostatitis, caused by Escherichia coli, Pr. mirabilis, and Klebsiella sp.

Note—Culture and susceptibility tests should be initiated prior to and during therapy. Renal function studies should be performed when indicated.

CONTRAINDICATIONS

Cephradine is contraindicated in patients with known hypersensitivity to the cephalosporin group of antibiotics.

WARNINGS

BEFORE CEPHRADINE THERAPY IS INSTITUTED, CAREFUL INQUIRY SHOULD BE MADE CONCERNING PREVIOUS HYPERSENSITIVITY REACTIONS TO CEPHALOSPORINS AND PENICILLIN. CEPHALOSPORIN C DERIVATIVES SHOULD BE GIVEN CAUTIOUSLY IN PENICILLIN-SENSITIVE PATIENTS.

SERIOUS ACUTE HYPERSENSITIVITY REACTIONS MAY REQUIRE EPINEPHRINE AND OTHER EMERGENCY MEASURES.

There is some clinical and laboratory evidence of partial cross-allergenicity of the penicillins and the cephalosporins.

Patients have been reported to have had severe reactions (including anaphylaxis) to both drugs.

Any patient who has demonstrated some form of allergy, particularly to drugs, should receive antibiotics cautiously. No exception should be made with regard to Anspor (cephradine, SK&F).

Pseudomembranous colitis has been reported with the use of cephalosporins (and other broad-spectrum antibiotics); therefore, it is important to consider its diagnosis in patients who develop diarrhea in association with antibiotic use.

Treatment with broad-spectrum antibiotics alters normal flora of the colon and may permit overgrowth of clostridia. Studies indicate a toxin produced by Clostridium difficile is one primary cause of antibiotic-associated colitis. Cholestyramine and colestipol resins have been shown to bind the toxin in vitro.

Mild cases of colitis may respond to drug discontinuance alone.

Moderate to severe cases should be managed with fluid, electrolyte and protein supplementation as indicated.

When the colitis is not relieved by drug discontinuance or when it is severe, oral vancomycin is the treatment of choice for antibiotic-associated pseudomembranous colitis produced by C. difficile. Other causes of colitis should also be considered.

PRECAUTIONS

General—Patients should be followed carefully so that any side effects or unusual manifestations of drug idiosyncrasy may be detected. If a hypersensitivity reaction occurs, the drug should be discontinued and the patient treated with the usual agents, e.g., pressor amines, antihistamines, or corticosteroids.

Administer cephradine with caution in the presence of markedly impaired renal function. In patients with known or suspected renal impairment, careful clinical observation and appropriate laboratory studies should be made prior to and during therapy as cephradine accumulates in the serum and tissues. See DOSAGE AND ADMINISTRATION section for information on treatment of patients with impaired renal function.

Prolonged use of antibiotics may promote the overgrowth of nonsusceptible organisms. Should superinfection occur during therapy, appropriate measures should be taken.

Anspor (cephradine, SK&F), as with all cephalosporins, should be prescribed with caution in individuals with a history of gastrointestinal disease, particularly colitis.

Information for Patients—Cephradine may be taken without regard to meals, unless gastrointestinal irritation occurs. Diabetic patients receiving 'Anspor' should be cautioned to check with physicians before changing diet or dosage of diabetes medication. A false positive reaction for glucose in the urine may occur with Benedict's solution, Fehling's solution, or with Clinitest® tablets, but not with enzyme-based tests such as Clinistix® and Tes-Tape®.

Laboratory Tests—In chronic urinary tract infections, frequent bacteriologic tests are necessary during drug therapy and may be necessary for several months afterwards.

Drug Interactions—Probenecid may decrease renal tubular secretion of cephalosporins when used concurrently, resulting in increased and more prolonged cephalosporin blood levels.

Drug/Laboratory Test Interactions—After treatment with cephradine, a false positive reaction for glucose in the urine may occur with Benedict's solution, Fehling's solution, or with Clinitest® tablets, but not with enzyme-based tests such as Clinistix® and Tes-Tape®.

A false positive direct Coombs test has been reported after treatment with other cephalosporins; therefore, it should be recognized that a positive Coombs test may be due to the drug.

Carcinogenesis/Mutagenesis — Mutagenicity studies and long-term studies in animals to determine the carcinogenic potential of Anspor (cephradine, SK&F) have not been performed.

Pregnancy—Teratogenic Effects —Pregnancy Category B. Reproduction studies have been performed in mice and rats receiving doses up to four times the maximum human dose and have revealed no evidence of impaired fertility or harm to the fetus due to cephradine. There are, however, no adequate and well-controlled studies in pregnant women. Because animal reproduction studies are not always predictive of human response, this drug should be used during pregnancy only if clearly needed.

Nursing Mothers—Cephradine is present in very low concentrations in the milk of nursing mothers. Caution should be exercised when cephradine is administered to a nursing woman.

Pediatric Use—Safety and effectiveness for use in infants under nine months of age have not been established. See DOSAGE AND ADMINISTRATION section for recommended dosage in children over nine months.

ADVERSE REACTIONS

As with other cephalosporins, untoward reactions are limited essentially to gastrointestinal disturbances and to hy-

persensitivity phenomena. The latter are more likely to occur in individuals who have previously demonstrated hypersensitivity and those with a history of allergy, asthma, hay fever, or urticaria.

The following adverse reactions have been reported following the use of cephradine:

Gastrointestinal: Diarrhea or loose stools, vomiting, glossitis, nausea, abdominal pain and heartburn.

Symptoms of pseudomembranous colitis can appear during antibiotic treatment.

Nausea and vomiting have been reported rarely.

Allergic: Anaphylaxis, mild urticaria or skin rash, pruritus, joint pains.

Hematologic: Mild, transient eosinophilia, leukopenia and neutropenia.

Liver: Transient mild rise of SGOT, SGPT, and total bilirubin has been observed with no evidence of hepatocellular damage.

Renal: Transitory rises in BUN have been observed in some patients treated with cephalosporins; their frequency increases in patients over 50 years old. In adults for whom serum creatinine determinations were performed, the rise in BUN was not accompanied by a rise in serum creatinine.

Other: Dizziness and tightness in the chest and candidal vaginitis.

DOSAGE AND ADMINISTRATION

Anspor (cephradine, SK&F) may be given without regard to meals.

Adults: For skin and soft-tissue and respiratory tract infections (other than lobar pneumonia), the usual dose is 250 mg. every 6 hours or 500 mg. every 12 hours. For acute infections of the urinary tract, including prostatitis, and pneumococcal lobar pneumonia, the usual dose is 500 mg. every 6 hours or 1 gram every 12 hours. Severe or chronic infections may require larger doses.

Children: No adequate information is available on the efficacy of b.i.d. regimens in children under nine months of age. The usual dose in children over nine months of age is 25 to 50 mg./kg./day administered in equally divided doses every 6 or 12 hours. For otitis media due to H. influenzae, doses are from 75 to 100 mg./kg./day administered in equally divided doses every 6 or 12 hours. Doses for children should not exceed doses recommended for adults. The maximum dose should not exceed 4 grams per day.

All patients, regardless of age and weight: Larger doses (up to 1 gram, q.i.d.) may be given for severe or chronic infections.

As with antibiotic therapy generally, therapy should be continued for a minimum of 48 to 72 hours after the patient becomes asymptomatic or evidence of bacterial eradication has been obtained. In infections caused by group A beta-hemolytic streptococci, a minimum of 10 days of treatment is recommended to guard against the risk of rheumatic fever or glomerulonephritis. In the treatment of chronic urinary tract infection, frequent bacteriologic and clinical appraisal is necessary during therapy and may be necessary for several months afterwards. Persistent infections may require treatment for several weeks. Prolonged intensive therapy is recommended for prostatitis. Doses smaller than those indicated are not recommended.

Patients with Impaired Renal Function

Not on Dialysis: The following initial dosage schedule is suggested as a guideline based on creatinine clearance. Further modification in the dosage schedule may be required because of individual variations in absorption.

Creatinine Clearance	Dose	Time Interval
> 20 ml./min.	500 mg.	6 hours
5–20 ml./min.	250 mg.	6 hours
< 5 ml./min.	250 mg.	12 hours

On Chronic, Intermittent Hemodialysis:

250 mg.	Start	
250 mg.	at 12 hours	
250 mg.	36–48 hours (after start)	

Children may require dosage modification proportional to their weight and severity of infection.

HOW SUPPLIED

Anspor (cephradine, SK&F) Capsules: 250 mg. in bottles of 100 and in Single Unit Packages of 100 (intended for institutional use only); 500 mg. in bottles of 20 and 100 and in Single Unit Packages of 100 (intended for institutional use only). 'Anspor' for Oral Suspension after reconstitution provides 125 mg. or 250 mg. of cephradine per 5 ml. (one teaspoonful) in 100 ml. bottles.

NOTES ON STABILITY

Anspor (cephradine, SK&F) Capsules—Do not store above 86°F.; keep bottle tightly closed. 'Anspor' for Oral Suspension—Prior to reconstitution, do not store above 86°F. After reconstitution, suspensions retain their potency for seven days at room temperature and for 14 days if refrigerated.

AN:L14

Shown in Product Identification Section, page 430

Continued on next page

Smith Kline & French—Cont.

CEFIZOX®   Rx
[sef'eh-zocks]
(brand of sterile ceftizoxime sodium)

PRODUCT OVERVIEW

KEY FACTS

'Cefizox' is a sterile, semisynthetic cephalosporin antibiotic for parenteral (I.V., I.M.) administration. 'Cefizox' is highly resistant to a broad spectrum of beta-lactamases, and is active against a wide range of both aerobic and anaerobic gram-positive and gram-negative organisms.

MAJOR USES

'Cefizox' is indicated in the treatment of infections due to susceptible microorganisms listed below in the full prescribing information. In particular, because of its mixed aerobic /anaerobic coverage, 'Cefizox' has proven to be useful for treating intra-abdominal infections.

SAFETY INFORMATION

'Cefizox' is contraindicated in patients who have shown hypersensitivity to ceftizoxime. Careful inquiry should be made concerning previous hypersensitivity reactions to cephalosporins, penicillins or other drugs. 'Cefizox' should be administered with caution to penicillin-sensitive patients. Serious acute hypersensitivity reactions may require epinephrine and other emergency measures. Because pseudomembranous colitis has been reported with the use of cephalosporins, it is important to consider its diagnosis in patients who develop diarrhea in association with antibiotic use.

PRESCRIBING INFORMATION

CEFIZOX®   Rx
[sef'eh-zocks]
(brand of sterile ceftizoxime sodium and ceftizoxime sodium injection)

DESCRIPTION

Cefizox (sterile ceftizoxime sodium, FSK) is a sterile, semisynthetic, broad-spectrum, beta-lactamase resistant cephalosporin antibiotic for parenteral (I.V., I.M.) administration. It is the sodium salt of [6R-[6α, 7 β(Z)]]-7-[[(2,3-dihydro-2-imino-4-thiazolyl) (methoxyimino) acetyl] amino]-8-oxo-5-thia-1-azabicyclo [4.2.0] oct-2-ene-2-carboxylic acid. Its sodium content is approximately 60 mg. (2.6 mEq.) per gram of ceftizoxime activity.

Sterile ceftizoxime sodium is a white to pale yellow crystalline powder.

'Cefizox' is supplied in vials equivalent to 1 gram, 2 grams or 10 grams of ceftizoxime, and in "Piggyback" Vials for intravenous admixture equivalent to 1 gram or 2 grams of ceftizoxime.

'Cefizox', equivalent to 1 gram or 2 grams of ceftizoxime, is also supplied as a frozen, sterile, nonpyrogenic solution of ceftizoxime sodium in an iso-osmotic diluent in plastic containers. After thawing, the solution is intended for intravenous use.

The plastic container is fabricated from specially formulated polyvinyl chloride. Solutions in contact with the plastic container can leach out certain of its chemical components in very small amounts within the expiration period, e.g., di 2-ethylhexyl phthalate (DEHP), up to 5 parts per million. However, the safety of the plastic has been confirmed in tests in animals according to the USP biological tests for plastic containers as well as by tissue culture toxicity studies.

CLINICAL PHARMACOLOGY

The table below demonstrates the serum levels and duration of Cefizox (sterile ceftizoxime sodium, FSK) following intramuscular administration of 500 mg. and 1.0 gram doses respectively to normal volunteers.
[See table below].
Following intravenous administration of 1.0, 2.0 and 3.0 gram doses of 'Cefizox' to normal volunteers, the following serum levels were obtained:
[See table above].
ND = Not Done
A serum half-life of approximately 1.7 hours was observed after intravenous or intramuscular administration.
'Cefizox' is 30% protein bound.
'Cefizox' is not metabolized, and is excreted virtually unchanged by the kidneys in 24 hours. This provides a high urinary concentration. Concentrations greater than 6,000 mcg./mL. have been achieved in the urine by 2 hours after a

1 gram dose of 'Cefizox' intravenously. Probenecid slows tubular secretion and produces even higher serum levels, increasing the duration of measurable serum concentrations.

'Cefizox' achieves therapeutic levels in various body fluids, e.g., cerebrospinal fluid (in patients with inflamed meninges), bile, surgical wound fluid, pleural fluid, aqueous humor, ascitic fluid, peritoneal fluid, prostatic fluid and saliva, and the following body tissues: heart, gallbladder, bone, biliary, peritoneal, prostatic and uterine.

In clinical experience to date, no disulfiram-like reactions have been reported with Cefizox (sterile ceftizoxime sodium, FSK).

Microbiology

The bactericidal action of 'Cefizox' results from inhibition of cell-wall synthesis. 'Cefizox' is highly resistant to a broad spectrum of beta-lactamases (penicillinase and cephalosporinase), including Richmond types I, II, III, TEM, and IV, produced by both aerobic and anaerobic gram-positive and gram-negative organisms. 'Cefizox' is active against a wide range of gram-positive and gram-negative organisms, and is usually active against the following organisms in vitro and in clinical situations (see Indications and Usage):

Gram-Positive Aerobes:

Staphylococcus sp. including penicillinase and nonpenicillinase producing *S. aureus* and *S. epidermidis*. Note: Methicillin-resistant staphylococci are resistant to cephalosporins, including ceftizoxime.
Streptococcus sp. including *S. pneumoniae* (formerly *D. pneumoniae*) and *S. pyogenes*.
Note: 'Cefizox' is usually inactive in vitro against most strains of enterococci, e.g., *S. faecalis*.

Gram-Negative Aerobes:

Klebsiella sp. including *K. pneumoniae*	*Enterobacter* sp.
	Pseudomonas sp. including
Escherichia coli	*Ps. aeruginosa*
Proteus mirabilis	*Haemophilus* sp.
Proteus vulgaris	including ampicillin-resistant strains
Morganella morganii (formerly *Proteus morganii*) and	of *H. influenzae*
Providencia rettgeri (formerly *Proteus rettgeri*)	*Neisseria gonorrhoeae*
Serratia sp. including *S. marcescens*	

Anaerobes:

Bacteroides sp. including *B. fragilis*
Anaerobic cocci including
  Peptococcus sp.
  Peptostreptococcus sp.
'Cefizox' is usually active against strains of *Acinetobacter* sp.

Cefizox (sterile ceftizoxime sodium, FSK) is usually active against the following organisms in vitro, but the clinical significance of these data has not been established:

Gram-Positive Aerobes:

Corynebacterium diphtheriae

Gram-Negative Aerobes:

Shigella sp.	*Moraxella* sp.
Providencia stuartii	*Pasteurella multocida*
Salmonella sp.	
Aeromonas hydrophila	*Neisseria meningitidis*
Yersinia enterocolitica	*Citrobacter* sp.

Anaerobes:

Actinomyces sp.	*Fusobacterium* sp.
Veillonella sp.	*Bifidobacterium* sp.
Eubacterium sp.	*Propionibacterium* sp.
Clostridium sp.	
(Note: Most strains of *C. difficile* are resistant.)	

Susceptibility Testing

Quantitative methods that require measurement of zone diameters give the most precise estimate of antibiotic susceptibility. One such procedure* has been recommended for use with disks to test susceptibility to ceftizoxime.

Reports from the laboratory giving results of the standard single-disk susceptibility test with a 30 mcg. ceftizoxime disk should be interpreted according to the following criteria (with the exception of *Ps. aeruginosa*):

Susceptible organisms produce zones of 20 mm. or greater, indicating that the test organism is likely to respond to therapy.

Organisms that produce zones of 15 to 19 mm. are expected to be susceptible if high dosage is used or if the infection is confined to tissues and fluids (e.g., urine) in which high antibiotic levels are attained.

Resistant organisms produce zones of 14 mm. or less, indicating that other therapy should be selected.

Organisms should be tested with the 'Cefizox' disk, since 'Cefizox' has been shown by in vitro tests to be active against certain strains found resistant when other beta-lactam disks are used.

Susceptibility Testing for Pseudomonas in Urinary Tract Infections

Most strains of *Ps. aeruginosa* are moderately susceptible to Cefizox (sterile ceftizoxime sodium, FSK). 'Cefizox' achieves high levels in the urine (greater than 6,000 mcg./mL. at 2 hours with 1 gram I.V.) and therefore the following zone sizes should be used when testing 'Cefizox' for treatment of urinary tract infections caused by *Ps. aeruginosa*:

Susceptible organisms produce zones of 20 mm. or greater, indicating that the test organism is likely to respond to therapy.

Organisms that produce zones of 11 to 19 mm. are expected to be susceptible when the infection is confined to the urinary tract in which high antibiotic levels are attained.

Resistant organisms produce zones of 10 mm. or less, indicating that other therapy should be selected.

A bacterial isolate may be considered susceptible if the MIC value for 'Cefizox' is equal to or less than 16 mcg./mL. Organisms are considered moderately susceptible if the MIC is greater than 16 mcg./mL. but less than 64 mcg./mL. Organisms are considered resistant if the MIC is 64 mcg./mL. or greater. For most organisms the MBC value for 'Cefizox' is the same as the MIC value.

The standardized quality control procedure requires use of control organisms. The 30 mcg. ceftizoxime disk should give the zone diameters listed below for the quality control strains.

Organism	ATCC	Zone Size Range
E. coli	25922	30–36 mm.
S. aureus	25923	27–35 mm.
Ps. aeruginosa	27853	12–17 mm.

INDICATIONS AND USAGE

Cefizox (sterile ceftizoxime sodium, FSK) is indicated in the treatment of infections due to susceptible strains of the microorganisms listed below:

LOWER RESPIRATORY TRACT INFECTIONS caused by *Streptococcus* sp. including *S. pneumoniae* (formerly *D. pneumoniae*), but excluding enterococci; *Klebsiella* sp.; *Proteus mirabilis*; *Escherichia coli*; *Haemophilus influenzae* including ampicillin-resistant strains; *Staphylococcus aureus* (penicillinase and nonpenicillinase producing); *Serratia* sp.; *Enterobacter* sp.; and *Bacteroides* sp.

URINARY TRACT INFECTIONS caused by *Staphylococcus aureus* (penicillinase and nonpenicillinase producing); *Escherichia coli*; *Pseudomonas* sp. including *Ps. aeruginosa*; *Proteus mirabilis*; *P. vulgaris*; *Providencia rettgeri* (formerly *Proteus rettgeri*) and *Morganella morganii* (formerly *Proteus morganii*); *Klebsiella* sp.; *Serratia* sp. including *S. marcescens*; *Enterobacter* sp.

GONORRHEA. Uncomplicated cervical and urethral gonorrhea caused by *Neisseria gonorrhoeae*.

INTRA-ABDOMINAL INFECTIONS caused by *Escherichia coli*; *Staphylococcus epidermidis*; *Streptococcus* sp. (excluding enterococci); *Enterobacter* sp.; *Klebsiella* sp.; *Bacteroides* sp. including *B. fragilis*; and anaerobic cocci, including *Peptococcus* sp. and *Peptostreptococcus* sp.

SEPTICEMIA caused by *Streptococcus* sp. including *S. pneumoniae* (formerly *D. pneumoniae*), but excluding enterococci; *Staphylococcus aureus* (penicillinase and nonpenicillinase

Serum Concentrations After Intravenous Administration
Serum Concentration (mcg./mL.)

Dose	5 mins.	10 mins.	30 mins.	1 hr.	2 hrs.	4 hrs.	8 hrs.
1.0 gram	ND	ND	60.5	38.9	21.5	8.4	1.4
2.0 grams	131.8	110.9	77.5	53.6	33.1	12.1	2.0
3.0 grams	221.1	174.0	112.7	83.9	47.4	26.2	4.8

Serum Concentrations After Intramuscular Administration
Serum Concentration (mcg./mL.)

Dose	½ hr.	1 hr.	2 hrs.	4 hrs.	6 hrs.	8 hrs.
500 mg.	13.3	13.7	9.2	4.8	1.9	0.7
1.0 gram	36.0	39.0	31.0	15.0	6.0	3.0

producing); *Escherichia coli; Bacteroides* sp. including *B. fragilis; Klebsiella* sp.; and *Serratia* sp.

SKIN AND SKIN STRUCTURE INFECTIONS caused by *Staphylococcus aureus* (penicillinase and nonpenicillinase producing); *Staphylococcus epidermidis; Escherichia coli; Klebsiella* sp.; *Streptococcus* sp. including *Streptococcus pyogenes* (group A beta-hemolytic), but excluding enterococci; *Proteus mirabilis; Serratia* sp.; *Enterobacter* sp.; *Bacteroides* sp. including *B. fragilis;* and anaerobic cocci, including *Peptococcus* sp. and *Peptostreptococcus* sp.

BONE AND JOINT INFECTIONS caused by *Staphylococcus aureus* (penicillinase and nonpenicillinase producing); *Streptococcus* sp. (excluding enterococci); *Proteus mirabilis; Bacteroides* sp.; and anaerobic cocci, including *Peptococcus* sp. and *Peptostreptococcus* sp.

MENINGITIS caused by *Haemophilus influenzae.* 'Cefizox' has also been used successfully in the treatment of a limited number of pediatric and adult cases of meningitis caused by *Streptococcus pneumoniae.*

'Cefizox' has been effective in the treatment of seriously ill, compromised patients, including those who were debilitated, immunosuppressed or neutropenic.

Infections caused by aerobic gram-negative and by mixtures of organisms resistant to other cephalosporins, aminoglycosides, or penicillins have responded to treatment with 'Cefizox'.

Because of the serious nature of some urinary tract infections due to *Ps. aeruginosa* and because many strains of *Pseudomonas* species are only moderately susceptible to 'Cefizox', higher dosage is recommended. Other therapy should be instituted if the response is not prompt.

Susceptibility studies on specimens obtained prior to therapy should be used to determine the response of causative organisms to 'Cefizox'. Therapy with 'Cefizox' may be initiated pending results of the studies; however, treatment should be adjusted according to study findings. In serious infections 'Cefizox' has been used concomitantly with aminoglycosides (see Precautions). Before using 'Cefizox' concomitantly with other antibiotics, the prescribing information for those agents should be reviewed for contraindications, warnings, precautions and adverse reactions. Renal function should be carefully monitored.

CONTRAINDICATIONS

Cefizox (sterile ceftizoxime sodium, FSK) is contraindicated in patients who have known allergy to the drug.

WARNINGS

BEFORE THERAPY WITH CEFIZOX (STERILE CEFTIZOXIME SODIUM, FSK) IS INSTITUTED, CAREFUL INQUIRY SHOULD BE MADE TO DETERMINE WHETHER THE PATIENT HAS HAD PREVIOUS HYPERSENSITIVITY REACTIONS TO CEPHALOSPORINS, PENICILLINS, OR OTHER DRUGS. THIS PRODUCT SHOULD BE GIVEN CAUTIOUSLY TO PENICILLIN-SENSITIVE PATIENTS. ANTIBIOTICS SHOULD BE ADMINISTERED WITH CAUTION TO ANY PATIENT WHO HAS DEMONSTRATED SOME FORM OF ALLERGY, PARTICULARLY TO DRUGS. SERIOUS ACUTE HYPERSENSITIVITY REACTIONS MAY REQUIRE EPINEPHRINE AND OTHER EMERGENCY MEASURES.

Pseudomembranous colitis has been reported with the use of cephalosporins (and other broad-spectrum antibiotics); therefore, it is important to consider its diagnosis in patients who developed diarrhea in association with antibiotic use. Treatment with broad-spectrum antibiotics alters normal flora of the colon and may permit overgrowth of *Clostridia.* Studies indicate a toxin produced by *Clostridium difficile* is one primary cause of antibiotic-associated colitis. Cholestyramine and colestipol resins have been shown to bind the toxin *in vitro.*

Mild cases of colitis may respond to drug discontinuance alone.

Moderate to severe cases should be managed with fluid, electrolyte and protein supplementation as indicated.

When the colitis is not relieved by drug discontinuance or when it is severe, oral vancomycin is the treatment of choice for antibiotic-associated pseudomembranous colitis produced by *C. difficile.* Other causes of colitis should also be considered.

PRECAUTIONS

General: As with all broad-spectrum antibiotics, Cefizox (sterile ceftizoxime sodium, FSK) should be prescribed with caution in individuals with a history of gastrointestinal disease, particularly colitis.

Although 'Cefizox' has not been shown to produce an alteration in renal function, renal status should be evaluated, especially in seriously ill patients receiving maximum dose therapy. As with any antibiotic, prolonged use may result in overgrowth of nonsusceptible organisms. Careful observation is essential; appropriate measures should be taken if superinfection occurs.

Drug Interactions: Although the occurrence has not been reported with 'Cefizox', nephrotoxicity has been reported following concomitant administration of other cephalosporins and aminoglycosides.

General Guidelines for Dosage of 'Cefizox'

Type of Infection	Daily Dose (Grams)	Frequency and Route
Uncomplicated Urinary Tract	1	500 mg. q12h I.M. or I.V.
Other Sites	2–3	1 gram q8–12h I.M. or I.V.
Severe or Refractory	3–6	1 gram q8h I.M. or I.V. 2 grams q8–12h I.M.* or I.V.
Life-Threatening†	9–12	3–4 grams q8h I.V.

*When administering 2 gram I.M. doses, the dose should be divided and given in different large muscle masses.
†In life-threatening infections dosages up to 2 grams every 4 hours have been given.

Pregnancy: (Category B.) Reproduction studies have been performed in rats and rabbits and have revealed no evidence of impaired fertility or harm to the fetus due to 'Cefizox'. There are, however, no adequate and well-controlled studies in pregnant women. Because animal reproduction studies are not always predictive of human response, this drug should be used during pregnancy only if clearly needed.

Labor and Delivery: Safety of 'Cefizox' use during labor and delivery has not been established.

Nursing Mothers: 'Cefizox' is excreted in human milk in low concentrations. Caution should be exercised when 'Cefizox' is administered to a nursing woman.

Infants and Children: Safety and efficacy in infants from birth to six months of age have not been established. In children six months of age and older, treatment with 'Cefizox' has been associated with transient elevated levels of eosinophils, SGOT, SGPT and CPK (creatine phosphokinase). The CPK elevation may be related to I.M. administration.

ADVERSE REACTIONS

Ceftizoxime is generally well tolerated. The *most* frequent adverse reactions (*greater than* 1% but less than 5%) are:

Hypersensitivity—Rash, pruritus, fever.

Hepatic—Transient elevation in SGOT, SGPT and alkaline phosphatase.

Hematologic—Transient eosinophilia, thrombocytosis. Some individuals have developed a positive Coombs test.

Local—Injection site—Burning, cellulitis, phlebitis with I.V. administration, pain, induration, tenderness, paresthesia.

The *less* frequent adverse reactions (*less than* 1%) are:

Hypersensitivity—Numbness has been reported rarely.

Hepatic—Elevation of bilirubin has been reported rarely.

Renal—Transient elevations of BUN and creatinine have been occasionally observed with ceftizoxime.

Hematologic—Anemia, leukopenia, neutropenia and thrombocytopenia have been reported rarely.

Genitourinary—Vaginitis has rarely occurred.

Gastrointestinal—Diarrhea; nausea and vomiting have been reported occasionally.

Symptoms of pseudomembranous colitis can appear during or after antibiotic treatment. (See Warnings section.)

DOSAGE AND ADMINISTRATION

The usual adult dosage is 1 or 2 grams of Cefizox (sterile ceftizoxime sodium, FSK) every 8 to 12 hours. Proper dosage and route of administration should be determined by the condition of the patient, severity of the infection and susceptibility of the causative organisms.

[See table above.]

Because of the serious nature of urinary tract infections due to *Ps. aeruginosa* and because many strains of *Pseudomonas* species are only moderately susceptible to 'Cefizox', higher dosage is recommended. Other therapy should be instituted if the response is not prompt.

A single, 1 gram I.M. dose is the usual dose for treatment of uncomplicated gonorrhea.

The intravenous route may be preferable for patients with bacterial septicemia, localized parenchymal abscesses (such as intra-abdominal abscess), peritonitis, or other severe or life-threatening infections.

In those with normal renal function, the intravenous dosage for such infections is 2 to 12 grams of Cefizox (sterile ceftizoxime sodium, FSK) daily. In conditions such as bacterial septicemia, 6 to 12 grams/day may be given initially by the intravenous route for several days, and the dosage may then be gradually reduced according to clinical response and laboratory findings.

Pediatric Dosage Schedule

	Unit Dose	Frequency
Children 6 months and older	50 mg./kg.	q6-8h

Dosage may be increased to a total daily dose of 200 mg./kg. (not to exceed the maximum adult dose for serious infection).

Impaired Renal Function

Modification of 'Cefizox' dosage is necessary in patients with impaired renal function. Following an initial loading dose of 500 mg.–1.0 gram I.M. or I.V., the maintenance dosing schedule shown below should be followed. Further dosing should be determined by therapeutic monitoring, severity of the infection and susceptibility of the causative organisms. When only the serum creatinine level is available, creatinine clearance may be calculated from the following formula. The serum creatinine level should represent current renal function at the steady state.

Males

$$Clcr = \frac{Weight\ (kg.) \times (140 - age)}{72 \times serum\ creatinine\ (mg./100\ mL.)}$$

Females 0.85 of the above values

In patients undergoing hemodialysis no additional supplemental dosing is required following hemodialysis; however, dosing should be timed so that the patient receives the dose (according to the table below) at the end of the dialysis.

Dosage in Adults with Reduced Renal Function

Creatinine Clearance mL./min.	Renal Function	Less Severe Infections	Life-Threatening Infections
79–50	Mild impairment	500 mg. q8h	0.75 gram– 1.5 grams q8h
49–5	Moderate to severe impairment	250 mg.– 500 mg. q12h	0.5 gram– 1.0 gram q12h
4–0	Dialysis patients	500 mg. q48h or 250 mg. q24h	0.5 gram– 1.0 gram q48h or 0.5 gram q24h

Preparation of Parenteral Solution
RECONSTITUTION

I.M. Administration: Reconstitute with Sterile Water for Injection. SHAKE WELL.

Vial Size	Diluent to Be Added	Approx. Avail. Vol.	Approx. Avg. Concentration
1 gram	3.0 mL.	3.7 mL.	270 mg./mL.
2 grams*	6.0 mL.	7.4 mL.	270 mg./mL.

*When administering 2 gram I.M. doses, the dose should be divided and given in different large muscle masses.

I.V. Administration: Reconstitute with Sterile Water for Injection. SHAKE WELL.

Vial Size	Diluent to Be Added	Approx. Avail. Vol.	Approx. Avg. Concentration
1 gram	10 mL.	10.7 mL.	95 mg./mL.
2 grams	20 mL.	21.4 mL.	95 mg./mL.

These solutions of Cefizox (sterile ceftizoxime sodium, FSK) are stable 24 hours at room temperature or 96 hours if refrigerated (5°C.).

Parenteral drug products should be inspected visually for particulate matter prior to administration. If particulate matter is evident in reconstituted fluids, then the drug solution should be discarded. Reconstituted solutions may range from yellow to amber without changes in potency.

Pharmacy Bulk Vials: For I.M. or I.V. direct injection, add Sterile Water for Injection according to table below. SHAKE WELL. For I.V. intermittent or continuous infusion, add

Continued on next page

Smith Kline & French—Cont.

Sterile Water for Injection according to table below. SHAKE WELL. Add to parenteral fluids listed below under I.V. Administration.

Vial Size	Diluent to Be Added	Approx. Avail. Vol.	Approx. Avg. Concentration
10 grams	30 mL	37 mL	1 gram/3.5 mL
	45 mL	51 mL	1 gram/5 mL

These reconstituted solutions of Cefizox are stable 24 hours at room temperature or 96 hours if refrigerated (5°C.).

"Piggyback" Vials: Reconstitute with 50 to 100 mL. of Sodium Chloride Injection or any other I.V. solution listed below. SHAKE WELL.

Administer with primary I.V. fluids, as a single dose. These solutions of 'Cefizox' are stable 24 hours at room temperature or 96 hours if refrigerated (5°C.).

A solution of 1 gram 'Cefizox' in 13 mL. Sterile Water for Injection is isotonic.

I.M. Injection: Inject well within the body of a relatively large muscle. Aspiration is necessary to avoid inadvertent injection into a blood vessel. When administering 2 gram I.M. doses, the dose should be divided and given in different large muscle masses.

I.V. Administration: Direct (bolus) injection, slowly over 3 to 5 minutes, directly or through tubing for patients receiving parenteral fluids (see list below). Intermittent or continuous infusion, dilute reconstituted 'Cefizox' in 50 to 100 mL. of one of the following solutions:

Sodium Chloride Injection
5% or 10% Dextrose Injection
5% Dextrose and 0.9%, 0.45%, or 0.2% Sodium Chloride Injection
Ringer's Injection
Lactated Ringer's Injection
Invert Sugar 10% in Sterile Water for Injection
5% Sodium Bicarbonate in Sterile Water for Injection
5% Dextrose in Lactated Ringer's Injection (only when reconstituted with 4% Sodium Bicarbonate Injection)

In these fluids 'Cefizox' is stable 24 hours at room temperature or 96 hours if refrigerated (5°C.).

DIRECTIONS FOR USE OF CEFIZOX (CEFTIZOXIME SODIUM INJECTION, FSK) PLASTIC CONTAINERS

'Cefizox' supplied as a frozen, sterile, nonpyrogenic solution in plastic containers is to be administered either as a continuous or intermittent infusion.

Thaw container at room temperature. After thawing, check for minute leaks by squeezing bag firmly. If leaks are found, discard solution as sterility may be impaired. Additives should not be introduced into this solution. Do not use if the solution is cloudy or precipitated or if the seal is not intact. After thawing, the solution is stable for 24 hours at room temperature or 10 days if stored under refrigeration (5°C.). DO NOT REFREEZE.

Use sterile equipment. It is recommended that the intravenous administration apparatus be replaced at least once every 48 hours.

CAUTION: Do not use plastic containers in series connections. Such use could result in air embolism due to residual air being drawn from the primary container before administration of the fluid from the secondary container is complete.

Preparation for administration:
1. Suspend container from eyelet support.
2. Remove plastic protector from outlet port at bottom of container.
3. Attach administration set. Refer to complete directions accompanying set.

HOW SUPPLIED

Cefizox (sterile ceftizoxime sodium, FSK)—supplied in vials equivalent to 1 gram or 2 grams of ceftizoxime; in Pharmacy Bulk Vials equivalent to 10 grams of ceftizoxime; and in "Piggyback" Vials for I.V. admixture equivalent to 1 gram or 2 grams of ceftizoxime.

Note: Unreconstituted Cefizox (sterile ceftizoxime sodium, FSK) should be protected from excessive light, and stored at controlled room temperature (59°-86°F.) in the original package until used.

Cefizox (ceftizoxime sodium injection, FSK) as a frozen, sterile, nonpyrogenic solution in plastic containers—supplied in 50 mL. single-dose containers equivalent to 1 gram or 2 grams of ceftizoxime in 5% Dextrose (D5W). Do not store above −20°C.

'Cefizox' supplied as a frozen, sterile, nonpyrogenic solution in plastic containers is manufactured for Fujisawa Smith-Kline Corporation by Baxter Healthcare Corporation, Deerfield, IL 60015.

* Am. J. Clin. Pathol. 45:493, 1966; Federal Register 39:19182–19184, 1974.

CF:L17

Shown in Product Identification Section, page 430

COMPAZINE® ℞
[komp'ah-zeen]
(brand of prochlorperazine)

PRODUCT OVERVIEW

KEY FACTS

'Compazine' is a phenothiazine derivative of the piperazine group, available in 13 dosage forms and strengths for oral, rectal, IV or IM parenteral administration. The Spansule® sustained release capsule dosage form provides an equivalent milligram dose of tablets given in divided doses.

MAJOR USES

'Compazine' is indicated for control of severe nausea and vomiting. 'Compazine' is also indicated in the management of the manifestations of psychotic disorders, as well as the short-term treatment of generalized non-psychotic anxiety, where it is considered second-line therapy.

SAFETY INFORMATION

'Compazine' is contraindicated in comatose states, pediatric surgery, children under 2 years of age or under 20 pounds, and in the presence of large amounts of CNS depressants. EPS, which can occur secondary to 'Compazine', may be confused with the CNS signs of Reye's syndrome or other encephalopathy. Avoid using in children and adolescents whose signs and symptoms suggest Reye's syndrome. Use 'Compazine' in children with acute illnesses or dehydration only under close supervision, since they appear much more susceptible to EPS, particularly dystonias, than adults. Pregnant patients, patients with bone marrow depression or with previous hypersensitivity reactions to a phenothiazine should not receive 'Compazine' unless the potential benefits outweigh possible hazards. (See full prescribing information.)

PRESCRIBING INFORMATION

COMPAZINE® ℞
[komp'ah-zeen]
(brand of prochlorperazine)

DESCRIPTION

Tablets—Each round, yellow-green, coated tablet contains prochlorperazine maleate equivalent to prochlorperazine as follows: 5 mg. imprinted SKF and C66; 10 mg. imprinted SKF and C67; 25 mg. imprinted SKF and C69. Inactive ingredients consist of acacia, calcium sulfate, D&C Green No. 5, D&C Yellow No. 10, FD&C Blue No. 1, FD&C Blue No. 2, FD&C Yellow No. 6, FD&C Red No. 40, gelatin, iron oxide, mineral oil, starch, stearic acid, sucrose, talc and trace amounts of other inactive ingredients.

Spansule® sustained release capsules—Each 'Compazine' *Spansule* capsule is so prepared that an initial dose is released promptly and the remaining medication is released gradually over a prolonged period.

Each capsule, with black cap and natural body, contains prochlorperazine maleate equivalent to prochlorperazine as follows: 10 mg. imprinted SKF and C44; 15 mg. imprinted SKF and C46; 30 mg. imprinted SKF and C47. Inactive ingredients consist of benzyl alcohol, cetylpyridinium chloride, D&C Green No. 5, D&C Yellow No. 10, FD&C Blue No. 1, FD&C Red No. 40, FD&C Yellow No. 6, gelatin, glyceryl monostearate, sodium lauryl sulfate, starch, sucrose, wax and trace amounts of other inactive ingredients.

Ampuls, 2 mL. (5 mg./mL.)—Each mL. contains, in aqueous solution, 5 mg. prochlorperazine as the edisylate, 1 mg. sodium sulfite, 1 mg. sodium bisulfite, 8 mg. sodium phosphate and 12 mg. sodium biphosphate.

Multiple-dose Vials, 10 mL. (5 mg./mL.)—Each mL. contains, in aqueous solution, 5 mg. prochlorperazine as the edisylate, 5 mg. sodium biphosphate, 12 mg. sodium tartrate, 0.9 mg. sodium saccharin, and 0.75% benzyl alcohol as preservative.

Disposable Syringes, 2 mL. (5 mg./mL.)—Each mL. contains, in aqueous solution, 5 mg. prochlorperazine as the edisylate, 5 mg. sodium biphosphate, 12 mg. sodium tartrate, 0.9 mg. sodium saccharin, and 0.75% benzyl alcohol as preservative.

Suppositories—Each suppository contains 2½ mg., 5 mg., or 25 mg. of prochlorperazine; with glycerin, glyceryl monopalmitate, glyceryl monostearate, hydrogenated cocoanut oil fatty acids and hydrogenated palm kernel oil fatty acids.

Syrup—Each 5 mL. (one teaspoonful) of clear, yellow-orange, fruit-flavored liquid contains 5 mg. of prochlorperazine as the edisylate. Inactive ingredients consist of FD&C Yellow No. 6, flavors, polyoxyethylene polyoxypropylene glycol, sodium benzoate, sodium citrate, sucrose and water.

INDICATIONS

For control of severe nausea and vomiting.
For management of the manifestations of psychotic disorders.
Compazine (prochlorperazine, SK&F) is effective for the short-term treatment of generalized non-psychotic anxiety. However, 'Compazine' is not the first drug to be used in therapy for most patients with non-psychotic anxiety, because certain risks associated with its use are not shared by common alternative treatments (e.g., benzodiazepines).

When used in the treatment of non-psychotic anxiety, 'Compazine' should not be administered at doses of more than 20 mg. per day or for longer than 12 weeks, because the use of 'Compazine' at higher doses or for longer intervals may cause persistent tardive dyskinesia that may prove irreversible (see Warnings).

The effectiveness of 'Compazine' as treatment for non-psychotic anxiety was established in four-week clinical studies of outpatients with generalized anxiety disorder. This evidence does not predict that 'Compazine' will be useful in patients with other non-psychotic conditions in which anxiety, or signs that mimic anxiety, are found (e.g., physical illness, organic mental conditions, agitated depression, character pathologies, etc.).

'Compazine' has not been shown effective in the management of behavioral complications in patients with mental retardation.

CONTRAINDICATIONS

Do not use in comatose states or in the presence of large amounts of central nervous system depressants (alcohol, barbiturates, narcotics, etc.).
Do not use in pediatric surgery.
Do not use in children under 2 years of age or under 20 lbs.
Do not use in children for conditions for which dosage has not been established.

WARNINGS

The extrapyramidal symptoms which can occur secondary to Compazine (prochlorperazine, SK&F) may be confused with the central nervous system signs of an undiagnosed primary disease responsible for the vomiting, e.g., Reye's syndrome or other encephalopathy. The use of 'Compazine' and other potential hepatotoxins should be avoided in children and adolescents whose signs and symptoms suggest Reye's syndrome.

Tardive Dyskinesia: Tardive dyskinesia, a syndrome consisting of potentially irreversible, involuntary, dyskinetic movements, may develop in patients treated with neuroleptic (antipsychotic) drugs. Although the prevalence of the syndrome appears to be highest among the elderly, especially elderly women, it is impossible to rely upon prevalence estimates to predict, at the inception of neuroleptic treatment, which patients are likely to develop the syndrome. Whether neuroleptic drug products differ in their potential to cause tardive dyskinesia is unknown.

Both the risk of developing the syndrome and the likelihood that it will become irreversible are believed to increase as the duration of treatment and the total cumulative dose of neuroleptic drugs administered to the patient increase. However, the syndrome can develop, although much less commonly, after relatively brief treatment periods at low doses. There is no known treatment for established cases of tardive dyskinesia, although the syndrome may remit, partially or completely, if neuroleptic treatment is withdrawn. Neuroleptic treatment itself, however, may suppress (or partially suppress) the signs and symptoms of the syndrome and thereby may possibly mask the underlying disease process. The effect that symptomatic suppression has upon the long-term course of the syndrome is unknown.

Given these considerations, neuroleptics should be prescribed in a manner that is most likely to minimize the occurrence of tardive dyskinesia. Chronic neuroleptic treatment should generally be reserved for patients who suffer from a chronic illness that, 1) is known to respond to neuroleptic drugs, and, 2) for whom alternative, equally effective, but potentially less harmful treatments are *not* available or appropriate. In patients who do require chronic treatment, the smallest dose and the shortest duration of treatment producing a satisfactory clinical response should be sought. The need for continued treatment should be reassessed periodically.

If signs and symptoms of tardive dyskinesia appear in a patient on neuroleptics, drug discontinuation should be considered. However, some patients may require treatment despite the presence of the syndrome.

For further information about the description of tardive dyskinesia and its clinical detection, please refer to the sections on Precautions and Adverse Reactions.

Neuroleptic Malignant Syndrome (NMS): A potentially fatal symptom complex sometimes referred to as Neuroleptic Malignant Syndrome (NMS) has been reported in association with antipsychotic drugs. Clinical manifestations of NMS are hyperpyrexia, muscle rigidity, altered mental status and evidence of autonomic instability (irregular pulse or blood pressure, tachycardia, diaphoresis, and cardiac dysrhythmias).

The diagnostic evaluation of patients with this syndrome is complicated. In arriving at a diagnosis, it is important to identify cases where the clinical presentation includes both serious medical illness (e.g., pneumonia, systemic infection, etc.) and untreated or inadequately treated extrapyramidal signs and symptoms (EPS). Other important considerations in the differential diagnosis include central anticholinergic toxicity, heat stroke, drug fever and primary central nervous system (CNS) pathology.

The management of NMS should include 1) immediate discontinuation of antipsychotic drugs and other drugs not essential to concurrent therapy, 2) intensive symptomatic treatment and medical monitoring, and 3) treatment of any concomitant serious medical problems for which specific treatments are available. There is no general agreement about specific pharmacological treatment regimens for uncomplicated NMS.

If a patient requires antipsychotic drug treatment after recovery from NMS, the potential reintroduction of drug therapy should be carefully considered. The patient should be carefully monitored, since recurrences of NMS have been reported.

'Compazine' ampuls contain sodium bisulfite and sodium sulfite, sulfites that may cause allergic-type reactions including anaphylactic symptoms and life-threatening or less severe asthmatic episodes in certain susceptible people. The overall prevalence of sulfite sensitivity in the general population is unknown and probably low. Sulfite sensitivity is seen more frequently in asthmatic than in non-asthmatic people.

Patients with bone marrow depression or who have previously demonstrated a hypersensitivity reaction (e.g., blood dyscrasias, jaundice) with a phenothiazine should not receive any phenothiazine, including 'Compazine', unless in the judgment of the physician the potential benefits of treatment outweigh the possible hazards.

Compazine (prochlorperazine, SK&F) may impair mental and/or physical abilities, especially during the first few days of therapy. Therefore, caution patients about activities requiring alertness (e.g., operating vehicles or machinery).

Phenothiazines may intensify or prolong the action of central nervous system depressants (e.g., alcohol, anesthetics, narcotics).

Usage in Pregnancy: Safety for the use of 'Compazine' during pregnancy has not been established. Therefore, 'Compazine' is not recommended for use in pregnant patients except in cases of severe nausea and vomiting that are so serious and intractable that, in the judgment of the physician, drug intervention is required and potential benefits outweigh possible hazards.

There have been reported instances of prolonged jaundice, extrapyramidal signs, hyperreflexia or hyporeflexia in newborn infants whose mothers received phenothiazines.

Nursing Mothers: There is evidence that phenothiazines are excreted in the breast milk of nursing mothers.

PRECAUTIONS

The antiemetic action of Compazine (prochlorperazine, SK&F) may mask the signs and symptoms of overdosage of other drugs and may obscure the diagnosis and treatment of other conditions such as intestinal obstruction, brain tumor and Reye's syndrome (see Warnings).

When 'Compazine' is used with cancer chemotherapeutic drugs, vomiting as a sign of the toxicity of these agents may be obscured by the antiemetic effect of 'Compazine'.

Because hypotension may occur, large doses and parenteral administration should be used cautiously in patients with impaired cardiovascular systems. To minimize the occurrence of hypotension after injection, keep patient lying down and observe for at least ½ hour. If hypotension occurs after parenteral or oral dosing, place patient in head-low position with legs raised. If a vasoconstrictor is required, Levophed®* and Neo-Synephrine®† are suitable. Other pressor agents, including epinephrine, should not be used because they may cause a paradoxical further lowering of blood pressure.

Aspiration of vomitus has occurred in a few post-surgical patients who have received 'Compazine' as an antiemetic. Although no causal relationship has been established, this possibility should be borne in mind during surgical aftercare. Deep sleep, from which patients can be aroused, and coma have been reported, usually with overdosage.

Neuroleptic drugs elevate prolactin levels; the elevation persists during chronic administration. Tissue culture experiments indicate that approximately one-third of human breast cancers are prolactin-dependent *in vitro*, a factor of potential importance if the prescribing of these drugs is contemplated in a patient with a previously detected breast cancer. Although disturbances such as galactorrhea, amenorrhea, gynecomastia and impotence have been reported, the clinical significance of elevated serum prolactin levels is unknown for most patients. An increase in mammary neoplasms has been found in rodents after chronic administration of neuroleptic drugs. Neither clinical nor epidemiologic studies conducted to date, however, have shown an association between chronic administration of these drugs and mammary tumorigenesis; the available evidence is considered too limited to be conclusive at this time.

Chromosomal aberrations in spermatocytes and abnormal sperm have been demonstrated in rodents treated with certain neuroleptics.

As with all drugs which exert an anticholinergic effect, and/or cause mydriasis, prochlorperazine should be used with caution in patients with glaucoma.

Because phenothiazines may interfere with thermoregulatory mechanisms, use with caution in persons who will be exposed to extreme heat.

Phenothiazines can diminish the effect of oral anticoagulants.

Phenothiazines can produce alpha-adrenergic blockade.

Thiazide diuretics may accentuate the orthostatic hypotension that may occur with phenothiazines.

Antihypertensive effects of guanethidine and related compounds may be counteracted when phenothiazines are used concomitantly.

Concomitant administration of propranolol with phenothiazines results in increased plasma levels of both drugs.

Phenothiazines may lower the convulsive threshold; dosage adjustments of anticonvulsants may be necessary. Potentiation of anticonvulsant effects does not occur. However, it has been reported that phenothiazines may interfere with the metabolism of Dilantin®‡ and thus precipitate 'Dilantin' toxicity.

The presence of phenothiazines may produce false positive phenylketonuria (PKU) test results.

Long-Term Therapy: Given the likelihood that some patients exposed chronically to neuroleptics will develop tardive dyskinesia, it is advised that all patients in whom chronic use is contemplated be given, if possible, full information about this risk. The decision to inform patients and/or their guardians must obviously take into account the clinical circumstances and the competency of the patient to understand the information provided.

To lessen the likelihood of adverse reactions related to cumulative drug effect, patients with a history of long-term therapy with Compazine (prochlorperazine, SK&F) and/or other neuroleptics should be evaluated periodically to decide whether the maintenance dosage could be lowered or drug therapy discontinued.

Children with acute illnesses (e.g., chickenpox, C.N.S. infections, measles, gastroenteritis) or dehydration seem to be much more susceptible to neuromuscular reactions, particularly dystonias, than are adults. In such patients, the drug should be used only under close supervision.

Drugs which lower the seizure threshold, including phenothiazine derivatives, should not be used with Amipaque®§. As with other phenothiazine derivatives, Compazine (prochlorperazine, SK&F) should be discontinued at least 48 hours before myelography, should not be resumed for at least 24 hours postprocedure, and should not be used for the control of nausea and vomiting occurring either prior to myelography with 'Amipaque', or postprocedure.

ADVERSE REACTIONS

Drowsiness, dizziness, amenorrhea, blurred vision, skin reactions and hypotension may occur.

Cholestatic jaundice has occurred. If fever with grippe-like symptoms occurs, appropriate liver studies should be conducted. If tests indicate an abnormality, stop treatment. There have been a few observations of fatty changes in the livers of patients who have died while receiving the drug. No causal relationship has been established.

Leukopenia and agranulocytosis have occurred. Warn patients to report the sudden appearance of sore throat or other signs of infection. If white blood cell and differential counts indicate leukocyte depression, stop treatment and start antibiotic and other suitable therapy.

Neuromuscular (Extrapyramidal) Reactions

These symptoms are seen in a significant number of hospitalized mental patients. They may be characterized by motor restlessness, be of the dystonic type, or they may resemble parkinsonism.

Depending on the severity of symptoms, dosage should be reduced or discontinued. If therapy is reinstituted, it should be at a lower dosage. Should these symptoms occur in children or pregnant patients, the drug should be stopped and not reinstituted. In most cases barbiturates by suitable route of administration will suffice. (Or, injectable Benadryl®ǁ may be useful.) In more severe cases, the administration of an anti-parkinsonism agent, except levodopa, usually produces rapid reversal of symptoms. Suitable supportive measures such as maintaining a clear airway and adequate hydration should be employed.

Motor Restlessness: Symptoms may include agitation or jitteriness and sometimes insomnia. These symptoms often disappear spontaneously. At times these symptoms may be similar to the original neurotic or psychotic symptoms. Dosage should not be increased until these side effects have subsided.

If this phase becomes too troublesome, the symptoms can usually be controlled by a reduction of dosage or change of drug. Treatment with anti-parkinsonian agents, benzodiazepines or propranolol may be helpful.

Dystonias: Symptoms may include: spasm of the neck muscles, sometimes progressing to torticollis; extensor rigidity of back muscles, sometimes progressing to opisthotonos; carpopedal spasm, trismus, swallowing difficulty, oculogyric crisis and protrusion of the tongue.

These usually subside within a few hours, and almost always within 24 to 48 hours, after the drug has been discontinued.

In mild cases, reassurance or a barbiturate is often sufficient. *In moderate cases,* barbiturates will usually bring rapid relief. *In more severe adult cases,* the administration of an anti-parkinsonism agent, except levodopa, usually produces rapid reversal of symptoms. *In children,* reassurance and barbiturates will usually control symptoms. (Or, injectable 'Benadryl' may be useful. Note: See 'Benadryl' prescribing information for appropriate *children's* dosage.) If appropriate treatment with anti-parkinsonism agents or 'Benadryl' fails to reverse the signs and symptoms, the diagnosis should be reevaluated.

Pseudo-parkinsonism: Symptoms may include: mask-like facies; drooling; tremors; pillrolling motion; cogwheel rigidity; and shuffling gait. Reassurance and sedation are important. In most cases these symptoms are readily controlled when an anti-parkinsonism agent is administered concomitantly. Anti-parkinsonism agents should be used only when required. Generally, therapy of a few weeks to two or three months will suffice. After this time patients should be evaluated to determine their need for continued treatment. (Note: Levodopa has not been found effective in pseudo-parkinsonism.) Occasionally it is necessary to lower the dosage of Compazine (prochlorperazine, SK&F) or to discontinue the drug.

Tardive Dyskinesia: As with all antipsychotic agents, tardive dyskinesia may appear in some patients on long-term therapy or may appear after drug therapy has been discontinued. The syndrome can also develop, although much less frequently, after relatively brief treatment periods at low doses. This syndrome appears in all age groups. Although its prevalence appears to be highest among elderly patients, especially elderly women, it is impossible to rely upon prevalence estimates to predict at the inception of neuroleptic treatment which patients are likely to develop the syndrome. The symptoms are persistent and in some patients appear to be irreversible. The syndrome is characterized by rhythmical involuntary movements of the tongue, face, mouth or jaw (e.g., protrusion of tongue, puffing of cheeks, puckering of mouth, chewing movements). Sometimes these may be accompanied by involuntary movements of extremities. In rare instances, these involuntary movements of the extremities are the only manifestations of tardive dyskinesia. A variant of tardive dyskinesia, tardive dystonia, has also been described.

There is no known effective treatment for tardive dyskinesia; anti-parkinsonism agents do not alleviate the symptoms of this syndrome. It is suggested that all antipsychotic agents be discontinued if these symptoms appear. Should it be necessary to reinstitute treatment, or increase the dosage of the agent, or switch to a different antipsychotic agent, the syndrome may be masked.

It has been reported that fine vermicular movements of the tongue may be an early sign of the syndrome and if the medication is stopped at that time the syndrome may not develop.

Contact Dermatitis: Avoid getting the Injection solution on hands or clothing because of the possibility of contact dermatitis.

Adverse Reactions Reported with Compazine (prochlorperazine, SK&F) or Other Phenothiazine Derivatives: Adverse reactions with different phenothiazines vary in type, frequency, and mechanism of occurrence, i.e., some are dose-related, while others involve individual patient sensitivity. Some adverse reactions may be more likely to occur, or occur with greater intensity, in patients with special medical problems, e.g., patients with mitral insufficiency or pheochromocytoma have experienced severe hypotension following recommended doses of certain phenothiazines.

Not all of the following adverse reactions have been observed with every phenothiazine derivative, but they have been reported with one or more and should be borne in mind when drugs of this class are administered: extrapyramidal symptoms (opisthotonos, oculogyric crisis, hyperreflexia, dystonia, akathisia, dyskinesia, parkinsonism) some of which have lasted months and even years—particularly in elderly patients with previous brain damage; grand mal and petit mal convulsions, particularly in patients with EEG abnormalities or history of such disorders; altered cerebrospinal fluid proteins; cerebral edema; intensification and prolongation of the action of central nervous system depressants (opiates, analgesics, antihistamines, barbiturates, alcohol), atropine, heat, organophosphorus insecticides; autonomic reactions (dryness of mouth, nasal congestion, headache, nausea, constipation, obstipation, adynamic ileus, ejaculatory disorders/impotence, priapism, atonic colon, urinary retention, miosis and mydriasis); reactivation of psychotic processes, catatonic-like states; hypotension (sometimes fatal); cardiac arrest; blood dyscrasias (pancytopenia, thrombocytopenic purpura, leukopenia, agranulocytosis, eosinophilia, hemolytic anemia, aplastic anemia); liver damage (jaundice, biliary stasis); endocrine disturbances (hyperglycemia, hypoglycemia, glycosuria, lactation, galactorrhea, gynecomastia, menstrual irregularities, false positive pregnancy tests); skin disorders (photosensitivity, itching, erythema, urticaria, eczema up to exfoliative dermatitis); other allergic reactions

Continued on next page

Smith Kline & French—Cont.

(asthma, laryngeal edema, angioneurotic edema, anaphylactoid reactions); peripheral edema; reversed epinephrine effect; hyperpyrexia; mild fever after large I.M. doses; increased appetite; increased weight; a systemic lupus erythematosus-like syndrome; pigmentary retinopathy; with prolonged administration of substantial doses, skin pigmentation, epithelial keratopathy, and lenticular and corneal deposits.

EKG changes—particularly nonspecific, usually reversible Q and T wave distortions—have been observed in some patients receiving phenothiazine tranquilizers.

Although phenothiazines cause neither psychic nor physical dependence, sudden discontinuance in long-term psychiatric patients may cause temporary symptoms, e.g., nausea and vomiting, dizziness, tremulousness.

Note: There have been occasional reports of sudden death in patients receiving phenothiazines. In some cases, the cause appeared to be cardiac arrest or asphyxia due to failure of the cough reflex.

DOSAGE AND ADMINISTRATION

Notes on Injection: *Stability*—This solution should be protected from light. Slight yellowish discoloration will not alter potency. If markedly discolored, solution should be discarded.

Compatibility—It is recommended that Compazine (prochlorperazine, SK&F) Injection not be mixed with other agents in the syringe. Do not dilute the contents of 'Compazine' ampuls with any diluent that contains parabens as a preservative.

DOSAGE AND ADMINISTRATION—ADULTS

(For children's dosage and administration, see below.) Dosage should be increased more gradually in debilitated or emaciated patients.

Elderly Patients: In general, dosages in the lower range are sufficient for most elderly patients. Since they appear to be more susceptible to hypotension and neuromuscular reactions, such patients should be observed closely. Dosage should be tailored to the individual, response carefully monitored, and dosage adjusted accordingly. Dosage should be increased more gradually in elderly patients.

1. To Control Severe Nausea and Vomiting: Adjust dosage to the response of the individual. Begin with the lowest recommended dosage.

Oral Dosage—Tablets: Usually one 5 mg. or 10 mg. tablet 3 or 4 times daily. Daily dosages above 40 mg. should be used only in resistant cases.

'Spansule' capsules: Initially, usually one 15 mg. capsule on arising or one 10 mg. capsule q12h. Some patients may subsequently require one 30 mg. capsule in the morning. Daily doses above 40 mg. should be used only in resistant cases.

Rectal Dosage: 25 mg. twice daily.

I.M. Dosage: Initially 5 to 10 mg. (1–2 mL.) injected *deeply* into the upper outer quadrant of the buttock. If necessary, repeat every 3 or 4 hours. Total I.M. dosage should not exceed 40 mg. per day.

I.V. Dosage: $2\frac{1}{2}$ to 10 mg. ($\frac{1}{2}$ to 2 mL.) by slow I.V. injection or infusion at a rate not to exceed 5 mg. per minute. 'Compazine' Injection may be administered either undiluted or diluted in isotonic solution. A single dose of the drug should not exceed 10 mg.; total I.V. dosage should not exceed 40 mg. per day. When administered I.V., do not use bolus injection. Hypotension is a possibility if the drug is given by I.V. injection or infusion.

Subcutaneous administration is not advisable because of local irritation.

2. Adult Surgery (for severe nausea and vomiting): Total parenteral dosage should not exceed 40 mg. per day. Hypotension is a possibility if the drug is given by I.V. injection or infusion.

I.M. Dosage: 5 to 10 mg. (1–2 mL.) 1 to 2 hours before induction of anesthesia (repeat once in 30 minutes, if necessary), or to control acute symptoms during and after surgery (repeat once if necessary).

I.V. Dosage: 5 to 10 mg. (1–2 mL.) as a slow I.V. injection or infusion 15 to 30 minutes before induction of anesthesia, or to control acute symptoms during or after surgery. Repeat once if necessary. Compazine (prochlorperazine, SK&F) may be administered either undiluted or diluted in isotonic solution, but a single dose of the drug should not exceed 10 mg. The rate of administration should not exceed 5 mg. per minute. When administered I.V., do not use bolus injection.

3. In Adult Psychiatric Disorders: Adjust dosage to the response of the individual and according to the severity of the condition. Begin with the lowest recommended dose. Although response ordinarily is seen within a day or two, longer treatment is usually required before maximal improvement is seen.

Oral Dosage: *Non-Psychotic Anxiety*—Usual dosage is 5 mg. 3 or 4 times daily; by 'Spansule' capsule, usually one 15 mg. capsule on arising or one 10 mg. capsule q12h. Do not

administer in doses of more than 20 mg. per day or for longer than 12 weeks.

Psychotic Disorders—*In relatively mild conditions,* as seen in private psychiatric practice or in outpatient clinics, dosage is 5 or 10 mg. 3 or 4 times daily.

In moderate to severe conditions, for hospitalized or adequately supervised patients, usual starting dosage is 10 mg. 3 or 4 times daily. Increase dosage gradually until symptoms are controlled or side effects become bothersome. When dosage is increased by small increments every 2 or 3 days, side effects either do not occur or are easily controlled. Some patients respond satisfactorily on 50 to 75 mg. daily.

In more severe disturbances, optimum dosage is usually 100 to 150 mg. daily.

I.M. Dosage: For immediate control of severely disturbed adults, inject an initial dose of 10 to 20 mg. (2–4 mL.) *deeply* into the upper outer quadrant of the buttock. Many patients respond shortly after the first injection. If necessary, however, repeat the initial dose every 2 to 4 hours (or, in resistant cases, every hour) to gain control of the patient. More than 3 or 4 doses are seldom necessary. After control is achieved, switch patient to an oral form of the drug at the same dosage level or higher. If, in rare cases, parenteral therapy is needed for a prolonged period, give 10 to 20 mg. (2–4 mL.) every 4 to 6 hours. Pain and irritation at the site of injection have seldom occurred.

Subcutaneous administration is not advisable because of local irritation.

DOSAGE AND ADMINISTRATION—CHILDREN

Do not use in pediatric surgery.

Children are more prone to develop extrapyramidal reactions, even on moderate doses. Therefore, use lowest effective dosage. Tell parents not to exceed prescribed dosage, since the possibility of adverse reactions increases as dosage rises. Occasionally the patient may react to the drug with signs of restlessness and excitement; if this occurs, do not administer additional doses. Take particular precaution in administering the drug to children with acute illnesses or dehydration (see under Dystonias).

When writing a prescription for the $2\frac{1}{2}$ mg. size suppository, write "$2\frac{1}{2}$," not "2.5"; this will help avoid confusion with the 25 mg. adult size.

1. Severe Nausea and Vomiting in Children: Compazine (prochlorperazine, SK&F) should not be used in children under 20 pounds in weight or two years of age. It should not be used in conditions for which children's dosages have not been established. Dosage and frequency of administration should be adjusted according to the severity of the symptoms and the response of the patient. The duration of activity following intramuscular administration may last up to 12 hours. Subsequent doses may be given by the same route if necessary.

Oral or Rectal Dosage: More than one day's therapy is seldom necessary.

Weight	Usual Dosage	Not to Exceed
under 20 lbs.	not recommended	
20–29 lbs.	$2\frac{1}{2}$ mg. 1 or 2 times a day	7.5 mg. per day
30–39 lbs.	$2\frac{1}{2}$ mg. 2 or 3 times a day	10 mg. per day
40–85 lbs.	$2\frac{1}{2}$ mg. 3 times a day or 5 mg. 2 times a day	15 mg. per day

I.M. Dosage: Calculate each dose on the basis of 0.06 mg. of the drug per lb. of body weight; give by deep I.M. injection. Control is usually obtained with one dose.

2. In Psychotic Children:

Oral or Rectal Dosage: For children 2 to 12 years, starting dosage is $2\frac{1}{2}$ mg. 2 or 3 times daily. Do not give more than 10 mg. the first day. Then increase dosage according to patient's response.

FOR AGES 2–5, total daily dosage usually does not exceed 20 mg.

FOR AGES 6–12, total daily dosage usually does not exceed 25 mg.

I.M. Dosage: For ages under 12, calculate each dose on the basis of 0.06 mg. of Compazine (prochlorperazine, SK&F) per lb. of body weight; give by deep I.M. injection. Control is usually obtained with one dose. After control is achieved, switch the patient to an oral form of the drug at the same dosage level or higher.

OVERDOSAGE

(See also Adverse Reactions.)

SYMPTOMS—Primarily involvement of the extrapyramidal mechanism producing some of the dystonic reactions described above.

Symptoms of central nervous system depression to the point of somnolence or coma. Agitation and restlessness may also

occur. Other possible manifestations include convulsions, EKG changes and cardiac arrhythmias, fever, and autonomic reactions such as hypotension, dry mouth and ileus.

TREATMENT—It is important to determine other medications taken by the patient since multiple dose therapy is common in overdosage situations. Treatment is essentially symptomatic and supportive. Early gastric lavage is helpful. Keep patient under observation and maintain an open airway, since involvement of the extrapyramidal mechanism may produce dysphagia and respiratory difficulty in severe overdosage. **Do not attempt to induce emesis because a dystonic reaction of the head or neck may develop that could result in aspiration of vomitus.** Extrapyramidal symptoms may be treated with anti-parkinsonism drugs, barbiturates, or 'Benadryl'. See prescribing information for these products. Care should be taken to avoid increasing respiratory depression.

If administration of a stimulant is desirable, amphetamine, dextroamphetamine, or caffeine with sodium benzoate is recommended. Stimulants that may cause convulsions (e.g., picrotoxin or pentylenetetrazol) should be avoided.

If hypotension occurs, the standard measures for managing circulatory shock should be initiated. If it is desirable to administer a vasoconstrictor, 'Levophed' and 'Neo-Synephrine' are most suitable. Other pressor agents, including epinephrine, are not recommended because phenothiazine derivatives may reverse the usual elevating action of these agents and cause a further lowering of blood pressure.

Limited experience indicates that phenothiazines are *not* dialyzable.

Special note on 'Spansule' capsules—Since much of the 'Spansule' capsule medication is coated for gradual release, therapy directed at reversing the effects of the ingested drug and at supporting the patient should be continued for as long as overdosage symptoms remain. Saline cathartics are useful for hastening evacuation of pellets that have not already released medication.

HOW SUPPLIED

Tablets—5 and 10 mg., in bottles of 100 and 1000; in Single Unit Packages of 100 (intended for institutional use only). For use in severe neuropsychiatric conditions, 25 mg., in bottles of 100 and 1000.

'Spansule' capsules—10, 15 and 30 mg., in bottles of 50 and 500; in Single Unit Packages of 100 (intended for institutional use only).

Ampuls—2 mL. (5 mg./mL.), in boxes of 10 and 100.

Multiple-dose Vials—10 mL. (5 mg./mL.), in boxes of 1, 20 and 100.

Disposable Syringes—2 mL. (5 mg./mL.), in individual cartons.

Suppositories—$2\frac{1}{2}$ mg. (for young children), 5 mg. (for older children) and 25 mg. (for adults), in boxes of 12.

Syrup—5 mg./5 mL. (1 teaspoonful) in 4 fl. oz. bottles.

Veterans Administration—Injection, 10 mL., 100's, 6505-00-684-9630; 'Spansule' Capsules, 15 mg., 500's, 6505-00-014-1188.

Military—Suppositories, $2\frac{1}{2}$ mg., 12's, 6505-00-133-5213; 5 mg., 12's, 6505-01-153-2894; 25 mg., 12's, 6505-00-133-5214; Tablets, 5 mg., SUP 100's 6505-00-118-2563.

* norepinephrine bitartrate, Winthrop Pharmaceuticals.
† phenylephrine hydrochloride, Winthrop Pharmaceuticals.
‡ phenytoin, Parke-Davis.
§ metrizamide, Winthrop Pharmaceuticals.
ꟾ diphenhydramine hydrochloride, Parke-Davis.

CZ:L74

Shown in Product Identification Section, page 430

CYTOMEL®   ℞

[sigh "toe'mel]
brand of liothyronine sodium
Tablets

PRODUCT OVERVIEW

KEY FACTS

'Cytomel' contains liothyronine, a synthetic form of a natural thyroid hormone. It is available in tablets in three strengths: 5 mcg., 25 mcg. and 50 mcg. tablets.

MAJOR USES

'Cytomel' is indicated as replacement or supplemental therapy in patients with hypothyroidism of any etiology, except transient hypothyroidism during the recovery phase of subacute thyroiditis; as a pituitary thyroid-stimulating hormone (TSH) suppressant, and as a diagnostic agent in suppression tests.

SAFETY INFORMATION

Thyroid hormone preparations are generally contraindicated in patients with diagnosed but as yet uncorrected adrenal cortical insufficiency, untreated thyrotoxicosis and apparent hypersensitivity to any of their active or extraneous constituents. There is no well-documented evidence from the literature, however, of true allergic or idiosyncratic reactions to thyroid hormone.

Drugs with thyroid hormone activity, alone or with other therapeutic agents, have been used for treatment of obesity. In euthyroid patients, doses within range of daily hormonal requirements are ineffective for weight reduction. Larger doses may produce serious or even life-threatening manifestations of toxicity. (See full prescribing information, below.)

PRESCRIBING INFORMATION

CYTOMEL®

[sigh "toe 'mel]

brand of liothyronine sodium

Tablets

DESCRIPTION

Thyroid hormone drugs are natural or synthetic preparations containing tetraiodothyronine (T_4, levothyroxine) sodium or triiodothyronine (T_3, liothyronine) sodium or both. T_4 and T_3 are produced in the human thyroid gland by the iodination and coupling of the amino acid tyrosine. T_4 contains four iodine atoms and is formed by the coupling of two molecules of diiodotyrosine (DIT). T_3 contains three atoms of iodine and is formed by the coupling of one molecule of DIT with one molecule of monoiodotyrosine (MIT). Both hormones are stored in the thyroid colloid as thyroglobulin.

Thyroid hormone preparations belong to two categories: (1) natural hormonal preparations derived from animal thyroid, and (2) synthetic preparations. Natural preparations include desiccated thyroid and thyroglobulin. Desiccated thyroid is derived from domesticated animals that are used for food by man (either beef or hog thyroid), and thyroglobulin is derived from thyroid glands of the hog. The United States Pharmacopeia (USP) has standardized the total iodine content of natural preparations. Thyroid USP contains not less than (NLT) 0.17 percent and not more than (NMT) 0.23 percent iodine, and thyroglobulin contains not less than (NLT) 0.7 percent of organically bound iodine. Iodine content is only an indirect indicator of true hormonal biologic activity.

Cytomel (liothyronine sodium, SK&F) Tablets contain liothyronine (L-triiodothyronine or LT_3), a synthetic form of a natural thyroid hormone, and is available as the sodium salt. Twenty-five mcg. of liothyronine is equivalent to approximately 1 grain of desiccated thyroid or thyroglobulin and 0.1 mg. of L-thyroxine.

Each round, white Cytomel (liothyronine sodium, SK&F) tablet contains liothyronine sodium equivalent to liothyronine as follows: 5 mcg. debossed SKF and D14; 25 mcg. scored and debossed SKF and D16; 50 mcg. scored and debossed SKF and D17. Inactive ingredients consist of calcium sulfate, gelatin, starch, stearic acid, sucrose and talc.

CLINICAL PHARMACOLOGY

The mechanisms by which thyroid hormones exert their physiologic action are not well understood. These hormones enhance oxygen consumption by most tissues of the body, increase the basal metabolic rate and the metabolism of carbohydrates, lipids and proteins. Thus, they exert a profound influence on every organ system in the body and are of particular importance in the development of the central nervous system.

Pharmacokinetics

Since liothyronine sodium (T_3) is not firmly bound to serum protein, it is readily available to body tissues. The onset of activity of liothyronine sodium is rapid, occurring within a few hours. Maximum pharmacologic response occurs within two or three days, providing early clinical response. The biological half-life is about 2-½ days.

T_3 is almost totally absorbed, 95 percent in four hours. The hormones contained in the natural preparations are absorbed in a manner similar to the synthetic hormones.

Liothyronine sodium has a rapid cutoff of activity which permits quick dosage adjustment and facilitates control of the effects of overdosage, should they occur.

The higher affinity of levothyroxine (T_4) for both thyroid-binding globulin and thyroid-binding prealbumin as compared to triiodothyronine (T_3) partially explains the higher serum levels and longer half-life of the former hormone. Both protein-bound hormones exist in reverse equilibrium with minute amounts of free hormone, the latter accounting for the metabolic activity.

INDICATIONS AND USAGE

Thyroid hormone drugs are indicated:

1. As replacement or supplemental therapy in patients with hypothyroidism of any etiology, except transient hypothyroidism during the recovery phase of subacute thyroiditis. This category includes cretinism, myxedema and ordinary hypothyroidism in patients of any age (children, adults, the elderly), or state (including pregnancy); primary hypothyroidism resulting from functional deficiency, primary atrophy, partial or total absence of thyroid gland, or the effects of surgery, radiation, or drugs, with or without the presence of goiter; and secondary (pituitary) or tertiary (hypothalamic) hypothyroidism (See WARNINGS).

2. As pituitary thyroid-stimulating hormone (TSH) suppressants, in the treatment or prevention of various types of euthyroid goiters, including thyroid nodules, subacute or chronic lymphocytic thyroiditis (Hashimoto's) and multinodular goiter.

3. As diagnostic agents in suppression tests to differentiate suspected mild hyperthyroidism or thyroid gland autonomy.

Cytomel (liothyronine sodium, SK&F) Tablets can be used in patients allergic to desiccated thyroid or thyroid extract derived from pork or beef.

CONTRAINDICATIONS

Thyroid hormone preparations are generally contraindicated in patients with diagnosed but as yet uncorrected adrenal cortical insufficiency, untreated thyrotoxicosis and apparent hypersensitivity to any of their active or extraneous constituents. There is no well-documented evidence from the literature, however, of true allergic or idiosyncratic reactions to thyroid hormone.

WARNINGS

> Drugs with thyroid hormone activity, alone or together with other therapeutic agents, have been used for the treatment of obesity. In euthyroid patients, doses within the range of daily hormonal requirements are ineffective for weight reduction. Larger doses may produce serious or even life-threatening manifestations of toxicity, particularly when given in association with sympathomimetic amines such as those used for their anorectic effects.

The use of thyroid hormones in the therapy of obesity, alone or combined with other drugs, is unjustified and has been shown to be ineffective. Neither is their use justified for the treatment of male or female infertility unless this condition is accompanied by hypothyroidism.

Thyroid hormones should be used with great caution in a number of circumstances where the integrity of the cardiovascular system, particularly the coronary arteries, is suspected. These include patients with angina pectoris or the elderly, in whom there is a greater likelihood of occult cardiac disease. In these patients, liothyronine sodium therapy should be initiated with low doses, with due consideration for its relatively rapid onset of action. Starting dosage of Cytomel (liothyronine sodium, SK&F) Tablets is 5 mcg. daily, and should be increased by no more than 5 mcg. increments at two-week intervals. When, in such patients, a euthyroid state can only be reached at the expense of an aggravation of the cardiovascular disease, thyroid hormone dosage should be reduced.

Morphologic hypogonadism and nephrosis should be ruled out before the drug is administered. If hypopituitarism is present, the adrenal deficiency must be corrected prior to starting the drug.

Myxedematous patients are very sensitive to thyroid; dosage should be started at a very low level and increased gradually. Severe and prolonged hypothyroidism can lead to a decreased level of adrenocortical activity commensurate with the lowered metabolic state. When thyroid-replacement therapy is administered, the metabolism increases at a greater rate than adrenocortical activity. This can precipitate adrenocortical insufficiency. Therefore, in severe and prolonged hypothyroidism, supplemental adrenocortical steroids may be necessary.

In rare instances the administration of thyroid hormone may precipitate a hyperthyroid state or may aggravate existing hyperthyroidism.

PRECAUTIONS

General—Thyroid hormone therapy in patients with concomitant diabetes mellitus or insipidus or adrenal cortical insufficiency aggravates the intensity of their symptoms. Appropriate adjustments of the various therapeutic measures directed at these concomitant endocrine diseases are required.

The therapy of myxedema coma requires simultaneous administration of glucocorticoids.

Hypothyroidism decreases and hyperthyroidism increases the sensitivity to oral anticoagulants. Prothrombin time should be closely monitored in thyroid-treated patients on oral anticoagulants and dosage of the latter agents adjusted on the basis of frequent prothrombin time determinations. In infants, excessive doses of thyroid hormone preparations may produce craniosynostosis.

Information for the Patient—Patients on thyroid hormone preparations and parents of children on thyroid therapy should be informed that:

1. Replacement therapy is to be taken essentially for life, with the exception of cases of transient hypothyroidism, usually associated with thyroiditis, and in those patients receiving a therapeutic trial of the drug.

2. They should immediately report during the course of therapy any signs or symptoms of thyroid hormone toxicity, e.g., chest pain, increased pulse rate, palpitations, excessive sweating, heat intolerance, nervousness, or any other unusual event.

3. In case of concomitant diabetes mellitus, the daily dosage of antidiabetic medication may need readjustment as thyroid hormone replacement is achieved. If thyroid medication is stopped, a downward readjustment of the dosage of insulin or oral hypoglycemic agent may be necessary to avoid hypoglycemia. At all times, close monitoring of urinary glucose levels is mandatory in such patients.

4. In case of concomitant oral anticoagulant therapy, the prothrombin time should be measured frequently to determine if the dosage of oral anticoagulants is to be readjusted.

5. Partial loss of hair may be experienced by children in the first few months of thyroid therapy, but this is usually a transient phenomenon and later recovery is usually the rule.

Laboratory Tests—Treatment of patients with thyroid hormones requires the periodic assessment of thyroid status by means of appropriate laboratory tests besides the full clinical evaluation. The TSH suppression test can be used to test the effectiveness of any thyroid preparation, bearing in mind the relative insensitivity of the infant pituitary to the negative feedback effect of thyroid hormones. Serum T_4 levels can be used to test the effectiveness of all thyroid medications except products containing liothyronine sodium. When the total serum T_4 is low but TSH is normal, a test specific to assess unbound (free) T_4 levels is warranted. Specific measurements of T_4 and T_3 by competitive protein binding or radioimmunoassay are not influenced by blood levels of organic or inorganic iodine and have essentially replaced older tests of thyroid hormone measurements, i.e., PBI, BEI and T_4 by column.

Drug Interactions

Oral Anticoagulants—Thyroid hormones appear to increase catabolism of vitamin K-dependent clotting factors. If oral anticoagulants are also being given, compensatory increases in clotting factor synthesis are impaired. Patients stabilized on oral anticoagulants who are found to require thyroid replacement therapy should be watched very closely when thyroid is started. If a patient is truly hypothyroid, it is likely that a reduction in anticoagulant dosage will be required. No special precautions appear to be necessary when oral anticoagulant therapy is begun in a patient already stabilized on maintenance thyroid replacement therapy.

Insulin or Oral Hypoglycemics—Initiating thyroid replacement therapy may cause increases in insulin or oral hypoglycemic requirements. The effects seen are poorly understood and depend upon a variety of factors such as dose and type of thyroid preparations and endocrine status of the patient. Patients receiving insulin or oral hypoglycemics should be closely watched during initiation of thyroid replacement therapy.

Cholestyramine—Cholestyramine binds both T_4 and T_3 in the intestine, thus impairing absorption of these thyroid hormones. *In vitro* studies indicate that the binding is not easily removed. Therefore, four to five hours should elapse between administration of cholestyramine and thyroid hormones.

Estrogen, Oral Contraceptives—Estrogens tend to increase serum thyroxine-binding globulin (TBg). In a patient with a nonfunctioning thyroid gland who is receiving thyroid replacement therapy, free levothyroxine may be decreased when estrogens are started thus increasing thyroid requirements. However, if the patient's thyroid gland has sufficient function, the decreased free thyroxine will result in a compensatory increase in thyroxine output by the thyroid. Therefore, patients without a functioning thyroid gland who are on thyroid replacement therapy may need to increase their thyroid dose if estrogens or estrogen-containing oral contraceptives are given.

Tricyclic Antidepressants—Use of thyroid products with imipramine and other tricyclic antidepressants may increase receptor sensitivity and enhance antidepressant activity; transient cardiac arrhythmias have been observed. Thyroid hormone activity may also be enhanced.

Digitalis—Thyroid preparations may potentiate the toxic effects of digitalis. Thyroid hormonal replacement increases metabolic rate, which requires an increase in digitalis dosage.

Ketamine—When administered to patients on a thyroid preparation, this parenteral anesthetic may cause hypertension and tachycardia. Use with caution and be prepared to treat hypertension, if necessary.

Levarterenol—Thyroxine increases the adrenergic effect of catecholamines such as epinephrine and norepinephrine. Therefore, injection of these agents into patients receiving thyroid preparations increases the risk of precipitating coronary insufficiency, especially in patients with coronary artery disease. Careful observation is required.

Drug/Laboratory Test Interactions—The following drugs or moieties are known to interfere with laboratory tests performed in patients on thyroid hormone therapy: androgens,

Continued on next page

Smith Kline & French—Cont.

corticosteroids, estrogens, oral contraceptives containing estrogens, iodine-containing preparations and the numerous preparations containing salicylates.

1. Changes in TBg concentration should be taken into consideration in the interpretation of T_4 and T_3 values. In such cases, the unbound (free) hormone should be measured. Pregnancy, estrogens and estrogen-containing oral contraceptives increase TBg concentrations. TBg may also be increased during infectious hepatitis. Decreases in TBg concentrations are observed in nephrosis, acromegaly and after androgen or corticosteroid therapy. Familial hyper- or hypo-thyroxine-binding-globulinemias have been described. The incidence of TBg deficiency approximates 1 in 9000. The binding of thyroxine by thyroxine-binding prealbumin (TBPA) is inhibited by salicylates.
2. Medicinal or dietary iodine interferes with all *in vivo* tests of radioiodine uptake, producing low uptakes which may not be reflective of a true decrease in hormone synthesis.
3. The persistence of clinical and laboratory evidence of hypothyroidism in spite of adequate dosage replacement indicates either poor patient compliance, poor absorption, excessive fecal loss, or inactivity of the preparation. Intracellular resistance to thyroid hormone is quite rare.

Carcinogenesis, Mutagenesis and Impairment of Fertility—A reportedly apparent association between prolonged thyroid therapy and breast cancer has not been confirmed and patients on thyroid for established indications should not discontinue therapy. No confirmatory long-term studies in animals have been performed to evaluate carcinogenic potential, mutagenicity, or impairment of fertility in either males or females.

Pregnancy—Category A. Thyroid hormones do not readily cross the placental barrier. The clinical experience to date does not indicate any adverse effect on fetuses when thyroid hormones are administered to pregnant women. On the basis of current knowledge, thyroid replacement therapy to hypothyroid women should not be discontinued during pregnancy.

Nursing Mothers—Minimal amounts of thyroid hormones are excreted in human milk. Thyroid is not associated with serious adverse reactions and does not have a known tumorigenic potential. However, caution should be exercised when thyroid is administered to a nursing woman.

Pediatric Use—Pregnant mothers provide little or no thyroid hormone to the fetus. The incidence of congenital hypothyroidism is relatively high (1:4000) and the hypothyroid fetus would not derive any benefit from the small amounts of hormone crossing the placental barrier. Routine determinations of serum T_4 and/or TSH is strongly advised in neonates in view of the deleterious effects of thyroid deficiency on growth and development.

Treatment should be initiated immediately upon diagnosis and maintained for life, unless transient hypothyroidism is suspected, in which case, therapy may be interrupted for two to eight weeks after the age of three years to reassess the condition. Cessation of therapy is justified in patients who have maintained a normal TSH during those two to eight weeks.

ADVERSE REACTIONS

Adverse reactions, other than those indicative of hyperthyroidism because of therapeutic overdosage, either initially or during the maintenance period are rare (See OVERDOSAGE).

In rare instances, allergic skin reactions have been reported with Cytomel (liothyronine sodium, SK&F) Tablets.

OVERDOSAGE

Signs and Symptoms—Headache, irritability, nervousness, sweating, tachycardia, increased bowel motility and menstrual irregularities. Angina pectoris or congestive heart failure may be induced or aggravated. Shock may also develop. Massive overdosage may result in symptoms resembling thyroid storm. Chronic excessive dosage will produce the signs and symptoms of hyperthyroidism.

Treatment of Overdosage—Dosage should be reduced or therapy temporarily discontinued if signs and symptoms of overdosage appear. Treatment may be reinstituted at a lower dosage. In normal individuals, normal hypothalamic-pituitary-thyroid axis function is restored in six to eight weeks after thyroid suppression.

Treatment of acute massive thyroid hormone overdosage is aimed at reducing gastrointestinal absorption of the drugs and counteracting central and peripheral effects, mainly those of increased sympathetic activity. Vomiting may be induced initially if further gastrointestinal absorption can reasonably be prevented and barring contraindications such as coma, convulsions, or loss of the gagging reflex. Treatment is symptomatic and supportive. Oxygen may be administered and ventilation maintained. Cardiac glycosides may be indicated if congestive heart failure develops. Measures to control fever, hypoglycemia, or fluid loss should be instituted if needed. Antiadrenergic agents, particularly propranolol,

have been used advantageously in the treatment of increased sympathetic activity. Propranolol may be administered intravenously at a dosage of 1 to 3 mg. over a 10-minute period or orally, 80 to 160 mg./day, especially when no contraindications exist for its use.

DOSAGE AND ADMINISTRATION

The dosage of thyroid hormones is determined by the indication and must in every case be individualized according to patient response and laboratory findings.

Thyroid hormones are given orally. In acute, emergency conditions, injectable levothyroxine sodium may be given intravenously when oral administration is not feasible or desirable, as in the treatment of myxedema coma or during total parenteral nutrition. Injectable liothyronine sodium is also available from Smith Kline & French Laboratories upon request, under investigational status, for the treatment of myxedema coma. Intramuscular administration of these two preparations is not advisable because of reported poor absorption.

With Cytomel (liothyronine sodium, SK&F) Tablets once-a-day dosage is recommended; although liothyronine sodium has a rapid cutoff, its metabolic effects persist for a few days following discontinuance.

Mild Hypothyroidism: Recommended starting dosage is 25 mcg. daily. Daily dosage then may be increased by 12.5 or 25 mcg. every one or two weeks. Usual maintenance dose is 25-75 mcg. daily. Smaller doses may be fully effective in some patients, while dosage of 100 mcg. daily may be required in others.

The rapid onset and dissipation of action of liothyronine sodium (T_3), as compared with levothyroxine sodium (T_4), has led some clinicians to prefer its use in patients who might be more susceptible to the untoward effects of thyroid medication. However, the wide swings in serum T_3 levels that follow its administration and the possibility of more pronounced cardiovascular side effects tend to counterbalance the stated advantages.

Cytomel (liothyronine sodium, SK&F) Tablets may be used in preference to levothyroxine (T_4) during radioisotope scanning procedures, since induction of hypothyroidism in those cases is more abrupt and can be of shorter duration. It may also be preferred when impairment of peripheral conversion of T_4 and T_3 is suspected.

Myxedema: Recommended starting dosage is 5 mcg. daily. This may be increased by 5 to 10 mcg. daily every one or two weeks. When 25 mcg. daily is reached, dosage may often be increased by 12.5 or 25 mcg. every one or two weeks. Usual maintenance dose is 50 to 100 mcg. daily.

Myxedema Coma: Myxedema coma is usually precipitated in the hypothyroid patient of long standing by intercurrent illness or drugs such as sedatives and anesthetics and should be considered a medical emergency. A 'Cytomel' Injection Kit for the emergency treatment of myxedema coma is available from Smith Kline & French Laboratories upon request, under investigational status. Instructions which accompany this kit provide information on administration.

Congenital Hypothyroidism: Recommended starting dosage is 5 mcg. daily, with a 5 mcg. increment every three to four days until the desired response is achieved. Infants a few months old may require only 20 mcg. daily for maintenance. At one year, 50 mcg. daily may be needed. Above three years, full adult dosage may be necessary (See PRECAUTIONS, Pediatric Use).

Simple (non-toxic) Goiter: Recommended starting dosage is 5 mcg. daily. This dosage may be increased by 5 to 10 mcg. daily every one or two weeks. When 25 mcg. daily is reached, dosage may be increased every week or two by 12.5 or 25 mcg. Usual maintenance dosage is 75 mcg. daily.

In the elderly or in children, therapy should be started with 5 mcg. daily and increased only by 5 mcg. increments at the recommended intervals.

When switching a patient to Cytomel (liothyronine sodium, SK&F) Tablets from thyroid, L-thyroxine or thyroglobulin, discontinue the other medication, initiate 'Cytomel' at a low dosage, and increase gradually according to the patient's response. When selecting a starting dosage, bear in mind that this drug has a rapid onset of action, and that residual effects of the other thyroid preparation may persist for the first several weeks of therapy.

Thyroid Suppression Therapy: Administration of thyroid hormone in doses higher than those produced physiologically by the gland results in suppression of the production of endogenous hormone. This is the basis for the thyroid suppression test and is used as an aid in the diagnosis of patients with signs of mild hyperthyroidism in whom baseline laboratory tests appear normal or to demonstrate thyroid gland autonomy in patients with Graves' ophthalmopathy. [131]I uptake is determined before and after the administration of the exogenous hormone. A 50 percent or greater suppression of uptake indicates a normal thyroid-pituitary axis and thus rules out thyroid gland autonomy.

Cytomel (liothyronine sodium, SK&F) Tablets are given in doses of 75-100 mcg./day for seven days, and radioactive iodine uptake is determined before and after administration of

the hormone. If thyroid function is under normal control, the radioiodine uptake will drop significantly after treatment. Cytomel (liothyronine sodium, SK&F) Tablets should be administered cautiously to patients in whom there is a strong suspicion of thyroid gland autonomy, in view of the fact that the exogenous hormone effects will be additive to the endogenous source.

HOW SUPPLIED

Cytomel (liothyronine sodium, SK&F) tablets: 5 mcg. in bottles of 100; 25 mcg. in bottles of 100 and 1000; and 50 mcg. in bottles of 100.

CY:L30

Shown in Product Identification Section, page 430

DARBID® TABLETS, 5 mg.   ℞

[dahr'bid]
(brand of isopropamide iodide)

DESCRIPTION

Darbid (brand of isopropamide iodide) is available as a tablet for oral administration. Each tablet contains isopropamide iodide equivalent to 5 mg. of isopropamide. Inactive ingredients consist of acacia, calcium sulfate, FD&C Red No. 3, FD&C Yellow No. 6, gelatin, iron oxide, mineral oil, starch, stearic acid, sucrose, talc, titanium dioxide and trace amounts of other inactive ingredients.

Chemically, isopropamide iodide is (3-carbamoyl-3, 3-diphenylpropyl) diisopropylmethyl ammonium iodide. The empirical formula is $C_{23}H_{33}IN_2O$, representing a molecular weight of 480.42:

'Darbid' is an anticholinergic.

Solubility Characteristics: Isopropamide iodide is freely soluble in chloroform, soluble in alcohol and sparingly soluble in water.

CLINICAL PHARMACOLOGY

Isopropamide iodide is a synthetic quaternary ammonium compound of the anticholinergic drug class that can inhibit vagal activity by blocking the actions of acetylcholine and nerve stimulation to those effector organs innervated by postganglionic cholinergic fibers. By this mechanism, it produces both gastric acid antisecretory effect and inhibition of gastrointestinal motility in man. These effects may last as long as 10 to 12 hours, depending upon the dose administered.

Because of its physicochemical characteristics, attempts to make accurate determinations of the drug's metabolism in man have not been successful.

The ability of 'Darbid' to inhibit gastrointestinal motility in man has been demonstrated by both radiographic and kymograph balloon techniques, although the clinical significance of this activity has not been established. The duration of motor inhibition appears to be dose-related.

INDICATIONS

Darbid (brand of isopropamide iodide) is effective as adjunctive therapy in the treatment of peptic ulcer.

'DARBID' HAS NOT BEEN SHOWN TO BE EFFECTIVE AS SOLE THERAPY IN CONTRIBUTING TO THE HEALING OF PEPTIC ULCER, DECREASING THE RATE OF RECURRENCE OR PREVENTING COMPLICATIONS.

CONTRAINDICATIONS

Glaucoma; obstructive uropathy (e.g., bladder neck obstruction due to prostatic hypertrophy); obstructive disease of the gastrointestinal tract (e.g., pyloroduodenal stenosis), paralytic ileus, intestinal atony of the elderly or debilitated patient; unstable cardiovascular status in acute hemorrhage; severe ulcerative colitis; toxic megacolon complicating inflammatory bowel disease; myasthenia gravis.

WARNINGS

In inflammatory bowel disease, Darbid (brand of isopropamide iodide) may suppress intestinal motility to the point of producing a paralytic ileus and, for this reason, precipitate "toxic megacolon," a serious complication of the disease. Diarrhea may be an early symptom of intestinal obstruction, especially in patients with ileostomy or colostomy. Gastrointestinal obstruction should be ruled out before 'Darbid' is prescribed. In this instance, treatment with 'Darbid' would be inappropriate and possibly harmful.

With overdosage, a curare-like action may occur, i.e., a neuromuscular blockade leading to muscular weakness and possible paralysis.

'Darbid' may cause increased heart rate and, therefore, should be used with caution in patients with heart disease.

PRECAUTIONS

General
Use Darbid (brand of isopropamide iodide) with caution in the elderly and in all patients with:

Autonomic neuropathy.

Hyperthyroidism, coronary heart disease, congestive heart failure, cardiac arrhythmia, hypertension and prostatic hypertrophy.

Reflux esophagitis (anticholinergic drugs may aggravate this condition).

Investigate any tachycardia before giving anticholinergic drugs, since they may increase the heart rate.

The use of anticholinergic drugs in the treatment of gastric ulcer may produce a delay in gastric emptying and, thus, complicate therapy.

Information for Patients
The patient should be advised that in the presence of a high environmental temperature, heat prostration (fever and heat stroke due to decreased sweating) can occur with the use of 'Darbid'.

'Darbid' may produce drowsiness or blurred vision. The patient should be cautioned regarding activities requiring mental alertness such as operating a motor vehicle or other machinery or performing hazardous work while taking this drug.

Drug Interactions
Anticholinergics may delay absorption of other medication given concomitantly.

Excessive cholinergic blockade may occur if Darbid (brand of isopropamide iodide) is given concomitantly with belladonna alkaloids, synthetic or semisynthetic anticholinergic agents, narcotic analgesics such as meperidine, Type 1 antiarrhythmic drugs (e.g., disopyramide, procainamide, or quinidine), antihistamines, phenothiazines, tricyclic antidepressants, or other psychoactive drugs. 'Darbid' may also potentiate the sedative effect of phenothiazines.

Increased intraocular pressure may result from concurrent administration of anticholinergics and corticosteroids.

Drug/Laboratory Test Interactions
Effect on PBI Determination and I^{131} Uptake: The iodine in isopropamide iodide may alter the PBI determination and will suppress I^{131} uptake. Therefore, thyroid function tests unaffected by exogenous iodides should be substituted.

Carcinogenicity, Mutagenicity and Impairment of Fertility: No long-term carcinogenicity, mutagenicity or fertility studies have been done with 'Darbid'.

Pregnancy
Teratogenic Effects—Pregnancy Category C: Animal reproduction studies have not been conducted with 'Darbid'. It is also not known whether 'Darbid' can cause fetal harm when administered to a pregnant woman or can affect reproductive capacity. 'Darbid' should be given to a pregnant woman only if clearly needed.

Nursing Mothers
As with all anticholinergic drugs, suppression of lactation may occur.

It is not known whether this drug is excreted in human milk. Because many drugs are excreted in human milk, caution should be exercised when 'Darbid' is administered to a nursing woman.

Pediatric Use
Safety and effectiveness in children below the age of 12 have not been established.

ADVERSE REACTIONS
The following adverse reactions have been observed with Darbid (brand of isopropamide iodide) and/or other anticholinergics, but there is insufficient data to support an estimate of their frequency. Within each category, adverse reactions are listed in decreasing order of severity:

Hypersensitivity: Severe allergic reactions or drug idiosyncrasies, including anaphylaxis; urticaria and other dermal manifestations; fever.

Autonomic: Increased ocular tension; blurred vision; mydriasis; cycloplegia; xerostomia; decreased sweating; loss of taste; nasal congestion.

CNS: Some degree of mental confusion and/or excitement, especially in elderly patients; headache; dizziness; drowsiness; nervousness; weakness; insomnia.

Renal: Urinary retention and hesitancy.

Cardiovascular: Tachycardia and palpitations.

Gastrointestinal: Constipation; dysphagia; vomiting; nausea; bloated feeling.

Endocrine: Impotence and suppression of lactation.

OVERDOSAGE
The symptoms of overdosage with anticholinergic agents can range from an intensification of the usual side effects to CNS disturbances (from restlessness and excitement to psychotic behavior); circulatory changes (flushing, fall in blood pressure, circulatory failure; respiratory failure; paralysis and coma.

Oral LD$_{50}$—The oral LD$_{50}$ of Darbid (brand of isopropamide iodide) in mice is 1109 mg./kg.

Treatment—Suggestions for treatment of anticholinergic overdosage include the following measures:

General Measures—1) Emesis should be initiated unless the patient is comatose, convulsing or has lost the gag reflex. If any of these contraindications are present, endotracheal intubation should precede gastric lavage with a large-bore tube.

2) Maintenance of an adequate airway, using artificial respiration if needed.

3) Administration of I.V. fluids, and

4) For fever, alcohol sponging or ice packs.

Specific Measures—1) Antidote: Physostigmine. *In children*, a therapeutic trial dose of 0.5 mg. should be administered slowly I.V. If toxic effects persist and no cholinergic effects are produced, the drug should be readministered at 5-minute intervals until a maximum dose of 2 mg. is attained. If life-threatening symptoms recur, the lowest total effective trial dose should be repeated, no more frequently than once per hour.

In adults, the therapeutic trial dose of physostigmine is 2 mg. administered slowly I.V. A second dose of 1 to 2 mg. may be attempted in 20 minutes if no reversal has occurred. One to 4 mg. slowly I.V. should be repeated as life-threatening symptoms recur. **Do not use as continuous drip.**

2) Levarterenol or metaraminol infusions may be used against hypotension and circulatory collapse.

3) Peritoneal dialysis and hemodialysis are ineffective.

DOSAGE AND ADMINISTRATION
Adults and Children 12 and over—Usual starting dose is one 5 mg. Darbid (brand of isopropamide iodide) tablet, b.i.d. (every 12 hours). Some patients may require two 5 mg. tablets, b.i.d. or more.

Not recommended for use in children under 12.

Dosage should be individualized and titrated to the patient's therapeutic response.

HOW SUPPLIED
Round, pink, coated tablets, 5 mg., imprinted SKF and D62; in bottles of 50. NDC 0007-3462-15.

Store at controlled room temperature. Dispense in a tight, light-resistant container.

DB:L18

Shown in Product Identification Section, page 430

DEXEDRINE®   Ⓒ
[*dex'eh-dreen*]
(brand of dextroamphetamine sulfate)
SPANSULE® CAPSULES,
TABLETS and ELIXIR

WARNING

> AMPHETAMINES HAVE A HIGH POTENTIAL FOR ABUSE. THEY SHOULD THUS BE TRIED ONLY IN WEIGHT REDUCTION PROGRAMS FOR PATIENTS IN WHOM ALTERNATIVE THERAPY HAS BEEN INEFFECTIVE. ADMINISTRATION OF AMPHETAMINES FOR PROLONGED PERIODS OF TIME IN OBESITY MAY LEAD TO DRUG DEPENDENCE AND MUST BE AVOIDED. PARTICULAR ATTENTION SHOULD BE PAID TO THE POSSIBILITY OF SUBJECTS OBTAINING AMPHETAMINES FOR NONTHERAPEUTIC USE OR DISTRIBUTION TO OTHERS, AND THE DRUGS SHOULD BE PRESCRIBED OR DISPENSED SPARINGLY.

DESCRIPTION
Dexedrine (dextroamphetamine sulfate, SK&F) is the dextro isomer of the compound *d,l*-amphetamine sulfate, a sympathomimetic amine of the amphetamine group. Chemically, dextroamphetamine is *d*-alpha-methylphenethylamine, and is present in all forms of 'Dexedrine' as the neutral sulfate.

Spansule® capsules
Each 'Spansule' sustained release capsule is so prepared that an initial dose is released promptly and the remaining medication is released gradually over a prolonged period.

Each capsule, with brown cap and natural body, contains dextroamphetamine sulfate as follows: 5 mg. imprinted SKF and E12; 10 mg. imprinted SKF and E13, 15 mg. imprinted SKF and E14. Inactive ingredients consist of acacia, benzyl alcohol, calcium sulfate, cetylpyridinium chloride, FD&C Blue No. 1, FD&C Red No. 40, FD&C Yellow No. 5 (tartrazine), FD&C Yellow No. 6, gelatin, glyceryl distearate, glyceryl monostearate, sodium lauryl sulfate, starch, sucrose, wax and trace amounts of other inactive ingredients.

Tablets
Each triangular, orange, scored tablet is debossed SKF and E19 and contains dextroamphetamine sulfate, 5 mg. Inactive ingredients consist of calcium sulfate, FD&C Yellow No. 5 (tartrazine), FD&C Yellow No. 6, gelatin, lactose, mineral oil, starch, stearic acid, sucrose, talc and trace amounts of other inactive ingredients.

Elixir
Each 5 ml. (one teaspoonful) of clear, orange-colored, orange-flavored liquid contains dextroamphetamine sulfate, 5 mg., and alcohol, 10%. Inactive ingredients consist of benzoic acid, citric acid, FD&C Yellow No. 5 (tartrazine), FD&C Yellow No. 6, flavor, sucrose, water and wine.

CLINICAL PHARMACOLOGY
Amphetamines are non-catecholamine, sympathomimetic amines with CNS stimulant activity. Peripheral actions include elevations of systolic and diastolic blood pressures and weak bronchodilator and respiratory stimulant action.

There is neither specific evidence which clearly establishes the mechanism whereby amphetamines produce mental and behavioral effects in children, nor conclusive evidence regarding how these effects relate to the condition of the central nervous system.

Drugs of this class used in obesity are commonly known as "anorectics" or "anorexigenics." It has not been established, however, that the action of such drugs in treating obesity is primarily one of appetite suppression. Other central nervous system actions, or metabolic effects, may be involved, for example.

Adult obese subjects instructed in dietary management and treated with "anorectic" drugs lose more weight on the average than those treated with placebo and diet, as determined in relatively short-term clinical trials.

The magnitude of increased weight loss of drug-treated patients over placebo-treated patients is only a fraction of a pound a week. The rate of weight loss is greatest in the first weeks of therapy for both drug and placebo subjects and tends to decrease in succeeding weeks. The origins of the increased weight loss due to the various possible drug effects are not established. The amount of weight loss associated with the use of an "anorectic" drug varies from trial to trial, and the increased weight loss appears to be related in part to variables other than the drug prescribed, such as the physician-investigator, the population treated, and the diet prescribed. Studies do not permit conclusions as to the relative importance of the drug and nondrug factors on weight loss. The natural history of obesity is measured in years, whereas the studies cited are restricted to a few weeks' duration; thus, the total impact of drug-induced weight loss over that of diet alone must be considered clinically limited.

Dexedrine (dextroamphetamine sulfate, SK&F) *Spansule* capsules are formulated to release the active drug substance *in vivo* in a more gradual fashion than the standard formulation, as demonstrated by blood levels. The formulation has not been shown superior in effectiveness over the same dosage of the standard, noncontrolled-release formulations given in divided doses.

Pharmacokinetics
Elixir—Ingestion of 10 mg. of dextroamphetamine sulfate in elixir form by healthy volunteers produced an average peak dextroamphetamine blood level of 33.2 ng./ml. The half-life was 11.75 hours. The average urinary recovery was 38% in 48 hours.

Tablet—The single ingestion of two 5 mg. tablets by healthy volunteers produced an average peak dextroamphetamine blood level of 29.2 ng./ml. at 2 hours post-administration. The average half-life was 10.25 hours. The average urinary recovery was 45% in 48 hours.

'Spansule' capsule—Ingestion of a 'Spansule' capsule containing 15 mg. radiolabeled dextroamphetamine sulfate by healthy volunteers produced a peak blood level of radioactivity, on the average, at 8-10 hours post-administration with peak urinary recovery seen at 12–24 hours.

INDICATIONS AND USAGE
Dexedrine (dextroamphetamine sulfate, SK&F) is indicated:

1. In Narcolepsy.

2. **In Attention Deficit Disorder with Hyperactivity,** as an integral part of a total treatment program which typically includes other remedial measures (psychological, educational, social) for a stabilizing effect in children with a behavioral syndrome characterized by the following group of developmentally inappropriate symptoms: moderate to severe distractibility, short attention span, hyperactivity, emotional lability, and impulsivity. The diagnosis of this syndrome should not be made with finality when these symptoms are only of comparatively recent origin. Nonlocalizing (soft) neurological signs, learning disability, and abnormal EEG may or may not be present, and a diagnosis of central nervous system dysfunction may or may not be warranted.

3. **In Exogenous Obesity,** as a short-term (a few weeks) adjunct in a regimen of weight reduction based on caloric restriction, for patients refractory to alternative therapy, e.g., repeated diets, group programs, and other drugs. The limited usefulness of amphetamines (see CLINICAL PHARMACOLOGY) should be weighed against possible risks inherent in use of the drug, such as those described below.

Continued on next page

Smith Kline & French—Cont.

CONTRAINDICATIONS

Advanced arteriosclerosis, symptomatic cardiovascular disease, moderate to severe hypertension, hyperthyroidism, known hypersensitivity or idiosyncrasy to the sympathomimetic amines, glaucoma.

Agitated states.

Patients with a history of drug abuse.

During or within 14 days following the administration of monoamine oxidase inhibitors (hypertensive crises may result).

WARNING

When tolerance to the "anorectic" effect develops, the recommended dose should not be exceeded in an attempt to increase the effect; rather, the drug should be discontinued.

PRECAUTIONS

General: Caution is to be exercised in prescribing amphetamines for patients with even mild hypertension.

The least amount feasible should be prescribed or dispensed at one time in order to minimize the possibility of overdosage.

These products contain FD&C Yellow No. 5 (tartrazine), which may cause allergic-type reactions (including bronchial asthma) in certain susceptible individuals. Although the overall incidence of FD&C Yellow No. 5 (tartrazine) sensitivity in the general population is low, it is frequently seen in patients who also have aspirin hypersensitivity.

Information for Patients: Amphetamines may impair the ability of the patient to engage in potentially hazardous activities such as operating machinery or vehicles; the patient should therefore be cautioned accordingly.

Drug Interactions

Acidifying agents—Gastrointestinal acidifying agents (guanethidine, reserpine, glutamic acid HCl, ascorbic acid, fruit juices, etc.) lower absorption of amphetamines. Urinary acidifying agents (ammonium chloride, sodium acid phosphate, etc.) increase the concentration of the ionized species of the amphetamine molecule, thereby increasing urinary excretion. Both groups of agents lower blood levels and efficacy of amphetamines.

Adrenergic blockers—Adrenergic blockers are inhibited by amphetamines.

Alkalinizing agents—Gastrointestinal alkalinizing agents (sodium bicarbonate, etc.) increase absorption of amphetamines. Urinary alkalinizing agents (acetazolamide, some thiazides) increase the concentration of the non-ionized species of the amphetamine molecule, thereby decreasing urinary excretion. Both groups of agents increase blood levels and therefore potentiate the actions of amphetamines.

Antidepressants, tricyclic—Amphetamines may enhance the activity of tricyclic or sympathomimetic agents; d-amphetamine with desipramine or protriptyline and possibly other tricyclics cause striking and sustained increases in the concentration of d-amphetamine in the brain; cardiovascular effects can be potentiated.

MAO inhibitors—MAOI antidepressants, as well as a metabolite of furazolidone, slow amphetamine metabolism. This slowing potentiates amphetamines, increasing their effect on the release of norepinephrine and other monoamines from adrenergic nerve endings; this can cause headaches and other signs of hypertensive crisis. A variety of neurological toxic effects and malignant hyperpyrexia can occur, sometimes with fatal results.

Antihistamines—Amphetamines may counteract the sedative effect of antihistamines.

Antihypertensives—Amphetamines may antagonize the hypotensive effects of antihypertensives.

Chlorpromazine—Chlorpromazine blocks dopamine and norepinephrine reuptake, thus inhibiting the central stimulant effects of amphetamines, and can be used to treat amphetamine poisoning.

Ethosuximide—Amphetamines may delay intestinal absorption of ethosuximide.

Haloperidol—Haloperidol blocks dopamine and norepinephrine reuptake, thus inhibiting the central stimulant effects of amphetamines.

Lithium carbonate—The antiobesity and stimulatory effects of amphetamines may be inhibited by lithium carbonate.

Meperidine—Amphetamines potentiate the analgesic effect of meperidine.

Methenamine therapy—Urinary excretion of amphetamines is increased, and efficacy is reduced, by acidifying agents used in methenamine therapy.

Norepinephrine—Amphetamines enhance the adrenergic effect of norepinephrine.

Phenobarbital—Amphetamines may delay intestinal absorption of phenobarbital; co-administration of phenobarbital may produce a synergistic anticonvulsant action.

Phenytoin—Amphetamines may delay intestinal absorption of phenytoin; co-administration of phenytoin may produce a synergistic anticonvulsant action.

Propoxyphene—In cases of propoxyphene overdosage, amphetamine CNS stimulation is potentiated and fatal convulsions can occur.

Veratrum alkaloids—Amphetamines inhibit the hypotensive effect of veratrum alkaloids.

Drug/Laboratory Test Interactions

- Amphetamines can cause a significant elevation in plasma corticosteroid levels. This increase is greatest in the evening.
- Amphetamines may interfere with urinary steroid determinations.

Carcinogenesis/Mutagenesis: Mutagenicity studies and long-term studies in animals to determine the carcinogenic potential of Dexedrine (dextroamphetamine sulfate, SK&F) have not been performed.

Pregnancy—Teratogenic Effects: Pregnancy Category C. 'Dexedrine' has been shown to have embryotoxic and teratogenic effects when administered to A/Jax mice and C57BL mice in doses approximately 41 times the maximum human dose. Embryotoxic effects were not seen in New Zealand white rabbits given the drug in doses 7 times the human dose nor in rats given 12.5 times the maximum human dose. There are no adequate and well-controlled studies in pregnant women. 'Dexedrine' should be used during pregnancy only if the potential benefit justifies the potential risk to the fetus.

Nonteratogenic Effects: Infants born to mothers dependent on amphetamines have an increased risk of premature delivery and low birth weight. Also, these infants may experience symptoms of withdrawal as demonstrated by dysphoria, including agitation, and significant lassitude.

Nursing Mothers: Amphetamines are excreted in human milk. Mothers taking amphetamines should be advised to refrain from nursing.

Pediatric Use: Long-term effects of amphetamines in children have not been well established.

Amphetamines are not recommended for use as anorectic agents in children under 12 years of age, or in children under 3 years of age with Attention Deficit Disorder with Hyperactivity described under INDICATIONS AND USAGE.

Clinical experience suggests that in psychotic children, administration of amphetamines may exacerbate symptoms of behavior disturbance and thought disorder.

Amphetamines have been reported to exacerbate motor and phonic tics and Tourette's syndrome. Therefore, clinical evaluation for tics and Tourette's syndrome in children and their families should precede use of stimulant medications.

Data are inadequate to determine whether chronic administration of amphetamines may be associated with growth inhibition; therefore, growth should be monitored during treatment.

Drug treatment is not indicated in all cases of Attention Deficit Disorder with Hyperactivity and should be considered only in light of the complete history and evaluation of the child. The decision to prescribe amphetamines should depend on the physician's assessment of the chronicity and severity of the child's symptoms and their appropriateness for his/her age. Prescription should not depend solely on the presence of one or more of the behavioral characteristics.

When these symptoms are associated with acute stress reactions, treatment with amphetamines is usually not indicated.

ADVERSE REACTIONS

Cardiovascular: Palpitations, tachycardia, elevation of blood pressure. There have been isolated reports of cardiomyopathy associated with chronic amphetamine use.

Central Nervous System: Psychotic episodes at recommended doses (rare), overstimulation, restlessness, dizziness, insomnia, euphoria, dyskinesia, dysphoria, tremor, headache, exacerbation of motor and phonic tics and Tourette's syndrome.

Gastrointestinal: Dryness of the mouth, unpleasant taste, diarrhea, constipation, other gastrointestinal disturbances. Anorexia and weight loss may occur as undesirable effects when amphetamines are used for other than the anorectic effect.

Allergic: Urticaria.

Endocrine: Impotence, changes in libido.

DRUG ABUSE AND DEPENDENCE

Dextroamphetamine sulfate is a Schedule II controlled substance.

Amphetamines have been extensively abused. Tolerance, extreme psychological dependence, and severe social disability have occurred. There are reports of patients who have increased the dosage to many times that recommended. Abrupt cessation following prolonged high dosage administration results in extreme fatigue and mental depression; changes are also noted on the sleep EEG.

Manifestations of chronic intoxication with amphetamines include severe dermatoses, marked insomnia, irritability, hyperactivity, and personality changes. The most severe manifestation of chronic intoxication is psychosis, often clinically indistinguishable from schizophrenia. This is rare with oral amphetamines.

OVERDOSAGE

Individual patient response to amphetamines varies widely. While toxic symptoms occasionally occur as an idiosyncrasy at doses as low as 2 mg., they are rare with doses of less than 15 mg.; 30 mg. can produce severe reactions, yet doses of 400 to 500 mg. are not necessarily fatal.

In rats, the oral LD_{50} of dextroamphetamine sulfate is 96.8 mg./kg.

Manifestations of acute overdosage with amphetamines include restlessness, tremor, hyperreflexia, rhabdomyolysis, rapid respiration, hyperpyrexia, confusion, assaultiveness, hallucinations, panic states.

Fatigue and depression usually follow the central stimulation.

Cardiovascular effects include arrhythmias, hypertension or hypotension and circulatory collapse. Gastrointestinal symptoms include nausea, vomiting, diarrhea, and abdominal cramps. Fatal poisoning is usually preceded by convulsions and coma.

TREATMENT—Management of acute amphetamine intoxication is largely symptomatic and includes gastric lavage and sedation with a barbiturate. Experience with hemodialysis or peritoneal dialysis is inadequate to permit recommendation in this regard. Acidification of the urine increases amphetamine excretion. If acute, severe hypertension complicates amphetamine overdosage, administration of intravenous phentolamine (Regitine®, CIBA) has been suggested. However, a gradual drop in blood pressure will usually result when sufficient sedation has been achieved. Chlorpromazine antagonizes the central stimulant effects of amphetamines and can be used to treat amphetamine intoxication.

Since much of the 'Spansule' capsule medication is coated for gradual release, therapy directed at reversing the effects of the ingested drug and at supporting the patient should be continued for as long as overdosage symptoms remain. Saline cathartics are useful for hastening the evacuation of pellets that have not already released medication.

DOSAGE AND ADMINISTRATION

Regardless of indication, amphetamines should be administered at the lowest effective dosage and dosage should be individually adjusted. Late evening doses—particularly with the 'Spansule' capsule form—should be avoided because of the resulting insomnia.

Narcolepsy: Usual dose 5 to 60 milligrams per day in divided doses, depending on the individual patient response. Narcolepsy seldom occurs in children under 12 years of age; however, when it does, Dexedrine (dextroamphetamine sulfate, SK&F) may be used. The suggested initial dose for patients aged 6–12 is 5 mg. daily; daily dose may be raised in increments of 5 mg. at weekly intervals until optimal response is obtained. In patients 12 years of age and older, start with 10 mg. daily; daily dosage may be raised in increments of 10 mg. at weekly intervals until optimal response is obtained. If bothersome adverse reactions appear (e.g., insomnia or anorexia), dosage should be reduced. 'Spansule' capsules may be used for once-a-day dosage wherever appropriate. With tablets or elixir, give first dose on awakening; additional doses (1 or 2) at intervals of 4 to 6 hours.

Attention Deficit Disorder with Hyperactivity: Not recommended for children under 3 years of age.

In children from 3 to 5 years of age, start with 2.5 mg. daily, by tablet or elixir; daily dosage may be raised in increments of 2.5 mg. at weekly intervals until optimal response is obtained.

In children 6 years of age and older, start with 5 mg. once or twice daily; daily dosage may be raised in increments of 5 mg. at weekly intervals until optimal response is obtained. Only in rare cases will it be necessary to exceed a total of 40 milligrams per day.

'Spansule' capsules may be used for once-a-day dosage wherever appropriate.

With tablets or elixir, give first dose on awakening; additional doses (1 or 2) at intervals of 4 to 6 hours.

Where possible, drug administration should be interrupted occasionally to determine if there is a recurrence of behavioral symptoms sufficient to require continued therapy.

Exogenous Obesity: Usual dosage is one 10 or 15 mg. 'Spansule' capsule daily, taken in the morning, or up to 30 mg. daily by tablets or elixir, taken in divided doses of 5 to 10 mg. 30 to 60 minutes before meals. Not recommended for this use in children under 12 years of age.

HOW SUPPLIED

'Spansule' capsules available: 5 mg., in bottles of 50; 10 mg. and 15 mg., in bottles of 50 and 500.

Tablets, 5 mg., available in bottles of 100 and 1000.

Elixir, 5 mg./5 ml., available in 16 fl. oz. (473 ml.) bottles.

Military–'Spansule' Capsules, 5 mg., 50's, 6505-01-153-4029.

DX:L37

Shown in Product Identification Section, page 430

DIBENZYLINE® Capsules   ℞
[di-benz'eh-leen]
(brand of phenoxybenzamine hydrochloride)

DESCRIPTION
Each 'DIBENZYLINE' capsule, with red cap and red body, is imprinted SKF and E33 and contains phenoxybenzamine hydrochloride, 10 mg. Inactive ingredients consist of benzyl alcohol, cetylpyridinium chloride, D&C Red No. 33, FD&C Red No. 3, FD&C Yellow No. 6, gelatin, lactose, sodium lauryl sulfate and trace amounts of other inactive ingredients. 'Dibenzyline' is N-(2-Chloroethyl)-N-(1-methyl-2-phenoxyethyl)benzylamine hydrochloride.
Phenoxybenzamine hydrochloride is a colorless, crystalline powder with a molecular weight of 340.3 which melts between 136° and 141°C. It is soluble in water, alcohol and chloroform; insoluble in ether.

CLINICAL PHARMACOLOGY
Dibenzyline (phenoxybenzamine hydrochloride, SK&F) is a long-acting, adrenergic, *alpha*-receptor blocking agent which can produce and maintain "chemical sympathectomy" by oral administration. It increases blood flow to the skin, mucosa and abdominal viscera, and lowers both supine and erect blood pressures. It has no effect on the parasympathetic system.
Twenty to thirty percent of orally administered phenoxybenzamine appears to be absorbed in the active form.[1]
The half-life of orally administered phenoxybenzamine hydrochloride is not known; however, the half-life of intravenously administered drug is approximately 24 hours. Demonstrable effects with intravenous administration persist for at least three to four days, and the effects of daily administration are cumulative for nearly a week.[1]

INDICATION AND USAGE
Pheochromocytoma, to control episodes of hypertension and sweating. If tachycardia is excessive, it may be necessary to use a beta-blocking agent concomitantly.

CONTRAINDICATIONS
Conditions where a fall in blood pressure may be undesirable.

WARNING
'Dibenzyline'-induced *alpha*-adrenergic blockade leaves *beta*-adrenergic receptors unopposed. Compounds that stimulate both types of receptors may therefore produce an exaggerated hypotensive response and tachycardia.

PRECAUTIONS
General—Administer with caution in patients with marked cerebral or coronary arteriosclerosis or renal damage. Adrenergic blocking effect may aggravate symptoms of respiratory infections.
Drug Interactions[2]—Dibenzyline (phenoxybenzamine hydrochloride, SK&F) may interact with compounds that stimulate both *alpha*- and *beta*-adrenergic receptors (i.e., epinephrine) to produce an exaggerated hypotensive response and tachycardia. (See WARNING.)
'Dibenzyline' blocks hyperthermia production by levarterenol, and blocks hypothermia production by reserpine.
Carcinogenesis, Mutagenesis, Impairment of Fertility—Phenoxybenzamine hydrochloride has shown *in vitro* mutagenic activity in the Ames test and in the mouse lymphoma assay; it has not shown mutagenic activity in the micronucleus test in mice. In rats and mice repeated intraperitoneal administration of phenoxybenzamine hydrochloride resulted in peritoneal sarcomas. Chronic oral dosing in rats has produced malignant tumors in the gastrointestinal tract. The majority of these tumors were found in the nonglandular stomach of the rats.
In chronic oral studies in rats, ulcerative and/or erosive gastritis of the glandular stomach occurred which was probably drug related.
Pregnancy-Teratogenic Effects—Pregnancy Category C. Adequate reproductive studies have not been performed with Dibenzyline (phenoxybenzamine hydrochloride, SK&F). It is also not known whether 'Dibenzyline' can cause fetal harm when administered to a pregnant woman. 'Dibenzyline' should be given to a pregnant woman only if clearly needed.
Nursing Mothers—It is not known whether this drug is excreted in human milk. Because many drugs are excreted in human milk, and because of the potential for serious adverse reactions from phenoxybenzamine hydrochloride, a decision should be made whether to discontinue nursing or to discontinue the drug, taking into account the importance of the drug to the mother.
Pediatric Use—Safety and effectiveness in children have not been established.

ADVERSE REACTIONS
The following adverse reactions have been observed, but there are insufficient data to support an estimate of their frequency:

Autonomic Nervous System*: Postural hypotension, tachycardia, inhibition of ejaculation, nasal congestion, miosis.
Miscellaneous: Gastrointestinal irritation, drowsiness, fatigue.

*These so-called "side effects" are actually evidence of adrenergic blockade and vary according to the degree of blockade.

OVERDOSAGE
SYMPTOMS—These are largely the result of block of the sympathetic nervous system and of the circulating epinephrine. They may include postural hypotension resulting in dizziness or fainting; tachycardia, particularly postural; vomiting; lethargy; shock.
TREATMENT—When symptoms and signs of overdosage exist, discontinue the drug. Treatment of circulatory failure, if present, is a prime consideration. In cases of mild overdosage, recumbent position with legs elevated usually restores cerebral circulation. In the more severe cases, the usual measures to combat shock should be instituted. Usual pressor agents are *not* effective. Epinephrine is contraindicated because it stimulates both *alpha* and *beta* receptors; since *alpha* receptors are blocked, the net effect of epinephrine administration is vasodilation and a further drop in blood pressure (epinephrine reversal).
The patient may have to be kept flat for 24 hours or more in the case of overdose, as the effect of the drug is prolonged. Leg bandages and an abdominal binder may shorten the period of disability.
I.V. infusion of levarterenol bitartrate* may be used to combat severe hypotensive reactions, because it stimulates *alpha* receptors primarily. Although Dibenzyline (phenoxybenzamine hydrochloride, SK&F) is an *alpha* adrenergic blocking agent, a sufficient dose of levarterenol bitartrate will overcome this effect.
The oral LD_{50} for phenoxybenzamine hydrochloride is approximately 2000 mg./kg. in rats and approximately 500 mg./kg. in guinea pigs.

DOSAGE AND ADMINISTRATION
The dosage should be adjusted to fit the needs of each patient. Small initial doses should be *slowly* increased until the desired effect is obtained or the side effects from blockade become troublesome. *After each increase, the patient should be observed on that level before instituting another increase.* The dosage should be carried to a point where symptomatic relief and/or objective improvement are obtained, but not so high that the side effects from blockade become troublesome. Initially, 10 mg. of Dibenzyline (phenoxybenzamine hydrochloride, SK&F) twice a day. Dosage should be increased every other day, usually to 20 to 40 mg. two or three times a day, until an optimal dosage is obtained, as judged by blood pressure control.

HOW SUPPLIED
Dibenzyline (phenoxybenzamine hydrochloride, SK&F) capsules, 10 mg., in bottles of 100 (*NDC* 0007-3533-20).
Military—Capsules, 10 mg., 100's, 6505-00-890-1193.

REFERENCES
1. Weiner, N.: Drugs That Inhibit Adrenergic Nerves and Block Adrenergic Receptors, in Goodman, L., and Gilman, A., *The Pharmacological Basis of Therapeutics*, ed. 6, New York, Macmillan Publishing Co., 1980, p. 179; p. 182.
2. Martin, E.W.: *Drug Interactions Index 1978/1979*, Philadelphia, J.B. Lippincott Co., 1978, pp. 209–210.

*Available as Levophed® Bitartrate (brand of norepinephrine bitartrate) from Winthrop-Breon.

DI:L23

Shown in Product Identification Section, page 430

DYAZIDE® Capsules   ℞
[dye-uh-zide']

PRODUCT OVERVIEW
KEY FACTS
'Dyazide' is a diuretic/antihypertensive product that combines natriuretic and antikaliuretic effects. It has a once-daily-dosing regimen to help foster patient compliance.

MAJOR USES
This fixed combination drug is not indicated for the initial therapy of edema or hypertension except in individuals in whom the development of hypokalemia cannot be risked.
'Dyazide' is indicated for (1) the treatment of hypertension or edema in patients who develop hypokalemia on hydrochlorothiazide alone; (2) those patients who require a thiazide diuretic and in whom the development of hypokalemia cannot be risked.
'Dyazide' may be used alone or as an adjunct to other antihypertensive drugs. Since 'Dyazide' may enhance the action of these agents, dosage adjustments may be necessary.

SAFETY INFORMATION
'Dyazide' should not be given to patients taking other potassium-sparing agents or potassium containing salt substitutes. Potassium supplementation should not be used with 'Dyazide' except in severe cases of hypokalemia. If potassium supplementation is used, careful monitoring of the serum potassium level is necessary. 'Dyazide' is contraindicated in patients with anuria, acute and chronic renal insufficiency or significant renal impairment, hypersensitivity to either drug in the preparation or to other sulfonamide-derived drugs or preexisting elevated serum potassium.
Abnormal elevation of serum potassium levels (≥ 5.5 mEq/liter) can occur with all potassium-conserving diuretic combinations, including 'Dyazide'. Since uncorrected hyperkalemia may be fatal, serum potassium levels must be monitored at frequent intervals especially in patients first receiving 'Dyazide', when dosages are changed or with any illness that may influence renal function. Potassium-conserving therapy should be avoided in severely ill patients in whom respiratory or metabolic acidosis may occur. Acidosis may be associated with rapid elevations in serum potassium levels. If 'Dyazide' is employed, frequent evaluations of acid/base balance and serum electrolytes are necessary. (See full prescribing information.)

PRESCRIBING INFORMATION
DYAZIDE® Capsules   ℞
[dye-uh-zide']

('Dyazide' is a product of SK&F Co., Cidra, P.R. 00639, Subsidiary of SmithKline Beckman Corporation, Philadelphia, Pa.)

DESCRIPTION
Each 'Dyazide' capsule for oral use, with opaque red cap and opaque white body, contains hydrochlorothiazide 25 mg. and triamterene 50 mg., and is imprinted with the product name DYAZIDE and SKF. Hydrochlorothiazide is a diuretic/antihypertensive agent and triamterene is an antikaliuretic agent.
Hydrochlorothiazide is slightly soluble in water. It is soluble in dilute ammonia, dilute aqueous sodium hydroxide and dimethylformamide. It is sparingly soluble in methanol.
Hydrochlorothiazide is 6-chloro-3,4-dihydro-2H-1,2,4-benzothiadiazine-7-sulfonamide 1,1-dioxide and its structural formula is:

At 50°C., triamterene is practically insoluble in water (less than 0.1%). It is soluble in formic acid, sparingly soluble in methoxyethanol and very slightly soluble in alcohol.
Triamterene is 2,4,7-triamino-6-phenylpteridine and its structural formula is:

Inactive ingredients consist of benzyl alcohol, cetylpyridinium chloride, D&C Red No. 33, FD&C Yellow No. 6, gelatin, lactose, magnesium stearate, povidone, sodium lauryl sulfate, titanium dioxide and trace amounts of other inactive ingredients.

CLINICAL PHARMACOLOGY
'Dyazide' is a diuretic/antihypertensive drug product that combines natriuretic and antikaliuretic effects. Each component complements the action of the other. The hydrochlorothiazide component blocks the reabsorption of sodium and chloride ions, and thereby increases the quantity of sodium traversing the distal tubule and the volume of water excreted. A portion of the additional sodium presented to the distal tubule is exchanged there for potassium and hydrogen ions. With continued use of hydrochlorothiazide and depletion of sodium, compensatory mechanisms tend to increase this exchange and may produce excessive loss of potassium, hydrogen and chloride ions. Hydrochlorothiazide also decreases the excretion of calcium and uric acid, may increase the excretion of iodide and may reduce glomerular filtration rate. The exact mechanism of the antihypertensive effect of hydrochlorothiazide is not known.
The triamterene component of 'Dyazide' exerts its diuretic effect on the distal renal tubule to inhibit the reabsorption of sodium in exchange for potassium and hydrogen ions. Its natriuretic activity is limited by the amount of sodium reaching its site of action. Although it blocks the increase in this exchange that is stimulated by mineralocorticoids

Continued on next page

Smith Kline & French—Cont.

(chiefly aldosterone) it is not a competitive antagonist of aldosterone and its activity can be demonstrated in adrenalectomized rats and patients with Addison's disease. As a result, the dose of triamterene required is not proportionally related to the level of mineralocorticoid activity, but is dictated by the response of the individual patients, and the kaliuretic effect of concomitantly administered drugs. By inhibiting the distal tubular exchange mechanism, triamterene maintains or increases the sodium excretion and reduces the excess loss of potassium, hydrogen, and chloride ions induced by hydrochlorothiazide. As with hydrochlorothiazide, triamterene may reduce glomerular filtration and renal plasma flow. Via this mechanism it may reduce uric acid excretion although it has no tubular effect on uric acid reabsorption or secretion. Triamterene does not affect calcium excretion. No predictable antihypertensive effect has been demonstrated for triamterene.

Duration of diuretic activity and effective dosage range of the hydrochlorothiazide and triamterene components of 'Dyazide' are similar. Onset of diuresis with 'Dyazide' takes place within one hour, peaks at two to three hours and tapers off during the subsequent seven to nine hours.

The bioavailability of the hydrochlorothiazide and the triamterene components of 'Dyazide' is, in each case, about 50% of that observed with an aqueous suspension of the components. (See PRECAUTIONS, Bioavailability.)

INDICATIONS AND USAGE

This fixed combination drug is not indicated for the initial therapy of edema or hypertension except in individuals in whom the development of hypokalemia cannot be risked.

'Dyazide' is indicated for the treatment of hypertension or edema in patients who develop hypokalemia on hydrochlorothiazide alone.

'Dyazide' is also indicated for those patients who require a thiazide diuretic and in whom the development of hypokalemia cannot be risked.

'Dyazide' may be used alone or as an adjunct to other antihypertensive drugs, such as beta-blockers. Since 'Dyazide' may enhance the action of these agents, dosage adjustments may be necessary.

Usage in Pregnancy: The routine use of diuretics in an otherwise healthy woman is inappropriate and exposes mother and fetus to unnecessary hazard. Diuretics do not prevent development of toxemia of pregnancy, and there is no satisfactory evidence that they are useful in the treatment of developed toxemia.

Edema during pregnancy may arise from pathological causes or from the physiologic and mechanical consequences of pregnancy. Diuretics are indicated in pregnancy when edema is due to pathologic causes, just as they are in the absence of pregnancy. Dependent edema in pregnancy resulting from restriction of venous return by the expanded uterus is properly treated through elevation of the lower extremities and use of support hose; use of diuretics to lower intravascular volume in this case is illogical and unnecessary. There is hypervolemia during normal pregnancy which is harmful to neither the fetus nor the mother (in the absence of cardiovascular disease), but which is associated with edema, including generalized edema in the majority of pregnant women. If this edema produces discomfort, increased recumbency will often provide relief. In rare instances this edema may cause extreme discomfort which is not relieved by rest. In these cases a short course of diuretics may provide relief and may be appropriate.

CONTRAINDICATIONS

Antikaliuretic Therapy and Potassium Supplementation

'Dyazide' should not be given to patients receiving other potassium-conserving agents such as spironolactone, amiloride or other formulations containing triamterene. Concomitant potassium-containing salt substitutes should also not be used.

Potassium supplementation should not be used with 'Dyazide' except in severe cases of hypokalemia. Such concomitant therapy can be associated with rapid increases in serum potassium levels. If potassium supplementation is used, careful monitoring of the serum potassium level is necessary.

Impaired Renal Function

'Dyazide' is contraindicated in patients with anuria, acute and chronic renal insufficiency or significant renal impairment.

Hypersensitivity

Hypersensitivity to either drug in the preparation or to other sulfonamide-derived drugs is a contraindication.

Hyperkalemia

'Dyazide' should not be used in patients with preexisting elevated serum potassium.

WARNINGS: Hyperkalemia

Abnormal elevation of serum potassium levels (greater than or equal to 5.5 mEq/liter) can occur with all potassium-conserving diuretic combinations, including 'Dyazide'. Hyperkalemia is more likely to occur in patients with renal impairment, diabetes (even without evidence of renal impairment), elderly or severely ill patients. Since uncorrected hyperkalemia may be fatal, serum potassium levels must be monitored at frequent intervals especially in patients first receiving 'Dyazide', when dosages are changed or with any illness that may influence renal function.

If hyperkalemia is suspected (warning signs include paresthesia, muscular weakness, fatigue, flaccid paralysis of the extremities, bradycardia and shock), an electrocardiogram (ECG) should be obtained. However, it is important to monitor serum potassium levels because hyperkalemia may not be associated with ECG changes.

If hyperkalemia is present, 'Dyazide' should be discontinued immediately and a thiazide alone should be substituted. If the serum potassium exceeds 6.5 mEq/liter, more vigorous therapy is required. The clinical situation dictates the procedures to be employed. These include the intravenous administration of calcium chloride solution, sodium bicarbonate solution and/or the oral or parenteral administration of glucose with a rapid-acting insulin preparation. Cationic exchange resins such as sodium polystyrene sulfonate may be orally or rectally administered. Persistent hyperkalemia may require dialysis.

The development of hyperkalemia associated with potassium-sparing diuretics is accentuated in the presence of renal impairment (see Contraindications section). Patients with mild renal functional impairment should not receive this drug without frequent and continuing monitoring of serum electrolytes. Cumulative drug effects may be observed in patients with impaired renal function. The renal clearances of hydrochlorothiazide and the pharmacologically active metabolite of triamterene, the sulfate ester of hydroxytriamterene, have been shown to be reduced and the plasma levels increased following 'Dyazide' administration to elderly patients and patients with impaired renal function. Hyperkalemia has been reported in diabetic patients with the use of potassium-conserving agents even in the absence of apparent renal impairment. Accordingly, serum electrolytes must be frequently monitored if 'Dyazide' is used in diabetic patients.

Metabolic or Respiratory Acidosis

Potassium-conserving therapy should also be avoided in severely ill patients in whom respiratory or metabolic acidosis may occur. Acidosis may be associated with rapid elevations in serum potassium levels. If 'Dyazide' is employed, frequent evaluations of acid/base balance and serum electrolytes are necessary.

PRECAUTIONS

General

Bioavailability: The bioavailability of the hydrochlorothiazide and triamterene components of 'Dyazide' is about 50% of the maximum obtainable with oral therapy. Theoretically, a patient transferred from therapy with hydrochlorothiazide with or without triamterene might show an increase in blood pressure, fluid retention, or change in serum potassium. Extensive clinical experience with 'Dyazide', however, suggests that these conditions have not been commonly observed in clinical practice. (See CLINICAL PHARMACOLOGY.)

Impaired Hepatic Function

Thiazides should be used with caution in patients with impaired hepatic function. They can precipitate hepatic coma in patients with severe liver disease. Potassium depletion induced by the thiazide may be important in this connection. Administer 'Dyazide' cautiously and be alert for such early signs of impending coma as confusion, drowsiness and tremor; if mental confusion increases discontinue 'Dyazide' for a few days. Attention must be given to other factors that may precipitate hepatic coma, such as blood in the gastrointestinal tract or preexisting potassium depletion.

Hypokalemia

Hypokalemia is uncommon with 'Dyazide'; but, should it develop, corrective measures should be taken such as potassium supplementation or increased intake of potassium-rich foods. Institute such measures cautiously with frequent determinations of serum potassium levels, especially in patients receiving digitalis or with a history of cardiac arrhythmias. If serious hypokalemia (serum potassium less than 3.0 mEq/L) is demonstrated by repeat serum potassium determinations, 'Dyazide' should be discontinued and potassium chloride supplementation initiated. Less serious hypokalemia should be evaluated with regard to other coexisting conditions and treated accordingly.

Electrolyte Imbalance

Electrolyte imbalance, often encountered in such conditions as heart failure, renal disease or cirrhosis of the liver, may also be aggravated by diuretics and should be considered during 'Dyazide' therapy when using high doses for prolonged periods or in patients on a salt-restricted diet. Serum determinations of electrolytes should be performed, and are particularly important if the patient is vomiting excessively or receiving fluids parenterally. Possible fluid and electrolyte imbalance may be indicated by such warning signs as: dry mouth, thirst, weakness, lethargy, drowsiness, restlessness, muscle pain or cramps, muscular fatigue, hypotension, oliguria, tachycardia and gastrointestinal symptoms.

Hypochloremia

Although any chloride deficit is generally mild and usually does not require specific treatment except under extraordinary circumstances (as in liver disease or renal disease), chloride replacement may be required in the treatment of metabolic alkalosis. Dilutional hyponatremia may occur in edematous patients in hot weather; appropriate therapy is water restriction, rather than administration of salt, except in rare instances when the hyponatremia is life threatening. In actual salt depletion, appropriate replacement is the therapy of choice.

Renal Stones

Triamterene has been found in renal stones in association with the other usual calculus components. 'Dyazide' should be used with caution in patients with a history of renal stones.

Laboratory Tests

Serum Potassium: The normal adult range of serum potassium is 3.5 to 5.0 mEq per liter with 4.5 mEq often being used for a reference point. If hypokalemia should develop, corrective measures should be taken such as potassium supplementation or increased dietary intake of potassium-rich foods. Institute such measures cautiously with frequent determinations of serum potassium levels. Potassium levels persistently above 6 mEq per liter require careful observation and treatment. Serum potassium levels do not necessarily indicate true body potassium concentration. A rise in plasma pH may cause a decrease in plasma potassium concentration and an increase in the intracellular potassium concentration. Discontinue corrective measures for hypokalemia immediately if laboratory determinations reveal an abnormal elevation of serum potassium. Discontinue 'Dyazide' and substitute a thiazide diuretic alone until potassium levels return to normal.

Serum Creatinine and BUN: 'Dyazide' may produce an elevated blood urea nitrogen level, creatinine level or both. This apparently is secondary to a reversible reduction of glomerular filtration rate or a depletion of intravascular fluid volume (prerenal azotemia) rather than renal toxicity; levels usually return to normal when 'Dyazide' is discontinued. If azotemia increases, discontinue 'Dyazide'. Periodic BUN or serum creatinine determinations should be made, especially in elderly patients and in patients with suspected or confirmed renal insufficiency.

Serum PBI: Thiazide may decrease serum PBI levels without sign of thyroid disturbance.

Parathyroid Function: Thiazides should be discontinued before carrying out tests for parathyroid function. Calcium excretion is decreased by thiazides. Pathologic changes in the parathyroid glands with hypercalcemia and hypophosphatemia have been observed in a few patients on prolonged thiazide therapy. The common complications of hyperparathyroidism such as bone resorption and peptic ulceration have not been seen.

Drug Interactions

Angiotensin-converting enzyme inhibitors: Potassium-sparing agents should be used with caution in conjunction with angiotensin-converting enzyme (ACE) inhibitors due to an increased risk of hyperkalemia.

Oral hypoglycemic drugs: Concurrent use with chlorpropamide may increase the risk of severe hyponatremia.

Nonsteroidal anti-inflammatory drugs: A possible interaction resulting in acute renal failure has been reported in a few patients on 'Dyazide' when treated with indomethacin, a nonsteroidal anti-inflammatory agent. Caution is advised in administering nonsteroidal anti-inflammatory agents with 'Dyazide'.

Lithium: Lithium generally should not be given with diuretics because they reduce its renal clearance and increase the risk of lithium toxicity. Read circulars for lithium preparations before use of such concomitant therapy with 'Dyazide'.

Surgical considerations: Thiazides have been shown to decrease arterial responsiveness to norepinephrine (an effect attributed to loss of sodium). This diminution is not sufficient to preclude effectiveness of the pressor agent for therapeutic use. Thiazides have also been shown to increase the paralyzing effect of nondepolarizing muscle relaxants such as tubocurarine (an effect attributed to potassium loss); consequently caution should be observed in patients undergoing surgery.

Other Considerations: Concurrent use of hydrochlorothiazide with amphotericin B or corticosteroids or corticotropin (ACTH) may intensify electrolyte imbalance, particularly hypokalemia, although the presence of triamterene minimizes the hypokalemic effect.

Thiazides may add to or potentiate the action of other antihypertensive drugs. See Indications and Usage for concomitant use with other antihypertensive drugs.

The effect of oral anticoagulants may be decreased when used concurrently with hydrochlorothiazide; dosage adjustments may be necessary.

'Dyazide' may raise the level of blood uric acid; dosage adjustments of antigout medication may be necessary to control hyperuricemia and gout.

The following agents given together with triamterene may promote serum potassium accumulation and possibly result in hyperkalemia because of the potassium-sparing nature of triamterene, especially in patients with renal insufficiency: blood from blood bank (may contain up to 30 mEq of potassium per liter of plasma or up to 65 mEq per liter of whole blood when stored for more than 10 days); low-salt milk (may contain up to 60 mEq of potassium per liter); potassium-containing medications (such as parenteral penicillin G potassium); salt substitutes (most contain substantial amounts of potassium).

Exchange resins, such as sodium polystyrene sulfonate, whether administered orally or rectally, reduce serum potassium levels by sodium replacement of the potassium; fluid retention may occur in some patients because of the increased sodium intake.

Chronic or overuse of laxatives may reduce serum potassium levels by promoting excessive potassium loss from the intestinal tract; laxatives may interfere with the potassium-retaining effects of triamterene.

The effectiveness of methenamine may be decreased when used concurrently with hydrochlorothiazide because of alkalinization of the urine.

Drug/Laboratory Test Interactions

Triamterene and quinidine have similar fluorescence spectra; thus, 'Dyazide' will interfere with the fluorescent measurement of quinidine.

Pregnancy: Category C

Teratogenic Effects—The safe use of 'Dyazide' in pregnancy has not been established. Animal reproduction studies have not been conducted with 'Dyazide'. It is also not known if 'Dyazide' can cause fetal harm when administered to a pregnant woman or can affect reproductive capacity. 'Dyazide' should be given to a pregnant woman only if clearly needed. *Nonteratogenic Effects*—Thiazides cross the placental barrier and appear in cord blood. The use of thiazides in pregnant women requires that the anticipated benefit be weighed against possible hazards to the fetus. These hazards include fetal or neonatal jaundice, thrombocytopenia, and possible other adverse reactions which have occurred in the adult. Triamterene has been shown to cross the placental barrier and appear in the cord blood of animals. The use of triamterene in pregnant women requires that the anticipated benefit be weighed against possible hazards to the fetus. These possible hazards include adverse reactions which have occurred in the adult.

Nursing Mothers—Thiazides appear and triamterene may appear in breast milk. If use of the drug product is deemed essential, the patient should stop nursing.

Pediatric Use—Safety and effectiveness in children have not been established.

ADVERSE REACTIONS

Adverse effects are listed in decreasing order of frequency; however, the most serious adverse effects are listed first regardless of frequency. The serious adverse effects associated with 'Dyazide' have commonly occurred in less than 0.1% of patients treated with this product.

Hypersensitivity: anaphylaxis, rash, urticaria, photosensitivity.

Cardiovascular: arrhythmia, postural hypotension.

Metabolic: diabetes mellitus, hyperkalemia, hyperglycemia, glycosuria, hyperuricemia, hypokalemia, hyponatremia, acidosis, hypochloremia.

Gastrointestinal: jaundice and/or liver enzyme abnormalities, pancreatitis, nausea and vomiting, diarrhea, constipation, abdominal pain.

Renal: acute renal failure, interstitial nephritis, renal stones composed primarily of triamterene, elevated BUN and serum creatinine, abnormal urinary sediment.

Hematologic: leukopenia, thrombocytopenia and purpura, megaloblastic anemia.

Musculoskeletal: muscle cramps.

Central Nervous System: weakness, fatigue, dizziness, headache, dry mouth.

Miscellaneous: impotence, sialadenitis.

Thiazides alone have been shown to cause the following additional adverse reactions.

Central Nervous System: paresthesias, vertigo.

Ophthalmic: xanthopsia, transient blurred vision.

Respiratory: allergic pneumonitis, pulmonary edema, respiratory distress.

Other: necrotizing vasculitis, exacerbation of lupus.

Hematologic: aplastic anemia, agranulocytosis, hemolytic anemia.

Neonate and infancy: thrombocytopenia and pancreatitis—rarely, in newborns whose mothers have received thiazides during pregnancy.

DOSAGE AND ADMINISTRATION

The usual dose of 'Dyazide' is one or two capsules given once daily, with appropriate monitoring of serum potassium and of the clinical effect. (See WARNINGS, Hyperkalemia and PRECAUTIONS, Bioavailability.)

OVERDOSAGE

Electrolyte imbalance is the major concern (see Warnings section). Symptoms reported include: polyuria, nausea, vomiting, weakness, lassitude, fever, flushed face, and hyperactive deep tendon reflexes. If hypotension occurs, it may be treated with pressor agents such as levarterenol to maintain blood pressure. Carefully evaluate the electrolyte pattern and fluid balance. Induce immediate evacuation of the stomach through emesis or gastric lavage. There is no specific antidote.

Reversible acute renal failure following ingestion of 50 tablets of a product containing a combination of 50 mg. triamterene and 25 mg. hydrochlorothiazide has been reported. Although triamterene is largely protein-bound (approximately 67%), there may be some benefit to dialysis in cases of overdosage.

HOW SUPPLIED

Capsules containing 25 mg. hydrochlorothiazide and 50 mg. triamterene, in bottles of 1000 capsules; in Single Unit Packages (unit-dose) of 100 (intended for institutional use only); in Patient-Pak™ unit-of-use bottles of 100.

They are supplied as follows:

NDC 0484-3590-21—Single Unit Packages (unit-dose) of 100 (intended for institutional use only).

NDC 0484-3590-22—in Patient-Pak™ unit-of-use bottles of 100.

NDC 0484-3590-30—bottles of 1000.

Store at controlled room temperature (15°–30°C [59°–86°F]). Protect from light. Dispense in a tight, light-resistant container.

Military—Capsules, 100's (SUP), 6505-00-524-7060.

Veterans Administration—Capsules, 100's (SUP), 6505-00-524-7060.

DZ:L58

Shown in Product Identification Section, page 430

DYRENIUM®   ℞

[di-ren 'ee-um]
(brand of triamterene)

('Dyrenium' is a product of SK&F Co., Cidra, P.R. 00639, Subsidiary of SmithKline Beckman Corporation, Philadelphia, Pa.)

DESCRIPTION

Dyrenium (triamterene, SK&F CO.) is a potassium-conserving diuretic.

Triamterene is 2,4,7-triamino-6-phenylpteridine. Its molecular weight is 253.27. At 50°C., triamterene is slightly soluble in water. It is soluble in dilute ammonia, dilute aqueous sodium hydroxide and dimethylformamide. It is sparingly soluble in methanol.

Each capsule, with opaque red cap and body, contains triamterene, 50 or 100 mg., and is imprinted with the product name DYRENIUM, strength (50 or 100) and SKF. Inactive ingredients consist of benzyl alcohol, cetylpyridinium chloride, D&C Red No. 33, FD&C Yellow No. 6, gelatin, lactose, magnesium stearate, povidone, sodium lauryl sulfate, titanium dioxide and trace amounts of other inactive ingredients.

CLINICAL PHARMACOLOGY

Triamterene has a unique mode of action; it inhibits the reabsorption of sodium ions in exchange for potassium and hydrogen ions at that segment of the distal tubule under the control of adrenal mineralocorticoids (especially aldosterone). This activity is not directly related to aldosterone secretion or antagonism; it is a result of a direct effect on the renal tubule.

The fraction of filtered sodium reaching this distal tubular exchange site is relatively small, and the amount which is exchanged depends on the level of mineralocorticoid activity. Thus, the degree of natriuresis and diuresis produced by inhibition of the exchange mechanism is necessarily limited. Increasing the amount of available sodium and the level of mineralocorticoid activity by the use of more proximally acting diuretics will increase the degree of diuresis and potassium conservation.

Triamterene occasionally causes increases in serum potassium which can result in hyperkalemia. It does not produce alkalosis because it does not cause excessive excretion of titratable acid and ammonium.

Triamterene has been shown to cross the placental barrier and appear in the cord blood of animals.

Pharmacokinetics

Onset of action is two to four hours after ingestion. In normal volunteers the mean peak serum levels were 30 ng./mL. at three hours. The average percent of drug recovered in the urine (0–48 hours) was 21%. Triamterene is primarily metabolized to the sulfate conjugate of hydroxytriamterene. Both the plasma and urine levels of this metabolite greatly exceed triamterene levels. Triamterene is rapidly absorbed, with somewhat less than 50% of the oral dose reaching the urine. Most patients will respond to Dyrenium (triamterene, SK&F CO.) during the first day of treatment. Maximum therapeutic effect, however, may not be seen for several days. Duration of diuresis depends on several factors, especially renal function, but it generally tapers off seven to nine hours after administration.

INDICATIONS AND USAGE

Dyrenium (triamterene, SK&F CO.) is indicated in the treatment of edema associated with congestive heart failure, cirrhosis of the liver, and the nephrotic syndrome; also in steroid-induced edema, idiopathic edema, and edema due to secondary hyperaldosteronism.

'Dyrenium' may be used alone or with other diuretics either for its added diuretic effect or its potassium-conserving potential. It also promotes increased diuresis when patients prove resistant or only partially responsive to thiazides or other diuretics because of secondary hyperaldosteronism.

Usage in Pregnancy. The routine use of diuretics in an otherwise healthy woman is inappropriate and exposes mother and fetus to unnecessary hazard. Diuretics do not prevent development of toxemia of pregnancy, and there is no satisfactory evidence that they are useful in the treatment of developed toxemia.

Edema during pregnancy may arise from pathological causes or from the physiologic and mechanical consequences of pregnancy. Diuretics are indicated in pregnancy when edema is due to pathologic causes, just as they are in the absence of pregnancy (however, see Precautions below). Dependent edema in pregnancy, resulting from restriction of venous return by the expanded uterus, is properly treated through elevation of the lower extremities and use of support hose; use of diuretics to lower intravascular volume in this case is illogical and unnecessary. There is hypervolemia during normal pregnancy which is harmful to neither the fetus nor the mother (in the absence of cardiovascular disease), but which is associated with edema, including generalized edema, in the majority of pregnant women. If this edema produces discomfort, increased recumbency will often provide relief. In rare instances, this edema may cause extreme discomfort which is not relieved by rest. In these cases, a short course of diuretics may provide relief and may be appropriate.

CONTRAINDICATIONS

Anuria. Severe or progressive kidney disease or dysfunction with the possible exception of nephrosis. Severe hepatic disease. Hypersensitivity to the drug.

Dyrenium (triamterene, SK&F CO.) should not be used in patients with preexisting elevated serum potassium, as is sometimes seen in patients with impaired renal function or azotemia, or in patients who develop hyperkalemia while on the drug. Patients should not be placed on dietary potassium supplements, potassium salts, or potassium-containing salt substitutes in conjunction with 'Dyrenium'.

'Dyrenium' should not be given to patients receiving other potassium-conserving agents such as spironolactone, amiloride hydrochloride, or other formulations containing triamterene. Two deaths have been reported in patients receiving concomitant spironolactone and 'Dyrenium' or Dyazide®. Although dosage recommendations were exceeded in one case and in the other serum electrolytes were not properly monitored, these two drugs should not be given concomitantly.

WARNINGS

There have been isolated reports of hypersensitivity reactions; therefore, patients should be observed regularly for the possible occurrence of blood dyscrasias, liver damage, or other idiosyncratic reactions.

Periodic BUN and serum potassium determinations should be made to check kidney function, especially in patients with suspected or confirmed renal insufficiency. It is particularly important to make serum potassium determinations in elderly or diabetic patients receiving the drug; these patients should be observed carefully for possible serum potassium increases.

If hyperkalemia is present or suspected, an electrocardiogram should be obtained. If the ECG shows no widening of the QRS or arrhythmia in the presence of hyperkalemia, it is usually sufficient to discontinue Dyrenium (triamterene, SK&F CO.) and any potassium supplementation and substitute a thiazide alone. Sodium polystyrene sulfonate (Kayexalate®, Winthrop) may be administered to enhance the excretion of excess potassium. **The presence of a widened QRS complex or arrhythmia in association with hyperkalemia requires prompt additional therapy.** For tachyarrhythmia, infuse 44 mEq. of sodium bicarbonate or 10 mL. of 10% calcium gluconate or calcium chloride over several minutes. For asystole, bradycardia, or A-V block transvenous pacing is also recommended.

Continued on next page

Smith Kline & French—Cont.

The effect of calcium and sodium bicarbonate is transient and repeated administration may be required. When indicated by the clinical situation, excess K^+ may be removed by dialysis or oral or rectal administration of Kayexalate®. Infusion of glucose and insulin has also been used to treat hyperkalemia.

PRECAUTIONS

General

Dyrenium (triamterene, SK&F CO.) tends to conserve potassium rather than to promote the excretion as do many diuretics and, occasionally, can cause increases in serum potassium which, in some instances, can result in hyperkalemia. In rare instances, hyperkalemia has been associated with cardiac irregularities.

Electrolyte imbalance often encountered in such diseases as congestive heart failure, renal disease, or cirrhosis may be aggravated or caused independently by any effective diuretic agent including 'Dyrenium'. The use of full doses of a diuretic when salt intake is restricted can result in a low-salt syndrome.

Triamterene can cause mild nitrogen retention which is reversible upon withdrawal of the drug and is seldom observed with intermittent (every-other-day) therapy.

Triamterene may cause a decreasing alkali reserve with the possibility of metabolic acidosis.

By the very nature of their illness, cirrhotics with splenomegaly sometimes have marked variations in their blood pictures. Since triamterene is a weak folic acid antagonist, it may contribute to the appearance of megaloblastosis in cases where folic acid stores have been depleted. Therefore, periodic blood studies in these patients are recommended. They should also be observed for exacerbations of underlying liver disease.

Triamterene has elevated uric acid, especially in persons predisposed to gouty arthritis.

Triamterene has been reported in renal stones in association with other calculus components. 'Dyrenium' should be used with caution in patients with histories of renal stones.

Information for Patients

To help avoid stomach upset, it is recommended that the drug be taken after meals.

If a single daily dose is prescribed, it may be preferable to take it in the morning to minimize the effect of increased frequency of urination on nighttime sleep.

If a dose is missed, the patient should not take more than the prescribed dose at the next dosing interval.

Laboratory Tests

Hyperkalemia will rarely occur in patients with adequate urinary output, but it is a possibility if large doses are used for considerable periods of time. If hyperkalemia is observed, Dyrenium (triamterene, SK&F CO.) should be withdrawn. The normal adult range of serum potassium is 3.5 to 5.0 mEq. per liter with 4.5 mEq. often being used for a reference point. Potassium levels persistently above 6 mEq. per liter require careful observation and treatment. Normal potassium levels tend to be higher in neonates (7.7 mEq. per liter) than in adults.

Serum potassium levels do not necessarily indicate true body potassium concentration. A rise in plasma pH may cause a decrease in plasma potassium concentration and an increase in the intracellular potassium concentration. Because 'Dyrenium' conserves potassium, it has been theorized that in patients who have received intensive therapy or been given the drug for prolonged periods, a rebound kaliuresis could occur upon abrupt withdrawal. In such patients withdrawal of 'Dyrenium' should be gradual.

Drug Interactions

Caution should be used when lithium and diuretics are used concomitantly because diuretic-induced sodium loss may reduce the renal clearance of lithium and increase serum lithium levels with risk of lithium toxicity. Patients receiving such combined therapy should have serum lithium levels monitored closely and the lithium dosage adjusted if necessary.

A possible interaction resulting in acute renal failure has been reported in a few subjects when indomethacin, a nonsteroidal anti-inflammatory agent, was given with triamterene. Caution is advised in administering nonsteroidal anti-inflammatory agents with triamterene.

The effects of the following drugs may be potentiated when given together with triamterene: antihypertensive medication, other diuretics, preanesthetic and anesthetic agents, skeletal muscle relaxants (nondepolarizing).

Potassium-sparing agents should be used with caution in conjunction with angiotensin-converting enzyme (ACE) inhibitors due to an increased risk of hyperkalemia.

The following agents, given together with triamterene, may promote serum potassium accumulation and possibly result in hyperkalemia because of the potassium-sparing nature of triamterene, especially in patients with renal insufficiency: blood from blood bank (may contain up to 30 mEq. of potassium per liter of plasma or up to 65 mEq. per liter of whole blood when stored for more than 10 days); low-salt milk (may contain up to 60 mEq. of potassium per liter); potassium-containing medications (such as parenteral penicillin G potassium); salt substitutes (most contain substantial amounts of potassium).

Dyrenium (triamterene, SK&F CO.) may raise blood glucose levels; for adult-onset diabetes, dosage adjustments of hypoglycemic agents may be necessary during and after therapy; concurrent use with chlorpropamide may increase the risk of severe hyponatremia.

Drug/Laboratory Test Interactions

Triamterene and quinidine have similar fluorescence spectra; thus, triamterene will interfere with the fluorescent measurement of quinidine.

Carcinogenesis, Mutagenesis, Impairment of Fertility

Long-term studies to determine the carcinogenic potential of triamterene are not available. Studies to determine the mutagenic potential of triamterene are not available. Reproductive studies have been performed in rats at doses up to 30 times the human dose and have revealed no evidence of impaired fertility.

Pregnancy

Teratogenic Effects: Pregnancy Category B: Reproduction studies have been performed in rats at doses up to 30 times the human dose and have revealed no evidence of impaired fertility or harm to the fetus due to triamterene. There are, however, no adequate and well-controlled studies in pregnant women. Because animal reproductive studies are not always predictive of human response, this drug should be used during pregnancy only if clearly needed.

Nonteratogenic Effects: Triamterene has been shown to cross the placental barrier and appear in the cord blood of animals; this may occur in humans. The use of 'Dyrenium' in pregnant women requires that the anticipated benefit be weighed against possible hazards to the fetus. These possible hazards include adverse reactions which have occurred in the adult.

Nursing Mothers: Triamterene appears in animal milk; this may occur in humans. If use of the drug is deemed essential, the patient should stop nursing.

Pediatric Use: Safety and effectiveness in children have not been established.

ADVERSE REACTIONS

Adverse effects are listed in decreasing order of frequency; however, the most serious adverse effects are listed first regardless of frequency. All adverse effects occur rarely (that is, one in 1000, or less).

Hypersensitivity: anaphylaxis, rash, photosensitivity.
Metabolic: hyperkalemia, hypokalemia.
Renal: azotemia, elevated BUN and creatinine, renal stones, acute interstitial nephritis (rare).
Gastrointestinal: jaundice and/or liver enzyme abnormalities, nausea and vomiting, diarrhea.
Hematologic: thrombocytopenia, megaloblastic anemia.
Central Nervous System: weakness, fatigue, dizziness, headache, dry mouth.

OVERDOSAGE

In the event of overdosage it can be theorized that electrolyte imbalance would be the major concern, with particular attention to possible hyperkalemia. Other symptoms that might be seen would be nausea and vomiting, other g.i. disturbances, and weakness. It is conceivable that some hypotension could occur. As with an overdose of any drug, immediate evacuation of the stomach should be induced through emesis and gastric lavage. Careful evaluation of the electrolyte pattern and fluid balance should be made. There is no specific antidote.

Reversible acute renal failure following ingestion of 50 tablets of a product containing a combination of 50 mg. triamterene and 25 mg. hydrochlorothiazide has been reported.

The oral LD_{50} in mice is 380 mg./kg. The amount of drug in a single dose ordinarily associated with symptoms of overdose or likely to be life-threatening is not known.

Although triamterene is 67% protein-bound, there may be some benefit to dialysis in cases of overdosage.

DOSAGE AND ADMINISTRATION

Adult Dosage

Dosage should be titrated to the needs of the individual patient. When used alone, the usual starting dose is 100 mg. twice daily after meals. When combined with another diuretic or antihypertensive agent, the total daily dosage of each agent should usually be lowered initially and then adjusted to the patient's needs. The total daily dosage should not exceed 300 mg. Please refer to Precautions—General. When Dyrenium (triamterene, SK&F CO.) is added to other diuretic therapy or when patients are switched to 'Dyrenium' from other diuretics, all potassium supplementation should be discontinued.

HOW SUPPLIED

Capsules: 50 mg. in bottles of 100 and in Single Unit Packages of 100 (intended for institutional use only); 100 mg. in bottles of 100 and 1000 and in Single Unit Packages of 100 (intended for institutional use only).

Veterans Administration–Capsules, 100 mg., 100's, 6505-00-982-9143.
Military–Capsules, 100 mg., 100's, 6505-00-982-9143.

DY:L36

Shown in Product Identification Section, page 430

ESKALITH®   ℞
[*ess-kah 'lith*]
(brand of lithium carbonate)
Capsules, 300 mg.
Tablets, 300 mg.

ESKALITH CR®   ℞
(brand of lithium carbonate)
Controlled Release Tablets, 450 mg.

PRODUCT OVERVIEW

KEY FACTS

'Eskalith' contains lithium carbonate, and is available in 300 mg. capsules and tablets. It is also available in 450 mg. Controlled Release tablets.

MAJOR USES

'Eskalith' is indicated in the treatment of the manic episodes of manic depressive illness and for maintenance therapy to prevent or diminish the intensity of subsequent episodes in those manic depressive patients with a history of mania.

SAFETY INFORMATION

Lithium toxicity is closely related to serum lithium levels and can occur at doses close to therapeutic levels. 'Eskalith' should not be given to patients with significant renal or cardiovascular disease, severe debilitation or dehydration, or sodium depletion, since the risk of lithium toxicity is very high in such patients. (See full prescribing information, below.)

PRESCRIBING INFORMATION

ESKALITH®   ℞
[*ess-kah 'lith*]
(brand of lithium carbonate)
Capsules, 300 mg.
Tablets, 300 mg.

ESKALITH CR®   ℞
(brand of lithium carbonate)
Controlled Release Tablets, 450 mg.

WARNING

Lithium toxicity is closely related to serum lithium levels, and can occur at doses close to therapeutic levels. Facilities for prompt and accurate serum lithium determinations should be available before initiating therapy (see DOSAGE AND ADMINISTRATION).

DESCRIPTION

'Eskalith' contains lithium carbonate, a white, light alkaline powder with molecular formula Li_2CO_3 and molecular weight 73.89. Lithium is an element of the alkali-metal group with atomic number 3, atomic weight 6.94 and an emission line at 671 nm on the flame photometer.

'Eskalith' Capsules: Each capsule, with opaque gray cap and opaque yellow body, is imprinted with the product name ESKALITH and SKF and contains lithium carbonate, 300 mg. Inactive ingredients consist of benzyl alcohol, cetylpyridinium chloride, D&C Yellow No. 10, FD&C Green No. 3, FD&C Red No. 40, FD&C Yellow No. 6, gelatin, lactose, magnesium stearate, povidone, sodium lauryl sulfate, titanium dioxide and trace amounts of other inactive ingredients.

'Eskalith' Tablets: Each round, gray, scored tablet is debossed SKF and J09 and contains lithium carbonate, 300 mg. Inactive ingredients consist of cellulose, iron oxide, lactose, magnesium stearate and sodium lauryl sulfate.

'Eskalith CR' Controlled Release Tablets: Each round, buff, scored tablet is debossed SKF and J10 and contains lithium carbonate, 450 mg. Inactive ingredients consist of alginic acid, gelatin, iron oxide, magnesium stearate and sodium starch glycolate.

'Eskalith CR' tablets 450 mg. are designed to release a portion of the dose initially and the remainder gradually; the release pattern of the controlled release tablets reduces the variability in lithium blood levels seen with the immediate release dosage forms.

ACTIONS

Preclinical studies have shown that lithium alters sodium transport in nerve and muscle cells and effects a shift toward intraneuronal metabolism of catecholamines, but the specific biochemical mechanism of lithium action in mania is unknown.

INDICATIONS

Eskalith (lithium carbonate, SK&F) is indicated in the treatment of manic episodes of manic-depressive illness. Maintenance therapy prevents or diminishes the intensity of subsequent episodes in those manic-depressive patients with a history of mania.

Typical symptoms of mania include pressure of speech, motor hyperactivity, reduced need for sleep, flight of ideas, grandiosity, elation, poor judgment, aggressiveness, and possibly hostility. When given to a patient experiencing a manic episode, 'Eskalith' may produce a normalization of symptomatology within 1 to 3 weeks.

WARNINGS

Lithium should generally not be given to patients with significant renal or cardiovascular disease, severe debilitation or dehydration, or sodium depletion, since the risk of lithium toxicity is very high in such patients. If the psychiatric indication is life-threatening, and if such a patient fails to respond to other measures, lithium treatment may be undertaken with extreme caution, including daily serum lithium determinations and adjustment to the usually low doses ordinarily tolerated by these individuals. In such instances, hospitalization is a necessity.

Chronic lithium therapy may be associated with diminution of renal concentrating ability, occasionally presenting as nephrogenic diabetes insipidus, with polyuria and polydipsia. Such patients should be carefully managed to avoid dehydration with resulting lithium retention and toxicity. This condition is usually reversible when lithium is discontinued. Morphologic changes with glomerular and interstitial fibrosis and nephron atrophy have been reported in patients on chronic lithium therapy. Morphologic changes have also been seen in manic-depressive patients never exposed to lithium. The relationship between renal functional and morphologic changes and their association with lithium therapy have not been established.

When kidney function is assessed, for baseline data prior to starting lithium therapy or thereafter, routine urinalysis and other tests may be used to evaluate tubular function (e.g., urine specific gravity or osmolality following a period of water deprivation, or 24-hour urine volume) and glomerular function (e.g., serum creatinine or creatinine clearance). During lithium therapy, progressive or sudden changes in renal function, even within the normal range, indicate the need for reevaluation of treatment.

An encephalopathic syndrome (characterized by weakness, lethargy, fever, tremulousness and confusion, extrapyramidal symptoms, leukocytosis, elevated serum enzymes, BUN and FBS) has occurred in a few patients treated with lithium plus a neuroleptic. In some instances, the syndrome was followed by irreversible brain damage. Because of a possible causal relationship between these events and the concomitant administration of lithium and neuroleptics, patients receiving such combined therapy should be monitored closely for early evidence of neurologic toxicity and treatment discontinued promptly if such signs appear. This encephalopathic syndrome may be similar to or the same as neuroleptic malignant syndrome (NMS).

Lithium toxicity is closely related to serum lithium levels, and can occur at doses close to therapeutic levels (see DOSAGE AND ADMINISTRATION).

Outpatients and their families should be warned that the patient must discontinue lithium carbonate therapy and contact his physician if such clinical signs of lithium toxicity as diarrhea, vomiting, tremor, mild ataxia, drowsiness, or muscular weakness occur.

Lithium carbonate may impair mental and/or physical abilities. Caution patients about activities requiring alertness (e.g., operating vehicles or machinery).

Lithium may prolong the effects of neuromuscular blocking agents. Therefore, neuromuscular blocking agents should be given with caution to patients receiving lithium.

Usage in Pregnancy: Adverse effects on implantation in rats, embryo viability in mice, and metabolism *in vitro* of rat testes and human spermatozoa have been attributed to lithium, as have teratogenicity in submammalian species and cleft palates in mice.

In humans, lithium carbonate may cause fetal harm when administered to a pregnant woman. Data from lithium birth registries suggest an increase in cardiac and other anomalies, especially Ebstein's anomaly. If this drug is used in women of childbearing potential, or during pregnancy, or if a patient becomes pregnant while taking this drug, the patient should be apprised of the potential hazard to the fetus.

Usage in Nursing Mothers: Lithium is excreted in human milk. Nursing should not be undertaken during lithium therapy except in rare and unusual circumstances where, in the view of the physician, the potential benefits to the mother outweigh possible hazards to the child.

Usage in Children: Since information regarding the safety and effectiveness of lithium carbonate in children under 12 years of age is not available, its use in such patients is not recommended at this time.

There has been a report of a transient syndrome of acute dystonia and hyperreflexia occurring in a 15 kg. child who ingested 300 mg. of lithium carbonate.

Usage in the Elderly: Elderly patients often require lower lithium dosages to achieve therapeutic serum levels. They may also exhibit adverse reactions at serum levels ordinarily tolerated by younger patients.

PRECAUTIONS

The ability to tolerate lithium is greater during the acute manic phase and decreases when manic symptoms subside (see DOSAGE AND ADMINISTRATION).

Caution should be used when lithium and diuretics are used concomitantly because diuretic-induced sodium loss may reduce the renal clearance of lithium and increase serum lithium levels with risk of lithium toxicity. Patients receiving such combined therapy should have serum lithium levels monitored closely and the lithium dosage adjusted if necessary.

The distribution space of lithium approximates that of total body water. Lithium is primarily excreted in urine with insignificant excretion in feces. Renal excretion of lithium is proportional to its plasma concentration. The half-life of elimination of lithium is approximately 24 hours. Lithium decreases sodium reabsorption by the renal tubules which could lead to sodium depletion. Therefore, it is essential for the patient to maintain a normal diet, including salt, and an adequate fluid intake (2500–3000 ml.) at least during the initial stabilization period. Decreased tolerance to lithium has been reported to ensue from protracted sweating or diarrhea and, if such occur, supplemental fluid and salt should be administered under careful medical supervision and lithium intake reduced or suspended until the condition is resolved. In addition to sweating and diarrhea, concomitant infection with elevated temperatures may also necessitate a temporary reduction or cessation of medication.

Previously existing underlying thyroid disorders do not necessarily constitute a contraindication to lithium treatment; where hypothyroidism exists, careful monitoring of thyroid function during lithium stabilization and maintenance allows for correction of changing thyroid parameters, if any; where hypothyroidism occurs during lithium stabilization and maintenance, supplemental thyroid treatment may be used.

Indomethacin and piroxicam have been reported to increase significantly, steady state plasma lithium levels. In some cases, lithium toxicity has resulted from such interactions. There is also some evidence that other nonsteroidal antiinflammatory agents may have a similar effect. When such combinations are used, increased plasma lithium level monitoring is recommended. Concurrent use of metronidazole with lithium may provoke lithium toxicity due to reduced renal clearance. Patients receiving such combined therapy should be monitored closely.

The following drugs can lower serum lithium concentrations by increasing urinary lithium excretion: acetazolamide, urea, xanthine preparations and alkalinizing agents such as sodium bicarbonate.

ADVERSE REACTIONS

The occurrence and severity of adverse reactions are generally directly related to serum lithium concentrations as well as to individual patient sensitivity to lithium, and generally occur more frequently and with greater severity at higher concentrations.

Adverse reactions may be encountered at serum lithium levels below 1.5 mEq./l. Mild to moderate adverse reactions may occur at levels from 1.5 to 2.5 mEq./l., and moderate to severe reactions may be seen at levels of 2.0 mEq./l. and above.

Fine hand tremor, polyuria, and mild thirst may occur during initial therapy for the acute manic phase, and may persist throughout treatment. Transient and mild nausea and general discomfort may also appear during the first few days of lithium administration.

These side effects usually subside with continued treatment or a temporary reduction or cessation of dosage. If persistent, cessation of lithium therapy may be required.

Diarrhea, vomiting, drowsiness, muscular weakness, and lack of coordination may be early signs of lithium intoxication, and can occur at lithium levels below 2.0 mEq./l. At higher levels, ataxia, giddiness, tinnitus, blurred vision, and a large output of dilute urine may be seen. Serum lithium levels above 3.0 mEq./l. may produce a complex clinical picture, involving multiple organs and organ systems. Serum lithium levels should not be permitted to exceed 2.0 mEq./l. during the acute treatment phase.

The following reactions have been reported and appear to be related to serum lithium levels, including levels within the therapeutic range: **Neuromuscular/Central Nervous System**—tremor, muscle hyperirritability (fasciculations, twitching, clonic movements of whole limbs), hypertonicity, ataxia, choreo-athetotic movements, hyperactive deep tendon reflex, extrapyramidal symptoms including acute dystonia, cogwheel rigidity, blackout spells, epileptiform seizures, slurred speech, dizziness, vertigo, downbeat nystagmus, incontinence of urine or feces, somnolence, psychomotor retardation, restlessness, confusion, stupor, coma, tongue movements, tics, tinnitus, hallucinations, poor memory, slowed intellectual functioning, startled response, worsening of organic brain syndromes; **Cardiovascular**—cardiac arrhyth-

mia, hypotension, peripheral circulatory collapse, bradycardia, sinus node dysfunction with severe bradycardia (which may result in syncope); **Gastrointestinal**—anorexia, nausea, vomiting, diarrhea, gastritis, salivary gland swelling, abdominal pain, excessive salivation, flatulence, indigestion; **Genitourinary**—glycosuria, decreased creatinine clearance, albuminuria, oliguria, and symptoms of nephrogenic diabetes insipidus including polyuria, thirst, and polydipsia; **Dermatologic**—drying and thinning of hair, alopecia, anesthesia of skin, acne, chronic folliculitis, xerosis cutis, psoriasis or its exacerbation, generalized pruritus with or without rash, cutaneous ulcers, angioedema; **Autonomic**—blurred vision, dry mouth, impotence/sexual dysfunction; **Thyroid Abnormalities**—euthyroid goiter and/or hypothyroidism (including myxedema) accompanied by lower T_3 and T_4. I^{131} uptake may be elevated. (See Precautions.) Paradoxically, rare cases of hyperthyroidism have been reported; **EEG Changes**—diffuse slowing, widening of the frequency spectrum, potentiation and disorganization of background rhythm; **EKG Changes**—reversible flattening, isoelectricity or inversion of T-waves; **Miscellaneous**—fatigue, lethargy, transient scotomata, dehydration, weight loss, leukocytosis, headache, transient hyperglycemia, hypercalcemia, hyperparathyroidism, excessive weight gain, edematous swelling of ankles or wrists, metallic taste, dysgeusia/taste distortion, salty taste, thirst, swollen lips, tightness in chest, swollen and/or painful joints, fever, polyarthralgia, dental caries. Some reports of nephrogenic diabetes insipidus, hyperparathyroidism and hypothyroidism which persist after lithium discontinuation have been received.

A few reports have been received of the development of painful discoloration of fingers and toes and coldness of the extremities within one day of the starting of treatment with lithium. The mechanism through which these symptoms (resembling Raynaud's syndrome) developed is not known. Recovery followed discontinuance.

Cases of pseudotumor cerebri (increased intracranial pressure and papilledema) have been reported with lithium use. If undetected, this condition may result in enlargement of the blind spot, constriction of visual fields and eventual blindness due to optic atrophy.

Lithium should be discontinued, if clinically possible, if this syndrome occurs.

DOSAGE AND ADMINISTRATION

Immediate release capsules and tablets are usually given t.i.d. or q.i.d. Doses of controlled release tablets are usually given b.i.d. (approximately 12-hour intervals). When initiating therapy with immediate release or controlled release lithium, dosage must be individualized according to serum levels and clinical response.

When switching a patient from immediate release capsules or tablets to the Eskalith CR (lithium carbonate, SK&F) Controlled Release Tablets, give the same total daily dose when possible. Most patients on maintenance therapy are stabilized on 900 mg. daily, e.g., 450 mg. 'Eskalith CR' b.i.d. When the previous dosage of immediate release lithium is not a multiple of 450 mg., for example, 1500 mg., initiate 'Eskalith CR' dosage at the multiple of 450 mg. nearest to, but *below*, the original daily dose, i.e., 1350 mg. When the two doses are unequal, give the larger dose in the evening. In the above example, with a total daily dosage of 1350 mg., generally 450 mg. 'Eskalith CR' should be given in the morning and 900 mg. 'Eskalith CR' in the evening. If desired, the total daily dosage of 1350 mg. can be given in three equal 450 mg. 'Eskalith CR' doses. These patients should be monitored in 1–2 week intervals, and dosage adjusted if necessary, until stable and satisfactory serum levels and clinical state are achieved. When patients require closer titration than that available with 'Eskalith CR' doses in increments of 450 mg., immediate release capsules or tablets should be used.

Acute Mania—Optimal patient response to Eskalith (lithium carbonate, SK&F) can usually be established and maintained with 1800 mg. per day in divided doses. Such doses will normally produce the desired serum lithium level ranging between 1.0 and 1.5 mEq./l.

Dosage must be individualized according to serum levels and clinical response. Regular monitoring of the patient's clinical state and serum lithium levels is necessary. Serum levels should be determined twice per week during the acute phase, and until the serum level and clinical condition of the patient have been stabilized.

Long-Term Control—The desirable serum lithium levels are 0.6 to 1.2 mEq./l. Dosage will vary from one individual to another, but usually 900 mg. to 1200 mg. per day in divided doses will maintain this level. Serum lithium levels in uncomplicated cases receiving maintenance therapy during remission should be monitored at least every two months. Patients unusually sensitive to lithium may exhibit toxic signs at serum levels below 1.0 mEq./l.

N.B.: Blood samples for serum lithium determinations should be drawn immediately prior to the next dose when lithium concentrations are relatively stable (i.e., 8–12 hours after the previous dose). Total reliance must not be placed on

Continued on next page

Smith Kline & French—Cont.

serum levels alone. Accurate patient evaluation requires both clinical and laboratory analysis.

Elderly patients often respond to reduced dosage, and may exhibit signs of toxicity at serum levels ordinarily tolerated by younger patients.

OVERDOSAGE

The toxic levels for lithium are close to the therapeutic levels. It is therefore important that patients and their families be cautioned to watch for early toxic symptoms and to discontinue the drug and inform the physician should they occur. Toxic symptoms are listed in detail under ADVERSE REACTIONS.

Treatment

No specific antidote for lithium poisoning is known. Early symptoms of lithium toxicity can usually be treated by reduction or cessation of dosage of the drug and resumption of the treatment at a lower dose after 24 to 48 hours. In severe cases of lithium poisoning, the first and foremost goal of treatment consists of elimination of this ion from the patient. Treatment is essentially the same as that used in barbiturate poisoning: 1) gastric lavage, 2) correction of fluid and electrolyte imbalance, and 3) regulation of kidney function. Urea, mannitol, and aminophylline all produce significant increases in lithium excretion. Hemodialysis is an effective and rapid means of removing the ion from the severely toxic patient. Infection prophylaxis, regular chest X-rays, and preservation of adequate respiration are essential.

HOW SUPPLIED

Capsules containing 300 mg. lithium carbonate per capsule, in bottles of 100 and 500.

Tablets containing 300 mg. lithium carbonate per tablet, in bottles of 100.

Controlled Release Tablets containing 450 mg. lithium carbonate per tablet, in bottles of 100.

EL:L34

Shown in Product Identification Section, page 430

MONOCID® ℞
[mon 'oh-sid]
brand of sterile cefonicid sodium

PRODUCT OVERVIEW

KEY FACTS

'Monocid' is a sterile, lyophilized, semisynthetic, broad-spectrum cephalosporin antibiotic for parenteral (I.V., I.M.) administration. The 4.5 hour serum half-life of 'Monocid', combined with therapeutic serum and tissue levels, allows dosing once daily (every 24 hours).

MAJOR USES

'Monocid' is indicated in the treatment of infections due to susceptible strains of the microorganisms listed below in the full prescribing information. In particular, 'Monocid' has been proven to be clinically effective in lower respiratory tract infections, including ampicillin-sensitive and ampicillin-resistant *H. influenzae*, and as single-dose prophylaxis in surgical procedures classified as contaminated or potentially contaminated.

SAFETY INFORMATION

'Monocid' is contraindicated in patients who have shown hypersensitivity to cephalosporin antibiotics. Careful inquiry should be made concerning previous hypersensitivity reactions to cephalosporins, penicillins, or other drugs. 'Monocid' should be administered with caution to penicillin-sensitive patients. Serious acute hypersensitivity reactions may require epinephrine and other emergency measures. Because pseudomembranous colitis has been reported with the use of cephalosporins, it is important to consider its diagnosis in patients who develop diarrhea in association with antibiotic use.

PRESCRIBING INFORMATION

MONOCID® ℞
[mon 'oh-sid]
brand of sterile cefonicid sodium
(lyophilized)

DESCRIPTION

Monocid (sterile cefonicid sodium, SK&F), a sterile, lyophilized, semisynthetic, broad-spectrum cephalosporin antibiotic for intravenous and intramuscular administration, is 5-Thia-1-azabicyclo [4.2.0] oct-2-ene-2-carboxylic acid, 7-[(hydroxyphenyl-acetyl)-amino]-8-oxo-3-[[[1-(sulfomethyl)-

1*H*-tetrazol-5-yl]thio] methyl]-disodium salt, [6*R* -[6α, 7β(*R* *)]].

Cefonicid sodium contains 85 mg. (3.7 mEq.) sodium per gram of cefonicid activity.

CLINICAL PHARMACOLOGY

Human Pharmacology

The table below demonstrates the levels and duration of Monocid (sterile cefonicid sodium, SK&F) in serum following intravenous and intramuscular administration of 1 gram to normal volunteers.

[See table below].

Serum half-life is approximately 4.5 hours with intravenous and intramuscular administration. 'Monocid' is highly (greater than 90%) and reversibly protein bound.

'Monocid' is not metabolized; 99% is excreted unchanged in the urine in 24 hours. A 500 mg. I.M. dose provides a high (384 mcg./mL.) urinary concentration at 6–8 hours. Probenecid, given concurrently with 'Monocid', slows renal excretion, produces higher peak serum levels and significantly increases the serum half-life of the drug (8.2 hours).

'Monocid' reaches therapeutic levels in the following tissues and fluids:

[See table above].

Note: Although 'Monocid' reaches therapeutic levels in bile, those levels are lower than those seen with other cephalosporins, and amounts of 'Monocid' released into the gastrointestinal tract are minute. This small amount of 'Monocid' in the gastrointestinal tract is thought to be the reason for the low incidence of gastrointestinal reactions following therapy with 'Monocid'.

No disulfiram-like reactions were reported in a crossover study conducted in healthy volunteers receiving 'Monocid' and alcohol.

Microbiology

The bactericidal action of Monocid (sterile cefonicid sodium, SK&F) results from inhibition of cell-wall synthesis. 'Monocid' is highly resistant to beta-lactamases produced by *Staphylococcus aureus, Hemophilus influenzae, Neisseria gonorrhoeae* and Richmond type I beta-lactamases. 'Monocid' is resistant to degradation by beta-lactamases from certain members of *Enterobacteriaceae*. Active against a wide range of gram-positive and gram-negative organisms, 'Monocid' is usually active against the following organisms *in vitro* and in clinical situations:

Gram-Positive Aerobes: Staphylococcus aureus (beta-lactamase producing and non-beta-lactamase producing) and *S. epidermidis* (Note: Methicillin-resistant staphylococci are resistant to cephalosporins, including cefonicid.); *Streptococcus pneumoniae, S. pyogenes* (Group A beta-hemolytic *Streptococcus*), and *S. agalactiae* (Group B *Streptococcus*).

Gram-Negative Aerobes: Escherichia coli; Klebsiella pneumoniae; Providencia rettgeri (formerly *Proteus rettgeri*); *Proteus vulgaris; Morganella morganii* (formerly *Proteus morganii*); *Proteus mirabilis;* and *Hemophilus influenzae* (ampicillin-sensitive and -resistant).

In addition to the preceding, 'Monocid' is usually active against the following organisms *in vitro*, but the clinical significance of these data has not been established:

Gram-Negative Aerobes: Klebsiella oxytoca; Enterobacter aerogenes; Neisseria gonorrhoeae (penicillin-sensitive and -resistant); *Citrobacter freundii* and *C. diversus.*

Gram-Positive Anaerobes: Clostridium perfringens; Peptostreptococcus anaerobius; Peptococcus magnus; P. prevotii; and *Propionibacterium acnes.*

Gram-Negative Anaerobes: Fusobacterium nucleatum.

Monocid (sterile cefonicid sodium, SK&F) is usually inactive *in vitro* against most strains of *Pseudomonas, Serratia, En-*

terococcus and *Acinetobacter*. Most strains of *B. fragilis* are resistant.

Susceptibility Testing

Results from standardized single-disk susceptibility tests using a 30 mcg. 'Monocid' disk should be interpreted according to the following criteria:

Zones of 18 mm. or greater indicate that the tested organism is susceptible to 'Monocid' and is likely to respond to therapy.

Zones from 15 to 17 mm. indicate that the tested organism is of intermediate (moderate) susceptibility, and is likely to respond to therapy if a higher dosage is used or if the infection is confined to tissues and fluids in which high antibiotic levels are attained.

Zones of 14 mm. or less indicate that the organism is resistant.

Only the 'Monocid' disk should be used to determine susceptibility, since *in vitro* tests show that 'Monocid' has activity against certain strains not susceptible to other cephalosporins. The 'Monocid' disk should not be used for testing susceptibility to other cephalosporins.

A bacterial isolate may be considered susceptible if the MIC value for 'Monocid' is equal to or less than 8 mcg./mL. in accordance with the National Committee for Clinical Laboratory Standards (NCCLS) guidelines. Organisms are considered resistant if the MIC is equal to or greater than 32 mcg./mL. For most organisms the MBC value for 'Monocid' is the same as the MIC value.

The standardized quality control procedure requires use of control organisms. The 30 mcg. 'Monocid' disk should give the zone diameters listed below for the quality control strains.

Organism	ATCC	Zone Size Range
E. coli	25922	25–29 mm.
S. aureus	25923	22–28 mm.

INDICATIONS AND USAGE

Due to the long half-life of 'Monocid', a 1 gram dose results in therapeutic serum levels which provide coverage against susceptible organisms (listed below) for 24 hours.

Studies on specimens obtained prior to therapy should be used to determine the susceptibility of the causative organisms to 'Monocid'. Therapy with 'Monocid' may be initiated pending results of the studies; however, treatment should be adjusted according to study findings.

Treatment

Monocid (sterile cefonicid sodium, SK&F) is indicated in the treatment of infections due to susceptible strains of the microorganisms listed below:

LOWER RESPIRATORY TRACT INFECTIONS, due to *Streptococcus pneumoniae* (formerly *D. pneumoniae*); *Klebsiella pneumoniae**; *Escherichia coli;* and *Hemophilus influenzae* (ampicillin-resistant and ampicillin-sensitive).

URINARY TRACT INFECTIONS, due to *Escherichia coli; Proteus mirabilis* and *Proteus* spp. (which may include the organisms now called *Proteus vulgaris,** *Providencia rettgeri* and *Morganella morganii*); and *Klebsiella pneumoniae.**

SKIN AND SKIN STRUCTURE INFECTIONS, due to *Staphylococcus aureus* and *S. epidermidis; Streptococcus pyogenes* (Group A *Streptococcus*) and *S. agalactiae* (Group B *Streptococcus*).

SEPTICEMIA, due to *Streptococcus pneumoniae* (formerly *D. pneumoniae*) and *Escherichia coli.**

BONE AND JOINT INFECTIONS, due to *Staphylococcus aureus.*

*Efficacy for this organism in this organ system has been demonstrated in fewer than 10 infections.

Surgical Prophylaxis

Administration of a single 1 gram dose of 'Monocid' before surgery may reduce the incidence of postoperative infections in patients undergoing surgical procedures classified as contaminated or potentially contaminated (e.g., colorectal surgery, vaginal hysterectomy, or cholecystectomy in high-risk patients), or in patients in whom infection at the operative site would present a serious risk (e.g., prosthetic arthroplasty, open heart surgery). Although cefonicid has been shown to be as effective as cefazolin in prevention of infec-

Tissue and Body Fluid Levels

Tissue or Body Fluid	Dosage and Route (No. of Patients Sampled)		Time of Sampling After Dose	Average Tissue or Fluid Levels (mcg./g. or/mL.)
Bone	1 g. I.M.	(7)	60–90 min.	6.8
	1 g. I.V.	(10)	44–99 min.	14.0
Gallbladder	1 g. I.M.	(10)	60–70 min.	15.5
Bile	1 g. I.M.	(10)	60–70 min.	7.5
Prostate	1 g. I.M.	(10)	50–115 min.	13.0
Uterine Tissue	1 g. I.M.	(6)	60–90 min.	17.5
Wound Fluid	1 g. I.M.	(10)	60–75 min.	37.7
Purulent Wound	1 g. I.M.	(9)	60 min.	11.5
Adipose Tissue	1 g. I.M.	(5)	60 min.	4.0
Atrial Appendage	1 g. I.M.	(7)	77–170 min.	7.5
	2 g. I.M.	(7)	105–170 min.	8.7
	15 mg./kg. I.V.	(10)	53–160 min.	15.4

Serum Concentrations After 1 Gram Administration
(mcg./mL.)

Interval	5 min.	15 min.	30 min.	1 hr.	2 hr.	4 hr.	6 hr.	8 hr.	10 hr.	12 hr.	24 hr.
I.V.	221.3	176.4	147.6	124.2	88.9	61.4	40.0	29.3	20.6	15.2	2.6
I.M.	13.5	45.9	73.1	98.6	97.1	77.8	54.9	38.5	28.9	20.6	4.5

tion following coronary artery bypass surgery, no placebo-controlled trials have been conducted to evaluate any cephalosporin antibiotic in the prevention of infection following coronary artery bypass surgery or prosthetic heart valve replacement.

In cesarean section, the use of 'Monocid' (after the umbilical cord has been clamped) may reduce the incidence of certain postoperative infections.

When administered one hour prior to surgical procedures for which it is indicated, a single 1 gram dose of 'Monocid' provides protection from most infections due to susceptible organisms throughout the course of the procedure. Intraoperative and/or postoperative administrations of 'Monocid' are not necessary. Daily doses of 'Monocid' may be administered for two additional days in patients undergoing prosthetic arthroplasty or open heart surgery.

If there are signs of infection, the causative organisms should be identified and appropriate therapy determined through susceptibility testing.

Before using 'Monocid' concomitantly with other antibiotics, the prescribing information for those agents should be reviewed for contraindications, warnings, precautions and adverse reactions. Renal function should be carefully monitored.

CONTRAINDICATIONS

Monocid (sterile cefonicid sodium, SK&F) is contraindicated in persons who have shown hypersensitivity to cephalosporin antibiotics.

WARNINGS

BEFORE THERAPY WITH MONOCID (STERILE CEFONICID SODIUM, SK&F) IS INSTITUTED, CAREFUL INQUIRY SHOULD BE MADE TO DETERMINE WHETHER THE PATIENT HAS HAD PREVIOUS HYPERSENSITIVITY REACTIONS TO CEPHALOSPORINS, PENICILLINS, OR OTHER DRUGS. THIS PRODUCT SHOULD BE GIVEN CAUTIOUSLY TO PENICILLIN-SENSITIVE PATIENTS. ANTIBIOTICS SHOULD BE ADMINISTERED WITH CAUTION TO ANY PATIENT WHO HAS DEMONSTRATED SOME FORM OF ALLERGY, PARTICULARLY TO DRUGS. SERIOUS ACUTE HYPERSENSITIVITY REACTIONS MAY REQUIRE EPINEPHRINE AND OTHER EMERGENCY MEASURES.

Pseudomembranous colitis has been reported with the use of cephalosporins (and other broad-spectrum antibiotics); therefore, it is important to consider that diagnosis in patients who develop diarrhea in association with antibiotic use.

Treatment with broad-spectrum antibiotics alters normal flora of the colon and may permit overgrowth of Clostridia. Studies indicate a toxin produced by *Clostridium difficile* is one primary cause of antibiotic-associated colitis. Cholestyramine and colestipol resins have been shown to bind the toxin *in vitro*.

Mild cases of colitis may respond to drug discontinuance alone.

Moderate to severe cases should be managed with fluid, electrolyte and protein supplementation as indicated.

When the colitis is not relieved by drug discontinuance and when it is severe, oral vancomycin is the treatment of choice for antibiotic-associated pseudomembranous colitis produced by *C. difficile*. Other causes of colitis should also be considered.

PRECAUTIONS

General: With any antibiotic, prolonged use may result in overgrowth of nonsusceptible organisms. Careful observation is essential, and appropriate measures should be taken if superinfection occurs.

Drug Interactions: Nephrotoxicity has been reported following concomitant administration of other cephalosporins and aminoglycosides.

Pregnancy: (Category B.) Reproduction studies have been performed in mice, rabbits and rats at doses up to an equivalent of 40 times the usual adult human dose and have revealed no evidence of impaired fertility or harm to the fetus due to Monocid (sterile cefonicid sodium, SK&F). There are, however, no adequate and well-controlled studies in pregnant women. Because animal reproduction studies are not always predictive of human response, this drug should be used in pregnancy only if clearly needed.

Labor and Delivery: In cesarean section, 'Monocid' should be administered only after the umbilical cord has been clamped.

Nursing Mothers: 'Monocid' is excreted in human milk in low concentrations. Caution should be exercised when 'Monocid' is administered to a nursing woman.

Pediatric Use: Safety and effectiveness in children have not been established.

Beta-lactam antibiotics with methyl-thio-tetrazole side chains have been shown to cause testicular atrophy in prepubertal rats, which persisted into adulthood and resulted in decreased spermatogenesis and decreased fertility. Cefonicid, which contains a methylsulfonic-thio-tetrazole moiety, has no adverse effect on the male reproductive system of

Dosage of 'Monocid' in Adults with Reduced Renal Function

(Monitor renal function and adjust accordingly.)

Creatinine Clearance (ml./min. per 1.73 M^2)	Dosage Regimen	
	Mild to Moderate Infections	Severe Infections
79–60	10 mg./kg. (every 24 hours)	25 mg./kg. (every 24 hours)
59–40	8 mg./kg. (every 24 hours)	20 mg./kg. (every 24 hours)
39–20	4 mg./kg. (every 24 hours)	15 mg./kg. (every 24 hours)
19–10	4 mg./kg. (every 48 hours)	15 mg./kg. (every 48 hours)
9–5	4 mg./kg. (every 3 to 5 days)	15 mg./kg. (every 3 to 5 days)
<5	3 mg./kg. (every 3 to 5 days)	4 mg./kg. (every 3 to 5 days)

prepubertal, juvenile or adult rats when given under identical conditions.

ADVERSE REACTIONS

Monocid (sterile cefonicid sodium, SK&F) is generally well tolerated and adverse reactions have occurred infrequently. The most common adverse reaction has been pain on I.M. injection. On-therapy conditions occurring in greater than 1% of 'Monocid'-treated patients were:

Injection Site Phenomena (5.7%): Pain and/or discomfort on injection; less often, burning, phlebitis at I.V. site.
Increased Platelets (1.7%).
Increased Eosinophils (2.9%).
Liver Function Test Alterations (1.6%): Increased alkaline phosphatase, increased SGOT, increased SGPT, increased GGTP, increased LDH.

Less frequent on-therapy conditions occurring in less than 1% of 'Monocid'-treated patients were:

Hypersensitivity Reactions: Fever, rash, pruritus, erythema, myalgia and anaphylactoid-type reactions have been reported.
Hematology: Decreased WBC, neutropenia, thrombocytopenia, positive Coombs' test.
Renal: Increased BUN and creatinine levels have occasionally been seen. Rare reports of acute renal failure associated with interstitial nephritis, observed with other beta-lactam antibiotics, have also occurred with 'Monocid'.
Diarrhea.

DOSAGE AND ADMINISTRATION

General

The usual adult dosage is 1 gram of Monocid (sterile cefonicid sodium, SK&F) given once every 24 hours, intravenously or by deep intramuscular injection. Doses in excess of 1 gram daily are rarely necessary; however, in exceptional cases dosage of up to 2 grams given once daily have been well tolerated. When administering 2 gram I.M. doses once daily, one-half the dose should be administered in different large muscle masses.

Outpatient Use

'Monocid' has been used (once daily I.M. or I.V.) on an outpatient basis. Individuals responsible for outpatient administration of 'Monocid' should be instructed thoroughly in appropriate procedures for storage, reconstitution and administration.

Surgical Prophylaxis

When administered one hour prior to appropriate surgical procedures (see INDICATIONS AND USAGE), a 1 gram dose of 'Monocid' provides protection from most infections due to susceptible organisms throughout the course of the procedure. Intraoperative and/or postoperative administrations of 'Monocid' are not necessary. Daily doses of 'Monocid' may be administered for two additional days in patients undergoing prosthetic arthroplasty or open heart surgery.

In cesarean section 'Monocid' should be administered only after the umbilical cord has been clamped.

General Guidelines for Dosage of 'Monocid', I.V. or I.M.

Type of Infection	Daily Dose (grams)	Frequency
Uncomplicated Urinary Tract	0.5	once every 24 hours
Mild to Moderate	1	once every 24 hours
Severe or Life-Threatening	2*	once every 24 hours
Surgical Prophylaxis	1	1 hour preoperatively

* When administering 2 gram I.M. doses once daily, one-half the dose should be administered in different large muscle masses.

Impaired Renal Function

Modification of Monocid (sterile cefonicid sodium, SK&F) dosage is necessary in patients with impaired renal function. Following an initial loading dosage of 7.5 mg./kg. I.M. or I.V., the maintenance dosing schedule shown below should be followed. Further dosing should be determined by severity of the infection and susceptibility of the causative organism. [See table above].

Note: It is not necessary to administer additional dosage following dialysis.

Preparation of Parenteral Solution

Parenteral drug products should be SHAKEN WELL when reconstituted, and inspected visually for particulate matter prior to administration. If particulate matter is evident in reconstituted fluids, the drug solutions should be discarded.

RECONSTITUTION

Single-Dose Vials

For I.M. injection, I.V. direct (bolus) injection, or I.V. infusion, reconstitute with Sterile Water for Injection according to the following table. SHAKE WELL.

Vial Size	Diluent to Be Added	Approx. Avail. Volume	Approx. Avg. Concentration
500 mg.	2.0 mL.	2.2 mL.	225 mg./mL.
1 gram	2.5 mL.	3.1 mL.	325 mg./mL.

These solutions of Monocid (sterile cefonicid sodium, SK&F) are stable 24 hours at room temperature or 72 hours if refrigerated (5℃.). Slight yellowing does not affect potency.

For I.V. infusion, dilute reconstituted solution in 50 to 100 mL. of the parenteral fluids listed under ADMINISTRATION.

Pharmacy Bulk Vials (10 grams)

For I.M. injection, I.V. direct (bolus) injection or I.V. infusion, reconstitute with Sterile Water for Injection, Bacteriostatic Water for Injection, or Sodium Chloride Injection according to the following table:

Amount of Diluent	Approx. Concentration	Approx. Avail. Volume
25 mL.	1 gram/3 mL.	31 mL.
45 mL.	1 gram/5 mL.	51 mL.

These solutions of 'Monocid' are stable 24 hours at room temperature or 72 hours if refrigerated (5℃.). Slight yellowing does not affect potency.

For I.V. infusion add to parenteral fluids listed under ADMINISTRATION.

"Piggyback" Vials

Reconstitute with 50 to 100 mL. of Sodium Chloride Injection or other I.V. solution listed under ADMINISTRATION. Administer with primary I.V. fluids, as a single dose. These solutions of 'Monocid' are stable 24 hours at room temperature or 72 hours if refrigerated (5℃.). Slight yellowing does not affect potency.

A solution of 1 gram of 'Monocid' in 18 mL. of Sterile Water for Injection is isotonic.

ADMINISTRATION

I.M. Injection: Inject well within the body of a relatively large muscle. Aspiration is necessary to avoid inadvertent injection into a blood vessel. When administering 2 gram I.M. doses once daily, one-half the dose should be given in different large muscle masses.

Continued on next page

Smith Kline & French—Cont.

I.V. Administration: For direct (bolus) injection, administer reconstituted 'Monocid' slowly over 3 to 5 minutes, directly or through tubing for patients receiving parenteral fluids (see list below). For infusion, dilute reconstituted 'Monocid' in 50 to 100 mL. of one of the following solutions:

0.9% Sodium Chloride Injection, USP
5% Dextrose Injection, USP
5% Dextrose and 0.9% Sodium Chloride Injection, USP
5% Dextrose and 0.45% Sodium Chloride Injection, USP
5% Dextrose and 0.2% Sodium Chloride Injection, USP
10% Dextrose Injection, USP
Ringer's Injection, USP
Lactated Ringer's Injection, USP
5% Dextrose and Lactated Ringer's Injection
10% Invert Sugar in Sterile Water for Injection
5% Dextrose and 0.15% Potassium Chloride Injection
Sodium Lactate Injection, USP

In these fluids 'Monocid' is stable 24 hours at room temperature or 72 hours if refrigerated (5°C.). Slight yellowing does not affect potency.

HOW SUPPLIED

Monocid (sterile cefonicid sodium, SK&F) is supplied in vials equivalent to 500 mg. and 1 gram of cefonicid; in "Piggyback" Vials for I.V. admixture equivalent to 1 gram of cefonicid; and in Pharmacy Bulk Vials equivalent to 10 grams of cefonicid.

MC:L22

Shown in Product Identification Section, page 430

ORNADE® SPANSULE® CAPSULES   ℞
[or 'naid]

PRODUCT OVERVIEW

KEY FACTS

'Ornade' *Spansule* capsules contain phenylpropanolamine HCl, a decongestant that provides vasoconstriction similar to that of ephedrine but with less CNS stimulation, and chlorpheniramine maleate, an antihistamine. *Spansule* capsules are prepared so that an initial dose is released promptly and the remaining dose is released gradually over a prolonged period of time, thus permitting b.i.d. dosing.

MAJOR USES

'Ornade' *Spansule* capsules are for symptomatic relief of nasal congestion, runny nose, sneezing, itchy nose or throat, and itchy and watery eyes due, for example, to the common cold or allergic rhinitis.

SAFETY INFORMATION

'Ornade' *Spansule* capsules are contraindicated in patients with: hypersensitivity to either phenylpropanolamine HCl, or chlorpheniramine maleate; severe hypertension; coronary artery disease; stenosing peptic ulcer; pyloroduodenal or bladder neck obstruction; concurrent MAO inhibitor therapy. They should not be used to treat lower respiratory tract conditions including asthma. They should not be used in nursing mothers, or in newborn or premature infants or in children under 12. Further, patients should be cautioned about activities requiring alertness and about the possible additive effects of alcohol and other CNS depressants. (See full prescribing information.)

PRESCRIBING INFORMATION

ORNADE® SPANSULE® CAPSULES   ℞
[or 'naid]

DESCRIPTION

'Ornade' is a combination of an oral nasal decongestant and an antihistamine.

Each 'Ornade' *Spansule* capsule contains phenylpropanolamine hydrochloride, 75 mg. and chlorpheniramine maleate, 12 mg. Inactive ingredients consist of benzyl alcohol, cetylpyridinium chloride, FD&C Blue No. 1, FD&C Red No. 3, FD&C Yellow No. 6, gelatin, glyceryl distearate, iron oxide, polyethylene glycol, povidone, silicon dioxide, sodium lauryl sulfate, starch, sucrose, titanium dioxide, wax and trace amounts of other inactive ingredients.

Each 'Ornade' *Spansule* capsule is so prepared that an initial dose is released promptly and the remaining medication is released gradually over a prolonged period.

CLINICAL PHARMACOLOGY

Phenylpropanolamine Hydrochloride

Phenylpropanolamine hydrochloride is a sympathomimetic agent which is closely related to ephedrine in chemical structure and pharmacologic action, but produces less central nervous system stimulation than ephedrine. It is a vasoconstrictor with decongestant action on nasal and upper respiratory tract mucosal membranes.

Chlorpheniramine Maleate

Chlorpheniramine maleate is an antihistamine with anticholinergic (drying) and sedative side effects. Antihista-

mines appear to compete with histamine for H_1 cell receptor sites on effector cells.

Pharmacokinetics

A single 'Ornade' *Spansule* capsule produces blood levels comparable to those produced by administration of three 25 mg. doses of phenylpropanolamine hydrochloride and three 4 mg. doses of chlorpheniramine maleate in conventional release form given at four-hour intervals. At steady-state conditions, the following peak levels are reached after the oral administration of an 'Ornade' *Spansule* capsule: 21 ng./mL. chlorpheniramine maleate in 7.7 hours; 173 ng./mL. phenylpropanolamine hydrochloride in 6.1 hours; under these circumstances, the half-lives are approximately 21 and 7 hours, respectively.

INDICATIONS AND USAGE

For the treatment of the symptoms of seasonal and perennial allergic rhinitis and vasomotor rhinitis, including nasal obstruction (congestion); also for the treatment of runny nose, sneezing and nasal congestion associated with the common cold.

CONTRAINDICATIONS

Hypersensitivity to either phenylpropanolamine hydrochloride or chlorpheniramine maleate and other antihistamines of similar chemical structure; severe hypertension; coronary artery disease.

This drug should NOT be used in newborn or premature infants.

Because of the higher risk of antihistamines for infants generally, and for newborns and prematures in particular, antihistamine therapy is contraindicated in nursing mothers.

As with any product containing a sympathomimetic, 'Ornade' *Spansule* capsules should NOT be used in patients taking monoamine oxidase (MAO) inhibitors.

WARNINGS

'Ornade' *Spansule* capsules may potentiate the effects of alcohol and other CNS depressants. Also, this product should not be taken simultaneously with other products containing phenylpropanolamine hydrochloride or amphetamines.

'Ornade' *Spansule* capsules should be used with considerable caution in patients with narrow-angle glaucoma, stenosing peptic ulcer, pyloroduodenal obstruction, symptomatic prostatic hypertrophy, or bladder neck obstruction.

Use in Children: In infants and children, especially, antihistamines in *overdosage* may cause hallucinations, convulsions, or death. As in adults, antihistamines may diminish mental alertness in children. In the young child, particularly, they may produce excitation.

Use in the Elderly (approximately 60 years or older): Antihistamines are more likely to cause dizziness, sedation and hypotension in elderly patients.

PRECAUTIONS

General: Use with caution in patients with lower respiratory disease including asthma, hypertension, cadiovascular disease, hyperthyroidism, increased intraocular pressure, or diabetes.

Information for Patients: Caution patients about activities requiring alertness (e.g., operating vehicles or machinery). Also caution patients about the possible additive effects of alcohol and other CNS depressants (hypnotics, sedatives, tranquilizers, etc.), and not to take simultaneously other products containing phenylpropanolamine hydrochloride or amphetamines. Patients should not take 'Ornade' *Spansule* capsules in conjunction with a monoamine oxidase inhibitor or an oral anticoagulant.

Drug Interactions: 'Ornade' *Spansule* capsules may interact with alcohol and other CNS depressants to potentiate their effects.

This product may have additive effects when taken simultaneously with other products containing phenylpropanolamine hydrochloride or amphetamines.

MAO inhibitors prolong and intensify the anticholinergic (drying) effects of antihistamines and potentiate the pressor effects of sympathomimetics such as phenylpropanolamine hydrochloride (see CONTRAINDICATIONS).

Phenylpropanolamine hydrochloride should not be used with ganglionic blocking drugs—such as mecamylamine—which potentiate reactions of sympathomimetics. It also should not be used with adrenergic blocking drugs, such as guanethidine sulfate or bethanidine, since it antagonizes the hypotensive action of these drugs.

The action of oral anticoagulants may be inhibited by antihistamines.

The CNS depressant and atropine-like effects of anticholinergics may be potentiated by concomitant administration of antihistamines. Concomitant administration of anticholinergics such as trihexyphenidyl, and other drugs with anticholinergic action (such as imipramine), with antihistamines may result in xerostomia.

β-adrenergic blockers may be antagonized by antihistamines.

Concomitant administration of corticosteroids and antihistamines may decrease the effects of the corticosteroids by enzyme induction.

Antihistamines inhibit norepinephrine reuptake by tissues and therefore potentiate the cardiovascular effects of norepinephrine.

Concomitant use of antihistamines with phenothiazines may produce an additive CNS depressant effect; concomitant use also may cause urinary retention or glaucoma.

Carcinogenesis, Mutagenesis, Impairment of Fertility: A long-term oncogenic study in rats with the chlorpheniramine maleate component of 'Ornade' *Spansule* capsules did not produce an increase in the incidence of tumors in the drug-treated groups, as compared with the controls. No evidence of mutagenicity was found when chlorpheniramine maleate was evaluated in a battery of mutagenic studies, including the Ames test.

In an early study in rats with chlorpheniramine maleate a reduction in fertility was observed in female rats at doses approximately 67 times the human dose. More recent studies in rabbits and rats, using more appropriate methodology and doses up to approximately 50 and 85 times the human dose, showed no reduction in fertility.

There are no studies available which indicate whether phenylpropanolamine hydrochloride has carcinogenic or mutagenic effects or impairs fertility.

Pregnancy, Teratogenic Effects, Pregnancy Category B: Reproduction studies have been performed with the components of 'Ornade' *Spansule* capsules. Studies with chlorpheniramine maleate in rabbits and rats at doses up to 50 times and 85 times the human dose, respectively, revealed no evidence of harm to the fetus. A study with phenylpropanolamine hydrochloride in rats at doses up to 7 times the human dose revealed no evidence of harm to the fetus. There are, however, no adequate and well-controlled studies in pregnant women. Because animal reproduction studies are not always predictive of human response, 'Ornade' *Spansule* capsules should be used during pregnancy only if clearly needed.

Nonteratogenic Effects: Studies of chlorpheniramine maleate in rats showed a decrease in the postnatal survival rate of offspring of animals dosed with 33 and 67 times the human dose.

Nursing Mothers: Small amounts of antihistamines are excreted in breast milk. Because of the higher risk with antihistamines in infants generally, and for newborns and prematures in particular, 'Ornade' *Spansule* capsules should not be administered to a nursing mother (see CONTRAINDICATIONS).

Pediatric Use: The safety and effectiveness of 'Ornade' *Spansule* capsules in children under 12 years of age have not been established.

In infants and children, especially, antihistamines in *overdosage* may cause hallucinations, convulsions, or death.

As in adults, antihistamines may diminish mental alertness in children. In the young child, particularly, they may produce excitation. (See WARNINGS.)

ADVERSE REACTIONS

The following adverse reactions have been reported following the use of antihistamines and/or sympathomimetic amines:

General: Anaphylactic shock; chills; drug rash; excessive dryness of mouth, nose and throat; increased intraocular pressure; excessive perspiration; photosensitivity; urticaria; weakness.

Cardiovascular System: Angina pain; extrasystoles; headache; hypertension; hypotension; palpitations; tachycardia.

Hematologic: Agranulocytosis; hemolytic anemia; leukopenia; thrombocytopenia.

Nervous System: Blurred vision; confusion; convulsions; diplopia; disturbed coordination; dizziness; drowsiness; euphoria; excitation; fatigue; hysteria; insomnia; irritability; acute labyrinthitis; nervousness; neuritis; paresthesia; restlessness; sedation; tinnitus; tremor; vertigo.

GI System: Abdominal pain; anorexia; constipation; diarrhea; epigastric distress; nausea; vomiting.

GU System: Dysuria; early menses; urinary frequency; urinary retention.

Respiratory System: Thickening of bronchial secretions; tightness of chest and wheezing; nasal stuffiness.

OVERDOSAGE

In the event of overdosage, emergency treatment should be started immediately.

Symptoms: Effects of antihistamine overdosage may vary from central nervous system depression (sedation, apnea, diminished mental alertness, cardiovascular collapse) to stimulation (insomnia, hallucinations, tremors, or convulsions) to death.

Other signs and symptoms may be dizziness, tinnitus, ataxia, blurred vision and hypotension. Stimulation is particularly likely in children, as are atropine-like signs and symptoms (dry mouth; fixed, dilated pupils; flushing; hyperthermia; and gastrointestinal symptoms). In large doses, sympathomimetics may cause giddiness, headache, nausea, vomiting, sweating, thirst, tachycardia, precordial pain, palpitations, difficulty in micturition, muscular weakness and tenseness, anxiety, restlessness and insomnia. Many patients can present a toxic psychosis with delusions and hallucinations. Some may develop cardiac arrhythmias, circulatory collapse, convulsions, coma and respiratory failure.

Toxicity: In acute oral toxicity tests in rats, the LD_{50} for the ratio of 75 mg. phenylpropanolamine hydrochloride and 12 mg. chlorpheniramine maleate was 774.2 mg./kg.; in mice, the LD_{50} for the formulation was 757.4 mg./kg.

Treatment: The patient should be induced to vomit even if emesis has occurred spontaneously. Pharmacologically induced vomiting by the administration of ipecac syrup is a preferred method. But vomiting should not be induced in patients with impaired consciousness. The action of ipecac is facilitated by physical activity and by the administration of 8 to 12 fluid ounces of water. If emesis does not occur within 15 minutes, the dose of ipecac should be repeated. Precautions against aspiration must be taken, especially in infants and children.

Following emesis, any drug remaining in the stomach may be adsorbed by activated charcoal administered as a slurry with water. If vomiting is unsuccessful or contraindicated, gastric lavage should be performed. Isotonic and one-half isotonic saline are the lavage solutions of choice. Since much of the 'Spansule' capsule medication is coated for gradual release, saline cathartics should be administered to hasten evacuation of pellets that have not already released medication. Saline cathartics, such as milk of magnesia, draw water into the bowel by osmosis and therefore may be valuable for their action in rapid dilution of bowel content. Dialysis has not been reported to be effective in the treatment of phenylpropanolamine hydrochloride and chlorpheniramine maleate overdosage. After emergency treatment, the patient should continue to be medically monitored.

Treatment of the signs and symptoms of overdosage is symptomatic and supportive. *Stimulants* (analeptic agents) should *not* be used. Vasopressors may be used to treat hypotension. Short-acting barbiturates, diazepam, or paraldehyde may be administered to control seizures. Hyperpyrexia, especially in children, may require treatment with tepid water sponge baths or a hypothermic blanket. Apnea is treated with ventilatory support.

DOSAGE AND ADMINISTRATION
Adults and children over 12 years of age—one capsule every 12 hours.
'Ornade' *Spansule* capsules should NOT be used in children under 12.

HOW SUPPLIED
In gelatin capsules with opaque red cap and natural body. Each capsule is imprinted with the product name ORNADE and SKF, and filled with small red, white and gray pellets; in bottles of 50 and 500 capsules, and in Single Unit Packages of 100 capsules (intended for institutional use only). Each capsule contains 75 mg. phenylpropanolamine hydrochloride and 12 mg. chlorpheniramine maleate. Capsules should be stored at controlled room temperature (59°–86°F.).
Veterans Administration–Capsules, 500's, 6505-01-108-9574.
Military–Capsules, 500's, 6505-01-108-9574.

OR:L35

Shown in Product Identification Section, page 431

PARNATE®
[*pahr'naight*]
(brand of tranylcypromine sulfate)

℞

Before prescribing, the physician should be familiar with the entire contents of this prescribing information.

DESCRIPTION
Chemically, tranylcypromine sulfate is (±)-*trans* -2-phenylcyclopropylamine sulfate (2:1).
Each round, rose-red, coated tablet is imprinted with the product name PARNATE and SKF and contains tranylcypromine sulfate equivalent to 10 mg of tranylcypromine. Inactive ingredients consist of acacia, calcium sulfate, cellulose, ethylcellulose, FD&C Red No. 3, FD&C Yellow No. 6, gelatin, iron oxide, magnesium stearate, starch, sucrose and trace amounts of other inactive ingredients.

ACTION
Tranylcypromine is a non-hydrazine monoamine oxidase inhibitor with a rapid onset of activity. It increases the concentration of epinephrine, norepinephrine, and serotonin in storage sites throughout the nervous system, and in theory, this increased concentration of monoamines in the brain stem is the basis for its antidepressant activity. When tranylcypromine is withdrawn, monoamine oxidase activity is recovered in 3 to 5 days, although the drug is excreted in 24 hours.

INDICATIONS
For the treatment of Major Depressive Episode Without Melancholia.
Parnate (tranylcypromine sulfate, SK&F) should be used in adult patients who can be closely supervised. It should rarely be the first antidepressant drug given. Rather, the drug is suited for patients who have failed to respond to the drugs more commonly administered for depression.

The effectiveness of 'Parnate' has been established in adult outpatients, most of whom had a depressive illness which would correspond to a diagnosis of Major Depressive Episode Without Melancholia. As described in the American Psychiatric Association's Diagnostic and Statistical Manual, third edition (DSM III), Major Depressive Episode implies a prominent and relatively persistent (nearly every day for at least two weeks) depressed or dysphoric mood that usually interferes with daily functioning and includes at least four of the following eight symptoms: change in appetite, change in sleep, psychomotor agitation or retardation, loss of interest in usual activities or decrease in sexual drive, increased fatigability, feelings of guilt or worthlessness, slowed thinking or impaired concentration, and suicidal ideation or attempts. The effectiveness of 'Parnate' in patients who meet the criteria for Major Depressive Episode with Melancholia (endogenous features) has not been established.

SUMMARY OF CONTRAINDICATIONS
Parnate (tranylcypromine sulfate, SK&F) should not be administered in combination with any of the following: MAO inhibitors or dibenzazepine derivatives; sympathomimetics (including amphetamines); some central nervous system depressants (including narcotics and alcohol); antihypertensive, diuretic, antihistaminic, sedative or anesthetic drugs; buspirone HCl; dextromethorphan; cheese or other foods with a high tyramine content; or excessive quantities of caffeine.
Parnate (tranylcypromine sulfate, SK&F) should not be administered to any patient beyond 60 years of age or with a confirmed or suspected cerebrovascular defect or to any patient with cardiovascular disease, hypertension or history of headache.
(For complete discussion of contraindications and warnings, see below.)

CONTRAINDICATIONS
Parnate (tranylcypromine sulfate, SK&F) is contraindicated:
1. In patients with cerebrovascular defects or cardiovascular disorders
'Parnate' should not be administered to any patient with a confirmed or suspected cerebrovascular defect or to any patient with cardiovascular disease or hypertension. The drug should also be withheld from individuals beyond the age of 60 because of the possibility of existing cerebral sclerosis with damaged vessels.
2. In the presence of pheochromocytoma
'Parnate' should not be used in the presence of pheochromocytoma since such tumors secrete pressor substances.
3. In combination with MAO inhibitors or with dibenzazepine-related entities
Parnate (tranylcypromine sulfate, SK&F) should not be administered together or in rapid succession with other MAO inhibitors or with dibenzazepine-related entities. Hypertensive crises or severe convulsive seizures may occur in patients receiving such combinations.
In patients being transferred to 'Parnate' from another MAO inhibitor or from a dibenzazepine-related entity, allow a medication-free interval of at least a week, then initiate 'Parnate' using half the normal starting dosage for at least the first week of therapy. Similarly, at least a week should elapse between the discontinuance of 'Parnate' and the administration of another MAO inhibitor or a dibenzazepine-related entity, or the readministration of 'Parnate'.

Other MAO Inhibitors

Generic Name	Trademark
Furazolidone	Furoxone®
	(Norwich Eaton)
Isocarboxazid	Marplan®
	(Roche Laboratories)
Pargyline HCl	Eutonyl®
	(Abbott Laboratories)
Pargyline HCl and	Eutron®
methyclothiazide	(Abbott Laboratories)
Phenelzine sulfate	Nardil®
	(Parke-Davis)
Procarbazine HCl	Matulane®
	(Roche Laboratories)

Dibenzazepine-Related and Other Tricyclics

Generic Name	Trademark
Amitriptyline HCl	Elavil®
	(Merck Sharp & Dohme)
	Endep®
	(Roche Products)
Perphenazine and	Etrafon®
amitriptyline HCl	(Schering)
	Triavil®
	(Merck Sharp & Dohme)
Clomipramine hydrochloride	Anafranil®
	(CIBA-GEIGY)
Desipramine HCl	Norpramin®
	(Merrell Dow)
	Pertofrane®
	(Rorer Pharmaceuticals)
Imipramine HCl	Janimine®
	(Abbott Laboratories)
	Tofranil®
	(Geigy Pharmaceuticals)
Nortriptyline HCl	Aventyl®
	(Eli Lilly & Co.)
	Pamelor®
	(Sandoz)
Protriptyline HCl	Vivactil®
	(Merck Sharp & Dohme)
Doxepin HCl	Adapin®
	(Pennwalt)
	Sinequan®
	(Roerig)
Carbamazepine	Tegretol®
	(Geigy Pharmaceuticals)
Cyclobenzaprine HCl	Flexeril®
	(Merck Sharp & Dohme)
Amoxapine	Asendin®
	(Lederle)
Maprotiline HCl	Ludiomil®
	(CIBA)
Trimipramine maleate	Surmontil®
	(Wyeth-Ayerst Laboratories)

4. In combination with fluoxetine
Although a causal relationship has not been established, death has been reported to occur following the initiation of MAOI therapy shortly after discontinuation of fluoxetine. Therefore, 'Parnate' should not be used in combination with fluoxetine. Allow at least five weeks between discontinuation of fluoxetine and initiation of 'Parnate'.
5. In combination with buspirone
Parnate (tranylcypromine sulfate, SK&F) should not be used in combination with buspirone HCl, since several cases of elevated blood pressure have been reported in patients taking MAO inhibitors who were then given buspirone HCl. At least 10 days should elapse between the discontinuation of 'Parnate' and the institution of buspirone HCl.
6. In combination with sympathomimetics
Parnate (tranylcypromine sulfate, SK&F) should not be administered in combination with sympathomimetics, including amphetamines, and over-the-counter drugs such as cold, hay fever or weight-reducing preparations that contain vasoconstrictors.
During 'Parnate' therapy, it appears that certain patients are particularly vulnerable to the effects of sympathomimetics when the activity of certain enzymes is inhibited. Use of sympathomimetics and compounds such as guanethidine, methyldopa, reserpine, dopamine, levodopa and tryptophane with 'Parnate' may precipitate hypertension, headache, and related symptoms. In addition, use with tryptophane may precipitate disorientation, memory impairment, and other neurologic and behavioral signs.
7. In combination with meperidine
Do not use meperidine concomitantly with MAO inhibitors or within two or three weeks following MAOI therapy. Serious reactions have been precipitated with concomitant use, including coma, severe hypertension or hypotension, severe respiratory depression, convulsions, malignant hyperpyrexia, excitation, peripheral vascular collapse and death. It is thought that these reactions may be mediated by accumulation of 5-HT (serotonin) consequent to MAO inhibition.
8. In combination with dextromethorphan
The combination of MAO inhibitors and dextromethorphan has been reported to cause brief episodes of psychosis or bizarre behavior.
9. In combination with cheese or other foods with a high tyramine content
Hypertensive crises have sometimes occurred during 'Parnate' therapy after ingestion of foods with a high tyramine content. In general, the patient should avoid protein foods in which aging or protein breakdown is used to increase flavor. In particular, patients should be instructed not to take foods such as cheese (particularly strong or aged varieties), sour cream, Chianti wine, sherry, beer (including nonalcoholic beer), liqueurs, pickled herring, anchovies, caviar, liver, canned figs, raisins, bananas or avocados (particularly if overripe), chocolate, soy sauce, the pods of broad beans (fava beans), yeast extracts, yogurt, meat extracts or meat prepared with tenderizers.
10. In patients undergoing elective surgery
Patients taking 'Parnate' should not undergo elective surgery requiring general anesthesia. Also, they should not be given cocaine or local anesthesia containing sympathomimetic vasoconstrictors. The possible combined hypotensive effects of 'Parnate' and spinal anesthesia should be kept in mind. 'Parnate' should be discontinued at least 10 days prior to elective surgery. (Withdrawal should be gradual.)

Continued on next page

Smith Kline & French—Cont.

ADDITIONAL CONTRAINDICATIONS

In general, the physician should bear in mind the possibility of a lowered margin of safety when Parnate (tranylcypromine sulfate, SK&F) is administered in combination with potent drugs.

1. 'Parnate' should not be used in combination with some central nervous system depressants such as narcotics and alcohol, or with hypotensive agents. A marked potentiating effect on these classes of drugs has been reported.

2. Anti-parkinsonism drugs should be used with caution in patients receiving 'Parnate' since severe reactions have been reported.

3. 'Parnate' should not be used in patients with a history of liver disease or in those with abnormal liver function tests.

4. Excessive use of caffeine in any form should be avoided in patients receiving 'Parnate'.

WARNING TO PHYSICIANS

Parnate (tranylcypromine sulfate, SK&F) is a potent agent with the capability of producing serious side effects. 'Parnate' is not recommended in those depressive reactions where other antidepressant drugs may be effective. It should be reserved for patients who can be closely supervised and who have not responded satisfactorily to the drugs more commonly administered for depression.

Before prescribing, the physician should be completely familiar with the full material on dosage, side effects, and contraindications on these pages, with the principles of MAO inhibitor therapy and the side effects of this class of drugs. Also, the physician should be familiar with the symptomatology of mental depressions and alternate methods of treatment to aid in the careful selection of patients for 'Parnate' therapy. In depressed patients, the possibility of suicide should always be considered and adequate precautions taken.

Pregnancy Warning: Use of any drug in pregnancy, during lactation, or in women of childbearing age requires that the potential benefits of the drug be weighed against its possible hazards to mother and child.

Animal reproductive studies show that 'Parnate' passes through the placental barrier into the fetus of the rat, and into the milk of the lactating dog. The absence of a harmful action of 'Parnate' on fertility or on postnatal development by either prenatal treatment or from the milk of treated animals has not been demonstrated. Tranylcypromine is excreted in human milk.

WARNING TO THE PATIENT

Patients should be instructed to report promptly the occurrence of headache or other unusual symptoms, i.e., palpitation and/or tachycardia, a sense of constriction in the throat or chest, sweating, dizziness, neck stiffness, nausea or vomiting.

Patients should be warned against eating the foods listed in Section 9 under Contraindications while on Parnate (tranylcypromine sulfate, SK&F) therapy. Also, they should be told not to drink alcoholic beverages. The patient should also be warned about the possibility of hypotension and faintness, as well as drowsiness sufficient to impair performance of potentially hazardous tasks such as driving a car or operating machinery.

Patients should also be cautioned not to take concomitant medications, whether prescription or over-the-counter drugs such as cold, hay fever or weight-reducing preparations, without the advice of a physician. They should be advised not to consume excessive amounts of caffeine in any form. Likewise, they should inform other physicians, and their dentist, about their use of 'Parnate'.

WARNINGS

HYPERTENSIVE CRISES: The most important reaction associated with Parnate (tranylcypromine sulfate, SK&F) is the occurrence of hypertensive crises which have sometimes been fatal.

These crises are characterized by some or all of the following symptoms: occipital headache which may radiate frontally, palpitation, neck stiffness or soreness, nausea or vomiting, sweating (sometimes with fever and sometimes with cold, clammy skin) and photophobia. Either tachycardia or bradycardia may be present, and associated constricting chest pain and dilated pupils may occur. **Intracranial bleeding, sometimes fatal in outcome, has been reported in association with the paradoxical increase in blood pressure.**

In all patients taking 'Parnate' blood pressure should be followed closely to detect evidence of any pressor response. It is emphasized that full reliance should not be placed on blood pressure readings, but that the patient should also be observed frequently.

Therapy should be discontinued immediately upon the occurrence of palpitation or frequent headaches during 'Parnate' therapy. These signs may be prodromal of a hypertensive crisis.

Important:
Recommended treatment in
hypertensive crises

If a hypertensive crisis occurs, Parnate (tranylcypromine sulfate, SK&F) should be discontinued and therapy to lower blood pressure should be instituted immediately. Headache tends to abate as blood pressure is lowered. On the basis of present evidence, phentolamine (available as Regitine®*) is recommended. (The dosage reported for phentolamine is 5 mg i.v.) Care should be taken to administer this drug slowly in order to avoid producing an excessive hypotensive effect. Fever should be managed by means of external cooling. Other symptomatic and supportive measures may be desirable in particular cases. Do not use parenteral reserpine.

PRECAUTIONS

Hypotension

Hypotension has been observed during Parnate (tranylcypromine sulfate, SK&F) therapy. Symptoms of postural hypotension are seen most commonly but not exclusively in patients with pre-existent hypertension; blood pressure usually returns rapidly to pretreatment levels upon discontinuation of the drug. At doses above 30 mg daily, postural hypotension is a major side effect and may result in syncope. Dosage increases should be made more gradually in patients showing a tendency toward hypotension at the beginning of therapy. Postural hypotension may be relieved by having the patient lie down until blood pressure returns to normal. Also, when 'Parnate' is combined with those phenothiazine derivatives or other compounds known to cause hypotension, the possibility of additive hypotensive effects should be considered.

OTHER PRECAUTIONS

There have been reports of drug dependency in patients using doses of tranylcypromine significantly in excess of the therapeutic range. Some of these patients had a history of previous substance abuse. The following withdrawal symptoms have been reported: restlessness, anxiety, depression, confusion, hallucinations, headache, weakness and diarrhea. Drugs which lower the seizure threshold, including MAO inhibitors, should not be used with Amipaque®†. As with other MAO inhibitors, Parnate (tranylcypromine sulfate, SK&F) should be discontinued at least 48 hours before myelography (Withdrawal should be gradual.) and should not be resumed for at least 24 hours postprocedure.

In depressed patients, the possibility of suicide should always be considered and adequate precautions taken. Exclusive reliance on drug therapy to prevent suicidal attempts is unwarranted, as there may be a delay in the onset of therapeutic effect or an increase in anxiety and agitation. Also, some patients fail to respond to drug therapy or may respond only temporarily.

MAO inhibitors may have the capacity to suppress anginal pain that would otherwise serve as a warning of myocardial ischemia. The usual precautions should be observed in patients with impaired renal function since there is a possibility of cumulative effects in such patients.

Although excretion of 'Parnate' is rapid, inhibition of MAO may persist up to 10 days following discontinuation.

Because the influence of 'Parnate' on the convulsive threshold is variable in animal experiments, suitable precautions should be taken if epileptic patients are treated.

Some MAO inhibitors have contributed to hypoglycemic episodes in diabetic patients receiving insulin or oral hypoglycemic agents. Therefore, 'Parnate' should be used with caution in diabetics using these drugs.

'Parnate' may aggravate coexisting symptoms in depression, such as anxiety and agitation.

Use 'Parnate' with caution in hyperthyroid patients because of their increased sensitivity to pressor amines.

'Parnate' should be administered with caution to patients receiving Antabuse®‡. In a single study, rats given high intraperitoneal doses of d or l isomers of tranylcypromine sulfate plus disulfiram experienced severe toxicity including convulsions and death. Additional studies in rats given high oral doses of racemic tranylcypromine sulfate ('Parnate') and disulfiram produced no adverse interaction.

ADVERSE REACTIONS

Overstimulation which may include increased anxiety, agitation and manic symptoms is usually evidence of excessive therapeutic action. Dosage should be reduced, or a phenothiazine tranquilizer should be administered concomitantly.

Patients may experience restlessness or insomnia; may notice some weakness, drowsiness, episodes of dizziness, or dry mouth; or may report nausea, diarrhea, abdominal pain, or constipation. Most of these effects can be relieved by lowering the dosage or by giving suitable concomitant medication. Tachycardia, significant anorexia, edema, palpitation, blurred vision, chills, and impotence have each been reported.

Headaches without blood pressure elevation have occurred.

Rare instances of hepatitis and skin rash have been reported. Impaired water excretion compatible with the syndrome of inappropriate secretion of antidiuretic hormone (SIADH) has been reported.

Tinnitus, muscle spasm, tremors, myoclonic jerks, numbness, paresthesia, urinary retention and retarded ejaculation have been reported.

Hematologic disorders including anemia, leukopenia, agranulocytosis, and thrombocytopenia have been reported.

DOSAGE AND ADMINISTRATION

Dosage should be adjusted to the requirements of the individual patient. Improvement should be seen within 48 hours to three weeks after starting therapy.

The usual effective dosage is 30 mg per day, usually given in divided doses. If there are no signs of improvement after a reasonable period (up to two weeks), then the dosage may be increased in 10 mg per day increments at intervals of one to three weeks; the dosage range may be extended to a maximum of 60 mg per day from the usual 30 mg per day. Withdrawal from Parnate (tranylcypromine sulfate, SK&F) should be gradual.

OVERDOSAGE

SYMPTOMS: The characteristic symptoms that may be caused by overdosage are usually those described on the preceding pages.

However, an intensification of these symptoms and sometimes severe additional manifestations may be seen, depending on the degree of overdosage and individual susceptibility. Some patients exhibit insomnia, restlessness and anxiety, progressing in severe cases to agitation, mental confusion and incoherence. Hypotension, dizziness, weakness and drowsiness may occur, progressing in severe cases to extreme dizziness and shock. A few patients have displayed hypertension with severe headache and other symptoms. Rare instances have been reported in which hypertension was accompanied by twitching or myoclonic fibrillation of skeletal muscles with hyperpyrexia, sometimes progressing to generalized rigidity and coma.

TREATMENT: Gastric lavage is helpful if performed early. Treatment should normally consist of general supportive measures, close observation of vital signs and steps to counteract specific symptoms as they occur, since MAO inhibition may persist. The management of hypertensive crises is described under WARNINGS in the HYPERTENSIVE CRISES section.

External cooling is recommended if hyperpyrexia occurs. Barbiturates have been reported to help relieve myoclonic reactions, but frequency of administration should be controlled carefully because Parnate (tranylcypromine sulfate, SK&F) may prolong barbiturate activity. When hypotension requires treatment, the standard measures for managing circulatory shock should be initiated. If pressor agents are used, the rate of infusion should be regulated by careful observation of the patient because an exaggerated pressor response sometimes occurs in the presence of MAO inhibition. Remember that the toxic effect of Parnate (tranylcypromine sulfate, SK&F) may be delayed or prolonged following the last dose of the drug. Therefore, the patient should be closely observed for at least a week. It is not known if tranylcypromine is dialyzable.

HOW SUPPLIED

Tablets, containing tranylcypromine sulfate equivalent to 10 mg of tranylcypromine, in bottles of 100 and 1000.

* phentolamine mesylate, U.S.P., CIBA.
† metrizamide, Winthrop Pharmaceuticals.
‡ disulfiram, Wyeth-Ayerst Laboratories.

PT:L52
Shown in Product Identification Section, page 431

RIDAURA®   ℞
[ri-door'ah]
(brand of auranofin)
Capsules

PRODUCT OVERVIEW

KEY FACTS

Ridaura (auranofin, SK&F) is an oral form (3 mg. capsules) of gold therapy for adult rheumatoid arthritis. 'Ridaura' may modify disease activity as manifested by synovitis and associated symptoms, and reflected by laboratory parameters such as ESR. Gold therapy cannot reverse structural damage to joint cartilage and bone caused by previous disease. The greatest potential benefit occurs in patients with active synovitis, particularly in its early stage.

The usual adult dosage is 6 mg. daily in a single or divided dose.

MAJOR USES

'Ridaura' is indicated in the management of adults with active classical or definite rheumatoid arthritis (ARA criteria) who have had an insufficient therapeutic response to, or are intolerant of, baseline therapy with nonsteroidal anti-inflammatory drugs. 'Ridaura' should be added to a comprehensive baseline program for rheumatoid arthritis patients, including NSAIDS and non-drug therapies.

SAFETY INFORMATION

See complete list of CONTRAINDICATIONS, WARNINGS, PRECAUTIONS and ADVERSE REACTIONS below.

PRESCRIBING INFORMATION

RIDAURA® ℞
[ri-door'ah]
(brand of auranofin)
Capsules

Ridaura (auranofin, SK&F) contains gold and, like other gold-containing drugs, can cause gold toxicity, signs of which include: fall in hemoglobin, leukopenia below 4,000 WBC/cu mm, granulocytes below 1,500/cu mm, decrease in platelets below 150,000/cu mm, proteinuria, hematuria, pruritus, rash, stomatitis or persistent diarrhea. Therefore, the results of recommended laboratory work (See PRECAUTIONS) should be reviewed before writing each 'Ridaura' prescription. Like other gold preparations, 'Ridaura' is only indicated for use in selected patients with active rheumatoid arthritis. Physicians planning to use 'Ridaura' should be experienced with chrysotherapy and should thoroughly familiarize themselves with the toxicity and benefits of 'Ridaura'.
In addition, the following precautions should be routinely employed:
1. The possibility of adverse reactions should be explained to patients before starting therapy.
2. Patients should be advised to report promptly any symptoms suggesting toxicity. (See PRECAUTIONS —Information for Patients.)

DESCRIPTION

Ridaura (auranofin, SK&F) is available in oral form as capsules containing 3 mg. auranofin.
Auranofin is (2,3,4,6-tetra-O-acetyl-1-thio-β-D-glucopyranosato-S-) (triethylphosphine) gold.
Auranofin contains 29% gold and has the following chemical structure:

Each 'Ridaura' capsule, with opaque brown cap and opaque tan body, contains auranofin, 3 mg., and is imprinted with the product name RIDAURA and SKF. Inactive ingredients consist of benzyl alcohol, cellulose, cetylpyridinium chloride, D&C Red No. 33, FD&C Blue No. 1, FD&C Red No. 40, FD&C Yellow No. 6, gelatin, lactose, magnesium stearate, povidone, sodium lauryl sulfate, sodium starch glycolate, starch, titanium dioxide and trace amounts of other inactive ingredients.

CLINICAL PHARMACOLOGY

The mechanism of action of Ridaura (auranofin, SK&F) is not understood. In patients with adult rheumatoid arthritis, 'Ridaura' may modify disease activity as manifested by synovitis and associated symptoms, and reflected by laboratory parameters such as ESR. There is no substantial evidence, however, that gold-containing compounds induce remission of rheumatoid arthritis.
Pharmacokinetics: Pharmacokinetic studies were performed in rheumatoid arthritis patients, not in normal volunteers. Auranofin is rapidly metabolized and intact auranofin has never been detected in the blood. Thus, studies of the pharmacokinetics of auranofin have involved measurement of gold concentrations. Approximately 25% of the gold in auranofin is absorbed.
The mean terminal plasma half-life of auranofin gold at steady state was 26 days (range 21 to 31 days; n=5). The mean terminal body half-life was 80 days (range 42 to 128; n=5). Approximately 60% of the absorbed gold (15% of the administered dose) from a single dose of auranofin is excreted in urine; the remainder is excreted in the feces.
In clinical studies, steady state blood-gold concentrations are achieved in about three months. In patients on 6 mg. auranofin/day, mean steady state blood-gold concentrations were 0.68 ± 0.45 mcg./mL. (n=63 patients). In blood, approximately 40% of auranofin gold is associated with red cells, and 60% associated with serum proteins. In contrast, 99% of injectable gold is associated with serum proteins.
Mean blood-gold concentrations are proportional to dose; however, no correlation between blood-gold concentrations and safety or efficacy has been established.

INDICATIONS AND USAGE

Ridaura (auranofin, SK&F) is indicated in the management of adults with active classical or definite rheumatoid arthritis (ARA criteria) who have had an insufficient therapeutic response to, or are intolerant of, an adequate trial of full doses of one or more nonsteroidal anti-inflammatory drugs. 'Ridaura' should be added to a comprehensive baseline program, including non-drug therapies.
Unlike anti-inflammatory drugs, 'Ridaura' does not produce an immediate response. Therapeutic effects may be seen after three to four months of treatment, although improvement has not been seen in some patients before six months. When cartilage and bone damage has already occurred, gold cannot reverse structural damage to joints caused by previous disease. The greatest potential benefit occurs in patients with active synovitis, particularly in its early stage.
In controlled clinical trials comparing 'Ridaura' with injectable gold, 'Ridaura' was associated with fewer dropouts due to adverse reactions, while injectable gold was associated with fewer dropouts for inadequate or poor therapeutic effect. Physicians should consider these findings when deciding on the use of 'Ridaura' in patients who are candidates for chrysotherapy.

CONTRAINDICATIONS

Ridaura (auranofin, SK&F) is contraindicated in patients with a history of any of the following gold-induced disorders: anaphylactic reactions, necrotizing enterocolitis, pulmonary fibrosis, exfoliative dermatitis, bone marrow aplasia or other severe hematologic disorders.

WARNINGS

Danger signs of possible gold toxicity include fall in hemoglobin, leukopenia below 4,000 WBC/cu mm, granulocytes below 1,500/cu mm, decrease in platelets below 150,000/cu mm, proteinuria, hematuria, pruritus, rash, stomatitis or persistent diarrhea.
Thrombocytopenia has occurred in 1–3% of patients (See ADVERSE REACTIONS) treated with Ridaura (auranofin, SK&F), some of whom developed bleeding. The thrombocytopenia usually appears to be peripheral in origin and is usually reversible upon withdrawal of 'Ridaura'. Its onset bears no relationship to the duration of 'Ridaura' therapy and its course may be rapid. While patients' platelet counts should normally be monitored at least monthly (See PRECAUTIONS—Laboratory Tests), the occurrence of a precipitous decline in platelets or a platelet count less than 100,000/cu mm or signs and symptoms (e.g., purpura, ecchymoses or petechiae) suggestive of thrombocytopenia indicates a need to immediately withdraw 'Ridaura' and other therapies with the potential to cause thrombocytopenia, and to obtain additional platelet counts. No additional 'Ridaura' should be given unless the thrombocytopenia resolves and further studies show it was not due to gold therapy.
Proteinuria has developed in 3–9% of patients (See ADVERSE REACTIONS) treated with 'Ridaura'. If clinically significant proteinuria or microscopic hematuria is found (See PRECAUTIONS—Laboratory Tests), 'Ridaura' and other therapies with the potential to cause proteinuria or microscopic hematuria should be stopped immediately.

PRECAUTIONS

General: The safety of concomitant use of Ridaura (auranofin, SK&F) with injectable gold, hydroxychloroquine, penicillamine, immunosuppressive agents (e.g., cyclophosphamide, azathioprine, or methotrexate) or high doses of corticosteroids has not been established.
Medical problems that might affect the signs or symptoms used to detect 'Ridaura' toxicity should be under control before starting Ridaura (auranofin, SK&F).
The potential benefits of using 'Ridaura' in patients with progressive renal disease, significant hepatocellular disease, inflammatory bowel disease, skin rash or history of bone marrow depression should be weighed against 1) the potential risks of gold toxicity on organ systems previously compromised or with decreased reserve, and 2) the difficulty in quickly detecting and correctly attributing the toxic effect. The following adverse reactions have been reported with the use of gold preparations and require modification of 'Ridaura' treatment or additional monitoring. See ADVERSE REACTIONS for the approximate incidence of those reactions specifically reported with 'Ridaura'.
Gastrointestinal Reactions: Gastrointestinal reactions reported with gold therapy include diarrhea/loose stools, nausea, vomiting, anorexia and abdominal cramps. The most common reaction to 'Ridaura' is diarrhea/loose stools reported in approximately 50% of the patients. This is generally manageable by reducing the dosage (e.g., from 6 mg. daily to 3 mg.) and in only 6% of the patients is it necessary to discontinue 'Ridaura' permanently.
Ulcerative enterocolitis is a rare serious gold reaction. Therefore, patients with gastrointestinal symptoms should be monitored for the appearance of gastrointestinal bleeding.
Cutaneous Reactions: Dermatitis is the most common reaction to injectable gold therapy and the second most common

reaction to 'Ridaura'. *Any eruption, especially if pruritic, that develops during treatment should be considered a gold reaction until proven otherwise.* Pruritus often exists before dermatitis becomes apparent, and therefore should be considered to be a warning signal of a cutaneous reaction. Gold dermatitis may be aggravated by exposure to sunlight or an actinic rash may develop. The most serious form of cutaneous reaction reported with injectable gold is generalized exfoliative dermatitis.
Mucous Membrane Reactions: Stomatitis, another common gold reaction, may be manifested by shallow ulcers on the buccal membranes, on the borders of the tongue, and on the palate or in the pharynx. Stomatitis may occur as the only adverse reaction or with a dermatitis. Sometimes diffuse glossitis or gingivitis develops. A metallic taste may precede these oral mucous membrane reactions and should be considered a warning signal.
Renal Reactions: Gold can produce a nephrotic syndrome or glomerulitis with proteinuria and hematuria. These renal reactions are usually relatively mild and subside completely if recognized early and treatment is discontinued. They may become severe and chronic if treatment is continued after the onset of the reaction. *Therefore it is important to perform urinalyses regularly and to discontinue treatment promptly if proteinuria or hematuria develops.*
Hematologic Reactions: Blood dyscrasias including leukopenia, granulocytopenia, thrombocytopenia and aplastic anemia have all been reported as reactions to injectable gold and 'Ridaura'. These reactions may occur separately or in combination at anytime during treatment. Because they have potentially serious consequences, *blood dyscrasias should be constantly watched for through regular monitoring (at least monthly) of the formed elements of the blood throughout treatment.*
Miscellaneous Reactions: Rare reactions attributed to gold include cholestatic jaundice; gold bronchitis and interstitial pneumonitis and fibrosis; peripheral neuropathy; partial or complete hair loss; fever.
Information for Patients: Patients should be advised of the possibility of toxicity from 'Ridaura' and of the signs and symptoms that they should report promptly. (Patient information sheets are available.)
Women of childbearing potential should be warned of the potential risks of 'Ridaura' therapy during pregnancy (See PRECAUTIONS—Pregnancy).
Laboratory Tests: CBC with differential, platelet count, urinalysis, and renal and liver function tests should be performed prior to Ridaura (auranofin, SK&F) therapy to establish a baseline and to identify any preexisting conditions. CBC with differential, platelet count and urinalysis should then be monitored at least monthly; other parameters should be monitored as appropriate.
Drug Interactions: In a single patient-report, there is the suggestion that concurrent administration of 'Ridaura' and phenytoin may have increased phenytoin blood levels.
Carcinogenesis/Mutagenesis: In a 24-month study in rats, animals treated with auranofin at 0.4, 1.0 or 2.5 mg./kg./day orally (3, 8 or 21 times the human dose) or gold sodium thiomalate at 2 or 6 mg./kg. injected twice weekly (4 or 12 times the human dose) were compared to untreated control animals.
There was a significant increase in the frequency of renal tubular cell karyomegaly and cytomegaly and renal adenoma in the animals treated with 1.0 or 2.5 mg./kg./day of auranofin and 2 or 6 mg./kg. twice weekly of gold sodium thiomalate. Malignant renal epithelial tumors were seen in the 1.0 mg./kg./day and the 2.5 mg./kg./day auranofin and in the 6 mg./kg. twice weekly gold sodium thiomalate-treated animals.
In a 12-month study, rats treated with auranofin at 23 mg./kg./day (192 times the human dose) developed tumors of the renal tubular epithelium, whereas those treated with 3.6 mg./kg./day (30 times the human dose) did not.
In an 18-month study in mice given oral auranofin at doses of 1, 3 and 9 mg./kg./day (8, 24 and 72 times the human dose), there was no statistically significant increase above controls in the instances of tumors.
In the mouse lymphoma forward mutation assay, auranofin at high concentrations (313 to 700 ng./mL.) induced increases in the mutation frequencies in the presence of a rat liver microsomal preparation. Auranofin produced no mutation effects in the Ames test (Salmonella), in the in vitro assay (Forward and Reverse Mutation Inducement Assay with Saccharomyces), in the in vitro transformation of BALB/T3 cell mouse assay or in the Dominant Lethal Assay.
Pregnancy: Teratogenic Effects—Pregnancy Category C. Use of Ridaura (auranofin, SK&F) by pregnant women is not recommended. Furthermore, women of childbearing potential should be warned of the potential risks of 'Ridaura' therapy during pregnancy. (See below.)
Pregnant rabbits given auranofin at doses of 0.5, 3 or 6 mg./kg./day (4.2 to 50 times the human dose) had impaired food intake, decreased maternal weights, decreased fetal

Continued on next page

Smith Kline & French—Cont.

weights and an increase above controls in the incidence of resorptions, abortions and congenital abnormalities, mainly abdominal defects such as gastroschisis and umbilical hernia.

Pregnant rats given auranofin at a dose of 5 mg./kg./day (42 times the human dose) had an increase above controls in the incidence of resorptions and a decrease in litter size and weight linked to maternal toxicity. No such effects were found in rats given 2.5 mg./kg./day (21 times the human dose).

Pregnant mice given auranofin at a dose of 5 mg./kg./day (42 times the human dose) had no teratogenic effects.

There are no adequate and well-controlled 'Ridaura' studies in pregnant women.

Nursing Mothers: Nursing during 'Ridaura' therapy is not recommended. Following auranofin administration to rats and mice, gold is excreted in milk. Following the administration of injectable gold, gold appears in the milk of nursing women; human data on auranofin are not available.

Pediatric Use: Ridaura (auranofin, SK&F) is not recommended for use in children because its safety and effectiveness have not been established.

ADVERSE REACTIONS

The adverse reactions incidences listed below are based on observations of 1) 4,784 'Ridaura'-treated patients in clinical trials (2,474 U.S., 2,310 foreign), of whom 2,729 were treated more than one year and 573 for more than three years; and 2) postmarketing experience. The highest incidence is during the first six months of treatment; however, reactions can occur after many months of therapy. With rare exceptions, all patients were on concomitant nonsteroidal anti-inflammatory therapy; some of them were also taking low dosages of corticosteroids.

Reactions occurring in more than 1% of 'Ridaura'-treated patients

Gastrointestinal: loose stools or diarrhea (47%); abdominal pain (14%); nausea with or without vomiting (10%); constipation; anorexia*; flatulence*; dyspepsia*; dysgeusia.

Dermatological: rash (24%); pruritus (17%); hair loss; urticaria.

Mucous Membrane: stomatitis (13%); conjunctivitis*; glossitis.

Hematological: anemia; leukopenia; thrombocytopenia; eosinophilia.

Renal: proteinuria*; hematuria.

Hepatic: elevated liver enzymes.

---

* Reactions marked with an asterisk occurred in 3–9% of the patients. The other reactions listed occurred in 1–3%.

Reactions occurring in less than 1% of 'Ridaura'-treated patients

Gastrointestinal: dysphagia; gastrointestinal bleeding†; melena†; positive stool for occult blood†; ulcerative enterocolitis.

Dermatological: angioedema.

Mucous Membrane: gingivitis†.

Hematological: aplastic anemia; neutropenia†; agranulocytosis; pure red cell aplasia; pancytopenia.

Hepatic: jaundice.

Respiratory: interstitial pneumonitis.

Neurological: peripheral neuropathy.

---

† Reactions marked with a dagger occurred in 0.1–1% of the patients. The other reactions listed occurred in less than 0.1%.

Reactions reported with injectable gold preparations, but not with Ridaura (auranofin, SK&F) (based on clinical trials and on postmarketing experience)

Cutaneous Reactions: generalized exfoliative dermatitis.

Incidence of Adverse Reactions for Specific Categories—18 Comparative Trials

	'Ridaura' (445 patients)	Injectable Gold (445 patients)
Proteinuria	0.9%	5.4%
Rash	26 %	39 %
Diarrhea	42.5%	13 %
Stomatitis	13 %	18 %
Anemia	3.1%	2.7%
Leukopenia	1.3%	2.2%
Thrombocytopenia	0.9%	2.2%
Elevated liver function tests	1.9%	1.7%
Pulmonary	0.2%	0.2%

OVERDOSAGE

The acute oral LD$_{50}$ for auranofin is 310 mg./kg. in adult mice and 265 mg./kg. in adult rats. The minimum lethal dose in rats is 30 mg./kg.

In case of acute overdosage, immediate induction of emesis or gastric lavage and appropriate supportive therapy are recommended.

'Ridaura' overdosage experience is limited. A 50-year-old female, previously on 6 mg. 'Ridaura' daily, took 27 mg. (9 capsules) daily for 10 days and developed an encephalopathy and peripheral neuropathy. 'Ridaura' was discontinued and she eventually recovered.

There has been no experience with treating 'Ridaura' overdosage with modalities such as chelating agents. However, they have been used with injectable gold and may be considered for 'Ridaura' overdosage.

DOSAGE AND ADMINISTRATION

Usual Adult Dosage: The usual adult dosage of Ridaura (auranofin, SK&F) is 6 mg. daily, given either as 3 mg. twice daily or 6 mg. once daily. Initiation of therapy at dosages exceeding 6 mg. daily is not recommended because it is associated with an increased incidence of diarrhea. If response is inadequate after six months, an increase to 9 mg. (3 mg. three times daily) may be tolerated. If response remains inadequate after a three-month trial of 9 mg. daily, 'Ridaura' therapy should be discontinued. Safety at dosages exceeding 9 mg. daily has not been studied.

Transferring from Injectable Gold: In controlled clinical studies, patients on injectable gold have been transferred to Ridaura (auranofin, SK&F) by discontinuing the injectable agent and starting oral therapy with 'Ridaura', 6 mg. daily. When patients are transferred to 'Ridaura', they should be informed of its adverse reaction profile, in particular the gastrointestinal reactions. (See PRECAUTIONS—Information for Patients.) At six months, control of disease activity of patients transferred to 'Ridaura' and those maintained on the injectable agent was not different. Data beyond six months are not available.

HOW SUPPLIED

Capsules, containing 3 mg. auranofin, in bottles of 60.

STORAGE AND HANDLING

Store at controlled room temperature. Dispense in a tight, light-resistant container.

RI:L27

Shown in Product Identification Section, page 431

STELAZINE® ℞
[stel 'ah-zeen]
(brand of trifluoperazine hydrochloride)

PRODUCT OVERVIEW

KEY FACTS

'Stelazine' is a phenothiazine derivative of the piperazine group, available in 6 dosage forms and strengths for oral and parenteral administration.

MAJOR USES

'Stelazine' is indicated for the management of manifestations of psychotic disorders as well as the short-term treatment of non-psychotic anxiety, where it is considered second-line therapy.

SAFETY INFORMATION

'Stelazine' is contraindicated for use in comatose or greatly depressed states due to CNS depressants, and in cases of existing blood dyscrasias, bone marrow depression and pre-existing liver damage. (See full prescribing information.)

PRESCRIBING INFORMATION

STELAZINE® ℞
[stel 'ah-zeen]
(brand of trifluoperazine hydrochloride)

('Stelazine' is a product of SK&F Co., Cidra, P.R. 00639, Subsidiary of SmithKline Beckman Corporation, Philadelphia, Pa.)

DESCRIPTION

Tablets: Each round, blue, film-coated tablet contains trifluoperazine hydrochloride equivalent to trifluoperazine as follows: 1 mg. imprinted SKF and S03; 2 mg. imprinted SKF and S04; 5 mg. imprinted SKF and S06; 10 mg. imprinted SKF and S07. Inactive ingredients consist of cellulose, croscarmellose sodium, FD&C Blue No. 2, FD&C Yellow No. 6, gelatin, lactose, magnesium stearate, talc, titanium dioxide and trace amounts of other inactive ingredients.

NOTE: Stelazine (trifluoperazine HCl, SK&F) tablets have been changed from blue, sugar-coated tablets to blue, film-coated tablets. The film-coated tablets differ in size from the corresponding sugar-coated tablets, but the drug content remains unchanged.

Multiple-dose Vials, 10 mL. (2 mg./mL.)—Each mL. contains, in aqueous solution, trifluoperazine, 2 mg., as the hydrochloride; sodium tartrate, 4.75 mg.; sodium biphosphate, 11.6 mg.; sodium saccharin, 0.3 mg.; benzyl alcohol, 0.75%, as preservative.

Concentrate —Each mL. of clear, yellow, banana-vanilla flavored liquid contains 10 mg. of trifluoperazine as the hy-

drochloride. Inactive ingredients consist of D&C Yellow No. 10, FD&C Yellow No. 6, flavor, sodium benzoate, sodium bisulfite, sucrose and water.

N.B.: The Concentrate is for use in severe neuropsychiatric conditions when oral medication is preferred and other oral forms are considered impractical.

INDICATIONS

For the management of the manifestations of psychotic disorders.

Stelazine (trifluoperazine HCl, SK&F) is effective for the short-term treatment of generalized non-psychotic anxiety. However, 'Stelazine' is not the first drug to be used in therapy for most patients with non-psychotic anxiety because certain risks associated with its use are not shared by common alternative treatments (i.e., benzodiazepines).

When used in the treatment of non-psychotic anxiety, 'Stelazine' should not be administered at doses of more than 6 mg. per day or for longer than 12 weeks because the use of 'Stelazine' at higher doses or for longer intervals may cause persistent tardive dyskinesia that may prove irreversible (see Warnings section).

The effectiveness of 'Stelazine' as a treatment for non-psychotic anxiety was established in a four-week clinical multicenter study of outpatients with generalized anxiety disorder (DSM-III). This evidence does not predict that 'Stelazine' will be useful in patients with other non-psychotic conditions in which anxiety, or signs that mimic anxiety, are found (i.e., physical illness, organic mental conditions, agitated depression, character pathologies, etc.).

Stelazine (trifluoperazine HCl, SK&F) has not been shown effective in the management of behavioral complications in patients with mental retardation.

CONTRAINDICATIONS

Comatose or greatly depressed states due to central nervous system depressants, and in cases of existing blood dyscrasias, bone marrow depression and pre-existing liver damage.

WARNINGS

Tardive Dyskinesia: Tardive dyskinesia, a syndrome consisting of potentially irreversible, involuntary, dyskinetic movements, may develop in patients treated with neuroleptic (antipsychotic) drugs. Although the prevalence of the syndrome appears to be highest among the elderly, especially elderly women, it is impossible to rely upon prevalence estimates to predict, at the inception of neuroleptic treatment, which patients are likely to develop the syndrome. Whether neuroleptic drug products differ in their potential to cause tardive dyskinesia is unknown.

Both the risk of developing the syndrome and the likelihood that it will become irreversible are believed to increase as the duration of treatment and the total cumulative dose of neuroleptic drugs administered to the patient increase. However, the syndrome can develop, although much less commonly, after relatively brief treatment periods at low doses.

There is no known treatment for established cases of tardive dyskinesia, although the syndrome may remit, partially or completely, if neuroleptic treatment is withdrawn. Neuroleptic treatment itself, however, may suppress (or partially suppress) the signs and symptoms of the syndrome and thereby may possibly mask the underlying disease process. The effect that symptomatic suppression has upon the long-term course of the syndrome is unknown.

Given these considerations, neuroleptics should be prescribed in a manner that is most likely to minimize the occurrence of tardive dyskinesia. Chronic neuroleptic treatment should generally be reserved for patients who suffer from a chronic illness that 1) is known to respond to neuroleptic drugs, and, 2) for whom alternative, equally effective, but potentially less harmful treatments are not available or appropriate. In patients who do require chronic treatment, the smallest dose and the shortest duration of treatment producing a satisfactory clinical response should be sought. The need for continued treatment should be reassessed periodically.

If signs and symptoms of tardive dyskinesia appear in a patient on neuroleptics, drug discontinuation should be considered. However, some patients may require treatment despite the presence of the syndrome.

For further information about the description of tardive dyskinesia and its clinical detection, please refer to the sections on Precautions and Adverse Reactions.

Neuroleptic Malignant Syndrome (NMS)

A potentially fatal symptom complex sometimes referred to as Neuroleptic Malignant Syndrome (NMS) has been reported in association with antipsychotic drugs. Clinical manifestations of NMS are hyperpyrexia, muscle rigidity, altered mental status and evidence of autonomic instability (irregular pulse or blood pressure, tachycardia, diaphoresis, and cardiac dysrhythmias).

The diagnostic evaluation of patients with this syndrome is complicated. In arriving at a diagnosis, it is important to identify cases where the clinical presentation includes both serious medical illness (e.g., pneumonia, systemic infection, etc.) and untreated or inadequately treated extrapyramidal signs and symptoms (EPS). Other important considerations in the differential diagnosis include central anticholinergic toxicity, heat stroke, drug fever and primary central nervous system (CNS) pathology.

The management of NMS should inlude 1) immediate discontinuation of antipsychotic drugs and other drugs not essential to concurrent therapy, 2) intensive symptomatic treatment and medical monitoring, and 3) treatment of any concomitant serious medical problems for which specific treatments are available. There is no general agreement about specific pharmacological treatment regimens for uncomplicated NMS.

If a patient requires antipsychotic drug treatment after recovery from NMS, the potential reintroduction of drug therapy should be carefully considered. The patient should be carefully monitored, since recurrences of NMS have been reported.

Patients who have demonstrated a hypersensitivity reaction (e.g., blood dyscrasias, jaundice) with a phenothiazine should not be re-exposed to any phenothiazine, including Stelazine (trifluoperazine HCl, SK&F), unless in the judgment of the physician the potential benefits of treatment outweigh the possible hazard.

'Stelazine' Concentrate contains sodium bisulfite, a sulfite that may cause allergic-type reactions including anaphylactic symptoms and life-threatening or less severe asthmatic episodes in certain susceptible people. The overall prevalence of sulfite sensitivity in the general population is unknown and probably low. Sulfite sensitivity is seen more frequently in asthmatic than in non-asthmatic people.

Stelazine (trifluoperazine HCl, SK&F) may impair mental and/or physical abilities, especially during the first few days of therapy. Therefore, caution patients about activities requiring alertness (e.g., operating vehicles or machinery).

If agents such as sedatives, narcotics, anesthetics, tranquilizers, or alcohol are used either simultaneously or successively with the drug, the possibility of an undesirable additive depressant effect should be considered.

Usage in Pregnancy: Safety for the use of 'Stelazine' during pregnancy has not been established. Therefore, it is not recommended that the drug be given to pregnant patients except when, in the judgment of the physician, it is essential. The potential benefits should clearly outweigh possible hazards. There are reported instances of prolonged jaundice, extrapyramidal signs, hyperreflexia or hyporeflexia in newborn infants whose mothers received phenothiazines.

Reproductive studies in rats given over 600 times the human dose showed an increased incidence of malformations above controls and reduced litter size and weight linked to maternal toxicity. These effects were not observed at half this dosage. No adverse effect on fetal development was observed in rabbits given 700 times the human dose nor in monkeys given 25 times the human dose.

Nursing Mothers: There is evidence that phenothiazines are excreted in the breast milk of nursing mothers.

PRECAUTIONS

Given the likelihood that some patients exposed chronically to neuroleptics will develop tardive dyskinesia, it is advised that all patients in whom chronic use is contemplated be given, if possible, full information about this risk. The decision to inform patients and/or their guardians must obviously take into account the clinical circumstances and the competency of the patient to understand the information provided.

Thrombocytopenia and anemia have been reported in patients receiving the drug. Agranulocytosis and pancytopenia have also been reported—warn patients to report the sudden appearance of sore throat or other signs of infection. If white blood cell and differential counts indicate cellular depression, stop treatment and start antibiotic and other suitable therapy.

Jaundice of the cholestatic type of hepatitis or liver damage has been reported. If fever with grippe-like symptoms occurs, appropriate liver studies should be conducted. If tests indicate an abnormality, stop treatment.

One result of therapy may be an increase in mental and physical activity. For example, a few patients with angina pectoris have complained of increased pain while taking the drug. Therefore, angina patients should be observed carefully and, if an unfavorable response is noted, the drug should be withdrawn.

Because hypotension has occurred, large doses and parenteral administration should be avoided in patients with impaired cardiovascular systems. To minimize the occurrence of hypotension after injection, keep patient lying down and observe for at least ½ hour. If hypotension occurs from parenteral or oral dosing, place patient in head-low position with legs raised. If a vasoconstrictor is required, Levophed®* and Neo-Synephrine®† are suitable. Other pressor agents, including epinephrine, should not be used as they may cause a paradoxical further lowering of blood pressure.

Since certain phenothiazines have been reported to produce retinopathy, the drug should be discontinued if ophthalmoscopic examination or visual field studies should demonstrate retinal changes.

An antiemetic action of Stelazine (trifluoperazine HCl, SK&F) may mask the signs and symptoms of toxicity or overdosage of other drugs and may obscure the diagnosis and treatment of other conditions such as intestinal obstruction, brain tumor and Reye's syndrome.

With prolonged administration at high dosages, the possibility of cumulative effects, with sudden onset of severe central nervous system or vasomotor symptoms, should be kept in mind.

Neuroleptic drugs elevate prolactin levels; the elevation persists during chronic administration. Tissue culture experiments indicate that approximately one-third of human breast cancers are prolactin-dependent in vitro, a factor of potential importance if the prescribing of these drugs is contemplated in a patient with a previously detected breast cancer. Although disturbances such as galactorrhea, amenorrhea, gynecomastia and impotence have been reported, the clinical significance of elevated serum prolactin levels is unknown for most patients. An increase in mammary neoplasms has been found in rodents after chronic administration of neuroleptic drugs. Neither clinical nor epidemiologic studies conducted to date, however, have shown an association between chronic administration of these drugs and mammary tumorigenesis; the available evidence is considered too limited to be conclusive at this time.

Chromosomal aberrations in spermatocytes and abnormal sperm have been demonstrated in rodents treated with certain neuroleptics.

Because phenothiazines may interfere with thermoregulatory mechanisms, use with caution in persons who will be exposed to extreme heat.

As with all drugs which exert an anticholinergic effect, and/or cause mydriasis, trifluoperazine should be used with caution in patients with glaucoma.

Phenothiazines may diminish the effect of oral anticoagulants.

Phenothiazines can produce alpha-adrenergic blockade.

Concomitant administration of propranolol with phenothiazines results in increased plasma levels of both drugs.

Antihypertensive effects of guanethidine and related compounds may be counteracted when phenothiazines are used concurrently.

Thiazide diuretics may accentuate the orthostatic hypotension that may occur with phenothiazines.

Phenothiazines may lower the convulsive threshold; dosage adjustments of anticonvulsants may be necessary. Potentiation of anticonvulsant effects does not occur. However, it has been reported that phenothiazines may interfere with the metabolism of Dilantin®‡ and thus precipitate 'Dilantin' toxicity.

Drugs which lower the seizure threshold, including phenothiazine derivatives, should not be used with Amipaque®§. As with other phenothiazine derivatives, 'Stelazine' should be discontinued at least 48 hours before myelography, should not be resumed for at least 24 hours postprocedure, and should not be used for the control of nausea and vomiting occurring either prior to myelography or postprocedure with 'Amipaque'.

The presence of phenothiazines may produce false positive phenylketonuria (PKU) test results.

Long-Term Therapy: To lessen the likelihood of adverse reactions related to cumulative drug effect, patients with a history of long-term therapy with Stelazine (trifluoperazine HCl, SK&F) and/or other neuroleptics should be evaluated periodically to decide whether the maintenance dosage could be lowered or drug therapy discontinued.

ADVERSE REACTIONS

Drowsiness, dizziness, skin reactions, rash, dry mouth, insomnia, amenorrhea, fatigue, muscular weakness, anorexia, lactation, blurred vision and neuromuscular (extrapyramidal) reactions.

Neuromuscular (Extrapyramidal) Reactions

These symptoms are seen in a significant number of hospitalized mental patients. They may be characterized by motor restlessness, be of the dystonic type, or they may resemble parkinsonism.

Depending on the severity of symptoms, dosage should be reduced or discontinued. If therapy is reinstituted, it should be at a lower dosage. Should these symptoms occur in children or pregnant patients, the drug should be stopped and not reinstituted. In most cases barbiturates by suitable route of administration will suffice. (Or, injectable Benadryl®‖ may be useful.) In more severe cases, the administration of an anti-parkinsonism agent, except levodopa, usually produces rapid reversal of symptoms. Suitable supportive measures such as maintaining a clear airway and adequate hydration should be employed.

Motor Restlessness: Symptoms may include agitation or jitteriness and sometimes insomnia. These symptoms often disappear spontaneously. At times these symptoms may be similar to the original neurotic or psychotic symptoms. Dosage should not be increased until these side effects have subsided.

If this phase becomes too troublesome, the symptoms can usually be controlled by a reduction of dosage or change of

drug. Treatment with anti-parkinsonian agents, benzodiazepines or propranolol may be helpful.

Dystonias: Symptoms may include: spasm of the neck muscles, sometimes progressing to torticollis; extensor rigidity of back muscles, sometimes progressing to opisthotonos; carpopedal spasm, trismus, swallowing difficulty, oculogyric crisis and protrusion of the tongue.

These usually subside within a few hours, and almost always within 24 to 48 hours, after the drug has been discontinued. In mild cases, reassurance or a barbiturate is often sufficient. In moderate cases, barbiturates will usually bring rapid relief. In more severe adult cases, the administration of an anti-parkinsonism agent, except levodopa, usually produces rapid reversal of symptoms. Also, intravenous caffeine with sodium benzoate seems to be effective. In children, reassurance and barbiturates will usually control symptoms. (Or, injectable 'Benadryl' may be useful.) Note: See 'Benadryl' prescribing information for appropriate children's dosage. If appropriate treatment with anti-parkinsonism agents or 'Benadryl' fails to reverse the signs and symptoms, the diagnosis should be reevaluated.

Pseudo-parkinsonism: Symptoms may include: mask-like facies; drooling; tremors; pill-rolling motion; cogwheel rigidity; and shuffling gait. Reassurance and sedation are important. In most cases these symptoms are readily controlled when an anti-parkinsonism agent is administered concomitantly. Anti-parkinsonism agents should be used only when required. Generally, therapy of a few weeks to two or three months will suffice. After this time patients should be evaluated to determine their need for continued treatment. (Note: Levodopa has not been found effective in pseudo-parkinsonism.) Occasionally it is necessary to lower the dosage of Stelazine (trifluoperazine HCl, SK&F) or to discontinue the drug.

Tardive Dyskinesia: As with all antipsychotic agents, tardive dyskinesia may appear in some patients on long-term therapy or may appear after drug therapy has been discontinued. The syndrome can also develop, although much less frequently, after relatively brief treatment periods at low doses. This syndrome appears in all age groups. Although its prevalence appears to be highest among elderly patients, especially elderly women, it is impossible to rely upon prevalence estimates to predict at the inception of neuroleptic treatment which patients are likely to develop the syndrome. The symptoms are persistent and in some patients appear to be irreversible. The syndrome is characterized by rhythmical involuntary movements of the tongue, face, mouth or jaw (e.g., protrusion of tongue, puffing of cheeks, puckering of mouth, chewing movements). Sometimes these may be accompanied by involuntary movements of extremities. In rare instances, these involuntary movements of the extremities are the only manifestations of tardive dyskinesia. A variant of tardive dyskinesia, tardive dystonia, has also been described.

There is no known effective treatment for tardive dyskinesia; anti-parkinsonism agents do not alleviate the symptoms of this syndrome. If clinically feasible, it is suggested that all antipsychotic agents be discontinued if these symptoms appear. Should it be necessary to reinstitute treatment, or increase the dosage of the agent, or switch to a different antipsychotic agent, the syndrome may be masked.

It has been reported that fine vermicular movements of the tongue may be an early sign of the syndrome and if the medication is stopped at that time the syndrome may not develop.

Adverse Reactions Reported with Stelazine (trifluoperazine HCl, SK&F) or Other Phenothiazine Derivatives: Adverse effects with different phenothiazines vary in type, frequency, and mechanism of occurrence, i.e., some are dose-related, while others involve individual patient sensitivity. Some adverse effects may be more likely to occur, or occur with greater intensity, in patients with special medical problems, e.g., patients with mitral insufficiency or pheochromocytoma have experienced severe hypotension following recommended doses of certain phenothiazines.

Not all of the following adverse reactions have been observed with every phenothiazine derivative, but they have been reported with one or more and should be borne in mind when drugs of this class are administered: extrapyramidal symptoms (opisthotonos, oculogyric crisis, hyperreflexia, dystonia, akathisia, dyskinesia, parkinsonism) some of which have lasted months and even years—particularly in elderly patients with previous brain damage; grand mal and petit mal convulsions, particularly in patients with EEG abnormalities or history of such disorders; altered cerebrospinal fluid proteins; cerebral edema; intensification and prolongation of the action of central nervous system depressants (opiates, analgesics, antihistamines, barbiturates, alcohol), atropine, heat, organophosphorus insecticides; autonomic reactions (dryness of mouth, nasal congestion, headache, nausea, constipation, obstipation, adynamic ileus, ejaculatory disorders/impotence, priapism, atonic colon, urinary retention, miosis and mydriasis); reactivation of psychotic processes, catatonic-like states; hypotension (sometimes fatal); cardiac arrest; blood dyscrasias (pancytopenia, thrombocytopenic

Continued on next page

Smith Kline & French—Cont.

purpura, leukopenia, agranulocytosis, eosinophilia, hemolytic anemia, aplastic anemia); liver damage (jaundice, biliary stasis); endocrine disturbances (hyperglycemia, hypoglycemia, glycosuria, lactation, galactorrhea, gynecomastia, menstrual irregularities, false positive pregnancy tests); skin disorders (photosensitivity, itching, erythema, urticaria, eczema up to exfoliative dermatitis); other allergic reactions (asthma, laryngeal edema, angioneurotic edema, anaphylactoid reactions); peripheral edema; reversed epinephrine effect; hyperpyrexia; mild fever after large I.M. doses; increased appetite; increased weight; a systemic lupus erythematosus-like syndrome; pigmentary retinopathy; with prolonged administration of substantial doses, skin pigmentation, epithelial keratopathy, and lenticular and corneal deposits.

EKG changes—particularly nonspecific, usually reversible Q and T wave distortions—have been observed in some patients receiving phenothiazine tranquilizers. Although phenothiazines cause neither psychic nor physical dependence, sudden discontinuance in long-term psychiatric patients may cause temporary symptoms, e.g., nausea and vomiting, dizziness, tremulousness.

Note: There has been occasional reports of sudden death in patients receiving phenothiazines. In some cases, the cause appeared to be cardiac arrest or asphyxia due to failure of the cough reflex.

DOSAGE AND ADMINISTRATION—ADULTS

Dosage should be adjusted to the needs of the individual. The lowest effective dosage should always be used. Dosage should be increased more gradually in debilitated or emaciated patients. When maximum response is achieved, dosage may be reduced gradually to a maintenance level. Because of the inherent long action of the drug, patients may be controlled on convenient b.i.d. administration; some patients may be maintained on once-a-day administration.

When Stelazine (trifluoperazine HCl, SK&F) is administered by intramuscular injection, equivalent oral dosage may be substituted once symptoms have been controlled.

Note: Although there is little likelihood of contact dermatitis due to the drug, persons with known sensitivity to phenothiazine drugs should avoid direct contact.

Elderly Patients: In general, dosages in the lower range are sufficient for most elderly patients. Since they appear to be more susceptible to hypotension and neuromuscular reactions, such patients should be observed closely. Dosage should be tailored to the individual, response carefully monitored, and dosage adjusted accordingly. Dosage should be increased more gradually in elderly patients.

Non-psychotic Anxiety

Usual dosage is 1 or 2 mg. twice daily. Do not administer at doses of more than 6 mg. per day or for longer than 12 weeks.

Psychotic Disorders

Oral: Usual starting dosage is 2 mg. to 5 mg. b.i.d. (Small or emaciated patients should always be started on the lower dosage.)

Most patients will show optimum response on 15 mg. or 20 mg. daily, although a few may require 40 mg. a day or more. Optimum therapeutic dosage levels should be reached within two or three weeks.

When the Concentrate dosage form is to be used, it should be added to 60 mL. (2 fl. oz.) or more of diluent *just prior to administration* to insure palatability and stability. Vehicles suggested for dilution are: tomato or fruit juice, milk, simple syrup, orange syrup, carbonated beverages, coffee, tea, or water. Semisolid foods (soup, puddings, etc.) may also be used.

Intramuscular (for prompt control of severe symptoms): Usual dosage is 1 mg. to 2 mg. ($\frac{1}{2}$-1 mL.) by deep intramuscular injection q4-6h, p.r.n. More than 6 mg. within 24 hours is rarely necessary.

Only in very exceptional cases should intramuscular dosage exceed 10 mg. within 24 hours. Injections should not be given at intervals of less than 4 hours because of a possible cumulative effect.

Note: Stelazine (trifluoperazine HCl, SK&F) Injection has been usually well tolerated and there is little, if any, pain and irritation at the site of injection.

The Injection should be protected from light. Exposure may cause discoloration. Slight yellowish discoloration will not alter potency or efficacy. If markedly discolored, the solution should be discarded.

DOSAGE AND ADMINISTRATION—PSYCHOTIC CHILDREN

Dosage should be adjusted to the weight of the child and severity of the symptoms. These dosages are for children, ages 6 to 12, who are hospitalized or under close supervision.

Oral: The starting dosage is 1 mg. administered once a day or b.i.d. Dosage may be increased gradually until symptoms are controlled or until side effects become troublesome.

While it is usually not necessary to exceed dosages of 15 mg. daily, some older children with severe symptoms may require higher dosages.

Intramuscular: There has been little experience with the use of Stelazine (trifluoperazine HCl, SK&F) Injection in children. However, if it is necessary to achieve rapid control of severe symptoms, 1 mg. ($\frac{1}{2}$ mL.) of the drug may be administered intramuscularly once or twice a day.

OVERDOSAGE

(See also under Adverse Reactions.)

Symptoms—Primarily involvement of the extrapyramidal mechanism producing some of the dystonic reactions described above. Symptoms of central nervous system depression to the point of somnolence or coma. Agitation and restlessness may also occur. Other possible manifestations include convulsions, EKG changes and cardiac arrhythmias, fever, and autonomic reactions such as hypotension, dry mouth and ileus.

Treatment—It is important to determine other medications taken by the patient since multiple dose therapy is common in overdosage situations. Treatment is essentially symptomatic and supportive. Early gastric lavage is helpful. Keep patient under observation and maintain an open airway, since involvement of the extrapyramidal mechanism may produce dysphagia and respiratory difficulty in severe overdosage. **Do not attempt to induce emesis because a dystonic reaction of the head or neck may develop that could result in aspiration of vomitus.** Extrapyramidal symptoms may be treated with anti-parkinsonism drugs, barbiturates, or 'Benadryl'. See prescribing information for these products. Care should be taken to avoid increasing respiratory depression. If administration of a stimulant is desirable, amphetamine, dextroamphetamine, or caffeine with sodium benzoate is recommended. Stimulants that may cause convulsions (e.g., picrotoxin or pentylenetetrazol) should be avoided.

If hypotension occurs, the standard measures for managing circulatory shock should be initiated. If it is desirable to administer a vasoconstrictor, 'Levophed'* and 'Neo-Synephrine'† are most suitable. Other pressor agents, including epinephrine, are not recommended because phenothiazine derivatives may reverse the usual elevating action of these agents and cause a further lowering of blood pressure.

Limited experience indicates that phenothiazines are *not* dialyzable.

HOW SUPPLIED

Tablets, 1 mg. and 2 mg., in bottles of 100 and 1000; in Single Unit Packages of 100 (intended for institutional use only). For psychiatric patients who are hospitalized or under close supervision:

Tablets, 5 mg. and 10 mg., in bottles of 100 and 1000; in Single Unit Packages of 100 (intended for institutional use only). **Multiple-dose Vials**, 10 mL. (2 mg./mL.), in boxes of 1 and 20. **Concentrate**, 10 mg./mL., in 2 fl. oz. bottles and in cartons of 12 bottles.

Each bottle is packaged with a graduated dropper.

The Concentrate form is light-sensitive. For this reason, it should be protected from light and dispensed in amber bottles. *Refrigeration is not required.*

---

* norepinephrine bitartrate, Winthrop Pharmaceuticals.
† phenylephrine hydrochloride, Winthrop Pharmaceuticals.
‡ phenytoin, Parke-Davis.
§ metrizamide, Winthrop Pharmaceuticals.
ǁ diphenhydramine hydrochloride, Parke-Davis.

SZ:L63

Shown in Product Identification Section, page 431

TAGAMET®   ℞
[*tag 'ah-met*]
**(brand of cimetidine tablets
cimetidine hydrochloride liquid and
cimetidine hydrochloride injection)**

PRODUCT OVERVIEW

KEY FACTS

'Tagamet' is a histamine H_2 receptor antagonist which inhibits both daytime and nocturnal basal gastric acid secretion. 'Tagamet' also inhibits gastric acid secretion stimulated by food, histamine, pentagastrin, caffeine and insulin.

MAJOR USES

'Tagamet' is indicated in the short-term treatment of active duodenal ulcer, and promotes healing in most patients within 4 weeks. It offers a variety of dosage regimens that are very effective in healing duodenal ulcers and in providing rapid pain relief: 300 mg. q.i.d., 400 mg. b.i.d. and 800 mg. h.s. After healing of active ulcer, patients have been maintained on continued treatment with 'Tagamet' 400 mg. at bedtime for periods of up to five years. 'Tagamet' 300 mg. q.i.d. or 800 mg. h.s. have proven effective in the treatment of active benign gastric ulcer. 'Tagamet' 300 mg. q.i.d. has proven effective in the treatment of pathological hypersecretory conditions (i.e., Zollinger-Ellison Syndrome). In some

pathologic hypersecretory patients it may be necessary to administer 'Tagamet' 300 mg. doses more frequently. Doses should be adjusted to individual patient needs, but should not usually exceed 2400 mg. per day and should continue as long as clinically indicated.

In hospitalized patients with pathological hypersecretory conditions or intractable ulcers, or in patients who are unable to take oral medication, 'Tagamet' may be administered parenterally up to every 8 hours.

SAFETY INFORMATION

'Tagamet' is contraindicated for patients known to have hypersensitivity to the product.

PRESCRIBING INFORMATION

TAGAMET®   ℞
[*tag 'ah-met*]
**(brand of cimetidine tablets
cimetidine hydrochloride liquid and
cimetidine hydrochloride injection)**

('Tagamet' is a product of SK&F Lab Co., Cidra, P.R. 00639, Subsidiary of SmithKline Beckman Corporation, Philadelphia, Pa.)

DESCRIPTION

'Tagamet' (brand of cimetidine) is a histamine H_2 receptor antagonist. Chemically it is N''-cyano-$\underline{N}$-methyl-N'-[2-[[(5-methyl-1$\underline{H}$-imidazol-4-yl) methyl] thio]-ethyl]-guanidine. The empirical formula for cimetidine is $C_{10}H_{16}N_6S$ and for cimetidine hydrochloride, $C_{10}H_{16}N_6S$HCl; these represent molecular weights of 252.34 and 288.80, respectively.

Cimetidine

Cimetidine contains an imidazole ring, and is chemically related to histamine.

(The liquid and injection dosage forms contain cimetidine as the hydrochloride.)

Cimetidine has a bitter taste and characteristic odor.

Solubility Characteristics: Cimetidine is soluble in alcohol, slightly soluble in water, very slightly soluble in chloroform, and insoluble in ether. Cimetidine hydrochloride is freely soluble in water, soluble in alcohol, very slightly soluble in chloroform, and practically insoluble in ether.

Tablets for Oral Administration: Each light green, film-coated tablet contains cimetidine as follows: 200 mg.—round, imprinted with the product name TAGAMET, SKF and 200; 300 mg.—round, imprinted with the product name TAGAMET, SKF and 300; 400 mg.—capsule-shaped, imprinted with the product name TAGAMET, SKF and 400; 800 mg.—oval Tiltab® tablets, imprinted with the product name TAGAMET, SKF and 800. Inactive ingredients consist of cellulose, D&C Yellow No. 10, FD&C Blue No. 2, FD&C Red No. 40, FD&C Yellow No. 6, hydroxypropyl methylcellulose, iron oxides, magnesium stearate, povidone, propylene glycol, sodium lauryl sulfate, sodium starch glycolate, starch, titanium dioxide and trace amounts of other inactive ingredients.

Liquid for Oral Administration: Each 5 mL. (one teaspoonful) of clear, light orange, mint-peach flavored liquid contains cimetidine hydrochloride equivalent to cimetidine, 300 mg.; alcohol, 2.8%. Inactive ingredients consist of FD&C Yellow No. 6, flavors, methylparaben, polyoxyethylene polyoxypropylene glycol, propylene glycol, propylparaben, saccharin sodium, sodium chloride, sodium phosphate, sorbitol and water.

Injection:

Single-Dose Vials for Intramuscular or Intravenous Administration: Each 2 mL. contains, in sterile aqueous solution (pH range 3.8-6), cimetidine hydrochloride equivalent to cimetidine, 300 mg.; phenol, 10 mg.

Multiple-Dose Vials for Intramuscular or Intravenous Administration: 8 mL. (300 mg./2 mL.): Each 2 mL. contains, in sterile aqueous solution (pH range 3.8-6), cimetidine hydrochloride equivalent to cimetidine, 300 mg.; phenol, 10 mg.

Single-Dose Prefilled Disposable Syringes for Intramuscular or Intravenous Administration: Each 2 mL. contains, in sterile aqueous solution (pH range 3.8-6), cimetidine hydrochloride equivalent to cimetidine, 300 mg.; phenol, 10 mg.

Single-Dose Premixed Plastic Containers for Intravenous Administration: Each 50 mL. of sterile aqueous solution (pH range 5–7) contains cimetidine hydrochloride equivalent to 300 mg. cimetidine and 0.45 grams sodium chloride. No preservative has been added.

The plastic container is fabricated from specially formulated polyvinyl chloride. The amount of water that can permeate from inside the container into the overwrap is insufficient to affect the solution significantly. Solutions in contact with the plastic container can leach out certain of its chemical components in very small amounts within the expiration period, e.g., di 2-ethylhexyl phthalate (DEHP), up to 5 parts per million. However, the safety of the plastic has been confirmed in tests in animals according to the USP biological tests for plastic containers as well as by tissue culture toxicity studies.

ADD-Vantage® * Vials for Intravenous Administration: Each 2 mL. contains, in sterile aqueous solution (pH range 3.8-6), cimetidine hydrochloride equivalent to cimetidine, 300 mg.; phenol, 10 mg.

All of the above injection formulations are pyrogen free, and sodium hydroxide N.F. is used as an ingredient to adjust the pH.

* ADD-Vantage® is a trademark of Abbott Laboratories.

CLINICAL PHARMACOLOGY

'Tagamet' (brand of cimetidine) competitively inhibits the action of histamine at the histamine H_2 receptors of the parietal cells and thus is a histamine H_2-receptor antagonist. 'Tagamet' is not an anticholinergic agent. Studies have shown that 'Tagamet' inhibits both daytime and nocturnal basal gastric acid secretion. 'Tagamet' also inhibits gastric acid secretion stimulated by food, histamine, pentagastrin, caffeine and insulin.

Antisecretory Activity

1) Acid Secretion: *Nocturnal:* 'Tagamet' 800 mg. at bedtime reduces mean hourly H^+ activity by greater than 85% over an eight-hour period in duodenal ulcer patients, with no effect on daytime acid secretion. 'Tagamet' 1600 mg. h.s. produces 100% inhibition of mean hourly H^+ activity over an eight-hour period in duodenal ulcer patients, but also reduces H^+ activity by 35% for an additional five hours into the following morning. 'Tagamet' 400 mg. b.i.d. and 300 mg. q.i.d. decrease nocturnal acid secretion in a dose-related manner, i.e., 47%–83% over a six- to eight-hour period and 54% over a nine-hour period, respectively.

Food Stimulated: During the first hour after a standard experimental meal, oral 'Tagamet' 300 mg. inhibited gastric acid secretion in duodenal ulcer patients by at least 50%. During the subsequent two hours 'Tagamet' inhibited gastric acid secretion by at least 75%.

The effect of a 300 mg. breakfast dose of 'Tagamet' continued for at least four hours and there was partial suppression of the rise in gastric acid secretion following the luncheon meal in duodenal ulcer patients. This suppression of gastric acid output was enhanced and could be maintained by another 300 mg. dose of 'Tagamet' given with lunch.

In another study, 'Tagamet' 300 mg. given with the meal increased gastric pH as compared with placebo.

	Mean Gastric pH	
	'Tagamet'	**Placebo**
1 hour	3.5	2.6
2 hours	3.1	1.6
3 hours	3.8	1.9
4 hours	6.1	2.2

24-Hour Mean H^+ Activity: 'Tagamet' 800 mg. h.s., 400 mg. b.i.d. and 300 mg. q.i.d. all provide a similar, moderate (less than 60%) level of 24-hour acid suppression. However, the 800 mg. h.s. regimen exerts its entire effect on nocturnal acid, and does not affect daytime gastric physiology.

Chemically Stimulated: Oral 'Tagamet' (brand of cimetidine) significantly inhibited gastric acid secretion stimulated by betazole (an isomer of histamine), pentagastrin, caffeine and insulin as follows:

Stimulant	Stimulant Dose	'Tagamet'	% Inhibition
Betazole	1.5mg/kg (sc)	300mg (po)	85% at 2½ hours
Penta-gastrin	6mcg/kg/ hr (iv)	100mg/hr (iv)	60% at 1 hour
Caffeine	5mg/kg/ hr (iv)	300mg (po)	100% at 1 hour
Insulin	0.03 units/ kg/hr (iv)	100mg/hr (iv)	82% at 1 hour

When food and betazole were used to stimulate secretion, inhibition of hydrogen ion concentration usually ranged from 45–75% and the inhibition of volume ranged from 30–65%.

2) Pepsin: Oral 'Tagamet' 300 mg. reduced total pepsin output as a result of the decrease in volume of gastric juice.

3) Intrinsic Factor: Intrinsic factor secretion was studied with betazole as a stimulant. Oral 'Tagamet' 300 mg. inhibited the rise in intrinsic factor concentration produced by betazole, but some intrinsic factor was secreted at all times.

Other

Lower Esophageal Sphincter Pressure and Gastric Emptying

'Tagamet' has no effect on lower esophageal sphincter (LES) pressure or the rate of gastric emptying.

Pharmacokinetics

'Tagamet' is rapidly absorbed after oral administration and peak levels occur in 45–90 minutes. The half-life of 'Tagamet' is approximately 2 hours. Both oral and parenteral (IV or IM) administration provide comparable periods of therapeutically effective blood levels; blood concentrations remain above that required to provide 80% inhibition of basal gastric acid secretion for 4–5 hours following a dose of 300 mg.

The principal route of excretion of 'Tagamet' is the urine. Following parenteral administration, most of the drug is excreted as the parent compound; following oral administration, the drug is more extensively metabolized, the sulfoxide being the major metabolite. Following a single oral dose, 48% of the drug is recovered from the urine after 24 hours as the parent compound. Following IV or IM administration, approximately 75% of the drug is recovered from the urine after 24 hours as the parent compound.

CLINICAL TRIALS

Duodenal Ulcer

'Tagamet' (brand of cimetidine) has been shown to be effective in the treatment of active duodenal ulcer and, at reduced dosage, in maintenance therapy following healing of active ulcers.

Active Duodenal Ulcer: 'Tagamet' accelerates the rate of duodenal ulcer healing. Healing rates reported in U.S. and foreign controlled trials with 'Tagamet' are summarized below, beginning with the regimen providing the lowest nocturnal dose.

Duodenal Ulcer Healing Rates with Various 'Tagamet' Dosage Regimens*

Regimen	300 mg. q.i.d.	400 mg. b.i.d.	800 mg. h.s.	1600 mg. h.s.
week 4	68%	73%	80%	86%
week 6	80%	80%	89%	—
week 8	—	92%	94%	—

* Averages from controlled clinical trials.

A U.S., double-blind, placebo-controlled, dose-ranging study demonstrated that all once-daily at bedtime (h.s.) 'Tagamet' regimens were superior to placebo in ulcer healing and that 'Tagamet' 800 mg. h.s. healed 75% of patients at four weeks. The healing rate with 800 mg. h.s. was significantly superior to 400 mg. h.s. (66%) and not significantly different from 1600 mg. h.s. (81%).

In the U.S. dose-ranging trial, over 80% of patients receiving 'Tagamet' 800 mg. h.s. experienced nocturnal pain relief after one day. Relief from daytime pain was reported in approximately 70% of patients after two days. As with ulcer healing, the 800 mg. h.s. dose was superior to 400 mg. h.s. and not different from 1600 mg. h.s.

In foreign, double-blind studies with 'Tagamet' 800 mg. h.s., 79–85% of patients were healed at four weeks.

While short-term treatment with 'Tagamet' (brand of cimetidine) can result in complete healing of the duodenal ulcer, acute therapy will not prevent ulcer recurrence after 'Tagamet' has been discontinued. Some follow-up studies have reported that the rate of recurrence once therapy was discontinued was slightly higher for patients healed on 'Tagamet' than for patients healed on other forms of therapy; however, the 'Tagamet'-treated patients generally had more severe disease.

Maintenance Therapy in Duodenal Ulcer: Treatment with a reduced dose of 'Tagamet' has been proven effective as maintenance therapy following healing of active duodenal ulcers.

In numerous placebo-controlled studies conducted worldwide, the percent of patients with observed ulcers at the end of one year's therapy with 'Tagamet' 400 mg. h.s. was significantly lower (10%–45%) than in patients receiving placebo (44%–70%). Thus, from 55% to 90% of patients were maintained free of observed ulcers at the end of one year with 'Tagamet' 400 mg. h.s.

Factors such as smoking, duration and severity of disease, gender, and genetic traits may contribute to variations in actual percentages.

Trials of other anti-ulcer therapy, whether placebo-controlled, positive-controlled or open, have demonstrated a range of results similar to that seen with 'Tagamet'.

Active Benign Gastric Ulcer

'Tagamet' has been shown to be effective in the short-term treatment of active benign gastric ulcer.

In a multicenter, double-blind U.S. study, patients with endoscopically confirmed benign gastric ulcer were treated with 'Tagamet' 300 mg. four times a day or with placebo for six weeks. Patients were limited to those with ulcers ranging from 0.5-2.5 cm. in size. Endoscopically confirmed healing at six weeks was seen in significantly*

more 'Tagamet'-treated patients than in patients receiving placebo, as shown below:

	'Tagamet'	**Placebo**
week 2	14/63 (22%)	7/63 (11%)
total at week 6	43/65 (66%)*	30/67 (45%)

*p < 0.05

In a similar multicenter U.S. study of the 800 mg. h.s. oral regimen, the endoscopically confirmed healing rates were:

	'Tagamet'	**Placebo**
total at week 6	63/83 (76%)*	44/80 (55%)

*p = 0.005

Similarly, in worldwide double-blind clinical studies, endoscopically evaluated benign gastric ulcer healing rates were consistently higher with 'Tagamet' than with placebo.

Pathological Hypersecretory Conditions (such as Zollinger-Ellison Syndrome)

'Tagamet' significantly inhibited gastric acid secretion and reduced occurrence of diarrhea, anorexia and pain in patients with pathological hypersecretion associated with Zollinger-Ellison Syndrome, systemic mastocytosis and multiple endocrine adenomas. Use of 'Tagamet' was also followed by healing of intractable ulcers.

INDICATIONS AND USAGE

'Tagamet' (brand of cimetidine) is indicated in:

(1) Short-term treatment of active duodenal ulcer. Most patients heal within 4 weeks and there is rarely reason to use 'Tagamet' at full dosage for longer than 6–8 weeks (see Dosage and Administration–Duodenal Ulcer). Concomitant antacids should be given as needed for relief of pain. However, simultaneous administration of 'Tagamet' and antacids is not recommended, since antacids have been reported to interfere with the absorption of 'Tagamet'.

(2) Maintenance therapy for duodenal ulcer patients at reduced dosage after healing of active ulcer. Patients have been maintained on continued treatment with 'Tagamet' 400 mg. h.s. for periods of up to five years.

(3) Short-term treatment of active benign gastric ulcer. There is no information concerning usefulness of treatment periods of longer than 8 weeks.

(4) The treatment of pathological hypersecretory conditions (i.e., Zollinger-Ellison Syndrome, systemic mastocytosis, multiple endocrine adenomas).

CONTRAINDICATIONS

'Tagamet' is contraindicated for patients known to have hypersensitivity to the product.

PRECAUTIONS

General: Rare instances of cardiac arrhythmias and hypotension have been reported following the rapid administration of 'Tagamet' HCl (brand of cimetidine hydrochloride) Injection by intravenous bolus.

Symptomatic response to 'Tagamet' therapy does not preclude the presence of a gastric malignancy. There have been rare reports of transient healing of gastric ulcers despite subsequently documented malignancy.

Reversible confusional states have been observed on occasion, predominantly, but not exclusively, in severely ill patients. Advancing age (50 or more years) and preexisting liver and/or renal disease appear to be contributing factors. In some patients these confusional states have been mild and have not required discontinuation of 'Tagamet' therapy. In cases where discontinuation was judged necessary, the condition usually cleared within 3-4 days of drug withdrawal.

Drug Interactions: 'Tagamet', apparently through an effect on certain microsomal enzyme systems, has been reported to reduce the hepatic metabolism of warfarin-type anticoagulants, phenytoin, propranolol, chlordiazepoxide, diazepam, certain tricyclic antidepressants, lidocaine, theophylline and metronidazole, thereby delaying elimination and increasing blood levels of these drugs.

Clinically significant effects have been reported with the warfarin anticoagulants; therefore, close monitoring of prothrombin time is recommended, and adjustment of the anticoagulant dose may be necessary when 'Tagamet' is administered concomitantly. Interaction with phenytoin, lidocaine and theophylline has also been reported to produce adverse clinical effects.

However, a crossover study in healthy subjects receiving either 'Tagamet' 300 mg. q.i.d. or 800 mg. h.s. concomitantly with a 300 mg. b.i.d. dosage of theophylline (Theo-Dur®, Key Pharmaceuticals, Inc.) demonstrated less alteration in steady-state theophylline peak serum levels with the 800 mg. h.s. regimen, particularly in subjects aged 54 years and older. Data beyond ten days are not available. (Note: All patients receiving theophylline should be monitored appropriately, regardless of concomitant drug therapy.)

Dosage of the drugs mentioned above and other similarly metabolized drugs, particularly those of low therapeutic ratio or in patients with renal and/or hepatic impairment, may require adjustment when starting or stopping concomitantly administered 'Tagamet' to maintain optimum therapeutic blood levels.

Continued on next page

Smith Kline & French—Cont.

Additional clinical experience may reveal other drugs affected by the concomitant administration of 'Tagamet'.

Carcinogenesis, Mutagenesis, Impairment of Fertility: In a 24-month toxicity study conducted in rats, at dose levels of 150, 378 and 950 mg./kg./day (approximately 8 to 48 times the recommended human dose), there was a small increase in the incidence of benign Leydig cell tumors in each dose group; when the combined drug-treated groups and control groups were compared, this increase reached statistical significance. In a subsequent 24-month study, there were no differences between the rats receiving 150 mg./kg./day and the untreated controls. However, a statistically significant increase in benign Leydig cell tumor incidence was seen in the rats that received 378 and 950 mg./kg./day. These tumors were common in control groups as well as treated groups and the difference became apparent only in aged rats. 'Tagamet' (brand of cimetidine) has demonstrated a weak antiandrogenic effect. In animal studies this was manifested as reduced prostate and seminal vesicle weights. However, there was no impairment of mating performance or fertility, nor any harm to the fetus in these animals at doses 8 to 48 times the full therapeutic dose of 'Tagamet', as compared with controls. The cases of gynecomastia seen in patients treated for one month or longer may be related to this effect. In human studies, 'Tagamet' has been shown to have no effect on spermatogenesis, sperm count, motility, morphology or *in vitro* fertilizing capacity.

Pregnancy: Teratogenic Effects. Pregnancy Category B: Reproduction studies have been performed in rats, rabbits and mice at doses up to 40 times the normal human dose and have revealed no evidence of impaired fertility or harm to the fetus due to 'Tagamet'. There are, however, no adequate and well-controlled studies in pregnant women. Because animal reproductive studies are not always predictive of human response, this drug should be used during pregnancy only if clearly needed.

Nursing Mothers: Cimetidine is secreted in human milk and, as a general rule, nursing should not be undertaken while a patient is on a drug.

Pediatric Use: Clinical experience in children is limited. Therefore, 'Tagamet' therapy cannot be recommended for children under 16, unless, in the judgment of the physician, anticipated benefits outweigh the potential risks. In very limited experience, doses of 20–40 mg./kg. per day have been used.

ADVERSE REACTIONS

Adverse effects reported in patients taking 'Tagamet' are described below by body system. Incidence figures of 1 in 100 and greater are generally derived from controlled clinical studies.

Gastrointestinal: Diarrhea (usually mild) has been reported in approximately 1 in 100 patients.

CNS: Dizziness and somnolence (usually mild) have been reported in approximately 1 in 100 patients. Headache, ranging from mild to severe, has been reported.

Reversible confusional states, e.g., mental confusion, agitation, psychosis, depression, anxiety, hallucinations, disorientation, have been reported predominantly, but not exclusively, in severely ill patients. They have usually developed within 2-3 days of initiation of 'Tagamet' therapy and have cleared within 3-4 days of discontinuation of the drug.

Endocrine: Gynecomastia has been reported in patients treated for one month or longer. In patients being treated for pathological hypersecretory states, this occurred in about 4 percent of cases while in all others the incidence was 0.3% to 1% in various studies. No evidence of induced endocrine dysfunction was found, and the condition remained unchanged or returned toward normal with continuing 'Tagamet' (brand of cimetidine) treatment.

Reversible impotence has been reported in patients with pathological hypersecretory disorders, e.g., Zollinger-Ellison Syndrome, receiving 'Tagamet', particularly in high doses, for at least 12 months (range 12–79 months, mean 38 months). However, in large-scale surveillance studies at regular dosage, the incidence has not exceeded that commonly reported in the general population.

Hematologic: Decreased white blood cell counts in 'Tagamet'-treated patients (approximately 1 per 100,000 patients), including agranulocytosis (approximately 3 per million patients), have been reported, including a few reports of recurrence on rechallenge. Most of these reports were in patients who had serious concomitant illnesses and received drugs and/or treatment known to produce neutropenia. Thrombocytopenia (approximately 3 per million patients) and, very rarely, cases of aplastic anemia have also been reported.

Hepatobiliary: Increases in serum transaminase have been reported. In most cases they did not progress with continued therapy and returned to normal at the end of therapy. There have been rare reports of cholestatic or mixed cholestatic-hepatocellular effects. These were usually reversible. Because of the predominance of cholestatic features, severe parenchymal injury is considered highly unlikely.

There has been reported a single case of biopsy-proven periportal hepatic fibrosis in a patient receiving 'Tagamet'. Rare cases of pancreatitis, which cleared on withdrawal of the drug, have been reported.

Hypersensitivity: Rare cases of fever and allergic reactions including anaphylaxis and hypersensitivity vasculitis, which cleared on withdrawal of the drug, have been reported.

Renal: Small increases in plasma creatinine, presumably due to competition for renal tubular secretion, have been observed. Rare cases of interstitial nephritis and urinary retention, which cleared on withdrawal of the drug, have been reported.

Cardiovascular: Rare cases of bradycardia, tachycardia and A-V heart block have been reported with H$_2$-receptor antagonists.

Musculoskeletal: There have been rare reports of reversible arthralgia and myalgia; exacerbation of joint symptoms in patients with preexisting arthritis has also been reported. Such symptoms have usually been alleviated by a reduction in 'Tagamet' (brand of cimetidine) dosage. Rare cases of polymyositis have been reported, but no causal relationship has been established.

Integumental: Mild rash and, very rarely, cases of severe generalized skin reactions including Stevens-Johnson syndrome, epidermal necrolysis, erythema multiforme, exfoliative dermatitis and generalized exfoliative erythroderma have been reported with H$_2$-receptor antagonists. Reversible alopecia has been reported very rarely.

OVERDOSAGE

The usual measures to remove unabsorbed material from the gastrointestinal tract, clinical monitoring and supportive therapy should be employed. Studies in animals indicate that toxic doses are associated with respiratory failure and tachycardia which may be controlled by assisted respiration and the administration of a beta-blocker.

Human experience with gross overdosage is limited. However, in the few cases which have been reported, doses up to 10 grams have not been associated with any untoward effects.

DOSAGE AND ADMINISTRATION

Duodenal Ulcer

Active Duodenal Ulcer: Clinical studies have indicated that suppression of nocturnal acid is the most important factor in duodenal ulcer healing (see Clinical Pharmacology—Acid Secretion). This is supported by recent clinical trials (see Clinical Trials—Active Duodenal Ulcer). Therefore, there is no apparent rationale, except for familiarity with use, for treating with anything other than a once-daily at bedtime dosage regimen (h.s.).

In a U.S. dose-ranging study of 400 mg. h.s., 800 mg. h.s. and 1600 mg. h.s., a continuous dose response relationship for ulcer healing was demonstrated.

However, 800 mg. h.s. is the dose of choice for most patients, as it provides a high healing rate (the difference between 800 mg. h.s. and 1600 mg. h.s. being small), maximal pain relief, a decreased potential for drug interactions (see Precautions—Drug Interactions) and maximal patient convenience. Patients unhealed at four weeks, or those with persistent symptoms, have been shown to benefit from two to four weeks of continued therapy.

It has been shown that patients who both have an endoscopically demonstrated ulcer larger than 1.0 cm. and are also heavy smokers (i.e., smoke one pack of cigarettes or more per day) are more difficult to heal. There is some evidence which suggests that more rapid healing can be achieved in this subpopulation with 'Tagamet' 1600 mg. at bedtime. While early pain relief with either 800 mg. h.s. or 1600 mg. h.s. is equivalent in all patients, 1600 mg. h.s. provides an appropriate alternative when it is important to ensure healing within four weeks for this subpopulation. Alternatively, approximately 94% of all patients will also heal in eight weeks with 'Tagamet' 800 mg. h.s.

Other 'Tagamet' regimens in the U.S. which have been shown to be effective are: 300 mg. four times daily, with meals and at bedtime, the original regimen with which U.S. physicians have the most experience, and 400 mg. twice daily, in the morning and at bedtime (see Clinical Trials—Active Duodenal Ulcer).

Concomitant antacids should be given as needed for relief of pain. However, simultaneous administration of 'Tagamet' and antacids is not recommended, since antacids have been reported to interfere with the absorption of 'Tagamet' (brand of cimetidine).

While healing with 'Tagamet' often occurs during the first week or two, treatment should be continued for 4–6 weeks unless healing has been demonstrated by endoscopic examination.

Maintenance Therapy for Duodenal Ulcer: In those patients requiring maintenance therapy, the recommended adult oral dose is 400 mg. at bedtime.

Active Benign Gastric Ulcer

The recommended adult oral dosage for short-term treatment of active benign gastric ulcer is 800 mg. h.s., or 300 mg. four times a day with meals and at bedtime. Controlled clinical studies were limited to six weeks of treat-

ment (see Clinical Trials). 800 mg. h.s. is the preferred regimen for most patients based upon convenience and reduced potential for drug interactions. Symptomatic response to 'Tagamet' does not preclude the presence of a gastric malignancy. It is important to follow gastric ulcer patients to assure rapid progress to complete healing.

Pathological Hypersecretory Conditions (such as Zollinger-Ellison Syndrome)

Recommended adult oral dosage: 300 mg. four times a day with meals and at bedtime. In some patients it may be necessary to administer 'Tagamet' 300 mg. doses more frequently. Doses should be adjusted to individual patient needs, but should not usually exceed 2400 mg. per day and should continue as long as clinically indicated.

Parenteral Administration

In hospitalized patients with pathological hypersecretory conditions or intractable ulcers, or in patients who are unable to take oral medication, 'Tagamet' may be administered parenterally.

All parenteral drug products should be inspected visually for particulate matter and discoloration prior to administration.

Recommendations for parenteral administration:

Intramuscular injection: 300 mg. q 6–8 hours (no dilution necessary). Transient pain at the site of injection has been reported.

Intravenous injection: 300 mg. q 6–8 hours. Dilute 'Tagamet' HCl (brand of cimetidine hydrochloride) Injection, 300 mg., in Sodium Chloride Injection (0.9%) or another compatible i.v. solution (see Stability of 'Tagamet' HCl Injection) to a total volume of 20 mL. and inject over a period of not less than 2 minutes (see Precautions).

Intermittent intravenous infusion: 300 mg. q 6–8 hours, infused over 15–20 minutes. Vials: Dilute 'Tagamet' HCl Injection, 300 mg., in at least 50 mL. of 5% Dextrose Injection, or another compatible i.v. solution (see Stability of 'Tagamet' HCl Injection). Plastic containers: Use premixed 'Tagamet' HCl Injection, 300 mg., in 0.9% Sodium Chloride in 50 mL. plastic containers. ADD-Vantage® Vials: Dilute contents of one vial in an ADD-Vantage® Diluent Container, available in 50 mL. and 100 mL. sizes of 0.9% Sodium Chloride Injection, and 5% Dextrose Injection.

DIRECTIONS FOR USE OF 'TAGAMET' HCl (brand of cimetidine hydrochloride) INJECTION IN PLASTIC CONTAINERS

To open: Tear overwrap down side at slit and remove solution containers.

Some opacity of the plastic due to moisture absorption during the sterilization process may be observed. This is normal and does not affect solution quality or safety. The opacity will diminish gradually.

Do not add other drugs to premixed 'Tagamet' HCl Injection in plastic containers.

CAUTION: Check for minute leaks by squeezing inner bag firmly. If leaks are found, discard solution as sterility may be impaired. Additives should not be introduced into this solution. Do not use if the solution is cloudy or precipitated or if the seal is not intact.

Do not use plastic containers in series connections. Such use could result in air embolism due to residual air being drawn from the primary container before administration of the fluid from the secondary container is complete. Use sterile equipment.

Preparation for administration:

1. Suspend container from eyelet support.
2. Remove plastic protector from outlet port at bottom of container.
3. Attach administration set. Refer to complete directions accompanying set.

DIRECTIONS FOR USE OF 'TAGAMET' HCl INJECTION IN ADD-VANTAGE® VIALS are enclosed in ADD-Vantage® Vial packaging.

Stability of 'Tagamet' HCl Injection

When added to or diluted with most commonly used intravenous solutions, e.g., Sodium Chloride Injection (0.9%), Dextrose Injection (5% or 10%), Lactated Ringer's Solution, 5% Sodium Bicarbonate Injection, 'Tagamet' HCl (brand of cimetidine hydrochloride) Injection should not be used after more than 48 hours of storage at room temperature.

'Tagamet' HCl Injection premixed in plastic containers is stable through the labeled expiration date when stored under the recommended conditions.

In some patients it may be necessary to increase dosage. When this is necessary, the increases should be made by more frequent administration of a 300 mg. dose but should not exceed 2400 mg. per day.

Dosage Adjustment for Patients with Impaired Renal Function

Patients with severely impaired renal function have been treated with 'Tagamet'. However, such usage has been very limited. On the basis of this experience the recommended dosage is 300 mg. q 12 hours orally or by intravenous injection. Should the patient's condition require, the frequency of dosing may be increased to q 8 hours or even further with caution. In severe renal failure, accumulation may occur and the lowest frequency of dosing compatible with an adequate patient response should be used. When liver impairment is also present, further reductions in dosage may be necessary. Hemodialysis reduces the level of circulating 'Tagamet'. Ideally, the dosage schedule should be adjusted so that the timing of a scheduled dose coincides with the end of hemodialysis.

HOW SUPPLIED

Tablets: Light green, film-coated as follows: 200 mg.—round, imprinted with the product name TAGAMET, SKF and 200—tablets in bottles of 100; 300 mg.—round, imprinted with the product name TAGAMET, SKF and 300—tablets in bottles of 100 and Single Unit Packages of 100 (intended for institutional use only); 400 mg.—capsule-shaped, imprinted with the product name TAGAMET, SKF and 400—tablets in bottles of 60 and Single Unit Packages of 100 (intended for institutional use only); 800 mg.—oval-shaped Tiltab®, imprinted with the product name TAGA-MET, SKF and 800—tablets in bottles of 30 and Single Unit Packages of 100 (intended for institutional use only).
Store at controlled room temperature; dispense in a tight light-resistant container.
200 mg. 100's: NDC 0108-5012-20
300 mg. 100's: NDC 0108-5013-20
300 mg. SUP 100's: NDC 0108-5013-21
400 mg. 60's: NDC 0108-5026-18
400 mg. SUP 100's: NDC 0108-5026-21
800 mg. 30's: NDC 0108-5027-13
800 mg. SUP 100's: NDC 0108-5027-21
Liquid: Clear, light orange, mint-peach flavored, as follows: 300 mg./5 mL., in 8 fl. oz. (237 mL.) amber glass bottles and in single-dose units (300 mg./5 mL.), in packages of 10 (intended for institutional use only).
Store at controlled room temperature; dispense in a tight light-resistant container.
300 mg./5 mL. 8 fl. oz.: NDC 0108-5014-48
300 mg./5 mL. SUP 10's: NDC 0108-5014-10
Injection:
Vials: 300 mg./2 mL. in single-dose vials, in packages of 10 and 30, and in 8 mL. multiple-dose vials, in packages of 10 and 25.
Store at controlled room temperature; do not refrigerate.
300 mg./2 mL. Single-Dose Vials:
   NDC 0108-5017-11 (package of 10 vials)
   NDC 0108-5017-13 (package of 30 vials)
300 mg./2 mL. in 8 mL. Multiple-Dose Vials:
   NDC 0108-5022-11 (package of 10 vials)
   NDC 0108-5022-16 (package of 25 vials)
Prefilled Syringes: 300 mg./2 mL. in single-dose prefilled disposable syringes.
Store at controlled room temperature; do not refrigerate.
300 mg./2 mL.: NDC 0108-5020-01
Single-Dose Premixed Plastic Containers: 300 mg. in 50 mL. of 0.9% Sodium Chloride in single-dose plastic containers, in packages of 4 units. No preservative has been added.
Store at controlled room temperature; do not refrigerate.
Exposure of the premixed product to excessive heat should be avoided. It is recommended the product be stored at controlled room temperature. Brief exposure up to 40°C does not adversely affect the premixed product.
300 mg./50 mL. SUP's: NDC 0108-5029-04
ADD-Vantage® Vials: 300 mg./2 mL. in single-dose ADD-Vantage® Vials, in packages of 25.
Store at controlled room temperature; do not refrigerate.
300 mg./2 mL.: NDC 0108-5031-16 (package of 25 vials)
'Tagamet' HCl (brand of cimetidine hydrochloride) Injection premixed in single-dose plastic containers is manufactured for SK&F Lab Co. by Baxter Healthcare Corporation, Deerfield, IL 60015.
Military—Tablets, 200 mg., 100's, 6505-01-103-6335; 300 mg., SUP, 100's, 6505-01-050-3546, and 300 mg., 100's, 6505-01-050-3547; 400 mg., 60's, 6505-01-176-0712; Injection, 300 mg./2 mL., 10's, 6505-01-051-4698; 8 mL., 300 mg./2 mL., 10's, 6505-01-069-1661; Liquid, 300 mg./5 mL., 8 fl. oz., 6505-01-119-0616.
Veterans Administration—Tablets, 200 mg., 100's, 6505-01-103-6335; 300 mg., 100's, 6505-01-050-3547; 300 mg., SUP, 100's, 6505-01-050-3546; 400 mg., 60's, 6505-01-176-0712; Liquid, 300 mg./5 mL., 8 fl. oz., 6505-01-119-0616; Injection, 300 mg./2 mL., 10's, 6505-01-051-4698; 8 mL., 300 mg./2 mL., 10's, 6505-01-069-1661.   TG:L78
Shown in Product Identification Section, page 431

TAZICEF®   ℞
[taz 'i-sef]
(brand of ceftazidime for injection)

PRODUCT OVERVIEW

KEY FACTS

'Tazicef' is a cephalosporin with enhanced anti-pseudomonal activity. A wide range of gram-negative organisms, including strains resistant to gentamicin and other aminoglycosides, are susceptible to ceftazidime *in vitro*. Ceftazidime has also been shown to be active against gram-positive organisms.

Table 2. Ceftazidime Concentrations in Body Tissues and Fluids

Tissue or Fluid	Dose/Route	No. Patients	Time of Sample Post-Dose	Average Tissue or Fluid Level (mcg./mL.)
Urine	500 mg. I.M.	6	0–2 hours	2,100
	2 g. I.V.	6	0–2 hours	12,000
Bile	2 g. I.V.	3	90 min.	36.4
Synovial fluid	2 g. I.V.	13	2 hours	25.6
Peritoneal fluid	2 g. I.V.	8	2 hours	48.6
Sputum	1 g. I.V.	8	1 hour	9
Cerebrospinal fluid (inflamed meninges)	2 g. q8h I.V.	5	120 min.	9.8
	2 g. q8h I.V.	6	180 min.	9.4
Aqueous humor	2 g. I.V.	13	1–3 hours	11
Blister fluid	1 g. I.V.	7	2–3 hours	19.7
Lymphatic fluid	1 g. I.V.	7	2–3 hours	23.4
Bone	2 g. I.V.	8	0.67 hour	31.1
Heart muscle	2 g. I.V.	35	30–280 min.	12.7
Skin	2 g. I.V.	22	30–180 min.	6.6
Skeletal muscle	2 g. I.V.	35	30–280 min.	9.4
Myometrium	2 g. I.V.	31	1–2 hours	18.7

MAJOR USES

'Tazicef' is indicated for the treatment of patients with infections caused by susceptible strains of the designated organisms in the diseases listed in the full prescribing information below. In particular, ceftazidime has been proven to be clinically effective against *Pseudomonas* in skin and skin structure infections, respiratory tract infections, urinary tract infections, and in infections in neutropenic patients.

SAFETY INFORMATION

'Tazicef' is contraindicated in patients who have shown hypersensitivity to ceftazidime or the cephalosporin group of antibiotics. Careful inquiry should be made concerning previous hypersensitivity reactions to ceftazidime, cephalosporins, penicillins or other drugs. 'Tazicef' should be administered with caution to penicillin-sensitive patients. Serious acute hypersensitivity reactions may require epinephrine and other emergency measures. Because pseudomembranous colitis has been reported with the use of cephalosporins, it is important to consider its diagnosis in patients who develop diarrhea in association with antibiotic use.

PRESCRIBING INFORMATION

TAZICEF®   ℞
[taz 'i-sef]
(brand of ceftazidime for injection)
For Intravenous or Intramuscular Use

('Tazicef' is manufactured for Smith Kline & French Laboratories, Division of SmithKline Beckman Corporation, Philadelphia, Pa. by Merck & Co., Inc., Rahway, N.J.)

DESCRIPTION

Ceftazidime is a semisynthetic, broad-spectrum, beta-lactam antibiotic for parenteral administration. It is the pentahydrate of Pyridinium, 1-[[7-[[(2-amino-4-thiazolyl)][(1-carboxy-1-methylethoxy) imino]acetyl]amino]-2-carboxy-8-oxo-5-thia-1-azabicyclo (4.2.0.)oct-2-en-3-yl] methyl]-,hydroxide,inner salt, [6R-[6α,7β(Z)]].
Tazicef (ceftazidime for injection, SK&F) is a sterile, dry, powdered mixture of ceftazidime pentahydrate and sodium carbonate. The sodium carbonate at a concentration of 118 mg./g. of ceftazidime activity has been admixed to facilitate dissolution. The total sodium content of the mixture is approximately 54 mg. (2.3 mEq.)/g. of ceftazidime activity. Solutions of 'Tazicef' range in color from light yellow to amber, depending upon the diluent and volume used. The pH of freshly reconstituted solutions usually ranges from 5.0 to 8.0.

CLINICAL PHARMACOLOGY

After intravenous administration of 500 mg. and 1 g. doses of ceftazidime over five minutes to normal adult male volunteers, mean peak serum concentrations of 45 mcg./mL. and 90 mcg./mL., respectively, were achieved. After intravenous infusion of 500 mg., 1 g. and 2 g. doses of ceftazidime over 20 to 30 minutes to normal adult male volunteers, mean peak serum concentrations of 42 mcg./mL., 69 mcg./mL. and 170 mcg./mL., respectively, were achieved. The average serum concentrations following intravenous infusion of 500 mg., 1 g. and 2 g. doses to these volunteers over an eight-hour interval are given in Table 1.

Table 1

Ceftazidime I.V. Dosage	Serum Concentrations (mcg./mL.)				
	0.5 hr.	1 hr.	2 hr.	4 hr.	8 hr.
500 mg.	42	25	12	6	2
1 g.	60	39	23	11	3
2 g.	129	75	42	13	5

The absorption and elimination of ceftazidime were directly proportional to the size of the dose. The half-life following intravenous administration was approximately 1.9 hours. Less than 10% of ceftazidime was protein bound. The degree of protein binding was independent of concentration. There was no evidence of accumulation of ceftazidime in the serum in individuals with normal renal function following multiple intravenous doses of 1 g. and 2 g. every eight hours for ten days.

Following intramuscular administration of 500 mg. and 1 g. doses of ceftazidime to normal adult volunteers, the mean peak serum concentrations were 17 mcg./mL. and 39 mcg./mL., respectively, at approximately one hour. Serum concentrations remained above 4 mcg./mL. for six and eight hours after the intramuscular administration of 500 mg. and 1 g. doses, respectively. The half-life of ceftazidime in these volunteers was approximately two hours.

The presence of hepatic dysfunction had no effect on the pharmacokinetics of ceftazidime in individuals administered 2 g. intravenously every eight hours for five days. Therefore, a dosage adjustment from the normal recommended dosage is not required for patients with hepatic dysfunction, provided renal function is not impaired.

Approximately 80%–90% of an intramuscular or intravenous dose of ceftazidime is excreted unchanged by the kidneys over a 24-hour period. After the intravenous administration of single 500 mg. or 1 g. doses, approximately 50% of the dose appeared in the urine in the first two hours. An additional 20% was excreted between two and four hours after dosing, and approximately another 12% of the dose appeared in the urine between four and eight hours later. The elimination of ceftazidime by the kidneys resulted in high therapeutic concentrations in the urine.

The mean renal clearance of ceftazidime was approximately 100 mL./min. The calculated plasma clearance of approximately 115 mL./min. indicated nearly complete elimination of ceftazidime by the renal route. Administration of probenecid prior to dosing had no effect on the elimination kinetics of ceftazidime. This suggests that ceftazidime is eliminated by glomerular filtration and is not actively secreted by renal tubular mechanisms.

Since ceftazidime is eliminated almost solely by the kidneys, its serum half-life is significantly prolonged in patients with impaired renal function. Consequently, dosage adjustments in such patients as described in the DOSAGE AND ADMINISTRATION section are suggested.

Therapeutic concentrations of ceftazidime are achieved in the following body tissues and fluid.

[See table above].

Microbiology

Ceftazidime is bactericidal in action, exerting its effect by inhibition of enzymes responsible for cell-wall synthesis. A wide range of gram-negative organisms is susceptible to ceftazidime *in vitro*, including strains resistant to gentamicin and other aminoglycosides. In addition, ceftazidime has been shown to be active against gram-positive organisms. It is highly stable to most clinically important beta-lactamases, plasmid or chromosomal, which are produced by both gram-negative and gram-positive organisms, and consequently is active against many strains resistant to ampicillin and other cephalosporins.

Ceftazidime has been shown to be active against the following organisms both *in vitro* and in clinical infections (see INDICATIONS AND USAGE).

Continued on next page

Smith Kline & French—Cont.

Aerobes, Gram-Negative: *Pseudomonas* species (including *Pseudomonas aeruginosa*); *Klebsiella* species (including *Klebsiella pneumoniae*); *Proteus mirabilis; Proteus vulgaris; Escherichia coli; Enterobacter* species, including *Enterobacter cloacae* and *Enterobacter aerogenes; Citrobacter* species, including *Citrobacter freundii* and *Citrobacter diversus; Serratia* species; *Haemophilus influenzae,* including ampicillin-resistant strains; and *Neisseria meningitidis.*
Aerobes, Gram-Positive: *Staphylococcus aureus,* including penicillinase- and non-penicillinase-producing strains; *Streptococcus pyogenes* (group A beta-hemolytic streptococci); *Streptococcus agalactiae* (group B streptococci); and *Streptococcus pneumoniae.*
Anaerobes: *Bacteroides* species (NOTE: Many strains of *Bacteroides fragilis* are resistant).
Ceftazidime has also been shown to demonstrate *in vitro* activity against the following microorganisms, although its clinical significance is not known: *Staphylococcus epidermidis; Morganella morganii* (formerly *Proteus morganii*); *Providencia* species (including *Providencia rettgeri,* formerly *Proteus rettgeri*); *Acinetobacter* species; *Salmonella* species; *Clostridium* species (not including *Clostridium difficile*); *Peptococcus* species; *Peptostreptococcus* species; *Neisseria gonorrhoeae; Haemophilus parainfluenzae; Yersinia enterocolitica;* and *Shigella* species.
Ceftazidime and the aminoglycosides have been shown to be synergistic *in vitro* against *P. aeruginosa* and the *Enterobacteriaceae.* Ceftazidime and carbenicillin have also been shown to be synergistic *in vitro* against *P. aeruginosa.*
Ceftazidime is not active *in vitro* against: methicillin-resistant staphylococci; *Streptococcus faecalis* and many other enterococci; *Listeria monocytogenes; Campylobacter* species; or *Clostridium difficile.*

Susceptibility Tests
Quantitative methods that require measurement of zone diameters give the most precise estimate of antibiotic susceptibility. One such procedure[1-3] has been recommended for use with disks to test susceptibility to ceftazidime.
Reports from the laboratory giving results of the standard single-disk susceptibility test with a 30 mcg. ceftazidime disk should be interpreted according to the following criteria:
Susceptible organisms produce zones of 18 mm. or greater, indicating that the test organism is likely to respond to therapy.
Organisms that produce zones of 15 mm. to 17 mm. are expected to be susceptible if high dosage is used or if the infection is confined to tissues and fluids (e.g., urine) in which high antibiotic levels are attained.
Resistant organisms produce zones of 14 mm. or less, indicating that other therapy should be selected.
Organisms should be tested with the ceftazidime disk, since ceftazidime has been shown by *in vitro* tests to be active against certain strains found resistant when other beta-lactam disks are used.
Standardized procedures require the use of laboratory control organisms. The 30 mcg. ceftazidime disk should give zone diameters between 25 mm. and 32 mm. for *E. coli* ATCC 25922. For *P. aeruginosa* ATCC 27853, the zone diameters should be between 22 mm. and 29 mm. For *S. aureus* ATCC 25923, the zone diameters should be between 16 mm. and 20 mm.
In other susceptibility testing procedures, e.g., ICS agar dilution or the equivalent, a bacterial isolate may be considered susceptible if the MIC value for ceftazidime is not more than 16 mcg./mL. Organisms are considered resistant to ceftazidime if the MIC is equal to or greater than 64 mcg./mL. Organisms having an MIC value of less than 64 mcg./mL. but greater than 16 mcg./mL. are expected to be susceptible if high dosage is used or if the infection is confined to tissues and fluids (e.g., urine) in which high antibiotic levels are attained.
As with standard diffusion methods, dilution procedures require the use of laboratory control organisms. Standard ceftazidime powder should give MIC values in the range of 4 mcg./mL. and 16 mcg./mL. for *S. aureus* ATCC 25923. For *E. coli* ATCC 25922, the MIC range should be between 0.125 mcg./mL. and 0.5 mcg./mL. For *P. aeruginosa* ATCC 27853, the MIC range should be between 0.5 mcg./mL. and 2 mcg./mL.

INDICATIONS AND USAGE
Tazicef (ceftazidime for injection, SK&F) is indicated for the treatment of patients with infections caused by susceptible strains of the designated organisms in the diseases listed below:
LOWER RESPIRATORY TRACT INFECTIONS, including pneumonia, caused by *P. aeruginosa* and other *Pseudomonas* species; *H. influenzae,* including ampicillin-resistant strains; *Klebsiella* species; *Enterobacter* species, *P. mirabilis; E. coli; Serratia* species; *Citrobacter* species; *S. pneumoniae;* and *S. aureus* (methicillin-susceptible strains).
SKIN AND SKIN STRUCTURE INFECTIONS, caused by *P. aeruginosa, Klebsiella* species; *E. coli; Proteus* species including *P. mirabilis* and indole-positive *Proteus, Enterobacter* species; *Serratia* species; *S. aureus* (methicillin-susceptible strains) and *S. pyogenes* (group A beta-hemolytic streptococci.
URINARY TRACT INFECTIONS, both complicated and uncomplicated, caused by *P. aeruginosa; Enterobacter* species; *Proteus* species, including *P. mirabilis* and indole-positive *Proteus; Klebsiella* species and *E. coli.*
BACTERIAL SEPTICEMIA, caused by *P. aeruginosa, Klebsiella* species; *H. influenzae; E. coli, Serratia* species, *S. pneumoniae* and *S. aureus* (methicillin-susceptible strains).
BONE AND JOINT INFECTIONS, caused by *P. aeruginosa; Klebsiella* species; *Enterobacter* species; and *S. aureus* (methicillin-susceptible strains).
GYNECOLOGICAL INFECTIONS, including endometritis, pelvic cellulitis and other infections of the female genital tract caused by *E. coli.*
INTRA-ABDOMINAL INFECTIONS, including peritonitis caused by *E. coli, Klebsiella* species; *S. aureus* (methicillin-susceptible strains), and polymicrobial infections caused by aerobic and anaerobic organisms, and *Bacteroides* species (many strains of *B. fragilis* are resistant).
CENTRAL NERVOUS SYSTEM INFECTIONS, including meningitis caused by *H. influenzae* and *Neisseria meningitidis.* Ceftazidime has also been used successfully in a limited number of cases of meningitis due to *P. aeruginosa* and *S. pneumoniae.*
Specimens for bacterial cultures should be obtained prior to therapy in order to isolate and identify causative organisms and to determine their susceptibility to ceftazidime. Therapy may be instituted before results of susceptibility studies are known; however, once these results become available, the antibiotic treatment should be adjusted accordingly.
Tazicef (ceftazidime for injection, SK&F) may be used alone in cases of confirmed or suspected sepsis. Ceftazidime has been used successfully in clinical trials as empiric therapy in cases where various concomitant therapies with other antibiotics have been used.
'Tazicef' may also be used concomitantly with other antibiotics, such as aminoglycosides, vancomycin and clindamycin, in severe and life-threatening infections and in the immunocompromised patient. When such concomitant treatment is appropriate, prescribing information in the labeling for the other antibiotics should be followed. The dose depends on the severity of the infection and the patient's condition.

CONTRAINDICATIONS
'Tazicef' is contraindicated in patients who have shown hypersensitivity to ceftazidime or the cephalosporin group of antibiotics.

WARNINGS
BEFORE THERAPY WITH 'TAZICEF' IS INSTITUTED, CAREFUL INQUIRY SHOULD BE MADE TO DETERMINE WHETHER THE PATIENT HAS HAD PREVIOUS HYPERSENSITIVITY REACTIONS TO CEFTAZIDIME, CEPHALOSPORINS, PENICILLINS, OR OTHER DRUGS. ANTIBIOTICS SHOULD BE ADMINISTERED WITH CAUTION TO ANY PATIENT WHO HAS DEMONSTRATED SOME FORM OF ALLERGY, PARTICULARLY TO DRUGS. THIS PRODUCT SHOULD BE GIVEN WITH CAUTION TO PATIENTS WITH TYPE 1 HYPERSENSITIVITY REACTIONS TO PENICILLIN. IF AN ALLERGIC REACTION TO 'TAZICEF' OCCURS, DISCONTINUE TREATMENT WITH THE DRUG. SERIOUS ACUTE HYPERSENSITIVITY REACTIONS MAY REQUIRE EPINEPHRINE AND OTHER EMERGENCY MEASURES.

Pseudomembranous colitis has been reported with the use of cephalosporins (and other broad-spectrum antibiotics); therefore, it is important to consider its diagnosis in patients who develop diarrhea in association with antibiotic use.
Treatment with broad-spectrum antibiotics alters normal flora of the colon and may permit overgrowth of clostridia. Studies indicate a toxin produced by *C. difficile* is one primary cause of antibiotic-associated colitis.
Mild cases of colitis may respond to drug discontinuance alone. Moderate to severe cases should be managed with fluid, electrolyte and protein supplementation as indicated. When the colitis is not relieved by drug discontinuance or when it is severe, oral vancomycin is the treatment of choice for antibiotic-associated pseudomembranous colitis produced by *C. difficile.* Other causes of colitis should also be considered.

PRECAUTIONS
Ceftazidime has not been shown to be nephrotoxic; however, because high and prolonged serum antibiotic concentrations can occur from usual doses in patients with transient or persistent reduction of urinary output because of renal insufficiency, the total daily dosage should be reduced when ceftazidime is administered to such patients (see DOSAGE AND ADMINISTRATION). Continued dosage should be determined by degree of renal impairment, severity of infection and susceptibility of the causative organisms.

As with other antibiotics, prolonged use of Tazicef (ceftazidime for injection, SK&F) may result in overgrowth of nonsusceptible organisms. Repeated evaluation of the patient's condition is essential. If superinfection occurs during therapy, appropriate measures should be taken.
'Tazicef' should be prescribed with caution in individuals with a history of gastrointestinal disease, particularly colitis.
Drug Interactions: Nephrotoxicity has been reported following concomitant administration of cephalosporins with aminoglycoside antibiotics or potent diuretics, such as furosemide. Renal function should be carefully monitored, especially if higher dosages of the aminoglycosides are to be administered or if therapy is prolonged, because of the potential nephrotoxicity and ototoxicity of aminoglycoside antibiotics. Nephrotoxicity and ototoxicity were not noted when ceftazidime was given alone in clinical trials.
Carcinogenesis, Mutagenesis, Impairment of Fertility: Longterm studies in animals have not been performed to evaluate carcinogenic potential. However, a mouse micronucleus test and an Ames test were both negative for mutagenic effects.
Usage in Pregnancy: Pregnancy Category B. Reproduction studies have been performed in mice and rats at doses up to 40 times the human dose and have revealed no evidence of impaired fertility or harm to the fetus due to ceftazidime. There are, however, no adequate and well-controlled studies in pregnant women. Because animal reproduction studies are not always predictive of human response, this drug should be used during pregnancy only if clearly needed.
Nursing Mothers: Ceftazidime is excreted in human milk in low concentrations. Caution should be exercised when 'Tazicef' is administered to a nursing woman.

ADVERSE REACTIONS
Ceftazidime is generally well tolerated. The incidence of adverse reactions associated with the administration of ceftazidime was low in clinical trials. The most common were local reactions following intravenous injection, and allergic and gastrointestinal reactions. Other adverse reactions were encountered infrequently. No disulfiram-like reactions were reported. The following adverse effects from premarketing clinical trials were considered to be either related to ceftazidime therapy or were of uncertain etiology.

Local Effects, reported in less than 2% of patients, were phlebitis and inflammation at the site of injection (1 in 69 patients).
Hypersensitivity Reactions, reported in 2% of patients, were pruritus, rash and fever. Immediate hypersensitivity reactions occurred in 1 in 285 patients.
Gastrointestinal Symptoms, reported in less than 2% of patients, were diarrhea (1 in 78), nausea (1 in 156), vomiting (1 in 500) and abdominal pain (1 in 416).
Symptoms of pseudomembranous colitis can appear during or after antibiotic treatment (See WARNINGS section).
Less Frequent Adverse Events (less than 1%) were candidiasis and vaginitis; central nervous system events which included headache, dizziness and paresthesia.
Laboratory Test Changes noted during ceftazidime clinical trials were transient and included: eosinophilia (1 in 13), positive Coombs' test without hemolysis (1 in 23), thrombocytosis (1 in 45), and slight elevations in one or more of the hepatic enzymes, SGOT (1 in 16), SGPT (1 in 15), LDH (1 in 18) and alkaline phosphatase (1 in 23). As with some other cephalosporins, transient elevations of blood urea, blood urea nitrogen and/or serum creatinine were observed occasionally. Transient leukopenia, neutropenia, thrombocytopenia and lymphocytosis were seen very rarely.

DOSAGE AND ADMINISTRATION
Dosage: The usual adult dosage is 1 g. administered intravenously or intramuscularly every eight or 12 hours. The dosage and route should be determined by the susceptibility of the causative organisms, the severity of infection and the condition and renal function of the patient.

The guidelines for dosage of 'Tazicef' are listed in Table 3. The following dosage schedule is recommended.
[See table on next page].

Impaired Hepatic Function: No adjustment in dosage is required for patients with hepatic dysfunction.

Impaired Renal Function: Ceftazidime is excreted by the kidneys, almost exclusively by glomerular filtration. Therefore, in patients with impaired renal function (GFR < 50 mL./min.), it is recommended that the dosage of ceftazidime be reduced to compensate for its slower excretion. In patients with suspected renal insufficiency, an initial loading dose of 1 g. of ceftazidime may be given. An estimate of GFR should be made to determine the appropriate maintenance dose. The recommended dosage is presented in Table 4.

Table 4. Recommended Maintenance Doses of Tazicef (ceftazidime for injection, SK&F) in Renal Insufficiency

Creatinine Clearance (mL./min.)	Recommended Unit Dose of Ceftazidime	Frequency of Dosing
50–31	1 g.	q12h
30–16	1 g.	q24h
15–6	500 mg.	q24h
<5	500 mg.	q48h

When only serum creatinine is available, the following formula (Cockcroft's equation)[4] may be used to estimate creatinine clearance. The serum creatinine should represent a steady state of renal function:

Males:

$$\text{Creatinine clearance (mL./min.)} = \frac{\text{Weight (kg.)} \times (140 - \text{age})}{72 \times \text{serum creatinine (mg./dl.)}}$$

Females:
$0.85 \times$ above value

In patients with severe infections who would normally receive 6 g. of ceftazidime daily were it not for renal insufficiency, the unit dose given in the table above may be increased by 50% or the dosing frequency increased appropriately. Further dosing should be determined by therapeutic monitoring, severity of the infection and susceptibility of the causative organism.

In children as for adults, the creatinine clearance should be adjusted for body surface area or lean body mass and the dosing frequency reduced in cases of renal insufficiency.

In patients undergoing hemodialysis, a loading dose of 1 g. is recommended, followed by 1 g. after each hemodialysis period.

Tazicef (ceftazidime for injection, SK&F) can also be used in patients undergoing intra-peritoneal dialysis (IPD) and continuous ambulatory peritoneal dialysis (CAPD). In such patients, a loading dose of 'Tazicef' 1 g. may be given, followed by 500 mg. every 24 hours. In addition to intravenous use, 'Tazicef' can be incorporated in the dialysis fluid at a concentration of 250 mg. for 2 liters of dialysis fluid.

NOTE: Generally, 'Tazicef' should be continued for two days after the signs and symptoms of infection have disappeared, but in complicated infections longer therapy may be required.

RECONSTITUTION

Single Dose Vials:

For I.M. injection, I.V. direct (bolus) injection, or I.V. infusion, reconstitute with Sterile Water for Injection according to the following table. The vacuum may assist entry of the diluent. SHAKE WELL.

Table 5

Vial Size	Diluent to Be Added	Approx. Avail. Volume	Approx. Avg. Concentration
Intramuscular or Intravenous Direct (bolus) Injection			
1 gram	3.0 mL.	3.6 mL.	280 mg./mL.
Intravenous Infusion			
1 gram	10 mL.	10.6 mL.	95 mg./mL.
2 gram	10 mL.	11.2 mL.	180 mg./mL.

Withdraw the total volume of solution into the syringe (the pressure in the vial may aid withdrawal). The withdrawn solution may contain some bubbles of carbon dioxide.

NOTE: As with the administration of all parenteral products, accumulated gases should be expressed from the syringe immediately before injection of 'Tazicef'.

These solutions of 'Tazicef' are stable for 18 hours at room temperature or seven days if refrigerated (5℃.). Slight yellowing does not affect potency.

For I.V. infusion, dilute reconstituted solution in 50 to 100 mL. of one of the parenteral fluids listed under COMPATIBILITY AND STABILITY.

Pharmacy Bulk Vials:

Reconstitute with Sterile Water for Injection according to the following table. **Table 6**

Diluent to Be Added	Approx. Avail. Volume	Approx. Avg. Concentration
26 mL.	30 mL.	1 gram/5 mL.
53 mL.	60 mL.	1 gram/10 mL.

The vacuum may assist entry of the diluent. SHAKE WELL. Insert a gas relief needle through the vial closure to relieve the internal pressure. Remove the gas relief needle before extracting any solution.

NOTE: To preserve product sterility, it is important that a gas relief needle is not inserted through the vial closure before the product has dissolved.

These solutions of 'Tazicef' are stable for 18 hours at room temperature or seven days if refrigerated (5℃.). Slight yellowing does not affect potency. For I.V. infusion add to one of the parenteral fluids listed under COMPATIBILITY AND STABILITY.

"Piggyback" Vials:

For I.V. infusion, reconstitute with 10 mL. of Sodium Chloride Injection according to the following table. The vacuum may assist entry of the diluent. SHAKE WELL.

Table 7

Vial Size	Diluent to Be Added	Approx. Avail. Volume	Approx. Avg. Concentration
1 gram	100 mL.*	100 mL.	10 mg./mL.
2 gram	100 mL.*	100 mL.	20 mg./mL.

*Addition should be in two stages.

Insert a gas relief needle through the vial closure to relieve the internal pressure. With the gas relief needle in position, add the remaining 90 mL. of Sodium Chloride Injection. Remove the gas relief needle and syringe needle; shake the vial and set up for infusion in the normal way.

NOTE: To preserve product sterility, it is important that a gas relief needle is not inserted through the vial closure before the product has dissolved.

These solutions of Tazicef (ceftazidime for injection, SK&F) are stable for 18 hours at room temperature or seven days if refrigerated (5℃.). Slight yellowing does not affect potency.

Administration: 'Tazicef' may be given intravenously or by deep intramuscular injection into a large muscle mass such as the upper outer quadrant of the gluteus maximus or lateral part of the thigh.

Intramuscular Administration: For intramuscular administration, 'Tazicef' should be reconstituted with Sterile Water for Injection. Refer to Table 5.

Intravenous Administration: The I.V. route is preferable for patients with bacterial septicemia, bacterial meningitis, peritonitis, or other severe or life-threatening infections, or for patients who may be poor risks because of lowered resistance resulting from such debilitating conditions as malnutrition, trauma, surgery, diabetes, heart failure or malignancy, particularly if shock is present or pending.

For direct intermittent intravenous administration, reconstitute 'Tazicef' as directed in Table 5 with Sterile Water for Injection. Slowly inject directly into the vein over a period of three to five minutes or give through the tubing of an administration set while the patient is also receiving one of the compatible intravenous fluids (See COMPATIBILITY AND STABILITY).

For intravenous infusion, reconstitute the 1 or 2 g. piggyback vial with 100 mL. of Sodium Chloride Injection or one of the compatible intravenous fluids listed under the COMPATIBILITY AND STABILITY section. Alternatively, reconstitute the 1 g. or 2 g. vial and add an appropriate quantity of the resulting solution to an I.V. container with one of the compatible intravenous fluids.

Intermittent intravenous infusion with a Y-type administration set can be accomplished with compatible solutions. However, during infusion of a solution containing 'Tazicef' it is advisable to discontinue the other solution.

All vials of 'Tazicef' as supplied are under reduced pressure. When 'Tazicef' is dissolved, carbon dioxide is released and a positive pressure develops. See RECONSTITUTION.

Solutions of 'Tazicef', like those of most beta-lactam antibiotics, should not be added to solutions of aminoglycoside antibiotics because of potential interaction.

However, if concurrent therapy with 'Tazicef' and an aminoglycoside is indicated, each of these antibiotics can be administered separately to the same patient.

Table 3. Recommended Dosage Schedule

	Dose	Frequency
Adults		
Usual recommended dose	1 g. I.V. or I.M.	q8–12h
Uncomplicated urinary tract infections	250 mg. I.V. or I.M.	q12h
Bone and joint infections	2 g. I.V.	q12h
Complicated urinary tract infections	500 mg. I.V. or I.M.	q8–12h
Uncomplicated pneumonia; mild skin and skin structure infections	500 mg.–1 g. I.V. or I.M.	q8h
Serious gynecological and intra-abdominal infections	2 g. I.V.	q8h
Meningitis	2 g. I.V.	q8h
Very severe life-threatening infections, especially in immunocompromised patients	2 g. I.V.	q8h
Pseudomonal lung infections in patients with cystic fibrosis with normal renal function*	30–50 mg./kg. I.V. to a maximum of 6 g./day	q8h
Neonates (0–4 weeks)	30 mg./kg. I.V.	q12h
Infants and children (1 month–12 years)	30–50 mg./kg. I.V. to a maximum of 6 g./day†	q8h

* Although clinical improvement has been shown, bacteriological cures cannot be expected in patients with chronic respiratory disease and cystic fibrosis.
† The higher dose should be reserved for immunocompromised children or children with cystic fibrosis or meningitis.

COMPATIBILITY AND STABILITY

Intramuscular: 'Tazicef', when reconstituted as directed with Sterile Water for Injection, maintains satisfactory potency for 18 hours at room temperature or for seven days under refrigeration (5℃.). Solutions in Sterile Water for Injection that are frozen immediately after reconstitution in the original container are stable for three months when stored at −20℃. Once thawed, solutions should not be refrozen. Thawed solutions may be stored for up to eight hours at room temperature or for four days in a refrigerator (5℃.).

Intravenous: Tazicef (ceftazidime for injection, SK&F), when reconstituted as directed with Sterile Water for Injection, maintains satisfactory potency for 18 hours at room temperature or for seven days under refrigeration (5℃.). Solutions in Sterile Water for Injection in the original container or in 0.9% Sodium Chloride Injection in Viaflex® small volume containers that are frozen immediately after reconstitution are stable for three months when stored at −20℃. For larger volumes where it may be necessary to warm the frozen product (to a maximum of 40℃.), care should be taken to avoid heating after thawing is complete. Once thawed, solutions should not be refrozen. Thawed solutions may be stored for up to eight hours at room temperature or for four days in a refrigerator (5℃.).

'Tazicef' is compatible with the more commonly used intravenous infusion fluids. Solutions at concentrations between 1 mg./mL. and 40 mg./mL. in the following infusion fluids may be stored for up to 18 hours at room temperature or seven days if refrigerated: 0.9% Sodium Chloride Injection; Ringer's Injection USP; Lactated Ringer's Injection USP; 5% Dextrose Injection; 5% Dextrose and 0.225% Sodium Chloride Injection; 5% Dextrose and 0.45% Sodium Chloride Injection; 5% Dextrose and 0.9% Sodium Chloride Injection; 10% Dextrose Injection.

'Tazicef' is less stable in Sodium Bicarbonate Injection than in other intravenous fluids. It is not recommended as a diluent. Solutions of 'Tazicef' in 5% Dextrose and 0.9% Sodium Chloride Injection are stable for at least six hours at room temperature in plastic tubing, drip chambers and volume control devices of common intravenous infusion sets.

Ceftazidime at a concentration of 20 mg./mL. has been found compatible for 18 hours at room temperature or seven days under refrigeration in Sterile Water for Injection when admixed with: cefazolin sodium (Ancef®) 330 mg./mL.; heparin 1000 units/mL.; and cimetidine HCl (Tagamet® HCl) 150 mg./mL.

Ceftazidime at a concentration of 20 mg./mL. has been found compatible for 18 hours at room temperature or seven days under refrigeration in 5% Dextrose Injection when admixed with Potassium Chloride 40 mEq/l.

Note: Parenteral drug products should be inspected visually for particulate matter prior to administration wherever solution and container permit.

As with other cephalosporins, 'Tazicef' powder as well as solutions tend to darken depending on storage conditions; within the stated recommendations, however, product potency is not adversely affected.

HOW SUPPLIED

Tazicef (ceftazidime for injection, SK&F) is supplied in vials equivalent to 1 gram and 2 grams of ceftazidime; in "Piggyback" Vials for I.V. admixture equivalent to 1 gram and 2

Continued on next page

Smith Kline &French—Cont.

grams of ceftazidime; and in Pharmacy Bulk Vials equivalent to 6 grams of ceftazidime.

REFERENCES

1. Bauer, A.W.; Kirby, W.M.M., and Sherris, J.C., et al.: Antibiotic susceptibility testing by a standardized single disc method, Am. J. Clin. Pathol. 45:493, 1966. 2. National Committee for Clinical Laboratory Standards, Approved Standard: Performance Standards for Antimicrobial Disc Susceptibility Tests (M2-A3), December, 1984. 3. Standardized disc susceptibility test, Federal Register 39:19182–19184, 1974. 4. Cockcroft, D.W., and Gault, M.H.: Prediction of creatinine clearance from serum creatinine, Nephron 16:31–41, 1976.

TF:L7

Shown in Product Identification Section, page 431

THORAZINE® ℞
[thor'ah-zeen]
(brand of chlorpromazine)

PRODUCT OVERVIEW

KEY FACTS

'Thorazine' is a dimethylamine derivative of phenothiazine of the aliphatic group, available in 18 dosage forms and strengths for oral, rectal or parenteral administration. The Spansule® sustained release capsule dosage form provides an equivalent milligram dose of tablets given in divided doses.

MAJOR USES

'Thorazine' is indicated for the management of manifestations of psychotic disorders, to control nausea and vomiting, for the relief of restlessness and apprehension before surgery, for acute intermittent porphyria, as an adjunct in the treatment of tetanus, to control the manifestations of the manic type of manic-depressive illness, for the relief of intractable hiccups, and for the treatment of severe behavioral problems in children marked by combativeness and/or explosive hyperexcitable behavior.

SAFETY INFORMATION

'Thorazine' is contraindicated for use in comatose states or in the presence of large amounts of CNS depressants. EPS, which can occur secondary to 'Thorazine', may be confused with the CNS signs of Reye's syndrome. Use of 'Thorazine' and other potential hepatotoxins should be avoided in children and adolescents whose signs and symptoms suggest Reye's syndrome. (See full prescribing information.)

PRESCRIBING INFORMATION

THORAZINE® ℞
[thor'ah-zeen]
(brand of chlorpromazine)

DESCRIPTION

Thorazine (chlorpromazine, SK&F) is 10 - (3 - dimethylaminopropyl) -2-chlorphenothiazine, a dimethylamine derivative of phenothiazine. It is present in oral and injectable forms as the hydrochloride salt, and in the suppositories as the base.

Tablets—Each round, orange, coated tablet contains chlorpromazine hydrochloride as follows: 10 mg. imprinted SKF and T73; 25 mg. imprinted SKF and T74; 50 mg. imprinted SKF and T76; 100 mg. imprinted SKF and T77; 200 mg. imprinted SKF and T79. Inactive ingredients consist of benzoic acid, croscarmellose sodium, D&C Yellow No. 10, FD&C Blue No. 2, FD&C Yellow No. 6, gelatin, hydroxypropyl methylcellulose, lactose, magnesium stearate, methylparaben, polyethylene glycol, propylparaben, talc, titanium dioxide, and trace amounts of other inactive ingredients.

Spansule® sustained release capsules—Each 'Thorazine' *Spansule* capsule is so prepared that an initial dose is released promptly and the remaining medication is released gradually over a prolonged period.

Each capsule, with opaque orange cap and natural body, contains chlorpromazine hydrochloride as follows: 30 mg. imprinted SKF and T63; 75 mg. imprinted SKF and T64; 150 mg. imprinted SKF and T66; 200 mg. imprinted SKF and T67; 300 mg. imprinted SKF and T69. Inactive ingredients consist of benzyl alcohol, calcium sulfate, cetylpyridinium chloride, FD&C Yellow No. 6, gelatin, glyceryl distearate, glyceryl monostearate, iron oxide, povidone, silicon dioxide, sodium lauryl sulfate, starch, sucrose, titanium dioxide, wax and trace amounts of other inactive ingredients.

Ampuls—Each mL. contains, in aqueous solution, chlorpromazine hydrochloride, 25 mg.; ascorbic acid, 2 mg.; sodium bisulfite, 1 mg.; sodium chloride, 6 mg.; sodium sulfite, 1 mg.

Multiple-dose Vials—Each mL. contains, in aqueous solution, chlorpromazine hydrochloride, 25 mg.; ascorbic acid, 2 mg.; sodium bisulfite, 1 mg.; sodium chloride, 1 mg.; sodium sulfite, 1 mg.; benzyl alcohol, 2%, as a preservative.

Syrup—Each 5 mL. (one teaspoonful) of clear, orange-custard flavored liquid contains chlorpromazine hydrochloride,

10 mg. Inactive ingredients consist of citric acid, flavors, sodium benzoate, sucrose and water.

Suppositories—Each suppository contains chlorpromazine, 25 or 100 mg., glycerin, glyceryl monopalmitate, glyceryl monostearate, hydrogenated coconut oil fatty acids, and hydrogenated palm kernel oil fatty acids.

Concentrate—Each mL. of clear, custard flavored liquid contains chlorpromazine hydrochloride, 30 or 100 mg. Inactive ingredients consist of calcium disodium edetate, citric acid, flavors, hydroxypropyl methylcellulose, propylene glycol, saccharin sodium, sodium benzoate, water and trace amounts of other inactive ingredients.

ACTIONS

The precise mechanism whereby the therapeutic effects of chlorpromazine are produced is not known. The principal pharmacological actions are psychotropic. It also exerts sedative and antiemetic activity. Chlorpromazine has actions at all levels of the central nervous system—primarily at subcortical levels—as well as on multiple organ systems. Chlorpromazine has strong antiadrenergic and weaker peripheral anticholinergic activity; ganglionic blocking action is relatively slight. It also possesses slight antihistaminic and antiserotonin activity.

INDICATIONS

For the management of manifestations of psychotic disorders.
To control nausea and vomiting.
For relief of restlessness and apprehension before surgery.
For acute intermittent porphyria.
As an adjunct in the treatment of tetanus.
To control the manifestations of the manic type of manic-depressive illness.
For relief of intractable hiccups.
For the treatment of severe behavioral problems in children marked by combativeness and/or explosive hyperexcitable behavior (out of proportion to immediate provocations), and in the short-term treatment of hyperactive children who show excessive motor activity with accompanying conduct disorders consisting of some or all of the following symptoms: impulsivity, difficulty sustaining attention, aggressivity, mood lability and poor frustration tolerance.

CONTRAINDICATIONS

Do not use in comatose states or in the presence of large amounts of central nervous system depressants (alcohol, barbiturates, narcotics, etc.).

WARNINGS

The extrapyramidal symptoms which can occur secondary to Thorazine (chlorpromazine, SK&F) may be confused with the central nervous system signs of an undiagnosed primary disease responsible for the vomiting, e.g., Reye's syndrome or other encephalopathy. The use of 'Thorazine' and other potential hepatotoxins should be avoided in children and adolescents whose signs and symptoms suggest Reye's syndrome.

Tardive Dyskinesia: Tardive dyskinesia, a syndrome consisting of potentially irreversible, involuntary, dyskinetic movements, may develop in patients treated with neuroleptic (antipsychotic) drugs. Although the prevalence of the syndrome appears to be highest among the elderly, especially elderly women, it is impossible to rely upon prevalence estimates to predict, at the inception of neuroleptic treatment, which patients are likely to develop the syndrome. Whether neuroleptic drug products differ in their potential to cause tardive dyskinesia is unknown.

Both the risk of developing the syndrome and the likelihood that it will become irreversible are believed to increase as the duration of treatment and the total cumulative dose of neuroleptic drugs administered to the patient increase. However, the syndrome can develop, although much less commonly, after relatively brief treatment periods at low doses.

There is no known treatment for established cases of tardive dyskinesia, although the syndrome may remit, partially or completely, if neuroleptic treatment is withdrawn. Neuroleptic treatment itself, however, may suppress (or partially suppress) the signs and symptoms of the syndrome and thereby may possibly mask the underlying disease process. The effect that symptomatic suppression has upon the long-term course of the syndrome is unknown.

Given these considerations, neuroleptics should be prescribed in a manner that is most likely to minimize the occurrence of tardive dyskinesia. Chronic neuroleptic treatment should generally be reserved for patients who suffer from a chronic illness that, 1) is known to respond to neuroleptic drugs, and, 2) for whom alternative, equally effective, but potentially less harmful treatments are *not* available or appropriate. In patients who do require chronic treatment, the smallest dose and the shortest duration of treatment producing a satisfactory clinical response should be sought. The need for continued treatment should be reassessed periodically.

If signs and symptoms of tardive dyskinesia appear in a patient on neuroleptics, drug discontinuation should be consid-

ered. However, some patients may require treatment despite the presence of the syndrome.

For further information about the description of tardive dyskinesia and its clinical detection, please refer to the sections on Precautions and Adverse Reactions.

Neuroleptic Malignant Syndrome (NMS): A potentially fatal symptom complex sometimes referred to as Neuroleptic Malignant Syndrome (NMS) has been reported in association with antipsychotic drugs. Clinical manifestations of NMS are hyperpyrexia, muscle rigidity, altered mental status and evidence of autonomic instability (irregular pulse or blood pressure, tachycardia, diaphoresis, and cardiac dysrhythmias).

The diagnostic evaluation of patients with this syndrome is complicated. In arriving at a diagnosis, it is important to identify cases where the clinical presentation includes both serious medical illness (e.g., pneumonia, systemic infection, etc.) and untreated or inadequately treated extrapyramidal signs and symptoms (EPS). Other important considerations in the differential diagnosis include central anticholinergic toxicity, heat stroke, drug fever and primary central nervous system (CNS) pathology.

The management of NMS should include 1) immediate discontinuation of antipsychotic drugs and other drugs not essential to concurrent therapy, 2) intensive symptomatic treatment and medical monitoring, and 3) treatment of any concomitant serious medical problems for which specific treatments are available. There is no general agreement about specific pharmacological treatment regimens for uncomplicated NMS.

If a patient requires antipsychotic drug treatment after recovery from NMS, the potential reintroduction of drug therapy should be carefully considered. The patient should be carefully monitored, since recurrences of NMS have been reported.

Thorazine (chlorpromazine, SK&F) ampuls and multiple-dose vials contain sodium bisulfite and sodium sulfite, sulfites that may cause allergic-type reactions including anaphylactic symptoms and life-threatening or less severe asthmatic episodes in certain susceptible people. The overall prevalence of sulfite sensitivity in the general population is unknown and probably low. Sulfite sensitivity is seen more frequently in asthmatic than in nonasthmatic people.

Patients with bone marrow depression or who have previously demonstrated a hypersensitivity reaction (e.g., blood dyscrasias, jaundice) with a phenothiazine should not receive any phenothiazine, including 'Thorazine', unless in the judgment of the physician the potential benefits of treatment outweigh the possible hazard.

'Thorazine' may impair mental and/or physical abilities, especially during the first few days of therapy. Therefore, caution patients about activities requiring alertness (e.g., operating vehicles or machinery).

The use of alcohol with this drug should be avoided due to possible additive effects and hypotension.

'Thorazine' may counteract the antihypertensive effect of guanethidine and related compounds.

Usage in Pregnancy: Safety for the use of Thorazine (chlorpromazine, SK&F) during pregnancy has not been established. Therefore, it is not recommended that the drug be given to pregnant patients except when, in the judgment of the physician, it is essential. The potential benefits should clearly outweigh possible hazards. There are reported instances of prolonged jaundice, extrapyramidal signs, hyperreflexia or hyporeflexia in newborn infants whose mothers received phenothiazines.

Reproductive studies in rodents have demonstrated potential for embryotoxicity, increased neonatal mortality and nursing transfer of the drug. Tests in the offspring of the drug-treated rodents demonstrate decreased performance. The possibility of permanent neurological damage cannot be excluded.

Nursing Mothers: There is evidence that chlorpromazine is excreted in the breast milk of nursing mothers.

PRECAUTIONS

Given the likelihood that some patients exposed chronically to neuroleptics will develop tardive dyskinesia, it is advised that all patients in whom chronic use is contemplated be given, if possible, full information about this risk. The decision to inform patients and/or their guardians must obviously take into account the clinical circumstances and the competency of the patient to understand the information provided.

Thorazine (chlorpromazine, SK&F) should be administered cautiously to persons with cardiovascular or liver disease. There is evidence that patients with a history of hepatic encephalopathy due to cirrhosis have increased sensitivity to the C.N.S. effects of 'Thorazine' (i.e., impaired cerebration and abnormal slowing of the EEG).

Because of its C.N.S. depressant effect, 'Thorazine' should be used with caution in patients with chronic respiratory disorders such as severe asthma, emphysema and acute respiratory infections, particularly in children.

Because 'Thorazine' can suppress the cough reflex, aspiration of vomitus is possible.

Thorazine (chlorpromazine, SK&F) prolongs and intensifies the action of C.N.S. depressants such as anesthetics, barbiturates and narcotics. When 'Thorazine' is administered concomitantly, about $\frac{1}{4}$ to $\frac{1}{2}$ the usual dosage of such agents is required. When 'Thorazine' is not being administered to reduce requirements of C.N.S. depressants, it is best to stop such depressants before starting 'Thorazine' treatment. These agents may subsequently be reinstated at low doses and increased as needed.

Note: 'Thorazine' does *not* intensify the anticonvulsant action of barbiturates. Therefore, dosage of anticonvulsants, including barbiturates, should *not* be reduced if 'Thorazine' is started. Instead, start 'Thorazine' at low doses and increase as needed.

Use with caution in persons who will be exposed to extreme heat, organophosphorus insecticides, and in persons receiving atropine or related drugs.

Neuroleptic drugs elevate prolactin levels; the elevation persists during chronic administration. Tissue culture experiments indicate that approximately one-third of human breast cancers are prolactin-dependent *in vitro*, a factor of potential importance if the prescribing of these drugs is contemplated in a patient with a previously detected breast cancer. Although disturbances such as galactorrhea, amenorrhea, gynecomastia and impotence have been reported, the clinical significance of elevated serum prolactin levels is unknown for most patients. An increase in mammary neoplasms has been found in rodents after chronic administration of neuroleptic drugs. Neither clinical nor epidemiologic studies conducted to date, however, have shown an association between chronic administration of these drugs and mammary tumorigenesis; the available evidence is considered too limited to be conclusive at this time.

Chromosomal aberrations in spermatocytes and abnormal sperm have been demonstrated in rodents treated with certain neuroleptics.

As with all drugs which exert an anticholinergic effect, and/or cause mydriasis, chlorpromazine should be used with caution in patients with glaucoma.

Chlorpromazine diminishes the effect of oral anticoagulants. Phenothiazines can produce alpha-adrenergic blockade.

Chlorpromazine may lower the convulsive threshold; dosage adjustments of anticonvulsants may be necessary. Potentiation of anticonvulsant effects does not occur. However, it has been reported that chlorpromazine may interfere with the metabolism of Dilantin®* and thus precipitate 'Dilantin' toxicity.

Concomitant administration with propranolol results in increased plasma levels of both drugs.

Thiazide diuretics may accentuate the orthostatic hypotension that may occur with phenothiazines.

The presence of phenothiazines may produce false positive phenylketonuria (PKU) test results.

Drugs which lower the seizure threshold, including phenothiazine derivatives, should not be used with Amipaque®†. As with other phenothiazine derivatives, 'Thorazine' should be discontinued at least 48 hours before myelography, should not be resumed for at least 24 hours postprocedure, and should not be used for the control of nausea and vomiting occurring either prior to myelography or postprocedure with 'Amipaque'.

Long-Term Therapy: To lessen the likelihood of adverse reactions related to cumulative drug effect, patients with a history of long-term therapy with 'Thorazine' and/or other neuroleptics should be evaluated periodically to decide whether the maintenance dosage could be lowered or drug therapy discontinued.

Antiemetic Effect: The antiemetic action of 'Thorazine' may mask the signs and symptoms of overdosage of other drugs and may obscure the diagnosis and treatment of other conditions such as intestinal obstruction, brain tumor and Reye's syndrome. (See Warnings.)

When 'Thorazine' is used with cancer chemotherapeutic drugs, vomiting as a sign of the toxicity of these agents may be obscured by the antiemetic effect of 'Thorazine'.

Abrupt Withdrawal: Like other phenothiazines, Thorazine (chlorpromazine, SK&F) is not known to cause psychic dependence and does not produce tolerance or addiction. There may be, however, following abrupt withdrawal of high-dose therapy, some symptoms resembling those of physical dependence such as gastritis, nausea and vomiting, dizziness and tremulousness. These symptoms can usually be avoided or reduced by gradual reduction of the dosage or by continuing concomitant anti-parkinsonism agents for several weeks after 'Thorazine' is withdrawn.

ADVERSE REACTIONS

Note: Some adverse effects of 'Thorazine' may be more likely to occur, or occur with greater intensity, in patients with special medical problems, e.g., patients with mitral insufficiency or pheochromocytoma have experienced severe hypotension following recommended doses.

Drowsiness, usually mild to moderate, may occur, particularly during the first or second week, after which it generally disappears. If troublesome, dosage may be lowered.

Jaundice: Overall incidence has been low, regardless of indication or dosage. Most investigators conclude it is a sensitivity reaction. Most cases occur between the second and fourth weeks of therapy. The clinical picture resembles infectious hepatitis, with laboratory features of obstructive jaundice, rather than those of parenchymal damage. It is usually promptly reversible on withdrawal of the medication; however, chronic jaundice has been reported.

There is no conclusive evidence that preexisting liver disease makes patients more susceptible to jaundice. Alcoholics with cirrhosis have been successfully treated with Thorazine (chlorpromazine, SK&F) without complications. Nevertheless, the medication should be used cautiously in patients with liver disease. Patients who have experienced jaundice with a phenothiazine should not, if possible, be reexposed to 'Thorazine' or other phenothiazines.

If fever with grippe-like symptoms occurs, appropriate liver studies should be conducted. If tests indicate an abnormality, stop treatment.

Liver function tests in jaundice induced by the drug may mimic extrahepatic obstruction; withhold exploratory laparotomy until extrahepatic obstruction is confirmed.

Hematological Disorders, including agranulocytosis, eosinophilia, leukopenia, hemolytic anemia, aplastic anemia, thrombocytopenic purpura and pancytopenia have been reported.

Agranulocytosis—Warn patients to report the sudden appearance of sore throat or other signs of infection. If white blood cell and differential counts indicate cellular depression, stop treatment and start antibiotic and other suitable therapy.

Most cases have occurred between the 4th and 10th weeks of therapy; patients should be watched closely during that period.

Moderate suppression of white blood cells is not an indication for stopping treatment unless accompanied by the symptoms described above.

Cardiovascular:

Hypotensive Effects—Postural hypotension, simple tachycardia, momentary fainting and dizziness may occur after the first injection; occasionally after subsequent injections; rarely, after the first oral dose. Usually recovery is spontaneous and symptoms disappear within $\frac{1}{2}$ to 2 hours. Occasionally, these effects may be more severe and prolonged, producing a shock-like condition.

To minimize hypotension after injection, keep patient lying down and observe for at least $\frac{1}{2}$ hour. To control hypotension, place patient in head-low position with legs raised. If a vasoconstrictor is required, Levophed®‡ and Neo-Synephrine®§ are the most suitable. Other pressor agents, including epinephrine, should not be used as they may cause a paradoxical further lowering of blood pressure.

EKG Changes—particularly nonspecific, usually reversible Q and T wave distortions—have been observed in some patients receiving phenothiazine tranquilizers, including Thorazine (chlorpromazine, SK&F).

Note: Sudden death, apparently due to cardiac arrest, has been reported.

C.N.S. Reactions:

Neuromuscular (Extrapyramidal) Reactions— Neuromuscular reactions include dystonias, motor restlessness, pseudo-parkinsonism and tardive dyskinesia, and appear to be dose-related. They are discussed in the following paragraphs:

Dystonias: Symptoms may include spasm of the neck muscles, sometimes progressing to acute, reversible torticollis; extensor rigidity of back muscles, sometimes progressing to opisthotonos; carpopedal spasm, trismus, swallowing difficulty, oculogyric crisis and protrusion of the tongue.

These usually subside within a few hours, and almost always within 24 to 48 hours after the drug has been discontinued.

In mild cases, reassurance or a barbiturate is often sufficient. *In moderate cases,* barbiturates will usually bring rapid relief. *In more severe adult cases,* the administration of an anti-parkinsonism agent, except levodopa, usually produces rapid reversal of symptoms. *In children,* reassurance and barbiturates will usually control symptoms. (Or, parenteral Benadryl‖ may be useful. See 'Benadryl' prescribing information for appropriate children's dosage.) If appropriate treatment with anti-parkinsonism agents or 'Benadryl' fails to reverse the signs and symptoms, the diagnosis should be reevaluated.

Suitable supportive measures such as maintaining a clear airway and adequate hydration should be employed when needed. If therapy is reinstituted, it should be at a lower dosage. Should these symptoms occur in children or pregnant patients, the drug should not be reinstituted.

Motor Restlessness: Symptoms may include agitation or jitteriness and sometimes insomnia. These symptoms often disappear spontaneously. At times these symptoms may be similar to the original neurotic or psychotic symptoms. Dosage should not be increased until these side effects have subsided.

If these symptoms become too troublesome, they can usually be controlled by a reduction of dosage or change of drug. Treatment with anti-parkinsonian agents, benzodiazepines or propranolol may be helpful.

Pseudo-parkinsonism: Symptoms may include: mask-like facies, drooling, tremors, pillrolling motion, cogwheel rigidity and shuffling gait. In most cases these symptoms are readily controlled when an anti-parkinsonism agent is administered concomitantly. Anti-parkinsonism agents should be used only when required. Generally, therapy of a few weeks to two or three months will suffice. After this time patients should be evaluated to determine their need for continued treatment. (Note: Levodopa has not been found effective in neuroleptic-induced pseudo-parkinsonism.) Occasionally it is necessary to lower the dosage of Thorazine (chlorpromazine, SK&F) or to discontinue the drug.

Tardive Dyskinesia: As with all antipsychotic agents, tardive dyskinesia may appear in some patients on long-term therapy or may appear after drug therapy has been discontinued. The syndrome can also develop, although much less frequently, after relatively brief treatment periods at low doses. This syndrome appears in all age groups. Although its prevalence appears to be highest among elderly patients, especially elderly women, it is impossible to rely upon prevalence estimates to predict at the inception of neuroleptic treatment which patients are likely to develop the syndrome. The symptoms are persistent and in some patients appear to be irreversible. The syndrome is characterized by rhythmical involuntary movements of the tongue, face, mouth or jaw (e.g., protrusion of tongue, puffing of cheeks, puckering of mouth, chewing movements). Sometimes these may be accompanied by involuntary movements of extremities. In rare instances, these involuntary movements of the extremities are the only manifestations of tardive dyskinesia. A variant of tardive dyskinesia, tardive dystonia, has also been described.

There is no known effective treatment for tardive dyskinesia; anti-parkinsonism agents do not alleviate the symptoms of this syndrome. If clinically feasible, it is suggested that all antipsychotic agents be discontinued if these symptoms appear. Should it be necessary to reinstitute treatment, or increase the dosage of the agent, or switch to a different antipsychotic agent, the syndrome may be masked.

It has been reported that fine vermicular movements of the tongue may be an early sign of the syndrome and if the medication is stopped at that time the syndrome may not develop.

Adverse Behavioral Effects—Psychotic symptoms and catatonic-like states have been reported rarely.

Other C.N.S. Effects—Cerebral edema has been reported. Convulsive seizures (*petit mal* and *grand mal*) have been reported, particularly in patients with EEG abnormalities or history of such disorders.

Abnormality of the cerebrospinal fluid proteins has also been reported.

Allergic Reactions of a mild urticarial type or photosensitivity are seen. Avoid undue exposure to sun. More severe reactions, including exfoliative dermatitis, have been reported occasionally.

Contact dermatitis has been reported in nursing personnel; accordingly, the use of rubber gloves when administering 'Thorazine' liquid or injectable is recommended.

In addition, asthma, laryngeal edema, angioneurotic edema and anaphylactoid reactions have been reported.

Endocrine Disorders: Lactation and moderate breast engorgement may occur in females on large doses. If persistent, lower dosage or withdraw drug. False-positive pregnancy tests have been reported, but are less likely to occur when a serum test is used. Amenorrhea and gynecomastia have also been reported. Hyperglycemia, hypoglycemia and glycosuria have been reported.

Autonomic Reactions: Occasional dry mouth; nasal congestion; nausea; obstipation; constipation; adynamic ileus; urinary retention; priapism; miosis and mydriasis, atonic colon, ejaculatory disorders/impotence.

Special Considerations in Long-Term Therapy: Skin pigmentation and ocular changes have occurred in some patients taking substantial doses of Thorazine (chlorpromazine, SK&F) for prolonged periods.

Skin Pigmentation—Rare instances of skin pigmentation have been observed in hospitalized mental patients, primarily females who have received the drug usually for three years or more in dosages ranging from 500 mg. to 1500 mg. daily. The pigmentary changes, restricted to exposed areas of the body, range from an almost imperceptible darkening of the skin to a slate gray color, sometimes with a violet hue. Histological examination reveals a pigment, chiefly in the dermis, which is probably a melanin-like complex. The pigmentation may fade following discontinuance of the drug.

Ocular Changes—Ocular changes have occurred more frequently than skin pigmentation and have been observed both in pigmented and nonpigmented patients receiving Thorazine (chlorpromazine, SK&F) usually for two years or more in dosages of 300 mg. daily and higher. Eye changes are characterized by deposition of fine particulate matter in the lens and cornea. In more advanced cases, star-shaped opacities have also been observed in the anterior portion of the lens. The nature of the eye deposits has not yet been deter-

Continued on next page

Smith Kline & French—Cont.

mined. A small number of patients with more severe ocular changes have had some visual impairment. In addition to these corneal and lenticular changes, epithelial keratopathy and pigmentary retinopathy have been reported. Reports suggest that the eye lesions may regress after withdrawal of the drug.

Since the occurrence of eye changes seems to be related to dosage levels and/or duration of therapy, it is suggested that long-term patients on moderate to high dosage levels have periodic ocular examinations.

Etiology—The etiology of both of these reactions is not clear, but exposure to light, along with dosage/duration of therapy, appears to be the most significant factor. If either of these reactions is observed, the physician should weigh the benefits of continued therapy against the possible risks and, on the merits of the individual case, determine whether or not to continue present therapy, lower the dosage, or withdraw the drug.

Other Adverse Reactions: Mild fever may occur after large I.M. doses. Hyperpyrexia has been reported. Increases in appetite and weight sometimes occur. Peripheral edema and a systemic lupus erythematosus-like syndrome have been reported.

Note: There have been occasional reports of sudden death in patients receiving phenothiazines. In some cases, the cause appeared to be cardiac arrest or asphyxia due to failure of the cough reflex.

DOSAGE AND ADMINISTRATION—ADULTS

Adjust dosage to individual and the severity of his condition, recognizing that the milligram for milligram potency relationship among all dosage forms has not been precisely established clinically. It is important to increase dosage until symptoms are controlled. Dosage should be increased more gradually in debilitated or emaciated patients. In continued therapy, gradually reduce dosage to the lowest effective maintenance level, after symptoms have been controlled for a reasonable period.

In general, dosage recommendations for other oral forms of the drug may be applied to Spansule® brand sustained release capsules on the basis of total daily dosage in milligrams.

The 100 mg. and 200 mg. tablets and the 300 mg. 'Spansule' capsules are for use in severe neuropsychiatric conditions. Increase parenteral dosage only if hypotension has not occurred. Before using I.M., see Important Notes on Injection.

Elderly Patients—In general, dosages in the lower range are sufficient for most elderly patients. Since they appear to be more susceptible to hypotension and neuromuscular reactions, such patients should be observed closely. Dosage should be tailored to the individual, response carefully monitored, and dosage adjusted accordingly. Dosage should be increased more gradually in elderly patients.

Psychotic Disorders—Increase dosage gradually until symptoms are controlled. Maximum improvement may not be seen for weeks or even months. Continue optimum dosage for 2 weeks; then gradually reduce dosage to the lowest effective maintenance level. Daily dosage of 200 mg. is not unusual. Some patients require higher dosages (e.g., 800 mg. daily is not uncommon in discharged mental patients).

HOSPITALIZED PATIENTS: ACUTELY DISTURBED OR MANIC—*I.M.:* 25 mg. (1 mL.). If necessary, give additional 25 to 50 mg. injection in 1 hour. Increase subsequent I.M. doses gradually over several days—up to 400 mg. q4-6h in exceptionally severe cases—until patient is controlled. Usually patient becomes quiet and cooperative within 24 to 48 hours and oral doses may be substituted and increased until the patient is calm. 500 mg. a day is generally sufficient. While gradual increases to 2,000 mg. a day or more may be necessary, there is usually little therapeutic gain to be achieved by exceeding 1,000 mg. a day for extended periods. In general, dosage levels should be lower in the elderly, the emaciated and the debilitated. LESS ACUTELY DISTURBED—*Oral:* 25 mg. t.i.d. Increase gradually until effective dose is reached—usually 400 mg. daily. OUTPATIENTS—*Oral:* 10 mg. t.i.d. or q.i.d., or 25 mg. b.i.d. or t.i.d. MORE SEVERE CASES—*Oral:* 25 mg. t.i.d. After 1 or 2 days, daily dosage may be increased by 20–50 mg. at semiweekly intervals until patient becomes calm and cooperative. PROMPT CONTROL OF SEVERE SYMPTOMS—*I.M.:* 25 mg. (1 mL.). If necessary, repeat in 1 hour. Subsequent doses should be oral, 25–50 mg. t.i.d.

Nausea and Vomiting—*Oral:* 10 to 25 mg. q4–6h, p.r.n., increased, if necessary. *I.M.:* 25 mg. (1 mL.). If no hypotension occurs, give 25 to 50 mg. q3–4h, p.r.n., until vomiting stops. Then switch to oral dosage. *Rectal:* One 100 mg. suppository q6–8h, p.r.n. In some patients, half this dose will do. DURING SURGERY—*I.M.:* 12.5 mg. (0.5 mL.). Repeat in ½ hour if necessary and if no hypotension occurs. *I.V.:* 2 mg. per fractional injection, at 2-minute intervals. Do not exceed 25 mg. Dilute to 1 mg./mL., i.e., 1 mL. (25 mg.) mixed with 24 mL. of saline.

Presurgical Apprehension—*Oral:* 25 to 50 mg., 2 to 3 hours before the operation. *I.M.:* 12.5 to 25 mg. (0.5-1 mL.), 1 to 2 hours before operation.

Intractable Hiccups—*Oral:* 25 to 50 mg. t.i.d. or q.i.d. If symptoms persist for 2-3 days, give 25 to 50 mg. (1-2 mL.) I.M. Should symptoms persist, use *slow* I.V. infusion with patient flat in bed: 25 to 50 mg. (1-2 mL.) in 500 to 1,000 mL. of saline. Follow blood pressure closely.

Acute Intermittent Porphyria—*Oral:* 25 to 50 mg. t.i.d. or q.i.d. Can usually be discontinued after several weeks, but maintenance therapy may be necessary for some patients. *I.M.:* 25 mg. (1 mL.) t.i.d. or q.i.d. until patient can take oral therapy.

Tetanus—*I.M.:* 25 to 50 mg. (1-2 mL.) given 3 or 4 times daily, usually in conjunction with barbiturates. Total doses and frequency of administration must be determined by the patient's response, starting with low doses and increasing gradually. *I.V.:* 25 to 50 mg. (1-2 mL.). Dilute to at least 1 mg. per mL. and administer at a rate of 1 mg. per minute.

DOSAGE AND ADMINISTRATION—CHILDREN

Thorazine (chlorpromazine, SK&F) should generally not be used in children under 6 months of age except where potentially lifesaving. It should not be used in conditions for which specific children's dosages have not been established.

Severe Behavioral Problems—OUTPATIENTS—Select route of administration according to severity of patient's condition and increase dosage gradually as required. *Oral:* ¼ mg./lb. body weight q4-6h, p.r.n. (e.g., for 40 lb. child—10 mg. q4-6h). *Rectal:* ½ mg./lb. body weight q6-8h, p.r.n. (e.g., for 20-30 lb. child—half a 25 mg. suppository q6-8h). *I.M.:* ¼ mg./lb. body weight q6-8h, p.r.n.

HOSPITALIZED PATIENTS—As with outpatients, start with low doses and increase dosage gradually. In severe behavior disorders or psychotic conditions, higher dosages (50-100 mg. daily, and in older children, 200 mg. daily or more) may be necessary. There is little evidence that behavior improvement in severely disturbed mentally retarded patients is further enhanced by doses beyond 500 mg. per day. *Maximum I.M. Dosage:* Children up to 5 years (or 50 lbs.), not over 40 mg./day; 5-12 years (or 50-100 lbs.), not over 75 mg./day except in unmanageable cases.

Nausea and Vomiting—Dosage and frequency of administration should be adjusted according to the severity of the symptoms and response of the patient. The duration of activity following intramuscular administration may last up to 12 hours. Subsequent doses may be given by the same route if necessary. *Oral:* ¼ mg./lb. body weight (e.g., 40 lb. child—10 mg. q4-6h). *Rectal:* ½ mg./lb. body weight q6-8h, p.r.n. (e.g., 20-30 lb. child—half of a 25 mg. suppository q6-8h). *I.M.:* ¼ mg./lb. body weight q6-8h, p.r.n. *Maximum I.M. Dosage:* Children up to 5 yrs. (or 50 lbs.), not over 40 mg./day; 5-12 yrs. (or 50-100 lbs.), not over 75 mg./day except in severe cases. DURING SURGERY—*I.M.:* ⅛ mg./lb. body weight. Repeat in ½ hour if necessary and if no hypotension occurs. *I.V.:* 1 mg. per fractional injection at 2-minute intervals and not exceeding recommended I.M. dosage. Always dilute to 1 mg./mL., i.e., 1 mL. (25 mg.) mixed with 24 mL. of saline. **Presurgical Apprehension**—¼ mg./lb. body weight, either *orally* 2 to 3 hours before operation, or *I.M.* 1 to 2 hours before.

Tetanus—*I.M.* or *I.V.:* ¼ mg./lb. body weight q6-8h. When given I.V., dilute to at least 1 mg./mL. and administer at rate of 1 mg. per 2 minutes. In children up to 50 lbs., do not exceed 40 mg. daily; 50 to 100 lbs., do not exceed 75 mg., except in severe cases.

IMPORTANT NOTES ON INJECTION

Inject slowly, deep into upper outer quadrant of buttock. Because of possible hypotensive effects, reserve parenteral administration for bedfast patients or for acute ambulatory cases, and keep patient lying down for at least ½ hour after injection. If irritation is a problem, dilute Injection with saline or 2% procaine; mixing with other agents in the syringe is not recommended. Subcutaneous injection is not advised. Avoid injecting undiluted Thorazine (chlorpromazine, SK&F) into vein. I.V. route is only for severe hiccups, surgery and tetanus.

Because of the possibility of contact dermatitis, avoid getting solution on hands or clothing. Protect from light, or discoloration may occur. Slight yellowing will not alter potency. Discard if markedly discolored. For information on sulfite sensitivity, see the Warnings section of this labeling.

Note on Concentrate: When the Concentrate is to be used, add the desired dosage of Concentrate to 60 mL. (2 fl. oz.) or more of diluent *just prior to administration.* This will insure palatability and stability. Vehicles suggested for dilution are: tomato or fruit juice, milk, simple syrup, orange syrup, carbonated beverages, coffee, tea, or water. Semisolid foods (soups, puddings, etc.) may also be used. The Concentrate is light sensitive; it should be protected from light and dispensed in amber glass bottles. *Refrigeration is not required.*

OVERDOSAGE
(See also Adverse Reactions.)

SYMPTOMS—Primarily symptoms of central nervous system depression to the point of somnolence or coma. Hypotension and extrapyramidal symptoms.

Other possible manifestations include agitation and restlessness, convulsions, fever, autonomic reactions such as dry mouth and ileus, EKG changes and cardiac arrhythmias.

TREATMENT—It is important to determine other medications taken by the patient since multiple drug therapy is common in overdosage situations. Treatment is essentially symptomatic and supportive. Early gastric lavage is helpful. Keep patient under observation and maintain an open airway, since involvement of the extrapyramidal mechanism may produce dysphagia and respiratory difficulty in severe overdosage. **Do not attempt to induce emesis because a dystonic reaction of the head or neck may develop that could result in aspiration of vomitus.** Extrapyramidal symptoms may be treated with anti-parkinsonism drugs, barbiturates, or 'Benadryl'. See prescribing information for these products. Care should be taken to avoid increasing respiratory depression.

If administration of a stimulant is desirable, amphetamine, dextroamphetamine, or caffeine with sodium benzoate is recommended. Stimulants that may cause convulsions (e.g., picrotoxin or pentylenetetrazol) should be avoided.

If hypotension occurs, the standard measures for managing circulatory shock should be initiated. If it is desirable to administer a vasoconstrictor, 'Levophed' and 'Neo-Synephrine' are most suitable. Other pressor agents, including epinephrine, are not recommended because phenothiazine derivatives may reverse the usual elevating action of these agents and cause a further lowering of blood pressure.

Limited experience indicates that phenothiazines are *not* dialyzable.

Special note on 'Spansule' capsules—Since much of the 'Spansule' capsule medication is coated for gradual release, therapy directed at reversing the effects of the ingested drug and at supporting the patient should be continued for as long as overdosage symptoms remain. Saline cathartics are useful for hastening evacuation of pellets that have not already released medication.

HOW SUPPLIED

Tablets: 10 mg., 25 mg. or 50 mg., in bottles of 100 and 1000; in Single Unit Packages of 100 (intended for institutional use only). For use in severe neuropsychiatric conditions, 100 mg. and 200 mg., in bottles of 100 and 1000; in Single Unit Packages of 100 (intended for institutional use only).

Spansule® brand of sustained release capsules: 30 mg., 75 mg., 150 mg. or 200 mg., in bottles of 50 and 500; in Single Unit Packages of 100 (intended for institutional use only). For use in severe neuropsychiatric conditions, 300 mg., in bottles of 50; in Single Unit Packages of 100 (intended for institutional use only).

Ampuls: 1 mL. and 2 mL. (25 mg./mL.), in boxes of 10, 100 and 500.

Multiple-dose Vials: 10 mL. (25 mg./mL.), in boxes of 1, 20 and 100.

Syrup: 10 mg./5 mL. in 4 fl. oz. bottles.

Suppositories: 25 mg. or 100 mg., in boxes of 12.

Concentrate: 30 mg./mL., in 4 fl. oz. bottles, and in cartons of 36 bottles. 100 mg./mL., in 8 fl. oz. bottles, in cartons of 12.

Veterans Administration—Tablets, 50 mg., 1000's, 6505-01-212-0639; Tablets, 100 mg., 1000's, 6505-01-212-0637; Tablets, 200 mg., 1000's, 6505-00-014-1186; 'Spansule' Capsules, 150 mg., 500's, 6505-00-022-1324; Injection, 2 mL., 100's, 6505-00-619-8639.

Military—Tablets, 25 mg., SUP, 100's, 6505-00-118-2529; Tablets, 50 mg., SUP, 100's, 6505-00-132-0371; Tablets, 100 mg., SUP, 100's, 6505-00-132-0372; Tablets, 50 mg., 1000's, 6505-01-212-0639; Tablets, 100 mg., 1000's, 6505-01-212-0637.

---

* phenytoin, Parke-Davis.
† metrizamide, Winthrop Pharmaceuticals.
‡ norepinephrine bitartrate, Winthrop Pharmaceuticals.
§ phenylephrine hydrochloride, Winthrop Pharmaceuticals.
‖ diphenhydramine hydrochloride, Parke-Davis.

TZ:L72

Shown in Product Identification Section, page 431

TUSS-ORNADE®   ℞

[*tuss 'or-naid '*]
LIQUID

DESCRIPTION

Each 5 mL. (one teaspoonful) of clear, fruit-flavored 'Tuss-Ornade' Liquid contains caramiphen edisylate, 6.7 mg.; phenylpropanolamine hydrochloride, 12.5 mg.; and alcohol, 5.0%. Inactive ingredients consist of citric acid, flavors, glycerin, menthol, methylparaben, propylparaben, sodium citrate, sorbitol and water.

ACTIONS

The 'Tuss-Ornade' formula contains caramiphen edisylate, a synthetic, non-narcotic cough suppressant, and phenylpropanolamine hydrochloride, a vasoconstrictor with decongestant action on nasal and upper respiratory tract mucosal membranes.

INDICATIONS

For the symptomatic relief of coughs and nasal congestion associated with common colds.
N.B.: A final determination has not been made on the effectiveness of this drug combination in accordance with efficacy requirements of the 1962 Amendments to the Food, Drug and Cosmetic Act.

CONTRAINDICATIONS

Hypersensitivity to either of the components; concurrent MAO inhibitor therapy; severe hypertension; bronchial asthma; coronary artery disease.
Do not use 'Tuss-Ornade' Liquid in children under 15 pounds or in children less than six months of age.

PRECAUTIONS

Use with caution in patients with cardiovascular disease, glaucoma, prostatic hypertrophy, thyroid disease or diabetes. Use with caution in patients in whom productive cough is desirable to clear excessive secretions from the bronchial tree. Patients taking this medication should be cautioned not to take simultaneously other products containing phenylpropanolamine HCl or amphetamines.
Usage in Pregnancy: Safe use in pregnancy has not been established. This drug should not be used in pregnancy, nursing mothers, or women of childbearing potential unless, in the judgment of the physician, the anticipated benefits outweigh the potential risks.

ADVERSE REACTIONS

Adverse effects associated with products containing a centrally acting antitussive or sympathomimetic amine may occur and include: nausea, gastrointestinal upset, diarrhea, constipation, dizziness, drowsiness, nervousness, insomnia, anorexia, weakness, tightness of chest, angina pain, irritability, palpitations, headache, incoordination, tremor, difficulty in urination, dysuria, hypertension, hypotension, visual disturbances.

DOSAGE AND ADMINISTRATION

Adults and children over 12 years—2 teaspoonfuls every 4 hours; do not exceed 12 teaspoonfuls in 24 hours. Children 6 to 12 years—1 teaspoonful every 4 hours; do not exceed 6 teaspoonfuls in 24 hours. Children 2 to 6 years—½ teaspoonful every 4 hours; do not exceed 3 teaspoonfuls in 24 hours. Data are not available on which to base dosage recommendations for children under 2 years of age. **Do not use in children under 15 pounds or less than 6 months old.**

OVERDOSAGE

Symptoms—May include dryness of mouth, dysphagia, thirst, blurred vision, dilated pupils, photophobia, fever, rapid pulse and respiration, disorientation, dizziness, nausea, fainting, tachycardia, and either excitation or depression of the central nervous system.
Treatment—Immediate evacuation of the stomach should be induced by emesis and gastric lavage, repeated as necessary. Respiratory depression should be treated promptly with oxygen and respiratory stimulants. Do not treat respiratory or CNS depression with analeptics that might precipitate convulsions. If marked excitement occurs, a short-acting barbiturate or chloral hydrate may be used.

SUPPLIED

Liquid containing caramiphen edisylate 6.7 mg.; phenylpropanolamine hydrochloride 12.5 mg.; and alcohol 5.0% per 5 mL. (one teaspoonful), in 16 fl. oz. bottles.

TOL:L16

TUSS-ORNADE®   ℞
[tuss'or-naid']
SPANSULE® CAPSULES

PRODUCT OVERVIEW

KEY FACTS

Tuss-Ornade® Spansule® capsules contain caramiphen edisylate, a non-narcotic cough suppressant, and phenylpropanolamine HCl, a decongestant that provides vasoconstriction similar to that of ephedrine but with less CNS stimulation. Spansule® capsules are prepared so that an initial dose is released promptly and the remaining medication is released gradually over a prolonged period of time, thus permitting b.i.d. dosing.

MAJOR USE

Tuss-Ornade® Spansule® capsules are for symptomatic relief of cough and nasal congestion associated with the common cold.

SAFETY INFORMATION

Tuss-Ornade® Spansule® capsules are contraindicated in patients with: hypersensitivity to either component; concurrent MAO inhibitor therapy; severe hypertension; bronchial asthma; coronary artery disease. Do not use 'Tuss-Ornade' Spansule capsules in children under the age of 12 years. Further, patients should be cautioned not to take simultaneously other products containing phenylpropanolamine HCl or amphetamines.

PRESCRIBING INFORMATION

TUSS-ORNADE®   ℞
[tuss'or-naid']
SPANSULE® CAPSULES

DESCRIPTION

Each 'Tuss-Ornade' Spansule capsule, with opaque light blue cap and natural body, is imprinted with the product name TUSS-ORNADE and SKF and contains caramiphen edisylate, 40 mg. and phenylpropanolamine hydrochloride, 75 mg. Inactive ingredients consist of benzyl alcohol, cetylpyridinium chloride, D&C Red No. 33, FD&C Blue No. 1, FD&C Red No. 3, FD&C Yellow No. 6, gelatin, glyceryl distearate, polyethylene glycol, povidone, silicon dioxide, sodium lauryl sulfate, starch, sucrose, titanium dioxide, wax and trace amounts of other inactive ingredients.
Each 'Tuss-Ornade' Spansule capsule is so prepared that an initial dose is released promptly and the remaining medication is released gradually over a prolonged period.

ACTIONS

The 'Tuss-Ornade' formula contains caramiphen edisylate, a synthetic, non-narcotic cough suppressant, and phenylpropanolamine hydrochloride, a vasoconstrictor with decongestant action on nasal and upper respiratory tract mucosal membranes.
Pharmacokinetics: At steady-state conditions, the following peak levels are reached after the oral administration of a 'Spansule' capsule: 24 ng./mL. caramiphen in 4.6 hours; 200 ng./mL. phenylpropanolamine in 5.5 hours; the half-lives are approximately 11 and 8 hours, respectively.

INDICATIONS

For the symptomatic relief of coughs and nasal congestion associated with common colds.
N.B.: A final determination has not been made on the effectiveness of this drug combination in accordance with efficacy requirements of the 1962 Amendments to the Food, Drug and Cosmetic Act.

CONTRAINDICATIONS

Hypersensitivity to either of the components; concurrent MAO inhibitor therapy; severe hypertension; bronchial asthma; coronary artery disease.
Do not use 'Tuss-Ornade' Spansule capsules in children under 12 years of age.

PRECAUTIONS

Use with caution in persons with cardiovascular disease, glaucoma, prostatic hypertrophy, thyroid disease or diabetes. Use with caution in patients in whom productive cough is desirable to clear excessive secretions from the bronchial tree. Patients taking this medication should be cautioned not to take simultaneously other products containing phenylpropanolamine HCl or amphetamines.
Usage in Pregnancy: Safe use in pregnancy has not been established. This drug should not be used in pregnancy, nursing mothers, or women of childbearing potential unless, in the judgment of the physician, the anticipated benefits outweigh the potential risks.

ADVERSE REACTIONS

Adverse effects associated with products containing a centrally acting antitussive or sympathomimetic amine may occur and include: nausea, gastrointestinal upset, diarrhea, constipation, dizziness, drowsiness, nervousness, insomnia, anorexia, weakness, tightness of chest, angina pain, irritability, palpitation, headache, incoordination, tremor, difficulty in urination, dysuria, hypertension, hypotension, visual disturbances.

DOSAGE AND ADMINISTRATION

'Tuss-Ornade' Spansule capsules: Adults and children over 12 years of age—one 'Tuss-Ornade' Spansule capsule every 12 hours. **Do not use in children under 12 years of age.**

OVERDOSAGE

Symptoms—May include dryness of mouth, dysphagia, thirst, blurred vision, dilated pupils, photophobia, fever, rapid pulse and respiration, disorientation, dizziness, nausea, fainting, tachycardia, and either excitation or depression of the central nervous system.

Treatment—Immediate evacuation of the stomach should be induced by emesis and gastric lavage, repeated as necessary. Respiratory depression should be treated promptly with oxygen and respiratory stimulants. Do not treat respiratory or CNS depression with analeptics that might precipitate convulsions. If marked excitement occurs, a short-acting barbiturate or chloral hydrate may be used.
Since much of the 'Spansule' capsule medication is coated for gradual release, saline cathartics should be administered to hasten evacuation of pellets that have not already released medication.

SUPPLIED

'Spansule' capsules (brand of sustained release capsules) containing caramiphen edisylate 40 mg. and phenylpropanolamine hydrochloride 75 mg., in bottles of 50 and 500.

TO:L33

Shown in Product Identification Section, page 431

URISPAS®   ℞
[yore'eh-spaz]
(brand of flavoxate HCl)
100 mg. tablets
Urinary tract spasmolytic

DESCRIPTION

Urispas (flavoxate HCl, SK&F) tablets contain flavoxate hydrochloride, a synthetic urinary tract spasmolytic.
Chemically, flavoxate hydrochloride is 2-piperidinoethyl 3-methyl-4-oxo-2-phenyl-4$\underline{H}$-1-benzopyran-8-carboxylate hydrochloride. The empirical formula of flavoxate hydrochloride is $C_{24}H_{25}NO_4 \cdot HCl$. The molecular weight is 427.94. 'Urispas' is supplied in tablets for oral administration. Each round, white, film-coated 'Urispas' tablet is debossed URISPAS SKF and contains flavoxate hydrochloride, 100 mg. Inactive ingredients consist of calcium phosphate, castor oil, cellulose acetate phthalate, magnesium stearate, polyethylene glycol, starch and talc.

CLINICAL PHARMACOLOGY

Flavoxate hydrochloride counteracts smooth muscle spasm of the urinary tract and exerts its effect directly on the muscle.
In a single study of 11 normal male subjects, the time to onset of action was 55 minutes. The peak effect was observed at 112 minutes. 57% of the flavoxate HCl was excreted in the urine within 24 hours.

INDICATIONS AND USAGE

Urispas (flavoxate HCl, SK&F) is indicated for symptomatic relief of dysuria, urgency, nocturia, suprapubic pain, frequency and incontinence as may occur in cystitis, prostatitis, urethritis, urethrocystitis/urethrotrigonitis. 'Urispas' is not indicated for definitive treatment, but is compatible with drugs used for the treatment of urinary tract infections.

CONTRAINDICATIONS

Urispas (flavoxate HCl, SK&F) is contraindicated in patients who have any of the following obstructive conditions: pyloric or duodenal obstruction, obstructive intestinal lesions or ileus, achalasia, gastrointestinal hemorrhage, and obstructive uropathies of the lower urinary tract.

WARNINGS

Urispas (flavoxate HCl, SK&F) should be given cautiously in patients with suspected glaucoma.

PRECAUTIONS

Information for Patients: Patients should be informed that if drowsiness and blurred vision occur, they should not operate a motor vehicle or machinery or participate in activities where alertness is required.
Carcinogenesis, Mutagenesis, Impairment of Fertility: Mutagenicity studies and long-term studies in animals to determine the carcinogenic potential of Urispas (flavoxate HCl, SK&F) have not been performed.
Pregnancy: Teratogenic Effects—Pregnancy Category B. Reproduction studies have been performed in rats and rabbits at doses up to 34 times the human dose and revealed no evidence of impaired fertility or harm to the fetus due to flavoxate HCl. There are, however, no well-controlled studies in pregnant women. Because animal reproduction studies are not always predictive of human response, this drug should be used during pregnancy only if clearly needed.
Nursing Mothers: It is not known whether this drug is excreted in human milk. Because many drugs are excreted in human milk, caution should be exercised when 'Urispas' is administered to a nursing woman.
Pediatric Use: Safety and effectiveness in children below the age of 12 years have not been established.

ADVERSE REACTIONS

The following adverse reactions have been observed, but there are not enough data to support an estimate of their frequency.

Continued on next page

Smith Kline & French—Cont.

Gastrointestinal: Nausea, vomiting, dry mouth.

CNS: Vertigo, headache, mental confusion, especially in the elderly, drowsiness, nervousness.

Hematologic: Leukopenia (one case which was reversible upon discontinuation of the drug).

Cardiovascular: Tachycardia and palpitation.

Allergic: Urticaria and other dermatoses, eosinophilia and hyperpyrexia.

Ophthalmic: Increased ocular tension, blurred vision, disturbance in eye accommodation.

Renal: Dysuria.

OVERDOSAGE

The oral LD_{50} for flavoxate HCl in rats is 4273 mg./kg. The oral LD_{50} for flavoxate HCl in mice is 1837 mg./kg. It is not known whether flavoxate HCl is dialyzable.

DOSAGE AND ADMINISTRATION

Adults and children over 12 years of age: One or two 100 mg. tablets three or four times a day. With improvement of symptoms, the dose may be reduced. This drug cannot be recommended for infants and children under 12 years of age because safety and efficacy have not been demonstrated in this age group.

HOW SUPPLIED

Urispas (flavoxate HCl, SK&F) tablets, 100 mg., in bottles of 100 and in Single Unit Packages of 100 (intended for institutional use only).

Military—Tablets, 100 mg., 100's, 6505-00-172-3420.

UR:L14

Shown in Product Identification Section, page 431

VONTROL®   ℞

[*vohn 'trole*]

(brand of diphenidol)

'Vontrol' may cause hallucinations, disorientation, or confusion. For this reason, its use is limited to patients who are hospitalized or under comparable, continuous, close, professional supervision. Even then, the physician should carefully weigh the benefits against the possible risks and give due consideration to alternate therapeutic measures.

DESCRIPTION

Diphenidol, α, α-diphenyl-1-piperidinebutanol, is a compound not related to the antihistamines, phenothiazines, barbiturates, or other agents with antivertigo or antiemetic action.

Each round, orange 'Vontrol' tablet is debossed SKF and 25 and contains diphenidol hydrochloride equivalent to diphenidol, 25 mg. Inactive ingredients consist of acacia, calcium sulfate, cellulose, FD&C Yellow No. 5 (tartrazine), FD&C Yellow No. 6, magnesium stearate and starch.

ACTIONS

'Vontrol' (diphenidol, SK&F) apparently exerts a specific antivertigo effect on the vestibular apparatus to control vertigo and inhibits the chemoreceptor trigger zone to control nausea and vomiting.

INDICATIONS (SEE WARNINGS)

1) VERTIGO—'Vontrol' is indicated in peripheral (labyrinthine) vertigo and associated nausea and vomiting, as seen in such conditions as: Meniere's disease, middle- and inner-ear surgery (labyrinthitis).

2) NAUSEA AND VOMITING—'Vontrol' is indicated in the control of nausea and vomiting, as seen in such conditions as: postoperative states, malignant neoplasms and labyrinthine disturbances.

CONTRAINDICATIONS

Known hypersensitivity to the drug is a contraindication. Anuria is a contraindication. (Since approximately 90% of the drug is excreted in the urine, renal shutdown could cause systemic accumulation.)

WARNINGS

'Vontrol' (diphenidol, SK&F) may cause hallucinations, disorientation or confusion. For this reason, its use is limited to patients who are hospitalized or under comparable, continuous, close, professional supervision. Even then, the physician should carefully weigh the benefits against the possible risks and give due consideration to alternate therapeutic measures.

The incidence of auditory and visual hallucinations, disorientation and confusion appears to be less than ½% or approximately one in 350 patients. The reaction has usually occurred within three days of starting the drug in recommended dosage and has subsided spontaneously usually within three days after discontinuation of the drug. Patients on 'Vontrol' should be observed closely and in the event of such a reaction the drug should be stopped.

Usage in Pregnancy: Use of any drug in pregnancy, lactation or in women of childbearing age requires that the poten-

tial benefits of the drug be weighed against its possible hazards to the mother and child.

In animal teratogenesis and reproduction studies of 'Vontrol' (diphenidol, SK&F), there were no significant differences between drug-treated groups and untreated control groups, except as noted under animal Reproduction Studies (see "Pharmacology [animal]").

In 936 patients who received 'Vontrol' during pregnancy, the incidences of normal and abnormal birth were comparable to those reported in the literature for the average population of pregnant patients. And in no instance was there any evidence that 'Vontrol' played a part in birth abnormality (see "In Pregnancy").

'Vontrol' is not indicated for use in nausea and vomiting of pregnancy, since the therapeutic value and safety in this indication have not yet been determined.

PRECAUTIONS

The antiemetic action of 'Vontrol' (diphenidol, SK&F) may mask signs of overdose of drugs (e.g., digitalis) or may obscure diagnosis of conditions such as intestinal obstruction and brain tumor.

Although there have been no reports of blood dyscrasias with 'Vontrol', patients should be observed regularly for any idiosyncratic reactions.

'Vontrol' has a weak peripheral anticholinergic effect and should be used with care in patients with glaucoma, obstructive lesions of the gastrointestinal and genitourinary tracts, such as stenosing peptic ulcer, prostatic hypertrophy, pyloric and duodenal obstruction, and organic cardiospasm.

'Vontrol' Tablets contain FD&C Yellow No. 5 (tartrazine) which may cause allergic-type reactions (including bronchial asthma) in certain susceptible individuals. Although the overall incidence of FD&C Yellow No. 5 (tartrazine) sensitivity in the general population is low, it is frequently seen in patients who also have aspirin hypersensitivity.

Usage in Children

'Vontrol' is not recommended for use in children under 50 pounds. (See Dosage and Administration—Children.)

ADVERSE REACTIONS

Auditory and visual hallucinations, disorientation and confusion have been reported. Drowsiness, overstimulation, depression, sleep disturbance, dry mouth, g.i. irritation (nausea and indigestion), or blurred vision may occur.

Rarely, slight dizziness, skin rash, malaise, headache, or heartburn may occur. Mild jaundice of questionable relationship to the use of 'Vontrol' (diphenidol, SK&F) has been reported. Slight, transient lowering of blood pressure has been reported in a few patients.

(See laboratory studies under "Pharmacology [human]".)

DOSAGE AND ADMINISTRATION (SEE WARNINGS)

ADULTS—FOR VERTIGO OR NAUSEA AND VOMITING: The usual dose is one tablet (25 mg.) every four hours as needed. Some patients may require two tablets (50 mg.).

CHILDREN—FOR NAUSEA AND VOMITING: These recommendations are for nausea and vomiting only. There has been no experience with 'Vontrol' in vertigo in children. Unit doses in children are best calculated by body weight: usually 0.4 mg./lb.

Children's doses usually should not be given more often than every four hours. However, if symptoms persist after the first dose, administration may be repeated after one hour. Thereafter, doses may be given every four hours as needed. The total dose in 24 hours should not exceed 2.5 mg./lb.

NOTE: The drug is not recommended for use in children under 50 pounds. The dosage for children 50 to 100 pounds is one tablet (25 mg.).

OVERDOSAGE

In the event of overdosage, the patient should be managed according to his symptoms. Treatment is essentially supportive, with maintenance of blood pressure and respiration, plus careful observation. Early gastric lavage may be indicated depending on the amount of overdose and nature of symptoms.

HOW SUPPLIED

Tablets containing 25 mg. diphenidol, as the hydrochloride, in bottles of 100.

PHARMACOLOGY (animal): 'Vontrol' (diphenidol, SK&F) exerts its antiemetic effect primarily by inhibiting the chemoreceptor trigger zone, as evidenced by its activity in blocking emesis induced by apomorphine in dogs. In this regard 'Vontrol', as the hydrochloride salt, has a potency equal to the potent phenothiazine antiemetic, chlorpromazine hydrochloride. In animals 'Vontrol' has only weak parasympatholytic activity and no significant sedative, tranquilizing or antihistaminic action or effects on blood pressure, heart rate, respiration or the electrocardiogram.

Subacute and chronic toxicity studies in rats and dogs, in which large doses of 'Vontrol', as the hydrochloride salt, were administered orally and intramuscularly for periods up to one year, revealed no significant effects on hematology, liver function, kidney function or blood glucose determinations. Histological examination of the animals' tissues did

not reveal any significant lesions attributable to administration of 'Vontrol'.

Reproduction Studies: Teratogenesis and reproduction studies were carried out in rats and rabbits. In rats, 'Vontrol' (diphenidol, SK&F), as the hydrochloride salt, was fed daily to male and female animals in doses of 20 mg./kg. and 40 mg./kg. (approximately three and six times the maximum recommended daily dose in adult humans) for 60 days before mating, and during mating, gestation and lactation for each of two litters. There were no significant differences between drug-treated and untreated control groups with regard to conception rate, litter size, live birth or viability in either of the two litters. There was no congenital anomaly among the offspring. In rabbits, 'Vontrol', as the hydrochloride salt, was fed in the diets in doses of 5 mg./kg. or 75 mg./kg. (approximately equal to, and 12 times as much as, the maximum recommended daily dose in adult humans) from the first day of gestation through the 26th or 27th day of gestation, when the young were delivered by Cesarean section. There were no significant differences between drug-treated and control groups with regard to number and weight of fetuses, numbers of resorption sites or viable fetuses. There was also no statistically significant difference between drug-treated and control groups with regard to the total percentage of underdeveloped fetuses. However, when data were calculated on the basis of a ratio between underdeveloped fetuses and number of pregnant does, an adverse dose-related effect was observed in the high-dose test group.

PHARMACOLOGY (human): Three double-blind controlled studies comparing 'Vontrol' (diphenidol, SK&F) to placebo were carried out: one in 32 male volunteers over a four-week period; one in 45 volunteers of whom 15 were studied for 12 weeks and 17 for 24 weeks; and one in 48 volunteers of whom 36 were studied for 12 weeks.

In the first study 'Vontrol', as the hydrochloride salt, was given orally in daily doses that were started at 75 mg. during the first week and graduated up to 200 mg. by the fourth week. In the second study, one group received 'Vontrol' orally, as the hydrochloride salt, titrated up to 500 mg. daily, then down to 200 mg. daily; another group received a maximum of 200 mg. daily. In the third study, patients received oral doses of 200 mg. to 300 mg. of 'Vontrol' daily, as the hydrochloride or pamoate salts.

The studies included these laboratory determinations: complete blood counts (including hemoglobin and hematocrit determinations), urinalyses (including microscopic examination), serum alkaline phosphatase, serum bilirubin, and bromsulphalein retention. The studies also included records of weight and blood pressure and, in one, electrocardiograms.

In two of these studies, clinical laboratory changes were seen among volunteers in both treated and control groups. The changes included: extrasystoles, white cells in the urine, increase in prothrombin time, rise in hematocrit, rise in leucocytes, rise in eosinophils, and rise or reduction in neutrophils. At no time in any study did changes in the treated group differ significantly from those in the control group. 'Vontrol', as the hydrochloride salt, was given orally to 17 children (aged five to 15). Total daily doses ranged from 90 to 240 mg. Complete blood counts and, in some patients, urinalyses were done before treatment and after approximately four days of treatment. There was no significant difference between pre- and post-treatment laboratory determinations in any child. No side effects were seen.

EXCRETION: Following oral administration of 'Vontrol' (diphenidol, SK&F) to dogs, as the hydrochloride or pamoate salts, and to humans, as the hydrochloride salt, peak blood concentration of the drug generally occurs in one and a half to three hours. In dogs and rats, virtually all of an oral dose of C^{14}-labeled 'Vontrol' is excreted in the urine and feces within three to four days, as determined by radioactivity counts. Approximately the same percentage of an administered dose appeared in the urine of dogs following either oral administration of the hydrochloride salt or rectal administration of the free base.

IN PREGNANCY: Investigators kept follow-up records on 936 patients who had received 'Vontrol' (diphenidol, SK&F) at some time during pregnancy, primarily during the first trimester.

Of the 936 women, 864 (92%) had normal births of normal infants.

Seventy-two (8%) of the women experienced some birth abnormality. Of the 72, six patients had premature but otherwise normal infants, 40 patients aborted, 10 had stillbirths, and 16 had infants with miscellaneous defects. These included hernias, congenital heart defects, hydrocephalus, internal strabismus, anencephalus, enlarged thyroid, and hypospadia.

These incidences of abnormal birth are lower than those generally reported in the literature for the average population of pregnant patients. And in no instance was there any evidence that the administration of 'Vontrol' played a part in birth abnormality.

VN:L15

Shown in Product Identification Section, page 431

EDUCATIONAL MATERIAL

BOOKLETS

"Essentials of Immune Response, Inflammation and the Pathogenesis of Rheumatoid Arthritis," a 63-page booklet (6½" × 8½"). Reviews current thinking on the pathogenesis of rheumatoid arthritis and, briefly, the basic terminology and principles of immunology and inflammation. Free to physicians and allied health personnel.

"Essentials of a Differential Diagnosis of Rheumatoid Arthritis," a 66-page booklet (6½" × 8½"). Provides a logical stepwise approach to rheumatoid arthritis diagnosis. Free to physicians and allied health personnel.

"Essentials of Managing Rheumatoid Arthritis," a 64-page booklet (6½" × 8½"). Examines the drug and nondrug therapies used to manage rheumatoid arthritis. Free to physicians and allied health personnel.

PATIENT I.D. CARDS

"I am taking Eskalith®/ Eskalith CR® (brand of lithium carbonate)." Packet of 10 wallet-size (2½" × 3½") cards. Provides information to emergency room or other medical personnel about the patient and attending physician and about possible drug-related side effects and their management. Free to physicians.

"I am taking Stelazine® (brand of trifluoperazine hydrochloride)." Packet of 10 wallet-size (2½" × 3½") cards. Provides information to emergency room or other medical personnel about the patient and attending physician and about possible drug-related side effects and their management. Free to physicians.

"I am taking Parnate® (brand of tranylcypromine sulfate)." Packet of 10 wallet-size (2½" × 3½") cards. Provides information to emergency room or other medical personnel about the patient and attending physician and about possible drug-related side effects and their management. Free to physicians.

PATIENT INFORMATION

Patient information on Dyazide® (triamterene and hydrochlorothiazide). Pad (8½" × 11") of 50 sheets. Provides basic information about high blood pressure and 'Dyazide', including special considerations about diet, possible drug interactions, and side effects. Free to physicians. Patient I.D. Card.

Instruction sheets for patients on Parnate® (brand of tranylcypromine sulfate). Pad (4¼" × 8") of 24 sheets. Serves as a reminder of principal instructions about 'Parnate' therapy, e.g.: the importance of following dosage instructions exactly; the need for consulting before taking any other drugs; what foods and beverages must be avoided; what symptoms should be reported promptly. A carbon copy is provided for the physician's records. Free to physicians.

Patient information on Ridaura® (brand of auranofin). "Understanding Your Treatment of Rheumatoid Arthritis," a 12-page booklet (3" × 6½"). Describes and depicts rheumatoid arthritis and its effects on the body, and discusses how the disease is typically managed. Provides information on what to expect from 'Ridaura' therapy with regard to disease control and potential side effects. Emphasizes the importance of cooperating with physician instructions. Free to physicians and other health professionals.

Solgar Vitamin Company, Inc.
410 OCEAN AVENUE
LYNBROOK, NY 11563

BCAA PLUS CAPSULES
BRANCHED-CHAIN AMINO ACIDS

Each capsule provides L-Leucine 270 mg, L-Isoleucine 180 mg and L-Valine 150 mg. plus 10 mg. of vitamin B₆.

SUPPLIED
Bottles of 50 and 100 capsules.

STRESS FORMULA
B-COMPLEX WITH C

Provides dietary supplementation for Vitamin C and B-Complex.

SUPPLIED
Bottles of 100, 250 and 500 tablets.

BETA CAROTENE CAPSULES (Natural)
(PROVITAMIN A)

Available in 11,000 IU and 25,000 IU (Vitamin A Activity) dosages, from 100% Natural Beta Carotene.

SUPPLIED
Bottles of 50 and 100 capsules.

BIOTIN TABLETS AND CAPSULES
300 mcg, 600 mcg Tablets, 1000 mcg Capsules

SUPPLIED
Bottles of 100 and 250 tablets or capsules.

CALCIUM 600
From Oyster Shells

Two tablets provide 1200 mg of calcium (calcium carbonate) with 400 IU of Vitamin D.

SUPPLIED
Bottles of 60 and 120 tablets.

CHROMIUM PICOLINATE CAPSULES AND TABLETS
(YEAST-FREE GTF)

Provides a yeast-free source of (Trivalent) GTF Chromium as Chromium Picolinate. 100 mcg tablets or 200 mcg capsules.

SUPPLIED
Bottles of 90 and 180 tablets or capsules.

CoQ-10 CAPSULES
(COENZYME Q-10)
15 mg, 30 mg and 60 mg Capsules

SUPPLIED
Bottles of 30, 60 and 90 capsules.

DAILY GOLD PACK
HIGH POTENCY MULTIVITAMIN
MULTIMINERAL SUPPLEMENT PACKET

SUPPLIED
Boxes of 30 packets.

FORMULA B-50 CAPSULES
HIGH POTENCY B-COMPLEX
FORMULA

A balanced proportion of all the recognized B-Complex factors.
Each Capsule Provides:

Vitamin B-1	50 mg
Vitamin B-2	50 mg
Vitamin B-6	50 mg
Vitamin B-12	50 mcg
Niacinamide	50 mg
Folic Acid	400 mcg
Pantothenic Acid	50 mg
Para Aminobenzoic Acid	50 mg
Choline Bitartrate	50 mg
Inositol	50 mg
Biotin	50 mcg

SUPPLIED
Bottles of 50, 100 and 250 capsules.

FORMULA VM-75 MULTIVITAMIN & MINERAL TABLETS
EXTRA HIGH POTENCY—
BALANCED B-COMPLEX WITH
CHELATED MINERALS

Each Tablet Daily Provides:

Vitamin C (with Rose Hips)	250 mg
Vitamin E (d-Alpha Tocopherol)	150 IU
Vitamin A (Palmitate and Beta-Carotene)	25,000 IU
Vitamin D	1,000 IU
Vitamin B-1 (Thiamine)	75 mg
Vitamin B-2 (Riboflavin)	75 mg
Vitamin B-6 (Pyridoxine)	75 mg
Vitamin B-12	75 mcg
Niacinamide	75 mg
Choline Bitartrate	75 mg
Inositol	75 mg
Para Aminobenzoic Acid	75 mg
Pantothenic Acid	75 mg
Biotin	75 mcg
Folic Acid	400 mcg
Rutin	25 mg
Citrus Bioflavonoid Complex	25 mg
Hesperidin Complex	5 mg
Betaine HCl	25 mg
Glutamic Acid	25 mg

Iodine (Kelp)	150 mcg
Calcium Amino Acid Chelate	50 mg
Potassium Amino Acid Complex	10 mg
Iron Amino Acid Chelate	10 mg
Magnesium Amino Acid Chelate	7.2 mg
Manganese Amino Acid Chelate	6.1 mg
Zinc Amino Acid Chelate	15 mg
Selenium (L-selenomethionine)	10 mcg

SUPPLIED
Bottles of 30, 60, 90 and 180 tablets.

GINKGO BILOBA CAPSULES

Each capsule provides 65 mg. of Ginkgo biloba leaf 8:1 extract equivalent to 520 mg. of Ginkgo biloba leaf.

SUPPLIED
Bottles of 50, 100 and 250 capsules.

HY-C TABLETS
HIGH POTENCY VITAMIN C
SUPPLEMENT

Vitamin C with Rose Hips and Citrus Bioflavonoid Complex. Rutin and Hesperidin Complex.
Each Tablet Contains:

Vitamin C	600 mg
Citrus Bioflavonoid Complex	100 mg
Rutin	50 mg
Hesperidin Complex	25 mg

SUPPLIED
Bottles of 50, 100, 250, 500 and 1000 tablets.

LIVER TABLETS
11 GRAINS

Natural Desiccated and Defatted Argentinian Liver fortified with Vitamin B-12 and Red Bone Marrow. Provides the naturally occurring B-Complex Factors and Amino Acids found in Dried Beef Liver.

SUPPLIED
Bottles of 100, 250, 500 and 1000 tablets.

MaxEPA™ SOFTGELS

MaxEPA™ is a natural triglyceride fish oil concentrate providing a dietary source of the omega-3 polyunsaturates eicosapentaenoic acid (EPA) and docosahexaenoic acid (DHA). Each MaxEPA softgel supplies 180 mg of EPA and 120 mg of DHA from 1000 mg of MaxEPA™ fish oil concentrate. A 1275 mg potency (Mega-MaxEPA) is also available.

SUPPLIED
Bottles of 60 and 120 softgels.
Shown in Product Identification Section, page 431

MILK THISTLE (70% SILYMARIN)
100 mg. CAPSULES

Each capsule provides 100 mg of milk thistle extract (Silybum marianum) which supplies 70 mg of silymarin.

SUPPLIED
Bottles of 50, 100 and 250 capsules.

NIACIN (BUFFERED) 500 mg Tablets
(VITAMIN B-3)

A Buffered Niacin Supplement especially formulated to reduce or eliminate flushing and gastrointestinal irritation. Each tablet provides 500 mg of Buffered nictotinic acid (Niacin).

SUPPLIED
Bottles of 100 and 250 Tablets.

PYRIDOXAL-5-PHOSPHATE (P-5-P)
50 mg Enteric Coated Tablets

Provides the coenzyme form of Vitamin B-6.

SUPPLIED
Bottles of 50 and 100 Tablets.

THREONINE 500 mg CAPSULES

SUPPLIED
Bottles of 50, 100 and 250 capsules

Continued on next page

Solgar—Cont.

L–TRYPTOPHAN CAPSULES
(Free-form)
500 mg and 1000 mg.

SUPPLIED
Bottles of 30, 60 and 90 capsules.

VITA–KID WAFERS
CHILDREN'S CHEWABLE MULTIVITAMIN
Contains No Refined Sugars, Natural Orange Flavor

Each wafer provides:
Vitamin A	5000 IU
Vitamin D	400 IU
Vitamin E	10 IU
Vitamin C (w/Rose Hips)	100 mg.
Vitamin B-1	2 mg.
Vitamin B-2	2 mg.
Niacinamide	10 mg.
Vitamin B-6	2 mg.
Vitamin B-12	5 mcg.
Folic Acid	300 mcg.

SUPPLIED
Bottles of 50 and 100 Wafers.

VITAMIN B–1 TABLETS AND CAPSULES
(Thiamine)
25 mg, 50 mg, 100 mg and 500 mg

SUPPLIED
Bottles of 100, 250 and 500 tablets or capsules.

VITAMIN B–2 TABLETS AND CAPSULES
(Riboflavin)
25 mg, 50 mg and 100 mg

SUPPLIED
Bottles of 100, 250 and 500 tablets or capsules.

VITAMIN B–6 TABLETS AND CAPSULES
(Pyridoxine)
25 mg, 50 mg, 100 mg and 500 mg

SUPPLIED
Bottles of 100, 250 and 500 tablets or capsules.

VITAMIN B–12 TABLETS AND CAPSULES
50 mcg, 100 mcg, 250 mcg, 500 mcg
and 1000 mcg

SUPPLIED
Bottles of 100, 250 and 500 tablets or capsules.

VITAMIN C TABLETS OR CAPSULES
(Ascorbic Acid)
500 mg and 1000 mg.

SUPPLIED
Bottles of 100, 250 and 500 tablets or capsules.

VITAMIN E CAPSULES (Natural)
100 IU, 200 IU, 400 IU and 1000 IU
D-ALPHA TOCOPHEROL plus
MIXED TOCOPHEROLS

SUPPLIED
Bottles of 50, 100, 250, 500 and 1000 capsules.

ZINC "50" TABLETS

Each Tablet Provides:
Zinc Gluconate (Organically
  Complexed) ....409 mg
providing elemental Zinc .... 50 mg

SUPPLIED
Bottles of 100, 250 and 500 tablets.

Somerset Pharmaceuticals, Inc.
400 MORRIS AVENUE
SUITE 7S
DENVILLE, NJ 07834

ELDEPRYL®   ℞
(selegiline hydrochloride)
Tablets

DESCRIPTION
ELDEPRYL (selegiline hydrochloride) is a levorotatory acetylenic derivative of phenethylamine. It is commonly referred to in the clinical and pharmacological literature as L-deprenyl.

The chemical name is (R)-(-)-N,2-dimethyl-N-2-propynylphenethylamine hydrochloride. It is a white to near white crystalline powder, freely soluble in water, chloroform, and methanol, and has a molecular weight of 223.75. The structural formula is as follows:

Each round white tablet, debossed on one side with "JU", contains 5 mg selegiline hydrochloride. Inactive ingredients are lactose, starch, povidone, magnesium stearate, and talc.

CLINICAL PHARMACOLOGY
The mechanisms accounting for selegiline's beneficial adjunctive action in the treatment of Parkinson's Disease are not fully understood. Inhibition of monoamine oxidase, type B, activity is generally considered to be of primary importance; in addition, there is evidence that selegiline may act through other mechanisms to increase dopaminergic activity.

Selegiline is best known as an irreversible inhibitor of monoamine oxidase (MAO), an intracellular enzyme associated with the outer membrane of mitochondria. Selegiline inhibits MAO by acting as a 'suicide' substrate for the enzyme; that is, it is converted by MAO to an active moiety, which combines irreversibly with the active site and/or the enzyme's essential FAD cofactor. Because selegiline has greater affinity for type B than for type A active sites, it can serve as a selective inhibitor of MAO type B if it is administered at the recommended dose.

MAOs are widely distributed throughout the body; their concentration is especially high in liver, kidney, stomach, intestinal wall, and brain. MAOs are currently subclassified into two types, A and B, which differ in their substrate specificity and tissue distribution. In humans, intestinal MAO is predominantly type A, while most of that in brain is type B. In CNS neurons, MAO plays an important role in the catabolism of catecholamines (dopamine, norepinephrine and epinephrine) and serotonin. MAOs are also important in the catabolism of various exogenous amines found in a variety of foods and drugs. MAO in the GI tract and liver (primarily type A), for example, is thought to provide vital protection from exogenous amines (e.g., tyramine) that have the capacity, if absorbed intact, to cause a 'hypertensive crisis,' the so-called 'cheese reaction.' (If large amounts of certain exogenous amines gain access to the systemic circulation—e.g., from fermented cheese, red wine, herring, over-the-counter cough/cold medications, etc.—they are taken up by adrenergic neurons and displace norepinephrine from storage sites within membrane bound vesicles. Subsequent release of the displaced norepinephrine causes the rise in systemic blood pressure, etc.)

In theory, therefore, because MAO A of the gut is not inhibited, patients treated with selegiline at a dose of 10 mg a day can take medications containing pharmacologically active amines and consume tyramine-containing foods without risk of uncontrolled hypertension. To date, clinical experience appears to confirm this prediction; cheese reactions have not been reported in selegiline treated patients. The pathophysiology of the 'cheese reaction' is complicated and, in addition to its ability to inhibit MAO B selectively, selegiline's apparent freedom from this reaction has been attributed to an ability to prevent tyramine and other indirect acting sympathomimetics from displacing norepinephrine from adrenergic neurons.

However, until the pathophysiology of the cheese reaction is more completely understood, it seems prudent to assume that selegiline can only be used safely without dietary restrictions at doses where it presumably selectively inhibits MAO B (e.g., 10 mg/day). **In short, attention to the dose dependent nature of selegiline's selectivity is critical if it is to be used without elaborate restrictions being placed on diet and concomitant drug use. (See WARNINGS and PRECAUTIONS).**

It is important to be aware that selegiline may have pharmacological effects unrelated to MAO B inhibition. As noted above, there is some evidence that it may increase dopaminergic activity by other mechanisms, including interfering with dopamine re-uptake at the synapse. Effects resulting from selegiline administration may also be mediated through its metabolites. Two of its three principal metabolites, amphetamine and methamphetamine, have pharmacological actions of their own; they interfere with neuronal uptake and enhance release of several neurotransmitters (e.g., norepinephrine, dopamine, serotonin). However, the extent to which these metabolites contribute to the effects of selegiline are unknown.

Rationale for the Use of a Selective Monoamine Oxidase Type B Inhibitor in Parkinson's Disease
Many of the prominent symptoms of Parkinson's Disease are due to a deficiency of striatal dopamine that is the consequence of a progressive degeneration and loss of a population of dopaminergic neurons which originate in the substantia nigra of the midbrain and project to the basal ganglia or striatum. Early in the course of Parkinson's, the deficit in the capacity of these neurons to synthesize dopamine can be overcome by administration of exogenous levodopa, usually given in combination with a peripheral decarboxylase inhibitor (carbidopa).

With the passage of time, due to the progression of the disease and/or the effect of sustained treatment, the efficacy and quality of the therapeutic response of levodopa diminishes. Thus, after several years of levodopa treatment, the response, for a given dose of levodopa, is shorter, has less predictable onset and offset (i.e., there is 'wearing off'), and is often accompanied by side effects (e.g., dyskinesia, akinesias, on-off phenomena, freezing, etc.)

This deteriorating response is currently interpreted as a manifestation of the inability of the ever decreasing population of intact nigrostriatal neurons to synthesize and release adequate amounts of dopamine.

MAO B inhibition may be useful in this setting because, by blocking the catabolism of dopamine, it would increase the net amount of dopamine available (i.e., it would increase the pool of dopamine). Whether or not this mechanism or an alternative one actually accounts for the observed beneficial effects of adjunctive selegiline is unknown.

Selegiline's benefit in Parkinson's Disease has only been documented as an adjunct to levodopa/carbidopa. Whether or not it might be effective as a sole treatment is unknown, but past attempts to treat Parkinson's Disease with non-selective MAOI monotherapy are reported to have been unsuccessful. It is important to note that attempts to treat Parkinsonian patients with combinations of levodopa and currently marketed non-selective MAO inhibitors were abandoned because of multiple side effects including hypertension, increase in involuntary movement and toxic delirium.

Pharmacokinetic Information (Absorption, Distribution, Metabolism and Elimination—ADME)
Only preliminary information about the details of the pharmacokinetics of selegiline and its metabolites is available. Data obtained in a study of 12 healthy subjects that was intended to examine the effects of selegiline on the ADME of an oral hypoglycemic agent, however, provides some information. Following the oral administration of a single dose of 10 mg of selegiline hydrochloride to these subjects, serum levels of intact selegiline were below the limit of detection (less than 10 ng/ml). Three metabolites, N-desmethyldeprenyl, the major metabolite (mean half-life 2.0 hours), amphetamine (mean half-life 17.7 hours), and methamphetamine (mean half-life 20.5 hours), were found in serum and urine. Over a period of 48 hours, 45% of the dose administered appeared in the urine as these 3 metabolites.

In an extension of this study intended to examine the effects of steady state conditions, the same subjects were given a 10 mg dose of selegiline hydrochloride for seven consecutive days. Under these conditions, the mean trough serum levels for amphetamine were 3.5 ng/ml and 8.0 ng/ml for methamphetamine; trough levels of N-desmethyldeprenyl were below the levels of detection.

The rate of MAO B regeneration following discontinuation of treatment has not been quantitated. It is this rate, dependent upon de novo protein synthesis, which seems likely to determine how fast normal MAO B activity can be restored.

INDICATIONS AND USAGE
ELDEPRYL is indicated as an adjunct in the management of Parkinsonian patients being treated with levodopa/carbidopa who exhibit deterioration in the quality of their response to this therapy. There is no evidence from controlled studies that selegiline has any beneficial effect in the absence of concurrent levodopa therapy.

Evidence supporting this claim was obtained in randomized controlled clinical investigations that compared the effects of added selegiline or placebo in patients receiving levodopa/carbidopa. Selegiline was significantly superior to placebo on all three principal outcome measures employed; change from baseline in daily levodopa/carbidopa dose, the amount of 'off' time, and patient self-rating of treatment success. Beneficial effects were also observed on other measures of treatment success (e.g., measures of reduced end of dose akinesia, decreased tremor and sialorrhea, improved speech and dressing ability and improved overall disability as assessed by walking and comparison to previous state).

CONTRAINDICATIONS

ELDEPRYL is contraindicated in patients with a known hypersensitivity to this drug.

WARNING

Selegiline should not be used at daily doses exceeding those recommended (10 mg/day) because of the risks associated with non-selective inhibition of MAO. (See CLINICAL PHARMACOLOGY.)

The selectivity of selegiline for MAO B may not be absolute even at the recommended daily dose of 10 mg a day and selectivity is further diminished with increasing daily doses. The precise dose at which selegiline becomes a non-selective inhibitor of all MAO is unknown, but may be in the range of 30 to 40 mg a day.

Because of reports of fatal interactions, MAOIs are ordinarily contraindicated for use with meperidine (DEMEROL & other tradenames). This warning is often extended to other opioids. Because the mechanism of interaction between MAOIs and meperidine is unknown, it seems prudent, in general, to avoid this combination.

PRECAUTIONS

General

Some patients given selegiline may experience an exacerbation of levodopa associated side effects, presumably due to the increased amounts of dopamine reacting with supersensitive post-synaptic receptors. These effects may often be mitigated by reducing the dose of levodopa/carbidopa by approximately 10 to 30%.

The decision to prescribe selegiline should take into consideration that the MAO system of enzymes is complex and incompletely understood and there is only a limited amount of carefully documented clinical experience with selegiline. Consequently, the full spectrum of possible responses to selegiline may not have been observed in pre-marketing evaulation of the drug. It is advisable, therefore, to observe patients closely for atypical responses.

Information for Patients

Patients should be advised of the possible need to reduce levodopa dosage after the initiation of ELDEPRYL therapy. Patients (or their families if the patient is incompetent) should be advised not to exceed the daily recommended dose of 10 mg. The risk of using higher daily doses of selegiline should be explained, and a brief description of the 'cheese reaction' provided. While hypertensive reactions with selegiline have not been reported, documented experience is limited. Consequently, it may be useful to inform patients (or their families) about the signs and symptoms associated with MAOI induced hypertensive reactions. In particular, patients should be urged to report, immediately, any severe headache or other atypical or unusual symptoms not previously experienced.

Laboratory Tests

No specific laboratory tests are deemed essential for the management of patients on ELDEPRYL. Periodic routine evaluation of all patients, however, is appropriate.

Drug Interactions

No interactions attributed to the combined use of selegiline and other drugs have been reported. However, because the database of documented clinical experience is limited, the level of reassurance provided by this lack of adverse reporting is uncertain. (See WARNINGS and PRECAUTIONS.)

Carcinogenesis, Mutagenesis, and Impairment of Fertility

Studies have not been performed to date to evaluate the carcinogenic potential of selegiline hydrochloride.

Pregnancy

Pregnancy category C. Insufficient animal reproduction studies have been done with selegiline to conclude that selegiline poses no teratogenic risk. However, one rat study carried out at doses as much as 180 fold the recommended human dose revealed no evidence of a teratogenic effect. It is not known whether selegiline can cause fetal harm when administered to a pregnant woman or can affect reproduction capacity. Selegiline should be given to a pregnant woman only if clearly needed.

Nursing Mothers

It is not known whether selegiline hydrochloride is excreted in human milk. Because many drugs are excreted in human milk, consideration should be given to discontinuing the use of all but absolutely essential drug treatments in nursing women.

Pediatric Use

The use of selegiline hydrochloride in children have not been evaluated.

ADVERSE REACTIONS

Introduction

The number of patients who received selegiline in prospectively monitored pre-marketing studies is limited. While other sources of information about the use of selegiline are available (e.g., literature reports, foreign post-marketing reports, etc.) they do not provide the kind of information necessary to estimate the incidence of adverse events. Thus, overall incidence figures for adverse reactions associated

with the use of selegiline cannot be provided. Many of the adverse reactions seen have been also reported as symptoms of dopamine excess.

Moreover, the importance and severity of various reactions reported often cannot be ascertained. One index of relative importance, however, is whether or not a reaction caused treatment discontinuation. In prospective pre-marketing studies, the following events led, in decreasing order of frequency, to discontinuation of treatment with selegiline: nausea, hallucinations, confusion, depression, loss of balance, insomnia, orthostatic hypotension, increased akinetic involuntary movements, agitation, arrhythmia, bradykinesia, chorea, delusions, hypertension, new or increased angina pectoris and syncope. Events reported only once as a cause of discontinuation are ankle edema, anxiety, burning lips/mouth, constipation, drowsiness/lethargy, dystonia, excess perspiration, increased freezing, gastrointestinal bleeding, hair loss, increased tremor, nervousness, weakness and weightloss.

Experience with ELDEPRYL obtained in parallel, placebo controlled, randomized studies provides only a limited basis for estimates of adverse reaction rates. The following reactions that occurred with greater frequency among the 49 patients assigned to selegiline as compared to the 50 patients assigned to placebo in the only parallel, placebo controlled trial performed in patients with Parkinson's Disease are shown in the following Table. None of these adverse reactions led to a discontinuation of treatment.

INCIDENCE OF TREATMENT-EMERGENT ADVERSE EXPERIENCES IN THE PLACEBO-CONTROLLED CLINICAL TRIAL

Adverse Event	Number of Patients Reporting Events	
	selegiline hydrochloride N=49	placebo N=50
Nausea	10	3
Dizziness/Lightheaded/ Fainting	7	1
Abdominal Pain	4	2
Confusion	3	0
Hallucinations	3	1
Dry mouth	3	1
Vivid Dreams	2	0
Dyskinesias	2	5
Headache	2	1

The following events were reported once in either or both groups:

Ache, generalized	1	0
Anxiety/Tension	1	1
Anemia	0	1
Diarrhea	1	0
Hair Loss	0	1
Insomnia	1	1
Lethargy	1	0
Leg pain	1	0
Low back pain	1	0
Malaise	0	1
Palpitations	1	0
Urinary Retention	1	0
Weight Loss	1	0

In all prospectively monitored clinical investigations, enrolling approximately 920 patients, the following adverse events, classified by body system, were reported.

CENTRAL NERVOUS SYSTEM

Motor/Coordination/Extrapyramidal: increased tremor, chorea, loss of balance, restlessness, blephorospasm, increased bradykinesia, facial grimace, falling down, heavy leg, muscle twitch*, myoclonic jerks*, stiff neck, tardive dyskinesia, dystonic symptoms, dyskinesia, involuntary movements, freezing, festination, increased apraxia, muscle cramps.

Mental Status Behavioral/Psychiatric: hallucinations, dizziness, confusion, anxiety, depression, drowsiness, behavior/mood change, dreams/nightmares, tiredness, delusions, disorientation, lightheadedness, impaired memory*, increased energy*, transient high*, hollow feeling, lethargy/malaise, apathy, overstimulation, vertigo, personality change, sleep disturbance, restlessness, weakness, transient irritability.

Pain/Altered Sensation: headache, back pain, leg pain, tinnitus, migraine, supraorbital pain, throat burning, generalized ache, chills, numbness of toes/fingers, taste disturbance.

AUTONOMIC NERVOUS SYSTEM

dry mouth, blurred vision, sexual dysfunction.

CARDIOVASCULAR

orthostatic hypotension, hypertension, arrhythmia, palpitations, new or increased angina pectoris, hypotension, tachycardia, peripheral edema, sinus bradycardia, syncope.

GASTROINTESTINAL

nausea/vomiting, constipation, weight loss, anorexia, poor appetite, dysphagia, diarrhea, heartburn, rectal bleeding, bruxism*.

GENITOURINARY/GYNECOLOGIC/ENDOCRINE

slow urination, transient anorgasmia*, nocturia, prostatic hypertrophy, urinary hesitancy, urinary retention, decreased penile sensation*, urinary frequency.

SKIN AND APPENDAGES

increased sweating, diaphoresis, facial hair, hematoma, rash, photosensitivity.

MISCELLANEOUS

asthma, diplopia, shortness of breath, speech affected.
*indicates events reported only at doses greater than 10 mg/day.

OVERDOSAGE

Selegiline

No specific information is available about clinically significant overdoses with ELDEPRYL. However, experience gained during selegiline's development reveals that some individuals exposed to doses of 600 mg d l selegiline suffered severe hypotension and psychomotor agitation.

Since the selective inhibition of MAO B by selegiline hydrochloride is achieved only at doses in the range recommended for the treatment of Parkinson's Disease (e.g., 10 mg/day), overdoses are likely to cause significant inhibition of both MAO A and MAO B. Consequently, the signs and symptoms of overdose may resemble those observed with marketed non-selective MAO inhibitors [e.g., tranylcypromine (PARNATE), isocarboxazide (MARPLAN), and phenelzine (NARDIL)].

Overdose with Non-Selective MAO Inhibition

NOTE: This section is provided for reference; it does not describe events that have actually been observed with selegiline in overdose.

Characteristically, signs and symptoms of non-selective MAOI overdose may not appear immediately. Delays of up to 12 hours between ingestion of drug and the appearance of signs may occur. Importantly, the peak intensity of the syndrome may not be reached for upwards of a day following the overdose. Death has been reported following overdosage. Therefore, immediate hospitalization, with continuous patient observation and monitoring for a period of at least two days following the ingestion of such drugs in overdose is strongly recommended.

The clinical picture of MAOI overdose varies considerably; its severity may be a function of the amount of drug consumed. The central nervous and cardiovascular systems are prominently involved.

Signs and symptoms of overdosage may include, alone or in combination, any of the following: drowsiness, dizziness, faintness, irritability, hyperactivity, agitation, severe headache, hallucinations, trismus, opisthotonus, convulsions, and coma; rapid and irregular pulse, hypertension, hypotension and vascular collapse; precordial pain, respiratory depression and failure, hyperpyrexia, diaphoresis, and cool, clammy skin.

Treatment Suggestions for Overdose

NOTE: Because there is no recorded experience with selegiline overdose, the following suggestions are offered based upon the assumption that selegiline overdose may be modeled by non-selective MAOI poisoning. In any case, up-to-date information about the treatment of overdose can often be obtained from a certified Regional Poison Control Center. Telephone numbers of certified Poison Control Centers are listed in the Physician's Desk Reference (PDR).

Treatment of overdose with non-selective MAOIs is symptomatic and supportive. Induction of emesis or gastric lavage with instillation of charcoal slurry may be helpful in early poisoning, provided the airway has been protected against aspiration. Signs and symptoms of central nervous system stimulation, including convulsions, should be treated with diazepam, given slowly intravenously. Phenothiazine derivatives and central nervous system stimulants should be avoided. Hypotension and vascular collapse should be treated with intravenous fluids and, if necessary, blood pressure titration with an intravenous infusion of a dilute pressor agent. It should be noted that adrenergic agents may produce a markedly increased pressor response.

Respiration should be supported by appropriate measures, including management of the airway, use of supplemental oxygen, and mechanical ventilatory assistance, as required. Body temperature should be monitored closely. Intensive management of hyperpyrexia may be required. Maintenance of fluid and electrolyte balance is essential.

DOSAGE AND ADMINISTRATION

ELDEPRYL is intended for administration to Parkinsonian patients receiving levodopa/carbidopa therapy who demonstrate a deteriorating response to this treatment. The recommended regimen for the administration of ELDEPRYL is 10

Continued on next page

Somerset—Cont.

mg per day administered as divided doses of 5 mg each taken at breakfast and lunch. There is no evidence that additional benefit will be obtained from the administration of higher doses. Moreover, higher doses should ordinarily be avoided because of the increased risk of side effects.

After two to three days of selegiline treatment, an attempt may be made to reduce the dose of levodopa/carbidopa. A reduction of 10 to 30% was achieved with the typical participant in the domestic placebo controlled trials who was assigned to selegiline treatment. Further reductions of levodopa/carbidopa may be possible during continued selegiline therapy.

HOW SUPPLIED

Tablets:

5 mg, bottles of 60 tablets, NDC 39506-011-25

Store at controlled room temperature, 59° to 86°F (15° to 30°C).

Caution—Federal (USA) law prohibits dispensing without prescription.

Literature issued June, 1989

011-25-P-100

E. R. Squibb & Sons, Inc.

GENERAL OFFICES
P.O. BOX 4000
PRINCETON, NJ 08543-4000

For listing of standard, purified, and human insulins, see Squibb–Novo, Inc.

UNILOG®
(Tablet and Capsule Identification Code)
NUMERICAL INDEX

Unilog Number	Product
F16	Principen with Probenecid (Ampicillin-Probenecid Capsules)
113	Velosef '250' Capsules (Cephradine Capsules USP) 250 mg
114	Velosef '500' Capsules (Cephradine Capsules USP) 500 mg
133	Clorazepate Dipotassium Tablets 3.75 mg
138	SMZ-TMP Tablets (Sulfamethoxazole and Trimethoprim Tablets USP) 400 mg-80 mg
139	Chlorpropamide Tablets USP 100 mg
152	Chlorpropamide Tablets USP 250 mg
157	Chlorazepate Dipotassium Tablets 7.5 mg
159	Oxazepam Capsules USP 30 mg
162	Chlorthalidone Tablets USP 25 mg
163	Clorazepate Dipotassium Tablets 15 mg
164	Pentids '500' Tablets (Penicillin G Potassium Tablets USP) 200,000 u.
165	Pentids '400' Tablets (Penicillin G Potassium Tablets USP) 400,000 u.
168	Pentids '800' Tablets (Penicillin G Potassium Tablets USP) 800,000 u.
171	SMZ-TMP Tablets (Sulfamethoxazole and Trimethoprim Tablets USP) 800 mg-160 mg
180	Chlorthalidone Tablets USP 50 mg
181	Cephalexin Capsules USP 250 mg
185	Diazepam Tablets USP 2 mg
193	Perphenazine and Amitriptyline HCl Tablets 2 mg-10 mg
195	Tolazamide Tablets USP 100 mg
196	Vitamin C Tablets 250 mg
197	Vitamin C Tablets 500 mg
201	Aspirin Tablets USP, 5 gr. (324 mg)
202	Dicloxacillin Sodium Capsules USP 250 mg
203	Dicloxacillin Sodium Capsules USP 500 mg
211	Cloxacillin Sodium Capsules USP 250 mg
212	Cloxacillin Sodium Capsules USP 500 mg
230	Trimox '250' Capsules (Amoxicillin Capsules USP) 250 mg
231	Trimox '500' Capsules (Amoxicillin Capsules USP) 500 mg
238	Diazepam Tablets USP 5 mg
239	Cephalexin Capsules USP 500 mg
245	Diazepam Tablets USP 10 mg
259	Perphenazine and Amitriptyline HCl Tablets 2 mg-25 mg
267	Perphenazine and Amitriptyline HCl Tablets 4 mg-10 mg
271	Perphenazine and Amitriptyline HCl Tablets 4 mg-25 mg
274	Trazodone Hydrochloride Tablets 50 mg
277	Tolazamide Tablets USP 250 mg
280	Indomethacin Capsules USP 25 mg
286	Quinidine Gluconate Sustained-Release Tablets 324 mg
288	Allopurenol Tablets 300 mg
289	Clonidine Tablets 0.1 mg
295	Indomethacin Capsules USP 50 mg
298	Lorazepam Tablets USP 0.5 mg
316	Triamterene/Hydrochlorothiazide Capsules 50 mg/25 mg
338	Capozide (Captopril-Hydrochlorothiazide Tablets) 25 mg–15 mg
348	Indomethacin Sustained-Release Capsules 75 mg
349	Capozide (Captopril-Hydrochlorothiazide Tablets) 25 mg–25 mg
355	Valadol Tablets (Acetaminophen Tablets USP) 325 mg (5 gr.)
359	Furosemide Tablets USP 20 mg
360	Furosemide Tablets USP 40 mg
384	Capozide (Captopril-Hydrochlorothiazide Tablets) 50 mg–15 mg
390	Capozide (Captopril-Hydrochlorothiazide Tablets) 50 mg–25 mg
408	Lorazepam Tablets USP 1.0 mg
429	Florinef Acetate (Fludrocortisone Acetate Tablets USP) 0.1 mg
433	Methyldopa Tablets USP 500 mg
447	Methyldopa Tablets USP 250 mg
450	Capoten (Captopril Tablets) 12.5 mg
452	Capoten (Captopril Tablets) 25 mg
455	Oragrafin Sodium Capsules (Ipodate Sodium Capsules USP) 500 mg
457	Mycostatin Vaginal Tablets (Nystatin Vaginal Tablets USP) 100,000 u.
478	Engran-HP Tablets (Multi-Vitamin and Multi-Mineral Supplement)
482	Capoten (Captopril Tablets) 50 mg
485	Capoten (Captopril Tablets) 100 mg
487	Lorazepam Tablets USP 2.0 mg
488	Metronidazole Tablets USP 250 mg
512	Kenacort (Triamcinolone Tablets USP) 4 mg
518	Kenacort (Triamcinolone Tablets USP) 8 mg
520	Clonidine Tablets 0.2 mg
534	Clonidine Tablets 0.3 mg
535	Theragran Hematinic (Therapeutic Formula Vitamin Tablets with Hematinics)
537	Niacin Tablets USP, 500 mg
549	Iron and Vitamin C Tablets
572	Metronidazole Tablets USP 500 mg
573	'Ora-Testryl' (Fluoxymesterone Tablets USP) 5 mg
574	Oxazepam Capsules USP 10 mg
580	Mycostatin Oral Tablets (Nystatin Tablets USP) 500,000 u.
599	Oxazepam Capsules USP 15 mg
603	Sumycin '500' Tablets (Tetracycline Hydrochloride Tablets USP) 500 mg
611	Niacin Tablets USP, 50 mg
612	Niacin Tablets USP, 100 mg
622	Meclofenamate Capsules 50 mg
623	Noctec Capsules (Chloral Hydrate Capsules USP) 250 mg (3¾ grains)
626	Noctec Capsules (Chloral Hydrate Capsules USP) 500 mg (7½ grains)
629	Meclofenamate Capsules 100 mg
630	Methyldopa/Hydrochlorothiazide Tablets USP 250 mg/15 mg
645	Methyldopa/Hydrochlorothiazide Tablets USP 250 mg/25 mg
648	Veetids '500' Tablets (Penicillin V Potassium Tablets USP) 500 mg (800,000 u.)
655	Sumycin '250' Capsules (Tetracycline Hydrochloride Capsules USP) 250 mg
663	Sumycin '250' Tablets (Tetracycline Hydrochloride Tablets USP) 250 mg
674	Doxycycline Hyclate Capsules USP 50 mg
684	Veetids '250' Tablets (Penicillin V Potassium Tablets USP) 250 mg (400,000 u.)
690	Teslac Tablets (Testolactone Tablets USP) 50 mg
693	Metoclopramide Hydrochloride Tablets USP 10 mg
723	Phenytoin Capsules 100 mg
726	Procainamide Hydrochloride Sustained-Release Tablets 250 mg
729	Propranolol Hydrochloride Tablets USP 10 mg
731	Propranolol Hydrochloride Tablets USP 20 mg
738	Temazepam Capsules 15 mg
742	Procainamide Hydrochloride Sustained-Release Tablets 500 mg
745	Propranolol Hydrochloride Tablets USP 40 mg
747	Temazepam Capsules 30 mg
750	Propranolol Hydrochloride Tablets USP 60 mg
763	Sumycin '500' Capsules (Tetracycline Hydrochloride Capsules USP) 500 mg
765	Propranolol Hydrochloride Tablets USP 80 mg
777	Procainamide Hydrochloride Sustained-Release Tablets 750 mg
812	Doxycycline Hyclate Tablets USP 100 mg
830	Hydrea Capsules (Hydroxyurea Capsules USP) 500 mg
834	Theragran Stress Formula Tablets (High Potency Multivitamin with Iron and Biotin)
842	Theragran Tablets (High Potency Multivitamin Formula)
845	Allopurinol Tablets 100 mg
849	Theragran-M Tablets (High Potency Multivitamin Formula with Minerals)
851	Triamterene/Hydrochlorothiazide Tablets 75 mg/50 mg
876	Trigesic Tablets (Analgesic Compound)
940	Doxycycline Hyclate Capsules USP 100 mg
963	Trazodone Hydrochloride Tablets 100 mg
971	Principen '250' Capsules (Ampicillin Capsules USP) 250 mg
974	Principen '500' Capsules (Ampicillin Capsules USP) 500 mg
1175	Loxapine Succinate Capsules 5 mg
1235	Loxapine Succinate Capsules 10 mg
1455	Loxapine Succinate Capsules 25 mg
1535	Loxapine Succinate Capsules 50 mg
9550	Fenoprofen Tablets USP 600 mg

AZACTAM® FOR INJECTION ℞

[a-zak 'tam]

Aztreonam For Injection

DESCRIPTION

AZACTAM (aztreonam, Squibb) is the first member of a new class of antibiotics developed by the Squibb Institute for Medical Research and classified as monobactams. These agents were originally isolated from *Chromobacterium violaceum*. AZACTAM is a totally synthetic bactericidal antibiotic with activity against a wide spectrum of gram-negative aerobic pathogens.

The monobactams, having a unique monocyclic beta-lactam nucleus, are structurally different from other beta-lactam antibiotics (e.g., penicillins, cephalosporins, cephamycins). The sulfonic acid substituent in the 1-position of the ring activates the beta-lactam moiety; an aminothiazolyl oxime side chain in the 3-position and a methyl group in the 4-position confer the specific antibacterial spectrum and beta-lactamase stability.

Aztreonam is designated chemically as (Z)-2-[[[(2-amino-4-thiazolyl)][[(2S,3S)-2-methyl-4-oxo-1-sulfo-3-azetidinyl]carbamoyl]methylene]amino]oxy]-2-methylpropionic acid.

AZACTAM For Injection (Aztreonam For Injection) is a sterile, nonpyrogenic, sodium-free, white to yellowish-white lyophilized cake containing approximately 780 mg arginine per gram of aztreonam. Following constitution, the product is for intramuscular or intravenous use. Aqueous solutions of aztreonam have a pH in the range of 4.5 to 7.5.

CLINICAL PHARMACOLOGY

Single 30-minute intravenous infusions of 500 mg, 1 g and 2 g doses of AZACTAM in healthy subjects produced peak serum levels of 54, 90 and 204 μg/mL, respectively, immediately after administration; at eight hours, serum levels were 1, 3 and 6 μg/mL, respectively (Figure 1). Single 3-minute intravenous injections of the same doses resulted in serum levels of 58, 125 and 242 μg/mL at five minutes following completion of injection.

Serum concentrations of aztreonam in healthy subjects following completion of single intramuscular injections of 500 mg and 1 g doses are depicted in Figure 1; maximum serum concentrations occur at about one hour. After identical single intravenous or intramuscular doses of AZACTAM, the serum concentrations of aztreonam are comparable at one hour (1.5 hours from start of intravenous infusion) with similar slopes of serum concentrations thereafter.

FIGURE 1

The serum levels of aztreonam following single 500 mg, or 1 g (intramuscular or intravenous) or 2 g (intravenous) doses of AZACTAM (aztreonam) exceed the MIC_{90} for *Neisseria* sp., *H. influenzae* and most genera of the *Enterobacteriaceae* for eight hours (*Enterobacter* sp., the eight hour serum levels exceed the MIC for 80 percent of strains). For *Ps. aeruginosa*, a single 2 g intravenous dose produces serum levels that exceed the MIC_{90} for approximately four to six hours. All of the above doses of AZACTAM result in average urine levels of aztreonam that exceed the MIC_{90} for the same pathogens for up to 12 hours.

The serum half-life of aztreonam averaged 1.7 hour (1.5 to 2.0) in subjects with normal renal function, independent of the dose and route of administration. In healthy subjects, based on a 70 kg person, the serum clearance was 91 mL/min and renal clearance was 56 mL/min; the apparent mean volume of distribution at steady-state averaged 12.6 liters, approximately equivalent to extracellullar fluid volume.

In a study of healthy elderly male subjects (65 to 75 years of age), the average elimination half-life of aztreonam was slightly longer than in young healthy males.

In patients with impaired renal function, the serum half-life of aztreonam is prolonged (see DOSAGE AND ADMINISTRATION, Renal Impairment). The serum half-life of aztreonam is only slightly prolonged in patients with hepatic impairment since the liver is a minor pathway of excretion.

Average urine concentrations of aztreonam were approximately 1100, 3500 and 6600 µg/mL within the first two hours following single 500 mg, 1 g and 2 g intravenous doses of AZACTAM (30-minute infusions), respectively. The range of average concentrations for aztreonam in the 8 to 12 hour urine specimens in these studies was 25 to 120 µg/mL. After intramuscular injection of single 500 mg and 1 g doses of AZACTAM, urinary levels were approximately 500 and 1200 µg/mL, respectively, within the first two hours, declining to 180 and 470 µg/mL in the six to eight hour specimens. In healthy subjects, aztreonam is excreted in the urine about equally by active tubular secretion and glomerular filtration. Approximately 60 to 70 percent of an intravenous or intramuscular dose was recovered in the urine by eight hours. Urinary excretion of a single parenteral dose was essentially complete by 12 hours after injection. About 12 percent of a single intravenous radiolabeled dose was recovered in the feces. Unchanged aztreonam and the inactive beta-lactam ring hydrolysis product of aztreonam were present in feces and urine.

Intravenous or intramuscular administration of a single 500 mg or 1 g dose of AZACTAM (aztreonam) every eight hours for seven days to healthy subjects produced no apparent accumulation of aztreonam or modification of its disposition characteristics; serum protein binding averaged 56 percent and was independent of dose. An average of about 6 percent of a 1 g intramuscular dose was excreted as a microbiologically inactive open beta-lactam ring hydrolysis product (serum half-life approximately 26 hours) of aztreonam in the zero to eight hour urine collection on the last day of multiple dosing.

Renal function was monitored in healthy subjects given aztreonam; standard tests (serum creatinine, creatinine clearance, BUN, urinalysis and total urinary protein excretion) as well as special tests (excretion of N-acetyl-β-glucosaminidase, alanine aminopeptidase and $β_2$-microglobulin) were used. No abnormal results were obtained.

Aztreonam achieves measurable concentrations in the following body fluids and tissues:

[See table above].

The concentration of aztreonam in saliva at 30 minutes after a single 1 g intravenous dose (9 patients) was 0.2 µg/mL; in breast milk at two hours after a single 1 g intravenous dose (6 patients), 0.2 µg/mL, and at six hours after a single 1 g intramuscular dose (6 patients), 0.3 µg/mL; in amniotic fluid at

EXTRAVASCULAR CONCENTRATIONS OF AZTREONAM AFTER A SINGLE PARENTERAL DOSE[1]

Fluid or Tissue	Dose (g)	Route	Hours Post-Injection	Number of Patients	Mean Concentration (µg/mL or µg/g)
Fluids					
bile	1	IV	2	10	39
blister fluid	1	IV	1	6	20
bronchial secretion	2	IV	4	7	5
cerebrospinal fluid (inflamed meninges)	2	IV	0.9–4.3	16	3
pericardial fluid	2	IV	1	6	33
pleural fluid	2	IV	1.1–3.0	3	51
synovial fluid	2	IV	0.8–1.9	11	83
Tissues					
atrial appendage	2	IV	0.9–1.6	12	22
endometrium	2	IV	0.7–1.9	4	9
fallopian tube	2	IV	0.7–1.9	8	12
fat	2	IV	1.3–2.0	10	5
femur	2	IV	1.0–2.1	15	16
gallbladder	2	IV	0.8–1.3	4	23
kidney	2	IV	2.4–5.6	5	67
large intestine	2	IV	0.8–1.9	9	12
liver	2	IV	0.9–2.0	6	47
lung	2	IV	1.2–2.1	6	22
myometrium	2	IV	0.7–1.9	9	11
ovary	2	IV	0.7–1.9	7	13
prostate	1	IM	0.8–3.0	8	8
skeletal muscle	2	IV	0.3–0.7	6	16
skin	2	IV	0.0–1.0	8	25
sternum	2	IV	1	6	6

[1] Tissue penetration is regarded as essential to therapeutic efficacy, but specific tissue levels have not been correlated with specific therapeutic effects.

six to eight hours after a single 1 g intravenous dose (5 patients), 2 µg/mL. The concentration of aztreonam in peritoneal fluid obtained one to six hours after multiple 2 g intravenous doses ranged between 12 and 90 µg/mL in 7 of 8 patients studied.

Aztreonam given intravenously rapidly reaches therapeutic concentrations in peritoneal dialysis fluid; conversely, aztreonam given intraperitoneally in dialysis fluid rapidly produces therapeutic serum levels.

Concomitant administration of probenecid or furosemide and AZACTAM (aztreonam) causes clinically insignificant increases in the serum levels of aztreonam. Single-dose intravenous pharmacokinetic studies have not shown any significant interaction between aztreonam and concomitantly administered gentamicin, nafcillin sodium, cephradine, clindamycin or metronidazole. No reports of disulfiram-like reactions with alcohol ingestion have been noted; this is not unexpected since aztreonam does not contain a methyl-tetrazole side chain.

The implications of the following information for predicting the occurrence of hypersensitivity reactions to AZACTAM have not been established. The number of patients included in immunologic studies is too small to draw firm conclusions with regard to clinical practice:

A study in rabbits suggests that antibodies produced in response to benzylpenicillin and to cephalothin show little cross-reactivity with aztreonam, and antibodies produced in response to aztreonam show little cross-reactivity with benzylpenicillin and cephalothin.

In a group of 22 subjects with positive skin tests to penicillin reagents, three also had positive skin tests to aztreonam. One was negative on retesting, one was confirmed as positive, and the third subject refused further evaluation. The 20 subjects with negative aztreonam skin tests were given one injection of AZACTAM 1 g IM. There were no immediate hypersensitivity reactions, but one subject later developed a localized rash that was compatible with a fixed drug eruption.

In 36 subjects receiving multiple doses of AZACTAM over a seven-day period, no IgE antibody response was detectable and only one subject demonstrated an IgG response.

Microbiology

Aztreonam exhibits potent and specific activity *in vitro* against a wide spectrum of gram-negative aerobic pathogens including *Pseudomonas aeruginosa*. The bactericidal action of aztreonam results from the inhibition of bacterial cell wall synthesis due to a high affinity of aztreonam for penicillin binding protein 3 (PBP3). Aztreonam, unlike the majority of beta-lactam antibiotics, does not induce beta-lactamase activity and its molecular structure confers a high degree of resistance to hydrolysis by beta-lactamases (i.e., penicillinases and cephalosporinases) produced by most gram-negative and gram-positive pathogens; it is therefore usually active against gram-negative aerobic organisms that are resistant to antibiotics hydrolyzed by beta-lactamases. Aztreonam maintains its antimicrobial activity over a pH range of 6 to 8 *in vitro*, as well as in the presence of human serum and under anaerobic conditions. Aztreonam is active *in vitro* and

is effective in laboratory animal models and clinical infections against most strains of the following organisms, including many that are multiply-resistant to other antibiotics (i.e., certain cephalosporins, penicillins, and aminoglycosides):

Escherichia coli
Enterobacter species
Klebsiella pneumoniae and *K. oxytoca*
Proteus mirabilis
Pseudomonas aeruginosa
Serratia marcescens
Haemophilus influenzae (including ampicillin-resistant and other penicillinase-producing strains)
Citrobacter species

While *in vitro* studies have demonstrated the susceptibility to aztreonam of most strains of the following organisms, clinical efficacy for infections other than those included in the INDICATIONS AND USAGE section has not been documented:

Neisseria gonorrhoeae (including penicillinase-producing strains)
Proteus vulgaris
Morganella morganii (formerly *Proteus morganii*)
Providencia species, including *P. stuartii* and *P. rettgeri* (formerly *Proteus rettgeri*)
Pseudomonas species
Shigella species
Pasteurella multocida
Yersinia enterocolitica
Aeromonas hydrophila
Neisseria meningitidis

Aztreonam and aminoglycosides have been shown to be synergistic *in vitro* against most strains of *Ps. aeruginosa*, many strains of *Enterobacteriaceae*, and other gram-negative aerobic bacilli.

Alterations of the anaerobic intestinal flora by broad spectrum antibiotics may decrease colonization resistance, thus permitting overgrowth of potential pathogens, e.g., *Candida* and Clostridia species. Aztreonam has little effect on the aerobic intestinal microflora in *in vitro* studies. *Clostridium difficile* and its cytotoxin were not found in animal models following administration of aztreonam (see ADVERSE REACTIONS, Gastrointestinal).

Susceptibility Testing

Diffusion Technique: Quantitative procedures that require measurement of zone diameters give precise estimates of microbial susceptibility to antibiotics. One such method, recommended for use with the aztreonam 30 µg disk, is the National Committee of Clinical Laboratory Standards (NCCLS) approved procedure. Only a 30 µg aztreonam disk should be used; there are no suitable surrogate disks.

Continued on next page

Squibb—Cont.

Results of laboratory tests using 30 μg aztreonam disks should be interpreted using the following criteria:

Zone Diameter (mm)	Interpretation
≥ 22	(S) Susceptible
16–21	(I) Intermediate (Moderate Susceptibility)
≤ 15	(R) Resistant

Dilution Technique: Broth or agar dilution methods may be used to determine the minimal inhibitory concentration (MIC) of aztreonam.

MIC test results should be interpreted according to the concentrations of aztreonam that can be attained in serum, tissues and body fluids.

MIC (μg/mL)	Interpretation
≤ 8	(S) Susceptible
16	(I) Intermediate (Moderate Susceptibility)
≥ 32	(R) Resistant

For any susceptibility test, a report of "susceptible" indicates that the pathogen is likely to respond to AZACTAM therapy; a report of "resistant" indicates that the pathogen is not likely to respond. A report of "intermediate" (moderate susceptibility) indicates that the pathogen is expected to be susceptible to AZACTAM (aztreonam) if high dosages are used, or if the infection is confined to tissues and fluids (e.g., urine, bile) in which high aztreonam levels are attained.

The quality control cultures should have the following assigned daily ranges for aztreonam:

	Disks	Mode MIC (μg/mL)
E. coli (ATCC 25922)	28–36 mm	0.06–0.25
Ps. aeruginosa (ATCC 27853)	23–29 mm	2.0–8.0

INDICATIONS AND USAGE

Before initiating treatment with AZACTAM, appropriate specimens should be obtained for isolation of the causative organism(s) and for determination of susceptibility to aztreonam. Treatment with AZACTAM may be started empirically before results of the susceptibility testing are available; subsequently, appropriate antibiotic therapy should be continued.

AZACTAM For Injection (Aztreonam For Injection) is indicated for the treatment of the following infections caused by susceptible gram-negative microorganisms:

Urinary Tract Infections (complicated and uncomplicated), including pyelonephritis and cystitis (initial and recurrent) caused by *Escherichia coli, Klebsiella pneumoniae, Proteus mirabilis, Pseudomonas aeruginosa, Enterobacter cloacae, Klebsiella oxytoca*, Citrobacter* species* and *Serratia marcescens**.

Lower Respiratory Tract Infections, including pneumonia and bronchitis caused by *Escherichia coli, Klebsiella pneumoniae, Pseudomonas aeruginosa, Haemophilus influenzae, Proteus mirabilis, Enterobacter* species and *Serratia marcescens**.

Septicemia caused by *Escherichia coli, Klebsiella pneumoniae, Pseudomonas aeruginosa, Proteus mirabilis*, Serratia marcescens** and *Enterobacter* species.

Skin and Skin-Structure Infections, including those associated with post-operative wounds, ulcers and burns caused by *Escherichia coli, Proteus mirabilis, Serratia marcescens, Enterobacter* species, *Pseudomonas aeruginosa, Klebsiella pneumoniae* and *Citrobacter* species*.

Intra-abdominal Infections, including peritonitis caused by *Escherichia coli, Klebsiella* species including *K. pneumoniae, Enterobacter* species including *E. cloacae*, Pseudomonas aeruginosa, Citrobacter* species* including *C. freundii** and *Serratia* species* including *S. marcescens**.

Gynecologic Infections, including endometritis and pelvic cellulitis caused by *Escherichia coli, Klebsiella pneumoniae*, Enterobacter* species* including *E. cloacae** and *Proteus mirabilis**.

---

*Efficacy for this organism in this organ system was studied in fewer than ten infections.

AZACTAM (aztreonam) is indicated for adjunctive therapy to surgery in the management of infections caused by susceptible organisms, including abscesses, infections complicating hollow viscus perforations, cutaneous infections and infections of serous surfaces. AZACTAM is effective against most of the commonly encountered gram-negative aerobic pathogens seen in general surgery.

Concurrent Therapy

Concurrent initial therapy with other antimicrobial agents and AZACTAM is recommended before the causative organism(s) is known in seriously ill patients who are also at risk of having an infection due to gram-positive aerobic pathogens. If anaerobic organisms are also suspected as etiologic agents, therapy should be initiated using an anti-anaerobic agent concurrently with AZACTAM (see DOSAGE AND ADMINISTRATION). Certain antibiotics (e.g., cefoxitin, imipenem) may induce high levels of beta-lactamase *in vitro* in some gram-negative aerobes such as *Enterobacter* and *Pseudomonas* species, resulting in antagonism to many beta-lactam antibiotics including aztreonam. These *in vitro* findings suggest that such beta-lactamase inducing antibiotics

not be used concurrently with aztreonam. Following identification and susceptibility testing of the causative organism(s), appropriate antibiotic therapy should be continued.

CONTRAINDICATIONS

Aztreonam is contraindicated in patients with known allergy to this antibiotic.

WARNINGS

Careful inquiry should be made for a history of hypersensitivity reaction to any antibiotic or other drugs. Antibiotics should be given with caution to any patient who has had some form of allergy, particularly to drugs. It is recommended that patients who have had immediate hypersensitivity reactions (e.g., anaphylactic or urticarial) to penicillins and/or cephalosporins should be followed with special care. If an allergic reaction to aztreonam occurs, discontinue the drug and institute supportive treatment as appropriate (e.g., maintenance of ventilation, pressor amines, antihistamines, corticosteroids). Serious hypersensitivity reactions may require epinephrine and other emergency measures.

PRECAUTIONS

General

In patients with impaired hepatic or renal function, appropriate monitoring is recommended during therapy.

If an aminoglycoside is used concurrently with aztreonam, especially if high dosages of the former are used or if therapy is prolonged, renal function should be monitored because of the potential nephrotoxicity and ototoxicity of aminoglycoside antibiotics.

The use of antibiotics may promote the overgrowth of non-susceptible organisms, including gram-positive organisms (*Staphylococcus aureus* and *Streptococcus faecalis*) and fungi. Should superinfection occur during therapy, appropriate measures should be taken.

Carcinogenesis, Mutagenesis, Impairment of Fertility

Carcinogenicity studies in animals have not been performed. Genetic toxicology studies performed *in vivo* and *in vitro* with aztreonam in several standard laboratory models revealed no evidence of mutagenic potential at the chromosomal or gene level.

Two-generation reproduction studies in rats at daily doses up to 20 times the maximum recommended human dose, prior to and during gestation and lactation, revealed no evidence of impaired fertility. There was a slightly reduced survival rate during the lactation period in the offspring of rats that received the highest dosage, but not in offspring of rats that received five times the maximum recommended human dose.

Pregnancy

Pregnancy Category B

Aztreonam crosses the placenta and enters the fetal circulation.

Studies in pregnant rats and rabbits, with daily doses up to 15 and 5 times, respectively, the maximum recommended human dose, revealed no evidence of embryo- or fetotoxicity or teratogenicity. No drug induced changes were seen in any of the maternal, fetal, or neonatal parameters that were monitored in rats receiving 15 times the maximum recommended human dose of aztreonam during late gestation and lactation.

There are no adequate and well-controlled studies in pregnant women. Because animal reproduction studies are not always predictive of human response, aztreonam should be used during pregnancy only if clearly needed.

Nursing Mothers

Aztreonam is excreted in breast milk in concentrations that are less than 1 percent of concentrations determined in simultaneously obtained maternal serum; consideration should be given to temporary discontinuation of nursing and use of formula feedings.

Pediatric Use

Safety and effectiveness have not been established in infants and children.

ADVERSE REACTIONS

Local reactions such as phlebitis/thrombophlebitis following IV administration, and discomfort/swelling at the injection site following IM administration, occurred at rates of approximately 1.9 percent and 2.4 percent, respectively.

Systemic reactions (considered to be related to therapy or of uncertain etiology) occurring at an incidence of 1 to 1.3 percent include diarrhea, nausea and/or vomiting, and rash. Reactions occurring at an incidence of less than 1 percent are listed within each body system in order of decreasing severity:

Hypersensitivity —anaphylaxis.

Hematologic —pancytopenia, neutropenia, thrombocytopenia, anemia, leukocytosis, thrombocytosis.

Gastrointestinal —abdominal cramps; rare cases of *C. difficile*-associated diarrhea, including pseudomembranous colitis, or gastrointestinal bleeding have been reported.

Dermatologic —purpura, erythema multiforme, urticaria, exfoliative dermatitis, petechiae, pruritus, diaphoresis.

Cardiovascular —hypotension, transient ECG changes (ventricular bigeminy and PVC).

Respiratory —one patient experienced flushing, chest pain, and dyspnea.

Hepatobiliary —hepatitis, jaundice.

Nervous System —seizure, confusion, vertigo, paresthesia, insomnia, dizziness.

Musculoskeletal —muscular aches.

Special Senses —tinnitus, diplopia, mouth ulcer, altered taste, numb tongue, sneezing and nasal congestion, halitosis.

Other —vaginal candidiasis, vaginitis, breast tenderness.

Body as a Whole —weakness, headache, fever, malaise.

Adverse Laboratory Changes

Adverse laboratory changes without regard to drug relationship that were reported during clinical trials were:

Hepatic —elevations of AST (SGOT), ALT (SGPT), and alkaline phosphatase; signs or symptoms of hepatobiliary dysfunction occurred in less than 1 percent of recipients (see above).

Hemic —increases in prothrombin and partial thromboplastin times, eosinophilia, positive Coombs test.

Renal —increases in serum creatinine.

OVERDOSAGE

If necessary, aztreonam may be cleared from the serum by hemodialysis and/or peritoneal dialysis.

DOSAGE AND ADMINISTRATION

AZACTAM (aztreonam) For Injection may be administered intravenously or by intramuscular injection. Dosage and route of administration should be determined by susceptibility of the causative organisms, severity and site of infection, and the condition of the patient.

AZACTAM DOSAGE GUIDE (ADULTS)		
Type of Infection	Dose*	Frequency (hours)
Urinary tract infection	500 mg or 1 g	8 or 12
Moderately severe systemic infection	1 g or 2 g	8 or 12
Severe systemic or life-threatening infections	2 g	6 or 8

* Maximum recommended dose is 8 g per day.

The intravenous route is recommended for patients requiring single doses greater than 1 g or those with bacterial septicemia, localized parenchymal abscess (e.g., intra-abdominal abscess), peritonitis or other severe systemic or life-threatening infections. Because of the serious nature of infections due to *Pseudomonas aeruginosa,* dosage of 2 g every six or eight hours is recommended, at least upon initiation of therapy, in systemic infections caused by this organism.

The duration of therapy depends on the severity of infection. Generally, AZACTAM should be continued for at least 48 hours after the patient becomes asymptomatic or evidence of bacterial eradication has been obtained. Persistent infections may require treatment for several weeks. Doses smaller than those indicated should not be used.

Renal Impairment

Prolonged serum levels of aztreonam may occur in patients with transient or persistent renal insufficiency. Therefore, the dosage of AZACTAM should be halved in patients with estimated creatinine clearances between 10 and 30 mL/min/1.73 m^2 after an initial loading dose of 1 g or 2 g. When only the serum creatinine concentration is available, the following formula (based on sex, weight, and age of the patient) may be used to approximate the creatinine clearance (Clcr). The serum creatinine should represent a steady state of renal function.

Males: $\quad$ Clcr = $\dfrac{\text{weight (kg)} \times (140 - \text{age})}{72 \times \text{serum creatinine (mg/dL)}}$

Females: $\quad 0.85 \times$ above value

In patients with severe renal failure (creatinine clearance less than 10 mL/min/1.73 m^2), such as those supported by hemodialysis, the usual dose of 500 mg, 1 g or 2 g should be given initially. The maintenance dose should be one-fourth of the usual initial dose given at the usual fixed interval of 6, 8 or 12 hours. For serious or life-threatening infections, in addition to the maintenance doses, one-eighth of the initial dose should be given after each hemodialysis session.

Dosage In The Elderly

Renal status is a major determinant of dosage in the elderly; these patients in particular may have diminished renal function. Serum creatinine may not be an accurate determinant of renal status. Therefore, as with all antibiotics eliminated by the kidneys, estimates of creatinine clearance should be obtained, and appropriate dosage modifications made if necessary.

Preparation of Parenteral Solutions

General

Upon the addition of the diluent to the container, contents should be shaken **immediately** and **vigorously**. Constituted solutions are not for multiple-dose use; should the entire volume in the container not be used for a single dose, the unused solution must be discarded.

Depending upon the concentration of aztreonam and diluent used, constituted AZACTAM (aztreonam) For Injection yields a colorless to light straw yellow solution which may develop a slight pink tint on standing (potency is not affected). Parenteral drug products should be inspected visually for particulate matter and discoloration whenever solution and container permit.

Admixtures With Other Antibiotics

Intravenous infusion solutions of AZACTAM (Aztreonam For Injection) not exceeding 2% w/v prepared with Sodium Chloride Injection USP 0.9% or Dextrose Injection USP 5%, to which clindamycin phosphate, gentamicin sulfate, tobramycin sulfate, or cefazolin sodium have been added at concentrations usually used clinically, are stable for up to 48 hours at room temperature or seven days under refrigeration. Ampicillin sodium admixtures with aztreonam in Sodium Chloride Injection USP 0.9% are stable for 24 hours at room temperature and 48 hours under refrigeration; stability in Dextrose Injection USP 5% is two hours at room temperature and eight hours under refrigeration.

Aztreonam-cloxacillin sodium and aztreonam-vancomycin hydrochloride admixtures are stable in Dianeal® 137 (Peritoneal Dialysis Solution) with 4.25% Dextrose for up to 24 hours at room temperature.

Aztreonam is incompatible with nafcillin sodium, cephradine, and metronidazole.

Other admixtures are not recommended since compatibility data are not available.

Intravenous (IV) Solutions

For Bolus Injection: The contents of an AZACTAM (aztreonam) For Injection 15 mL or 30mL capacity vial should be constituted with 6 to 10 mL Sterile Water for Injection USP.

For Infusion: Contents of the 100 mL capacity bottle should be constituted to a final concentration not exceeding 2 percent w/v (at least 50 mL of any appropriate infusion solution listed below per gram aztreonam). These solutions may be frozen immediately after constitution in the original container (see Stability below).

If the contents of a 15 mL or 30 mL capacity vial are to be transferred to an appropriate infusion solution, each gram of aztreonam should be initially constituted with at least 3 mL Sterile Water for Injection USP. Further dilution may be obtained with one of the following intravenous infusion solutions:

Sodium Chloride Injection USP, 0.9%
Ringer's Injection USP
Lactated Ringer's Injection USP
Dextrose Injection USP, 5% or 10%
Dextrose and Sodium Chloride Injection USP, (5%:0.9%), (5%:0.45%) or (5%:0.2%)
Sodium Lactate Injection USP (M/6 Sodium Lactate)
Ionosol® B and 5% Dextrose
Isolyte® E
Isolyte® E with 5% Dextrose
Isolyte® M with 5% Dextrose
Normosol®-R
Normosol®-R and 5% Dextrose
Normosol®-M and 5% Dextrose
Mannitol Injection USP, 5% or 10%
Lactated Ringer's and 5% Dextrose Injection
Plasma-Lyte® M and 5% Dextrose
10% Travert® Injection
10% Travert® and Electrolyte No. 1 Injection
10% Travert® and Electrolyte No. 2 Injection
10% Travert® and Electrolyte No. 3 Injection

Intramuscular (IM) Solutions

The contents of an AZACTAM (aztreonam) For Injection 15 mL or 30 mL capacity vial should be constituted with at least 3 mL of an appropriate diluent per gram aztreonam. The following diluents may be used:

Sterile Water for Injection USP
Bacteriostatic Water for Injection USP (with benzyl alcohol or with methyl- and propylparabens)
Sodium Chloride Injection USP, 0.9%
Bacteriostatic Sodium Chloride Injection USP (with benzyl alcohol)

Stability of IV And IM Solutions

AZACTAM (aztreonam) solutions for IV infusion at concentrations not exceeding 2% w/v, must be used within 48 hours following constitution if kept at controlled room temperature (59°–86°F/15°–30°C) or within seven days if refrigerated (36°–46°F/2°–8°C).

Frozen aztreonam infusion solution may be stored for up to three months at −4°F/−20°C; frozen solutions may be thawed at controlled room temperature or by overnight refrigeration. Solutions that have been thawed and maintained at controlled room temperature or under refrigeration should be used within 24 or 72 hours after removal from the freezer, respectively. Solutions should not be refrozen.

AZACTAM solutions at concentrations exceeding 2% w/v, except those prepared with Sterile Water for Injection USP or Sodium Chloride Injection USP, should be used promptly after preparation; the two excepted solutions must be used

within 48 hours if stored at controlled room temperature or within seven days if refrigerated.

Intravenous Administration

Bolus Injection: A bolus injection may be used to initiate therapy. The dose should be **slowly** injected directly into the vein, or the tubing of a suitable administration set, over a period of three to five minutes (see next paragraph regarding flushing of tubing).

Infusion: With any intermittent infusion of aztreonam and another drug with which it is not pharmaceutically compatible, the common delivery tube should be flushed before and after delivery of aztreonam with any appropriate infusion solution compatible with both drug solutions; the drugs should not be delivered simultaneously. Any AZACTAM infusion should be completed within a 20 to 60 minute period. With use of a *Y-type administration set,* careful attention should be given to the calculated volume of aztreonam solution required so that the entire dose will be infused. A *volume control administration set* may be used to deliver an initial dilution of AZACTAM (aztreonam) For Injection (see Preparation of Parenteral Solutions, For Infusion) into a compatible infusion solution during administration; in this case, the final dilution of aztreonam should provide a concentration not exceeding 2% w/v.

Intramuscular Administration

The dose should be given by deep injection into a large muscle mass (such as the upper outer quadrant of the gluteus maximus or lateral part of the thigh). Aztreonam is well tolerated and should not be admixed with any local anesthetic agent.

HOW SUPPLIED

AZACTAM For Injection (Aztreonam For Injection)—Lyophilized

Single-dose 15 mL capacity vials:
500 mg/vial: Packages of 10 (NDC 0003-2550-10) and 25 (NDC 0003-2550-15)
1 g/vial: Packages of 10 (NDC 0003-2560-10) and 25 (NDC 0003-2560-15)

Single-dose 30 mL capacity vials:
2 g/vial: Packages of 10 (NDC 0003-2570-10) and 25 (NDC 0003-2570-15)

Single-dose 100 mL capacity intravenous infusion bottles with bail bands:
500 mg/bottle: Packages of 10 (NDC 0003-2550-20)
1 g/bottle: Packages of 10 (NDC 0003-2560-20)
2 g/bottle: Packages of 10 (NDC 0003-2570-20)

Storage
Store original packages at room temperature; avoid excessive heat.
(J4-231A)

AZACTAM®   ℞
Aztreonam Injection
Intravenous Solution

DESCRIPTION

AZACTAM (Aztreonam, Squibb) is the first member of a new class of antibiotics developed by the Squibb Institute for Medical Research and classified as monobactams. These agents were originally isolated from *Chromobacterium violaceum.* AZACTAM is a totally synthetic bactericidal antibiotic with activity against a wide spectrum of gram-negative aerobic pathogens.

The monobactams, having a unique monocyclic beta-lactam nucleus, are structurally different from other beta-lactam antibiotics (e.g., penicillins, cephalosporins, cephamycins). The sulfonic acid substituent in the 1-position of the ring activates the beta-lactam moiety; an aminothiazolyl oxime side chain in the 3-position and a methyl group in the 4-position confer the specific antibacterial spectrum and beta-lactamase stability.

Aztreonam is designated chemically as (Z)-2-[[[(2-amino-4-thiazolyl)[[(2S,3S)-2-methyl -4- oxo -1- sulfo -3- azetidinyl] carbamoyl]methylene]amino]oxy]-2-methylpropionic acid.

AZACTAM (Aztreonam Injection) is a frozen, iso-osmotic, sterile, sodium-free, nonpyrogenic intravenous solution. Each 50 mL of solution contains 500 mg, 1 g, or 2 g aztreonam with approximately 2.3 g, 1.7 g, or 700 mg dextrose hydrous added to adjust osmolality, and approximately 390 mg, 780 mg, or 1.6 g of arginine added for pH adjustment, respectively. Thawed solutions have a pH in the range of 4.5 to 7.5. The solution is for intravenous administration following thawing at room temperature or under refrigeration.

The plastic container is fabricated from a specially formulated polyvinyl chloride (PL 146® Plastic). Solutions in contact with the plastic container can leach out certain of its chemical components in very small amounts within the expiration period, e.g., di-2-ethylhexyl phthalate (DEHP), up to 5 parts per million. The suitability of the plastic has been confirmed in tests in animals according to USP biological tests for plastic containers as well as by tissue culture toxicity studies.

CLINICAL PHARMACOLOGY

Single 30-minute intravenous infusions of 500 mg, 1 g and 2 g doses of AZACTAM in healthy subjects produced peak serum levels of 54, 90 and 204 µg/mL, respectively, immediately after administration; at eight hours, serum levels were 1, 3 and 6 µg/mL, respectively (Figure 1). Single 3-minute intravenous injections of the same doses resulted in serum levels of 58, 125 and 242 µg/mL at five minutes following completion of injection.

Serum concentrations of aztreonam following completion of single intravenous infusions of 500 mg, 1 g, and 2 g doses are depicted in Figure 1.

FIGURE 1

The serum levels of aztreonam following single 500 mg, 1 g or 2 g intravenous doses of AZACTAM (aztreonam) exceed the MIC₉₀ for *Neisseria* sp., *H. influenzae* and most genera of the *Enterobacteriaceae* for eight hours (*Enterobacter* sp., the eight hour serum levels exceed the MIC for 80 percent of strains). For *Ps. aeruginosa,* a single 2 g intravenous dose produces serum levels that exceed the MIC₉₀ for approximately four to six hours. All of the above doses of AZACTAM result in average urine levels of aztreonam that exceed the MIC₉₀ for the same pathogens for up to 12 hours.

The serum half-life of aztreonam averaged 1.7 hours (1.5 to 2.0) in subjects with normal renal function, independent of the dose. In healthy subjects, based on a 70 kg person, the serum clearance was 91 mL/min and renal clearance was 56 mL/min; the apparent mean volume of distribution at steady-state averaged 12.6 liters, approximately equivalent to extracellular fluid volume.

In a study of healthy elderly male subjects (65 to 75 years of age), the average elimination half-life of aztreonam was slightly longer than in young healthy males.

In patients with impaired renal function, the serum half-life of aztreonam is prolonged (see DOSAGE AND ADMINISTRATION, Renal Impairment). The serum half-life of aztreonam is only slightly prolonged in patients with hepatic impairment since the liver is a minor pathway of excretion.

Average urine concentrations of aztreonam were approximately 1100, 3500 and 6600 µg/mL within the first two hours following single 500 mg, 1 g and 2 g intravenous doses of AZACTAM (30-minute infusions), respectively. The range of average concentrations for aztreonam in the 8 to 12 hour urine specimens in these studies was 25 to 120 µg/mL. In healthy subjects, aztreonam is excreted in the urine about equally by active tubular secretion and glomerular filtration. Approximately 60 to 70 percent of an intravenous dose was recovered in the urine by eight hours. Urinary excretion of a single intravenous dose was essentially complete by 12 hours after injection. About 12 percent of a single intravenous radiolabeled dose was recovered in the feces. Unchanged aztreonam and the inactive beta-lactam ring hydrolysis product of aztreonam were present in feces and urine.

Intravenous administration of a single 500 mg or 1 g dose of AZACTAM (aztreonam) every eight hours for seven days to healthy subjects produced no apparent accumulation of aztreonam or modification of its disposition characteristics; serum protein binding averaged 56 percent and was independent of dose.

Renal function was monitored in healthy subjects given aztreonam; standard tests (serum creatinine, creatinine clearance, BUN, urinalysis and total urinary protein excretion) as well as special tests (excretion of N-acetyl-β-glucosaminidase, alanine aminopeptidase and β₂-microglobulin) were used. No abnormal results were obtained. Aztreonam achieves measurable concentrations in the following body fluids and tissues:

[See table on next page]

The concentration of aztreonam in saliva at 30 minutes after a single 1 g intravenous dose (9 patients) was 0.2 µg/mL; in breast milk at two hours after a single 1 g intravenous dose (6 patients), 0.2 µg/mL; in amniotic fluid at six to eight hours after a single 1 g intravenous dose (5 patients), 2 µg/mL. The concentration of aztreonam in peritoneal fluid obtained one

Continued on next page

Squibb—Cont.

to six hours after multiple 2 g intravenous doses ranged between 12 and 90 μg/mL in 7 of 8 patients studied.

Aztreonam given intravenously rapidly reaches therapeutic concentrations in peritoneal dialysis fluid; conversely, aztreonam given intraperitoneally in dialysis fluid rapidly produces therapeutic serum levels.

Concomitant administration of probenecid or furosemide and AZACTAM (aztreonam) causes clinically insignificant increases in the serum levels of aztreonam. Single-dose intravenous pharmacokinetic studies have not shown any significant interaction between aztreonam and concomitantly administered gentamicin, nafcillin sodium, cephradine, clindamycin or metronidazole. No reports of disulfiram-like reactions with alcohol ingestion have been noted; this is not unexpected since aztreonam does not contain a methyl-tetrazole side chain.

The implications of the following information for predicting the occurrence of hypersensitivity reactions to AZACTAM have not been established. The number of patients included in immunologic studies is too small to draw firm conclusions with regard to clinical practice:

A study in rabbits suggests that antibodies produced in response to benzylpenicillin and to cephalothin show little cross-reactivity with aztreonam, and antibodies produced in response to aztreonam show little cross-reactivity with benzylpenicillin and cephalothin.

In a group of 22 subjects with positive skin tests to penicillin reagents, three also had positive skin tests to aztreonam. One was negative on retesting, one was confirmed as positive, and the third subject refused further evaluation. The 20 subjects with negative aztreonam skin tests were given one injection of AZACTAM 1 g IM. There were no immediate hypersensitivity reactions, but one subject later developed a localized rash that was compatible with a fixed drug eruption.

In 36 subjects receiving multiple doses of AZACTAM over a seven-day period, no IgE antibody response was detectable and only one subject demonstrated an IgG response.

Microbiology

Aztreonam exhibits potent and specific activity in vitro against a wide spectrum of gram-negative aerobic pathogens including *Pseudomonas aeruginosa*. The bactericidal action of aztreonam results from the inhibition of bacterial cell wall synthesis due to a high affinity of aztreonam for penicillin binding protein 3 (PBP3). Aztreonam, unlike the majority of beta-lactam antibiotics, does not induce beta-lactamase activity and its molecular structure confers a high degree of resistance to hydrolysis by beta-lactamases (i.e., penicillinases and cephalosporinases) produced by most gram-negative and gram-positive pathogens; it is therefore usually active against gram-negative aerobic organisms that are resistant to antibiotics hydrolyzed by beta-lactamases. Aztreonam maintains its antimicrobial activity over a pH range of 6 to 8 in vitro, as well as in the presence of human serum and under anaerobic conditions. Aztreonam is active in vitro and is effective in laboratory animal models and clinical infec-

tions against most strains of the following organisms, including many that are multiply-resistant to other antibiotics (i.e., certain cephalosporins, penicillins, and aminoglycosides):

Escherichia coli
Enterobacter species
Klebsiella pneumoniae and *K. oxytoca*
Proteus mirabilis
Pseudomonas aeruginosa
Serratia marcescens
Haemophilus influenzae (including ampicillin-resistant and other penicillinase-producing strains)
Citrobacter species

While in vitro studies have demonstrated the susceptibility to aztreonam of most strains of the following organisms, clinical efficacy for infections other than those included in the INDICATIONS AND USAGE section has not been documented:

Neisseria gonorrhoeae (including penicillinase-producing strains)
Proteus vulgaris
Morganella morganii (formerly *Proteus morganii*)
Providencia species, including *P. stuartii* and *P. rettgeri* (formerly *Proteus rettgeri*)
Pseudomonas species
Shigella species
Pasteurella multocida
Yersinia enterocolitica
Aeromonas hydrophila
Neisseria meningitidis

Aztreonam and aminoglycosides have been shown to be synergistic in vitro against most strains of *Ps. aeruginosa*, many strains of *Enterobacteriaceae*, and other gram-negative aerobic bacilli.

Alterations of the anaerobic intestinal flora by broad spectrum antibiotics may decrease colonization resistance, thus permitting overgrowth of potential pathogens, e.g., *Candida* and *Clostridia* species. Aztreonam has little effect on the anaerobic intestinal microflora in in vitro studies. *Clostridium difficile* and its cytotoxin were not found in animal models following administration of aztreonam (see ADVERSE REACTIONS, Gastrointestinal).

Susceptibility Testing

Diffusion Technique: Quantitative procedures that require measurement of zone diameters give precise estimates of microbial susceptibility to antibiotics. One such method, recommended for use with the aztreonam 30 μg disk, is the National Committee of Clinical Laboratory Standards (NCCLS) approved procedure. Only a 30 μg aztreonam disk should be used; there are no suitable surrogate disks.

Results of laboratory tests using 30 μg aztreonam disks should be interpreted using the following criteria:

Zone Diameter (mm)	Interpretation
≥ 22	(S) Susceptible
16–21	(I) Intermediate (Moderate Susceptibility)
≤ 15	(R) Resistant

Dilution Technique: Broth or agar dilution methods may be used to determine the minimal inhibitory concentration (MIC) of aztreonam.

MIC test results should be interpreted according to the concentrations of aztreonam that can be attained in serum, tissues and body fluids.

MIC (μg/mL)	Interpretation
≤ 8	(S) Susceptible
16	(I) Intermediate (Moderate Susceptibility)
≥ 32	(R) Resistant

For any susceptibility test, a report of "susceptible" indicates that the pathogen is likely to respond to AZACTAM therapy; a report of "resistant" indicates that the pathogen is not likely to respond. A report of "intermediate" (moderate susceptibility) indicates that the pathogen is expected to be susceptible to AZACTAM (aztreonam) if high dosages are used, or if the infection is confined to tissues and fluids (e.g., urine, bile) in which high aztreonam levels are attained.

The quality control cultures should have the following assigned daily ranges for aztreonam:

	Disks	Mode MIC (μg/mL)
E. coli (ATCC 25922)	28–36 mm	0.06–0.25
Ps. aeruginosa (ATCC 27853)	23–29 mm	2.0–8.0

INDICATIONS AND USAGE

Before initiating treatment with AZACTAM, appropriate specimens should be obtained for isolation of the causative organism(s) and for determination of susceptibility to aztreonam. Treatment with AZACTAM may be started empirically before results of the susceptibility testing are available; subsequently, appropriate antibiotic therapy should be continued.

AZACTAM (Aztreonam Injection) is indicated for the treatment of the following infections caused by susceptible gram-negative microorganisms:

Urinary Tract Infections (complicated and uncomplicated), including pyelonephritis and cystitis (initial and recurrent) caused by *Escherichia coli, Klebsiella pneumoniae, Proteus mirabilis, Pseudomonas aeruginosa, Enterobacter cloacae, Klebsiella oxytoca*, Citrobacter* species* and *Serratia marcescens**.

Lower Respiratory Tract Infections, including pneumonia and bronchitis caused by *Escherichia coli, Klebsiella pneumoniae, Pseudomonas aeruginosa, Haemophilus influenzae, Proteus mirabilis, Enterobacter* species, and *Serratia marcescens**.

Septicemia caused by *Escherichia coli, Klebsiella pneumoniae, Pseudomonas aeruginosa, Proteus mirabilis*, Serratia marcescens*,* and *Enterobacter* species.

Skin and Skin-Structure Infections, including those associated with post-operative wounds, ulcers, and burns caused by *Escherichia coli, Proteus mirabilis, Serratia marcescens, Enterobacter* species, *Pseudomonas aeruginosa, Klebsiella pneumoniae* and *Citrobacter* species*.

Intra-abdominal Infections, including peritonitis caused by *Escherichia coli, Klebsiella* species including *K. pneumoniae, Enterobacter* species including *E. cloacae*, Pseudomonas aeruginosa, Citrobacter* species* including *C. freundii** and *Serratia* species* including *S. marcescens**.

Gynecologic Infections, including endometritis and pelvic cellulitis caused by *Escherichia coli, Klebsiella pneumoniae*, Enterobacter* species* including *E. cloacae** and *Proteus mirabilis**.

* Efficacy for this organism in this organ system was studied in fewer than ten infections.

AZACTAM (aztreonam) is indicated for adjunctive therapy to surgery in the management of infections caused by susceptible organisms, including abscesses, infections complicating hollow viscus perforations, cutaneous infections and infections of serous surfaces. AZACTAM is effective against most of the commonly encountered gram-negative aerobic pathogens seen in general surgery.

Concurrent Therapy

Concurrent initial therapy with other antimicrobial agents and AZACTAM is recommended before the causative organism(s) is known in seriously ill patients who are also at risk of having an infection due to gram-positive aerobic pathogens. If anaerobic organisms are also suspected as etiologic agents, therapy should be initiated using an anti-anaerobic agent concurrently with AZACTAM (see DOSAGE AND ADMINISTRATION). Certain antibiotics (e.g., cefoxitin, imipenem) may induce high levels of beta-lactamase in vitro in some gram-negative aerobes such as *Enterobacter* and *Pseudomonas* species, resulting in antagonism to many beta-lactam antibiotics including aztreonam. These in vitro findings suggest that such beta-lactamase inducing antibiotics not be used concurrently with aztreonam. Following identification and susceptibility testing of the causative organism(s), appropriate antibiotic therapy should be continued.

CONTRAINDICATIONS

Aztreonam is contraindicated in patients with known allergy to this antibiotic.

WARNINGS

Careful inquiry should be made for a history of hypersensitivity reaction to any antibiotic or other drugs. Antibiotics

EXTRAVASCULAR CONCENTRATIONS OF AZTREONAM AFTER A SINGLE INTRAVENOUS DOSE[1]

Fluid or Tissue	Dose (g)	Route	Hours Post-Injection	Number of Patients	Mean Concentration (μg/mL or μg/g)
Fluids					
bile	1	IV	2	10	39
blister fluid	1	IV	1	6	20
bronchial secretion	2	IV	4	7	5
cerebrospinal fluid (inflamed meninges)	2	IV	0.9–4.3	16	3
pericardial fluid	2	IV	1	6	33
pleural fluid	2	IV	1.1–3.0	3	51
synovial fluid	2	IV	0.8–1.9	11	83
Tissues					
atrial appendage	2	IV	0.9–1.6	12	22
endometrium	2	IV	0.7–1.9	4	9
fallopian tube	2	IV	0.7–1.9	8	12
fat	2	IV	1.3–2.0	10	5
femur	2	IV	1.0–2.1	15	16
gallbladder	2	IV	0.8–1.3	4	23
kidney	2	IV	2.4–5.6	5	67
large intestine	2	IV	0.8–1.9	9	12
liver	2	IV	0.9–2.0	6	47
lung	2	IV	1.2–2.1	6	22
myometrium	2	IV	0.7–1.9	9	11
ovary	2	IV	0.7–1.9	7	13
skeletal muscle	2	IV	0.3–0.7	6	16
skin	2	IV	0.0–1.0	8	25
sternum	2	IV	1	6	6

[1] Tissue penetration is regarded as essential to therapeutic efficacy, but specific tissue levels have not been correlated with specific therapeutic effects.

should be given with caution to any patient who has had some form of allergy, particularly to drugs. It is recommended that patients who have had immediate hypersensitivity reactions (e.g., anaphylactic or urticarial) to penicillins and/or cephalosporins should be followed with special care. If an allergic reaction to aztreonam occurs, discontinue the drug and institute supportive treatment as appropriate (e.g., maintenance of ventilation, pressor amines, antihistamines, corticosteroids). Serious hypersensitivity reactions may require epinephrine and other emergency measures.

PRECAUTIONS

General

In patients with impaired hepatic or renal function, appropriate monitoring is recommended during therapy.

If an aminoglycoside is used concurrently with aztreonam, especially if high dosages of the former are used or if therapy is prolonged, renal function should be monitored because of the potential nephrotoxicity and ototoxicity of aminoglycoside antibiotics.

The use of antibiotics may promote the overgrowth of non-susceptible organisms, including gram-positive organisms (*Staphylococcus aureus* and *Streptococcus faecalis*) and fungi. Should superinfection occur during therapy, appropriate measures should be taken.

Carcinogenesis, Mutagenesis, Impairment of Fertility

Carcinogenicity studies in animals have not been performed. Genetic toxicology studies performed *in vivo* and *in vitro* with aztreonam in several standard laboratory models revealed no evidence of mutagenic potential at the chromosomal or gene level.

Two-generation reproduction studies in rats at daily doses up to 20 times the maximum recommended human dose, prior to and during gestation and lactation, revealed no evidence of impaired fertility. There was a slightly reduced survival rate during the lactation period in the offspring of rats that received the highest dosage, but not in offspring of rats that received five times the maximum recommended human dose.

Pregnancy Category C. Animal reproduction studies have not been conducted with Aztreonam Injection. It is also not known whether Aztreonam Injection can cause fetal harm when administered to a pregnant woman or can affect reproduction capacity. Aztreonam Injection should be given to a pregnant woman only if clearly needed.

Nursing Mothers

Aztreonam is excreted in breast milk in concentrations that are less than 1 percent of concentrations determined in simultaneously obtained maternal serum; consideration should be given to temporary discontinuation of nursing and use of formula feedings.

Pediatric Use

Safety and effectiveness have not been established in infants and children.

ADVERSE REACTIONS

Local reactions (e.g., phlebitis/thrombophlebitis; discomfort/swelling) following IV administration occurred at a rate of approximately 1.9 percent.

Systemic reactions (considered to be related to therapy or of uncertain etiology) occurring at an incidence of 1 to 1.3 percent include diarrhea, nausea and/or vomiting, and rash. Reactions occurring at an incidence of less than 1 percent are listed within each body system in order of decreasing severity:

Hypersensitivity —anaphylaxis.

Hematologic —pancytopenia, neutropenia, thrombocytopenia, anemia, leukocytosis, thrombocytosis.

Gastrointestinal —abdominal cramps; rare cases of *C. difficile*-associated diarrhea, including pseudomembranous colitis, or gastrointestinal bleeding have been reported.

Dermatologic —purpura, erythema multiforme, urticaria, exfoliative dermatitis, petechiae, pruritus, diaphoresis.

Cardiovascular —hypotension, transient ECG changes (ventricular bigeminy and PVC).

Respiratory —one patient experienced flushing, chest pain, and dyspnea.

Hepatobiliary —hepatitis, jaundice.

Nervous System —seizure, confusion, vertigo, paresthesia, insomnia, dizziness.

Musculoskeletal —muscular aches.

Special Senses —tinnitus, diplopia, mouth ulcer, altered taste, numb tongue, sneezing and nasal congestion, halitosis.

Other —vaginal candidiasis, vaginitis, breast tenderness.

Body as a Whole —weakness, headache, fever, malaise.

Adverse Laboratory Changes

Adverse laboratory changes without regard to drug relationship that were reported during clinical trials were:

Hepatic —elevations of AST (SGOT), ALT (SGPT), and alkaline phosphatase; signs or symptoms of hepatobiliary dysfunction occurred in less than 1 percent of recipients (see above).

Hematologic —increases in prothrombin and partial thromboplastin times, eosinophilia, positive Coombs test.

Renal —increases in serum creatinine.

OVERDOSAGE

If necessary, aztreonam may be cleared from the serum by hemodialysis and/or peritoneal dialysis.

DOSAGE AND ADMINISTRATION

AZACTAM (Aztreonam Injection), an intravenous solution in plastic containers, is intended for intravenous use only. Dosage should be determined by susceptibility of the causative organisms, severity and site of infection, and the condition of the patient.

AZACTAM DOSAGE GUIDELINES ADULTS

Type of Infection	Dose*	Frequency (hours)
Urinary tract infections	500 mg or 1 g	8 or 12
Moderately severe systemic infections	1 g or 2 g	8 or 12
Severe systemic or life-threatening infections	2 g	6 or 8

*Maximum recommended dose is 8 g per day.

The intravenous route is recommended for patients with bacterial septicemia, localized parenchymal abscess (e.g., intra-abdominal abscess), peritonitis or other severe systemic or life-threatening infections. Because of the serious nature of infections due to *Pseudomonas aeruginosa*, dosage of 2 g every six or eight hours is recommended, at least upon initiation of therapy, in systemic infections caused by this organism.

The duration of therapy depends on the severity of infection. Generally, AZACTAM should be continued for at least 48 hours after the patient becomes asymptomatic or evidence of bacterial eradication has been obtained. Persistent infections may require treatment for several weeks. Doses smaller than those indicated should not be used.

Renal Impairment

Prolonged serum levels of aztreonam may occur in patients with transient or persistent renal insufficiency. Therefore, the dosage of AZACTAM should be halved in patients with estimated creatinine clearances between 10 and 30 mL/min/1.73 m^2 after an initial loading dose of 1 g or 2 g. When only the serum creatinine concentration is available, the following formula (based on sex, weight, and age of the patient) may be used to approximate the creatinine clearance (Clcr). The serum creatinine should represent a steady state of renal function.

Males: $\quad$ Clcr = $\dfrac{\text{weight (kg)} \times (140 - \text{age})}{72 \times \text{serum creatinine (mg/dL)}}$

Females: $\quad 0.85 \times$ above value

In patients with severe renal failure (creatinine clearance less than 10 mL/min/1.73 m^2), such as those supported by hemodialysis, the usual dose of 500 mg, 1 g or 2 g should be given initially. The maintenance dose should be one-fourth of the usual initial dose given at the usual fixed interval of 6, 8 or 12 hours. For serious or life-threatening infections, in addition to the maintenance doses, one-eighth of the initial dose should be given after each hemodialysis session.

Dosage In The Elderly

Renal status is a major determinant of dosage in the elderly; these patients in particular may have diminished renal function. Serum creatinine may not be an accurate determinant of renal status. Therefore, as with all antibiotics eliminated by the kidneys, estimates of creatinine clearance should be obtained, and appropriate dosage modifications made if necessary.

Directions for Use of AZACTAM (Aztreonam Injection) in Plastic Containers

AZACTAM (Aztreonam Injection) is to be administered as an intermittent intravenous infusion only.

Storage

Use an appropriate storage module in order to avoid unnecessary handling and to prevent surface contact between bags. Store in a freezer capable of maintaining a temperature of −20° C (−4° F).

Thawing of Plastic Containers

Thaw frozen bag at room temperature, 25° C (77° F) or in a refrigerator, 2° to 8° C (36° to 46° F). After thawing is complete, invert the container to assure a well-mixed solution. **(DO NOT FORCE THAW BY IMMERSION IN WATER BATHS OR BY MICROWAVE IRRADIATION.)** Check for minute leaks by squeezing bag firmly. If leaks are detected, discard solution as sterility may be impaired.

The bag should be visually inspected. Thawed solutions should not be used unless clear; solutions will be light yellow to amber in color. Components of the solution may precipitate in the frozen state and will dissolve upon reaching room temperature with little or no agitation. If after visual inspection the solution remains discolored, cloudy, or if an insolu-

ble precipitate is noted or if any seals or outlet parts are not intact, the bag should be discarded.

Additives or other medication should not be added to AZACTAM (Aztreonam Injection) or infused simultaneously through the same intravenous line. If the same intravenous line is used for sequential infusion of several different drugs, it should be flushed before and after infusion of AZACTAM (Aztreonam Injection) with an infusion solution compatible with Aztreonam for Injection* and any other drug(s) administered via this common line.

Use sterile equipment. It is recommended that the intravenous administration apparatus be replaced at least once every 48 hours.

Infusion of AZACTAM (Aztreonam Injection) should be completed within a 20 to 60 minute period. Plastic containers are single-dose units; discard any unused portion remaining in the container.

The thawed solution is stable for either 14 days under refrigeration (2° to 8° C/36° to 46° F) or for 48 hours at room temperature (25° C/77° F). Do not refreeze thawed antibiotics.

CAUTION: Do not use plastic containers in series connections. Such use could result in an embolism due to residual air being drawn from the primary container before administration of the fluid from the secondary container is complete.

Preparation for Administration

a. Suspend container(s) from eyelet support.

b. Remove protector from outlet part at bottom of container.

c. Attach administration set. Refer to complete directions accompanying set.

*The following infusion solutions are compatible with Aztreonam for Injection:

Sodium Chloride Injection USP, 0.9%
Ringer's Injection USP
Lactated Ringer's Injection USP
Dextrose Injection USP, 5% or 10%
Dextrose and Sodium Chloride Injection USP, (5%:0.9%), (5%:0.45%) or (5%:0.2%)
Sodium Lactate Injection USP (M/6 Sodium Lactate)
Ionosol® B and 5% Dextrose
Isolyte® E
Isolyte® E with 5% Dextrose
Isolyte® M with 5% Dextrose
Normosol®-R
Normosol®-R and 5% Dextrose
Normosol®-M and 5% Dextrose
Mannitol Injection USP, 5% or 10%
Lactated Ringer's and 5% Dextrose Injection
Plasma-Lyte® M and 5% Dextrose
10% Travert® Injection
10% Travert® and Electrolyte No. 1 Injection
10% Travert® and Electrolyte No. 2 Injection
10% Travert® and Electrolyte No. 3 Injection

HOW SUPPLIED

AZACTAM (Aztreonam Injection) Intravenous Solution Frozen single-dose 50 mL Viaflex® (PL 146®) plastic containers:

1 g/container: Packages of 24 (NDC 0003-2230-51)
2 g/container: Packages of 24 (NDC 0003-2240-51)
Do not store above −20° C/−4° F [See Directions for Use of AZACTAM (Aztreonam Injection) in Plastic Containers].

AZACTAM and Squibb logo are registered trademarks of E.R. Squibb & Sons, Inc.
VIAFLEX and (PL 146) are registered trademarks of Baxter International, Inc.
Aztreonam Injection is manufactured to SQUIBB specifications by

Baxter Healthcare Corporation
Deerfield, IL 60015
for
E. R. Squibb & Sons, Inc.
Princeton, NJ 08540

(J4-269BB)

CAPOTEN® TABLETS   ℞
[*kap 'o-ten "*]
Captopril Tablets

DESCRIPTION

CAPOTEN (captopril) is the first of a new class of antihypertensive agents, a specific competitive inhibitor of angiotensin I-converting enzyme (ACE), the enzyme responsible for the conversion of angiotensin I to angiotensin II. Captopril is also effective in the management of heart failure.

CAPOTEN (captopril) is designated chemically as 1-[(2S)-3-mercapto-2-methylpropionyl]-L-proline [MW 217.29]. Captopril is a white to off-white crystalline powder that may have a slight sulfurous odor; it is soluble in water (approx. 160 mg/mL), methanol, and ethanol and sparingly soluble in chloroform and ethyl acetate.

CAPOTEN (captopril) is available in potencies of 12.5 mg, 25 mg, 50 mg, and 100 mg as scored tablets for oral administra-

Continued on next page

Squibb—Cont.

tion. Inactive ingredients: microcrystalline cellulose, corn starch, lactose, and stearic acid.

CLINICAL PHARMACOLOGY

Mechanism of Action

The mechanism of action of CAPOTEN (captopril) has not yet been fully elucidated. Its beneficial effects in hypertension and heart failure appear to result primarily from suppression of the renin-angiotensin-aldosterone system. However, there is no consistent correlation between renin levels and response to the drug. Renin, an enzyme synthesized by the kidneys, is released into the circulation where it acts on a plasma globulin substrate to produce angiotensin I, a relatively inactive decapeptide. Angiotensin I is then converted by angiotensin converting enzyme (ACE) to angiotensin II, a potent endogenous vasoconstrictor substance. Angiotensin II also stimulates aldosterone secretion from the adrenal cortex, thereby contributing to sodium and fluid retention. CAPOTEN (captopril) prevents the conversion of angiotensin I to angiotensin II by inhibition of ACE, a peptidyldipeptide carboxy hydrolase. This inhibition has been demonstrated in both healthy human subjects and in animals by showing that the elevation of blood pressure caused by exogenously administered angiotensin I was attenuated or abolished by captopril. In animal studies, captopril did not alter the pressor responses to a number of other agents, including angiotensin II and norepinephrine, indicating specificity of action.

ACE is identical to "bradykininase," and CAPOTEN (captopril) may also interfere with the degradation of the vasodepressor peptide, bradykinin. Increased concentrations of bradykinin or prostaglandin E_2 may also have a role in the therapeutic effect of CAPOTEN.

Inhibition of ACE results in decreased plasma angiotensin II and increased plasma renin activity (PRA), the latter resulting from loss of negative feedback on renin release caused by reduction in angiotensin II. The reduction of angiotensin II leads to decreased aldosterone secretion, and, as a result, small increases in serum potassium may occur along with sodium and fluid loss.

The antihypertensive effects persist for a longer period of time than does demonstrable inhibition of circulating ACE. It is not known whether the ACE present in vascular endothelium is inhibited longer than the ACE in circulating blood.

Pharmacokinetics

After oral administration of therapeutic doses of CAPOTEN (captopril), rapid absorption occurs with peak blood levels at about one hour. The presence of food in the gastrointestinal tract reduces absorption by about 30 to 40 percent; captopril therefore should be given one hour before meals. Based on carbon-14 labeling, average minimal absorption is approximately 75 percent. In a 24-hour period, over 95 percent of the absorbed dose is eliminated in the urine; 40 to 50 percent is unchanged drug; most of the remainder is the disulfide dimer of captopril and captopril-cysteine disulfide.

Approximately 25 to 30 percent of the circulating drug is bound to plasma proteins. The apparent elimination half-life for total radioactivity in blood is probably less than 3 hours. An accurate determination of half-life of unchanged captopril is not, at present, possible, but it is probably less than 2 hours. In patients with renal impairment, however, retention of captopril occurs (see DOSAGE AND ADMINISTRATION).

Pharmacodynamics

Administration of CAPOTEN (captopril) results in a reduction of peripheral arterial resistance in hypertensive patients with either no change, or an increase, in cardiac output. There is an increase in renal blood flow following administration of CAPOTEN (captopril) and glomerular filtration rate is usually unchanged.

Reductions of blood pressure are usually maximal 60 to 90 minutes after oral administration of an individual dose of CAPOTEN (captopril). The duration of effect is dose related. The reduction in blood pressure may be progressive, so to achieve maximal therapeutic effects, several weeks of therapy may be required. The blood pressure lowering effects of captopril and thiazide-type diuretics are additive. In contrast, captopril and beta-blockers have a less than additive effect.

Blood pressure is lowered to about the same extent in both standing and supine positions. Orthostatic effects and tachycardia are infrequent but may occur in volume-depleted patients. Abrupt withdrawal of CAPOTEN has not been associated with a rapid increase in blood pressure.

In patients with heart failure, significantly decreased peripheral (systemic vascular) resistance and blood pressure (afterload), reduced pulmonary capillary wedge pressure (preload) and pulmonary vascular resistance, increased cardiac output, and increased exercise tolerance time (ETT) have been demonstrated. These hemodynamic and clinical effects occur after the first dose and appear to persist for the duration of therapy. Placebo controlled studies of 12 weeks

duration in patients who did not respond adequately to diuretics and digitalis show no tolerance to beneficial effects on ETT; open studies, with exposure up to 18 months in some cases, also indicate that ETT benefit is maintained. Clinical improvement has been observed in some patients where acute hemodynamic effects were minimal.

Studies in rats and cats indicate that CAPOTEN (captopril) does not cross the blood-brain barrier to any significant extent.

INDICATIONS AND USAGE

Hypertension: CAPOTEN (captopril) is indicated for the treatment of hypertension.

In using CAPOTEN, consideration should be given to the risk of neutropenia/agranulocytosis (see WARNINGS).

CAPOTEN may be used as initial therapy for patients with normal renal function, in whom the risk is relatively low. In patients with impaired renal function, particularly those with collagen vascular disease, captopril should be reserved for hypertensives who have either developed unacceptable side effects on other drugs, or have failed to respond satisfactorily to drug combinations.

CAPOTEN is effective alone and in combination with other antihypertensive agents, especially thiazide-type diuretics. The blood pressure lowering effects of captopril and thiazides are approximately additive.

Heart Failure: CAPOTEN is indicated in the treatment of congestive heart failure in patients who have not responded adequately to treatment with diuretics and digitalis. Although the beneficial effect of captopril in heart failure does not require the presence of digitalis, most controlled clinical trial experience with captopril has been in patients receiving digitalis, as well as diuretic treatment. Consequently, CAPOTEN should generally be added to both of these agents except when digitalis use is poorly tolerated or otherwise not feasible.

CONTRAINDICATIONS

CAPOTEN is contraindicated in patients who are hypersensitive to this product.

WARNINGS

Angioedema

Angioedema involving the extremities, face, lips, mucous membranes, tongue, glottis or larynx has been seen in patients treated with ACE inhibitors, including captopril. If angioedema involves the tongue, glottis or larynx, airway obstruction may occur and be fatal. Emergency therapy, including but not necessarily limited to, subcutaneous administration of a 1:1000 solution of epinephrine should be promptly instituted.

Swelling confined to the face, mucous membranes of the mouth, lips and extremities has usually resolved with discontinuation of captopril; some cases required medical therapy. (See PRECAUTIONS: Information for Patients and ADVERSE REACTIONS.)

Neutropenia/Agranulocytosis

Neutropenia ($<1000/mm^3$) with myeloid hypoplasia has resulted from use of captopril. About half of the neutropenic patients developed systemic or oral cavity infections or other features of the syndrome of agranulocytosis.

The risk of neutropenia is dependent on the clinical status of the patient:

In clinical trials in patients with hypertension who have normal renal function (serum creatinine less than 1.6 mg/dL and no collagen vascular disease), neutropenia has been seen in one patient out of over 8,600 exposed.

In patients with some degree of renal failure (serum creatinine at least 1.6 mg/dL) but no collagen vascular disease, the risk of neutropenia in clinical trials was about 1 per 500, a frequency over 15 times that for uncomplicated hypertension. Daily doses of captopril were relatively high in these patients, particularly in view of their diminished renal function. In foreign marketing experience in patients with renal failure, use of allopurinol concomitantly with captopril has been associated with neutropenia but this association has not appeared in U.S. reports.

In patients with collagen vascular diseases (e.g., systemic lupus erythematosus, scleroderma) and impaired renal function, neutropenia occurred in 3.7 percent of patients in clinical trials.

While none of the over 750 patients in formal clinical trials of heart failure developed neutropenia, it has occurred during the subsequent clinical experience. About half of the reported cases had serum creatinine $\geq$ 1.6 mg/dL and more than 75 percent were in patients also receiving procainamide. In heart failure, it appears that the same risk factors for neutropenia are present.

The neutropenia has usually been detected within three months after captopril was started. Bone marrow examinations in patients with neutropenia consistently showed myeloid hypoplasia, frequently accompanied by erythroid hypoplasia and decreased numbers of megakaryocytes (e.g., hypoplastic bone marrow and pancytopenia); anemia and thrombocytopenia were sometimes seen.

In general, neutrophils returned to normal in about two weeks after captopril was discontinued, and serious infections were limited to clinically complex patients. About 13 percent of the cases of neutropenia have ended fatally, but almost all fatalities were in patients with serious illness, having collagen vascular disease, renal failure, heart failure or immunosuppressant therapy, or a combination of these complicating factors.

Evaluation of the hypertensive or heart failure patient should always include assessment of renal function.

If captopril is used in patients with impaired renal function, white blood cell and differential counts should be evaluated prior to starting treatment and at approximately two-week intervals for about three months, then periodically.

In patients with collagen vascular disease or who are exposed to other drugs known to affect the white cells or immune response, particularly when there is impaired renal function, captopril should be used only after an assessment of benefit and risk, and then with caution.

All patients treated with captopril should be told to report any signs of infection (e.g., sore throat, fever). If infection is suspected, white cell counts should be performed without delay.

Since discontinuation of captopril and other drugs has generally led to prompt return of the white count to normal, upon confirmation of neutropenia (neutrophil count $< 1000/mm^3$) the physician should withdraw captopril and closely follow the patient's course.

Proteinuria

Total urinary proteins greater than 1 g per day were seen in about 0.7 percent of patients receiving captopril. About 90 percent of affected patients had evidence of prior renal disease or received relatively high doses of captopril (in excess of 150 mg/day), or both. The nephrotic syndrome occurred in about one-fifth of proteinuric patients. In most cases, proteinuria subsided or cleared within six months whether or not captopril was continued. Parameters of renal function, such as BUN and creatinine, were seldom altered in the patients with proteinuria.

Since most cases of proteinuria occurred by the eighth month of therapy with captopril, patients with prior renal disease or those receiving captopril at doses greater than 150 mg per day, should have urinary protein estimations (dipstick on first morning urine) prior to treatment, and periodically thereafter.

Hypotension

Excessive hypotension was rarely seen in hypertensive patients but is a possible consequence of captopril use in severely salt/volume depleted persons such as those treated vigorously with diuretics, for example, patients with severe congestive heart failure (see PRECAUTIONS [Drug Interactions]).

In heart failure, where the blood pressure was either normal or low, transient decreases in mean blood pressure greater than 20 percent were recorded in about half of the patients. This transient hypotension may occur after any of the first several doses and is usually well tolerated, producing either no symptoms or brief mild lightheadedness, although in rare instances it has been associated with arrhythmia or conduction defects. Hypotension was the reason for discontinuation of drug in 3.6 percent of patients with heart failure.

BECAUSE OF THE POTENTIAL FALL IN BLOOD PRESSURE IN THESE PATIENTS, THERAPY SHOULD BE STARTED UNDER VERY CLOSE MEDICAL SUPERVISION. A starting dose of 6.25 or 12.5 mg tid may minimize the hypotensive effect. Patients should be followed closely for the first two weeks of treatment and whenever the dose of captopril and/or diuretic is increased.

Hypotension is not *per se* a reason to discontinue captopril. Some decrease of systemic blood pressure is a common and desirable observation upon initiation of CAPOTEN (captopril) treatment in heart failure. The magnitude of the decrease is greatest early in the course of treatment; this effect stabilizes within a week or two, and generally returns to pretreatment levels, without a decrease in therapeutic efficacy, within two months.

PRECAUTIONS

General

Impaired Renal Function

Hypertension—Some patients with renal disease, particularly those with severe renal artery stenosis, have developed increases in BUN and serum creatinine after reduction of blood pressure with captopril. Captopril dosage reduction and/or discontinuation of diuretic may be required. For some of these patients, it may not be possible to normalize blood pressure and maintain adequate renal perfusion.

Heart Failure—About 20 percent of patients develop stable elevations of BUN and serum creatinine greater than 20 percent above normal or baseline upon long-term treatment with captopril. Less than 5 percent of patients, generally those with severe preexisting renal disease, required discontinuation of treatment due to progressively increasing creatinine; subsequent improvement probably depends upon the severity of the underlying renal disease.

See CLINICAL PHARMACOLOGY, DOSAGE AND ADMINISTRATION, ADVERSE REACTIONS [Altered Laboratory Findings].

Valvular Stenosis: There is concern, on theoretical grounds, that patients with aortic stenosis might be at particular risk of decreased coronary perfusion when treated with vasodilators because they do not develop as much afterload reduction as others.

Surgery/Anesthesia: In patients undergoing major surgery or during anesthesia with agents that produce hypotension, captopril will block angiotensin II formation secondary to compensatory renin release. If hypotension occurs and is considered to be due to this mechanism, it can be corrected by volume expansion.

Information for Patients

Patients should be advised to immediately report to their physician any signs or symptoms suggesting angioedema (e.g., swelling of face, eyes, lips, tongue, larynx and extremities; difficulty in swallowing or breathing; hoarseness) and to discontinue therapy. (See WARNINGS.)

Patients should be told to report promptly any indication of infection (e.g., sore throat, fever), which may be a sign of neutropenia, or of progressive edema which might be related to proteinuria and nephrotic syndrome.

All patients should be cautioned that excessive perspiration and dehydration may lead to an excessive fall in blood pressure because of reduction in fluid volume. Other causes of volume depletion such as vomiting or diarrhea may also lead to a fall in blood pressure; patients should be advised to consult with the physician.

Patients should be warned against interruption or discontinuation of medication unless instructed by the physician. Heart failure patients on captopril therapy should be cautioned against rapid increases in physical activity.

Patients should be informed that CAPOTEN (captopril) should be taken one hour before meals (see DOSAGE AND ADMINISTRATION).

Drug Interactions

Hypotension—Patients on Diuretic Therapy: Patients on diuretics and especially those in whom diuretic therapy was recently instituted, as well as those on severe dietary salt restriction or dialysis, may occasionally experience a precipitous reduction of blood pressure usually within the first hour after receiving the initial dose of captopril.

The possibility of hypotensive effects with captopril can be minimized by either discontinuing the diuretic or increasing the salt intake approximately one week prior to initiation of treatment with CAPOTEN (captopril) or initiating therapy with small doses (6.25 or 12.5 mg). Alternatively, provide medical supervision for at least one hour after the initial dose. If hypotension occurs, the patient should be placed in a supine position and, if necessary, receive an intravenous infusion of normal saline. This transient hypotensive response is not a contraindication to further doses which can be given without difficulty once the blood pressure has increased after volume expansion.

Agents Having Vasodilator Activity: Data on the effect of concomitant use of other vasodilators in patients receiving CAPOTEN (captopril) for heart failure are not available; therefore, nitroglycerin or other nitrates (as used for management of angina) or other drugs having vasodilator activity should, if possible, be discontinued before starting CAPOTEN. If resumed during CAPOTEN therapy, such agents should be administered cautiously, and perhaps at lower dosage.

Agents Causing Renin Release: Captopril's effect will be augmented by antihypertensive agents that cause renin release. For example, diuretics (e.g., thiazides) may activate the renin-angiotensin-aldosterone system.

Agents Affecting Sympathetic Activity: The sympathetic nervous system may be especially important in supporting blood pressure in patients receiving captopril alone or with diuretics. Therefore, agents affecting sympathetic activity (e.g., ganglionic blocking agents or adrenergic neuron blocking agents) should be used with caution. Beta-adrenergic blocking drugs add some further antihypertensive effect to captopril, but the overall response is less than additive.

Agents Increasing Serum Potassium: Since captopril decreases aldosterone production, elevation of serum potassium may occur. Potassium-sparing diuretics such as spironolactone, triamterene, or amiloride, or potassium supplements should be given only for documented hypokalemia, and then with caution, since they may lead to a significant increase of serum potassium. Salt substitutes containing potassium should also be used with caution.

Inhibitors Of Endogenous Prostaglandin Synthesis: It has been reported that indomethacin may reduce the antihypertensive effect of captopril, especially in cases of low renin hypertension. Other nonsteroidal anti-inflammatory agents (e.g., aspirin) may also have this effect.

Lithium: Increased serum lithium levels and symptoms of lithium toxicity have been reported in patients receiving concomitant lithium and ACE inhibitor therapy. These drugs should be coadministered with caution and frequent monitoring of serum lithium levels is recommended. If a diuretic is also used, it may increase the risk of lithium toxicity.

Drug/Laboratory Test Interaction

Captopril may cause a false-positive urine test for acetone.

Carcinogenesis, Mutagenesis and Impairment of Fertility

Two-year studies with doses of 50 to 1350 mg/kg/day in mice and rats failed to show any evidence of carcinogenic potential.

Studies in rats have revealed no impairment of fertility.

Animal Toxicology

Chronic oral toxicity studies were conducted in rats (2 years), dogs (47 weeks; 1 year), mice (2 years), and monkeys (1 year). Significant drug related toxicity included effects on hematopoiesis, renal toxicity, erosion/ulceration of the stomach, and variation of retinal blood vessels.

Reductions in hemoglobin and/or hematocrit values were seen in mice, rats, and monkeys at doses 50 to 150 times the maximum recommended human dose (MRHD). Anemia, leukopenia, thrombocytopenia, and bone marrow suppression occurred in dogs at doses 8 to 30 times MRHD. The reductions in hemoglobin and hematocrit values in rats and mice were only significant at 1 year and returned to normal with continued dosing by the end of the study. Marked anemia was seen at all dose levels (8 to 30 times MRHD) in dogs, whereas moderate to marked leukopenia was noted only at 15 and 30 times MRHD and thrombocytopenia at 30 times MRHD. The anemia could be reversed upon discontinuation of dosing. Bone marrow suppression occurred to a varying degree, being associated only with dogs that died or were sacrificed in a moribund condition in the 1 year study. However, in the 47-week study at a dose 30 times MRHD, bone marrow suppression was found to be reversible upon continued drug administration.

Captopril caused hyperplasia of the juxtaglomerular apparatus of the kidneys at doses 7 to 200 times the MRHD in rats and mice, at 20 to 60 times MRHD in monkeys, and at 30 times the MRHD in dogs.

Gastric erosions/ulcerations were increased in incidence at 20 and 200 times MRHD in male rats and at 30 and 65 times MRHD in dogs and monkeys, respectively. Rabbits developed gastric and intestinal ulcers when given oral doses approximately 30 times MRHD for only 5 to 7 days.

In the two-year rat study, irreversible and progressive variations in the caliber of retinal vessels (focal sacculations and constrictions) occurred at all dose levels (7 to 200 times MRHD) in a dose-related fashion. The effect was first observed in the 88th week of dosing, with a progressively increased incidence thereafter, even after cessation of dosing.

Pregnancy: Category C

Captopril was embryocidal in rabbits when given in doses about 2 to 70 times (on a mg/kg basis) the maximum recommended human dose, and low incidences of craniofacial malformations were seen. These effects in rabbits were most probably due to the particularly marked decrease in blood pressure caused by the drug in this species.

Captopril given to pregnant rats at 400 times the recommended human dose continuously during gestation and lactation caused a reduction in neonatal survival.

No teratogenic effects (malformations) have been observed after large doses of captopril in hamsters and rats.

Human Experience: There are no adequate and well-controlled studies of captopril in pregnant women. Data, however, are available that show captopril crosses the human placenta. Because the risk of fetal toxicity with the use of ACE inhibitors has not been defined, captopril should be used during pregnancy only if the potential benefit justifies the potential risk to the fetus.

Based on post-marketing experience with all ACE inhibitors, the following information has been collected with regard to pregnancy outcome. Inadvertent exposure limited to the first trimester of pregnancy does not appear to affect fetal outcome adversely. Fetal exposure during the second and third trimester of pregnancy has been associated with fetal and neonatal morbidity and mortality.

When ACE inhibitors are used during the later stages of pregnancy, there have been reports of hypotension and decreased renal perfusion in the newborn. Oligohydramnios in the mother has also been reported, presumably representing decreased renal function in the fetus. Infants exposed *in utero* to ACE inhibitors should be closely observed for hypotension, oliguria and hyperkalemia. If oliguria occurs, attention should be directed toward support of blood pressure and renal perfusion with the administration of fluids and pressors as appropriate. Problems associated with prematurity such as patent ductus arteriosus have occurred in association with maternal use of ACE inhibitors but it is not clear whether they are related to ACE inhibition, maternal hypertension or the underlying prematurity.

While captopril may be removed from the circulation of adults by hemodialysis, there is no experience with exchange transfusion, hemodialysis or peritoneal dialysis for removing captopril from the neonatal circulation.

Nursing Mothers

Concentrations of captopril in human milk are approximately one percent of those in maternal blood. The effect of low levels of captopril on the nursing infant has not been determined. Caution should be exercised when captopril is administered to a nursing woman, and, in general, nursing should be interrupted.

Pediatric Use

Safety and effectiveness in children have not been established although there is limited experience with the use of captopril in children from 2 months to 15 years of age with secondary hypertension and varying degrees of renal insufficiency. Dosage, on a weight basis, was comparable to that used in adults. CAPOTEN (captopril) should be used in children only if other measures for controlling blood pressure have not been effective.

ADVERSE REACTIONS

Reported incidences are based on clinical trials involving approximately 7000 patients.

Renal—About one of 100 patients developed proteinuria (see WARNINGS).

Each of the following has been reported in approximately 1 to 2 of 1000 patients and are of uncertain relationship to drug use: renal insufficiency, renal failure, polyuria, oliguria, and urinary frequency.

Hematologic—Neutropenia/agranulocytosis has occurred (see WARNINGS). Cases of anemia, thrombocytopenia, and pancytopenia have been reported.

Dermatologic—Rash, often with pruritus, and sometimes with fever, arthralgia, and eosinophilia, occurred in about 4 to 7 (depending on renal status and dose) of 100 patients, usually during the first four weeks of therapy. It is usually maculopapular, and rarely urticarial. The rash is usually mild and disappears within a few days of dosage reduction, short-term treatment with an antihistaminic agent, and/or discontinuing therapy; remission may occur even if captopril is continued. Pruritus, without rash, occurs in about 2 of 100 patients. Between 7 and 10 percent of patients with skin rash have shown an eosinophilia and/or positive ANA titers. A reversible associated pemphigoid-like lesion, and photosensitivity, have also been reported. Flushing or pallor has been reported in 2 to 5 of 1000 patients.

Cardiovascular—Hypotension may occur; see WARNINGS and PRECAUTIONS [Drug Interactions] for discussion of hypotension on initiation of captopril therapy.

Tachycardia, chest pain, and palpitations have each been observed in approximately 1 of 100 patients.

Angina pectoris, myocardial infarction, Raynaud's syndrome, and congestive heart failure have each occurred in 2 to 3 of 1000 patients.

Dysgeusia—Approximately 2 to 4 (depending on renal status and dose) of 100 patients developed a diminution or loss of taste perception. Taste impairment is reversible and usually self-limited (2 to 3 months) even with continued drug administration. Weight loss may be associated with the loss of taste.

Angioedema—Angioedema involving the extremities, face, lips, mucous membranes, tongue, glottis or larynx has been reported in approximately one in 1000 patients. Angioedema involving the upper airways has caused fatal airway obstruction. (See WARNINGS and PRECAUTIONS: Information for patients.)

The following have been reported in about 0.5 to 2 percent of patients but did not appear at increased frequency compared to placebo or other treatments used in controlled trials; gastric irritation, abdominal pain, nausea, vomiting, diarrhea, anorexia, constipation, aphthous ulcers, peptic ulcer, dizziness, headache, malaise, fatigue, insomnia, dry mouth, dyspnea, cough, alopecia, paresthesias.

Other clinical adverse effects reported since the drug was marketed are listed below by body system. In this setting, an incidence or causal relationship cannot be accurately determined.

General: Asthenia, gynecomastia.
Cardiovascular: Cardiac arrest, cerebrovascular accident, syncope.
Dermatologic: Bullous pemphigus.
Gastrointestinal: Pancreatitis, glossitis.
Hematologic: Anemia, including aplastic and hemolytic.
Hepatobiliary: Hepatitis, including rare cases of necrosis, cholestasis.
Metabolic: Symptomatic hyponatremia.
Musculoskeletal: Myalgia, myasthenia.
Nervous/Psychiatric: Ataxia, confusion, depression, nervousness, somnolence.
Respiratory: Bronchospasm, eosinophilic pneumonitis, rhinitis.
Special Senses: Blurred vision.
Urogenital: Impotence.

As with other ACE inhibitors, a syndrome has been reported which includes: fever, myalgia, arthralgia, rash or other dermatologic manifestations, eosinophilia and an elevated ESR. Findings have usually resolved with discontinuation of treatment.

Continued on next page

Squibb—Cont.

Altered Laboratory Findings

Serum Electrolytes: Hyperkalemia: small increases in serum potassium, especially in patients with renal impairment (see PRECAUTIONS).

Hyponatremia: particularly in patients receiving a low sodium diet or concomitant diuretics.

BUN/Serum Creatinine: Transient elevations of BUN or serum creatinine especially in volume or salt depleted patients or those with renovascular hypertension may occur. Rapid reduction of longstanding or markedly elevated blood pressure can result in decreases in the glomerular filtration rate and, in turn, lead to increases in BUN or serum creatinine.

Hematologic: A positive ANA has been reported.

Liver Function Tests: Elevations of liver transaminases, alkaline phosphatase, and serum bilirubin have occurred.

OVERDOSAGE

Correction of hypotension would be of primary concern. Volume expansion with an intravenous infusion of normal saline is the treatment of choice for restoration of blood pressure.

Captopril may be removed from the general circulation by hemodialysis.

DOSAGE AND ADMINISTRATION

CAPOTEN (captopril) should be taken one hour before meals. Dosage must be individualized.

Hypertension—Initiation of therapy requires consideration of recent antihypertensive drug treatment, the extent of blood pressure elevation, salt restriction, and other clinical circumstances. If possible, discontinue the patient's previous antihypertensive drug regimen for one week before starting CAPOTEN.

The initial dose of CAPOTEN (captopril) is 25 mg bid or tid. If satisfactory reduction of blood pressure has not been achieved after one or two weeks, the dose may be increased to 50 mg bid or tid. Concomitant sodium restriction may be beneficial when CAPOTEN is used alone.

The dose of CAPOTEN in hypertension usually does not exceed 50 mg tid. Therefore, if the blood pressure has not been satisfactorily controlled after one to two weeks at this dose (and the patient is not already receiving a diuretic), a modest dose of a thiazide-type diuretic (e.g., hydrochlorothiazide, 25 mg daily) should be added. The diuretic dose may be increased at one- to two-week intervals until its highest usual antihypertensive dose is reached.

If CAPOTEN (captopril) is being started in a patient already receiving a diuretic, CAPOTEN therapy should be initiated under close medical supervision (see WARNINGS and PRECAUTIONS [Drug Interactions] regarding hypotension), with dosage and titration of CAPOTEN as noted above.

If further blood pressure reduction is required, the dose of CAPOTEN may be increased to 100 mg bid or tid and then, if necessary, to 150 mg bid or tid (while continuing the diuretic). The usual dose range is 25 to 150 mg bid or tid. A maximum daily dose of 450 mg CAPOTEN should not be exceeded.

For patients with severe hypertension (e.g., accelerated or malignant hypertension), when temporary discontinuation of current antihypertensive therapy is not practical or desirable, or when prompt titration to more normotensive blood pressure levels is indicated, diuretic should be continued but other current antihypertensive medication stopped and CAPOTEN dosage promptly initiated at 25 mg bid or tid, under close medical supervision.

When necessitated by the patient's clinical condition, the daily dose of CAPOTEN may be increased every 24 hours or less under continuous medical supervision until a satisfactory blood pressure response is obtained or the maximum dose of CAPOTEN (captopril) is reached. In this regimen, addition of a more potent diuretic, e.g., furosemide, may also be indicated.

Beta-blockers may also be used in conjunction with CAPOTEN therapy (see PRECAUTIONS [Drug Interactions]), but the effects of the two drugs are less than additive.

Heart Failure—Initiation of therapy requires consideration of recent diuretic therapy and the possibility of severe salt/volume depletion. In patients with either normal or low blood pressure, who have been vigorously treated with diuretics and who may be hyponatremic and/or hypovolemic, a starting dose of 6.25 or 12.5 mg tid may minimize the magnitude or duration of the hypotensive effect (see WARNINGS, [Hypotension]); for these patients, titration to the usual daily dosage can then occur within the next several days.

For most patients the usual initial daily dosage is 25 mg tid. After a dose of 50 mg tid is reached, further increases in dosage should be delayed, where possible, for at least two weeks to determine if a satisfactory response occurs. Most patients studied have had a satisfactory clinical improvement at 50 or 100 mg tid. A maximum daily dose of 450 mg of CAPOTEN (captopril) should not be exceeded.

CAPOTEN should generally be used in conjunction with a diuretic and digitalis. CAPOTEN therapy must be initiated under very close medical supervision.

Dosage Adjustment in Renal Impairment—Because CAPOTEN (captopril) is excreted primarily by the kidneys, excretion rates are reduced in patients with impaired renal function. These patients will take longer to reach steady-state captopril levels and will reach higher steady-state levels for a given daily dose than patients with normal renal function. Therefore, these patients may respond to smaller or less frequent doses.

Accordingly, for patients with significant renal impairment, initial daily dosage of CAPOTEN (captopril) should be reduced, and smaller increments utilized for titration, which should be quite slow (one- to two-week intervals). After the desired therapeutic effect has been achieved, the dose should be slowly back-titrated to determine the minimal effective dose. When concomitant diuretic therapy is required, a loop diuretic (e.g., furosemide), rather than a thiazide diuretic, is preferred in patients with severe renal impairment.

HOW SUPPLIED

12.5 mg tablets in bottles of 100 (NDC 0003-0450-54) and 1000 (NDC 0003-0450-75), **25 mg tablets** in bottles of 100 (NDC 0003-0452-50) and 1000 (DCN 0003-0452-75), **50 mg tablets** in bottles of 100 (NDC 0003-0482-50) and 1000 (NDC 0003-0482-75), and **100 mg tablets** in bottles of 100 (NDC 0003-0485-50). Bottles contain a desiccant-charcoal canister. Unimatic® unit-dose packs containing 100 tablets are also available for each potency: **12.5 mg** (NDC 0003-0450-51), **25 mg,** (NDC 0003-0452-51), **50 mg,** (NDC 0003-0482-51), and **100 mg** (NDC 0003-0485-51).

The **12.5 mg tablet** is a flat oval with a partial bisect bar; the **25 mg tablet** is a biconvex rounded square with a quadrisect bar; the **50 and 100 mg tablets** are biconvex ovals with a bisect bar.

All captopril tablets are white and may exhibit a slight sulfurous odor. Tablet identification numbers: **12.5 mg,** 450; **25 mg,** 452; **50 mg,** 482; and **100 mg,** 485.

Storage

Do not store above 86°F. Keep bottles tightly closed (protect from moisture).

(J3-658R)

Shown in Product Identification Section, page 431

CAPOZIDE® 25/15   ℞
CAPOZIDE® 25/25   ℞
CAPOZIDE® 50/15   ℞
CAPOZIDE® 50/25   ℞

[*kap'o-zīd"*]

Captopril-Hydrochlorothiazide Tablets

DESCRIPTION

CAPOZIDE (Captopril-Hydrochlorothiazide Tablets) for oral administration combines two antihypertensive agents: CAPOTEN® (captopril) and hydrochlorothiazide. Captopril, the first of a new class of antihypertensive agents, is a specific competitive inhibitor of angiotensin I-converting enzyme (ACE), the enzyme responsible for the conversion of angiotensin I to angiotensin II. Hydrochlorothiazide is a benzothiadiazide (thiazide) diuretic-antihypertensive.

CAPOZIDE tablets are available in four combinations of captopril with hydrochlorothiazide: 25 mg with 15 mg, 25 mg with 25 mg, 50 mg with 15 mg, and 50 mg with 25 mg. Inactive ingredients: microcrystalline cellulose, colorant (FD&C Yellow No. 6), lactose, magnesium stearate, pregelatinized starch, and stearic acid.

Captopril is designated chemically as 1-[(2S)-3-mercapto-2-methylpropionyl]-L-proline; hydrochlorothiazide is 6-Chloro-3,4-dihydro-2H-1, 2, 4-benzothiadiazine-7-sulfonamide 1,1-dioxide.

Captopril is a white to off-white crystalline powder that may have a slight sulfurous odor; it is soluble in water (approx. 160 mg/mL), methanol, and ethanol and sparingly soluble in chloroform and ethyl acetate.

Hydrochlorothiazide is a white crystalline powder slightly soluble in water but freely soluble in sodium hydroxide solution.

CLINICAL PHARMACOLOGY

Captopril

Mechanism of Action

The mechanism of action of captopril has not yet been fully elucidated. Its beneficial effects in hypertension and heart failure appear to result primarily from suppression of the renin-angiotensin-aldosterone system. However, there is no consistent correlation between renin levels and response to the drug. Renin, an enzyme synthesized by the kidneys, is released into the circulation where it acts on a plasma globulin substrate to produce angiotensin I, a relatively inactive decapeptide. Angiotensin I is then converted by angiotensin converting enzyme (ACE) to angiotensin II, a potent endogenous vasoconstrictor substance. Angiotensin II also stimulates aldosterone secretion from the adrenal cortex, thereby contributing to sodium and fluid retention.

Captopril prevents the conversion of angiotensin I to angiotensin II by inhibition of ACE, a peptidyldipeptide carboxy hydrolase. This inhibition has been demonstrated in both healthy human subjects and in animals by showing that the elevation of blood pressure caused by exogenously administered angiotensin I was attenuated or abolished by captopril. In animal studies, captopril did not alter the pressor responses to a number of other agents, including angiotensin II and norepinephrine, indicating specificity of action.

ACE is identical to "bradykininase" and captopril may also interfere with the degradation of the vasodepressor peptide, bradykinin. Increased concentrations of bradykinin or prostaglandin E_2 may also have a role in the therapeutic effect of captopril.

Inhibition of ACE results in decreased plasma angiotensin II and increased plasma renin activity (PRA), the latter resulting from loss of negative feedback on renin release caused by reduction in angiotensin II. The reduction of angiotensin II leads to decreased aldosterone secretion, and, as a result, small increases in serum potassium may occur along with sodium and fluid loss.

The antihypertensive effects persist for a longer period of time than does demonstrable inhibition of circulating ACE. It is not known whether the ACE present in vascular endothelium is inhibited longer than the ACE in circulating blood.

Pharmacokinetics

After oral administration of therapeutic doses of captopril, rapid absorption occurs with peak blood levels at about one hour. The presence of food in the gastrointestinal tract reduces absorption by about 30 to 40 percent; captopril therefore should be given one hour before meals. Based on carbon-14 labeling, average minimal absorption is approximately 75 percent. In a 24-hour period, over 95 percent of the absorbed dose is eliminated in the urine; 40 to 50 percent is unchanged drug; most of the remainder is the disulfide dimer of captopril and captopril-cysteine disulfide.

Approximately 25 to 30 percent of the circulating drug is bound to plasma proteins. The apparent elimination half-life for total radioactivity in blood is probably less than three hours. An accurate determination of half-life of unchanged captopril is not, at present, possible, but it is probably less than two hours. In patients with renal impairment, however, retention of captopril occurs (see DOSAGE AND ADMINISTRATION).

Pharmacodynamics

Administration of captopril results in a reduction of peripheral arterial resistance in hypertensive patients with either no change, or an increase, in cardiac output. There is an increase in renal blood flow following administration of captopril and glomerular filtration rate is usually unchanged. In patients with heart failure, significantly decreased peripheral (systemic vascular) resistance and blood pressure (afterload), reduced pulmonary capillary wedge pressure (preload) and pulmonary vascular resistance, increased cardiac output, and increased exercise tolerance time (ETT) have been demonstrated.

Reductions of blood pressure are usually maximal 60 to 90 minutes after oral administration of an individual dose of captopril. The duration of effect is dose related. The reduction in blood pressure may be progressive, so to achieve maximal therapeutic effects, several weeks of therapy may be required. The blood pressure lowering effects of captopril and thiazide-type diuretics are additive. In contrast, captopril and beta-blockers have a less than additive effect.

Blood pressure is lowered to about the same extent in both standing and supine positions. Orthostatic effects and tachycardia are infrequent but may occur in volume-depleted patients. Abrupt withdrawal of captopril has not been associated with a rapid increase in blood pressure.

Studies in rats and cats indicate that captopril does not cross the blood-brain barrier to any significant extent.

Hydrochlorothiazide

Thiazides affect the renal tubular mechanism of electrolyte reabsorption. At maximal therapeutic dosage all thiazides are approximately equal in their diuretic potency.

Thiazides increase excretion of sodium and chloride in approximately equivalent amounts. Natriuresis causes a secondary loss of potassium and bicarbonate.

The mechanism of the antihypertensive effect of thiazides is unknown. Thiazides do not affect normal blood pressure.

The mean plasma half-life of hydrochlorothiazide in fasted individuals has been reported to be approximately 2.5 hours. Onset of diuresis occurs in two hours and the peak effect at about four hours. Its action persists for approximately six to twelve hours. Hydrochlorothiazide is eliminated rapidly by the kidney.

INDICATIONS AND USAGE

CAPOZIDE (Captopril-Hydrochlorothiazide Tablets) is indicated for the treatment of hypertension. The blood pressure lowering effects of captopril and thiazides are approximately additive.

This fixed combination drug is not indicated for initial therapy of hypertension. If the fixed combination represents the

dose titrated to the individual patient's needs, it may be more convenient than the separate components.

In using CAPOZIDE, consideration should be given to the risk of neutropenia/agranulocytosis (see WARNINGS). CAPOZIDE may be used for patients with normal renal function, in whom the risk is relatively low. In patients with impaired renal function, particularly those with collagen vascular disease, CAPOZIDE should be reserved for hypertensives who have either developed unacceptable side effects on other drugs, or have failed to respond satisfactorily to other drug combinations.

CONTRAINDICATIONS

Captopril—This product is contraindicated in patients who are hypersensitive to captopril.

Hydrochlorothiazide—Hydrochlorothiazide is contraindicated in anuria. It is also contraindicated in patients who have previously demonstrated hypersensitivity to hydrochlorothiazide or other sulfonamide-derived drugs.

WARNINGS

Captopril

Angioedema

Angioedema involving the extremities, face, lips, mucous membranes, tongue, glottis or larynx has been seen in patients treated with ACE inhibitors, including captopril. If angioedema involves the tongue, glottis or larynx, airway obstruction may occur and be fatal. Emergency therapy, including but not necessarily limited to, subcutaneous administration of a 1:1000 solution of epinephrine should be promptly instituted.

Swelling confined to the face, mucous membranes of the mouth, lips and extremities has usually resolved with discontinuation of treatment; some cases required medical therapy. (See PRECAUTIONS: Information for Patients and ADVERSE REACTIONS: Captopril.)

Neutropenia/Agranulocytosis

Neutropenia ($<1000/mm^3$) with myeloid hypoplasia has resulted from use of captopril. About half of the neutropenic patients developed systemic or oral cavity infections or other features of the syndrome of agranulocytosis.

The risk of neutropenia is dependent on the clinical status of the patient:

In clinical trials in patients with hypertension who have normal renal functions (serum creatinine less than 1.6 mg/dL and no collagen vascular disease), neutropenia has been seen in one patient out of over 8,600 exposed.

In patients with some degree of renal failure (serum creatinine at least 1.6 mg/dL) but no collagen vascular disease, the risk of neutropenia in clinical trials was about 1 per 500, a frequency over 15 times that for uncomplicated hypertension. Daily doses of captopril were relatively high in these patients, particularly in view of their diminished renal function. In foreign marketing experience in patients with renal failure, use of allopurinol concomitantly with captopril has been associated with neutropenia but this association has not appeared in U.S. reports.

In patients with collagen vascular diseases (e.g., systemic lupus erythematosus, scleroderma) and impaired renal function, neutropenia occurred in 3.7 percent of patients in clinical trials.

While none of the over 750 patients in formal clinical trials of heart failure developed neutropenia, it has occurred during the subsequent clinical experience. About half of the reported cases had serum creatinine ≥ 1.6 mg/dL and more than 75 percent were in patients also receiving procainamide. In heart failure, it appears that the same risk factors for neutropenia are present.

The neutropenia has usually been detected within three months after captopril was started. Bone marrow examinations in patients with neutropenia consistently showed myeloid hypoplasia, frequently accompanied by erythroid hypoplasia and decreased numbers of megakaryocytes (e.g., hypoplastic bone marrow and pancytopenia); anemia and thrombocytopenia were sometimes seen.

In general, neutrophils returned to normal in about two weeks after captopril was discontinued, and serious infections were limited to clinically complex patients. About 13 percent of the cases of neutropenia have ended fatally, but almost all fatalities were in patients with serious illness, having collagen vascular disease, renal failure, heart failure or immunosuppressant therapy, or a combination of these complicating factors.

Evaluation of the hypertensive or heart failure patient should always include assessment of renal function.

If captopril is used in patients with impaired renal function, white blood cell and differential counts should be evaluated prior to starting treatment and at approximately two-week intervals for about three months, then periodically.

In patients with collagen vascular disease or who are exposed to other drugs known to affect the white cells or immune response, particularly when there is impaired renal function, captopril should be used only after an assessment of benefit and risk, and then with caution.

All patients treated with captopril should be told to report any signs of infection (e.g., sore throat, fever). If infection is suspected, white cell counts should be performed without delay.

Since discontinuation of captopril and other drugs has generally led to prompt return of the white count to normal, upon confirmation of neutropenia (neutrophil count $<1000/mm^3$) the physician should withdraw captopril and closely follow the patient's course.

Proteinuria

Total urinary proteins greater than 1 g per day were seen in about 0.7 percent of patients receiving captopril. About 90 percent of affected patients had evidence of prior renal disease or received relatively high doses of captopril (in excess of 150 mg/day), or both. The nephrotic syndrome occurred in about one-fifth of proteinuric patients. In most cases, proteinuria subsided or cleared within six months whether or not captopril was continued. Parameters of renal function, such as BUN and creatinine, were seldom altered in the patients with proteinuria.

Since most cases of proteinuria occurred by the eighth month of therapy with captopril, patients with prior renal disease or those receiving captopril at doses greater than 150 mg per day, should have urinary protein estimations (dipstick on first morning urine) prior to treatment, and periodically thereafter.

Hypotension

Excessive hypotension was rarely seen in hypertensive patients but is a possible consequence of captopril use in severely salt/volume depleted persons such as those treated vigorously with diuretics, for example, patients with severe congestive heart failure (see PRECAUTIONS [Drug Interactions]).

Hydrochlorothiazide

Thiazides should be used with caution in severe renal disease. In patients with renal disease, thiazides may precipitate azotemia. Cumulative effects of the drug may develop in patients with impaired renal function.

Thiazides should be used with caution in patients with impaired hepatic function or progressive liver disease, since minor alterations of fluid and electrolyte balance may precipitate hepatic coma.

Sensitivity reactions may occur in patients with or without a history of allergy or bronchial asthma.

The possibility of exacerbation or activation of systemic lupus erythematosus has been reported.

In general, lithium should not be given with diuretics (see PRECAUTIONS, Drug Interactions, Hydrochlorothiazide).

PRECAUTIONS

General

Captopril

Impaired Renal Function—Some patients with renal disease, particularly those with severe renal artery stenosis, have developed increases in BUN and serum creatinine after reduction of blood pressure with captopril. Captopril dosage reduction and/or discontinuation of diuretic may be required. For some of these patients, it may not be possible to normalize blood pressure and maintain adequate renal perfusion (see CLINICAL PHARMACOLOGY, DOSAGE AND ADMINISTRATION, ADVERSE REACTIONS [Altered Laboratory Findings]).

Surgery/Anesthesia—In patients undergoing major surgery or during anesthesia with agents that produce hypotension, captopril will block angiotensin II formation secondary to compensatory renin release. If hypotension occurs and is considered to be due to this mechanism, it can be corrected by volume expansion.

Hydrochlorothiazide

All patients receiving thiazide therapy should be observed for clinical signs of fluid or electrolyte imbalance; namely hyponatremia, hypochloremic alkalosis, and hypokalemia. Serum and urine electrolyte determinations are particularly important when the patient is vomiting excessively or receiving parenteral fluids. Warning signs, irrespective of cause include dryness of mouth, thirst, weakness, lethargy, drowsiness, restlessness, muscle pains or cramps, muscular fatigue, hypotension, oliguria, tachycardia, and gastrointestinal disturbances such as nausea and vomiting.

Hypokalemia may develop, especially with brisk diuresis, when severe cirrhosis is present. Interference with adequate oral electrolyte intake will also contribute to hypokalemia. Hypokalemia can sensitize or exaggerate the response of the heart to the toxic effects of digitalis (e.g., increased ventricular irritability). Because captopril reduces the production of aldosterone, concomitant therapy with captopril reduces the diuretic-induced hypokalemia. Fewer patients may require potassium supplements and/or foods with a high potassium content (see Drug Interactions, Agents Increasing Serum Potassium).

Any chloride deficit is generally mild and usually does not require specific treatment except under extraordinary circumstances (as in liver disease or renal disease). Dilutional hyponatremia may occur in edematous patients in hot weather; appropriate therapy is water restriction, rather than administration of salt except in rare instances when the hyponatremia is life-threatening. In actual salt depletion, appropriate replacement is the therapy of choice.

Hyperuricemia may occur or frank gout may be precipitated in certain patients receiving thiazide therapy.

Diabetes mellitus which has been latent may become manifest during thiazide administration.

The antihypertensive effects of the drug may be enhanced in the postsympathectomy patient.

If progressive renal impairment becomes evident, as indicated by rising nonprotein nitrogen or blood urea nitrogen, a careful reappraisal of therapy is necessary with consideration given to withholding or discontinuing diuretic therapy.

Thiazides may decrease serum PBI levels without signs of thyroid disturbance.

Calcium excretion is decreased by thiazides. Pathologic changes in the parathyroid gland with hypercalcemia and hypophosphatemia have been observed in a few patients on prolonged thiazide therapy. The common complications of hyperparathyroidism have not been seen.

Information for Patients

Patients should be advised to immediately report to their physician any signs or symptoms suggesting angioedema (e.g., swelling of face, eyes, lips, tongue, larynx and extremities; difficulty in swallowing or breathing; hoarseness) and to discontinue therapy. (See WARNINGS: Captopril)

Patients should be told to report promptly any indication of infection (e.g., sore throat, fever), which may be a sign of neutropenia, or of progressive edema which might be related to proteinuria and nephrotic syndrome.

All patients should be cautioned that excessive perspiration and dehydration may lead to an excessive fall in blood pressure because of reduction in fluid volume. Other causes of volume depletion such as vomiting or diarrhea may also lead to a fall in blood pressure; patients should be advised to consult with the physician.

Patients should be warned against interruption or discontinuation of medication unless instructed by the physician. Heart failure patients on captopril therapy should be cautioned against rapid increases in physical activity.

Patients should be informed that CAPOZIDE (Captopril-Hydrochlorothiazide Tablets) should be taken one hour before meals (see DOSAGE AND ADMINISTRATION).

Laboratory Tests

Serum and urine electrolyte levels should be regularly monitored (see WARNINGS [Captopril and Hydrochlorothiazide], also PRECAUTIONS [General, Hydrochlorothiazide]).

Drug Interactions

Captopril

Hypotension—Patients on Diuretic Therapy: Patients on diuretics and especially those in whom diuretic therapy was recently instituted, as well as those on severe dietary salt restrictions or dialysis, may occasionally experience a precipitous reduction of blood pressure usually within the first hour after receiving the initial dose of captopril.

The possibility of hypotensive effects with captopril can be minimized by either discontinuing the diuretic or increasing the salt intake approximately one week prior to initiation of treatment with captopril or initiating therapy with small doses (6.25 or 12.5 mg). Alternatively, provide medical supervision for at least one hour after the initial dose. If hypotension occurs, the patient should be placed in a supine position and, if necessary, receive an intravenous infusion of normal saline. This transient hypotensive response is not a contraindication to further doses which can be given without difficulty once the blood pressure has increased after volume expansion.

Agents Having Vasodilator Activity: Data on the effect of concomitant use of other vasodilators in patients receiving captopril for heart failure are not available; therefore, nitroglycerin or other nitrates (as used for management of angina) or other drugs having vasodilator activity should, if possible, be discontinued before starting captopril. If resumed during captopril therapy, such agents should be administered cautiously, and perhaps at lower dosage.

Agents Causing Renin Release: Captopril's effect will be augmented by antihypertensive agents that cause renin release. For example, diuretics (e.g., thiazides) may activate the renin-angiotensin-aldosterone system.

Agents Affecting Sympathetic Activity: The sympathetic nervous system may be especially important in supporting blood pressure in patients receiving captopril alone or with diuretics. Therefore, agents affecting sympathetic activity (e.g., ganglionic blocking agents or adrenergic neuron blocking agents) should be used with caution. Beta-adrenergic blocking drugs add some further antihypertensive effect to captopril, but the overall response is less than additive.

Agents Increasing Serum Potassium: Since captopril decreases aldosterone production, elevation of serum potassium may occur. Potassium-sparing diuretics such as spironolactone, triamterene, or amiloride, or potassium supplements, should be given only for documented hypokalemia, and then with caution, since they may lead to a significant increase of serum potassium. Salt substitutes containing potassium should also be used with caution.

Continued on next page

Squibb—Cont.

Inhibitors Of Endogenous Prostaglandin Synthesis: It has been reported that indomethacin may reduce the antihypertensive effect of captopril, especially in cases of low renin hypertension. Other nonsteroidal anti-inflammatory agents (e.g., aspirin) may also have this effect.

Lithium: Increased serum lithium levels and symptoms of lithium toxicity have been reported in patients receiving concomitant lithium and ACE inhibitor therapy. These drugs should be coadministered with caution and frequent monitoring of serum lithium levels is recommended. If a diuretic is also used, it may increase the risk of lithium toxicity (see PRECAUTIONS, Drug Interactions, Hydrochlorothiazide: Lithium).

Hydrochlorothiazide

When administered concurrently the following drugs may interact with thiazide diuretics:

Alcohol, barbiturates, or narcotics—potentiation of orthostatic hypotension may occur.

Antidiabetic drugs (oral agents and insulin)—hyperglycemia induced by thiazides may require dosage adjustment of the antidiabetic drug.

Other antihypertensive drugs—additive effect or potentiation. Potentiation occurs with ganglionic or peripheral adrenergic blocking drugs.

Corticosteroids, ACTH—intensified electrolyte depletion, particularly hypokalemia.

Preanesthetic and anesthetic agents—effects of preanesthetic and anesthetic agents may be potentiated; adjust dosage of these agents accordingly.

Pressor amines (e.g., norepinephrine)—possible decreased response to pressor amines but not sufficient to preclude their use.

Skeletal muscle relaxants, nondepolarizing (e.g., tubocurarine)—possible increased responsiveness to the muscle relaxant.

Lithium—diuretic agents reduce the renal clearance of lithium and increase the risk of lithium toxicity. These drugs should be coadministered with caution and frequent monitoring of serum lithium levels is recommended (see PRECAUTIONS, Drug Interactions, Captopril: Lithium).

Drug/Laboratory Test Interactions

Captopril

Captopril may cause a false-positive urine test for acetone.

Hydrochlorothiazide

Thiazides should be discontinued before carrying out tests for parathyroid function (see PRECAUTIONS [General, Hydrochlorothiazide]).

Carcinogenesis, Mutagenesis, Impairment of Fertility

Captopril

Two-year studies with doses of 50 to 1350 mg/kg/day in mice and rats failed to show any evidence of carcinogenic potential.

Studies in rats have revealed no impairment of fertility.

Animal Toxicology

Chronic oral toxicity studies were conducted in rats (2 years), dogs (47 weeks; 1 year), mice (2 years), and monkeys (1 year). Significant drug-related toxicity included effects on hematopoiesis, renal toxicity, erosion/ulceration of the stomach, and variation of retinal blood vessels.

Reductions in hemoglobin and/or hematocrit values were seen in mice, rats, and monkeys at doses 50 to 150 times the maximum recommended human dose (MRHD). Anemia, leukopenia, thrombocytopenia, and bone marrow suppression occurred in dogs at doses 8 to 30 times MRHD. The reductions in hemoglobin and hematocrit values in rats and mice were only significant at 1 year and returned to normal with continued dosing by the end of the study. Marked anemia was seen at all dose levels (8 to 30 times MRHD) in dogs, whereas moderate to marked leukopenia was noted only at 15 and 30 times MRHD and thrombocytopenia at 30 times MRHD. The anemia could be reversed upon discontinuation of dosing. Bone marrow suppression occurred to a varying degree, being associated only with dogs that died or were sacrificed in a moribund condition in the 1 year study. However, in the 47-week study at a dose 30 times MRHD, bone marrow suppression was found to be reversible upon continued drug administration.

Captopril caused hyperplasia of the juxtaglomerular apparatus of the kidneys at doses 7 to 200 times the MRHD in rats and mice, at 20 to 60 times MRHD in monkeys, and at 30 times the MRHD in dogs.

Gastric erosions/ulcerations were increased in incidence at 20 and 200 times MRHD in male rats and at 30 and 65 times MRHD in dogs and monkeys, respectively. Rabbits developed gastric and intestinal ulcers when given oral doses approximately 30 times MRHD for only five to seven days.

In the two-year rat study, irreversible and progressive variations in the caliber of retinal vessels (focal sacculations and constrictions) occurred at all dose levels (7 to 200 times MRHD) in a dose-related fashion. The effect was first observed in the 88th week of dosing, with a progressively increased incidence thereafter, even after cessation of dosing.

Hydrochlorothiazide

Long-term studies in animals have not been performed to evaluate carcinogenic potential, mutagenesis, or whether this drug affects fertility in males or females.

Pregnancy—Category C

Captopril

Captopril was embryocidal in rabbits when given in doses about 2 to 70 times (on a mg/kg basis) the maximum recommended human dose, and low incidences of craniofacial malformations were seen. These effects in rabbits were most probably due to the particularly marked decrease in blood pressure caused by the drug in this species.

Captopril given to pregnant rats at 400 times the recommended human dose continuously during gestation and lactation caused a reduction in neonatal survival.

No teratogenic effects (malformations) have been observed after large doses of captopril in hamsters and rats.

Human Experience: There are no adequate and well-controlled studies of captopril in pregnant women. Data, however, are available that show captopril crosses the human placenta. Because the risk of fetal toxicity with the use of ACE inhibitors has not been defined, captopril should be used during pregnancy only if the potential benefit justifies the potential risk to the fetus.

Based on post-marketing experience with all ACE inhibitors, the following information has been collected with regard to pregnancy outcome. Inadvertent exposure limited to the first trimester of pregnancy does not appear to affect fetal outcome adversely. Fetal exposure during the second and third trimester of pregnancy has been associated with fetal and neonatal morbidity and mortality.

When ACE inhibitors are used during the later stages of pregnancy, there have been reports of hypotension and decreased renal perfusion in the newborn. Oligohydramnios in the mother has also been reported, presumably representing decreased renal function in the fetus. Infants exposed *in utero* to ACE inhibitors should be closely observed for hypotension, oliguria and hyperkalemia. If oliguria occurs, attention should be directed toward support of blood pressure and renal perfusion with the administration of fluids and pressors as appropriate. Problems associated with prematurity such as patent ductus arteriosus have occurred in association with maternal use of ACE inhibitors but it is not clear whether they are related to ACE inhibition, maternal hypertension or the underlying prematurity.

While captopril may be removed from the circulation of adults by hemodialysis, there is no experience with exchange transfusion, hemodialysis or peritoneal dialysis for removing captopril from the neonatal circulation.

Hydrochlorothiazide

Teratology studies have been performed in pregnant rats using captopril and hydrochlorothiazide individually and in combination; each agent was administered in doses up to 1350 mg/kg (400 times the maximum recommended human dose for hydrochlorothiazide). No evidence of embryotoxicity, fetotoxicity, or teratogenicity was found in any group. There are no adequate and well-controlled studies with captopril and hydrochlorothiazide in pregnant women. Because animal reproduction studies are not always predictive of human response, CAPOZIDE should be used during pregnancy, or for patients likely to become pregnant, only if the potential benefit justifies a potential risk to the fetus (see PRECAUTIONS, Pregnancy—Category C, Captopril).

Pregnancy—Nonteratogenic Effects

Hydrochlorothiazide

Thiazides cross the placental barrier and appear in cord blood. The use of thiazides in pregnant women requires that the anticipated benefit be weighed against possible hazards to the fetus. These hazards include fetal or neonatal jaundice, thrombocytopenia, and possibly other adverse reactions which have occurred in the adult.

Nursing Mothers

Both captopril and hydrochlorothiazide are excreted in human milk. Because of the potential for serious adverse reactions in nursing infants from both drugs, a decision should be made whether to discontinue nursing or to discontinue therapy taking into account the importance of CAPOZIDE (Captopril-Hydrochlorothiazide Tablets) to the mother.

Pediatric Use

Safety and effectiveness in children have not been established although there is limited experience with the use of captopril in children from 2 months to 15 years of age with secondary hypertension and varying degrees of renal insufficiency. Dosage, on a weight basis, was comparable to that used in adults. CAPOZIDE (Captopril-Hydrochlorothiazide Tablets) should be used in children only if other measures for controlling blood pressure have not been effective.

ADVERSE REACTIONS

Captopril

Reported incidences are based on clinical trials involving approximately 7000 patients.

Renal—About one of 100 patients developed proteinuria (see WARNINGS).

Each of the following has been reported in approximately 1 to 2 of 1000 patients and are of uncertain relationship to

drug use: renal insufficiency, renal failure, polyuria, oliguria, and urinary frequency.

Hematologic—Neutropenia/agranulocytosis has occurred (see WARNINGS). Cases of anemia, thrombocytopenia, and pancytopenia have been reported.

Dermatologic—Rash, often with pruritus, and sometimes with fever, arthralgia, and eosinophilia, occurred in about 4 to 7 (depending on renal status and dose) of 100 patients, usually during the first four weeks of therapy. It is usually maculopapular, and rarely urticarial. The rash is usually mild and disappears within a few days of dosage reduction, short-term treatment with an antihistaminic agent, and/or discontinuing therapy; remission may occur even if captopril is continued. Pruritus, without rash, occurs in about 2 of 100 patients. Between 7 and 10 percent of patients with skin rash have shown an eosinophilia and/or positive ANA titers. A reversible associated pemphigoid-like lesion, and photosensitivity, have also been reported. Flushing or pallor has been reported in 2 to 5 of 1000 patients.

Cardiovascular—Hypotension may occur; see WARNINGS and PRECAUTIONS (Drug Interactions) for discussion of hypotension on initiation of captopril therapy.

Tachycardia, chest pain, and palpitations have each been observed in approximately 1 of 100 patients.

Angina pectoris, myocardial infarction, Raynaud's syndrome, and congestive heart failure have each occurred in 2 to 3 of 1000 patients.

Dysgeusia—Approximately 2 to 4 (depending on renal status and dose) of 100 patients developed a diminution or loss of taste perception. Taste impairment is reversible and usually self-limited (2 to 3 months) even with continued drug administration. Weight loss may be associated with the loss of taste.

Angioedema—Angioedema involving the extremities, face, lips, mucous membranes, tongue, glottis or larynx has been reported in approximately one in 1000 patients. Angioedema involving the upper airways has caused fatal airway obstruction. (See WARNINGS: Captopril and PRECAUTIONS: Information for Patients.)

The following have been reported in about 0.5 to 2 percent of patients but did not appear at increased frequency compared to placebo or other treatments used in controlled trials: gastric irritation, abdominal pain, nausea, vomiting, diarrhea, anorexia, constipation, aphthous ulcers, peptic ulcer, dizziness, headache, malaise, fatigue, insomnia, dry mouth, dyspnea, cough, alopecia, paresthesias.

Other clinical adverse effects reported since the drug was marketed are listed below by body system. In this setting, an incidence or causal relationship cannot be accurately determined.

General: Asthenia, gynecomastia.

Cardiovascular: Cardiac arrest, cerebrovascular accident, syncope.

Dermatologic: Bullous pemphigus.

Gastrointestinal: Pancreatitis, glossitis.

Hematologic: Anemia, including aplastic and hemolytic.

Hepatobiliary: Hepatitis, including rare cases of necrosis, cholestasis.

Metabolic: Symptomatic hyponatremia.

Musculoskeletal: Myalgia, myasthenia.

Nervous/Psychiatric: Ataxia, confusion, depression, nervousness, somnolence.

Respiratory: Bronchospasm, eosinophilic pneumonitis, rhinitis.

Special Senses: Blurred vision.

Urogenital: Impotence.

As with other ACE inhibitors, a syndrome has been reported which includes: fever, myalgia, arthralgia, rash or other dermatologic manifestations, eosinophilia and an elevated ESR. Findings have usually resolved with discontinuation of treatment.

Hydrochlorothiazide

Gastrointestinal System—anorexia, gastric irritation, nausea, vomiting, cramping, diarrhea, constipation, jaundice (intrahepatic cholestatic jaundice), pancreatitis, and sialadenitis.

Central Nervous System—dizziness, vertigo, paresthesias, headache, and xanthopsia.

Hematologic—Leukopenia, agranulocytosis, thrombocytopenia, aplastic anemia, and hemolytic anemia.

Cardiovascular—orthostatic hypotension.

Hypersensitivity—purpura, photosensitivity, rash, urticaria, necrotizing angiitis (vasculitis; cutaneous vasculitis), fever, respiratory distress including pneumonitis, and anaphylactic reactions.

Other—hyperglycemia, glycosuria, hyperuricemia, muscle spasm, weakness, restlessness, and transient blurred vision. Whenever adverse reactions are moderate or severe, thiazide dosage should be reduced or therapy withdrawn.

Altered Laboratory Findings

Serum Electrolytes: Hyperkalemia: small increases in serum potassium, especially in patients with renal impairment (see PRECAUTIONS).

Hyponatremia: particularly in patients receiving a low sodium diet or concomitant diuretics.

BUN/Serum Creatinine: Transient elevations of BUN or serum creatinine especially in volume or salt depleted patients or those with renovascular hypertension may occur. Rapid reduction of longstanding or markedly elevated blood pressure can result in decreases in the glomerular filtration rate and, in turn, lead to increases in BUN or serum creatinine.

Hematologic: A positive ANA has been reported.

Liver Function Tests: Elevations of liver transaminases, alkaline phosphatase, and serum bilirubin have occurred.

OVERDOSAGE

Captopril

Correction of hypotension would be of primary concern. Volume expansion with an intravenous infusion of normal saline is the treatment of choice for restoration of blood pressure.

Captopril may be removed from the general circulation by hemodialysis.

Hydrochlorothiazide

In addition to the expected diuresis, overdosage of thiazides may produce varying degrees of lethargy which may progress to coma within a few hours, with minimal depression of respiration and cardiovascular function and without evidence of serum electrolyte changes or dehydration. The mechanism of thiazide-induced CNS depression is unknown. Gastrointestinal irritation and hypermotility may occur. Transitory increase in BUN has been reported, and serum electrolyte changes may occur, especially in patients with impaired renal function.

In addition to gastric lavage and supportive therapy for stupor or coma, symptomatic treatment of gastrointestinal effects may be needed. The degree to which hydrochlorothiazide is removed by hemodialysis has not been clearly established. Measures as required to maintain hydration, electrolyte balance, respiration, and cardiovascular and renal function should be instituted.

DOSAGE AND ADMINISTRATION

DOSAGE MUST BE INDIVIDUALIZED (SEE INDICATIONS AND USAGE).

CAPOZIDE (Captopril-Hydrochlorothiazide Tablets) should be taken one hour before meals.

The usual initial dose of captopril is 25 mg bid or tid. Hydrochlorothiazide is usually given at a total daily dose of 25 to 100 mg.

The approximate daily dose of captopril and hydrochlorothiazide, as determined by titration of the individual components (see INDICATIONS AND USAGE), may be administered by utilizing an appropriate potency of CAPOZIDE bid. For example, CAPOZIDE may be administered beginning with the 25 mg/15 mg combination tablet bid. Increased captopril dosage may be obtained by utilizing the 50 mg/15 mg combination tablet bid or increased hydrochlorothiazide dosage may be obtained by utilizing the 25 mg/25 mg combination tablet bid. CAPOZIDE 25 mg/15 mg and 50 mg/15 mg tablets may also be utilized in tid dosage regimens to provide higher daily dosages.

If additional control beyond that provided by the 50 mg/15 mg tid CAPOZIDE dose is indicated, it is recommended that other antihypertensive agents be added to the regimen.

A maximum daily dose of 450 mg captopril should not be exceeded.

Beta-blockers may be used in conjunction with CAPOZIDE therapy (see PRECAUTIONS [Drug Interactions]), but the effects are less than additive. Other agents may be added gradually beginning with 50 percent of the usual recommended starting dose to avoid an excessive fall in blood pressure.

For patients with severe hypertension (e.g., accelerated or malignant hypertension), the dosage increments may be made more frequently than every two weeks with the patient under continuous medical supervision until a satisfactory blood pressure response is obtained or the maximal dose of captopril is reached.

Dosage Adjustment in Renal Impairment—Because captopril and hydrochlorothiazide are excreted primarily by the kidneys, excretion rates are reduced in patients with impaired renal function. These patients will take longer to reach steady-state captopril levels and will reach higher steady-state levels for a given daily dose than patients with normal renal function. Therefore, these patients may respond to smaller or less frequent doses of CAPOZIDE.

After the desired therapeutic effect has been achieved, the dose intervals should be increased or the total daily dose reduced until the minimal effective dose is achieved. When concomitant diuretic therapy is required in patients with severe renal impairment, a loop diuretic (e.g., furosemide), rather than a thiazide diuretic is preferred for use with captopril; therefore, for patients with severe renal dysfunction the captopril-hydrochlorothiazide combination tablet is not usually recommended.

HOW SUPPLIED

CAPOZIDE (Captopril-Hydrochlorothiazide Tablets)

25 mg captopril combined with 15 mg hydrochlorothiazide in bottles of 100 (NDC 0003-0338-50). Tablets are white with distinct orange mottling; they are biconvex rounded squares with quadrisect bars. Tablet identification no. **338**.

25 mg captopril combined with 25 mg hydrochlorothiazide in bottles of 100 (NDC 0003-0349-50). Tablets are peach-colored and may show slight mottling; they are biconvex rounded squares with quadrisect bars. Tablet identification no. **349**.

50 mg. captopril combined with 15 mg hydrochlorothiazide in bottles of 100 (NDC 0003-0384-50). Tablets are white with distinct orange mottling; they are biconvex ovals with a bisect bar. Tablet identification no. **384**.

50 mg captopril combined with 25 mg hydrochlorothiazide in bottles of 100 (NDC 0003-0390-50). Tablets are peach-colored and may show slight mottling; they are biconvex ovals with a bisect bar. Tablet identification no. **390**.

STORAGE

Keep bottles tightly closed (protect from moisture); do not store above 86°F.

(J4-005K)

Shown in Product Identification Section, page 431

FUNGIZONE® Cream   ℞
Amphotericin B Cream USP
FUNGIZONE® Lotion   ℞
Amphotericin B Lotion USP
FUNGIZONE® Ointment   ℞
Amphotericin B Ointment USP

DESCRIPTION

FUNGIZONE Cream (Amphotericin B Cream) for dermatologic use contains the antifungal antibiotic amphotericin B at a concentration of 3% (30 mg/g) in a pleasantly tinted aqueous vehicle, which also contains titanium dioxide, thimerosal, propylene glycol, cetearyl alcohol (and) ceteareth-20, white petrolatum, methylparaben, propylparaben, sorbitol solution, glyceryl monostearate, polyethylene glycol monostearate, simethicone, and sorbic acid.

FUNGIZONE Lotion (Amphotericin B Lotion) contains the antifungal antibiotic amphotericin B at a concentration of 3% (30 mg/mL) in a tinted aqueous lotion vehicle, which is pleasantly scented, and also contains thimerosal, titanium dioxide, guar gum, propylene glycol, cetyl alcohol, stearyl alcohol, sorbitan monopalmitate, polysorbate 20, glyceryl monostearate, polyethylene glycol monostearate, simethicone, sorbic acid, sodium citrate, methylparaben, and propylparaben.

FUNGIZONE Ointment (Amphotericin B Ointment) contains the antifungal antibiotic amphotericin B at a concentration of 3% (30 mg/g) in a tinted form of Plastibase® (Plasticized Hydrocarbon Gel), a polyethylene and mineral oil gel base with titanium dioxide.

CLINICAL PHARMACOLOGY

Amphotericin B is an antibiotic with antifungal activity which is produced by a strain of *Streptomyces nodosus*. It has been shown to exhibit greater *in vitro* activity than nystatin against *Candida* (Monilia) *albicans*. In clinical studies involving cutaneous and mucocutaneous candidal infections, results with topical preparations of amphotericin B were comparable to those obtained with nystatin in similar formulations.

Although amphotericin B exhibits some *in vitro* activity against the superficial dermatophytes (ringworm organisms), it has not demonstrated an effectiveness *in vivo* on topical application. Amphotericin B has no significant effect either *in vitro* or clinically against gram-positive or gram-negative bacteria, or viruses.

INDICATIONS AND USAGE

FUNGIZONE (Amphotericin B) topical preparations are indicated in the treatment of cutaneous and mucocutaneous mycotic infections caused by Candida (Monilia) species.

CONTRAINDICATIONS

These preparations are contraindicated in patients with a history of hypersensitivity to any of their components.

PRECAUTIONS

Should a reaction of hypersensitivity occur the drug should be immediately withdrawn and appropriate measures taken. These preparations are not for ophthalmic use.

ADVERSE REACTIONS

FUNGIZONE Cream (Amphotericin B Cream)

No evidence of any systemic toxicity or side effects has been observed during or following the use of FUNGIZONE Cream. The preparation is usually well tolerated by all age groups. It is not a primary irritant and apparently has only a slight sensitizing potential. It may have a "drying" effect on some skin, and local irritation characterized by erythema, pruritus, or a burning sensation sometimes occurs, particularly in intertriginous areas.

FUNGIZONE Lotion (Amphotericin B Lotion)

No evidence of any systemic toxicity or side effects has been observed during or following even prolonged, intensive and extensive application of FUNGIZONE Lotion.

The preparation is extremely well tolerated by all age groups, including infants, even when therapy must be continued for many months. It is not a primary irritant and apparently has only a slight sensitizing potential. Local intolerance, which seldom occurs, has included increased pruritus with or without other subjective or objective evidence of local irritation, or exacerbation of preexisting candidal lesions. Allergic contact dermatitis is rare.

FUNGIZONE Ointment (Amphotericin B Ointment)

No evidence of any systemic toxicity or side effects has been observed during or following even prolonged, intensive and extensive application of FUNGIZONE Ointment.

The preparation is usually well tolerated by all age groups. It is not a primary irritant and apparently has only a slight sensitizing potential. However, it is well to remember that any oleaginous ointment vehicle may occasionally irritate when applied to moist, intertriginous areas.

DOSAGE AND ADMINISTRATION

FUNGIZONE (Amphotericin B) Cream, Lotion, or Ointment should be applied liberally to the candidal lesions two to four times daily. Duration of therapy depends on individual patient response. Intertriginous lesions usually respond within a few days, and treatment may be completed in one to three weeks. Similarly, candidiasis of the diaper area, perleche, and glabrous skin lesions usually clear in one to two weeks. Interdigital (erosio) lesions may require two to four weeks of intensive therapy, paronychias also require relatively prolonged therapy, and those onychomycoses which respond may require several months or more of treatment. (Relapses are frequently encountered in the last three clinical conditions.)

NOTE: When rubbed into the lesion, the Cream discolors the skin minimally. The Lotion and Ointment do not stain the skin when thoroughly rubbed into the lesion although nail lesions may be stained. The patient should be informed that any discoloration of fabrics from the Cream may be removed by hand-washing the fabric with soap and warm water, that any discoloration of fabrics from the Lotion is readily removed with soap and warm water, or that any discoloration of fabrics from the Ointment may be removed by applying a standard cleaning fluid.

HOW SUPPLIED

FUNGIZONE Cream (Amphotericin B Cream USP) is supplied in 20 gram tubes (NDC 0003-0411-20) providing 3% amphotericin B (30 mg/g).

FUNGIZONE Lotion (Amphotericin B Lotion USP) in 30 mL plastic squeeze bottles (NDC 0003-0412-30) providing 30 mg amphotericin B per mL.

FUNGIZONE Ointment (Amphotericin B Ointment USP) is supplied in 20 gram tubes (NDC 0003-0426-20) providing 3% amphotericin B (30 mg/g).

Storage

Store the Cream and Lotion at room temperature; avoid freezing. Store the Ointment at room temperature.

(J2-224G/J3-521B/J2-151D)

FUNGIZONE® INTRAVENOUS   ℞

[*fun 'ji-zōn*]

Amphotericin B for Injection USP

> **WARNING**
>
> This drug should be used primarily for treatment of patients with progressive and potentially fatal fungal infections; it should not be used to treat the common clinically inapparent forms of fungal disease which show only positive skin or serologic tests.

DESCRIPTION

FUNGIZONE Intravenous (Amphotericin B for Injection) contains amphotericin B, an antimycotic polyene antibiotic obtained from a strain of *Streptomyces nodosus*. Amphotericin B is designated chemically as [1R-(1R*, 3S*,5R*,6R*,-9R*, 11R*, 15S*, 16R*, 17R*,18S*, 19E, 21E, 23E,25E,27E,-29E,31E,33R*,35S*,36R*,37S*)] -33- [(3-Amino-3, 6-dideoxy-β-D-mannopyranosyl)-oxy]- 1,3,5,6,9,11,17,37 -octahydroxy-15,16, 18-trimethyl-13-oxo-14, 39-dioxabicyclo[33.3.1]nona-triaconta-19,21,23,25,27,29,31-heptaene-36-carboxylic acid.

Each vial contains a sterile, nonpyrogenic, lyophilized cake (which may partially reduce to powder following manufacture) providing 50 mg amphotericin B and 41 mg sodium desoxycholate with 20.2 mg sodium phosphates as a buffer. Crystalline amphotericin B is insoluble in water; therefore, the antibiotic is "solubilized" by the addition of sodium desoxycholate to form a mixture which provides a colloidal dispersion for intravenous infusion following reconstitution. At the time of manufacture the air in the vial is replaced by nitrogen.

Continued on next page

Squibb—Cont.

CLINICAL PHARMACOLOGY

Microbiology

Amphotericin B shows a high order of *in vitro* activity against many species of fungi. *Histoplasma capsulatum, Coccidioides immitis, Candida species, Blastomyces dermatitidis, Rhodotorula, Cryptococcus neoformans, Sporothrix schenckii, Mucor mucedo,* and *Aspergillus fumigatus* are all inhibited by concentrations of amphotericin B ranging from 0.03 to 1.0 mcg/mL *in vitro*. The antibiotic is without effect on bacteria, rickettsiae, and viruses.

Susceptibility Testing

Standard techniques for determining the minimal inhibitory concentration (MIC) have not been established for antifungal agents, and values will vary with the method employed. The broth and agar dilution methods as described by Shadomy *et al,* Manual of Clinical Microbiology, 4th edition provide quantitative procedures for determining MICs for amphotericin B.

Pharmacokinetics

Amphotericin B is fungistatic or fungicidal depending on the concentration obtained in body fluids and the susceptibility of the fungus. The drug acts by binding to sterols in the cell membrane of sensitive fungi with a resultant change in membrane permeability allowing leakage of intracellular components. Mammalian cell membranes also contain sterols and it has been suggested that the damage to human cells and fungal cells may share common mechanisms.

An initial intravenous infusion of 1 to 5 mg of amphotericin B per day, gradually increased to 0.4 to 0.6 mg/kg daily, produces peak plasma concentrations ranging from approximately 0.5 to 2 mcg/mL. Following a rapid initial fall, plasma concentrations plateau at about 0.5 mcg/mL. An elimination half-life of approximately 15 days follows an initial plasma half-life of about 24 hours. It has been reported that amphotericin B circulating in plasma is highly bound (>90%) to plasma proteins and is poorly dialyzable; also that approximately two thirds of concurrent plasma concentrations have been detected in fluids from inflamed pleura, peritoneum, synovium, and aqueous humor; concentrations in the cerebrospinal fluid seldom exceed 2.5 percent of those in the plasma; little amphotericin B penetrates into vitreous humor or normal amniotic fluid. Complete details of tissue distribution are not known.

Amphotericin B is excreted very slowly by the kidneys with two to five percent of a given dose being excreted in the biologically active form. Details of possible metabolic pathways are not known. After treatment is discontinued, the drug can be detected in the urine for at least seven weeks due to the slow disappearance of the drug. The cumulative urinary output over a seven day period amounts to approximately 40 percent of the amount of drug infused.

INDICATIONS AND USAGE

FUNGIZONE Intravenous (Amphotericin B for Injection USP) should be administered primarily to patients with progressive, potentially fatal infections. This potent drug should not be used to treat the common inapparent forms of fungal disease which show only positive skin or serologic tests.

FUNGIZONE Intravenous is specifically intended to treat cryptococcosis (*torulosis*); North American blastomycosis; the disseminated forms of moniliasis, coccidioidomycosis, and histoplasmosis; mucormycosis (phycomycosis) caused by species of the genera *Mucor, Rhizopus, Absidia, Entomophthora,* and *Basidiobolus;* sporotrichosis (*Sporothrix schenckii* [formerly *Sporotrichum schenckii*]); aspergillosis (*Aspergillus fumigatus*).

Amphotericin B may be helpful in the treatment of American mucocutaneous leishmaniasis, but is not the drug of choice in primary therapy.

CONTRAINDICATIONS

This product is contraindicated in those patients who have shown hypersensitivity to it unless, in the opinion of the physician, the condition requiring treatment is life-threatening and amenable only to amphotericin B therapy.

WARNINGS

Amphotericin B is frequently the only effective treatment available for potentially fatal fungal disease. In each case, its possible life-saving benefit must be balanced against its untoward and dangerous side effects.

PRECAUTIONS

General

Prolonged therapy with amphotericin B is usually necessary. Unpleasant reactions are quite common when the drug is given intravenously at therapeutic dosage levels. **Some of these reactions are potentially dangerous.** Hence, amphotericin B should be used intravenously only in hospitalized patients or those under close clinical observation by medically trained personnel, and should be reserved for those patients in whom a diagnosis of the progressive, potentially fatal forms of susceptible mycotic infections has been firmly established, preferably by positive culture or histologic study.

Whenever medication is interrupted for a period longer than seven days, therapy should be resumed by starting with the lowest dosage level, e.g., 0.25 mg/kg of body weight, and increased gradually as outlined under DOSAGE AND ADMINISTRATION.

Laboratory Tests

Laboratory facilities must be available to perform blood urea nitrogen and serum creatinine or endogenous creatinine clearance tests. These determinations should be made at least weekly during therapy. If the BUN exceeds 40 mg per 100 mL or the serum creatinine exceeds 3.0 mg per 100 mL, the drug should be discontinued or the dosage markedly reduced until renal function improves. Weekly hemograms and serum potassium determinations are also advisable. Low serum magnesium levels have also been noted during treatment with amphotericin B. Therapy should be discontinued if liver function test results (i.e., elevated bromsulphalein, alkaline phosphatase, and bilirubin) are abnormal.

Drug Interactions

When administered concurrently, the following drugs may interact with amphotericin B:

Antineoplastic agents (e.g., nitrogen mustard) —may enhance the potential for renal toxicity. Antineoplastic agents such as nitrogen mustard should be given concomitantly only with great caution.

Corticosteroids and Corticotropin (ACTH) —may potentiate amphotericin B-induced hypokalemia (see ADVERSE REACTIONS).

Digitalis glycosides —amphotericin B-induced hypokalemia may potentiate digitalis toxicity.

Flucytosine —while a synergistic relationship with amphotericin B has been reported, concomitant use may increase the toxicity of flucytosine by increasing its cellular uptake and impairing its renal excretion.

Other nephrotoxic medications —may enhance the potential for renal toxicity, and should be used concomitantly only with great caution.

Skeletal muscle relaxants (e.g., tubocurarine) —amphotericin B-induced hypokalemia may enhance curariform effect.

Carcinogenesis, Mutagenesis, Impairmemt of Fertility

No long-term studies in animals have been performed to evaluate carcinogenic potential. There have also been no studies to determine mutagenicity or whether this medication affects fertility in males or females.

Pregnancy; Teratogenic Effects, Pregnancy Category B

Reproduction studies in animals have revealed no evidence of harm to the fetus due to Amphotericin B for Injection. Systemic fungal infections have been successfully treated in pregnant women with Amphotericin B for Injection without obvious effects to the fetus, but the number of cases reported has been small. Because animal reproduction studies are not always predictive of human response, and adequate and well-controlled studies have not been conducted in pregnant women, this drug should be used during pregnancy only if clearly needed.

Nursing Mothers

It is not known whether amphotericin B is excreted in human milk. Because many drugs are excreted in human milk, consideration should be given to discontinuation of nursing during treatment with and elimination of intravenously administered amphotericin B.

Pediatric Use

Safety and effectiveness in pediatric patients have not been established through adequate and well-controlled studies. Systemic fungal infections have been successfully treated in pediatric patients without reports of unusual side effects. Amphotericin B for Injection when administered to pediatric patients should be limited to the least amount compatible with an effective therapeutic regimen.

ADVERSE REACTIONS

While some few patients may tolerate full intravenous doses of amphotericin B without difficulty, most will exhibit some intolerance, often at less than the full therapeutic dosage. They may be made less severe by giving aspirin, antipyretics (e.g., acetaminophen), antihistamines, and antiemetics. Administration of the drug on alternate days may decrease anorexia and phlebitis. Intravenous administration of small doses of adrenal corticosteroids just prior to or during the amphotericin B infusion may decrease febrile reactions. The dosage and duration of such corticosteroid therapy should be kept to a minimum (see PRECAUTIONS, Drug Interactions). Addition of heparin (1000 units per infusion), and the use of a pediatric scalp-vein needle may lessen the incidence of thrombophlebitis. Extravasation may cause chemical irritation.

The adverse reactions that are most commonly observed are: fever (sometimes with shaking chills which, because they usually occur within 15 to 20 minutes after treatment is initiated, can be differentiated from chills due to bacterial infection); headache; anorexia; weight loss; nausea and vomiting; malaise, dyspepsia; diarrhea; generalized pain including muscle and joint pains, cramping epigastric pain, and local venous pain at the injection site with phlebitis and thrombophlebitis; and normochromic, normocytic anemia. Abnormal renal function including hypokalemia, azotemia, hyposthe-

nuria, renal tubular acidosis and nephrocalcinosis is also commonly observed, and usually improves upon interruption of therapy; however, some permanent impairment often occurs, especially in those patients receiving large amounts (over 5 g) of amphotericin B. Supplemental alkali medication may decrease renal tubular acidosis complications.

The following adverse reactions occur less frequently or rarely; anuria; anaphylactoid reactions; acute liver failure; and flushing.

DOSAGE AND ADMINISTRATION

FUNGIZONE Intravenous (Amphotericin B for Injection USP) should be administered by *slow* intravenous infusion. Intravenous infusion should be given over a period of approximately six hours observing the usual precautions for intravenous therapy. The recommended concentration for intravenous infusion is 0.1 mg/mL (1 mg/10 mL).

Dosage must be adjusted to the specific requirements of each patient since tolerance to amphotericin B varies individually. Therapy is usually instituted with a daily dose of 0.25 mg/kg of body weight and **gradually** increased as tolerance permits. An initial test dose of 1 mg in 20 mL of 5% dextrose solution administered intravenously over 20 to 30 minutes may be preferred. The patient's temperature, pulse, respiration, and blood pressure should be recorded every 30 minutes for 4 hours. A patient with a severe and rapidly progressing fungal infection, with good cardiopulmonary function and a mild reaction to the test dose may then receive 0.3 mg/kg amphotericin B intravenously over a period of 2 to 6 hours. A smaller second dose, i.e., 5 to 10 mg, is recommended for the patient with cardiopulmonary impairment or a severe reaction to the test dose. In patients with normal renal function, doses may then be increased by 5 to 10 mg per day to a final daily dosage of 0.5 to 0.7 mg/kg. There are insufficient data presently available to define total dosage requirements and duration of treatment necessary for eradication of mycoses such as phycomycosis. The optimal dose is unknown. Total daily dosage may range up to 1.0 mg/kg of body weight or alternate day dosages ranging up to 1.5 mg/kg. Several months of therapy are usually necessary; a shorter period of therapy may produce an inadequate response and lead to relapse.

CAUTION: Under no circumstances should a total daily dosage of 1.5 mg/kg be exceeded.

Therapy with intravenous amphotericin B for sporotrichosis has ranged up to nine months. The usual dose per injection is 20 mg.

Aspergillosis has been treated with amphotericin B intravenously for a period up to 11 months with a total dose up to 3.6 g.

Rhinocerebral phycomycosis, a fulminating disease, generally occurs in association with diabetic ketoacidosis. It is, therefore, imperative that rapid restoration of diabetic control be instituted before successful treatment with FUNGIZONE Intravenous (Amphotericin B for Injection USP) can be accomplished. In contradistinction, pulmonary phycomycosis, which is more common in association with hematologic malignancies, is often an incidental finding at autopsy. A cumulative dose of at least 3 g of amphotericin B is recommended. Although a total dose of 3 to 4 g will infrequently cause lasting renal impairment, this would seem a reasonable minimum where there is clinical evidence of invasion of the deep tissues; since rhinocerebral phycomycosis usually follows a rapidly fatal course, the therapeutic approach must necessarily be more aggressive than that used in more indolent mycoses.

PREPARATION OF SOLUTIONS

Reconstitute as follows: An initial concentrate of 5 mg amphotericin B per mL is first prepared by rapidly expressing 10 mL Sterile Water for Injection USP *without a bacteriostatic agent* directly into the lyophilized cake, using a sterile needle (minimum diameter: 20 gauge) and syringe. Shake the vial immediately until the colloidal solution is clear. The infusion solution, providing 0.1 mg amphotericin B per mL is then obtained by further dilution (1:50) with 5% Dextrose Injection USP *of pH above 4.2*. The pH of each container of Dextrose Injection should be ascertained before use. Commercial Dextrose Injection usually has a pH above 4.2; however, if it is below 4.2, then 1 or 2 mL of buffer should be added to the Dextrose Injection before it is used to dilute the concentrated solution of amphotericin B. The recommended buffer has the following composition:

Dibasic sodium phosphate (anhydrous)	1.59 g
Monobasic sodium phosphate (anhydrous)	0.96 g
Water for Injection USP	qs 100.0 mL

The buffer should be sterilized before it is added to the Dextrose Injection, either by filtration through a bacterial retenapplied or by briefly wetting the affected area with water immediately prior to applying the medication. The frequency of changing dressings is best determined on an individual basis. It may be convenient to apply the preparation under an occlusive dressing in the evening and to remove the dressing in the morning (i.e., 12-hour occlusion). When utilizing the 12-hour occlusion regimen, additional preparation should be applied, without occlusion, during the day. Reapplication is essential at each dressing change.

If an infection develops, the use of occlusive dressings should be discontinued and appropriate antimicrobial therapy instituted.

KENALOG Ointment (Triamcinolone Acetonide Ointment) 0.025%, 0.1% and 0.5% and KENALOG Spray (Triamcinolone Acetonide Topical Aerosol): Occlusive dressings may be used for the management of psoriasis or other recalcitrant conditions. Apply a thin coating of the preparation onto the lesion, cover with a pliable nonporous film, and seal the edges. If needed, additional moisture may be provided by covering the lesion with a dampened clean cotton cloth before the nonporous film is applied or by briefly wetting the affected area with water immediately prior to applying the medication. The frequency of changing dressings is best determined on an individual basis. It may be convenient to apply the preparation under an occlusive dressing in the evening and to remove the dressing in the morning (i.e., 12-hour occlusion). When utilizing the 12-hour occlusion regimen, additional preparation should be applied, without occlusion, during the day. Reapplication is essential at each dressing change.

If an infection develops, the use of occlusive dressings should be discontinued and appropriate antimicrobial therapy instituted.

HOW SUPPLIED

KENALOG Cream (Triamcinolone Acetonide Cream USP)
0.025%: tubes containing 15 g (NDC 0003-0172-22) and 80 g (NDC 0003-0172-68); and jars containing 240 g (NDC 0003-0172-70) and 2.38 kg (NDC 0003-0172-80) of cream.
0.1%: tubes containing 15 g (NDC 0003-0506-20), 60 g (NDC 0003-0506-46) and 80 g (NDC 0003-0506-49); and jars containing 240 g (NDC 0003-0506-60) and 2.38 kg (NDC 0003-0506-89) of cream.
0.5%: tubes containing 20 g (NDC 0003-1483-20) of cream.
KENALOG Lotion (Triamcinolone Acetonide Lotion USP)
0.025%: plastic squeeze bottles containing 60 mL (NDC 0003-0173-60) of lotion.
0.1%: plastic squeeze bottles containing 15 mL (NDC 0003-0502-20) and 60 mL (NDC 0003-0502-70) of lotion.
KENALOG Ointment (Triamcinolone Acetonide Ointment USP)
0.025%: tubes containing 15 g (NDC 0003-0495-22) and 80 g (NDC 0003-0495-60); and jars containing 240 g (NDC 0003-0495-70) of ointment.
0.1%: tubes containing 15 g (NDC 0003-0508-20), 60 g (NDC 0003-0508-56) and 80 g (NDC 0003-0508-58); and jars containing 240 g (NDC 0003-0508-60) of ointment.
0.5%: tubes containing 20 g (NDC 0003-1484-20) of ointment.
KENALOG Spray (Triamcinolone Acetonide Topical Aerosol USP)
23 g (NDC 0003-0501-42 and 63 g (NDC 0003-0501-62) aerosol cans.
Storage
KENALOG Cream (Triamcinolone Acetonide Cream USP)
Store at room temperature; avoid freezing.
KENALOG Lotion (Triamcinolone Acetonide Lotion USP)
Store at room temperature; avoid freezing.
KENALOG Ointment (Triamcinolone Acetonide Ointment USP)
Store at room temperature
KENALOG Spray (Triamcinolone Acetonide Topical Aerosol USP)
Store at room temperature; avoid excessive heat.
(J3-584F/528E/585E/232G)

KENALOG®-40 INJECTION   ℞
[ken'ah-log"]
Sterile Triamcinolone Acetonide Suspension
USP
NOT FOR INTRAVENOUS OR
INTRADERMAL USE

DESCRIPTION
KENALOG-40 Injection (Sterile Triamcinolone Acetonide Suspension USP) provides a synthetic corticosteroid with marked anti-inflammatory action. Each mL of the sterile aqueous suspension provides 40 mg of triamcinolone acetonide, with sodium chloride for isotonicity, 0.9% (w/v) benzyl alcohol as a preservative, 0.75% carboxymethylcellulose sodium and 0.04% polysorbate 80. Sodium hydroxide or hydrochloric acid may be present to adjust pH to 5.0–7.5. At the time of manufacture, the air in the container is replaced by nitrogen.

ACTIONS
Naturally occurring glucocorticoids (hydrocortisone), which also have salt-retaining properties, are used as replacement therapy in adrenocortical deficiency states. Their synthetic analogs are primarily used for their potent anti-inflammatory effects in disorders of many organ systems. Glucocorticoids cause profound and varied metabolic effects. In addition, they modify the body's immune responses to diverse stimuli.

KENALOG-40 Injection has an extended duration of effect which may be permanent, or sustained over a period of several weeks. Studies indicate that following a single intramuscular dose of 60 to 100 mg of triamcinolone acetonide, adrenal suppression occurs within 24 to 48 hours and then gradually returns to normal, usually in 30 to 40 days. This finding correlates closely with the extended duration of therapeutic action achieved with the drug.

INDICATIONS
Intramuscular
Where oral therapy is not feasible or is temporarily undesirable in the judgment of the physician, KENALOG-40 Injection is indicated for intramuscular use as follows:
1. *Endocrine disorders*—Nonsuppurative thyroiditis.
2. *Rheumatic disorders*—As adjunctive therapy for short-term administration (to tide the patient over an acute episode or exacerbation) in: post-traumatic osteoarthritis; synovitis of osteoarthritis; rheumatoid arthritis; acute and subacute bursitis; epicondylitis; acute nonspecific tenosynovitis; acute gouty arthritis; psoriatic arthritis; ankylosing spondylitis; juvenile rheumatoid arthritis.
3. *Collagen diseases*—During an exacerbation or as maintenance therapy in selected cases of: systemic lupus erythematosus; acute rheumatic carditis.
4. *Dermatologic diseases*—Pemphigus; severe erythema multiforme (Stevens-Johnson syndrome); exfoliative dermatitis; bullous dermatitis herpetiformis; severe seborrheic dermatitis; severe psoriasis.
5. *Allergic states*—Control of severe or incapacitating allergic conditions intractable to adequate trials of conventional treatment in: bronchial asthma; contact dermatitis; atopic dermatitis; seasonal or perennial allergic rhinitis.
6. *Ophthalmic diseases*—Severe chronic allergic and inflammatory processes involving the eye, such as: herpes zoster ophthalmicus; iritis; iridocyclitis; chorioretinitis; diffuse posterior uveitis and choroiditis; optic neuritis; sympathetic ophthalmia; anterior segment inflammation.
7. *Gastrointestinal diseases*—To tide the patient over a critical period of disease in: ulcerative colitis (systemic therapy); regional enteritis (systemic therapy).
8. *Respiratory diseases*—Symptomatic sarcoidosis; berylliosis; aspiration pneumonitis.
9. *Hematologic disorders*—Acquired (autoimmune) hemolytic anemia.
10. *Neoplastic diseases*—For palliative management of: leukemias and lymphomas in adults; acute leukemia of childhood.
11. *Edematous state*—To induce diuresis or remission of proteinuria in the nephrotic syndrome, without uremia, of the idiopathic type or that due to lupus erythematosus.
Intra-Articular
KENALOG-40 Injection (Sterile Triamcinolone Acetonide Suspension USP) is indicated for intra-articular or intrabursal administration, and for injections into tendon sheaths, as adjunctive therapy for short-term administration (to tide the patient over an acute episode or exacerbation) in: synovitis of osteoarthritis; rheumatoid arthritis; acute and subacute bursitis; acute gouty arthritis; epicondylitis; acute nonspecific tenosynovitis; post-traumatic osteoarthritis.

CONTRAINDICATIONS
Corticosteroids are contraindicated in patients with systemic fungal infections. Intramuscular corticosteroid preparations are contraindicated for idiopathic thrombocytopenic purpura.

WARNINGS
Because it is a suspension, the preparation should **not** be administered intravenously. Strict aseptic technique is mandatory. This preparation is not recommended for children under six years of age.

Adequate studies to demonstrate the safety of administration of KENALOG-40 Injection (Sterile Triamcinolone Acetonide Suspension USP) by intraturbinal, subconjunctival, subtenon and retrobulbar injections have not been performed. Several instances of blindness have been reported following injection of corticosteroid suspensions into the nasal turbinates and intralesional injection about the head.

When patients who are receiving corticosteroid therapy are subjected to unusual stress, increased dosage of rapidly acting corticosteroids is indicated before, during and after the stressful situation.

Corticosteroids may mask some signs of infection, and new infections may appear during their use. There may be decreased resistance and inability to localize infection when corticosteroids are used. If an infection occurs during cortico-

steroid therapy, it should be promptly controlled by suitable antimicrobial therapy (see PRECAUTIONS).

Prolonged use of corticosteroids may produce posterior subcapsular cataracts, glaucoma with possible damage to the optic nerves, and may enhance the establishment of secondary ocular infections due to fungi or viruses.

Average and large doses of hydrocortisone or cortisone can cause elevation of blood pressure, salt and water retention and increased excretion of potassium. These effects are less likely to occur with the synthetic derivatives except when they are used in large doses; dietary salt restriction and potassium supplementation may be necessary (see PRECAUTIONS). All corticosteroids increase calcium excretion.

Patients should not be vaccinated against smallpox while on corticosteroid therapy. Other immunization procedures should not be undertaken in patients who are on corticosteroids, especially on high dose, because of possible hazards of neurological complications and a lack of antibody response.

The use of corticosteroids in patients with active tuberculosis should be restricted to those cases of fulminating or disseminated tuberculosis in which the corticosteroid is used for the management of the disease in conjunction with an appropriate antituberculous regimen. If corticosteroids are indicated in patients with latent tuberculosis or tuberculin reactivity, close observation is necessary since reactivation of the disease may occur. During prolonged corticosteroid therapy, these patients should receive chemoprophylaxis.

Because rare instances of anaphylactoid reactions have occurred in patients receiving parenteral corticosteroid therapy, appropriate precautionary measures should be taken prior to administration, especially when the patient has a history of allergy to any drug.

Unless a **deep** intramuscular injection is given, local atrophy is likely to occur. (For recommendations on injection techniques, see DOSAGE AND ADMINISTRATION.) Due to the significantly higher incidence of local atrophy when the material is injected into the deltoid area, this injection site should be avoided in favor of the gluteal area. Only very unusual circumstances would warrant injection into the deltoid area.

USAGE IN PREGNANCY
Since adequate human reproduction studies have not been done with corticosteroids, the use of these drugs in pregnancy, nursing mothers, or women of childbearing potential requires that the possible benefits of the drug be weighed against the potential hazards to the mother and the embryo, fetus, or nursing infant. Infants born of mothers who have received substantial doses of corticosteroids during pregnancy should be carefully observed for signs of hypoadrenalism.

PRECAUTIONS
Drug-induced secondary adrenocortical insufficiency may be minimized by a gradual reduction of dosage. This type of relative insufficiency may persist for months after discontinuation of therapy; therefore, in any situation of stress (such as trauma, surgery, or severe illness) occurring during that period, hormone therapy should be reinstituted. Since mineralocorticoid secretion may be impaired, salt and/or a mineralocorticoid should be administered concurrently.

There is an enhanced corticosteroid effect in patients with hypothyroidism and in those with cirrhosis.

Corticosteroids should be used cautiously in patients with ocular herpes simplex because of possible corneal perforation.

The lowest possible dose of corticosteroid should be used to control the condition being treated. A gradual reduction in dosage should be made when possible.

Psychic derangements may appear when corticosteroids are used. These may range from euphoria, insomnia, mood swings, personality changes and severe depression to frank psychotic manifestations. Existing emotional instability or psychotic tendencies may also be aggravated by corticosteroids.

Aspirin should be used cautiously in conjunction with corticosteroids in patients with hypoprothrombinemia.

Corticosteroids should be used with caution in patients with nonspecific ulcerative colitis if there is a probability of impending perforation, abscess, or other pyogenic infection. Corticosteroids should also be used cautiously in patients with diverticulitis, fresh intestinal anastomoses, active or latent peptic ulcer, renal insufficiency, hypertension, osteoporosis, acute glomerulonephritis, vaccinia, varicella, exanthema, Cushing's syndrome, antibiotic resistant infections, diabetes mellitus, congestive heart failure, chronic nephritis, thromboembolitic tendencies, thrombophlebitis, convulsive disorders, metastatic carcinoma, and myasthenia gravis.

Growth and development of infants and children on prolonged corticosteroid therapy should be carefully observed. Although therapy with KENALOG-40 Injection (Sterile Triamcinolone Acetonide Suspension USP) will ameliorate symptoms, it is in no sense a cure and the hormone has no

Continued on next page

Squibb—Cont.

effect on the cause of the inflammation. Therefore, this method of treatment does not obviate the need for the conventional measures usually employed.

Intra-articular injection of a corticosteroid may produce systemic as well as local effects. The inadvertent injection of the suspension into the soft tissues surrounding a joint is not harmful, but may lead to the occurrence of systemic effects, and is the most common cause of failure to achieve the desired local results.

Following intra-articular steroid therapy, patients should be specifically warned to avoid overuse of joints in which symptomatic benefit has been obtained. Negligence in this matter may permit an increase in joint deterioration that will more than offset the beneficial effects of the steroid. To detect deterioration, follow-up x-ray examination is suggested in selected cases.

Overdistention of the joint capsule and deposition of steroid along the needle track should be avoided in intra-articular injection since this may lead to subcutaneous atrophy.

Corticosteroids should not be injected into unstable joints. Repeated intra-articular injection may in some cases result in instability of the joint. In selected cases, particularly when repeated injections are given, x-ray follow-up is suggested.

An increase in joint discomfort has seldom occurred. A marked increase in pain accompanied by local swelling, further restriction of joint motion, fever and malaise are suggestive of a septic arthritis. If these complications should appear, and the diagnosis of septic arthritis is confirmed, administration of triamcinolone acetonide should be stopped, and antimicrobial therapy should be instituted immediately and continued for 7 to 10 days after all evidence of infection has disappeared. Appropriate examination of any joint fluid present is necessary to exclude a septic process. Local injection of a steroid into a previously infected joint is to be avoided.

KENALOG-40 Injection (Sterile Triamcinolone Acetonide Suspension USP) should be administered only with full knowledge of characteristic activity of, and varied responses to, adrenocortical hormones. Like other potent corticosteroids, triamcinolone acetonide should be used under close clinical supervision. Triamcinolone acetonide can cause elevation of blood pressure, salt and water retention, and increased potassium and calcium excretion necessitating dietary salt restriction and potassium supplementation. Edema may occur in the presence of renal disease with a fixed or decreased glomerular filtration rate.

During prolonged therapy, **a liberal protein intake is essential** for counteracting the tendency to gradual weight loss sometimes associated with negative nitrogen balance, wasting and weakness of skeletal muscles.

When local or systemic microbial infections are present, therapy with triamcinolone acetonide is not recommended, but may be employed with caution and only in conjunction with appropriate antibiotic or chemotherapeutic medication. Triamcinolone acetonide may mask signs of infection and enhance dissemination of the infecting organism. Hence, all patients receiving triamcinolone acetonide should be watched for evidence of intercurrent infection. Should infection occur, vigorous, appropriate anti-infective therapy should be initiated. If possible, abrupt cessation of steroids should be avoided because of the danger of superimposing adrenocortical insufficiency on the infectious process.

Menstrual irregularities may occur, and this possibility should be mentioned to female patients past menarche.

In peptic ulcer, recurrence may be asymptomatic until perforation or hemorrhage occurs. Long-term adrenocorticoid therapy may evoke hyperacidity or peptic ulcer; therefore, as a prophylactic measure, an ulcer regimen and the administration of an antacid are highly recommended. X-rays should be taken in peptic ulcer patients complaining of gastric distress, or when therapy is prolonged. Whether or not changes are observed, an ulcer regimen is recommended.

As with other corticosteroids, the possibility of other severe reactions should be considered. If such reactions should occur, appropriate corrective measures should be instituted and use of the drug discontinued.

Continued supervision of the patient after termination of triamcinolone acetonide therapy is essential, since there may be a sudden reappearance of severe manifestations of the disease for which the patient was treated.

ADVERSE REACTIONS

Following Administration by Any Route — Patients should be watched closely for the following adverse reactions which may be associated with any corticosteroid therapy:

Fluid and electrolyte disturbances — sodium retention, fluid retention, congestive heart failure in susceptible patients, potassium loss, cardiac arrhythmias or ECG changes due to potassium deficiency, hypokalemic alkalosis and hypertension.

Musculoskeletal — muscle weakness, fatigue, steroid myopathy, loss of muscle mass, osteoporosis, vertebral compression

fractures, delayed healing of fractures, aseptic necrosis of femoral and humeral heads, pathologic fractures of long bones, and spontaneous fractures.

Gastrointestinal — peptic ulcer with possible subsequent perforation and hemorrhage, pancreatitis, abdominal distention, and ulcerative esophagitis.

Dermatologic — impaired wound healing, thin fragile skin, petechiae and ecchymoses, facial erythema, increased sweating, purpura, striae, hirsutism, acneiform eruptions, lupus erythematosus-like lesions and suppressed reactions to skin tests.

Neurological — convulsions, increased intracranial pressure with papilledema (pseudo-tumor cerebri) usually after treatment, vertigo, headache, neuritis or paresthesias, and aggravation of preexisting psychiatric conditions.

Endocrine — menstrual irregularities; development of the cushingoid state; suppression of growth in children; secondary adrenocortical and pituitary unresponsiveness, particularly in times of stress (e.g., trauma, surgery, or illness); decreased carbohydrate tolerance; manifestations of latent diabetes mellitus and increased requirements for insulin or oral hypoglycemic agents in diabetics.

Ophthalmic — posterior subcapsular cataracts, increased intraocular pressure, glaucoma, and exophthalmos.

Metabolic — hyperglycemia, glycosuria and negative nitrogen balance due to protein catabolism.

Others — necrotizing angiitis, thrombophlebitis, thromboembolism, aggravation or masking of infections, insomnia, syncopal episodes, and anaphylactoid reactions.

Following Intramuscular Administration — Severe pain has been reported in a few cases. Sterile abscess formation, subcutaneous and cutaneous atrophy, hyperpigmentation and hypopigmentation and charcot-like arthropathy have also occurred.

Following Intra-Articular Administration — Undesirable reactions have included postinjection flare, transient pain, occasional irritation at the injection site, sterile abscess formation, hyperpigmentation and hypopigmentation, charcot-like arthropathy and occasional brief increase in joint discomfort.

DOSAGE AND ADMINISTRATION

General

The initial dose of KENALOG-40 Injection (Sterile Triamcinolone Acetonide Suspension USP) may vary from 2.5 to 60 mg per day depending on the specific disease entity being treated (see **Dosage** section below). In situations of less severity, lower doses will generally suffice while in selected patients higher initial doses may be required. Usually the parenteral dosage ranges are one-third to one-half the oral dose given every 12 hours. However, in certain overwhelming, acute, life-threatening situations, administration of dosages exceeding the usual dosages may be justified and may be in multiples of the oral dosages.

The initial dosage should be maintained or adjusted until a satisfactory response is noted. If after a reasonable period of time there is a lack of satisfactory clinical response, KENALOG-40 Injection should be discontinued and the patient transferred to other appropriate therapy. **IT SHOULD BE EMPHASIZED THAT DOSAGE REQUIREMENTS ARE VARIABLE AND MUST BE INDIVIDUALIZED ON THE BASIS OF THE DISEASE UNDER TREATMENT AND THE RESPONSE OF THE PATIENT.** After a favorable response is noted, the proper maintenance dosage should be determined by decreasing the initial drug dosage in small increments at appropriate time intervals until the lowest dosage which will maintain an adequate clinical response is reached. It should be kept in mind that constant monitoring is needed in regard to drug dosage. Included in the situations which may make dosage adjustments necessary are changes in clinical status secondary to remissions or exacerbations in the disease process, the patient's individual drug responsiveness, and the effect of patient exposure to stressful situations not directly related to the disease entity under treatment; in this latter situation it may be necessary to increase the dosage of KENALOG-40 Injection for a period of time consistent with the patient's condition. If after long-term therapy the drug is to be stopped, it is recommended that it be withdrawn gradually rather than abruptly.

Dosage

Systemic

Although KENALOG-40 Injection may be administered intramuscularly for initial therapy, most physicians prefer to adjust the dose orally until adequate control is attained. Intramuscular administration provides a sustained or depot action which can be used to supplement or replace initial oral therapy. With intramuscular therapy, greater supervision of the amount of steroid used is made possible in the patient who is inconsistent in following an oral dosage schedule. In maintenance therapy, the patient-to-patient response is not uniform and, therefore, the dose must be individualized for optimal control.

For **adults and children over 12 years of age,** the suggested initial dose is 60 mg, **injected deeply into the gluteal muscle.** Subcutaneous fat atrophy may occur if care is not taken to inject the preparation intramuscularly. Dosage is usually

adjusted within the range of 40 to 80 mg, depending upon patient response and duration of relief. However, some patients may be well controlled on dosages as low as 20 mg or less. Patients with hay fever or pollen asthma who are not responding to pollen administration and other conventional therapy may obtain a remission of symptoms lasting throughout the pollen season after one injection of 40 to 100 mg.

For **children from 6 to 12 years of age,** the suggested initial dose is 40 mg, although dosage depends more on the severity of symptoms than on age or weight. There is insufficient clinical experience with KENALOG-40 Injection (Sterile Triamcinolone Acetonide Suspension USP) to recommend its use in children under six years of age.

Local: For intra-articular or intrabursal administration and for injection into tendon sheaths, the initial dose of KENALOG-40 Injection may vary from 2.5 to 5 mg for smaller joints and from 5 to 15 mg for larger joints depending on the specific disease entity being treated. (A more dilute form of Sterile Triamcinolone Acetonide Suspension USP is available—see ALSO AVAILABLE.) For adults, doses up to 10 mg for smaller areas and up to 40 mg for larger areas have usually been sufficient to alleviate symptoms. Single injections into several joints for multiple locus involvement, up to a total of 80 mg, have been given without undue reactions. A single local injection of triamcinolone acetonide is frequently sufficient, but several injections may be needed for adequate relief of symptoms. The lower dosages in the initial dosage range of triamcinolone acetonide may produce the desired effect when the corticosteroid is administered to provide a localized concentration. The site of the injection and the volume of the injection should be carefully considered when triamcinolone acetonide is administered for this purpose.

Administration

General

Shake the vial before use to insure a uniform suspension. Prior to withdrawal, inspect suspension for clumping or granular appearance (agglomeration). An agglomerated product results from exposure to freezing temperatures and should not be used. After withdrawal, inject without delay to prevent settling in the syringe. Careful technique should be employed to avoid the possibility of entering a blood vessel or introducing infection.

Routine laboratory studies, such as urinalysis, two-hour postprandial blood sugar, determination of blood pressure and body weight and a chest x-ray should be made at regular intervals during prolonged therapy. Upper GI x-rays are desirable in patients with an ulcer history or significant dyspepsia.

Systemic

For systemic therapy, injection should be made **deeply into the gluteal muscle** to insure intramuscular delivery (see WARNINGS). For adults, a minimum needle length of 1 ½ inches is recommended. In obese patients, a longer needle may be required. Use alternate sites for subsequent injections.

Local

For treatment of joints, the usual intra-articular injection technique, as described in standard textbooks, should be followed. If an excessive amount of synovial fluid is present in the joint, some, but not all, should be aspirated to aid in the relief of pain and to prevent undue dilution of the corticosteroid.

With intra-articular or intrabursal administration, and with injection of the drug into tendon sheaths, the use of a local anesthetic may often be desirable. When a local anesthetic is used, its package insert should be read with care and all the precautions connected with its use should be observed. It should be injected into the surrounding soft tissues prior to the injection of the corticosteroid. A small amount of the anesthetic solution may be instilled into the joint. Care should be taken with intra-articular and intrabursal injections (particularly in the deltoid region) and with injection into tendon sheaths to avoid injecting the suspension into the tissues surrounding the site since this may lead to tissue atrophy.

In treating acute nonspecific tenosynovitis, care should be taken to insure that the injection of the corticosteroid is made into the tendon sheath rather than the tendon substance. Epicondylitis (tennis elbow) may be treated by infiltrating the preparation into the area of greatest tenderness.

HOW SUPPLIED

KENALOG-40 Injection (Sterile Triamcinolone Acetonide Suspension USP) is supplied in vials providing 40 mg triamcinolone acetonide per mL.

Also Available: KENALOG-10 Injection (Sterile Triamcinolone Acetonide Suspension USP) providing 10 mg triamcinolone acetonide per mL, with sodium chloride for isotonicity, 0.9% (w/v) benzyl alcohol as a preservative, 0.75% sodium carboxymethylcellulose, and 0.04% polysorbate 80. See package insert for full information.

Storage

Store at room temperature; avoid freezing. Protect from light.

(J3-064F)

KENALOG® -10 INJECTION ℞

[*ken'ah-log "*]

Sterile Triamcinolone Acetonide Suspension

USP

For Intra-articular, Intrabursal or Intradermal

Use

NOT FOR INTRAVENOUS OR

INTRAMUSCULAR USE

DESCRIPTION

KENALOG-10 Injection (Sterile Triamcinolone Acetonide Suspension USP) provides triamcinolone acetonide, a synthetic corticosteroid with marked anti-inflammatory action, in a sterile aqueous suspension suitable for intradermal, intra-articular, and intrabursal injection and for injection into tendon sheaths. This preparation is NOT suitable for intravenous or intramuscular use. Each mL of the sterile aqueous suspension provides 10 mg triamcinolone acetonide, with sodium chloride for isotonicity, 0.9% (w/v) benzyl alcohol as a preservative, 0.75% carboxymethylcellulose sodium, and 0.04% polysorbate 80; sodium hydroxide or hydrochloric acid may have been added to adjust pH between 5.0 and 7.5. At the time of manufacture, the air in the container is replaced by nitrogen.

The chemical name for triamcinolone acetonide is 9-fluoro-11β, 16α, 17, 21-tetrahydroxypregna-1,4-diene-3,20-dione cyclic 16, 17-acetal with acetone.

CLINICAL PHARMACOLOGY

Naturally occurring glucocorticoids (hydrocortisone), which also have salt-retaining properties, are used as replacement therapy in adrenocortical deficiency states. Their synthetic analogs are primarily used for their potent anti-inflammatory effects in disorders of many organ systems.

Glucocorticoids cause profound and varied metabolic effects. In addition, they modify the body's immune responses to diverse stimuli.

INDICATIONS AND USAGE

Intra-Articular

KENALOG-10 Injection (Sterile Triamcinolone Acetonide Suspension USP) is indicated for intra-articular or intrabursal administration, and for injection into tendon sheaths, as adjunctive therapy for short-term administration (to tide the patient over an acute episode or exacerbation) in: synovitis of osteoarthritis, rheumatoid arthritis, acute and subacute bursitis, acute gouty arthritis, epicondylitis, acute nonspecific tenosynovitis, and post-traumatic osteoarthritis.

Intradermal

Intralesional administration of KENALOG-10 Injection is indicated for the treatment of keloids, discoid lupus erythematosus, necrobiosis lipoidica diabeticorum, alopecia areata, and localized hypertrophic, infiltrated, inflammatory lesions of: lichen planus, psoriatic plaques, granuloma annulare, and lichen simplex chronicus (neurodermatitis). KENALOG-10 Injection also may be useful in cystic tumors of an aponeurosis or tendon (ganglia).

CONTRAINDICATIONS

Corticosteroids are contraindicated in patients with systemic fungal infections.

WARNINGS

Because it is a suspension, the preparation should *not* be administered intravenously. Strict aseptic technique is mandatory.

When patients who are receiving corticosteroid therapy are subjected to unusual stress, increased dosage of rapidly acting corticosteroids is indicated before, during, and after the stressful situation. KENALOG-10 Injection (Sterile Triamcinolone Acetonide Suspension USP), as a long-acting preparation, is *not* suitable for use in acute stress situations.

Corticosteroids may mask some signs of infection, and new infections may appear during their use. There may be decreased resistance and inability to localize infection when corticosteroids are used. If an infection occurs during corticosteroid therapy, it should be promptly controlled by suitable antimicrobial therapy (see PRECAUTIONS).

Prolonged use of corticosteroids may produce posterior subcapsular cataracts, glaucoma with possible damage to the optic nerves, and may enhance the establishment of secondary ocular infections due to fungi or viruses.

Average and large doses of hydrocortisone or cortisone can cause elevation of blood pressure, salt and water retention, and increased excretion of potassium. These effects are less likely to occur with the synthetic derivatives except when they are used in large doses; dietary salt restriction and potassium supplementation may be necessary (see PRECAUTIONS). All corticosteroids increase calcium excretion.

Patients should not be vaccinated against smallpox while on corticosteroid therapy. Other immunization procedures should not be undertaken in patients who are on corticosteroids, especially on high dose, because of possible hazards of neurological complications and a lack of antibody response.

The use of triamcinolone acetonide in patients with active tuberculosis should be restricted to those cases of fulminating or disseminated tuberculosis in which the corticosteroid is used for the management of the disease in conjunction with an appropriate antituberculous regimen. If corticosteroids are indicated in patients with latent tuberculosis or tuberculin reactivity, close observation is necessary since reactivation of the disease may occur. During prolonged corticosteroid therapy these patients should receive chemoprophylaxis.

Because rare instances of anaphylactoid reactions have occurred in patients receiving parenteral corticosteroid therapy, appropriate precautionary measures should be taken prior to administration, especially when the patient has a history of allergy to any drug.

Safety of use of KENALOG-10 Injection (Sterile Triamcinolone Acetonide Suspension USP) by intraturbinal, subconjunctival, subtenons, and retrobulbar injection has not been established.

Usage in Pregnancy

Since adequate human reproduction studies have not been done with corticosteroids, the use of these drugs in pregnancy, nursing mothers, or women of child-bearing potential requires that the possible benefits of the drug be weighed against the potential hazards to the mother and the embryo, fetus, or nursing infant. Infants born of mothers who have received substantial doses of corticosteroids during pregnancy should be carefully observed for signs of hypoadrenalism.

PRECAUTIONS

Drug-induced secondary adrenocortical insufficiency may be minimized by a gradual reduction of dosage. This type of relative insufficiency may persist for months after discontinuation of therapy; therefore, in any situation of stress (such as trauma, surgery, or severe illness) occurring during that period, hormone therapy should be reinstituted. Since mineralocorticoid secretion may be impaired, salt and/or a mineralocorticoid should be administered concurrently.

There is an enhanced corticosteroid effect in patients with hypothyroidism and in those with cirrhosis.

Corticosteroids should be used cautiously in patients with ocular herpes simplex because of possible corneal perforation.

The lowest possible dose of corticosteroid should be used to control the condition being treated. A gradual reduction in dosage should be made when possible.

Psychic derangements may appear when corticosteroids are used. These may range from euphoria, insomnia, mood swings, personality changes, and severe depression, to frank psychotic manifestations. Existing emotional instability or psychotic tendencies may also be aggravated by corticosteroids.

Aspirin should be used cautiously in conjunction with corticosteroids in patients with hypoprothrombinemia.

Corticosteroids should be used with caution in patients with nonspecific ulcerative colitis if there is a probability of impending perforation, abscess, or other pyogenic infection. Corticosteroids should also be used cautiously in patients with diverticulitis, fresh intestinal anastomoses, active or latent peptic ulcer, renal insufficiency, hypertension, osteoporosis, and myasthenia gravis.

Growth and development of infants and children on prolonged corticosteroid therapy should be carefully observed. Although therapy with KENALOG-10 Injection (Sterile Triamcinolone Acetonide Suspension USP) may ameliorate symptoms, it is in no sense a cure and the hormone has no effect on the cause of the inflammation. Therefore, this method of treatment does not obviate the need for the conventional measures usually employed.

Intra-articular injection of a corticosteroid may produce systemic as well as local effects. The inadvertent injection of the suspension into the soft tissues surrounding a joint is not harmful, but is the most common cause of failure to achieve the desired local results.

Following intra-articular steroid therapy, patients should be specifically warned to avoid overuse of joints in which symptomatic benefit has been obtained. Negligence in this matter may permit an increase in joint deterioration that will more than offset the beneficial effects of the steroid. To detect deterioration follow-up x-ray examination is suggested in selected cases.

Overdistention of the joint capsule and deposition of steroid along the needle track should be avoided in intra-articular injection since this may lead to subcutaneous atrophy.

Corticosteroids should not be injected into unstable joints. Repeated intra-articular injection may in some cases result in instability of the joint. In selected cases, particularly when repeated injections are given, x-ray follow-up is suggested.

An increase in joint discomfort has seldom occurred. A marked increase in pain accompanied by local swelling, further restriction of joint motion, fever, and malaise are suggestive of a septic arthritis. If these complications should appear, and the diagnosis of septic arthritis is confirmed, administration of triamcinolone acetonide should be stopped, and antimicrobial therapy should be instituted immediately and continued for 7 to 10 days after all evidence of infection has disappeared. Appropriate examination of any joint fluid present is necessary to exclude a septic process. Local injection of a steroid into a previously infected joint is to be avoided.

KENALOG-10 Injection (Sterile Triamcinolone Acetonide Suspension USP) should be administered only with full knowledge of characteristic activity of, and varied responses to, adrenocortical hormones. Like other potent corticosteroids, triamcinolone acetonide should be used under close clinical supervision. Triamcinolone acetonide can cause elevation of blood pressure, salt and water retention, and increased potassium and calcium excretion necessitating dietary salt restriction and potassium supplementation. Edema may occur in the presence of renal disease with a fixed or decreased glomerular filtration rate.

During prolonged therapy, *a liberal protein intake is essential* for counteracting the tendency to gradual weight loss sometimes associated with negative nitrogen balance, wasting and weakness of skeletal muscles.

When local or systemic microbial infections are present, therapy with triamcinolone acetonide is not recommended, but may be employed with caution and only in conjunction with appropriate antibiotic or chemotherapeutic medication. Triamcinolone acetonide may mask signs of infection and enhance dissemination of the infecting organism. Hence, all patients receiving triamcinolone acetonide should be watched for evidence of intercurrent infection. Should infection occur, vigorous, appropriate anti-infective therapy should be initiated. If possible, abrupt cessation of steroids should be avoided because of the danger of superimposing adrenocortical insufficiency on the infectious process.

Menstrual irregularities may occur, and this possibility should be mentioned to female patients past menarche.

In peptic ulcer, recurrence may be asymptomatic until perforation or hemorrhage occurs. X-rays should be taken in peptic ulcer patients complaining of gastric distress, or when therapy is prolonged. Whether or not changes are observed, an ulcer regimen is recommended.

As with other corticosteroids, the possibility of other severe reactions should be considered. If such reactions should occur, appropriate corrective measures should be instituted and use of the drug discontinued.

Continued supervision of the patient after termination of triamcinolone acetonide therapy is essential, since there may be a sudden reappearance of severe manifestations of the disease for which the patient was treated.

ADVERSE REACTIONS

Undesirable reactions following intra-articular administration of the preparation have included postinjection flare, transient pain, occasional local irritation at the injection site, sterile abscesses, hyper- and hypopigmentation, charcot-like arthropathy, and occasional brief increase in joint discomfort; following intradermal administration, rare instances of blindness associated with intralesional therapy around the face and head, transient local discomfort, sterile abscesses, hyper- and hypopigmentation, and subcutaneous and cutaneous atrophy (which usually disappears, unless the basic disease process is itself atrophic) have occurred.

Since systemic absorption may occasionally occur with intra-articular or other local administration, patients should be watched closely for the following adverse reactions which may be associated with any corticosteroid therapy:

Fluid and electrolyte disturbances —sodium retention, fluid retention, congestive heart failure in susceptible patients, potassium loss, cardiac arrythmias or ECG changes due to potassium deficiency, hypokalemic alkalosis, and hypertension.

Musculoskeletal —muscle weakness, fatigue, steroid myopathy, loss of muscle mass, osteoporosis, vertebral compression fractures, delayed healing of fractures, aseptic necrosis of femoral and humeral heads, pathologic fractures of long bones, and spontaneous fractures.

Gastrointestinal —peptic ulcer with possible subsequent perforation and hemorrhage, pancreatitis, abdominal distention, and ulcerative esophagitis.

Dermatologic —impaired wound healing, thin fragile skin, petechiae and ecchymoses, facial erythema, increased sweating, purpura, striae, hirsutism, acneiform eruptions, lupus erythematosus-like lesions and suppressed reactions to skin tests.

Neurological —convulsions, increased intracranial pressure with papilledema (pseudo-tumor cerebri) usually after treatment, vertigo, headache, neuritis or paresthesias, and aggravation of pre-existing psychiatric conditions.

Endocrine —menstrual irregularities; development of the cushingoid state; suppression of growth in children; secondary adrenocortical and pituitary unresponsiveness, particularly in times of stress (e.g., trauma, surgery, or illness); de-

Continued on next page

Squibb—Cont.

creased carbohydrate tolerance; manifestations of latent diabetes mellitus; and increased requirements for insulin or oral hypoglycemic agents in diabetics.

Ophthalmic —posterior subcapsular cataracts, increased intraocular pressure, glaucoma, and exophthalmos.

Metabolic —hyperglycemia, glycosuria, and negative nitrogen balance due to protein catabolism.

Others —necrotizing angiitis, thrombophlebitis, thromboembolism, aggravation or masking of infections, insomnia, syncopal episodes, and anaphylactoid reactions.

DOSAGE AND ADMINISTRATION

Dosage

The initial dose of KENALOG-10 Injection (Sterile Triamcinolone Acetonide Suspension USP) for intra-articular or intrabursal administration and for injection into tendon sheaths may vary from 2.5 mg to 5 mg for smaller joints and from 5 to 15 mg for larger joints depending on the specific disease entity being treated. Single injections into several joints for multiple locus involvement, up to a total of 20 mg or more, have been given without incident. For intradermal administration, the initial dose of triamcinolone acetonide will vary depending upon the specific disease entity being treated but should be limited to 1.0 mg (0.1 mL) per injection site, since larger volumes are more likely to produce cutaneous atrophy. Multiple sites (separated by one centimeter or more) may be so injected, keeping in mind that the greater the *total* volume employed the more corticosteroid becomes available for possible systemic absorption and subsequent corticosteroid effects. Such injections may be repeated, if necessary, at weekly or less frequent intervals.

The lower dosages in the initial dosage range of triamcinolone acetonide may produce the desired effect when the corticosteroid is administered to provide a localized concentration. The site of the injection and the volume of the injection should be carefully considered when triamcinolone acetonide is administered for this purpose. The inital dosage should be maintained or adjusted until a satisfactory response is noted. If after a reasonable period of time there is a lack of satisfactory clinical response, KENALOG-10 Injection should be discontinued and the patient transferred to other appropriate therapy. IT SHOULD BE EMPHASIZED THAT DOSAGE REQUIREMENTS ARE VARIABLE AND MUST BE INDIVIDUALIZED ON THE BASIS OF THE DISEASE UNDER TREATMENT AND THE RESPONSE OF THE PATIENT. After a favorable response is noted, the proper maintenance dosage should be determined by decreasing the initial drug dosage in small increments at appropriate time intervals until the lowest dosage which will maintain an adequate clinical response is reached. It should be kept in mind that constant monitoring is needed in regard to drug dosage. Included in the situations which may make dosage adjustments necessary are changes in clinical status secondary to remissions or exacerbations in the disease process, the patient's individual drug responsiveness, and the effect of patient exposure to stressful situations not directly related to the disease entity under treatment; in this latter situation it may be necessary to increase the dosage of KENALOG-10 Injection (Sterile Triamcinolone Acetonide Suspension USP) for a period of time consistent with the patient's condition. If the drug is to be stopped after long-term therapy, it is recommended that it be withdrawn gradually rather than abruptly.

Administration

Shake the vial before use to insure a uniform suspension. Prior to withdrawal, inspect suspension for clumping or granular appearance (agglomeration). An agglomerated product results from exposure to freezing temperatures and should not be used. After withdrawal, inject without delay to prevent settling in the syringe. Careful technique should be employed to avoid the possibility of entering a blood vessel or introducing infection.

Routine laboratory studies, such as urinalysis, two-hour postprandial blood sugar, determination of blood pressure and body weight, and a chest x-ray should be made at regular intervals during prolonged therapy. Upper GI x-rays are desirable in patients with an ulcer history or significant dyspepsia.

For treatment of joints, the usual intra-articular injection technique, as described in standard textbooks, should be followed. If an excessive amount of synovial fluid is present in the joint, some, but not all, should be aspirated to aid in the relief of pain and to prevent undue dilution of the steroid. With intra-articular or intrabursal administration, and with injection of KENALOG-10 Injection into tendon sheaths, the use of a local anesthetic may often be desirable. When a local anesthetic is used, its package insert should be read with care and all the precautions connected with its use should be observed. It should be injected into the surrounding soft tissue prior to the injection of the corticosteroid. A small amount of the anesthetic solution may be instilled into the joint.

In treating acute nonspecific tenosynovitis, care should be taken to insure that the injection of KENALOG-10 Injection is made into the tendon sheath rather than the tendon substance. Epicondylitis (tennis elbow) may be treated by infiltrating the preparation into the area of greatest tenderness. For treatment of dermal lesions, KENALOG-10 Injection is injected directly into the lesion, i.e., intradermally or sometimes subcutaneously. For accuracy of dosage measurement and ease of administration, it is preferable to employ a tuberculin syringe and a small bore needle (23 to 25 gauge). Ethyl chloride spray may be used to alleviate the discomfort of the injection.

HOW SUPPLIED

KENALOG-10 Injection (Sterile Triamcinolone Acetonide Suspension USP) is supplied in 5 mL multiple dose vials (NDC 0003-0494-20) providing 10 mg triamcinolone acetonide per mL.

Storage

Store at room temperature; avoid freezing; protect from light.

(J3-526A)

KENALOG® IN ORABASE®   ℞

[*ken'ah-log" in or'a-bās"*]
Triamcinolone Acetonide Dental Paste USP

DESCRIPTION

Each gram of KENALOG IN ORABASE provides 1 mg (0.1%) triamcinolone acetonide in emollient dental paste containing gelatin, pectin, and carboxymethylcellulose sodium in Plastibase® (Plasticized Hydrocarbon Gel), a polyethylene and mineral oil gel base.

ACTIONS

KENALOG® (Triamcinolone Acetonide) is a synthetic corticosteroid which possesses anti-inflammatory, antipruritic, and antiallergic action. The emollient dental paste acts as an adhesive vehicle for applying the active medication to the oral tissues. The vehicle provides a protective covering which may serve to temporarily reduce the pain associated with oral irritation.

INDICATIONS

KENALOG IN ORABASE is indicated for adjunctive treatment and for the temporary relief of symptoms associated with oral inflammatory lesions and ulcerative lesions resulting from trauma.

CONTRAINDICATIONS

This preparation is contraindicated in patients with a history of hypersensitivity to any of its components.

Because it contains a corticosteroid, the preparation is contraindicated in the presence of fungal, viral, or bacterial infections of the mouth or throat.

WARNING

Usage In Pregnancy

Safe use of this preparation during pregnancy has not been established with respect to possible adverse reactions upon fetal development; therefore, it should not be used in women of childbearing potential and particularly during early pregnancy unless, in the judgment of the physician or dentist, the potential benefits outweigh the possible hazards.

PRECAUTIONS

Patients with tuberculosis, peptic ulcer or diabetes mellitus should not be treated with any corticosteroid preparation without the advice of the patient's physician.

It should be borne in mind that the normal defensive responses of the oral tissues are depressed in patients receiving topical corticosteroid therapy. Virulent strains of oral microorganisms may multiply without producing the usual warning symptoms of oral infections.

The small amount of steroid released when the preparation is used as recommended makes systemic effects very unlikely; however, they are a possibility when topical corticosteroid preparations are used over a long period of time.

If local irritation or sensitization should develop, the preparation should be discontinued and appropriate therapy instituted.

If significant regeneration or repair of oral tissues has not occurred in seven days, additional investigation into the etiology of the oral lesion is advised.

ADVERSE REACTIONS

Prolonged administration may elicit the adverse reactions known to occur with systemic steroid preparations; for example, adrenal suppression, alteration of glucose metabolism, protein catabolism, peptic ulcer activations, and others. These are usually reversible and disappear when the hormone is discontinued.

DOSAGE AND ADMINISTRATION

Press a small dab (about ¼ inch) to the lesion until a thin film develops. A larger quantity may be required for coverage of some lesions. For optimal results use only enough to coat the lesion with a thin film. Do not rub in. Attempting to

spread this preparation may result in a granular, gritty sensation and cause it to crumble. After application, however, a smooth, slippery film develops.

The preparation should be applied at bedtime to permit steroid contact with the lesion throughout the night. Depending on the severity of symptoms, it may be necessary to apply the preparation two or three times a day, preferably after meals. If significant repair or regeneration has not occurred in seven days, further investigation is advisable.

HOW SUPPLIED

KENALOG IN ORABASE (Triamcinolone Acetonide Dental Paste USP) is available in 5 g tubes.

Storage

Store at room temperature. Keep tightly closed.

(J2-482F)

MYCOLOG®-II   ℞

[*mĭk'ō-log"*]
Nystatin and Triamcinolone Acetonide Cream USP
Nystatin and Triamcinolone Acetonide Ointment
For Dermatologic Use Only; Not for Ophthalmic Use

DESCRIPTION

MYCOLOG-II Cream and Ointment (Nystatin and Triamcinolone Acetonide Cream and Ointment) for dermatologic use contains the antifungal agent nystatin and the synthetic corticosteroid triamcinolone acetonide.

Nystatin is a polyene antimycotic obtained from *Streptomyces noursei*. It is a yellow to light tan powder with a cereal-like odor, very slightly soluble in water, and slightly to sparingly soluble in alcohol.

Triamcinolone acetonide is designated chemically as 9-fluoro-11β,16α,17,21-tetrahydroxypregna-1,4-diene-3,20-dione cyclic 16,17-acetal with acetone. The white to cream crystalline powder has a slight odor, is practically insoluble in water, and very soluble in alcohol.

MYCOLOG-II Cream (Nystatin and Triamcinolone Acetonide Cream) is a soft, smooth, cream having a light yellow to buff color. Each gram provides 100,000 units nystatin and 1 mg triamcinolone acetonide in an aqueous perfumed vanishing cream base with aluminum hydroxide concentrated wet gel, titanium dioxide, glyceryl monostearate, polyethylene glycol monostearate, simethicone, sorbic acid, propylene glycol, white petrolatum, cetearyl alcohol (and) ceteareth-20, and sorbitol solution.

MYCOLOG-II Ointment (Nystatin and Triamcinolone Acetonide Ointment) provides, in each gram, 100,000 units nystatin and 1 mg triamcinolone acetonide in a protective ointment base, Plastibase® (Plasticized Hydrocarbon Gel), a polyethylene and mineral oil gel base.

CLINICAL PHARMACOLOGY

Nystatin

Nystatin exerts its antifungal activity against a variety of pathogenic and nonpathogenic yeasts and fungi by binding to sterols in the cell membrane. The binding process renders the cell membrane incapable of functioning as a selective barrier. Nystatin provides specific anticandidal activity to *Candida* (Monilia) *albicans* and other *Candida* species, but is not active against bacteria, protozoa, trichomonads, or viruses.

Nystatin is not absorbed from intact skin or mucous membranes.

Triamcinolone Acetonide

Triamcinolone acetonide is primarily effective because of its anti-inflammatory, antipruritic and vasoconstrictive actions, characteristic of the topical corticosteroid class of drugs. The pharmacologic effects of the topical corticosteroids are well-known; however, the mechanisms of their dermatologic actions are unclear. Various laboratory methods, including vasoconstrictor assays, are used to compare and predict potencies and/or clinical efficacies of the topical corticosteroids. There is some evidence to suggest that a recognizable correlation exists between vasoconstrictor potency and therapeutic efficacy in man.

Pharmacokinetics

The extent of percutaneous absorption of topical corticosteroids is determined by many factors including the vehicle, the integrity of the epidermal barrier, and the use of occlusive dressings (see DOSAGE AND ADMINISTRATION). Topical corticosteroids can be absorbed from normal intact skin. Inflammation and/or other disease processes in the skin increase percutaneous absorption. Occlusive dressings substantially increase the percutaneous absorption of topical corticosteroids (see DOSAGE AND ADMINISTRATION). Once absorbed through the skin, topical corticosteroids are handled through pharmacokinetic pathways similar to systemically administered corticosteroids. Corticosteroids are bound to plasma proteins in varying degrees. Corticosteroids are metabolized primarily in the liver and are then excreted by the kidneys. Some of the topical corticosteroids and their metabolites are also excreted into the bile.

Nystatin and Triamcinolone Acetonide

During clinical studies of mild to severe manifestations of cutaneous candidiasis, patients treated with combined nystatin and triamcinolone acetonide showed a faster and more pronounced clearing of erythema and pruritus than patients treated with nystatin or triamcinolone acetonide alone.

INDICATIONS AND USAGE

MYCOLOG-II Cream and Ointment (Nystatin and Triamcinolone Acetonide Cream and Ointment) are indicated for the treatment of cutaneous candidiasis; it has been demonstrated that the nystatin-steroid combination provides greater benefit than the nystatin component alone during the first few days of treatment.

CONTRAINDICATIONS

These preparations are contraindicated in those patients with a history of hypersensitivity to any of their components.

PRECAUTIONS

General

Systemic absorption of topical corticosteroids has produced reversible hypothalamic-pituitary-adrenal (HPA) axis suppression, manifestations of Cushing's syndrome, hyperglycemia, and glucosuria in some patients.

Conditions that augment systemic absorption include application of the more potent steroids, use over large surface areas, prolonged use, and the addition of occlusive dressings (see DOSAGE AND ADMINISTRATION).

Therefore, patients receiving a large dose of any potent topical steroid applied to a large surface area should be evaluated periodically for evidence of HPA axis suppression by using the urinary free cortisol and ACTH stimulation tests, and for impairment of thermal homeostasis. If HPA axis suppression or elevation of the body temperature occurs, an attempt should be made to withdraw the drug, to reduce the frequency of application, or to substitute a less potent steroid.

Recovery of HPA axis function and thermal homeostasis are generally prompt and complete upon discontinuation of the drug. Infrequently, signs and symptoms of steroid withdrawal may occur, requiring supplemental systemic corticosteroids.

Children may absorb proportionally larger amounts of topical corticosteroids and thus be more susceptible to systemic toxicity (see PRECAUTIONS, Pediatric Use).

If irritation or hypersensitivity develops with the combination nystatin and triamcinolone acetonide, treatment should be discontinued and appropriate therapy instituted.

Information for the Patient

Patients using these medications should receive the following information and instructions:

1. These medications are to be used as directed by the physician. They are for dermatologic use only. Avoid contact with the eyes.
2. Patients should be advised not to use these medication for any disorder other than for which it was prescribed.
3. The treated skin area should not be bandaged or otherwise covered or wrapped as to be occluded (see DOSAGE AND ADMINISTRATION).
4. Patients should report any signs of local adverse reactions.
5. When using these medication in the inguinal area, patients should be advised to apply the cream or ointment sparingly and to wear loosely fitting clothing.
6. Parents of pediatric patients should be advised not to use tight-fitting diapers or plastic pants on a child being treated in the diaper area, as these garments may constitute occlusive dressings.
7. Patients should be advised on preventive measures to avoid reinfection.

Laboratory Tests

If there is a lack of therapeutic response, appropriate microbiological studies (e.g., KOH smears and/or cultures) should be repeated to confirm the diagnosis and rule out other pathogens, before instituting another course of therapy.

A urinary free cortisol test and ACTH stimulation test may be helpful in evaluating hypothalamic-pituitary-adrenal (HPA) axis suppression due to corticosteroid.

Carcinogenesis, Mutagenesis, and Impairment of Fertility

Long-term animal studies have not been performed to evaluate carcinogenic or mutagenic potential, or possible impairment of fertility in males or females.

Pregnancy Category C

There are no teratogenic studies with combined nystatin and triamcinolone acetonide. Corticosteroids are generally teratogenic in laboratory animals when administered systemically at relatively low dosage levels. The more potent corticosteroids have been shown to be teratogenic after dermal application in laboratory animals. Therefore, any topical corticosteroid preparation should be used during pregnancy only if the potential benefit justifies the potential risk to the fetus.

Topical preparations containing corticosteroids should not be used extensively on pregnant patients, in large amounts, or for prolonged periods of time.

Nursing Mothers

It is not known whether any component of these preparations are excreted in human milk. Because many drugs are excreted in human milk, caution should be exercised during use of these preparations by a nursing woman.

Pediatric Use

In clinical studies of a limited number of pediatric patients ranging in age from two months through 12 years, nystatin-triamcinolone cream formulation cleared or significantly ameliorated the disease state in most patients.

Pediatric patients may demonstrate greater susceptibility to topical corticosteroid-induced hypothalamic-pituitary-adrenal (HPA) axis suppression and Cushing's syndrome than mature patients because of a larger skin surface area to body weight ratio.

HPA axis suppression, Cushing's syndrome, and intracranial hypertension have been reported in children receiving topical corticosteroids. Manifestations of adrenal suppression in children include linear growth retardation, delayed weight gain, low plasma cortisol levels, and absence of response to ACTH stimulation. Manifestations of intracranial hypertension include bulging fontanelles, headaches, and bilateral papilledema.

Administration of topical corticosteroids to children should be limited to the least amount compatible with an effective therapeutic regimen. Chronic corticosteroid therapy may interfere with the growth and development of children.

ADVERSE REACTIONS

A single case (approximately one percent of patients studied) of acneform eruption occurred with use of combined nystatin and triamcinolone acetonide in clinical studies.

Nystatin is virtually nontoxic and nonsensitizing and is well tolerated by all age groups, even during prolonged use. Rarely, irritation may occur.

The following local adverse reactions are reported infrequently with topical corticosteroids (reactions are listed in an approximate decreasing order of occurrence): burning, itching, irritation, dryness, folliculitis, hypertrichosis, acneform eruptions, hypopigmentation, perioral dermatitis, allergic contact dermatitis, maceration of the skin, secondary infection, skin atrophy, striae, and miliaria.

OVERDOSAGE

Topically applied corticosteroids can be absorbed in sufficient amounts to produce systemic effects (see PRECAUTIONS, General); however, acute overdosage and serious adverse effects with dermatologic use are unlikely.

DOSAGE AND ADMINISTRATION

MYCOLOG-II Cream (Nystatin and Triamcinolone Acetonide Cream) is usually applied to the affected areas twice daily in the morning and evening by gently and thoroughly massaging the preparation into the skin. The cream should be discontinued if symptoms persist after 25 days of therapy (see PRECAUTIONS, Laboratory Tests).

MYCOLOG-II Cream should *not* be used with occlusive dressings.

A thin film of MYCOLOG-II Ointment (Nystatin and Triamcinolone Acetonide Ointment) is usually applied to the affected areas twice daily in the morning and evening.

The preparation should be discontinued if symptoms persist after 25 days of therapy (see PRECAUTIONS, Laboratory Tests).

MYCOLOG-II Ointment should *not* be used with occlusive dressings.

HOW SUPPLIED

MYCOLOG-II Cream (Nystatin and Triamcinolone Acetonide Cream USP) is supplied in 15 g (NDC 0003-0566-30), 30 g (NDC 0003-0566-60), and 60 g (NDC 0003-0566-65) tubes and 120 g (NDC 0003-0566-50) jars.

MYCOLOG-II Ointment (Nystatin and Triamcinolone Acetonide Ointment) is supplied in 15 g (NDC 0003-0466-30), 30 g (NDC 0003-0466-60), and 60 g (NDC 0003-0466-65) tubes and 120 g (NDC 0003-0466-50) jars.

Storage

Store at room temperature; avoid freezing cream. (J4-019B/J4-024)

MYCOSTATIN® CREAM   ℞
[mĭk´ō-stat˝in]
Nystatin Cream USP
MYCOSTATIN TOPICAL POWDER   ℞
Nystatin Topical Powder USP
MYCOSTATIN OINTMENT   ℞
Nystatin Ointment USP

DESCRIPTION

MYCOSTATIN Cream (Nystatin Cream), MYCOSTATIN Topical Powder (Nystatin Topical Powder), and MYCOSTATIN Ointment (Nystatin Ointment) are for dermatologic use.

MYCOSTATIN Cream contains the antifungal antibiotic nystatin at a concentration of 100,000 units per gram in an aqueous, perfumed vanishing cream base containing aluminum hydroxide concentrated wet gel, titanium dioxide, propylene glycol, cetearyl alcohol (and) ceteareth-20, white petrolatum, sorbitol solution, glyceryl monostearate, polyethylene glycol monostearate, sorbic acid and simethicone.

MYCOSTATIN Topical Powder provides, in each gram, 100,000 units nystatin dispersed in Talc.

MYCOSTATIN Ointment provides 100,000 units nystatin per gram in Plastibase® (Plasticized Hydrocarbon Gel), a polyethylene and mineral oil gel base.

CLINICAL PHARMACOLOGY

Nystatin is an antifungal antibiotic which is both fungistatic and fungicidal *in vitro* against a wide variety of yeasts and yeast-like fungi. It probably acts by binding to sterols in the cell membrane of the fungus with a resultant change in membrane permeability allowing leakage of intracellular components. Nystatin is a polyene antibiotic of undetermined structural formula that is obtained from *Streptomyces noursei*, and is the first well tolerated antifungal antibiotic of dependable efficacy for the treatment of cutaneous, oral and intestinal infections caused by *Candida* (Monilia) *albicans* and other Candida species. It exhibits no appreciable activity against bacteria.

Nystatin provides specific therapy for all localized forms of candidiasis. Symptomatic relief is rapid, often occurring within 24 to 72 hours after the initiation of treatment. Cure is effected both clinically and mycologically in most cases of localized candidiasis.

INDICATIONS AND USAGE

MYCOSTATIN (nystatin) topical preparations are indicated in the treatment of cutaneous or mucocutaneous mycotic infections caused by *Candida* (Monilia) *albicans* and other Candida species.

CONTRAINDICATIONS

MYCOSTATIN topical preparations are contraindicated in patients with a history of hypersensitivity to any of their components.

PRECAUTIONS

Should a reaction of hypersensitivity occur the drug should be immediately withdrawn and appropriate measures taken. These preparations are not for ophthalmic use.

ADVERSE REACTIONS

Nystatin is virtually nontoxic and nonsensitizing and is well tolerated by all age groups including debilitated infants, even on prolonged administration. If irritation on topical application should occur, discontinue medication.

DOSAGE AND ADMINISTRATION

The cream and the ointment should be applied liberally to affected areas twice daily or as indicated until healing is complete. The powder should be applied to candidal lesions two or three times daily until lesions have healed. For fungal infection of the feet caused by Candida species, the powder should be dusted freely on the feet as well as in shoes and socks. The cream is usually preferred to the ointment in candidiasis involving intertriginous areas; very moist lesions, however, are best treated with the topical dusting powder. The preparations do not stain skin or mucous membranes and they provide a simple, convenient means of treatment.

HOW SUPPLIED

MYCOSTATIN Cream (Nystatin Cream USP) is supplied in tubes providing 100,000 units nystatin per gram in an aqueous, perfumed vanishing cream base.

MYCOSTATIN Topical Powder (Nystatin Topical Powder USP) is supplied in plastic squeeze bottles providing, in each gram, 100,000 units nystatin.

MYCOSTATIN Ointment (Nystatin Ointment USP) is supplied in tubes providing 100,000 units nystatin per gram.

Store

Store the cream at room temperature; avoid freezing. Store the ointment at room temperature. Store the topical powder at room temperature; avoid excessive heat; keep bottle tightly closed.

(J3-331E)

MYCOSTATIN® ORAL SUSPENSION   ℞
[mĭk´ō-stat˝in]
Nystatin Oral Suspension USP

DESCRIPTION

Nystatin is an antifungal antibiotic which is both fungistatic and fungicidal *in vitro* against a wide variety of yeasts and yeast-like fungi. It is a polyene antibiotic of undetermined structural formula that is obtained from *Streptomyces noursei*. MYCOSTATIN Oral Suspension is provided for oral administration containing 100,000 units nystatin per mL. Inactive ingredients: alcohol (not > 1% v/v), carboxymethylcellulose sodium, flavors, glycerin, methylparaben,

Continued on next page

Squibb—Cont.

propylparaben, saccharin sodium, sodium phosphate, sucrose (50% w/v), and purified water.

CLINICAL PHARMACOLOGY

Nystatin probably acts by binding to sterols in the cell membrane of the fungus with a resultant change in membrane permeability allowing leakage of intracellular components. It exhibits no appreciable activity against bacteria or trichomonads.

Following oral administration, nystatin is sparingly absorbed with no detectable blood levels when given in the recommended doses. Most of the orally administered nystatin is passed unchanged in the stool.

INDICATIONS AND USAGE

MYCOSTATIN Oral Suspension is indicated for the treatment of candidiasis in the oral cavity.

CONTRAINDICATION

The preparation is contraindicated in patients with a history of hypersensitivity to any of its components.

PRECAUTIONS

Usage in Pregnancy

No adverse effects or complications have been attributed to nystatin in infants born to women treated with nystatin.

ADVERSE REACTIONS

Nystatin is virtually nontoxic and nonsensitizing and is well tolerated by all age groups including debilitated infants, even on prolonged administration. Large oral doses have occasionally produced diarrhea, gastrointestinal distress, nausea, and vomiting.

DOSAGE AND ADMINISTRATION

INFANTS: 2 mL (200,000 units nystatin) four times daily (1 mL in each side of mouth).

NOTE: Limited clinical studies in premature and low birth weight infants indicate that 1 mL four times daily is effective.

CHILDREN AND ADULTS: 4-6 mL (400,000 to 600,000 units nystatin) four times daily (one-half of dose in each side of mouth). The preparation should be retained in the mouth as long as possible before swallowing.

Continue treatment for at least 48 hours after perioral symptoms have disappeared and cultures returned to normal.

HOW SUPPLIED

MYCOSTATIN Oral Suspension (Nystatin Oral Suspension USP), 100,000 units per mL, is available as a pleasant-tasting, light creamy yellow, ready-to-use suspension in 5 mL bottles (NDC 0003-0588-50), 60 mL bottles (NDC 0003-0588-60), and 473 mL bottles (NDC 0003-0588-10).

Storage

Store at room temperature; avoid freezing.

(J3-208K)

MYCOSTATIN® ORAL TABLETS   ℞

[mĭk'ō-stat"in]
Nystatin Tablets USP

DESCRIPTION

Nystatin is an antifungal antibiotic which is both fungistatic and fungicidal *in vitro* against a wide variety of yeasts and yeast-like fungi. It is a polyene antibiotic of undetermined structural formula that is obtained from *Streptomyces noursei.* MYCOSTATIN Oral Tablets are provided for oral administration as coated tablets containing 500,000 units nystatin. Inactive ingredients: cellulose, colorants (FD&C Blue No. 2, Red No. 3, and Yellow No. 6), cornstarch, flavor, lactose, magnesium stearate, povidone, stearic acid and other ingredients.

CLINICAL PHARMACOLOGY

Nystatin probably acts by binding to sterols in the cell membrane of the fungus with a resultant change in membrane permeability allowing leakage of intracellular components. It exhibits no appreciable activity against bacteria or trichomonads.

Following oral administration, nystatin is sparingly absorbed with no detectable blood levels when given in the recommended doses. Most of the orally administered nystatin is passed unchanged in the stool.

INDICATIONS AND USAGE

MYCOSTATIN Oral Tablets are intended for the treatment of intestinal candidiasis.

CONTRAINDICATIONS

MYCOSTATIN Oral Tablets are contraindicated in patients with a history of hypersensitivity to any of their components.

PRECAUTIONS

Usage in Pregnancy

No adverse effects or complications have been attributed to nystatin in infants born to women treated with nystatin.

ADVERSE REACTIONS

Nystatin is virtually nontoxic and nonsensitizing and is well tolerated by all age groups including debilitated infants, even on prolonged administration. Large oral doses have occasionally produced diarrhea, gastrointestinal distress, nausea and vomiting.

DOSAGE AND ADMINISTRATION

The usual therapeutic dosage is one to two tablets (500,000 to 1,000,000 units nystatin) three times daily. Treatment should generally be continued for at least 48 hours after clinical cure to prevent relapse.

HOW SUPPLIED

MYCOSTATIN Oral Tablets (Nystatin Tablets USP, 500,000 units nystatin each) are available in cartons of 100 single dose UNIMATIC® packs (NDC 0003-0580-54) and bottles of 100 tablets (NDC 0003-0580-53).

Each FILMLOK® tablet is imprinted with identification number 580.

ALSO AVAILABLE

Mycostatin (Nystatin USP) is also available as Vaginal Tablets, Topical Powder, Cream, Ointment, and as a ready-to-use Oral Suspension (see package inserts for complete information).

Storage

Store at room temperature; avoid excessive heat. Dispense in tight, light-resistant containers.

* FILMLOK is a Squibb trademark for veneer-coated tablets. (J3-513B)

Shown in Product Identification Section, page 431

MYCOSTATIN® PASTILLES   ℞

[mĭk'ō-stat"in]
Nystatin

DESCRIPTION

Nystatin is a polyene antifungal antibiotic obtained from *Streptomyces noursei.*

MYCOSTATIN (nystatin) Pastilles are round, light to dark gold-colored troches designed to dissolve slowly in the mouth. Each pastille provides 200,000 units nystatin. Inactive ingredients: anise oil, cinnamon oil, gelatin, sucrose, and other ingredients.

CLINICAL PHARMACOLOGY

Nystatin is both fungistatic and fungicidal *in vitro* against a wide variety of yeasts and yeast-like fungi. *Candida albicans* demonstrates no significant resistance to nystatin *in vitro* on repeated subculture in increasing levels of nystatin; other *Candida* species become quite resistant. Generally, resistance does not develop *in vivo*. Nystatin acts by binding to sterols in the cell membrane of susceptible fungi with a resultant change in membrane permeability allowing leakage of intracellular components. Nystatin exhibits no activity against bacteria, protozoa, trichomonads, or viruses.

Pharmacokinetics

Gastrointestinal absorption of nystatin is insignificant. Most orally administered nystatin is passed unchanged in the stool. Significant concentrations of nystatin may appear occasionally in the plasma of patients with renal insufficiency during oral therapy with conventional dosage forms. Mean nystatin concentrations in excess of those required *in vitro* to inhibit growth of clinically significant *Candida* persisted in saliva for approximately two hours after the start of oral dissolution of two nystatin pastilles (400,000 units nystatin) administered simultaneously to 12 healthy volunteers.

INDICATIONS AND USAGE

MYCOSTATIN (nystatin) Pastilles are indicated for the treatment of candidiasis in the oral cavity.

CONTRAINDICATIONS

The pastille is contraindicated in those patients with a history of hypersensitivity to any of its components.

PRECAUTIONS

General

This medication is not to be used for the treatment of systemic mycoses.

In order to achieve maximum effect from the medication, pastilles must be allowed to dissolve slowly in the mouth; therefore, patients for whom the pastille is prescribed, including children and the elderly, must be competent to utilize the dosage form as intended.

If irritation or hypersensitivity develops with nystatin pastilles, treatment should be discontinued and appropriate therapy instituted.

Information for the Patient

Patients taking this medication should receive the following information and instructions:

1. Use as directed; the medication is not for any disorder other than for which it was prescribed.
2. Allow pastille to dissolve slowly in the mouth; **do not chew or swallow the pastille.**

3. The patient should be advised regarding replacement of any missed doses.
4. There should be no interruption or discontinuation of medication until the prescribed course of treatment is completed even though symptomatic relief may occur within a few days.
5. If symptoms of local irritation develop, the physician should be notified promptly.
6. Good oral hygiene, including proper care of dentures, is particularly important for denture wearers.

Laboratory Tests

If there is a lack of therapeutic response, appropriate microbiological studies (e.g., KOH smears and/or cultures) should be repeated to confirm the diagnosis of candidiasis and rule out other pathogens before instituting another course of therapy.

Carcinogenesis, Mutagenesis, Impairment of Fertility

Studies have not been performed to evaluate carcinogenic or mutagenic potential, or possible impairment of fertility in males or females.

Pregnancy: Teratogenic Effects

Category C. Animal reproduction studies have not been conducted with nystatin pastilles. It is also not known whether nystatin pastilles can cause fetal harm when administered to a pregnant woman or can affect reproduction capacity. Nystatin pastilles should be dispensed to a pregnant woman only if clearly needed.

Pediatric Use

See PRECAUTIONS, General.

ADVERSE REACTIONS

Nystatin is virtually nontoxic and nonsensitizing and is well-tolerated by all age groups, even during prolonged use. Rarely, oral irritation or sensitization may occur. Nausea has been reported occasionally during therapy.

Large oral doses of nystatin have occasionally produced diarrhea, gastrointestinal distress, nausea and vomiting.

OVERDOSAGE

Oral doses of nystatin in excess of five million units daily have caused nausea and gastrointestinal upset. There have been no reports of serious toxic effects or superinfections (see CLINICAL PHARMACOLOGY, Pharmacokinetics).

DOSAGE AND ADMINISTRATION

Children and Adults: The recommended dose is one or two pastilles (200,000 or 400,000 units nystatin) four or five times daily for as long as 14 days if necessary. The dosage regimen should be continued for at least 48 hours after disappearance of oral symptoms.

Dosage should be discontinued if symptoms persist after the initial 14 day period of treatment (see PRECAUTIONS, Laboratory Tests).

Administration: Pastilles must be allowed to dissolve slowly in the mouth, and should not be chewed or swallowed whole.

HOW SUPPLIED

MYCOSTATIN (nystatin) Pastilles, 200,000 units nystatin each, in packages containing 30 pleasant-tasting pastilles (NDC 0003-0543-20).

ALSO AVAILABLE

MYCOSTATIN (Nystatin USP) is also available as a ready-to-use oral suspension, oral tablets, vaginal tablets, and topical powder, cream, and ointment (see package inserts accompanying those products for complete information).

Storage

Refrigerate between 2° and 8°C (36° and 46°F).

(J4-030)

Shown in Product Identification Section, page 431

MYCOSTATIN® VAGINAL TABLETS   ℞

[mĭk'ō-stat"in]
(Nystatin Vaginal Tablets USP)

DESCRIPTION

Nystatin is an antimycotic polyene antibiotic obtained from *Streptomyces noursei.*

MYCOSTATIN Vaginal Tablets (Nystatin Vaginal Tablets USP) are available as diamond-shaped compressed tablets for intravaginal administration, providing 100,000 units of nystatin dispersed in lactose with ethyl cellulose, stearic acid, and starch.

CLINICAL PHARMACOLOGY

Nystatin is both fungistatic and fungicidal *in vitro* against a wide variety of yeasts and yeast-like fungi. Nystatin acts by binding to sterols in the cell membrane of sensitive fungi with a resultant change in membrane permeability allowing leakage of intracellular components. Nystatin exhibits no appreciable activity against bacteria, protozoa, trichomonads, or viruses.

Nystatin is not absorbed from intact skin or mucous membranes.

INDICATIONS AND USAGE

MYCOSTATIN Vaginal Tablets (Nystatin Vaginal Tablets USP) are effective for the local treatment of vulvovaginal candidiasis (moniliasis). The diagnosis should be confirmed, prior to therapy, by KOH smears and/or cultures. Other pathogens commonly associated with vulvovaginitis (Trichomonas and *Haemophilus vaginalis*) do not respond to nystatin and should be ruled out by appropriate laboratory methods.

CONTRAINDICATIONS

This preparation is contraindicated in patients with a history of hypersensitivity to any of its components.

PRECAUTIONS

General

Discontinue treatment if sensitization or irritation is reported during use.

Information for Patients

The patient should be informed of symptoms of sensitization or irritation and told to report them promptly.

The patient should be warned against interruption or discontinuation of medication even during menstruation and even though symptomatic relief may occur within a few days.

The patient should be advised that adjunctive measures such as therapeutic douches are unnecessary and sometimes inadvisable, but cleansing douches may be used by nonpregnant women, if desired, for esthetic purposes.

Laboratory Tests

If there is a lack of response to MYCOSTATIN Vaginal Tablets (Nystatin Vaginal Tablets USP), appropriate microbiological studies should be repeated to confirm the diagnosis and rule out other pathogens, before instituting another course of antimycotic therapy (see INDICATIONS AND USAGE).

Carcinogenesis, Mutagenesis, Impairment of Fertility

Long-term studies in animals have not been performed to evaluate carcinogenic potential, mutagenesis, or whether this medication affects fertility in females.

Pregnancy: Teratogenic Effects

Category A. There have been no reports that use of nystatin vaginal tablets by pregnant women increases the risk of fetal abnormalities or affects later growth, development, and functional maturation of the child. Nevertheless, because the possibility of harm cannot be ruled out, nystatin vaginal tablets should be used during pregnancy only if the physician considers it essential to the welfare of the patient.

Animal reproduction studies have not been conducted with nystatin vaginal tablets.

Pediatric Use

Safety and effectiveness in children have not been established.

ADVERSE REACTIONS

Nystatin is virtually nontoxic and nonsensitizing and is well tolerated by all age groups, even on prolonged administration. Rarely, irritation or sensitization may occur (see PRECAUTIONS).

DOSAGE AND ADMINISTRATION

The usual dosage is one tablet (100,000 units nystatin) daily for two weeks. The tablets should be deposited high in the vagina by means of the applicator. "Instructions for the Patient" are enclosed in each package.

HOW SUPPLIED

MYCOSTATIN Vaginal Tablets (Nystatin Vaginal Tablets USP) are available in packages of individually foil wrapped tablets with applicator as follows: package of 15 (NSN 6505-00-616-9128); and package of 30.

UNIMATIC® cartons of 50 celloprotected unit-dose packs contain one individually foil wrapped tablet, one applicator, and one "Instructions for the Patient" leaflet.

Each diamond-shaped tablet is imprinted with identification number **457**.

Storage

Store in refrigerator below 15° C (59° F).

(J3-635)

Shown in Product Identification Section, page 431

PENTIDS® FOR SYRUP   ℞
[pen'tidz]
PENTIDS® '400' FOR SYRUP   ℞
Penicillin G Potassium for Oral Solution USP

DESCRIPTION

PENTIDS For Syrup (Penicillin G Potassium for Oral Solution) contain penicillin G potassium in flavored powder forms for preparation as syrups for oral administration. Penicillin G potassium is chemically designated as monopotassium (2S,5R,6R)-3,3-dimethyl-7-oxo-6-(2-phenylacetamido)-4-thia-1-azabicyclo[3.2.0]heptane-2-carboxylate.

PENTIDS For Syrup and PENTIDS '400' For Syrup contain 125 mg (200,000 u) and 250 mg (400,000 u) of penicillin G potassium, respectively, per 5 mL after constitution. Inactive ingredients: colorants [FD&C Yellow No. 5 (tartrazine) and Yellow No. 6], flavors, saccharin sodium, sodium phosphate, and sucrose.

CLINICAL PHARMACOLOGY

Penicillin G is bactericidal against penicillin-susceptible microorganisms during the stage of active multiplication. It acts by inhibiting biosynthesis of cell-wall mucopeptide. It is not active against the penicillinase-producing bacteria, which include many strains of staphylococci.

Oral preparations of penicillin G are only slightly affected by normal gastric acidity (pH 2.0 to 3.5); however, a pH below 2.0 may partially or totally inactivate penicillin G. Oral penicillin G is absorbed in the upper small intestine, chiefly the duodenum; however, serum level and urinary excretion data indicate that only approximately 30 percent of the dose is absorbed. For this reason four to five times the dose of oral penicillin G must be given to obtain a blood level comparable to that obtained with parenteral penicillin G. Since gastric acidity, stomach emptying time, and other factors affecting absorption may vary considerably, serum levels may be appreciably reduced to nontherapeutic levels in certain individuals.

Approximately 60 percent of penicillin G is bound to serum protein. The drug is distributed throughout the body tissues in widely varying amounts. Highest levels are found in the kidneys with lesser amounts in the liver, skin, and intestines. Penicillin G penetrates into all other tissues to a lesser degree with very limited amounts found in the cerebrospinal fluid. The drug is excreted rapidly by tubular excretion in patients with normal kidney function. In neonates and young infants, and in individuals with impaired kidney function, excretion is considerably delayed. Normally, approximately 20 percent of a dose of oral penicillin G is excreted in the urine.

Microbiology

While *in vitro* studies have demonstrated the susceptibility of most strains of the following organisms, clinical efficacy for infections other than those included in the INDICATIONS AN USAGE section has not been documented.

Penicillin G is highly active *in vitro* against staphylococci (except penicillinase-producing strains), streptococci (groups A,C,G,H,L, and M), except group D enterococcus which is resistant, and pneumococci. Other organisms susceptible *in vitro* to penicillin G are *Neisseria gonorrhoeae* (nonpenicillinase producing strains), *Corynebacterium diphtheriae, Bacillus anthracis,* Clostridia, *Actinomyces bovis, Streptobacillus moniliformis, Listeria monocytogenes,* and Leptospira; *Treponema pallidum* is extremely susceptible.

Some species of gram-negative bacilli are susceptible to moderate to high concentrations of penicillin G obtained with intravenous administration. These include most strains of *Escherichia coli,* all strains of *Proteus mirabilis,* Salmonella and Shigella and some strains of *Enterobacter aerogenes* (formerly *Aerobacter aerogenes*) and *Alcaligenes fecalis.*

INDICATIONS AND USAGE

PENTIDS For Syrup and PENTIDS '400' For Syrup (Penicillin G Potassium for Oral Solution) are indicated in the treatment of infections caused by susceptible strains of the designated organisms in the diseases or conditions listed below. Therapy should be guided by bacteriological studies, including susceptibility tests, and by clinical response. Note: For severe pneumonia, empyema, streptococcal and other infections with bacteremia, pericarditis, meningitis, and septic arthritis, treatment with aqueous penicillin G is recommended during the acute stage.

Oral penicillin G is not recommended for short-term prevention of bacterial endocarditis in patients with valvular heart disease undergoing dental or surgical procedures.

Therapy of susceptible infections should be accompanied by any indicated surgical procedures.

The following infections will usually respond to adequate dosage:

Upper Respiratory Tract Infections—Including otitis media caused by group A streptococci and oral pharyngeal infections caused by fusobacteria.

NOTE: Necessary dental care should be accomplished in infections involving gum tissue.

Lower Respiratory Tract Infections—Due to *S. pneumoniae.*

Skin and Skin Structure Infections—Due to group A streptococci and susceptible strains of staphylococci.

NOTE: There are a number of strains of staphylococci resistant to penicillin G, emphasizing the need for culture and susceptibility studies in treating suspected staphylococcal infections.

Other—Scarlet fever due to group A streptococci; prevention of recurrence following rheumatic fever and/or chorea.

CONTRAINDICATIONS

Contraindicated in patients with a history of hypersensitivity to any penicillin.

WARNINGS

Serious and occasionally fatal hypersensitivity (anaphylactoid) reactions have been reported in patients on penicillin therapy. Although anaphylaxis is more frequent following parenteral administration, it has occurred in patients on oral penicillins. These reactions are more apt to occur in individuals with a history of penicillin hypersensitivity and/or a history of sensitivity to multiple allergens.

There have been well-documented reports of individuals with a history of penicillin hypersensitivity who have experienced severe hypersensitivity reactions when treated with cephalosporins. Before initiating therapy with any penicillin, careful inquiry should be made concerning previous hypersensitivity reactions to penicillins, cephalosporins, and other allergens. If an allergic reaction occurs, the drug should be discontinued and the appropriate therapy instituted. Serious anaphylactoid reactions require immediate emergency treatment with epinephrine. Oxygen, intravenous steroids, and airway management, including intubation, should also be administered as indicated.

PRECAUTIONS

General

Penicillin should be used with caution in individuals with histories of significant allergies and/or asthma.

The oral route of administration should not be relied upon in patients with severe illness, or with nausea, vomiting, gastric dilatation, cardiospasm or intestinal hypermotility.

Occasional patients will not absorb therapeutic amounts of orally administered penicillin.

Prolonged use of antibiotics may promote the overgrowth of nonsusceptible organisms, including fungi. Should superinfection occur, appropriate measures should be taken.

PENTIDS For Syrup and PENTIDS '400' For Syrup (Penicillin G Potassium for Oral Solution) contain FD&C Yellow No. 5 (tartrazine) which may cause allergic-type reactions (including bronchial asthma) in certain susceptible individuals. Although the overall incidence of FD&C Yellow No. 5 (tartrazine) sensitivity in the general population is low, it is frequently seen in patients who also have aspirin hypersensitivity.

Information for Patients

1. Penicillin G Potassium is best taken on an empty stomach one-half hour before or at least two hours after meals. Acidic fruit juices or other acidic beverages should be avoided within one hour of drug administration since they interfere with absorption.
2. The patient should inform the physician of any history of sensitivity to allergens, including previous hypersensitivity reactions to penicillins and cephalosporins (see WARNINGS).
3. The patient should discontinue the drug and contact the physician immediately if any side effect occurs (see WARNINGS).
4. Diabetic patients should consult with the physician before changing diet or dosage of diabetes medication (see PRECAUTIONS, Drug/Laboratory Test Interactions).

Laboratory Tests

In streptococcal infections, therapy must be sufficient to eliminate the organism (10 days minimum); otherwise the sequelae of streptococcal disease may occur. Cultures should be taken following completion of treatment to determine whether streptococci have been eradicated.

In prolonged therapy with penicillin, and particularly with high dosage regimens, periodic evaluation of the renal and hematopoietic systems is recommended.

Drug Interactions

When administered concurrently, the following drugs may interact with penicillins:

Aspirin or phenylbutazone—Drugs capable of displacing bound penicillin from plasma protein binding sites may elevate the level of free penicillin in the serum; however, the clinical significance of this interaction is not well documented.

Bacteriostatic antibiotics—Chloramphenicol, erythromycins, sulfonamides, or tetracyclines may interfere with the bactericidal effect of penicillins. This has been documented *in vitro;* however, the clinical significance of this interaction is not well documented.

Probenecid—May decrease renal tubular secretion of penicillin resulting in increased blood levels and/or penicillin toxicity.

Drug/Laboratory Test Interactions

After treatment with penicillin, a false-positive reaction for glucose in the urine may occur with copper sulfate tests (Benedict's solution, Fehling's solution or Clinitest® tablets) but not with enzyme based tests such as Clinistix® and Tes-Tape®.

Carcinogenesis, Mutagenesis, Impairment of Fertility

Long-term studies in animals have not been performed to evaluate carcinogenesis, mutagenesis, or impairment of fertility in males or females.

Pregnancy: Teratogenic Effects

Category B

Reproduction studies performed in the mouse, rat, and rabbit have revealed no evidence of impaired fertility or harm to the fetus due to penicillin. Human experience with the penicillins during pregnancy has not shown any positive evidence of adverse effects on the fetus. There are, however, no adequate and well-controlled studies in pregnant women

Continued on next page

Squibb—Cont.

showing conclusively that harmful effects of these drugs on the fetus can be excluded. Because animal reproduction studies are not always predictive of human response, penicillin should be used during pregnancy only if clearly needed.

Nursing Mothers
Since penicillins are excreted in breast milk during lactation, penicillin use by nursing mothers may lead to sensitization of infants; therefore, a decision should be made whether to discontinue nursing or to discontinue the drug, taking into account, the importance of the drug to the mother.

Pediatric Use
Penicillins are excreted primarily unchanged by the kidney; therefore, the incompletely developed renal function in neonates and young infants will delay the excretion of penicillin. Administration to neonates and young infants should be limited to the lowest dosage compatible with an effective therapeutic regimen (see DOSAGE AND AMINISTRATION).

ADVERSE REACTIONS
Although the incidence of reactions to oral penicillins has been reported with much less frequency than following parenteral therapy, it should be remembered that all degrees of hypersensitivity, including fatal anaphylaxis, have been reported with oral penicillin.

The most common reactions to oral penicillin are nausea, vomiting, epigastric distress, diarrhea, and black hairy tongue. The hypersensitivity reactions reported are skin rashes ranging from maculopapular to exfoliative dermatitis; urticaria; serum sickness-like reactions including chills, fever, edema, arthralgia, and prostration; laryngeal edema; and anaphylaxis. Fever and eosinophilia may frequently be the only reactions observed. Hemolytic anemia, leukopenia, thrombocytopenia, neuropathy, and nephropathy are infrequent reactions usually associated with high doses of parenteral penicillin. Urticaria, other skin rashes, and serum sickness-like reactions may be controlled by antihistamines and, if necessary, corticosteroids. Whenever such reactions occur, penicillin should be discontinued unless, in the opinion of the physician, the condition being treated is life-threatening and amenable only to penicillin therapy. Serious anaphylactoid reactions require emergency measures (see WARNINGS). An occasional patient may complain of sore mouth or tongue, as with any oral penicillin preparation.

OVERDOSAGE
In case of overdosage, discontinue medication, treat symptomatically and institute supportive measures as required. Penicillin G may be removed from the blood by hemodialysis.

DOSAGE AND ADMINISTRATION
The dosage of penicillin G should be determined according to the susceptibility of the causative microorganisms and the severity of infection, and adjusted to the clinical response of the patient.

Therapy for children under 12 years of age is calculated on the basis of body weight. For infants and small children the suggested dose is 15 to 56 mg (25,000 to 90,000 u) per kg/day in three to six divided doses.

For maximum absorption of penicillin, dosage should be given on an empty stomach. Thus, a dose of 200,000 u should be administered one-half hour before or at least two hours after meals. The blood concentration with a dose of 400,000 u is sufficiently high to inhibit susceptible bacteria when the antibiotic is given without regard to meals but, as can be expected, the resultant concentration will be higher when it is given before meals.

The usual dosage recommendation for adults and children 12 years and over is as follows:

Streptococcal infections—mild to moderately severe—of the upper respiratory tract and including otitis media, scarlet fever and mild erysipelas: 125 mg (200,000 u) tid or qid for 10 days for mild infections; 250 mg (400,000 u) tid for 10 days for moderately severe infections; alternatively, 500 mg (800,000 u) may be given bid (see PRECAUTIONS, Laboratory Tests).

Pneumococcal infections—mild to moderately severe—of the respiratory tract, including otitis media: 250 mg (400,000 u) qid until the patient has been afebrile for at least two days.

Staphylococcal infections—mild infections of skin and skin structures (culture and susceptibility tests should be performed): 125 to 250 mg (200,000 to 400,000 u) tid or qid until infection is cured.

Vincent's gingivitis and pharyngitis (fusospirochetosis)—mild to moderately severe infections of the oropharynx: 250 mg (400,000 u) tid or qid.

For the prevention of recurrence following rheumatic fever and/or chorea: 125 mg (200,000 u) twice daily on a continuing basis.

HOW SUPPLIED
PENTIDS For Syrup
(Penicillin G Potassium for Oral Solution USP)
125 mg (200,000 u)/   When constituted as directed on

5 mL teaspoonful: the container label, a fruit-flavored syrup in 100 mL (NDC 0003-0746-38) size bottles.

PENTIDS '400' For Syrup
250 mg (400,000 u)/   When constituted as directed on
5 mL teaspoonful: the container label, a fruit-flavored syrup in 100 mL (NDC 0003-0743-39) and 200 mL (NDC 0003-0743-54) size bottles.

Storage
Store at room temperature prior to constitution. After constitution, store syrup in refrigerator and discard unused portion after 14 days. Keep bottle tightly closed.
(J4-158A)

PENTIDS® TABLETS   ℞
[pen 'tidz]
PENTIDS® '400' TABLETS   ℞
PENTIDS® '800' TABLETS   ℞
Penicillin G Potassium Tablets USP

DESCRIPTION
PENTIDS Tablets (Penicillen G Potassium Tablets) contain crystalline penicillin G potassium for oral administration. Penicillin G potassium is chemically designated as monopotassium (2S,5R,6R)-3,3-dimethyl-7-oxo-6-(2-phenylacetamido)-4-thia-1-azabicyclo[3.2.0]heptane-2-carboxylate.
PENTIDS Tablets contain 125 mg (200,000 u) crystalline penicillin G potassium. Inactive ingredients: calcium carbonate, corn starch, lactose, magnesium stearate, and sodium benzoate.
PENTIDS '400' Tablets contain 250 mg (400,000 u) crystalline penicillin G potassium. Inactive ingredients: calcium carbonate, corn starch, lactose, magnesium stearate, and povidone.
PENTIDS '800' Tablets contain 500 mg (800,000 u) crystalline penicillin G potassium. Inactive ingredients: calcium carbonate, colorants [FD&C Blue No. 1 and FD&C Yellow No. 5 (tartrazine)], corn starch, lactose, magnesium stearate, and povidone.

CLINICAL PHARMACOLOGY
Penicillin G is bactericidal against penicillin-susceptible microorganisms during the stage of active multiplication. It acts by inhibiting biosynthesis of cell-wall mucopeptide. It is not active against the penicillinase-producing bacteria, which include many strains of staphylococci.
Oral preparations of penicillin G are only slightly affected by normal gastric acidity (pH 2.0 to 3.5); however, a pH below 2.0 may partially or totally inactivate penicillin G. Oral penicillin G is absorbed in the upper small intestine, chiefly the duodenum; however, serum level and urinary excretion data indicate that only approximately 30 percent of the dose is absorbed. For this reason four to five times the dose of oral penicillin G must be given to obtain a blood level comparable to that obtained with parenteral penicillin G. Since gastric acidity, stomach emptying time, and other factors affecting absorption may vary considerably, serum levels may be appreciably reduced to nontherapeutic levels in certain individuals.
Approximately 60 percent of penicillin G is bound to serum protein. The drug is distributed throughout the body tissues in widely varying amounts. Highest levels are found in the kidneys with lesser amounts in the liver, skin, and intestines. Penicillin G penetrates into all other tissues to a lesser degree with very limited amounts found in the cerebrospinal fluid. The drug is excreted rapidly by tubular excretion in patients with normal kidney function. In neonates and young infants, and in individuals with impaired kidney function, excretion is considerably delayed. Normally, approximately 20 percent of a dose of oral penicillin G is excreted in the urine.

Microbiology
While *in vitro* studies have demonstrated the susceptibility of most strains of the following organisms, clinical efficacy for infections other than those included in the INDICATIONS AN USAGE section has not been documented.
Penicillin G is highly active *in vitro* against staphylococci (except penicillinase-producing strains), streptococci (groups A,C,G,H,L, and M), except group D enterococcus which is resistant, and pneumococci. Other organisms susceptible *in vitro* to penicillin G are *Neisseria gonorrhoeae* (nonpenicillinase-producing strains), *Corynebacterium diphtheriae, Bacillus anthracis,* Clostridia, *Actinomyces bovis, Streptobacillus moniliformis, Listeria monocytogenes,* and Leptospira; *Treponema pallidum* is extremely susceptible.
Some species of gram-negative bacilli are susceptible to moderate to high concentrations of penicillin G obtained with intravenous administration. These include most strains of *Escherichia coli,* all strains of *Proteus mirabilis, Salmonella* and *Shigella* and some strains of *Enterobacter aerogenes* (formerly *Aerobacter aerogenes*) and *Alcaligenes fecalis.*

INDICATIONS AND USAGE
PENTIDS, PENTIDS '400', and PENTIDS '800' Tablets (Penicillin G Potassium Tablets) are indicated in the treatment of infections caused by susceptible strains of the designated organisms in the diseases or conditions listed below. Therapy should be guided by bacteriological studies, including susceptibility tests, and by clinical response. Note: For severe pneumonia, empyema, streptococcal and other infections with bacteremia, pericarditis, meningitis, and septic arthritis, treatment with aqueous penicillin G is recommended during the acute stage.
Oral penicillin G is not recommended for short-term prevention of bacterial endocarditis in patients with valvular heart disease undergoing dental or surgical procedures.
Therapy of susceptible infections should be accompanied by any indicated surgical procedures.
The following infections will usually respond to adequate dosage:
Upper Respiratory Tract Infections—Including otitis media caused by group A streptococcus and oral pharyngeal infections caused by fusobacteria.
NOTE: Necessary dental care should be accomplished in infections involving gum tissue.
Lower Respiratory Tract Infections—Due to *S. pneumoniae.*
Skin and Skin Structure Infections—Due to group A streptococci and susceptible strains of staphylococci.
NOTE: There are a number of strains of staphylococci resistant to penicillin G, emphasizing the need for culture and susceptibility studies in treating suspected staphylococcal infections.
Other—Scarlet fever due to group A streptococci; prevention of recurrence following rheumatic fever and/or chorea.

CONTRAINDICATIONS
Contraindicated in patients with a history of hypersensitivity to any penicillin.

WARNINGS
Serious and occasionally fatal hypersensitivity (anaphylactoid) reactions have been reported in patients on penicillin therapy. Although anaphylaxis is more frequent following parenteral administration, it has occurred in patients on oral penicillins. These reactions are more apt to occur in individuals with a history of penicillin hypersensitivity and/or a history of sensitivity to multiple allergens.
There have been well-documented reports of individuals with a history of penicillin hypersensitivity who have experienced severe hypersensitivity reactions when treated with cephalosporins. Before initiating therapy with any penicillin, careful inquiry should be made concerning previous hypersensitivity reactions to penicillins, cephalosporins, and other allergens. If an allergic reaction occurs, the drug should be discontinued and the appropriate therapy instituted. Serious anaphylactoid reactions require immediate emergency treatment with epinephrine. Oxygen, intravenous steroids, and airway management, including intubation, should also be administered as indicated.

PRECAUTIONS
General
Penicillin should be used with caution in individuals with histories of significant allergies and/or asthma.
The oral route of administration should not be relied upon in patients with severe illness, or with nausea, vomiting, gastric dilatation, cardiospasm or intestinal hypermotility.
Occasional patients will not absorb therapeutic amounts of orally administered penicillin.
Prolonged use of antibiotics may promote the overgrowth of nonsusceptible organisms, including fungi. Should superinfection occur, appropriate measures should be taken.
PENTIDS '800' Tablets (Penicillin G Potassium Tablets) contain FD&C Yellow No. 5 (tartrazine) which may cause allergic-type reactions (including bronchial asthma) in certain susceptible individuals. Although the overall incidence of FD&C Yellow No. 5 (tartrazine) sensitivity in the general population is low, it is frequently seen in patients who also have aspirin hypersensitivity.
Information for Patients
1. Penicillin G Potassium tablets are best taken with a full glass (8 oz) of water on an empty stomach one-half hour before or at least two hours after meals. Acidic fruit juices or other acidic beverages should be avoided within one hour of drug administration since they interfere with absorption.
2. The patient should inform the physician of any history of sensitivity to allergens, including previous hypersensitivity reactions to penicillins and cephalosporins (see WARNINGS).
3. The patient should discontinue penicillin G potassium tablets and contact the physician immediately if any side effect occurs (see WARNINGS).
4. Diabetic patients should consult with the physician before changing diet or dosage of diabetes medication (see PRECAUTIONS, Drug/Laboratory Test Interactions).
Laboratory Tests
In streptococcal infections, therapy must be sufficient to eliminate the organism (10 days minimum); otherwise the

sequelae of streptococcal disease may occur. Cultures should be taken following completion of treatment to determine whether streptococci have been eradicated.

In prolonged therapy with penicillin, and particularly with high dosage regimens, periodic evaluation of the renal and hematopoietic systems is recommended.

Drug Interactions

When administered concurrently, the following drugs may interact with penicillins:

Aspirin or phenylbutazone—Drugs capable of displacing bound penicillin from plasma protein binding sites may elevate the level of free penicillin in the serum; however, the clinical significance of this interaction is not well documented.

Bacteriostatic antibiotics—Chloramphenicol, erythromycins, sulfonamides, or tetracyclines may interfere with the bactericidal effect of penicillins. This has been documented *in vitro*; however, the clinical significance of this interaction is not well documented.

Probenecid—May decrease renal tubular secretion of penicillin resulting in increased blood levels and/or penicillin toxicity.

Drug/Laboratory Test Interactions

After treatment with penicillin, a false-positive reaction for glucose in the urine may occur with copper sulfate tests (Benedict's solution, Fehling's solution, or Clinitest® tablets) but not with enzyme based tests such as Clinistix® and Tes-Tape®.

Carcinogenesis, Mutagenesis, Impairment of Fertility

Long-term studies in animals have not been performed to evaluate carcinogenesis, mutagenesis, or impairment of fertility in males or females.

Pregnancy: Teratogenic Effects

Category B

Reproduction studies performed in the mouse, rat, and rabbit have revealed no evidence of impaired fertility or harm to the fetus due to penicillin. Human experience with the penicillins during pregnancy has not shown any positive evidence of adverse effects on the fetus. There are, however, no adequate and well-controlled studies in pregnant women showing conclusively that harmful effects of these drugs on the fetus can be excluded. Because animal reproduction studies are not always predictive of human response, penicillin should be used during pregnancy only if clearly needed.

Nursing Mothers

Since penicillins are excreted in breast milk during lactation, penicillin use by nursing mothers may lead to sensitization of infants; therefore, a decision should be made whether to discontinue nursing or to discontinue the drug, taking into account the importance of the drug to the mother.

Pediatric Use

Penicillins are excreted primarily unchanged by the kidney (see CLINICAL PHARMACOLOGY). Administration should be limited to the lowest dosage compatible with an effective therapeutic regimen (see DOSAGE AND ADMINISTRATION).

ADVERSE REACTIONS

Although the incidence of reactions to oral penicillins has been reported with much less frequency than following parenteral therapy, it should be remembered that all degrees of hypersensitivity, including fatal anaphylaxis, have been reported with oral penicillin.

The most common reactions to oral penicillin are nausea, vomiting, epigastric distress, diarrhea, and black hairy tongue. The hypersensitivity reactions reported are skin rashes ranging from maculopapular to exfoliative dermatitis; urticaria; serum sickness-like reactions including chills, fever, edema, arthralgia, and prostration; laryngeal edema; and anaphylaxis. Fever and eosinophilia may frequently be the only reactions observed. Hemolytic anemia, leukopenia, thrombocytopenia, neuropathy, and nephropathy are infrequent reactions usually associated with high doses of parenteral penicillin. Urticaria, other skin rashes, and serum sickness-like reactions may be controlled by antihistamines and, if necessary, corticosteroids. Whenever such reactions occur, penicillin should be discontinued unless, in the opinion of the physician, the condition being treated is life-threatening and amenable only to penicillin therapy. Serious anaphylactoid reactions require emergency measures (see WARNINGS).

An occasional patient may complain of sore mouth or tongue, as with any oral penicillin preparation.

OVERDOSAGE

In case of overdosage, discontinue medication, treat symptomatically and institute supportive measures as required. Penicillin G may be removed from the blood by hemodialysis.

DOSAGE AND ADMINISTRATION

The dosage of penicillin G should be determined according to the susceptibility of the causative microorganisms and the severity of infection, and adjusted to the clinical response of the patient.

Therapy for children under 12 years of age who are able to swallow tablets is calculated on the basis of body weight. The suggested dose is 15 to 56 mg (25,000 to 90,000 u) per kg/day in three to six divided doses.

For maximum absorption of penicillin, dosage should be given on an empty stomach. Thus, a dose of 200,000 u should be administered one-half hour before or at least two hours after meals. The blood concentration with a dose of 400,000 u is sufficiently high to inhibit susceptible bacteria when the antibiotic is given without regard to meals but, as can be expected, the resultant concentration will be higher when it is given before meals.

The usual dosage recommendation for adults and children 12 years and over is as follows:

Streptococcal infections—mild to moderately severe—of the upper respiratory tract and including otitis media, scarlet fever and mild erysipelas: 125 mg (200,000 u) tid or qid for 10 days for mild infections; 250 mg (400,000 u) tid for 10 days for moderately severe infections; alternatively, 500 mg (800,000 u) may be given bid (see PRECAUTIONS, Laboratory Tests).

Pneumococcal infections—mild to moderately severe—of the respiratory tract, including otitis media: 250 mg (400,000 u) qid until the patient has been afebrile for at least two days.

Staphylococcal infections—mild infections of skin and skin structures (culture and susceptibility tests should be performed): 125 to 250 mg (200,000 to 400,000 u) tid or qid until infection is cured.

Vincent's gingivitis and pharyngitis (fusospirochetosis) —mild to moderately severe infections of the oropharynx: 250 mg (400,000 u) tid or qid.

For the prevention of recurrence following rheumatic fever and/or chorea: 125 mg (200,000 u) twice daily on a continuing basis.

HOW SUPPLIED

PENTIDS Tablets
(Penicillin G Potassium Tablets USP)

125 mg (200,000 u) per tablet:	White, oval, scored, uncoated tablets in bottles of 100 (NDC 0003-0164-50); identification no. **164**.
PENTIDS '400' Tablets	
250 mg (400,000 u) per tablet:	White, oval, scored, uncoated tablets in bottles of 100 (NDC 0003-0165-50); identification no. **165**.
PENTIDS '800' Tablets	
500 mg (800,000 u) per tablet:	Yellow (buff), oval, scored, uncoated tablets in bottles of 100 (NDC 0003-0168-50); identification no. **168**.

Storage

Store at room temperature; avoid excessive heat. Keep tightly closed.
(J4-157A)

PRINCIPEN® '250' CAPSULES ℞
[prin 'si-pen ″]
PRINCIPEN® '500' CAPSULES ℞
Ampicillin Capsules USP

PRINCIPEN® '125' FOR ORAL SUSPENSION ℞
PRINCIPEN® '250' FOR ORAL SUSPENSION ℞
Ampicillin for Oral Suspension USP

DESCRIPTION

Ampicillin trihydrate is a semisynthetic penicillin derived from the basic penicillin nucleus, 6-aminopenicillanic acid. Ampicillin is designated chemically as (2S,5R,6R)-6-[(R)-2-Amino-2-phenylacetamido] -3, 3-dimethyl-7-oxo-4-thia-1-aza-bicyclo [3.2.0] heptane-2-carboxylic acid.

PRINCIPEN capsules (Ampicillin Capsules) for oral administration provide ampicillin trihydrate equivalent to 250 mg and 500 mg ampicillin. Inactive ingredients: gelatin, iron oxide colorant, lactose, magnesium stearate, and titanium dioxide. PRINCIPEN for oral suspensions (Ampicillin for Oral Suspension) provide, after constitution, ampicillin trihydrate equivalent to 125 mg and 250 mg ampicillin per 5 mL. Inactive ingredients: colorants (FD&C Red No. 3, FD&C Blue No. 1 in '125' only; FD&C Yellow No. 6 in '250' only), flavors, guar gum, saccharin, sodium citrate, and sucrose.

CLINICAL PHARMACOLOGY

Ampicillin is bactericidal at low concentrations and is clinically effective not only against the gram-positive organisms usually susceptible to penicillin G but also against a variety of gram-negative organisms. It is stable in the presence of gastric acid and is well absorbed from the gastrointestinal tract. It diffuses readily into most body tissues and fluids; however, penetration into the cerebrospinal fluid and brain occurs only with meningeal inflammation. Ampicillin is excreted largely unchanged in the urine; its excretion can be delayed by concurrent administration of probenecid which inhibits the renal tubular secretion of ampicillin. In blood serum, ampicillin is the least bound of all the penicillins; an average of about 20 percent of the drug is bound to the plasma proteins as compared to 60 to 90 percent for other penicillins. The administration of a 500 mg dose of ampicillin trihydrate capsules results in an average peak blood serum level of approximately 3.0 mcg/mL; the average peak serum

level for the same dose of ampicillin trihydrate for oral suspension is approximately 3.4 mcg/mL.

Microbiology: While *in vitro* studies have demonstrated the susceptibility of most strains of the following organisms, clinical efficacy for infections other than those included in the INDICATIONS AND USAGE section has not been documented.

GRAM-POSITIVE—strains of alpha- and beta-hemolytic streptococci, *Streptococcus pneumoniae*, those strains of staphylococci which do not produce penicillinase, *Clostridium* sp., *Bacillus anthracis*, *Corynebacterium xerose*, and most strains of enterococci.

GRAM-NEGATIVE—*Hemophilus influenzae*; *Neisseria gonorrhoeae* and *N. meningitidis*; *Proteus mirabilis*; and many strains of *Salmonella* (including *S. typhosa*), *Shigella*, and *Escherichia coli*.

NOTE: Ampicillin is inactivated by penicillinase and therefore is ineffective against penicillinase-producing organisms including certain strains of staphylococci, *Pseudomonas aeruginosa*, *P. vulgaris*, *Klebsiella pneumoniae*, *Enterobacter aerogenes*, and some strains of *E. coli*. Ampicillin is not active against Rickettsia, Mycoplasma, and "large viruses" (Miyagawanella).

TESTING FOR SUSCEPTIBILITY: The invading organism should be cultured and its susceptibility demonstrated as a guide to therapy. If the Kirby-Bauer method of disc susceptibility is used, a 10 mcg ampicillin disc should be used to determine the relative *in vitro* susceptibility.

INDICATIONS AND USAGE

PRINCIPEN Capsules (Ampicillin Capsules) and PRINCIPEN for Oral Suspension (Ampicillin for Oral Suspension) are indicated in the treatment of infections caused by susceptible strains of the designated organisms listed below:

Infections of the genitourinary tract including gonorrhea—*E. coli*, *P. mirabilis*, enterococci, *Shigella*, *S. typhosa* and other *Salmonella*, and nonpenicillinase-producing *N. gonorrhoeae*.

Infections of the respiratory tract—Nonpenicillinase-producing *H. influenzae* and staphylococci, and streptococci including *streptococcus pneumoniae*.

Infections of the gastrointestinal tract—*Shigella*, *S. typhosa* and other *Salmonella*, *E. coli*, *P. mirabilis*, and enterococci.

Meningitis—*N. Meningitidis*.

Bacteriology studies to determine the causative organisms and their sensitivity to ampicillin should be performed. Therapy may be instituted prior to the results of susceptibility testing.

CONTRAINDICATIONS

A history of a previous hypersensitivity reaction to any of the penicillins is a contraindication. Ampicillin is also contraindicated in infections caused by penicillinase-producing organisms.

WARNINGS

Serious and occasional fatal hypersensitivity (anaphylactoid) reactions have been reported in patients on penicillin therapy. Although anaphylaxis is more frequent following parenteral administration, it has occurred in patients on oral penicillins. These reactions are more apt to occur in individuals with a history of penicillin hypersensitivity and/or a history of sensitivity to multiple allergens.

There have been well-documented reports of individuals with a history of penicillin hypersensitivity who have experienced severe hypersensitivity reactions when treated with cephalosporins. Before initiating therapy with any penicillin, careful inquiry should be made concerning previous hypersensitivity reactions to penicillins, cephalosporins, and other allergens. If an allergic reaction occurs, the drug should be discontinued and appropriate therapy instituted. **Serious anaphylactoid reactions require immediate emergency treatment with epinephrine. Oxygen, intravenous steroids and airway management, including intubation, should also be administered as indicated.**

PRECAUTIONS

General

Prolonged use of antibiotics may promote the overgrowth of nonsusceptible organisms, including fungi. Should superinfection occur, appropriate measures should be taken.

Patients with gonorrhea who also have syphilis should be given additional appropriate parenteral penicillin treatment.

Treatment with ampicillin does not preclude the need for surgical procedures, particularly in staphylococcal infections.

Information for the Patient

1. The patient should inform the physician of any history of sensitivity to allergens, including previous hypersensitivity reactions to penicillins and cephalosporins (see WARNINGS).

Continued on next page

Squibb—Cont.

2. The patient should discontinue ampicillin and contact the physician immediately if any side effect occurs (see WARNINGS).

3. Ampicillin should be taken with a full glass (8 oz) of water, one-half hour before or two hours after meals.

4. Diabetic patients should consult with the physician before changing diet or dosage of diabetes medication (see PRECAUTIONS Drug/Laboratory Test Interactions).

Laboratory Tests

In prolonged therapy, and particularly with high dosage regimens, periodic evaluation of the renal, hepatic, and hematopoietic systems is recommended.

In streptococcal infections, therapy must be sufficient to eliminate the organism (10 days minimum); otherwise the sequelae of streptococcal disease may occur. Cultures should be taken following completion of treatment to determine whether streptococci have been eradicated.

Cases of gonococcal infection with a suspected lesion of syphilis should have darkfield examinations ruling out syphilis before receiving ampicillin. Patients who do not have suspected lesions of syphilis and are treated with ampicillin should have a follow-up serologic test for syphilis each month for four months to detect syphilis that may have been masked by treatment for gonorrhea.

Drug Interactions

When administered concurrently, the following drugs may interact with ampicillin:

Allopurinol—Increased possibility of skin rash, particularly in hyperuricemic patients may occur.

Bacteriostatic antibiotics—Chloramphenicol, erythromycins, sulfonamides, or tetracyclines may interfere with the bactericidal effect of penicillins. This has been demonstrated *in vitro*; however, the clinical significance of this interaction is not well-documented.

Oral contraceptives—May be less effective and increased breakthrough bleeding may occur.

Probenecid—May decrease renal tubular secretion of ampicillin resulting in increased blood levels and/or ampicillin toxicity.

Drug/Laboratory Test Interaction

After treatment with ampicillin, a false-positive reaction for glucose in the urine may occur with copper sulfate tests (Benedict's solution, Fehling's solution, or Clinitest® tablets) but not with enzyme based tests such as Clinistix® and Tes-Tape®.

Carcinogenesis, Mutagenesis, Impairment of Fertility

Long-term studies in animals have not been performed to evaluate carcinogenesis, mutagenesis, or impairment of fertility in males or females.

Pregnancy: Teratogenic Effects

Category B

Reproduction studies in animals have revealed no evidence of impaired fertility or harm to the fetus due to penicillin. There are, however, no adequate and well-controlled studies in pregnant women. Because animal reproduction studies are not always predictive of human response, penicillin should be used during pregnancy only if clearly needed.

Labor and Delivery

Oral ampicillin-class antibiotics are poorly absorbed during labor. Studies in guinea pigs showed that intravenous administration of ampicillin slightly decreased the uterine tone and frequency of contractions, but moderately increased the height and duration of contractions. However, it is not known whether use of these drugs in humans during labor or delivery has immediate or delayed adverse effects on the fetus, prolongs the duration of labor, or increases the likelihood that forceps delivery or other obstetrical intervention or resuscitation of the newborn will be necessary.

Nursing Mothers

Ampicillin-class antibiotics are excreted in milk. Ampicillin use by nursing mothers may lead to sensitization of infants; therefore, a decision should be made whether to discontinue nursing or to discontinue ampicillin, taking into account the importance of the drug to the mother.

Pediatric Use

Penicillins are excreted primarily unchanged by the kidney; therefore, the incompletely developed renal function in neonates and young infants will delay the excretion of penicillin. Administration to neonates and young infants should be limited to the lowest dosage compatible with an effective therapeutic regimen (see DOSAGE AND ADMINISTRATION).

ADVERSE REACTIONS

As with other penicillins, it may be expected that untoward reactions will be essentially limited to sensitivity phenomena. They are more likely to occur in individuals who have previously demonstrated hypersensitivity to penicillin and in those with a history of allergy, asthma, hay fever, or urticaria.

The following adverse reactions have been reported as associated with the use of ampicillin:

Gastrointestinal: glossitis, stomatitis, nausea, vomiting, enterocolitis, pseudomembranous colitis, and diarrhea. These reactions are usually associated with oral dosage forms of the drug.

Hypersensitivity Reactions: an erythematous, mildly pruritic, maculopapular skin rash has been reported fairly frequently. The rash, which usually does not develop within the first week of therapy, may cover the entire body including the soles, palms, and oral mucosa. The eruption usually disappears in three to seven days. Other hypersensitivity reactions that have been reported are: skin rash, pruritus, urticaria, erythema multiforme, and an occasional case of exfoliative dermatitis. Anaphylaxis is the most serious reaction experienced and has usually been associated with the parenteral dosage form of the drug.

NOTE: Urticaria, other skin rashes, and serum sickness-like reactions may be controlled by antihistamines, and, if necessary, systemic corticosteroids. Whenever such reactions occur, ampicillin should be discontinued unless, in the opinion of the physician, the condition being treated is life-threatening and amenable only to ampicillin therapy. Serious anaphylactoid reactions require emergency measures (see WARNINGS).

Liver: moderate elevation in serum glutamic oxaloacetic transaminase (SGOT) has been noted, but the significance of this finding is unknown.

Hemic and Lymphatic Systems: anemia, thrombocytopenia, thrombocytopenic purpura, eosinophilia, leukopenia, and agranulocytosis have been reported during therapy with penicillins. These reactions are usually reversible on discontinuation of therapy and are believed to be hypersensitivity phenomena.

Other adverse reactions that have been reported with the use of ampicillin are laryngeal stridor and high fever. An occasional patient may complain of sore mouth or tongue as with any oral penicillin preparation.

OVERDOSAGE

In case of overdosage, discontinue medication, treat symptomatically and institute supportive measures as required. In patients with renal function impairment, ampicillin-class antibiotics can be removed by hemodialysis but not by peritoneal dialysis.

DOSAGE AND ADMINISTRATION

Adults and children weighing over 20 kg: For **genitourinary or gastrointestinal tract infections other than gonorrhea in men and women,** the usual dose is 500 mg qid in equally spaced doses; severe or chronic infections may require larger doses. For the treatment of gonorrhea in both men and women, a single oral dose of 3.5 grams of ampicillin administered simultaneously with 1.0 gram of probenecid is recommended. Physicians are cautioned to use no less than the above recommended dosage for the treatment of gonorrhea. Follow-up cultures should be obtained from the original site(s) of infection 7 to 14 days after therapy. In women, it is also desirable to obtain culture test-of-cure from both the endocervical and anal canals. Prolonged intensive therapy is needed for complications such as prostatitis and epididymitis. For **respiratory tract infections,** the usual dose is 250 mg qid in equally spaced doses.

Children weighing 20 kg or less: For **genitourinary or gastrointestinal tract infections,** the usual dose is 100 mg/kg/day total, qid in equally divided and spaced doses. For **respiratory infections,** the usual dose is 50 mg/kg/day total, in equally divided and spaced doses three to four times daily. Doses for children should not exceed doses recommended for adults.

All patients, irrespective of age and weight: Larger doses may be required for severe or chronic infections. Although ampicillin is resistant to degradation by gastric acid, it should be administered at least one-half hour before or two hours after meals for maximal absorption. Except for the single dose regimen for gonorrhea referred to above, therapy should be continued for a minimum of 48 to 72 hours after the patient becomes asymptomatic or evidence of bacterial eradication has been obtained. In infections caused by hemolytic strains of streptococci, a minimum of 10 days' treatment is recommended to guard against the risk of rheumatic fever or glomerulonephritis (see PRECAUTIONS, Laboratory Tests). In the treatment of chronic urinary or gastrointestinal infections, frequent bacteriologic and clinical appraisal is necessary during therapy and may be necessary for several months afterwards. Stubborn infections may require treatment for several weeks. Smaller doses than those indicated above should not be used.

HOW SUPPLIED

PRINCIPEN Capsules (Ampicillin Capsules USP)

PRINCIPEN '250' 250 mg/capsule:	bottles of 100 (NDC 0003-0971-51) and 500 (NDC 0003-0971-60) and Unimatic® unit-dose packs of 100 (NDC 0003-0971-50). Each two-piece, grey, hard gelatin capsule is imprinted with identification no. 971.
PRINCIPEN '500' 500 mg/capsule:	bottles of 100 (NDC 0003-0974-50) and 500 (NDC 0003-0974-61) and Unimatic unit-dose packs of 100 (NDC 0003-0974-51). Each two-piece, dark grey/light grey, hard gelatin capsule is imprinted with identification no. 974.

PRINCIPEN for Oral Suspension (Ampicillin for Oral Suspension USP)

PRINCIPEN '125'	When constituted as directed on the container label, a pleasant fruit-flavored suspension containing **125 mg per 5 mL,** in bottle sizes for preparation of 100 mL (NDC 0003-0969-09), 150 mL (NDC 0003-0969-52), and 200 mL (NDC 0003-0969-61). **125 mg/bottle:** packs of 100 Unimatic unit-dose bottles (NDC 0003-0969-15).
PRINCIPEN '250'	When constituted as directed on the container label, a pleasant fruit-flavored suspension containing **250 mg per 5 mL,** in bottle sizes for preparation of 100 mL (NDC 0003-0972-52), 150 mL (NDC 0003-0972-47), and 200 mL (NDC 0003-0972-61). **250 mg/bottle:** packs of 100 Unimatic unit-dose bottles (NDC 0003-0072-20).

Storage

Principen Capsules: Store at room temperature; avoid excessive heat; keep bottles tightly closed.

PRINCIPEN for Oral Suspension: Store at room temperature; after constitution, discard unused portion after 7 days if kept at room temperature or after 14 days if refrigerated; keep bottles tightly closed.

(J4-177A)

Shown in Product Identification Section, page 431

PRINCIPEN® with PROBENECID   ℞

[*prin'si-pen" with pro"ben'e-sid"*]

Ampicillin and Probenecid Capsules USP

DESCRIPTION

Ampicillin trihydrate is a semisynthetic penicillin antibiotic derived from the basic penicillin nucleus, 6-aminopenicillanic acid. Ampicillin is designated chemically as (2S,5R,6R)-6-[(R)-2-Amino-2-phenylacetamido]-3, 3-dimethyl-7-oxo-4-thia-1-azabicyclo[3.2.0]heptane-2-carboxylic acid.

Probenecid, as used with ampicillin, is a renal tubular blocking agent. Probenecid is designated chemically as *p*-(Dipropylsulfamoyl) benzoic acid.

Each PRINCIPEN with Probenecid (ampicillin and probenecid) capsule for oral administration contains ampicillin trihydrate equivalent to 389 mg ampicillin, and 111 mg probenecid. Nine capsules (single dose) contain ampicillin trihydrate equivalent to 3.5 g ampicillin and 1 g probenecid. Inactive ingredients: colorants (D&C Red No. 33, D&C Yellow No. 10; FD&C Blue No. 1, FD&C Red No. 3, FD&C Yellow No. 6), gelatin, magnesium stearate, and titanium dioxide.

CLINICAL PHARMACOLOGY

Ampicillin is stable in the presence of gastric acid and is well absorbed from the gastrointestinal tract. It diffuses readily into most body tissues and fluids; however, penetration into the cerebrospinal fluid and brain occurs only with meningeal inflammation. Ampicillin is excreted largely unchanged in the urine; its excretion is delayed by concurrent administration of probenecid which inhibits the renal tubular secretion of ampicillin. In blood serum, ampicillin is the least bound of all the penicillins; an average of about 20 percent of the drug is bound to the plasma proteins as compared to 60 to 90 percent for the other penicillins. Probenecid inhibits the tubular reabsorption of urate, thus increasing the urinary excretion of uric acid and decreasing serum uric acid levels. As an adjuvant to ampicillin therapy, it also inhibits the tubular secretion of ampicillin and usually increases ampicillin plasma levels by any route the antibiotic is given. A two-fold to four-fold elevation has been demonstrated for various penicillins. Probenecid is metabolized by the liver and excreted in the urine principally as the monoacyl glucuronide and, following hydroxylation, as metabolites retaining their carboxyl function; 85 to 95 percent of the drug is bound to plasma protein.

Microbiology

While *in vitro* studies have demonstrated the susceptibility of most strains of the following organisms, clinical efficacy for infections other than those included in the INDICATIONS AND USAGE section has not been documented.

GRAM-POSITIVE—strains of alpha- and beta-hemolytic streptococci, *Streptococcus pneumoniae,* those strains of staphylococci which do not produce penicillinase, *Clostridium sp., Bacillus anthracis, Corynebacterium xerose,* and most strains of enterococci.

GRAM-NEGATIVE—*Hemophilus influenzae; Neisseria gonorrhoeae* and *N. memingitidis; Proteus mirabilis;* and many strains of *Salmonella* (including *S. typhosa*), *Shigella*, and *Escherichia coli.*

NOTE: Ampicillin is inactivated by penicillinase and therefore is ineffective against penicillinase-producing organisms including certain strains of staphylococci, *Pseudomonas aeruginosa, P. vulgaris, Klebsiella pneumoniae, Enterobacter aerogenes,* and some strains of *E. coli.* Ampicillin is not active against *Rickettsia, Mycoplasma,* and "large viruses" (*Miyagawanella*).

TESTING FOR SUSCEPTIBILITY: The invading organism should be cultured and its susceptibility demonstrated as a guide to therapy. If the Kirby-Bauer method of disc susceptibility is used, a 10 mcg ampicillin disc should be used to determine the relative *in vitro* susceptibility.

INDICATIONS AND USAGE

PRINCIPEN with Probenecid (Ampicillin and Probenecid Capsules) is indicated for the treatment of uncomplicated infection (urethral, endocervical, or rectal) caused by non-penicillinase-producing *N. gonorrhoeae* in men and women. Urethritis and the presence of gram-negative diplococci in urethral smears is strong presumptive evidence of gonorrhea. Culture or fluorescent antibody studies will confirm the diagnosis.

Susceptibility studies should be performed with recurrent infections or when resistant strains are encountered. Therapy may be instituted prior to obtaining results of susceptibility testing.

CONTRAINDICATIONS

A history of a previous hypersensitivity reaction to any of the penicillins or to probenecid is a contraindication.

Probenecid is not recommended in persons with known blood dyscrasias or uric acid kidney stones or during an acute attack of gout. It is not recommended in conjunction with ampicillin in the presence of known renal impairment.

WARNINGS

Serious and occasional fatal hypersensitivity (anaphylactoid) reactions have been reported in patients on penicillin therapy. Although anaphylaxis is more frequent following parenteral administration, it has occurred in patients on oral penicillins. These reactions are more apt to occur in individuals with a history of penicillin hypersensitivity and/or a history of sensitivity to multiple allergens.

There have been well-documented reports of individuals with a history of penicillin hypersensitivity who have experienced severe hypersensitivity reactions when treated with cephalosporins. Before initiating therapy with any penicillin, careful inquiry should be made concerning previous hypersensitivity reactions to penicillins, cephalosporins, and other allergens. If an allergic reaction occurs, the drug should be discontinued and appropriate therapy instituted. **Serious anaphylactoid reactions require immediate emergency treatment with epinephrine. Oxygen, intravenous steroids, and airway management, including intubation, should also be administered as indicated.**

PRECAUTIONS

General

Patients with gonorrhea who also have syphilis should be given additional appropriate parenteral penicillin treatment.

Information for the Patient

1. The patient should inform the physician of any history of sensitivity to allergens, including previous hypersensitivity reactions to penicillins and cephalosporins (see WARNINGS).
2. The patient should discontinue ampicillin and contact the physician immediately if any side effect occurs (see WARNINGS).
3. Ampicillin should be taken with a full glass (8 oz) of water, one-half hour before or two hours after meals.
4. Diabetic patients should consult with the physician before changing diet or dosage of diabetes medication (see PRECAUTIONS Drug/Laboratory Test Interactions).

Laboratory Tests

Follow-up cultures should be obtained from the original site(s) of infection 7 to 14 days after therapy. In women, it is also desirable to obtain culture test-of-cure from both the endocervical and anal canals.

Cases of gonococcal infection with a suspected lesion of syphilis should have darkfield examinations ruling out syphilis before receiving ampicillin. Patients who do not have suspected lesions of syphilis and are treated with ampicillin should have a follow-up serologic test for syphilis each month for four months to detect syphilis that may have been masked by treatment for gonorrhea.

Probenecid has been reported to inhibit the renal transport of many compounds including aminohippuric acid (PAH), sodium iodomethamate and related iodinated organic acids, 17-ketosteroids, and phenolsulfonphthalein (PSP). Probenecid decreases both hepatic and renal excretion of sulfobromophthalein (BSP).

Drug Interactions

When administered concurrently, the following drugs may interact with ampicillin or probenecid:

Ampicillin

Allopurinol—Increased possibility of skin rash, particularly in hyperuricemic patients, may occur.

Bacteriostatic antibiotics—Chloramphenicol, erthromycins, sulfonamides, or tetracyclines may interfere with the bactericidal effect of penicillins. This has been demonstrated *in vitro*; however, the clinical significance of this interaction is not well-documented.

Oral contraceptives—May be less effective and increased breakthrough bleeding may occur.

Probenecid

Inhibits the renal excretion and may increase plasma levels of conjugated *sulfonamides, dapsone, rifampin, aminosalicyclic acid, indomethacin,* and *methotrexate.*

Antidiabetics, oral—Hypoglycemic effect may be potentiated (see also Drug/Laboratory Test Interactions).

Naproxen—Probenecid given concurrently increases naproxen anion plasma levels and extends its plasma half-life significantly.

Salicylates, pyrazinamide—Probenecid antagonists.

Drug/Laboratory Test Interactions

After treatment with both ampicillin and probenecid, a false-positive reaction for glucose in the urine may occur with copper sulfate tests (Benedict's solution, Fehling's solution, or Clinitest® tablets) but not with enzyme based tests such as Clinistix® and Tes-Tape®.

Carcinogenesis, Mutagenesis, Impairment of Fertility

Long-term studies in animals have not been performed to evaluate carcinogenesis, mutagenesis, or impairment of fertility in males or females.

Pregnancy: Teratogenic Effects

Category C

Animal reproduction studies have not been conducted with PRINCIPEN with Probenecid (Ampicillin and Probenecid Capsules). Ampicillin and probenecid cross the placental barrier and appear in cord blood; it is not known whether Ampicillin and Probenecid Capsules can cause fetal harm when administered to a pregnant woman or can affect reproduction capacity. Ampicillin and Probenecid Capsules should be given to a pregnant woman only if clearly needed.

Labor and Delivery

Oral ampicillin-class antibiotics are poorly absorbed during labor. Studies in guinea pigs showed that intravenous administration of ampicillin slightly decreased the uterine tone and frequency of contractions, but moderately increased the height and duration of contractions. However, it is not known whether use of these drugs in humans during labor or delivery has immediate or delayed adverse effects on the fetus, prolongs the duration of labor, or increases the likelihood that forceps delivery or other obstetrical intervention or resuscitation of the newborn will be necessary.

Nursing Mothers

Ampicillin is excreted in milk. It is not known whether probenecid is excreted in human milk. Ampicillin use by nursing mothers may lead to sensitization of infants; therefore, caution should be exercised when Ampicillin and Probenecid Capsules are administered to a nursing woman.

Pediatric Use

Safety and effectiveness in children have not been established.

ADVERSE REACTIONS

Ampicillin

As with other penicillins, it may be expected that untoward reactions will be essentially limited to sensitivity phenomena. They are more likely to occur in individuals who have previously demonstrated hypersensitivity to penicillin and in those with a history of allergy, asthma, hay fever, or urticaria.

The following adverse reactions have been reported as associated with the use of ampicillin:

Gastrointestinal: glossitis, stomatitis, nausea, vomiting, enterocolitis, pseudomembranous colitis, and diarrhea. These reactions are usually associated with oral dosage forms of the drug.

Hypersensitivity Reactions: An erythematous, mildly pruritic, maculopapular skin rash has been reported fairly frequently. The rash, which usually does not develop within the first week of therapy, may cover the entire body including the soles, palms, and oral mucosa. The eruption usually disappears in three to seven days. Other hypersensitivity reactions that have been reported are: skin rash, pruritus, urticaria, erythema multiforme, and an occasional case of exfoliative dermatitis. Anaphylaxis is the most serious reaction experienced and has usually been associated with the parenteral dosage form of the drug.

NOTE: Urticaria, other skin rashes, and serum sickness-like reactions may be controlled by antihistamines and, if necessary, systemic corticosteroids. Serious anaphylactoid reactions require emergency measures (see WARNINGS).

Liver: Moderate elevation in serum glutamic oxaloacetic transaminase (SGOT) has been noted, but the significance of this finding is unknown.

Hemic and Lymphatic Systems: Anemia, thrombocytopenia, thrombocytopenic purpura, eosinophilia, leukopenia, and agranulocytosis have been reported during therapy with penicillins. These reactions are usually reversible on discontinuation of therapy and are believed to be hypersensitivity phenomena.

Probenecid

The following are the principal adverse reactions which have been reported as associated with the use of probenecid, generally with more prolonged or repeated administration: headache, gastrointestinal symptoms (e.g., anorexia, nausea, vomiting), urinary frequency, hypersensitivity reactions (including anaphylaxis, dermatitis, pruritus, and fever), sore gums, flushing, dizziness, and anemia have occurred.

In patients with gout, exacerbation of gout, and uric acid stones with or without hematuria, renal colic, or costovertebral pain have been observed. The nephrotic syndrome, hepatic necrosis, and aplastic anemia occur rarely. Hemolytic anemia which in some instances could be related to genetic deficiency of glucose-6-phosphate dehydrogenase in red blood cells has been reported.

DOSAGE AND ADMINISTRATION

For the treatment of gonorrhea in both men and women—3.5 g ampicillin and 1 g probenecid (9 capsules) are administered as a single dose.

Physicians are cautioned to use no less than the above recommended dosage.

HOW SUPPLIED

PRINCIPEN with Probenecid (Ampicillin and Probenecid Capsules USP)

Single-unit bottles of 9 capsules (NDC 0003-1616-10).

Each two piece, orange/red, hard gelatin capsule is imprinted with identification no. **F16.**

Storage

Store at room temperature; avoid excessive heat.

J4-178A

SUMYCIN® '250' TABLETS　　　　℞

[*sū "mī'sin*]

SUMYCIN® '500' TABLETS　　　　℞

Tetracycline Hydrochloride Tablets USP

SUMYCIN® '250' CAPSULES　　　　℞

SUMYCIN® '500' CAPSULES　　　　℞

Tetracycline Hydrochloride Capsules USP

SUMYCIN® SYRUP　　　　℞

Tetracycline Oral Suspension USP

DESCRIPTION

SUMYCIN '250' and SUMYCIN '500' Tablets (Tetracycline Hydrochloride Tablets) are available for oral administration as FILMLOK®* tablets providing 250 mg and 500 mg tetracycline hydrochloride, respectively. Inactive ingredients: microcrystalline cellulose, colorant (D&C Red No. 30), lactose, magnesium stearate, povidone, pregelatinized starch, stearic acid, and other ingredients.

SUMYCIN '250' and SUMYCIN '500' Capsules (Tetracycline Hydrochloride Capsules) contain 250 mg and 500 mg crystalline tetracycline hydrochloride, respectively. Inactive ingredients: colorants (FD&C Blue No. 1 and Red No. 3), gelatin, lactose, magnesium stearate, mineral oil, and titanium dioxide.

Symycin Syrup (Tetracycline Oral Suspension) is a suspension containing, in each 5 mL teaspoonful, tetracycline equivalent to 125 mg tetracycline hydrochloride. Inactive ingredients: citric acid, colorant (D&C Yellow No. 10), flavor, potassium citrate, potassium metaphosphate, purified water, saccharin sodium, sodium benzoate, sodium citrate, sodium metabisulfite, sorbitol solution, sucrose, and tragacanth.

CLINICAL PHARMACOLOGY

The tetracyclines are primarily bacteriostatic antibiotics and are thought to exert their antimicrobial effect by the inhibition of protein synthesis. Tetracyclines are active against a wide range of gram-negative and gram-positive organisms.

The drugs in the tetracycline class have closely similar antimicrobial spectra. Microorganisms that have become insensitive to one tetracycline invariably exhibit cross-resistance to other tetracyclines. In addition, gram-negative bacilli made tetracycline-resistant may also show cross-resistance to chloramphenicol. Microorganisms may be considered susceptible if the MIC (minimum inhibitory concentration) is not more than 4 mcg/mL and intermediate if the MIC is 4 to 12.5 mcg/mL.

Susceptibility plate testing: A tetracycline disc may be used to determine microbial susceptibility to drugs in the tetracycline class. If the Kirby-Bauer method of disc sensitivity is used, a 30 mcg tetracycline disc should give a zone of at least

Continued on next page

Squibb—Cont.

19 mm when tested against a tetracycline-susceptible bacterial strain.

Tetracyclines are readily absorbed and are bound to plasma proteins in varying degree. They are concentrated by the liver in the bile and excreted in the urine and feces at high concentrations and in a biologically active form.

INDICATIONS AND USAGE

Tetracycline is indicated in infections caused by the following microorganisms.

Rickettsiae: Rocky mountain spotted fever, typhus fever and the typhus group, Q fever, rickettsialpox, tick fevers, *Mycoplasma pneumoniae* (PPLO, Eaton agent), agents of psittacosis and ornithosis, agents of *Lymphogranuloma, venereum* and *Granuloma inguinale,* and the spirochetal agent of relapsing fever *(B. recurrentis).*

The following gram-negative organisms: *H. ducreyi* (chancroid), *Pasteurella pestis* and *Past. tularensis, Bartonella bacilliformis,* Bacteroides, *Vibrio comma* and *V. fetus,* and Brucella organisms (in conjunction with streptomycin).

Because many strains of the following groups of microorganisms have been shown to be resistant to tetracyclines, culture and susceptibility testing are recommended.

The following gram-negative organisms, when bacteriologic testing indicates appropriate susceptibility to the drug: *E. coli, Enterobacter aerogenes* (formerly *A. aerogenes*), Shigella, Mima, Herellea, *H. influenzae* (respiratory infections), and Klebsiella infections (respiratory and urinary).

The following gram-positive organisms when bacteriologic testing indicates appropriate susceptibility to the drug:
1) Streptococcus species: Up to 44 percent of strains of *Streptococcus pyogenes* and 74 percent of *Streptococcus faecalis* have been found to be resistant to tetracycline drugs. Therefore, tetracyclines should not be used for streptococcal disease unless the organism has been demonstrated to be sensitive.

(For upper respiratory infections due to group A beta-hemolytic streptococci, penicillin is the usual drug of choice including prophylaxis of rheumatic fever.)
2) *D. pneumoniae.*
3) *Staphylococcus aureus* (skin and soft tissue infections). Tetracyclines are not the drugs of choice in the treatment of any type of staphylococcal infections.

When penicillin is contraindicated, tetracyclines are alternative drugs in the treatment of infections due to: *N. gonorrhoeae, T. pallidum* and *T. pertenue* (syphilis and yaws), *Listeria monocytogenes,* Clostridia, *B. anthracis, Fusobacterium fusiforme* (Vincent's infection), and *Actinomyces.*

Tetracycline hydrochloride is indicated for the treatment of uncomplicated urethral, endocervical, or rectal infections in adults caused by *Chlamydia trachomatis.*[1]

In acute intestinal amebiasis, the tetracyclines may be a useful adjunct to amebicides.

In severe acne the tetracyclines may be useful adjunctive therapy.

Tetracyclines are indicated in the treatment of trachoma, although the infectious agent is not always eliminated, as judged by immunofluorescence.

Inclusion conjunctivitis may be treated with oral tetracyclines or with a combination of oral and topical agents.

CONTRAINDICATIONS

This drug is contraindicated in persons who have shown hypersensitivity to any of the tetracyclines.

WARNINGS

THE USE OF DRUGS OF THE TETRACYCLINE CLASS DURING TOOTH DEVELOPMENT (LAST HALF OF PREGNANCY, INFANCY AND CHILDHOOD TO AGE OF EIGHT YEARS) MAY CAUSE PERMANENT DISCOLORATION OF THE TEETH (YELLOW-GRAY-BROWN). This reaction is more common during long-term use of the drugs but has been observed following repeated short-term courses. Enamel hypoplasia has also been reported. TETRACYCLINE DRUGS, THEREFORE, SHOULD NOT BE USED IN THIS AGE GROUP UNLESS OTHER DRUGS ARE NOT LIKELY TO BE EFFECTIVE OR ARE CONTRAINDICATED.

If renal impairment exists, even usual oral or parenteral doses may lead to excessive systemic accumulation of the drug and possible liver toxicity. Under such conditions, lower than usual doses are indicated and, if therapy is prolonged, serum level determinations of the drug may be advisable. The antianabolic action of tetracycline may cause an increase in BUN. While this is not a problem in those with normal renal function, in patients with significantly impaired function, higher serum levels of tetracycline may lead to azotemia, hyperphosphatemia, and acidosis.

Photosensitivity, manifested by an exaggerated sunburn reaction, has been observed in some individuals taking tetracyclines. Patients apt to be exposed to direct sunlight or ultra-violet light should be advised that this reaction can occur with tetracycline drugs, and treatment should be discontinued at the first evidence of skin erythema. NOTE: Photosen-

sitization reactions have occurred most frequently with demeclocycline, less with chlortetracycline, and very rarely with oxytetracycline and tetracycline.

SUMYCIN Syrup (Tetracycline Oral Suspension) contains sodium metabisulfite, a sulfite that may cause allergic-type reactions including anaphylactic symptoms and life-threatening or less severe asthmatic episodes in certain susceptible people. The overall prevalence of sulfite sensitivity in the general population is unknown and probably low. Sulfite sensitivity is seen more frequently in asthmatic than in non-asthmatic people.

Usage in Pregnancy
(See WARNINGS about use during tooth development.)
Results of animal studies indicate that tetracyclines cross the placenta, are found in fetal tissues and can have toxic effects on the developing fetus (often related to retardation of skeletal development). Evidence of embryo-toxicity has also been noted in animals treated early in pregnancy.

Usage in Newborns, Infants, and Children
(See WARNINGS about use during tooth development.)
Tetracyclines form a stable calcium complex in any bone-forming tissue. A decrease in the fibula growth rate has been observed in prematures given oral tetracycline in doses of 25 mg/kg every six hours. This reaction was shown to be reversible when the drug was discontinued.

Tetracyclines are present in the milk of lactating women who are taking a drug in this class.

PRECAUTIONS

As with other antibiotics, use of this drug may result in overgrowth of nonsusceptible organisms, including fungi. If superinfection occurs, the antibiotic should be discontinued and appropriate therapy instituted. Note: Superinfection of the bowel by staphylococci may be life-threatening.

In venereal diseases when coexistent syphilis is suspected, patients should have darkfield examinations before treatment is started and the blood serology should be repeated monthly for at least four months.

Because the tetracyclines have been shown to depress plasma prothrombin activity, patients who are on anticoagulant therapy may require downward adjustment of their anticoagulant dosage.

During long-term therapy, periodic laboratory evaluation of organ systems, including hematopoietic, renal and hepatic studies should be performed.

All infections due to group A beta-hemolytic streptococci should be treated for at least 10 days.

Since bacteriostatic drugs may interfere with the bactericidal action of penicillin, it is advisable to avoid giving tetracycline in conjunction with penicillin.

Since sensitivity reactions are more likely to occur in persons with a history of allergy, asthma, hay fever, or urticaria, the preparation should be used with caution in such individuals.

ADVERSE REACTIONS

Gastrointestinal: anorexia, epigastric distress, nausea, vomiting, diarrhea, bulky loose stools, stomatitis, sore throat, glossitis, black hairy tongue, dysphagia, hoarseness, enterocolitis, and inflammatory lesions (with candidal overgrowth) in the anogenital region, including proctitis and pruritus ani. These reactions have been caused by both the oral and parenteral administration of tetracyclines but are less frequent after parenteral use.

Skin: maculopapular and erythematous rashes. Exfoliative dermatitis has been reported but is uncommon. Onycholysis and discoloration of the nails have been reported rarely. Photosensitivity has occurred (see WARNINGS).

Renal toxicity: rise in BUN has been reported and is apparently dose-related (see WARNINGS).

Hepatic cholestasis has been reported rarely, and is usually associated with high dosage levels of tetracycline.

Hypersensitivity reactions: urticaria, angioneurotic edema, anaphylaxis, anaphylactoid purpura, pericarditis, exacerbation of systemic lupus erythematosus, and serum sickness-like reactions, as fever, rash, and arthralgia.

When given over prolonged periods, tetracyclines have been reported to produce brown-black microscopic discoloration of thyroid glands. No abnormalities of thyroid function studies are known to occur.

Bulging fontanels have been reported in young infants following full therapeutic dosage. This sign disappeared rapidly when the drug was discontinued.

Blood: anemia, hemolytic anemia, thrombocytopenia, thrombocytopenic purpura, neutropenia and eosinophilia have been reported.

Dizziness and headache have been reported.

DOSAGE AND ADMINISTRATION

Adults: usual daily dose is 1 to 2 g; for mild to moderate infections: 500 mg bid or 250 mg qid; higher dosages such as 500 mg qid may be required for severe infections.

For children above eight years of age: usual daily dose is 10 to 20 mg/lb (25 to 50 mg/kg) body weight divided in four equal doses.

Representative pediatric dosages for the syrup on a qid basis are as follows: 20 lbs—½ teaspoonful; 40 lbs—1 teaspoonful; 60 lbs—1½ teaspoonfuls; and 80 lbs—2 teaspoonfuls.

Therapy should be continued for at least 24 to 48 hours after symptoms and fever have subsided.

The treatment of brucellosis, 500 mg tetracycline four times daily for three weeks should be accompanied by streptomycin, 1 g intramuscularly twice daily the first week and once daily the second week.

For treatment of gonorrhea, the recommended dose is 1.5 g initially, then 0.5 g every six hours until a total of 9 g have been given.

For treatment of syphilis, a total of 30 to 40 g in equally divided doses over a period of 10 to 15 days should be given. Close followup, including laboratory tests, is recommended.

Uncomplicated urethral, endocervical, or rectal infection in adults caused by *Chlamydia trachomatis:* 500 mg, by mouth, four times a day for at least seven days.[1]

In cases of severe acne which, in the judgment of the clinician, require long-term treatment, the recommended initial dosage is 1 g daily in divided doses. When improvement is noted, usually within one week, dosage should be gradually reduced to maintenance levels ranging from 125 mg to 500 mg daily. In some patients it may be possible to maintain adequate remission of lesions with alternate-day or intermittent therapy. Tetracycline therapy of acne should augment the other standard measures known to be of value.

In patients with renal impairment (see WARNINGS) total dosage should be decreased by reduction of recommended individual doses and/or by extending time intervals between doses.

In the treatment of streptococcal infections, a therapeutic dose of tetracycline should be administered for at least 10 days.

Concomitant therapy: Antacids containing aluminum, calcium, or magnesium impair absorption and should not be given to patients taking oral tetracycline.

Foods and some dairy products also interfere with absorption. Oral forms of tetracycline should be given one hour before or two hours after meals. Pediatric oral dosage forms should not be given with milk formulas and should be given at least one hour prior to feeding.

HOW SUPPLIED

*Sumycin '250' *Sumycin '500' Tablets (Tetracycline Hydrochloride Tablets USP) are available for oral administration as tablets containing 250 mg and 500 mg tetracycline hydrochloride, respectively.

*Sumycin '250' and *Sumycin '500' Capsules (Tetracycline Hydrochloride Capsules USP) are available for oral administration as capsules containing 250 mg and 500 mg tetracycline hydrochloride, respectively.

Sumycin Syrup (Tetracycline Oral Suspension USP) is available as a fruit-flavored suspension containing, in each 5 mL teaspoonful, tetracycline equivalent to 125 mg tetracycline hydrochloride.

Storage
Store the tablets and capsules at room temperature; avoid excessive heat. Store the syrup below 30° C (86° F); avoid freezing; protect from light; keep bottle tightly closed.

REFERENCE
1. CDC Sexually Transmitted Diseases Treatment Guidelines 1982.
(J3-291G)

Shown in Product Identification Section, page 432

TESLAC® TABLETS   ℞
[*tez 'lak*]
Testolactone Tablets USP

DESCRIPTION
TESLAC (Testolactone Tablets) is available for oral administration as tablets providing 50 mg testolactone per tablet. Testolactone is a synthetic antineoplastic agent that is structurally distinct from the androgen steroid nucleus in possessing a six-membered lactone ring in place of the usual five-membered carbocyclic D-ring. Testolactone is chemically designated as 13-hydroxy-3-oxo-13,17-secoandrosta-1,4-dien-17-oic acid δ-lactone.

Inactive ingredients: calcium stearate, cornstarch, gelatin, and lactose.

Testolactone is a white, odorless, crystalline solid, soluble in ethanol and slightly soluble in water.

CLINICAL PHARMACOLOGY
Although the precise mechanism by which testolactone produces its clinical antineoplastic effects has not been established, its principal action is reported to be inhibition of steroid aromatase activity and consequent reduction in estrone synthesis from adrenal androstenedione, the major source of estrogen in postmenopausal women. Based on *in vitro* studies, the aromatase inhibition may be noncompetitive and irreversible. This phenomenon may account for the persistence of testolactone's effect on estrogen synthesis after drug withdrawal.

Despite some similarity to testosterone, testolactone has no *in vivo* androgenic effect. No other hormonal effects have been reported in clinical studies in patients receiving testolactone. In one study, testolactone administered orally (1000 mg/day) was reported to increase renal tubular reabsorption of calcium but to have no effect on serum calcium concentration. The mechanism of the hypocalciuric effect is unknown. No clinical effects in humans of testolactone on adrenal function have been reported; however, one study noted an increase in urinary excretion of 17-ketosteroids in most of the patients treated with 150 mg/day orally.

Testolactone is well absorbed from the gastrointestinal tract. It is metabolized to several derivatives in the liver, all of which preserve the lactone D-ring. These metabolites, as well as some unmetabolized drug, are excreted in the urine. Additional pharmacokinetic data in humans are unavailable.

For information concerning carcinogenesis, mutagenesis, pregnancy, and lactation, see the corresponding PRECAUTIONS sections.

In animals, parenteral but not oral testolactone reduced cortisone acetate induced hepatic glycogen deposits. In animal tests conducted to detect any hormonal activity for testolactone, some evidence of antiandrogenic and antiglucocorticoid activity was seen; increased growth rate in the newborn was suggested. However there was no clear manifestation of androgenic, estrogenic or antiestrogenic, progestational or antiprogestational, gonadotropin-like or antigonadotropic effects. Testolactone did not demonstrate anti-inflammatory, mineralocorticoid-like, or glucocorticoid-like properties.

INDICATIONS AND USAGE

TESLAC (Testolactone Tablets) is recommended as adjunctive therapy in the palliative treatment of advanced or disseminated breast cancer in postmenopausal women when hormonal therapy is indicated. It may also be used in women who were diagnosed as having had disseminated breast carcinoma when premenopausal, in whom ovarian function has been subsequently terminated.

TESLAC (Testolactone Tablets) was found to be effective in approximately 15 percent of patients with advanced or disseminated mammary cancer evaluated according to the following criteria: 1) those with a measurable decrease in size of all demonstrable tumor masses; 2) those in whom more than 50 percent of non-osseous lesions decreased in size although all bone lesions remained static; and 3) those in whom more than 50 percent of total lesions improved while the remainder were static.

CONTRAINDICATIONS

Testolactone is contraindicated in the treatment of breast cancer in men and in patients with a history of hypersensitivity to the drug.

PRECAUTIONS

Information for Patients
The physician should be consulted regarding missed doses. Notify the physician if adverse reactions occur or become more pronounced.

Laboratory Tests
Plasma calcium levels should be routinely determined in any patient receiving therapy for mammary cancer, particularly during periods of active remission of bony metastases. If hypercalcemia occurs, appropriate measures should be instituted.

Drug Interactions
When administered concurrently, testolactone may increase the effects of oral anticoagulants; monitor and adjust anticoagulant dosage accordingly.

Drug/Laboratory Test Interactions
Physiologic effects of testolactone may result in decreased estradiol concentrations with radioimmunoassays for estradiol, increased plasma calcium concentrations (see PRECAUTIONS, Laboratory Tests), and increased 24-hour urinary excretion of creatine and 17-ketosteroids.

Carcinogenesis, Mutagenesis, Impairment of Fertility
No long-term animal studies have been performed to evaluate carcinogenic potential or mutagenesis. Testolactone did not affect fertility in male or female rats.

Pregnancy: Teratogenic Effects, Category C
In rats, testolactone has been shown to produce increased fetal mortality, increased abnormal fetal development, and increased mortality in growing pups when given at doses 5 to 15 times the recommended human dose. In rabbits, no teratologic effects were observed at doses 2.5 to 7.5 times the recommended human dose. There are no adequate and well controlled studies in pregnant women. Testolactone is intended for use only in postmenopausal women and should not be used during pregnancy.

Nursing Mothers
It is not known whether this drug is excreted in human milk. Because many drugs are excreted in human milk, a decision should be made whether or not to discontinue nursing.

Pediatric Use
Safety and effectiveness in children have not been established.

ADVERSE REACTIONS

Certain signs and symptoms have been reported in association with the use of this drug but, in these instances, it is often impossible to determine the relationship of the underlying disease and drug administration to the reported reaction. Such reactions include maculopapular erythema, increase in blood pressure, paresthesia, aches and edema of the extremities, glossitis, anorexia and nausea and vomiting. Alopecia alone and with associated nail growth disturbance have been reported rarely; these side effects subsided without interruption of treatment.

OVERDOSAGE

There have ben no reports of acute overdosage with testolactone tablets.

DOSAGE AND ADMINISTRATION

The recommended oral dose is 250 mg qid.
In order to evaluate the response, therapy with testolactone should be continued for a minimum of three months unless there is active progression of the disease.

HOW SUPPLIED

TESLAC (Testolactone Tablets USP), **50 mg/tablet:** bottles of 100 (NDC 0003-0690-50). Each round, white, biconvex tablet is imprinted with the identification number **690**.
Storage
Store at room temperature; avoid excessive heat.
(J4-184)

THERAGRAN HEMATINIC®   ℞

[*ther'ah-gran" hē mah-tin'ik*]
Therapeutic Formula Vitamin Tablets with Hematinics

DESCRIPTION

THERAGRAN HEMATINIC is a therapeutic iron-containing multivitamin with minerals tablet for oral administration.
Graphic formulas and physical/chemical information for the vitamins may be found in the US Pharmacopeia XX. THERAGRAN HEMATINIC Tablets supply:

Active Ingredients		Each Tablet	3 Tablets (usual daily dose)
Vitamin A (as Acetate)	(8,333 IU)	2.5mg	25,000IU
Vitamin D (Ergocalciferol)	(133 IU)	3.3mcg	400IU
Thiamine Mononitrate		3.3mg	10mg
Riboflavin		3.3mg	10mg
Pyridoxine Hydrochloride		3.3mg	10mg
Niacinamide		33.3mg	100mg
Calcium Pantothenate		11.7mg	35mg
Vitamin E (dl-α-Tocopheryl Acetate)	(5 IU)	5mg	15IU
Copper (as Sulfate)		0.67mg	2mg
Magnesium (as Carbonate)		41.7mg	125mg
Iron, elemental (as Ferrous Fumarate)		66.7mg	200mg
Vitamin B$_{12}$ (as Cyanocobalamin)		50mcg	150mcg
Folic Acid		0.33mg	1mg
Vitamin C (as Sodium Ascorbate)		100mg	300mg

Inactive ingredients: acacia, calcium carbonate, carnauba wax, castor oil, cellulose, colorants [FD&C Red No. 3 and Yellow No. 5 (tartrazine)], ethylcellulose, flavor, gelatin, lactose, magnesium stearate, povidone, shellac, sodium bisulfite, sodium starch glycolate, sucrose, talc, titanium dioxide, and white wax.

CLINICAL PHARMACOLOGY

Vitamins and dietary minerals are fundamentally involved in vital metabolic processes, where they usually serve as oxidizing and reducing agents and as factors in various enzyme systems. These essential micronutrients are so closely interrelated that the lack of any one may affect the body requirements of others.
Metabolic Functions of Inorganic Ions—*Iron* plays an important role in oxygen and electron transport. Iron may be functional (in hemoglobin, myoglobin, heme enzymes, and cofactor and transport iron) or stored as ferritin and hemosiderin in the liver, spleen, bone marrow, and reticuloendothelial system. The hemoglobin (0.34 percent iron) content of blood is about 14 to 17 g per 100 mL in adult males; in adult females it ranges between 12 and 14 g. Following ingestion, ferrous iron forms low molecular chelates with amino acids, ascorbic acid, and sugars which may be solubilized and absorbed before they reach the distal small intestine. Iron is probably absorbed passively into the mucosal layer of the small intestine, then transferred actively to transferrin where it is incorporated into red blood cells in bone marrow or into all body cells. Transferrin iron may also be stored in bone marrow, liver and spleen. Iron is removed from the

body in the urine, bile, sweat, feces, and via desquamation of cells.
Copper: an essential enzyme cofactor in the utilization of iron in hemoglobin synthesis.
Magnesium: an enzyme activator—certain peptidases and phosphatases require magnesium for maximal activity as do virtually all reactions involving adenosine triphosphate.
Metabolic Functions of the Vitamins—*Fat Soluble Vitamins*—These tend to be stored in the body; their precise mode of action is largely unknown.
Vitamin A: essential to the production and regeneration of the visual purple of the retina; maintenance of the integrity of epithelial tissue; lysosome stability.
Vitamin D: functions in bone metabolism by regulating the intestinal absorption of calcium and phosphorus.
Vitamin E: intracellular antioxidant, important to the stability of biologic membranes.
Water Soluble Vitamins: except for vitamin B$_{12}$, these micronutrients are not stored in the body.
B Complex Vitamins (thiamine, riboflavin, pyridoxine, niacinamide, pantothenic acid, vitamin B$_{12}$, folic acid): these function, either alone or as structural components of more complex molecules, in catalytic systems where they usually function as coenzymes in carbohydrate, protein, or amino acid metabolism, synthesis of DNA and other molecules, maturation of RBCs, nerve cell function, or oxidation-reduction reactions.
Vitamin C: a coenzyme, essential to osteoid tissue; collagen formation; vascular function; tissue respiration and wound healing; facilitates absorption of iron.

INDICATIONS AND USAGE

THERAGRAN HEMATINIC (Therapeutic Formula Vitamin Tablets with Hematinics) Tablets are indicated in the treatment of many of the common iron-deficiency anemias, particularly those associated with nutritional deficiency states or when nutritional requirements are high, and tropical and nontropical sprue. These iron-deficiency states include anemias associated with dietary inadequacy, convalescence, those frequently encountered in late childhood, early adolescence and old age, menorrhagia, and the anemias of women from menarche to menopause including macrocytic or microcytic anemia of pregnancy.
Iron deficiency may result in fatigue, palpitation, smooth and sore tongue, angular stomatitis, dysphagia, gastritis, enteropathy, and koilonychia, as well as anemia. In young children, depressed growth and impaired mental performance occur.

CONTRAINDICATIONS

Hemochromatosis and hemosiderosis are contraindications to iron therapy.

WARNINGS

Folic acid alone is improper therapy in the treatment of pernicious anemia and other megaloblastic anemias where vitamin B$_{12}$ is deficient.

PRECAUTIONS

General
The use of niacin-containing preparations in patients with gastritis, peptic ulcer, or asthma should be undertaken carefully.
Since iron-deficiency anemia may be a manifestation of a basic systemic disturbance such as recurrent blood loss, the underlying cause of the anemia should be determined and corrected if possible.
The ingredients in THERAGRAN HEMATINIC are not sufficient nor are they intended for the treatment of pernicious anemia. Folic acid in doses above 0.1 mg daily may obscure pernicious anemia in that hematologic remission can occur while neurological manifestations remain progressive; therefore, the possibility of pernicious anemia should be excluded before treatment with this preparation. Parenteral use of vitamin B$_{12}$ is recommended to assure essential medical supervision of the patient (see WARNINGS).
This product contains FD&C Yellow No. 5 (tartrazine) which may cause allergic-type reactions (including bronchial asthma) in certain susceptible individuals. Although the overall incidence of FD&C Yellow No. 5 (tartrazine) sensitivity in the general population is low, it is frequently seen in patients who also have aspirin hypersensitivity.
Information for the Patient
Keep THERAGRAN HEMATINIC (Therapeutic Formula Vitamin Tablets with Hematinics) and all other medication out of the reach of children.
Patients should be informed of symptoms of intolerance to components of this preparation; if any of these symptoms appear the patient should be advised to discontinue dosing, and to notify the physician.
Recommended dosage should not be exceeded unless directed by the physician.

Continued on next page

Squibb—Cont.

Laboratory Tests
Periodic hematologic studies should be performed.
Drug Interactions
Since oral iron products interfere with absorption of oral tetracyclines, these products should not be taken within two hours of each other.
Mineral oil and bile-acid sequestrants such as cholestyramine and colestipol hydrochloride in long-term therapy have been shown to decrease the absorption of fat-soluble vitamins.
Pyridoxine hydrochloride may act as an antagonist to levodopa.
Hydralazine hydrochloride, penicillamine, isoniazid, and cycloserine may antagonize pyridoxine hydrochloride.
Phenytoin, methotrexate, and pyrimethamine may interfere with folic acid absorption.
Colestipol hydrochloride may decrease the bioavailability of niacin.
Vitamin C may decrease the hypoprothrombinemic effect of oral anticoagulants; prothrombin levels should be monitored.
Neomycin and colchicine may impair cyanocobalamin absorption.
Carcinogenesis, Mutagenesis, Impairment of Fertility
Long-term studies in animals have not been performed.
Pregnancy Category C
Animal reproduction studies have not been conducted with therapeutic formula vitamin tablets with hematinics. Controlled clinical studies have not been performed to determine if therapeutic formula vitamin tablets with hematinics can cause fetal harm when administered to a pregnant woman or can affect reproduction capacity. THERAGRAN HEMATINIC should be given to a pregnant woman only if clearly needed.
Nursing Mothers
It is not known whether components of this product are excreted in human milk. Because many substances are excreted in human milk, caution should be exercised when THERAGRAN HEMATINIC is administered to a nursing woman.
Pediatric Use
Safety and effectiveness in children have not been established.

ADVERSE REACTIONS

Allergic reactions, skin rashes, and gastrointestinal disturbances, such as nausea, vomiting, diarrhea, or constipation may occur.
A generalized flushing and a feeling of warmth has been reported following niacinamide therapy.
Allergic sensitization has been reported following both oral and parenteral administration of folic acid.

DOSAGE AND ADMINISTRATION

The usual adult dose is one THERAGRAN HEMATINIC Tablet three times daily. When prescribed in late childhood and early adolescence, dosage reduction according to the size and weight of the child should be considered by the physician. Dosage may be adjusted according to the response of the patient. Since ferrous fumarate is not likely to cause gastric upsets, dosage need not be given at mealtime.

HOW SUPPLIED

THERAGRAN HEMATINIC (Therapeutic Formula Vitamin Tablets with Hematinics) is supplied in bottles of 90 tablets (NDC 0003-0535-40).
Storage
Store at room temperature; avoid excessive heat.
(J2-574H)
Shown in Product Identification Section, page 432

THERAGRAN JR.™
[*ther'ah-gran"*]
(Children's Chewable Vitamin Formula)

(See PDR For Nonprescription Drugs)

THERAGRAN® LIQUID
[*ther'ah-gran"*]
(High Potency Vitamin Supplement)

(See PDR For Nonprescription Drugs)

THERAGRAN® TABLETS
[*ther'ah-gran"*]
(High Potency Multivitamin Formula)
ADVANCED FORMULA

(See PDR For Nonprescription Drugs)

THERAGRAN–M® TABLETS
[*ther'ah-gran"em*]
(High Potency Multivitamin Formula with Minerals)
ADVANCED FORMULA

(See PDR For Nonprescription Drugs)

THERAGRAN® STRESS FORMULA
(High Potency Multivitamin Formula with Iron and Biotin)

(See PDR For Nonprescription Drugs)

TRIMOX® '250' CAPSULES ℞
[*tri'mokz*]
TRIMOX® '500' CAPSULES ℞
Amoxicillin Capsules USP
TRIMOX® '125' FOR ORAL ℞
SUSPENSION
TRIMOX® '250' FOR ORAL ℞
SUSPENSION
Amoxicillin for Oral Suspension USP

DESCRIPTION

Amoxicillin trihydrate is a semisynthetic antibiotic, an analog of ampicillin, with a broad spectrum of bactericidal activity against many gram-positive and gram-negative microorganisms. Amoxicillin is designated chemically as (2S,5R,6R)-6-[(R)-(—)-2-Amino-2-(p-hydroxyphenyl) acetamido]-3,3-dimethyl -7- oxo -4- thia-1-azabicyclo [3.2.0] heptane-2-carboxylic acid trihydrate.
TRIMOX '250' and TRIMOX '500' Capsules (Amoxicillin Capsules) are available for oral administration as capsules providing amoxicillin trihydrate equivalent to 250 and 500 mg amoxicillin, respectively. Inactive ingredients: colorants (D&C Yellow No. 10, FD&C Blue No. 1 and FD&C Yellow No. 6), gelatin, magnesium stearate, and titanium dioxide.
TRIMOX '125' and TRIMOX '250' for Oral Suspension (Amoxicillin for Oral Suspension) provide, after constitution, amoxicillin trihydrate equivalent to 125 mg and 250 mg amoxicillin per 5 mL, respectively. Inactive ingredients: calcium carrageenan, citric acid, colorant (FD&C Red. No. 3), flavor, potassium sorbate, silica gel, sucrose, and xanthan gum.

CLINICAL PHARMACOLOGY

Amoxicillin is stable in the presence of gastric acid and may be given without regard to meals. It is rapidly absorbed after oral administration. It diffuses readily into most body tissues and fluids, with the exception of brain and spinal fluid, except when meninges are inflamed. The half-life of amoxicillin is 61.3 minutes. Most of the amoxicillin is excreted unchanged in the urine; its excretion can be delayed by concurrent administration of probenecid. Amoxicillin is not highly protein-bound. In blood serum, amoxicillin is approximately 20 percent protein-bound as compared to 60 percent for penicillin G.
Orally administered doses of 250 mg and 500 mg amoxicillin capsules result in average peak blood levels one to two hours after administration in the range of 3.5 mcg/mL to 5.0 mcg/mL and 5.5 mcg/mL to 7.5 mcg/mL, respectively.
Orally administered doses of amoxicillin suspension 125 mg/5 mL and 250 mg/5 mL result in average peak blood levels one to two hours after administration in the range of 1.5 mcg/mL to 3.0 mcg/mL and 3.5 mcg/mL to 5.0 mcg/mL, respectively.
Detectable serum levels are observed up to 8 hours after an orally administered dose of amoxicillin. Following a 1 g dose and utilizing a special skin window technique to determine levels of the antibiotic, it was noted that therapeutic levels were found in the interstitial fluid. Approximately 60 percent of an orally administered dose of amoxicillin is excreted in the urine within six to eight hours.
Microbiology
TRIMOX (amoxicillin) is similar to ampicillin in its bactericidal action against susceptible organisms during the stage of active multiplication. It acts through the inhibition of biosynthesis of cell wall mucopeptides. While *in vitro* studies have demonstrated the susceptibility of most strains of the following organisms, clinical efficacy for infections other than those included in the INDICATIONS AND USAGE SECTION has not been documented: gram-positive bacteria: alpha- and beta-hemolytic streptococci, *Streptococcus pneumoniae* (formerly *Diplococcus pneumoniae*), nonpenicillinase-producing staphylococci, and *Streptococcus faecalis*. It is active *in vitro* against many strains of *Haemophilus influenzae*, *Neisseria gonorrhoeae*, *Escherichia coli* and *Proteus mirabilis*. Because it does not resist destruction by penicillinase, it is *not* effective against penicillinase-producing bacteria, particularly resistant staphylococci. All strains of *Pseudomonas* and most strains of *Klebsiella* and *Enterobacter* are resistant.
Disc Susceptibility Tests
Quantitative methods that require measurement of the diameters of zones of inhibition of microbial growth give the most precise estimates of antibiotic susceptibility. One recommended procedure (21 CFR §460.1) uses discs for testing susceptibility to ampicillin-class antibiotics. Interpretations correlate diameters of the disc test with MIC values for amoxicillin. With this procedure, a report from the laboratory of "susceptible" indicates that the infecting organism is likely to respond to therapy. A report of "resistant" indicates that the infecting organism is not likely to respond to therapy. A report of "intermediate susceptibility" suggests that the organism would be susceptible if high dosage is used, or if the infection is confined to tissues and fluids (e.g., urine), in which high antibiotic levels are attained.

INDICATIONS AND USAGE

TRIMOX (amoxicillin) is indicated in the treatment of infections caused by susceptible strains of the designated organisms listed below:
Infections of the ear, nose, and throat —streptococci, pneumococci, and nonpenicillinase-producing staphylococci and *H. influenzae*.
Infections of the genitourinary tract —E. coli, P. mirabilis, and S. faecalis.
Infections of the skin and skin structures —streptococci, nonpenicillinase-producing staphylococci, and *E. coli.*
Infections of the lower respiratory tract —streptococci, pneumococci, and nonpenicillinase-producing staphylococci and *H. influenzae.*
Gonorrhea, acute uncomplicated ano-genital and urethral infections —nonpenicillinase-producing N. gonorrhoeae.
Therapy may be instituted prior to obtaining results from bacteriological and susceptibility studies to determine the causative organisms and their susceptibility to amoxicillin. Indicated surgical procedures should be performed.

CONTRAINDICATIONS

The use of this drug is contraindicated in individuals with a history of an allergic reaction to any of the penicillins.

WARNINGS

Serious and occasionally fatal hypersensitivity (anaphylactoid) reactions have been reported in patients on penicillin therapy. Although anaphylaxis is more frequent following parenteral therapy, it has occurred in patients on oral penicillins. These reactions are more likely to occur in persons with a history of penicillin hypersensitivity and/or a history of sensitivity to multiple allergens. There have been reports of individuals with a history of penicillin hypersensitivity who have experienced severe reactions when treated with a cephalosporin. Before initiating therapy with any penicillin, careful inquiry should be made concerning previous hypersensitivity reactions to penicillins, cephalosporins, or other allergens. If an allergic reaction occurs, amoxicillin should be discontinued and appropriate therapy should be instituted. **Serious anaphylactoid reactions require immediate emergency treatment with epinephrine. Oxygen, intravenous steroids, and airway management, including intubation, should also be administered as indicated.**

PRECAUTIONS

General
The possibility of superinfections with mycotic or bacterial pathogens should be kept in mind during therapy. If superinfections occur (usually involving *Enterobacter, Pseudomonas* or *Candida*), amoxicillin should be discontinued and/or appropriate therapy instituted.
Information for the Patient
1. The patient should inform the physician of any history of sensitivity to allergens, including previous hypersensitivity reactions to penicillins and cephalosporins (see WARNINGS).
2. The patient should discontinue amoxicillin and contact the physician immediately if any side effect occurs (see WARNINGS).
3. Diabetic patients should consult with the physician before changing diet or dosage of diabetes medication (see PRECAUTIONS, Drug/Laboratory Test Interactions).
Laboratory Tests
As with any potent drug, periodic assessment of renal, hepatic and hematopoietic function should be made during prolonged therapy.
In streptococcal infections, therapy must be sufficient to eliminate the organism (10 days minimum); otherwise the sequelae of streptococcal disease may occur. Cultures should be taken following completion of treatment to determine whether streptococci have been eradicated.
Cases of gonorrhea with a suspected lesion of syphilis should have darkfield examinations before receiving amoxicillin and monthly serological tests for a minimum of four months.
Drug Interactions
When administered concurrently, the following drugs may interact with amoxicillin:
Bacteriostatic antibiotics—Chloramphenicol, erythromycins, sulfonamides, or tetracyclines may interfere with the bactericidal effects of penicillins. This has been demonstrated *in vitro*; however, the clinical significance of this interaction is not well-documented.

Probenecid—May decrease renal tubular secretion of amoxicillin resulting in increased blood levels and/or amoxicillin toxicity.

Drug/Laboratory Test Interactions

After treatment with amoxicillin, a false-positive reaction for glucose in the urine may occur with copper sulfate tests (Benedict's solution, Fehling's solution, or Clinitest® tablets) but not with enzyme based tests such as Clinistix® and Tes-Tape®.

Carcinogenesis, Mutagenesis, Impairment of Fertility

Long-term studies in animals have not been performed to evaluate carcinogenesis, mutagenesis, or impairment of fertility in males or females.

Pregnancy: Teratogenic Effects
Category B

Reproduction studies in animals have revealed no evidence of impaired fertility or harm to the fetus due to amoxicillin. There are, however, no adequate and well-controlled studies in pregnant women. Because animal reproduction studies are not always predictive of human response, amoxicillin should be used during pregnancy only if clearly needed.

Labor and Delivery

Oral ampicillin-class antibiotics are poorly absorbed during labor. Studies in guinea pigs showed that intravenous administration of ampicillin slightly decreased the uterine tone and frequency of contractions, but moderately increased the height and duration of contractions. However, it is not known whether use of these drugs in humans during labor or delivery has immediate or delayed adverse effects on the fetus, prolongs the duration of labor, or increases the likelihood that forceps delivery or other obstetrical intervention or resuscitation of the newborn will be necessary.

Nursing Mothers

Since penicillins are excreted in breast milk during lactation, penicillin use by nursing mothers may lead to sensitization of infants; therefore, a decision should be made whether to discontinue nursing or to discontinue amoxicillin, taking into account the importance of the drug to the mother.

Pediatric Use

Penicillins are excreted primarily unchanged by the kidney; therefore, the incompletely developed renal function in neonates and young infants will delay the excretion of penicillins. Guidelines for administration of this antibiotic to pediatric patients are presented in DOSAGE AND ADMINISTRATION.

ADVERSE REACTIONS

As with other penicillins, it may be expected that untoward reactions will be essentially limited to sensitivity phenomena. They are more likely to occur in individuals who have previously demonstrated hypersensitivity to penicillin and in those with a history of allergy, asthma, hay fever or urticaria. The following adverse reactions have been reported as associated with the use of penicillins:

Gastrointestinal: Glossitis, stomatitis, black "hairy" tongue, nausea, vomiting, diarrhea, and pseudomembranous colitis.

Hypersensitivity Reactions: Erythematous maculopapular rashes, urticaria, and a few cases of exfoliative dermatitis and erythema multiforme have been reported. Anaphylaxis is the most serious reaction experienced and has usually been associated with parenteral dosage forms (See WARNINGS).

NOTE: Urticaria, other skin rashes and serum sickness-like reactions may be controlled with antihistamines and, if necessary, systemic corticosteroids. Whenever such reactions occur, amoxicillin should be discontinued unless, in the opinion of the physician, the condition being treated is life-threatening and amenable only to amoxicillin therapy.

Liver: A moderate rise in serum glutamic oxaloacetic transaminase (SGOT) has been noted, but the significance of this finding is unknown.

Hemic and Lymphatic Systems: Anemia, thrombocytopenia, thrombocytopenic purpura, eosinophilia, leukopenia and agranulocytosis have been reported during therapy with the penicillins. These reactions are usually reversible on discontinuation of therapy and are believed to be hypersensitivity phenomena.

OVERDOSAGE

In case of overdosage, discontinue medication, treat symptomatically and institute supportive measures as required. Amoxicillin can be removed from the circulation by hemodialysis.

DOSAGE AND ADMINISTRATION

Infections of the ear, nose and throat due to streptococci, pneumococci, and nonpenicillinase-producing staphylococci and *H. influenzae:*

Infections of the genitourinary tract due to *E. coli, P. mirabilis* and *S. faecalis:*

Infections of the skin and skin structures due to streptococci, nonpenicillinase-producing staphylococci and susceptible *E. coli:*

USUAL DOSAGE:

Adults: 250 mg every 8 hours

Children: 20 mg/kg/day in divided doses every 8 hours

Children weighing 20 kg or more should be dosed according to the adult recommendations.

In severe infections or those caused by less susceptible organisms:

500 mg every 8 hours for adults and 40 mg/kg/day in divided doses every 8 hours for children may be needed.

Infections of the lower respiratory tract due to streptococci, pneumococci, and nonpenicillinase-producing staphylococci and *H. influenzae.*

USUAL DOSAGE:

Adults: 500 mg every 8 hours

Children: 40 mg/kg/day in divided doses every 8 hours

Children weighing 20 kg or more should be dosed according to the adult recommendations.

Gonorrhea, acute uncomplicated ano-genital and urethral infections due to nonpenicillinase-producing *N. gonorrhoeae* (males and females):

3 grams as a single oral dose

Cases of gonorrhea with a suspected lesion of syphilis should have darkfield examinations before receiving amoxicillin, and monthly serological tests for a minimum of four months.

General

Larger doses may be required for stubborn or severe infections.

The children's dosage is intended for individuals whose weight will not cause a dosage to be calculated greater than that recommended for adults.

It should be recognized that in the treatment of chronic urinary tract infections, frequent bacteriological and clinical appraisals are necessary. Smaller doses than those recommended above should not be used. Even higher doses may be needed at times. Except for gonorrhea, treatment should be continued for a minimum of 48 to 72 hours beyond the time that the patient becomes asymptomatic or evidence of bacterial eradication has been obtained. It is recommended that there be at least 10 days' treatment for any infection caused by hemolytic streptococci to prevent the occurrence of acute rheumatic fever or glomerulonephritis (see PRECAUTIONS, Laboratory Tests).

Preparation and Storage of Oral Suspensions

Prepare the suspension at the time of dispensing. Follow the directions for constitution on the label of the package. Discard any unused suspension after 14 days. The suspension may be kept at room temperature; refrigeration is not required. **Shake well before using.**

HOW SUPPLIED

TRIMOX Capsules (Amoxicillin Capsules USP)

TRIMOX '250'	bottles of 100 (NDC 0003-0230-50)
250 mg/capsule:	and 500 (NDC 0003-0230-60), and cartons of 100 Unimatic® unit-dose packs (NDC 0003-0230-51).
	Each two-piece, green, hard gelatin capsule is imprinted with identification no. **230.**
TRIMOX '500'	bottles of 50 (NDC 0003-0231-45) and
500 mg/capsule:	500 (NDC 0003-0231-60), and cartons of 100 Unimatic unit-dose packs (NDC 0003-0231-51).
	Each two-piece, light green/dark green, hard gelatin capsule is imprinted with identification number **231.**

TRIMOX for Oral Suspension (Amoxicillin for Oral Suspension USP)

TRIMOX '125'	When constituted as directed on the container label, a pleasantly flavored suspension containing **125 mg per 5 mL,** in bottle sizes for preparation of 80 mL (NDC 0003-1737-30), 100 mL (NDC 0003-1737-40), and 150 mL (NDC 0003-1737-45). **125 mg/bottle:** packs of 100 Unimatic unit-dose bottles (NDC 0003-1737-25).
TRIMOX '250'	When constituted as directed on the container label, a pleasantly flavored suspension containing **250 mg per 5 mL,** in bottle sizes for preparation of 80 mL (NDC 0003-1738-30), 100 mL (NDC 0003-1738-40), and 150 mL (NDC 0003-1738-45). **250 mg/bottle:** packs of 100 Unimatic unit-dose bottles (NDC 0003-1738-25).

Storage

Store TRIMOX Capsules and TRIMOX for Oral Suspension at room temperature.

(J4-176A)

Shown in Product Identification Section, page 432

VEETIDS® '250' TABLETS   ℞

[vē'tidz]

VEETIDS® '500' TABLETS   ℞

Penicillin V Potassium Tablets USP

VEETIDS® '125' FOR ORAL SOLUTION   ℞

VEETIDS® '250' FOR ORAL SOLUTION   ℞

Penicillin V Potassium for Oral Solution USP

DESCRIPTION

VEETIDS (Penicillin V Potassium) oral dosage forms contain the potassium salt of semi-synthetically-produced penicillin V. Penicillin V potassium is designated chemically as Monopotassium (2S,5R,6R)-3,3-dimethyl-7-oxo-6-(2-phenoxyacetamido)-4-thia -1- azabicyclo [3.2.0] heptane-2-carboxylate.

VEETIDS tablets provide penicillin V potassium equivalent to 250 mg (400,000 u) and 500 mg (800,000 u), of penicillin V. Inactive ingredients: carnauba wax, microcrystalline cellulose, colorants (for '250' only, D&C Red No. 30 and FD&C Yellow No. 6), flavor, lactose, magnesium stearate, povidone, talc, and other ingredients.

VEETIDS for oral solution are available as powders that, when constituted, provide solutions containing penicillin V potassium equivalent to 125 mg (200,000 u) and 250 mg (400,000 u) penicillin V per 5 mL, respectively. Inactive ingredients: colorants [FD&C Red No. 40, and, for '125' only, Yellow No. 5 (tartrazine)], dibasic sodium phosphate, flavors, monobasic sodium phosphate, saccharin sodium, and sucrose.

CLINICAL PHARMACOLOGY

Penicillin V is more resistant to inactivation by gastric acid than penicillin G; however, it has the same bacterial spectrum as penicillin G. It may be given with meals; however, blood levels are slightly higher when the drug is given on an empty stomach. Average blood levels are two to five times higher than the levels following the same dose of oral penicillin G and also show much less individual variation.

About 60 percent of a given dose of penicillin V is absorbed. Once absorbed, penicillin V is about 80 percent bound to serum protein. Highest levels are found in the kidneys, with lesser amounts in the liver, skin, and intestines. Penicillin V penetrates into all other tissues to a lesser degree with a very small level found in the cerebrospinal fluid. It has been reported that penicillin V crosses the placental barrier and can be detected in cord serum and amniotic fluid. The drug is rapidly excreted by glomerular filtration and tubular secretion in patients with normal kidney function. In neonates and young infants, and in individuals with impaired kidney function, excretion is considerably delayed.

Microbiology

Penicillin V is bactericidal against penicillin G-susceptible microorganisms during the stage of active multiplication. It acts by inhibiting biosynthesis of cell-wall mucopeptide. It is not active against the penicillinase-producing bacteria, which include many strains of staphylococci. While *in vitro* studies have demonstrated the susceptibility of most strains of the following organisms, clinical efficacy for infections other than those included in the INDICATIONS AND USAGE section has not been documented. Penicillin V is highly active *in vitro* against staphylococci (except penicillinase-producing strains), streptococci (groups A, C, G, H, L, and M) and pneumococci. Other organisms susceptible *in vitro* to penicillin V are *Corynebacterium diphtheriae, Bacillus anthracis,* Clostridia, Actinomyces bovis, Streptobacillus moniliformis, Listeria monocytogenes, Leptospira and *Neisseria gonorrhoeae; Treponema pallidum* is extremely susceptible.

Susceptibility Testing

Diffusion Technique: Quantitative procedures that require measurement of zone diameters give precise estimates of microbial susceptibility to antibiotics. One such method, recommended for use with the penicillin G 10 unit disk (used for testing susceptibility to phenoxymethyl penicillin), is the National Committee of Clinical Laboratory Standards (NCCLS) approved procedure.

Dilution Technique: Broth or agar dilution methods may be used to determine the minimal inhibitory concentration (MIC) of penicillin V.

MIC test results should be interpreted according to the concentrations of penicillin V that can be obtained in serum, tissues and body fluids.

For any susceptibility test, a report of "susceptible" indicates that the pathogen is likely to respond to penicillin V therapy; a report of "resistant" indicates that the pathogen is not likely to respond. A report of "intermediate" (moderate susceptibility) indicates that the pathogen is expected to be susceptible to penicillin V if high dosages are used, or if the infection is confined to tissues and fluids in which high penicillin V levels are attained.

Continued on next page

Squibb—Cont.

INDICATIONS AND USAGE

VEETIDS (Penicillin V Potassium) are indicated in the treatment of infections caused by susceptible strains of the designated organisms in the conditions listed below. Therapy should be guided by bacteriological studies, including susceptibility tests, and by clinical response. Note: severe pneumonia, empyema, bacteremia, pericarditis, meningitis, and septic arthritis should not be treated with penicillin V during the acute stage.

Indicated surgical procedures should be performed.

Treatment

Upper Respiratory Tract Infections [including a) otitis media and b) Vincent's gingivitis and pharyngitis (fusospirochetosis)]—Mild to moderately severe infections without bacteremia caused by penicillin-susceptible group A streptococci and *Fusobacteria*, respectively.

NOTE: Streptococci in groups A, C, G, H, L, and M are very susceptible to penicillin; other groups including group D (*Enterococcus*) are resistant. Necessary dental care should be accomplished in infections involving gum tissue.

Lower Respiratory Tract Infections (pneumococcal infections)—Mild to moderately severe infections caused by penicillin-susceptible streptococci (formerly diplococci).

Skin and Skin Structure Infections (including erysipelas)—Mild infections caused by penicillin-susceptible staphylococci and streptococci.

NOTE: Reports indicate an increasing number of strains of staphylococci resistant to penicillin, emphasizing the need for culture and susceptibility studies in treating suspected staphylococcal infections.

Scarlet Fever—Mild to moderate infections without bacteremia caused by penicillin-susceptible group A streptococci.

Prophylaxis

Prevention of recurrence following rheumatic fever and/or chorea—Prophylaxis with oral penicillin on a continuing basis is effective in preventing recurrence of these conditions.

Prevention of bacterial endocarditis—Although no controlled clinical efficacy studies have been conducted penicillin V has been suggested by the American Heart Association and the American Dental Association for use in a standard regimen (oral) and a special regimen (parenteral-oral) for prophylaxis against bacterial endocarditis in patients with congenital heart disease or rheumatic or other acquired valvular heart disease when they undergo dental procedures and surgical procedures of the respiratory tract.[1] Since it may happen that *alpha* hemolytic streptococci relatively resistant to penicillin may be found when patients are receiving continuous oral penicillin for secondary prevention of rheumatic fever, prophylactic agents other than penicillin may be chosen for these patients and prescribed in addition to their continuous rheumatic fever prophylactic regimen. Oral penicillin should not be used as adjunctive prophylaxis for genitourinary instrumentation or surgery, lower intestinal tract surgery, sigmoidoscopy, and childbirth. NOTE: When selecting antibiotics for the prevention of bacterial endocarditis the physician or dentist should read the full joint statement of the American Heart Association and the American Dental Association.[1]

CONTRAINDICATIONS

Contraindicated in patients with a history of hypersensitivity to any penicillin.

WARNINGS

Serious and occasionally fatal hypersensitivity (anaphylactoid) reactions have been reported in patients on penicillin therapy. These reactions are more likely to occur in individuals with a history of penicillin hypersensitivity and/or a history of sensitivity to multiple allergens. There have been reports of individuals with a history of penicillin hypersensitivity who have experienced severe reactions when treated with cephalosporins. Before initiating therapy with any penicillin, careful inquiry should be made concerning previous hypersensitivity reactions to penicillin, cephalosporins, or other allergens. If an allergic reaction occurs, the drug should be discontinued and the appropriate therapy instituted. Serious anaphylactoid reactions require immediate emergency treatment with epinephrine. Oxygen, intravenous steroids, and airway management, including intubation, should also be administered as indicated.

PRECAUTIONS

General

Penicillin should be used with caution in individuals with histories of significant allergies and/or asthma.

The oral route of administration should not be relied upon in patients with severe illness, or with nausea, vomiting, gastric dilatation, cardiospasm or intestinal hypermotility.

Occasional patients will not absorb therapeutic amounts of orally administered penicillin.

Prolonged use of antibiotics may promote the overgrowth of nonsusceptible organisms, including fungi. Should superinfection occur, appropriate measures should be taken.

VEETIDS '125' for Oral Solution contains FD&C Yellow No. 5 (tartrazine) which may cause allergic-type reactions (including bronchial asthma) in certain susceptible individuals. Although the overall incidence of FD&C Yellow No. 5 (tartrazine) sensitivity in the general population is low, it is frequently seen in patients who also have aspirin hypersensitivity.

Information for the Patient

1. The patient should inform the physician of any history of sensitivity to allergens, including previous hypersensitivity reactions to penicillins and cephalosporins (see WARNINGS).

2. The patient should discontinue penicillin V and contact the pyhsician immediately if any side effect occurs (see WARNINGS).

3. Penicillin V should be taken one hour before or two hours after meals.

Laboratory Tests

In streptococcal infections, therapy must be sufficient to eliminate the organism (10 days minimum); otherwise the sequelae of streptococcal disease may occur. Cultures should be taken following completion of treatment to determine whether streptococci have been eradicated.

In prolonged therapy with penicillin, and particularly with high dosage regimens, periodic evaluation of the renal and hematopoietic systems is recommended.

Drug Interactions

When adminsitered concurrently the following drugs may interact with penicillin V:

Aspirin or phenylbutazone—Drugs capable of displacing bound penicillin from plasma protein binding sites may elevate the level of free penicilin in the serum; however, the clinical significance of this interaction is not well documented.

Bacteriostatic antibiotics (e.g., *chloramphenicol, erythromycins, sulfonamides, or tetracyclines*)—May interfere with the bactericidal effect of penicillins. This has been documented *in vitro*; however, the clinical significance of this interaction is not well-documented.

Oral contraceptives—Oral contraceptives may be less effective and increased breakthrough bleeding may occur.

Oral Neomycin—Reports indicate oral neomycin may result in malabsorption of penicillin V potassium.

Probenecid—May decrease renal tubular secretion of penicillin resulting in increased blood levels and/or penicillin toxicity.

Carcinogensis, Mutagenesis, Impairment of Fertility

Long-term studies in animals have not been performed to evaluate carcinogenic or mutagenic potential, or whether this medication affects fertility in males or females.

Pregnancy: Teratogenic Effects

Category B. Reproduction studies performed in the mouse, rat and rabbit have revealed no evidence of impaired fertility or harm to the fetus due to penicillin V. Human experience with the penicillins during pregnancy has not shown any positive evidence of adverse effects on the fetus. There are, however, no adequate and well-controlled studies in pregnant women showing conclusively that harmful effects of these drugs on the fetus can be excluded. Because animal reproductions studies are not always predictive of human response, penicillin should be used during pregnancy only if clearly needed.

Labor and Delivery

It is not known whether use of penicillin V prolongs the duration of labor or delivery, increases the likelihood that obstetrical intervention will be necessary, or has immediate or delayed adverse effects on the fetus.

Nursing Mothers

Since penicillins are excreted in breast milk during lactation, penicillin use by nursing mothers may lead to sensitization of infants; therefore, a decision should be made whether to discontinue nursing or to discontinue the drug, taking into account the importance of the drug to the mother.

Pediatric Use

Penicillins are excreted primarily unchanged by the kidney; therefore, the incompletely developed renal function in neonates and young infants will delay the excretion of penicillin. Administration to neonates and young infants should be limited to the lowest dosage compatible with an effective therapuetic regimen (see DOSAGE AND ADMINISTRATION).

ADVERSE REACTIONS

Although the incidence of reactions to oral penicillins has been reported with much less frequency than following parenteral therapy, it should be remembered that all degrees of hypersensitivity, including fatal anaphylaxis, have been reported with oral penicillin.

The most common reactions to oral penicillin are nausea, vomiting, epigastric distress, diarrhea, and black hairy tongue. The hypersensitivity reactions reported are skin rashes ranging from maculopapular to exfoliative dermatitis; urticaria; serum sickness-like reactions including chills, fever, edema, arthralgia, and prostration; laryngeal edema; and anaphylaxis. Fever and eosinophilia may frequently be the only reactions observed. Hemolytic anemia, leukopenia, thrombocytopenia, neuropathy, and nephropathy are infrequent reactions usually associated with high doses of parenteral penicillin. Urticaria, other skin rashes, and serum sickness-like reactions may be controlled by antihistamines and, if necessary, corticosteroids. Whenever such reactions occur, penicillin should be discontinued unless, in the opinion of the physician, the condition being treated is life-threatening and amenable only to penicillin therapy. Serious anaphylactoid reactions require emergency measures (see WARNINGS). An occasional patient may complain of sore mouth or tongue, as with any oral penicillin preparation.

OVERDOSAGE

In case of overdosage, discontinue medication, treat symptomatically and institute supportive measures as required.

DOSAGE AND ADMINISTRATION

The dosage of VEETIDS (Penicillin V Potassium) should be determined according to the susceptibility of the causative microorganism and the severity of infection, and adjusted to the clinical response of the patient.

For Therapeutic Use

Dosage for *children under 12 years* of age is calculated on the basis of body weight. For *infants and small children* the suggested dose is 15 to 56 mg (25,000 to 90,000 u) per kg/day in three to six divided doses.

The usual dosage recommendations for *adults and children 12 years and over* are as follows:

Streptococcal infections—mild to moderately severe—of the upper respiratory tract and including otitis media, scarlet fever and mild erysipelas: 125 mg (200,000 u) tid or qid for 10 days for mild infections; 250 mg (400,000 u) tid for 10 days for moderately severe infections; for mild to moderately severe streptococcal pharyngitis: 500 mg (800,000 u) bid may be used as an alternative regimen (see PRECAUTIONS, Laboratory Tests).

Pneumococcal infections—mild to moderately severe—of the respiratory tract, including otitis media: 250 to 500 mg (400,000 to 800,000 u) qid until the patient has been afebrile for at least two days.

Staphylococcal infections—mild infections of skin and skin structures (culture and susceptibility tests should be performed): 250 mg (400,000 u) tid or qid, or 500 mg (800,000 u) tid.

Vincent's gingivitis and pharyngitis (fusospirochetosis)—mild to moderately severe infections of the oropharynx: 250 mg (400,000 u) tid or qid, or 500 mg tid.

For Prophylactic Use

For the prevention of recurrence following rheumatic fever and/or chorea:

Adults—125 mg (200,000 u) bid on a continuing basis. Dosage for *children under 12 years* of age is calculated on the basis of body weight. For *infants and small children* the suggested dose is 15 to 56 mg (25,000 to 90,000 u) per kg/day in three to six divided doses.

To prevent bacterial endocarditis. For prophylaxis against bacterial endocarditis[1] in patients with congenital heart disease or rheumatic or other acquired valvular heart disease when undergoing dental procedures or surgical procedures of the upper respiratory tract, one of two regimens may be selected:

(1) Standard regimen—administer 2 g of penicillin V orally (1 g for children under 60 lb) one hour before the procedure, and then 1 g (500 mg for children under 60 lb) six hours later.

(2) Special regimen—ampicillin 1 to 2 g (50 mg/kg for children) intramuscularly or intravenously, plus gentamicin 1.5 mg/kg (2 mg/kg for children) intramuscularly or intravenously, one-half hour before procedure, followed by 1 g (500 mg for children under 60 lb) oral penicillin V six hours later. Alternatively, omit the oral penicillin V and repeat the parenteral regimen eight hours later. Doses for children should not exceed recommendations for adults for a single dose or for a 24-hour period.

HOW SUPPLIED

*VEETIDS Tablets (Penicillin V Potassium Tablets USP)	
*VEETIDS '250' 250 mg/tablet:	bottles of 100 (NDC 0003-0684-60) and 1000 (NDC 0003-0684-75), and cartons of 100 UNIMATIC® unit-dose packs (NDC 0003-0684-61). Each peach-orange, biconvex, capsule-shaped FILMLOK®* tablet is imprinted with identification number **684**.
*VEETIDS '500' 500 mg/tablet:	bottles of 100 (NDC 0003-0648-50) and 1000 (NDC 0003-0648-75), and cartons of 100 UNIMATIC unit-dose packs (NDC 0003-0648-51). Each white, biconvex, capsule-shaped FILMLOK tablet is imprinted with identification number **648**.

VEETIDS for Oral Solution
(Penicillin V Potassium for Oral Solution USP)

VEETIDS '125' 125 mg/5 mL: teaspoonful:	When constituted as directed on the container label, a pleasant berry-like flavored solution in 100 mL (NDC 0003-0681-44) and 200 mL (NDC 0003-0681-54) sizes.
VEETIDS '250' 250 mg/5 mL: teaspoonful:	When constituted as directed on the container label, a pleasant berry-like flavored solution in 100 mL (NDC 0003-0682-44) and 200 mL (NDC 0003-0682-54) sizes.

Storage

VEETIDS Tablets: Store at room temperature; avoid excessive heat. Bottled tablets should be kept and dispensed in tightly closed containers.

VEETIDS for Oral Solution: Store at room temperature prior to constitution. Following constitution, solution should be refrigerated; discard any unused portion after 14 days.

REFERENCE

1. American Heart Association: Prevention of bacterial endocarditis. Circulation 70:1123A–1127A, 1984

---

*FILMLOK is a Squibb trademark for veneer-coated tablets. (J4-116B)

*Shown in Product Identification Section, page 432

VELOSEF® '250' CAPSULES   ℞
[vel´ō-sef]
VELOSEF® '500' CAPSULES   ℞
Cephradine Capsules USP
VELOSEF® '125' FOR ORAL
SUSPENSION   ℞
VELOSEF® '250' FOR ORAL
SUSPENSION   ℞
Cephradine for Oral Suspension USP

DESCRIPTION

VELOSEF (Cephradine, Squibb) is a semisynthetic cephalosporin antibiotic; oral dosage forms include capsules containing 250 mg and 500 mg cephradine, and cephradine for oral suspension containing, after constitution, 125 mg and 250 mg per 5 mL dose.

Cephradine is designated chemically as (6R,7R)-7-[(R)-2-amino-2-(1,4-cyclohexadien-1-yl) acetamido]-3-methyl-8-oxo-5-thia-1-azabicyclo[4.2.0]oct-2-ene-2-carboxylic acid.

Inactive ingredients: VELOSEF Capsules—colorants (D&C Red No. 33 and Yellow No. 10; FD&C Blue No. 1, and, for '250' only, Red No. 3), gelatin, lactose, magnesium stearate, talc, and titanium dioxide. VELOSEF for Oral Suspension—citric acid, colorants (FD&C Red No. 40 for '250' only; FD&C Yellow No. 6 for '125' only), flavors, guar gum, methylcellulose, sodium citrate, and sucrose.

CLINICAL PHARMACOLOGY

VELOSEF (Cephradine, Squibb) is acid stable. It is rapidly absorbed after oral administration in the fasting state. Following single doses of 250 mg, 500 mg, and 1 g in normal adult volunteers, average peak serum concentrations within one hour were approximately 9 mcg/mL, 16.5 mcg/mL, and 24.2 mcg/mL, respectively. *In vitro* studies by an ultracentrifugation technique show that at therapeutic serum antibiotic concentrations, cephradine is minimally bound (8 to 17 percent) to normal serum protein. Cephradine does not pass across the blood-brain barrier to any appreciable extent. The presence of food in the gastrointestinal tract delays absorption but does not affect the total amount of cephradine absorbed. Over 90 percent of the drug is excreted unchanged in the urine within six hours. Peak urine concentrations are approximately 1600 mcg/mL, 3200 mcg/mL, and 4000 mcg/mL following single doses of 250 mg, 500 mg, and 1 g, respectively.

Microbiology: In vitro tests demonstrate that the cephalosporins are bactericidal because of their inhibition of cell-wall synthesis. Cephradine is active against the following organisms *in vitro:*

Group A beta-hemolytic streptococci
Staphylococci, including coagulase-positive, coagulase-negative, and penicillinase-producing strains
Streptococcus pneumoniae (formerly *Diplococcus pneumoniae*)
Escherichia coli
Proteus mirabilis
Klebsiella species
Hemophilus influenzae

Cephradine is not active against most strains of *Enterobacter* species, *P. morganii*, and *P. vulgaris*. It has no activity against *Pseudomonas* or *Herellea* species. When tested by *in vitro* methods, staphylococci exhibit cross-resistance between cephradine and methicillin-type antibiotics.

Note—Most strains of enterococci (*Streptococcus faecalis*) are resistant to cephradine.

Disc Susceptibility Tests—Quantitative methods that require measurement of zone diameters give the most precise esti-mates of antibiotic susceptibility. One recommended procedure (21 CFR §460.1) uses cephalosporin class discs for testing susceptibility; interpretations correlate zone diameters of this disc test with MIC values for cephradine. With this procedure, a report from the laboratory of "resistant" indicates that the infecting organism is not likely to respond to therapy. A report of "intermediate susceptibility" suggests that the organism would be susceptible if the infection is confined to the urinary tract, as high antibiotic levels can be obtained in the urine, or if high dosage is used in other types of infection.

INDICATIONS AND USAGE

VELOSEF (Cephradine, Squibb) Capsules and VELOSEF for Oral Suspension are indicated in the treatment of the following infections when caused by susceptible strains of the designated microorganisms:

RESPIRATORY TRACT INFECTIONS (e.g., tonsillitis, pharyngitis, and lobar pneumonia) caused by group A beta-hemolytic streptococci and *S. pneumoniae* (formerly *D. pneumoniae*).

(Penicillin is the usual drug of choice in the treatment and prevention of streptococcal infections, including the prophylaxis of rheumatic fever. VELOSEF is generally effective in the eradication of streptococci from the nasopharynx; substantial data establishing the efficacy of VELOSEF in the subsequent prevention of rheumatic fever are not available at present.)

OTITIS MEDIA caused by group A beta-hemolytic streptococci, *S. pneumoniae* (formerly *D. pneumoniae*), *H. influenzae*, and staphylococci.

SKIN AND SKIN STRUCTURE INFECTIONS caused by staphylococci (penicillin-susceptible and penicillin-resistant) and beta-hemolytic streptococci.

URINARY TRACT INFECTIONS, including prostatitis, caused by *E. coli, P. mirabilis, Klebsiella* species, and enterococci (*S. faecalis*). The high concentrations of cephradine achievable in the urinary tract will be effective against many strains of enterococci for which disc susceptibility studies indicate relative resistance. It is to be noted that among beta-lactam antibiotics, ampicillin is the drug of choice for enterococcal urinary tract (*S. faecalis*) infection.

Note—Culture and susceptibility tests should be initiated prior to and during therapy.

Following clinical improvement achieved with parenteral therapy, oral cephradine may be utilized for continuation of treatment of persistent or severe conditions where prolonged therapy is indicated.

CONTRAINDICATIONS

Cephradine is contraindicated in patients with known hypersensitivity to the cephalosporin group of antibiotics.

WARNINGS

In penicillin-sensitive patients, cephalosporin derivatives should be used with great caution. There is clinical and laboratory evidence of partial cross-allergenicity of the penicillins and the cephalosporins, and there are instances of patients who have had reactions to both drug classes (including anaphylaxis after parenteral use).

Any patient who has demonstrated some form of allergy, particularly to drugs, should receive antibiotics, including cephradine, cautiously and then only when absolutely necessary.

Pseudomembranous colitis has been reported with the use of cephalosporins (and other broad spectrum antibiotics); therefore, it is important to consider its diagnosis in patients who develop diarrhea in association with antibiotic use. Treatment with broad spectrum antibiotics alters normal flora of the colon and may permit overgrowth of clostridia. Studies indicate a toxin produced by *Clostridium difficile* is one primary cause of antibiotic-associated colitis. Cholestyramine and colestipol resins have been shown to bind the toxin *in vitro*. Mild cases of colitis may respond to drug discontinuance alone. Moderate to severe cases should be managed with fluid, electrolyte and protein supplementation as indicated. When the colitis is not relieved by drug discontinuance or when it is severe, oral vancomycin is the treatment of choice for antibiotic-associated pseudomembranous colitis produced by *C. difficile*. Other causes of colitis should also be considered.

PRECAUTIONS

General

Patients should be followed carefully so that any side effects or unusual manifestations of drug idiosyncrasy may be detected. If a hypersensitivity reaction occurs, the drug should be discontinued and the patient treated with the usual agents, e.g., pressor amines, antihistamines, or corticosteroids.

Administer cephradine with caution in the presence of markedly impaired renal function. In patients with known or suspected renal impairment, careful clinical observation and appropriate laboratory studies should be made prior to and during therapy as cephradine accumulates in the serum and tissues. See DOSAGE AND ADMINISTRATION section for information on treatment of patients with impaired renal function.

Cephradine should be prescribed with caution in individuals with a history of gastrointestinal disease, particularly colitis. Prolonged use of antibiotics may promote the overgrowth of nonsusceptible organisms. Should superinfection occur during therapy, appropriate measures should be taken.

Indicated surgical procedures should be performed in conjunction with antibiotic therapy.

Information for Patients

Caution diabetic patients that false results may occur with urine glucose tests (see PRECAUTIONS, Drug/Laboratory Test Interactions).

Advise the patient to comply with the full course of therapy even if he begins to feel better and to take a missed dose as soon as possible. Inform the patient that this medication may be taken with food or milk since gastrointestinal upset may be a factor in compliance with the dosage regimen. The patient should report current use of any medicines and should be cautioned not to take other medications unless the physician knows and approves of their use (see PRECAUTIONS, Drug Interactions).

Laboratory Tests

In patients with known or suspected renal impairment, it is advisable to monitor renal function (see DOSAGE AND ADMINISTRATION).

Drug Interactions

When administered concurrently, the following drugs may interact with cephalosporins:

Other antibacterial agents—Bacteriostats may interfere with the bactericidal action of cephalosporins in acute infection; other agents, e.g., aminoglycosides, colistin, polymyxins, vancomycin, may increase the possibility of nephrotoxicity.

Diuretics (potent "loop diuretics," e.g., furosemide and ethacrynic acid)—Enhanced possibility for renal toxicity.

Probenecid—Increased and prolonged blood levels of cephalosporins, resulting in increased risk of nephrotoxicity.

Drug/Laboratory Test Interactions

After treatment with cephradine, a false-positive reaction for glucose in the urine may occur with Benedict's solution, Fehling's solution, or with Clinitest® tablets, but not with enzyme-based tests such as Clinistix® and Tes-Tape®.

False-positive Coombs test results may occur in newborns whose mothers received a cephalosporin prior to delivery.

Cephalosporins have been reported to cause false-positive reactions in tests for urinary proteins which use sulfosalicylic acid, false elevations of urinary 17-ketosteroid values, and prolonged prothrombin times.

Carcinogenesis, Mutagenesis

Long-term studies in animals have not been performed to evaluate carcinogenic potential or mutagenesis.

Pregnancy—Category B

Reproduction studies have been peformed in mice and rats at doses up to four times the maximum indicated human dose and have revealed no evidence of impaired fertility or harm to the fetus due to cephradine. There are, however, no adequate and well-controlled studies in pregnant women. Because animal reproduction studies are not always predictive of human response, this drug should be used during pregnancy only if clearly needed.

Nursing Mothers

Since cephradine is excreted in breast milk during lactation, caution should be exercised when cephradine is administered to a nursing woman.

Pediatric Use

See DOSAGE AND ADMINISTRATION. Adequate information is unavailable on the efficacy of b.i.d. regimens in children under nine months of age.

ADVERSE REACTIONS

As with other cephalosporins, untoward reactions are limited essentially to gastrointestinal disturbances and, on occasion, to hypersensitivity phenomena. The latter are more likely to occur in individuals who have previously demonstrated hypersensitivity and those with a history of allergy, asthma, hay fever, or urticaria.

The following adverse reactions have been reported following the use of cephradine:

Gastrointestinal: Symptoms of pseudomembranous colitis can appear during antibiotic treatment. Nausea and vomiting have been reported rarely.

Skin and Hypersensitivity Reactions: Mild urticaria or skin rash, pruritus, and joint pains were reported by very few patients.

Hematologic: Mild, transient eosinophilia, leukopenia, and neutropenia have been reported.

Liver: Transient mild rise of SGOT, SGPT, and total bilirubin have been observed with no evidence of hepatocellular damage.

Renal: Transitory rises in BUN have been observed in some patients treated with cephalosporins; their frequency increases in patients over 50 years old. In adults for whom

Continued on next page

Squibb—Cont.

serum creatinine determinations were performed, the rise in BUN was not accompanied by a rise in serum creatinine. Other adverse reactions have included dizziness and tightness in the chest and candidal vaginitis.

DOSAGE AND ADMINISTRATION

VELOSEF (Cephradine, Squibb) may be given without regard to meals.

Adults: *For respiratory tract infections (other than lobar pneumonia) and skin and skin structure infections,* the usual dose is 250 mg every 6 hours or 500 mg every 12 hours.

For lobar pneumonia, the usual dose is 500 mg every 6 hours or 1 g every 12 hours.

For uncomplicated urinary tract infections, the usual dose is 500 mg every 12 hours. In more serious urinary tract infections, including prostatitis, 500 mg every 6 hours or 1 g every 12 hours may be administered.

Larger doses (up to 1 g every 6 hours) may be given for severe or chronic infections.

Children: No adequate information is available on the efficacy of b.i.d. regimens in children under nine months of age. The usual dose in children over nine months of age is 25 to 50 mg/kg/day administered in equally divided doses every 6 or 12 hours. For otitis media due to *H. influenzae,* doses are from 75 to 100 mg/kg/day administered in equally divided doses every 6 or 12 hours, but should not exceed 4 g per day. Dosage for children should not exceed dosage recommended for adults.

All patients, regardless of age and weight: Larger doses (up to 1 gram q.i.d.) may be given for severe or chronic infections. As with antibiotic therapy in general, treatment should be continued for a minimum of 48 to 72 hours after the patient becomes asymptomatic or evidence of bacterial eradication has been obtained. In infections caused by group A beta-hemolytic streptococci, a minimum of 10 days of treatment is recommended to guard against the risk of rheumatic fever or glomerulonephritis. In the treatment of chronic urinary tract infection, frequent bacteriologic and clinical appraisal is necessary during therapy and may be necessary for several months afterwards. Persistent infections may require treatment for several weeks. Prolonged intensive therapy is recommended for prostatitis. Doses smaller than those indicated are not recommended.

Patients With Impaired Renal Function

Not on Dialysis: The following initial dosage schedule is suggested as a guideline based on creatinine clearance. Further modification in the dosage schedule may be required because of individual variations in absorption.

Creatinine Clearance	Dose	Time Interval
> 20 mL/min.	500 mg	6 hours
5–20 mL/min.	250 mg	6 hours
< 5 mL/min.	250 mg	12 hours

On Chronic, Intermittent Hemodialysis:
   250 mg Start
   250 mg at 12 hours
   250 mg 36–48 hours (after start)

Children may require dosage modification proportional to their weight and severity of infection.

HOW SUPPLIED

VELOSEF Capsules (Cephradine Capsules USP)

*VELOSEF '250' 250 mg/capsule: bottles of 24 (NDC 0003-0113-24) and 100 (NDC 0003-0113-50) and 100 Unimatic® unit-dose packs (NDC 0003-0113-52). Capsule identification no. **113**.

*VELOSEF '500' 500 mg/capsule: bottles of 24 (NDC 0003-0114-26) and 100 (NDC 0003-0114-50) and 100 Unimatic unit-dose packs (NDC 0003-0114-52). Capsule identification no. **114**.

VELOSEF for Oral Suspension (Cephradine for Oral Suspension USP)

VELOSEF '125'   When constituted as directed on the container label, a pleasant fruit-flavored suspension containing **125 mg per 5 mL**, in bottle sizes for preparation of 100 mL (NDC 0003-1193-50) and 200 mL (NDC 0003-1193-80). 125 mg/bottle: packs of 100 Unimatic unit-dose bottles (NDC 0003-1193-20).

VELOSEF '250'   When constituted as directed on the container label, a pleasant fruit-flavored suspension containing **250 mg per 5 mL**, in bottle sizes for preparation of 100 mL (NDC 0003-1194-50) and 200 mL (NDC 0003-1194-80). 250 mg/bottle: packs of 100 Unimatic unit-dose bottles (NDC 0003-1194-20).

Storage

VELOSEF Capsules—Keep tightly closed. Do not store above 86°F.

VELOSEF for Oral Suspension— Prior to constitution, store at room temperature; avoid excessive heat. After constitution, when the suspension stored at room temperature, discard unused portion after seven days; when stored in refrigerator, discard unused portion after 14 days. Keep tightly closed.

(J4-092A)

    Shown in Product Identification Section, page 432

VELOSEF® for INJECTION   ℞

[*vel 'ō-sef*]

Cephradine for Injection USP

DESCRIPTION

VELOSEF (Cephradine, Squibb) is a semisynthetic cephalosporin antibiotic. Cephradine is designated chemically as (6R, 7R)-7-[(R)- 2-amino-2-(1, 4-cyclohexadien-1-yl) acetamido]-3- methyl-8-oxo-5-thia-1-azabicyclo-[4.2.0] oct-2-ene-2-carboxylic acid.

VELOSEF for Injection is a sterile powder for constitution available in vials containing 250 mg, 500 mg, or 1 g cephradine; and bottles containing 2 g cephradine; the preparations also contain 79 mg, 157 mg, 315 mg, or 630 mg anhydrous sodium carbonate, respectively. The sodium content is approximately 136 mg (6 mEq) per gram of cephradine. At the time of manufacture, the air in the container is replaced by nitrogen.

CLINICAL PHARMACOLOGY

Table I indicates the blood levels following intramuscular administration of a 500 mg or 1 g dose to normal adults. [See table below].

Figure I depicts representative mean serum concentrations after administration of a 500 mg and 1 g IM dose, and a 500 mg oral dose of cephradine. Areas beneath the curves for the 500 mg oral and IM dose are equivalent.

Figure I
VELOSEF FOR INJECTION
(Cephradine for Injection USP)

A single intravenous dose of 1 g cephradine resulted in serum levels of approximately 86 mcg/mL at 5 minutes, 50 mcg/mL at 15 minutes, 26 mcg/mL at 30 minutes, and 12 mcg/mL at 60 minutes; these levels declined to 1 mcg/mL at four hours.

In vitro studies by an ultracentrifugation technique show that, at therapeutic serum antibiotic concentrations, cephradine is minimally bound (8 to 17 percent) to normal human serum protein. Cephradine does not pass across the blood-brain barrier to any appreciable extent.

VELOSEF (Cephradine) is excreted unchanged in the urine. The kidneys excrete 57 to 80 percent of an intramuscular dose in the first six hours; this results in a high urine concentration, e.g., a mean urine concentration of 313 mcg/mL within a six hour period following a 500 mg IM dose. Probenecid slows tubular excretion and increases serum concentration.

Assays of bone and cardiac tissue (atrial appendage) obtained at surgery have shown that cephradine penetrates these tissues.

Microbiology: In vitro tests demonstrate that the cephalosporins are bactericidal because of their inhibition of cell-wall synthesis. Cephradine is active against the following organisms *in vitro:* group A beta-hemolytic streptococci; staphylococci, including coagulase-positive, coagulase-negative, and p icillinase-producing strains; *Escherichia coli; Streptococcus pneumoniae* (formerly *Diplococcus pneumoniae); Proteus mirabilis; Klebsiella* species; and *Hemophilus influenzae.*

It is not active against most strains of *Enterobacter* species, *Proteus morganii,* and *Proteus vulgaris.* It has no activity against *Pseudomonas* or *Herellea* species. When tested by *in vitro* methods, staphylococci exhibit cross-resistance between cephradine and methicillin-type antibiotics.

NOTE—Most strains of enterococci (*Streptococcus faecalis*) are resistant to cephradine.

Disc Susceptibility Tests: Quantitative methods that require measurement of zone diameters give the most precise estimates of antibiotic susceptibility. One recommended procedure (21 CFR § 460.1) uses cephalosporin class discs for testing susceptibility; interpretations correlate zone diameters of this disc test with MIC values for cephradine. With this procedure, a report from the laboratory of "resistant" indicates that the infecting organism is not likely to respond to therapy. A report of "intermediate susceptibility" suggests that the organism would be susceptible if the infection is confined to the urinary tract, as high antibiotic levels can be obtained in the urine, or if high dosage is used in other types of infection.

INDICATIONS AND USAGE

Treatment

VELOSEF for Injection (Cephradine for Injection USP) is indicated in the treatment of the following serious infections caused by susceptible strains of the designated microorganisms:

RESPIRATORY TRACT INFECTIONS due to *Streptococcus pneumoniae* (formerly *Diplococcus pneumoniae), Klebsiella* species, *H. influenzae, Staphylococcus aureus* (penicillin-susceptible and penicillin-resistant), and group A beta-hemolytic streptococci.

(Penicillin is the usual drug of choice in the treatment and prevention of streptococcal infections, including the prophylaxis of rheumatic fever. VELOSEF is generally effective in the eradication of streptococci from the nasopharynx; substantial data establishing the efficacy of VELOSEF in the subsequent prevention of rheumatic fever are not available at present.)

URINARY TRACT INFECTIONS due to *E. coli, P. mirabilis,* and *Klebsiella* species.

SKIN AND SKIN STRUCTURE INFECTIONS due to *S. aureus* (penicillin-susceptible and penicillin-resistant) and group A beta-hemolytic streptococci.

BONE INFECTIONS due to *S. aureus* (penicillin-susceptible and penicillin-resistant).

SEPTICEMIA due to *Streptococcus pneumoniae* (formerly *Diplococcus pneumoniae), S. aureus* (penicillin-susceptible and penicillin-resistant), *P. mirabilis,* and *E. coli.*

NOTE—Culture and susceptibility tests should be initiated prior to and during therapy.

Prevention

When compared to placebo in randomized controlled studies in patients undergoing vaginal hysterectomy and cesarean section, the prophylactic use of VELOSEF (cephradine) resulted in a significant reduction in the number of postoperative infections.

The prophylactic administration of VELOSEF perioperatively (preoperatively, intraoperatively, and postoperatively) may reduce the incidence of certain postoperative infections in patients undergoing surgical procedures (e.g., vaginal hysterectomy) that are classified as contaminated or potentially contaminated.

In patients undergoing cesarean section, intraoperative (after clamping the umbilical cord) and postoperative use of VELOSEF may reduce the incidence of certain postoperative infections.

Effective perioperative use depends on the time of administration. VELOSEF usually should be given 30 to 90 minutes before surgery, which is sufficient time to achieve effective

---

TABLE I
VELOSEF FOR INJECTION
(Cephradine for Injection USP)

	MEAN TIME TO PEAK SERUM LEVELS Minutes		MEAN PEAK SERUM CONCENTRATION mcg/mL		MEAN SERUM CONCENTRATION AT 1 HR. - mcg/mL	
	500 mg IM	1 g IM	500 mg IM	1 g IM	500 mg IM	1 g IM
MALES	49 (41–59)*	52 (45–61)	6.3 (5.5–7.2)	13.6 (12.2–15.1)	6.2 (5.5–6.9)	12.4 (11.0–14.0)
FEMALES	98 (87–111)	128 (103–157)	5.8 (5.1–6.6)	9.9 (8.7–11.2)	4.3 (3.5–5.2)	6.0 (4.4–8.1)

*Figures in parentheses are 95% confidence limits.

tissue levels. Prophylactic administration should usually be stopped within 24 hours since continuing administration of any antibiotic increases the possibility of adverse reactions but, in the majority of surgical procedures, does not reduce the incidence of subsequent infection.

If there are signs of infection, specimens for culture should be obtained for identification of the causative organism so that appropriate therapy may be instituted.

CONTRAINDICATIONS

Cephradine is contraindicated in patients with known hypersensitivity to the cephalosporin group of antibiotics.

WARNINGS

In penicillin-sensitive patients, cephalosporin derivatives should be used with great caution. There is clinical and laboratory evidence of partial cross-allergenicity of the penicillins and the cephalosporins, and there are instances of patients who have had reactions to both drug classes (including fatal anaphylaxis after parenteral use).

Any patient who has demonstrated some form of allergy, particularly to drugs, should receive antibiotics, including cephradine, cautiously and then only when absolutely necessary. Serious anaphylactoid reactions require immediate emergency treatment with epinephrine. Oxygen, intravenous steroids, and airway management, including intubation, should also be administered as indicated.

Pseudomembranous colitis has been reported with the use of cephalosporins (and other broad spectrum antibiotics); therefore, it is important to consider its diagnosis in patients who develop diarrhea in association with antibiotic use. Treatment with broad spectrum antibiotics alters normal flora of the colon and may permit overgrowth of clostridia. Studies indicate a toxin produced by *Clostridium difficile* is one primary cause of antibiotic-associated colitis. Cholestyramine and colestipol resins have been shown to bind the toxin *in vitro*. Mild cases of colitis may respond to drug discontinuance alone. Moderate to severe cases should be managed with fluid, electrolyte and protein supplementation as indicated. When the colitis is not relieved by drug discontinuance or when it is severe, oral vancomycin is the treatment of choice for antibiotic-associated pseudomembranous colitis produced by *C. difficile*. Other causes of colitis should also be considered.

PRECAUTIONS

General

Prolonged use of antibiotics may promote the overgrowth of nonsusceptible organisms. Should superinfection occur during therapy, appropriate measures should be taken.

When cephradine is administered to patients with markedly impaired renal function lower daily dosage is required (see DOSAGE AND ADMINISTRATION). In patients with known or suspected renal impairment, careful clinical observation and appropriate laboratory studies should be conducted because cephradine in the usual recommended dosage will accumulate in the serum and tissues.

Cephradine should be prescribed with caution in individuals with a history of gastrointestinal disease, particularly colitis. Patients should be followed carefully so that any side effects or unusual manifestations of drug idiosyncrasy may be detected. If a hypersensitivity reaction occurs, the drug should be discontinued and the patient treated with the usual agents, e.g., pressor amines, antihistamines, or corticosteroids.

VELOSEF for Injection (Cephradine for Injection USP) is physically compatible with most commonly used intravenous fluids and electrolyte solutions (such as 5% Dextrose Injection or Sodium Chloride Injection or M/6 sodium lactate); however, it is *not* compatible with Lactated Ringer's Injection because of the incompatibility between calcium ions and the sodium carbonate present in VELOSEF for Injection.

Information for Patients

Caution diabetic patients that false test results may occur with urine glucose tests (see PRECAUTIONS, Drug/Laboratory Test Interactions). The patient should report current use of any medicines and should be cautioned not to take other medications unless the physician knows and approves of their use (see PRECAUTIONS, Drug Interactions).

Laboratory Tests

In patients with known or suspected renal impairment, it is advisable to monitor renal function (see DOSAGE AND ADMINISTRATION).

Drug Interactions

When administered concurrently, the following drugs may interact with cephalosporins:

Other antibacterial agents—Bacteriostats may interfere with the bactericidal action of cephalosporins in acute infection; other agents, e.g., aminoglycosides, colistin, polymyxins, vancomycin, may increase the possibility of nephrotoxicity.

Diuretics (potent "loop diuretics," e.g., furosemide and ethacrynic acid)—Enhanced possibility for renal toxicity.

Probenecid—Increased and prolonged blood levels of cephalosporins, resulting in increased risk of nephrotoxicity.

Drug/Laboratory Test Interactions

After treatment with cephradine, a false-positive reaction for glucose in the urine may occur with Benedict's solution, Fehling's solution, or with Clinitest® tablets, but not with enzyme-based tests such as Clinistix® and Tes-Tape®. False-positive Coombs test results may occur in newborns whose mothers received a cephalosporin prior to delivery. Cephalosporins have been reported to cause false-positive reactions in tests for urinary proteins which use sulfosalicylic acid, false elevations of urinary 17-ketosteroid values, and prolonged prothrombin times.

Carcinogenesis, Mutagenesis

Long-term studies in animals have not been performed to evaluate carcinogenic potential or mutagenesis.

Pregnancy Category B

Reproduction studies have been performed in mice and rats at doses up to four times the maximum indicated human dose and have revealed no evidence of impaired fertility or harm to the fetus due to cephradine. There are, however, no adequate and well-controlled studies in pregnant women. Because animal reproduction studies are not always predictive of human response, this drug should be used during pregnancy only if clearly needed.

Nursing Mothers

Since cephradine is excreted in breast milk during lactation, caution should be exercised when cephradine is administered to a nursing woman.

Pediatric Use

See DOSAGE AND ADMINISTRATION. Cephradine has been effectively used in infants, but all laboratory parameters have not been extensively studied in infants one month to one year of age; therefore, in the treatment of children in this age group, the benefits of the drug to the risk involved must be considered.

Since safety for use in premature infants and in infants under one month of age has not been established, the use of cephradine by injection or infusion should be based on careful consideration of the benefits of the drug against the risk involved.

ADVERSE REACTIONS

As with other cephalosporins, untoward reactions are limited essentially to gastrointestinal disturbances and, on occasion, to hypersensitivity phenomena. The latter are more likely to occur in individuals who have previously demonstrated hypersensitivity and those with a history of allergy, asthma, hay fever, or urticaria.

The following adverse reactions have been reported following the use of cephradine:

Gastrointestinal: Symptoms of pseudomembranous colitis can appear during antibiotic treatment. Nausea and vomiting have been reported rarely.

Skin and Hypersensitivity Reactions: Mild urticaria or skin rash, edema, erythema, pruritus, joint pains and drug fever.

Hematologic: Mild, transient eosinophilia, leukopenia and neutropenia.

Liver: Instances of elevated SGOT and SGPT of approximately 10 percent and 2 percent of patients, respectively, have been observed; also, a few cases of elevated total bilirubin, alkaline phosphatase and LDH have been observed. In most patients, values tended to return to normal after the end of therapy.

Renal: Mild elevations in BUN have been observed in some patients treated with cephalosporins; their frequency increases in patients over 50 years old and in children under three. In adults for whom serum creatinine determinations were performed, the rise in BUN was not accompanied by a rise in serum creatinine.

Other adverse reactions are headache, dizziness, dyspnea, paresthesia, candidal overgrowth, candidal vaginitis, isolated instances of hepatomegaly, and thrombophlebitis at the site of injection.

Pain on intramuscular injection has been experienced by some patients. Since sterile abscesses have been reported following accidental subcutaneous injection, the preparation should be administered by deep intramuscular injection.

VELOSEF FOR INJECTION
(Cephradine for Injection USP)

PEDIATRIC DOSAGE GUIDE

		50 mg/kg/day			100 mg/kg/day	
Weight lbs	kg	Approx. single dose mg q 6 h	Volume needed @ 208 mg/mL dilution		Approx. single dose mg q 6 h	Volume needed @ 227 mg/mL dilution
10	4.5	56 mg	0.27 mL		112 mg	0.5 mL
20	9.1	114 mg	0.55 mL		227 mg	1 mL
30	13.6	170 mg	0.82 mL		340 mg	1.5 mL
40	18.2	227 mg	1.1 mL		455 mg	2 mL
50	22.7	284 mg	1.4 mL		567 mg	2.5 mL

DOSAGE AND ADMINISTRATION

Adults

Treatment: The usual daily dosage of VELOSEF for Injection (Cephradine for Injection) is 2 to 4 g of cephradine given in equally divided doses four times a day intramuscularly or intravenously (e.g., 500 mg to 1 g qid). In bone infections the usual dosage is 1 g qid administered intravenously. A dosage of 500 mg qid is adequate in uncomplicated pneumonia, skin and skin structure infections and most urinary tract infections. In severe infections, the total daily dose may be increased by using a q 4 h dosage regimen or by increasing the dose given qid; the maximum dose should not exceed 8 g per day.

Prevention: To prevent postoperative infection in contaminated or potentially contaminated surgery, recommended doses are as follows:

a. 1 g IV or IM administered 30 to 90 minutes prior to start of surgery.

b. 1 g every 4 to 6 hours after the first dose for one or two doses, or for up to 24 hours postoperatively.

Cesarean Section Patients: The first dose of 1 g is administered intravenously as soon as the umbilical cord is clamped. The second and third doses should be given as 1 g intravenously or intramuscularly at 6 and 12 hours after the first dose.

Infants and Children

The usual dosage range of VELOSEF is 50 to 100 mg/kg/day (approximately 23 to 45 mg/lb/day) in equally divided doses four times a day and should be regulated by age, weight of the patient and severity of the infection being treated.

All laboratory parameters have not been extensively studied in infants under one year of age; therefore, in the treatment of children in this age group, the benefits of the drug to the risk involved must be considered. In newborn infants, accumulation of other cephalosporin-class antibiotics (with resultant prolongation of drug half-life) has been reported.

The maximum daily pediatric dose should not exceed doses recommended for adults.

[See table above].

As with antibiotic therapy generally: therapy should be continued for a minimum of 48 to 72 hours after the patient becomes asymptomatic or evidence of bacterial eradication has been obtained; in infections caused by group A beta-hemolytic streptococci, a minimum of 10 days of treatment is recommended to guard against the risk of rheumatic fever or glomerulonephritis; in the treatment of chronic urinary tract infection, frequent bacteriologic and clinical appraisal is necessary during therapy and may be necessary for several months afterwards; persistent infections may require treatment for several weeks; doses smaller than those indicated above should not be used.

Parenteral therapy may be followed by oral VELOSEF either as capsules or as an oral suspension.

VELOSEF for Injection (Cephradine for Injection) may be given intravenously or by deep intramuscular injection. To minimize pain and induration, intramuscular injections should be made into a large muscle mass, such as the gluteus or lateral aspect of the thigh.

Patients With Impaired Renal Function

Not on Dialysis: The following initial dosage schedule is suggested as a guideline based on creatinine clearance. Further modification in the dosage schedule may be required because of individual variations in absorption.

Creatinine Clearance	Dose	Time Interval
> 20 mL/min	500 mg	6 hours
5–20 mL/min	250 mg	6 hours
< 5 mL/min	250 mg	12 hours

On Chronic Intermittent Hemodialysis:
250 mg Start
250 mg at 12 hours
250 mg 36–48 hours (after start)

Continued on next page

Squibb—Cont.

Children may require dosage modification proportional to their weight and severity of infection.

Constitution and Storage

Parenteral drug products should be inspected visually for particulate matter and discoloration prior to administration, whenever solution and container permit.

For I.M. Use: Aseptically add Sterile Water for Injection or Bacteriostatic Water for Injection (containing 0.9% [w/v] benzyl alcohol, or 0.12% methylparaben and 0.014% propylparaben) according to the following table [i.e., the table entitled "IM Dilution Table"].
[See table below].

Intramuscular solutions should be used within two hours at room temperature; if stored in the refrigerator at 5° C., solutions retain full potency for 24 hours. Constituted solutions may vary in color from light straw to yellow; however, this does not affect the potency.

For IV Use: VELOSEF may also be administered by direct intravenous injection or by continuous or intermittent infusion. A 3 mcg/mL serum concentration can be maintained for each mg of cephradine per kg body weight per hour of infusion.

For Direct IV Administration: Suitable diluents are Sterile Water for Injection, 5% Dextrose Injection, or Sodium Chloride Injection. **Do not use Lactated Ringer's Injection.**
Aseptically add 5 mL of diluent to the 250 mg or 500 mg vials, 10 mL of diluent to the 1 g vial, or 20 mL of diluent to the 2 g bottle; withdraw entire contents. The solution may be slowly injected directly into a vein over a three to five minute period or may be given as a supplementary injection through the injection site on the administration set when the infusion solution is compatible with cephradine. These VELOSEF solutions should be used within two hours when held at room temperature; if stored at 5° C, the solutions retain full potency for 24 hours.

For Continuous or Intermittent IV Infusion: Suitable intravenous infusion solutions for VELOSEF are 5% or 10% Dextrose Injection; Sodium Chloride Injection; Sodium Lactate Injection (M/6 sodium lactate); Dextrose and Sodium Chloride Injection (5% : 0.9%) or (5% : 0.45%); 10% Invert Sugar in Water for Injection; Normosol®-R, and Ionosol® B with Dextrose 5%. Sterile Water for Injection may be used as an IV infusion solution for VELOSEF at a concentration of 30 to 50 mg/mL (30 mg/mL is approximately isotonic). **Do not use Lactated Ringer's Injection.**

a) To prepare a VELOSEF solution for transfer into an IV infusion bottle, aseptically add 10 mL or 20 mL of Sterile Water for Injection or a suitable infusion solution, respectively, to the 1 g vial, or 2 g bottles. Promptly withdraw the entire contents of the resulting solution and aseptically transfer to an IV infusion bottle. Intravenous infusion solutions containing VELOSEF at a concentration of five percent (50 mg/mL) or less retain potency as noted under (b) below. The choice of IV infusion solution and the volume to be employed are dictated by fluid and electrolyte management.

b) VELOSEF may be infused directly from the 2 g IV bottle. Constitute the 2 g bottle with 40 mL of a suitable intravenous infusion solution; attach an IV administration set directly to the VELOSEF IV infusion bottle. The 2 g IV bottles are designed to be suspended from an IV stand.
Intravenous infusion solutions containing VELOSEF retain full potency for 10 hours at room temperature or 48 hours at 5° C; infusion solutions of VELOSEF in Sterile Water for Injection that are frozen immediately after reconstitution in the original container are stable for as long as six weeks when stored at −20° C.
For prolonged infusions, replace the infusion every 10 hours with a freshly prepared solution.
Extemporaneous mixtures of VELOSEF with other antibiotics are not recommmended.
Protect solutions of VELOSEF from concentrated light or direct sunlight. VELOSEF for Injection may be stored at room temperature prior to constitution; avoid excessive heat; protect from light.

HOW SUPPLIED

Velosef for Injection (Cephradine for Injection USP) is available for intramuscular or intravenous use in vials containing 250 mg (NDC 0003-1476-10), 500 mg (NDC 0003-1198-10), or 1 g (NDC 0003-1199-10) cephradine; and for intravenous use in 100 mL infusion bottles containing 2 g (NDC 0003-1197-20) cephradine.
(J3-508E)

For information on Squibb products, write to: Squibb Professional Services Department, P.O. Box 4500, Princeton, N.J. 08543-4500.

Squibb Derm
CN 5271
PRINCETON, NJ 08543-5271

DERMATOLOGY PRODUCTS

For information on Squibb Derm dermatology products, consult the PDR for E.R. Squibb & Sons, Inc. and Princeton Pharmaceutical Products.

Squibb-Novo, Inc.
211 CARNEGIE CENTER
PRINCETON, NJ 08540-6213

STANDARD INSULIN
REGULAR INSULIN
Insulin Injection
USP (Pork) 100 units/ml

DESCRIPTION

Regular Insulin, Insulin Injection USP, 100 units of insulin per milliliter, is a clear, colorless solution which has a short duration of action. The effect of **Regular Insulin** begins approximately ½ hour after injection. The effect is maximal between 2½ and 5 hours and ends approximately 8 hours after injection. The time course of action of any insulin may vary considerably in different individuals, or at different times in the same individual. Because of this variation, the time periods listed here should be considered as general guidelines only.

SEMILENTE® INSULIN
Prompt Insulin Zinc Suspension
USP (Beef) 100 units/ml

DESCRIPTION

Semilente® Insulin, Prompt Insulin Zinc Suspension USP, 100 units of insulin per milliliter, is a cloudy or milky suspension of amorphous beef insulin. The insulin substance (the cloudy material) settles at the bottom of the vial, therefore, the vial must be gently agitated or rotated so that the contents are uniformly mixed before a dose is withdrawn. The effect of **Semilente® Insulin** begins approximately 1½ hours after injection. The effect is maximal between 5 and 10 hours and ends approximately 16 hours after injection. The time course of action of any insulin may vary considerably in different individuals, or at different times in the same individual. Because of this variation, the time periods listed here should be considered as general guidelines only.

LENTE® INSULIN
Insulin Zinc Suspension
USP (Beef) 100 units/ml

DESCRIPTION

LENTE® Insulin, Insulin Zinc Suspension USP, 100 units of insulin per milliliter, is a cloudy or milky suspension of 70% crystalline and 30% amorphous beef insulin. The Insulin substance (the cloudy material) settles at the bottom of the vial, therefore, the vial must be gently agitated or rotated so

that the contents are uniformly mixed before a dose is withdrawn. **Lente® Insulin** has an intermediate duration of action. The effect of **Lente® Insulin** begins approximately 2½ hours after injection. The effect is maximal between 7 and 15 hours and ends approximately 24 hours after injection. The time course of action of any insulin may vary considerably in different individuals, or at different times in the same individual. Because of this variation, the time periods listed here should be considered as general guidelines only.

NPH INSULIN
Isophane Insulin Suspension USP (Beef) 100 units/ml

DESCRIPTION

NPH Insulin, Isophane Insulin Suspension USP, 100 units of insulin per milliliter, is a cloudy or milky suspension of beef insulin with protamine and zinc. The insulin substance (the cloudy material) settles at the bottom of the vial, therefore, the vial must be gently agitated or rotated so that the contents are uniformly mixed before a dose is withdrawn. **NPH Insulin** has an intermediate duration of action. The effect of **NPH Insulin** begins approximately 1½ hours after injection. The effect is maximal between 4 and 12 hours and ends approximately 24 hours after injection. The time course of action of any insulin may vary considerably in different individuals, or at different times in the same individual. Because of this variation, the time periods listed here should be considered as general guidelines only.

ULTRALENTE® INSULIN
Extended Insulin Zinc
Suspension USP (Beef) 100 units/ml

DESCRIPTION

Ultralente® Insulin, Extended Insulin Zinc Suspension USP, 100 units of insulin per milliliter, is a cloudy or milky suspension of crystalline beef insulin. The insulin substance (the cloudy material) settles at the bottom of the vial, therefore, the vial must be gently agitated or rotated so that the contents are uniformly mixed before a dose is withdrawn. The effect of **Ultralente® Insulin** begins approximately 4 hours after injection. The effect is maximal between 10 and 30 hours and ends approximately 36 hours after injection. The time course of action of any insulin may vary considerably in different individuals, or at different times in the same individual. Because of this variation, the time periods listed here should be considered as general guidelines only.

PURIFIED INSULIN
REGULAR PURIFIED PORK INSULIN
INJECTION USP 100 units/ml

DESCRIPTION

Regular Purified Pork Insulin Injection, USP, 100 units of insulin per milliliter, is a clear, colorless solution which has a short duration of action. The effect of Regular Purified Insulin begins approximately ½ hour after injection. The effect is maximal between 2½ and 5 hours and ends approximately 8 hours after injection. The time course of action of any insulin may vary considerably in different individuals, or at different times in the same individual. Because of this variation, the time periods listed here should be considered as general guidelines only.
The word "purified" on the label indicates that this insulin differs from standard insulin in that it has undergone additional purification steps (i.e., molecular sieve and ion-exchange chromatography).

SEMILENTE® PURIFIED PORK PROMPT INSULIN ZINC SUSPENSION USP 100 units/ml

DESCRIPTION

Semilente® Purified Pork Prompt Insulin Zinc Suspension, USP, 100 units of insulin per milliliter, is a cloudy or milky suspension of amorphous purified pork insulin. The insulin substance (the cloudy material) settles at the bottom of the vial, therefore, the vial must be gently agitated or rotated so that the contents are uniformly mixed before a dose is withdrawn. The effect of Semilente® Purified Insulin begins approximately 1½ hours after injection. The effect is maximal between 5 and 10 hours and ends approximately 16 hours after injection. The time course of action of any insulin may vary considerably in different individuals, or at different times in the same individual. Because of this variation, the time periods listed here should be considered as general guidelines only.
The word "purified" on the label indicates that this insulin differs from standard insulin in that it has undergone additional purification steps (i.e., molecular sieve and ion-exchange chromatography).

VELOSEF FOR INJECTION
(Cephradine for Injection USP)

IM DILUTION TABLE

Vial Size	Volume of Diluent	Approximate Available Volume	Approximate Available Concentration
250 mg	1.2 mL	1.2 mL	208 mg/mL
500 mg	2.0 mL	2.2 mL	227 mg/mL
1 g	4.0 mL	4.5 mL	222 mg/mL

LENTE® PURIFIED PORK INSULIN ZINC SUSPENSION USP 100 units/ml

DESCRIPTION

Lente® Purified Pork Insulin Zinc Suspension, USP, 100 units of insulin per milliliter, is a cloudy or milky suspension of 70% crystalline and 30% amorphous purified pork insulin. The insulin substance (the cloudy material) settles at the bottom of the vial, therefore, the vial must be gently agitated or rotated so that the contents are uniformly mixed before a dose is withdrawn. Lente® Purified Insulin has an intermediate duration of action. The effect of Lente® Purified Insulin begins approximately 2½ hours after injection. The effect is maximal between 7 and 15 hours and ends approximately 22 hours after injection. The time course of action of any insulin may vary considerably in different individuals, or at different times in the same individual. Because of this variation, the time periods listed here should be considered as general guidelines only. The word "purified" on the label indicates that this insulin differs from standard insulin in that it has undergone additional purification steps (i.e., molecular sieve and ion-exchange chromatography).

NPH PURIFIED PORK ISOPHANE INSULIN SUSPENSION USP 100 units/ml

DESCRIPTION

NPH Purified Pork Isophane Insulin Suspension, USP, 100 units of insulin per milliliter, is a cloudy or milky suspension of purified pork insulin with protamine and zinc. The insulin substance (the cloudy material) settles at the bottom of the vial, therefore, the vial must be gently agitated or rotated so that the contents are uniformly mixed before a dose is withdrawn. NPH Purified Insulin has an intermediate duration of action. The effect of NPH Purified Insulin begins approximately 1½ hours after injection. The effect is maximal between 4 and 12 hours and ends approximately 24 hours after injection. The time course of action of any insulin may vary considerably in different individuals, or at different times in the same individual. Because of this variation, the time periods listed here should be considered as general guidelines only.
The word "purified" on the label indicates that this insulin differs from standard insulin in that it has undergone additional purification steps (i.e., molecular sieve and ion-exchange chromatography).

ULTRALENTE® PURIFIED BEEF EXTENDED INSULIN ZINC SUSPENSION USP 100 units/ml

DESCRIPTION

Ultralente® Purified Beef Insulin Zinc Suspension, USP, 100 units of insulin per milliliter, is a cloudy or milky suspension of crystalline purified beef insulin. The insulin substance (the cloudy material) settles at the bottom of the vial, therefore, the vial must be gently agitated or rotated so that the contents are uniformly mixed before a dose is withdrawn. The effect of Ultralente® Purified Insulin begins approximately 4 hours after injection. The effect is maximal between 10 and 30 hours and ends approximately 36 hours after injection. The time course of action of any insulin may vary considerably in different individuals, or at different times in the same individual. Because of this variation, the time periods listed here should be considered as general guidelines only.
The word "purified" on the label indicates that this insulin differs from standard insulin in that it has undergone additional purification steps (i.e., molecular sieve and ion-exchange chromatography).

HUMAN INSULIN

NOVOLIN® R
Regular Human Insulin Injection (semi-synthetic) USP
100 units/ml

NOVOLIN® R is generically known as Regular Human Insulin Injection (semi-synthetic) USP. The concentration of this product is 100 Units per milliliter. It is a clear, colorless solution which has a short duration of action. The effects of NOVOLIN® R begins approximately ½ hour after injection. The effect is maximal between 2½ and 5 hours and ends approximately 8 hours after injection. The time course of action of any insulin may vary considerably in different individuals or a different times in the same individual. Because of this variation, the time periods listed here should be considered as general guidelines only.
This human insulin (semi-synthetic) is structurally identical to the insulin produced by the human pancreas and has undergone a special purification process. A naturally occurring enzyme is used in a process which converts pork insulin into human insulin. By this enzymatic transpeptidation process the amino acid alanine in pork insulin is selectively sub-

stituted by the amino acid threonine thus forming the human insulin molecule.
Shown in Product Identification Section, page 432

NOVOLIN® L
Lente® Human Insulin Zinc Suspension (semi-synthetic)
100 units/ml

NOVOLIN® L is generically known as Lente® Human Insulin Zinc Suspension (semi-synthetic). The concentration of this product is 100 units of insulin per milliliter. It is a cloudy or milky suspension of 70% crystalline and 30% amorphous human insulin. The insulin substance (the cloudy material) settles at the bottom of the vial, therefore, the vial must be gently agitated or rotated so that the contents are uniformly mixed before a dose is withdrawn. NOVOLIN® L has an intermediate duration of action. The effect of NOVOLIN® L begins approximately 2½ hours after injection. The effect is maximal between 7 and 15 hours and ends approximately 22 hours after injection. The time course of action for any insulin may vary considerably in different individuals or at different times in the same individual. Because of this variation, the periods listed here should be considered as general guidelines only.
This human insulin (semi-synthetic) is structurally identical to the insulin produced by the human pancreas and has undergone a special purification process. A naturally occurring enzyme is used in a process which converts pork insulin into human insulin. By this enzymatic-transpeptidation process the amino acid alanine in pork insulin is selectively substituted by the amino acid threonine thus forming the human insulin molecule.
Shown in Product Identification Section, page 432

NOVOLIN® N
NPH Human Insulin Isophane Suspension (semi-synthetic)
100 units/ml

NOVOLIN® N is generically known as NPH Human Insulin Isophane Suspension (semi-synthetic). The concentration of this product is 100 units of insulin per milliliter. It is a cloudy or milky suspension of human insulin with protamine and zinc. The insulin substance (the cloudy material) settles at the bottom of the vial, therefore, the vial must be gently agitated or rotated so that the contents are uniformly mixed before a dose is withdrawn. NOVOLIN® N has an intermediate duration of action. The effect of NOVOLIN® N begins approximately 1½ hours after injection. The effect is maximal between 4 and 12 hours. The full duration of action may last up to 24 hours after injection. The time course of action for any insulin may vary considerably in different individuals, or at different times in the same individual. Because of this variation, the periods listed here should be considered as general guidelines only.
This human insulin (semi-synthetic) is structurally identical to the insulin produced by the human pancreas and has undergone a special purification process. A naturally occurring enzyme is used in a process which converts pork insulin into human insulin. By this enzymatic-transpeptidation process the amino acid alanine in pork insulin is selectively substituted by the amino acid threonine thus forming the human insulin molecule.
Shown in Product Identification Section, page 432

NOVOLIN® 70/30
70% NPH
Human Insulin Isophane Suspension &
30% Regular
Human Insulin Injection
(semi-synthetic)
100 units/ml

DESCRIPTION

Novolin® 70/30 is a mixture of 70% NPH Human Insulin Isophane Suspension (semi-synthetic) and 30% Regular Human Insulin Injection (semi-synthetic) USP. The concentration of this product is 100 units of insulin per milliliter. It is a cloudy or milky suspension of human insulin with protamine and zinc. The insulin substance (the cloudy material) settles at the bottom of the vial, therefore, the vial must be gently agitated or rotated so that the contents are uniformly mixed before a dose is withdrawn. Novolin® 70/30 has an intermediate duration of action. The effect of Novolin® 70/30 begins approximately ½ hour after injection. The effect is maximal between 2 and approximately 12 hours. The full duration of action may last up to 24 hours after injection. The time course of action of any insulin may vary considerably in different individuals, or at different times in the same individual. Because of this variation, the time periods listed here should be considered as general guidelines only.
This human insulin (semi-synthetic) is structurally identical to the insulin produced by the human pancreas and has undergone a special purification process. A naturally-occurring

enzyme is used in a process which converts pork insulin into human insulin. By this enzymatic transpeptidation process the amino acid alanine in pork insulin is selectively substituted by the amino acid threonine thus forming the human insulin molecule.
Shown in Product Identification Section, page 432

HUMAN INSULIN DELIVERY SYSTEM

NOVOLIN® R PenFill
Regular Human Insulin Injection (semi-synthetic)
100 units/ml
5 x 1.5 ml cartridges

Novolin® R PenFill® cartridges contain *Novolin® R*, generically known as Regular Human Insulin Injection (semi-synthetic). The concentration of this product is 100 units of insulin per milliliter. It is a clear, colorless solution which has a short duration of action. The effect of *Novolin® R* begins approximately ½ hour after injection. The effect is maximal between 2½ and 5 hours and ends approximately 8 hours after injection. The time course of action of any insulin may vary considerably in different individuals, or at different times in the same individual. Because of this variation, the time periods listed here should be considered as general guidelines only.
This human insulin (semi-synthetic) is structurally identical to the insulin produced by the human pancreas and has undergone a special purification process. A naturally occurring enzyme is used in a process which converts pork insulin into human insulin. By this enzymatic transpeptidation process the amino acid alanine in pork insulin is selectively substituted by the amino acid threonine thus forming the human insulin molecule.

NOVOLIN® N PenFill
NPH Human Insulin Isophane Suspension (semi-synthetic)
100 units/ml
5 × 1.5 ml cartridges

Novolin® N PenFill® cartridges contain Novolin® N, generically known as NPH Human Insulin Isophane Suspension (semi-synthetic).
The concentration of this product is 100 units of insulin per milliliter. It is a cloudy or milky suspension of human insulin with protamine and zinc. The insulin substance (the cloudy material) settles at the bottom of the cartridge.
Therefore the cartridge must be turned up and down at least 10 times or until the liquid appears uniformly white and cloudy (a glass ball inside the cartridge facilitates mixing). Novolin® N has an intermediate duration of action. The effect of Novolin® N begins approximately 1½ hours after injection. The effect is maximal between 4 and 12 hours and ends approximately 24 hours after injection. The time course of action for any insulin may vary considerably in different individuals, or at different times in the same individual. Because of this variation, the periods listed here should be considered as general guidelines only.
This human insulin (semi-synthetic) is structurally identical to the insulin produced by the human pancreas and has undergone a special purification process. A naturally occurring enzyme is used in a process which converts pork insulin into human insulin. By this enzymatic transpeptidation process the amino acid alanine in pork insulin is selectively substituted by the amino acid threonine thus forming the human insulin molecule.

NOVOLIN® 70/30 PenFill
70% NPH Human Insulin Isophane Suspension & 30% Regular Human Insulin Injection (semi-synthetic)
100 units/ml
5 × 1.5 ml cartridges

Novolin® 70/30 PenFill® cartridges contain Novolin® 70/30, a mixture of 70% NPH Human Insulin Isophane Suspension and 30% Regular Human Insulin Injection (semi-synthetic).
The concentration of this product is 100 units of insulin per milliliter. It is a cloudy or milky suspension of human insulin with protamine and zinc. The insulin substance (the cloudy material) settles at the bottom of the cartridge.
Therefore the cartridge must be turned up and down at least 10 times or until the liquid appears uniformly white and cloudy (a glass ball inside the cartridge facilitates mixing). Novolin® 70/30 has an intermediate duration of action. The effect of Novolin® 70/30 begins approximately ½ hour after injection. The effect is maximal between 2 and approximately 12 hours and ends approximately 24 hours after injection. The time course of action for any insulin may vary considerably in different individuals, or at different times in the same individual. Because of this variation, the time pe-

Continued on next page

Squibb-Novo—Cont.

riods listed here should be considered as general guidelines only.

This human insulin (semi-synthetic) is structurally identical to the insulin produced by the human pancreas and has undergone a special purification process. A naturally occurring enzyme is used in a process which converts pork insulin into human insulin. By this enzymatic-transpeptidation process the amino acid alanine in pork insulin is selectively substituted by the amino acid threonine thus forming the human insulin molecule.

NOVOPEN®
Insulin Delivery Device

NovoPen® Insulin Delivery Device is made of nickel and chromium-plated brass, is 6 inches in length and 7 ounces in weight, designed to utilize a replaceable 1.5 ml cartridge of human insulin (PenFill®) and a single-use disposable needle (PenNeedle™) to deliver 2 or more units of insulin by a push-button mechanism. Dosage accuracy was evaluated over a wide range of units and resulted in a standard deviation for a dose from the test cartridges which was 0.12 units. NovoPen® should not be stored in the refrigerator or exposed to extremely hot temperatures. NovoPen® can be cleaned by wiping it with a moistened clean cloth. NovoPen® should be used with PenFill® and PenNeedle™ only.

PENNEEDLE™
Disposable Needle

The self-contained disposable needle consists of protective plastic outer cap, a smooth plastic needle cap and a protective tab. (The needle should not be used if the protective tab is missing or damaged.)

Each PenNeedle™ is bevelled and siliconized throughout its length to ensure minimal friction with the skin. Each PenNeedle™ is 27 gauge, one-half (½) inch (12.5mm) in length and is intended for single use only.

The product is sold in boxes containing 100 single-use PenNeedle™ needles.

NOVOLINPEN™
Dial-A-Dose Insulin Delivery Device

NovolinPen™ is a lightweight dial-a-dose insulin delivery system which injects Novolin® Human Insulin (semi synthetic) in 2 unit increments. The maximum dose is 36 units and the minimum dose is 2 units. NovolinPen™ should only be used with Novolin® Penfill® cartridges and PenNeedle™ disposable needles.

Dosage accuracy is 99.5% and the coefficient of variation is 2.5% for a single dose.

NovolinPen™ must not be stored in a refrigerator. NovolinPen™ should be stored without the needle attached and with the pen cap in position.

NOVOLINPEN™
Assembly and Injection

[See table below].

NovolinPen™

1 Clear cartridge casing
2 Barrel
3 Locking ring
4 Dose indicator window
5 Serial number location
6 Dial-a-dose selector
7 Push button

PenNeedle™

8 Plastic outer cap
9 Plastic needle cap
10 Needle
11 Protective tab

Novolin® PenFill®

12 Rubber stopper
13 Metal cap
14 Glass ball (suspensions only)
15 Plunger

Fig. 1.
Remove NovolinPen™ from case.
Twist and remove pen cap.

Fig. 2.
Be sure the locking ring (A) is in the "unlocked" position (raised circles in lines with open circle).
Unscrew and remove clear cartridge casing (B) from barrel.

Fig. 3.
If the cartridge contains a Novolin® insulin suspension, turn it up and down between positions A and B as shown above. This mixing step must be performed at least 10 times or until the liquid appears uniformly white and cloudy. (A glass ball inside the cartridge facilitates mixing.)

Fig. 4.
A   Insert Novolin® PenFill® cartridge into the clear cartridge casing, metal cap first. Push cartridge until it is fully inserted.
B   Hold barrel in vertical position and lower barrel onto casing. Screw together securely, keeping the pen in vertical position.
Wipe rubber stopper on cartridge with alcohol swab.

Fig. 5.
Remove protective tab from PenNeedle™ and screw needle securely onto NovolinPen™.
Never place a PenNeedle™ single-use disposable needle on your NovolinPen™ until you are ready to give an injection. The needle should be removed immediately after each injection. If the needle is not removed, some liquid may be expelled from the cartridge causing a change in insulin concentration (strength) in insulin suspensions.

Fig. 6.
Giving the air shot prior to each injection:
A   Be sure dial-a-dose selector is set at zero and locking ring is in "unlocked" position (raised circles in line with open circle and window).
B   Dial 2 units.
C   Twist locking ring ¼ turn into "locked" position (raised circles in line with raised circle on barrel). This sets the mechanism for insulin delivery.
Remove both plastic outer and needle caps.

Fig. 7.
Small amounts of air may collect in PenNeedle™ and the Novolin® PenFill® cartridge during normal use. To avoid injection of air and ensure proper dosing, hold the pen with the needle pointing upward; tap the clear cartridge casing gently with the finger a few times; press push button. A drop of insulin should appear at the needle tip; if it does not, return locking ring to "unlocked" position and repeat procedure as in Fig. 6 until a drop of insulin appears.
A small air bubble may remain but it will not be injected, because the operating mechanism prevents the cartridge from being emptied completely.

Fig. 8.
Giving the injection:
Return locking ring to "unlocked" position. (See Fig. 6)
If cartridge contains an insulin suspension, remix by turning pen up and down as shown in Fig. 11.
A   Set dial-a-dose selector to zero to reset.
B   Dial the number of units you wish to inject.
C   Twist locking ring ¼ turn to "locked" position.
NOTE:
The dial-a-dose selector should <u>not</u> be turned when pen is in "locked" position. If the wrong dose has been selected, return the locking ring to "unlocked" position, then proceed from A above.

Fig. 9.
Use the injection technique recommended by your physician. (If you have questions, contact your physician.)
Press push button as far as it will go.
If you need more than 36 units, 2 injections will be necessary.
If locking ring is not in "locked" position, no insulin will be delivered even though push button can be depressed.

Fig. 10.
After injection, return locking ring to "unlocked" position.
Replace needle caps, hold pen firmly, unscrew PenNeedle™ and discard it carefully.
Replace pen cap.

Fig. 11.
Before each subsequent injection:
Twist and remove pen cap.
If you are using more than one type of insulin, check that NovolinPen™ contains the correct insulin cartridge.
If cartridge contains an insulin suspension, turn pen up and down between positions A and B as shown above, at least 10 times to ensure adequate mixing.
Wipe rubber stopper on cartridge with alcohol swab, then proceed from Figs. 5–10.

Continued on next page

Squibb-Novo—Cont.

Fig. 12.
When your injection has been completed the locking ring should be returned to the "unlocked" position.
To change PenFill® cartridge:
Be sure the locking ring is in the "unlocked" position. Unscrew clear cartridge casing and remove cartridge. Proceed as in Figs. 3–10. Be sure to complete all steps.

Fig. 13.
NovolinPen™ is designed to ensure that you cannot select a dose of insulin greater than the amount of insulin remaining in the cartridge.
The number in the dose indicator window will not advance beyond the number of units remaining, even though the dial-a-dose selector can be forced to turn.
If you are using a Novolin® suspension, do not initiate a new injection with fewer than 12 units in the cartridge. The glass ball must have adequate room for movement to mix the suspension. If your dose is lower than 12, be sure the dial will advance to 12 before starting the injection; then mix and redial your proper dose.

Function check

Fig. 14.
You should check the functioning of your NovolinPen™ regularly (once a month or before starting a new pack of PenFill™ cartridges).
Always check the functioning of NovolinPen™ if you suspect it has been damaged. To check:
- Assemble NovolinPen™ as previously described. Remove both the plastic outer cap and plastic needle cap.
- Expel air as shown in Figs. 6, 7.
- The lower cylindrical part of the plastic outer cap holds 20 units of insulin (Fig. 14).

Fig. 15.
- Be sure there is sufficient insulin in the cartridge to complete the test.
- Place the plastic outer cap securely over the exposed needle (Fig. 15).
- Set dial-a-dose selector to zero to reset and then dial 20 units. Twist locking ring ¼ turn to "locked" position. Press push button to deliver 20 units of insulin.

Fig. 16.
The insulin should fill the lower cylindrical portion of the plastic outer cap (Fig. 16).
- If the insulin does not fill or overfills the lower cylindrical part of the plastic outer cap, repeat the test with a new PenNeedle™ and plastic outer cap.
- If the second test also shows under- or over-filling, do not use your NovolinPen™.
Do not try to repair a defective NovolinPen™. [See table below].

Fig. 17.
One spare cartridge and three spare needles can be kept with NovolinPen™ in the carrying case.
For information on storage conditions for Novolin® PenFill® cartridges, see the PenFill® package insert.
NovolinPen™ must not be stored in a refrigerator when a cartridge is in place. NovolinPen™ should be stored without the needle and with the pen cap in position.
NovolinPen™ can be cleaned by wiping it with a soft cloth moistened with alcohol. It should not be soaked in alcohol, washed or lubricated as this may damage the mechanism. Even though made of durable materials, NovolinPen™ must not be exposed to excessive pressure or blows, or dropped, and it should be protected from dust and dirt when not in its case.

Important Notes
- Always check before each injection that NovolinPen™ contains the correct insulin cartridge.
- Before each injection, always expel air with needle pointing upward. (See Figs. 6, 7).
- Always check that the locking ring is in "locked" position before injection.
- Do not turn the dial-a-dose selector when the pen is in "locked" position.
- Perform the function check if you suspect your NovolinPen™ is not functioning properly.
- When using Novolin® insulin suspensions, never initiate an injection if there are fewer than 12 units in the cartridge. (See Fig. 13).
- Never place a PenNeedle™ on your NovolinPen™ until you are ready to give an injection; remove it immediately after injection. If the needle is not removed, some liquid may be expelled from the cartridge causing a change in insulin concentration (strength) in insulin suspensions.
- Protect NovolinPen™ from dust and dirt, from moisture and from extremes of temperature. Care should be taken not to drop it or subject it to impact.
- The compact size of NovolinPen™ makes it easy to use and convenient to carry. Rememeber to keep it with you; don't leave it in a car or other location where extremes of temperature can occur.

EDUCATIONAL MATERIAL

Patient Education Materials
"Keeping Well With Diabetes"
A 36 page, four color booklet explaining the basics of diabetes and insulin therapy. Suitable for both Type I and Type II diabetics.

Storage and Maintenance

Star Pharmaceuticals, Inc.
1990 N.W. 44TH STREET
POMPANO BEACH, FL 33064-8712

APHRODYNE®   ℞
[af"ro-din']
brand of yohimbine hydrochloride

Each scored aqua caplet contains 5.4 mg yohimbine hydrochloride.

HOW SUPPLIED
Bottles of 100 and 1000.
NDC 0076-0401-03 and 04
Shown in Product Identification Section, page 432

URO–KP–NEUTRAL®   OTC
[ū'ro-kp-nū'tral]
Phosphorus Supplement

Each peach capsule-shaped, film coated tablet contains:
Phosphorus ....250 mg.
Potassium ....49.25 mg.
Sodium ....250 mg.
Derived from Disodium Phosphate Anhydrous, Dipotassium Phosphate Anhydrous, and Sodium Monobasic Anhydrous.

HOW SUPPLIED
Bottles of 100.
NDC 0076-0109-03

UROLENE BLUE®   ℞
[ū'ro-lene blue]
Methylene Blue Tablets

Each blue coated tablet contains: Methylene blue USP 65 mg.

HOW SUPPLIED
Bottles of 100 and 1000.
NDC 0076-0501-03 & 04

VIRILON®   ℞
[vir'i-lon]
Methyltestosterone Macro-Beads Capsules
Oral Androgen Macro-Beads

Each capsule contains: Methyltestosterone........USP 10 mg.
In a special base. Look for the grey and white seeds in the black and transparent capsule, available only from Star Pharmaceuticals.

HOW SUPPLIED
Bottles of 100 and 1000.
NDC 0076-0301-03 & 04
Write for complete prescribing information and samples.
Shown in Product Identification Section, page 432

VIRILON® IM   ℞
brand of testosterone cypionate
injection sterile solution
200 mg/ml
For Intramuscular Use Only

HOW SUPPLIED
Multiple dose vials of 10 ml containing 200 mg/ml.
NDC 0076-0301-10
Shown in Product Identification Section, page 432

EDUCATIONAL MATERIAL

Samples Available to Physicians
APHRODYNE® CAPLETS—4's
  Yohimbine Hydrochloride 5.4 mg
URO-KP-NEUTRAL CAPLETS—4's
  Orthophosphate Formula
UROLENE® BLUE TABLETS—4's
  Methylene Blue 65 mg
VIRILON® CAPSULES—4's
  Methyltestosterone Macro-Beads 10 mg

Products are cross-indexed by
generic and chemical names in the
YELLOW SECTION

Stellar Pharmacal Corp.
1990 N.W. 44TH STREET
POMPANO BEACH, FL 33064-8712

STAR–OTIC®

(See PDR For Nonprescription Drugs)

Stiefel Laboratories, Inc.
2801 PONCE DE LEON BLVD.
CORAL GABLES, FL 33134

DUOFILM®   ℞
[du'ō-film]

DESCRIPTION
Duofilm is a topical preparation containing 16.7% Salicylic Acid, U.S.P., and 16.7% Lactic Acid, U.S.P., as the active ingredients in a base of Flexible Collodion, U.S.P. Duofilm's pharmacologic activity is generally attributed to the keratolytic action of Salicylic Acid and Lactic Acid. The structural formula of Salicylic Acid is:

The structural formula of Lactic Acid is:

CLINICAL PHARMACOLOGY
The exact mode of action of Salicylic Acid and Lactic Acid in the treatment of warts is not known. Their activity appears to be associated with keratolytic action which results in mechanical removal of epidermal cells infected with wart viruses.

INDICATIONS AND USAGE
Duofilm is indicated in the treatment of benign epithelial tumors such as common warts. See Dosage and Administration section for information on frequency and duration of use.

CONTRAINDICATIONS
Duofilm should not be used by diabetics or patients with impaired blood circulation. Do not use on moles, birthmarks, or unusual warts with hair growing from them.

PRECAUTIONS
Duofilm is for external use only. Do not permit Duofilm to contact eyes or mucosal membranes. If spilled in eyes or on mucosal membranes, flush with water, remove precipitated collodion, and flush with water for an additional 15 minutes. Duofilm should not be allowed to contact normal skin surrounding wart. Treatment should be discontinued if excessive irritation occurs. Duofilm is highly flammable and should be kept away from fire or flame. Keep bottle tightly capped when not in use. Store at controlled room temperature.

ADVERSE REACTIONS
A localized irritant reaction will occur if Duofilm is applied to the normal skin surrounding the wart. The irritation will normally be controlled by temporarily discontinuing use of Duofilm, and by applying the medication only to the wart site when treatment is resumed.

DOSAGE AND ADMINISTRATION
Prior to the application of Duofilm, soak affected area in hot water for at least five minutes. Dry thoroughly with a clean towel.
Apply a thin layer of Duofilm directly to wart once a day using the brush applicator. Duofilm should be applied with care to avoid contact with normal skin surrounding wart. Treated area may be covered with a lightly applied Band-Aid® or adhesive tape.
Clinically visible improvement will normally occur during the first two to four weeks of therapy. Maximum resolution may be expected after six to twelve weeks of drug use.

HOW SUPPLIED
Duofilm is supplied in a ½ oz. bottle with brush applicator, NDC 0145-6788-05.
See Precautions section for special handling and storage conditions.

DUOPLANT®   ℞
[du'ō-plant]
(Salicylic Acid 27%)

DESCRIPTION
Duoplant is a topical preparation containing 27% Salicylic Acid in a vehicle of flexible collodion, hydroxypropylcellulose, lactic acid and 50% (w/w) alcohol.
The pharmacologic activity of Duoplant is generally attributed to the keratolytic action of Salicylic Acid.
The structural formula of Salicylic Acid is:

CLINICAL PHARMACOLOGY
The exact mode of action of Salicylic Acid in the treatment of warts is not known. Activity appears to be associated with keratolytic action which results in mechanical removal of epidermal cells associated with wart viruses.

INDICATIONS AND USAGE
Duoplant is indicated in the treatment and removal of plantar and common warts.

CONTRAINDICATIONS
Duoplant should not be used by diabetics or patients with impaired blood circulation. Do not use on moles, birthmarks, or unusual warts with hair growing from them.

PRECAUTIONS
Duoplant is for external use only. Do not permit Duoplant to contact eyes or mucous membranes. If spilled in eyes or on mucous membranes, flush with water, remove precipitated collodion, and flush with water for an additional 15 minutes. Duoplant should not be allowed to contact normal skin surrounding the wart. Treatment should be discontinued if excessive irritation occurs. Duoplant is highly flammable and should be kept away from fire or flame. Keep tube tightly capped when not in use. Store at controlled room temperature (59°–86°F).

ADVERSE REACTIONS
A localized irritant reaction will occur if Duoplant is applied to the normal skin surrounding the wart. The irritation will normally be controlled by temporarily discontinuing use of Duoplant and by applying the medication only to the wart site when treatment is resumed.

DOSAGE AND ADMINISTRATION
Prior to the application of Duoplant, soak affected area in warm water for at least five minutes. Dry thoroughly with a clean towel.
Apply a thin layer of Duoplant directly to wart once a day. Duoplant should be applied with care to avoid contact with normal skin surrounding wart. Cover treated area with adhesive tape.
Visible improvement will normally occur during the first two to four weeks of therapy. Maximum resolution may be expected after six to twelve weeks of drug use.

HOW SUPPLIED
Duoplant is supplied in a 14 gram tube, NDC 0145-6790-05. See PRECAUTIONS section for special handling and storage conditions.

CAUTION
Federal law prohibits dispensing without prescription.

LACTICARE®–HC Lotion 1%, 2½%   ℞
[lăk'tĭ-kār"]
(hydrocortisone lotion, USP)

CONTAINS
Each ml of LactiCare-HC Lotion 1% and 2½% (hydrocortisone lotion, USP) contains 10 mg and 25 mg respectively of hydrocortisone in a vehicle consisting of carbomer 940, sodium PCA, lactic acid, sodium hydroxide, stearyl alcohol (and) ceteareth-20, glyceryl stearate (and) PEG-100 stearate, cetyl alcohol, isopropyl palmitate, light mineral oil, myristyl lactate, DMDM hydantoin, dehydroacetic acid, fragrance and purified water.

HOW SUPPLIED
2½%—2 fl. oz. bottle NDC 0145-2538-02
1%—4 fl. oz. bottle NDC 0145-2537-04

Continued on next page

Stiefel—Cont.

PANOXYL® 5   ℞
[pan 'ăhx-il]
(benzoyl peroxide 5%)
PANOXYL® 10   ℞
(benzoyl peroxide 10%)

CONTAINS

PanOxyl 5 and PanOxyl 10 are topical preparations containing benzoyl peroxide as the active ingredient.
PanOxyl 5 contains: 5% benzoyl peroxide in a gel base formulated with 20% alcohol, polyoxyethylene lauryl ether, colloidal magnesium aluminum silicate, hydroxypropylmethylcellulose, citric acid and purified water.
PanOxyl 10 contains: 10% benzoyl peroxide in a gel base formulated with 20% alcohol, polyoxyethylene lauryl ether, colloidal magnesium aluminum silicate, hydroxypropylmethylcellulose, citric acid and purified water.

HOW SUPPLIED

PanOxyl 5 and PanOxyl 10 are supplied in 2.0 ounce and 4.0 ounce plastic tubes.

PanOxyl 5
2.0 oz. tube NDC 0145-2372-06
4.0 oz. tube NDC 0145-2372-08
PanOxyl 10
2.0 oz. tube NDC 0145-2373-06
4.0 oz. tube NDC 0145-2373-08
U.S. Patent 4056611

PANOXYL® AQ 2½   ℞
[pan 'ăhx-il]
(benzoyl peroxide 2½%)
PANOXYL® AQ 5   ℞
(benzoyl peroxide 5%)
PANOXYL® AQ 10   ℞
(benzoyl peroxide 10%)

CONTAINS

PanOxyl AQ 2½, PanOxyl AQ 5, and PanOxyl AQ 10 are topical preparations containing benzoyl peroxide as the active ingredient.
PanOxyl AQ 2½ contains: 2½% benzoyl peroxide in a gel base formulated with purified water, polyoxyethylene lauryl ether, carbomer, sodium hydroxide and methyl paraben.
PanOxyl AQ 5 contains: 5% benzoyl peroxide in a gel base formulated with purified water, polyoxyethylene lauryl ether, carbomer, sodium hydroxide and methyl paraben.
PanOxyl AQ 10 contains: 10% benzoyl peroxide in a gel base formulated with purified water, polyoxyethylene lauryl ether, carbomer, sodium hydroxide and methyl paraben.

HOW SUPPLIED

PanOxyl AQ 2½, PanOxyl AQ 5, and PanOxyl AQ 10 are supplied in 2.0 ounce and 4.0 ounce plastic tubes.
PanOxyl AQ 2½
2.0 oz. tube NDC 0145-2375-06
4.0 oz. tube NDC 0145-2375-08
PanOxyl AQ 5
2.0 oz. tube NDC 0145-2376-06
4.0 oz. tube NDC 0145-2376-08
PanOxyl AQ 10
2.0 oz. tube NDC 0145-2377-06
4.0 oz. tube NDC 0145-2377-08

SULFOXYL® Lotion Regular   ℞
SULFOXYL® Lotion Strong   ℞
[sul 'fox-ul]

CONTAINS

Sulfoxyl Lotion Regular and Sulfoxyl Lotion Strong are topical preparations containing benzoyl peroxide and sulfur as the active ingredients.
Sulfoxyl Lotion Regular contains: 5% benzoyl peroxide and 2% sulfur in a lotion base formulated with PEG-20 stearate, stearic acid, glycerol stearate, isopropyl palmitate, propylene glycol, zinc laurate, chloroxylenol and purified water.
Sulfoxyl Lotion Strong contains: 10% benzoyl peroxide and 5% sulfur in a lotion base formulated with PEG-20 stearate, stearic acid, glycerol stearate, isopropyl palmitate, propylene glycol, zinc laurate, chloroxylenol and purified water.

HOW SUPPLIED

Sulfoxyl Lotion Regular and Sulfoxyl Lotion Strong are supplied in 2.0 ounce plastic bottles.
Sulfoxyl Lotion Regular   **Sulfoxyl Lotion Strong**
NDC 0145-3518-07   NDC 0145-3519-07

Stuart Pharmaceuticals
A business unit of ICI Americas Inc.
WILMINGTON, DE 19897 USA

ALternaGEL®
[al-tern 'a-jel]
Liquid
High-Potency Aluminum Hydroxide Antacid

DESCRIPTION

ALternaGEL is available as a white, pleasant-tasting, high-potency aluminum hydroxide liquid antacid. Each 5 mL teaspoonful contains: Active: 600 mg aluminum hydroxide (equivalent to dried gel, USP) providing 16 milliequivalents (mEq) of acid-neutralizing capacity (ANC), and less than 2.5 mg (0.109 mEq) of sodium and no sugar. Inactive: butylparaben, flavors, propylparaben, purified water, simethicone, and other ingredients.

INDICATIONS

ALternaGEL is indicated for the symptomatic relief of hyperacidity associated with peptic ulcer, gastritis, peptic esophagitis, gastric hyperacidity, hiatal hernia, and heartburn.
ALternaGEL will be of special value to those patients for whom magnesium-containing antacids are undesirable, such as patients with renal insufficiency, patients requiring control of attendant GI complications resulting from steroid or other drug therapy, and patients experiencing the laxation which may result from magnesium or combination antacid regimens.

DIRECTIONS

One to two teaspoonfuls, as needed, between meals and at bedtime, or as directed by a physician: May be followed by a sip of water if desired. Concentrated product. Shake well before using. Keep tightly closed.

WARNINGS

As with all medications, ALternaGEL should be kept out of the reach of children. ALternaGEL may cause constipation. Except under the advice and supervision of a physician: do not take more than 18 teaspoonfuls in a 24-hour period, or use the maximum dose of ALternaGEL for more than two weeks. ALternaGEL may cause constipation.

DRUG INTERACTION PRECAUTION

ALternaGEL should not be taken concurrently with an antibiotic containing any form of tetracycline.

HOW SUPPLIED

ALternaGEL is available in bottles of 12 fluid ounces and 5 fluid ounces, and 1 fluid ounce hospital unit doses. NDC 0038-0860.
Shown in Product Identification Section, page 432

BUCLADIN®-S SOFTAB® Chewable Tablets   ℞
[bu 'cla-din]
(buclizine hydrochloride)

DESCRIPTION

Buclizine hydrochloride is 1-(p-tert-Butylbenzyl) -4- (p-chloro- α -phenylbenzyl) piperazine dihydrochloride. Each tablet contains 50 mg buclizine hydrochloride.
Inactive Ingredients: citric acid, flavor, magnesium stearate, mannitol, microcrystalline cellulose, povidone, starch, Yellow 5 (tartrazine).

ACTIONS

BUCLADIN-S (buclizine hydrochloride) acts centrally to suppress nausea and vomiting.

INDICATIONS

BUCLADIN-S is effective in the management of nausea, vomiting, and dizziness associated with motion sickness.

CONTRAINDICATIONS

Buclizine hydrochloride, when administered to the pregnant rat, induced fetal abnormalities at doses above the human therapeutic range. Clinical data are not adequate to establish nonteratogenicity in early pregnancy. Until such data are available, buclizine hydrochloride is contraindicated for use in early pregnancy.
Buclizine hydrochloride is contraindicated in individuals who have shown a previous hypersensitivity to it.

WARNINGS

Since drowsiness may occur with use of this drug, patients should be warned of this possibility and cautioned against engaging in activities requiring mental alertness, such as driving a car, or operating heavy machinery or appliances. Safe and effective dosage in children has not been established.

PRECAUTION

This product contains Yellow 5 (tartrazine) which may cause allergic-type reactions (including bronchial asthma) in certain susceptible individuals. Although the overall incidence of Yellow 5 (tartrazine) sensitivity in the general population is low, it is frequently seen in patients who also have aspirin hypersensitivity.

ADVERSE REACTIONS

Occasionally drowsiness, dryness of mouth, headache, and jitteriness are encountered.

DOSAGE AND ADMINISTRATION

BUCLADIN-S (buclizine hydrochloride) SOFTAB Tablets can be taken without swallowing water. Place the SOFTAB tablet in the mouth and allow it to dissolve, or the tablet may be chewed.
Adults: One tablet usually serves to alleviate nausea. In severe cases, three tablets a day may be taken. The usual maintenance dosage is one tablet twice daily. In the prevention of motion sickness, one tablet taken at least ½ hour before beginning travel usually suffices. For extended travel, a second tablet may be taken after 4 to 6 hours.

HOW SUPPLIED

Bottles of 100 scored, yellow, SOFTAB Tablets, embossed front "STUART," reverse "864." NDC 0038-0864.
Shown in Product Identification Section, page 432
Rev E 6/87

CEFOTAN®   ℞
[cef 'o-tan "]
(cefotetan disodium)
For Intravenous or Intramuscular Use

PRODUCT OVERVIEW

KEY FACTS

CEFOTAN (cefotetan disodium) is a semisynthetic, broad-spectrum, beta-lactamase stable, cephalosporin (cephamycin) antibiotic for parenteral administration. The bactericidal action of cefotetan results from inhibition of cell wall synthesis. Therefore, CEFOTAN is exquisitely active against a wide range of gram-negative aerobes. Like other cephamycins, CEFOTAN exhibits good activity against *Bacteroides fragilis* and many other anaerobic organisms. The plasma elimination half-life of CEFOTAN is 3 to 4.6 hours after either intravenous or intramuscular administraion allowing twice-daily dosing for the treatment of indicated infections and single dose prophylaxis in appropriate surgical procedures.

MAJOR USES

CEFOTAN is indicated for the treatment of the following infections caused by susceptible organisms:
Gynecologic Infections
Intra-abdominal Infections
Skin and Skin Structure Infections
The preoperative administration of CEFOTAN may reduce the incidence of certain postoperative infections in patients undergoing surgical procedures that are classified as clean contaminated or potentially contaminated (eg, cesarean section, abdominal or vaginal hysterectomy, transurethral surgery, biliary tract surgery, and gastrointestinal surgery).

SAFETY INFORMATION

CEFOTAN is contraindicated in patients with known allergy to the cephalosporin group of antibiotics. In patients with renal impairment, dosage adjustment is necessary.

PRESCRIBING INFORMATION

CEFOTAN®   ℞
[cefo 'tan]
(cefotetan disodium)
For Intravenous or Intramuscular Use

DESCRIPTION

CEFOTAN (cefotetan disodium) is a sterile, semisynthetic, broad-spectrum, beta-lactamase resistant, cephalosporin (cephamycin) antibiotic for parenteral administration. It is the disodium salt of [6R -(6α, 7α)]-7-[[[4-(2-amino-1-carboxy-2-oxoethylidene)-1,3-dithietan-2-yl]carbonyl]amino]-7-methoxy-3-[[(1-methyl-1H -tetrazol-5-yl)thio]methyl]-8-oxo-5-thia-1-azabicyclo [4.2.0]oct-2-ene-2-carboxylic acid. Its molecular formula is $C_{17}H_{15}N_7Na_2O_8S_4$ with a molecular weight of 619.56.

STRUCTURAL FORMULA

CEFOTAN contains approximately 80 mg (3.5 mEq) of sodium per gram of cefotetan activity. It is a white to pale yellow powder which is very soluble in water. The solution varies from colorless to yellow depending on the concentration. The pH of freshly reconstituted solutions is usually between 4.5 to 6.5.

PHARMACY BULK PACKAGE

Pharmacy bulk package is not for direct infusion.
This is a container of sterile powder for reconstitution intended for parenteral use and contains many single doses. The contents are intended for use in a pharmacy admixture program and are restricted to the preparation of admixtures for intravenous infusion or the filling of empty sterile syringes for intravenous injection for patients with individualized dosing requirements.

CLINICAL PHARMACOLOGY

High plasma levels of cefotetan are attained after intravenous and intramuscular administration of single doses to normal volunteers.

PLASMA CONCENTRATIONS AFTER 1.0 GRAM IV* or IM DOSE
Mean Plasma Concentration (µg/mL)

Route	Time After Injection						
	15 min	30 min	1 h	2 h	4 h	8 h	12 h
IV	92	158	103	72	42	18	9
IM	34	56	71	68	47	20	9

*30-minute infusion

PLASMA CONCENTRATIONS AFTER 2.0 GRAM IV* or IM DOSE
Mean Plasma Concentration (µg/mL)

Route	Time After Injection						
	5 min	10 min	1 h	3 h	5 h	9 h	12 h
IV	237	223	135	74	48	22	12†
IM	–	20	75	91	69	33	19

* Injected over 3 minutes
† Concentrations estimated from regression line

The plasma elimination half-life of cefotetan is 3 to 4.6 hours after either intravenous or intramuscular administration. Repeated administration of CEFOTAN does not result in accumulation of the drug in normal subjects.
Cefotetan is 88% plasma protein bound.
No active metabolites of cefotetan have been detected; however, small amounts (less than 7%) of cefotetan in plasma and urine may be converted to its tautomer, which has antimicrobial activity similar to the parent drug.
In normal patients, from 51% to 81% of an administered dose of CEFOTAN is excreted unchanged by the kidneys over a 24 hour period, which results in high and prolonged urinary concentrations. Following intravenous doses of 1 gram and 2 grams, urinary concentrations are highest during the first hour and reach concentrations of approximately 1700 and 3500 µg/mL respectively.
In patients with reduced renal function, the plasma half-life of cefotetan is prolonged.
Therapeutic levels of cefotetan are achieved in many body tissues and fluids including:

skin	ureter
muscle	bladder
fat	maxillary sinus mucosa
myometrium	tonsil
endometrium	bile
cervix	peritoneal fluid
ovary	umbilical cord serum
kidney	amniotic fluid

MICROBIOLOGY

The bactericidal action of cefotetan results from inhibition of cell wall synthesis. Cefotetan has in vitro activity against a wide range of gram-positive and gram-negative organisms. The methoxy group in the 7-alpha position provides cefotetan with a high degree of stability in the presence of beta-lactamases, both penicillinases and cephalosporinases of gram-negative bacteria. Cefotetan is usually active against the following organisms in vitro and in clinical infections:

GRAM-NEGATIVE:

Escherichia coli
Klebsiella species (including K pneumoniae)
Enterobacter aerogenes
Enterobacter agglomerans
Enterobacter cloacae
Proteus mirabilis
Proteus vulgaris
Morganella morganii (formerly *Proteus morganii*)
Providencia rettgeri (formerly *Proteus rettgeri*)
Providencia stuartii
Haemophilus influenzae (including ampicillin-resistant strains)
Neisseria gonorrhoeae
NOTE: Approximately one-half of the strains of *Enterobacter* species, and *Citrobacter* species are resistant to cefotetan.

Most strains of *Pseudomonas aeruginosa* and *Acinetobacter* species are resistant to cefotetan.

GRAM-POSITIVE:

Staphylococcus aureus (including penicillinase- and non-penicillinase-producing strains)
Staphylococcus epidermidis
Streptococcus pyogenes (group A beta-hemolytic streptococci)
Streptococcus agalactiae (group B beta-hemolytic streptococci)
Streptococcus pneumoniae (formerly *Diplococcus pneumoniae*)
NOTE: Methicillin-resistant staphylococci are resistant to cephalosporins. Some strains of *Staphylococcus epidermidis* and most strains of enterococci, eg, *S faecalis*, are resistant to cefotetan.

ANAEROBES:

Bacteroides fragilis subsp *fragilis*
Bacteroides bivius
Bacteroides disiens
Bacteroides melaninogenicus
Bacteroides vulgatus
Fusobacterium species
Gram-positive bacilli (including *Clostridium* species)
Peptococcus and *Peptostreptococcus* species
NOTE: Most strains of *B distasonis, B ovatus,* and *B thetaiotaomicron* are resistant to cefotetan.
Cefotetan also demonstrates in vitro activity against the following microorganisms, although its clinical significance is unknown: *Citrobacter* species (including *C diversus* and *C freundii*), *Serratia* species (including *S marcescens*), *Salmonella* species, *Shigella* species, *Yersinia enterocolitica, Clostridium difficile, B asaccharolyticus, B oralis, B splanchnicus, Veillonella* species, and *Propionibacterium* species.
NOTE: Many strains of *C difficile* are resistant.

SUSCEPTIBILITY TESTS

Diffusion Technique: Quantitative methods that require measurement of zone diameters give the most precise estimate of antibiotic susceptibility. One such procedure[1] has been recommended for use with disks to test susceptibility to cefotetan. Organisms should be tested with the cefotetan 30 µg disk since cefotetan has been shown to be active in vitro against organisms which were found to be resistant to other beta-lactam antibiotics.
Reports from the laboratory with results of standardized single-disk susceptibility tests with a 30 µg cefotetan disk should be interpreted according to the following criteria:
Susceptible organisms produce zone sizes of 16 mm or greater, indicating that the tested organism is likely to respond to therapy.
Moderately susceptible organisms produce zones of 13 to 15 mm indicating the test organism would be susceptible if high dosage is used or if the infection is confined to tissues and fluids (eg, urine) in which high antibiotic levels are attained. Resistant organisms produce zones of 12 mm or less, indicating that other therapy should be selected.
Standardized procedures require the use of laboratory control organisms. The 30 µg cefotetan disk should give zone diameters between 17 and 22 mm for *S aureus* ATCC 25923. For *E coli* ATCC 25922, the zone diameters should be between 29 and 34 mm.
Dilution Techniques: Broth or agar dilution methods, eg, ICS agar dilution[2] or an equivalent method such as that recommended by the National Committee for Clinical Laboratory Standards (NCCLS)[3], may be used to determine the minimal inhibitory concentration (MIC) of cefotetan.
Organisms inhibited by cefotetan at 16 µg/mL or less are considered susceptible. Organisms with MIC values 64 µg/mL or more are considered resistant to cefotetan.
As with standard diffusion methods, dilution procedures require the use of laboratory control organisms. Standard cefotetan powder should give MIC values in the range of 4 µg/mL and 16 µg/mL for *S aureus* ATCC 25923. For *E coli* ATCC 25922, the MIC range should be between 0.06 µg/mL and 0.25 µg/mL.

INDICATIONS AND USAGE

TREATMENT

CEFOTAN is indicated for the therapeutic treatment of the following infections when caused by susceptible strains of the designated organisms:
Urinary Tract Infections caused by *E coli, Klebsiella* species (including *K pneumoniae), Proteus mirabilis* and *Proteus* sp (which may include the organisms now called *Proteus vulgaris, Providencia rettgeri,* and *Morganella morganii*).
Lower Respiratory Tract Infections caused by *Streptococcus pneumoniae* (formerly *D pneumoniae*), *Staphylococcus aureus* (penicillinase- and nonpenicillinase-producing strains), *Haemophilus influenzae* (including ampicillin-resistant strains), *Klebsiella* species (including *K pneumoniae),* and *E coli.*
Skin and Skin Structure Infections caused by *Staphylococcus aureus* (penicillinase- and nonpenicillinase-producing strains), *Staphylococcus epidermidis, Streptococcus pyogenes* and *Streptococcus* species (excluding enterococci), and *E. coli.*

Gynecologic Infections caused by *Staphylococcus aureus‡* (including penicillinase- and nonpenicillinase-producing strains), *Staphylococcus epidermidis, Streptococcus* species (excluding enterococci), *E. coli, Proteus mirabilis, Neisseria gonorrhoeae, Bacteroides* species (excluding *B distasonis, B ovatus, B thetaiotaomicron*), *Fusobacterium species‡,* and gram-positive anaerobic cocci (including *Peptococcus* and *Peptostreptococcus species‡*).
Intra-abdominal Infections caused by *E coli, Klebsiella* species (including *K pneumoniae‡), Streptococcus* species (excluding enterococci), and *Bacteroides* species (excluding *B distasonis, B ovatus, B thetaiotaomicron*).
Bone and Joint Infections caused by *Staphylococcus aureus.‡*
‡ Efficacy for this organism in this organ system was studied in fewer than ten infections.
Specimens for bacteriological examination should be obtained in order to isolate and identify causative organisms and to determine their susceptibilities to cefotetan. Therapy may be instituted before results of susceptibility studies are known; however, once these results become available, the antibiotic treatment should be adjusted accordingly.
In cases of confirmed or suspected gram-positive or gram-negative sepsis or in patients with other serious infections in which the causative organism has not been identified, it is possible to use CEFOTAN concomitantly with an aminoglycoside. Cefotetan combinations with aminoglycosides have been shown to be synergistic in vitro against many Enterobacteriaceae and also some other gram-negative bacteria. The dosage recommended in the labeling of both antibiotics may be given and depends on the severity of the infection and the patient's condition.
NOTE: If CEFOTAN and an aminoglycoside are used concomitantly, renal function should be carefully monitored, especially if higher dosages of the aminoglycoside are to be administered or if therapy is prolonged, because of the potential nephrotoxicity and ototoxicity of aminoglycosidic antibiotics. Although, to date, nephrotoxicity has not been noted when CEFOTAN was given alone, it is possible that nephrotoxicity may be potentiated if CEFOTAN is used concomitantly with an aminoglycoside.

PROPHYLAXIS

The preoperative administration of CEFOTAN may reduce the incidence of certain postoperative infections in patients undergoing surgical procedures that are classified as clean contaminated or potentially contaminated (eg, cesarean section, abdominal or vaginal hysterectomy, transurethral surgery, biliary tract surgery, and gastrointestinal surgery). The prophylactic dose of CEFOTAN should be administered 30 to 60 minutes prior to surgery. In patients undergoing cesarean section, CEFOTAN should be administered intravenously after the clamping of the umbilical cord.
If there are signs and symptoms of infection, specimens for culture should be obtained for identification of the causative organism so that appropriate therapeutic measures may be initiated.

CONTRAINDICATIONS

CEFOTAN is contraindicated in patients with known allergy to the cephalosporin group of antibiotics.

WARNINGS

Before therapy with CEFOTAN is instituted, careful inquiry should be made to determine whether the patient has had previous hypersensitivity reactions to cefotetan disodium, cephalosporins, penicillins, or other drugs. This product should be given cautiously to penicillin-sensitive patients. Antibiotics should be administered with caution to any patient who has demonstrated some form of allergy, particularly to drugs. If an allergic reaction to CEFOTAN occurs, discontinue the drug. Serious acute hypersensitivity reactions may require epinephrine and other emergency measures.

Pseudomembranous colitis has been reported with the use of cephalosporins (and other broad-spectrum antibiotics); therefore, it is important to consider its diagnosis in patients who develop diarrhea in association with antibiotic use.
Treatment with broad-spectrum antibiotics may alter normal flora of the colon and may permit overgrowth of clostridia. Studies indicate a toxin produced by *Clostridium difficile* is one primary cause of antibiotic-associated colitis. Cholestyramine and colestipol resins have been shown to bind the toxin in vitro.
Mild cases of colitis may respond to drug discontinuance alone. Moderate to severe cases should be managed with fluid, electrolyte, and protein supplementation as indicated. When the colitis is not relieved by drug discontinuance or when it is severe, oral vancomycin is the treatment of choice for antibiotic-associated pseudomembranous colitis produced by *C difficile.* Other causes should also be considered.

PRECAUTIONS

General: As with other broad-spectrum antibiotics, prolonged use of CEFOTAN may result in overgrowth of nonsusceptible organisms. Careful observation of the patient is es-

Continued on next page

Stuart—Cont.

sential. If superinfection does occur during therapy, appropriate measures should be taken.

In common with many other broad-spectrum antibiotics, CEFOTAN may be associated with a fall in prothrombin activity. Those at risk include patients with renal or hepatic impairment, or poor nutritional state, the elderly, and patients with cancer. Prothrombin times should be monitored in patients at risk and exogenous vitamin K administered as indicated.

CEFOTAN should be used with caution in individuals with a history of gastrointestinal disease, particularly colitis.

Information for Patients: As with some other cephalosporins, a disulfiram-like reaction characterized by flushing, sweating, headache, and tachycardia may occur when alcohol (beer, wine, etc) is ingested within 72 hours after CEFOTAN administration. Patients should be cautioned about the ingestion of alcoholic beverages following the administration of CEFOTAN.

Drug Interactions: Although to date nephrotoxicity has not been noted when CEFOTAN was given alone, it is possible that nephrotoxicity may be potentiated if CEFOTAN is used concomitantly with an aminoglycoside.

Drug/Laboratory Test Interactions: A false positive reaction for glucose in urine may occur with Benedict's or Fehling's solution.

As with other cephalosporins, high concentrations of cefotetan may intefere with measurement of serum and urine creatinine levels of Jaffe reaction and produce false increases in the levels of creatinine reported.

Carcinogenesis, Mutagenesis, Impairment of Fertility: Although long-term studies in animals have not been performed to evaluate carcinogenic potential, no mutagenic potential of cefotetan was found in standard laboratory tests. Cefotetan has adverse effects on the testes of prepubertal rats. Subcutaneous administration of 500 mg/kg/day (approximately 8–16 times the usual adult human dose) on days 6–35 of life (thought to be developmentally analogous to late childhood and prepuberty in humans) resulted in reduced testicular weight and seminiferous tubule degeneration in 10 of 10 animals. Affected cells included spermatogonia and spermatocytes; Sertoli and Leydig cells were unaffected. Incidence and severity of lesions were dose-dependent; at 120 mg/kg/day (approximately 2–4 times the usual human dose), only 1 of 10 treated animals was affected, and the degree of degeneration was mild.

Similar lesions have been observed in experiments of comparable design with other methylthiotetrazole-containing antibiotics and impaired fertility has been reported, particularly at high dose levels. No testicular effects were observed in 7-week-old rats treated with up to 1000 mg/kg/day SC for 5 weeks, or in infant dogs (3 weeks old) that received up to 300 mg/kg/day IV for 5 weeks. The relevance of these findings to humans is unknown.

Usage in Pregnancy: Pregnancy Category B: Reproduction studies have been performed in rats and monkeys at doses up to 20 times the human dose and have revealed no evidence of impaired fertility or harm to the fetus due to cefotetan. There are, however, no adequate and well-controlled studies in pregnant women. Because animal reproductive studies are not always predictive of human response, this drug should be used during pregnancy only if clearly needed.

Usage in Nursing Mothers: Cefotetan is excreted in human milk in very low concentrations. Caution should be exercised when cefotetan is administered to a nursing woman.

Pediatric Use: Safety and effectiveness in children have not been established.

ADVERSE REACTIONS

In clinical studies the following adverse effects were considered related to CEFOTAN therapy.

Gastrointestinal symptoms occurred in 1.5% of patients, the most frequent were diarrhea (1 in 80) and nausea (1 in 700).

Hematologic laboratory abnormalities occurred in 1.4% of patients and included eosinophilia (1 in 200), positive direct Coomb's test (1 in 250), and thrombocytosis (1 in 300).

Hepatic enzyme elevations occurred in 1.2% of patients and included a rise in SGPT (1 in 150), SGOT (1 in 300), alkaline phosphatase (1 in 700), and LDH (1 in 700).

DOSAGE GUIDELINES FOR PATIENTS WITH IMPAIRED RENAL FUNCTION

Creatinine Clearance mL/min	Dose	Frequency
>30	Usual Recommended Dosage*	Every 12 hours
10–30	Usual Recommended Dosage*	Every 24 hours
<10	Usual Recommended Dosage*	Every 48 hours

*Dose determined by the type and severity of infection, and susceptibility of the causative organism.

Hypersensitivity reactions were reported in 1.2% of patients and included rash (1 in 150) and itching (1 in 700).

Local effects were reported in less than 1.0% of patients and included phlebitis at the site of injection (1 in 300), and discomfort (1 in 500).

During postmarketing experience with CEFOTAN, anaphylactic reactions and transient thrombocytopenia have been reported.

DOSAGE AND ADMINISTRATION

TREATMENT

The usual adult dosage is 1 or 2 grams of CEFOTAN administered intravenously or intramuscularly every 12 hours for 5 to 10 days. Proper dosage and route of administration should be determined by the condition of the patient, severity of the infection, and susceptibility of the causative organism. [See table below].

PROPHYLAXIS

To prevent postoperative infection in clean contaminated or potentially contaminated surgery in adults, the recommended dosage is 1 or 2 g of CEFOTAN administered once, intravenously 30 to 60 minutes prior to surgery. In patients undergoing cesarean section, the dose should be administered as soon as the umbilical cord is clamped.

IMPAIRED RENAL FUNCTION

When renal function is impaired, a reduced dosage schedule must be employed. the following dosage guidelines may be used. [See table above].

Alternatively, the dosing interval may remain constant at 12 hour intervals, but the dose reduced to one-half the usual recommended dose for patients with a creatinine clearance of 10–30 mL/min, and one-quarter the usual recommended dose for patients with a creatinine clearance of less than 10 mL/min.

When only serum creatinine levels are available, creatinine clearance may be calculated from the following formula. The serum creatinine level should represent a steady state of renal function.

Males:
$$\frac{\text{Weight (kg)} \times (140 - \text{age})}{72 \times \text{serum creatinine (mg/100 mL)}}$$

Females: $0.9 \times$ value for males

Cefotetan is dialyzable and it is recommended that for patients undergoing intermittent hemodialysis, one-quarter of the usual recommended dose be given every 24 hours on days between dialysis and one-half the usual recommended dose on the day of dialysis.

PREPARATION OF SOLUTION

For Intravenous Use: Reconstitute with Sterile Water for Injection. Shake to dissolve and let stand until clear.

Vial Size	Amount of Diluent To Be Added (mL)	Approximate Withdrawable Vol (mL)	Approximate Average Concentration (mg/mL)
1 gram	10	10.5	95
2 gram	10–20	11.0–21.0	182–95

Infusion bottles (100 mL) may be reconstituted with 50 to 100 mL of 5% Dextrose Solution or 0.9% Sodium Chloride Solution.

For Intramuscular Use: Reconstitute with Sterile Water for Injection; Bacteriostatic Water for Injection; Normal Saline, USP; 0.5% Lidocaine HCl; or 1.0% Lidocaine HCl. Shake to dissolve and let stand until clear.

Vial Size	Amount of Diluent To Be Added (mL)	Approximate Withdrawable Vol (mL)	Approximate Average Concentration (mg/mL)
1 gram	2	2.5	400
2 gram	3	4.0	500

For Pharmacy Bulk Package: Reconstitute with Sterile Water for Injection; 5% Dextrose Solution; or 0.9% Sodium Chloride Solution. Shake to dissolve and let stand until clear. (See PROPER USE OF PHARMACY BULK PACKAGE.)

Vial Size	Amount of Diluent To Be Added (mL)	Approximate Withdrawable Vol (mL)	Approximate Average Concentration (mg/mL)
10 g Pharmacy Bulk	50	55	180
10 g Pharmacy Bulk	100	105	95

INTRAVENOUS ADMINISTRATION

The intravenous route is preferable for patients with bacteremia, bacterial septicemia, or other severe or life-threatening infections, or for patients who may be poor risks because of lowered resistance resulting from such debilitating conditions as malnutrition, trauma, surgery, diabetes, heart failure, or malignancy, particularly if shock is present or impending.

For intermittent intravenous administration, a solution containing 1 gram or 2 grams of CEFOTAN in Sterile Water for Injection can be injected over a period of three to five minutes. Using an infusion system, the solution may also be given over a longer period of time through the tubing system by which the patient may be receiving other intravenous solutions. Butterfly® or scalp vein-type needles are preferred for this type of infusion. However, during infusion of the solution containing CEFOTAN, it is advisable to discontinue temporarily the administration of other solutions at the same site.

NOTE: Solutions of CEFOTAN must not be admixed with solutions containing aminoglycosides. If CEFOTAN and aminoglycosides are to be administered to the same patient, they must be administered separately and not as a mixed injection.

INTRAMUSCULAR ADMINISTRATION

As with all intramuscular preparations, CEFOTAN should be injected well within the body of a relatively large muscle such as the upper outer quadrant of the buttock (ie, gluteus maximus); aspiration is necessary to avoid inadvertent injection into a blood vessel.

Compatability and Stability: CEFOTAN reconstituted as described above (Preparation of Solution) maintains satisfactory potency for 24 hours at room temperature (25°C), for 96 hours under refrigeration (5°C), and for at least 1 week in the frozen state. After reconstitution and subsequent storage in disposable glass or plastic syringes, CEFOTAN is stable for 24 hours at room temperature and 96 hours under refrigeration.

Frozen samples should be thawed at room temperature before use. After the periods mentioned above, any unused solutions or frozen materials should be discarded. Do not refreeze.

NOTE: Parenteral drug products should be inspected visually for particulate matter and discoloration prior to administration whenever solution and container permit.

PROPER USE OF PHARMACY BULK PACKAGE

The closure may be penetrated only one time after reconstitution. If necessary, the use of a suitable sterile transfer device or dispensing set which allows measured dispensing of the contents should be considered.

Use of this package is restricted to a suitable work area, such as a laminar flow hood.

The aliquotting operation should be completed promptly after reconstitution of the contents (see PREPARATION OF SOLUTION). Product dispensed in this manner should be administered within 24 hours if stored at room temperature, 96 hours if stored under refrigeration (5°C), and 1 week if stored in the frozen state. Any unused portion must be discarded within 24 hours after initial entry.

HOW SUPPLIED

CEFOTAN is a dry, white to pale yellow powder supplied in vials containing cefotetan disodium equivalent to 1 g and 2 g cefotetan activity for intravenous and intramuscular administration. The 1 g dose is available in 10 mL and 100 mL vials, and the 2 g dose is available in 20 mL and 100 mL vials. CEFOTAN is also available in a pharmacy bulk package of 10 g in 100 mL vials. The vials should not be stored at temperatures above 22°C and should be protected from light.

GENERAL GUIDELINES FOR DOSAGE OF CEFOTAN

Type of Infection	Daily Dose	Frequency and Route
Urinary Tract	1–4 grams	500 mg every 12 hours IV or IM 1 or 2 g every 24 hours IV or IM 1 or 2 g every 12 hours IV or IM
Other Sites	2–4 grams	1 or 2 g every 12 hours IV or IM
Severe	4 grams	2 g every 12 hours IV
Life-Threatening	6* grams	3 g every 12 hours IV

*Maximum daily dosage should not exceed 6 grams.

1 g in 10 mL vial (NDC 0038-0376-10)
2 g in 20 mL vial (NDC 0038-0377-20)
1 g in 100 mL vial (NDC 0038-0376-11)
2 g in 100 mL vial (NDC 0038-0377-21)
10 g in 100 mL vial (NDC 0038-0375-10)

1. Am J Clin Pathol 1966:45:493.
   Federal Register 1974:39:19182–19184.
2. Ericson HM, Sherris JC: Acta Pathol Microbiol Immunol Scand (B) 1971; (suppl No. 217).
3. Thornsberry C, et al: Methods for Dilution: Antimicrobial Susceptibility Tests for Bacteria that Grow Aerobically. 1983, Vol 3, No. 2.

Rev. J 11/88

Shown in Product Identification Section, page 432

DIALOSE® Capsules
[di′a-lose]
Stool Softener Laxative

DESCRIPTION
DIALOSE is a sodium-free, nonhabit forming, stool softener containing docusate potassium in capsules of 100 mg.
The docusate in DIALOSE is a highly efficient surfactant which facilitates absorption of water by the stool to form a soft, easily evacuated mass. Unlike stimulant laxatives, DIALOSE does not interfere with normal peristalsis, neither does it cause griping nor sensations of urgency.

INGREDIENTS
Each capsule contains: Active: docusate potassium. Inactive: Blue 1, gelatin, lactose, magnesium stearate, Red 28, Red 40, silicon dioxide, titanium dioxide.

INDICATIONS
DIALOSE is indicated for the relief of occasional constipation (irregularity).
DIALOSE is an effective aid to soften or prevent formation of hard stools in a wide range of conditions that may lead to constipation. DIALOSE helps to eliminate straining associated with obstetric, geriatric, cardiac, surgical, anorectal, or proctologic conditions. In cases of mild constipation, the fecal softening action of DIALOSE can prevent constipation from progressing and relieve painful defecation.

DIRECTIONS
Adults: Adjust dosage as needed, one capsule one to three times daily. *Children:* 6 years and over—One capsule at bedtime, or as directed by physician. *Children:* under 6 years —As directed by physician. It is helpful to increase the daily intake of fluids by taking a glass of water with each dose.

WARNINGS
As with any drug, if you are pregnant or nursing a baby, seek the advice of a health professional before using this product. Keep out of the reach of children.

HOW SUPPLIED
Bottles of 36 and 100 pink capsules, identified "STUART 470." Also available in 100 capsule unit dose boxes (10 strips of 10 capsules each). NDC-0038-0470.
Shown in Product Identification Section, page 432

DIALOSE® PLUS Capsules
[di′a-lose Plus]
Stool Softener/Stimulant Laxative

DESCRIPTION
DIALOSE PLUS provides a sodium-free formulation of docusate potassium in capsules of 100 mg and casanthranol, 30 mg.

INGREDIENTS
Each capsule contains: Active: docusate potassium, casanthranol. Inactive: gelatin, lactose, magnesium stearate, Red 33, silicon dioxide, titanium dioxide, Yellow 10.

INDICATIONS
DIALOSE PLUS is indicated for the treatment of constipation characterized by lack of moisture in the intestinal contents, resulting in hardness of stool and decreased intestinal motility.
DIALOSE PLUS combines the advantages of the stool softener, docusate potassium, with the peristaltic activating effect of casanthranol.

DIRECTIONS
Adults:—Initially, one capsule two times a day. *Children* —As directed by physician. When adequate bowel function is restored, the dose may be adjusted to meet individual needs. It is helpful to increase the daily intake of fluids by taking a glass of water with each dose.

WARNINGS
As with any drug, if you are pregnant or nursing a baby, seek the advice of a health professional before using this product. And, as with any laxative, DIALOSE PLUS should not be used when abdominal pain, nausea, or vomiting are present.

Frequent or prolonged use may result in dependence on laxatives. Keep out of the reach of children.

HOW SUPPLIED
Bottles of 36, 100, and 500 yellow capsules, identified "STUART 475." Also available in 100 capsule unit dose boxes (10 strips of 10 capsules each). NDC 0038-0475.
Shown in Product Identification Section, page 432

EFFER-SYLLIUM®
[ef′fer-sil′lium]
Natural Fiber Bulking Agent

DESCRIPTION
EFFER-SYLLIUM is an effervescent granular powder. Each rounded teaspoonful, or individual packet (7 g) contains psyllium hydrocolloid, 3 g.

INGREDIENTS
Active: psyllium hydrocolloid. Inactive: citric acid, ethyl vanillin, lemon and lime flavors, potassium bicarbonate, potassium citrate, saccharin calcium, starch, sucrose.
EFFER-SYLLIUM contains less than 5 mg sodium per rounded teaspoonful and is considered dietetically sodium free.

INDICATIONS
EFFER-SYLLIUM is indicated to restore normal bowel habits in chronic constipation, to promote normal elimination in irritable bowel syndrome, and to ease passage of stools in presence of anorectal disorders. EFFER-SYLLIUM produces a soft, lubricating bulk which promotes natural elimination. EFFER-SYLLIUM is not a one-dose, fast-acting bowel regulator. Administration for several days may be needed to establish regularity.

DIRECTIONS
Adults: One rounded teaspoonful, or one packet, in a glass of water one to three times a day, or as directed by physician. *Children, 6 years and over:* One level teaspoonful, or one-half packet (3.5 g) in one-half glass of water at bedtime, or as directed by physician. *Children, under 6 years:* As directed by physician.

INSTRUCTIONS
Pour EFFER-SYLLIUM into a *dry* glass, add water and stir briskly. Drink immediately. To avoid caking, always use a *dry* spoon to remove EFFER-SYLLIUM from its container. Replace cap tightly. Keep in a dry place.

WARNING
Avoid inhalation. May cause a potentially severe reaction when inhaled by persons sensitive to psyllium powder or suffering from respiratory disorders. As with all medications, keep out of the reach of children.

HOW SUPPLIED
Bottles of 9 oz and 16 oz tan, granular instant mix powder. Convenient pouch package (7 g per packet) in boxes of 12 or 24.
NDC 0038-0440.
Shown in Product Identification Section, page 432

FERANCEE®
[fer′an-see]
Chewable Hematinic

INGREDIENTS
TWO TABLETS DAILY PROVIDE:

	US RDA*	
Iron	744%	134 mg
Vitamin C	500%	300 mg

*Percentage of US Recommended Daily Allowances for adults and children 4 or more years of age.
Active: ferrous fumarate, sodium ascorbate, ascorbic acid.
Inactive: confectioner's sugar, flavors, magnesium stearate, mannitol, povidone, saccharin calcium, starch, Yellow 5 (tartrazine), Yellow 6.

INDICATIONS
A pleasant-tasting hematinic for iron deficiency anemias, well-tolerated FERANCEE is particularly useful when chronic blood loss, onset of menses, or pregnancy create additional demands for iron supplementation. Available information indicates a low incidence of staining of the teeth by ferrous fumarate, alone or in combination with ascorbic acid. The peach-cherry flavored chewable tablets dissolve quickly in the mouth and may be either chewed or swallowed.

DIRECTIONS
Adults: Two tablets daily, or as directed by physician.
Children over 6 years of age: One tablet daily, or as directed by physician.
Children under 6 years of age: As directed by physician.
IMPORTANT: KEEP IN DRY PLACE. REPLACE CAP TIGHTLY.

WARNINGS
As with any drug, if you are pregnant or nursing a baby, seek the advice of a health professional before using this product. Keep out of the reach of children. In case of accidental overdose, seek professional assistance or contact a Poison Control Center immediately.

HOW SUPPLIED
Bottles of 100 brown and yellow, two-layer tablets identified "STUART 650" on brown layer. A child-resistant cap is standard on each bottle as a safeguard against accidental ingestion by children. Keep in a dry place. Replace cap tightly. NDC 0038-0650.
Shown in Product Identification Section, page 432

FERANCEE®-HP Tablets
[fer′an-see-hp]
High Potency Hematinic

INGREDIENTS
ONE TABLET DAILY PROVIDES:

	US RDA*	
Iron	611%	110 mg
Vitamin C	1000%	600 mg

*Percentage of US Recommended Daily Allowances for adults and children 4 or more years of age.
Active: ascorbic acid, ferrous fumarate, sodium ascorbate.
Inactive: flavor, hydrogenated vegetable oil, microcrystalline cellulose, povidone, Red 40, and other ingredients.

INDICATIONS
FERANCEE-HP is a high potency formulation of iron and vitamin C and is intended for use as either:
(1) a maintenance hematinic for those patients needing a daily iron supplement to maintain normal hemoglobin levels, or
(2) intensive therapy for the acute and/or severe iron deficiency anemia where a high intake of elemental iron is required.
The use of well-tolerated ferrous fumarate provides high levels of elemental iron with a low incidence of gastric distress. The inclusion of 600 mg of vitamin C per tablet serves to maintain more of the iron in the absorbable ferrous state.

PRECAUTIONS
Because FERANCEE-HP contains 110 mg of elemental iron per tablet, it is recommended that its use be limited to adults, ie over age 12 years.

DIRECTIONS
One tablet per day taken after a meal or as directed by a physician, should be sufficient to maintain normal hemoglobin levels in most patients with a history of recurring iron deficiency anemia. Not recommended for children under 12 years of age.
For acute and/or severe iron deficiency anemia, two or three tablets per day taken one tablet per dose after meals. (Each tablet provides 110 mg elemental iron).

WARNINGS
As with all medications, keep out of the reach of children. In case of accidental overdose, seek professional assistance or contact a Poison Control Center immediately.

HOW SUPPLIED
FERANCEE-HP is supplied in bottles of 60 red, film-coated, oval-shaped tablets.
NDC 0038-0863.
Note: A child-resistant safety cap is standard on each bottle of 60 tablets as a safeguard against accidental ingestion by children.
Shown in Product Identification Section, page 432

HIBICLENS® Antiseptic Antimicrobial
[hi′bi-klenz]
Skin Cleanser
(chlorhexidine gluconate)

DESCRIPTION
HIBICLENS is an antiseptic antimicrobial skin cleanser possessing bactericidal activities. HIBICLENS contains 4% w/v HIBITANE® (chlorhexidine gluconate), a chemically unique hexamethylenebis biguanide with inactive ingredients: fragrance, isopropyl alcohol 4%, purified water, Red 40, and other ingredients, in a mild, sudsing base adjusted to pH 5.0–6.5 for optimal activity and stability as well as compatability with the normal pH of the skin.

ACTION
HIBICLENS is bactericidal on contact. It has antiseptic activity and a persistent antimicrobial effect with rapid bactericidal activity against a wide range of microorganisms, including gram-positive bacteria, and gram-negative bacteria such as *Pseudomonas aeruginosa*. The effectiveness of

Continued on next page

Stuart—Cont.

HIBICLENS is not signficantly reduced by the presence of organic matter, such as blood.[1]

In a study[2] simulating surgical use, the immediate bactericidal effect of HIBICLENS after a single six-minute scrub resulted in a 99.9% reduction in resident bacterial flora, with a reduction of 99.98% after the eleventh scrub. Reductions on surgically gloved hands were maintained over the six-hour test period.

HIBICLENS displays persistent antimicrobial action. In one study[2], 93% of a radiolabeled formulation of HIBICLENS remained present on uncovered skin after five hours.

HIBICLENS prevents skin infection thereby reducing the risk of cross-infection.

INDICATIONS

HIBICLENS is indicated for use as a surgical scrub, as a health-care personnel handwash, for patient preoperative showering and bathing, as a patient preoperative skin preparation, and as a skin wound cleanser and general skin cleanser.

SAFETY

The extensive use of chlorhexidine gluconate for over 20 years outside the United States has produced no evidence of absorption of the compound through intact skin. The potential for producing skin reactions is extremely low. HIBICLENS can be used many times a day without causing irritation, dryness, or discomfort. Experimental studies indicate that when used for cleaning superficial wounds, HIBICLENS will neither cause additional tissue injury nor delay healing.

WARNINGS

FOR EXTERNAL USE ONLY. KEEP OUT OF EYES, EARS AND MOUTH. HIBICLENS SHOULD NOT BE USED AS A PREOPERATIVE SKIN PREPARATION OF THE FACE OR HEAD. MISUSE OF HIBICLENS HAS BEEN REPORTED TO CAUSE SERIOUS AND PERMANENT EYE INJURY WHEN IT HAS BEEN PERMITTED TO ENTER AND REMAIN IN THE EYE DURING SURGICAL PROCEDURES. IF HIBICLENS SHOULD CONTACT THESE AREAS, RINSE OUT PROMPTLY AND THOROUGHLY WITH WATER. Avoid contact with meninges. HIBICLENS should not be used by persons who have a sensitivity to it or its components. Chlorhexidine gluconate has been reported to cause deafness when instilled in the middle ear through perforated ear drums. Irritation, sensitization and generalized allergic reactions have been reported with chlorhexidine-containing products, especially in the genital areas. If adverse reactions occur, discontinue use immediately and if severe, contact a physician. Keep this and all drugs out of the reach of children. In case of accidental ingestion, seek professional assistance or contact a Poison Control Center immediately.

Accidental ingestion: Chlorhexidine gluconate taken orally is poorly absorbed. Treat with gastric lavage using milk, egg white, gelatin or mild soap. Employ supportive measures as appropriate.

Avoid excessive heat (above 104°F).

DIRECTIONS FOR USE

Patient preoperative skin preparation

Apply HIBICLENS liberally to surgical site and swab for at least two minutes. Dry with a sterile towel. Repeat procedure for an additional two minutes and dry with a sterile towel.

Preoperative showering and whole-body bathing

The patient should be instructed to wash the entire body, including the scalp, on two consecutive occasions immediately prior to surgery. Each procedure should consist of two consecutive thorough applications of HIBICLENS followed by thorough rinsing. If the patient's condition allows, showering is recommended for whole-body bathing. The recommended procedure is: Wet the body, including hair. Wash the hair using 25 mL of HIBICLENS and the body with another 25 mL of HIBICLENS. Rinse. Repeat. Rinse thoroughly after second application.

Skin wound and general skin cleansing

Wounds which involve more than the superficial layers of the skin should not be routinely treated with HIBICLENS. HIBICLENS should not be used for repeated general skin cleansing of large body areas except in those patients whose underlying skin condition makes it necessary to reduce the bacterial population of the skin. To use, thoroughly rinse the area to be cleansed with water. Apply the minimum amount of HIBICLENS necessary to cover the skin or wound area and wash gently. Rinse again thoroughly.

Health-care personnel use

SURGICAL HAND SCRUB

Directions for use of HIBICLENS Liquid: Wet hands and forearms to the elbows with warm water. (Avoid using very cold or very hot water.) Dispense about 5 mL of HIBICLENS into cupped hands. Spread over both hands. Scrub hands and forearms for 3 minutes without adding water, using a brush or sponge. (Avoid using extremely hard-bristled brushes.) While scrubbing, pay particular attention to fingernails, cuticles, and interdigital spaces. (Do not use excessive pressure to produce additional lather.) Rinse thoroughly with warm water. Dispense about 5 mL of HIBICLENS into cupped hands. Wash for an additional 3 minutes. (No need to use brush or sponge.) Then rinse thoroughly. Dry thoroughly.

HAND WASH

Wet hands with warm water. (Avoid using very cold or very hot water.) Dispense about 5 mL of HIBICLENS into cupped hands. Wash for 15 seconds. (Do not use excessive pressure to produce additional lather.) Rinse thoroughly with warm water. Dry thoroughly.

Directions for use of HIBICLENS® Sponge/Brush: Open package and remove nail cleaner. Wet hands. Use nail cleaner under fingernails and to clean cuticles. Wet hands and forearms to the elbow with warm water. (Avoid using very cold or very hot water.) Wet sponge side of sponge/brush. Squeeze and pump immediately to work up adequate lather. Apply lather to hands and forearms using *sponge* side of the product. *Start 3 minute scrub* by using the brush side of the product to scrub *only* nails, cuticles, and interdigital areas. Use sponge side for scrubbing hands and forearms. (Avoid using brush on these more sensitive areas.) Rinse thoroughly with warm water. Scrub for an additional 3 minutes *using sponge side* only. To produce additional lather, add a small amount of water and pump the sponge. (While scrubbing, do not use excessive pressure to produce lather—a small amount of lather is all that is required to adequately cleanse skin with HIBICLENS.) Rinse and dry thoroughly, blotting hands and forearms with a soft sterile towel.

IMPORTANT LAUNDERING ADVICE FOR HOSPITAL STAFF AND OTHER USERS OF ANTISEPTIC PATIENT SKIN PREPARATIONS CONTAINING CHLORHEXIDINE GLUCONATE

Chlorhexidine gluconate is a unique agent that most closely fits the definition of an ideal antimicrobial agent, having (among others) one of the most important characteristics of persistent activity. This persistence is due to chlorhexidine gluconate binding to the protein of the skin and, thus, being available for residual activity over a relatively long period of time.

Chlorhexidine gluconate, however, binds not only to protein of the skin, but also to many fabrics, particularly cotton. Thus, special laundering procedures should be considered when such products contact these fabrics. As a result of such contact, chlorhexidine gluconate may become adsorbed onto the fabric and not be removed by washing. If sufficient available chlorine is present during the washing procedure, a fast brown stain may develop due to a chemical reaction between chlorhexidine gluconate and chlorine.

SUGGESTED LAUNDERING PROCEDURES TO LIMIT STAINING

1. **Not Aging.** Avoid allowing the product to age (set) on unwashed linens.
2. **Flushing and Washing.** A flush operation as the initial step in the wash process is helpful in the laundering of linen exposed to chlorhexidine gluconate. Such flushing is also important in the laundering of linen which contains organic materials such as blood or pus. For best results,

warm water flushes (90°–100°F) are recommended. After a number of initial flushings followed by a washing with a low alkaline/nonchlorine detergent, most articles which come in contact with chlorhexidine gluconate should have an acceptable level of whiteness. If a rewash process using bleach is necessary to achieve a greater degree of whiteness, the bleach used should be a nonchlorine bleach.

3. **Not Using Chlorine Bleach.** Modern laundering methods often make the use of chlorine bleach unnecessary. It is worthwhile trying to wash without chlorine to ascertain if the resulting degree of whiteness is acceptable. Omission of chlorine from the laundering process can extend the useful life of cotton articles since oxidizing bleaches such as chlorine may cause some damage to cellulose even when used in low concentration.
4. **Changing to a Peroxide-Type Bleach, Such as Sodium Perborate, Sodium Percarbonate or Hydrogen Peroxide.** This should eliminate the reaction which could occur with the use of chlorine bleaches. If a chlorine bleach must be used, a concentration of less than 7 ppm available chlorine ($\frac{1}{10}$ the normal bleach level) is suggested to minimize possible staining.

A NOTE ON LAUNDERING OF PERSONAL CLOTHING

The laundering procedures set forth above using low alkaline, nonchlorinated laundry detergents are also applicable to laundering of uniforms and lab coats. Commercially available laundry detergents which do not contain chlorine include Borax, Borateem, Dreft, Oxydol, and Ivory Snow. These products, however, will not remove stains previously set into the fabric.

RECLAMATION OF STAINED LINENS

For those linens which previously have been stained due to the chemical reaction between chlorhexidine gluconate and chlorine, the following laundering procedure may be helpful in reducing the visible stain:

[See table below].

HOW SUPPLIED

For general handwashing locations: pocket-size, 15 mL foil Packettes; plastic disposable bottles of 4 oz and 8 oz with dispenser caps; and 16 oz filled globes. *For surgical scrub areas:* disposable, unit-of-use 22 mL impregnated Sponge/Brushes with nail cleaner; plastic disposable bottles of 32 oz and 1 gal. The 32-oz bottle is designed for a special foot-operated wall dispenser. A hand-operated wall dispenser is available for the 16-oz globe. Hand pumps are available for 16 oz, 32 oz, and 1 gal sizes. Liquid: NDC 0038-0575. Sponge/Brush: NDC 0038-0577.

REFERENCES

1. Lowbury, EJL and Lilly, HA: The effect of blood on disinfection of surgeons' hands, Brit. J. Surg. 61:19–21 (Jan.) 1974.
2. Peterson AF, Rosenberg A, Alatary SD: Comparative evaluation of surgical scrub preparations, Surg. Gynecol. Obstet. 146:63–65 (Jan.) 1978.
Shown in Product Identification Section, page 432

HIBISTAT® Germicidal Hand Rinse
HIBISTAT® TOWELETTE
Germicidal Hand Wipe
[hi 'bi-stat]
(chlorhexidine gluconate)

DESCRIPTION

HIBISTAT is a germicidal hand rinse which provides rapid bactericidal action and has a persistent antimicrobial effect against a wide range of microorganisms. HIBISTAT is a clear, colorless liquid containing 0.5% w/w HIBITANE® (chlorhexidine gluconate) with inactive ingredients: emollients, isopropyl alcohol 70%, purified water.

INDICATIONS

HIBISTAT is indicated for health-care personnel use as a germicidal hand rinse. HIBISTAT is for hand hygiene on physically clean hands. It is used in those situations where hands are physically clean, but in need of degerming, when routine handwashing is not convenient or desirable. HIBISTAT provides rapid germicidal action and has a persistent effect.

HIBISTAT should be used in-between patients and procedures where there are no sinks available or continued return to the sink area is inconvenient. HIBISTAT can be used as an alternative to detergent-based products when hands are physically clean. Also, HIBISTAT is an effective germicidal hand rinse following a soap and water handwash.

WARNINGS

Flammable. This product is alcohol based. Alcohol is extremely flammable. It should be kept away from flame or devices which may generate an electrical spark.

FOR EXTERNAL USE ONLY. KEEP OUT OF EYES, EARS AND MOUTH. HIBISTAT SHOULD NOT BE USED AS A PREOPERATIVE SKIN PREPARATION OF THE FACE OR HEAD. MISUSE OF CHLORHEXIDINE-CONTAINING PRODUCTS HAS BEEN REPORTED TO CAUSE SERIOUS

Operation	Water Level	Temperature	Time (Min)	Supplies/ 100 lb
Break	Low	180°F	20	1.5 lb oxalic acid
Flush	High	Cold	1	
Emulsify	Low	160°F	5	18 oz emulsifier
Flush	High	Cold	1	
Bleach	Low	180°F	20	2 lb alkali builder and 1 lb organic bleach
Rinse	High	Cold	1	—
Antichlor	High	Cold	2	4 oz antichlor
Rinse	High	Cold	1	—
Rinse	High	Cold	1	—
Sour	Low	Cold	4	2 oz rust removing sour

AND PERMANENT EYE INJURY WHEN IT HAS BEEN PERMITTED TO ENTER AND REMAIN IN THE EYE DURING SURGICAL PROCEDURES. IF HIBISTAT SHOULD CONTACT THESE AREAS, RINSE OUT PROMPTLY AND THOROUGHLY WITH WATER. Avoid contact with meninges. HIBISTAT should not be used by persons who have a sensitivity to it or its components. Chlorhexidine gluconate has been reported to cause deafness when instilled in the middle ear through perforated ear drums. Irritation, sensitization, and generalized allergic reactions have been reported with chlorhexidine-containing products, especially in the genital areas. If adverse reactions occur, discontinue use immediately and if severe, contact a physician. Keep this and all drugs out of the reach of children. In case of accidental ingestion, seek professional assistance or contact a Poison Control Center immediately. Avoid excessive heat (above 104°F).

Accidental ingestion: Chlorhexidine gluconate taken orally is poorly absorbed. Treat with gastric lavage using milk, egg white, gelatin or mild soap avoiding pulmonary aspiration. Do not use apomorphine. Assist respiration if necessary and keep patient warm. Intravenous levulose can accelerate alcohol metabolism. In severe cases, hemodialysis or peritoneal dialysis may be appropriate.

DIRECTIONS FOR USE

HIBISTAT Towelette: Rub hands vigorously with the HIBISTAT Towelette for approximately 15 seconds, paying particular attention to nails and interdigital spaces. HIBISTAT dries rapidly in use. No water or towel drying are necessary. The emollients contained in the HIBISTAT Towelette protect the hands from the potential drying effect of alcohol.

HIBISTAT Liquid: Dispense about 5 mL of HIBISTAT into cupped hands and rub vigorously until dry (about 15 seconds), paying particular attention to nails and interdigital spaces. HIBISTAT dries rapidly in use. No water or toweling are necessary. The emollients contained in HIBISTAT protect the hands from the potential drying effect of alcohol.

LAUNDERING

Chlorhexidine gluconate chemically reacts with chlorine to form a brown stain on fabric. Fabric which has come in contact with chlorhexidine gluconate should be rinsed well and washed without the addition of chlorine products. If bleach is desired, only nonchlorine bleach should be used. Full laundering instructions are packed with each case of HIBISTAT. (Please see HIBICLENS® for full laundering instructions).

HOW SUPPLIED

In plastic disposable bottles of 4 oz and 8 oz with flip-top cap, and in disposable towelettes containing 5 mL, packaged 50 towelettes to a carton.
NDC 0038-0585 (bottles)
NDC 0038-0587 (towelettes)

Shown in Product Identification Section, page 432

KASOF® Capsules
[*kay 'sof*]
High Strength Stool Softener Laxative

DESCRIPTION

KASOF provides a highly efficient wetting action to restore moisture to the bowel, thus softening the stool to prevent straining. The action of KASOF does not interfere with normal peristalsis and generally does not cause griping or extreme sensation of urgency: KASOF is sodium-free, containing a unique potassium formulation, without the problems associated with sodium intake.

INGREDIENTS

Each capsule contains: Active: docusate potassium, 240 mg. Inactive: Blue 1, gelatin, glycerin, methylparaben, polyethylene glycol, propylparaben, purified water, Red 40, sorbitol, Yellow 10.

INDICATIONS

KASOF is indicated for the relief of occasional constipation (irregularity).
KASOF is especially valuable for the severely constipated, as well as for patients with anorectal disorders, such as hemorrhoids and anal fissures. KASOF is ideal for patients with any condition that can be complicated by straining at stool, for example, cardiac patients. The simple, one-a-day dosage helps assure patient compliance in maintaining normal bowel function.

DIRECTIONS

Adults: One KASOF capsule daily for several days, or until bowel movements are normal and gentle. It is helpful to increase the daily intake of fluids by drinking a glass of water with each dose.
Store in a closed container, protect from freezing and avoid excessive heat (104°F).

WARNINGS

As with any drug, if you are pregnant or nursing a baby, seek the advice of a health professional before using this product. Keep out of the reach of children.

HOW SUPPLIED

KASOF is available in bottles of 30 and 60 brown, gelatin capsules, identified "Stuart 380."
NDC 0038-0380.

Shown in Product Identification Section, page 432

KINESED® Tablets   ℞
[*kin 'e-sed*]
(belladonna alkaloids and phenobarbital)

DESCRIPTION

Each chewable, fruit-flavored, scored, oval KINESED tablet contains:

Phenobarbital	16 mg

    (Warning: May be habit forming)

Hyoscyamine Sulfate ⎞	
Atropine Sulfate ⎬	0.12 mg
Scopolamine Hydrobromide	0.007 mg

Inactive ingredients: calcium silicate, citric acid, confectioner's sugar, flavors, glyceryl monostearate, lactose, mannitol, povidone, saccharin calcium, sodium citrate, starch, stearic acid.

ACTIONS

This drug combination provides natural belladonna alkaloids in a specific, fixed ratio combined with phenobarbital to provide peripheral anticholinergic/antispasmodic action and mild sedation.

INDICATIONS

Based on a review of this drug by the National Academy of Sciences—National Research Council and/or other information, FDA has classified the following indications as "possibly" effective:
For use as adjunctive therapy in the treatment of irritable bowel syndrome (irritable colon, spastic colon, mucous colitis) and acute enterocolitis.
May also be useful as adjunctive therapy in the treatment of duodenal ulcer. IT HAS NOT BEEN SHOWN CONCLUSIVELY WHETHER ANTICHOLINERGIC/ANTISPASMODIC DRUGS AID IN THE HEALING OF A DUODENAL ULCER, DECREASE THE RATE OF RECURRENCES, OR PREVENT COMPLICATIONS.

CONTRAINDICATIONS

Glaucoma, obstructive uropathy (for example, bladder neck obstruction due to prostatic hypertrophy); obstructive disease of the gastrointestinal tract (as in achalasia, pyloroduodenal stenosis, etc.); paralytic ileus, intestinal atony of the elderly or debilitated patient; unstable cardiovascular status in acute hemorrhage; severe ulcerative colitis, especially if complicated by toxic megacolon; myasthenia gravis; hiatal hernia associated with reflux esophagitis.
KINESED is contraindicated in patients with known hypersensitivity to any of the ingredients. Phenobarbital is contraindicated in acute intermittent porphyria and in those patients in whom phenobarbital produces restlessness and/or excitement.

WARNINGS

In the presence of a high environmental temperature, heat prostration can occur with belladonna alkaloids (fever and heatstroke due to decreased sweating). Diarrhea may be an early symptom of incomplete intestinal obstruction, especially in patients with ileostomy or colostomy. In this instance treatment with this drug would be inappropriate and possibly harmful.
KINESED may produce drowsiness or blurred vision. The patient should be warned, should these occur, not to engage in activities requiring mental alertness, such as operating a motor vehicle or other machinery, and not to perform hazardous work.
Phenobarbital may decrease the effect of anticoagulants, and necessitate larger doses of the anticoagulant for optimal effect. When the phenobarbital is discontinued, the dose of the anticoagulant may have to be decreased.
Phenobarbital may be habit forming and should not be administered to individuals known to be addiction prone or those with a history of physical and/or psychological dependence upon drugs.
Since barbiturates are metabolized in the liver, they should be used with caution and initial doses should be small in patients with hepatic dysfunction.

PRECAUTIONS

Use with caution in patients with: autonomic neuropathy, hepatic or renal disease, hyperthyroidism, coronary heart disease, congestive heart failure, cardiac arrhythmias, tachycardia, and hypertension.
Belladonna alkaloids may produce a delay in gastric emptying (antral stasis) which would complicate the management of gastric ulcer. Theoretically, with overdosage, a curare-like action may occur.
Carcinogenesis, mutagenesis. Long-term studies in animals have not been performed to evaluate carcinogenic potential.
Pregnancy Category C. Animal reproduction studies have not been conducted with KINESED. It is not known whether KINESED can cause fetal harm when administered to a pregnant woman or can affect reproductive capacity. KINESED should be given to a pregnant woman only if clearly needed.
Nursing mothers. Because belladonna alkaloids and phenobarbital are excreted in human milk, caution should be exercised when KINESED is administered to a nursing mother.

ADVERSE REACTIONS

Adverse reactions may include xerostomia; urinary hesitancy and retention; blurred vision; tachycardia; palpitation; mydriasis; cycloplegia; increased ocular tension; loss of taste sense; headache; nervousness; drowsiness; weakness; dizziness; insomnia; nausea; vomiting; impotence; suppression of lactation; constipation; bloated feeling; severe allergic reaction or drug idiosyncrasies, including anaphylaxis, urticaria and other dermal manifestations; and decreased sweating. Elderly patients may react with symptoms of excitement, agitation, drowsiness, and other untoward manifestations to even small doses of the drug.
Phenobarbital may produce excitement in some patients, rather than a sedative effect. In patients habituated to barbiturates, abrupt withdrawal may produce delirium or convulsions.

DOSAGE AND ADMINISTRATION

The dosage of KINESED chewable tablets should be adjusted to the needs of the individual patient to assure symptomatic control with a minimum of adverse effects.
ADULTS: One or two KINESED tablets, three or four times daily, chewed or swallowed with liquids.
CHILDREN, 2 to 12 years: One-half to one KINESED tablet, three or four times daily, chewed or swallowed with liquids.

OVERDOSAGE

The signs and symptoms of overdose are headache, nausea, vomiting, blurred vision, dilated pupils, hot and dry skin, dizziness, dryness of the mouth, difficulty in swallowing and CNS stimulation. Treatment should consist of gastric lavage, emetics, and activated charcoal. If indicated, parenteral cholinergic agents such as physostigmine or bethanechol chloride should be added.

HOW SUPPLIED

Bottles of 100 white scored, oval, fruit-flavored, chewable tablets (embossed front "STUART," reverse "220"). Store at room temperature; avoid excessive heat (above 104°F/40°C). Dispense in well-closed, light-resistant container. NDC 0038-0220.

Shown in Product Identification Section, page 432
C/10/85

MULVIDREN®–F SOFTAB® Tablets   ℞
[*mul 'vi-dren*]
(fluoride with multivitamins)

DESCRIPTION

MULVIDREN-F SOFTAB Tablets are formulated to provide daily, oral supplementation of fluoride and multivitamins. The unique design of the tablet assures delivery of all ingredients whether swallowed whole, chewed, allowed to dissolve in the mouth or crushed and mixed with food.

EACH TABLET CONTAINS

Fluoride (from 2.2 mg sodium fluoride)	1 mg
Vitamin A	4,000 USP units
Vitamin D (ergocalciferol)	400 USP units
Vitamin C (ascorbic acid and	
sodium ascorbate)	75 mg
Thiamin Mononitrate	1.6 mg
Riboflavin	2 mg
Vitamin B_6 (as pyridoxine hydrochloride)	1.0 mg
Vitamin B_{12} (cyanocobalamin)	3 mcg
Niacinamide	10 mg
Pantothenic Acid	2.8 mg

Inactive ingredients: flavors, mannitol, saccharin calcium, starch, Yellow 6 (Sunset Yellow).

CLINICAL PHARMACOLOGY

Soluble fluorides such as sodium fluoride are efficiently absorbed from the gastrointestinal tract of man, and some topical absorption occurs on tooth surfaces. The major route of fluoride excretion is by way of the kidneys. Fluoride is also excreted in small amounts in sweat, breast milk and feces.

Continued on next page

Stuart—Cont.

Fluoride provides much of its protective action against dental caries by combining with apatite crystals in the tooth structure, thus, forming the less acid soluble compound fluorapatite.

Controlled studies show a decrease in the incidence of dental caries in children receiving an optimal nutritional supply of fluoride. To achieve maximal anticariogenic effect, fluoride must be provided throughout the stages of tooth formation and calcification. Thus, fluoride should be provided in adequate amounts from birth through the first 15 years of life. If natural sources are deficient, fluoride should be made available throughout this period by daily dietary supplementation. MULVIDREN-F SOFTAB is a well-accepted and convenient form of administering fluoride for both topical and systemic effects.

INDICATIONS AND USAGE

As an aid in promoting the development of caries-resistant teeth in children from birth through the first 15 years of life. MULVIDREN-F provides a source of daily fluoride supplementation in addition to full nutritional amounts of vitamins.

CONTRAINDICATIONS

Patients living in areas where the drinking water is fluoridated at a concentration of greater than 0.7 ppm and those persons with a known sensitivity to fluoride should not take MULVIDREN-F.

WARNINGS

Dental fluorosis (mottling) may result from exceeding the recommended dose (see Dosage and Administration).

PRECAUTIONS

When prescribing MULVIDREN-F, the physician should make sure the child is not receiving significant amounts of fluoride from other sources (ie, medications, drinking water) (see Dosage and Administration).

ADVERSE REACTIONS

In hypersensitive individuals, fluorides occasionally cause skin eruptions such as atropic dermatitis, eczema or urticaria. Gastric distress, headache and weakness have also been reported. These hypersensitivity reactions usually disappear promptly after discontinuation of the fluoride. In rare cases, a delay in the eruption of teeth has been reported.

DOSAGE AND ADMINISTRATION

The daily fluoride intake from dietary supplements such as MULVIDREN-F must be adjusted according to the fluoride intake from other sources such as drinking water. The following dosage schedules are recommended.

Less than 0.3 ppm fluoride in drinking water:
Infants, birth to 2 years of age—0.25 mg of fluoride daily.
Children 2 to 3 years of age—0.5 mg of fluoride daily or one-half MULVIDREN-F tablet daily.
Children 3 to 16 years of age—1.0 mg of fluoride daily or one MULVIDREN-F tablet daily.

0.3 to 0.7 ppm fluoride in drinking water:
Infants, birth to 2 years of age—no fluoride supplementation recommended.
Children 2 to 3 years of age—0.25 mg of fluoride daily
Children 3 to 16 years of age—0.5 mg of fluoride daily or one-half MULVIDREN-F tablet daily

Greater than 0.7 ppm fluoride in drinking water:
No fluoride supplementation recommended.
MULVIDREN-F tablets may be swallowed, chewed and swallowed, allowed to dissolve in the mouth or crushed and mixed with food.

HOW SUPPLIED

In bottles of 100 orange colored, scored SOFTAB tablets, identified front "Stuart," reverse "710." A child-resistant safety cap is standard on each 100 tablet bottle as a safeguard against accidental ingestion. NDC 0038-0710.

Rev. C 9/87

Shown in Product Identification Section, page 432

MYLANTA®
[my-lan'ta]
Liquid and Tablets
Antacid/Anti-Gas

INGREDIENTS

Each chewable tablet or each 5 mL (one teaspoonful) of liquid contains:
Active: Aluminum hydroxide
(Dried Gel, USP in tablet and equiv.
to Dried Gel, USP in liquid) .... 200 mg
Magnesium hydroxide .... 200 mg
Simethicone .... 20 mg
Inactive: Tablets: dextrates, flavors, magnesium stearate, mannitol, sorbitol, starch, Yellow 10. Liquid: butylparaben, carboxymethylcellulose sodium, flavors, hydroxypropyl methylcellulose, microcrystalline cellulose, propylparaben, purified water, sorbitol solution with no added sugar.
Sodium Content: MYLANTA contains an insignificant amount of sodium per daily dose and is considered dietetically sodium free. Typical values are 0.68 mg (0.03 mEq) sodium per 5 mL teaspoonful of liquid and 0.77 mg (0.03 mEq) per tablet.
Acid Neutralizing Capacity: Two teaspoonfuls of MYLANTA Liquid will neutralize 25.4 mEq of acid. Two MYLANTA tablets will neutralize 23.0 mEq.

INDICATIONS

MYLANTA, a well-balanced combination of two antacids and simethicone, provides consistently dependable relief of symptoms associated with gastric hyperacidity, and mucus-entrapped air or "gas". These indications include:

Common heartburn (pyrosis)
Hiatal hernia
Peptic esophagitis
Gastritis
Peptic ulcer

The exceptionally pleasant tasting liquid and soft, easy-to-chew tablets encourage patients' acceptance, thereby minimizing the skipping of prescribed doses. MYLANTA is appropriate whenever there is a need for effective relief of temporary gastric hyperacidity and mucus-entrapped gas.

DIRECTIONS

Liquid: Shake well, 2–4 teaspoonfuls between meals and at bedtime or as directed by a physician.
Tablets: 2–4 tablets, well chewed, between meals and at bedtime or as directed by a physician.

WARNINGS

Keep this and all other drugs out of the reach of children. Except under the advice and supervision of a physician: Do not take more than 24 tsps/tablets in a 24 hour period or use the maximum dose of this product for more than two weeks. Do not use this product if you have kidney disease.
Magnesium hydroxide and other magnesium salts, in the presence of renal insufficiency, may cause central nervous system depression and other symptoms of hypermagnesemia.

DRUG INTERACTION PRECAUTION

Do not use this product for any patient receiving a prescription antibiotic containing any form of tetracycline.

HOW SUPPLIED

MYLANTA is available as a white, pleasant-tasting liquid suspension, and as a two-layer yellow and white chewable tablet, identified on yellow layer "STUART 620." Liquid supplied in bottles of 5 oz, 12 oz, and 24 oz. Tablets supplied in boxes of individually wrapped 40s and 100s, economy size bottles of 180, consumer convenience pocket packs of 48, roll packs of 12 tablets each and 3-roll packs containing 36 tablets. Also available for hospital use in liquid unit dose bottles of 1 oz, and bottles of 5 oz.
NDC 0038-0610 (liquid). NDC 0038-0620 (tablets).

Shown in Product Identification Section, page 432

MYLANTA®–II
[my-lan'ta]
Liquid and Tablets
Double Strength Antacid/Anti-Gas

INGREDIENTS

Each chewable tablet or each 5 mL (one teaspoonful) of liquid contains:
Active: Aluminum hydroxide
(Dried Gel, USP in tablet and equiv.
to Dried Gel, USP in liquid) .... 400 mg
Magnesium hydroxide .... 400 mg
Simethicone .... 40 mg
Inactive: Liquid: butylparaben, carboxymethylcellulose sodium, flavors, hydroxypropyl methylcellulose, microcrystalline cellulose, potassium citrate, propylparaben, purified water, sorbitol solution with no added sugar.
Tablets: Blue 1, cereal solids, confectioner's sugar, flavors, glycerin, lactose, mannitol, starch, Yellow 10.
Sodium Content: MYLANTA-II contains an insignificant amount of sodium per daily dose. Typical values are 1.14 mg (0.05 mEq) sodium per 5 mL teaspoonful of liquid and 1.3 mg (0.06 mEq) per tablet.
Acid Neutralizing Capacity: Two teaspoonfuls of MYLANTA-II liquid will neutralize 50.8 mEq of acid. Two MYLANTA-II tablets will neutralize 46.0 mEq.

INDICATIONS

MYLANTA-II is a double strength antacid with an anti-gas ingredient for the relief of heartburn, acid indigestion, sour stomach, and accompanying gas. The exceptionally pleasant tasting liquid and soft, easy-to-chew tablets encourage patient acceptance, thereby minimizing the skipping of prescribed doses. MYLANTA-II provides consistently dependable relief of the symptoms of peptic ulcer and other problems related to acid hypersecretion. The high potency of MYLANTA-II is achieved through its concentration of non-calcium antacid ingredients. Thus MYLANTA-II can produce both rapid and long lasting neutralization without the acid rebound associated with calcium carbonate. The balanced formula of aluminum and magnesium hydroxides minimizes undesirable bowel effects. Simethicone is effective for the relief of concomitant distress caused by mucus-entrapped gas and swallowed air.

DIRECTIONS

Liquid: Shake well, 2–4 teaspoonfuls between meals and at bedtime, or as directed by a physician.
Tablets: 2–4 tablets, well chewed, between meals and at bedtime, or as directed by a physician.
Because patients with peptic ulcer vary greatly in both acid output and gastric emptying time, the amount and schedule of dosages should be varied accordingly.

WARNINGS

Keep this and all drugs out of the reach of children. Except under the advice and supervision of a physician: Do not take more than 12 tsps/tablets in a 24 hour period or use the maximum dose of this product for more than two weeks. Do not use this product if you have kidney disease.
Magnesium hydroxide and other magnesium salts, in the presence of renal insufficiency, may cause central nervous system depression and other symptoms of hypermagnesemia.

DRUG INTERACTION PRECAUTION

Do not use this product for any patient receiving a prescription antibiotic containing any form of tetracycline.

HOW SUPPLIED

MYLANTA-II is available as a white, pleasant-tasting liquid suspension and a two-layer green and white chewable tablet, identified on green layer "STUART 651." Liquid supplied in 2 oz, 5 oz, 12 oz, and 24 oz bottles. Tablets supplied in boxes of 60 individually wrapped chewable tablets and consumer convenience pocket packs of 24, 8 tablet roll packs and 3-roll packs containing 24 tablets. Also available for hospital use in liquid unit dose bottles of 1 oz, and bottles of 5 oz.
NDC 0038-0652 (liquid). NDC 0038-0651 (tablets).

Shown in Product Identification Section, page 432

MYLICON® Tablets and Drops
[my'li-con]
Antiflatulent

INGREDIENTS

Each tablet or 0.6 mL of drops contains: Active: simethicone, 40 mg. Inactive: Tablets: calcium silicate, lactose, povidone, saccharin calcium. Drops: carbomer 934P, citric acid, flavors, hydroxypropyl methylcellulose, purified water, Red 3, saccharin calcium, sodium benzoate, sodium citrate.

INDICATIONS

For relief of the painful symptoms of excess gas in the digestive tract. Such gas is frequently caused by excessive swallowing of air or by eating foods that disagree. If condition persists, consult your physician. MYLICON is a valuable adjunct in the treatment of many conditions in which the retention of gas may be a problem, such as: postoperative gaseous distention, air swallowing, functional dyspepsia, peptic ulcer, spastic or irritable colon, diverticulosis.
The defoaming action of MYLICON relieves flatulence by dispersing and preventing the formation of mucus-surrounded gas pockets in the gastrointestinal tract. MYLICON acts in the stomach and intestines to change the surface tension of gas bubbles enabling them to coalesce; thus the gas is freed and is eliminated more easily by belching or passing flatus.
Infants: MYLICON Drops are also useful for relief of the painful symptoms of excess gas associated with such conditions as colic, lactose intolerance, or air swallowing.

DIRECTIONS

Tablets—One or two tablets four times daily after meals and at bedtime. May also be taken as needed up to 12 tablets daily or as directed by a physician. TABLETS SHOULD BE CHEWED THOROUGHLY.
Drops—Adults and Children: 0.6 mL four times daily after meals and at bedtime or as directed by a physician. Infants (under 2 years): Initially, 0.3 mL four times daily, after meals and at bedtime, or as directed by a physician.
The dosage can also be mixed with 1 oz of cool water, infant formula, or other suitable liquids to ease administration. Dosage should not exceed 12 doses per day. Shake well before using.

WARNINGS

Keep this and all drugs out of the reach of chldren.

HOW SUPPLIED

Bottles of 100 and 500 white, scored, chewable tablets, identified front "STUART," reverse "450," and dropper bottles of 30 mL (1 fl. oz.) pink, pleasant tasting liquid. Also available in 100 tablet unit dose boxes (10 strips of 10 tablets each).

NDC 0038-0450 (tablets).
NDC 0038-0630 (drops).
Shown in Product Identification Section, page 432

MYLICON®-80 Tablets
[*my'li-con*]
High-Capacity Antiflatulent

INGREDIENTS
Each tablet contains: Active: simethicone, 80 mg. Inactive: cereal solids, flavor, lactose, mannitol, povidone, Red 3, talc.

INDICATIONS
For relief of the painful symptoms of excess gas in the digestive tract. Such gas is frequently caused by excessive swallowing of air or by eating foods that disagree. If condition persists, consult your physician. MYLICON-80 is a high capacity antiflatulent for adjunctive treatment of many conditions in which the retention of gas may be a problem, such as the following: air swallowing, functional dyspepsia, postoperative gaseous distention, peptic ulcer, spastic or irritable colon, diverticulosis.
MYLICON-80 has a defoaming action that relieves flatulence by dispersing and preventing the formation of mucussurrounded gas pockets in the gastrointestinal tract. MYLICON-80 acts in the stomach and intestines to change the surface tension of gas bubbles enabling them to coalesce; thus, the gas is freed and is eliminated more easily by belching or passing flatus.

DIRECTIONS
One tablet four times daily after meals and at bedtime. May also be taken as needed up to 6 tablets daily or as directed by a physician. TABLETS SHOULD BE CHEWED THOROUGHLY.

WARNINGS
Keep this and all drugs out of the reach of children.

HOW SUPPLIED
Economical bottles of 100 and convenience packages of individually wrapped 12 and 48 pink, scored, chewable tablets identified "STUART 858." Also available in 100 tablet unit dose boxes (10 strips of 10 tablets each).
NDC 0038-0858.
Shown in Product Identification Section, page 432

MYLICON®-125 Tablets
[*my'li-con*]
Maximum Strength Antiflatulent

INGREDIENTS
Each tablet contains: Active: simethicone, 125 mg. Inactive: cereal solids, flavor, lactose, mannitol, povidone, Red 3, talc.

INDICATIONS
MYLICON-125 is useful for relief of the painful symptoms of excess gas in the digestive tract. Such gas is frequently caused by excessive swallowing of air or by eating foods that disagree. If condition persists, consult your physician. MYLICON-125 is the strongest antiflatulent for adjunctive treatment of many conditions in which the retention of gas may be a problem such as the following: air swallowing, functional dyspepsia, postoperative gaseous distention, peptic ulcer, spastic or irritable colon, diverticulosis. MYLICON-125 has a defoaming action that relieves flatulence by dispensing and preventing the formation of mucus-surrounded gas pockets in the gastrointestinal tract. MYLICON-125 acts in the stomach and intestines to change the surface tension of gas bubbles enabling them to coalesce; thus, the gas is freed and is eliminated more easily by belching or passing flatus.

DIRECTIONS
One tablet four times daily after meals and at bedtime or as directed by physician. TABLETS SHOULD BE CHEWED THOROUGHLY.

WARNINGS
Keep this and all drugs out of the reach of children.

HOW SUPPLIED
Convenience packages of individually wrapped 12 and 60 dark pink, scored, chewable tablets, identified "STUART 455." Also available in 100 tablet unit dose boxes (10 strips of 10 tablets each). NDC 0038-0455.
Shown in Product Identification Section, page 432

OREXIN® SOFTAB® Tablets
[*o-rex'in*]
High Potency Vitamin Supplement

INGREDIENTS
Each tablet contains: Active: vitamin B_1, (thiamin mononitrate) 8.1 mg; vitamin B_6 (as pyridoxine hydrochloride), 4.1 mg; and vitamin B_{12} (cyanocobalamin), 25 mcg. Inactive: flavor, mannitol, saccharin calcium, sodium chloride, starch.

INDICATIONS
OREXIN is a high-potency vitamin supplement providing vitamins B_1, B_6, and B_{12}.
OREXIN SOFTAB tablets are specially formulated to dissolve quickly in the mouth. They may be chewed or swallowed. Dissolve tablet in a teaspoonful of water or fruit juice if liquid is preferred.

DIRECTIONS
One tablet daily or as directed by physician.

WARNINGS
Keep this and all drugs out of the reach of children.

HOW SUPPLIED
Bottles of 100 pale pink SOFTAB tablets, identified "STUART."
NDC 0038-0280.

PROBEC®-T Tablets
[*pro'bec-t*]
Vitamin B Complex Supplement

INGREDIENTS
Each tablet contains: Active: vitamin C (as ascorbic acid, 67 mg and sodium ascorbate, 600 mg); 600 mg; thiamin mononitrate, 12.2 mg; riboflavin, 10 mg; vitamin B_6 (as pyridoxine hydrochloride), 4.1 mg; vitamin B_{12} (cyanocobalamin), 5 mcg; niacinamide, 100 mg; calcium pantothenate, 18.4 mg.
Inactive: calcium sulfate, carnauba wax, magnesium oxide, pharmaceutical glaze, povidone, Red 30, sucrose, titanium dioxide, white wax, Yellow 10.

INDICATIONS
PROBEC-T is a high-potency B complex supplement with 600 mg of vitamin C in easy to swallow odorless tablets.

DIRECTIONS
One tablet a day with a meal, or as directed by physician.

WARNING
As with all medications, keep out of the reach of children.

HOW SUPPLIED
Bottles of 60, peach colored, capsule-shaped tablets.
NDC 0038-0840.
Shown in Product Identification Section, page 432

THE STUART FORMULA® Tablets
Multivitamin/Multimineral Supplement

ONE TABLET DAILY PROVIDES:

VITAMINS:	US RDA*		
A	100%		5,000 IU
D	100%		400 IU
E	50%		15 IU
C	100%		60 mg
Folic Acid	100%		0.4 mg
Thiamin	80%		1.2 mg
Riboflavin	100%		1.7 mg
Niacin	100%		20 mg
B_6	100%		2 mg
B_{12}	100%		6 mcg
MINERALS:	**US RDA**		
Calcium	16%		160 mg
Phosphorus	12%		125 mg
Iodine	100%		150 mcg
Iron	100%		18 mg
Magnesium	25%		100 mg

*Percentage of US Recommended Daily Allowances for adults and children 4 or more years of age.

INGREDIENTS
Active: dibasic calcium phosphate, magnesium oxide, ascorbic acid, ferrous fumarate, dl-alpha tocopheryl acetate, folic acid, niacinamide, vitamin A palmitate, cyanocobalamin, pyridoxine hydrochloride, riboflavin, thiamin mononitrate, ergocalciferol, potassium iodide. Inactive: calcium sulfate, carnauba wax, pharmaceutical glaze, povidone, sodium starch glycolate, starch, sucrose, titanium dioxide, white wax.

INDICATIONS
The STUART FORMULA tablet provides a well-balanced multivitamin/multimineral formula intended for use as a daily dietary supplement for adults and children over age four.

DIRECTIONS
One tablet daily or as directed by physician.

WARNINGS
Keep this and all drugs out of the reach of children. In case of accidental overdose, seek professional assistance or contact a Poison Control Center immediately.

HOW SUPPLIED
Bottles of 100 and 250 white, round tablets. Child-resistant safety caps are standard on both bottles as a safeguard against accidental ingestion by children.
NDC 0038-0866.
Shown in Product Identification Section, page 432

STUART PRENATAL® Tablets
Multivitamin/Multimineral Supplement

ONE TABLET DAILY PROVIDES:

Vitamins	RDA*	
A	100%	4,000 IU
D	100%	400 IU
E	100%	11 mg
C	100%	100 mg
Folic acid	100%	0.8 mg
Thiamin mononitrate	100%	1.5 mg
Riboflavin	100%	1.7 mg
Niacinamide	100%	18 mg
B_6 (pyridoxine)	100%	2.6 mg
B_{12}	100%	4 mcg
Minerals		
Calcium	17%	200 mg
Iron	330%**	60 mg
Zinc	100%	25 mg

*Recommended Dietary Allowances (Food and Nutrition Board, NAS/NRC-1980) for pregnant and lactating women.
**Recommended Dietary Allowances (Food and Nutrition Board, NAS/NRC-1980) for adults, not pregnant and lactating women.

Ingredients:
Active: calcium sulfate, ferrous fumarate, ascorbic acid, dl-alpha tocopheryl acetate, zinc oxide, niacinamide, vitamin A acetate, pyridoxine hydrochloride, riboflavin, thiamin, mononitrate, folic acid, cholecalciferol, cyanocobalamin. Inactive: croscarmellose sodium, hydroxpropyl methylcellulose, microcrystalline cellulose, pregelatinized starch, red iron oxide, titanium dioxide.

INDICATIONS
STUART PRENATAL is a nonprescription multivitamin/multimineral supplement for use before, during, and after pregnancy. It provides vitamins equal to 100% or more of the RDA for pregnant and lactating women, plus essential minerals, including 60 mg of elemental iron as well-tolerated ferrous fumarate, 200 mg of elemental calcium (non-alkalizing and phosphorus-free), and 25 mg zinc.

DIRECTIONS
Before, during and after pregnancy, one tablet daily, or as directed by a physician.

WARNINGS
As with all medications, keep out of the reach of children. In case of accidental overdose, seek professional assistance or contact a Poison Control Center immediately.

HOW SUPPLIED
Bottles of 100 light pink capsule-shaped tablets imprinted "Stuart 071." A child-resistant safety cap is standard on 100 tablet bottles as a safeguard against accidental ingestion by children.
NDC 0038-0071.
Shown in Product Identification Section, page 432

STUARTINIC® Tablets
[*stu"are-tin'ic*]
Hematinic

ONE TABLET DAILY PROVIDES:

	US RDA*		
Iron	556%		100 mg
VITAMINS:			
C	833%		500 mg
Thiamin	327%		4.9 mg
Riboflavin	353%		6 mg
Niacin	100%		20 mg
B_6	40%		0.8 mg
B_{12}	417%		25 mcg
Pantothenic Acid	92%		9.2 mg

*Percentage of US Recommended Daily Allowances for adults and children 4 or more years of age.

INGREDIENTS
Active: ferrous fumarate, ascorbic acid, sodium ascorbate, niacinamide, calcium pantothenate, thiamin mononitrate, riboflavin, pyridoxine hydrochloride, cyanocobalamin. Inactive: flavor, hydrogenated vegetable oil, microcrystalline cellulose, povidone, Yellow 6, Yellow 10, and other ingredients.

Continued on next page

Stuart—Cont.

INDICATIONS

STUARTINIC is a complete hematinic for patients with history of iron deficiency anemia who also lack proper amounts of vitamin C and B-complex vitamins due to inadequate diet.

The use of well-tolerated ferrous fumarate in STUARTINIC provides a high level of elemental iron with a low incidence of gastric distress. The inclusion of 500 mg of vitamin C per tablet serves to maintain more of the iron in the absorbable ferrous state. The B-complex vitamins improve nutrition where B-complex deficient diets contribute to the anemia.

WARNINGS

As with any drug, if you are pregnant or nursing a baby, seek the advice of a health professional before using this product. Keep out of the reach of children. In case of accidental overdose, seek professional assistance or contact a Poison Control Center immediately.

DOSAGE

One tablet daily taken after a meal or as directed by physician. Because of the high amount of iron per tablet, STUARTINIC is not recommended for children under 12 years of age.

HOW SUPPLIED

STUARTINIC is supplied in bottles of 60 yellow, film-coated, oval-shaped tablets. NDC 0038-0862.
Note: A child-resistant safety cap is standard on each 60 tablet bottle as a safeguard against accidental ingestion by children.

Shown in Product Identification Section, page 432

STUARTNATAL® 1+1 Tablets ℞
[stu 'art na 'tal]
Multivitamin/Multimineral Supplement

COMPOSITION

One tablet daily provides:

Vitamins	RDA*	
A	100%	4,000 IU
D (cholecalciferol)	100%	400 IU
E	100%	11 mg
C (ascorbic acid)	120%	120 mg
Folic acid	125%	1 mg
Thiamin mononitrate	100%	1.5 mg
Riboflavin	175%	3 mg
Niacinamide	110%	20 mg
B₆ (pyridoxine)	385%	10 mg
B₁₂ (cyanocobalamin)	300%	12 mcg
Minerals		
Calcium	17%	200 mg
Copper	100%	2 mg
Iron	360%**	65 mg
Zinc	100%	25 mg

*Recommended Dietary Allowances (Food and Nutrition Board, NAS/NRC-1980) for pregnant and lactating women.

**Recommended Dietary Allowances (Food and Nutrition Board, NAS/NRC-1980) for adults, not pregnant and/or lactating women.

INDICATIONS

STUARTNATAL 1+1 is indicated to provide potent vitamin and mineral supplementation throughout pregnancy and during the postnatal period—for both the lactating and non-lactating mother. It is also useful for improving nutritional status prior to conception.

Each tablet provides vitamins equal to 100% or more of RDA for pregnant and lactating women plus essential minerals, including 1 full grain of elemental iron and 200 mg. of elemental calcium (non-alkalizing and phosphorus-free), and 25 mg zinc. STUARTNATAL 1+1 also offers 1 mg folic acid to aid in the prevention of megaloblastic anemia.

PRECAUTION

Federal law prohibits dispensing without prescription. Folic acid may partially correct the hematological damage due to vitamin B₁₂ deficiency of pernicious anemia, while the associated neurological damage progresses.
Store at room temperature; avoid excess heat. Dispense in well-closed, light-resistant container.

DIRECTIONS

Before, during and after pregnancy, one tablet daily, or as directed by a physician.

WARNING

As with all medications, keep out of the reach of children. In case of accidental overdose, seek professional assistance or contact a Poison Control Center immediately.

HOW SUPPLIED

Bottles of 100 and 500 light yellow, capsule-shaped tablets identified "Stuart 021." A child-resistant safety cap is stan-

dard on 100 tablet bottles as a safeguard against accidental ingestion by children.
NDC 0038-0021.
Shown in Product Identification Section, page 432

ZESTORETIC® ℞
(lisinopril and hydrochlorothiazide)

DESCRIPTION

ZESTORETIC® (Lisinopril and Hydrochlorothiazide) combines an angiotensin converting enzyme inhibitor, lisinopril, and a diuretic, hydrochlorothiazide.

Lisinopril, a synthetic peptide derivative, is an oral long-acting angiotensin converting enzyme inhibitor. It is chemically described as (S)-1-[N^2-(1-Carboxy-3-phenylpropyl)-L-lysyl]-L-proline dihydrate. Its empirical formula is $C_{21}H_{31}N_3O_5 \cdot 2H_2O$ and its structural formula is:

Lisinopril is a white to off-white, crystalline powder, with a molecular weight of 441.53. It is soluble in water, sparingly soluble in methanol, and practically insoluble in ethanol. Hydrochlorothiazide is 6-chloro-3,4-dihydro-2H-1,2,4-benzothiadiazine-7-sulfonamide 1,1-dioxide. Its empirical formula is $C_7H_8ClN_3O_4S_2$ and its structural formula is:

Hydrochlorothiazide is a white, or practically white, crystalline powder with a molecular weight of 297.72, which is slightly soluble in water, but freely soluble in sodium hydroxide solution.
ZESTORETIC is available for oral use in two tablet combinations of lisinopril with hydrochlorothiazide: ZESTORETIC 20-12.5 containing 20 mg lisinopril and 12.5 mg hydrochlorothiazide; and, ZESTORETIC 20-25 containing 20 mg lisinopril and 25 mg hydrochlorothiazide.
Inactive Ingredients:
20-12.5 tablets—calcium phosphate, magnesium stearate, mannitol, starch.
20-25 tablets—calcium phosphate, magnesium stearate, mannitol, red ferric oxide, starch, yellow ferric oxide.

CLINICAL PHARMACOLOGY

Lisinopril and Hydrochlorothiazide: As a result of its diuretic effects, hydrochlorothiazide increases plasma renin activity, increases aldosterone secretion, and decreases serum potassium. Administration of lisinopril blocks the renin-angiotensin aldosterone axis and tends to reverse the potassium loss associated with the diuretic.
In clinical studies, the extent of blood pressure reduction seen with the combination of lisinopril and hydrochlorothiazide was approximately additive. The combination appeared somewhat less effective in black patients, but relatively few black patients were studied. In most patients, the antihypertensive effect of ZESTORETIC was sustained for at least 24 hours.
In a randomized, controlled comparison, the mean antihypertensive effects of ZESTORETIC 20-12.5 and ZESTORETIC 20-25 were similar, suggesting that many patients who respond adequately to the latter combination may be controlled with ZESTORETIC 20-12.5. (See DOSAGE AND ADMINISTRATION.)
Concomitant administration of lisinopril and hydrochlorothiazide has little or no effect on the bioavailability of either drug. The combination tablet is bioequivalent to concomitant administration of the separate entities.
Lisinopril
Mechanism of Action: Lisinopril inhibits angiotensin-converting enzyme (ACE) in human subjects and animals. ACE is a peptidyl dipeptidase that catalyzes the conversion of angiotensin I to the vasoconstrictor substance, angiotensin II. Angiotensin II also stimulates aldosterone secretion by the adrenal cortex. Inhibition of ACE results in decreased plasma angiotensin II which leads to decreased vasopressor activity and to decreased aldosterone secretion. The latter decrease may result in a small increase of serum potassium. Removal of angiotensin II negative feedback on renin secretion leads to increased plasma renin activity. In hypertensive patients with normal renal function treated with lisinopril alone for up to 24 weeks, the mean increase in serum potassium was less than 0.1 mEq/L; however, approximately 15 percent of patients had increases greater than 0.5 mEq/L and approximately six percent had a decrease greater than 0.5 mEq/L. In the same study, patients treated with lisino-

pril plus a thiazide diuretic showed essentially no change in serum potassium. (See PRECAUTIONS.)
ACE is identical to kininase, an enzyme that degrades bradykinin. Whether increased levels of bradykinin, a potent vasodepressor peptide, play a role in the therapeutic effects of lisinopril remains to be elucidated.
While the mechanism through which lisinopril lowers blood pressure is believed to be primarily suppression of the renin-angiotensin-aldosterone system, lisinopril is antihypertensive even in patients with low-renin hypertension. Although lisinopril was antihypertensive in all races studied, black hypertensive patients (usually a low-renin hypertensive population) had a smaller average response to lisinopril monotherapy than nonblack patients.
Pharmacokinetics and Metabolism: Following oral administration of lisinopril, peak serum concentrations occur within about 7 hours. Declining serum concentrations exhibit a prolonged terminal phase which does not contribute to drug accumulation. This terminal phase probably represents saturable binding to ACE and is not proportional to dose. Lisinopril does not appear to be bound to other serum proteins.
Lisinopril does not undergo metabolism and is excreted unchanged entirely in the urine. Based on urinary recovery, the mean extent of absorption of lisinopril is approximately 25 percent, with large intersubject variability (6%–60%) at all doses tested (5–80 mg). Lisinopril absorption is not influenced by the presence of food in the gastrointestinal tract. Upon multiple dosing, lisinopril exhibits an effective half-life of accumulation of 12 hours.
Impaired renal function decreases elimination of lisinopril, which is excreted principally through the kidneys, but this decrease becomes clinically important only when the glomerular filtration rate is below 30 mL/min. Above this glomerular filtration rate, the elimination half-life is little changed. With greater impairment, however, peak and trough lisinopril levels increase, time to peak concentration increases and time to attain steady state is prolonged. Older patients, on average, have (approximately doubled) higher blood levels and area under the plasma concentration time curve (AUC) than younger patients. (See DOSAGE AND ADMINISTRATION.) Lisinopril can be removed by hemodialysis.
Studies in rats indicate that lisinopril crosses the blood-brain barrier poorly. Multiple doses of lisinopril in rats do not result in accumulation in any tissues. However, milk of lactating rats contains radioactivity following administration of ¹⁴C lisinopril. By whole body autoradiography, radioactivity was found in the placenta following administration of labeled drug to pregnant rats, but none was found in the fetuses.
Pharmacodynamics: Administration of lisinopril to patients with hypertension results in a reduction of supine and standing blood pressure to about the same extent with no compensatory tachycardia. Symptomatic postural hypotension is usually not observed although it can occur and should be anticipated in volume and/or salt-depleted patients. (See WARNINGS.)
In most patients studied, onset of antihypertensive activity was seen at one hour after oral administration of an individual dose of lisinopril, with peak reduction of blood pressure achieved by six hours.
In some patients achievement of optimal blood pressure reduction may require two to four weeks of therapy.
At recommended single daily doses, antihypertensive effects have been maintained for at least 24 hours, after dosing, although the effect at 24 hours was substantially smaller than the effect six hours after dosing.
The antihypertensive effects of lisinopril have continued during long term therapy. Abrupt withdrawal of lisinopril has not been associated with a rapid increase in blood pressure; nor with a significant overshoot of pretreatment blood pressure.
In hemodynamic studies in patients with essential hypertension, blood pressure reduction was accompanied by a reduction in peripheral arterial resistance with little or no change in cardiac output and in heart rate. In a study in nine hypertensive patients, following administration of lisinopril, there was an increase in mean renal blood flow that was not significant. Data from several small studies are inconsistent with respect to the effect of lisinopril on glomerular filtration rate in hypertensive patients with normal renal function, but suggest that changes, if any, are not large.
In patients with renovascular hypertension lisinopril has been shown to be well tolerated and effective in controlling blood pressure. (See PRECAUTIONS.)
Hydrochlorothiazide
The mechanism of the antihypertensive effect of thiazides is unknown. Thiazides do not usually affect normal blood pressure.
Hydrochlorothiazide is a diuretic and antihypertensive. It affects the distal renal tubular mechanism of electrolyte reabsorption. Hydrochlorothiazide increases excretion of sodium and chloride in approximately equivalent amounts. Natriuresis may be accompanied by some loss of potassium and bicarbonate.

After oral use diuresis begins within two hours, peaks in about four hours and lasts about 6 to 12 hours. Hydrochlorothiazide is not metabolized but is eliminated rapidly by the kidney. When plasma levels have been followed for at least 24 hours, the plasma half-life has been observed to vary between 5.6 and 14.8 hours. At least 61 percent of the oral dose is eliminated unchanged within 24 hours. Hydrochlorothiazide crosses the placental but not the blood-brain barrier.

INDICATIONS AND USAGE

ZESTORETIC is indicated for the treatment of hypertension in patients for whom combination therapy is appropriate. **This fixed dose combination is not indicated for initial therapy. Patients already receiving a diuretic when lisinopril is initiated, or given a diuretic and lisinopril simultaneously, can develop symptomatic hypotension. In the initial titration of the individual entities, it is important, if possible, to stop the diuretic for several days before starting lisinopril or, if this is not possible, begin lisinopril at a low initial dose. (See DOSAGE AND ADMINISTRATION.)**

In using ZESTORETIC, consideration should be given to the fact that an angiotensin converting enzyme inhibitor, captopril, has caused agranulocytosis, particularly in patients with renal impairment or collagen vascular disease, and that available data are insufficient to show that lisinopril does not have a similar risk. (See WARNINGS.)

CONTRAINDICATIONS

ZESTORETIC is contraindicated in patients who are hypersensitive to any component of this product and in patients with a history of angioedema related to previous treatment with an angiotensin converting enzyme inhibitor. Because of the hydrochlorothiazide component, this product is contraindicated in patients with anuria or hypersensitivity to other sulfonamide-derived drugs.

WARNINGS

Lisinopril

Angioedema: Angioedema of the face, extremities, lips, tongue, glottis and/or larynx has been reported rarely in patients treated with angiotensin converting enzyme inhibitors, including lisinopril. In such cases ZESTORETIC should be promptly discontinued and the patient carefully observed until the swelling disappears. In instances where swelling has been confined to the face and lips the condition has generally resolved without treatment, although antihistamines have been useful in relieving symptoms. Angioedema associated with laryngeal edema may be fatal. **Where there is involvement of the tongue, glottis or larynx, likely to cause airway obstruction, subcutaneous epinephrine solution 1:1000 (0.3 mL to 0.5 mL) should be promptly administered and/or other appropriate therapy should be instituted. (See ADVERSE REACTIONS.)**

Hypotension and Related Effects: Excessive hypotension was rarely seen in uncomplicated hypertensive patients but is a possible consequence of lisinopril use in salt/volume-depleted persons such as those treated vigorously with diuretics or patients on dialysis. (See PRECAUTIONS, Drug Interactions and ADVERSE REACTIONS.)

Syncope has been reported in 0.8 percent of patients receiving ZESTORETIC. In patients with hypertension receiving lisinopril alone, the incidence of syncope was 0.1 percent. The overall incidence of syncope may be reduced by proper titration of the individual components. (See PRECAUTIONS, Drug Interactions, ADVERSE REACTIONS and DOSAGE AND ADMINISTRATION.)

In patients with severe congestive heart failure, with or without associated renal insufficiency, excessive hypotension has been observed and may be associated with oliguria and/or progressive azotemia, and rarely with acute renal failure and/or death. Because of the potential fall in blood pressure in these patients, therapy should be started under very close medical supervision. Such patients should be followed closely for the first two weeks of treatment and whenever the dose of lisinopril and/or diuretic is increased. Similar considerations apply to patients with ischemic heart or cerebrovascular disease in whom an excessive fall in blood pressure could result in a myocardial infarction or cerebrovascular accident.

If hypotension occurs, the patient should be placed in supine position and, if necessary, receive an intravenous infusion of normal saline. A transient hypotensive response is not a contraindication to further doses which usually can be given without difficulty once the blood pressure has increased after volume expansion.

Neutropenia/Agranulocytosis: Another angiotensin converting enzyme inhibitor, captopril, has been shown to cause agranulocytosis and bone marrow depression, rarely in uncomplicated patients but more frequently in patients with renal impairment, especially if they also have a collagen vascular disease. Available data from clinical trials of lisinopril are insufficient to show that lisinopril does not cause agranulocytosis at similar rates. Periodic monitoring of white blood cell counts in patients with collagen vascular disease and renal disease should be considered.

Hydrochlorothiazide

Thiazides should be used with caution in severe renal disease. In patients with renal disease, thiazides may precipitate azotemia. Cumulative effects of the drug may develop in patients with impaired renal function.

Thiazides should be used with caution in patients with impaired hepatic function or progressive liver disease, since minor alterations of fluid and electrolyte balance may precipitate hepatic coma.

Sensitivity reactions may occur in patients with or without a history of allergy or bronchial asthma.

The possibility of exacerbation or activation of systemic lupus erythematosus has been reported.

Lithium generally should not be given with thiazides. (See PRECAUTIONS, Drug Interactions, Lisinopril and Hydrochlorothiazide.)

PRECAUTIONS

General

Lisinopril

Impaired Renal Function: As a consequence of inhibiting the renin-angiotensin-aldosterone system, changes in renal function may be anticipated in susceptible individuals. In patients with severe congestive heart failure whose renal function may depend on the activity of the renin-angiotensin-aldosterone system, treatment with angiotensin converting enzyme inhibitors, including lisinopril, may be associated with oliguria and/or progressive azotemia and rarely with acute renal failure and/or death.

In hypertensive patients with unilateral or bilateral renal artery stenosis, increases in blood urea nitrogen and serum creatinine may occur. Experience with another angiotensin converting enzyme inhibitor suggests that these increases are usually reversible upon discontinuation of lisinopril and/or diuretic therapy. In such patients renal function should be monitored during the first few weeks of therapy.

Some hypertensive patients with no apparent pre-existing renal vascular disease have developed increases in blood urea and serum creatinine, usually minor and transient, especially when lisinopril has been given concomitantly with a diuretic. This is more likely to occur in patients with pre-existing renal impairment. Dosage reduction of lisinopril and/or discontinuation of the diuretic may be required.

Evaluation of the hypertensive patient should always include assessment of renal function. (See DOSAGE and ADMINISTRATION.)

Hyperkalemia: In clinical trials hyperkalemia (serum potassium greater than 5.7 mEq/L) occurred in approximately 1.4 percent of hypertensive patients treated with lisinopril plus hydrochlorothiazide. In most cases these were isolated values which resolved despite continued therapy. Hyperkalemia was not a cause of discontinuation of therapy. Risk factors for the development of hyperkalemia include renal insufficiency, diabetes mellitus, and the concomitant use of potassium-sparing diuretics, potassium supplements and/or potassium-containing salt substitutes, which should be used cautiously if at all with ZESTORETIC. (See Drug Interactions.)

Surgery/Anesthesia: In patients undergoing major surgery or during anesthesia with agents that produce hypotension, lisinopril may block angiotensin II formation secondary to compensatory renin release. If hypotension occurs and is considered to be due to this mechanism, it can be corrected by volume expansion.

Hydrochlorothiazide

Periodic determination of serum electrolytes to detect possible electrolyte imbalance should be performed at appropriate intervals.

All patients receiving thiazide therapy should be observed for clinical signs of fluid or electrolyte imbalance: namely, hyponatremia, hypochloremic alkalosis, and hypokalemia. Serum and urine electrolyte determinations are particularly important when the patient is vomiting excessively or receiving parenteral fluids. Warning signs or symptoms of fluid and electrolyte imbalance, irrespective of cause, include dryness of mouth, thirst, weakness, lethargy, drowsiness, restlessness, muscle pains or cramps, muscular fatigue, hypotension, oliguria, tachycardia, and gastrointestinal disturbances such as nausea and vomiting.

Hypokalemia may develop, especially with brisk diuresis, when severe cirrhosis is present, or after prolonged therapy. Interference with adequate oral electrolyte intake will also contribute to hypokalemia. Hypokalemia may cause cardiac arrhythmia and may also sensitize or exaggerate the response of the heart to the toxic effects of digitalis (eg, increased ventricular irritability). Because lisinopril reduces the production of aldosterone, concomitant therapy with lisinopril attenuates the diuretic-induced potassium loss. (See Drug Interactions, Agents Increasing Serum Potassium.)

Although any chloride deficit is generally mild and usually does not require specific treatment, except under extraordinary circumstances (as in liver disease or renal disease), chloride replacement may be required in the treatment of metabolic alkalosis.

Dilutional hyponatremia may occur in edematous patients in hot weather; appropriate therapy is water restriction, rather than administration of salt except in rare instances when the hyponatremia is life-threatening. In actual salt depletion, appropriate replacement is the therapy of choice. Hyperuricemia may occur or frank gout may be precipitated in certain patients receiving thiazide therapy.

In diabetic patients dosage adjustments of insulin or oral hypoglycemic agents may be required. Hyperglycemia may occur with thiazide diuretics. Thus latent diabetes mellitus may become manifest during thiazide therapy.

The antihypertensive effects of the drug may be enhanced in the postsympathectomy patient.

If progressive renal impairment becomes evident consider withholding or discontinuing diuretic therapy.

Thiazides have been shown to increase the urinary excretion of magnesium; this may result in hypomagnesemia.

Thiazides may decrease urinary calcium excretion. Thiazides may cause intermittent and slight elevation of serum calcium in the absence of known disorders of calcium metabolism. Marked hypercalcemia may be evidence of hidden hyperparathyroidism. Thiazides should be discontinued before carrying out tests for parathyroid function.

Increases in cholesterol and triglyceride levels may be associated with thiazide diuretic therapy.

Information for Patients

Angioedema: Angioedema, including laryngeal edema, may occur especially following the first dose of lisinopril. Patients should be so advised and told to report immediately any signs or symptoms suggesting angioedema (swelling of face, extremities, eyes, lips, tongue, difficulty in swallowing or breathing) and to take no more drug until they have consulted with the prescribing physician.

Symptomatic Hypotension: Patients should be cautioned to report lightheadedness especially during the first few days of therapy. If actual syncope occurs, the patients should be told to discontinue the drug until they have consulted with the prescribing physician.

All patients should be cautioned that excessive perspiration and dehydration may lead to an excessive fall in blood pressure because of reduction in fluid volume. Other causes of volume depletion such as vomiting or diarrhea may also lead to a fall in blood pressure; patients should be advised to consult with their physician.

Hyperkalemia: Patients should be told not to use salt substitutes containing potassium without consulting their physician.

Neutropenia: Patients should be told to report promptly any indication of infection (eg, sore throat, fever) which may be a sign of neutropenia.

NOTE: As with many other drugs, certain advice to patients being treated with ZESTORETIC is warranted. This information is intended to aid in the safe and effective use of this medication. It is not a disclosure of all possible adverse or intended effects.

Drug Interactions

Lisinopril

Hypotension—Patients on Diuretic Therapy: Patients on diuretics and especially those in whom diuretic therapy was recently instituted, may occasionally experience an excessive reduction of blood pressure after initiation of therapy with lisinopril. The possibility of hypotensive effects with lisinopril can be minimized by either discontinuing the diuretic or increasing the salt intake prior to initiation of treatment with lisinopril. If it is necessary to continue the diuretic, initiate therapy with lisinopril at a dose of 5 mg daily, and provide close medical supervision after the initial dose for at least two hours and until blood pressure has stabilized for at least an additional hour. (See WARNINGS, and DOSAGE AND ADMINISTRATION.) When a diuretic is added to the therapy of a patient receiving lisinopril, an additional antihypertensive effect is usually observed. (See DOSAGE AND ADMINISTRATION.)

Indomethacin: In a study in 36 patients with mild to moderate hypertension where the antihypertensive effects of lisinopril alone were compared to lisinopril given concomitantly with indomethacin, the use of indomethacin was associated with a reduced effect, although the difference between the two regimens was not significant.

Other Agents: Lisinopril has been used concomitantly with nitrates and/or digoxin without evidence of clinically significant adverse interactions. No meaningful clinically important pharmacokinetic interactions occurred when lisinopril was used concomitantly with propranolol, digoxin, or hydrochlorothiazide. The presence of food in the stomach does not alter the bioavailability of lisinopril.

Agents Increasing Serum Potassium: Lisinopril attenuates potassium loss caused by thiazide-type diuretics. Use of lisinopril with potassium-sparing diuretics (eg, spironolactone, triamterene, or amiloride), potassium supplements, or potassium-containing salt substitutes may lead to significant increases in serum potassium. Therefore, if concomitant use of these agents is indicated, because of demonstrated hypo-

Continued on next page

Stuart—Cont.

kalemia, they should be used with caution and with frequent monitoring of serum potassium.

Lithium: Lithium toxicity has been reported in patients receiving lithium concomitantly with drugs which cause elimination of sodium, including ACE inhibitors. Lithium toxicity was usually reversible upon discontinuation of lithium and the ACE inhibitor. It is recommended that serum lithium levels be monitored frequently if lisinopril is administered concomitantly with lithium.

Hydrochlorothiazide

When administered concurrently the following drugs may interact with thiazide diuretics.

Alcohol, barbiturates, or narcotics—potentiation of orthostatic hypotension may occur.

Antidiabetic drugs (oral agents and insulin)—dosage adjustment of the antidiabetic drug may be required.

Other antihypertensive drugs—additive effect or potentiation.

Corticosteroids, ACTH—intensified electrolyte depletion, particularly hypokalemia.

Pressor amines (eg, norepinephrine)—possible decreased response to pressor amines but not sufficient to preclude their use.

Skeletal muscle relaxants, nondepolarizing (eg, tubocurarine)—possible increased responsiveness to the muscle relaxant.

Lithium—should not generally be given with diuretics. Diuretic agents reduce the renal clearance of lithium and add a high risk of lithium toxicity. Refer to the package insert for lithium preparations before use of such preparations with ZESTORETIC.

Non-Steroidal Anti-inflammatory Drugs—In some patients, the administration of a non-steroidal anti-inflammatory agent can reduce the diuretic, natriuretic, and antihypertensive effects of loop, potassium-sparing and thiazide diuretics. Therefore, when ZESTORETIC and non-steroidal anti-inflammatory agents are used concomitantly, the patient should be observed closely to determine if the desired effect of ZESTORETIC is obtained.

Carcinogenesis, Mutagenesis, Impairment of Fertility

Lisinopril and Hydrochlorothiazide: Lisinopril in combination with hydrochlorothiazide was not mutagenic in a microbial mutagen test using *Salmonella typhimurium* (Ames test) or *Escherichia coli* with or without metabolic activation or in a forward mutation assay using Chinese hamster lung cells. Lisinopril and hydrochlorothiazide did not produce DNA single strand breaks in an in vitro alkaline elution rat hepatocyte assay. In addition, it did not produce increases in chromosomal aberrations in an in vitro test in Chinese hamster ovary cells or in an in vivo study in mouse bone marrow.

Lisinopril: There was no evidence of a tumorigenic effect when lisinopril was administered for 105 weeks to male and female rats at doses up to 90 mg/kg/day (about 56 times* the maximum recommended daily human dose). Lisinopril has also been administered for 92 weeks to (male and female) mice at doses up to 135 mg/kg/day (about 84 times* the maximum recommended daily human dose) and showed no evidence of carcinogenicity.

*Based on patient weight of 50 kg.

Lisinopril was not mutagenic in the Ames microbial mutagen test with or without metabolic activation. It was also negative in a forward mutation assay using Chinese hamster lung cells. Lisinopril did not produce single strand DNA breaks in an in vitro alkaline elution rat hepatocyte assay. In addition, lisinopril did not produce increases in chromosomal aberrations in an in vitro test in Chinese hamster ovary cells or in an in vivo study in mouse bone marrow.

There were no adverse effects on reproductive performance in male and female rats treated with up to 300 mg/kg/day of lisinopril.

Hydrochlorothiazide: Hydrochlorothiazide is currently under study in the US Carcinogenesis Testing Program. Hydrochlorothiazide was not mutagenic in the in vitro Ames mutagenicity assay of *Salmonella typhimurium* strains TA 98, TA 100, TA 1535, TA 1537 and TA 1538 or in in vitro mutagenicity assays of mouse germinal cell chromosomes and Chinese hamster bone marrow cell chromosomes. It was, however, mutagenic in inducing nondisjunction (96% frequency) in diploid strains of *Aspergillus nidulans*.

Hydrochlorothiazide had no adverse effect on fertility of male or female mice or rats in studies in which these species were exposed to doses of up to 4 and 100 mg/kg/day, respectively.

Pregnancy

Lisinopril and Hydrochlorothiazide

Pregnancy Category C: Teratogenicity studies were conducted in mice and rats with up to 90 mg/kg/day of lisinopril (56 times the maximum recommended human dose) in combination with 10 mg/kg/day of hydrochlorothiazide (2.5 times the maximum recommended human dose). Maternal or fetotoxic effects were not seen in mice with the combination. In rats decreased maternal weight gain and decreased fetal weight occurred down to 3/10 mg/kg/day (the lowest dose tested). Associated with the decreased fetal weight was a delay in fetal ossification. The decreased fetal weight and delay in fetal ossification were not seen in saline-supplemented animals given 90/10 mg/kg/day.

There are no adequate and well-controlled studies of ZESTORETIC in pregnant women. ZESTORETIC should be used during pregnancy only if the potential benefit justifies the potential risk to the fetus.

Lisinopril

Lisinopril was not teratogenic in mice treated on days 6–15 of gestation with up to 1,000 mg/kg/day (625 times the maximum recommended human dose). There was an increase in fetal resorptions at doses down to 100 mg/kg; at doses of 1,000 mg/kg this was prevented by saline supplementation. By whole body autoradiography, radioactivity was found in the placenta following administration of labeled drug to pregnant rats, but none was found in the fetuses. There was no fetotoxicity or teratogenicity in rats treated with up to 300 mg/kg/day (188 times the maximum recommended dose) of lisinopril on days 6–17 of gestation. However, in rats receiving lisinopril from day 15 of gestation through day 21 postpartum, there was an increased incidence of pup deaths on days 2–7 postpartum and a lower average body weight of pups on day 21 postpartum. The increase in pup deaths and decrease in pup weight did not occur with maternal saline supplementation.

Lisinopril, at doses up to 1 mg/kg/day, was not teratogenic when given throughout the organogenic period in the saline supplemented rabbits. Saline supplementation (physiologic saline in place of tap water) was used to eliminate maternotoxic effects and enable evaluation of the teratogenic potential at the highest possible dosage level. The rabbit has been shown to be extremely sensitive to angiotensin converting enzyme inhibitors (captopril and enalapril) with maternal and fetotoxic effects apparent at or below the recommended therapeutic dosage levels in man.

Fetotoxicity was demonstrated in rabbits by an increased incidence of fetal resorptions at a dose of lisinopril of 1 mg/kg/day and by an increased incidence of incomplete ossification at 0.1 mg/kg/day (the lowest dose tested). A single intravenous dose of 15 mg/kg of lisinopril administered to pregnant rabbits on gestation days 16, 21 or 26 resulted in 88 percent to 100 percent fetal death.

By whole body autoradiography, radioactivity was found in the placenta following administration of labeled lisinopril to pregnant rats, but none was found in the fetuses.

Human Experience: There are no adequate and well-controlled studies of lisinopril in pregnant women. However, data are available that show drugs of this class cross the human placenta. Because the risk of fetal toxicity with the use of ACE inhibitors has not been clearly defined (see below), lisinopril should be used during pregnancy only if the potential benefit justifies the potential risk to the fetus.

Postmarketing experience with all ACE inhibitors thus far suggests the following with regard to pregnancy outcome. Inadvertent exposure limited to the first trimester of pregnancy has not been reported to affect fetal outcome adversely. Fetal exposure during the second and third trimesters of pregnancy has been associated with fetal and neonatal morbidity and mortality.

When ACE inhibitors are used during the later stages of pregnancy, there have been reports of hypotension and decreased renal perfusion in the newborn. Oligohydramnios in the mother has also been reported, presumably representing decreased renal function in the fetus. Infants exposed in utero to ACE inhibitors should be closely observed for hypotension, oliguria and hyperkalemia. If oliguria occurs, attention should be directed toward support of blood pressure and renal perfusion with the administration of fluids and pressors as appropriate. Problems associated with prematurity such as patent ductus arteriosus have occurred in association with maternal use of ACE inhibitors, but it is not clear whether they are related to ACE inhibition, maternal hypertension or the underlying prematurity.

Another ACE inhibitor, enalapril, has been removed from the neonatal circulation by peritoneal dialysis and theoretically may be removed by exchange transfusion, although there is no experience with the latter procedure. There is no experience with either of these procedures for removing lisinopril or other ACE inhibitors from the neonatal circulation.

Hydrochlorothiazide

There was no evidence of harm to the fetus when hydrochlorothiazide was administered to pregnant mice and rats during organogenesis at doses up to 3,000 and 1,350 mg/kg/day, respectively.

Thiazides cross the placental barrier and appear in cord blood. They may cause fetal or neonatal jaundice, thrombocytopenia, and possibly other adverse reactions which have occurred in the adult.

Nursing Mothers

It is not known whether lisinopril is excreted in human milk. However, milk of lactating rats contains radioactivity following administration of ^{14}C lisinopril. In another study, lisinopril was present in rat milk at levels similar to plasma levels in the dams. Thiazides do appear in human milk. Because of the potential for serious reactions in nursing infants from hydrochlorothiazide and the unknown effects of lisinopril in infants, a decision should be made whether to discontinue nursing or to discontinue ZESTORETIC, taking into account the importance of the drug to the mother.

Pediatric Use

Safety and effectiveness in children have not been established.

ADVERSE REACTIONS

ZESTORETIC has been evaluated for safety in 930 patients including 100 patients treated for 50 weeks or more.

In clinical trials with ZESTORETIC no adverse experiences peculiar to this combination drug have been observed. Adverse experiences that have occurred have been limited to those that have been previously reported with lisinopril or hydrochlorothiazide.

The most frequent clinical adverse experiences in controlled trials (including open label extensions) with any combination of lisinopril and hydrochlorothiazide were: dizziness (7.5%), headache (5.2%), cough (3.9%), fatigue (3.7%) and orthostatic effects (3.2%) all of which were more common than in placebo-treated patients. Generally, adverse experiences were mild and transient in nature, but see WARNINGS regarding angioedema and excessive hypotension or syncope. Discontinuation of therapy due to adverse effects was required in 4.4% of patients principally because of dizziness, cough, fatigue and muscle cramps.

Adverse experiences occurring in greater than one percent of patients treated with lisinopril plus hydrochlorothiazide in controlled clinical trials are shown below.

[See table left].

Clinical adverse experiences occurring in 0.3% to 1.0% of patients in controlled trials included:

Body as a Whole: Chest pain, abdominal pain, syncope, chest discomfort, fever, trauma, virus infection.

Cardiovascular: Palpitation, orthostatic hypotension.

Digestive: Gastrointestinal cramps, dry mouth, constipation, heartburn.

Musculoskeletal: Back pain, shoulder pain, knee pain, back strain, myalgia, foot pain.

Nervous/Psychiatric: Decreased libido, vertigo, depression, somnolence.

Percent of Patients in Controlled Studies

	Lisinopril and Hydrochlorothiazide (n=930) Incidence (discontinuation)	Placebo (n=207) Incidence
Dizziness	7.5 (0.8)	1.9
Headache	5.2 (0.3)	1.9
Cough	3.9 (0.6)	1.0
Fatigue	3.7 (0.4)	1.0
Orthostatic Effects	3.2 (0.1)	1.0
Diarrhea	2.5 (0.2)	2.4
Nausea	2.2 (0.1)	2.4
Upper Respiratory Infection	2.2 (0.0)	0.0
Muscle Cramps	2.0 (0.4)	0.5
Asthenia	1.8 (0.2)	1.0
Paresthesia	1.5 (0.1)	0.0
Hypotension	1.4 (0.3)	0.5
Vomiting	1.4 (0.1)	0.5
Dyspepsia	1.3 (0.0)	0.0
Rash	1.2 (0.1)	0.5
Impotence	1.2 (0.3)	0.0

Respiratory: Common cold, nasal congestion, influenza, bronchitis, pharyngeal pain, dyspnea, pulmonary congestion, chronic sinusitis, allergic rhinitis, pharyngeal discomfort.

Skin: Flushing, pruritus, skin inflammation, hyperhidrosis.

Special Senses: Blurred vision, tinnitus, otalgia.

Urogenital: Urinary tract infection.

Angioedema: Angioedema of the face, extremities, lips, tongue, glottis and/or larynx has been reported rarely. (See WARNINGS.)

Hypotension: In clinical trials, adverse effects relating to hypotension occurred as follows: hypotension (1.4%), orthostatic hypotension (0.5%), other orthostatic effects (3.2%). In addition syncope occurred in 0.8% of patients. (See WARNINGS.)

Clinical Laboratory Test Findings

Serum Electrolytes: (See PRECAUTIONS.)

Creatinine, Blood Urea Nitrogen: Minor reversible increases in blood urea nitrogen and serum creatinine were observed in patients with essential hypertension treated with ZESTORETIC. More marked increases have also been reported and were more likely to occur in patients with renal stenosis. (See PRECAUTIONS.)

Serum Uric Acid, Glucose, Magnesium, Cholesterol, Triglycerides and Calcium: (See PRECAUTIONS.)

Hemoglobin and Hematocrit: Small decreases in hemoglobin and hematocrit (mean decreases of approximately 0.5 g% and 1.5 vol%, respectively) occurred frequently in hypertensive patients treated with ZESTORETIC but were rarely of clinical importance unless another cause of anemia coexisted. In clinical trials, 0.4% of patients discontinued therapy due to anemia.

Other (Causal Relationship Unknown): Rarely, elevations of liver enzymes and/or serum bilirubin have occurred.

Other adverse reactions that have been reported with the individual components are listed below:

Lisinopril—Lisinopril has been evaluated for safety in 2003 patients. In clinical trials adverse reactions which occurred with lisinopril were also seen with ZESTORETIC. In addition, the following were reported: **Cardiovascular:** Angina pectoris, rhythm disturbances, tachycardia, peripheral edema; **Digestive:** Anorexia, flatulence; **Metabolism:** Gout; **Musculoskeletal:** Joint pain; **Nervous System/Psychiatric:** Insomnia, stroke; **Urogenital:** Oliguria, progressive azotemia, acute renal failure. **Other:** Vasculitis.

Hydrochlorothiazide—Body as a Whole: Weakness; **Digestive:** Anorexia, gastric irritation, cramping, jaundice (intrahepatic cholestatic jaundice), pancreatitis, sialadenitis, constipation; **Hematologic:** Leukopenia, agranulocytosis, thrombocytopenia, aplastic anemia, hemolytic anemia; **Musculoskeletal:** Muscle spasm; **Nervous System/Psychiatric:** Restlessness; **Renal:** Renal failure, renal dysfunction, interstitial nephritis (see WARNINGS); **Special Senses:** Xanthopsia; **Hypersensitivity:** Purpura, photosensitivity, urticaria, necrotizing angiitis (vasculitis and cutaneous vasculitis), respiratory distress including pneumonitis and pulmonary edema, anaphylactic reactions.

OVERDOSAGE

No specific information is available on the treatment of overdosage with ZESTORETIC. Treatment is symptomatic and supportive. Therapy with ZESTORETIC should be discontinued and the patient observed closely. Suggested measures include induction of emesis and/or gastric lavage, and correction of dehydration, electrolyte imbalance and hypotension by established procedures.

Lisinopril: The oral LD_{50} of lisinopril is greater than 20 g/kg in mice and rats. The most likely manifestations of overdosage would be hypotension, for which the usual treatment would be intravenous infusion of normal saline solution.

Lisinopril can be removed by hemodialysis.

Hydrochlorothiazide: The oral LD_{50} of hydrochlorothiazide is greater than 10.0 g/kg in both mice and rats. The most common signs and symptoms observed are those caused by electrolyte depletion (hypokalemia, hypochloremia, hyponatremia) and dehydration resulting from excessive diuresis. If digitalis has also been administered, hypokalemia may accentuate cardiac arrhythmias.

DOSAGE AND ADMINISTRATION

DOSAGE MUST BE INDIVIDUALIZED. THE FIXED COMBINATION IS NOT FOR INITIAL THERAPY. IT MAY BE SUBSTITUTED FOR THE TITRATED INDIVIDUAL COMPONENTS. ALTERNATIVELY, PATIENTS WHO HAVE RECEIVED LISINOPRIL MONOTHERAPY 20 OR 40 MG MAY BE GIVEN ZESTORETIC 20-12.5, THEN ZESTORETIC 20-25, THUS TITRATING THE HYDROCHLOROTHIAZIDE COMPONENT USING THE COMBINATION.

The usual dose is one or two tablets of ZESTORETIC 20-12.5 or ZESTORETIC 20-25 once daily. (See INDICATIONS and USAGE and WARNINGS.) However, because data from a clinical trial suggest that the mean group antihypertensive response is similar when lisinopril 20 mg is combined with hydrochlorothiazide 12.5 mg or 25 mg, patients whose blood

pressure is controlled with lisinopril 20 mg plus hydrochlorothiazide 25 mg ordinarily should be given a trial of ZESTORETIC 20-12.5 before ZESTORETIC 20-25 is used. (See CLINICAL PHARMACOLOGY, Lisinopril and Hydrochlorothiazide.)

Patients usually do not require doses in excess of 50 mg of hydrochlorothiazide daily, particularly when it is combined with other antihypertensive agents.

For lisinopril monotherapy the recommended initial dose in patients not on diuretics is 10 mg of lisinopril once a day. Dosage should be adjusted according to blood pressure response. The usual dosage range of lisinopril is 20 to 40 mg administered in a single daily dose; the maximum recommended dose is 80 mg in a single daily dose. Blood pressure should be measured at the interdosing interval to ensure that there is an adequate antihypertensive response at that time. If blood pressure is not controlled with lisinopril alone, a diuretic may be added. Hydrochlorothiazide 12.5 mg has been shown to provide an additive effect. After addition of the diuretic it may be possible to reduce the dose of lisinopril. In patients who are currently being treated with a diuretic, symptomatic hypotension occasionally may occur following the initial dose of lisinopril. The diuretic should, if possible, be discontinued for two to three days before beginning therapy with lisinopril to reduce the likelihood of hypotension. (See WARNINGS.) If the patient's blood pressure is not controlled with lisinopril alone, diuretic therapy may be resumed.

If the diuretic cannot be discontinued, an initial dose of 5 mg of lisinopril should be used under medical supervision for at least two hours and until blood pressure has stabilized for at least an additional hour. (See WARNINGS AND PRECAUTIONS, Drug Interactions.)

Concomitant administration of ZESTORETIC with potassium supplements, potassium salt substitutes or potassium-sparing diuretics may lead to increases of serum potassium. (See PRECAUTIONS.)

Dosage Adjustment in Renal Impairment: The usual dose of ZESTORETIC is recommended for patients with a creatinine clearance > 30 mL/min (serum creatinine of up to approximately 3 mg/dL).

When concomitant diuretic therapy is required in patients with severe renal impairment, a loop diuretic, rather than a thiazide diuretic is preferred for use with lisinopril; therefore, for patients with severe renal dysfunction the lisinopril and hydrochlorothiazide combination tablet is not recommended.

HOW SUPPLIED

20-12.5 Tablets (NDC 0038-0142) White, round, biconvex, uncoated tablets identified with "STUART" and "142" debossed on one side, are supplied in bottles of 100 tablets.

20-25 Tablets (NDC 0038-0145) Peach, round, biconvex, uncoated tablets identified with "STUART" and "145" debossed on one side, are supplied in bottles of 100 tablets.

Avoid storage at temperatures above 40°C (104°F). Dispense in a well-closed container.

Rev 6 05/89

SIC 63994-03

Stuart Pharmaceuticals

Division of ICI Americas Inc.

Wilmington, DE 19897

These tablets are distributed by Stuart Pharmaceuticals.

Shown in Product Identification Section, page 432

ZESTRIL®   ℞
(lisinopril-Stuart)

DESCRIPTION

ZESTRIL® (lisinopril), a synthetic peptide derivative, is an oral long-acting angiotensin converting enzyme inhibitor. Lisinopril is chemically described as (S)-1-[N^2-(1-carboxy-3-phenylpropyl)-L-lysyl-proline dihydrate. Its empirical formula is $C_{21}H_{31}N_3O_5 \cdot 2H_2O$ and its structural formula is:

Lisinopril is a white to off-white, crystalline powder, with a molecular weight of 441.53. It is soluble in water and sparingly soluble in methanol and practically insoluble in ethanol.

ZESTRIL is supplied as 5 mg, 10 mg, 20 mg and 40 mg tablets for oral administration.

Inactive Ingredients:

5, 10 and 20 mg tablets—calcium phosphate, magnesium stearate, mannitol, red ferric oxide, starch.

40 mg tablets—calcium phosphate, magnesium stearate, mannitol, starch, yellow ferric oxide.

CLINICAL PHARMACOLOGY

Mechanism of Action: Lisinopril inhibits angiotensin converting enzyme (ACE) in human subjects and animals. ACE is a peptidyl dipeptidase that catalyzes the conversion of angiotensin I to the vasoconstrictor substance, angiotensin II. Angiotensin II also stimulates aldosterone secretion by the adrenal cortex. Inhibition of ACE results in decreased plasma angiotensin II which leads to decreased vasopressor activity and to decreased aldosterone secretion. The latter decrease may result in a small increase of serum potassium. In hypertensive patients with normal renal function treated with ZESTRIL alone for up to 24 weeks, the mean increase in serum potassium was approximately 0.1 mEq/L; however, approximately 15% of patients had increases greater than 0.5 mEq/L and approximately 6% had a decrease greater than 0.5 mEq/L. In the same study, patients treated with ZESTRIL and hydrochlorothiazide for up to 24 weeks had a mean decrease in serum potassium of 0.1 mEq/L; approximately 4% of patients had increases greater than 0.5 mEq/L and approximately 12% had a decrease greater than 0.5 mEq/L. (See PRECAUTIONS.) Removal of angiotensin II negative feedback on renin secretion leads to increased plasma renin activity.

ACE is identical to kininase, an enzyme that degrades bradykinin. Whether increased levels of bradykinin, a potent vasodepressor peptide, play a role in the therapeutic effects of ZESTRIL remains to be elucidated.

While the mechanism through which ZESTRIL lowers blood pressure is believed to be primarily suppression of the renin-angiotensin-aldosterone system, ZESTRIL is antihypertensive even in patients with low-renin hypertension. Although ZESTRIL was antihypertensive in all races studied, black hypertensive patients (usually a low-renin hypertensive population) had a smaller average response to monotherapy than nonblack patients.

Concomitant administration of ZESTRIL and hydrochlorothiazide further reduced blood pressure in black and nonblack patients and any racial differences in blood pressure response were no longer evident.

Pharmacokinetics and Metabolism: Following oral administration of ZESTRIL, peak serum concentrations of lisinopril occur within about 7 hours. Declining serum concentrations exhibit a prolonged terminal phase which does not contribute to drug accumulation. This terminal phase probably represents saturable binding to ACE and is not proportional to dose. Lisinopril does not appear to be bound to other serum proteins.

Lisinopril does not undergo metabolism and is excreted unchanged entirely in the urine. Based on urinary recovery, the mean extent of absorption of lisinopril is approximately 25%, with large intersubject variability (6–60%) at all doses tested (5–80 mg). Lisinopril absorption is not influenced by the presence of food in the gastrointestinal tract.

Upon multiple dosing, lisinopril exhibits an effective half-life of accumulation of 12 hours.

Impaired renal function decreases elimination of lisinopril, which is excreted principally through the kidneys, but this decrease becomes clinically important only when the glomerular filtration rate is below 30 mL/min. Above this glomerular filtration rate, the elimination half-life is little changed. With greater impairment, however, peak and trough lisinopril levels increase, time to peak concentration increases and time to attain steady state is prolonged. Older patients, on average, have (approximately doubled) higher blood levels and the area under the plasma concentration time curve (AUC) than younger patients. (See DOSAGE AND ADMINISTRATION.) Lisinopril can be removed by hemodialysis.

Studies in rats indicate that lisinopril crosses the blood-brain barrier poorly. Multiple doses of lisinopril in rats do not result in accumulation in any tissues. Milk of lactating rats contains radioactivity following administration of ^{14}C lisinopril. By whole body autoradiography, radioactivity was found in the placenta following administration of labeled drug to pregnant rats, but none was found in the fetuses.

Pharmacodynamics: Administration of ZESTRIL to patients with hypertension results in a reduction of both supine and standing blood pressure to about the same extent with no compensatory tachycardia. Symptomatic postural hypotension is usually not observed although it can occur and should be anticipated in volume and/or salt-depleted patients. (See WARNINGS.) When given together with thiazide-type diuretics, the blood pressure lowering effects of the two drugs are approximately additive.

In most patients studied, onset of antihypertensive activity was seen at one hour after oral administration of an individual dose of ZESTRIL, with peak reduction of blood pressure achieved by 6 hours. Although an antihypertensive effect was observed 24 hours after dosing with recommended single daily doses, the effect was more consistent and the mean effect was considerably larger in some studies with doses of 20 mg or more than with lower doses. However, at all doses studied, the mean antihypertensive effect was substantially

Continued on next page

Stuart—Cont.

smaller 24 hours after dosing than it was 6 hours after dosing.

In some patients achievement of optimal blood pressure reduction may require two to four weeks of therapy.

The antihypertensive effects of ZESTRIL are maintained during long-term therapy. Abrupt withdrawal of ZESTRIL has not been associated with a rapid increase in blood pressure, or a significant increase in blood pressure compared to pretreatment levels.

Two dose-response studies utilizing a once daily regimen were conducted in 438 mild to moderate hypertensive patients not on a diuretic. Blood pressure was measured 24 hours after dosing. An antihypertensive effect of ZESTRIL was seen with 5 mg in some patients. However, in both studies blood pressure reduction occurred sooner and was greater in patients treated with 10, 20 or 80 mg of ZESTRIL. In controlled clinical studies, ZESTRIL 20–80 mg has been compared in patients with mild to moderate hypertension to hydrochlorothiazide 12.5–50 mg and with atenolol 50–200 mg; and in patients with moderate to severe hypertension to metoprolol 100–200 mg. It was superior to hydrochlorothiazide in effects on systolic and diastolic pressure in a population that was ¾ Caucasian. ZESTRIL was approximately equivalent to atenolol and metoprolol in effects on diastolic blood pressure, and had somewhat greater effects on systolic blood pressure.

ZESTRIL had similar effectiveness and adverse effects in younger and older (> 65 years) patients. It was less effective in blacks than in Caucasians.

In hemodynamic studies in patients with essential hypertension, blood pressure reduction was accompanied by a reduction in peripheral arterial resistance with little or no change in cardiac output and in heart rate. In a study in nine hypertensive patients, following administration of ZESTRIL, there was an increase in mean renal blood flow that was not significant. Data from several small studies are inconsistent with respect to the effect of lisinopril on glomerular filtration rate in hypertensive patients with normal renal function, but suggest that changes, if any, are not large.

In patients with renovascular hypertension ZESTRIL has been shown to be well tolerated and effective in controlling blood pressure. (See PRECAUTIONS.)

INDICATIONS AND USAGE

ZESTRIL is indicated for the treatment of hypertension. It may be used alone as initial therapy or concomitantly with other classes of antihypertensive agents.

In using ZESTRIL, consideration should be given to the fact that another angiotensin converting enzyme inhibitor, captopril, has caused agranulocytosis, particularly in patients with renal impairment or collagen vascular disease, and that available data are insufficient to show that ZESTRIL does not have a similar risk. (See WARNINGS.)

CONTRAINDICATIONS

Zestril is contraindicated in patients who are hypersensitive to this product and in patients with a history of angioedema related to previous treatment with an angiotensin converting enzyme inhibitor.

WARNINGS

Angioedema: Angioedema of the face, extremities, lips, tongue, glottis and/or larynx has been reported in patients treated with angiotensin converting enzyme inhibitors, including ZESTRIL. In such cases, ZESTRIL should be promptly discontinued, and the patient carefully observed until the swelling disappears. In instances where swelling has been confined to the face and lips the condition has generally resolved without treatment, although antihistamines have been useful in relieving symptoms. Angioedema associated with laryngeal edema may be fatal. **Where there is involvement of the tongue, glottis or larynx, likely to cause airway obstruction, appropriate therapy, eg, subcutaneous epinephrine solution 1:1000 (0.3 mL to 0.5 mL) should be promptly administered. (See ADVERSE REACTIONS.)**

Hypotension: Excessive hypotension was rarely seen in uncomplicated hypertensive patients but is a possible consequence of use with ZESTRIL in salt/volume-depleted persons, such as those treated vigorously with diuretics or patients on dialysis. (See PRECAUTIONS, Drug Interactions and ADVERSE REACTIONS.) In patients with severe congestive heart failure, with or without associated renal insufficiency, excessive hypotension has been observed and may be associated with oliguria and/or progressive azotemia, and rarely with acute renal failure and/or death. Because of the potential fall in blood pressure in these patients, therapy should be started under very close medical supervision. Such patients should be followed closely for the first two weeks of treatment and whenever the dose of ZESTRIL and/or diuretic is increased. Similar considerations apply to patients with ischemic heart or cerebrovascular disease in whom an excessive fall in blood pressure could result in a myocardial infarction or cerebrovascular accident.

If hypotension occurs, the patient should be placed in supine position and, if necessary, receive an intravenous infusion of normal saline. A transient hypotensive response is not a contraindication to further doses which usually can be given without difficulty once the blood pressure has increased after volume expansion.

Neutropenia/Agranulocytosis: Another angiotensin converting enzyme inhibitor, captopril, has been shown to cause agranulocytosis and bone marrow depression, rarely in uncomplicated patients but more frequently in patients with renal impairment especially if they also have a collagen vascular disease. Available data from clinical trials of ZESTRIL are insufficient to show that ZESTRIL does not cause agranulocytosis at similar rates. Periodic monitoring of white blood cell counts in patients with collagen vascular disease and renal disease should be considered.

PRECAUTIONS

General

Impaired Renal Function: As a consequence of inhibiting the renin-angiotensin-aldosterone system, changes in renal function may be anticipated in susceptible individuals. In patients with severe congestive heart failure whose renal function may depend on the activity of the renin-angiotensin-aldosterone system, treatment with angiotensin converting enzyme inhibitors, including ZESTRIL, may be associated with oliguria and/or progressive azotemia and rarely with acute renal failure and/or death.

In hypertensive patients with unilateral or bilateral renal artery stenosis, increases in blood urea nitrogen and serum creatinine may occur. Experience with another angiotensin converting enzyme inhibitor suggests that these increases are usually reversible upon discontinuation of ZESTRIL and/or diuretic therapy. In such patients, renal function should be monitored during the first few weeks of therapy. Some hypertensive patients with no apparent pre-existing renal vascular disease have developed increases in blood urea nitrogen and serum creatinine, usually minor and transient, especially when ZESTRIL has been given concomitantly with a diuretic. This is more likely to occur in patients with pre-existing renal impairment. Dosage reduction of ZESTRIL and/or discontinuation of the diuretic may be required.

Evaluation of the hypertensive patient should always include assessment of renal function. (See DOSAGE AND ADMINISTRATION.)

Hyperkalemia: In clinical trials hyperkalemia (serum potassium greater than 5.7 mEq/L) occurred in approximately 2.2% of hypertensive patients and 4.0% of patients with congestive heart failure. In most cases these were isolated values which resolved despite continued therapy. Hyperkalemia was a cause of discontinuation of therapy in approximately 0.1% of hypertensive patients. Risk factors for the development of hyperkalemia include renal insufficiency, diabetes mellitus, and the concomitant use of potassium-sparing diuretics, potassium supplements and/or potassium-containing salt substitutes, which should be used cautiously, if at all, with ZESTRIL. (See Drug Interactions.)

Surgery/Anesthesia: In patients undergoing major surgery or during anesthesia with agents that produce hypotension, ZESTRIL may block angiotensin II formation secondary to compensatory renin release. If hypotension occurs and is considered to be due to this mechanism, it can be corrected by volume expansion.

Information for Patients

Angioedema: Angioedema, including laryngeal edema, may occur especially following the first dose of ZESTRIL. Patients should be so advised and told to report immediately any signs or symptoms suggesting angioedema (swelling of face, extremities, eyes, lips, tongue, difficulty in swallowing or breathing) and to take no more drug until they have consulted with the prescribing physician.

Symptomatic Hypotension: Patients should be cautioned to report lightheadedness especially during the first few days of therapy. If actual syncope occurs, the patient should be told to discontinue the drug until they have consulted with the prescribing physician.

All patients should be cautioned that excessive perspiration and dehydration may lead to an excessive fall in blood pressure because of reduction in fluid volume. Other causes of volume depletion such as vomiting or diarrhea may also lead to a fall in blood pressure; patients should be advised to consult with their physician.

Hyperkalemia: Patients should be told not to use salt substitutes containing potassium without consulting their physician.

Neutropenia: Patients should be told to report promptly any indication of infection (eg, sore throat, fever) which may be a sign of neutropenia.

NOTE: As with many other drugs, certain advice to patients being treated with ZESTRIL is warranted. This information is intended to aid in the safe and effective use of this medication. It is not a disclosure of all possible adverse or intended effects.

DRUG INTERACTIONS

Hypotension—Patients on Diuretic Therapy: Patients on diuretics and especially those in whom diuretic therapy was recently instituted, may occasionally experience an excessive reduction of blood pressure after initiation of therapy with ZESTRIL. The possibility of hypotensive effects with ZESTRIL can be minimized by either discontinuing the diuretic or increasing the salt intake prior to initiation of treatment with ZESTRIL. If it is necessary to continue the diuretic, initiate therapy with ZESTRIL at a dose of 5 mg daily, and provide close medical supervision after the initial dose for at least two hours and until blood pressure has stabilized for at least an additional hour. (See WARNINGS, and DOSAGE AND ADMINISTRATION.) When a diuretic is added to the therapy of a patient receiving ZESTRIL, an additional antihypertensive effect is usually observed. Studies with ACE inhibitors in combination with diuretics indicate that the dose of the ACE inhibitor can be reduced when it is given with a diuretic. (See DOSAGE AND ADMINISTRATION.)

Indomethacin: In a study in 36 patients with mild to moderate hypertension where the antihypertensive effects of ZESTRIL alone were compared to ZESTRIL given concomitantly with indomethacin, the use of indomethacin was associated with a reduced effect, although the difference between the two regimens was not significant.

Other Agents: ZESTRIL has been used concomitantly with nitrates and/or digoxin without evidence of clinically significant adverse interactions.

No clinically important pharmacokinetic interactions occurred when ZESTRIL was used concomitantly with propranolol or hydrochlorothiazide. The presence of food in the stomach does not alter the bioavailability of ZESTRIL.

Agents Increasing Serum Potassium: ZESTRIL attenuates potassium loss caused by thiazide-type diuretics. Use of ZESTRIL with potassium-sparing diuretics (eg, spironolactone, triamterene or amiloride), potassium supplements, or potassium-containing salt substitutes may lead to significant increases in serum potassium. Therefore, if concomitant use of these agents is indicated because of demonstrated hypokalemia, they should be used with caution and with frequent monitoring of serum potassium.

Lithium: Lithium toxicity has been reported in patients receiving lithium with drugs which cause elimination of sodium, including ACE inhibitors. Lithium toxicity was usually reversible upon discontinuation of both drugs. It is recommended that serum lithium levels be monitored frequently if ZESTRIL is administered concomitantly with lithium.

Carcinogenesis, Mutagenesis, Impairment of Fertility: There was no evidence of a tumorigenic effect when lisinopril was administered for 105 weeks to male and female rats at doses up to 90 mg/kg/day (about 56 times* the maximum recommended daily human dose) or when lisinopril was administered for 92 weeks to (male and female) mice at doses up to 135 mg/kg/day (about 84 times* the maximum recommended daily human dose).

*Based on patient weight of 50 kg.

Lisinopril was not mutagenic in the Ames microbial mutagen test with or without metabolic activation. It was also negative in a forward mutation assay using Chinese hamster lung cells. Lisinopril did not produce single strand DNA breaks in an in vitro alkaline elution rat hepatocyte assay. In addition, lisinopril did not produce increases in chromosomal aberrations in an in vitro test in Chinese hamster ovary cells or in an in vivo study in mouse bone marrow. There were no adverse effects on reproductive performance in male and female rats treated with up to 300 mg/kg/day of lisinopril.

Pregnancy

Pregnancy Category C: Lisinopril was not teratogenic in mice treated on days 6–15 of gestation with up to 1,000 mg/kg/day (625 times the maximum recommended human dose). There was an increase in fetal resorptions at doses down to 100 mg/kg; at doses of 1,000 mg/kg this was prevented by saline supplementation. There was no fetotoxicity or teratogenicity in rats treated with up to 300 mg/kg/day (188 times the maximum recommended dose) of lisinopril at days 6–17 of gestation. In rats receiving lisinopril from day 15 of gestation through day 21 postpartum, there was an increased incidence in pup deaths on days 2–7 postpartum and a lower average body weight of pups on day 21 postpartum. The increase in pup deaths and decrease in pup weight did not occur with maternal saline supplementation.

Lisinopril, at doses up to 1 mg/kg/day, was not teratogenic when given throughout the organogenic period in saline supplemented rabbits. Saline supplementation (physiologic saline in place of tap water) was used to eliminate maternotoxic effects and enable evaluation of the teratogenic potential at the highest possible dosage level. The rabbit has been shown to be extremely sensitive to angiotensin converting enzyme inhibitors (captopril and enalapril) with maternal and fetotoxic effects apparent at or below the recommended therapeutic dosage levels in man.

Fetotoxicity was demonstrated in rabbits by an increased incidence of fetal resorptions at an oral dose of lisinopril of 1 mg/kg/day and by an increased incidence of incomplete ossification at the lowest dose tested (0.1 mg/kg/day). A single intravenous dose of 15 mg/kg of lisinopril administered to pregnant rabbits on gestation days 16, 21 or 26 resulted in 88% to 100% fetal death.

By whole body autoradiography, radioactivity was found in the placenta following administration of labeled lisinopril to pregnant rats, but none was found in the fetuses.

Human Experiences: There are no adequate and well-controlled studies of lisinopril in pregnant women. However, data are available that show drugs of this class cross the human placenta. Because the risk of fetal toxicity with the use of ACE inhibitors has not been clearly defined (see below), lisinopril should be used during pregnancy only if the potential benefit justifies the potential risk to the fetus.

Postmarketing experience with all ACE inhibitors thus far suggests the following with regard to pregnancy outcome. Inadvertent exposure limited to the first trimester of pregnancy has not been reported to affect fetal outcome adversely. Fetal exposure during the second and third trimesters of pregnancy has been associated with fetal and neonatal morbidity and mortality.

When ACE inhibitors are used during the later stages of pregnancy, there have been reports of hypotension and decreased renal perfusion in the newborn. Oligohydramnios in the mother has also been reported, presumably representing decreased renal function in the fetus. Infants exposed in utero to ACE inhibitors should be closely observed for hypotension, oliguria and hyperkalemia. If oliguria occurs, attention should be directed toward support of blood pressure and renal perfusion with the administration of fluids and pressors as appropriate. Problems associated with prematurity such as patent ductus arteriosus have occurred in association with maternal use of ACE inhibition, but it is not clear whether they are related to ACE inhibition, maternal hypertension or the underlying prematurity.

Another ACE inhibitor, enalapril, has been removed from the neonatal circulation by peritoneal dialysis and theoretically may be removed by exchange transfusion, although there is no experience with the latter procedure. There is no experience with either of these procedures for removing lisinopril or other ACE inhibitors from the neonatal circulation.

Nursing Mothers: Milk of lactating rats contains radioactivity following administration of ^{14}C lisinopril. It is not known whether this drug is excreted in human milk. Because many drugs are excreted in human milk, caution should be exercised when ZESTRIL is given to a nursing mother.

Pediatric Use: Safety and effectiveness in children have not been established.

ADVERSE REACTIONS

ZESTRIL has been found to be generally well tolerated in controlled clinical trials involving 2003 patients and subjects.

The most frequent clinical adverse experiences in controlled trials with ZESTRIL were dizziness (6.3%), headache (5.3%), fatigue (3.3%), diarrhea (3.2%), upper respiratory symptoms (3.0%), and cough (2.9%), all of which were more frequent than in placebo-treated patients. For the most part, adverse experiences were mild and transient in nature. Discontinuation of therapy was required in 6.0% of patients. In clinical trials, the overall frequency of adverse experiences could not be related to total daily dosage within the recommended therapeutic dosage range.

For adverse experiences which occurred in more than 1% of patients and subjects treated with ZESTRIL or ZESTRIL plus hydrochlorothiazide in controlled clinical trials, comparative incidence data are listed in the table below. [See table above].

Clinical adverse experiences occurring in 0.3% to 1.0% of patients in the controlled trials and rarer, serious, possibly drug-related events reported in uncontrolled studies or marketing experience included:

BODY AS A WHOLE: Chest discomfort, fever, flushing.
CARDIOVASCULAR: Angina pectoris, orthostatic hypotension, rhythm disturbances, tachycardia, peripheral edema, palpitation.
DIGESTIVE: Abdominal pain, anorexia, constipation, flatulence.
METABOLISM: Gout.
MUSCULOSKELETAL: Joint pain, shoulder pain.
NERVOUS SYSTEM/PSYCHIATRIC: Depression, somnolence, insomnia, stroke.
RESPIRATORY SYSTEM: Bronchitis, sinusitis, pharyngeal pain.
UROGENITAL: Oliguria, progressive azotemia, acute renal failure.
OTHER: Blurred vision, pruritus, urinary tract infection, vasculitis of the legs.
ANGIOEDEMA: Angioedema has been reported in patients receiving ZESTRIL (0.1%). Angioedema associated with laryngeal edema may be fatal. If angioedema of the

Percent of Patients in Controlled Studies

	ZESTRIL (n=2003†) Incidence (discontinuation)	ZESTRIL/ Hydrochlorothiazide (n=644) Incidence (discontinuation)	Placebo (n=207) Incidence
Dizziness	6.3 (0.6)	9.0 (0.9)	1.9
Headache	5.3 (0.2)	4.3 (0.5)	1.9
Fatigue	3.3 (0.2)	3.9 (0.5)	1.0
Diarrhea	3.2 (0.3)	2.6 (0.3)	2.4
Upper Respiratory Symptoms	3.0 (0.0)	4.5 (0.0)	0.0
Cough	2.9 (0.4)	4.5 (0.8)	1.0
Nausea	2.3 (0.3)	2.5 (0.2)	2.4
Hypotension	1.8 (0.8)	1.6 (0.5)	0.5
Rash	1.5 (0.4)	1.6 (0.2)	0.5
Orthostatic Effects	1.4 (0.0)	3.4 (0.2)	1.0
Asthenia	1.3 (0.4)	2.0 (0.2)	1.0
Chest Pain	1.3 (0.1)	1.2 (0.2)	1.4
Vomiting	1.3 (0.2)	1.4 (0.0)	0.5
Dyspnea	1.1 (0.0)	0.5 (0.2)	1.4
Dyspepsia	1.0 (0.0)	1.9 (0.0)	0.0
Paresthesia	0.8 (0.0)	2.0 (0.2)	0.0
Impotence	0.7 (0.2)	1.6 (0.3)	0.0
Muscle Cramps	0.6 (0.0)	2.8 (0.6)	0.5
Back Pain	0.5 (0.0)	1.1 (0.0)	1.4
Nasal Congestion	0.3 (0.0)	1.2 (0.0)	0.0
Decreased Libido	0.2 (0.1)	1.2 (0.0)	0.0
Vertigo	0.1 (0.0)	1.1 (0.2)	0.0

† Includes 420 patients treated for congestive heart failure who were receiving concomitant digitalis and/or diuretic therapy.

face, extremities, lips, tongue, glottis and/or larynx occurs, treatment with ZESTRIL should be discontinued and appropriate therapy instituted immediately. (See WARNINGS.)

HYPOTENSION: In hypertensive patients, hypotension occurred in 1.2% and syncope occurred in 0.1% of patients. Hypotension or syncope was a cause of discontinuation of therapy in 0.5% of hypertensive patients. (See WARNINGS.) In patients with congestive heart failure, hypotension occurred in 5.0% and syncope occurred in 1.0% of patients. These adverse experiences were causes for discontinuation of therapy in 1.3% of these patients.

Clinical Laboratory Test Findings

Serum Electrolytes: Hyperkalemia (See PRECAUTIONS.)
Creatinine, Blood Urea Nitrogen: Minor increases in blood urea nitrogen and serum creatinine, reversible upon discontinuation of therapy, were observed in about 2.0% of patients with essential hypertension treated with ZESTRIL alone. Increases were more common in patients receiving concomitant diuretics and in patients with renal artery stenosis. (See PRECAUTIONS.) Reversible minor increases in blood urea nitrogen and serum creatinine were observed in approximately 9.1% of patients with congestive heart failure on concomitant diuretic therapy. Frequently, these abnormalities resolved when the dosage of the diuretic was decreased.
Hemoglobin and Hematocrit: Small decreases in hemoglobin and hematocrit (mean decreases of approximately 0.4 g% and 1.3 vol%, respectively) occurred frequently in patients treated with ZESTRIL but were rarely of clinical importance in patients without some other cause of anemia. In clinical trials, less than 0.1% of patients discontinued therapy due to anemia.
Other (Causal Relationship Unknown): Rarely, elevations of liver enzymes and/or serum bilirubin have occurred.
Overall, 2.0% of patients discontinued therapy due to laboratory adverse experiences, principally elevations in blood urea nitrogen (0.6%), serum creatinine (0.5%), and serum potassium (0.4%).

OVERDOSAGE

The oral LD$_{50}$ of lisinopril is greater than 20 g/kg in mice and rats. The most likely manifestation of overdosage would be hypotension, for which the usual treatment would be intravenous infusion of normal saline solution.
Lisinopril can be removed by hemodialysis.

DOSAGE AND ADMINISTRATION

Initial Therapy: In patients with uncomplicated essential hypertension not on diuretic therapy, the recommended initial dose is 10 mg once a day. Dosage should be adjusted according to blood pressure response. The usual dosage range is 20–40 mg per day administered in a single daily dose. The antihypertensive effect may diminish toward the end of the dosing interval regardless of the administered dose, but most commonly with a dose of 10 mg daily. This can be evaluated by measuring blood pressure just prior to dosing to determine whether satisfactory control is being maintained for 24 hours. If it is not, an increase in dose should be considered. Doses up to 80 mg have been used but do not appear to give greater effect. If blood pressure is not controlled with ZESTRIL alone, a low dose of a diuretic may be added. Hydrochlorothiazide, 12.5 mg has been shown to provide an

additive effect. After the addition of a diuretic, it may be possible to reduce the dose of ZESTRIL.

Diuretic Treated Patients: In hypertensive patients who are currently being treated with a diuretic, symptomatic hypotension may occur occasionally following the initial dose of ZESTRIL. The diuretic should be discontinued, if possible, for two or three days before beginning therapy with ZESTRIL to reduce the likelihood of hypotension. (See WARNINGS.) The dosage of ZESTRIL should be adjusted according to blood pressure response. If the patient's blood pressure is not controlled with ZESTRIL alone, diuretic therapy may be resumed as described above.

If the diuretic cannot be discontinued, an initial dose of 5 mg should be used under medical supervision for at least two hours and until blood pressure has stabilized for at least an additional hour. (See WARNINGS and PRECAUTIONS, Drug Interactions.)

Concomitant administration of ZESTRIL with potassium supplements, potassium salt substitutes, or potassium-sparing diuretics may lead to increases of serum potassium. (See PRECAUTIONS.)

Use in Elderly: In general, blood pressure response and adverse experiences were similar in younger and older patients given similar doses of ZESTRIL. Pharmacokinetic studies, however, indicate that maximum blood levels and area under the plasma concentration time curve (AUC) are doubled in older patients so that dosage adjustments should be made with particular caution.

Dosage Adjustment in Renal Impairment: The usual dose of ZESTRIL (10 mg) is recommended for patients with creatinine clearance > 30 mL/min (serum creatinine of up to approximately 3 mg/dL). For patients with creatinine clearance ≥ 10 mL/min ≤ 30 mL/min (serum creatinine ≥ 3 mg/dL), the first dose is 5 mg once daily. For patients with creatinine clearance < 10 mL/min (usually on hemodialysis) the recommended initial dose is 2.5 mg. The dosage may be titrated upward until blood pressure is controlled or to a maximum of 40 mg daily.

Renal Status	Creatinine-Clearance mL/min	Initial Dose mg/day
Normal Renal Function to Mild Impairment	> 30	10
Moderate to Severe Impairment	≥ 10 ≤ 30	5
Dialysis Patients	< 10	2.5‡

‡ Dosage or dosing interval should be adjusted depending on the blood pressure response.

HOW SUPPLIED

5 mg Tablets (NDC 0038-0130) pink, round, biconvex, uncoated, scored tablets, identified "ZESTRIL 5" debossed on

Continued on next page

Stuart—Cont.

one side, and "130" debossed and scored on the other side are supplied in bottles of 100 tablets and unit dose packages of 100 tablets.

10 mg Tablets (NDC 0038-0131) pink, round, biconvex, uncoated tablets identified "ZESTRIL 10" debossed on one side, and "131" debossed on the other side are supplied in bottles of 100 tablets and unit dose packages of 100 tablets.

20 mg Tablets (NDC 0038-0132) red, round, biconvex, uncoated tablets identified "ZESTRIL 20" debossed on one side, and "132" debossed on the other side are supplied in bottles of 100 tablets and unit dose packages of 100 tablets.

40 mg Tablets (NDC 0038-0134) yellow, round, biconvex, uncoated tablets identified "ZESTRIL 40" debossed on one side, and "134" debossed on the other side are supplied in bottles of 100 tablets and unit dose packages of 100 tablets. Store at room temperature. Protect from moisture, freezing and excessive heat. Dispense in a tight container.

Rev. J 04/89
SIC 63986-07

Shown in Product Identification Section, page 432

Summit Pharmaceuticals
Division of CIBA-GEIGY Corporation
SUMMIT, NJ 07901

To provide a convenient and accurate means of identifying Summit Pharmaceuticals' solid dosage form products, a code number has been imprinted on all tablets and capsules. To help you quickly identify a Summit Tablet or Capsule by its code number, a numerical listing of codes (with corresponding product names) and an alphabetical listing of products (with corresponding codes and list numbers) have been compiled below.

Summit Product Identification Number	ALPHABETICAL LISTING	National Drug Code Number
	Actigall™ ursodiol	
153	CAPSULES, 300 mg (white and pink, hard gelatin)	
	100s	57267-153-30
	Slow-K® potassium chloride USP	
165	TABLETS (round, buff-colored, sugar-coated), each containing 8 mEq (600 mg) potassium chloride	
	100s	57267-165-30
	1000s	57267-165-40
	Accu-Pak®	
	100s	57267-165-32
	Consumer Pack	
	100s	57267-165-65
	Ten-K® potassium chloride TABLETS, 750 mg (10 mEq) (white, capsule-shaped, scored)	
146	100s	57267-146-30
	500s	57267-146-35
	100s Unit Dose Pkg.	57267-146-32

[See table below].

Summit Product Identification Number	NUMERICAL LISTING	
	Actigall™ ursodiol	
153	Capsules, 300 mg (white and pink, hard gelatin)	
	Slow-K® potassium chloride USP	

165	TABLETS (buff colored, sugar-coated), each containing 8 mEq (600 mg) potassium chloride	
	Ten-K® potassium chloride TABLETS, 750 mg (10 mEq) (white, capsule-shaped, scored)	
146	100s	57267-146-30
	500s	57267-146-35
	100s Unit Dose Pkg.	57267-146-32
	Transderm-Nitro® nitroglycerin	
902	2.5 mg	30 systems
		*100 systems
905	5 mg	30 systems
		*100 systems
910	10 mg	30 systems
		*100 systems
915	15 mg	30 systems
		*100 systems
		*Hospital Pack 100's

ACTIGALL™   ℞
ursodiol
Capsules

Caution: Federal law prohibits dispensing without prescription.

SPECIAL NOTE

Gallbladder stone dissolution with Actigall treatment requires months of therapy. Complete dissolution does not occur in all patients and recurrence of stones within 5 years has been observed in up to 50% of patients who do dissolve their stones on bile acid therapy. Patients should be carefully selected for therapy with ursodiol, and alternative therapies should be considered.

DESCRIPTION

Actigall is an agent intended for dissolution of radiolucent gallstones. It is available as 300 mg capsules suitable for oral administration.

Actigall is ursodiol (ursodeoxycholic acid), a naturally-occurring bile acid found in small quantities in normal human bile and in larger quantities in the biles of certain species of bears. It is a bitter-tasting, white powder freely soluble in ethanol, and in glacial acetic acid, slightly soluble in chloroform, sparingly soluble in ether, and practically insoluble in water. The chemical name for ursodiol is $3\alpha,7\beta$-dihydroxy-5β-cholan-24-oic acid ($C_{24}H_{40}O_4$). Ursodiol has a molecular weight of 392.56.

Inactive Ingredients: Gelatin; iron oxide; magnesium stearate; colloidal silicon dioxide; starch; and titanium dioxide.

CLINICAL PHARMACOLOGY

About 90% of a therapeutic dose of Actigall is absorbed in the small bowel after oral administration. After absorption, ursodiol enters the portal vein and undergoes efficient extraction from portal blood by the liver (i.e., there is a large "first pass" effect) where it is conjugated with either glycine or taurine and is then secreted into the hepatic bile ducts. Ursodiol in bile is concentrated in the gallbladder and expelled into the duodenum in gallbladder bile via the cystic and common ducts by gallbladder contractions provoked by physiologic responses to eating. Only small quantities of ursodiol appear in the systemic circulation and very small amounts are excreted into urine. The sites of the drug's therapeutic actions are in the liver, bile and gut lumen.

Beyond conjugation, ursodiol is not altered or catabolized appreciably by the liver or intestinal mucosa. A small proportion of orally administered drug undergoes bacterial degradation with each cycle of enterohepatic circulation. Ursodiol can be both oxidized and reduced at the 7-carbon, yielding either 7-keto-lithocholic acid or lithocholic acid, respectively. Further, there is some bacterially catalyzed deconjugation of glyco- and tauro-ursodeoxycholic acid in the small bowel. Free ursodiol, 7-keto-lithocholic acid and lithocholic acid are relatively insoluble in aqueous media and larger proportions of these compounds are lost from the distal gut into the feces. Reabsorbed free ursodiol is reconju-

gated by the liver. Eighty percent of lithocholic acid formed in the small bowel is excreted in the feces, but the 20% that is absorbed is sulfated at the 3-hydroxyl group in the liver to relatively insoluble lithocholyl conjugates which are excreted into bile and lost in feces. Absorbed 7-keto-lithocholic acid is stereospecifically reduced in the liver to chenodiol. Lithocholic acid causes cholestatic liver injury and can cause death from liver failure in certain species unable to form sulfate conjugates. Lithocholic acid is formed by 7-dehydroxylation of the dihydroxy bile acids (ursodiol and chenodiol) in the gut lumen. The 7-dehydroxylation reaction appears to be alpha-specific, i.e., chenodiol is more efficiently 7-dehydroxylated than ursodiol and for equimolar doses of ursodiol and chenodiol, levels of lithocholic acid appearing in bile are lower with the former. Man has the capacity to sulfate lithocholic acid. Although liver injury has not been associated with ursodiol therapy, a reduced capacity to sulfate may exist in some individuals, but such a deficiency has not yet been clearly demonstrated.

Pharmacodynamics

Ursodiol suppresses hepatic synthesis and secretion of cholesterol, and also inhibits intestinal absorption of cholesterol. It appears to have little inhibitory effect on synthesis and secretion into bile of endogenous bile acids, and does not appear to affect secretion of phospholipids into bile.

With repeated dosing, bile ursodeoxycholic acid concentrations reach a steady state in about 3 weeks. Although insoluble in aqueous media, cholesterol can be solubilized in at least two different ways in the presence of dihydroxy bile acids. In addition to solubilizing cholesterol in micelles, ursodiol acts by an apparently unique mechanism to cause dispersion of cholesterol as liquid crystals in aqueous media. Thus, even though administration of high doses (e.g., 15–18 mg/kg/day) does not result in a concentration of ursodiol higher than 60% of the total bile acid pool, ursodiol-rich bile effectively solubilizes cholesterol. The overall effect of ursodiol is to increase the concentration level at which saturation of cholesterol occurs.

The various actions of ursodiol combine to change the bile of patients with gallstones from cholesterol-precipitating to cholesterol-solubilizing, thus resulting in bile conducive to cholesterol stone dissolution.

After ursodiol dosing is stopped, the concentration of the bile acid in bile falls exponentially, declining to about 5–10% of its steady state level in about 1 week.

Clinical Results

On the basis of clinical trial results in a total of 868 patients with radiolucent gallstones treated in 8 studies (three in the U.S. involving 282 patients, one in the U.K. involving 130 patients and four in Italy involving 456 patients) for periods ranging from 6–78 months with Actigall doses ranging from about 5 to 20 mg/kg/day, an Actigall dose of about 8–10 mg/kg/day appeared to be the best dose. With an Actigall dose of about 10 mg/kg/day, complete stone dissolution can be anticipated in about 30% of unselected patients with uncalcified gallstones < 20 mm in maximal diameter treated for up to two years. Patients with calcified gallstones prior to treatment, or patients who develop stone calcification or gallbladder non-visualization on treatment, and patients with stones larger than 20 mm in maximal diameter rarely dissolve their stones. The chance of gallstone dissolution is increased up to 50% in patients with floating or floatable stones (i.e., those with high cholesterol content), and is inversely related to stone size for those less than 20 mm in maximal diameter. Complete dissolution was observed in 81% of patients with stones up to 5 mm in diameter. Age, sex, weight, degree of obesity and serum cholesterol level are not related to the chance of stone dissolution with Actigall. A non-functioning (i.e., non-visualizing) gallbladder by oral cholecystogram prior to the initiation of therapy is not a contraindication to Actigall therapy (the group of patients with non-visualizing gallbladders in the Actigall studies had complete stone dissolution rates similar to the group of patients with visualizing gallbladders). However, gallbladder non-visualization developing during ursodiol treatment predicts failure of complete stone dissolution and in such cases therapy should be discontinued.

Partial stone dissolution occurring within 6 months of beginning therapy with Actigall appears to be associated with a > 70% chance of eventual complete stone dissolution with further treatment; partial dissolution observed within one year of starting therapy indicates a 40% probability of complete dissolution.

Stone recurrence after dissolution with Actigall therapy was seen within 2 years in 8/27 (30%) of patients in the U.K. studies. Of 16 patients in the U.K. study whose stones had previously dissolved on chenodiol but later recurred, 11 had complete dissolution on Actigall. Stone recurrence has been observed in up to 50% of patients within 5 years of complete stone dissolution on ursodiol therapy. Serial ultrasonographic examinations should be obtained to monitor for recurrence of stones, bearing in mind that radiolucency of the stones should be established before another course of Actigall is instituted. A prophylactic dose of Actigall has not been established.

	Transderm-Nitro® nitroglycerin				
Code	Transderm-Nitro System Rated Release *in vivo*	Total Nitroglycerin in System	System Size	National Drug Code Number	Carton Size
902	2.5 mg/24 hr	12.5 mg	5 cm²	57267-902-26	30 Systems
				57267-902-30	*100 Systems
905	5 mg/24 hr	25 mg	10 cm²	57267-905-26	30 Systems
				57267-905-30	*100 Systems
910	10 mg/24 hr	50 mg	20 cm²	57267-910-26	30 Systems
				57267-910-30	*100 Systems
915	15 mg/24 hr	75 mg	30 cm²	57267-915-26	30 Systems
				57267-915-30	*100 Systems
				*Hospital Pack 100's	

ALTERNATIVE THERAPIES

Watchful Waiting

Watchful waiting has the advantage that no therapy may ever be required. For patients with silent or minimally symptomatic stones, the rate of development of moderate to severe symptoms or gallstone complications is estimated to be between 2% and 6% per year, leading to a cumulative rate of 7% to 27% in five years. Presumably the rate is higher for patients already having symptoms.

Cholecystectomy

Surgery offers the advantage of immediate and permanent stone removal, but carries a high risk in some patients. About 5% of cholecystectomized patients have residual symptoms or retained common duct stones. The spectrum of surgical risk varies as a function of age and the presence of disease other than cholelithiasis.

Mortality Rates for Cholecystectomy in the U.S.
(National Halothane Study, JAMA 1966; 197:775–8)
27,600 Cholecystectomies (Smoothed Rates)
Deaths/1000 Operations***

Low Risk Patients* Age (Yrs)	Cholecystectomy	Cholecystectomy + Common Duct Exploration
Women 0–49	.54	2.13
50–69	2.80	10.10
Men 0–49	1.04	4.12
50–69	5.41	19.23
High Risk Patients**		
Women 0–49	12.66	47.62
50–69	17.24	58.82
Men 0–49	24.39	90.91
50–69	33.33	111.11

* In good health or with moderate systemic disease.
** With severe or extreme systemic disease.
*** Includes both elective and emergency surgery.
Women in good health or who have only moderate systemic disease, and are under 49 years of age have the lowest surgical mortality rate (0.054); men in all categories have a surgical mortality rate twice that of women. Common duct exploration quadruples the rates in all categories. The rates rise with each decade of life and increase tenfold or more in all categories with severe or extreme systemic disease.

INDICATIONS AND USAGE

Actigall is indicated for patients with radiolucent, non-calcified, gallbladder stones < 20 mm in greatest diameter in whom elective cholecystectomy would be undertaken except for the presence of increased surgical risk due to systemic disease, advanced age, idiosyncratic reaction to general anesthesia, or for those patients who refuse surgery. Safety of use of Actigall beyond 24 months is not established.

CONTRAINDICATIONS

1. Actigall will not dissolve calcified cholesterol stones, radio-opaque stones or radiolucent bile pigment stones. Hence, patients with such stones are not candidates for Actigall therapy.
2. Patients with compelling reasons for cholecystectomy including unremitting acute cholecystitis, cholangitis, biliary obstruction, gallstone pancreatitis or biliary-gastrointestinal fistula are not candidates for Actigall therapy.
3. Allergy to bile acids.
4. Chronic liver disease. Data currently available are insufficient to allow recommendation of use of Actigall in patients with chronic liver disease.

PRECAUTIONS

Liver Tests

Ursodiol therapy has not been associated with liver damage. Lithocholic acid, a naturally occurring bile acid, is known to be a liver-toxic metabolite. This bile acid is formed in the gut from ursodiol less efficiently and in smaller amounts than that seen from chenodiol. Lithocholic acid is detoxified in the liver by sulfation and although man appears to be an efficient sulfater, it is possible that some patients may have a congenital or acquired deficiency in sulfation, thereby predisposing them to lithocholic-induced liver damage. For these reasons, patients given Actigall should have SGOT (AST) and SGPT (ALT) measured at the initiation of therapy, after one and three months of therapy, and every six months thereafter.
Patients found to have significant abnormalities in liver tests at any point should be monitored frequently and should be evaluated carefully for worsening gallstone disease which, in the controlled clinical trials, has been the only identified cause of significant liver test abnormality. Therapy with ursodiol should be discontinued if increased levels persist.

Drug Interactions

Bile acid sequestering agents such as cholestyramine and colestipol may interfere with the action of Actigall by reducing its absorption. Aluminum-based antacids have been shown to adsorb bile acids in vitro and may be expected to interfere with Actigall in the same manner as the bile acid sequestering agents. Estrogens, oral contraceptives and clofibrate (and perhaps other lipid-lowering drugs) increase hepatic cholesterol secretion, and encourage cholesterol gallstone formation and hence may counteract the effectiveness of Actigall.

Carcinogenesis, Mutagenesis, and Impairment of Fertility

Carcinogenicity studies with Actigall in animals are in progress. A 78-week rat study employing intrarectal instillation of lithocholic acid and tauro-deoxycholic acid, metabolites of ursodiol and chenodiol, has been conducted. These bile acids alone did not produce any tumors. A tumor-promoting effect of both metabolites was observed when they were co-administered with a carcingenic agent. Results of epidemiologic studies suggest that bile acids might be involved in the pathogenesis of human colon cancer in patients who had undergone a cholecystectomy, but direct evidence is lacking. Ursodiol is not mutagenic in the Ames test. Dietary administration of lithocholic acid to chickens is reported to cause hepatic adenomatous hyperplasia.

Pregnancy Category B

Reproduction studies have been performed in rats and rabbits with ursodiol doses up to 200-fold the therapeutic dose and have revealed no evidence of impaired fertility or harm to the fetus at doses of 20 to 100-fold the human dose in rats and at 5-fold the human dose (highest dose tested) in rabbits. Studies employing 100 to 200-fold the human dose in rats have shown some reduction in fertility rate and litter size. There have been no adequate and well-controlled studies of the use of ursodiol in pregnant women, but inadvertent exposure of 4 women to therapeutic doses of the drug in the first trimester of pregnancy during the Actigall trials led to no evidence of effects on the fetus or newborn baby. Although it seems unlikely, the possibility that ursodiol can cause fetal harm cannot be ruled out; hence, the drug is not recommended for use during pregnancy.

Nursing Mothers

It is not known whether ursodiol is excreted in human milk. Because many drugs are excreted in human milk, caution should be exercised when Actigall is administered to a nursing mother.

Pediatric Use

The safety and effectiveness of Actigall in children have not been established.

ADVERSE REACTIONS

Gastrointestinal

Actigall given in doses of 8–10 mg/kg/day rarely causes diarrhea (< 1%). One study in which a placebo control was not used was associated with a 6% incidence of mild, transient diarrhea not requiring termination of therapy or lowering of Actigall dose. One patient with ulcerative colitis in the Actigall studies developed diarrhea on therapy. In the National Cooperative Gallstone Study, the incidence of diarrhea was 27.1% in the placebo group.

Dermatological

One patient in the Actigall studies with pre-existing psoriasis apparently developed exacerbation of itching on Actigall, which remitted on withdrawal of the drug.

Other

In two ongoing double-blind, placebo-controlled ursodiol studies in the U.S., for which the treatment codes have not yet been broken, the following minor events have been reported:

Pruritus, rash, urticaria, dry skin, sweating, hair thinning, nausea, vomiting, dyspepsia, metallic taste, abdominal pain, biliary pain, cholecystitis, diarrhea, constipation, stomatitis, flatulence, headache, fatigue, anxiety, depression, sleep disorder, arthralgia, myalgia, back pain, cough, rhinitis.

Since these studies are ongoing and blinded, incidence rates in the ursodiol and placebo groups cannot be calculated, nor has it been established whether the reactions listed are associated with ursodiol.

Overdosage

Neither accidental nor intentional overdosing with Actigall has been reported. Doses of Actigall in the range of 16–20 mg/kg/day have been tolerated for 6–37 months without symptoms by 7 patients. The LD_{50} for ursodiol in rats is over 5,000 mg/kg given over 7–10 days and over 7,500 mg/kg for mice. The most likely manifestation of severe overdose with Actigall would probably be diarrhea, which should be treated symptomatically.

DOSAGE AND ADMINISTRATION

The recommended dose for Actigall treatment of radiolucent gallbladder stones is 8–10 mg/kg/day given in 2 or 3 divided doses.
Ultrasound images of the gallbladder should be obtained at six month intervals for the first year of Actigall therapy to monitor gallstone response. If gallstones appear to have dissolved, Actigall therapy should be continued and dissolution confirmed on a repeat ultrasound examination within one to three months. Most patients who eventually achieve complete stone dissolution will show partial or complete dissolution at the first on-treatment re-evaluation. If partial stone dissolution is not seen by 12 months of Actigall therapy, the likelihood of success is greatly reduced.

HOW SUPPLIED

Actigall capsules brand of ursodiol are supplied in a strength of 300 mg. The hard-gelatin capsules are white and pink and printed with the product name and strength. They are supplied as follows:
Capsules 300 mg
Bottles of 100 .... NDC 57267-153-30
Do not store above 86°F (30°C).
Samples, when available, are identified by the word *SAMPLE* appearing on each capsule.
Dispense in tight container, USP.

C89-3 (Rev. 2/89)

Dist. by:
Summit Pharmaceuticals
Division of CIBA-GEIGY Corporation
Summit, New Jersey 07901
Shown in Product Identification Section, page 433

SLOW-K®   ℞

[sloe-kay]
potassium chloride USP
slow–release tablets

DESCRIPTION

Slow-K, potassium chloride USP, is a sugar-coated (not enteric-coated) tablet for oral administration, containing 600 mg of potassium chloride (equivalent to 8 mEq) in a wax matrix. This formulation is intended to provide a controlled release of potassium from the matrix to minimize the likelihood of producing high, localized concentrations of potassium within the gastrointestinal tract.
Slow-K is an electrolyte replenisher. Its chemical name is potassium chloride, and its structural formula is KCl. Potassium chloride USP is a white, granular powder or colorless crystals. It is odorless and has a saline taste. Its solutions are neutral to litmus. It is freely soluble in water and insoluble in alcohol.
Inactive Ingredients. Acacia, cetostearyl alcohol, gelatin, iron oxide, magnesium stearate, polyvinylpyrrolidone, parabens, sodium benzoate, starch, sucrose, talc, and titanium dioxide.

CLINICAL PHARMACOLOGY

The potassium ion is the principal intracellular cation of most body tissues. Potassium ions participate in a number of essential physiological processes, including the maintenance of intracellular tonicity, the transmission of nerve impulses, the contraction of cardiac, skeletal, and smooth muscle, and the maintenance of normal renal function.
In adults normal plasma potassium concentration is 3.5–5.0 mEq/L.
Potassium depletion may occur whenever the rate of potassium loss through renal excretion and/or loss from the gastrointestinal tract exceeds the rate of potassium intake. Such depletion usually develops slowly as a consequence of prolonged therapy with oral diuretics, primary or secondary hyperaldosteronism, diabetic ketoacidosis, severe diarrhea, or inadequate replacement of potassium in patients on prolonged parenteral nutrition. Potassium depletion due to these causes is usually accompanied by a concomitant deficiency of chloride and is manifested by hypokalemia and metabolic alkalosis. Potassium depletion may produce weakness, fatigue, disturbances of cardiac rhythm (primarily ectopic beats), prominent U-waves in the electrocardiogram, and in advanced cases flaccid paralysis and/or impaired ability to concentrate urine.
Potassium depletion associated with metabolic alkalosis is managed by correcting the fundamental causes of the deficiency whenever possible and administering supplemental potassium chloride in the form of high potassium food or potassium chloride solution or tablets.
In rare circumstances (e.g., patients with renal tubular acidosis) potassium depletion may be associated with metabolic acidosis and hyperchloremia. In such patients potassium replacement should be accomplished with potassium salts other than the chloride, such as potassium bicarbonate, potassium citrate, or potassium acetate.
The potassium chloride in Slow-K is completely absorbed before it leaves the small intestine. The wax matrix is not absorbed and is excreted in the feces; in some instances the empty matrices may be noticeable in the stool. When the bioavailability of the potassium ion from Slow-K is compared to that of a true solution the extent of absorption is similar. The slow-release properties of Slow-K are demonstrated by the finding that a significant increase in time is required for renal excretion of the first 50% of the Slow-K dose as compared to the solution.

Continued on next page

Summit Pharm.—Cont.

Increased urinary potassium excretion is first observed 1 hour after administration of Slow-K, reaches a peak at 4 hours, and extends up to 8 hours. Mean daily steady-state plasma levels of potassium following daily administration of Slow-K cannot be distinguished from those following administration of a potassium chloride solution or from control plasma levels of potassium ion.

INDICATIONS AND USAGE

BECAUSE OF REPORTS OF INTESTINAL AND GASTRIC ULCERATION AND BLEEDING WITH SLOW-RELEASE POTASSIUM CHLORIDE PREPARATIONS, THESE DRUGS SHOULD BE RESERVED FOR THOSE PATIENTS WHO CANNOT TOLERATE OR REFUSE TO TAKE LIQUID OR EFFERVESCENT POTASSIUM PREPARATIONS OR FOR PATIENTS IN WHOM THERE IS A PROBLEM OF COMPLIANCE WITH THESE PREPARATIONS.

1. For therapeutic use in patients with hypokalemia with or without metabolic alkalosis; in digitalis intoxication and in patients with hypokalemic familial periodic paralysis.

2. For prevention of potassium depletion when the dietary intake of potassium is inadequate in the following conditions: patients receiving digitalis and diuretics for congestive heart failure; hepatic cirrhosis with ascites; states of aldosterone excess with normal renal function; potassium-losing nephropathy, and certain diarrheal states.

3. The use of potassium salts in patients receiving diuretics for uncomplicated essential hypertension is often unnecessary when such patients have a normal dietary pattern. Serum potassium should be checked periodically, however, and, if hypokalemia occurs, dietary supplementation with potassium-containing foods may be adequate to control milder cases. In more severe cases supplementation with potassium salts may be indicated.

CONTRAINDICATIONS

Potassium supplements are contraindicated in patients with hyperkalemia, since a further increase in serum potassium concentration in such patients can produce cardiac arrest. Hyperkalemia may complicate any of the following conditions: chronic renal failure, systemic acidosis such as diabetic acidosis, acute dehydration, extensive tissue breakdown as in severe burns, adrenal insufficiency, or the administration of a potassium-sparing diuretic (e.g., spironolactone, triamterene) (see OVERDOSAGE).

All solid dosage forms of potassium supplements are contraindicated in any patient in whom there is cause for arrest or delay in tablet passage through the gastrointestinal tract. In these instances, potassium supplementation should be with a liquid preparation. Wax-matrix potassium chloride preparations have produced esophageal ulceration in certain cardiac patients with esophageal compression due to an enlarged left atrium.

WARNINGS

Hyperkalemia (See OVERDOSAGE.)
In patients with impaired mechanisms for excreting potassium, the administration of potassium salts can produce hyperkalemia and cardiac arrest. This occurs most commonly in patients given potassium by the intravenous route but may also occur in patients given potassium orally. Potentially fatal hyperkalemia can develop rapidly and be asymptomatic.

The use of potassium salts in patients with chronic renal disease, or any other condition which impairs potassium excretion, requires particularly careful monitoring of the serum potassium concentration and appropriate dosage adjustment.

Interaction with Potassium-Sparing Diuretics
Hypokalemia should not be treated by the concomitant administration of potassium salts and a potassium-sparing diuretic (e.g., spironolactone or triamterene), since the simultaneous administration of these agents can produce severe hyperkalemia.

Gastrointestinal lesions
Potassium chloride tablets have produced stenotic and/or ulcerative lesions of the small bowel and deaths. These lesions are caused by a high localized concentration of potassium ion in the region of a rapidly dissolving tablet, which injures the bowel wall and thereby produces obstruction, hemorrhage, or perforation. Slow-K is a wax-matrix tablet formulated to provide a controlled rate of release of potassium chloride and thus to minimize the possibility of a high local concentration of potassium ion near the bowel wall. While the reported frequency of small-bowel lesions is much less with wax-matrix tablets (less than one per 100,000 patient-years) than with enteric-coated potassium chloride tablets (40–50 per 100,000 patient-years) cases associated with wax-matrix tablets have been reported both in foreign countries and in the United States. In addition, perhaps because the wax-matrix preparations are not enteric-coated and release potassium in the stomach, there have been reports of upper gastrointestinal bleeding associated with

these products. The total number of gastrointestinal lesions remains approximately one per 100,000 patient-years. Slow-K should be discontinued immediately and the possibility of bowel obstruction or perforation considered if severe vomiting, abdominal pain, distention, or gastrointestinal bleeding occurs.

Metabolic acidosis
Hypokalemia in patients with metabolic *acidosis* should be treated with an alkalinizing potassium salt such as potassium bicarbonate, potassium citrate, or potassium acetate.

PRECAUTIONS

General: The diagnosis of potassium depletion is ordinarily made by demonstrating hypokalemia in a patient with a clinical history suggesting some cause for potassium depletion. In interpreting the serum potassium level, the physician should bear in mind that acute alkalosis *per se* can produce hypokalemia in the absence of a deficit in total body potassium, while acute acidosis *per se* can increase the serum potassium concentration into the normal range even in the presence of a reduced total body potassium.

Information for Patients
Physicians should consider reminding the patient of the following:
To take each dose without crushing, chewing, or sucking the tablets.
To take this medicine only as directed. This is especially important if the patient is also taking both diuretics and digitalis preparations.
To check with the physician if there is trouble swallowing tablets or if the tablets seem to stick in the throat.
To check with the doctor at once if tarry stools or other evidence of gastrointestinal bleeding is noticed.

Laboratory Tests
Regular serum potassium determinations are recommended. In addition, during the treatment of potassium depletion, careful attention should be paid to acid-base balance, other serum electrolyte levels, the electrocardiogram, and the clinical status of the patient, particularly in the presence of cardiac disease, renal disease, or acidosis.

Drug Interactions
Potassium-sparing diuretics: see **WARNINGS.**

Carcinogenesis, Mutagenesis, Impairment of Fertility
Long-term carcinogenicity studies in animals have not been performed.

Pregnancy Category C
Animal reproduction studies have not been conducted with Slow-K. It is also not known whether Slow-K can cause fetal harm when administered to a pregnant woman or can affect reproduction capacity. Slow-K should be given to a pregnant woman only if clearly needed.

Nursing Mothers
The normal potassium ion content of human milk is about 13 mEq/L. It is not known if Slow-K has an effect on this content. Caution should be exercised when Slow-K is administered to a nursing woman.

Pediatric Use
Safety and effectiveness in children have not been established.

ADVERSE REACTIONS

One of the most severe adverse effects is hyperkalemia (see **CONTRAINDICATIONS, WARNINGS** and **OVERDOSAGE**). There also have been reports of upper and lower gastrointestinal conditions including obstruction, bleeding, ulceration and perforation (see **CONTRAINDICATIONS** and **WARNINGS**); other factors known to be associated with such conditions were present in many of these patients.

The most common adverse reactions to oral potassium salts are nausea, vomiting, abdominal discomfort, and diarrhea. These symptoms are due to irritation of the gastrointestinal tract and are best managed by taking the dose with meals or reducing the dose.

Skin rash has been reported rarely.

OVERDOSAGE

The administration of oral potassium salts to persons with normal excretory mechanisms for potassium rarely causes serious hyperkalemia. However, if excretory mechanisms are impaired or if potassium is administered too rapidly intravenously, potentially fatal hyperkalemia can result (see **CONTRAINDICATIONS and WARNINGS**). It is important to recognize that hyperkalemia is usually asymptomatic and may be manifested only by an increased serum potassium concentration (6.5–8.0 mEq/L) and characteristic electrocardiographic changes (peaking of T waves, loss of P wave, depression of S-T segment, and prolongation of the Q-T interval). Late manifestations include muscle paralysis and cardiovascular collapse from cardiac arrest (9–12 mEq/L).

Treatment measures for hyperkalemia include the following: (1) elimination of foods and medications containing potassium and of potassium-sparing diuretics; (2) intravenous administration of 300–500 ml/hr of 10% dextrose solution containing 10–20 units of insulin per 1,000 ml; (3) correction of acidosis, if present, with intravenous sodium bicarbonate; (4) use of exchange resins, hemodialysis, or peritoneal dialysis.

In treating hyperkalemia in patients who have been stabilized on digitalis, too rapid a lowering of the serum potassium concentration can produce digitalis toxicity.

DOSAGE AND ADMINISTRATION

The usual dietary intake of potassium by the average adult is 40–80 mEq per day. Potassium depletion sufficient to cause hypokalemia usually requires the loss of 200 or more mEq of potassium from the total body store. Dosage must be adjusted to the individual needs of each patient but is typically in the range of 20 mEq per day for the prevention of hypokalemia to 40–100 mEq or more per day for the treatment of potassium depletion. Large numbers of tablets should be given in divided doses.

NOTE: Slow-K slow-release tablets must be swallowed whole and never crushed, chewed, or sucked.

HOW SUPPLIED

Tablets 600 mg potassium chloride (equivalent to 8 mEq)
round, buff colored, sugar-coated (imprinted Slow-K)
  Bottles of 100 ....NDC 57267-165-30
  Bottles of 1000 ....NDC 57267-165-40
  Consumer Pack—One Unit
    12 Bottles—100 tablets each ....NDC 57267-165-65
  Accu-Pak® Unit Dose (Blister pack)
    Box of 100 (strips of 10) ....NDC 57267-165-32
Samples, when available, are identified by the word *SAMPLE* appearing on each tablet.
Do not store above 86°F (30°C). Protect from moisture. Protect from light.
Dispense in tight, light-resistant container (USP).
Dist. by:
Summit Pharmaceuticals
Division of CIBA-GEIGY Corporation
Summit, NJ 07901

C89-5 (Rev. 3/89)
Shown in Product Identification Section, page 433

TEN-K®   ℞
potassium chloride USP
Controlled-Release Multiple-Unit Tablets

DESCRIPTION

Ten-K, potassium chloride (KCl), is a controlled-release, multiple-unit tablet for oral administration. Each tablet contains 750 mg of potassium chloride as polymeric-coated crystals (equivalent to 10 mEq of potassium) in a rice starch binder. After ingestion, the tablets disintegrate and disperse rapidly into small particles, each with a polymeric coating, which allows for controlled release of potassium and chloride ions over approximately an 8- to 10-hour period. The dispersibility of the coated crystals and the controlled release of ions are intended to minimize the likelihood of high localized concentrations of potassium chloride in the gastrointestinal tract.

Potassium chloride has an empirical formula of KCl and a molecular weight of 74.55.

Ten-K as a multiple-unit tablet can be subdivided without significant changes in the release characteristics to improve swallowability. The polymeric coating functions as a water-permeable membrane. Fluids pass through the membrane and gradually dissolve the potassium chloride within the polymeric-coated crystals. The resulting potassium chloride solution slowly diffuses outward through the membrane.

Inactive Ingredients. Acetyl tributyl citrate, cellulose compounds, colloidal silicone dioxide, magnesium stearate, rice starch, talc, and wax.

CLINICAL PHARMACOLOGY

Potassium ion is the principal intracellular cation of most body tissues. Potassium ions participate in a number of essential physiological processes, including the maintenance of intracellular tonicity, the transmission of nerve impulses, the contraction of cardiac, skeletal, and smooth muscle, and the maintenance of normal renal function.

Potassium depletion may occur whenever the rate of potassium loss through renal excretion and/or loss from the gastrointestinal tract exceeds the rate of potassium intake. Such depletion usually develops slowly as a consequence of prolonged therapy with oral diuretics, primary or secondary hyperaldosteronism, diabetic ketoacidosis, severe diarrhea, or inadequate replacement of potassium in patients on prolonged parenteral nutrition. Potassium depletion due to these causes is usually accompanied by a concomitant deficiency of chloride and is manifested by hypokalemia and metabolic alkalosis.

Potassium depletion may produce weakness, fatigue, disturbances of cardiac rhythm (primarily ectopic beats), prominent U waves in the electrocardiogram, and in advanced cases, flaccid paralysis and/or impaired ability to concentrate urine.

Potassium depletion associated with metabolic alkalosis is managed by correcting the fundamental causes of the deficiency whenever possible and administering supplemental potassium chloride in the form of high potassium food or potassium chloride solution, capsules, or tablets. In rare circumstances (e.g., in patients with renal tubular acidosis) potassium depletion may be associated with metabolic acidosis and hyperchloremia. In such patients, potassium replacement should be accomplished with potassium salts other than the chloride, such as potassium bicarbonate, potassium citrate, or potassium acetate.

INDICATIONS AND USAGE

BECAUSE OF REPORTS OF INTESTINAL AND GASTRIC ULCERATION AND BLEEDING WITH SLOW-RELEASE POTASSIUM CHLORIDE PREPARATIONS, THESE DRUGS SHOULD BE RESERVED FOR THOSE PATIENTS WHO CANNOT TOLERATE OR REFUSE TO TAKE LIQUID OR EFFERVESCENT POTASSIUM PREPARATIONS OR FOR PATIENTS IN WHOM THERE IS A PROBLEM OF COMPLIANCE WITH THESE PREPARATIONS.

1. For therapeutic use in patients with hypokalemia with or without metabolic alkalosis; in digitalis intoxication and in patients with hypokalemic familial periodic paralysis.
2. For prevention of potassium depletion when the dietary intake of potassium is inadequate in the following conditions: patients receiving digitalis and diuretics for congestive heart failure; hepatic cirrhosis with ascites; states of aldosterone excess with normal renal function; potassium-losing nephropathy; and certain diarrheal states.
3. The use of potassium salts in patients receiving diuretics for uncomplicated essential hypertension is often unnecessary when such patients have a normal dietary pattern. Serum potassium should be checked periodically, however, and if hypokalemia occurs, dietary supplementation with potassium-containing foods may be adequate to control milder cases. In more severe cases, supplementation with potassium salts may be indicated.

CONTRAINDICATIONS

Potassium supplements are contraindicated in patients with hyperkalemia, since a further increase in serum potassium concentration in such patients can produce cardiac arrest. Hyperkalemia may complicate any of the following conditions: chronic renal failure, systemic acidosis such as diabetic acidosis, acute dehydration, extensive tissue breakdown as in severe burns, adrenal insufficiency, or the administration of a potassium-sparing diuretic (e.g., spironolactone, triamterene, amiloride).

Wax-matrix potassium chloride preparations have produced esophageal ulceration in certain cardiac patients with esophageal compression due to an enlarged left atrium.

All solid dosage forms of potassium supplements are contraindicated in any patients in whom there is cause for arrest or delay in tablet passage through the gastrointestinal tract. In these instances, potassium supplementation should be with a liquid preparation.

WARNINGS

Hyperkalemia

In patients with impaired mechanisms for excreting potassium, the administration of potassium salts can produce hyperkalemia and cardiac arrest. This occurs most commonly in patients given potassium by the intravenous route but may also occur in patients given potassium orally. Potentially fatal hyperkalemia can develop rapidly and be asymptomatic.

The use of potassium salts in patients with chronic renal disease, or any other condition which impairs potassium excretion, requires particularly careful monitoring of the serum potassium concentration and appropriate dosage adjustments.

Interaction With Potassium-Sparing Diurectics

Hypokalemia should not be treated by the concomitant administration of potassium salts and a potassium-sparing diuretic (e.g., spironolactone, triamterene, amiloride), since the simultaneous administration of these agents can produce severe hyperkalemia.

Gastrointestinal Lesions

Potassium chloride tablets have produced stenotic and/or ulcerative lesions of the small bowel and deaths, in addition to upper gastrointestinal bleeding. These lesions are caused by a high localized concentration of potassium ion in the region of a rapidly dissolving tablet, which injures the bowel wall and thereby produces obstruction, hemorrhage, or perforation.

Ten-K tablets consist of polymeric-coated crystals. After ingestion the tablets disintegrate and disperse rapidly in the stomach into subunits, which are formulated to provide a controlled release of potassium chloride. The dispersibility of the subunits and the controlled release of potassium ions from the subunits are intended to minimize the possibility of a high local concentration near the gastrointestinal mucosa and the ability of the potassium chloride to cause stenosis or ulceration. Other means of accomplishing this (e.g., incorporation of potassium chloride into a wax matrix) have reduced the frequency of such lesions to less than one per 100,000 patient-years (compared to 40-50 per 100,000 patient-years with enteric-coated potassium chloride) but have not eliminated them. The frequency of gastrointestinal lesions with Ten-K is at present unknown. Ten-K should be discontinued

immediately and the possibility of bowel obstruction or perforation considered if severe vomiting, abdominal pain, distention, or gastrointestinal bleeding occurs.

Metabolic Acidosis

Hypokalemia in patients with metabolic *acidosis* should be treated with an alkalinizing potassium salt such as potassium bicarbonate, potassium citrate, or potassium acetate.

PRECAUTIONS

The diagnosis of potassium depletion is ordinarily made by demonstrating hypokalemia in a patient with a clinical history suggesting some cause for potassium depletion. In interpreting the serum potassium level, the physician should bear in mind that acute alkalosis per se can produce hypokalemia in the absence of a deficit in total body potassium, while acute acidosis per se can increase the serum potassium concentration into the normal range even in the presence of a reduced total body potassium. The treatment of potassium depletion, particularly in the presence of cardiac disease, renal disease, or acidosis, requires careful attention to acid-base balance and appropriate monitoring of serum electrolytes, the electrocardiogram, and the clinical status of the patient.

Carcinogenesis, Mutagenesis, Impairment of Fertility

Long-term carcinogenicity studies in animals have not been performed.

Pregnancy Category C

Animal reproduction studies have not been conducted with Ten-K. It is also not known whether Ten-K can cause fetal harm when administered to a pregnant woman or can affect reproduction capacity. Ten-K should be given to a pregnant woman only if clearly needed.

Nursing Mothers

The normal potassium ion content of human milk is about 13 mEg/L. It is not known if Ten-K has an effect on this content. Caution should be exercised when Ten-K is administered to a nursing woman.

Pediatric Use

Safety and effectiveness in children have not been established.

ADVERSE REACTIONS

The most common adverse reactions to oral potassium salts are nausea, vomiting, abdominal discomfort, and diarrhea. These symptoms are due to irritation of the gastrointestinal tract and may be minimized by taking the dose with meals or by reducing the dose.

Intestinal bleeding, ulceration, perforation, and obstruction have been reported in patients treated with solid dosage forms of potassium salts and may occur with Ten-K (see CONTRAINDICATIONS and WARNINGS). One of the most severe adverse effects of potassium supplementation is hyperkalemia (see CONTRAINDICATIONS, WARNINGS, and OVERDOSAGE).

Skin rash has been reported rarely with potassium preparations.

OVERDOSAGE

The administration of oral potassium salts to persons with normal excretory mechanisms for potassium rarely causes serious hyperkalemia. However, if excretory mechanisms are impaired or if potassium is administered too rapidly intravenously, potentially fatal hyperkalemia can result (see CONTRAINDICATIONS and WARNINGS). It is important to recognize that hyperkalemia is usually asymptomatic and may be manifested only by an increased serum potassium concentration and characteristic electrocardiogram changes (peaking of T-waves, loss of P-wave, depression of S-T segment, and prolongation of the Q-T interval). Late manifestations include muscle paralysis and cardiovascular collapse from cardiac arrest.

Treatment measures for hyperkalemia include the following: (1) elimination of foods and medications containing potassium and of potassium-sparing diuretics; (2) intravenous administration of 300–500 ml/hr of 10% dextrose solution containing 10–20 units of insulin per 1,000 ml; (3) correction of acidosis, if present with intravenous sodium bicarbonate; (4) use of exchange resins, hemodialysis, or peritoneal dialysis.

In treating hyperkalemia, it should be recalled that in patients who have been stabilized on digitalis, too rapid a lowering of the serum potassium concentration can produce digitalis toxicity.

DOSAGE AND ADMINISTRATION

The usual dietary intake of potassium by the average adult is 40–80 mEq per day. Potassium depletion sufficient to cause hyperkalemia usually requires the loss of 200 or more mEq of potassium from the total body store.

Dosage must be adjusted to the individual needs of each patient, but typically is in the range of two to three tablets of Ten-K per day (20–30 mEq of potassium) for the prevention of hypokalemia and four to ten tablets of Ten-K (40–100 mEq of potassium) or more per day for the treatment of potassium depletion. If more than two Ten-K mEq tablets are prescribed per day, the total daily dosage should be divided into two or more separate doses and any single dose should not exceed 20 mEq.

Because Ten-K tablets can be subdivided without a significant change in the dissolution profile and since each crystal of potassium chloride has a polymeric coating, the tablets can be broken in half or crushed without an unpleasant taste. This mode of administration may be preferred for patients with difficulty in swallowing tablets.

HOW SUPPLIED

Tablets —750 mg of potassium chloride (equivalent to 10 mEq) capsule-shaped, white, scored

    Bottles of 100 ....NDC 57267-146-30
    Unit Dose (blister pack)
      Box of 100 (strips of 10)......................NDC 57267-146-32
    Bottles of 500 ....NDC 57267-146-35

Do not store above 86°F (30°C). Protect from moisture.

ANIMAL TOXICITY

The ulcerogenic potential of polymeric-coated crystals of potassium chloride was studied in monkeys. In monkeys receiving 2400 mEq of potassium chloride as Ten-K for 8½ days, Ten-K showed no tendency to cause intestinal ulceration.

Dist. by:
Summit Pharmaceuticals   C89-6 (Rev. 3/89)
Division of CIBA-GEIGY Corporation
Summit, NJ 07901

    Shown in Product Identification Section, page 433

TRANSDERM–NITRO®   ℞
[*trans'derm nye'trow*]
nitroglycerin
Transdermal Therapeutic System

DESCRIPTION

Transderm-Nitro (nitroglycerin) transdermal therapeutic system is a flat unit designed to provide controlled release of nitroglycerin through a semipermeable membrane continuously for 24 hours following application to intact skin. Nitroglycerin (glyceryl trinitrate) is a prompt-acting vasodilator for the relief and prevention of anginal attacks. Systems are rated to release *in vivo* 2.5, 5, 10 and 15 mg nitroglycerin over 24 hours and are in sizes of 5, 10, 20 and 30 cm² respectively. One-fifth of the total nitroglycerin in the system is delivered transdermally to the patient over 24 hours; the remainder serves as the reservoir to release the drug and remains in the system. The rated release of drug is dependent upon the area of the system; 0.5 mg nitroglycerin is delivered *in vivo* for every cm² of system size.

The Transderm-Nitro system comprises four layers as shown below. Proceeding from the visible surface towards the surface attached to the skin, these layers are: 1) a tan-colored backing layer (aluminized plastic) that is impermeable to nitroglycerin; 2) a drug reservoir containing nitroglycerin adsorbed on lactose, colloidal silicon dioxide, and silicone medical fluid; 3) an ethylene/vinyl acetate copolymer membrane that is permeable to nitroglycerin; and 4) a layer of hypoallergenic silicone adhesive. Prior to use, a protective peel strip is removed from the adhesive surface.

Cross section of the system:

Backing
Drug Reservoir
Semipermeable Membrane
Adhesive
Protective Peel Strip

ACTIONS

When the Transderm-Nitro system is applied to the skin, nitroglycerin is absorbed continuously through the skin into the systemic circulation. This results in active drug reaching the target organs (heart, extremities) before being inactivated by the liver. Nitroglycerin is a smooth muscle relaxant with vascular effects manifested predominantly by venous dilatation and pooling. The major beneficial effect of nitroglycerin in angina pectoris is a reduction in myocardial oxygen consumption secondary to vascular smooth muscle relaxation and consequent reduced cardiac preload and afterload. In recent years there has been an increasing recognition of a direct vasodilator effect of nitroglycerin on the coronary vessels.

In healthy volunteers transdermal absorption of nitroglycerin from a nitroglycerin system occurred in a continuous and well-controlled manner for a minimum of 24 hours. Steady-state plasma levels are attained within 2 hours after application, and continue for the duration of wearing the system. Precise definition of "therapeutic plasma level" is not known at this time. Plasma levels of nitroglycerin fall to approximately one-half the steady-state values 1 hour after system removal and are undetectable after 2 hours.

The amount of nitroglycerin released (2.5 mg, 5 mg, 10 mg, or 15 mg per 24 hours) represents the mean release rate of nitroglycerin from the system as determined from healthy volunteers, and hence, the amount potentially available for absorption through the skin. Absorption will vary among individuals.

Continued on next page

Summit Pharm.—Cont.

INDICATIONS AND USAGE

This drug product has been conditionally approved by the FDA for the prevention and treatment of angina pectoris due to coronary artery disease. The conditional approval reflects a determination that the drug may be marketed while further investigation of its effectiveness is undertaken. A final evaluation of the effectiveness of the product will be announced by the FDA.

CONTRAINDICATIONS

Intolerance of organic nitrate drugs, marked anemia, increased intraocular pressure or increased intracranial pressure.

WARNINGS

In patients with acute myocardial infarction or congestive heart failure, Transderm-Nitro system should be used under careful clinical and/or hemodynamic monitoring.

In terminating treatment of anginal patients, both the dosage and frequency of application must be gradually reduced over a period of 4 to 6 weeks to prevent sudden withdrawal reactions, which are characteristic of all vasodilators in the nitroglycerin class.

Transdermal nitroglycerin systems should be removed before attempting defibrillation or cardioversion because of the potential for altered electrical conductivity which may enhance the possibility of arcing, a phenomenon associated with the use of defibrillators.

PRECAUTIONS

Symptoms of hypotension, such as faintness, weakness or dizziness, particularly orthostatic hypotension may be due to overdosage. When these symptoms occur, the dosage should be reduced or use of the product discontinued.

Transderm-Nitro system is not intended for immediate relief of anginal attacks. For this purpose occasional use of the sublingual preparations may be necessary.

ADVERSE REACTIONS

Transient headaches are the most common side effect, especially when higher doses of the drug are used. These headaches should be treated with mild analgesics while Transderm-Nitro therapy is continued. When such headaches are unresponsive to treatment, the nitroglycerin dosage should be reduced or use of the product discontinued. Adverse reactions reported less frequently include hypotension, increased heart rate, faintness, flushing, dizziness, nausea and vomiting. These symptoms are attributable to the known pharmacologic effects of nitroglycerin, but may be symptoms of overdosage. When they persist the dose should be reduced or use of the product discontinued. In some patients, dermatitis may occur.

DOSAGE AND ADMINISTRATION

Therapy should be initiated with application of one Transderm-Nitro 5 mg/24 hr system to the desired area of skin. Many patients prefer the chest; if hair is likely to interfere with system adhesion or removal, it can be clipped prior to placement of the system. Each system is designed to remain in place for 24 hours, and each successive application should be to a different skin area. Transderm-Nitro should not be applied to the distal parts of the extremities. The usual dosage is one Transderm-Nitro 5 mg/24 hr system. Some patients, however, may require the Transderm-Nitro 10 mg/24 hr system. If a single Transderm-Nitro 5 mg/24 hr system fails to provide adequate clinical response, the patient should be instructed to remove it and apply either two Transderm-Nitro 5 mg/24 hr systems or one Transderm-Nitro 10 mg/24 hr system. More systems may be added as indicated by continued careful monitoring of clinical response. The Transderm-Nitro 2.5 mg/24 hr system is useful principally for decreasing the dosage gradually, though it may provide adequate therapy for some patients when used alone.

The optimal dosage should be selected based upon the clinical response, side effects, and the effects of therapy upon blood pressure. The greatest attainable decrease in resting blood pressure that is not associated with clinical symptoms of hypotension especially during orthostasis indicates the optimal dosage. To decrease adverse reactions, the size and/or number of systems should be tailored to the individual patient's needs.

Do not store above 86°F (30°C).

PATIENT INSTRUCTIONS FOR APPLICATIONS

A patient leaflet is supplied with the systems.

HOW SUPPLIED

[See table below].

C89-8 (Rev. 3/89)

Dist. by:
Summit Pharmaceuticals
Division of CIBA-GEIGY Corporation
Summit, New Jersey 07901
How to use.

TRANSDERM–NITRO®

nitroglycerin
Transdermal Therapeutic System
for the prevention of angina

Transderm-Nitro is easy to use—it has a clear plastic backing, and a special adhesive that keeps the system firmly in place for 24 hours.

Where to place Transderm-Nitro

Select any area of skin on the body, EXCEPT the extremities below the knee or elbow. The chest is the preferred site. The area should be clean, dry, and hairless. If hair is likely to interfere with system adhesion or removal, it can be clipped, but not shaved. Take care to avoid areas with cuts or irritations. Do NOT apply the system immediately after showering or bathing. It is best to wait until you are certain the skin is completely dry.

How to apply Transderm-Nitro® nitroglycerin

1. Open the package by tearing at the indicated indentations. Carefully pick up the system lengthwise with the tab up, and the clear plastic backing facing you. You should be able to see the white cream containing nitroglycerin. (On very rare occasions, you may find a system without any white medication in it. Do not use it. Simply apply another system.)

Figure A

2. Firmly bend the tab forward with the thumb (Figure A). With both thumbs, begin to remove the clear plastic backing from the system at the tab (Figure B). Do not touch the inside of the exposed system, because the adhesive covers the entire surface.

Figure B

3. Continue to remove the clear plastic backing slowly along the length of the system, allowing the system to rest on the outside of your fingers (Figure C).

Figure C

4. Place the exposed, adhesive side of the system on the chosen skin site. Press firmly in place with the palm of your hand (Figure D). Once the system is in place, do not test the adhesion by pulling on it.

Figure D

When Transderm-Nitro is applied to your body, the nitroglycerin contained in the system begins to flow onto your skin through a unique rate-controlling membrane. This membrane allows the nitroglycerin to be released and available for absorption through your skin at a uniform rate for 24 hours.

5. Remove and discard the system after 24 hours. Place a new system on a different skin site, following steps 1–4.

Please note:

Contact with water, as in bathing, swimming, or showering will not affect the system. In the unlikely event that a system falls off, discard it and put a new one on a different skin site.

PRECAUTIONS

The most common side effect is headache, which often decreases as therapy is continued, but may require treatment with a mild analgesic. Although uncommon, faintness, flushing, and dizziness may occur, especially when suddenly rising from the recumbent (lying horizontal) position. If these symptoms occur, remove the system and notify your physician.

Skin irritation may occur. If it persists, consult your physician.

Keep these systems and all drugs out of the reach of children.

Important: Your doctor may decide to increase or decrease the size of the system, or prescribe a combination of systems, to suit your particular needs. The dose may vary depending on your individual response to the system.

This system is to be used for preventing angina, not for treating an acute attack.

DO NOT STORE ABOVE 86°F (30°C).

Dist. by:
Summit Pharmaceuticals
Div. of CIBA-GEIGY Corp.
Summit, NJ 07901

C89-9 (Rev. 3/89)

Shown in Product Identification Section, page 433

Transderm-Nitro System Rated Release *in vivo*	Total Nitroglycerin in System	System Size	Carton Size		
2.5 mg/24 hr	12.5 mg	5 cm²	30 Systems	NDC 57267-902-26	
			*30 Systems	NDC 57267-902-42	
			*100 Systems	NDC 57267-902-30	
5 mg/24 hr	25 mg	10 cm²	30 Systems	NDC 57267-905-26	
			*30 Systems	NDC 57267-905-42	
			*100 Systems	NDC 57267-905-30	
10 mg/24 hr	50 mg	20 cm²	30 Systems	NDC 57267-910-26	
			*30 Systems	NDC 57267-910-42	
			*100 Systems	NDC 57267-910-30	
15 mg/24 hr	75 mg	30 cm²	30 Systems	NDC 57267-915-26	
			*30 Systems	NDC 57267-915-42	
			*100 Systems	NDC 57267-915-30	

*Institutional Pack

Sween Corporation
1940 COMMERCE DRIVE
P.O. BOX 8300
N. MANKATO, MN 56001

ATRAC–TAIN™
[ŭtrăc′tān]
Moisturizing
CREAM
with 10% Urea

DESCRIPTION
ATRAC-TAIN CREAM is a moisturizing vanishing cream consisting of Water, Urea (10%), Lactic Acid, Isopropyl Palmitate, Octyl Palmitate, Stearyl Alcohol, Glyceryl Stearte, Sorbitol, Stearic Acid, Ceteareth-25, Ceteareth-6, and Methylbenzethonium Chloride.

INDICATIONS AND USAGE
ATRAC-TAIN CREAM's dual-action urea formula moisturizes and softens severely dry, rough skin and thereby, relieves the itching and associated discomforts of many dry skin conditions. Urea increases the water binding capacity of the stratum corneum by attracting water to the dry skin cells. It also causes a physical softening of the desquamating layer of the epidermis by opening up more areas for H-bonding to water thus partially solubilizing the hard keratins that cause dry skin to feel rough. ATRAC-TAIN CREAM is non-occlusive, contains no petrolatum, mineral oil, parabens, dyes or perfumes.

CONTRAINDICATIONS
Hypersensitivity to any components of the preparation.

PRECAUTIONS AND ADVERSE REACTIONS
For External Use Only. Avoid Contact with eyes. Keep out of reach of children. If irritation occurs, temporarily discontinue use.

DOSAGE AND ADMINISTRATION
1. Cleanse affected area with gentle cleanser and pat dry.
2. Apply ATRAC-TAIN CREAM evenly to affected skin area—massage until absorbed.
3. Reapply CREAM 2–3 times daily.

HOW SUPPLIED
2 oz. tubes, ½ oz. tube.

ATRAC–TAIN™
[ŭtrăc′tān]
Moisturizing
LOTION

DESCRIPTION
ATRAC-TAIN LOTION is a moisturizing Lotion containing Water, Urea (5%), Sorbitol, Glyceryl Stearate, Lactic Acid, Isopropyl Palmitate, Octyl Palmitate, Stearyl Alcohol, Stearic Acid, Ceteareth-25, Ceteareth-6, PEG-40 Jojoba Oil, EDTA, Quaternium-15 and Methylbenzethonium Chloride.

INDICATIONS AND USAGE
ATRAC-TAIN LOTION's formula enhances the body's normal remoisturizing system offering relief to mild dry skin conditions. ATRAC-TAIN LOTION also aids in maintaining healthy integrity of the skin once a dry skin condition has improved. Urea increases the water-binding capacity of the stratum corneum by opening up more areas for H-bonding to water thus attracting mosisture to the dry skin cells. It also causes a physical softening of the desquamating layer of the epidermis by partially solubilizing the hard keratins that cause dry skin to feel rough.
ATRAC-TAIN LOTION is non-occlusive, contains no petrolatum, mineral oil, parabens, dyes or perfumes.

CONTRAINDICATIONS
Hypersensitivity to any components of the preparation.

PRECAUTIONS AND ADVERSE REACTIONS
For External Use Only. Avoid contact with eyes. Keep out of reach of children. If irritation occurs, temporarily discontinue use.

DOSAGE AND ADMINISTRATION
1. Apply ATRAC-TAIN LOTION evenly to affected area and massage until absorbed.
2. Reapply LOTION as required for soothing relief.

HOW SUPPLIED
4 fl.oz. and 8 fl. oz. bottles with disk-top caps

MICRO–GUARD™
[mī′crŏ-gūard]
Antiseptic, Antifungal Skin Cream

DESCRIPTION
MICRO-GUARD Skin Cream contains the antimicrobial agent Chloroxylenol (PCMX) in a water washable, vanishing cream base. National Drug Code (NDC) 11701-012.

INDICATIONS AND USAGE
MICRO-GUARD is a soothing antiseptic and antifungal cream. MICRO-GUARD's antifungal action is effective treatment for conditions such as athlete's foot, jock itch and ringworm, while its antiseptic activity helps prevent skin infection. MICRO-GUARD can be used for adjunctive topical treatment of superficial skin infections when oral antibiotic agents are concurrently being administered.

CONTRAINDICATIONS
Hypersensitivity to any components of the preparation.

WARNINGS
MICRO-GUARD is not for ophthalmic, otic or vaginal use.

PRECAUTIONS
For External Use Only. Do not use near eyes. If contact with eye occurs, rinse thoroughly with water and consult physician. Keep out of reach of children. If skin irritation occurs, or if there is no improvement within two weeks, discontinue use and consult physician. In case of accidental ingestion, seek professional assistance or contact a Poison Control Center immediately. Do not use on children under 2 years of age without consulting a physician.

ADVERSE REACTIONS
MICRO-GUARD is not considered a primary skin irritant or sensitizer, but occasional erythema, stinging and eczematous reactions have occurred following its use. If irritation or sensitivity develops with the use of MICRO-GUARD, treatment should be discontinued and appropriate therapy instituted.

DOSAGE AND ADMINISTRATION
Gently and thoroughly cleanse affected area and pat dry. Apply a thin layer of MICRO-GUARD over involved area. Repeat application 2 to 3 times daily or as directed by physician.

HOW SUPPLIED
½ oz. tubes and 2 oz. jars.

MICRO–GUARD™
[mī′crŏ gūard]
Antifungal Powder

DESCRIPTION
MICRO-GUARD Powder contains Chloroxylenol (2.5%) in a Corn Starch base, with Sodium Bicarbonate, Silica and Methybenzethonium Chloride. NDC 11701-026.

INDICATIONS AND USAGE
MICRO-GUARD Powder is a soothing antifungal powder. MICRO-GUARD'S antifungal action is an effective treatment for conditions such as jock itch, athletes foot, ring worm and diaper rash. MICRO-GUARD Powder can be used for adjunctive topical treatment of superficial skin infections when oral antibiotic agents are concurrently being administered.

CONTRAINDICATIONS
Hypersensitivity to any components of the preparation.

WARNINGS
MICRO-GUARD Powder is not for ophthalmic, otic or vaginal use.

PRECAUTIONS
For external use only. If irritation occurs or if there is no improvement within two weeks, discontinue use and consult a physician. Keep out of reach of children. In case of accidental ingestion, seek professional assistance or contact a poison control center immediately. Do not use on children under 2 years of age except under the advice and supervision of a physician. Children under 12 years of age should be supervised in the use of this product. This product is not effective on the scalp or nails.

ADVERSE REACTIONS
MICRO-GUARD Powder is not considered a primary skin irritant or sensitizer. If irritation or sensitivity develops with the use of MICRO-GUARD Powder, treatment should be discontinued and appropriate therapy instituted.

DOSAGE AND ADMINISTRATION
Cleanse area and dry. Apply MICRO-GUARD Powder. Smooth over entire area including skin creases and folds. Repeat application 2-3 times daily or as directed by physician.

HOW SUPPLIED
3 oz. container with dispensing top.

PURI-CLENS™
[pūri-clĕns]
Wound Deodorizer and Cleanser

DESCRIPTION
PURI-CLENS contains a safe and effective, non-irritating, antimicrobial ingredient, Methylbenzethonium Chloride, in a water washable, soothing base. National Drug Code (NDC) 11701-008.

INDICATIONS AND USAGE
PURI-CLENS deodorizes wounds and aids in the removal of foreign materials and exudates. Will not delay wound healing.

CONTRAINDICATIONS
Hypersensitivity to any components of the preparation.

PRECAUTIONS AND ADVERSE REACTIONS
For External Use Only. Do not use on animal bites or puncture wounds. Do not use for more than ten days without consulting physician. PURI-CLENS is not toxic by oral ingestion and is not considered a primary eye or skin irritant under normal use conditions. Keep out of the reach of children.

DOSAGE AND ADMINISTRATION
Apply PURI-CLENS liberally to a sterile 4″ × 4″ pad. Gently and thoroughly cleanse wound and surrounding area. To aid in removing foreign material and exudates, dab wound carefully with clean 4″ × 4″ pad saturated with PURI-CLENS. May be rinsed with sterile saline, water or hydrogen peroxide solution.

DEODORIZATION
Apply PURI-CLENS directly to wound and cover with a sterile absorbent pad. Do not use solution with occlusive dressing. Repeat one to three times daily to control odors.

HOW SUPPLIED
2 fl. oz. unit dose and 8 fl. oz bottles with flip top caps.

SWEEN-A-PEEL™
Wafer Skin Protectant

DESCRIPTION
SWEEN-A-PEEL is a hydrophilic, hydrocolloidal wafer skin protectant containing the following: WA4 hydrophilic polymer—to provide moisture absorption; high molecular weight synthetic rubber polymers—to provide elasticity and strength; low molecular weight synthetic rubber polymers—to provide adhesion to dry surface; karaya gum powder—to provide adhesion to moist surfaces.

INDICATIONS AND USAGE
SWEEN-A-PEEL wafers applied to the peristomal area in ostomy care or to the area surrounding draining wounds, aid in protecting the skin against contact with exudates. SWEEN-A-PEEL may also be applied to pressure points of immobile patients to help preserve skin integrity and reduce the possible occurrence of decubitus ulcers. SWEEN-A-PEEL has also proven effective when incorporated into a decubitus ulcer treatment procedure.

CONTRAINDICATIONS
Hypersensitivity to any components of the preparation.

PRECAUTIONS
Avoid excess heat and humidity. Store below 77°F (25°C). Reseal container after each use.

ADMINISTRATION
Preparation. 1. Cleanse entire area thoroughly. 2. Remove any residue from weeping, excoriated areas as effectively as possible to assure maximum adherence of SWEEN-A-PEEL. **Ostomy Care.** 1. Use measuring guide to accurately measure stoma base. Transfer pattern to wafer using pencil, then cut. 2. Remove backing paper. Position wafer carefully onto skin. 3. Mold over entire area from stoma base to outer edges. **Wound Care.** 1. Cleanse wound and surrounding area. 2. Measure wound accurately. Use Sween-A-Peel piece large enough to extend 1½″ beyond edge of wound. 3. Remove backing and center over wound. 4. Mold over area from center to outer edges.

HOW SUPPLIED
Individually sealed 4″ × 4″ in cartons of five or twenty, 6″ × 8″ wafers in cartons of three and 12″ × 12″ squares in packages of two and twelve.

SWEEN CREAM®
[Swĕēn Crĕam]
Protective Cream

DESCRIPTION
A vanishing cream consisting of Water, Lanolin Oil, Cetyl Alcohol, Propylene Glycol, Ichthyo Liver Oil (Natural Vita-

Continued on next page

Sween—Cont.

mins A & D), Sodium Lauryl Sulfate, Beeswax, Fragrance, Quaternium-15, Methylbenzethonium Chloride and BHT. Health Related Item (HRI) 11701-002. Fragrance-Free formulation is also available. Health Related Item (HRI) 11701-019.

INDICATIONS AND USAGE

SWEEN CREAM is an effective preparation for use on skin conditions such as urine scald, diaper rash, rectal itch, psoriasis, minor burns, diarrheal breakdown, chafing and itching. Applied on skin before taping, SWEEN CREAM aids in the prevention of tape burns. SWEEN CREAM is used in long-term care of incontinent, geriatric and para/quadraplegic skin conditions. Also apply to folds of skin subject to perspiration irritation, to dry or cracked skin and to pressure sensitive areas. For ostomy care, apply a small amount on peristomal skin for protection before attaching appliance. This relieves itching and improves adhesion.

CONTRAINDICATIONS

Hypersensitivity to any components of the preparation.

PRECAUTIONS AND ADVERSE REACTIONS

For External Use Only. Avoid contact with eyes. SWEEN CREAM is not toxic by oral ingestion and is not considered a primary eye or skin irritant under normal use conditions.

DOSAGE AND ADMINISTRATION

Apply liberally as required.

HOW SUPPLIED

½ oz., 2 oz. and 5 oz. tubes; 2-oz. and 9 oz. jars, 3 oz. pump.

SWEEN PREP™
[Swēen Prĕp]
Protective Skin Barrier Film

DESCRIPTION

SWEEN PREP is a medicated, liquid skin barrier which contains Chloroxylenol (PCMX), a well known antimicrobial agent, in a protective film forming base.

INDICATIONS AND USAGE

SWEEN PREP applies to the skin as a liquid, with the aid of the special "Dab-O-Matic" applicator, the non-aerosol sprayer or the single use wipe. It dries rapidly to form a tough film which provides a visible shield on the skin. . . a barrier between the skin and irritants. This protective film creates a surface other than the skin itself for the application of tapes, cements and doublefaced adhesives.

CONTRAINDICATIONS

Hypersensitivity to any components of the preparation.

PRECAUTIONS AND ADVERSE REACTIONS

For External Use Only. Do not use near eyes. Will cause eye irritation. If contact occurs, flush with water for 15 minutes and consult physician. Keep out of the reach of children. In case of accidental ingestion, seek professional assistance or contact a Poison Control Center immediately.
Flammable. Do not use near open flame or while smoking.

DOSAGE AND ADMINISTRATION

Cleanse the skin area thoroughly, rinse and pat dry. Apply SWEEN PREP liberally to the entire area to be protected (slight stinging may be experienced if the skin is excoriated). Allow to dry (approximately 2 minutes) and apply tapes, adhesives, etc., in the normal manner to the SWEEN PREPPED skin. SWEEN PREP may be removed from the skin with soap and water or for easier removal, with isopropyl alcohol. Removal is, however, not necessary and the skin may be recoated as frequently as required.

HOW SUPPLIED

Unit dose wipes (NDC 11701-007-20), 2 fl. oz. "Dab-O-Matic" applicator (NDC 11701-007-03) and 4 fl. oz. non-aerosol spray (NDC 11701-006-04).

IDENTIFICATION PROBLEM?
Consult PDR's
Product Identification Section
where you'll find over 1700
products pictured actual size
and in full color.

Syntex (F.P.) Inc.
HUMACAO, PUERTO RICO 00661

Syntex Laboratories, Inc
3401 HILLVIEW AVE.
P.O. BOX 10850
PALO ALTO, CA 94303

Syntex Puerto Rico, Inc.
HUMACAO, PUERTO RICO 00661

ANADROL®-50   ℞
[an 'ă-drawl]
(oxymetholone)
50 mg. Tablets
A product of Syntex Laboratories, Inc.

DESCRIPTION

ANADROL (oxymetholone) tablets for oral administration each contain 50 mg of the steroid oxymetholone, a potent anabolic and androgenic drug.
The chemical name for oxymetholone is 17β-hydroxy-2-(hydroxymethylene)-17-methyl-5α-androstan-3-one.
Inactive Ingredients—lactose, magnesium stearate, povidone, starch

CLINICAL PHARMACOLOGY

Anabolic steroids are synthetic derivatives of testosterone. Nitrogen balance is improved with anabolic agents but only when there is sufficient intake of calories and protein. Whether this positive nitrogen balance is of primary benefit in the utilization of protein-building dietary substances has not been established. Oxymetholone enhances the production and urinary excretion of erythropoietin in patients with anemias due to bone marrow failure and often stimulates erythropoiesis in anemias due to deficient red cell production.
Certain clinical effects and adverse reactions demonstrate the androgenic properties of this class of drugs. Complete dissociation of anabolic and androgenic effects has not been achieved. The actions of anabolic steroids are therefore similar to those of male sex hormones with the possibility of causing serious disturbances of growth and sexual development if given to young children. They suppress the gonadotropic functions of the pituitary and may exert a direct effect upon the testes.

INDICATIONS AND USAGE

ANADROL-50 is indicated in the treatment of anemias caused by deficient red cell production. Acquired aplastic anemia, congenital aplastic anemia, myelofibrosis and the hypoplastic anemias due to the administration of myelotoxic drugs often respond.
ANADROL-50 should not replace other supportive measures such as transfusion, correction of iron, folic acid, vitamin B$_{12}$ or pyridoxine deficiency, antibacterial therapy and the appropriate use of corticosteroids.

CONTRAINDICATIONS

1. Carcinoma of the prostate or breast in male patients.
2. Carcinoma of the breast in females with hypercalcemia; androgenic anabolic steroids may stimulate osteolytic resorption of bones.
3. Oxymetholone can cause fetal harm when administered to pregnant women. It is contraindicated in women who are or may become pregnant. If the patient becomes pregnant while taking the drug, she should be apprised of the potential hazard to the fetus.
4. Nephrosis or the nephrotic phase of nephritis.
5. Hypersensitivity to the drug.

WARNINGS

The following conditions have been reported in patients receiving androgenic, anabolic steroids as a general class of drugs:

Peliosis hepatis, a condition in which liver and sometimes splenic tissue is replaced with blood-filled cysts, has been reported in patients receiving androgenic anabolic steroid therapy. These cysts are sometimes present with minimal hepatic dysfunction, but at other times they have been associated with liver failure. They are often not recognized until life-threatening liver failure or intra-abdominal hemorrhage develops. Withdrawal of drug usually results in complete disappearance of lesions.
Liver cell tumors are also reported. Most often these tumors are benign and androgen-dependent, but fatal malignant tumors have been reported. Withdrawal of drug often results in regression or cessation of progression of the tumor. However, hepatic tumors associated

with androgens or anabolic steroids are much more vascular than other hepatic tumors and may be silent until life-threatening intra-abdominal hemorrhage develops. Blood lipid changes that are known to be associated with increased risk of atherosclerosis are seen in patients treated with androgens and anabolic steroids. These changes include decreased high density lipoprotein and sometimes increased low density lipoprotein. The changes may be very marked and could have a serious impact on the risk of atheroclerosis and coronary artery disease.

Cholestatic hepatitis and jaundice occur with 17-alpha-alkylated androgens at relatively low doses. If cholestatic hepatitis with jaundice appears, the anabolic steroid should be discontinued. If liver function tests become abnormal, the patient should be monitored closely and the etiology determined. Generally the anabolic steroid should be discontinued, although in cases of mild abnormalities, the physician may elect to follow the patient carefully at a reduced drug dosage.
In patients with breast cancer, anabolic steroid therapy may cause hypercalcemia by stimulating osteolysis. In this case, the drug should be discontinued.
Edema with or without congestive heart failure may be a serious complication in patients with pre-existing cardiac, renal or hepatic disease.
Geriatric male patients treated with androgenic anabolic steroids may be at an increased risk for the development of prostate hypertrophy and prostatic carcinoma.
Anabolic steroids have not been shown to enhance athletic ability.

PRECAUTIONS
General:
Women should be observed for signs of virilization (deepening of the voice, hirsutism, acne, and clitoromegaly). To prevent irreversible change, drug therapy must be discontinued, when mild virilism is first detected. Such virilization is usual following androgenic anabolic steroid use at high doses. Some virilizing changes in women are irreversible even after prompt discontinuance of therapy and are not prevented by concomitant use of estrogens. Menstrual irregularities may also occur.
The insulin or oral hypoglycemic dosage may need adjustment in diabetic patients who receive anabolic steroids.
Anabolic steroids may cause suppression of clotting factors II, V, VII, and X, and an increase in prothrombin time.
Information for the patient:
The physician should instruct patients to report any of the following side effects of androgens.
Adult or Adolescent Males: Too frequent or persistent erections of the penis, appearance or aggravation of acne.
Women: Hoarseness, acne, changes in menstrual periods, or more hair on the face.
All Patients: Any nausea, vomiting, changes in skin color or ankle swelling.
Laboratory Tests:
Women with disseminated breast carcinoma should have frequent determination of urine and serum calcium levels druing the course of androgenic anabolic steroid therapy (see WARNINGS).
Because of the hepatotoxicity associated with the use of 17-alpha-alkylated androgens, liver function tests should be obtained periodically.
Periodic (every 6 months) x-ray examinations of bone age should be made during treatment of prepubertal patients to determine the rate of bone maturation and the effects of androgenic anabolic steroid therapy on the epiphyseal centers.
Anabolic steroids have been reported to lower the level of high-density lipoproteins and raise the level of low-density lipoproteins. These changes usually revert to normal on discontinuation of treatment. Increased low-density lipoproteins and decreased high-density lipro proteins are considered cardiovascular risk factors. Serum lipids and high-density lipoprotein cholesterol should be determined periodically.
Hemoglobin and hematocrit should be checked periodically for polycythemia in patients who are receiving high doses of anabolics.
Drug Interaction:
Anabolic steroids may increase sensitivity to anticoagulants; therefore dosage of an anticoagulant may have to be decreased in order to maintain the prothrombin time at the desired therapeutic level.
Drug/Laboratory Test Interferences: Therapy with androgenic anabolic steroids may decrease levels of thyroxine-binding globulin resulting in decreased total T$_4$ serum levels and increased resin uptake of T$_3$ and T$_4$. Free thyroid hormone levels remain unchanged and there is no clinical evidence of thyroid dysfunction.
Anabolic steroids may cause an increase in prothrombin time.
Carcinogenesis, Mutagenesis, Impairment of Fertility:
Long-term studies in animals have not been performed to evaluate the carcinogenic potential of oxymetholone. There

are rare reports of hepatocellular carcinoma in patients receiving long-term therapy with anabolics in high doses. Withdrawal of the drugs did not lead to regression of the tumors in all cases.

Pregnancy:
Pregnancy category X. See CONTRAINDICATIONS.

Nursing Mothers:
It is not known whether anabolics are excreted in human milk. Because of the potential for serious adverse reactions in nursed infants from anabolics, women who take oxymetholone should not nurse.

Pediatric Use:
Anabolic/androgenic steroids should be used very cautiously in children and only by specialists who are aware of their effects on bone maturation.

Anabolic agents may accelerate epiphyseal maturation more rapidly than linear growth in children, and the effect may continue for 6 months after the drug has been stopped. Therefore, therapy should be monitored by x-ray studies at 6-month intervals in order to avoid the risk of compromising the adult height.

ADVERSE REACTIONS

Hepatic:
Cholestatic jaundice with, rarely, hepatic necrosis and death. Hepatocellular neoplasms and peliosis hepatis have been reported in association with long-term androgenic-anabolic steroid therapy (see WARNINGS).

Genitourinary System:
In Men:
Prepubertal: Phallic enlargement and increased frequency of erections.
Postpubertal: Inhibition of testicular function, testicular atrophy and oligospermia, impotence, chronic priapism, epididymitis and bladder irritability.
In Women:
Clitoral enlargement, menstrual irregularities.
In both sexes:
Increased or decreased libido.
CNS: Excitation, insomnia.
Gastrointestinal: Nausea, vomiting, diarrhea.
Hematologic: Bleeding in patients on concomitant anticoagulant therapy, iron-deficiency anemia.

Leukemia has been observed in patients with aplastic anemia treated with oxymetholone. The role, if any, of oxymetholone is unclear because malignant transformation has been seen in blood dyscrasias and leukemia has been reported in patients with aplastic anemia who have not been treated with oxymetholone.

Breast: Gynecomastia.
Larynx: Deepening of the voice in women.
Hair: Hirsutism and male-pattern baldness in women.
Skin: Acne (especially in women and prepubertal boys.)
Skeletal: Premature closure of epiphyses in children (see PRECAUTIONS, Pediatric Use.)
Fluid and Electrolytes: Edema, retention of serum electrolytes (sodium, chloride, potassium, phosphate, calcium).
Metabolic/Endocrine: Decreased glucose tolerance (see PRECAUTIONS), increased serum levels of low-density lipoproteins and decreased levels of high-density lipoproteins (see PRECAUTIONS, Laboratory tests), increased creatine and creatinine excretion, increased serum levels of creatinine phosphokinase (CPK). Reversible changes in liver function tests also occur including increased bromsulphalein (BSP) retention and increases in serum bilirubin, glutamic oxaloacetic transaminase (SGOT), and alkaline phosphatase.

OVERDOSAGE

There have been no reports of acute overdosage with anabolics.

DOSAGE AND ADMINISTRATION

The recommended daily dose in children and adults is 1–5 mg/kg body weight per day. The usual effective dose is 1–2 mg/kg/day but higher doses may be required and the dose should be individualized. Response is not often immediate and a minimum trial of three to six months should be given. Following remission, some patients may be maintained without the drug; others may be maintained on an established lower daily dosage. A continued maintenance dose is usually necessary in patients with congenital aplastic anemia.

HOW SUPPLIED

ANADROL-50 (oxymetholone) is supplied in bottles of 100 white scored tablets imprinted with "2902" and "SYNTEX" (NDC 0033-2902-42).

CAUTION: Federal law prohibits dispensing without prescription.

02-2902-42-5 © Revised April 1986
Shown in Product Identification Section, page 433

ANAPROX® ℞
[an'ă-prox]
ANAPROX® DS ℞
(naproxen sodium)
Tablets

A product of Syntex Puerto Rico, Inc.

DESCRIPTION

ANAPROX® (naproxen sodium) filmcoated tablets for oral administration each contain 275 mg of naproxen sodium, which is equivalent to 250 mg naproxen with 25 mg (about 1 mEq) sodium. ANAPROX® DS (naproxen sodium) filmcoated tablets for oral administration each contain 550 mg of naproxen sodium, which is equivalent to 500 mg naproxen with 50 mg (about 2 mEq) sodium. Naproxen sodium is a member of the arylacetic acid group of nonsteroidal anti-inflammatory drugs.

The chemical name of naproxen sodium is 2-naphthaleneacetic acid, 6-methoxy-α-methyl-, sodium salt, (−).

Naproxen sodium is a white to creamy white crystalline solid, freely soluble in water.

Each ANAPROX 275 mg tablet contains naproxen sodium, the active ingredient, with lactose, magnesium stearate, and microcrystalline cellulose. The coating suspension may contain hydroxypropyl methycellulose, Opaspray® K-1-4210A, polyethylene glycol 8000 or Opadry® YS-1-4215. Each ANAPROX DS 550 mg tablet contains naproxen sodium, the active ingredient, with magnesium stearate, microcrystalline celluose, povidone, and talc. The coating suspension may contain hydroxypropyl methylcellulose 2910, Opaspray® K-1-4227, polyethylene glycol 8000 or Opadry® YS-1-4216.

CLINICAL PHARMACOLOGY

The sodium salt of naproxen has been developed as an analgesic because it is more rapidly absorbed. Naproxen is a nonsteroidal anti-inflammatory drug with analgesic and antipyretic properties. Naproxen anion inhibits prostaglandin synthesis but beyond this its mode of action is unknown.

Naproxen sodium is rapidly and completely absorbed from the gastrointestinal tract. After administration of naproxen sodium, peak plasma levels of naproxen anion are attained at 1–2 hours with steady-state conditions normally achieved after 4–5 doses. The mean biological half-life of the anion in humans is approximately 13 hours, and at therapeutic levels it is greater than 99% albumin bound. Approximately 95% of the dose is excreted in the urine, primarily as naproxen, 6-0-desmethyl naproxen or their conjugates. The rate of excretion has been found to coincide closely with the rate of drug disappearance from the plasma. The drug does not induce metabolizing enzymes.

In children of 5 to 16 years of age with arthritis, plasma naproxen levels following a 5 mg/kg single dose of naproxen suspension (see Dosage and Administration) were found to be similar to those found in normal adults following a 500 mg dose. The terminal half-life appears to be similar in children and adults. Pharmacokinetic studies of naproxen were not performed in children of less than 5 years of age.

The drug was studied in patients with mild to moderate pain, and pain relief was obtained within 1 hour. It is not a narcotic and is not a CNS-acting drug. Controlled double-blind studies have demonstrated the analgesic properties of the drug in, for example, post-operative, post-partum, orthopedic and uterine contraction pain and dysmenorrhea. In dysmenorrheic patients, the drug reduces the level of prostaglandins in the uterus, which correlates with a reduction in the frequency and severity of uterine contractions. Analgesic action has been shown by such measures as reduction of pain intensity scores, increase in pain relief scores, decrease in numbers of patients requiring additional analgesic medication, and delay in time for required remedication. The analgesic effect has been found to last for up to 7 hours.

The drug was studied in patients with rheumatoid arthritis, osteoarthritis, juvenile arthritis, ankylosing spondylitis, tendinitis and bursitis, and acute gout. It is not a corticosteroid. Improvement in patients treated for rheumatoid arthritis has been demonstrated by a reduction in joint swelling, a reduction in pain, a reduction in duration of morning stiffness, a reduction in disease activity as assessed by both the investigator and patient, and by increased mobility as demonstrated by a reduction in walking time.

In patients with osteoarthritis, the therapeutic action of the drug has been shown by a reduction in joint pain or tenderness, an increase in range of motion in knee joints, increased mobility as demonstrated by a reduction in walking time, and improvement in capacity to perform activities of daily living impaired by the disease.

In clinical studies in patients with rheumatoid arthritis, osteoarthritis, and juvenile arthritis, the drug has been shown to be comparable to aspirin and indomethacin in controlling the aforementioned measures of disease activity, but the frequency and severity of the milder gastrointestinal adverse effects (nausea, dyspepsia, heartburn) and nervous system adverse effects (tinnitus, dizziness, lightheadeness) were less than in both the aspirin- and indomethacin-treated

---

patients. It is not known whether the drug causes less peptic ulceration than aspirin.

In patients with ankylosing spondylitis, the drug has been shown to decrease night pain, morning stiffness and pain at rest. In double-blind studies the drug was shown to be as effective as aspirin, but with fewer side effects.

In patients with acute gout, a favorable response to the drug was shown by significant clearing of inflammatory changes (e.g., decrease in swelling, heat) within 24–48 hours, as well as by relief of pain and tenderness.

The drug may be used safely in combination with gold salts and/or corticosteroids; however, in controlled clinical trials, when added to the regimen of patients receiving corticosteroids it did not appear to cause greater improvement over that seen with corticosteroids alone. Whether the drug could be used in conjunction with partially effective doses of corticosteroids for a "steroid-sparing" effect has not been adequately studied. When added to the regimen of patients receiving gold salts, the drug did result in greater improvement. Its use in combination with salicylates is not recommended because data are inadequate to demonstrate that the drug produces greater improvement over that achieved with aspirin alone. Further, there is some evidence that aspirin increases the rate of excretion of the drug.

Generally, improvement due to the drug has not been found to be dependent on age, sex, severity or duration of disease. In clinical trials in patients with osteoarthritis and rheumatoid arthritis comparing treatments of 825 mg per day with 1,650 mg per day, there were trends toward increased efficacy with the higher dose and a more clearcut increase in adverse reactions, particularly gastrointestinal reactions severe enough to cause the patient to leave the trial, which approximately doubled.

In ^{51}Cr blood loss and gastroscopy studies with normal volunteers, daily administration of 1,100 mg of naproxen sodium has been demonstrated to cause statistically significantly less gastric bleeding and erosion than 3,250 mg of aspirin.

INDICATIONS AND USAGE

Naproxen sodium is indicated in the relief of mild to moderate pain and for the treatment of primary dysmenorrhea. It is also indicated for the treatment of rheumatoid arthritis, osteoarthritis, juvenile arthritis, ankylosing spondylitis, tendinitis and bursitis, and acute gout.

CONTRAINDICATIONS

The drug is contraindicated in patients who have had allergic reactions to ANAPROX® (naproxen sodium), ANAPROX® DS or to NAPROSYN® (naproxen). It is also contraindicated in patients in whom aspirin or other nonsteroidal anti-inflammatory/analgesic drugs induce the syndrome of asthma, rhinitis, and nasal polyps. Both types of reactions have the potential of being fatal. Anaphylactoid reactions to ANAPROX, ANAPROX DS or NAPROSYN, whether of the true allergic type or the pharmacologic idiosyncratic (e.g., aspirin syndrome) type, usually but not always occur in patients with a known history of such reactions. Therefore, careful questioning of patients for such things as asthma, nasal polyps, urticaria, and hypotension associated with nonsteroidal anti-inflammatory drugs before starting therapy is important. In addition, if such symptoms occur during therapy, treatment should be discontinued.

WARNINGS

Risk of GI Ulceration, Bleeding and Perforation with NSAID Therapy:
Serious gastrointestinal toxicity such as bleeding, ulceration, and perforation, can occur at any time, with or without warning symptoms, in patients treated chronically with NSAID therapy. Although minor upper gastrointestinal problems, such as dyspepsia, are common, usually developing early in therapy, physicians should remain alert for ulceration and bleeding in patients treated chronically with NSAIDs even in the absence of previous GI tract symptoms. In patients observed in clinical trials of several months to two years duration, symptomatic upper GI ulcers, gross bleeding or perforation appear to occur in approximately 1% of patients treated for 3–6 months, and in about 2–4% of patients treated for one year. Physicians should inform patients about the signs and/or symptoms of serious GI toxicity and what steps to take if they occur.

Studies to date have not identified any subset of patients not at risk of developing peptic ulceration and bleeding. Except for a prior history of serius GI events and other risk factors known to be associated with peptic ulcer disease, such as alcoholism, smoking, etc., no risk factors (e.g., age, sex) have been associated with increased risk. Elderly or debilitated patients seem to tolerate ulceration or bleeding less well than other individuals and most spontaneous reports of fatal GI events are in this population. Studies to date are inconclusive concerning the relative risk of various NSAIDs in causing such reactions. High doses of any NSAID probably carry a greater risk of these reactions, although controlled clinical trials showing this do not exist in most cases. In considering the use of relatively large doses (within the recommended

Continued on next page

Syntex—Cont.

dosage range), sufficient benefit should be anticipated to offset the potential increased risk of GI toxicity.

PRECAUTIONS
General:
ANAPROX (NAPROXEN SODIUM) or *ANAPROX DS* (NA-PROXEN SODIUM) SHOULD NOT BE USED CONCOMI-TANTLY WITH THE RELATED DRUG *NAPROSYN* (NA-PROXEN) SINCE THEY BOTH CIRCULATE IN PLASMA AS THE NAPROXEN ANION.

Renal Effects: As with other nonsteroidal anti-inflammatory drugs, long-term administration of naproxen to animals has resulted in renal papillary necrosis and other abnormal renal pathology. In humans, there have been reports of acute interstitial nephritis with hematuria, proteinuria, and occasionally nephrotic syndrome.

A second form of renal toxicity has been seen in patients with prerenal conditions leading to a reduction in renal blood flow or blood volume, where the renal prostaglandins have a supportive role in the maintenance of renal perfusion. In these patients, administration of a nonsteroidal anti-inflammatory drug may cause a dose-dependent reduction in prostaglandin formation and may precipitate overt renal decompensation. Patients at greatest risk of this reaction are those with impaired renal function, heart failure, liver dysfunction, those taking diuretics, and the elderly. Discontinuation of nonsteroidal anti-inflammatory therapy is typically followed by recovery to the pretreatment state.

Naproxen sodium and its metabolites are eliminated primarily by the kidneys, therefore the drug should be used with great caution in patients with significantly impaired renal function and the monitoring of serum creatinine and/or creatinine clearance is advised in these patients. Caution should be used if the drug is given to patients with creatinine clearance of less than 20 mL/minute because accumulation of naproxen metabolites has been seen in such patients.

Chronic alcoholic liver disease and probably other forms of cirrhosis reduce the total plasma concentration of naproxen, but the plasma concentration of unbound naproxen is increased. Caution is advised when high doses are required and some adjustment of dosage may be required in these patients. It is prudent to use the lowest effective dose.

One study indicates that although total plasma concentration of naproxen is unchanged, the unbound plasma fraction of naproxen is increased in the elderly. Caution is advised when high doses are required and some adjustment of dosage may be required in elderly patients. As with other drugs used in the elderly, it is prudent to use the lowest effective dose.

As with other nonsteroidal anti-inflammatory drugs, borderline elevations of one or more liver tests may occur in up to 15% of patients. These abnormalities may progress, may remain essentially unchanged, or may be transient with continued therapy. The SGPT (ALT) test is probably the most sensitive indicator of liver dysfunction. Meaningful (3 times the upper limit of normal) elevations of SGPT or SGOT (AST) occurred in controlled clinical trials in less than 1% of patients. A patient with symptoms and/or signs suggesting liver dysfunction, or in whom an abnormal liver test has occurred, should be evaluated for evidence of the development of more severe hepatic reaction while on therapy with this drug. Severe hepatic reactions, including jaundice and cases of fatal hepatitis, have been reported with this drug as with other nonsteroidal anti-inflammatory drugs. Although such reactions are rare, if abnormal liver tests persist or worsen, if clinical signs and symptoms consistent with liver disease develop, or if systemic manifestations occur (e.g., eosinophilia, rash, etc.), this drug should be discontinued.

If steroid dosage is reduced or eliminated during therapy, the steroid dosage should be reduced slowly and the patients must be observed closely for any evidence of adverse effects, including adrenal insufficiency and exacerbation of symptoms of arthritis.

Patients with initial hemoglobin values of 10 grams or less who are to receive long-term therapy should have hemoglobin values determined periodically.

Peripheral edema has been observed in some patients. Since each naproxen sodium tablet contains approximately 25 mg or 50 mg (about 1 or 2 mEq) of sodium, this should be considered in patients whose overall intake of sodium must be markedly restricted. For these reasons, the drug should be used with caution in patients with fluid retention, hypertension or heart failure.

The antipyretic and anti-inflammatory activities of the drug may reduce fever and inflammation, thus diminishing their utility as diagnostic signs in detecting complications of presumed non-infectious, non-inflammatory painful conditions. Because of adverse eye findings in animal studies with drugs of this class it is recommended that ophthalmic studies be carried out if any change or disturbance in vision occurs.
Information for Patients:
Naproxen sodium, like other drugs of its class, is not free of side effects. The side effects of these drugs can cause discomfort and, rarely, there are more serious side effects, such as gastrointestinal bleeding, which may result in hospitalization and even fatal outcomes.

NSAIDs (Nonsteroidal Anti-Inflammatory Drugs) are often essential agents in the management of arthritis and have a major role in the treatment of pain, but they also may be commonly employed for conditions which are less serious. Physicians may wish to discuss with their patients the potential risks (see Warnings, Precautions, and Adverse Reactions sections) and likely benefits of NSAID treatment, particularly when the drugs are used for less serious conditions where treatment without NSAIDs may represent an acceptable alternative to both the patient and physician.

Caution should be exercised by patients whose activities require alertness if they experience drowsiness, dizziness, vertigo or depression during therapy with the drug.
Laboratory Tests:
Because serious GI tract ulceration and bleeding can occur without warning symptoms, physicians should follow chronically treated patients for the signs and symptoms of ulceration and bleeding and should inform them of the importance of this follow-up (see Risk of GI Ulcerations, Bleeding and Perforation with NSAID Therapy).
Drug Interactions:
In vitro studies have shown that naproxen anion, because of its affinity for protein, may displace from their binding sites other drugs which are also albumin-bound. Theoretically, the naproxen anion itself could likewise be displaced. Short-term controlled studies failed to show that taking the drug significantly affects prothrombin times when administered to individuals with coumarin-type anticoagulants. Caution is advised nonetheless, since interactions have been seen with other nonsteroidal agents of this class. Similarly, patients receiving the drug and a hydantoin, sulfonamide or sulfonylurea should be observed for signs of toxicity to these drugs. The natriuretic effect of furosemide has been reported to be inhibited by some drugs of this class. Inhibition of renal lithium clearance leading to increases in plasma lithium concentrations has also been reported.

This and other nonsteroidal anti-inflammatory drugs can reduce the antihypertensive effect of propranolol and other beta-blockers.

Probenecid given concurrently increases naproxen anion plasma levels and extends its plasma half-life significantly.

Caution should be used if this drug is administered concomitantly with methotrexate. Naproxen and other nonsteroidal anti-inflammatory drugs have been reported to reduce the tubular secretion of methotrexate in an animal model, possibly enhancing the toxicity of that drug.
Drug/Laboratory Test Interactions:
The drug may decrease platelet aggregation and prolong bleeding time. This effect should be kept in mind when bleeding times are determined.

The administration of the drug may result in increased urinary values for 17-ketogenic steroids because of an interaction between the drug and/or its metabolites with m-dinitrobenzene used in this assay. Although 17-hydroxy-corticosteroid measurements (Porter-Sibler test) do not appear to be artifactually altered, it is suggested that therapy with the drug be temporarily discontinued 72 hours before adrenal function tests are performed.

The drug may interfere with some urinary assays of 5-hydroxy indoleacetic acid (5HIAA).
Carcinogenesis:
A two-year study was performed in rats to evaluate the carcinogenic potential of the drug. No evidence of carcinogenicity was found.
Pregnancy:
Teratogenic Effects: Pregnancy Category B. Reproduction studies have been performed in rats, rabbits and mice at doses up to six times the human dose and have revealed no evidence of impaired fertility or harm to the fetus due to the drug. There are, however, no adequate and well-controlled studies in pregnant women. Because animal reproduction studies are not always predictive of human response, the drug should not be used during pregnancy unless clearly needed. Because of the known effect of drugs of this class on the human fetal cardiovascular system (closure of ductus arteriosus), use during late pregnancy should be avoided.

Non-teratogenic Effects: As with other drugs known to inhibit prostaglandin synthesis, an increased incidence of dystocia and delayed parturition occurred in rats.
Nursing Mothers:
The naproxen anion has been found in the milk of lactating women at a concentration of approximately 1% of that found in the plasma. Because of the possible adverse effects of prostaglandin-inhibiting drugs on neonates, use in nursing mothers should be avoided.
Pediatric Use:
Safety and effectiveness in children below the age of 2 years have not been established. Pediatric dosing recommendations for juvenile arthritis are based on well-controlled studies. There are no adequate effectiveness or dose-response data for other pediatric conditions, but the experience in juvenile arthritis and other use experience have established that single doses of 2.5–5 mg/kg (as naproxen suspension, see Dosage and Administration), with total daily dose not exceeding 15 mg/kg/day, are safe in children over 2 years of age.

ADVERSE REACTIONS
The following adverse reactions are divided into three parts based on frequency and likelihood of causal relationship to naproxen sodium.
Incidence greater than 1%
Probable Causal Relationship:
Adverse reactions reported in controlled clinical trials in 960 patients treated for rheumatoid arthritis or osteoarthritis are listed below. In general, these reactions were reported 2 to 10 times more frequently than they were in studies in the 962 patients treated for mild to moderate pain or for dysmenorrhea.

A clinical study found gastrointestinal reactions to be more frequent and more severe in rheumatoid arthritis patients taking 1,650 mg naproxen sodium daily compared to those taking 825 mg daily (see Clinical Pharmacology).

In controlled clinical trials with about 80 children and in well monitored open studies with about 400 children with juvenile arthritis, the incidences of rash and prolonged bleeding times were increased, the incidences of gastrointestinal and central nervous system reactions were about the same, and the incidences of other reactions were lower in children than in adults.

Gastrointestinal: The most frequent complaints reported related to the gastrointestinal tract. They were constipation*, heartburn*, abdominal pain*, nausea*, dyspepsia, diarrhea, stomatitis.

Central Nervous System: Headache*, dizziness*, drowsiness*, lightheadedness, vertigo.

Dermatologic: Itching (pruritus)*, skin eruptions*, ecchymoses*, sweating, purpura.

Special Senses: Tinnitus*, hearing disturbances, visual disturbances.

Cardiovascular: Edema*, dyspnea*, palpitations.

General: Thirst.

*Incidence of reported reaction between 3% and 9%. Those reactions occurring in less than 3% of the patients are unmarked.
Incidence less than 1%
Probable Causal Relationship:
The following adverse reactions were reported less frequently than 1% during controlled clinical trials and through voluntary reports since marketing. The probability of a causal relationship exists between the drug and these adverse reactions.

Gastrointestinal: Abnormal liver function tests, colitis, gastrointestinal bleeding and/or perforation, hematemesis, jaundice, melena, peptic ulceration with bleeding and/or perforation, vomiting.

Renal: Glomerular nephritis, hematuria, interstitial nephritis, nephrotic syndrome, renal disease.

Hematologic: Agranulocytosis, eosinophilia, granulocytopenia, leukopenia, thrombocytopenia.

Central Nervous System: Depression, dream abnormalties, inability to concentrate, insomnia, malaise, myalgia and muscle weakness.

Dermatologic: Alopecia, photosensitive dermatitis, skin rashes.

Special Senses: Hearing impairment.

Cardiovascular: Congestive heart failure.

Respiratory: Eosinophilic pneumonitis.

General: Anaphylactoid reactions, menstrual disorders, pyrexia (chills and fever).
Casual Relationship Unknown:
Other reactions have been reported in circumstances in which a causal relationship could not be established. However, in these rarely reported events, the possibility cannot be excluded. Therefore these observations are being listed to serve as alerting information to the physicians.

Hematologic: Aplastic anemia, hemolytic anemia.

Central Nervous System: Cognitive dysfunction.

Dermatologic: Epidermal necrolysis, erythema multiforme, Stevens-Johnson syndrome, urticaria.

Gastrointestinal: Non-peptic gastrointestinal ulceration, ulcerative stomatitis.

Cardiovascular: Vasculitis.

General: Angioneurotic edema, hyperglycemia, hypoglycemia.

OVERDOSAGE
Significant overdosage may be characterized by drowsiness, heartburn, indigestion, nausea or vomiting. Because naproxen sodium may be rapidly absorbed, high and early blood levels should be anticipated. No evidence of toxicity or late sequelae have been reported 5 to 15 months after ingestion for three to seven days of doses equivalent to up to 3,300 mg of naproxen sodium. One patient ingested a single dose of 27.5 g of naproxen sodium and experienced mild nausea and indigestion. It is not known what dose of the drug would be life threatening. The oral LD_{50} of the drug is 543 mg/kg in rats, 1,234 mg/kg in mice, 4,110 mg/kg in hamsters and greater than 1,000 mg/kg in dogs.

Should a patient ingest a large number of tablets, accidentally or purposefully, the stomach may be emptied and usual supportive measures employed. In animals 0.5 g/kg of activated charcoal was effective in reducing plasma levels of naproxen. Hemodialysis does not decrease the plasma concentration of naproxen because of the high degree of its protein binding.

DOSAGE AND ADMINISTRATION
For Mild to Moderate Pain, Primary Dysmenorrhea and Acute Tendinitis and Bursitis:
The recommended starting dose is 550 mg, followed by 275 mg every 6 to 8 hours, as required. The total daily dose should not exceed 1,375 mg.
For Rheumatoid Arthritis, Osteoarthritis, and Ankylosing Spondylitis:
The recommended dose in adults is 275 mg or 550 mg twice daily (morning and evening). During long-term administration, the dose may be adjusted up or down depending on the clinical response of the patient. A lower daily dose may suffice for long-term administration. The morning and evening doses do not have to be equal in size and the administration of the drug more frequently than twice daily is not necessary.
In patients who tolerate lower doses well, the dose may be increased to 1,650 mg per day for limited periods when a higher level of anti-inflammatory/analgesic activity is required. When treating such patients with the 1,650 mg/day dose, the physician should observe sufficient increased clinical benefits to offset the potential increased risk (see Clinical Pharmacology).
Symptomatic improvement in arthritis usually begins within two weeks. However, if improvement is not seen within this period, a trial for an additional two weeks should be considered.
For Acute Gout:
The recommended starting dose is 825 mg, followed by 275 mg every eight hours until the attack has subsided.
For Juvenile Arthritis:
The recommended total daily dose is approximately 10 mg/kg given in two divided doses. The 275 mg ANAPROX tablets is not well suited to this dosage so use of the related drug NAPROSYN® (naproxen) as the 250 mg scored tablet or the 125 mg/5mL suspension is recommended for this indication.

HOW SUPPLIED
ANAPROX® (naproxen sodium) is available in filmcoated tablets of 275 mg (light blue), in bottles of 100 tablets (NDC 18393-274-42) and 500 tablets (NDC 18393-274-62) (NSN 6505-01-130-6832) or in cartons of 100 individually blister packed tablets (NDC 18393-274-53). ANAPROX® DS (naproxen sodium) is available in filmcoated tablets of 550 mg (dark blue), in bottles of 100 tablets (NDC 18393-276-42). Store at room temperature in well-closed containers.
CAUTION: Federal law prohibits dispensing without prescription.
U.S. Patent Nos. 4,009,197; 3,998,966 and others.
©Revised OCTOBER 1988

Shown in Product Indentification Section, page 433

BREVICON® Tablets ℞
[brev 'ĭ-kahn]
(norethindrone and
    ethinyl estradiol)

NORINYL® 1 + 35 Tablets ℞
[nor 'ĭ-nil]
(norethindrone and
    ethinyl estradiol)

NORINYL® 1 + 50 Tablets ℞
(norethindrone and mestranol)

NOR–Q.D® ℞
(norethindrone)
Tablets 0.35 mg.

TRI–NORINYL® Tablets ℞
(norethindrone and
ethinyl estradiol)
Oral Contraceptives

PRODUCT OVERVIEW

KEY FACTS
The Syntex line of oral contraceptives includes a triphasic "combination" oral contraceptive (TRI-NORINYL) in which the ethinyl estradiol dose is constant (0.035 mg.) but the norethindrone dose is 0.5 mg. on pill-taking days 1–7, increases to 1.0 mg. on days 8–16, and returns to 0.5 mg. on days 17–21, five constant-dose "combination" oral contraceptives (BREVICON, NORINYL 1 + 35, NORINYL 1 + 50) containing norethindrone (0.5 mg. or 1.0 mg.) and either ethinyl estradiol (0.035 mg) or mestranol (0.05 mg.) and a constant-dose oral contraceptive containing norethindrone (0.35 mg) alone (NOR-Q.D.). Except for NOR-Q.D., each of the oral con-

traceptive products is available in both 28-day (including 7 days of inert tablets) and 21-day dosage regimens and is packaged in the Wallette® pill dispenser.

MAJOR USES
Each of the Syntex oral contraceptive products is highly effective in the prevention of pregnancy.

SAFETY INFORMATION
See complete safety information set forth below.

PRESCRIBING INFORMATION

BREVICON® Tablets ℞
[brev 'ĭ-kahn]
(norethindrone and
    ethinyl estradiol)

NORINYL® 1 + 35 Tablets ℞
[nor 'ĭ-nil]
(norethindrone and
    ethinyl estradiol)

NORINYL® 1 + 50 Tablets ℞
(norethindrone and mestranol)

NOR–Q.D® ℞
(norethindrone)
Tablets 0.35 mg.

TRI–NORINYL® Tablets ℞
(norethindrone and
ethinyl estradiol)
Oral Contraceptives
Products of Syntex (F.P.) Inc.

DESCRIPTION
BREVICON 21-DAY Tablets provide an oral contraceptive regimen consisting of 21 blue tablets containing norethindrone 0.5 mg. with ethinyl estradiol 0.035 mg.
BREVICON 28-DAY Tablets provide a continuous oral contraceptive regimen consisting of 21 blue tablets containing norethindrone 0.5 mg. with ethinyl estradiol 0.035 mg. and 7 orange tablets containing inert ingredients.
NORINYL 1 + 35 21-DAY Tablets provide an oral contraceptive regimen consisting of 21 yellow/green tablets containing norethindrone 1 mg. with ethinyl estradiol 0.035 mg.
NORINYL 1 + 35 28-DAY Tablets provide a continuous oral contraceptive regimen consisting of 21 yellow/green tablets containing norethindrone 1 mg. with ethinyl estradiol 0.035 mg. and 7 orange tablets containing inert ingredients.
NORINYL 1 + 50 21-DAY Tablets provide an oral contraceptive regimen consisting of 21 white tablets containing norethindrone 1 mg. with mestranol 0.05 mg.
NORINYL 1 + 50 28-DAY Tablets provide a continuous oral contraceptive regimen consisting of 21 white tablets containing norethindrone 1 mg. with mestranol 0.05 mg. and 7 orange tablets containing inert ingredients.
NOR-QD (norethindrone) Tablets provide a continuous oral contraceptive regimen of one yellow norethindrone 0.35 mg. tablet daily.
TRI-NORINYL 21-DAY Tablets provide an oral contraceptive regimen of 7 blue tablets followed by 9 yellow/green tablets and 5 more blue tablets. Each blue tablet contains norethindrone 0.5 mg with ethinyl estradiol 0.035 mg and each yellow/green tablet contains norethindrone 1.0 mg with ethinyl estradiol 0.035 mg.
TRI-NORINYL 28-DAY Tablets provide a continuous oral contraceptive regimen of 7 blue tablets, 9 yellow/green tablets, 5 more blue tablets, and then 7 orange tablets. Each blue tablet contains norethindrone 0.5 mg with ethinyl estradiol 0.035 mg, each yellow/green tablet contains norethindrone 1.0 mg with ethinyl estradiol 0.035 mg, and each orange tablet contains inert ingredients.
Norethindrone is a potent progestational agent with the chemical name 17-hydroxy-19-nor-17α-pregn-4-en-20-yn-3-one. Ethinyl estradiol is an estrogen with the chemical name 19-nor-17α-pregna-1, 3, 5(10) -trien-20-yne-3, 17-diol. Mestranol is an estrogen with the chemical name 3-methoxy-19-nor-17α-pregna-1, 3, 5(10) -trien-20-yn-17-ol.
Inactive Ingredients: Each tablet contains the following inactive ingredients: lactose, magnesium stearate, povidone, starch, and one or more of the following FDA certified dyes; D&C Green No. 5, D&C Yellow No. 10, FD&C Blue No. 1, FD&C Yellow No. 6.

CLINICAL PHARMACOLOGY
Combination oral contraceptives act by suppression of gonadotrophins. Although the primary mechanism of this action is inhibition of ovulation, other alterations include changes in the cervical mucus (which increase the difficulty of sperm entry into the uterus) and the endometrium (which may reduce the likelihood of implantation).
The primary mechanism through which NOR-Q.D. prevents conception is not known, but progestogen-only contraceptives are known to alter the cervical mucus, exert a progestational effect on the endometrium, interfering with implantation, and, in some patients, suppress ovulation.

INDICATIONS AND USAGE
Oral contraceptives are indicated for the prevention of pregnancy in women who elect to use these products as a method of contraception.
Oral contraceptives are highly effective. Table I lists the typical accidental pregnancy rates for users of combination oral contraceptives and other methods of contraception.[1] The efficacy of these contraceptive methods, except sterilization, depends upon the reliability with which they are used. Correct and consistent use of methods can result in lower failure rates.

TABLE I: LOWEST EXPECTED AND TYPICAL
FAILURE RATES DURING THE FIRST YEAR OF
CONTINUOUS USE OF A METHOD
% of Women Experiencing an Accidental Pregnancy
in the First Year of Continuous Use

Method	Lowest Expected[a]	Typical[b]
(No contraception)	(89)	(89)
Oral contraceptives		
combined	0.1	N/A[c]
progestogen only	0.5	N/A[c]
Diaphragm with spermicidal cream or jelly	3	18
Spermicides alone (foam, creams, jellies and vaginal suppositories)	3	21
Vaginal sponge		
Nulliparous	5	18
Multiparous	>8	>28
IUD (medicated)	1	6[d]
Condom without spermicides	2	12
Periodic abstinence (all methods)	2–10	20
Female sterilization	0.2	0.4
Male sterilization	0.1	0.15

Adapted from J. Trussell and K. Kost, Table II [1]
[a] The authors' best guess of the percentage of women expected to experience an accidental pregnancy among couples who initiate a method (not necessarily for the first time) and who use it consistently and correctly during the first year if they do not stop for any other reason.
[b] This term represents "typical" couples who initiate use of a method (not necessarily for the first time), who experience an accidental pregnancy during the first year if they do not stop for any other reason. The authors derive these data largely from the National Surveys of Family Growth (NSFG), 1976 and 1982.
[c] N/A—Data not available from the NSFG, 1976 and 1982.
[d] Combined typical rate for both medicated and non-medicated IUD. The rate for medicated IUD alone is not available.

CONTRAINDICATIONS
Oral contraceptives should not be used in women who have the following conditions:
● Thrombophlebitis or thromboembolic disorders
● A past history of deep vein thrombophlebitis or thromboembolic disorders
● Cerebral vascular or coronary artery disease
● Known or suspected carcinoma of the breast
● Carcinoma of the endometrium, and known or suspected estrogen-dependent neoplasia
● Undiagnosed abnormal genital bleeding
● Cholestatic jaundice of pregnancy or jaundice with prior pill use
● Hepatic adenomas, carcinomas or benign liver tumors
● Known or suspected pregnancy

WARNINGS

> Cigarette smoking increases the risk of serious cardiovascular side effects from oral contraceptive use. This risk increases with age and with heavy smoking (15 or more cigarettes per day) and is quite marked in women over 35 years of age. Women who use oral contraceptives should be strongly advised not to smoke.

The use of oral contraceptives is associated with increased risks of several serious conditions including myocardial infarction, thromboembolism, stroke, hepatic neoplasia and gallbladder disease, although the risk of serious morbidity and mortality increases significantly in the presence of other underlying risk factors such as hypertension, hyperlipidemias, hypercholesterolemia, obesity and diabetes.[2-5] Practitioners prescribing oral contraceptives should be familiar with the following information relating to these risks.

Continued on next page

Syntex—Cont.

The information contained in this package insert is principally based on studies carried out in patients who used oral contraceptives with formulations containing 0.05 mg or higher of estrogen.[6-11] The effects of long-term use with lower dose formulations of both estrogens and progestogens remain to be determined.

Throughout this labeling, epidemiological studies reported are of two types: retrospective or case control studies and prospective or cohort studies. Case control studies provide a measure of the relative risk of a disease. Relative risk, the *ratio* of the incidence of a disease among oral contraceptive users to that among nonusers, cannot be assessed directly from case control studies, but the odds ratio obtained is a measure of relative risk. The relative risk does not provide information on the actual clinical occurrence of a disease. Cohort studies provide not only a measure of the relative risk but a measure of attributable risk, which is the *difference* in the incidence of disease between oral contraceptive users and nonusers. The attributable risk does provide information about the actual occurrence of a disease in the population.[12-13]

1. THROMBOEMBOLIC DISORDERS AND OTHER VASCULAR PROBLEMS

a. Myocardial Infarction

An increased risk of myocardial infarction has been attributed to oral contraceptive use. This risk is primarily in smokers or women with other underlying risk factors for coronary artery disease such as hypertension, hypercholesterolemia, morbid obesity, and diabetes.[2-5,13] The relative risk of heart attack for current oral contraceptive users has been estimated to be 2 to 6.[2,14-19] The risk is very low under the age of 30. However, there is the possibility of a risk of cardiovascular disease even in very young women who take oral contraceptives.

Smoking in combination with oral contraceptive use has been shown to contribute substantially to the incidence of myocardial infarctions in women 35 or older, with smoking accounting for the majority of excess cases.[20]

Mortality rates associated with circulatory disease have been shown to increase substantially in smokers over the age of 35 and non-smokers over the age of 40 among women who use oral contraceptives (See Table II).[16]

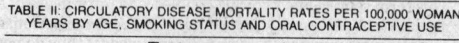

TABLE II: CIRCULATORY DISEASE MORTALITY RATES PER 100,000 WOMAN YEARS BY AGE, SMOKING STATUS AND ORAL CONTRACEPTIVE USE

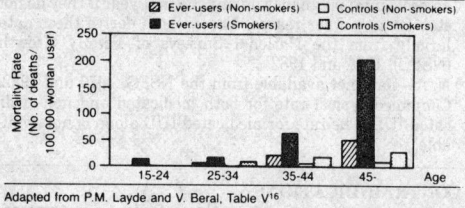

Adapted from P.M. Layde and V. Beral, Table V[16]

Oral contraceptives may compound the effects of well-known risk factors for coronary artery disease, such as hypertension, diabetes, hyperlipidemias, hypercholesterolemia, age and obesity.[3,13,21] In particular, some progestogens are known to decrease HDL cholesterol and impair oral glucose tolerance, while estrogens may create a state of hyperinsulinism.[21-25] Oral contraceptives have been shown to increase blood pressure among users (see **WARNINGS**, section 9). Similar effects on risk factors have been associated with an increased risk of heart disease. Oral contraceptives must be used with caution in women with cardiovascular disease risk factors.

b. Thromboembolism

An increased risk of thromboembolic and thrombotic disease associated with the use of oral contraceptives is well established. Case control studies have found the relative risk of users compared to non-users to be 3 for the first episode of superficial venous thrombosis, 4 to 11 for deep vein thrombosis or pulmonary embolism, and 1.5 to 6 for women with predisposing conditions for venous thromboembolic disease.[12,13,26-31] One cohort study has shown the relative risk to be somewhat lower, about 3 for new cases (subjects with no past history of venous thrombosis or varicose veins) and about 4.5 for new cases requiring hospitalization.[32] The risk of thromboembolic disease due to oral contraceptives is not related to length of use and disappears after pill use is stopped.[12]

A 2-to 6 fold increase in relative risk of post-operative thromboembolic complications has been reported with the use of oral contraceptives.[18] If feasible, oral contraceptives should be discontinued at least 4 weeks prior to and for 2 weeks after elective surgery and during and following prolonged immobilization. Since the immediate postpartum period is also associated with an increased risk of thromboembolism, oral contraceptives should be started no earlier than 4 to 6 weeks after delivery in women who elect not to breast feed.[33]

c. Cerebrovascular diseases

An increase in both the relative and attributable risks of cerebrovascular events (thrombotic and hemorrhagic strokes) has been shown in users of oral contraceptives. In general, the risk is greatest among older (> 35 years), hypertensive women who also smoke. Hypertension was found to be a risk factor for both users and non-users for both types of strokes while smoking interacted to increase the risk for hemorrhagic strokes.[34]

In a large study, the relative risk of thrombotic strokes has been shown to range from 3 for normotensive users to 14 for users with severe hypertension.[35] The relative risk of hemorrhagic stroke is reported to be 1.2 for non-smokers who used oral contraceptives, 2.6 for smokers who did not use oral contraceptives, 7.6 for smokers who used oral contraceptives, 1.8 for normotensive users and 25.7 for users with severe hypertension.[35] The attributable risk is also greater in women 35 or older and among smokers.[13]

d. Dose-related risk of vascular disease from oral contraceptives

A positive association has been observed between the amount of estrogen and progestogen in oral contraceptives and the risk of vascular disease.[36-38] A decline in serum high density lipoproteins (HDL) has been reported with some progestational agents.[22-24] A decline in serum high density lipoproteins has been associated with an increased incidence of ischemic heart disease.[39] Because estrogens increase HDL cholesterol, the net effect of an oral contraceptive depends on a balance achieved between doses of estrogen and progestogen and the nature and absolute amount of progestogens used in the contraceptives. The amount of both hormones should be considered in the choice of an oral contraceptive.[37] Minimizing exposure to estrogen and progestogen is in keeping with good principles of therapeutics. For any particular estrogen/progestogen combination, the dosage regimen prescribed should be one which contains the least amount of estrogen and progestogen that is compatible with a low failure rate and the needs of the individual patient. New acceptors of oral contraceptive agents should be started on preparations containing the lowest estrogen content that produces satisfactory results for the individual.

e. Persistence of risk of vascular disease

There are three studies which have shown persistence of risk of vascular disease for ever-users of oral contraceptives.[17,34,40] In a study in the United States, the risk of developing myocardial infarction after discontinuing oral contraceptives persists for at least 9 years for women 40–49 years who had used oral contraceptives for 5 or more years, but this increased risk was not demonstrated in other age groups.[17] In another study in Great Britain, the risk of developing cerebrovascular disease persisted for at least 6 years after discontinuation of oral contraceptives, although excess risk was very small.[40] Subarachnoid hemorrhage also has a significantly increased relative risk after termination of use of oral contraceptives.[34] However, these studies were performed with oral contraceptive formulations containing 0.05 mg or higher of estrogen.

2. ESTIMATES OF MORTALITY FROM CONTRACEPTIVE USE

One study gathered data from a variety of sources which have estimated the mortality rates associated with different methods of contraception at different ages (see Table III).[41] These estimates include the combined risk of death associated with contraceptive methods plus the risk attributable to pregnancy in the event of method failure. Each method of contraception has its specific benefits and risks. The study concluded that with the exception of oral contraceptive users 35 and older who smoke and 40 and older who do not smoke, mortality associated with all methods of birth control is low and below that associated with childbirth. However, smokers 35 and older and non-smokers 40 and older who use oral contraceptives have an increase in mortality greater than those using other methods of birth control. These facts must be weighed in conjunction with failure rates for other methods and the risk associated with subsequent pregnancy. (see Table I).

[See table below].

3. CARCINOMA OF THE BREAST AND REPRODUCTIVE ORGANS

Numerous epidemiological studies have been performed on the incidence of breast, endometrial, ovarian and cervical cancer in women using oral contraceptives. The evidence in the literature suggests that use of oral contraceptives is not associated with an increase in the risk of developing breast cancer, regardless of the age and parity of first use or with most of the marketed brands and doses.[42,43] The Cancer and Steroid Hormone study also showed no latent effect on the risk of breast cancer for at least a decade following long-term use.[43] A few studies have shown a slightly increased relative risk of developing breast cancer,[44-47] although the methodology of these studies, which included differences in examination of users and non-users and differences in age at start of use, has been questioned.[47-49]

Some studies suggest that oral contraceptive use has been associated with an increase in the risk of cervical intraepithelial neoplasia in some populations of women.[50-53] However, there continues to be controversy about the extent to which such findings may be due to differences in sexual behavior and other factors.

In spite of many studies of the relationship between oral contraceptive use and breast and cervical cancers, a cause and effect relationship has not been established.

4. HEPATIC NEOPLASIA

Benign hepatic adenomas are associated with oral contraceptive use although the incidence of benign tumors is rare in the United States. Indirect calculations have estimated the attributable risk to be in the range of 3.3 cases per 100,000 for users, a risk that increases after 4 or more years of use.[54] Rupture of rare, benign, hepatic adenomas may cause death through intra-abdominal hemorrhage.[55-56]

Studies in the United States and Britain have shown an increased risk of developing hepatocellular carcinoma in long-term (> 8 years) oral contraceptive users.[57-59] However, these cancers extremely rare in the United States and the attributable risk (the excess incidence) of liver cancers in oral contraceptive users is less than 1 per 1,000,000 users.

5. OCULAR LESIONS

There have been clinical case reports of retinal thrombosis associated with the use of oral contraceptives. Oral contraceptives should be discontinued if there is unexplained partial or complete loss of vision; onset of proptosis or diplopia; papilledema; or retinal vascular lesions. Appropriate diagnostic and therapeutic measures should be undertaken immediately.

6. ORAL CONTRACEPTIVE USE BEFORE OR DURING EARLY PREGNANCY

Extensive epidemiological studies have revealed no increased risk of birth defects in women who have used oral contraceptives prior to pregnancy.[60-62] More recent studies do not suggest a teratogenic effect, particularly insofar as cardiac anomalies and limb reduction defects are concerned, when taken inadvertently during early pregnancy.[60,61,63,64] The administration of oral contraceptives to induce withdrawal bleeding should not be used as a test for pregnancy. Oral contraceptives should not be used during pregnancy to treat threatened or habitual abortion.

It is recommended that for any patient who has missed 2 consecutive periods, pregnancy should be ruled out before continuing oral contraceptive use. If the patient has not adhered to the prescribed schedule, the possibility of pregnancy should be considered at the time of the first missed period. Oral contraceptive use should be discontinued if pregnancy is confirmed.

TABLE III: ESTIMATED ANNUAL NUMBER OF BIRTH-RELATED OR METHOD-RELATED DEATHS ASSOCIATED WITH CONTROL OF FERTILITY PER 100,000 NONSTERILE WOMEN, BY FERTILITY CONTROL METHOD ACCORDING TO AGE

Method of control and outcome	15–19	20–24	25–29	30–34	35–39	40–44
No fertility control methods*	7.0	7.4	9.1	14.8	25.7	28.2
Oral contraceptives non-smoker**	0.3	0.5	0.9	1.9	13.8	31.6
Oral contraceptives smoker**	2.2	3.4	6.6	13.5	51.1	117.2
IUD**	0.8	0.8	1.0	1.0	1.4	1.4
Condom*	1.1	1.6	0.7	0.2	0.3	0.4
Diaphragm/Spermicide*	1.9	1.2	1.2	1.3	2.2	2.8
Periodic abstinence*	2.5	1.6	1.6	1.7	2.9	3.6

* Deaths are birth related
** Deaths are method related

Estimates adapted from H.W. Ory, Table 3[41]

7. GALLBLADDER DISEASE

Earlier studies have reported an increased lifetime relative risk of gallbladder surgery in users of oral contraceptives and estrogens.[65-66] More recent studies, however, have shown that the relative risk of developing gallbladder disease among oral contraceptive users may be minimal.[67] The recent findings of minimal risk may be related to the use of oral contraceptive formulations containing lower hormonal doses of estrogens and progestogens.[68]

8. CARBOHYDRATE AND LIPID METABOLIC EFFECTS

Oral contraceptives have been shown to impair oral glucose tolerance.[69] Oral contraceptives containing greater than 0.075 mg of estrogen cause glucose intolerance with impaired insulin secretion, while lower doses of estrogen may produce less glucose intolerance.[70] Progestogens increase insulin secretion and create insulin resistance, this effect varying with different progestational agents.[25,71] However, in the non-diabetic woman, oral contraceptives appear to have no effect on fasting blood glucose.[69] Because of these demonstrated effects, prediabetic and diabetic women should be carefully observed while taking oral contraceptives.

Some women may develop persistent hypertriglyceridemia while on the pill.[72] As discussed earlier (see **WARNINGS** sections 1a. and 1d.), changes in serum triglycerides and lipoprotein levels have been reported in oral contraceptive users.[23]

9. ELEVATED BLOOD PRESSURE

An increase in blood pressure has been reported in women taking oral contraceptives. The incidence of risk also was reported to increase with continued use and among older women.[66] Data from the Royal College of General Practitioners and subsequent randomized trials have shown that the incidence of hypertension increases with increasing concentrations of progestogens.

Women with a history of hypertension or hypertension-related diseases, or renal disease should be encouraged to use another method of contraception. If women elect to use oral contraceptives, they should be monitored closely and if significant elevation of blood pressure occurs, oral contraceptives should be discontinued. For most women, elevated blood pressure will return to normal after stopping oral contraceptives, and there is no difference in the occurrence of hypertension among ever-and never-users.[73-75]

10. HEADACHE

The onset or exacerbation of migraine or development of headache with a new pattern which is recurrent, persistent or severe requires discontinuation of oral contraceptives and evaluation of the cause.

11. BLEEDING IRREGULARITIES

Breakthrough bleeding and spotting are sometimes encountered in patients on oral contraceptives, especially during the first 3 months of use. Non-hormonal causes should be considered and adequate diagnostic measures taken to rule out malignancy or pregnancy in the event of breakthrough bleeding, as in the case of any abnormal vaginal bleeding. If pathology has been excluded, time or a change to another formulation may solve the problem. In the event of amenorrhea, pregnancy should be ruled out.

Some women may encounter post-pill amenorrhea or oligomenorrhea, especially when such a condition was pre-existent.

PRECAUTIONS

1. PHYSICAL EXAMINATION AND FOLLOW UP

A complete medical history and physical examination should be taken prior to the initiation or reinstitution of oral contraceptives and at least annually during use of oral contraceptives. These physical examinations should include special reference to blood pressure, breasts, abdomen and pelvic organs, including cervical cytology, and relevant laboratory tests. In case of undiagnosed, persistent or recurrent abnormal vaginal bleeding, appropriate diagnostic measures should be conducted to rule out malignancy. Women with a strong family history of breast cancer or who have breast nodules should be monitored with particular care.

2. LIPID DISORDERS

Women who are being treated for hyperlipidemias should be followed closely if they elect to use oral contraceptives. Some progestogens may elevate LDL levels and may render the control of hyperlipidemias more difficult.

3. LIVER FUNCTION

If jaundice develops in any woman receiving oral contraceptives, the medication should be discontinued. Steroid hormones may be poorly metabolized in patients with impaired liver function.

4. FLUID RETENTION

Oral contraceptives may cause some degree of fluid retention. They should be prescribed with caution, and only with careful monitoring, in patients with conditions which might be aggravated by fluid retention.

5. EMOTIONAL DISORDERS

Women with a history of depression should be carefully observed and the drug discontinued if depression recurs to a serious degree.

6. CONTACT LENSES

Contact lens wearers who develop visual changes or changes in lens tolerance should be assessed by an ophthalmologist.

7. DRUG INTERACTIONS

Reduced efficacy and increased incidence of breakthrough bleeding and menstrual irregularities have been associated with concomitant use of rifampin. A similar assocation, though less marked, has been suggested with barbiturates, phenylbutazone, phenytoin sodium, and possibly with griseofulvin, ampicillin and tetracyclines.[76]

8. INTERACTIONS WITH LABORATORY TESTS

Certain endocrine and liver function tests and blood components may be affected by oral contraceptives:

a. Increased prothrombin and factors VII, VIII, IX, and X; decreased antithrombin 3; increased norepinephrine-induced platelet aggregability.

b. Increased thyroid binding globulin (TBG) leading to increased circulating total thyroid hormone, as measured by protein-bound iodine (PBI), T4 by column or by radio-immunoassay. Free T3 resin uptake is decreased, reflecting the elevated TBG. Free T4 concentration is unaltered.

c. Other binding proteins may be elevated in serum.

d. Sex steroid binding globulins are increased and result in elevated levels of total circulating sex steroids and corticoids; however, free or biologically active levels remain unchanged.

e. Triglycerides may be increased.

f. Glucose tolerance may be decreased.

g. Serum folate levels may be depressed by oral contraceptive therapy. This may be of clinical significance if a woman becomes pregnant shortly after discontinuing oral contraceptives.

9. CARCINOGENESIS

See **WARNINGS** section.

10. PREGNANCY

Pregnancy Category X. See **CONTRAINDICATIONS** and **WARNINGS** sections.

11. NURSING MOTHERS

Small amounts of oral contraceptive steroids have been identified in the milk of nursing mothers and a few adverse effects on the child have been reported, including jaundice and breast enlargement. In addition, oral contraceptives given in the postpartum period may interfere with lactation by decreasing the quantity and quality of breast milk. If possible, the nursing mother should be advised not to use oral contraceptives but to use other forms of contraception until she has completely weaned her child.

INFORMATION FOR THE PATIENT

See **Patient Labeling** printed below

ADVERSE REACTIONS

An increased risk of the following serious adverse reactions has been associated with the use of oral contraceptives (see **WARNINGS** section):

- Thrombophlebitis
- Arterial thromboembolism
- Pulmonary embolism
- Myocardial infarction
- Cerebral hemorrhage
- Cerebral thrombosis
- Hypertension
- Gallbladder disease
- Hepatic adenomas, carcinomas or benign liver tumors

There is evidence of an association between the following conditions and the use of oral contraceptives, although additional confirmatory studies are needed:

- Mesenteric thrombosis
- Retinal thrombosis

The following adverse reactions have been reported in patients receiving oral contraceptives and are believed to be drug-related:

- Nausea
- Vomiting
- Gastrointestinal symptoms (such as abdominal cramps and bloating)
- Breakthrough bleeding
- Spotting
- Change in menstrual flow
- Amenorrhea
- Temporary infertility after discontinuation of treatment
- Edema
- Melasma which may persist
- Breast changes: tenderness, enlargement, secretion
- Change in weight (increase or decrease)
- Change in cervical erosion and secretion
- Diminution in lactation when given immediately postpartum
- Cholestatic jaundice
- Migraine
- Rash (allergic)
- Mental depression
- Reduced tolerance to carbohydrates
- Vaginal candidiasis

- Change in corneal curvature (steepening)
- Intolerance to contact lenses

The following adverse reactions have been reported in users of oral contraceptives and the association has been neither confirmed nor refuted:

- Pre-menstrual syndrome
- Cataracts
- Changes in appetite
- Cystitis-like syndrome
- Headache
- Nervousness
- Dizziness
- Hirsutism
- Loss of scalp hair
- Erythema multiforme
- Erythema nodosum
- Hemorrhagic eruption
- Vaginitis
- Porphyria
- Impaired renal function
- Hemolytic uremic syndrome
- Budd-Chiari syndrome
- Acne
- Changes in libido
- Colitis

OVERDOSAGE

Serious ill effects have not been reported following acute ingestion of large doses of oral contraceptives by young children. Overdosage may cause nausea, and withdrawal bleeding may occur in females.

NON-CONTRACEPTIVE HEALTH BENEFITS

The following non-contraceptive health benefits related to the use of oral contraceptives are supported by epidemiological studies which largely utilized oral contraceptive formulations containing estrogen doses exceeding 0.035 mg of ethinyl estradiol or 0.05 mg of mestranol.[6-11]

Effects on menses:

- Increased menstrual cycle regularity
- Decreased blood loss and decreased incidence of iron deficiency anemia
- Decreased incidence of dysmenorrhea

Effects related to inhibition of ovulation:

- Decreased incidence of functional ovarian cysts
- Decreased incidence of ectopic pregnancies

Effects from long-term use:

- Decreased incidence of fibroadenomas and fibrocystic disease of the breast
- Decreased incidence of acute pelvic inflammatory disease
- Decreased incidence of endometrial cancer
- Decreased incidence of ovarian cancer

DOSAGE AND ADMINISTRATION

To achieve maximum contraceptive effectiveness, oral contraceptives must be taken exactly as described and at intervals not exceeding 24 hours.

21-Day Regimen Dosage Schedule for BREVICON, NORINYL 1 + 35, NORINYL 1 + 50, For the initial cycle of therapy the first tablet may be taken on Day 5 of the menstrual cycle, counting the first day of menstrual flow as Day 1 (DAY 5 START), or the first tablet may be taken on the first Sunday after menstrual flow begins (SUNDAY START). For SUNDAY START when menstrual flow begins on Sunday, the first tablet is taken on that day. With either DAY 5 START or SUNDAY START, one tablet is taken each evening at bedtime for 21 days. No tablets are taken for 7 days, then, whether bleeding has stopped or not, a new course is started of one tablet a day for 21 days. This institutes a three weeks on, one week off dosage regimen.

28-Day Regimen Dosage Schedule for BREVICON, NORINYL 1 + 35, NORINYL 1 + 50, For the initial cycle of therapy the first tablet may be taken on Day 5 of the menstrual cycle, counting the first day of menstrual flow as Day 1 (DAY 5 START), or the first tablet may be taken on the first Sunday after menstrual flow begins (SUNDAY START). For SUNDAY START when menstrual flow begins on Sunday, the first tablet is taken on that day. With either DAY 5 START or SUNDAY START, one white, blue, or yellow/green tablet is taken each evening at bedtime for 21 days. Then the orange tablets are taken, one each evening at bedtime for 7 days. After all 28 tablets have been taken, whether bleeding has stopped or not, repeat the same dosage schedule beginning on the following day.

21-Day Regimen Dosage Schedule for TRI-NORINYL: The first blue tablet is taken on the first Sunday after menstrual flow begins. If menstrual flow begins on Sunday, the first blue tablet is taken on that day. One blue tablet is taken each evening at bedtime for 7 days, then one yellow/green tablet each evening for 9 days, then one blue tablet each evening for 5 days. No tablets are taken for 7 days; then, whether bleeding has stopped or not, a new sequence of tablets is started for 21 days. This institutes a three weeks on, one week off dosage regimen.

Continued on next page

Syntex—Cont.

28-Day Regimen Dosage Schedule for TRI-NORINYL: The first blue tablet is taken on the first Sunday after menstrual flow begins. If menstrual flow begins on Sunday, the first blue tablet is taken on that day. One blue tablet is taken each evening at bedtime for 7 days, then one yellow/green tablet each evening for 9 days, then one blue tablet each evening for 5 days, then one orange (inert) tablet each evening for 7 days. After all 28 tablets have been taken, whether bleeding has stopped or not, the same dosage schedule is repeated beginning on the following day.

NOR-QD® (norethindrone) is administered as a continuous daily dosage regimen starting on the first day of menstruation, i.e., one tablet each day, every day of the year. Tablets should be taken at the same time each day and continued daily, without interruption, whether bleeding occurs or not. This is especially important for patients new to progestogen alone oral contraception. The patient should be advised that if prolonged bleeding occurs, she should consult her physician.

The risk of pregnancy increases with each tablet missed. If the patient misses one tablet, she should be instructed to take it as soon as she remembers and also to take her next tablet at the regular time which means she will be taking two tablets on that day. If she misses two tablets in a row, she should take one of the missed tablets as soon as she remembers, discard the other missed tablet, and take her regular tablet for that day at the proper time. Furthermore, she should use an additional method of contraception in addition to taking NOR-QD until menses has appeared or pregnancy has been excluded. If more than two tablets in a row have been missed, NOR-QD should be discontinued immediately and an additional method of contraception should be used until menses has appeared or pregnancy has been excluded. Whether or not the patient has adhered to the prescribed schedule, if she does not have a period within 45 days of her last period, she should stop taking NOR-QD and depend upon a method of nonhormonal contraception until pregnancy has been ruled out.

HOW SUPPLIED

BREVICON® 21-Day Tablets and BREVICON® 28-Day Tablets (norethindrone and ethinyl estradiol) are available in 21-pill or 28-pill blister cards with a WALLETTE® pill dispenser. Each 28-pill card contains 7 orange inert pills.
NORINYL® 1 + 35 21-Day Tablets and NORINYL® 1 + 35 28-Day Tablets (norethindrone and ethinyl estradiol) are available in 21-pill or 28-pill blister cards with a WALLETTE® pill dispenser. Each 28-pill card contains 7 orange inert pills.
NORINYL® 1 + 50 21-Day Tablets and NORINYL® 1 + 50 28-Day Tablets (norethindrone and mestranol) are available in 21-pill or 28-pill blister cards with a WALLETTE® pill dispenser. Each 28-pill card contains 7 orange inert pills.
TRI-NORINYL® 21-DAY Tablets and TRI-NORINYL 28-DAY Tablets (norethindrone and ethinyl estradiol) are each available in 21-pill or 28-pill blister cards with a WALLETTE pill dispenser. Each 28-pill card contains 7 orange inert pills.
CAUTION: Federal law prohibits dispensing without prescription.

INSTRUCTIONS TO PATIENTS

- To achieve maximum contraceptive effectiveness, the oral contraceptive pill must be taken exactly as directed and at intervals not exceeding 24 hours.
- Important: Women utilizing a SUNDAY START schedule should be instructed to use an additional method of protection until after the first 7 days of administration *in the initial cycle.*
- Due to the normally increased risk of thromboembolism occurring postpartum, women should be instructed not to initiate treatment with oral contraceptives earlier than 4 weeks after a full-term delivery. If pregnancy is terminated in the first 12 weeks, the patient should be instructed to start oral contraceptives immediately or within 7 days. If pregnancy is terminated after 12 weeks, the patient should be instructed to start oral contraceptives after 2 weeks.[33,77]
- If spotting or breakthrough bleeding should occur, the patient should continue the medication according to the schedule. Should spotting or breakthrough bleeding persist, the patient should notify her physician.
- If the patient misses 1 pill, she should be instructed to take it as soon as she remembers and then take the next pill at the regular time. If the patient has missed 2 pills, she should take 1 of the missed pills as soon as she remembers and discard the other missed pill. She should then take her next pill at the regular time. Furthermore, she should use an additional method of contraception in addition to taking her pills for the remainder of the cycle.
- If the patient has missed more than 2 pills, she should be instructed to discontinue taking the remaining pills and to

use an alternative method of contraception until pregnancy has been ruled out.
- Use of oral contraceptives in the event of a missed menstrual period:
  1. If the patient has not adhered to the prescribed dosage regimen, the possibility of pregnancy should be considered after the first missed period and oral contraceptives should be withheld until pregnancy has been ruled out.
  2. If the patient has adhered to the prescribed regimen and misses 2 consecutive periods, pregnancy should be ruled out before continuing the contraceptive regimen.

REFERENCES

1. Trussell, J., et al: *Stud Fam Plann* 18(5):237–283, 1987. **2.** Mann, J., et al.: *Br Med J* 2(5956):241–245, 1975. **3.** Knopp, R.H.: *J Reprod Med* 31(9):913–921, 1986. **4.** Mann, J.I., et al.: *Br Med J* 2:445–447, 1976. **5.** Ory, H.: *JAMA* 237:2619–2622, 1977. **6.** The Cancer and Steroid Hormone Study of the Centers for Disease Control: *JAMA* 249(2):1596–1599, 1983. **7.** The Cancer and Steroid Hormone Study of the Centers for Disease Control: *JAMA* 257(6):796–800, 1987. **8.** Ory, H.W.: *JAMA* 228(1):68–69, 1974. **9.** Ory, H.W., et al.: *N Engl J Med* 294:419–422, 1976. **10.** Ory, H.W.: *Fam Plann Perspect* 14:182–184, 1982. **11.** Ory, H.W., et al.: *Making Choices*, New York, The Alan Guttmacher Institute, 1983. **12.** Stadel, B.: *N Engl J Med* 305(11):612–618, 1981. **13.** Stadel, B: *N Engl J Med* 305(12):672–677, 1981. **14.** Adam, S., et al.: *Br J Obstet Gynaecol* 88:838–845, 1981. **15.** Mann, J., et al.: *Br Med J* 2(5965):245–248, 1975. **16.** Royal College of General Practitioners' Oral Contraceptive Study: *Lancet* 1:541–546, 1981. **17.** Slone, D., et al.: *N Engl J Med* 305(8):420–424, 1981. **18.** Vessey, M.P.: *Br J Fam Plann* 6 (supplement:1–12, 1980. **19.** Russell-Briefel, R., et al.: *Prev Med* 15:352–362, 1986. **20.** Goldbaum, G., et al.: *JAMA* 258(10):1339–1342, 1987. **21.** LaRosa, J.C.: *J Reprod Med* 31(9):906–912, 1986. **22.** Krauss, R.M., et al.: *Am J Obstet Gynecol* 145:446–452, 1983. **23.** Wahl, P., et al.: *N Engl J Med* 308(15):862–867, 1983. **24.** Wynn, V., et al.: *Am J Obstet Gynecol* 142(6):766–771, 1982. **25.** Wynn V., et al.: *J Reprod Med* 31(9):892–897, 1986. **26.** Inman, W.H., et al.: *Br Med J* 2(5599):193–199, 1968. **27.** Maguire, M.G., et al.: *Am J Epidemiol* 110(2):188–195, 1979. **28.** Petitti, D., et al.: *JAMA* 242(11):1150–1154, 1979. **29.** Vessey, M.P., et al.: *Br Med J* 2(5599):199–205, 1968. **30.** Vessey, M.P., et al.: *Br Med J* 2(5658):651–657, 1969. **31.** Porter, J.B., et al.: *Obstet Gynecol* 59(3):299–302, 1982. **32.** Vessey, M.P., et al.: *J Biosoc Sci* 8:373–427, 1976. **33.** Mishell, D.R., et al.: *Reproductive Endocrinology*, Philadelphia, F.A. Davis Co., 1979. **34.** Petitti, D.B., et al.: *Lancet* 2:234–236, 1978. **35.** Collaborative Group for the Study of Stroke in Young Women: *JAMA* 231(7):718–722, 1975. **36.** Inman, W.H., et al.: *Br Med J* 2:203–209, 1970. **37.** Meade, T.W., et al.: *Br Med J* 280 (6224):1157–1161, 1980. **38.** Kay, C.R.: *Am J Obstet Gynecol* 142(6):762–765, 1982. **39.** Gordon, T., et al.: *Am J Med* 62:707–714, 1977. **40.** Royal College of General Practitioners' Oral Contraceptive Study: *J Coll Gen Pract* 33:75–82, 1983. **41.** Ory, H.W.: *Fam Plann Perspect* 15(2):57–63, 1983. **42.** Paul, C., et al.: *Br Med J* 293:723–725, 1986. **43.** The Cancer and Steroid Hormone Study of the Centers for Disease Control: *N Engl J Med* 315(7):405–411, 1986. **44.** Pike, M.C., et al.: *Lancet* 2:926–929, 1983. **45.** Miller, D.R., et al.: *Obstet Gynecol* 68:863–868, 1986. **46.** Olsson, H., et al.: *Lancet* 2:748–749, 1985. **47.** McPherson, K., et al.: *Br J Cancer* 56:653–660, 1987. **48.** Huggins, G.R., et al.: *Fertil Steril* 47(5):733–761, 1987. **49.** McPherson, K., et al.: *Br Med J* 293:709–710, 1986. **50.** Ory, H., et al.: *Am J Obstet Gynecol* 124(6):573–577, 1976. **51.** Vessey, M.P., et al.: *Lancet*, 2:930, 1983. **52.** Brinton, L.A., et al.: *Int J Cancer* 38:339–344, 1986. **53.** WHO Collaborative Study of Neoplasia and Steroid Contraceptives: *Br Med J* 290:961–965, 1985. **54.** Rooks, J.B., et al.: *JAMA* 242(7):644–648, 1979. **55.** Bein, N.N., et al.: *Br J Surg* 64:433–435, 1977. **56.** Klatskin, G.: *Gastroenterology* 73:386–394, 1977. **57.** Henderson, B.E., et al.: *Br J Cancer* 48:437–440, 1983. **58.** Neuberger, J., et al.: *Br Med J* 292:1355–1357, 1986. **59.** Forman, D., et al.: *Br Med J* 292:1357–1361, 1986. **60.** Harlap, S., et al.: *Obstet Gynecol* 55(4):447–452, 1980. **61.** Savolainen, E., et al.: *Am J Obstet Gynecol* 140(5):521–524, 1981. **62.** Janerich, D.T., et al.: *Am J Epidemiol* 112(1):73–79, 1980. **63.** Ferencz, C., et al.: *Teratology* 21:225–239, 1980. **64.** Rothman, K.J., et al.: *Am J Epidemiol* 109(4):433–439, 1979. **65.** Boston Collaborative Drug Surveillance Program: *Lancet* 1:1399–1404, 1973. **66.** Royal College of General Practitioners: *Oral contraceptives and health.* New York, Pittman, 1974. **67.** Rome Group for the Epidemiology and Prevention of Cholelithiasis: *Am J Epidemiol* 119(5):796–805, 1984. **68.** Strom, B.L., et al.: *Clin Pharmacol Ther* 39(3):335–341, 1986. **69.** Perlman, J.A., et al.: *J Chornic Dis* 38(10):857–864, 1985. **70.** Wynn, V., et al.: *Lancet* 1:1045–1049, 1979. **71.** Wynn, V: *Progesterone and Progestin*, New York, Raven Press, 1983. **72.** Wynn, V., et al.: *Lancet* 2:720–723, 1966. **73.** Fisch, I.R., et al.: *JAMA* 237(23):2499–2503, 1977. **74.** Laragh, J.J.: *Am J Obstet Gynecol* 126(1):141–147, 1976. **75.** Ramcharan, S., et al.: *Pharmacology of Steroid Contraceptive Drugs*, New York, Raven Press, 1977. **76.** Stockley, I.: *Pharm J* 216:140–143, 1976. **77.** Dickey, R.P.: *Managing Contraceptive Pill Patients*, Oklahoma, Creative Informatics Inc., 1984.

DETAILED PATIENT LABELING

INTRODUCTION

Any woman who considers using oral contraceptives ("birth control pills" or "the pill") should understand the benefits and risks of using this form of birth control. This leaflet will give you much of the information you will need to make this decision and will also help you determine if you are at risk of developing any of the serious side effects of the pill. It will tell you how to use the pill properly so that it will be as effective as possible. However, this leaflet is not a replacement for a careful discussion between you and your health care provider. You should discuss the information provided in this leaflet with him or her, both when you first start taking the pill and during your revisits. You also should follow the advice of your health care provider with regard to regular check-ups while you are on the pill.

EFFECTIVENESS OF ORAL CONTRACEPTIVES

Oral contraceptives are used to prevent pregnancy and are more effective than other non-surgical methods of birth control. When they are taken correctly, without missing any pills, the chance of becoming pregnant is less than 1% (1 pregnancy per 100 women per year of use). Typical failure rates are actually 3% per year. The chance of becoming pregnant increases with each missed pill during a menstrual cycle.

In comparison, typical failure rates for other non-surgical methods of birth control during the first year of use are as follows:
IUD: 6%
Diaphragm with spermicides: 18%
Spermicides alone: 21%
Vaginal sponge: 18% to 30%
Condom alone: 12%
Periodic abstinence: 20%
No methods: 89%

WHO SHOULD NOT TAKE ORAL CONTRACEPTIVES

> **Cigarette smoking increases the risk of serious cardiovascular side effects from oral contraceptive use. This risk increases with age and with heavy smoking (15 or more cigarettes per day) and is quite marked in women over 35 years of age. Women who use oral contraceptives are strongly advised not to smoke.**

Some women should not use the pill. For example, you should not take the pill if you are pregnant or think you may be pregnant. You should also not use the pill if you have any of the following conditions:
- A history of heart attack or stroke
- Blood clots in the legs (thrombophlebitis), brain (stroke), lungs (pulmonary embolism), or eyes
- A history of blood clots in the deep veins of your legs
- Chest pain (angina pectoris)
- Known or suspected breast cancer or cancer of the lining of the uterus, cervix or vagina
- Unexplained vaginal bleeding (until a diagnosis is reached by your doctor)
- Yellowing of the whites of the eyes or of the skin (jaundice) during pregnancy or during previous use of the pill
- Liver tumor (benign or cancerous)
- Known or suspected pregnancy
Tell your health care provider if you have ever had any of these conditions. Your health care provider can recommend a safer method of birth control.

OTHER CONSIDERATIONS BEFORE TAKING ORAL CONTRACEPTIVES

Tell your health care provider if you have or have had:
- Breast nodules, fibrocystic disease of the breast, an abnormal breast x-ray or mammogram
- Diabetes
- Elevated cholesterol or triglycerides
- High blood pressure
- Migraine or other headaches or epilepsy
- Mental depression
- Gallbladder, heart or kidney disease
- History of scanty or irregular menstrual periods
Women with any of these conditions should be checked often by their health care provider if they choose to use oral contraceptives.
Also, be sure to inform your doctor or health care provider if you smoke or are on any medications.

RISKS OF TAKING ORAL CONTRACEPTIVES
1. Risk of developing blood clots
Blood clots and blockage of blood vessels are the most serious side effects of taking oral contraceptives. In particular, a clot in the legs can cause thrombophlebitis and a clot that travels to the lungs can cause a sudden blocking of the vessel carrying blood to the lungs. Rarely, clots occur in the blood vessels of the eye and may cause blindness, double vision, or impaired vision.
If you take oral contraceptives and need elective surgery, need to stay in bed for a prolonged illness or have recently

delivered a baby, you may be at risk of developing blood clots. You should consult your doctor about stopping oral contraceptives three to four weeks before surgery and not taking oral contraceptives for two weeks after surgery or during bed rest. You should also not take oral contraceptives soon after delivery of a baby. It is advisable to wait for at least four weeks after delivery if you are not breast feeding. If you are breast feeding, you should wait until you have weaned your child before using the pill (see **GENERAL PRECAUTIONS, While Breast Feeding**).

2. Heart attacks and strokes

Oral contraceptives may increase the tendency to develop strokes (stoppage or rupture of blood vessels in the brain) and angina pectoris and heart attacks (blockage of blood vessels in the heart). Any of these conditions can cause death or temporary or permanent disability.

Smoking greatly increases the possibility of suffering heart attacks and strokes. Furthermore, smoking and the use of oral contraceptives greatly increase the chances of developing and dying of heart disease.

3. Gallbladder disease

Oral contraceptive users may have a greater risk than nonusers of having gallbladder disease, although this risk may be related to pills containing high doses of estrogen.

4. Liver tumors

In rare cases, oral contraceptives can cause benign but dangerous liver tumors. These benign liver tumors can rupture and cause fatal internal bleeding. In addition, a possible but not definite association has been found with the pill and liver cancers in 2 studies, in which a few women who developed these very rare cancers were found to have used oral contraceptives for long periods. However, liver cancers are extremely rare.

5. Cancer of the breast and reproductive organs

There is, at present, no confirmed evidence that oral contraceptives increase the risk of cancer of the reproductive organs in human studies. Several studies have found no overall increase in the risk of developing breast cancer. However, women who use oral contraceptives and have a strong family history of breast cancer or who have breast nodules or abnormal mammograms should be followed closely by their doctors.

Some studies have found an increase in the incidence of cancer of the cervix in women who use oral contraceptives. However, this finding may be related to factors other than the use of oral contraceptives.

ESTIMATED RISK OF DEATH FROM A BIRTH CONTROL METHOD OR PREGNANCY

All methods of birth control and pregnancy are associated with a risk of developing certain diseases which may lead to disability or death. An estimate of the number of deaths associated with different methods of birth control and pregnancy has been calculated and is shown in the following table. [See table above].

In the above table, the risk of death from any birth control method is less than the risk of the childbirth except for oral contraceptive users over the age of 35 who smoke and pill users over the age of 40 even if they do not smoke. It can be seen from the table that for women aged 15 to 39 the risk of death is highest with pregnancy (7–26 deaths per 100,000 women, depending on age). Among pill users who do not smoke the risk of death is always lower than that associated with pregnancy for any age group, although over the age of 40 the risk increases to 32 deaths per 100,000 women compared to 28 associated with pregnancy at that age. However, for pill users who smoke and are over the age of 35 the estimated number of deaths exceeds those for other methods of birth control. If a woman is over the age of 40 and smokes, her estimated risk of death is 4 times higher (117/100,000 women) than the estimated risk associated with pregnancy (28/100,000 women) in that age group.

According to this table, for women who do not smoke and are under the age of 35, the possible risk of death from oral contraceptive use is low compared to the pregnancy-related risk of death associated with no fertility control method or the failure of other methods of contraception.

WARNING SIGNALS

If any of these adverse effects occur while you are taking oral contraceptives, call your doctor immediately:

- Sharp chest pain, coughing of blood or sudden shortness of breath (indicating a possible clot in the lung)
- Pain in the calf (indicating a possible clot in the leg)
- Crushing chest pain or heaviness in the chest (indicating a possible heart attack)
- Sudden severe headache or vomiting, dizziness or fainting, disturbances of vision or speech, weakness, or numbness in an arm or leg (indicating a possible stroke)
- Sudden partial or complete loss of vision (indicating a possible clot in the eye)
- Breast lumps (indicating possible breast cancer or fibrocystic disease of the breast: ask your doctor or health care provider to show you how to examine your breasts)
- Severe pain or tenderness in the stomach area (indicating a possible ruptured liver tumor)

ESTIMATED ANNUAL NUMBER OF BIRTH-RELATED OR METHOD-RELATED DEATHS ASSOCIATED WITH CONTROL OF FERTILITY PER 100,000 NONSTERILE WOMEN, BY FERTILITY CONTROL METHOD ACCORDING TO AGE

Method of control and outcome	15–19	20–24	25–29	30–34	35–39	40–44
No fertility control methods*	7.0	7.4	9.1	14.8	25.7	28.2
Oral contraceptives non-smoker**	0.3	0.5	0.9	1.9	13.8	31.6
Oral contraceptives smoker**	2.2	3.4	6.6	13.5	51.1	117.2
IUD**	0.8	0.8	1.0	1.0	1.4	1.4
Condom*	1.1	1.6	0.7	0.2	0.3	0.4
Diaphragm/Spermicide*	1.9	1.2	1.2	1.3	2.2	2.8
Periodic abstinence*	2.5	1.6	1.6	1.7	2.9	3.6

*Deaths are birth-related
**Deaths are method-related

- Difficulty in sleeping, weakness, lack of energy, fatigue or change in mood (possibly indicating severe depression)
- Jaundice or a yellowing of the skin or eyeballs, accompanied frequently by fever, fatigue, loss of appetite, dark colored urine or light colored bowel movements (indicating possible liver problems)

SIDE EFFECTS OF ORAL CONTRACEPTIVES

1. Vaginal bleeding

Irregular vaginal bleeding or spotting may occur while you are taking the pill. Irregular bleeding may vary from slight staining between menstrual periods to breakthrough bleeding which is a flow much like a regular period. Irregular bleeding occurs most often during the first few months of oral contraceptive use but may also occur after you have been taking the pill for some time. Such bleeding may be temporary and usually does not indicate any serious problem. It is important to continue taking your pills on schedule. If the bleeding occurs in more than 1 cycle or lasts for more than a few days, talk to your doctor or health care provider.

2. Contact lenses

If you wear contact lenses and notice a change in vision or an inability to wear your lenses, contact your doctor or health care provider.

3. Fluid retention

Oral contraceptives may cause edema (fluid retention) with swelling of the fingers or ankles and may raise your blood pressure. If you experience fluid retention, contact your doctor or health care provider.

4. Melasma (Mask of Pregnancy)

A spotty darkening of the skin is possible, particularly of the face.

5. Other side effects

Other side effects may include change in appetite, headache, nervousness, depression, dizziness, loss of scalp hair, rash, and vaginal infections.

If any of these side effects occur, contact your doctor or health care provider.

GENERAL PRECAUTIONS

1. Missed periods and use of oral contraceptives before or during early pregnancy

At times you may not menstruate regularly after you have completed taking a cycle of pills. If you have taken your pills regularly and miss 1 menstrual period, continue taking your pills for the next cycle but be sure to inform your health care provider before doing so. If you have not taken the pills daily as instructed and miss 1 menstrual period, or if you miss 2 consecutive menstrual periods, you may be pregnant. You should stop taking oral contraceptives until you are sure you are not pregnant and continue to use another method of contraception.

There is no conclusive evidence that oral contraceptive use is associated with an increase in birth defects when taken inadvertently during early pregnancy. Previously, a few studies had reported that oral contraceptives might be associated with birth defects but these studies have not been confirmed. Nevertheless, oral contraceptives or any other drugs should not be used during pregnancy unless clearly necessary and prescribed by your doctor. You should check with your doctor about risks to your unborn child from any medication taken during pregnancy.

2. While breast feeding

If you are breast feeding, consult your doctor before starting oral contraceptives. Some of the drug will be passed on to the child in the milk. A few adverse effects on the child have been reported, including yellowing of the skin (jaundice) and breast enlargement. In addition, oral contraceptives may decrease the amount and quality of your milk. If possible, use another method of contraception while breast feeding. You should consider starting oral contraceptives only after you have weaned your child completely.

3. Laboratory tests

If you are scheduled for any laboratory tests, tell your doctor you are taking birth control pills. Certain blood tests may be affected by birth control pills.

4. Drug interactions

Certain drugs may interact with birth control pills to make them less effective in preventing pregnancy or cause an increase in breakthrough bleeding. Such drugs include rifampin, drugs used for epilepsy such as barbiturates (for example, phenobarbital) and phenytoin (Dilantin is one brand of this drug), phenylbutazone (Butazolidin is one brand of this drug) and possibly certain antibiotics. You may need to use additional contraception when you take drugs which can make oral contraceptives less effective.

HOW TO TAKE ORAL CONTRACEPTIVES

1. General instructions

- You must take your pill every day according to the instructions. Oral contraceptives are most effective if taken no more than 24 hours apart. Take your pill at the same time every day so that you are less likely to forget to take it. You will then maintain the proper amount of drug in your body.
- If you are scheduled for surgery or you need prolonged bed rest you should advise your doctor that you are on the pill and stop taking the pill 4 weeks before surgery to avoid an increased risk of blood clots. It is also advisable not to start oral contraceptives sooner than 4 weeks after delivery of a baby.
- When you first begin to use the pill, you should use an additional method of protection until you have taken your first 7 pills.

Your physician has prescribed one of the following dosage schedules. Please follow the instructions appropriate for your schedule.

- 21-Day Schedule: Take the first blue pill on the first Sunday after menstrual flow begins. If menstrual flow begins on Sunday, take the first blue pill on that day. Take 1 blue pill the same time each day, preferably at bedtime, for the first 7 days, 1 yellow-green pill daily for the next 9 days, and then 1 blue pill each day for 5 days. Wait for 7 days, during which time a menstrual period usually occurs, then begin a new cycle of pills on the eighth day after you took your last pill, whether or not the menstrual flow has stopped. This cycle of 21 days on pills and 7 days off pills is repeated until the time for your visit with your physician or health care provider.
- 28-Day Schedule: Take the first blue pill on the first Sunday after the menstrual flow begins. If menstrual flow begins on Sunday, take the blue pill on that day. Take 1 blue pill the same time each day, preferably at bedtime, for the first 7 days, 1 yellow-green pill daily for the next 9 days, and then 1 blue pill each day for 5 days. Take 1 orange pill daily for the next 7 days and expect a menstrual period during this week. The orange pills contain no active drug and are included simply for your convenience—to eliminate the need for counting days. After all 28 pills have been taken, whether bleeding has stopped or not, take the first blue pill of the next cycle without any interruption. With the 28-day package, a pill is taken every day with no gap between cycles until the time for your visit with your physician or health care provider.

2. Missed periods/breakthrough bleeding

At times, there may be no menstrual period after you complete a cycle of pills. If you miss 1 menstrual period but have taken the pills *exactly as you were supposed to*, continue as usual into the next cycle. If you have not taken the pills correctly, and have missed a menstrual period, *you may be pregnant* and you should stop taking oral contraceptives until your doctor determines whether or not you are pregnant. Until you can get to your doctor, use another form of contraception. If you miss 2 consecutive menstrual periods, you should stop taking the pills until it is determined that you are not pregnant.

Even if spotting or breakthrough bleeding should occur, continue the medication according to the schedule. Should spotting or breakthrough bleeding persist, you should notify your physician.

Continued on next page

Syntex—Cont.

3. If you forget to take your pill

If you miss only 1 pill in a cycle, the chance of becoming pregnant is small. Take the missed pill as soon as you realize that you have forgotten it. Since the risk of pregnancy increases with each additional pill you skip, it is very important that you take each pill according to schedule.

If you miss 2 pills in a row, you should take 1 of the missed pills as soon as you remember, discard the other missed pill and take your regular pill for that day at the proper time. Furthermore, you should use an additional method of contraception in addition to taking your pills for the remainer of the cycle. If more than 2 pills in a row have been missed, discontinue taking your pills immediately and use an additional method of contraception until you have a period or your doctor determines that you are not pregnant. Missing orange pills in the 28-day schedule does not increase your chances of becoming pregnant.

4. Pregnancy due to pill failure

When taken correctly, the incidence of pill failure resulting in pregnancy is approximately 1% (i.e., 1 pregnancy per 100 women per year). If failure occurs, the risk to the fetus is minimal. The typical failure rate of large numbers of pill users is less than 3% when women who miss pills are included. If you become pregnant, you should discuss your pregnancy with your doctor.

5. Pregnancy after stopping the pill

There may be some delay in becoming pregnant after you stop using oral contraceptives, especially if you had irregular menstrual cycles before you used oral contraceptives. It may be advisable to postpone conception until you begin menstruating regularly once you have stopped taking the pill and desire pregnancy.

There does not appear to be any increase in birth defects in newborn babies when pregnancy occurs soon after stopping the pill.

6. Overdosage

Serious ill effects have not been reported following ingestion of large doses of oral contraceptives by young children. Overdosage may cause nausea and withdrawal bleeding in females. In case of overdosage, contact your health care provider or pharmacist.

7. Other information

Your health care provider will take a medical and family history and will examine you before prescribing oral contraceptives. You should be reexamined at least once a year. Be sure to inform your health care provider if there is a family history of any of the conditions listed previously in this leaflet. Be sure to keep all appointments with your health care provider because this is a time to determine if there are early signs of side effects of oral contraceptive use.

Do not use the drug for any condition other than the one for which it was prescribed. This drug has been prescribed specifically for you: do not give it to others who may want birth control pills.

If you want more information about birth control pills, ask your doctor or health care provider. They have a more technical leaflet called **PHYSICIAN LABELING** which you may wish to read.

NON-CONTRACEPTIVE HEALTH BENEFITS

In addition to preventing pregnancy, use of oral contraceptives may provide certain non-contraceptive benefits:
- Menstrual cycles may become more regular
- Blood flow during menstruation may be lighter and less iron may be lost. Therefore, anemia due to iron deficiency is less likely to occur.
- Pain or other symptoms during menstruation may be encountered less frequently
- Ectopic (tubal) pregnancy may occur less frequently
- Non-cancerous cysts or lumps in the breast may occur less frequently
- Acute pelvic inflammatory disease may occur less frequently
- Oral contraceptive use may provide some protection against developing two forms of cancer: cancer of the ovaries and cancer of the lining of the uterus.

BRIEF SUMMARY
PATIENT PACKAGE INSERT

Oral contraceptives, also known as "birth control pills" or "the pill," are taken to prevent pregnancy and, when taken correctly, have a failure rate of about 1% per year when used without missing any pills. The typical failure rate of large numbers of pill users is less than 3% per year when women who miss pills are included. For most women, oral contraceptives are also free of serious or unpleasant side effects. However, forgetting to take oral contraceptives considerably increases the chances of pregnancy.

For the majority of women, oral contraceptives can be taken safely, but there are some women who are at high risk of developing certain serious diseases that can be life-threatening or may cause temporary or permanent disability. The risks associated with taking oral contraceptives increase significantly if you:
- Smoke
- Are over the age of 40
- Have high blood pressure, diabetes, or high cholesterol
- Have or have had clotting disorders, heart attack, stroke, angina pectoris, cancer of the breast or sex organs, jaundice or malignant or benign liver tumors

You should not take the pill if you suspect you are pregnant or have unexplained vaginal bleeding.

> Cigarette smoking increases the risk of serious cardiovascular side effects from oral contraceptive use. This risk increases with age and with heavy smoking (15 or more cigarettes per day) and is quite marked in women over 35 years of age. Women who use oral contraceptives are strongly advised not to smoke.

Most side effects of the pill are not serious. The most common such effects are nausea, vomiting, bleeding between menstrual periods, weight gain, breast tenderness, and difficulty wearing contact lenses. These side effects, especially nausea and vomiting, may subside within the first 3 months of use. The serious side effects of the pill occur very infrequently, especially if you are in good health and are young. However, you should know that the following medical conditions have been associated with or made worse by the pill:

1. Blood clots in the legs (thrombophlebitis) or lungs (pulmonary embolism), stoppage or rupture of a blood vessel in the brain (stroke), blockage of blood vessels in the heart (heart attack or angina pectoris), eye or other organs of the body. As mentioned above, smoking increases the risk of heart attacks and strokes and subsequent serious medical consequences.
2. Liver tumors, which may rupture and cause severe bleeding. A possible but not definite association has been found with the pill and liver cancer. However, liver cancers are extremely rare.
3. High blood pressure, although blood pressure usually returns to normal when the pill is stopped.

The symptoms associated with these serious side effects are discussed in the detailed leaflet given to you with your supply of pills. Notify your doctor or health care provider if you notice any unusual physical disturbances while taking the pill. In addition, drugs such as rifampin, as well as some anticonvulsants and some antibiotics, may decrease oral contraceptive effectiveness.

Studies to date of women taking the pill have not shown an increase in the incidence of cancer of the breast or cervix. There is, however, insufficient evidence to rule out the possibility that the pill may cause such cancers.

Taking the pill may provide some important non-contraceptive benefits. These include less painful menstruation, less menstrual blood loss and anemia, fewer acute pelvic infections, and fewer cancers of the ovary and the lining of the uterus.

Be sure to discuss any medical condition you may have with your health care provider. Your health care provider will take a medical and family history before prescribing oral contraceptives and will examine you. You should be reexamined at least once a year while taking oral contraceptives. The detailed patient information leaflet gives you further information which you should read and discuss with your health care provider.

U.S. Patent No. 4,390,531
SYNTEX (F.P.) Inc.

02-0115-97-03   © Syntex Revised MARCH 1989
Shown in Product Identification Section, page 433

CARDENE®   ℞

[kar'deen]
(nicardipine hydrochloride)
Capsules

DESCRIPTION

CARDENE® capsules for oral administration each contain 20 mg or 30 mg of nicardipine hydrochloride. CARDENE is a calcium ion influx inhibitor (slow channel blocker or calcium channel blocker).

Nicardipine hydrochloride is a dihydropyridine structure with the IUPAC (International Union of Pure and Applied Chemistry) chemical name 2-(benzyl-methyl amino) ethyl methyl 1,4-dihydro-2,6-dimethyl-4-(m-nitrophenyl)-3,5-pyridinedicarboxylate monohydrochloride.

Nicardipine hydrochloride is a greenish-yellow, odorless, crystalline powder that melts at about 169°C. It is freely soluble in chloroform, methanol, and glacial acetic acid, sparingly soluble in anhydrous ethanol, slightly soluble in n-butanol, water, 0.01 M potassium dihydrogen phosphate, acetone, and dioxane, very slightly soluble in ethyl acetate, and practically insoluble in benzene, ether and hexane. It has a molecular weight of 515.99.

CARDENE is available in hard gelatin capsules containing 20 mg or 30 mg nicardipine hydrochloride with magnesium stearate and pregelatinized starch as the inactive ingredients. The 20 mg strength is provided in opaque white-white capsules made tamper evident by a brilliant blue gelatin band while the 30 mg capsules are opaque light blue-powder blue with a brilliant blue gelatin band. The colorants used in the 20 mg capsules are titanium dioxide, D& C Red #7 Calcium Lake and FD&C Blue #1 and the 30 mg capsules use titanium dioxide, FD&C Blue #1, D&C Yellow #10 Aluminum Lake, D&C Red #7 Calcium Lake, and FD&C Blue #2.

CLINICAL PHARMACOLOGY
Mechanism of Action

CARDENE is a calcium entry blocker (slow channel blocker or calcium ion antagonist) which inhibits the transmembrane influx of calcium ions into cardiac muscle and smooth muscle without changing serum calcium concentrations. The contractile processes of cardiac muscle and vascular smooth muscle are dependent upon the movement of extracellular calcium ions into these cells through specific ion channels. The effects of CARDENE are more selective to vascular smooth muscle than cardiac muscle. In animal models, CARDENE produces relaxation of coronary vascular smooth muscle at drug levels which cause little or no negative inotropic effect.

Pharmacokinetics and Metabolism

CARDENE is completely absorbed following oral doses administered as capsules. Plasma levels are detectable as early as 20 minutes following an oral dose and maximal plasma levels are observed within 30 minutes to two hours (mean $T_{max} = 1$ hour). While CARDENE is completely absorbed, it is subject to saturable first pass metabolism and the systemic bioavailability is about 35% following a 30 mg oral dose at steady state.

When CARDENE was administered one (1) or three (3) hours after a high fat meal, the mean Cmax and mean AUC were lower (20% to 30%) than when CARDENE was given to fasting subjects. These decreases in plasma levels observed following a meal may be significant but the clinical trials establishing the efficacy and safety of CARDENE were done in patients without regard to the timing of meals. Thus the results of these trials reflect the effects of meal-induced variability.

The pharmacokinetics of CARDENE are nonlinear due to saturable hepatic first pass metabolism. Following oral administration, increasing doses result in a disproportionate increase in plasma levels. Steady state Cmax values following 20, 30, and 40 mg doses every 8 hours averaged 36, 88, and 133 ng/mL, respectively. Hence, increasing the dose from 20 to 30 mg every 8 hours more than doubled Cmax and increasing the dose from 20 to 40 mg every 8 hours increased Cmax more than 3-fold. A similar disproportionate increase in AUC with dose was observed. Considerable inter-subject variability in plasma levels was also observed.

Post-absorption kinetics of CARDENE are also non-linear, although there is a reproducible terminal plasma half-life that averaged 8.6 hours following 30 and 40 mg doses at steady state (TID). The terminal half-life represents the elimination of less than 5% of the absorbed drug (measured by plasma concentrations). Elimination over the first 8 hours after dosing is much faster with a half-life of 2–4 hours. Steady state plasma levels are achieved after 2 to 3 days of TID dosing (every 8 hours) and are 2-fold higher than after a single dose.

CARDENE is highly protein bound (>95%) in human plasma over a wide concentration range.

CARDENE is metabolized extensively by the liver; less than 1% of intact drug is detected in the urine. Following a radioactive oral dose in solution, 60% of the radioactivity was recovered in the urine and 35% in feces. Most of the dose (over 90%) was recovered within 48 hours of dosing. CARDENE does not induce its own metabolism and does not induce hepatic microsomal enzymes.

The steady-state pharmacokinetics of CARDENE in elderly hypertensive patients (≥65 years) are similar to those obtained in young normal adults. After one week of CARDENE dosing at 20 mg three times a day, the Cmax, Tmax, AUC, terminal plasma half-life, and the extent of protein binding of CARDENE observed in healthy elderly hypertensive patients did not differ significantly from those observed in young normal volunteers.

CARDENE plasma levels were higher in patients with mild renal impairment (baseline serum creatinine concentration ranged from 1.2 to 5.5 mg/dl) than in normal subjects. After 30 mg CARDENE TID at steady state, Cmax and AUC were approximately 2-fold higher in these patients.

Because CARDENE is extensively metabolized by the liver, the plasma levels of the drug are influenced by changes in hepatic function. CARDENE plasma levels were higher in patients with severe liver disease (hepatic cirrhosis confirmed by liver biopsy or presence of endoscopically-confirmed esophageal varices) than in normal subjects. After 20 mg CARDENE BID at steady state, Cmax and AUC were 1.8 and 4-fold higher, and the terminal half-life was prolonged to 19 hours in these patients.

Hemodynamics

In man, CARDENE produces a significant decrease in systemic vascular resistance. The degree of vasodilation and the resultant hypotensive effects are more prominent in hypertensive patients. In hypertensive patients, nicardipine reduces the blood pressure at rest and during isometric and dynamic exercise. In normotensive patients, a small decrease of about 9 mmHg in systolic and 7 mmHg in diastolic blood pressure may accompany this fall in peripheral resistance. An increase in heart rate may occur in response to the vasodilation and decrease in blood pressure, and in a few patients this heart rate increase may be pronounced. In clinical studies mean heart rate at time of peak plasma levels was usually increased by 5–10 beats per minute compared to placebo, with the greater increases at higher doses, while there was no difference from placebo at the end of the dosing interval. Hemodynamic studies following intravenous dosing in patients with coronary artery disease and normal or moderately abnormal left ventricular function have shown significant increases in ejection fraction and cardiac output with no significant change, or a small decrease, in left ventricular end-diastolic pressure (LVEDP). Although there is evidence that CARDENE increases coronary blood flow, there is no evidence that this property plays any role in its effectiveness in stable angina. In patients with coronary artery disease, intracoronary administration of nicardipine caused no direct myocardial depression. CARDENE does, however, have a negative inotropic effect in some patients with severe left ventricular dysfunction and could, in patients with very impaired function, lead to worsened failure.

"Coronary Steal", the detrimental redistribution of coronary blood flow in patients with coronary artery disease (diversion of blood from underperfused areas toward better perfused areas), has not been observed during nicardipine treatment. On the contrary, nicardipine has been shown to improve systolic shortening in normal and hypokinetic segments of myocardial muscle, and radio-nuclide angiography has confirmed that wall motion remained improved during an increase in oxygen demand. Nonetheless, occasional patients have developed increased angina upon receiving nicardipine. Whether this represents steal in those patients, or is the result of increased heart rate and decreased diastolic pressure, is not clear.

In patients with coronary artery disease nicardipine improves L.V. diastolic distensibility during the early filling phase, probably due to a faster rate of myocardial relaxation in previously underperfused areas. There is little or no effect on normal myocardium, suggesting the improvement is mainly by indirect mechanisms such as afterload reduction, and reduced ischemia. Nicardipine has no negative effect on myocardial relaxation at therapeutic doses. The clinical consequences of these properties are as yet undemonstrated.

Electrophysiologic Effects

In general, no detrimental effects on the cardiac conduction system were seen with the use of CARDENE.

CARDENE increased the heart rate when given intravenously during acute electrophysiologic studies, and prolonged the corrected QT interval to a minor degree. The sinus node recovery times and SA conduction times were not affected by the drug. The PA, AH, and HV intervals* and the functional and effective refractory periods of the atrium were not prolonged by CARDENE and the relative and effective refractory periods of the His-Purkinje system were slightly shortened after intravenous CARDENE.

*PA = conduction time from high to low right atrium, AH = conduction time from low right atrium to His bundle deflection, or AV nodal conduction time, HV = conduction time through the His bundle and the bundle branch-Purkinje system.

Renal Function

There is a transient increase in electrolyte excretion, including sodium. CARDENE does not cause generalized fluid retention, as measured by weight changes, although 7–8% of the patients experience pedal edema.

Effects in Angina Pectoris

In controlled clinical trials of up to 12 weeks duration in patients with chronic stable angina, CARDENE increased exercise tolerance and reduced nitroglycerin consumption and the frequency of anginal attacks. The antianginal efficacy of CARDENE (20–40 mg) has been demonstrated in four placebo-controlled studies involving 258 patients with chronic stable angina. In exercise tolerance testing, CARDENE significantly increased time to angina, total exercise duration and time to 1 mm ST segment depression. Included among these four studies was a dose-definition study in which dose-related improvements in exercise tolerance at one and four hours post-dosing and reduced frequency of anginal attacks were seen at doses of 10, 20 and 30 mg TID. Effectiveness at 10 mg TID was, however, marginal. In a fifth placebo-controlled study, the antianginal efficacy of CARDENE was demonstrated at 8 hours post-dose (trough). The sustained efficacy of CARDENE has been demonstrated over long-term dosing. Blood pressure fell in patients with angina by about 10/8 mmHg at peak blood levels and was little different from placebo at trough blood levels.

Dose	SYSTOLIC BP (mmHg)				Dose	DIASTOLIC BP (mmHg)			
	Number of Patients	Mean Peak Response	Mean Trough Response	Trough/ Peak		Number of Patients	Mean Peak Response	Mean Trough Response	Trough/ Peak
20 mg	50	−10.3	−4.9	48%	20 mg	50	−10.6	−4.6	43%
	52	−17.6	−7.9	45%		52	−9.0	−2.9	32%
30 mg	45	−14.5	−7.2	50%	30 mg	45	−12.8	−4.9	38%
	44	−14.6	−7.5	51%		44	−14.2	−4.3	30%
40 mg	50	−16.3	−9.5	58%	40 mg	50	−15.4	−5.9	38%
	38	−15.9	−6.0	38%		38	−14.8	−3.7	25%

Effects in Hypertension

CARDENE produced dose-related decreases in both systolic and diastolic blood pressure in clinical trials. The antihypertensive efficacy of CARDENE administered three times daily has been demonstrated in three placebo-controlled studies involving 517 patients with mild to moderate hypertension. The blood pressure responses in the three studies were statistically significant from placebo at peak (1 hour post-dosing) and trough (8 hours post-dosing) although it is apparent that well over half of the antihypertensive effect is lost by the end of the dosing interval. The results from placebo controlled studies of CARDENE given three times daily are shown in the following table:

[See table above].

The responses are shown as differences from the concurrent placebo control group. The large changes between peak and trough effects were not accompanied by observed side effects at peak response times. In a study using 24 hour intra-arterial blood pressure monitoring, the circadian variation in blood pressure remained unaltered, but the systolic and diastolic blood pressures were reduced throughout the whole 24 hours.

When added to beta-blocker therapy, CARDENE further lowers both systolic and diastolic blood pressure.

INDICATIONS AND USAGE

I. Stable Angina

CARDENE is indicated for the management of patients with chronic stable angina (effort-associated angina). CARDENE may be used alone or in combination with beta-blockers.

II. Hypertension

CARDENE is indicated for the treatment of hypertension. CARDENE may be used alone or in combination with other antihypertensive drugs. In administering nicardipine it is important to be aware of the relatively large peak to trough differences in blood pressure effect. (See DOSAGE AND ADMINISTRATION.)

CONTRAINDICATIONS

CARDENE is contraindicated in patients with hypersensitivity to the drug.

Because part of the effect of CARDENE is secondary to reduced afterload, the drug is also contraindicated in patients with advanced aortic stenosis. Reduction of diastolic pressure in these patients may worsen rather than improve myocardial oxygen balance.

WARNINGS

Increased Angina

About 7% of patients in short term placebo-controlled angina trials have developed increased frequency, duration or severity of angina on starting CARDENE or at the time of dosage increases, compared with 4% of patients on placebo. Comparisons with beta-blockers also show a greater frequency of increased angina, 4% vs 1%. The mechanism of this effect has not been established. (See ADVERSE REACTIONS.)

Use in Patients with Congestive Heart Failure

Although preliminary hemodynamic studies in patients with congestive heart failure have shown that CARDENE reduced afterload without impairing myocardial contractility, it has a negative inotropic effect *in vitro* and in some patients. Caution should be exercised when using the drug in congestive heart failure patients, particularly in combination with a beta-blocker.

Beta-Blocker Withdrawal

CARDENE is not a beta-blocker and therefore gives no protection against the dangers of abrupt beta-blocker withdrawal; any such withdrawal should be by gradual reduction of the dose of beta-blocker, preferably over 8–10 days.

PRECAUTIONS

GENERAL

Blood Pressure: Because CARDENE decreases peripheral resistance, careful monitoring of blood pressure during the initial administration and titration of CARDENE is suggested. CARDENE, like other calcium channel blockers, may occasionally produce symptomatic hypotension. Caution is advised to avoid systemic hypotension when administering the drug to patients who have sustained an acute cerebral infarction or hemorrhage. Because of prominent effects at the time of peak blood levels, initial titration should be performed with measurements of blood pressure at peak effect (1–2 hours after dosing) and just before the next dose.

Use in patients with impaired hepatic function: Since the liver is the major site of biotransformation and since CARDENE is subject to first pass metabolism, the drug should be used with caution in patients having impaired liver function or reduced hepatic blood flow. Patients with severe liver disease developed elevated blood levels (4-fold increase in AUC) and prolonged half-life (19 hours) of CARDENE. (See DOSAGE AND ADMINISTRATION.)

Use in patients with impaired renal function: When CARDENE 20 mg or 30 mg TID was given to hypertensive patients with mild renal impairment, mean plasma concentrations, AUC and Cmax were approximately 2-fold higher in renally impaired patients than in healthy controls. Doses in these patients must be adjusted. (See CLINICAL PHARMACOLOGY and DOSAGE AND ADMINISTRATION.)

DRUG INTERACTIONS

Beta-Blockers

In controlled clinical studies, adrenergic beta-receptor blockers have been frequently administered concomitantly with CARDENE. The combination is well tolerated.

Cimetidine

Cimetidine increases CARDENE plasma levels. Patients receiving the two drugs concomitantly should be carefully monitored.

Digoxin

Some calcium blockers may increase the concentration of digitalis preparations in the blood. CARDENE usually does not alter the plasma levels of digoxin, however, serum digoxin levels should be evaluated after concomitant therapy with CARDENE is initiated.

Maalox

Co-administration of Maalox TC had no effect on CARDENE absorption.

Fentanyl Anesthesia

Severe hypotension has been reported during fentanyl anesthesia with concomitant use of a beta-blocker and a calcium channel blocker. Even though such interactions were not seen during clinical studies with CARDENE, an increased volume of circulating fluids might be required if such an interaction were to occur.

Cyclosporine

Concomitant administration of nicardipine and cyclosporine results in elevated plasma cyclosporine levels. Plasma concentrations of cyclosporine should therefore be closely monitored, and its dosage reduced accordingly, in patients treated with nicardipine.

When therapeutic concentrations of *furosemide, propranolol, dipyridamole, warfarin, quinidine,* or *naproxen* were added to human plasma (*in vitro*), the plasma protein binding of CARDENE was not altered.

Carcinogenesis, Mutagenesis, Impairment of Fertility

Rats treated with nicardipine in the diet (at concentrations calculated to provide daily dosage levels of 5, 15 or 45 mg/kg/day) for two years showed a dose-dependent increase in thyroid hyperplasia and neoplasia (follicular adenoma/carcinoma). One and three month studies in the rat have suggested that these results are linked to a nicardipine-induced reduction in plasma thyroxine (T4) levels with a consequent increase in plasma levels of thyroid stimulating hormone (TSH). Chronic elevation of TSH is known to cause hyperstimulation of the thyroid. In rats on an iodine deficient diet, nicardipine administration for one month was associated with thyroid hyperplasia that was prevented by T4 supplementation. Mice treated with nicardipine in the diet (at concentrations calculated to provide daily dosage levels of up to 100 mg/kg/day) for up to 18 months showed no evidence of neoplasia of any tissue and no evidence of thyroid changes. There was no evidence of thyroid pathology in dogs treated with up to 25 mg nicardipine/kg/day for one year and no evidence of effects of nicardipine on thyroid function (plasma T4 and TSH) in man.

There was no evidence of a mutagenic potential of nicardipine in a battery of genotoxicity tests conducted on microbial indicator organisms, in micronucleus tests in mice and hamsters, or in a sister chromatid exchange study in hamsters. No impairment of fertility was seen in male or female rats administered nicardipine at oral doses as high as 100 mg/kg/day (50 times the 40 mg TID maximum recommended antianginal or antihypertensive dose in man, assuming a patient weight of 60 kg).

Continued on next page

Syntex—Cont.

Pregnancy Pregnancy Category C

Nicardipine was embryocidal when administered orally to pregnant Japanese White rabbits, during organogenesis, at 150 mg/kg/day (a dose associated with marked body weight gain suppression in the treated doe) but not at 50 mg/kg/day (25 times the maximum recommended antianginal or antihypertensive dose in man). No adverse effects on the fetus were observed when New Zealand albino rabbits were treated, during organogenesis, with up to 100 mg nicardipine/kg/day (a dose associated with significant mortality in the treated doe). In pregnant rats administered nicardipine orally at up to 100 mg/kg/day (50 times the maximum recommended human dose) there was no evidence of embryolethality or teratogenicity. However, dystocia, reduced birth weights, reduced neonatal survival and reduced neonatal weight gain were noted. There are no adequate and well-controlled studies in pregnant women. CARDENE® should be used during pregnancy only if the potential benefit justifies the potential risk to the fetus.

Nursing Mothers

Studies in rats have shown significant concentrations of CARDENE in maternal milk following oral administration. For this reason it is recommended that women who wish to breast-feed should not take this drug.

Pediatric Use

Safety and efficacy in patients under the age of 18 have not been established.

Use in the Elderly

Pharmacokinetic parameters did not differ between elderly hypertensive patients (≥ 65 years) and healthy controls after one week of CARDENE treatment at 20 mg TID. Plasma CARDENE concentrations in elderly hypertensive patients were similar to plasma concentrations in healthy young adult subjects when CARDENE was administered at doses of 10, 20 and 30 mg TID, suggesting that the pharmacokinetics of CARDENE are similar in young and elderly hypertensive patients. No significant differences in responses to CARDENE have been observed in elderly patients and the general adult population of patients who participated in clinical studies.

ADVERSE REACTIONS

In multiple-dose U.S. and foreign controlled short-term (up to three months) studies 1,910 patients received CARDENE alone or in combination with other drugs. In these studies adverse events were reported spontaneously; adverse experiences were generally not serious but occasionally required dosage adjustment and about 10% of patients left the studies prematurely because of them. Peak responses were not observed to be associated with adverse effects during clinical trials, but physicians should be aware that adverse effects associated with decreases in blood pressure (tachycardia, hypotension, etc.) could occur around the time of the peak effect. Most adverse effects were expected consequences of the vasodilator effects of CARDENE.

Angina

The incidence rates of adverse effects in anginal patients were derived from multicenter, controlled clinical trials. Following are the rates of adverse effects for CARDENE (N = 520) and placebo (N = 310), respectively, that occurred in 0.4% of patients or more. These represent events considered probably drug-related by the investigator (except for certain cardiovascular events which were recorded in a different category). Where the frequency of adverse effects for CARDENE and placebo is similar, causal relationship is uncertain. The only dose-related effects were pedal edema and increased angina.

Percent of Patients with Adverse Effects in
Controlled Studies (Incidence of
discontinuations shown in parentheses)

Adverse Experience	CARDENE (N=520)	PLACEBO (N=310)
Pedal Edema	7.1 (0)	0.3 (0)
Dizziness	6.9 (1.2)	0.6 (0)
Headache	6.4 (0.6)	2.6 (0)
Asthenia	5.8 (0.4)	2.6 (0)
Flushing	5.6 (0.4)	1.0 (0)
Increased Angina	5.6 (3.5)	4.2 (1.9)
Palpitations	3.3 (0.4)	0.0 (0)
Nausea	1.9 (0)	0.3 (0)
Dyspepsia	1.5 (0.6)	0.6 (0.3)
Dry Mouth	1.4 (0)	0.3 (0)
Somnolence	1.4 (0)	1.0 (0)
Rash	1.2 (0.2)	0.3 (0)
Tachycardia	1.2 (0.2)	0.6 (0)
Myalgia	1.0 (0)	0.0 (0)
Other edema	1.0 (0)	0.0 (0)
Paresthesia	1.0 (0.2)	0.3 (0)
Sustained Tachycardia	0.8 (0.6)	0.0 (0)
Syncope	0.8 (0.2)	0.0 (0)
Constipation	0.6 (0.2)	0.6 (0)
Dyspnea	0.6 (0)	0.0 (0)
Abnormal ECG	0.6 (0.6)	0.0 (0)
Malaise	0.6 (0)	0.0 (0)
Nervousness	0.6 (0)	0.3 (0)
Tremor	0.6 (0)	0.0 (0)

In addition, adverse events were observed which are not readily distinguishable from the natural history of the atherosclerotic vascular disease in these patients. Adverse events in this category each occurred in < 0.4% of patients receiving CARDENE and included myocardial infarction, atrial fibrillation, exertional hypotension, pericarditis, heart block, cerebral ischemia and ventricular tachycardia. It is possible that some of these events were drug-related.

Hypertension

The incidence rates of adverse effects in hypertensive patients were derived from multicenter, controlled clinical trials. Following are the rates of adverse effects for CARDENE (N = 1390) and placebo (N = 211), respectively, that occurred in 0.4% of patients or more. These represent events considered probably drug-related by the investigator. Where the frequency of adverse effects for CARDENE and placebo is similar, causal relationship is uncertain. The only dose-related effect was pedal edema.

Percent of Patients with Adverse Effects in
Controlled Studies (Incidence of
discontinuations shown in parentheses)

Adverse Experience	CARDENE (N=1390)	PLACEBO (N=211)
Flushing	9.7 (2.1)	2.8 (0)
Headache	8.2 (2.6)	4.7 (0)
Pedal Edema	8.0 (1.8)	0.9 (0)
Asthenia	4.2 (1.7)	0.5 (0)
Palpitations	4.1 (1.0)	0.0 (0)
Dizziness	4.0 (1.8)	0.0 (0)
Tachycardia	3.4 (1.2)	0.5 (0)
Nausea	2.2 (0.9)	0.9 (0)
Somnolence	1.1 (0.1)	0.0 (0)
Dyspepsia	0.8 (0.3)	0.5 (0)
Insomnia	0.6 (0.1)	0.0 (0)
Malaise	0.6 (0.1)	0.0 (0)
Other edema	0.6 (0.3)	1.4 (0)
Abnormal dreams	0.4 (0)	0.0 (0)
Dry mouth	0.4 (0.1)	0.0 (0)
Nocturia	0.4 (0)	0.0 (0)
Rash	0.4 (0)	0.0 (0)
Vomiting	0.4 (0.4)	0.0 (0)

Rare Events

The following rare adverse events have been reported in clinical trials or the literature:

Body as a Whole: infection, allergic reaction

Cardiovascular: hypotension, postural hypotension, atypical chest pain, peripheral vascular disorder, ventricular extrasystoles, ventricular tachycardia

Digestive: sore throat, abnormal liver chemistries

Musculoskeletal: arthralgia

Nervous: hot flashes, vertigo, hyperkinesia,, impotence, depression, confusion, anxiety

Respiratory: rhinitis, sinusitis

Special Senses: tinnitus, abnormal vision, blurred vision

Urogenital: increased urinary frequency

OVERDOSAGE

Overdosage with a 600 mg single dose (15 to 30 times normal clinical dose) has been reported. Marked hypotension (blood pressure unobtainable) and bradycardia (heart rate 20 bpm in normal sinus rhythm) occurred, along with drowsiness, confusion and slurred speech. Supportive treatment with a vasopressor resulted in gradual improvement with normal vital signs approximately 9 hours post treatment.

Based on results in laboratory animals, overdosage may cause systemic hypotension, bradycardia (following initial tachycardia) and progressive atrioventricular conduction block. Reversible hepatic function abnormalities and sporadic focal hepatic necrosis were noted in some animal species receiving very large doses of nicardipine.

For treatment of overdose standard measures (for example, evacuation of gastric contents, elevation of extremities, attention to circulating fluid volume and urine output) including monitoring of cardiac and respiratory functions should be implemented. The patient should be positioned so as to avoid cerebral anoxia. Frequent blood pressure determinations are essential. Vasopressors are clinically indicated for patients exhibiting profound hypotension. Intravenous calcium gluconate may help reverse the effects of calcium entry blockade.

DOSAGE AND ADSMINISTRATION

Angina

The dose should be individually titrated for each patient beginning with 20 mg three times daily. Doses in the range of 20–40 mg three times a day have been shown to be effective. At least three days should be allowed before increasing the CARDENE dose to ensure achievement of steady state plasma drug concentrations.

Concomitant Use With Other Antianginal Agents

1. Sublingual NTG may be taken as required to abort acute anginal attacks during CARDENE therapy.
2. Prophylactic Nitrate Therapy—CARDENE may be safely coadministered with short- and long-acting nitrates.
3. Beta-blockers—CARDENE may be safely coadministered with beta-blockers. (See DRUG INTERACTIONS.)

Hypertension

The dose of CARDENE should be individually adjusted according to the blood pressure response beginning with 20 mg three times daily. The effective doses in clinical trials have ranged from 20 mg to 40 mg three times daily. The maximum blood pressure lowering effect occurs approximately 1–2 hours after dosing. **To assess the adequacy of blood pressure response, the blood pressure should be measured at trough (8 hours after dosing). Because of the prominent peak effects of nicardipine, blood pressure should be measured 1–2 hours after dosing, particularly during initiation of therapy.** (See PRECAUTIONS: Blood Pressures, INDICATIONS and CLINICAL PHARMACOLOGY—Peak/Trough Effects in Hypertension.) At least three days should be allowed before increasing the CARDENE dose to ensure achievement of steady state plasma drug concentrations.

Concomitant use with other Antihypertensive Agents

1. Diuretics—CARDENE may be safely coadministered with thiazide diuretics.
2. Beta-blockers—CARDENE may be safely coadministered with beta-blockers (See DRUG INTERACTIONS.)

Special Patient Populations

Renal Insufficiency—although there is no evidence that CARDENE impairs renal function, careful dose titration beginning with 20 mg TID is advised. (See PRECAUTIONS.)

Hepatic Insufficiency—CARDENE should be administered cautiously in patients with severely impaired hepatic function. A suggested starting dose of 20 mg twice a day is advised with individual titration based on clinical findings maintaining the twice a day schedule. (See PRECAUTIONS.)

Congestive Heart Failure—Caution is advised when titrating CARDENE dosage in patients with congestive heart failure. (See WARNINGS.)

HOW SUPPLIED

CARDENE® 20 mg capsules are available in opaque white-white hard gelatin capsules with a brilliant blue band and printed "CARDENE 20 mg" on the cap and "SYNTEX 2437" on the capsule body. These are supplied in bottles of 100 (NDC 0033-2437-42), bottles of 500 (NDC 0033-2437-62) and in foil wrapped cartons of 100 unit dose blister packages (NDC 0033-2437-53).

CARDENE® 30 mg capsules are available in opaque light blue-powder blue hard gelatin capsules with a brilliant blue band and printed "CARDENE 30 mg" on the cap and "SYNTEX 2438" on the capsule body. These are supplied in bottles of 100 (NDC 0033-2438-42), bottles of 500 (NDC 0033-2438-62) and in foil wrapped cartons of 100 unit dose blister packages (NDC 0033-2438-53).

Store bottles at room temperature and dispense in light resistant containers.

Store blister packages at room tempertaure and protect from excessive humidity and light. To protect from light, product should remain in manufacturer's package until consumed.

CAUTION: Fedral law prohibits dispensing without prescription.

U.S. Patent No. 3,985,758   ©DECEMBER 1988
02-2437-42-00

Shown in Product Identification Section, page 433

CARMOL® 10   OTC
[kahr'mawl]
**10% urea lotion
for total body
dry skin care.**

A product of Syntex Laboratories, Inc.

(See PDR For Nonprescription Drugs)

CARMOL® 20   OTC
[kahr'mawl]
**20% Urea Cream
Extra strength for
rough, dry skin**

A product of Syntex Laboratories, Inc.

(See PDR For Nonprescription Drugs)

CARMOL® HC   ℞
[kahr'mawl]
**(hydrocortisone acetate)
Cream 1%**

Refer to entry under LIDEX® (fluocinonide) Cream 0.05%.

CYTOVENE® ℞

[si'tō-veen]
(ganciclovir sodium)

THE CLINICAL TOXICITY OF CYTOVENE INCLUDES GRANULOCYTOPENIA AND THROMBOCYTOPENIA. IN ANIMAL STUDIES CYTOVENE WAS CARCINOGENIC, TERATOGENIC, AND CAUSED ASPERMATOGENESIS. CYTOVENE IS INDICATED FOR USE *ONLY* IN IMMUNOCOMPROMISED PATIENTS WITH CYTOMEGALOVIRUS (CMV) RETINITIS.

DESCRIPTION

CYTOVENE is the brand name for ganciclovir sodium, an antiviral drug active against cytomegalovirus. Reconstituted CYTOVENE Sterile Powder is for intravenous administration only. Each vial of CYTOVENE Sterile Powder contains the equivalent of 500 mg ganciclovir as the sodium salt (46 mg sodium). All doses in this insert are specified in terms of ganciclovir. The chemical name of ganciclovir sodium is 9-(1,3-dihydroxy-2-propoxymethyl) guanine, monosodium salt. CYTOVENE is manufactured as a sterile lyophilized powder. Reconstitution with 10 mL of Sterile Water for Injection, USP, yields a solution with pH 11 and a ganciclovir concentration of approximately 50 mg/mL. Further dilution in an appropriate intravenous solution must be performed before infusion (see **DOSAGE AND ADMINISTRATION**).

CLINICAL PHARMACOLOGY

Virology

Ganciclovir is a synthetic nucleoside analogue of 2'-deoxyguanosine that inhibits replication of herpes viruses both *in vitro* and *in vivo*. Sensitive human viruses include cytomegalovirus (CMV), herpes simplex virus -1 and -2 (HSV-1, HSV-2), Epstein-Barr virus (EBV) and varicella zoster virus (VZV). Clinical studies have been limited to assessment of efficacy in patients with CMV infection.

Median effective inhibitory doses (ED_{50}) of ganciclovir for human CMV isolates tested *in vitro* in several cell lines ranged from 0.2 to 3.0 μg/mL. The relationship between *in vitro* sensitivity of CMV to ganciclovir and clinical response has not been established. CYTOVENE inhibits mammalian cell proliferation *in vitro* at higher concentrations (10 to 60 μg/mL) with bone marrow colony forming cells being the most sensitive ($ID_{50} \geq 10$ μg/mL) of those cell types tested. Available evidence indicates that upon entry into host cells, cytomegaloviruses induce one or more cellular kinases that phosphorylate ganciclovir to its triphosphate. It has been shown that there is approximately a 10-fold greater concentration of ganciclovir-triphosphate in CMV-infected cells than in uninfected cells, indicating a preferential phosphorylation of ganciclovir in virus-infected cells. *In vitro*, ganciclovir-triphosphate is catabolized slowly, with 60 to 70% of the original level remaining in the infected cells 18 hours after removal of ganciclovir from the extracellular medium.[1] The antiviral activity of ganciclovir-triphosphate is believed to be the result of inhibition of viral DNA synthesis by two known modes: (1) competitive inhibition of viral DNA polymerases (2) direct incorporation into vial DNA, resulting in eventual termination of viral DNA elongation. The cellular DNA polymerase alpha is also inhibited, but at a higher concentration than required for viral DNA polymerase.

Ganciclovir has shown antiviral activity *in vivo* in several animal CMV infection models. Both normal and immunosuppressed mice had reduced titers of murine CMV when treated with ganciclovir at 5 to 50 mg/kg/day.[2] Normal mice had increased survival as well, when treated with doses of 3 mg/kg/day. Immunosuppressed mice did not show increased survival until they received doses of at least 10 mg/kg/day.[3] In guinea pigs infected with cavian CMV and treated with ganciclovir at 50 mg/kg/day for 7 days, viral titers in the salivary glands were reduced approximately 50% at day 28 post-infection as compared to sham-treated controls.[4] Of 314 immunocompromised patients enrolled in an open label study of the treatment of life- or sight-threatening CMV disease, 121 patients were identified who had a positive culture for CMV within 7 days prior to treatment and had sequential viral cultures after treatment with CYTOVENE.[5] Post-treatment virologic response was defined as conversion to culture negativity, or a greater than 100-fold decrease in CMV infectious units, as shown in the following table:

Virologic Response

Culture Source	No. Patients Cultured	No. (%) Patients Responding	Median Days to Responses
Urine	107	93 (87)	8
Blood	41	34 (83)	8
Throat	21	19 (90)	7
Semen	6	6 (100)	15

Emergence of viral resistance has been reported based on *in vitro* sensitivity testing of CMV isolates from patients receiving CYTOVENE treatment.[6] The prevalence of resistant isolates is unknown, and there is a possibility that some patients may be infected with strains of CMV resistant to ganciclovir. Therefore, the possibility of viral resistance should be considered in patients who show poor clinical response or experience persistent viral excretion during therapy.

Pharmacokinetics

The pharmacokinetics of CYTOVENE have been evaluated in immunocompromised patients with serious CMV disease. Twenty-two such patients with normal renal function received 5 mg/kg doses of CYTOVENE, each dose infused intravenously over one hour. The plasma level of ganciclovir at the end of the first one hour infusion (Cmax) was 8.3 ± 4.0 μg/mL (mean ± SD) and the plasma level 11 hours after the start of infusion (Cmin) was 0.56 ± 0.66 μg/mL. The plasma half-life was 2.9 ± 1.3 hours and the systemic clearance was 3.64 ± 1.86 mL/kg/min (approximately 250 mL/1.73M^2/min). Dose-independent kinetics were demonstrated over the range of 1.6 to 5.0 mg/kg. Multiple-dose kinetics were measured in eight patients with normal renal function who received CYTOVENE® (ganciclovir sodium) Sterile Powder, 5 mg/kg twice daily for 12–14 days. After the first dose and after multiple dosing, plasma levels of ganciclovir at the end of infusion were 7.1 μg/mL (3.1 to 14.0 μg/mL) and 9.5 μg/mL (2.7 to 24.2 μg/mL), respectively. At 7 hours after infusion, plasma levels after the first dose were 0.85 μg/mL (0.2 to 1.8 μg/mL) and were 1.2 μg/mL (0.6 to 1.8 μg/mL) after multiple dosing.

Renal excretion of unchanged drug by glomerular filtration is the major route of elimination of CYTOVENE. In patients with normal renal function, more than 90% of the administered CYTOVENE was recovered unmetabolized in the urine. The pharmacokinetic analysis in 10 patients with renal impairment showed that in 4 patients with mild impairment (creatinine clearance 50 to 79 mL/1.73M^2/min) the systemic clearance of CYTOVENE was 128 ± 63 mL/1.73M^2/min, and the plasma half-life was 4.6 ± 1.4 hours. In 3 patients with moderate impairment (creatinine clearance 25 to 49 mL/1.73M^2/min) the systemic clearance of CYTOVENE was 57 ± 8 mL/1.73M^2/min, and the plasma half-life was 4.4 ± 0.4 hours. In 3 patients with severe impairment (creatinine clearance less than 25 mL/1.73M^2/min) the systemic clearance was 30 ± 13 mL/1.73M^2/min, and the plasma half-life was 10.7 ± 5.7 hours. There was positive correlation between systemic clearance of CYTOVENE and creatinine clearance (r = 0.90).

Data from 4 patients with severe renal impairment showed that hemodialysis reduced plasma drug levels by approximately 50%.

BECAUSE THE MAJOR EXCRETION PATHWAY FOR CYTOVENE IS RENAL, DOSAGE MUST BE REDUCED ACCORDING TO CREATININE CLEARANCE. FOR DOSING INSTRUCTIONS IN RENAL IMPAIRMENT, REFER TO THE SECTION ON DOSAGE AND ADMINISTRATION.

There is limited evidence to suggest that ganciclovir crosses the blood-brain barrier. Cerebrospinal fluid (CSF) concentrations have been measured in three patients, with the results shown in the following table:

CSF Concentrations[7,8]

Patients	CSF Conc. (μg/mL)	Plasma Conc. (μg/mL)	Hr after dose	CSF/Plasma Ratio
1	0.62	0.92*	5.67	.67
	0.68	2.20*	3.5	.31
	0.51	1.96*	2.75	.26
2	0.50	2.05*	0.25	.24
3	0.31	0.44	5.5	.70

* Estimation (model-predicted values)

Binding of CYTOVENE to plasma proteins is 1–2%. Drug interactions involving binding site displacement are not expected.

INDICATIONS AND USAGE

CYTOVENE is indicated for the treatment of CMV retinitis in immunocompromised individuals, including patients with acquired immunodeficiency syndrome (AIDS). SAFETY AND EFFICACY OF CYTOVENE HAVE NOT BEEN ESTABLISHED FOR CONGENITAL OR NEONATAL CMV DISEASE; NOR FOR TREATMENT OF OTHER CMV INFECTIONS (E.G., PNEUMONITIS, COLITIS); NOR FOR USE IN NON-IMMUNOCOMPROMISED INDIVIDUALS. The diagnosis of CMV retinitis is ophthalmologic and should be made by indirect ophthalmoscopy. Other conditions in the differential diagnosis of CMV retinitis include candidiasis, toxoplasmosis, and cotton wool spots, any of which may produce a retinal appearance similar to CMV. For this reason it is essential that the diagnosis of CMV be established by an ophthalmologist familiar with the retinal presentation of these conditions. The diagnosis of CMV retinitis may be supported by culture of CMV from urine, blood, throat, or other sites, but a negative CMV culture does not rule out CMV retinitis.

In most studies conducted with CYTOVENE, treatment was begun with a BID dosage regimen (5 mg/kg/dose) for the first 2 to 3 weeks, followed by a once-daily regimen (maintenance treatment) to maintain viral suppression. Patients who experienced progression of retinitis while receiving maintenance treatment were retreated with the BID regimen (see **DOSAGE AND ADMINISTRATION**).

In a retrospective, non-randomized, single-center analysis[9,10] of 41 patients with AIDS and CMV retinitis, treatment with CYTOVENE resulted in a significant delay in median time to first retinitis progression compared to untreated controls (71 days from diagnosis versus 29 days from diagnosis). Patients in this series received induction treatment of CYTOVENE 5 mg/kg BID for 14–21 days followed by maintenance treatment with either 5 mg/kg once per day, seven days per week or 6 mg/kg one per day, five days each week.

CONTRAINDICATIONS

CYTOVENE is contraindicated in patients with hypersensitivity to ganciclovir or acyclovir.

WARNINGS

Approximately 40% of 522 immunocompromised patients with serious CMV infections who received intravenous CYTOVENE developed granulocytopenia (neutropenia, i.e., neutrophil count less than 1,000 cells/mm^3). CYTOVENE should, therefore, be used with caution in patients with pre-existing cytopenias, or with a history of cytopenic reactions to other drugs, chemicals or irradiation. Granulocytopenia usually occurs during the first or second week of treatment, but may occur at any time during treatment. Cell counts usually begin to recover within 3 to 7 days of discontinuing drug. *CYTOVENE should not be administered if the absolute neutrophil count is less than 500 cells/min*[3] *or the platelet count is less than 25,000/mm*[3].

Thrombocytopenia (platelet count < 50,000/mm^3) was observed in approximately 20% of the same 522 patients treated with CYTOVENE. Patients with iatrogenic immunosuppression were more likely to develop thrombocytopenia than patients with AIDS (46% versus 14% of cases).

Animal data indicate that administration of CYTOVENE causes inhibition of spermatogenesis and subsequent infertility. These effects were reversible at lower doses and irreversible at higher doses (see **Carcinogenesis, Mutagenesis, Impairment of Fertility** section in **PRECAUTIONS**). Although data in humans have not been obtained regarding this effect, *it is considered probable that intravenous CYTOVENE at the recommended doses causes temporary or permanent inhibition of spermatogenesis. Animal data also indicate that suppression of fertility in females may occur.*

Because of the mutagenic potential of CYTOVENE, women of childbearing potential should be advised to use effective contraception during treatment. Similarly, male patients should be advised to practice barrier contraception during and for at least 90 days following treatment with CYTOVENE.

PRECAUTIONS

General

In clinical studies with CYTOVENE, the maximum single dose administered was 6 mg/kg by intravenous infusion over one hour. It is likely that larger doses, or more rapid infusions, would result in increased toxicity.

Administration of CYTOVENE by intravenous infusion should be accompanied by adequate hydration, since CYTOVENE is excreted by the kidneys and normal clearance depends on adequate renal function. IF RENAL FUNCTION IS IMPAIRED, DOSAGE ADJUSTMENTS ARE REQUIRED. Such adjustments should be based on measured or estimated creatinine clearance (see **DOSAGE AND ADMINISTRATION**).

Initially reconstituted CYTOVENE solutions have a high pH (range 9 to 11). Despite further dilution in intravenous fluids, phlebitis and/or pain may occur at the site of intravenous infusion. Care must be taken to infuse solutions containing CYTOVENE only into veins with adequate blood flow to permit rapid dilution and distribution (see **DOSAGE AND ADMINISTRATION**).

Information for Patients

CYTOVENE® (ganciclovir sodium) Sterile Powder is not a cure for CMV retinitis, and immunocompromised patients may continue to experience progession of retinitis during or following treatment. Patients should be advised to have regular ophthalmologic examinations. They should be informed that the major toxicities of ganciclovir are granulocytopenia and thrombocytopenia and that dose modifications may be required, including possible discontinuation. The importance of close monitoring of blood counts while on therapy should be emphasized.

Patients with AIDS may be receiving zidovudine (Retrovir). They should be counseled that treatment with zidovudine or CYTOVENE, and especially the combination, can result in severe granulocytopenia. Therefore, it is recommended that the two drugs not be given concomitantly.

Continued on next page

Syntex—Cont.

Patients should be advised that CYTOVENE has caused decreased sperm production in animals and may cause infertility in humans. Women of childbearing potential should be advised that CYTOVENE causes birth defects in animals and should not be used during pregnancy. Women of childbearing potential should be advised to use effective contraception during CYTOVENE treatment. Similarly, men should be advised to practice barrier contraception during and for at least 90 days following CYTOVENE treatment. Patients should be advised that CYTOVENE causes tumors in animals. Although there is no information from human studies, CYTOVENE should be considered a potential carcinogen.

Laboratory Testing

Due to the frequency of granulocytopenia and thrombocytopenia in patients receiving CYTOVENE (see **ADVERSE REACTIONS**), it is recommended that neutrophil counts and platelet counts be performed every two days during BID dosing of CYTOVENE and at least weekly thereafter. Neutrophil counts should be monitored daily in patients in whom CYTOVENE or other nucleoside analogues have previously resulted in leukopenia, or in whom neutrophil counts are less than 1,000 cells/mm^3 at the beginning of treatment. Because dosing must be modified in patients with renal impairment, patients should have serum creatinine or creatinine clearance monitored at least once every two weeks.

Drug Interactions

It is possible that probenecid, as well as other drugs that inhibit renal tubular secretion or resorption, may reduce renal clearance of CYTOVENE. It is also possible that drugs that inhibit replication of rapidly dividing cell populations such as bone marrow, spermatogonia, and germinal layers of skin and gastrointestinal mucosa may have additive toxicity when administered concomitantly with CYTOVENE. Therefore, drugs such as dapsone, pentamidine, flucytosine, vincristine, vinblastine, adriamycin, amphotericin B, trimethoprim/sulfa combinations or other nucleoside analogues, should be considered for concomitant use with CYTOVENE only if the potential benefits are judged to outweigh the risks.

Patients with AIDS may be receiving, or have received, treatment with zidovudine (Retrovir). *Because both zidovudine and CYTOVENE can cause granulocytopenia, it is recommended that these two drugs not be given concomitantly.* Data from a small number of patients indicate that treatment with ganciclovir plus zidovudine at the recommended doses is not tolerated.

Generalized seizures have been reported in six patients who received CYTOVENE and imipenem-cilastatin. These drugs should not be used concomitantly with CYTOVENE unless the potential benefits outweigh the risks.

Carinogenesis, Mutagenesis, Impairment of Fertility

The carcinogenic potential of ganciclovir is currently under evaluation in an 18-month bioassaay in mice. In mice given daily oral doses of 1,000 mg/kg, interim findings revealed an increased incidence of tumors in the preputial gland of males, nonglandular mucosa of the stomach of males and females, and ovary, vagina and liver of females. A slightly increased incidence of tumors occurred in the preputial gland (males) and nonglandular mucosa (males and females) of the stomach in mice given daily oral doses of 20 mg/kg. The preputial gland and nonglandular mucosa of the stomach of mice do not have human counterparts. However, CYTOVENE should be considered a potential carcinogen in humans.

Ganciclovir caused point mutations and chromosomal damage in mammalian cells *in vitro* and *in vivo*.

Ganciclovir caused decreased mating behavior, decreased fertility, and increased embryolethality in female mice at doses approximately equivalent to the recommended human dose (calculated on the basis of body surface area). Ganciclovir caused decreased fertility in male mice and hypospermatogenesis in rats and dogs at doses equivalent to or less than the recommended human dose.

Pregnancy: Category C

CYTOVENE has been shown to be teratogenic in rabbits and embryotoxic in mice when given in doses approximately equivalent to the recommended human dose (calculated on the basis of body surface area). The adverse effects observed in mice were maternal/fetal toxicity and embryolethality. In rabbits, the effects were: fetal growth retardation, embryolethality, teratogenicity, and/or maternal toxicity. Teratogenic changes included cleft palate, anophthalmia/microphthalmia, aplastic organs (kidney and pancreas), hydrocephaly, and brachygnathia.

It is therefore expected that CYTOVENE may be teratogenic and/or embryotoxic at the dose levels recommended for human use. There are no adequate and well-controlled studies in pregnant women. CYTOVENE should be used during pregnancy only if the potential benefit justifies the potential risk to the fetus.

Nursing Mothers

It is not known if CYTOVENE is excreted in human milk. Carcinogenicity and teratogenicity occurred in animals treated with ganciclovir. Because many drugs are excreted in human milk and because of the potential for serious adverse reactions from ganciclovir in nursing infants, mothers should be instructed to discontinue nursing if they are receiving CYTOVENE. Nursing should not be resumed until at least 72 hours after the last dose of CYTOVENE.

Daily intravenous doses of 90 mg/kg administered to female mice prior to mating, during gestation, and during lactation caused hypoplasia of the testes and seminal vesicles in the month-old male offspring, as well as pathologic changes in the non-glandular region of the stomach.

Pediatric Use

THE USE OF CYTOVENE IN CHILDREN WARRANTS EXTREME CAUTION DUE TO THE PROBABILITY OF LONG-TERM CARCINOGENICITY AND REPRODUCTIVE TOXICITY. ADMINISTRATION TO CHILDREN SHOULD BE UNDERTAKEN ONLY AFTER CAREFUL EVALUATION AND ONLY IF THE POTENTIAL BENEFITS OF TREATMENT OUTWEIGH THE RISKS.

There has been very limited clinical experience in treating cytomegalovirus retinitis in patients under the age of 12 years. Two children (ages 9 and 5 years) showed improvement or stabilization of retinitis for 23 and 9 months, respectively. These children received induction treatment with 2.5 mg/kg TID followed by maintenance therapy with 6–6.5 mg/kg once per day, five to seven days per week. When retinitis progressed during once daily maintenance therapy, both children were treated with the 5 mg/kg BID regimen. Two other children (ages 2.5 and 4 years) who received similar induction regimens showed only partial or no response to treatment. Another child, a six year old with T-cell dysfunction, showed stabilization of retinitis for 3 months while receiving continuous infusions of CYTOVENE at doses of 2–5 mg/kg/24 hours. Continuous infusion treatment was discontinued due to granulocytopenia. Pharmacokinetic data have not been obtained in pediatric patients.

Adverse events reported in 120 immunocompromised children with serious CMV infections receiving ganciclovir were similar to those reported in adults. Granulocytopenia (17%) and thrombocytopenia (10%) were the most common adverse events reported.

Use in Patients with Renal Impairment

CYTOVENE should be used with caution in patients with impaired renal function because the plasma half-life and peak plasma levels of CYTOVENE will be increased due to reduced renal clearance (see **DOSAGE AND ADMINISTRATION**).

Data from 4 patients indicate that CYTOVENE plasma levels are reduced approximately 50% following hemodialysis.

Use in the Elderly

No studies of the efficacy or safety of CYTOVENE in elderly patients have been conducted. Since elderly individuals frequently have reduced glomerular filtration, particular attention should be paid to assessing renal function before and during CYTOVENE administration (see **DOSAGE AND ADMINISTRATION**).

ADVERSE REACTIONS

During clinical trials, CYTOVENE® (ganciclovir sodium) Sterile Powder was withdrawn or interrupted in approximately 32% of patients because of adverse events. In some instances treatment was restarted and the reappearance of adverse events again necessitated withdrawal or interruption.

The most frequent adverse events seen in patients treated with CYTOVENE involved the hematopoietic system. Granulocytopenia (defined as an absolute neutrophil count less than 1,000 cell/mm^3) occurred in approximately 40% and thrombocytopenia (defined as a platelet count below 50,000/mm^3) occurred in approximately 20% of the patients. In most cases, withdrawal of CYTOVENE resulted in increased neutrophil or platelet counts.

While granulocytopenia was generally reversible with discontinuation of treatment, patients may experience irreversible neutropenia or sepsis during neutropenic episodes. In an open label study fo 522 immunocompromised patients with sight-threatening or life-threatening CMV disease, five neutropenic patients died with severe bacterial or fungal infections.

Adverse events other than granulocytopenia and thrombocytopenia were reported as "probably related", "probably not related", and "unknown" in relationship to CYTOVENE therapy. Evaluation of these reports was difficult because of the protean manifestations of the underlying disease, and because most patients received numerous concomitant medications.

Other than leukopenia and thrombocytopenia, the most frequent adverse events observed in over 5,000 patients who received CYTOVENE were anemia, fever, rash, and abnormal liver function values, each of which was reported in approximately 2% of treated patients. Adverse events that were thought to be possibly related to drug and occurred in 1% or fewer patients who received CYTOVENE were:

Body as a Whole: chills, edema, infections, malaise

Cardiovascular System: arrhythmia, hypertension, hypotension

Central Nervous System: abnormal thoughts or dreams, ataxia, coma, confusion, dizziness, headache, nervousness, paresthesia, psychosis, somnolence, tremor. (Overall, neurologic system events occurred in 5% of patients.)

Digestive System: nausea, vomiting, anorexia, diarrhea, hemorrhage, abdominal pain

Hematologic System: eosinophilia

Labortory Abnormalities: decrease in blood glucose

Respiratory System: dyspnea

Skin and Appendages: alopecia, pruritus, urticaria

Special Senses: retinal detachment in patients with CMV retinitis

Urogenital System: hematuria, increased serum creatinine, increased blood urea nitrogen (BUN)

Injection Site: Inflammation, pain, phlebitis

OVERDOSAGE

Overdosage with CYTOVENE has been reported in five patients. In three of these patients, no adverse events were observed after the overdosage. (The doses received were: 7 doses of 22 mg/kg over a 3-day period, 9 mg/kg BID for 3 days, and 2 doses of 500 mg to a 21 month old child.) Neutropenia was reported following overdoses in two patients: one who had a history of bone marrow suppression prior to treatment and who received CYTOVENE 5 mg/kg BID for 14 days followed by treatment with 8 mg/kg given as single daily doses for 4 days, and one patient who received a single dose of 1,675 mg (approximately 24 mg/kg). In both cases the neutropenia was reversible (17 days and 1 day, respectively), following discontinuation of CYTOVENE.

Toxic manifestations observed in animals given very high single doses of CYTOVENE (500 mg/kg) included emesis, hypersalivation, anorexia, bloody diarrhea, inactivity, cytopenia, elevated liver function test results, elevated blood urea nitrogen, testicular atrophy and death.

Hemodialysis and hydration may be of benefit in reducing drug plasma levels in patients who receive an overdosage of CYTOVENE.

DOSAGE AND ADMINISTRATION

CAUTION—DO NOT ADMINISTER CYTOVENE BY RAPID OR BOLUS INTRAVENOUS INJECTION. THE TOXICITY OF CYTOVENE MAY BE INCREASED AS A RESULT OF EXCESSIVE PLASMA LEVELS.

CAUTION—INTRAMUSCULAR OR SUBCUTANEOUS INJECTION OF RECONSTITUTED CYTOVENE MAY RESULT IN SEVERE TISSUE IRRITATION DUE TO HIGH PH (~11).

Dosage

THE RECOMMENDED DOSAGE, FREQUENCY, OR INFUSION RATES SHOULD NOT BE EXCEEDED.

Induction Treatment. The recommended initial dose of CYTOVENE for patients with normal renal function is 5 mg/kg (given intravenously at a constant rate over 1 hour) every 12 hours for 14–21 days.

Maintenance Treatment. Following induction treatment the recommended dose of CYTOVENE is 5 mg/kg given as an intravenous infusion over one hour once per day on seven days each week, or 6 mg/kg once per day on five days each week. Patients who experience progression of retinitis while receiving maintenance therapy may be retreated with the BID regimen.

Patients should have frequent hematologic monitoring throughout treatment. CYTOVENE should not be administered if the neutrophil count falls below 500 cells/mm^3 or the platelet count falls below 25,000/mm^3.

RENAL IMPAIRMENT

For patients with impairment of renal function, refer to the table below for recommended doses during the induction phase of treatment, and adjust the dosing interval as indicated.

Creatinine Clearance* (mL/1.73M^2/min)	CYTOVENE Dose (mg/kg)	Dosing Interval (hours)
≥ 80	5.0	12
50–79	2.5	12
25–49	2.5	24
< 25	1.25	24

*Creatinine clearance can be related to serum creatinine by the following formulae:

[See table on next page].

The optimal maintenance dose for patients with renal impairment is not known. Physicians may elect to reduce the dose to 50% of the induction dose and monitor the patient for disease progression.

Only limited data are available on CYTOVENE® (ganciclovir sodium) Sterile Powder elimination in patients undergoing hemodialysis. Dosing for these patients should not exceed 1.25 mg/kg/24 hours. On days when hemodialysis is performed, the dose should be given shortly after the completion of the hemodialysis session, since hemodialysis has been shown to reduce plasma levels by approximately 50%. Neutrophil and platelet counts should be monitored daily.

PATIENT MONITORING

Due to the frequency of granulocytopenia and thrombocytopenia in patients receiving CYTOVENE (see **ADVERSE REACTIONS**), it is recommended that neutrophil counts and platelet counts be performed every two days during BID dosing of CYTOVENE and at least weekly thereafter. In patients in whom CYTOVENE or other nucleoside analogues have previously resulted in leukopenia, or in whom neutrophil counts are less than 1,000 cells/mm^3 at the beginning of treatment, neutrophil counts should be monitored daily. Because dosing must be modified in patients with renal impairment, all patients should have serum creatinine or creatinine clearance monitored at least once every two weeks.

REDUCTION OF DOSE

The most frequently reported adverse event following treatment with CYTOVENE is leukopenia/neutropenia, which occurs in approximately 40% of patients. Therefore, frequent white blood cell counts should be performed. Severe neutropenia (ANC less than 500/mm^3) or severe thrombocytopenia (platelets less than 25,000/mm^3) requires a dose interruption until evidence of marrow recovery is observed (ANC $\geq$ 750/mm^3).

Method of Preparation

Each 10 mL clear glass vial contains ganciclovir sodium equivalent to 500 mg of the free base form of CYTOVENE and 46 mg of sodium. The contents of the vial should be prepared for administration in the following manner:

1. Lyophilized CYTOVENE should be reconstituted by injecting 10 mL of Sterile Water for Injection, USP, into the vial.
DO NOT USE BACTERIOSTATIC WATER FOR INJECTION CONTAINING PARABENS. IT IS INCOMPATIBLE WITH CYTOVENE STERILE POWDER AND MAY CAUSE PRECIPITATION.
2. The vial should be shaken to dissolve the drug.
3. Reconstituted solution should be inspected visually for particulate matter and discoloration prior to proceeding with admixture preparation. If particulate matter or discoloration is observed, the vial should be discarded.
4. Reconstituted solution in the vial is stable at room temperature for 12 hours. It should not be refrigerated.

Admixture Preparation and Administration

Based on patient weight, the appropriate calculated dose volume should be removed from the vial (ganciclovir concentration 50 mg/mL) and added to an acceptable (see below) infusion fluid (typically 100 mL) for delivery over the course of one hour. Infusion concentrations greater than 10 mg/mL are not recommended. The following infusion fluids have been determined to be chemically and physically compatible with CYTOVENE: 0.9% Sodium Chloride, 5% Dextrose, Ringer's Injection, and Lactated Ringer's Injection, USP. Note: Because non-bacteriostatic infusion fluid must be used with CYTOVENE, the infusion solution must be used within 24 hours of dilution to reduce the risk of bacterial contamination. The infusion solution should be refrigerated. Freezing is not recommended.

HANDLING AND DISPOSAL

Caution should be exercised in the handling and preparation of CYTOVENE solution. CYTOVENE solutions are alkaline (pH approximately 11). The use of latex gloves and safety glasses is recommended to avoid exposure in case of breakage of the vial or other accidental spillage. If the solution contacts the skin or mucous membranes, wash thoroughly with soap and water; rinse eyes thoroughly with plain water. Since CYTOVENE has the potential to cause cancer, avoid exposure by inhalation or by direct contact of the skin or mucous membranes.

Procedures for proper handling and disposal of CYTOVENE should be considered. Because CYTOVENE is a nucleoside analogue, consideration should be given to handling and disposal according to guidelines issued for cytotoxic drugs. Several guidelines on this subject have been published.[11-16] There is no general agreement that all of the procedures recommended in the guidelines are necessary or appropriate.

HOW SUPPLIED

CYTOVENE® (ganciclovir sodium) Sterile Powder is supplied in 10 mL sterile vials, each containing ganciclovir sodium equivalent to 500 mg of ganciclovir, in cartons of 25 (NDC 0033-2903-48).

Store at room temperature. Avoid excessive heat, above 40°C (104°F).

CAUTION: Federal law prohibits dispensing without prescription.

REFERENCES

1. Smee D.F., Boehme R., Chernow M., et al: Intracellular metabolism and enzymatic phosphorylation of 9-(1,3-dihydroxy-2-propoxymethyl) guanine and acyclovir in herpes simplex virus-infected and uninfected cells. *Biochemical Pharmacol* 1985; 34:1049–1056.

Creatinine clearance for males $= \dfrac{(140 - \text{age [yrs]}) (\text{body wt [kg]})}{(72) (\text{serum creatinine [mg/dL]})} \times 1.73/\text{body surface [sq M]}$

Creatinine clearance for females $= 0.85 \times$ male value

2. Shanley J.D., Morningstar J., Jordan M.C.: Inhibition of murine cytomegalovirus lung infection and interstitial pneumonitis by acyclovir and 9-(1,3-dihydroxy-2-propoxymethyl) guanine. *Antimicrob Agents Chemother* 1985; 28: 172–175.
3. Wilson E. J., Medearis D.N. Jr., Hansen L.A., et al: 9-(1,3-dihydroxy-2-propoxymethyl) guanine prevents death but not immunity in murine cytomegalovirus-infected normal and immunosuppressed BALB/c mice, *Antimicrob Agents Chemother* 1987; 31:1017–1020.
4. Fong C.K.Y., Cohen S.D., McCormick S., Hsiung G.D.: Antiviral Effect of 9-(1,3-dihydroxy-2-propoxymethyl) guanine against cytomegalovirus infection in a guinea pig model. *Antiviral Res* 1987; 7: 11–23.
5. Buhles W.C., Mastre B.J., Tinker A.J., et al: Ganciclovir Treatment of Life- or Sight-Threatening Cytomegalovirus Infection: Experience in 314 immunocompromised Patients. *Rev Inf Dis* 1988; 10:495–506.
6. Erice A., Chou S., Byron K.K., et al: Progressive disease due to ganciclovir-resistant cytomegalovirus in immunocompromised patients. *N Eng J Med* 1989; 320:289–293.
7. Fletcher C., Balfour H.: Evaluation of ganciclovir for cytomegalovirus disease. *DICP, Ann Pharmacother* 1989; 23:5–12.
8. Fletcher C., Sawchuk R., Chinnock B., et al: Human pharmacokinetics of the antiviral drug DHPG. *Clin Pharmacol Ther* 1986; 40:281–286.
9. Jabs D., Enger E., Bartlett J.: Cytomegalovirus retinitis and acquired immunodeficiency syndrome. *Arch Ophthalmol* 1989; 107:75–80.
10. Updated unpublished data on file with Syntex Corp.
11. Recommendations for the Safe Handling of Parenteral Antineoplastic Drugs. NIH Publication No. 83-2621. For sale by the Superintendent of Documents, U.S. Government Printing Office, Washington, D.C. 20402.
12. AMA Council Report. Guidelines for Handling Parenteral Antineoplastics. *JAMA*, March 15, 1985.
13. National Study Commission on Cytotoxic Exposure-Recommendations for Handling Cytotoxic Agents. Available from Louis P. Jeffrey, Sc. D., Director of Pharmacy Services, Rhode Island Hospital, 593 Eddy Street, Providence, Rhode Island 02902.
14. Clinical Oncological Society of Australia: Guidelines and recommendations for safe handling of antineoplastic agents. *Med J Australia* 1:426–428 1983.
15. Jones R.B., et al. Safe handling of chemotherapeutic agents: A report from the Mount Sinai Medical Center, CA—*A Cancer Journal for Clinicians* Sept/Oct, 258–263 1983.
16. American Society of Hospital Pharmacists technical assistance bulletin on handling cytotoxic drugs in hospitals. *Am J Hosp Pharm* 42:131–137, 1985.

U.S. Patent No. 4,355,032; 4,507,305 and others.
© Syntex June 1989

FEMSTAT®   ℞
[fem 'stat]
(butoconazole nitrate)
Vaginal Cream 2%

PRODUCT OVERVIEW

KEY FACTS

FEMSTAT Vaginal Cream contains as its active ingredient butoconazole nitrate 2%, an imidazole derivative that is clinically highly effective against vaginal infections induced by *Candida* species. The primary site of action of imidazoles appears to be the fungal cell membrane, although the exact mechanism of antifungal activity of butoconazole nitrate is unknown. FEMSTAT is unique in being a cream anticandidiasis preparation that is typically effective in 3 days (an additional 3 days of treatment is recommended for pregnant patients). It is packaged with three disposable applicators.

MAJOR USES

FEMSTAT Vaginal Cream is indicated for the local treatment of vulvovaginal mycotic infections caused by *Candida* species. It can be used concomitantly with oral contraceptives and antibiotics, and is effective in both non-pregnant and pregnant women (second and third trimesters). The recommended treatment regimen is 3 days in non-pregnant women and 6 days in pregnant women.

SAFETY INFORMATION

See complete safety information set forth below.

PRESCRIBING INFORMATION

FEMSTAT®   ℞
[fem 'stat]
(butoconazole nitrate)
Vaginal Cream 2%

DESCRIPTION

FEMSTAT Vaginal Cream contains butoconazole nitrate 2%, an imidazole derivative with antifungal activity. Its chemical name is ($\pm$)-1-[4-(p -Chlorophenyl)-2-[(2,6-dichlorophenyl) thio]butyl] imidazole mononitrate.

Butoconazole nitrate is a white to off-white crystalline powder with a molecular weight of 474.79. It is sparingly soluble in methanol; slightly soluble in chloroform, methylene chloride, acetone and ethanol; very slightly soluble in ethyl acetate; and practically insoluble in water. It melts at about 159°C with decomposition.

FEMSTAT Vaginal Cream contains butoconazole nitrate 2% in a water-washable emollient cream of stearyl alcohol, propylene glycol, cetyl alcohol, sorbitan monostearate, glyceryl stearate (and) PEG-100 stearate, mineral oil, polysorbate 60, purified water, with methylparaben and propylparaben as preservatives.

CLINICAL PHARMACOLOGY

Butoconazole nitrate is an imidazole derivative that has fungicidal activity *in vitro* against *Candida, Trichophyton, Microsporum,* and *Epidermophyton.* It is also active *in vitro* against some gram positive bacteria. Clinically, it is highly effective against vaginal infections induced by strains of *Candida albicans, Candida tropicalis,* and other species of this genus.

The primary site of action of imidazoles appears to be the cell membrane. The permeablilty of the cell membrane is altered, resulting in a reduced osmotic resistance and viability of the fungus. The exact mechanism of the antifungal activity of butoconazole nitrate is not known.

Following vaginal administration of butoconazole nitrate, 5.5% of the dose is absorbed on average. After vaginal administration peak plasma levels of the drug and its metabolites are attained at 24 hours and the plasma half-life is approximately 21–24 hours.

INDICATIONS AND USAGE

FEMSTAT Vaginal Cream is indicated for the local treatment of vulvovaginal mycotic infections caused by Candida species. The diagnosis should be confirmed by KOH smears and/or cultures.

FEMSTAT Vaginal Cream can be used in association with oral contraceptive and antibiotic therapy. FEMSTAT is effective in both non-pregnant and pregnant women, but in pregnant women it should be used only during the second and third trimesters.

CONTRAINDICATIONS

FEMSTAT Vaginal Cream 2% is contraindicated in patients with a history of hypersensitivity to any of the components of the cream.

PRECAUTIONS

General

If clinical symptoms persist, microbiological tests should be repeated to rule out other pathogens and to confirm the diagnosis.

If sensitization or irritation is reported during use, the treatment should be discontinued.

Information for the Patient

The patient should be cautioned against premature discontinuation of the medication during menstruation or in response to relief of symptoms.

Carcinogenesis

Long-term studies in animals have not been performed to evaluate the carcinogenic potential of this drug.

Mutagenesis

Butoconazole nitrate was not mutagenic when tested on microbial indicator organisms.

Impairment of Fertility

No impairment of fertility was seen in rabbits or rats administered butoconazole nitrate in oral doses up to 30 mg/kg/day or 100 mg/kg/day respectively.

Pregnancy

Pregnancy Category C.

In pregnant rats administered 6 mg/kg/day (3–7 times the human dose) butoconazole nitrate intravaginally during the period of organogenesis, there was an increase in resorption rate and decrease in litter size, but no teratogenicity. Butoconazole nitrate had no apparent adverse effect when administered orally to pregnant rats throughout organogenesis, at dose levels up to 50 mg/kg/day. Daily oral doses of 100, 300, or 750 mg/kg resulted in fetal malformations (abdominal wall defects, cleft palate), but maternal stress was evident at these higher dose levels. There were no adverse effects on litters of rabbits receiving butoconazole nitrate orally, even at maternally stressful dose levels (e.g., 150

Continued on next page

Syntex—Cont.

mg/kg). There are no adequate and well-controlled studies in pregnant women during the first trimester.

Butoconazole nitrate, like other azole antimycotic agents, causes dystocia in rats when treatment is extended through parturition. However, this effect was not apparent in rabbits treated with as much as 100 mg/kg/day orally.

In clinical studies, over 200 pregnant patients have used butoconazole nitrate cream 2% for 3 or 6 days during the second or third trimester and the drug had no adverse effect on the course of pregnancy. Follow-up reports available on infants born to these women reveal no adverse effects or complications that were attributable to the drug.

Nursing Mothers

It is not known whether this drug is excreted in human milk. Because many drugs are excreted in human milk, caution should be exercised when butoconazole nitrate is administered to a nursing woman.

Pediatric Use

Safety and effectiveness in children have not been established.

ADVERSE REACTIONS

Of the 561 patients treated with butoconazole nitrate cream 2% for 3 or 6 days in controlled clinical trials, 13 (2.3%) reported complaints probably related to therapy. Vulvar/vaginal burning occurred in 2.3%, vulvar itching in 0.9%, and discharge, soreness, swelling, and itching of the fingers each occurred in 0.2%. Nine patients (1.6%) discontinued because of these complaints.

DOSAGE AND ADMINISTRATION

Non-pregnant Patients: The recommended dose is one applicatorful of cream (approximately 5 grams) intravaginally at bedtime for three days. Treatment can be extended for an additional three days if necessary.

Pregnant Patients (2nd and 3rd trimesters only): The recommended dose is one applicatorful of cream (approximately 5 grams) intravaginally at bedtime for six days.

HOW SUPPLIED

FEMSTAT® (butoconazole nitrate) Vaginal Cream 2% is available in a 28-gram tube with 3 disposable measured-dose applicators (NDC 0033-2280-14).

Store at room temperature. Avoid excessive heat, above 40°C (104°F), and avoid freezing.

Caution: Federal law prohibits dispensing without prescription.

U.S. Patent No. 4,078,071   © MAY 1988
Shown in Product Identification Section, page 433

FEMSTAT® PREFILL   ℞
(butoconazole nitrate)
Vaginal Cream 2%
Prefilled Applicator

DESCRIPTION

FEMSTAT Vaginal Cream contains butoconazole nitrate 2%, an imidazole derivative with antifungal activity. Its chemical name is (±)-1-[4-(p-Chlorophenyl)-2-[(2,6-dichlorophenyl) thio]butyl] imidazole mononitrate.

Butoconazole nitrate is a white to off-white crystalline powder with a molecular weight of 474.79. It is sparingly soluble in methanol; slightly soluble in chloroform, methylene chloride, acetone and ethanol; very slightly soluble in ethyl acetate; and practically insoluble in water. It melts at about 159°C with decomposition.

FEMSTAT Vaginal Cream contains butoconazole nitrate 2% in a water-washable emollient cream of stearyl alcohol, propylene glycol, cetyl alcohol, sorbitan monostearate, glyceryl stearate (and) PEG-100 stearate, mineral oil, polysorbate 60, purified water, with methylparaben and propylparaben as preservatives.

CLINICAL PHARMACOLOGY

Butoconazole nitrate is an imidazole derivative that has fungicidal activity *in vitro* against *Candida, Trichophyton, Microsporum,* and *Epidermophyton.* It is also active against some gram positive bacteria. Clinically, it is highly effective against vaginal infections induced by strains of *Candida albicans, Candida tropicalis,* and other species of this genus. The primary site of action of imidazoles appears to be the cell membrane. The permeability of the cell membrane is altered, resulting in a reduced osmotic resistance and viability of the fungus. The exact mechanism of antifungal activity of butoconazole nitrate is not known.

Following vaginal administration of butoconazole nitrate, 5.5% of the dose is absorbed on average. After vaginal administration peak plasma levels of the drug and its metabolites are attained at 24 hours and the plasma half-life is approximately 21–24 hours.

INDICATIONS AND USAGE

FEMSTAT Vaginal Cream is indicated for the local treatment of vulvovaginal mycotic infections caused by *Candida*

species. The diagnosis should be confirmed by KOH smears and/or cultures.

FEMSTAT Vaginal Cream can be used in association with oral contraceptive and antibiotic therapy. FEMSTAT is effective in both non-pregnant and pregnant women, but in pregnant women it should be used only during the second and third trimesters.

CONTRAINDICATIONS

FEMSTAT Vaginal Cream 2% is contraindicated in patients with a history of hypersensitivity to any of the components of the cream.

PRECAUTIONS

General:
If clinical symptoms persist, microbiological tests should be repeated to rule out other pathogens and to confirm the diagnosis.

If sensitization or irritation is reported during use, the treatment should be discontinued.

Information for the Patient:
The patient should be cautioned against premature discontinuation of the medication during menstruation or in response to relief of symptoms.

Carcinogenesis:
Long-term studies in animals have not been performed to evaluate the carcinogenic potential of this drug.

Mutagenesis:
Butoconazole nitrate was not mutagenic when tested on microbial indicator organisms.

Impairment of Fertility:
No impairment of fertility was seen in rabbits or rats administered butoconazole nitrate in oral doses up to 30 mg/kg/day or 100 mg/kg/day respectively.

Pregnancy:
Pregnancy Category C. In pregnant rats administered 6 mg/kg/day (3–7 times the human dose) butoconazole nitrate intravaginally during the period of organogenesis, there was an increase in resorption rate and decrease in litter size, but no teratogenicity. Butoconazole nitrate had no apparent adverse effect when administered orally to pregnant rats throughout organogenesis, at dose levels up to 50 mg/kg/day. Daily oral doses of 100, 300, or 750 mg/kg resulted in fetal malformations (abdominal wall defects, cleft palate), but maternal stress was evident at these higher dose levels. There were no adverse effects on litters of rabbits receiving butoconazole nitrate orally, even at maternally stressful dose levels (e.g., 150 mg/kg). There are no adequate and well-controlled studies in pregnant women during the first trimester.

Butoconazole nitrate, like other azole antimycotic agents, causes dystocia in rats when treatment is extended through parturition. However, this effect was not apparent in rabbits treated with as much as 100 mg/kg/day orally.

In clinical studies, over 200 pregnant patients have used butoconazole nitrate cream 2% for 3 or 6 days during the second or third trimester and the drug had no adverse effect on the course of pregnancy. Follow-up reports available on infants born to these women reveal no adverse effects or complications that were attributable to the drug.

Nursing Mothers:
It is not known whether this drug is excreted in human milk. Because many drugs are excreted in human milk, caution should be exercised when butoconazole nitrate is administered to a nursing woman.

Pediatric Use:
Safety and effectiveness in children have not been established.

ADVERSE REACTIONS

Of the 561 patients treated with butoconazole nitrate cream 2% for 3 or 6 days in controlled clinical trials, 13 (2.3%) reported complaints probably related to therapy. Vulvar/vaginal burning occurred in 2.3%, vulvar itching in 0.9%, and discharge, soreness, swelling, and itching of the fingers each occurred in 0.2%. Nine patients (1.6%) discontinued because of these complaints.

DOSAGE AND ADMINISTRATION

Non-pregnant Patients: The recommended dose is one applicatorful of cream (approximately 5 grams) intravaginally at bedtime for three days. Treatment can be extended for an additional three days if necessary.

Pregnant Patients (2nd and 3rd trimesters only): The recommended dose is one applicatorful of cream (approximately 5 grams) intravaginally at bedtime for six days.

HOW SUPPLIED

FEMSTAT® PREFILL (butoconazole nitrate) Vaginal Cream 2% is available in cartons containing 3 single dose prefilled disposable applicators (NDC 0033-2280-16).

Store at room temperature. Avoid excessive heat, above 40°C (104°F), and avoid freezing.

CAUTION: Federal law prohibits dispensing without prescription.

U.S. Patent Nos. 4,078,071 and 4,636,202   © March 1988
Shown in Product Identification Section, page 433

LIDEX®   ℞
[li'dex]
(fluocinonide)
Cream 0.05%
Gel 0.05%
Ointment 0.05%
Topical Solution 0.05%

LIDEX®–E   ℞
(fluocinonide)
Cream 0.05%

CARMOL® HC   ℞
[kahr'mawl]
(hydrocortisone acetate)
Cream 1%

NEO-SYNALAR® Cream   ℞
[ne"o sin'ă-lahr]
[neomycin sulfate 0.5% (0.35% neomycin base),
fluocinolone acetonide 0.025%]

SYNACORT®   ℞
[sin'ă-cort]
(hydrocortisone)
Cream 1%
Cream 2.5%

SYNALAR®   ℞
[sin'ă-lahr]
(fluocinolone acetonide)
Cream 0.025%
Cream 0.01%
Ointment 0.025%
Topical Solution 0.01%

SYNALAR–HP®   ℞
(fluocinolone acetonide)
Cream 0.2%

SYNEMOL®   ℞
[sin'ĕ-mol]
(fluocinolone acetonide)
Cream 0.025%

Products of Syntex Laboratories, Inc.

DESCRIPTION

These preparations are all intended for topical administration.

LIDEX preparations have as their active component the corticosteroid fluocinonide, which is the 21-acetate ester of fluocinolone acetonide and has the chemical name pregna-1,4-diene-3,20-dione, 21-(acetyloxy)-6, 9-difluoro-11-hydroxy - 16,17- ((1-methylethylidene)bis(oxy))-, (6α,11β, 16α).

LIDEX cream contains fluocinonide 0.5 mg/g in FAPG® cream, a specially formulated cream base consisting of stearyl alcohol, polyethylene glycol 8000, propylene glycol, 1,2,6-hexanetriol and citric acid. This white cream vehicle is greaseless, non-staining, anhydrous and completely water miscible. The base provides emollient and hydrophilic properties. In this formulation the active ingredient is totally in solution.

LIDEX gel contains fluocinonide 0.5 mg/g in a specially formulated gel base consisting of propylene glycol, propyl gallate, edetate disodium, and carbomer 940, with NaOH and /or HCl added to adjust the pH. This clear, colorless thixotropic vehicle is greaseless, non-staining and completely water miscible. In this formulation the active ingredient is totally in solution.

LIDEX ointment contains fluocinonide 0.5 mg/g in a specially formulated ointment base consisting of Amerchol CAB (mixture of sterols and higher alcohols), white petrolatum, propylene carbonate and propylene glycol. It provides the occlusive and emollient effects desirable in an ointment. In this formulation the active ingredient is totally in solution.

LIDEX topical solution contains fluocinonide 0.5 mg/ml in a solution of alcohol (35%), diisopropyl adipate, citric acid and propylene glycol. In this formulation the active ingredient is totally in solution.

LIDEX-E cream contains fluocinonide 0.5 mg/g in a water-washable aqueous emollient base of stearyl alcohol, cetyl alcohol, mineral oil, propylene glycol, sorbitan monostearate, polysorbate 60, citric acid and purified water.

CARMOL HC Cream has the corticosteroid hydrocortisone acetate, which has the chemical name pregn-4-ene-3,20-dione,21-(acetyloxy)-11,17-dihydroxy-,(11β)-, as its active component. CARMOL HC contains micronized hydrocortisone acetate, USP, 10 mg/g, in a water-washable vanishing cream containing urea (10%), purified water, stearic acid, isopropyl myristate, PPG-26 oleate, isopropyl palmitate, propylene glycol, trolamine, cetyl alcohol, carbomer 940, sodium bisulfite, sodium laureth sulfate, edetate disodium, xanthan gum; scented with hypoallergenic perfume.

CARMOL HC is non-lipid, non-occlusive and hypoallergenic; it contains no mineral oil, petrolatum, lanolin or parabens.

NEO-SYNALAR cream contains neomycin sulfate 5 mg/g (3.5 mg/g neomycin base) and fluocinolone acetonide 0.25 mg/g in a water-washable aqueous base of stearyl alcohol, propylene glycol, cetyl alcohol, polyoxyl 20 cetostearyl ether, mineral oil, white wax, simethicone, butylated hydroxytoluene, edetate disodium, citric acid, and purified water, with methylparaben and propylparaben as preservatives.

SYNACORT creams have as their active component the corticosteroid hydrocortisone, which has the chemical name pregn-4-ene-3,20-dione, 11,17,21-trihydroxy-,(11β)-.

SYNACORT creams contain hydrocortisone, USP, 10 mg/g or 25 mg/g in a cream containing propylene glycol, stearyl alcohol, mineral oil, cetyl alcohol, sorbitan monostearate, polysorbate 60, citric acid and purified water.

SYNALAR preparations, SYNALAR-HP cream, and SYNEMOL cream have as their active component the corticosteroid fluocinolone acetonide, which has the chemical name pregna-1,4-diene-3,20-dione,6,9-difluoro-11,21-dihydroxy-16,17-[(1-methylethylidene)bis(oxy)]-,(6α,11β, 16α)-.

SYNALAR creams contains fluocinolone acetonide 0.25 mg/g or 0.1 mg/g in a water-washable aqueous base of stearyl alcohol, propylene glycol, cetyl alcohol, polyoxyl 20 cetostearyl ether, mineral oil, white wax, simethicone, butylated hydroxytoluene, edetate disodium, citric acid, and purified water, with methylparaben and propylparaben as preservatives.

SYNALAR ointment contains fluocinolone acetonide 0.25 mg/g in a white petrolatum USP vehicle.

SYNALAR solution contains fluocinolone acetonide 0.1 mg/ml in a water-washable base of propylene glycol with citric acid.

SYNALAR-HP cream contains fluocinolone acetonide 2 mg/g in a water-washable aqueous base of stearyl alcohol, cetyl alcohol, mineral oil, propylene glycol, sorbitan monostearate, polysorbate 60, purified water and citric acid with methylparaben and propylparaben as preservatives.

SYNEMOL cream contains fluocinolone acetonide 0.25 mg/g in a water-washable aqueous emollient base of stearyl alcohol, cetyl alcohol, mineral oil, propylene glycol, sorbitan monostearate, polysorbate 60, purified water and citric acid.

CLINICAL PHARMACOLOGY

Topical corticosteroids share anti-inflammatory, anti-pruritic and vasoconstrictive actions.

The mechanism of anti-inflammatory activity of the topical corticosteroids is unclear. Various laboratory methods, including vasoconstrictor assays, are used to compare and predict potencies and/or clinical efficacies of the topical corticosteroids. There is some evidence to suggest that a recognizable correlation exists between vasoconstrictor potency and therapeutic efficacy in man.

PHARMACOKINETICS

The extent of percutaneous absorption of topical corticosteroids is determined by many factors including the vehicle, the integrity of the epidermal barrier, and the use of occlusive dressings. A significantly greater amount of fluocinonide is absorbed from the solution than from the cream or gel formulations.

Topical corticosteroids can be absorbed from normal intact skin. Inflammation and/or other disease processes in the skin increase percutaneous absorption. Occlusive dressings substantially increase the percutaneous absorption of topical corticosteroids. Thus, occlusive dressings may be a valuable therapeutic adjunct for treatment of resistant dermatoses. (See DOSAGE AND ADMINISTRATION).

Once absorbed through the skin, topical corticosteroids are handled through pharmacokinetic pathways similar to systemically administered corticosteroids. Corticosteroids are bound to plasma proteins in varying degrees. Corticosteroids are metabolized primarily in the liver and are then excreted by the kidneys. Some of the topical corticosteroids and their metabolites are also excreted into the bile.

INDICATIONS AND USAGE

Relief of the inflammatory and pruritic manifestations of corticosteroid-responsive dermatoses.

NEO-SYNALAR is indicated for the treatment of corticosteroid-responsive dermatoses with secondary infection. It has not been demonstrated that this steroid-antibiotic combination provides greater benefit then the steroid component alone after 7 days of treatment (see WARNINGS).

CONTRAINDICATIONS

Topical corticosteroids are contraindicated in those patients with a history of hypersensitivity to any of the components of the preparation. NEO-SYNALAR should not be used in the external auditory canal if the eardrum is perforated.

Warnings for NEO-SYNALAR: If local infection should continue or become severe, or in the presence of systemic infection, appropriate systemic antibacterial therapy, based on susceptibility testing, should be considered.

Because of the concern of nephrotoxicity and ototoxicity associated with neomycin, this combination should not be used over a wide area or for extended periods of time.

There are articles in the current medical literature that indicate an increase in the prevalence of persons sensitive to neomycin.

Warnings for CARMOL HC: Contains sodium bisulfite, a sulfite that may cause allergic-type reactions including anaphylactic symptoms and life-threatening or less severe asthmatic episodes in certain susceptible people. The overall prevalence of sulfite sensitivity in the general population is unknown and probably low. Sulfite sensitivity is seen more frequently in asthmatic than in nonasthmatic people.

PRECAUTIONS

General: It is recommended that NEO-SYNALAR cream not be used under occlusive dressing.

Systemic absorption of topical corticosteroids has produced reversible hypothalamic-pituitary-adrenal (HPA) axis suppression, manifestations of Cushing's syndrome, hyperglycemia, and glucosuria in some patients.

Conditions which augment systemic absorption include the application of the more potent steroids, use over large surface areas, prolonged use, the addition of occlusive dressings, and dosage form.

Therefore, patients receiving a large dose of a potent topical steroid applied to a large surface area or under an occlusive dressing should be evaluated periodically for evidence of HPA axis suppression by using the urinary free cortisol and ACTH stimulation tests. If HPA axis suppression is noted, an attempt should be made to withdraw the drug, to reduce the frequency of application, or to substitute a less potent steroid.

Recovery of HPA axis function is generally prompt and complete upon discontinuation of the drug. Infrequently, signs and symptoms of steroid withdrawal may occur, requiring supplemental systemic corticosteroids.

Children may absorb proportionally larger amounts of topical corticosteroids and thus be more susceptible to systemic toxicity. (See PRECAUTIONS—Pediatric Use).

Not for ophthalmic use. Severe irritation is possible if fluocinonide solution contacts the eye. If that should occur, immediate flushing of the eye with a large volume of water is recommended.

If irritation develops, topical corticosteroids should be discontinued and appropriate therapy instituted.

In the presence of dermatological infections, the use of an appropriate antifungal or antibacterial agent should be instituted. If a favorable response does not occur promptly, the corticosteroid should be discontinued until the infection has been adequately controlled.

As with all antibiotics, prolonged use of NEO-SYNALAR may result in over-growth of nonsusceptible organisms. If superinfection occurs, appropriate measures should be taken.

SYNALAR-HP cream should not be used for prolonged periods and the quantity per day should not exceed 2 g. of formulated material.

Information for the Patient: Patients using topical corticosteroids should receive the following information and instructions:

1. This medication is to be used as directed by the physician. It is for external use only. Avoid contact with the eyes. If there is contact with the eyes and severe irritation occurs, immediately flush with a large volume of water.

2. Patients should be advised not to use this medication for any disorder other than for which it was prescribed.

3. The treated skin area should not be bandaged or otherwise covered or wrapped as to be occlusive unless directed by the physician.

4. Patients should report any signs of local adverse reactions especially under occlusive dressing.

5. Parents of pediatric patients should be advised not to use tight-fitting diapers or plastic pants on a child being treated in the diaper area, as these garments may constitute occlusive dressings.

Laboratory Tests: The following tests may be helpful in evaluating HPA axis suppression: Urinary free cortisol test and ACTH stimulation test.

Carcinogenesis, Mutagenesis, and Impairment of Fertility: Long-term animal studies have not been performed to evaluate the carcinogenic potential or the effect on fertility of topical corticosteroids.

Studies to determine mutagenicity with prednisolone and hydrocortisone have revealed negative results.

Pregnancy Category C: Corticosteroids are generally teratogenic in laboratory animals when administered systemically at relatively low dosage levels. The more potent corticosteroids have been shown to be teratogenic after dermal application in laboratory animals. There are no adequate and well-controlled studies in pregnant women on teratogenic effects from topically applied corticosteroids. Therefore, topical corticosteroids should be used during pregnancy only if the potential benefit justifies the potential risk to the fetus. Drugs of this class should not be used extensively on pregnant patients, in large amounts, or for prolonged periods of time.

Nursing Mothers: It is not known whether topical administration of corticosteroids could result in sufficient systemic absorption to produce detectable quantities in breast milk. Systemically administered corticosteroids are secreted into breast milk in quantities *not* likely to have a deleterious effect on the infant. Nevertheless, caution should be exercised when topical corticosteroids are administered to a nursing woman.

Pediatric Use: SYNALAR-HP® (fluocinolone acetonide) cream 0.2% should not be used on infants up to 2 years of age.

Pediatric patients may demonstrate greater susceptibility to topical corticosteroid-induced HPA axis suppression and Cushing's syndrome than mature patients because of a larger skin surface area to body weight ratio.

Hypothalamic-pituitary-adrenal (HPA) axis suppression, Cushing's syndrome, and intracranial hypertension have been reported in children receiving topical corticosteroids. Manifestations of adrenal suppression in children include linear growth retardation, delayed weight gain, low plasma cortisol levels, and absence of response to ACTH stimulation. Manifestations of intracranial hypertension include bulging fontanelles, headaches, and bilateral papilledema.

Administration of topical corticosteroids to children should be limited to the least amount compatible with an effective therapeutic regimen. Chronic corticosteroid therapy may interfere with the growth and development of children.

ADVERSE REACTIONS

The following local adverse reactions are reported infrequently with topical corticosteroids, but may occur more frequently with the use of occlusive dressings. These reactions are listed in an approximate decreasing order of occurrence: burning, itching, irritation, dryness, folliculitis, hypertrichosis, acneiform eruptions, hypopigmentation, perioral dermatitis, allergic contact dermatitis, maceration of the skin, secondary infection, skin atrophy, striae, miliaria. The following reactions have been reported with the topical use of neomycin: ototoxicity and nephrotoxicity.

OVERDOSAGE

Topically applied corticosteroids can be absorbed in sufficient amounts to produce systemic effects (See PRECAUTIONS).

DOSAGE AND ADMINISTRATION

Topical corticosteroids are generally applied to the affected area as a thin film from two to four times daily depending on the severity of the condition. In hairy sites, the hair should be parted to allow direct contact with the lesion.

Occlusive dressings may be used for the management of psoriasis or recalcitrant conditions. Some plastic films may be flammable and due care should be exercised in their use. Similarly, caution should be employed when such films are used on children or left in their proximity, to avoid the possibility of accidental suffocation.

If an infection develops, the use of occlusive dressings should be discontinued and appropriate antimicrobial therapy instituted.

HOW SUPPLIED

LIDEX® (fluocinonide) cream 0.05%—15 g Tube (NDC 0033-2511-13), 30 g Tube (NDC 0033-2511-14), 60 g Tube (NDC 0033-2511-17), and 120 g Tube (NDC 0033-2511-22). Store at room temperature. Avoid excessive heat, above 40℃ (104°F).

LIDEX® (fluocinonide) gel 0.05%—15 g Tube (NDC 0033-2507-13), 30 g Tube (NDC 0033-2507-14), 60 g Tube (NDC 0033-2507-17), and 120 g Tube (NDC 0033-2507-22). Store at controlled room temperature, 15–30℃ (59–86°F).

LIDEX® (fluocinonide) ointment 0.05%—15 g Tube (NDC 0033-2514-13), 30 g Tube (NDC 0033-2514-14), 60 g Tube (NDC 0033-2514-17), and 120 g Tube (NDC 0033-2514-22). Store at room temperature. Avoid excessive heat, above 40℃ (104°F).

LIDEX® (fluocinonide) topical solution 0.05%—Plastic squeeze bottles: 20 cc (NDC 0033-2517-44) and 60 cc (NDC 0033-2517-46). Store at room temperature. Avoid excessive heat, above 40℃ (104°F).

LIDEX-E® (fluocinonide) cream 0.05%—15 g Tube (NDC 0033-2513-13), 30 g Tube (NDC 0033-2513-14), 60 g Tube (NDC 0033-2513-17), and 120 g Tube (NDC 0033-2513-22). Store at room temperature. Avoid excessive heat, above 40℃ (104°F).

CARMOL® HC (hydrocortisone acetate) cream 1%—1 oz. Tube (NDC 0033-2550-15) and 4 oz. Jar (NDC 0033-2550-11). Avoid excessive heat, above 40℃ (104°F).

NEO-SYNALAR cream—15 g Tube (NDC 0033-2505-13), 30 g Tube (NDC 0033-2505-14), 60 g Tube (NDC 0033-2505-17). Store at room temperature. Avoid freezing and excessive heat, above 40℃ (104°F).

SYNACORT® (hydrocortisone) cream 1%—15 g Tube (NDC 0033-2519-13), 30 g Tube (NDC 0033-2519-14), and 60 g Tube (NDC 0033-2519-17). SYNACORT® (hydrocortisone) cream 2.5%—30 g Tube (NDC 0033-2520-14). Store at room temperature. Avoid excessive heat, above 40℃ (104°F).

Continued on next page

Syntex—Cont.

SYNALAR® (fluocinolone acetonide) cream 0.025%—15 g Tube (NDC 0033-2501-13), 30 g Tube (NDC 0033-2501-14), 60 g Tube—(NDC 0033-2501-17), and 425 g Jar (NDC 0033-2501-23). Store tubes at room temperature. Avoid freezing and excessive heat, above 40°C (104°F). Store jars at controlled room temperature, 15°-30°C (59°-86°F).

SYNALAR® (fluocinolone acetonide) cream 0.01%—15 g Tube (NDC 0033-2502-13), 30 g Tube (NDC 0033-2502-14), 60 g Tube (NDC 0033-2502-17), and 425 g Jar (NDC 0033-2502-23). Store tubes at room temperature. Avoid freezing and excessive heat, above 40°C (104°F). Store jars at controlled room temperature, 15°-30°C (59°-86°F).

SYNALAR® (fluocinolone acetonide) ointment 0.025%—15 g Tube (NDC 0033-2504-13), 30 g Tube (NDC 0033-2504-14), 60 g Tube (NDC 0033-2504-17), 120 g Tube (NDC 0033-2504-22), and 425 g Jar (NDC 0033-2504-23). Store at room temperature. Avoid excessive heat, above 40°C (104°F).

SYNALAR® (fluocinolone acetonide) topical solution 0.01%—Plastic squeeze bottles: 20 cc (NDC 0033-2506-44) and 60 cc (NDC 0033-2506-46). Store at room temperature. Avoid freezing.

SYNALAR-HP® (fluocinolone acetonide) cream 0.2%—12 g Tube (NDC 0033-2503-12). Store at room temperature. Avoid excessive heat, above 40°C (104°F).

SYNEMOL® (fluocinolone acetonide) cream 0.025%—15 g Tube (NDC 0033-2509-13), 30 g Tube (NDC 0033-2509-14), 60 g Tube (NDC 0033-2509-17). Store at room temperature. Avoid excessive heat, above 40°C (104°F).

CAUTION: Federal law prohibits dispensing without a prescription.

LIDEX ointment: U.S. Patent No. 4,017,615

LIDEX cream: U.S. Patent Nos. 3,592,930 and 3,888,995

Revised 1/87

© 1985 Syntex Laboratories, Inc.

NAPROSYN®   ℞

[nă'pro-sin]
(naproxen)
Tablets and Suspension

PRODUCT OVERVIEW

KEY FACTS

NAPROSYN (naproxen) is an orally administered nonsteroidal anti-inflammatory drug (arylacetic acid group) with analgesic and antipyretic properties. The naproxen anion inhibits prostaglandin synthesis but beyond this its mode of action is unknown.

MAJOR USES

NAPROSYN has proved to be clinically effective for rheumatoid arthritis, osteoarthritis, juvenile arthritis, ankylosing spondylitis, tendinitis and bursitis, and acute gout. It is also indicated in the relief of mild to moderate pain and the treatment of primary dysmenorrhea.

SAFETY INFORMATION

See complete safety information set forth below.

PRESCRIBING INFORMATION

NAPROSYN®   ℞

[nă'pro-sin]
(naproxen)
Tablets and Suspension
A product of Syntex Puerto Rico, Inc.

DESCRIPTION

NAPROSYN® (naproxen) tablets for oral administration each contain 250 mg, 375 mg or 500 mg of naproxen. NAPROSYN suspension for oral administration contains 125 mg/5 mL of naproxen. NAPROSYN is a member of the arylacetic acid group of nonsteroidal anti-inflammatory drugs.

The chemical name for naproxen is 2-naphthaleneacetic acid, 6-methoxy-α-methyl-,(+).

Naproxen is an odorless, white to off-white crystalline substance. It is lipid soluble, practically insoluble in water at low pH and freely soluble in water at high pH.

Each NAPROSYN tablet contains naproxen, the active ingredient, with D&C Yellow #10 (the 375 mg tablet does not contain this color additive), FD&C Yellow #6, lactose, magnesium stearate, povidone and starch.

NAPROSYN suspension for oral administration contains 125 mg/5 mL of naproxen, the active ingredient, in a vehicle of FD&C Yellow #6, fumaric acid, imitation orange flavor, imitation pineapple flavor, magnesium aluminum silicate, methyl paraben, purified water, sodium chloride, sorbitol solution and sucrose.

CLINICAL PHARMACOLOGY

NAPROSYN (naproxen) is a nonsteroidal anti-inflammatory drug with analgesic and antipyretic properties. Naproxen sodium, the sodium salt of naproxen, has been developed as an analgesic because it is more rapidly absorbed. The naproxen anion inhibits prostaglandin synthesis but beyond this its mode of action is unknown.

Naproxen is rapidly and completely absorbed from the gastrointestinal tract. After administration of naproxen, peak plasma levels of naproxen anion are attained in 2 to 4 hours, with steady-state conditions normally achieved after 4–5 doses. The mean biological half-life of the anion in humans is approximately 13 hours, and at therapeutic levels it is greater than 99% albumin bound. At doses of naproxen greater than 500 mg/day there is a lack of dose proportionality due to an increase in clearance caused by saturation of plasma proteins at higher doses. Approximately 95% of the dose is excreted in the urine, primarily as naproxen, 6-0-desmethyl naproxen or their conjugates. The rate of excretion has been found to coincide closely with the rate of drug disappearance from the plasma. The drug does not induce metabolizing enzymes.

In children of 5 to 16 years of age with arthritis, plasma naproxen levels following a 5 mg/kg single dose of suspension were found to be similar to those found in normal adults following a 500 mg dose. The terminal half-life appears to be similar in children and adults. Pharmacokinetic studies of naproxen were not performed in children of less than 5 years of age.

The drug was studied in patients with rheumatoid arthritis, osteoarthritis, juvenile arthritis, ankylosing spondylitis, tendinitis and bursitis, and acute gout. It is not a corticosteroid. Improvement in patients treated for rheumatoid arthritis has been demonstrated by a reduction in joint swelling, a reduction in pain, a reduction in duration of morning stiffness, a reduction in disease activity as assessed by both the investigator and patient, and by increased mobility as demonstrated by a reduction in walking time.

In patients with osteoarthritis, the therapeutic action of the drug has been shown by a reduction in joint pain or tenderness, an increase in range of motion in knee joints, increased mobility as demonstrated by a reduction in walking time, and improvement in capacity to perform activities of daily living impaired by the disease.

In clinical studies in patients with rheumatoid arthritis, osteoarthritis, and juvenile arthritis, the drug has been shown to be comparable to aspirin and indomethacin in controlling the aforementioned measures of disease activity, but the frequency and severity of the milder gastrointestinal adverse effects (nausea, dyspepsia, heartburn) and nervous system adverse effects (tinnitus, dizziness, lightheadedness) were less than in both the aspirin- and indomethacin-treated patients. It is not known whether the drug causes less peptic ulceration than aspirin.

In patients with ankylosing spondylitis, the drug has been shown to decrease night pain, morning stiffness and pain at rest. In double-blind studies the drug was shown to be as effective as aspirin, but with fewer side effects.

In patients with acute gout, a favorable response to the drug was shown by significant clearing of inflammatory changes (e.g., decrease in swelling, heat) within 24–48 hours, as well as by relief of pain and tenderness.

The drug may be used safely in combination with gold salts and/or corticosteroids; however, in controlled clinical trials, when added to the regimen of patients receiving corticosteroids it did not appear to cause greater improvement over that seen with corticosteroids alone. Whether the drug could be used in conjunction with partially effective doses of corticosteroid for a "steroid-sparing" effect has not been adequately studied. When added to the regimen of patients receiving gold salts the drug did result in greater improvement. Its use in combination with salicylates is not recommended because data are inadequate to demonstrate that the drug produces greater improvement over that achieved with aspirin alone. Further, there is some evidence that aspirin increases the rate of excretion of the drug.

Generally, improvement due to the drug has not been found to be dependent on age, sex, severity or duration of disease. In clinical trials in patients with osteoarthritis and rheumatoid arthritis comparing treatments of 750 mg per day with 1,500 mg per day, there were trends toward increased efficacy with the higher dose and a more clearcut increase in adverse reactions, particularly gastrointestinal reactions severe enough to cause the patient to leave the trial, which approximately doubled.

The drug was studied in patients with mild to moderate pain, and pain relief was obtained within 1 hour. It is not a narcotic and is not a CNS-acting drug. Controlled double-blind studies have demonstrated the analgesic properties of the drug in, for example, post-operative, post-partum, orthopedic and uterine contraction pain and dysmenorrhea. In dysmenorrheic patients, the drug reduces the level of prostaglandins in the uterus, which correlates with a reduction in the frequency and severity of uterine contractions. Analgesic action has been shown by such measures as a reduction of pain intensity scores, increase in pain relief scores, decrease in numbers of patients requiring additional analgesic medication, and delay in time for required remedication. The analgesic effect has been found to last for up to 7 hours.

In ^{51}Cr blood loss and gastroscopy studies with normal volunteers, daily administration of 1000 mg of the drug has been demonstrated to cause statistically significantly less gastric bleeding and erosion than 3250 mg of aspirin.

INDICATIONS AND USAGE

NAPROSYN (naproxen) is indicated for the treatment of rheumatoid arthritis, osteoarthritis, juvenile arthritis, ankylosing spondylitis, tendinitis and acute gout. It is also indicated in the relief of mild to moderate pain and for the treatment of primary dysmenorrhea.

CONTRAINDICATIONS

The drug is contraindicated in patients who have had allergic reactions to NAPROSYN® (naproxen) or to ANAPROX® (naproxen sodium). It is also contraindicated in patients in whom aspirin or other nonsteroidal anti-inflammatory/analgesic drugs induce the syndrome of asthma, rhinitis, and nasal polyps. Both types of reactions have the potential of being fatal. Anaphylactoid reactions to NAPROSYN or ANAPROX, whether of the true allergic type or the pharmacologic idiosyncratic (e.g., aspirin syndrome) type, usually but not always occur in patients with a known history of such reactions. Therefore, careful questioning of patients for such things as asthma, nasal polyps, urticaria, and hypotension associated with nonsteroidal anti-inflammatory drugs before starting therapy is important. In addition, if such symptoms occur during therapy, treatment should be discontinued.

WARNINGS

Risk of GI Ulceration, Bleeding and Perforation with NSAID Therapy:

Serious gastrointestinal toxicity such as bleeding, ulceration, and perforation, can occur at any time, with or without warning symptoms, in patients treated chronically with NSAID therapy. Although minor upper gastrointestinal problems, such as dyspepsia, are common, usually developing early in therapy, physicians should remain alert for ulceration and bleeding in patients treated chronically with NSAIDs even in the absence of previous GI tract symptoms. In patients observed in clinical trials of several months to two years duration, symptomatic upper GI ulcers, gross bleeding or perforation appear to occur in approximately 1% of patients treated for 3–6 months, and in about 2–4% of patients treated for one year. Physicians should inform patients about the signs and/or symptoms of serious GI toxicity and what steps to take if they occur.

Studies to date have not identified any subset of patients not at risk of developing peptic ulceration and bleeding. Except for a prior history of serious GI events and other risk factors known to be associated with peptic ulcer disease, such as alcoholism, smoking, etc., no risk factors (e.g., age, sex) have been associated with increased risk. Elderly or debilitated patients seem to tolerate ulceration or bleeding less well than other individuals and most spontaneous reports of fatal GI events are in this population. Studies to date are inconclusive concerning the relative risk of various NSAIDs in causing such reactions. High doses of any NSAID probably carry a greater risk of these reactions, although controlled clinical trials showing this do not exist in most cases. In considering the use of relatively large doses (within the recommended dosage range), sufficient benefit should be anticipated to offset the potential increased risk of GI toxicity.

PRECAUTIONS

General:

NAPROSYN (NAPROXEN) SHOULD NOT BE USED CONCOMITANTLY WITH THE RELATED DRUG ANAPROX (NAPROXEN SODIUM) SINCE THEY BOTH CIRCULATE IN PLASMA AS THE NAPROXEN ANION.

Renal Effects: As with other nonsteroidal anti-inflammatory drugs, long-term administration of naproxen to animals has resulted in renal papillary necrosis and other abnormal renal pathology. In humans, there have been reports of acute interstitial nephritis with hematuria, proteinuria, and occasionally nephrotic syndrome.

A second form of renal toxicity has been seen in patients with prerenal conditions leading to the reduction in renal blood flow or blood volume, where the renal prostaglandins have a supportive role in the maintenance of renal perfusion. In these patients, administration of a nonsteroidal anti-inflammatory drug may cause a dose-dependent reduction in prostaglandin formation and may precipitate overt renal decompensation. Patients at greatest risk of this reaction are those with impaired renal function, heart failure, liver dysfunction, those taking diuretics, and the elderly. Discontinuation of nonsteroidal anti-inflammatory therapy is typically followed by recovery to the pretreatment state.

NAPROSYN and its metabolites are eliminated primarily by the kidneys, therefore the drug should be used with great caution in patients with significantly impaired renal function and the monitoring of serum creatinine and/or creatinine clearance is advised in these patients. Caution should be used if the drug is given to patients with creatinine clearance of less than 20 mL/minute because accumulation of naproxen metabolites has been seen in such patients. Chronic alcoholic liver disease and probably other forms of cirrhosis reduce the total plasma concentration of naproxen, but the plasma concentration of unbound naproxen is increased. Caution is advised when high doses are required and some adjustment of dosage may be required in these patients. It is prudent to use the lowest effective dose.

One study indicates that although total plasma concentration of naproxen is unchanged, the unbound plasma fraction of naproxen is increased in the elderly. Caution is advised when high doses are required and some adjustment of dosage may be required in elderly patients. As with other drugs used in the elderly, it is prudent to use the lowest effective dose. As with other nonsteroidal anti-inflammatory drugs, borderline elevations of one or more liver tests may occur in up to 15% of patients. These abnormalities may progress, may remain essentially unchanged, or may be transient with continued therapy. The SGPT (ALT) test is probably the most sensitive indicator of liver dysfunction. Meaningful (3 times the upper limit of normal) elevations of SGPT or SGOT (AST) occurred in controlled clinical trials in less than 1% of patients. A patient with symptoms and/or signs suggesting liver dysfunction, or in whom an abnormal liver test has occurred, should be evaluated for evidence of the development of more severe hepatic reaction while on therapy with this drug. Severe hepatic reactions, including jaundice and cases of fatal hepatitis, have been reported with this drug as with other nonsteroidal anti-inflammatory drugs. Although such reactions are rare, if abnormal liver tests persist or worsen, if clinical signs and symptoms consistent with liver disease develop, or if systemic manifestations occur (e.g. eosinophilia, rash, etc.), this drug should be discontinued.

If steroid dosage is reduced or eliminated during therapy, the steroid dosage should be reduced slowly and the patients must be observed closely for any evidence of adverse effects, including adrenal insufficiency and exacerbation of symptoms of arthritis.

Patients with initial hemoglobin values of 10 grams or less who are to receive long-term therapy should have hemoglobin values determined periodically.

Peripheral edema has been observed in some patients. For this reason, the drug should be used with caution in patients with fluid retention, hypertension or heart failure.

Naprosyn suspension contains 8 mg/mL of sodium. This should be considered in patients whose overall intake of sodium must be restricted.

The antipyretic and anti-inflammatory activities of the drug may reduce fever and inflammation, thus diminishing their utility as diagnostic signs in detecting complications of presumed non-infectious, non-inflammatory painful conditions. Because of adverse eye findings in animal studies with drugs of this class, it is recommended that ophthalmic studies be carried out if any change or disturbance in vision occurs.

Information for Patients:
Naproxen, like other drugs of its class, is not free of side effects. The side effects of these drugs can cause discomfort and, rarely, there are more serious side effects, such as gastrointestinal bleeding, which may result in hospitalization and even fatal outcomes.

NSAIDs (Nonsteroidal Anti-Inflammatory Drugs) are often essential agents in the management of arthritis and have a major role in the treatment of pain, but they also may be commonly employed for conditions which are less serious. Physicians may wish to discuss with their patients the potential risks (see Warnings, Precautions, and Adverse Reactions sections) and likely benefits of NSAID treatment, particularly when the drugs are used for less serious conditions where treatment without NSAIDs may represent an acceptable alternative to both the patient and physician.

Caution should be exercised by patients whose activities require alertness if they experience drowsiness, dizziness, vertigo or depression during therapy with the drug.

Laboratory Tests:
Because serious GI tract ulceration and bleeding can occur without warning symptoms, physicians should follow chronically treated patients for the signs and symptoms of ulceration and bleeding and should inform them of the importance of this follow-up (see Risk of GI Ulcerations, Bleeding and Perforation with NSAID Therapy).

Drug Interactions:
In vitro studies have shown that naproxen anion, because of its affinity for protein, may displace from their binding sites other drugs which are also albumin-bound. Theoretically, the naproxen anion itself could likewise be displaced. Short-term controlled studies failed to show that taking the drug significantly affects prothrombin times when administered to individuals on coumarin-type anticoagulants. Caution is advised nonetheless, since interactions have been seen with other nonsteroidal agents of this class. Similarly, patients receiving the drug and a hydantoin, sulfonamide or sulfonylurea should be observed for signs of toxicity to these drugs. The natriuretic effect of furosemide has been reported to be inhibited by some drugs of this class. Inhibition of renal lithium clearance leading to increases in plasma lithium concentrations has also been reported.

This and other nonsteroidal anti-inflammatory drugs can reduce the antihypertensive effect of propranolol and other beta-blockers.

Probenecid given concurrently increases naproxen anion plasma levels and extends its plasma half-life significantly. Caution should be used if this drug is administered concomitantly with methotrexate. Naproxen and other nonsteroidal anti-inflammatory drugs have been reported to reduce the tubular secretion of methotrexate in an animal model, possibly enhancing the toxicity of that drug.

Drug/Laboratory Test Interactions:
The drug may decrease platelet aggregation and prolong bleeding time. This effect should be kept in mind when bleeding times are determined.

The administration of the drug may result in increased urinary values for 17-ketogenic steroids because of an interaction between the drug and/or its metabolites with m-dinitrobenzene used in this assay. Although 17-hydroxy-corticosteroid measurements (Porter-Silber test) do not appear to be artifactually altered, it is suggested that therapy with the drug be temporarily discontinued 72 hours before adrenal function tests are performed.

The drug may interfere with some urinary assays of 5-hydroxy indoleacetic acid (5HIAA).

Carcinogenesis:
A two-year study was performed in rats to evaluate the carcinogenic potential of the drug. No evidence of carcinogenicity was found.

Pregnancy:
Teratogenic Effects: Pregnancy Category B. Reproduction studies have been performed in rats, rabbits and mice at doses up to six times the human dose and have revealed no evidence of impaired fertility or harm to the fetus due to the drug. There are, however, no adequate and well-controlled studies in pregnant women. Because animal reproduction studies are not always predictive of human response, the drug should not be used during pregnancy unless clearly needed. Because of the known effect of drugs of this class on the human fetal cardiovascular system (closure of ductus arteriosus), use during late pregnancy should be avoided.

Non-teratogenic Effects: As with other drugs known to inhibit prostaglandin synthesis, an increased incidence of dystocia and delayed parturition occurred in rats.

Nursing Mothers:
The naproxen anion has been found in the milk of lactating women at a concentration of approximately 1% of that found in the plasma. Because of the possible adverse effects of prostaglandin-inhibiting drugs on neonates, use in nursing mothers should be avoided.

Pediatric Use:
Safety and effectiveness in children below the age of 2 years have not been established. Pediatric dosing recommendations for juvenile arthritis are based on well-controlled studies (see Dosage and Administration). There are no adequate effectiveness or dose-response data for other pediatric conditions, but the experience in juvenile arthritis and other use experience have established that single doses of 2.5–5 mg/kg, with total daily dose not exceeding 15 mg/kg/day, are safe in children over 2 years of age.

ADVERSE REACTIONS

The following adverse reactions are divided into 3 parts based on frequency and likelihood of causal relationship to naproxen.

Incidence greater than 1%

Probable Causal Relationship:
Adverse reactions reported in controlled clinical trials in 960 patients treated for rheumatoid arthritis or osteoarthritis are listed below. In general, these reactions were reported 2 to 10 times more frequently than they were in studies in the 962 patients treated for mild to moderate pain or for dysmenorrhea.

A clinical study found gastrointestinal reactions to be more frequent and more severe in rheumatoid arthritis patients taking 1,500 mg naproxen daily compared to those taking 750 mg daily (see Clinical Pharmacology).

In controlled clinical trials with about 80 children and in well-monitored open studies with about 400 children with juvenile arthritis, the incidences of rash and prolonged bleeding times were increased, the incidences of gastrointestinal and central nervous system reactions were about the same, and the incidences of other reactions were lower in children than in adults.

Gastrointestinal: The most frequent complaints reported related to the gastrointestinal tract. They were: constipation*, heartburn*, abdominal pain*, nausea*, dyspepsia, diarrhea, stomatitis.

Central Nervous System: Headache*, dizziness*, drowsiness*, lightheadedness, vertigo.

Dermatologic: Itching (pruritus)*, skin eruptions*, ecchymoses*, sweating, purpura.

Special Senses: Tinnitus*, hearing disturbances, visual disturbances.

Cardiovascular: Edema*, dyspnea*, palpitations.

General: Thirst.

* Incidence of reported reactions between 3% and 9%. Those reactions occurring in less than 3% of the patients are unmarked.

Incidence less than 1%

Probable Causal Relationship:
The following adverse reactions were reported less frequently than 1% during controlled clinical trials and through voluntary reports since marketing. The probability of a causal relationship exists between the drug and these adverse reactions:

Gastrointestinal: Abnormal liver function tests, gastrointestinal bleeding and/or perforation, hematemesis, jaundice, melena, peptic ulceration with bleeding and/or perforation, vomiting.

Renal: Glomerular nephritis, hematuria, interstitial nephritis, nephrotic syndrome, renal disease.

Hematologic: Agranulocytosis, eosinophilia, granulocytopenia, leukopenia, thrombocytopenia.

Central Nervous System: Depression, dream abnormalities, inability to concentrate, insomnia, malaise, myalgia and muscle weakness.

Dermatologic: Alopecia, photosensitive dermatitis, skin rashes.

Special Senses: Hearing impairment.

Cardiovascular: Congestive heart failure.

Respiratory: Eosinophilic pneumonitis.

General: Anaphylactoid reactions, menstrual disorders, pyrexia (chills and fever).

Causal Relationship Unknown:
Other reactions have been reported in circumstances in which a causal relationship could not be established. However, in these rarely reported events, the possibility cannot be excluded. Therefore, these observations are being listed to serve as alerting information to the physicians:

Hematologic: Aplastic anemia, hemolytic anemia.

Central Nervous System: Cognitive dysfunction.

Dermatologic: Epidermal necrolysis, erythema multiforme, Stevens-Johnson syndrome, urticaria.

Gastrointestinal: Non-peptic gastrointestinal ulceration, ulcerative stomatitis.

Cardiovascular: Vasculitis.

General: Angioneurotic edema, hyperglycemia, hypoglycemia.

OVERDOSAGE

Significant overdosage may be characterized by drowsiness, heartburn, indigestion, nausea or vomiting. No evidence of toxicity or late sequelae have been reported 5 to 15 months after ingestion for three to seven days of doses up to 3,000 mg of naproxen. One patient ingested a single dose of 25 g of naproxen and experienced mild nausea and indigestion. It is not known what dose of the drug would be life threatening. The oral LD$_{50}$ of the drug is 543 mg/kg in rats, 1234 mg/kg in mice, 4110 mg/kg in hamsters and greater than 1000 mg/kg in dogs.

Should a patient ingest a large number of tablets or a large volume of suspension, accidentally or purposefully, the stomach may be emptied and usual supportive measures employed. In animals 0.5 g/kg of activated charcoal was effective in reducing plasma levels of naproxen. Hemodialysis does not decrease the plasma concentration of naproxen because of the high degree of its protein binding.

DOSAGE AND ADMINISTRATION

A measuring cup marked in $\frac{1}{2}$ teaspoon and 2.5 milliliter increments is provided with the suspension. This cup or a teaspoon may be used to measure the appropriate dose.

For Rheumatoid Arthritis, Osteoarthritis, and Ankylosing Spondylitis:
The recommended dose of NAPROSYN® (naproxen) in adults is 250 mg (10 mL or 2 tsp of suspension), 375 mg (15 mL or 3 tsp), or 500 mg (20 mL or 4 tsp) twice daily (morning and evening). During long-term administration, the dose may be adjusted up or down depending on the clinical response of the patient. A lower daily dose may suffice for long-term administration. The morning and evening doses do not have to be equal in size and the administration of the drug more frequently than twice daily is not necessary. In patients who tolerate lower doses well, the dose may be increased to 1,500 mg per day for limited periods when a higher level of anti-inflammatory/analgesic activity is required. When treating such patients with the 1,500 mg/day dose, the physician should observe sufficient increased clinical benefits to offset the potential increased risk (see Clinical Pharmacology).

Symptomatic improvement in arthritis usually begins within 2 weeks. However, if improvement is not seen within this period, a trial for an additional 2 weeks should be considered.

For Juvenile Arthritis:
The recommended total daily dose of NAPROSYN is approximately 10 mg/kg given in 2 divided doses. The scored 250 mg tablet may be used to approximate this dose. The following table may be used as a guide for the suspension:

Child's Weight	Dose
13 kg (29 lb)	2.5 mL ($\frac{1}{2}$ tsp) b.i.d.
25 kg (55 lb)	5 mL (1 tsp) b.i.d.
38 kg (84 lb)	7.5 mL (1$\frac{1}{2}$ tsp) b.i.d.

Continued on next page

Syntex—Cont.

For Acute Gout:
The recommended starting dose of NAPROSYN is 750 mg (30 mL or 6 tsp), followed by 250 mg (10 mL or 2 tsp) every 8 hours until the attack has subsided.

For Mild to Moderate Pain, Primary Dysmenorrhea and Acute Tendinitis and Bursitis:
The recommended starting dose of NAPROSYN is 500 mg (20 mL or 4 tsp), followed by 250 mg (10 mL or 2 tsp) every 6 to 8 hours as required. The total daily dose should not exceed 1,250 mg (50 mL or 10 tsp).

HOW SUPPLIED

NAPROSYN® (naproxen) is available in scored tablets of 250 mg (yellow) in light-resistant bottles of 100 tablets (NDC 18393-272-42) (NSN 6505-01-026-9730) and 500 tablets (NDC 18393-272-62) (NSN 6505-01-046-0126) or in cartons of 100 individually blister packed tablets (NDC 18393-272-53) (NSN 6505-01-097-9611) and in 375 mg (peach) tablets in light-resistant bottles of 100 tablets (NDC 18393-273-42) (NSN 6505-01-135-8462) and 500 tablets (NDC 18393-273-62) (NSN 6505-01-204-5297) or in cartons of 100 individually blister packed tablets (NDC 18393-273-53) (NSN 6505-01-204-5298). The 500 mg (yellow) tablets are available in light-resistant bottles of 100 tablets (NDC 18393-277-42) (NSN 6505-01-200-2474) and 500 tablets (NDC 18393-277-62) (NSN 6505-01-186-8758). Store at room temperature in well-closed containers; dispense in light-resistant containers.

NAPROSYN® suspension is available in 1 pint (474 mL) light-resistant bottles (NDC 18393-278-20). Measuring cups are provided so that one can be dispensed with each prescription. Store at room temperature; avoid excessive heat, above 40°C (104° F). Dispense in light-resistant container.

CAUTION: Federal law prohibits dispensing without prescription.

U.S. Patent Nos. 3,904,682; 3,998,966 and others.

© 1985 Syntex Puerto Rico, Inc.   Revised 10/88

Shown in Product Identification Section, page 433

NASALIDE®   ℞
[na'ză-lide]
(flunisolide)
Nasal Solution
0.025%
For Nasal Use Only

PRODUCT OVERVIEW

KEY FACTS

NASALIDE Nasal Solution, intended for administration as a spray to the nasal mucosa, contains the active ingredient flunisolide, an anti-inflammatory topical steroid. Clinical studies with flunisolide have shown local therapeutic activity on nasal mucous membranes, including reduction of symptoms of stuffy nose, runny nose and sneezing, with minimal evidence of systemic activity at the recommended doses.

MAJOR USES

NASALIDE is indicated for the topical treatment of the symptoms of seasonal or perennial rhinitis when effectiveness of or tolerance to conventional treatment is unsatisfactory. Symptomatic relief is usually seen within a few days after starting NASALIDE, but may not occur in some patients for as long as two weeks.

SAFETY INFORMATION

See complete safety information set forth below.

PRESCRIBING INFORMATION

NASALIDE®   ℞
[na'ză-lide]
(flunisolide)
Nasal Solution
0.025%
For Nasal Use Only

A product of Syntex Laboratories, Inc.

DESCRIPTION

NASALIDE® (flunisolide) nasal solution is intended for administration as a spray to the nasal mucosa. Flunisolide, the active component of NASALIDE nasal solution, is an anti-inflammatory steroid with the chemical name: 6α-fluoro-11β, 16α, 17,21-tetrahydroxypregna-1,4-diene-3,20-dione cyclic 16,17-acetal with acetone (USAN).

Flunisolide is a white to creamy white crystalline powder with a molecular weight of 434.49. It is soluble in acetone, sparingly soluble in chloroform, slightly soluble in methanol, and practically insoluble in water. It has a melting point of about 245°C.

Each 25 ml spray bottle contains flunisolide 6.25 mg (0.25 mg/mL) in a solution of propylene glycol, polyethylene glycol 3350, citric acid, sodium citrate, butylated hydroxyanisole, edetate disodium, benzalkonium chloride, and puri-

fied water, with NaOH and/or HCl added to adjust the pH to approximately 5.3. It contains no fluorocarbons.

After priming the delivery system for NASALIDE, each actuation of the unit delivers a metered droplet spray containing approximately 25 mcg of flunisolide. The size of the droplets produced by the unit is in excess of 8 microns to facilitate deposition on the nasal mucosa. The contents of one nasal spray bottle deliver at least 200 sprays.

CLINICAL PHARMACOLOGY

NASALIDE® (flunisolide) has demonstrated potent glucocorticoid and weak mineralocorticoid activity in classical animal test systems. As a glucocorticoid it is several hundred times more potent than the cortisol standard. Clinical studies with flunisolide have shown therapeutic activity on nasal mucous membranes with minimal evidence of systemic activity at the recommended doses.

A study in approximately 100 patients which compared the recommended dose of flunisolide nasal solution with an oral dose providing equivalent systemic amounts of flunisolide has shown that the clinical effectiveness of NASALIDE, when used topically as recommended, is due to its direct local effect and not to an indirect effect through systemic absorption.

Following administration of flunisolide to man, approximately half of the administered dose is recovered in the urine and half in the stool; 65–70% of the dose recovered in urine is the primary metabolite, which has undergone loss of the 6α fluorine and addition of a 6β hydroxy group. Flunisolide is well absorbed but is rapidly converted by the liver to the much less active primary metabolite and to glucuronate and/or sulfate conjugates. Because of first-pass liver metabolism, only 20% of the flunisolide reaches the systemic circulation when it is given orally whereas 50% of the flunisolide administered intranasally reaches the systemic circulation unmetabolized. The plasma half-life of flunisolide is 1–2 hours.

The effects of flunisolide on hypothalamic-pituitary-adrenal (HPA) axis function have been studied in adult volunteers. NASALIDE was administered intranasally as a spray in total doses over 7 times the recommended dose (2200 mcg, equivalent to 88 sprays/day) in 2 subjects for 4 days, about 3 times the recommended dose (800 mcg, equivalent to 32 sprays/day) in 4 subjects for 4 days, and over twice the recommended dose (700 mcg, equivalent to 28 sprays/day) in 6 subjects for 10 days. Early morning plasma cortisol concentrations and 24-hour urinary 17-ketogenic steroids were measured daily. There was evidence of decreased endogenous cortisol production at all three doses.

In controlled studies, NASALIDE was found to be effective in reducing symptoms of stuffy nose, runny nose and sneezing in most patients. These controlled clinical studies have been conducted in 488 adult patients at doses ranging from 8 to 16 sprays (200–400 mcg) per day and 127 children at doses ranging from 6 to 8 sprays (150–200 mcg) per day for periods as long as 3 months. In 170 patients who had cortisol levels evaluated at baseline and after 3 months or more of flunisolide treatment, there was no unequivocal flunisolide-related depression of plasma cortisol levels.

The mechanisms responsible for the anti-inflammatory action of corticosteroids and for the activity of the aerosolized drug on the nasal mucosa are unknown.

INDICATIONS

NASALIDE® (flunisolide) is indicated for the topical treatment of the symptoms of seasonal or perennial rhinitis when effectiveness of or tolerance to conventional treatment is unsatisfactory.

Clinical studies have shown that improvement is based on a local effect rather than systemic absorption, and is usually apparent within a few days after starting NASALIDE. However, symptomatic relief may not occur in some patients for as long as two weeks. Although systemic effects are minimal at recommended doses, NASALIDE should not be continued beyond 3 weeks in the absence of significant symptomatic improvement.

NASALIDE should not be used in the presence of untreated localized infection involving nasal mucosa.

CONTRAINDICATIONS

Hypersensitivity to any of the ingredients.

WARNINGS

The replacement of a systemic corticosteroid with a topical corticoid can be accompanied by signs of adrenal insufficiency, and in addition some patients may experience symptoms of withdrawal, e.g., joint and/or muscular pain, lassitude and depression. Patients previously treated for prolonged periods with systemic corticosteroids and transferred to NASALIDE® (flunisolide) should be carefully monitored to avoid acute adrenal insufficiency in response to stress.

When transferred to NASALIDE, careful attention must be given to patients previously treated for prolonged periods with systemic corticosteroids. This is particularly important in those patients who have associated asthma or other clinical conditions, where too rapid a decrease in systemic corticosteroids may cause a severe exacerbation of their symptoms.

The use of NASALIDE with alternate-day prednisone systemic treatment could increase the likelihood of HPA suppression compared to a therapeutic dose of either one alone. Therefore, NASALIDE treatment should be used with caution in patients already on alternate-day prednisone regimens for any disease.

PRECAUTIONS

General: In clinical studies with flunisolide administered intranasally, the development of localized infections of the nose and pharynx with *Candida albicans* has occurred only rarely. When such an infection develops it may require treatment with appropriate local therapy or discontinuance of treatment with NASALIDE® (flunisolide).

Flunisolide is absorbed into the circulation. Use of excessive doses of NASALIDE may suppress hypothalamic-pituitary-adrenal function.

Flunisolide should be used with caution, if at all, in patients with active or quiescent tuberculosis infections of the respiratory tract or in untreated fungal, bacterial or systemic viral infections or ocular herpes simplex.

Because of the inhibitory effect of corticosteroids on wound healing, in patients who have experienced recent nasal septal ulcers, recurrent epistaxis, nasal surgery or trauma, a nasal corticosteroid should be used with caution until healing has occurred.

Although systemic effects have been minimal with recommended doses, this potential increases with excessive dosages. Therefore, larger than recommended doses should be avoided.

Information for Patients: Patients should use NASALIDE at regular intervals since its effectiveness depends on its regular use. The patient should take the medication as directed. It is not acutely effective and the prescribed dosage should not be increased. Instead, nasal vasoconstrictors or oral antihistamines may be needed until the effects of NASALIDE are fully manifested. One to two weeks may pass before full relief is obtained. The patient should contact the physician if symptoms do not improve, or if the condition worsens, or if sneezing or nasal irritation occurs.

For the proper use of this unit and to attain maximum improvement, the patient should read and follow the accompanying Patient Instructions carefully.

Carcinogenesis: Long-term studies were conducted in mice and rats using oral administration to evaluate the carcinogenic potential of the drug. There was an increase in the incidence of pulmonary adenomas in mice, but not in rats.

Female rats receiving the highest oral dose had an increased incidence of mammary adenocarcinoma compared to control rats. An increased incidence of this tumor type has been reported for other corticosteroids.

Impairment of fertility: Female rats receiving high doses of flunisolide (200 mcg/kg/day) showed some evidence of impaired fertility. Reproductive performance in the low (8 mcg/kg/day) and mid-dose (40 mcg/kg/day) groups was comparable to controls.

Pregnancy: Teratogenic effects: Pregnancy Category C. As with other corticosteroids, flunisolide has been shown to be teratogenic in rabbits and rats at doses of 40 and 200 mcg/kg/day respectively. It was also fetotoxic in these animal reproductive studies. There are no adequate and well-controlled studies in pregnant women. Flunisolide should be used during pregnancy only if the potential benefit justifies the potential risk to the fetus.

Nursing Mothers: It is not known whether this drug is excreted in human milk. Because other corticosteroids are excreted in human milk, caution should be exercised when flunisolide is administered to nursing women.

ADVERSE REACTIONS

Adverse reactions reported in controlled clinical trials and long-term open studies in 595 patients treated with NASALIDE are described below. Of these patients, 409 were treated for 3 months or longer, 323 for 6 months or longer, 259 for 1 year or longer, and 91 for 2 years or longer.

In general, side effects elicited in the clinical studies have been primarily associated with the nasal mucous membranes. The most frequent complaints were those of mild transient nasal burning and stinging, which were reported in approximately 45% of the patients treated with NASALIDE in placebo-controlled and long-term studies. These complaints do not usually interfere with treatment; in only 3% of patients was it necessary to decrease dosage or stop treatment because of these symptoms. Approximately the same incidence of mild transient nasal burning and stinging was reported in patients on placebo as was reported in patients treated with NASALIDE in controlled studies, implying that these complaints may be related to the vehicle or the delivery system. The incidence of complaints of nasal burning and stinging decreased with increasing duration of treatment.

Other side effects reported at a frequency of 5% or less were: nasal congestion, sneezing, epistaxis and/or bloody mucus, nasal irritation, watery eyes, sore throat, nausea and/or vomiting, headaches and loss of sense of smell and taste. As is the case with other nasally inhaled corticosteroids, nasal septal perforations have been observed in rare instances. Systemic corticosteroid side effects were not reported during the controlled clinical trials. If recommended doses are exceeded, or if individuals are particularly sensitive, symptoms of hypercorticism, i.e., Cushing's syndrome, could occur.

OVERDOSAGE

I.V. flunisolide in animals at doses up to 4 mg/kg showed no effect. One spray bottle contains 6.25 mg of NASALIDE; therefore acute overdosage is unlikely.

DOSAGE AND ADMINISTRATION

The therapeutic effects of corticosteroids, unlike those of decongestants, are not immediate. This should be explained to the patient in advance in order to ensure cooperation and continuation of treatment with the prescribed dosage regimen. Full therapeutic benefit requires regular use, and is usually evident within a few days. However, a longer period of therapy may be required for some patients to achieve maximum benefit (up to 3 weeks). If no improvement is evident by that time, NASALIDE® (flunisolide) should not be continued.

Patients with blocked nasal passages should be encouraged to use a decongestant just before NASALIDE administration to ensure adequate penetration of the spray. Patients should also be advised to clear their nasal passages of secretions prior to use.

Adults: The recommended starting dose of NASALIDE is 2 sprays (50 mcg) in each nostril 2 times a day (total dose 200 mcg/day). If needed, this dose may be increased to 2 sprays in each nostril 3 times a day (total dose 300 mcg/day).

Children 6 to 14 years: The recommended starting dose of NASALIDE is one spray (25 mcg) in each nostril 3 times a day or two sprays (50 mcg) in each nostril 2 times a day (total dose 150-200 mcg/day). NASALIDE is not recommended for use in children less than 6 years of age as safety and efficacy studies, including possible adverse effects on growth, have not been conducted.

Maximum total daily doses should not exceed 8 sprays in each nostril for adults (total dose 400 mcg/day) and 4 sprays in each nostril for children under 14 years of age (total dose 200 mcg/day). Since there is no evidence that exceeding the maximum recommended dosage is more effective and increased systemic absorption would occur, higher doses should be avoided.

After the desired clinical effect is obtained, the maintenance dose should be reduced to the smallest amount necessary to control the symptoms. Approximately 15% of patients with perennial rhinitis may be maintained on as little as 1 spray in each nostril per day.

HOW SUPPLIED

Each 25 ml NASALIDE® (flunisolide) nasal solution spray bottle (NDC 0033-2906-40) (NSN 6505-01-132-9979) contains 6.25 mg (0.25 mg/mL) of flunisolide and is supplied in a nasal pump dispenser with dust cover and a patient leaflet of instructions.

Store at controlled room temperature, 15°–30°C (59°–86°F)

Revised 12/88

© Syntex Laboratories, Inc.

NORINYL® 1+35 Tablets   ℞
(norethindrone and ethinyl estradiol)
NORINYL® 1+50 Tablets   ℞
(norethindrone and mestranol)

Refer to entry under BREVICON® Tablets (norethindrone and ethinyl estradiol).

Shown in Product Identification Section, page 433

NOR–QD®   ℞
(norethindrone)
Tablets 0.35 mg.

Refer to entry under BREVICON® Tablets (norethindrone and ethinyl estradiol).

Shown in Product Identification Section, page 433

SYNACORT®   ℞
(hydrocortisone)
Cream 1%
Cream 2.5%
SYNALAR®   ℞
(fluocinolone acetonide)
Cream 0.025%
Cream 0.01%
Ointment 0.025%
Topical Solution 0.01%
SYNALAR–HP®   ℞
(fluocinolone acetonide)
Cream 0.2%
SYNEMOL®   ℞
(fluocinolone acetonide)
Cream 0.025%

Refer to entry under LIDEX® (fluocinonide) Cream 0.05%.

TAP Pharmaceuticals
NORTH CHICAGO, IL 60064

LUPRON®   ℞
[lu 'pron]
leuprolide acetate injection

DESCRIPTION

LUPRON (leuprolide acetate) Injection is a synthetic nonapeptide analog of naturally occurring gonadotropin releasing hormone (GnRH or LH-RH). The analog possesses greater potency than the natural hormone. The chemical name is 5-Oxo-L-prolyl-L-histidyl-L-tryptophyl-L-seryl-L-tyrosyl-D-leucyl-L-leucyl-L-arginyl-N-ethyl-L-prolinamide acetate (salt) with the following structural formula:
[See structural formula above].

LUPRON is a sterile, aqueous solution intended for subcutaneous injection. It is available in a 2.8 ml multiple-dose vial containing 5 mg/ml of leuprolide acetate, sodium chloride for tonicity adjustment, 9 mg/ml of benzyl alcohol as a preservative and water for injection. The pH may have been adjusted with sodium hydroxide and/or acetic acid.

CLINICAL PHARMACOLOGY

Leuprolide acetate, an LH-RH agonist, acts as a potent inhibitor of gonadotropin secretion when given continuously and in therapeutic doses. Animal and human studies indicate that following an initial stimulation, chronic administration of leuprolide acetate results in suppression of ovarian and testicular steroidogenesis. This effect is reversible upon discontinuation of drug therapy. Administration of leuprolide acetate has resulted in inhibition of the growth of certain hormone dependent tumors (prostatic tumors in Noble and Dunning male rats and DMBA-induced mammary tumors in female rats) as well as atrophy of the reproductive organs. In humans, subcutaneous administration of single daily doses of leuprolide acetate results in an initial increase in circulating levels of luteinizing hormone (LH) and follicle stimulating hormone (FSH), leading to a transient increase in levels of the gonadal steroids (testosterone and dihydrotestosterone in males, and estrone and estradiol in pre-menopausal females). However, continuous daily administration of leuprolide acetate results in decreased levels of LH and FSH in all patients. In males, testosterone is reduced to castrate levels. In pre-menopausal females, estrogens are reduced to post-menopausal levels. These decreases occur within two to four weeks after initiation of treatment, and castrate levels of testosterone in prostatic cancer patients have been demonstrated for periods of up to three years. Leuprolide acetate is not active when given orally. Bioavailability by subcutaneous administration is comparable to that by intravenous administration. Leuprolide acetate has a plasma half-life of approximately three hours. The metabo-

lism, distribution and excretion of leuprolide acetate in man have not been determined.

INDICATIONS AND USAGE

LUPRON (leuprolide acetate) Injection is indicated in the palliative treatment of advanced prostatic cancer. It offers an alternative treatment of prostatic cancer when orchiectomy or estrogen administration are either not indicated or unacceptable to the patient. In a controlled study comparing LUPRON 1 mg/day given subcutaneously to DES (diethylstilbestrol), 3 mg/day, the survival rate for the two groups was comparable after two years treatment. The objective response to treatment was also similar for the two groups.

CONTRAINDICATIONS

There are no known contraindications to the use of LUPRON.

WARNINGS

Isolated cases of worsening of signs and symptoms during the first weeks of treatment have been reported. Worsening of symptoms may contribute to paralysis with or without fatal complications.

PRECAUTIONS

Patients with metastatic vertebral lesions and/or with urinary tract obstruction should be closely observed during the first few weeks of therapy (see "ADVERSE REACTIONS" section).

Patients with known allergies to benzyl alcohol, an ingredient of the drug's vehicle, may present symptoms of hypersensitivity, usually local, in the form of erythema and induration at the injection site.

Information for Patients: See Information for Patients which appears after the "HOW SUPPLIED" section.

Laboratory Tests: Response to leuprolide acetate should be monitored by measuring serum levels of testosterone and acid phosphatase. In the majority of patients, testosterone levels increased above baseline during the first week, declining thereafter to baseline levels or below by the end of the second week of treatment. Castrate levels were reached within two to four weeks and once attained were maintained for as long as drug administration continued. Transient increases in acid phosphatase levels occurred sometimes early in treatment. However, by the fourth week, the elevated levels usually decreased to values at or near baseline.

Drug Interactions: None have been reported.

Carcinogenesis, Mutagenesis, Impairment of Fertility: Two-year carcinogenicity studies were conducted in rats and mice. In rats, a dose-related increase of benign pituitary hyperplasia and benign pituitary adenomas was noted at 24 months when the drug was administered subcutaneously at high daily doses (0.6 to 4 mg/kg). In mice no pituitary abnormalities were observed at a dose as high as 60 mg/kg for two years. Patients have been treated with leuprolide acetate for up to three years with doses as high as 10 mg/day and for two years with doses as high as 20 mg/day without demonstrable pituitary abnormalities.

Mutagenicity studies have been performed with leuprolide acetate using bacterial and mammalian systems. These studies provided no evidence of a mutagenic potential.

Clinical and pharmacologic studies with analogs similar to leuprolide acetate have shown full reversibility of fertility suppression when the drug is discontinued after continuous administration for periods of up to 20 weeks. However, no clinical studies have been conducted with leuprolide acetate to assess the reversibility of fertility suppression.

ADVERSE REACTIONS

In the majority of patients testosterone levels increased above baseline during the first week, declining thereafter to baseline levels or below by the end of the second week of treatment. This transient increase was occasionally associated with a temporary worsening of signs and symptoms, usually manifested by an increase in bone pain (See "WARN-

Continued on next page

TAP Pharmaceuticals—Cont.

INGS" section). In a few cases a temporary worsening of existing hematuria and urinary tract obstruction occurred during the first week. Temporary weakness and paresthesia of the lower limbs have been reported in a few cases.

Potential exacerbations of signs and symptoms during the first few weeks of treatment is a concern in patients with vertebral metastases and/or urinary obstruction which, if aggravated, may lead to neurological problems or increase the obstruction.

In a comparative trial of LUPRON (leuprolide acetate) Injection versus DES, in 5% or more of the patients receiving either drug, the following adverse reactions were reported to have a possible or probable relationship to drug as ascribed by the treating physician. Reactions considered not drug related are excluded.

	LUPRON (N = 98)	DES (N = 101)
	Number of Reports	
Cardiovascular System		
Congestive heart failure	1	5
ECG changes/ischemia	19	22
High blood pressure	8	5
Murmur	3	8
Peripheral edema	12	30
Phlebitis/thrombosis	2	10
Gastrointestinal System		
Anorexia	6	5
Constipation	7	9
Nausea/vomiting	5	17
Endocrine System		
Decreased testicular size	7	11
Gynecomastia/breast tenderness		
or pain	7	63
Hot flashes	55	12
Impotence	4	12
Hemic and Lymphatic System		
Anemia	5	5
Musculoskeletal System		
Bone pain	5	2
Myalgia	3	9
Central/Peripheral Nervous System		
Dizziness/lightheadedness	5	7
General pain	13	13
Headache	7	4
Insomnia/sleep disorders	7	5
Respiratory System		
Dyspnea	2	8
Sinus congestion	5	6
Integumentary System		
Dermatitis	5	8
Urogenital System		
Frequency/urgency	6	8
Hematuria	6	4
Urinary tract infection	3	7
Miscellaneous		
Asthenia	10	10

In this same study, the following adverse reactions were reported in less than 5% of the patients on Lupron.
Cardiovascular System —Angina, Cardiac arrhythmias, Myocardial infarction, Pulmonary emboli; *Gastrointestinal System* —Diarrhea, Dysphagia, Gastrointestinal bleeding, Gastrointestinal disturbance, Peptic ucler, Rectal polyps; *Endocrine System* —Libido decrease, Thyroid enlargement; *Musculoskeletal System* —Joint pain; *Central/Peripheral Nervous System* —Anxiety, Blurred vision, Lethargy, Memory disorder, Mood swings, Nervousness, Numbness, Paresthesia, Peripheral neuropathy, Syncope/blackouts, Taste disorders; *Respiratory System* —Cough, Pleural rub, Pneumonia, Pulmonary fibrosis; *Integumentary System* —Carcinoma of skin/ear, Dry skin, Ecchymosis, Hair loss, Itching, Local skin reactions, Pigmentation, Skin lesions; *Urogenital System* —Bladder spasms, Dysuria, Incontinence, Testicular pain, Urinary obstruction; *Miscellaneous* —Depression, Diabetes, Fatigue, Fever/chills, Hypoglycemia, Increased BUN, Increased calcium, Increased creatinine, Infection/inflammation, Ophthalmologic disorders, Swelling (temporal bone).

The following additional adverse reactions have been reported with Lupron in another clinical trial and/or during postmarketing surveillance. Reactions considered by the treating physician as nondrug related are not included.
Cardiovascular System —Hypotension, Transient ischemic attack/stroke; *Gastrointestinal System* —Hepatic dysfunction; *Endocrine System* —Libido increase; *Hemic and Lymphatic System* —Decreased WBC, Hemoptysis; *Musculoskeletal System* —Ankylosing spondylosis, Pelvic fibrosis; *Central/Peripheral Nervous System* —Hearing disorder, Peripheral neuropathy, Spinal fracture/paralysis; *Respiratory System* —Pulmonary infiltrate, Respiratory disorders; *Urogenital System* —Penile swelling, Prostate pain; *Miscellaneous* —Hypoproteinemia.

OVERDOSAGE

In rats subcutaneous administration of 250 to 500 times the recommended human dose, expressed on a per body weight basis, resulted in dyspnea, decreased activity, and local irritation at the injection site. There is no evidence at present that there is a clinical counterpart of this phenomenon. In early clinical trials with leuprolide acetate doses as high as 20 mg/day for up to two years caused no adverse effects differing from those observed with the 1 mg/day dose.

DOSAGE AND ADMINISTRATION

The recommended dose is 1 mg (0.2 ml) administered as a single daily subcutaneous injection. As with other drugs administered chronically by subcutaneous injection, the injection site should be be varied periodically.
NOTE: As with all parenteral products, inspect container's solution for discoloration and particulate matter before each use.

HOW SUPPLIED

LUPRON (leuprolide acetate) Injection is a sterile solution supplied in a 2.8 ml multiple-dose vial, **NDC** 0300-3626-28. Refrigerate until dispensed. Patient may store unrefrigerated below 86°F. Avoid freezing. Protect from light—store vial in carton until use.
Each 0.2 ml contains 1 mg of leuprolide acetate, sodium chloride for tonicity adjustment, 1.8 mg of benzyl alcohol as preservative and water for injection. The pH may have been adjusted with sodium hydroxide and/or acetic acid.
Caution: Federal (U.S.A.) law prohibits dispensing without a prescription.
Revised: November, 1986.
U.S. Patent Nos. 4,005,063 and 4,005,194.

INFORMATION FOR PATIENTS

NOTE: Be sure to consult your physician with any questions you may have or for information about LUPRON (leuprolide acetate) Injection and its use.

WHAT IS CANCER?

Cancer is a disease characterized by uncontrolled growth and spread of abnormal body cells. Normally, the cells that make up all parts of the body reproduce themselves in an orderly manner so that growth occurs, worn out tissues are replaced and injuries repaired. Occasionally, certain cells grow into a mass of tissue called a tumor. Some tumors are benign; others are malignant, or cancerous.
Benign tumors may interfere with body function and may require surgical treatment but they do not invade neighboring tissue and seldom threaten life. However, malignant tumors invade and destroy normal tissue. By a process called metastasis, cells break away from a malignant tumor and spread through the blood and lymphatic systems to other parts of the body where they form new tumors. Sometimes cancer grows and spreads rapidly; sometimes the process takes years.
One very common place for cancer to develop in men is the prostate gland.

WHAT IS THE PROSTATE?

The prostate is a male sex gland about the size of a chestnut. It lies just below the urinary bladder and surrounds the first inch of the urethra, the canal that carries urine from the bladder during urination. The secretion of the prostate provides part of the fluid for ejaculation.

TREATMENT OF PROSTATIC CANCER

Your doctor has a choice of treatments for prostatic cancer including surgery, radiation and drugs. The best choice for a particular patient usually depends on whether the cancer was found early or in an advanced stage.
The growth and function of the normal prostate gland is dependent upon the male hormone testosterone. If you have a prostatic tumor, its growth is usually stimulated by testosterone as well. For this reason, decreasing the body's supply of testosterone often controls tumor growth and relieves pain and difficulty in urinating.
The primary source of testosterone is the testes; therefore, one way to reduce production of testosterone is to remove the testes by surgery.
Another way is for men to take a female hormone, estrogen. This also causes the body to stop making testosterone. Estrogens have potential side effects such as swelling of the breasts, fluid retention, blood clotting problems, and decrease in libido and impotence.
Another choice is LUPRON which will also decrease testosterone production LUPRON has potential side effects, such as hot flashes and decrease in libido and impotence. It may also initially aggravate signs and symptoms of your disease by temporary stimulation of the tumor during the first one to two weeks of treatment.

WHAT IS LUPRON?

LUPRON (leuprolide acetate) Injection is chemically similar to gonadotropin releasing hormone (GnRH or LH-RH), a hormone which occurs naturally in your body.

Normally, your body releases small amounts of LH-RH, and this leads to events which stimulate the production of testosterone.
However, when you inject LUPRON Injection, the normal events that lead to testosterone production are interrupted and testosterone is no longer produced by the testes.
LUPRON must be injected because, like insulin which is injected by diabetics, LUPRON is inactive when taken by mouth.
If you were to discontinue the drug for any reason, your body would begin making testosterone again.

DIRECTIONS FOR USING LUPRON

1. Wash hands thoroughly with soap and water.
2. If using a new bottle for the first time, flip off the plastic cover to expose the gray rubber stopper. Wipe metal ring and rubber stopper with an alcohol wipe each time you use LUPRON. Check the liquid in the container. If it is not clear or has particles in it, DO NOT USE IT. Exchange it at your pharmacy for another container.
3. Remove outer wrapping from one syringe. Pull plunger back until the tip of the plunger is at the .2 mark.
4. Take cover off needle and push the cover into the appropriate hole in the Daily Dose Reminder area. Push the needle through the center of the rubber stopper on the LUPRON bottle.
5. Push the plunger all the way in to inject air into the bottle.
6. Keep the needle in the bottle and turn the bottle upside down. Check to make sure the tip of the needle is in the liquid. Slowly pull back on the plunger, until the syringe fills to the .2 mark.
7. Toward the end of a two-week period, the amount of LUPRON left in the bottle will be small. Take special care to hold the bottle straight and to keep the needle tip in liquid while pulling back on the plunger.
8. Keeping the needle in the bottle and the bottle upside down, check for air bubbles in the syringe. If you see any, push the plunger *slowly* in to push the air bubble back into the bottle. Keep the tip of the needle in the liquid and pull the plunger back again to fill to the .2 mark.
9. Do this again if necessary to eliminate air bubbles. Remove needle from bottle and lay syringe down on the syringe rest. DO NOT TOUCH THE NEEDLE OR ALLOW THE NEEDLE TO TOUCH ANY SURFACE.
10. To protect your skin, inject each daily dose at a different body spot.
11. Choose an injection spot. Cleanse the injection spot with another alcohol wipe.
12. Hold the syringe in one hand. Hold the skin taut, or pull up a little flesh with the other hand, as you were instructed.
13. Hold the syringe alongside the skin and slide the needle quickly just under the skin as far as it will go. Inject the drug by pushing in the plunger as far as it will go.
14. Hold an alcohol wipe down on your skin where the needle is inserted and withdraw the needle at the same angle it was inserted.
15. Use the disposable syringe only once and dispose of it properly as you were instructed. A waste area is provided in the LUPRON Patient Administration Kit. Needles thrown into a garbage bag could accidentally stick someone. NEVER LEAVE SYRINGES, NEEDLES OR DRUGS WHERE CHILDREN CAN REACH THEM.

SOME SPECIAL ADVICE

- You may experience hot flashes when using LUPRON (leuprolide acetate) Injection. During the first few weeks of treatment you may experience increased bone pain, increased difficulty in urinating, and less commonly but most importantly, you may experience the onset or aggravation of nerve symptoms. In any of these events, discuss the symptoms with your doctor.
- You may experience some irritation at the injection site, such as burning, itching or swelling. These reactions are usually mild and go away. If they do not, tell your doctor.
- Do not stop taking your injections because you feel better. You need an injection every day to make sure LUPRON keeps working for you.
- Use only the syringes provided in the kit, as other types may dispense an incorrect dose. If for any reason you cannot use one of the syringes, contact your doctor or pharmacist for advice.
- When the drug level gets low, take special care to hold the bottle straight and down and to keep the needle tip in liquid while pulling back on the plunger.
- Do not try to get every last drop out of the bottle. This will increase the possibility of drawing air into the syringe and getting an incomplete dose. Some extra drug has been provided so that you can withdraw the recommended number of doses.
- Tell your pharmacist when you will need your next LUPRON kit so it will be at the pharmacy when you need it.

- This drug may be stored at room temperature (not above 86°F). Do not store near a radiator or other very warm place.
- Do not leave your drug or hypodermic syringes where anyone can pick them up.
- Keep this and all other medications out of reach of children.

Manufactured for TAP Pharmaceuticals
North Chicago, IL 60064, U.S.A.
by Abbott Laboratories
North Chicago, IL 60064

LUPRON DEPOT® ℞
[*lu 'pron dē 'pō*]
(leuprolide acetate for depot suspension)

DESCRIPTION
Leuprolide acetate is a synthetic nonapeptide analog of naturally occurring gonadotropin releasing hormone (GnRH or LH-RH). The analog possesses greater potency than the natural hormone. The chemical name is 5-Oxo-L-prolyl-L-histidyl-L-tryptophyl-L-seryl-L-tyrosyl-D-leucyl-L- leucyl-L-arginyl-N-ethyl-L-prolinamide acetate (salt) with the following structural formula:
[See structural formula above right].

LUPRON DEPOT is available in a vial containing sterile lyophilized microspheres, which when mixed with diluent, become a suspension, which is intended as a monthly intramuscular injection.
The single-dose vial of LUPRON DEPOT contains leuprolide acetate (7.5 mg), purified gelatin (1.3 mg), DL-lactic and glycolic acids copolymer (66.2 mg), and D-mannitol (13.2 mg). The accompanying ampule of diluent contains carboxymethylcellulose sodium (7.5 mg), D-mannitol (75 mg), polysorbate 80 (1.5 mg), and water for injection, USP.

CLINICAL PHARMACOLOGY
Leuprolide acetate, an LH-RH agonist, acts as a potent inhibitor of gonadotropin secretion when given continuously and in therapeutic doses. Animal and human studies indicate that following an initial stimulation, chronic administration of leuprolide acetate results in suppression of ovarian and testicular steroidogenesis. This effect is reversible upon discontinuation of drug therapy. Administration of leuprolide acetate has resulted in inhibition of the growth of certain hormone dependent tumors (prostatic tumors in Noble and Dunning male rats and DMBA-induced mammary tumors in female rats) as well as atrophy of the reproductive organs.
In humans, administration of leuprolide acetate results in an initial increase in circulating levels of luteinizing hormone (LH) and follicle stimulating hormone (FSH), leading to a transient increase in levels of the gonadal steroids (testosterone and dihydrotestosterone in males, and estrone and estradiol in pre-menopausal females). However, continuous administration of leuprolide acetate results in decreased levels of LH and FSH. In males, testosterone is reduced to castrate levels. In pre-menopausal females, estrogens are reduced to post-menopausal levels. These decreases occur within two to four weeks after initiation of treatment, and castrate levels of testosterone in prostatic cancer patients have been demonstrated for periods of up to five years.
Leuprolide acetate is not active when given orally. Following a single LUPRON DEPOT injection to patients, mean peak leuprolide acetate plasma concentration was almost 20 ng/mL at 4 hours and 0.36 ng/mL at 4 weeks. Nondetectable leuprolide acetate plasma concentrations have been observed during chronic LUPRON DEPOT administration, but testosterone levels appear to be maintained at castrate levels. The metabolism, distribution, and excretion of leuprolide acetate in humans have not been determined.

INDICATIONS AND USAGE
LUPRON DEPOT is indicated in the palliative treatment of advanced prostatic cancer. It offers an alternative treatment of prostatic cancer when orchiectomy or estrogen administration are either not indicated or unacceptable to the patient. In clinical trials, the safety and efficacy of LUPRON DEPOT does not differ from that of the original daily subcutaneous injection.

CONTRAINDICATIONS
A report of an anaphylactic reaction to synthetic GnRH (Factrel) has been reported in the medical literature.[1]
LUPRON DEPOT is contraindicated in women who are or may become pregnant while receiving the drug. When administered on day 6 of pregnancy at test dosages of 0.00024, 0.0024, and 0.024 mg/kg ($\frac{1}{600}$ to $\frac{1}{6}$ the human dose) to rabbits, LUPRON DEPOT produced a dose related increase in major fetal abnormalities. Similar studies in rats failed to demonstrate an increase in fetal malformations. There was increased fetal mortality and decreased fetal weights with the two higher doses of LUPRON DEPOT (leuprolide acetate for depot suspension) in rabbits and with the highest dose in rats. The effects on fetal mortality are logical consequences of the alterations in hormonal levels brought about by this drug. Therefore, the possibility exists that spontaneous abortion may occur if the drug is administered during pregnancy.

WARNINGS
Isolated cases of worsening of signs and symptoms during the first weeks of treatment have been reported with LH-RH analogs. Worsening of symptoms may contribute to paralysis with or without fatal complications. For patients at risk, the physician may consider initiating therapy with daily LUPRON® (leuprolide acetate) Injection for the first two weeks to facilitate withdrawal of treatment if that is considered necessary.

PRECAUTIONS
Patients with metastatic vertebral lesions and/or with urinary tract obstruction should be closely observed during the first few weeks of therapy (see "WARNINGS" section).
Laboratory Tests: Response to leuprolide acetate should be monitored by measuring serum levels of testosterone and acid phosphatase. In the majority of patients, testosterone levels increased above baseline during the first week, declining thereafter to baseline levels or below by the end of the second week. Castrate levels were reached within two to four weeks and once achieved were maintained for as long as the patients received their monthly injection on time. Transient increases in acid phosphatase levels may occur sometime early in treatment. However, by the fourth week, the elevated levels can be expected to decrease to values at or near baseline.
Drug Interactions: None have been reported.
Carcinogenesis, Mutagenesis, Impairment of Fertility: Two-year carcinogenicity studies were conducted in rats and mice. In rats, a dose-related increase of benign pituitary hyperplasia and benign pituitary adenomas was noted at 24 months when the drug was administered subcutaneously at high daily doses (0.6 to 4 mg/kg). In mice no pituitary abnormalities were observed at a dose as high as 60 mg/kg for two years. Patients have been treated with leuprolide acetate for up to three years with doses as high as 10 mg/day and for two years with doses as high as 20 mg/day without demonstrable pituitary abnormalities.
Mutagenicity studies have been performed with leuprolide acetate using bacterial and mammalian systems. These studies provided no evidence of a mutagenic potential.
Clinical and pharmacologic studies with leuprolide acetate and similar analogs have shown reversibility of fertility suppression when the drug is discontinued after continuous administration for periods of up to 24 weeks.
Pregnancy Category X. See "CONTRAINDICATIONS" section.

ADVERSE REACTIONS
In the majority of patients testosterone levels increased above baseline during the first week, declining thereafter to baseline levels or below by the end of the second week of treatment.
Potential exacerbations of signs and symptoms during the first few weeks of treatment is a concern in patients with vertebral metastases and/or urinary obstruction or hematuria which, if aggravated, may lead to neurological problems such as temporary weakness and/or paresthesia of the lower limbs or worsening of urinary symptoms (see "WARNINGS" section).
In a clinical trial of LUPRON DEPOT, the following adverse reactions were reported to have a possible or probable relationship to drug as ascribed by the treating physician in 5% or more of the patients receiving the drug. Often, causality is difficult to assess in patients with metastatic prostate cancer. Reactions considered not drug related are excluded.

	LUPRON DEPOT	
	N = 56	(Percent)
Cardiovascular System		
Edema	7	(12.5%)
Gastrointestinal System		
Nausea/vomiting	3	(5.4%)
Endocrine System		
*Decreased testicular size	3	(5.4%)
*Hot flashes/sweats	33	(58.9%)
*Impotence	3	(5.4%)
Central/Peripheral Nervous System		
General pain	4	(7.1%)
Respiratory System		
Dyspnea	3	(5.4%)
Miscellaneous		
Asthenia	3	(5.4%)

*Physiologic effect of decreased testosterone.
Laboratory: Elevations of certain parameters were observed, but it is difficult to assess these abnormalities in this population.

SGOT (> 2N)	4	(5.4%)
LDH (> 2N)	11	(19.6%)
Alkaline phos (> 1.5N)	4	(5.4%)

In this same study, the following adverse reactions were reported in less than 5% of the patients on LUPRON DEPOT.
Cardiovascular System —Angina, Cardiac arrhythmia; *Gastrointestinal System* —Anorexia, Diarrhea; *Endocrine System* —Gynecomastia, Libido decrease; *Musculoskeletal System* —Bone pain, Myalgia; *Central/Peripheral Nervous System* —Paresthesia, Insomnia; *Respiratory System* —Hemoptysis; *Integumentary System* —Dermatitis, Local skin reactions, hair growth; *Urogenital System* —Dysuria, Frequency/urgency, Hematuria, Testicular pain; *Miscellaneous* —Diabetes, Fever/chills, hard nodule in throat, Increased calcium, Weight gain, Increased uric acid.
The following additional adverse reactions have been reported with LUPRON (leuprolide acetate) Injection. Reactions considered by the treating physician as nondrug related are not included.
Cardiovascular System —Congestive heart failure, ECG changes/ischemia, High blood pressure, Hypotension, Myocardial infarction, Murmur, Phlebitis/thrombosis, Pulmonary emboli, Transient ischemic attack/stroke; *Gastrointestinal System* —Constipation, Dysphagia, Gastrointestinal bleeding, Gastrointestinal disturbance, Hepatic dysfunction, Peptic ulcer, Rectal polyps; *Endocrine System* —Breast tenderness or pain, Libido increase, Thyroid enlargement; *Hemic and Lymphatic System* —Anemia, Decreased WBC; *Musculoskeletal System* —Ankylosing spondylosis, Joint pain, Pelvic fibrosis; *Central/Peripheral Nervous System* —Anxiety, Blurred vision, Dizziness/lightheadedness, Headache, Hearing disorder, Sleep disorders, Lethargy, Memory disorder, Mood swings, Nervousness, Numbness, Peripheral neuropathy, Spinal fracture/paralysis, Syncope/blackouts, Taste disorders; *Respiratory System* —Cough, Pleural rub, Pneumonia, Pulmonary fibrosis, Pulmonary infiltrate, Respiratory disorders, Sinus congestion; *Integumentary System* —Carcinoma of skin/ear, Dry skin, Ecchymosis, Hair loss, Itching, Pigmentation, Skin lesions; *Urogenital System* —Bladder spasms, Incontinence, Penile swelling, Prostate pain, Urinary obstruction, Urinary tract infection; *Miscellaneous* —Depression, Hypoglycemia, Hypoproteinemia, Increased BUN, Increased creatinine, Infection/inflammation, Ophthalmologic disorders, Swelling (temporal bone).

OVERDOSAGE
In rats, subcutaneous administration of 250 to 500 times the recommended human dose, expressed on a per body weight basis, resulted in dyspnea, decreased activity, and local irritation at the injection site. There is no evidence at present that there is a clinical counterpart of this phenomenon. In early clinical trials with daily subcutaneous leuprolide acetate, doses as high as 20 mg/day for up to two years caused no adverse effects differing from those observed with the 1 mg/day dose.

DOSAGE AND ADMINISTRATION
LUPRON DEPOT Must Be Administered Under The Supervision Of A Physician.
The recommended dose of LUPRON DEPOT is 7.5 mg, incorporated in a depot formulation. The lyophilized micros-

Continued on next page

TAP Pharmaceuticals—Cont.

pheres are to be reconstituted and administered monthly as a single intramuscular injection, in accord with the following directions:

1. Using a syringe with a 22 gauge needle, withdraw 1 mL of diluent from the ampule, and inject it into the vial. (Extra diluent is provided; any remaining should be discarded.)
2. Shake well to thoroughly disperse particles to obtain a uniform suspension. The suspension will appear milky.
3. Withdraw the entire contents of the vial into the syringe and inject it at the time of reconstitution.

Although the solution has been shown to be stable for 24 hours following reconstitution, since the product does not contain a preservative, the suspension should be discarded if not used immediately.

As with other drugs administered by injection, the injection site should be varied periodically.

The vial of LUPRON DEPOT and the ampule of diluent may be stored at room temperature.

HOW SUPPLIED

LUPRON DEPOT (NDC 0300-3629-01) is available in a vial containing sterile lyophilized microspheres which is leuprolide acetate incorporated in a biodegradable copolymer of lactic and glycolic acids. The single-dose vial of LUPRON DEPOT contains leuprolide acetate (7.5 mg), purified gelatin (1.3 mg), DL-lactic & glycolic acids copolymer (66.2 mg), and D-mannitol (13.2 mg). The accompanying ampule of diluent contains carboxymethylcellulose sodium (7.5 mg), D-mannitol (75 mg), polysorbate 80 (1.5 mg), and water for injection, USP. When mixed with 1 mL of diluent, LUPRON DEPOT is administered as a single monthly IM injection. Caution: Federal (U.S.A.) law prohibits dispensing without a prescription.

U.S. Patent Nos. 4,005,063; 4,005,194 and patent pending (LUPRON DEPOT).

Reference:

1. MacLeod TL, Eisen A, Sussman GL, et al: Anaphylactic reaction to synthetic luteinizing hormone-releasing hormone. *Fertil Steril* 1987 Sept;48(3):500-502.

TAP Pharmaceuticals
North Chicago, IL 60064 U.S.A.
LUPRON DEPOT manufactured
by Takeda Chemical Industries, Ltd.
Osaka, Japan
R-Registered
© 1989, TAP Pharmaceuticals

EDUCATIONAL MATERIAL

All Free to the medical profession
Lupron® Injection
"Introduction to Lupron® (leuprolide acetate) Injection"—product monograph.
"Information for Patient Instruction"—a brochure to help professionals answer patients' questions about Lupron and to aid in subcutaneous self-injection.
Lupron Depot®
"An Introduction: Lupron Depot the Next Generation of GnRH Agonist Analogs"—product monograph.
"Questions and Answers on Lupron Depot the First Once-a-Month GnRH Agonist"—a bruchure that answers many common questions posed by the health professional.
"Treatment with Lupron Depot"—a brochure for the patient that briefly describes prostate cancer and how Lupron Depot is used to treat it.

ToppMed, Inc.
5015 BIRCH STREET
NEWPORT BEACH, CA 92660

TOPPFAST™
Physician-Formulated Diet Supplement

DESCRIPTION

Each serving delivers 120 calories consisting of 10 grams of protein, 19 grams of carbohydrate, 1 gram of fat, 1 gram of fiber, 240 mg. of sodium, 545 mg. of potassium and at least ⅕ of the RDA for vitamins.

USE

ToppFast is used as a meal substitute or as a total dietary intake supplement (5 servings per day) which is to be physician monitored per published protocol.

NUTRITION INFORMATION

	1 Serving	5 Servings
Serving Size	1 scoop (33.5 g)	
Servings per container	21	
Calories	120	600
Protein	10 g	50 g
Carbohydrate	19 g	95 g
Fat	1.0 g	5.0 g
*Sodium (715 mg/100 g)	240 mg	1200 mg**
*Potassium	545 mg	2725 mg**
Fiber	1.0 g	5.0 g

Percentage of U.S. Recommended Daily Allowances
For Adults and Children Over 12 Years of Age

	1 Serving	5 Servings
Protein	20%	100%
Vitamin A	40%	200%
Vitamin C	40%	200%
Thiamine	35%	175%
Riboflavin	35%	175%
Niacin	40%	200%
Calcium	20%	100%
Iron	40%	200%
Vitamin D	20%	100%
Vitamin E	40%	200%
Vitamin B6	40%	200%
Folic Acid	20%	100%
Vitamin B12	40%	200%
Phosphorus	20%	100%
Iodine	20%	100%
Magnesium	20%	100%
Zinc	20%	100%
Copper	30%	150%
Biotin	20%	100%
Pantothenic Acid	20%	100%
*Vitamin K	20 mcg	100 mcg**
*Manganese	0.8 mg	4 mg**
*Chromium	40 mcg	200 mcg**
*Selenium	40 mcg	200 mcg**
**Molybdate	100 mcg	500 mcg**

*U.S. RDA HAS NOT BEEN ESTABLISHED.
**THE FOOD AND NUTRITION BOARD OF THE NATIONAL RESEARCH COUNCIL RECOMMENDS THESE QUANTITIES OF THESE ESSENTIAL TRACE MINERALS AS BEING WITHIN THE RANGE REQUIRED IN THE DIET OF AN ADULT.

INGREDIENTS

Calcium sodium caseinate, fructose, nonfat milk, natural and artificial flavors, calcium sulfate, cellulose, partially hydrogenated soybean oil, guar gum, corn syrup solids, potassium chloride, salt, potassium and sodium citrate, magnesium oxide, ascorbic acid, ferrous fumarate, alpha tocopheryl acetate, niacinamide, dipotassium phosphate, vitamin A palmitate, zinc oxide, mono- and di-glycerides, d-calcium pantothenate, manganese sulfate, cupric sulfate, artificial color (including FD&C yellow #5), pyridoxine hydrochloride, riboflavin, thiamine hydrochloride, sodium molybdate, folic acid, chromium chloride, vitamin D₃, sodium selenite, biotin, potassium iodide, vitamin K, cyanocobalamin.

Tyson and Associates, Inc.
1661 LINCOLN BLVD.
SUITE 300
SANTA MONICA, CA 90404

PRODUCTS

L-Alanine	(600mg)	50c
L-Arginine	(700mg)	100c
L-Aspartic Acid	(600mg)	50c
L-Carnitine	(250mg)	30c
L-Cysteine Mono HCl	(750mg)	50c
L-Cystine	(700mg)	100c
L-Citrulline	(600mg)	50c
GABA	(500mg)	100c
L-Glutamic Acid	(500mg)	100c
L-Glutamine	(500mg)	100c
Glycine	(600mg)	100c
L-Histidine	(600mg)	50c
L-Isoleucine	(600mg)	50c
L-Leucine	(600mg)	50c
L-Lysine	(500mg)	100c
L-Methionine	(500mg)	30c
L-Ornithine	(600mg)	100c
Alphaketoglutaric Acid	(500mg)	100c
D-Phenylalanine	(500mg)	100c
L-Phenylalanine	(600mg)	100c
Proline	(600mg)	50c
L-Serine	(600mg)	50c
Taurine	(500mg)	100c
L-Threonine	(500mg)	60c
L-Tryptophan	(500mg)	100c
L-Tyrosine	(800mg)	100c
L-Valine	(600mg)	50c
Riboflavin 5 ' Phosphate	(5mg)	100t
Adenosine Triphosphate	(20mg)	100t

ALPHA PLUS™
(Urea Cycle Intermediates)

U.S.P. Crystalline Amino Acid Formulation. 700 mg Capsules

DOSAGE AND ADMINISTRATION
1–2 capsules daily.

HOW SUPPLIED
Bottles of 100 capsules—NDC 53335-1232-1

AMINOLETE™

U.S.P. Crystalline Amino Acid Formulation. 700 mg Capsules

DOSAGE AND ADMINISTRATION
1–3 capsules half an hour before meals.

HOW SUPPLIED
Bottles of 100 capsules—NDC 53335-1205-1

AMINOMINE™
(Excitatory neurotransmitters and L-Glutamine)

U.S.P. Crystalline Amino Acid Formulation. 700 mg Capsules

DOSAGE AND ADMINISTRATION
1–3 capsules half an hour before meals.

HOW SUPPLIED
Bottles of 100 capsules—NDC 53335-1129-1

AMINOPLEX®

DESCRIPTION
U.S.P. crystalline amino acid formulation. Formula contains 740 mg Anhydrous of 19 crystalline L-amino acids including neurotransmitter precursors and sulfur amino acids, and supplies 130 mg Nitrogen per capsule. Balanced formulation replacement based on quantitative Amino Acid Fractionation.

COMPOSITION
L-Lysine, L-Tryptophan, L-Arginine, L-Isoleucine, L-Leucine, L-Alanine, L-Threonine, L-Histidine, L-Cystine, L-Methionine, L-Glutamine, L-Tyrosine, L-Aspartic Acid, L-Valine, L-Glutamic Acid, L-Phenylalanine, Glycine, L-Serine, L-Cysteine HCl.

DOSAGE AND ADMINISTRATION
1–3 capsules half an hour before meals.

HOW SUPPLIED
Bottles of 100 capsules—NDC 53335-1116-1

AMINOSINE™
(Arginine-free Amino Acid Formulation)

U.S.P. Crystalline Amino Acid Formulation. 700 mg Capsules

DOSAGE AND ADMINISTRATION
1–3 capsules half an hour before meals.

HOW SUPPLIED
Bottles of 100 capsules—NDC 53335-1207-1

AMINOSTASIS™
(Branched Chain Amino Acid Formulation)

DESCRIPTION
U.S.P. crystalline amino acid formulation. Formula contains 700 mg of 12 crystalline L-amino acids supplying 107 mg Nitrogen per capsule. Formula is a rich source of the branched chain amino acids.

COMPOSITION
L-Lysine, Glycine, L-Leucine, L-Methionine, L-Arginine, L-Phenylalanine, L-Valine, L-Isoleucine, L-Histidine, L-Threonine, L-Tyrosine, L-Tryptophan.

DOSAGE AND ADMINISTRATION
2–6 capsules three times a day half an hour before meals.

HOW SUPPLIED
Bottles of 100 capsules—NDC 53335-1200-1

AMINOTATE®
(Glycogenic Amino Acid Formulation)

U.S.P. Crystalline Amino Acid Formulation. 700 mg Capsules

DOSAGE AND ADMINISTRATION

2–6 capsules three times a day half an hour before meals.

HOW SUPPLIED

Bottles of 100 capsules—NDC 53335-1209-1

AMINOXIN™
(Pyridoxal-5′-Phosphate)

DESCRIPTION

Each Aminoxin tablet contains 20 mg of pyridoxal-5′-phosphate, the co-enzymatic form of vitamin B_6. Enterically coated to protect the pyridoxal-5′-phosphate from dephosphorylization in the stomach acids, and enhancing molecular absorption.

ACTIONS AND USES

Required in transamination and decarboxylation reactions.

DOSAGE AND ADMINISTRATION

1–2 tablets 45–60 minutes before meals.

HOW SUPPLIED

Bottles of 100 tablets—NDC 53335-1120-1

L–CARNITINE

U.S.P. Crystalline L-Carnitine 250 mg Capsules

DOSAGE AND ADMINISTRATION

1–3 capsules mid a.m. and p.m.

HOW SUPPLIED

Bottles of 30 capsules—NDC 53335-1124-1

CATEMINE™
(Catecholamine Precursor)

DESCRIPTION

Enterically coated preparation of 800 mg L-Tyrosine and 10 mg pyridoxal-5′-phosphate.

ACTIONS AND USES

Biochemical precursor of dopamine and norepinephrine.

DOSAGE AND ADMINISTRATION

2 tablets b.i.d. in between meals.

HOW SUPPLIED

Bottles of 60—NDC 53335-1244-3
Samples upon request.

COMPLEX–CHO™
(Complex Carbohydrate Formulation from rice with minerals and fiber)

DOSAGE AND ADMINISTRATION

1–4 heaping teaspoons per day mixed with juice or water.

EFA PLUS Liquid
(Omega 3, 6, and essential fatty acids)

DOSAGE AND ADMINISTRATION

4–8 drops before meals.

HOW SUPPLIED

2 oz bottles —NDC 53335-1223-1

ENDORPHAN™
(D-Phenylalanine, D-Leucine, L-Tryptophan)

U.S.P. Crystalline Powder 530 mg Capsules

DOSAGE AND ADMINISTRATION

1–3 capsules twice daily.

HOW SUPPLIED

Bottles of 50 capsules—NDC 53335-1183-1

ENDORPHENYL™
(D-Phenylalanine U.S.P.)

U.S.P. Crystalline D-Phenylalanine 200 mg and 500 mg Capsules

DOSAGE AND ADMINISTRATION

1–5 capsules daily.

HOW SUPPLIED

Bottles of 50 capsules—NDC 53335-1226-1

ISO–B™
(B-complex free of common allergens)

DOSAGE AND ADMINISTRATION

2 capsules daily.

HOW SUPPLIED

Bottles of 60 capsules—NDC 53335-1185-1

M.V.M.™
(Multi-vitamin/mineral formula free of common allergens)

DOSAGE AND ADMINISTRATION

5 capsules daily in divided doses.

HOW SUPPLIED

Bottles of 150 capsules—NDC 53335-1184-1

MAXOVITE™
(Pre-Menstrual Syndrome—Multiple-Vitamin/Mineral)

DOSAGE AND ADMINISTRATION

2–6 tablets daily with breakfast.

HOW SUPPLIED

Bottles of 120 tablets—NDC 53335-1148-1

NIAPLUS™
(400 mg sustained release Niacin)

DOSAGE AND ADMINISTRATION

One capsule daily.

HOW SUPPLIED

Bottles of 60 capsules—NDC 53335-1218-1

NUTROX™
(Antioxidant Formulation free of common allergens)

DOSAGE AND ADMINISTRATION

1–3 capsules daily with meals.

HOW SUPPLIED

Bottles of 90 capsules—NDC 53335-1186-1

RIBO-2™
(co-enzymatic Vitamin B-2)

DESCRIPTION

Enteric coated preparation of 5 mg Riboflavin 5′ Phosphate.

DOSAGE AND ADMINISTRATION

1 tablet 60 minutes before breakfast and lunch or as directed.

HOW SUPPLIED

Bottles of 100 tablets—NDC# 53335-044-14

THIAMILATE™
(co-enzymatic vitamin B-1)

DESCRIPTION

Enteric coated preparation of 20 mg Thiamine Pyrophosphate.

DOSAGE AND ADMINISTRATION

1 to 2 tablets 60 minutes prior to meals or as directed.

HOW SUPPLIED

Bottles of 100 tablets—NDC# 53335-102-14

THREOSTAT™
(L-Threonine USP)

DESCRIPTION

Encapsulated U.S.P. Crystalline powder of 500 mg L-Threonine.

ACTIONS AND USES

May be helpful in reducing some symptoms of ALS.

DOSAGE AND ADMINISTRATION

4 to 8 capsules per day divided t.i.d. taken 60 minutes before meals or as directed.

HOW SUPPLIED

Bottles of 60 capsules—NDC# 53335-101-12

TRIO-DOPHILUS™
(L. acidophilus, B. bifidus, S. faecalis)

DESCRIPTION

Specially cloned and cultured strains of L. acidophilus, B. bifidus, S. faecalis in a base of potato complex carbohydrate. Each capsule provides 350 mgs., equivalent to 1.7 billion live cells.

DOSAGE AND ADMINISTRATION

1 capsule within an hour after breakfast and dinner or as directed.

HOW SUPPLIED

Bottles of 90 capsules—NDC# 53335-105-13

TRYPTOPLEX™
(Serotoninergic Precursor)

DESCRIPTION

Encapsulated pure U.S.P. crystalline powder of 400 mg L-Tryptophan, and the essential coenzymes. 4 mg nicotinic acid, 1 mg pyridoxine HCl.

ACTIONS AND USES

Biochemical precursor of serotonin.

DOSAGE AND ADMINISTRATION

2–5 capsules at bedtime or as directed.

HOW SUPPLIED

Bottles of 60—NDC 53335-1243-1
Samples upon request.

TRYPTO-SOM™ USP
(L-Tryptophan USP)

U.S.P. Crystalline Powder 500 mg Capsules
(See also Tryptoplex™)

DOSAGE AND ADMINISTRATION

1–2 capsules daily.

HOW SUPPLIED

Bottles of 100 capsules—NDC 53335-1173-1
Unit dose 100's

ULTRACHOLINE™
(Phosphatidylcholine and phospholipid)

Biologically active forms of choline and phospholipids.

DOSAGE AND ADMINISTRATION

1–2 capsules two times a day after meals.

HOW SUPPLIED

Bottles of 120 capsules—NDC 53335-1202-1

UAD Laboratories, Inc.
8339 HIGHWAY 18
JACKSON, MS 39209

BUCET™   ℞
[bu 'set]

DESCRIPTION

Each capsule contains:
Butalbital .... 50 mg
  (WARNING: May be habit forming.)
Acetaminophen .... 650 mg

HOW SUPPLIED

Bucet capsules are opaque white capsules imprinted Bucet/UAD 307 and are supplied in bottles of 100 capsules. Each capsule contains Butalbital 50 mg. (WARNING: May be habit forming.) and Acetaminophen 650 mg. The NDC number for 100 capsules is 0785-2307-01.

LORCET®-HD   © ℞
[lōr-sét h d]

DESCRIPTION

Each Lorcet-HD capsule contains 5 mg. of Hydrocodone Bitartrate (WARNING: May be habit forming) and 500 mg. of Acetaminophen.

HOW SUPPLIED

Lorcet-HD Capsules are opaque maroon capsules imprinted with the UAD logo, 1120 and are supplied in bottles of 100 capsules. Each capsule contains Hydrocodone Bitartrate, 5 mg. (WARNING: May be habit forming) and Acetaminophen (APAP), 500 mg. The NDC number for containers of 100 capsules is 0785-1120-01.

Continued on next page

UAD Laboratories—Cont.

LORCET® PLUS   Ⓒ Ⓡ
[lōr-sét plus]

DESCRIPTION
Each Lorcet Plus tablet contains:
Hydrocodone Bitartrate .... 7.5 mg
    WARNING: May be habit forming
Acetaminophen .... 650 mg

HOW SUPPLIED
Lorcet Plus, each tablet of which contains hydrocodone bitartrate 7.5 mg (WARNING: May be habit forming) and acetaminophen 650 mg, are white, capsule-shaped, scored tablets, debossed "U" on one side and "201" on the other side, and are supplied in containers of 100 tablets, NDC #0785-1122-01.

ZONE–A CREAM 1%   Ⓡ
[zōn 'a]

DESCRIPTION
A topical preparation containing Hydrocortisone acetate 1% and Pramoxine HCl 1% in a hydrophilic cream base containing stearic acid, cetyl alcohol, aquaphor, isopropylpalmitate, polyoxyl-40-stearate, propylene glycol, potassium sorbate 0.1%, sorbic acid 0.1%, triethanolamine lauryl sulfate and water.

HOW SUPPLIED
1 oz. tube.

ZONE–A LOTION 1%   Ⓡ
[zōn 'ā]

DESCRIPTION
Zone-A Lotion is a topical preparation containing Hydrocortisone acetate 1% and Pramoxine HCl 1% in a hydrophilic lotion base containing stearic acid, cetyl alcohol, forlan-L, glycerine, Triethanolamine, Myrj-52, Di-isopropyl adipate, polyvinyl-pyrrolidone, silicone, potassium sorbate 0.1% and sorbic acid 0.1% and water. Topical corticosteroids are anti-inflammatory and anti-pruritic agents.

HOW SUPPLIED
2 fl. oz.

U.S. Pharmaceutical Corporation
2500 PARK CENTRAL BLVD.
DECATUR, GA 30035

HEMOCYTE™ Tablets   OTC
(ferrous fumarate 324 mg.)

HOW SUPPLIED
Bottles of 100 NDC 52747-307-60

HEMOCYTE PLUS™ Tabules   Ⓡ
Iron-Vitamin-Mineral Complex

DESCRIPTION
Each tabule contains:
Ferrous Fumarate
   (anhydrous) 324   mg.
   [Equivalent to about 106 mg. of Elemental Iron]
Sodium Ascorbate (Vit. C) 200   mg.
Vit. B-1—Thiamine
   Mononitrate 10   mg.
Vit. B-2—Riboflavin 6   mg.
Vit. B-6—Pyridoxine HCl 5   mg.
Vit. B-12—Cyanocobalamin
   Concentrate 15   mcg.
Folic Acid 1   mg.
Niacinamide 30   mg.
Calcium Pantothenate 10   mg.
Zinc Sulfate 80   mg.
Magnesium Sulfate 70   mg.
Manganese Sulfate 4   mg.
Copper Sulfate 2   mg.

HOW SUPPLIED
Bottles of 100 NDC 52747-308-60

HEMOCYTE–F TABLETS   Ⓡ

DESCRIPTION
Each tablet contains:
Ferrous Fumarate .... 324 mg.
Folic Acid .... 1 mg.

HOW SUPPLIED
Bottles of 100 NDC 52747-306-60

ISOVEX® Capsules   Ⓡ
(ethaverine hydrochloride 100 mg.)

HOW SUPPLIED
Bottles of 100 NDC 52747-204-60
Bottles of 1000 NDC 52747-204-80

MAGSAL™ TABLETS   Ⓡ

DESCRIPTION
Each tablet contains:
Magnesium Salicylate .... 600 mg.
Phenyltoloxamine Citrate .... 25 mg.

HOW SUPPLIED
Bottles of 100 NDC 52747-321-60

MEDIGESIC® Capsules/Tablets   Ⓡ

DESCRIPTION
Each capsule or tablet contains:
Butalbital* .... 50 mg
     *WARNING: May be habit forming.
Acetaminophen .... 325 mg
Caffeine .... 40 mg

HOW SUPPLIED
Capsules: Bottles of 100 NDC 52747-212-60
Tablets: Bottles of 100 NDC 52747-311-60

The Upjohn Company
KALAMAZOO, MI 49001

UPJOHN PRODUCT IDENTIFICATION
Most capsules and tablets manufactured by The Upjohn Company are imprinted with one or a combination of the following: (1) Product trademark (2) Dosage strength (3) "Upjohn" or "U" (4) That portion of the National Drug Code (NDC) number which indicates product and strength.
A complete list of oral solid dosage forms with their assigned NDC numbers is provided below.

Code #	Product	Strength
10	HALCION® Tablets (triazolam) *See Product Identification Section*	0.125 mg
11	FEMINONE® Tablets (ethinyl estradiol tablets, USP)	0.05 mg
12	CORTEF® Tablets (hydrocortisone tablets, USP)	5 mg
14	HALOTESTIN® Tablets (fluoxymesterone tablets, USP) *See Product Identification Section*	2 mg
15	CORTISONE ACETATE Tablets, USP	5 mg
17	HALCION® Tablets (triazolam) *See Product Identification Section*	0.25 mg
18	DIDREX® Tablets Ⓒ (benzphetamine hydrochloride) *See Product Identification Section*	25 mg
19	HALOTESTIN® Tablets (fluoxymesterone tablets, USP) *See Product Identification Section*	5 mg
22	MEDROL® Tablets (methylprednisolone tablets, USP) *See Product Identification Section*	8 mg
23	CORTISONE ACETATE Tablets, USP	10 mg
24	DIDREX® Tablets (benzphetamine hydrochloride) *See Product Identification Section*	50 mg
25	DELTA-CORTEF® Tablets (prednisolone tablets, USP)	5 mg
29	XANAX® Tablets (alprazolam) *See Product Identification Section*	0.25 mg
31	CORTEF® Tablets (hydrocortisone tablets, USP)	10 mg
32	DELTASONE® Tablets (prednisone tablets, USP) *See Product Identification Section*	2.5 mg.
34	CORTISONE ACETATE Tablets, USP	25 mg
36	HALOTESTIN® Tablets (fluoxymesterone tablets, USP) *See Product Identification Section*	10 mg
38	HALODRIN® Tablets (fluoxymesterone and ethinyl estradiol)	
44	CORTEF® Tablets (hydrocortisone tablets, USP)	20 mg
45	DELTASONE® Tablets (prednisone tablets, USP) *See Product Identification Section*	5 mg
49	MEDROL® Tablets (methylprednisolone tablets, USP) *See Product Identification Section*	2 mg
50	PROVERA® Tablets (medroxyprogesterone acetate tablets, USP) *See Product Identification Section*	10 mg
55	XANAX® Tablets (alprazolam) *See Product Identification Section*	0.5 mg
56	MEDROL® Tablets (methylprednisolone tablets, USP) *See Product Identification Section*	4 mg
61	PAMINE® Tablets (methscopolamine bromide tablets, USP) *See Product Identification Section*	2.5 mg
64	PROVERA® Tablets (medroxyprogesterone acetate tablets, USP) *See Product Identification Section*	2.5 mg
70	TOLINASE® Tablets (tolazamide tablets, USP) *See Product Identification Section*	100 mg
73	MEDROL® Tablets (methylprednisolone tablets, USP) *See Product Identification Section*	16 mg
81	ADEFLOR CHEWABLE® Tablets Fluoride and vitamins *See Product Identification Section*	0.5 mg
90	XANAX® Tablets (alprazolam) *See Product Identification Section*	1 mg
92	ADEFLOR CHEWABLE® Tablets Fluoride and vitamins *See Product Identification Section*	1 mg
100	ORINASE® Tablets (tolbutamide tablets, USP) *See Product Identification Section*	0.5 Gm
101	ALBAMYCIN® Capsules (novobiocin sodium)	250 mg
106	DIOSTATE D® Tablets Vitamin, calcium and phosphorus supplement	
114	TOLINASE® Tablets (tolazamide tablets, USP) *See Product Identification Section*	250 mg
115	ADEFLOR M® Tablets Vitamins and minerals with fluoride	
121	LONITEN® Tablets (minoxidil) *See Product Identification Section*	2.5 mg
131	MICRONASE® Tablets (glyburide) *See Product Identification Section*	1.25 mg
137	LONITEN® Tablets (minoxidil) *See Product Identification Section*	10 mg
138	UNICAP® Capsules Multivitamin Supplement	
141	MICRONASE® Tablets (glyburide) *See Product Identification Section*	2.5 mg
155	MEDROL® Tablets (methylprednisolone tablets, USP) *See Product Identification Section*	24 mg
165	DELTASONE® Tablets (prednisone tablets, USP) *See Product Identification Section*	20 mg
170	ANSAID® Tablets (flurbiprofen)	50 mg
171	MICRONASE® Tablets (glyburide) *See Product Identification Section*	5.0 mg
176	MEDROL® Tablets (methylprednisolone tablets, USP) *See Product Identification Section*	32 mg
193	DELTASONE® Tablets (prednisone tablets, USP) *See Product Identification Section*	10 mg

ADEFLOR CHEWABLE® ℞
brand of fluoride with vitamins tablets

COMPOSITION

Each 0.5 mg or 1 mg tablet contains:

Fluoride (as sodium fluoride)	0.5 mg
	or 1 mg
Vitamin A	4000 Int. Units
Vitamin D (cholecalciferol)	400 Int. Units
Ascorbic Acid (as sodium ascorbate)	75 mg
Thiamine Mononitrate	2 mg
Riboflavin	2 mg
Niacinamide	18 mg
Pyridoxine Hydrochloride	1 mg
Calcium Pantothenate	5 mg
Cyanocobalamin	2 mcg

INACTIVE INGREDIENTS

artificial flavors, calcium phosphate, corn starch, erythrosine sodium, FD & C Blue No. 1, lactose, mannitol, saccharin sodium, sorbitol.

The palatable cherry-flavored ADEFLOR CHEWABLE Tablets 0.5 mg or raspberry-flavored 1 mg tablets may be chewed, dissolved in the mouth or swallowed whole.

HOW SUPPLIED

0.5 mg (round, pink) Bottles of 100   NDC 0009-0081-01
1 mg (round, purple) Bottles of 100   NDC 0009-0092-01
Shown in Product Identification Section, page 433

ADEFLOR® ℞
brand of fluoride with vitamins A, C, D and B₆ drops

COMPOSITION

Each 0.6 ml contains:

Fluoride (as sodium fluoride)	0.5 mg
Vitamin A	2000 Int. Units
Vitamin D (cholecalciferol)	400 Int. Units
Ascorbic Acid (C)	50 mg
Pyridoxine Hydrochloride (B₆)	1 mg

INACTIVE INGREDIENTS

caramel, corn oil, flavors, glycerin, methylparaben, nonionic oxyalkene polymer, propylene glycol, propylparaben, saccharin sodium, sorbitan monooleate and purified water.

HOW SUPPLIED

50 ml bottles with dropper calibrated for 0.3 and 0.6 ml.
NDC 0009-0211-02

ANSAID® ℞
brand of flurbiprofen tablets

DESCRIPTION

ANSAID Tablets contain flurbiprofen, a nonsteroidal anti-flammatory agent. Flurbiprofen is a phenylalkanoic acid derivative designated chemically as [1,1′-biphenyl]-4-acetic acid, 2-fluoro-alphamethyl-, (±)-. The empirical formula is $C_{15}H_{13}FO_2$, with a molecular weight of 244.26. Flurbiprofen is a white or slightly yellow crystalline powder. It is slightly soluble in water at pH 7.0 and readily soluble in most polar solvents. Its structural formula is:

ANSAID is available as 50 mg and 100 mg tablets for oral administration. Inactive ingredients for both strengths are carnauba wax, colloidal silicon dioxide, croscarmellose sodium, hydroxypropyl methylcellulose, lactose, magnesium stearate, microcrystalline cellulose, propylene glycol, and titanium dioxide. In addition, the 100 mg tablet contains FD&C blue No. 2.

CLINICAL PHARMACOLOGY

Flurbiprofen is a nonsteroidal anti-inflammatory agent which has shown anti-inflammatory, analgesic, and antipyretic properties in pharmacologic studies. As with other such drugs, its mode of action is not known. However, it is a potent prostaglandin synthesis inhibitor, and this property may be involved in its anti-inflammatory effect.

Flurbiprofen is well absorbed after oral administration, reaching peak blood levels in approximately 1.5 hours (range 0.5 to 4 hours). Administration with food alters the rate of absorption but does not affect the extent of drug availability. The elimination half-life is 5.7 hours with 90% of the half-life values from 3 to 9 hours. Individual half-life values ranged from 2.8 to 12 hours. There is no evidence of drug accumulation and flurbiprofen does not induce enzymes that alter its metabolism. Excretion of flurbiprofen is 88% to 98% complete 24 hours after the last dose.

Flurbiprofen is extensively metabolized and excreted primarily in the urine, about 20% as free and conjugated drug and about 50% as hydroxylated metabolites. About 90% of the flurbiprofen in urine is present as conjugates. The major metabolite, 4′-hydroxyl-flurbiprofen, has been detected in human plasma, but in animal models of inflammation this metabolite showed little anti-inflammatory activity. Flurbiprofen is more than 99% bound to human serum proteins. The average maximum serum concentration of flurbiprofen, following a 100 mg oral dose of ANSAID Tablets in normal volunteers (n=184), was 15.2 μg/ml, with 90% of the values between 10 and 22 μg/ml. In geriatric subjects (n=7) be-

tween the ages of 58 and 77 years, 100 mg ANSAID Tablets resulted in an average peak drug level of 18.0 μg/ml and an average elimination half-life of 6.5 hours (range 3–10 hours). In geriatric rheumatoid arthritis patients (n=13) between the ages of 65 and 83 years receiving 100 mg ANSAID Tablets, the average maximum blood level was 12.7 μg/ml and the average elimination half-life was 5.6 hours (range 4–10 hours).

In a study assessing flurbiprofen pharmacokinetics in end stage renal disease (ESRD), mean urinary recovery of a 100 mg dose was 73% in 48 hours for 9 normal subjects and 17% in 96 hours for 8 ESRD patients undergoing continuous ambulatory peritoneal dialysis. Plasma concentrations of flurbiprofen were about 40% lower in the ESRD patients; the elimination half-life of flurbiprofen was unchanged. Elimination of the 4′-hydroxy-flurbiprofen metabolite was markedly reduced in the ESRD patients. The pharmacokinetics of flurbiprofen in patients with decreased renal function but not ESRD have not been determined.

The pharmacokinetics of flurbiprofen in patients with hepatic disease have not been determined.

The efficacy of ANSAID has been demonstrated in patients with rheumatoid arthritis and osteoarthritis. Using standard assessments of therapeutic response, ANSAID (200–300 mg/day) demonstrated effectiveness comparable to aspirin (2000–4000 mg/day), ibuprofen (2400–3200 mg/day), and indomethacin (75–150 mg/day).

In patients with rheumatoid arthritis, ANSAID may be used in combination with gold salts or corticosteroids.

INDICATIONS AND USAGE

ANSAID Tablets are indicated for the acute or long-term treatment of the signs and symptoms of rheumatoid arthritis and osteoarthritis.

CONTRAINDICATIONS

ANSAID Tablets are contraindicated in patients who have previously demonstrated hypersensitivity to it. ANSAID should not be given to patients in whom ANSAID, aspirin, or other nonsteroidal anti-inflammatory drugs induce asthma, urticaria, or other allergic-type reactions. Fatal asthmatic reactions have been reported in such patients receiving this type of drug.

WARNINGS

Risk of Gastrointestinal (GI) Ulcerations, Bleeding and Perforation with Nonsteroidal Anti-inflammatory Therapy

Serious gastrointestinal toxicity, such as bleeding, ulceration, and perforation, can occur at any time, with or without warning symptoms, in patients treated chronically with nonsteroidal anti-inflammatory drugs. Although minor upper GI problems, such as dyspepsia, are common, usually developing early in therapy, physicians should remain alert for ulceration and bleeding in patients treated chronically with nonsteroidal anti-inflammatory drugs, even in the absence of previous GI tract symptoms. In patients observed in clinical trials of such agents for several months to two years, symptomatic upper GI ulcers, gross bleeding, or perforation appear to occur in approximately 1% of patients treated for 3–6 months, and in about 2–4% of patients treated for one year. Physicians should inform patients about the signs and/or symptoms of serious GI toxicity and what steps to take if they occur.

Studies to date have not identified any subset of patients not at risk of developing peptic ulceration and bleeding. Except for a prior history of serious GI events and other risk factors known to be associated with peptic ulcer disease, such as alcoholism, smoking, etc., no risk factors (e.g., age, sex) have been associated with increased risk. Elderly or debilitated patients seem to tolerate ulceration or bleeding less well than other individuals and most spontaneous reports of fatal GI events are in this population. Studies to date are inconclusive concerning the relative risk of various nonsteroidal anti-inflammatory agents in causing such reactions. High doses of any such agent probably carry a greater risk of these reactions, although controlled clinical trials showing this do not exist in most cases. In considering the use of relatively large doses (within the recommended dosage range), sufficient benefit should be anticipated to off-set the potential increased risk of GI toxicity.

Because serious GI tract ulceration and bleeding can occur without warning symptoms, physicians should follow chronically treated patients for the signs and symptoms of ulceration and bleeding and should inform the patients of the importance of this follow-up.

Continued on next page

Information on these Upjohn products is based on labeling in effect September 1, 1989. Further information concerning these and other Upjohn products may be obtained by direct inquiry to Medical Information, The Upjohn Company, Kalamazoo, Michigan 49001.

Upjohn—Cont.

PRECAUTIONS

General Precautions

Impaired Renal or Hepatic Function: As with other nonsteroidal anti-inflammatory drugs, ANSAID Tablets should be used with caution in patients with impaired renal or hepatic function, or a history of kidney or liver disease. Studies to assess the pharmacokinetics of ANSAID in patients with decreased liver function have not been done.

Renal Effects: Toxicology studies in rats have shown renal papillary necrosis at dosage levels equivalent on a mg/kg basis to those used clinically in humans. Similar findings were seen in monkeys given high doses (50–100 mg/kg, or approximately 20–40 times the human therapeutic dose) for 90 days.

In Upjohn clinical studies, kidney function tests were done at least monthly in patients taking ANSAID. In these studies, renal effects of ANSAID were similar to those seen with other nonsteroidal anti-inflammatory drugs.

A second form of renal toxicity has been seen in patients with prerenal conditions leading to a reduction in renal blood flow or blood volume, where the renal prostaglandins have a supportive role in the maintenance of renal perfusion. In these patients administration of a nonsteroidal anti-inflammatory drug may cause a dose-dependent reduction in prostaglandin formation, which may precipitate overt renal decompensation. Patients at greatest risk of this reaction are those with renal function, heart failure, liver dysfunction, those taking diuretics, and the elderly. Discontinuation of nonsteroidal anti-inflammatory drug therapy is typically followed by recovery of the pretreatment state. Those patients at high risk who chronically take ANSAID should have renal function monitored if they have signs or symptoms that may be consistent with renal azotemia, such as malaise, fatigue, loss of appetite, etc. Occasional patients may develop some elevation of serum creatinine and BUN levels without signs or symptoms.

The elimination half-life of flurbiprofen was unchanged in patients with end stage renal disease (ESRD). Flurbiprofen metabolites are primarily eliminated by the kidneys and elimination of 4-hydroxy-flurbiprofen was markedly reduced in ESRD patients. Therefore, patients with significantly impaired renal function may require a reduction of dosage to avoid accumulation of flurbiprofen metabolites and should be monitored. (See also the CLINICAL PHARMACOLOGY section.)

Liver Tests: As with other nonsteroidal anti-inflammatory drugs, borderline elevations of one or more liver tests may occur in up to 15% of patients. These abnormalities may progress, may remain essentially unchanged, or may disappear with continued therapy. The ALT (SGPT) test is probably the most sensitive indicator of liver injury. Meaningful (3 times the upper limit of normal) elevations of ALT or AST (SGOT) have been reported in controlled clinical trials in less than 1% of patients. A patient with symptoms and/or signs suggesting liver dysfunction, or in whom an abnormal liver test has occurred, should be evaluated for evidence of the development of a more severe hepatic reaction while on therapy with flurbiprofen.

Anemia: Anemia is commonly observed in rheumatoid arthritis and is sometimes aggravated by nonsteroidal anti-inflammatory drugs, which may produce fluid retention or minor gastrointestinal blood loss in some patients. Therefore, patients who have initial hemoglobin values of 10 g/dL or less, and who are to receive long-term therapy, should have hemoglobin values determined periodically.

Fluid Retention and Edema: Fluid retention and edema have been reported; therefore, ANSAID should be used with caution in patients with cardiac decompensation, hypertension, or similar conditions.

Vision Changes: Blurred and/or diminished vision has been reported with the use of ANSAID and other nonsteroidal anti-inflammatory drugs. Patients experiencing eye complaints should have ophthalmologic examinations.

Effect on Platelets and Coagulation: Flurbiprofen inhibits collagen-induced platelet aggregation. Prolongation of bleeding time by flurbiprofen has been demonstrated in humans after single and multiple oral doses. Patients who may be adversely affected by prolonged bleeding time should be carefully observed when ANSAID is administered.

Information for Patients: ANSAID, like other drugs of its class, is not free of side effects. The side effects of these drugs can cause discomfort and, rarely, there are more serious side effects, such as gastrointestinal bleeding, which may result in hospitalization and even fatal outcomes. Nonsteroidal anti-inflammatory drugs are often essential agents in the management of arthritis, but they also may be commonly employed for conditions which are less serious. Physicians may wish to discuss with their patients the potential risks (see WARNINGS, PRECAUTIONS, and ADVERSE REACTIONS sections) and likely benefits of nonsteroidal anti-inflammatory drug treatment, particularly when the drugs are used for less serious conditions where treatment without

such agents may represent an acceptable alternative to both the patient and the physician.

Drug Interactions

Antacids: Administration of ANSAID to volunteers under fasting conditions, or with antacid suspension, yielded similar serum flurbiprofen-time profiles in young subjects (n=12). In geriatric subjects (n=7) there was a reduction in the rate but not the extent of flurbiprofen absorption.

Anticoagulants: Flurbiprofen, like other nonsteroidal anti-inflammatory drugs, has been shown to affect bleeding parameters in patients receiving anticoagulants, and serious clinical bleeding has been reported. The physician should be cautious when administering ANSAID to patients taking anticoagulants.

Aspirin: Concurrent administration of aspirin and flurbiprofen resulted in 50% lower serum flurbiprofen concentrations. This effect of aspirin (which also lowers serum concentrations of other nonsteroidal anti-inflammatory drugs given with it) has been demonstrated in patients with rheumatoid arthritis (n=15) as well as normal volunteers (n=16). Concurrent use of ANSAID and aspirin is therefore not recommended.

Beta-adrenergic Blocking Agents: The effect of flurbiprofen on blood pressure response to propranolol and atenolol was evaluated in men with mild uncomplicated hypertension (n=10). Flurbiprofen pretreatment attenuated the hypotensive effect of a single dose of propranolol but not atenolol. Flurbiprofen did not appear to affect the beta-blocker-mediated reduction in heart rate. Flurbiprofen did not affect the pharmacokinetic profile of either drug, and the mechanism underlying the interference with propranolol's hypotensive effect is unknown. Patients taking both flurbiprofen and a beta-blocker should be monitored to ensure that a satisfactory hypotensive effect is achieved.

Cimetidine, Ranitidine: In normal volunteers (n=9), pretreatment with cimetidine or ranitidine did not affect flurbiprofen pharmacokinetics, except that a small (13%) but statistically significant increase in the area under the serum concentration curve of flurbiprofen resulted with cimetidine.

Digoxin: Studies of concomitant administration of flurbiprofen and digoxin to healthy men (n=14) did not show a change in the steady state serum levels of either drug.

Diuretics: Studies in normal volunteers have shown that flurbiprofen, like other nonsteroidal anti-inflammatory drugs, can interfere with the effects of furosemide. Although results have varied from study to study, effects have been shown on furosemide-stimulated diuresis, natriuresis, and kaliuresis. Other nonsteroidal anti-inflammatory drugs that inhibit prostaglandin synthesis have been shown to interfere with thiazide diuretics in some studies, and with potassium-sparing diuretics. Patients receiving ANSAID and furosemide or other diuretics should be observed closely to determine if the desired effect is obtained.

Oral Hypoglycemia Agents: In one study, flurbiprofen was given to adult diabetics who were already receiving glyburide (n=4), metformin (n=2), chlorpropamide with phenformin (n=3), or glyburide with phenformin (n=6). Although there was a slight reduction in blood sugar concentrations during concomitant administration of flurbiprofen and hypoglycemic agents, there were no signs or symptoms of hypoglycemia.

Carcinogenesis, Mutagenesis, impairment of Fertility

An 80-week study in mice at doses of 2, 5, and 12/mg/kg/day and a 2-year study in rats at doses of 0.5, 2, and 4 mg/kg/day did not show evidence of carcinogenicity at maximum tolerated doses of flurbiprofen.

Flurbiprofen did not impair the fertility of male or female rats treated orally at 2.25 mg/kg/day for 65 days and 16 days, respectively, before mating.

Teratogenic Effects: Pregnancy Category B

In teratology studies flurbiprofen, given to mice in doses up to 12 mg/kg/day, to rats in doses up to 25 mg/kg/day, and to rabbits in doses up to 7.5 mg/kg/day, showed no teratogenic effects.

Because there re no adequate and well-controlled studies in pregnant women, and animal teratology studies do not always predict human response, ANSAID is not recommended for use in pregnancy.

Labor and Delivery: The effects of ANSAID on labor and delivery in women are not known. As with other drugs known to inhibit prostaglandin synthesis, an increased incidence of dystocia and delayed parturition occurred in rats treated throughout pregnancy. Because of the known effects of prostaglandin-inhibiting drugs on the fetal cardiovascular system (closure of the ductus arteriosus), use of ANSAID during late pregnancy is not recommended.

Nursing Mothers: Concentrations of flurbiprofen in breast milk and plasma of nursing mothers suggested that a nursing infant could receive approximately 0.10 mg flurbiprofen per day in the established milk of a woman taking 200 mg/day. Because of possible adverse effects of prostaglandin-inhibiting drugs on neonates, ANSAID is not recommended for use in nursing mothers.

Pediatric Use: Safety and effectiveness in children have not been established.

ADVERSE REACTIONS

Adverse reaction information was derived from patients who received flurbiprofen in blinded-controlled and open-label clinical trials, and from worldwide marketing experience and from publications. In the description below, rates of the more common events (greater than 1%) and many of the less common events (less than 1%) represent clinical study results. For rarer events that were derived principally from worldwide marketing experience and the literature (printed in *italics*), accurate rate estimates are generally impossible. Of the 4123 patients in premarketing studies, 2954 were treated for at least 1 month, 1448 for at least 3 months, 948 for at least 6 months, 356 for at least 1 year, and 100 for at least 2 years. Of the 4123 patients, 9.4% dropped out of the studies because of an adverse drug reaction, principally involving the gastrointestinal tract (5.8%) central nervous system and special senses (1.4%), skin (0.6%) and genitourinary tract (0.5%).

Incidence Greater Than 1%

An asterisk after a reaction identifies reactions which occurred in 3–9% of patients treated with flurbiprofen. Reactions occurring in 1–3% of the patients are unmarked.

Gastrointestinal: Dyspepsia*, diarrhea*, abdominal pain*, nausea*, constipation, GI bleeding, flatulence, elevated liver enzymes, and vomiting.

Central Nervous System: Headache*, nervousness, and other manifestations of CNS "stimulation" (e.g., anxiety, insomnia, reflexes increased, and tremor), and symptoms associated with CNS "inhibition" (e.g., amnesia, asthenia, somnolence, malaise, and depression).

Respiratory: Rhinitis.

Dermatological: Rash.

Special Senses: Dizziness, tinnitus, and changes in vision.

Genitourinary: Signs and symptoms suggesting urinary tract infection*.

Body as a Whole: Edema*.

Metabolic/Nutritional: Body weight changes.

Incidence Less than 1%

(Causal Relationship Probable)

The reactions listed in this category occurred in <1% of patients in the clinical trials or were reported during postmarketing experience from other countries. Adverse reactions reported only in worldwide postmarketing experience or the literture (which presumably indicates that they are rarer) are italicized.

Gastrointestinal: Peptic ulcer disease (see also WARNINGS, Risk of Gastrointestinal (GI) Ulcerations, Bleeding and Perforation with Nonsteroidal Anti-inflammatory Therapy), gastritis, bloody diarrhea, stomatitis, esophageal disease, hematemesis, and hepatitis; *cholestatic and non-cholestatic jaundice.*

Central Nervous System: Ataxia, cerebrovascular ischemia, confusion, parethesia, and twitching.

Hematologic: Decrease in hemoglobin and hematocrit, iron deficiency anemia, *hemolytic anemia* and *aplastic anemia;* leukopenia; eosinophilia; ecchymosis and *thrombocytopenia.* (See also PRECAUTIONS, Effect On Platelets and Coagulation.)

Respiratory: Asthma and epistaxis.

Dermatological: Angioedema, urticaria, eczema, and pruritus; *photosensitivity, toxic epidermal necrolysis,* and *exfoliative dermatitis.*

Special Senses: Conjunctivitis and parosmia.

Genitourinary: Hematuria and renal failure; *interstititial nephritis.*

Body as a Whole: Chills and fever; *anaphylactic reaction.*

Metabolic/Nutritional: Hyperuricemia.

Cardiovascular: Heart failure, hypertension, vascular diseases and vasodilation.

Incidence Less than 1% (Causal Relationship Unknown)

The following reactions have been reported in patients taking flurbiprofen under circumstances that do not permit a clear attribution of the reaction to flurbiprofen. These reactions are being included as alerting information for physicians. Adverse reactions reported only in worldwide postmarketing experience or the literature (which presumably indicates that they are rarer) are italicized.

Gastrointestinal: Periodontal abscess, appetite changes, cholecystitis, and dry mouth.

Central Nervous System: Convulsion, meningitis, hypertonia, cerebrovascular accident, emotional lability, and subarachnoid hemorrhage.

Hematologic: Lymphadenopathy.

Respiratory: Bronchitis, laryngitis, dyspnea, pulmonary embolism, pulmonary infarct, and hyperventilation.

Dermatological: Alopecia, nail disorder, herpes simplex, zoster, dry skin, and sweating.

Special Senses: Ear disease, corneal opacity, glaucoma, retrobulbar neuritis, changes in taste, and transient hearing loss; *retinal hemorrhage.*

Genitourinary: Menstrual disturbances, vaginal and uterine hemorrhage, vulvovaginitis, and prostate disease.

Metabolic/Nutritional: Hyperkalemia.

Cardiovascular: Arrhythmias, angina pectoris, and myocardial infarction.

Musculoskeletal: Myasthenia.

DRUG ABUSE AND DEPENDENCE

No drug abuse or drug dependence has been observed with ANSAID.

OVERDOSAGE

Information on overdosage is available for 13 children and 12 adults. Nine of the 13 children were less than 6 years old. Drowsiness occurred after doses of 150 to 800 mg in 3 of these young children (with dilated pupils in 1), and in a 2-year-old who also had semi-consciousness, pinpoint pupils, diminished tone, and elevated liver enzymes. Other children who ingested doses of 200 mg to 2.5 g showed no symptoms.

Among the adults, a 70-year-old man with a history of chronic obstructive airway disease died. Toxicological analysis showed acute flurbiprofen overdose and a blood ethanol concentration of 100 mg/dL. In the other cases, symptoms were as follows: coma and respiratory depression after 3–6 g; drowsiness, nausea and epigastric pain after 2.5–5 g; epigastric pain and dizziness after 3 g; headache and nausea after ≤2 g; agitation after 1.5 g; and drowsiness after 1.0 g. One patient, who took 200–400 mg flurbiprofen and 2.4 g fenoprofen, had disorientation and diplopia. Three adults had no symptoms after 3–5 g flurbiprofen.

Treatment of an overdose: the stomach should be emptied by vomiting or lavage, though little drug will likely be recovered if more than an hour has elapsed since ingestion. Supportive treatment should be instituted as necessary. Some patients have been given supplemental oral or intravenous fluids and required no other treatment.

In mice, the flurbiprofen LD_{50} was 750 mg/kg when administered orally and 200 mg/kg when administered intraperitoneally. The primary signs of toxicity were prostration, ataxia, loss of righting reflex, labored respiration, twitches, convulsions, CNS depression, and splayed hind limbs. In rats, the flurbiprofen LD_{50} was 160 mg/kg when administered orally and 400 mg/kg when administered intraperitoneally. The primary signs of toxicity were tremors, convulsions, labored respiration, and prostration. These were observed mostly in the intraperitoneal studies.

DOSAGE AND ADMINISTRATION

ANSAID Tablets are administered orally.

Rheumatoid arthritis and osteoarthritis: Recommended starting dose is 200 to 300 mg total daily dose administered BID, TID, or QID. (Most experience in rheumatoid arthritis has been with TID or QID dosage.) The largest recommended single dose in a multiple-dose daily regimen is 100 mg. The dose should be tailored to each patient according to the severity of the symptoms and the response to therapy.

Although a few patients have received higher doses, doses above 300 mg per day are not recommended until more clinical experience with ANSAID is obtained.

HOW SUPPLIED

ANSAID Tablets 50 mg (white)
- Bottles of 100   NDC 0009-0170-07
- Bottles of 500   NDC 0009-0170-09
- Unit Dose (blister pack)
  packages of 100   NDC 0009-0170-08

ANSAID Tablets 100 mg (blue)
- Bottles of 100   NDC 0009-0305-03
- Bottles of 500   NDC 0009-0305-05
- Unit Dose (blister pack)
  packages of 100   NDC 0009-0305-06

Store at controlled room temperature 15°-30°C (59°-86°F).

Code 813 094 001

Shown in Product Identification Section, page 433

BACIGUENT® Antibiotic Ointment

(See PDR For Nonprescription Drugs)

CHERACOL D® Cough Formula

(See PDR For Nonprescription Drugs)

CHERACOL PLUS® Head Cold/Cough Formula

(See PDR For Nonprescription Drugs)

CITROCARBONATE® Antacid

(See PDR For Nonprescription Drugs)

CLEOCIN HCl®   ℞
brand of clindamycin hydrochloride capsules, USP

    150 mg (100's):
    NSN 6505-00-159-4892 (M)

<table>
<tr><td>

WARNING

Clindamycin therapy has been associated with severe colitis which may end fatally. Therefore, it should be reserved for serious infections where less toxic antimicrobial agents are inappropriate, as described in the Indications section. It should not be used in patients with nonbacterial infections, such as most upper respiratory tract infections. Studies indicate a toxin(s) produced by *Clostridia* is one primary cause of antibiotic associated colitis. Cholestyramine and colestipol resins have been shown to bind the toxin *in vitro*. See WARNINGS section. The colitis is usually characterized by severe, persistent diarrhea and severe abdominal cramps and may be associated with the passage of blood and mucus. Endoscopic examination may reveal pseudomembranous colitis. Stool culture for *Clostridium difficile* and stool assay for *C. difficile* toxin may be helpful diagnostically.

When significant diarrhea occurs, the drug should be discontinued or, if necessary, continued only with close observation of the patient. Large bowel endoscopy has been recommended.

Antiperistaltic agents such as opiates and diphenoxylate with atropine (Lomotil) may prolong and/or worsen the condition. Vancomycin has been found to be effective in the treatment of antibiotic associated pseudomembranous colitis produced by *Clostridium difficile*. The usual adult dosage is 500 milligrams to 2 grams of vancomycin orally per day in three to four divided doses administered for 7 to 10 days. Cholestyramine or colestipol resins bind vancomycin *in vitro*. If both a resin and vancomycin are to be administered concurrently, it may be advisable to separate the time of administration of each drug.

Diarrhea, colitis, and pseudomembranous colitis have been observed to begin up to several weeks following cessation of therapy with clindamycin.

</td></tr>
</table>

DESCRIPTION

Clindamycin hydrochloride is the hydrated hydrochloride salt of clindamycin. Clindamycin is a semisynthetic antibiotic produced by a 7(S)-chloro-substitution of the 7(R)-hydroxyl group of the parent compound lincomycin.

CLEOCIN HCL Capsules contain clindamycin hydrochloride equivalent to 75 mg, 150 mg or 300 mg of clindamycin. Inactive ingredients: **75 mg**—corn starch, erythrosine sodium, FD&C blue no. 1, FD&C yellow no. 5, gelatin, lactose, magnesium stearate and talc; **150 mg**—corn starch, erythrosine sodium, FD&C blue no. 1, FD&C yellow no. 5, gelatin, lactose, magnesium stearate, talc and titanium dioxide; **300 mg**—corn starch, erythrosine sodium, FD&C blue no. 1, gelatin, lactose, magnesium, stearate, talc and titanium dioxide. The chemical name for clindamycin hydrochloride is Methyl 7-chloro-6, 7, 8-trideoxy-6-(1-methyl-*trans*-4-propyl-L-2-pyrrolidinecarboxamido)-1-thio-L-*threo*-α-D-galacto-octopyranoside monohydrochloride.

CLINICAL PHARMACOLOGY

Microbiology: Clindamycin has been shown to have *in vitro* activity against isolates of the following organisms:
Aerobic gram-positive cocci, including:
    Staphylococcus aureus
    Staphylococcus epidermidis
    (penicillinase and nonpenicillinase producing strains). When tested by *in vitro* methods some staphylococcal strains originally resistant to erythromycin rapidly develop resistance to clindamycin.
    Streptococci (except *Streptococcus faecalis*)
    Pneumococci
Anaerobic gram-negative bacilli, including:
    Bacteroides species (including *Bacteroides fragilis* group and *Bacteroides melaninogenicus* group)
    Fusobacterium species
Anaerobic gram-positive nonsporeforming bacilli, including;
    Propionibacterium
    Eubacterium
    Actinomyces species
Anaerobic and microaerophilic gram-positive cocci, including:
    Peptococcus species
    Peptostreptococcus species
    Microaerophilic streptococci
    Clostridia: Clostridia are more resistant than most anaerobes to clindamycin. Most *Clostridium perfringens* are susceptible, but other species, eg, *Clostridium sporogenes* and *Clostridium tertium*, are frequently resistant to clindamycin. Susceptibility testing should be done.

Cross resistance has been demonstrated between clindamycin and lincomycin.

Antagonism has been demonstrated between clindamycin and erythromycin.

Human Pharmacology. Serum level studies with a 150 mg oral dose of clindamycin hydrochloride in 24 normal adult volunteers showed that clindamycin was rapidly absorbed after oral administration. An average peak serum level of 2.50 mcg/ml was reached in 45 minutes; serum levels averaged 1.51 mcg/ml at 3 hours and 0.70 mcg/ml at 6 hours. Absorption of an oral dose is virtually complete (90%), and the concomitant administration of food does not appreciably modify the serum concentrations; serum levels have been uniform and predictable from person to person and dose to dose. Serum level studies following multiple doses of CLEOCIN HCL Capsules (clindamycin hydrochloride) for up to 14 days show no evidence of accumulation or altered metabolism of drug.

Serum half-life of clindamycin is increased slightly in patients with markedly reduced renal function. Hemodialysis and peritoneal dialysis are not effective in removing clindamycin from the serum.

Concentrations of clindamycin in the serum increased linearly with increased dose. Serum levels exceed the MIC (minimum inhibitory concentration) for most indicated organisms for at least six hours following administration of the usually recommended doses. Clindamycin is widely distributed in body fluids and tissues (including bones). The average biological half-life is 2.4 hours. Approximately 10% of the bio-activity is excreted in the urine and 3.6% in the feces; the remainder is excreted as bio-inactive metabolites.

Doses of up to 2 grams of clindamycin per day for 14 days have been well tolerated by healthy volunteers, except that the incidence of gastrointestinal side effects is greater with the higher doses.

No significant levels of clindamycin are attained in the cerebrospinal fluid, even in the presence of inflamed meninges.

INDICATIONS AND USAGE

Clindamycin is indicated in the treatment of serious infections caused by susceptible anaerobic bacteria.

Clindamycin is also indicated in the treatment of serious infections due to susceptible strains of streptococci, pneumococci, and staphylococci. Its use should be reserved for penicillin-allergic patients or other patients for whom, in the judgment of the physician, a penicillin is inappropriate. Because of the risk of colitis, as described in the WARNING box, before selecting clindamycin the physician should consider the nature of the infection and the suitability of less toxic alternatives (eg, erythromycin).

Anaerobes: Serious respiratory tract infections such as empyema, anaerobic pneumonitis and lung abscess; serious skin and soft tissue infections; septicemia; intra-abdominal infections such as peritonitis and intra-abdominal abscess (typically resulting from anaerobic organisms resident in the normal gastrointestinal tract); infections of the female pelvis and genital tract such as endometritis, nongonococcal tubo-ovarian abscess, pelvic cellulitis and postsurgical vaginal cuff infection.

Streptococci: Serious respiratory tract infections; serious skin and soft tissue infections.

Staphylococci: Serious respiratory tract infections; serious skin and soft tissue infections.

Pneumococci: Serious respiratory tract infections.

Bacteriologic studies should be performed to determine the causative organisms and their susceptibility to clindamycin.

In Vitro Susceptibility Testing: A standardized disk testing procedure[*] is recommended for determining susceptibility of aerobic bacteria to clindamycin. A description is contained in the CLEOCIN® Susceptibility Disk (clindamycin) insert. Using this method, the laboratory can designate isolates as resistant, intermediate, or susceptible. Tube or agar dilution methods may be used for both anaerobic and aerobic bacteria. When the directions in the CLEOCIN® Susceptibility Powder insert are followed, an MIC of 1.6 mcg/ml may be considered susceptible; MICs of 1.6 to 4.8 mcg/ml may be considered intermediate and MICs greater than 4.8 mcg/ml may be considered resistant.

[*]Bauer, AW, Kirby, WMM, Sherris, JC, et al; Antibiotic susceptibility testing by a standardized single disc method, *Am J Clin Path* 45:493-496, 1966. Standardized disc susceptibility test, *Federal Register* 37:20527-29, 1972.

CLEOCIN Susceptibility Disks 2 mcg. See package insert for use.

CLEOCIN Susceptibility Powder 20 mg. See package insert for use.

For anaerobic bacteria the minimal inhibitory concentration (MIC) of clindamycin can be determined by agar dilution and broth dilution (including microdilution) techniques. If MICs are not determined routinely, the disk broth method is recommended for routine use. THE KIRBY-BAUER DISK DIFFUSION METHOD AND ITS INTERPRETIVE STANDARDS ARE NOT RECOMMENDED FOR ANAEROBES.

Continued on next page

Information on these Upjohn products is based on labeling in effect September 1, 1989. Further information concerning these and other Upjohn products may be obtained by direct inquiry to Medical Information, The Upjohn Company, Kalamazoo, Michigan 49001.

Upjohn—Cont.

CONTRAINDICATIONS

CLEOCIN HCL Capsules (clindamycin hydrochloride) are contraindicated in individuals with a history of hypersensitivity to preparations containing clindamycin or lincomycin.

WARNINGS

See WARNING box. Studies indicate a toxin(s) produced by *Clostridia* is one primary cause of antibiotic associated colitis.[1-5] Cholestyramine and colestipol resins have been shown to bind the toxin *in vitro*. Mild cases of colitis may respond to drug discontinuance alone. Moderate to severe cases should be managed with fluid, electrolyte and protein supplementation as indicated. Vancomycin has been found to be effective in the treatment of antibiotic associated pseudomembranous colitis produced by *Clostridial difficile*. The usual adult dosage is 500 milligrams to 2 grams of vancomycin orally per day in three to four divided doses administered for 7 to 10 days. Cholestyramine or colestipol resins bind vancomycin *in vitro*. If both a resin and vancomycin are to be administered concurrently, it may be advisable to separate the time of administration of each drug. Systemic corticoids and corticoid retention enemas may help relieve the colitis. Other causes of colitis should also be considered.

A careful inquiry should be made concerning previous sensitivities to drugs and other allergens.

Usage in Pregnancy - Safety for use in pregnancy has not been established.

Usage in Newborns and Infants: When CLEOCIN HCL Capsules (clindamycin hydrochloride) are administered to newborns and infants, appropriate monitoring of organ system functions is desirable.

Nursing Mothers—Clindamycin has been reported to appear in breast milk in ranges of 0.7 to 3.8 mcg/ml.

Usage in Meningitis: Since clindamycin does not diffuse adequately into the cerebrospinal fluid, the drug should not be used in the treatment of meningitis.

Antagonism has been demonstrated between clindamycin and erythromycin *in vitro*. Because of possible clinical significance, these two drugs should not be administered concurrently.

1. Bartlett JG, et al: Antibiotic associated Pseudomembranous Colitis Due to Toxin-producing *Clostridia. N Engl J Med* 298(10):531-534, 1978.
2. George RH, et al: Identification of *Clostridium difficile* as a cause of Pseudomembranous Colitis. *Br Med J* 6114:669-671, 1978.
3. Larson HE, Price AB: Pseudomembranous Colitis Presence of Clostridial Toxin, *Lancet* 8052/3:1312-1314, 1977.
4. Rifkin GD, Fekety FR, Silva J: Antibiotic-induced Colitis Implication of a Toxin Neutralized by *Clostridium sordellii* Antitoxin. *Lancet* 8048:1103-1106, 1977.
5. Bailey WR, Scott EG: Diagnostic Microbiology. The CV Mosby Company, St. Louis, 1978.

PRECAUTIONS

Review of experience to date suggests that a subgroup of older patients with associated severe illness may tolerate diarrhea less well. When clindamycin is indicated in these patients, they should be carefully monitored for change in bowel frequency.

CLEOCIN HCL Capsules (clindamycin hydrochloride) should be prescribed with caution in individuals with a history of gastrointestinal disease, particularly colitis.

CLEOCIN HCL should be prescribed with caution in atopic individuals.

During prolonged therapy, periodic liver and kidney function tests and blood counts should be performed.

Indicated surgical procedures should be performed in conjunction with antibiotic therapy.

The use of CLEOCIN HCL occasionally results in overgrowth of nonsusceptible organisms—particularly yeasts. Should superinfections occur, appropriate measures should be taken as indicated by the clinical situation.

Patients with very severe renal disease and/or very severe hepatic disease accompanied by severe metabolic aberrations should be dosed with caution, and serum clindamycin levels monitored during high-dose therapy.

Clindamycin has been shown to have neuromuscular blocking properties that may enhance the action of other neuromuscular blocking agents. Therefore, it should be used with caution in patients receiving such agents.

The 75 mg and 150 mg capsules contain FD&C Yellow No. 5 (tartrazine) which may cause allergic-type reactions (including bronchial asthma) in certain susceptible individuals. Although the overall incidence of FD&C Yellow No. 5 (tartrazine) sensitivity in the general population is low, it is frequently seen in patients who also have aspirin hypersensitivity.

ADVERSE REACTIONS

The following reactions have been reported with the use of clindamycin.

Gastrointestinal: Abdominal pain, esophagitis, nausea, vomiting and diarrhea. (See **Warning** Box)

Hypersensitivity Reactions: Maculopapular rash and urticaria have been observed during drug therapy. Generalized mild to moderate morbilliform-like skin rashes are the most frequently reported of all adverse reactions. Rare instances of erythema multiforme, some resembling Stevens-Johnson syndrome, have been associated with clindamycin. A few cases of anaphylactoid reactions have been reported. If a hypersensitivity reaction occurs, the drug should be discontinued. The usual agents (epinephrine, corticosteroids, antihistamines) should be available for emergency treatment of serious reactions.

Liver: Jaundice and abnormalities in liver function tests have been observed during clindamycin therapy.

Renal: Although no direct relationship of clindamycin to renal damage has been established, renal dysfunction as evidenced by azotemia, oliguria, and/or proteinuria has been observed in rare instances.

Hematopoietic: Transient neutropenia (leukopenia) and eosinophilia have been reported. Reports of agranulocytosis and thrombocytopenia have been made. No direct etiologic relationship to concurrent clindamycin therapy could be made in any of the foregoing.

Musculoskeletal: Rare instances of polyarthritis have been reported.

DOSAGE AND ADMINISTRATION

If significant diarrhea occurs during therapy, this antibiotic should be discontinued. (See **Warning** box).

Adults: *Serious infections*—150 to 300 mg every 6 hours. *More severe infections*—300 to 450 mg every 6 hours.

Children: *Serious infections*—8 to 16 mg/kg/day (4 to 8 mg/lb/day) divided into three or four equal doses. *More severe infections*—16 to 20 mg/kg/day (8 to 10 mg/lb/day) divided into three or four equal doses.

To avoid the possibility of esophageal irritation, CLEOCIN HCL Capsules (clindamycin hydrochloride) should be taken with a full glass of water.

Serious infections due to anaerobic bacteria are usually treated with CLEOCIN PHOSPHATE® Sterile Solution (clindamycin phosphate). However, in clinically appropriate circumstances, the physician may elect to initiate treatment or continue treatment with CLEOCIN HCl Capsules.

In cases of β-hemolytic streptococcal infections, treatment should continue for at least 10 days.

HOW SUPPLIED

CLEOCIN HCL Capsules (clindamycin hydrochloride) are available in the following strengths, colors and sizes:

75 mg Lavender:

Bottles of 100	NDC 0009-0331-02

150 mg Lavender and Maroon:

Bottles of 16	NDC 0009-0225-01
Bottles of 100	NDC 0009-0225-02
Unit Dose Package (100)	NDC 0009-0225-03

300 mg Maroon:

Bottles of 16	NDC 0009-0395-13
Bottles of 100	NDC 0009-0395-14
Unit dose package of 100	NDC 0009-0395-02

Store at controlled room temperature 15°–30°C (59°–86°F).

TOXICOLOGY

Animal toxicity studies showed the following:

LD_{50} I.P. Administration—	
Mouse	361 mg/kg
LD_{50} I.V. Administration—	
Mouse	245 mg/kg
LD_{50} Oral Administration—	
Rat	2,618 mg/kg

One year oral toxicity studies in Spartan Sprague-Dawley rats and Beagle dogs at levels of 30, 100 and 300 mg/kg/day (3 grams/day per dog) have shown CLEOCIN HCL to be well tolerated. No appreciable difference in pathological findings has been obtained in CLEOCIN HCL treated groups of animals from comparable control groups. Rats receiving CLEOCIN HCL Capsules (clindamycin hydrochloride) at 600 mg/kg/day for six months tolerated the drug well; however, dogs dosed at this level vomited, would not eat, and lost weight.

Code 810 570 313

Shown in Product Identification Section, page 433

CLEOCIN PEDIATRIC® ℞
brand of clindamycin palmitate hydrochloride flavored granules
(clindamycin palmitate hydrochloride for oral solution, USP)
Not for Injection

crobial agents are inappropriate, as described in the Indications Section. It should not be used in patients with nonbacterial infections, such as most upper respiratory tract infections. Studies indicate a toxin(s) produced by *Clostridia* is one primary cause of antibiotic associated colitis. Cholestyramine and colestipol resins have been shown to bind the toxin *in vitro*. See WARNINGS section. The colitis is usually characterized by severe, persistent diarrhea and severe abdominal cramps and may be associated with the passage of blood and mucus. Endoscopic examination may reveal pseudomembranous colitis. Stool culture for *Clostridium difficile* and stool assay for *C. difficile* toxin may be helpful diagnostically.

When significant diarrhea occurs, the drug should be discontinued or, if necessary, continued only with close observation of the patient. Large bowel endoscopy has been recommended.

Antiperistaltic agents such as opiates and diphenoxylate with atropine (Lomotil) may prolong and/or worsen the condition. Vancomycin has been found to be effective in the treatment of antibiotic associated pseudomembranous colitis produced by *Clostridium difficile*. The usual adult dosage is 500 milligrams to 2 grams of vancomycin orally per day in three to four divided doses administered for 7 to 10 days. Cholestyramine or colestipol resins bind vancomycin *in vitro*. If both a resin and vancomycin are to be administered concurrently, it may be advisable to separate the time of administration of each drug.

Diarrhea, colitis, and pseudomembranous colitis have been observed to begin up to several weeks following cessation of therapy with clindamycin.

DESCRIPTION

Clindamycin palmitate hydrochloride is a water soluble hydrochloride salt of the ester of clindamycin and palmitic acid. Clindamycin is a semisynthetic antibiotic produced by a 7(S)-chloro-substitution of the 7(R)-hydroxyl group of the parent compound lincomycin.

The chemical name for clindamycin palmitate hydrochloride is Methyl 7-chloro-6,7,8-trideoxy-6-(1-methyl-*trans*-4-propyl-L-2-pyrrolidinecarboxamido)-1-thio-L-*threo*-α-D-*galacto*-octopyranoside 2-palmitate monohydrochloride.

CLEOCIN PEDIATRIC Flavored Granules contain clindamycin palmitate hydrochloride for reconstitution. Each 5 ml contains the equivalent of 75 mg clindamycin. Inactive ingredients: artificial cherry flavor, dextrin, ethylparaben, pluronic F68, polymethylsiloxane, sucrose.

CLINICAL PHARMACOLOGY

Microbiology: Although clindamycin palmitate HCl is inactive *in vitro*, rapid *in vivo* hydrolysis converts this compound to the antibacterially active clindamycin.

Clindamycin has been shown to have *in vitro* activity against isolates of the following organisms:

Aerobic gram positive cocci, including:

Staphylococcus aureus
Staphylococcus epidermidis
(penicillinase and non-penicillinase producing strains). When tested by *in vitro* methods some staphylococcal strains originally resistant to erythromycin rapidly develop resistance to clindamycin.
Streptococci (except *Streptococcus faecalis*)
Pneumococci

Anaerobic gram negative bacilli, including:
Bacteroides species (including *Bacteroides fragilis* group and *Bacteroides melaninogenicus* group)
Fusobacterium species

Anaerobic gram positive nonsporeforming bacilli, including:
Propionibacterium
Eubacterium
Actinomyces species

Anaerobic and microaerophilic gram positive cocci, including:
Peptococcus species
Peptostreptococcus species
Microaerophilic streptococci

Clostridia: Clostridia are more resistant than most anaerobes to clindamycin. Most *Clostridium perfringens* are susceptible, but other species, eg, *Clostridium sporogenes* and *Clostridium tertium* are frequently resistant to clindamycin. Susceptibility testing should be done.

Cross resistance has been demonstrated between clindamycin and lincomycin.

Antagonism has been demonstrated between clindamycin and erythromycin.

Human Pharmacology: Blood level studies comparing clindamycin palmitate HCl with clindamycin hydrochloride show that both products reach their peak active serum levels at the same time, indicating a rapid hydrolysis of the palmitate to the clindamycin.

Clindamycin is widely distributed in body fluids and tissues (including bones). Approximately 10% of the biological activity is excreted in the urine. The average biological half-life after doses of clindamycin is approximately two hours in children.

Serum half-life of clindamycin is increased slightly in patients with markedly reduced renal function. Hemodialysis and peritoneal dialysis do not appreciably affect the half-life of clindamycin in the serum.

Serum level studies with clindamycin palmitate HCl in normal children weighing 50-100 lbs given 2, 3 or 4 mg/kg every 6 hours (8, 12 or 16 mg/kg/day) demonstrated mean peak clindamycin serum levels of 1.24, 2.25 and 2.44 mcg/ml respectively, one hour after the first dose. By the fifth dose, the 6-hour serum concentration had reached equilibrium. Peak serum concentrations after this time would be about 2.46, 2.98 and 3.79 mcg/ml with doses of 8, 12, 16 mg/kg/day, respectively. Serum levels have been uniform and predictable from person to person and dose to dose. Multiple-dose studies in newborns and infants up to 6 months of age show that the drug does not accumulate in the serum and is excreted rapidly. Serum levels exceed the MICs for most indicated organisms for at least six hours following administration of the usually recommended doses of CLEOCIN PEDIATRIC in adults and children.

No significant levels of clindamycin are attained in the cerebrospinal fluid, even in the presence of inflamed meninges.

INDICATIONS AND USAGE

CLEOCIN PEDIATRIC Flavored Granules (clindamycin palmitate HCl) are indicated in the treatment of serious infections caused by susceptible anaerobic bacteria.

Clindamycin is also indicated in the treatment of serious infections due to susceptible strains of streptococci, pneumococci, and staphylococci. Its use should be reserved for penicillin-allergic patients or other patients for whom, in the judgment of the physician, a penicillin is inappropriate. Because of the risk of colitis, as described in the WARNING box, before selecting clindamycin the physician should consider the nature of the infection and the suitability of less toxic alternatives (eg, erythromycin).

Anaerobes: Serious respiratory tract infections such as empyema, anaerobic pneumonitis and lung abscess; serious skin and soft tissue infections; septicemia; intra-abdominal infections such as peritonitis and intra-abdominal abscess (typically resulting from anaerobic organisms resident in the normal gastrointestinal tract); infections of the female pelvis and genital tract such as endometritis, nongonococcal tubo-ovarian abscess, pelvic cellulitis and postsurgical vaginal cuff infection.

Streptococci: Serious respiratory tract infections; serious skin and soft tissue infections.

Staphylococci: Serious respiratory tract infections; serious skin and soft tissue infections.

Pneumococci: Serious respiratory tract infections.

Bacteriologic studies should be performed to determine the causative organisms and their susceptibility to clindamycin.

In Vitro Susceptibility Testing: A standardized disk testing procedure* is recommended for determining susceptibility of aerobic bacteria to clindamycin. A description is contained in the CLEOCIN® Susceptibility Disk (clindamycin) insert. Using this method, the laboratory can designate isolates as resistant, intermediate, or susceptible. Tube or agar dilution methods may be used for both anaerobic and aerobic bacteria. When the directions in the CLEOCIN Susceptibility Powder insert are followed, an MIC (minimal inhibitory concentration) of 1.6 mcg/ml may be considered susceptible; MICs of 1.6 to 4.8 mcg/ml may be considered intermediate and MICs greater than 4.8 mcg/ml may be considered resistant.

CLEOCIN Susceptibility Disks 2 mcg. See package insert for use.

CLEOCIN Susceptibility Powder 20 mg. See package insert for use.

For anaerobic bacteria the minimal inhibitory concentration (MIC) of clindamycin can be determined by agar dilution and broth dilution (including microdilution) techniques. If MICs are not determined routinely, the disk broth method is recommended for routine use. THE KIRBY-BAUER DISK DIFFUSION METHOD AND ITS INTERPRETIVE STANDARDS ARE NOT RECOMMENDED FOR ANAEROBES.

*Bauer, AW, Kirby, WMM, Sherris, JC, Turck, M.: Antibiotic susceptibility testing by a standardized single disc method, *Am J Clin Path*, **45**:493-496, 1966. Standardized Disc Susceptibility Test, *Federal Register* **37**:20527-29, 1972.

CONTRAINDICATIONS

This drug is contraindicated in individuals with a history of hypersensitivity to preparations containing clindamycin or lincomycin.

WARNINGS

See WARNING box. Studies indicate a toxin(s) produced by *Clostridia* is one primary cause of antibiotic associated colitis.[1-5] Cholestyramine and colestipol resins have been shown to bind the toxin *in vitro*. Mild cases of colitis may respond to drug discontinuance alone. Moderate to severe cases should be managed promptly with fluid, electrolyte and protein supplementation as indicated. Vancomycin has been found

to be effective in the treatment of antibiotic associated pseudomembranous colitis produced by *Clostridium difficile*. The usual adult dosage is 500 milligrams to 2 grams of vancomycin orally per day in three to four divided doses administered for 7 to 10 days. Cholestyramine or colestipol resins bind vancomycin *in vitro*. If both a resin and vancomycin are to be administered concurrently, it may be advisable to separate the time of administration of each drug. Systemic corticoids and corticoid retention enemas may help relieve the colitis. Other causes of colitis should also be considered.

A careful inquiry should be made concerning previous sensitivities to drugs and other allergens.

Usage in Pregnancy—Safety for use in pregnancy has not been established.

Usage in Newborns and Infants: When CLEOCIN PEDIATRIC Flavored Granules (clindamycin palmitate HCl) are administered to newborns and infants, appropriate monitoring of organ system functions is desirable.

Nursing Mothers—Clindamycin has been reported to appear in breast milk in ranges of 0.7 to 3.8 mcg/ml.

Usage in Meningitis: Since clindamycin does not diffuse adequately into the cerebrospinal fluid, the drug should not be used in the treatment of meningitis.

Antagonism has been demonstrated between clindamycin and erythromycin *in vitro*. Because of possible clinical significance, these two drugs should not be administered concurrently.

1. Bartlett JG, et al: Antibiotic associated Pseudomembranous Colitis Due to Toxin-producing *Clostridia*. *N Engl J Med* 298(10):531-534, 1978.
2. George RH, et al: Identification of *Clostridium difficile* as a cause of Pseudomembranous Colitis. *Br Med J* 6114:669-671, 1978.
3. Larson HE, Price AB: Pseudomembranous Colitis Presence of Clostridial Toxin. *Lancet* 8052/3:1312-1314, 1977.
4. Rifkin GD, Fekety FR, Silva J: Antibiotic-induced Colitis Implication of a Toxin Neutralized by *Clostridium sordellii* Antitoxin. *Lancet* 8048:1103-1106, 1977.
5. Bailey WR, Scott EG: Diagnostic Microbiology. The CV Mosby Company, St. Louis, 1978.

PRECAUTIONS

Review of experience to date suggests that a subgroup of older patients with associated severe illness may tolerate diarrhea less well. When clindamycin is indicated in these patients, they should be carefully monitored for change in bowel frequency.

CLEOCIN PEDIATRIC Flavored Granules (clindamycin palmitate HCl) should be prescribed with caution in individuals with a history of gastrointestinal disease, particularly colitis.

CLEOCIN PEDIATRIC should be prescribed with caution in atopic individuals.

During prolonged therapy periodic liver and kidney function tests and blood counts should be performed.

Indicated surgical procedures should be performed in conjunction with antibiotic therapy.

The use of CLEOCIN PEDIATRIC may result in overgrowth of nonsusceptible organisms—particularly yeasts. Should superinfections occur, appropriate measures should be taken as indicated by the clinical situation.

Patients with very severe renal disease and/or very severe hepatic disease accompanied by severe metabolic aberrations should be dosed with caution, and serum clindamycin levels monitored during high-dose therapy.

Clindamycin has been shown to have neuromuscular blocking properties that may enhance the action of other neuromuscular blocking agents. Therefore, it should be used with caution in patients receiving such agents.

ADVERSE REACTIONS

The following reactions have been reported with the use of clindamycin.

Gastrointestinal: Abdominal pain, nausea, vomiting and diarrhea. (See **Warning** box)

Hypersensitivity Reactions: Maculopapular rash and urticaria have been observed during drug therapy. Generalized mild to moderate morbilliform-like skin rashes are the most frequently reported of all adverse reactions. Rare instances of erythema multiforme, some resembling Stevens-Johnson syndrome, have been associated with clindamycin. A few cases of anaphylactoid reactions have been reported. If a hypersensitivity reaction occurs, the drug should be discontinued. The usual agents (epinephrine, corticosteroids, antihistamines) should be available for emergency treatment of serious reactions.

Liver: Jaundice and abnormalities in liver function tests have been observed during clindamycin therapy.

Renal: Although no direct relationship of clindamycin to renal damage has been established, renal dysfunction as evidenced by azotemia, oliguria, and/or proteinuria has been observed in rare instances.

Hematopoietic: Transient neutropenia (leukopenia) and eosinophilia have been reported. Reports of agranulocytosis and thrombocytopenia have been made. No direct etiologic

relationship to concurrent clindamycin therapy could be made in any of the foregoing.

Musculoskeletal: Rare instances of polyarthritis have been reported.

DOSAGE AND ADMINISTRATION

If significant diarrhea occurs during therapy, this antibiotic should be discontinued. (See **Warning** box.) Concomitant administration of food does not adversely affect the absorption of clindamycin palmitate HCl contained in CLEOCIN PEDIATRIC Flavored Granules.

Serious infections: 8-12 mg/kg/day (4-6 mg/lb/day) divided into 3 or 4 equal doses.

Severe infections: 13-16 mg/kg/day (6.5-8 mg/lb/day) divided into 3 or 4 equal doses.

More severe infections: 17-25 mg/kg/day (8.5-12.5 mg/lb/day) divided into 3 or 4 equal doses.

In children weighing 10 kg or less, ½ teaspoon (37.5 mg) three times a day should be considered the minimum recommended dose.

Serious infections due to anaerobic bacteria are usually treated with CLEOCIN PHOSPHATE® Sterile Solution (clindamycin phosphate). However, in clinically appropriate circumstances, the physician may elect to initiate treatment or continue treatment with CLEOCIN PEDIATRIC.

NOTE: In cases of β-hemolytic streptococcal infections, treatment should be continued for at least 10 days.

Reconstitution instructions:

When reconstituted with water as follows, each 5 ml (teaspoon) of solution contains clindamycin palmitate HCl equivalent to 75 mg clindamycin.

Reconstitute bottles of 100 ml with **75 ml** of water. Add a large portion of the water and shake vigorously; add the remainder of the water and shake until the solution is uniform.

Storage conditions:

Store unreconstituted product at controlled room temperature 15°-30°C (59°-86°F).

Do **NOT** refrigerate the reconstituted solution; when chilled, the solution may thicken and be difficult to pour. The solution is stable for 2 weeks at room temperature.

HOW SUPPLIED

CLEOCIN PEDIATRIC Flavored Granules (clindamycin palmitate HCl) for oral solution is available in bottles of 100 ml *NDC* 0009-0760-04

When reconstituted as directed, each bottle yields a solution containing 75 mg of clindamycin per 5 ml.

Code 810 568 009

CLEOCIN PHOSPHATE®   ℞

brand of clindamycin phosphate sterile solution and clindamycin phosphate IV Solution)

(clindamycin phosphate injection, USP and clindamycin phosphate injection in 5% dextrose)

Sterile Solution is for Intramuscular and Intravenous Use

CLEOCIN PHOSPHATE in the ADD-Vantage™Vial is For Intravenous Use Only

---

WARNING

Clindamycin therapy has been associated with severe colitis which may end fatally. Therefore, it should be reserved for serious infections where less toxic antimicrobial agents are inappropriate, as described in the Indications and Usage Section. It should not be used in patients with nonbacterial infections, such as most upper respiratory tract infections. Studies indicate a toxin(s) produced by *Clostridia* is one primary cause of antibiotic-associated colitis. Cholestyramine and colestipol resins have been shown to bind the toxin *in vitro*. See WARNINGS section. The colitis is usually characterized by severe, persistent diarrhea and severe abdominal cramps and may be associated with the passage of blood and mucus. Endoscopic examination may reveal pseudomembranous colitis. Stool culture for *Clostridium difficile* and stool assay for *C. difficile* toxin may be helpful diagnostically.

When significant diarrhea occurs, the drug should be discontinued or, if necessary, continued only with close observation of the patient. Large bowel endoscopy has been recommended.

Antiperistaltic agents such as opiates and diphenoxylate with atropine (Lomotil) may prolong and/or worsen the condition. Vancomycin has been found to be effective in the treatment of antibiotic associated pseudomembranous colitis produced by *Clostridium difficile*.

Continued on next page

Information on these Upjohn products is based on labeling in effect September 1, 1989. Further information concerning these and other Upjohn products may be obtained by direct inquiry to Medical Information, The Upjohn Company, Kalamazoo, Michigan 49001.

Upjohn—Cont.

The usual adult dosage is 500 milligrams to 2 grams of vancomycin orally per day in three to four divided doses administered for 7 to 10 days. Cholestyramine or colestipol resins bind vancomycin in vitro. If both a resin and vancomycin are to be administered concurrently, it may be advisable to separate the time of administration of each drug.

Diarrhea, colitis, and pseudomembranous colitis have been observed to begin up to several weeks following cessation of therapy with clindamycin.

DESCRIPTION

CLEOCIN PHOSPHATE Sterile Solution in vials contains clindamycin phosphate, a water soluble ester of clindamycin and phosphoric acid. Each mL contains the equivalent of 150 mg clindamycin, 0.5 mg disodium edetate and 9.45 mg benzyl alcohol added as preservative in each mL. Clindamycin is a semisynthetic antibiotic produced by a 7(S)-chloro-substitution of the 7(R)-hydroxyl group of the parent compound lincomycin.

The chemical name of clindamycin phosphate is L-threo-α-D-galacto-octopyranoside, methyl 7-chloro-6,7,8-trideoxy-6-[[(1-methyl-4-propyl-2-pyrrolidinyl) carbonyl] amino]-1-thio-, 2-(dihydrogen phosphate, (2s-trans)-.

The molecular formula is $C_{18}H_{34}ClN_2O_8PS$ and the molecular weight is 504.96.

CLEOCIN PHOSPHATE in the ADD-Vantage Vial is intended for intravenous use only after further dilution with appropriate volume of ADD-Vantage diluent base solution.

CLEOCIN PHOSPHATE IV Solution in the Viaflex†† Plus plastic container for intravenous use is composed of clindamycin phosphate equivalent to 300 and 600 mg of clindamycin premixed with 5% dextrose as a sterile solution. Disodium edetate has been added at a concentration of 0.04 mg/mL. The pH has been adjusted with sodium hydroxide and/or hydrochloric acid.

The plastic container is fabricated from a specially designed multilayer plastic, PL 2501. Solutions in contact with the plastic container can leach out certain of its chemical components in very small amounts within the expiration period. The suitability of the plastic has been confirmed in tests in animals according to the USP biological tests for plastic containers, as well as by tissue culture toxicity studies.

CLINICAL PHARMACOLOGY

Biologically inactive clindamycin phosphate is rapidly converted to active clindamycin.

By the end of short-term intravenous infusion, peak serum levels of active clindamycin are reached. Biologically inactive clindamycin phosphate disappears rapidly from the serum; the average disappearance half-life is 6 minutes; however, the serum disappearance half-life of active clindamycin is about 3 hours in adults and 2 ½ hours in children.

After intramuscular injection of clindamycin phosphate, peak levels of active clindamycin are reached within 3 hours in adults and 1 hour in children. Serum level curves may be constructed from IV peak serum levels as given in Table 1 by application of disappearance half-lives listed above.

Serum levels of clindamycin can be maintained above the in vitro minimum inhibitory concentrations for most indicated organisms by administration of clindamycin phosphate every 8-12 hours in adults and every 6-8 hours in children, or by continuous intravenous infusion. An equilibrium state is reached by the third dose.

The disappearance half-life of clindamycin is increased slightly in patients with markedly reduced renal or hepatic function. Hemodialysis and peritoneal dialysis are not effective in removing clindamycin from the serum. Dosage schedules need not be modified in the presence of mild or moderate renal or hepatic disease.

No significant levels of clindamycin are attained in the cerebrospinal fluid, even in the presence of inflamed meninges. Serum assays for active clindamycin require an inhibitor to prevent in vitro hydrolysis of clindamycin phosphate. [See table below].

Microbiology: Although clindamycin phosphate is inactive in vitro, rapid in vivo hydrolysis converts this compound to the antibacterially active clindamycin.

Clindamycin has been shown to have in vitro activity against isolates of the following organisms:

Aerobic gram positive cocci, including:
     Staphylococcus aureus
     Staphylococcus epidermidis
     (penicillinase and nonpenicillinase producing strains). When tested by in vitro methods some staphylococcal strains originally resistant to erythromycin rapidly develop resistance to clindamycin.
     Streptococci (except S. faecalis)
     Pneumococci

Anaerobic gram negative bacilli, including:
     Bacteroides species (including Bacteroides fragilis group and Bacteroides melaninogenicus group)
     Fusobacterium species

Anaerobic gram positive nonsporeforming bacilli, including:
     Propionibacterium
     Eubacterium
     Actinomyces species

Anaerobic and microaerophilic gram positive cocci, including:
     Peptococcus species
     Peptostreptococcus species
     Microaerophilic streptococci
     Clostridia: Clostridia are more resistant than most anaerobes to clindamycin. Most Clostridium perfringens are susceptible, but other species, eg, Clostridium sporogenes and Clostridium tertium are frequently resistant to clindamycin. Susceptibility testing should be done.

Cross resistance has been demonstrated between clindamycin and lincomycin.

Antagonism has been demonstrated between clindamycin and erythromycin.

In vitro Susceptibility Testing:

Disk diffusion technique—Quantitative methods that require measurement of zone diameters give the most precise estimates of antibiotic susceptibility. One such procedure[1] has been recommended for use with disks to test susceptibility to clindamycin.

Reports from a laboratory using the standardized single-disk susceptibility test[1] with a 2 mcg clindamycin disk should be interpreted according to the following criteria:

Susceptible organisms produce zones of 17 mm or greater, indicating that the tested organism is likely to respond to therapy.

Organisms of intermediate susceptibility produce zones of 15–16 mm, indicating that the tested organism would be susceptible if a high dosage is used or if the infection is confined to tissues and fluids (e.g., urine), in which high antibiotic levels are attained.

Resistant organisms produce zones of 14 mm or less, indicating that other therapy should be selected.

Standardized procedures require the use of control organisms. The 2 mcg clindamycin disk should give a zone diameter between 24 and 30 mm for S. aureus ATCC 25923.

Dilution techniques—A bacterial isolate may be considered susceptible if the minimum inhibitory concentration (MIC) for clindamycin is not more than 1.6 mcg/mL. Organisms are considered moderately susceptible if the MIC is greater than 1.6 mcg/mL and less than or equal to 4.8 mcg/mL. Organisms are considered resistant if the MIC is greater than 4.8 mcg per mL.

The range of MIC's for the control strains are as follows:
     S. aureus ATCC 29213, 0.06–0.25 mcg/mL.
     S. faecalis ATCC 29212, 4.0–16 mcg/mL.

For anaerobic bacteria the minimum inhibitory concentration (MIC) of clindamycin can be determined by agar dilution

and broth dilution (including microdilution) techniques. If MICs are not determined routinely, the disk broth method is recommended for routine use. THE KIRBY-BAUER DISK DIFFUSION METHOD AND ITS INTERPRETIVE STANDARDS ARE NOT RECOMMENDED FOR ANAEROBES. National Committee for Clinical Lab. Standards. Methods for Antimicrobial Susceptibility Testing of Anaerobic Bacteria—Second Edition; Tentative Standard. NCCLS publication M11-T2. Villanova, PA; NCCLS; 1988.

INDICATIONS AND USAGE

CLEOCIN PHOSPHATE products are indicated in the treatment of serious infections caused by susceptible anaerobic bacteria.

CLEOCIN PHOSPHATE products are also indicated in the treatment of serious infections due to susceptible strains of streptococci, pneumococci, and staphylococci. Its use should be reserved for penicillin-allergic patients or other patients for whom, in the judgment of the physician, a penicillin is inappropriate. Because of the risk of colitis, as described in the WARNING box, before selecting clindamycin the physician should consider the nature of the infection and the suitability of less toxic alternatives (e.g., erythromycin).

Bacteriologic studies should be performed to determine the causative organisms and their susceptibility to clindamycin. Indicated surgical procedures should be performed in conjunction with antibiotic therapy.

CLEOCIN PHOSPHATE is indicated in the treatment of serious infections caused by susceptible strains of the designated organisms in the conditions listed below:

Lower respiratory tract infections including pneumonia, empyema, and lung abscess caused by anaerobes, Streptococcus pneumoniae, other streptococci (except S faecalis), and Staphylococcus aureus.

Skin and skin structure infections caused by Streptococcus pyogenes, Staphylococcus aureus, and anaerobes.

Gynecological infections including endometritis, nongonococcal tubo-ovarian abscess, pelvic cellulitis, and postsurgical vaginal cuff infection caused by susceptible anaerobes.

Intra-abdominal infections including peritonitis and intra-abdominal abscess caused by susceptible anaerobic organisms.

Septicemia caused by Staphylococcus aureus, streptococci (except Streptococcus faecalis), and susceptible anaerobes.

Bone and joint infections including acute hematogenous osteomyelitis caused by Staphylococcus aureus and as adjunctive therapy in the surgical treatment of chronic bone and joint infections due to susceptible organisms.

CONTRAINDICATIONS

This drug is contraindicated in individuals with a history of hypersensitivity to preparations containing clindamycin or lincomycin.

WARNINGS

See WARNING box. Studies indicate a toxin(s) produced by Clostridia is one primary cause of antibiotic associated colitis.[1-5] Cholestyramine and colestipol resins have been shown to bind the toxin in vitro. Mild cases of colitis may respond to drug discontinuance alone. Moderate to severe cases should be managed promptly with fluid, electrolyte and protein supplementation as indicated. Vancomycin has been found to be effective in the treatment of antibiotic-associated pseudomembranous colitis produced by Clostridium difficile. The usual adult dosage is 500 milligrams to 2 grams of vancomycin orally per day in three to four divided doses administered for 7 to 10 days. Cholestyramine or colestipol resins bind vancomycin in vitro. If both a resin and vancomycin are to be administered concurrently, it may be advisable to separate the time of administration of each drug. Systemic corticoids and corticoid retention enemas may help relieve the colitis. Other causes of colitis should also be considered.

A careful inquiry should be made concerning previous sensitivities to drugs and other allergens.

Usage in Newborns and infants: This product contains benzyl alcohol as a preservative. Benzyl alcohol has been associated with a fatal "Gasping Syndrome" in premature infants.

Usage in Meningitis: Since clindamycin does not diffuse adequately into the cerebrospinal fluid, the drug should not be used in the treatment of meningitis.

SERIOUS ANAPHYLACTOID REACTIONS REQUIRE IMMEDIATE EMERGENCY TREATMENT WITH EPINEPHRINE. OXYGEN AND INTRAVENOUS CORTICOSTEROIDS SHOULD ALSO BE ADMINISTERED AS INDICATED.

1. Bartlett JG, et al: Antibiotic associated pseudomembranous colitis due to toxin-producing Clostridia. N Engl J Med 298(10):531-534, 1978.
2. George RH, et al: Identification of Clostridium difficile as a cause of pseudomembranous colitis. Br Med J 6114:669-671, 1978.
3. Larson HE, Price AB: Pseudomembranous colitis presence of clostridial toxin. Lancet 8052/3:1312-1314, 1977.

Table 1. Average Peak Serum Concentrations After Dosing with Clindamycin Phosphate

CLEOCIN PHOSPHATE Dosage Regimen	Clindamycin mcg/ml	Clindamycin Phosphate mcg/ml
Healthy Adult Males (Post equilibrium)		
300 mg IV in 10 min, q8h	7	15
600 mg IV in 20 min, q8h**	10	23
900 mg IV in 30 min, q12h**	11	29
1200 mg IV in 45 min, q12h	14	49
300 mg IM q8h	6	3
600 mg IM q12h*	9	3
Children (first dose)*		
5-7 mg/kg IV in 1 hr	10	
3-5 mg/kg IM	4	
5-7 mg/kg IM	8	

*Data in this group from patients being treated for infection
**CLEOCIN PHOSPHATE in the ADD-Vantage Vial is For Intravenous Use Only.

4. Rifkin GD, Fekety FR, Silva J: Antibiotic-induced colitis implication of a toxin neutralized by *Clostridium sordellii* antitoxin. *Lancet* 8048:1103-1106, 1977.

5. Bailey WR, Scott EG: Diagnostic Microbiology. The CV Mosby Company, St. Louis, 1978.

PRECAUTIONS

General

Review of experience to date suggests that a subgroup of older patients with associated severe illness may tolerate diarrhea less well. When clindamycin is indicated in these patients, they should be carefully monitored for change in bowel frequency.

CLEOCIN PHOSPHATE products should be prescribed with caution in individuals with a history of gastrointestinal disease, particularly colitis.

CLEOCIN PHOSPHATE should be prescribed with caution in atopic individuals.

Certain infections may require incision and drainage or other indicated surgical procedures in addition to antibiotic therapy.

The use of CLEOCIN PHOSPHATE may result in overgrowth of nonsusceptible organisms—particularly yeasts. Should superinfections occur, appropriate measures should be taken as indicated by the clinical situation.

CLEOCIN PHOSPHATE should not be injected intravenously undiluted as a bolus, but should be infused over at least 10–60 minutes as directed in the DOSAGE AND ADMINISTRATION section.

Patients with very severe renal disease and/or very severe hepatic disease accompanied by severe metabolic aberrations should be dosed with caution, and serum clindamycin levels monitored during high-dose therapy (see OVERDOSAGE).

Laboratory Tests

During prolonged therapy periodic liver and kidney function tests and blood counts should be performed.

Drug Interactions

Clindamycin has been shown to have neuromuscular blocking properties that may enhance the action of other neuromuscular blocking agents. Therefore, it should be used with caution in patients receiving such agents.

Antagonism has been demonstrated between clindamycin and erythromycin *in vitro*. Because of possible clinical significance, the two drugs should not be administered concurrently.

Usage in Pregnancy: Safety for use in pregnancy has not been established.

Nursing Mothers

Clindamycin has been reported to appear in breast milk in the range of 0.7 to 3.8 mcg/mL at dosages of 150 mg orally to 600 mg intravenously. Because of the potential for adverse reactions due to clindamycin in neonates (see Pediatric Use), the decision to discontinue the drug should be made, taking into account the importance of the drug to the mother.

Pediatric Use

When CLEOCIN PHOSPHATE Sterile Solution is administered to newborns, infants, and children, appropriate monitoring of organ system functions is desirable.

The product contains benzyl alcohol as a preservative. Benzyl alcohol has been associated with a fatal "Gasping Syndrome" in premature infants.

The potential for the toxic effect in children from chemicals that may leach from the single dose premixed IV preparation in plastic has not been evaluated.

ADVERSE REACTIONS

The following reactions have been reported with the use of clindamycin.

Gastrointestinal: Abdominal pain, nausea, vomiting and diarrhea (See **Warnings**). An unpleasant or metallic taste occasionally has been reported after intravenous administration of the higher doses of clindamycin phosphate.

Hypersensitivity Reactions: Maculopapular rash and urticaria have been observed during drug therapy. Generalized mild to moderate morbilliform-like skin rashes are the most frequently reported of all adverse reactions. Rare instances of erythema multiforme, some resembling Stevens-Johnson syndrome, have been associated with clindamycin. A few cases of anaphylactoid reactions have been reported.

If a hypersensitivity reaction occurs, the drug should be discontinued. The usual agents (epinephrine, corticosteroids, antihistamines) should be available for emergency treatment of serious reactions.

Liver: Jaundice and abnormalities in liver function tests have been observed during clindamycin therapy.

Renal: Although no direct relationship of clindamycin to renal damage has been established, renal dysfunction as evidenced by azotemia, oliguria, and/or proteinuria has been observed in rare instances.

Hematopoietic: Transient neutropenia (leukopenia) and eosinophilia have been reported. Reports of agranulocytosis and thrombocytopenia have been made. No direct etiologic relationship to concurrent clindamycin therapy could be made in any of the foregoing.

CLEOCIN PHOSPHATE

To maintain serum clindamycin levels	Rapid infusion rate	Maintenance infusion rate
Above 4 mcg/ml	10 mg/min for 30 min	0.75 mg/min
Above 5 mcg/ml	15 mg/min for 30 min	1.00 mg/min
Above 6 mcg/ml	20 mg/min for 30 min	1.25 mg/min

Local Reactions: Pain, induration and sterile abscess have been reported after intramuscular injection and thrombophlebitis after intravenous infusion. Reactions can be minimized or avoided by giving deep intramuscular injections and avoiding prolonged use of indwelling intravenous catheters.

Musculoskeletal: Rare instances of polyarthritis have been reported.

Cardiovascular: Rare instances of cardiopulmonary arrest and hypotension have been reported following too rapid intravenous administration. (See DOSAGE AND ADMINISTRATION Section)

OVERDOSAGE

Hemodialysis and peritoneal dialysis are not effective in removing clindamycin from the serum.

DOSAGE AND ADMINISTRATION

If diarrhea occurs during therapy, this antibiotic should be discontinued. (See **Warning** box).

Adults

Parenteral (IM or IV Administration):
Serious infections due to aerobic gram-positive cocci and the more susceptible anaerobes (NOT generally including *Bacteroides fragilis, Peptococcus* species and *Clostridium* species other than *Clostridium perfringens*):
1200–2700 mg/day in 2, 3 or 4 equal doses
For more serious infections, these doses may have to be increased. In life threatening situations due to aerobes or anaerobes, these doses may be increased. Doses of as much as 4800 mg daily have been given intravenously to adults. See **Dilution and Infusion Rates** section below.

Single intramuscular injections of greater than 600 mg are not recommended. Alternatively, drug may be administered in the form of a single rapid infusion of the first dose followed by continuous IV infusion as follows:
[See table above].

Neonates (less than 1 month):
15 to 20 mg/kg/day in 3 to 4 equal doses. The lower dosage may be adequate for small prematures.

Children (over 1 month of age): Parenteral (IM or IV) administration: 20 to 40 mg/kg/day in 3 or 4 equal doses. The higher doses would be used for more severe infections. As an alternative to dosing on a body weight basis, children may be dosed on the basis of square meters body surface: 350 mg/m^2/day for serious infections and 450 mg/m^2/day for more severe infections.

Parenteral therapy may be changed to oral CLEOCIN PEDIATRIC® Flavored Granules (clindamycin palmitate hydrochloride) or CLEOCIN HCl® Capsules (clindamycin hydrochloride) when the condition warrants and at the discretion of the physician.

In cases of β-hemolytic streptococcal infections, treatment should be continued for at least 10 days.

Dilution and Infusion Rates

Clindamycin phosphate must be diluted prior to IV administration. The concentration of clindamycin in diluent for infusion should not exceed 12 mg per mL and infusion rates should not exceed 30 mg per minute. The usual infusion dilutions and rates are as follows:

Dose	Diluent	Time
300 mg	50 ml	10 min
600 mg	50 ml	20 min
900 mg	100 ml	30 min
1200 mg	100 ml	40 min

Administration of more than 1200 mg in a single 1-hour infusion is not recommended.

Parenteral drug products should be inspected visually for particulate matter and discoloration prior to administration, whenever solution and container permit.

Dilution and Compatibility. Physical and biological compatibility studies monitored for 24 hours at room temperature have demonstrated no inactivation or incompatibility with the use of CLEOCIN PHOSPHATE Sterile Solution (clindamycin phosphate) in IV solutions containing sodium chloride, glucose, calcium or potassium, and solutions containing vitamin B complex in concentrations usually used clinically. No incompatibility has been demonstrated with the antibiotics cephalothin, kanamycin, gentamicin, penicillin or carbenicillin.

The following drugs are physically incompatible with clindamycin phosphate: ampicillin sodium, phenytoin sodium, barbiturates, aminophylline, calcium gluconate, and magnesium sulfate.

The compatibility and duration of stability of drug admixtures will vary depending on concentration and other condi-

tions. For current information regarding compatibilities of clindamycin phosphate under specific conditions, please contact the Medical Correspondence Unit, The Upjohn Company.

Physico-Chemical Stability of diluted solutions of CLEOCIN PHOSPHATE

Room temperature: 6, 9 and 12 mg/ml (equivalent to clindamycin base) in dextrose 5% in water, sodium chloride 0.9%, or Lactated Ringers in glass bottles or minibags, demonstrated physical and chemical stability for at least 16 days at 25°C.

Refrigeration: 6, 9 and 12 mg/mL (equivalent to clindamycin base) in dextrose 5% in water, sodium chloride 0.9%, or Lactated Ringers in glass bottles or minibags, demonstrated physical and chemical stability for at least 32 days at 4°C.

Frozen: 6,9 and 12 mg/mL (equivalent to clindamycin base) in dextrose 5% in water, sodium chloride 0.9%, or Lactated Ringers in minibags demonstrated physical and chemical stability for at least eight weeks at −10°C.

Frozen solutions should be thawed at room temperature and not refrozen.

DIRECTIONS FOR DISPENSING:

Pharmacy Bulk Package—Not for Direct Infusion
The Pharmacy Bulk Package is for use in a Pharmacy Admixture Service only under a laminar flow hood. Entry into the vial should be made with a small diameter sterile transfer set or other small diameter sterile dispensing device, and contents dispensed in aliquots using aseptic technique. Multiple entries with a needle and syringe are not recommended. AFTER ENTRY USE ENTIRE CONTENTS OF VIAL PROMPTLY. ANY UNUSED PORTION MUST BE DISCARDED WITHIN 24 HOURS AFTER INITIAL ENTRY.

DIRECTIONS FOR USE

CLEOCIN PHOSPHATE IV Solution in Viaflex†† Plus Plastic Container

Premixed CLEOCIN PHOSPHATE IV Solution is for intravenous administration using sterile equipment. Check for minute leaks prior to use by squeezing bag firmly. If leaks are found, discard solution as sterility may be impaired. Do not add supplementary medication. Parenteral drug products should be inspected visually for particulate matter and discoloration prior to administration whenever solution and container permit. Do not use unless solution is clear and seal is intact.

Caution: Do not use plastic containers in series connections. Such use cculd result in air embolism due to residual air being drawn from the primary container before administration of the fluid from the secondary container is complete.

Preparation for Administration:

1. Suspend container from eyelet support.
2. Remove protector from outlet port at bottom of container.
3. Attach administration set. Refer to complete directions accompanying set.

Preparation of CLEOCIN PHOSPHATE in ADD-Vantage‡ System-For IV Use Only. CLEOCIN PHOSPHATE 600 mg and 900 mg may be reconstituted in 50 ml or 100 ml, respectively, of 5% Dextrose or 0.9% Sodium Chloride in the ADD-diluent container. Refer to separate instructions for ADD-Vantage System.

HOW SUPPLIED

Each ml of CLEOCIN PHOSPHATE Sterile Solution contains clindamycin phosphate equivalent to 150 mg clindamycin; 0.5 mg disodium edetate; 9.45 mg benzyl alcohol added as preservative. When necessary, pH is adjusted with sodium hydroxide and/or hydrochloric acid.

CLEOCIN PHOSPHATE is available in the following packages:

25-2 mL vials	NDC 0009-0870-21
100-2 mL vials	NDC 0009-0870-22
25-4 mL vials	NDC 0009-0775-20
100-4 mL vials	NDC 0009-0775-21
25-6 mL vials	NDC 0009-0902-11
100-6 mL vials	NDC 0009-0902-12

Continued on next page

Information on these Upjohn products is based on labeling in effect September 1, 1989. Further information concerning these and other Upjohn products may be obtained by direct inquiry to Medical Information, The Upjohn Company, Kalamazoo, Michigan 49001.

Upjohn—Cont.

1–60 mL Pharmacy
Bulk Package   NDC 0009-0728-05
CLEOCIN PHOSPHATE is supplied in ADD-Vantage vials as follows:

NDC#	Vial Size	Total Clindamycin Phosphate/vial	Amount of Diluent
0009-3124-01	4 mL	600 mg	50 mL
0009-3447-01	6 mL	900 mg	100 mL

Store at controlled room temperature 15°–30°C (59°–86°F).
CLEOCIN PHOSPHATE IV Solution in Viaflex Plus plastic containers is a sterile solution of clindamycin phosphate with 5% dextrose. The single dose Viaflex Plus plastic containers are available as follows:
24—300 mg/50 mL containers   NDC 0009-3381-01
24—600 mg/50 mL containers   NDC 0009-3375-01
Exposure of pharmaceutical products to heat should be minimized. It is recommended that Viaflex Plus plastic containers be stored at room temperature (25° C). Avoid temperatures above 30° C.
Code 810 020 123

[1] Bauer, AW, Kirby, WMM, Sherris, JC, Turck, M: Antibiotic susceptibility testing by a standardized single disc method, *Am J Clin Path*, **45**:493–496, 1966. Standardized Disc Susceptibility Test, *Federal Register* **37**:20527–29, 1972.
‡ ADD-Vantage is a registered trademark of Abbott Laboratories.
CLEOCIN PHOSPHATE IV Solution in the Viaflex Plus plastic containers is manufactured for The Upjohn Company by Baxter-Healthcare Corporation, Deerfield, IL 60015.
††Viaflex is a registered trademark of Baxter Travenol Laboratories, Inc.
Shown in Product Identification Section, page 433

CLEOCIN T®   ℞
brand of clindamycin phosphate topical solution, topical gel and topical lotion
For External Use

30 ml bottle
NSN 6505-01-140-6450(M)
60 ml bottle
NSN 6505-01-116-5655 (M & VA)

DESCRIPTION
CLEOCIN T Topical Solution , CLEOCIN T Topical Gel and CLEOCIN T Topical Lotion contain clindamycin phosphate, USP, at a concentration equivalent to 10 mg clindamycin per milliliter.
Clindamycin phosphate is a water soluble ester of the semisynthetic antibiotic produced by a 7(S)-chloro-substitution of the 7(R)-hydroxyl group of the parent antibiotic lincomycin. The solution contains isopropyl alcohol 50% v/v, propylene glycol, and water.
The gel contains allantoin, carbomer 934P, methylparaben, polyethylene glycol 400, propylene glycol, sodium hydroxide, and purified water.
The lotion contains clindamycin equivalent to clindamycin 10mg/mL. Also cetostearyl alcohol (2.5%); glycerin; glyceryl stearate SE (with potassium monostearate); isostearyl alcohol (2.5%); methylparaben (0.3%); sodium lauroyl sarcosinate; stearic acid; and purified water.
The chemical name for clindamycin phosphate is 7(S)-chloro-7-deoxylincomycin-2-phosphate. (MW = 504.96.)

CLINICAL PHARMACOLOGY
Although clindamycin phosphate is inactive *in vitro*, rapid *in vivo* hydrolysis converts this compound to the antibacterially active clindamycin.
Clindamycin has been shown to have *in vivo* activity against isolates of *Propionibacterium acnes*. This may account for its usefulness in acne.
Cross resistance has been demonstrated between clindamycin and lincomycin.
Antagonism has been demonstrated between clindamycin and erythromycin.
Following multiple topical applications of clindamycin phosphate at a concentration equivalent to 10 mg clindamycin per ml in an isopropyl alcohol and water solution, very low levels of clindamycin are present in the serum (0–3 ng/mL) and less than 0.2% of the dose is recovered in urine as clindamycin.
Clindamycin activity has been demonstrated in comedones from acne patients. The mean concentration of antibiotic activity in extracted comedones after application of CLEOCIN T Topical Solution for 4 weeks was 597 mcg/g of comedonal material (range 0–1490). Clindamycin *in vitro* inhibits all *Propionibacterium acnes* cultures tested (MICs 0.4 mcg/mL). Free fatty acids on the skin surface have been de-

creased from approximately 14% to 2% following application of clindamycin.

INDICATIONS AND USAGE
CLEOCIN T Topical Solution, CLEOCIN T Topical Gel and CLEOCIN T Topical Lotion are indicated in the treatment of acne vulgaris. In view of the potential for diarrhea, bloody diarrhea and pseudomembranous colitis, the physician should consider whether other agents are more appropriate. (See CONTRAINDICATIONS, WARNINGS and ADVERSE REACTIONS.)

CONTRAINDICATIONS
CLEOCIN T Topical Solution, CLEOCIN T Topical Gel and CLEOCIN T Topical Lotion are contraindicated in individuals with a history of hypersensitivity to preparations containing clindamycin or lincomycin, a history of regional enteritis or ulcerative colitis, or a history of antibiotic-associated colitis.

WARNINGS
Orally and parenterally administered clindamycin has been associated with severe colitis which may end fatally. Use of the topical formulation results in absorption of the antibiotic from the skin surface. Diarrhea, bloody diarrhea, and colitis (including pseudomembranous colitis) have been reported with the use of topical and systemic clindamycin. Symptoms can occur after a few days, weeks or months following initiation of clindamycin therapy. They have also been observed to begin up to several weeks after cessation of therapy with clindamycin. Studies indicate a toxin(s) produced by *Clostridium difficile* is one primary cause of antibiotic-associated colitis. The colitis is usually characterized by severe persistent diarrhea and severe abdominal cramps and may be associated with the passage of blood and mucus. Endoscopic examination may reveal pseudomembranous colitis.
When significant diarrhea occurs, the drug should be discontinued. Large bowel endoscopy should be considered in cases of severe diarrhea.
Antiperistaltic agents such as opiates and diphenoxylate with atropine (Lomotil) may prolong and /or worsen the condition. Vancomycin has been found to be effective in the treatment of antibiotic-associated pseudomembranous colitis produced by *Clostridium difficile*. The usual adult dosage is 500 mg to 2 grams of vancomycin orally per day in three to four divided doses administered for 7 to 10 days.
Mild cases of colitis may respond to discontinuance of clindamycin. Moderate to severe cases should be managed promptly with fluid, electrolyte, and protein supplementation as indicated. Cholestyramine and colestipol resins have been shown to bind the toxin *in vitro*. If both a resin and vancomycin are to be administered concurrently, it may be advisable to separate the time of administration of each drug. Systemic corticoids and corticoid retention enemas may help relieve the colitis. Other causes of colitis should also be considered. A careful inquiry should be made concerning previous sensitivities to drugs and other allergens.

PRECAUTIONS
CLEOCIN T Topical Solution contains an alcohol base which will cause burning and irritation of the eye. In the event of accidental contact with sensitive surfaces (eye, abraded skin, mucous membranes), bathe with copious amounts of cool tap water. The solution has an unpleasant taste and caution should be exercised when applying medication around the mouth.
CLEOCIN T should be prescribed with caution in atopic individuals.
Pregnancy Category B
Reproduction studies have been performed in rats and mice using subcutaneous and oral doses of clindamycin ranging from 100 to 600 mg/kg/day and have revealed no evidence of impaired fertility or harm to the fetus due to clindamycin. There are, however, no adequate and well-controlled studies in pregnant women. Because animal reproduction studies are not always predictive of human response, this drug should be used during pregnancy only if clearly needed.
Nursing Mothers
It is not known whether clindamycin is excreted in human milk following use of CLEOCIN T. However, orally and parenterally administered clindamycin has been reported to appear in breast milk. As a general rule, nursing should not be undertaken while a patient is on a drug since many drugs are excreted in human milk.
Pediatric Use
Safety and effectiveness in children under the age of 12 has not been established.

ADVERSE REACTIONS
Skin dryness is the most common adverse reaction seen with the solution.
Clindamycin has been associated with severe colitis which may end fatally (See WARNINGS).
Cases of diarrhea, bloody diarrhea and colitis (including pseudomembranous colitis) have been reported as adverse reactions in patients treated with topical formulations of clindamycin.

Other effects which have been reported in association with the use of topical formulations of clindamycin include:

Local Effects	Systemic Effects
Contact dermatitis	Abdominal pain
Irritation (e.g., erythema, peeling, and burning)	Gastrointestinal disturbances
Oily skin	
Gram-negative folliculitis	

DOSAGE AND ADMINISTRATION
Apply a thin film of CLEOCIN T Topical Solution, CLEOCIN T Topical Lotion or CLEOCIN T Topical Gel twice daily to affected area.
Lotion: Shake well immediately before using. Keep all dosage form containers tightly closed.

HOW SUPPLIED
CLEOCIN T Topical Solution containing clindamycin phosphate equivalent to 10 mg clindamycin per milliliter is available in the following sizes:
30 mL applicator bottle—NDC 0009-3116-01
60 mL applicator bottle—NDC 0009-3116-02
16 oz (473 mL) bottle—NDC 0009-3116-04
CLEOCIN T Topical Gel containing clindamycin phosphate equivalent to 10 mg clindamycin per milliliter is available in the following sizes:
7.5 gram tube—NDC 0009-3331-03
30 gram tube—NDC 0009-3331-02
CLEOCIN T Topical Lotion containing clindamycin phosphate equivalent to 10 mg clindamycin per milliliter is available in the following size:
60 mL plastic squeeze bottle—NDC 0009-3329-01
Store at controlled room temperature 15°–30°C (59°–86°F). Protect from freezing.
Code 811 373 119
CLEOCIN T Topical Gel is manufactured for
The Upjohn Company
Kalamazoo, MI 49001, USA
by Paco
Pharmaceutical Services, Inc.
Lakewood, NJ 08701
Shown in Product Identification Section, page 433

COLESTID®   ℞
brand of colestipol hydrochloride granules
(colestipol hydrochloride for oral suspension, USP)

Box of 30-5 gram packets
                    NSN 6505-01-051-4697 (M & VA)
500 gram   NSN 6505-01-244-5511 (M & VA)

DESCRIPTION
COLESTID Granules consist of colestipol hydrochloride, which is a hyperlipidemia agent for oral use. COLESTID is an insoluble, high molecular weight basic anion-exchange copolymer of diethylenetriamine and 1-chloro-2,3-epoxypropane, with approximately 1 out of 5 amine nitrogens protonated (chloride form). It is a light yellow resin which is hygroscopic and swells when placed in water or aqueous fluids. COLESTID is tasteless and odorless. Inactive ingredient: Silicon dioxide.

CLINICAL PHARMACOLOGY
Cholesterol is the major, and probably the sole precursor of bile acids. During normal digestion, bile acids are secreted via the bile from the liver and gall bladder into the intestines. Bile acids emulsify the fat and oily materials present in food, thus facilitating absorption. A major portion of the bile acids secreted is reabsorbed from the intestines and returned via the portal circulation to the liver, thus completing the enterohepatic cycle. Only very small amounts of bile acids are found in normal serum.
COLESTID Granules (colestipol hydrochloride) bind bile acids in the intestine forming a complex that is excreted in the feces. This nonsystemic action results in a partial removal of the bile acids from the enterohepatic circulation, preventing their reabsorption. Since colestipol hydrochloride is an anion exchange resin, the chloride anions of the resin can be replaced by other anions, usually those with a greater affinity for the resin than chloride ion.
Colestipol hydrochloride is hydrophilic, but it is virtually water insoluble (99.75%) and it is not hydrolyzed by digestive enzymes. The high molecular weight polymer in COLESTID apparently is not absorbed. Less than 0.05% of ^{14}C-labeled colestipol hydrochloride is excreted in the urine.
The increased fecal loss of bile acids due to COLESTID administration leads to an increased oxidation of cholesterol to bile acids, a decrease in beta lipoprotein or low density lipoprotein serum levels, and a decrease in serum cholesterol levels. Although COLESTID produces an increase in the hepatic synthesis of cholesterol in man, serum cholesterol levels fall.
There is evidence to show that this fall in cholesterol is secondary to an increased rate of cholesterol rich lipoproteins (beta or low density lipoproteins) from the plasma. Serum triglyceride levels may increase or remain unchanged in colestipol treated patients.

The decline in serum cholesterol levels with treatment with COLESTID is usually evident by one month. When COLESTID is discontinued, serum cholesterol levels usually return to baseline levels within one month. Cholesterol may rise even with continued use of COLESTID, and serum levels should be determined periodically to confirm that a favorable initial response is maintained.

COLESTID is more effective than clofibrate in lowering total serum cholesterol and low density lipoprotein cholesterol in Frederickson type IIa hyperlipoproteinemia (pure hypercholesterolemia without hypertriglyceridemia) without affecting high density lipoprotein cholesterol.

In patients with heterozygous familial hypercholesterolemia who have not obtained an optimal response to colestipol hydrochloride alone in maximal doses, the combination of colestipol hydrochloride and nicotinic acid has been shown to provide effective further lowering of serum cholesterol, triglyceride, and LDL cholesterol values. Simultaneously, HDL cholesterol values increased significantly. In many such patients it is possible to normalize serum lipid values.[1-3]

INDICATIONS AND USAGE

Since no drug is innocuous, strict attention should be paid to the indications and contraindications, particularly when selecting drugs for chronic long-term use.

COLESTID Granules (colestipol hydrochloride) are indicated as adjunctive therapy to diet for the reduction of elevated serum cholesterol in patients with primary hypercholesterolemia (elevated low density lipoproteins). COLESTID has been shown to have no effect on or to increase triglyceride levels.

In a large, placebo-controlled, multiclinic study, the LRC-CPPT[4], hypercholesterolemic subjects treated with cholestyramine, a bile acid sequestrant with an effect on serum cholesterol similar to that of COLESTID, had reductions in total and low-density lipoprotein cholesterol (LDL-C). Over the seven-year study period the cholestyramine group experienced a 19% reduction in the combined rate of coronary heart disease death plus non-fatal myocardial infarction (cumulative incidences of 7% cholestyramine and 8.6% placebo). The subjects included in the study were middle-aged men (age 35-59) with serum cholesterol levels above 265 mg/dl and no history of heart disease. It is not clear to what extent these findings can be extrapolated to other segments of the hypercholesterolemic population not studied.

Dietary therapy specific for the type of hyperlipoproteinemia is in the initial treatment of choice. Excess body weight may be an important factor and caloric restriction for weight normalization should be addressed prior to drug therapy in the overweight. The use of drugs should be considered only when reasonable attempts have been made to obtain satisfactory results with non-drug methods. If the decision ultimately is to use drugs, the patient should be instructed that this does not reduce the importance of adhering to diet.

CONTRAINDICATIONS

COLESTID Granules (colestipol hydrochloride) are contraindicated in those individuals who have shown hypersensitivity to any of its components.

WARNINGS

TO AVOID ACCIDENTAL INHALATION OR ESOPHAGEAL DISTRESS, COLESTID GRANULES (colestipol hydrochloride) SHOULD NOT BE TAKEN IN ITS DRY FORM. ALWAYS MIX COLESTID WITH WATER OR OTHER FLUIDS BEFORE INGESTING.

PRECAUTIONS

Before instituting therapy with COLESTID Granules (colestipol hydrochloride), diseases contributing to increased blood cholesterol such as hypothyroidism, diabetes mellitus, nephrotic syndrome, dysproteinemias and obstructive liver disease should be looked for and specifically treated.

Because it sequesters bile acids, COLESTID may interfere with normal fat absorption and thus may prevent absorption of fat soluble vitamins such as A, D, and K. If COLESTID resin is to be given for long periods of time, supplemental vitamin A and D should be considered.

Chronic use of COLESTID may be associated with an increased bleeding tendency due to hypoprothrombinemia from vitamin K deficiency. This will usually respond promptly to parenteral vitamin K_1 and recurrences can be prevented by oral administration of vitamin K_1.

Serum cholesterol and triglyceride levels should be measured periodically to detect significant changes. COLESTID may raise the serum triglycerides in long term use and, in some patients, the cholesterol levels return to baseline or rise above baseline.

COLESTID may produce or severely worsen pre-existing constipation. The dosage should be decreased in these patients since impaction may occur. Particular effort should be made to avoid constipation in patients with symptomatic coronary artery disease. Constipation associated with COLESTID may aggravate hemorrhoids.

While there have been no reports of hypothyroidism induced in individuals with normal thyroid function, the theoretical possibility exists, particularly in patients with limited thyroid reserve.

Carcinogenesis, mutagenesis and impairment of fertility

In studies conducted in rats in which cholestyramine resin (a bile acid sequestering agent similar to colestipol hydrochloride) was used as a tool to investigate the role of various intestinal factors, such as fat, bile salts and microbial flora, in the development of intestinal tumors induced by potent carcinogens, the incidence of such tumors was observed to be greater in cholestyramine resin treated rats than in control rats.

The relevance of this laboratory observation from studies in rats with cholestyramine resin to the clinical use of COLESTID is not known. In the LRC-CPPT study referred to above, the total incidence of fatal and non-fatal neoplasms was similar in both treatment groups. When the many different categories of tumors are examined, various alimentary system cancers were somewhat more prevalent in the cholestyramine group. The small numbers and the multiple categories prevent conclusions from being drawn. Further follow-up of the LRC-CPPT participants by the sponsors of that study is planned for cause-specific mortality and cancer morbidity. When COLESTID was administered in the diet to rats for 18 months, there was no evidence of any drug related intestinal tumor formation. In the Ames assay, COLESTID was not mutagenic.

Use in Pregnancy

The use of COLESTID in pregnancy or lactation or by women of childbearing age requires that the potential benefits of drug therapy be weighed against the possible hazards to the mother and child. The safe use of COLESTID resin by pregnant women has not been established.

Use in Children

Safety and effectiveness in children have not been established.

DRUG INTERACTIONS

Since colestipol hydrochloride is an anion exchange resin, it may have a strong affinity for anions other than the bile acids. Therefore, colestipol hydrochloride resin may delay or reduce the absorption of concomitant oral medication. The interval between the administration of COLESTID and any other medication should be as long as possible. Patients should take other drugs at least one hour before or four hours after COLESTID to avoid impeding their absorption. Human studies have demonstrated that COLESTID may decrease propranolol absorption. Effects on the absorption of other beta-blockers have not been determined. Therefore, patients on propranolol should be observed when COLESTID is either added or deleted from a therapeutic regimen.

In vitro studies have indicated that COLESTID binds a number of drugs. Studies in humans show that the absorption of chlorothiazide as reflected in urinary excretion is markedly decreased even when administered one hour before COLESTID. The absorption of tetracycline and of penicillin G was significantly decreased when either one was given at the same time as COLESTID; these drugs were not tested to determine the effect of administration one hour before COLESTID.

No depressant effect on blood levels in humans was noted when COLESTID was administered with any of the following drugs: aspirin, clindamycin, clofibrate, methyldopa, tolbutamide or warfarin. Particular caution should be observed with digitalis preparations since there are conflicting results for the effect of COLESTID on the availability of digoxin and digitoxin. The potential for binding of these drugs if given concomitantly is present. Discontinuing COLESTID could pose a hazard to health if a potentially toxic drug that is significantly bound to the resin has been titrated to a maintenance level while the patient was taking COLESTID.

ADVERSE REACTIONS

1. *Gastrointestinal*

The most common adverse reactions are confined to the gastrointestinal tract. Constipation, reported by about one patient in 10, is the major single complaint and at times is severe and occasionally accompanied by fecal impaction. Hemorrhoids may be aggravated. Most instances of constipation are mild, transient, and controlled with standard treatment. Some patients require decreased dosage or discontinuation of therapy.

Less frequent gastrointestinal complaints occurring in about one in 30 to one in 100 patients, are abdominal discomfort (abdominal pain and distention), belching, flatulence, nausea, vomiting, and diarrhea. Peptic ulceration, gastrointestinal irritation and bleeding, cholecystitis, and cholelithiasis have been reported by fewer than one in 500 patients and are not necessarily drug related.

2. *Hypersensitivity*

Urticaria and dermatitis were noted in fewer than one in 1,000 patients. Asthma and wheezing were not reported in the studies with COLESTID but have been noted during treatment with other cholesterol-lowering agents.

3. *Musculoskeletal*

Muscle and joint pains, and arthritis have had a reported incidence of less than one in 1,000 patients.

4. *Neurologic*

Headache and dizziness were noted in about one in 300 patients; anxiety, vertigo, and drowsiness were reported in fewer than one in 1,000.

5. *Miscellaneous*

Anorexia, fatigue, weakness, and shortness of breath have been seen in 1–3 patients in 1,000. Transient and modest elevations of serum glutamic oxaloacetic transaminase and of alkaline phosphatase were observed in one or more occasions in various patients treated with COLESTID Granules (colestipol hydrochloride). Some patients have shown an increase in serum phosphorus and chloride with a decrease in sodium and potassium.

OVERDOSE

Overdosage of COLESTID Granules (colestipol hydrochloride) has not been reported. Should overdosage occur, however, the chief potential harm would be obstruction of the gastrointestinal tract. The location of such potential obstruction, the degree of obstruction and the presence or absence of normal gut motility would determine treatment.

DOSAGE AND ADMINISTRATION

For adults, COLESTID Granules (colestipol hydrochloride) are recommended in doses of 15–30 grams/day taken in divided doses two to four times daily. To avoid accidental inhalation or esophageal distress, COLESTID should not be taken in its dry form. COLESTID should always be mixed with water or other fluids before ingesting. Patients should take other drugs at least one hour before or four hours after COLESTID to minimize possible interference with their absorption. (See DRUG INTERACTIONS).

Before Administration of COLESTID

1. Define the type of hyperlipoproteinemia.
2. Institute a trial of diet and weight reduction.
3. Establish baseline serum cholesterol and triglyceride levels.

During Administration of COLESTID

1. The patient should be carefully monitored clinically, including serum cholesterol and triglyceride levels.
2. Failure of cholesterol to fall or significant rise in triglyceride level should be considered as indications to discontinue medication.

Mixing and Administration Guide

COLESTID Granules (colestipol hydrochloride) should always be taken mixed in a liquid such as orange or tomato juice, water, milk, or carbonated beverage. It may also be taken in soups or with cereals or pulpy fruits. COLESTID *should never be taken in its dry form.*

With beverages

1. Add the prescribed amount of COLESTID to a glassful (three ounces or more) of water, milk, flavored drink, or a favorite juice (orange, tomato, pineapple, or other fruit juice).
2. Stir the mixture until the medication is completely mixed. (COLESTID will not dissolve in the liquid.) COLESTID may also be mixed with carbonated beverages, slowly stirred in a large glass.

Rinse the glass with a small amount of additional beverage to make sure all the medication is taken.

With cereals, soups, and fruits

COLESTID may be taken mixed with milk in hot or regular breakfast cereals, or even mixed in soups that have a high fluid content (tomato or chicken noodle soup). It may also be added to fruits that are pulpy such as crushed pineapple, pears, peaches, or fruit cocktail.

HOW SUPPLIED

COLESTID Granules (colestipol hydrochloride) are available as follows:

Cartons of 30 foil packets—	NDC 0009-0260-01
Cartons of 90 foil packets—	NDC 0009-0260-04
Bottles of 500 grams with scoop—	NDC 0009-0260-02

Each packet or each level scoop supplies 5 grams of COLESTID.
Store at controlled room temperature 15°-30°C (59°-86°F).

REFERENCES

1. Kane JP, Malloy MJ, Tun P et al: Normalization of low-density-lipoprotein levels in heterozygous familial hypercholesterolemia with a combined drug regimen. *N. Engl J Med* 304:251–258, 1981.
2. Illingworth DR, Phillipson BE, JH Rapp et al: Colestipol plus nicotinic acid in treatment of heterozygous familial hypercholesterolemia. *Lancet* 1:296–298, 1981.
3. Kuo PT, Kostis JB, Moreyra AE et al: Familial type II hyperlipoproteinemia with coronary heart disease: Effect of

Continued on next page

Information on these Upjohn products is based on labeling in effect September 1, 1989. Further information concerning these and other Upjohn products may be obtained by direct inquiry to Medical Information, The Upjohn Company, Kalamazoo, Michigan 49001.

Upjohn—Cont.

diet-colestipol-nicotinic acid treatment. *Chest* 79:286–291, 1981.

4. Lipid Metabolism-Atherogenesis Branch, National Heart, Lung, and Blood Institute, Bethesda, MD: The Lipid Research Clinics Coronary Primary Prevention Trial Results. I. Reduction in Incidence of Coronary Heart Disease, *JAMA* 251:351–364, 1984.

Code 810 307 004

CORTAID® Cream with Aloe

(See PDR For Nonprescription Drugs)

CORTAID® Lotion

(See PDR For Nonprescription Drugs)

CORTAID® Ointment with Aloe

(See PDR For Nonprescription Drugs)

CORTAID® Spray

(See PDR For Nonprescription Drugs)

CORTEF® Feminine Itch Cream

(See PDR For Nonprescription Drugs)

CYTOSAR-U®   ℞
brand of cytarabine sterile powder
(sterile cytarabine, USP)
For intravenous, Intrathecal and Subcutaneous Use Only

100 mg vial	NDC 6505-00-434-0733 (M)
500 mg vial	NDC 6505-01-077-5690 (M)

WARNING

Only physicians experienced in cancer chemotherapy should use CYTOSAR-U Sterile Powder.

For induction therapy patients should be treated in a facility with laboratory and supportive resources sufficient to monitor drug tolerance and protect and maintain a patient compromised by drug toxicity. The main toxic effect of CYTOSAR-U is bone marrow suppression with leukopenia, thrombocytopenia and anemia. Less serious toxicity includes nausea, vomiting, diarrhea and abdominal pain, oral ulceration, and hepatic dysfunction.

The physician must judge possible benefit to the patient against known toxic effects of this drug in considering the advisability of therapy with CYTOSAR-U. Before making this judgment or beginning treatment, the physician should be familiar with the following text.

DESCRIPTION

CYTOSAR-U Sterile Powder (cytarabine), commonly known as ara-C, an antineoplastic, is a sterile lyophilized material for reconstitution and intravenous, intrathecal or subcutaneous administration. It is available in multi-dose vials containing 100 mg, 500 mg, 1 g or 2 g sterile cytarabine. The pH of CYTOSAR-U was adjusted, when necessary, with hydrochloric acid and/or sodium hydroxide.

Cytarabine is chemically 4-amino-1-β-D-arabinofuranosyl-2(1H)-pyrimidinone.

Cytarabine is an odorless, white to off-white, crystalline powder which is freely soluble in water and slightly soluble in alcohol and in chloroform.

PHARMACOLOGY

Cell Culture Studies

Cytarabine is cytotoxic to a wide variety of proliferating mammalian cells in culture. It exhibits cell phase specificity, primarily killing cells undergoing DNA synthesis (S-phase) and under certain conditions blocking the progression of cells from the G_1 phase to the S-phase. Although the mechanism of action is not completely understood, it appears that cytarabine acts through the inhibition of DNA polymerase. A limited, but significant, incorporation of cytarabine into both DNA and RNA has also been reported. Extensive chromosomal damage, including chromatoid breaks, have been produced by cytarabine and malignant transformation of rodent cells in culture has been reported. Deoxycytidine prevents or delays (but does not reverse) the cytotoxic activity. Cell culture studies have shown an antiviral effect.[1] However, efficacy against herpes zoster or smallpox could not be demonstrated in controlled clinical trials.[2–4]

Cellular Resistance and Sensitivity

Cytarabine is metabolized by deoxycytidine kinase and other nucleotide kinases to the nucleotide triphosphate, an effective inhibitor of DNA polymerase; it is inactivated by a pyrimidine nucleoside deaminase which converts it to the nontoxic uracil derivative. It appears that the balance of kinase and deaminase levels may be an important factor in determining sensitivity or resistance of the cell to cytarabine.

Animal Studies

In experimental studies with mouse tumors, cytarabine was most effective in those tumors with a high growth fraction. The effect was dependent on the treatment schedule; optimal effects were achieved when the schedule (multiple closely spaced doses or constant infusion) ensured contact of the drug with the tumor cells when the maximum number of cells were in the susceptible S-phase. The best results were obtained when courses of therapy were separated by intervals sufficient to permit adequate host recovery.

Human Pharmacology

Cytarabine is rapidly metabolized and is not effective orally; less than 20 percent of the orally administered dose is absorbed from the gastrointestinal tract.

Following rapid intravenous injection of cytarabine with tritium, the disappearance from plasma is biphasic. There is an initial distributive phase with a half-life of about 10 minutes, followed by a second elimination phase with a half-life of about 1 to 3 hours. After the distributive phase, more than 80 percent of plasma radioactivity can be accounted for by the inactive metabolite 1-β-D-arabinofuranosyluracil (ara-U). Within 24 hours about 80 percent of the administered radioactivity can be recovered in the urine, approximately 90 percent of which is excreted as ara-U.

Relatively constant plasma levels can be achieved by continuous intravenous infusion.

After subcutaneous or intramuscular administration of cytarabine labeled with tritium, peak-plasma levels of radioactivity are achieved about 20 to 60 minutes after injection and are considerably lower than those after intravenous administration.

A reversible decrease in steady-state plasma digoxin concentrations and renal glycoside excretion followed one cytostatic dose of CYTOSAR-U.[39] Digoxin levels should be closely monitored during cytostatic drug therapy. Steady-state digitoxin plasma concentrations did not appear to change. The utilization of digitoxin for such patients may be considered as an alternative.

An *in vitro* interaction study between gentamicin and cytarabine showed a cytarabine related antagonism for the susceptibility of *K. pneumoniae* strains. This study suggests that in patients on cytarabine being treated with gentamicin for a *K. pneumoniae* infection, the lack of a prompt therapeutic response may indicate the need for reevaluation of antibacterial therapy.[40]

Clinical evidence in one patient showed possible inhibition of fluorocytosine efficacy during therapy with CYTOSAR-U.[41] This may be due to potential competitive inhibition of its uptake.[42]

Cerebrospinal fluid levels of cytarabine are low in comparison to plasma levels after single intravenous injection. However, in one patient in whom cerebrospinal levels were examined after 2 hours of constant intravenous infusion, levels approached 40 percent of the steady state plasma level. With intrathecal administration, levels of cytarabine in the cerebrospinal fluid declined with a first order half-life of about 2 hours. Because cerebrospinal fluid levels of deaminase are low, little conversion to ara-U was observed.

Immunosuppressive Action

CYTOSAR-U Sterile Powder is capable of obliterating immune responses in man during administration with little or no accompanying toxicity.[5,6] Suppression of antibody responses to E-coli-VI antigen and tetanus toxoid have been demonstrated. This suppression was obtained during both primary and secondary antibody responses.

CYTOSAR-U also suppressed the development of cell-mediated immune responses such as delayed hypersensitivity skin reaction to dinitrochlorobenzene. However, it had no effect on already established delayed hypersensitivity reactions.

Following 5-day courses of intensive therapy with CYTOSAR-U the immune response was suppressed, as indicated by the following parameters: macrophage ingress into skin windows; circulating antibody response following primary antigenic stimulation; lymphocyte blastogenesis with phytohemagglutinin. A few days after termination of therapy there was a rapid return to normal.[7]

INDICATIONS AND USAGE

CYTOSAR-U Sterile Powder in combination with other approved anticancer drugs is indicated for remission induction in acute non-lymphocytic leukemia of adults and children. It has also been found useful in the treatment of acute lymphocytic leukemia and the blast phase of chronic myelocytic leukemia. Intrathecal administration of CYTOSAR-U is indicated in the prophylaxis and treatment of meningeal leukemia.

CONTRAINDICATIONS

CYTOSAR-U Sterile Powder is contraindicated in those patients who are hypersensitive to the drug.

WARNINGS (See boxed WARNING)

Cytarabine is a potent bone marrow suppressant. Therapy should be started cautiously in patients with pre-existing drug-induced bone marrow suppression. Patients receiving this drug must be under close medical supervision and, during induction therapy, should have leukocyte and platelet counts performed daily. Bone marrow examinations should be performed frequently after blasts have disappeared from the peripheral blood. Facilities should be available for management of complications, possibly fatal, of bone marrow suppression (infection resulting from granulocytopenia and other impaired body defenses, and hemorrhage secondary to thrombocytopenia). One case of anaphylaxis that resulted in acute cardiopulmonary arrest and required resuscitation has been reported. This occurred immediately after the intravenous administration of CYTOSAR-U Sterile Powder. Severe and at times fatal CNS, GI and pulmonary toxicity (different from that seen with conventional therapy regimens of CYTOSAR-U) has been reported following some experimental dose schedules of CYTOSAR-U.[8–11] These reactions include reversible corneal toxicity, and hemorrhagic conjunctivitis, which may be prevented or diminished by prophylaxis with a local corticosteroid eye drop; cerebral and cerebellar dysfunction, including personality changes, somnolence and coma, usually reversible; severe gastrointestinal ulceration, including pneumatosis cystoides intestinalis leading to peritonitis; sepsis and liver abscess; pulmonary edema, liver damage with increased hyperbilirubinemia; bowel necrosis; and necrotizing colitis. Rarely, severe skin rash, leading to desquamation has been reported. Complete alopecia is more commonly seen with experimental high dose therapy than with standard treatment programs for CYTOSAR-U. If experimental high dose therapy is used, do not use a diluent containing benzyl alcohol.

An increase in cardiomyopathy with subsequent death has been reported following experimental high dose therapy with cytarabine in combination with cyclophosphamide when used for bone marrow transplant preparation.[12]

A syndrome of sudden respiratory distress, rapidly progressing to pulmonary edema and radiographically pronounced cardiomegaly has been reported following experimental high dose therapy with cytarabine used for the treatment of relapsed leukemia from one institution in 16/72 patients. The outcome of this syndrome can be fatal.[13]

Benzyl alcohol is contained in the diluent for this product. Benzyl alcohol has been reported to be associated with a fatal "Gasping Syndrome" in premature infants.

Two patients with childhood acute myelogenous leukemia who received intrathecal and intravenous CYTOSAR-U at conventional doses (in addition to a number of other concomitantly administered drugs) developed delayed progressive ascending paralysis resulting in death in one of the two patients.[14]

Use in Pregnancy

CYTOSAR-U can cause fetal harm when administered to a pregnant woman. (See ANIMAL TOXICOLOGY). There are no adequate and well-controlled studies in pregnant women. If CYTOSAR-U is used during pregnancy, or if the patient becomes pregnant while taking CYTOSAR-U, the patient should be apprised of the potential hazard to the fetus. Women of childbearing potential should be advised to avoid becoming pregnant.

PRECAUTIONS

1. General Precautions

Patients receiving CYTOSAR-U Sterile Powder must be monitored closely. Frequent platelet and leukocyte counts and bone marrow examinations are mandatory. Consider suspending or modifying therapy when drug-induced marrow depression has resulted in a platelet count under 50,000 or a polymorphonuclear granulocyte count under 1000/mm³. Counts of formed elements in the peripheral blood may continue to fall after the drug is stopped and reach lowest values after drug-free intervals of 12 to 24 days. When indicated, restart therapy when definite signs of marrow recovery appear (on successive bone marrow studies). Patients whose drug is withheld until "normal" peripheral blood values are attained may escape from control.

When large intravenous doses are given quickly, patients are frequently nauseated and may vomit for several hours postinjection. This problem tends to be less severe when the drug is infused.

The human liver apparently detoxifies a substantial fraction of an administered dose. Use the drug with caution and at reduced dose in patients whose liver function is poor.

Periodic checks of bone marrow, liver and kidney functions should be performed in patients receiving CYTOSAR-U.

Like other cytotoxic drugs, CYTOSAR-U may induce hyperuricemia secondary to rapid lysis of neoplastic cells.

The clinician should monitor the patient's blood uric acid level and be prepared to use such supportive and pharmacologic measures as might be necessary to control this problem.

Acute pancreatitis has been reported to occur in patients being treated with CYTOSAR-U who have had prior treatment with L-asparaginase.[15]

In patients who develop abdominal tenderness (peritonitis), early aggressive surgical or conservative close medical management may be appropriate depending upon the clinical status of the patient.[43,44]

2. Information for patient
Not applicable

3. Laboratory tests
See General Precautions

4. Drug Interactions
Not applicable

5. Carcinogenesis, mutagenesis, impairment of fertility
Extensive chromosomal damage, including chromatoid breaks have been produced by cytarabine and malignant transformation of rodent cells in culture has been reported.

6. Pregnancy
Pregnancy Category D. See WARNINGS.

A review of the literature has shown 32 reported cases where CYTOSAR-U was given during pregnancy, either alone or in combination with other cytotoxic agents: Eighteen normal infants were delivered. Four of these had first trimester exposure. Five infants were premature or low birth weight. Twelve of the 18 normal infants were followed up at ages ranging from six weeks to seven years, and showed no abnormalities. One apparently normal infant died at 90 days of gastroenteritis.

Two cases of congenital abnormalities have been reported, one with upper and lower distal limb defects,[16] and the other with extremity and ear deformities.[17] Both of these cases had first trimester exposure.

There were seven infants with various problems in the neonatal period, including pancytopenia; transient depression of WBC, hematocrit or platelets; electrolyte abnormalities; transient eosinophilia; and one case of increased IgM levels and hyperpyrexia possibly due to sepsis. Six of the seven infants were also premature. The child with pancytopenia died at 21 days of sepsis.

Therapeutic abortions were done in five cases. Four fetuses were grossly normal, but one had an enlarged spleen and another showed Trisomy C chromosome abnormality in the chorionic tissue.

Because of the potential for abnormalities with cytotoxic therapy, particularly during the first trimester, a patient who is or who may become pregnant while on CYTOSAR-U should be apprised of the potential risk to the fetus and the advisability of pregnancy continuation. There is a definite, but considerably reduced risk if therapy is initiated during the second or third trimester. Although normal infants have been delivered to patients treated in all three trimesters of pregnancy, follow-up of such infants would be advisable.

7. Labor and deliver
Not applicable

8. Nursing mothers
It is now known whether this drug is excreted in human milk. Because many drugs are excreted in human milk and because of the potential for serious adverse reactions in nursing infants from cytarabine, a decision should be made whether to discontinue nursing or to discontinue the drug, taking into account the importance of the drug to the mother.

9. Pediatric use
See INDICATIONS AND USAGE

ADVERSE REACTIONS

Expected Reactions
Because cytarabine is a bone marrow suppressant, anemia, leukopenia, thrombocytopenia, megaloblastosis and reduced reticulocytes can be expected as a result of administration with CYTOSAR-U Sterile Powder. The severity of these reactions are dose and schedule dependent.[18] Cellular changes in the morphology of bone marrow and peripheral smears can be expected.[19]

Following 5-day constant infusions or acute injections of 50 mg/m^2 to 600 mg/m^2, white cell depression follows a biphasic course. Regardless of initial count, dosage level, or schedule, there is an initial fall starting the first 24 hours with a nadir at days 7–9. This is followed by a brief rise which peaks around the twelfth day. A second and deeper fall reaches nadir at days 15–24. Then there is rapid rise to above baseline in the next 10 days. Platelet depression is noticeable at 5 days with a peak depression occurring between days 12–15. Thereupon, a rapid rise to above baseline occurs in the next 10 days.[20]

The Cytarabine (Ara-C) Syndrome
A cytarabine syndrome has been described by Castleberry.[21] It is characterized by fever, myalgia, bone pain, occasionally chest pain, maculopapular rash, conjunctivitis and malaise. It usually occurs 6–12 hours following drug administration.

Corticosteroids have been shown to be beneficial in treating or preventing this syndrome. If the symptoms of the syndrome are deemed treatable, corticosteroids should be contemplated as well as continuation of therapy with CYTOSAR-U.

Most Frequent Adverse Reactions
anorexia
nausea
vomiting
diarrhea
oral and anal inflammation or ulceration
hepatic dysfunction
fever
rash
thrombophlebitis
bleeding (all sites)
Nausea and vomiting are most frequent following rapid intravenous injection.

Less Frequent Adverse Reactions
sepsis
pneumonia
cellulitis at injection site
skin ulceration
urinary retention
renal dysfunction
neuritis
neural toxicity
sore throat
esophageal ulceration
esophagitis
chest pain
bowel necrosis
abdominal pain
freckling
jaundice
conjunctivitis (may occur with rash)
dizziness
alopecia
anaphylaxis (See WARNINGS)
allergic edema
pruritus
shortness of breath
urticaria
headache

Experimental Doses
Severe and at times fatal CNS, GI and pulmonary toxicity (different from that seen with conventional therapy regimens of CYTOSAR-U) has been reported following some experimental dose schedules of CYTOSAR-U.[8–11] These reactions include reversible corneal toxicity and hemorrhagic conjunctivitis, which may be prevented or diminished by prophylaxis with a local corticosteroid eye drop; cerebral and cerebellar dysfunction, including personality changes, somnolence and coma, usually reversible; severe gastrointestinal ulceration, including pneumatosis cystoides intestinalis leading to peritonitis; sepsis and liver abscess; pulmonary edema, liver damage with increased hyperbilirubinemia; bowel necrosis; and necrotizing colitis. Rarely, severe skin rash, leading to desquamation has been reported. Complete alopecia is more commonly seen with experimental high dose therapy than with standard treatment programs of CYTOSAR-U. If experimental high dose therapy is used, do not use a diluent containing benzyl alcohol.

An increase in cardiomyopathy with subsequent death has been reported following experimental high dose therapy with cytarabine in combination with cyclophosphamide when used for bone marrow transplant preparation.[12]

A syndrome of sudden respiratory distress, rapidly progressing to pulmonary edema and radiographically pronounced cardiomegaly has been reported following experimental high dose therapy with cytarabine used for the treatment of relapsed leukemia from one institution in 16/72 patients. The outcome of this syndrome can be fatal.[13]

Two patients with adult acute non-lymphocytic leukemia developed peripheral motor and sensory neuropathies after consolidation with high-dose CYTOSAR-U, daunorubicin, and asparaginase. Patients treated with high-dose CYTOSAR-U should be observed for neuropathy since dose schedule alterations may be needed to avoid irreversible neurologic disorders.[22]

Ten patients treated with experimental intermediate doses of CYTOSAR-U (1 g/m^2) with and without other chemotherapeutic agents (meta-AMSA, daunorubicin, etoposide) at various dose regimes developed a diffuse interstitial pneumonitis without clear cause that may have been related to the CYTOSAR-U.[45]

Two cases of pancreatitis have been reported following experimental doses of CYTOSAR-U and numerous other drugs. CYTOSAR-U could have been the causative agent.[46]

OVERDOSAGE

There is no antidote for overdosage of CYTOSAR-U. Doses of 4.5 g/m^2 by intravenous infusion over 1 hour every 12 hours for 12 doses has caused an unacceptable increase in irreversible CNS toxicity and death.[9]

Single doses as high as 3 g/m^2 have been administered by rapid intravenous infusion without apparent toxicity.[23]

DOSAGE AND ADMINISTRATION

CYTOSAR-U Sterile Powder is not active orally. The schedule and method of administration varies with the program of therapy to be used. CYTOSAR-U may be given by intravenous infusion or injection, subcutaneously or intrathecally. Thrombophlebitis has occurred at the site of drug injection or infusion in some patients, and rarely patients have noted pain and inflammation at subcutaneous injection sites. In most instances, however, the drug has been well tolerated. Patients can tolerate higher total doses when they receive the drug by rapid intravenous injection as compared with slow infusion. This phenomenon is related to the drug's rapid inactivation and brief exposure of susceptible normal and neoplastic cells to significant levels after rapid injection. Normal and neoplastic cells seem to respond in somewhat parallel fashion to these different modes of administration and no clear-cut clinical advantage has been demonstrated for either.

In the induction therapy of acute non-lymphocytic leukemia, the usual cytarabine dose in combination with other anticancer drugs is 100 mg/m^2 day by continuous IV infusion (Days 1–7) or 100 mg/m^2 IV every 12 hours (Days 1–7). The literature should be consulted for the current recommendations for use in acute lymphocytic leukemia.

Intrathecal Use in Meningeal Leukemia
CYTOSAR-U has been used intrathecally in acute leukemia in doses ranging from 5 mg/m^2 to 75 mg/m^2 of body surface area. The frequency of administration varied from once a day for 4 days to once every 4 days. The most frequently used dose was 30 mg/m^2 every 4 days until cerebrospinal fluid findings were normal, followed by one additional treatment.[24–28] The dosage schedule is usually governed by the type and severity of central nervous system manifestations and the response to previous therapy.

If used intrathecally, do not use a diluent containing benzyl alcohol. Many clinicians reconstitute with autologous spinal fluid or preservative-free 0.9% Sodium Chloride, USP, for Injection and use immediately.

CYTOSAR-U given intrathecally may cause systemic toxicity and careful monitoring of the hemopoietic system is indicated. Modification of other anti-leukemia therapy may be necessary. Major toxicity is rare. The most frequently reported reactions after intrathecal administration were nausea, vomiting and fever; these reactions are mild and self-limiting. Paraplegia has been reported.[29] Necrotizing leukoencephalopathy occurred in 5 children; these patients had also been treated with intrathecal methotrexate and hydrocortisone, as well as by central nervous system radiation.[30] Isolated neurotoxicity has been reported.[31] Blindness occurred in two patients in remission whose treatment had consisted of combination systemic chemotherapy, prophylactic central nervous system radiation and intrathecal CYTOSAR-U.[32]

Focal leukemic involvement of the central nervous system may not respond to intrathecal CYTOSAR-U and may better be treated with radiotherapy.

The 100 mg vial may be reconstituted with 5 ml of Bacteriostatic Water for Injection with Benzyl Alcohol 0.945% w/v added as preservative. The resulting solution contains 20 mg of cytarabine per ml. (Do not use Bacteriostatic Water for Injection with Benzyl Alcohol 0.945% w/v as a diluent for intrathecal use. See WARNINGS).

The 500 mg vial may be reconstituted with 10 ml Bacteriostatic Water for Injection with Benzyl Alcohol 0.945% w/v added as preservative. The resulting solution contains 50 mg of cytarabine per ml. (Do not use Bacteriostatic Water for Injection with Benzyl Alcohol 0.945% w/v as a diluent for intrathecal use. See WARNINGS).

The 1 gram vial may be reconstituted with 10 ml of Bacteriostatic Water for Injection with Benzyl Alcohol 0.945% w/v added as preservative. The resulting solution contains 100 mg of cytarabine per ml. (Do not use Bacteriostatic Water for Injection with Benzyl Alcohol 0.945% w/v as a dilient for intrathecal use. See WARNINGS).

The 2 gram vial may be reconstituted with 20 ml of Bacteriostatic Water for Injection with Benzyl Alcohol 0.945% w/v added as preservative. The resulting solution contains 100 mg of cytarabine per ml. (Do not use Bacteriostatic Water for Injection with Benzyl Alcohol 0.945% w/v as a diluent for intrathecal use. See WARNINGS).

If used intrathecally many clinicians reconstitute with preservative-free 0.9% Sodium Chloride for Injection and use immediately.

Continued on next page

Information on these Upjohn products is based on labeling in effect September 1, 1989. Further information concerning these and other Upjohn products may be obtained by direct inquiry to Medical Information, The Upjohn Company, Kalamazoo, Michigan 49001.

Upjohn—Cont.

The pH of the reconstituted solutions is about 5. Solutions reconstituted with Bacteriostatic Water for Injection with Benzyl Alcohol 0.945% w/v may be stored at controlled room temperature, 15°–30°C (59°–86°F) for 48 hours. Discard any solutions in which a slight haze develops.

Solutions reconstituted without a preservative should be used immediately.

Chemical Stability of Infusion Solutions:

Chemical stability studies were performed by ultraviolet assay on infusion solutions of CYTOSAR-U. These studies showed that when reconstituted CYTOSAR-U was added to Water for Injection, 5% Dextrose in Water or Sodium Chloride Injection, 94 to 96 percent of the cytarabine was present after 192 hours storage at room temperature.

Parenteral drugs should be inspected visually for particulate matter and discoloration, prior to administration, whenever solution and container permit.

Procedures for proper handling and disposal of anticancer drugs should be considered. Several guidelines on this subject have been published.[33–38] There is no general agreement that all of the procedures recommended in the guidelines are necessary or appropriate.

HOW SUPPLIED

CYTOSAR-U Sterile Powder (sterile cytarabine) is available in multi-dose vials of four sizes:

100 mg vial, NDC 0009-3063-01
500 mg vial, NDC 0009-3070-01
1 g vial, NDC 0009-3295-01
2 g vial, NDC 0009-3296-01

Store the product at controlled room temperature 15°–30°C (59°–86°F.)

REFERENCES

1. Zaky DA, Betts RF, Douglas RG, et al: Varicella-Zoster Virus and Subcutaneous Cytarabine: Correlation of In Vitro Sensitivities to Blood Levels, *Antimicrob Agents Chemother* 1975; 7:229–232
2. Davis CM, VanDersarl JV, Coltman CA Jr: Failure of Cytarabine in Varicella-Zoster Infections, *JAMA* 1973; 224:122–123
3. Betts RF, Zaky DA, Douglas RG, et al: Ineffectiveness of Subcutaneous Cytosine Arabinoside in Localized Herpes Zoster, *Ann Intern Med* 1975; 82:778–783
4. Dennis DT, Doberstyn EB, Awoke S, et al: Failure of Cytosine Arabinoside in Treatment Smallpox; A Double-blind Study, *Lancet* 1974; 2:377–379
5. Gray GD: ARA-C and Derivatives as Examples of Immunosuppressive Nucleoside Analogs, *Ann NY Acad Sci* 1975; 255:372–379
6. Mitchell MS, Wade ME, DeConti RC, et al: Immunosuppressive Effects of Cytosine Arabinoside and Methotrexate in Man, *Ann Intern Med* 1969; 70:535–547
7. Frei E, Ho DHW, Bodey GP, et al: Pharmacologic and Cytokinetic Studies of Arabinosyl Cytosine. In *Unifying Concepts of Leukemia*, Bibl. Hematol. No. 39. Karger, Basel 1973, pp 1085–1097
8. Hopen G, Mondino BJ, Johnson BL, et al: Corneal Toxicity with Systemic Cytarabine, *Am J Ophthalmol* 1981; 91:500–504
9. Lazarus HM, Herzig RH, Herzig GP, et al; Central Nervous System Toxicity of High-Dose Systemic Cytosine Arabinoside, *Cancer* 1981; 48:2577–2582
10. Slavin RE, Dias MA, Soral R: Cytosine Arabinoside Induced Gastrointestinal Toxic Alterations in Sequential Chemotherapeutic Protocols—A Clinical Pathologic Study of 33 Patients, *Cancer* 1978; 42:1747–1759
11. Haupt HM, Hutchins GM, Moore GW; Ara-C Lung: Noncardiogenic Pulmonary Edema Complicating Cytosine Arabinoside Therapy of Leukemia, *Am J Med* 1981; 70:256–261
12. Takvorian T, Anderson K, Ritz J: A Fatal Cardiomyopathy Associated with High Dosage Ara-C (HIDAC) and Cyclophosphamide (CTX) in Bone Marrow Transplantation (BMTx). (Abstract submitted for 1985 AACR Meetings in Houston, Texas.)
13. Andersson BS, Cogan B, Keating MJ, Estey EH, et al: Subacute Pulmonary Failure Complicating Therapy with High-Dose Ara-C in Acute Leukemia, *Cancer* 1985; 56:2181–2184
14. Dunton SF, Ruprecht N, Spruce W, et al: Progressive Ascending Paralysis Following Administration of Intra-thecal and Intravenous Cytosine Arabinoside, *Cancer* 1986; 57:1083–1088
15. Altman AJ, Dinndorf P, Quinn JJ: Acute Pancreatitis in Association with Cytosine Arabinoside Therapy, *Cancer* 1982; 49:1384–1386
16. Shafer AI: Teratogenic Effects of Antileukemic Chemotherapy, *Arch Intern Med* 1981; 141:514–515
17. Wagner VM, et al: Congenital Abnormalities in Baby Born to Cytarabine Treated Mother, *Lancet* 1980; 2:98–99
18. Frei E III, Bickers JN, Hewlett JS, et al: Dose Schedule and Antitumor Studies of Arabinosyl Cytosine (NSC 63878), *Cancer Res* 1969; 29:1325–1332
19. Bell WR, Wang JJ, Carbone PP, et al: Cytogenetic and Morphologic Abnormalities in Human Bone Marrow Cells during Cytosine Arabinoside Therapy, *J Hematol* 1966; 27:771–781
20. Burke PJ, Serpick AA, Carbone PP, et al: A Clinical Evaluation of Dose and Schedule of Administration of Cytosine Arabinoside (NSC 63878), *Cancer Res* 1968; 28:274–279
21. Castleberry RP, Crist WM, Holbrook T, et al: The Cytosine Arabinoside (Ara-C) Syndrome, *Med Pediatr Oncol* 1981; 9:257–264
22. Powell BL, Capizzi RL, Lyerly EW, et al: Peripheral Neuropathy After High-Dose Cytosine Arabinoside, Daunorubicin, and Asparaginase Consolidation for Acute Nonlymphocytic Leukemia, *J Clin Oncol* 1986; 4(1):95–97
23. Rudnick SA, et al: High Dose Cytosine Arabinoside (HDARAC) in Refractory Acute Leukemia, *Cancer* 1979; 44:1189–1193
24. Proceedings of the Chemotherapy Conference on ARA-C: Development and Application (Cytosine Arabinoside Hydrochloride—NSC 63878), Oct. 10, 1969
25. Lay HN, Colebatch JH, Ekert H: Experiences with Cytosine Arabinoside in Childhood Leukaemia and Lymphoma, *Med J Aust* 1971; 2:187–192
26. Halikowski B, Cyklis R, Armata J, et al: Cytosine Arabinoside Administered Intrathecally in Cerebromeningeal Leukemia, *Acta Paediat Scand* 1970; 59:164–168
27. Wang JJ, Pratt CB: Intrathecal Arabinosyl Cytosine in Meningeal Leukemia, *Cancer* 1970; 25:531–534
28. Band PR, Holland JF, Bernard J, et al: Treatment of Central Nervous System Leukemia with Intrathecal Cytosine Arabinoside, *Cancer* 1973; 32:744–748
29. Saiki JH, Thompson S, Smith F, et al: Paraplegia Following Intrathecal Chemotherapy, *Cancer* 1972; 29:370–374
30. Rubinstein LJ, Herman MM, Long TF, et al: Disseminated Necrotizing Leukoencephalopathy: A Complication of Treated Central System Leukemia and Lymphoma, *Cancer* 1975; 35:291–305
31. Marmont AM, Damasio EE: Neurotoxicity of Intrathecal Chemotherapy for Leukaemia, *Brit Med J* 1973; 4:47
32. Margileth DA, Poplack DG, Pizzo PA, et al: Blindness During Remission in Two Patients with Acute Lymphoblastic Leukemia, *Cancer* 1977; 39:58–61
33. Recommendations for the Safe Handling of Parenteral Antineoplastic Drugs. NIH Publication No. 83-2621. For sale by the Superintendent of Documents, US Government Printing Office, Washington, DC 20402.
34. AMA Council Report. Guidelines for Handling Parenteral Antineoplastics. *JAMA*, March 15, 1985.
35. National Study Commission on Cytotoxic Exposure-Recommendations for Handling Cytotoxic Agents. Available from Louis P. Jeffrey, ScD, Director of Pharmacy Services, Rhode Island Hospital, 593 Eddy Street, Providence, Rhode Island 02902.
36. Clinical Oncological Society of Australia: Guidelines and recommendations for safe handling of antineoplastic agents. *Med J Australia* 1983; 1:426–428.
37. Jones, RB, et al. Safe handling of chemotherapeutic agents: A report from the Mount Sinai Medical Center CA-A *Cancer Journal for Clinicians* Sept/Oct., 1983, pp. 258–263.
38. American Society of Hospital Pharmacists Technical assistance bulletin on handling cytotoxic drugs in hospitals. *Am J Hosp Pharm* 1985; 42:131–137.
39. Kuhlman J: Inhibition of Digoxin Absorption but not of Digitoxin During Cytostatic Drug Therapy. *Arzneim Forsch* 1982; 32:698–704.
40. Moody MR, Morris JJ, Yang VM, et al: Effect of Two Cancer Chemotherapeutic Agents on the Antibacterial Activity of Three Antimicrobial Agents. *Antimicrob Agents Chemother* 1978; 14:737–742.
41. Holt RJ: Clinical Problems with 5-Fluorocytosine. *Mykosen* 1978; 21(11):363–369.
42. Polak A, Grenson M: Interference Between the Uptake of Pyrimidines and Purines in Yeasts. *Path Microbiol* 1973; 39:37–38.
43. Johnson H, Smith TJ, Desforges J: Cytosine-Arabinoside-Induced Colitis and Peritonitis: Nonoperative Management. *J Clin Oncol* 1985; 3(5):607–612.
44. Martell RW, Jacobs P: Surgery for the acute abdomen in adults with leukemia. *Postgraduate Med J* 1986; 62:915–918.
45. Peters WG, Willemze R, Colly LP: Results of Induction and Consolidation Treatment with Intermediate and High-Dose Ara-C and m-AMSA Containing Regimens in Patients with Primarily Failed or Relapsed Acute Leukemia and Non-Hodgkin's Lymphoma. *Scan J Hemat* 1986; 36 (Suppl 44):7–16.
46. Siemers RF, Friedenberg WR, Norfleet RG: High-Dose Cytosine Arabinoside-Associated Pancreatitis. *Cancer* 1985; 56:1940–1942.

ANIMAL TOXICOLOGY

Toxicity of cytarabine in experimental animals, as well as activity, is markedly influenced by the schedule of administration. For example, in mice the LD_{10} for single intraperitoneal administration is greater than 6000 mg/m². However, when administered in 8 doses, each separated by 3 hours, the LD_{10} is less than 750 mg/m² total dose. Similarly, although a total dose of 1920 mg/m² administered as 12 injections at 6-hour intervals was lethal to beagle dogs (severe bone marrow hypoplasia with evidence of liver and kidney damage), dogs receiving the same total dose administered in 8 injections (again at 6-hour intervals) over a 48-hour period survived with minimal signs of toxicity. The most consistent observation in surviving dogs was elevated transaminase levels. In all experimental species the primary limiting toxic effect is marrow suppression with leukopenia. In addition, cytarabine causes abnormal cerebellar development in the neonatal hamster and is teratogenic to the rat fetus.

Code 810 126 114

DELTASONE®   ℞

brand of prednisone tablets, USP

HOW SUPPLIED

Scored tablets in the following strengths and sizes:

2.5 mg	Bottles of 100	NDC 0009-0032-01
5 mg	Bottles of 100	NDC 0009-0045-01
	Bottles of 500	NDC 0009-0045-02
Dosepak ™	Unit of use (21)	NDC 0009-0045-04
	Unit Dose Package (100)	NDC 0009-0045-05
10 mg	Bottles of 100	NDC 0009-0193-01
	Bottles of 500	NDC 0009-0193-02
	Unit Dose Packages (100)	NDC 0009-0193-03
20 mg	Bottles of 100	NDC 0009-0165-01
	Bottles of 500	NDC 0009-0165-02
	Unit dose Packages (100)	NDC 0009-0165-03
50 mg	Bottles of 100	NDC 0009-0388-01

Shown in Product Identification Section, page 433

DEPO-MEDROL®   ℞

brand of methylprednisolone acetate
sterile aqueous suspension
(sterile methylprednisolone acetate
suspension, USP)
Not for Intravenous Use

40 mg/ml (1 ml vial):
NSN 6505-00-952-0267 (M)

DESCRIPTION

DEPO-MEDROL Sterile Aqueous Suspension contains methylprednisolone acetate which is the 6-methyl derivative of prednisolone. Methylprednisolone acetate is a white or practically white, odorless, crystalline powder which melts at about 215° with some decomposition. It is soluble in dioxane, sparingly soluble in acetone, in alcohol, in chloroform, and in methanol, and slightly soluble in ether. It is practically insoluble in water.

The chemical name for methylprednisolone acetate is pregna-1,4-diene-3,20-dione,21-(acetyloxy)- 11, 17-dihydroxy-6-methyl-,(6α, 11β)- and the molecular weight is 416.51.

DEPO-MEDROL is an anti-inflammatory glucocorticoid for intramuscular, intrasynovial, soft tissue or intralesional injection. It is available in three strengths: 20 mg/ml; 40 mg/ml; 80 mg/ml.

[See table below].

ACTIONS

Naturally occurring glucocorticoids (hydrocortisone), which also have salt retaining properties, are used in replacement therapy in adrenocortical deficiency states. Their synthetic analogs are used primarily for their potent anti-inflammatory effects in disorders of many organ systems.

DEPO-MEDROL

Each ml of these preparations contains:

	20 mg	40 mg	80 mg
Methylprednisolone Acetate	20 mg	40 mg	80 mg
Polyethylene Glycol 3350	29.6 mg	29 mg	28 mg
Sodium Chloride	8.9 mg	8.7 mg	8.5 mg
Myristyl-gamma-picolinium Chloride	0.198 mg	0.195 mg	0.189 mg

added as preservative
When necessary, pH was adjusted with sodium hydroxide and/or hydrochloric acid.
The pH of the finished product remains within the USP specified range; ie, 3.5 to 7.0.

Glucocorticoids cause profound and varied metabolic effects. In addition, they modify the body's immune response to diverse stimuli.

INDICATIONS

A. FOR INTRAMUSCULAR ADMINISTRATION

When oral therapy is not feasible and the strength, dosage form, and route of administration of the drug reasonably lend the preparation to the treatment of the condition, the intramuscular use of DEPO-MEDROL Sterile Aqueous Suspension (methylprednisolone acetate) is indicated as follows:

1. **Endocrine Disorders**
   Primary or secondary adrenocortical insufficiency (hydrocortisone or cortisone is the drug of choice; synthetic analogs may be used in conjunction with mineralocorticoids where applicable; in infancy, mineralocorticoid supplementation is of particular importance)
   Acute adrenocortical insufficiency (hydrocortisone or cortisone is the drug of choice; mineralocorticoid supplementation may be necessary, particularly when synthetic analogs are used)
   Preoperatively and in the event of serious trauma or illness, in patients with known adrenal insufficiency or when adrenocortical reserve is doubtful
   Congenital adrenal hyperplasia
   Hypercalcemia associated with cancer
   Nonsuppurative thyroiditis

2. **Rheumatic Disorders**
   As adjunctive therapy for short-term administration (to tide the patient over an acute episode or exacerbation) in:
   Post-traumatic osteoarthritis
   Synovitis of osteoarthritis
   Rheumatoid arthritis, including juvenile rheumatoid arthritis (selected cases may require low-dose maintenance therapy)
   Acute and subacute bursitis
   Epicondylitis
   Acute nonspecific tenosynovitis
   Acute gouty arthritis
   Psoriatic arthritis
   Ankylosing spondylitis

3. **Collagen Diseases**
   During an exacerbation or as maintenance therapy in selected cases of:
   Systemic lupus erythematosus
   Systemic dermatomyositis (polymyositis)
   Acute rheumatic carditis

4. **Dermatologic Diseases**
   Pemphigus
   Severe erythema multiforme (Stevens-Johnson syndrome)
   Exfoliative dermatitis
   Bullous dermatitis herpetiformis
   Severe seborrheic dermatitis
   Severe psoriasis
   Mycosis fungoides

5. **Allergic States**
   Control of severe or incapacitating allergic conditions intractable to adequate trials of conventional treatment in:
   Bronchial asthma
   Contact dermatitis
   Atopic dermatitis
   Serum sickness
   Seasonal or perennial allergic rhinitis
   Drug hypersensitivity reactions
   Urticarial transfusion reactions
   Acute noninfectious laryngeal edema (epinephrine is the drug of first choice)

6. **Ophthalmic Diseases**
   Severe acute and chronic allergic and inflammatory processes involving the eye, such as:
   Herpes zoster ophthalmicus
   Iritis, iridocyclitis
   Chorioretinitis
   Diffuse posterior uveitis and choroiditis
   Optic neuritis
   Sympathetic ophthalmia
   Anterior segment inflammation
   Allergic conjunctivitis
   Allergic corneal marginal ulcers
   Keratitis

7. **Gastrointestinal Diseases**
   To tide the patient over a critical period of the disease in:
   Ulcerative colitis (systemic therapy)
   Regional enteritis (systemic therapy)

8. **Respiratory Diseases**
   Symptomatic sarcoidosis
   Berylliosis
   Fulminating or disseminated pulmonary tuberculosis when used concurrently with appropriate antituberculous chemotherapy
   Loeffler's syndrome not manageable by other means
   Aspiration pneumonitis

9. **Hematologic Disorders**
   Acquired (autoimmune) hemolytic anemia
   Secondary thrombocytopenia in adults
   Erythroblastopenia (RBC anemia)
   Congenital (erythroid) hypoplastic anemia

10. **Neoplastic Diseases**
    For palliative management of:
    Leukemias and lymphomas in adults
    Acute leukemia of childhood

11. **Edematous States**
    To induce diuresis or remission of proteinuria in the nephrotic syndrome, without uremia, of the idiopathic type or that due to lupus erythematosus

12. **Nervous System**
    Acute exacerbations of multiple sclerosis

13. **Miscellaneous**
    Tuberculous meningitis with subarachnoid block or impending block when used concurrently with appropriate antituberculous chemotherapy
    Trichinosis with neurologic or myocardial involvement

B. FOR INTRASYNOVIAL OR SOFT TISSUE ADMINISTRATION (see WARNINGS)

DEPO-MEDROL is indicated as adjunctive therapy for short-term administration (to tide the patient over an acute episode or exacerbation) in:
Synovitis of osteoarthritis
Rheumatoid arthritis
Acute and subacute bursitis
Acute gouty arthritis
Epicondylitis
Acute nonspecific tenosynovitis
Post-traumatic osteoarthritis

C. FOR INTRALESIONAL ADMINISTRATION

DEPO-MEDROL is indicated for intralesional use in the following conditions:
Keloids
Localized hypertrophic, infiltrated, inflammatory lesions of:
   lichen planus, psoriatic plaques, granuloma annulare, and lichen simplex chronicus (neurodermatitis)
Discoid lupus erythematosus
Necrobiosis lipodica diabeticorum
Alopecia areata
DEPO-MEDROL also may be useful in cystic tumors of an aponeurosis or tendon (ganglia).

CONTRAINDICATIONS

Systemic fungal infections and known hypersensitivity to components.

WARNINGS

Multidose use of DEPO-MEDROL Sterile Aqueous Suspension from a single vial requires special care to avoid contamination

Although initially sterile, any multidose use of vials may lead to contamination unless strict aseptic technique is observed. The preservative in DEPO-MEDROL Sterile Aqueous Suspension (methylprednisolone acetate) will prevent growth of most pathogenic organisms, but certain ones (eg Serratia marcescens) may remain viable. Particular care, such as use of disposable sterile syringes and needles is necessary. Multidose use of DEPO-MEDROL from vials is not recommended for intrasynovial injection.

While crystals of adrenal steroids in the dermis suppress inflammatory reactions, their presence may cause disintegration of the cellular elements and physiochemical changes in the ground substance of the connective tissue. The resultant infrequently occurring dermal and/or subdermal changes may form depressions in the skin at the injection site. The degree to which this reaction occurs will vary with the amount of adrenal steroid injected. Regeneration is usually complete within a few months or after all crystals of the adrenal steroid have been absorbed.

In order to minimize the incidence of dermal and subdermal atrophy, care must be exercised not to exceed recommended doses in injections. Multiple small injections into the area of the lesion should be made whenever possible. The technique of intrasynovial and intramuscular injection should include precautions against injection or leakage into the dermis. Injection into the deltoid muscle should be avoided because of a high incidence of subcutaneous atrophy.

DEPO-MEDROL is Not Recommended For Intrathecal Administration.

In patients on corticosteroid therapy subjected to any unusual stress, increased dosage of rapidly acting corticosteroids before, during, and after the stressful situation is indicated.

Corticosteroids may mask some signs of infection, and new infections may appear during their use. There may be decreased resistance and inability to localize infection when corticosteroids are used. Do not use intra-articularly, intrabursally or for intratendinous administration for *local* effect in the presence of acute infection.

Prolonged use of corticosteroids may produce posterior subcapsular cataracts, glaucoma with possible damage to the optic nerves, and may enhance the establishment of secondary ocular infections due to fungi or viruses.

Usage in pregnancy. Since adequate human reproduction studies have not been done with corticosteroids, the use of these drugs in pregnancy, nursing mothers, or women of childbearing potential requires that the possible benefits of the drug be weighed against the potential hazards to the mother and embryo or fetus. Infants born of mothers who have received substantial doses of corticosteroids during pregnancy should be carefully observed for signs of hypoadrenalism.

Average and large doses of cortisone or hydrocortisone can cause elevation of blood pressure, salt and water retention, and increased excretion of potassium. These effects are less likely to occur with the synthetic derivatives except when used in large doses. Dietary salt restriction and potassium supplementation may be necessary. All corticosteroids increase calcium excretion.

While on corticosteroid therapy patients should not be vaccinated against smallpox. Other immunization procedures should not be undertaken in patients who are on corticosteroids, especially in high doses, because of possible hazards of neurological complications and lack of antibody response.

The use of DEPO-MEDROL in active tuberculosis should be restricted to those cases of fulminating or disseminated tuberculosis in which the corticosteroid is used for the management of the disease in conjunction with appropriate antituberculous regimen.

If corticosteroids are indicated in patients with latent tuberculosis or tuberculin reactivity, close observation is necessary as reactivation of the disease may occur. During prolonged corticosteroid therapy, these patients should receive chemoprophylaxis.

Because rare instances of anaphylactoid reactions have occurred in patients receiving parenteral corticosteroid therapy, appropriate precautionary measures should be taken prior to administration especially when the patient has a history of allergy to any drug.

PRECAUTIONS

Drug-induced secondary adrenocortical insufficiency may be minimized by gradual reduction of dosage. This type of relative insufficiency may persist for months after discontinuation of therapy; therefore, in any situation of stress occurring during that period, hormone therapy should be reinstituted. Since mineralocorticoid secretion may be impaired, salt and/or a mineralocorticoid should be administered concurrently.

When multidose vials are used, special care to prevent contamination of the contents is essential. There is some evidence that benzalkonium chloride is not an adequate antiseptic for sterilizing DEPO-MEDROL Sterile Aqueous Suspension multidose vials. A povidone-iodine solution or similar product is recommended to cleanse the vial top prior to aspiration of contents. (See WARNINGS).

There is an enhanced effect of corticosteroids in patients with hypothyroidism and in those with cirrhosis.

Corticosteroids should be used cautiously in patients with ocular herpes simplex for fear of corneal perforation.

The lowest possible dose of corticosteroid should be used to control the condition under treatment, and when reduction in dosage is possible, the reduction must be gradual.

Psychic derangements may appear when corticosteroids are used, ranging from euphoria, insomnia, mood swings, personality changes, and severe depression to frank psychotic manifestations. Also, existing emotional instability or psychotic tendencies may be aggravated by corticosteroids.

Aspirin should be used cautiously in conjunction with corticosteroids in hypoprothrombinemia.

Steroids should be used with caution in nonspecific ulcerative colitis, if there is a probability of impending perforation, abscess or other pyogenic infection. Caution must also be used in diverticulitis, fresh intestinal anastomoses, active or latent peptic ulcer, renal insufficiency, hypertension, osteoporosis, and myasthenia gravis, when steroids are used as direct or adjunctive therapy.

Growth and development of infants and children on prolonged corticosteroid therapy should be carefully followed.

The following additional precautions apply for parenteral corticosteroids. Intrasynovial injection of a corticosteroid may produce systemic as well as local effects.

Appropriate examination of any joint fluid present is necessary to exclude a septic process.

A marked increase in pain accompanied by local swelling, further restriction of joint motion, fever, and malaise are suggestive of septic arthritis. If this complication occurs and

Continued on next page

Information on these Upjohn products is based on labeling in effect September 1, 1989. Further information concerning these and other Upjohn products may be obtained by direct inquiry to Medical Information, The Upjohn Company, Kalamazoo, Michigan 49001.

Upjohn—Cont.

the diagnosis of sepsis is confirmed, appropriate antimicrobial therapy should be instituted.

Local injection of a steroid into a previously infected joint is to be avoided.

Corticosteroids should not be injected into unstable joints. The slower rate of absorption by intramuscular administration should be recognized.

Although controlled clinical trials have shown corticosteroids to be effective in speeding the resolution of acute exacerbations of multiple sclerosis, they do not show that corticosteroids affect the ultimate outcome or natural history of the disease. The studies do show that relatively high doses of corticosteroids are necessary to demonstrate a significant effect. (See **Dosage And Administration**).

Since complications of treatment with glucocorticoids are dependent on the size of the dose and the duration of treatment, a risk/benefit decision must be made in each individual case as to dose and duration of treatment and as to whether daily or intermittent therapy should be used.

ADVERSE REACTIONS

Fluid and electrolyte disturbances:
Sodium retention
Fluid retention
Congestive heart failure in susceptible patients
Potassium loss
Hypokalemic alkalosis
Hypertension

Musculoskeletal:
Muscle weakness
Steroid myopathy
Loss of muscle mass
Osteoporosis
Vertebral compression fractures
Aseptic necrosis of femoral and humeral heads
Pathologic fracture of long bones

Gastrointestinal:
Peptic ulcer with possible subsequent perforation and hemorrhage
Pancreatitis
Abdominal distention
Ulcerative esophagitis

Dermatologic:
Impaired wound healing
Thin fragile skin
Petechiae and ecchymoses
Facial erythema
Increased sweating
May suppress reactions to skin tests

Neurological:
Convulsions
Increased intracranial pressure with papilledema (pseudotumor cerebri) usually after treatment
Vertigo
Headache

Endocrine:
Menstrual irregularities
Development of Cushingoid state
Suppression of growth in children
Secondary adrenocortical and pituitary unresponsiveness, particularly in times of stress, as in trauma, surgery or illness
Decreased carbohydrate tolerance
Manifestations of latent diabetes mellitus
Increased requirements for insulin or oral hypoglycemic agents in diabetes

Ophthalmic:
Posterior subcapsular cataracts
Increased intraocular pressure
Glaucoma
Exophthalmos

Metabolic:
Negative nitrogen balance due to protein catabolism
The following *additional* adverse reactions are related to parenteral corticosteroid therapy:
Rare instances of blindness associated with intralesional therapy around the face and head
Anaphylactic reaction
Allergic or hypersensitivity reactions
Urticaria
Hyperpigmentation or hypopigmentation
Subcutaneous and cutaneous atrophy
Sterile abscess
Injection site infections following non-sterile administration (see WARNINGS)
Postinjection flare, following intra-articular use
Charcot-like arthropathy
Arachnoiditis has been reported following intrathecal administration

DOSAGE AND ADMINISTRATION

Because of possible physical incompatibilities, DEPO-MEDROL Sterile Aqueous Suspension (methylprednisolone acetate) should not be diluted or mixed with other solutions.

A. Administration for Local Effect

Therapy with DEPO-MEDROL does not obviate the need for the conventional measures usually employed. Although this method of treatment will ameliorate symptoms, it is in no sense a cure and the hormone has no effect on the cause of the inflammation.

1. Rheumatoid and Osteoarthritis. The dose for intra-articular administration depends upon the size of the joint and varies with the severity of the condition in the individual patient. In chronic cases, injections may be repeated at intervals ranging from one to five or more weeks depending upon the degree of relief obtained from the initial injection. The doses in the following table are given as a general guide:

Size of Joint	Examples	Range of Dosage
Large	Knees Ankles Shoulders	20 to 80 mg
Medium	Elbows Wrists	10 to 40 mg
Small	Metacarpophalangeal Interphalangeal Sternoclavicular Acromioclavicular	4 to 10 mg

Procedure: It is recommended that the anatomy of the joint involved be reviewed before attempting intra-articular injection. In order to obtain the full anti-inflammatory effect it is important that the injection be made into the synovial space. Employing the same sterile technique as for a lumbar puncture, a sterile 20 to 24 gauge needle (on a dry syringe) is quickly inserted into the synovial cavity. Procaine infiltration is elective. The aspiration of only a few drops of joint fluid proves the joint space has been entered by the needle. *The injection site for each joint is determined by that location where the synovial cavity is most superficial and most free of large vessels and nerves.* With the needle in place, the aspirating syringe is removed and replaced by a second syringe containing the desired amount of DEPO-MEDROL Sterile Aqueous Suspension. The plunger is then pulled outward slightly to aspirate synovial fluid and to make sure the needle is still in the synovial space. After injection, the joint is moved gently a few times to aid mixing of the synovial fluid and the suspension. The site is covered with a small sterile dressing. Suitable sites for intra-articular injection are the knee, ankle, wrist, elbow, shoulder, phalangeal, and hip joints. Since difficulty is not infrequently encountered in entering the hip joint, precautions should be taken to avoid any large blood vessels in the area. Joints not suitable for injection are those that are anatomically inaccessible such as the spinal joints and those like the sacroiliac joints that are devoid of synovial space. Treatment failures are most frequently the result of failure to enter the joint space. Little or no benefit follows injection into surrounding tissue. If failures occur when injections into the synovial spaces are certain, as determined by aspiration of fluid, repeated injections are usually futile. Local therapy does not alter the underlying disease process, and whenever possible comprehensive therapy including physiotherapy and orthopedic correction should be employed.

Following intra-articular steroid therapy, care should be taken to avoid overuse of joints in which symptomatic benefit has been obtained. Negligence in this matter may permit an increase in joint deterioration that will more than offset the beneficial effects of the steroid.

Unstable joints should not be injected. Repeated intra-articular injection may in some cases result in instability of the joint. X-ray follow-up is suggested in selected cases to detect deterioration.

If a local anesthetic is used prior to injection of DEPO-MEDROL the anesthetic package insert should be read carefully and all the precautions observed.

2. Bursitis. The area around the injection site is prepared in a sterile way and a wheal at the site made with 1 percent procaine hydrochloride solution. A 20 to 24 gauge needle attached to a dry syringe is inserted into the bursa and the fluid aspirated. The needle is left in place and the aspirating syringe changed for a small syringe containing the desired dose. After injection, the needle is withdrawn and a small dressing applied.

3. Miscellaneous: Ganglion, Tendinitis, Epicondylitis. In the treatment of conditions such as tendinitis or tenosynovitis, care should be taken, following application of a suitable antiseptic to the overlying skin, to inject the suspension into the tendon sheath rather than into the substance of the tendon. The tendon may be readily palpated when placed on a stretch. When treating conditions such as epicondylitis, the area of greatest tenderness should be outlined carefully and the suspension infiltrated into the area. For ganglia of the tendon sheaths, the suspension is injected directly into the cyst. In many cases, a single injection causes a marked decrease in the size of the cystic tumor and may effect disappearance. The usual sterile precautions should be observed, of course, with each injection.

The dose in the treatment of the various conditions of the tendinous or bursal structures listed above varies with the condition being treated and ranges from 4 to 30 mg. In recurrent or chronic conditions, repeated injections may be necessary.

4. Injections for Local Effect in Dermatologic Conditions. Following cleansing with an appropriate antiseptic such as 70% alcohol, 20 to 60 mg of the suspension is injected into the lesion. It may be necessary to distribute doses ranging from 20 to 40 mg by repeated local injections in the case of large lesions. Care should be taken to avoid injection of sufficient material to cause blanching since this may be followed by a small slough. One to four injections are usually employed, the intervals between injections varying with the type of lesion being treated and the duration of improvement produced by the initial injection.

When multidose vials are used, special care to prevent contamination of the contents is essential (See WARNINGS).

B. Administration for Systemic Effect

The intramuscular dosage will vary with the condition being treated. When employed as a temporary substitute for oral therapy, a single injection during each 24-hour period of a dose of the suspension equal to the total daily oral dose of MEDROL® Tablets (methylprednisolone) is usually sufficient. When a prolonged effect is desired, the weekly dose may be calculated by multiplying the daily oral dose by 7 and given as a single intramuscular injection.

Dosage must be individualized according to the severity of the disease and response of the patient. For infants and children, the recommended dosage will have to be reduced, but dosage should be governed by the severity of the condition rather than by strict adherence to the ratio indicated by age or body weight.

Hormone therapy is an adjunct to, and not a replacement for, conventional therapy. Dosage must be decreased or discontinued gradually when the drug has been administered for more than a few days. The severity, prognosis and expected duration of the disease and the reaction of the patient to medication are primary factors in determining dosage. If a period of spontaneous remission occurs in a chronic condition, treatment should be discontinued. Routine laboratory studies, such as urinalysis, two-hour postprandial blood sugar, determination of blood pressure and body weight, and a chest X-ray should be made at regular intervals during prolonged therapy. Upper GI X-rays are desirable in patients with an ulcer history or significant dyspepsia.

In patients with the **adrenogenital syndrome**, a single intramuscular injection of 40 mg every two weeks may be adequate. For maintenance of patients with **rheumatoid arthritis**, the weekly intramuscular dose will vary from 40 to 120 mg. The usual dosage for patients with **dermatologic lesions** benefited by systemic corticoid therapy is 40 to 120 mg of methylprednisolone acetate administered intramuscularly at weekly intervals for one to four weeks. In acute severe dermatitis due to poison ivy, relief may result within 8 to 12 hours following intramuscular administration of a single dose of 80 to 120 mg. In chronic contact dermatitis repeated injections at 5 to 10 day intervals may be necessary. In seborrheic dermatitis, a weekly dose of 80 mg may be adequate to control the condition.

Following intramuscular administration of 80 to 120 mg to asthmatic patients, relief may result within 6 to 48 hours and persist for several days to two weeks. Similarly in patients with allergic rhinitis (hay fever) an intramuscular dose of 80 to 120 mg may be followed by relief of coryzal symptoms within six hours persisting for several days to three weeks.

If signs of stress are associated with the condition being treated, the dosage of the suspension should be increased. If a rapid hormonal effect of maximum intensity is required, the intravenous administration of highly soluble methylprednisolone sodium succinate is indicated.

Multiple Sclerosis

In treatment of acute exacerbations of multiple sclerosis daily doses of 200 mg of prednisolone for a week followed by 80 mg every other day for 1 month have been shown to be effective (4 mg of methylprednisolone is equivalent to 5 mg of prednisolone).

HOW SUPPLIED

DEPO-MEDROL Sterile Aqueous Suspension (methylprednisolone acetate) is available in the following strengths and package sizes:

20 mg/ml   5 ml vial   NDC 0009-0274-01
                 25–5 ml vials   NDC 0009-0274-05

40 mg/ml	1 ml vial	NDC 0009-0280-01
	25-1 ml vials	NDC 0009-0280-23
	5 ml vial	NDC 0009-0280-02
	25-5 ml vials	NDC 0009-0280-32
	10 ml vial	NDC 0009-0280-03
	25-10 vials	NDC 0009-0280-33
80 mg/ml	1 ml vial	NDC 0009-0306-01
	25-1 ml vials	NDC 0009-0306-09
	1 ml U-Ject®	NDC 0009-0306-04
	Disposable Syringe	
	5 ml vial	NDC 0009-0306-02
	25-5 ml vials	NDC 0009-0306-10

Store at controlled room temperature 15°–30° C (59°–86° F)
Code 810 341 011

Shown in Product Identification Section, page 433

DEPO–PROVERA®   ℞

brand of medroxyprogesterone sterile aqueous suspension
(sterile medroxyprogesterone acetate suspension, USP)

| 100 mg/ml, 5 ml | NSN 6505-00-207-7965 (M) |
| 400 mg/ml, 2.5 ml | NSN 6505-01-059-9006 (M) |

WARNING

THE USE OF PROGESTATIONAL AGENTS DURING THE FIRST FOUR MONTHS OF PREGNANCY IS NOT RECOMMENDED Progestational agents have been used beginning with the first trimester of pregnancy in an attempt to prevent habitual abortion or treat threatened abortion. There is no adequate evidence that such use is effective and there is evidence of potential harm to the fetus when such drugs are given during the first four months of pregnancy. Furthermore, in the vast majority of women, the cause of abortion is a defective ovum, which progestational agents could not be expected to influence. In addition, the use of progestational agents, with their uterine-relaxant properties, in patients with fertilized defective ova may cause a delay in spontaneous abortion. Therefore, the use of such drugs during the first four months of pregnancy is not recommended. Several reports suggest an association between intrauterine exposure to female sex hormones and congenital anomalies, including congenital heart defects and limb reduction defects[1-5]. One study[4] estimated a 4.7-fold increased risk of limb reduction defects in infants exposed in utero to sex hormones (oral contraceptives, hormone withdrawal tests for pregnancy, or attempted treatment for threatened abortion). Some of these exposures were very short and involved only a few days of treatment. The data suggest that the risk of limb reduction defects in exposed fetuses is somewhat less than 1 in 1000.
If the patient is exposed to DEPO-PROVERA Sterile Aqueous Suspension (medroxyprogesterone acetate) during the first four months of pregnancy or if she becomes pregnant while taking this drug, she should be apprised of the potential risks to the fetus.

DESCRIPTION

DEPO-PROVERA Sterile Aqueous Suspension contains medroxyprogesterone acetate which is a derivative of progesterone and is active by the parenteral and oral routes of administration. It is a white to off-white, odorless crystalline powder, stable in air, melting between 200 and 210° C. It is freely soluble in chloroform, soluble in acetone and dioxane, sparingly soluble in alcohol and methanol, slightly soluble in ether and insoluble in water.
The chemical name for medroxyprogesterone acetate is Pregn-4-ene-3,20-dione, 17-(acetyloxy)-6-methyl-, (6α).
DEPO-PROVERA for intramuscular injection is available in 2 strengths, 100 mg/ml and 400 mg/ml medroxyprogesterone acetate.
Each ml of the **100 mg/ml** suspension contains:
Medroxyprogesterone Acetate ....100 mg
Also
Polyethylene Glycol 3350 ....27.6 mg
Polysorbate 80 ....1.84 mg
Sodium Chloride ....8.3 mg
with
Methylparaben ....1.75 mg
Propylparaben ....0.194 mg
added as preservatives
Each ml of the **400 mg/ml** suspension contains:
Medroxyprogesterone Acetate ....400 mg
Polyethylene Glycol 3350 ....20.3 mg
Sodium Sulfate Anhydrous ....11 mg
with
Myristyl-gamma-picolinium
  Chloride ....1.69 mg
added as preservative
When necessary, pH was adjusted with sodium hydroxide and/or hydrochloric acid.

ACTIONS

Medroxyprogesterone acetate administered parenterally in the recommended doses to women with adequate endoge-

nous estrogen transforms proliferative endometrium into secretory endometrium.
Medroxyprogesterone acetate inhibits (in the usual dose range) the secretion of pituitary gonadotropin which, in turn, prevents follicular maturation and ovulation.
Because of its prolonged action and the resulting difficulty in predicting the time of withdrawal bleeding following injection, medroxyprogesterone acetate is not recommended in secondary amenorrhea or dysfunctional uterine bleeding. In these conditions oral therapy is recommended.

INDICATIONS

Adjunctive therapy and palliative treatment of inoperable, recurrent, and metastatic endometrial carcinoma or renal carcinoma.

CONTRAINDICATIONS

1. Thrombophlebitis, thromboembolic disorders, cerebral apoplexy or patients with a past history of these conditions.
2. Carcinoma of the breast.
3. Undiagnosed vaginal bleeding.
4. Missed abortion.
5. As a diagnostic test for pregnancy.
6. Known sensitivity to DEPO-PROVERA Sterile Aqueous Suspension (medroxyprogesterone acetate).

WARNINGS

1. The physician should be alert to the earliest manifestations of thrombotic disorders (thrombophlebitis, cerebrovascular disorders, pulmonary embolism, and retinal thrombosis). Should any of these occur or be suspected, the drug should be discontinued immediately.
2. Long term toxicology studies in the monkey, dog and rat disclose:
   1) Beagle dogs receiving 75 mg/kg and 3 mg/kg every 90 days developed mammary nodules, as did some of the control animals. The nodules appearing in the control animals were intermittent in nature, whereas the nodules in the drug treated animals were larger, more numerous, persistent, and there were two high dose animals that developed breast malignancies.
   2) Two of the monkeys receiving 150 mg/kg every 90 days developed undifferentiated carcinoma of the uterus. No uterine malignancies were found in monkeys receiving 30 mg/kg, 3 mg/kg, or placebo every 90 days. Transient mammary nodules were found during the study in the control, 3 mg/kg and 30 mg/kg groups, but not in the 150 mg/kg group. At sacrifice, the only nodules extant were in three of the monkeys in the 30 mg/kg group. Upon histopathologic examination these nodules have been determined to be hyperplastic.
   3) No uterine or breast abnormalities were revealed in the rat.
   The relevance of any of these findings with respect to humans has not been established.
3. The use of DEPO-PROVERA Sterile Aqueous Suspension (medroxyprogesterone acetate) for contraception is investigational since there are unresolved questions relating to its safety for this indication. Therefore, this is not an approved indication.
4. Discontinue medication pending examination if there is sudden partial or complete loss of vision, or if there is a sudden onset of proptosis, diplopia or migraine. If examination reveals papilledema or retinal vascular lesions, medication should be withdrawn.
5. Usage in pregnancy (See WARNING Box).
6. Retrospective studies of morbidity and mortality in Great Britain and studies of morbidity in the United States have shown a statistically significant association between thrombophlebitis, pulmonary embolism, and cerebral thrombosis and embolism and the use of oral contraceptives.[6-9] The estimate of the relative risk of thromboembolism in the study by Vessey and Doll[8] was about sevenfold, while Sartwell and associates[9] in the United States found a relative risk of 4.4, meaning that the users are several times as likely to undergo thromboembolic disease without evident cause as non-users. The American study also indicated that the risk did not persist after discontinuation of administration, and that it was not enhanced by long continued administration. The American study was not designed to evaluate a difference between products.
7. Following repeated injections, amenorrhea and infertility may persist for periods up to 18 months and occasionally longer.
8. The physician should be alert to the earliest manifestations of impaired liver function. Should these occur or be suspected, the drug should be discontinued and the patient's status re-evaluated.

PRECAUTIONS

1. The pretreatment physical examination should include special reference to breast and pelvic organs, as well as Papanicolaou smear.

2. Because progestogens may cause some degree of fluid retention, conditions which might be influenced by this factor, such as epilepsy, migraine, asthma, cardiac or renal dysfunction, require careful observation.
3. In cases of breakthrough bleeding, as in all cases of irregular bleeding per vaginum, nonfunctional causes should be borne in mind. In cases of undiagnosed vaginal bleeding, adequate diagnostic measures are indicated.
4. Patients who have a history of psychic depression should be carefully observed and the drug discontinued if the depression recurs to a serious degree.
5. Any possible influence of prolonged progestin therapy on pituitary, ovarian, adrenal, hepatic or uterine functions awaits further study.
6. A decrease in glucose tolerance has been observed in a small percentage of patients on estrogen-progestin combination drugs. The mechanism of this decrease is obscure. For this reason, diabetic patients should be carefully observed while receiving progestin therapy.
7. The age of the patient constitutes no absolute limiting factor although treatment with progestins may mask the onset of the climacteric.
8. The pathologist should be advised of progestin therapy when relevant specimens are submitted.
9. Because of the occasional occurrence of thrombotic disorders, (thrombophlebitis, pulmonary embolism, retinal thrombosis, and cerebrovascular disorders) in patients taking estrogen-progestin combinations and since the mechanism is obscure, the physician should be alert to the earliest manifestation of these disorders.

Information for the Patient
See Patient Information at the end of the insert.
The patient insert should be given to all premenopausal women, except those in whom childbearing is impossible.

ADVERSE REACTIONS

(See WARNING Box for possible adverse effects on the fetus).
In a few instances there have been undesirable sequelae at the site of injection, such as residual lump, change in color of skin or sterile abscess.
The following adverse reactions have been associated with the use of DEPO-PROVERA Sterile Aqueous Suspension (medroxyprogesterone acetate).
Breast—In a few instances, breast tenderness or galactorrhea have occurred.
Psychic—An occasional patient has experienced nervousness, insomnia, somnolence, fatigue or dizziness.
Thromboembolic Phenomena—Thromboembolic phenomena including thrombophlebitis and pulmonary embolism have been reported.
Skin and Mucous Membranes—Sensitivity reactions ranging from pruritus, urticaria, angioneurotic edema to generalized rash and anaphylaxis and/or anaphylactoid reactions have occasionally been reported. Acne, alopecia, or hirsutism have been reported in a few cases.
Gastrointestinal—Rarely, nausea has been reported. Jaundice, including neonatal jaundice, has been noted in a few instances.
Miscellaneous—Rare cases of headache and hyperpyrexia have been reported.
The following adverse reactions have been observed in women taking progestins including DEPO-PROVERA:
breakthrough bleeding
spotting
change in menstrual flow
amenorrhea
edema
change in weight
  (increase or decrease)
changes in cervical erosion and
  cervical secretions
cholestatic jaundice
rash (allergic) with and
  without pruritus
melasma or chloasma
mental depression
A statistically significant association has been demonstrated between use of estrogen-progestin combination drugs and the following serious adverse reactions: thrombophlebitis; pulmonary embolism and cerebral thrombosis and embolism. For this reason patients on progestin therapy should be carefully observed.
Although available evidence is suggestive of an association, such a relationship has been neither confirmed nor refuted

Continued on next page

Information on these Upjohn products is based on labeling in effect September 1, 1989. Further information concerning these and other Upjohn products may be obtained by direct inquiry to Medical Information, The Upjohn Company, Kalamazoo, Michigan 49001.

Upjohn—Cont.

for the following serious adverse reactions: neuro-ocular lesions, eg, retinal thrombosis and optic neuritis.

The following adverse reactions have been observed in patients receiving estrogen-progestin combination drugs:

rise in blood pressure in susceptible individuals
premenstrual-like syndrome
changes in libido
changes in appetite
cystitis-like syndrome
headache
nervousness
dizziness
fatigue
backache
hirsutism
loss of scalp hair
erythema multiforme
erythema nodosum
hemorrhagic eruption
itching

In view of these observations, patients on progestin therapy should be carefully observed.

The following laboratory results may be altered by the use of estrogen-progestin combination drugs:

Increased sulfobromophthalein retention and other hepatic function tests.

Coagulation tests: increase in prothrombin factors VII, VIII, IX and X.

Metyrapone test.

Pregnanediol determination.

Thyroid function: increase in PBI, and butanol extractable protein bound iodine and decrease in T^3 uptake values.

DOSAGE AND ADMINISTRATION

The suspension is intended for intramuscular administration only.

Endometrial or renal carcinoma—doses of 400 mg to 1000 mg of DEPO-PROVERA Sterile Aqueous Suspension (medroxyprogesterone acetate) per week are recommended initially. If improvement is noted within a few weeks or months and the disease appears stabilized, it may be possible to maintain improvement with as little as 400 mg per month. Medroxyprogesterone acetate is not recommended as primary therapy, but as adjunctive and palliative treatment in advanced inoperable cases including those with recurrent or metastatic disease.

HOW SUPPLIED

DEPO-PROVERA Sterile Aqueous Suspension (medroxyprogesterone acetate) is available in 2 strengths:

100 mg/ml: 5 ml vials   NDC 0009-0248-02
400 mg/ml:
  1 ml U-JECT® Disposable Syringe   NDC 0009-0626-03
  2.5 ml vial   NDC 0009-0626-01
  10 ml vial   NDC 0009-0626-02

REFERENCES

1. Gal I, Kirman B, Stern J: Hormonal pregnancy tests and congenital malformation. Nature 216:83, 1967.
2. Levy EP, Cohen A, Fraser FC: Hormone treatment during pregnancy and congenital heart defects. Lancet 1:611, 1973.
3. Nora JJ, Nora AH: Birth defects and oral contraceptives. Lancet 1:941-942, 1973.
4. Janerich DT, Piper JM, Glebatis DM: Oral contraceptives and congenital limb-reduction defects. N Engl J Med 291:697-700, 1974.
5. Heinonen OP, Slone D, Monson RR, et al: Cardiovascular birth defects and antenatal exposure to female sex hormones. N Engl J Med 296:67-70, 1977.
6. Royal College of General Practitioners: Oral contraception and thromboembolic disease. J Coll Gen Pract 13:267-279, 1967.
7. Inman WHW, Vessey MP: Investigation of deaths from pulmonary, coronary, and cerebral thrombosis and embolism in women of child-bearing age. Br Med J 2:193-199, 1968.
8. Vessey MP, Doll R: Investigation of relation between use of oral contraceptives and thromboembolic disease. A further report. Br Med J 2:651-657, 1969.
9. Sartwell PE, Masi AT, Arthes FG, et al: Thromboembolism and oral contraceptives: An epidemiological case-control study. Am J Epidemiol 90:365-380, 1969.

The text of the patient insert for progesterone and progesterone-like drugs is set forth below.

Patient Information: DEPO-PROVERA Sterile Aqueous Suspension contains medroxyprogesterone acetate. The information below is that which the U.S. Food and Drug Administration requires be provided for all patients taking progesterones. The information below relates only to the risk to the unborn child associated with use of progesterone during pregnancy. For further information on the use, side effects and other risks associated with this product, ask your doctor.

WARNING FOR WOMEN

There is an increased risk of birth defects in children whose mothers take this drug during the first four months of pregnancy.

Medroxyprogesterone acetate is similar to the progesterone hormones naturally produced by the body. Progesterone and progesterone-like drugs are used to treat menstrual disorders, to test if the body is producing certain hormones, and to treat some forms of cancer in women.

They have been used as a test for pregnancy but such use is no longer considered safe because of possible damage to a developing baby. Also, more rapid methods for testing for pregnancy are now available.

These drugs have also been used to prevent miscarriage in the first few months of pregnancy. No adequate evidence is available to show that they are effective for this purpose. Furthermore, most cases of early miscarriage are due to causes which could not be helped by these drugs.

There is an increased risk of birth defects, such as heart or limb defects, if progesterone and progesterone-like drugs are taken during the first four months of pregnancy. The exact risk of taking this drug early in pregnancy and having a baby with a birth defect is not known. However, one study found that babies born to women who had taken sex hormones (such as progesterone-like drugs) during the first three months of pregnancy were 4 to 5 times more likely to have abnormalities of the arms or legs than if their mothers had not taken such drugs. Some of these women had taken these drugs for only a few days. The chance that an infant whose mother had taken this drug will have this type of defect is about 1 in 1,000.

If you take DEPO-PROVERA Sterile Aqueous Suspension and later find you were pregnant when you took it, be sure to discuss this with your doctor as soon as possible.

Code 810 597 003

DEPO®-Testosterone   ℞

brand of testosterone cypionate sterile solution
(testosterone cypionate injection, USP)
For Intramuscular Use Only

HOW SUPPLIED

DEPO-Testosterone Sterile Solution is available in the following packages:

100 mg per ml. Each ml contains 100 mg testosterone cypionate, also 0.1 ml benzyl benzoate, 9.45 mg benzyl alcohol in 736 mg cottonseed oil.
  1 ml vial   NDC 0009-0347-01
  10 ml vial NDC 0009-0347-02

200 mg per ml. Each ml contains 200 mg testosterone cypionate, also 0.2 ml benzyl benzoate, 9.45 mg benzyl alcohol, in 560 mg cottonseed oil.
  1 ml vial   NDC 0009-0417-01
  10 ml vial NDC 0009-0417-02

DIDREX®   ⓒ ℞

brand of benzphetamine hydrochloride tablets

DESCRIPTION

DIDREX Tablets contain the anorectic agent benzphetamine hydrochloride. Benzphetamine hydrochloride is a white crystalline powder readily soluble in water and 95% ethanol. The chemical name for benzphetamine hydrochloride is d-N,α-Dimethyl-N-(phenylmethyl)-benzeneethanamine hydrochloride and its molecular weight is 275.82.

Each DIDREX tablet, for oral administration, contains 25 or 50 mg of benzphetamine hydrochloride.

Inactive Ingredients

25 mg—Calcium Stearate, Corn Starch, FD & C Yellow #5, Lactose, Povidone, Sorbital.

50 mg—Calcium Stearate, Corn Starch, Erythrosine Sodium, FD & C Yellow #6, Lactose, Povidone, Sorbital.

CLINICAL PHARMACOLOGY

Benzphetamine hydrochloride is a sympathomimetic amine with pharmacologic activity similar to the prototype drugs of this class used in obesity, the amphetamines. Actions include central nervous system stimulation and elevation of blood pressure. Tachyphylaxis and tolerance have been demonstrated with all drugs of this class in which these phenomena have been looked for.

Drugs of this class used in obesity are commonly known as "anorectics" or "anorexigenics." It has not been established, however, that the action of such drugs in treating obesity is primarily one of appetite suppression. Other central nervous system actions, or metabolic effects, may be involved.

Adult obese subjects instructed in dietary management and treated with "anorectic" drugs, lose more weight on the average than those treated with placebo and diet, as determined in relatively short term clinical trials.

The magnitude of increased weight loss of drug treated patients over placebo treated patients is only a fraction of a pound a week. The rate of weight loss is greatest in the first weeks of therapy for both drug and placebo subjects and

tends to decrease in succeeding weeks. The possible origins of the increased weight loss due to the various drug effects are not established. The amount of weight loss associated with the use of an "anorectic" drug varies from trial to trial, and the increased weight loss appears to be related in part to variables other than the drug prescribed, such as the physician-investigator, the population treated, and the diet prescribed. Studies do not permit conclusions as to the relative importance of the drug and nondrug factors on weight loss. The natural history of obesity is measured in years, whereas the studies cited are restricted to a few weeks duration; thus, the total impact of drug induced weight loss over that of diet alone must be considered to be clinically limited.

Pharmacokinetic data in humans are not available.

INDICATIONS AND USAGE

DIDREX Tablets (benzphetamine hydrochloride) are indicated in the management of exogenous obesity as a short term adjunct (a few weeks) in a regimen of weight reduction based on caloric restriction. The limited usefulness of agents of this class (see **Clinical Pharmacology**) should be weighed against possible risks inherent in their use such as those described below.

CONTRAINDICATIONS

DIDREX Tablets (benzphetamine hydrochloride) are contraindicated in patients with advanced arteriosclerosis, symptomatic cardiovascular disease, moderate to severe hypertension, hyperthyroidism, known hypersensitivity or idiosyncrasy to sympathomimetic amines, and glaucoma. Benzphetamine should not be given to patients who are in an agitated state or who have a history of drug abuse.

Hypertensive crises have resulted when sympathomimetic amines have been used concomitantly or within 14 days following use of monamine oxidase inhibitors. DIDREX should not be used concomitantly with other CNS stimulants.

DIDREX may cause fetal harm when administered to a pregnant woman. Amphetamines have been shown to be teratogenic and embryotoxic in mammals at high multiples of the human dose. DIDREX is contraindicated in women who are or may become pregnant. If this drug is used during pregnancy, or if the patient becomes pregnant while taking this drug, the patient should be apprised of the potential hazard to the fetus.

WARNINGS

When tolerance to the anorectic effect develops, the recommended dose should not be exceeded in an attempt to increase the effect; rather, the drug should be discontinued.

PRECAUTIONS

General: Insulin requirements in diabetes mellitus may be altered in association with use of anorexigenic drugs and the concomitant dietary restrictions.

Psychological disturbances have been reported in patients who receive an anorectic agent together with a restrictive dietary regime.

Caution is to be exercised in prescribing amphetamines for patients with even mild hypertension. The least amount feasible should be prescribed or dispensed at one time in order to minimize the possibility of overdosage.

DIDREX Tablets, 25 mg, contain FD&C Yellow No. 5 (tartrazine) which may cause allergic-type reactions (including bronchial asthma) in certain susceptible individuals. Although the overall incidence of FD&C Yellow No. 5 (tartrazine) sensitivity in the general population is low, it is frequently seen in patients who also have aspirin hypersensitivity.

INFORMATION FOR PATIENTS

Amphetamines may impair the ability of the patient to engage in potentially hazardous activities such as operating machinery or driving a motor vehicle; the patient should therefore be cautioned accordingly.

DRUG INTERACTIONS

Hypertensive crises have resulted when sympathomimetic amines have been used concomitantly or within 14 days following use of monoamine oxidase inhibitors. DIDREX should not be used concomitantly with other CNS stimulants.

Amphetamines may decrease the hypotensive effect of antihypertensives. Amphetamines may enhance the effects of tricyclic antidepressants.

Urinary alkalinizing agents increase blood levels and decrease excretion of amphetamines. Urinary acidifying agents decrease blood levels and increase excretion of amphetamines.

Carcinogenesis, Mutagenesis, Impairment of Fertility: Animal studies to evaluate the potential for carcinogenesis, mutagenesis or impairment of fertility have not been performed by The Upjohn Company.

Pregnancy: Pregnancy Category X. (See CONTRAINDICATIONS section.)

Nursing Mothers: Amphetamines are excreted in human milk. Mothers taking amphetamines should be advised to refrain from nursing.

Pediatric Use: Use of benzphetamine hydrochloride is not recommended in children under 12 years of age.

ADVERSE REACTIONS

The following have been associated with the use of benzphetamine hydrochloride:

Cardiovascular
Palpitation, tachycardia, elevation of blood pressure. There have been isolated reports of cardiomyopathy associated with chronic amphetamine use.

CNS
Overstimulation, restlessness, dizziness, insomnia, tremor, sweating, headache; rarely, psychotic episodes at recommended doses; depression following withdrawal of the drug.

Gastrointestinal
Dryness of the mouth, unpleasant taste, nausea, diarrhea, other gastrointestinal disturbances.

Allergic
Urticaria and other allergic reactions involving the skin.

Endocrine
Changes in libido.

DRUG ABUSE AND DEPENDENCE

Benzphetamine is a controlled substance under the Controlled Substance Act by the Drug Enforcement Administration and has been assigned to Schedule III.

Benzphetamine hydrochloride is related chemically and pharmacologically to the amphetamines. Amphetamines and related stimulant drugs have been extensively abused and the possibility of abuse of DIDREX Tablets should be kept in mind when evaluating the desirability of including a drug as part of a weight reduction program. Abuse of amphetamines and related drugs may be associated with intense psychological dependence and severe social dysfunction. There are reports of patients who have increased the dosage to many times that recommended. Abrupt cessation following prolonged high dosage administration results in extreme fatigue and mental depression; changes are also noted on the sleep EEG. Manifestations of chronic intoxication with anorectic drugs include severe dermatoses, marked insomnia, irritability, hyperactivity, and personality changes. The most severe manifestation of chronic intoxication is psychosis, often clinically indistinguishable from schizophrenia.

OVERDOSAGE

Manifestations of Overdosage:
Acute overdosage with amphetamines may result in restlessness, tremor, tachypnea, confusion, assaultiveness and panic states. Fatigue and depression usually follow the central stimulation. Cardiovascular effects include arrhythmias, hypertension or hypotension, and circulatory collapse. Gastrointestinal symptoms include nausea, vomiting, diarrhea, and abdominal cramps. Hyperpyrexia and rhabdomyolysis have been reported and can lead to a number of associated complications. Fatal poisoning is usually preceded by convulsions and coma.

TREATMENT OF OVERDOSAGE

(See **Warnings**) Information concerning the effects of overdosage with DIDREX Tablets (benzphetamine hydrochloride) is extremely limited. The following is based on experience with other anorexiants.
Management of acute amphetamine intoxication is largely symptomatic and includes sedation with a barbiturate. If hypertension is marked, the use of a nitrite or rapidly acting alpha receptor blocking agent should be considered. Experience with hemodialysis or peritoneal dialysis is inadequate to permit recommendations in this regard.
Acidification of the urine increases amphetamine excretion. The oral LD$_{50}$ is 174 mg/kg in mice and 104 mg/kg in rats. The intraperitoneal LD$_{50}$ in mice is 153 mg/kg.

DOSAGE AND ADMINISTRATION

Dosage should be individualized according to the response of the patient. The suggested dosage ranges from 25 to 50 mg one to three times daily. Treatment should begin with 25 to 50 mg once daily with subsequent increase in individual dose or frequency according to response. A single daily dose is preferably given in mid-morning or mid-afternoon, according to the patient's eating habits. In an occasional patient it may be desirable to avoid late afternoon administration. Use of benzphetamine hydrochloride is not recommended in children under 12 years of age.

HOW SUPPLIED

DIDREX Tablets (benzphetamine hydrochloride) are available in the following strengths and colors:
25 mg (yellow)
Bottles of 100 *NDC 0009-0018-01*
50 mg (peach, scored)
Bottles of 100 *NDC 0009-0024-01*
Bottles of 500 *NDC 0009-0024-02*
Store at controlled room temperature 15°–30°C (59°–86°F).
Code 810 735 309

Shown in Product Identification Section, page 433

GELFOAM®
brand of absorbable gelatin sterile sponge
(absorbable gelatin sponge, USP)

Size 12-7 mm:	NSN 6510-00-080-2053 (M & VA)
Size 100:	NSN 6510-00-080-2054 (M & VA)
Size 200:	NSN 6510-00-655-8522 (VA)
Size 100 Compressed:	NSN 6510-01-066-8966 (VA)
Dental Packs, Size 4:	NSN 6510-00-064-4858 (M)

DESCRIPTION

GELFOAM Sterile Sponge is a medical device intended for application to bleeding surfaces as a hemostatic. It is a water-insoluble, off-white, nonelastic, porous, pliable product prepared from purified pork Skin Gelatin USP Granules and Water for Injection, USP. It may be cut without fraying and is able to absorb and hold within its interstices, many times its weight of blood and other fluids.

ACTION

GELFOAM Sterile Sponge has hemostatic properties. While its mode of action is not fully understood, its effect appears to be more physical than the result of altering the blood clotting mechanism.
When not used in excessive amounts, GELFOAM is absorbed completely, with little tissue reaction. This absorption is dependent on several factors, including the amount used, degree of saturation with blood or other fluids, and the site of use. When placed in soft tissues, GELFOAM is usually absorbed completely in from four to six weeks, without inducing excessive scar tissue. When applied to bleeding nasal, rectal or vaginal mucosa, it liquefies within two to five days.
HEMOSTASIS: GELFOAM Sterile Sponge, used dry or saturated with sterile sodium chloride solution, is indicated in surgical procedures as a hemostatic device, when control of capillary, venous, and arteriolar bleeding by pressure, ligature, and other conventional procedures is either ineffective or impractical.

DIRECTIONS FOR USE

Sterile technique should always be used to remove GELFOAM Sterile Sponge from its packaging. Cut to the desired size, a piece of GELFOAM, either dry or saturated with sterile, isotonic sodium chloride solution (sterile saline), can be applied with pressure directly to the bleeding site. When applied dry, a single piece of GELFOAM should be manually compressed before application to the bleeding site, and then held in place with moderate pressure until hemostasis results. When used with sterile saline, GELFOAM should be first immersed in the solution and then withdrawn, squeezed between gloved fingers to expel air bubbles, and then replaced in saline until needed. The GELFOAM sponge should promptly return to its original size and shape in the solution. If it does not, it should be removed again and kneaded vigorously until all air is expelled and it does expand to its original size and shape when returned to the sterile saline.
GELFOAM is used wet or blotted to dampness on gauze before application to the bleeding site. It should be held in place with moderate pressure, using a pledget of cotton or small gauze sponge until hemostasis results. Removal of the pledget or gauze is made easier by wetting it with a few drops of sterile saline, to prevent pulling up the GELFOAM which by then should enclose a firm clot. Use of suction applied over the pledget of cotton or gauze to draw blood into the GELFOAM is unnecessary, as the GELFOAM will draw up sufficient blood by capillary action. The first application of GELFOAM will usually control bleeding, but if not, additional applications may be made using fresh pieces, prepared as described above.
Use only the minimum amount of GELFOAM, cut to appropriate size, necessary to produce hemostasis. The GELFOAM may be left in place at the bleeding site, when necessary. Since GELFOAM causes little more cellular reaction than does the blood clot, the wound may be closed over it. GELFOAM may be left in place when applied to mucosal surfaces until it liquifies.

CONTRAINDICATIONS

GELFOAM Sterile Sponge should not be used in closure of skin incisions because it may interfere with healing of the skin edges. This is due to mechanical interposition of gelatin and is not secondary to intrinsic interference with wound healing.
GELFOAM should not be placed in intravascular compartments, because of the risk of embolization.

WARNINGS

GELFOAM Sterile Sponge is not intended as a substitute for meticulous surgical technique and the proper application of ligatures, or other conventional procedures for hemostasis.
GELFOAM is supplied as a sterile product and cannot be resterilized. Unused, opened envelopes of GELFOAM should be discarded.
Only the minimum amount of GELFOAM necessary to achieve hemostatis should be used. Once hemostatis is attained, excess GELFOAM should be carefully removed.

The use of GELFOAM is not recommended in the presence of infection. GELFOAM should be used with caution in contaminated areas of the body. If signs of infection or abscess develop where GELFOAM has been positioned, reoperation may be necessary in order to remove the infected material and allow drainage.
The hemostatic property of GELFOAM has not been shown to be enhanced by the addition of exogenous thrombin. Because thrombin is antigenic, it should not be combined with GELFOAM.
While packing a cavity for hemostasis is sometimes surgically indicated, GELFOAM should not be used in this manner unless excess product not needed to maintain hemostasis is removed.
Whenever possible, it should be removed after use in laminectomy procedures and from foramina in bone, once hemostasis is achieved. This is because GELFOAM may swell to its original size on absorbing fluids, and produce nerve damage by pressure within confined bony spaces.
The packing or wadding of GELFOAM, particularly within bony cavities, should be avoided, since swelling to original size may interfere with normal function and/or possibly result in compression necrosis of surrounding tissues.

PRECAUTIONS

Use only the minimum amount of GELFOAM Sterile Sponge needed for hemostasis, holding it at the site until bleeding stops, then removing the excess.
GELFOAM should **not** be used for controlling postpartum hemorrhage or menorrhagia.
It has been demonstrated that fragments of microfibrillar collagen pass through the 40µ transfusion filters of blood scavenging systems. Although not the same product, GELFOAM should also not be used in conjunction with autologous blood salvage circuits.
Microfibrillar collagen has been reported to reduce the strength of methylmethacrylate adhesives used to attach prosthetic devices to bone surfaces. As a precaution, GELFOAM should not be used in conjunction with such adhesives.
GELFOAM is not recommended for the primary treatment of coagulation disorders.
It is not recommended that GELFOAM be saturated with an antibiotic solution or dusted with antibiotic powder.

ADVERSE REACTIONS

There have been reports of fever associated with the use of GELFOAM, without demonstrable infection. GELFOAM Sterile Sponge may serve as a nidus for infection and abscess formation[1], and has been reported to potentiate bacterial growth. Giant-cell granuloma has been reported at the implantation site of absorbable gelatin product in the brain[2], as has compression of the brain and spinal cord resulting from the accumulation of sterile fluid.[3]
Foreign body reactions, "encapsulation" of fluid and hematoma have also been reported.
When GELFOAM was used in laminectomy operations, multiple neurologic events were reported, including but not limited to cauda equina syndrome, spinal stenosis, meningitis, arachnoiditis, headaches, paresthesias, pain, bladder and bowel dysfunction, and impotence.
Excessive fibrosis and prolonged fixation of a tendon have been reported when absorbable gelatin products were used in severed tendon repair.
Toxic shock syndrome has been reported in association with the use of GELFOAM in nasal surgery.
Fever, failure of absorption, and hearing loss have been reported in association with the use of GELFOAM during tympanoplasty.

ADVERSE REACTIONS REPORTED FROM UNAPPROVED USES

GELFOAM is not recommended for use other than as an adjunct for hemostasis.
While some adverse medical events following the unapproved use of GELFOAM have been reported to The Upjohn Company (see Adverse Reactions), other hazards associated with such use may not have been reported.
When GELFOAM has been used during intravascular catheterization for the purpose of producing vessel occlusion, the following adverse events have been reported; fever, duodenal and pancreatic infarct, embolization of lower extremity vessels, pulmonary embolization, splenic abscess, necrosis of specific anatomic areas, asterixis, and death.
These adverse medical events have been associated with the use of GELFOAM for repair of dural defects encountered during laminectomy and craniotomy operations: fever, infection, leg paresthesias, neck and back pain, bladder and bowel

Continued on next page

Information on these Upjohn products is based on labeling in effect September 1, 1989. Further information concerning these and other Upjohn products may be obtained by direct inquiry to Medical Information, The Upjohn Company, Kalamazoo, Michigan 49001.

Upjohn—Cont.

incontinence, cauda equina syndrome, neurogenic bladder, impotence, and paresis.

DOSAGE AND ADMINISTRATION

Sterile technique should always be used in removing the inner envelope containing the GELFOAM Sterile Sponge from the outer printed sealed envelope. The minimum amount of GELFOAM of appropriate size and shape should be applied (dry or wet, see DIRECTIONS FOR USE) to the bleeding site and held firmly in place until hemostasis is observed. Opened envelopes of unused GELFOAM should always be discarded.

HOW SUPPLIED

GELFOAM Sterile Sponge (absorbable gelatin sponge) is available in the following sizes:

Size 12—3 mm 20 mm × 60 mm (12 sq cm) × 3 mm [¾ in × 2⅜ in (1¾ sq in) × ⅛ in] *in boxes of 4 sponges in individual envelopes.*

NDC 0009-0301-01

Size 12—7 mm 20 mm × 60 mm (12 sq cm) × 7 mm [¾ in × 2⅜ in (1¾ sq in) × ¼ in] *in boxes of 12 sponges in individual envelopes, and in jars of 4 sponges.*

Box NDC 0009-0315-03
Jar NDC 0009-0315-02

Size 50, 80 mm × 62.5 mm (50 sq cm) × 10 mm [3⅛ in × 2½ in (7⅞ sq in) × ⅜ in] *in boxes of 4 sponges in individual envelopes.*

NDC 0009-0323-01

Size 100, 80 mm × 125 mm (100 sq cm) × 100 mm [3⅛ in × 5 in (15⅝ sq in) × ⅜ in] *in boxes of 6 sponges in individual envelopes.*

NDC 0009-0342-01

Size 200, 80 mm × 250 mm (200 sq cm) × 10 mm (3⅛ in × 10 in (31¼ sq in) × ⅜ in] *in boxes of 6 sponges in individual envelopes.*

NDC 0009-0349-01

Size 2 cm (approximately 40 cm × 2 cm) [15¾ in × ¾ in] *packaged in individual jars.*

NDC 0009-0364-01

Size 6 cm (approximately 40 cm × 6 cm) [15¾ in × 2⅜ in] *packaged in cartons of six sponges in individual envelopes.*

NDC 0009-0371-01

STORAGE AND HANDLING

GELFOAM Sterile Sponge (absorbable gelatin sponge) should be stored at controlled room temperature 15°–30°C (59°–86°F). Once the package is opened, contents are subject to contamination. It is recommended that GELFOAM be used as soon as the package is opened and unused contents discarded.

CAUTION

Federal law restricts this device to sale by or on the order of a physician.

CLINICAL STUDIES

GELFOAM Sterile Sponge is a water-soluble, hemostatic device prepared from purified skin gelatin, and capable of absorbing up to 45 times its weight of whole blood.[4] The absorptive capacity of GELFOAM is a function of its physical size, increasing as the size of the gelatin sponge increases.[5] The mechanism of action of surface-mediated hemostatic devices is supportive and mechanical.[5] Surface-acting devices, when applied directly to bleeding surfaces, arrest bleeding by the formation of an artifical clot and by producing a mechanical matrix that facilitates clotting.[6] Jenkins et al[7] have theorized that the clotting effect of GELFOAM may be due to release of thromboplastin from platelets, occurring when platelets entering the sponge become damaged by contact with the walls of its myriad of interstices. Thromboplastin interacts with prothrombin and calcium to produce thrombin, and this sequence of events initiates the clotting reaction. The authors suggest that the physiologic formation of thrombin in the sponge is sufficient to produce formation of a clot, by its action on the fibrinogen in blood.[7] The spongy physical properties of the gelatin sponge hasten clot formation and provide structural support for the forming clot.[6,8] Several investigators have claimed that GELFOAM becomes liquefied within a week or less and is completely absorbed in four to six weeks, without inducing excessive scar formation.[4,7,9,10,11] Barnes[10] reviewed experiences with GELFOAM in gynecologic surgery. No excessive scar tissue, attributable to the absorption of GELFOAM, could be palpated at postoperative examination.

ANIMAL PHARMACOLOGY

Surface-acting hemostatic devices, when applied directly to bleeding surfaces, arrest bleeding by providing a mechanical matrix that facilitates clotting.[6,8,15,16] Due to their bulk, surface-acting hemostatic agents slow the flow of blood, protect the forming clot, and offer a framework for deposition of the cellular elements of blood.[6,7,8,15]

MacDonald and Mathews[14] studied GELFOAM implants in canine kidneys and reported that it assisted in healing, with no marked inflammatory or foreign-body reactions.
Jenkins and Janda[15] studied the use of GELFOAM in canine liver resections and noted that the gelatin sponge appeared to offer a protective cover and provide structural support for the reparative process.
Correll et al[16] studied the histology of GELFOAM Sterile Sponge when implanted in rat muscle and reported no significant tissue reaction.

REFERENCES

1. Lindstrom, PA: Complications from the use of absorbable hemostatic sponges. *AMA Arch Surg* 1956;73:133–141.
2. Knowlson GTG: Gel-foam granuloma in the brain. *J Neuro Neurosurg Psychiatry* 1974;37:971–973.
3. Herndon JH, Grillo HC, Riseborough EJ, et al: Compression of the brain and spinal cord following use of GELFOAM. *Arch Surg* 1972;104:107.
4. Council on Pharmacy and Chemistry: Absorbable Gelatin sponge—new and nonofficial remedies. *JAMA* 1947;135:921.
5. Goodman LS, Gilman A: Surface-acting drugs, in The Pharmacologic Basis of Therapeutics, ed 6. *New York, MacMillan Publishing Co.* 1980, p955.
6. Guralnick W, Berg L: GELFOAM in oral surgery. *Oral Surg* 1948;1:629–632.
7. Jenkins HP, Senz EH, Owen H, et al: Present status of gelatin sponge for control of hemorrhage. *JAMA* 1946;132:614–619.
8. Jenkins HP, Janda R, Clarke J: Clinical and experimental observations on the use of gelatin sponge or foam. *Surg* 1946;20 :124–132.
9. Treves N: Prophylaxis of post mammectomy lymphedema by the use of GELFOAM laminated rolls. *Cancer* 1952;5:73–83.
10. Barnes AC: The use of gelatin foam sponges in obstetrics and gynecology. *Am J Obstet Gynecol* 1963;86:105–107.
11. Rarig HR: Successful use of gelatin foam sponge in surgical restoration of fertility. *Am J Obstet Gynecol* 1963;86:136.
12. Jacobs BJ, Rafel SS: Pharmacology and Therapeutics: Absorbable hemostatic agents. *Oral Surg* 1950;2:356–377.
13. Nishimura S: The fate of a gelatin sponge introduced into the fourth ventricle: Experiments in dogs. *Arch Jap Chir* 1954; 23:310–319.
14. MacDonald SA, Mathews WH: Fibrin foam and GELFOAM in experimental kidney wounds. *Annual American Urological Association,* July 1946.
15. Jenkins HP, Janda R: Studies on the use of gelatin sponge or foam as a hemostatic agent in experimental liver resections and injuries to large veins. *Ann Surg* 1946;124:952–961.
16. Correll JT, Prentice HR, Wise EC: Biologic investigations of a new absorbable sponge. *Surg Gynecol Obstet* 1945;181:585–589.

Code 812 250 005

Also available:

GELFOAM Sterile Compressed Sponge (absorbable gelatin sponge, USP) Size 100. For application in dry state. Sponges measure 80 mm × 125 mm and are available in boxes of 6 sponges in individual envelopes.

NDC 0009-0353-01

GELFOAM Sterile Dental Packs (absorbable gelatin sponge, USP), Size 2 or 4. Each measures 10 × 20 × 7 mm or 20 × 20 × 7 mm, respectively; packaged in jars of 15 packs.

Size 2 NDC 0009-0379-01
Size 4 NDC 0009-0396-01

GELFOAM Sterile Prostatectomy Cones, (absorbable gelatin sponge, USP) Size 13 cm or 18 cm (for use with Foley bag catheter). Each cone diameter measures 13 cm or 18 cm, respectively; packaged in boxes of 6 cones in individual envelopes.

Size 13 cm NDC 0009-0449-01
Size 18 cm NDC 0009-0457-01

GELFOAM®
brand of absorbable gelatin sterile powder
(absorbable gelatin powder)

HOW SUPPLIED

GELFOAM Sterile Powder (absorbable gelatin powder) is supplied in jars containing 1 gram.

NDC 0009-0433-01

HALCION®   © ℞
brand of triazolam tablets, USP

0.125 mg, 100's	NSN 6505-01-220-5833 (VA)
0.125 mg, 4-25's	
Visipak:	NSN 6505-01-241-3591 (VA)
0.25 mg, 30's:	NSN 6505-01-243-6438 (VA)
0.25 mg, 100's:	NSN 6505-01-161-5036 (M&VA)
0.25 mg, 100's Unit Dose:	
	NSN 6505-01-184-1576 (VA)
0.25 mg, 4-25's Visipak:	NSN 6505-01-179-4968 (M)
0.25 mg, 500's:	NSN 6505-01-260-0904 (VA)

DESCRIPTION

HALCION Tablets contain triazolam, a triazolobenzodiazepine hypnotic agent.
Triazolam is a white crystalline powder, soluble in alcohol and poorly soluble in water. It has a molecular weight of 343.21.
The chemical name for triazolam is 8-chloro- 6- (o-chlorophenyl) -1- methyl-4H-s-triazolo- [4,3-a] [1,4] benzodiazepine.
Each HALCION tablet, for oral administration, contains 0.125 mg, 0.25 mg or 0.5 mg of triazolam. Inactive ingredients: **0.125 mg**—cellulose, corn starch, docusate sodium, FD&C red no. 3, FD&C blue no. 2, lactose, magnesium stearate, sodium benzoate; **0.25 mg**—cellulose, corn starch, docusate sodium, FD&C blue no. 2, lactose, magnesium stearate, silicon dioxide, sodium benzoate.

CLINICAL PHARMACOLOGY

Triazolam is a hypnotic with a short mean plasma half-life reported to be in the range of 1.5 to 5.5 hours. In normal subjects treated for seven days with four times the recommended dose, there was no evidence of altered systemic bioavailability, rate of elimination, or accumulation. Peak plasma levels are reached within 2 hours following oral administration. Following recommended doses of HALCION, triazolam peak plasma levels in the range of 1 to 6 ng/ml are seen. The plasma levels achieved are proportional to the dose given.
Triazolam and its metabolites, principally as conjugated glucuronides which are presumably inactive, are excreted primarily in the urine. Only small amounts of unmetabolized triazolam appear in the urine. The two primary metabolites accounted for 79.9% of urinary excretion. Urinary excretion appeared to be biphasic in its time course.
HALCION Tablets (triazolam) 0.5 mg, in two separate studies, did not affect the prothrombin times or plasma warfarin levels in male volunteers administered sodium warfarin orally.
Extremely high concentrations of triazolam do not displace bilirubin bound to human serum albumin *in vitro.*
Triazolam ^{14}C was administered orally to pregnant mice. Drug-related material appeared uniformly distributed in the fetus with ^{14}C concentrations approximately the same as in the brain of the mother.
In sleep laboratory studies, HALCION Tablets significantly decreased sleep latency, increased the duration of sleep and decreased the number of nocturnal awakenings. After two weeks of consecutive nightly administration, the drug's effect on total wake time is decreased, and the values recorded in the last third of the night approach baseline levels. On the first and/or second night after drug discontinuance (first or second post-drug night), total time asleep, percentage of time spent sleeping, and rapidity of falling asleep frequently were significantly less than on baseline (pre-drug) nights. This effect is often called "rebound" insomnia.
The type and duration of hypnotic effects and the profile of unwanted effects during administration of benzodiazepine drugs may be influenced by the biologic half-life of administered drug and any active metabolites formed. When half-lives are long, drug or metabolites may accumulate during periods of nightly administration and be associated with impairments of cognitive and motor performance during waking hours; the possibility of interaction with other psychoactive drugs or alcohol will be enhanced. In contrast, if half-lives are short, drug and metabolites will be cleared before the next dose is ingested, and carry-over effects related to excessive sedation or CNS depression should be minimal or absent. However, during nightly use for an extended period, pharmacodynamic tolerance or adaptation to some effects of benzodiazepine hypnotics may develop. If the drug has a short half-life of elimination, it is possible that a relative deficiency of the drug or its active metabolites (ie, in relationship to the receptor site) may occur at some point in the interval between each night's use. This sequence of events may account for two clinical findings reported to occur after several weeks of nightly use of rapidly eliminated benzodiazepine hypnotics: 1) increased wakefulness during the last third of the night, and 2) the appearance of increased signs of day-time anxiety reported by one author in a selected group of patients.

INDICATIONS AND USAGE

HALCION Tablets contain triazolam which is a hypnotic agent useful in the short-term management of insomnia characterized by difficulty in falling asleep, frequent nocturnal awakenings, and/or early morning awakenings.
In polysomnographic studies in man of 1 to 42 days duration, triazolam decreased sleep latency, increased duration of sleep, and decreased the number of nocturnal awakenings. It is recommended that HALCION not be prescribed in quantities exceeding a one-month supply.

CONTRAINDICATIONS

HALCION Tablets (triazolam) are contraindicated in patients with known hypersensitivity to this drug or other benzodiazepines.

Benzodiazepines may cause fetal damage when administered during pregnancy. An increased risk of congenital malformations associated with the use of diazepam and chlordiazepoxide during the first trimester of pregnancy has been suggested in several studies. Transplacental distribution has resulted in neonatal CNS depression following the ingestion of therapeutic doses of a benzodiazepine hypnotic during the last weeks of pregnancy.

HALCION is contraindicated in pregnant women. If there is a likelihood of the patient becoming pregnant while receiving HALCION she should be warned of the potential risk to the fetus. Patients should be instructed to discontinue the drug prior to becoming pregnant. The possibility that a woman of childbearing potential may be pregnant at the time of institution of therapy should be considered.

WARNINGS

Overdosage may occur at four times the maximum recommended therapeutic dose (see DOSAGE AND ADMINISTRATION section). Patients should be cautioned not to exceed prescribed dosage.

Because of its depressant CNS effects, patients receiving triazolam should be cautioned against engaging in hazardous occupations requiring complete mental alertness such as operating machinery or driving a motor vehicle. For the same reason, patients should be cautioned about the simultaneous ingestion of alcohol and other CNS depressant drugs during treatment with HALCION Tablets (triazolam).

As with some but not all benzodiazepines, anterograde amnesia of varying severity and paradoxical reactions have been reported following therapeutic doses of HALCION.

PRECAUTIONS

General: In elderly and/or debilitated patients, it is recommended that treatment with HALCION Tablets be initiated at 0.125 mg to decrease the possibility of development of oversedation, dizziness, or impaired coordination.

Some side effects reported in association with the use of HALCION appear to be dose related. These include drowsiness, dizziness, lightheadedness, and amnesia.

The relationship between dose and what may be more serious behavioral phenomena is less certain. Specifically, some evidence, based on spontaneous marketing reports, suggests that confusion, bizarre or abnormal behavior, agitation and hallucinations may also be dose related, but this evidence is inconclusive. In accordance with good medical practice it is recommended that therapy be initiated at the lowest effective dose. (See DOSAGE AND ADMINISTRATION)

Caution should be exercised if HALCION is prescribed to patients with signs or symptoms of depression which could be intensified by hypnotic drugs. Suicidal tendencies may be present in such patients and protective measures may be required. Intentional overdosage is more common in these patients, and the least amount of drug that is feasible should be available to the patient at any one time.

The usual precautions should be observed in patients with impaired renal or hepatic function and chronic pulmonary insufficiency.

Information for Patients: To assure safe and effective use of HALCION Tablets (triazolam), the following information and instructions should be given to patients:

1. Inform your physician about any alcohol consumption and medicine you are taking now, including drugs you may buy without a prescription. Alcohol should generally not be used during treatment with hypnotics.
2. Inform your physician if you are planning to become pregnant, if you are pregnant, or if you become pregnant while you are taking this medicine.
3. Inform your physician if you are nursing.
4. Until you experience how this medication affects you, do not drive a car or operate potentially dangerous machinery, etc.
5. Do not increase prescribed dosage.
6. Patients should also be advised that they may experience an increase in sleep complaints (rebound insomnia) on the first night or two after discontinuing the drug.

Laboratory Tests: Laboratory tests are not ordinarily required in otherwise healthy patients.

Drug Interactions: Both pharmacodynamic and pharmacokinetic interactions have been reported with benzodiazepines. In particular, triazolam produces additive CNS depressant effects when co-administered with other psychotropic medications, anticonvulsants, antihistamines, ethanol, and other drugs which themselves produce CNS depression.

Pharmacokinetic interactions can occur when triazolam is administered along with drugs that interfere with its metabolism. Specific examples, documented with evidence from controlled trials, show that the co-administration of either cimetidine or erythromycin with triazolam cause an approximate doubling of the elimination half-life and plasma levels of triazolam. Consequently, consideration of dose reduction

Number of patients	HALCION 380		Placebo 361	
% of Patients Reporting:	Low	High	Low	High
Hematology				
Hematocrit	*	*	*	*
Hemoglobin	*	*	*	*
Total WBC Count	1.7	2.1	*	1.3
Neutrophil Count	1.5	1.5	3.3	1.0
Lymphocyte Count	2.3	4.0	3.1	3.8
Monocyte Count	3.6	*	4.4	1.5
Eosinophil Count	10.2	3.2	9.8	3.4
Basophil Count	1.7	2.1	*	1.8
Urinalysis				
Albumin	—	1.1	—	*
Sugar		*		*
RBC/HPF	—	2.9	—	2.9
WBC/HPF	—	11.7	—	7.9
Blood Chemistry				
Creatinine	2.4	1.9	3.6	1.5
Bilirubin	*	1.5	1.0	*
SGOT	*	5.3	*	4.5
Alkaline Phosphatase	*	2.2	*	2.6

*Less than 1%

may be appropriate in patients treated concomitantly with either cimetidine or erythromycin and triazolam.

Carcinogenesis, Mutagenesis, Impairment of Fertility: No evidence of carcinogenic potential was observed in mice during a 24-month study with HALCION in doses up to 4000 times the human dose.

Pregnancy:

1. Teratogenic Effects: Pregnancy Category X. See CONTRAINDICATIONS.
2. Non-Teratogenic Effects: It is to be considered that the child born of a mother who is on benzodiazepines may be at some risk for withdrawal symptoms from the drug, during the postnatal period. Also, neonatal flaccidity has been reported in an infant born of a mother who had been receiving benzodiazepines.

Nursing Mothers: Human studies have not been performed; however, studies in rats have indicated that HALCION and its metabolites are secreted in milk. Therefore, administration of HALCION to nursing mothers is not recommended.

Pediatric Use: Safety and efficacy of HALCION in children below the age of 18 have not been established.

ADVERSE REACTIONS

During placebo-controlled clinical studies in which 1003 patients received HALCION Tablets (triazolam), the most troublesome side effects were extensions of the pharmacologic activity of triazolam, eg, drowsiness, dizziness, or lightheadedness.

The figures cited below are estimates of untoward clinical event incidence among subjects who participated in the relatively short duration (ie, 1 to 42 days) placebo-controlled clinical trials of HALCION. The figures cannot be used to predict precisely the incidence of untoward events in the course of usual medical practice where patient characteristics and other factors often differ from those in the clinical trials. These figures cannot be compared with those obtained from other clinical studies involving related drug products and placebo as each group of drug trials are conducted under a different set of conditions.

Comparison of the cited figures, however, can provide the prescriber with some basis for estimating the relative contributions of drug and non-drug factors to the untoward event incidence rate in the population studied. Even this use must be approached cautiously, as a drug may relieve a symptom in one patient while inducing it in others. [For example, an anticholinergic, anxiolytic drug may relieve dry mouth (a sign of anxiety) in some subjects but induce it (an untoward event) in others.]

	HALCION	Placebo
Number of Patients	1003	997
% of Patients Reporting:		
Central Nervous System		
Drowsiness	14.0	6.4
Headache	9.7	8.4
Dizziness	7.8	3.1
Nervousness	5.2	4.5
Lightheadedness	4.9	0.9
Coordination Disorders/Ataxia	4.6	0.8
Gastrointestinal		
Nausea/Vomiting	4.6	3.7

In addition to the relatively common (ie, 1% or greater) untoward events enumerated above, the following adverse events have been reported less frequently (ie, 0.9–0.5%): euphoria, tachycardia, tiredness, confusional states/memory impairment, cramps/pain, depression, visual disturbances.

Rare (ie, less than 0.5%) adverse reactions included constipation, taste alterations, diarrhea, dry mouth, dermatitis/allergy, dreaming/nightmares, insomnia, paresthesia, tinnitus,

dysesthesia, weakness, congestion, death from hepatic failure in a patient also receiving diuretic drugs.

In addition to these untoward events for which estimates of incidence are available, the following adverse events have been reported in association with the use of HALCION and other benzodiazepines: amnestic symptoms (anterograde amnesia with appropriate or inappropriate behavior), confusional states (disorientation, derealization, depersonalization, and/or clouding of consciousness), dystonia, anorexia, fatigue, sedation, slurred speech, jaundice, pruritus, dysarthria, changes in libido, menstrual irregularities, incontinence and urinary retention. Other factors may contribute to some of these reactions, eg, concomitant intake of alcohol or other drugs, sleep deprivation, an abnormal premorbid state, etc.

Other events reported include: paradoxical reactions such as stimulation, an agitational state (restlessness, irritability and excitation), increased muscle spasticity, sleep disturbances, hallucinations, aggressiveness, falling, somnambulism, inappropriate behavior and other adverse behavioral effects. Should these occur, use of the drug should be discontinued.

Laboratory analyses were performed on all patients participating in the clinical program for HALCION. The following incidences of abnormalities were observed in patients receiving HALCION and the corresponding placebo group. None of these changes were considered to be of physiological significance.

[See table above].

When treatment with HALCION is protracted, periodic blood counts, urinalysis and blood chemistry analyses are advisable.

Minor changes in EEG patterns, usually low-voltage fast activity have been observed in patients during therapy with HALCION and are of no known significance.

DRUG ABUSE AND DEPENDENCE

Controlled Substance: Triazolam is a controlled substance under the Controlled Substance Act and HALCION Tablets have been assigned to Schedule IV.

Abuse and Dependence: Withdrawal symptoms similar in character to those noted with barbiturates and alcohol have occurred following abrupt discontinuance of benzodiazepine drugs. These can range from mild dysphoria to a major syndrome which may include abdominal and muscle cramps, vomiting, sweating, tremor, and convulsions.

Patients with a history of seizures should not be abruptly withdrawn from any CNS depressant agent, including HALCION. Addiction-prone individuals, such as drug addicts and alcoholics, should be under careful surveillance when receiving triazolam because of the predisposition of such patients to habituation and dependence. As with all hypnotics, repeat prescriptions should be limited to those who are under medical supervision.

OVERDOSAGE

Because of the potency of triazolam, overdosage may occur at 2 mg, four times the maximum recommended therapeutic dose (0.5 mg).

Manifestations of overdosage with HALCION Tablets (triazolam) include somnolence, confusion, impaired coordination, slurred speech, and ultimately, coma. As in all cases

Continued on next page

Information on these Upjohn products is based on labeling in effect September 1, 1989. Further information concerning these and other Upjohn products may be obtained by direct inquiry to Medical Information, The Upjohn Company, Kalamazoo, Michigan 49001.

Upjohn—Cont.

of drug overdosage, respiration, pulse, and blood pressure should be monitored and supported by general measures when necessary. Immediate gastric lavage should be performed. An adequate airway should be maintained. Intravenous fluids may be administered.

Experiments in animals have indicated that cardiopulmonary collapse can occur with massive intravenous doses of HALCION (over 100 mg/kg, more than 10,000 times the maximum daily human dose). This could be reversed with positive mechanical respiration and the intravenous infusion of norepinephrine bitartrate or metaraminol bitartrate. Hemodialysis and forced diuresis are probably of little value. As with the management of intentional overdosage with any drug, the physician should bear in mind that multiple agents may have been ingested by the patient.

The oral LD_{50} in mice is greater than 1000 mg/kg and in rats is greater than 5000 mg/kg.

DOSAGE AND ADMINISTRATION

It is important to individualize the dosage of HALCION Tablets for maximum beneficial effect and to help avoid significant adverse effects.

The recommended dose for most adults is 0.25 mg before retiring. A dose of 0.125 mg may be found to be sufficient for selected patients. A dose of 0.5 mg should be reserved for those patients who do not respond adequately to a lower dose since the risk of several adverse reactions increases with the size of the dose administered.

In geriatric and/or debilitated patients, the recommended dosage range is 0.125 mg to 0.25 mg. Therapy should be initiated at 0.125 mg in this group.

As with all medications, the lowest effective dose should be used.

HOW SUPPLIED

HALCION Tablets (triazolam) scored, are available in the following strengths and package sizes:

0.125 mg (pale lavender):

Bottles of 100	NDC 0009-0010-01
Unit Dose Pkg (100)	NDC 0009-0010-22
VISIPAK®	
Reverse Numbered Pack (100)	NDC 0009-0010-04
Bottles of 500	NDC 0009-0010-11

0.25 mg (powder blue, scored):

Bottles of 100	NDC 0009-0017-01
Unit Dose Pkg (100)	NDC 0009-0017-08
VISIPAK®	
Reverse Numbered Pack (100)	NDC 0009-0017-17
Bottles of 500	NDC 0009-0017-02

Store at controlled room temperature 15°–30°C (59°–86°F).
Code 812 110 217

Shown in Product Identification Section, page 433

HALOTESTIN®   ℞
brand of fluoxymesterone tablets, USP

10 mg-100s
NSN 6505-01-041-8165 (M & VA)

DESCRIPTION

HALOTESTIN Tablets contain fluoxymesterone, an androgenic hormone.

Fluoxymesterone is a white or practically white odorless, crystalline powder, melting at about 240° C. with some decomposition. It is practically insoluble in water, sparingly soluble in alcohol and slightly soluble in chloroform.

The chemical name for fluoxymesterone is androst-4-en-3-one, 9-fluoro -11, 17- dihydroxy-17- methyl-,(11β,17β). The molecular formula is $C_{20}H_{29}FO_3$ and the molecular weight 336.45.

Each HALOTESTIN tablet, for oral administration, contains 2 mg, 5 mg or 10 mg fluoxymesterone. Inactive ingredients: calcium stearate, corn starch, FD&C yellow no. 5, lactose, sorbic acid, sucrose, tragacanth. In addition, the **2 mg** tablet contains FD&C yellow no. 6 and the **5 mg** and **10 mg** contain FD&C blue no. 2.

CLINICAL PHARMACOLOGY

Endogenous androgens are responsible for normal growth and development of the male sex organs and for maintenance of secondary sex characteristics. These effects include growth and maturation of the prostate, seminal vesicles, penis, and scrotum; development of male hair distribution, such as beard, pubic, chest, and axillary hair; laryngeal enlargement, vocal cord thickening, and alterations in body musculature and fat distribution. Drugs in this class also cause retention of nitrogen, sodium, potassium, and phosphorus, and decreased urinary excretion of calcium. Androgens have been reported to increase protein anabolism and decrease protein catabolism. Nitrogen balance is improved only when there is sufficient intake of calories and protein. Androgens are responsible for the growth spurt of adolescence and for eventual termination of linear growth, brought about by fusion of the epiphyseal growth centers. In chil-

dren, exogenous androgens accelerate linear growth rates, but may cause disproportionate advancement in bone maturation. Use over long periods may result in fusion of the epiphyseal growth centers and termination of the growth process. Androgens have been reported to stimulate production of red blood cells by enhancing production of erythropoietic stimulation factor.

During exogenous administration of androgens, endogenous testosterone release is inhibited through feedback inhibition of pituitary luteinizing hormone (LH). At large doses of exogenous androgen, spermatogenesis may also be suppressed through feedback inhibition of pituitary follicle stimulating hormone (FSH).

Inactivation of testosterone occurs primarily in the liver. The half-life of fluoxymesterone after oral administration is approximately 9.2 hours.

INDICATIONS AND USAGE

In the male—HALOTESTIN Tablets (fluoxymesterone) are indicated for:

1. Replacement therapy in conditions associated with symptoms of deficiency or absence of endogenous testosterone:

   a. Primary hypogonadism (congenital or acquired)—testicular failure due to cryptorchidism, bilateral torsion, orchitis, vanishing testis syndrome; or orchidectomy.

   b. Hypogonadotropic hypogonadism (congenital or acquired)—idiopathic gonadotropin or LHRH deficiency, or pituitary-hypothalamic injury from tumors, trauma, or radiation.

2. Delayed puberty, provided it has been definitely established as such, and is not just a familial trait.

In the female—HALOTESTIN Tablets are indicated for palliation of androgen-responsive recurrent mammary cancer in women who are more than one year but less than five years postmenopausal, or who have been proven to have a hormone-dependent tumor as shown by previous beneficial response to castration.

CONTRAINDICATIONS

1. Known hypersensitivity to the drug
2. Males with carcinoma of the breast
3. Males with known or suspected carcinoma of the prostate gland
4. Women known or suspected to be pregnant
5. Patients with serious cardiac, hepatic or renal disease

WARNINGS

Hypercalcemia may occur in immobilized patients and in patients with breast cancer. If this occurs, the drug should be discontinued.

Prolonged use of high doses of androgens (principally the 17-α alkyl-androgens) has been associated with development of hepatic adenomas, hepatocellular carcinoma, and peliosis hepatis—all potentially life-threatening complications.

Cholestatic hepatitis and jaundice may occur with 17-α-alkyl-androgens. Should this occur, the drug should be discontinued. This is reversible with discontinuation of the drug.

Geriatric patients treated with androgens may be at an increased risk of developing prostatic hypertrophy and prostatic carcinoma although conclusive evidence to support this concept is lacking.

Edema, with or without congestive heart failure, may be a serious complication in patients with pre-existing cardiac, renal or hepatic disease.

Gynecomastia may develop and occasionally persists in patients being treated for hypogonadism.

Androgen therapy should be used cautiously in males with delayed puberty. Androgens can accelerate bone maturation without producing compensatory gain in linear growth. The effect on bone maturation should be monitored by assessing bone age of the wrist and hand every six months.

PRECAUTIONS

General

Women should be observed for signs of virilization which is usual following androgen use at high doses. Discontinuation of drug therapy at the time of evidence of mild virilism is necessary to prevent irreversible virilization. A decision may be made by the patient and the physician that some virilization will be tolerated during treatment for breast carcinoma. Patients with benign prostatic hypertrophy may develop acute urethral obstruction. Priapism or excessive sexual stimulation may develop. Oligospermia may occur after prolonged administration or excessive dosage. If any of these effects appear, the androgen should be stopped and if restarted, a lower dosage should be utilized.

This product contains FD&C Yellow No. 5 (tartrazine) which may cause allergic-type reactions (including bronchial asthma) in certain susceptible individuals. Although the overall incidence of FD&C Yellow No. 5 (tartrazine) sensitivity in the general population is low, it is frequently seen in patients who also have aspirin hypersensitivity.

Information for patients

Patients should be instructed to report any of the following: nausea, vomiting, changes in skin color, and ankle swelling. Males should be instructed to report too frequent or persis-

tent erections of the penis and females any hoarseness, acne, changes in menstrual periods or increase in facial hair.

Laboratory tests

Women with disseminated breast carcinoma should have frequent determination of urine and serum calcium levels during the course of androgen therapy (See WARNINGS).

Because of the hepatotoxicity associated with the use of 17-alpha-alkylated androgens, liver function tests should be obtained periodically.

Periodic (every six months) x-ray examinations of bone age should be made during treatment of prepubertal males to determine the rate of bone maturation and the effects of androgen therapy on the epiphyseal centers.

Hemoglobin and hematocrit levels (to detect polycythemia) should be checked periodically in patients receiving long-term androgen administration.

Serum cholesterol may increase during androgen therapy.

DRUG INTERACTIONS

Androgens may increase sensitivity to oral anticoagulants. Dosage of the anticoagulant may require reduction in order to maintain satisfactory therapeutic hypoprothrombinemia. Concurrent administration of oxyphenbutazone and androgens may result in elevated serum levels of oxyphenbutazone.

In diabetic patients, the metabolic effects of androgens may decrease blood glucose and, therefore, insulin requirements.

Drug/Laboratory test interferences

Androgens may decrease levels of thyroxine-binding globulin, resulting in decreased total T_4 serum levels and increased resin uptake of T_3 and T_4. Free thyroid hormone levels remain unchanged, however, and there is no clinical evidence of thyroid dysfunction.

Carcinogenesis

Animal data: Testosterone has been tested by subcutaneous injection and implantation in mice and rats. The implant induced cervical-uterine tumors in mice, which metastasized in some cases. There is suggestive evidence that injection of testosterone into some strains of female mice increases their susceptibility to hepatoma. Testosterone is also known to increase the number of tumors and decrease the degree of differentiation of chemically-induced carcinomas of the liver in rats.

Human data: There are rare reports of hepatocellular carcinoma in patients receiving long-term therapy with androgens in high doses. Withdrawal of the drugs did not lead to regression of the tumors in all cases.

Geriatric patients treated with androgens may be at an increased risk of developing prostatic hypertrophy and prostatic carcinoma although conclusive evidence to support this concept is lacking.

Pregnancy

Teratogenic effects: Pregnancy Category X. (See CONTRA-INDICATIONS).

Nursing mothers

HALOTESTIN Tablets (fluoxymesterone) are not recommended for use in nursing mothers.

Pediatric use

Androgen therapy should be used very cautiously in children and only by specialists aware of the adverse effects on bone maturation. Skeletal maturation must be monitored every six months by an x-ray of the hand and wrist (See WARNINGS).

ADVERSE REACTIONS

Endocrine and urogenital

Female: The most common side effects of androgen therapy are amenorrhea and other menstrual irregularities; inhibition of gonadotropin secretion; and virilization, including deepening of the voice and clitoral enlargement. The latter usually is not reversible after androgens are discontinued. When administered to a pregnant woman, androgens can cause virilization of external genitalia of the female fetus.

Male: Gynecomastia, and excessive frequency and duration of penile erections. Oligospermia may occur at high dosage.

Skin and appendages

Hirsutism, male pattern of baldness, seborrhea, and acne.

Fluid and electrolyte disturbances

Retention of sodium, chloride, water, potassium, calcium, and inorganic phosphates.

Gastrointestinal

Nausea, cholestatic jaundice, alterations in liver function tests, rarely hepatocellular neoplasms and peliosis hepatis (see WARNINGS).

Hematologic

Suppression of clotting factors II, V, VII, and X, bleeding in patients on concomitant anticoagulant therapy, and polycythemia.

Nervous system

Increased or decreased libido, headache, anxiety, depression, and generalized paresthesia.

Allergic

Hypersensitivity, including skin manifestations and anaphylactoid reactions.

OVERDOSAGE

There have been no reports of acute overdosage with the androgens.

DOSAGE AND ADMINISTRATION

The dosage will vary depending upon the individual, the condition being treated, and its severity. The total daily oral dose may be administered singly or in divided (three or four) doses.

Male hypogonadism: For complete replacement in the hypogonadal male, a daily dose of 5 to 20 mg will suffice in the majority of patients. It is usually preferable to begin treatment with full therapeutic doses which are later adjusted to individual requirements. Priapism is indicative of excessive dosage and is indication for temporary withdrawal of the drug.

Delayed puberty: Dosage should be carefully titrated utilizing a low dose, appropriate skeletal monitoring, and by limiting the duration of therapy to four to six months.

Inoperable carcinoma of the breast in the female: The recommended total daily dose for palliative therapy in advanced inoperable carcinoma of the breast is 10 to 40 mg. Because of its short action, fluoxymesterone should be administered to patients in divided, rather than single, daily doses to ensure more stable blood levels. In general, it appears necessary to continue therapy for at least one month for a satisfactory subjective response, and for two to three months for an objective response.

HOW SUPPLIED

HALOTESTIN Tablets (fluoxymesterone), scored, are available in the following strengths and colors:

2 mg (peach)
Bottles of 100   NDC 0009-0014-01
5 mg (light green)
Bottles of 100   NDC 0009-0019-06
10 mg (green)
Bottles of 30   NDC 0009-0036-03
Bottles of 100   NDC 0009-0036-04
Code 810 804 203

Shown in Product Identification Section, page 434

HEPARIN SODIUM INJECTION, USP   ℞
Sterile Solution

DESCRIPTION

Heparin is a heterogenous group of straight-chain anionic mucopolysaccharides, called glycosaminoglycans having anticoagulant properties. Although others may be present, the main sugars occurring in heparin are: (1) α-L-iduronic acid 2-sulfate, (2) 2-deoxy-2-sulfamino-α-D-glucose 6-sulfate, (3) β-D-glucoronic acid, (4) 2-acetamido-2-deoxy-α-D-glucose, and (5) α-L-iduronic acid. These sugars are present in decreasing amounts, usually in the order (2) > (1) > (4) > (3) > (5), and are joined by glycosidic linkages, forming polymers of varying sizes. Heparin is strongly acidic because of its content of covalently linked sulfate and carboxylic acid groups. In heparin sodium, the acidic protons of the sulfate units are partially replaced by sodium ions.

Heparin Sodium Injection, USP is a sterile solution of heparin sodium derived from bovine lung tissue, standardized for anticoagulant activity. It is to be administered by intravenous or deep subcutaneous routes. The potency is determined by a biological assay using a USP reference standard based on units of heparin activity per milligram. Heparin is pyrogen-free.

Each ml of the 1,000 and 5,000 USP Units per ml preparations contains: Heparin sodium 1,000 or 5,000 USP Units; 9 mg sodium chloride; 9.45 mg benzyl alcohol added as preservative. Each ml of the 10,000 USP Units per ml preparations contains: heparin sodium 10,000 USP Units; 9.45 mg benzyl alcohol added as preservative.

When necessary, the pH of Heparin Sodium Injection, USP was adjusted with hydrochloric acid and/or sodium hydroxide. The pH range is 5.0-7.5.

CLINICAL PHARMACOLOGY

Heparin inhibits reactions that lead to the clotting of blood and the formation of fibrin clots both *in vitro* and *in vivo*. Heparin acts at multiple sites in the normal coagulation system. Small amounts of heparin in combination with antithrombin III (heparin cofactor) can inhibit thrombosis by inactivating activated Factor X and inhibiting the conversion of prothrombin to thrombin. Once active thrombosis has developed, larger amounts of heparin can inhibit further coagulation by inactivating thrombin and preventing the conversion of fibrinogen to fibrin. Heparin also prevents the formation of a stable fibrin clot by inhibiting the activation of the fibrin stabilizing factor.

Bleeding time is usually unaffected by heparin. Clotting time is prolonged by full therapeutic doses of heparin; in most cases, it is not measurably affected by low doses of heparin. Peak plasma levels of heparin are achieved 2-4 hours following subcutaneous administration, although there are considerable individual variations. Loglinear plots of heparin plasma concentrations with time for a wide range of dose levels are linear which suggests the absence of zero order processes. Liver and the reticulo-endothelial system are the site of biotransformation. The biphasic elimination curve, a rapidly declining alpha phase ($t\frac{1}{2} = 10$ minutes) and after the age of 40 a slower beta phase, indicates uptake in organs. The absence of a relationship between anticoagulant half-life and concentration half-life may reflect factors such as protein binding of heparin.

Heparin does not have fibrinolytic activity; therefore, it will not lyse existing clots.

INDICATIONS AND USAGE

Heparin Sodium Injection is indicated for:
Anticoagulant therapy in prophylaxis and treatment of venous thrombosis and its extension;
(In a low-dose regimen) for prevention of postoperative deep venous thrombosis and pulmonary embolism in patients undergoing major abdomino-thoracic surgery or who for other reasons are at risk of developing thromboembolic disease (see DOSAGE AND ADMINISTRATION);
Prophylaxis and treatment of pulmonary embolism;
Atrial fibrillation with embolization;
Diagnosis and treatment of acute and chronic consumption coagulopathies (disseminated intravascular coagulation);
Prevention of clotting in arterial and heart surgery;
Prophylaxis and treatment of peripheral arterial embolism;
As an anticoagulant in blood transfusions, extracorporeal circulation, and dialysis procedures and in blood samples for laboratory purposes.

CONTRAINDICATIONS

Heparin sodium should not be used in patients:
With severe thrombocytopenia;
In whom suitable blood coagulation tests—e.g., the whole-blood clotting time, partial thromboplastin time, etc.—cannot be performed at appropriate intervals (this contraindication refers to full-dose heparin; there is usually no need to monitor coagulation parameters in patients receiving low-dose heparin);
With an uncontrollable active bleeding state (see WARNINGS), except when this is due to disseminated intravascular coagulation.

WARNINGS

Heparin is not intended for intramuscular use.
Hypersensitivity: Patients with documented hypersensitivity to heparin should be given the drug only in clearly life-threatening situations.
Hemorrhage: Hemorrhage can occur at virtually any site in patients receiving heparin. An unexplained fall in hematocrit, fall in blood pressure, or any other unexplained symptom should lead to serious consideration of a hemorrhagic event.
Heparin sodium should be used with extreme caution in disease states in which there is increased danger of hemorrhage. Some of the conditions in which increased danger of hemorrhage exists are:
Cardiovascular—Subacute bacterial endocarditis. Severe hypotension.
Surgical—During and immediately following (a) spinal tap or spinal anesthesia or (b) major surgery, especially involving the brain, spinal cord, or eye.
Hematologic—Conditions associated with increased bleeding tendencies, such as hemophilia, thrombocytopenia, and some vascular purpuras.
Gastrointestinal—Ulcerative lesions and continuous tube drainage of the stomach or small intestine.
Other—Menstruation, liver disease with impaired hemostasis.
Coagulation Testing: When heparin sodium is administered in therapeutic amounts, its dosage should be regulated by frequent blood coagulation tests. If the coagulation test is unduly prolonged or if hemorrhage occurs, heparin sodium should be discontinued promptly (see OVERDOSAGE).
Thrombocytopenia: Thrombocytopenia has been reported to occur in patients receiving heparin with a reported incidence of 0 to 30%. Mild thrombocytopenia (count greater than 100,000/mm³) may remain stable or reverse even if heparin is continued. However, thrombocytopenia of any degree should be monitored closely. If the count falls below 100,000/mm³ or if recurrent thrombosis develops (see White Clot Syndrome, PRECAUTIONS), the heparin product should be discontinued. If continued heparin therapy is essential, administration of heparin from a different organ source can be reinstituted with caution.
Miscellaneous: This product contains benzyl alcohol as preservative: Benzyl alcohol has been reported to be associated with a fatal "Gasping Syndrome" in premature infants.

PRECAUTIONS

1. General
   a. White Clot Syndrome
   It has been reported that patients on heparin may develop new thrombus formation in association with thrombocytopenia resulting from irreversible aggregation of platelets induced by heparin, the so-called "white clot syndrome."

The process may lead to severe thromboembolic complications like skin necrosis, gangrene of the extremities that may lead to amputation, myocardial infarction, pulmonary embolism, stroke, and possibly death. Therefore, heparin administration should be promptly discontinued if a patient develops new thrombosis in association with thrombocytopenia.
   b. Heparin Resistance
   Increased resistance to heparin is frequently encountered in fever, thrombosis, thrombophlebitis, infections with thrombosing tendencies, myocardial infarction, cancer and in postsurgical patients.
   c. Increased Risk in Older Women:
   A higher incidence of bleeding has been reported in women over 60 years of age.
2. Laboratory Tests: Periodic platelet counts, hematocrits, and tests for occult blood in stool are recommended during the entire course of heparin therapy, regardless of the route of administration (see DOSAGE AND ADMINISTRATION).
3. Drug Interactions:
Oral anticoagulants: Heparin sodium may prolong the one-stage prothrombin time. Therefore, when heparin sodium is given with dicumarol or warfarin sodium, a period of at least 5 hours after the last intravenous dose or 24 hours after the last subcutaneous dose should elapse before blood is drawn if a valid prothrombin time is to be obtained.
Platelet inhibitors: Drugs such as acetylsalicylic acid, dextran, phenylbutazone, ibuprofen, indomethacin, dipyridamole, hydroxychloroquine and others that interfere with platelet-aggregation reactions (the main hemostatic defense of heparinized patients) may induce bleeding and should be used with caution in patients receiving heparin sodium.
Other interactions: Digitalis, tetracyclines, nicotine, or antihistamines may partially counteract the anticoagulant action of heparin sodium.
4. Drug/Laboratory Tests Interactions:
Hyperaminotransferasemia: Significant elevations of aminotransferase (SGOT [S-AST] and SPT [S-ALT])levels have occurred in a high percentage of patients (and healthy subjects) who have received heparin. Since aminotransferase determinations are important in the differential diagnosis of myocardial infarction, liver disease, and pulmonary emboli, rises that might be caused by drugs (like heparin) should be interpreted with caution.
5. Carcinogenesis, Mutagenesis, Impairment of Fertility: No long-term studies in animals have been performed to evaluate carcinogenic potential of heparin. Also, no reproduction studies in animals have been performed concerning mutagenesis or impairment of fertility.
6. Pregnancy:
Teratogenic Effects: Pregnancy Category C. Animal reproduction studies have not been conducted with heparin sodium. It is also not known whether heparin sodium can cause fetal harm when administered to a pregnant woman or can affect reproduction capacity. Heparin sodium should be given to a pregnant woman only if clearly needed.
Nonteratogenic Effects: Heparin does not cross the placental barrier.
7. Nursing Mothers: Heparin is not excreted in human milk.
8. Pediatric Use: See DOSAGE AND ADMINISTRATION.

ADVERSE REACTIONS

1. Hemorrhage. Hemorrhage is the chief complication that may result from heparin therapy (see WARNINGS). An overly prolonged clotting time or minor bleeding during therapy can usually be controlled by withdrawing the drug (see OVERDOSAGE). **It should be appreciated that gastrointestinal or urinary tract bleeding during anticoagulant therapy may indicate the presence of an underlying occult lesion.** Bleeding can occur at any site but certain specific hemorrhagic complications may be difficult to detect.
   a. Adrenal hemorrhage, with resultant acute adrenal insufficiency, has occurred during anticoagulant therapy. Therefore, such treatment should be discontinued in patients who develop signs and symptoms of acute adrenal hemorrhage and insufficiency. Initiation of corrective therapy should not depend on laboratory confirmation of the diagnosis, since any delay in an acute situation may result in the patient's death.
   b. Ovarian (corpus luteum) hemorrhage developed in a number of women of reproductive age receiving short- or long-term anticoagulant therapy. This complication if unrecognized may be fatal.
   c. Retroperitoneal hemorrhage.

Continued on next page

Information on these Upjohn products is based on labeling in effect September 1, 1989. Further information concerning these and other Upjohn products may be obtained by direct inquiry to Medical Information, The Upjohn Company, Kalamazoo, Michigan 49001.

Upjohn—Cont.

2. Local irritation. Local irritation, erythema, mild pain, hematoma or ulceration may follow deep subcutaneous (intrafat) injection of heparin sodium. These complications are much more common after intramuscular use, and such use is not recommended.

3. Hypersensitivity. Generalized hypersensitivity reactions have been reported, with chills, fever, and urticaria as the most usual manifestations, and asthma, rhinitis, lacrimation, headache, nausea and vomiting, and anaphylactoid reactions, including shock, occurring more rarely. Itching and burning, especially on the plantar site of the feet, may occur.

Thrombocytopenia has been reported to occur in patients receiving heparin with a reported incidence of 0–30%. While often mild and of no obvious clinical significance, such thrombocytopenia can be accompanied by severe thromboembolic complications such as skin necrosis, gangrene of the extremities, that may lead to amputation, myocardial infarction, pulmonary embolism, stroke, and possibly death. (See WARNINGS, PRECAUTIONS.)

Certain episodes of painful, ischemic, and cyanosed limbs have in the past been attributed to allergic vasospastic reactions. Whether these are in fact identical to the thrombocytopenia associated complications remains to be determined.

4. Miscellaneous. Osteoporosis following long-term administration of high doses of heparin, cutaneous necrosis after systemic administration, supression of aldosterone synthesis, delayed transient alopecia, priapism, and rebound hyperlipemia on discontinuation of heparin sodium have also been reported.

Significant elevations of aminotransferase (SGOT [S-AST] and SGPT [S-ALT]) levels have occurred in a high percentage of patients (and healthy subjects) who have received heparin.

OVERDOSAGE

Symptoms: Bleeding is the chief sign of heparin overdosage. Nosebleeds, blood in urine or tarry stools may be noted as the first sign of bleeding. Easy bruising or petechial formations may precede frank bleeding.

Treatment: Neutralization of heparin effect. When clinical circumstances (bleeding) require reversal of heparinization, protamine sulfate (1% solution) by slow infusion will neutralize heparin effect. **No more than 50 mg** should be administered, **very slowly,** in any 10 minute period. Each mg of protamine sulfate neutralizes approximately 100 USP heparin units. The amount of protamine required decreases over time as heparin is metabolized. Although the metabolism of heparin is complex, it may, for the purpose of choosing a protamine dose, be assumed to have a half-life of about $\frac{1}{2}$ hour after intravenous injection.

Administration of protamine sulfate can cause severe hypotensive and anaphylactoid reactions. Because fatal reactions often resembling anaphylaxis have been reported, the drug should be given only when resuscitation techniques and treatment of anaphylactoid shock are readily available.

For additional information the labeling of Protamine Sulfate Injection, USP products should be consulted.

DOSAGE AND ADMINISTRATION

Parenteral drug products should be inspected visually for particulate matter and discoloration prior to administration, whenever solution and container permit. Slight discoloration does not alter potency.

When heparin is added to an infusion solution for continuous intravenous administration, the container should be inverted at least six times to insure adequate mixing and prevent pooling of the heparin in the solution.

Heparin sodium is not effective by oral administration and should be given by intermittent intravenous injection, intravenous infusion, or deep subcutaneous (intrafat, i.e., above the iliac crest or abdominal fat layer) injection. **The intramuscular route of administration should be avoided because of the frequent occurrence of hematoma at the injection site.** The dosage of heparin sodium should be adjusted according to the patient's coagulation test results. When heparin is given by continuous intravenous infusion, the coagulation time should be determined approximately every 4 hours in the early stages of treatment. When the drug is administered intermittently by intravenous injection, coagulation tests should be performed before each injection during the early stages of treatment and at appropriate intervals thereafter. Dosage is considered adequate when the activated partial thromboplastin time (APTT) is 1.5 to 2 times normal or when the whole blood clotting time is elevated approximately 2.5 to 3 times the control value. After deep subcutaneous (intrafat) injections, tests for adequacy of dosage are best performed on samples drawn 4–6 hours after the injection. Periodic platelet counts, hematocrits, and tests for occult blood in stool are recommended during the entire course of heparin therapy, regardless of the route of administration.

Heparin Sodium Injection should not be mixed with Adriamycin (doxorubicin) or Inapsine (droperidol) since it has been reported that these drugs are incompatible with heparin and a precipitate may form.

Converting to Oral Anticoagulant: When an oral anticoagulant of the coumarin or similar type is to be begun in patients already receiving heparin sodium, baseline and subsequent tests of prothrombin activity must be determined at a time when heparin activity is too low to affect the prothrombin time. This is about 5 hours after the last I.V. bolus and 24 hours after the last subcutaneous dose. If continuous I.V. heparin infusion is used, prothrombin time can usually be measured at any time.

In converting from heparin to an oral anticoagulant, the dose of the oral anticoagulant should be the usual initial amount and thereafter prothrombin time should be determined at the usual intervals. To ensure continuous anticoagulation, it is advisable to continue full heparin therapy for several days after the prothrombin time has reached the therapeutic range. Heparin therapy may then be discontinued without tapering.

Therapeutic Anticoagulant Effect with Full-Dose Heparin. Although dosage must be adjusted for the individual patient according to the results of suitable laboratory tests, the following dosage schedules may be used as guidelines: [See table below].

Pediatric Use: Follow recommendations of appropriate pediatric reference texts. In general, the following dosage schedule may be used as a guideline:

Initial Dose: 50 units/kg (I.V., drip)
Maintenance Dose: 100 units/kg (I.V., drip) every four hours, or 20,000 units/M²/24 hours continuously

Surgery of the Heart and Blood Vessels: Patients undergoing total body perfusion for open-heart surgery should receive an initial dose of not less than 150 units of heparin sodium per kilogram of body weight. Frequently, a dose of 300 units per kilogram is used for procedures estimated to last less than 60 minutes or 400 units per kilogram for those estimated to last longer than 60 minutes.

Low-Dose Prophylaxis of Postoperative Thromboembolism: A number of well-controlled clinical trials have demonstrated that low-dose heparin prophylaxis, given just prior to and after surgery, will reduce the incidence of postoperative deep vein thrombosis in the legs (as measured by the I-125 fibrinogen technique and venography) and of clinical pulmonary embolism. The most widely used dosage has been 5,000 units 2 hours before surgery and 5,000 units every 8 to 12 hours thereafter for 7 days or until the patient is fully ambulatory, whichever is longer. The heparin is given by deep subcutaneous (intrafat, i.e., above the iliac crest or abdominal fat layer, arm or thigh) injection with a fine (25 to 26 - gauge) needle to minimize tissue trauma. A concentrated solution of heparin sodium is recommended. Such prophylaxis should be reserved for patients over the age of 40 who are undergoing major surgery. Patients with bleeding disorders and those having brain or spinal cord surgery, spinal anesthesia, eye surgery, or potentially sanguineous operations should be excluded, as should patients receiving oral anticoagulants or platelet-active drugs (see WARNINGS). The value of such prophylaxis in hip surgery has not been established. The possibility of increased bleeding during surgery or postoperatively should be borne in mind. If such bleeding occurs, discontinuance of heparin and neutralization with protamine sulfate are advisable. If clinical evidence of thromboembolism develops despite low-dose prophylaxis, full therapeutic doses of anticoagulants should be given unless contraindicated. Prior to initiating heparinization the physician should rule out bleeding disorders by appropriate history and laboratory tests, and appropriate coagulations tests should be repeated just prior to surgery. Coagulation tests values should be normal or only slightly elevated at these times.

Extracorporeal Dialysis: Follow equipment manufacturers' operating directions carefully.

Blood Transfusion: Addition of 400 to 600 USP units per 100 ml of whole blood is usually employed to prevent coagulation. Usually, 7,500 USP units of heparin sodium are added to 100 ml of 0.9% Sodium Chloride Injection, USP (or 75,000 USP units per 1,000 ml of 0.9% Sodium Chloride Injection, USP) and mixed; from this sterile solution, 6 to 8 ml are added per 100 ml of whole blood.

Laboratory Samples: Addition of 70 to 150 units of heparin sodium per 10 to 20 ml sample of whole blood is usually employed to prevent coagulation of the sample. Leukoycte counts should be performed on heparinized blood within 2 hours after addition of the heparin. Heparinized blood should not be used for isoagglutinin, complement, or erythrocyte fragility tests or platelet counts.

HOW SUPPLIED

Heparin Sodium Injection, USP derived **from beef lung** is available in the following strengths and package sizes:

1,000 units per ml
   10 ml vials   NDC 0009-0268-01
   25–10 ml vials   NDC 0009-0268-07
   30 ml vials   NDC 0009-0268-02
5,000 units per ml
   1 ml vials   NDC 0009-0291-02
   10 ml vials   NDC 0009-0291-01
10,000 units per ml
   1 ml vials   NDC 0009-0317-01
   25–1 ml vials   NDC 0009-0317-08
   4 ml vials   NDC 0009-0317-02
   25–4 ml vials   NDC 0009-0317-09

Store the product at controlled room temperature 15°–30°C (59°–86°F).
Code 810 670 016

KAOPECTATE® Tablets
Anti-Diarrhea Medicine

(See PDR For Nonprescription Drugs)

METHOD OF ADMINISTRATION	FREQUENCY	RECOMMENDED DOSE*
Deep Subcutaneous (Intrafat) Injection A different site should be used for each injection to prevent the development of massive hematoma.	Initial Dose	5,000 units by I.V. injection, followed by 10,000–20,000 units of a concentrated solution, subcutaneously
	Every 8 hours	8,000 –10,000 units of a concentrated solution
	or Every 12 hours	15,000–20,000 units of a concentrated solution
Intermittent Intravenous Injection	Initial Dose	10,000 units, either undiluted or in 50–100 ml of 0.9% Sodium Chloride Injection, USP
	Every 4 to 6 hours	5,000–10,000 units, either diluted or in 50–100 ml of 0.9% Sodium Chloride Injection, USP
Continuous intravenous Infusion	Initial Dose	5,000 units by I.V. injection
	Continuous	20,000–40,000 units/24 hours in 1,000 ml of 0.9% Sodium Chloride Injection, USP (or in any compatible solution) for infusion

*Based on 150-lb. (68-kg) patient.

Advanced Formula
KAOPECTATE®
Concentrated Anti-Diarrheal

(See PDR For Nonprescription Drugs)

LINCOCIN® ℞
brand of lincomycin hydrochloride capsules and
lincomycin hydrochloride sterile solution
(lincomycin hydrochloride capsules, USP, and
lincomycin hydrochloride injection, USP)

WARNING

Lincomycin therapy has been associated with severe colitis which may end fatally. Therefore, it should be reserved for serious infections where less toxic antimicrobial agents are inappropriate, as described in the Indications Section. It should not be used in patients with nonbacterial infections, such as most upper respiratory tract infections. Studies indicate a toxin(s) produced by Clostridia is one primary cause of antibiotic associated colitis. The colitis is usually characterized by severe, persistent diarrhea and severe abdominal cramps and may be associated with the passage of blood and mucus. Endoscopic examination may reveal pseudomembranous colitis.

When significant diarrhea occurs, the drug should be discontinued or, if necessary, continued only with close observation of the patient. Large bowel endoscopy has been recommended.

Antiperistaltic agents such as opiates and diphenoxylate with atropine (Lomotil) may prolong and/or worsen the condition. Vancomycin has been found to be effective in the treatment of antibiotic associated pseudomembranous colitis produced by Clostridium difficile. The usual adult dose is 500 milligrams to 2 grams of vancomycin orally per day in three to four divided doses administered for 7 to 10 days. Cholestyramine or colestipol resins bind vancomycin in vitro. If both a resin and vancomycin are to be administered concurrently, it may be advisable to separate the time of administration of each drug.

Diarrhea, colitis, and pseudomembranous colitis have been observed to begin up to several weeks following cessation of therapy with lincomycin.

DESCRIPTION

LINCOCIN Capsules and LINCOCIN Sterile Solution contain lincomycin hydrochloride which is the monohydrated salt of lincomycin, a substance produced by the growth of a member of the *lincolnensis* group of *Streptomyces lincolnensis* (Fam. *Streptomycetaceae*). It is a white, or practically white, crystalline powder and is odorless or has a faint odor. Its solutions are acid and are dextrorotatory. Lincomycin hydrochloride is freely soluble in water; soluble in dimethylformamide and very slightly soluble in acetone.

LINCOCIN Capsules contain the following inactive ingredients: erythrosine sodium, FD&C blue No. 1, gelatin, lactose, magnesium stearate, talc and titanium dioxide.

CLINICAL PHARMACOLOGY

Microbiology—Lincomycin has been shown to be effective against most of the common gram-positive pathogens. Depending on the sensitivity of the organism and concentration of the antibiotic, it may be either bactericidal or bacteriostatic. Cross resistance has not been demonstrated with penicillin, chloramphenicol, ampicillin, cephalosporins or the tetracyclines. Despite chemical differences, lincomycin exhibits antibacterial activity similar but not identical to the macrolide antibiotics (eg erythromycin). Some cross resistance (with erythromycin) including a phenomenon known as dissociated cross resistance or macrolide effect has been reported. Microorganisms have not developed resistance to lincomycin rapidly when tested by in vitro or in vivo methods. Staphylococci develop resistance to lincomycin in a slow, step-wise manner based on in vitro, serial subculture experiments. This pattern of resistance development is unlike that shown for streptomycin.

Studies indicate that lincomycin does not share antigenicity with penicillin compounds.

Biological Studies—*In vitro* studies indicate that the spectrum of activity includes *Staphylococcus aureus, Staphylococcus albus, β-hemolytic Streptococcus, Streptococcus viridans, Diplococcus pneumoniae, Clostridium tetani, Clostridium perfringens, Corynebacterium diphtheriae* and *Corynebacterium acnes.*

NOTE: The drug is not active against most strains of *Streptococcus faecalis*, nor against *Neisseria gonorrhoeae, Neisseria meningitidis, Hemophilus influenzae,* or other gram-negative organisms or yeasts.

Human Pharmacology—Lincomycin is absorbed rapidly after a 500 mg oral dose, reaching peak levels in 2 to 4 hours. Levels are maintained above the MIC (minimum inhibitory concentration) for most gram-positive organisms for 6 to 8 hours. Urinary recovery of drug in a 24-hour period ranges from 1.0 to 31 percent (mean: 4.0) after a single oral dose of 500 mg of lincomycin. Tissue level studies indicate that bile is an important route of excretion. Significant levels have been demonstrated in the majority of body tissues. Although the drug is not present in significant amounts in the spinal fluid of normal volunteers, it has been demonstrated in the spinal fluid of one patient with pneumococcal meningitis. Intramuscular administration of a single dose of 600 mg produces a peak serum level at 30 minutes with detectable levels persisting for 24 hours. Urinary excretion after this dose ranges from 1.8 to 24.8 percent (mean: 17.3).

The intravenous infusion over a 2-hour interval of 600 mg of lincomycin hydrochloride in 500 ml of 5 percent glucose in distilled water yields therapeutic levels for 14 hours. Urinary excretion ranges from 4.9 to 30.3 percent (mean: 13.8). The biological half-life, after oral, intramuscular or intravenous administration is 5.4 ± 1.0 hours.

Hemodialysis and peritoneal dialysis do not effectively remove lincomycin from the blood.

INDICATIONS AND USAGE

LINCOCIN preparations (lincomycin) are indicated in the treatment of serious infections due to susceptible strains of streptococci, pneumococci, and staphylococci. Its use should be reserved for penicillin-allergic patients or other patients for whom, in the judgment of the physician, a penicillin is inappropriate. Because of the risk of colitis, as described in the WARNING box, before selecting lincomycin the physician should consider the nature of the infection and the suitability of less toxic alternatives (eg, erythromycin).

Lincomycin has been demonstrated to be effective in the treatment of staphylococcal infections resistant to other antibiotics and susceptible to lincomycin. Staphylococcal strains resistant to LINCOCIN have been recovered; culture and susceptibility studies should be done in conjunction with therapy with LINCOCIN. In the case of macrolides, partial but not complete cross resistance may occur (see **Microbiology**). The drug may be administered concomitantly with other antimicrobial agents when indicated.

CONTRAINDICATIONS

This drug is contraindicated in patients previously found to be hypersensitive to lincomycin or clindamycin. It is not indicated in the treatment of minor bacterial infections or viral infections.

WARNINGS

(See WARNING box). Studies indicate a toxin(s) produced by *Clostridia* is one primary cause of antibiotic associated colitis.[1-5] Mild cases of colitis may respond to drug discontinuance alone. Moderate to severe cases should be managed promptly with fluid, electrolyte and protein supplementation as indicated. Vancomycin has been found to be effective in the treatment of antibiotic associated pseudomembranous colitis produced by *Clostridium difficile.* The usual adult dosage is 500 milligrams to 2 grams of vancomycin orally per day in three to four divided doses administered for 7 to 10 days. Cholestyramine or colestipol resins bind vancomycin *in vitro.* If both a resin and vancomycin are to be administered concurrently, it may be advisable to separate the time of administration of each drug. Systemic corticoids and corticoid retention enemas may help relieve the colitis. Other causes of colitis should also be considered.

A careful inquiry should be made concerning previous sensitivities to drugs and other allergens.

Usage in Pregnancy—Safety for use in pregnancy has not been established.

Usage in Newborn—Until further clinical experience is obtained, LINCOCIN preparations (lincomycin) are not indicated in the newborn.

Nursing Mothers—LINCOCIN has been reported to appear in breast milk in ranges of 0.5 to 2.4 mcg/ml.

LINCOCIN Sterile Solution contains benzyl alcohol which has been associated with a fatal gasping syndrome in infants.

1. Bailey, WR, Scott, EG, *Diagnostic Microbiology* CV Mosby Company, St. Louis, 1978.
2. Bartlett, JG, et al, "Clindamycin-associated Colitis due to a Toxin-producing Species of *Clostridium* in Hamsters" *J. Inf. Dis.* **136**(5): 701–705, (November) 1977.
3. Larson, HE, Price, AB, "Pseudomembranous Colitis: Presence of Clostridial Toxin," *Lancet,* 1312–1314 (December) 24 and 31, 1977.
4. Lusk, RH, et al, "Clindamycin-Induced Enterocolitis in Hamsters", *J. Inf. Dis.* **137**(4): 464–474 (April) 1978.
5. "Antibiotic-associated Colitis: A Progress Report", *British Med. J.* 1:669–671 (March 18) 1978.

PRECAUTIONS

Review of experience to date suggests that a subgroup of older patients with associated severe illness may tolerate diarrhea less well. When LINCOCIN preparations (lincomycin) are indicated in these patients, they should be carefully monitored for change in bowel frequency.

LINCOCIN should be prescribed with caution in individuals with a history of gastrointestinal disease, particularly colitis. LINCOCIN, like any drug, should be used with caution in patients with a history of asthma or significant allergies. The use of antibiotics occasionally results in overgrowth of nonsusceptible organisms—particularly yeasts. Should superinfections occur, appropriate measures should be taken. When patients with pre-existing monilial infections require therapy with LINCOCIN, concomitant antimonilial treatment should be given.

During prolonged therapy with LINCOCIN, periodic liver and renal function studies and blood counts should be performed.

Since adequate data are not yet available in patients with pre-existing liver disease, its use in such patients is not recommended at this time unless special clinical circumstances so indicate.

Lincomycin has been shown to have neuromuscular blocking properties that may enhance the action of other neuromuscular blocking agents. Therefore, it should be used with caution in patients receiving such agents.

Indicated surgical procedures should be performed in conjunction with antibiotic therapy.

ADVERSE REACTIONS

Gastrointestinal—Glossitis, stomatitis, nausea, vomiting. Persistent diarrhea, enterocolitis and pruritus ani. (See **Warning** box)

Hematopoietic: Neutropenia, leukopenia, agranulocytosis and thrombocytopenic purpura have been reported. There have been rare reports of aplastic anemia and pancytopenia in which LINCOCIN preparations (lincomycin hydrochloride) could not be ruled out as the causative agent.

Hypersensitivity Reactions—Hypersensitivity reactions such as angioneurotic edema, serum sickness and anaphylaxis have been reported, some of these in patients known to be sensitive to penicillin. Rare instances of erythema multiforme, some resembling Stevens-Johnson syndrome, have been associated with LINCOCIN. If an allergic reaction should occur, the drug should be discontinued and the usual agents (epinephrine, corticosteroids, antihistamines) should be available for emergency treatment.

Skin and Mucous Membranes—Skin rashes, urticaria and vaginitis and rare instances of exfoliative and vesiculobullous dermatitis have been reported.

Liver—Although no direct relationship of LINCOCIN to liver dysfunction has been established, jaundice and abnormal liver function tests (particularly elevations of serum transaminase) have been observed in a few instances.

Renal—Although no direct relationship of lincomycin to renal damage has been established, renal dysfunction as evidenced by azotemia, oliguria, and/or proteinuria has been observed in rare instances.

Cardiovascular—After too rapid intravenous administration, rare instances of cardiopulmonary arrest and hypotension have been reported. (See **Dosage and Administration**).

Special Senses—Tinnitus and vertigo have been reported occasionally.

Local Reactions—Patients have demonstrated excellent local tolerance to intramuscularly administered LINCOCIN. Reports of pain following injection have been infrequent. Intravenous administration of LINCOCIN in 250 to 500 ml of 5 percent glucose in distilled water or normal saline produced no local irritation or phlebitis.

DOSAGE AND ADMINISTRATION

If significant diarrhea occurs during therapy, this antibiotic should be discontinued. (See **Warning** box).

Oral—**Adults:** *Serious infections* —500 mg 3 times per day (500 mg approximately every 8 hours). *More severe infections* —500 mg or more 4 times per day (500 mg or more approximately every 6 hours). **Children over 1 month of age:** *Serious infections* —30 mg/kg/day (15 mg/lb/day) divided into 3 or 4 equal doses. *More severe infections* —60 mg/kg/day (30 mg/lb/day) divided into 3 or 4 equal doses. With β-hemolytic streptococcal infections, treatment should continue for at least 10 days to diminish the likelihood of subsequent rheumatic fever or glomerulonephritis.

NOTE: For optimal absorption it is recommended that nothing be given by mouth except water for a period of one to two hours before and after oral administration of LINCOCIN preparations (lincomycin).

Intramuscular—**Adults:** *Serious infections* —600 mg (2 ml) intramuscularly every 24 hours. *More severe infections* —600 mg (2 ml) intramuscularly every 12 hours or more often. **Children over 1 month of age:** *Serious infections* —one intramuscular injection of 10 mg/kg (5 mg/lb) every 24 hours.

Continued on next page

Information on these Upjohn products is based on labeling in effect September 1, 1989. Further information concerning these and other Upjohn products may be obtained by direct inquiry to Medical Information, The Upjohn Company, Kalamazoo, Michigan 49001.

Upjohn—Cont.

More severe infections —one intramuscular injection of 10 mg/kg (5 mg/lb) every 12 hours or more often.

Intravenous —**Adults:** The intravenous dose will be determined by the severity of the infection. For serious infections doses of 600 mg of lincomycin (2 ml of LINCOCIN Sterile Solution) to 1 gram are given every 8-12 hours. For more severe infections these doses may have to be increased. In life-threatening situations daily intravenous doses of as much as 8 grams may be given. **Intravenous doses are given on the basis of 1 gram of lincomycin diluted in not less than 100 ml of appropriate solution (see PHYSICAL COMPATIBILITIES) and infused over a period of not less than one hour.**

Dose	Vol. Diluent	Time
600 mg	100 ml	1 hr
1 gram	100 ml	1 hr
2 grams	200 ml	2 hr
3 grams	300 ml	3 hr
4 grams	400 ml	4 hr

These doses may be repeated as often as required to the limit of the maximum recommended daily dose of 8 grams of lincomycin.

Children over 1 month of age: 10-20 mg/kg/day (5-10 mg/lb/day) depending on the severity of the infection may be infused in divided doses as described above for adults.

NOTE: Severe cardiopulmonary reactions have occurred when this drug has been given at greater than the recommended concentration and rate.

Subconjunctival Injection—0.25 ml (75 mg) injected subconjunctivally will result in ocular fluid levels of antibiotic (lasting for at least 5 hours) with MIC's sufficient for most susceptible pathogens.

Patients with diminished renal function: *When therapy with LINCOCIN is required in individuals with severe impairment of renal function, an appropriate dose is 25 to 30% of that recommended for patients with normally functioning kidneys.*

HOW SUPPLIED

LINCOCIN Capsules (lincomycin) are available in the following strengths and package sizes:

250 mg Pediatric (blue):
Bottles of 24   NDC 0009-0336-01

500 mg (powder blue and dark blue):
Bottles of 24   NDC 0009-0500-01
Bottles of 100   NDC 0009-0500-02

LINCOCIN Capsules contain lincomycin hydrochloride equivalent to 250 mg or 500 mg of lincomycin.

LINCOCIN Sterile Solution is available in the following strength and package sizes:

300 mg
2 ml Syringe—NDC 0009-0600-01
2 ml Vials—NDC 0009-0555-01
10 ml Vials—NDC 0009-0555-02

Each ml of LINCOCIN Sterile Solution contains lincomycin hydrochloride equivalent to lincomycin 300 mg; also benzyl alcohol, 9.45 mg added as preservative.

Store at controlled room temperature 15°–30°C (59°–86°F).

ANIMAL PHARMACOLOGY

In vivo experimental animal studies demonstrated the effectiveness of LINCOCIN preparations (lincomycin) in protecting animals infected with *Streptococcus viridans*, β-hemolytic *Streptococcus*, *Staphylococcus aureus*, *Diplococcus pneumoniae* and *Leptospira pomona*. It was ineffective in *Klebsiella*, *Pasteurella*, *Pseudomonas*, *Salmonella* and *Shigella* infections.

CLINICAL STUDIES

Experience with 345 obstetrical patients receiving this drug revealed no ill effects related to pregnancy.

Physical Compatibilities:
Physically compatible for 24 hours at room temperature unless otherwise indicated.

Infusion Solutions
Dextrose in Water, 5% and 10%
Dextrose in Saline, 5% and 10%
Ringer's Solution
Sodium Lactate 1/6 Molar
Travert 10%—Electrolyte No. 1
Dextran in Saline 6% w/v

Vitamins in Infusion Solutions
B-Complex
B-Complex with Ascorbic Acid

Antibiotics in Infusion Solutions
Penicillin G Sodium (Satisfactory for 4 hours)
Cephalothin
Tetracycline HCl
Cephaloridine
Colistimethate (Satisfactory for 4 hours)
Ampicillin
Methicillin
Chloramphenicol
Polymyxin B Sulfate

Physically Incompatible with:
Novobiocin
Kanamycin

IT SHOULD BE EMPHASIZED THAT THE COMPATIBLE AND INCOMPATIBLE DETERMINATIONS ARE PHYSICAL OBSERVATIONS ONLY, NOT CHEMICAL DETERMINATIONS. ADEQUATE CLINICAL EVALUATION OF THE SAFETY AND EFFICACY OF THESE COMBINATIONS HAS NOT BEEN PERFORMED.
Code 810 174 006

LONITEN®   ℞
brand of minoxidil tablets, USP

WARNINGS

LONITEN Tablets contain the powerful antihypertensive agent, minoxidil, which may produce serious adverse effects. It can cause pericardial effusion, occasionally progressing to tamponade, and angina pectoris may be exacerbated. LONITEN should be reserved for hypertensive patients who do not respond adequately to maximum therapeutic doses of a diuretic and two other antihypertensive agents.

In experimental animals, minoxidil caused several kinds of myocardial lesions as well as other adverse cardiac effects (see Cardiac Lesions in Animals).

LONITEN must be administered under close supervision, usually concomitantly with therapeutic doses of a beta-adrenergic blocking agent to prevent tachycardia and increased myocardial workload. It must also usually be given with a diuretic, frequently one acting in the ascending limb of the loop of Henle, to prevent serious fluid accumulation. Patients with malignant hypertension and those already receiving guanethidine (see Warnings) should be hospitalized when LONITEN is first administered so that they can be monitored to avoid too rapid, or large orthostatic, decreases in blood pressure.

DESCRIPTION

LONITEN Tablets contain minoxidil, an antihypertensive peripheral vasodilator. Minoxidil occurs as a white or off-white, odorless, crystalline solid that is soluble in water to the extent of approximately 2 mg/ml; is readily soluble in propylene glycol or ethanol; and is almost insoluble in acetone, chloroform or ethyl acetate. The chemical name for minoxidil is 2,4-pyrimidinediamine, 6-(1-piperidinyl)-, 3-oxide (mw = 209.25).

LONITEN Tablets for oral administration contain either 2.5 mg or 10 mg of minoxidil. Inactive ingredients: cellulose, corn starch, lactose, magnesium stearate, silicon dioxide.

CLINICAL PHARMACOLOGY

1. General Pharmacologic Properties
Minoxidil is an orally effective direct acting peripheral vasodilator that reduces elevated systolic and diastolic blood pressure by decreasing peripheral vascular resistance. Microcirculatory blood flow in animals is enhanced or maintained in all systemic vascular beds. In man, forearm and renal vascular resistance decline; forearm blood flow increases while renal blood flow and glomerular filtration rate are preserved.

Because it causes peripheral vasodilation, minoxidil elicits a number of predictable reactions. Reduction of peripheral arteriolar resistance and the associated fall in blood pressure trigger sympathetic, vagal inhibitory, and renal homeostatic mechanisms, including an increase in renin secretion, that lead to increased cardiac rate and output and salt and water retention. These adverse effects can usually be minimized by concomitant administration of a diuretic and a beta-adrenergic blocking agent or other sympathetic nervous system suppressant.

Minoxidil does not interfere with vasomotor reflexes and therefore does not produce orthostatic hypotension. The drug does not enter the central nervous system in experimental animals in significant amounts, and it does not affect CNS function in man.

2. Effects on Blood Pressure and Target Organs
The extent and time-course of blood pressure reduction by minoxidil do not correspond closely to its concentration in plasma. After an effective single oral dose, blood pressure usually starts to decline within one-half hour, reaches a minimum between 2 and 3 hours and recovers at an arithmetically linear rate of about 30%/day. The total duration of effect is approximately 75 hours. When minoxidil is administered chronically, once or twice a day, the time required to achieve maximum effect on blood pressure with a given daily dose is inversely related to the size of the dose. Thus, maximum effect is achieved on 10 mg/day within 7 days, on 20 mg/day within 5 days, and on 40 mg/day within 3 days.

The blood pressure response to minoxidil is linearly related to the logarithm of the dose administered. The slope of this log-linear dose-response relationship is proportional to the

extent of hypertension and approaches zero at a supine diastolic blood pressure of approximately 85 mmHg.

When used in severely hypertensive patients resistant to other therapy, frequently with an accompanying diuretic and beta-blocker, LONITEN Tablets (minoxidil) usually decreased the blood pressure and reversed encephalopathy and retinopathy."

3. Absorption and Metabolism
Minoxidil is at least 90% absorbed from the GI tract in experimental animals and man. Plasma levels of the parent drug reach maximum within the first hour and decline rapidly thereafter. The average plasma half-life in man is 4.2 hours. Approximately 90% of the administered drug is metabolized, predominantly by conjugation with glucuronic acid at the N-oxide position in the pyrimidine ring, but also by conversion to more polar products. Known metabolites exert much less pharmacologic effect than minoxidil itself; all are excreted principally in the urine. Minoxidil does not bind to plasma proteins, and its renal clearance corresponds to the glomerular filtration rate. In the absence of functional renal tissue, minoxidil and its metabolites can be removed by hemodialysis.

4. Cardiac Lesions in Animals
Minoxidil produced two types of cardiac lesions in non-primate species:

(a) Dog atrial lesion—
Daily oral doses of 0.5 mg/kg for several days to 1 month or longer produced a grossly visible hemorrhagic lesion of the right atrium of the dog. This lesion has not been seen in other species. Microscopic examination showed replacement of myocardial cells by proliferating fibroblasts and angioblasts; phagocytosis; and hemosiderin accumulation in macrophages.

(b) Papillary muscle lesion—
Short term treatment (about 3 days) in several species (dog, rat, minipig) produced necrosis of the papillary muscles, and, in some cases subendocardial areas of the left ventricle, lesions similar to those produced by other peripheral dilators and by beta-adrenergic receptor agonists such as isoproterenol and epinephrine. These are thought to result from myocardial ischemia resulting from reflex sympathetic or vagal withdrawal-induced tachycardia in combination with hypotension. These lesions were reduced in incidence and severity by beta-adrenergic receptor blockade.

(c) *Hemorrhagic lesions* were seen in many parts of the heart, mainly in the epicardium, endocardium, and walls of small coronary arteries and arterioles, after acute minoxidil treatment in dogs, and left atrial hemorrhagic lesions were seen in minipigs.

In addition to these lesions, longer term studies in rats, dogs, and monkeys showed cardiac hypertrophy and (in rats) cardiac dilation. In monkeys, hydrochlorothiazide partly reversed the increased heart weight, suggesting it may be related to fluid overload. In a one-year dog study, serosanguinous pericardial fluid was seen.

Autopsies of 79 patients who died from various causes and who had received minoxidil did not reveal right atrial or other hemorrhagic pathology of the kind seen in dogs. Instances of necrotic areas in the papillary muscles were seen, but these occurred in the presence of known pre-existing ischemic heart disease and did not appear different from, or more common than, lesions seen in patients never exposed to minoxidil. Studies to date cannot rule out the possibility that minoxidil can be associated with cardiac damage in humans.

INDICATIONS AND USAGE

Because of the potential for serious adverse effects, LONITEN Tablets (minoxidil) are indicated only in the treatment of hypertension that is symptomatic or associated with target organ damage and is not manageable with maximum therapeutic doses of a diuretic plus two other antihypertensive drugs. At the present time use in milder degrees of hypertension is not recommended because the benefit-risk relationship in such patients has not been defined.

LONITEN reduced supine diastolic blood pressure by 20 mm Hg or to 90 mm Hg or less in approximately 75% of patients, most of whom had hypertension that could not be controlled by other drugs.

CONTRAINDICATIONS

LONITEN Tablets (minoxidil) are contraindicated in pheochromocytoma, because minoxidil may stimulate secretion of catecholamines from the tumor through its antihypertensive action.

WARNINGS

1. Salt and Water Retention; Congestive Heart Failure—concomitant use of an adequate diuretic is required—
LONITEN Tablets (minoxidil) must usually be administered concomitantly with a diuretic adequate to prevent fluid retention and possible congestive heart failure; a high ceiling (loop) diuretic is *almost always* required. Body weight should be monitored closely. If LONITEN is used without a diuretic, retention of several hundred milli-equivalents of salt and corresponding volumes of water can occur within a few days, leading to increased plasma and interstitial fluid volume and

local or generalized edema. Diuretic treatment alone, or in combination with restricted salt intake, will usually minimize fluid retention, although reversible edema did develop in approximately 10% of nondialysis patients so treated. Ascites has also been reported. Diuretic effectiveness was limited mostly by disease-related impaired renal function. The condition of patients with preexisting congestive heart failure occasionally deteriorated in association with fluid retention although because of the fall in blood pressure (reduction of afterload), more than twice as many improved than worsened. Rarely, refractory fluid retention may require discontinuation of LONITEN. Provided that the patient is under close medical supervision, it may be possible to resolve refractory salt retention by discontinuing LONITEN for 1 or 2 days and then resuming treatment in conjunction with vigorous diuretic therapy.

2. Concomitant Treatment to Prevent Tachycardia is Usually Required—LONITEN increases the heart rate. Angina may worsen or appear for the first time during treatment with LONITEN, probably because of the increased oxygen demands associated with increased heart rate and cardiac output. The increase in rate and the occurrence of angina generally can be prevented by the concomitant administration of a beta-adrenergic blocking drug or other sympathetic nervous system suppressant. The ability of beta-adrenergic blocking agents to minimize papillary muscle lesions in animals is further reason to utilize such an agent concomitantly. Round-the-clock effectiveness of the sympathetic suppressant should be ensured.

3. Pericarditis, Pericardial Effusion and Tamponade— There have been reports of pericarditis occurring in association with the use of LONITEN. The relationship of this association to renal status is uncertain. Pericardial effusion, occasionally with tamponade, has been observed in about 3% of treated patients not on dialysis, especially those with inadequate or compromised renal function. Although in many cases, the pericardial effusion was associated with a connective tissue disease, the uremic syndrome, congestive heart failure, or marked fluid retention, there have been instances in which these potential causes of effusion were not present. Patients should be observed closely for any suggestion of a pericardial disorder, and echocardiographic studies should be carried out if suspicion arises. More vigorous diuretic therapy, dialysis, pericardiocentesis, or surgery may be required. If the effusion persists, withdrawal of LONITEN should be considered in light of other means of controlling the hypertension and the patient's clinical status.

4. *Interaction with Guanethidine:*
Although minoxidil does not itself cause orthostatic hypotension, its administration to patients already receiving guanethidine can result in profound orthostatic effects. If at all possible, guanethidine should be discontinued well before minoxidil is begun. Where this is not possible, minoxidil therapy should be started in the hospital and the patient should remain institutionalized until severe orthostatic effects are no longer present or the patient has learned to avoid activities that provoke them.

5. *Hazard of Rapid Control of Blood Pressure:*
In patients with very severe blood pressure elevation, too rapid control of blood pressure, especially with intravenous agents, can precipitate syncope, cerebrovascular accidents, myocardial infarction and ischemia of special sense organs with resulting decrease or loss of vision or hearing. Patients with compromised circulation or cryoglobulinemia may also suffer ischemic episodes of the affected organs. Although such events have not been unequivocally associated with minoxidil use, total experience is limited at present.
Any patient with malignant hypertension should have initial treatment with minoxidil carried out in a hospital setting, both to assure that blood pressure is falling and to assure that it is not falling more rapidly than intended.

PRECAUTIONS

1. General Precautions—(a) **Monitor fluid and electrolyte balance and body weight** (see **Warnings:** Salt and Water Retention).
(b) **Observe patients for signs and symptoms of pericardial effusion** (see **Warnings:** Pericardial Effusion and Tamponade).
(c) **Use after myocardial infarction**—LONITEN Tablets (minoxidil) have not been used in patients who have had a myocardial infarction within the preceding month. It is possible that a reduction of arterial pressure with LONITEN might further limit blood flow to the myocardium, although this might be compensated by decreased oxygen demand because of lower blood pressure.
(d) **Hypersensitivity**—Possible hypersensitivity to LONITEN, manifested as a skin rash, has been seen in less than 1% of patients; whether the drug should be discontinued when this occurs depends on treatment alternatives.
(e) **Renal failure or dialysis patients** may require smaller doses of LONITEN and should have close medical supervision to prevent exacerbation of renal failure or precipitation of cardiac failure.

2. **Information for patient**—The patient should be made fully aware of the importance of continuing all of his antihypertensive medications and of the nature of symptoms that would suggest fluid overload. A patient brochure has been prepared and is included with each package of LONITEN. The text of this brochure is reprinted at the end of the insert.

3. **Laboratory tests**
Those laboratory tests which are abnormal at the time of initiation of minoxidil therapy, such as urinalysis, renal function tests, EKG, chest x-ray, echocardiogram, etc., should be repeated at intervals to ascertain whether improvement or deterioration is occuring under minoxidil therapy. Initially, such tests should be performed frequently, eg, 1–3 month intervals; later as stabilization occurs, at intervals of 6–12 months.

4. **Drug Interactions**
See "Interaction with guanethidine" under **WARNINGS.**

5. **Carcinogenesis, Mutagenesis and Impairment of Fertility**—Twenty-two month carcinogenicity studies in rats at doses 15 times the human dose did not provide evidence of tumorigenicity. The drug was not mutagenic in the Salmonella (Ames) test.
Rats receiving up to five times the human dose of minoxidil had a reduction in conception rate, possibly related to drug treatment. There was no evidence of increased fetal resorptions in rats but they did occur in rabbits.

6. **Pregnancy-Teratogenic Effects**—Pregnancy Category C. Minoxidil has been shown to reduce the conception rate in rats and to show evidence of increased fetal absorption in rabbits when administered at five times the human dose. There was no evidence of teratogenic effects in rats and rabbits. There are no adequate and well controlled studies in pregnant women. LONITEN should be used during pregnancy only if the potential benefit justifies the potential risk to the fetus.

7. **Labor and delivery**
The effects on labor and delivery are unknown.

8. **Nursing Mothers**—Minoxidil has been reported to be secreted in human milk. As a general rule, nursing should not be undertaken while a patient is on LONITEN.

9. **Pediatric Use**—Use in children has been limited to date, particularly in infants. The recommendations under **Dosage and Administration** can be considered only a rough guide at present and careful titration is essential.

10. **Unapproved Use**—Use of LONITEN Tablets, in any formulation, to promote hair growth is not an approved indication. Clinical trials are in progress and are designed to determine efficacy, dosage, duration of treatment, and actual side effects. Pending completion and analysis of these trials, efficacy, dose and duration of the therapy are not known. Because systemic absorption of topically applied drug may occur and is dependent on vehicle and/or method of use, extemporaneous topical formulations made from LONITEN should be considered to share in the full range of CONTRAINDICATIONS, WARNINGS, PRECAUTIONS, and ADVERSE REACTIONS listed in this insert. In addition, skin intolerance to drug and/or vehicle may occur.

ADVERSE REACTIONS

1. **Salt and Water Retention** (see **Warnings:** Concomitant Use of Adequate Diuretic is Required)—Temporary edema developed in 7% of patients who were not edematous at the start of therapy.
2. **Pericarditis, Pericardial Effusion and Tamponade** (see **Warnings**).
3. **Dermatologic** - Hypertrichosis—Elongation, thickening, and enhanced pigmentation of fine body hair are seen in about 80% of patients taking LONITEN Tablets (minoxidil). This develops within 3 to 6 weeks after starting therapy. It is usually first noticed on the temples, between the eyebrows, between the hairline and the eyebrows, or in the side-burn area of the upper lateral cheek, later extending to the back, arms, legs, and scalp. Upon discontinuation of LONITEN, new hair growth stops, but 1 to 6 months may be required for restoration to pretreatment appearance. No endocrine abnormalities have been found to explain the abnormal hair growth; thus, it is hypertrichosis without virilism. Hair growth is especially disturbing to children and women and such patients should be thoroughly informed about this effect before therapy with LONITEN is begun.
Allergic—Rashes have been reported, including rare reports of bullous eruptions, and Stevens-Johnson Syndrome.
4. **Hematologic**—Thrombocytopenia and leukopenia (WBC < 3000/mm³) have rarely been reported.
5. **Gastrointestinal**—Nausea and/or vomiting has been reported. In clinical trials the incidence of nausea and vomiting associated with the underlying disease has shown a decrease from pretrial levels.
6. **Miscellaneous**—Breast tenderness—This developed in less than 1% of patients.
7. **Altered Laboratory Findings**—(a) ECG changes— changes in direction and magnitude of the ECG T-waves occur in approximately 60% of patients treated with LONITEN. In rare instances a large negative amplitude of the T-wave may encroach upon the S-T segment, but the S-T segment is not independently altered. These changes usually

disappear with continuance of treatment and revert to the pretreatment state if LONITEN is discontinued. No symptoms have been associated with these changes, nor have there been alterations in blood cell counts or in plasma enzyme concentrations that would suggest myocardial damage. Long-term treatment of patients manifesting such changes has provided no evidence of deteriorating cardiac function. At present the changes appear to be nonspecific and without identifiable clinical significance. (b) Effects of hemodilution—hematocrit, hemoglobin and erythrocyte count usually fall about 7% initially and then recover to pretreatment levels. (c) Other—Alkaline phosphatase increased varyingly without other evidence of liver or bone abnormality. Serum creatinine increased an average of 6% and BUN slightly more, but later declined to pretreatment levels.

OVERDOSAGE

There have been only a few instances of deliberate or accidental overdosage with LONITEN Tablets (minoxidil). One patient recovered after taking 50 mg of minoxidil together with 500 mg of a barbiturate. When exaggerated hypotension is encountered, it is most likely to occur in association with residual sympathetic nervous system blockade from previous therapy (guanethidine-like effects or alpha-adrenergic blockage), which prevents the usual compensatory maintenance of blood pressure. Intravenous administration of normal saline will help to maintain blood pressure and facilitate urine formation in these patients. Sympathomimetic drugs such as norepinephrine or epinephrine should be avoided because of their excessive cardiac stimulating action. Phenylephrine, angiotensin II, vasopressin, and dopamine all reverse hypotension due to LONITEN, but should only be used if underperfusion of a vital organ is evident. Radioimmunoassay can be performed to determine the concentration of minoxidil in the blood. At the maximum adult dosage of 100 mg/day, peak blood levels of 1641 ng/ml and 2441 ng/ml were observed in two patients, respectively. Due to patient-to-patient variation in blood levels, it is difficult to establish an overdosage warning level. In general, a substantial increase above 2000 ng/ml should be regarded as overdosage, unless the physician is aware that the patient has taken no more than the maximum dose.
Oral LD_{50} in rats has ranged from 1321–3492 mg/kg; in mice, 2456-2648 mg/kg.

DOSAGE AND ADMINISTRATION

Patients over 12 years of age: The recommended initial dosage of LONITEN Tablets (minoxidil) is 5 mg given as a single daily dose. Daily dosage can be increased to 10, 20 and then to 40 mg in single or divided doses if required for optimum blood pressure control. The effective dosage range is usually 10 to 40 mg per day. The maximum recommended dosage is 100 mg per day.
Patients under 12 years of age: The initial dosage is 0.2 mg/kg minoxidil as a single daily dose. The dosage may be increased in 50 to 100% increments until optimum blood pressure control is achieved. The effective dosage range is usually 0.25 to 1.0 mg/kg/day. The maximum recommended dosage is 50 mg daily. (see **9. Pediatric Use** under Precautions).
Dose frequency: The magnitude of within-day fluctuation of arterial pressure during therapy with LONITEN is directly proportional to the extent of pressure reduction. If supine diastolic pressure has been reduced less than 30 mmHg, the drug need be administered only once a day; if supine diastolic pressure has been reduced more than 30 mmHg, the daily dosage should be divided into two equal parts.
Frequency of dosage adjustment: Dosage must be titrated carefully according to individual response. Intervals between dosage adjustments normally should be at least 3 days since the full response to a given dose is not obtained for at least that amount of time. **Where a more rapid management of hypertension is required, dose adjustments can be made every 6 hours if the patient is carefully monitored.**
Concomitant therapy: Diuretic and beta-blocker or other sympathetic nervous system suppressant.
Diuretics: LONITEN must be used in conjunction with a diuretic in patients relying on renal function for maintaining salt and water balance. Diuretics have been used at the following dosages when starting therapy with LONITEN: hydrochlorothiazide (50 mg, b.i.d.) or other thiazides at equieffective dosage; chlorthalidone (50 to 100 mg, once daily); furosemide (40 mg, b.i.d.). If excessive salt and water retention results in a weight gain of more than 5 pounds, diuretic therapy should be changed to furosemide; if the pa-

Continued on next page

Information on these Upjohn products is based on labeling in effect September 1, 1989. Further information concerning these and other Upjohn products may be obtained by direct inquiry to Medical Information, The Upjohn Company, Kalamazoo, Michigan 49001.

Upjohn—Cont.

tient is already taking furosemide, dosage should be increased in accordance with the patient's requirements.

Beta-blocker or other sympathetic nervous system suppressants: When therapy with LONITEN is begun, the dosage of a beta-adrenergic receptor blocking drug should be the equivalent of 80 to 160 mg of propranolol per day in divided doses.

If beta-blockers are contraindicated, methyldopa (250 to 750 mg, b.i.d.) may be used instead. Methyldopa must be given for at least 24 hours before starting therapy with LONITEN because of the delay in the onset of methyldopa's action. Limited clinical experience indicates that clonidine may also be used to prevent tachycardia induced by LONITEN; the usual dosage is 0.1 to 0.2 mg twice daily.

Sympathetic nervous system suppressants may not completely prevent an increase in heart rate due to LONITEN but usually do prevent tachycardia. Typically, patients receiving a beta-blocker prior to initiation of therapy with LONITEN have a bradycardia and can be expected to have an increase in heart rate toward normal when LONITEN is added. When treatment with LONITEN and beta-blocker or other sympathetic nervous system suppressant are begun simultaneously, their opposing cardiac effects usually nullify each other, leading to little change in heart rate.

HOW SUPPLIED

LONITEN Tablets (minoxidil) are available as round, scored, white tablets. Dosage strengths are imprinted on one convex surface. The following strengths and container sizes are available:

Strength	Container and Size	NDC Number
2.5 mg	Unit of Use bottles of 100,	0009-0121-01
10 mg	Unit of Use bottles of 100,	0009-0137-01
	bottles of 500	0009-0137-02

Store at controlled room temperature 15°–30°C (59°–86°F).

Patient Information: LONITEN Tablets contain minoxidil, a medicine for the treatment of high blood pressure in the patient who has not been controlled or is experiencing unacceptable side effects with other medications. It must usually be taken with other medicines.

Be absolutely sure to take all of your medicines for high blood pressure according to your doctor's instructions. Do not stop taking LONITEN unless your doctor tells you to. Do not give any of your medicine to other people.

It is important that you look for the warning signals of certain undesired effects of LONITEN. Call your doctor if they occur. Your doctor will need to see you regularly while you are taking LONITEN. Be sure to keep all your appointments or to arrange for new ones if you must miss one.

Do not hesitate to call your doctor if any discomforts or problems occur.

The information here is intended to help you take LONITEN properly. It does not tell you all there is to know about LONITEN. There is a more technical leaflet that you may request from the pharmacist; you may need your doctor's help in understanding parts of that leaflet.

What is LONITEN?

LONITEN Tablets contain minoxidil which is a drug for lowering the blood pressure. It works by relaxing and enlarging certain small blood vessels so that blood flows through them more easily.

Why lower blood pressure?

Your doctor has prescribed LONITEN to lower your blood pressure and protect vital parts of your body. Uncontrolled blood pressure can cause stroke, heart failure, blindness, kidney failure, and heart attacks.

Most people with high blood pressure need to take medicines to treat it for their whole lives.

Who should take LONITEN?

There are many people with high blood pressure, but most of them do not need LONITEN. LONITEN is used ONLY when your doctor decides that:

1. your high blood pressure is severe;
2. your high blood pressure is causing symptoms or damage to vital organs; and
3. other medicines did not work well enough or had very disturbing side effects.

LONITEN should be taken only when a doctor prescribes it. Never give any of your LONITEN Tablets, or any other high blood pressure medicine, to a friend or relative.

Pregnancy: In some cases doctors may prescribe LONITEN for women who are pregnant or who are planning to have children. However, its safe use in pregnancy has not been established. Laboratory animals had a reduced ability to become pregnant and a reduced survival of offspring while taking LONITEN. If you are pregnant or are planning to become pregnant, be sure to tell your doctor.

How to take LONITEN.

Usually, your doctor will prescribe two other medicines along with LONITEN. These will help lower blood pressure and will help prevent undesired effects of LONITEN.

Often, when a medicine like LONITEN lowers blood pressure, your body tries to return the blood pressure to the original, higher level. It does this by holding on to water and salt (so there will be more fluid to pump) and by making your heart beat faster. To prevent this, your doctor will usually prescribe a water tablet to remove the extra salt and water from your body (a diuretic dye-u-RET-tic) and another medicine to slow your heart beat.

You must follow your doctor's instructions exactly, taking all the prescribed medicines, in the right amounts, each day. These medicines will help keep your blood pressure down. The water tablet and heart beat medicine will help prevent the undesired effects of LONITEN.

LONITEN Tablets come in two strengths (2 ½ milligrams and 10 milligrams) that are marked on each tablet. Pay close attention to the tablet markings to be sure you are taking the correct strength. Your doctor may prescribe half a tablet; the tablets are scored (partly cut on one side) so that you can easily break them.

When you first start taking LONITEN, your doctor may need to see you often in order to adjust your dosage. Take all your medicine according to the schedule prescribed by your doctor. **Do not skip any doses. If you should forget a dose of LONITEN, wait until it is time for your next dose, then continue with your regular schedule. Remember: do not stop taking LONITEN, or any of your other high blood pressure medicines, without checking with your doctor.** Make sure that any doctor treating or examining you knows that you are taking high blood pressure medicines, including LONITEN.

WARNING SIGNALS

Even if you take all your medicines correctly, LONITEN Tablets may cause undesired effects. Some of these are serious and you should be on the lookout for them. **If any of the following warning signals occur, you must call your doctor immediately:**

1. **Increase in heart rate** —You should measure your heart rate by counting your pulse rate **while you are resting.** If you have an increase of 20 beats or more a minute over your normal pulse, contact your doctor immediately. If you do not know how to take your pulse rate, ask your doctor. Also ask your doctor how often to check your pulse.

2. **Rapid weight gain of more than 5 pounds** —You should weigh yourself daily. If you quickly gain five or more pounds, or if there is any swelling or puffiness in the face, hands, ankles, or stomach area, this could be a sign that you are retaining body fluids. Your doctor may have to change your drugs or change the dose of your drugs. You may also need to reduce the amount of salt you eat. A smaller weight gain (2 to 3 pounds) often occurs when treatment is started. You may lose this extra weight with continued treatment.

3. **Increased difficulty in breathing,** especially when lying down. This too may be due to an increase of body fluids. It can also happen because your high blood pressure is getting worse. In either case, you might require treatment with other medicines.

4. **New or worsening of pain in the chest, arm, or shoulder or signs of severe indigestion** — These could be signs of serious heart problems.

5. **Dizziness, lightheadedness or fainting** — These can be signs of high blood pressure or they may be side effects from one of the medicines. Your doctor may need to change or adjust the dosage of the medicines you are taking.

OTHER UNDESIRED EFFECTS

LONITEN Tablets can cause other undesired effects such as nausea and/or vomiting that are annoying but not dangerous. Do not stop taking the drug because of these other undesired effects without talking to your doctor.

Hair growth: About 8 out of every 10 patients who have taken LONITEN noticed that fine **body hair grew darker or longer** on certain parts of the body. This happened about three to six weeks after beginning treatment. The hair may first be noticed on the forehead and temples, between the eyebrows, or on the upper part of the cheeks. Later, hair may grow on the back, arms, legs, or scalp. Although hair growth may not be noticeable to some patients, it often is bothersome in women and children. **Unwanted hair can be controlled with a hair remover or by shaving.** The extra hair is not permanent, it disappears within 1 to 6 months of stopping LONITEN. Nevertheless, **you should not stop taking LONITEN without first talking to your doctor.**

A few patients have developed a rash or breast tenderness while taking LONITEN Tablets (minoxidil), but this is unusual.

Code 810 384 212

Shown in Product Identification Section, page 434

MAOLATE®   ℞
brand of chlorphenesin carbamate tablets

500's
NSN 6505-00-998-7143 (M & VA)

HOW SUPPLIED

Scored tablets containing 400 mg chlorphenesin carbamate are available in the following packages.

Bottles of 50	NDC 0009-0412-01
Bottles of 500	NDC 0009-0412-02

Shown in Product Identification Section, page 434

MEDROL®   ℞
brand of methylprednisolone acetate topical
For External Use Only

HOW SUPPLIED

In two concentrations-2.5 mg (0.25%) or 10 mg (1.0%) methylprednisolone acetate per gram.

0.25%	30 gram tubes	NDC 0009-0483-02
1%	30 gram tubes	NDC 0009-0505-02

MEDROL®   ℞
brand of methylprednisolone tablets, USP

4 mg, 21's Dosepak	NSN 6505-01-131-5619 (M)
4 mg, 100's	NSN 6505-01-134-6647 (M)
4 mg, 500's	NSN 6505-00-050-3068 (M)

DESCRIPTION

MEDROL Tablets contain methylprednisolone which is a glucocorticord. Glucocorticoids are adrenocortical steroids, both naturally occurring and synthetic, which are readily absorbed from the gastrointestinal tract. Methylprednisolone occurs as a white to practically white, odorless, crystalline powder. It is sparingly soluble in alcohol, in dioxane, and in methanol, slightly soluble in acetone, and in chloroform, and very slightly soluble in ether. It is practically insoluble in water.

The chemical name for methylprednisolone is pregna-1, 4-diene-3, 20-dione,11, 17, 21-trihydroxy-6-methyl-,(6α, 11β)- and the molecular weight is 374.48.

Each MEDROL tablet for oral administration contains 2 mg, 4 mg, 8 mg, 16 mg, 24 mg, or 32 mg of methylprednisolone. Inactive ingredients:

2 mg	4 and 16 mg
Calcium Stearate	Calcium Stearate
Corn Starch	Corn Starch
Erythrosine Sodium	Lactose
Lactose	Mineral Oil
Mineral Oil	Sorbic Acid
Sorbic Acid	Sucrose
Sucrose	

8 and 32 mg	24 mg
Calcium Stearate	Calcium Stearate
Corn Starch	Corn Starch
F D & C Yellow No. 6	F D & C Yellow No. 5
Lactose	Lactose
Mineral Oil	Mineral Oil
Sorbic Acid	Sorbic Acid
Sucrose	Sucrose

ACTIONS

Naturally occurring glucocorticoids (hydrocortisone and cortisone), which also have salt-retaining properties, are used as replacement therapy in adrenocortical deficiency states. Their synthetic analogs are primarily used for their potent anti-inflammatory effects in disorders of many organ systems.

Glucocorticoids cause profound and varied metabolic effects. In addition, they modify the body's immune responses to diverse stimuli.

INDICATIONS

MEDROL Tablets (methylprednisolone) are indicated in the following conditions:

1. **Endocrine Disorders**
   Primary or secondary adrenocortical insufficiency (hydrocortisone or cortisone is the first choice; synthetic analogs may be used in conjunction with mineralocorticoids where applicable; in infancy mineralocorticoid supplementation is of particular importance).
   Congenital adrenal hyperplasia
   Nonsuppurative thyroiditis
   Hypercalcemia associated with cancer

2. **Rheumatic Disorders**
   As adjunctive therapy for short-term administration (to tide the patient over an acute episode or exacerbation) in:
   Psoriatic arthritis
   Rheumatoid arthritis, including juvenile rheumatoid arthritis (selected cases may require low-dose maintenance therapy)

Ankylosing spondylitis
Acute and subacute bursitis
Acute nonspecific tenosynovitis
Acute gouty arthritis
Post-traumatic osteoarthritis
Synovitis of osteoarthritis
Epicondylitis

3. **Collagen Diseases**
During an exacerbation or as maintenance therapy
in selected cases of:
Systemic lupus erythematosus
Acute rheumatic carditis
Systemic dermatomyositis (polymyositis)

4. **Dermatologic Diseases**
Pemphigus
Bullous dermatitis herpetiformis
Severe erythema multiforme (Stevens-Johnson syndrome)
Exfoliative dermatitis
Mycosis fungoides
Severe psoriasis
Severe seborrheic dermatitis

5. **Allergic States**
Control of severe or incapacitating allergic conditions intractable to adequate trials of conventional treatment:
Seasonal or perennial allergic rhinitis
Serum sickness
Bronchial asthma
Drug hypersensitivity reactions
Contact dermatitis
Atopic dermatitis

6. **Ophthalmic Diseases**
Severe acute and chronic allergic and inflammatory
processes involving the eye and its adnexa such as:
Allergic corneal marginal ulcers
Herpes zoster ophthalmicus
Anterior segment inflammation
Diffuse posterior uveitis and choroiditis
Sympathetic ophthalmia
Allergic conjunctivitis
Keratitis
Chorioretinitis
Optic neuritis
Iritis and iridocyclitis

7. **Respiratory Diseases**
Symptomatic sarcoidosis
Loeffler's syndrome not manageable by other means
Berylliosis
Fulminating or disseminated pulmonary tuberculosis when used concurrently with appropriate antituberculous chemotherapy
Aspiration pneumonitis

8. **Hematologic Disorders**
Idiopathic thrombocytopenic purpura in adults
Secondary thrombocytopenia in adults
Acquired (autoimmune) hemolytic anemia
Erythroblastopenia (RBC anemia)
Congenital (erythroid) hypoplastic anemia

9. **Neoplastic Diseases**
For palliative management of:
Leukemias and lymphomas in adults
Acute leukemia of childhood

10. **Edematous States**
To induce a diuresis or remission of proteinuria in
the nephrotic syndrome, without uremia, of the
idiopathic type or that due to lupus erythematosus.

11. **Gastrointestinal diseases**
To tide the patient over a critical period of the disease in:
Ulcerative colitis
Regional enteritis

12. **Nervous System**
Acute exacerbations of multiple sclerosis

13. **Miscellaneous**
Tuberculous meningitis with subarachnoid block or
impending block when used concurrently with
appropriate antituberculous chemotherapy.
Trichinosis with neurologic or myocardial involvement

CONTRAINDICATIONS
Systemic fungal infections and known hypersensitivity to
components.

WARNINGS
In patients on corticosteroid therapy subjected to unusual
stress, increased dosage of rapidly acting corticosteroids before, during, and after the stressful situation is indicated.
Corticosteroids may mask some signs of infection and new
infections may appear during their use. There may be decreased resistance and inability to localize infection when
corticosteroids are used.
Prolonged use of corticosteroids may produce posterior subcapsular cataracts, glaucoma with possible damage to the

optic nerves, and may enhance the establishment of secondary ocular infections due to fungi or viruses.
Usage in pregnancy: Since adequate human reproduction
studies have not been done with corticosteroids, the use of
these drugs in pregnancy, nursing mothers or women of
childbearing potential requires that the possible benefits of
the drug be weighed against the potential hazards to the
mother and embryo or fetus. Infants born of mothers who
have received substantial doses of corticosteroids during
pregnancy should be carefully observed for signs of hypoadrenalism.
Average and large doses of hydrocortisone or cortisone can
cause elevation of blood pressure, salt and water retention,
and increased excretion of potassium. These effects are less
likely to occur with the synthetic derivatives except when
used in large doses. Dietary salt restriction and potassium
supplementation may be necessary. All corticosteroids increase calcium excretion.
**While on corticosteroid therapy patients should not be vaccinated against smallpox. Other immunization procedures
should not be undertaken in patients who are on corticosteroids, especially on high dose, because of possible hazards of
neurological complications and a lack of antibody response.**
The use of MEDROL Tablets (methylprednisolone) in active
tuberculosis should be restricted to those cases of fulminating or disseminated tuberculosis in which the corticosteroid
is used for the management of the disease in conjunction
with an appropriate antituberculous regimen.
If corticosteroids are indicated in patients with latent tuberculosis or tuberculin reactivity, close observation is necessary as reactivation of the disease may occur. During prolonged corticosteroid therapy, these patients should receive
chemoprophylaxis.

PRECAUTIONS
Drug-induced secondary adrenocortical insufficiency may be
minimized by gradual reduction of dosage. This type of relative insufficiency may persist for months after discontinuation of therapy; therefore, in any situation of stress occurring
during that period, hormone therapy should be reinstituted.
Since mineralocorticoid secretion may be impaired, salt and/
or a mineralocorticoid should be administered concurrently.
There is an enhanced effect of corticosteroids on patients
with hypothyroidism and in those with cirrhosis.
Corticosteroids should be used cautiously in patients with
ocular herpes simplex because of possible corneal perforation.
The lowest possible dose of corticosteroid should be used to
control the condition under treatment, and when reduction
in dosage is possible, the reduction should be gradual.
Psychic derangements may appear when corticosteroids are
used, ranging from euphoria, insomnia, mood swings, personality changes and severe depression, to frank psychotic
manifestations. Also, existing emotional instability or psychotic tendencies may be aggravated by corticosteroids.
Aspirin should be used cautiously in conjunction with corticosteroids in hypoprothrombinemia.
Steroids should be used with caution in nonspecific ulcerative colitis, if there is a probability of impending perforation, abscess or other pyogenic infection; diverticulitis; fresh
intestinal anastomoses; active or latent peptic ulcer; renal
insufficiency; hypertension; osteoporosis; and myasthenia
gravis.
Growth and development of infants and children on prolonged corticosteroid therapy should be carefully observed.
Although controlled clinical trials have shown corticosteroids to be effective in speeding the resolution of acute exacerbations of multiple sclerosis, they do not show that corticosteroids affect the ultimate outcome or natural history of the
disease. The studies do show that relatively high doses of
corticosteroids are necessary to demonstrate a significant
effect. (See **Dosage and Administration**)
Since complications of treatment with glucocorticoids are
dependent on the size of the dose and the duration of treatment, a risk/benefit decision must be made in each individual case as to dose and duration of treatment and as to
whether daily or intermittent therapy should be used.
The 24 mg tablet contains FD&C Yellow No. 5 (tartrazine)
which may cause allergic-type reactions (including bronchial
asthma) in certain susceptible individuals. Although the
overall incidence of FD&C Yellow No. 5 (tartrazine) sensitivity in the general population is low, it is frequently seen in
patients who also have aspirin hypersensitivity.

ADVERSE REACTIONS
Fluid and Electrolyte Disturbances
Sodium retention
Fluid retention
Congestive heart failure in susceptible patients
Potassium loss
Hypokalemic alkalosis
Hypertension
Musculoskeletal
Muscle weakness
Steroid myopathy
Loss of muscle mass

Osteoporosis
Vertebral compression fractures
Aseptic necrosis of femoral and humeral heads
Pathologic fracture of long bones
Gastrointestinal
Peptic ulcer with possible perforation and hemorrhage
Pancreatitis
Abdominal distention
Ulcerative esophagitis
Dermatologic
Impaired wound healing
Thin fragile skin
Petechiae and ecchymoses
Facial erythema
Increased sweating
May suppress reactions to skin tests
Neurological
Increased intracranial pressure with papilledema (pseudotumor cerebri) usually after treatment
Convulsions
Vertigo
Headache
Endocrine
Development of Cushingoid state
Suppression of growth in children
Secondary adrenocortical and pituitary unresponsiveness,
particularly in times of stress, as in trauma, surgery or
illness
Menstrual irregularities
Decreased carbohydrate tolerance
Manifestations of latent diabetes mellitus
Increased requirements for insulin or oral hypoglycemic
agents in diabetics
Ophthalmic
Posterior subcapsular cataracts
Increased intraocular pressure
Glaucoma
Exophthalmos
Metabolic
Negative nitrogen balance due to protein catabolism
The following additional reactions have been reported
following oral as well as parenteral therapy: Urticaria and
other allergic, anaphylactic or hypersensitivity reactions.

DOSAGE AND ADMINISTRATION
The initial dosage of MEDROL Tablets (methylprednisolone)
may vary from 4 mg to 48 mg per day depending on the specific disease entity being treated. In situations of less severity lower doses will generally suffice while in selected patients higher initial doses may be required. The initial dosage should be maintained or adjusted until a satisfactory
response is noted. If after a reasonable period of time there is
a lack of satisfactory clinical response, MEDROL should be
discontinued and the patient transferred to other appropriate therapy. IT SHOULD BE EMPHASIZED THAT DOSAGE
REQUIREMENTS ARE VARIABLE AND MUST BE INDIVIDUALIZED ON THE BASIS OF THE DISEASE UNDER TREATMENT AND THE RESPONSE OF THE PATIENT. After a favorable response is noted, the proper maintenance dosage
should be determined by decreasing the initial drug dosage
in small decrements at appropriate time intervals until the
lowest dosage which will maintain an adequate clinical response is reached. It should be kept in mind that constant
monitoring is needed in regard to drug dosage. Included in
the situations which may make dosage adjustments necessary are changes in clinical status secondary to remissions or
exacerbations in the disease process, the patient's individual
drug responsiveness, and the effect of patient exposure to
stressful situations not directly related to the disease entity
under treatment; in this latter situation it may be necessary
to increase the dosage of MEDROL for a period of time consistent with the patient's condition. If after long-term therapy the drug is to be stopped, it is recommended that it be
withdrawn gradually rather than abruptly.

Multiple Sclerosis
In treatment of acute exacerbations of multiple sclerosis
daily doses of 200 mg of prednisolone for a week followed by
80 mg every other day for 1 month have been shown to be
effective (4 mg of methylprednisolone is equivalent to 5 mg of
prednisolone).

ADT® (Alternate Day Therapy)
Alternate day therapy is a corticosteroid dosing regimen in
which twice the usual daily dose of corticoid is administered
every other morning. The purpose of this mode of therapy is
to provide the patient requiring long-term pharmacologic
dose treatment with the beneficial effects of corticoids while
minimizing certain undesirable effects, including pituitary-

Continued on next page

Information on these Upjohn products is based on labeling in
effect September 1, 1989. Further information concerning
these and other Upjohn products may be obtained by direct
inquiry to Medical Information, The Upjohn Company,
Kalamazoo, Michigan 49001.

Upjohn—Cont.

adrenal suppression, the Cushingoid state, corticoid withdrawal symptoms, and growth suppression in children.

The rationale for this treatment schedule is based on two major premises: (a) the anti-inflammatory or therapeutic effect of corticoids persists longer than their physical presence and metabolic effects and (b) administration of the corticosteroid every other morning allows for re-establishment of more nearly normal hypothalamic-pituitary-adrenal (HPA) activity on the off-steroid day.

A brief review of the HPA physiology may be helpful in understanding this rationale. Acting primarily through the hypothalamus a fall in free cortisol stimulates the pituitary gland to produce increasing amounts of corticotropin (ACTH) while a rise in free cortisol inhibits ACTH secretion. Normally the HPA system is characterized by diurnal (circadian) rhythm. Serum levels of ACTH rise from a low point about 10 pm to a peak level about 6 am. Increasing levels of ACTH stimulate adrenal cortical activity resulting in a rise in plasma cortisol with maximal levels occurring between 2 am and 8 am. This rise in cortisol dampens ACTH production and in turn adrenal cortical activity. There is a gradual fall in plasma corticoids during the day with lowest levels occurring about midnight.

The diurnal rhythm of the HPA axis is lost in Cushing's disease, a syndrome of adrenal cortical hyperfunction characterized by obesity with centripetal fat distribution, thinning of the skin with easy bruisability, muscle wasting with weakness, hypertension, latent diabetes, osteoporosis, electrolyte imbalance, etc. The same clinical findings of hyperadrenocorticism may be noted during long-term pharmacologic dose corticoid therapy administered in conventional daily divided doses. It would appear, then, that a disturbance in the diurnal cycle with maintenance of elevated corticoid values during the night may play a significant role in the development of undesirable corticoid effects. Escape from these constantly elevated plasma levels for even short periods of time may be instrumental in protecting against undesirable pharmacologic effects.

During conventional pharmacologic dose corticosteroid therapy, ACTH production is inhibited with subsequent suppression of cortisol production by the adrenal cortex. Recovery time for normal HPA activity is variable depending upon the dose and duration of treatment. During this time the patient is vulnerable to any stressful situation. Although it has been shown that there is considerably less adrenal suppression following a single morning dose of prednisolone (10 mg) as opposed to a quarter of that dose administered every 6 hours, there is evidence that some suppressive effect on adrenal activity may be carried over into the following day when pharmacologic doses are used. Further, it has been shown that a single dose of certain corticosteroids will produce adrenal cortical suppression for two or more days. Other corticoids, including methylprednisolone, hydrocortisone, prednisone, and prednisolone, are considered to be short acting (producing adrenal cortical suppression for $1\frac{1}{4}$ to $1\frac{1}{2}$ days following a single dose) and thus are recommended for alternate day therapy.

The following should be kept in mind when considering alternate day therapy:

1) Basic principles and indications for corticosteroid therapy should apply. The benefits of ADT should not encourage the indiscriminate use of steroids.

2) ADT is a therapeutic technique primarily designed for patients in whom long-term pharmacologic corticoid therapy is anticipated.

3) In less severe disease processes in which corticoid therapy is indicated, it may be possible to initiate treatment with ADT. More severe disease states usually will require daily divided high dose therapy for initial control of the disease process. The initial suppressive dose level should be continued until satisfactory clinical response is obtained, usually four to ten days in the case of many allergic and collagen diseases. It is important to keep the period of initial suppressive dose as brief as possible particularly when subsequent use of alternate day therapy is intended.

Once control has been established, two courses are available: (a) change to ADT and then gradually reduce the amount of corticoid given every other day *or* (b) following control of the disease process reduce the daily dose of corticoid to the lowest effective level as rapidly as possible and then change over to an alternate day schedule. Theoretically, course (a) may be preferable.

4) Because of the advantages of ADT, it may be desirable to try patients on this form of therapy who have been on daily corticoids for long periods of time (eg, patients with rheumatoid arthritis). Since these patients may already have a suppressed HPA axis, establishing them on ADT may be difficult and not always successful. However, it is recommended that regular attempts be made to change them over. It may be helpful to triple or even quadruple the daily maintenance dose and administer this every other day rather than just doubling the daily dose if difficulty is encountered. Once the

patient is again controlled, an attempt should be made to reduce this dose to a minimum.

5) As indicated above, certain corticosteroids, because of their prolonged suppressive effect on adrenal activity, are not recommended for alternate day therapy (eg, dexamethasone and betamethasone).

6) The maximal activity of the adrenal cortex is between 2 am and 8 am, and it is minimal between 4 pm and midnight. Exogenous corticosteroids suppress adrenocortical activity the least, when given at the time of maximal activity (am).

7) In using ADT it is important, as in all therapeutic situations, to individualize and tailor the therapy to each patient. Complete control of symptoms will not be possible in all patients. An explanation of the benefits of ADT will help the patient to understand and tolerate the possible flare-up in symptoms which may occur in the latter part of the off-steroid day. Other symptomatic therapy may be added or increased at this time if needed.

8) In the event of an acute flare-up of the disease process, it may be necessary to return to a full suppressive daily divided corticoid dose for control. Once control is again established alternate day therapy may be reinstituted.

9) Although many of the undesirable features of corticosteroid therapy can be minimized by ADT, as in any therapeutic situation, the physician must carefully weigh the benefit-risk ratio for each patient in whom corticoid therapy is being considered.

HOW SUPPLIED

MEDROL Tablets (methylprednisolone) are available in the following strengths and sizes:

2 mg	Bottles of 100	*NDC 0009-0049-02*
4 mg	Bottles of 30	*NDC 0009-0056-01*
	Bottles of 100	*NDC 0009-0056-02*
	Bottles of 500	*NDC 0009-0056-03*
	Unit Dose Package (100)	*NDC 0009-0056-05*
	Dosepak ™ Unit of Use (21 tablets)	*NDC 0009-0056-04*
8 mg	Bottles of 25	*NDC 0009-0022-01*
16 mg	Bottles of 50	*NDC 0009-0073-01*
	ADT Pak ® (14 tablets) Unit of Use	
		NDC 0009-0073-02
24 mg	Bottles of 25	*NDC 0009-0155-01*
32 mg	Bottles of 25	*NDC 0009-0176-01*

Code 810 487 309

Shown in Product Identification Section, page 434

MICRONASE®   ℞
brand of glyburide tablets
(1.25, 2.5, and 5 mg)

2.5 mg, 100's	NSN 6505-01-216-6289 (M & VA)
5 mg, 30's	NSN 6505-01-259-7117 (VA)
5 mg, 60's	NSN 6505-01-263-4532 (VA)
5 mg, 90's	NSN 6505-01-263-4533 (VA)
5 mg, 100's	NSN 6505-01-204-5417 (M & VA)
5 mg, 100's, Unit Dose	NSN 6505-01-243-4103 (VA)
5 mg, 500's	NSN 6505-01-216-6288 (M & VA)
5 mg, 1000's	NSN 6505-01-219-7968 (M & VA)

DESCRIPTION

MICRONASE Tablets contain glyburide, which is an oral blood-glucose-lowering drug of the sulfonylurea class. Glyburide is a white, crystalline compound, formulated as MICRONASE Tablets of 1.25, 2.5, and 5 mg strengths for oral administration. Inactive ingredients: colloidal silicon dioxide, dibasic calcium phosphate, magnesium stearate, microcrystalline cellulose, sodium alginate, talc. In addition, the **2.5 mg** contains aluminum oxide and FD&C red no. 40 and the **5 mg** contains aluminum oxide and FD&C blue no. 1. The chemical name for glyburide is 1-[[p-[2-(5-chloro-o-anisamido)ethyl]phenyl]-sulfonyl]-3-cyclohexylurea and the molecular weight is 493.99.

CLINICAL PHARMACOLOGY

Actions

Glyburide appears to lower the blood glucose acutely by stimulating the release of insulin from the pancreas, an effect dependent upon functioning beta cells in the pancreatic islets. The mechanism by which glyburide lowers blood glucose during long-term administration has not been clearly established. With chronic administration in Type II diabetic patients, the blood glucose lowering effect persists despite a gradual decline in the insulin secretory response to the drug. Extrapancreatic effects may be involved in the mechanism of action of oral sulfonylurea hypoglycemic drugs.

Some patients who are initially responsive to oral hypoglycemic drugs, including MICRONASE Tablets (glyburide), may become unresponsive or poorly responsive over time. Alternatively, MICRONASE may be effective in some patients who have become unresponsive to one or more other sulfonylurea drugs.

In addition to its blood glucose lowering actions, glyburide produces a mild diuresis by enhancement of renal free water

clearance. Disulfiram-like reactions have very rarely been reported in patients treated with MICRONASE Tablets.

Pharmacokinetics

Single dose studies with MICRONASE Tablets in normal subjects demonstrate significant absorption of glyburide within one hour, peak drug levels at about four hours, and low but detectable levels at twenty-four hours. Mean serum levels of glyburide, as reflected by areas under the serum concentration-time curve, increase in proportion to corresponding increases in dose. Multiple dose studies with MICRONASE in diabetic patients demonstrate drug level concentration-time curves similar to single dose studies, indicating no buildup of drug in tissue depots. The decrease of glyburide in the serum of normal healthy individuals is biphasic; the terminal half-life is about 10 hours. In single dose studies in fasting normal subjects, the degree and duration of blood glucose lowering is proportional to the dose administered and to the area under the drug level concentration-time curve. The blood glucose lowering effect persists for 24 hours following single morning doses in nonfasting diabetic patients. Under conditions of repeated administration in diabetic patients, however, there is no reliable correlation between blood drug levels and fasting blood glucose levels. A one year study of diabetic patients treated with MICRONASE showed no reliable correlation between administered dose and serum drug level.

The major metabolite of glyburide is the 4-trans-hydroxy derivative. A second metabolite, the 3-cis-hydroxy derivative, also occurs. These metabolites probably contribute no significant hypoglycemic action in humans since they are only weakly active (1/400th and 1/40th as active, respectively, as glyburide) in rabbits.

Glyburide is excreted as metabolites in the bile and urine, approximately 50% by each route. This dual excretory pathway is qualitatively different from that of other sulfonylureas, which are excreted primarily in the urine.

Sulfonylurea drugs are extensively bound to serum proteins. Displacement from protein binding sites by other drugs may lead to enhanced hypoglycemic action. *In vitro*, the protein binding exhibited by glyburide is predominantly non-ionic, whereas that of other sulfonylureas (chlorpropamide, tolbutamide, tolazamide) is predominantly ionic. Acidic drugs such as phenylbutazone, warfarin, and salicylates displace the ionic-binding sulfonylureas from serum proteins to a far greater extent than the non-ionic binding glyburide. It has not been shown that this difference in protein binding will result in fewer drug-drug interactions with MICRONASE Tablets in clinical use.

INDICATIONS AND USAGE

MICRONASE Tablets (glyburide) are indicated as an adjunct to diet to lower the blood glucose in patients with non-insulin-dependent diabetes mellitus (type II) whose hyperglycemia cannot be satisfactorily controlled by diet alone.

In initiating treatment for non-insulin-dependent diabetes, diet should be emphasized as the primary form of treatment. Caloric restriction and weight loss are essential in the obese diabetic patient. Proper dietary management alone may be effective in controlling the blood glucose and symptoms of hyperglycemia. The importance of regular physical activity should also be stressed, and cardiovascular risk factors should be identified and corrective measures taken where possible. If this treatment program fails to reduce symptoms and/or blood glucose, the use of an oral sulfonylurea or insulin should be considered. Use of MICRONASE must be viewed by both the physician and patient as a treatment in addition to diet and not as a substitution or as a convenient mechanism for avoiding dietary restraint. Furthermore, loss of blood glucose control on diet alone may be transient, thus requiring only short-term administration of MICRONASE. During maintenance programs, MICRONASE should be discontinued if satisfactory lowering of blood glucose is no longer achieved. Judgment should be based on regular clinical and laboratory evaluations.

In considering the use of MICRONASE in asymptomatic patients, it should be recognized that controlling blood glucose in non-insulin-dependent diabetes has not been definitely established to be effective in preventing the long-term cardiovascular or neural complications of diabetes.

CONTRAINDICATIONS

MICRONASE Tablets (glyburide) are contraindicated in patients with:

1. Known hypersensitivity or allergy to the drug.

2. Diabetic ketoacidosis, with or without coma. This condition should be treated with insulin.

3. Type I diabetes mellitus, as sole therapy.

Special Warning on Increased Risk of Cardiovascular Mortality: The administration of oral hypoglycemic drugs has been reported to be associated with increased cardiovascular mortality as compared to treatment with diet alone or diet plus insulin. This warning is based on the study conducted by the University Group Diabetes Program (UGDP), a long-term prospective clinical trial designed to evaluate the effectiveness of glucose-lowering drugs in preventing or delaying vascular complications in patients with non-insulin-dependent diabetes. The study involved 823 patients who were randomly assigned to one of four treatment groups (*Diabetes*, 19 (Suppl. 2):747–830, 1970).

UGDP reported that patients treated for 5 to 8 years with diet plus a fixed dose of tolbutamide (1.5 grams per day) had a rate of cardiovascular mortality approximately 2½ times that of patients treated with diet alone. A significant increase in total mortality was not observed, but the use of tolbutamide was discontinued based on the increase in cardiovascular mortality, thus limiting the opportunity for the study to show an increase in overall mortality. Despite controversy regarding the interpretation of these results, the findings of the UGDP study provide an adequate basis for this warning. The patient should be informed of the potential risks and advantages of MICRONASE and of alternative modes of therapy.

Although only one drug in the sulfonylurea class (tolbutamide) was included in this study, it is prudent from a safety standpoint to consider that this warning may also apply to other oral hypoglycemic drugs in this class, in view of their close similarities in mode of action and chemical structure.

PRECAUTIONS

General

Hypoglycemia: All sulfonylureas are capable of producing severe hypoglycemia. Proper patient selection and dosage and instructions are important to avoid hypoglycemic episodes. Renal or hepatic insufficiency may cause elevated drug levels of glyburide and the latter may also diminish gluconeogenic capacity, both of which increase the risk of serious hypoglycemic reactions. Elderly, debilitated or malnourished patients, and those with adrenal or pituitary insufficiency, are particularly susceptible to the hypoglycemic action of glucose-lowering drugs. Hypoglycemia may be difficult to recognize in the elderly and in people who are taking beta-adrenergic blocking drugs. Hypoglycemia is more likely to occur when caloric intake is deficient, after severe or prolonged exercise, when alcohol is ingested, or when more than one glucose lowering drug is used.

Loss of Control of Blood Glucose: When a patient stabilized on any diabetic regimen is exposed to stress such as fever, trauma, infection or surgery, a loss of control may occur. At such times it may be necessary to discontinue MICRONASE Tablets (glyburide) and administer insulin.

The effectiveness of any hypoglycemic drug, including MICRONASE, in lowering blood glucose to a desired level decreases in many patients over a period of time which may be due to progression of the severity of diabetes or to diminished responsiveness to the drug. This phenomenon is known as secondary failure, to distinguish it from primary failure in which the drug is ineffective in an individual patient when MICRONASE is first given. Adequate adjustment of dose and adherence to diet should be assessed before classifying a patient as a secondary failure.

Information for Patients: Patients should be informed of the potential risks and advantages of MICRONASE and of alternative modes of therapy. They also should be informed about the importance of adherence to dietary instructions, of a regular exercise program, and of regular testing of urine and/or blood glucose.

The risks of hypoglycemia, its symptoms and treatment, and conditions that predispose to its development should be explained to patients and responsible family members. Primary and secondary failure also should be explained.

Laboratory Tests

Therapeutic response to MICRONASE Tablets should be monitored by frequent urine glucose tests and periodic blood glucose tests. Measurement of glycosylated hemoglobin levels may be helpful in some patients.

Drug Interactions

The hypoglycemic action of sulfonylureas may be potentiated by certain drugs including nonsteroidal anti-inflammatory agents and other drugs that are highly protein bound, salicylates, sulfonamides, chloramphenicol, probenecid, coumarins, monoamine oxidase inhibitors, and beta adrenergic blocking agents. When such drugs are administered to a patient receiving MICRONASE, the patient should be observed closely for hypoglycemia. When such drugs are withdrawn from a patient receiving MICRONASE, the patient should be observed closely for loss of control.

Certain drugs tend to produce hyperglycemia and may lead to loss of control. These drugs include the thiazides and other diuretics, corticosteroids, phenothiazines, thyroid products, estrogens, oral contraceptives, phenytoin, nicotinic acid, sympathomimetics, calcium channel blocking drugs, and isoniazid. When such drugs are administered to a patient receiving MICRONASE, the patient should be closely observed for loss of control. When such drugs are withdrawn from a patient receiving MICRONASE, the patient should be observed closely for hypoglycemia.

A potential interaction between oral miconazole and oral hypoglycemic agents leading to severe hypoglycemia has been reported. Whether this interaction also occurs with the intravenous, topical or vaginal preparations of miconazole is not known.

Carcinogenesis, Mutagenesis, and Impairment of Fertility

Studies in rats at doses to 300 mg/kg/day for 18 months showed no carcinogenic effects. Glyburide is non-mutagenic when studied in the Salmonella microsome test (Ames test) and in the DNA damage/alkaline elution assay.

Pregnancy

Teratogenic Effects: Pregnancy Category B

Reproduction studies have been performed in rats and rabbits at doses up to 500 times the human dose and have revealed no evidence of impaired fertility or harm to the fetus due to glyburide. There are, however, no adequate and well controlled studies in pregnant women. Because animal reproduction studies are not always predictive of human response, this drug should be used during pregnancy only if clearly needed.

Because recent information suggests that abnormal blood glucose levels during pregnancy are associated with a higher incidence of congenital abnormalities, many experts recommend that insulin be used during pregnancy to maintain blood glucose as close to normal as possible.

Nonteratogenic Effects: Prolonged severe hypoglycemia (4 to 10 days) has been reported in neonates born to mothers who were receiving a sulfonylurea drug at the time of delivery. This has been reported more frequently with the use of agents with prolonged half-lives. If MICRONASE is used during pregnancy, it should be discontinued at least two weeks before the expected delivery date.

Nursing Mothers

Although it is not known whether glyburide is excreted in human milk, some sulfonylurea drugs are known to be excreted in human milk. Because the potential for hypoglycemia in nursing infants may exist, a decision should be made whether to discontinue nursing or to discontinue the drug, taking into account the importance of the drug to the mother. If the drug is discontinued, and if diet alone is inadequate for controlling blood glucose, insulin therapy should be considered.

Pediatric Use

Safety and effectiveness in children have not been established.

ADVERSE REACTIONS

Hypoglycemia: See Precautions and Overdosage Sections.

Gastrointestinal Reactions: Cholestatic jaundice and hepatitis may occur rarely; MICRONASE Tablets (glyburide) should be discontinued if this occurs.

Liver function abnormalities, including isolated transaminase elevations, have been reported.

Gastrointestinal disturbances, e.g., nausea, epigastric fullness, and heartburn are the most common reactions, having occurred in 1.8% of treated patients during clinical trials. They tend to be dose related and may disappear when dosage is reduced.

Dermatologic Reactions: Allergic skin reactions, e.g., pruritus, erythema, urticaria, and morbilliform or maculopapular eruptions occurred in 1.5% of treated patients during clinical trials. These may be transient and may disappear despite continued use of MICRONASE; if skin reactions persist, the drug should be discontinued.

Porphyria cutanea tarda and photosensitivity reactions have been reported with sulfonylureas.

Hematologic Reactions: Leukopenia, agranulocytosis, thrombocytopenia, hemolytic anemia, aplastic anemia, and pancytopenia have been reported with sulfonylureas.

Metabolic Reactions: Hepatic porphyria and disulfiram-like reactions have been reported with sulfonylureas; however, hepatic porphyria has not been reported with MICRONASE and disulfiram-like reactions have been reported very rarely.

Cases of hyponatremia have been reported with glyburide and all other sulfonylureas, most often in patients who are on other medications or have medical conditions known to cause hyponatremia or increase release of antidiuretic hormone. The syndrome of inappropriate antidiuretic hormone (SIADH) secretion has been reported with certain other sulfonylureas, and it has been suggested that these sulfonylureas may augment the peripheral (antidiuretic) action of ADH and/or increase release of ADH.

OVERDOSAGE

Overdosage of sulfonylureas, including MICRONASE Tablets (glyburide), can produce hypoglycemia. Mild hypoglycemic symptoms, without loss of consciousness or neurological findings, should be treated aggressively with oral glucose and adjustments in drug dosage and/or meal patterns. Close monitoring should continue until the physician is assured that the patient is out of danger. Severe hypoglycemic reactions with coma, seizure, or other neurological impairment occur infrequently, but constitute medical emergencies requiring immediate hospitalization. If hypoglycemic coma is diagnosed or suspected, the patient should be given a rapid intravenous injection of concentrated (50%) glucose solution. This should be followed by a continuous infusion of a more dilute (10%) glucose solution at a rate which will maintain the blood glucose at a level above 100 mg/dL. Patients should be closely monitored for a minimum of 24 to 48 hours,

since hypoglycemia may recur after apparent clinical recovery.

DOSAGE AND ADMINISTRATION

There is no fixed dosage regimen for the management of diabetes mellitus with MICRONASE Tablets (glyburide) or any other hypoglycemic agent. In addition to the usual monitoring of urinary glucose, the patient's blood glucose must also be monitored periodically to determine the minimum effective dose for the patient; to detect primary failure, i.e., inadequate lowering of blood glucose at the maximum recommended dose of medication; and to detect secondary failure, i.e., loss of adequate blood glucose lowering response after an initial period of effectiveness. Glycosylated hemoglobin levels may also be of value in monitoring the patient's response to therapy.

Short-term administration of MICRONASE may be sufficient during periods of transient loss of control in patients usually controlled well on diet.

Usual Starting Dose

The usual starting dose of MICRONASE Tablets is 2.5 to 5.0 mg daily, administered with breakfast or the first main meal. Those patients who may be more sensitive to hypoglycemic drugs should be started at 1.25 mg daily. (See Precautions Sections for patients at increased risk.) Failure to follow an appropriate dosage regimen may precipitate hypoglycemia. Patients who do not adhere to their prescribed dietary and drug regimen are more prone to exhibit unsatisfactory response to therapy.

Transfer From Other Hypoglycemic Therapy

Patients Receiving Other Oral Antidiabetic Therapy: Transfer of patients from other oral antidiabetic regimens to MICRONASE should be done conservatively and the initial daily dose should be 2.5 to 5 mg. When transferring patients from oral hypoglycemic agents other than chlorpropamide to MICRONASE, no transition period and no initial or priming dose are necessary. When transferring patients from chlorpropamide, particular care should be exercised during the first two weeks because the prolonged retention of chlorpropamide in the body and subsequent overlapping drug effects may provoke hypoglycemia.

Patients Receiving Insulin: Some type II diabetic patients being treated with insulin may respond satisfactorily to MICRONASE. If the insulin dose is less than 20 units daily, substitution of MICRONASE Tablets 2.5 to 5.0 mg as a single daily dose may be tried. If the insulin dose is between 20 and 40 units daily, the patient may be placed directly on MICRONASE Tablets 5.0 mg daily as a single dose. If the insulin dose is more than 40 units daily, a transition period is required for conversion to MICRONASE. In these patients, insulin dosage is decreased by 50% and MICRONASE Tablets 5 mg daily is started. Please refer to Titration to Maintenance Dose for further explanation.

Titration to Maintenance Dose

The usual maintenance dose is in the range of 1.25 to 20 mg daily, which may be given as a single dose or in divided doses (See Dosage Interval Section). Dosage increases should be made in increments of no more than 2.5 mg at weekly intervals based upon the patient's blood glucose response.

No exact dosage relationship exists between MICRONASE and the other oral hypoglycemic agents. Although patients may be transferred from the maximum dose of other sulfonylureas, the maximum starting dose of 5.0 mg of MICRONASE Tablets should be observed. A maintenance dose of 5 mg of MICRONASE Tablets provides approximately the same degree of blood glucose control as 250 to 375 mg chlorpropamide, 250 to 375 mg tolazamide, 500 to 750 mg acetohexamide, or 1000 to 1500 mg tolbutamide.

When transferring patients receiving more than 40 units of insulin daily, they may be started on a daily dose of MICRONASE Tablets 5 mg concomitantly with a 50% reduction in insulin dose. Progressive withdrawal of insulin and increase of MICRONASE in increments of 1.25 to 2.5 mg every 2 to 10 days is then carried out. During this conversion period when both insulin and MICRONASE are being used, hypoglycemia may rarely occur. During insulin withdrawal, patients should test their urine for glucose and acetone at least three times daily and report results to their physician. The appearance of persistent acetonuria with glycosuria indicates that the patient is a type I diabetic who requires insulin therapy.

Maximum Dose

Daily doses of more than 20 mg are not recommended.

Dosage Interval

Once-a-day therapy is usually satisfactory. Some patients, particularly those receiving more than 10 mg daily, may have a more satisfactory response with twice-a-day dosage.

Continued on next page

Information on these Upjohn products is based on labeling in effect September 1, 1989. Further information concerning these and other Upjohn products may be obtained by direct inquiry to Medical Information, The Upjohn Company, Kalamazoo, Michigan 49001.

Upjohn—Cont.

Specific Patient Populations

MICRONASE is not recommended for use in pregnancy or for use in children.

In elderly patients, debilitated or malnourished patients, and patients with impaired renal or hepatic function, the initial and maintenance dosing should be conservative to avoid hypoglycemic reactions. (See Precautions Section.)

HOW SUPPLIED

MICRONASE Tablets (glyburide) are supplied as follows:

MICRONASE Tablets 1.25 mg (White, Round, Scored)

Bottles of 100	NDC 0009-0131-01

MICRONASE Tablets 2.5 mg (Dark Pink, Round, Scored)

Bottles of 30	NDC 0009-0141-06
Bottles of 60	NDC 0009-0141-07
Bottles of 100	NDC 0009-0141-01
Unit Dose Pkg of 100	NDC 0009-0141-02

MICRONASE Tablets 5 mg (Blue, Round, Scored)

Glass bottles of 30	NDC 0009-0171-08
Plastic bottles of 30	NDC 0009-0171-11
Glass bottles of 60	NDC 0009-0171-09
Plastic bottles of 60	NDC 0009-0171-12
Glass bottles of 90	NDC 0009-0171-10
Plastic bottles of 90	NDC 0009-0171-13
Glass bottles of 100	NDC 0009-0171-01
Plastic bottles of 100	NDC 0009-0171-05
Glass bottles of 500	NDC 0009-0171-02
Plastic bottles of 500	NDC 0009-0171-06
Glass bottles of 1000	NDC 0009-0171-04
Plastic bottles of 1000	NDC 0009-0171-07
Unit Dose Pkg of 100	NDC 0009-0171-03

Caution: Federal law prohibits dispensing without prescription. Store at controlled room temperature 15°–30° C (59°–86° F). Dispensed in well closed containers with safety closures. Keep container tightly closed.

Code 811 985 314

Shown in Product Identification Section, page 434

MOTRIN®   ℞
brand of ibuprofen tablets, USP

DESCRIPTION

MOTRIN Tablets contain the active ingredient ibuprofen, which is (±)-2-(p-isobutylphenyl) propionic acid. Ibuprofen is a white powder with a melting point of 74–77°C and is very slightly soluble in water (< 1 mg/ml) and readily soluble in organic solvents such as ethanol and acetone.

The structural formula is represented below:

MOTRIN, a nonsteroidal anti-inflammatory agent, is available in 300 mg, 400 mg, 600 mg, and 800 mg tablets for oral administration.

Inactive ingredients: **300 mg**—acacia, acetylated monoglyceride, calcium sulfate, carboxymethylcellulose sodium, carnauba wax, colloidal silicon dioxide, corn starch, povidone, pregelatinized starch, sesame oil, shellac, stearic acid, sucrose, white wax; **400 mg**—acacia, acetylated monoglyceride, calcium sulfate, carboxymethylcellulose sodium, carnauba wax, colloidal silicon dioxide, corn starch, FD&C yellow no. 6, pregelatinized starch, povidone, sesame oil, shellac, sodium benzoate, stearic acid, sucrose, titanium dioxide, white wax; **600 mg**—carnauba wax, colloidal silicon dioxide, corn starch, FD&C yellow no. 6, hydroxypropyl cellulose, hydroxypropyl methylcellulose, pregelatinized starch, propylene glycol, stearic acid, titanium dioxide; **800 mg**—carnauba wax, colloidal silicon dioxide, croscarmellose sodium, FD&C yellow no. 6, hydroxypropyl methylcellulose, magnesium stearate, microcrystalline cellulose, propylene glycol, talc, titanium dioxide.

CLINICAL PHARMACOLOGY

MOTRIN Tablets contain ibuprofen which possesses analgesic and antipyretic activities. Its mode of action, like that of other nonsteroidal anti-inflammatory agents, is not completely understood, but may be related to prostaglandin synthetase inhibition.

In clinical studies in patients with rheumatoid arthritis and osteoarthritis, MOTRIN has been shown to be comparable to aspirin in controlling pain and inflammation and to be associated with a statistically significant reduction in the milder gastrointestinal side effects (see ADVERSE REACTIONS). MOTRIN may be well tolerated in some patients who have had gastrointestinal side effects with aspirin, but these patients when treated with MOTRIN should be carefully followed for signs and symptoms of gastrointestinal ulceration

and bleeding. Although it is not definitely known whether MOTRIN causes less peptic ulceration than aspirin, in one study involving 885 patients with rheumatoid arthritis treated for up to one year, there were no reports of gastric ulceration with MOTRIN whereas frank ulceration was reported in 13 patients in the aspirin group (statistically significant p < .001).

Gastroscopic studies at varying doses show an increased tendency toward gastric irritation at higher doses. However, at comparable doses, gastric irritation is approximately half that seen with aspirin. Studies using ^{51}Cr-tagged red cells indicate that fecal blood loss associated with MOTRIN Tablets in doses up to 2400 mg daily did not exceed the normal range, and was significantly less than that seen in aspirin-treated patients.

In clinical studies in patients with rheumatoid arthritis, MOTRIN has been shown to be comparable to indomethacin in controlling the signs and symptoms of disease activity and to be associated with a statistically significant reduction of the milder gastrointestinal (see ADVERSE REACTIONS) and CNS side effects.

MOTRIN may be used in combination with gold salts and/or corticosteroids.

Controlled studies have demonstrated that MOTRIN is a more effective analgesic than propoxyphene for the relief of episiotomy pain, pain following dental extraction procedures, and for the relief of the symptoms of primary dysmenorrhea.

In patients with primary dysmenorrhea, MOTRIN has been shown to reduce elevated levels of prostaglandin activity in the menstrual fluid and to reduce resting and active intrauterine pressure, as well as the frequency of uterine contractions. The probable mechanism of action is to inhibit prostaglandin synthesis rather than simply to provide analgesia.

The ibuprofen in MOTRIN is rapidly absorbed when administered orally. Peak serum ibuprofen levels are generally attained one to two hours after administration. With single doses up to 800 mg, a linear relationship exists between amount of drug administered and the integrated area under the serum drug concentration vs time curve. Above 800 mg, however, the area under the curve increases less than proportional to increases in dose. There is no evidence of drug accumulation or enzyme induction.

The administration of MOTRIN Tablets either under fasting conditions or immediately before meals yields quite similar serum ibuprofen concentration-time profiles. When MOTRIN is administered immediately after a meal, there is a reduction in the rate of absorption but no appreciable decrease in the extent of absorption. The bioavailability of the drug is minimally altered by the presence of food.

A bioavailability study has shown that there was no interference with the absorption of ibuprofen when MOTRIN was given in conjunction with an antacid containing both aluminum hydroxide and magnesium hydroxide.

Ibuprofen is rapidly metabolized and eliminated in the urine. The excretion of ibuprofen is virtually complete 24 hours after the last dose. The serum half-life is 1.8 to 2.0 hours.

Studies have shown that following ingestion of the drug, 45% to 79% of the dose was recovered in the urine within 24 hours as metabolite A (25%), (+) - 2 - [p - (2hydroxymethylpropyl)- phenyl] propionic acid and metabolite B (37%), (+)- 2-[p-(2carboxypropyl)-phenyl] propionic acid; the percentages of free and conjugated ibuprofen were approximately 1% and 14%, respectively.

INDICATIONS AND USAGE

MOTRIN Tablets (ibuprofen) are indicated for relief of the signs and symptoms of rheumatoid arthritis and osteoarthritis.

MOTRIN is indicated for relief of mild to moderate pain.

MOTRIN is also indicated for the treatment of primary dysmenorrhea.

Since there have been no controlled clinical trials to demonstrate whether or not there is any beneficial effect or harmful interaction with the use of MOTRIN in conjunction with aspirin, the combination cannot be recommended (see **Drug Interactions**).

Controlled clinical trials to establish the safety and effectiveness of MOTRIN in children have not been conducted.

CONTRAINDICATIONS

MOTRIN Tablets (ibuprofen) should not be used in patients who have previously exhibited hypersensitivity to the drug, or in individuals with the syndrome of nasal polyps, angioedema and bronchospastic reactivity to aspirin or other nonsteroidal anti-inflammatory agents. Anaphylactoid reactions have occurred in such patients.

WARNINGS

Risk of GI Ulceration, Bleeding and Perforation with Nonsteroidal Anti-inflammatory Therapy:

Serious gastrointestinal toxicity such as bleeding, ulceration, and perforation, can occur at any time, with or without warning symptoms, in patients treated chronically with nonsteroidal anti-inflammatory drugs. Although minor upper gastrointestinal problems, such as dyspepsia, are com-

mon, usually developing early in therapy, physicians should remain alert for ulceration and bleeding in patients treated chronically with nonsteroidal anti-inflammatory drugs even in the absence of previous GI tract symptoms. In patients observed in clinical trials of several months to two years duration, symptomatic upper GI ulcers, gross bleeding or perforation appear to occur in approximately 1% of patients treated for 3–6 months, and in about 2–4% of patients treated for one year. Physicians should inform patients about the signs and/or symptoms of serious GI toxicity and what steps to take if they occur.

Studies to date have not identified any subset of patients not at risk of developing peptic ulceration and bleeding. Except for a prior history of serious GI events and other risk factors known to be associated with peptic ulcer disease, such as alcoholism, smoking, etc., no risk factors (eg, age, sex) have been associated with increased risk. Elderly or debilitated patients seem to tolerate ulceration or bleeding less well than other individuals and most spontaneous reports of fatal GI events are in this population. Studies to date are inconclusive concerning the relative risk of various nonsteroidal anti-inflammatory agents in causing such reactions. High doses of any such agents probably carry a greater risk of these reactions, although controlled clinical trials showing this do not exist in most cases. In considering the use of relatively large doses (within the recommended dosage range), sufficient benefit should be anticipated to offset the potential increased risk of GI toxicity.

PRECAUTIONS

Blurred and/or diminished vision, scotomata, and/or changes in color vision have been reported. If a patient develops such complaints while receiving MOTRIN Tablets (ibuprofen), the drug should be discontinued and the patient should have an ophthalmologic examination which includes central visual fields and color vision testing.

Fluid retention and edema have been reported in association with MOTRIN; therefore, the drug should be used with caution in patients with a history of cardiac decompensation or hypertension.

MOTRIN, like other nonsteroidal anti-inflammatory agents, can inhibit platelet aggregation but the effect is quantitatively less and of shorter duration than that seen with aspirin. MOTRIN has been shown to prolong bleeding time (but within the normal range) in normal subjects. Because this prolonged bleeding effect may be exaggerated in patients with underlying hemostatic defects, MOTRIN should be used with caution in persons with intrinsic coagulation defects and those on anticoagulant therapy.

Patients on MOTRIN should report to their physicians signs or symptoms of gastrointestinal ulceration or bleeding, blurred vision or other eye symptoms, skin rash, weight gain, or edema.

In order to avoid exacerbation of disease or adrenal insufficiency, patients who have been on prolonged corticosteroid therapy should have their therapy tapered slowly rather than discontinued abruptly when MOTRIN is added to the treatment program.

The antipyretic and anti-inflammatory activity of ibuprofen may reduce fever and inflammation, thus diminishing their utility as diagnostic signs in detecting complications of presumed noninfectious noninflammatory painful conditions.

As with other nonsteroidal anti-inflammatory drugs, borderline elevations of one or more liver tests may occur in up to 15% of patients. These abnormalities may progress, may remain essentially unchanged, or may be transient with continued therapy. The SGPT (ALT) test is probably the most sensitive indicator of liver dysfunction. Meaningful (3 times the upper limit of normal) elevations of SGPT or SGOT (AST) occurred in controlled clinical trials in less than 1% of patients. A patient with symptoms and/or signs suggesting liver dysfunction, or in whom an abnormal liver test has occurred, should be evaluated for evidence of the development of more severe hepatic reaction while on therapy with MOTRIN. Severe hepatic reactions, including jaundice and cases of fatal hepatitis, have been reported with ibuprofen as with other nonsteroidal anti-inflammatory drugs. Although such reactions are rare, if abnormal liver tests persist or worsen, if clinical signs and symptoms consistent with liver disease develop, or if systemic manifestations occur (eg, eosinophilia, rash, etc.), MOTRIN should be discontinued.

In cross-study comparisons with doses ranging from 1200 mg to 3200 mg daily for several weeks, a slight dose-response decrease in hemoglobin/hematocrit was noted. This has been observed with other nonsteroidal anti-inflammatory drugs; the mechanism is unknown. With daily doses of 3200 mg, the total decrease in hemoglobin may exceed 1 gram; if there are no signs of bleeding, it is probably not clinically important. In two postmarketing clinical studies the incidence of a decreased hemoglobin level was greater than previously reported. Decrease in hemoglobin of 1 gram or more was observed in 17.1% of 193 patients on 1600 mg ibuprofen daily (osteoarthritis), and in 22.8% of 189 patients taking 2400 mg of ibuprofen daily (rheumatoid arthritis). Positive stool occult blood tests and elevated serum creatinine levels were also observed in these studies.

MOTRIN

Incidence Greater than 1% (but less than 3%) Probable Causal Relationship	Precise Incidence Unknown (but less than 1%) Probable Causal Relationship**	Precise Incidence Unknown (but less than 1%) Causal Relationship Unknown**
GASTROINTESTINAL Nausea*, epigastric pain*, heartburn*, diarrhea, abdominal distress, nausea and vomiting, indigestion, constipation, abdominal cramps or pain, fullness of GI tract (bloating and flatulence)	Gastric or duodenal ulcer with bleeding and/or perforation, gastrointestinal hemorrhage, melena, gastritis, hepatitis, jaundice, abnormal liver function tests; pancreatis	
CENTRAL NERVOUS SYSTEM Dizziness*, headache, nervousness	Depression, insomnia, confusion, emotional lability, somnolence, aseptic meningitis with fever and coma	Paresthesias, hallucinations, dream abnormalities, pseudotumor cerebri
DERMATOLOGIC Rash* (including maculopapular type), pruritis	Vesiculobullous eruptions, urticaria, erythema multiforme, Stevens-Johnson syndrome, alopecia	Toxic epidermal necrolysis, photoallergic skin reactions
SPECIAL SENSES Tinnitus	Hearing loss, amblyopia (blurred and/or diminished vision, scotomata and/or changes in color vision) (see PRECAUTIONS)	Conjunctivitis, diplopia, optic neuritis, cataracts
HEMATOLOGIC	Neutropenia, agranulocytosis, aplastic anemia, hemolytic anemia (sometimes Coombs positive), thrombocytopenia with or without purpura, eosinophilia, decreases in hemoglobin and hematocrit (see PRECAUTIONS)	Bleeding episodes (eg epistaxis, menorrhagia)
METABOLIC/ENDOCRINE Decreased appetite		Gynecomastia, hypoglycemic reaction, acidosis
CARDIOVASCULAR Edema, fluid retention (generally responds promptly to drug discontinuation; see PRECAUTIONS)	Congestive heart failure in patients with marginal cardiac function, elevated blood pressure, palpitations	Arrhythmias (sinus tachycardia, sinus bradycardia)
ALLERGIC	Syndrome of abdominal pain, fever, chills, nausea and vomiting; anaphylaxis; bronchospasm (see CONTRAINDICATIONS)	Serum sickness, lupus erythematosus syndrome, Henoch-Schönlein vasculitis, angioedema
RENAL	Acute renal failure (see PRECAUTIONS), decreased creatinine clearance, polyuria, azotemia, cystitis, hematuria	Renal papillary necrosis
MISCELLANEOUS	Dry eyes and mouth, gingival ulcer, rhinitis	

*   Reactions occurring in 3% to 9% of patients treated with MOTRIN. (Those reactions occurring in less than 3% of the patients are unmarked).

**   Reactions are classified under "*Probable Causal Relationship (PCR)*" if there has been one positive rechallenge or if three or more cases occur which might be causally related. Reactions are classified under "*Causal Relationship Unknown*" if seven or more events have been reported but the criteria for PCR have not been met.

Aseptic Meningitis: Aseptic meningitis with fever and coma has been observed on rare occasions in patients on ibuprofen therapy. Although it is probably more likely to occur in patients with systemic lupus erythematosus and related connective tissue diseases, it has been reported in patients who do not have an underlying chronic disease. If signs or symptoms of meningitis develop in a patient on MOTRIN, the possibility of its being related to MOTRIN should be considered.

Renal Effects: As with other nonsteroidal anti-inflammatory drugs, long term administration of ibuprofen to animals has resulted in renal papillary necrosis and other abnormal renal pathology. In humans, there have been reports of acute interstitial nephritis with hematuria, proteinuria, and occasionally nephrotic syndrome.

A second form of renal toxicity has been seen in patients with prerenal conditions leading to a reduction in renal blood flow or blood volume, where the renal prostaglandins have a supportive role in the maintenance of renal perfusion. In these patients administration of a nonsteroidal anti-inflammatory drug may cause a dose dependent reduction in prostaglandin formation and may precipitate overt renal decompensation. Patients at greatest risk of this reaction are those with impaired renal function, heart failure, liver dysfunction, those taking diuretics and the elderly. Discontinuation of nonsteroidal anti-inflammatory drug therapy is typically followed by recovery to the pretreatment state. Those patients at high risk who chronically take MOTRIN should have renal function monitored if they have signs or symptoms which may be consistent with mild azotemia, such as malaise, fatigue, loss of appetite, etc. Occasional patients may develop some elevation of serum creatinine and BUN levels without signs or symptoms.

Since ibuprofen is eliminated primarily by the kidneys, patients with significantly impaired renal function should be closely monitored; and a reduction in dosage should be anticipated to avoid drug accumulation. Prospective studies on the safety of ibuprofen in patients with chronic renal failure have not been conducted.

Information for Patients

MOTRIN, like other drugs of its class, is not free of side effects. The side effects of these drugs can cause discomfort and, rarely, there are more serious side effects, such as gastrointestinal bleeding, which may result in hospitalization and even fatal outcomes.

Nonsteroidal anti-inflammatory drugs are often essential agents in the management of arthritis and have a major role in the treatment of pain, but they also may be commonly employed for conditions which are less serious.

Physicians may wish to discuss with their patients the potential risks (see WARNINGS, PRECAUTIONS, and ADVERSE REACTIONS) and likely benefits of nonsteroidal anti-inflammatory drug treatment, particularly when the drugs are used for less serious conditions where treatment without such agents may represent an acceptable alternative to both the patient and physician.

Laboratory Tests

Because serious GI tract ulcerations and bleeding can occur without warning symptoms, physicians should follow chronically treated patients for the signs and symptoms of ulcerations and bleeding and should inform them of importance of this follow-up (see Risk of GI Ulceration, Bleeding and Perforation with Nonsteroidal Anti-inflammatory therapy).

Drug Interactions: *Coumarin-type anticoagulants.* Several short-term controlled studies failed to show that MOTRIN significantly affected prothrombin times or a variety of other clotting factors when administered to individuals on coumarin-type anticoagulants. However, because bleeding has been reported when MOTRIN and other nonsteroidal anti-inflammatory agents have been administered to patients on coumarin-type anticoagulants, the physician should be cautious when administering MOTRIN to patients on anticoagulants.

Aspirin: Animal studies show that aspirin given with nonsteroidal anti-inflammatory agents, including MOTRIN, yields a net decrease in anti-inflammatory activity with lowered blood levels of the non-aspirin drug. Single dose bioavailability studies in normal volunteers have failed to show an effect of aspirin on ibuprofen blood levels. Correlative clinical studies have not been done.

Methotrexate: Ibuprofen, as well as other nonsteroidal anti-inflammatory drugs, probably reduces the tubular secretion of methotrexate based on *in-vitro* studies in rabbit kidney slices. This may indicate that ibuprofen could enhance the toxicity of methotrexate. Caution should be used if MOTRIN is administered concomitantly with methotrexate.

H-2 Antagonists: In studies with human volunteers, co-administration of cimetidine or ranitidine with ibuprofen had no substantive effect on ibuprofen serum concentrations.

Furosemide: Clinical studies, as well as random observations, have shown that ibuprofen can reduce the natriuretic effect of furosemide and thiazides in some patients. This response has been attributed to inhibition of renal prostaglandin synthesis. During concomitant therapy with ibuprofen, the patient should be observed closely for signs of renal failure (See **PRECAUTIONS, Renal Effects**) as well as to assure diuretic efficacy.

Lithium: Ibuprofen produced an elevation of plasma lithium levels and a reduction in renal lithium clearance in a study of eleven normal volunteers. The mean minimum lithium concentration increased 15% and the renal clearance of lithium was decreased by 19% during this period of concomitant drug administration. This effect has been attributed to inhibition of renal prostaglandin synthesis by ibuprofen. Thus, when ibuprofen and lithium are administered concurrently, subjects should be observed carefully for signs of lithium toxicity. (Read circulars for lithium preparation before use of such concurrent therapy.)

Pregnancy: Reproductive studies conducted in rats and rabbits at doses somewhat less than the maximal clinical dose did not demonstrate evidence of developmental abnormalities. However, animal reproduction studies are not always predictive of human response. As there are no adequate and well-controlled studies in pregnant women, this drug should be used during pregnancy only if clearly needed. Be-

Continued on next page

Information on these Upjohn products is based on labeling in effect September 1, 1989. Further information concerning these and other Upjohn products may be obtained by direct inquiry to Medical Information, The Upjohn Company, Kalamazoo, Michigan 49001.

Upjohn—Cont.

cause of the known effects of nonsteroidal anti-inflammatory drugs on the fetal cardiovascular system (closure of ductus arteriosus), use during late pregnancy should be avoided. As with other drugs known to inhibit prostaglandin synthesis, an increased incidence of dystocia and delayed parturition occurred in rats. Administration of MOTRIN is not recommended during pregnancy.

Nursing Mothers: In limited studies, an assay capable of detecting 1 mcg/ml did not demonstrate ibuprofen in the milk of lactating mothers. However, because of the limited nature of the studies, and the possible adverse effects of prostaglandin-inhibiting drugs on neonates, MOTRIN is not recommended for use in nursing mothers.

ADVERSE REACTIONS

The most frequent type of adverse reaction occurring with MOTRIN Tablets (ibuprofen) is gastrointestinal. In controlled clinical trials the percentage of patients reporting one or more gastrointestinal complaints ranged from 4% to 16%.

In controlled studies when MOTRIN was compared to aspirin and indomethacin in equally effective doses, the overall incidence of gastrointestinal complaints was about half that seen in either the aspirin- or indomethacin-treated patients. Adverse reactions observed during controlled clinical trials at an incidence greater than 1% are listed in the table. Those reactions listed in Column one encompass observations in approximately 3,000 patients. More than 500 of these patients were treated for periods of at least 54 weeks.

Still other reactions occurring less frequently than 1 in 100 were reported in controlled clinical trials and from marketing experience. These reactions have been divided into two categories: Column two of the following table lists reactions with therapy with MOTRIN where the probability of a causal relationship exists: for the reactions in Column three, a causal relationship with MOTRIN has not been established. Reported side effects were higher at doses of 3200 mg/day than at doses of 2400 mg or less per day in clinical trials of patients with rheumatoid arthritis. The increases in incidence were slight and still within the ranges reported in the following table.

[See table on preceding page].

OVERDOSAGE

Approximately 1½ hours after the reported ingestion of from 7 to 10 MOTRIN Tablets (ibuprofen) (400 mg), a 19-month old child weighing 12 kg was seen in the hospital emergency room, apneic and cyanotic, responding only to painful stimuli. This type of stimulus, however, was sufficient to induce respiration. Oxygen and parenteral fluids were given; a greenish-yellow fluid was aspirated from the stomach with no evidence to indicate the presence of ibuprofen. Two hours after ingestion the child's condition seemed stable; she still responded only to painful stimuli and continued to have periods of apnea lasting from 5 to 10 seconds. She was admitted to intensive care and sodium bicarbonate was administered as well as infusions of dextrose and normal saline. By four hours post-ingestion she could be aroused easily, sit by herself and respond to spoken commands. Blood level of ibuprofen was 102.9 μg/ml approximately 8½ hours after accidental ingestion. At 12 hours she appeared to be completely recovered.

In two other reported cases where children (each weighing approximately 10 kg) accidentally, acutely ingested approximately 120 mg/kg, there were no signs of acute intoxication or late sequelae. Blood level in one child 90 minutes after ingestion was 700 μg/ml—about 10 times the peak levels seen in absorption-excretion studies.

A 19-year old male who had taken 8,000 mg of ibuprofen over a period of a few hours complained of dizziness, and nystagmus was noted. After hospitalization, parenteral hydration and three days' bed rest, he recovered with no reported sequelae.

In cases of acute overdosage, the stomach should be emptied by vomiting or lavage, though little drug will likely be recovered if more than an hour has elapsed since ingestion. Because the drug is acidic and is excreted in the urine, it is theoretically beneficial to administer alkali and induce diuresis. In addition to supportive measures the use of oral activated charcoal may help to reduce the absorption and reabsorption of MOTRIN.

DOSAGE AND ADMINISTRATION

Do not exceed 3200 mg total daily dose. If gastrointestinal complaints occur, administer MOTRIN Tablets (ibuprofen) with meals or milk.

Rheumatoid arthritis and osteoarthritis, including flare-ups of chronic disease:

Suggested Dosage: 1200 mg-3200 mg daily (300 mg qid; 400 mg, 600 mg or 800 mg tid or qid). Individual patients may show a better response to 3200 mg daily, as compared with 2400 mg, although in well-controlled clinical trials patients

on 3200 mg did not show a better mean response in terms of efficacy. Therefore, when treating patients with 3200 mg/day, the physician should observe sufficient increased clinical benefits to offset potential increased risk.

The dose should be tailored to each patient, and may be lowered or raised depending on the severity of symptoms either at time of initiating drug therapy or as the patient responds or fails to respond.

In general, patients with rheumatoid arthritis seem to require higher doses of MOTRIN than do patients with osteoarthritis.

The smallest dose of MOTRIN that yields acceptable control should be employed. A linear blood level dose-response relationship exists with single doses up to 800 mg (See CLINICAL PHARMACOLOGY for effects of food on rate of absorption).

The availability of four tablet strengths facilitates dosage adjustment.

In chronic conditions, a therapeutic response to therapy with MOTRIN is sometimes seen in a few days to a week but most often is observed by two weeks. After a satisfactory response has been achieved, the patient's dose should be reviewed and adjusted as required.

Mild to moderate pain:

400 mg every 4 to 6 hours as necessary for relief of pain. In controlled analgesic clinical trials, doses of MOTRIN greater than 400 mg were no more effective than the 400 mg dose.

Dysmenorrhea:

For the treatment of dysmenorrhea, beginning with the earliest onset of such pain, MOTRIN should be given in a dose of 400 mg every 4 hours as necessary for the relief of pain.

HOW SUPPLIED

MOTRIN Tablets (ibuprofen) are supplied as follows:

MOTRIN Tablets, 300 mg (white)

Unit of Use bottles of 60	NDC 0009-0733-01
Bottles of 500	NDC 0009-0733-02

MOTRIN Tablets, 400 mg (orange)

Unit of Use bottles of 30	NDC 0009-0750-31
Unit of Use bottles of 50	NDC 0009-0750-32
Unit of Use bottles of 100	NDC 0009-0750-25
Unit-dose package of 100	NDC 0009-0750-06
Unit of Use bottles of 120	NDC 0009-0750-26
Bottles of 500	NDC 0009-0750-02

MOTRIN Tablets, 600 mg (peach)

Unit of Use bottles of 30	NDC 0009-0742-19
Unit of Use bottles of 50	NDC 0009-0742-20
Unit of Use bottles of 90	NDC 0009-0742-08
Unit of Use bottles of 100	NDC 0009-0742-03
Unit-dose package of 100	NDC 0009-0742-05
Bottles of 500	NDC 0009-0742-02

MOTRIN Tablets, 800 mg (apricot)

Unit of Use bottles of 30	NDC 0009-0725-06
Unit of Use bottles of 50	NDC 0009-0725-07
Unit of Use bottles of 90	NDC 0009-0725-08
Unit of Use bottles of 100	NDC 0009-0725-01
Unit-dose package of 100	NDC 0009-0725-02
Bottles of 500	NDC 0009-0725-03

Code 810 015 227

Shown in Product Identification Section, page 434

MYCIGUENT® Antibiotic Ointment

(See PDR For Nonprescription Drugs)

MYCITRACIN® Triple Antibiotic Ointment

(See PDR For Nonprescription Drugs)

ORINASE®   ℞

brand of tolbutamide tablets, USP
0.5 gram, 100's, Unit Dose   NSN 6505-00-131-9268 (M)

DESCRIPTION

ORINASE Tablets contain tolbutamide, an oral blood glucose lowering drug of the sulfonylurea category. Tolbutamide is a pure white crystalline compound practically insoluble in water but forming water-soluble salts with alkalies. The chemical names for tolbutamide are (1) Benzenesulfonamide, N-[(butylamino) carbonyl]-4-methyl; (2) 1-Butyl-3-(p-tolylsulfonyl)urea and its molecular weight is 270.35. Each ORINASE Tablet for oral administration contains 250 mg or 500 mg tolbutamide. Inactive ingredients: colloidal silicon dioxide, crosscarmellose sodium, magnesium stearate, pregelatinized starch.

CLINICAL PHARMACOLOGY

Actions

Tolbutamide appears to lower blood glucose acutely by stimulating the release of insulin from the pancreas, an effect dependent upon functioning beta cells in the pancreatic islets. The mechanism by which tolbutamide lowers blood glu-

cose during long-term administration has not been clearly established. With chronic administration in Type II diabetic patients, the blood glucose lowering effect persists despite a gradual decline in the insulin secretory response to the drug. Extrapancreatic effects may be involved in the mechanism of action of oral sulfonylurea hypoglycemic drugs.

Some patients who are initially responsive to oral hypoglycemic drugs, including ORINASE, may become unresponsive or poorly responsive over time. Alternatively, ORINASE may be effective in some patients who have become unresponsive to one or more other sulfonylurea drugs.

Pharmacokinetics

When administered orally, the tolbutamide in ORINASE Tablets is readily absorbed from the gastrointestinal tract. Absorption is not impaired and glucose lowering and insulin releasing effects are not altered if the drug is taken with food. Detectable levels are present in the plasma within twenty minutes after oral ingestion of a 500 mg ORINASE tablet, with peak levels occurring at three to four hours and only small amounts detectable at 24 hours. The half-life of tolbutamide is 4.5 to 6.5 hours. As tolbutamide has no p-amino group, it cannot be acetylated, which is one of the common modes of metabolic degradation for the antibacterial sulfonamides. However, the presence of the p-methyl group renders tolbutamide susceptible to oxidation, and this appears to be the principal manner of its metabolic degradation in man. The p-methyl group is oxidized to form a carboxyl group, converting tolbutamide into the totally inactive metabolite 1-butyl-3-p-carboxy-phenylsulfonylurea, which can be recovered in the urine within 24 hours in amounts accounting for up to 75% of the administered dose.

The major tolbutamide metabolite has been found to have no hypoglycemic or other action when administered orally and IV to both normal and diabetic subjects. This tolbutamide metabolite is highly soluble over the critical acid range of urinary pH values, and its solubility increases with increase in pH. Because of the marked solubility of the tolbutamide metabolite, crystalluria does not occur. A second metabolite, 1-butyl-3-(p-hydroxymethyl) phenyl sulfonylurea also occurs to a limited extent. It is an inactive metabolite.

The administration of 3 grams of tolbutamide to either nondiabetic or tolbutamide-responsive diabetic subjects will, in both instances, occasion a gradual lowering of blood glucose. Increasing the dose to 6 grams does not usually cause a response which is significantly different from that produced by the 3 gram dose. Following the administration of a 3 gram dose of ORINASE solution, nondiabetic fasting adults exhibit a 30% or greater reduction in blood glucose within one hour, following which the blood glucose gradually returns to the fasting level over six to twelve hours. Following the administration of a 3 gram dose of ORINASE solution, tolbutamide responsive diabetic patients show a gradually progressive blood glucose lowering effect, the maximal response being reached between five to eight hours after ingestion of a single 3 gram dose. The blood glucose then rises gradually and by the 24th hour has usually returned to pretest levels. The magnitude of the reduction, when expressed in terms of percent of the protest blood glucose, tends to be similar to the response seen in the nondiabetic subject.

INDICATIONS AND USAGE

ORINASE Tablets (tolbutamide) are indicated as an adjunct to diet to lower the blood glucose in patients with noninsulin-dependent diabetes whose hyperglycemia cannot be satisfactorily controlled by diet alone. In initiating treatment for noninsulin-dependent diabetes, diet should be emphasized as the primary form of treatment. Caloric restriction and weight loss are essential in the obese diabetic patient. Proper dietary management alone may be effective in controlling the blood glucose and symptoms of hyperglycemia. The importance of regular physical activity should also be stressed and cardiovascular risk factors should be identified and corrective measures taken where possible.

If this treatment program fails to reduce symptoms and/or blood glucose, the use of an oral sulfonylurea or insulin should be considered. Use of ORINASE must be viewed by both the physician and patient as a treatment in addition to diet, and not as a substitute for diet or as a convenient mechanism for avoiding dietary restraint. Furthermore, loss of blood glucose control on diet alone may be transient, thus requiring only short-term administration of ORINASE. During maintenance programs, ORINASE should be discontinued if satisfactory lowering of blood glucose is no longer achieved. Judgments should be based on regular clinical and laboratory evaluations.

In considering the use of ORINASE in asymptomatic patients, it should be recognized that controlling the blood glucose in noninsulin-dependent diabetes has not been definitely established to be effective in preventing the long-term cardiovascular or neural complications of diabetes.

CONTRAINDICATIONS

ORINASE Tablets (tolbutamide) are contraindicated in patients with: 1) known hypersensitivity or allergy to ORINASE; 2) diabetic ketoacidosis, with or without coma. This condition should be treated with insulin. 3) Type I diabetes, as sole therapy.

Special Warning on Increased Risk of Cardiovascular Mortality: The administration of oral hypoglycemic drugs has been reported to be associated with increased cardiovascular mortality as compared to treatment with diet alone or diet plus insulin. This warning is based on the study conducted by the University Group Diabetes Program (UGDP), a long-term prospective clinical trial designed to evaluate the effectiveness of glucose-lowering drugs in preventing or delaying vascular complications in patients with noninsulin-dependent diabetes. The study involved 823 patients who were randomly assigned to one of four treatment groups (Diabetes, 19 (supp. 2):747-830, 1970.)

UGDP reported that patients treated for five to eight years with diet plus a fixed dose of tolbutamide (1.5 grams per day) had a rate of cardiovascular mortality approximately 2½ times that of patients with diet alone. A significant increase in total mortality was not observed, but the use of tolbutamide was discontinued based on the increase in cardiovascular mortality, thus limiting the opportunity for the study to show an increase in overall mortality. Despite controversy regarding the interpretation of these results, the findings of the UGDP study provide an adequate basis for this warning. The patient should be informed of the potential risks and advantages of ORINASE and of alternative modes of therapy.

Although only one drug in the sulfonylurea class (tolbutamide) was included in this study, it is prudent from a safety standpoint to consider that this warning may also apply to other oral hypoglycemic drugs in this class, in view of their close similarities in mode of action and chemical structure.

PRECAUTIONS

General

Hypoglycemia—All sulfonylurea drugs are capable of producing severe hypoglycemia. Proper patient selection and dosage and instructions are important to avoid hypoglycemic episodes. Renal or hepatic insufficiency may cause elevated blood levels of tolbutamide and the latter may also diminish gluconeogenic capacity, both of which increase the risk of serious hypoglycemic reactions. Elderly, debilitated or malnourished patients and those with adrenal or pituitary insufficiency are particularly susceptible to the hypoglycemic action of glucose lowering drugs. Hypoglycemia may be difficult to recognize in the elderly and people who are taking beta-adrenergic blocking drugs. Hypoglycemia is more likely to occur when caloric intake is deficient, after severe or prolonged exercise, when alcohol is ingested, or when more than one glucose lowering drug is used.

Loss of Control of Blood Glucose—When a patient stabilized on any diabetic regimen is exposed to stress such as fever, trauma, infection, or surgery, loss of blood glucose control may occur. At such times it may be necessary to discontinue ORINASE and administer insulin.

The effectiveness of any hypoglycemic drug, including ORINASE, in lowering blood glucose to a desired level decreases in patients over a period of time, which may be due to progression of the severity of the diabetes or to diminished responsiveness to the drug. This phenomenon is known as secondary drug failure to distinguish it from primary failure in which the drug is ineffective in an individual patient when first given. Adequate adjustment of dose and adherence to diet should be assessed before classifying a patient as a secondary failure.

Information for Patients

Patients should be informed of the potential risks and advantages of ORINASE Tablets (tolbutamide) and of alternative modes of therapy. They should also be informed about the importance of adherence to dietary instructions, of a regular exercise program, and of regular testing of urine and/or blood glucose.

The risks of hypoglycemia, its symptoms and treatment, and conditions that predispose to its development should be explained to patients and responsible family members. Primary and secondary failure should also be explained.

Laboratory Tests

Blood and urine glucose should be monitored periodically. Measurement of glycosylated hemoglobin may be useful in some patients.

A metabolite of tolbutamide in urine may give a false positive reaction for albumin if measured by the acidification-after-boiling test, which causes the metabolite to precipitate. There is no interference with the sulfosalicylic acid test.

Drug Interactions

The hypoglycemic action of sulfonylureas may be potentiated by certain drugs including nonsteroidal anti-inflammatory agents and other drugs that are highly protein bound, salicylates, sulfonamides, chloramphenicol, probenecid, coumarins, monoamine oxidase inhibitors, and beta adrenergic blocking agents. When such drugs are administered to a patient receiving ORINASE, the patient should be closely observed for hypoglycemia. When such drugs are withdrawn from a patient receiving ORINASE, the patient should be observed closely for loss of control.

Certain drugs tend to produce hyperglycemia and may lead to loss of control. These drugs include the thiazides and other diuretics, corticosteroids, phenothiazines, thyroid products, estrogens, oral contraceptives, phenytoin, nicotinic acid, sympathomimetics, calcium channel blocking drugs and isoniazid. When such drugs are administered to a patient receiving ORINASE, the patient should be closely observed for loss of control of blood glucose. When such drugs are withdrawn from a patient receiving ORINASE, the patient should be observed closely for hypoglycemia.

A potential interaction between oral miconazole and oral hypoglycemic agents leading to severe hypoglycemia has been reported. Whether this interaction also occurs with the intravenous, topical or vaginal preparations of miconazole is not known.

Carcinogenesis and Mutagenicity

Bioassay for carcinogenicity was performed in both sexes of rats and mice following ingestion of tolbutamide for 78 weeks. No evidence of carcinogenicity was found.

Tolbutamide has also been demonstrated to be nonmutagenic in the Ames salmonella/mammalian microsome mutagenicity test.

Pregnancy

Teratogenic Effects

Pregnancy Category C. ORINASE has been shown to be teratogenic in rats given in doses 25 to 100 times the human dose. In some studies, pregnant rats given high doses of tolbutamide have shown increased mortality in offspring and ocular and bony abnormalities. Repeat studies in other species (rabbits) have not demonstrated a teratogenic effect. There are no adequate and well controlled studies in pregnant women. ORINASE is not recommended for the treatment of pregnant diabetic patients. Serious consideration should also be given to the possible hazards of the use of ORINASE in women of child-bearing age and in those who might become pregnant while using the drug.

Because recent information suggests that abnormal blood glucose levels during pregnancy are associated with a higher incidence of congenital abnormalities, many experts recommend that insulin be used during pregnancy to maintain blood glucose levels as close to normal as possible.

Nonteratogenic Effects

Prolonged severe hypoglycemia (four to ten days) has been reported in neonates born to mothers who were receiving a sulfonylurea drug at the time of delivery. This has been reported more frequently with the use of agents with prolonged half lives. if ORINASE is used during pregnancy, it should be discontinued at least two weeks before the expected delivery date.

Nursing Mothers

Although it is not known whether tolbutamide is excreted in human milk, some sulfonylurea drugs are known to be excreted in human milk. Because the potential for hypoglycemia in nursing infants may exist, a decision should be made whether to discontinue nursing or to discontinue the drug, taking into account the importance of the drug to the mother. If the drug is discontinued and if diet alone is inadequate for controlling blood glucose, insulin therapy should be considered.

Pediatric Use

Safety and effectiveness in children have not been established.

ADVERSE REACTIONS

Hypoglycemia—See **Precautions** and **Overdosage** sections.

Gastrointestinal Reactions: Cholestatic jaundice may occur rarely; ORINASE Tablets (tolbutamide) should be discontinued if this occurs. Gastrointestinal disturbances, eg, nausea, epigastric fullness, and heartburn, are the most common reactions and occurred in 1.4% of patients treated during clinical trials. They tend to be dose-related and may disappear when dosage is reduced.

Dermatologic Reactions: Allergic skin reactions, eg, pruritus, erythema, urticaria, and morbilliform or maculopapular eruptions, occurred in 1.1% of patients treated during clinical trials. These may be transient and may disappear despite continued use of ORINASE; if skin reactions persist, the drug should be discontinued.

Porphyria cutanea tarda and photosensitivity reactions have been reported with sulfonylureas.

Hematologic Reactions: Leukopenia, agranulocytosis, thrombocytopenia, hemolytic anemia, aplastic anemia, and pancytopenia have been reported with sulfonylureas.

Metabolic Reactions: Hepatic porphyria and disulfiram-like reactions have been reported with sulfonylureas.

Endocrine Reactions: Cases of hyponatremia and the syndrome of inappropriate antidiuretic hormone (SIADH) secretion have been reported with this and other sulfonylureas.

Miscellaneous Reactions: Headache and taste alterations have occasionally been reported with tolbutamide administration.

OVERDOSAGE

Overdosage of sulfonylureas, including ORINASE Tablets, can produce symptoms of hypoglycemia.

Mild hypoglycemic symptoms without loss of consciousness or neurologic findings should be treated aggressively with oral glucose and adjustments in drug dosage and/or meal patterns. Close monitoring should continue until the physician is assured the patient is out of danger. Severe hypoglycemic reactions with coma, seizure, or other neurological impairment occur infrequently but constitute medical emergencies requiring immediate hospitalization. If hypoglycemic coma is suspected or diagnosed, the patient should be given a rapid intravenous injection of concentrated (50%) glucose solution. This should be followed by a continuous infusion of a more dilute (10%) glucose solution at a rate which will maintain the blood glucose level above 100 mg/dl. Patients should be closely monitored for a minimum of 24 to 48 hours, since hypoglycemia may recur after apparent clinical recovery.

DOSAGE AND ADMINISTRATION

There is no fixed dosage regimen for the management of diabetes mellitus with ORINASE Tablets (tolbutamide) or any other hypoglycemic agent. In addition to the usual monitoring of urinary glucose, the patient's blood glucose must also be monitored periodically to determine the minimum effective dose for the patient; to detect primary failure, ie, inadequate lowering of blood glucose at the maximum recommended dose of medication; and to detect secondary failure, ie, loss of adequate blood glucose response after an initial period of effectiveness. Glycosylated hemoglobin levels may also be of value in monitoring the patient's response to therapy.

Short-term administration of ORINASE may be sufficient during periods of transient loss of control in patients usually controlled well on diet.

Usual Starting Dose

The usual starting dose is 1 to 2 grams daily. This may be increased or decreased depending on individual patient response. Failure to follow an appropriate dosage regimen may precipitate hyoglycemia. Patients who do not adhere to their prescribed dietary regimens are more prone to exhibit unsatisfactory response to drug therapy.

Transfer From Other Hypoglycemic Therapy

Patients Receiving Other Oral Antidiabetic Therapy—Transfer of patients from other oral antidiabetes regimens to ORINASE should be done conservatively. When transferring patients from oral hypoglycemic agents other than chlorpropamide to ORINASE, no transition period and no initial or priming doses are necessary. When transferring patients from chlorpropamide, however, particular care should be exercised during the first two weeks because of the prolonged retention of chlorpropamide in the body and the possibility that subsequent overlapping drug effects might provoke hypoglycemia.

Patients Receiving Insulin—Patients requiring 20 units or less of insulin daily may be placed directly on ORINASE and insulin abruptly discontinued. Patients whose insulin requirement is between 20 and 40 units daily may be started on therapy with ORINASE with a concurrent 30 to 50% reduction in insulin dose, with further daily reduction of the insulin when response to tolbutamide is observed. In patients requiring more than 40 units of insulin daily, therapy with ORINASE may be initiated in conjunction with a 20% reduction in insulin dose the first day, with further careful reduction of insulin as response is observed. Occasionally, conversion to ORINASE in the hospital may be advisable in candidates who require more than 40 units of insulin daily. During this conversion period when both insulin and ORINASE are being used, hypoglycemia may rarely occur. During insulin withdrawal, patients should test their urine for glucose and acetone at least three times daily and report results to their physician. The appearance of persistent acetonuria with glycosuria indicates that the patient is a type 1 diabetic patient who requires insulin therapy.

Maximum Dose

Daily doses of greater than 3 grams are not recommended.

Usual Maintenance Dose

The maintenance dose is in the range of 0.25 - 3 grams daily. Maintenance doses above 2 grams are seldom required.

Dosage Interval

The total daily dose may be taken either in the morning or in divided doses through the day. While either schedule is usually effective, the divided dose system is preferred by some clinicians from the standpoint of digestive tolerance.

In elderly, debilitated or malnourished patients and patients with impaired renal or hepatic function, the initial and maintenance dosing should be conservative to avoid hypoglycemic reactions (see **Precautions** section).

HOW SUPPLIED

ORINASE Tablets (tolbutamide) are available in the following strengths and package sizes:

Continued on next page

Information on these Upjohn products is based on labeling in effect September 1, 1989. Further information concerning these and other Upjohn products may be obtained by direct inquiry to Medical Information, The Upjohn Company, Kalamazoo, Michigan 49001.

Upjohn—Cont.

250 mg (scored, round, white)
Unit-of-Use bottles of 100   NDC 0009-0701-01
500 mg (scored, round, white)
Bottles of 200   NDC 0009-0100-02
Bottles of 500   NDC 0009-0100-03
Bottles of 1000   NDC 0009-0100-05
Unit-of-Use bottles of 50   NDC 0009-0100-11
Unit-of-Use bottles of 100   NDC 0009-0100-11
Unit-Dose package of 100   NDC 0009-0100-06
Store at controlled room temperature 15–30°C (59–86°F).
Code 811 646 008
Shown in Product Identification Section, page 434

PAMINE® ℞
brand of methscopolamine bromide tablets, USP

HOW SUPPLIED
Each tablet contains 2.5 mg methscopolamine bromide.
   Bottles of 100   NDC 0009-0061-01

PROSTIN VR PEDIATRIC® ℞
brand of alprostadil sterile solution
(alprostadil injection, USP)
500 micrograms per ml

WARNING
Apnea is experienced by about 10 to 12% of neonates with congenital heart defects treated with PROSTIN VR PEDIATRIC Sterile Solution (alprostadil). Apnea is most often seen in neonates weighing less than 2 kg at birth and usually appears during the first hour of drug infusion. Therefore, respiratory status should be monitored throughout treatment, and PROSTIN VR PEDIATRIC should be used where ventilatory assistance is immediately available.

DESCRIPTION
PROSTIN VR PEDIATRIC Sterile Solution for intravascular infusion contains 500 micrograms alprostadil, more commonly known as prostaglandin E₁, in 1.0 ml dehydrated alcohol.
The chemical name for alprostadil is (11α, 13E, 15S)-11,15 dihydroxy-9-oxoprost-13-en-1-oic acid, and the molecular weight is 354.49.
Alprostadil is a white to off-white crystalline powder with a melting point between 110° and 116°C. Its solubility at 35°C is 8000 micrograms per 100 ml double distilled water.

CLINICAL PHARMACOLOGY
Alprostadil (prostaglandin E₁) is one of a family of naturally occurring acidic lipids with various pharmacologic effects. Vasodilation, inhibition of platelet aggregation, and stimulation of intestinal and uterine smooth muscle are among the most notable of these effects. Intravenous doses of 1 to 10 micrograms of alprostadil per kilogram of body weight lower the blood pressure in mammals by decreasing peripheral resistance. Reflex increases in cardiac output and rate accompany the reduction in blood pressure.
Smooth muscle of the ductus arteriosus is especially sensitive to alprostadil, and strips of lamb ductus markedly relax in the presence of the drug. In addition, administration of alprostadil reopened the closing ductus of newborn rats, rabbits, and lambs. These observations led to the investigation of alprostadil in infants who had congenital defects which restricted the pulmonary or systemic blood flow and who depended on a patent ductus arteriosus for adequate blood oxygenation and lower body perfusion.
In infants with restricted pulmonary blood flow, about 50% responded to alprostadil infusion with at least a 10 torr increase in blood pO₂ (mean increase about 14 torr and mean increase in oxygen saturation about 23%). In general, patients who responded best had low pretreatment blood pO₂ and were 4 days old or less.
In infants with restricted systemic blood flow, alprostadil often increased pH in those having acidosis, increased systemic blood pressure, and decreased the ratio of pulmonary artery pressure to aortic pressure.
Alprostadil must be infused continuously because it is very rapidly metabolized. As much as 80% of the circulating alprostadil may be metabolized in one pass through the lungs, primarily by β- and w-oxidation. The metabolites are excreted primarily by the kidney, and excretion is essentially complete within 24 hours after administration. No unchanged alprostadil has been found in the urine, and there is no evidence of tissue retention of alprostadil or its metabolites.

INDICATIONS AND USAGE
PROSTIN VR PEDIATRIC Sterile Solution (alprostadil) is indicated for palliative, not definitive, therapy to temporarily maintain the patency of the ductus arteriosus until corrective or palliative surgery can be performed in neonates who have congenital heart defects and who depend upon the patent ductus for survival. Such congenital heart defects include pulmonary atresia, pulmonary stenosis, tricuspid atresia, tetralogy of Fallot, interruption of the aortic arch, coarctation of the aorta, or transposition of the great vessels with or without other defects.
In infants with restricted pulmonary blood flow, the increase in blood oxygenation is inversely proportional to pretreatment pO₂ values; that is, patients with low pO₂ values respond best, and patients with pO₂ values of 40 torr or more usually have little response.
PROSTIN VR PEDIATRIC should be administered only by trained personnel in facilities that provide pediatric intensive care.

CONTRAINDICATIONS
None.

WARNINGS
See WARNING box.
Note: PROSTIN VR PEDIATRIC Sterile Solution (alprostadil) must be diluted before it is administered. See dilution instructions in DOSAGE AND ADMINISTRATION section.

PRECAUTIONS
General Precautions
Cortical proliferation of the long bones, first observed in dogs, has also been observed in infants during long-term infusions of alprostadil. The cortical proliferation in infants regressed after withdrawal of the drug.
PROSTIN VR PEDIATRIC Sterile Solution (alprostadil) should be infused for the shortest time and at the lowest dose that will produce the desired effects. The risks of long-term infusion of PROSTIN VR PEDIATRIC should be weighed against the possible benefits that critically ill infants may derive from its administration.
Because alprostadil inhibits platelet aggregation, use PROSTIN VR PEDIATRIC cautiously in neonates with bleeding tendencies.
PROSTIN VR PEDIATRIC should not be used in neonates with respiratory distress syndrome. A differential diagnosis should be made between respiratory distress syndrome (hyaline membrane disease) and cyanotic heart disease (restricted pulmonary blood flow). If full diagnostic facilities are not immediately available, cyanosis (pO₂ less than 40 torr) and restricted pulmonary blood flow apparent on an X-ray are appropriate indicators of congenital defects.
Necessary Monitoring: In all neonates, arterial pressure should be monitored intermittently by umbilical artery catheter, auscultation, or with a Doppler transducer. *Should arterial pressure fall significantly, decrease the rate of infusion immediately.*
In infants with restricted pulmonary blood flow, measure efficacy of PROSTIN VR PEDIATRIC by monitoring improvement in blood oxygenation. In infants with restricted systemic blood flow, measure efficacy by monitoring improvement of systemic blood pressure and blood pH.
Drug Interactions: No drug interactions have been reported between PROSTIN VR PEDIATRIC and the therapy standard in neonates with restricted pulmonary or systemic blood flow. Standard therapy includes antibiotics, such as penicillin and gentamicin; vasopressors, such as dopamine and isoproterenol; cardiac glycosides; and diuretics, such as furosemide.
Carcinogenesis, Mutagenesis, and Impairment of Fertility: Long-term carcinogenicity studies and fertility studies have not been done. The Ames and Alkaline Elution assays reveal no potential for mutagenesis.

ADVERSE REACTIONS
Central Nervous System: Apnea has been reported in about 12% of the neonates treated. (See WARNING box.) Other common adverse reactions reported have been fever in about 14% of the patients treated and seizures in about 4%. The following reactions have been reported in less than 1% of the patients: cerebral bleeding, hyperextension of the neck, hyperirritability, hypothermia, jitteriness, lethargy, and stiffness.
Cardiovascular System: The most common adverse reactions reported have been flushing in about 10% of patients (more common after intraarterial dosing), bradycardia in about 7%, hypotension in about 4%, tachycardia in about 3%, cardiac arrest in about 1%, and edema in about 1%. The following reactions have been reported in less than 1% of the patients: congestive heart failure, hyperemia, second degree heart block, shock, spasm of the right ventricle infundibulum, supraventricular tachycardia, and ventricular fibrillation.
Respiratory System: The following reactions have been reported in less than 1% of the patients: bradypnea, bronchial wheezing, hypercapnia, respiratory depression, respiratory distress, and tachypnea.

Gastrointestinal System: The most common adverse reaction reported has been diarrhea in about 2% of the patients. The following reactions have been reported in less than 1% of the patients; gastric regurgitation, and hyperbilirubinemia.
Hematologic System: The most common hematologic event reported has been disseminated intravascular coagulation in about 1% of the patients. The following events have been reported in less than 1% of the patients: anemia, bleeding, and thrombocytopenia.
Excretory System: Anuria and hematuria have been reported in less than 1% of the patients.
Skeletal System: Cortical proliferation of the long bones has been reported. See PRECAUTIONS.
Miscellaneous: Sepsis has been reported in about 2% of the patients. Peritonitis has been reported in less than 1% of the patients. Hypokalemia has been reported in about 1%, and hypoglycemia and hyperkalemia have been reported in less than 1% of the patients.

OVERDOSAGE
Apnea, bradycardia, pyrexia, hypotension, and flushing may be signs of drug overdosage. If apnea or bradycardia occurs, discontinue the infusion, and provide appropriate medical treatment. Caution should be used in restarting the infusion. If pyrexia or hypotension occurs, reduce the infusion rate until these symptoms subside. Flushing is usually a result of incorrect intraarterial catheter placement, and the catheter should be repositioned.

DOSAGE AND ADMINISTRATION
The preferred route of administration for PROSTIN VR PEDIATRIC Sterile Solution (alprostadil) is continuous intravenous infusion into a large vein. Alternatively, PROSTIN VR PEDIATRIC may be administered through an umbilical artery catheter placed at the ductal opening. Increases in blood pO₂ (torr) have been the same in neonates who received the drug by either route of administration.
Begin infusion with 0.05 to 0.1 micrograms alprostadil per kilogram of body weight per minute. A starting dose of 0.1 micrograms per kilogram of body weight per minute is the recommended starting dose based on clinical studies; however, adequate clinical response has been reported using a starting dose of 0.05 micrograms per kilogram of body weight per minute. After a therapeutic response is achieved (increased pO₂ in infants with restricted pulmonary blood flow or increased systemic blood pressure and blood pH in infants with restricted systemic blood flow), reduce the infusion rate to provide the lowest possible dosage that maintains the response. This may be accomplished by reducing the dosage from 0.1 to 0.05 to 0.025 to 0.01 micrograms per kilogram of body weight per minute. If response to 0.05 micrograms per kilogram of body weight per minute is inadequate, dosage can be increased up to 0.4 micrograms per kilogram of body weight per minute although, in general, higher infusion rates do not produce greater effects.
Dilution instructions: To prepare infusion solutions, dilute 1 ml of PROSTIN VR PEDIATRIC Sterile Solution with Sodium Chloride Injection USP or Dextrose Injection USP. Dilute to volumes appropriate for the pump delivery system available. Prepare fresh infusion solutions every 24 hours. *Discard any solution more than 24 hours old.*

Sample Dilutions and Infusion Rates to
Provide a Dosage of 0.1 Micrograms per
Kilogram of Body Weight per Minute

Add 1 ampoule (500 micrograms) alprostadil to:	Approximate concentration of resulting solution (micrograms/ml)	Infusion rate (ml/min per kg of body weight)
250 ml	2	0.05
100 ml	5	0.02
50 ml	10	0.01
25 ml	20	0.005

Example: To provide 0.1 micrograms/kilogram of body weight per minute to an infant weighing 2.8 kilograms using a solution of 1 ampoule PROSTIN VR PEDIATRIC in 100 ml of saline or dextrose: INFUSION RATE = 0.02 ml/min per kg × 2.8 kg = 0.056 ml/min or 3.36 ml/hr.

HOW SUPPLIED
PROSTIN VR PEDIATRIC Sterile Solution (alprostadil) is available in packages of 5—1 ml ampoules (NDC 0009-3169-01). Each ml contains 500 micrograms alprostadil in dehydrated alcohol.
Store PROSTIN VR PEDIATRIC Sterile Solution in a refrigerator at 2°–8°C (36°–46°F).
Code 811 987 003

PROVERA®   ℞

brand of medroxyprogesterone acetate tablets, USP

2.5 mg, 25's
NSN 6505-01-184-1249 (M)
10 mg, Dosepak of 10, Box of 10
NSN 6505-01-071-5605 (M)
10 mg, 100's
NSN 6505-00-890-1355 (M & VA)

WARNING:

THE USE OF PROGESTATIONAL AGENTS DURING THE FIRST FOUR MONTHS OF PREGNANCY IS NOT RECOMMENDED

Progestational agents have been used beginning with the first trimester of pregnancy in an attempt to prevent habitual abortion or treat threatened abortion. There is no adequate evidence that such use is effective and there is evidence of potential harm to the fetus when such drugs are given during the first four months of pregnancy. Furthermore, in the vast majority of women, the cause of abortion is a defective ovum, which progestational agents could not be expected to influence. In addition, the use of progestational agents with their uterine-relaxant properties, in patients with fertilized defective ova may cause a delay in spontaneous abortion. Therefore, the use of such drugs during the first four months of pregnancy is not recommended. Several reports suggest an association between intrauterine exposure to female sex hormones and congenital anomalies, including congenital heart defects and limb reduction defects[1-5]. One study[4] estimated a 4.7-fold increased risk of limb reduction defects in infants exposed in utero to sex hormones (oral contraceptives, hormone withdrawal tests for pregnancy, or attempted treatment for threatened abortion). Some of these exposures were very short and involved only a few days of treatment. The data suggest that the risk of limb reduction defects in exposed fetuses is somewhat less than 1 in 1,000.

If the patient is exposed to PROVERA Tablets (medroxyprogesterone acetate) during the first four months of pregnancy or if she becomes pregnant while taking this drug, she should be apprised of the potential risks to the fetus.

DESCRIPTION

PROVERA Tablets contain medroxyprogesterone acetate, which is a derivative of progesterone. It is a white to off-white, odorless crystalline powder, stable in air, melting between 200 and 210° C. It is freely soluble in chloroform, soluble in acetone and in dioxane, sparingly soluble in alcohol and in methanol, slightly soluble in ether, and insoluble in water.

The chemical name for medroxyprogesterone acetate is Pregn-4-ene-3,20-dione, 17-(acetyloxy)-6-methyl-, (6α)-.

Each PROVERA tablet for oral administration contains 2.5 mg, 5 mg or 10 mg of medroxyprogesterone acetate. Inactive ingredients: calcium stearate, corn starch, lactose, mineral oil, sorbic acid, sucrose, talc. The 2.5 mg tablet contains FD&C Yellow no. 6.

ACTIONS

Medroxyprogesterone acetate, administered orally or parenterally in the recommended doses to women with adequate endogenous estrogen, transforms proliferative into secretory endometrium. Androgenic and anabolic effects have been noted, but the drug is apparently devoid of significant estrogenic activity. While parenterally administered medroxyprogesterone acetate inhibits gonadotropin production, which in turn prevents follicular maturation and ovulation, available data indicate that this does not occur when the usually recommended oral dosage is given as single daily doses.

INDICATIONS AND USAGE

Secondary amenorrhea; abnormal uterine bleeding due to hormonal imbalance in the absence of organic pathology, such as fibroids or uterine cancer.

CONTRAINDICATIONS

1. Thrombophlebitis, thromboembolic disorders, cerebral apoplexy or patients with a past history of these conditions.
2. Liver dysfunction or disease.
3. Known or suspected malignancy of breast or genital organs.
4. Undiagnosed vaginal bleeding.
5. Missed abortion.
6. As a diagnostic test for pregnancy.
7. Known sensitivity to PROVERA Tablets (medroxyprogesterone acetate).

WARNINGS

1. The physician should be alert to the earliest manifestations of thrombotic disorders (thrombophlebitis, cerebrovascular disorders, pulmonary embolism, and retinal thrombosis). Should any of these occur or be suspected, the drug should be discontinued immediately.

2. Beagle dogs treated with medroxyprogesterone acetate developed mammary nodules some of which were malignant. Although nodules occasionally appeared in control animals, they were intermittent in nature, whereas the nodules in the drug-treated animals were larger, more numerous, persistent, and there were some breast malignancies with metastases. Their significance with respect to humans has not been established.

3. Discontinue medication pending examination if there is sudden partial or complete loss of vision, or if there is a sudden onset of proptosis, diplopia or migraine. If examination reveals papilledema or retinal vascular lesions, medication should be withdrawn.

4. Detectable amounts of progestin have been identified in the milk of mothers receiving the drug. The effect of this on the nursing infant has not been determined.

5. Usage in pregnancy is not recommended (See WARNING Box).

6. Retrospective studies of morbidity and mortality in Great Britain and studies of morbidity in the United States have shown a statistically significant association between thrombophlebitis, pulmonary embolism, and cerebral thrombosis and embolism and the use of oral contraceptives.[6-9] The estimate of the relative risk of thromboembolism in the study by Vessey and Doll[8] was about sevenfold, while Sartwell and associates[9] in the United States found a relative risk of 4.4, meaning that the users are several times as likely to undergo thromboembolic disease without evident cause as nonusers. The American study also indicated that the risk did not persist after discontinuation of administration, and that it was not enhanced by long continued administration. The American study was not designed to evaluate a difference between products.

PRECAUTIONS

1. The pretreatment physical examination should include special reference to breast and pelvic organs, as well as Papanicolaou smear.

2. Because progestogens may cause some degree of fluid retention, conditions which might be influenced by this factor, such as epilepsy, migraine, asthma, cardiac or renal dysfunction, require careful observation.

3. In cases of breakthrough bleeding, as in all cases of irregular bleeding per vaginum, nonfunctional causes should be borne in mind. In cases of undiagnosed vaginal bleeding, adequate diagnostic measures are indicated.

4. Patients who have a history of psychic depression should be carefully observed and the drug discontinued if the depression recurs to a serious degree.

5. Any possible influence of prolonged progestin therapy on pituitary, ovarian, adrenal, hepatic or uterine functions awaits further study.

6. A decrease in glucose tolerance has been observed in a small percentage of patients on estrogen-progestin combination drugs. The mechanism of this decrease is obscure. For this reason, diabetic patients should be carefully observed while receiving progestin therapy.

7. The age of the patient constitutes no absolute limiting factor although treatment with progestins may mask the onset of the climacteric.

8. The pathologist should be advised of progestin therapy when relevant specimens are submitted.

9. Because of the occasional occurrence of thrombotic disorders, (thrombophlebitis, pulmonary embolism, retinal thrombosis, and cerebrovascular disorders) in patients taking estrogen-progestin combinations and since the mechanism is obscure, the physician should be alert to the earliest manifestation of these disorders.

Information for the Patient

See Patient Information at the end of insert.

ADVERSE REACTIONS

Pregnancy—(See WARNING Box for possible adverse effects on the fetus)

Breast—Breast tenderness or galactorrhea has been reported rarely.

Skin—Sensitivity reactions consisting of urticaria, pruritus, edema and generalized rash have occurred in an occasional patient. Acne, alopecia and hirsutism have been reported in a few cases.

Thromboembolic Phenomena—Thromboembolic phenomena including thrombophlebitis and pulmonary embolism have been reported.

The following adverse reactions have been observed in women taking progestins including PROVERA Tablets (medroxyprogesterone acetate):

  breakthrough bleeding
  spotting
  change in menstrual flow
  amenorrhea
  edema
  change in weight
   (increase or decrease)
  changes in cervical erosion
   and cervical secretions

  cholestatic jaundice
  anaphylactoid reactions and
   anaphylaxis
  rash (allergic) with and
   without pruritus
  mental depression
  pyrexia
  insomnia
  nausea
  somnolence

A statistically significant association has been demonstrated between use of estrogen-progestin combination drugs and the following serious adverse reactions: thrombophlebitis; pulmonary embolism and cerebral thrombosis and embolism. For this reason patients on progestin therapy should be carefully observed.

Although available evidence is suggestive of an association, such a relationship has been neither confirmed nor refuted for the following serious adverse reactions:

  neuro-ocular lesions, eg, retinal thrombosis and optic neuritis.

The following adverse reactions have been observed in patients receiving estrogen-progestin combination drugs:

  rise in blood pressure in susceptible individuals
  premenstrual-like syndrome
  changes in libido
  changes in appetite
  cystitis-like syndrome
  headache
  nervousness
  dizziness
  fatigue
  backache
  hirsutism
  loss of scalp hair
  erythema multiforme
  erythema nodosum
  hemorrhagic eruption
  itching

In view of these observations, patients on progestin therapy should be carefully observed.

The following laboratory results may be altered by the use of estrogen-progestin combination drugs:

Increased sulfobromophthalein retention and other hepatic function tests.

Coagulation tests: increase in prothrombin factors VII, VIII, IX and X.

Metyrapone test.

Pregnanediol determination.

Thyroid function: increase in PBI, and butanol extractable protein bound iodine and decrease in T[3] uptake values.

DOSAGE AND ADMINISTRATION

Secondary Amenorrhea—PROVERA Tablets (medroxyprogesterone acetate) may be given in dosages of 5 to 10 mg daily for from 5 to 10 days. A dose for inducing an optimum secretory transformation of an endometrium that has been adequately primed with either endogenous or exogenous estrogen is 10 mg of PROVERA Tablets daily for 10 days. In cases of secondary amenorrhea, therapy may be started at any time. Progestin withdrawal bleeding usually occurs within three to seven days after discontinuing therapy with PROVERA.

Abnormal Uterine Bleeding Due to Hormonal Imbalance in the Absence of Organic Pathology—Beginning on the calculated 16th or 21st day of the menstrual cycle, 5 to 10 mg of PROVERA Tablets may be given daily for from 5 to 10 days. To produce an optimum secretory transformation of an endometrium that has been adequately primed with either endogenous or exogenous estrogen, 10 mg of PROVERA Tablets daily for 10 days beginning on the 16th day of the cycle is suggested. Progestin withdrawal bleeding usually occurs within three to seven days after discontinuing therapy with PROVERA. Patients with a past history of recurrent episodes of abnormal uterine bleeding may benefit from planned menstrual cycling with PROVERA.

HOW SUPPLIED

PROVERA Tablets are available in the following strengths and package sizes:

2.5 mg (scored, round, orange)

Bottles of 25	NDC 0009-0064-01
Bottles of 30	NDC 0009-0064-06
Bottles of 100	NDC 0009-0064-04

5 mg (scored, hexagonal, white)

Bottles of 25	NDC 0009-0286-02
Bottles of 30	NDC 0009-0286-32
Bottles of 100	NDC 0009-0286-03

Continued on next page

Information on these Upjohn products is based on labeling in effect September 1, 1989. Further information concerning these and other Upjohn products may be obtained by direct inquiry to Medical Information, The Upjohn Company, Kalamazoo, Michigan 49001.

Upjohn—Cont.

10 mg (scored, round, white)

Bottles of 25	NDC 0009-0050-01
Bottles of 30	NDC 0009-0050-09
Bottles of 100	NDC 0009-0050-02
Bottles of 500	NDC 0009-0050-11
DOSEPAK™ Unit of Use (10)	NDC 0009-0050-12

Store at controlled room temperature 15°–30°C (59°–86°F).

REFERENCES

1. Gal I, Kirman B, Stern J: Hormonal pregnancy tests and congenital malformation. Nature 216:83, 1967.
2. Levy EP, Cohen A, Fraser FC: Hormone treatment during pregnancy and congenital heart defects. Lancet 1:611, 1973.
3. Nora JJ, Nora AH: Birth defects and oral contraceptives. Lancet 1:941–942, 1973.
4. Janerich DT, Piper JM, Glebatis DM: Oral contraceptives and congenital limb-reduction defects. N Engl J Med 291:697–700, 1974.
5. Heinonen OP, Slone D, Monson RR, et al: Cardiovascular birth defects and antenatal exposure to female sex hormones. N Engl J Med 296:67–70, 1977.
6. Royal College of General Practitioners: Oral contraception and thromboembolic disease. J Coll Gen Pract 13:267–279, 1967.
7. Inman WHW, Vessey MP: Investigation of deaths from pulmonary, coronary, and cerebral thrombosis and embolism in women of child-bearing age. Br Med J 2:193–199, 1968.
8. Vessey MP, Doll R: Investigation of relation between use of oral contraceptives and thromboembolic disease. A further report. Br Med J 2:651–657, 1969.
9. Sartwell PE, Masi AT, Arthes FG, et al: Thromboembolism and oral contraceptives: An epidemiological case-control study. Am J Epidemiol 90:365–380, 1969.

The text of the patient insert for progesterone and progesterone-like drugs is set forth below.

Patient Information: PROVERA Tablets contain medroxyprogesterone acetate, a progesterone. The information below is that which the U.S. Food and Drug Administration requires be provided for all patients taking progesterones. The information below relates only to the risk to the unborn child associated with use of progesterone during pregnancy. For further information on the use, side effects and other risks associated with this product, ask your doctor.

WARNING FOR WOMEN

There is an increased risk of birth defects in children whose mothers take this drug during the first four months of pregnancy.

Medroxyprogesterone acetate is similar to the progesterone hormones naturally produced by the body. Progesterone and progesterone-like drugs are used to treat menstrual disorders, to test if the body is producing certain hormones, and to treat some forms of cancer in women.

They have been used as a test for pregnancy but such use is no longer considered safe because of possible damage to a developing baby. Also, more rapid methods for testing for pregnancy are now available.

These drugs have also been used to prevent miscarriage in the first few months of pregnancy. No adequate evidence is available to show that they are effective for this purpose. Furthermore, most cases of early miscarriage are due to causes which could not be helped by these drugs.

There is an increased risk of birth defects, such as heart or limb defects if progesterone and progesterone-like drugs are taken during the first four months of pregnancy. The exact risk of taking this drug early in pregnancy and having a baby with a birth defect is not known. However, one study found that babies born to women who had taken sex hormones (such as progesterone-like drugs) during the first three months of pregnancy were 4 to 5 times more likely to have abnormalities of the arms or legs than if their mothers had not taken such drugs. Some of these women had taken these drugs for only a few days. The chance that an infant whose mother had taken this drug will have this type of defect is about 1 in 1,000.

If you take PROVERA Tablets and later find you were pregnant when you took it, be sure to discuss this with your doctor as soon as possible.
Code 812 584 206

Shown in Product Identification Section, page 434

PYRROXATE® Capsules

(See PDR For Nonprescription Drugs)

ROGAINE®   ℞
brand of minoxidil topical solution
2%
For Topical Use

DESCRIPTION

ROGAINE Topical Solution is a hair growth stimulant. ROGAINE contains the active ingredient minoxidil. Minoxidil appears as a white or off-white, odorless crystalline solid that is soluble in water to the extent of approximately 2 mg/ml, is readily soluble in propylene glycol or ethanol, and is almost insoluble in acetone, choroform or ethyl acetate. The chemical name for minoxidil is 2,4-pyrimidinediamine, 6-(l-piperidinyl)-, 3-oxide (MW = 209.25). The structural formula is represented below:

ROGAINE Topical Solution is available at a concentration of 2% (20 mg minoxidil per milliliter) in a solution of alcohol 60% v/v, propylene glycol, and water.

CLINICAL PHARMACOLOGY

Pharmacologic Properties and Pharmacokinetics

ROGAINE Topical Solution stimulates vertex hair growth in individuals with male pattern baldness (alopecia androgenetica). No effect has been seen in patients with predominantly frontal hair loss. The mechanism by which minoxidil stimulates hair growth is not known but like minoxidil some other arterial dilating drugs also stimulate hair growth when given systemically.

Because of its serious side effects oral minoxidil is indicated only for the treatment of hypertension that is symptomatic or associated with target organ damage and is not manageable with maximum therapeutic doses of a diuretic plus two other antihypertensive drugs. It is a direct acting peripheral arterial dilator that reduces blood pressure by decreasing peripheral vascular resistance. Reduction of peripheral arteriolar resistance and the resulting fall in blood pressure trigger sympathetic, vagal inhibitory, and renal homeostatic mechanisms, including increased renin secretion, that lead to increased heart rate and cardiac output and salt and water retention.

The major side effects of oral minoxidil, aside from unwelcome generalized hair growth, result from fluid retention, often profound, and tachycardia, and require that minoxidil be administered in most cases with a beta-blocker or other agent to reduce heart rate and a diuretic, almost always a high ceiling (loop) diuretic. Fluid retention can lead to marked weight gain, local or generalized edema, heart failure, and pleural or pericardial effusion, including cardiac tamponade. Pericarditis has been reported, usually in patients with renal failure or collagen vascular disease, but in some cases these causes of pericarditis do not seem to have been present. The tachycardia and increased cardiac output caused by minoxidil can lead to exacerbation of existing angina or the onset of angina in persons with compromised coronary circulation. It is these serious side effects that have restricted use of oral minoxidil to patients with severe hypertension not controllable with other agents.

In placebo controlled trials involving over 3500 patients given topical minoxidil for 4 months (longer treatment was given after the placebo group was discontinued) the typical systemic effects of oral minoxidil (weight gain, edema, tachycardia, fall in blood pressure, and their more serious consequences) were not seen more frequently in patients given topical minoxidil than in those given topical placebo (See ADVERSE REACTIONS). The mean changes from baseline in weight, heart rate, and blood pressure in the treated and placebo groups were similar, and the number of patients experiencing significant changes, such as a blood pressure decrease of 15 mmHg or more diastolic or 30 mmHg or more systolic, a heart rate increase of 15 beats/minute or more, or weight gain of at least 5 pounds, was also similar.

In an effort to explore the potential for systemic effects of topical minoxidil, three concentrations of topical minoxidil (1, 2 and 5%) applied twice daily were compared to low oral doses (2.5 and 5 mg given once daily), and placebo in hypertensive patients (normotensive patients have little or no blood pressure response to minoxidil at dose of 10 mg per day) in a double-blind controlled trial. The 5 mg oral dose had readily detectable effects, a fall in diastolic pressure of about 5 mmHg and an increase in heart rate of 7 beats/minute. No other group had a clear effect, although there was some evi-

---

dence of a weak and inconsistent effect in the 2.5 mg oral, and possibly the 5% topical, treatments.

The failure to detect evidence of systemic effects during treatment with topical minoxidil reflects the poor absorption of topical minoxidil, which averages about 1.4% (range 0.3 to 4.5%) from normal intact scalp, and was about 2% in the hypertensive patients, whose scalps were shaved.

In a comparison of topical and oral absorption, peak serum levels of unchanged minoxidil after 1 ml b.i.d. of 2% minoxidil solution (the maximum recommended dose) averaged 5.8% (range 1.4% to 12.7%) of the level observed after 2.5 mg b.i.d. oral doses (5 mg is the recommended starting dose of oral minoxidil). Similarly, in the hypertension study, where patients had shaved scalps, mean minoxidil concentrations after 1 ml b.i.d. of 2% topical minoxidil (1.7 ng/ml) were 1/20 the concentrations seen after daily oral doses of 2.5 mg (32.8 ng/ml) or 5 mg (59.2 ng/ml). Blood levels obtained in the large controlled hair growth trials averaged less than 2 ng/ml for the 2% solution. There were, however, occasional values that were higher; about 1% of the patients on 2% minoxidil had serum levels of 5 ng/ml or greater and a few approached 30 ng/ml. It is possible, therefore, that if more than the recommended dose were applied to inflamed skin in an individual with relatively high absorption, blood levels with systemic effects might rarely be obtained. Physicians and patients need to be aware of the possibility.

Serum minoxidil levels resulting from administration of ROGAINE are governed by the drug's percutaneous absorption rate. Following cessation of topical dosing of ROGAINE approximately 95% of systemically absorbed minoxidil is eliminated within four days. The metabolic biotransformation of minoxidil absorbed following administration of ROGAINE has not been fully determined.

Minoxidil absorbed following oral administration is metabolized predominantly by conjugation with glucoronic acid at the N-oxide position in the pyrimidine ring but also by conversion to more polar products. Known metabolites exert much less pharmacologic effect than the parent compound. Minoxidil and its metabolites are excreted principally in the urine. Minoxidil does not bind to plasma proteins and its renal clearance corresponds to the glomerular filtration rate. Minoxidil does not enter the central nervous system (CNS) of experimental animals in significant amounts and it does not affect CNS function in man.

Cardiac Lesions in Animals

Minoxidil produces several cardiac lesions in animals. Some are characteristic of agents that cause tachycardia and diastolic hypotension (beta-agonists like isoproterenol, arterial dilators like hydralazine) while others are produced by a narrower range of agents with arterial dilating properties. The significance of these lesions for humans is not clear, as they have not been recognized in patients treated with oral minoxidil at systemically active doses, despite formal review of over 150 autopsies of treated patients.

(a) Papillary muscle/subendocardial necrosis

The most characteristic lesion of minoxidil, seen in rat, dog, and minipig (but not monkeys) is focal necrosis of the papilliary muscle and subendocardial areas of the left ventricle. These lesions appear rapidly, within a few days of treatment with doses of 0.5 to 10 mg/kg/day in the dog and minipig, and are not progressive, although they leave residual scars. They are similar to lesions produced by other peripheral arterial dilators, by theobromine, and by beta-adrenergic receptor agonists such as isoproterenol, epinephrine, and albuterol. The lesions are thought to reflect ischemia provoked by increased oxygen demand (tachycardia, increased cardiac output) and relative decrease in coronary flow (decreased diastolic pressure and decreased time in diastole) caused by the vasodilatory effects of these agents coupled with reflex or directly induced tachycardia.

(b) Hemorrhagic lesions

After acute oral minoxidil treatment (0.5 to 10 mg/kg/day) in dogs and minipigs, hemorrhagic lesions are seen in many parts of the heart, mainly in the epicardium, endocardium, and walls of small coronary arteries and arterioles. In minipigs the lesions occur primarily in the left atrium while in dogs they are most prominent in the right atrium, frequently appearing as grossly visible hemorrhagic lesions. With exposure of 1–20 mg/kg/day in the dog for 30 days or longer, there is replacement of myocardial cells by proliferating fibroblasts and angioblasts, hemorrhage and hemosiderin accumulation. These lesions can be produced by topical minoxidil administration that gives systemic absorption of 0.5 to 1 mg/kg/day. Other peripheral dilators, including an experimental agent, nicorandil, and theobromine, have produced similar lesions.

(c) Epicarditis

A less fully studied lesion is focal epicarditis, seen in dogs after 2 days of oral minoxidil. More recently, chronic proliferative epicarditis was observed in dogs treated topically twice a day for 90 days. In one year oral dog study, serosanguinous percardial fluid was seen.

(d) Hypertrophy and Dilation

Oral and topical studies in rats, dogs, monkeys (oral only), and rabbits (dermal only) show cardiac hypertrophy and dilation. This is presumed to represent the consequences of prolonged fluid overload; there is preliminary evidence in monkeys that diuretics partly reverse these effects.

Autopsies of over 150 patients who died of various causes after receiving oral minoxidil for hypertension have not revealed the characteristics hemorrhagic (especially atrial) lesions seen in dogs and minipigs. While areas of papillary muscle and subendocardial necrosis were occasionally seen, they occurred in the presence of known pre-existing coronary artery disease and were also seen in patients never exposed to minoxidil in another series using similar, but not identical, autopsy methods.

CLINICAL TRIAL EXPERIENCE

In clinical trials, three main parameters of efficacy were used: hair counts in a one inch diameter circle on the vertex of the scalp; investigator evaluation of terminal hair regrowth; and patient evaluation of hair regrowth. At the end of four-month placebo-controlled portions of 12-month clinical studies (ie, baseline to Month 4), ROGAINE Topical Solution (20 mg minoxidil per ml) demonstrated the following efficacy:

A. Hair Counts
ROGAINE was significantly more effective than placebo in producing hair regrowth as assessed by hair counts. Patients using ROGAINE had a mean increase from baseline of 72 non-vellus hairs in the one inch diameter circle compared with a mean increase of 39 non-vellus hairs in patients using the placebo (P <0.0005).

B. Investigator Evaluation
Based on the investigators' evaluation, there was no statistically significant difference in terminal hair regrowth between treatment groups. Eight percent (8%) of the patients using ROGAINE demonstrated moderate to dense terminal hair regrowth compared with 4% using the placebo. During the initial four months of treatment, however, very little regrowth of terminal hair can be expected. Although most patients did not demonstrate cosmetically significant regrowth of hair, 26% of the patients showed minimal terminal hair regrowth using ROGAINE compared with 16% of those using placebo as assessed by the investigator.

C. Patient Evaluation
Based on the patients' self-evaluation, 26% using ROGAINE demonstrated moderate to dense hair regrowth compared with 11% using the placebo (P <0.0005).
Patients who continued on ROGAINE during the remaining eight months of the 12-month clinical studies (ie, the non-placebo-controlled portion of the studies) continued to sustain a regrowth response as evaluated by hair counts, investigator evaluation, and patient evaluation.
At the end of the eight month non-placebo-controlled portion of the 12-month clinical studies (ie, Months 4 to 12), the following results were obtained.

A. Hair Count
Patients using ROGAINE had a mean increase of 112 non-vellus hairs in the same one inch diameter circle as compared to Month 4 (P <0.0005).

B. Investigator Evaluation
Based on the investigators' evaluation, 39% of the patients achieved moderate to dense terminal hair by Month 12.

C. Patient Evaluation
Based on the patients' assessment, 48% felt they had achieved moderate to dense hair regrowth at Month 12.

INDICATIONS AND USAGE
ROGAINE Topical Solution is indicated for the treatment of male pattern baldness (alopecia androgenetica) of the vertex of the scalp. No effect has been seen on frontal baldness. At least four months of continuous use is generally required before evidence of hair growth can be expected and further growth continues through one year of treatment. The new growth of hair is not permanent; cessation of treatment with ROGAINE will lead to its loss within a few months.

CONTRAINDICATIONS
ROGAINE Topical Solution is contraindicated in those patients with a history of hypersensitivity to any of the components of the preparation.

WARNINGS
1. Need for normal scalp
The majority of clinical studies included only healthy men with normal scalps and no cardiovascular disease. Before starting a patient on ROGAINE, the physician should ascertain that the patient has a healthy, normal scalp. Local abrasion or dermatitis may increase absorption and hence increase the risk of side effects.
2. Potential adverse effects
Although extensive use of topical minoxidil has not revealed evidence that enough minoxidil is absorbed to have systemic effects, greater absorption because of misuse or individual

variability or unusual sensitivity could lead, at least theoretically, to a systemic effect, and physicians and patients need to be aware of this.
Experience with oral minoxidil has shown the following major cardiovascular effects (the package insert for LONITEN®, minoxidil tablets, should be reviewed for details):
—salt and water retention, generalized and local edema
—pericardial effusion, pericarditis, tamponade
—tachycardia
—increased frequency of angina or new onset of angina
If systemic effects were to occur, patients with underlying heart disease, including coronary artery disease and congestive heart failure, would be at particular risk. Minoxidil could also have additive effects with other therapy in patients being treated for hypertension.
Patients being considered for ROGAINE Topical Solution should have a history and physical examination. Patients should be advised of the potential risk and a decision should be made by the patient and physician that the benefits outweigh the risks. Patients with a history of underlying heart disease should be aware that adverse effects in them might be especially serious. Patients should be alerted to the possibility of tachycardia and fluid retention and should watch for, and be monitored for, increased heart rate and weight gain or other systemic effects.

PRECAUTIONS
General Precautions
Patients treated with ROGAINE Topical Solution should be monitored one month after starting ROGAINE and at least every six months thereafter. If systemic effects should occur, discontinue use of ROGAINE.
ROGAINE contains an alcohol base which will cause burning and irritation of the eye. In the event of accidental contact with sensitive surfaces (eye, abraded skin, and mucous membranes), the area should be bathed with large amounts of cool tap water.
Inhalation of the spray mist should be avoided.
ROGAINE should not be used in conjunction with other topical agents including topical corticosteroids, retinoids, and petrolatum or agents that are known to enhance cutaneous drug absorption.
ROGAINE is for Topical Use Only. Each milliliter of ROGAINE contains 20 mg minoxidil. Accidental ingestion of the solution could lead to possible adverse systemic effects (see OVERDOSAGE.)
As is the case with other topically applied drugs, decreased integrity of the epidermal barrier caused by inflammation or disease processes in the skin (eg, excoriations of the scalp, scalp psoriasis, or severe sunburn) may increase percutaneous absorption of minoxidil.

Information for the Patient
A patient information leaflet has been prepared and is included with each package of ROGAINE. The text of the leaflet is printed at the end of this insert.

Drug Interactions
There are currently no known drug interactions associated with the use of ROGAINE Topical Solution. Although it has not been clinically demonstrated, there exists the theoretical possibility of absorbed minoxidil potentiating orthostatic hypotension in patients concurrently taking guanethidine.

Carcinogenesis, Mutagenesis, and Impairment of Fertility
No evidence of carcinogenicity was detected in rats and rabbits when ROGAINE Topical Solution was applied to the skin for up to one year. Dietary administration of minoxidil to mice for up to 24 months was associated with an increased incidence of malignant lymphomas in females and an increased incidence of hepatic nodules in males. The lymphoma incidence was unrelated to dose levels and at all doses was within the range seen in control groups from other studies employing mice from the same colony. The incidence of hepatic nodules was dose dependent, with a significant increase observed at 63 but not at 25 or 10 mg/kg/day. There was no effect of drug on the incidence of malignant tumors of the liver. As with the lymphomas, the incidence of hepatic nodules was within the historical control range for the subject mouse colony. No evidence of carcinogenic potential was obtained from a dietary administration study of minoxidil in rats. However, the rat study involved only $\frac{1}{3}$ the number of animals and half the maximum dosage level evaluated in the mouse experiment, and shorter durations of administration (up to 15 months in males and up to 22 months in females). Minoxidil was not mutagenic in the salmonella (Ames) test, the DNA damage/alkaline elution assay or the rat micronucleus test.
In a study in which male and female rats received one or five times the maximum recommended human oral antihypertensive dose of minoxidil (multiples based on a 50 kg patient) there was a dose-dependent reduction in conception rate.

Pregnancy
Pregnancy Category C. Adequate and well-controlled studies have not been conducted in pregnant women treated with ROGAINE Topical Solution nor in pregnant women treated with oral minoxidil for hypertension. Oral administration of minoxidil has been associated with evidence of increased

fetal resorption in rabbits, but not rats, when administered at five times the oral antihypertensive human dose. There was no evidence of teratogenic effects of ORALLY administered minoxidil in rats or rabbits. Subcutaneous administration of minoxidil to pregnant rats at 80 mg/kg/day (approximately 2000 times the maximal systemic human exposure from daily topical administration) was maternally toxic but not teratogenic. Higher subcutaneous doses produced evidence of developmental toxicity. ROGAINE should not be administered to pregnant women.

Labor and Delivery
The effects on labor and delivery are unknown.

Nursing Mothers
There has been one report of minoxidil excretion in the breast milk of a woman treated with 5 mg oral minoxidil twice daily for hypertension. Because of the potential for adverse effects in nursing infants from minoxidil absorption, ROGAINE should not be administered to a nursing woman.

Pediatric Use
Safety and effectiveness in patients under 18 years of age have not been established.

ADVERSE REACTIONS
ROGAINE Topical Solution was utilized by 3,510 patients enrolled in placebo-controlled trials. The rate of adverse events, grouped by body system, is shown in the following table. Except dermatologic events, which were more common in the minoxidil group, no individual reaction or body system grouping seemed to be increased in the minoxidil-treated group.
[See table on next page].
Patients have been followed for up to 5 years and there has been no change in incidence or severity of reported reactions. Additional events reported in postmarketing clinical experience include:
eczema, hypertrichosis, local erythema, pruritus, dry skin/scalp flaking, sexual dysfunction, visual disturbances including decreased visual acuity, exacerbation of hair loss, alopecia.

OVERDOSAGE
Increased systemic absorption of minoxidil may potentially occur if more frequent or larger doses of ROGAINE (than directed) are used or if ROGAINE is applied to large surface areas of the body or areas other than the scalp. There are no known cases of minoxidil overdosage resulting from topical administration of ROGAINE.
In a 14-day controlled clinical trial, 1 ml of 3% minoxidil solution was applied eight times daily (six times the recommended dose) to the scalp of 11 normal male volunteers and to the chest of 11 other volunteers. No significant systemic effects were observed in these subjects when compared with a similar number of placebo-treated subjects. All subjects in the study were monitored for vital sign, electrocardiographic, and echocardiographic changes.
In a reported case of accidental ingestion, a 3-year-old male swallowed 1 to 2 ml of a 3% concentration of topical minoxidil solution. After vomiting he was treated in an emergency room. The child was found to be alert and active with no obvious signs of distress. His temperature was 37° C, pulse 152 bpm, respiration 32, and systolic blood pressure 110 by palpation. Cardiovascular, chest, lungs, abdomen, head, skin, and neurological examinations were normal. Blood levels taken indicated a total minoxidil level (glucuronide and unchanged) of 320.6 ng/ml. The child was discharged without sequelae.
Because of the high concentration of minoxidil in ROGAINE Topical Solution, accidental ingestion has the potential of producing systemic effects related to the pharmacologic action of the drug (5 ml of ROGAINE Topical Solution contains 100 mg minoxidil, the maximum adult dose for oral minoxidil administration when used to treat hypertension). Signs and symptoms of minoxidil overdosage would most likely be cardiovascular effects associated with fluid retention and tachycardia. Fluid retention can be managed with appropriate diuretic therapy. Clinically significant tachycardia can be controlled by administration of a beta-adrenergic blocking agent. If encountered, hypotension should be treated by intravenous administration of normal saline. Sympathomimetic drugs, such as norepinephrine and epinephrine, should be avoided because of their excessive cardiac stimulating activity.
Oral LD_{50} in rats has ranged from 1321 to 3492 mg/kg; in mice 2457 to 2648 mg/kg. Minoxidil and its metabolites are hemodialyzable.

Continued on next page

Information on these Upjohn products is based on labeling in effect September 1, 1989. Further information concerning these and other Upjohn products may be obtained by direct inquiry to Medical Information, The Upjohn Company, Kalamazoo, Michigan 49001.

Upjohn—Cont.

DOSAGE AND ADMINISTRATION

Hair and scalp should be dry prior to topical application of ROGAINE Topical Solution. A dose of 1 ml ROGAINE Topical Solution should be applied to the total affected areas of the scalp twice daily. The total daily dosage should not exceed 2 ml. If finger tips are used to facilitate drug application, hands should be washed afterwards. Twice daily application for four months or longer may be required before evidence of hair regrowth is observed. Onset and degree of hair regrowth may be variable among patients. If hair regrowth is realized, twice daily applications of ROGAINE are necessary for additional and continued hair regrowth. Some anecdotal patient reports indicate that regrown hair and the balding process return to their untreated state three to four months following cessation of the drug.

HOW SUPPLIED

ROGAINE Topical Solution is a clear, colorless to light yellow solution containing 20 mg minoxidil per ml and is available as a 60 ml bottle with multiple applicators NDC 0009-3367-05.

Store at controlled room temperature: 15° to 30° C (59°–86° F)

CAUTION

Federal law prohibits dispensing without a prescription.

IMPORTANT INFORMATION ABOUT—
ROGAINE® Topical Solution (minoxidil 2%)

Your doctor has prescribed ROGAINE Topical Solution for you to use as a hair regrowth stimulant to treat male pattern baldness. ROGAINE is a prescription medication and therefore should be used only as directed by your doctor.

Please read this booklet thoroughly. It will help you to understand ROGAINE Topical Solution and what to expect from its use. If you have any questions after reading this booklet, or anytime during treatment with ROGAINE, you should consult your doctor or ask your pharmacist.

What is ROGAINE?

ROGAINE Topical Solution, discovered and made by The Upjohn Company, is a standardized topical (for use only on the skin) prescription medication proved effective for the long-term treatment of male pattern baldness.

ROGAINE is a topical solution of minoxidil. Minoxidil in tablet form has been used since 1980 to lower blood pressure. The use of *minoxidil tablets* is limited to treatment of patients with severe high blood pressure. When a high enough dosage in tablet form is used to lower blood pressure, certain effects that merit your attention may occur. These effects appear to be dose related. (See [What are the potential side effects on the heart and circulation when using ROGAINE?]) Persons who use ROGAINE Topical Solution have a low level of absorption of minoxidil, much lower than that of persons being treated with *minoxidil tablets* for high blood pressure. Therefore, the likelihood that a person using ROGAINE Topical Solution will develop the effects associated with *minoxidil tablets* is very small. In fact, none of these effects has been directly attributed to ROGAINE in clinical studies.

Exactly how ROGAINE works to stimulate hair regrowth in some people is not known. Upjohn scientists are doing research in this area.

How effective is ROGAINE?

Clinical studies with ROGAINE were conducted by physicians in 27 US medical centers involving over 2,300 patients with male pattern baldness involving the top (vertex) of the head. There is no evidence that ROGAINE is useful in causing hair to grow on the front of the scalp. At the end of four months, hair counts showed that on average, the patients using ROGAINE Topical Solution had significantly more hair regrowth than those who used placebo (a similar solution without the active medication).

Based on the patients' self evaluation at the end of four months, 26% using ROGAINE had moderate to dense hair growth compared with 11% using the placebo.

By the end of one year, 48% of the people who continued in the study using ROGAINE rated their hair growth as moderate or better.

How soon can I expect results from using ROGAINE?

Studies have shown that the response to treatment with ROGAINE may vary widely. If you respond to treatment, it usually will take four months or longer before there is evidence of hair growth.

Some people receiving ROGAINE may see faster results than others; others may respond with a slower rate of hair growth. You should not expect visible growth in less than four months.

If I respond to ROGAINE, what will the hair look like?

If you have very little hair and respond to treatment, your first hair growth may be soft, downy, colorless hair that is barely visible. After further treatment the new hair should be the same color and thickness as the other hair on your scalp. If you start with substantial hair, the new hair should be of the same color and thickness as the rest of your hair.

How long do I need to use ROGAINE?

ROGAINE is a treatment, not a cure. If you respond to treatment, you will need to continue using ROGAINE to maintain or increase hair growth. If you do not begin to show a response to treatment with ROGAINE after a reasonable period of time (at least four months or more), your doctor may advise you to discontinue using ROGAINE.

What happens if I stop using ROGAINE? Will I keep the new hair?

If you stop using ROGAINE, you will probably shed the new hair within a few months after stopping treatment.

What is the dosage of ROGAINE?

You should apply a 1 ml dose of ROGAINE two times a day, once in the morning and once at night, before bedtime. Each bottle should last about 30 days (one month). The applicators in each package of ROGAINE are designed to apply the correct amount of ROGAINE with each application. *Please refer to the Instructions for Use.*

What if I miss a dose or forget to use ROGAINE?

If you miss one or two daily applications of ROGAINE, you should restart your twice-daily application and return to your usual schedule. You should not attempt to make up for missed applications.

Can I use ROGAINE more than twice a day? Will it work faster?

No. Studies by The Upjohn Company have been carefully conducted to determine the correct amount of ROGAINE to use to obtain the most satisfactory results. More frequent applications or use of larger doses (more than one ml twice a day) have not been shown to speed up the process of hair growth and may increase the possibility of side effects.

What are the most common side effects reported in clinical studies with ROGAINE?

Studies of patients using ROGAINE have shown that the most common adverse effects directly attributable to ROGAINE Topical Solution were itching and other skin irritations of the treated area of the scalp.

Other side effects, including light-headedness, dizziness, and headaches were reported by patients using ROGAINE or placebo (a similar solution without the active medication). The frequency of these side effects was similar in the ROGAINE and placebo groups. For further information about side effects please ask your doctor.

ROGAINE Topical Solution contains alcohol, which could cause burning or irritation of the eyes, mucous membranes, or sensitive skin areas. If ROGAINE accidentally gets into these areas, bathe the area with large amounts of cool tap water. Contact your doctor if irritation persists.

What are the potential side effects on the heart and circulation when using ROGAINE?

Although serious side effects have not been attributed to ROGAINE in clinical studies, there is a possibility that they could occur because the active ingredient in ROGAINE Topical Solution is the same as in *minoxidil tablets.*

Minoxidil tablets are used to treat high blood pressure. *Minoxidil tablets* lower blood pressure by relaxing the arteries, an effect called vasodilation. Vasodilation leads to retention of fluid and increased heart rate. The following effects have occurred in some patients taking *minoxidil tablets* for high blood pressure:

1) Increased heart rate. Some patients have reported that their resting heart rate increased by more than 20 beats per minute.

2) Rapid weight gain of more than 5 pounds or swelling (edema) of the face, hands, ankles, or stomach area.

3) Difficulty in breathing, especially when lying down, a result of an increase in body fluids or fluid around the heart.

4) Worsening of, or new onset of, angina pectoris.

When ROGAINE Topical Solution is used on normal skin very little minoxidil is absorbed and these effects are not expected. If, however, you experience any of the above, discontinue use of ROGAINE and consult your doctor.

Presumably, such effects would be most likely if greater absorption occurred, eg, because ROGAINE was used on damaged or inflamed skin or in greater than recommended amounts.

MEDICAL EVENT PERCENT OCCURRENCE BY BODY SYSTEM IN THE PLACEBO CONTROL CLINICAL TRIALS INVOLVING MINOXIDIL TOPICAL SOLUTION—ALL PATIENTS ENROLLED

BODY SYSTEM	MINOXIDIL SOLN N=3510 (4–6 months)		PLACEBO N=2381 (4–6 months)	
	# PATS.	% OCC.	# PATS.	% OCC.
RESPIRATORY (bronchitis, upper respiratory infection, sinusitis)	209	5.95	155	6.51
DERMATOLOGICAL (irritant dermatitis, allergic contact dermatitis)	185	5.27	82	3.44
GASTROINTESTINAL (diarrhea, nausea, vomiting)	120	3.42	117	4.91
NEUROLOGY (headache, dizziness, faintness, lightheadedness)	90	2.56	71	2.98
MUSCULOSKELETAL (fractures, back pain, tendinitis)	76	2.17	43	1.81
CARDIOVASCULAR (edema, chest pain, blood pressure increases/decreases, palpitations, pulse rate increases/decreases)	45	1.28	28	1.18
ALLERGY (non-specific allergic reactions, hives, allergic rhinitis, facial swelling, and sensitivity)	36	1.03	15	0.63
SPECIAL SENSES (conjunctivitis, ear infections, vertigo)	33	0.94	26	1.09
METABOLIC-NUTRITIONAL (edema, weight gain)	21	0.60	19	0.80
URINARY TRACT (urinary tract infections, renal calculi, urethitis)	16	0.46	15	0.63
GENITAL TRACT (prostatitis, epididymitis)	16	0.46	10	0.42
PSYCHIATRIC (anxiety, depression, fatigue)	10	0.28	21	0.88
HEMATOLOGY (lymphadenopathy, thrombocytopenia)	8	0.23	6	0.25
ENDROCRINE	3	0.09	4	0.17

In animal studies, minoxidil, in doses higher than would be obtained from topical use in people, has caused important heart structure damage. This kind of damage has not been seen in humans given *minoxidil tablets* for high blood pressure at effective doses.

What factors may increase the risk of serious side effects with ROGAINE?

Individuals with known or suspected underlying coronary artery disease, or the presence of or predisposition to heart failure would be a particular risk if systemic effects (that is, increased heart rate or fluid retention) of minoxidil were to occur. Physicians, and patients with these kinds of underlying diseases, should be conscious of the potential risk of treatment if they choose to use ROGAINE.

Because absorption of minoxidil may be increased and the risk of side effects may become greater, ROGAINE should be applied only to the scalp and should not be used on other parts of the body. You should not use ROGAINE if your scalp becomes irritated or is sunburned, and you should not use it along with another topical treatment medication on your scalp.

Can men with high blood pressure use ROGAINE?

Individuals with hypertension, including those under treatment with antihypertensive agents, can use ROGAINE but should be monitored closely by their doctor. Patients taking guanethidine for high blood pressure should not use ROGAINE.

Instructions for Use

Please read this information before using ROGAINE Topical Solution. One ml (or 1 dose) of ROGAINE should be applied to the total affected areas of the scalp twice daily. The hair and scalp should be dry before application of ROGAINE. Each prescription of ROGAINE comes with three complimentary, disposable applicators to accommodate your individual preference and needs. You will receive a new set of these applicators with every prescription refill. You may wish to change the applicator if the condition of your hair changes.

Each special applicator included with a prescription for ROGAINE is designed to deliver a measured amount (1 ml, or 1 dose) of solution when used as directed. This amount of ROGAINE has been used in extensive clinical studies and determined to be the proper amount for the treatment of male pattern baldness.

You must understand that twice-daily application for four months or longer may be required before hair regrowth may be observed.

Like all medications, keep ROGAINE out of the reach of children. In the event of accidental ingestion, contact your doctor. If, after reading this information, you have any questions, consult your doctor or ask your pharmacist.

Complimentary Applicators

A. Metered Spray Attachment

for applying the solution to large areas of the scalp

B. Extender Spray Attachment

for applying the solution on small scalp areas or under hair

C. Rub-on Applicator Tip

for use in spreading the solution on scalp

DIRECTIONS FOR USE

Remove large outer cap; remove small inside child-resistant protective cap. Both caps should be retained for reuse:

A. Metered Spray Attachment

1. Insert spray assembly into bottle and screw on firmly. The spray attachment is now ready to use.
2. Pump the spray attachment six times (for one full dose of 1 ml), applying the solution to the scalp area to be treated. Be careful not to inhale the spray mist. Place large outer cap on bottle when not in use.

B. Extender Spray Attachment

1. The metered spray attachment (A) must be on the bottle to use the extender spray attachment. Follow steps under A. 1.
2. Remove small spray head from top of metered spray attachment; fit the extender spray attachment onto the spray shaft and push down firmly to seat the extender spray attachment. Remove the small cap on the end of the extender spray nozzle. The extender spray attachment is now ready to use.
3. Pump the spray attachment six times (for one full dose of 1 ml), applying solution to the scalp area to be treated. If desired, replace the small cap on end of nozzle tip when not in use.

C. Rub-on Applicator Tip

When used as directed, the special design of this rub-on applicator allows the chamber to be filled with one full dose of ROGAINE Topical Solution.

1. Fit the rub-on applicator tip onto the bottle and screw on firmly.
2. Holding the bottle upright, squeeze the bottle to fill the upper chamber to the black line. The metered applicator tip now contains one full dose (1 ml) and is ready to use.
3. Holding the bottle upside down, rub the applicator on the scalp area to be treated until the chamber is com-

pletely empty. Place large outer cap on bottle when not in use.

Code 813 264 004

Shown in Product Identification Section, page 434

SIGTAB® Tablets

(See PDR For Nonprescription Drugs)

SOLU–CORTEF®   ℞

brand of hydrocortisone sodium succinate sterile powder

(hydrocortisone sodium succinate

for injection, USP)

For Intravenous or Intramuscular

Administration

DESCRIPTION

SOLU-CORTEF Sterile Powder contains hydrocortisone sodium succinate as the active ingredient. Hydrocortisone sodium succinate is a white or nearly white, odorless, hygroscopic amorphous solid. It is very soluble in water and in alcohol, very slightly soluble in acetone and insoluble in chloroform. The chemical name is pregn-4-ene-3,20-dione,21-(3-carboxy-1-oxopropoxy)-11,17-dihydroxy-, monosodium salt, (11β)-and its molecular weight is 484.52.

Hydrocortisone sodium succinate is an anti-inflammatory adrenocortical steroid. This highly water-soluble sodium succinate ester of hydrocortisone permits the immediate intravenous administration of high doses of hydrocortisone in a small volume of diluent and is particularly useful where high blood levels of hydrocortisone are required rapidly.

SOLU-CORTEF Sterile Powder (hydrocortisone sodium succinate) is available in several packages for intravenous or intramuscular administration.

100 mg Plain—Vials containing hydrocortisone sodium succinate equivalent to 100 mg hydrocortisone, also 0.8 mg monobasic sodium phosphate anhydrous, 8.73 mg dibasic sodium phosphate dried.

[See table above].

ACTIONS

Hydrocortisone sodium succinate has the same metabolic and anti-inflammatory actions as hydrocortisone. When given parenterally and in equimolar quantities, the two compounds are equivalent in biologic activity. Following the intravenous injection of hydrocortisone sodium succinate, demonstrable effects are evident within one hour and persist for a variable period. Excretion of the administered dose is nearly complete within 12 hours. Thus, if constantly high blood levels are required, injections should be made every 4 to 6 hours. This preparation is also rapidly absorbed when administered intramuscularly and is excreted in a pattern similar to that observed after intravenous injection.

INDICATIONS

When oral therapy is not feasible, and the strength, dosage form and route of administration of the drug reasonably lend the preparation to the treatment of the condition, SOLU-CORTEF Sterile Powder (hydrocortisone sodium succinate) is indicated for intravenous or intramuscular use in the following conditions:

1. **Endocrine Disorders**

   Primary or secondary adrenocortical insufficiency (hydrocortisone or cortisone is the drug of choice; synthetic analogs may be used in conjunction with mineralocorticoids where applicable; in infancy, mineralocorticord supplementation is of particular importance)

   Acute adrenocortical insufficiency (hydrocortisone or cortisone is the drug of choice; mineralocorticoid supplementation may be necessary, particularly when synthetic analogs are used)

Preoperatively and in the event of serious trauma or illness, in patients with known adrenal insufficiency or when adrenocortical reserve is doubtful

Shock unresponsive to conventional therapy if adrenocortical insufficiency exists or is suspected

Congenital adrenal hyperplasia

Hypercalcemia associated with cancer

Nonsuppurative thyroiditis

2. **Rheumatic Disorders**

   As adjunctive therapy for short-term administration (to tide the patient over an acute episode or exacerbation) in:

   Post-traumatic osteoarthritis

   Synovitis of osteoarthritis

   Rheumatoid arthritis, including juvenile rheumatoid arthritis (selected cases may require low-dose maintenance therapy)

   Acute and subacute bursitis

   Epicondylitis

   Acute nonspecific tenosynovitis

   Acute gouty arthritis

   Psoriatic arthritis

   Ankylosing spondylitis

3. **Collagen Diseases**

   During an exacerbation or as maintenance therapy in selected cases of:

   Systemic lupus erythematosus

   Systemic dermatomyositis (polymyositis)

   Acute rheumatic carditis

4. **Dermatologic Diseases**

   Pemphigus

   Severe erythema multiforme (Stevens-Johnson syndrome)

   Exfoliative dermatitis

   Bullous dermatitis herpetiformis

   Severe seborrheic dermatitis

   Severe psoriasis

   Mycosis fungoides

5. **Allergic States**

   Control of severe or incapacitating allergic conditions intractable to adequate trials of conventional treatment in:

   Bronchial asthma

   Contact dermatitis

   Atopic dermatitis

   Serum sickness

   Seasonal or perennial allergic rhinitis

   Drug hypersensitivity reactions

   Urticarial transfusion reactions

   Acute noninfectious laryngeal edema (epinephrine is the drug of first choice)

6. **Ophthalmic Diseases**

   Severe acute and chronic allergic and inflammatory processes involving the eye, such as:

   Herpes zoster ophthalmicus

   Iritis, iridocyclitis

   Chorioretinitis

   Diffuse posterior uveitis and choroiditis

   Optic neuritis

   Sympathetic ophthalmia

   Anterior segment inflammation

   Allergic conjunctivitis

   Allergic corneal marginal ulcers

   Keratitis

Continued on next page

Information on these Upjohn products is based on labeling in effect September 1, 1989. Further information concerning these and other Upjohn products may be obtained by direct inquiry to Medical Information, The Upjohn Company, Kalamazoo, Michigan 49001.

SOLU-CORTEF	100 mg (MIX-O-VIAL)® (ACT-O-VIAL)® Each 2 ml contains: (when mixed)	250 mg (MIX-O-VIAL) (ACT-O-VIAL) Each 2 ml contains: (when mixed)	500 mg (MIX-O-VIAL) (ACT-O-VIAL) Each 4 ml contains: (when mixed)	1000 mg (MIX-O-VIAL) (ACT-O-VIAL) Each 8 ml contains: (when mixed)
Hydrocortisone sodium succinate	equiv. to 100 mg hydrocortisone	equiv. to 250 mg hydrocortisone	equiv. to 500 mg hydrocortisone	equiv. to 1000 mg hydrocortisone
Monobasic sodium phosphate anhydrous	0.8 mg	2 mg	4 mg	8 mg
Diabasic sodium phosphate dried	8.76 mg	21.8 mg	44 mg	88 mg
Benzyl alcohol added as preservative	18.1 mg	16.4 mg	33.4 mg	66.9 mg

When necessary, the pH of each formula was adjusted with sodium hydroxide so that the pH of the reconstituted solution is within the USP specified range of 7 to 8.

Upjohn—Cont.

7. **Gastrointestinal Diseases**
   To tide the patient over a critical period of the disease in:
   Ulcerative colitis (systemic therapy)
   Regional enteritis (systemic therapy)
8. **Respiratory Diseases**
   Symptomatic sarcoidosis
   Berylliosis
   Fulminating or disseminated pulmonary tuberculosis when used concurrently with appropriate antituberculous chemotherapy
   Loeffler's syndrome not manageable by other means
   Aspiration pneumonitis
9. **Hematologic Disorders**
   Acquired (autoimmune) hemolytic anemia
   Idiopathic thrombocytopenic purpura in adults (IV only; IM administration is contraindicated)
   Secondary thrombocytopenia in adults
   Erythroblastopenia (RBC anemia)
   Congenital (erythroid) hypoplastic anemia
10. **Neoplastic Diseases**
    For palliative mangement of:
    Leukemias and lymphomas in adults
    Acute leukemia of childhood
11. **Edematous States**
    To induce diuresis or remission of proteinuria in the nephrotic syndrome, without uremia, of the idiopathic type or that due to lupus erythematosus
12. **Nervous System**
    Acute exacerbations of multiple sclerosis
13. **Miscellaneous**
    Tuberculous meningitis with subarachnoid block or impending block when used concurrently with appropriate antituberculous chemotherapy
    Trichinosis with neurologic or myocardial involvement

CONTRAINDICATIONS

Systemic fungal infections and known hypersensitivity to components.

WARNINGS

In patients on corticosteroid therapy subjected to unusual stress, increased dosage of rapidly acting corticosteroids before, during, and after the stressful situation is indicated.
Corticosteroids may mask some signs of infection, and new infections may appear during their use. There may be decreased resistance and inability to localize infection when corticosteroids are used.
Prolonged use of corticosteroids may produce posterior subcapsular cataracts, glaucoma with possible damage to the optic nerves, and may enhance the establishment of secondary ocular infections due to fungi or viruses.
Usage in pregnancy. Since adequate human reproduction studies have not been done with corticosteroids, the use of these drugs in pregnancy, nursing mothers, or women of childbearing potential requires that the possible benefits of the drug be weighed against the potential hazards to the mother and embryo or fetus. Infants born of mothers who have received substantial doses of corticosteroids during pregnancy should be carefully observed for signs of hypoadrenalism.
Average and large doses of hydrocortisone can cause elevation of blood pressure, salt and water retention, and increased excretion of potassium. These effects are less likely to occur with the synthetic derivatives except when used in large doses. Dietary salt restriction and potassium supplementation may be necessary. All corticosteroids increase calcium excretion.
While on corticosteroid therapy patients should not be vaccinated against smallpox. Other immunization procedures should not be undertaken in patients who are on corticosteroids, especially on high dose, because of possible hazards of neurological complications and a lack of antibody response.
The use of SOLU-CORTEF Sterile Powder (hydrocortisone sodium succinate) in active tuberculosis should be restricted to those cases of fulminating or disseminated tuberculosis in which the corticosteroid is used for the management of the disease in conjunction with appropriate antituberculous regimen.
If corticosteroids are indicated in patients with latent tuberculosis or tuberculin reactivity, close observation is necessary as reactivation of the disease may occur. During prolonged corticosteroid therapy, these patients should receive chemoprophylaxis.
Because rare instances of anaphylactoid reactions (eg, bronchospasm) have occurred in patients receiving parenteral corticosteroid therapy, appropriate precautionary measures should be taken prior to administration, especially when the patient has a history of allergy to any drug.
The SOLU-CORTEF Sterile Powder 100 mg, 250 mg, 500 mg and 1000 mg MIX-O-VIAL Two-Compartment Vials contain

benzyl alcohol. Benzyl alcohol has been reported to be associated with a fatal "Gasping Syndrome" in premature infants.

PRECAUTIONS

Drug-induced secondary adrenocortical insufficiency may be minimized by gradual reduction of dosage. This type of relative insufficiency may persist for months after discontinuation of therapy; therefore, in any situation of stress occurring during that period, hormone therapy should be reinstituted. Since mineralocorticoid secretion may be impaired, salt and/or a mineralocorticoid should be administered concurrently. There is an enhanced effect of corticosteroids in patients with hypothyroidism and in those with cirrhosis.
Corticosteroids should be used cautiously in patients with ocular herpes simplex for fear of corneal perforation.
The lowest possible dose of corticosteroid should be used to control the condition under treatment, and when reduction in dosage is possible, the reduction must be gradual.
Psychic derangements may appear when corticosteroids are used, ranging from euphoria, insomnia, mood swings, personality changes, and severe depression to frank psychotic manifestations. Also, existing emotional instability or psychotic tendencies may be aggravated by corticosteroids.
Aspirin should be used cautiously in conjunction with corticosteroids in hypoprothrombinemia.
Steroids should be used with caution in nonspecific ulcerative colitis, if there is a probability of impending perforation, abscess or other pyogenic infection, also in diverticulitis, fresh intestinal anastomoses, active or latent peptic ulcer, renal insufficiency, hypertension, osteoporosis, and myasthenia gravis.
Growth and development of infants and children on prolonged corticosteroid therapy should be carefully followed.
Although controlled clinical trials have shown corticosteroids to be effective in speeding the resolution of acute exacerbations of multiple sclerosis, they do not show that corticosteroids affect the ultimate outcome or natural history of the disease. The studies do show that relatively high doses of corticosteroids are necessary to demonstrate a significant effect. (See **Administration and Dosage**).
Since complications of treatment with glucocorticoids are dependent on the size of the dose and the duration of treatment, a risk/benefit decision must be made in each individual case as to dose and duration of treatment and as to whether daily or intermittent therapy should be used.

ADVERSE REACTIONS

Fluid and Electrolyte Disturbances
Sodium retention
Fluid retention
Congestive heart failure in susceptible patients
Potassium loss
Hypokalemic alkalosis
Hypertension
Musculoskeletal
Muscle weakness
Steroid myopathy
Loss of muscle mass
Osteoporosis
Vertebral compression fractures
Aseptic necrosis of femoral and humeral heads
Pathologic fracture of long bones
Gastrointestinal
Peptic ulcer with possible perforation and hemorrhage
Pancreatitis
Abdominal distention
Ulcerative esophagitis
Dermatologic
Impaired wound healing
Thin fragile skin
Petechiae and ecchymoses
Facial erythema
Increased sweating
May suppress reactions to skin tests
Neurological
Convulsions
Increased intracranial pressure with papilledema (pseudotumor cerebri) usually after treatment
Vertigo
Headache
Endocrine
Menstrual irregularities
Development of Cushingoid state
Suppression of growth in children
Secondary adrenocortical and pituitary unresponsiveness, particularly in times of stress, as in trauma, surgery, or illness
Decreased carbohydrate tolerance
Manifestations of latent diabetes mellitus
Increased requirements for insulin or oral hypoglycemic agents in diabetics
Ophthalmic
Posterior subcapsular cataracts
Increased intraocular pressure
Glaucoma
Exophthalmos

Metabolic
Negative nitrogen balance due to protein catabolism
The following additional reactions are related to parenteral corticosteroid therapy:
Allergic, anaphylactic or other hypersensitivity reactions
Hyperpigmentation or hypopigmentation
Subcutaneous and cutaneous atrophy
Sterile abscess

ADMINISTRATION AND DOSAGE

This preparation may be administered by intravenous injection, by intravenous infusion, or by intramuscular injection, the preferred method for initial emergency use being intravenous injection. Following the initial emergency period, consideration should be given to employing a longer acting injectable preparation or an oral preparation.
Therapy is initiated by administering SOLU-CORTEF Sterile Powder (hydrocortisone sodium succinate) intravenously over a period of 30 seconds (eg, 100 mg) to 10 minutes (eg, 500 mg or more). In general, high dose corticosteroid therapy should be continued only until the patient's condition has stabilized—usually not beyond 48 to 72 hours. Although adverse effects associated with high dose, short-term corticoid therapy are uncommon, peptic ulceration may occur. Prophylactic anatacid therapy may be indicated.
When high dose hydrocortisone therapy must be continued beyond 48–72 hours, hypernatremia may occur. Under such circumstances it may be desirable to replace SOLU-CORTEF with a corticoid such as methylprednisolone sodium succinate which causes little or no sodium retention.
The initial dose of SOLU-CORTEF Sterile Powder is 100 mg to 500 mg, depending on the severity of the condition. This dose may be repeated at intervals of 2, 4 or 6 hours as indicated by the patient's response and clinical condition. While the dose may be reduced for infants and children, it is governed more by the severity of the condition and response of the patient than by age or body weight but should not be less than 25 mg daily.
Patients subjected to severe stress following corticosteroid therapy should be observed closely for signs and symptoms of adrenocortical insufficiency.
Corticoid therapy is an adjunct to, and not a replacement for, conventional therapy.
Preparation of Solutions
100 mg Plain—For intravenous or intramuscular injection, prepare solution by aseptically adding **not more than 2 ml** of Bacteriostatic Water for Injection or Bacteriostatic Sodium Chloride Injection to the contents of one vial. **For intravenous infusion,** first prepare solution by adding **not more than 2 ml** of Bacteriostatic Water for Injection to the vial; this solution may then be added to 100 to 1000 ml (but not less than 100 ml) of the following: 5% dextrose in water (or isotonic saline solution or 5% dextrose in isotonic saline solution if patient is not on sodium restriction).
Directions for using MIX-O-VIAL Two-Compartment Vial
1. Remove protective cap, give the plunger-stopper a quarter-turn and press to force diluent into the lower compartment.
2. Gently agitate to effect solution.
3. Sterilize top of plunger-stopper with a suitable germicide.
4. Insert needle **squarely through center** of plunger-stopper until tip is just visible. Invert vial and withdraw dose.
DIRECTIONS FOR USING THE ACT-O-VIAL SYSTEM
1. Press down on plastic activator to force diluent into the lower compartment.
2. Gently agitate to effect solution.
3. Remove plastic tab covering center of stopper.
4. Sterilize top of stopper with a suitable germicide.
5. Insert needle **squarely through center** of stopper until tip is just visible. Invert vial and withdraw dose.
Further dilution is not necessary for intravenous or intramuscular injection. For intravenous infusion, first prepare solution as just described. The **100 mg** solution may then be added to 100 to 1000 ml of 5% dextrose in water (or isotonic saline solution or 5% dextrose in isotonic saline solution if patient is not on sodium restriction). The **250 mg** solution may be added to 250 to 1000 ml, the **500 mg** solution may be added to 500 to 1000 ml and the **1000 mg** solution to 1000 ml of the same diluents. In cases where administration of a small volume of fluid is desirable, 100 mg to 3000 mg of SOLU-CORTEF Sterile Powder may be added to 50 ml of the above diluents. The resulting solutions are stable for at least 4 hours and may be administered either directly or by IV piggyback.
When reconstituted as directed, pH's of the solutions range from 7 to 8 and the tonicities are: 100 mg MIX-O-VIAL (ACT-O-VIAL), .36 osmolar; 250 mg MIX-O-VIAL (ACT-O-VIAL), 500 mg MIX-O-VIAL (ACT-O-VIAL), and the 1000 mg MIX-O-VIAL (ACT-O-VIAL), .57 osmolar. (Isotonic saline =.28 osmolar.)

HOW SUPPLIED

SOLU-CORTEF Sterile Powder (hydrocortisone sodium suc-

cinate) is available in the following packages:
100 mg Plain—NDC 0009-0825-01
100 mg MIX-O-VIAL
    2 ml—NDC 0009-0900-01
    25-2 ml—NDC 0009-0900-12
100 mg ACT-O-VIAL
    2 ml—NDC 0009-0900-13
    25-2 ml—NDC 0009-0900-15
250 mg MIX-O-VIAL
    2 ml—NDC 0009-0909-01
    25-2 ml—NDC 0009-0909-07
250 mg ACT-O-VIAL
    2 ml—NDC 0009-0909-08
    25-2 ml—NDC 0009-0909-09
500 mg MIX-O-VIAL—NDC 0009-0912-01
500 mg ACT-O-VIAL—NDC 0009-0912-05
1000 mg MIX-O-VIAL—NDC 0009-0920-01
1000 mg ACT-O-VIAL—NDC 0009-0920-03

STORAGE CONDITIONS
Store unreconstituted product at controlled room temperature 15°–30°C (59°–86°F).
Store solution at controlled room temperature 15°–30°C (59°–86°F) and protect from light. Use solution only if it is clear. Unused solution should be discarded after 3 days.
Code 810 379 011

SOLU–MEDROL®   ℞
brand of methylprednisolone sodium succinate sterile powder
(methylprednisolone sodium succinate for injection, USP)
For Intravenous or Intramuscular Administration

DESCRIPTION
SOLU-MEDROL Sterile Powder contains methylprednisolone sodium succinate as the active ingredient. Methylprednisolone sodium succinate, USP, occurs as a white, or nearly white, odorless powder. It is very soluble in water and in alcohol; it is insoluble in chloroform and is very slightly soluble in acetone.
The chemical name for methylprednisolone sodium succinate is pregna-1,4-diene-3,20-dione,21-(3-carboxy-1-oxopropoxy)-11,17-dihydroxy-6-methyl-,monosodium salt, (6α, 11β), and the molecular weight is 496.53.
Methylprednisolone sodium succinate is so extremely soluble in water that it may be administered in a small volume of diluent and is especially well suited for intravenous use in situations in which high blood levels of methylprednisolone are required rapidly.
SOLU-MEDROL is available in several strengths and packages for intravenous or intramuscular administration. **40 mg ACT-O-VIAL® System**—Each ml (when mixed) contains methylprednisolone sodium succinate equivalent to 40 mg methylprednisolone; also 1.6 mg monobasic sodium phosphate anhydrous; 17.46 mg dibasic sodium phosphate dried; 25 mg lactose hydrous; 8.8 mg benzyl alcohol added as preservative. **125 mg ACT-O-VIAL System**—Each 2 ml (when mixed) contains methylprednisolone sodium succinate equivalent to 125 mg methylprednisolone; also 1.6 mg monobasic sodium biphosphate anhydrous; 17.4 mg dibasic sodium phosphate dried; 17.6 mg benzyl alcohol added as preservative. **500 mg Vial**—Each 8 ml (when mixed as directed) contains methylprednisolone sodium succinate equivalent to 500 mg methylprednisolone; also 6.4 mg monobasic sodium biphosphate anhydrous; 69.6 mg dibasic sodium phosphate dried. **500 mg Vial with Diluent**—Each 8 ml (when mixed as directed) contains methylprednisolone sodium succinate equivalent to 500 mg methylprednisolone; also 6.4 mg monobasic sodium phosphate anhydrous; 69.6 mg dibasic sodium phosphate dried; 70.2 mg benzyl alcohol added as preservative. **1 gram Vial**—Each 16 ml (when mixed as directed) contains methylprednisolone sodium succinate equivalent to 1 gram methylprednisolone; also 12.8 mg monobasic sodium phosphate anhydrous; 139.2 mg dibasic sodium phosphate dried. **1 gram Vial with Diluent**—Each 16 ml (when mixed as directed) contains methylprednisolone sodium succinate equivalent to 1 gram methylprednisolone; also 12.8 mg monobasic sodium phosphate anhydrous; 139.2 mg dibasic sodium phosphate dried; 141 mg benzyl alcohol added as preservative. **2 gram Vial with Diluent**—Each 30.6 ml (when mixed as directed) contains methylprednisolone sodium succinate equivalent to 2 grams methylprednisolone; also 25.6 mg monobasic sodium phosphate anhydrous; 278 mg dibasic sodium phosphate dried; 273 mg benzyl alcohol added as preservative.
When necessary, the pH of each formula was adjusted with sodium hydroxide so that the pH of the reconstituted solution is within the USP specified range of 7 to 8 and the tonicities are, for the 40 mg per ml solution, 0.50 osmolar; for the 125 mg per 2 ml, 500 mg per 8 ml and 1 gram per 16 ml solutions, 0.40 osmolar; for the 2 gram per 30.6 ml solutions, 0.42 osmolar. (Isotonic saline = 0.28 osmolar).

IMPORTANT—Use only the accompanying diluent or Bacteriostac Water For Injection with Benzyl Alcohol when reconstituting SOLU-MEDROL.
    Use within 48 hours after mixing

ACTIONS
Methylprednisolone is a potent anti-inflammatory steroid synthesized in the Research Laboratories of The Upjohn Company. It has a greater anti-inflammatory potency than prednisolone and even less tendency than prednisolone to induce sodium and water retention.
Methylprednisolone sodium succinate has the same metabolic and anti-inflammatory actions as methylprednisolone. When given parenterally and in equimolar quantities, the two compounds are equivalent in biologic activity. The relative potency of SOLU-MEDROL Sterile Powder (methylprednisolone sodium succinate) and hydrocortisone sodium succinate, as indicated by depression of eosinophil count, following intravenous administration, is at least four to one. This is in good agreement with the relative oral potency of methylprednisolone and hydrocortisone.

INDICATIONS
When oral therapy is not feasible, and the strength, dosage form and route of administration of the drug reasonably lend the preparation to the treatment of the condition, SOLU-MEDROL Sterile Powder (methylprednisolone sodium succinate) is indicated for intravenous or intramuscular use in the following conditions:
1. **Endocrine Disorders**
Primary or secondary adrenocortical insufficiency (hydrocortisone or cortisone is the drug of choice; synthetic analogs may be used in conjunction with mineralocorticoids where applicable; in infancy, mineralocorticoid supplementation is of particular importance)
Acute adrenocortical insufficiency (hydrocortisone or cortisone is the drug of choice; mineralocorticoid supplementation may be necessary, particularly when synthetic analogs are used)
Preoperatively and in the event of serious trauma or illness, in patients with known adrenal insufficiency or when adrenocortical reserve is doubtful
Shock unresponsive to conventional therapy if adrenocortical insufficiency exists or is suspected
Congenital adrenal hyperplasia
Hypercalcemia associated with cancer
Nonsuppurative thyroiditis
2. **Rheumatic Disorders**
As adjunctive therapy for short-term administration (to tide the patient over an acute episode or exacerbation) in:
Post-traumatic osteoarthritis
Synovitis of osteoarthritis
Rheumatoid arthritis, including juvenile rheumatoid arthritis (selected cases may require low-dose maintenance therapy)
Acute and subacute bursitis
Epicondylitis
Acute nonspecific tenosynovitis
Acute gouty arthritis
Psoriatic arthritis
Ankylosing spondylitis
3. **Collagen Diseases**
During an exacerbation or as maintenance therapy in selected cases of:
Systemic lupus erythematosus
Systemic dermatomyositis (polymyositis)
Acute rheumatic carditis
4. **Dermatologic Diseases**
Pemphigus
Severe erythema multiforme (Stevens-Johnson syndrome)
Exfoliative dermatitis
Bullous dermatitis herpetiformis
Severe seborrheic dermatitis
Severe psoriasis
Mycosis fungoides
5. **Allergic States**
Control of severe or incapacitating allergic conditions intractable to adequate trials of conventional treatment in:
Bronchial asthma
Contact dermatitis
Atopic dermatitis
Serum sickness
Seasonal or perennial allergic rhinitis
Drug hypersensitivity reactions
Urticarial transfusion reactions
Acute noninfectious laryngeal edema (epinephrine is the drug of first choice)
6. **Ophthalmic Diseases**
Severe acute and chronic allergic and inflammatory processes involving the eye, such as:
Herpes zoster ophthalmicus
Iritis, iridocyclitis
Chorioretinitis

Diffuse posterior uveitis and choroiditis
Optic neuritis
Sympathetic ophthalmia
Anterior segment inflammation
Allergic conjunctivitis
Allergic corneal marginal ulcers
Keratitis
7. **Gastrointestinal Diseases**
To tide the patient over a critical period of the disease in:
Ulcerative colitis (systemic therapy)
Regional enteritis (systemic therapy)
8. **Respiratory Diseases**
Symptomatic sarcoidosis
Berylliosis
Fulminating or disseminated pulmonary tuberculosis when used concurrently with appropriate antituberculous chemotherapy
Loeffler's syndrome not manageable by other means
Aspiration pneumonitis
9. **Hematologic Disorders**
Acquired (autoimmune) hemolytic anemia
Idiopathic thrombocytopenic purpura in adults (IV only; IM administration is contraindicated)
Secondary thrombocytopenia in adults
Erythroblastopenia (RBC anemia)
Congenital (erythroid) hypoplastic anemia
10. **Neoplastic Diseases**
For palliative management of:
Leukemias and lymphomas in adults
Acute leukemia of childhood
11. **Edematous States**
To induce diuresis or remission of proteinuria in the nephrotic syndrome, without uremia, of the idiopathic type or that due to lupus erythematosus
12. **Nervous System**
Acute exacerbations of multiple sclerosis
13. **Miscellaneous**
Tuberculous meningitis with subarachnoid block or impending block when used concurrently with appropriate antituberculous chemotherapy
Trichinosis with neurologic or myocardial involvement

CONTRAINDICATIONS
Systemic fungal infections and known hypersensitivity to components.

WARNINGS
In patients on corticosteroid therapy subjected to any unusual stress, increased dosage of rapidly acting corticosteroids before, during, and after the stressful situation is indicated.
Corticosteroids may mask some signs of infection, and new infections may appear during their use. There may be decreased resistance and inability to localize infection when corticosteroids are used.
A study has failed to establish the efficacy of SOLU-MEDROL in the treatment of sepsis syndrome and septic shock. The study also suggests that treatment of these conditions with SOLU-MEDROL may increase the risk of mortality in certain patients (ie, patients with elevated serum creatinine levels or patients who develop secondary infections after SOLU-MEDROL).
Prolonged use of corticosteroids may produce posterior subcapsular cataracts, glaucoma with possible damage to the optic nerves, and may enhance the establishment of secondary ocular infections due to fungi or viruses.
Usage in pregnancy. Since adequate human reproduction studies have not been done with corticosteroids, the use of these drugs in pregnancy, nursing mothers, or women of childbearing potential requires that the possible benefits of the drug be weighed against the potential hazards to the mother and embryo or fetus. Infants born of mothers who have received substantial doses of corticosteroids during pregnancy should be carefully observed for signs of hypoadrenalism.
Average and large doses of cortisone or hydrocortisone can cause elevation of blood pressure, salt and water retention, and increased excretion of potassium. These effects are less likely to occur with the synthetic derivatives except when used in large doses. Dietary salt restriction and potassium supplementation may be necessary. All corticosteroids increase calcium excretion.
While on corticosteroid therapy patients should not be vaccinated against smallpox. Other immunization procedures should not be undertaken in patients who are on corticoster-

Continued on next page

Information on these Upjohn products is based on labeling in effect September 1, 1989. Further information concerning these and other Upjohn products may be obtained by direct inquiry to Medical Information, The Upjohn Company, Kalamazoo, Michigan 49001.

Upjohn—Cont.

oids, especially on high dose, because of possible hazards of neurological complications and a lack of antibody response.

The use of SOLU-MEDROL Sterile Powder (methylprednisolone sodium succinate) in active tuberculosis should be restricted to those cases of fulminating or disseminated tuberculosis in which the corticosteroid is used for the management of the disease in conjunction with appropriate antituberculous regimen.

If corticosteroids are indicated in patients with latent tuberculosis or tuberculin reactivity, close observation is necessary as reactivation of the disease may occur. During prolonged corticosteroid therapy, these patients should receive chemoprophylaxis.

Because rare instances of anaphylactic (eg, bronchospasm) reactions have occurred in patients receiving parenteral corticosteroid therapy, appropriate precautionary measures should be taken prior to administration, especially when the patient has a history of allergy to any drug.

There are reports of cardiac arrhythmias and/or circulatory collapse and/or cardiac arrest following the rapid administration of large IV doses of SOLU-MEDROL (greater than 0.5 gram administered over a period of less than 10 minutes). Bradycardia has been reported during or after the administration of large doses of methylprednisolone sodium succinate, and may be unrelated to the speed or duration of infusion.

Benzyl alcohol is contained in the **40 mg ACT-O-VIAL,** and the **125 mg ACT-O-VIAL,** and in the accompanying diluent for the 500 mg, 1 gram and 2 gram vials. Benzyl alcohol has been reported to be associated with a fatal "Gasping Syndrome" in premature infants.

PRECAUTIONS

Drug-induced secondary adrenocortical insufficiency may be minimized by gradual reduction of dosage. This type of relative insufficiency may persist for months after discontinuation of therapy; therefore, in any situation of stress occurring during that period, hormone therapy should be reinstituted. Since mineralocorticoid secretion may be impaired, salt and/or a mineralocorticoid should be administered concurrently.

There is an enhanced effect of corticosteroids on patients with hypothyroidism and in those with cirrhosis.

Corticosteroids should be used cautiously in patients with ocular herpes simplex because of possible corneal perforation.

The lowest possible dose of corticosteroid should be used to control the condition under treatment, and when reduction in dosage is possible, the reduction should be gradual.

Psychic derangements may appear when corticosteroids are used, ranging from euphoria, insomnia, mood swings, personality changes and severe depression, to frank psychotic manifestations. Also, existing emotional instability or psychotic tendencies may be aggravated by corticosteroids.

Aspirin should be used cautiously in conjunction with corticosteroids in hypoprothrombinemia.

Steroids should be used with caution in nonspecific ulcerative colitis, if there is a probability of impending perforation, abscess or other pyogenic infection; diverticulitis; fresh intestinal anastomoses; active or latent peptic ulcer; renal insufficiency; hypertension; osteoporosis; and myasthenia gravis.

Growth and development of infants and children on prolonged corticosteroid therapy should be carefully observed. Although controlled clinical trials have shown corticosteroids to be effective in speeding the resolution of acute exacerbations of multiple sclerosis, they do not show that corticosteroids affect the ultimate outcome or natural history of the disease. The studies do show that relatively high doses of corticosteroids are necessary to demonstrate a significant effect. (See DOSAGE AND ADMINISTRATION).

Since complications of treatment with glucocorticoids are dependent on the size of the dose and the duration of treatment, a risk/benefit decision must be made in each individual case as to dose and duration of treatment and as to whether daily or intermittent therapy should be used.

ADVERSE REACTIONS

Fluid and Electrolyte Disturbances
Sodium retention
Fluid retention
Congestive heart failure in susceptible patients
Potassium loss
Hypokalemic alkalosis
Hypertension
Musculoskeletal
Muscle weakness
Steroid myopathy
Loss of muscle mass
Severe arthralgia
Vertebral compression fractures
Aseptic necrosis of femoral and humeral heads
Pathologic fracture of long bones
Osteoporosis

Gastrointestinal
Peptic ulcer with possible perforation and hemorrhage
Pancreatitis
Abdominal distention
Ulcerative esophagitis
Dermatologic
Impaired wound healing
Thin fragile skin
Petechiae and ecchymoses
Facial erythema
Increased sweating
May suppress reactions to skin tests
Neurological
Increased intracranial pressure with papilledema (pseudotumor cerebri) usually after treatment
Convulsions
Vertigo
Headache
Endocrine
Development of Cushingoid state
Suppression of growth in children
Secondary adrenocortical and pituitary unresponsiveness, particularly in times of stress, as in trauma, surgery or illness
Menstrual irregularities
Decreased carbohydrate tolerance
Manifestations of latent diabetes mellitus
Increased requirements for insulin or oral hypoglycemic agents in diabetics
Ophthalmic
Posterior subcapsular cataracts
Increased intraocular pressure
Glaucoma
Exophthalmos
Metabolic
Negative nitrogen balance due to protein catabolism
The following *additional* adverse reactions are related to parenteral corticosteroid therapy:
Hyperpigmentation or hypopigmentation
Subcutaneous and cutaneous atrophy
Sterile abscess
Anaphylactic reaction with or without circulatory collapse, cardiac arrest, bronchospasm
Urticaria
Nausea and vomiting
Cardiac arrhythmias; hypotension or hypertension

DOSAGE AND ADMINISTRATION

When high dose therapy is desired, the recommended dose of SOLU-MEDROL Sterile Powder (methylprednisolone sodium succinate) is 30 mg/kg administered intravenously over at least 30 minutes. This dose may be repeated every 4 to 6 hours for 48 hours.

In general, high dose corticosteroid therapy should be continued only until the patient's condition has stabilized; usually not beyond 48 to 72 hours.

Although adverse effects associated with high dose short-term corticoid therapy are uncommon, peptic ulceration may occur. Prophylactic antacid therapy may be indicated.

In other indications initial dosage will vary from 10 to 40 mg of methylprednisolone depending on the clinical problem being treated. The larger doses may be required for short-term management of severe, acute conditions. The initial dose usually should be given intravenously over a period of one to several minutes. Subsequent doses may be given intravenously or intramuscularly at intervals dictated by the patient's response and clinical condition. Corticoid therapy is an adjunct to, and not replacement for conventional therapy.

Dosage may be reduced for infants and children but should be governed more by the severity of the condition and response of the patient than by age or size. It should not be less than 0.5 mg per kg every 24 hours.

Dosage must be decreased or discontinued gradually when the drug has been administered for more than a few days. If a period of spontaneous remission occurs in a chronic condition, treatment should be discontinued. Routine laboratory studies, such as urinalysis, two-hour postprandial blood sugar, determination of blood pressure and body weight, and a chest X-ray should be made at regular intervals during prolonged therapy. Upper GI X-rays are desirable in patients with an ulcer history or significant dyspepsia.

SOLU-MEDROL may be administered by intravenous or intramuscular injection or by intravenous infusion, the preferred method for initial emergency use being intravenous injection. To administer by intravenous (or intramuscular) injection, prepare solution as directed. The desired dose may be administered intravenously over a period of several minutes. Subsequent doses may be withdrawn and administered similarly. If desired, the medication may be administered in diluted solutions by adding Water for Injection or other suitable diluent (see below) to the **ACT-O-VIAL** and withdrawing the indicated dose.

To prepare solutions for intravenous infusion, first prepare the solution for injection as directed. This solution may then be added to indicated amounts of 5% dextrose in water, iso-

tonic saline solution or 5% dextrose in isotonic saline solution.

Multiple Sclerosis
In treatment of acute exacerbations of multiple sclerosis, daily doses of 200 mg of prednisolone for a week followed by 80 mg every other day for 1 month have been shown to be effective (4 mg of methylprednisolone is equivalent to 5 mg of prednisolone).

Directions for Using the ACT-O-VIAL System
1. Press down on plastic activator to force diluent into the lower compartment.
2. Gently agitate to effect solution.
3. Remove plastic tab covering center of stopper.
4. Sterilize top of stopper with a suitable germicide.
5. Insert needle squarely through center of stopper until tip is just visible. Invert vial and withdraw dose.

STORAGE CONDITIONS

Store unreconstituted product at controlled room temperature 15°–30°C (59°– 86°F).

Store solution at controlled room temperature 15°–30°C (59°– 86°F).

Use solution within 48 hours after mixing.

HOW SUPPLIED

SOLU-MEDROL Sterile Powder (methylprednisolone sodium succinate) is available in the following packages:

  40 mg ACT-O-VIAL System
    1 ml NDC 0009-0113-12
    25—1 ml NDC 0009-0113-13
  125 mg ACT-O-VIAL System
    2 ml NDC 0009-0190-09
    25—2 ml NDC 0009-0190-10
  500 mg Vial NDC 0009-0758-01
  500 mg Vial with Diluent NDC 0009-0887-01
  1 gram Vial NDC 0009-0698-01
  1 gram Vial with Diluent NDC 0009-0911-01
  1 gram Vial with Diluent and IV Administration Set
    NDC 0009-0911-05
  2 gram Vial with Diluent NDC 0009-0796-01

                          Code 810 431 116
Shown in Product Identification Section, page 434

TOLINASE®   ℞
brand of tolazamide tablets, USP

DESCRIPTION

TOLINASE Tablets contain tolazamide, an oral blood glucose lowering drug of the sulfonylurea class. Tolazamide is a white or creamy-white powder with a melting point of 165° to 173° C. The solubility of tolazamide at pH 6.0 (mean urinary pH) is 27.8 mg per 100 ml.

The chemical names for tolazamide are (1) Benzenesulfonamide, N-[[(hexahydro-1H -azepin-1-yl)amino]-carbonyl]-4-methyl-; (2) 1-(Hexahydro-1H-azepin-1-yl)-3-(p-tolylsulfonyl)-urea and its molecular weight is 311.40.

TOLINASE Tablets for oral administration are available as scored, white tablets containing 100 mg, 250 mg or 500 mg tolazamide. Inactive ingredients: calcium sulfate, docusate sodium, magnesium stearate, methylcellulose, sodium alginate.

CLINICAL PHARMACOLOGY

Actions

Tolazamide appears to lower the blood glucose acutely by stimulating the release of insulin from the pancreas, an effect dependent upon functioning beta cells in the pancreatic islets. The mechanism by which tolazamide lowers blood glucose during long-term administration has not been clearly established. With chronic administration in type II diabetic patients, the blood glucose lowering effect persists despite a gradual decline in the insulin secretory response to the drug. Extrapancreatic effects may be involved in the mechanism of action of oral sulfonylurea hypoglycemic drugs.

Some patients who are initially responsive to oral hypoglycemic drugs, including TOLINASE Tablets (tolazamide), may become unresponsive or poorly responsive over time. Alternatively, TOLINASE may be effective in some patients who have become unresponsive to one or more sulfonylurea drugs.

In addition to its blood glucose lowering actions, tolazamide produces a mild diuresis by enhancement of renal free water clearance.

Pharmacokinetics

Tolazamide is rapidly and well absorbed from the gastrointestinal tract. Peak serum concentrations occur at three to four hours following a single oral dose of the drug. The average biological half-life of the drug is seven hours. The drug does not continue to accumulate in the blood after the first four to six doses are administered. A steady or equilibrium state is reached during which the peak and nadir values do not change from day to day after the fourth to sixth doses. Tolazamide is metabolized to five major metabolites ranging in hypoglycemic activity from 0–70%. They are excreted principally in the urine. Following a single oral dose of tritiated tolazamide, 85% of the dose was excreted in the urine and 7% in the feces over a five-day period. Most of the urinary excretion of the drug occurred within the first 24 hours postadministration.

When nomal fasting nondiabetic subjects are given a single 500 mg dose of tolazamide orally, a hypoglycemic effect can be noted within 20 minutes after ingestion with a peak hypoglycemic effect occurring in two to four hours. Following a single oral dose of 500 mg tolazamide, a statistically significant hypoglycemic effect was demonstrated in fasted nondiabetic subjects 20 hours after administration. With fasting diabetic patients, the peak hypoglycemic effect occurs at four to six hours. The duration of maximal hypoglycemic effect in fed diabetic patients is about ten hours, with the onset occurring at four to six hours and with the blood glucose levels beginning to rise at 14 to 16 hours. Single dose potency of tolazamide in normal subjects has been shown to be 6.7 times that of tolbutamide on a milligram basis. Clinical experience in diabetic patients has demonstrated tolazamide to be approximately five times more potent than tolbutamide on a milligram basis, and approximately equivalent in milligram potency to chlorpropamide.

INDICATIONS AND USAGE

TOLINASE Tablets (tolazamide) are indicated as an adjunct to diet to lower the blood glucose in patients with noninsulin dependent diabetes mellitus (type II) whose hyperglycemia cannot be satisfactorily controlled by diet alone.

In initiating treatment for noninsulin-dependent diabetes, diet should be emphasized as the primary form of treatment. Caloric restriction and weight loss are essential in the obese diabetic patient. Proper dietary management alone may be effective in controlling the blood glucose and symptoms of hyperglycemia. The importance of regular physical activity should also be stressed and cardiovascular risk factors should be identified and corrective measures taken where possible.

If this treatment program fails to reduce symptoms and/or blood glucose, the use of an oral sulfonylurea or insulin should be considered. Use of TOLINASE must be viewed by both the physician and patient as a treatment in addition to diet and not as a substitute for diet or as a convenient mechanism for avoiding dietary restraint. Furthermore, loss of blood glucose control on diet alone may be transient thus requiring only short-term administration of TOLINASE.

During maintenance programs, TOLINASE should be discontinued if satisfactory lowering of blood glucose is no longer achieved. Judgments should be based on regular clinical and laboratory evaluations.

In considering the use of TOLINASE in asymptomatic patients, it should be recognized that controlling the blood glucose in noninsulin-dependent diabetes has not been definitely established to be effective in preventing the long-term cardiovascular or neural complications of diabetes.

CONTRAINDICATIONS

TOLINASE Tablets (tolazamide) are contraindicated in patients with: 1) known hypersensitivity or allergy to TOLINASE; 2) diabetic ketoacidosis, with or without coma. This condition should be treated with insulin; 3) Type I diabetes, as sole therapy.

Special Warning on Increased Risk of Cardiovascular Mortality: The administration of oral hypoglycemic drugs has been reported to be associated with increased cardiovascular mortality as compared to treatment with diet alone or diet plus insulin. This warning is based on the study conducted by the University Group Diabetes Program (UGDP), a long-term prospective clinical trial designed to evaluate the effectiveness of glucose-lowering drugs in preventing or delaying vascular complications in patients with noninsulin-dependent diabetes. The study involved 823 patients who were randomly assigned to one of four treatment groups (DIABETES, 19 (supp. 2):747–830, 1970.)

UGDP reported that patients treated for five to eight years with diet plus a fixed dose of tolbutamide (1.5 grams per day) had a rate of cardiovascular mortality approximately 2½ times that of patients with diet alone. A significant increase in total mortality was not observed, but the use of tolbutamide was discontinued based on the increase on cardiovascular mortality, thus limiting the opportunity for the study to show an increase in overall mortality. Despite controversy regarding the interpretation of these results, the findings of the UGDP study provide an adequate basis for this warning. The patient should be informed of the potential risks and advantages of TOLINASE and of alternative modes of therapy.

Although only one drug in the sulfonylurea class (tolbutamide) was included in this study, it is prudent from a safety standpoint to consider that this warning may also apply to other oral hypoglycemic drugs in this class, in view of their close similarities in mode of action and chemical structure.

PRECAUTIONS

General

Hypoglycemia—All sulfonylurea drugs are capable of producing severe hypoglycemia. Proper patient selection and dosage and instructions are important to avoid hypoglycemic episodes. Renal or hepatic insufficiency may cause elevated blood levels of TOLINASE Tablets (tolazamide) and the latter may also diminish gluconeogenic capacity, both of which increase the risk of serious hypoglycemic reactions. Elderly, debilitated, or malnourished patients and those with adrenal or pituitary insufficiency are particularly susceptible to the hypoglycemic action of glucose lowering drugs. Hypoglycemia may be difficult to recognize in the elderly and in people who are taking beta-adrenergic blocking drugs. Hypoglycemia is more likely to occur when caloric intake is deficient, after severe or prolonged exercise, when alcohol is ingested, or when more than one glucose-lowering drug is used.

Loss of Control of Blood Glucose—When a patient stabilized on any diabetic regimen is exposed to stress such as fever, trauma, infection, or surgery, loss of control of blood glucose may occur. At such times it may be necessary to discontinue TOLINASE and administer insulin.

The effectiveness of any hypoglycemic drug, including TOLINASE, in lowering blood glucose to a desired level decreases in many patients over a period of time, which may be due to progression of the severity of the diabetes or to diminished responsiveness to the drug. This phenomenon is known as secondary failure to distinguish it from primary failure in which the drug is ineffective in an individual patient when first given. Adequate adjustment of dose and adherence to diet should be assessed before classifying a patient as a secondary failure.

Information for Patients

Patients should be informed of the potential risks and advantages of TOLINASE Tablets (tolazamide) and of alternative modes of therapy. They should also be informed about the importance of adherence to dietary instructions, of a regular exercise program, and of regular testing of urine and/or blood glucose.

The risks of hypoglycemia, its symptoms and treatment, and conditions that predispose to its development should be explained to patients and responsible family members. Primary and secondary failure should also be explained.

Laboratory Tests

Blood and urine glucose should be monitored periodically. Measurement of glycosylated hemoglobin may be useful in some patients.

Drug Interactions

The hypoglycemic action of sulfonylureas may be potentiated by certain drugs including nonsteroidal anti-inflammatory agents and other drugs that are highly protein bound, salicylates, sulfonamides, chloramphenicol, probenecid, coumarins, monoamine oxidase inhibitors, and beta-adrenergic blocking agents. When such drugs are administered to a patient receiving TOLINASE, the patient should be closely observed for hypoglycemia. When such drugs are withdrawn from a patient receiving TOLINASE, the patient should be observed closely for loss of control.

Certain drugs tend to produce hyperglycemia and may lead to loss of control. These drugs include the thiazides and other diuretics, corticosteroids, phenothiazines, thyroid products, estrogens, oral contraceptives, phenytoin, nicotinic acid, sympathomimetics, calcium channel blocking drugs, and isoniazid. When such drugs are administered to a patient receiving TOLINASE, the patient should be closely observed for loss of control. When such drugs are withdrawn from a patient receiving TOLINASE, the patient should be observed closely for hypoglycemia.

A potential interaction between oral miconazole and oral hypoglycemic agents leading to severe hypoglycemia has been reported. Whether this interaction also occurs with the intravenous, topical or vaginal preparations of miconazole is not known.

Carcinogenicity

In a bioassay for carcinogenicity, rats and mice of both sexes were treated with tolazamide for 103 weeks at low and high doses. No evidence of carcinogenicity was found.

Pregnancy

Teratogenic Effects:

Pregnancy Category C. TOLINASE, administered to pregnant rats at ten times the human dose, decreased litter size but did not produce teratogenic effects in the offspring. In rats treated at a daily dose of 14 mg/kg no reproductive aberrations or drug related fetal anomalies were noted. At an elevated dose of 100 mg/kg per day there was a reduction in the number of pups born and an increased perinatal mortality. There are, however, no adequate and well-controlled studies in pregnant women. Because animal reproduction studies are not always predictive of human response, TOLINASE is not recommended for the treatment of the pregnant diabetic patient. Serious consideration should also be given to the possible hazards of the use of TOLINASE in women of child bearing age and in those who might become pregnant while using the drug.

Because recent information suggests that abnormal blood glucose levels during pregnancy are associated with a higher incidence of congenital abnormalities, many experts recommend that insulin be used during pregnancy to maintain blood glucose levels as close to normal as possible.

Nonteratogenic Effects:

Prolonged severe hypoglycemia (four to ten days) has been reported in neonates born to mothers who were receiving a sulfonylurea drug at the time of delivery. This has been reported more frequently with the use of agents with prolonged half-lives. If TOLINASE is used during pregnancy, it should be discontinued at least two weeks before the expected delivery date.

Nursing Mothers

Altough it is not known whether tolazamide is excreted in human milk, some sulfonylurea drugs are known to be excreted in human milk. Because the potential for hypoglycemia in nursing infants may exist, a decision should be made whether to discontinue nursing or to discontinue the drug, taking into account the importance of the drug to the mother. If the drug is discontinued and if diet alone is inadequate for controlling blood glucose, insulin therapy should be considered.

Pediatric Use

Safety and effectiveness in children have not been established.

ADVERSE REACTIONS

TOLINASE Tablets (tolazamide) have generally been well tolerated. In clinical studies in which more than 1,784 diabetic patients were specifically evaluated for incidence of side effects, only 2.1% were discontinued from therapy because of side effects.

Hypoglycemia: See **Precautions** and **Overdosage** sections.

Gastrointestinal Reactions: Cholestatic jaundice may occur rarely; TOLINASE Tablets should be discontinued if this occurs. Gastrointestinal disturbances, eg, nausea, epigastric fullness, and heartburn, are the most common reactions and occurred in 1% of patients treated during clinical trials. They tend to be dose-related and may disappear when dosage is reduced.

Dermatologic Reactions: Allergic skin reactions, eg, pruritus, erythema, urticaria, and morbilliform or maculopapular eruptions, occurred in 0.4% of patients treated during clinical trials. These may be transient and may disappear despite continued use of TOLINASE; if skin reactions persist, the drug should be discontinued.

Porphyria cutanea tarda and photosensitivity reactions have been reported with sulfonylureas.

Hematologic Reactions: Leukopenia, agranulocytosis, thrombocytopenia, hemolytic anemia, aplastic anemia, and pancytopenia have been reported with sulfonylureas.

Metabolic Reactions: Hepatic porphyria and disulfiram-like reactions have been reported with sulfonylureas; however, disulfiram-like reactions with TOLINASE have been reported very rarely.

Cases of hyponatremia have been reported with tolazamide and all other sulfonylureas, most often in patients who are on other medications or have medical conditions known to cause hyponatremia or increase release of antidiuretic hormone. The syndrome of inappropriate antidiuretic hormone (SIADH) secretion has been reported with certain other sylfonylureas, and it has been suggested that these sulfonylureas may augment the peripheral (antidiuretic) action of ADH and/or increase release of ADH.

Miscellaneous: Weakness, fatigue, dizziness, vertigo, malaise and headache were reported infrequently in patients treated during clinical trials. The relationship to therapy with TOLINASE is difficult to assess.

OVERDOSAGE

Overdosage of sulfonylureas, including TOLINASE Tablets (tolazamide), can produce hypoglycemia.

Mild hypoglycemic symptoms without loss of consciousness or neurologic findings should be treated aggressively with oral glucose and adjustment in drug dosage and/or meal patterns. Close monitoring should continue until the physician is assured the patient is out of danger. Severe hypoglycemic reactions with coma, seizure, or other neurological impairment occur infrequently, but constitute medical emergencies requiring immediate hospitalization. If hypoglycemic coma is suspected or diagnosed, the patient should be given a rapid intravenous injection of concentrated (50%) glucose solution. This should be followed by a continuous infusion of a more dilute (10%) glucose solution at a rate which will maintain the blood glucose at a level above 100 mg/dl. Patients should be closely monitored for a minimum of 24 to 48 hours since hypoglycemia may recur after apparent clinical recovery.

Continued on next page

Information on these Upjohn products is based on labeling in effect September 1, 1989. Further information concerning these and other Upjohn products may be obtained by direct inquiry to Medical Information, The Upjohn Company, Kalamazoo, Michigan 49001.

Upjohn—Cont.

DOSAGE AND ADMINISTRATION

There is no fixed dosage regimen for the management of diabetes mellitus with TOLINASE Tablets (tolazamide) or any other hypoglycemic agent. In addition to the usual monitoring of urinary glucose, the patient's blood glucose must also be monitored periodically to determine the minimum effective dose for the patient; to detect primary failure, ie, inadequate lowering of blood glucose at the maximum recommended dose of medication; and to detect secondary failure, ie, loss of adequate blood glucose response after an initial period of effectiveness. Glycosylated hemoglobin levels may also be of value in monitoring the patient's response to therapy.

Short-term administration of TOLINASE may be sufficient during periods of transient loss of control in patients usually controlled well on diet.

Usual Starting Dose

The usual starting dose of TOLINASE Tablets for the mild to moderately severe type II diabetic patient is 100–250 mg daily administered with breakfast or the first main meal. Generally, if the fasting blood glucose is less than 200 mg/dl, the starting dose is 100 mg/day as a single daily dose. If the fasting blood glucose value is greater than 200 mg/dl, the starting dose is 250 mg/day as a single dose. If the patient is malnourished, underweight, elderly, or not eating properly, the initial therapy should be 100 mg once a day. Failure to follow an appropriate dosage regimen may precipitate hypoglycemia. Patients who do not adhere to their prescribed dietary regimen are more prone to exhibit unsatisfactory response to drug therapy.

Transfer From Other Hypoglycemic Therapy

Patients Receiving Other Oral Antidiabetic Therapy—Transfer of patients from other oral antidiabetes regimens to TOLINASE should be done conservatively. When transferring patients from oral hypoglycemic agents other than chlorpropamide to TOLINASE, no transition period or initial or priming dose is necessary. When transferring from chlorpropamide, particular care should be exercised to avoid hypoglycemia.

Tolbutamide: If receiving less than 1 gm/day, begin at 100 mg of tolazamide per day. If receiving 1 gm or more per day, initiate at 250 mg of tolazamide per day as a single dose.

Chlorpropamide: 250 mg of chlorpropamide may be considered to provide approximately the same degree of blood glucose control as 250 mg of tolazamide. The patient should be observed carefully for hypoglycemia during the transition period from chlorpropamide to TOLINASE (one to two weeks) due to the prolonged retention of chlorpropamide in the body and the possibility of a subsequent overlapping drug effect.

Acetohexamide: 100 mg of tolazamide may be considered to provide approximately the same degree of blood glucose control as 250 mg of acetohexamide.

Patients Receiving Insulin—Some type II diabetic patients who have been treated only with insulin may respond satisfactorily to therapy with TOLINASE. If the patient's previous insulin dosage has been less than 20 units, substitution of 100 mg of tolazamide per day as a single daily dose may be tried. If the previous insulin dosage was less than 40 units, but more than 20 units, the patient should be placed directly on 250 mg of tolazamide per day as a single dose. If the previous insulin dosage was greater than 40 units, the insulin dosage should be decreased by 50% and 250 mg of tolazamide per day started. The dosage of TOLINASE should be adjusted weekly (or more often in the group previously requiring more than 40 units of insulin). During this conversion period when both insulin and TOLINASE are being used, hypoglycemia may rarely occur. During insulin withdrawal, patients should test their urine for glucose and acetone at least three times daily and report results to their physician. The appearance of persistent acetonuria with glycosuria indicates that the patient is a type I diabetic who requires insulin therapy.

Maximum Dose

Daily doses of greater than 1000 mg are not recommended. Patients will generally have no further response to doses larger than this.

Usual Maintenance Dose

The usual maintenance dose is in the range of 100–1000 mg/day with the average maintenance dose being 250–500 mg/day. Following initiation of therapy, dosage adjustment is made in increments of 100 mg to 250 mg at weekly intervals based on the patient's blood glucose response.

Dosage Interval

Once a day therapy is usually satisfactory. Doses up to 500 mg/day should be given as a single dose in the morning. 500 mg once daily is as effective as 250 mg twice daily. When a dose of more than 500 mg/day is required, the dose may be divided and given twice daily.

In elderly patients, debilitated or malnourished patients, and patients with impaired renal or hepatic function, the initial and maintenance dosing should be conservative to avoid hypoglycemic reactions (see PRECAUTIONS section).

HOW SUPPLIED

TOLINASE Tablets (tolazamide) are available in the following strengths and package sizes:

100 mg (scored, round, white)
    Unit-of-Use bottles of 100   NDC 0009-0070-02
250 mg (scored, round, white)
    Bottles of 200   NDC 0009-0114-04
    Bottles of 1000   NDC 0009-0114-02
    Unit-of-Use bottles of 100   NDC 0009-0114-05
    Unit-Dose package of 100   NDC 0009-0114-06
500 mg (scored, round, white)
    Unit-of-Use bottles of 100   NDC 0009-0477-06
Store at controlled room temperature 15–30° C (59–86° F).
Code 811 417 106

Shown in Product Identification Section, page 434

TROBICIN®   ℞
brand of spectinomycin hydrochloride sterile powder
(sterile spectinomycin hydrochloride for suspension, USP)
For Intramuscular Injection

2 Gm vial	NSN 6505-00-079-7611 (M)
4 Gm vial	NSN 6505-00-079-7643 (M)

DESCRIPTION

TROBICIN Sterile Powder contains spectinomycin hydrochloride which is an aminocyclitol antibiotic produced by a species of soil microorganism designated as *Streptomyces spectabilis*. Sterile spectinomycin hydrochloride is the pentahydrated dihydrochloride salt of spectinomycin.

Spectinomycin hydrochloride is isolated as a white to pale buff crystalline dihydrochloride pentahydrate powder, molecular weight 495, and is stable in the dry state for 36 months.

CLINICAL PHARMACOLOGY

Spectinomycin hydrochloride is an inhibitor of protein synthesis in the bacterial cell; the site of action is the 30S ribosomal subunit.

In vitro studies have shown spectinomycin hydrochloride to be active against most strains of *Neisseria gonorrhoeae* (minimum inhibitory concentration < 7.5 to 20 mcg/ml).

Definitive *in vitro* studies have shown no cross-resistance of *N. gonorrhoeae* between spectinomycin hydrochloride and penicillin. The antibiotic is not significantly bound to plasma protein.

INDICATIONS AND USAGE

TROBICIN Sterile Powder (spectinomycin hydrochloride) is indicated in the treatment of acute gonorrheal urethritis and proctitis in the male and acute gonorrheal cervicitis and proctitis in the female when due to susceptible strains of *Neisseria gonorrhoeae*. Men and women with known recent exposure to gonorrhea should be treated as those known to have gonorrhea.

The *in vitro* susceptibility of *Neisseria gonorrhoeae* to spectinomycin hydrochloride can be tested by agar dilution methods. TROBICIN Susceptibility Powder is available for this purpose, and its package insert should be consulted for details.

CONTRAINDICATIONS

The use of TROBICIN Sterile Powder (spectinomycin hydrochloride) is contraindicated in patients previously found hypersensitive to it.

WARNINGS

Spectinomycin hydrochloride is not effective in the treatment of syphilis. Antibiotics used in high doses for short periods of time to treat gonorrhea may mask or delay the symptoms of incubating syphilis. Since the treatment of syphilis demands prolonged therapy with any effective antibiotic, patients being treated for gonorrhea should be closely observed clinically. All patients with gonorrhea should have a serologic test for syphilis at the time of diagnosis. Patients treated with spectinomycin hydrochloride should have a follow-up serologic test for syphilis after three months.

Usage in pregnancy: Safety for use in pregnancy has not been established.

Usage in infants and children: Safety for use in infants and children has not been established.

The diluent provided with this product contains benzyl alcohol which has been associated with a fatal gasping syndrome in infants.

PRECAUTIONS

The usual precautions should be observed with atopic individuals.

The clinical effectiveness of TROBICIN Sterile Powder (spectinomycin hydrochloride) should be monitored to detect evidence of development of resistance by *Neisseria gonorrhoeae*.

ADVERSE REACTIONS

The following reactions were observed during the single dose clinical trials: soreness at the injection site, urticaria, dizziness, nausea, chills, fever and insomnia.

During multiple dose subchronic tolerance studies in normal human volunteers, the following were noted: a decrease in hemoglobin, hematocrit and creatinine clearance; elevation of alkaline phosphatase, BUN and SGPT. In single and multiple dose studies in normal volunteers, a reduction in urine output was noted. Extensive renal function studies demonstrated no consistent changes indicative of renal toxicity. Although no clearly defined case of anaphylaxis has been reported with TROBICIN Sterile Powder, the possibility of such reactions should be considered particularly when using antibiotics.

A few cases of anaphylaxis or anaphylactoid reactions have been reported. If serious allergic reactions occur, the usual agents (epinephrine, corticosteroids, and/or antihistamines) should be available for emergency use. In cases of severe anaphylaxis, airway support and oxygen may also be required.

DOSAGE AND ADMINISTRATION

Preparation of Drug for Intramuscular Injection
TROBICIN Sterile Powder, 2 grams (spectinomycin hydrochloride): reconstitute with 3.2 ml of the accompanying diluent.*

TROBICIN Sterile Powder, 4 grams: reconstitute with 6.2 ml of the accompanying diluent.*

*Bacteriostatic Water for Injection with Benzyl Alcohol 0.945% w/v added as preservative.

Shake vials vigorously immediately after adding diluent and before withdrawing dose. It is recommended that disposable syringes and needles be used to avoid contamination with penicillin residue, especially when treating patients known to be highly sensitive to penicillin. **Use of 20 gauge needle is recommended.**

Dosage

Intramuscular injections should be made deep into the upper outer quadrant of the gluteal muscle.

Adults (Men and Women)—Inject 5 ml intramuscularly for a 2 gram dose. This is also the recommended dose for patients being treated after failure of previous antibiotic therapy. In geographic areas where antibiotic resistance is known to be prevalent, initial treatment with 4 grams (10 ml) intramuscularly is preferred. The 10 ml injection may be divided between two gluteal injection sites.

STORAGE CONDITIONS

Store unreconstituted product at controlled room temperature 15°–30°C (59°–86°F). Store prepared suspension at controlled room temperature 15°–30°C (59°–86°F) and use within 24 hours.

HOW SUPPLIED

TROBICIN Sterile Powder (spectinomycin hydrochloride) is available as:

   TROBICIN Sterile Powder, 2 gram vial—with one ampoule of Bacteriostatic Water for Injection with Benzyl Alcohol 0.945% w/v added as preservative. When reconstituted with 3.2 ml of the accompanying diluent, each vial yields a sufficient quantity for withdrawal of 5 ml of a suspension containing 400 mg spectinomycin per ml (as the hydrochloride). 5 ml provides 2 grams spectinomycin. For intramuscular use only.

         NDC 0009-0566-01

   TROBICIN Sterile Powder 4 gram vial—with one ampoule of Bacteriostatic Water for Injection with Benzyl Alcohol 0.945% w/v added as preservative. When reconstituted with 6.2 ml of the accompanying diluent, each vial yields a sufficient quantity for withdrawal of 10 ml of a suspension containing spectinomycin hydrochloride equivalent to 400 mg spectinomycin per ml. 10 ml provides 4 grams spectinomycin. For intramuscular use only.

         NDC 0009-0592-01

   TROBICIN Susceptibility Powder—100 mg. See package insert for *in vitro* testing procedure.

HUMAN PHARMACOLOGY

TROBICIN Sterile Powder (spectinomycin hydrochloride) is rapidly absorbed after intramuscular injection. A single, two gram injection produces peak serum concentrations averaging about 100 mcg/ml at one hour; a single, four gram injection produces peak serum concentrations averaging 160 mcg/ml at two hours. Average serum concentrations of 15 mcg/ml for the two gram dose and 31 mcg/ml for the four gram dose were present eight hours after dosing.
Code 810 130 007

UNICAP® Capsules/Tablets

(See PDR For Nonprescription Drugs)

UNICAP JR™ Chewable Tablets

(See PDR For Nonprescription Drugs)

UNICAP M® Tablets

(See PDR For Nonprescription Drugs)

UNICAP® Plus Iron Tablets

(See PDR For Nonprescription Drugs)

UNICAP Sr.™ Tablets

(See PDR For Nonprescription Drugs)

UNICAP T® Tablets

(See PDR For Nonprescription Drugs)

XANAX®

Ⓒ ℞

brand of alprazolam tablets, USP

0.25 mg, 100's Unit Dose	NSN 6505-01-188-7936 (VA)
0.25 mg, 100's	NSN 6505-01-143-9269 (M & VA)
0.25 mg, 500's	NSN 6505-01-197-3966 (M & VA)
0.5 mg, 100's Unit Dose	
	NSN 6505-01-140-3201 (M & VA)
0.5 mg, 100's	NSN 6505-01-140-3199 (M & VA)
0.5 mg, 500's	NSN 6505-01-196-9501 (M & VA)
1.0 mg, 100's Unit Dose	NSN 6505-01-140-3202 (VA)
1.0 mg, 100's	NSN 6505-01-140-3200 (M & VA)
1.0 mg, 500's	NSN 6505-01-197-9003 (M & VA)

DESCRIPTION

XANAX Tablets contain alprazolam which is a triazolo analog of the 1,4 benzodiazepine class of central nervous system-active compounds.

The chemical name of alprazolam is 8- Chloro-1-methyl-6-phenyl-4H-s-triazolo[4,3-α] [1,4]benzodiazepine.

Alprazolam is a white crystalline powder, which is soluble in methanol or ethanol but which has no appreciable solublity in water at physiological pH.

Each XANAX tablet, for oral administration, contains, 0.25, 0.5 or 1.0 mg of alprazolam.

Inactive ingredients: cellulose, corn starch, docusate sodium, lactose, magnesium stearate, silicon dioxide and sodium benzoate. In addition, the 0.5 mg tablet contains FD&C Yellow No. 6 and the 1 mg tablet contains FD&C Blue No. 2 and FD&C Red No. 3.

CLINICAL PHARMACOLOGY

CNS agents of the 1,4 benzodiazepine class presumably exert their effects by binding at stereo specific receptors at several sites within the central nervous system. Their exact mechanism of action is unknown. Clinically, all benzodiazepines cause a dose-related central nervous system depressant activity varying from mild impairment of task performance to hypnosis.

Following oral administration, alprazolam is readily absorbed. Peak concentrations in the plasma occur in one to two hours following administration. Plasma levels are proportionate to the dose given; over the dose range of 0.5 to 3.0 mg, peak levels of 8.0 to 37 ng/ml were observed. The mean elimination half-life of alprazolam is 12–15 hours. The predominant metabolites are α-hydroxy-alprazolam and a benzophenone derived from alprazolam. The biological activity of α-hydroxy-alprazolam is approximately one-half that of alprazolam. The benzophenone metabolite is essentially inactive. Plasma levels of these metabolites are extremely low, thus precluding precise pharmacokinetic description. However, their half-lives appear to be of the same order of magnitude as that of alprazolam. Alprazolam and its metabolites are excreted primarily in the urine.

The ability of alprazolam to induce human hepatic enzyme systems has not yet been determined. However, this is not a property of benzodiazepines in general. Further, alprazolam did not affect the prothrombin or plasma warfarin levels in male volunteers administered sodium warfarin orally.

In vitro, alprazolam is bound (80 percent) to human serum protein.

Changes in the absorption, distribution, metabolism and excretion of benzodiazepines have been reported in a variety of disease states including alcoholism, impaired hepatic function and impaired renal function. Changes have also been demonstrated in geriatric patients. It has not yet been determined if similar changes occur in the pharmacokinetics of alprazolam.

Because of its similarity to other benzodiazepines, it is assumed that alprazolam undergoes transplacental passage and that it is excreted in human milk.

INDICATIONS AND USAGE

XANAX Tablets (alprazolam) are indicated for the management of anxiety disorders or for the short-term relief of the symptoms of anxiety. Anxiety or tension associated with the stress of everyday life usually does not require treatment with an anxiolytic.

Anxiety associated with depression is also responsive to XANAX.

The effectiveness of XANAX for long-term use, that is, more than four months, has not been established by systematic clinical trials. The physician should periodically reassess the usefulness of the drug for the individual patient.

CONTRAINDICATIONS

XANAX Tablets (alprazolam) are contraindicated in patients with known sensitivity to this drug or other benzodiazepines. XANAX may be used in patients with open angle glaucoma who are receiving appropriate therapy, but is contraindicated in patients with acute narrow angle glaucoma.

WARNINGS

XANAX Tablets (alprazolam) are not of value in the treatment of psychotic patients and should not be employed in lieu of appropriate treatment for psychosis. Because of its CNS depressant effects, patients receiving XANAX should be cautioned against engaging in hazardous occupations or activities requiring complete mental alertness such as operating machinery or driving a motor vehicle. For the same reason, patients should be cautioned about the simultaneous ingestion of alcohol and other CNS depressant drugs during treatment with XANAX.

Benzodiazepines can potentially cause fetal harm when administered to pregnant women. If XANAX is used during pregnancy, or if the patient becomes pregnant while taking this drug, the patient should be apprised of the potential hazard to the fetus. Because of experience with other members of the benzodiazepine class, XANAX is assumed to be capable of causing an increased risk of congenital abnormalities when administered to a pregnant woman during the first trimester. Because use of these drugs is rarely a matter of urgency, their use during the first trimester should almost always be avoided. The possibility that a woman of childbearing potential may be pregnant at the time of institution of therapy should be considered. Patients should be advised that if they become pregnant during therapy or intend to become pregnant they should communicate with their physicians about the desirability of discontinuing the drug.

In some patients receiving recommended (or higher) doses of XANAX Tablets (alprazolam) for relatively brief periods of time (eg, one week to four months), withdrawal seizures have been reported upon rapid decrease of dosage or abrupt discontinuation. Therefore, the dosage of XANAX should be reduced or discontinued gradually (see DRUG ABUSE AND DEPENDENCE and DOSAGE AND ADMINISTRATION.)

PRECAUTIONS

General: If XANAX Tablets are to be combined with other psychotropic agents or anticonvulsant drugs, careful consideration should be given to the pharmacology of the agents to be employed, particularly with compounds which might potentiate the action of benzodiazepines (See Drug Interactions).

As with other psychotropic medications, the usual precautions with respect to administration of the drug and size of the prescription are indicated for severely depressed patients or those in whom there is reason to expect concealed suicidal ideation or plans.

In elderly and debilitated patients, it is recommended that the dosage be limited to the smallest effective dose to preclude the development of ataxia or oversedation (See Dosage and Administration Section). The usual precautions in treating patients with impaired renal or hepatic function should be observed.

Episodes of hypomania and mania have been reported in association with the use of XANAX in patients with depression.

Information for Patients: To assure safe and effective use of benzodiazepines, the following information and instructions should be given to patients:

1. Inform your physician about any alcohol consumption and medicine you are taking now, including drugs you may buy without a prescription. Alcohol should generally not be used during treatment with benzodiazepines.

2. Not recommended for use in pregnancy. Therefore, inform your physician if you are pregnant, if you are planning to have a child, or if you become pregnant while you are taking this medication.

3. Inform your physician if you are nursing.

4. Until you experience how this medication affects you, do not drive a car or operate potentially dangerous machinery, etc.

5. If benzodiazepines are used in large doses and/or for extended periods of time, they may produce habituation and emotional and physical dependence. Therefore, do not increase the dose even if you think the drug "does not work anymore" without consulting your physician.

6 Do not stop taking the drug abruptly without consulting your physician, since withdrawal symptoms can occur.

Laboratory Tests: Laboratory tests are not ordinarily required in otherwise healthy patients.

Drug interactions: The benzodiazepines, including alprazolam, produce additive CNS depressant effects when co-administered with other psychotropic medications, anticonvulsants, anti-histaminics, ethanol and other drugs which themselves produce CNS depression.

The steady state plasma concentrations of imipramine and desipramine have been reported to be increased an average of 31% and 20%, respectively, by the concomitant administration of XANAX Tablets in doses up to 4 mg/day. The clinical significance of these changes is unknown.

Pharmacokinetic interactions of benzodiazepines with other drugs have been reported. For example, the clearance of alprazolam and certain other benzodiazepines can be delayed by the co-administration of cimetidine. The clinical significance of this is unclear.

Drug/Laboratory Test Interactions: Although interactions between benzodiazepines and commonly employed clinical laboratory tests have occasionally been reported, there is no consistent pattern for a specific drug or specific test.

Carcinogenesis, Mutagenesis, Impairment of Fertility: No evidence of carcinogenic potential was observed in rats during a 24-month study with alprazolam in doses up to 375 times the human dose.

Alprazolam was not mutagenic in the rat micronucleus test at doses up to 1250 times the human dose.

Alprazolam produced no impairment of fertility in rats at doses up to 62.5 times the human dose.

Pregnancy: Teratogenic Effects: Pregnancy Category D: (See Warnings Section)

Nonteratogenic Effects: It should be considered that the child born of a mother who is receiving benzodiazepines may be at some risk for withdrawal symptoms from the drug during the postnatal period. Also, neonatal flaccidity and respiratory problems have been reported in children born of mothers who have been receiving benzodiazepines.

Labor and Delivery: XANAX has no established use in labor or delivery.

Nursing Mothers: Benzodiazepines are known to be excreted in human milk. It should be assumed that alprazolam is as well. Chronic administration of diazepam to nursing mothers has been reported to cause their infants to become lethargic and to lose weight. As a general rule, nursing should not be undertaken by mothers who must use XANAX.

Pediatric Use: Safety and effectiveness in children below the age of 18 years have not been established.

ADVERSE REACTIONS

Side effects to XANAX Tablets (alprazolam), if they occur are generally observed at the beginning of therapy and usually disappear upon continued medication. In the usual patient, the most frequent side effects are likely to be an extension of the pharmacological activity of alprazolam, eg, drowsiness or lightheadedness.

The figures cited below are estimates of untoward clinical event incidence among subjects who participated in the relatively short duration (ie, four weeks) placebo-controlled clinical trials of XANAX. The figures cannot be used to predict precisely the incidence of untoward events in the course of usual medical practice where patient characteristics, and other factors often differ from those in clinical trials. These figures cannot be compared with those obtained from other clinical studies involving related drug products and placebo as each group of drug trials are conducted under a different set of conditions.

Comparison of the cited figures, however, can provide the prescriber with some basis for estimating the relative contributions of drug and non-drug factors to the untoward event incidence in the population studied. Even this use must be approached cautiously, as a drug may relieve a symptom in one patient but induce it in others. [For example, an anxiolytic drug may relieve dry mouth (a symptom of anxiety) in some subjects but induce it (an untoward event) in others.] Additionally, the cited figures can provide the prescriber with an indication as to the frequency with which physician intervention (eg increased surveillance, decreased dosage or discontinuation of drug therapy) may be necessary because of the untoward clinical event.

[See table on next page].

There have also been reports of withdrawal seizures upon rapid decrease or abrupt discontinuation of XANAX Tablets (See PRECAUTIONS—General).

In addition to the relatively common (i.e., greater than 1%) untoward events enumerated above, the following adverse events have been reported in association with the use of benzodiazepines: dystonia, irritability, concentration difficulties, anorexia, transient amnesia or memory impairment,

Continued on next page

Information on these Upjohn products is based on labeling in effect September 1, 1989. Further information concerning these and other Upjohn products may be obtained by direct inquiry to Medical Information, The Upjohn Company, Kalamazoo, Michigan 49001.

Upjohn—Cont.

loss of coordination, fatigue, seizures, sedation, slurred speech, jaundice, musculoskeletal weakness, pruritus, diplopia, dysarthria, changes in libido, menstrual irregularities, incontinence and urinary retention.

As with all benzodiazepines, paradoxical reactions such as stimulation, agitation, rage, increased muscle spasticity, sleep disturbances, hallucinations and other adverse behavioral effects may occur in rare instances and in a random fashion. Should these occur, use of the drug should be discontinued.

Laboratory analyses were performed on all patients participating in the clinical program for XANAX. The following incidences of abnormalities shown below were observed in patients receiving XANAX and in patients in the corresponding placebo group. None of these changes were considered to be of physiological significance.

	XANAX		Placebo	
	Low	High	Low	High
Hematology				
Hematocrit	*	*	*	*
Hemoglobin	*	*	*	*
Total WBC Count	1.4	2.3	1.0	2.0
Neutrophil Count	2.3	3.0	4.2	1.7
Lymphocyte Count	5.5	7.4	5.4	9.5
Monocyte Count	5.3	2.8	6.4	*
Eosinophil Count	3.2	9.5	3.3	7.2
Basophil Count	*	*	*	*
Urinalysis				
Albumin	—	*	—	*
Sugar	—	*	—	*
RBC/HPF	—	3.4	—	5.0
WBC/HPF	—	25.7	—	25.9
Blood Chemistry				
Creatinine	2.2	1.9	3.5	1.0
Bilirubin	*	1.6	*	*
SGOT	*	3.2	1.0	1.8
Alkaline Phosphatase	*	1.7	*	1.8

* Less than 1%

XANAX

	Treatment Symptom XANAX	Emergent Incidence Placebo	Incidence of Intervention Because of Symptoms XANAX
Number of Patients	565	505	565
% of Patients Reporting:			
Central Nervous System			
Drowsiness	41.0	21.6	15.1
Light-headedness	20.8	19.3	1.2
Depression	13.9	18.1	2.4
Headache	12.9	19.6	1.1
Confusion	9.9	10.0	0.9
Insomnia	8.9	18.4	1.3
Nervousness	4.1	10.3	1.1
Syncope	3.1	4.0	*
Dizziness	1.8	0.8	2.5
Akathisia	1.6	1.2	*
Tiredness/Sleepiness	*	*	1.8
Gastrointestinal			
Dry Mouth	14.7	13.3	0.7
Constipation	10.4	11.4	0.9
Diarrhea	10.1	10.3	1.2
Nausea/Vomiting	9.6	12.8	1.7
Increased Salivation	4.2	2.4	*
Cardiovascular			
Tachycardia/Palpitations	7.7	15.6	0.4
Hypotension	4.7	2.2	*
Sensory			
Blurred Vision	6.2	6.2	0.4
Musculoskeletal			
Rigidity	4.2	5.3	*
Tremor	4.0	8.8	0.4
Cutaneous			
Dermatitis/Allergy	3.8	3.1	0.6
Other			
Nasal Congestion	7.3	9.3	*
Weight Gain	2.7	2.7	*
Weight Loss	2.3	3.0	*

* None reported

When treatment with XANAX is protracted, periodic blood counts, urinalysis and blood chemistry analyses are advisable.

Minor changes in EEG patterns, usually low-voltage fast activity have been observed in patients during therapy with XANAX and are of no known significance.

Post Introduction Reports: Various adverse drug reactions have been reported in association with the use of XANAX since market introduction. The majority of these reactions were reported through the medical event voluntary reporting system. Because of the spontaneous nature of the reporting of medical events and the lack of controls, a causal relationship to the use of XANAX cannot be readily determined. Reported events include: liver enzyme elevations, gynecomastia and galactorrhea.

DRUG ABUSE AND DEPENDENCE

Physical and Psychological Dependence: Withdrawal symptoms (similar in character to those noted with barbiturates and alcohol) have occurred following abrupt discontinuance of benzodiazepines. (These can range from mild dysphoria and insomnia to a major syndrome which may include abdominal and muscle cramps, vomiting, sweating, tremor and convulsions). In addition, withdrawal seizures have occurred upon rapid decrease or abrupt discontinuation of therapy with XANAX Tablets (See PRECAUTIONS—General). It is recommended that all patients on XANAX who require a dosage reduction be gradually tapered under close supervision (See DOSAGE AND ADMINISTRATION).

Patients with a history of seizures or epilepsy, regardless of their concomitant anti-seizure drug therapy, should not be abruptly withdrawn from any CNS depressant agent, including XANAX Tablets (alprazolam). If benzodiazepines are used in large doses and/or for extended periods of time, they may produce psychological and physical dependence. Addiction-prone individuals (such as drug addicts or alcoholics) should be under careful surveillance when receiving alprazolam or other psychotropic agents because of the predisposition of such patients to habituation and dependence.

Controlled Substance Class:
XANAX is a controlled substance under the Controlled Substance Act by the Drug Enforcement Administration and has been assigned to Schedule IV.

OVERDOSAGE

Manifestations of alprazolam overdosage include somnolence, confusion, impaired coordination, diminished reflexes and coma.

The acute oral LD_{50} in rats is 331–2171 mg/kg. Other experiments in animals have indicated that cardiopulmonary collapse can occur following massive intravenous doses of alprazolam (over 195 mg/kg; 2000 times the maximum usual daily human dose). Animals could be resuscitated with positive mechanical ventilation and the intravenous infusion of levarterenol.

Animal experiments have suggested that forced diuresis or hemodialysis are probably of little value in treating overdosage.

General Treatment of Overdose: Overdosage reports with XANAX are limited. As in all cases of drug overdosage, respiration, pulse rate, and blood pressure should be monitored. General supportive measures should be employed, along with immediate gastric lavage. Intravenous fluids should be administered and an adequate airway maintained. If hypotension occurs, it may be combated by the use of vasopressors. Dialysis is of limited value. As with the management of intentional overdosing with any drug, it should be borne in mind that multiple agents may have been ingested.

DOSAGE AND ADMINISTRATION

Dosage should be individualized for maximum beneficial effect. While the usual daily dosages given below will meet the needs of most patients, there will be some who require higher doses. In such cases, dosage should be increased cautiously to avoid adverse effects. Dosage should be reduced gradually when discontinuing therapy or decreasing the daily dose. It is suggested that the daily dosage be decreased no more than 0.5 milligram every three days.

DAILY DOSAGE SCHEDULE

The usual starting dose is 0.25 to 0.5 mg, given three times daily. This dose may then be titrated according to the needs of the patient to a maximum total daily dose of 4 mg, given in divided doses.

In the elderly, or in the presence of debilitating disease, the usual starting dose is 0.25 mg, given two or three times daily. This may be gradually increased if needed and tolerated. If side effects occur with the starting dose, the dose should be lowered.

HOW SUPPLIED

XANAX Tablets (alprazolam), ovoid-shaped and scored, are available as follows:

0.25 mg (white)
Bottles of 30 **NDC** 00009-0029-17
Bottles of 90 **NDC** 00009-0029-03
Bottles of 100 **NDC** 0009-0029-01
Unit-Dose Pkg (100) **NDC** 0009-0029-09
VISIPAK® Reverse Numbered Pack (100) **NDC** 0009-0029-20
Bottles of 500 **NDC** 0009-0029-02

0.5 mg (peach)
Bottles of 30 **NDC** 0009-0055-18
Bottles of 90 **NDC** 0009-0055-04
Bottles of 100 **NDC** 0009-0055-01
Unit-Dose Pkg (100) **NDC** 0009-0055-02
VISIPAK® Reverse Numbered Pack (100) **NDC** 0009-0055-22
Bottles of 500 **NDC** 0009-0055-03

1 mg (lavender)
Bottles of 30 **NDC** 0009-0090-15
Bottles of 90 **NDC** 0009-0090-27
Bottles of 100 **NDC** 0009-0090-01
Unit-Dose Pkg (100) **NDC** 0009-0090-02
VISIPAK® Reverse Numbered Pack (100) **NDC** 0009-0090-17
Bottles of 500 **NDC** 0009-0090-04

Store at controlled room temperature 15°–30°C (59°–86°F).
Caution: Federal law prohibits dispensing without prescription.

ANIMAL STUDIES

When rats were treated with alprazolam at 3, 10, and 30 mg/kg/day (37.5 to 375 times the maximum recommended human dose) orally for 2 years, a tendency for a dose related increase in the number of cataracts was observed in females and a tendency for a dose related increase in corneal vascularization was observed in males. These lesions did not appear until after 11 months of treatment.

CLINICAL STUDIES

XANAX Tablets (alprazolam) were compared to placebo in double blind clinical trials in patients with a diagnosis of anxiety or anxiety with associated depressive symptomatology. XANAX was significantly better than placebo at each of the evaluation periods of these four week studies as judged by the following psychometric instruments: Physician's

Global Impressions, Hamilton Anxiety Rating Scale Target Symptoms, Patient's Global Impressions and Self-Rating Symptom Scale.
Code 811 557 416

Shown in Product Identification Section, page 434

Upsher-Smith Laboratories, Inc.
14905 23RD AVE., NORTH
MINNEAPOLIS, MN 55447

ACETAMINOPHEN UNISERTS®   OTC
[u'ni"sertz]
Rectal Suppositories

DESCRIPTION
Acetaminophen Uniserts suppositories are supplied in 120 mg. (pediatric), 325 mg. and 650 mg. strengths. Acetaminophen Uniserts are unit dose labeled.

INDICATIONS
For the temporary relief of fever, minor aches, pains and headaches.

DOSAGE
Adults—One 650 mg. suppository every 4 to 6 hours. No more than a total of 6 suppositories in any 24-hour period. Children (over 6)—One 325 mg. suppository every 4 to 6 hours. No more than a total of 8 suppositories in any 24-hour period.
Children (3 to 6)—One 120 mg. (pediatric) suppository every 4 to 6 hours. No more than a total of 6 suppositories in any 24-hour period. Children (under 3)—Consult a physician.

WARNING
Severe or recurrent pain or high or continued fever may be indicative of serious illness. Under these conditions, consult a physician. Do not use consistently for more than 2 days except on the advice of a physician. As with any drug, if you are pregnant or nursing a baby, seek the advice of a health professional before using this product.

HOW SUPPLIED
120 mg. 12's	NDC 0245-0121-12
120 mg. 50's	NDC 0245-0121-50
325 mg. 12's	NDC 0245-0123-12
325 mg. 50's	NDC 0245-0123-50
650 mg. 12's	NDC 0245-0122-12
650 mg. 50's	NDC 0245-0122-50
650 mg. 500's	NDC 0245-0122-05

CONDOM MATE® Lubricant   OTC
[cŏn'dŏm-māt]

List No.: 0245-0119-12

FEVERNOL™   OTC
[fĕ'ver-nol]
Acetaminophen Suppositories
120 mg Pediatric (Children's Strength)
325 mg Junior Strength

List No.: 0245-0116-06 (120 mg)
List No.: 0245-0117-06 (325 mg)

HOW SUPPLIED
Fevernol™ Suppositories are available in packages of 6 suppositories.

KLOR–CON® Powder   ℞
[klōr'kon]
Potassium Chloride for Oral Solution, USP
20 mEq. (1.5g) per packet

DESCRIPTION
Each packet contains 1.5g potassium chloride providing potassium 20 mEq and chloride 20 mEq. Fruit-flavored with artificial color and sweetener (saccharin) added.

HOW SUPPLIED
KLOR-CON Powder 20 mEq (1.5g Potassium Chloride). In cartons of 30 and 100 packets.
30's NDC 0245-0035-30, 100's NDC 0245-0035-01

KLOR–CON®/25 Powder   ℞
[klōr'kon]
Potassium Chloride for Oral Solution, USP
25 mEq. (1.875 g) per packet

DESCRIPTION
Each packet contains 1.875 g potassium chloride providing potassium 25 mEq. and chloride 25 mEq. Fruit-flavored with artificial color and sweetener (saccharin) added.

HOW SUPPLIED
Cartons of 30, 100 and 250 packets.
30's NDC 0245-0037-30, 100's NDC 0245-0037-01
250's NDC 0245-0037-25

KLOR–CON® 8/KLOR–CON® 10   ℞
[klōr'kon]
Potassium Chloride
Extended–release tablets, USP
8 mEq and 10 mEq

DESCRIPTION
KLOR-CON® Extended-release Tablets, U.S.P. are solid oral dosage form of potassium chloride. Each contains 600 mg or 750 mg of potassium chloride equivalent to 8mEq or 10 mEq of potassium in a wax matrix tablet. This formulation is intended to slow the release of potassium so that the likelihood of a high localized concentration of potassium chloride within the gastrointestinal tract is reduced.
Klor-Con® Extended-release Tablets are an electrolyte replenisher. The chemical name is potassium chloride, and the structural formula is KCl. Potassium chloride USP occurs as a white, granular powder or as colorless crystals. It is odorless and has a saline taste. Its solutions are neutral to litmus. It is freely soluble in water and insoluble in alcohol.
Inactive Ingredients: Castor oil, hydroxypropyl methylcellulose 2910, magnesium stearate, polyethylene glycol 3350, propylene glycol, synthetic iron oxide, titanium dioxide, and other ingredients. Yellow tablets also contain FD& C Yellow No. 10 aluminum lake and FD & C Yellow No. 6 aluminum lake. Blue tablets also contain FD & C Blue No. 1 aluminum lake.

CLINICAL PHARMACOLOGY
The potassium ion is the principal intracellular cation of most body tissues. Potassium ions participate in a number of essential physiological processes, including the maintenance of intracellular tonicity, the transmission of nerve impulses, the contraction of cardiac, skeletal, and smooth muscle, and the maintenance of normal renal function.
The intracellular concentration of potassium is approximately 150 to 160 mEq per liter. The normal adult plasma concentration is 3.5 to 5 mEq per liter. An active ion transport system maintains this gradient across the plasma membrane.
Potassium is a normal dietary constituent and under steady state conditions the amount of potassium absorbed from the gastrointestinal tract is equal to the amount excreted in the urine. The usual dietary intake of potassium is 50 to 100 mEq per day.
Potassium depletion will occur whenever the rate of potassium loss through renal excretion and/or loss from the gastrointestinal tract exceeds the rate of potassium intake. Such depletion usually develops as a consequence of therapy with diuretics, primary or secondary hyperaldosteronism, diabetic ketoacidosis, or inadequate replacement of potassium in patients on prolonged parenteral nutrition. Depletion can develop rapidly with severe diarrhea, especially if associated with vomiting. Potassium depletion due to these causes is usually accompanied by a concomitant loss of chloride and is manifested by hypokalemia and metabolic alkalosis. Potassium depletion may produce weakness, fatigue, disturbances of cardiac rhythm (primarily ectopic beats), prominent U-waves in the electrocardiogram, and, in advanced cases, flaccid paralysis and/or impaired ability to concentrate urine.
If potassium depletion associated with metabolic alkalosis cannot be managed by correcting the fundamental causes of the deficiency, e.g., where the patient requires long term diuretic therapy, supplemental potassium in the form of high potassium food or potassium chloride may be able to restore normal potassium levels.
In rare circumstances (e.g., patients with renal tubular acidosis) potassium depletion may be associated with metabolic acidosis and hyperchloremia. In such patients potassium replacement should be accomplished with potassium salts other than the chloride, such as potassium bicarbonate, potassium citrate, potassium acetate, or potassium gluconate.

INDICATIONS AND USAGE
BECAUSE OF REPORTS OF INTESTINAL AND GASTRIC ULCERATION AND BLEEDING WITH CONTROLLED RELEASE POTASSIUM CHLORIDE PREPARATIONS, THESE DRUGS SHOULD BE RESERVED FOR THOSE PATIENTS WHO CANNOT TOLERATE OR REFUSE TO TAKE LIQUIDS OR EFFERVESCENT POTASSIUM PREPARATIONS OR FOR PATIENTS IN WHOM THERE IS A PROBLEM OF COMPLIANCE WITH THESE PREPARATIONS.
1. For the treatment of patients with hypokalemia with or without metabolic alkalosis; in digitalis intoxication and patients with hypokalemic familial periodic paralysis. If hypokalemia is the result of diuretic therapy, consideration should be given to the use of a lower dose of diuretic, which may be sufficient without leading to hypokalemia.

---

2. For the prevention of hypokalemia in patients who would be at particular risk if hypokalemia were to develop, e.g., digitalized patients or patients with significant cardiac arrhythmias.
The use of potassium salts in patients receiving diuretics for uncomplicated essential hypertension is often unnecessary when such patients have a normal dietary pattern and when low doses of the diuretic are used. Serum potassium should be checked periodically, however, and, if hypokalemia occurs, dietary supplementation with potassium-containing foods may be adequate to control milder cases. In more severe cases, and if dose adjustment of the diuretic is ineffective or unwarranted, supplementation with potassium salts may be indicated.

CONTRAINDICATIONS
Potassium supplements are contraindicated in patients with hyperkalemia since a further increase in serum potassium concentration is such patients can produce cardiac arrest. Hyperkalemia may complicate any of the following conditions: chronic renal failure, systemic acidosis such as diabetic acidosis, acute dehydration, extensive tissue breakdown as in severe burns, adrenal insufficiency, or the administration of a potassium-sparing diuretic (e.g., spironolactone, triamterene or amiloride) (see OVERDOSAGE).
Controlled release formulations of potassium chloride have produced esophageal ulceration in certain cardiac patients with esophageal compression due to an enlarged left atrium. Potassium supplementation, when indicated in such patients, should be given as a liquid preparation.
All solid oral dosage forms of potassium chloride are contraindicated in any patients in whom there is structural, pathological (e.g., diabetic gastroparesis) or pharmacologic (use of anticholinergic agents or other agents with anticholinergic properties at sufficient doses to exert anticholinergic effects) cause for arrest or delay in tablet passage through the gastrointestinal tract.

WARNINGS
Hyperkalemia (see Overdosage):
In patients with impaired mechanisms for excreting potassium, the administration of potassium salts can produce hyperkalemia and cardiac arrest. This occurs most commonly in patients given potassium by the intravenous route but may also occur in patients given potassium orally. Potentially fatal hyperkalemia can develop rapidly and be asymptomatic. The use of potassium salts in patients with chronic renal disease, or any other condition which impairs potassium excretion, requires particularly careful monitoring of the serum potassium concentration and appropriate dosage adjustment.
Interaction with Potassium-Sparing Diuretics:
Hypokalemia should not be treated by the concomitant administration of potassium salts and a potassium-sparing diuretic (e.g., spironolactone, triamterene, or amiloride), since the simultaneous administration of these agents can produce severe hyperkalemia.
Interaction with Angiotensin Converting Enzyme Inhibitors:
Angiotensin coverting enzyme (ACE) inhibitors (e.g., captopril, enalapril) will produce some potassium retention by inhibiting aldosterone production). Potassium supplements should be given to patients receiving ACE inhibitors only with close monitoring.
Gastrointestinal Lesions: Solid oral dosage forms of potassium chloride can produce ulcerative and/or stenotic lesions of the gastrointestinal tract. Based on spontaneous adverse reaction reports, enteric coated preparations of potassium chloride are associated with an increased frequency of small bowel lesions (40–50 per 100,000 patient years) compared to sustained release wax matrix formulations (less than one per 100,000 patient years). Because of the lack of extensive marketing experience with microencapsulated products, a comparison between such products and wax matrix or enteric coated products is not available. KlorCon® Extended-release Tablets are wax matrix tablets formulated to provide a controlled rate of release of potassium chloride and thus to minimize the possibility of high local concentration of potassium near the gastrointestinal wall.
Prospective trials have been conducted in normal human volunteers in which the upper gastrointestinal tract was evaluated by endoscopic inspection before and after one week of solid oral potassium chloride therapy. The ability of this model to predict events occurring in usual clinical practice is unknown. Trials which approximated usual clinical practice did not reveal any clear differences between the wax matrix and microencapsulated dosage forms. In contrast, there was a higher incidence of gastric and duodenal lesions in subjects receiving a high dose of a wax matrix controlled release formulation under conditions which did not resemble usual or recommended clinical practice (i.e., 96 mEq per day in divided doses of potassium chloride administered to fasted patients, in the presence of an anticholinergic drug to delay gastric emptying). The upper gastrointestinal lesions observed by endoscopy were asymptomatic and were not ac-

Continued on next page

Upsher-Smith—Cont.

companied by evidence of bleeding (hemoccult testing). The relevance of these findings to the usual conditions (i.e., non-fasting, no anticholinergic agent, smaller doses) under which controlled release potassium chloride products are used is uncertain; epidemiologic studies have not identified an elevated risk, compared to microencapsulated products, for upper gastrointestinal lesions in patients receiving wax matrix formulations. Klor-Con® Extended-release Tablets should be discontinued immediately and the possibility of ulceration, obstruction, or perforation considered if severe vomiting, abdominal pain, distention, or gastrointestinal bleeding occurs.

Metabolic Acidosis:
Hypokalemia in patients with metabolic acidosis should be treated with an alkalinizing potassium salt such as potassium bicarbonate, potassium citrate, or potassium acetate, or potassium gluconate.

PRECAUTIONS

General: The diagnosis of potassium depletion is ordinarily made by demonstrating hypokalemia in a patient with a clinical history suggesting some cause for potassium depletion. In interpreting the serum potassium level, the physician should bear in mind that acute alkalosis per se can produce hypokalemia in the absence of a deficit in total body potassium, while acute acidosis per se can increase the serum potassium concentration into the normal range even in the presence of a reduced total body potassium. The treatment of potassium depletion, particularly in the presence of cardiac disease, renal disease, or acidosis, requires careful attention to acid-base balance and appropriate monitoring of serum electrolytes, the electrocardiogram, and the clinical status of the patient.

Information for Patients: Physicians should consider reminding the patient of the following:
To take each dose without crushing, chewing or sucking the tablets.
To take each dose with meals and with a full glass of water or other liquid.
To take this medicine following the frequency and amount prescribed by the physician. This is especially important if the patient is also taking diuretics and/or digitalis preparations.
To check with the physician if there is trouble swallowing the tablets or if the tablets seem to stick in the throat.
To check with the physician at once if tarry stools or other evidence of gastrointestinal bleeding is noticed.
To be aware that the expended matrix is not absorbed and may be excreted intact in the stool.

Laboratory Tests: When blood is drawn for analysis of plasma potassium it is important to recognize that artifactual elevations can occur after improper venipuncture technique or as a result of in vitro hemolysis of the sample.

Drug Interactions: Potassium-sparing diuretic, angiotensin converting enzyme inhibitors: see WARNINGS.

Carcinogenesis, Mutagenesis, Impairment of Fertility: Carcinogenicity, mutagenicity, and fertility studies in animals have not been performed. Potassium is a normal dietary constituent.

Pregnancy Catetory C: Animal reproduction studies have not been conducted with Klor-Con® Extended-release Tablets. It is unlikely that potassium supplementation that does not lead to hyperkalemia would have an adverse effect on the fetus or would affect reproductive capacity.

Nursing Mothers: The normal potassium ion content of human milk is about 13 mEq per liter. Since oral potassium becomes part of the body potassium pool, so long as body potassium is not excessive, the contribution of potassium chloride supplementation should have little or no effect on the level in human milk.

Pediatric Use: Safety and effectiveness in children have not been established.

ADVERSE REACTIONS

One of the most severe adverse effects is hyperkalemia (see CONTRAINDICATIONS, WARNINGS, and OVERDOSAGE). There also have been reports of upper and lower gastrointestinal conditions including obstruction, bleeding, ulceration, and perforation (see CONTRAINDICATIONS and WARNINGS).
The most common adverse reactions to the oral potassium salts are nausea, vomiting, abdominal pain/discomfort, and diarrhea. These symptoms are due to irritation of the gastrointestinal tract and are best managed by diluting the preparation further, taking the dose with meals, or reducing the amount taken at one time.

OVERDOSAGE

The administration of oral potassium salts to persons with normal excretory mechanisms for potassium rarely causes serious hyperkalemia. However, if excretory mechanisms are impaired, or if potassium is administered too rapidly intravenously, potentially fatal hyperkalemia can result (see CONTRAINDICATIONS and WARNINGS). It is important

---

to recognize that hyperkalemia is usually asymptomatic and may be manifested only by an increased serum potassium concentration 6.5–8.0 mEq/L) and characteristic electrocardiographic changes (peaking of T-waves, loss of P-wave, depression of S-T segment, and prolongation of the QT interval). Late manifestations include muscle paralysis and cardiovascular collapse from cardiac arrest (9–12 mEq./L).

Treatment measures for hyperkalemia include the following:

1. Elimination of foods and medications containing potassium and of any agents with potassium-sparing diuretics;
2. Intravenous administration of 300 to 500 ml/hr of 10% dextrose solution containing 10–20 units of crystalline insulin per 1,000 ml;
3. Correction of acidosis, if present, with intravenous sodium bicarbonate;
4. Use of exchange resins, hemodialysis, or peritoneal dialysis.

In treating hyperkalemia, it should be recalled that in patients who have been stabilized on digitalis, too rapid a lowering of the serum potassium concentration can produce digitalis toxicity.

DOSAGE AND ADMINISTRATION

The usual dietary potassium intake by the average adult is 50 to 100 mEq per day. Potassium depletion sufficient to cause hypokalemia usually requires the loss of 200 or more mEq of potassium from the total body store.
Dosage must be adjusted to the individual needs of each patient. The dose for the prevention of hypokalemia is typically in the range of 20 mEq per day. Doses of 40–100 mEq per day or more are used for the treatment of potassium depletion. Dosage should be divided if more than 20 mEq per day is given such that no more than 20 mEq is given in a single dose.
Each Klor-Con® Extended-release Tablet provides 8 mEq or 10 mEq of potassium chloride.
Klor-Con® Extended-release Tablets should be taken with meals and with a glass of water or other liquid. This product should not be taken on an empty stomach because of its potential for gastric irritation (see WARNINGS).
NOTE: Klor-Con® Extended-release Tablets must be swallowed whole. Take each dose without crushing, chewing or sucking the tablets.

HOW SUPPLIED

Film Coated, Klor-Con® 8 (blue), Klor-Con® 10 (yellow), imprinted round tablets containing:
  600 mg potassium chloride (equivalent to 8 mEq) in bottles of 100 (NDC 0245-0040-11), bottles of 500 (NDC 0245-0040-15), and unit-dose packages of 100 (NDC 0245-0040-01);
  750 mg potassium chloride (equivalent to 10 mEq) in bottles of 100 (NDC 0245-0041-11), bottles of 500 (NDC 0245-0041-15), and unit-dose packages of 100 (NDC 0245-0041-01).
Protect from light and moisture. Store at controlled room temperature 59°–86°F (15°–30°C). Dispense in container with child resistant closure.
Shown in Product Identification Section, page 434

KLOR-CON®/EF 25mEq   ℞
[klōr 'kon]
Potassium Bicarbonate Effervescent Tablets for Oral Solution, USP

DESCRIPTION

Each effervescent tablet in solution provides 25 mEq (978 mg) potassium as bicarbonate and citrate. KLOR-CON®/EF tablets are sugar free and orange flavored.

HOW SUPPLIED

KLOR-CON®/EF 25 mEq effervescent tablets in cartons of 30 and 100 individually wrapped tablets.
30's NDC 0245-0039-30, 100's NDC 0245-0039-01

LUBRIN® Vaginal Lubricating Inserts
[lu 'brin]

List No. 0245-0118-19

DESCRIPTION

Vaginal dryness can occur due to a variety of reasons including: menopause, stress, medication use or even after the use of a tampon. Lubrin® Inserts are the first premeasured, easy-to-use inserts specifically designed for vaginal dryness. Lubrin® Inserts are unscented, colorless, water-soluble inserts that provide long lasting lubrication. Lubrin Inserts quickly liquefy within the vagina to simulate natural lubrication for several hours.
Please see enclosed circular for complete instructions.

HOW SUPPLIED

Lubrin Inserts are available in packages of six inserts.

RMS® Suppositories   Ⓒ ℞
Rectal Morphine Sulfate

WARNING—MAY BE HABIT FORMING

DESCRIPTION

Suppositories contain 5, 10, 20, or 30 mg of morphine sulfate.

HOW SUPPLIED

RMS® suppositories are individually sealed and unit dose labeled. 12 suppositories per carton.
 5 mg   NDC 0245-0160-12, 10 mg NDC 0245-0161-12
20 mg   NDC 0245-0162-12, 30 mg NDC 0245-0163-12

SSKI®   ℞
Potassium Iodide Oral Solution, U.S.P.

DESCRIPTION

SSKI® (potassium iodide oral solution, U.S.P.) is a saturated solution of potassium iodide containing 1 g of potassium iodide per ml.

HOW SUPPLIED

SSKI® (potassium iodide oral solution, U.S.P.) is supplied in 1 fluid ounce (30 ml) bottles (NDC 0245-0003-31) with a calibrated dropper marked to deliver 0.3 ml and 0.6 ml; and 8 fluid ounces (237 ml) bottles (NDC 0245-0003-08).

SALSITAB®   ℞
[sal 'si "tab]
(salsalate)
Tablets

DESCRIPTION

Salsitab® (salsalate) is a nonsteroidal anti-inflammatory agent for oral administration.
Each round, blue, film coated Salsitab® tablet contains 500 mg salsalate. Each capsule-shaped, blue, scored, film coated Salsitab® tablet contains 750 mg salsalate.

HOW SUPPLIED

500 mg tablets in bottles of 100 (NDC 0245-0153-11)
500 mg tablets in bottles of 500 (NDC 0245-0153-15)
500 mg tablets in cartons of 100 unit dose (NDC 0245-0153-01)
750 mg tablets in bottles of 100 (NDC 0245-0154-11)
750 mg tablets in bottles of 500 (NDC 0245-0154-15)
750 mg tablets in cartons of 100 unit dose (NDC 0245-0154-01)

SLO–NIACIN®   OTC
[slō "nī '-a-sin]
Controlled-Release Niacin Tablets
(Nicotinic Acid)
250, 500, and 750 mg

DESCRIPTION

Each Slo-Niacin® Controlled-Release Tablet contains 250, 500, or 750 mg of niacin (nicotinic acid, vitamin B_3). Slo-Niacin® Tablets slowly release niacin over several hours.

USES

Slo-Niacin® Tablets are used in all those conditions in which niacin supplementation is indicated. It has the advantage of a slower release of niacin than conventional tablet dosage forms. This may permit its use by those who do not tolerate immediate-release tablets.

CAUTIONS

Slo-Niacin® Tablets should not be used by persons with a known sensitivity to niacin (nicotinic acid, vitamin B_3) and by persons with arterial bleeding, glaucoma, severe diabetes, impaired liver function, peptic ulcer, or by pregnant women.

SIDE EFFECTS

Temporary flushing and feeling of warmth may be expected. These seldom reach levels so as to necessitate discontinuance. If these symptoms persist, discontinue use and consult a physician. Temporary headache, itching and tingling, gastric disturbances, skin rash, and allergies may occur.

DOSAGE

Usual adult dose—One Slo-Niacin® Tablet morning and evening or as directed by physician.
NOTE: Slo-Niacin® Tablets may be broken on the score line but should not be crushed or chewed.

TROFAN®
[tro'fan]
L–Tryptophan Tablets, 0.5 Gm.

COMPOSITION
Each capsule shaped tablet contains L-tryptophan, 0.5 Gm.

HOW SUPPLIED
Trofan® tablets 0.5 Gm. in bottles of 30 and 100 and unit dose 100's.
List No.—30's 0245-0095-30, 100's 0245-0095-11, UD 100's 0245-0095-01

TROFAN®–DS
[tro'fan]
L–Tryptophan tablets, 1 gram

COMPOSITION
Each capsule shaped tablet contains L-tryptophan, 1 gram.

HOW SUPPLIED
Trofan® DS tablets 1 gram in bottles of 30 and 100 and unit dose 100.
List No.—30's 0245-0094-30, 100's 0245-0094-11, UD 100's 0245-0094-01

EDUCATIONAL MATERIAL

Brochures
Questions and Answers
Brochure addressing the issue of vaginal dryness and condom usage.
QUESTIONS YOU MIGHT HAVE BEEN AFRAID TO ASK... ABOUT A VERY COMMON PROBLEM
Brochure about vaginal dryness, a problem millions of women suffer from, but seldom talk about.

Vitaline Formulas
722 JEFFERSON AVE
ASHLAND, OR 97520

BIOTIN FORTE
and
Extra Strength 5mg BIOTIN FORTE

Medical Food Products for physicians who want their patients supplemented with high potency biotin and folic acid.

BIOTIN FORTE

Each Tablet Provides:

BIOTIN	3000 mcg (3 mg)
FOLIC ACID	800 mcg
VITAMIN B-1 (thiamine mononitrate)	10 mg
VITAMIN B-2 (riboflavin)	10 mg
NIACINAMIDE	40 mg
PANTOTHENIC ACID	10 mg
VITAMIN B-6 (pyridoxine hydrochloride)	25 mg
VITAMIN B-12 (cyanocobalamine on ion exchange resin)	10 mcg
VITAMIN C (ascorbic acid)	200 mg
ZINC (zinc acetate)	30 mg

Extra Strength—No Zinc
5mg BIOTIN FORTE

Each Tablet Provides:

BIOTIN	(5000 mcg) 5 mg
FOLIC ACID	800 mcg
VITAMIN B-1 (thiamine mononitrate)	10 mg
VITAMIN B-2 (riboflavin)	10 mg
NIACINAMIDE	40 mg
PANTOTHENIC ACID	10 mg
VITAMIN B-6 (pyridoxine hydrochloride)	25 mg
VITAMIN B-12 (cyanocobalamine on ion exchange resin)	10 mcg
VITAMIN C (ascorbic acid)	100 mg

Biotin Forte is a medical food product for use only under medical supervision to meet nutritional requirements in specific medical conditions.

DOSAGE AND ADMINISTRATION
Adults and children as directed by physician or Registered Dietician.

SIDE EFFECTS
None reported

HOW SUPPLIED
Biotin Forte—yellow coated tablets in bottles of 60 NDC 54022-1098-01 and 1000 NDC 54022-1098-02. Extra Strength 5mg Biotin Forte—light green coated tablets in bottles of 60 NDC 54022-1075-01 and 1000 NDC 54022-1075-02.

LITERATURE AND SAMPLES
On request by physicians or Registered Dieticians.

BORON 6mg (scored tablet)
Boron citrate/aspartate

DESCRIPTION
Each scored tablet contains 6mg elemental boron as 50% B citrate and 50% B aspartate. Boron has been shown to improve the metabolism of calcium and magnesium, increase concentrations of estrogen, assist in the synthesis of vitamin D, reduce urinary excretion of calcium and magnesium and plays a role in the prevention of osteoporosis. Boron appears to play an important role in human nutrition, particularly in relation to bone health.

INDICATIONS
As a source of boron for patients deficient in this essential nutrient.

ADMINISTRATION AND DOSAGE
As a dietary supplement, ½ tablet daily or as directed by physician.

ADVERSE REACTIONS
None Reported

HOW SUPPLIED
6mg (scored tablets) in bottles of 90 NDC 54022-2300-01
6mg (scored tablets) in bottles of 1000 NDC 54022-2300-02

LITERATURE AND SAMPLES
On request by physician

REFERENCES
Nutrition Reviews, Vol 46, Oct. 88
Nutrition Today, Jan./Feb. 88
USDA Agricultural Research Service, Apr. 87
USDA Agricultural Research Service, Apr. 89

COENZYME Q₁₀ (Ubiquinone)
25mg & 60mg

DESCRIPTION
Coenzyme Q_{10} is an essential nutrient that is a cofactor in the mitochondrial electron transport chain, the biochemical pathway in cellular respiration from which ATP and metabolic energy is derived. Since nearly all cellular functions are dependent on energy, Coenzyme Q_{10} is essential for the health of all human tissues and organs. The involvement of Coenzyme Q_{10} as a redox carrier of the respiratory chain is well established on the basis of both reconstitution studies and kinetic evidence.

INDICATIONS
As a source of coenzyme Q_{10} for patients deficient in this essential nutrient.

ADMINISTRATION AND DOSAGE
As a dietary supplement, adults—60mg–180mg daily or as directed by physician.

ADVERSE REACTIONS
None reported.

HOW SUPPLIED
25mg tablets in bottles of 60 NDC 54022-2055-01
60mg tablets in bottles of 30 NDC 54022-2081-01
60mg tablets in bottles of 60 NDC 54022-2080-01

LITERATURE AND SAMPLES
On request by physician.

REFERENCES
Elsevier Science Publishers NY (Biomedical Div.) 1986 Biomedical & Clinical Aspects of Coenzyme Q, Volumes 1–5, K. Folkers and Y. Yamamura, editors.
Coenzyme Q10: A Review Of The Supporting Literature, Kohl, RL, Universities Space Research Association, Div. of Space Biomedicine NASA/Johnson Space Center, Houston, TX 4/7/89

High Lipase
8X PANCREATIN 900mg USP
(non enteric coated)

Each Tablet Provides:

Lipase	22,500 USP Units
Protease	180,000 USP Units
Amylase	180,000 USP Units

Vitaline's 8X Pancreatin 900mg USP (High Lipase) tablets resist gastric inactivation and deliver predictable, high levels of biologically active enzymes into the duodenum. The enzymes catalyze the hydrolysis of fats into glycerol and fatty acids, proteoses and derived substances, and starch into dextrins and sugars. 8X Pancreatin 900mg USP tablets are effective in controlling steatorrhea and its consequences at low daily dosage levels.

Under conditions of the USP test method (in vitro) Vitaline's 8X Pancreatin 900mg USP has the following total digestive capacity:
Each Tablet

Dietary fat, grams	78gm
Dietary protein, grams	180gm
Dietary starch, grams	180gm

INDICATIONS AND USAGE
8X Pancreatin 900mg USP is indicated for patients with exocrine pancreatic enzyme deficiency as in:
* chronic pancreatitis
* pancreatectomy or gastrectomy
* cystic fibrosis

PRECAUTIONS
Use with caution in patients known to be allergic to pork protein.
Vitaline's 8X Pancreatin 900mg USP tablets contain no sugar, corn, wheat, soya, yeast, phenol, salicylates, preservatives or artificial coloring agents.

DOSAGE AND ADMINISTRATION
Usual dosage: One or two tablets during each meal and one tablet with snacks. Occasionally a third tablet with meals may be required depending upon individual requirements for control of steatorrhea.

HOW SUPPLIED
Uncoated tablets in bottles of 90 NDC 54022-1034-01 and 1000 NDC 54022-1034-02.

LITERATURE AVAILABLE
Complete literature available upon request by physician.

TOTAL FORMULA®
(High Potency Multivitamin/Multimineral Supplement with micro-trace elements; Chromium, Selenium and Molybdenum)

DESCRIPTION
TOTAL FORMULA utilizes a unique technique of microspheres within the tablet to protect the delicate nutrients from moisture, air and the incompatibilities of certain minerals. Vitaline's microsphere technique also protects those nutrients that are susceptible to acid hydrolysis.
Each tablet provides:

Vitamins			RDA %
A (Water Soluble, Palmitate)	10,000	I.U.	200%
D-3	400	I.U.	100%
E (d-alpha tocopherol succinate) Water Soluble)	30	I.U.	100%
K (Water Soluble)	70	mcg	70%
C (Ascorbic Acid, from Sago Palm)	100	mg	166%
B-1 (Thiamine)	15	mg	1000%
B-2 (Riboflavin)	15	mg	882%
B-3 (Niacinamide)	25	mg	400%
B-5 (Pantothenic Acid)	25	mg	250%
B-6 (Pyridoxine HCL)	25	mg	1250%
B-12 (on ion exchange resin)	25	mcg	416%
Folic Acid	400	mcg	100%
Biotin	300	mcg	100%
Choline (Bitartrate)	10	mg	**
Hesperidin Complex	10	mg	***
Citrus Bioflavinoids	10	mg	***
Rutin	10	mg	***
Inositol	10	mg	***
PABA (para amino benzoic acid)	8	mg	***

Minerals			
Calcium (oyster shell)	100	mg	10%
Magnesium (chelate)	100	mg	25%
Phosphorus	52	mg	5%
Potassium (chelate)	25	mg	**
Iron (Fumarate)	20	mg	111%
Zinc (Gluconate)	30	mg	200%
Copper (Gluconate)	2	mg	100%
Manganese (Gluconate)	6	mg	**
Iodine (kelp)	100	mcg	66%
Chromium (GTF factor)	500	mcg	**
Selenium (organically bound chelate)	10	mcg	**
Molybdenum (chelate)	100	mcg	**
Silicon (kelp)	2.4	mg	**
Vanadium (chelate)	25	mcg	**

Chlorophyll coloring in coating. *RDA—recommended daily allowance. **Need in human nutrition established, RDA not determined. ***Need in human nutrition not determined.
TOTAL FORMULA contains no yeast, corn, wheat, soya, sugar, phenol, preservatives, dairy products, artificial colors, or added salicylates.

Continued on next page

Vitaline—Cont.

Directions: Adults, 1 tablet daily as a dietary supplement ... children, as directed by physician.

HOW SUPPLIED

Bottles of 90 tablets NDC 54022-1042-01
Bottles of 1000 tablets NDC 54022-1042-02
Literature and Samples: On request by physician.

Wallace Laboratories
P.O. BOX 1001
CRANBURY, NJ 08512

AQUATENSEN®   ℞
(methyclothiazide, USP 5 mg)
Tablets

DESCRIPTION

AQUATENSEN (methyclothiazide), a diuretic-antihypertensive agent, is an analogue of hydrochlorothiazide and a member of the benzothiadiazine (thiazide) family of drugs. Chemically, methyclothiazide is 6-chloro-3-(chloromethyl)-3, 4-dihydro-2-methyl-2H-1, 2, 4-benzothiadiazine-7-sulfonamide 1,1-dioxide. It is a white or practically white, crystalline powder which is odorless or has a slight odor. It is very slightly soluble in water, chloroform and benzene; freely soluble in acetone and pyridine; sparingly soluble in methanol; and slightly soluble in alcohol. The molecular formula for methyclothiazide is $C_9H_{11}Cl_2N_3O_4S_2$ with a molecular weight of 360.23; the structural formula may be represented as follows:

Each AQUATENSEN tablet for oral administration contains 5 mg methyclothiazide. Other ingredients: corn starch, D&C Red No. 36, lactose, magnesium stearate, talc.

CLINICAL PHARMACOLOGY

The diuretic and saluretic effects of AQUATENSEN result from a drug-induced inhibition of the renal tubular reabsorption of electrolytes. Diuresis and the excretion of sodium and chloride are significantly enhanced within two hours after a single oral dose of methyclothiazide. These effects reach a peak in about six hours and persist for 24 hours. Potassium excretion is also enhanced to a variable degree, as it is with the other thiazides. In non-edematous patients the (maximum) natriuretic effect of a single dose is seen with 10 mg of methyclothiazide whereas the maximum kaliuretic effect is seen with a 5 mg dose. Thus, doubling a daily dose of 5 mg results in an increase of sodium output without significantly increasing potassium excretion. Although urinary excretion of bicarbonate is increased slightly, there is usually no significant change in urinary pH. Methyclothiazide has a per mg natriuretic activity approximately 100 times that of the prototype thiazide, chlorothiazide. At maximal therapeutic dosages, all thiazides are approximately equal in their diuretic/natriuretic effects.

Like other benzothiadiazines, AQUATENSEN also has antihypertensive properties, and may be used for this purpose either alone or to enhance the antihypertensive action of other drugs. The mechanism by which the benzothiadiazines, including methyclothiazide, produce a reduction of elevated blood pressure has not been definitely established. However, sodium depletion appears to be of primary importance.

AQUATENSEN is readily absorbed from the gastrointestinal tract and is excreted unchanged by the kidneys.

INDICATIONS AND USAGE

AQUATENSEN is indicated in the management of hypertension either as the sole therapeutic agent or to enhance the effect of other antihypertensive drugs in the more severe forms of hypertension.

AQUATENSEN is indicated as adjunctive therapy in edema associated with congestive heart failure, hepatic cirrhosis, and corticosteroid and estrogen therapy.

AQUATENSEN has also been found useful in edema due to various forms of renal dysfunction such as the nephrotic syndrome, acute glomerulonephritis and chronic renal failure.

Usage in pregnancy: The routine use of diuretics in an otherwise healthy woman is inappropriate and exposes the mother and fetus to unnecessary hazard. Diuretics do not prevent development of toxemia of pregnancy, and there is no satisfactory evidence that they are useful in the treatment of developed toxemia.

Edema during pregnancy may arise from pathological causes or from the physiological and mechanical consequences of pregnancy. Thiazides are indicated in pregnancy when edema is due to pathologic causes, just as they are in the absence of pregnancy (however, see Precautions, *Pregnancy* below). Dependent edema in pregnancy, resulting from restriction of venous return by the expanded uterus, is properly treated through elevation of the lower extremities and use of support hose; use of diuretics to lower intravascular volume in this case is illogical and unnecessary. There is hypervolemia during normal pregnancy which is harmful to neither the fetus nor the mother (in the absence of cardiovascular disease), but which is associated with edema, including generalized edema, in the majority of pregnant women. If this edema produces discomfort, increased recumbency will often provide relief. In rare instances, this edema may cause extreme discomfort which is not relieved by rest. In these cases, a short course of diuretics may provide relief and may be appropriate.

CONTRAINDICATIONS

Renal decompensation (anuria). Hypersensitivity to methyclothiazide or other sulfonamide-derived drugs.

WARNINGS

Thiazides should be used with caution in patients with severe renal disease or significant impairment of renal function, since azotemia may be precipitated and cumulative drug effects may occur.

Thiazides should be used with caution in patients with impaired hepatic function or progressive liver disease, since minor alterations of fluid and electrolyte balance may precipitate hepatic coma.

Sensitivity reactions are more likely to occur in patients with a history of allergy or bronchial asthma.

The possibility of exacerbation or activation of systemic lupus erythematosus has been reported.

PRECAUTIONS

General: All patients should be observed for clinical signs of fluid or electrolyte imbalances such as dryness of mouth, thirst, weakness, lethargy, drowsiness, restlessness, muscle pains or cramps, muscular fatigue, hypotension, oliguria, tachycardia, and gastrointestinal disturbances such as nausea and vomiting.

Hypokalemia may develop with thiazides as with any other potent diuretic, especially when brisk diuresis occurs or severe cirrhosis is present. Interference with the adequate oral intake of electrolytes will also contribute to the possible development of hypokalemia.

Any chloride deficit is generally mild and usually does not require specific treatment except under extraordinary circumstances (as in liver disease or renal disease). Dilutional hyponatremia may occur in edematous patients in hot weather; appropriate therapy is water restriction, rather than administration of salt except in rare instances when the hyponatremia is life threatening. In actual salt depletion, appropriate replacement is the therapy of choice.

Hyperuricemia may occur or frank gout may be precipitated in certain patients receiving thiazide therapy.

Insulin requirements in diabetic patients may be increased, decreased, or unchanged. Latent diabetes mellitus may become manifest during thiazide administration.

The antihypertensive effects of the drug may be enhanced in the postsympathectomy patient.

If progressive renal impairment becomes evident as indicated by a rising nonprotein nitrogen or blood urea nitrogen, a careful reappraisal of therapy is necessary with consideration given to withholding or discontinuing diuretic therapy. Thiazides have been shown to increase the urinary excretion of magnesium; this may result in hypomagnesemia.

Pathological changes in the parathyroid gland with hypercalcemia and hypophosphatemia have been observed in a few patients on prolonged thiazide therapy. The common complications of hyperparathyroidism such as renal lithiasis, bone resorption, and peptic ulceration have not been seen.

There have been isolated reports that certain nonedematous individuals developed severe fluid and electrolyte derangements after only brief exposure to normal doses of thiazide and non-thiazide diuretics. The condition is usually manifested as severe dilutional hypotatremia, hypokalemia, and hypochloremia. It has been reported to be due to inappropriately increased ADH secretion and appears to be idiosyncratic. Potassium replacement is apparently the most important therapy in the treatment of this syndrome along with removal of the offending drug.

Information for patients: Caution patients that thiazides cause the body to lose mineral salts such as sodium, chloride and especially potassium and advise them to report any of the following without delay: excessive thirst, tiredness, drowsiness, muscle pains or cramps, nausea, vomiting, increased heart rate or pulse.

Laboratory tests: Periodic determination of serum electrolytes should be performed at appropriate intervals for the purpose of detecting possible electrolyte imbalances such as hyponatremia, hypochloremic alkalosis and hypokalemia. Serum and urine electrolyte determinations are particularly important when a patient is vomiting excessively or receiving parenteral fluids.

Drug interactions: Thiazides may add to or potentiate the action of other antihypertensive drugs. Potentiation occurs with ganglionic or peripheral adrenergic blocking drugs. Thiazide drugs may increase the responsiveness to nondepolarizing muscle relaxants, such as tubocurarine.

Thiazides may decrease arterial responsiveness to norepinephrine. This diminution is not sufficient to preclude effectiveness of the pressor agent for therapeutic use.

Hypokalemia may develop during concomitant use of steroids or ACTH.

Hypokalemia may sensitize or exaggerate the response of the heart to the toxic effects of cardiac glycosides such as digitalis (e.g., increased ventricular irritability).

Lithium renal clearance is reduced by thiazides, increasing the risk of lithium toxicity.

In some patients, the administration of a non-steroidal anti-inflammatory agent can reduce the diuretic, natriuretic, and antihypertensive effects of loop, potassium sparing, and thiazide diuretics. Therefore, when methyclothiazide and non-steroidal anti-inflammatory agents are used concomitantly, the patient should be observed closely to determine if the desired effect of the diuretic is obtained.

Drug/laboratory test interactions: Thiazides may decrease serum PBI levels without signs of thyroid disturbance.

Thiazides decrease calcium excretion and, on rare occasions, serum calcium has been elevated to hypercalcemic levels. The serum calcium levels have returned to normal when the medication was stopped. Thiazides should be discontinued before carrying out tests for parathyroid function.

Carcinogenesis, mutagenesis: Studies to determine the carcinogenic or mutagenic potential of AQUATENSEN have not been performed.

Pregnancy: Teratogenic effects: Pregnancy Category C (see Indications and Usage Section). Animal reproduction studies have not been conducted with AQUATENSEN. It is not known whether AQUATENSEN can cause fetal harm when administered to a pregnant woman or can affect reproduction capacity. Aquatensen should be given to a pregnant woman only if clearly needed.

Non-Teratogenic effects: Fetal or neonatal jaundice, thrombocytopenia, and possibly other adverse reactions which have occurred in the adult are potential hazards in fetuses and neonates of thiazide-treated mothers.

Nursing mothers: Because of the potential for serious adverse reactions in nursing infants from AQUATENSEN, a decision should be made whether to discontinue nursing or to discontinue the drug, taking into account the importance of the drug to the mother.

Pediatric use: Safety and effectiveness in children have not been established.

ADVERSE REACTIONS

Gastrointestinal: Anorexia, gastric irritation, nausea, vomiting, cramping, diarrhea, constipation, jaundice (intrahepatic cholestatic), pancreatitis, sialadenitis.

Central nervous system: Dizziness, vertigo, paresthesia, headache, xanthopsia.

Hematologic: Leukopenia, agranulocytosis, thrombocytopenia, aplastic anemia.

Cardiovascular: Orthostatic hypotension (may be potentiated by alcohol, barbiturates, or narcotics).

Hypersensitivity: Purpura, photosensitivity, rash, urticaria, necrotizing angiitis, Stevens-Johnson syndrome and other hypersensitivity reactions.

Other: Hyperglycemia, glycosuria, hypercalcemia, hyperuricemia, muscle spasm, weakness, restlessness, and idiosyncratic reactions including inappropriate ADH secretion (see Precautions).

Whenever adverse reactions with AQUATENSEN are moderate or severe, dosage should be reduced or therapy withdrawn.

OVERDOSAGE

Signs and symptoms: Diuresis is to be expected. Lethargy of varying degree may appear and may progress to coma within a few hours, even in the absence of significant changes in serum electrolytes or dehydration and with minimal depression of respiration and cardiovacular function. The mechanism of CNS depression with thiazide overdosage is not known. GI irritation, hypermotility, and signs of potassium deficiency such as confusion, dizziness, and muscular weakness may occur. A temporary rise in BUN and changes in serum electrolytes could occur, especially in patients with compromised renal function.

Treatment: Evacuate stomach contents using appropriate caution and procedures to guard against aspiration and protect the airway, especially in the stuporous or comatose patient. Monitor serum electrolyte levels, blood gases, and renal function. Institute general supportive measures as required individually to maintain hydration, electrolyte balance, respiration, and cardiovascular-renal function. GI side effects are usually of short duration but may require symptomatic treatment.

DOSAGE AND ADMINISTRATION

Therapy should be individualized by titration according to patient response to gain the maximal therapeutic response at the minimum dose necessary to maintain that therapeutic response.

Usual adult dosage: 2.5 to 10 mg once daily.

To maintain an edema-free state or as an adjunct in the management of hypertension, 2.5 to 5.0 mg once daily is often adequate.

The maximum effective single dose is 10 mg; larger single doses do not accomplish greater diuresis, and are not recommended.

In the treatment of hypertension, methyclothiazide may be employed alone or concurrently with other antihypertensive drugs. Combined therapy may provide adequate control of hypertension with lower dosage of the component drugs and fewer or less severe side effects.

For treatment of moderately severe or severe hypertension, supplemental use of other more potent antihypertensive agents may be indicated.

When other antihypertensive agents are to be added to the regimen, this should be accomplished gradually. Ganglionic blocking agents should be given at only half the usual dose since their effect is potentiated by pre-treatment with AQUATENSEN.

HOW SUPPLIED

AQUATENSEN (methyclothiazide) Tablets—5 mg, peach colored, monogrammed, grooved, rectangular-shaped tablets in bottles of 100 (NDC 0037-0153-92) and 500 (NDC 0037-1053-96).

Storage: Avoid excessive heat—above 40°C (104°F).

CAUTION: Federal law prohibits dispensing without prescription.

WALLACE LABORATORIES
Division of
CARTER-WALLACE, INC.
Cranbury, New Jersey 08512
Rev. 10/87
Shown in Product Identification Section, page 434

BUTISOL SODIUM®   ⓒ ℞
(butabarbital sodium)
Tablets and Elixir

DESCRIPTION

BUTISOL SODIUM (butabarbital sodium) is a nonselective central nervous system depressant which is used as a sedative or hypnotic (WARNING: May be habit-forming). It is available for oral administration as *Tablets* containing 15 mg, 30 mg, 50 mg or 100 mg butabarbital sodium; and as *Elixir* containing 30 mg/5 mL, with alcohol (by volume) 7%. Other ingredients in the Tablets are: calcium stearate, corn starch, dibasic calcium phosphate, FD&C Blue No. 1 (15 mg and 30 mg only), FD&C Blue No. 2 (100 mg only); FD&C Red No. 3 (15 mg and 100 mg only), FD&C Yellow No. 5 (30 mg and 50 mg only)—see Precautions), FD&C Yellow No. 6 (100 mg only). Other ingredients in the Elixir are: D&C Green No. 5, edetate disodium, FD&C Yellow No. 5 (see Precautions), flavors (natural and artificial), propylene glycol, purified water, saccharin sodium, sodium benzoate. Butabarbital sodium occurs as a white, bitter powder which is freely soluble in water and alcohol, but practically insoluble in benzene and ether.

The structural formula for butabarbital sodium is:

Sodium 5-*sec*-butyl-5-ethylbarbiturate

CLINICAL PHARMACOLOGY

BUTISOL SODIUM (butabarbital sodium), like other barbiturates, is capable of producing all levels of CNS mood alteration from excitation to mild sedation, to hypnosis, and deep coma. Overdosage can produce death. Barbiturates depress the sensory cortex, decrease motor activity, alter cerebellar function, and produce drowsiness, sedation, and hypnosis.

Barbiturate-induced sleep differs from physiological sleep. Sleep laboratory studies have demonstrated that barbiturates reduce the amount of time spent in the rapid eye movement (REM) phase of sleep or dreaming stage. Also, Stages III and IV sleep are decreased. Following abrupt cessation of barbiturates used regularly, patients may experience markedly increased dreaming, nightmares, and/or insomnia. Therefore, withdrawal of a single therapeutic dose over 5 or 6 days has been recommended to lessen the REM rebound and disturbed sleep which contribute to drug withdrawal syndrome (for example, decrease the dose from 3 to 2 doses a day for 1 week).

In studies, secobarbital sodium and pentobarbital sodium have been found to lose most of their effectiveness for both inducing and maintaining sleep by the end of 2 weeks of continued drug administration even with the use of multiple doses. As with secobarbital sodium and pentobarbital sodium, other barbiturates might be expected to lose their effectiveness for inducing and maintaining sleep after about 2 weeks. The short-, intermediate-, and, to a lesser degree, long-acting barbiturates have been widely prescribed for treating insomnia. Although the clinical literature abounds with claims that the short-acting barbiturates are superior for producing sleep while the intermediate-acting compounds are more effective in maintaining sleep, controlled studies have failed to demonstrate these differential effects. Therefore, as sleep medications, the barbiturates are of limited value beyond the short-term use.

Barbiturates are respiratory depressants. The degree of respiratory depression is dependent upon dose. With hypnotic doses, respiratory depression produced by barbiturates is similar to that which occurs during physiologic sleep with slight decrease in blood pressure and heart rate.

Barbiturates do not impair normal hepatic function, but have been shown to induce liver microsomal enzymes, thus increasing and/or altering the metabolism of barbiturates and other drugs (see Precautions—*Drug interactions*).

Pharmacokinetics: BUTISOL SODIUM (butabarbital sodium) is the sodium salt of a weak acid. Barbiturates are weak acids that are absorbed and rapidly distributed to all tissues and fluids with high concentrations in the brain, liver, and kidneys. Barbiturates are bound to plasma and tissue proteins. The rate of absorption is increased if it is ingested as a dilute solution or taken on an empty stomach. Barbiturates are metabolized primarily by the hepatic microsomal enzyme system, and most metabolic products are excreted in the urine. The excretion of unchanged butabarbital in the urine is negligible. BUTISOL SODIUM (butabarbital sodium) is classified as an intermediate-acting barbiturate. The average plasma half-life for butabarbital is 100 hours in the adult.

Although variable from patient to patient, butabarbital has an onset of action of about ¾ to 1 hour, and a duration of action of about 6 to 8 hours.

INDICATIONS AND USAGE

BUTISOL SODIUM (butabarbital sodium) is indicated for use as a sedative or hypnotic.

Since barbiturates appear to lose their effectiveness for sleep induction and sleep maintenance after 2 weeks, use of BUTISOL SODIUM in treating insomnia should be limited to this time (see Clinical Pharmacology above).

CONTRAINDICATIONS

Barbiturates are contraindicated in patients with known barbiturate sensitivity. Barbiturates are also contraindicated in patients with a history of manifest or latent porphyria.

WARNINGS

Habit forming: Barbiturates may be habit forming. Tolerance, psychological and physical dependence may occur with continued use (see Drug Abuse and Dependence below). Patients who have psychological dependence on barbiturates may increase the dosage or decrease the dosage interval without consulting a physician and may subsequently develop a physical dependence on barbiturates. To minimize the possibility of overdosage or the development of dependence, the prescribing and dispensing of sedative-hypnotic barbiturates should be limited to the amount required for the interval until the next appointment. Abrupt cessation after prolonged use in the dependent person may result in withdrawal symptoms, including delirium, convulsions, and possibly death. Barbiturates should be withdrawn gradually from any patient known to be taking excessive dosage over long periods of time. (See Drug Abuse and Dependence below.)

Acute or chronic pain: Caution should be exercised when barbiturates are administered to patients with acute or chronic pain, because paradoxical excitement could be induced, or important symptoms could be masked. However, the use of barbiturates as sedatives in the postoperative surgical period, and as adjuncts to cancer chemotherapy, is well established.

Use in pregnancy: Barbiturates can cause fetal damage when administered to a pregnant woman. Retrospective, case-controlled studies have suggested a connection between the maternal consumption of barbiturates and a higher than expected incidence of fetal abnormalities. Following oral administration, barbiturates readily cross the placental barrier and are distributed throughout fetal tissues with highest concentrations found in the placenta, fetal liver, and brain. Withdrawal symptoms occur in infants born to mothers who receive barbiturates throughout the last trimester of pregnancy (see Drug Abuse and Dependence). If this drug is used during pregnancy, or if the patient becomes pregnant while taking this drug, the patient should be apprised of the potential hazard to the fetus.

PRECAUTIONS

General: Barbiturates should be administered with caution, if at all, to patients who are mentally depressed, have suicidal tendencies, or a history of drug abuse.

Elderly or debilitated patients may react to barbiturates with marked excitement, depression, and confusion. In some persons, barbiturates repeatedly produce excitement rather than depression.

In patients with hepatic damage, barbiturates should be administered with caution and initially in reduced doses. Barbiturates should not be administered to patients showing the premonitory signs of hepatic coma.

BUTISOL SODIUM (butabarbital sodium) Tablets, 30 mg and 50 mg, and Elixir contain FD&C Yellow No. 5 (tartrazine) which may cause allergic-type reactions (including bronchial asthma) in certain susceptible individuals. Although the overall incidence of FD&C Yellow No. 5 (tartrazine) sensitivity in the general population is low, it is frequently seen in patients who also have aspirin hypersensitivity.

Information for Patients: Practitioners should give the following information and instructions to patients receiving barbiturates.

The use of barbiturates carries with it an associated risk of psychological and/or physical dependence. The patient should be warned against increasing the dose of the drug without consulting a physician.

Barbiturates may impair mental and/or physical abilities required for the performance of potentially hazardous tasks, such as driving or operating machinery.

Alcohol should not be consumed while taking barbiturates. Concurrent use of the barbiturates with other CNS depressants, including other sedatives or hypnotics, alcohol, narcotics, tranquilizers, and antihistamines, may result in additional CNS depressant effects.

Laboratory tests: Prolonged therapy with barbiturates should be accompanied by periodic laboratory evaluation of organ systems, including hematopoietic, renal, and hepatic systems (see Precautions—*General* and Adverse Reactions).

Drug interactions: Most reports of clinically significant drug interactions occurring with the barbiturates have involved phenobarbital. However, the application of these data to other barbiturates appears valid and warrants serial blood level determinations of the relevant drugs when there are multiple therapies.

1. *Anticoagulants.* Phenobarbital lowers the plasma levels of dicumarol and causes a decrease in anticoagulant activity as measured by the prothrombin time. Barbiturates can induce hepatic microsomal enzymes resulting in increased metabolism and decreased anticoagulant response of oral anticoagulants (e.g., warfarin, acenocoumarol, dicumarol, and phenprocoumon). Patients stabilized on anticoagulant therapy may require dosage adjustments if barbiturates are added to or withdrawn from their dosage regimen.

2. *Corticosteroids.* Barbiturates appear to enhance the metabolism of exogenous corticosteroids probably through the induction of hepatic microsomal enzymes. Patients stabilized on corticosteroid therapy may require dosage adjustments if barbiturates are added to or withdrawn from their dosage regimen.

3. *Griseofulvin.* Phenobarbital appears to interfere with the absorption of orally administered griseofulvin, thus decreasing its blood level. The effect of the resultant decreased blood levels of griseofulvin on therapeutic response has not been established. However, it would be preferable to avoid concomitant administration of these drugs.

4. *Doxycycline.* Phenobarbital has been shown to shorten the half-life of doxycycline for as long as 2 weeks after barbiturate therapy is discontinued. The mechanism is probably through the induction of hepatic microsomal enzymes that metabolize the antibiotic. If phenobarbital and doxycycline are administered concurrently, the clinical response to doxycycline should be monitored closely.

5. *Phenytoin, sodium valproate, valproic acid.* The effect of barbiturates on the metabolism of phenytoin appears to be variable. Some investigators report an accelerating effect, while others report no effect. Because the effect of barbiturates on the metabolism of phenytoin is not predictable, phenytoin and barbiturate blood levels should be monitored more frequently if these drugs are given concurrently. Sodium valproate and valproic acid appear to decrease barbiturate metabolism; therefore, barbiturate blood levels should be monitored and appropriate adjustments made as indicated.

6. *Central nervous system.* The concomitant use of other central nervous system depressants, including other sedatives or hypnotics, antihistamines, tranquilizers, or alcohol, may produce additive depressant effects.

7. *Monoamine oxidase inhibitors (MAOI).* MAOI prolong the effects of barbiturates probably because metabolism of the barbiturate is inhibited.

Continued on next page

Wallace—Cont.

8. *Estradiol, estrone, progesterone and other steroid hormones.*
Pretreatment with or concurrent administration of phenobarbital may decrease the effect of estradiol by increasing
its metabolism. There have been reports of patients
treated with antiepileptic drugs (e.g. phenobarbital) who
become pregnant while taking oral contraceptives. An
alternate contraceptive method might be suggested to
women taking phenobarbital.

Carcinogenesis, mutagenesis, impairment of fertility: No
long-term studies in animals have been performed with butabarbital sodium to determine carcinogenic and mutagenic
potential, or effects on fertility.

Pregnancy: Teratogenic effects —Pregnancy Category D (See
Warnings—*Use in pregnancy* above).

Nonteratogenic effects —Infants suffering from long-term
barbiturate exposure *in utero* may have an acute withdrawal
syndrome of seizures and hyperirritability from birth to a
delayed onset of up to 14 days (see Drug Abuse and Dependence).

Labor and delivery: Hypnotic doses of barbiturates do not
appear to significantly impair uterine activity during labor.
Administration of sedative-hypnotic barbiturates to the
mother during labor may result in respiratory depression in
the newborn. Premature infants are particularly susceptible
to the depressant effects of barbiturates. If barbiturates are
used during labor and delivery, resuscitation equipment
should be available.

Nursing mothers: Caution should be exercised when a barbiturate is administered to a nursing woman since small
amounts of some barbiturates are excreted in the milk.

ADVERSE REACTIONS

The following adverse reactions have been observed with the
use of barbiturates in hospitalized patients. Because such
patients may be less aware of certain of the milder adverse
effects of barbiturates, the incidence of these reactions may
be somewhat higher in fully ambulatory patients.

More than 1 in 100 patients. The most common adverse
reaction, somnolence, is estimated to occur at a rate of 1 to 3
patients per 100.

Less than 1 in 100 patients. The most common adverse reactions estimated to occur at a rate of less than 1 in 100 patients listed below, grouped by organ system, and by decreasing order of occurrence are:

Central nervous system/psychiatric: Agitation, confusion,
hyperkinesia, ataxia, CNS depression, nightmares, nervousness, psychiatric disturbance, hallucinations, insomnia, anxiety, dizziness, thinking abnormality.

Respiratory: Hypoventilation, apnea.

Cardiovascular: Bradycardia, hypotension, syncope.

Gastrointestinal: Nausea, vomiting, constipation.

Other reported reactions: Headache, hypersensitivity (angioedema, skin rashes, exfoliative dermatitis), fever, liver damage.

DRUG ABUSE AND DEPENDENCE

Controlled substance: Schedule III.

Abuse and dependence: Barbiturates may be habit-forming.
Tolerance, psychological dependence, and physical dependence may occur especially following prolonged use of high
doses of barbiturates. Daily administration in excess of 400
milligrams (mg) of pentobarbital or secobarbital for approximately 90 days is likely to produce some degree of physical
dependence. A dosage of from 600 to 800 mg taken for at least
35 days is sufficient to produce withdrawal seizures. The
average daily dose for the barbiturate addict is usually about
1.5 grams. As tolerance to barbiturates develops, the amount
needed to maintain the same level of intoxication increases;
tolerance to a fatal dosage, however, does not increase more
than two-fold. As this occurs, the margin between an intoxicating dosage and fatal dosage becomes smaller.

Symptoms of acute intoxication with barbiturates include
unsteady gait, slurred speech, and sustained nystagmus.
Mental signs of chronic intoxication include confusion, poor
judgment, irritability, insomnia, and somatic complaints.
Symptoms of barbiturate dependence are similar to those of
chronic alcoholism.

If an individual appears to be intoxicated with alcohol to a
degree that is radically disproportionate to the amount of
alcohol in his or her blood, the use of barbiturates should be
suspected. The lethal dose of a barbiturate is far less if alcohol is also ingested.

The symptoms of barbiturate withdrawal can be severe and
may cause death. Minor withdrawal symptoms may appear 8
to 12 hours after the last dose of a barbiturate. These symptoms usually appear in the following order: anxiety, muscle
twitching, tremor of hands and fingers, progressive weakness, dizziness, distortion in visual perception, nausea, vomiting, insomnia, and orthostatic hypotension. Major withdrawal symptoms (convulsions and delirium) may occur
within 16 hours and last up to 5 days after abrupt cessation
of these drugs. Intensity of withdrawal symptoms gradually
declines over a period of approximately 15 days.

Drug dependence to barbiturates arises from repeated administration of a barbiturate or agent with barbiturate-like
effect on a continuous basis, generally in amounts exceeding
the therapeutic dose levels. The characteristics of drug dependence to barbiturates include: (a) a strong desire or need
to continue taking the drug; (b) a tendency to increase the
dose; (c) a psychic dependence on the effects of the drug related to subjective and individual appreciation for those effects; and (d) a physical dependence on the effects of the drug
requiring its presence for maintenance of homeostasis and
resulting in a definite, characteristic, and self-limited abstinence syndrome when the drug is withdrawn.

Treatment of barbiturate dependence consists of cautious
and gradual withdrawal of the drug. Barbiturate-dependent
patients can be withdrawn by using a number of different
withdrawal regimens. In all cases, withdrawal takes an extended period of time. One method involves initiating treatment at the patient's regular dosage level, in 3 to 4 divided
doses, and decreasing the daily dose by 10 percent if tolerated by the patient.

Infants physically dependent on barbiturates may be given
phenobarbital 3 to 10 mg/kg/day. After withdrawal symptoms (hyperactivity, disturbed sleep, tremors, hyperreflexia)
are relieved, the dosage of phenobarbital should be gradually
decreased and completely withdrawn over a 2-week period.

OVERDOSAGE

Signs and symptoms: The toxic dose of barbiturates varies
considerably. In general, an oral dose of 1 gram of most barbiturates produces serious poisoning in an adult. Death commonly occurs after 2 to 10 grams of ingested barbiturates.
Symptoms of acute intoxication with barbiturates include
unsteady gait, slurred speech, and sustained nystagmus.
Mental signs of chronic intoxication include confusion, poor
judgment, irritability, insomnia, and somatic complaints.
Barbiturate intoxication may be confused with alcoholism,
bromide intoxication, and with various neurological disorders.

Acute overdosage with barbiturates is manifested by CNS
and respiratory depression which may progress to Cheyne-
Stokes respiration, areflexia, constriction of the pupils to a
slight degree (though in severe poisoning they may show
paralytic dilation), oliguria, tachycardia, hypotension, lowered body temperature, and coma. Typical shock syndrome
(apnea, circulatory collapse, respiratory arrest, and death)
may occur.

In extreme overdose, all electrical activity in the brain may
cease, in which case a "flat" EEG normally equated with
clinical death cannot be accepted. This effect is fully reversible unless hypoxic damage occurs. Consideration should be
given to the possibility of barbiturate intoxication even in
situations that appear to involve trauma.

Complications: Pneumonia, pulmonary edema, cardiac
arrhythmias, congestive heart failure, and renal failure may
occur. Uremia may increase CNS sensitivity to barbiturates
if renal function is impaired. Differential diagnosis should
include hypoglycemia, head trauma, cerebrovascular accidents, convulsive states, and diabetic coma.

Treatment: Treatment of overdosage is mainly supportive
and consists of the following:

1. Maintenance of an adequate airway, with assisted respiration and oxygen administration as necessary.

2. Monitoring of vital signs and fluid balance.

3. If the patient is conscious and has not lost the gag reflex,
emesis may be induced with ipecac. Care should be taken
to prevent pulmonary aspiration of vomitus. After completion of vomiting, 30 grams activated charcoal in a glass of
water may be administered.

4. If emesis is contraindicated, gastric lavage may be performed with a cuffed endotracheal tube in place with the
patient in the face down position. Activated charcoal may
be left in the emptied stomach and a saline cathartic administered.

5. Fluid therapy and other standard treatment for shock, if
needed.

6. If renal function is normal, forced diuresis may aid in the
elimination of the barbiturate.

7. Although not recommended as a routine procedure, hemodialysis may be used in severe barbiturate intoxications or
if the patient is anuric or in shock.

8. Appropriate nursing care, including rolling patients from
side-to-side every 30 minutes, to prevent hypostatic pneumonia, decubiti, aspiration, and other complications of
patients with altered states of consciousness.

9. Antibiotics should be given if pneumonia is suspected.

DOSAGE AND ADMINISTRATION

Usual adult dosage:
Daytime sedative —15 to 30 mg, 3 or 4 times daily.
Bedtime hypnotic —50 to 100 mg.
Preoperative sedative —50 to 100 mg, 60 to 90 minutes be-
fore surgery.

Usual pediatric dosage:
Preoperative sedative —2 to 6 mg/kg maximum 100 mg.
Special patient population:
Dosage should be reduced in the elderly or debilitated be-
cause these patients may be more sensitive to barbiturates.
Dosage should be reduced for patients with impaired renal
function or hepatic disease (see Precautions).

HOW SUPPLIED

BUTISOL SODIUM® (butabarbital sodium) Tablets:
15 mg—colored lavender, scored, imprinted "BUTISOL SO-
DIUM" and [37]112 in bottles of 100 (NDC 0037-0112-60) and
1000 (NDC 0037-0112-80).
30 mg*—colored green, scored, imprinted "BUTISOL SO-
DIUM" and [37]113 in bottles of 100 (NDC 0037-0113-60) and
1000 (NDC 0037-0113-80).
50 mg*—colored orange, scored, imprinted "BUTISOL SO-
DIUM" and [37]114 in bottles of 100 (NDC 0037-0114-60).
100 mg—colored pink, scored, imprinted "BUTISOL SO-
DIUM" and [37]115 in bottles of 100 (NDC 0037-0115-60).
BUTISOL SODIUM® (butabarbital sodium) Elixir*: 30
mg/5 mL, alcohol (by volume) 7%—colored green in bottles
of one pint (NDC 0037-0110-16) and one gallon (NDC 0037-
0110-28).
*Contains FD&C Yellow No. 5 (see Precautions).
Storage: Tablets and *Elixir* —Store at room temperature.
Keep bottle tightly closed.

Rev. 2/85

Shown in Product Identification Section, page 434

DEPEN®   ℞
(Penicillamine, Wallace)
Titratable Tablets

Physicians planning to use penicillamine should thoroughly familiarize themselves with its toxicity, special
dosage considerations, and therapeutic benefits. Penicillamine should never be used casually. Each patient
should remain constantly under the close supervision of
the physician. Patients should be warned to report
promptly any symptoms suggesting toxicity.

DESCRIPTION

Penicillamine is 3-mercapto-D-valine. It is a white or practically white, crystalline powder, freely soluble in water,
slightly soluble in alcohol, and insoluble in chloroform and
ether. Although its configuration is D, it is levorotatory as
usually measured:

$$25°$$
$$[\alpha]\, D = -62.5° \pm 2° \,(C = 0.05\%,\, 1N\ \text{NaOH})$$

The empirical formula is $C_5H_{11}NO_2S$, giving it a molecular
weight of 149.21.
It reacts readily with formaldehyde or acetone to form a
thiazolidine-carboxylic acid.
Other ingredients: acetylated monoglycerides, edetate
disodium, hydroxypropyl cellulose, hydroxypropyl methylcellulose, lactose, magnesium stearate, magnesium trisilicate, povidone, starch, stearic acid, titanium dioxide.

CLINICAL PHARMACOLOGY

Penicillamine is a chelating agent recommended for the removal of excess copper in patients with Wilson's disease.
From *in vitro* studies which indicate that one atom of copper
combines with two molecules of penicillamine, it would appear that one gram of penicillamine should be followed by
the excretion of about 200 milligrams of copper; however, the
actual amount excreted is about one percent of this.
Penicillamine also reduces excess cystine excretion in cystinuria. This is done, at least in part, by disulfide interchange
between penicillamine and cystine, resulting in formation of
penicillamine-cysteine disulfide, a substance that is much
more soluble than cystine and is excreted readily.
Penicillamine interferes with the formation of cross-links
between tropocollagen molecules and cleaves them when
newly formed. The mechanism of action of penicillamine in
rheumatoid arthritis is unknown, although it appears to
suppress disease activity. Unlike cytotoxic immunosuppressants, penicillamine markedly lowers IgM rheumatoid factor
but produces no significant depression in absolute levels of
serum immunoglobulins. Also unlike cytotoxic immunosuppressants, which act on both, penicillamine *in vitro* depresses
T-cell activity but not B-cell activity. *In vitro*, penicillamine
dissociates macroglobulins (rheumatoid factor) although the
relationship of the activity to its effect in rheumatoid arthritis is not known.
In rheumatoid arthritis, the onset of therapeutic response to
DEPEN (Penicillamine, Wallace) may not be seen for two or
three months. In those patients who respond, however, the
first evidence of suppression of symptoms such as pain, tenderness, and swelling usually is apparent within three
months. The optimum duration of therapy has not been determined. If remissions occur, they may last from months to
years but usually require continued treatment (see DOSAGE
AND ADMINISTRATION).

In patients with rheumatoid arthritis, it is important that DEPEN be given on an empty stomach, at least one hour before meals and at least one hour apart from any other drug, food or milk. This permits maximum absorption and reduces the likelihood of metal binding.

Methodology for determining the bioavailability of penicillamine is not available; however, penicillamine is known to be a very soluble substance.

INDICATIONS

DEPEN is indicated in the treatment of Wilson's disease, cystinuria, and in patients with severe, active rheumatoid arthritis who have failed to respond to an adequate trial of conventional therapy. Available evidence suggests that DEPEN is not of value in ankylosing spondylitis.

Wilson's Disease—Wilson's disease (hepatolenticular degeneration) results from the interaction of an inherited defect and an abnormality in copper metabolism. The metabolic defect, which is the consequence of the autosomal inheritance of one abnormal gene from each parent, manifests itself in a greater positive copper balance than normal. As a result, copper is deposited in several organs and appears eventually to produce pathologic effects most prominently seen in the brain, where degeneration is widespread; in the liver, where fatty infiltration, inflammation, and hepatocellular damage progress to postnecrotic cirrhosis; in the kidney, where tubular and glomerular dysfunction results; and in the eye, where characteristic corneal copper deposits are known as Kayser-Fleischer rings.

Two types of patients require treatment for Wilson's disease: (1) the symptomatic, and (2) the asymptomatic in whom it can be assumed the disease will develop in the future if the patient is not treated.

Diagnosis, suspected on the basis of family or individual history, physical examination, or a low serum concentration of ceruloplasmin*, is confirmed by the demonstration of Kayser-Fleischer rings or, particularly in the asymptomatic patient, by the quantitative demonstration in a liver biopsy specimen of a concentration of copper in excess of 250 mcg/g dry weight.

---

* For quantitative test for serum ceruloplasmin see: Morell, A. G.; Windsor, J.; Sternlieb, I.; Scheinberg, I. H.: Measurement of the concentration of ceruloplasmin in serum by determination of its oxidase activity, in "Laboratory Diagnosis of Liver Disease," F. W. Sunderman; F. W Sunderman, Jr. (eds.), St. Louis, Warren H. Green, Inc., 1968, pp. 193–195.

Treatment has two objectives:
(1)   to minimize dietary intake and absorption of copper.
(2)   to promote excretion of copper deposited in tissues.
The first objective is attained by a daily diet that contains no more than one or two milligrams of copper. Such a diet should exclude, most importantly, chocolate, nuts, shellfish, mushrooms, liver, molasses, broccoli, and cereals enriched with copper, and be composed to as great an extent as possible of foods with a low copper content. Distilled or demineralized water should be used if the patient's drinking water contains more than 0.1 mg of copper per liter.

For the second objective, a copper chelating agent is used. Penicillamine is the only one of these agents that is orally effective.

In symptomatic patients, this treatment usually produces marked neurologic improvement, fading of Kayser-Fleischer rings, and gradual amelioration of hepatic dysfunction and psychic disturbances.

Clinical experience to date suggests that life is prolonged with the above regimen.

Noticeable improvement may not occur for one to three months. Occasionally, neurologic symptoms become worse during initiation of therapy with DEPEN. Despite this, the drug should not be discontinued permanently, although temporary interruption may result in clinical improvement of the neurological symptoms but it carries an increased risk of developing a sensitivity reaction upon resumption of therapy (See WARNINGS).

Treatment of asymptomatic patients has been carried out for over ten years. Symptoms and signs of the disease appear to be prevented indefinitely if daily treatment with DEPEN can be continued.

Cystinuria—Cystinuria is characterized by excessive urinary excretion of the dibasic amino acids, arginine, lysine, ornithine, and cystine, and the mixed disulfide of cysteine and homocysteine. The metabolic defect that leads to cystinuria is inherited as an autosomal, recessive trait. Metabolism of the affected amino acids is influenced by at least two abnormal factors: (1) defective gastrointestinal absorption and (2) renal tubular dysfunction.

Arginine, lysine, ornithine, and cysteine are soluble substances, readily excreted. There is no apparent pathology connected with their excretion in excessive quantities.

Cystine, however, is so slightly soluble at the usual range of urinary pH that it is not excreted readily, and so crystallizes and forms stones in the urinary tract. Stone formation is the only known pathology in cystinuria.

Normal daily output of cystine is 40 to 80 mg. In cystinuria, output is greatly increased and may exceed 1 g/day. At 500 to 600 mg/day, stone formation is almost certain. When it is more than 300 mg/day, treatment is indicated. Conventional treatment is directed at keeping urinary cystine diluted enough to prevent stone formation, keeping the urine alkaline enough to dissolve as much cystine as possible, and minimizing cystine production by a diet low in methionine (the major dietary precursor of cystine). Patients must drink enough fluid to keep urine specific gravity below 1.010, take enough alkali to keep urinary pH at 7.5 to 8, and maintain a diet low in methionine. This diet is not recommended in growing children and probably is contraindicated in pregnancy because of its low protein content (see PRECAUTIONS).

When these measures are inadequate to control recurrent stone formation, DEPEN may be used as additional therapy. When patients refuse to adhere to conventional treatment, DEPEN may be a useful substitute. It is capable of keeping cystine excretion to near normal values, thereby hindering stone formation and the serious consequences of pyelonephritis and impaired renal function that develop in some patients.

Bartter and colleagues depict the process by which penicillamine interacts with cystine to form penicillamine-cysteine mixed disulfide as:

$$
\begin{array}{lcl}
CSSC + PS' & \rightleftharpoons & CS' + CSSP \\
PSSP + CS' & \rightleftharpoons & PS' + CSSP \\
CSSC + PSSP & \rightleftharpoons & 2\ CSSP
\end{array}
$$

CSSC	= cystine
CS'	= deprotonated cysteine
PSSP	= penicillamine
PS'	= deprotonated penicillamine sulfhydryl
CSSP	= penicillamine-cysteine mixed disulfide

In this process, it is assumed that the deprotonated form of penicillamine, PS', is the active factor in bringing about the disulfide interchange.

Rheumatoid Arthritis—Because DEPEN can cause severe adverse reactions, its use in rheumatoid arthritis should be restricted to patients who have severe, active disease and who have failed to respond to an adequate trial of conventional therapy. Even then, benefit-to-risk ratio should be carefully considered. Other measures, such as rest, physiotherapy, salicylates and corticosteroids should be used, when indicated, in conjunction with DEPEN (see PRECAUTIONS).

CONTRAINDICATIONS

Penicillamine should not be administered to patients with rheumatoid arthritis who are pregnant (see PRECAUTIONS).

Patients with a history of penicillamine-related aplastic anemia or agranulocytosis should not be restarted on penicillamine (see WARNINGS and ADVERSE REACTIONS).

Because of its potential for causing renal damage, penicillamine should not be administered to rheumatoid arthritis patients with a history or other evidence of renal insufficiency.

WARNINGS

The use of penicillamine has been associated with fatalities due to certain diseases, such as aplastic anemia, agranulocytosis, thrombocytopenia, Goodpasture's syndrome, and myasthenia gravis.

Because of the potential for serious hematological and renal adverse reactions, routine urinalysis, white and differential blood cell count, hemoglobin determination, and direct platelet count must be done every two weeks for the first six months of penicillamine therapy and monthly thereafter. Patients should be instructed to report promptly signs and symptoms of granulocytopenia and/or thrombocytopenia such as fever, sore throat, chills, bruising or bleeding and the above laboratory studies should be promptly repeated.

Leukopenia and thrombocytopenia have been reported to occur in up to 5% of patients during penicillamine therapy. Leukopenia is of the granulocytic series and may or may not be associated with an increase in eosinophils. A confirmed reduction in WBC below 3500 mandates discontinuation of penicillamine therapy. Thrombocytopenia may be on an idiosyncratic basis with decreased or absent megakaryocytes in the marrow, when it is part of an aplastic anemia. In other cases the thrombocytopenia is presumably on an immune basis since the number of megakaryocytes in the marrow has been reported to be normal or sometimes increased. The development of a platelet count below 100,000, even in the absence of clinical bleeding, requires at least temporary cessation of penicillamine therapy. A progressive fall in either platelet count or WBC in three successive determinations, even though values are still within the normal range, likewise requires at least temporary cessation.

Proteinuria and/or hematuria may develop during therapy and may be warning signs of membranous glomerulopathy which can progress to a nephrotic syndrome. Close observation of these patients is essential. In some patients the proteinuria disappears with continued therapy; in others penicillamine must be discontinued. When a patient develops proteinuria or hematuria the physician must ascertain

whether it is a sign of drug-induced glomerulopathy or is unrelated to penicillamine.

Rheumatoid arthritis patients who develop moderate degrees of proteinuria may be continued cautiously on penicillamine therapy, provided that quantitative 24-hour urinary protein determinations are obtained at intervals of one to two weeks. Penicillamine dosage should not be increased under these circumstances. Proteinuria which exceeds 1 g/24 hours, or proteinuria which is progressively increasing requires either discontinuance of the drug or a reduction in the dosage. In some patients, proteinuria has been reported to clear following reduction in dosage.

In rheumatoid arthritis patients, penicillamine should be discontinued if unexplained gross hematuria or persistent microscopic hematuria develops.

In patients with Wilson's disease or cystinuria the risks of continued penicillamine therapy in patients manifesting potentially serious urinary abnormalities must be weighed against the expected therapeutic benefits.

When penicillamine is used in cystinuria, an annual x-ray for renal stones is advised. Cystine stones form rapidly, sometimes in six months.

Up to one year or more may be required for any urinary abnormalities to disappear after penicillamine has been discontinued.

Because of rare reports of intrahepatic cholestasis and toxic hepatitis, liver function tests are recommended every six months during therapy.

Goodpasture's syndrome has occurred rarely. The development of abnormal urinary findings associated with hemoptysis and pulmonary infiltrates on x-ray requires immediate cessation of penicillamine.

Myasthenic syndrome sometimes progressing to myasthenia gravis has been reported. In the majority of cases, symptoms of myasthenia have receded after withdrawal of penicillamine.

Pemphigoid-type reactions characterized by bullous lesions clinically indistinguishable from pemphigus have occurred and have required discontinuation of penicillamine and treatment with corticosteroids.

Once instituted for Wilson's disease or cystinuria, treatment with penicillamine should, as a rule, be continued on a daily basis. Interruptions for even a few days have been followed by sensitivity reactions after reinstitution of therapy.

PRECAUTIONS

Some patients may experience drug fever, a marked febrile response to penicillamine, usually in the second or third week following initiation of therapy. Drug fever may sometimes be accompanied by a macular cutaneous eruption.

In the case of drug fever in patients with Wilson's disease or cystinuria, because no alternative treatment is available, penicillamine should be temporarily discontinued until the reaction subsides. Then penicillamine should be reinstituted with a small dose that is gradually increased until the desired dosage is attained. Systemic steroid therapy may be necessary, and is usually helpful, in such patients in whom toxic reactions develop a second or third time.

In the case of drug fever in rheumatoid arthritis patients, because other treatments are available, penicillamine should be discontinued and another therapeutic alternative tried, since experience indicates that the febrile reaction will recur in a very high percentage of patients upon readministration of penicillamine.

The skin and mucous membranes should be observed for allergic reactions. Early and late rashes have occurred. Early rash occurs during the first few months of treatment and is more common. It is usually a generalized pruritic, erythematous, maculopapular or morbilliform rash and resembles the allergic rash seen with other drugs. Early rash usually disappears within days after stopping penicillamine and seldom recurs when the drug is restarted at a lower dosage. Pruritus and early rash may often be controlled by the concomitant administration of antihistamines. Less commonly, a late rash may be seen, usually after six months or more of treatment, and requires discontinuation of penicillamine. It is usually on the trunk, is accompanied by intense pruritus, and is usually unresponsive to topical corticosteroid therapy. Late rash may take weeks to disappear after penicillamine is stopped and usually recurs if the drug is restarted.

The appearance of drug eruption accompanied by fever, arthralgia, lymphadenopathy or other allergic manifestations usually requires discontinuation of penicillamine.

Certain patients will develop a positive antinuclear antibody (ANA) test and some of these may show a lupus erythematosus-like syndrome similar to drug-induced lupus associated with other drugs. The lupus erythematosus-like syndrome is not associated with hypocomplementemia and may be present without nephropathy. The development of a positive ANA test does not mandate discontinuation of the drug; however, the physician should be alerted to the possibility that a lupus erythematosus-like syndrome may develop in the future.

Continued on next page

Wallace—Cont.

Some patients may develop oral ulcerations which in some cases have the appearance of aphthous stomatitis. The stomatitis usually recurs on rechallenge but often clears on a lower dosage. Although rare, cheilosis, glossitis and gingivostomatitis have also been reported. These oral lesions are frequently dose-related and may preclude further increase in penicillamine dosage or require discontinuation of the drug.

Hypogeusia (a blunting or diminution in taste perception) has occurred in some patients. This may last two to three months or more and may develop into a total loss of taste; however, it is usually self-limited, despite continued penicillamine treatment. Such taste impairment is rare in patients with Wilson's disease.

Penicillamine should not be used in patients who are receiving concurrent gold therapy, antimalarial or cytotoxic drugs, oxyphenbutazone or phenylbutazone because these drugs are also associated with similar serious hematologic and/or renal adverse reactions. Patients who have had gold salt therapy discontinued due to a major toxic reaction may be at greater risk of serious side effects with penicillamine, but not necessarily of the same type. Patients who are allergic to penicillin may theoretically have cross-sensitivity to penicillamine. The possibility of reactions from contamination of penicillamine by trace amounts of penicillin has been precluded now that penicillamine is being produced synthetically rather than as a degradation product of penicillin.

Because of their dietary restrictions, patients with Wilson's disease and cystinuria should be given 25 mg/day of pyridoxine during therapy, since penicillamine increases the requirement for this vitamin. Patients also may receive benefit from a multivitamin preparation, although there is no evidence that deficiency of any vitamin other than pyridoxine is associated with penicillamine. In Wilson's disease, multivitamin preparations must be copper-free.

Rheumatoid arthritis patients whose nutrition is impaired should also be given a daily supplement of pyridoxine. Mineral supplements should not be given, since they may block the response to penicillamine.

Iron deficiency may develop, especially in children and in menstruating women. In Wilson's disease, this may be a result of adding the effects of the low copper diet, which is probably also low in iron, and the penicillamine to the effects of blood loss or growth. In cystinuria, a low methionine diet may contribute to iron deficiency, since it is necessarily low in protein. If necessary, iron may be given in short courses, but a period of two hours should elapse between administration of penicillamine and iron, since orally administered iron has been shown to reduce the effects of penicillamine.

Penicillamine causes an increase in the amount of soluble collagen. In the rat this results in inhibition of normal healing and also a decrease in tensile strength of intact skin. In man this may be the cause of increased skin friability at sites especially subject to pressure or trauma, such as shoulders, elbows, knees, toes, and buttocks. Extravasations of blood may occur and may appear as purpuric areas, with external bleeding if the skin is broken, or as vesicles containing dark blood. Neither type is progressive. There is no apparent association with bleeding elsewhere in the body and no associated coagulation defect has been found. Therapy with penicillamine may be continued in the presence of these lesions. They may disappear if dosage is reduced. Other reported effects probably due to the action of penicillamine on collagen are excessive wrinkling of the skin and development of small, white papules at venipuncture and surgical sites.

The effects of penicillamine on collagen and elastin make it advisable to consider a reduction in dosage to 250 mg/day when surgery is contemplated. Reinstitution of full therapy should be delayed until wound healing is complete.

Caution patients to report immediately any abrupt onset of pulmonary symptoms, such as exertional dyspnea, wheezing, or cough and have appropriate pulmonary function studies done to rule out obstructive bronchiolitis.

Carcinogenesis—Long-term animal carcinogenicity studies have not been done with penicillamine. There is a report that 5 of 10 autoimmune disease-prone NZB Hybrid mice developed lymphocytic leukemia after 6 months' intraperitoneal treatment with a dose of 400 mg/kg penicillamine 5 days per week.

Usage in Pregnancy—Penicillamine has been shown to be teratogenic in rats when given in doses several times higher than the highest dose recommended for human use. Skeletal defects, cleft palates and fetal toxicity (resorptions) have been reported.

Wilson's disease—There are no controlled studies in pregnant women with Wilson's disease, but experience does not include any positive evidence of adverse effects to the fetus. Reported experience* shows that continued treatment with penicillamine throughout pregnancy protects the mother against relapse of the Wilson's disease, and that discontinuation of penicillamine has deleterious effects on the mother. It indicates that the drug does not increase the risk of fetal abnormalities, but it does not exclude the possibility of infrequent or subtle damage to the fetus.

---

* Scheinberg, I. H., Sternlieb, I.: *N Engl J Med 293*: 1300–1302, Dec. 18, 1975.

If penicillamine is administered during pregnancy to patients with Wilson's disease, it is recommended that the daily dosage be limited to 1 g. If Caesarean section is planned, the daily dosage should be limited to 250 mg during the last six weeks of pregnancy and postoperatively until wound healing is complete.

Cystinuria—If possible, penicillamine should not be given during pregnancy to women with cystinuria. There is a report of a woman with cystinuria treated with 2 g/day of penicillamine during pregnancy who gave birth to a child with a generalized connective tissue defect that may have been caused by penicillamine. If stones continue to form in these patients, the benefits of therapy to the mother must be evaluated against the risk to the fetus.

Rheumatoid Arthritis—Penicillamine should not be administered to rheumatoid arthritis patients who are pregnant (see CONTRAINDICATIONS) and should be discontinued promptly in patients in whom pregnancy is suspected or diagnosed. Penicillamine should be used in women of childbearing potential only when the expected benefits outweigh possible hazards. Women of childbearing potential should be informed of the possible hazards of penicillamine to the developing fetus and should be advised to report promptly any missed menstrual periods or other indications of possible pregnancy.

There is a report that a woman with rheumatoid arthritis treated with less than 1 g/day of penicillamine during pregnancy gave birth (Caesarean delivery) to an infant with growth retardation, flattened face with broad nasal bridge, low set ears, short neck with loose skin folds, and unusually lax body skin.

Usage in Children—The efficacy of DEPEN in juvenile rheumatoid arthritis has not been established.

ADVERSE REACTIONS

Penicillamine is a drug with a high incidence of untoward reactions, some of which are potentially fatal. Therefore, it is mandatory that patients receiving penicillamine therapy remain under close medical supervision throughout the period of drug administration (see WARNINGS and PRECAUTIONS).

Reported incidences (%) for the most commonly occurring adverse reactions in rheumatoid arthritis patients are noted, based on 17 representative clinical trials reported in the literature (1270 patients).

Allergic—Generalized pruritus, early and late rashes (5%), pemphigoid-type reactions and drug eruptions which may be accompanied by fever, arthralgia or lymphadenopathy have occurred (see WARNINGS and PRECAUTIONS). Some patients may show a lupus erythematosus-like syndrome similar to drug induced lupus produced by other pharmacological agents (see PRECAUTIONS).

Urticaria and exfoliative dermatitis have occurred.

Thyroiditis has been reported but is extremely rare.

Some patients may develop a migratory polyarthralgia, often with objective synovitis (see DOSAGE AND ADMINISTRATION).

Gastrointestinal—Anorexia, epigastric pain, nausea, vomiting or occasional diarrhea may occur (17%).

Isolated cases of reactivated peptic ulcer have occurred, as have hepatic dysfunction, cholestatic jaundice and pancreatitis. There have been a few reports of increased serum alkaline phosphatase, lactic dehydrogenase, and positive cephalin flocculation and thymol turbidity tests.

Some patients may report a blunting, diminution or total loss of taste perception (12%) or may develop oral ulcerations. Although rare, cheilosis, glossitis and gingivostomatitis have been reported (see PRECAUTIONS).

Gastrointestinal side effects are usually reversible following cessation of therapy.

Hematological—Penicillamine can cause bone marrow depression (see WARNINGS). Leukopenia (2%) and thrombocytopenia (4%) have occurred. Fatalities have been reported as a result of thrombocytopenia, agranulocytosis and aplastic anemia.

Thrombotic thrombocytopenic purpura, hemolytic anemia, red cell aplasia, monocytosis, leukocytosis, eosinophilia and thrombocytosis have also been reported.

Renal—Patients on penicillamine therapy may develop proteinuria (6%) and/or hematuria which, in some, may progress to the development of the nephrotic syndrome as a result of an immune complex membranous glomerulopathy (see WARNINGS).

Central Nervous System—Tinnitus has been reported. Reversible optic neuritis has been reported with the administration of penicillamine and may be related to pyridoxine deficiency.

Neuromuscular—Myasthenia gravis (see WARNINGS).

Other—Adverse reactions that have been reported rarely include thrombophlebitis; hyperpyrexia (see PRECAU-TIONS); falling hair or alopecia; polymyositis; dermatomyositis; mammary hyperplasia; elastosis perforans serpiginosa; toxic epidermal necrolysis; anetoderma (cutaneous macular atrophy); Goodpasture's syndrome, a severe and ultimately fatal glomerulonephritis associated with intra-alveolar hemorrhage (see WARNINGS); and fatal renal vasculitis. Allergic alveolitis and obliterative bronchiolitis have been reported in patients with severe rheumatoid arthritis, some of whom were receiving penicillamine (see PRECAUTIONS).

Increased skin friability, excessive wrinkling of skin, and development of small, white papules at venipuncture and surgical sites have been reported (See PRECAUTIONS).

The chelating action of the drug may cause increased excretion of other heavy metals such as zinc, mercury and lead.

There have been reports associating penicillamine with leukemia. However, circumstances involved in these reports are such that a cause and effect relationship to the drug has not been established.

DOSAGE AND ADMINISTRATION

Wilson's Disease—DEPEN tablets should be given on an empty stomach, four times a day; one-half to one hour before meals and at bedtime—at least two hours after the evening meal.

Optimal dosage can be determined only by measurement of urinary copper excretion. The urine must be collected in copper-free glassware, and should be quantitatively analyzed for copper before and soon after initiation of therapy with DEPEN. Continued therapy should be monitored by doing a 24-hour urinary copper analysis every three months or so for the duration of therapy. Since a low copper diet should keep copper absorption down to less than one milligram a day, the patient probably will be in negative copper balance if 0.5 to one milligram of copper is present in a 24-hour collection of urine.

To achieve this, the suggested initial dosage of DEPEN in the treatment of Wilson's disease is 1 g/day for children or adults. This may be increased, as indicated by the urinary copper analyses, but it is seldom necessary to exceed a dosage of 2 g/day.

In patients who cannot tolerate as much as 1 g/day initially, initiating dosage with 250 mg/day, and increasing gradually to the requisite amount, gives closer control of the effects of the drug and may help to reduce the incidence of adverse reactions.

Cystinuria—It is recommended that DEPEN be used along with conventional therapy. By reducing urinary cystine, it decreases crystalluria and stone formation. In some instances, it has been reported to decrease the size of, and even to dissolve, stones already formed.

The usual dosage of DEPEN in the treatment of cystinuria is 2 g/day for adults; with a range of 1 to 4 g/day. For children, dosage can be based on 30 mg/kg/day. The total daily amount should be divided into four doses. If four equal doses are not feasible, give the larger portion at bedtime. If adverse reactions necessitate a reduction in dosage, it is important to retain the bedtime dose.

Initiating dosage with 250 mg/day, and increasing gradually to the requisite amount, gives closer control of the effects of the drug and may help to reduce the incidence of adverse reactions.

In addition to taking DEPEN, patients should drink copiously. It is especially important to drink about a pint of fluid at bedtime and another pint once during the night when urine is more concentrated and more acid than during the day. The greater the fluid intake, the lower the required dosage of DEPEN.

Dosage must be individualized to an amount that limits cystine excretion to 100–200 mg/day in those with no history of stones, and below 100 mg/day in those who have had stone formation and/or pain. Thus, in determining dosage, the inherent tubular defect, the patient's size, age, and rate of growth, and his diet and water intake all must be taken into consideration.

The standard nitroprusside cyanide test has been reported useful as a qualitative measure of the effective dose*: Add 2 ml of freshly prepared 5 percent sodium cyanide to 5 ml of a 24-hour aliquot of protein-free urine and let stand ten minutes. Add 5 drops of freshly prepared 5 percent sodium nitroprusside and mix. Cystine will turn the mixture magenta. If the result is negative, it can be assumed that cystine excretion is less than 100 mg/g creatinine.

---

* Lotz, M., Potts, J. T. and Bartter, F. C.: *Brit Med J 2*:521, Aug. 28, 1965 (in Medical Memoranda).

Although penicillamine is rarely excreted unchanged, it also will turn the mixture magenta. If there is any question as to which substance is causing the reaction, a ferric chloride test can be done to eliminate doubt: Add 3 percent ferric chloride dropwise to the urine. Penicillamine will turn the urine an immediate and quickly fading blue. Cystine will not produce any change in appearance.

Rheumatoid Arthritis—The principal rule of treatment with DEPEN in rheumatoid arthritis is patience. The onset of therapeutic response is typically delayed. Two or three months may be required before the first evidence of a clinical response is noted (see CLINICAL PHARMACOLOGY). When treatment with DEPEN has been interrupted because of adverse reactions or other reasons, the drug should be reintroduced cautiously by starting with a lower dosage and increasing slowly.

Initial Therapy—

The currently recommended dosage regimen in rheumatoid arthritis begins with a single daily dose of 125 mg or 250 mg which is thereafter increased at one to three month intervals, by 125 mg or 250 mg/day, as patient response and tolerance indicate. If a satisfactory remission of symptoms is achieved, the dose associated with the remission should be continued (see **Maintenance Therapy**). If there is no improvement and there are no signs of potentially serious toxicity after two to three months of treatment with doses of 500–750 mg/day, increases of 250 mg/day at two to three month intervals may be continued until a satisfactory remission occurs (see **Maintenance Therapy**) or signs of toxicity develop (see WARNINGS and PRECAUTIONS). If there is no discernible improvement after three to four months of treatment with 1000 to 1500 mg penicillamine/day, it may be assumed the patient will not respond and DEPEN should be discontinued.

It is important that DEPEN be given on an empty stomach at least one hour before meals and at least one hour apart from any other drug, food or milk (see CLINICAL PHARMACOLOGY).

Maintenance Therapy—

The maintenance dosage of DEPEN must be individualized, and may require adjustment during the course of treatment. Many patients respond satisfactorily to a dosage within the 500–750 mg/day range. Some need less.

Changes in maintenance dosage levels may not be reflected clinically or in the erythrocyte sedimentation rate for two to three months after each dosage adjustment.

Some patients will subsequently require an increase in the maintenance dosage to achieve maximal disease suppression. In those patients who do respond, but who evidence incomplete suppression of their disease after the first six to nine months of treatment, the daily dosage of DEPEN may be increased by 125 mg or 250 mg/day at three-month intervals. It is unusual in current practice to employ a dosage in excess of 1 g/day, but up to 1.5 g/day has sometimes been required.

Management of Exacerbations—

During the course of treatment some patients may experience an exacerbation of disease activity following an initial good response. These may be self-limited and can subside within twelve weeks. They are usually controlled by the addition of nonsteroidal anti-inflammatory drugs, and only if the patient has demonstrated a true "escape" phenomenon (as evidenced by failure of the flare to subside within this time period) should an increase in the maintenance dose ordinarily be considered.

In the rheumatoid patient, migratory polyarthralgia due to penicillamine is extremely difficult to differentiate from an exacerbation of the rheumatoid arthritis. Discontinuance or a substantial reduction in the dosage of DEPEN for up to several weeks will usually determine which of these processes is responsible for the arthralgia.

Duration of Therapy—

The optimum duration of DEPEN therapy in rheumatoid arthritis has not been determined. If the patient has been in remission for six months or more, a gradual, stepwise dosage reduction in decrements of 125 mg or 250 mg/day at approximately three month intervals may be attempted.

Concomitant Drug Therapy—

DEPEN should not be used in patients who are receiving gold therapy, antimalarial or cytotoxic drugs, oxyphenbutazone or phenylbutazone (see PRECAUTIONS). Other measures, such as salicylates, other nonsteroidal anti-inflammatory drugs or systemic corticosteroids may be continued when DEPEN is initiated. After improvement commences, analgesic and anti-inflammatory drugs may be slowly discontinued as symptoms permit. Steroid withdrawal must be done gradually, and many months of DEPEN treatment may be required before steroids can be completely eliminated.

Dosage Frequency—

Based on clinical experience, dosages up to 500 mg/day can be given as a single daily dose. Dosages in excess of 500 mg/day should be administered in divided doses.

HOW SUPPLIED

DEPEN® Titratable Tablets: 250 mg scored, oval, white tablets imprinted in red with 37-4401; available in bottles of 100 (NDC 0037-4401-01).

Manufactured under license from
HOMBURG (Degussa), West Germany.
Rev. 5/85

DEPROL®   © ℞

(meprobamate 400 mg + benactyzine hydrochloride 1 mg)

DESCRIPTION

'Deprol' is available as light pink, scored tablets, each containing meprobamate, U.S.P., 400 mg and benactyzine hydrochloride 1 mg.
Other ingredients: alginic acid, D&C Red #30 Aluminum Lake, FD&C Yellow #5 Aluminum Lake, purified stearic acid, starch, talc.

ACTIONS

'Deprol'* (meprobamate + benactyzine hydrochloride) combines the tranquilizing action of meprobamate with the antidepressant action of benactyzine hydrochloride.

* U.S. Patent No. 3,090,726 covers the ingredients combination.

Benactyzine hydrochloride
Benactyzine hydrochloride is a mild antidepressant and anticholinergic agent which in animals has been shown to reduce the autonomic response to emotion-provoking stress.

Meprobamate
Meprobamate is a carbamate derivative which has been shown in animal studies to have effects at multiple sites in the central nervous system, including the thalamus and limbic system.

> ### INDICATIONS
>
> Based on a review of this drug by the National Academy of Sciences—National Research Council and/or other information, FDA has classified the indication as follows:
> "Possibly" effective: in the management of depression, both acute (reactive) and chronic. It is particularly useful in the less severe depressions and where the depression is accompanied by anxiety, insomnia, agitation, or rumination. It is also useful for management of depression and associated anxiety accompanying or related to organic illnesses. Final classification of this indication requires further investigation.

CONTRAINDICATIONS

Benactyzine hydrochloride
Glaucoma and allergic or idiosyncratic reactions to benactyzine hydrochloride or related compounds.

Meprobamate
Acute intermittent porphyria as well as allergic or idiosyncratic reactions to meprobamate or related compounds such as carisoprodol, mebutamate, tybamate, or carbromal.

WARNINGS

The following information on meprobamate pertains to 'Deprol' (meprobamate + benactyzine hydrochloride):

Meprobamate
Drug Dependence—Physical dependence, psychological dependence, and abuse have occurred. When chronic intoxication from prolonged use occurs, it usually involves ingestion of greater than recommended doses and is manifested by ataxia, slurred speech, and vertigo. Therefore, careful supervision of dose and amounts prescribed is advised, as well as avoidance of prolonged administration, especially for alcoholics and other patients with a known propensity for taking excessive quantities of drugs.

Sudden withdrawal of the drug after prolonged and excessive use may precipitate recurrence of pre-existing symptoms, such as anxiety, anorexia, or insomnia, or withdrawal reactions, such as vomiting, ataxia, tremors, muscle twitching, confusional states, hallucinosis, and, rarely, convulsive seizures. Such seizures are more likely to occur in persons with central nervous system damage or pre-existent or latent convulsive disorders. Onset of withdrawal symptoms occurs usually within 12 to 48 hours after discontinuation of meprobamate; symptoms usually cease within the next 12 to 48 hours.

When excessive dosage has continued for weeks or months, dosage should be reduced gradually over a period of one or two weeks rather than abruptly stopped. Alternatively, a short-acting barbiturate may be substituted, then gradually withdrawn.

Potentially Hazardous Tasks—Patients should be warned that this drug may impair the mental and/or physical abilities required for the performance of potentially hazardous tasks such as driving a motor vehicle or operating machinery.

Additive Effects—Since the effects of meprobamate and alcohol or meprobamate and other CNS depressants or psychotropic drugs may be additive, appropriate caution should be exercised with patients who take more than one of these agents simultaneously.

Usage in Pregnancy and Lactation
An increased risk of congenital malformations associated with the use of minor tranquilizers (meprobamate, chlordiaz-

epoxide, and diazepam) during the first trimester of pregnancy has been suggested in several studies. Because use of these drugs is rarely a matter of urgency, their use during this period should almost always be avoided. The possibility that a woman of childbearing potential may be pregnant at the time of institution of therapy should be considered. Patients should be advised that if they become pregnant during therapy or intend to become pregnant they should communicate with their physicians about the desirability of discontinuing the drug.

Meprobamate passes the placental barrier. It is present both in umbilical cord blood at or near maternal plasma levels and in breast milk of lactating mothers at concentrations two to four times that of maternal plasma. When use of meprobamate is contemplated in breast-feeding patients, the drug's higher concentrations in breast milk as compared to maternal plasma levels should be considered.

Usage in Children—This combination is not intended for use in children.

PRECAUTIONS

Meprobamate—The lowest effective dose should be administered, particularly to elderly and/or debilitated patients, in order to preclude oversedation.

The possibility of suicide attempts should be considered and the least amount of drug feasible should be dispensed at any one time.

Meprobamate is metabolized in the liver and excreted by the kidney; to avoid its excess accumulation, caution should be exercised in administration to patients with compromised liver or kidney function.

Meprobamate occasionally may precipitate seizures in epileptic patients.

This product contains FD&C Yellow No. 5 (tartrazine) which may cause allergic-type reactions (including bronchial asthma) in certain susceptible individuals. Although the overall incidence of FD&C Yellow No. 5 (tartrazine) sensitivity in the general population is low, it is frequently seen in patients who also have aspirin hypersensitivity.

ADVERSE REACTIONS

Side effects have included nausea, dryness of mouth, and other gastrointestinal symptoms; syncope; and one case each of severe nervousness and loss of power of concentration.

The following side effects, which have occurred after administration of its components alone, have either occurred or might occur when the combination is taken.

Benactyzine Hydrochloride
Benactyzine hydrochloride alone, particularly in high dosage, may produce dizziness, thought-blocking, a sense of depersonalization, aggravation of anxiety, or disturbance of sleep patterns, and a subjective feeling of muscle relaxation. There may also be anticholinergic effects such as blurred vision, dryness of mouth, or failure of visual accommodation. Other reported side effects have included gastric distress, allergic response, ataxia, and euphoria.

Meprobamate
Central Nervous System—Drowsiness, ataxia, dizziness, slurred speech, headache, vertigo, weakness, paresthesias, impairment of visual accommodation, euphoria, overstimulation, paradoxical excitement, fast EEG activity.

Gastrointestinal—Nausea, vomiting, diarrhea.

Cardiovascular—Palpitations, tachycardia, various forms of arrhythmia, transient ECG changes, syncope; also, hypotensive crises (including one fatal case).

Allergic or Idiosyncratic—Allergic or idiosyncratic reactions are usually seen within the period of the first to fourth dose in patients having had no previous contact with the drug. Milder reactions are characterized by an itchy, urticarial, or erythematous maculopapular rash which may be generalized or confined to the groin. Other reactions have included leukopenia, acute nonthrombocytopenic purpura, petechiae, ecchymoses, eosinophilia, peripheral edema, adenopathy, fever, fixed drug eruption with cross reaction to carisoprodol, and cross sensitivity between meprobamate/mebutamate and meprobamate/carbromal.

More severe hypersensitivity reactions, rarely reported, include hyperpyrexia, chills, angioneurotic edema, bronchospasm, oliguria, and anuria. Also, anaphylaxis, erythema multiforme, exfoliative dermatitis, stomatitis, proctitis, Stevens-Johnson syndrome, and bullous dermatitis, including one fatal case of the latter following administration of meprobamate in combination with prednisolone.

In case of allergic or idiosyncratic reactions to meprobamate, discontinue the drug and initiate appropriate symptomatic therapy, which may include epinephrine, antihistamines, and in severe cases corticosteroids. In evaluating possible allergic reactions, also consider allergy to excipients (information on excipients is available to physicians on request).

Hematologic (See also **Allergic or Idiosyncratic.**)—Agranulocytosis and aplastic anemia have been reported, although no causal relationship has been established. These cases rarely were fatal. Rare cases of thrombocytopenic purpura have been reported.

Other—Exacerbation of porphyric symptoms.

Continued on next page

Wallace—Cont.

DOSAGE AND ADMINISTRATION

The usual adult starting dosage of 'Deprol' (meprobamate + benactyzine hydrochloride) is one tablet three or four times daily, which may be increased gradually to six tablets daily and gradually reduced to maintenance levels upon establishment of relief. Doses above six tablets daily are not recommended, even though higher doses have been used by some clinicians to control depression, and in chronic psychotic patients.

OVERDOSAGE

Overdosage of 'Deprol' (meprobamate + benactyzine hydrochloride) has not differed substantially from meprobamate overdosage:

Meprobamate

Suicidal attempts with meprobamate have resulted in drowsiness, lethargy, stupor, ataxia, coma, shock, vasomotor and respiratory collapse. Some suicidal attempts have been fatal. The following data on meprobamate tablets have been reported in the literature and from other sources. These data are not expected to correlate with each case (considering factors such as individual susceptibility and length of time from ingestion to treatment), but represent the *usual ranges* reported.

Acute simple overdose (meprobamate alone): Death has been reported with ingestion of as little as 12 gm meprobamate and survival with as much as 40 gm.

Blood Levels:

0.5–2.0 mg% represents the usual blood level range of meprobamate after therapeutic doses. The level may occasionally be as high as 3.0 mg%.

3–10 mg% usually corresponds to findings of mild to moderate symptoms of overdosage, such as stupor or light coma.

10–20 mg% usually corresponds to deeper coma, requiring more intensive treatment. Some fatalities occur.

At levels greater than 20 mg%, more fatalities than survivals can be expected.

Acute combined overdose (meprobamate with alcohol or other CNS depressants or psychotropic drugs): Since effects can be additive, a history of ingestion of a low dose of meprobamate plus any of these compounds (or of a relatively low blood or tissue level) cannot be used as a prognostic indicator. In cases where excessive doses have been taken, sleep means rapidly and blood pressure, pulse, and respiratory rates are reduced to basal levels. Any drug remaining in the stomach should be removed and symptomatic therapy given. Should respiration or blood pressure become compromised, respiratory assistance, central nervous system stimulants, and pressor agents should be administered cautiously as indicated. Meprobamate is metabolized in the liver and excreted by the kidney. Diuresis, osmotic (mannitol) diuresis, peritoneal dialysis, and hemodialysis have been used successfully. Careful monitoring of urinary output is necessary and caution should be taken to avoid overhydration. Relapse and death, after initial recovery, have been attributed to incomplete gastric emptying and delayed absorption. Meprobamate can be measured in biological fluids by two methods: colorimetric (Hoffman, A.J. and Ludwig, B.J.: *J Amer Pharm Assn* 48: 740, 1959) and gas chromatographic (Douglas, J.F. et al: *Anal Chem* 39: 956, 1967).

HOW SUPPLIED

Bottles of 100 (NDC 0037-3001-01). Bottles of 500 (NDC 0037-3001-03).

WALLACE LABORATORIES
Division of
CARTER-WALLACE, INC.
Cranbury, New Jersey 08512

Rev. 4/86

DIUTENSEN®-R   ℞
Tablets

> **WARNING**
> THIS FIXED COMBINATION DRUG IS NOT INDICATED FOR INITIAL THERAPY OF HYPERTENSION. HYPERTENSION REQUIRES THERAPY TITRATED TO THE INDIVIDUAL PATIENT. IF THE FIXED COMBINATION REPRESENTS THE DOSAGE SO DETERMINED, ITS USE MAY BE MORE CONVENIENT IN PATIENT MANAGEMENT. THE TREATMENT OF HYPERTENSION IS NOT STATIC, BUT MUST BE RE-EVALUATED AS CONDITIONS IN EACH PATIENT WARRANT.

DESCRIPTION

DIUTENSEN®-R is a two-component system of active ingredients containing 2.5 mg. methyclothiazide and 0.1 mg. reserpine per tablet. DIUTENSEN-R thus provides for easier titration of hypertensive patients than does a three-component system. DIUTENSEN-R tablets are round, white, pink-mottled tablets. NOTE: DIUTENSEN-R previously contained cryptenamine tannate as a third antihypertensive agent.

ACTIONS

Methyclothiazide—The predominant effects of methyclothiazide are diuresis, natriuresis, and chloruresis. The mechanism of action results in an interference with the renal tubular mechanism of electrolyte reabsorption. There is significant natriuresis and diuresis within two hours after administration of a single dose of methyclothiazide. These effects reach a peak in about six hours and persist for 24 hours following oral administration of a single dose.

In nonedematous patients the "peak" (maximum effective) natriuretic single dose of methyclothiazide is 10 mg., whereas the peak kaliuretic dose is 5 mg. Thus, doubling a daily dose of 5 mg. results in an increase of sodium output without significantly increasing potassium excretion.

Like other benzothiadiazines, methyclothiazide also has antihypertensive properties. It also may be used to enhance the antihypertensive action of other drugs. The mechanism by which benzothiadiazines, including methyclothiazide, produce a reduction of elevated blood pressure has not been definitely established. Sodium depletion, however, appears to be of primary importance.

Methyclothiazide is readily absorbed from the gastrointestinal tract and is excreted unchanged by the kidneys.

Reserpine—Reserpine is a pure crystalline alkaloid from the root of *Rauwolfia serpentina*. The drug has mild antihypertensive and bradycrotic effects in addition to sedative and tranquilizing properties.

Reserpine probably produces its antihypertensive effects through depletion of tissue stores of catecholamines (epinephrine and norepinephrine) from peripheral sites. By contrast, its sedative and tranquilizing properties are thought to be due to a depletion of 5-hydroxytryptamine from the brain. Reserpine is characterized by slow onset of action and sustained effect. Both its cardiovascular and central nervous system effects may persist following withdrawal of the drug.

INDICATIONS

Hypertension (see box warning).

CONTRAINDICATIONS

Methyclothiazide—This compound should not be used in anuric patients or those who exhibit a hypersensitivity to this or other sulfonamide derived drugs.

Reserpine—Reserpine is contraindicated in patients with known hypersensitivity, mental depression, especially with suicidal tendencies, active peptic ulcer, and ulcerative colitis. It is also contraindicated in patients receiving electroconvulsive therapy.

WARNINGS

Methyclothiazide—Thiazides should be used with caution in severe renal disease. In patients with renal disease, thiazides may precipitate azotemia. Cumulative effects of the drug may develop in patients with impaired renal function.

Thiazides should be used with caution in patients with impaired hepatic function or progressive liver disease, since minor alterations of fluid and electrolyte balance may precipitate hepatic coma.

Thiazides may be additive or potentiate the action of other antihypertensive drugs. Potentiation occurs with ganglionic or peripheral adrenergic blocking drugs.

Sensitivity reactions may occur in patients with a history of allergy or bronchial asthma. The possibility of exacerbation or activation of systemic lupus erythematosus has been reported.

Reserpine—Extreme caution should be exercised in treating patients with a history of mental depression. Discontinue the drug at the first sign of despondency, early morning insomnia, loss of appetite, impotence, or self-deprecation. Drug-induced depression may persist for several months after drug withdrawal and may be severe enough to result in suicide.

Electroshock therapy should not be given to patients under treatment with reserpine since severe and even fatal reactions to such therapy have been reported in patients receiving reserpine. Reserpine should be discontinued for two weeks before electroshock therapy is given.

Use in Pregnancy: USE OF ANY DRUG IN PREGNANCY, LACTATION, OR IN WOMEN OF CHILDBEARING AGE REQUIRES THAT THE POTENTIAL BENEFITS OF THE DRUG SHOULD BE WEIGHED AGAINST THE POSSIBLE HAZARDS TO THE MOTHER AND CHILD. DIUTENSEN-R SHOULD BE USED WITH CARE IN PREGNANT AND NURSING MOTHERS SINCE METHYCLOTHIAZIDE AND RESERPINE CROSS THE PLACENTAL BARRIER AND APPEAR IN CORD BLOOD AND BREAST MILK.

THE SAFETY OF RESERPINE FOR USE DURING PREGNANCY OR LACTATION HAS NOT BEEN ESTABLISHED. INCREASED RESPIRATORY SECRETIONS, NASAL CONGESTION, CYANOSIS, AND ANOREXIA MAY OCCUR IN INFANTS BORN TO RESERPINE-TREATED MOTHERS.

THIAZIDES MAY RESULT IN FETAL OR NEONATAL JAUNDICE, THROMBOCYTOPENIA, AND POSSIBLE OTHER ADVERSE REACTIONS WHICH HAVE OCCURRED IN THE ADULT.

PRECAUTIONS

Methyclothiazide—Periodic determinations of serum electrolytes to detect possible electrolyte imbalance should be performed at appropriate intervals.

All patients receiving thiazide therapy should be observed for clinical signs of fluid or electrolyte imbalance; namely, hyponatremia, hypochloremic alkalosis, and hypokalemia. Serum and urine electrolyte determinations are particularly important when the patient is vomiting excessively or receiving parenteral fluids. Medication such as digitalis may also influence serum electrolytes. Warning signs, irrespective of cause, are: Dryness of mouth, thirst, weakness, lethargy, drowsiness, restlessness, muscle pains or cramps, muscular fatigue, hypotension, oliguria, tachycardia, and gastrointestinal disturbances such as nausea and vomiting.

Hypokalemia may develop with thiazides as with any other potent diuretic, especially with brisk diuresis, when severe cirrhosis is present, or during concomitant use of corticosteroids or ACTH.

Interference with adequate oral electrolyte intake will also contribute to hypokalemia. Digitalis therapy may exaggerate metabolic effects of hypokalemia especially with reference to myocardial activity.

Any chloride deficit is generally mild and usually does not require specific treatment except under extraordinary circumstances (as in liver disease or renal disease). Dilutional hyponatremia may occur in edematous patients in hot weather; appropriate therapy is water restriction, rather than administration of salt except in rare instances when the hyponatremia is life threatening. In actual salt depletion, appropriate replacement is the therapy of choice.

Hyperuricemia may occur or frank gout may be precipitated in certain patients receiving thiazide therapy.

Insulin requirements in diabetic patients may be increased, decreased, or unchanged. Latent diabetes mellitus may become manifest during thiazide administration.

Thiazide drugs may increase the responsiveness of tubocurarine.

The antihypertensive effects of the drug may be enhanced in the postsympathectomy patient.

Thiazides may decrease arterial responsiveness to norepinephrine. This diminution is not sufficient to preclude effectiveness of the pressor agent for therapeutic use.

If progressive renal impairment becomes evident, as indicated by a rising non-protein nitrogen or blood urea nitrogen, a careful reappraisal of therapy is necessary with consideration given to withholding or discontinuing diuretic therapy.

Thiazides may decrease serum PBI levels without signs of thyroid disturbance.

Reserpine—Because reserpine preparations increase gastrointestinal motility and secretion, this drug should be used cautiously in patients with a history of peptic ulcer, ulcerative colitis, or gallstones, where biliary colic may be precipitated.

Caution should be exercised when treating hypertensive patients with renal insufficiency since they adjust poorly to lowered blood pressure levels.

Use reserpine cautiously with digitalis and quinidine since cardiac arrhythmias have occurred with the concurrent use of rauwolfia preparations.

Preoperative withdrawal of reserpine does not assure that circulatory instability will not occur. It is important that the anesthesiologist be aware of the patient's drug intake and consider this in the overall management, since hypotension has occurred in patients receiving rauwolfia preparations. Anticholinergic and/or adrenergic drugs (metaraminol, norepinephrine) have been employed to treat adverse vagocirculatory effects.

Animal tumorigenicity: Rodent studies have shown that reserpine is an animal tumorigen, causing an increased incidence of mammary fibroadenomas in female mice, malignant tumors of the seminal vesicles in male mice, and malignant adrenal medullary tumors in male rats. These findings arose in 2 year studies in which the drug was administered in the feed at concentrations of 5 and 10 ppm—about 100 to 300 times the usual human dose. The breast neoplasms are thought to be related to reserpine's prolactin-elevating effect. Several other prolactin-elevating drugs have also been associated with an increased incidence of mammary neoplasia in rodents.

The extent to which these findings indicate a risk to humans is uncertain. Tissue culture experiments show that about one-third of human breast tumors are prolactin-dependent in vitro, a factor of considerable importance if the use of the drug is contemplated in a patient with previously detected breast cancer. The possibility of an increased risk of breast cancer in reserpine users has been studied extensively; however, no firm conclusion has emerged. Although a few epidemiologic studies have suggested a slightly increased risk (less than twofold in all studies except one) in women who have used reserpine, other studies of generally similar design have not confirmed this. Epidemiologic studies conducted using other drugs (neuroleptic agents) that, like reserpine, increase prolactin levels and therefore would be considered rodent mammary carcinogens, have not shown an association between chronic administration of the drug and human mammary tumorigenesis. While long-term clinical observation has not suggested such an association, the available evidence is considered too limited to be conclusive at this time. An association of reserpine intake with pheochromocytoma or tumors of the seminal vesicles has not been explored.

ADVERSE REACTIONS

Methyclothiazide—The following adverse reactions have been associated with the use of thiazide diuretics.

Gastrointestinal: Anorexia, gastric irritation, nausea, vomiting, cramping, diarrhea, constipation, jaundice (intrahepatic cholestatic jaundice), pancreatitis.

Central nervous system: Dizziness, vertigo, paresthesia, headache, xanthopsia.

Dermatologic-Hypersensitivity: Purpura, photosensitivity, rash, urticaria, necrotizing angiitis (vasculitis) (cutaneous vasculitis).

Hematologic: Leukopenia, agranulocytosis, thrombocytopenia, aplastic anemia.

Cardiovascular: Orthostatic hypotension may occur and may be aggravated by alcohol, barbiturates or narcotics.

Miscellaneous: Hyperglycemia, glycosuria, hyperuricemia, muscle spasm, weakness, restlessness.

Reserpine—Reserpine preparations have caused gastrointestinal reactions including hypersecretion, nausea and vomiting, anorexia, and diarrhea; cardiovascular reactions including angina-like symptoms, arrhythmias particularly when used concurrently with digitalis or quinidine, and bradycardia; and central nervous system reactions including drowsiness, depression, nervousness, paradoxical anxiety, nightmares, rare parkinsonian syndrome, CNS sensitization manifested by dull sensorium, deafness, glaucoma, uveitis, and optic atrophy. Nasal congestion is a frequent complaint, and pruritus, rash, dryness of mouth, dizziness, headache, dyspnea, purpura, impotence or decreased libido, dysuria, muscular aches, conjunctival injection, and weight gain have been reported. Extrapyramidal tract symptoms have also occurred. These reactions are usually reversible and disappear when the drug is discontinued.

Whenever DIUTENSEN-R therapy results in adverse reactions which are moderate or severe, dosage should be reduced or therapy withdrawn.

DOSAGE AND ADMINISTRATION

As determined by individual titration (see box warning). The usual adult dosage of DIUTENSEN-R is 1 to 4 tablets a day depending on the individual patient response.

HOW SUPPLIED

NDC 0037-0274-92, bottle of 100
NDC 0037-0274-96, bottle of 500

CAUTION

Federal law prohibits dispensing without prescription.
Rev. 5/83

Shown in Product Identification Section, page 434

LUFYLLIN® ℞
(dyphylline)
Elixir

DESCRIPTION

LUFYLLIN (dyphylline) Elixir is a bronchodilator available for oral administration as a clear red liquid. Each 15 ml (one tablespoonful) contains dyphylline, 100 mg, and alcohol, 20% (by volume).

Other ingredients: FD&C Blue No. 1, FD&C Red No. 40, saccharin sodium, white port wine.

Chemically, dyphylline is 7-(2,3-dihydroxypropyl)-theophylline, a white, extremely bitter, amorphous powder that is freely soluble in water and soluble in alcohol to the extent of 2 g/100 ml. Dyphylline forms a neutral solution that is stable in gastrointestinal fluids over a wide range of pH.

The molecular formula for dyphylline is $C_{10}H_{14}N_4O_4$ with a molecular weight of 254.25.

CLINICAL PHARMACOLOGY

Dyphylline is a xanthine derivative with pharmacologic actions similar to theophylline and other members of this class of drugs. Its primary action is that of bronchodilation, but it also exhibits peripheral vasodilatory and other smooth muscle relaxant activity to a lesser degree. The bronchodilatory action of dyphylline, as with other xanthines, is thought to be mediated through competitive inhibition of phosphodiesterase with a resulting increase in cyclic AMP producing relaxation of bronchial smooth muscle.

Dyphylline is well tolerated and produces less nausea than aminophylline and other alkaline theophylline compounds

when administered orally. Unlike the hydrolyzable salts of theophylline, dyphylline is not converted to free theophylline *in vivo*. It is absorbed rapidly in therapeutically active form and in healthy volunteers reaches a mean peak plasma concentration of 17.1 mcg/ml in approximately 45 minutes following a single oral dose of 1000 mg.

Dyphylline exerts its bronchodilatory effects directly and, unlike theophylline, is excreted unchanged by the kidneys without being metabolized by the liver. Because of this, dyphylline pharmacokinetics and plasma levels are not influenced by various factors that affect liver function and hepatic enzyme activity, such as smoking, age, congestive heart failure or concomitant use of drugs which effect liver function.

The elimination half-life of dyphylline is approximately two hours (1.8–2.1 hr) and approximately 88% of a single oral dose can be recovered from the urine unchanged. The renal clearance would be correspondingly reduced in patients with impaired renal function. In anuric patients, the half-life may be increased 3 to 4 times normal.

Dyphylline plasma levels are dose-related and generally predictable. The range of plasma levels within which dyphylline can be expected to produce effective bronchodilation has not been determined.

Dyphylline plasma concentrations can be accurately determined using high pressure liquid chromatography (HPLC)* or gas-liquid chromatography (GLC).

* *See Valia, et al, J Chromatogr 221 :170 (1980).* Small quantities of pure dyphylline powder may be obtained from Wallace Laboratories, Cranbury, N.J. The internal standard, β-hydroxyethyltheophylline may be obtained from companies supplying analytic chemicals.

INDICATIONS AND USAGE

For relief of acute bronchial asthma and for reversible bronchospasm associated with chronic bronchitis and emphysema.

CONTRAINDICATIONS

Hypersensitivity to dyphylline or related xanthine compounds.

WARNINGS

LUFYLLIN Elixir is not indicated in the management of status asthmaticus which is a serious medical emergency. Although the relationship between plasma levels of dyphylline and appearance of toxicity is unknown, excessive doses may be expected to be associated with an increased risk of adverse effects.

PRECAUTIONS

General: Use LUFYLLIN Elixir with caution in patients with severe cardiac disease, hypertension, hyperthyroidism, or acute myocardial injury or peptic ulcer.

Drug interactions: Synergism between xanthine bronchodilators (e.g., theophylline), ephedrine and other sympathomimetic bronchodilators has been reported. This should be considered whenever these agents are prescribed concomitantly. Concurrent administration of dyphylline and probenecid, which competes for tubular secretion, has been shown to increase the plasma half-life of dyphylline (see CLINICAL PHARMACOLOGY).

Carcinogenesis, mutagenesis, impairment of fertility: No long-term animal studies have been performed with LUFYLLIN Elixir.

Pregnancy: Teratogenic effects—Pregnancy category C. Animal reproduction studies have not been conducted with LUFYLLIN Elixir. It is also not known if 'Lufyllin' Elixir can cause fetal harm when administered to a pregnant woman or can affect reproduction capacity. LUFYLLIN Elixir should be given to a pregnant woman only if clearly needed.

Nursing mothers: Dyphylline is present in human milk at approximately twice the maternal plasma concentration. Caution should be exercised when 'Lufyllin' Elixir is administered to a nursing woman.

Pediatric use: Safety and effectiveness in children have not been established.

ADVERSE REACTIONS

Adverse reactions with the use of LUFYLLIN Elixir have been infrequent, relatively mild, and rarely required reduction in dosage or withdrawal of therapy.

The following adverse reactions which have been reported with other xanthine bronchodilators, and which have most often been related to excessive drug plasma levels, should be considered as potential adverse effects when dyphylline is administered:

Gastrointestinal: nausea, vomiting, epigastric pain, hematemesis, diarrhea.

Central nervous system: headache, irritability, restlessness, insomnia, hyperexcitability, agitation, muscle twitching, generalized clonic and tonic convulsions.

Cardiovascular: palpitation, tachycardia, extrasystoles, flushing, hypotension, circulatory failure, ventricular arrhythmias.

Respiratory: tachypnea.

Renal: albuminuria, gross and microscopic hematuria, diuresis.

Others: hyperglycemia, inappropriate ADH syndrome.

OVERDOSAGE

There have been no reports, in the literature, of overdosage with LUFYLLIN Elixir. However, the following information based on reports of theophylline overdosage are considered typical of the xanthine class of drugs and should be kept in mind.

Signs and symptoms: Restlessness, anorexia, nausea, vomiting, diarrhea, insomnia, irritability, and headache. Marked overdosage with resulting severe toxicity has produced agitation, severe vomiting, dehydration, excessive thirst, tinnitus, cardiac arrhythmias, hyperthermia, diaphoresis, and generalized clonic and tonic convulsions. Cardiovascular collapse has also occurred, with some fatalities. Seizures have occured in some cases associated with very high theophylline plasma concentrations, without any premonitory symptoms of toxicity.

Treatment: There is no specific antidote for overdosage with drugs of the xanthine class. Symptomatic treatment and general supportive measures should be instituted with careful monitoring and maintenance of vital signs, fluids and electrolytes. The stomach should be emptied by inducing emesis if the patient is conscious and responsive, or by gastric lavage, taking care to protect against aspiration, especially in stuporous or comatose patients. Maintenance of an adequate airway is essential in case oxygen or assisted respiration is needed. Symptomatic agents should be avoided but sedatives such as short-acting barbiturates may be useful. Dyphylline is dialyzable and, although not recommended as a routine procedure in overdosage cases, hemodialysis may be of some benefit when severe intoxication is present or when the patient has not responded to general supportive and symptomatic treatment.

DOSAGE AND ADMINISTRATION

Dosage should be individually titrated according to the severity of the condition and the response of the patient.

Usual adult dosage: 2 to 4 tablespoonfuls every six hours. Appropriate dosage adjustments should be made in patients with impaired renal function (see CLINICAL PHARMACOLOGY).

HOW SUPPLIED

LUFYLLIN Elixir:
NDC 0037-0515-68, pint bottle.
NDC 0037-0515-69, gallon bottle.
Storage: Store below 30°C (86°F).
CAUTION: Federal law prohibits dispensing without prescription.
Rev. 2/85

LUFYLLIN® Injection ℞
(dyphylline injection USP)
FOR INTRAMUSCULAR USE ONLY

DESCRIPTION

Chemically, dyphylline is 7-(2,3-dihydroxypropyl)-theophylline, a white, extremely bitter, amorphous powder that is freely soluble in water and alcohol to the extent of 2 g/100 mL.

LUFYLLIN Injection is a clear, colorless, sterile aqueous solution of dyphylline, a xanthine derivative available as a bronchodilator *for intramuscular use only.*

Each mL of LUFYLLIN Injection contains 250 mg of dyphylline (pH adjusted with sodium hydroxide and/or hydrochloric acid).

The molecular formula for dyphylline is $C_{10}H_{14}N_4O_4$ with a molecular weight of 254.25. Its structural formula is:

CLINICAL PHARMACOLOGY

Dyphylline is a xanthine derivative with pharmacologic actions similar to theophylline and other members of this class of drugs. Its primary action is that of bronchodilation, but it also exhibits peripheral vasodilatory and other smooth muscle relaxant activity to a lesser degree. The bronchodilatory action of dyphylline, as with other xanthines, is thought to be mediated through competitive inhibition of phosphodiesterase with a resulting increase in cyclic AMP producing relaxation of bronchial smooth muscle.

LUFYLLIN Injection is well tolerated and causes little or no discomfort, by the intramuscular route, and produces less nausea than aminophylline and other alkaline theophylline compounds. Unlike the hydrolyzable salts of theophylline,

Continued on next page

Wallace—Cont.

dyphylline is not converted to free theophylline *in vivo*. It is absorbed rapidly in therapeutically active form and in healthy volunteers reaches a mean peak plasma concentration comparable to that achieved with equivalent oral doses in approximately 45 minutes (17.1 mg following a single oral dose of 1000 mg).

Dyphylline exerts it bronchodilatory effects directly and, unlike theophylline, is excreted unchanged by the kidneys without being metabolized by the liver. Because of this, dyphylline pharmacokinetics and plasma levels are not influenced by various factors that affect liver function and hepatic enzyme activity, such as smoking, age, congestive heart failure or concomitant use of drugs which effect liver function. The renal clearance would be correspondingly reduced in patients with impaired renal function. In anuric patients, the half-life may be increased 3 to 4 times normal.

The range of plasma levels within which dyphylline can be expected to produce effective bronchodilation has not been determined.

Dyphylline plasma concentrations can be accurately determined using high pressure liquid chromatography (HPLC)* or gas-liquid chromatography (GLC).

* See Valia, *et al: J. Chromatogr.* **221**:170 (1980). Small quantities of pure dyphylline powder may be obtained from Wallace Laboratories, Cranbury, N.J. The internal standard, β-hydroxyethyltheophylline, may be obtained from companies supplying analytical chemicals.

INDICATIONS AND USAGE

For relief of acute bronchial asthma and for reversible bronchospasm associated with chronic bronchitis and emphysema.

CONTRAINDICATIONS

Hypersensitivity to dyphylline or related xanthine compounds.

WARNINGS

LUFYLLIN Injection is not indicated in the management of status asthmaticus or apnea in the newborn, which are serious medical emergencies.

Although the relationship between plasma levels of dyphylline and appearance of toxicity is unknown, excessive doses may be expected to be associated with an increased risk of adverse effects.

PRECAUTIONS

General: Use LUFYLLIN Injection with caution in patients with severe cardiac disease, hypertension, hyperthyroidism, acute myocardial injury or peptic ulcer.

Drug interactions: Synergism between xanthine bronchodilators (e.g., theophylline), ephedrine and other sympathomimetic bronchodilators has been reported. This should be considered whenever these agents are prescribed concomitantly. Concurrent administration of dyphylline and probenecid, which competes for tubular secretion, has been shown to increase the plasma half-life of dyphylline (see Clinical Pharmacology).

Carcinogenesis, mutagenesis, impairment of fertility: No long-term animal studies have been performed with LUFYLLIN Injection.

Pregnancy: Teratogenic effects—Pregnancy Category C. Animal reproduction studies have not been conducted with LUFYLLIN Injection. It is also not known if LUFYLLIN Injection can cause fetal harm when administered to a pregnant woman or can affect reproduction capacity. LUFYLLIN Injection should be given to a pregnant woman only if clearly needed.

Nursing mothers: Dyphylline is present in human milk at approximately twice the maternal plasma concentration. Caution should be exercised when LUFYLLIN Injection is administered to a nursing woman.

Pediatric use: Safety and effectiveness in children have not been established.

ADVERSE REACTIONS

Adverse reactions with the use of LUFYLLIN Injection have been infrequent, relatively mild, and rarely required reduction in dosage or withdrawal of therapy.

The following adverse reactions which have been reported with other xanthine bronchodilators, and which have most often been related to excessive drug plasma levels, should be considered as potential adverse effects when dyphylline is administered:

Gastrointestinal: nausea, vomiting, epigastric pain, hematemesis, diarrhea.

Central nervous system: headache, irritability, restlessness, insomnia, hyperexcitability, agitation, muscle twitching, generalized clonic and tonic convulsions.

Cardiovascular: palpitation, tachycardia, extrasystoles, flushing, hypotension, circulatory failure, ventricular arrhythmias.

Respiratory: tachypnea.

Renal: albuminuria, gross and microscopic hematuria, diuresis.

Other: hyperglycemia, inappropriate ADH syndrome.

OVERDOSAGE

There have been no reports, in the literature, of overdosage with LUFYLLIN Injection. However, the following information based on reports of theophylline overdosage are considered typical of the xanthine class of drugs and should be kept in mind.

Signs and symptoms: Restlessness, anorexia, nausea, vomiting, diarrhea, insomnia, irritability, and headache. Marked overdosage with resulting severe toxicity has produced agitation, severe vomiting, dehydration, excessive thirst, tinnitus, cardiac arrhythmias, hyperthermia, diaphoresis, and generalized clonic and tonic convulsions. Cardiovascular collapse has also occurred, with some fatalities. Seizures have occurred in some cases associated with very high theophylline plasma concentrations, without any premonitory symptoms of toxicity.

Treatment: There is no specific antidote for overdosage with drugs of the xanthine class. Symptomatic treatment and general supportive measures should be instituted with careful monitoring and maintenance of vital signs, fluids and electrolytes. The stomach should be emptied by inducing emesis if the patient is conscious and responsive, or by gastric lavage, taking care to protect against aspiration, especially in stuporous or comatose patients. Maintenance of an adequate airway is essential in case oxygen or assisted respiration is needed. Sympathomimetic agents should be avoided but sedatives such as short-acting barbiturates may be useful.

Dyphylline is dialyzable and, although not recommended as a routine procedure in overdosage cases, hemodialysis may be of some benefit when severe intoxication is present or when the patient has not responded to general supportive and symptomatic treatment.

DOSAGE AND ADMINISTRATION

LUFYLLIN Injection is *for intramuscular use only.*

Usual adult dosage: 500 mg (2 mL) I.M. initially, followed by 250–500 mg (1 to 2 mL) every two to six hours, as indicated by the patient's response. Do not exceed total dosage of 15 mg/kg every six hours.

HOW SUPPLIED

Box of 25 × 2 mL ampuls (NDC 0037-0537-01).

Storage: Store below 40°C (104°F), preferably between 15° and 30°C (59° to 86°F). Excessive cold may cause formation of a precipitate. DO NOT USE if precipitate is present.

CAUTION: Federal law prohibits dispensing without prescription.

Distributed by
WALLACE LABORATORIES
Division of
CARTER-WALLACE, INC.
Cranbury, New Jersey 08512

Manufactured by:
Taylor Pharmacal Co.
Decatur, Illinois 62526

Rev. 2/85
Shown in Product Identification Section, page 434

LUFYLLIN® Tablets   ℞
(dyphylline tablets, USP, 200 mg)
LUFYLLIN®–400 Tablets   ℞
(dyphylline tablets, USP, 400 mg)

DESCRIPTION

LUFYLLIN (dyphylline), a xanthine derivative, is a bronchodilator available for oral administration as tablets containing 200 mg and 400 mg of dyphylline. Other ingredients: magnesium stearate, microcrystalline cellulose.

Chemically, dyphylline is 7-(2,3-dihydroxypropyl)-theophylline, a white, extremely bitter, amorphous powder that is freely soluble in water and soluble in alcohol to the extent of 2 g/100 ml. Dyphylline forms a neutral solution that is stable in gastrointestinal fluids over a wide range of pH.

The molecular formula for dyphylline is $C_{10}H_{14}N_4O_4$ with a molecular weight of 254.25. Its structural formula is:

CLINICAL PHARMACOLOGY

Dyphylline is a xanthine derivative with pharmacologic actions similar to theophylline and other members of this class of drugs. Its primary action is that of bronchodilation, but it also exhibits peripheral vasodilatory and other smooth muscle relaxant activity to a lesser degree. The bronchodilatory action of dyphylline, as with other xanthines, is thought to be mediated through competitive inhibition of phosphodiesterase with a resulting increase in cyclic AMP producing relaxation of bronchial smooth muscle.

LUFYLLIN is well tolerated and produces less nausea than aminophylline and other alkaline theophylline compounds when administered orally. Unlike the hydrolyzable salts of theophylline, dyphylline is not converted to free theophylline *in vivo*. It is absorbed rapidly in therapeutically active form and in healthy volunteers reaches a mean peak plasma concentration of 17.1 mcg/ml in approximately 45 minutes following a single oral dose of 1000 mg of LUFYLLIN.

Dyphylline exerts its bronchodilatory effects directly and, unlike theophylline, is excreted unchanged by the kidneys without being metabolized by the liver. Because of this, dyphylline pharmacokinetics and plasma levels are not influenced by various factors that affect liver function and hepatic enzyme activity, such as smoking, age, congestive heart failure or concomitant use of drugs which affect liver function.

The elimination half-life of dyphylline is approximately two hours (1.8–2.1 hr) and approximately 88% of a single oral dose can be recovered from the urine unchanged. The renal clearance would be correspondingly reduced in patients with impaired renal function. In anuric patients, the half-life may be increased 3 to 4 times normal.

Dyphylline plasma levels are dose-related and generally predictable. The range of plasma levels within which dyphylline can be expected to produce effective bronchodilation has not been determined.

Dyphylline plasma concentrations can be accurately determined using high pressure liquid chromatography (HPLC)* or gas-liquid chromatography (GLC).

*See Valia, *et al. J. Chromatogr.* **221**: 170 (1980). Small quantities of pure dyphylline powder may be obtained from Wallace Laboratories, Cranbury, N.J. The internal standard, β-hydroxyethyltheophylline, may be obtained from companies supplying analytical chemicals.

INDICATIONS AND USAGE

For relief of acute bronchial asthma and for reversible bronchospasm associated with chronic bronchitits and emphysema.

CONTRAINDICATIONS

Hypersensitivity to dyphylline or related xanthine compounds.

WARNINGS

LUFYLLIN is not indicated in the management of status asthmaticus, which is a serious medical emergency.

Although the relationship between plasma levels of dyphylline and appearance of toxicity is unknown, excessive doses may be expected to be associated with an increased risk of adverse effects.

PRECAUTIONS

General: Use LUFYLLIN with caution in patients with severe cardiac disease, hypertension, hyperthyroidism, acute myocardial injury or peptic ulcer.

Drug interactions: Synergism between xanthine bronchodilators (e.g., theophylline), ephedrine and other sympathomimetic bronchodilators has been reported. This should be considered whenever these agents are prescribed concomitantly. Concurrent administration of dyphylline and probenecid, which competes for tubular secretion, has been shown to increase the plasma half-life of dyphylline (see Clinical Pharmacology).

Carcinogenesis, mutagenesis, impairment of fertility: No long-term animal studies have been performed with LUFYLLIN.

Pregnancy: Teratogenic effects—Pregnancy Category C. Animal reproduction studies have not been conducted with LUFYLLIN. It is also not known if LUFYLLIN can cause fetal harm when administered to a pregnant woman or can affect reproduction capacity. LUFYLLIN should be given to a pregnant woman only if clearly needed.

Nursing mothers: Dyphylline is present in human milk at approximately twice the maternal plasma concentration. Caution should be exercised when LUFYLLIN is administered to a nursing woman.

Pediatric use: Safety and effectiveness in children have not been established.

ADVERSE REACTIONS

Adverse reactions with the use of LUFYLLIN have been infrequent, relatively mild, and rarely required reduction in dosage or withdrawal of therapy.

The following adverse reactions which have been reported with other xanthine bronchodilators, and which have most often been related to excessive drug plasma levels, should be considered as potential adverse effects when dyphylline is administered:

Gastrointestinal: nausea, vomiting, epigastric pain, hematemesis, diarrhea.

Central nervous system: headache, irritability, restlessness, insomnia, hyperexcitability, agitation, muscle twitching, generalized clonic and tonic convulsions.

Cardiovascular: palpitation, tachycardia, extrasystoles, flushing, hypotension, circulatory failure, ventricular arrhythmias.

Respiratory: tachypnea.

Renal: albuminuria, gross and microscopic hematuria, diuresis.

Other: hyperglycemia, inappropriate ADH syndrome.

OVERDOSAGE

There have been no reports, in the literature, of overdosage with LUFYLLIN. However, the following information based on reports of theophylline overdosage are considered typical of the xanthine class of drugs and should be kept in mind.

Signs and symptoms: Restlessness, anorexia, nausea, vomiting, diarrhea, insomnia, irritability, and headache. Marked overdosage with resulting severe toxicity has produced agitation, severe vomiting, dehydration, excessive thirst, tinnitus, cardiac arrhythmias, hyperthermia, diaphoresis, and generalized clonic and tonic convulsions. Cardiovascular collapse has also occcured, with some fatalities. Seizures have occurred in some cases associated with very high theophylline plasma concentrations, without any premonitory symptoms of toxicity.

Treatment: There is no specific antidote for overdosage with drugs of the xanthine class. Symptomatic treatment and general supportive measures should be instituted with careful monitoring and maintenance of vital signs, fluids and electrolytes. The stomach should be emptied by inducing emesis if the patient is conscious and responsive, or by gastric lavage, taking care to protect against aspiration, especially in stuporous or comatose patients. Maintenance of an adequate airway is essential in case oxygen or assisted respiration is needed. Sympathomimetic agents should be avoided but sedatives such as short-acting barbiturates may be useful.

Dyphylline is dialyzable and, although not recommended as a routine procedure in overdosage cases, hemodialysis may be of some benefit when severe intoxication is present or when the patient has not responded to general supportive and symptomatic treatment.

DOSAGE AND ADMINISTRATION

Dosage should be individually titrated according to the severity of the condition and the response of the patient.

Usual adult dosage: Up to 15 mg/kg every six hours. Appropriate dosage adjustments should be made in patients with impaired renal function (see Clinical Pharmacology).

HOW SUPPLIED

LUFYLLIN Tablets: Available as white, rectangular, monogrammed tablets containing 200 mg dyphylline in bottles of 100 (NDC 0037-0521-92) and 1000 (NDC 0037-0521-97), and individually film-sealed tablets in unit-dose boxes of 100 (NDC 0037-0521-85).

LUFYLLIN-400 Tablets: Available as white, capsule-shaped, monogrammed tablets containing 400 mg dyphylline in bottles of 100 (NDC 0037-0731-92) and 1000 (NDC 0037-0731-97), and individually film-sealed tablets in unit-dose boxes of 100 (NDC 0037-0731-85).

Storage: Store at controlled room temperature.

CAUTION: Federal law prohibits dispensing without prescription.

WALLACE LABORATORIES
Division of
CARTER-WALLACE, INC.
Cranbury, New Jersey 08512

8/87

Shown in Product Identification Section, page 434

LUFYLLIN®–GG   ℞
Tablets and Elixir

DESCRIPTION

LUFYLLIN®-GG is a bronchodilator/expectorant combination available for oral administration as *Tablets* and *Elixir.*
Each Tablet contains:
Dyphylline .... 200 mg
Guaifenesin .... 200 mg
Other ingredients: corn starch, D&C Yellow No. 10, magnesium aluminium silicate, magnesium stearate, microcrystalline cellulose.
Each 15 mL (one tablespoonful) of Elixir contains:
Dyphylline .... 100 mg
Guaifenesin .... 100 mg
Alcohol (by volume) 17%
Other ingredients: citric acid, FD&C Yellow No. 6, flavor (artificial), purified water, saccharin sodium, sodium citrate, sucrose.
Dyphylline is 7-(2,3-dihydroxypropyl)-theophylline, a white, extremely bitter, amorphous powder that is fully soluble in water and soluble in alcohol to the extent of 2 g/100 mL. Dyphylline forms a neutral solution that is stable in gastrointestinal fluids over a wide range of pH.

CLINICAL PHARMACOLOGY

Dyphylline is a xanthine derivative with pharmacologic actions similar to theophylline and other members of this class of drugs. Its primary action is that of bronchodilation, but it also exhibits peripheral vasodilatory and other smooth muscle relaxant activity to a lesser degree. The bronchodilatory action of dyphylline, as with as other xanthines, is thought to be mediated through competitive inhibition of phosphodiesterase with a resulting increase in cyclic AMP producing relaxation of bronchial smooth muscle.

Dyphylline in LUFYLLIN-GG is well tolerated and produces less nausea than aminophylline and other alkaline theophylline compounds when administered orally. Unlike the hydrolyzable salts of theophylline, dyphylline is not converted to free theophylline *in vivo.* It is absorbed rapidly in therapeutically active form and in healthy volunteers reaches a mean peak plasma concentration of 17.1 mcg/mL in approximately 45 minutes following a single oral dose of 1000 mg of dyphylline.

Dyphylline exerts its bronchodilatory effects directly and, unlike theophylline, is excreted unchanged by the kidneys without being metabolized by the liver. Because of this, dyphylline pharmacokinetics and plasma levels are not influenced by various factors that affect liver function and hepatic enzyme activity, such as smoking, age, or concomitant use of drugs which effect liver function.

The elimination half-life of dyphylline is approximately two hours (1.8–2.1 hr) and approximately 88% of a single oral dose can be recovered from the urine unchanged. The renal clearance would be correspondingly reduced in patients with impaired renal function. In anuric patients, the half-life may be increased 3 to 4 times normal.

Dyphylline plasma levels are dose-related and generally predictable. The therapeutic range of plasma levels within which dyphylline can be expected to produce effective bronchodilation has not been determined.

Dyphylline plasma concentrations can be accurately determined using high pressure liquid chromatography (HPLC)* or gas-liquid chromatography (GLC).

Guaifenesin is an expectorant whose action helps increase the output of thin respiratory tract fluid to facilitate mucociliary clearance and removal of inspissated mucus.

* *See* Valia, *et al, J Chromatogr.* **221:** 170 (1980). Small quantities of pure dyphylline powder may be obtained from Wallace Laboratories, Cranbury, N.J. The internal standard, β-hydroxyethyltheophylline, may be obtained from companies supplying analytical chemicals.

Guaifensin is an expectorant whose action helps increase the output of thin respiratory tract fluid to facilitate mucociliary clearance and removal of inspissated mucus.

INDICATIONS AND USAGE

For relief of acute bronchial asthma and for reversible bronchospasm associated with chronic bronchitis and emphysema.

CONTRAINDICATIONS

Hypersensitivity to any of the ingredients or related compounds.

WARNINGS

LUFYLLIN-GG is not indicated in the management of status asthmaticus, which is a serious medical emergency.

Although the relationship between plasma levels of dyphylline and appearance of toxicity is unknown, excessive doses may be expected to be associated with an increased risk of adverse effects.

PRECAUTIONS

General: Use LUFYLLIN-GG with caution in patients with severe cardiac disease, hypertension, hyperthyroidism, acute myocardial injury or peptic ulcer.

Drug interactions: Synergism between xanthine bronchodilators (e.g., theophylline), ephedrine and other sympathomimetic bronchodilators has been reported. This should be considered whenever these agents are prescribed concomitantly. Concurrent administration of dyphylline and probenecid, which competes for tubular secretion, has been shown to increase plasma half-life of dyphylline (see Clinical Pharmacology).

Carcinogenesis, mutagenesis, impairment of fertility: No long-term animal studies have been performed with LUFYLLIN-GG.

Pregnancy: Teratogenic effects—Pregnancy Category C. Animal reproduction studies have not been conducted with LUFYLLIN-GG. It is also not known whether the product can cause fetal harm when administered to a pregnant woman or can affect reproduction capacity. LUFYLLIN-GG should be given to a pregnant woman only if clearly needed.

Nursing mothers: Dyphylline is present in human milk at approximately twice the maternal plasma concentration. Caution should be exercised when LUFYLLIN-GG is administered to a nursing woman.

Pediatric use: Safety and effectiveness in children below the age of six have not been established. Use caution when administering to children six years of age or older.

ADVERSE REACTIONS

LUFYLLIN-GG may cause nausea, headache, cardiac palpitation and CNS stimulation. Postprandial administration may help avoid gastric discomfort.

The following adverse reactions which have been reported with other xanthine bronchodilators, and which have most often been related to excessive drug plasma levels, should be considered as potential adverse effects when dyphylline is administered:

Gastrointestinal: nausea, vomiting, epigastric pain, hematemesis, diarrhea.

Central nervous system: headache, irritability, restlessness, insomnia, hyperexcitability, agitation, muscle twitching, generalized clonic and tonic convulsions.

Cardiovascular: palpitation, tachycardia, extrasystoles, flushing, hypotension, circulatory failure, ventricular arrhythmias.

Respiratory: tachypnea.

Renal: albuminuria, gross and microscopic hematuria, diuresis.

Other: hyperglycemia, inappropriate ADH syndrome.

OVERDOSAGE

There have been no reports, in the literature, of overdosage with LUFYLLIN-GG. However, the following information based on reports of theophylline overdosage are considered typical of the xanthine class of drugs and should be kept in mind.

Signs and symptoms: Restlessness, anorexia, nausea, vomiting, diarrhea, insomnia, irritability, and headache. Marked overdosage with resulting severe toxicity has produced agitation, severe vomiting, dehydration, excessive thirst, tinnitus, cardiac arrhythmias, hyperthermia, diaphoresis, and generalized clonic and tonic convulsions. Cardiovascular collapse has also occured, with some fatalities. Seizures have occured in some cases associated with very high theophylline plasma concentrations, without any premonitory symptoms of toxicity.

Treatment: There is no specific antidote for overdosage with drugs of the xanthine class. Symptomatic treatment and general supportive measures should be instituted with careful monitoring and maintenance of vital signs, fluids and electrolytes. The stomach should be emptied by inducing emesis if the patient is conscious and responsive, or by gastric lavage, taking care to protect against aspiration, especially in stuporous or comatose patients. Maintenance of an adequate airway is essential in case oxygen or assisted respiration is needed. Sympathomimetic agents should be avoided but sedatives such as short-acting barbiturates may be useful.

Dyphylline is dialyzable and, although not recommended as a routine procedure in overdosage cases, hemodialysis may be of some benefit when severe intoxication is present or when the patient has not responded to general supportive and symptomatic treatment.

DOSAGE AND ADMINISTRATION

Dosage should be individually titrated according to the severity of the condition and the response of the patient.

Usual adult dosage:
One tablet or 30 mL (2 tablespoonfuls) elixir, four times daily.

Children above age six:
One-half to one tablet or 15 to 30 mL (one to two tablespoonfuls) elixir, three to four times daily.

Not recommended for use in children below age six: (see Precautions).

HOW SUPPLIED

LUFYLLIN-GG Tablets: round, light yellow, monogrammed tablets, scored on one side, in bottles of 100 (NDC 0037-0541-92) and 1000 (NDC 0037-0541-97) and boxes of 100 unit-dose, individually film-sealed tablets (NDC 0037-0541-85).

LUFYLLIN-GG Elixir: clear, light yellow-orange liquid with a mild wine-like odor and taste, in bottles of one pint (NDC 0037-0545-68) and one gallon (NDC 0037-0545-69).

Storage:
Tablets—Avoid excessive heat—above 40°C (104°F).
Elixir—Store below 30°C (86°F).

CAUTION: Federal law prohibits dispensing without prescription.

WALLACE LABORATORIES
Division of
CARTER-WALLACE, INC.
Cranbury, New Jersey 08512

Rev. 2/85

Shown in Product Identification Section, page 434

MALTSUPEX®   OTC
(malt soup extract)
Powder, Liquid, Tablets

(See PDR For Nonprescription Drugs)

Continued on next page

Wallace—Cont.

MEPROSPAN® ℂ ℞
(meprobamate, sustained-release capsules)

DESCRIPTION

Meprobamate is a white powder with a characteristic odor and a bitter taste. It is slightly soluble in water, freely soluble in acetone and alcohol, and sparingly soluble in ether. The structural formula of meprobamate is

$$NH_2COOCH_2-\underset{\underset{CH_2CH_2CH_3}{|}}{\overset{\overset{CH_3}{|}}{C}}-CH_2OOCNH_2$$

'Meprospan' 400 contains 400 mg meprobamate per capsule. Other ingredients: corn starch, FD&C Blue #1, FD&C Yellow #6, gelatin, sucrose and other ingredients.
'Meprospan' 200 contains 200 mg meprobamate per capsule. Other ingredients: corn starch, FD&C Yellow #6, gelatin, sucrose and other ingredients.

ACTIONS

Meprobamate is a carbamate derivative which has been shown in animal studies to have effects at multiple sites in the central nervous system, including the thalamus and limbic system.

INDICATIONS

'Meprospan' (meprobamate) is indicated for the management of anxiety disorders or for the short-term relief of the symptoms of anxiety. Anxiety or tension associated with the stress of everyday life usually do not require treatment with an anxiolytic.
The effectiveness of 'Meprospan' in long-term use, that is, more than 4 months, has not been assessed by systematic clinical studies. The physician should periodically reassess the usefulness of the drug for the individual patient.

CONTRAINDICATIONS

Acute intermittent porphyria as well as allergic or idiosyncratic reactions to meprobamate or related compounds such as carisoprodol, mebutamate, tybamate, or carbromal.

WARNINGS

Drug Dependence—Physical dependence, psychological dependence, and abuse have occurred. When chronic intoxication from prolonged use occurs, it usually involves ingestion of greater than recommended doses and is manifested by ataxia, slurred speech, and vertigo. Therefore, careful supervision of dose and amounts prescribed is advised, as well as avoidance of prolonged administration, especially for alcoholics and other patients with a known propensity for taking excessive quantities of drugs.
Sudden withdrawal of the drug after prolonged and excessive use may precipitate recurrence of pre-existing symptoms, such as anxiety, anorexia, or insomnia, or withdrawal reactions, such as vomiting, ataxia, tremors, muscle twitching, confusional states, hallucinosis, and, rarely, convulsive seizures. Such seizures are more likely to occur in persons with central nervous system damage or pre-existent or latent convulsive disorders. Onset of withdrawal symptoms occurs usually within 12 to 48 hours after discontinuation of meprobamate; symptoms usually cease within the next 12 to 48 hours.
When excessive dosage has continued for weeks or months, dosage should be reduced gradually over a period of one or two weeks rather than abruptly stopped. Alternatively, a short-acting barbiturate may be substituted, then gradually withdrawn.
Potentially Hazardous Tasks—Patients should be warned that this drug may impair the mental and/or physical abilities required for the performance of potentially hazardous tasks such as driving a motor vehicle or operating machinery.
Additive Effects—Since the effects of meprobamate and alcohol or meprobamate and other CNS depressants or psychotropic drugs may be additive, appropriate caution should be exercised with patients who take more than one of these agents simultaneously.
USAGE IN PREGNANCY AND LACTATION—An increased risk of congenital malformations associated with the use of minor tranquilizers (meprobamate, chlordiazepoxide, and diazepam) during the first trimester of pregnancy has been suggested in several studies. Because use of these drugs is rarely a matter of urgency, their use during this period should almost always be avoided. The possibility that a woman of childbearing potential may be pregnant at the time of institution of therapy should be considered. Patients should be advised that if they become pregnant during therapy or intend to become pregnant they should communicate with their physicians about the desirability of discontinuing the drug.

Meprobamate passes the placental barrier. It is present both in umbilical cord blood at or near maternal plasma levels and in breast milk of lactating mothers at concentrations two or four times that of maternal plasma. When use of meprobamate is contemplated in breast-feeding patients, the drug's higher concentration in breast milk as compared to maternal plasma levels should be considered.
Usage in Children—Meprobamate should not be administered to children under age six, since there is a lack of documented evidence for safety and effectiveness in this age group.

PRECAUTIONS

The lowest effective dose should be administered, particularly to elderly and/or debilitated patients, in order to preclude oversedation.
The possibility of suicide attempts should be considered and the least amount of drug feasible should be dispensed at any one time.
Meprobamate is metabolized in the liver and excreted by the kidney; to avoid its excess accumulation, caution should be exercised in administration to patients with compromised liver or kidney function.
Meprobamate occasionally may precipitate seizures in epileptic patients.

ADVERSE REACTIONS

Central Nervous System: Drowsiness, ataxia, dizziness, slurred speech, headache, vertigo, weakness, paresthesias, impairment of visual accommodation, euphoria, overstimulation, paradoxical excitement, fast EEG activity.
Gastrointestinal—Nausea, vomiting, diarrhea.
Cardiovascular—Palpitations, tachycardia, various forms of arrhythmia, transient ECG changes, syncope; also, hypotensive crises (including one fatal case).
Allergic or Idiosyncratic—Allergic or idiosyncratic reactions are usually seen within the period of the first to fourth dose in patients having had no previous contact with the drug. Milder reactions are characterized by an itchy, urticarial, or erythematous maculopapular rash which may be generalized or confined to the groin. Other reactions have included leukopenia, acute nonthrombocytopenic purpura, petechiae, ecchymoses, eosinophilia, peripheral edema, adenopathy, fever, fixed drug eruption with cross reaction to carisoprodol, and cross sensitivity between meprobamate/mebutamate and meprobamate/carbromal.
More severe hypersensitivity reactions, rarely reported, include hyperpyrexia, chills, angioneurotic edema, bronchospasm, oliguria, and anuria. Also, anaphylaxis, erythema multiforme, exfoliative dermatitis, stomatitis, proctitis, Stevens-Johnson syndrome, and bullous dermatitis, including one fatal case of the latter following administration of meprobamate in combination with prednisolone.
In case of allergic or idiosyncratic reactions to meprobamate, discontinue the drug and initiate appropriate symptomatic therapy, which may include epinephrine, antihistamines, and in severe cases corticosteroids. In evaluating possible allergic reactions, also consider allergy to excipients (information on excipients is available to physicians on request).
Hematologic—(See also *Allergic or Idiosyncratic*.) Agranulocytosis and aplastic anemia have been reported, although no causal relationship has been established. These cases rarely were fatal. Rare cases of thrombocytopenic purpura have been reported.
Other—Exacerbation of porphyric symptoms.

DOSAGE AND ADMINISTRATION

The usual adult dosage of 'Meprospan' (meprobamate, sustained-release capsules) is one to two 400 mg capsules in the morning and again at bedtime; doses above 2400 mg daily are not recommended. The usual dosage for children ages six to twelve is one 200 mg capsule in the morning and again at bedtime. Meprobamate is not recommended for children under age six.

OVERDOSAGE

Suicidal attempts with meprobamate have resulted in drowsiness, lethargy, stupor, ataxia, coma, shock, vasomotor and respiratory collapse. Some suicidal attempts have been fatal. Overdosage experience with 'Meprospan' (meprobamate, sustained-release capsules) is limited. However, the following data on meprobamate tablets have been reported in the literature and from other sources. These data are not expected to correlate with each case (considering factors such as individual susceptibility and length of time from ingestion to treatment), but represent the *usual ranges* reported.
Acute simple overdose (meprobamate alone): Death has been reported with ingestion of as little as 12 gm meprobamate and survival with as much as 40 gm.
Blood Levels:
0.5–2.0 mg% represents the usual blood level range of meprobamate after therapeutic doses. The level may occasionally be as high as 3.0 mg%.
3–10 mg% usually corresponds to findings of mild to moderate symptoms of overdosage, such as stupor or light coma.
10–20 mg% usually corresponds to deeper coma, requiring more intensive treatment. Some fatalities occur.

At levels greater than 20 mg%, more fatalities than survivals can be expected.
Acute combined overdose (meprobamate with alcohol or other CNS depressants or psychotropic drugs): Since effects can be additive, a history of ingestion of a low dose of meprobamate plus any of these compounds (or of a relatively low blood or tissue level) cannot be used as a prognostic indicator.
In cases where excessive doses have been taken, sleep ensues rapidly and blood pressure, pulse, and respiratory rates are reduced to basal levels. Any drug remaining in the stomach should be removed and symptomatic therapy given. Should respiration or blood pressure become compromised, respiratory assistance, central nervous system stimulants, and pressor agents should be administered cautiously as indicated. Meprobamate is metabolized in the liver and excreted by the kidney. Diuresis, osmotic (mannitol) diuresis, peritoneal dialysis, and hemodialysis have been used successfully. Careful monitoring of urinary output is necessary and caution should be taken to avoid overhydration. Relapse and death, after initial recovery, have been attributed to incomplete gastric emptying and delayed absorption. Meprobamate can be measured in biological fluids by two methods: colorimetric (Hoffman, A. J. and Ludwig, B. J.: *J Amer Pharm Assn 48:* 740, 1959) and gas chromatographic (Douglas, J. F. et al: *Anal Chem 39:* 956, 1967).

HOW SUPPLIED

'Meprospan' 400: Each sustained-release, blue-topped capsule contains meprobamate, U.S.P., 400 mg in bottles of 100 (NDC 0037-1301-01). 'Meprospan' 200: Each sustained-release, yellow-topped capsule contains meprobamate, U.S.P., 200 mg in bottles of 100 (NDC 0037-1401-01).

Distributed by WALLACE LABORATORIES
Division of CARTER-WALLACE, INC.
Cranbury, New Jersey 08512
Manufactured by KV Pharmacal, St. Louis, Mo. 63144
Rev. 8/85

MILTOWN® ℂ ℞
(meprobamate, U.S.P.)
Tablets

DESCRIPTION

Meprobamate is a white powder with a *characteristic odor* and a bitter taste. It is slightly soluble in water, freely soluble in acetone and alcohol, and sparingly soluble in ether.
'Miltown'-200 contains 200 mg meprobamate per tablet. Other ingredients: acacia, carnauba wax, corn starch, gelatin, magnesium carbonate, magnesium stearate, methylcellulose, shellac, sugar, talc, titanium dioxide, white wax and other ingredients.
'Miltown'-400 contains 400 mg meprobamate per tablet. Other ingredients: corn starch, magnesium stearate, methylcellulose.
'Miltown'-600 contains 600 mg meprobamate per tablet. Other ingredients: alginic acid, corn starch, ethylcellulose, magnesium stearate, purified stearic acid.

ACTIONS

Meprobamate is a carbamate derivative which has been shown in animal studies to have effects at multiple sites in the central nervous system, including the thalamus and limbic system.

INDICATIONS

'Miltown' (meprobamate) is indicated for the management of anxiety disorders or for the short-term relief of the symptoms of anxiety. Anxiety or tension associated with the stress of everyday life usually do not require treatment with an anxiolytic.
The effectiveness of 'Miltown' in long-term use, that is, more than 4 months, has not been assessed by systematic clinical studies. The physician should periodically reassess the usefulness of the drug for the individual patient.

CONTRAINDICATIONS

Acute intermittent porphyria as well as allergic or idiosyncratic reactions to meprobamate or related compounds such as carisoprodol, mebutamate, tybamate or carbromal.

WARNINGS

Drug Dependence
Physical dependence, psychological dependence, and abuse have occurred. When chronic intoxication from prolonged use occurs, it usually involves ingestion of greater than recommended doses and is manifested by ataxia, slurred speech, and vertigo. Therefore, careful supervision of dose and amounts prescribed is advised, as well as avoidance of prolonged administration, especially for alcoholics and other patients with a known propensity for taking excessive quantities of drugs.
Sudden withdrawal of the drug after prolonged and excessive use may precipitate recurrence of pre-existing symptoms, such as anxiety, anorexia, or insomnia, or withdrawal reactions, such as vomiting, ataxia, tremors, muscle twitching, confusional states, hallucinosis, and, rarely, convulsive seizures. Such seizures are more likely to occur in persons

with central nervous system damage or pre-existent or latent convulsive disorders. Onset of withdrawal symptoms occurs usually within 12 to 48 hours after discontinuation of meprobamate; symptoms usually cease within the next 12 to 48 hours.

When excessive dosage has continued for weeks or months, dosage should be reduced gradually over a period of one or two weeks rather than abruptly stopped. Alternatively, a short-acting barbiturate may be substituted, then gradually withdrawn.

Potentially Hazardous Tasks

Patients should be warned that this drug may impair the mental and/or physical abilities required for the performance of potentially hazardous tasks such as driving a motor vehicle or operating machinery.

Additive Effects

Since the effects of meprobamate and alcohol or meprobamate and other CNS depressants or psychotropic drugs may be additive, appropriate caution should be exercised with patients who take more than one of these agents simultaneously.

Usage in Pregnancy and Lactation

An increased risk of congenital malformations associated with the use of minor tranquilizers (meprobamate, chlordiazepoxide, and diazepam) during the first trimester of pregnancy has been suggested in several studies. Because use of these drugs is rarely a matter of urgency, their use during this period should almost always be avoided. The possibility that a woman of childbearing potential may be pregnant at the time of institution of therapy should be considered. Patients should be advised that if they become pregnant during therapy or intend to become pregnant they should communicate with their physician about the desirability of discontinuing the drug.

Meprobamate passes the placental barrier. It is present both in umbilical cord blood at or near maternal plasma levels and in breast milk of lactating mothers at concentrations two to four times that of maternal plasma. When use of meprobamate is contemplated in breast-feeding patients, the drug's higher concentration in breast milk as compared to maternal plasma levels should be considered.

Usage in Children

'Miltown'-200 and 'Miltown'-400 should not be administered to children under age six, since there is a lack of documented evidence for safety and effectiveness in this age group. 'Miltown'-600 is not intended for use in children.

PRECAUTIONS

The lowest effective dose should be administered, particularly to elderly and/or debilitated patients, in order to preclude oversedation.

The possibility of suicide attempts should be considered and the least amount of drug feasible should be dispensed at any one time.

Meprobamate is metabolized in the liver and excreted by the kidney; to avoid its excess accumulation, caution should be exercised in administration to patients with compromised liver or kidney function.

Meprobamate occasionally may precipitate seizures in epileptic patients.

ADVERSE REACTIONS

Central Nervous System

Drowsiness, ataxia, dizziness, slurred speech, headache, vertigo, weakness, paresthesias, impairment of visual accomodation, euphoria, overstimulation, paradoxical excitement, fast EEG activity.

Gastrointestinal

Nausea, vomiting, diarrhea.

Cardiovascular

Palpitations, tachycardia, various forms of arrhythmia, transient ECG changes, syncope; also, hypotensive crises (including one fatal case).

Allergic or Idiosyncratic

Allergic or idiosyncratic reactions are usually seen within the period of the first to fourth dose in patients having had no previous contact with the drug. Milder reactions are characterized by an itchy, urticarial, or erythematous maculopapular rash which may be generalized or confined to the groin. Other reactions have included leukopenia, acute non-thrombocytopenic purpura, petechiae, ecchymoses, eosinophilia, peripheral edema, adenopathy, fever, fixed drug eruption with cross reaction to carisoprodol, and cross sensitivity between meprobamate/mebutamate and meprobamate/carbromal.

More severe hypersensitivity reactions, rarely reported, include hyperpyrexia, chills, angioneurotic edema, bronchospasm, oliguria, and anuria. Also, anaphylaxis, erythema multiforme, exfoliative dermatitis, stomatitis, proctitis, Stevens-Johnson syndrome, and bullous dermatitis, including one fatal case of the latter following administration of meprobamate in combination with prednisolone.

In case of allergic or idiosyncratic reactions to meprobamate, discontinue the drug and initiate appropriate symptomatic therapy, which may include epinephrine, antihistamines, and in severe cases corticosteroids. In evaluating possible allergic reactions, also consider allergy to excipients.

Hematologic

(See also **Allergic or Idiosyncratic**.) Agranulocytosis and aplastic anemia have been reported. These cases rarely were fatal. Rare cases of thrombocytopenic purpura have been reported.

Other

Exacerbation of porphyric symptoms.

DOSAGE AND ADMINISTRATION

'Miltown'-200 and 400:

The usual adult daily dosage is 1200 mg to 1600 mg, in three or four divided doses; a daily dosage above 2400 mg is not recommended. The usual daily dosage for children ages six to twelve is 200 mg to 600 mg, in two or three divided doses.

Not recommended for children under age 6 (see **Usage in Children**).

'Miltown'-600:

Adults—One tablet twice a day. Doses of meprobamate above 2400 mg daily are not recommended.

Not recommended for use in children (see **Usage in Children**).

OVERDOSAGE

Suicidal attempts with meprobamate have resulted in drowsiness, lethargy, stupor, ataxia, coma, shock, vasomotor and respiratory collapse. Some suicidal attempts have been fatal. The following data on meprobamate tablets have been reported in the literature and from other sources. These data are not expected to correlate with each case (considering factors such as individual susceptibility and length of time from ingestion to treatment), but represent the usual ranges reported.

Acute simple overdose (meprobamate alone): Death has been reported with ingestion of as little as 12 gm meprobamate and survival with as much as 40 gm.

Blood Levels:

0.5–2.0 mg% represents the usual blood level range of meprobamate after therapeutic doses. The level may occasionally be as high as 3.0 mg%.

3–10 mg% usually corresponds to findings of mild to moderate symptoms of overdosage, such as stupor or light coma.

10–20 mg% usually corresponds to deeper coma, requiring more intensive treatment. Some fatalities occur.

At levels greater than 20%, more fatalities than survivals can be expected.

Acute combined overdeose (meprobamate with alcohol or other CNS depressants or psychotropic drugs): Since effects can be additive, a history of ingestion of a low dose of meprobamate plus any of these compounds (or of a relative low blood or tissue level) cannot be used as a prognostic indicator. In cases where excessive doses have been taken, sleep ensues rapidly and blood pressure, pulse, and respiratory rates are reduced to basal levels. Any drug remaining in the stomach should be removed and symptomatic therapy given. Should respiration or blood pressure become compromised, respiratory assistance, central nervous system stimulants, and pressor agents should be administered cautiously as indicated. Meprobamate is metabolized in the liver and excreted by the kidney. Diuresis, osmotic (mannitol) diuresis, peritoneal dialysis, and hemodialysis have been used successfully. Careful monitoring of urinary output is necessary and caution should be taken to avoid overhydration. Relapse and death, after initial recovery, have been attributed to incomplete gastric emptying and delayed absorption. Meprobamate can be measured in biological fluids by two methods: colorimetric (Hoffman, A.J. and Ludwig, B.J.: *J Amer Pharm Assn 48*: 740, 1959) and gas chromatographic (Douglas, J.F. et al.: *Anal Chem 39* : 956, 1967).

HOW SUPPLIED

'Miltown'-200: 200 mg white, sugar-coated tablets in bottles of 100 (NDC 0037-1101-01).

'Miltown'-400: 400 mg white, scored tablets in bottles of 100 (NDC 0037-1001-01), 500 (NDC 0037-1001-03), and 1000 (NDC 0037-1001-02).

'Miltown'-600: 600 mg white, capsule-shaped tablets in bottles of 100 (NDC 0037-1601-01).

WALLACE LABORATORIES
Division of
CARTER-WALLACE, INC.
Cranbury, New Jersey 08512

Rev. 2/87

Shown in Product Identification Section, page 434

ORGANIDIN®   ℞
(iodinated glycerol)
Solution, Tablets, Elixir

DESCRIPTION

Organidin® (iodinated glycerol), a mucolytic-expectorant, is an isomeric mixture formed by the interaction of iodine and glycerol, whose active ingredient is thought to be iodopropylidene glycerol but whose structural and chemical formulas have not been precisely established. Iodinated glycerol is a viscous, amber liquid stable in acid media, including

gastric juice, which contains virtually no inorganic iodide and no free iodine. ORGANIDIN is available for oral administration as:

Solution—5%, containing 50 mg ORGANIDIN (25 mg organically bound iodine) per mL. Other ingredients: caramel, glycerin, purified water.

Tablets—each containing 30 mg ORGANIDIN (15 mg organically bound iodine). Other ingredients: corn starch, dibasic calcium phosphate, FD&C Red No. 40, magnesium stearate, microcrystalline cellulose, tribasic calcium phosphate.

Elixir—1.2%, containing 60 mg ORGANIDIN (30 mg organically bound iodine) per 5 mL (teaspoonful); and alcohol, 21.75% by volume. Other ingredients: flavors (natural and artificial), liquid glucose, purified water, saccharin sodium.

CLINICAL PHARMACOLOGY

ORGANIDIN increases the output of thin respiratory tract fluid and helps liquefy tenacious mucus in the bronchial tree. Iodines are readily absorbed from the gastrointestinal tract and concentrated primarily in the secretions of the respiratory tract, but their mechanism of action as mucolytic-expectorants is not clear.

INDICATIONS AND USAGE

ORGANIDIN is indicated for adjunctive treatment as a mucolytic-expectorant in respiratory tract conditions such as bronchitis, bronchial asthma, pulmonary emphysema, cystic fibrosis, chronic sinusitis, or after surgery to help prevent atelectasis.

CONTRAINDICATIONS

History of marked sensitivity to inorganic iodides; hypersensitivity to any of the ingredients or related compounds; pregnancy; newborns; and nursing mothers.

The human fetal thyroid begins to concentrate iodine in the 12th to 14th week of gestation and the use of inorganic iodides in pregnant women during this period and thereafter has rarely been reported to induce fetal goiter (with or without hypothyroidism) with the potential for airway obstruction. If the patient becomes pregnant while taking ORGANIDIN, the drug should be discontinued and the patient should be apprised of the potential risk to the fetus.

WARNINGS

Discontinue use if rash or other evidence of hypersensitivity appears. Use with caution or avoid use in patients with history or evidence of thyroid disease.

PRECAUTIONS

General—Iodides have been reported to cause a flare-up of adolescent acne. Children with cystic fibrosis appear to have an exaggerated susceptibility to the goitrogenic effect of iodides.

Dermatitis and other reversible manifestations of iodism have been reported with chronic use of inorganic iodides. Although these have not been reported to be a problem clinically with ORGANIDIN, they should be kept in mind in patients receiving these preparations for prolonged periods.

Drug Interactions: Iodides may potentiate the hypothyroid effect of lithium and other antithyroid drugs.

Carcinogenesis, Mutagenesis, impairment of fertility: No long-term animal studies have been performed with ORGANIDIN.

Pregnancy Teratogenic Effects: Pregnancy Category X (see CONTRAINDICATIONS).

Nursing Mothers: ORGANIDIN should not be administered to a nursing woman.

ADVERSE REACTIONS

Reports of gastrointestinal irritation, rash, hypersensitivity, thyroid gland enlargement, and acute parotitis have been rare.

OVERDOSAGE

Acute overdosage experience with ORGANIDIN has been rare and there have been no reports of any serious problems.

DOSAGE AND ADMINISTRATION

Note: Add *Solution* to fruit juice or other liquid. One drop *Solution* equals approximately 3 mg ORGANIDIN.

Adults: *Solution* —20 drops 4 times a day.

Tablets —2 tablets 4 times a day, with liquid.

Elixir —1 teaspoonful 4 times a day.

Children: Up to one-half the adult dosage based on the child's weight.

HOW SUPPLIED

ORGANIDIN is available as—

Solution:	5%—clear amber liquid, in 30 ml dropper bottles (NDC 0037-4211-10).
Tablets:	30 mg—round, scored, rose-colored tablets, in bottles of 100 (NDC 0037-4224-40).
Elixir:	1.2%—clear amber liquid, in bottles of one pint (NDC 0037-4213-30) and one gallon (NDC 0037-4213-40).

Continued on next page

Wallace—Cont.

Storage: Store at room temperature; avoid excessive heat. Keep bottle tightly closed.

ORGANIDIN *Solution* and *Elixir* are
distributed by
WALLACE LABORATORIES
Division of
CARTER-WALLACE, Inc.
Cranbury, New Jersey 08512
Manufactured by
DENVER CHEMICAL (Puerto Rico), Inc.
Humacao, Puerto Rico 00661
ORGANIDIN *Tablets* are manufactured by
WALLACE LABORATORIES
Division of
CARTER-WALLACE, Inc.
Cranbury, New Jersey 08512

Rev. 3/85

Shown in Product Identification Section, page 434

RONDOMYCIN®   ℞
(methacycline HCl)

DESCRIPTION
'Rondomycin' (methacycline HCl) is a broad-spectrum antibiotic synthetically derived from oxytetracycline. Chemical dehydration at the 6-position yields a structural homologue which is a light-yellow crystalline powder with a chemical designation of 6-methylene-5-oxytetracycline.
'Rondomycin'-300 contains 300 mg methacycline HCl per capsule. Other ingredients: D&C Red #28. FD&C Blue #1, FD&C Red #40, gelatin. magnesium stearate, sodium lauryl sulfate, starch, titanium dioxide.
'Rondomycin'-150 contains 150 mg methacycline HCl per capsule.
Other ingredients: D&C Red #28. FD&C Blue #1, FD&C Red #40, gelatin. magnesium stearate, sodium lauryl sulfate, starch, titanium dioxide.

ACTIONS
The tetracyclines are primarily bacteriostatic and are thought to exert their antimicrobial effect by the inhibition of protein synthesis. Tetracyclines are active against a wide range of gram-negative and gram-positive organisms.
The drugs in the tetracycline class have closely similar antimicrobial spectra, and cross-resistance among them is common. Micro-organisms may be considered susceptible if the MIC (minimum inhibitory concentration) is not more than 4.0 mcg/ml and intermediate if the MIC is 4.0 to 12.5 mcg/ml.
Susceptibility plate testing: A tetracycline disc may be used to determine microbial susceptibility to drugs in the tetracycline class. If the Kirby-Bauer method of disc susceptibility testing is used, a 30 mcg tetracycline disc should give a zone of at least 19 mm when tested against a tetracycline-susceptible bacterial strain.
Tetracyclines are readily absorbed and are bound to plasma proteins in varying degree. They are concentrated by the liver in the bile and excreted in the urine and feces at high concentrations and in a biologically active form.

INDICATIONS
'Rondomycin' (methacycline HCl) is indicated in infections caused by the following micro-organisms:
Rickettsiae (Rocky Mountain spotted fever, typhus fever and the typhus group, Q fever, rickettsialpox and tick fevers),
Mycoplasma pneumoniae (PPLO, Eaton Agent),
Agents of psittacosis and ornithosis,
Agents of lymphogranuloma venereum and granuloma inguinale,
The spirochetal agent of relapsing fever (*Borrelia recurrentis*).
The following gram-negative micro-organisms:
Haemophilus ducreyi (chancroid),
Pasteurella pestis and *Pasteurella tularensis*,
Bartonella bacilliformis,
Bacteroides species,
Vibrio comma and *Vibrio fetus*,
Brucella species (in conjunction with streptomycin).
Because many strains of the following groups of micro-organisms have been shown to be resistant to tetracyclines, culture and susceptibility testing are recommended.
'Rondomycin' (methacycline HCl) is indicated for treatment of infections caused by the following gram-negative micro-organisms, when bacteriologic testing indicates appropriate susceptibility to the drug:
Escherichia coli,
Enterobacter aerogenes (formerly *Aerobacter aerogenes*),
Shigella species,
Mima species and *Herellea* species,
Haemophilus influenzae (respiratory infections),
Klebsiella species (respiratory and urinary infections).
'Rondomycin' (methacycline HCl) is indicated for treatment of infections caused by the following gram-positive micro-organisms when bacteriologic testing indicates appropriate susceptibility to the drug:
Streptococcus species: Up to 44 percent of strains of *streptococcus pyogenes* and 74 percent of *streptococcus faecalis* have been found to be resistant to tetracycline drugs. Therefore, tetracyclines should not be used for streptococcal disease unless the organism has been demonstrated to be sensitive.
For upper respiratory infections due to group A beta-hemolytic streptococci, penicillin is the usual drug of choice, including prophylaxis of rheumatic fever.
Diplococcus pneumoniae,
Staphylococcus aureus, skin and soft tissue infections. Tetracyclines are not the drugs of choice in the treatment of any type of staphylococcal infections.
When penicillin is contraindicated, tetracyclines are alternative drugs in the treatment of infections due to:
Neisseria gonorrhoeae,
Treponema pallidum and *Treponema pertenue* (syphilis and yaws),
Listeria monocytogenes,
Clostridium species,
Bacillus anthracis,
Fusobacterium fusiforme (Vincent's infection),
Actinomyces species.
In acute intestinal amebiasis, the tetracyclines may be a useful adjunct to amebicides.
In severe acne, the tetracyclines may be useful adjunctive therapy.
Tetracyclines are indicated in the treatment of trachoma, although the infectious agent is not always eliminated, as judged by immunofluorescence.
Inclusion conjunctivitis may be treated with oral tetracyclines or with a combination of oral and topical agents.

CONTRAINDICATIONS
This drug is contraindicated in persons who have shown hypersensitivity to any of the tetracyclines.

WARNINGS
THE USE OF DRUGS OF THE TETRACYCLINE CLASS DURING TOOTH DEVELOPMENT (LAST HALF OF PREGNANCY, INFANCY, AND CHILDHOOD TO THE AGE OF 8 YEARS) MAY CAUSE PERMANENT DISCOLORATION OF THE TEETH (YELLOW-GRAY-BROWN). This adverse reaction is more common during long-term use of the drugs but has been observed following repeated short-term courses. Enamel hypoplasia has also been reported. TETRACYCLINE DRUGS, THEREFORE, SHOULD NOT BE USED IN THIS AGE GROUP UNLESS OTHER DRUGS ARE NOT LIKELY TO BE EFFECTIVE OR ARE CONTRAINDICATED.
If renal impairment exists, even usual oral or parenteral doses may lead to excessive systemic accumulation of the drug and possible liver toxicity. Under such conditions, lower than usual total doses are indicated, and, if therapy is prolonged, serum level determinations of the drug may be advisable.
Photosensitivity manifested by an exaggerated sunburn reaction has been observed in some individuals taking tetracyclines. Patients apt to be exposed to direct sunlight or ultraviolet light should be advised that this reaction can occur with tetracycline drugs, and treatment should be discontinued at the first evidence of skin erythema.
The anti-anabolic action of the tetracyclines may cause an increase in BUN. While this is not a problem in those with normal renal function, in patients with significantly impaired function, higher serum levels of tetracyclines may lead to azotemia, hyperphosphatemia, and acidosis.
Usage in pregnancy. (See above "Warnings" about use during tooth development.)
Results of animal studies indicate that tetracyclines cross the placenta, are found in fetal tissues and can have toxic effects on the developing fetus (often related to retardation of skeletal development). Evidence of embryotoxicity has also been noted in animals treated early in pregnancy.
Usage in newborns, infants, and children. (See above "Warnings" about use during tooth development.)
All tetracyclines form a stable calcium complex in any bone-forming tissue. A decrease in the fibula growth rate has been observed in prematures given oral tetracycline in doses of 25 mg/kg every 6 hours. This reaction was shown to be reversible when the drug was discontinued.
Tetracyclines are present in the milk of lactating women who are taking a drug in this class.

PRECAUTIONS
As with other antibiotic preparations, use of this drug may result in overgrowth of nonsusceptible organisms, including fungi. If superinfection occurs, the antibiotic should be discontinued and appropriate therapy instituted.
In venereal diseases when coexistent syphilis is suspected, darkfield examination should be done before treatment is started and the blood serology repeated monthly for at least 4 months.
Because tetracyclines have been shown to depress plasma prothrombin activity, patients who are on anticoagulant therapy may require downward adjustment of their anticoagulant dosage.
In long-term therapy, periodic laboratory evaluation of organ systems, including hematopoietic, renal and hepatic studies should be performed.
All infections due to Group A beta-hemolytic streptococci should be treated for at least 10 days.
Since bacteriostatic drugs may interfere with the bactericidal action of penicillin, it is advisable to avoid giving tetracycline in conjunction with penicillin.

ADVERSE REACTIONS
Gastrointestinal: Anorexia, nausea, vomiting, diarrhea, glossitis, dysphagia, enterocolitis, and inflammatory lesions (with monilial overgrowth) in the anogenital region. These reactions have been caused by both the oral and parenteral administration of tetracyclines.
Skin: Maculopapular and erythematous rashes. Exfoliative dermatitis has been reported but is uncommon. Photosensitivity is discussed above. (See "Warnings".)
Renal toxicity: Rise in BUN has been reported and is apparently dose related. (See "Warnings".)
Hypersensitivity reactions: Urticaria, angioneurotic edema, anaphylaxis, anaphylactoid purpura, pericarditis and exacerbation of systemic lupus erythematosus.
Bulging fontanels in infants and benign intracranial hypertension in adults have been reported in individuals receiving full therapeutic dosages. These conditions disappeared rapidly when the drug was discontinued.
Blood: Hemolytic anemia, thrombocytopenia, neutropenia and eosinophilia have been reported.
When given over prolonged periods, tetracyclines have been reported to produce brown-black microscopic discoloration of thyroid glands. No abnormalities of thyroid function studies are known to occur.

DOSAGE AND ADMINISTRATION
The usual adult dosage of 'Rondomycin' (methacycline HCl) is 600 mg daily. This may be given in four divided doses of 150 mg each or two divided doses of 300 mg each. An initial dose of 300 mg followed by 150 mg every six hours or 300 mg every 12 hours may be used in the management of more severe infections.
In uncomplicated gonorrhea, when penicillin is contraindicated, 'Rondomycin' (methacycline HCl) may be used for treating both males and females in the following clinical dosage schedule: 900 mg initially, followed by 300 mg q.i.d. for a total of 5.4 grams.
For treatment of syphilis, when penicillin is contraindicated, a total of 18 to 24 grams of 'Rondomycin' (methacycline HCl) in equally divided doses over a period of 10–15 days should be given. Close follow-up, including laboratory tests, is recommended.
In Eaton Agent pneumonia, the usual adult dosage is 900 mg daily for 6 days.
The recommended dosage schedule for children above eight years of age is 3 to 6 mg/lb of body weight per day divided into two or four equally spaced doses.
Therapy should be continued for at least 24–48 hours after symptoms and fever have subsided. It should be noted, however, that antibacterial serum levels may usually be present from 24 to 36 hours following the discontinuation of 'Rondomycin' (methacycline HCl).
Concomitant therapy: Antacids containing aluminum, calcium, or magnesium impair absorption and should no be given to patients taking oral tetracyclines.
Food and some dairy products also interfere with absorption. Oral forms of tetracycline should be given 1 hour before or 2 hours after meals. Pediatric oral dosage forms should not be given with milk formulas and should be given at least 1 hour prior to feeding.
In patients with renal impairment (see "Warnings"): Total dosage should be decreased by reduction of recommended individual doses and/or by extending time intervals between doses.
In the treatment of streptococcal infections, a therapeutic dose of tetracycline should be administered for at least 10 days.

HOW SUPPLIED
'Rondomycin'-300 is available as blue and white capsules, each containing 300 mg methacycline HCl equivalent to 280 mg methacycline base, supplied in bottles of 50 (NDC 0037-4101-06).
'Rondomycin'-150 is available as blue and white capsules, each containing 150 mg methacycline HCl equivalent to 140 mg methacycline base, supplied in bottles of 100 (NDC 0037-4001-01).

Rev. 4/85

WALLACE LABORATORIES
Division of
CARTER-WALLACE, INC.
Cranbury, New Jersey 08512
Shown in Product Identification Section, page 434

RYNA™(Liquid)
RYNA-C®   ℂ
(Liquid)
RYNA-CX®   ℂ
(Liquid)

(See PDR For Nonprescription Drugs)

RYNATAN®   ℞
Tablets
Pediatric Suspension
RYNATAN®-S*
Pediatric Suspension

DESCRIPTION

RYNATAN® is an antihistaminic/decongestant combination available for oral administration as **Tablets** and as **Pediatric Suspension.** Each tablet contains:
Phenylephrine Tannate ....25 mg
Chlorpheniramine Tannate ....8 mg
Pyrilamine Tannate ....25 mg
Other ingredients: corn starch, dibasic calcium phosphate, magnesium stearate, methylcellulose, polygalacturonic acid, talc.
Each 5 mL (teaspoonful) of the Pediatric Suspension contains:
Phenylephrine Tannate ....5 mg
Chlorpheniramine Tannate ....2 mg
Pyrilamine Tannate ....12.5 mg
Other ingredients: benzoic acid, FD&C Red No. 3, flavors (natural and artificial), glycerin, kaolin, magnesium aluminum silicate, methylparaben, pectin, purified water, saccharin sodium, sucrose.

CLINICAL PHARMACOLOGY

RYNATAN combines the sympathomimetic decongestant effect of phenylephrine with the antihistaminic actions of chlorpheniramine and pyrilamine.

INDICATIONS AND USAGE

RYNATAN is indicated for symptomatic relief of the coryza and nasal congestion associated with the common cold, sinusitis, allergic rhinitis and other upper respiratory tract conditions. Appropriate therapy should be provided for the primary disease.

CONTRAINDICATIONS

RYNATAN is contraindicated for newborns, nursing mothers and patients sensitive to any of the ingredients or related compounds.

WARNINGS

Use with caution in patients with hypertension, cardiovascular disease, hyperthyroidism, diabetes, narrow angle glaucoma or prostatic hypertrophy. Use with caution or avoid use in patients taking monoamine (MAO) inhibitors. This product contains antihistamines which may cause drowsiness and may have additive central nervous system (CNS) effects with alcohol or other CNS depressants (e.g., hypnotics, sedatives, tranquilizers).

PRECAUTIONS

General: Antihistamines are more likely to cause dizziness, sedation and hypotension in elderly patients. Antihistamines may cause excitation, particularly in children, but their combination with sympathomimetics may cause either mild stimulation or mild sedation.
Information for Patients: Caution patients against drinking alcoholic beverages or engaging in potentially hazardous activities requiring alertness, such as driving a car or operating machinery, while using this product.
Drug Interactions: MAO inhibitors may prolong and intensify the anticholinergic effects of antihistamines and the overall effects of sympathomimetic agents.
Carcinogenesis, Mutagenesis, Impairment of Fertility: No long-term animal studies have been performed with RYNATAN®.
Pregnancy: Teratogenic Effects: Pregnancy Category C. Animal reproduction studies have not been conducted with RYNATAN. It is also not known whether RYNATAN can cause fetal harm when administered to a pregnant woman or can affect reproduction capacity. RYNATAN should be given to a pregnant woman only if clearly needed.
Nursing mothers: RYNATAN should not be administered to a nursing woman.

ADVERSE REACTIONS

Adverse effects associated with RYNATAN at recommended doses have been minimal. The most common have been drowsiness, sedation, dryness of mucous membranes, and gastrointestinal effects. Serious side effects with oral antihistamines or sympathomimetics have been rare.

OVERDOSAGE

Signs & Symptoms: May vary from CNS depression to stimulation (restlessness to convulsions). Antihistamine overdosage in young children may lead to convulsions and death. Atropine-like signs and symptoms may be prominent.

Treatment: Induce vomiting if it has not occurred spontaneously. Precautions must be taken against aspiration especially in infants, children and comatose patients. If gastric lavage is indicated, isotonic or half-isotonic saline solution is preferred. Stimulants should not be used. If hypotension is a problem, vasopressor agents may be considered.

DOSAGE AND ADMINISTRATION

Administer the recommended dose every 12 hours.
RYNATAN Tablets: Adults—1 or 2 tablets.
RYNATAN Pediatric Suspension: **Children over six years of age**—5 to 10 mL (1 to 2 teaspoonfuls); **Children two to six years of age**—2.5 to 5 mL (½ to 1 teaspoonful); **Children under two years of age**—Titrate dose individually.

HOW SUPPLIED

RYNATAN® Tablets: buff, capsule-shaped, compressed tablets in bottles of 100 (NDC 0037-0713-92) and 500 (NDC 0037-0713-96).
RYNATAN® Pediatric Suspension: pink with strawberry-currant flavor, in 4 fl. oz. bottles (NDC 0037-0715-67, labeled RYNATAN®-S*) and in pint bottles (NDC 0037-0715-68).
Storage
RYNATAN® Tablets—Store at room temperature; avoid excessive heat—(above 40°C (104°F).
RYNATAN® Pediatric Suspension—Store at controlled room temperature—between 15°C–30°C (59°F-86°F); protect from freezing.
* Patent Pending
RYNATAN®-S is the combination of RYNATAN Pediatric Suspension (4 fl. oz.) and a 10 mL, calibrated, oral syringe.
WALLACE LABORATORIES
Division of
CARTER-WALLACE, INC.
Cranbury, New Jersey 08512
Rev. 6/88
Shown in Product Identification Section, page 434

RYNATUSS®   ℞
Tablets
Pediatric Suspension

DESCRIPTION

RYNATUSS® is an antitussive/ antihistaminic/ decongestant/ bronchodilator combination available for oral administration as *Tablets* and as *Pediatric Suspension*.
Each tablet contains:
Carbetapentane Tannate ....60 mg
Chlorpheniramine Tannate ....5 mg
Ephedrine Tannate ....10 mg
Phenylephrine Tannate ....10 mg
Other ingredients: corn starch, dibasic calcium phosphate, FD&C Blue No. 1, FD&C Red No. 40, magnesium stearate, methylcellulose, polygalacturonic acid, povidone, talc.
Each 5 ml (one teaspoonful) of the Pediatric Suspension contains:
Carbetapentane Tannate ....30 mg
Chlorpheniramine Tannate ....4 mg
Ephedrine Tannate ....5 mg
Phenylephrine Tannate ....5 mg
Other ingredients: benzoic acid, FD&C Blue No. 1, FD&C Red No. 3, FD&C Red No. 40, FD&C Yellow #5, flavors (natural and artificial), glycerin, kaolin, magnesium aluminum silicate, methylparaben, pectin, purified water, saccharin sodium, sucrose.

CLINICAL PHARMACOLOGY

RYNATUSS combines the antitussive action of carbetapentane, the sympathomimetic decongestant effect of phenylephrine, the antihistaminic action of chlorpheniramine, and the bronchodilator action of ephedrine.

INDICATIONS AND USAGE

RYNATUSS is indicated for the symptomatic relief of cough associated with respiratory tract conditions such as the common cold, bronchial asthma, acute and chronic bronchitis. Appropriate therapy should be provided for the primary disease.

CONTRAINDICATIONS

RYNATUSS is contraindicated for newborns, nursing mothers and patients who are sensitive to any of the ingredients or related compounds.

WARNINGS

Use with caution in patients with hypertension, cardiovascular disease, hyperthyroidism, diabetes, narrow angle glaucoma or prostatic hypertrophy. Use with caution or avoid use in patients taking monoamine oxidase (MAO) Inhibitors. This product contains antihistamines which may cause drowsiness and may have additive central nervous system (CNS) effects with alcohol or other CNS depressants (e.g., hypnotics, sedatives, tranquilizers).

PRECAUTIONS

For RYNATUSS Pediatric Suspension only: This product contains FD&C Yellow No. 5 (tartrazine) which may cause allergic-type reactions (including bronchial asthma) in cer-

tain susceptible individuals. Although the overall incidence of FD&C Yellow No. 5 (tartrazine) sensitivity in the general population is low, it is frequently seen in patients who also have aspirin hypersensitivity.
General: Antihistamines are more likely to cause dizziness, sedation and hypotension in elderly patients. Antihistamines may cause excitation, particularly in children, but their combination with sympathomimetics may cause either mild stimulation or mild sedation.
Information for patients: Caution patients against drinking alcoholic beverages or engaging in potentially hazardous activities requiring alertness, such as driving a car or operating machinery, while using this product.
Drug interactions: MAO inhibitors may prolong and intensify the anticholinergic effects of antihistamines and the overall effects of sympathomimetic agents.
Carcinogenesis, mutagenesis, impairment of fertility: No long term animal studies have been performed with RYNATUSS.
Pregnancy: Teratogenic Effects: Pregnancy Category C. Animal reproduction studies have not been conducted with RYNATUSS. It is also not known whether RYNATUSS can cause fetal harm when administered to a pregnant woman or can affect reproduction capacity. RYNATUSS should be given to a pregnant woman only if clearly needed.
Nursing mothers: RYNATUSS should not be administered to a nursing woman.

ADVERSE REACTIONS

Adverse effects associated with RYNATUSS at recommended doses have been minimal. The most common have been drowsiness, sedation, dryness of mucous membranes, and gastrointestinal effects. Serious side effects with oral antihistamines or sympathomimetics have been rare.

OVERDOSAGE

Signs and Symptoms: May vary from CNS depression to stimulation (restlessness to convulsions). Antihistamine overdosage in young children may lead to convulsions and death. Atropine-like signs and symptoms may be prominent.
Treatment: Induce vomiting if it has not occurred spontaneously. Precautions must be taken against aspiration especially in infants, children and comatose patients. If gastric lavage is indicated, isotonic or half-isotonic saline solution is preferred. Stimulants should not be used. If hypotension is a problem, vasopressor agents may be considered.

DOSAGE AND ADMINISTRATION

Administer the recommended dose every 12 hours.
RYNATUSS Tablets: Adults—1 to 2 tablets.
RYNATUSS Pediatric Suspension: *Children over six years of age*—5 to 10 mL (1 to 2 teaspoonfuls); *Children two to six years of age*—2.5 to 5 mL (½ to 1 teaspoonful); *Children under two years of age*—Titrate dose individually.

HOW SUPPLIED

RYNATUSS® Tablets: mauve, capsule-shaped, compressed tablets in bottles of 100 (NDC 0037-0717-92) and bottles of 500 (NDC 0037-0717-96).
RYNATUSS® Pediatric Suspension: pink with strawberry-currant flavor, in bottles of 8 fl oz (NDC 0037-0718-67) and one pint (NDC 0037-0718-68).

STORAGE

RYNATUSS Tablets: Store at room temperature; avoid excessive heat—above 40°C (104°F).
RYNATUSS Pediatric Suspension: Store at controlled room temperature—between 15°C-30°C (59°F-86°F); protect from freezing.
WALLACE LABORATORIES
Division of
CARTER WALLACE, INC.
Cranbury, N.J. 08512   2/85
Shown in Product Identification Section, page 434

SOMA®   ℞
(carisoprodol tablets, USP)
350 mg

DESCRIPTION

'Soma' (carisoprodol) is available as 350 mg round, white tablets. Carisoprodol is N-isopropyl-2-methyl-2-propyl-1,3-propanediol dicarbamate.
Other ingredients: alginic acid, magnesium stearate, potassium sorbate, starch, tribasic calcium phosphate.

ACTIONS

Carisoprodol produces muscle relaxation in animals by blocking interneuronal activity in the descending reticular formation and spinal cord. The onset of action is rapid and effects last four to six hours.

INDICATIONS

Carisoprodol is indicated as an adjunct to rest, physical therapy, and other measures for the relief of discomfort associated with acute, painful musculoskeletal conditions. The

Continued on next page

Wallace—Cont.

mode of action of this drug has not been clearly identified, but may be related to its sedative properties. Carisoprodol does not directly relax tense skeletal muscles in man.

CONTRAINDICATIONS

Acute intermittent porphyria as well as allergic or idiosyncratic reactions to carisoprodol or related compounds such as meprobamate, mebutamate, or tybamate.

WARNINGS

Idiosyncratic Reactions—On very rare occasions, the first dose of carisoprodol has been followed by idiosyncratic symptoms appearing within minutes or hours. Symptoms reported include: extreme weakness, transient quadriplegia, dizziness, ataxia, temporary loss of vision, diplopia, mydriasis, dysarthria, agitation, euphoria, confusion, and disorientation. Symptoms usually subside over the course of the next several hours. Supportive and symptomatic therapy, including hospitalization, may be necessary.

Usage in Pregnancy and Lactation—Safe usage of this drug in pregnancy or lactation has not been established. Therefore, use of this drug in pregnancy, in nursing mothers, or in women of childbearing potential requires that the potential benefits of the drug be weighed against the potential hazards to mother and child. Carisoprodol is present in breast milk of lactating mothers at concentrations two to four times that of maternal plasma. This factor should be taken into account when use of the drug is contemplated in breast-feeding patients.

Usage in Children—Because of limited clinical experience, 'Soma' is not recommended for use in patients under 12 years of age.

Potentially Hazardous Tasks—Patients should be warned that this drug may impair the mental and/or physical abilities required for the performance of potentially hazardous tasks such as driving a motor vehicle or operating machinery.

Additive Effects—Since the effects of carisoprodol and alcohol or carisoprodol and other CNS depressants or psychotropic drugs may be additive, appropriate caution should be exercised with patients who take more than one of these agents simultaneously.

Drug Dependence—In dogs, no withdrawal symptoms occurred after abrupt cessation of carisoprodol from dosages as high as 1 gm/kg/day. In a study in man, abrupt cessation of 100 mg/kg/day (about five times the recommended daily adult dosage) was followed in some subjects by mild withdrawal symptoms such as abdominal cramps, insomnia, chilliness, headache, and nausea. Delirium and convulsions did not occur. In clinical use, psychological dependence and abuse have been rare, and there have been no reports of significant abstinence signs. Nevertheless, the drug should be used with caution in addiction-prone individuals.

PRECAUTIONS

Carisoprodol is metabolized in the liver and excreted by the kidney; to avoid its excess accumulation, caution should be exercised in administration to patients with compromised liver or kidney function.

ADVERSE REACTIONS

Central Nervous System —Drowsiness and other CNS effects may require dosage reduction. Also observed: dizziness, vertigo, ataxia, tremor, agitation, irritability, headache, depressive reactions, syncope, and insomnia. (See also Idiosyncratic Reactions under "Warnings".)

Allergic or Idiosyncratic —Allergic or idiosyncratic reactions occasionally develop. They are usually seen within the period of the first to fourth dose in patients having had no previous contact with the drug. Skin rash, erythema multiforme, pruritus, eosinophilia, and fixed drug eruption with cross reaction to meprobamate have been reported with carisoprodol. Severe reactions have been manifested by asthmatic episodes, fever, weakness, dizziness, angioneurotic edema, smarting eyes, hypotension, and anaphylactoid shock. (See also Idiosyncratic Reactions under "Warnings".) In case of allergic or idiosyncratic reactions to carisoprodol, discontinue the drug and initiate appropriate symptomatic therapy, which may include epinephrine, antihistamines, and in severe cases corticosteroids. In evaluating possible allergic reactions, also consider allergy to excipients (information on excipients is available to physicians on request).

Cardiovascular —Tachycardia, postural hypotension, and facial flushing.

Gastrointestinal —Nausea, vomiting, hiccup, and epigastric distress.

Hematologic —Leukopenia, in which other drugs or viral infection may have been responsible, and pancytopenia, attributed to phenylbutazone, have been reported. No serious blood dyscrasias have been attributed to carisoprodol.

DOSAGE AND ADMINISTRATION

The usual adult dosage of 'Soma' (carisoprodol) is one 350 mg tablet, three times daily and at bedtime. Usage in patients under age 12 is not recommended.

OVERDOSAGE

Overdosage of carisoprodol has produced stupor, coma, shock, respiratory depression, and, very rarely, death. The effects of an overdosage of carisoprodol and alcohol or other CNS depressants or psychotropic agents can be additive even when one of the drugs has been taken in the usual recommended dosage. Any drug remaining in the stomach should be removed and symptomatic therapy given. Should respiration or blood pressure become compromised, respiratory assistance, central nervous system stimulants, and pressor agents should be administered cautiously as indicated. Carisoprodol is metabolized in the liver and excreted by the kidney. Although carisoprodol overdosage experience is limited, the following types of treatment have been used successfully with the related drug meprobamate: diuresis, osmotic (mannitol) diuresis, peritoneal dialysis, and hemodialysis (carisoprodol is dialyzable). Careful monitoring of urinary output is necessary and caution should be taken to avoid overhydration. Observe for possible relapse due to incomplete gastric emptying and delayed absorption. Carisoprodol can be measured in biological fluids by gas chromatography (Douglas, J. F. et al: *J Pharm Sci* 58: 145, 1969).

HOW SUPPLIED

'Soma': Bottles of 100 (NDC 0037-2001-01) and 500 (NDC 0037-2001-03), and Unit Dose packages of 100 (NDC 0037-2001-85).

Rev. 5/87

WALLACE LABORATORIES
Division of CARTER-WALLACE, INC.
Cranbury, New Jersey 08512
Shown in Product Identification Section, page 434

SOMA COMPOUND† ℞
(carisoprodol and aspirin tablets, USP)
carisoprodol 200 mg + aspirin 325 mg
TABLETS

DESCRIPTION

'Soma' Compound is a combination product containing carisoprodol, a centrally-acting muscle relaxant, plus aspirin, an analgesic with antipyretic and anti-inflammatory properties. It is available as a two-layered, white and orange, round tablet for oral administration. Each tablet contains carisoprodol 200 mg and aspirin 325 mg. Chemically, carisoprodol is N-isopropyl-2-methyl-2,2-propyl-1,3-propanediol dicarbonate. Its empirical formula is $C_{12}H_{24}N_2O_4$, with a molecular weight of 260.33. The structural formula is:

$$H_2NCOOCH_2CCH_2OOCNHCH(CH_3)_2$$
$$CH_2CH_2CH_3$$
$$CH_3$$

Other Ingredients: croscarmellose sodium, FD&C Red #40, FD&C Yellow #6, hydroxypropyl methylcellulose, magnesium stearate, microcrystalline cellulose, povidone, starch, stearic acid.

CLINICAL PHARMACOLOGY

Carisoprodol: Carisoprodol is a centrally-acting muscle relaxant that does not directly relax tense skeletal muscles in man. The mode of action of carisoprodol in relieving acute muscle spasm of local origin has not been clearly identified, but may be related to its sedative properties. In animals, carisoprodol has been shown to produce muscle relaxation by blocking interneuronal activity and depressing transmission of polysynaptic neurons in the spinal cord and in the descending reticular formation of the brain. The onset of action is rapid and lasts four to six hours.

Carisoprodol is metabolized in the liver and is excreted by the kidneys. It is dialyzable by peritoneal and hemodialysis.

Aspirin: Aspirin is a non-narcotic analgesic with anti-inflammatory and antipyretic activity. Inhibition of prostaglandin biosynthesis appears to account for most of its anti-inflammatory and for at least part of its analgesic and antipyretic properties.

Aspirin is rapidly absorbed and almost totally hydrolyzed to salicylic acid following oral administration. Although aspirin has a half-life of only about 15 minutes, the apparent biologic half-life of salicylic acid in the therapeutic plasma concentration range is between 6 and 12 hours. Salicylic acid is eliminated by renal excretion and by biotransformation to inactive metabolites. Clearance of salicylic acid in the high-dose range is sensitive to urinary pH (see **Drug Interactions**) and is reduced by renal dysfunction.

INDICATIONS AND USAGE

'Soma' Compound is indicated as an adjunct to rest, physical therapy, and other measures for the relief of pain, muscle spasm, and limited mobility associated with acute, painful musculoskeletal conditions.

CONTRAINDICATIONS

Acute intermittent porphyria; bleeding disorders; allergic or idiosyncratic reactions to carisoprodol, aspirin or related compounds.

WARNINGS

On very rare occasions, the first dose of carisoprodol has been followed by an idiosyncratic reaction with symptoms appearing within minutes or hours. These may include extreme weakness, transient quadriplegia, dizziness, ataxia, temporary loss of vision, diplopia, mydriasis, dysarthia, agitation, euphoria, confusion, and disorientation. Although symptoms usually subside over the course of the next several hours, discontinue 'Soma' Compound and initiate appropriate supportive and symptomatic therapy, which may include epinephrine or antihistamines. In severe cases, corticosteroids may be necessary. Severe reactions have been manifested by asthmatic episodes, fever, weakness, dizziness, angioneurotic edema, smarting eyes, hypotension, and anaphylactoid shock.

The effects of carisoprodol with agents such as alcohol, other CNS depressants, or psychotropic drugs may be additive. Appropriate caution should be exercised with patients who may take one or more of these agents simultaneously with 'Soma' Compound.

PRECAUTIONS

General: To avoid excessive accumulation of carisoprodol, aspirin, or their metabolites, use 'Soma' Compound with caution in patients with compromised liver or kidney function, or in elderly or debilitated patients (see CLINICAL PHARMACOLOGY).

Use with caution in patients with history of gastritis or peptic ulcer, in patients on anticoagulant therapy, and in addiction-prone individuals.

Information for Patients: Caution patients that this drug may impair the mental and/or physical abilities required for the performance of potentially hazardous tasks such as driving a motor vehicle or operating machinery.

Caution patients with a predisposition for gastrointestinal bleeding that concomitant use of aspirin and alcohol may have an additive effect in this regard.

Caution patients that dosage of medications used for gout, arthritis, or diabetes may have to be adjusted when aspirin is administered or discontinued (see **Drug Interactions**).

Drug Interactions: Clinically important interactions may occur when certain drugs are administered concomitantly with aspirin or aspirin-containing drugs.

1. **Oral anticoagulants**—By interfering with platelet function or decreasing plasma prothrombin concentration, aspirin enhances the potential for bleeding in patients on anticoagulants.
2. **Methotrexate**—aspirin enhances the toxic effects of this drug.
3. **Probenecid and Sulfinpyrazone**—large doses of aspirin reduce the uricosuric effect of both drugs. Renal excretion of salicylate may also be reduced.
4. **Oral Antidiabetic Drugs**—enhancement of hypoglycemia may occur.
5. **Antacids**—to the extent that they raise urinary pH, antacids may substantially decrease plasma salicylate concentrations; conversely, their withdrawal can result in a substantial increase.
6. **Ammonium Chloride**—this and other drugs that acidify a relatively alkaline urine can elevate plasma salicylate concentrations.
7. **Ethyl Alcohol**—enhanced aspirin-induced fecal blood loss has been reported.
8. **Corticosteroids**—salicylate plasma levels may be decreased when adrenal corticosteroids are given, and may be increased substantially when they are discontinued.

Carcinogenesis, Mutagenesis, Impairment of Fertility: No long-term studies have been done with 'Soma' Compound.

Pregnancy—Teratogenic Effects: Pregnancy Category C. Adequate animal reproduction studies have not been conducted with 'Soma' Compound. It is also not known whether 'Soma' Compound can cause fetal harm when administered to a pregnant woman or can affect reproduction capacity. 'Soma' Compound should be given to a pregnant woman only if clearly needed.

Studies in rodents have shown salicylates to be teratogenic when given in early gestation, and embryocidal when given in later gestation in doses considerably greater than usual therapeutic doses in humans. Studies in women who took aspirin during pregnancy have not demonstrated an increased incidence of congenital abnormalities in the offspring.

Labor and Delivery: Ingestion of aspirin near term or prior to delivery may prolong delivery or lead to bleeding in mother, fetus, or neonate.

Nursing Mothers: Carisoprodol is excreted in human milk in concentrations two-to-four times that in maternal plasma. Aspirin is excreted in human milk in moderate amounts and can produce a bleeding tendency in nursing infants. Because of the potential for serious adverse reactions in nursing infants, a decision should be made whether to discontinue nursing or the drug, taking into account the importance of the drug to the mother.

Pediatric Use: Safety and effectiveness in children below the age of twelve have not been established.

ADVERSE REACTIONS

If severe reactions occur, discontinue 'Soma' Compound and initiate appropriate symptomatic and supportive therapy. The following side effects which have occurred with the administration of the individual ingredients alone may also occur with the combination.

Carisoprodol: Central Nervous System—Drowsiness is the most frequent complaint and along with other CNS effects may require dosage reduction. Observed less frequently are dizziness, vertigo and ataxia. Tremor, agitation, irritability, headache, depressive reactions, syncope, and insomnia have been infrequent or rare.

Idiosyncratic—Idiosyncratic reactions are very rare. They are usually seen within the period of the first to fourth dose in patients having had no previous contact with the drug (see WARNINGS).

Allergic—Skin rash, erythema multiforme, pruritus, eosinophilia, and fixed drug eruptions with cross-reaction to meprobamate have been reported. If allergic reactions occur, discontinue 'Soma' Compound and treat symptomatically. In evaluating possible allergic reactions, also consider allergy to excipients (information on excipients is available to physicians on request).

Cardiovascular—Tachycardia, postural hypotension, and facial flushing.

Gastrointestinal—Nausea, vomiting, epigastric distress and hiccup.

Hematologic—No serious blood dyscrasias have been attributed to carisoprodol alone. Leukopenia and pancytopenia have been reported, rarely, in situations in which other drugs or viral infections may have been responsible.

Aspirin: The most common adverse reactions associated with the use of aspirin have been gastrointestinal, including nausea, vomiting, gastritis, occult bleeding, constipation and diarrhea. Gastric erosion, angioedema, asthma, rash, pruritus and urticaria have been reported less commonly. Tinnitus is a sign of high serum salicylate levels (see OVERDOSAGE).

Aspirin Intolerance—Allergic type reactions in aspirin-sensitive individuals may involve the respiratory tract or the skin. Symptoms of the former range from rhinorrhea and shortness of breath to severe asthma, and the latter may consist of urticaria, edema, rash, or angioedema (giant hives). These may occur independently or in combination.

DRUG ABUSE AND DEPENDENCE

Abuse: In clinical use, abuse has been rare.

Dependence: In clinical use, dependence with 'Soma' Compound has been rare and there have been no reports of significant abstinence signs. Nevertheless, the following information on the individual ingredients should be kept in mind.

Carisoprodol—In dogs, no withdrawal symptoms occurred after abrupt cessation of carisoprodol from dosages as high as 1 gm/kg/day. In a study in man, abrupt cessation of 100 mg/kg/day (about five times the recommended daily adult dosage) was followed in some subjects by mild withdrawal symptoms such as abdominal cramps, insomnia, chills, headache, and nausea. Delirium and convulsions did not occur (see PRECAUTIONS).

OVERDOSAGE

Signs and Symptoms: Any of the following which have been reported with the individual ingredients may occur and may be modified to a varying degree by the effects of the other ingredients present in 'Soma' Compound.

Carisoprodol—Stupor, coma, shock, respiratory depression and, very rarely, death. Overdosage with carisoprodol in combination with alcohol, other CNS depressants, or psychotropic agents can have additive effects, even when one of the agents has been taken in the usually recommended dosage.

Aspirin—Headache, tinnitus, hearing difficulty, dim vision, dizziness, lassitude, hyperpnea, rapid breathing, thirst, nausea, vomiting, sweating and occasionally diarrhea are characteristic of mild to moderate salicylate poisoning. Salicylate poisoning should be considered in children with symptoms of vomiting, hyperpnea, and hyperthermia.

Hyperpnea is an early sign of salicylate poisoning, but dyspnea supervenes at plasma levels above 50 mg/dl. These respiratory changes eventually lead to serious acid-base disturbances. Metabolic acidosis is a constant finding in infants but occurs in older children only with severe poisoning; adults usually exhibit respiratory alkalosis initially and acidosis terminally.

Other symptoms of severe salicylate poisoning include hyperthermia, dehydration, delirium, and mental disturbances. Skin eruptions, GI hemorrhage, or pulmonary edema are less common. Early CNS stimulation is replaced by increasing depression, stupor, and coma. Death is usually due to respiratory failure or cardiovascular collapse.

Treatment: General: Provide symptomatic and supportive treatment, as indicated. Any drug remaining in the stomach should be removed using appropriate procedures and caution to protect the airway and prevent aspiration, especially in the stuporous or comatose patient. Incomplete gastric emptying with delayed absorption of carisoprodol has been reported as a cause for relapse. Should respiration or blood pressure become compromised, respiratory assistance, central nervous system stimulants, and pressor agents should be administered cautiously, as indicated.

Carisoprodol: The following have been used successfully in overdosage with the related drug meprobamate: diuretics, osmotic (mannitol) diuresis, peritoneal dialysis, and hemodialysis (see CLINICAL PHARMACOLOGY). Careful monitoring of urinary output is necessary and caution should be taken to avoid overhydration. Carisoprodol can be measured in biological fluid by gas chromatography (Douglas, J. F., et al: *J Pharm Sci 58:* 145, 1969).

Aspirin—Since there are no specific antidotes for salicylate poisoning, the aim of treatment is to enhance elimination of salicylate and prevent or reduce further absorption; to correct any fluid, electrolyte or metabolic imbalance; and to provide general and cardiorespiratory support. If acidosis is present, intravenous sodium bicarbonate must be given, along with adequate hydration, until salicylate levels decrease to within the therapeutic range. To enhance elimination, forced diuresis and alkalinization of the urine may be beneficial. The need for hemoperfusion or hemodialysis is rare and should be used only when other measures have failed.

DOSAGE AND ADMINISTRATION

Usual Adult Dosage: 1 or 2 tablets, four times daily.
Not recommended for use in children under age twelve (see PRECAUTIONS).

HOW SUPPLIED

'Soma' Compound Tablets: In bottles of 100 (NDC 0037-2103-01) and 500 (NDC 0037-2103-03) and Unit dose packages of 100 (NDC 0037-2103-85).

Storage: Store at controlled room temperature. Protect from excessive heat and moisture. Keep bottle tightly closed.
†Patent Pending

WALLACE LABORATORIES
Division of
CARTER-WALLACE, INC.
Cranbury, New Jersey 08512

Rev 8/87

Shown in Product Identification Section, page 434

SOMA® COMPOUND with CODEINE Ⓒ
(carisoprodol, aspirin, and codeine phosphate tablets, USP)
carisoprodol 200 mg + aspirin 325 mg + codeine phosphate 16 mg
Warning: May be habit-forming

DESCRIPTION

'SOMA' Compound with Codeine is a combination product containing carisoprodol, a centrally-acting muscle relaxant, plus aspirin, an analgesic with antipyretic and anti-inflammatory properties and codeine phosphate, a centrally-acting narcotic analgesic. It is available as a two-layered, white and yellow, oval shaped tablet for oral administration. Each tablet contains carisoprodol 200 mg, aspirin 325 mg, and codeine phosphate 16 mg. Chemically, carisoprodol is N-isopropyl-2-methyl-2-propyl-1,3-propanediol dicarbamate. Its empirical formula is $C_{12}H_{24}N_2O_4$, with a molecular weight of 260.33. The structural formula is:

$$CH_2CH_2CH_3$$
$$|$$
$$H_2NCOOCH_2CCH_2OOCNHCH(CH_3)_2$$
$$|$$
$$CH_3$$

Other Ingredients: croscarmellose sodium, D&C Yellow #10, hydroxypropyl methycellulose, magnesium stearate, microcrystalline cellulose, povidone, sodium metabisulfite, starch, stearic acid.

CLINICAL PHARMACOLOGY

Carisoprodol: Carisoprodol is a centrally-acting muscle relaxant that does not directly relax tense skeletal muscles in man. The mode of action of carisoprodol in relieving acute muscle spasm of local origin has not been clearly identified, but may be related to its sedative properties. In animals, carisoprodol has been shown to produce muscle relaxation by blocking interneuronal activity and depressing transmission of polysynaptic neurons in the spinal cord and in the descending reticular formation of the brain. The onset of action is rapid and lasts four to six hours.

Carisoprodol is metabolized in the liver and is excreted by the kidneys. It is dialyzable by peritoneal and hemodialysis.

Aspirin: Aspirin is a non-narcotic analgesic with anti-inflammatory and antipyretic activity. Inhibition of prostaglandin biosynthesis appears to account for most of its anti-inflammatory and for at least part of its analgesic and antipyretic properties.

Aspirin is rapidly absorbed and almost totally hydrolyzed to salicylic acid following oral administration. Although aspirin has a half-life of only about 15 minutes, the apparent biologic half-life of salicylic acid in the therapeutic plasma concentration range is between 6 and 12 hours. Salicylic acid is eliminated by renal excretion and by biotransformation to inactive metabolites. Clearance of salicylic acid in the high-dose range is sensitive to urinary pH (see *Drug Interactions*) and is reduced by renal dysfunction.

Codeine Phosphate: Codeine phosphate is a centrally-acting narcotic-analgesic. Its actions are qualitatively similar to morphine, but its potency is substantially less.

Clinical studies have shown that combining aspirin and codeine produces a significant additive effect in analgesic efficacy.

INDICATIONS AND USAGE

'Soma' Compound with Codeine is indicated as an adjunct to rest, physical therapy, and other measures for the relief of pain, muscle spasm, and limited mobility associated with acute, painful musculoskeletal conditions when the additional action of codeine is desired.

CONTRAINDICATIONS

Acute intermittent porphyria; bleeding disorders; allergic or idiosyncratic reactions to carisoprodol, aspirin, codeine, or related compounds.

WARNINGS

On very rare occasions, the first dose of carisoprodol has been followed by idiosyncratic reactions, with symptoms appearing within minutes or hours. These may include extreme weakness, transient quadriplegia, dizziness, ataxia, temporary loss of vision, diplopia, mydriasis, dysarthria, agitation, euphoria, confusion, and disorientation. Although symptoms usually subside over the course of the next several hours, discontinue 'Soma' Compound with Codeine and initiate appropriate supportive and symptomatic therapy, which may include epinephrine and/or antihistamines. In severe cases, corticosteroids may be necessary. Severe reactions have been manifested by asthmatic episodes, fever, weakness, dizziness, angioneurotic edema, smarting eyes, hypotension, and anaphylactoid shock.

The effects of carisoprodol with agents such as alcohol, other CNS depressants, or psychotropic drugs may be additive. Appropriate caution should be exercised with patients who may take one or more of these agents simultaneously with 'Soma' Compound with Codeine.

'Soma' Compound with Codeine contains sodium metabisulfite, a sulfite that may cause allergic-type reactions including anaphylactic symptoms and life-threatening or less severe asthmatic episodes in certain susceptible people. The overall prevalence of sulfite sensitivity in the general population is unknown and probably low. Sulfite sensitivity is seen more frequently in asthmatic than in nonasthmatic people.

PRECAUTIONS

General: To avoid excessive accumulation of carisoprodol, aspirin, or their metabolites, use 'Soma' Compound with Codeine with caution in patients with compromised liver or kidney function, or in elderly or debilitated patients (see CLINICAL PHARMACOLOGY).

Use with caution in patients with history of gastritis or peptic ulcer, in patients on anticoagulant therapy, and in addiction-prone individuals.

Information for Patients: Caution patients that this drug may impair the mental and/or physical abilities required for the performance of potentially hazardous tasks such as driving a motor vehicle or operating machinery. Caution patients with a predisposition for gastrointestinal bleeding that concomitant use of aspirin and alcohol may have an additive effect in this regard.

Caution patients that dosage of medications used for gout, arthritis, or diabetes may have to be adjusted when aspirin is administered or discontinued (see *Drug Interactions*).

Drug Interactions: Clinically important interactions may occur when certain drugs are administered concomitantly with aspirin or aspirin-containing drugs.

1. *Oral anticoagulants*—By interfering with platelet function or decreasing plasma prothrombin concentration, aspirin enhances the potential for bleeding in patients on anticoagulants.
2. *Methotrexate*—aspirin enhances the toxic effects of this drug.
3. *Probenecid and Sulfinpyrazone*—large doses of aspirin reduce the uricosuric effect of both drugs. Renal excretion of salicylate may also be reduced.
4. *Oral Antidiabetic Drugs*—enhancement of hypoglycemia may occur.
5. *Antacids*—to the extent that they raise urinary pH, antacids may substantially decrease plasma salicylate concentrations; conversely, their withdrawal can result in a substantial increase.
6. *Ammonium Chloride*—this and other drugs that acidify a relatively alkaline urine can elevate plasma salicylate concentrations.
7. *Ethyl Alcohol*—enhanced aspirin-induced fecal blood loss has been reported.

Continued on next page

Wallace—Cont.

8. *Corticosteroids* —salicylate plasma levels may be decreased when adrenal corticosteroids are given, and may be increased substantially when they are discontinued.

Carcinogenesis, Mutagenesis, Impairment of Fertility: No long-term studies have been done with 'Soma' Compound with Codeine.

Pregnancy—Teratogenic Effects: Pregnancy Category C. Adequate animal reproduction studies have not been conducted with 'Soma' Compound with Codeine. It is also not known whether 'Soma' Compound with Codeine can cause fetal harm when administered to a pregnant woman or can affect reproduction capacity. 'Soma' Compound with Codeine should be given to a pregnant woman only if clearly needed. Studies in rodents have shown salicylates to be teratogenic when given in early gestation, and embryocidal when given in later gestation in doses considerably greater than usual therapeutic doses in humans. Studies in women who took aspirin during pregnancy have not demonstrated an increased incidence of congenital abnormalities in the offspring.

Labor and Delivery: Ingestion of aspirin near term or prior to delivery may prolong delivery or lead to bleeding in mother, fetus, or neonate.

Nursing Mothers: Carisoprodol is excreted in human milk in concentrations two-to-four times that in maternal plasma. Aspirin is excreted in human milk in moderate amounts and can produce a bleeding tendency in nursing infants. Because of the potential for serious adverse reactions in nursing infants, a decision should be made whether to discontinue nursing or the drug, taking into account the importance of the drug to the mother.

Pediatric Use: Safety and effectiveness in children below the age of twelve have not been established.

ADVERSE REACTIONS

If severe reactions occur, discontinue 'Soma' Compound with Codeine and initiate appropriate symptomatic and supportive therapy.

The following side effects which have occurred with the administration of the individual ingredients alone may also occur with the combination.

Carisoprodol: Central Nervous System—Drowsiness is the most frequent complaint and along with other CNS effects may require dosage reduction. Observed less frequently are dizziness, vertigo and ataxia. Tremor, agitation, irritability, headache, depressive reactions, syncope, and insomnia have been infrequent or rare.

Idiosyncratic—Idiosyncratic reactions are very rare. They are usually seen within the period of the first to fourth dose in patients having had no previous contact with the drug (see WARNINGS).

Allergic—Skin rash, erythema multiforme, pruritus, eosinophilia, and fixed drug eruptions with cross-reaction to meprobamate have been reported. If allergic reactions occur, discontinue 'Soma' Compound with Codeine and treat symptomatically. In evaluating possible allergic reactions, also consider allergy to excipients (information on excipients is available to physicians on request).

Cardiovascular—Tachycardia, postural hypotension, and facial flushing.

Gastrointestinal—Nausea, vomiting, epigastric distress and hiccup.

Hematologic—No serious blood dyscrasias have been attributed to carisoprodol alone. Leukopenia and pancytopenia have been reported, very rarely, in situations in which other drugs or viral infections may have been responsible.

Aspirin: The most common adverse reactions associated with the use of aspirin have been gastrointestinal, including nausea, vomiting, gastritis, occult bleeding, constipation and diarrhea. Gastric erosion, angioedema, asthma, rash, pruritus and urticaria have been reported less commonly. Tinnitus is a sign of high serum salicylate levels (see OVERDOSAGE).

Aspirin Intolerance—Allergic type reactions in aspirin-sensitive individuals may involve the respiratory tract or the skin. Symptoms of the former range from rhinorrhea and shortness of breath to severe asthma, and the latter may consist of urticaria, edema, rash, or angioedema (giant hives). These may occur independently or in combination.

Codeine Phosphate: Nausea, vomiting, constipation, miosis, sedation, and dizziness have been reported.

DRUG ABUSE AND DEPENDENCE

Controlled Substance: Schedule C-III (see PRECAUTIONS).

Abuse: In clinical use, abuse has been rare.

Dependence: In clinical use, dependence with 'Soma' Compound with Codeine has been rare and there have been no reports of significant abstinence signs. Nevertheless, the following information on the individual ingredients should be kept in mind.

Carisoprodol—In dogs, no withdrawal symptoms occurred after abrupt cessation of carisoprodol from dosages as high

as 1 gm/kg/day. In a study in man, abrupt cessation of 100 mg/kg/day (about five times the recommended daily adult dosage) was followed in some subjects by mild withdrawal symptoms such as abdominal cramps, insomnia, chills, headache, and nausea. Delirium and convulsions did not occur (see PRECAUTIONS).

Codeine Phosphate: Drug dependence of the morphine type may result.

OVERDOSAGE

Signs and Symptoms: Any of the following which have been reported with the individual ingredients may occur and may be modified to a varying degree by the effects of the other ingredients present in 'Soma' Compound with Codeine.

Carisoprodol—Stupor, coma, shock, respiratory depression and, very rarely, death. Overdosage with carisoprodol in combination with alcohol, other CNS depressants, or psychotropic agents can have additive effects, even when one of the agents has been taken in the usually recommended dosage.

Aspirin—Headache, tinnitus, hearing difficulty, dim vision, dizziness, lassitude, hyperpnea, rapid breathing, thirst, nausea, vomiting, sweating and occasionally diarrhea are characteristic of mild to moderate salicylate poisoning. Salicylate poisoning should be considered in children with symptoms of vomiting, hyperpnea, and hyperthermia.

Hyperpnea is an early sign of salicylate poisoning, but dyspnea supervenes at plasma levels above 50 mg/dl. These respiratory changes eventually lead to serious acid-base disturbances. Metabolic acidosis is a constant finding in infants but occurs in older children only with severe poisoning; adults usually exhibit respiratory alkalosis initially and acidosis terminally.

Other symptoms of severe salicylate poisoning include hyperthermia, dehydration, delirium, and mental disturbances. Skin eruptions, GI hemorrhage, or pulmonary edema are less common. Early CNS stimulation is replaced by increasing depression, stupor, and coma. Death is usually due to respiratory failure or cardiovascular collapse.

Codeine Phosphate: pinpoint pupils, CNS depression, coma, respiratory depression, and shock.

Treatment: General—Provide symptomatic and supportive treatment, as indicated. Any drug remaining in the stomach should be removed using appropriate procedures and caution to protect the airway and prevent aspiration, especially in the stuporous or comatose patient. Incomplete gastric emptying with delayed absorption of carisoprodol has been reported as a cause for relapse. Should respiration or blood pressure become compromised, respiratory assistance, central nervous system stimulants, and pressor agents should be administered cautiously, as indicated.

Carisoprodol—The following have been used successfully in overdosage with the related drug meprobamate: diuretics, osmotic (mannitol) diuresis, peritoneal dialysis, and hemodialysis (see CLINICAL PHARMACOLOGY). Careful monitoring of urinary output is necessary and caution should be taken to avoid overhydration. Carisoprodol can be measured in biological fluid by gas chromatography (Douglas, J. F., et al.: *J Pharm Sci 58:* 145, 1969).

Aspirin—Since there are no specific antidotes for salicylate poisoning, the aim of treatment is to enhance elimination of salicylate and prevent or reduce further absorption; to correct any fluid, electrolyte or metabolic imbalance; and to provide general and cardiorespiratory support. If acidosis is present, intravenous sodium bicarbonate must be given, along with adequate hydration, until salicylate levels decrease to within the therapeutic range. To enhance elimination, forced diuresis and alkalinization of the urine may be beneficial. The need for hemoperfusion or hemodialysis is rare and should be used only when other measures have failed.

Codeine Phosphate: Narcotic antagonists, such as nalorphine and levallorphan, may be indicated.

DOSAGE AND ADMINISTRATION

Usual Adult Dosage: 1 or 2 tablets, four times daily. Not recommended for use in children under age twelve.

HOW SUPPLIED

'Soma' Compound with Codeine Tablets: In bottles of 100 (NDC 0037-2403-01).

Storage: Store at room temperature; avoid excessive heat and prolonged light exposure. Keep bottle tightly closed.

WALLACE LABORATORIES
Division of
CARTER-WALLACE, INC.
Cranbury, New Jersey 08512

Rev. 1/87

Shown in Product Identification Section, page 434

THEO–ORGANIDIN®   ℞
Elixir

DESCRIPTION

Theo-Organidin is a bronchodilator/mucolytic-expectorant combination available for oral administration as an *Elixir.* Each 15 ml (tablespoonful) contains theophylline (anhy-

drous), 120 mg; Organidin® (iodinated glycerol), 30 mg (15 mg organically bound iodine); and alcohol, 15% by volume. Other ingredients: citric acid, flavor, glycerin, purified water, saccharin sodium, sodium benzoate.

CLINICAL PHARMACOLOGY

Theo-Organidin combines the bronchodilator effects of theophylline, a xanthine derivative, and the mucolytic-expectorant action of Organidin. Therapeutic blood levels of theophylline are reached in approximately 15 minutes and peak blood levels in one hour.

INDICATIONS AND USAGE

Theo-Organidin is indicated for symptomatic treatment in bronchial asthma and other bronchospastic conditions such as bronchitis, bronchiolitis, and pulmonary emphysema; for the relief of wheezing and respiratory distress due to reversible bronchospasm and tenacious mucous secretions; and for daily maintenance therapy of patients with bronchial asthma and other chronic bronchospastic pulmonary disorders.

CONTRAINDICATIONS

History of marked sensitivity to inorganic iodides; hypersensitivity to any of the ingredients or related compounds; pregnancy; newborns; and nursing mothers.

The human fetal thyroid begins to concentrate iodine in the 12th to 14th week of gestation and the use of inorganic iodides in pregnant women during this period and thereafter has rarely been reported to induce fetal goiter (with or without hypothyroidism) with the potential for airway obstruction. If the patient becomes pregnant while taking Theo-Organidin, the drug should be discontinued and the patient should be apprised of the potential risk to the fetus.

WARNINGS

Discontinue use if rash or other evidence of hypersensitivity appears. Use with caution or avoid use in patients with history or evidence of thyroid disease. Do not exceed recommended dosage. Do not administer more often than every 6 hours or within 12 hours after rectal administration of any preparation containing theophylline or aminophylline. Use with caution or avoid use with other xanthine derivatives or CNS stimulants.

PRECAUTIONS

General —Children have been known to exhibit marked sensitivity to the CNS stimulant action of the xanthines. Toxic synergism (i.e., CNS stimulation) may occur with other sympathomimetic bronchodilator agents, particularly in children. Iodides have been reported to cause a flare-up of adolescent acne. Children with cystic fibrosis appear to have an exaggerated susceptibility to the goitrogenic effects of iodides.

Dermatitis and other reversible manifestations of iodism have been reported with chronic use of inorganic iodides. Although these have not been reported to be a problem clinically with Organidin formulations, they should be kept in mind in patients receiving these preparations for prolonged periods.

Drug Interactions —Iodides may potentiate the hypothyroid effect of lithium and other antithyroid drugs.

Carcinogenesis, Mutagenesis, Impairment of Fertility —No long-term animal studies have been performed with Theo-Organidin.

Pregnancy —Teratogenic Effects: Pregnancy Category X (see CONTRAINDICATIONS).

Nursing Mothers —Theo-Organidin should not be administered to a nursing woman.

ADVERSE REACTIONS

Side effects sometimes seen with individual ingredients may occur and may be modified as a result of their combination. *Theophylline* —Gastric irritation, nausea, and vomiting may occur; these can be minimized by taking Theo-Organidin after meals. Palpitations and mild central nervous system stimulation (e.g., restlessness, sleeplessness) have been reported, particularly in children. *Organidin* —Reports of gastrointestinal irritation, rash, hypersensitivity, thyroid enlargement, and acute parotitis have been rare.

OVERDOSAGE

There have been no reports of any serious problems from overdosage with Theo-Organidin. However, overdosage with theophylline has been reported and the following may be expected if overdosage with Theo-Organidin should occur:

Signs and Symptoms —Toxic overdosage with theophylline may produce severe gastrointestinal adverse effects including nausea, vomiting, epigastric pain, hematemesis and diarrhea; CNS effects including insomnia, headache, irritability, restlessness, severe agitation and convulsions; cardiovascular effects including hypotension, circulatory failure, and life-threatening arrhythmias; renal effects including diuresis and hypokalemia; and respiratory arrest. Serious toxicity leading to seizures and death can occur with serum concentrations of 40 mcg/ml or more.

Treatment —There is no specific antidote for theophylline toxicity. Discontinue drug immediately. Avoid sympathomimetic agents. Emetics and gastric lavage may be of value.

Provide general supportive measures to prevent hypotension, overcome hydration, and maintain adequate ventilation. Hemodialysis with the use of resin or charcoal hemoperfusion may be helpful in reducing theophylline serum levels.

DOSAGE AND ADMINISTRATION

Do not exceed recommended dosage. Acute attacks of asthma can usually be terminated fairly rapidly with the recommended dosage of Theo-Organidin; but in severe attacks, or when initiating treatment, the dose may be increased by ½ for up to 24 hours. The need for intravenous aminophylline and/or other regimens should also be considered in the management of severe episodes.

Usual Adult Dosage: For maintenance therapy: 1-2 tablespoonfuls 3 times a day (every 6-8 hours).

For the acute asthmatic attack: 3 tablespoonfuls initially, then reduce to maintenance dosage.

Children: 1 teaspoonful per 20 lbs. (9 kg) body weight, 2-3 times daily. Children over 99 lbs. (45 kg) may require adult dosage.

HOW SUPPLIED

Theo-Organidin Elixir —clear amber liquid, in bottles of one pint (NDC 0037-4611-10) and one gallon (NDC 0037-4611-20).

Storage: Store at room temperature; avoid excessive heat; protect from freezing. Keep bottle tightly closed.

Distributed by
WALLACE LABORATORIES
Division of
CARTER-WALLACE, INC.
Cranbury, New Jersey 08512
Manufactured by Denver Chemical (Puerto Rico), Inc.
Humacao, Puerto Rico 00661

Rev. 6/85

Shown in Product Identification Section, page 434

TUSSI–ORGANIDIN®   Ⓒ ℞
Liquid

DESCRIPTION

Tussi-Organidin is an antitussive/mucolytic-expectorant combination available for oral administration as a *Liquid.* Each 5 ml (teaspoonful) contains: Organidin® (iodinated glycerol), 30 mg (15 mg organically bound iodine); and codeine phosphate (*Warning:* May be habit forming), 10 mg. Other Ingredients: citric acid, FD&C Red #40, flavor (artificial), glycerin, propylene glycol, purified water, saccharin sodium, sodium benzoate, sorbitol solution.

CLINICAL PHARMACOLOGY

Tussi-Organidin combines the antitussive action of codeine with the mucolytic-expectorant action of Organidin.

INDICATIONS AND USAGE

Tussi-Organidin is indicated for the symptomatic relief of irritating, nonproductive cough associated with respiratory tract conditions such as chronic bronchitis, bronchial asthma, tracheobronchitis, and the common cold; also for the symptomatic relief of cough accompanying other respiratory tract conditions such as laryngitis, pharyngitis, croup, pertussis and emphysema. Appropriate therapy should be provided for the primary disease.

CONTRAINDICATIONS

History of marked sensitivity to inorganic iodides; hypersensitivity to any of the ingredients or related compounds; pregnancy; newborns; and nursing mothers.

The human fetal thyroid begins to concentrate iodine in the 12th to 14th week of gestation and the use of inorganic iodides in pregnant women during this period and thereafter has rarely been reported to induce fetal goiter (with or without hypothyroidism) with the potential for airway obstruction. If the patient becomes pregnant while taking Tussi-Organidin, the drug should be discontinued and the patient should be apprised of the potential risk to the fetus.

WARNINGS

Discontinue use if rash or other evidence of hypersensitivity appears. Use with caution or avoid use in patients with history or evidence of thyroid disease.

PRECAUTIONS

General —Iodides have been reported to cause a flare-up of adolescent acne. Children with cystic fibrosis appear to have an exaggerated susceptibility to the goitrogenic effect of iodides.

Dermatitis and other reversible manifestations of iodism have been reported with chronic use of inorganic iodides. Although these have not been a problem clinically with Organidin formulations, they should be kept in mind in patients receiving these preparations for prolonged periods.

Drug Interactions —Iodides may potentiate the hypothyroid effect of lithium and other antithyroid drugs.

Carcinogenesis, Mutagenesis, Impairment of Fertility —No long-term animal studies have been performed with Tussi-Organidin.

Pregnancy —Teratogenic effects: Pregnancy Category X (see CONTRAINDICATIONS).

Nursing Mothers —Tussi-Organidin should not be administered to a nursing woman.

ADVERSE REACTIONS

Side effects have been rare, including those which may occur with the individual ingredients and which may be modified as a result of their combination. *Organidin* —Rare side effects include gastrointestinal irritation, rash, hypersensitivity, thyroid gland enlargement, and acute parotitis. *Codeine* —Nausea, vomiting, constipation, drowsiness, and miosis have been reported.

DRUG ABUSE AND DEPENDENCE

Controlled Substance —Schedule V.

Dependence —Codeine may be habit-forming.

OVERDOSAGE

Acute overdosage experience with Organidin formulations has been rare and there have been no reports of any serious problems.

DOSAGE AND ADMINISTRATION

Adults: 1 to 2 teaspoonfuls every 4 hours.

Children: ½ to 1 teaspoonful every 4 hours.

HOW SUPPLIED

Tussi-Organidin Liquid —clear red liquid, in bottles of one pint (NDC 0037-4812-10) and one gallon (NDC 0037-4812-20).

Storage: Store at room temperature; avoid excessive heat. Keep bottle tightly closed.

Distributed by
WALLACE LABORATORIES
Division of
CARTER-WALLACE, INC.
Cranbury, New Jersey 08512
Manufactured by Denver Chemical (Puerto Rico) Inc.
Humacao, Puerto Rico 00661

Rev. 4/87

Shown in Product Identification Section, page 434

TUSSI–ORGANIDIN® DM   ℞
Liquid

DESCRIPTION

Tussi-Organidin DM is an antitussive/mucolytic-expectorant combination available for oral administration as a *Liquid.* Each 5 ml (teaspoonful) of Tussi-Organidin DM contains: Organidin® (iodinated glycerol), 30 mg (15 mg organically bound iodine); and dextromethorphan hydrobromide, 10 mg. Other Ingredients: citric acid, D&C Yellow #10, FD&C Red #40, flavor (artificial), glycerin, propylene glycol, purified water, saccharin sodium, sodium benzoate, sorbitol solution.

CLINICAL PHARMACOLOGY

Tussi-Organidin DM combines the non-narcotic antitussive action of dextromethorphan with the mucolytic-expectorant action of Organidin.

INDICATIONS AND USAGE

Tussi-Organidin DM is indicated for the symptomatic relief of irritating, nonproductive cough associated with respiratory tract conditions such as chronic bronchitis, bronchial asthma, tracheobronchitis, and the common cold; also for the symptomatic relief of cough accompanying other respiratory tract conditions such as laryngitis, pharyngitis, croup, pertussis and emphysema. Appropriate therapy should be provided for the primary disease.

CONTRAINDICATIONS

History of marked sensitivity to inorganic iodides; hypersensitivity to any of the ingredients or related compounds; pregnancy; newborns; and nursing mothers.

The human fetal thyroid begins to concentrate iodine in the 12th to 14th week of gestation and the use of inorganic iodides in pregnant women during this period and thereafter has rarely been reported to induce fetal goiter (with or without hypothyroidism) with the potential for airway obstruction. If the patient becomes pregnant while taking Tussi-Organidin DM, the drug should be discontinued and the patient should be apprised of the potential risk to the fetus.

WARNINGS

Discontinue use if rash or other evidence of hypersensitivity appears. Use with caution or avoid use in patients with history or evidence of thyroid disease.

PRECAUTIONS

General —Iodides have been reported to cause a flare-up of adolescent acne. Children with cystic fibrosis appear to have an exaggerated susceptibility to the goitrogenic effect of iodides.

Dermatitis and other reversible manifestations of iodism have been reported with chronic use of inorganic iodides. Although these have not been a problem clinically with Organidin formulations, they should be kept in mind in patients receiving these preparations for prolonged periods.

Drug Interactions —Iodides may potentiate the hypothyroid effect of lithium and other antithyroid drugs.

Carcinogenesis, Mutagenesis, Impairment of Fertility —No long-term animal studies have been performed with Tussi-Organidin DM

Pregnancy —Teratogenic effects: Pregnancy Category X (see CONTRAINDICATIONS).

Nursing Mothers —Tussi-Organidin DM should not be administered to a nursing woman.

ADVERSE REACTIONS

Side effects have been rare, including those which may occur with the individual ingredients and which may be modified as a result of their combination. *Organidin* —Rare side effects include gastrointestinal irritation, rash, hypersensitivity, thyroid gland enlargement, and acute parotitis. *Dextromethorphan* —Rarely produces drowsiness or gastrointestinal disturbances.

OVERDOSAGE

Acute overdosage experience with Organidin formulations has been rare and there have been no reports of any serious problems.

DOSAGE AND ADMINISTRATION

Adults: 1 to 2 teaspoonfuls every 4 hours.

Children: ½ to 1 teaspoonful every 4 hours.

HOW SUPPLIED

Tussi-Organidin DM Liquid —clear yellow liquid, in bottles of one pint (NDC 0037-4712-10) and one gallon (NDC 0037-4712-20).

Storage: Store at room temperature; avoid excessive heat. Keep bottle tightly closed.

Distributed by
WALLACE LABORATORIES
Division of
CARTER-WALLACE, INC.
Cranbury, New Jersey 08512
Manufactured by Denver Chemical (Puerto Rico) Inc.
Humacao, Puerto Rico 00661

Rev. 4/87

Shown in Product Identification Section, page 434

VoSoL®   ℞
(acetic acid otic solution, USP)
OTIC SOLUTION

VoSoL® HC   ℞
(hydrocortisone and acetic acid otic solution, USP)
OTIC SOLUTION

DESCRIPTION

VoSoL (acetic acid otic solution, USP) is a solution of acetic acid (2%), in a propylene glycol vehicle containing propylene glycol diacetate (3%), benzethonium chloride (0.02%), and sodium acetate (0.015%).

VoSoL HC (hydrocortisone and acetic acid otic solution, USP) also contains hydrocortisone (1%) and citric acid (0.05%). The empirical formulas for acetic acid and hydrocortisone are CH_3COOH and $C_{21}H_{30}O_5$, with a molecular weight of 60.05 and 362.46, respectively. The structural formulas are:

Acetic Acid

Chemically, hydrocortisone is:
Pregn-4-ene-3,20-dione,
11,17,21-trihydroxy-(11β)-.

VoSoL and VoSoL HC are available as nonaqueous otic solutions buffered at pH 3 for use in the external ear canal.

CLINICAL PHARMACOLOGY

Acetic acid is anti-bacterial and anti-fungal; propylene glycol is hydrophilic and provides a low surface tension; benzethonium chloride is a surface active agent that promotes contact of the solution with tissues; hydrocortisone (in VoSoL HC) is anti-inflammatory, anti-allergic and anti-pruritic.

Continued on next page

Wallace—Cont.

INDICATIONS AND USAGE

<u>VoSoL</u>—For the treatment of superficial infections of the external auditory canal caused by organisms susceptible to the action of the antimicrobial.

<u>VoSoL HC</u>—For the treatment of superficial infections of the external auditory canal caused by organisms susceptible to the action of the antimicrobial, complicated by inflammation.

CONTRAINDICATIONS

Hypersensitivity to any of the ingredients. VoSoL <u>HC</u> is contraindicated in herpes simplex, vaccinia and varicella. Perforated tympanic membrane is considered a contraindication to the use of any medication in the external ear canal.

WARNINGS

Discontinue promptly if sensitization or irritation occurs.

PRECAUTIONS

Transient stinging or burning may be noted occasionally when the solution is first instilled into the acutely inflamed ear.

ADVERSE REACTIONS

Stinging or burning may be noted occasionally; local irritation has occurred very rarely.

DOSAGE AND ADMINISTRATION

Carefully remove all cerumen and debris to allow solution to contact infected surfaces directly. To promote continuous contact, insert a wick saturated with VoSoL or VoSoL <u>HC</u> into the ear canal; the wick may also be saturated after insertion. Instruct the patient to keep the wick in for at least 24 hours and to keep it moist by adding 3 to 5 drops of VoSoL or VoSoL <u>HC</u> every 4 to 6 hours. The wick may be removed after 24 hours but the patient should continue to instill 5 drops of VoSoL 3 or 4 times daily thereafter, for as long as indicated.

HOW SUPPLIED

<u>VoSoL</u> Otic Solution, in 15 mL (NDC 0037-3611-10) and 30 mL (NDC 0037-3611-30) measured drop, safety-tip plastic bottles.

<u>VoSoL HC</u> Otic Solution, in 10 mL measured-drop, safety-tip plastic bottle (NDC 0037-3811-12).

Storage: Store at room temperature; avoid excessive heat. Keep container tightly closed.

Distributed by
WALLACE LABORATORIES
Division of
CARTER-WALLACE, INC.
Cranbury, New Jersey 08512
Manufactured by Denver Chemical (Puerto Rico), Inc.
Humacao, Puerto Rico 00661

Rev. 5/89

Shown in Product Identification Section, page 434

Warner Chilcott Laboratories
Division of Warner-Lambert Company
201 TABOR ROAD
MORRIS PLAINS, NJ 07950

NDC #	PRODUCT	
0640	Acetaminophen Tablets, USP 325 mg	OTC
0759	Acetaminophen Caplets 500 mg	OTC
0634	Acetaminophen with Codeine Phosphate Tablets No. 2	©/℞
0635	Acetaminophen with Codeine Phosphate Tablets No. 3	©/℞
0637	Acetaminophen with Codeine Phosphate Tablets No. 4	©/℞
2911	Allerhist™ Elixir (brompheniramine maleate, USP 2 mg/5 mL phenylpropanolamine HCl, USP 12.5 mg/5 mL)	OTC
0876	Allerhist Extended Release Tablets	OTC
0853	Amantadine HCl Capsules, USP 100 mg	℞
0272	Amitriptyline HCl Tablets, USP 10 mg	℞
0273	Amitriptyline HCl Tablets, USP 25 mg	℞
0274	Amitriptyline HCl Tablets, USP 50 mg	℞
0275	Amitriptyline HCl Tablets, USP 75 mg	℞
0271	Amitriptyline HCl Tablets, USP 100 mg	℞
0730	Amoxicillin Capsules, USP 250 mg	℞
0731	Amoxicillin Capsules, USP 500 mg	℞
2500	Amoxicillin for Oral Suspension, USP 125 mg/5 mL	℞
2501	Amoxicillin for Oral Suspension, USP 250 mg/5 mL	℞
0402	Ampicillin Capsules, USP 250 mg	℞
0404	Ampicillin Capsules, USP 500 mg	℞
2301	Ampicillin for Oral Suspension, USP 125 mg/5 mL	

2302	Ampicillin for Oral Suspension, USP 250 mg/5 mL	℞
0606	Aspirin Tablets, USP 5 gr	OTC
0725	Aspirin with Codeine Phosphate Tablets No. 2	©/℞
0726	Aspirin with Codeine Phosphate Tablets No. 3	©/℞
0727	Aspirin with Codeine Phosphate Tablets No. 4	©/℞
0611	Baclofen Tablets 10 mg	℞
0612	Baclofen Tablets 20 mg	℞
2910	Bromarest DC Cough Syrup (brompheniramine maleate 2 mg/5 mL phenylpropanolamine HCl 12.5 mg/5 mL codeine phosphate 10 mg/5 mL)	©/℞
2909	Bromarest DX Cough Syrup (brompheniramine maleate 2 mg/5 mL pseudoephedrine HCl 30 mg/5 mL dextromethorphan HBr 10 mg/5 mL)	OTC
2908	Bromarest Elixir (brompheniramine maleate elixir, USP) 2 mg/5 mL	℞
0976	Brompheril Tablets	OTC
4239	Calcium Gluconate Injection, USP	℞
0243	Carbamazepine Tablets, USP 200 mg	℞
0242	Carbamazepine Chewable Tablets, 100 mg	℞
0538	Cefadroxil Capsules 500 mg	℞
0938	Cephalexin Capsules, USP 250 mg	℞
0939	Cephalexin Capsules, USP 500 mg	℞
2375	Cephalexin for Oral Suspension, USP 125 mg/5 mL	℞
2376	Cephalexin for Oral Suspension, USP 250 mg/5 mL	℞
0548	Cephalexin Tablets 250 mg	℞
0549	Cephalexin Tablets 500 mg	℞
0808	Cephradine Capsules, USP 250 mg	℞
0809	Cephradine Capsules, USP 500 mg	℞
1810	Cherry Syrup	OTC
2892	Chlorpromazine HCl Concentrate 30 mg/mL	℞
2886	Chlorpromazine HCl Concentrate 100 mg/mL	℞
0123	Chlorthalidone Tablets, USP 25 mg	℞
0121	Chlorthalidone Tablets, USP 50 mg	℞
0443	Clonidine HCl Tablets, USP 0.1 mg	℞
0444	Clonidine HCl Tablets, USP 0.2 mg	℞
0445	Clonidine HCl Tablets, USP 0.3 mg	℞
0985	Clonidine HCl and Chlorthalidone Tablets, USP 0.1 mg/15 mg	℞
0986	Clonidine HCl and Chlorthalidone Tablets, USP 0.2 mg/15 mg	℞
0987	Clonidine HCl and Chlorthalidone Tablets, USP 0.3 mg/15 mg	℞
0451	Clorazepate Dipotassium Tablets 3.75 mg	℞
0452	Clorazepate Dipotassium Tablets 7.5 mg	℞
0453	Clorazepate Dipotassium Tablets 15 mg	℞
0949	Cloxacillin Sodium Capsules, USP 250 mg	℞
0950	Cloxacillin Sodium Capsules, USP 500 mg	℞
2995	Cloxacillin for Oral Solution 125 mg/5 mL	℞
2914	Codan™ Syrup (hydrocodone bitartrate 5 mg/5 mL homatropine methylbromide 1.5 mg/5 mL)	©/℞
4119	Cyanocobalamin Injection, USP	℞
0575	Danazol Capsules 200 mg	℞
3998	DermUspray™	℞
0594	Desipramine Tablets 25 mg	℞
0595	Desipramine Tablets 50 mg	℞
0596	Desipramine Tablets 75 mg	℞
4050	Diazepam Injection 5 mg/mL Ampoules and Vials	©/℞
0141	Diazepam Tablets, USP 2 mg	©/℞
0142	Diazepam Tablets, USP 5 mg	©/℞
0143	Diazepam Tablets, USP 10 mg	©/℞
0945	Dicloxacillin Sodium Capsules, USP 250 mg	℞
0946	Dicloxacillin Sodium Capsules, USP 500 mg	℞
0558	Disopyramide Phosphate CR Capsules 100 mg	℞
0720	Disopyramide Phosphate CR Capsules 150 mg	℞
4210	Dopamine HCl Injection, USP Ampoules and Vials	℞
0247	Docusate Sodium Capsules, USP (D-S-S)	OTC
0248	Docusate Sodium with Casanthranol Capsules (D-S-S Plus)	OTC
2623	Doxepin HCl Oral Solution 10 mg/mL	℞
0829	Doxycycline Hyclate Capsules, USP 50 mg	℞
0830	Doxycycline Hyclate Capsules, USP 100 mg	℞
0813	Doxycycline Hyclate Tablets, USP 100 mg	℞
0850	Duraquin® Tablets (quinidine gluconate)	
2330	Erythromycin Ethylsuccinate Suspension 200 mg/5 mL	℞
2331	Erythromycin Ethylsuccinate Suspension 400 mg/5 mL	℞

0672	Erythromycin Stearate Tablets, USP 250 mg	℞
0919	Erythromycin Stearate Tablets, USP 500 mg	℞
0081	Fenoprofen Calcium Capsules 300 mg	℞
0077	Fenoprofen Calcium Tablets 600 mg	℞
0796	Fluphenazine Tablets 1 mg	℞
0797	Fluphenazine Tablets 2.5 mg	℞
0798	Fluphenazine Tablets 5 mg	℞
0799	Fluphenazine Tablets 10 mg	℞
0988	Flurazepam HCl Capsules, USP 15 mg	©/℞
0989	Flurazepam HCl Capsules, USP 30 mg	©/℞
4143	Furosemide Injection, USP	℞
0440	Furosemide Tablets, USP 20 mg	℞
0441	Furosemide Tablets, USP 40 mg	℞
0442	Furosemide Tablets, USP 80 mg	℞
0981	Haloperidol Tablets, USP 0.5 mg	℞
0982	Haloperidol Tablets, USP 1 mg	℞
0983	Haloperidol Tablets, USP 2 mg	℞
0984	Haloperidol Tablets, USP 5 mg	℞
2913	Haloperidol Concentrate (haloperidol oral solution, USP) 2 mg/mL	℞
0702	Hydrochlorothiazide Tablets, USP 25 mg	℞
0710	Hydrochlorothiazide Tablets, USP 50 mg	℞
2917	Hydromine Syrup (hydrocodone bitartrate and phenylpropanolamine HCl)	©/℞
2991	Hydromine Pediatric Syrup (hydrocodone bitartrate and phenylpropanolamine HCl)	©/℞
2902	Hydroxyzine HCl Syrup, USP 10 mg/5 mL	℞
0887	Indomethacin Capsules, USP 25 mg	℞
0888	Indomethacin Capsules, USP 50 mg	℞
0875	Indomethacin Sustained Release Capsules, USP 75 mg	℞
0431	Lorazepam Tablets 0.5 mg	©/℞
0432	Lorazepam Tablets 1 mg	©/℞
0433	Lorazepam Tablets 2 mg	©/℞
0621	Loxapine Capsules 5 mg	℞
0632	Loxapine Capsules 10 mg	℞
0650	Loxapine Capsules 25 mg	℞
0651	Loxapine Capsules 50 mg	℞
0790	Maprotiline Tablets 25 mg	℞
0791	Maprotiline Tablets 50 mg	℞
0795	Maprotiline Tablets 75 mg	℞
2891	Medi-Tuss Syrup Brand of Guaifenesin Syrup, USP 100 mg/5 mL	OTC
2931	Medi-Tuss AC codeine phosphate 10 mg/5 mL guaifenesin 100 mg/5 mL	©/℞
2932	Medi-Tuss DAC guaifenesin, USP 100 mg/5 mL pseudoephedrine HCl, USP 30 mg/5 mL codeine phosphate 10 mg/5 mL	©/℞
2933	Medi-Tuss DM guaifenesin 100 mg/5 mL dextromethorphan HBr 15 mg/5 mL	OTC
0865	Methyldopa Tablets, USP 250 mg	℞
0866	Methyldopa Tablets, USP 500 mg	℞
0030	Methyldopa and Hydrochlorothiazide Tablets, USP 250 mg/15 mg	℞
0031	Methyldopa and Hydrochlorothiazide Tablets, USP 250 mg/25 mg	℞
0032	Methyldopa and Hydrochlorothiazide Tablets, USP 500 mg/30 mg	℞
0033	Methyldopa and Hydrochlorothiazide Tablets, USP 500 mg/50 mg	℞
2996	Metoclopramide HCl Syrup 5 mg/5 mL	℞
0878	Metoclopramide HCl Tablets 10 mg	℞
0930/0927	Nelova™ 1/35E (norethindrone 1 mg and ethinyl estradiol 35 mcg)	
0929/0926	Nelova™ 0.5/35E (norethindrone 0.5 mg and ethinyl estradiol 35 mcg)	
0941/0944	Nelova™ 10/11	℞
0942/0947	Nelova™ 1/50M	℞
0789	Nitrofurantoin Capsules 100 mg (macrocrystals)	℞
0788	Nitrofurantoin Capsules 50 mg (macrocrystals)	℞
2922	Nystatin Oral Suspension, USP	℞
0690	Oxazepam Capsules 10 mg	©/℞
0665	Oxazepam Capsules 15 mg	©/℞
0667	Oxazepam Capsules 30 mg	©/℞
0551	Oxazepam Tablets, USP 15 mg	©/℞
0648	Penicillin V Potassium Tablets, USP 250 mg	℞
0673	Penicillin V Potassium Tablets, USP 500 mg	℞
2449	Penicillin VK for Oral Solution, USP 125 mg/ 5 mL	℞
2506	Penicillin VK for Oral Solution, USP 250 mg/5 mL	℞

2923	Phena-Chlor Syrup (phenylpropanolamine HCl, 20 mg/5 mL phenylephrine HCl 5 mg/5 mL phenyltoloxamine citrate 7.5 mg/5 mL chlorpheniramine maleate 2.5 mg/5 mL)	℞
0699	Phenobarbital Tablets, USP 15 mg	©/℞
0700	Phenobarbital Tablets, USP 30 mg	©/℞
0607	Phenobarbital Tablets, USP 60 mg	©/℞
0698	Phenobarbital Tablets, USP 100 mg	©/℞
0951	Potassium Chloride Extended-Release Tablets, USP 8 mEq (600 mg)	℞
0539	Potassium Chloride Extended-Release Capsules l0 mEq (750 mg)	℞
0843	Prazosin Capsules 1 mg	℞
0844	Prazosin Capsules 2 mg	℞
0845	Prazosin Capsules 5 mg	℞
4186	Procainamide HCl Injection 100 mg/mL	℞
4187	Procainamide HCl Injection 500 mg/mL	℞
2924	Promethazine Syrup Plain (promethazine HCl syrup, USP) 6.25 mg/5 mL	℞
2928	Promethazine VC Plain (promethazine HCl 6.25 mg/5 mL and phenylephrine HCl 5 mg/5 mL)	©/℞
2890	Promethazine VC with Codeine (promethazine HCl 6.25 mg/5 mL phenylephrine HCl 5 mg/5 mL codeine phosphate 10 mg/5 mL)	©/℞
0979	Propoxyphene HCl and Acetaminophen Tablets, USP 65 mg/650 mg	©/℞
0980	Propoxyphene Napsylate and Acetaminophen Tablets, USP 100 mg/650 mg	©/℞
0070	Propranolol HCl Tablets, USP 10 mg	℞
0071	Propranolol HCl Tablets, USP 20 mg	℞
0072	Propranolol HCl Tablets, USP 40 mg	℞
0073	Propranolol HCl Tablets, USP 60 mg	℞
0074	Propranolol HCl Tablets, USP 80 mg	℞
0014	Propranolol HCl and Hydrochlorothiazide Tablets 40 mg/25 mg	℞
0015	Propranolol HCl and Hydrochlorothiazide Tablets 80 mg/25 mg	℞
0849	Quinidine Sulfate Tablets, USP	℞
0420	Quinine Sulfate Capsules, USP	OTC
2885	R-Tannate Pediatric Suspension	℞
0940	R-Tannate Tablets phenylephrine tannate 25 mg chlorpheniramine tannate 8 mg pyrilamine tannate 25 mg	℞
2899	Sinu-Clear Syrup triprolidine and pseudoephedrine HCl syrup, USP	OTC
0713	Spironolactone Tablets, USP 25 mg	℞
0712	Spironolactone with Hydrochlorothiazide Tablets, USP 25 mg/25 mg	℞
0977	Temazepam Capsules, 15 mg	©/℞
0978	Temazepam Capsules, 30 mg	©/℞
0407	Tetracycline HCl Capsules, USP 250 mg	℞
0697	Tetracycline HCl Capsules, USP 500 mg	℞
2912	Theophylline Elixir, 80 mg/15 mL	℞
2920	Thioridazine HCl Oral Solution, USP (concentrate) 30 mg/mL	℞
2889	Thioridazine HCl Oral Solution, USP (concentrate) 100 mg/mL	℞
0966	Thioridazine HCl Tablets, 10 mg	℞
0967	Thioridazine HCl Tablets, 25 mg	℞
0968	Thioridazine HCl Tablets, 50 mg	℞
0969	Thioridazine HCl Tablets, 100 mg	℞
0971	Thiothixene Capsules, USP 2 mg	℞
0972	Thiothixene Capsules, USP 5 mg	℞
0975	Thiothixene Capsules, USP 10 mg	℞
2877	Thiothixene HCl Oral Solution 5 mg/mL	℞
0729	Timolol Maleate Tablets 5 mg	℞
0728	Timolol Maleate Tablets l0 mg	℞
0724	Timolol Maleate Tablets 20 mg	℞
0835	Transdermal-NTG (nitroglycerin transdermal system) 5 mg/24 hour	℞
0837	Transdermal-NTG (nitroglycerin transdermal system) 10 mg/24 hour	℞
0577	Trazodone HCl Tablets 50 mg	℞
0578	Trazodone HCl Tablets 100 mg	℞
0716	Trazodone HCl Tablets 150 mg	℞
0834	Triamterene and Hydrochlorothiazide Capsules, 50 mg/25 mg	℞
0833	Triamterene and Hydrochlorothiazide Tablets, 75 mg/50 mg	℞
2897	Tri-Clear Expectorant phenylpropanolamine HCl 12.5 mg/5 mL guaifenesin 100 mg/5 mL	OTC
2898	Tri-Clear Syrup phenylpropanolamine HCl 12.5 mg/5 mL chlorpheniramine maleate 2 mg/5 mL	OTC
2935	Trifluoperazine HCl Syrup, USP (concentrate) 10 mg/mL	℞
0695	Trifluoperazine Tablets l mg	℞
0709	Trifluoperazine Tablets 2 mg	℞
0718	Trifluoperazine Tablets 5 mg	℞
0756	Trifluoperazine Tablets l0 mg	℞

2900	Triprolidine Pseudoephedrine with Codeine Syrup	©/℞
2903	Trisulfam Oral Suspension	℞
2905	Trisulfam Pediatric Oral Suspension	℞
3122	Unibase	OTC
0557	Verapamil HCl Tablets 80 mg	℞
0573	Verapamil HCl Tablets 120 mg	℞

Webcon Pharmaceuticals
Division of
ALCON (Puerto Rico) INC.
P.O. BOX 3000
HUMACAO, PUERTO RICO 00661

SUPPRETTES®, Webcon's identifying trademark for suppository medication in the NEOCERA® base, a unique blend of water-soluble Carbowaxes* that release drugs by hydrophilic action.
*TM Union Carbide.

ANESTACON®   ℞
[ăne'stăcon]
(2% lidocaine hydrochloride viscous solution for topical use)

DESCRIPTION
A sterile anesthetic for endourethral use. Each mL contains: Active: Lidocaine Hydrochloride 20 mg (2%). Vehicle: Hydroxypropyl Methylcellulose 10 mg (1%). Preservative: Benzalkonium Chloride 0.1 mg (0.01%). Inactive: Sodium Chloride, Hydrochloric Acid and/or Sodium Hydroxide (to adjust pH), Purified Water.   DM-00

$$\text{NHCOCH}_2\text{N}(C_2H_5)_2 \cdot \text{HCl} \cdot \text{H}_2\text{O}$$

with two CH_3 substituents on the ring.

Established Name:
Lidocaine Hydrocloride
Chemical Name:
2-(diethylamino)-
N-(2,6-dimethylphenyl) acetamide
monohydrochloride monohydrate

CLINICAL PHARMACOLOGY
Mechanism of Action: Lidocaine HCl acts on surface mucous membranes of the urethra to produce local anesthesia by altering the permeability of the nerve cell membrane to sodium and potassium ions, resulting in an increased threshold for electrical excitability and a decreased conduction of impulses whereby depolarization and ion exchanges are inhibited. The anesthetic effect usually begins within two to five minutes and lasts for at least 15 minutes.

HEMODYNAMICS
Excessive blood levels may cause changes in cardiac output, total peripheral resistance, and mean arterial pressure. These changes may be attributable to a direct depressant effect of the local anesthetic agent on various components of the cardiovascular system. The net effect is normally a modest hypotension when the recommended dosages are not exceeded.

PHARMACOKINETICS AND METABOLISM
Lidocaine is absorbed following topical administration to mucous membranes, its rate and extent of absorption being dependent upon concentration and total dose administered, the specific site of application, and duration of exposure. In general, the rate of absorption of local anesthetic agents following topical application occurs most rapidly after intratracheal administration. Lidocaine is also well-absorbed from the urethra, but little intact drug appears in the circulation because of biotransformation into the liver.
The plasma binding of lidocaine is dependent on drug concentration, and the fraction bound decreases with increasing concentration. At concentrations of 1 to 4 μg of free base per mL, 60 to 80 percent of lidocaine is protein bound. Binding is also dependent on the plasma concentration of the alpha-1-acid glycoprotein.
Lidocaine crosses the blood-brain and placental barriers, presumably by passive diffusion.
Lidocaine is metabolized rapidly by the liver, and metabolites and unchanged drug are excreted by the kidneys. Biotransformation includes oxidative N-dealkylation, ring hydroxylation, cleavage of the amide linkage, and conjugation. N-dealkylation, a major pathway of biotransformation, yields the metabolites monoethylglycinexylidide and glycinexylidide. The pharmacological/toxicological actions of these metabolites are similar to, but less potent than, those of lidocaine. Approximately 90% of lidocaine administered is excreted in the form of various metabolites, and less than

10% is excreted unchanged. The primary metabolite in urine is a conjugate of 4-hydroxy-2, 6-dimethylaniline.
The elimination half-life of lidocaine following an intravenous bolus injection is typically 1.5 to 2.0 hours. Because of the rapid rate at which lidocaine is metabolized, any condition that affects liver function may alter lidocaine kinetics. The half-life may be prolonged two-fold or more in patients with liver dysfunction. Renal dysfunction does not affect lidocaine kinetics but may increase the accumulation of metabolites.
Factors such as acidosis and the use of CNS stimulants and depressants affect the CNS levels of lidocaine required to produce overt systemic effects. Objective adverse manifestations become increasingly apparent with increasing venous plasma levels above 6.0 μg free base per mL. In the rhesus monkey arterial blood levels of 18–21 μg/mL have been shown to be threshold for convulsive activity.

INDICATIONS AND USAGE
For prevention and control of pain in procedures involving the male and female urethra and for topical treatment of painful urethritis.

CONTRAINDICATIONS
Contraindicated in patients with a known sensitivity (allergy) to lidocaine or other drugs of a similar chemical nature, or to other components of the formulation.

WARNINGS
EXCESSIVE DOSAGE, OR SHORT INTERVALS BETWEEN DOSES, CAN RESULT IN HIGH PLASMA LEVELS AND SERIOUS ADVERSE EFFECTS. PATIENTS SHOULD BE INSTRUCTED TO STRICTLY ADHERE TO THE RECOMMENDED DOSAGE AND ADMINISTRATION GUIDELINES AS SET FORTH IN THIS PACKAGE INSERT.
THE MANAGEMENT OF SERIOUS ADVERSE REACTIONS MAY REQUIRE THE USE OF RESUSCITATIVE EQUIPMENT, OXYGEN, AND OTHER RESUSCITATIVE DRUGS.
LIDOCAINE SHOULD BE USED WITH EXTREME CAUTION ON TRAUMATIZED MUCOSA OR IN A REGION OF SEPSIS. **NOT FOR OPHTHALMIC USE OR INJECTION.**
NOTE: After initial use of the 15 mL single-dose container, the remaining contents of the container should be discarded. The 240 mL container should be used for only an individual patient. See CAUTION under DOSAGE AND ADMINISTRATION.

PRECAUTIONS
General: The safety and effectiveness of lidocaine depend on proper dosage, correct technique, adequate precautions, and readiness for emergencies (See WARNINGS and ADVERSE REACTIONS). The lowest dosage that results in effective anesthesia should be used to avoid high plasma levels and serious adverse effects. Repeated doses of lidocaine may cause significant increases in blood levels with each repeated dose because of slow accumulation of the drug and/or its metabolites. Tolerance varies with the status of the patient. Debilitated, elderly patients, acutely ill patients, and children should be given reduced doses commensurate with their age, weight and physical condition. Lidocaine should also be used with caution in patients with severe shock or heart block. ANESTACON should be used with caution in persons with known drug sensitivities. Patients allergic to para-aminobenzoic acid derivatives (procaine, tetracaine, benzocaine, etc.) are not likely to show cross sensitivity to lidocaine.
PATIENTS SHOULD BE INSTRUCTED TO STRICTLY ADHERE TO DOSING INSTRUCTIONS, AND TO KEEP THE SUPPLY OF MEDICATION OUT OF THE REACH OF CHILDREN.
CARCINOGENESIS, MUTAGENESIS, IMPAIRMENT OF FERTILITY: Studies of lidocaine in animals to evaluate the carcinogenic and mutagenic potential or the effect on fertility have not been conducted.
PREGNANCY CATEGORY C: Animal reproduction studies have not been conducted with ANESTACON®. It is also not known whether ANESTACON can cause fetal harm when administered to a pregnant woman or can affect reproduction capacity. ANESTACON should be administered to a pregnant woman only if clearly needed.
NURSING MOTHERS: It is not known whether this drug is excreted in human milk. Because many drugs are excreted in human milk, caution should be exercised when ANESTACON is administered to a nursing mother.

ADVERSE REACTIONS
Adverse experiences following the administration of lidocaine are similar in nature to those observed with other amide local anesthetic agents. These adverse experiences are, in general, dose-related and may result from high plasma levels caused by excessive dosage or rapid absorption, or may result from a hypersensitivity, idiosyncrasy or diminished tolerance on the part of the patient. Serious adverse experiences

Continued on next page

Webcon—Cont.

are generally systemic in nature. The following types are those most commonly reported:

CENTRAL NERVOUS SYSTEM: CNS manifestations are excitatory and/or depressant and may be characterized by light-headedness, nervousness, apprehension, euphoria, confusion, dizziness, drowsiness, tinnitus, blurred or double vision, vomiting, sensations of heat, cold or numbness, twitching, tremors, convulsions, unconsciousness, respiratory depression and arrest. The excitatory manifestations may be very brief or may not occur at all, in which case manifestation of toxicity may be drowsiness merging into unconsciousness and respiratory arrest.

Drowsiness following the administration of lidocaine is usually an early sign of a high blood level of the drug and may occur as a consequence of rapid absorption.

CARDIOVASCULAR SYSTEM: Cardiovascular manifestations are usually depressant and are characterized by bradycardia, hypotension, and cardiovascular collapse, which may lead to cardiac arrest.

ALLERGIC: Allergic reactions are characterized by cutaneous lesions of delayed onset, urticaria, edema or other manifestations of allergy. Allergic reactions as a result of sensitivity to lidocaine are rare and, if they occur, should be managed by conventional means. The detection of sensitivity by skin testing is of doubtful value.

OVERDOSAGE

Acute emergencies from local anesthetics are generally related to high plasma levels encountered during therapeutic use of local anesthetics. (See ADVERSE REACTIONS, WARNINGS, and PRECAUTIONS.)

DOSAGE AND ADMINISTRATION

Dosage varies and depends upon the area to be anesthetized, vascularity of the tissues, individual tolerance, and the technique of anesthesia. The least volume of the drug needed to provide effective anesthesia should be administered. For specific techniques and procedures refer to standard texts. Avoid forceful injection in the presence of known stricture, as this may cause intravascular injection. THE USUAL ADULT DOSE SHOULD NOT EXCEED 600 mg OR 30 mL OF ANESTACON IN ANY TWELVE HOUR PERIOD. THE CHILD DOSE SHOULD BE REDUCED COMMENSURATE WITH AGE, WEIGHT AND PHYSICAL CONDITION.

15 ML SINGLE-DOSE CONTAINER: ADULT MALES: Immediately before use, remove the label and cap and firmly insert the sterile tip into the urethral orifice. Slowly instill 5 mL to 15 mL by exerting pressure on opposite sides of the container—the full dose should be administered in a single action without removing the tip. While waiting two to five minutes for induction of anesthesia, the urethra should be occluded with a penile clamp or by manual compression. ADULT FEMALES: The sterile tip may be used to insert about 1 mL.

240 ML CONTAINER: This is for use for an individual patient only. CAUTION: Care should be taken to prevent contamination of bottle contents (e.g., aspiration of urethral contents into the container when using insertion tip). ADULT MALES: Instill slowly into the urethra 5 mL to 15 mL and allow two to five minutes for induction of anesthesia. Optimal anesthesia is attained after 5 minutes. The medication is retained in the urethra by means of a penile clamp or by manual compression of the distal urethra. ADULT FEMALES: Apply liberal amount of medication on a cotton swab and insert into urethra for two to five minutes, or a dropper may be employed to insert about 1 mL.

STORAGE

Store at room temperature.

HOW SUPPLIED

In 15 mL single-dose and 240 mL multiple-dose disposable containers for single patient use.

STRENGTH: 2% (20 mg/mL) Lidocaine Hydrochloride
15 mL: **NDC** 0998-0300-10
240 mL: **NDC** 0998-0300-20

A URICEUTICAL® Specialty of
WEBCON™
Mfd. for: ALCON (Puerto Rico) INC.
Humacao, P.R. 00661
Mfd. by: Alcon Laboratories, Inc.
Fort Worth, Texas 76134 USA

B & O SUPPRETTES®   ℞
No. 15A and No. 16A
(belladonna and opium) rectal suppositories

DESCRIPTION

Each B&O SUPPRETTE® contains (in the water-soluble NEOCERA® Suppository Base for rectal administration):
B&O No. 15A: Powdered opium* 30 mg (½ gr) and Powdered Belladonna Extract 16.2 mg (equivalent to 0.21 mg or 0.0035 gr alkaloid of belladonna).

B&O No. 16A: Powdered opium* 60 mg (1 gr) and Powdered Belladonna Extract 16.2 mg (equivalent to 0.21 mg or 0.0035 gr alkaloid of belladonna).
NEOCERA® Base is a blend of Polyethylene Glycol 400, 1450, 8000 and Polysorbate 60.
This drug falls into the pharmacologic/therapeutic class of narcotic analgesic/antispasmotic agents.
The pharmacologically active principles present in the belladonna extract component of B&O SUPPRETTES are:

Established Name: Atropine
Chemical Name: dl Tropyl Tropate

Established Name: Scopolamine
Chemical Name: dl Scopolamine

Opium contains more than a score of alkaloids, the principal ones being morphine (10%), narcotine (6%), papaverine (1%) and codeine (0.5%). The major pharmacologically active principle of the powdered opium component of B&O SUPPRETTES, however is:

Established Name: Morphine
Chemical Name:
7,8-Didehydro-4,5-epoxy-
17-methyl-morphinan-3,6-diol

CLINICAL PHARMACOLOGY

Through its parasympatholytic action, atropine relaxes smooth muscle resulting from parasympathetic stimulation. It is the dl isomer of l-hyoscyamine and therefore exhibits the same clinical effects. It is, however, approximately one-half as active peripherally as l-hyoscyamine, the latter being the major active plant principle. The dl isomer atropine is formed during the process of isolation of the belladonna extract.[1]

Morphine, the major active principle of powdered opium, is responsible for the action of powdered opium although the other alkaloids present also contribute to it. The sedative and analgesic action of morphine, the effect desired by inclusion in B&O SUPPRETTES of powdered opium, are thought to be due to its depressant effect on the cerebral cortex, hypothalamus and medullary centers. In large doses, the opiates and their analogs also inhibit synaptic conduction in the spinothalamic tracts, depress the function of the reticular formation, the lemniscus and the thalamic relays, and inhibit spinal synaptic reflexes; but these inhibitor actions are not elicited with therapeutic doses of the drug. Moderate doses of powdered opium do not alter the electroencepahalogram.

The action of morphine consists mainly of a descending depression of the central nervous system. It exerts its analgesic action by increasing the pain threshold or the magnitude of stimulus required to evoke pain and by dulling the sensibility or reaction to pain. In addition to its action in abolishing pain, morphine induces a sense of well-being (euphoria) facilitating certain mental processes while retarding others. Upon absorption of morphine, oxidative dealkylation to produce nor-compounds appears to be the first step in the reaction sequence which imparts analgesia. Morphine is conjugated in the liver to form the 3-glucuronide which passes into the bile and is reabsorbed and excreted in the urine. The atropine effect of the belladonna extract serves to eliminate morphine induced smooth muscle spasm without affecting the sedative analgesic action of powdered opium.[2]

INDICATIONS AND USAGE

B&O SUPPRETTES are used for relief of moderate to severe pain associated with ureteral spasm not responsive to non-narcotic analgesics and to space intervals between injections of opiates.

CONTRAINDICATIONS

Do not use B&O SUPPRETTES in patients suffering from glaucoma, severe hepatic or renal disease, bronchial asthma, narcotic idiosyncrasies, respiratory depression, convulsive

disorders, acute alcoholism, delirium tremens and premature labor.

*WARNINGS

True addiction may result from opium usage. These preparations are not recommended for use in children.

PRECAUTIONS

Administer with caution to persons with a known idiosyncrasy to atropine or atropine-like compounds; to persons known to be sensitive to or addicted to morphine or morphine-like drugs; to persons with cardiac disease, incipient glaucoma or prostatic hypertrophy. Caution should be used in the administration of this drug to old and debilitated patients and patients with increased intracranial pressure, toxic psychosis and myxedema.

Pregnancy Category C. Animal studies have not been conducted with B&O SUPPRETTES. It is also not known whether B&O SUPPRETTES 15A and 16A can affect reproduction capacity. The active principles of B&O SUPPRETTES, atropine and morphine, are known to enter the fetal circulation. Regular use of opium alkaloids during pregnancy has resulted in addiction of the fetus leading to withdrawal symptoms in the neonate. B&O SUPPRETTES therefore should be used by a pregnant woman with caution and only when clearly indicated.

Nursing Mothers: It is not known whether this drug is excreted in human milk. Because many drugs are excreted in human milk, caution should be exercised when B&O SUPPRETTES are administered to a nursing woman.

ADVERSE REACTIONS

Belladonna may cause drowsiness, dry mouth, urinary retention, photophobia, rapid pulse, dizziness and blurred vision. Opium usage may result in constipation, nausea or vomiting. Pruritis and urticaria may occasionally occur.

DRUG ABUSE AND DEPENDENCE

Because of their content of opium, B&O SUPPRETTES are considered as Schedule II drugs by the Drug Enforcement Administration. No data exists on chronic abuse effects or dependence characteristics of B&O SUPPRETTES.

OVERDOSAGE

As with morphine and related narcotics, overdosage is characterized by respiratory depression, pinpoint pupils and coma. Respiratory depression may be reversed by intravenous administration of naloxone hydrochloride. In addition, supportive measures such as oxygenation, intravenous fluids and vasopressors should be used as indicated. As with atropine derivatives, hot, dry, flushed skin, dry mouth and hyperpyrexia may occur.

DOSAGE AND ADMINISTRATION

Adults: One B&O SUPPRETTE No. 15A or No. 16A rectally once or twice daily, not to exceed four doses daily or, as recommended by the physician. Moisten finger and SUPPRETTE with water before inserting. Not recommended for use in children. Absorption is dependent on body hydration and not on body temperature.

HOW SUPPLIED

In strip packaged units of 12 (scored for ½ dosage), DEA order required (Schedule II).
B&O SUPPRETTES No. 15A NDC 0998-5015-75.
B&O SUPPRETTES No. 16A NDC 0998-5016-75.

1. Gilman, A. G., Goodman, L. S. & Gilman, A. 6th Edition, *The Pharmacological Basis of Therapeutics*, MacMillan Pub. Co., N.Y. 1980, pp. 121–127.
2. Ibid, pp. 494-513.

WEBCON
ALCON (Puerto Rico) INC.
Humacao, Puerto Rico 00661

CYSTOSPAZ®   ℞
(Hyoscyamine) Tablets
CYSTOSPAZ–M®   ℞
(hyoscyamine sulfate) Timed-Release Capsules

DESCRIPTION

CYSTOSPAZ® is a pale blue uncoated compressed tablet for oral administration. It contains the parasympatholytic agent hyoscyamine as the free base. Each tablet contains: Active hyoscyamine 0.15 mg. Inactive: FD&C Blue No. 2, Lactose, Magnesium Stearate, Povidone, Starch and Talc. CYSTOSPAZ-M® is a light blue timed-release capsule containing hyoscyamine sulfate 0.375 mg.

Established name:
Hyoscyamine
Chemical name:
λ tropyl tropate

CLINICAL PHARMACOLOGY

Through its parasympatholytic action, hyoscyamine relaxes smooth muscle spasm resulting from parasympathetic stimulation. It is the λ-isomer of atropine and therefore exhibits the same clinical effects as atropine. It is, however, approximately twice as active peripherally as atropine, since the latter is the racemic (dλ) form of hyoscyamine and d-hyoscyamine possesses only a very weak anti-cholinergic action. Since only one-half the atropine dose is required for λ-hyoscyamine, it has only one-half the unwanted central effects of atropine.[1]

INDICATIONS AND USAGE

In the management of disorders of the lower urinary tract associated with hypermotility. Although specific therapy is often required to remove the underlying cause of spasm, Cystospaz Tablets and Cystospaz-M Capsules are offered as antispasmodic agent dosage forms which may be combined with other forms of therapy where indicated.

CONTRAINDICATIONS

Glaucoma, urinary bladder neck or pyloric obstruction, duodenal obstruction and cardiospasm. Hypersensitivity to any of the ingredients.

PRECAUTIONS

Administer with caution to persons with known idiosyncrasy to atropine-like compounds and to patients suffering cardiac disease.

Pregnancy Category C. Animal reproduction studies have not been conducted with Cystospaz Tablets or Cystospaz-M Capsules. It is also not known whether Cystospaz Tablets or Cystospaz-M Capsules can cause fetal harm when administered to a pregnant woman or can affect reproduction capacity. Cystospaz Tablets and Cystospaz-M Capsules should be taken by a pregnant woman only if clearly needed.

Nursing Mothers—It is not known whether this drug is excreted in human milk. Because many drugs are excreted in human milk, caution should be exercised when Cystospaz Tablets or Cystospaz-M Capsules are administered to a nursing woman.

ADVERSE REACTIONS

Through rarely a problem, the side effects encountered with this class of antispasmodic-antisecretory agents (drowsiness, dryness of the mouth, photophobia, constipation, urinary retention) may also be seen with this drug. If rapid pulse, dizziness or blurring of vision occurs, discontinue use immediately. Acute urinary retention may be precipitated in prostatic hypertrophy. **Note:** Slight dryness of the mouth is an indication that parasympathetic blockage is effective. The patient should be warned that this may occur.

DRUG ABUSE AND DEPENDENCE

A dependence on the use of Cystospaz Tablets or Cystospaz-M Capsules has not been reported and due to the nature of their ingredients, abuse of Cystospaz Tablets or Cystospaz-M Capsules is not expected.

OVERDOSAGE

Symptoms of overdosage include severe dryness of the mouth, nose, throat, and hot dry flushed skin, hyperpyrexia (especially in children), difficulty or inability to swallow, difficult speech, dilated pupils until iris almost disappears, restlessness and garrulity indicating an irritability of the brain, marked tremors, convulsions, respiratory failure, death.[2] In adults, symptoms of overdosage may begin in the range of ingestion of 0.6 to 1 mg with doses exceeding 1–2 mg eliciting more profound toxicity.

DOSAGE AND ADMINISTRATION

Adults: Cystospaz® Tablets—One or two tablets four times daily or fewer if needed. Cystospaz-M Capsules—One capsule every twelve hours.

Children (12 and under): Reduce dosage in proportion to age and weight.

HOW SUPPLIED

Cystospaz Tablets— Bottles of 100 light blue tablets **NDC** 0998-2225-10. Tablets are imprinted with a "**W 2225**". Cystospaz-M Capsules—Bottles of 100 light blue timed-release capsules **NDC** 0998-2260-10. Capsules are identified with "**W 2260**" printed in black.

REFERENCES

1. Gilman, A. L., Goodman, L.S. & Gilman, A., *The Pharmacological Basis of Therapeutics*, 6th Edition, p. 125.
2. Ibid, p. 127.

Cystospaz-M Capsules are manufactured by:
K. V. Pharmaceutical Company
St. Louis, Mo. 63144

A URICEUTICAL® Specialty of
WEBCON™
ALCON (Puerto Rico) INC.
Humacao, Puerto Rico 00661

URISED® ℞

DESCRIPTION

URISED® is a purple, round, sugar coated tablet for oral administration. It is a combination of antiseptics (Methenamine, Methylene Blue, Phenyl Salicylate, Benzoic Acid) and parasympatholytics (Atropine Sulfate, Hyoscyamine). The active ingredients are represented by the chemical structures:

Established name:
Methanamine
Chemical name:
Hexamethylenetetramine

Established name:
Phenyl Salicylate
Chemical name:
2-Hydroxybenzoic acid phenyl ester

Established name:
Methylene Blue
Chemical name:
Methylthionine chloride

Established name:
Benzoic Acid
Chemical name:
Benzenecarboxylic acid

Established name:
AtropineSulfate
Chemical name:
dl tropyl tropate

Established name:
Hyoscyamine
Chemical name:
l-tropyl tropate

Each tablet contains: Methenamine 40.8 mg, Phenyl Salicylate 18.1 mg, Methylene Blue 5.4 mg, Benzoic Acid 4.5 mg, Atropine Sulfate 0.03 mg and Hyoscyamine 0.03 mg.

CLINICAL PHARMACOLOGY

Methenamine itself does not have antiseptic, irritant, or toxic properties in the urine. Methenamine, in an acid urine (pH 6 or below), hydrolyzes into formaldehyde within the urinary tract providing mild antiseptic activity[1]. When given as directed and the daily urine volume is 1000 to 1500 mL, a daily dose of 2 grams will yield a urine concentration of 18–60 mcg/mL of free formaldehyde in the urine. This is more than the minimal inhibitory dose of formaldehyde which must be available for most urinary tract pathogens. Methenamine is readily absorbed from the gastrointestinal tract and is rapidly excreted almost entirely in the urine.

Methylene Blue and Benzoic Acid are mild but effective antiseptics which contribute to the antiseptic properties of Methenamine. Phenyl Salicylate is a mild analgesic and antipyretic with weak antiseptic activity. All of these compounds are readily absorbed from the gastrointestinal tract and excreted in the urine. Through parasympatholytic action, atropine and hyoscyamine relax smooth muscle spasms resulting from parasympathetic stimulation.[2]

INDICATIONS AND USAGE

URISED is indicated for the relief of discomfort of the lower urinary tract caused by hypermotility resulting from inflammation or diagnostic procedures and in the treatment of cystitis, urethritis, and trigonitis when caused by organisms which maintain or produce an acid urine and are susceptible to formaldehyde.

CONTRAINDICATIONS

Glaucoma, urinary bladder neck obstruction, pyloric or duodenal obstruction, or cardiospasm. Hypersensitivity to any of the ingredients.

WARNINGS

Do not exceed recommended dose. Methenamine may combine with sulfonamides in the urine to give mutual antagonism and should not be used with sulfonamides.

PRECAUTIONS

Administer with caution to persons with known idiosyncrasy to atropine-like compounds and to patients suffering from cardiac disease. Bacteriological studies of the urine may be helpful in following the patient response. Methylene Blue interferes with the analysis for some urinary components such as free formaldehyde. Drugs and/or foods which produce an alkaline urine should be restricted.[3]

Patient should be advised that the urine may become blue to blue-green and the feces may be discolored as a result of excretion of Methylene Blue. Methenamine preparations should not be given to patients taking sulfonamides since insoluble precipitates may form with formaldehyde in the urine. No known long-term animal studies have been performed to evaluate carcinogenic potential.

Pregnancy Category C. Animal reproduction studies have not been conducted with URISED® tablets. It is also not known whether URISED tablets can cause fetal harm when administered to a pregnant woman or can affect reproduction capacity. URISED tablets should be given to a pregnant woman only if clearly needed.

Nursing Mothers: It is not known whether this drug is excreted in human milk. Because many drugs are excreted in human milk, caution should be exercised when URISED tablets are administered to a nursing woman.

Prolonged Use: There have been no studies to establish the safety of prolonged use in humans.

ADVERSE REACTIONS

Prolonged use may result in a generalized skin rash, pronounced dryness of the mouth, flushing, difficulty in initiating micturition, rapid pulse, dizziness or blurring of vision. If any of these reactions occurs, discontinue use immediately. Acute urinary retention may be precipitated in prostatic hypertrophy. See "OVERDOSAGE."

DRUG ABUSE AND DEPENDENCE

A dependence on the use of URISED has not been reported and due to the nature of its ingredients, abuse of URISED is not expected.

OVERDOSAGE

By exceeding the recommended dosage of URISED, symptomology related to the overdose of its individual active ingredients may be expected as follows:

Atropine Sulfate, Hyoscyamine: Symptoms associated with an overdosage of URISED will most probably be manifested in the symptoms related to overdosage of the alkaloids Atropine Sulfate and Hyoscyamine. Such symptoms as dryness of mucous membranes; dilatation of pupils; hot, dry, flushed skin; hyperpyrexia; tachycardia; palpitations; elevated blood pressure; coma; circulatory collapse and death from respiratory failure can occur due to overdosage of these alkaloids.

Methenamine: If large amounts of the drug (2–8 gm daily) are used over extended periods (3–4 weeks), bladder and gastrointestinal irritation, painful and frequent micturition, albuminuria and gross hematuria may be expected.

Methylene Blue: Symptoms of Methylene Blue overdosage associated with the overdosage of URISED are not expected to be discernible from those associated with the other active ingredients in URISED.

Benzoic Acid: Symptoms of Benzoic Acid overdosage associated with the overdosage of URISED are not expected to be discernible from those associated with the other active ingredients in URISED.

Phenyl Salicylate: Symptoms of Phenyl Salicylate overdosage include burning pain in throat and mouth, white necrotic lesions in the mouth, abdominal pain, vomiting, bloody diarrhea, pallor, sweating, weakness, headache, dizziness and tinnitus. The symptoms, however, are not expected to be

Continued on next page

Webcon—Cont.

discernible from those associated with the other active ingredients in URISED.

DOSAGE AND ADMINISTRATION

Adults: Two tablets four times daily. See "PRECAUTIONS."
Usual pediatric dosage: Children up to 6 years of age—Use is not recommended. Children 6 years of age and older—Dosage must be individualized by physician.

HOW SUPPLIED

Bottles of 100 (NDC 0998-2183-10), 500 (NDC 0998-2183-20) and 1000 (NDC 0998-2183-30) tablets. Tablets are imprinted with a "**W 2183**".

STORAGE

Store in a dry place at room temperature.

REFERENCES

[1] Gollamudi, R., Straughn, A.B., and Meyer, M.C., "Urinary Excretion of Methenamine and Formaldehyde: Evaluation of 10 Methenamine Products in Humans," J. Pharm. Sci., 70, 596, 1981.

[2] Goodman, L. S. and Gilman, G., *The Pharmacological Basis of Therapeutics*, Sixth Edition, Macmillan Pub. Co. 121, 971, 980, 1119 (1980).

[3] *AMA Drug Evaluation*, Fifth Edition, 1745 (1983).

A URICEUTICAL® Specialty of
WEBCON™
Alcon (Puerto Rico) Inc.
Humacao, Puerto Rico 00661

Westwood Pharmaceuticals Inc.
100 FOREST AVENUE
BUFFALO, NY 14213

ALPHA KERI®
Moisture Rich Body Oil

COMPOSITION

Contains mineral oil, Hydroloc™ brand of Westwood's PEG-4 dilaurate, lanolin oil, fragrance, benzophenone-3, D&C green 6.

ACTION AND USES

ALPHA KERI is a water-dispersible, antipruritic oil for the care of dry skin. ALPHA KERI effectively deposits a thin, uniform, emulsified film of oil over the skin. This film helps relieve itching, lubricates and softens the skin. ALPHA KERI Moisture Rich Body Oil is an all-over skin moisturizer. Only Alpha Keri contains Hydroloc™ — the unique emulsifier that provides a more uniform distribution of the therapeutic oils to moisturize dry skin. ALPHA KERI is valuable as an aid in the treatment of dry, pruritic skin and mild skin irritations such as chronic atopic dermatitis; pruritus senilis and hiemalis; contact dermatitis; "bath-itch"; xerosis or asteatosis; ichthyosis; soap dermatitis; psoriasis.

ADMINISTRATION AND DOSAGE

ALPHA KERI *should always be used with water, either added to water or rubbed on to wet skin.* Because of its inherent cleansing properties it is not necessary to use soap when ALPHA KERI is being used.
For exact dosage, label directions should be followed.
BATH: Added as directed to bathtub of water. For optimum relief: 10 to 20 minute soak.
SHOWER: Dispense a small amount into hand and rub onto wet skin. Rinse as desired and pat dry.
SPONGE BATH: Added as directed to a basin of warm water then rubbed over entire body with washcloth.
SITZ BATH: Added as directed to tub water. Soak should last for 10 to 20 minutes.
INFANT BATH: Added as directed to basin or bathinette of water.
SKIN CLEANSING OTHER THAN BATH OR SHOWER: A small amount is rubbed onto wet skin. Rinse. Pat dry.

PRECAUTION

The patient should be warned to guard against slipping in tub or shower.

HOW SUPPLIED

4 fl. oz. (NDC 0072-3600-04), 8 fl. oz. (NDC 0072-3600-08), 12 fl. oz. (NDC 0072-3600-12) and 16 fl. oz. (NDC 0072-3600-16) plastic bottles. Also available in non-aerosol pump spray, 3.5 oz. (NDC 0072-3601-35)

ALPHA KERI®
Moisture Rich Cleansing Bar
Non-detergent Soap

COMPOSITION

Sodium tallowate, sodium cocoate, water, mineral oil, fragrance, PEG-75, glycerin, titanium dioxide, lanolin oil, sodium chloride, BHT, trisodium HEDTA, D&C Green 5, D&C Yellow 10.

ACTION AND USES

ALPHA KERI Moisture Rich Cleansing Bar, rich in emollient oils, thoroughly cleanses as it soothes and softens the skin.

INDICATIONS

Adjunctive use in dry skin care.

ADMINISTRATION AND DOSAGE

To be used as any other soap.

HOW SUPPLIED

4 oz. (NDC 0072-3500-04) bar.

BALNETAR®
Water-dispersible Emollient Tar

COMPOSITION

Contains WESTWOOD® TAR (equivalent to 2.5% Coal Tar USP) in mineral oil, laureth-4, lanolin oil, PEG-4 dilaurate, fragrance, and sodium dioctyl sulfosuccinate.

ACTION AND USES

For temporary relief of itching and scaling due to psoriasis, eczema, and other tar-responsive dermatoses. Tar ingredient is chemically and biologically standardized to insure uniform therapeutic activity. BALNETAR exerts keratoplastic, antieczematous, antipruritic, and emollient actions. It deposits microfine particles of tar over the skin in a lubricant-moisturizing film that helps soften and remove scales and crusts, making the skin smoother and more supple. BALNETAR is an important adjunct in a wide range of dermatoses, including: psoriasis, atopic dermatitis; chronic eczematoid dermatitis; seborrheic dermatitis.

CONTRAINDICATIONS

Not indicated when acute inflammation is present.

ADMINISTRATION AND DOSAGE

BALNETAR *should always be used with water.... either added to water or rubbed onto wet skin.* For exact dosage label directions are to be followed.
IN THE TUB—Add as directed to a bathtub of water. Soap is not used. The patient soaks for 10 to 20 minutes and then pats dry.
FOR DIRECT APPLICATION—A small amount is rubbed onto the wet skin. Excess is wiped off with tissue to help prevent staining of clothes or linens.
FOR SCALP APPLICATION —A small amount is rubbed onto the wet scalp with fingertips.

CAUTION

If irritation persists, discontinue use. May temporarily discolor blond, bleached or tinted hair. In rare cases BALNETAR may cause allergic sensitization attributable to coal tar. For external use only. Keep this and all drugs out of reach of children.

PRECAUTION

After use of BALNETAR, patient should avoid exposure to direct sunlight unless sunlight is being used therapeutically in a supervised, modified Goeckerman regimen. Contact with the eyes should be avoided. Patient should be cautioned against slipping when BALNETAR is used in bathtub. Also advise patient that use in a plastic or fiberglass tub may cause staining of the tub.

HOW SUPPLIED

8 fl. oz. (NDC 0072-4200-08) plastic shatterproof bottle.

New Formula
CAPITROL®   ℞
(chloroxine 2%)
Shampoo

CAUTION

Federal law prohibits dispensing without a prescription.

DESCRIPTION

CAPITROL is an antibacterial shampoo containing 2% (w/w) chloroxine (each gram contains 20 mg chloroxine) suspended in a base of sodium octoxynol-2 ethane sulfonate, water, PEG-6 lauramide, dextrin, sodium lauryl sulfoacetate, sodium dioctyl sulfosuccinate, 1% benzyl alcohol, PEG-14M, magnesium aluminum silicate, fragrance, EDTA, citric acid and color. The pH of the shampoo is 7.0.

Chloroxine is a synthetic antibacterial compound that is effective in the treatment of dandruff and seborrheic dermatitis when incorporated in a shampoo.
The chemical name of chloroxine is 5,7-dichloro-8-hydroxyquinoline. The chemical structure of chloroxine is:

CLINICAL PHARMACOLOGY

Well controlled studies demonstrate Capitrol effectively reduces the excess scaling in patients with dandruff or seborrheic dermatitis. Though the cause of dandruff is not known, it is thought to be the result of accelerated mitotic activity in the epidermis. The presumed mechanism of action to reduce scaling would be to slow down the mitotic activity.
The role of microbes in seborrheic dermatitis is not known; however, *Staphylococcus aureus* and *Pityrosporon* species are often present in increased numbers during the course of the disease. Chloroxine is antibacterial, inhibiting the growth of Gram-positive as well as some Gram-negative organisms. Antifungal activity against some dermatophytes and yeasts also has been shown.
The absorption, metabolism and pharmacokinetics of Capitrol in humans have not been studied.

INDICATIONS AND USAGE

Capitrol is indicated in the treatment of dandruff and mild-to-moderately severe seborrheic dermatitis of the scalp. Clinical studies indicate that improvement may be observed after 14 days of therapy.

CONTRAINDICATIONS

Capitrol is contraindicated in those patients with a history of hypersensitivity to any of the listed ingredients.

WARNINGS

Capitrol should not be used on acutely inflamed (exudative) lesions of the scalp.

PRECAUTIONS

Information for patients: Exercise care to prevent Capitrol from entering the eyes. If contact occurs, the patient should flush eyes with cool water. Discoloration of light-colored hair (e.g. blond, gray or bleached) may follow use of this preparation.
Irritation and a burning sensation on the scalp and adjacent areas have been reported.
Drug/Laboratory Test Interactions: There is no known interference of Capitrol with laboratory tests.
Carcinogenesis, Mutagenesis: No long term studies in animals have been performed to evaluate the carcinogenic potential of Capitrol.
Results of in vitro Ames Salmonella/Microsome Plate test show that Capitrol does not demonstrate genetic activity and is considered non-mutagenic.
Pregnancy Category C: Animal reproduction studies have not been conducted with Capitrol. It is also not known whether Capitrol can cause fetal harm when administered to a pregnant woman or can affect reproduction capacity. Capitrol should be given to a pregnant woman only if clearly needed.
Nursing Mothers: It is not known whether this drug is excreted in human milk. Because many drugs are excreted in human milk, caution should be exercised when Capitrol is administered to a nursing woman.
Pediatric Use: Specific studies to demonstrate the safety and effectiveness for use of Capitrol in children have not been conducted.

ADVERSE REACTION

One patient out of 225 in clinical studies was reported to have contact dermatitis.

OVERDOSAGE

The acute oral LD_{50} in mice was found to be 200 mg/kg and in rats 450 mg/kg. On the basis of these animal studies, Capitrol may be considered practically non-toxic.

DOSAGE AND ADMINISTRATION

Capitrol should be massaged thoroughly onto the wet scalp, avoiding contact with the eyes. Lather should remain on the scalp for approximately three minutes, then rinsed. The application should be repeated and the scalp rinsed thoroughly. Two treatments per week are usually sufficient.

HOW SUPPLIED

Capitrol shampoo contains 2% (w/w) chloroxine (20 mg chloroxine per gram) and is supplied in 4 oz. plastic bottles (NDC 0072-6850-04).
Store at room temperature.

WATERBASE
DESQUAM–E™ 2.5 Emollient Gel   ℞
(2.5% benzoyl peroxide)

WATERBASE
DESQUAM–E™ 5 Emollient Gel   ℞
(5% benzoyl peroxide)

WATERBASE
DESQUAM–E™ 10 Emollient Gel   ℞
(10% benzoyl peroxide)

CAUTION
Federal law prohibits dispensing without prescription.

DESCRIPTION
DESQUAM-E 2.5, DESQUAM-E 5 and DESQUAM-E 10 brand topical anti-acne gels contain benzoyl peroxide (2.5, 5 and 10%) in a waterbase vehicle of carbomer 940, diisopropanolamine, disodium edetate, docusate sodium, methyl gluceth-20 and polyquaternium-7.

Benzoyl Peroxide

CLINICAL PHARMACOLOGY
The effectiveness of benzoyl peroxide in the treatment of acne vulgaris is primarily attributable to its antibacterial activity, especially with respect to *Propionibacterium acnes*, the predominant organism in sebaceous follicles and comedones. The antibacterial activity of this compound is presumably due to the release of active or free-radical oxygen capable of oxidizing bacterial proteins. In acne patients treated topically with benzoyl peroxide, resolution of the acne usually coincides with reduction in the level of *P. acnes* and free fatty acids (FFA). Mild desquamation is another observed action of topically applied benzoyl peroxide and may also play a role in the drug's effectiveness in acne. Studies also indicate that topical benzoyl peroxide may exert a sebostatic effect with a resultant reduction of skin surface lipids. Benzoyl peroxide has been shown to be absorbed by the skin, where it is metabolized to benzoic acid and then excreted as benzoate in the urine.

INDICATIONS AND USAGE
DESQUAM-E (2..5, 5 or 10) EMOLLIENT GEL is indicated for the topical treatment of mild to moderate acne vulgaris and as an adjunct in therapeutic regimens including antibiotics, retinoic acid products and sulfur/salicylic acid-containing preparations. DESQUAM-E EMOLLIENT GEL has been shown effective in the treatment of the following acne lesion types: papules, pustules, open and closed comedones. Clinical studies have demonstrated therapeutic response after two to three weeks.

CONTRAINDICATIONS
This product should not be used in patients known to be sensitive to benzoyl peroxide or any of the other listed ingredients.

PRECAUTIONS
General: Avoid contact with eyes and other mucous membranes. For external use only. In patients known to be sensitive to the following substances, there is a possibility of cross-sensitization: benzoic acid derivatives (including certain topical anesthetics) and cinnamon.
Information for Patients: This product may bleach colored fabric or hair. Concurrent use with PABA-containing sunscreens may result in transient discoloration of the skin.
Carcinogenesis, Mutagenesis, Impairment of Fertility: Based upon considerable evidence, benzoyl peroxide is not considered to be a carcinogen. However, in one study, using mice known to be highly susceptible to cancer, there was evidence for benzoyl peroxide as a tumor promoter. Benzoyl peroxide has been found to be inactive as a mutagen in the *Ames Salmonella* and other assays, including the mouse dominant lethal assay. This assay is frequently used to assess the effect of substances on spermatogenesis.
Pregnancy (Category C): Animal reproduction studies have not been conducted with benzoyl peroxide (DESQUAM-E EMOLLIENT GEL). It is also not known whether benzoyl peroxide (DESQUAM-E EMOLLIENT GEL) can cause fetal harm when administered to a pregnant woman or can affect reproductive capacity. Benzoyl peroxide (DESQUAM-E EMOLLIENT GEL) should be given to a pregnant woman only if clearly needed.
Nursing Mothers: It is not known whether this drug is excreted in human milk. Caution should be exercised when benzoyl peroxide is administered to a nursing woman.
Pediatric Use: Safety and effectiveness in children below the age of 12 have not been established.

ADVERSE REACTIONS
Adverse reactions which may be encountered with topical benzoyl peroxide include excessive drying (manifested by marked peeling, erythema and possible edema), and allergic contact sensitization.
Excessive dryness would appear to occur in approximately 2 patients in 50.
Pertinent literature indicates that allergic sensitization to benzoyl peroxide may occur in 10 to 25 patients in 1,000. There is one reference that reports an occurrence of sensitization in 5 of 100 patients.

OVERDOSAGE
In the event that excessive scaling, erythema or edema occur, the use of this preparation should be discontinued. If the reaction is judged to be due to excessive use and not allergenicity, after symptoms and signs subside, a reduced dosage schedule may be cautiously tried.
To hasten resolution of the adverse effects, emollients, cool compresses and/or topical corticosteroid preparations may be used.

DOSAGE AND ADMINISTRATION
DESQUAM-E EMOLLIENT GEL should be gently rubbed into all affected areas once or twice daily. Suitable cleansing of the affected area should precede application. In fair-skinned individuals or under excessively drying conditions, it is suggested that therapy be initiated with one application daily. The degree of drying or peeling may be controlled by modification of dose frequency or drug concentration. The use of DESQUAM-E EMOLLIENT GEL may be continued as long as deemed necessary.

HOW SUPPLIED
DESQUAM-E 2.5 EMOLLIENT GEL
1.5 oz. (42.5g)   Plastic Tubes   NDC 0072-6003-45
DESQUAM-E 5 EMOLLIENT GEL
1.5 oz. (42.5g)   Plastic Tubes   NDC 0072-6103-45
DESQUAM-E 10 EMOLLIENT GEL
1.5 oz. (42.5g)   Plastic Tubes   NDC 0072-6203-45
   Store at controlled room temperature (59°–86°F).

DESQUAM-X10® Bar   ℞
10% benzoyl peroxide

CAUTION
Federal law prohibits dispensing without prescription.

DESCRIPTION
DESQUAM-X10 brand therapeutic anti-acne BAR contains 10% benzoyl peroxide, boric acid, cellulose gum, dextrin (may contain wheat starch), disodium EDTA, docusate sodium, lactic acid, PEG-14M, sodium lauryl sulfoacetate (or sodium dodecyl benzene sulfonate and trisodium sulfosuccinate), sorbitol, urea and water.

O=C–O–O–C=O

Benzoyl Peroxide

CLINICAL PHARMACOLOGY
The effectiveness of benzoyl peroxide in the treatment of acne vulgaris is primarily attributable to its antibacterial activity, especially with respect to *Propionibacterium acnes*, the predominant organism in sebaceous follicles and comedones. The antibacterial activity of this compound is presumably due to the release of active or free-radical oxygen capable of oxidizing bacterial proteins. In acne patients treated topically with benzoyl peoxide, resolution of the acne usually coincides with reduction in the levels of *P. acnes* and free fatty acids (FFA). Mild desquamation is another observed action of topically applied benzoyl peroxide and may also play a role in the drug's effectiveness in acne. Studies also indicate that topical benzoyl peroxide may exert a sebostatic effect with a resultant reduction of skin surface lipids. Benzoyl peroxide has been shown to be absorbed by the skin, where it is metabolized to benzoic acid and then excreted as benzoate in the urine.

INDICATIONS AND USAGE
DESQUAM-X10 BAR is indicated for the topical treatment of acne. It may be used as an adjunct in therapeutic regimens including benzoyl peroxide gels, antibiotics, retinoic acid products and sulfur/salicylic acid-containing preparations. The improvement of the treated condition is dependent on the degree and type of acne, the frequency of use of DESQUAM-X10 BAR and the nature of other therapies employed.

CONTRAINDICATIONS
This product should not be used in patients known to be sensitive to benzoyl peroxide or any other of the listed ingredients.

PRECAUTIONS
General: Avoid contact with eyes and other mucous membranes. For external use only. In patients known to be sensitive to the following substances, there is a possibility of cross-sensitization: benzoic acid derivatives (including certain topical anesthetics) and cinnamon.
Information for Patients: This product may bleach colored fabric or hair. Concurrent use with PABA-containing sunscreens may result in transient discoloration of the skin.
Carcinogenesis, Mutagenesis, Impairment of Fertility: Based upon considerable evidence, benzoyl peroxide is not considered to be a carcinogen. However, in one study, using mice known to be highly susceptible to cancer, there was evidence for benzoyl peroxide as a tumor promoter. Benzoyl peroxide has been found to be inactive as a mutagen in the Ames Salmonella and other assays, including the mouse dominant lethal assay. This assay is frequently used to assess the effect of substances on spermatogenesis.
Pregnancy (Category C): Animal reproduction studies have not been conducted with benzoyl peroxide (DESQUAM-X10 BAR). It is also not known whether benzoyl peroxide can cause fetal harm when administered to a pregnant woman or can affect reproductive capacity. Benzoyl peroxide should be given to a pregnant woman only if clearly needed.
Nursing Mothers: It is not known whether this drug is excreted in human milk. Caution should be exercised when benzoyl peoxide is administered to a nursing woman.
Pediatric Use: Safety and effectiveness in children below the age of 12 have not been established.

ADVERSE REACTIONS
Adverse reactions which may be encountered with topical benzoyl peroxide include excessive drying (manifested by marked peeling, erythema and possible edema) and allergic contact sensitization.
Excessive dryness would appear to occur in approximately 2 patients in 50.
Pertinent literature would seem to indicate that allergic sensitization to benzoyl peroxide may occur in 10 to 25 patients in 1,000. There is one reference that reports an occurrence of sensitization in 5 of 100 patients.

OVERDOSAGE
In the event that excessive scaling, erythema or edema occur, the use of this preparation should be discontinued. If the reaction is judged to be due to excessive use and not allergenicity, after symptoms and signs subside, a reduced dosage schedule may be cautiously tried.
To hasten resolution of the adverse effects, emollients, cool compresses and/or topical corticosteroid preparations may be used.

DOSAGE AND ADMINISTRATION
Wash entire area gently with fingertips for 1 to 2 minutes 2 or 3 times daily or as physician directs. Rinse well. The desired degree of dryness and peeling may be obtained by regulating frequency of use.

HOW SUPPLIED
DESQUAM-X BAR (10%):
3.75 oz.   carton   NDC 0072-2000-04
   Store at controlled room temperature (59°–86°F).

DESQUAM-X 2.5® Gel   ℞
2.5% Benzoyl Peroxide, 6% Laureth-4

DESQUAM-X 5® Gel   ℞
5% Benzoyl Peroxide, 6% Laureth-4

DESQUAM-X 10® Gel   ℞
10% Benzoyl Peroxide, 6% Laureth-4

CAUTION
Federal law prohibits dispensing without prescription.

DESCRIPTION
DESQUAM-X2.5, DESQUAM-X5 and DESQUAM-X10 brand topical anti-acne gels contain benzoyl peroxide (2.5, 5 and 10%) and laureth-4 (6%), in a water-base vehicle of carbomer 940, diisopropanolamine and disodium edetate.
benzoyl peroxide

laureth-4

CLINICAL PHARMACOLOGY
The effectiveness of benzoyl peroxide in the treatment of acne vulgaris is primarily attributable to its antibacterial activity, especially with respect to *Propionibacterium acnes*, the predominant organism in sebaceous follicles and comedones. The antibacterial activity of this compound is presumably due to the release of active or free-radical oxygen capable of oxidizing bacterial proteins. In acne patients treated topically with benzoyl peroxide, resolution of the acne usually coincides with reduction in the levels of *P. acnes* and free

Continued on next page

Westwood—Cont.

fatty acids (FFA). Mild desquamation is another observed action of topically applied benzoyl peroxide and may also play a role in the drug's effectiveness in acne. Studies also indicate that topical benzoyl peroxide may exert a sebostatic effect with a resultant reduction of skin surface lipids. Benzoyl peroxide has been shown to be absorbed by the skin, where it is metabolized to benzoic acid and then excreted as benzoate in the urine.

Laureth-4 is a non-toxic surfactant which exerts its action through cleansing and mild desquamation. The result of these actions is a drying and degreasing of the skin.

INDICATIONS AND USAGE

DESQUAM-X (2.5, 5 or 10) GEL is indicated for the topical treatment of mild to moderate acne vulgaris and as an adjunct in therapeutic regimens including antibiotics, retinoic acid products and sulfur/salicylic acid-containing preparations. DESQUAM-X GEL has been shown effective in the treatment of the following acne lesion types: papules, pustules, open and closed comedones. Clinical studies have demonstrated therapeutic response after two to three weeks. DESQUAM-X GEL may also be used as adjunctive treatment for nodulo-cystic acne (acne conglobata), although its effectiveness for this condition has not been proven.

CONTRAINDICATIONS

This product should not be used in patients known to be sensitive to benzoyl peroxide or any of the other listed ingredients.

PRECAUTIONS

General: Avoid contact with eyes and other mucous membranes. For external use only. In patients known to be sensitive to the following substances, there is a possibility of cross-sensitization: benzoic acid derivatives (including certain topical anesthetics) and cinnamon.

Information for Patients: This product may bleach colored fabric or hair. Concurrent use with PABA-containing sunscreens may result in transient discoloration of the skin.

Carcinogenesis, Mutagenesis, Impairment of Fertility: Based upon considerable evidence, benzoyl peroxide is not considered to be a carcinogen. However, in one study, using mice known to be highly susceptible to cancer, there was evidence for benzoyl peroxide as a tumor promoter. Benzoyl peroxide has been found to be inactive as a mutagen in the *Ames Salmonella* and other assays, including the mouse dominant lethal assay. This assay is frequently used to assess the effect of substances on spermatogenesis.

Pregnancy (Category C): Animal reproduction studies have not been conducted with benzoyl peroxide (DESQUAM-X GEL). It is also not known whether benzoyl peroxide (DESQUAM-X GEL) can cause fetal harm when administered to a pregnant woman or can affect reproductive capacity. Benzoyl peroxide (DESQUAM-X GEL) should be given to a pregnant woman only if clearly needed.

Nursing Mothers: It is not known whether this drug is excreted in human milk. Caution should be exercised when benzoyl peroxide is administered to a nursing woman.

Pediatric Use: Safety and effectiveness in children below the age of 12 have not been established.

ADVERSE REACTIONS

Adverse reactions which may be encountered with topical benzoyl peroxide include excessive drying (manifested by marked peeling, erythema and possibly edema), and allergic contact sensitization.

Excessive dryness appears to occur in approximately 2 patients in 50.

Pertinent literature seems to indicate that allergic sensitization to benzoyl peroxide may occur in 10 to 25 patients in 1,000. There is one reference that reports an occurrence of sensitization in 5 of 100 patients.

OVERDOSAGE

In the event that excessive scaling, erythema or edema occur, the use of this preparation should be discontinued. If the reaction is judged to be due to excessive use and not allergenicity, after symptoms and signs subside, a reduced dosage schedule may be cautiously tried.

To hasten resolution of the adverse effects, emollients, cool compresses and/or topical corticosteroid preparations may be used.

DOSAGE AND ADMINISTRATION

DESQUAM-X GEL should be gently rubbed into all affected areas once or twice daily. Suitable cleansing of the affected area should precede application. In fair-skinned individuals or under excessively drying conditions, it is suggested that therapy be initiated with one application daily. The degree of drying or peeling may be controlled by modification of dose frequency or drug concentration. The use of DESQUAM-X GEL may be continued as long as deemed necessary.

HOW SUPPLIED

DESQUAM-X 2.5 GEL

1.5 oz. (42.5 g)	Plastic Tubes	NDC 0072-6300-01

DESQUAM-X 5 GEL

1.5 oz. (42.5 g)	Plastic Tubes	NDC 0072-6621-01
3 oz. (85 g)	Plastic Tubes	NDC 0072-6621-03

DESQUAM-X 10 GEL

1.5 oz. (42.5 g)	Plastic Tubes	NDC 0072-6721-01
3 oz. (85 g)	Plastic Tubes	NDC 0072-6721-03

Store at controlled room temperature (59°–86° F).

WATER BASE
DESQUAM–X® 5 WASH   ℞
(5% benzoyl peroxide)
WATER BASE
DESQUAM–X® 10 WASH   ℞
(10% benzoyl peroxide)

CAUTION

Federal law prohibits dispensing without prescription.

DESCRIPTION

DESQUAM-X[5] and DESQUAM-X[10] brand topical therapeutic anti-acne cleansers contain benzoyl peroxide (5% and 10%) in a lathering water base of sodium octoxynol-3 sulfonate, dioctyl sodium sulfosuccinate, magnesium aluminum silicate, methylcellulose and EDTA.

benzoyl peroxide

CLINICAL PHARMACOLOGY

The effectiveness of benzoyl peroxide in the treatment of acne vulgaris is primarily attributable to its antibacterial activity, especially with respect to *Propionibacterium acnes*, the predominant organism in sebaceous follicles and comedones. The antibacterial activity of this compound is presumably due to the release of active or free-radical oxygen capable of oxidizing bacterial proteins. In acne patients treated topically with benzoyl peroxide, resolution of the acne usually coincides with reduction in the levels of *P. acnes* and free fatty acids (FFA). Mild desquamation is another observed action of topically applied benzoyl peroxide and may also play a role in the drug's effectiveness in acne. Studies also indicate that topical benzoyl peroxide may exert a sebostatic effect with a resultant reduction of skin surface lipids.

Benzoyl peroxide has been shown to be absorbed by the skin, where it is metabolized to benzoic acid and then excreted as benzoate in the urine.

INDICATIONS AND USAGE

DESQUAM-X (5 or 10) WASH is indicated for the topical treatment of mild to moderate acne. In more severe cases, it may be used as an adjunct in therapeutic regimens including benzoyl peroxide gels, antibiotics, retinoic acid products and sulfur/salicylic acid-containing preparations. The improvement of the treated condition is dependent on the degree and type of acne, the frequency of use of DESQUAM-X WASH and the nature of other therapies employed.

CONTRAINDICATIONS

This product should not be used in patients known to be sensitive to benzoyl peroxide or any other of the listed ingredients.

PRECAUTIONS

General: Avoid contact with eyes and other mucous membranes. For external use only. In patients known to be sensitive to the following substances, there is a possibility of cross-sensitization: benzoic acid derivatives (including certain topical anesthetics) and cinnamon.

Information for Patients: This product may bleach colored fabric or hair. Concurrent use with PABA-containing sunscreens may result in transient discoloration of the skin.

Carcinogenesis, Mutagenesis, Impairment of Fertility: Based upon considerable evidence, benzoyl peroxide is not considered to be a carcinogen. However, in one study, using mice known to be highly susceptible to cancer, there was evidence for benzoyl peroxide as a tumor promoter. Benzoyl peroxide has been found to be inactive as a mutagen in the *Ames Salmonella* and other assays, including the mouse dominant lethal assay. This assay is frequently used to assess the effect of substances on spermatogenesis.

Pregnancy (Category C): Animal reproduction studies have not been conducted with benzoyl peroxide (DESQUAM-X WASH). It is also not known whether benzoyl peroxide can cause fetal harm when administered to a pregnant woman or can affect reproductive capacity. Benzoyl peroxide should be given to a pregnant woman only if clearly needed.

Nursing Mothers: It is not known whether this drug is excreted in human milk. Caution should be exercised when benzoyl peroxide is administered to a nursing woman.

Pediatric Use: Safety and effectiveness in children below the age of 12 have not been established.

ADVERSE REACTIONS

Adverse reactions which may be encountered with topical benzoyl peroxide include excessive drying (manifested by marked peeling, erythema and possible edema), and allergic contact sensitization.

Excessive dryness would appear to occur in approximately 2 patients in 50.

Pertinent literature would seem to indicate that allergic sensitization to benzoyl peroxide may occur in 10 to 25 patients in 1,000. There is one reference that reports an occurrence of sensitization in 5 of 100 patients.

OVERDOSAGE

In the event that excessive scaling, erythema or edema occur, the use of this preparation should be discontinued. If the reaction is judged to be due to excessive use and not allergenicity, after symptoms and signs subside, a reduced dosage schedule may be cautiously tried.

To hasten resolution of the adverse effects, emollients, cool compresses and/or topical corticosteroid preparations may be used.

DOSAGE AND ADMINISTRATION

Shake well before use. Wash affected areas once or twice daily, avoiding contact with eyes or mucous membranes. Wet skin areas to be treated prior to administration; apply DESQUAM-X WASH, work to a full lather, rinse thoroughly and pat dry. The amount of drying or peeling may be controlled by modification of dose frequency or drug concentration.

HOW SUPPLIED

Desquam-X Wash (5%): 5 oz. plastic bottle, NDC 0072-6905-05.

Desquam-X Wash (10%): 5 oz. plastic bottle, NDC 0072-7000-05.

Store at controlled room temperature (59°-86°F; 15°-30°C).

ESTAR®
Therapeutic Tar Gel

ACTIVE INGREDIENT

Westwood tar (biologically equivalent to 5% coal tar USP). Also contains: B-alanine, benzyl alcohol, carbomer 940, glycereth-7 coconate, polysorbate 80, 15.6% SD alcohol 40, simethicone, sorbitol and water.

ACTIONS AND USES

A therapeutic aid in the treatment of eczema, psoriasis, and other tar-responsive dermatoses such as atopic dermatitis, lichen simplex chronicus, and nummular eczema. ESTAR exerts keratoplastic, antieczematous, and antipruritic actions. It is equivalent in its photodynamic activity to 5% crude coal tar in either hydrophilic ointment or petrolatum. ESTAR provides the characteristic benefits of tar therapy in a form that is readily accepted by patients and nursing staff, due to its negligible tar odor and staining potential, and the superior cosmetic qualities of its gel base. ESTAR is suitable for use in a modified Goeckerman regimen, either in the hospital or on an outpatient basis; it also can be used in follow-up treatment to help maintain remissions. Substantivity to the skin can be demonstrated by examination with a Wood's light, which shows residual microfine particles of tar on the skin several days after application.

CONTRAINDICATIONS

ESTAR should not be applied to acutely inflamed skin or used by individuals who are known to be sensitive to coal tar.

ADMINISTRATION AND DOSAGE

Psoriasis: ESTAR can be applied at bedtime in the following manner: the patient should massage ESTAR into affected areas, allowing the gel to remain for five minutes, and then remove excess by patting with tissues. This procedure minimizes staining of skin and clothing, leaving behind an almost invisible layer of the active tar. If any staining of fabric should occur, it can be removed easily by standard laundry procedures.

The same technique of application may be used the following morning. If dryness occurs, an emollient may be applied one hour after ESTAR.

Because of ESTAR's superior substantivity and cosmetic qualities, patients who might otherwise be hospitalized for tar/UV therapy can now be treated as outpatients. The patient can easily apply ESTAR at bedtime and the following morning, then report for UV treatment that day. Laboratory tests and clinical experience to date suggest that it may be advisable to carefully regulate the length of UV exposure. *Chronic atopic dermatitis, lichen simplex chronicus, nummular eczema, and seborrheic dermatitis:* One or two applications per day, as described above, are suggested. If dryness occurs, an emollient may be applied one hour after ESTAR and between applications as needed.

CAUTION

PROTECT TREATED AREAS FROM DIRECT SUNLIGHT, FOR AT LEAST 24 HOURS AFTER APPLICATION, UNLESS DIRECTED BY A PHYSICIAN. AVOID USE ON IN-

FECTED, HIGHLY INFLAMED OR BROKEN SKIN. DO NOT APPLY TO GENITAL AREA. If used on the scalp, temporary discoloration of blond, bleached, or tinted hair may occur. If undue irritation develops or increases, the usage schedule should be changed or ESTAR discontinued. Contact with the eyes should be avoided. In case of contact, flush eyes with water.

Slight staining of clothing may occur. Standard laundry procedures will usually remove stains. For external use only.

HOW SUPPLIED
3 oz. (NDC 0072-7603-03) plastic tube.

EURAX®
(crotamiton USP)
Lotion/Cream
Scabicide/Antipruritic

     ℞

CAUTION
Federal law prohibits dispensing without prescription.

DESCRIPTION
EURAX, crotamiton USP, is a scabicidal and antipruritic agent available as a cream or lotion for topical use only. EURAX provides 10% (w/w) of the synthetic, crotamiton USP, in a vanishing-cream or emollient-lotion base containing: water, petrolatum, propylene glycol, steareth-2, cetyl alcohol, dimethicone, laureth-23, fragrance, magnesium aluminum silicate, carbomer-934, sodium hydroxide, diazolidinyl urea, methylchloroisothiazolinone, methylisothiazolinone and magnesium nitrate. In addition, the cream contains glyceryl stearate. Crotamiton is N-ethyl-N-(o-methylphenyl)-2-butenamide and its structural formula is:

Crotamiton USP is a colorless to slightly yellowish oil, having a faint amine-like odor. It is miscible with alcohol and with methanol. Crotamiton is a mixture of the *cis* and *trans* isomers. Its molecular weight is 203.28.

CLINICAL PHARMACOLOGY
EURAX has scabicidal and antipruritic actions. The mechanisms of these actions are not known.

INDICATIONS AND USAGE
For eradication of scabies (*Sarcoptes scabiei*) and for symptomatic treatment of pruritic skin.

CONTRAINDICATIONS
EURAX should not be applied topically to patients who develop a sensitivity or are allergic to it or who manifest a primary irritation response to topical medications.

WARNINGS
If severe irritation or sensitization develops, treatment with this product should be discontinued and appropriate therapy instituted.

PRECAUTIONS
General: EURAX should not be applied in the eyes or mouth because it may cause irritation. It should not be applied to acutely inflamed skin or raw or weeping surfaces until the acute inflammation has subsided.
Information for Patients: See "Directions for patients with scabies".
Drug Interactions: None known.
Carcinogenesis, Mutagenesis, Impairment of Fertility: Long-term carcinogenicity studies in animals have not been conducted.
Pregnancy (Category C): Animal reproduction studies have not been conducted with EURAX. It is also not known whether EURAX can cause fetal harm when applied topically to a pregnant woman or can affect reproduction capacity. EURAX should be given to a pregnant woman only if clearly needed.
Pediatric Use: Safety and effectiveness in children have not been established.

ADVERSE REACTIONS
Allergic sensitivity or primary irritation reactions may occur in some patients.

OVERDOSAGE
There is no specific information on the effect of overtreatment with repeated topical applications in humans. Acute toxicity (after accidental oral administration in children): Highest known doses ingested: Cream: children—2g (age 1½ years); Lotion: 1 ounce (age 2 years). A death was reported but cause was not confirmed.
Oral LD$_{50}$ in animals (mg/kg): rats, 2212; mice, 2011.
Signs and symptoms (of oral ingestion): Burning sensation in the mouth, irritation of the buccal, esophageal and gastric mucosa, nausea, vomiting, abdominal pain.
Treatment: There is no specific antidote if taken orally. General measures to eliminate the drug and reduce its ab-

sorption, combined with symptomatic treatment, are recommended.

DOSAGE AND ADMINISTRATION
LOTION: Shake well before using—*In Scabies:* Thoroughly massage into the skin of the whole body from the chin down, paying particular attention to all folds and creases. A second application is advisable 24 hours later. Clothing and bed linen should be changed the next morning. A cleansing bath should be taken 48 hours after the last application. *In Pruritus:* Massage gently into affected areas until medication is completely absorbed. Repeat as needed.

DIRECTIONS FOR PATIENTS WITH SCABIES
1. Take a routine bath or shower. Thoroughly massage EURAX cream or lotion into the skin from the chin to the toes including folds and creases.
2. A second application is advisable 24 hours later.
3. This 60 gram tube or bottle is sufficient for two applications.
4. Clothing and bed linen should be changed the next day. Contaminated clothing and bed linen may be dry-cleaned, or washed in the hot cycle of the washing machine.
5. A cleansing bath should be taken 48 hours after the last application.

HOW SUPPLIED
Cream: 60g tubes (NDC 0072-2103-60; NSN 6505-00-116-0200).
Lotion: 60g (2 oz.) bottles (NDC 0072-2203-60, NSN 6505-01-153-4423).
  454 g (16 oz.) bottles (NDC 0072-2203-16).
Store at room temperature.

EXELDERM®
(sulconazole nitrate)
Cream, 1.0% For Topical Use Only

     ℞

CAUTION
Federal law prohibits dispensing without prescription.

DESCRIPTION
EXELDERM (sulconazole nitrate) CREAM, 1.0% is a broad-spectrum antifungal agent intended for topical application. Sulconazole nitrate, the active ingredient in EXELDERM CREAM, is an imidazole derivative with in vitro antifungal and antiyeast activity. Its chemical name is (±)-1-[2.4-dichloro-β-[(p-chlorobenzyl)-thio]-phenethyl] imidazole mononitrate and it has the following chemical structure:

Sulconazole nitrate is a white to off-white crystalline powder with a molecular weight of 460.77. It is freely soluble in pyridine: slightly soluble in ethanol, acetone, and chloroform: and very slightly soluble in water. It has a melting point of about 130°C.

EXELDERM CREAM contains sulconazole nitrate 10 mg/g in an emollient cream base consisting of propylene glycol, stearyl alcohol, isopropyl myristate, cetyl alcohol, polysorbate 60, sorbitan monostearate, glyceryl stearate (and) PEG-100 stearate, ascorbyl palmitate, and purified water, with sodium hydroxide and/or nitric acid added to adjust the pH.

CLINICAL PHARMACOLOGY
Sulconazole nitrate is an imidazole derivative with broad-spectrum antifungal activity that inhibits the growth in vitro of the common pathogenic dermatophytes including *Trichophyton rubrum, Trichophyton mentagrophytes, Epidermophyton floccosum* and *Microsporum canis.* It also inhibits (*in vitro*) the organism responsible for tinea versicolor, *Malassezia furfur.* Sulconazole nitrate has been shown to be active *in vitro* against the following microorganisms, although clinical efficacy has not been established: *Candida albicans* and certain gram positive bacteria.

A modified Draize test showed no allergic contact dermatitis and a phototoxicity study showed no phototoxic or photoallergic reaction to sulconazole nitrate cream. Maximization tests with sulconazole nitrate cream showed no evidence of contact sensitization or irritation.

INDICATIONS AND USAGE
EXELDERM (sulconazole nitrate) CREAM, 1.0% is an antifungal agent indicated for the treatment of tinea pedis (athlete's foot), tinea cruris, and tinea corporis caused by *Trichophyton rubrum, Trichophyton mentagrophytes, Epidermophyton floccosum* and *Microsporum canis,** and for the treatment of tinea versicolor.
*Efficacy for this organism in the organ system was studied in fewer than ten infections.

CONTRAINDICATIONS
EXELDERM (sulconazole nitrate) CREAM, 1.0% is contraindicated in patients who have a history of hypersensitivity to any of its ingredients.

PRECAUTIONS
General: EXELDERM (sulconazole nirate) CREAM, 1.0% is for external use only. Avoid contact with the eyes. If irritation develops, the cream should be discontinued and appropriate therapy instituted.
Information for Patients: Patients should be told to use EXELDERM CREAM as directed by the physician, to use it externally only, and to avoid contact with the eyes.
Carcinogenesis, Mutagenesis, Impairment of Fertility: Long-term animal studies to determine carcinogenic potential have not been performed. In vitro studies have shown no mutagenic activity.
Pregnancy (Category C): There are no adequate and well controlled studies in pregnant women. Sulconazole nitrate should be used during pregnancy only if clearly needed. Sulconazole nitrate has been shown to be embryotoxic in rats when given in doses of 125 times the adult human dose (in mg/kg). The drug was not teratogenic in rats or rabbits at oral doses of 50 mg/kg/day.
Sulconazole nitrate given orally to rats at a dose 125 times the human dose resulted in prolonged gestation and dystocia. Several females died during the prenatal period, most likely due to labor complications.
Nursing Mothers: It is not known whether sulconazole nitrate is excreted in human milk. Caution should be exercised when sulconazole nitrate is administered to a nursing woman.
Pediatric Use: Safety and effectiveness in children have not been established.

ADVERSE REACTIONS
There were no systemic effects and only infrequent cutaneous adverse reactions in 1185 patients treated with sulconazole nitrate cream in controlled clinical trials. Approximately 3% of these patients reported itching, 3% burning or stinging, and 1% redness. These complaints did not usually interfere with treatment.

CLINICAL STUDIES
In a vehicle-controlled study for the treatment of tinea pedis (moccasin type) due to *T. rubrum*, after 4–6 weeks of treatment 69% of patients on the active drug and 19% of patients on the drug vehicle had become KOH and culture negative. In addition, 68% of patients on the active drug and 20% of patients on the drug vehicle showed a good or excellent clinical response.

DOSAGE AND ADMINISTRATION
A small amount of cream should be gently massaged into the affected and surrounding skin areas once or twice daily, except in tinea pedis, where administration should be twice daily.

Early relief of symptoms is experienced by the majority of patients and clinical improvement may be seen fairly soon after treatment is begun; however, tinea corporis/cruris and tinea versicolor should be treated for 3 weeks and tinea pedis for 4 weeks to reduce the possibility of recurrence.

If significant clinical improvement is not seen after 4 to 6 weeks of treatment, an alternate diagnosis should be considered.

HOW SUPPLIED
EXELDERM (sulconazole nitrate) CREAM, 1.0%:
15 g tube—NDC 0072-8200-15
30 g tube—NDC 0072-8200-30
60 g tube—NDC 0072-8200-60
Avoid excessive heat, above 40°C (104°F).

EXELDERM®
(sulconazole nitrate)
Solution, 1.0%

     ℞

CAUTION
Federal law prohibits dispensing without prescription.

DESCRIPTION
EXELDERM (sulconazole nitrate) SOLUTION, 1.0% is a broad-spectrum antifungal agent intended for topical application. Sulconazole nitrate, the active ingredient in EXELDERM SOLUTION, is an imidazole derivative with antifungal and antiyeast activity. Its chemical name is (±)-1-[2.4-dichloro-β-[(p-chlorobenzyl)-thio]-phenethyl] imidazole mononitrate and it has the following chemical structure:
[See Chemical Formula at top of next page].
Sulconazole nitrate is a white to off-white crystalline powder with a molecular weight of 460.77. It is freely soluble in pyridine; slightly soluble in ethanol, acetone, and chloroform; and very slightly soluble in water. It has a melting point of about 130°C.

Continued on next page

Westwood—Cont.

EXELDERM SOLUTION contains sulconazole nitrate 10 mg/ml in a solution of propylene glycol, poloxamer 407, polysorbate 20, butylated hydroxyanisole, and purified water, with sodium hydroxide and, if necessary, nitric acid added to adjust the pH.

CLINICAL PHARMACOLOGY

Sulconazole nitrate is an imidazole derivative that inhibits the growth of the common pathogenic dermatophytes including *Trichophyton mentagrophytes, Epidermophyton floccosum,* and *Microsporum canis.* It also inhibits the organism responsible for tinea versicolor, *Malassezia furfur,* and certain gram positive bacteria.

A maximization test with sulconazole nitrate solution showed no evidence of irritation or contact sensitization.

INDICATIONS AND USAGE

EXELDERM (sulconazole nitrate) SOLUTION, 1.0% is a broad-spectrum antifungal agent indicated for the treatment of tinea cruris and tinea corporis caused by *Trichophyton mentagrophytes, Epidermophyton floccosum,* and *Microsporum canis;* and for the treatment of tinea versicolor. Effectiveness has not been proven in tinea pedis (athlete's foot). Symptomatic relief usually occurs within a few days after starting EXELDERM SOLUTION and clinical improvement usually occurs within one week.

CONTRAINDICATIONS

EXELDERM (sulconazole nitrate) SOLUTION, 1.0% is contraindicated in patients who have a history of hypersensitivity to any of the ingredients.

PRECAUTIONS

General: EXELDERM (sulconazole nitrate) SOLUTION, 1.0% is for external use only. Avoid contact with the eyes. If irritation develops, the solution should be discontinued and appropriate therapy instituted.

Information for Patients: Patients should be told to use EXELDERM SOLUTION as directed by the physician, to use it externally only, and to avoid contact with the eyes.

Carcinogenesis, Mutagenesis, Impairment of Fertility: Long-term animal studies to determine carcinogenic potential have not been performed. In vitro studies have shown no mutagenic activity.

Pregnancy (Category C): There are no adequate and well controlled studies in pregnant women. Sulconazole nitrate should be used during pregnancy only if clearly needed. Sulconazole nitrate has been shown to be embryotoxic in rats when given in doses of 125 times the adult human dose (in mg/kg). The drug was not teratogenic in rats or rabbits at oral doses of 50 mg/kg/day.

Sulconazole nitrate given orally to rats at a dose 125 times the human dose resulted in prolonged gestation and dystocia. Several females died during the perinatal period, most likely due to labor complications.

Nursing Mothers: Use with caution in nursing mothers since it is not known if sulconazole nitrate appears in breast milk.

Pediatric Use: Safety and effectiveness in children have not been established.

ADVERSE REACTIONS

There were no systemic effects and only infrequent cutaneous adverse reactions in 370 patients treated with sulconazole nitrate solution in controlled clinical trials. Approximately 1% of these patients reported itching and 1% burning or stinging. These complaints did not usually interfere with treatment.

DOSAGE AND ADMINISTRATION

A small amount of the solution should be gently massaged into the affected and surrounding skin areas once or twice daily.

Symptomatic relief usually occurs within a few days after starting EXELDERM (sulconazole nitrate) SOLUTION, 1.0%, and clinical improvement usually occurs within one week. To reduce the possibility of recurrence, tinea cruris, tinea corporis, and tinea versicolor should be treated for 3 weeks.

If significant clinical improvement is not seen after 4 weeks of treatment, an alternate diagnosis should be considered.

HOW SUPPLIED

EXELDERM SOLUTION, 1.0%

30 ml   Plastic Bottle   NDC 0072-8400-30

Avoid excessive heat, above 40°C (104°F), and protect from light.

HALOTEX®   ℞

(Haloprogin)

Cream 1%, Solution 1%

Antifungal Agent for Topical Use

CAUTION

Federal law prohibits dispensing without a prescription.

DESCRIPTION

HALOTEX (brand of haloprogin) Cream/Solution for topical use. Each gram of the cream contains 10 mg haloprogin in a water-dispersible base composed of polyethylene glycol 400, polyethylene glycol 4000, diethyl sebacate and polyvinylpyrrolidone.

Each ml of the solution contains 10 mg haloprogin in a clear, colorless vehicle composed of 75% alcohol and diethyl sebacate.

These preparations are effective topical antifungal agents. The chemical name for haloprogin is: 1,2,4-trichloro-5[(3-iodo-2-propynyl)oxy]benzene. The structure is:

CLINICAL PHARMACOLOGY

The mechanism of antifungal activity for haloprogin in yeast cells is believed to be inhibition of respiration and disruption of the yeast cell membrane. The mechanism of antifungal activity in dermatophytes is unknown.

Dermal penetration studies utilizing single applications of ^{14}C ring-labeled haloprogin formulated as creams, or dissolved in acetone or alcoholic solutions, were performed in 18 male subjects. Urinary recovery from 3 subjects ranged from 9.47% (0.25% cream) to 14.89% (1% cream) over 5 days. The 0.25% and 1% alcoholic solutions were associated with lesser recoveries of 3% and 6%, respectively. Subtotal inunction studies have been conducted with both the cream and the solution. Fifteen grams of HALOTEX Cream (n=8) and 15 ml of HALOTEX Solution (n=14) were administered to the entire body for 10 consecutive days. Physical examinations and clinical laboratory tests conducted throughout the study showed no abnormalities. Repeat patch testing for contact sensitization and photosensitivity also were negative.

The following *in-vitro* data on haloprogin are available, but their clinical significance is not known.

Organism (# Strains Tested)	MIC[1] (µg/ml) Range Found
Microsporum audouini (2)	< 0.0470 – 0.390
M. canis (2)	< 0.0470 – 0.390
M. gypseum (2)	0.0950 – 0.190
Other *Microsporum* spp (3)	0.0030 – 0.190
Trichophyton mentagrophytes (5)	0.0950 – 0.780
T. rubrum (4)	0.0120 – 0.780
Other *Trichophyton* spp (9)	0.0015 – 0.095
Candida albicans (3)	0.0500 – 0.400
Other *Candida* spp (2)	0.4000 – 0.800
Other Yeasts/yeast-like fungi (8)	0.0500 – 0.400
Staphylococcus aureus (5)	1.5600 – 3.120
Streptococcus pyogenes (3)	0.7800 –50.000
Other gram pos. organisms (6)	25.00 – > 100.000
Gram neg. organisms	> 100

[1]Minimal Inhibitory Concentration

INDICATIONS AND USAGE

HALOTEX Cream and Solution are indicated for the treatment of superficial mycotic infections including tinea pedis, tinea cruris, tinea corporis and tinea manuum due to infection with *Tricophyton rubrum, T. tonsurans, T. mentaprophytes, Microsporum canis* and *Epidermophyton floccosum.* HALOTEX also is indicated for the treatment of tinea versicolor caused by *Malassezia furfur.*

CONTRAINDICATIONS

HALOTEX Cream and Solution should not be used by patients known to have hypersensitivity to any of the listed ingredients.

WARNINGS

See Contraindications and Precautions.

PRECAUTIONS

General: Treatment with HALOTEX Cream or Solution should be discontinued in case of sensitization or persistent irritation and appropriate therapy instituted. The diagnosis in patients showing no improvement after four weeks of treatment with HALOTEX should be reconsidered.

In mixed infections, where bacteria or nonsusceptible fungi are present, supplementary antiinfective therapy may be indicated.

Information for Patients: HALOTEX is for topical use only. Contact of this drug with the eyes should be avoided.

Use of HALOTEX should be discontinued and a physician contacted in the event of increased irritation.

In order to minimize the risk of recurrence, use the prescribed medication for the full duration even if symptoms have abated.

Laboratory Tests: KOH preparations of the afflicted areas may be useful to verify the diagnosis of fungal infection prior to treatment. Periodic repeat KOH preparations at 2-week intervals during treatment and at 2–4 weeks after treatment will document the beneficial response to treatment. Cultures for bacteria or fungi of specimens from affected area, not responding to treatment may help to elucidate the lack of response.

In the event of a suspected irritation or sensitization, patch testing with components of the formulation used may help verify the reaction and identify its cause.

Carcinogenesis, Mutagenesis, Impairment of Fertility: The carcinogenic potential of haloprogin in laboratory animals has not been evaluated. HALOTEX was shown to be non-mutagenic in The Ames-Salmonella/Microsome Plate Assay.

Pregnancy: Pregnancy Category B: Reproduction studies have been performed in rats and rabbits, each group being given 10 daily topical applications, representing up to 3 times the estimated total human dose needed for a 30-day course of therapy. No evidence of impaired fertility or harm to the fetus due to haloprogin was revealed. There are, however, no adequate and well-controlled studies in pregnant women. Because animal reproduction studies are not always predictive of human response, this drug should be used during pregnancy only if clearly needed.

Nursing Mothers: It is not known whether this drug is excreted in human milk. Because many drugs are excreted in human milk, caution should be exercised when HALOTEX formulations are applied to a nursing mother.

Pediatric Use: Safety and efficacy studies in children have not been performed.

ADVERSE REACTIONS

In clinical studies with the cream and the solution 26 adverse reactions were noted out of a total 1796 patients treated. These reactions are tabulated below for each formulation.

REACTION	FORMULATION Cream (n=977)	Solution (n=819)
Burning and/or irritation on application	8	14
Erythema and Scaling	1	—
Erythema and Itching	1	—
Folliculitis	1	—
Pruritus and Vesicle Formation	—	1

Reactions noted did not always require interruption of treatment.

OVERDOSAGE

The oral LD_{50} of haloprogin is > 3000 mg/kg in mice, rats, dogs and rabbits. The maximum haloprogin in any single package is 300 mg total. There is no experience to allow extrapolation of acute toxicity and expected symptoms in man.

DOSAGE AND ADMINISTRATION

HALOTEX Cream and Solution should be applied liberally to the affected areas twice daily for 2–3 weeks. Intertriginous areas may require 4 weeks of treatment.

HOW SUPPLIED

HALOTEX (haloprogin) cream 1% is supplied in 15 g (NDC 0072-7130-15); and 30 g (NDC 0072-7130-02; NSN 6505-00-118-2318) tubes. Store below 45°C (113°F). HALOTEX (haloprogin) Solution 1% is supplied in 10 ml (NDC 0072-7200-10; NSN 6505-00-118-2211) and 30 ml (NDC 0072-7200-30; NSN 6505-00-118-2308) bottles with controlled drop tip.

KERALYT® GEL   ℞

6% Salicylic Acid

CAUTION

Federal law prohibits dispensing without prescription.

DESCRIPTION

KERALYT is a gel for topical administration containing 6% salicylic acid in a vehicle composed of propylene glycol, alcohol (19.4%), hydroxypropylcellulose and water. Salicylic acid is the 2-hydroxy derivative of benzoic acid having the following structure:

[See Chemical Formula at top of next column].

CLINICAL PHARMACOLOGY

Salicylic acid has been shown to produce desquamation of the horny layer of skin while not effecting qualitative or quantitative changes in the structure of the viable epidermis. The mechanism of action has been attributed to a dissolution of intercellular cement substance. In a study of the percutaneous absorption of salicylic acid from KERALYT GEL in four patients with extensive active psoriasis, Taylor and Halprin showed that the peak serum salicylate levels never exceeded 5 mg/100 ml even though more than 60% of the applied salicylic acid was absorbed. Systemic toxic reactions are usually associated with much higher serum levels (30 to 40 mg/100 ml). Peak serum levels occurred within 5 hours of the topical application under occlusion. The sites were occluded for 10 hours over the entire body surface below the neck. Since salicylates are distributed in the extracellular space, patients with a contracted extracellular space due to dehydration or diuretics have higher salicylate levels than those with a normal extracellular space. (See PRECAUTIONS.)

The major metabolites identified in the urine after topical administration are salicyluric acid (52%), salicylate glucuronides (42%) and free salicylic acid (6%). The urinary metabolites after percutaneous absorption differ from those after oral salicylate administration; those derived from percutaneous absorption contain more salicylate glucuronides and less salicyluric and salicylic acid. Almost 95% of a single dose of salicylate is excreted within 24 hours of its entrance into the extracellular space.

Fifty to eighty percent of salicylate is protein bound to albumin. Salicylates compete with the binding of several drugs and can modify the action of these drugs; by similar competitive mechanisms other drugs can influence the serum levels of salicylate. (See PRECAUTIONS.)

INDICATIONS AND USAGE

For Dermatologic Use: KERALYT GEL is a topical aid in the removal of excessive keratin in hyperkeratotic skin disorders, including verrucae, and the various ichthyoses (vulgaris, sex-linked and lamellar), keratosis palmaris and plantaris, keratosis pilaris, pityriasis rubra pilaris, psoriasis (including body, scalp, palms and soles).

For Podiatric Use: KERALYT GEL is a topical aid in the removal of excessive keratin on dorsal and plantar hyperkeratotic lesions. KERALYT has been reported to be useful adjunctive therapy for verrucae plantares.

CONTRAINDICATIONS

KERALYT GEL should not be used in any patient known to be sensitive to salicylic acid or any other listed ingredients. KERALYT should not be used in children under 2 years of age.

WARNINGS

Prolonged use over large areas, especially in children and those patients with significant renal or hepatic impairment, could result in salicylism. Concomitant use of other drugs which may contribute to elevated serum salicylate levels should be avoided where the potential for toxicity is present. In children under 12 years of age and those patients with renal or hepatic impairment, the area to be treated should be limited and the patient monitored closely for signs of salicylate toxicity: nausea, vomiting, dizziness, loss of hearing, tinnitus, lethargy, hyperpnea, diarrhea, psychic disturbances. In the event of salicylic acid toxicity, the use of KERALYT GEL should be discontinued. Fluids should be administered to promote urinary excretion. Treatment with sodium bicarbonate (oral or intravenous) should be instituted as appropriate.

PRECAUTIONS

For external use only. Avoid contact with eyes and other mucous membranes.

DRUG INTERACTIONS

(The following interactions are from a published review and include reports concerning both oral and topical salicylate administration. The relationship of these interactions to the use of KERALYT GEL is not known.)

I. Due to the competition of salicylate with other drugs for binding to serum albumin the following drug interactions may occur:

DRUG	DESCRIPTION OF INTERACTION
Tolbutamide	Hypoglycemia potentiated.
Methotrexate	Decreases tubular reabsorption; clinical toxicity from methotrexate can result.

II. Drugs changing salicylate levels by altering renal tubular reabsorption:

DRUG	DESCRIPTION
Corticosteroids	Decreases plasma salicylate level; tapering doses of steroids may promote salicylism.
Ammonium Sulfate	Increases plasma salicylate level.

III. Drugs with Complicated Interactions with Salicylates

DRUG	DESCRIPTION
Heparin	Salicylate decreases platelet adhesiveness and interferes with hemostasis in heparin-treated patients.
Pyrazinamide	Inhibits pyrazinamide-induced hyperuricemia.
Uricosuric Agents	Effect of probenemide, sulfinpyrazone and phenylbutazone inhibited.

The following alterations of laboratory tests have been reported during salicylate therapy.

LABORATORY TESTS	EFFECT OF SALICYLATES
Thyroid Function	Decreased PBI; increased T_3 uptake.
Urinary Sugar	False negative with glucose oxidase; false positive with Clinitest with high-dose salicylate therapy (2-5g q.d.).
5-Hydroxyindole acetic acid	False negative with fluorometric test.
Acetone, ketone bodies	False positive FeCl₃ in Gerhardt reaction; red color persists with boiling.
17-OH corticosteroids	False reduced values with >4.8g q.d. salicylate.
Vanilmandelic acid	False reduced values.
Uric acid	May increase or decrease depending on dose.
Prothrombin	Decreased levels; slightly increased prothrombin time.

Pregnancy (Category C): Salicylic acid has been shown to be teratogenic in rats and monkeys. It is difficult to extrapolate from oral doses of acetylsalicylic acid used in these studies to topical administration as the oral dose to monkeys may represent 6 times the maximal daily human dose of salicylic acid (as supplied in one tube, 28 g, of Keralyt) when applied topically over a large body surface. There are no adequate and well-controlled studies in pregnant women. KERALYT GEL should be used during pregnancy only if the potential benefit justifies the potential risk to the fetus.

Nursing Mothers: Because of the potential for serious adverse reactions in nursing infants from the mother's use of KERALYT GEL, a decision should be made whether to discontinue nursing or to discontinue the drug, taking into account the importance of the drug to the mother.

Carcinogenesis, Mutagenesis, Impairment of Fertility: No data are available concerning potential carcinogenic or reproductive effects of KERALYT GEL. It has been shown to lack mutagenic potential in the Ames Salmonella test.

ADVERSE REACTIONS

Excessive erythema and scaling conceivably could result from use on open skin lesions.

OVERDOSAGE

See **Warnings.**

DOSAGE AND ADMINISTRATION

The preferable method of use is to apply KERALYT GEL thoroughly to the affected area and occlude the area at night. Preferably, the skin should be hydrated for at least five minutes prior to application. The medication is washed off in the morning and if excessive drying and/or irritation is observed a bland cream or lotion may be applied. Once clearing is apparent, the occasional use of KERALYT GEL will usually maintain the remission. In those areas where occlusion is difficult or impossible, application may be made more frequently; hydration by wet packs or baths prior to application apparently enhances the effect. Unless hands are being treated, hands should be rinsed thoroughly after application.

HOW SUPPLIED

1 oz. (28.4g) (NDC 0072-6500-01) plastic tube.

LAC–HYDRIN®   ℞
(ammonium lactate)
12%* Lotion

PRODUCT OVERVIEW

KEY FACTS

Lac-Hydrin® is a therapeutic lotion which is active in the treatment of moderate to severe xerosis and ichthyosis vulgaris. The active ingredient, ammonium lactate, helps improve the stratum corneum to provide a sustained effect in the treatment of dry skin.

MAJOR USES

Lac-Hydrin has been shown to be clinically effective for cases of moderate to severe xerosis and ichthyosis vulgaris.

SAFETY INFORMATION

Contact with eyes, lips or mucous membranes should be avoided. A mild transient stinging may occur on application to abraded or inflamed areas or in individuals with sensitive skin.

PRESCRIBING INFORMATION

LAC–HYDRIN®   ℞
(ammonium lactate)
12%* Lotion

CAUTION

Federal law prohibits dispensing without a prescription.

DESCRIPTION*

LAC-HYDRIN, specially formulates 12% lactic acid neutralized with ammonium hydroxide, as ammonium lactate to provide a lotion pH of 4.5–5.5. LAC-HYDRIN also contains light mineral oil, glyceryl stearate, PEG-100 stearate, propylene glycol, polyoxyl 40 stearate, glycerin, magnesium aluminum silicate, laureth-4, cetyl alcohol, methyl and propylparabens, methylcellulose, fragrance, quaternium-15 and water. Lactic acid is a racemic mixture of 2-hydroxypropanoic acid and has the following structural formula:

$$\begin{array}{c} \text{COOH} \\ | \\ \text{CHOH} \\ | \\ \text{CH}_3 \end{array}$$

CLINICAL PHARMACOLOGY

It is generally accepted that the water content of the stratum corneum is a controlling factor in maintaining skin flexibility. When the stratum corneum contains more than 10% water it remains soft and pliable; however, when the water content drops below 10% the stratum corneum becomes less flexible and rough, and may exhibit scaling and cracking and the underlying skin may become irritated.

Symptomatic relief of dry skin is provided by skin protectants containing hygroscopic substances (humectants) which increase skin moisture. Lactic acid, an α-hydroxy acid, is reported to be one of the most effective naturally occurring humectants in the skin. The α-hydroxy acids (and their salts), in addition to having beneficial effects on dry skin, have also been shown to reduce excessive epidermal keratinization in patients with hyperkeratotic conditions (e.g., ichthyosis).

Pharmacokinetics: The mechanism of action of topically applied neutralized lactic acid is not yet known.

INDICATIONS AND USAGE

LAC-HYDRIN is indicated for the treatment of dry, scaly skin (xerosis) and ichthyosis vulgaris and for temporary relief of itching associated with these conditions.

CONTRAINDICATIONS

Known hypersensitivity to any of the label ingredients.

PRECAUTIONS

General: For external use only. Avoid contact with eyes, lips or mucous membranes. Caution is advised when used on the face of fair-skinned individuals since irritation may occur. A mild, transient stinging may occur on application to abraded or inflamed areas or in individuals with sensitive skin.

Carcinogenesis, Mutagenesis, Impairment of Fertility: LAC-HYDRIN was nonmutagenic in the Ames/Salmonella/Microsome Plate Assay. Reproductive studies in rats given lactic acid orally showed no effect on the sex ratio of the offspring.

Pregnancy (Category C): Animal reproduction studies have not been conducted with LAC-HYDRIN. It is also not known whether LAC-HYDRIN can cause fetal harm when administered to a pregnant woman or can affect reproduction capacity. LAC-HYDRIN should be given to a pregnant woman only if clearly needed.

Nursing Mothers: Although lactic acid is a normal constituent of blood and tissues, it is not known to what extent this drug affects normal lactic acid levels in human milk. Because many drugs are excreted in human milk, caution should be exercised when LAC-HYDRIN is administered to a nursing woman.

Pediatric Use: Safety and effectiveness of LAC-HYDRIN have been demonstrated in infants and children. No unusual toxic effects were reported.

ADVERSE REACTIONS

The most frequent adverse experiences in patients with xerosis are transient stinging (1 in 30 patients), burning (1 in 30 patients), erythema (1 in 50 patients) and peeling (1 in 60 patients). Other adverse reactions which occur less fre-

Continued on next page

Westwood—Cont.

quently are irritation, eczema, petechiae, dryness and hyperpigmentation.

Due to the more severe initial skin conditions associated with ichthyosis, there was a higher incidence of transient stinging, burning and erythema (each occurring in 1 in 10 patients).

OVERDOSAGE

The oral administration of LAC-HYDRIN to rats and mice showed this drug to be practically non-toxic (LD$_{50}$ > 15 ml/kg).

DOSAGE AND ADMINISTRATION

Shake well. Apply to the affected areas and rub in thoroughly. Use twice daily or as directed by a physician.

HOW SUPPLIED

5 oz. (NDC 0072-5712-05; NSN 6505-01-216-6274) plastic tube and 12 oz. (NDC 0072-5712-12) plastic bottle.
Store at controlled room temperature (15°–30°C; 59°–86°F).

LOWILA® CAKE
Soap-free Skin Cleanser

COMPOSITION

Contains dextrin, sodium lauryl sulfoacetate, water, boric acid, urea, sorbitol, mineral oil, PEG-14 M, lactic acid, dioctyl sodium sulfosuccinate, cellulose gum, fragrance.

ACTION AND USES

LOWILA CAKE is indicated when soap should not be used, for cleansing skin that is sensitive or irritated, or in dermatitic and eczematous conditions. Used for general bathing, infant bathing, routine washing of hands and face and shampooing. The pH of LOWILA CAKE helps protect the skin's normal acid mantle and create an environment favorable to therapy and healing.

ADMINISTRATION AND DOSAGE

LOWILA CAKE is used in place of soap. Lathers well in both hard and soft water.

HOW SUPPLIED

3¾ oz. (NDC 0072-2300-01) bar.

MAXIVATE™   ℞
(betamethasone dipropionate)
0.05%
For topical use. Not for use in eyes.

DESCRIPTION

Maxivate™ contains Betamethasone Dipropionate U.S.P. (Pregna-1, 4-diene-3, 20-dione, 9-fluoro-11-hydroxy-16-methyl-17, 21-bis (1-oxopropoxy)-,(11B, 16B)-); it has an empirical formula of $C_{28}H_{37}FO_7$ and a molecular weight of 504.59 (CAS Registry Number 5593-20-4).

Cream

Each gram of the 0.05% Cream contains 0.64 mg Betamethasone Dipropionate (equivalent to 0.5 mg Betamethasone) in a soft, white, hydrophilic cream of Purified Water, Mineral Oil, White Petrolatum, Polyethylene Glycol 1000 Monocetyl Ether, Cetostearyl Alcohol, Monobasic Sodium Phosphate and Phosphoric Acid or Sodium Hydroxide. Chlorocresol is present as a preservative. Maxivate™ Cream contains no parabens.

Ointment

Each gram of the 0.05% Ointment contains 0.64 mg Betamethasone Dipropionate (equivalent to 0.5 mg Betamethasone) in an ointment base of Mineral Oil and White Petrolatum. Maxivate™ Ointment contains no parabens.

Lotion

Each gram of the 0.05% Lotion contains 0.64 mg Betamethasone Dipropionate (equivalent to 0.5 mg Betamethasone) in a vehicle of Isopropyl Alcohol and Purified Water slightly thickened with Carbomer 934P. Phosphoric Acid or Sodium Hydroxide are used to adjust pH.

CLINICAL PHARMACOLOGY

Topical corticosteroids share anti-inflammatory, anti-pruritic and vasoconstrictive actions. The mechanism of anti-inflammatory activity of the topical corticosteroids is unclear. Various laboratory methods, including vasoconstrictor assays, are used to compare and predict potencies and/or clinical efficacies of the topical corticosteroids. There is some evidence to suggest that a recognizable correlation exists between vasoconstrictor potency and therapeutic efficacy in man.

Pharmacokinetics: The extent of percutaneous absorption of topical corticosteroids is determined by many factors including the vehicle, the integrity of the epidermal barrier, and the use of occlusive dressings. Topical corticosteroids can be absorbed from normal intact skin. Inflammation and/or other disease processes in the skin increase percutaneous absorption. Occlusive dressings substantially increase the percutaneous absorption of topical corticosteroids. (See DOSAGE AND ADMINISTRATION). Once absorbed through the skin, topical corticosteroids are handled through pharmacokinetic pathways similar to systemically administered corticosteroids. Corticosteroids are bound to plasma proteins in varying degrees. Corticosteroids are metabolized primarily in the liver and are then excreted by the kidneys. Some of the topical corticosteroids and their metabolites are also excreted into the bile.

INDICATIONS AND USAGE

Topical corticosteroids are indicated for the relief of the inflammatory and pruritic manifestations of corticosteroid-responsive dermatoses.

CONTRAINDICATIONS

Topical corticosteroids are contraindicated in those patients with a history of hypersensitivity to any of the components of the preparation.

PRECAUTIONS

General: Systemic absorption of topical corticosteroids has produced reversible hypothalamic-pituitary-adrenal (HPA) axis suppression, manifestations of Cushing's syndrome, hyperglycemia, and glucosuria in some patients. Conditions which augment systemic absorption include the application of the more potent steroids, use over large surface areas, prolonged use, and the addition of occlusive dressings. (See DOSAGE AND ADMINISTRATION). Therefore, patients receiving a large dose of a potent topical steroid applied to a large surface area should be evaluated periodically for evidence of HPA axis suppression by using the urinary free cortisol and ACTH stimulation tests. If HPA axis suppression is noted, an attempt should be made to withdraw the drug, to reduce the frequency of application, or to substitute a less potent steroid. Recovery of HPA axis function is generally prompt and complete upon discontinuation of the drug. Infrequently, signs and symptoms of steroid withdrawal may occur, requiring supplemental systemic corticosteroids. Children may absorb proportionally larger amounts of topical corticosteroids and thus be more susceptible to systemic toxicity. (See PRECAUTIONS—Pediatric Use). If irritation develops, topical corticosteroids should be discontinued and appropriate therapy instituted. In the presence of dermatological infections, the use of an appropriate antifungal or antibacterial agent should be instituted. If a favorable response does not occur promptly, the corticosteroid should be discontinued until the infection has been adequately controlled.

Information for the Patient: Patients using topical corticosteroids should receive the following information and instructions:
1. This medication is to be used as directed by the physician. It is for external use only. Avoid contact with the eyes.
2. Patients should be advised not to use this medication for any disorder other than for which it was prescribed.
3. The treated skin area should not be bandaged or otherwise covered or wrapped as to be occlusive. (See DOSAGE AND ADMINISTRATION).
4. Patients should report any signs of local adverse reactions.
5. Parents of pediatric patients should be advised not to use tight fitting diapers or plastic pants on a child being treated in the diaper area, as these garments may constitute occlusive dressings. (See DOSAGE AND ADMINISTRATION).

Laboratory Tests: The following test may be helpful in evaluating the HPA axis suppression: Urinary free cortisol test; ACTH stimulation test.

Carcinogenesis, Mutagenesis, and Impairment of Fertility: Long-term animal studies have not been performed to evaluate the carcinogenic potential or the effect on fertility of topical corticosteroids. Studies to determine mutagenicity with prednisolone and hydrocortisone have revealed negative results.

Pregnancy Category C: Corticosteroids are generally teratogenic in laboratory animals when administered systemically at relatively low dosage levels. The more potent corticosteroids have been shown to be teratogenic after dermal application in laboratory animals. There are no adequate and well-controlled studies in pregnant women on teratogenic effects from topically applied corticosteroids. Therefore, topical corticosteroids should be used during pregnancy only if the potential benefit justifies the potential risk to the fetus. Drugs of this class should not be used extensively on pregnant patients, in large amounts, or for prolonged periods of time.

Nursing Mothers: It is not known whether topical administration of corticosteroids could result in sufficient systemic absorption to produce detectable quantities in breast milk. Systemically administered corticosteroids are secreted into breast milk in quantities not likely to have a deleterious effect on the infant. Nevertheless, caution should be exercised when topical corticosteroids are administered to a nursing woman.

Pediatric Use: *Pediatric patients may demonstrate greater susceptibility to topical corticosteroid-induced HPA axis suppression and Cushing's syndrome than mature patients because of a larger skin surface to body weight ratio.* Hypothalamic-pituitary-adrenal (HPA) axis suppression, Cushing's syndrome, and intracranial hypertension have been reported in children receiving topical corticosteroids. Manifestations of adrenal suppression in children include linear growth retardation, delayed weight gain, low plasma cortisol levels, and absence of response to ACTH stimulation. Manifestations of intracranial hypertension include bulging fontanelles, headaches, and bilateral papilledema. Administration of topical corticosteroids to children should be limited to the least amount compatible with an effective therapeutic regimen. Chronic corticosteroid therapy may interfere with the growth and development of children.

ADVERSE REACTIONS

The following local adverse reactions are reported infrequently when Maxivate™ is used as recommended in the DOSAGE AND ADMINISTRATION section. These reactions are listed in an approximate decreasing order of occurrence; burning, itching, irritation, dryness, folliculitis, hypertrichosis, acneiform eruptions, hypopigmentation, perioral dermatitis, allergic contact dermatitis, maceration of the skin, secondary infection, skin atrophy, striae and miliaria. Systemic absorption of topical corticosteroids has produced reversible hypothalmic-pituitary-adrenal (HPA) axis suppression, manifestations of Cushing's syndrome, hyperglycemia and glucosuria in some patients.

OVERDOSAGE

Topically applied corticosteroids can be absorbed in sufficient amounts to produce systemic effects. (See PRECAUTIONS).

DOSAGE AND ADMINISTRATION

Ointment/Cream: Apply to the affected skin areas as a thin film once daily. In some cases, twice daily dosage may be necessary. If an infection develops, appropriate antimicrobial therapy should be instituted. Maxivate™ should not be used with occlusive dressings.

Lotion: Apply a few drops to the affected skin areas and massage lightly until it disappears. Apply twice daily, in the morning and at night. If an infection develops, appropriate antimicrobial therapy should be instituted. Maxivate™ Lotion should not be used with occlusive dressings.

HOW SUPPLIED

Maxivate™ Ointment, 0.05% in 15 gram tubes, NDC 0072-9450-15 and 45 gram tubes, NDC 0072-9450-45; NSN 6505-01-035-6358.
Maxivate™ Cream, 0.05% in 15 gram tubes, NDC 0072-9410-15 and 45 gram tubes, NDC 0072-9410-45; NSN 6505-01-011-8518.
Maxivate™ Lotion, 0.05% in 60 ml bottles, NDC 0072-9490-60. Shake well before using.
Store at controlled room temperature 15°–30°C (59°–86°F).

CAUTION

Federal law prohibits dispensing without prescription.

MOISTUREL® CREAM
Skin Lubricant—Moisturizer

COMPOSITION

Water, petrolatum, glycerin, PG dioctanoate, cetyl alcohol, steareth-2, dimethicone, PVP/hexadecene copolymer, laureth-23, Mg Al silicate, diazolidinyl urea, carbomer-934, sodium hydroxide, methylchloroisothiazolinone and methylisothiazolinone.

ACTIONS AND USES

A highly effective concentrated formula clinically proven to relieve dry skin and designed not to cause acne or blemishes. Free of lanolins, fragrances, and parabens that can sensitize or irritate skin. Indicated for generalized dry skin, chapped or chafed skin, diaper rash, sunburn, windburn, heat rash, itching and dryness associated with eczema.

ADMINISTRATION AND DOSAGE

Apply a small amount as often as needed.

HOW SUPPLIED

4 oz. (NDC 0072-9500-04) and 16 oz. (NDC 0072-9500-16) plastic jars.

MOISTUREL® LOTION
Skin Lubricant—Moisturizer

COMPOSITION
Water, petrolatum, glycerin, dimethicone, steareth-2, cetyl alcohol, benzyl alcohol, laureth-23, Mg Al silicate, carbomer-934, sodium hydroxide, quaternium-15.

ACTION AND USES
MOISTUREL is a non-greasy formula that leaves the skin feeling smooth and soft. Clinically proven to relieve dry skin and designed not to cause acne or blemishes. Free of parabens and fragrances that can sensitize or irritate skin. Indicated for generalized dry skin, chapped or chafed skin, diaper rash, sunburn, heat rash, itching and dryness associated with eczema.

ADMINISTRATION AND DOSAGE
Apply liberally as often as needed.

HOW SUPPLIED
8 oz. (NDC 0072-9100-08) and 12 oz. (NDC 0072-9100-12) plastic bottles.

MOISTUREL®
SENSITIVE SKIN CLEANSER
Pure, Clear and Soap-Free

COMPOSITION
Sodium laureth sulfate and laureth 6 carboxylic acid and disodium laureth sulfosuccinate, methyl gluceth-20, cocamidopropyl betaine, water, diazolidinyl urea, and methylchloroisothiazolinone and methylisothiazolinone.

ACTIONS AND USES
Moisturel Sensitive Skin Cleanser is a crystal clear, lathering, soap-free cleanser. It cleans thoroughly without stinging, irritating, or drying. Unlike soaps, Moisturel Sensitive Skin Cleanser rinses refreshingly clean without leaving a film or residue. Its pure and gentle formula makes it ideal for facial use. Its non-drying, non-comedogenic, and fragrance-free formula makes it ideal for cleansing:
- Sensitive skin—even a baby's
- Dry, itchy skin caused by cold and wind, or overexposure to sun
- Skin robbed of moisture by use and removal of cosmetics
- Irritated, allergic skin
- Skin that breaks out
- Skin dried by harsh acne medications

ADMINISTRATION AND DOSAGE
With skin wet, gently work Moisturel Sensitive Skin Cleanser into a rich lather by massaging in a circular motion. Rinse thoroughly and pat dry with a soft cloth.

CAUTION
Avoid contact with eyes. For external use only.

HOW SUPPLIED
8.75 oz. (NDC 0072-6420-08) plastic bottle with pump.

PRESUN® FOR KIDS
Children's Sunscreen

ACTIVE INGREDIENTS
Octyl methoxycinnamate, oxybenzone, octyl salicylate. Also contains: Carbomer-940, cetyl alcohol, diazolidinyl urea, dimethicone, methylchloroisothiazolinone and methylisothiazolinone, stearic acid, triethanolamine, water and other ingredients.

ACTIONS AND USES
29 TIMES NATURAL PROTECTION: Used as directed, PRESUN for Kids provides 29 times your child's natural sunburn protection and may help reduce the chance of premature aging and wrinkling of skin. Clinical research indicates that regular use of sunscreen (SPF 15) during the first 18 years of life may reduce the risk of developing the two most common forms of skin cancer by as much as 78%.
NON-STINGING: A non-PABA, fragrance-free formula that is designed not to sting sensitive skin. (Avoid contact with eyes since all sunscreens can cause irritation and stinging of the eye.)
HYPOALLERGENIC: PRESUN For Kids is hypoallergenic and, because the known sensitizers common to most sunscreens have been removed, is suitable for your child's sensitive skin.
WATERPROOF 29: PRESUN For Kids maintains its degree of protection (SPF 29) even after 80 minutes in the water.

WARNINGS
For external use only. Protect from freezing. *As with all sunscreens:* Apply to small area; check after 24 hours. Discontinue use if irritation or rash appears. Avoid contact with eyes. In case of contact, flush eyes with water. Keep out of the reach of children. Use on children under six months of age only with the advice of a physician.

ADMINISTRATION AND DOSAGE
For maximum protection, smooth evenly and liberally onto dry skin before sun exposure. Massage in gently. Reapplication to dry skin after prolonged swimming, excessive perspiration or towel drying is recommended for all day protection.

HOW SUPPLIED
4 oz (NDC 0072-9399-04) plastic bottle.

PRESUN® 8, 15 and 39 CREAMY SUNSCREENS

ACTIVE INGREDIENTS
Octyl dimethyl PABA, oxybenzone. Also contains: Carbomer-940, cetyl alcohol, diazolidinyl urea, dimethicone, fragrance, methylchloroisothiazolinone and methylisothiazolinone, stearic acid, triethanolamine, water, and other ingredients.

ACTION AND USES
8, 15 or 39 TIMES NATURAL PROTECTION: Used as directed, PRESUN 8, 15 or 39 Sunscreens provide 8, 15 or 39 times your natural *sunburn* protection and may help reduce the chance of premature aging and wrinkling of the skin as well as skin cancer caused by overexposure to the sun.
UVA/UVB PROTECTION: PRESUN Suncreen is formulated to provide protection from the harmful effects of both UVA and UVB rays.
WATERPROOF: PRESUN Creamy Sunscreen maintains its degree of protection even after 80 minutes in the water.

WARNINGS
For external use only. Protect from freezing. Do not use if sensitive to P-aminobenzoic acid (PABA) or related compounds. *As with all sunscreens:* Apply to a small area; check after 24 hours. Discontinue use if irritation or rash appears. Avoid contact with eyes. In case of contact, flush eyes with water. Keep out of the reach of children. Use on children under six months of age only with the advice of a physician.

ADMINISTRATION AND DOSAGE
Smooth evenly onto dry skin before sun exposure. Massage in gently. Reapply to dry skin after prolonged swimming, excessive perspiration or towel drying. Repeated applications during prolonged sun exposure are recommended.

HOW SUPPLIED
8 Creamy: 4 oz. (NDC 0072-8506-04) plastic bottle. 15 Creamy: 4 oz. (NDC 0072-8906-04) plastic bottle. 39 Creamy: 4 oz. (NDC 0072-9600-04) plastic bottle.

PRESUN® 8 AND 15 LOTION SUNSCREENS

ACTIVE INGREDIENTS
8 Lotion: 7.3% (w/w) Octyl dimethyl PABA, 2.3% (w/w) oxybenzone. Also contains: Choleth-24, hydroxypropylcellulose, PG dioctanoate, PPG-15 stearyl ether, 60% (w/w) SD alcohol 40 and water.
15 Lotion: 5% Aminobenzoic acid (PABA), 5% Octyl dimethyl PABA, 3% oxybenzone. Also contains: hydroxypropylcellulose, PPG-15 stearyl ether, 58% SD alcohol 40 and water.

ACTION AND USES
8 or 15 TIMES NATURAL PROTECTION: Used as directed, PRESUN 8 or 15 Sunscreens provide 8 or 15 times your natural *sunburn* protection and may help reduce the chance of premature aging and wrinkling of the skin as well as skin cancer caused by overexposure to the sun.
UVA/UVB PROTECTION: PRESUN Suncreen is formulated to provide protection from the harmful effects of both UVA and UVB rays.
PRESUN Lotion Sunscreen is a clear formula containing a PABA ester—an ingredient widely recommended by physicians.

WARNINGS
For external use only. Do not use if sensitive to P-aminobenzoic acid (PABA) or related compounds. Transient facial stinging may occur in hot, humid weather. Avoid flame. *As with all sunscreens:* Apply to a small area; check after 24 hours. Discontinue use if irritation or rash appears. Avoid contact with eyes. In case of contact, flush eyes with water. Keep out of the reach of children. Use on children under six months of age only with the advice of a physician.
15 Lotion: Avoid contact with fabric or other materials as staining may result.

ADMINISTRATION AND DOSAGE
Shake well. Apply evenly to dry skin before sun exposure; let dry before dressing. Reapply to dry skin after swimming, excessive perspiration or towel drying. Repeated applications during prolonged sun exposure are recommended.

HOW SUPPLIED
8 Lotion: 4 fl. oz. (NDC 0072-5403-04) plastic bottle. 15 Lotion: 4 fl. oz. (NDC 0072-8800-04) plastic bottle.

PRESUN® 15 FACIAL STICK/LIP PROTECTOR SUNSCREEN

ACTIVE INGREDIENTS
8% Octyl dimethyl PABA, 3% oxybenzone. Also contains: Flavoring, lanolin oil, mineral oil, ozokerite, PEG-4 dilaurate, petrolatum and propylparaben.

ACTIONS AND USES
15 TIMES NATURAL PROTECTION: Used as directed, PRESUN 15 Facial Sunscreen Stick and Sunscreen Lip Protector provide 15 times your natural *sunburn* protection and may help reduce the chance of premature aging and wrinkling of the skin as well as skin cancer caused by overexposure to the sun.
UVA/UVB PROTECTION: PRESUN 15 Facial Sunscreen Stick and Sunscreen Lip Protector are formulated to provide protection from the harmful effects of both UVA and UVB rays.
MOISTURIZES: PRESUN 15 Facial Sunscreen Stick helps keep your skin soft and smooth—even after long hours in the sun.
PRESUN 15 Sunscreen Lip Protector helps prevent drying, cracking and chapping from the sun, wind or cold.

WARNINGS
For external use only. Do not use if sensitive to P-aminobenzoic acid (PABA) or related compounds. *As with all sunscreens:* Apply to a small area; check after 24 hours. Discontinue use if irritation or rash appears. Avoid contact with eyes. In case of contact, flush eyes with water. Keep out of the reach of children. Use on children under six months of age only with the advice of a physician.

ADMINISTRATION AND DOSAGE
Facial Stick: Apply evenly to dry skin before sun exposure. Reapply to dry skin after swimming, excessive perspiration or towel drying. Repeated applications during prolonged sun exposure are recommended.
Lip Protector: Apply to lips as needed. Repeated applications during prolonged exposure to the sun, wind or cold are recommended.

HOW SUPPLIED
.42 oz. (NDC 0072-8703-04) plastic facial stick, .15 oz. (NDC 0072-8703-01) plastic lip stick.

PRESUN® 15 FACIAL SUNSCREEN
Ultra Sunscreen Protection

ACTIVE INGREDIENTS
8% Octyl dimethyl PABA, 3% oxybenzone. Also contains: Benzyl alcohol, carbomer-934, cetyl alcohol, dimethicone, glyceryl stearate, laureth-23, magnesium aluminum silicate, petrolatum, propylene glycol dioctanoate, quaternium-15, sodium hydroxide, stearth-2 and water.

ACTION AND USES
15 TIMES NATURAL PROTECTION: Used as directed, PRESUN 15 Facial Sunscreen provides 15 times your natural *sunburn* protection and may help reduce the chance of premature aging and wrinkling of the skin as well as skin cancer caused by overexposure to the sun.
UVA/UVB PROTECTION: PRESUN 15 Facial Sunscreen is formulated to provide protection from the harmful effects of both UVA and UVB rays.
MOISTURIZES: PRESUN 15 Facial Sunscreen was developed especially for use on the face. The special moisturizers soften and smooth your skin while protecting it from the drying effects of the sun.
SUITABLE UNDER MAKE-UP: A non-greasy cream made especially for daily use under facial make-up and designed not to clog pores or cause acne or blemishes.

ADMINISTRATION AND DOSAGE
Gently smooth evenly onto dry skin before sun exposure. Reapply to dry skin after swimming, excessive perspiration or towel drying. Repeated applications during prolonged sun exposure are recommended.

WARNINGS
For external use only. Do not use if sensitive to P-aminobenzoic acid (PABA) or related compounds. *As with all sunscreens:* Apply to a small area; check after 24 hours. Discontinue use if irritation or rash appears. Avoid contact with eyes. In case of contact, flush eyes with water. Keep out of reach of children. Use on children under six months of age only with the advice of a physician.

Continued on next page

Westwood—Cont.

PRESUN® 15 and 29 SENSITIVE SKIN SUNSCREENS
PABA-FREE Sunscreen Protection

HOW SUPPLIED
2 oz. (NDC 0072-9200-02) plastic tube.

PRESUN® 15 and 29 SENSITIVE SKIN SUNSCREENS
PABA-FREE Sunscreen Protection

ACTIVE INGREDIENTS
Octyl methoxycinnamate, oxybenzone, octyl salicylate. Also contains: Carbomer-940, cetyl alcohol, diazolidinyl urea, dimethicone, methylchloroisothiazolinone and methylisothiazolinone, stearic acid, triethanolamine, water, and other ingredients.

ACTIONS AND USES
15 or 29 TIMES NATURAL PROTECTION
Used as directed, PRESUN 15 or 29 Sensitive Skin Sunscreen provides 15 or 29 times your natural *sunburn* protection and may help reduce the chance of premature aging and wrinkling of the skin as well as skin cancer caused by overexposure to the sun.
UVA/UVB PROTECTION
PRESUN 15 or 29 Sensitive Skin Sunscreen is formulated to provide protection from the harmful effects of both UVA and UVB rays.
PABA-FREE FORMULA
A PABA- and fragrance-free formula that provides a very high degree of sunburn protection and, because the known sensitizers common to most sunscreens have been removed, is suitable for sensitive skin.
WATERPROOF:
PRESUN Sensitive Skin Sunscreen maintains its degree of protection even after 80 minutes in the water.

ADMINISTRATION AND DOSAGE
For maximum protection, smooth evenly and liberally onto dry skin before sun exposure. Massage in gently. Reapplication to dry skin after prolonged swimming, excessive perspiration or towel drying is recommended for all day protection.

WARNINGS
For external use only. Protect from freezing. *As with all sunscreens:* Apply to a small area; check after 24 hours. Discontinue use if irritation or rash appears. Avoid contact with eyes. In case of contact, flush eyes with water. Keep out of the reach of children. Use on children under six months of age only with the advice of a physician.

HOW SUPPLIED
29 Sensitive Skin: 4 oz. (NDC 0072-9300-04; 6505-01-267-1483) plastic bottle.
15 Sensitive Skin: 4 oz. (NDC 0072-9370-04) plastic bottle.

SEBULEX®
Antiseborrheic Treatment Shampoo

ACTIVE INGREDIENTS
2% sulfur and 2% salicylic acid. Also contains: D&C yellow #10, docusate sodium, EDTA, FD&C blue #1, fragrance, PEG-6 lauramide, PEG-14M, sodium dodecyl benzene sulfonate, sodium octoxynol-2 ethane sulfonate and water.

ACTION AND USES
A penetrating therapeutic shampoo for the temporary relief of itchy scalp and the scaling of dandruff, SEBULEX helps relieve itching, remove dandruff, excess oil. It penetrates and softens the crusty, matted layers of scales adhering to the scalp, and leaves the hair soft and manageable.

ADMINISTRATION AND DOSAGE
SEBULEX liquid should be shaken before use. SEBULEX is massaged into wet scalp. Lather should be allowed to remain on scalp for about 5 minutes and then rinsed. Application is repeated, followed by a thorough rinse. Initially, SEBULEX can be used daily, or every other day, or as directed, depending on the condition. Once symptoms are under control, one or two treatments a week usually will maintain control of itching, oiliness and scaling.

CAUTION
If undue skin irritation develops or increases, discontinue use. For external use only. Contact with eyes should be avoided. In case of contact, flush eyes thoroughly with water. Keep this and all drugs out of reach of children.

HOW SUPPLIED
SEBULEX in 4 oz. (NDC 0072-2700-04) and 8 oz. (NDC 0072-2700-08) plastic bottles.

SEBULEX® SHAMPOO WITH CONDITIONERS
Antiseborrheic Treatment and Conditioning Shampoo

ACTIVE INGREDIENTS
2% sulfur, 2% salicylic acid. Also contains: water, sodium octoxynol-3 sulfonate, sodium lauryl sulfate, lauramide DEA, acetamide MEA, amphoteric-2, hydrolyzed animal protein, magnesium aluminum silicate, propylene glycol, methylcellulose, PEG-14 M, fragrance, disodium EDTA, dioctyl sodium sulfosuccinate, FD & C blue 1, D & C yellow 10.

ACTION AND USES
SEBULEX SHAMPOO WITH CONDITIONERS provides effective temporary control of the scaling and itching of dandruff and seborrheic dermatitis, while adding protein to the hair shaft to increase its manageability.

ADMINISTRATION AND DOSAGE
SEBULEX SHAMPOO WITH CONDITIONERS should be shaken well before use. Shampoo five minutes. For optimum dandruff control and conditioning leave lather on scalp for the full five minutes. Rinse. Repeat. Use daily until control is achieved. Use two to three times weekly to maintain control, although daily use may be continued. Consult physician for severe or unresponsive scalp conditions.

CAUTION
If undue skin irritation develops or increases, discontinue use and consult physician. Contact with eyes should be avoided. In cases of contact, eyes should be flushed thoroughly with water. For external use only. Keep this and all drugs out of reach of children.

HOW SUPPLIED
4 oz. (NDC 0072-2600-04) and 8 oz. (NDC 0072-2600-08) plastic bottles.

SEBUTONE® and SEBUTONE® CREAM
Antiseborrheic Tar Shampoo

ACTIVE INGREDIENTS
Coal tar 0.5%, salicylic acid 2%, sulfur 2%. SEBUTONE also contains: D&C yellow #10, docusate sodium, EDTA, FD&C blue #1, fragrance, lanolin oil, PEG-6 lauramide, PEG-90M, sodium dodecyl benzene sulfonate, sodium octoxynol-2 ethane sulfonate, titanium dioxide, and water. SEBUTONE CREAM also contains: Ceteareth-20, D&C yellow #10, dextrin, docusate sodium, EDTA, FD&C blue #1, fragrance, laureth-4, lanolin oil, magnesium aluminum silicate, PEG-6 lauramide, PEG-14 M, sodium dodecyl benzene sulfonate, sodium octoxynol-2 ethane sulfonate, stearyl alcohol, titanium dioxide and water.

ACTION AND USES
A surface-active, penetrating therapeutic shampoo for the temporary relief of itchy scalp and the scaling of stubborn dandruff and psoriasis. Provides prompt and prolonged relief of itching, helps control oiliness and rid the scalp of scales and crust. Tar ingredient is chemically and biologically standardized to produce uniform therapeutic activity. Wood's light demonstrates residual microfine particles of tar on the scalp several days after a course of SEBUTONE shampoo. In addition to its antipruritic and antiseborrheic actions, SEBUTONE also helps offset excessive scalp dryness with a special moisturizing emollient.

ADMINISTRATION AND DOSAGE
SEBUTONE liquid should be well shaken before use. A liberal amount of SEBUTONE or SEBUTONE CREAM is massaged into the wet scalp for 5 minutes and the scalp is then rinsed. Application is repeated, followed by a thorough rinse. Use as often as necessary to keep the scalp free from itching and scaling or as directed. No other shampoo or soap washings are required.

CAUTION
If undue skin irritation develops or increases, discontinue use. In rare instances, temporary discoloration of white, blond, bleached or tinted hair may occur. Contact with the eyes is to be avoided. In case of contact flush eyes with water. For external use only. Keep this and all drugs out of reach of children.

HOW SUPPLIED
SEBUTONE in 4 oz. (NDC 0072-5000-04) and 8 oz. (NDC 0072-5000-08) plastic bottles.
SEBUTONE CREAM in 4 oz. (NDC 0072-5100-01) tubes.

TACARYL® Chewable Tablets ℞
(Methdilazine)
TACARYL® Hydrochloride Tablets/Syrup ℞
(Methdilazine HCl)

CAUTION
FEDERAL LAW PROHIBITS DISPENSING WITHOUT PRESCRIPTION

DESCRIPTION
TACARYL is an antihistamine antipruritic with the following chemical structure:
10 [(1-methyl-3-pyrrolidinyl) methyl] phenothiazine

Methdilazine and its hydrochloride salt occur as light tan, crystalline powders with respectively poor and free solubility in water.
TACARYL (methdilazine or methdilazine HCl) is a phenothiazine derivative available as
Tablets—Each tablet contains 8 mg methdilazine HCl. Also contains acacia, ascorbic acid, dibasic calcium phosphate, corn starch, D&C red #27 lake, ethyl cellulose, lactose, magnesium stearate and tablet brown;
Syrup—Each 5 ml (one teaspoonful) contains 4 mg methdilazine HCl in a syrup base of benzoic acid, citric acid, ethyl alcohol (7.37%), ethyl vanillin, flavoring, menthol, sodium bisulfite, sodium citrate, sorbitol, sucrose and water; and
Chewable Tablets—Each table contains methdilazine equivalent to 4 mg methdilazine HCl. Also contains acacia, D&C red #21 lake, D&C red #27 lake, flavoring, hydrogenated cottonseed oil, magnesium stearate, mannitol, sodium chloride, sodium saccharin and talc.

CLINICAL PHARMACOLOGY
No information is currently available which assesses the disposition of methdilazine.

INDICATIONS AND USAGE
TACARYL and TACARYL HCl are indicated for the treatment of pruritic symptoms in urticaria, symptomatic relief in the management of nasal allergies (hayfever, allergic rhinitis, etc.), relief of pruritic symptoms in a variety of allergic and non-allergic conditions including: atopic dermatitis, neurodermatitis, contact dermatitis, pityriasis rosea, poison ivy dermatitis, eczematous dermatitis, pruritus ani and vulvae, and drug rash.

CONTRAINDICATIONS
TACARYL is contraindicated in patients who are comatose, those who have received large amounts of CNS depressants, patients with bone marrow depression, jaundice or those who have demonstrated an idiosyncrasy or hypersensitivity to methdilazine or other phenothiazines.
This drug is contraindicated in newborn or premature infants and nursing mothers as well as in children who are acutely ill and dehydrated, since there may be an increased susceptibility to dystonias.

WARNINGS
Phenothiazines with antihistaminic and anticholinergic effects, including methdilazine and methdilazine HCl, should be used with extreme caution in patients with: asthmatic attack, narrow-angle glaucoma, prostatic hypertrophy, stenosing peptic ulcer, pyloroduodenal obstruction, bladder neck obstruction, as well as in patients receiving monoamine oxidase inhibitors. Phenothiazine should **not** be used with alcohol ingestion.
TACARYL syrup contains sodium bisulfite, a sulfite that may cause allergic-type reactions including anaphylactic symptoms and life-threatening or less severe asthmatic episodes in certain susceptible people. The overall prevalence of sulfite sensitivity in the general population is unknown and probably low. Sulfite sensitivity is seen more frequently in asthmatic than in nonasthmatic people.
Usage in Pregnancy: There are reports of jaundice and prolonged extrapyramidal symptoms in infants whose mothers received phenothiazines during pregnancy.
Hyperreflexia has been reported in the newborn when a phenothiazine was used during pregnancy.
Use in Children: TACARYL should be used with caution, as administration in the young child may result in excitation. Overdosage may produce hallucinations, convulsions, and sudden death.
Use in the Elderly (60 years or older): The elderly are more prone to develop the following side effects from phenothia-

zines: hypotension, syncope, toxic confusional states, excessive sedation, extrapyramidal signs (especially parkinsonism), akathisia and persistent dyskinesia.

PRECAUTIONS

General: Phenothiazines may block and even reverse some of the actions of epinephrine. TACARYL should be used cautiously in persons with acute or chronic respiratory impairment, particularly in children, as it may suppress the cough reflex.

The drug should be used cautiously in persons with cardiovascular disease, impairment of liver function or those with a history of ulcer disease.

Information for Patients: Patients should be cautioned that methdilazine or methdilazine HCl may impair the mental and/or physical ability required for the performance of potentially hazardous tasks, such as driving a vehicle or operating machinery. Similarly, it may impair mental alertness in children. The concomitant use of alcohol or other central nervous system depressants may have an additive effect.

DRUG INTERACTIONS

- CNS Depressants/Narcotics—Phenothiazines may increase, prolong or intensify the sedative action of nervous system depressants such as anesthetics, barbiturates or alcohol. The dose of a narcotic or barbiturate may be reduced to ¼ or ½ the usual amount when TACARYL is administered concomitantly. Excessive amounts of TACARYL, relative to a narcotic, may lead to restlessness and motor hyperactivity in the patient with pain.
- Epinephrine—Phenothiazines may block and even reverse some of the actions of epinephrine.
- MAO Inhibitors—Combined use of MAO inhibitors and phenthiazines may result in hypotension and extrapyramidal reactions.
- Thiazide Diuretics—The anticholinergic effects of phenothiazines may be prolonged and intensified by the concomitant use of thiazide diuretics.
- Oral Contraceptives, Progesterone, Reserpine, Nylidrin Hydrochloride—These drugs potentiate the effects of phenothiazines.

DRUG/LABORATORY TEST INTERACTIONS

The following changes in laboratory determinations have been reported in patients taking phenothiazines:
- increased serum cholesterol, blood glucose, spinal fluid protein, and urinary urobilinogen levels
- decreased protein bound iodine (PBI)
- false positives in urine bilirubin tests
- interference with urinary ketone determinations, pregnancy tests and steroid determinations.

Carcinogenesis/Mutagenesis/Impairment of Fertility: Mutagenicity and long-term carcinogenicity studies in animals have not been evaluated. Mutagenicity has been evaluated using the Ames Salmonella/Microsome Plate test. TACARYL tablets and syrup were found to be non-mutagenic.

Pregnancy Category B: Reproduction studies have been performed in rats at doses up to 70 times the usual human dose and have revealed no evidence of impaired fertility or harm to the fetus due to TACARYL. There are, however, no adequate and well controlled studies in pregnant women. Because animal reproduction studies are not always predictive of human response, this drug should be used during pregnancy only if clearly needed.

Nonteratogenic Effects: There are reports of jaundice and prolonged extrapyramidal symptoms in infants whose mothers received phenothiazines during pregnancy.

Nursing Mothers: It is not known whether this drug is excreted in human milk. Because many drugs are excreted in human milk, caution should be exercised when methdilazine is administered to a nursing woman. (See CONTRAINDICATIONS).

Pediatric Usage: Safety and effectiveness in children below the age of 3 years have not been established. (See CONTRAINDICATIONS, WARNINGS and DOSAGE and ADMINISTRATION.)

ADVERSE REACTIONS

This drug may produce adverse reactions common to both phenothiazines and antihistamines.

Note: Not all of the following adverse reactions have been reported with this specific drug; however, pharmacological similarities among the phenothiazine derivatives require that each be considered when TACARYL is administered. There have been occasional reports of sudden death in patients receiving phenothiazine derivatives chronically.

CNS: Drowsiness is the most prominent CNS effect of this drug. Extrapyramidal reactions occur, particularly with high doses. Other reported reactions include dizziness, lassitude, tinnitus, incoordination, fatigue, blurred vision, euphoria, diplopia, nervousness, insomnia, tremors and grand mal seizures, excitation, catatonic-like states, neuritis and hysteria.

Cardiovascular: Postural hypotension is the most common cardiovascular effect of the phenothiazines. Reflex tachycardia may be seen. Bradycardia, faintness, dizziness and car-

diac arrest have been reported. ECG changes, including blunting of T waves and prolongation of the Q-T interval may be seen.

Gastrointestinal: Anorexia, nausea, vomiting, epigastric distress, constipation and dry mouth may occur. Diarrhea has also been reported as well as increased appetite and weight gain.

Genitourinary: Urinary frequency, dysuria and urinary retention have been reported.

Respiratory: Thickening of bronchial secretions, tightness of the chest, wheezing and nasal stuffiness may occur.

Allergic Reactions: These include urticaria, dermatitis, asthma, laryngeal edema, angioneurotic edema, photosensitivity, lupus erythematosus-like syndrome and anaphylactoid reactions.

Other reported reactions: Leukopenia, agranulocytosis, thrombocytopenic purpura and jaundice of the obstructive type have been reported. The jaundice is usually reversible, but chronic jaundice has been reported.

Long-term therapy considerations: After prolonged administration at high dosage, pigmentation of the skin has occurred, chiefly in the exposed areas. Ocular changes consist of the appearance of lenticular and corneal opacities, epithelial keratopathies and pigmentary retinopathy. Vision may be impaired.

Endocrine: Early menses, induced lactation, gynecomastia, decreased libido and inhibition of ejaculation have been reported.

OVERDOSAGE

Signs and symptoms of overdosage range from mild depression of the central nervous system and cardiovascular system, to profound hypotension, respiratory depression and unconsciousness. Stimulation may be evident, especially in children and geratric patients. Atropine-like signs and symptoms—dry mouth, fixed dilated pupils, flushing, etc.—as well as gastrointestinal symptoms may occur. The treatment of overdosage is essentially symptomatic and supportive. Early gastric lavage may be beneficial. Centrally acting emetics are of little use.

Avoid analeptics, which may cause convulsions. Severe hypotension usually responds to the administration of levarterenol or phenylephrine. **EPINEPHRINE SHOULD NOT BE USED,** since its use in the patient with partial adrenergic blockade may further lower the blood pressure. Additional measures include oxygen and intravenous fluids. Limited experience with dialysis indicates that it is not helpful. The oral LD_{50} of methdilazine HCl is approximately 225 mg/kg in mice, 448 mg/kg in rats and 269 mg/kg in guinea pigs.

DOSAGE AND ADMINISTRATION

TACARYL® Hydrochloride Tablets (methdilazine HCl) Adults: 1 tablet (8 mg) 2 to 4 times daily. Children over 3 years: ½ tablet (4 mg) 2 to 4 times daily.

TACARYL® Hydrochloride Syrup (methdilazine HCl) Adults: 2 teaspoons (8 mg) 2 to 4 times daily. Children over 3 years: 1 teaspoon (4 mg) 2 to 4 times daily.

TACARYL® Chewable Tablets (methdilazine) Adults: 2 tablets (7.2 mg) 2 to 4 times daily. Children over 3 years: 1 tablet (3.6 mg) 2 to 4 times daily. This product form should be chewed and swallowed promptly.

HOW SUPPLIED

TACARYL® Hydrochloride (methdilazine HCl) Tablets 8 mg: a scored, peach colored tablet (W logo)

  NDC 0072-7400-01   Bottles of 100
      (with child-resistant closures)

TACARYL® Hydrochloride (methdilazine HCl) Syrup 4 mg/5ml:

  NDC 0072-7500-01   Bottles of 16 fl. oz. (1 pint)
      (with child-resistant closures)

TACARYL® (methdilazine) Chewable Tablets 3.6 mg each (equivalent to 4 mg. methdilazine HCl) a pink unscored table (W logo)

  NDC 0072-7300-01   Bottles of 100
      (with child-resistant closures)

Dispense in tight, light-resistant container. Store at room temperature away from strong light.

Shown in Product Identification Section, page 435

T-STAT® ℞
(erythromycin) 2.0% Topical Solution and Pads

CAUTION
Federal law prohibits dispensing without prescription.

DESCRIPTION
Erythromycin is an antibiotic produced from a strain of Streptomyces erythraeus. It is basic and readily forms salts with acids. Each ml of T-STAT (erythromycin). 2.0% Topical Solution contains 20 mg of erythromycin base in a vehicle consisting of alcohol (71.2%), propylene glycol and fragrance. It may contain citric acid to adjust pH.

ACTIONS
Although the mechanism by which T-STAT Solution acts in reducing inflammatory lesions of acne vulgaris is unknown, it is presumably due to its antibiotic action.

INDICATIONS
T-STAT Solution is indicated for the topical control of acne vulgaris.

CONTRAINDICATIONS
T-STAT Solution is contraindicated in persons who have shown hypersentivity to any of its ingredients.

WARNING
The safe use of T-STAT (erythromycin) 2.0% Solution during pregnancy or lactation has not been established.

PRECAUTIONS

General—The use of antibiotic agents may be associated with the overgrowth of antibiotic-resistant organisms. If this occurs, administration of this drug should be discontinued and appropriate measures taken.

Information for Patients—T-STAT Solution is for external use only and should be kept away from the eyes, nose, mouth, and other mucous membranes. Concomitant topical acne therapy should be used with caution because a cumulative irritant effect may occur, especially with the use of peeling, desquamating, or abrasive agents.

Carcinogensis, Mutagenesis, Impairment of Fertility—Long-term animal studies to evaluate carcinogenic potential, mutagenicity, or the effect on fertility of erythromycin have not been performed.

Pregnancy: Pregnancy Category C.—Animal reproduction studies have not been conducted with erythromycin. It is also not known whether erythromycin can cause fetal harm when administered to a pregnant woman or can affect reproduction capacity. Erythromycin should be given to a pregnant woman only if clearly needed.

Nursing Mothers—Erythromycin is excreted in breast milk. Caution should be exercised when erythromycin is administered to a nursing woman.

ADVERSE REACTIONS
Adverse conditions reported include dryness, tenderness, pruritis, desquamation, erythema, oiliness, and burning sensation. Irritation of the eyes has also been reported. A case of generalized urticarial reaction, possibly related to the drug, which required the use of systemic steroid therapy has been reported.

DOSAGE AND ADMINISTRATION
T-STAT Solution or Pads should be applied over the affected area twice a day after the skin is thoroughly washed with warm water and soap and patted dry. Acne lesions on the face, neck, shoulder, chest, and back may be treated in this manner. Additional pads may be used, if needed.

This medication should be applied with applicator top or the disposable applicator pads. If fingertips or pads are used, wash hands after application. Drying and peeling may be controlled by reducing the frequency of applications.

HOW SUPPLIED
T-STAT Solution, 60 ml plastic bottle with optional applicator, NDC 0072-8300-60. T-STAT Pads, 60 disposable premoistened applicator pads in a plastic jar. NDC-0072-8300-61. Store at controlled room temperature—15°–30°C (59°–86°F).

WESTCORT® ℞
(hydrocortisone valerate)
Cream/Ointment, 0.2%

Caution: Federal law prohibits dispensing without a prescription.

DESCRIPTION
WESTCORT is a topical formulation containing hydrocortisone valerate, a non-fluorinated steroid. It has the chemical name Pregn-4-ene-3, 20-dione, 11, 21-dihydroxy-17-[(1-oxopentyl) oxy]-, (11β)-; the empirical formula is: $C_{26}H_{38}O_6$; the molecular weight is 446.58, and the CAS registry number is: 57524-89-7. The structural formula is:

Each gram of WESTCORT CREAM contains 2.0 mg hydrocortisone valerate in a hydrophilic base composed of white petrolatum, stearyl alcohol, propylene glycol, amphoteric-9,

Continued on next page

Westwood—Cont.

carbomer-940, dried sodium phosphate, sodium lauryl sulfate, sorbic acid and water.

Each gram of Westcort Ointment contains 2.0 mg hydrocortisone valerate in a hydrophilic base composed of white petrolatum, stearyl alcohol, propylene glycol, sorbic acid, sodium lauryl sulfate, carbomer-934, dried sodium phosphate, mineral oil, steareth-2, steareth-100, and water.

CLINICAL PHARMACOLOGY

Topical corticosteroids share anti-inflammatory, anti-pruritic and vasoconstrictive actions.

The mechanism of anti-inflammatory activity of the topical corticosteroids is unclear. Various laboratory methods, including vasoconstrictor assays, are used to compare and predict potencies and/or clinical efficacies of the topical corticosteroids. There is some evidence to suggest that a recognizable correlation exists between vasoconstrictor potency and therapeutic efficacy in man.

Pharmacokinetics: The extent of percutaneous absorption of topical corticosteroids is determined by many factors including the vehicle, the integrity of the epidermal barrier, and the use of occlusive dressings.

Topical corticosteroids can be absorbed from normal intact skin. Inflammation and/or other disease processes in the skin increase percutaneous absorption. Occlusive dressings substantially increase the percutaneous absorption of topical corticosteroids. Thus, occlusive dressings may be a valuable therapeutic adjunct for treatment of resistant dermatoses (see DOSAGE AND ADMINISTRATION).

Once absorbed through the skin, topical corticosteroids are handled through pharmacokinetic pathways similar to systemically administered corticosteroids. Corticosteroids are bound to plasma proteins in varying degrees. Corticosteroids are metabolized primarily in the liver and are then excreted by the kidneys. Some of the topical corticosteroids and their metabolites are also excreted into the bile.

INDICATIONS AND USAGE

WESTCORT is indicated for the relief of the inflammatory and pruritic manifestations of the corticosteroid-responsive dermatoses.

CONTRAINDICATIONS

Topical corticosteroids are contraindicated in those patients with a history of hypersensitivity to any of the components of the preparation.

PRECAUTIONS

General: Systemic absorption of topical corticosteroids has produced reversible hypothalamic-pituitary-adrenal (HPA) axis suppression, manifestations of Cushing's syndrome, hyperglycemia, and glucosuria in some patients. Conditions which augment systemic absorption include the application of the more potent steroids, use over large surface areas, prolonged use, and the addition of occlusive dressings.

Therefore, patients receiving a large dose of a potent topical steroid applied to a large surface area or under an occlusive dressing should be evaluated periodically for evidence of HPA axis suppression by using the urinary free cortisol and ACTH stimulation tests. If HPA axis suppression is noted, an attempt should be made to withdraw the drug, to reduce the frequency of application, or to substitute a less potent steroid.

Recovery of HPA axis function is generally prompt and complete upon discontinuation of the drug. Infrequently, signs and symptoms of steroid withdrawal may occur, requiring supplemental systemic corticosteroids.

Children may absorb proportionally larger amounts of topical corticosteroids and thus be more susceptible to systemic toxicity (see PRECAUTIONS—Pediatric Use).

If irritation develops, topical corticosteroids should be discontinued and appropriate therapy instituted.

In the presence of dermatological infections, the use of an appropriate antifungal or antibacterial agent should be instituted. If a favorable response does not occur promptly, the corticosteroids should be discontinued until the infection has been adequately controlled.

Information for the Patient: Patients using topical corticosteroids should receive the following information and instructions:

1. This medication is to be used as directed by the physician. It is for external use only. Avoid contact with the eyes.
2. Patients should be advised not to use this medication for any disorder other than for which it was prescribed.
3. The treated skin area should not be bandaged or otherwise covered or wrapped as to be occlusive unless directed by the physician.
4. Patients should report any signs of local adverse reactions especially under occlusive dressing.
5. Parents of pediatric patients should be advised not to use tight-fitting diapers or plastic pants on a child being treated in the diaper area, as these garments may constitute occlusive dressing.

Laboratory Tests: The following tests may be helpful in evaluating the HPA axis suppression:
   Urinary free cortisol test
   ACTH stimulation test

Carcinogenesis, Mutagenesis, and Impairment of Fertility: Long-term animal studies have not been performed to evaluate the carcinogenic potential or the effect on fertility of topical corticosteroids.

Studies to determine mutagenicity with prednisolone and hydrocortisone have revealed negative results.

Pregnancy Category C: Corticosteroids are generally teratogenic in laboratory animals when administered systemically at relatively low dosage levels. The more potent corticosteroids have been shown to be teratogenic after dermal application in laboratory animals. There are no adequate and well-controlled studies in pregnant women on teratogenic effects from topically applied corticosteroids. Therefore, topical corticosteroids should be used during pregnancy only if the potential benefit justifies the potential risk to the fetus. Drugs of this class should not be used extensively on pregnant patients, in large amounts, or for prolonged periods of time.

Nursing Mothers: It is not known whether topical administration of corticosteroids could result in sufficient systemic absorption to produce detectable quantities in breast milk. Systemically administered corticosteroids are secreted into breast milk in quantities *not* likely to have a deleterious effect on the infant. Nevertheless, caution should be exercised when topical corticosteroids are administered to a nursing woman.

Pediatric Use: Pediatric patients may demonstrate greater susceptibility to topical corticosteroid-induced HPA axis suppression and Cushing's syndrome than mature patients because of a larger skin surface area to body weight ratio.

Hypothalamic-pituitary-adrenal (HPA) axis suppression, Cushing's syndrome, and intracranial hypertension have been reported in children receiving topical corticosteroids. Manifestations of adrenal suppression in children include linear growth retardation, delayed weight gain, low plasma cortisol levels, and absence of response to ACTH stimulation. Manifestations of intracranial hypertension include bulging fontanelles, headaches, and bilateral papilledema.

Administration of topical corticosteroids to children should be limited to the least amount compatible with an effective therapeutic regimen. Chronic corticosteroid therapy may interfere with the growth and development of children.

ADVERSE REACTIONS

The following local adverse reactions are reported infrequently with topical corticosteroids, but may occur more frequently with the use of occlusive dressings. These reactions are listed in an approximate decreasing order of occurrence: burning; itching; irritation; dryness; folliculitis; hypertrichosis; acneiform eruptions; hypopigmentation; perioral dermatitis; allergic contact dermatitis; maceration of the skin; secondary infection; skin atrophy; striae; miliaria.

OVERDOSAGE

Topically applied corticosteroids can be absorbed in sufficient amounts to produce systemic effects (see PRECAUTIONS).

DOSAGE AND ADMINISTRATION

WESTCORT should be applied to the affected area as a thin film two or three times daily depending on the severity of the condition.

Occlusive dressings may be used for the management of psoriasis or recalcitrant conditions.

If an infection develops, the use of occlusive dressings should be discontinued and appropriate antimicrobial therapy instituted.

HOW SUPPLIED

WESTCORT CREAM, 0.2% is supplied in the following tube sizes:
  15 g NDC 0072-8100-15; 6505-01-093-9901.
  45 g NDC 0072-8100-45; 6505-01-083-9395.
  60 g NDC 0072-8100-60; 6505-01-121-0118.
120 g NDC 0072-8100-12.
WESTCORT OINTMENT, 0.2% is supplied in the following tube sizes:
  15 g NDC 0072-7800-15; 6505-01-224-0178
  45 g NDC 0072-7800-45; 6505-01-204-1835
  60 g NDC 0072-7800-60; 6505-01-224-0177
Store below 78°F (26°C).

Products are
listed alphabetically
in the
PINK SECTION.

Whitehall Laboratories Inc.

Division of American Home
Products Corporation
685 THIRD AVENUE
NEW YORK, NY 10017

CHILDREN'S ADVIL® SUSPENSION   ℞
(ibuprofen 100mg/5mL)

SHAKE WELL BEFORE USE

DESCRIPTION

CHILDREN'S ADVIL® SUSPENSION contains ibuprofen which is (±)-2-(p-isobutylphenyl) propionic acid. Ibuprofen is a white powder with a melting point of 74-77°C and is very slightly soluble in water (1 mg/mL) and readily soluble in organic solvents such as ethanol and acetone.

Ibuprofen's structural formula is:

CHILDREN'S ADVIL® SUSPENSION is a nonsteroidal anti-inflammatory agent. It is available for oral administration as a sucrose-sweetened, fruit-flavored liquid suspension containing 100mg of ibuprofen per 5mL.

Inactive Ingredients: Cellulose Gum, Citric Acid, Disodium EDTA, FD&C Red No. 40, Flavors, Glycerin, Microcrystalline Cellulose, Polysorbate 80, Sodium Benzoate, Sorbitol, Sucrose, Water, Xanthan Gum.

CLINICAL PHARMACOLOGY

CHILDREN'S ADVIL® SUSPENSION is a nonsteroidal anti-inflammatory agent that possesses analgesic and antipyretic activities. Its mode of action, like that of other nonsteroidal anti-inflammatory agents, is not completely understood, but may be related to prostaglandin synthetase inhibition.

In clinical studies in adult patients with rheumatoid arthritis and osteoarthritis, ibuprofen has been shown to be comparable to aspirin in controlling pain and inflammation and to be associated with a statistically significant reduction in the milder gastrointestinal side effects (see ADVERSE REACTIONS). CHILDREN'S ADVIL® SUSPENSION may be well tolerated in some patients who have had gastrointestinal side effects with aspirin, but these patients, when treated with CHILDREN'S ADVIL® SUSPENSION, should be carefully followed for signs and symptoms of gastrointestinal ulceration and bleeding. CHILDREN'S ADVIL® SUSPENSION did display a statistically significant lower incidence of adverse effects than aspirin, particularly with respect to the incidence of liver function test elevation, in a controlled clinical study of children with juvenile arthritis.

Although it is not definitely known whether ibuprofen causes less peptic ulceration than aspirin, in one study involving 885 adult patients with rheumatoid arthritis treated for up to one year, there were no reports of gastric ulceration with ibuprofen whereas frank ulceration was reported in 13 patients in the aspirin group (statistically significant $p < .001$). Gastroscopic studies at varying doses show an increased tendency toward gastric irritation at higher doses. However, at comparable doses, gastric irritation is approximately half that seen with aspirin. Studies using ^{51}Cr-tagged red cells indicate that fecal blood loss associated with ibuprofen in doses up to 2400mg daily did not exceed the normal range, and was significantly less than that seen in aspirin-treated patients.

In clinical studies in patients with rheumatoid arthritis, ibuprofen has been shown to be comparable to indomethacin in controlling the signs and symptoms of disease activity and to be associated with a statistically significant reduction of the milder gastrointestinal (see ADVERSE REACTIONS), and CNS side effects.

CHILDREN'S ADVIL® SUSPENSION may be used in combination with gold salts and/or corticosteroids.

In clinical studies in patients aged 2 to 15 with juvenile arthritis, CHILDREN'S ADVIL® SUSPENSION in doses of 20 to 50 mg/kg/day divided into 3 or 4 daily doses, has been shown to be similar to aspirin in controlling the signs and symptoms of their disease. In these trials, there was a significantly lower incidence of liver test abnormalities associated with CHILDREN'S ADVIL® SUSPENSION than with aspirin. Although ibuprofen may be better tolerated in terms of liver test abnormalities in children treated with CHILDREN'S ADVIL® SUSPENSION, they should be carefully followed for signs and symptoms suggesting liver dysfunction particularly with doses above 30mg/kg/day, or if abnormal liver tests have occurred with previous NSAID treatment (see PRECAUTIONS).

Controlled studies in adults have demonstrated that ibuprofen is a more effective analgesic than propoxyphene for the relief of episiotomy pain, pain following dental extraction procedures, and for the relief of the symptoms of primary dysmenorrhea.

In patients with primary dysmenorrhea, ibuprofen has been shown to reduce elevated levels of prostaglandin activity in the menstrual fluid and to reduce resting and active intrauterine pressure, as well as the frequency of uterine contractions. The probable mechanism of action is to inhibit prostaglandin synthesis rather than simply to provide analgesia. Controlled clinical trials comparing doses of 5 to 10mg/kg ibuprofen and 10–15 mg/kg of acetaminophen have been conducted in children 6 months to 12 years of age with fever primarily due to viral illnesses. In these studies there were no differences between treatments in fever reduction for the first hour and maximum fever reduction occurred between 2 and 4 hours. Response after 1 hour was dependent on both the level of temperature elevation as well as the treatment. In children with baseline temperatures at or below 102.5°F both ibuprofen doses and acetaminophen were equally effective in their maximum effect. In those children with temperatures above 102.5°F, the ibuprofen 10mg/kg dose was more effective. By 6 hours children treated with ibuprofen 5mg/kg tended to have recurrence of fever, whereas children treated with ibuprofen 10 mg/kg still had significant fever reduction at 8 hours. In control groups treated with 10mg/kg acetaminophen, fever reduction resembled that seen in children treated with 5mg/kg of ibuprofen, with the exception that temperature elevation tended to return 1–2 hours earlier.

Pharmacokinetics: Ibuprofen is rapidly absorbed when administered orally. As is true with most tablet and suspension formulations, CHILDREN'S ADVIL® SUSPENSION is absorbed somewhat faster than the tablet with a time to peak serum level generally within one hour. Peak serum ibuprofen levels are generally attained one to two hours after administration of ibuprofen tablets and within about 1 hour after the suspension. With single, oral, solid doses up to 800mg in adults, a linear relationship exists between the amount of drug administered and the integrated area under the serum drug concentration vs. time curve. Above 800mg, however, the area under the curve increase is less than proportional to the increase in dose. There is no evidence of age-dependent kinetics in patients 2 to 11 years old. With single doses of CHILDREN'S ADVIL® SUSPENSION ranging up to 10mg/kg, a dose/response relationship exists between the amount of drug administered to febrile children and the serum concentration vs. time curve. There is also a correlation between reduction of fever and drug concentration over time, although the peak reduction in fever occurs 2–4 hours after dosing.

No absorption differences are noticeable when ibuprofen tablets or suspension are given under fasting conditions or immediately before meals. When either product is taken with food, however, the peak levels are somewhat lower (up to 30%) and the time to reach peak levels is slightly prolonged (up to 30 min.) although the extent of absorption is unchanged.

A bioavailability study has shown that there was no interference with the absorption of ibuprofen when given in conjunction with an antacid containing both aluminum hydroxide and magnesium hydroxide.

Ibuprofen is rapidly metabolized and eliminated in the urine. The excretion of ibuprofen is virtually complete 24 hours after the last dose. The serum half-life of ibuprofen is 1.8 to 2.0 hours.

Studies have shown that following ingestion of the drug, 45% to 79% of the dose was recovered in the urine within 24 hours as metabolite A (25%), (+)-2-4′-(2-hydroxy-2-methylpropyl)-phenyl propionic acid and metabolite B (37%), (+)-2-4′-(2-carboxypropyl)-phenyl propionic acid; the percentages of free and conjugated ibuprofen were approximately 1% and 14%, respectively.

INDICATIONS AND USAGE

CHILDREN'S ADVIL® SUSPENSION is indicated for relief of the signs and symptoms of juvenile arthritis, rheumatoid arthritis and osteoarthritis.

CHILDREN'S ADVIL® SUSPENSION is indicated for relief of mild to moderate pain in adults and of primary dysmenorrhea.

CHILDREN'S ADVIL® SUSPENSION is also indicated for the reduction of fever in patients ages 12 months and older. Since there have been no controlled trials to demonstrate whether there is any beneficial effect or harmful interaction with the use of ibuprofen in conjunction with aspirin, the combination cannot be recommended (see **Drug Interactions**).

CONTRAINDICATIONS

CHILDREN'S ADVIL® SUSPENSION should not be used in patients who have previously exhibited hypersensitivity to ibuprofen, or in individuals with all or part of the syndrome of nasal polyps, angioedema and bronchospastic reactivity to aspirin or other nonsteroidal anti-inflammatory

agents. Anaphylactoid reactions have occurred in such patients.

WARNINGS

Risk of GI Ulceration, Bleeding and Perforation with NSAID Therapy. Serious gastrointestinal toxicity such as bleeding, ulceration, and perforation, can occur at any time, with or without warning symptoms, in patients treated chronically with NSAID therapy. Although minor upper gastrointestinal problems, such as dyspepsia, are common, usually developing early in therapy, physicians should remain alert for ulceration and bleeding in patients treated chronically with NSAIDs even in the absence of previous GI tract symptoms. In patients observed in clinical trials of several months to two years duration, symptomatic upper GI ulcers, gross bleeding or perforation appear to occur in approximately 1% of patients treated for 3–6 months, and in about 2–4% of patients treated for one year. Physicians should inform patients about the signs and/or symptoms of serious GI toxicity and what steps to take if they occur. Studies to date have not identified any subset of patients not at risk of developing peptic ulceration and bleeding. Except for a prior history of serious GI events and other risk factors known to be associated with peptic ulcer disease, such as alcoholism, smoking, etc., no risk factors (e.g., age, sex) have been associated with increased risk. Elderly or debilitated patients seem to tolerate ulceration or bleeding less well than other individuals and most spontaneous reports of fatal GI events are in this population. Studies to date are inconclusive concerning the relative risk of various NSAID agents in causing such reactions. High doses of any NSAID probably carry a greater risk of these reactions, although controlled clinical trials showing this do not exist in most cases. In considering the use of relatively large doses (within the recommended dosage range), sufficient benefit should be anticipated to offset the potential increased risk of GI toxicity.

PRECAUTIONS

General: Blurred and/or diminished vision, scotomata, and/or changes in color vision have been reported. If a patient develops such complaints while receiving CHILDREN'S ADVIL® SUSPENSION (ibuprofen), the drug should be discontinued and the patient should have an ophthalmologic examination which includes central visual fields and color vision testing.

Fluid retention and edema have been reported in association with ibuprofen; therefore, the drug should be used with caution in patients with a history of cardiac decompensation or hypertension.

Ibuprofen, like other nonsteroidal anti-inflammatory agents, can inhibit platelet aggregation, but the effect is quantitatively less and of shorter duration than that seen with aspirin. Ibuprofen has been shown to prolong bleeding time (but within the normal range), in normal subjects. Because this prolonged bleeding effect may be exaggerated in patients with underlying hemostatic defects, CHILDREN'S ADVIL® SUSPENSION should be used with caution in persons with intrinsic coagulation defects and those on anticoagulant therapy.

Patients on ibuprofen should report to their physicians signs or symptoms of gastrointestinal ulceration or bleeding, blurred vision or other eye symptoms, skin rash, weight gain, or edema.

In order to avoid exacerbation of disease or adrenal insufficiency, patients who have been on prolonged corticosteroid therapy should have their therapy tapered slowly rather than discontinued abruptly when ibuprofen is added to the treatment program.

The antipyretic and anti-inflammatory activity of ibuprofen may reduce fever and inflammation, thus diminishing their utility as diagnostic signs in detecting complications of presumed noninfectious noninflammatory painful conditions.

Liver Effects: As with other nonsteroidal anti-inflammatory drugs, borderline elevations of one or more liver tests may occur in up to 15% of patients. These abnormalities may progress, may remain essentially unchanged, or may be transient with continued therapy. The SGPT (ALT) test is probably the most sensitive indicator of liver dysfunction. Meaningful (3 times the upper limit of normal) elevations of SGPT or SGOT (AST) occurred in controlled clinical trials in less than 1% of patients. A patient with symptoms and/or signs suggesting liver dysfunction, or in whom an abnormal liver test has occurred, should be evaluated for evidence of the development of more severe hepatic reactions while on therapy with ibuprofen. Severe hepatic reactions, including jaundice and cases of fatal hepatitis, have been reported with ibuprofen as with other nonsteroidal anti-inflammatory drugs. Although such reactions are rare, if abnormal liver tests persist or worsen, if clinical signs and symptoms consistent with liver disease develop, or if systemic manifestations occur (e.g., eosinophilia, rash, etc.), CHILDREN'S ADVIL® SUSPENSION should be discontinued.

Hemoglobin Levels: In cross-study comparisons with doses ranging from 1200mg to 3200mg daily for several weeks, a slight dose-response decrease in hemoglobin/hematocrit was noted. This has been observed with other nonsteroidal anti-

inflammatory drugs; the mechanism is unknown. However, even with daily doses of 3200mg, the total decrease in hemoglobin usually does not exceed 1 gram; if there are no signs of bleeding, it is probably not clinically important.

In two postmarketing clinical studies with ibuprofen the incidence of a decreased hemoglobin level was greater than previously reported. Decrease in hemoglobin of 1 gram or more was observed in 17.1% of 193 patients on 1600mg ibuprofen daily (osteoarthritis), and in 22.8% of 189 patients taking 2400mg of ibuprofen daily (rheumatoid arthritis). Positive stool occult blood tests and elevated serum creatinine levels were also observed in these studies.

Aseptic Meningitis: Aseptic meningitis with fever and coma has been observed on rare occasions in patients on ibuprofen therapy. Although it is probably more likely to occur in patients with systemic lupus erythematosus and related connective tissue diseases, it has been reported in patients who do not have an underlying chronic disease. If signs or symptoms of meningitis develop in a patient on CHILDREN'S ADVIL® SUSPENSION, the possibility of its being related to ibuprofen should be considered.

Renal Effects: As with other nonsteroidal anti-inflammatory drugs, long-term administration of ibuprofen to animals has resulted in renal papillary necrosis and other abnormal renal pathology. In humans, there have been reports of acute interstitial nephritis with hematuria, proteinuria, and occasionally nephrotic syndrome.

A second form of renal toxicity has been seen in patients with prerenal conditions leading to a reduction in renal blood flow or blood volume, where the renal prostaglandins have a supportive role in the maintenance of renal perfusion. In these patients administration of a nonsteroidal anti-inflammatory drug may cause a dose dependent reduction in prostaglandin formation and may precipitate overt renal decompensation. Patients at greatest risk of this reaction are those with impaired renal function, heart failure, liver dysfunction, those taking diuretics and the elderly. Discontinuation of nonsteroidal anti-inflammatory drug therapy is typically followed by recovery to the pretreatment state.

Those patients at high risk who chronically take ibuprofen should have renal function monitored if they have signs or symptoms which may be consistent with mild azotemia, such as malaise, fatigue, loss of appetite, etc. Occasional patients may develop some elevation of serum creatinine and BUN levels without signs or symptoms.

Since ibuprofen is eliminated primarily by the kidneys, patients with significantly impaired renal function should be closely monitored, and a reduction in dosage should be anticipated to avoid drug accumulation. Prospective studies on the safety of ibuprofen in patients with chronic renal failure have not been conducted.

Information for Patients: Ibuprofen, like other drugs of its class, is not free of side effects. The side effects of these drugs can cause discomfort and, rarely, there are more serious side effects, such as gastrointestinal bleeding, which may result in hospitalization and even fatal outcomes. NSAIDs (Nonsteroidal Anti-Inflammatory Drugs) are often essential agents in the management of arthritis and have a major role in the treatment of pain, but they also may be commonly employed for conditions which are less serious. Physicians may wish to discuss with their patients the potential risks (see **WARNINGS, PRECAUTIONS,** and **ADVERSE REACTIONS**) and likely benefits of NSAID treatment, particularly when the drugs are used for less serious conditions where treatment without NSAIDs may represent an acceptable alternative to both the patient and physician.

Laboratory Tests: Because serious GI tract ulceration and bleeding can occur without warning symptoms, physicians should follow chronically treated patients for the signs and symptoms of ulceration and bleeding and should inform them of the importance of this follow-up (see **WARNINGS**).

Drug Interactions: Coumarin-type anticoagulants. Several short-term controlled studies failed to show that ibuprofen significantly affected prothrombin times or a variety of other clotting factors when administered to individuals on coumarin-type anticoagulants. However, because bleeding has been reported when ibuprofen and other nonsteroidal anti-inflammatory agents have been administered to patients on coumarin-type anticoagulants, the physician should be cautious when administering CHILDREN'S ADVIL® SUSPENSION to patients on anticoagulants.

Aspirin: Animal studies show that aspirin given with nonsteroidal anti-inflammatory agents, including ibuprofen, yields a net decrease in anti-inflammatory activity with lowered blood levels of the non-aspirin drug. Single dose bioavailability studies in normal volunteers have failed to show an effect of aspirin on ibuprofen blood levels. Correlative clinical studies have not been performed.

Methotrexate: Ibuprofen, as well as other nonsteroidal anti-inflammatory drugs, has been reported to competitively inhibit methotrexate accumulation in rabbit kidney slices. This may indicate that ibuprofen could enhance the toxicity of methotrexate. Caution should be used if CHILDREN'S

Continued on next page

Whitehall—Cont.

ADVIL® SUSPENSION is administered concomitantly with methotrexate.

H-2 Antagonists: In studies with human volunteers, co-administration of cimetidine or ranitidine with ibuprofen had no substantive effect on ibuprofen serum concentrations.

Furosemide: Clinical studies, as well as random observations, have shown that ibuprofen can reduce the natriuretic effect of furosemide and thiazides in some patients. This response has been attributed to inhibition of renal prostaglandin synthesis. During concomitant therapy with ibuprofen, patients should be observed closely for signs of renal failure (See **PRECAUTIONS, Renal Effects**), as well as to assure diuretic efficacy.

Lithium: Ibuprofen produced an elevation of plasma lithium levels and a reduction in renal lithium clearance in a study of eleven normal volunteers. The mean minimum lithium concentration increased 15% and the renal clearance of lithium was decreased by 19% during this period of concomitant drug administration. This effect has been attributed to inhibition of renal prostaglandin synthesis by ibuprofen. Thus, when ibuprofen and lithium are administered concurrently, patients should be observed carefully for signs of lithium toxicity. (Read package insert for lithium preparation before use of such concurrent therapy.)

Diabetes: Each 5mL of CHILDREN'S ADVIL® SUSPENSION contians approximately 2.5g of sucrose, which should be taken into consideration when treating patients with impaired glucose tolerance. It also contains 350mg of sorbitol per 5mL. Although in clinical trials CHILDREN'S ADVIL® SUSPENSION was not associated with more diarrhea than control treatments, should a patient develop diarrhea, the physician may wish to review the patient's dietary intake of sorbitol from other sources.

Pregnancy. Reproductive studies conducted in rats and rabbits at doses somewhat less than the maximal clinical dose did not demonstrate evidence of developmental abnormalities. However, animal reproduction studies are not always predictive of human response. As there are no adequate and well-controlled studies in pregnant women, this drug should be used during pregnancy only if clearly needed. Because of the known effects of nonsteroidal anti-inflammatory drugs on the fetal cardiovascular system (closure of ductus arteriosus), use during late pregnancy should be avoided. As with other drugs known to inhibit prostaglandin synthesis, an increased incidence of dystocia and delayed parturition occurred in rats. Administration of CHILDREN'S ADVIL® SUSPENSION is not recommended during pregnancy.

Nursing Mothers: In limited studies, an assay capable of detecting 1mcg/mL did not demonstrate ibuprofen in the milk of lactating mothers. However, because of the limited nature of the studies, and the possible adverse effects of prostaglandin-inhibiting drugs on neonates, CHILDREN'S ADVIL® SUSPENSION is not recommended for use by nursing mothers.

Infants: Safety and efficacy of CHILDREN'S ADVIL® SUSPENSION in children below the age of 12 months has not been established.

ADVERSE REACTIONS

The most frequent type of adverse reaction occurring with ibuprofen is gastrointestinal. In controlled clinical trials, the percentage of adult patients reporting one or more gastrointestinal complaints ranged from 4% to 16%.

In controlled studies in adults when ibuprofen was compared to aspirin and indomethacin in equally effective doses, the overall incidence of gastrointestinal complaints was about half that seen in either the aspirin- or indomethacin-treated patients.

In a 12-week comparison of CHILDREN'S ADVIL® SUSPENSION (n=45) and aspirin (n=47) in children with juvenile arthritis, the most common adverse experiences were also gastrointestinal in nature, usually of mild severity. Abdominal pain of possible drug relationship was reported in about 25% of patients on ibuprofen and/or aspirin; other possibly drug-related effects associated with the digestive system were reported in 42% of the children taking ibuprofen and in 70% of those taking aspirin.

Adverse reactions observed during controlled clinical trials in adults at an incidence greater than 1% are listed in the table. Those reactions listed in column one encompass observations in approximately 3,000 adult patients. More than 500 of these patients were treated for periods of at least 54 weeks.

Still other reactions occurring less frequently than 1 in 100 were reported in controlled clinical trials and from marketing experience. These reactions have been divided into two categories: column two of the table lists reactions with therapy with ibuprofen where the probability of a causal relationship exists; for the reactions in column three, a causal relationship with ibuprofen has not been established.

Reported side effects were higher at doses of 3200mg/day than at doses of 2400mg or less per day in clinical trials of adults patients with rheumatoid arthritis. The increases in incidence were slight and still within the ranges reported in the table below.

[See table below].

OVERDOSAGE

Approximately 1½ hours after the reported ingestion of from 7 to 10 ibuprofen tablets (400mg), a 19-month old child weighing 12 kg was seen in the hospital emergency room, apneic and cyanotic, responding only to painful stimuli. This type of stimulus, however, was sufficient to induce respiration. Oxygen and parenteral fluids were given; a greenish-yellow fluid was aspirated from the stomach with no evidence to indicate the presence of ibuprofen. Two hours after ingestion the child's condition seemed stable; she still responded only to painful stimuli and continued to have periods of apnea lasting from 5 to 10 seconds. She was admitted to intensive care and sodium bicarbonate was administered as well as infusions of dextrose and normal saline. By four hours post-ingestion she could be aroused easily, sit by herself and respond to spoken commands. Blood level of ibuprofen was 102.9 mcg/mL approximately 8½ hours after accidental ingestion. At 12 hours she appeared to be completely recovered.

In two other reported cases where children (each weighing approximately 10kg) accidentally, acutely ingested approximately 120mg/kg, there were no signs of acute intoxication or late sequelae. Blood level in one child 90 minutes after

Children's Advil® (ibuprofen) Suspension Incidence Greater than 1% (but less than 3%) Probable Causal Relationship	Precise Incidence Unknown (but less than 1%) Probable Causal Relationship**	Precise Incidence Unknown (but less than 1%) Causal Relationship Unknown**
GASTROINTESTINAL Nausea*, epigastric pain*, heartburn*, diarrhea, abdominal distress, nausea and vomiting, indigestion, constipation, abdominal cramps or pain, fullness of GI tract (bloating and flatulence)	Gastric or duodenal ulcer with bleeding and/or perforation, gastrointestinal hemorrhage, melena, gastritis, hepatitis, jaundice, abnormal liver function tests; pancreatitis	
CENTRAL NERVOUS SYSTEM Dizziness*, headache, nervousness	Depression, insomnia, confusion, emotional lability, somnolence, aseptic meningitis with fever and coma	Paresthesias, hallucinations, dream abnormalities, pseudo-tumor cerebri
DERMATOLOGIC Rash* (including maculopapular type), pruritus	Vesiculobullous eruptions, urticaria, erythema multiforme, Stevens-Johnson syndrome, alopecia	Toxic epidermal necrolysis, photoallergic skin reactions
SPECIAL SENSES Tinnitus	Hearing loss, amblyopia (blurred and/or diminished vision, scotomata and/or changes in color vision) (see PRECAUTIONS)	Conjunctivitis, diplopia, optic neuritis, cataracts
HEMATOLOGIC	Neutropenia, agranulocytosis, aplastic anemia, hemolytic anemia (sometimes Coombs positive), thrombocytopenia with or without purpura, eosinophilia, decreases in hemoglobin and hematocrit (see PRECAUTIONS)	Bleeding episodes (eg epistaxis, menorrhagia)
METABOLIC/ENDOCRINE Decreased appetite		Gynecomastia, hypoglycemic reaction, acidosis
CARDIOVASCULAR Edema, fluid retention (generally responds promptly to drug discontinuation; see PRECAUTIONS)	Congestive heart failure in patients with marginal cardiac function, elevated blood pressure, palpitations	Arrhythmias (sinus tachycardia, sinus bradycardia)
ALLERGIC	Syndrome of abdominal pain, fever, chills, nausea and vomiting; anaphylaxis; bronchospasm (see CONTRAINDICATIONS)	Serum sickness, lupus erythematosus syndrome, Henoch-Schönlein vasculitis, angioedema
RENAL	Acute renal failure (see PRECAUTIONS), decreased creatinine clearance, polyuria, azotemia, cystitis, hematuria	Renal papillary necrosis
MISCELLANEOUS	Dry eyes and mouth, gingival ulcer, rhinitis	

*Reactions occurring in 3% to 9% of adult patients treated with ibuprofen. (Those reactions occurring in less than 3% of the patients are unmarked).

**Reactions are classified under "*Probable Causal Relationship (PCR)*" if there has been one positive rechallenge or if three or more cases occur which might be causally related. Reactions are classified under "*Causal Relationship Unknown*" if seven or more events have been reported but the criteria for PCR have not been met.

ingestion was 700 mcg/mL, about 10 times the peak levels seen in absorption-excretion studies.

A 19-year old male who had taken 8,000mg of ibuprofen over a period of a few hours complained of dizziness, and nystagmus was noted. After hospitalization, parenteral hydration and three days' bed rest, he recovered with no reported sequelae.

In cases of acute overdosage, the stomach should be emptied by vomiting or lavage, though little drug will likely be recovered if more than an hour has elapsed since ingestion. Because the drug is acidic and is excreted in the urine, it is theoretically beneficial to administer alkali and induce diuresis. In addition to supportive measures the use of oral activated charcoal may help to reduce the absorption and reabsorption of ibuprofen.

DOSAGE AND ADMINISTRATION

Shake well prior to administration.

Do not exceed 3200mg total daily dose. If gastrointestinal complaints occur, administer ibuprofen with meals or milk.

Juvenile Arthritis: The usual dose is 30 to 40mg/kg/day divided into 3 or 4 doses. Patients with milder disease may be adequately treated with 20mg/kg/day.

Doses above 50mg/kg/day are nor recommended because they have not been studied and because side effects appear to be dose related.

Therapeutic response may require from a few days to several weeks to be achieved. Once a clinical response is obtained, dosage can be lowered to the smallest dose of CHILDREN'S ADVIL® SUSPENSION needed to maintain adequate control of disease.

Rheumatoid arthritis and osteoarthritis, including flare-ups of chronic disease: Suggested Adult Dosage: 1200–3200mg daily (300mg qid, or 400mg, 600mg or 800mg t.i.d. or q.i.d.). Individual patients may show a better response to 3200mg daily, as compared with 2400mg, although in well-controlled clinical trials patients on 3200mg did not show a better mean response in terms of efficacy. Therefore, when treating patients with 3200mg/day, the physician should observe sufficient increased clinical benefits to offset potential increased risk.

The dose of CHILDREN'S ADVIL® SUSPENSION should be tailored to each patient, and may be lowered or raised from the suggested doses depending on the severity of symptoms either at the time of initiating drug therapy or as the patient responds or fails to respond.

In general, patients with rheumatoid arthritis seem to require higher doses of ibuprofen than do patients with osteoarthritis.

The smallest dose of CHILDREN'S ADVIL® SUSPENSION that yields acceptable control should be employed. A linear blood level dose-response relationship exists with single doses up to 800mg (see CLINICAL PHARMACOLOGY, **Pharmacokinetics** for effects of food on rate of absorption). In chronic conditions, a therapeutic response to ibuprofen therapy is sometimes seen in a few days to a week but most often is observed by two weeks. After a satisfactory response has been achieved, the patient's dose should be reviewed and adjusted as required.

Mild to moderate pain: 400mg every 4 to 6 hours as necessary for relief of pain in adults.

In controlled analgesic clinical trials, doses of ibuprofen greater than 400mg were no more effective than the 400mg dose.

Dysmenorrhea: For the treatment of dysmenorrhea, beginning with the earliest onset of such pain, CHILDREN'S ADVIL® SUSPENSION should be given in a dose of 400mg every 4 hours as necessary for the relief of pain.

FEVER REDUCTION IN CHILDREN 12 months to 12 years of age: Dosage should be adjusted on the basis of the initial temperature level (see CLINICAL PHARMACOLOGY for a description of the controlled clinical trial results). The recommended dose is 5mg/kg if the baseline temperature is 102.5°F or below or 10mg/kg if the baseline temperature is greater than 102.5°F. The duration of fever reduction is generally 6–8 hours and is longer with the higher dose. The recommended maximum daily dose is 40mg/kg.

Age	Weight (lb)	5mg/kg (Fever ≤102.5°F) (mg)	(tsp)	10mg/kg (Fever >102.5°F) (mg)	(tsp)
12–23 mos	18–23	50	½	100	1
2–3 yrs	24–35	75	¾	150	1½
4–5 yrs	36–47	100	1	200	2
6–8 yrs	48–59	125	1¼	250	2½
9–10 yrs	60–71	150	1½	300	3
11–12 yrs	72–95	200	2	400	4

FEVER REDUCTION IN ADULTS: 400mg every 4–6 hours as necessary.

HOW SUPPLIED

CHILDREN'S ADVIL® SUSPENSION is supplied as a sucrose-sweetened, fruit-flavored, aqueous suspension of ibuprofen 100mg/5mL in 4 and 16-ounce (119 and 473mL) bottles.

4 Ounce Bottles	NDC 0573-0710-20
16 Ounce Bottles	NDC 0573-0170-40

CHILDREN'S ADVIL® SUSPENSION should be stored at room temperature; 15°C to 30°C (59°F to 86°F).

Shake well before use. Keep container tightly closed.

Caution: Federal law prohibits dispensing without prescription.

Manufactured by:
WHITEHALL LABORATORIES INC.
New York, N.Y. 10017

Rev. 9/7/89

Shown in Product Identification Section, page 435

ADVIL®
Ibuprofen Tablets, USP
Ibuprofen Caplets
Pain Reliever/Fever Reducer

WARNING

ASPIRIN SENSITIVE PATIENTS. Do not take this product if you have had a severe allergic reaction to aspirin, e.g. —asthma, swelling, shock or hives, because even though this product contains no aspirin or salicylates, cross-reactions may occur in patients allergic to aspirin.

INDICATIONS

For the temporary relief of minor aches and pains associated with the common cold, headache, toothache, muscular aches, backache, for the minor pain of arthritis, for the pain of menstrual cramps and for reduction of fever.

DOSAGE AND ADMINISTRATION

Adults: Take one tablet every 4 to 6 hours while symptoms persist. If pain or fever does not respond to one tablet, two tablets may be used but do not exceed six tablets in 24 hours unless directed by a doctor. The smallest effective dose should be used. Take with food or milk if occasional and mild heartburn, upset stomach, or stomach pain occurs with use. Consult a doctor if these symptoms are more than mild or if they persist. Children: Do not give this product to children under 12 except under the advice and supervision of a doctor.

WARNINGS

Do not take for pain for more than 10 days or for fever for more than 3 days unless directed by a doctor. If pain or fever persists or gets worse, if new symptoms occur, or if the painful area is red or swollen, consult a doctor. These could be signs of serious illness. If you are under a doctor's care for any serious condition, consult a doctor before taking this product. As with aspirin and acetaminophen, if you have any condition which requires you to take prescription drugs or if you have had any problems or serious side effects from taking any non-prescription pain reliever, do not take this product without first discussing it with your doctor. If you experience any symptoms which are unusual or seem unrelated to the condition for which you took ibuprofen, consult a doctor before taking any more of it. Although ibuprofen is indicated for the same conditions as aspirin and acetaminophen, it should not be taken with them except under a doctor's direction. Do not combine this product with any other ibuprofen-containing product. As with any drug, if you are pregnant or nursing a baby, seek the advice of a health professional before using this product. IT IS ESPECIALLY IMPORTANT NOT TO USE IBUPROFEN DURING THE LAST 3 MONTHS OF PREGNANCY UNLESS SPECIFICALLY DIRECTED TO DO SO BY A DOCTOR BECAUSE IT MAY CAUSE PROBLEMS IN THE UNBORN CHILD OR COMPLICATIONS DURING DELIVERY.

Keep this and all drugs out of the reach of children. In case of accidental overdose, seek professional assistance or contact a poison control center immediately.

ACTIVE INGREDIENT

Each tablet contains Ibuprofen 200 mg.

INACTIVE INGREDIENTS

Acacia, Acetylated Monoglycerides, Beeswax or Carnauba Wax, Calcium Sulfate, Colloidal Silicon Dioxide, Dimethicone, Iron Oxide, Lecithin, Pharmaceutical Glaze, Povidone, Sodium Benzoate, Sodium Carboxymethylcellulose, Starch, Stearic Acid, Sucrose, Titanium Dioxide.

PROFESSIONAL LABELING

Same as stated under Indications.

HOW SUPPLIED

Coated tablets in bottles of 8, 24, 50, 100, 165 and 250.
Coated caplets in bottles of 8, 24, 50, 100 and 165.
Coated tablets in thermoform packaging of 8.

STORAGE

Store at room temperature; avoid excessive heat 40°C (104°F).

Shown in Product Identification Section, page 435

ANACIN®
[an 'a-sin]
Analgesic Coated Tablets and Coated Caplets

DESCRIPTION

Each tablet or caplet contains: Aspirin 400 mg., Caffeine 32 mg. Anacin® has a special protective coating that makes each tablet or caplet easy to swallow.

INDICATIONS AND ACTIONS

Anacin provides relief from the pain of headaches, neuralgia, neuritis, sprains, muscular aches, sinus pressure. . . discomforts and fever of colds. . . pain caused by tooth extraction and toothache. . . menstrual discomfort. Anacin also temporarily relieves the minor aches and pains of arthritis and rheumatism.

WARNINGS

Children and teenagers should not use this medicine for chicken pox or flu symptoms before a doctor is consulted about Reye syndrome, a rare but serious illness reported to be associated with aspirin. As with any drug, if you are pregnant or nursing a baby, seek the advice of a health professional before using this product. Keep this and all medicines out of children's reach. In case of accidental overdose, contact a physician immediately.

PRECAUTIONS

If pain persists for more than 10 days, or redness is present, or in arthritic or rheumatic conditions affecting children under 12 years of age, consult a physician immediately.

DOSAGE AND ADMINISTRATION

Two tablets or caplets with water every 4 hours as needed. Do not exceed 10 tablets or 10 caplets daily. For children 6–12, administer half the adult dosage.

INACTIVE INGREDIENTS

Tablets contain Hydroxypropyl Methylcellulose, Microcrystalline Cellulose, Polyethylene Glycol, Starch, Surfactant. Caplets contain Hydroxypropyl Methylcellulose, Iron Oxide, Microcrystalline Cellulose, Polyethylene Glycol, Starch, Surfactant.

HOW SUPPLIED

Tablets: In tins of 12's and bottles of 30's, 50's, 100's, 200's and 300's. Caplets: In bottles of 30's, 50's and 100's. Professional Samples: Available upon request. Write Whitehall Laboratories, New York, New York 10017.

Shown in Product Identification Section, page 435

Children's
ANACIN–3®
[an 'a-sin thre]
Acetaminophen
Chewable Tablets, Liquid
Infants'
ANACIN–3®
Acetaminophen Drops

DESCRIPTION

Chewable Tablets: Each Children's ANACIN-3 Chewable Tablet is cherry flavored and contains 80 mg acetaminophen.

Liquid: Children's Anacin-3 Liquid is stable, cherry flavored, red in color. It contains no alcohol or saccharin. Each 5 mL contains 160 mg of acetaminophen.

Infants' Drops: Infant Anacin-3 Drops are stable, fruit flavored, red in color and contain no alcohol. Each 0.8 mL (one calibrated dropperful) contains 80 mg acetaminophen.

ACTIONS

Children's Anacin-3 Chewable Tablets, Liquid and Infants' Drops are safe and effective 100% aspirin-free products designed for treatment of infants and children with conditions requiring reduction of fever or relief of pain.

INDICATIONS

Children's Anacin-3 is used for the treatment of fever and pain which may accompany conditions such as mild upper respiratory infections (tonsillitis, common cold, "grippe"), headache, myalgia, post-immunization reactions, post-tonsillectomy discomfort and gastroenteritis. Anacin-3 acetaminophen is useful as an analgesic and antipyretic in many bacterial or viral infections, such as bronchitis, pharyngitis, tracheobronchitis, sinusitis, pneumonia, otitis media and cervical adenitis, and can be used in conjunction with antibiotics.

PRECAUTIONS

If fever persists for more than 3 days or recurs, or if pain continues for more than 5 days, consult your physician immediately.

Phenylketonurics: tablets contain Phenylalanine 3.1 mg per tablet.

Continued on next page

Whitehall—Cont.

WARNINGS

Keep this and all medicines out of the reach of children. In case of accidental overdose contact a physician immediately.

DOSAGE AND ADMINISTRATION

All dosages may be repeated every 4 hours. Do not exceed 5 dosages in any 24 hour period.

		DOSE	
Age (yr)	Wt (lb)	Tablet	Liquid
1–2	18–23	1–1½	¾ teaspoon
2–3	24–35	2	1 "
4–5	36–47	3	1½ "
6–8	48–59	4	2 "
9–10	60–71	5	2½ "
11–12	72–95	6	3 "

Infants' Anacin-3 Drops: 0–3 months, 6 to 11 lbs: one-half dropperful. 4–11 months, 12 to 17 lbs: one dropperful. 12–23 months, 18 to 23 lbs: one and one-half droppersful. 2–3 years, 24 to 35 lbs: 2 droppersful. 4–5 years, 36 to 47 lbs: 3 droppersful.

OVERDOSAGE

Acetaminophen in massive overdosage may cause hepatic toxicity in some patients. In all cases of suspected overdose, immediately call your regional poison center for assistance in diagnosis and for directions in the use of N-acetylcysteine as an antidote. Adverse effects are rare when acetaminophen is used as recommended.

INACTIVE INGREDIENTS

Chewable Tablets: Aspartame, Cetyl Alcohol, Colloidal Silicon Dioxide, Dibutyl Sebacate, Ethyl Cellulose, FD&C Red No. 40 Lake, Flavor, Hydrogenated Vegetable Oil, Magnesium Stearate, Mannitol, Microcrystalline Cellulose, Simethicone, Sucrose and Surfactant.
Liquid: Citric Acid, D&C Red No. 33, Disodium Edetate, FD&C Red No. 40, Flavor, Glycerin, Methylparaben, Polyethylene Glycol, Propylene Glycol, Sorbitol, Sodium Benzoate, Sucrose and Water.
Infant Drops: FD&C Red No. 40, FD&C Yellow No. 6, Flavors, Glycerin, Polyethylene Glycol, Propylene Glycol, Saccharin, Sodium Benzoate, Sorbitol and Water.

HOW SUPPLIED

Chewable Tablets (colored pink, scored, imprinted "CHILDREN A-3")—Bottles of 30. Liquid (colored red)—bottles of 2 and 4 fl. oz. Drops (colored red)—bottles of ½ oz. (15 mL.) with calibrated plastic dropper.
All packages listed above have child-resistant safety caps and tamper resistant packaging.

Shown in Product Identification Section, page 435

MAXIMUM STRENGTH ANACIN®
Analgesic Coated Tablets

DESCRIPTION

Each tablet contains: Aspirin 500 mg, Caffeine 32 mg.

INDICATIONS AND ACTIONS

Maximum Strength Anacin provides fast relief from the pain of headaches, neuralgia, neuritis, sprains, muscular aches, sinus pressure... discomforts and fever of colds... pain caused by tooth extraction and toothache... menstrual discomfort. Maximum Strength Anacin also temporarily relieves the minor aches and pains of arthritis and rheumatism.

WARNINGS

Children and teenagers should not use this medicine for chicken pox or flu symptoms before a doctor is consulted about Reye syndrome, a rare but serious illness reported to be associated with aspirin. As with any drug, if you are pregnant or nursing a baby, seek the advice of a health professional before using this product. Keep this and all medicines out of children's reach. In case of accidental overdose, contact a physician immediately.

PRECAUTIONS

If pain persists for more than 10 days, or redness is present, or in arthritic or rheumatic conditions affecting children under 12 years of age, consult a physician immediately.

DOSAGE AND ADMINISTRATION

Adults: Two tablets with water 3 or 4 times a day. Do not exceed 8 tablets in any 24-hour period. Not recommended for children under 12 years of age.

INACTIVE INGREDIENTS

Tablets contain Hydroxypropyl Methylcellulose, Microcrystalline Cellulose, Polyethylene Glycol, Starch, Surfactant.

HOW SUPPLIED

Tablets: Tins of 12's and bottles of 20's, 40's, 75's and 150's.
Shown in Product Identification Section, page 435

Maximum Strength
ANACIN-3®
[an 'a-sin thre]
Film Coated Acetaminophen Tablets and Caplets

Regular Strength
ANACIN-3®
Film Coated Acetaminophen Tablets

DESCRIPTION

Maximum Strength Tablets and Caplets: Each film coated tablet and caplet contains acetaminophen 500 mg.
Regular Strength Tablets: Each film coated tablet contains acetaminophen 325 mg.

INDICATIONS AND ACTIONS

Anacin-3 is a safe and effective 100% aspirin-free analgesic product that acts fast to provide temporary relief from pain of headache, colds or "flu", sinusitis, muscle aches, bursitis, sprains, overexertion, backache, menstrual discomfort, minor arthritis pain, toothaches and to reduce fever.

WARNINGS

Keep this and all medicines out of children's reach. In case of accidental overdose, contact a physician immediately. As with any drug, if you are pregnant or nursing a baby, seek the advice of a health professional before using this product.

PRECAUTIONS

If pain persists for more than 10 days or redness is present or in arthritic or rheumatic conditions affecting children under 12, consult a physician immediately.

DOSAGE AND ADMINISTRATION

Maximum Strength—Adults: Two tablets or caplets 3 or 4 times a day. Do not exceed 8 tablets or caplets in any 24-hour period. Regular Strength—Adults: 2 or 3 tablets every 4 hours not to exceed 12 tablets in a 24-hour period. Children (6-12): ½ to 1 tablet 3 to 4 times daily. Consult a physician for use by children under 6 or for use longer than 10 days.

OVERDOSAGE

Acetaminophen in massive overdosage may cause hepatic toxicity in some patients. In all cases of suspected overdose, immediately call your regional poison center for assistance in diagnosis and for directions in the use of N-acetylcysteine as an antidote. Adverse effects are rare when acetaminophen is used as recommended.

INACTIVE INGREDIENTS

Maximum and Regular Strength Tablets:
Calcium Stearate, Croscarmellose Sodium, FD&C Blue No. 1 Lake, Hydroxypropyl Methylcellulose, Microcrystalline Cellulose, Polyethylene Glycol, Povidone, Propylene Gylcol, Starch, Stearic Acid and Titanium Dioxide.
Maximum Strength Caplets:
Calcium Stearate, Croscarmellose Sodium, D&C Red No. 7 Lake, FD&C Blue No. 1 Lake, Hydroxypropyl Methylcellulose, Microcrystalline Cellulose, Polyethylene Glycol, Povidone, Propylene Glycol, Starch, Stearic Acid and Titanium Dioxide.

HOW SUPPLIED

Maximum Strength Film Coated—Tablets (colored white, imprinted "A-3" and "500")—tins of 12 and bottles of 30, 60, and 100: Caplets (colored white, imprinted "Anacin-3")—bottles of 24's, 50's, and 100's. Regular Strength Film Coated—Tablets (colored white, scored, imprinted "A-3") in bottles of 24, 50, and 100.
Shown in Product Identification Section, page 435

Maximum Strength
ANBESOL® Gel and Liquid
Antiseptic Anesthetic
Regular Strength
ANBESOL® Gel and Liquid
Antiseptic Anesthetic
[an 'ba-sol "]

DESCRIPTION

Anbesol is an antiseptic-anesthetic which is available in a Maximum Strength and Regular Strength gel and liquid product.
The Maximum Strength formulations contain Benzocaine 20% and Alcohol 60%.
The Regular Strength formulations contain Benzocaine 6.3%, Phenol 0.5%, and Alcohol 70%.

INDICATIONS

Maximum Strength and Regular Strength Anbesol are indicated for the fast temporary relief of pain due to toothache, braces, denture and orthodontic irritation, sore gums, cold and canker sores and fever blisters. Regular Strength Anbesol is also indicated for the fast temporary relief of teething pain.

ACTIONS

Temporarily deadens sensations of nerve endings to provide relief of pain and discomfort; reduces oral bacterial flora temporarily as an aid in oral hygiene.

WARNINGS

Flammable. Keep away from fire or flame. Avoid smoking during application and until product has dried. Do not use near eyes. Keep this and all medicines out of the reach of children.

PRECAUTIONS

Not for prolonged use. If the condition persists or irritation develops, discontinue use and consult a physician or dentist. Not for use under dental work.

DOSAGE AND ADMINISTRATION

Apply topically to the affected area on or around the lips, or within the mouth. FOR DENTURE IRRITATION: Apply thin layer of gel to affected area and do not reinsert dental work until irritation/pain is relieved. Rinse mouth before reinserting dentures. If irritation/pain persists, contact a physician.

INACTIVE INGREDIENTS

Maximum Strength Gel: Carbomer 934P, D&C Yellow #10, FD&C Red #40, Flavor, Polyethylene Glycol, Saccharin. Maximum Strength Liquid: D&C Yellow #10, FD&C Red #40, Flavor, Polyethylene Glycol, Saccharin. Regular Gel: Carbomer 934P, D&C Red #33, Yellow #10, FD&C Blue #1, Yellow #6, Flavor, Glycerin. Regular Liquid: Camphor, Glycerin, Menthol, Potassium Iodide, Povidone Iodine.

HOW SUPPLIED

Maximum Strength Gel in .25 oz (7.2 gram) tube, Maximum Strength Liquid in .31 fl oz (9 mL) bottle.
Regular Gel in .25 oz. (7.2 gram) tube. Regular Liquid in two sizes—.31 fl. oz. (9 mL) and .74 fl. oz. (22 mL) bottles.
Shown in Product Identification Section, page 435

BABY ANBESOL®
[an 'ba-sol "]
Anesthetic Gel

DESCRIPTION

Baby Anbesol Gel contains Benzocaine 7.5%, a safe and effective anesthetic which soothes the sore gums of an infant by providing temporary relief from teething pain.

INDICATIONS

Baby Anbesol Gel is indicated for fast, temporary relief from the pain and irritation associated with teething.

ACTIONS

A topical anesthetic that temporarily inhibits the conduction of nerve impulses from sensory nerves in the gums to provide relief of pain and discomfort.

WARNINGS

Avoid getting into eyes. For persistent or excessive teething pain, consult a physician or dentist. Localized allergic reactions may occur after prolonged or repeated use. Keep this and all medicines out of the reach of children.

PRECAUTIONS

For persistent or excessive teething pain, consult a pediatrician.

DOSAGE AND ADMINISTRATION

Apply a small amount of Baby Anbesol on the infant's irritated gums with cotton swab or finger tip.

INACTIVE INGREDIENTS

Carbomer 934, D&C Red No. 33, Disodium Edetate, Flavor, Glycerin, Polyethylene Glycol, Saccharin, Water.

HOW SUPPLIED

Clear gel in .25 oz. (7.2 grams) tube.
Shown in Product Identification Section, page 435

ARTHRITIS PAIN FORMULA™
[ar 'thrit-is 'pān 'for-mye-la]
By the Makers of Anacin® Analgesic
Tablets

DESCRIPTION

Each caplet contains 500 mg microfined aspirin and two buffers, 27 mg Aluminum Hydroxide and 100 mg Magnesium Hydroxide. Arthritis Pain Formula is a buffered analgesic and antipyretic that is formulated with microfined aspirin, which means the aspirin particles are so fine that they dissolve more readily. The buffering agents help provide protection against stomach upset that could be associated with large antiarthritic doses of aspirin.

INDICATIONS AND ACTIONS

Arthritis Pain Formula provides hours of relief from minor aches and pain of arthritis and rheumatism and low back pain. Also relieves the pain of headache, neuralgia, neuritis, sprains, muscular aches, discomforts and fever of colds, pain caused by tooth extraction and toothache, and menstrual discomfort.

WARNINGS
Children and teenagers should not use this medicine for chicken pox or flu symptoms before a doctor is consulted about Reye syndrome, a rare but serious illness reported to be associated with aspirin.

As with any drug, if you are pregnant or nursing a baby, seek the advice of a health professional before using this product. Keep this and all medications out of children's reach. In case of accidental overdose, contact a physician immediately.

PRECAUTIONS
If pain persists for more than 10 days, or redness is present or in arthritic or rheumatic conditions affecting children under 12, consult a physician immediately.

DOSAGE AND ADMINISTRATION
Adult Dosage: 2 caplets, 3 or 4 times a day. Do not exceed 8 caplets in any 24-hour period. For children under 12, consult a physician.

INACTIVE INGREDIENTS
Hydrogenated Vegetable Oil, Microcrystalline Cellulose, Starch, Surfactant.

HOW SUPPLIED
In plastic bottles of 40, 100 and 175 caplets.
Shown in Product Identification Section, page 435

CoADVIL™
Ibuprofen/Pseudoephedrine Caplets*
Pain Reliever/Fever Reducer/Nasal Decongestant
*Oval-Shaped tablets

WARNING
ASPIRIN SENSITIVE PATIENTS. Do not take this product if you have had a severe allergic reaction to aspirin, e.g. —asthma, swelling, shock or hives, because even though this product contains no aspirin or salicylates, cross-reactions may occur in patients allergic to aspirin.

INDICATIONS
For temporary relief of symptoms associated with the common cold, sinusitis or flu including nasal congestion, headache, fever, body aches, and pains.

DIRECTIONS
Adults: Take 1 caplet every 4 to 6 hours while symptoms persist. If symptoms do not respond to 1 caplet, 2 caplets may be used but do not exceed 6 caplets in 24 hours unless directed by a doctor. The smallest effective dose should be used. Take with food or milk if occasional and mild heartburn, upset stomach, or stomach pain occurs with use. Consult a doctor if these symptoms are more than mild or if they persist. Children: Do not give this product to children under 12 years of age except under the advice and supervision of a doctor.

WARNINGS
Do not take for colds for more than 7 days or for fever for more than 3 days unless directed by a doctor. If the cold or fever persists or gets worse, or if new symptoms occur, consult a doctor. These could be signs of serious illness. As with aspirin and acetaminophen, if you have any condition which requires you to take prescription drugs or if you have had any problems or serious side effects from taking any nonprescription pain reliever, do not take this product without first discussing it with your doctor. IF YOU EXPERIENCE ANY SYMPTOMS WHICH ARE UNUSUAL OR SEEM UNRELATED TO THE CONDITION FOR WHICH YOU TOOK THIS PRODUCT, CONSULT A DOCTOR BEFORE TAKING ANY MORE OF IT. If you are under a doctor's care for any serious condition, consult a doctor before taking this product.

Do not exceed recommended dosage because at higher doses nervousness, dizziness or sleeplessness may occur. Do not take this product if you have high blood pressure, heart disease, diabetes, thyroid disease or difficulty in urination due to enlargement of the prostate gland, except under the advice and supervision of a doctor. Drug Interaction Precaution: Do not take this product if you are presently taking a prescription drug for high blood pressure or depression without first consulting your doctor. Do not combine this product with other non-prescription pain relievers. Do not combine this product with any other ibuprofen-containing product. As with any drug, if you are pregnant or nursing a baby, seek the advice of a health professional before using this product. IT IS ESPECIALLY IMPORTANT NOT TO USE THIS PRODUCT DURING THE LAST 3 MONTHS OF PREGNANCY UNLESS SPECIFICALLY DIRECTED TO DO SO BY A DOCTOR BECAUSE IT MAY CAUSE PROBLEMS IN THE UNBORN CHILD OR COMPLICATIONS DURING DELIVERY. Keep this and all drugs out of the reach of children. In case of accidental overdose, seek professional assis-

tance or contact a poison control center immediately. Store at room temperature; avoid excessive heat (40°C, 104°F).
ACTIVE INGREDIENTS: Each caplet contains Ibuprofen 200 mg and Pseudoephedrine HCl 30 mg.
INACTIVE INGREDIENTS: Carnauba or Equivalent Wax, Croscarmellose Sodium, Iron Oxides, Methylparaben, Microcrystalline Cellulose, Propylparaben, Silicon Dioxide, Sodium Benzoate, Sodium Lauryl Sulfate, Starch, Stearic Acid, Sucrose, Titanium Dioxide.

HOW SUPPLIED
CoAdvil is an oval-shaped tan-colored caplet supplied in consumer bottles of 6, 48, and 100, and Blister Packs of 20. Medical samples are available in 6's bottle and a 2's Pouch Dispenser.
Shown in Product Identification Section, page 435

COMPOUND W®
[kam-paund w]
Solution and Gel

DESCRIPTION
Compound W is a salicylic acid (17% W/W) preparation available as a solution or gel.

INDICATION
Compound W is indicated for the removal of common warts.

ACTIONS
Warts are common benign skin lesions which appear mainly on the back of hands and on fingers, but can also appear on other parts of the body. The common wart exhibits a rough, raised cauliflower-like surface. They are caused by an infectious virus which stimulates mitosis in the basal cell layer of the skin resulting in the production of elevated epithelial growths. The keratolytic action of salicylic acid in a flexible collodion vehicle causes the cornified epithelium to swell, soften, macerate and then desquamate.

WARNINGS
Highly Flammable. Keep away from fire or flame. Avoid smoking during application and until product has dried. This product should not be used by diabetics or those who have poor blood circulation as serious complications may result. Do not use on moles, birthmarks, unusual warts with hair growing from them, genital warts, or warts on the face or mucous membranes (inside mouth, nose, anus, genitals, or on lips). If pain should develop or if infection is present, consult a physician. Do not use near eyes. If product accidentally comes in contact with eyes flush with water to remove film and continue to flush with water for 15 minutes. Do not inhale. Keep bottle tightly capped. For external use only. In case of accidental ingestion, contact a physician or a Poison Control Center immediately. Keep this and all medicines out of the reach of children.

PRECAUTIONS
If redness or irritation occurs, discontinue product for 2 days and then reapply. Should stinging or irritation recur, discontinue use. Covering the treated wart with a bandage will increase effectiveness but may also increase the change of irritation. If a bandage is used, first allow the solution or gel to dry thoroughly.

DOSAGE AND ADMINISTRATION
Use on common warts once daily. 1. Soak affected area in hot water for 5 minutes. If any tissue has loosened, remove by rubbing with a washcloth or soft brush. Do not rub hard enough to cause bleeding. Dry thoroughly. 2. Using the plastic rod provided with the solution or by squeezing the tube to apply, completely cover the wart with solution or gel. To avoid irritating the skin surrounding the wart, confine the solution or gel to the wart only. To help achieve this, circle the wart with a ring of petrolatum. The area covered with the medicine will appear white. 3. Follow this procedure once daily for the next 6 to 7 days. Most warts should clear within this time period. However, if the wart still remains, continue the treatment for up to 12 weeks. If the wart shows no improvement, see a physician.

INACTIVE INGREDIENTS
Solution: Acetone Collodion, Alcohol 1.83% w/w, Camphor, Castor Oil, Ether 63.5%, Menthol, Polysorbate 80. Gel: Alcohol 67.5% by vol., Camphor, Castor Oil, Collodion, Colloidal Silicon Dioxide, Hydroxypropyl Cellulose, Hypophosphorous Acid, Polysorbate 80.

HOW SUPPLIED
Compound W is available in .31 fluid oz. clear bottles with plastic applicators. Compound W Gel is available in .25 oz. tubes. Store at room temperature.

DENOREX®
[děn'ō-reks]
Medicated Shampoo
DENOREX®
Mountain Fresh Herbal Scent
Medicated Shampoo
DENOREX®
Medicated Shampoo and Conditioner
DENOREX®
Extra Strength Medicated Shampoo

DESCRIPTION
The Shampoo (Regular and Mt. Fresh Herbal) and the Shampoo with Conditioner contain Coal Tar Solution 9.0% and Menthol 1.5%. The Extra Strength Shampoo contains Coal Tar Solution 12.5% and Menthol 1.5%.

ACTIONS
Denorex Shampoo is an antiseborrheic and antipruritic which loosens and softens scales and crusts. Coal tar helps correct abnormalities of keratinization by decreasing epidermal proliferation and dermal infiltration. Denorex also contains the antipruritic agent, menthol.

INDICATIONS
Relieves scaling, itching, and flaking of dandruff, seborrhea and psoriasis. Regular use promotes cleaner, healthier hair and scalp.

WARNINGS
For external use only. Discontinue treatment if irritation develops. Avoid contact with eyes. Keep this and all medicines out of children's reach.

DIRECTIONS
For best results, use regularly, but at least twice per week. For severe scalp problems use daily. Wet hair thoroughly and briskly massage until you obtain a rich lather. Rinse thoroughly and repeat. The scalp may tingle slightly during treatment.

INACTIVE INGREDIENTS
Shampoo: Also contains Chloroxylenol, Hydroxypropyl Methylcellulose, Lauramide DEA, Stearic Acid, TEA-Lauryl Sulfate, Water, Alcohol 7.5%.
Shampoo and Conditioner: Chloroxylenol, Citric Acid, Fragrance, Hydroxypropyl Methylcellulose, Lauramide DEA, PEG-27 Lanolin, Polyquaternium-11, TEA-Lauryl Sulfate, Water, Alcohol 7.5%.
Extra Strength: Chloroxylenol, FD&C Red #40, Fragrance, Glycol Distearate, Lauramide DEA, Methylcellulose, TEA-Lauryl Sulfate, Water, Alcohol 10.4%.

HOW SUPPLIED
Lotion: 4 oz., 8 oz. and 12 oz. bottles in Regular Scent, Mountain Fresh Herbal Scent, Shampoo and Conditioner, and Extra Strength Shampoo.
Shown in Product Identification Section, page 435

DERMOPLAST®
[der'mō-plăst]
Anesthetic Pain Relief Lotion

DESCRIPTION
Dermoplast Lotion contains benzocaine 8% and menthol 0.5%.

ACTIONS
Dermoplast is a topical anesthetic and antipruritic.

INDICATIONS
Dermoplast is indicated for the fast, temporary relief of pain and itching from sunburn, insect bites, minor cuts, abrasions, minor burns, and minor skin irritations.

WARNINGS
FOR EXTERNAL USE ONLY.
In case of accidental ingestion, seek professional assistance or contact a Poison Control Center. Avoid contact with eyes. If symptoms persist, discontinue use and consult physician. Keep this and all drugs out of the reach of children.

DIRECTIONS
Apply freely over sunburned or irritated skin. Repeat three or four times daily, as needed.

INACTIVE INGREDIENTS
Aloe Vera Gel, Carbomer 934P, Ceteth-16, Glycerin, Glyceryl Stearate, Laneth-16, Methylparaben, Oleth-16, Propylparaben, Simethicone, Steareth-16, Triethanolamine, Water.

HOW SUPPLIED
DERMOPLAST Anesthetic Pain Relief Lotion, in Net Wt 3 fl oz.

Continued on next page

Whitehall—Cont.

DERMOPLAST®
[der 'mō-plăst]
Anesthetic Pain Relief Spray

DESCRIPTION
DERMOPLAST is an aerosol containing benzocaine 20% and menthol 0.5%.

INDICATIONS
DERMOPLAST is indicated for the fast, temporary relief of skin pain and itching due to sunburn, minor cuts, insect bites, abrasions, minor burns, and minor skin irritations. May be applied without touching sensitive affected areas. Used in hospitals for pain and itch of episiotomy, pruritus vulvae and postpartum hemorrhoids.

WARNINGS
FOR EXTERNAL USE ONLY. Avoid spraying in eyes. Contents under pressure. Do not puncture or incinerate. Do not use near open flame. Use only as directed. Intentional misuse by deliberately concentrating and inhaling the contents can be harmful or fatal.
Do not take orally. Not for prolonged use. If the condition for which this preparation is used persists, or if a rash or irritation develops, discontinue use and consult physician.

DIRECTIONS FOR USE
Hold can in a comfortable position, 6-12 inches away from affected area. Point spray nozzle and press button. To apply to face, spray in palm of hand. May be administered three or four times daily, or as directed by physician.

INACTIVE INGREDIENTS
Acetylated Lanolin Alcohol, Aloe Vera Oil, Butane, Cetyl Acetate, Hydrofluorocarbon, Methylparaben, PEG-8 Laurate, Polysorbate 85.

HOW SUPPLIED
DERMOPLAST Anesthetic Pain Relief Spray, in Net Wt 2 oz (57 g) and Net Wt 2¾ oz (78 g).
Do not expose to heat or temperatures above 120°F.

DRISTAN®
[drĭs 'tăn]
Nasal Spray
DRISTAN®
Menthol Nasal Spray

DESCRIPTION
Dristan Nasal Spray contains Phenylephrine HCl 0.5%, Pheniramine Maleate 0.2%.

ACTIONS
Phenylephrine HCl is a sympathomimetic agent that constricts the smaller arterioles of the nasal passages producing a gentle and predictable decongesting effect. Pheniramine Maleate is an antihistamine that controls rhinorrhea, sneezing, and lacrimation associated with elevated histamine levels in disorders of the respiratory tract.

INDICATIONS
Dristan Nasal Spray provides prompt temporary relief of nasal congestion due to colds, sinusitis, hay fever or other upper respiratory allergies.

WARNINGS
Do not exceed recommended dosage because symptoms may occur such as burning, stinging, sneezing, or increase of nasal discharge. Do not use this product for more than 3 days. If symptoms persist, consult a physician. The use of this dispenser by more than one person may spread infection. For adult use only. Do not give this product to children under 12 years except under the advice and supervision of a physician. Keep these and all medicines out of children's reach. In case of accidental ingestion, seek professional assistance or contact a Poison Control Center immediately.

DOSAGE AND ADMINISTRATION
(Squeeze bottle) with head upright, insert nozzle in nostril. Spray quickly, firmly and sniff deeply. (Metered Dose Pump) prime the metered dose pump by depressing pump firmly several times. With head upright, insert nozzle in nostril. Depress pump 2 or 3 times, all the way down, with a firm even stroke and sniff deeply. Adults: Spray 2 or 3 times into each nostril. Repeat every 4 hours as needed. Children under 12 years: As directed by a physician.

INACTIVE INGREDIENTS
Dristan Nasal Spray: Benzalkonium Chloride 1:5000 in buffered isotonic aqueous solution, Eucalyptol, Hydroxypropyl Methylcellulose, Menthol, Sodium Chloride, Sodium Phosphate, Thimerosal 0.002%, Water, and Alcohol 0.4%.
Dristan Menthol Nasal Spray: Benzalkonium Chloride 1:5000 in buffered isotonic aqueous solution, Camphor, Eucalyptol, Hydroxypropyl Methylcellulose, Menthol, Methyl

Salicylate; Polysorbate 80, Sodium Chloride, Sodium Phosphate, Thimerosal 0.002% and Water.

HOW SUPPLIED
Dristan Nasal Spray: 15 mL and 30 mL plastic squeeze bottles, and 15 mL metered dose pumps.
Dristan Menthol Nasal Spray: 15 mL and 30 mL plastic squeeze bottles.
Shown in Product Identification Section, page 435

DRISTAN®
[drĭs 'tăn]
Long Lasting Nasal Spray
DRISTAN®
Long Lasting Menthol Nasal Spray

DESCRIPTION
Dristan Long Lasting Nasal Spray contains Oxymetazoline HCl 0.05%.

ACTIONS
The sympathomimetic action of Dristan Long Lasting Nasal Spray and Dristan Long Lasting Menthol Nasal Spray constricts the smaller arterioles of the nasal passages, producing a prolonged (up to 12 hours), gentle and predictable decongesting effect.

INDICATIONS
Dristan Long Lasting Nasal Spray and Dristan Long Lasting Menthol Nasal Spray provide prompt temporary relief of nasal congestion due to colds, sinusitis, hay fever, or other upper respiratory allergies for up to 12 hours.

WARNINGS
Do not exceed recommended dosage because symptoms may occur, such as burning, stinging, sneezing, or increase of nasal discharge. Do not use this product for more than 3 days. If symptoms persist, consult a physician. The use of the dispenser by more than one person may spread infection. Keep these and all medicines out of children's reach. In case of accidental ingestion, seek professional assistance or contact a Poison Control Center immediately.

DOSAGE AND ADMINISTRATION
(Squeeze bottle) with head upright, insert nozzle in nostril. Spray quickly, firmly and sniff deeply. (Metered Dose Pump) prime the metered dose pump by depressing pump firmly several times. With head upright, insert nozzle in nostril. Depress pump 2 or 3 times, all the way down, with a firm even stroke and sniff deeply. Adults and children 6 years of age and over, spray 2 or 3 times into each nostril. Repeat twice daily—morning and evening. Not recommended for children under six.

INACTIVE INGREDIENTS
Dristan Long Lasting Nasal Spray—Benzalkonium Chloride 1:5000 in buffered isotonic aqueous solution, Hydroxypropyl Methylcellulose, Potassium Phosphate, Sodium Chloride, Sodium Phosphate, Thimerosal Preservative 0.002%, and Water.
Dristan Long Lasting Menthol Nasal Spray—Benzalkonium Chloride 1:5000 in buffered isotonic aqueous solution, Camphor, Eucalyptol, Hydroxypropyl Methylcellulose Menthol, Potassium Phosphate, Sodium Chloride, Sodium Phosphate, Thimerosal 0.002%, Water, and Alcohol 0.4%.

HOW SUPPLIED
Dristan Long Lasting Nasal Spray: 15 mL and 30 mL plastic squeeze bottles, and 15 mL metered dose pump.
Dristan Long Lasting Menthol Nasal Spray: 15 mL plastic squeeze bottle.
Shown in Product Identification Section, page 435

DRISTAN®
[drĭs 'tăn]
Decongestant/Antihistamine/Analgesic Coated Tablets and Coated Caplets

DESCRIPTION
Each Dristan Coated Tablet or Coated Caplet contains: Phenylephrine HCl 5 mg, Chlorpheniramine Maleate 2 mg, Acetaminophen 325 mg.

ACTIONS
Acetaminophen is both an analgesic and an antipyretic. Therapeutic doses of acetaminophen will effectively reduce an elevated body temperature. Also, acetaminophen is effective in reducing the discomfort of pain associated with headache.
Phenylephrine HCl is an oral nasal decongestant (Sympathomimetic Amine), effective as a vasoconstrictor to help reduce nasal/sinus congestion. Phenylephrine produces little or no Central Nervous System stimulation.
Chlorpheniramine maleate is an antihistamine effective in the control of rhinorrhea, sneezing and lacrimation associated with elevated histamine levels in disorders of the respiratory tract.

INDICATIONS
Dristan is indicated for effective multi-symptom relief of colds/flu, sinusitis, hay fever, or other upper respiratory allergies: nasal congestion, sneezing, runny nose, fever, headache and minor aches and pains.

WARNINGS
Avoid alcoholic beverages and driving a motor vehicle or operating heavy machinery while taking this product. May cause drowsiness or excitability, especially in children. Persons with asthma, glaucoma, high blood pressure, diabetes, heart or thyroid disease, difficulty in urination due to enlarged prostate gland, or taking an antidepressant drug, should use only as directed by a physician. Do not exceed recommended dosage because at higher doses nervousness, dizziness, or sleeplessness may occur. If symptoms do not improve within 7 days or are accompanied by high fever, discontinue use and see a physician. As with any drug, if you are pregnant or nursing a baby, seek the advice of a health professional before using this product.
Do not give to children under 6. Keep this and all medication out of children's reach. In case of accidental overdose contact a physician immediately.

DOSAGE AND ADMINISTRATION
Adults: Two tablets or caplets every four hours, not to exceed 12 tablets or caplets in 24 hours. Children 6–12: One tablet or caplet every four hours, not to exceed six tablets or caplets in 24 hours.

INACTIVE INGREDIENTS
Tablets or Caplets—Calcium Stearate, Croscarmellose Sodium, D&C Yellow #10 Lake, FD&C Yellow #6 Lake, Hydroxypropyl Methylcellulose, Microcrystalline Cellulose, Polyethylene Glycol, Povidone, Starch, Stearic Acid.

HOW SUPPLIED
Yellow/White coated tablets in tins of 12 and blister packages of 24, and bottles of 48, and 100. Yellow/White coated caplets in blister packages of 24 and bottles of 48.
Shown in Product Identification Section, page 435

Maximum Strength DRISTAN®
[drĭs 'tăn]
Decongestant/Analgesic Coated Caplets

DESCRIPTION
Each Maximum Strength Dristan Coated Caplet contains: Acetaminophen 500 mg and Pseudoephedrine HCl 30 mg.

ACTIONS
Acetaminophen is both an analgesic and an antipyretic. This maximum strength non-aspirin pain reliever effectively reduces headache pain and the pain of a sinus cold. Acetaminophen also reduces an elevated body temperature. Pseudoephedrine HCl is an oral nasal decongestant and is effective in reducing nasal/sinus congestion.

INDICATIONS
Maximum Strength Dristan is indicated for effective relief without drowsiness from nasal and sinus congestion, sinus pressure and sinus pain due to colds, sinusitis, and upper respiratory allergies.

WARNINGS
Do not exceed recommended dosage because at higher doses nervousness, dizziness or sleeplessness may occur. Persons with high blood pressure, heart disease, diabetes, thyroid disease, difficulty in urination due to an enlarged prostate gland, or taking an antidepressant drug should use only as directed by a physician. If symptoms do not improve within 7 days, or are accompanied by high fever, discontinue use and see a physician. Do not give to children under 12. As with any drug, if you are pregnant or nursing a baby, seek the advice of a health professional before using this product. Keep this and all medication out of children's reach. In case of accidental overdose, contact a physician immediately.

DOSAGE AND ADMINISTRATION
Adults and children over 12: Two caplets every 6 hours, not to exceed 8 caplets in any 24-hour period. Children under 12 should use only as directed by a physician.

PROFESSIONAL LABELING
Same as those outlined under Indications.

INACTIVE INGREDIENTS
Calcium Stearate, Croscarmellose Sodium, D&C Yellow #10 Lake, FD&C Yellow #6 Lake, Hydrogenated Vegetable Oil, Hydroxypropyl Methylcellulose, Microcrystalline Cellulose, Polyethylene Glycol, Povidone, Starch, Stearic Acid, Titanium Dioxide.

HOW SUPPLIED
Yellow coated caplets in blister packages of 24, 48 and bottles of 100.
Shown in Product Identification Section, page 435

POSTURE®

[pos'tūr]
600 mg
High Potency Calcium Supplement

DESCRIPTION

Each film-coated tablet of POSTURE® contains Tribasic Calcium Phosphate 1565.2 mg which provides 600 mg of elemental calcium. Posture is specially formulated not to produce gas.

	For Adults—
Two tablets	% U.S.
contain:	RDA*
Elemental Calcium .... 1200 mg 120%	
(as calcium phosphate)	

*Percentage of U.S. Recommended Daily Allowance

INDICATION

POSTURE® Tablets provide a daily source of calcium to help maintain healthy bones or to supplement dietary calcium intake when directed by a physician.

DIRECTIONS FOR USE

One or two tablets daily, or as recommended by a physician.

INACTIVE INGREDIENTS

Croscarmellose Sodium, Ethylcellulose, Magnesium Stearate, Microcrystalline Cellulose, Polyethylene Glycol, Povidone, Sodium Lauryl Sulfate.

HOW SUPPLIED

In bottles of 60 scored tablets.

POSTURE®–D

[pos'tūr d]
600 mg
High Potency Calcium Supplement with Vitamin D

DESCRIPTION

Each film-coated tablet of POSTURE®–D contains Tribasic Calcium Phosphate 1565.2 mg which provides 600 mg of elemental calcium and 125 IU of Vitamin D. Posture-D is specially formulated not to produce gas.

	For Adults—
Two tablets	% U.S.
contain:	RDA*
Elemental Calcium .... 1200 mg 120%	
(as calcium phosphate)	
Vitamin D .... 250 IU 63%	

*Percentage of U.S. Recommended Daily Allowance.

INDICATION

POSTURE®-D Tablets provide a daily source of calcium and Vitamin D to help maintain healthy bones or to supplement dietary calcium and Vitamin D intake when directed by a physician.

DIRECTIONS FOR USE

One or two tablets daily, or as recommended by a physician.

INACTIVE INGREDIENTS

Croscarmellose Sodium, Ethylcellulose, Magnesium Stearate, Microcrystalline Cellulose, Polyethylene Glycol, Povidone, Sodium Lauryl Sulfate.

HOW SUPPLIED

In bottles of 60 scored tablets.

PREPARATION H®

[prep-e'rā-shen āch]
Hemorrhoidal Ointment and Cream
PREPARATION H®
Hemorrhoidal Suppositories

DESCRIPTION

Preparation H is available in ointment, cream and suppository product forms.
The ointment contains Live Yeast Cell Derivative supplying 2,000 units Skin Respiratory Factor per ounce of Ointment and Shark Liver Oil 3.0% in a specially prepared Rectal Petrolatum Base.
The suppositories contain Live Yeast Cell Derivative supplying 2,000 units Skin Respiratory Factor per ounce of Cocoa Butter Suppository Base and Shark Liver Oil 3.0%.
The cream contains Live Yeast Cell Derivative supplying 2,000 units Skin Respiratory Factor per ounce of Cream and Shark Liver Oil 3.0% in a specially prepared Rectal Cream Base containing Petrolatum.

ACTIONS

The Live Yeast Cell Derivative acts by increasing the oxygen uptake of dermal tissues and facilitating collagen formation. Shark Liver Oil has been incorporated to act as a protectant which softens and soothes the tissues. Preparation H also lubricates inflamed, irritated surfaces to help make bowel movements less painful.

INDICATIONS

Preparation H helps shrink swelling of hemorrhoidal tissues caused by inflammation and gives prompt, temporary relief in many cases from pain and itch in tissues.

PRECAUTIONS

In case of bleeding, or if the condition persists, a physician should be consulted.

DOSAGE AND ADMINISTRATION

Ointment/Cream: Before applying, remove protective cover from applicator. Lubricate applicator before each application and thoroughly cleanse after use. It is recommended that Preparation H Hemorrhoidal ointment/cream be applied freely to the affected rectal area whenever symptoms occur, from three to five times per day, especially at night, in the morning and after each bowel movement. Frequent application with Preparation H ointment/cream provides continual therapy which leads to more rapid improvement of rectal conditions. Suppositories: Whenever symptoms occur, remove wrapper, insert one suppository rectally from three to five times per day, especially at night, in the morning and after each bowel movement. Frequent application with Preparation H suppositories provides continual therapy which leads to more rapid improvement of rectal conditions.
Inactive Ingredients: Ointment—Beeswax, Glycerin, Lanolin, Lanolin Alcohol, Mineral Oil, Paraffin, Phenylmercuric Nitrate (1:10,000 as a preservative), Thyme Oil.
Suppositories—Beeswax, Glycerin, Phenylmercuric Nitrate 1:10,000 (as a preservative), Polyethylene Glycol 600 Dilaurate.
Cream—Beeswax, BHA, Citric Acid, Glycerin, Glyceryl Oleate, Lanolin, Lanolin Alcohol, Magnesium Aluminum Silicate, Mineral Oil, Paraffin, Phenylmercuric Nitrate 1:10,000 (as a preservative), Polysorbate 80, Propyl Gallate, Propylene Glycol, Silica, Water. May also contain Methylparaben and Propylparaben.

HOW SUPPLIED

Ointment: Net Wt. 1 oz. and 2 oz.
Cream: Net Wt. 0.9 oz. and 1.8 oz.
Suppositories: 12's, 24's, 36's, and 48's.
Store at controlled room temperature in cool place but not over 80°F.
Shown in Product Identification Section, page 435

PRIMATENE®

[prīm'a-tēn]
Mist
(Epinephrine Inhalation Aerosol)
Bronchodilator

DESCRIPTION

Primatene Mist contains Epinephrine 5.5 mg/mL.

ACTION

Epinephrine is a sympathomimetic agent which relaxes bronchial smooth muscle during an acute asthmatic attack.

INDICATIONS

Primatene Mist is indicated for temporary relief of shortness of breath, tightness of chest, and wheezing due to bronchial asthma. Eases breathing for asthma patients by reducing spasms of bronchial muscles.

DOSAGE AND ADMINISTRATION

Inhalation dosage for adults and children 4 years of age and older: Start with one inhalation, then wait at least 1 minute. If not relieved, use once more. Do not use again for at least 3 hours. The use of this product by children should be supervised by an adult. Children under 4 years of age: Consult a physician. Each inhalation delivers 0.22 mg of epinephrine.

WARNINGS

Do not use this product unless a diagnosis of asthma has been made by a physician. Do not use this product if you have heart disease, high blood pressure, thyroid disease, diabetes, or difficulty in urination due to enlargement of the prostate gland unless directed by a physician. As with any drug, if you are pregnant or nursing a baby, seek the advice of a health professional before using this product. Do not use this product if you have ever been hospitalized for asthma or if you are taking any prescription drug for asthma unless directed by a physician.
Keep this and all drugs out of the reach of children. In case of accidental overdose, seek professional assistance or contact a poison control center immediately.
DO NOT CONTINUE TO USE THIS PRODUCT, BUT SEEK MEDICAL ASSISTANCE IMMEDIATELY IF SYMPTOMS ARE NOT RELIEVED WITHIN 20 MINUTES OR BECOME WORSE. DO NOT USE THIS PRODUCT MORE FREQUENTLY OR AT HIGHER DOSES THAN RECOMMENDED UNLESS DIRECTED BY A PHYSICIAN. EXCESSIVE USE MAY CAUSE NERVOUSNESS AND RAPID HEART BEAT AND POSSIBLY, ADVERSE EFFECTS ON THE HEART.

DRUG INTERACTION PRECAUTION: Do not use this product if you are presently taking a prescription drug for high blood pressure or depression, without first consulting your physician.

PRECAUTIONS

Contents under pressure. Do not puncture or throw container into incinerator. Using or storing near open flame or heating above 120° F may cause bursting.

DIRECTIONS FOR USE OF THE MOUTHPIECE

The Primatene Mist mouthpiece, which is enclosed in the Primatene Mist 15cc size (not the refill size), should be used for inhalation only with Primatene Mist.
1. Take plastic cap off mouthpiece. (For refills, use mouthpiece from previous purchase.)
2. Take plastic mouthpiece off bottle.
3. Place other end of mouthpiece on bottle.
4. Turn bottle upside down. Place thumb on bottom of mouthpiece over circular button and forefinger on top of vial. Empty the lungs as completely as possible by exhaling.
5. Place mouthpiece in mouth with lips closed around opening. Inhale deeply while squeezing mouthpiece and bottle together. Release immediately and remove unit from mouth, then complete taking the deep breath, drawing medication into your lungs, holding breath as long as comfortable.
6. Then exhale slowly keeping the lips nearly closed. This distributes the medication in the lungs.
7. Replace plastic cap on mouthpiece.
8. The Primatene Mist mouthpiece should be washed once daily with soap and hot water, and rinsed thoroughly. Then it should be dried with a clean, lint-free cloth.

INACTIVE INGREDIENTS

Alcohol 34%, Ascorbic Acid, Fluorocarbons (Propellant), Water. Contains no Sulphites.

HOW SUPPLIED

½ Fl. oz. (15 cc) With Mouthpiece.
½ Fl. oz. (15 cc) Refill
¾ Fl. oz. (22.5cc) Refill
Shown in Product Identification Section, page 435

PRIMATENE®

[prīm'a-tēn]
Mist Suspension
(Epinephrine Bitartrate Inhalation Aerosol)
Bronchodilator

DESCRIPTION

Primatene Mist Suspension contains Epinephrine Bitartrate 7.0 mg/mL.

ACTION

Epinephrine is a sympathomimetic agent which relaxes bronchial smooth muscle and thereby eases breathing during an acute asthmatic attack.

INDICATIONS

Primatene Mist Suspension is indicated for temporary relief of shortness of breath, tightness of chest, and wheezing due to bronchial asthma.

DOSAGE AND ADMINISTRATION

Shake before using.
Inhalation dosage for adults and children 4 years of age and older: Start with one inhalation, then wait at least 1 minute. If not relieved, use once more. Do not use again for at least 3 hours. The use of this product by children should be supervised by an adult. Children under 4 years of age: Consult a physician. Each inhalation delivers 0.3 mg Epinephrine Bitartrate equivalent to 0.16 mg Epinephrine Base.

WARNINGS

Do not use this product unless a diagnosis of asthma has been made by a physician. Do not use this product if you have heart disease, high blood pressure, thyroid disease, diabetes, or difficulty in urination due to enlargement of the prostate gland unless directed by a physician. As with any drug, if you are pregnant or nursing a baby, seek the advice of a health professional before using this product. Do not use this product if you have ever been hospitalized for asthma or if you are taking any prescription drug for asthma unless directed by a physician.
Keep this and all drugs out of the reach of children. In case of accidental overdose, seek professional assistance or contact a poison control center immediately.
DO NOT CONTINUE TO USE THIS PRODUCT, BUT SEEK MEDICAL ASSISTANCE IMMEDIATELY IF SYMPTOMS ARE NOT RELIEVED WITHIN 20 MINUTES OR BECOME WORSE. DO NOT USE THIS PRODUCT MORE FREQUENTLY OR AT HIGHER DOSES THAN RECOMMENDED UNLESS DIRECTED BY A PHYSICIAN. EXCESSIVE USE MAY CAUSE NERVOUSNESS AND RAPID

Continued on next page

Whitehall—Cont.

HEART BEAT AND POSSIBLY, ADVERSE EFFECTS ON THE HEART.
DRUG INTERACTION PRECAUTION: Do not use this product if you are presently taking a prescription drug for high blood pressure or depression, without first consulting your physician.

PRECAUTIONS

Contents under pressure. Do not puncture or throw container into incinerator. Using or storing near open flame or heating above 120° F may cause bursting.

DIRECTIONS FOR USE OF THE INHALER

1. SHAKE WELL BEFORE USING.
2. HOLD INHALER WITH NOZZLE DOWN WHILE USING. Empty the lungs as completely as possible by exhaling.
3. Purse the lips, as in saying "O" and hold the nozzle up to the lips keeping the tongue flat. As you start to take a deep breath, squeeze nozzle and can together, releasing one full application. Complete taking deep breath, drawing medication into your lungs.
4. Hold breath for as long as comfortable. Then exhale slowly keeping the lips nearly closed. This distributes the medication in the lungs.
5. The Primatene Mist Suspension nozzle should be washed once daily. After removing the nozzle from the vial, wash it with soap and hot water, and rinse thoroughly. Then it should be dried with a clean, lint-free cloth.

INACTIVE INGREDIENTS

Fluorocarbons (Propellant), Sorbitan Trioleate. Contains No Sulfites.

HOW SUPPLIED

⅓ Fl. oz. (10cc) pocket-size aerosol inhaler.

PRIMATENE®
[prĭm'a-tēn]
Tablets

DESCRIPTION

Depending upon the state (see HOW SUPPLIED), Primatene Tablets are available in 3 formulations:
(regular formula): Theophylline Anhydrous 130 mg, Ephedrine Hydrochloride 24 mg.
P Formula: Theophylline Hydrous 130 mg, Ephedrine Hydrochloride 24 mg, Phenobarbital 8 mg. (⅛ gr.) per tablet. (Warning: May be habit forming.)
M Formula: Theophylline Hydrous 130 mg, Ephedrine Hydrochloride 24 mg, Pyrilamine Maleate 16.6 mg. per tablet.

INDICATIONS

Primatene Tablets are indicated for relief and control of attacks of bronchial asthma and associated hay fever.

ACTIONS

Primatene Tablets contain two bronchodilators, theophylline, a methylxanthine, and ephedrine, a sympathomimetic amine. The pharmacologic action of theophylline may be mediated through inhibition of phosphodiesterase with a resulting increase in intracellular cyclic AMP. The B-adrenergic ephedrine acts by a different mechanism to produce cyclic AMP. The combination of a xanthine and a sympathomimetic appears to produce more smooth muscle relaxation than when either drug is used alone. Phenobarbital (present in the P formula) counteracts the possible stimulation produced by ephedrine and acts as a mild sedative. Pyrilamine maleate (present in the M Formula) is an antihistamine with mild sedating action.

WARNINGS

If symptoms persist, consult your physician. Some people are sensitive to ephedrine and, in some cases, temporary sleeplessness and nervousness may occur. These reactions will disappear if the use of the medication is discontinued. Do not exceed recommended dosage.
People who have heart disease, high blood pressure, diabetes thyroid trouble, or difficulty in urination due to enlarged prostate gland, should take this preparation only on the advice of a physician. Both "M" and "P" formula may cause drowsiness. People taking the "M" or "P" formula should not drive or operate machinery.
As with any drug, if you are pregnant or nursing a baby, seek the advice of a health professional before using this product. Keep this and all medicines out of reach of children.

DOSAGE AND ADMINISTRATION

Adults: 1 or 2 tablets initially and then one every 4 hours, as needed, not to exceed 6 tablets in 24 hours. Children (6–12): One half adult dose. For children under 6, consult a physician.

INACTIVE INGREDIENTS

(regular formula): FD&C Yellow No. 6 Lake, D&C Yellow No. 10 Lake, Hydrogenated Vegetable Oil, Magnesium Stearate, Microcrystalline Cellulose, Sodium Starch Glycolate, Surfactant, Talc.
P Formula (Phenobarbital): Colloidal Silicon Dioxide, D&C Yellow No. 10, FD&C Yellow No. 6, Magnesium Stearate, Sodium Starch Glycolate, Starch, Surfactant.
M Formula (Pyrilamine Maleate): D&C Yellow No. 10 Lake, FD&C Yellow No. 6 Lake, Hydrogenated Vegetable Oil, Magnesium Stearate, Microcrystalline Cellulose, Sodium Starch Glycolate, Surfactant.
Contains No Sulfites.

HOW SUPPLIED

Available in three forms (regular) Primatene Tablets, "M" Formula, and "P" Formula. In those states where Phenobarbital is Rx only, "M" Formula, containing pyrilamine maleate, is available.
"P" Formula, containing phenobarbital, is available in other states.
(Regular) Primatene Tablets are currently available in the West and Southwest only. Both "M" and "P" formulas are supplied in glass bottles of 24 and 60 tablets. (Regular) Primatene Tablets are supplied in 24 and 60 tablet thermoform blister cartons.
Shown in Product Identification Section, page 435

RIOPAN®
[rī'o pan]
magaldrate
Antacid

DESCRIPTION

RIOPAN is a buffer antacid containing the unique chemical entity Magaldrate. Each teaspoonful (5 mL) of suspension contains Magaldrate, 540 mg. Each Chew Tablet or Swallow Tablet contains Magaldrate, 480 mg. RIOPAN is considered dietetically sodium-free (not more than 0.004 mEq, 0.1 mg sodium per teaspoonful or tablet).

ACTIONS

The active ingredient in RIOPAN, Magaldrate demonstrates a rapid and uniform buffering action. The acid-neutralizing capacity of RIOPAN is 15.0 mEq/5mL and 13.5 mEq/tablet. RIOPAN does not produce acid rebound or alkalinization.

INDICATIONS

RIOPAN is indicated for the relief of heartburn, sour stomach and acid indigestion. For symptomatic relief of hyperacidity associated with the diagnosis of peptic ulcer, gastritis, peptic esophagitis, gastric hyperacidity, and hiatal hernia.

DOSAGE AND ADMINISTRATION

RIOPAN (magaldrate) Antacid *Suspension*—Take one or two teaspoonfuls, between meals and at bedtime, or as directed by the physician. RIOPAN Antacid *Chew Tablets*—Chew one or two tablets, between meals and at bedtime, or as directed by the physician. RIOPAN Antacid *Swallow Tablets* -—Take one or two tablets, between meals and at bedtime, or as directed by the physician.

WARNINGS

Patients should not take more than 18 teaspoonfuls or 20 tablets in a 24-hour period or use the maximum dosage for more than two weeks, except under the advice and supervision of a physician. If you have kidney disease, do not use this product except under the advice and supervision of a physician.

DRUG INTERACTION PRECAUTION

Do not use in patients presently taking a prescription antibiotic drug containing any form of tetracycline.

INACTIVE INGREDIENTS

Chew Tablets: Flavor, Magnesium Stearate, Polyethylene Glycol, Sorbitol, Starch, Sucrose, Titanium Dioxide. Swallow Tablets: Flavor, Magnesium Stearate, Menthol, Microcrystalline Cellulose, Polyethylene Glycol, Starch, Talc, Titanium Dioxide. Suspension: Acacia, Flavor, Hydroxypropyl Methylcellulose, Menthol, Saccharin, Water.

HOW SUPPLIED

RIOPAN Antacid *Suspension* in 12 fl oz (355 mL) plastic bottles. Individual Cups, 1 fl oz (30 mL) ea., tray of 10—10 trays per packer. Store at room temperature (approximately 25°C). Avoid freezing. RIOPAN Antacid *Chew Tablets*—in bottles of 60 and 100. Also, single rollpacks of 12 tablets and 3-roll rollpacks of 36 tablets. RIOPAN Antacid *Swallow Tablets*—Boxes of 60 and 100 in individual film strips (6 × 10 and 10 × 10, respectively).
Shown in Product Identification Section, page 435

RIOPAN PLUS®
[rī'opan]
magaldrate and simethicone
Antacid Plus Anti-Gas

DESCRIPTION

Riopan Plus is a buffer antacid plus anti-gas combination product containing the unique chemical entity Magaldrate. Each teaspoonful (5mL) of suspension contains Magaldrate, 540 mg and Simethicone, 20 mg. Each Chew Tablet contains Magaldrate, 480 mg and Simethicone, 20 mg. Riopan Plus is considered dietetically sodium-free (not more than 0.004 mEq, 0.1 mg sodium per teaspoonful or tablet).

ACTIONS

The active antacid ingredient in Riopan Plus, Magaldrate, demonstrates a rapid and uniform buffering action. The acid-neutralizing capacity of Riopan Plus is 15.0 mEq/5mL and 13.5 mEq/tablet. Riopan Plus does not produce acid rebound or alkalinization. Simethicone reduces the surface tension of gas bubbles so that the gas is more easily eliminated.

INDICATIONS

RIOPAN Plus is indicated for the relief of heartburn, sour stomach and acid indigestion accompanied by the symptoms of gas. For symptomatic relief of hyperacidity associated with the diagnosis of peptic ulcer, gastritis, peptic esophagitis, gastric hyperacidity, hiatal hernia, and postoperative gas pain.

DOSAGE AND ADMINISTRATION

RIOPAN PLUS (magaldrate and simethicone) Antacid Plus Anti-Gas *Suspension*—Take one or two teaspoonfuls between meals and at bedtime, or as directed by the physician. RIOPAN PLUS Antacid Plus Anti-Gas *Chew Tablets*—Chew one or two tablets, between meals and at bedtime, or as directed by the physician.

WARNINGS

Patients should not take more than 18 teaspoonfuls, or 20 tablets, in a 24-hour period or use the maximum dosage for more than two weeks, except under the advice and supervision of a physician. If you have kidney disease, do not use this product except under the advice and supervision of a physician.

DRUG INTERACTION PRECAUTION

Do not use in patients presently taking a prescription antibiotic drug containing any form of tetracycline.

INACTIVE INGREDIENTS

Chew Tablets: Flavor, Magnesium Stearate, Methylcellulose, Polyethylene Glycol, Silica, Sorbitol, Starch, Sucrose, Titanium Dioxide. Suspension: Acacia, Flavor, Hydroxypropyl Methylcellulose, Menthol, PEG-8 Stearate, Saccharin, Sorbitan Stearate, Water.

HOW SUPPLIED

RIOPAN PLUS Antacid Plus Anti-Gas *Suspension*—in 12 fl oz (355 mL) plastic bottles and 6 fl oz (176 mL) plastic bottles. Individual Cups, 1 fl oz (30 mL) ea., tray of 10—10 trays per packer.
Store at room temperature (approximately 25°C). Avoid freezing.
RIOPAN PLUS Antacid Plus Anti-Gas *Chew Tablets*—in bottles of 60 and 100. Also single rollpacks of 12 tablets and 3-roll rollpacks of 36 tablets.
Shown in Product Identification Section, page 435

RIOPAN PLUS® 2
[rī'opan plus 2]
magaldrate and simethicone Double Strength Antacid plus Anti-Gas

DESCRIPTION

Riopan Plus 2 is a double strength buffer antacid plus anti-gas combination product containing the unique chemical entity Magaldrate. Each teaspoonful (5 mL) of suspension contains Magaldrate, 1080 mg and Simethicone, 30 mg. Each Chew Tablet contains Magaldrate, 1080 mg and Simethicone, 20 mg. Riopan Plus 2 is considered dietetically sodium-free (not more than 0.013 mEq, 0.3 mg per teaspoonful or 0.021 mEq, 0.5 mg per tablet).

ACTIONS

The active antacid ingredient in Riopan Plus 2, Magaldrate, demonstrates a rapid and uniform buffering action. The acid-neutralizing capacity of Double Strength Riopan Plus 2 is 30 mEq/5mL and 30.0 mEq/tablet. Riopan Plus 2 does not produce acid rebound or alkalinization. Simethicone reduces the surface tension of gas bubbles so that the gas is more easily eliminated.

INDICATIONS

RIOPAN PLUS 2 is indicated for the relief of heartburn, sour stomach and acid indigestion accompanied by the symptoms of gas. For symptomatic relief of hyperacidity associated with the diagnosis of peptic ulcer, gastritis, peptic esophagitis, gastric hyperacidity, hiatal hernia, and postoperative gas pain.

DOSAGE AND ADMINISTRATION

RIOPAN PLUS 2 (magaldrate and simethicone) Antacid plus Anti-Gas *Suspension*—Take one or two teaspoonfuls between meals and at bedtime, or as directed by the physician.

RIOPAN PLUS 2 Antacid plus Anti-Gas *Chew Tablets*—Chew one or two tablets, between meals and at bedtime, or as directed by physician.

WARNINGS

Patients should not take more than 9 teaspoonfuls (or 9 tablets) in a 24-hour period nor use the maximum dosage for more than two weeks, nor use if they have kidney disease, except under the advice and supervision of a physician.

DRUG INTERACTION PRECAUTION

Do not use in patients presently taking a prescription antibiotic drug containing any form of tetracycline.

INACTIVE INGREDIENTS

Chew Tablets: Flavor, Magnesium Stearate, Methylcellulose, Polyethylene Glycol, Saccharin, Silica, Sorbitol, Starch, Sucrose, Titanium Dioxide. Suspension: Flavor, Glycerin, PEG-8 Stearate, Potassium Citrate, Saccharin, Sorbitan Stearate, Sorbitol, Xanthan Gum, Water.

HOW SUPPLIED

RIOPAN PLUS 2 *Suspension*—in 12 fl oz (355 mL) plastic bottles and 6 fl oz (176 mL) plastic bottles.
Store at room temperature (approximately 25°C). Avoid freezing.
RIOPAN PLUS 2 Chew Tablets—in bottles of 60.
Shown in Product Identification Section, page 435

SEMICID®
[sĕm′ē-sĭd]
Vaginal Contraceptive Inserts

DESCRIPTION

Semicid is a safe and effective, non-systemic, reversible method of birth control. Each vaginal contraceptive insert contains 100 mg of the spermicide nonoxynol-9. It contains no hormones and is odorless and non-messy.
When used consistently and according to directions, the effectiveness of Semicid is approximately equal to vaginal foam contraceptives, but less than the pill or diaphragm. Semicid requires no applicator and has no unpleasant taste. Unlike foams, creams and jellies, Semicid does not drip or run, and Semicid inserts are easier to use than the diaphragm. Also, Semicid does not effervesce like some inserts, so it is not as likely to cause a burning feeling.

ACTIONS

Semicid dissolves in the vagina and blends with natural vaginal secretions to provide double birth control protection: an effective sperm killing barrier plus a physical barrier that covers the cervical opening and adjoining vaginal walls.

INDICATION

For the prevention of pregnancy.

WARNINGS

Do not insert in urethra. Do not take orally. If irritation occurs, discontinue use. If irritation persists, consult a physician. Keep this and all contraceptives out of the reach of children.

PRECAUTIONS

As with all spermicides, some Semicid users may experience irritation in using the product, but most women can use Semicid safely and without irritation.
If douching is desired, one should wait at least six hours after intercourse before douching. If either partner experiences irritation, discontinue use. If irritation persists, consult a physician.
If a menstrual period is missed, a physician should be consulted.

DOSAGE AND ADMINISTRATION

To use, unwrap one insert and insert it deeply into the vagina. It is essential that Semicid be inserted at least 15 minutes before intercourse. However, Semicid is also effective when inserted up to 1 hour before intercourse. If intercourse is delayed for more than 1 hour after Semicid is inserted, or if intercourse is repeated, then another insert must be inserted. Semicid can be used as frequently as needed.

INACTIVE INGREDIENTS

Benzethonium Chloride, Citric Acid, D&C Red #21 Lake, D&C Red #33 Lake, Methylparaben, Polyethylene Glycol, Water.

HOW SUPPLIED

Individually-wrapped inserts in Strip packaging of 10's and 20's.
Store at room temperature (not over 86°F or 30°C).
Shown in Product Identification Section, page 435

TODAY®
[tü-dā]
Vaginal Contraceptive Sponge

DESCRIPTION

Today Vaginal Contraceptive Sponge is a soft polyurethane foam sponge containing nonoxynol-9, a spermicide used by millions of women for over 25 years.
Today Sponge is Effective, Safe, and Convenient. Today Sponge provides 24-hour contraceptive protection without hormones, allowing spontaneity. Today Sponge is easy to use, non-messy, and disposable.

ACTIVE INGREDIENT

Each Today Sponge contains nonoxynol-9, one gram.

INACTIVE INGREDIENTS

Benzoic acid, citric acid, sodium dihydrogen citrate, sodium metabisulfite, sorbic acid, water in a polyurethane foam sponge.

INDICATION

For the prevention of pregnancy.

ACTIONS

Used as directed, Today Vaginal Contraceptive Sponge prevents pregnancy in three ways: 1) the spermicide nonoxynol-9 kills sperm before they can reach the egg; 2) Today Sponge traps and absorbs sperm; 3) Today Sponge blocks the cervix so that sperm cannot enter.
Today Sponge is designed for easy insertion into the vagina. It is positioned against the cervix, and while in place provides protection against pregnancy for 24 hours. The soft polyurethane foam sponge is formulated to feel like normal vaginal tissue and has a specially-designed ribbon loop attached to an interior web for maximum strength.
In clinical trials of Today Sponge in over 1,800 women worldwide who completed over 12,000 cycles of use, the method-effectiveness, i.e., the level of effectiveness seen in women who followed the printed instructions exactly and who used Today Sponge every time that they had intercourse, was 89 to 91%.

INSTRUCTIONS

Remove one Today Sponge from airtight inner pack, wet thoroughly with clean tap water, and squeeze gently until it becomes very sudsy. The water activates the spermicide. Fold the sides of Today Sponge upward until it looks long and narrow and then insert it deeply into the vagina with the string loop dangling below. Protection begins immediately and continues for 24 hours. It is not necessary to add creams, jellies, foams, or any other additional spermicide as long as Today Sponge is in place, no matter how many acts of intercourse may occur during a 24-hour period. Always wait 6 hours after your last act of intercourse before removing Today Sponge. If you have intercourse when Today Sponge has been in place for 24 hours, it must be left in place an additional 6 hours after intercourse before removing it.
To remove Today Sponge, place a finger in the vagina and reach up and back to find the string loop. Hook a finger around the loop. Slowly and gently pull the Sponge out. Some women, especially first-time users, may have difficulty removing the Sponge. This situation may be due to tension or unusually strong muscular pressure. Simple relaxation of the vaginal muscles and bearing down should make it possible to remove the Sponge without difficulty. See User Instruction Booklet (Section 7) for details on removing Today Sponge or call the Today TalkLine 1-800-223-2329.

WARNINGS

For best protection against pregnancy, follow instructions exactly. Any delay in your menstrual period may be an early sign of pregnancy. If this happens, consult your physician or clinic as soon as possible. A small number of men and women may be sensitive to the spermicide in this product (nonoxynol-9) or any of its other components and should not use this product if irritation occurs and persists. If genital burning or itching occurs in either partner, stop using Today Sponge and contact your physician. If you have ever had Toxic Shock Syndrome, do not use Today Sponge. If you experience two or more of the warning signs of Toxic Shock Syndrome (TSS), including fever, vomiting, diarrhea, muscular pain, dizziness, and rash similar to sunburn, consult your physician or clinic immediately. Today Sponge should not be used during the menstrual period. After childbirth, miscarriage, other termination of pregnancy, or if you are nursing a baby, it is important to consult your physician or clinic before using this product. Today Sponge should be removed within the specified time limit (maximum wear time is 30 hours). In clinical trials, approximately one-half of all unintended pregnancies occurred during the first three months of Today Sponge use. A back-up contraceptive, such as Today Condom, is recommended for additional contraceptive protection dur-

ing this time, until the user becomes familiar with Today Sponge.
Keep this and all drugs out of reach of children. In case of accidental ingestion of Today Sponge, call a poison control center, emergency medical facility, or doctor.

HOW TO STORE

Store at normal room temperature.

HOW SUPPLIED

Packages of 3s, 6s, and 12s.
Shown in Product Identification Section, page 435

EDUCATIONAL MATERIAL

Books—Booklets—Brochures
Today Sponge patient pamphlet available to physicians, pharmacists, and patients.
Pictures—Charts
8½ × 11 laminated Instructions for Use chart available to physicians.
Write to: TalkLine, Whitehall Laboratories, 685 Third Ave., New York, NY 10017, or call toll-free 1-800-223-2329.

Willen Drug Company
18 NORTH HIGH STREET
BALTIMORE, MD 21202

BICITRA®—Sugar-Free   ℞
[bye″si-trah]
(Sodium Citrate & Citric Acid
Oral Solution USP)

DESCRIPTION

BICITRA is a pleasant tasting and effective oral alkalinizing agent useful for conditions where long term maintenance of an alkaline urine is desirable. BICITRA is also a fast acting and effective nonparticulate neutralizing buffer useful in raising gastric pH.
BICITRA contains in each tablespoonful (15 mL):
SODIUM CITRATE Dihydrate ....1500 mg (0.34 Molar)
CITRIC ACID Monohydrate ....1002 mg (0.32 Molar)
Each mL contains 1 mEq Sodium ion and is equivalent to 1 mEq Bicarbonate (HCO₃).
BICITRA is sugar free and nonalcoholic. BICITRA is the highly palatable, improved SHOHL'S Solution.

CLINICAL PHARMACOLOGY

Sodium Citrate is absorbed and metabolized to sodium bicarbonate, thus acting as a systemic alkalizer. The effects are essentially those of chlorides before absorption and those of bicarbonates subsequently. Oxidation is virtually complete so that less than 5% of the citrate is excreted in the urine unchanged. BICITRA is a useful antacid for effectively buffering and neutralizing gastric acid.

INDICATIONS AND ADVANTAGES

BICITRA is an effective alkalinizing agent and a nonparticulate neutralizing buffer.
BICITRA is useful for conditions requiring long term maintenance of an alkaline urine, as in patients where dissolution and control of uric acid and cystine calculi of the urinary tract is indicated, especially when the administration of potassium salts is undesirable or contraindicated. It is highly valuable in preventing uric acid nephropathy when administered to patients with hyperuricosuria due to underlying metabolic defects (e.g. gout), or who are receiving drugs (e.g. cancer chemotherapy or uricosuric agents), resulting in acute or chronic increases in urinary uric acid excretion. BICITRA is also effective for alleviating chronic metabolic acidosis, particularly when caused by conditions which may result from renal insufficiency or renal tubular acidosis, where the administration of sodium citrate may be preferable.
BICITRA is concentrated, and when administered after meals and before bedtime, maintains an alkaline pH without the need for a 2 A.M. dose. In the recommended dosage, BICITRA alkalinizes the urine without producing systemic alkalosis. BICITRA is a fast acting buffering agent, and is useful in rapidly neutralizing gastric acid and raising the pH of stomach contents. In vitro tests have shown that 15 mL BICITRA will neutralize 117 mL of 0.1N HCl and raise gastric pH to 2.5, with no decrease of the pH value after 2 hours. BICITRA offers a maximum buffering capacity due to the equimolar ratio of sodium citrate to citric acid on a 1:1 basis. BICITRA is a nonparticulate buffer and, therefore, is decidedly advantageous over particulate aluminum-magnesium containing antacids, as a preanesthesia medication. BICITRA is pleasant tasting and tolerable, even when adminis-

Continued on next page

Willen—Cont.

tered over long periods. BICITRA offers these advantages over Shohl's Solution, while supplying equivalent alkalinizing effect and sodium content.

CONTRAINDICATIONS
Patients on sodium-restricted diets or with severe renal impairment. POLYCITRA-K or POLYCITRA-K CRYSTALS is recommended in those clinical situations where administration of potassium citrate is preferred.

PRECAUTIONS
Should be used with caution by patients with low urinary output unless under the supervision of a physician. Patients with renal insufficiency should not ingest BICITRA concurrently with aluminum-based gels (e.g. aluminum hydroxide or aluminum carbonate) used as phosphate binders. Patients should be directed to dilute adequately with water and preferably to take each dose after meals to avoid saline laxative effect. Sodium salts should be used cautiously in patients with cardiac failure, hypertension, impaired renal function, peripheral and pulmonary edema and toxemia of pregnancy. Periodic examinations of serum electrolytes, particularly serum bicarbonate level, should be carried out in those patients with renal disease in order to avoid these complications.

ADVERSE REACTIONS
BICITRA is generally well tolerated without any unpleasant side effects when given in recommended doses to patients with normal renal function and urinary output. However, as with any alkalinizing agent, caution must be used in certain patients with abnormal renal mechanisms to avoid development of alkalosis, especially in the presence of hypocalcemia.

DOSAGE AND ADMINISTRATION
BICITRA should be taken diluted in water followed by additional water, if desired.
For Systemic Alkalization: Usual Adult Prescribing Limits: Up to 150 mL daily. Occassional patients will require more or less to achieve the desired alkalinizing effect, and since 1 mEq Sodium and 1 mEq. Citrate is supplied per each mL, dosage is easy to regulate. To check urinary pH, HYDRION Paper (pH 6.0-8.0) or NITRAZINE Paper (pH 4.5-7.5) are available and easy to use.
Usual Adult Dose: 10 to 30 mL, diluted in 1 to 3 ounces of water or juice, after meals and at bedtime.
Usual Pediatric Dose: 5 to 15 mL diluted in 1 to 3 ounces of water or juice, after meals and at bedtime.
As a Neutralizing Buffer: 15 mL to 30 mL, taken as a single dose, or diluted, if desired, with 15 mL to 30 mL water, or as directed by physician.

OVERDOSAGE
Overdosage with sodium salts may cause diarrhea, nausea and vomiting, hypernoea, and convulsions.

HOW SUPPLIED
BICITRA—
   16 fl oz. (473 ml) (NDC 11414-207-01);
   1 gallon (3785 ml) (NDC 11414-207-08);
   4 fl oz (120 mL) (NDC 11414-207-04);
   15mL Unit-dose (NDC 11414-207-15);
   30 mL Unit-dose (NDC 11414-207-30).

NEUTRA–PHOS® Powder & Capsules
NEUTRA–PHOS®–K Powder & Capsules
[new "trah foss"]
Oral Phosphorus Dietary Supplement

NEUTRA-PHOS and NEUTRA-PHOS-K supply the physiologically important element—PHOSPHORUS—as inorganic orthophosphate, in a well tolerated oral compound. Each contains a chemically balanced combination of readily soluble inorganic phosphates, affording a very high source of elemental Phosphorus. Both products supply equal concentration of elemental Phosphorus.
NEUTRA-PHOS is a stable powder combination of monobasic and dibasic Sodium and Potassium Phosphates.
NEUTRA-PHOS-K is a stable sodium-free powder combination of monobasic and dibasic Potassium Phosphates intended for oral use in low sodium diets.
Both products form an oral solution by reconstitution with water and are neutral (pH 7.3), isotonic, pleasant tasting sources of Phosphorus. There is less than 1 calorie per average dose.

INDICATIONS
NEUTRA-PHOS and NEUTRA-PHOS-K are recommended as oral Phosphorus supplements, particularly if the diet supplies an insufficient quantity of Phosphorus, or if metabolic requirements for Phosphorus are increased. In addition, NEUTRA-PHOS and NEUTRA-PHOS-K are useful in the treatment of children and adults with conditions associated with excessive renal phosphate loss or inadequate gastrointestinal absorption of phosphate. They are also useful as an adjunct supplement in the management of phosphate diabetes.

ADVANTAGES
NEUTRA-PHOS and NEUTRA-PHOS-K, reconstituted to an oral liquid, provide a chemically balanced supply of Phosphorus in a pH neutral solution that shows rapid absorption and utilization from the alimentary tract. These liquid products have the advantage over coated or uncoated tablet dosage supplies, as slowly dissolving tablets may cause local gastrointestinal irritation or inflammation in sensitive individuals. Both products are highly concentrated and thus economically provide inorganic Phosphate. They are especially useful for long term maintenance of an adequate daily supply of Phosphorus. NEUTRA-PHOS also supplies Sodium and Potassium in equimolar proportions- a decided advantage over products which supply a high amount of sodium and a low amount of potassium per dose. NEUTRA-PHOS-K supplies only Potassium and is recommended when a low sodium intake is indicated.

ELECTROLYTES SUPPLIED
2½ fluid ounces (75 mL) of the reconstituted solution or contents of 1 capsule* supplies:

NEUTRA-PHOS

Electrolyte	mg	mEq	mg/ mL
Phosphorus	250	14.25	3.33
Phosphate (PO_4)	765	—	10.20
Sodium	164	7.125	2.18
Potassium	278	7.125	3.70

NEUTRA-PHOS-K

Electrolyte	mg	mEq	mg/ mL
Phosphorus	250	14.25	3.33
Phosphate (PO_4)	765	—	10.20
Sodium	none	none	none
Potassium	556	14.25	7.41

OSMOLALITY
NEUTRA-PHOS Solution*: 223–236 milliosmols per kg (mOsm/kg)
NEUTRA-PHOS-K Solution*: 240–244 milliosmols per kg (mOsm/kg)
(*reconstituted in water as per label directions. Refer to Capsules description.)

AVERAGE DIRECTIONS FOR ADULTS AND CHILDREN
4 or more years of age: 2½ fl. oz. (75 mL) of the oral solution, or contents of 1 capsule, equivalent to 250 mg Phosphorus, taken 4 times a day. (See Capsules description).

PEDIATRIC DOSE
Infants and children under 4 years of age: 2 fl. oz. (60 mL) of the oral solution, equivalent to 200 mg of Phosphorus, taken 4 times a day.

USUAL DOSE RANGE
2½ fl. oz. to 20 fl. oz. (75 mL to 600 mL) of the oral solution, or contents of 1 to 8 capsules (equivalent from 250 mg to 2 grams of Phosphorus) taken daily in divided doses, after meals and at bedtime.*
2½ fl. oz. (75 mL) or 1 capsule, 4 times a day supplies 1 g Phosphorus. 5 fl. oz. (150 mL) or 2 capsules, 3 times a day supplies 1.5 g Phosphorus. 5 fl. oz. (150 mL) or 2 capsules, 4 times a day supplies 2 g Phosphorus. (See Capsules description).*
(* This affords 100% of the R.D.A. of Phosphorus for adults and children 4 or more years of age. The U.S. R.D.A. for Phosphorus is 1.0 gram for adults and children 4 or more years of age ; 0.8 gram for infants and children under 4 years of age; and, 1.3 grams for pregnant or lactating women.)

PRECAUTIONS AND SIDE EFFECTS
Reconstitute powder and contents of capsules as directed before taking. Occasionally some individuals may experience a mild laxative effect for the first day or two when beginning to use NEUTRA-PHOS. If this persists to an unpleasant degree, reduce the daily intake until this effect subsides or, if necessary, discontinue its use.

HOW SUPPLIED
NEUTRA-PHOS and NEUTRA-PHOS-K are powder concentrates, to be reconstituted with water or other desirable liquids and are supplied in multiple bulk dose packages or single dose capsules.
MULTIPLE DOSE POWDER CONCENTRATE: For patient convenience, bulk powder concentrates are supplied in a package size sufficient to make 1 gallon (3.785 Liters) and are intended for use while at home. This is the most economical dosage form and is prepared by the patient, who is instructed to dissolve the entire contents of one bottle in one gallon of water or other desirable liquid. This solution is not to be further diluted, but can be chilled, if desired, to increase palat-

ability, and can be stored for up to 60 days. 2½ fluid ounces (75 mL) of this solution supplies 250 mg Phosphorus (refer to electrolyte chart).
SINGLE DOSE CAPSULES: NEUTRA-PHOS and NEUTRA-PHOS-K are also supplied in pre-measured single-dose capsules, which are intended for use if the above multiple dose form precludes transportation of liquid. The contents of 1 capsule makes 2½ fluid ounces (75 mL) of an oral suspension equal to the oral solution prepared above. To use, empty the contents of one capsule into ⅓ glassful water (approximately 2½ fluid ounces) and stir well before taking. *NOTE: All active components will dissolve rapidly while the excipients will remain in suspension.* If desired, the contents of 1 or 2 capsules can be mixed into the same amount of water or other liquid, depending on dosage requirements. Any palatable juice or beverage may be used in place of water. Each capsule supplies 250 mg Phosphorus (refer to electrolyte chart).
NEUTRA-PHOS POWDER CONCENTRATE (Potassium and Sodium Phosphates for Oral Use)—2¼ oz. (64 gm) per bottle. Each bottle reconstitutes to make 1 gallon of solution. (Stock No. 201-01)
NEUTRA-PHOS SINGLE DOSE CAPSULES—Each capsule contains 1.25 gam NEUTRA-PHOS POWDER CONCENTRATE, and makes 2½ fluid ounces (75 mL) of oral solution, Packaged 100 capsules per bottle (Stock No. 202-05).
NEUTRA-PHOS-K POWDER CONCENTRATE (Potassium Phosphates for Oral Use)—2½ oz. (71 gm) per bottle. Each bottle reconstitutes to make 1 gallon (Stock No. 203-01).
NEUTRA-PHOS-K SINGLE DOSE CAPSULES—Each capsule contains 1.45 gm NEUTRA-PHOS-K POWDER CONCENTRATE, and makes 2½ fluid ounces (75 mL) of oral solution. Packaged 100 capsules per bottle (Stock No. 204-05).

IS THIS PRODUCT O.T.C.
Yes.

POLYCITRA® Syrup   ℞
POLYCITRA®–LC–Sugar–Free   ℞
[polly "si-trah"]
(Tricitrates Oral Solution USP)

DESCRIPTION
Syrup POLYCITRA and POLYCITRA-LC are pleasant tasting and effective oral alkalinizing agents useful for conditions where long term maintenance of an alkaline urine is desirable. POLYCITRA-LC is also a fast acting and effective nonparticulate neutralizing buffer useful in raising gastric pH.
Syrup POLYCITRA and POLYCITRA-LC contain in each teaspoonful (5 mL):
POTASSIUM CITRATE Monohydrate ....550 mg
                                          (0.34 Molar)
SODIUM CITRATE Dihydrate...............500 mg (0.34 Molar)
CITRIC ACID Monohydrate...................334 mg (0.32 Molar)
Each mL contains 1 mEq Potassium and 1 mEq Sodium and is equivalent to 2 mEq Bicarbonate (HCO_3).
Syrup POLYCITRA is a sugar based solution.
POLYCITRA-LC is a sugar free solution.
Both products contain the identical amounts of active ingredients and are nonalcoholic.

CLINICAL PHARMACOLOGY
Potassium Citrate and Sodium Citrate are absorbed and metabolized to potassium bicarbonate and sodium bicarbonate, thus acting as systemic alkalizers. The effects are essentially those of chlorides before absorption and those of bicarbonates subsequently. Oxidation is virtually complete so that less than 5% of the citrates are excreted in the urine unchanged.

INDICATIONS AND ADVANTAGES
Syrup POLYCITRA and POLYCITRA-LC are effective alkalinizing agents useful for conditions where long term maintenance of an alkaline urine is desirable, as in patients where dissolution and control of uric acid and cystine calculi of the urinary tract is indicated. They are highly valuable in preventing uric acid nephropathy when administered to patients with hyperuricosuria (e.g. gout), or who are receiving drugs (e.g. cancer chemotherapy or uricosuric agents), resulting in acute or chronic increases in urinary uric acid excretion. They are also effective for alleviating chronic metabolic acidosis, which may result from renal insufficiency or renal tubular acidosis.
Syrup POLYCITRA and POLYCITRA-LC are highly concentrated, and when administered after meals and before bedtime, allows one to maintain an alkaline urine pH without the need for a 2 A.M. dose. In recommended dosage, Syrup POLYCITRA and POLYCITRA-LC alkalinize the urine without producing systemic alkalosis. POLYCITRA-LC is a fast acting buffering agent and is useful in rapidly neutralizing gastric acid and raising the pH of stomach contents. In vitro tests have shown that 15 mL POLYCITRA-LC will neutralize and buffer 235 mL of 0.1N HCl and raise gastric pH to 2.5, with no decrease of the pH value after 2 hours. POLYCITRA-LC is a nonparticulate buffer and, therefore, is decid-

edly advantageous over particulate aluminum-magnesium containing antacids, as a preanesthesia medication.

CONTRAINDICATIONS

Severe renal impairment with oliguria or azotemia, untreated Addison's disease or severe myocardial damage. In certain situations, when patients are on a sodium-restricted diet, the use of Potassium Citrate, as contained in POLYCITRA-K or POLYCITRA-K Crystals, may be preferable; or when patients are on a potassium-restricted diet, the use of Sodium Citrate, as contained in BICITRA, may be preferable.

PRECAUTIONS AND WARNINGS

Should be used with caution by patients with low urinary output or reduced glomerular filtration rates, unless under the supervision of a physician. Patients with renal insufficiency should not ingest POLYCITRA or POLYCITRA-LC concurrently with aluminum-based gels. Patients should be directed to dilute adequately with water and preferably to take each dose after meals, to minimize the possibility of gastrointestinal injury associated with oral ingestion of potassium salt preparations and to avoid saline laxative effect. Sodium salts should be used cautiously in patients with cardiac failure, hypertension, peripheral and pulmonary edema and toxemia of pregnancy. Concurrent administration of potassium-containing medication, potassium-sparing diuretics, angiotensin converting enzyme (ACE) inhibitors, or cardiac glycosides may lead to toxicity. Periodic examination and determinations of serum electrolytes, particularly serum levels of potassium and bicarbonate, should be carried out in those patients with renal disease in order to avoid these complications.

ADVERSE REACTIONS

Syrup POLYCITRA and POLYCITRA-LC are generally well tolerated without any unpleasant side effects when given in recommended doses to patients with normal renal function and urinary output. However, as with any alkalinizing agent, caution must be used in certain patients with abnormal renal mechanisms to avoid development of hyperkalemia or alkalosis, especially in the presence of hypocalcemia. Potassium intoxication causes listlessness, weakness, mental confusion and tingling of extremities.

DOSAGE AND ADMINISTRATION

Syrup POLYCITRA and POLYCITRA-LC should be taken diluted in water, followed by additional water if desired.
Usual Dosage: Adults: 15 to 30 mL diluted in water, four times a day after meals and at bedtime, or as directed by physician.
Children: 5 to 15 mL diluted in water, four times a day after meals and at bedtime, or as directed by physician.
Usual Dosage Range: 10 to 15 mL diluted with water, four times a day, will usually maintain a urine pH of 6.5-7.4. 15 to 20 mL diluted with water, taken four times a day, will usually maintain a urine pH of 7.0-7.6 throughout most of the 24 hours without unpleasant side effects.
As a Neutralizing Buffer: 15 mL POLYCITRA-LC taken as a single dose, or diluted, if desired, with 15 mL water, or as directed by physician.

OVERDOSAGE

Overdosage with sodium salts may cause diarrhea, nausea and vomiting, hypernoea, and convulsions. Overdosage with potassium salts may cause hyperkalemia and alkalosis, especially in the presence of renal disease.

HOW SUPPLIED

Syrup POLYCITRA—16 fl oz (473 mL) (NDC 11414-205-01)
POLYCITRA-LC—16 fl oz (473 mL) (NDC 11414-208-01)

POLYCITRA®-K Oral Solution
POLYCITRA®-K CRYSTALS   ℞
[polly "si-trah-ka 'y]
(Potassium Citrate and Citric Acid)
Sugar-Free

DESCRIPTION

POLYCITRA-K Oral Solution and POLYCITRA-K CRYSTALS are pleasant tasting and effective oral alkalinizing agents useful for conditions where long term maintenance of an alkaline urine is desirable.
POLYCITRA-K Oral Solution contains in each teaspoonful (5 mL):

POTASSIUM CITRATE Monohydrate ....1100 mg
CITRIC ACID Monohydrate ....334 mg
Each mL contains 2 mEq Potassium and is equivalent to 2 mEq Bicarbonate (HCO$_3$).
POLYCITRA-K Oral Solution (Potassium Citrate and Citric Acid Oral Solution USP) is sugar free and nonalcoholic.
POLYCITRA-K CRYSTALS—each unit dose packet contains:
POTASSIUM CITRATE Monohydrate ....3300 mg
CITRIC ACID Monohydrate ....1002 mg
Each unit dose packet, when reconstituted, supplies the same amount of active, ingredients as is contained in 15 mL (one tablespoonful) POLYCITRA-K Oral Solution and pro-

vides 30 mEq Potassium and is equivalent to 30 mEq Bicarbonate (HCO$_3$).
POLYCITRA-K CRYSTALS is sugar free and nonalcoholic.

CLINICAL PHARMACOLOGY

Potassium Citrate is absorbed and metabolized to potassium bicarbonate, thus acting as a systemic alkalizer. The effects are essentially those of chlorides before absorption and those of bicarbonates, subsequently. Oxidation is virtually complete so that less than 5% of the citrate is excreted in the urine unchanged.

INDICATIONS AND ADVANTAGES

POLYCITRA-K Oral Solution and POLYCITRA-K CRYSTALS are effective alkalinizing agent useful in those conditions where long term maintenance of an alkaline urine is desirable, as in patients where dissolution and control of uric acid and cystine calculi of the urinary tract is indicated, especially when the administration of sodium salts is undesirable or contraindicated. They are highly valuable in preventing uric acid nephrophathy when administered to patients with hyperuricosuria (e.g. gout), or who are receiving drugs (e.g. cancer chemotherapy or uricosuric agents), resulting in acute or chronic increases in urinary uric acid excretion. They are also effective for alleviating chronic metabolic acidosis, which may result from renal insufficiency or renal tubular acidosis, where the administration of Potassium Citrate may be preferable. Potassium Citrate has been reported to be effective in controlling mixed calcium oxalate/uric acid calculi.
POLYCITRA-K Oral Solution and POLYCITRA-K CRYSTALS are highly concentrated and when administered after meals and before bedtime, allows one to maintain an alkaline urine pH without the need for a 2 A.M. dose. In recommended dosage, these products alkalinize the urine without producing systemic alkalosis. They are pleasant tasting and tolerable, even when administered over long periods.
POLYCITRA-K is an oral liquid. POLYCITRA-K CRYSTALS, when constituted, becomes an oral liquid. Thus, both products provide rapid absorption from the alimentary tract. This is very advantageous compared to the use of tablet dosage forms. (The patient ingests a liquid rather than a slowly dissolving tablet which may cause local irritation or inflammation in sensitive individuals).

CONTRAINDICATIONS

Severe renal impairment with oliguria or azotemia, untreated Addison's disease, adynamia episodica hereditaria, acute dehydration, heat cramps, anuria, severe myocardial damage, and hyperkalemia from any cause.

WARNING

Large doses may cause hyperkalemia and alkalosis, especially in the presence of renal disease. Patients with renal insufficiency or uremia should not ingest POLYCITRA-K concurrently with aluminum-based gels. Concurrent administration of potassium-containing medication, potassium sparing diuretics, angiotensin converting enzyme (ACE) inhibitors, or cardiac glycosides may lead to toxicity.

PRECAUTIONS

Should be used with caution by patients with low urinary output unless under the supervision of a physician. As with all liquids containing a high concentration of potassium, patients should be directed to dilute adequately with water or other liquids to minimize the possibility of gastrointestinal injury associated with the oral ingestion of concentrated potassium salt preparations; and preferably, to take each dose after meals to avoid saline laxative effect.
Pregnancy: POLYCITRA-K Oral Solution and POLYCITRA-K CRYSTALS are not expected to cause fetal harm when administered in dosages which will not result in hyperkalemia.
Nursing Mothers: Caution should be exercised when administered to a nursing woman.
Pediatric Use: POLYCITRA-K Oral Solution (not POLYCITRA-K CRYSTALS Packets) is recommended for pediatric administration since dosage can be more easily regulated.

ADVERSE REACTIONS

POLYCITRA-K Oral Solution and POLYCITRA-K CRYSTALS are generally well tolerated without any unpleasant side effects when given in recommended doses to patients with normal renal function and urinary output. However, as with any alkalinizing agent, caution must be used in certain patients with abnormal renal mechanisms to avoid development of hyperkalemia or alkalosis. Potassium intoxication causes listlessness, weakness, mental confusion, tingling of extremities, and other symptoms associated with a high concentration of potassium in the serum. Periodic determinations of serum electrolytes should be carried out in those patients with renal disease in order to avoid these complications.

DOSAGE AND ADMINISTRATION

POLYCITRA-K Oral Solution and POLYCITRA-K CRYSTALS should be taken with water or juice according to directions, followed by additional water or juice if desired.

Usual Adult Dose: POLYCITRA-K Oral Solution—3 teaspoonfuls (15 mL), diluted with 6 ounces of water or juice, after meals and at bedtime, or as directed by physician.
POLYCITRA-K CRYSTALS—Contents of 1 packet reconstituted with at least 6 ounces of cool water or juice, after meals and at bedtime, or as directed by physician.
Usual Pediatric Dose: POLYCITRA-K Oral Solution—1 to 3 teaspoonfuls (5 to 15 mL), diluted with 6 ounces of water, after meals and at bedtime, or as directed by physician. (POLYCITRA-K CRYSTALS not recommended for pediatric use since dosage can be more easily regulated using POLYCITRA-K Oral Solution).
Usual Dosage Range: 10 to 15 mL POLYCITRA-K Oral Solution, diluted and taken four times a day, or contents of 1 packet POLYCITRA-K CRYSTALS, reconstituted as directed and taken four times a day, will usually maintain a urinary pH of 6.5 to 7.4.

OVERDOSAGE

The administration of oral potassium salts to persons with normal excretory mechanisms for potassium rarely causes serious hyperkalemia. However, if excretory mechanisms are impaired, hyperkalemia can result (see Contraindications and Warnings). Hyperkalemia, when detected, must be treated immediately because lethal levels can be reached in a few hours.
Treatment of Hyperkalemia: Should hyperkalemia occur, treatment measures include the following: (1) elimination of foods or medications containing potassium. (2) The intravenous administration of 300 to 500 mL/hr of dextrose solution (10 to 25%), containing 10 units of insulin/20 gm dextrose. (3) The use of exchange resins, hemodialysis, or peritoneal dialysis. In treating hyperkalemia, it should be recalled that in patients who have been stabilized on digitalis, too rapid a lowering of the plasma potassium concentration can produce digitalis toxicity.

HOW SUPPLIED

POLYCITRA-K—16 fl oz (473 mL) (NDC 11414-209-01)
POLYCITRA-K CRYSTALS—Unit Dose packets, 100/box (NDC 11414-215-01).

Winthrop Consumer Products
Division of Sterling Drug Inc.
90 PARK AVENUE
NEW YORK, NY 10016

BRONKAID® Mist
(Epinephrine)

DESCRIPTION

BRONKAID Mist, brand of epinephrine inhalation aerosol. Contains: Epinephrine, USP, 0.5% (w/w) (as nitrate and hydrochloric salts). Also contains: Alcohol 33% (w/w), ascorbic acid dichlorodifluoromethane, dichlorotetrafluroethane, purified water. Each spray delivers 0.25 mg epinephrine. Contains no sulfites.

INDICATION

For temporary relief of shortness of breath, tightness of chest and wheezing due to Bronchial Asthma.

WARNINGS

FOR ORAL INHALATION ONLY. Do not use this product unless a diagnosis of asthma has been made by a doctor, or if you have heart disease, high blood pressure, thyroid disease, diabetes, or difficulty in urination due to enlargement of the prostate gland, if you have ever been hospitalized for asthma or if you are taking any prescription drug for asthma. **Do not use this product more frequently or at higher doses than recommended, unless directed by a doctor.** Keep this and all drugs out of the reach of children. In case of accidental overdose, seek professional assistance or contact a poison control center immediately. As with any drug, if you are pregnant or nursing a baby, seek the advice of a health professional before using this product.
Excessive use may cause nervousness and rapid heart beat, and, possibly, adverse effects on the heart. **Do not continue to use this product, but seek medical assistance immediately if symptoms are not relieved within 20 minutes or become worse.**

DRUG INTERACTION PRECAUTION

Do not use this product if you are presently taking a prescription drug for high blood pressure or depression, without first consulting your doctor.
WARNING: Avoid spraying in eyes. Contents under pressure. Do not break or incinerate. Using or storing near open flame or heating above 120°F may cause bursting.

DOSAGE

Inhalation dosage for adults and children 4 years of age and older. Start with one inhalation, then wait at least one (1)

Continued on next page

Winthrop Consumer—Cont.

minute. If not relieved, use once more. Do not use again for at least 3 hours. The use of this product by children should be supervised by an adult. Children under 4 years of age, consult a doctor.

DIRECTIONS FOR USE

1. Remove cap and mouthpiece from bottle.
2. Remove cap from mouthpiece.
3. Turn mouthpiece sideways and fit metal stem of nebulizer into hole in flattened end of mouthpiece.
4. Exhale, as completely as possible. Now, hold bottle **upside down** between thumb and forefinger and close lips loosely around end of mouthpiece.
5. Inhale deeply while pressing down firmly on bottle, once only.
6. Remove mouthpiece and hold your breath a moment to allow for maximum absorption of medication. Then exhale slowly through nearly closed lips.

After use, remove mouthpiece from bottle and replace cap. Slide mouthpiece over bottle for protection. When possible rinse mouthpiece with tap water immediately after use. Soap and water will not hurt it. A clean mouthpiece always works better.

HOW SUPPLIED

Bottles of ½ fl. oz. (15 ml) NDC 0024-4082-15 with actuator. Also available—refills (no mouthpiece) in 15 ml (½ fl. oz.) NDC 0024-4083-16 and 22.5 ml (¾ fl. oz.) NDC 0024-4083-22.

BRONKAID® Mist Suspension
(Epinephrine Bitartrate)

ACTIVE INGREDIENTS

Each spray delivers 0.3 mg Epinephrine Bitartrate equivalent to 0.16 mg Epinephrine base. Contains Epinephrine Bitartrate 7.0 mg per cc. Also contains: Cetylpyridinium Chloride, Dichlorodifluoromethane, Dichlorotetrafluoroethane, Sorbitan Trioleate, Trichloromonofluoromethane, Contains no Sulfites.

INDICATION

Provides temporary relief of shortness of breath, tightness of chest, and wheezing due to Bronchial Asthma.

WARNINGS

FOR ORAL INHALATION ONLY. Do not use this product unless a diagnosis of asthma has been made by a doctor, or if you have heart disease, high blood pressure, thyroid disease, diabetes, or difficulty in urination due to enlargement of the prostate gland, if you have ever been hospitalized for asthma or if you are taking any prescription drug for asthma. **Do not use this product more frequently or at higher doses than recommended, unless directed by a doctor.** Keep this and all drugs out of the reach of children. In case of accidental overdose, seek professional assistance or contact a poison control center immediately. As with any drug, if you are pregnant or nursing a baby, seek the advice of a health professional before using this product.

Excessive use may cause nervousness and rapid heart beat, and, possibly, adverse effects on the heart. **Do not continue to use this product, but seek medical assistance immediately if symptoms are not relieved within 20 minutes or become worse.**

DRUG INTERACTION PRECAUTION

Do not use this product if you are presently taking a prescription drug for high blood pressure or depression, without first consulting your doctor.

WARNING

Avoid spraying in eyes. Contents under pressure. Do not break or incinerate. Using or storing near open flame or heating above 120°F may cause bursting.

ADMINISTRATION

(1) SHAKE WELL. (2) HOLD INHALER WITH NOZZLE DOWN WHILE USING. Empty the lungs as completely as possible by exhaling. (3) Purse the lips as in saying the letter "O" and hold the nozzle up to the lips, keeping the tongue flat. As you start to take a deep breath, squeeze nozzle and can together, releasing one full application. Complete taking deep breath, drawing medication into your lungs. (4) Hold breath for as long as comfortable. This distributes the medication in the lungs. Then exhale slowly keeping the lips nearly closed. (5) Rinse nozzle daily with soap and hot water after removing from vial. Dry with clean cloth. Before each use, remove dust cap and inspect mouthpiece for foreign objects. Replace dust cap after each use.

DOSAGE

Inhalation dosage for adults and children 4 years of age and older. Start with one inhalation, then wait at least one (1) minute. If not relieved, use once more. Do not use again for at least 3 hours. The use of this product by children should be

supervised by an adult. Children under 4 years of age; consult a doctor.

PROFESSIONAL LABELING

Same as stated under Indication.

HOW SUPPLIED

⅓ fl. oz. (10 cc) pocketsize aerosol inhaler NDC 0024-4082-10 with actuator.

BRONKAID® Tablets

DESCRIPTION

Each tablet contains ephedrine sulfate 24 mg, guaifenesin (glyceryl guaiacolate) 100 mg, and theophylline 100 mg. Also contains: magnesium stearate, magnesium trisilicate, microcrystalline cellulose, starch.

INDICATION

For symptomatic control of bronchial congestion and bronchial asthma. Clears bronchial passages. Helps relieve shortness of breath, plus helps loosen phlegm.

PRECAUTIONS

Do not use this product unless a diagnosis of asthma has been made by a doctor, or if you have heart disease, diabetes, difficulty in urination due to enlargement of the prostate gland, if you have ever been hospitalized for asthma or if you are taking any prescription drug for asthma unless directed by a doctor, do not continue to use this product, but seek medical assistance immediately if symptoms are not relieved within an hour or become worse. Some users of this product may experience nervousness, tremor, sleeplessness, nausea, and loss of appetite. If these symptoms persist or become worse, consult your doctor. Do not use this product if you are presently taking a prescription drug for high blood pressure or depression. Do not exceed recommended dosage unless directed by a physician.

WARNINGS

As with any drug, if you are pregnant or nursing a baby, seek the advice of a health professional before using this product. Keep this and all drugs out of the reach of children. In case of accidental overdose, seek professional assistance or contact a poison control center immediately.

DOSAGE AND ADMINISTRATION

Adult Dosage: 1 tablet every four hours. Do not take more than 5 tablets in a 24-hour period. Swallow tablets whole with water.

Children under 12 years of age: Consult a doctor.

Morning Dose: An early dose of 1 tablet (for adults) can relieve the coughing and wheezing caused by the night's accumulation of mucus, and can help you start the day with better breathing capacity.

Before an Attack: Many persons feel an attack of asthma coming on. One BRONKAID tablet beforehand may stop the attack before it starts.

During the Day: The precise dose of BRONKAID tablets can be varied to meet your individual needs as you gain experience with this product. It is advisable to take 1 tablet before going to bed, for nighttime relief. However, be sure not to exceed recommended daily dosage.

HOW SUPPLIED

Boxes of 24 (NDC 0024-4081-02)
Boxes of 60 (NDC 0024-4081-06)

CAMPHO-PHENIQUE®
[kam 'fo-finēk]
COLD SORE GEL

DESCRIPTION

Contains phenol 4.7% (w/w) and camphor 10.8% (w/w). Also contains: Colloidal silicon dioxide, eucalyptus oil, glycerin, light mineral oil.

ACTIONS

Use at the first sign of cold sore, fever blister and sun blister symptoms (tingling, pain, itching).

INDICATIONS

For relief of pain and itching due to cold sores, fever blisters and sun blisters. To combat infection from minor injuries and skin lesions.

Also effective for:

Minor Skin Injuries: abrasions, cuts, scrapes, burns, razor nicks and chafed or irritated skin.

Insect bites: Mosquitoes, black flies, sandfleas, chiggers.

WARNINGS

Not for prolonged use. Not to be used on large areas. In case of deep or puncture wounds, serious burns, or persisting redness, swelling or pain, or if rash or infection develops, discontinue use and consult physician. Do not bandage if applied to fingers or toes.

Avoid using near eyes. If product gets into the eye, flush thoroughly with water and obtain medical attention. Keep

this and all drugs out of the reach of children. In case of accidental ingestion, seek professional assistance or contact a poison control center immediately.

DIRECTIONS FOR USE

For external use. Apply directly to cold sore, fever blister or injury three or four times a day.

HOW SUPPLIED

Tubes of .23 oz. (6.5 g) NDC 0024-0212-01 and .50 oz. (14 g) NDC 0024-0212-02.

CAMPHO-PHENIQUE® Liquid
[kam 'fo-finēk]

DESCRIPTION

Contains phenol 4.7% (w/w) and camphor 10.8% (w/w). Also contains: Eucalyptus oil, light mineral oil.

ACTIONS

Pain-relieving antiseptic for scrapes, cuts, burns, insect bites, fever blisters, and cold sores.

INDICATIONS

For relief of pain and to combat infection from minor injuries and skin lesions.

WARNINGS

Not for prolonged use. Not to be used on large areas or in or near the eyes. In case of deep or puncture wounds, serious burns, or persisting redness, swelling or pain, or if rash or infection develops, discontinue use and consult physician. Do not bandage if applied to fingers or toes.

Keep this and all drugs out of the reach of children. In case of accidental ingestion, seek professional assistance or contact a poison control center immediately.

DIRECTIONS FOR USE

For external use. Apply with cotton three or four times daily. 4 oz size only:

Do not use more than ½ the contents of the 4 fl. oz. bottle in any 24-hour period.

HOW SUPPLIED

Bottles of   ¾ fl. oz. (NDC 0024-5150-05)
             1 ½ fl. oz. (NDC 0024-5150-06)
             4 fl. oz. (NDC 0024-5150-04)

CAMPHO-PHENIQUE®
[kam 'fo-finēk]
**TRIPLE ANTIBIOTIC OINTMENT
PLUS PAIN RELIEVER**

DESCRIPTION

Contains Bacitracin 400 units, Neomycin Sulfate 5 mg (equiv. to 3.5 mg Neomycin Base), Polymyxin B Sulfate 5000 units, Diperodon HCl 10mg (Pain Reliever). Also contains mineral oil and white petrolatum.

ACTIONS

Pain-relieving triple antibiotic with anesthetic to help prevent infection in minor cuts, scrapes, burns and other minor wounds.

INDICATIONS

Helps prevent infections in minor cuts, burns, and other minor wounds. Provides soothing, non-stinging temporary relief of pain and itching associated with these conditions.

WARNINGS

For external use only. In case of deep or puncture wounds, animal bites or serious burns, consult physician. If redness, irritation, swelling or pain persists or increases, or if infection occurs, discontinue use and consult physician. Do not use in eyes or over large areas. Keep this and all drugs out of children's reach. In case of accidental ingestion seek professional assistance or contact a poison control center immediately.

DIRECTIONS

Apply directly to the affected area and cover with a sterile gauze if necessary. May be applied 1 to 3 times daily as the condition indicates.

HOW SUPPLIED

Tubes of .50 oz. (NDC 0024-2015-05) and 1.0 oz. (NDC 0024-2015-01).

FERGON® TABLETS
[fur-gone]
brand of ferrous gluconate
FERGON® ELIXIR

COMPOSITION

FERGON (ferrous gluconate, USP) is stabilized to maintain a minimum of ferric ions. It contains not less than 11.5 percent iron.

Each FERGON tablet contains 320 mg (5 grains) ferrous gluconate equal to approximately 36 mg ferrous iron. Also contains: Acacia, Carnauba Wax, Dextrose Excipient, FD&C Red #40, D & C Yellow #10, FD & C Blue #1, Gelatin, Kaolin, Magnesium Stearate, Parabens, Povidone, Precipitated Calcium Carbonate, Sodium Benzoate, Starch, Sucrose, Talc, Titanium Dioxide, Yellow Wax. Not USP for dissolution. FERGON Elixir contains: Ferrous Gluconate 6%. Also contains: Alcohol 7%, Flavor, Glycerin, Liquid Glucose, Purified Water, Saccharin Sodium. Each teaspoon (5 ml) contains 300 mg (5 grains) Ferrous Gluconate equivalent to approximately 34 mg Ferrous Iron.

ACTION AND USES

FERGON preparations produce rapid hemoglobin regeneration in patients with iron deficiency anemias. FERGON is better utilized and better tolerated than other forms of iron because of its low ionization constant and solubility in the entire pH range of the gastrointestinal tract. It does not precipitate proteins or have the astringency of more ionizable forms of iron, does not interfere with proteolytic or diastatic activities of the digestive system, and will not produce nausea, abdominal cramps, constipation or diarrhea in the great majority of patients.

FERGON preparations are for use in the prevention and treatment of iron deficiency. They should be taken when the need for iron supplement therapy has been determined by a physician.

WARNINGS

Since oral iron products interfere with absorption of oral tetracycline antibiotics, these products should not be taken within two hours of each other. Keep this and all drugs out of the reach of children. As with any drug, if you are pregnant or nursing a baby, seek the advice of a health professional before using this product. In case of accidental overdose, seek professional assistance or contact a poison control center immediately.

DOSAGE AND ADMINISTRATION

Adults—One to two FERGON tablets or one to two teaspoonsful of FERGON Elixir daily. *For children and infants,* as prescribed by physician.

HOW SUPPLIED

FERGON Tablets of 320 mg (5 grains) bottle of 100 (NDC 0024-1015-10), bottle of 500 (NDC 0024-1015-50), and bottle of 1,000 (NDC 0024-1015-00). FERGON Elixir, 6% (5 grains per teaspoonful) bottle of 1 pint (NDC 0024-1019-16).

FERGON® IRON PLUS CALCIUM CAPLETS
[*fur-gone*]

DESCRIPTION

Each Caplet contains Ferrous Fumarate in a time-released system (yielding 18 mg of elemental iron), 1500 mg Calcium Carbonate (yielding 600 mg of elemental Calcium) and 125 IU of Vitamin D.

Also contains: Diethyl Phthalate, Ethylcellulose, Hydroxypropyl Methylcellulose, Magnesium Stearate, Microcrystalline Cellulose, Pharmaceutical Glaze, Povidone, FD&C Red 40, Colloidal Silicon Dioxide, Sodium Starch Glycolate, Stearic Acid, Talc, Titanium Dioxide and other ingredients. May also contain crospovidone.

ACTIONS AND USES

Fergon Iron Plus Calcium contains pure calcium and time-released iron for diets deficient in both minerals.

INDICATIONS

For use in the prevention of iron and/or calcium deficiency when the need for such therapy has been determined by a physician.

WARNINGS

Since oral iron products interfere with absorption of oral tetracycline antibiotics, these products should not be taken within two hours of each other. Keep this and all drugs out of the reach of children. As with any drug, if you are pregnant or nursing a baby, seek the advice of a health professional before using this product. In case of accidental overdose, seek professional assistance or contact a poison control center immediately. The treatment of any anemic condition should be under the advice and supervision of a physician.

DIRECTIONS

Adults, one to two caplets daily. For children and infants, consult physician.

HOW SUPPLIED

Fergon® Iron Plus Calcium Caplets (bottle of 60) NDC 0024-0596-60.

NaSal™
Saline (buffered)
0.65% Sodium chloride
Nasal Spray
Nose Drops

DESCRIPTION

Both the nasal spray and nose drops contain Sodium Chloride 0.65%. Also contains: Benzalkonium Chloride and Thimerosal 0.001% as preservative, Mono- and Dibasic Sodium Phosphates as buffers, Purified Water.
Contains No Alcohol.

ACTIONS

Immediate relief for dry nose. Formulated to match the pH of normal nasal secretions to help prevent stinging or burning.

INDICATIONS

Provides soothing relief for clogged nasal passages—without stinging or burning. Provides immediate relief for dry, inflamed nasal membranes due to colds, low humidity, allergies, minor nose bleeds, overuse of topical nasal decongestants, and other nasal irritations. As an ideal nasal moisturizer, it can be used in conjunction with oral decongestants.

ADVERSE REACTIONS

No associated side effects.

WARNINGS

Keep this and all drugs out of the reach of children. In case of accidental ingestion seek professional assistance or contact a poison control center immediately. The use of the dispenser by more than one person may spread infection.

DOSAGE AND ADMINISTRATION

Spray—For adults and children six years of age and over: with head upright, spray in each nostril as needed or as directed by physician. To spray, squeeze bottle quickly and firmly. *Nose Drops*—For infants and adults: 2 to 6 drops in each nostril as needed or as directed by physician.

HOW SUPPLIED

Nasal Spray—plastic squeeze bottles of 15 ml (½ fl. oz.) NDC 0024-1316-01.
Nose Drops—MonoDrop® bottles of 15 ml (½ fl. oz.) NDC 0024-1315-01.

NEO-SYNEPHRINE®
phenylephrine hydrochloride

DESCRIPTION

This line of Nasal Spray, Nose Drops and Nasal Spray Pumps contain Phenylephrine Hydrochloride in strengths ranging from .125% (drops only) to 1%. Also contains: Benzalkonium Chloride and Thimerosal 0.001% as preservatives, Citric Acid, Purified Water, Sodium Chloride, Sodium Citrate.

ACTION

Rapid-acting nasal decongestant.

INDICATIONS

For temporary relief of nasal congestion due to common cold, hay fever or other upper respiratory allergies, or associated with sinusitis.

PRECAUTIONS

Some hypersensitive individuals may experience a mild stinging sensation. This is usually transient and often disappears after a few applications.

Do not exceed recommended dosage. Follow directions for use carefully. If symptoms are not relieved after several applications, a physician should be consulted. Frequent and continued usage of the higher concentrations (especially the 1% solution) occasionally may cause a rebound congestion of the nose. Therefore, long-term or frequent use of this solution is not recommended without the advice of a physician. Prolonged exposure to air or strong light will cause oxidation and some loss of potency. Do not use if brown in color or contains a precipitate.

ADVERSE REACTIONS

Generally very well tolerated; systemic side effects such as tremor, insomnia, or palpitation rarely occur.

WARNINGS

Keep these and all drugs out of the reach of children. In case of accidental ingestion, seek professional assistance or contact a poison control center immediately. The use of this dispenser by more than one person may spread infection.
Do not use this product if you have heart disease, high blood pressure, thyroid disease, diabetes, or difficulty in urination due to enlargement of the prostate gland unless directed by a doctor.

DOSAGE AND ADMINISTRATION

Topical—dropper or spray. The *0.25% solution* is adequate in most cases (*0.125% for children 2 to 6 years*). In resistant cases, or if more powerful decongestion is desired, the *0.5% or 1% solution* should be used. Also used as *0.5% jelly.*

HOW SUPPLIED

Nasal spray 0.25%—15 ml (for children and for adults who prefer a mild nasal spray)—NDC 0024-1348-03; nasal spray 0.5%—15 ml (for adults)—NDC 0024-1353-01 and 30 ml (1 fl. oz.) NDC 0024-1353-05; nasal spray 1%—15 ml (extra strength for adults)—NDC 0024-1352-02; nasal spray pump 0.5%—15 ml bottle (½ fl. oz.) NDC 0024-1353-04; nasal solution 0.125% (for infants and small children), 15 ml bottles—NDC 0024-1345-05; nasal solution 0.25% (for children and adults who prefer a mild solution), 15 ml bottles—NDC 0024-1347-05; nasal solution 0.5% (for adults), 15 ml bottles—NDC 0024-1351-05; nasal solution 1% (extra strength for adults), 15 ml bottles—NDC 0024-1355-05; and 16 fl. oz. bottles—NDC 0024-1355-06; and water soluble nasal jelly 0.5%, ⅝ oz. tubes—NDC 0024-1367-01.

NEO-SYNEPHRINE® 12 HOUR
oxymetazoline hydrochloride

Nasal Spray 0.05%
Vapor Nasal Spray 0.05%
Nose Drops 0.05%

DESCRIPTION

Adult Strength Nasal Spray, and *Nose Drops* and *Nasal Spray Pump* contain: Oxymetazoline Hydrochloride 0.05%. Also contains: Benzalkonium Chloride and Phenylmercuric Acetate 0.002% as preservatives, Glycine, Purified Water, Sorbitol, may also contain Sodium Chloride. *Adult Strength Vapor Nasal Spray* contains Oxymetazoline Hydrochloride 0.05%. Also contains: Benzalkonium Chloride and Thimerosal 0.001% as preservatives, Camphor, Citric Acid, Eucalyptol, Menthol, Methyl Salicylate, Purified Water, Sodium Chloride, Sodium Citrate, Tyloxapol.

ACTION

12 HOUR Nasal Decongestant.

INDICATIONS

Provides temporary relief, for up to 12 HOURS, of nasal congestion due to colds, hay fever, sinusitis, or allergies. NEO-SYNEPHRINE 12-HOUR Nasal Sprays, Nose Drops and Nasal Spray Pump contain oxymetazoline which provides the longest-lasting relief of nasal congestion available.

WARNINGS

Do not exceed recommended dosage because symptoms may occur such as burning, stinging, sneezing, or increase of nasal discharge. (Nasal Spray 0.05%, Vapor Nasal Spray 0.05%, Nasal Spray Pump 0.05%, Nose Drops 0.05%) not recommended for children under 6. Do not use these products for more than 3 days. If symptoms persist, consult a physician. The use of the dispenser by more than one person may spread infection.
Do not use this product if you have heart disease, high blood pressure, thyroid disease, diabetes, or difficulty in urination due to enlargement of the prostate gland unless directed by a doctor.
Keep this and all drugs out of the reach of children. In case of accidental ingestion, seek professional assistance or contact a poison control center immediately.

DOSAGE AND ADMINISTRATION

Adult Strength Nasal Spray and Vapor Nasal Spray—For adults and children 6 years of age and over: With head upright, spray two or three times in each nostril twice daily—morning and evening. To spray, squeeze bottle quickly and firmly.
Nasal Spray Pump—For adults and children 6 to under 12 years of age (with adult supervision): spray 2 or 3 times in each nostril daily—morning and evening. Do not exceed 2 applications in any 24 hour period. Children under 6 years of age consult a doctor. Hold bottle with thumb at base and nozzle between first and second fingers. With head upright insert spray nozzle in nostril. Depress pump 2 or 3 times all the way down, with a firm even stroke and sniff deeply. Repeat in other nostril. Do not tilt head backward while spraying.
Adult Strength Nose Drops—For adults and children 6 years of age and over: two or three drops in each nostril twice daily—morning and evening.

HOW SUPPLIED

Nasal Spray Adult Strength—plastic squeeze bottles of 15 ml (½ fl. oz.) NDC 0024-1390-03 and 30 ml (1 fl. oz.) NDC 0024-1394-01; Nasal Spray Pump—15 ml bottle (½ fl. oz.) NDC 0024-1389-01; *Vapor Nasal Spray Adult Strength*—squeeze bottles of 15 ml (½ fl. oz.) NDC 0024-1391-03; *Nose Drops Adult Strength*—bottles of 15 ml (½ fl. oz.) with dropper NDC 0024-1392-01.

Continued on next page

Winthrop Consumer—Cont.

NTZ®
Long Acting
Oxymetazoline hydrochloride
Nasal Spray 0.05%
Nose Drops 0.05%

DESCRIPTION
Both the nasal spray and nose drops contain Oxymetazoline Hydrochloride 0.05%. Also contains: Benzalkonium Chloride and Phenylmercuric Acetate 0.002% as preservatives, Glycine, Purified Water, Sorbitol, and may also contain Sodium Chloride.

ACTIONS
12 Hour Nasal Decongestant

INDICATIONS
Provides temporary relief, for up to 12 hours, of nasal congestion due to colds, hay fever, sinusitis, or allergies. Oxymetazoline hydrochloride provides the longest-lasting relief of nasal congestion available. It decongests nasal passages up to 12 hours, reduces swelling of nasal passages, and temporarily restores freer breathing through the nose.

WARNINGS
Not recommended for children under six. Do not exceed recommended dosage because symptoms may occur such as burning, stinging, sneezing, or increase of nasal discharge. Do not use these products for more than 3 days. If symptoms persist, consult a physician. The use of the dispenser by more than one person may spread infection. Do not use this product if you have heart disease, high blood pressure, thyroid disease, diabetes, or difficulty in urination due to enlargement of the prostate gland unless directed by a doctor. Keep these and all drugs out of the reach of children. In case of accidental ingestion seek professional assistance or contact a poison control center immediately.

DOSAGE AND ADMINISTRATION
Intranasally by spray and dropper. *Nasal Spray*—For adults and children 6 years of age and over: With head upright, spray 2 or 3 times in each nostril twice daily—morning and evening. To spray, squeeze bottle quickly and firmly. *Nose Drops*—For adults and children 6 years of age and over: 2 or 3 drops in each nostril twice daily—morning and evening.

HOW SUPPLIED
Nasal Spray—plastic squeeze bottles of 15 ml (½ fl. oz.) NDC 0024-1312-02
Nose Drops—bottles of 15 ml (½ fl. oz.) with dropper NDC 0024-1311-03

pHisoDerm®
[fi-zo-derm]
Skin Cleanser and Conditioner

DESCRIPTION
pHisoDerm, a nonsoap emollient skin cleanser, is a unique liquid emulsion containing Sodium Octoxynol-2 Ethane Sulfonate Solution, Water, Petrolatum, Octoxynol-3, Mineral Oil (with Lanolin Alcohol and Oleyl Alcohol), Cocamide MEA, Imidazolidinyl Urea, Sodium Benzoate, Tetrasodium EDTA, and Methylcellulose. Adjusted to normal skin pH with Hydrochloric Acid. Contains no hexachlorophene. pHisoDerm contains no soap, perfumes, or irritating alkali. Its pH value, unlike that of soap, lies within the pH range of normal skin.

ACTIONS
pHisoDerm is well tolerated and can be used frequently by those persons whose skin may be irritated by the use of soap or other alkaline cleansers, or by those who are sensitive to the fatty acids contained in soap. pHisoDerm contains an effective detergent for removing soil and acts as an active emulsifier of all types of oil—animal, vegetable, and mineral.
pHisoDerm produces suds when used with any kind of water—hard or soft, hot or cold (even cold sea water)—at any temperature and under acid, alkaline, or neutral conditions. pHisoDerm deposits a fine film of lanolin components and petrolatum on the skin during the washing process and, thereby, helps protect against the dryness that soap can cause.

INDICATIONS
A sudsing emollient cleanser for use on skin of infants, children, and adults.
Useful for removal of ointments and cosmetics from the skin.

DIRECTIONS
For external use only.
HANDS. Squeeze a few drops of pHisoDerm into the palm, add a little water, and work up a lather. Rinse thoroughly.

FACE. After washing your hands, squeeze a small amount of pHisoDerm into the palm or onto a small sponge or washcloth, and work up a lather by adding a little water. Massage the suds onto the face for approximately one minute. Rinse thoroughly. Avoid getting suds into the eyes.
BATHING. First wet the body. Work a small amount of pHisoDerm into a lather with hands or a soft wet sponge, gradually adding small amounts of water to make more lather. Rinse thoroughly.

CAUTION
pHisoDerm suds that get into the eyes accidentally during washing should be rinsed out promptly with a sufficient amount of water.
pHisoDerm is intended for external use only. pHisoDerm should not be poured into measuring cups, medicine bottles, or similar containers since it may be mistaken for baby formula or medications. If swallowed, pHisoDerm may cause gastrointestinal irritation.
pHisoDerm should not be used on persons with sensitivity to any of its components.

HOW SUPPLIED
pHisoDerm is supplied in two formulations for regular and oily skin. It is packaged in sanitary squeeze bottles of 5 and 16 ounces. The regular formula is also supplied in squeeze bottles of 9 ounces and plastic bottles of 1 gallon.

pHisoDerm® FOR BABY
[fi'zo-derm]
Skin Cleanser

DESCRIPTION
pHisoDerm FOR BABY, a nonsoap emollient skin cleanser, is a unique liquid emulsion containing Sodium Octoxynol-2 Ethane Sulfonate Solution, Water, Petrolatum, Octoxynol-3, Mineral Oil (with Lanolin Alcohol and Oleyl Alcohol), Cocamide MEA, Fragrance, Imidazolidinyl Urea, Sodium Benzoate, Tetrasodium EDTA, and Methylcellulose. Adjusted to normal skin pH with Hydrochloric Acid. Contains no hexachlorophene or irritating alkali. Its pH value, unlike that of soap, lies within the pH range of normal skin.

ACTIONS
pHisoDerm FOR BABY gently cleans babies' delicate skin without irritating. Petrolatum and lanolin leave skin soft and smooth and protect against dryness.
pHisoDerm FOR BABY rinses easily without leaving a soapy film. The powder fragrance leaves skin smelling fresh and clean.

PRECAUTIONS
pHisoDerm FOR BABY suds that get into babies' eyes accidentally during washing should be rinsed out promptly with a sufficient amount of water.
pHisoDerm FOR BABY is intended for external use only. It should not be poured into measuring cups, medicine bottles, or similar containers since it may be mistaken for baby formula or medications. If swallowed, pHisoDerm FOR BABY may cause gastrointestinal irritation.
pHisoDerm FOR BABY should not be used on babies with sensitivity to any of its components.

ADMINISTRATION
First wet the baby's body. Work a small amount of pHisoDerm FOR BABY into a lather with hands or a soft wet sponge, gradually adding small amounts of water to make more lather. Spread the lather over all parts of the baby's body, including the head. Avoid getting suds into the baby's eyes. Wash the diaper area last. Be sure to carefully cleanse all folds and creases. Rinse thoroughly. Pat the baby dry with a soft towel.

HOW SUPPLIED
pHisoDerm FOR BABY is packaged in soft plastic, sanitary, squeeze bottles of 5 and 9 ounces and can be opened and closed with one hand.

WinGel®
[win'jel]
Liquid and Tablets

DESCRIPTION
Each teaspoon (5 ml) of liquid contains a specially processed, short polymer, hexitol stabilized aluminum-magnesium hydroxide equivalent to 180 mg of aluminum hydroxide and 160 mg of magnesium hydroxide. Also contains: Benzoic acid, flavor, methylcellulose, purified water, red ferric oxide, saccharin sodium, sodium hypochlorite solution, sorbitol solution.
Each tablet contains a specially processed, short polymer, hexitol stabilized aluminum-magnesium hydroxide equivalent to 180 mg of aluminum hydroxide and 160 mg of magnesium hydroxide. Also contains: D&C Red #28, FD&C Red #40, flavor, magnesium stearate, mannitol, saccharin sodium, starch. Smooth, easy-to-chew tablets.

ACTION
Antacid.

INDICATIONS
An antacid for the relief of acid indigestion, heartburn, and sour stomach. Nonconstipating. For the symptomatic relief of hyperacidity associated with the diagnosis of peptic ulcer, gastritis, peptic esophagitis, gastric hyperacidity, and hiatal hernia.

WARNINGS
Adults and children over 6—Patients should not take more than eight teaspoonfuls or eight tablets in a 24-hour period or use the maximum dosage of the product for more than 2 weeks, except under the advice and supervision of a physician.
Keep this and all drugs out of the reach of children. In case of accidental overdose, seek professional assistance or contact a poison control center immediately.

DRUG INTERACTION PRECAUTIONS
Antacids may react with certain prescription drugs. Do not take this product if you are presently taking a prescription antibiotic drug containing any form of tetracycline. If the patient is presently taking a prescription drug, this product should not be taken without checking with the physician.

DOSAGE AND ADMINISTRATION
Adults and children over 6—1 to 2 teaspoonfuls or 1 to 2 tablets up to four times daily, or as directed by a physician.
Acid Neutralization: The acid neutralization capacity of WINGEL liquid and tablets is not less than 10 mEq/5 ml.

HOW SUPPLIED
Liquid—bottles of 6 fl. oz. (NDC 0024-2247-03) and 12 fl. oz. (NDC 0024-2247-05).
Tablets—boxes of 50 (NDC 0024-2249-05) and 100 (NDC 0024-2249-06).

Winthrop Pharmaceuticals
90 PARK AVENUE
NEW YORK, NY 10016

ARALEN® Hydrochloride   ℞
brand of chloroquine hydrochloride
injection, USP

> **For Malaria and**
> **Extraintestinal Amebiasis**

> **WARNING: PHYSICIANS SHOULD COMPLETELY FAMILIARIZE THEMSELVES WITH THE COMPLETE CONTENTS OF THIS LEAFLET BEFORE PRESCRIBING ARALEN.**

DESCRIPTION
Parenteral solution, each mL containing 50 mg of the dihydrochloride salt equivalent to 40 mg of chloroquine base. ARALEN hydrochloride, a 4-aminoquinoline compound, is chemically 7-(Chloro-4-[[4-diethylamino)-1-methylbutyl]amino]-quinoline dihydrochloride, a white, crystalline substance, freely soluble in water.

ACTIONS
The compound is a highly active antimalarial and amebicidal agent.
ARALEN hydrochloride has been found to be highly active against the erythrocytic forms of *Plasmodium vivax* and *malariae* and most strains of *Plasmodium falciparum* (but not the gametocytes of *P. falciparum)*. The precise mechanism of action of the drug is not known.
ARALEN hydrochloride does not prevent relapses in patients with vivax or malariae malaria because it is not effective against exoerythrocytic forms of the parasite, nor will it prevent vivax or malariae infection when administered as a prophylactic. It is highly effective as a suppressive agent in patients with vivax or malariae malaria, in terminating acute attacks, and significantly lengthening the interval between treatment and relapse. In patients with falciparum malaria it abolishes the acute attack and effects complete cure of the infection, unless due to a resistant strain of *P. falciparum.*

INDICATIONS
ARALEN hydrochloride is indicated for the treatment of extraintestinal amebiasis and for treatment of acute attacks of malaria due to *P. vivax, P. malariae, P. ovale,* and susceptible strains of *P. falciparum* when oral therapy is not feasible.

CONTRAINDICATIONS
Use of this drug is contraindicated in the presence of retinal or visual field changes either attributable to 4-aminoquin-

oline compounds or to any other etiology, and in patients with known hypersensitivity to 4-aminoquinoline compounds. However, in the treatment of acute attacks of malaria caused by susceptible strains of plasmodia, the physician may elect to use this drug after carefully weighing the possible benefits and risks to the patient.

WARNINGS

Children and infants are extremely susceptible to adverse effects from an overdose of parenteral ARALEN and sudden deaths have been recorded after such administration. In no instance should the single dose of parenteral ARALEN administered to infants or children exceed 5 mg base per kg.

In recent years it has been found that certain strains of *P. falciparum* have become resistant to 4-aminoquinoline compounds (including chloroquine and hydroxychloroquine) as shown by the fact that normally adequate doses have failed to prevent or cure clinical malaria or parasitemia. Treatment with quinine or other specific forms of therapy is therefore advised for patients infected with a resistant strain of parasites.

Use of ARALEN should be avoided in patients with psoriasis, for it may precipitate a severe attack of psoriasis. Some authors consider the use of 4-aminoquinoline compounds contraindicated in patients with porphyria since the condition may be exacerbated.

Irreversible retinal damage has been observed in some patients who had received long-term or high-dosage 4-aminoquinoline therapy. Retinopathy has been reported to be dose related.

If there is any indication (past or present) of abnormality in the visual acuity, visual field, or retinal macular areas (such as pigmentary changes, loss of foveal reflex), or any visual symptoms (such as light flashes and streaks) which are not fully explainable by difficulties of accommodation or corneal opacities, the drug should be discontinued immediately and the patient closely observed for possible progression. Retinal changes (and visual disturbances) may progress even after cessation of therapy.

Usage in Pregnancy. Usage of this drug during pregnancy should be avoided except in the suppression or treatment of malaria when in the judgment of the physician the benefit outweighs the possible hazard. It should be noted that radioactively tagged chloroquine administered intravenously to pregnant pigmented CBA mice passed rapidly across the placenta, accumulated selectively in the melanin structures of the fetal eyes and was retained in the ocular tissues for five months after the drug had been eliminated from the rest of the body.[1]

PRECAUTIONS

Since the drug is known to concentrate in the liver, it should be used with caution in patients with hepatic disease or alcoholism or in conjunction with known hepatotoxic drugs. The drug should be administered with caution to patients having G-6-PD (glucose-6- phosphate dehydrogenase) deficiency.

ADVERSE REACTIONS

Respiratory depression, cardiovascular collapse, shock, convulsions, and death have been reported with overdoses of ARALEN hydrochloride, brand of chloroquine hydrochloride injection, especially in infants and children.

Any of the adverse reactions associated with short-term oral administration of chloroquine phosphate must be considered a possibility with chloroquine hydrochloride. Cardiovascular effects, such as hypotension and electrocardiographic changes (particularly inversion or depression of the T-wave, widening of the QRS complex), have rarely been noted in patients receiving usual antimalarial doses of the drug. Mild and transient headache, pruritus, psychic stimulation, visual disturbances (blurring of vision and difficulty of focusing or accommodation), pleomorphic skin eruptions, and gastrointestinal complaints (anorexia, nausea, vomiting, diarrhea, abdominal cramps) have been observed.

Instances of convulsive seizures associated with oral chloroquine therapy in patients with extraintestinal amebiasis have been reported.

A few cases of a nerve type of deafness have been reported after prolonged therapy, usually in high doses. Tinnitus and reduced hearing have been reported, in a patient with preexistent auditory damage, after administration of only 500 mg once a week for a few months. Since neuromyopathy, blood dyscrasias, lichen planus-like eruptions, and skin and mucosal pigmentary changes have been noted during prolonged oral therapy, their occurrence with this dosage form is possible.

Patients with retinal changes may be asymptomatic, especially in early cases, or may complain of nyctalopia and scotomatous vision with field defects of paracentral, pericentral ring types, and typically temporal scotomas, eg, difficulty in reading with words tending to disappear, seeing only half an object, misty vision, and fog before the eyes. Rarely scotomatous vision may occur without observable retinal changes.

DOSAGE AND ADMINISTRATION

Malaria —**Adult Dose.** An initial dose of 4 mL or 5 mL (160 mg to 200 mg chloroquine base) may be injected intramuscularly and repeated in 6 hours if necessary. The total parenteral dosage in the first 24 hours should not exceed 800 mg chloroquine base. Treatment by mouth should be started as soon as practicable and continued until a course of approximately 1.5 g of base in 3 days is completed.

Pediatric Dose. Infants and children are extremely susceptible to overdosage of parenteral ARALEN. Severe reactions and deaths have occurred. In the pediatric age range, parenteral ARALEN dosage should be calculated in proportion to the adult dose based upon body weight. The recommended single dose in infants and children is 5 mg base per kg. This dose may be repeated in 6 hours; however, the total dose in any 24 hour period should not exceed 10 mg base per kg of body weight. Parenteral administration should be terminated and oral therapy instituted as soon as possible.

Extraintestinal Amebiasis—In adult patients not able to tolerate oral therapy, from 4 mL to 5 mL (160 mg to 200 mg chloroquine base) may be injected daily for 10 to 12 days. Oral administration should be substituted or resumed as soon as possible.

OVERDOSAGE

Inadvertent toxic doses may produce respiratory depression or shock with hypotension. Respiratory depression is treated by artificial respiration and administration of oxygen. In shock with hypotension, a potent vasopressor, such as NEO-SYNEPHRINE® hydrochloride, brand of phenylephrine hydrochloride, USP, should be given intramuscularly in doses of 2 mg to 5 mg.

HOW SUPPLIED

Ampuls of 5 mL, box of 5 (NDC 0024-0074-01)

REFERENCE

Ullberg S, Lindquist N G, Sjostrand S E: Accumulation of chorio-retinotoxic drugs in the foetal eye. *Nature* 1970; 227:1257.

AW-100-H

ARALEN® Phosphate   ℞
brand of chloroquine phosphate tablets, USP

**For Malaria and
Extraintestinal Amebiasis**

WARNING: PHYSICIANS SHOULD COMPLETELY FAMILIARIZE THEMSELVES WITH THE COMPLETE CONTENTS OF THIS LEAFLET BEFORE PRESCRIBING ARALEN.

DESCRIPTION

ARALEN phosphate, a 4-aminoquinoline compound, is chemically 7-Chloro- 4-[[4- (diethylamino) -1-methylbutyl]amino]-quinoline phosphate (1:2), a white, crystalline substance, freely soluble in water.

Inactive Ingredients: Acacia, Carnauba Wax, Dibasic Calcium Phosphate, FD&C Red #3, Gelatin, Kaolin, Liquid Glucose, Magnesium Stearate, Pharmaceutical Glaze, Starch, Sucrose, Talc, Yellow Wax.

ACTIONS

ARALEN phosphate has been found to be highly active against the erythrocytic forms of *Plasmodium vivax* and *malariae* and most strains of *Plasmodium falciparum* (but not the gametocytes of *P. falciparum*). The precise mechanism of action of the drug is not known.

ARALEN phosphate does not prevent relapses in patients with vivax or malariae malaria because it is not effective against exo-erythrocytic forms of the parasite, nor will it prevent vivax or malariae infection when administered as a prophylactic. It is highly effective as a suppressive agent in patients with vivax or malariae malaria, in terminating acute attacks, and significantly lengthening the interval between treatment and relapse. In patients with falciparum malaria it abolishes the acute attack and effects complete cure of the infection, unless due to a resistant strain of *P. falciparum.*

In vitro studies with trophozoites of *Entamoeba histolytica* have demonstrated that ARALEN phosphate also possesses amebicidal activity comparable to that of emetine.

INDICATIONS

ARALEN phosphate is indicated for the suppressive treatment and for acute attacks of malaria due to *P. vivax, P. malariae, P. ovale,* and susceptible strains of *P. falciparum.* The drug is also indicated for treatment of extraintestinal amebiasis.

CONTRAINDICATIONS

Use of this drug is contraindicated in the presence of retinal or visual field changes either attributable to 4- aminoquinoline compounds or to any other etiology, and in patients with known hypersensitivity to 4-aminoquinoline compounds. However, in the treatment of acute attacks of malaria caused by susceptible strains of plasmodia, the physician may elect to use this drug after carefully weighing the possible benefits and risks to the patient.

WARNINGS

In recent years it has been found that certain strains of *P. falciparum* have become resistant to 4-aminoquinoline compounds (including chloroquine and hydroxychloroquine) as shown by the fact that normally adequate doses have failed to prevent or cure clinical malaria or parasitemia. Treatment with quinine or other specific forms of therapy is therefore advised for patients infected with a resistant strain of parasites.

Irreversible retinal damage has been observed in some patients who had received long-term or high-dosage 4-aminoquinoline therapy. Retinopathy has been reported to be dose related.

When prolonged therapy with any antimalarial compound is contemplated, initial (base line) and periodic ophthalmologic examinations (including visual acuity, expert slit-lamp, funduscopic, and visual field tests) should be performed.

If there is any indication (past or present) of abnormality in the visual acuity, visual field, or retinal macular areas (such as pigmentary changes, loss of foveal reflex), or any visual symptoms (such as light flashes and streaks) which are not fully explainable by difficulties of accommodation or corneal opacities, the drug should be discontinued immediately and the patient closely observed for possible progression. Retinal changes (and visual disturbances) may progress even after cessation of therapy.

All patients on long-term therapy with this preparation should be questioned and examined periodically, including testing knee and ankle reflexes, to detect any evidence of muscular weakness. If weakness occurs, discontinue the drug.

A number of fatalities have been reported following the accidental ingestion of chloroquine, sometimes in relatively small doses (0.75 or 1 g chloroquine phosphate in one 3-year-old child). Patients should be strongly warned to keep this drug out of the reach of children because they are especially sensitive to the 4- aminoquinoline compounds.

Use of ARALEN phosphate, brand of chloroquine phosphate tablets, in patients with psoriasis may precipitate a severe attack of psoriasis. When used in patients with porphyria the condition may be exacerbated. The drug should not be used in these conditions unless in the judgment of the physician the benefit to the patient outweighs the possible hazard.

Usage in Pregnancy. Usage of this drug during pregnancy should be avoided except in the suppression or treatment of malaria when in the judgment of the physician the benefit outweighs the possible hazard. It should be noted that radioactively tagged chloroquine administered intravenously to pregnant pigmented CBA mice passed rapidly across the placenta, accumulated selectively in the melanin structures of the fetal eyes and was retained in the ocular tissues for five months after the drug had been eliminated from the rest of the body.

PRECAUTIONS

Since the drug is known to concentrate in the liver, it should be used with caution in patients with hepatic disease or alcoholism or in conjunction with known hepatotoxic drugs.

Complete blood cell counts should be made periodically if patients are given prolonged therapy. If any severe blood disorder appears which is not attributable to the disease under treatment, discontinuance of the drug should be considered. The drug should be administered with caution to patients having G-6-PD (glucose-6-phosphate dehydrogenase) deficiency.

ADVERSE REACTIONS

Following the administration of ARALEN phosphate in doses adequate for the treatment of an acute malarial attack or extraintestinal amebiasis, mild and transient headache, pruritus, gastrointestinal complaints (anorexia, nausea, vomiting, diarrhea, abdominal cramps), psychic stimulation, and rarely psychotic episodes or convulsions have been observed. Cardiovascular effects, such as hypotension and electrocardiographic changes (particularly inversion or depression of the T wave, widening of the QRS complex), have rarely been noted in patients receiving usual antimalarial

Continued on next page

This product information was prepared in August, 1989. On these and other products of Winthrop Pharmaceuticals, detailed information may be obtained on a current basis by direct inquiry to the Professional Services Department, 90 Park Avenue, New York, NY 10016 (800) 446-6267.

Winthrop Pharm.—Cont.

doses of the drug. A few cases of a nerve type of deafness have been reported after prolonged therapy, usually in high doses. Tinnitus and reduced hearing have been reported, in a patient with preexistent auditory damage, after administration of only 500 mg once a week for a few months. Neuromyopathy, blood dyscrasias, lichen planus-like eruptions, and skin and mucosal pigmentary changes have also been noted during prolonged therapy.

When employed for the indications (malaria and extraintestinal amebiasis) and in the dosages recommended in this leaflet, visual disturbances, consisting of blurring of vision or difficulty in focusing or accommodation, occasionally may be noted; they are reversible and disappear on discontinuation of therapy. Other types of visual disturbances and ocular complications have been reported during the use of chloroquine for long-term therapy usually in daily doses exceeding 250 mg of chloroquine phosphate. These consisted of (1) reversible corneal changes (transient edema or opaque deposits in the epithelium) which may be asymptomatic or cause visual halos, focusing difficulties, or blurred vision and (2) generally irreversible, sometimes progressive, or, rarely delayed, retinal changes, such as narrowing of the arterioles, macular lesions (loss of foveal reflex, areas of edema, atrophy, and abnormal pigmentation), pallor of the optic disc, optic atrophy, and patchy retinal pigmentation.

Patients with retinal changes may be asymptomatic, especially in early cases, or may complain of nyctalopia and scotomatous vision with field defects of paracentral, pericentral ring types, and typically temporal scotomas, eg, difficulty in reading with words tending to disappear, seeing only half an object, misty vision, and fog before the eyes. Rarely scotomatous vision may occur without observable retinal changes.

DOSAGE AND ADMINISTRATION

The dosage of chloroquine phosphate is often expressed or calculated as the base. Each 500 mg tablet of ARALEN phosphate, brand of chloroquine phosphate tablets, is equivalent to 300 mg base. In infants and children the dosage is preferably calculated on the body weight.

Malaria: Suppression — **In adults,** 500 mg (= 300 mg base) on exactly the same day of each week. **In infants and children** the weekly suppressive dosage is 5 mg calculated as base, per kg of body weight, but should not exceed the adult dose regardless of weight.

If circumstances permit, suppressive therapy should begin two weeks prior to exposure. However, failing this in adults, an initial double (loading) dose of 1 g (= 600 mg base), or in children 10 mg base/kg may be taken in two divided doses, six hours apart. The suppressive therapy should be continued for eight weeks after leaving the endemic area.

Treatment of the acute attack—**In adults,** an initial dose of 1 g (= 600 mg base) followed by an additional 500 mg (= 300 mg base) after six to eight hours and a single dose of 500 mg (= 300 mg base) on each of two consecutive days. This represents a total dose of 2.5 g chloroquine phosphate or 1.5 g base in three days.

The dosage for adults may also be calculated on the basis of body weight; this method is preferred for infants and children. A total dose representing 25 mg of base per kg of body weight is administered in three days, as follows:

First dose: 10 mg base per kg (but not exceeding a single dose of 600 mg base).

Second dose: 5 mg base per kg (but not exceeding a single dose of 300 mg base) 6 hours after first dose.

Third dose: 5 mg base per kg 18 hours after second dose.

Fourth dose: 5 mg base per kg 24 hours after third dose.

For radical cure of *vivax* and *malariae* malaria concomitant therapy with an 8- aminoquinoline compound is necessary.

Extraintestinal Amebiasis: Adults, 1 g (600 mg base) daily for two days, followed by 500 mg (300 mg base) daily for at least two to three weeks. Treatment is usually combined with an effective intestinal amebicide.

OVERDOSAGE

Chloroquine is very rapidly and completely absorbed after ingestion, and in accidental overdosage, or rarely with lower doses in hypersensitive patients, toxic symptoms may occur within thirty minutes. These consist of headache, drowsiness, visual disturbances, cardiovascular collapse, and convulsions followed by sudden and early respiratory and cardiac arrest. The electrocardiogram may reveal atrial standstill, nodal rhythm, prolonged intraventricular conduction time, and progressive bradycardia leading to ventricular fibrillation and/or arrest. Treatment is symptomatic and must be prompt with immediate evacuation of the stomach by emesis (at home, before transportation to the hospital) or gastric lavage until the stomach is completely emptied. If finely powdered, activated charcoal is introduced by stomach tube, after lavage, and within 30 minutes after ingestion of the antimalarial, it may inhibit further intestinal absorption of the drug. To be effective, the dose of activated charcoal should be at least five times the estimated dose of chloroquine ingested.

Convulsions, if present, should be controlled before attempting gastric lavage. If due to cerebral stimulation, cautious administration of an ultrashort-acting barbiturate may be tried but, if due to anoxia, it should be corrected by oxygen administration, artificial respiration or, in shock with hypotension, by vasopressor therapy. Because of the importance of supporting respiration, tracheal intubation or tracheostomy, followed by gastric lavage, may also be necessary. Peritoneal dialysis and exchange transfusions have also been suggested to reduce the level of the drug in the blood.

A patient who survives the acute phase and is asymptomatic should be closely observed for at least six hours. Fluids may be forced, and sufficient ammonium chloride (8 g daily in divided doses for adults) may be administered for a few days to acidify the urine to help promote urinary excretion in cases of both overdosage or sensitivity.

HOW SUPPLIED

Tablets of 500 mg (= 300 mg base), bottle of 25 (NDC 0024-0077-01)

Shown in Product Identification Section, page 435

ARALEN® Phosphate   ℞
brand of chloroquine phosphate, USP
with
PRIMAQUINE Phosphate, USP

For Malaria Prophylaxis Only

> **WARNING: PHYSICIANS SHOULD COMPLETELY FAMILIARIZE THEMSELVES WITH THE COMPLETE CONTENTS OF THIS LEAFLET BEFORE PRESCRIBING ARALEN PHOSPHATE WITH PRIMAQUINE PHOSPHATE.**

DESCRIPTION

Each tablet contains ARALEN phosphate, brand of chloroquine phosphate, USP, 500 mg (equivalent to 300 mg base) and primaquine phosphate 79 mg (equivalent to 45 mg base). *Inactive Ingredients:* Dibasic Calcium Phosphate, FD&C Yellow #6, Lactose, Magnesium Stearate, Povidone, Starch, Stearic Acid, Talc, Titanium Dioxide, Triacetin, Zein.

ACTIONS

ARALEN is a 4-aminoquinoline compound which is highly active against the erythrocytic forms of *Plasmodium vivax* and most strains of *Plasmodium falciparum* (but not the gametocytes of *P. falciparum).*

Primaquine is an 8-aminoquinoline compound which eliminates tissue (exo-erythrocytic) infection. Thereby, it prevents the development of the blood (erythrocytic) forms of the parasite which are responsible for relapses in vivax malaria. Primaquine phosphate is active against gametocytes of *P. falciparum.*

ARALEN phosphate with primaquine phosphate demonstrates antimalarial activity against all stages of human malaria parasites, except for certain strains of *P. falciparum* resistant to chloroquine.

INDICATION

ARALEN phosphate with primaquine phosphate is intended solely for use in the prophylaxis of malaria, regardless of species, in all areas where this disease is endemic.

CONTRAINDICATIONS

The drug is contraindicated in acutely ill patients suffering from systemic disease manifested by tendency to granulocytopenia, such as rheumatoid arthritis and lupus erythematosus. The drug is also contraindicated in those patients receiving concurrently other potentially hemolytic drugs or depressants of myeloid elements of the bone marrow.

Primaquine should not be administered to patients who have received quinacrine recently, as toxicity is increased.

WARNINGS

Children are especially sensitive to 4-aminoquinoline compounds. A number of fatalities have been reported following the accidental ingestion of chloroquine, sometimes in relatively small doses (0.75 or 1 g in one 3- year-old child). Patients should be strongly warned to keep these drugs out of the reach of children.

Hemolytic reactions (moderate to severe) may occur after even a weekly dose of this preparation in glucose-6-phosphate dehydrogenase (G-6-PD) deficient Caucasians (particularly, in Sardinians and in individuals with a family or personal history of favism).

Usage in Pregnancy. Safe usage of this preparation in pregnancy has not been established. Therefore, use of it during pregnancy should be avoided except when in the judgment of the physician the benefit outweighs the possible hazard. It should be noted that radioactively tagged chloroquine administered intravenously to pregnant pigmented CBA mice passed rapidly across the placenta, accumulated selectively

in the melanin structures of the fetal eyes and was retained in the ocular tissues for five months after the drug had been eliminated from the rest of the body.[1]

PRECAUTIONS

ARALEN phosphate, brand of chloroquine phosphate, with primaquine phosphate is intended for malaria prophylaxis only; it should not be used for the treatment of clinical malaria. The recommended dosage (one tablet weekly, on the same day each week) should not be exceeded. The drug should not be taken more often than once every seven days to minimize danger of toxicity.

If the combination is prescribed for (1) an individual who has shown a previous idiosyncrasy to either chloroquine or primaquine (as manifested by dermatitis, hemolytic anemia, methemoglobinemia, or leukopenia), (2) an individual with a family or personal history of favism, or (3) an individual with erythrocytic glucose-6-phosphate dehydrogenase (G-6-PD) deficiency or nicotinamide adenine dinucleotide (NADH) methemoglobin reductase deficiency, the person should be observed closely for tolerance. The drug should be discontinued immediately if marked darkening of the urine, sudden decrease in hemoglobin concentration or leukocyte count, or severe skin reaction occurs.

In areas with endemic falciparum malaria due to strains that are resistant to the 4-aminoquinolines (chloroquine, amodiaquine, hydroxychloroquine), chemoprophylaxis with this combination alone may not be effective.

ADVERSE REACTIONS

Gastrointestinal reactions: anorexia, nausea, vomiting, epigastric distress, and abdominal cramps. *Hematologic reactions:* leukopenia, hemolytic anemia in glucose-6-phosphate dehydrogenase (G-6-PD) deficient individuals, methemoglobinemia in nicotinamide adenine dinucleotide (NADH) methemoglobin reductase deficient individuals.

Cardiovascular effects, such as hypotension and electrocardiographic changes (particularly inversion or depression of the T wave, widening of the QRS complex), have rarely been noted in patients receiving usual antimalarial doses of the drug.

Visual disturbances, consisting of blurring of vision or difficulty in focusing or accommodation, have occasionally been noted when chloroquine has been employed for malaria. These symptoms are reversible and disappear on discontinuation of therapy. Other types of visual disturbances (reversible corneal changes) and ocular complications including retinal changes (narrowing of the arterioles, macular lesions, pallor of the optic disc, optic atrophy, and patchy retinal pigmentation) have been reported during the use of chloroquine for long-term therapy usually in daily doses exceeding 250 mg of chloroquine phosphate. These changes have not been reported with the use of ARALEN phosphate, brand of chloroquine phosphate, with primaquine phosphate for malaria prophylaxis.

Auditory disturbances: tinnitus and reduced hearing have been reported, in a patient with preexistent auditory damage, after administration of only 500 mg of ARALEN phosphate, brand of chloroquine phosphate, once a week for a few months.

DOSAGE AND ADMINISTRATION

Adults—Starting at least one day before entering the malarious area, one tablet weekly, taken on the same day each week. This schedule (one tablet weekly) should be continued for eight weeks after leaving the endemic area.

Children—Table 1 gives suggested dosage based on body weight.

Table 1

Weight (lb)	ARALEN base (mg)	Primaquine base (mg)	Dose* (mL)
10-15	20	3	2.5
16-25	40	6	5.0
26-35	60	9	7.5
36-45	80	12	10.0
46-55	100	15	12.5
56-100	150	22.5	½ tab
100†	300	45	1 tab

*Dose based on liquid containing approximately 40 mg of chloroquine base and 6 mg of primaquine base per 5 mL (1 teaspoon) prepared from ARALEN phosphate, brand of chloroquine phosphate, with primaquine phosphate tablets. Chocolate syrup could be used to prepare a suspension (one tablet crushed and suspended in 40 mL of liquid). Shake well before use.

OVERDOSAGE

Symptoms of overdosage are due to the two drug components.

Chloroquine is very rapidly and completely absorbed after ingestion, and in accidental overdosage, or rarely with lower doses in hypersensitive patients, toxic symptoms may occur within thirty minutes. These consist of headache, drowsiness, visual disturbances, cardiovascular collapse, and convulsions followed by sudden and early respiratory and cardiac arrest. The electrocardiogram may reveal atrial standstill, nodal rhythm, prolonged intraventricular conduction time, and progressive bradycardia leading to ventricular fibrillation and/or arrest.

Symptoms of overdosage of primaquine are similar to those seen after overdosage of pamaquine. They include abdominal cramps, vomiting, burning epigastric distress, central nervous system and cardiovascular disturbances, cyanosis, methemoglobinemia, moderate leukocytosis or leukopenia, and anemia. The most striking symptoms are granulocytopenia and acute hemolytic anemia in sensitive persons. Acute hemolysis occurs, but patients recover completely if the dosage is discontinued.

Treatment is symptomatic and must be prompt with immediate evacuation of the stomach by emesis (at home, before transportation to the hospital) or gastric lavage until the stomach is completely emptied. Finely powdered, activated charcoal in a dose not less than five times the estimated dose of chloroquine ingested, if introduced by the stomach tube after lavage within thirty minutes after ingestion of the antimalarial, may inhibit further intestinal absorption of the drug.

Convulsions, if present, should be controlled before attempting gastric lavage. If due to cerebral stimulation, cautious administration of an ultrashort-acting barbiturate may be tried but, if due to anoxia, it should be corrected by oxygen administration, artificial respiration or, in shock with hypotension, by vasopressor therapy. Because of the importance of supporting respiration, tracheal intubation or tracheostomy, followed by gastric lavage, may also be necessary. Exchange transfusions have also been suggested to reduce the level of the drug in the blood.

The patient should be kept in bed and warm. If methemoglobinemia and cyanosis occur, oxygen may be administered and use of methylene blue may be considered. If collapse and hypotension or shock occur, vasopressors may be used. The patient should be observed for the possible development of leukopenia or hemolytic anemia.

A patient who survives the acute stage and is asymptomatic should be closely observed for at least six hours. Fluids may be forced, and sufficient ammonium chloride (8 g daily in divided doses for adults) may be administered for a few days to acidify the urine to help promote urinary excretion in cases of both overdosage or sensitivity.

HOW SUPPLIED

Tablets, bottles of 100 (NDC 0024-0079-04)

CLINICAL STUDIES

On the basis of carefully controlled preliminary clinical trials, Alving and his associates[2] found that the weekly administration of 300 mg chloroquine base and 45 mg primaquine base (administered as the phosphate salts) proved highly effective as a prophylactic against severe *P. vivax* infections with the Chesson strain and did not produce clinical hemolysis even among primaquine-sensitive American Negro adult volunteers. A weekly dose of primaquine phosphate equivalent to 45 mg primaquine base cured 90 percent of infections. The studies of these workers indicate that the toxicity of primaquine phosphate, as regards the production of hemolysis, is markedly diminished when administered in weekly doses. When administered with standard suppressive doses of chloroquine phosphate, its therapeutic effectiveness in the radical cure of Chesson vivax malaria is increased. Thus, a weekly dose equivalent to 60 mg of primaquine base is less toxic than 15 mg base administered daily; and a dose equivalent to 45 mg base administered weekly was found to be practically without demonstrable toxicity. A dose equivalent to 45 mg base weekly for 8 weeks was more effective in the radical cure of infections than 15 mg base daily for 14 days. Wittmer[3] conducted a double-blind study in 24 Caucasian male adults who received ARALEN phosphate, brand of chloroquine phosphate, with primaquine phosphate once each week (Friday) for 15 weeks to determine its safety and suitability for use in Armed Forces flying personnel. The author concluded that there appear to be no contraindications to the long-term use of the combination in flying personnel since there was no effect on vision, time of useful consciousness, or psychomotor performance. No deleterious synergistic effect of the two drugs was demonstrated. Charles[4] investigated the effects of 5 weekly doses of primaquine phosphate (1 mg to 1.5 mg base per kg body weight) in combination with a 4-aminoquinoline antimalarial agent on the parasitemia and blood picture of 100 Ghanaian children from 2½ to 8 years old. Although the enzyme-deficiency trait (glucose-6-phosphate dehydrogenase deficiency) for primaquine sensitivity occurred in approximately 25 percent of the group, no general evidence of hemolysis was observed. Eight of the treated subjects were positive for the glucose-6-phosphate dehydrogenase deficiency test but maintained their pretreatment hemoglobin values.

However, Ziai and his associates[5] noted that serious hematologic reactions can occur in persons with a glucose-6-phosphate dehydrogenase (G-6-PD) deficiency used for malaria

suppressive therapy. This has been reported primarily in patients with a family history and/or personal history of favism.

Methemoglobinemia has been discovered in individuals with nicotinamide adenine dinucleotide methemoglobin reductase deficiency.[6]

The susceptibility of primaquine-sensitive children to hemolysis by primaquine phosphate is considered to be of the same order of magnitude as that of adults on an equal drug/body weight basis.

REFERENCES

1. Ullberg S, Lindquist N G, Sjostrand S E: Accumulation of chorio-retinotoxic drugs in the foetal eye. *Nature* 1970; 227:1257.
2. Alving A S, et al: Mitigation of the haemolytic effect of primaquine and enhancement of its action against exo-erythrocytic forms of the Chesson strain of *Plasmodium vivax* by intermittent regimens of drug administration. *Bull WHO* 1960; 22:621.
3. Wittmer J F: Aeromedical aspects of malaria prophylaxis with chloroquine-primaquine. *Aerospace Med* 1963; 34:944.
4. Charles L J: Observations on the haemolytic effect of primaquine in 100 Ghanaian children. *Ann Trop Med* 1960; 54:460.
5. Ziai M, et al: Malaria prophylaxis and treatment in G-6-PD deficiency. *Clin Pediat* 1967; 6:242.
6. Cohen R, et al: Methemoglobinemia provoked by malarial chemoprophylaxis in Vietnam. *New Eng J Med* 1968; 279:1127-1131.

AW-109-J

ATABRINE® Hydrochloride   ℞
brand of quinacrine hydrochloride tablets, USP

DESCRIPTION

Each tablet contains 100 mg of quinacrine hydrochloride, a bright yellow, odorless, bitter crystalline powder that is water soluble (1:35), and bears identifying number A 82.
Inactive Ingredients: Pharmaceutical Glaze, Starch, Stearic Acid, Talc.

HOW SUPPLIED

Tablets of 100 mg (bright yellow, shellac-coated), bottle of 100 (NDC 0024-0082-04)

For complete prescribing information see package insert or contact Professional Services Department.

AW-91-K

BREONESIN®   OTC
brand of guaifenesin capsules, USP

(See PDR For Nonprescription Drugs)

BRONKEPHRINE®   ℞
**brand of ethylnorepinephrine hydrochloride injection, USP
IN AQUEOUS SOLUTION**

DESCRIPTION

BRONKEPHRINE is ethylnorepinephrine hydrochloride injection, USP. Each mL contains 2 mg ethylnorepinephrine HCl in a sterile isotonic solution of 0.7% sodium chloride with acetone sodium bisulfite 0.2% as preservative. The pH is adjusted to 2.9 to 4.5 with NaOH or HCl. BRONKEPHRINE is a synthetic sympathomimetic amine intended for subcutaneous or intramuscular injection. The chemical name is 1,2-Benzenediol,4-(2-amino-1-hydroxybutyl)-,hydrochloride.

CLINICAL PHARMACOLOGY

BRONKEPHRINE is primarily a beta-adrenergic agonist. Its actions are similar to those of isoproterenol, although it is less potent. Its bronchodilating properties closely simulate those of epinephrine but without significant pressor effects. It thus may be safer than epinephrine for hypertensive patients and severely ill patients in whom such effects are undesirable. It is particularly adapted for use in children because of its relative lack of adverse effects, especially central nervous system excitation. It also may be of value in diabetic asthmatics due to its lack of glycogenolytic activity.
Metabolic and pharmacokinetic data are unavailable.

INDICATIONS AND USAGE

BRONKEPHRINE is indicated for use as a bronchodilator for bronchial asthma and for reversible bronchospasm that may occur in association with bronchitis and emphysema.

CONTRAINDICATIONS

BRONKEPHRINE is contraindicated in patients who are hypersensitive to any of its ingredients or with idiosyncrasy to sympathomimetic drugs.

WARNINGS

BRONKEPHRINE should not be administered along with epinephrine or other sympathomimetic amines because these drugs are direct cardiac stimulants and may cause excessive tachycardia.

Contains acetone sodium bisulfite, a sulfite that may cause allergic-type reactions including anaphylactic symptoms and life-threatening or less severe asthmatic episodes in certain susceptible people. The overall prevalence of sulfite sensitivity in the general population is unknown and probably low. Sulfite sensitivity is seen more frequently in asthmatic than in nonasthmatic people.

PRECAUTIONS

BRONKEPHRINE should be used with caution in persons with cardiovascular disease, a history of stroke or coronary artery disease. It is a potent drug and may cause toxic symptoms through idiosyncratic response or overdosage.

Care should be taken in anatomical selection of injection sites to avoid inadvertent intraneural or intravascular injection.

Carcinogenesis, Mutagenesis, Impairment of Fertility: Long-term animal studies of BRONKEPHRINE to evaluate carcinogenic potential and reproduction studies in animals have not been performed. There is no evidence from human data that BRONKEPHRINE may be carcinogenic or mutagenic or that it impairs fertility.

Pregnancy Category C: Animal reproduction studies have not been conducted with BRONKEPHRINE. It is not known whether BRONKEPHRINE can cause fetal harm when administered to a pregnant woman or can affect reproduction capacity. BRONKEPHRINE should be given to a pregnant woman only if clearly needed and the potential benefits outweigh the risk.

Nursing Mothers: It is not known whether BRONKEPHRINE is excreted in human milk; however, because many drugs are excreted in human milk, caution should be exercised when BRONKEPHRINE is administered to a nursing woman.

ADVERSE REACTIONS

BRONKEPHRINE, brand of ethylnorepinephrine hydrochloride injection, is generally well tolerated. It may, however, produce changes in blood pressure (elevation or depression) or pulse rate (elevation), palpitation, headache, dizziness or nausea; as with other sympathomimetic amines.

OVERDOSAGE

The signs and symptoms of overdosage with BRONKEPHRINE are those typical of any sympathomimetic amine. Treatment should be symptomatic.

DOSAGE AND ADMINISTRATION

The usual adult dose by subcutaneous or intramuscular injection is 0.5 mL to 1 mL. Depending on severity of the asthmatic attack, smaller doses (0.3 mL to 0.5 mL) may suffice. Dosage in children varies according to age and weight; usually 0.1 mL to 0.5 mL is sufficient.

HOW SUPPLIED

Uni-Nest ™—Sterile single-dose ampuls of 1 mL, box of 25. NDC 0024-1001-25)
PROTECT AMPULS FROM LIGHT.

BW-96 B

BRONKODYL®   ℞
**brand of theophylline anhydrous capsules
100 mg and 200 mg**

DESCRIPTION

Theophylline is a bronchodilator structurally classified as a xanthine derivative. It occurs as a white, odorless, crystalline powder having a bitter taste. Theophylline anhydrous has the chemical name 1*H*-Purine-2, 6-dione, 3, 7-dihydro-1, 3-dimethyl-.

BRONKODYL is available as 100 mg, brown and white capsules and 200 mg, green and white capsules intended for oral administration, containing 100 mg of theophylline anhydrous and 200 mg of theophylline anhydrous respectively.
Inactive Ingredients: Benzyl Alcohol, Gelatin, Lactose, Magnesium Stearate, Parabens, Silicon Dioxide, Sodium Propionate, Sodium Starch Glycolate. Capsule **100 mg** contains FD&C Blue #1, Red #3, Yellow #6. Capsule **200 mg** contains D&C Yellow #10, FD&C Blue #1, Yellow #6.

HOW SUPPLIED

100 mg brown and white, hard gelatin capsules, bottles of 100 **NDC** 0024-1036-10

Continued on next page

This product information was prepared in August, 1989. On these and other products of Winthrop Pharmaceuticals, detailed information may be obtained on a current basis by direct inquiry to the Professional Services Department, 90 Park Avenue, New York, NY 10016 (800) 446-6267.

Winthrop Pharm.—Cont.

200 mg green and white, hard gelatin capsules, bottles of 100
NDC 0024-1037-10
Distributed by
Winthrop Pharmaceuticals
Division of Sterling Drug Inc. New York, NY 10016
Mfd. by KV Pharmaceutical Co., St. Louis, Missouri 63144
For complete prescribing information, see package insert or
contact Professional Services Department.

BW 98-C

BRONKOLIXIR®   OTC

(See PDR For Nonprescription Drugs)

BRONKOSOL®   R

brand of isoetharine inhalation solution, USP, 1%
BRONCHODILATOR SOLUTION FOR ORAL INHALATION

DESCRIPTION
Isoetharine hydrochloride, USP, 1% also contains: Acetone
Sodium Bisulfite, Glycerin, Parabens, Purified Water, So-
dium Chloride, and Sodium Citrate.

BRONKOMETER®   R

brand of isoetharine mesylate inhalation aerosol, USP

DESCRIPTION
BRONKOMETER is a complete pocket nebulizer containing
isoetharine mesylate 0.61% (w/w). BRONKOMETER also
contains: alcohol 30% (w/w), ascorbic acid 0.1% (w/w) as a
preservative, dichlorodifluoromethane and dichlorotetrafluoroethane as propellants, menthol, and saccharin.
Isoetharine is 1-(3,4 dihydroxyphenyl)-2-isopropylamino-
1-butanol. The BRONKOMETER unit delivers approximately 20 metered doses per mL of solution. Each average 56
mg delivery contains 340 mcg isoetharine.

CLINICAL PHARMACOLOGY
Isoetharine is a sympathomimetic amine with preferential
affinity for Beta₂ adrenergic receptor sites of bronchial and
certain arteriolar musculature, and a lower order of affinity
for Beta₁ adrenergic receptors. Its activity in symptomatic
relief of bronchospasm is rapid and of relatively long duration. By relieving bronchospasm, BRONKOSOL and
BRONKOMETER help give prompt relief and significantly
increase vital capacity.

INDICATIONS AND USAGE
BRONKOSOL and BRONKOMETER are indicated for use
as bronchodilators for bronchial asthma and for reversible
bronchospasm that may occur in association with bronchitis
and emphysema.

CONTRAINDICATION
BRONKOSOL and BRONKOMETER should not be administered to patients who are hypersensitive to any of their ingredients.

WARNINGS
BRONKOSOL contains acetone sodium bisulfite, a sulfite
that may cause allergic-type reactions including anaphylactic symptoms and life-threatening or less severe asthmatic
episodes in certain susceptible people. The overall prevalence of sulfite sensitivity in the general population is unknown and probably low. Sulfite sensitivity is seen more
frequently in asthmatic than in nonasthmatic people.
Excessive use of an adrenergic aerosol should be discouraged
as it may lose its effectiveness. Occasional patients have been
reported to develop severe paradoxical airway resistance
with repeated excessive use of an aerosol adrenergic inhalation preparation. The cause of this refractory state is unknown. It is advisable that in such instances the use of the
aerosol adrenergic be discontinued immediately and alternative therapy instituted, since in the reported cases the patients did not respond to other forms of therapy until the
drug was withdrawn. Cardiac arrest has been noted in several instances.

to sympathomimetic amines, since overdosage may result in
tachycardia, palpitation, nausea, headache, or epinephrine-
like side effects.

ADVERSE REACTIONS
Although BRONKOSOL and BRONKOMETER are relatively free of toxic side effects, too frequent use may cause
tachycardia, palpitation, nausea, headache, changes in blood
pressure, anxiety, tension, restlessness, insomnia, tremor,
weakness, dizziness, and excitement, as is the case with other
sympathomimetic amines.

DOSAGE AND ADMINISTRATION
BRONKOSOL can be administered by hand nebulizer, oxygen aerosolization, or intermittent positive pressure breathing (IPPB). Usually treatment need not be repeated more
often than every four hours, although in severe cases more
frequent administration may be necessary.

Method of Administration	Usual Dose	Usual Range	Usual Dilution
Hand nebulizer	4 inha-lations	3-7 inha-lations	undiluted
Oxygen aerosoli-zation*	½ mL	¼-½ mL	1:3 with saline or other diluent
IPPB†	½ mL	¼-1 mL	1:3 with saline or other diluent

* Administered with oxygen flow adjusted to 4 to 6
liters/minute over a period of 15 to 20 minutes.
† Usually an inspiratory flow rate of 15 liters/minute at a
cycling pressure of 15 cm H₂O is recommended. It may be
necessary, according to patient and type of IPPB apparatus, to adjust flow rate to 6 to 30 liters per minute, cycling
pressure to 10 to 15 cm H₂0, and further dilution according
to needs of patient.

BRONKOMETER®

DOSAGE AND ADMINISTRATION
The average adult dose is one or two inhalations. Occasionally, more may be required. It is important, however, to wait
one full minute after the initial one or two inhalations in
order to be certain whether another is necessary. In most
cases, inhalations need not be repeated more often than every four hours, although more frequent administration may
be necessary in severe cases.

HOW SUPPLIED
BRONKOMETER, brand of isoetharine mesylate inhalation
aerosol
Vial of 10 mL, with oral nebulizer (NDC 0024-1040-01)
Refill only, 10 mL (NDC 0024-1041-01)
Vial of 15 mL, with oral nebulizer (NDC 0024-1040-03)
Refill only, 15 mL (NDC 0024-1041-03)
The bronchodilator isoetharine is also available in a conve-
nient solution for use with conventional nebulizers, by oxy-
gen aerosolization, and in IPPB machines as BRONKOSOL,
brand of isoetharine inhalation solution, 1%. It is supplied as
follows:
Bottle of 10 mL (NDC 0024-1071-10)
Bottle of 30 mL (NDC 0024-1071-30)

BRONKOSOL and BRONKOMETER should not be administered along with epinephrine or other sympathomimetic
amines, since these drugs are direct cardiac stimulants and
may cause excessive tachycardia. They may, however, be
alternated if desired.
Usage in Pregnancy: Although there has been no evidence
of teratogenic effects with this drug, use of any drug in pregnancy, lactation, or in women of childbearing potential requires that the potential benefit of the drug be weighed
against its possible hazard to the mother or child.

PRECAUTIONS
Dosage must be carefully adjusted in patients with hyperthyroidism, hypertension, acute coronary disease, cardiac
asthma, limited cardiac reserve, and in individuals sensitive

Distributed by Winthrop-Breon Laboratories
Division of Sterling Drug Inc
New York, NY 10016
Manufactured by
Sterling Pharmaceuticals Inc
Barceloneta, Puerto Rico 00617

BRONKOTABS®   OTC

(See PDR For Nonprescription Drugs)

CARBOCAINE® HYDROCHLORIDE   R

brand of mepivacaine hydrochloride
injection, USP

THESE SOLUTIONS ARE NOT INTENDED FOR SPINAL
ANESTHESIA OR DENTAL USE

DESCRIPTION
Mepivacaine hydrochloride is 2-Piperidinecarboxamide, N-
(2,6-dimethylphenyl)-1-methyl-, monohydrochloride.
It is a white crystalline odorless powder, soluble in water, but
very resistant to both acid and alkaline hydrolysis.
CARBOCAINE hydrochloride is a local anesthetic available
as sterile isotonic solutions in concentrations of 1%, 1.5%,
and 2% for injection via local infiltration, peripheral nerve
block, and caudal and lumbar epidural blocks.
Mepivacaine hydrochloride is related chemically and pharmacologically to the amide-type local anesthetics. It contains
an amide linkage between the aromatic nucleus and the
amino group.
[See table below].
The pH of the solutions is adjusted between 4.5 and 6.8 with
sodium hydroxide or hydrochloric acid.

CLINICAL PHARMACOLOGY
Local anesthetics block the generation and the conduction of
nerve impulses, presumably by increasing the threshold for
electrical excitation in the nerve, by slowing the propagation
of the nerve impulse, and by reducing the rate of rise of the
action potential. In general, the progression of anesthesia is
related to the diameter, myelination, and conduction velocity of affected nerve fibers. Clinically, the order of loss of
nerve function is as follows: pain, temperature, touch, proprioception, and skeletal muscle tone.
Systemic absorption of local anesthetics produces effects on
the cardiovascular and central nervous systems. At blood
concentrations achieved with normal therapeutic doses,
changes in cardiac conduction, excitability, refractoriness,
contractility, and peripheral vascular resistance are minimal. However, toxic blood concentrations depress cardiac
conduction and excitability, which may lead to atrioventricular block and ultimately to cardiac arrest. In addition, myocardial contractility is depressed and peripheral vasodilation
occurs, leading to decreased cardiac output and arterial
blood pressure.
Following systemic absorption, local anesthetics can produce
central nervous system stimulation, depression, or both.
Apparent central stimulation is manifested as restlessness,
tremors, and shivering, progressing to convulsions, followed
by depression and coma progressing ultimately to respiratory arrest. However, the local anesthetics have a primary
depressant effect on the medulla and on higher centers. The
depressed stage may occur without a prior excited stage.
Pharmacokinetics
The rate of systemic absorption of local anesthetics is dependent upon the total dose and concentration of drug administered, the route of administration, the vascularity of the administration site, and the presence or absence of epinephrine
in the anesthetic solution. A dilute concentration of epinephrine (1:200,000 or 5 μg/mL) usually reduces the rate of absorption and plasma concentration of CARBOCAINE, however, it has been reported that vasoconstrictors do not significantly prolong anesthesia with CARBOCAINE.
Onset of anesthesia with CARBOCAINE is rapid, the time of
onset for sensory block ranging from about 3 to 20 minutes
depending upon such factors as the anesthetic technique, the
type of block, the concentration of the solution, and the individual patient. The degree of motor blockade produced is
dependent on the concentration of the solution. A 0.5% solution will be effective in small superficial nerve blocks while
the 1% concentration will block sensory and sympathetic
conduction without loss of motor function. The 1.5% solution
will provide extensive and often complete motor block and
the 2% concentration of CARBOCAINE will produce complete sensory and motor block of any nerve group.
The duration of anesthesia also varies depending upon the
technique and type of block, the concentration, and the individual. Mepivacaine will normally provide anesthesia which
is adequate for 2 to 2½ hours of surgery.
Local anesthetics are bound to plasma proteins in varying
degrees. Generally, the lower the plasma concentration of
drug, the higher the percentage of drug bound to plasma.
Local anesthetics appear to cross the placenta by passive
diffusion. The rate and degree of diffusion is governed by the
degree of plasma protein binding, the degree of ionization,
and the degree of lipid solubility. Fetal/maternal ratios of

Composition of Available Solutions*

	1% Single-Dose 30 mL Vial mg/mL	1% Multiple-Dose 50 mL Vial mg/mL	1.5% Single-Dose 30 mL Vial mg/mL	2% Single-Dose 20 mL Vial mg/mL	2% Multiple-Dose 50 mL Vial mg/mL
Mepivacaine hydrochloride	10	10	15	20	20
Sodium chloride	6.6	7	5.6	4.6	5
Potassium chloride	0.3		0.3	0.3	
Calcium chloride	0.33		0.33	0.33	
Methylparaben		1			1

*In Water for Injection

local anesthetics appear to be inversely related to the degree of plasma protein binding, because only the free, unbound drug is available for placental transfer. CARBOCAINE is approximately 75% bound to plasma proteins. The extent of placental transfer is also determined by the degree of ionization and lipid solubility of the drug. Lipid soluble, nonionized drugs readily enter the fetal blood from the maternal circulation.

Depending upon the route of administration, local anesthetics are distributed to some extent to all body tissues, with high concentrations found in highly perfused organs such as the liver, lungs, heart, and brain.

Various pharmacokinetic parameters of the local anesthetics can be significantly altered by the presence of hepatic or renal disease, addition of epinephrine, factors affecting urinary pH, renal blood flow, the route of drug administration, and the age of the patient. The half-life of CARBOCAINE in adults is 1.9 to 3.2 hours and in neonates 8.7 to 9 hours. Mepivacaine, because of its amide structure, is not detoxified by the circulating plasma esterases. It is rapidly metabolized, with only a small percentage of the anesthetic (5 percent to 10 percent) being excreted unchanged in the urine. The liver is the principal site of metabolism, with over 50% of the administered dose being excreted into the bile as metabolites. Most of the metabolized mepivacaine is probably resorbed in the intestine and then excreted into the urine since only a small percentage is found in the feces. The principal route of excretion is via the kidney. Most of the anesthetic and its metabolites are eliminated within 30 hours. It has been shown that hydroxylation and N-demethylation, which are detoxification reactions, play important roles in the metabolism of the anesthetic. Three metabolites of mepivacaine have been identified from human adults: two phenols, which are excreted almost exclusively as their glucuronide conjugates, and the N-demethyleted compound (2', 6'-pipecoloxylidide).

Mepivacaine does not ordinarily produce irritation or tissue damage, and does not cause methemoglobinemia when administered in recommended doses and concentrations.

INDICATIONS AND USAGE

CARBOCAINE, brand of mepivacaine hydrochloride, is indicated for production of local or regional analgesia and anesthesia by local infiltration, peripheral nerve block techniques, and central neural techniques including epidural and caudal blocks.

The routes of administration and indicated concentrations for CARBOCAINE are:

local infiltration	0.5% (via dilution) or 1%
peripheral nerve blocks	1% and 2%
epidural block	1%, 1.5%, 2%
caudal block	1%, 1.5%, 2%

See DOSAGE AND ADMINISTRATION for additional information. Standard textbooks should be consulted to determine the accepted procedures and techniques for the administration of CARBOCAINE.

CONTRAINDICATIONS

CARBOCAINE is contraindicated in patients with a known hypersensitivity to it or to any local anesthetic agent of the amide-type or to other components of CARBOCAINE solutions.

WARNINGS

LOCAL ANESTHETICS SHOULD ONLY BE EMPLOYED BY CLINICIANS WHO ARE WELL VERSED IN DIAGNOSIS AND MANAGEMENT OF DOSE-RELATED TOXICITY AND OTHER ACUTE EMERGENCIES WHICH MIGHT ARISE FROM THE BLOCK TO BE EMPLOYED, AND THEN ONLY AFTER INSURING THE IMMEDIATE AVAILABILITY OF OXYGEN, OTHER RESUSCITATIVE DRUGS, CARDIOPULMONARY RESUSCITATIVE EQUIPMENT, AND THE PERSONNEL RESOURCES NEEDED FOR PROPER MANAGEMENT OF TOXIC REACTIONS AND RELATED EMERGENCIES. (See also ADVERSE REACTIONS and PRECAUTIONS.) DELAY IN PROPER MANAGEMENT OF DOSE-RELATED TOXICITY, UNDERVENTILATION FROM ANY CAUSE, AND/OR ALTERED SENSITIVITY MAY LEAD TO THE DEVELOPMENT OF ACIDOSIS, CARDIAC ARREST AND, POSSIBLY, DEATH.

Local anesthetic solutions containing antimicrobial preservatives (ie, those supplied in multiple-dose vials) should not be used for epidural or caudal anesthesia because safety has not been established with regard to intrathecal injection, either intentionally or inadvertently, of such preservatives. It is essential that aspiration for blood or cerebrospinal fluid (where applicable) be done prior to injecting any local anesthetic, both the original dose and all subsequent doses, to avoid intravascular or subarachnoid injection. However, a negative aspiration does not ensure against an intravascular or subarachnoid injection.

Reactions resulting in fatality have occurred on rare occasions with the use of local anesthetics.

CARBOCAINE with epinephrine or other vasopressors should not be used concomitantly with ergot-type oxytocic drugs, because a severe persistent hypertension may occur. Likewise, solutions of CARBOCAINE containing a vasoconstrictor, such as epinephrine, should be used with extreme caution in patients receiving monoamine oxidase inhibitors (MAOI) or antidepressants of the triptyline or imipramine types, because severe prolonged hypertension may result. Local anesthetic procedures should be used with caution when there is inflammation and/or sepsis in the region of the proposed injection.

Mixing or the prior or intercurrent use of any local anesthetic with CARBOCAINE cannot be recommended because of insufficient data on the clinical use of such mixtures.

PRECAUTIONS

General

The safety and effectiveness of local anesthetics depend on proper dosage, correct technique, adequate precautions, and readiness for emergencies. Resuscitative equipment, oxygen, and other resuscitative drugs should be available for immediate use. (See WARNINGS and ADVERSE REACTIONS.) During major regional nerve blocks, the patient should have IV fluids running via an indwelling catheter to assure a functioning intravenous pathway. The lowest dosage of local anesthetic that results in effective anesthesia should be used to avoid high plasma levels and serious adverse effects. Injections should be made slowly, with frequent aspirations before and during the injection to avoid intravascular injection. Current opinion favors fractional administration with constant attention to the patient, rather than rapid bolus injection. Syringe aspirations should also be performed before and during each supplemental injection in continuous (intermittent) catheter techniques. An intravascular injection is still possible even if aspirations for blood are negative. During the administration of epidural anesthesia, it is recommended that a test dose be administered initially and the effects monitored before the full dose is given. When using a "continuous" catheter technique, test doses should be given prior to both the original and all reinforcing doses, because plastic tubing in the epidural space can migrate into a blood vessel or through the dura. When clinical conditions permit, an effective test dose should contain epinephrine (10 μg to 15 μg have been suggested) to serve as a warning of unintended intravascular injection. If injected into a blood vessel, this amount of epinephrine is likely to produce an "epinephrine response" within 45 seconds, consisting of an increase of pulse and blood pressure, circumoral pallor, palpitations, and nervousness in the unsedated patient. The sedated patient may exhibit only a pulse rate increase of 20 or more beats per minute for 15 or more seconds. Therefore, following the test dose, the heart rate should be monitored for a heart rate increase. The test dose should also contain 45 mg to 50 mg of CARBOCAINE to detect an unintended intrathecal administration. This will be evidenced within a few minutes by signs of spinal block (eg, decreased sensation of the buttocks, paresis of the legs, or, in the sedated patient, absent knee jerk).

Injection of repeated doses of local anesthetics may cause significant increases in plasma levels with each repeated dose due to slow accumulation of the drug or its metabolites or to slow metabolic degradation. Tolerance to elevated blood levels varies with the status of the patient. Debilitated, elderly patients, and acutely ill patients should be given reduced doses commensurate with their age and physical status. Local anesthetics should also be used with caution in patients with severe disturbances of cardiac rhythm, shock, heart block, or hypotension.

Careful and constant monitoring of cardiovascular and respiratory (adequacy of ventilation) vital signs, and the patient's state of consciousness should be performed after each local anesthetic injection. It should be kept in mind at such times that restlessness, anxiety, incoherent speech, lightheadedness, numbness and tingling of the mouth and lips, metallic taste, tinnitus, dizziness, blurred vision, tremors, twitching, depression, or drowsiness may be early warning signs of central nervous system toxicity.

Local anesthetic solutions containing a vasoconstrictor should be used cautiously and in carefully restricted quantities in areas of the body supplied by end arteries or having otherwise compromised blood supply such as digits, nose, external ear, penis. Patients with hypertensive vascular disease may exhibit exaggerated vasoconstrictor response. Ischemic injury or necrosis may result.

Mepivacaine should be used with caution in patients with known allergies and sensitivities.

Because amide-type local anesthetics such as CARBOCAINE, brand of mepivacaine hydrochloride, are metabolized by the liver and excreted by the kidneys, these drugs, especially repeat doses, should be used cautiously in patients with hepatic and renal disease. Patients with severe hepatic disease, because of their inability to metabolize local anesthetics normally, are at a greater risk of developing toxic plasma concentrations. Local anesthetics should also be used with caution in patients with impaired cardiovascular function because they may be less able to compensate for

functional changes associated with the prolongation of AV conduction produced by these drugs.

Serious dose-related cardiac arrhythmias may occur if preparations containing a vasoconstrictor such as epinephrine are employed in patients during or following the administration of potent inhalation anesthetics. In deciding whether to use these products concurrently in the same patient, the combined action of both agents upon the myocardium, the concentration and volume of vasoconstrictor used, and the time since injection, when applicable, should be taken into account.

Many drugs used during the conduct of anesthesia are considered potential triggering agents for familial malignant hyperthermia. Because it is not known whether amide-type local anesthetics may trigger this reaction and because the need for supplemental general anesthesia cannot be predicted in advance, it is suggested that a standard protocol for management should be available. Early unexplained signs of tachycardia, tachypnea, labile blood pressure, and metabolic acidosis may precede temperature elevation. Successful outcome is dependent on early diagnosis, prompt discontinuance of the suspect triggering agent(s), and institution of treatment, including oxygen therapy, indicated supportive measures, and dantrolene. (Consult dantrolene sodium intravenous package insert before using.)

Use in Head and Neck Area

Small doses of local anesthetics injected into the head and neck area may produce adverse reactions similar to systemic toxicity seen with unintentional intravascular injections of larger doses. The injection procedures require the utmost care.

Confusion, convulsions, respiratory depression, and/or respiratory arrest, and cardiovascular stimulation or depression have been reported. These reactions may be due to intraarterial injection of the local anesthetic with retrograde flow to the cerebral circulation. Patients receiving these blocks should have their circulation and respiration monitored and be constantly observed. Resuscitative equipment and personnel for treating adverse reactions should be immediately available. Dosage recommendations should not be exceeded.

Information for Patients

When appropriate, patients should be informed in advance that they may experience temporary loss of sensation and motor activity, usually in the lower half of the body, following proper administration of caudal or epidural anesthesia. Also, when appropriate, the physician should discuss other information including adverse reactions listed in the package insert on CARBOCAINE, brand of mepivacaine hydrochloride.

Clinically Significant Drug Interactions

The administration of local anesthetic solutions containing epinephrine or norepinephrine to patients receiving monoamine oxidase inhibitors or tricyclic antidepressants may produce severe, prolonged hypertension. Concurrent use of these agents should generally be avoided. In situations when concurrent therapy is necessary, careful patient monitoring is essential.

Concurrent administration of vasopressor drugs and of ergot-type oxytocic drugs may cause severe, persistent hypertension or cerebrovascular accidents.

Phenothiazines and butyrophenones may reduce or reverse the pressor effect of epinephrine.

Carcinogenesis, Mutagenesis, and Impairment of Fertility

Long-term studies in animals of most local anesthetics including mepivacaine to evaluate the carcinogenic potential have not been conducted. Mutagenic potential or the effect on fertility have not been determined. There is no evidence from human data that CARBOCAINE may be carcinogenic or mutagenic or that it impairs fertility.

Pregnancy Category C

Animal reproduction studies have not been conducted with mepivacaine. There are no adequate and well-controlled studies in pregnant women of the effect of mepivacaine on the developing fetus. Mepivacaine hydrochloride should be used during pregnancy only if the potential benefit justifies the potential risk to the fetus. This does not preclude the use of CARBOCAINE at term for obstetrical anesthesia or analgesia. (See *Labor and Delivery*.)

CARBOCAINE has been used for obstetrical analgesia by the epidural, caudal, and paracervical routes without evidence of adverse effects on the fetus when no more than the maximum safe dosages are used and strict adherence to technique is followed.

Labor and Delivery

Local anesthetics rapidly cross the placenta, and when used for epidural, paracervical, caudal, or pudendal block anes-

Continued on next page

This product information was prepared in August, 1989. On these and other products of Winthrop Pharmaceuticals, detailed information may be obtained on a current basis by direct inquiry to the Professional Services Department, 90 Park Avenue, New York, NY 10016 (800) 446-6267.

Winthrop Pharm.—Cont.

thesia, can cause varying degrees of maternal, fetal, and neonatal toxicity. (See *Pharmacokinetics* —CLINICAL PHARMACOLOGY.) The incidence and degree of toxicity depend upon the procedure performed, the type and amount of drug used, and the technique of drug administration. Adverse reactions in the parturient, fetus, and neonate involve alterations of the central nervous system, peripheral vascular tone, and cardiac function.

Maternal hypotension has resulted from regional anesthesia. Local anesthetics produce vasodilation by blocking sympathetic nerves. Elevating the patient's legs and positioning her on her left side will help prevent decreases in blood pressure. The fetal heart rate also should be monitored continuously and electronic fetal monitoring is highly advisable.

Epidural, paracervical, caudal, or pudendal anesthesia may alter the forces of parturition through changes in uterine contractility or maternal expulsive efforts. In one study, paracervical block anesthesia was associated with a decrease in the mean duration of first stage labor and facilitation of cervical dilation. Epidural anesthesia has been reported to prolong the second stage of labor by removing the parturient's reflex urge to bear down or by interfering with motor function. The use of obstetrical anesthesia may increase the need for forceps assistance.

The use of some local anesthetic drug products during labor and delivery may be followed by diminished muscle strength and tone for the first day or two of life. The long-term significance of these observations is unknown.

Fetal bradycardia may occur in 20 to 30 percent of patients receiving paracervical block anesthesia with the amide-type local anesthetics and may be associated with fetal acidosis. Fetal heart rate should always be monitored during paracervical anesthesia. Added risk appears to be present in prematurity, postmaturity, toxemia of pregnancy, and fetal distress. The physician should weigh the possible advantages against dangers when considering paracervical block in these conditions. Careful adherence to recommended dosage is of the utmost importance in obstetrical paracervical block. Failure to achieve adequate analgesia with recommended doses should arouse suspicion of intravascular or fetal intracranial injection.

Cases compatible with unintended fetal intracranial injection of local anesthetic solution have been reported following intended paracervical or pudendal block or both. Babies so affected present with unexplained neonatal depression at birth which correlates with high local anesthetic serum levels and usually manifest seizures within six hours. Prompt use of supportive measures combined with forced urinary excretion of the local anesthetic has been used successfully to manage this complication.

Case reports of maternal convulsions and cardiovascular collapse following use of some local anesthetics for paracervical block in early pregnancy (as anesthesia for elective abortion) suggest that systemic absorption under these circumstances may be rapid. The recommended maximum dose of the local anesthetic should not be exceeded. Injection should be made slowly and with frequent aspiration. Allow a five-minute interval between sides.

It is extremely important to avoid aortocaval compression by the gravid uterus during administration of regional block to parturients. To do this, the patient must be maintained in the left lateral decubitus position or a blanket roll or sandbag may be placed beneath the right hip and the gravid uterus displaced to the left.

Nursing Mothers

It is not known whether local anesthetic drugs are excreted in human milk. Because many drugs are excreted in human milk, caution should be exercised when local anesthetics are administered to a nursing woman.

Pediatric Use

Guidelines for the administration of mepivacaine to children are presented in DOSAGE AND ADMINISTRATION.

ADVERSE REACTIONS

Reactions to CARBOCAINE, brand of mepivacaine hydrochloride, are characteristic of those associated with other amide-type local anesthetics. A major cause of adverse reactions to this group of drugs is excessive plasma levels, which may be due to overdosage, inadvertent intravascular injection, or slow metabolic degradation.

Systemic

The most commonly encountered acute adverse experiences which demand immediate countermeasures are related to the central nervous system and the cardiovascular system. These adverse experiences are generally dose related and due to high plasma levels which may result from overdosage, rapid absorption from the injection site, diminished tolerance, or from unintentional intravascular injection of the local anesthetic solution. In addition to systemic dose-related toxicity, unintentional subarachnoid injection of drug during the intended performance of caudal or lumbar epidural block or nerve blocks near the vertebral column (especially in the head and neck region) may result in underventilation

or apnea ("Total or High Spinal"). Also, hypotension due to loss of sympathetic tone and respiratory paralysis or underventilation due to cephalad extension of the motor level of anesthesia may occur. This may lead to secondary cardiac arrest if untreated. Factors influencing plasma protein binding, such as acidosis, systemic diseases which alter protein production, or competition of other drugs for protein binding sites, may diminish individual tolerance.

Central Nervous System Reactions

These are characterized by excitation and/or depression. Restlessness, anxiety, dizziness, tinnitus, blurred vision, or tremors may occur, possibly proceeding to convulsions. However, excitement may be transient or absent, with depression being the first manifestation of an adverse reaction. This may quickly be followed by drowsiness merging into unconsciousness and respiratory arrest. Other central nervous system effects may be nausea, vomiting, chills, and constriction of the pupils.

The incidence of convulsions associated with the use of local anesthetics varies with the procedure used and the total dose administered. In a survey of studies of epidural anesthesia, overt toxicity progressing to convulsions occurred in approximately 0.1% of local anesthetic administrations.

Cardiovascular Reactions

High doses or, inadvertent intravascular injection, may lead to high plasma levels and related depression of the myocardium, decreased cardiac output, heart block, hypotension (or sometimes hypertension), bradycardia, ventricular arrhythmias, and possibly cardiac arrest. (See WARNINGS, PRECAUTIONS, and OVERDOSAGE sections.)

Allergic

Allergic-type reactions are rare and may occur as a result of sensitivity to the local anesthetic or to other formulation ingredients, such as the antimicrobial preservative methylparaben, contained in multiple-dose vials. These reactions are characterized by signs such as urticaria, pruritus, erythema, angioneurotic edema (including laryngeal edema), tachycardia, sneezing, nausea, vomiting, dizziness, syncope, excessive sweating, elevated temperature, and possibly, anaphylactoid-like symptomatology (including severe hypotension). Cross sensitivity among members of the amide-type local anesthetic group has been reported. The usefulness of screening for sensitivity has not been definitely established.

Neurologic

The incidences of adverse neurologic reactions associated with the use of local anesthetics may be related to the total dose of local anesthetic administered and are also dependent upon the particular drug used, the route of administration, and the physical status of the patient. Many of these effects may be related to local anesthetic techniques, with or without a contribution from the drug.

In the practice of caudal or lumbar epidural block, occasional unintentional penetration of the subarachnoid space by the catheter or needle may occur. Subsequent adverse effects may depend partially on the amount of drug administered intrathecally and the physiological and physical effects of a dural puncture. A high spinal is characterized by paralysis of the legs, loss of consciousness, respiratory paralysis, and bradycardia.

Neurologic effects following epidural or caudal anesthesia may include spinal block of varying magnitude (including high or total spinal block); hypotension secondary to spinal block; urinary retention; fecal and urinary incontinence; loss of perineal sensation and sexual function; persistent anesthesia, paresthesia, weakness, paralysis of the lower extremities, and loss of sphincter control all of which may have slow, incomplete, or no recovery; headache; backache; septic meningitis; meningismus; slowing of labor; increased incidence of forceps delivery; cranial nerve palsies due to traction on nerves from loss of cerebrospinal fluid.

OVERDOSAGE

Acute emergencies from local anesthetics are generally related to high plasma levels encountered during therapeutic use of local anesthetics or to unintended subarachnoid injection of local anesthetic solution. (See ADVERSE REACTIONS, WARNINGS, and PRECAUTIONS.)

Management of Local Anesthetic Emergencies

The first consideration is prevention, best accomplished by careful and constant monitoring of cardiovascular and respiratory vital signs and the patient's state of consciousness after each local anesthetic injection. At the first sign of change, oxygen should be administered.

The first step in the management of systemic toxic reactions, as well as underventilation or apnea due to unintentional subarachnoid injection of drug solution, consists of immediate attention to the establishment and maintenance of a patent airway and effective assisted or controlled ventilation with 100% oxygen with a delivery system capable of permitting immediate positive airway pressure by mask. This may prevent convulsions if they have not already occurred.

If necessary, use drugs to control the convulsions. A 50 mg to 100 mg bolus IV injection of succinylcholine will paralyze the patient without depressing the central nervous or cardiovascular systems and facilitate ventilation. A bolus IV dose

of 5 mg to 10 mg of diazepam or 50 mg to 100 mg of thiopental will permit ventilation and counteract central nervous system stimulation, but these drugs also depress central nervous system, respiratory, and cardiac function, add to postictal depression and may result in apnea. Intravenous barbiturates, anticonvulsant agents, or muscle relaxants should only be administered by those familiar with their use. Immediately after the institution of these ventilatory measures, the adequacy of the circulation should be evaluated. Supportive treatment of circulatory depression may require administration of intravenous fluids, and when appropriate, a vasopressor dictated by the clinical situation (such as ephedrine or epinephrine to enhance myocardial contractile force).

Endotracheal intubation, employing drugs and techniques familiar to the clinician may be indicated after initial administration of oxygen by mask, if difficulty is encountered in the maintenance of a patent airway or if prolonged ventilatory support (assisted or controlled) is indicated.

Recent clinical data from patients experiencing local anesthetic induced convulsions demonstrated rapid development of hypoxia, hypercarbia, and acidosis within a minute of the onset of convulsions. These observations suggest that oxygen consumption and carbon dioxide production are greatly increased during local anesthetic convulsions and emphasize the importance of immediate and effective ventilation with oxygen which may avoid cardiac arrest.

If not treated immediately, convulsions with simultaneous hypoxia, hypercarbia, and acidosis, plus myocardial depression from the direct effects of the local anesthetic may result in cardiac arrhythmias, bradycardia, asystole, ventricular fibrillation, or cardiac arrest. Respiratory abnormalities, including apnea, may occur. Underventilation or apnea due to unintentional subarachnoid injection of local anesthetic solution may produce these same signs and also lead to cardiac arrest if ventilatory support is not instituted. If cardiac arrest should occur, standard cardiopulmonary resuscitative measures should be instituted and maintained for a prolonged period if necessary. Recovery has been reported after prolonged resuscitative efforts.

The supine position is dangerous in pregnant women at term because of aortocaval compression by the gravid uterus. Therefore during treatment of systemic toxicity, maternal hypotension, or fetal bradycardia following regional block, the parturient should be maintained in the left lateral decubitus position if possible, or manual displacement of the uterus off the great vessels be accomplished.

The mean seizure dosage of mepivacaine in rhesus monkeys was found to be 18.8 mg/kg with mean arterial plasma concentration of 24.4 μg/mL. The intravenous and subcutaneous LD_{50} in mice is 23 mg/kg to 35 mg/kg and 280 mg/kg respectively.

DOSAGE AND ADMINISTRATION

The dose of any local anesthetic administered varies with the anesthetic procedure, the area to be anesthetized, the vascularity of the tissues, the number of neuronal segments to be blocked, the depth of anesthesia and degree of muscle relaxation required, the duration of anesthesia desired, individual tolerance and the physical condition of the patient. The smallest dose and concentration required to produce the desired result should be administered. Dosages of CARBOCAINE should be reduced for elderly and debilitated patients and patients with cardiac and/or liver disease. The rapid injection of a large volume of local anesthetic solution should be avoided and fractional doses should be used when feasible.

For specific techniques and procedures, refer to standard textbooks.

The recommended single **adult** dose (or the total of a series of doses given in one procedure) of CARBOCAINE, brand of mepivacaine hydrochloride, for unsedated, healthy, normal-sized individuals should not usually exceed 400 mg. The recommended dosage is based on requirements for the average adult and should be reduced for elderly or debilitated patients.

While maximum doses of 7 mg/kg (550 mg) have been administered without adverse effect, these are not recommended, except in exceptional circumstances and under no circumstances should the administration be repeated at intervals of less than 1½ hours. The total dose for any 24-hour period should not exceed 1,000 mg because of a slow accumulation of the anesthetic or its derivatives or slower than normal metabolic degradation or detoxification with repeat administration (See CLINICAL PHARMACOLOGY and PRECAUTIONS).

Children tolerate the local anesthetic as well as adults. However, the pediatric dose should be *carefully measured* as a percentage of the total adult dose *based on weight*, and should not exceed 5 mg/kg to 6 mg/kg (2.5 mg/lb to 3 mg/lb) in children, especially those weighing less than 30 lb. In children *under 3 years of age or weighing less than 30 lb* concentrations less than 2% (eg, 0.5% to 1.5%) should be employed. **Unused portions of solutions not containing preservatives, ie, those supplied in single-dose vials, should be discarded following initial use.**

Recommended Concentrations and Doses of CARBOCAINE

Procedure	Concentration	mL	Total Dose mg	Comments
Cervical, brachial, intercostal, pudendal nerve block	1% 2%	5–40 5–20	50–400 100–400	Pudendal block: one half of total dose injected each side.
Transvaginal block (paracervical plus pudendal)	1%	up to 30 (both sides)	up to 300 (both sides)	One half of total dose injected each side. See PRECAUTIONS.
Paracervical block	1%	up to 20 (both sides)	up to 200 (both sides)	One half of total dose injected each side. This is maximum recommended dose per 90-minute period in obstetrical and non-obstetrical patients. Inject slowly, 5 minutes between sides. See PRECAUTIONS.
Caudal and Epidural block	1% 1.5% 2%	15–30 10–25 10–20	150–300 150–375 200–400	Use only single-dose vials which do not contain a preservative.
Infiltration	1%	up to 40	up to 400	An equivalent amount of a 0.5% solution (prepared by diluting the 1% solution with Sodium Chloride Injection, USP) may be used for large areas.
Therapeutic block (pain management)	1% 2%	1–5 1–5	10–50 20–100	

Unused portions of solutions not containing preservatives should be discarded.

This product should be inspected visually for particulate matter and discoloration prior to administration whenever solution and container permit. Solutions which are discolored or which contain particulate matter should not be administered.
[See table above].

HOW SUPPLIED
Single-dose vials and multiple-dose vials of CARBOCAINE may be sterilized by autoclaving at 15 pound pressure, 121°C (250°F) for 15 minutes. Solutions of CARBOCAINE may be reautoclaved when necessary. Do not administer solutions which are discolored or which contain particulate matter. THESE SOLUTIONS ARE NOT INTENDED FOR SPINAL ANESTHESIA OR DENTAL USE
1% Single-dose vials of 30 mL (NDC 0024-0231-01)
1% Multiple-dose vials of 50 mL (NDC 0024-0232-01)
1.5% Single-dose vials of 30 mL (NDC 0024-0234-01)
2% Single-dose vials of 20 mL (NDC 0024-0236-01)
2% Multiple-dose vials of 50 mL (NDC 0024-0237-01)
Store at controlled room temperature between 15°C to 30°C (59°F to 86°F); brief exposure up to 40°C (104°F) does not adversely affect the product.

> For full prescribing information on the dental use of CARBOCAINE see Cook-Waite Laboratories, Inc. product listing in this publication.

CW-60-S

CARPUJECT® Sterile Cartridge-Needle Unit   ℞

Winthrop Pharmaceuticals offers a broad line of injectable drug products in unit of use pre-filled cartridges. Each cartridge is clearly labelled by medication name and dosage calibrations. In addition each individual cartridge label and outer package is specially color-coded allowing for ease of identification, making the system easily adaptable to any hospital setting.
The cartridges are packaged in a unique DETECTO-SEAL® tamper detection package specially designed to discourage narcotic diversion and allow for easy inventory analysis. This package contains a sturdy aluminum shield to prevent plunger end diversion.
Prior to injection the pre-filled cartridges are placed in a unique sturdy plastic holder. This full-length holder provides secure, stable injections and is lightweight, durable, and reusable in design.
In addition, the holder utilized for CARPUJECT has an open-ended barrel allowing for release of used needles into most any disposal bin. This holder is designed with nursing personnel in mind to eliminate the need for recapping needles and minimize the potential for needle stick injuries. The following products are currently available in CARPUJECT Sterile Cartridge-Needle Unit.

Product	Units/Package
atropine and DEMEROL® Injection **atropine sulfate and** **meperidine HCl, USP** 0.4 mg and 50 mg (22 G × 1¼″) 0024-0021-01	10 (1 mL fill in 2 mL)
0.4 mg and 75 mg (22 G × 1¼″) 0024-0022-02	10 (1 mL fill in 2 mL)
CODEINE Phosphate Injection, USP 30 mg (22 G × 1¼″) 0024-0272-02	10 (2 mL)
60 mg (22 G × 1¼″) 0024-0274-02	10 (2 mL)
DEMEROL® Hydrochloride brand of meperidine HCl injection, USP 25 mg (22 G × 1¼″) 0024-0324-02	10 (1 mL fill in 2 mL)
50 mg (22 G × 1¼″) 0024-0325-02	10 (1 mL fill in 2 mL)
75 mg (22 G × 1¼″) 0024-0326-02	10 (1 mL fill in 2 mL)
100 mg (22 G × 1¼″) 0024-0328-02	10 (1 mL fill in 2 mL)
DIAZEPAM Injection, USP 10 mg/2 mL (22 G × 1¼″) 0024-0376-02	10 (2 mL)
FUROSEMIDE Injection, USP 10 mg/mL (22 G × 1¼″) 0024-0611-03	10 (2 mL)
HEPARIN LOCK FLUSH Solution, USP 10 USP heparin U/mL (25 G × ⅝″) 0024-0721-12	50 (1 mL fill in 2 mL)
100 USP heparin U/mL (25 G × ⅝″) 0024-0722-12	50 (1 mL fill in 2 mL)
HEPARIN LOCK FLUSH Solution, USP 10 USP heparin U/mL (25 G × ⅝″) 0024-0721-13	50 (2 mL fill in 2 mL)
100 USP heparin U/mL (25 G × ⅝″) 0024-0722-13	50 (2 mL fill in 2 mL)

Product	Units/Package
HEP-PAK® Convenience Package[1] 10 USP heparin U/mL (25 G × ⅝″) 0024-0725-03	50 × 3
100 USP heparin U/mL (25 G × ⅝″) 0024-0736-03	50 × 3
HEP-PAK® 2 Convenience Package[2] 10 USP heparin U/mL (25 G × ⅝″) 0024-0741-12	50 × 2
100 USP heparin U/mL (25 G × ⅝″) 0024-0742-12	50 × 2
HEP-PAK® CVC Convenience Package[3] 10 USP heparin U/2 mL (25 G × ⅝″) 0024-0725-02	30 × 3
100 USP heparin U/2 mL (25 G × ⅝″) 0024-0736-02	30 × 3
HEPARIN Sodium Injection, USP 5,000 USP heparin U/mL (25 G × ⅝″) 0024-0793-02	10 (1 mL fill in 2 mL)
HEPARIN Sodium Injection, USP **Preservative-Free** 5,000 USP heparin U/0.5 mL (25 G × ⅝″) 0024-0733-05	10 (0.5 mL fill in 2 mL)
HEPARIN Sodium Injection, USP **Preservative-Free** 10,000 USP heparin U/1 mL (25 G × ⅝″) 0024-0733-02	10 (1 mL fill in 2 mL)
HYDROMORPHONE Hydrochloride Injection, USP 1 mg (22 G × 1¼″) 0024-0726-02	10 (1 mL fill in 2 mL)
2 mg (22 G × 1¼″) 0024-0728-02	10 (1 mL fill in 2 mL)
4 mg (22 G × 1¼″) 0024-0727-02	10 (1 mL fill in 2 mL)
HYDROXYZINE Hydrochloride Injection, USP 25 mg (22 G × 1¼″) 0024-0711-02	10 (1 mL fill in 2 mL)
50 mg (22 G × 1¼″) 0024-0712-02	10 (1 mL fill in 2 mL)
100 mg (22 G × 1¼″) 0024-0713-02	10 (2 mL)
MORPHINE Sulfate Injection, USP 2 mg (25 G × ⅝″) 0024-1257-02	10 (1 mL fill in 2 mL)
4 mg (25 G × ⅝″) 0024-1258-02	10 (1 mL fill in 2 mL)
8 mg (22 G × 1¼″) 0024-1259-02	10 (1 mL fill in 2 mL)
8 mg (25 G × ⅝″) 0024-1260-02	10 (1 mL fill in 2 mL)
10 mg (22 G × 1¼″) 0024-1261-02	10 (1 mL fill in 2 mL)
10 mg (25 G × ⅝″) 0024-1263-02	10 (1 mL fill in 2 mL)
15 mg (22 G × 1¼″) 0024-1262-02	10 (1 mL fill in 2 mL)
15 mg (25 G × ⅝″) 0024-1264-02	10 (1 mL fill in 2 mL)
NEO-SYNEPHRINE® Hydrochloride brand of phenylephrine HCl injection, USP 10 mg (22 G × 1¼″) 0024-1340-02	50 (1 mL fill in 2 mL)
PHENYTOIN Sodium Injection, USP 100 mg/2 mL (22 G × 1¼″) 0024-1549-01	10 (2 mL)
PROCAINAMIDE Hydrochloride, USP 500 mg/mL (22 G × 1¼″) 0024-1526-02	10 (2 mL)
PROCHLORPERAZINE Edisylate Injection, USP 10 mg/2 mL (22 G × 1¼″) 0024-1598-01	10 (2 mL)

Continued on next page

This product information was prepared in August, 1989. On these and other products of Winthrop Pharmaceuticals, detailed information may be obtained on a current basis by direct inquiry to the Professional Services Department, 90 Park Avenue, New York, NY 10016 (800) 446-6267.

Winthrop Pharm.—Cont.

SODIUM Chloride Injection, USP, 0.9%

(22 G × 1¼″)	50 (2 mL)
0024-1811-02	
(25 G × ⅝″)	50 (2 mL)
0024-1815-02	

TALWIN® Injection
brand of **pentazocine lactate injection, USP**

30 mg (22 G × 1¼″)	10 (1 mL fill in 2 mL)
0024-1917-02	
45 mg (22 G × 1¼″)	10 (1.5 mL fill in 2 mL)
0024-1918-02	
60 mg (22 G × 1¼″)	10 (2 mL)
0024-1919-02	

TRIMETHOBENZAMIDE
Hydrochloride Injection, USP

200 mg (22 G × 1¼″)	10 (2 mL)
0024-1955-03	

VERAPAMIL Hydrochloride

5 mg (22 G × 1¼″)	10 (2 mL)
0024-2110-03	

EMPTY STERILE CARPUJECT

(22 G × 1¼″)	10 (2 mL)
(25 G × ⅝″)	10 (2 mL)

[1] Each HEP-PAK® contains one cartridge of Heparin Lock Flush Solution, USP (10 U/mL or 100 U/mL) with two cartridges of Sodium Chloride Injection, USP, 0.9% (2 mL).

[2] Each HEP-PAK® 2 contains one cartridge of Heparin Lock Flush Solution (10 U/mL or 100 U/mL) with one cartridge of Sodium Chloride Injection, USP, 0.9% (2 mL).

[3] Each HEP-PAK® CVC Convenience Package contains one cartridge of Heparin Lock Flush Solution 2 mL fill (20 or 200 U/2 mL) with two cartridges of Sodium Chloride Injection, USP, 0.9% (2 mL).

DANOCRINE®
brand of **danazol capsules, USP**   ℞

DESCRIPTION
DANOCRINE, brand of danazol, is a synthetic androgen derived from ethisterone. Chemically, danazol is 17α-Pregna-2,4-dien-20-yno[2,3-*d*]-isoxazol-17-ol.

Inactive Ingredients: Benzyl Alcohol, Gelatin, Lactose, Magnesium Stearate, Parabens, Sodium Propionate, Starch, Talc. CAPSULES 50 mg and 200 mg contain D&C Yellow #10, FD&C Red #3. CAPSULE 100 mg contains D&C Yellow #10, FD&C Yellow #6.

CLINICAL PHARMACOLOGY
DANOCRINE suppresses the pituitary-ovarian axis by inhibiting the output of gonadotropins from the pituitary gland. The only other demonstrable hormonal effect is weak androgenic activity which is dose related. Studies have established that the drug is neither estrogenic nor progestational. DANOCRINE depresses the output of both follicle-stimulating hormone (FSH) and luteinizing hormone (LH).

Recent evidence suggests a direct inhibitory effect at gonadal sites and a binding of DANOCRINE to receptors of gonadal steroids at target organs.

Bioavailability studies indicate that blood levels do not increase proportionally with increases in the administered dose. When the dose of DANOCRINE is doubled the increase in plasma levels is only about 35% to 40%.

In the treatment of endometriosis, DANOCRINE alters the normal and ectopic endometrial tissue so that it becomes inactive and atrophic. Complete resolution of endometrial lesions occurs in the majority of cases.

Changes in vaginal cytology and cervical mucus reflect the suppressive effect of DANOCRINE on the pituitary-ovarian axis.

In the treatment of fibrocystic breast disease, DANOCRINE usually produces partial to complete disappearance of nodularity and complete relief of pain and tenderness. Changes in the menstrual pattern may occur.

Generally the pituitary-suppressive action of DANOCRINE is reversible. Ovulation and cyclic bleeding usually return within 60 to 90 days when therapy with DANOCRINE is discontinued.

In the treatment of hereditary angioedema, DANOCRINE at effective doses prevents attacks of the disease characterized by episodic edema of the abdominal viscera, extremities, face, and airway which may be disabling and, if the airway is involved, fatal. In addition, DANOCRINE corrects partially or completely the primary biochemical abnormality of hereditary angioedema by increasing the levels of the deficient C1 esterase inhibitor (C1EI). As a result of this action the serum levels of the C4 component of the complement system are also increased.

INDICATIONS AND USAGE
Endometriosis. DANOCRINE is indicated for the treatment of endometriosis amenable to hormonal management.

Fibrocystic Breast Disease. Most cases of symptomatic fibrocystic breast disease may be treated by simple measures (eg, padded brassieres and analgesics).

In infrequent patients, symptoms of pain and tenderness may be severe enough to warrant treatment by suppression of ovarian function. DANOCRINE is usually effective in decreasing nodularity, pain, and tenderness. It should be stressed to the patient that this treatment is not innocuous in that it involves considerable alterations of hormone levels and that recurrence of symptoms is very common after cessation of therapy.

Hereditary Angioedema. DANOCRINE is indicated for the prevention of attacks of angioedema of all types (cutaneous, abdominal, laryngeal) in males and females.

CONTRAINDICATIONS
DANOCRINE should not be administered to patients with:
1. Undiagnosed abnormal genital bleeding.
2. Markedly impaired hepatic, renal, or cardiac function.
3. Pregnancy.
4. Breast feeding.

WARNINGS
Safe use of the drug in pregnancy has not been established clinically. Therefore, a nonhormonal method of contraception should be recommended. If a patient becomes pregnant during treatment, administration of the drug should be discontinued. Continuing treatment may result in an androgenic effect on the fetus, which to date has been limited to clitoral hypertrophy and labial fusion of the external genitalia in the female fetus. If the patient becomes pregnant while taking DANOCRINE, she should be apprised of the potential risk to the fetus.

Before initiating therapy of fibrocystic breast disease with DANOCRINE, carcinoma of the breast should be excluded. However, nodularity, pain, tenderness due to fibrocystic breast disease may prevent recognition of underlying carcinoma before treatment is begun. Therefore, if any nodule persists or enlarges during treatment, carcinoma should be considered and ruled out.

Long-term experience with danazol is limited. Therapy with other steroids alkylated at the 17 position has been associated with serious toxicity (cholestatic jaundice, peliosis hepatis). The physician therefore should be alert to the possibility that similar toxicity may develop after therapy with danazol. Attempts should be made to determine the lowest dose that will provide adequate protection. If the drug was begun at a time of exacerbation of angioneurotic edema due to trauma, stress or other cause, periodic attempts to decrease or withdraw therapy should be considered.

Patients should be watched closely for signs of virilization. Some androgenic effects may not be reversible even when drug administration is stopped.

PRECAUTIONS
Because DANOCRINE may cause some degree of fluid retention, conditions that might be influenced by this factor, such as epilepsy, migraine, or cardiac or renal dysfunction, require careful observation.

Since hepatic dysfunction has been reported in patients treated with DANOCRINE, periodic liver function tests should be performed (see ADVERSE REACTIONS section).

Decreased high density lipoproteins and possibly increased low density lipoproteins have been reported during danazol therapy. While the clinical implications remain unclear, prescribers should consider this in accordance with the medical needs and related health concerns of the patient.

Check semen for volume, viscosity, sperm count, and motility every 3 to 4 months, especially in adolescents.

ADVERSE REACTIONS
The following androgenic effects have occurred in patients receiving DANOCRINE: acne, edema, mild hirsutism, decrease in breast size, deepening of the voice, oiliness of the skin or hair, weight gain, and rarely, clitoral hypertrophy, or testicular atrophy.

Also hypoestrogenic manifestations such as flushing, sweating, vaginitis including itching, dryness, burning and vaginal bleeding, nervousness, and emotional lability have been reported.

Hepatic dysfunction, as evidenced by elevated serum enzymes and/or jaundice, has been reported in patients receiving a daily dosage of DANOCRINE of 400 mg or more. It is recommended that patients receiving DANOCRINE, brand of danazol capsules, be monitored for hepatic dysfunction by laboratory tests and clinical observation. Prolongation of prothrombin time in patients stabilized on warfarin has also been reported.

Although the following reactions have also been reported, a causal relationship to the administration of DANOCRINE has neither been confirmed nor refuted: *allergic:* urticaria and rarely, nasal congestion; *CNS effects:* headache, dizziness, depression, fatigue, sleep disorders, tremor, paresthesias, visual disturbances, and rarely, benign intracranial

hypertension, anxiety, changes in appetite, chills, and Guillain-Barré syndrome; *gastrointestinal:* gastroenteritis, nausea, vomiting, constipation, and rarely, pancreatitis; *musculoskeletal:* muscle cramps or spasms, joint lock-up, joint swelling, pain in back, neck, or extremities, and rarely, carpal tunnel syndrome; *genitourinary:* hematuria, prolonged posttherapy amenorrhea; *hematologic:* thrombocytopenia and rarely, eosinophilia, leukocytosis; *skin:* rashes (maculopapular, vesicular, papular, purpuric, petechial), hair loss, and rarely, sun sensitivity, Stevens-Johnson syndrome; *other:* abnormal glucose tolerance test and increased insulin requirements in diabetic patients, changes in libido, elevation in blood pressure, and rarely, cataracts, bleeding gums, fever, pelvic pain, nipple discharge.

DOSAGE AND ADMINISTRATION
Endometriosis. In moderate to severe disease, or in patients infertile due to endometriosis, a starting dose of 800 mg given in two divided doses is recommended. Amenorrhea and a rapid response to painful symptoms is best achieved at this dosage level. Gradual downward titration to a dose sufficient to maintain amenorrhea may be considered depending upon patient response. For mild cases, an initial daily dose of 200 mg to 400 mg given in two divided doses is recommended and may be adjusted depending on patient response. **Therapy should begin during menstruation. Otherwise, appropriate tests should be performed to ensure that the patient is not pregnant while on therapy with DANOCRINE. (See WARNINGS.) It is essential that therapy continue uninterrupted for 3 to 6 months but may be extended to 9 months if necessary.** After termination of therapy, if symptoms recur, treatment can be reinstituted.

Fibrocystic Breast Disease. The total daily dosage of DANOCRINE for fibrocystic breast disease ranges from 100 mg to 400 mg given in two divided doses depending upon patient response. **Therapy should begin during menstruation. Otherwise, appropriate tests should be performed to ensure that the patient is not pregnant while on therapy with DANOCRINE.** A nonhormonal method of contraception is recommended when DANOCRINE is administered at this dose, since ovulation may not be suppressed.

In most instances, breast pain and tenderness are significantly relieved by the first month and eliminated in 2 to 3 months. Usually elimination of nodularity requires 4 to 6 months of uninterrupted therapy. Regular menstrual patterns, irregular menstrual patterns, and amenorrhea each occur in approximately one-third of patients treated with 100 mg of DANOCRINE, brand of danazol capsules. Irregular menstrual patterns and amenorrhea are observed more frequently with higher doses. Clinical studies have demonstrated that 50% of patients may show evidence of recurrence of symptoms within one year. In this event, treatment may be reinstated.

Hereditary Angioedema. The dosage requirements for continuous treatment of hereditary angioedema with DANOCRINE should be individualized on the basis of the clinical response of the patient. It is recommended that the patient be started on 200 mg, two or three times a day. After a favorable initial response is obtained in terms of prevention of episodes of edematous attacks, the proper continuing dosage should be determined by decreasing the dosage by 50% or less at intervals of one to three months or longer if frequency of attacks prior to treatment dictates. If an attack occurs the daily dosage may be increased by up to 200 mg. During the dose adjusting phase, close monitoring of the patient's response is indicated, particularly if the patient has a history of airway involvement.

HOW SUPPLIED
Capsules of 200 mg (orange), bottles of 60 (NDC 0024-0305-60).
Capsules of 200 mg (orange), bottles of 100 (NDC 0024-0305-06).
Capsules of 200 mg (orange), bottles of 250 (NDC 0024-0305-25).
Capsules of 100 mg (yellow), bottles of 100 (NDC 0024-0304-06).
Capsules of 50 mg (orange and white), bottles of 100 (NDC 0024-0303-06).

Distributed by Winthrop Pharmaceuticals
Division of Sterling Drug Inc.
New York, NY 10016
Manufactured by
Sterling Pharmaceuticals Inc.
Barceloneta, Puerto Rico 00617
Shown in Product Identification Section, page 435
DW-254 T(O)

DEMEROL® Hydrochloride
brand of **meperidine hydrochloride, USP**   ℞

DESCRIPTION
Meperidine hydrochloride is ethyl 1-methyl-4-phenylisonipecotate hydrochloride, a white crystalline substance with a melting point of 186°C to 189°C. It is readily

soluble in water and has a neutral reaction and a slightly bitter taste. The solution is not decomposed by a short period of boiling.

The syrup is a pleasant-tasting, nonalcoholic, banana-flavored solution containing 50 mg of DEMEROL hydrochloride, brand of meperidine hydrochloride, per 5 mL teaspoon (25 drops contain 13 mg of DEMEROL hydrochloride). The tablets contain 50 mg or 100 mg of the analgesic.

DEMEROL hydrochloride injectable is supplied in Carpuject® Sterile Cartridge-Needle Unit of 2.5% (25 mg/1 mL), 5% (50 mg/1 mL), 7.5% (75 mg/ 1 mL), and 10% (100 mg/1 mL). Uni-Amp® Unit Dose Pak—ampuls of 5% solution (25 mg/0.5 mL), (50 mg/1 mL), (75 mg/1.5 mL), 100 mg/2 mL), and 10% solution (100 mg/1 mL). Uni-Nest™ Pak —ampuls of 5% solution (25 mg/0.5 mL), (50 mg/1 mL), (75 mg/1.5 mL), (100 mg/2 mL), and 10% solution (100 mg/1 mL). Multiple-dose vials of 5% and 10% solutions contain metacresol 0.1% as preservative.

The pH of DEMEROL solution is adjusted between 3.5 and 6 with sodium hydroxide or hydrochloric acid.

DEMEROL hydrochloride, brand of meperidine hydrochloride, 5 percent solution has a specific gravity of 1.0086 at 20°C and 10 percent solution, a specific gravity of 1.0165 at 20°C.

Inactive Ingredients—TABLETS: Calcium Sulfate, Dibasic Calcium Phosphate, Starch, Stearic Acid, Talc.
SYRUP: Benzoic Acid, Flavor, Liquid Glucose, Purified Water, Saccharin Sodium.

CLINICAL PHARMACOLOGY

Meperidine hydrochloride is a narcotic analgesic with multiple actions qualitatively similar to those of morphine; the most prominent of these involve the central nervous system and organs composed of smooth muscle. The principal actions of therapeutic value are analgesia and sedation.

There is some evidence which suggests that meperidine may produce less smooth muscle spasm, constipation, and depression of the cough reflex than equianalgesic doses of morphine. Meperidine, in 60 mg to 80 mg parenteral doses, is approximately equivalent in analgesic effect to 10 mg of morphine. The onset of action is slightly more rapid than with morphine, and the duration of action is slightly shorter. Meperidine is significantly less effective by the oral than by the parenteral route, but the exact ratio of oral to parenteral effectiveness is unknown.

INDICATIONS AND USAGE

For the relief of moderate to severe pain (parenteral and oral forms)
For preoperative medication (parenteral form only)
For support of anesthesia (parenteral form only)
For obstetrical analgesia (parenteral form only)

CONTRAINDICATIONS

Hypersensitivity to meperidine.
Meperidine is contraindicated in patients who are receiving monoamine oxidase (MAO) inhibitors or those who have recently received such agents. Therapeutic doses of meperidine have occasionally precipitated unpredictable, severe, and occasionally fatal reactions in patients who have received such agents within 14 days. The mechanism of these reactions is unclear, but may be related to a preexisting hyperphenylalaninemia. Some have been characterized by coma, severe respiratory depression, cyanosis, and hypotension, and have resembled the syndrome of acute narcotic overdose. In other reactions the predominant manifestations have been hyperexcitability, convulsions, tachycardia, hyperpyrexia, and hypertension. Although it is not known that other narcotics are free of the risk of such reactions, virtually all of the reported reactions have occurred with meperidine. If a narcotic is needed in such patients, a sensitivity test should be performed in which repeated, small, incremental doses of morphine are administered over the course of several hours while the patient's condition and vital signs are under careful observation. (Intravenous hydrocortisone or prednisolone have been used to treat severe reactions, with the addition of intravenous chlorpromazine in those cases exhibiting hypertension and hyperpyrexia. The usefulness and safety of narcotic antagonists in the treatment of these reactions is unknown.)
Solutions of DEMEROL and barbiturates are chemically incompatible.

WARNINGS

Drug Dependence. Meperidine can produce drug dependence of the morphine type and therefore has the potential for being abused. Psychic dependence, physical dependence, and tolerance may develop upon repeated administration of meperidine, and it should be prescribed and administered with the same degree of caution appropriate to the use of morphine. Like other narcotics, meperidine is subject to the provisions of the Federal narcotic laws.
Interaction with Other Central Nervous System Depressants. MEPERIDINE SHOULD BE USED WITH GREAT CAUTION AND IN REDUCED DOSAGE IN PATIENTS WHO ARE CONCURRENTLY RECEIVING OTHER NARCOTIC ANALGESICS, GENERAL ANESTHETICS, PHENOTHIA-

ZINES, OTHER TRANQUILIZERS (SEE DOSAGE AND ADMINISTRATION), SEDATIVE-HYPNOTICS (INCLUDING BARBITURATES), TRICYCLIC ANTIDEPRESSANTS, AND OTHER CNS DEPRESSANTS (INCLUDING ALCOHOL). RESPIRATORY DEPRESSION, HYPOTENSION, AND PROFOUND SEDATION OR COMA MAY RESULT.
Head Injury and Increased Intracranial Pressure. The respiratory depressant effects of meperidine and its capacity to elevate cerebrospinal fluid pressure may be markedly exaggerated in the presence of head injury, other intracranial lesions, or a preexisting increase in intracranial pressure. Furthermore, narcotics produce adverse reactions which may obscure the clinical course of patients with head injuries. In such patients, meperidine must be used with extreme caution and only if its use is deemed essential.
Intravenous Use. If necessary, meperidine may be given intravenously, but the injection should be given very slowly, preferably in the form of a diluted solution. Rapid intravenous injection of narcotic analgesics, including meperidine, increases the incidence of adverse reactions; severe respiratory depression, apnea, hypotension, peripheral circulatory collapse, and cardiac arrest have occurred. Meperidine should not be administered intravenously unless a narcotic antagonist and the facilities for assisted or controlled respiration are immediately available. When meperidine is given parenterally, especially intravenously, the patient should be lying down.
Asthma and Other Respiratory Conditions. Meperidine should be used with extreme caution in patients having an acute asthmatic attack, patients with chronic obstructive pulmonary disease or cor pulmonale, patients having a substantially decreased respiratory reserve, and patients with preexisting respiratory depression, hypoxia, or hypercapnia. In such patients, even usual therapeutic doses of narcotics may decrease respiratory drive while simultaneously increasing airway resistance to the point of apnea.
Hypotensive Effect. The administration of meperidine may result in severe hypotension in the postoperative patient or any individual whose ability to maintain blood pressure has been compromised by a depleted blood volume or the administration of drugs such as the phenothiazines or certain anesthetics.
Usage in Ambulatory Patients. Meperidine may impair the mental and/or physical abilities required for the performance of potentially hazardous tasks such as driving a car or operating machinery. The patient should be cautioned accordingly.
Meperidine, like other narcotics, may produce orthostatic hypotension in ambulatory patients.
Usage in Pregnancy and Lactation. Meperidine should not be used in pregnant women prior to the labor period, unless in the judgment of the physician the potential benefits outweigh the possible hazards, because safe use in pregnancy prior to labor has not been established relative to possible adverse effects on fetal development.
When used as an obstetrical analgesic, meperidine crosses the placental barrier and can produce depression of respiration and psychophysiologic functions in the newborn. Resuscitation may be required (see section on **OVERDOSAGE**).
Meperidine appears in the milk of nursing mothers receiving the drug.

PRECAUTIONS

As with all intramuscular preparations DEMEROL intramuscular injection should be injected well within the body of a large muscle.
Supraventricular Tachycardias. Meperidine should be used with caution in patients with atrial flutter and other supraventricular tachycardias because of a possible vagolytic action which may produce a significant increase in the ventricular response rate.
Convulsions. Meperidine may aggravate preexisting convulsions in patients with convulsive disorders. If dosage is escalated substantially above recommended levels because of tolerance development, convulsions may occur in individuals without a history of convulsive disorders.
Acute Abdominal Conditions. The administration of meperidine or other narcotics may obscure the diagnosis or clinical course in patients with acute abdominal conditions.
Special Risk Patients. Meperidine should be given with caution and the initial dose should be reduced in certain patients such as the elderly or debilitated, and those with severe impairment of hepatic or renal function, hypothyroidism, Addison's disease, and prostatic hypertrophy or urethral stricture.

ADVERSE REACTIONS

The major hazards of meperidine, as with other narcotic analgesics, are respiratory depression and, to a lesser degree, circulatory depression; respiratory arrest, shock, and cardiac arrest have occurred.

The most frequently observed adverse reactions include lightheadedness, dizziness, sedation, nausea, vomiting, and sweating. These effects seem to be more prominent in ambulatory patients and in those who are not experiencing severe pain. In such individuals, lower doses are advisable. Some

adverse reactions in ambulatory patients may be alleviated if the patient lies down.
Other adverse reactions include:
Nervous System. Euphoria, dysphoria, weakness, headache, agitation, tremor, uncoordinated muscle movements, severe convulsions, transient hallucinations and disorientation, visual disturbances. Inadvertent injection about a nerve trunk may result in sensory-motor paralysis which is usually, though not always, transitory.
Gastrointestinal. Dry mouth, constipation, biliary tract spasm.
Cardiovascular. Flushing of the face, tachycardia, bradycardia, palpitation, hypotension (see Warnings), syncope, phlebitis following intravenous injection.
Genitourinary. Urinary retention.
Allergic. Pruritus, urticaria, other skin rashes, wheal and flare over the vein with intravenous injection.
Other. Pain at injection site; local tissue irritation and induration following subcutaneous injection, particularly when repeated; antidiuretic effect.

DOSAGE AND ADMINISTRATION

For Relief of Pain
Dosage should be adjusted according to the severity of the pain and the response of the patient. While subcutaneous administration is suitable for occasional use, intramuscular administration is preferred when repeated doses are required. If intravenous administration is required, dosage should be decreased and the injection made very slowly, preferably utilizing a diluted solution. Meperidine is less effective orally than on parenteral administration. The dose of DEMEROL should be proportionately reduced (usually by 25 to 50 percent) when administered concomitantly with phenothiazines and many other tranquilizers since they potentiate the action of DEMEROL, brand of meperidine.
Adults. The usual dosage is 50 mg to 150 mg intramuscularly, subcutaneously, or orally, every 3 or 4 hours as necessary.
Children. The usual dosage is 0.5 mg/lb to 0.8 mg/lb intramuscularly, subcutaneously, or orally up to the adult dose, every 3 or 4 hours as necessary.
Each dose of the syrup should be taken in one-half glass of water, since if taken undiluted, it may exert a slight topical anesthetic effect on mucous membranes.
For Preoperative Medication
Adults. The usual dosage is 50 mg to 100 mg intramuscularly or subcutaneously, 30 to 90 minutes before the beginning of anesthesia.
Children. The usual dosage is 0.5 mg/lb to 1 mg/lb intramuscularly or subcutaneously up to the adult dose, 30 to 90 minutes before the beginning of anesthesia.
For Support of Anesthesia
Repeated slow intravenous injections of fractional doses (eg, 10 mg/mL) or continuous intravenous infusion of a more dilute solution (eg, 1 mg/mL) should be used. The dose should be titrated to the needs of the patient and will depend on the premedication and type of anesthesia being employed, the characteristics of the particular patient, and the nature and duration of the operative procedure.
For Obstetrical Analgesia
The usual dosage is 50 mg to 100 mg intramuscularly or subcutaneously when pain becomes regular, and may be repeated at 1- to 3-hour intervals.

OVERDOSAGE

Symptoms. Serious overdosage with meperidine is characterized by respiratory depression (a decrease in respiratory rate and/or tidal volume, Cheyne-Stokes respiration, cyanosis), extreme somnolence progressing to stupor or coma, skeletal muscle flaccidity, cold and clammy skin, and sometimes bradycardia and hypotension. In severe overdosage, particularly by the intravenous route, apnea, circulatory collapse, cardiac arrest, and death may occur.
Treatment. Primary attention should be given to the reestablishment of adequate respiratory exchange through provision of a patent airway and institution of assisted or controlled ventilation. The narcotic antagonist, naloxone hydrochloride, is a specific antidote against respiratory depression which may result from overdosage or unusual sensitivity to narcotics, including meperidine. Therefore, an appropriate dose of this antagonist should be administered, preferably by the intravenous route, simultaneously with efforts at respiratory resuscitation.
An antagonist should not be administered in the absence of clinically significant respiratory or cardiovascular depression.

Continued on next page

This product information was prepared in August, 1989. On these and other products of Winthrop Pharmaceuticals, detailed information may be obtained on a current basis by direct inquiry to the Professional Services Department, 90 Park Avenue, New York, NY 10016 (800) 446-6267.

Winthrop Pharm.—Cont.

Oxygen, intravenous fluids, vasopressors, and other supportive measures should be employed as indicated.

In cases of overdosage with DEMEROL, brand of meperidine, tablets, the stomach should be evacuated by emesis or gastric lavage.

NOTE: In an individual physically dependent on narcotics, the administration of the usual dose of a narcotic antagonist will precipitate an acute withdrawal syndrome. The severity of this syndrome will depend on the degree of physical dependence and the dose of antagonist administered. The use of narcotic antagonists in such individuals should be avoided if possible. If a narcotic antagonist must be used to treat serious respiratory depression in the physically dependent patient, the antagonist should be administered with extreme care and only one-fifth to one-tenth the usual initial dose administered.

HOW SUPPLIED
For Parenteral Use

Detecto-Seal ® — *Carpuject* ® **Sterile Cartridge-Needle Unit**—*2.5 percent* (25 mg per 1 mL) **NDC** 0024-0324-02, *5 percent* (50 mg per 1 mL) **NDC** 0024-0325-02, *7.5 percent* (75 mg per 1 mL) **NDC** 0024-0326-02; and *10 percent* (100 mg per 1 mL) **NDC** 0024-0328-02 all in boxes of 10.

Each cartridge is only partially-filled based upon product volume to permit mixture with other sterile materials in accordance with the best judgment of the physician.

Uni-Amp ®—*5 percent solution;* ampuls of 0.5 mL (25 mg) **NDC** 0024-0361-04, 1 mL (50 mg) **NDC** 0024-0362-04, 1½ mL (75 mg) **NDC** 0024-0363-04, and 2 mL (100 mg) **NDC** 0024-0364-04 all in boxes of 25; and *10 percent solution,* ampuls of 1 mL (100 mg) **NDC** 0024-0365-04 in boxes of 25.

Uni-Nest ™—*5 percent solution;* ampuls of 0.5 mL (25 mg) **NDC** 0024-0371-04, 1 mL (50 mg) **NDC** 0024-0372-04, 1½ mL (75 mg) **NDC** 0024-0373-04, and 2 mL (100 mg) **NDC** 0024-0374-04 all in boxes of 25; and *10 percent solution,* ampuls of 1 mL (100 mg) **NDC** 0024-0375-04 in boxes of 25.

Vials—*5 percent* multiple-dose vials of 30 mL **NDC** 0024-0329-01, and *10 percent* multiple-dose vials of 20 mL **NDC** 0024-0331-01 all in boxes of 1.

Note: The pH of DEMEROL solutions is adjusted between 3.5 and 6 with sodium hydroxide or hydrochloric acid. Multiple-dose vials contain metacresol 0.1 percent as preservative. No preservatives are added to the ampuls or CARPUJECT Sterile Cartridge-Needle Units.

For Oral Use

Tablets of 50 mg, bottles of 100 (**NDC** 0024-0335-04) and 500 (**NDC** 0024-0335-06); Hospital Blister Pak of 25 (**NDC** 0024-0335-02); 100 mg, bottles of 100 (**NDC** 0024-0337-04) and 500 (**NDC** 0024-0337-06); Hospital Blister Pak of 25 (**NDC** 0024-0337-02).

Syrup, nonalcoholic, banana-flavored 50 mg per 5 mL teaspoon, bottles of 16 fl oz (**NDC** 0024-0332-06).

Shown in Product Identification Section, page 435

DW-55-HH

INOCOR® LACTATE INJECTION ℞
brand of amrinone lactate
Sterile Intravenous Solution

DESCRIPTION

INOCOR lactate injection, brand of amrinone lactate, represents a new class of cardiac inotropic agents distinct from digitalis glycosides or catecholamines. Amrinone lactate is designated chemically as 5-Amino[3,4'-bipyridin]-6(1*H*)-one lactate.

Amrinone is a pale yellow crystalline compound with a molecular weight of 187.2 and an empirical formula of $C_{10}H_9N_3O$. Each mole of lactic acid has a molecular weight of 90.08 and an empirical formula of $C_3H_6O_3$. The solubilities of amrinone at pH's 4.1, 6.0, and 8.0 are 25, 0.9, and 0.7 mg/mL, respectively.

INOCOR lactate injection is available as a sterile solution in 20 mL ampuls for intravenous administration. Each mL contains INOCOR lactate equivalent to 5 mg of base and 0.25 mg of sodium metabisulfite added as a preservative in Water for Injection. All dosages expressed in the package insert are expressed in terms of the base, amrinone. The pH is adjusted to between 3.2 to 4.0 with lactic acid or sodium hydroxide. The total concentration of lactic acid can vary between 5.0 mg/mL and 7.5 mg/mL.

CLINICAL PHARMACOLOGY

INOCOR lactate injection is a positive inotropic agent with vasodilator activity, different in structure and mode of action from either digitalis glycosides or catecholamines. The mechanism of its inotropic and vasodilator effects has not been fully elucidated.

With respect to its inotropic effect, experimental evidence indicates that it is not a beta-adrenergic agonist. It inhibits myocardial cyclic adenosine monophosphate (c-AMP) phosphodiesterase activity and increases cellular levels of c-

AMP. Unlike digitalis, it does not inhibit sodium-potassium adenosine triphosphatase activity.

With respect to its vasodilatory activity, INOCOR reduces afterload and preload by its direct relaxant effect on vascular smooth muscle.

Pharmacokinetics

Following intravenous bolus (1 to 2 minutes) injection of 0.68 mg/kg to 1.2 mg/kg to normal volunteers, INOCOR had a volume of distribution of 1.2 liters/kg, and following a distributive phase half-life of about 4.6 minutes in plasma, had a mean apparent first-order terminal elimination half-life of about 3.6 hours. In patients with congestive heart failure receiving infusions of INOCOR the mean apparent first-order terminal elimination half-life was about 5.8 hours.

Amrinone has been shown in one study to be 10% to 22% bound to human plasma protein by ultrafiltration in vitro, and in another study 35% to 49% bound by either ultrafiltration or equilibrium dialysis.

The primary route of excretion in man is *via* the urine as both amrinone and several metabolites (N-glycolyl, N-acetate, O-glucuronide and N-glucuronide). In normal volunteers, approximately 63% of an oral dose of ^{14}C-labelled amrinone was excreted in the urine over a 96-hour period. In the first 8 hours, 51% of the radioactivity in the urine was amrinone with 5% as the N-acetate, 8% as the N-glycolate, and less than 5% for each glucuronide. Approximately 18% of the administered dose was excreted in the feces in 72 hours. In a 24-hour nonradioactive intravenous study, 10% to 40% of the dose was excreted in urine as unchanged amrinone with the N-acetyl metabolite representing less than 2% of the dose.

In congestive heart failure patients, after a loading bolus dose, steady-state plasma levels of about 2.4 μg/mL were able to be maintained by an infusion of 5 μg/kg/min to 10 μg/kg/min. In some congestive heart failure patients, with associated compromised renal and hepatic perfusion, it is possible that plasma levels of amrinone may rise during the infusion period; therefore, in these patients, it may be necessary to monitor the hemodynamic response and/or drug level. The principal measures of patient response include cardiac index, pulmonary capillary wedge pressure, central venous pressure, and their relationship to plasma concentrations. Additionally, measurements of blood pressure, urine output, and body weight may prove useful, as may such clinical symptoms as orthopnea, dyspnea, and fatigue.

Pharmacodynamics

In patients with depressed myocardial function, INOCOR lactate injection produces a prompt increase in cardiac output due to its inotropic and vasodilator actions.

Following a single intravenous bolus dose of INOCOR of 0.75 mg/kg to 3 mg/kg in patients with congestive heart failure, dose-related maximum increases in cardiac output occur (of about 28% at 0.75 mg/kg to about 61% at 3 mg/kg). The peak effect occurs within 10 minutes at all doses. The duration of effect depends upon dose, lasting about ½ hour at 0.75 mg/kg and approximately 2 hours at 3 mg/kg.

Over the same range of doses, pulmonary capillary wedge pressure and total peripheral resistance show dose-related decreases (mean maximum decreases of 29% in pulmonary capillary wedge pressure and 29% in systemic vascular resistance). At doses up to 3.0 mg/kg dose-related decreases in diastolic pressure (up to 13%) have been observed. Mean arterial pressure decreases (9.7%) at a dose of 3.0 mg/kg. The heart rate is generally unchanged.

The changes in hemodynamic parameters are maintained during continuous intravenous infusion and for several hours thereafter.

INOCOR lactate injection, brand of amrinone lactate, is effective in fully digitalized patients without causing signs of cardiac glycoside toxicity. Its inotropic effects are additive to those of digitalis. In cases of atrial flutter/fibrillation, it is possible that INOCOR may increase ventricular response rate because of its slight enhancement of A/V conduction. In these cases, prior treatment with digitalis is recommended. Improvement in left ventricular function and relief of congestive heart failure in patients with ischemic heart disease have been observed. The improvement has occurred without inducing symptoms or electrocardiographic signs of myocardial ischemia.

At constant heart rate and blood pressure, increases in cardiac output occur without measurable increases in myocardial oxygen consumption or changes in arterio-venous oxygen difference.

Inotropic activity is maintained following repeated intravenous doses of INOCOR. INOCOR administration produces hemodynamic and symptomatic benefits to patients not satisfactorily controlled by conventional therapy with diuretics and cardiac glycosides.

INDICATIONS AND USAGE

INOCOR lactate injection is indicated for the short-term management of congestive heart failure. Because of limited experience and potential for serious adverse effects (see ADVERSE REACTIONS), INOCOR should be used only in patients who can be closely monitored and who have not responded adequately to digitalis, diuretics, and/or vasodi-

lators. Although most patients have been studied hemodynamically for periods only up to 24 hours, some patients were studied for longer periods and demonstrated consistent hemodynamic and clinical effects. The duration of therapy should depend on patient responsiveness.

CONTRAINDICATIONS

INOCOR lactate injection is contraindicated in patients who are hypersensitive to it.

It is also contraindicated in those patients known to be hypersensitive to bisulfites.

WARNING

Contains sodium metabisulfite, a sulfite that may cause allergic-type reactions including anaphylactic symptoms and life-threatening or less severe asthmatic episodes in certain susceptible people. The overall prevalence of sulfite sensitivity in the general population is unknown and probably low. Sulfite sensitivity is seen more frequently in asthmatic than in nonasthmatic people.

PRECAUTIONS

General: INOCOR lactate injection should not be used in patients with severe aortic or pulmonic valvular disease in lieu of surgical relief of the obstruction. Like other inotropic agents, it may aggravate outflow tract obstruction in hypertrophic subaortic stenosis.

During intravenous therapy with INOCOR lactate injection, blood pressure and heart rate should be monitored and the rate of infusion slowed or stopped in patients showing excessive decreases in blood pressure.

Patients who have received vigorous diuretic therapy may have insufficient cardiac filling pressure to respond adequately to INOCOR lactate injection, in which case cautious liberalization of fluid and electrolyte intake may be indicated.

Supraventricular and ventricular arrhythmias have been observed in the very high-risk population treated. While amrinone per se has not been shown to be arrhythmogenic, the potential for arrhythmia, present in congestive heart failure itself, may be increased by any drug or combination of drugs.

Thrombocytopenia and hepatotoxicity have been noted (see ADVERSE REACTIONS).

USE IN ACUTE MYOCARDIAL INFARCTION: No clinical trials have been carried out in patients in the acute phase of postmyocardial infarction. Therefore, INOCOR lactate injection, brand of amrinone lactate, is not recommended in these cases.

Laboratory Tests

Fluid and Electrolytes: Fluid and electrolyte changes and renal function should be carefully monitored during amrinone lactate therapy. Improvement in cardiac output with resultant diuresis may necessitate a reduction in the dose of diuretic. Potassium loss due to excessive diuresis may predispose digitalized patients to arrhythmias. Therefore, hypokalemia should be corrected by potassium supplementation in advance of or during amrinone use.

Drug Interactions

In a relatively limited experience, no untoward clinical manifestations have been observed in patients in which INOCOR lactate injection was used concurrently with the following drugs: digitalis glycosides; lidocaine, quinidine; metoprolol, propranolol; hydralazine, prazosin; isosorbide dinitrate, nitroglycerine; chlorthalidone; ethacrynic acid, furosemide, hydrochlorothiazide, spironolactone; captopril; heparin, warfarin; potassium supplements; insulin; diazepam.

One case report of excessive hypotension has been reported when amrinone was used concurrently with disopyramide. Until additional experience is available, concurrent administration with NORPACE® (disopyramide) should be undertaken with caution.

Chemical Interactions

A chemical interaction occurs slowly over a 24-hour period when the intravenous solution of INOCOR lactate injection is mixed directly with dextrose(glucose)-containing solutions. **THEREFORE, INOCOR LACTATE INJECTION SHOULD NOT BE DILUTED WITH SOLUTIONS THAT CONTAIN DEXTROSE (GLUCOSE) PRIOR TO INJECTION.**

A chemical interaction occurs immediately, which is evidenced by the formation of a precipitate when furosemide is injected into an intravenous line of an infusion of amrinone. Therefore, furosemide should not be administered in intravenous lines containing amrinone.

Carcinogenesis, Mutagenesis, Impairment of Fertility

There was no suggestion of a carcinogenic potential with amrinone when administered orally for up to two years to rats and mice at dose levels up to 80 mg/kg/day.

The mouse micronucleus test (at 7.5 to 10 times the maximum human dose) and the Chinese hamster ovary chromosome aberration assay were positive indicating both clastogenic potential and suppression of the number of polychromatic erythrocytes. However, the Ames Salmonella assay, mouse lymphoma study, and cultured human lymphocyte metaphase analysis were all negative. The clastogenic effects are in contrast to negative results obtained in the rat male and female fertility studies, and a three-generation study in rats, both with oral dosing.

Slight prolongation of the rat gestation period was seen in these studies at dose levels of 50 mg/kg/day and 100 mg/kg/day. Dystocia occurred in dams receiving 100 mg/kg/day resulting in increased numbers of stillbirths, decreased litter size, and poor pup survival.

Pregnancy Category C

In New Zealand white rabbits, amrinone has been shown to produce fetal skeletal and gross external malformations at oral doses of 16 mg/kg and 50 mg/kg which were toxic for the rabbit. Studies in French Hy/Cr rabbits using oral doses up to 32 mg/kg/day did not confirm this finding. No malformations were seen in rats receiving amrinone intravenously at the maximum dose used, 15 mg/kg/day (approximately the recommended daily intravenous dose for patients with congestive heart failure). There are no adequate and well-controlled studies in pregnant women. Amrinone should be used during pregnancy only if the potential benefit justifies the potential risk to the fetus.

Nursing Mothers

Caution should be exercised when amrinone is administered to nursing women, since it is not known whether it is excreted in human milk.

Pediatric Use

Safety and effectiveness in children have not been established.

ADVERSE REACTIONS

Thrombocytopenia: Intravenous INOCOR lactate injection, brand of amrinone lactate, resulted in platelet count reductions to below 100,000/mm³ or normal limits in 2.4 percent of the patients.

It is more common in patients receiving prolonged therapy. To date, in closely-monitored clinical trials, in patients whose platelet counts were not allowed to remain depressed, no bleeding phenomena have been observed.

Platelet reduction is dose dependent and appears due to a decrease in platelet survival time. Several patients who developed thrombocytopenia while receiving amrinone had bone marrow examinations which were normal. There is no evidence relating platelet reduction to immune response or to a platelet activating factor.

Gastrointestinal Effects: Gastrointestinal adverse reactions reported with INOCOR lactate injection during clinical use included nausea (1.7%), vomiting (0.9%), abdominal pain (0.4%), and anorexia (0.4%).

Cardiovascular Effects: Cardiovascular adverse reactions reported with INOCOR lactate injection include arrhythmia (3%) and hypotension (1.3%).

Hepatic Toxicity: In dogs, at IV doses between 9 mg/kg/day and 32 mg/kg/day, amrinone showed dose-related hepatotoxicity manifested either as enzyme elevation or hepatic cell necrosis or both. Hepatotoxicity has been observed in man following long-term oral dosing and has been observed, in a limited experience (0.2%), following intravenous administration of amrinone.

Hypersensitivity: There have been reports of several apparent hypersensitivity reactions in patients treated with oral amrinone for about two weeks. Signs and symptoms were variable but included pericarditis, pleuritis and ascites (1 case), myositis with interstitial shadowing on chest x-ray and elevated sedimentation rate (1 case) and vasculitis with nodular pulmonary densities, hypoxemia, and jaundice (1 case). The first patient died, not necessarily of the possible reaction, while the last two resolved with discontinuation of therapy. None of the cases were rechallenged so that attribution to amrinone is not certain, but possible hypersensitivity reactions should be considered in any patient maintained for a prolonged period on amrinone.

General: Additional adverse reactions observed in intravenous amrinone clinical studies include fever (0.9%), chest pain (0.2%), and burning at the site of injection (0.2%).

Management of Adverse Reactions

Platelet Count Reductions: Asymptomatic platelet count reduction (to < 150,000/mm³) may be reversed within one week of a decrease in drug dosage. Further, with no change in drug dosage, the count may stabilize at lower than predrug levels without any clinical sequelae. Pre-drug platelet counts and frequent platelet counts during therapy are recommended to assist in decisions regarding dosage modifications.

Should a platelet count less than 150,000/mm³ occur, the following actions may be considered:

- Maintain total daily dose unchanged, since in some cases counts have either stabilized or returned to pretreatment levels.
- Decrease total daily dose.
- Discontinue amrinone if, in the clinical judgment of the physician, risk exceeds the potential benefit.

Gastrointestinal Side Effects: While gastrointestinal side effects were seen infrequently with intravenous therapy, should severe or debilitating ones occur, the physician may wish to reduce dosage or discontinue the drug based on the usual benefit-to-risk considerations.

Hepatic Toxicity: In clinical experience to date with intravenous administration, hepatotoxicity has been observed rarely. If acute marked alterations in liver enzymes occur together with clinical symptoms suggesting an idiosyncratic hypersensitivity reaction, amrinone therapy should be promptly discontinued.

If less than marked enzyme alterations occur without clinical symptoms, these nonspecific changes should be evaluated on an individual basis. The clinician may wish to continue amrinone, reduce dosage, or discontinue the drug based on the usual benefit/risk considerations.

OVERDOSAGE

A death has been reported with a massive accidental overdose (840 mg over three hours by initial bolus and infusion) of amrinone, although causal relation is uncertain. Diligence should be exercised during product preparation and administration.

Doses of INOCOR lactate injection may produce hypotension because of its vasodilator effect. If this occurs, amrinone administration should be reduced or discontinued. No specific antidote is known, but general measures for circulatory support should be taken.

In rats, the LD₅₀ of amrinone, as the lactate salt, was 102 mg/kg or 130 mg/kg intravenously in two different studies and 132 mg/kg orally (intragastrically); as a suspension in aqueous gum tragacanth the oral LD₅₀ was 239 mg/kg.

DOSAGE AND ADMINISTRATION

INOCOR lactate injection may be administered as supplied or diluted in normal, or half normal saline solution to a concentration of 1 mg/mL to 3 mg/mL. Diluted solutions should be used within 24 hours.

INOCOR lactate injection, brand of amrinone lactate, may be injected into running dextrose (glucose) infusions through a Y-Connector or directly into the tubing where preferable.

Chemical Interactions

A chemical interaction occurs slowly over a 24-hour period when the intravenous solution of INOCOR lactate injection is mixed <u>directly</u> with dextrose (glucose)-containing solutions. **THEREFORE, INOCOR LACTATE INJECTION SHOULD NOT BE DILUTED WITH SOLUTIONS THAT CONTAIN DEXTROSE (GLUCOSE) PRIOR TO INJECTION.**

A chemical interaction occurs immediately, which is evidenced by the formation of a precipitate when furosemide is injected into an intravenous line of an infusion of amrinone. Therefore, furosemide should not be administered in intravenous lines containing amrinone.

The following procedure is recommended for the administration of INOCOR lactate injection:

1. Initiate therapy with a 0.75 mg/kg bolus given slowly over 2 to 3 minutes.
2. Continue therapy with a maintenance infusion between 5 µg/kg/min and 10 µg/kg/min.
3. Based on clinical response, an additional bolus injection of 0.75 mg/kg may be given 30 minutes after the initiation of therapy.
4. The rate of infusion usually ranges from 5 µg/kg/min to 10 µg/kg/min such that the recommended total daily dose (including boluses) does not exceed 10 mg/kg. A limited number of patients studied at higher doses support a dosage regimen up to 18 mg/kg/day for shortened durations of therapy.
5. The rate of administration and the duration of therapy should be adjusted according to the response of the patient. The physician may wish to reduce or titrate the infusion downward based on clinical responsiveness or untoward effects.

The above dosing regimens can be expected to place most patients' plasma concentration of amrinone at approximately 3 µg/mL. Increases in cardiac index show a linear relationship to plasma concentration of a range of 0.5 µg/mL to 7 µg/mL. No observations have been made at greater plasma concentrations.

Patient improvement may be reflected by increases in cardiac output, reduction in pulmonary capillary wedge pressure, and such clinical responses as a lessening of dyspnea and an improvement in other symptoms of heart failure, such as orthopnea and fatigue.

Monitoring central venous pressure (CVP) may be valuable in the assessment of hypotension and fluid balance management. Prior correction or adjustment of fluid/electrolytes is essential to obtain satisfactory response with amrinone.

Parenteral drug products should be inspected visually and should not be used if particulate matter or discoloration is observed.

HOW SUPPLIED

Ampuls of 20 mL sterile, clear yellow solution containing INOCOR 5 mg/mL, box of 5 (NDC 0024-0888-20). Each 1 mL contains INOCOR lactate equivalent to 5 mg base and 0.25 mg sodium metabisulfite in Water for Injection. The pH of INOCOR lactate injection, brand of amrinone lactate, is adjusted to a range of 3.2 to 4.0 with lactic acid or sodium hydroxide.

Protect INOCOR lactate ampuls from light. Ampul packaging is light resistant for protection during storage. Store at room temperature.

NOTE: Parenteral drug products should be inspected visually and should not be used if particulate matter or discoloration is observed.

NORPACE, trademark, G. D. Searle & Co.
Distributed by Winthrop Pharmaceuticals
Division of Sterling Drug Inc.
New York, NY 10016
Manufactured by SK&F LAB CO.
Cidra, Puerto Rico 00639

IW-161-L

FOR MEDICAL INFORMATION ON INOCOR CALL TOLL FREE 1-800-446-6267

ISUPREL® ℞

brand of isoproterenol hydrochloride injection, USP
Sterile Injection 1:5000

DESCRIPTION

Isoproterenol hydrochloride is 3,4-Dihydroxy-α-[(isopropylamino)methyl] benzyl alcohol hydrochloride, a synthetic sympathomimetic amine that is structurally related to epinephrine but acts almost exclusively on beta receptors.

Each milliliter of the sterile 1:5000 solution contains ISUPREL, brand of isoproterenol hydrochloride injection, USP, 0.2 mg, lactic acid 0.12 mg, sodium chloride 7.0 mg, sodium lactate 1.8 mg, sodium metabisulfite (as preservative) 1.0 mg, and Water for Injection qs ad 1.0 mL.

The pH is adjusted between 3.5 and 4.5 with hydrochloric acid. The air in the ampuls has been displaced by nitrogen gas.

The sterile 1:5000 solution can be administered by the intravenous, intramuscular, subcutaneous, or intracardiac routes.

CLINICAL PHARMACOLOGY

Isoproterenol hydrochloride injection acts primarily on the heart and on smooth muscle of bronchi, skeletal muscle vasculature, and alimentary tract. The positive inotropic and chronotropic actions of the drug result in an increase in minute blood flow. There is an increase in heart rate, an approximately unchanged stroke volume, and an increase in ejection velocity. The rate of discharge of cardiac pacemakers is increased with isoproterenol hydrochloride injection. Venous return to the heart is increased through a decreased compliance of the venous bed. Systemic resistance and pulmonary vascular resistance are decreased, and there is an increase in coronary and renal blood flow. Systolic blood pressure may increase and diastolic blood pressure may decrease. Mean arterial blood pressure is usually unchanged or reduced. The peripheral and coronary vasodilating effects of the drug may aid tissue perfusion.

Isoproterenol hydrochloride injection relaxes most smooth muscle, the most pronounced effect being on bronchial and gastrointestinal smooth muscle. It produces marked relaxation in the smaller bronchi and may even dilate the trachea and main bronchi past the resting diameter.

Isoproterenol hydrochloride injection is metabolized primarily in the liver by COMT. The duration of action of isoproterenol hydrochloride injection may be longer than epinephrine, but it is still brief.

INDICATIONS AND USAGE

Isoproterenol hydrochloride injection is indicated:

- For mild or transient episodes of heart block that do not require electric shock or pacemaker therapy.
- For serious episodes of heart block and Adams-Stokes attacks (except when caused by ventricular tachycardia or fibrillation). (See CONTRAINDICATIONS.)
- For use in cardiac arrest until electric shock or pacemaker therapy, the treatments of choice, is available. (See CONTRAINDICATIONS.)
- For bronchospasm occurring during anesthesia.
- As an adjunct to fluid and electrolyte replacement therapy and the use of other drugs and procedures in the treatment of hypovolemic and septic shock, low cardiac output (hypoperfusion) states, congestive heart failure, and cardiogenic shock. (See WARNINGS.)

Continued on next page

This product information was prepared in August, 1989. On these and other products of Winthrop Pharmaceuticals, detailed information may be obtained on a current basis by direct inquiry to the Professional Services Department, 90 Park Avenue, New York, NY 10016 (800) 446-6267.

Winthrop Pharm.—Cont.

CONTRAINDICATIONS

Use of isoproterenol hydrochloride injection is contraindicated in patients with tachyarrhythmias; tachycardia or heartblock caused by digitalis intoxication; ventricular arrhythmias which require inotropic therapy; and angina pectoris.

WARNINGS

Isoproterenol hydrochloride injection, by increasing myocardial oxygen requirements while decreasing effective coronary perfusion, may have a deleterious effect on the injured or failing heart. Most experts discourage its use as the initial agent in treating cardiogenic shock following myocardial infarction. However, when a low arterial pressure has been elevated by other means, isoproterenol hydrochloride injection may produce beneficial hemodynamic and metabolic effects.

In a few patients, presumably with organic disease of the AV node and its branches, isoproterenol hydrochloride injection has paradoxically been reported to worsen heart block or to precipitate Adams-Stokes attacks during normal sinus rhythm or transient heart block.

Contains sodium metabisulfite, a sulfite that may cause allergic-type reactions including anaphylactic symptoms and life-threatening or less severe asthmatic episodes in certain susceptible people. The overall prevalence of sulfite sensitivity in the general population is unknown and probably low. Sulfite sensitivity is seen more frequently in asthmatic than in nonasthmatic people.

PRECAUTIONS

General

Isoproterenol hydrochloride injection should generally be started at the lowest recommended dose. This may be gradually increased, if necessary, while carefully monitoring the patient. Doses sufficient to increase the heart rate to more than 130 beats per minute may increase the likelihood of inducing ventricular arrhythmias. Such increases in heart rate will also tend to increase cardiac work and oxygen requirements which may adversely affect the failing heart or the heart with a significant degree of arteriosclerosis.

Particular caution is necessary in administering isoproterenol hydrochloride injection to patients with coronary artery disease, coronary insufficiency, diabetes, hyperthyroidism, and sensitivity to sympathomimetic amines.

Adequate filling of the intravascular compartment by suitable volume expanders is of primary importance in most cases of shock, and should precede the administration of vasoactive drugs. In patients with normal cardiac function, determination of central venous pressure is a reliable guide during volume replacement. If evidence of hypoperfusion persists after adequate volume replacement, isoproterenol hydrochloride injection may be given.

In addition to the routine monitoring of systemic blood pressure, heart rate, urine flow, and the electrocardiograph, the response to therapy should also be monitored by frequent determination of the central venous pressure and blood gases. Patients in shock should be closely observed during isoproterenol hydrochloride injection administration. If the heart rate exceeds 110 beats per minute, it may be advisable to decrease the infusion rate or temporarily discontinue the infusion. Determinations of cardiac output and circulation time may also be helpful. Appropriate measures should be taken to ensure adequate ventilation. Careful attention should be paid to acid-base balance and to the correction of electrolyte disturbances. In cases of shock associated with

bacteremia, suitable antimicrobial therapy is, of course, imperative.

Drug Interactions

Isoproterenol hydrochloride injection and epinephrine should not be administered simultaneously because both drugs are direct cardiac stimulants and their combined effects may induce serious arrhythmias. The drugs may, however, be administered alternately provided a proper interval has elapsed between doses.

ISUPREL, brand of isoproterenol, should be used with caution, if at all, when potent inhalational anesthetics such as halothane are employed because of potential to sensitize the myocardium to effects of sympathomimetic amines.

Carcinogenesis, Mutagenesis, Impairment of Fertility

Long-term studies in animals to evaluate the carcinogenic potential of isoproterenol hydrochloride have not been done. Mutagenic potential and effect on fertility have not been determined. There is no evidence from human experience that isoproterenol hydrochloride injection may be carcinogenic or mutagenic or that it impairs fertility.

Pregnancy Category C

Animal reproduction studies have not been conducted with isoproterenol hydrochloride. It is also not known whether isoproterenol hydrochloride can cause fetal harm when administered to a pregnant woman or can affect reproduction capacity. Isoproterenol hydrochloride should be given to a pregnant woman only if clearly needed.

Nursing Mothers

It is not known whether this drug is excreted in human milk. Because many drugs are excreted in human milk, caution should be exercised when isoproterenol hydrochloride injection is administered to a nursing woman.

ADVERSE REACTIONS

The following reactions to isoproterenol hydrochloride injection have been reported:

CNS: Nervousness, headache, dizziness.

Cardiovascular: Tachycardia, palpitations, angina, Adams-Stokes attacks, pulmonary edema, hypertension, hypotension, ventricular arrhythmias, tachyarrhythmias.

In a few patients, presumably with organic disease of the AV node and its branches, isoproterenol hydrochloride injection has been reported to precipitate Adams-Stokes seizures during normal sinus rhythm or transient heart block.

Other: Flushing of the skin, sweating, mild tremors, weakness.

OVERDOSAGE

The acute toxicity of isoproterenol hydrochloride in animals is much less than that of epinephrine. Excessive doses in animals or man can cause a striking drop in blood pressure, and repeated large doses in animals may result in cardiac enlargement and focal myocarditis.

In case of accidental overdosage as evidenced mainly by tachycardia or other arrhythmias, palpitations, angina, hypotension, or hypertension, reduce rate of administration or discontinue isoproterenol hydrochloride injection until patient's condition stabilizes. Blood pressure, pulse, respiration, and EKG should be monitored.

It is not known whether isoproterenol hydrochloride is dialyzable.

The oral LD_{50} of isoproterenol hydrochloride in mice is 3,850 mg/kg $\pm$ 1,190 mg/kg of pure drug in solution.

DOSAGE AND ADMINISTRATION

ISUPREL injection 1:5000 should generally be started at the lowest recommended dose and the rate of administration gradually increased if necessary while carefully monitoring the patient. The usual route of administration is by intravenous infusion or bolus intravenous injection. In dire emergencies, the drug may be administered by intracardiac injection. If time is not of the utmost importance, initial therapy by intramuscular or subcutaneous injection is preferred. [See table below].

There are no well-controlled studies in children to establish appropriate dosing; however, the American Heart Association recommends an initial infusion rate of 0.1µg/kg/min, with the usual range being 0.1µg/kg/min to 1.0µg/kg/min. [See table above].

Parenteral drug products should be inspected visually for particulate matter and discoloration prior to administration, whenever solution and container permit. Such solution should not be used.

HOW SUPPLIED

Ampuls of 1 mL (0.2 mg) UNI-NEST™ PAK of 25 (NDC 0024-0866-25)
Ampuls of 5 mL (1 mg) box of 10 (NDC 0024-0866-02)
Protect from light. Keep in opaque container until used.
Store in a cool place between 8°C to 15°C (46° F to 59° F).
Do not use if the injection is pinkish to brownish in color or contains a precipitate.

IW-33-X

ISUPREL®   ℞
brand of isoproterenol hydrochloride inhalation aerosol, USP
MISTOMETER®

Potent Bronchodilator

DESCRIPTION

ISUPREL MISTOMETER is a beta agonist sympathomimetic bronchodilator. It is a complete nebulizing unit consisting of a plastic-coated vial of aerosol solution, detachable plastic mouthpiece with built-in nebulizer, and protective cap. The vial contains isoproterenol hydrochloride 0.25% (w/w) with inert ingredients of alcohol 33% (w/w) and ascorbic acid 0.1% (w/w) and, as propellants, dichlorodifluoromethane and dichlorotetrafluoroethane.

Chemically, isoproterenol hydrochloride is 3,4-Dihydroxy-α-[(isopropylamino)methyl]benzyl alcohol hydrochloride.

The contents permit the delivery of not less than 200 actuations from the 11.2 g (10 mL) vial and not less than 300 actuations from the 16.8 g (15 mL) vial. THE MISTOMETER deliv-

---

Recommended dosage for adults with shock and hypoperfusion states:

Route of Administration	Preparation of Dilution†	Infusion Rate††
Intravenous infusion	Dilute 5 mL (1 mg) in 500 mL of 5% Dextrose Injection, USP	0.5 µg to 5 µg per minute (0.25 mL to 2.5 mL of diluted solution)

† Concentrations up to 10 times greater have been used when limitation of volume is essential.
†† Rates over 30 µg per minute have been used in advanced stages of shock. The rate of infusion should be adjusted on the basis of heart rate, central venous pressure, systemic blood pressure, and urine flow. If the heart rate exceeds 110 beats per minute, it may be advisable to decrease or temporarily discontinue the infusion.

Recommended dosage for adults with bronchospasm occurring during anesthesia:

Route of Administration	Preparation of Dilution	Initial Dose	Subsequent Dose
Bolus intravenous injection	Dilute 1 mL (0.2 mg) to 10 mL with Sodium Chloride Injection, USP, or 5% Dextrose Injection, USP	0.01 mg to 0.02 mg (0.5 mL to 1 mL of diluted solution)	The initial dose may be repeated when necessary

---

Recommended dosage for adults with heart block, Adams-Stokes attacks, and cardiac arrest:

Route of Administration	Preparation of Dilution	Initial Dose	Subsequent Dose Range*
Bolus intravenous injection	Dilute 1 mL (0.2 mg) to 10 mL with Sodium Chloride Injection, USP, or 5% Dextrose Injection, USP	0.02 mg to 0.06 mg (1 mL to 3 mL of diluted solution)	0.01 mg to 0.2 mg (0.5 mL to 10 mL of diluted solution)
Intravenous infusion	Dilute 10 mL (2 mg) in 500 mL of 5% Dextrose Injection, USP	5 µg/min. (1.25 mL of diluted solution per minute)	
Intramuscular	Use Solution 1:5000 undiluted	0.2 mg (1 mL)	0.02 mg to 1 mg (0.1 mL to 5 mL)
Subcutaneous	Use Solution 1:5000 undiluted	0.2 mg (1 mL)	0.15 mg to 0.2 mg (0.75 mL to 1 mL)
Intracardiac	Use Solution 1:5000 undiluted	0.02 mg (0.1 mL)	

*Subsequent dosage and method of administration depend on the ventricular rate and the rapidity with which the cardiac pacemaker can take over when the drug is gradually withdrawn.

ers a measured dose of 131 µg of the bronchodilator in a fine, even mist for inhalation.

CLINICAL PHARMACOLOGY

ISUPREL relaxes bronchial spasm and facilitates expectoration of pulmonary secretions by acting almost exclusively on beta receptors. It is frequently effective when epinephrine and other drugs fail, and it has a wide margin of safety. ISUPREL is readily absorbed when given as an aerosol. It is metabolized primarily in the liver and other tissues by catechol-O-methyltransferase (COMT).

Recent studies in laboratory animals (minipigs, rodents, and dogs) recorded the occurrence of cardiac arrhythmias and sudden death (with histologic evidence of myocardial necrosis) when beta agonists and methylxanthines were concomitantly administered. The significance of these findings when applied to human usage is currently unknown.

INDICATIONS AND USAGE

ISUPREL is indicated for the relief of bronchospasm associated with acute and chronic asthma and reversible bronchospasm which may be associated with chronic bronchitis or emphysema.

CONTRAINDICATIONS

Use of isoproterenol in patients with preexisting cardiac arrhythmias associated with tachycardia is generally considered contraindicated because the cardiac stimulant effect of the drug may aggravate such disorders. The use of this medication is contraindicated in those patients who have a known hypersensitivity to isoproterenol or to any of the other components of this drug.

WARNINGS

Excessive use of an adrenergic aerosol should be discouraged as it may lose its effectiveness.

In patients with status asthmaticus and abnormal blood gas tensions, improvement in vital capacity and in blood gas tensions may not accompany apparent relief of bronchospasm. Facilities for administering oxygen mixtures and ventilatory assistance are necessary for such patients.

Occasional patients have been reported to develop severe paradoxical airway resistance with repeated, excessive use of isoproterenol inhalation preparations. The cause of this refractory state is unknown. It is advisable that in such instances the use of this preparation be discontinued immediately and alternative therapy instituted, since in the reported cases the patients did not respond to other forms of therapy until the drug was withdrawn.

Deaths have been reported following excessive use of isoproterenol inhalation preparations and the exact cause is unknown. Cardiac arrest was noted in several instances.

PRECAUTIONS

General

Isoproterenol should be used with caution in patients with cardiovascular disorders including coronary insufficiency, diabetes, or hyperthyroidism, and in persons sensitive to sympathomimetic amines.

A single treatment with the ISUPREL MISTOMETER is usually sufficient for controlling isolated attacks of asthma. Any patient who requires more than three aerosol treatments within a 24-hour period should be under the close supervision of a physician. Further therapy with the bronchodilator aerosol alone is inadvisable when three to five treatments within six to twelve hours produce minimal or no relief.

Information for Patients

Do not inhale more often than directed by your physician. Read enclosed instructions before using (see attachment or insert). Do not exceed the dose prescribed by your physician. If difficulty in breathing persists, contact your physician immediately. Avoid spraying in eyes. Contents under pressure. Do not break or incinerate. Do not store at temperatures above 120°F. Keep out of reach of children.

Drug Interactions

Epinephrine should not be administered concomitantly with ISUPREL, as both drugs are direct cardiac stimulants and their combined effects may induce serious arrhythmia. If desired they may, however, be alternated, provided an interval of at least four hours has elapsed.

Carcinogenesis, Mutagenesis, Impairment of Fertility

Long-term chronic toxicity studies in animals have not been done to evaluate isoproterenol in these areas.

Pregnancy Category C

Animal reproduction studies have not been conducted with isoproterenol hydrochloride. It is also not known whether isoproterenol hydrochloride can cause fetal harm when administered to a pregnant woman or can affect reproduction capacity. Isoproterenol hydrochloride should be given to a pregnant woman only if clearly needed.

Nursing Mothers

It is not known whether this drug is excreted in human milk. Because many drugs are excreted in human milk, caution should be exercised when isoproterenol hydrochloride is administered to a nursing woman.

Pediatric Use

In general, the technique of ISUPREL MISTOMETER in administration to children is similar to that of adults, since children's smaller ventilatory exchange capacity automatically provides proportionally smaller aerosol intake.

ADVERSE REACTIONS

The mist from the ISUPREL MISTOMETER contains alcohol but is generally very well tolerated. An occasional patient may experience some transient throat irritation which has been attributed to the alcohol content.

Serious reactions to ISUPREL, brand of isoproterenol hydrochloride inhalation aerosol, are infrequent. The following reactions, however, have been reported:

CNS: Nervousness, headache, dizziness, weakness.

Gastrointestinal: Nausea, vomiting.

Cardiovascular: Tachycardia, palpitations, precordial distress, anginal-type pain.

Other: Flushing of the skin, tremor, and sweating.

The inhalation route is usually accompanied by a minimum of side effects. These untoward reactions disappear quickly and do not, as a rule, inconvenience the patient to the extent that the drug must be discontinued. No cumulative effects have been reported.

OVERDOSAGE

Overdosage of ISUPREL may produce signs and symptoms typical of excessive sympathomimetic effects, including tachycardia, palpitations, nervousness, nausea, and vomiting. Excessive use of adrenergic aerosols may result in loss of effectiveness or severe paradoxical airway resistance. Cardiac arrest has been noted in several instances. In all cases of overdose or excessive use of ISUPREL, the drug should be discontinued immediately and vital functions supported until the patient is stabilized. It is not known whether isoproterenol hydrochloride is dialyzable.

The acute oral LD_{50} in mice is 3,850 mg/kg $\pm$ 1,190 mg/kg of pure drug in solution (isoproterenol hydrochloride). In dogs, the toxic dose is 1,000 times the therapeutic dose. Converted to the amount used clinically in man, this would be about 2,500 times the therapeutic dose.

DOSAGE AND ADMINISTRATION

This drug may not be dispensed without a prescription.

Acute Bronchial Asthma: Hold the MISTOMETER in an inverted position. Close lips and teeth around open end of mouthpiece. Breathe out, expelling as much air from the lungs as possible; then inhale deeply while pressing down on the bottle to activate spray mechanism. Try to hold breath for a few seconds before exhaling. Wait one full minute in order to determine the effect before considering a second inhalation. A treatment may be repeated up to 5 times daily if necessary. (See PRECAUTIONS.) If carefully instructed, children quickly learn to keep the stream of mist clear of the teeth and tongue, thereby assuring inhalation into the lungs. Occlusion of the nares of very young children may be advisable to make inhalation certain.

Warm water should be run through the mouthpiece once daily to wash it and prevent clogging.

The mouthpiece may also be sanitized by immersion in alcohol.

Bronchospasm in Chronic Obstructive Lung Disease: The MISTOMETER provides a convenient aerosol method for delivering ISUPREL, brand of isoproterenol hydrochloride inhalation aerosol. The treatment described above for Acute Bronchial Asthma may be repeated at not less than 3 to 4 hour intervals as part of a programmed regimen of treatment of obstructive lung disease complicated by a reversible bronchospastic component. One application from the MISTOMETER may be regarded as equivalent in effectiveness to 5 to 7 operations of a hand-bulb nebulizer using a 1:100 solution.

Children's Dosage

In general, the technique of ISUPREL MISTOMETER in administration to children is similar to that of adults, since children's smaller ventilatory exchange capacity automatically provides proportionally smaller aerosol intake.

HOW SUPPLIED

ISUPREL MISTOMETER is supplied as a metered dose aerosol providing 131 µg of isoproterenol hydrochloride per actuation.

   Vial of 11.2 g (10 mL) with oral nebulizer
   (NDC 0024-0878-05)
   Vial of 16.8 g (15 mL) with oral nebulizer
   (NDC 0024-0878-01)
   Refill only, 16.8 g (15 mL)
   (NDC 0024-0879-01)

Store at controlled room temperature 15°C to 30°C (59°F to 86°F).

Distributed by Winthrop Pharmaceuticals
Division of Sterling Drug Inc.
New York, NY 10016
Manufactured by Sterling Pharmaceuticals Inc.
Barceloneta, Puerto Rico 00617

IW-67-DD

ISUPREL® Hydrochloride   ℞
brand of isoproterenol
inhalation solution, USP
SOLUTION 1:200
SOLUTION 1:100

Potent Bronchodilator

DESCRIPTION

ISUPREL hydrochloride, brand of isoproterenol inhalation solution, is a beta agonist sympathomimetic bronchodilator.

Solution 1:200 contains isoproterenol hydrochloride 5 mg/mL.

Inactive Ingredients: Chlorobutanol 0.5 percent and Sodium Metabisulfite 0.3 percent as preservatives, Citric Acid, Glycerin, Purified Water, and Sodium Chloride.

Solution 1:100 contains isoproterenol hydrochloride 10 mg/mL.

Inactive Ingredients: Chlorobutanol 0.5 percent and Sodium Metabisulfite 0.3 percent as preservatives, Citric Acid, Purified Water, Saccharin Sodium, Sodium Chloride, and Sodium Citrate.

Isoproterenol hydrochloride is soluble in water (1 g isoproterenol hydrochloride dissolves in 3 mL H_2O). The solutions have a pH range of 3 to 4.5

Chemically, isoproterenol hydrochloride is 3,4-Dihydroxy-α-[(isopropylamino)methyl]benzyl alcohol hydrochloride.

The air in the bottles has been displaced by nitrogen gas.

CLINICAL PHARMACOLOGY

ISUPREL relaxes bronchial spasm and facilitates expectoration of pulmonary secretions by acting almost exclusively on beta receptors. It is frequently effective when epinephrine and other drugs fail, and it has a wide margin of safety. ISUPREL is readily absorbed when given as an aerosol. It is metabolized primarily in the liver and other tissues by catechol-0 methyltransferase (COMT).

Recent studies in laboratory animals (minipigs, rodents, and dogs) recorded the occurrence of cardiac arrhythmias and sudden death (with histologic evidence of myocardial necrosis) when beta agonists and methylxanthines were concomitantly administered. The significance of these findings when applied to human usage is currently unknown.

INDICATIONS AND USAGE

ISUPREL is indicated for the relief of bronchospasm associated with acute and chronic asthma and reversible bronchospasm which may be associated with chronic bronchitis or emphysema.

CONTRAINDICATION

Use of isoproterenol in patients with preexisting cardiac arrhythmias associated with tachycardia is generally considered contraindicated because the cardiac stimulant effect of the drug may aggravate such disorders.

WARNINGS

Excessive use of an adrenergic aerosol should be discouraged as it may lose its effectiveness.

In patients with status asthmaticus and abnormal blood gas tensions, improvement in vital capacity and in blood gas tensions may not accompany apparent relief of bronchospasm. Facilities for administering oxygen mixtures and ventilatory assistance are necessary for such patients.

Occasional patients have been reported to develop severe paradoxical airway resistance with repeated, excessive use of isoproterenol inhalation preparations. The cause of this refractory state is unknown. It is advisable that in such instances the use of this preparation be discontinued immediately and alternative therapy instituted, since in the reported cases the patients did not respond to other forms of therapy until the drug was withdrawn.

Deaths have been reported following excessive use of isoproterenol inhalation preparations and the exact cause is unknown. Cardiac arrest was noted in several instances.

Contains sodium metabisulfite, a sulfite that may cause allergic-type reactions including anaphylactic symptoms and life-threatening or less severe asthmatic episodes in certain susceptible people. The overall prevalence of sulfite sensitivity in the general population is unknown and probably low. Sulfite sensitivity is seen more frequently in asthmatic than in nonasthmatic people.

PRECAUTIONS

General: Isoproterenol should be used with caution in patients with cardiovascular disorders including coronary insufficiency, diabetes, or hyperthyroidism, and in persons sensitive to sympathomimetic amines.

Continued on next page

This product information was prepared in August, 1989. On these and other products of Winthrop Pharmaceuticals, detailed information may be obtained on a current basis by direct inquiry to the Professional Services Department, 90 Park Avenue, New York, NY 10016 (800) 446-6267.

Winthrop Pharm.—Cont.

Any patient who requires more than three aerosol treatments within a 24-hour period should be under the close supervision of his physician. Further therapy with the bronchodilator aerosol alone is inadvisable when three to five treatments within six to twelve hours produce minimal or no relief.

When compressed oxygen is employed as the aerosol propellant, the percentage of oxygen used should be determined by the patient's individual requirements to avoid depression of respiratory drive.

Drug Interactions: Epinephrine should not be administered concomitantly with ISUPREL, as both drugs are direct cardic stimulants and their combined effects may induce serious arrhythmia. If desired they may, however, be alternated, provided an interval of at least four hours has elapsed.

Carcinogenesis, Mutagenesis, Impairment of Fertility: Long-term chronic toxicity studies in animals have not been done to evaluate isoproterenol in these areas.

Pregnancy Category C: Animal reproduction studies have not been conducted with isoproterenol hydrochloride. It is also not known whether isoproterenol hydrochloride can cause fetal harm when administered to a pregnant woman or can affect reproduction capacity. Isoproterenol hydrochloride should be given to a pregnant woman only if clearly needed.

Nursing Mothers: It is not known whether this drug is excreted in human milk. Because many drugs are excreted in human milk, caution should be exercised when isoproterenol hydrochloride is administered to a nursing woman.

Pediatric Use: In general, the technique of isoproterenol hydrochloride solution in administration to children is similar to that of adults, since children's smaller ventilatory exchange capacity automatically provides proportionally smaller aerosol intake. However, it is generally recommended that the 1:200 solution (rather than the 1:100) be used for an acute attack of bronchospasm, and no more than 0.25 mL of the 1:200 solution should be used for each 10 to 15 minute programmed treatment in chronic bronchospastic disease.

ADVERSE REACTIONS

Serious reactions to ISUPREL are infrequent. The following reactions, however, have been reported:

CNS: Nervousness, headache, dizziness, weakness.
Gastrointestinal: Nausea, vomiting.
Cardiovascular: Tachycardia, palpitations, precordial distress, anginal-type pain.
Other: Flushing of the skin, tremor, and sweating.

The inhalation route is usually accompanied by a minimum of side effects. These untoward reactions disappear quickly and do not as a rule, inconvenience the patient to the extent that the drug must be discontinued. No cumulative effects have been reported.

OVERDOSAGE

Overdosage of ISUPREL may produce signs and symptoms typical of excessive sympathomimetic effects, including tachycardia, palpitations, nervousness, nausea, and vomiting. Excessive use of adrenergic aerosols may result in loss of effectiveness or severe paradoxical airway resistance. Cardiac arrest has been noted in several instances. In all cases of overdose or excessive use of ISUPREL, the drug should be discontinued immediately and vital functions supported until the patient is stabilized. It is not known whether isoproterenol hydrochloride is dialyzable.

The acute oral LD_{50} in mice is 3.850 mg/kg $\pm$ 1,190 mg/kg of pure drug in solution (isoproterenol hydrochloride). In dogs, the toxic dose is 1,000 times the therapeutic dose. Converted to the amount used clinically in man, this would be about 2,500 times the therapeutic dose.

DOSAGE AND ADMINISTRATION

ISUPREL hydrochloride solutions can be administered as an aerosol mist by hand-bulb nebulizer, compressed air or oxygen operated nebulizer, or by intermittent positive pressure breathing (IPPB) devices. The method of delivery, and the treatment regimen employed in the management of the reversible bronchospastic element accompanying bronchial asthma, chronic bronchitis, and chronic obstructive lung diseases, will depend on such factors as the severity of the bronchospasm, patient age, tolerance to the medication, complicating cardiopulmonary conditions, and whether therapy is for an intermittent acute attack of bronchospasm or is part of a programmed treatment regimen for constant bronchospasm.

Acute Bronchial Asthma. Hand-Bulb Nebulizer—Depending on the frequency of treatment and the type of nebulizer used, a volume of solution of ISUPREL, sufficient for not more than one day's treatment, should be placed in the nebulizer using the dropper provided. In time, the patient can learn to adjust the volume required. For adults and children, the 1:200 solution is administered by hand-bulb nebulization in a dosage of 5 to 15 deep inhalations (using an all glass or plastic nebulizer). In adults, the 1:100 solution may be used if

a stronger solution seems to be indicated. The dose is 3 to 7 deep inhalations. If after about 5 to 10 minutes inadequate relief is observed, these doses may be repeated one more time. If the acute attack recurs, treatments may be repeated up to 5 times daily if necessary. (See PRECAUTIONS.)

Bronchospasm in Chronic Obstructive Lung Disease. Hand-Bulb Nebulizer—A solution of 1:200 or 1:100 of ISUPREL may be administered daily at not less than 3 to 4 hour intervals for subacute bronchospastic attacks or as part of a programmed treatment regimen in patients with chronic obstructive lung disease with a reversible bronchospastic component. An adequate dose is usually 5 to 15 deep inhalations, using the 1:200 solution. Some patients with severe attacks of bronchospasm may require 3 to 7 deep inhalations using the 1:100 solution of ISUPREL.

Nebulization by Compressed Air or Oxygen—A method often used in patients with severe chronic obstructive lung disease is to deliver the isoproterenol mist *in more dilute form over a longer period of time.* The purpose is, not so much to increase the dose supplied, as to achieve progressively deeper bronchodilatation and thus insure that the mist achieves maximum penetration of the finer bronchioles. In this method, 0.5 mL of a 1:200 solution of ISUPREL is diluted to 2 mL to 2.5 mL with water or isotonic saline to achieve a use concentration of 1:800 to 1:1000. If desired, 0.25 mL of the 1:100 solution may be similarly diluted to achieve the same use concentration. The diluted solution is placed in a nebulizer (eg, DeVilbiss #640 unit) connected to either a source of compressed air or oxygen. The flow rate is regulated to suit the particular nebulizer so that the diluted solution of ISUPREL will be delivered over approximately 10 to 20 minutes. A treatment may be repeated up to 5 times daily if necessary. Although the total delivered dose of ISUPREL is somewhat higher than with the treatment regimen employing the hand-bulb nebulizer, patients usually tolerate it well because of the greater dilution and longer application-time factors.

Intermittent Positive Pressure Breathing (IPPB)—Diluted solutions of 1:200 or 1:100 of ISUPREL are used in a programmed regimen for the treatment of reversible bronchospasm in patients with chronic obstructive lung disease who require intermittent positive pressure breathing therapy. These devices generally have a small nebulizer, usually of 3 mL to 5 mL capacity, on a patient-operated side arm. The effectiveness of IPPB therapy is greatly enhanced by the simultaneous use of aerosolized bronchodilators. As with compressed air or oxygen operated nebulizers, the usual regimen is to place 0.5 mL of 1:200 solution of ISUPREL diluted to 2 mL to 2.5 mL with water or isotonic saline in the nebulizer cup and follow the IPPB manufacturer's operating instructions. IPPB-bronchodilator treatments are usually administered over 15 to 20 minutes, up to 5 times daily if necessary.

Children's Dosage: In general, the technique of isoproterenol hydrochloride solution in administration to children is similar to that of adults, since children's smaller ventilatory exchange capacity automatically provides proportionally smaller aerosol intake. However, it is generally recommended that the 1:200 solution (rather than the 1:100) be used for an acute attack of bronchospasm, and no more than 0.25 mL of the 1:200 solution should be used for each 10 to 15 minute programmed treatment in chronic bronchospastic disease.

HOW SUPPLIED

Solution 1:100 contains isoproterenol hydrochloride 1% (10 mg/mL).

Solution 1:200 contains isoproterenol hydrochloride 0.5% (5 mg/mL).

Solution 1:100
  bottle of 10 mL   **NDC** 0024-0873-01
Solution 1:200
  bottle of 10 mL   **NDC** 0024-0871-01
  bottle of 60 mL   **NDC** 0024-0871-03

Protect from light. Do not use the solutions if they are pinkish to brownish in color or contain a precipitate. Although solutions of ISUPREL left in nebulizers will remain clear and potent for many days, for sanitary reasons it is recommended that they be changed daily.

Store at controlled room temperature 15°C to 30°C (59°F to 86°F).

Distributed by Winthrop Pharmaceuticals
Division of Sterling Drug Inc.
New York, NY 10016
Manufactured by Sterling Pharmaceuticals Inc.
Barceloneta, Puerto Rico 00617

IW-154-F

ISUPREL® Hydrochloride   ℞
brand of isoproterenol hydrochloride tablets, USP
GLOSSETS®

DESCRIPTION

Each tablet contains 10 mg or 15 mg isoproterenol hydrochloride in a rapidly disintegrating base consisting of lactose,

saccharin sodium, sodium metabisulfite 2 mg per tablet as antioxidant, starch, and talc.

HOW SUPPLIED

ISUPREL GLOSSETS 10 mg, bottle of 50
(NDC 0024-0875-02)
ISUPREL GLOSSETS 15 mg, bottle of 50
(NDC 0024-0877-02)
For complete prescribing information, see package insert or contact Professional Services Department.

IW-121-I

KAYEXALATE®   ℞
brand of sodium polystyrene sulfonate, USP

> **Cation-Exchange Resin**

DESCRIPTION

The drug is a light brown to brown, finely ground, powdered form of sodium polystyrene sulfonate, a cation-exchange resin prepared in the sodium phase with an in vitro exchange capacity of approximately 3.1 mEq (in vivo approximately 1 mEq) of potassium per gram. The sodium content is approximately 100 mg (4.1 mEq) per gram of the drug.

CLINICAL PHARMACOLOGY

As the resin passes along the intestine or is retained in the colon after administration by enema, the sodium ions are partially released and are replaced by potassium ions. For the most part, this action occurs in the large intestine, which excretes potassium ions to a greater degree than does the small intestine. The efficiency of this process is limited and unpredictably variable. It commonly approximates the order of 33 percent but the range is so large that definitive indices of electrolyte balance must be clearly monitored.

INDICATION

KAYEXALATE is indicated for the treatment of hyperkalemia.

WARNINGS

Since effective lowering of serum potassium with KAYEXALATE may take hours to days, treatment with this drug alone may be insufficient to rapidly correct severe hyperkalemia associated with states of rapid tissue breakdown (eg, burns and renal failure) or hyperkalemia so marked as to constitute a medical emergency. Therefore, other definitive measures, including dialysis, should always be considered and may be imperative.

Serious potassium deficiency can occur from therapy with KAYEXALATE. The effect must be carefully controlled by frequent serum potassium determinations within each 24-hour period. Since intracellular potassium deficiency is not always reflected by serum potassium levels, the level at which treatment with KAYEXALATE should be discontinued must be determined individually for each patient. Important aids in making this determination are the patient's clinical condition and electrocardiogram. Early clinical signs of severe hypokalemia include a pattern of irritable confusion and delayed thought processes. Electrocardiographically, severe hypokalemia is often associated with a lengthened Q-T interval, widening, flattening, or inversion of the T wave, and prominent U waves. Also, cardiac arrhythmias may occur, such as premature atrial, nodal, and ventricular contractions, and supraventricular and ventricular tachycardias. The toxic effects of digitalis are likely to be exaggerated. Marked hypokalemia can also be manifested by severe muscle weakness, at times extending into frank paralysis. Like all cation-exchange resins, KAYEXALATE is not totally selective (for potassium) in its actions, and small amounts of other cations such as magnesium and calcium can also be lost during treatment. Accordingly, patients receiving KAYEXALATE should be monitored for all applicable electrolyte disturbances. Systemic alkalosis has been reported after cation-exchange resins were administered orally in combination with nonabsorbable cation-donating antacids and laxatives such as magnesium hydroxide and aluminum carbonate. Magnesium hydroxide should not be administered with KAYEXALATE. One case of grand mal seizure has been reported in a patient with chronic hypocalcemia of renal failure who was given KAYEXALATE with magnesium hydroxide as laxative. Also, the simultaneous oral administration of KAYEXALATE with nonabsorbable cation-donating antacids and laxatives may reduce the resin's potassium exchange capability.

PRECAUTIONS

Caution is advised when KAYEXALATE is administered to patients who cannot tolerate even a small increase in sodium loads (ie, severe congestive heart failure, severe hypertension, or marked edema). In such instances compensatory restriction of sodium intake from other sources may be indicated.

If constipation occurs, patients should be treated with sorbitol (from 10 mL to 20 mL of 70 percent syrup every two hours or as needed to produce one or two watery stools daily), a measure which also reduces any tendency to fecal impaction.

ADVERSE REACTIONS

KAYEXALATE may cause some degree of gastric irritation. Anorexia, nausea, vomiting, and constipation may occur especially if high doses are given. Also, hypokalemia, hypocalcemia, and significant sodium retention may occur. Occasionally diarrhea develops. Large doses in elderly individuals may cause fecal impaction (see PRECAUTIONS). This effect may be obviated through usage of the resin in enemas as described under DOSAGE AND ADMINISTRATION. Intestinal obstruction due to concretions of aluminum hydroxide, when used in combination with KAYEXALATE, has been reported.

DOSAGE AND ADMINISTRATION

Suspension of this drug should be freshly prepared and not stored beyond 24 hours.

The average daily adult dose of the resin is 15 g to 60 g. This is best provided by administering 15 g (approximately 4 *level* teaspoons) of KAYEXALATE one to four times daily. One gram of KAYEXALATE contains 4.1 mEq of sodium; one level teaspoon contains approximately 3.5 g of KAYEXALATE and 15 mEq of sodium. (A heaping teaspoon may contain as much as 10 g to 12 g of KAYEXALATE, brand of sodium polystyrene sulfonate.) Since the in vivo efficiency of sodium-potassium exchange resins is approximately 33 percent, about one third of the resin's actual sodium content is being delivered to the body.

In smaller children and infants lower doses should be employed by using as a guide a rate of 1 mEq of potassium per gram of resin as the basis for calculation.

Each dose should be given as a suspension in a small quantity of water or, for greater palatability, in syrup. The amount of fluid usually ranges from 20 mL to 100 mL, depending on the dose, or may be simply determined by allowing 3 mL to 4 mL per gram of resin. Sorbitol may be administered in order to combat constipation.

The resin may be introduced into the stomach through a plastic tube and, if desired, mixed with a diet appropriate for a patient in renal failure.

The resin may also be given, although with less effective results, in an enema consisting (for adults) of 30 g to 50 g every six hours. Each dose is administered as a warm emulsion (at body temperature) in 100 mL of aqueous vehicle, such as sorbitol. The emulsion should be agitated gently during administration. The enema should be retained as long as possible and followed by a cleansing enema.

After an initial cleansing enema, a soft, large size (French 28) rubber tube is inserted into the rectum for a distance of about 20 cm, with the tip well into the sigmoid colon, and taped in place. The resin is then suspended in the appropriate amount of aqueous vehicle at body temperature and introduced by gravity, while the particles are kept in suspension by stirring. The suspension is flushed with 50 mL or 100 mL of fluid, following which the tube is clamped and left in place. If back leakage occurs, the hips are elevated on pillows or a knee-chest position is taken temporarily. A somewhat thicker suspension may be used, but care should be taken that no paste is formed, because the latter has a greatly reduced exchange surface and will be particularly ineffective if deposited in the rectal ampulla. The suspension is kept in the sigmoid colon for several hours, if possible. Then, the colon is irrigated with nonsodium containing solution at body temperature in order to remove the resin. Two quarts of flushing solution may be necessary. The returns are drained constantly through a Y tube connection.

The intensity and duration of therapy depend upon the severity and resistance of hyperkalemia.

KAYEXALATE, brand of sodium polystyrene sulfonate, should not be heated for to do so may alter the exchange properties of the resin.

HOW SUPPLIED

Jar of 1 pound (453.6 g)
NDC 0024-1075-01

KW 2-M

LEVOPHED® Bitartrate   ℞
brand of norepinephrine bitartrate injection, USP

DESCRIPTION

Levarterenol (sometimes referred to as *l-arterenol* or as *l-norepinephrine*) is a primary amine which differs from epinephrine by the absence of a methyl group on the nitrogen atom.

LEVOPHED is supplied in sterile aqueous solution in the form of the bitartrate. Each 1 mL of norepinephrine bitartrate solution contains 1 mg of norepinephrine bitartrate base, sodium chloride for isotonicity, and not more than 2 mg of sodium metabisulfite as preservative. The air in the ampuls has been displaced by nitrogen gas.

CLINICAL PHARMACOLOGY

LEVOPHED functions as a powerful peripheral vasoconstrictor (alpha-adrenergic action) and as a potent inotropic stimulator of the heart and dilator of coronary arteries (beta-adrenergic action). Both of these actions result in an increase in systemic blood pressure and coronary artery blood flow. Cardiac output will vary reflexly in response to systemic hypertension but is usually increased in hypotensive man when the blood pressure is raised to an optimal level. In myocardial infarction accompanied by hypotension, LEVOPHED usually increases aortic blood pressure, coronary artery blood flow, and myocardial oxygenation, thereby helping to limit the area of myocardial ischemia and infarction. Venous return is increased and the heart tends to resume a more normal rate and rhythm than in the hypotensive state.

In hypotension that persists after correction of blood volume deficits, LEVOPHED helps raise the blood pressure to an optimal level and establish a more adequate circulation.

INDICATIONS AND USAGE

For the restoration of blood pressure in controlling certain acute hypotensive states (eg, pheochromocytomectomy, sympathectomy, poliomyelitis, spinal anesthesia, myocardial infarction, septicemia, blood transfusion, and drug reactions).

As an adjunct in the treatment of cardiac arrest and profound hypotension.

CONTRAINDICATIONS

LEVOPHED should not be given to patients who are hypotensive from blood volume deficits except as an emergency measure to maintain coronary and cerebral artery perfusion until blood volume replacement therapy can be completed. If LEVOPHED is continuously administered to maintain blood pressure in the absence of blood volume replacement, the following may occur: severe peripheral and visceral vasoconstriction, decreased renal perfusion and urine output, poor systemic blood flow despite "normal" blood pressure, tissue hypoxia, and lactate acidosis.

LEVOPHED should also not be given to patients with mesenteric or peripheral vascular thrombosis (because of the risk of increasing ischemia and extending the area of infarction) unless, in the opinion of the attending physician, the administration of LEVOPHED is necessary as a life-saving procedure.

Cyclopropane and halothane anesthetics increase cardiac autonomic irritability and therefore seem to sensitize the myocardium to the action of intravenously administered epinephrine or levarterenol. Hence, the use of LEVOPHED during cyclopropane and halothane anesthesia is generally considered contraindicated because of the risk of producing ventricular tachycardia or fibrillation. The same type of cardiac arrhythmias may result from the use of LEVOPHED in patients with profound hypoxia or hypercarbia.

WARNING

LEVOPHED should be used with extreme caution in patients receiving monoamine oxidase (MAO) inhibitors or antidepressants of the triptyline or imipramine types, because severe, prolonged hypertension may result.

Contains sodium metabisulfite, a sulfite that may cause allergic-type reactions including anaphylactic symptoms and life-threatening or less severe asthmatic episodes in certain susceptible people. The overall prevalence of sulfite sensitivity in the general population is unknown and probably low. Sulfite sensitivity is seen more frequently in asthmatic than in nonasthmatic people.

PRECAUTIONS

Avoid Hypertension: Because of the potency of LEVOPHED and because of varying response to pressor substances, the possibility always exists that dangerously high blood pressure may be produced with overdoses of this pressor agent. It is desirable, therefore, to record the blood pressure every two minutes from the time administration is started until the desired blood pressure is obtained, then every five minutes if administration is to be continued. The rate of flow must be watched constantly, and the patient should never be left unattended while receiving LEVOPHED. Headache may be a symptom of hypertension due to overdosage.

Site of Infusion: Whenever possible, LEVOPHED should be given into a large vein, particularly an antecubital vein because, when administered into this vein, the risk of necrosis of the overlying skin from prolonged vasoconstriction is apparently very slight. Some authors have indicated that the femoral vein is also an acceptable route of administration. A catheter tie-in technique should be avoided, if possible, since the obstruction to blood flow around the tubing may cause stasis and increased local concentration of the drug. Occlusive vascular diseases (for example, atherosclerosis, arteriosclerosis, diabetic endarteritis, Buerger's disease) are more likely to occur in the lower than in the upper extremity. Therefore, one should avoid the veins of the leg in elderly patients or in those suffering from such disorders. Gangrene has been reported in a lower extremity when LEVOPHED was given in an ankle vein.

Extravasation: The infusion site should be checked frequently for free flow. Care should be taken to avoid extravasation of LEVOPHED (norepinephrine) into the tissues, as local necrosis might ensue due to the vasoconstrictive action of the drug. Blanching along the course of the infused vein, sometimes without obvious extravasation, has been attributed to vasa vasorum constriction with increased permeability of the vein wall, permitting some leakage. This also may progress on rare occasions to superficial slough, particularly during infusion into leg veins in elderly patients or in those suffering from obliterative vascular disease. Hence, if blanching occurs, consideration should be given to the advisability of changing the infusion site at intervals to allow the effects of local vasoconstriction to subside.

> **IMPORTANT—Antidote for Extravasation Ischemia:** To prevent sloughing and necrosis in areas in which extravasation has taken place, the area should be infiltrated as soon as possible with 10 mL to 15 mL of saline solution containing from 5 mg to 10 mg of **Regitine® (brand of phentolamine)**, an adrenergic blocking agent. A syringe with a fine hypodermic needle is used, and the solution is infiltrated liberally throughout the area, which is easily identified by its cold, hard, and pallid appearance. Sympathetic blockade with phentolamine causes immediate and conspicuous local hyperemic changes if the area is infiltrated within 12 hours. Therefore, phentolamine should be given as soon as possible after the extravasation is noted.

Some investigators add phentolamine (5 mg to 10 mg) directly to the infusion flask because it is believed that the drug used in this manner is an effective antidote against sloughing should extravasation occur, whereas the systemic vasopressor activity of the LEVOPHED is not impaired.

Two investigators stated that, in the treatment of patients with severe hypotension following *myocardial infarction*, thrombosis in the infused vein and perivenous reactions and necrosis may usually be prevented if 10 mg of heparin are added to each 500 mL of infusion fluid (5 percent dextrose) containing LEVOPHED.

Sympathetic nerve block has also been suggested.

ADVERSE REACTIONS

When used as directed, LEVOPHED is more certain in action and better tolerated systemically than other pressor amines. Its therapeutic index is four times that of epinephrine. Bradycardia sometimes occurs, probably as a reflex result of a rise in blood pressure. Headache may indicate overdosage and extreme hypertension.

Overdosage with LEVOPHED may also result in severe hypertension, reflex bradycardia, marked increase in peripheral resistance, and decreased cardiac output.

Prolonged administration of any potent vasopressor may result in plasma volume depletion which should be continuously corrected by appropriate fluid and electrolyte replacement therapy. If plasma volumes are not corrected, hypotension may recur when LEVOPHED is discontinued, or blood pressure may be maintained at the risk of severe peripheral vasoconstriction with diminution in blood flow and tissue perfusion.

DOSAGE AND ADMINISTRATION

Restoration of Blood Pressure in Acute Hypotensive States

Blood volume depletion should always be corrected as fully as possible before any vasopressor is administered. When, as an emergency measure, intra-aortic pressures must be maintained to prevent cerebral or coronary artery ischemia, LEVOPHED bitartrate, brand of norepinephrine bitartrate injection, can be administered before and concurrently with blood volume replacement.

Diluent: Norepinephrine bitartrate solution should be administered in 5 percent dextrose solution in distilled water or 5 percent dextrose in saline solution. These fluids containing dextrose are protection against significant loss of potency due to oxidation. Administration in saline solution alone is not recommended. Whole blood or plasma, if indicated to increase blood volume, should be administered separately (for example, by use of a Y-tube and individual flasks if given simultaneously).

Average Dosage: Add 4 mL of norepinephrine bitartrate solution to 1000 mL of 5 percent dextrose solution. Each 1 mL of this dilution contains 4 µg of norepinephrine bitartrate base. Give this dilution intravenously. Insert a plastic intravenous catheter through a suitable bore needle well advanced centrally into the vein and securely fixed with

Continued on next page

This product information was prepared in August, 1989. On these and other products of Winthrop Pharmaceuticals, detailed information may be obtained on a current basis by direct inquiry to the Professional Services Department, 90 Park Avenue, New York, NY 10016 (800) 446-6267.

Winthrop Pharm.—Cont.

adhesive tape, avoiding, if possible, a catheter tie-in technique as this promotes stasis. A drip bulb is necessary to permit an accurate estimation of the rate of flow in drops per minute. After observing the response to an initial dose of 2 mL to 3 mL (from 8 μg to 12 μg of base) per minute, adjust the rate of flow to establish and maintain a low normal blood pressure (usually 80 mm Hg to 100 mm Hg systolic) sufficient to maintain the circulation to vital organs. In previously hypertensive patients, it is recommended that the blood pressure should be raised no higher than 40 mm Hg below the preexisting systolic pressure. The average maintenance dose ranges from 0.5 mL to 1 mL per minute (from 2 μg to 4 μg of base).

High Dosage: Great individual variation occurs in the dose required to attain and maintain an adequate blood pressure. In all cases, dosage of LEVOPHED should be titrated according to the response of the patient. Occasionally much larger or even enormous daily doses (as high as 68 mg base or 17 ampuls) may be necessary if the patient remains hypotensive, but occult blood volume depletion should always be suspected and corrected when present. Central venous pressure monitoring is usually helpful in detecting and treating this situation.

Fluid Intake: The degree of dilution depends on clinical fluid volume requirements. If large volumes of fluid (dextrose) are needed at a flow rate that would involve an excessive dose of the pressor agent per unit of time, a more dilute solution than 4 μg per mL should be used. On the other hand, when large volumes of fluid are clinically undesirable, a concentration greater than 4 μg per mL may be used.

Duration of Therapy: The infusion should be continued until adequate blood pressure and tissue perfusion are maintained without therapy. Norepinephrine bitartrate infusion should be reduced gradually, avoiding abrupt withdrawal. In some of the reported cases of vascular collapse due to acute myocardial infarction, treatment was required for up to six days.

Adjunctive Treatment in Cardiac Arrest

LEVOPHED is usually administered intravenously during cardiac resuscitation to restore and maintain an adequate blood pressure after an effective heartbeat and ventilation have been established by other means. [The powerful beta-adrenergic stimulating action of LEVOPHED is also thought to increase the strength and effectiveness of systolic contractions once they occur.]

Average Dosage: To maintain systemic blood pressure during the management of cardiac arrest, LEVOPHED bitartrate, brand of norepinephrine bitartrate injection, is used in the same manner as described under Restoration of Blood Pressure in Acute Hypotensive States.

HOW SUPPLIED

Ampuls of 4 mL containing 4 mg norepinephrine bitartrate base, box of 10 (NDC 0024-1123-02)
Store at room temperature.

Regitine, trademark, CIBA Pharmaceutical Company

LW-34-S

LOTUSATE® Caplets®   ℂⅢ ℞
brand of talbutal tablets, USP

DESCRIPTION

Each caplet contains 120 mg of 5-Allyl-5-*sec*-butylbarbituric acid, is white in color, and bears identifying number L 53.
Inactive Ingredients: Lactose, Magnesium Stearate, Starch, Talc.

HOW SUPPLIED

CAPLETS of 120 mg, (white) bottle of 100
(NDC 0024-1150-01)
For complete prescribing information, see package insert or contact Professional Services Department.

LW-87-S

MARCAINE® HYDROCHLORIDE   ℞
brand of bupivacaine hydrochloride injection, USP

MARCAINE® HYDROCHLORIDE   ℞
WITH EPINEPHRINE 1:200,000 (AS BITARTRATE)
brand of bupivacaine and epinephrine injection, USP

DESCRIPTION

Bupivacaine hydrochloride is 2-Piperidinecarboxamide, 1-butyl-*N*-(2,6-dimethylphenyl)-, monohydrochloride, monohydrate, a white crystalline powder that is freely soluble in 95 percent ethanol, soluble in water, and slightly soluble in chloroform or acetone.
Epinephrine is (-)-3, 4-Dihydroxy-α-[(methylamino)methyl] benzyl alcohol.
MARCAINE hydrochloride is available in sterile isotonic solutions with and without epinephrine (as bitartrate)

1:200,000 for injection via local infiltration, peripheral nerve block, and caudal and lumbar epidural blocks. Solutions of MARCAINE may be autoclaved if they do not contain epinephrine.

Bupivacaine is related chemically and pharmacologically to the aminoacyl local anesthetics. It is a homologue of mepivacaine and is chemically related to lidocaine. All three of these anesthetics contain an amide linkage between the aromatic nucleus and the amino, or piperidine group. They differ in this respect from the procaine-type local anesthetics, which have an ester linkage.

MARCAINE hydrochloride—Sterile isotonic solutions containing sodium chloride. In multiple-dose vials, each 1 mL also contains 1 mg methylparaben as antiseptic preservative. The pH of these solutions is adjusted to between 4 and 6.5 with sodium hydroxide or hydrochloric acid.

MARCAINE hydrochloride with epinephrine 1:200,000 (as bitartrate)—Sterile isotonic solutions containing sodium chloride. Each 1 mL contains bupivacaine hydrochloride and 0.0091 mg epinephrine bitartrate, with 0.5 mg sodium metabisulfite, 0.001 mL monothioglycerol, and 2 mg ascorbic acid as antioxidants, 0.0017 mL 60% sodium lactate buffer, and 0.1 mg edetate calcium disodium as stabilizer. In multiple-dose vials, each 1 mL also contains 1 mg methylparaben as antiseptic preservative. The pH of these solutions is adjusted to between 3.4 and 4.5 with sodium hydroxide or hydrochloric acid. The specific gravity of MARCAINE 0.5% with epinephrine 1:200,000 (as bitartrate) at 25°C is 1.008 and at 37°C is 1.008.

CLINICAL PHARMACOLOGY

Local anesthetics block the generation and the conduction of nerve impulses, presumably by increasing the threshold for electrical excitation in the nerve, by slowing the propagation of the nerve impulse, and by reducing the rate of rise of the action potential. In general, the progression of anesthesia is related to the diameter, myelination, and conduction velocity of affected nerve fibers. Clinically, the order of loss of nerve function is as follows: (1) pain, (2) temperature, (3) touch, (4) proprioception, and (5) skeletal muscle tone.

Systemic absorption of local anesthetics produces effects on the cardiovascular and central nervous systems (CNS). At blood concentrations achieved with normal therapeutic doses, changes in cardiac conduction, excitability, refractoriness, contractility, and peripheral vascular resistance are minimal. However, toxic blood concentrations depress cardiac conduction and excitability, which may lead to atrioventricular block, ventricular arrhythmias, and cardiac arrest, sometimes resulting in fatalities. In addition, myocardial contractility is depressed and peripheral vasodilation occurs, leading to decreased cardiac output and arterial blood pressure. Recent clinical reports and animal research suggest that these cardiovascular changes are more likely to occur after unintended intravascular injection of bupivacaine. Therefore, incremental dosing is necessary.

Following systemic absorption, local anesthetics can produce central nervous system stimulation, depression, or both. Apparent central stimulation is manifested as restlessness, tremors and shivering progressing to convulsions, followed by depression and coma progressing ultimately to respiratory arrest. However, the local anesthetics have a primary depressant effect on the medulla and on higher centers. The depressed stage may occur without a prior excited state.

Pharmacokinetics: The rate of systemic absorption of local anesthetics is dependent upon the total dose and concentration of drug administered, the route of administration, the vascularity of the administration site, and the presence or absence of epinephrine in the anesthetic solution. A dilute concentration of epinephrine (1:200,000 or 5 μg/mL) usually reduces the rate of absorption and peak plasma concentration of MARCAINE, permitting the use of moderately larger total doses and sometimes prolonging the duration of action. The onset of action with MARCAINE is rapid and anesthesia is long lasting. The duration of anesthesia is significantly longer with MARCAINE than with any other commonly used local anesthetic. It has also been noted that there is a period of analgesia that persists after the return of sensation, during which time the need for strong analgesics is reduced.

The onset of action following dental injections is usually 2 to 10 minutes and anesthesia may last two or three times longer than lidocaine and mepivacaine for dental use, in many patients up to 7 hours. The duration of anesthetic effect is prolonged by the addition of epinephrine 1:200,000.

Local anesthetics are bound to plasma proteins in varying degrees. Generally, the lower the plasma concentration of drug the higher the percentage of drug bound to plasma proteins.

Local anesthetics appear to cross the placenta by passive diffusion. The rate and degree of diffusion is governed by (1) the degree of plasma protein binding, (2) the degree of ionization, and (3) the degree of lipid solubility. Fetal/maternal ratios of local anesthetics appear to be inversely related to the degree of plasma protein binding, because only the free, unbound drug is available for placental transfer. MARCAINE with a high protein binding capacity (95%) has

a low fetal/maternal ratio (0.2 to 0.4). The extent of placental transfer is also determined by the degree of ionization and lipid solubility of the drug. Lipid soluble, nonionized drugs readily enter the fetal blood from the maternal circulation. Depending upon the route of administration, local anesthetics are distributed to some extent to all body tissues, with high concentrations found in highly perfused organs such as the liver, lungs, heart, and brain.

Pharmacokinetic studies on the plasma profile of MARCAINE after direct intravenous injection suggest a three-compartment open model. The first compartment is represented by the rapid intravascular distribution of the drug. The second compartment represents the equilibration of the drug throughout the highly perfused organs such as the brain, myocardium, lungs, kidneys, and liver. The third compartment represents an equilibration of the drug with poorly perfused tissues, such as muscle and fat. The elimination of drug from tissue distribution depends largely upon the ability of binding sites in the circulation to carry it to the liver where it is metabolized.

After injection of MARCAINE for caudal, epidural, or peripheral nerve block in man, peak levels of bupivacaine in the blood are reached in 30 to 45 minutes, followed by a decline to insignificant levels during the next three to six hours.

Various pharmacokinetic parameters of the local anesthetics can be significantly altered by the presence of hepatic or renal disease, addition of epinephrine, factors affecting urinary pH, renal blood flow, the route of drug administration, and the age of the patient. The half-life of MARCAINE (bupivacaine) in adults is 2.7 hours and in neonates 8.1 hours.

Amide-type local anesthetics such as MARCAINE are metabolized primarily in the liver via conjugation with glucuronic acid. Patients with hepatic disease, especially those with severe hepatic disease, may be more susceptible to the potential toxicities of the amide-type local anesthetics. Pipecoloxylidine is the major metabolite of MARCAINE. The kidney is the main excretory organ for most local anesthetics and their metabolites. Urinary excretion is affected by urinary perfusion and factors affecting urinary pH. Only 6% of bupivacaine is excreted unchanged in the urine.

When administered in recommended doses and concentrations, MARCAINE does not ordinarily produce irritation or tissue damage and does not cause methemoglobinemia.

INDICATIONS AND USAGE

MARCAINE is indicated for the production of local or regional anesthesia or analgesia for surgery, dental and oral surgery procedures, diagnostic and therapeutic procedures, and for obstetrical procedures. Only the 0.25% and 0.5% concentrations are indicated for obstetrical anesthesia. (See WARNINGS.)

Experience with nonobstetrical surgical procedures in pregnant patients is not sufficient to recommend use of 0.75% concentration of MARCAINE in these patients.

MARCAINE is not recommended for intravenous regional anesthesia (Bier Block). See WARNINGS.

The routes of administration and indicated MARCAINE concentrations are:

• local infiltration	0.25%
• peripheral nerve block	0.25% and 0.5%
• retrobulbar block	0.75%
• sympathetic block	0.25%
• lumbar epidural	0.25%, 0.5%, and 0.75% (0.75% not for obstetrical anesthesia)
• caudal	0.25% and 0.5%
• epidural test dose	0.5% with epinephrine 1:200,000
• dental blocks	0.5% with epinephrine 1:200,000

(See **DOSAGE AND ADMINISTRATION** for additional information.)

Standard textbooks should be consulted to determine the accepted procedures and techniques for the administration of MARCAINE.

CONTRAINDICATIONS

MARCAINE is contraindicated in obstetrical paracervical block anesthesia. Its use in this technique has resulted in fetal bradycardia and death.

MARCAINE (bupivacaine) is contraindicated in patients with a known hypersensitivity to it or to any local anesthetic agent of the amide-type or to other components of MARCAINE solutions.

WARNINGS

THE 0.75% CONCENTRATION OF MARCAINE IS NOT RECOMMENDED FOR OBSTETRICAL ANESTHESIA. THERE HAVE BEEN REPORTS OF CARDIAC ARREST WITH DIFFICULT RESUSCITATION OR DEATH DURING USE OF MARCAINE FOR EPIDURAL ANESTHESIA IN OBSTETRICAL PATIENTS. IN MOST CASES, THIS HAS FOLLOWED USE OF THE 0.75% CONCEN-

TRATION. RESUSCITATION HAS BEEN DIFFICULT OR IMPOSSIBLE DESPITE APPARENTLY ADEQUATE PREPARATION AND APPROPRIATE MANAGEMENT. CARDIAC ARREST HAS OCCURRED AFTER CONVULSIONS RESULTING FROM SYSTEMIC TOXICITY, PRESUMABLY FOLLOWING UNINTENTIONAL INTRAVASCULAR INJECTION. THE 0.75% CONCENTRATION SHOULD BE RESERVED FOR SURGICAL PROCEDURES WHERE A HIGH DEGREE OF MUSCLE RELAXATION AND PROLONGED EFFECT ARE NECESSARY.

LOCAL ANESTHETICS SHOULD ONLY BE EMPLOYED BY CLINICIANS WHO ARE WELL VERSED IN DIAGNOSIS AND MANAGEMENT OF DOSE-RELATED TOXICITY AND OTHER ACUTE EMERGENCIES WHICH MIGHT ARISE FROM THE BLOCK TO BE EMPLOYED, AND THEN ONLY AFTER INSURING THE *IMMEDIATE* AVAILABILITY OF OXYGEN, OTHER RESUSCITATIVE DRUGS, CARDIOPULMONARY RESUSCITATIVE EQUIPMENT, AND THE PERSONNEL RESOURCES NEEDED FOR PROPER MANAGEMENT OF TOXIC REACTIONS AND RELATED EMERGENCIES. (See also ADVERSE REACTIONS, PRECAUTIONS, and OVERDOSAGE.) DELAY IN PROPER MANAGEMENT OF DOSE-RELATED TOXICITY, UNDERVENTILATION FROM ANY CAUSE, AND/OR ALTERED SENSITIVITY MAY LEAD TO THE DEVELOPMENT OF ACIDOSIS, CARDIAC ARREST AND, POSSIBLY, DEATH.

Local anesthetic solutions containing antimicrobial preservatives, ie, those supplied in multiple-dose vials, should not be used for epidural or caudal anesthesia because safety has not been established with regard to intrathecal injection, either intentionally or unintentionally, of such preservatives.

It is essential that aspiration for blood or cerebrospinal fluid (where applicable) be done prior to injecting any local anesthetic, both the original dose and all subsequent doses, to avoid intravascular or subarachnoid injection. However, a negative aspiration does *not* ensure against an intravascular or subarachnoid injection.

MARCAINE with epinephrine 1:200,000 or other vasopressors should not be used concomitantly with ergot-type oxytocic drugs, because a severe persistent hypertension may occur. Likewise, solutions of MARCAINE containing a vasoconstrictor, such as epinephrine, should be used with extreme caution in patients receiving monoamine oxidase inhibitors (MAOI) or antidepressants of the triptyline or imipramine types, because severe prolonged hypertension may result.

Until further experience is gained in children younger than 12 years, administration of MARCAINE in this age group is not recommended.

Mixing or the prior or intercurrent use of any other local anesthetic with MARCAINE cannot be recommended because of insufficient data on the clinical use of such mixtures.

There have been reports of cardiac arrest and death during the use of MARCAINE for intravenous regional anesthesia (Bier Block). Information on safe dosages and techniques of administration of MARCAINE in this procedure is lacking. Therefore, MARCAINE is not recommended for use in this technique.

MARCAINE hydrochloride with epinephrine 1:200,000 contains sodium metabisulfite, a sulfite that may cause allergic-type reactions including anaphylactic symptoms and life-threatening or less severe asthmatic episodes in certain susceptible people. The overall prevalence of sulfite sensitivity in the general population is unknown and probably low. Sulfite sensitivity is seen more frequently in asthmatic than in nonasthmatic people. Single-dose ampuls and single-dose vials of *MARCAINE hydrochloride* without epinephrine do not contain sodium metabisulfite.

PRECAUTIONS

General: The safety and effectiveness of local anesthetics depend on proper dosage, correct technique, adequate precautions, and readiness for emergencies. Resuscitative equipment, oxygen, and other resuscitative drugs should be available for immediate use. (See WARNINGS, ADVERSE REACTIONS, and OVERDOSAGE.) During major regional nerve blocks, the patient should have IV fluids running via an indwelling catheter to assure a functioning intravenous pathway. The lowest dosage of local anesthetic that results in effective anesthesia should be used to avoid high plasma levels and serious adverse effects. The rapid injection of a large volume of local anesthetic solution should be avoided and fractional (incremental) doses should be used when feasible.

Epidural Anesthesia: During epidural administration of MARCAINE, 0.5% and 0.75% solutions should be administered in incremental doses of 3 mL to 5 mL with sufficient time between doses to detect toxic manifestations of unintentional intravascular or intrathecal injection. Injections should be made slowly, with frequent aspirations before and during the injection to avoid intravascular injection. Syringe aspirations should also be performed before and during

each supplemental injection in continuous (intermittent) catheter techniques. An intravascular injection is still possible even if aspirations for blood are negative.

During the administration of epidural anesthesia, it is recommended that a test dose be administered initially and the effects monitored before the full dose is given. When using a "continuous" catheter technique, test doses should be given prior to both the original and all reinforcing doses, because plastic tubing in the epidural space can migrate into a blood vessel or through the dura. When clinical conditions permit, the test dose should contain epinephrine (10 μg to 15 μg has been suggested) to serve as a warning of unintended intravascular injection. If injected into a blood vessel, this amount of epinephrine is likely to produce a transient "epinephrine response" within 45 seconds, consisting of an increase in heart rate and/or systolic blood pressure, circumoral pallor, palpitations, and nervousness in the unsedated patient. The sedated patient may exhibit only a pulse rate increase of 20 or more beats per minute for 15 or more seconds. Therefore, following the test dose, the heart rate should be monitored for a heart rate increase. Patients on beta-blockers may not manifest changes in heart rate, but blood pressure monitoring can detect a transient rise in systolic blood pressure. The test dose should also contain 10 mg to 15 mg of MARCAINE or an equivalent amount of another local anesthetic to detect an unintended intrathecal administration. This will be evidenced within a few minutes by signs of spinal block (eg, decreased sensation of the buttocks, paresis of the legs, or, in the sedated patient, absent knee jerk). The Test Dose formulation of MARCAINE contains 15 mg of bupivacaine and 15 μg of epinephrine in a volume of 3 mL. An intravascular or subarachnoid injection is still possible even if results of the test dose are negative. The test dose itself may produce a systemic toxic reaction, high spinal or epinephrine-induced cardiovascular effects.

Injection of repeated doses of local anesthetics may cause significant increases in plasma levels with each repeated dose due to slow accumulation of the drug or its metabolites, or to slow metabolic degradation. Tolerance to elevated blood levels varies with the status of the patient. Debilitated, elderly patients and acutely ill patients should be given reduced doses commensurate with their age and physical status. Local anesthetics should also be used with caution in patients with hypotension or heartblock.

Careful and constant monitoring of cardiovascular and respiratory (adequacy of ventilation) vital signs and the patient's state of consciousness should be performed after each local anesthetic injection. It should be kept in mind at such times that restlessness, anxiety, incoherent speech, lightheadedness, numbness and tingling of the mouth and lips, metallic taste, tinnitus, dizziness, blurred vision, tremors, twitching, depression, or drowsiness may be early warning signs of central nervous system toxicity.

Local anesthetic solutions containing a vasoconstrictor should be used cautiously and in carefully restricted quantities in areas of the body supplied by end arteries or having otherwise compromised blood supply such as digits, nose, external ear, or penis. Patients with hypertensive vascular disease may exhibit exaggerated vasoconstrictor response. Ischemic injury or necrosis may result.

Because amide-type local anesthetics such as MARCAINE (bupivacaine) are metabolized by the liver, these drugs, especially repeat doses, should be used cautiously in patients with hepatic disease. Patients with severe hepatic disease, because of their inability to metabolize local anesthetics normally, are at a greater risk of developing toxic plasma concentrations. Local anesthetics should also be used with caution in patients with impaired cardiovascular function because they may be less able to compensate for functional changes associated with the prolongation of AV conduction produced by these drugs.

Serious dose-related cardiac arrhythmias may occur if preparations containing a vasoconstrictor such as epinephrine are employed in patients during or following the administration of potent inhalation anesthetics. In deciding whether to use these products concurrently in the same patient, the combined action of both agents upon the myocardium, the concentration and volume of vasoconstrictor used, and the time since injection, when applicable, should be taken into account.

Many drugs used during the conduct of anesthesia are considered potential triggering agents for familial malignant hyperthermia. Because it is not known whether amide-type local anesthetics may trigger this reaction and because the need for supplemental general anesthesia cannot be predicted in advance, it is suggested that a standard protocol for management should be available. Early unexplained signs of tachycardia, tachypnea, labile blood pressure, and metabolic acidosis may precede temperature elevation. Successful outcome is dependent on early diagnosis, prompt discontinuance of the suspect triggering agent(s) and prompt institution of treatment, including oxygen therapy, indicated supportive measures and dantrolene. (Consult dantrolene sodium intravenous package insert before using.)

Use in Head and Neck Area: Small doses of local anesthetics injected into the head and neck area, including retrobulbar,

dental, and stellate ganglion blocks, may produce adverse reactions similar to systemic toxicity seen with unintentional intravascular injections of larger doses. The injection procedures require the utmost care. Confusion, convulsions, respiratory depression, and/or respiratory arrest, and cardiovascular stimulation or depression have been reported. These reactions may be due to intra-arterial injection of the local anesthetic with retrograde flow to the cerebral circulation. They may also be due to puncture of the dural sheath of the optic nerve during retrobulbar block with diffusion of any local anesthetic along the subdural space to the midbrain. Patients receiving these blocks should have their circulation and respiration monitored and be constantly observed. Resuscitative equipment and personnel for treating adverse reactions should be immediately available. Dosage recommendations should not be exceeded. (See DOSAGE AND ADMINISTRATION.)

Use in Ophthalmic Surgery: Clinicians who perform retrobulbar blocks should be aware that there have been reports of respiratory arrest following local anesthetic injection. Prior to retrobulbar block, as with all other regional procedures, the immediate availability of equipment, drugs, and personnel to manage respiratory arrest or depression, convulsions, and cardiac stimulation or depression should be assured (see also WARNINGS and *Use in Head and Neck Area,* above). As with other anesthetic procedures, patients should be constantly monitored following ophthalmic blocks for signs of these adverse reactions, which may occur following relatively low total doses. A concentration of 0.75% bupivacaine is indicated for retrobulbar block; however, this concentration is not indicated for any other peripheral nerve block, including the facial nerve, and not indicated for local infiltration, including the conjunctiva (see INDICATIONS and PRECAUTIONS, *General*). Mixing MARCAINE with other local anesthetics is not recommended because of insufficient data on the clinical use of such mixtures.

When MARCAINE 0.75% is used for retrobulbar block, complete corneal anesthesia usually precedes onset of clinically acceptable external ocular muscle akinesia. Therefore, presence of akinesia rather than anesthesia alone should determine readiness of the patient for surgery.

Use in Dentistry: Because of the long duration of anesthesia, when MARCAINE 0.5% with epinephrine is used for dental injections, patients should be cautioned about the possibility of inadvertent trauma to tongue, lips, and buccal mucosa and advised not to chew solid foods or test the anesthetized area by biting or probing.

Information for Patients: When appropriate, patients should be informed in advance that they may experience temporary loss of sensation and motor activity, usually in the lower half of the body, following proper administration of caudal or epidural anesthesia. Also, when appropriate, the physician should discuss other information including adverse reactions in the package insert of MARCAINE. Patients receiving dental injections of MARCAINE (bupivacaine) should be cautioned not to chew solid foods or test the anesthetized area by biting or probing until anesthesia has worn off (up to 7 hours).

Clinically Significant Drug Interactions: The administration of local anesthetic solutions containing epinephrine or norepinephrine to patients receiving monoamine oxidase inhibitors or tricyclic antidepressants may produce severe, prolonged hypertension. Concurrent use of these agents should generally be avoided. In situations when concurrent therapy is necessary, careful patient monitoring is essential. Concurrent administration of vasopressor drugs and of ergot-type oxytocic drugs may cause severe, persistent hypertension or cerebrovascular accidents.

Phenothiazines and butyrophenones may reduce or reverse the pressor effect of epinephrine.

Carcinogenesis, Mutagenesis, Impairment of Fertility: Long-term studies in animals of most local anesthetics including bupivacaine to evaluate the carcinogenic potential have not been conducted. Mutagenic potential or the effect on fertility has not been determined. There is no evidence from human data that MARCAINE may be carcinogenic or mutagenic or that it impairs fertility.

Pregnancy Category C: Decreased pup survival in rats and an embryocidal effect in rabbits have been observed when bupivacaine hydrochloride was administered to these species in doses comparable to nine and five times respectively the maximum recommended daily human dose (400 mg). There are no adequate and well-controlled studies in pregnant women of the effect of bupivacaine on the developing fetus. Bupivacaine hydrochloride should be used during pregnancy only if the potential benefit justifies the potential risk to the

Continued on next page

This product information was prepared in August, 1989. On these and other products of Winthrop Pharmaceuticals, detailed information may be obtained on a current basis by direct inquiry to the Professional Services Department, 90 Park Avenue, New York, NY 10016 (800) 446-6267.

Winthrop Pharm.—Cont.

fetus. This does not exclude the use of MARCAINE at term for obstetrical anesthesia or analgesia. (See *Labor and Delivery*.)

Labor and Delivery: SEE BOXED WARNING REGARDING OBSTETRICAL USE OF 0.75% MARCAINE.

MARCAINE is contraindicated for obstetrical paracervical block anesthesia.

Local anesthetics rapidly cross the placenta, and when used for epidural, caudal, or pudendal block anesthesia, can cause varying degrees of maternal, fetal, and neonatal toxicity. (See *Pharmacokinetics* in CLINICAL PHARMACOLOGY.) The incidence and degree of toxicity depend upon the procedure performed, the type, and amount of drug used, and the technique of drug administration. Adverse reactions in the parturient, fetus, and neonate involve alterations of the central nervous system, peripheral vascular tone, and cardiac function.

Maternal hypotension has resulted from regional anesthesia. Local anesthetics produce vasodilation by blocking sympathetic nerves. Elevating the patient's legs and positioning her on her left side will help prevent decreases in blood pressure. The fetal heart rate also should be monitored continuously and electronic fetal monitoring is highly advisable.

Epidural, caudal, or pudendal anesthesia may alter the forces of parturition through changes in uterine contractility or maternal expulsive efforts. Epidural anesthesia has been reported to prolong the second stage of labor by removing the parturient's reflex urge to bear down or by interfering with motor function. The use of obstetrical anesthesia may increase the need for forceps assistance.

The use of some local anesthetic drug products during labor and delivery may be followed by diminished muscle strength and tone for the first day or two of life. This has not been reported with bupivacaine.

It is extremely important to avoid aortocaval compression by the gravid uterus during administration of regional block to parturients. To do this, the patient must be maintained in the left lateral decubitus position or a blanket roll or sandbag may be placed beneath the right hip and gravid uterus displaced to the left.

Nursing Mothers: It is not known whether local anesthetic drugs are excreted in human milk. Because many drugs are excreted in human milk, caution should be exercised when local anesthetics are administered to a nursing woman.

Pediatric Use: Until further experience is gained in children younger than 12 years, administration of MARCAINE in this age group is not recommended.

ADVERSE REACTIONS

Reactions to MARCAINE (bupivacaine) are characteristic of those associated with other amide-type local anesthetics. A major cause of adverse reactions to this group of drugs is excessive plasma levels, which may be due to overdosage, unintentional intravascular injection, or slow metabolic degradation.

The most commonly encountered acute adverse experiences which demand immediate countermeasures are related to the central nervous system and the cardiovascular system. These adverse experiences are generally dose related and due to high plasma levels which may result from overdosage, rapid absorption from the injection site, diminished tolerance, or from unintentional intravascular injection of the local anesthetic solution. In addition to systemic dose-related toxicity, unintentional subarachnoid injection of drug during the intended performance of caudal or lumbar epidural block or nerve blocks near the vertebral column (especially in the head and neck region) may result in underventilation or apnea ("Total or High Spinal"). Also, hypotension due to loss of sympathetic tone and respiratory paralysis or underventilation due to cephalad extension of the motor level of anesthesia may occur. This may lead to secondary cardiac arrest if untreated. Factors influencing plasma protein binding, such as acidosis, systemic diseases which alter protein production, or competition of other drugs for protein binding sites, may diminish individual tolerance.

Central Nervous System Reactions: These are characterized by excitation and/or depression. Restlessness, anxiety, dizziness, tinnitus, blurred vision, or tremors may occur, possibly proceeding to convulsions. However, excitement may be transient or absent, with depression being the first manifestation of an adverse reaction. This may quickly be followed by drowsiness merging into unconsciousness and respiratory arrest. Other central nervous system effects may be nausea, vomiting, chills, and constriction of the pupils. The incidence of convulsions associated with the use of local anesthetics varies with the procedure used and the total dose administered. In a survey of studies of epidural anesthesia, overt toxicity progressing to convulsions occurred in approximately 0.1% of local anesthetic administrations.

Cardiovascular System Reactions: High doses or unintentional intravascular injection may lead to high plasma levels and related depression of the myocardium, decreased cardiac output, heartblock, hypotension, bradycardia, ventricular arrhythmias, including ventricular tachycardia and ventricular fibrillation, and cardiac arrest. (See WARNINGS, PRECAUTIONS, and OVERDOSAGE sections.)

Allergic: Allergic-type reactions are rare and may occur as a result of sensitivity to the local anesthetic or to other formulation ingredients, such as the antimicrobial preservative methylparaben contained in multiple-dose vials or sulfites in epinephrine-containing solutions. These reactions are characterized by signs such as urticaria, pruritus, erythema, angioneurotic edema (including laryngeal edema), tachycardia, sneezing, nausea, vomiting, dizziness, syncope, excessive sweating, elevated temperature, and, possibly, anaphylactoid-like symptomatology (including severe hypotension). Cross sensitivity among members of the amide-type local anesthetic group has been reported. The usefulness of screening for sensitivity has not been definitely established.

Neurologic: The incidences of adverse neurologic reactions associated with the use of local anesthetics may be related to the total dose of local anesthetic administered and are also dependent upon the particular drug used, the route of administration, and the physical status of the patient. Many of these effects may be related to local anesthetic techniques, with or without a contribution from the drug.

In the practice of caudal or lumbar epidural block, occasional unintentional penetration of the subarachnoid space by the catheter or needle may occur. Subsequent adverse effects may depend partially on the amount of drug administered intrathecally and the physiological and physical effects of a dural puncture. A high spinal is characterized by paralysis of the legs, loss of consciousness, respiratory paralysis, and bradycardia.

Neurologic effects following epidural or caudal anesthesia may include spinal block of varying magnitude (including high or total spinal block); hypotension secondary to spinal block; urinary retention; fecal and urinary incontinence; loss of perineal sensation and sexual function; persistent anesthesia, paresthesia, weakness, paralysis of the lower extremities and loss of sphincter control all of which may have slow, incomplete, or no recovery; headache; backache; septic meningitis; meningismus; slowing of labor; increased incidence of forceps delivery; and cranial nerve palsies due to traction on nerves from loss of cerebrospinal fluid.

Neurologic effects following other procedures or routes of administration may include persistent anesthesia, paresthesia, weakness, paralysis, all of which may have slow, incomplete, or no recovery.

OVERDOSAGE

Acute emergencies from local anesthetics are generally related to high plasma levels encountered during therapeutic use of local anesthetics or to unintended subarachnoid injection of local anesthetic solution. (See ADVERSE REACTIONS, WARNINGS, and PRECAUTIONS.)

Management of Local Anesthetic Emergencies: The first consideration is prevention, best accomplished by careful and constant monitoring of cardiovascular and respiratory vital signs and the patient's state of consciousness after each local anesthetic injection. At the first sign of change, oxygen should be administered.

The first step in the management of systemic toxic reactions, as well as underventilation or apnea due to unintentional subarachnoid injection of drug solution, consists of immediate attention to the establishment and maintenance of a patent airway and effective assisted or controlled ventilation with 100% oxygen with a delivery system capable of permitting immediate positive airway pressure by mask. This may prevent convulsions if they have not already occurred.

If necessary, use drugs to control the convulsions. A 50 mg to 100 mg bolus IV injection of succinylcholine will paralyze the patient without depressing the central nervous or cardiovascular systems and facilitate ventilation. A bolus IV dose of 5 mg to 10 mg of diazepam or 50 mg to 100 mg of thiopental will permit ventilation and counteract central nervous system stimulation, but these drugs also depress central nervous system, respiratory, and cardiac function, add to postictal depression and may result in apnea. Intravenous barbiturates, anticonvulsant agents, or muscle relaxants should only be administered by those familiar with their use. Immediately after the institution of these ventilatory measures, the adequacy of the circulation should be evaluated. Supportive treatment of circulatory depression may require administration of intravenous fluids, and when appropriate, a vasopressor dictated by the clinical situation (such as ephedrine or epinephrine to enhance myocardial contractile force).

Endotracheal intubation, employing drugs and techniques familiar to the clinician, may be indicated after initial administration of oxygen by mask if difficulty is encountered in the maintenance of a patent airway, or if prolonged ventilatory support (assisted or controlled) is indicated.

Recent clinical data from patients experiencing local anesthetic-induced convulsions demonstrated rapid development of hypoxia, hypercarbia, and acidosis with bupivacaine within a minute of the onset of convulsions. These observations suggest that oxygen consumption and carbon dioxide production are greatly increased during local anesthetic convulsions and emphasize the importance of immediate and effective ventilation with oxygen which may avoid cardiac arrest.

If not treated immediately, convulsions with simultaneous hypoxia, hypercarbia, and acidosis plus myocardial depression from the direct effects of the local anesthetic may result in cardiac arrhythmias, bradycardia, asystole, ventricular fibrillation, or cardiac arrest. Respiratory abnormalities, including apnea, may occur. Underventilation or apnea due to unintentional subarachnoid injection of local anesthetic solution may produce these same signs and also lead to cardiac arrest if ventilatory support is not instituted. *If cardiac arrest should occur, successful outcome may require prolonged resuscitative efforts.*

The supine position is dangerous in pregnant women at term because of aortocaval compression by the gravid uterus. Therefore during treatment of systemic toxicity, maternal hypotension or fetal bradycardia following regional block, the parturient should be maintained in the left lateral decubitus position if possible, or manual displacement of the uterus off the great vessels be accomplished.

The mean seizure dosage of bupivacaine in rhesus monkeys was found to be 4.4 mg/kg with mean arterial plasma concentration of 4.5 μg/mL. The intravenous and subcutaneous LD$_{50}$ in mice is 6 mg/kg to 8 mg/kg and 38 mg/kg to 54 mg/kg respectively.

DOSAGE AND ADMINISTRATION

The dose of any local anesthetic administered varies with the anesthetic procedure, the area to be anesthetized, the vascularity of the tissues, the number of neuronal segments to be blocked, the depth of anesthesia and degree of muscle relaxation required, the duration of anesthesia desired, individual tolerance, and the physical condition of the patient. The smallest dose and concentration required to produce the desired result should be administered. Dosages of MARCAINE should be reduced for elderly and debilitated patients and patients with cardiac and/or liver disease. The rapid injection of a large volume of local anesthetic solution should be avoided and fractional (incremental) doses should be used when feasible.

For specific techniques and procedures, refer to standard textbooks.

In recommended doses, MARCAINE (bupivacaine) produces complete sensory block, but the effect on motor function differs among the three concentrations.

0.25%—when used for caudal, epidural, or peripheral nerve block, produces incomplete motor block. Should be used for operations in which muscle relaxation is not important, or when another means of providing muscle relaxation is used concurrently. Onset of action may be slower than with the 0.5% or 0.75% solutions.

0.5%—provides motor blockade for caudal, epidural, or nerve block, but muscle relaxation may be inadequate for operations in which complete muscle relaxation is essential.

0.75%—produces complete motor block. Most useful for epidural block in abdominal operations requiring complete muscle relaxation, and for retrobulbar anesthesia. Not for obstetrical anesthesia.

The duration of anesthesia with MARCAINE is such that for most indications, a single dose is sufficient.

Maximum dosage limit must be individualized in each case after evaluating the size and physical status of the patient, as well as the usual rate of systemic absorption from a particular injection site. Most experience to date is with single doses of MARCAINE up to 225 mg with epinephrine 1:200,000 and 175 mg without epinephrine; more or less drug may be used depending on individualization of each case. These doses may be repeated up to once every three hours. In clinical studies to date, total daily doses have been up to 400 mg. Until further experience is gained, this dose should not be exceeded in 24 hours. The duration of anesthetic effect may be prolonged by the addition of epinephrine.

The dosages in Table 1 have generally proved satisfactory and are recommended as a guide for use in the average adult. These dosages should be reduced for elderly or debilitated patients. Until further experience is gained, MARCAINE (bupivacaine) is not recommended for children younger than 12 years. MARCAINE is contraindicated for obstetrical paracervical blocks, and is not recommended for intravenous regional anesthesia (Bier Block).

Use in Epidural Anesthesia: During epidural administration of MARCAINE, 0.5% and 0.75% solutions should be administered in incremental doses of 3 mL to 5 mL with sufficient time between doses to detect toxic manifestatons of unintentional intravascular or intrathecal injection. In obstetrics, only the 0.5% and 0.25% concentrations should be used; incremental doses of 3 mL to 5 mL of the 0.5% solution not exceeding 50 mg to 100 mg at any dosing interval are recommended. Repeat doses should be preceded by a test dose containing epinephrine if not contraindicated. Use only the single-dose ampuls and single-dose vials for caudal or epidural anesthesia; the multiple-dose vials contain a preservative and therefore should not be used for these procedures.

Test Dose for Caudal and Lumbar Epidural Blocks:
The Test Dose of MARCAINE (0.5% bupivacaine with 1:200,000 epinephrine in a 3 mL ampul) is recommended for use as a test dose when clinical conditions permit prior to caudal and lumbar epidural blocks. This may serve as a warning of unintended intravascular or subarachnoid injection. (See **PRECAUTIONS**.) The pulse rate and other signs should be monitored carefully immediately following each test dose administration to detect possible intravascular injection, and adequate time for onset of spinal block should be allotted to detect possible intrathecal injection. An intravascular or subarachnoid injection is still possible even if results of the test dose are negative. The test dose itself may produce a systemic toxic reaction, high spinal or cardiovascular effects from the epinephrine. (See **WARNINGS** and **OVERDOSAGE**.)

Use in Dentistry: The 0.5% concentration with epinephrine is recommended for infiltration and block injection in the maxillary and mandibular area when a longer duration of local anesthetic action is desired, such as for oral surgical procedures generally associated with significant postoperative pain. The average dose of 1.8 mL (9 mg) per injection site will usually suffice; an occasional second dose of 1.8 mL (9 mg) may be used if necessary to produce adequate anesthesia after making allowance for 2 to 10 minutes onset time. (See **CLINICAL PHARMACOLOGY**.) The lowest effective dose should be employed and time should be allowed between injections; it is recommended that the total dose for all injection sites, *spread out* over a single dental sitting, should not ordinarily exceed 90 mg for a healthy adult patient (ten 1.8 mL injections of 0.5% MARCAINE with epinephrine, bupivacaine and epinephrine). Injections should be made slowly and with frequent aspirations. Until further experience is gained, MARCAINE in dentistry is not recommended for children younger than 12 years.

Unused portions of solution not containing preservatives, ie, those supplied in single-dose ampuls and single-dose vials, should be discarded following initial use.
This product should be inspected visually for particulate matter and discoloration prior to administration whenever solution and container permit. Solutions which are discolored or which contain particulate matter should not be administered.
[See table above].

HOW SUPPLIED

These solutions are not for spinal anesthesia.
Store at controlled room temperature, between 15°C and 30°C (59°F and 86°F).

MARCAINE hydrochloride — Solutions of MARCAINE (bupivacaine) that do not contain epinephrine may be autoclaved. Autoclave at 15-pound pressure, 121°C (250°F) for 15 minutes.
0.25%—Contains 2.5 mg bupivacaine hydrochloride per mL.
Single-dose ampuls of 50 mL, box of 5
            NDC 0024-1212-02
Single-dose vials of 10 mL, box of 10
            NDC 0024-1212-10
Single-dose vials of 30 mL, box of 10
            NDC 0024-1212-30
Multiple-dose vials of 50 mL, box of 1
            NDC 0024-1217-01
0.5%—Contains 5 mg bupivacaine hydrochloride per mL.
Single-dose ampuls of 30 mL, box of 5
            NDC 0024-1213-02
Single-dose vials of 10 mL, box of 10
            NDC 0024-1213-10
Single-dose vials of 30 mL, box of 10
            NDC 0024-1213-30
Multiple-dose vials of 50 mL, box of 1
            NDC 0024-1218-01
0.75%—Contains 7.5 mg bupivacaine hydrochloride per mL.
Single-dose ampuls of 30 mL, box of 5
            NDC 0024-1214-02
Single-dose vials of 10 mL, box of 10
            NDC 0024-1214-10
Single-dose vials of 30 mL, box of 10
            NDC 0024-1214-30

MARCAINE hydrochloride with epinephrine 1:200,000 (as bitartrate)—Solutions of MARCAINE that contain epinephrine should not be autoclaved and should be protected from light. Do not use if solution is discolored or contains a precipitate.
0.25%—with epinephrine 1:200,000
Contains 2.5 mg bupivacaine hydrochloride per mL.
Single-dose ampuls of 50 mL, box of 5
            NDC 0024-1222-02
Single-dose vials of 10 mL, box of 10
            NDC 0024-1222-10
Single-dose vials of 30 mL, box of 10
            NDC 0024-1222-30
Multiple-dose vials of 50 mL, box of 1
            NDC 0024-1227-01

Table 1. Recommended Concentrations and Doses of MARCAINE

Type of Block	Conc.	Each Dose (mL)	Each Dose (mg)	Motor Block[1]
Local infiltration	0.25%[4]	up to max.	up to max.	—
Epidural	0.75%[2,4]	10–20	75–150	complete
	0.5%[4]	10–20	50–100	moderate to complete
	0.25%[4]	10–20	25–50	partial to moderate
Caudal	0.5%[4]	15–30	75–150	moderate to complete
	0.25%[4]	15–30	37.5–75	moderate
Peripheral nerves	0.5%[4]	5 to max.	25 to max.	moderate to complete
	0.25%[4]	5 to max.	12.5 to max.	moderate to complete
Retrobulbar[3]	0.75%[4]	2–4	15–30	complete
Sympathetic	0.25%	20–50	50–125	—
Dental[3]	0.5% w/epi	1.8–3.6 per site	9–18 per site	—
Epidural[3] Test Dose	0.5% w/epi	2–3	10–15 (10–15 micrograms epinephrine)	—

[1]With continuous (intermittent) techniques, repeat doses increase the degree of motor block. The first repeat dose of 0.5% may produce complete motor block. Intercostal nerve block with 0.25% may also produce complete motor block for intra-abdominal surgery.
[2]For single-dose use, not for intermittent (catheter) epidural technique. Not for obstetrical anesthesia.
[3]See PRECAUTIONS.
[4]Solutions with or without epinephrine.

0.5%—with epinephrine 1:200,000
Contains 5 mg bupivacaine hydrochloride per mL.
Single-dose ampuls of 3 mL, box of 10
            NDC 0024-1223-03
Single-dose ampuls of 30 mL, box of 5
            NDC 0024-1223-02
Single-dose vials of 10 mL, box of 10
            NDC 0024-1223-10
Single-dose vials of 30 mL, box of 10
            NDC 0024-1223-30
Multiple-dose vials of 50 mL, box of 1
            NDC 0024-1228-01
0.75%—with epinephrine 1:200,000
Contains 7.5 mg bupivacaine hydrochloride per mL.
Single-dose ampuls of 30 mL, box of 5
            NDC 0024-1224-02
            MW-126-M

MARCAINE® Spinal   ℞
brand of bupivacaine in dextrose injection, USP

STERILE HYPERBARIC SOLUTION FOR SPINAL ANESTHESIA

DESCRIPTION

Bupivacaine hydrochloride is 2-Piperidinecarboxamide, 1-butyl-*N*-(2,6-dimethylphenyl)-, monohydrochloride, monohydrate, a white crystalline powder that is freely soluble in 95 percent ethanol, soluble in water, and slightly soluble in chloroform or acetone.
Dextrose is D-glucopyranose monohydrate.
MARCAINE Spinal is available in sterile hyperbaric solution for subarachnoid injection (spinal block).
Bupivacaine hydrochloride is related chemically and pharmacologically to the aminoacyl local anesthetics. It is a homologue of mepivacaine and is chemically related to lidocaine. All three of these anesthetics contain an amide linkage between the aromatic nucleus and the amino or piperidine group. They differ in this respect from the procaine-type local anesthetics, which have an ester linkage.
Each 1 mL of MARCAINE Spinal contains 7.5 mg bupivacaine hydrochloride and 82.5 mg dextrose. The pH of this solution is adjusted to between 4.0 and 6.5 with sodium hydroxide or hydrochloric acid.
The specific gravity of MARCAINE Spinal is between 1.030 and 1.035 at 25° C and 1.03 at 37° C.
MARCAINE Spinal does not contain any preservatives.

CLINICAL PHARMACOLOGY

Local anesthetics block the generation and the conduction of nerve impulses, presumably by increasing the threshold for electrical excitation in the nerve, by slowing the propagation of the nerve impulse, and by reducing the rate of rise of the action potential. In general, the progression of anesthesia is related to the diameter, myelination, and conduction velocity of affected nerve fibers. Clinically, the order of loss of nerve function is as follows: (1) pain, (2) temperature, (3) touch, (4) proprioception, and (5) skeletal muscle tone.
Systemic absorption of local anesthetics produces effects on the cardiovascular and central nervous systems (CNS). At blood concentrations achieved with normal therapeutic doses, changes in cardiac conduction, excitability, refractoriness, contractility, and peripheral vascular resistance are minimal. However, toxic blood concentrations depress cardiac conduction and excitability, which may lead to atrioventricular block, ventricular arrhythmias, and cardiac arrest, sometimes resulting in fatalities. In addition, myocardial contractility is depressed and peripheral vasodilation occurs, leading to decreased cardiac output and arterial blood pressure. Recent clinical reports and animal research suggest that these cardiovascular changes are more likely to occur after unintended direct intravascular injection of bupivacaine. Therefore, when epidural anesthesia with bupivacaine is considered, incremental dosing is necessary.
Following systemic absorption, local anesthetics can produce central nervous system stimulation, depression, or both. Apparent central stimulation is manifested as restlessness, tremors and shivering, progressing to convulsions, followed by depression and coma progressing ultimately to respiratory arrest. However, the local anesthetics have a primary depressant effect on the medulla and on higher centers. The depressed stage may occur without a prior excited stage.
Pharmacokinetics: The rate of systemic absorption of local anesthetics is dependent upon the total dose and concentration of drug administered, the route of administration, the vascularity of the administraton site, and the presence or absence of epinephrine in the anesthetic solution. A dilute concentration of epinephrine (1:200,000 or 5 μg/mL) usually reduces the rate of absorption and peak plasma concentration of MARCAINE, permitting the use of moderately larger total doses and sometimes prolonging the duration of action. The onset of action with MARCAINE is rapid and anesthesia is long lasting. The duration of anesthesia is significantly longer with MARCAINE than with any other commonly used local anesthetic. It has also been noted that there is a period of analgesia that persists after the return of sensation, during which time the need for strong analgesics is reduced.
The onset of sensory blockade following spinal block with MARCAINE Spinal is very rapid (within one minute); maximum motor blockade and maximum dermatome level are achieved within 15 minutes in most cases. Duration of sensory blockade (time to return of complete sensation in the operative site or regression of two dermatomes) following a 12 mg dose averages 2 hours with or without 0.2 mg epinephrine. The time to return of complete motor ability with 12 mg MARCAINE Spinal averages 3½ hours without the addition of epinephrine and 4½ hours if 0.2 mg epinephrine is added. When compared to equal milligram doses of hyperbaric tetracaine, the duration of sensory blockade was the same but the time to complete motor recovery was significantly longer for tetracaine. Addition of 0.2 mg epinephrine significantly prolongs the motor blockade and time to first postoperative narcotic with MARCAINE Spinal.

Continued on next page

This product information was prepared in August, 1989. On these and other products of Winthrop Pharmaceuticals, detailed information may be obtained on a current basis by direct inquiry to the Professional Services Department, 90 Park Avenue, New York, NY 10016 (800) 446-6267.

Winthrop Pharm.—Cont.

Local anesthetics appear to cross the placenta by passive diffusion. The rate and degree of diffusion is governed by (1) the degree of plasma protein binding, (2) the degree of ionization, and (3) the degree of lipid solubility. Fetal/maternal ratios of local anesthetics appear to be inversely related to the degree of plasma protein binding, because only the free, unbound drug is available for placental transfer. MARCAINE with a high protein binding capacity (95%) has a low fetal/maternal ratio (0.2 to 0.4). The extent of placental transfer is also determined by the degree of ionization and lipid solubility of the drug. Lipid soluble, nonionized drugs readily enter the fetal blood from the maternal circulation. Depending upon the route of administration, local anesthetics are distributed to some extent to all body tissues, with high concentrations found in highly perfused organs such as the liver, lungs, heart, and brain.

Pharmacokinetic studies on the plasma profiles of MARCAINE after direct intravenous injection suggest a three-compartment open model. The first compartment is represented by the rapid intravascular distribution of the drug. The second compartment represents the equilibration of the drug throughout the highly perfused organs such as the brain, myocardium, lungs, kidneys, and liver. The third compartment represents an equilibration of the drug with poorly perfused tissues, such as muscle and fat. The elimination of drug from tissue distribution depends largely upon the ability of binding sites in the circulation to carry it to the liver where it is metabolized.

Various pharmacokinetic parameters of the local anesthetics can be significantly altered by the presence of hepatic or renal disease, addition of epinephrine, factors affecting urinary pH, renal blood flow, the route of drug administration, and the age of the patient. The half-life of MARCAINE in adults is 2.7 hours and in neonates 8.1 hours.

Amide-type local anesthetics such as MARCAINE are metabolized primarily in the liver via conjugation with glucuronic acid. Patients with hepatic disease, especially those with severe hepatic disease, may be more susceptible to the potential toxicities of the amide-type local anesthetics. Pipecolylxylidine is the major metabolite of MARCAINE.

The kidney is the main excretory organ for most local anesthetics and their metabolites. Urinary excretion is affected by urinary perfusion and factors affecting urinary pH. Only 6% of bupivacaine is excreted unchanged in the urine.

When administered in recommended doses and concentrations, MARCAINE does not ordinarily produce irritation or tissue damage and does not cause methemoglobinemia.

INDICATIONS AND USAGE

MARCAINE Spinal, brand of bupivacaine in dextrose injection, is indicated for the production of subarachnoid block (spinal anesthesia).

Standard textbooks should be consulted to determine the accepted procedures and techniques for the administration of spinal anesthesia.

CONTRAINDICATIONS

MARCAINE Spinal is contraindicated in patients with a known hypersensitivity to it or to any local anesthetic agent of the amide-type.

The following conditions preclude the use of spinal anesthesia:

1. Severe hemorrhage, severe hypotension or shock and arrhythmias, such as complete heart block, which severely restrict cardiac output.
2. Local infection at the site of proposed lumbar puncture.
3. Septicemia.

WARNINGS

LOCAL ANESTHETICS SHOULD ONLY BE EMPLOYED BY CLINICIANS WHO ARE WELL VERSED IN DIAGNOSIS AND MANAGEMENT OF DOSE-RELATED TOXICITY AND OTHER ACUTE EMERGENCIES WHICH MIGHT ARISE FROM THE BLOCK TO BE EMPLOYED, AND THEN ONLY AFTER INSURING THE **IMMEDIATE** AVAILABILITY OF OXYGEN, OTHER RESUSCITATIVE DRUGS, CARDIOPULMONARY RESUSCITATIVE EQUIPMENT, AND THE PERSONNEL RESOURCES NEEDED FOR PROPER MANAGEMENT OF TOXIC REACTIONS AND RELATED EMERGENCIES. (See also ADVERSE REACTIONS and PRECAUTIONS.) DELAY IN PROPER MANAGEMENT OF DOSE-RELATED TOXICITY, UNDERVENTILATION FROM ANY CAUSE AND/OR ALTERED SENSITIVITY MAY LEAD TO THE DEVELOPMENT OF ACIDOSIS, CARDIAC ARREST, AND, POSSIBLY, DEATH.

Spinal anesthetics should not be injected during uterine contractions, because spinal fluid current may carry the drug further cephalad than desired.

A free flow of cerebrospinal fluid during the performance of spinal anesthesia is indicative of entry into the subarachnoid space. However, aspiration should be performed before the anesthetic solution is injected to confirm entry into the subarachnoid space and to avoid intravascular injection.

MARCAINE solutions containing epinephrine or other vasopressors should not be used concomitantly with ergot-type oxytocic drugs, because a severe persistent hypertension may occur. Likewise, solutions of MARCAINE containing a vasoconstrictor, such as epinephrine, should be used with extreme caution in patients receiving monoamine oxidase inhibitors (MAOI) or antidepressants of the triptyline or imipramine types, because severe prolonged hypertension may result.

Until further experience is gained in patients younger than 18 years, administration of MARCAINE in this age group is not recommended.

Mixing or the prior or intercurrent use of any other local anesthetic with MARCAINE cannot be recommended because of insufficient data on the clinical use of such mixtures.

PRECAUTIONS

General: The safety and effectiveness of spinal anesthetics depend on proper dosage, correct technique, adequate precautions, and readiness for emergencies. Resuscitative equipment, oxygen, and other resuscitative drugs should be available for immediate use. (See WARNINGS and ADVERSE REACTONS.) The patient should have IV fluids running via an indwelling catheter to assure a functioning intravenous pathway. The lowest dosage of local anesthetic that results in effective anesthesia should be used. Aspiration for blood should be performed before injection and injection should be made slowly. Tolerance varies with the status of the patient. Elderly patients and acutely ill patients may require reduced doses. Reduced doses may also be indicated in patients with increased intra-abdominal pressure (including obstetrical patients), if otherwise suitable for spinal anesthesia.

There should be careful and constant monitoring of cardiovascular and respiratory (adequacy of ventilation) vital signs and the patient's state of consciousness after local anesthetic injection. Restlessness, anxiety, incoherent speech, lightheadedness, numbness and tingling of the mouth and lips, metallic taste, tinnitus, dizziness, blurred vision, tremors, depression, or drowsiness may be early warning signs of central nervous system toxicity.

Spinal anesthetics should be used with caution in patients with severe disturbances of cardiac rhythm, shock, or heart block.

Sympathetic blockade occurring during spinal anesthesia may result in peripheral vasodilation and hypotension, the extent depending on the number of dermatomes blocked. Blood pressure should, therefore, be carefully monitored especially in the early phases of anesthesia. Hypotension may be controlled by vasoconstrictors in dosages depending on the severity of hypotension and response of treatment. The level of anesthesia should be carefully monitored because it is not always controllable in spinal techniques.

Because amide-type local anesthetics such as MARCAINE are metabolized by the liver, these drugs, especially repeat doses, should be used cautiously in patients with hepatic disease. Patients with severe hepatic disease, because of their inability to metabolize local anesthetics normally, are at a greater risk of developing toxic plasma concentrations. Local anesthetics should also be used with caution in patients with impaired cardiovascular function because they may be less able to compensate for functional changes associated with the prolongation of AV conduction produced by these drugs. However, dosage recommendations for spinal anesthesia are much lower than dosage recommendations for other major blocks and most experience regarding hepatic and cardiovascular disease dose-related toxicity is derived from these other major blocks.

Serious dose-related cardiac arrhythmias may occur if preparations containing a vasoconstrictor such as epinephrine are employed in patients during or following the administration of potent inhalation agents. In deciding whether to use these products concurrently in the same patient, the combined action of both agents upon the myocardium, the concentration and volume of vasoconstrictor used, and the time since injection, when applicable, should be taken into account.

Many drugs used during the conduct of anesthesia are considered potential triggering agents for familial malignant hyperthermia. Because it is not known whether amide-type local anesthetics may trigger this reaction and because the need for supplemental general anesthesia cannot be predicted in advance, it is suggested that a standard protocol for management should be available. Early unexplained signs of tachycardia, tachypnea, labile blood pressure, and metabolic acidosis may precede temperature elevation. Successful outcome is dependent on early diagnosis, prompt discontinuance of the suspect triggering agent(s) and institution of treatment, including oxygen therapy, indicated supportive measures, and dantrolene. (Consult dantrolene sodium intravenous package insert before using.)

The following conditions may preclude the use of spinal anesthesia, depending upon the physician's evaluation of the situation and ability to deal with the complications or complaints which may occur:

- Preexisting diseases of the central nervous system, such as those attributable to pernicious anemia, poliomyelitis, syphilis, or tumor.
- Hematological disorders predisposing to coagulopathies or patients on anticoagulant therapy. Trauma to a blood vessel during the conduct of spinal anesthesia may, in some instances, result in uncontrollable central nervous system hemorrhage or soft tissue hemorrhage.
- Chronic backache and preoperative headache.
- Hypotension and hypertension.
- Technical problems (persistent paresthesias, persistent bloody tap).
- Arthritis or spinal deformity.
- Extremes of age.
- Psychosis or other causes of poor cooperation by the patient.

Information for Patients: When appropriate, patients should be informed in advance that they may experience temporary loss of sensation and motor activity, usually in the lower half of the body, following proper administration of spinal anesthesia. Also, when appropriate, the physician should discuss other information including adverse reactions in the MARCAINE Spinal package insert.

Clinically Significant Drug Interactions: The administration of local anesthetic solutions containing epinephrine or norepinephrine to patients receiving monoamine oxidase inhibitors or tricyclic antidepressants may produce severe, prolonged hypertension. Concurrent use of these agents should generally be avoided. In situations when concurrent therapy is necessary, careful patient monitoring is essential. Concurrent administration of vasopressor drugs and of ergot-type oxytocic drugs may cause severe persistent hypertension or cerebrovascular accidents.

Phenothiazines and butyrophenones may reduce or reverse the pressor effect of epinephrine.

Carcinogenesis, Mutagenesis, and Impairment of Fertility: Long-term studies in animals of most local anesthetics including bupivacaine to evaluate the carcinogenic potential have not been conducted. Mutagenic potential or the effect on fertility have not been determined. There is no evidence from human data that MARCAINE Spinal, brand of bupivacaine in dextrose injection, may be carcinogenic or mutagenic or that it impairs fertility.

Pregnancy Category C: Decreased pup survival in rats and an embryocidal effect in rabbits have been observed when bupivacaine hydrochloride was administered to these species in doses comparable to 230 and 130 times respectively the maximum recommended human spinal dose. There are no adequate and well-controlled studies in pregnant women of the effect of bupivacaine on the developing fetus. Bupivacaine hydrochloride should be used during pregnancy only if the potential benefit justifies the potential risk to the fetus. This does not exclude the use of MARCAINE Spinal at term for obstetrical anesthesia. (See *Labor and Delivery.*)

Labor and Delivery: Spinal anesthesia has a recognized use during labor and delivery. Bupivacaine hydrochloride, when administered properly, via the epidural route in doses 10 to 12 times the amount used in spinal anesthesia has been used for obstetrical analgesia and anesthesia without evidence of adverse effects on the fetus.

Maternal hypotension has resulted from regional anesthesia. Local anesthetics produce vasodilation by blocking sympathetic nerves. Elevating the patient's legs and positioning her on her left side will help prevent decreases in blood pressure. The fetal heart rate also should be monitored continuously and electronic fetal monitoring is highly advisable.

It is extremely important to avoid aortocaval compression by the gravid uterus during administrations of regional block to parturients. To do this, the patient must be maintained in the left lateral decubitus position or a blanket roll or sandbag may be placed beneath the right hip and the gravid uterus displaced to the left.

Spinal anesthesia may alter the forces of parturition through changes in uterine contractility or maternal expulsive efforts. Spinal anesthesia has also been reported to prolong the second stage of labor by removing the parturient's reflex urge to bear down or by interfering with motor function. The use of obstetrical anesthesia may increase the need for forceps assistance.

The use of some local anesthetic drug products during labor and delivery may be followed by diminished muscle strength and tone for the first day or two of life. This has not been reported with bupivacaine.

There have been reports of cardiac arrest during use of MARCAINE 0.75% solution for epidural anesthesia in obstetrical patients. The package insert for MARCAINE hydrochloride for epidural, nerve block, etc, has a more complete discussion of preparation for, and management of, this problem. These cases are compatible with systemic toxicity following unintended intravascular injection of the much larger doses recommended for epidural anesthesia and have not occurred within the dose range of bupivacaine hydrochloride 0.75% recommended for spinal anesthesia in obstetrics. The 0.75% concentration of MARCAINE is therefore

not recommended for obstetrical epidural anesthesia. MARCAINE Spinal, brand of bupivacaine in dextrose injection, is recommended for spinal anesthesia in obstetrics.

Nursing Mothers: It is not known whether local anesthetic drugs are excreted in human milk. Because many drugs are excreted in human milk, caution should be exercised when local anesthetics are administered to a nursing woman.

Pediatric Use: Until further experience is gained in patients younger than 18 years, administration of MARCAINE Spinal in this age group is not recommended.

ADVERSE REACTIONS

Reactions to bupivacaine are characteristic of those associated with other amide-type local anesthetics.

The most commonly encountered acute adverse experiences which demand immediate countermeasures following the administration of spinal anesthesia are hypotension due to loss of sympathetic tone and respiratory paralysis or underventilation due to cephalad extension of the motor level of anesthesia. These may lead to cardiac arrest if untreated. In addition, dose-related convulsions and cardiovascular collapse may result from diminished tolerance, rapid absorption from the injection site, or from unintentional intravascular injection of a local anesthetic solution. Factors influencing plasma protein binding, such as acidosis, systemic diseases which alter protein production, or competition of other drugs for protein binding sites, may diminish individual tolerance.

Respiratory System: Respiratory paralysis or underventilation may be noted as a result of upward extension of the level of spinal anesthesia and may lead to secondary hypoxic cardiac arrest if untreated. Preanesthetic medication, intraoperative analgesics and sedatives, as well as surgical manipulation, may contribute to underventilation. This will usually be noted within minutes of the injection of spinal anesthetic solution, but because of differing maximal onset times, differing intercurrent drug usage and differing surgical manipulation, it may occur at any time during surgery or the immediate recovery period.

Cardiovascular System: Hypotension due to loss of sympathetic tone is a commonly encountered extension of the clinical pharmacology of spinal anesthesia. This is more commonly observed in patients with shrunken blood volume, shrunken interstitial fluid volume, cephalad spread of the local anesthetic, and/or mechanical obstruction of venous return. Nausea and vomiting are frequently associated with hypotensive episodes following the administration of spinal anesthesia. High doses, or inadvertent intravascular injection, may lead to high plasma levels and related depression of the myocardium, decreased cardiac output, bradycardia, heart block, ventricular arrhythmias, and, possibly, cardiac arrest. (See **WARNINGS, PRECAUTIONS,** and **OVERDOSAGE** sections.)

Central Nervous System: Respiratory paralysis or underventilation secondary to cephalad spread of the level of spinal anesthesia (See *Respiratory System*) and hypotension for the same reason (see *Cardiovascular System*) are the two most commonly encountered central nervous system-related adverse observations which demand immediate countermeasures.

High doses or inadvertent intravascular injection may lead to high plasma levels and related central nervous system toxicity characterized by excitement and/or depression. Restlessness, anxiety, dizziness, tinnitus, blurred vision, or tremors may occur, possibly proceeding to convulsions. However, excitement may be transient or absent, with depression being the first manifestation of an adverse reaction. This may quickly be followed by drowsiness merging into unconsciousness and respiratory arrest.

Neurologic: The incidences of adverse neurologic reactions associated with the use of local anesthetics may be related to the total dose of local anesthetic administered and are also dependent upon the particular drug used, the route of administration, and the physical status of the patient. Many of these effects may be related to local anesthetic techniques, with or without a contribution from the drug.

Neurologic effects following spinal anesthesia may include loss of perineal sensation and sexual function; persistent anesthesia, paresthesia, weakness and paralysis of the lower extremities, and loss of sphincter control all of which may have slow, incomplete, or no recovery; hypotension; high or total spinal block; urinary retention; headache; backache; septic meningitis; meningismus; arachnoiditis; slowing of labor; increased incidence of forceps delivery; shivering; cranial nerve palsies due to traction on nerves from loss of cerebrospinal fluid; and fecal and urinary incontinence.

Allergic: Allergic-type reactions are rare and may occur as a result of sensitivity to the local anesthetic. These reactions are characterized by signs such as urticaria, pruritus, erythema, angioneurotic edema (including laryngeal edema), tachycardia, sneezing, nausea, vomiting, dizziness, syncope, excessive sweating, elevated temperature, and, possibly, anaphylactoid-like symptomatology (including severe hypotension). Cross sensitivity among members of the amide-type local anesthetic group has been reported. The usefulness of screening for sensitivity has not been definitely established.

Other: Nausea and vomiting may occur during spinal anesthesia.

OVERDOSAGE

Acute emergencies from local anesthetics are generally related to high plasma levels encountered during therapeutic use or to underventilation (and perhaps apnea) secondary to upward extension of spinal anesthesia. Hypotension is commonly encountered during the conduct of spinal anesthesia due to relaxation of sympathetic tone, and sometimes, contributory mechanical obstruction of venous return.

Management of Local Anesthetic Emergencies: The first consideration is prevention, best accomplished by careful and constant monitoring of cardiovascular and respiratory vital signs and the patient's state of consciousness after each local anesthetic injection. At the first sign of change, oxygen should be administered.

*The first step in the management of systemic toxic reactions, as well as underventilation or apnea due to a high or total spinal, consists of **immediate** attention to the establishment and maintenance of a patent airway and effective assisted or controlled ventilation with 100% oxygen with a delivery system capable of permitting immediate positive airway pressure by mask.* This may prevent convulsions if they have not already occurred.

If necessary, use drugs to control the convulsions. A 50 mg to 100 mg bolus IV injection of succinylcholine will paralyze the patient without depressing the central nervous or cardiovascular systems and facilitate ventilation. A bolus IV dose of 5 mg to 10 mg of diazepam or 50 mg to 100 mg of thiopental will permit ventilation and counteract central nervous system stimulation, but these drugs also depress central nervous system, respiratory and cardiac function, add to postictal depression and may result in apnea. Intravenous barbiturates, anticonvulsant agents, or muscle relaxants should only be administered by those familiar with their use. Immediately after the institution of these ventilatory measures, the adequacy of the circulation should be evaluated. Supportive treatment of circulatory depression may require administration of intravenous fluids, and, when appropriate, a vasopressor dictated by the clinical situation (such as ephedrine or epinephrine to enhance myocardial contractile force).

Hypotension due to sympathetic relaxation may be managed by giving intravenous fluids (such as isotonic saline or lactated Ringer's solution), in an attempt to relieve mechanical obstruction of venous return, or by using vasopressors (such as ephedrine which increases the force of myocardial contractions) and, if indicated, by giving plasma expanders or whole blood.

Endotracheal intubation, employing drugs and techniques familiar to the clinician, may be indicated after initial administration of oxygen by mask if difficulty is encountered in the maintenance of a patent airway, or if prolonged ventilatory support (assisted or controlled) is indicated.

Recent clinical data from patients experiencing local anesthetic-induced convulsions demonstrated rapid development of hypoxia, hypercarbia, and acidosis with bupivacaine within a minute of the onset of convulsions. These observations suggest that oxygen consumption and carbon dioxide production are greatly increased during local anesthetic convulsions and emphasize the importance of immediate and effective ventilation with oxygen which may avoid cardiac arrest.

If not treated immediately, convulsions with simultaneous hypoxia, hypercarbia, and acidosis plus myocardial depression from the direct effects of the local anesthetic may result in cardiac arrhythmias, bradycardia, asystole, ventricular fibrillation, or cardiac arrest. Respiratory abnormalities, including apnea, may occur. Underventilation or apnea due to a high or total spinal may produce these same signs and also lead to cardiac arrest if ventilatory support is not instituted. If cardiac arrest should occur, standard cardiopulmonary resuscitative measures should be instituted and maintained for a prolonged period if necessary. Recovery has been reported after prolonged resuscitative efforts.

The supine position is dangerous in pregnant women at term because of aortocaval compression by the gravid uterus. Therefore during treatment of systemic toxicity, maternal hypotension, or fetal bradycardia following regional block, the parturient should be maintained in the left lateral decubitus position if possible, or manual displacement of the uterus off the great vessels be accomplished.

The mean seizure dosage of bupivacaine in rhesus monkeys was found to be 4.4 mg/kg with mean arterial plasma concentration of 4.5 μg/mL. The intravenous and subcutaneous LD_{50} in mice is 6 mg/kg to 8 mg/kg and 38 mg/kg to 54 mg/kg respectively.

DOSAGE AND ADMINISTRATION

The dose of any local anesthetic administered varies with the anesthetic procedure, the area to be anesthetized, the vascularity of the tissues, the number of neuronal segments to be blocked, the depth of anesthesia and degree of muscle relaxation required, the duration of anesthesia desired, individual tolerance, and the physical condition of the patient. The

smallest dose and concentration required to produce the desired result should be administered. Dosages of MARCAINE Spinal, brand of bupivacaine in dextrose injection, should be reduced for elderly and debilitated patients and patients with cardiac and/or liver disease.

For specific techniques and procedures, refer to standard textbooks.

The extent and degree of spinal anesthesia depend upon several factors including dosage, specific gravity of the anesthetic solution, volume of solution used, force of injection, level of puncture, and position of the patient during and immediately after injection.

Seven and one-half mg (7.5 mg or 1.0 mL) MARCAINE Spinal has generally proven satisfactory for spinal anesthesia for lower extremity and perineal procedures including TURP and vaginal hysterectomy. Twelve mg (12.0 mg or 1.6 mL) has been used for lower abdominal procedures such as abdominal hysterectomy, tubal ligation, and appendectomy. These doses are recommended as a guide for use in the average adult and may be reduced for the elderly or debilitated patients. Because experience with MARCAINE Spinal is limited in patients below the age of 18 years, dosage recommendations in this age group cannot be made.

Obstetrical Use: Doses as low as 6 mg bupivacaine hydrochloride have been used for vaginal delivery under spinal anesthesia. The dose range of 7.5 mg to 10.5 mg (1 mL to 1.4 mL) bupivacaine hydrochloride has been used for Cesarean section under spinal anesthesia.

In recommended doses, MARCAINE Spinal produces complete motor and sensory block.

Unused portions of solutions should be discarded following initial use.

MARCAINE Spinal should be inspected visually for discoloration and particulate matter prior to administration; solutions which are discolored or which contain particulate matter should not be administered.

HOW SUPPLIED

Single-dose ampuls of 2 mL (15 mg bupivacaine hydrochloride with 165 mg dextrose), in Uni-Nest™ Unit Dose Pak of 10 (NDC 0024-1229-10)

Store at controlled room temperature, between 15° C and 30° C (59° F and 86° F).

MARCAINE Spinal solution may be autoclaved once at 15 pound pressure, 121° C (250° F) for 15 minutes. Do not administer any solution which is discolored or contains particulate matter.

                                                    MW-246-B

MEASURIN®   OTC
Timed-Released Aspirin

(See PDR For Nonprescription Drugs)

MEBARAL®   C ⴽ
brand of mephobarbital tablets, USP

DESCRIPTION

Mephobarbital, 5-Ethyl-1-methyl-5-phenylbarbituric acid, is a barbiturate with sedative, hypnotic, and anticonvulsant properties. It occurs as a white, nearly odorless, tasteless powder and is slightly soluble in water and in alcohol. MEBARAL is available as tablets for oral administration. *Inactive Ingredients:* Lactose, Starch, Stearic Acid, Talc.

CLINICAL PHARMACOLOGY

Barbiturates are capable of producing all levels of CNS mood alteration from excitation to mild sedation, to hypnosis, and deep coma. Overdosage can produce death. In high enough therapeutic doses, barbiturates induce anesthesia.

Barbiturates depress the sensory cortex, decrease motor activity, alter cerebellar function, and produce drowsiness, sedation, and hypnosis.

Barbiturates are respiratory depressants. The degree of respiratory depression is dependent upon dose. With hypnotic doses, respiratory depression produced by barbiturates is similar to that which occurs during physiologic sleep with slight decrease in blood pressure and heart rate.

Studies in laboratory animals have shown that barbiturates cause reduction in the tone and contractility of the uterus, ureters, and urinary bladder. However, concentrations of the drugs required to produce this effect in humans are not reached with sedative-hypnotic doses.

Barbiturates do not impair normal hepatic function, but have been shown to induce liver microsomal enzymes, thus

Continued on next page

This product information was prepared in August, 1989. On these and other products of Winthrop Pharmaceuticals, detailed information may be obtained on a current basis by direct inquiry to the Professional Services Department, 90 Park Avenue, New York, NY 10016 (800) 446-6267.

Winthrop Pharm.—Cont.

increasing and/or altering the metabolism of barbiturates and other drugs. (See PRECAUTIONS—Drug Interactions.) MEBARAL exerts a strong sedative and anticonvulsant action but has a relatively mild hypnotic effect. It reduces the incidence of epileptic seizures in grand mal and petit mal. MEBARAL usually causes little or no drowsiness or lassitude. Hence, when it is used as a sedative or anticonvulsant, patients usually become more calm, more cheerful, and better adjusted to their surroundings without clouding of mental faculties. MEBARAL is reported to produce less sedation than does phenobarbital.

Barbiturates are weak acids that are absorbed and rapidly distributed to all tissues and fluids with high concentrations in the brain, liver, and kidneys. Lipid solubility of the barbiturates is the dominant factor in their distribution within the body. Barbiturates are bound to plasma and tissue proteins to a varying degree with the degree of binding increasing directly as a function of lipid solubility.

Approximately 50% of an oral dose of mephobarbital is absorbed from the gastrointestinal tract. Therapeutic plasma concentrations for mephobarbital have not been established nor has the half-life been determined. Following oral administration, the onset of action of the drug is 30 to 60 minutes and the duration of action is 10 to 16 hours. The primary route of mephobarbital metabolism is N-demethylation by the microsomal enzymes of the liver to form phenobarbital. Phenobarbital may be excreted in the urine unchanged or further metabolized to p-hydroxyphenobarbital and excreted in the urine as glucuronide or sulfate conjugates. About 75% of a single oral dose of mephobarbital is converted to phenobarbital in 24 hours.

Therefore, chronic administration of mephobarbital may lead to an accumulation of phenobarbital (not mephobarbital) in plasma. It has not been determined whether mephobarbital or phenobarbital is the active agent during long-time mephobarbital therapy.

INDICATIONS AND USAGE

MEBARAL is indicated for use as a sedative for the relief of anxiety, tension, and apprehension, and as an anticonvulsant for the treatment of grand mal and petit mal epilepsy.

CONTRAINDICATIONS

Hypersensitivity to any barbiturate. Manifest or latent porphyria.

WARNINGS

Habit Forming

Barbiturates may be habit forming. Tolerance, psychological, and physical dependence may occur with continued use. (See DRUG ABUSE AND DEPENDENCE and CLINICAL PHARMACOLOGY.) Patients who have psychological dependence on barbiturates may increase the dosage or decrease the dosage interval without consulting a physician and may subsequently develop a physical dependence on barbiturates. To minimize the possibility of overdosage or the development of dependence, the prescribing and dispensing of sedative-hypnotic barbiturates should be limited to the amount required for the interval until the next appointment. Abrupt cessation after prolonged use in the dependent person may result in withdrawal symptoms, including delirium, convulsions, and possibly death. Barbiturates should be withdrawn gradually from any patient known to be taking excessive dosage over long periods of time. (See DRUG ABUSE AND DEPENDENCE.)

Acute or Chronic Pain

Caution should be exercised when barbiturates are administered to patients with acute or chronic pain, because paradoxical excitement could be induced or important symptoms could be masked. However, the use of barbiturates as sedatives in the postoperative surgical period and as adjuncts to cancer chemotherapy is well established.

Use in Pregnancy

Barbiturates can cause fetal damage when administered to a pregnant woman. Retrospective, case-controlled studies have suggested a connection between the maternal consumption of barbiturates and a higher than expected incidence of fetal abnormalities. Following oral or parenteral administration, barbiturates readily cross the placental barrier and are distributed throughout fetal tissues with highest concentrations found in the placenta, fetal liver, and brain. Fetal blood levels approach maternal blood levels following parenteral administration.

Withdrawal symptoms occur in infants born to mothers who receive barbiturates throughout the last trimester of pregnancy. (See DRUG ABUSE AND DEPENDENCE.) If this drug is used during pregnancy, or if the patient becomes pregnant while taking this drug, the patient should be apprised of the potential hazard to the fetus.

Synergistic Effects

The concomitant use of alcohol or other CNS depressants may produce additive CNS depressant effects.

PRECAUTIONS

General

Barbiturates may be habit forming. Tolerance and psychological and physical dependence may occur with continuing use. (See DRUG ABUSE AND DEPENDENCE.) Barbiturates should be administered with caution, if at all, to patients who are mentally depressed, have suicidal tendencies, or a history of drug abuse.

Elderly or debilitated patients may react to barbiturates with marked excitement, depression, and confusion. In some persons, barbiturates repeatedly produce excitement rather than depression.

In patients with hepatic damage, barbiturates should be administered with caution and initially in reduced doses. Barbiturates should not be administered to patients showing the premonitory signs of hepatic coma.

Status epilepticus may result from the abrupt discontinuation of MEBARAL, even when administered in small daily doses in the treatment of epilepsy.

Caution and careful adjustment of dosage are required when MEBARAL, brand of mephobarbital tablets, is used in patients with impaired renal, cardiac, or respiratory function and in patients with myasthenia gravis and myxedema. The least quantity feasible should be prescribed or dispensed at any one time in order to minimize the possibility of acute or chronic overdosage.

Vitamin D Deficiency: MEBARAL may increase vitamin D requirements, possibly by increasing vitamin D metabolism via enzyme induction. Rarely, rickets and osteomalacia have been reported following prolonged use of barbiturates.

Vitamin K: Bleeding in the early neonatal period due to coagulation defects may follow exposure to anticonvulsant drugs in utero; therefore, vitamin K should be given to the mother before delivery or to the child at birth.

Information for the Patient

Practitioners should give the following information and instructions to patients receiving barbiturates.

1. The use of barbiturates carries with it an associated risk of psychological and/or physical dependence. The patient should be warned against increasing the dose of the drug without consulting a physician.

2. Barbiturates may impair mental and/or physical abilities required for the performance of potentially hazardous tasks (eg, driving, operating machinery, etc).

3. Alcohol should not be consumed while taking barbiturates. Concurrent use of the barbiturates with other CNS depressants (eg, alcohol, narcotics, tranquilizers, and antihistamines) may result in additional CNS depressant effects.

Laboratory Tests

Prolonged therapy with barbiturates should be accompanied by periodic laboratory evaluation of organ systems, including hematopoietic, renal, and hepatic systems. (See PRECAUTIONS [General] and ADVERSE REACTIONS.)

Drug Interactions

Most reports of clinically significant drug interactions occurring with the barbiturates have involved phenobarbital. However, the application of these data to other barbiturates appears valid and warrants serial blood level determinations of the relevant drugs when there are multiple therapies.

1. *Anticoagulants.* Phenobarbital lowers the plasma levels of dicumarol (name previously used: bishydroxycoumarin) and causes a decrease in anticoagulant activity as measured by the prothrombin time. Barbiturates can induce hepatic microsomal enzymes resulting in increased metabolism and decreased anticoagulant response of oral anticoagulants (eg, warfarin, acenocoumarol, dicumarol, and phenprocoumon). Patients stabilized on anticoagulant therapy may require dosage adjustments if barbiturates are added to or withdrawn from their dosage regimen.

2. *Corticosteroids.* Barbiturates appear to enhance the metabolism of exogenous corticosteroids probably through the induction of hepatic microsomal enzymes. Patients stabilized on corticosteroid therapy may require dosage adjustments if barbiturates are added to or withdrawn from their dosage regimen.

3. *Griseofulvin.* Phenobarbital appears to interfere with the absorption of orally administered griseofulvin, thus decreasing its blood level. The effect of the resultant decreased blood levels of griseofulvin on therapeutic response has not been established. However, it would be preferable to avoid concomitant administration of these drugs.

4. *Doxycycline.* Phenobarbital has been shown to shorten the half-life of doxycycline for as long as 2 weeks after barbiturate therapy is discontinued. This mechanism is probably through the induction of hepatic microsomal enzymes that metabolize the antibiotic. If phenobarbital and doxycycline are administered concurrently, the clinical response to doxycycline should be monitored closely.

5. *Phenytoin, Sodium Valproate, Valproic Acid.* The effect of barbiturates on the metabolism of phenytoin appears to be variable. Some investigators report an accelerating effect, while others report no effect. Because the effect of barbiturates on the metabolism of phenytoin is not predictable, phenytoin and barbiturate blood levels should be monitored

more frequently if these drugs are given concurrently. Sodium valproate and valproic acid appear to decrease barbiturate metabolism; therefore, barbiturate blood levels should be monitored and appropriate dosage adjustments made as indicated.

6. *Central Nervous System Depressants.* The concomitant use of other central nervous system depressants, including other sedatives or hypnotics, antihistamines, tranquilizers, or alcohol, may produce additive depressant effects.

7. *Monoamine Oxidase Inhibitors (MAOI).* MAOI prolong the effects of barbiturates probably because metabolism of the barbiturate is inhibited.

8. *Estradiol, Estone, Progesterone, and other Steroidal Hormones.* Pretreatment with or concurrent administration of phenobarbital may decrease the effect of estradiol by increasing its metabolism. There have been reports of patients treated with antiepileptic drugs (eg, phenobarbital) who become pregnant while taking oral contraceptives. An alternant contraceptive method might be suggested to women taking phenobarbital.

Carcinogenesis

Animal Data. Phenobarbital sodium is carcinogenic in mice and rats after lifetime administration. In mice, it produced benign and malignant liver cell tumors. In rats, benign liver cell tumors were observed very late in life. Phenobarbital is the major metabolite of MEBARAL.

Human Data. In a 29-year epidemiological study of 9,136 patients who were treated on an anticonvulsant protocol which included phenobarbital, results indicated a higher than normal incidence of hepatic carcinoma. Previously, some of these patients were treated with thorotrast, a drug which is known to produce hepatic carcinomas. Thus, this study did not provide sufficient evidence that phenobarbital sodium is carcinogenic in humans. Phenobarbital is the major metabolite of MEBARAL, brand of mephobarbital tablets.

A retrospective study of 84 children with brain tumors matched to 73 normal controls and 78 cancer controls (malignant disease other than brain tumors) suggested an association between exposure to barbiturates prenatally and an increased incidence of brain tumors.

Pregnancy

Teratogenic Effects. Pregnancy Category D—See WARNINGS—Use in Pregnancy.

Nonteratogenic Effects. Reports of infants suffering from long-term barbiturate exposure in utero included the acute withdrawal syndrome of seizures and hyperirritability from birth to a delayed onset of up to 14 days. (See DRUG ABUSE AND DEPENDENCE.)

Labor and Delivery.

Hypnotic doses of these barbiturates do not appear to significantly impair uterine activity during labor. Full anesthetic doses of barbiturates decrease the force and frequency of uterine contractions. Administration of sedative-hypnotic barbiturates to the mother during labor may result in respiratory depression in the newborn. Premature infants are particularly susceptible to the depressant effects of barbiturates. If barbiturates are used during labor and delivery, resuscitation equipment should be available.

Data are currently not available to evaluate the effect of these barbiturates when forceps delivery or other intervention is necessary. Also, data are not available to determine the effect of these barbiturates on the later growth, development, and functional maturation of the child.

Nursing Mothers.

Caution should be exercised when a barbiturate is administered to a nursing woman since small amounts of barbiturates are excreted in the milk.

ADVERSE REACTIONS

The following adverse reactions and their incidence were compiled from surveillance of thousands of hospitalized patients. Because such patients may be less aware of certain of the milder adverse effects of barbiturates, the incidence of these reactions may be somewhat higher in fully ambulatory patients.

More than 1 in 100 Patients. The most common adverse reaction estimated to occur at a rate of 1 to 3 patients per 100 is:

Nervous System: Somnolence.

Less than 1 in 100 Patients. Adverse reactions estimated to occur at a rate of less than 1 in 100 patients listed below, grouped by organ system, and by decreasing order of occurrence are:

Nervous System: Agitation, confusion, hyperkinesia, ataxia, CNS depression, nightmares, nervousness, psychiatric disturbance, hallucinations, insomnia, anxiety, dizziness, thinking abnormality.

Respiratory System: Hypoventilation, apnea.

Cardiovascular System: Bradycardia, hypotension, syncope.

Digestive System: Nausea, vomiting, constipation.

Other Reported Reactions: Headache, hypersensitivity reactions (angioedema, skin rashes, exfoliative dermatitis), fever, liver damage, megaloblastic anemia following chronic phenobarbital use.

DRUG ABUSE AND DEPENDENCE

Mephobarbital is a controlled substance in Narcotic Schedule IV. Barbiturates may be habit forming. Tolerance, psychological dependence, and physical dependence may occur especially following prolonged use of high doses of barbiturates. As tolerance to barbiturates develops, the amount needed to maintain the same level of intoxication increases; tolerance to a fatal dosage, however, does not increase more than two-fold. As this occurs, the margin between an intoxicating dosage and fatal dosage becomes smaller.

Symptoms of acute intoxication with barbiturates include unsteady gait, slurred speech, and sustained nystagmus. Mental signs of chronic intoxication include confusion, poor judgment, irritability, insomnia, and somatic complaints. Symptoms of barbiturate dependence are similar to those of chronic alcoholism. If an individual appears to be intoxicated with alcohol to a degree that is radically disproportionate to the amount of alcohol in his or her blood the use of barbiturates should be suspected. The lethal dose of a barbiturate is far less if alcohol is also ingested.

The symptoms of barbiturate withdrawal can be severe and may cause death. Minor withdrawal symptoms may appear 8 to 12 hours after the last dose of a barbiturate. These symptoms usually appear in the following order: anxiety, muscle twitching, tremor of hands and fingers, progressive weakness, dizziness, distortion in visual perception, nausea, vomiting, insomnia, and orthostatic hypotension. Major withdrawal symptoms (convulsions and delirium) may occur within 16 hours and last up to 5 days after abrupt cessation of these drugs. Intensity of withdrawal symptoms gradually declines over a period of approximately 15 days. Individuals susceptible to a barbiturate abuse and dependence include alcoholics and opiate abusers, as well as other sedative-hypnotic and amphetamine abusers.

Drug dependence to barbiturates arises from repeated administration of a barbiturate or agent with barbiturate-like effect on a continuous basis, generally in amounts exceeding therapeutic dose levels. The characteristics of drug dependence to barbiturates include: (a) a strong desire or need to continue taking the drug; (b) a tendency to increase the dose; (c) a psychic dependence on the effects of the drug related to subjective and individual appreciation of those effects; and (d) a physical dependence on the effects of the drug requiring its presence for maintenance of homeostasis and resulting in a definite, characteristic, and self-limited abstinence syndrome when the drug is withdrawn.

Treatment of barbiturate dependence consists of cautious and gradual withdrawal of the drug. Barbiturate-dependent patients can be withdrawn by using a number of different withdrawal regimens. In all cases withdrawal takes an extended period of time. One method involves substituting a 30 mg dose of phenobarbital for each 100 mg to 200 mg dose of barbiturate that the patient has been taking. The total daily amount of phenobarbital is then administered in 3 to 4 divided doses, not to exceed 600 mg daily. Should signs of withdrawal occur on the first day of treatment, a loading dose of 100 mg to 200 mg of phenobarbital may be administered IM in addition to the oral dose. After stabilization on phenobarbital, the total daily dose is decreased by 30 mg a day as long as withdrawal is proceeding smoothly. A modification of this regimen involves initiating treatment at the patient's regular dosage level and decreasing the daily dosage by 10% if tolerated by the patient.

Infants physically dependent on barbiturates may be given phenobarbital 3 mg/kg/day to 10 mg/kg/day. After withdrawal symptoms (hyperactivity, disturbed sleep, tremors, hyperreflexia) are relieved, the dosage of phenobarbital should be gradually decreased and completely withdrawn over a 2-week period.

OVERDOSAGE

The toxic dose of barbiturates varies considerably. In general, an oral dose of 1 g of most barbiturates produces serious poisoning in an adult. Death commonly occurs after 2 g to 10 g of ingested barbiturate. Barbiturate intoxication may be confused with alcoholism, bromide intoxication, and with various neurological disorders.

Acute overdosage with barbiturates is manifested by CNS and respiratory depression which may progress to Cheyne-Stokes respiration, areflexia, constriction of the pupils to a slight degree (though in severe poisoning they may show paralytic dilation), oliguria, tachycardia, hypotension, lowered body temperature, and coma. Typical shock syndrome (apnea, circulatory collapse, respiratory arrest, and death) may occur.

In extreme overdose, all electrical activity in the brain may cease, in which case a "flat" EEG normally equated with clinical death cannot be accepted. This effect is fully reversible unless hypoxic damage occurs. Consideration should be given to the possibility of barbiturate intoxication even in situations that appear to involve trauma.

Complications such as pneumonia, pulmonary edema, cardiac arrhythmias, congestive heart failure, and renal failure may occur. Uremia may increase CNS sensitivity to barbiturates if renal function is impaired. Differential diagnosis should include hypoglycemia, head trauma, cerebrovascular accidents, convulsive states, and diabetic coma.

Treatment of overdosage is mainly supportive and consists of the following:

1. Maintenance of an adequate airway, with assisted respiration and oxygen administration as necessary.
2. Monitoring of vital signs and fluid balance.
3. If the patient is conscious and has not lost the gag reflex, emesis may be induced with ipecac. Care should be taken to prevent pulmonary aspiration of vomitus. After completion of vomiting, 30 g activated charcoal in a glass of water may be administered.
4. If emesis is contraindicated, gastric lavage may be performed with a cuffed endotracheal tube in place with the patient in the face down position. Activated charcoal may be left in the emptied stomach and a saline cathartic administered.
5. Fluid therapy and other standard treatment for shock, if needed.
6. If renal function is normal, forced diuresis may aid in the elimination of the barbiturate. Alkalinization of the urine increases renal excretion of some barbiturates, including mephobarbital (which is metabolized to phenobarbital).
7. Although not recommended as a routine procedure, hemodialysis may be used in severe barbiturate intoxications or if the patient is anuric or in shock.
8. Patient should be rolled from side to side every 30 minutes.
9. Antibiotics should be given if pneumonia is suspected.
10. Appropriate nursing care to prevent hypostatic pneumonia, decubiti aspiration, and other complications of patients with altered states of consciousness.

DOSAGE AND ADMINISTRATION

Epilepsy: Average dose for adults: 400 mg to 600 mg (6 grains to 9 grains) daily; children under 5 years: 16 mg to 32 mg ($\frac{1}{4}$ grain to $\frac{1}{2}$ grain) three or four times daily; children over 5 years: 32 mg to 64 mg ($\frac{1}{2}$ grain to 1 grain) three or four times daily. MEBARAL is best taken at bedtime if seizures generally occur at night, and during the day if attacks are diurnal. Treatment should be started with a small dose which is gradually increased over four or five days until the optimum dosage is determined. If the patient has been taking some other antiepileptic drug, it should be tapered off as the doses of MEBARAL are increased, to guard against the temporary marked attacks that may occur when any treatment for epilepsy is changed abruptly. Similarly, when the dose is to be lowered to a maintenance level or to be discontinued, the amount should be reduced gradually over four or five days.

Special Patient Population. Dosage should be reduced in the elderly or debilitated because these patients may be more sensitive to barbiturates. Dosage should be reduced for patients with impaired renal function or hepatic disease.

Combination with Other Drugs: MEBARAL may be used in combination with phenobarbital, either in the form of alternating courses or concurrently. When the two drugs are used at the same time, the dose should be about one-half the amount of each used alone. The average daily dose for an adult is from 50 mg to 100 mg ($\frac{3}{4}$ grain to 1$\frac{1}{2}$ grains) of phenobarbital and from 200 mg to 300 mg (3 grains to 4$\frac{1}{2}$ grains) of MEBARAL, brand of mephobarbital tablets.

MEBARAL may also be used with phenytoin sodium; in some cases, combined therapy appears to give better results than either agent used alone, since phenytoin sodium is particularly effective for the psychomotor types of seizure but relatively ineffective for petit mal. When the drugs are employed concurrently, a reduced dose of phenytoin sodium is advisable, but the full dose of MEBARAL may be given. Satisfactory results have been obtained with an average daily dose of 230 mg (3$\frac{1}{2}$ grains) of phenytoin sodium plus about 600 mg (9 grains) of MEBARAL.

Sedation: Adults: 32 mg to 100 mg ($\frac{1}{2}$ grain to 1$\frac{1}{2}$ grains) —optimum dose, 50 mg ($\frac{3}{4}$ grain)—three to four times daily. Children: 16 mg to 32 mg ($\frac{1}{4}$ grain to $\frac{1}{2}$ grain) three to four times daily.

HOW SUPPLIED

Tablets

32 mg ($\frac{1}{2}$ grain), bottles of 250
(NDC 0024-1231-05)
32 mg ($\frac{1}{2}$ grain), bottles of 1,000
(NDC 0024-1231-08)
50 mg ($\frac{3}{4}$ grain), bottles of 250
(NDC 0024-1232-05)
100 mg (1$\frac{1}{2}$ grains), bottles of 250
(NDC 0024-1233-05)

MW-86-V

NegGram® Caplets®   ℞
brand of nalidixic acid tablets, USP
NegGram® Suspension   ℞
brand of nalidixic acid oral suspension, USP

DESCRIPTION

Nalidixic acid, an oral antibacterial agent, is 1-Ethyl-1,4-dihydro-7-methyl-4-oxo-1,8-naphthyridine-3-carboxylic acid. It is a pale yellow, crystalline substance and a very weak organic acid.

Inactive Ingredients.—SUSPENSION: Carbomer 934P, FD&C Red #40, Flavor, Parabens, Purified Water, Saccharin Sodium, Sodium Chloride, Sorbitol Solution. CAPLETS: Hydrogenated Vegetable Oil, Methylcellulose, Microcrystalline Cellulose, Sodium Lauryl Sulfate, Yellow Ferric Oxide.

CLINICAL PHARMACOLOGY

NegGram has marked antibacterial activity against gram-negative bacteria including *Proteus mirabilis, P. morganii, P. vulgaris,* and *P. rettgeri; Escherichia coli;* Enterobacter (Aerobacter), and Klebsiella. Pseudomonas strains are generally resistant to the drug. NegGram is bactericidal and is effective over the entire urinary pH range. Conventional chromosomal resistance to NegGram taken in full dosage has been reported to emerge in approximately 2 to 14 percent of patients during treatment; however, bacterial resistance to NegGram has not been shown to be transferable via R factor.

INDICATIONS AND USAGE

NegGram is indicated for the treatment of urinary tract infections caused by susceptible gram-negative microorganisms, including the majority of Proteus strains, Klebsiella, Enterobacter (Aerobacter), and *E. coli.* Disc susceptibility testing with the 30 μg disc should be performed prior to administration of the drug, and during treatment if clinical response warrants.

CONTRAINDICATIONS

NegGram is contraindicated in patients with known hypersensitivity to nalidixic acid and in patients with a history of convulsive disorders.

WARNINGS

CNS effects including brief convulsions, increased intracranial pressure, and toxic psychosis have been reported rarely. These have occurred in infants and children or in geriatric patients, usually from overdosage or in patients with predisposing factors, and have been completely and rapidly reversible upon discontinuation of the drug. If these reactions occur, NegGram should be discontinued and appropriate therapeutic measures instituted; only if rapid disappearance of CNS symptoms does not occur within 48 hours should diagnostic procedures involving risk to the patient be undertaken. (See ADVERSE REACTIONS and OVERDOSAGE.)

PRECAUTIONS

Blood counts and renal and liver function tests should be performed periodically if treatment is continued for more than two weeks. NegGram should be used with caution in patients with liver disease, epilepsy, or severe cerebral arteriosclerosis. While caution should be used in patients with severe renal failure, therapeutic concentrations of NegGram in the urine, without increased toxicity due to drug accumulation in the blood, have been observed in patients on full dosage with creatinine clearances as low as 2 mL/minute to 8 mL/minute.

Patients should be cautioned to avoid undue exposure to direct sunlight while receiving NegGram. Therapy should be discontinued if photosensitivity occurs.

If bacterial resistance to NegGram emerges during treatment, it usually does so within 48 hours, permitting rapid change to another antimicrobial. Therefore, if the clinical response is unsatisfactory or if relapse occurs, cultures and sensitivity tests should be repeated. Underdosage with NegGram during initial treatment (with less than 4 g per day for adults) may predispose to emergence of bacterial resistance. (See DOSAGE AND ADMINISTRATION.)

Drug Interactions. Nitrofurantoin interferes with the therapeutic action of nalidixic acid.

Cross resistance between NegGram and other antimicrobials has been observed only with oxolinic acid.

Nalidixic acid may enhance the effects of oral anticoagulants, warfarin or bishydroxycoumarin, by displacing significant amounts from serum albumin binding sites.

When Benedict's or Fehling's solutions or Clinitest® Reagent Tablets are used to test the urine of patients taking NegGram, a false-positive reaction for glucose may be obtained, due to the liberation of glucuronic acid from the me-

Continued on next page

This product information was prepared in August, 1989. On these and other products of Winthrop Pharmaceuticals, detailed information may be obtained on a current basis by direct inquiry to the Professional Services Department, 90 Park Avenue, New York, NY 10016 (800) 446-6267.

Winthrop Pharm.—Cont.

tabolites excreted. However, a colorimetric test for glucose based on an enzyme reaction (eg, with Clinistix® Reagent Strips or Tes-Tape®) does not give a false-positive reaction to the liberated glucuronic acid.

Incorrect values may be obtained for urinary 17-keto and ketogenic steroids in patients receiving NegGram, brand of nalidixic acid, because of an interaction between the drug and the *m*-dinitrobenzene used in the usual assay method. In such cases, the Porter-Silber test for 17-hydroxycorticoids may be used.

Usage in Prepubertal Children. Recent toxicological studies have shown that nalidixic acid and related drugs can produce erosions of the cartilage in weight-bearing joints and other signs of arthropathy in immature animals of most species tested. No such joint lesions have been reported in man to date. Nevertheless, until the significance of this finding is clarified, care should be exercised when prescribing this product for prepubertal children.

Usage in Pregnancy. Safe use of NegGram during the first trimester of pregnancy has not been established. However, the drug has been used during the last two trimesters without producing apparent ill effects in mother or child. Caution should be used in administering NegGram in the days prior to delivery because of the theoretical risk that exposure to maternal nalidixic acid in utero may lead to significant blood levels of nalidixic acid in the neonate immediately after birth. Patients using NegGram during pregnancy should be advised to discontinue use at the first sign of labor.

ADVERSE REACTIONS

Reactions reported after oral administration of NegGram include *CNS effects:* drowsiness, weakness, headache, and dizziness and vertigo. Reversible subjective visual disturbances without objective findings have occurred infrequently (generally with each dose during the first few days of treatment). These reactions include overbrightness of lights, change in color perception, difficulty in focusing, decrease in visual acuity, and double vision. They usually disappeared promptly when dosage was reduced or therapy was discontinued. Toxic psychosis or brief convulsions have been reported rarely, usually following excessive doses. In general, the convulsions have occurred in patients with predisposing factors such as epilepsy or cerebral arteriosclerosis. In infants and children receiving therapeutic doses of NegGram, increased intracranial pressure with bulging anterior fontanel, papilledema, and headache has occasionally been observed. A few cases of 6th cranial nerve palsy have been reported. Although the mechanisms of these reactions are unknown, the signs and symptoms usually disappeared rapidly with no sequelae when treatment was discontinued. *Gastrointestinal:* abdominal pain, nausea, vomiting, and diarrhea. *Allergic:* rash, pruritus, urticaria, angioedema, eosinophilia, arthralgia with joint stiffness and swelling, and rarely, anaphylactoid reaction. Photosensitivity reactions consisting of erythema and bullae on exposed skin surfaces usually resolve completely in 2 weeks to 2 months after NegGram is discontinued; however, bullae may continue to appear with successive exposures to sunlight or with mild skin trauma for up to 3 months after discontinuation of drug. (See PRECAUTIONS.) *Other:* rarely, cholestasis, paresthesia, metabolic acidosis, thrombocytopenia, leukopenia, or hemolytic anemia, sometimes associated with glucose-6-phosphate dehydrogenase deficiency.

DOSAGE AND ADMINISTRATION

Adults. The recommended dosage for initial therapy in adults is 1 g administered four times daily for one or two weeks (total daily dose, 4 g). For prolonged therapy, the total daily dose may be reduced to 2 g after the initial treatment period. Underdosage during initial treatment may predispose to emergence of bacterial resistance.

Children. Until further experience is gained, NegGram should not be administered to infants younger than three months. Dosage in children 12 years of age and under should be calculated on the basis of body weight. The recommended total daily dosage for initial therapy is 25 mg/lb/day (55 mg/kg/day), administered in four equally divided doses. For prolonged therapy, the total daily dose may be reduced to 15 mg/lb/day (33 mg/kg/day). NegGram Suspension or NegGram CAPLETS of 250 mg may be used. One 250 mg tablet is equivalent to one teaspoon (5 mL) of the Suspension.

OVERDOSAGE

Manifestations: Toxic psychosis, convulsions, increased intracranial pressure, or metabolic acidosis may occur in patients taking more than the recommended dosage. Vomiting, nausea, and lethargy may also occur following overdosage. *Treatment:* Reactions are short-lived (two to three hours) because the drug is rapidly excreted. If overdosage is noted early, gastric lavage is indicated. If absorption has occurred, increased fluid administration is advisable and supportive measures such as oxygen and means of artificial respiration should be available. Although anticonvulsant therapy has

not been used in the few instances of overdosage reported, it may be indicated in a severe case.

HOW SUPPLIED

Suspension (250 mg/5 mL tsp), raspberry flavored, bottles of 1 pint (NDC 0024-1318-06)
CAPLETS of 1 g, scored, bottles of 100 (NDC 0024-1323-04)
Unit Dose Pack of 100 (NDC 0024-1323-14)— 10 strips of ten—1 g CAPLETS each
CAPLETS of 500 mg, scored, bottles of 56 (NDC 0024-1322-03), 500 (NDC 0024-1322-06), and 1000 (NDC 0024-1322-08)
Unit Dose Pack of 100 (NDC 0024-1322-14)—10 strips of ten-500 mg CAPLETS each
CAPLETS of 250 mg, scored, bottles of 56 (NDC 0024-1321-03)

PHARMACOLOGY

Following oral administration, NegGram, brand of nalidixic acid, is rapidly absorbed from the gastrointestinal tract, partially metabolized in the liver, and rapidly excreted through the kidneys. Unchanged nalidixic acid appears in the urine along with an active metabolite, hydroxynalidixic acid, which has antibacterial activity similar to that of nalidixic acid. Other metabolites include glucuronic acid conjugates of nalidixic acid and hydroxynalidixic acid, and the dicarboxylic acid derivative. The hydroxy metabolite represents 30 percent of the biologically active drug in the blood and 85 percent in the urine. Peak serum levels of active drug average approximately 20 µg to 40 µg per mL (90 percent protein bound), one to two hours after administration of a 1 g dose to a fasting normal individual, with a half-life of about 90 minutes. Peak urine levels of active drug average approximately 150 µg to 200 µg per mL, three to four hours after administration, with a half-life of about six hours. Approximately four percent of NegGram is excreted in the feces. Traces of nalidixic acid were found in blood and urine of an infant whose mother had received the drug during the last trimester of pregnancy.

ANIMAL PHARMACOLOGY

NegGram (nalidixic acid) and related drugs have been shown to cause arthropathy in juvenile animals of most species tested. (See PRECAUTIONS.)

Hydroxynalidixic acid, the principal metabolite of NegGram, did not produce any oculotoxic effects at any dosage level in seven species of animals including three primate species. However, oral administration of this metabolite in high doses has been shown to have oculotoxic potential, namely in dogs and cats where it produced retinal degeneration upon prolonged administration leading, in some cases, to blindness.

In experiments with NegGram itself, little if any such activity could be elicited in either dogs or cats. Sensitivity to CNS side effects in these species limited the doses of NegGram that could be used; this factor, together with a low conversion rate to the hydroxy metabolite in these species, may explain the absence of these effects.

Shown in Product Identification Section, page 435

NW-375-N(O)

NEO-SYNEPHRINE® Hydrochloride ℞
brand of phenylephrine hydrochloride
injection, USP
1% INJECTION

Well-Tolerated Vasoconstrictor and Pressor

> **WARNING:** PHYSICIANS SHOULD COMPLETELY FAMILIARIZE THEMSELVES WITH THE COMPLETE CONTENTS OF THIS LEAFLET BEFORE PRESCRIBING NEO-SYNEPHRINE.

DESCRIPTION

NEO-SYNEPHRINE hydrochloride, brand of phenylephrine hydrochloride injection, is a vasoconstrictor and pressor drug chemically related to epinephrine and ephedrine. NEO-SYNEPHRINE hydrochloride is a synthetic sympathomimetic agent in sterile form for parenteral injection. Chemically, phenylephrine hydrochloride is (−)-*m*-Hydroxy-α-[(methylamino) methyl] benzyl alcohol hydrochloride.

CLINICAL PHARMACOLOGY

NEO-SYNEPHRINE hydrochloride produces vasoconstriction that lasts longer than that of epinephrine and ephedrine. Responses are more sustained than those to epinephrine, lasting 20 minutes after intravenous and as long as 50 minutes after subcutaneous injection. Its action on the heart contrasts sharply with that of epinephrine and ephedrine, in that it slows the heart rate and increases the stroke output, producing no disturbance in the rhythm of the pulse. Phenylephrine is a powerful postsynaptic alpha-receptor stimulant with little effect on the beta receptors of the heart. In therapeutic doses, it produces little if any stimulation of either the spinal cord or cerebrum. A singular advantage of

this drug is the fact that repeated injections produce comparable effects.

The predominant actions of phenylephrine are on the cardiovascular system. Parenteral administration causes a rise in systolic and diastolic pressures in man and other species. Accompanying the pressor response to phenylephrine is a marked reflex bradycardia that can be blocked by atropine; after atropine, large doses of the drug increase the heart rate only slightly. In man, cardiac output is slightly decreased and peripheral resistance is considerably increased. Circulation time is slightly prolonged, and venous pressure is slightly increased; venous constriction is not marked. Most vascular beds are constricted; renal splanchnic, cutaneous, and limb blood flows are reduced but coronary blood flow is increased. Pulmonary vessels are constricted, and pulmonary arterial pressure is raised.

The drug is a powerful vasoconstrictor, with properties very similar to those of norepinephrine but almost completely lacking the chronotropic and inotropic actions on the heart. Cardiac irregularities are seen only very rarely even with large doses.

INDICATIONS AND USAGE

NEO-SYNEPHRINE is intended for the maintenance of an adequate level of blood pressure during spinal and inhalation anesthesia and for the treatment of vascular failure in shock, shocklike states, and drug-induced hypotension, or hypersensitivity. It is also employed to overcome paroxysmal supraventricular tachycardia, to prolong spinal anesthesia, and as a vasoconstrictor in regional analgesia.

CONTRAINDICATIONS

NEO-SYNEPHRINE hydrochloride should not be used in patients with severe hypertension, ventricular tachycardia, or in patients who are hypersensitive to it.

WARNINGS

If used in conjunction with oxytocic drugs, the pressor effect of sympathomimetic pressor amines is potentiated (see Drug Interaction). The obstetrician should be warned that some oxytocic drugs may cause severe persistent hypertension and that even a rupture of a cerebral blood vessel may occur during the postpartum period.

Contains sodium metabisulfite, a sulfite that may cause allergic-type reactions including anaphylactic symptoms and life-threatening or less severe asthmatic episodes in certain susceptible people. The overall prevalence of sulfite sensitivity in the general population is unknown and probably low. Sulfite sensitivity is seen more frequently in asthmatic than in nonasthmatic people.

PRECAUTIONS

NEO-SYNEPHRINE hydrochloride should be employed only with extreme caution in elderly patients or in patients with hyperthyroidism, bradycardia, partial heart block, myocardial disease, or severe arteriosclerosis.

Drug Interactions—Vasopressors, particularly metaraminol, may cause serious cardiac arrhythmias during halothane anesthesia and therefore should be used only with great caution or not at all.

MAO Inhibitors—The pressor effect of sympathomimetic pressor amines is markedly potentiated in patients receiving monoamine oxidase inhibitors (MAOI). Therefore, when initiating pressor therapy in these patients, the initial dose should be small and used with due caution. The pressor response of adrenergic agents may also be potentiated by tricyclic antidepressants.

Carcinogenesis, Mutagenesis, Impairment of Fertility—No long-term animal studies have been done to evaluate the potential of NEO-SYNEPHRINE in these areas.

Pregnancy Category C—Animal reproduction studies have not been conducted with NEO-SYNEPHRINE. It is also not known whether NEO-SYNEPHRINE can cause fetal harm when administered to a pregnant woman or can affect reproduction capacity. NEO-SYNEPHRINE should be given to a pregnant woman only if clearly needed.

Labor and Delivery—If vasopressor drugs are either used to correct hypotension or added to the local anesthetic solution, the obstetrician should be cautioned that some oxytocic drugs may cause severe persistent hypertension and that even a rupture of a cerebral blood vessel may occur during the postpartum period (see WARNINGS).

Nursing Mother—It is not known whether this drug is excreted in human milk. Because many are excreted in human milk, caution should be exercised when NEO-SYNEPHRINE hydrochloride, brand of phenylephrine hydrochloride injection, is administered to a nursing woman.

Pediatric Use—To combat hypotension during spinal anesthesia in children, a dose of 0.5 mg to 1 mg per 25 pounds of body weight, administered subcutaneously or intramuscularly, is recommended.

ADVERSE REACTIONS

Headache, reflex bradycardia, excitability, restlessness, and rarely arrhythmias.

OVERDOSAGE

Overdosage may induce ventricular extrasystoles and short paroxysms of ventricular tachycardia, a sensation of fullness in the head and tingling of the extremities.

Should an excessive elevation of blood pressure occur, it may be immediately relieved by an α-adrenergic blocking agent, eg, phentolamine.

The oral LD_{50} in the rat is 350 mg/kg, in the mouse 120 mg/kg.

DOSAGE AND ADMINISTRATION

NEO-SYNEPHRINE is generally injected subcutaneously, intramuscularly, slowly intravenously, or in dilute solution as a continuous intravenous infusion. In patients with paroxysmal supraventricular tachycardia and, if indicated, in case of emergency, NEO-SYNEPHRINE is administered directly intravenously. The dose should be adjusted according to the pressor response.

Dosage Calculations

Dose Required	Use NEO-SYNEPHRINE 1%
10 mg	1 mL
5 mg	0.5 mL
1 mg	0.1 mL

For convenience in intermittent intravenous administration, dilute 1 mL NEO-SYNEPHRINE 1% with 9 mL Sterile Water for Injection, USP, to yield 0.1% NEO-SYNEPHRINE.

Dose Required	Use Diluted NEO-SYNEPHRINE (0.1%)
0.1 mg	0.1 mL
0.2 mg	0.2 mL
0.5 mg	0.5 mL

Mild or Moderate Hypotension
Subcutaneously or Intramuscularly: Usual dose, from 2 mg to 5 mg. Range, from 1 mg to 10 mg. Initial dose should not exceed 5 mg.
Intravenously: Usual dose, 0.2 mg. Range, from 0.1 mg to 0.5 mg. Initial dose should not exceed 0.5 mg.
Injections should not be repeated more often than every 10 to 15 minutes. A 5 mg intramuscular dose should raise blood pressure for one to two hours. A 0.5 mg intravenous dose should elevate the pressure for about 15 minutes.

Severe Hypotension and Shock—Including Drug-Related Hypotension
Blood volume depletion should always be corrected as fully as possible before any vasopressor is administered. When, as an emergency measure, intraaortic pressures must be maintained to prevent cerebral or coronary artery ischemia, NEO-SYNEPHRINE hydrochloride, brand of phenylephrine hydrochloride injection, can be administered before and concurrently with blood volume replacement.

Hypotension and occasionally severe shock may result from overdosage or idiosyncrasy following the administration of certain drugs, especially adrenergic and ganglionic blocking agents, rauwolfia and veratrum alkaloids, and phenothiazine tranquilizers. Patients who receive a phenothiazine derivative as preoperative medication are especially susceptible to these reactions. As an adjunct in the management of such episodes, NEO-SYNEPHRINE hydrochloride is a suitable agent for restoring blood pressure.

Higher initial and maintenance doses of NEO-SYNEPHRINE are required in patients with persistent or untreated severe hypotension or shock. Hypotension produced by powerful peripheral adrenergic blocking agents, chlorpromazine, or pheochromocytomectomy may also require more intensive therapy.

Continuous Infusion—Add 10 mg of the drug (1 mL of 1 percent solution) to 500 mL of Dextrose Injection, USP, or Sodium Chloride Injection, USP (providing a 1:50,000 solution). To raise the blood pressure rapidly, start the infusion at about 100 µg to 180 µg per minute (based on 20 drops per mL this would be 100 to 180 drops per minute). When the blood pressure is stabilized (at a low normal level for the individual), a maintenance rate of 40 µg to 60 µg per minute usually suffices (based on 20 drops per mL this would be 40 to 60 drops per minute). If the drop size of the infusion system varies from the 20 drops per mL, the dose must be adjusted accordingly.

If a prompt initial pressor response is not obtained, additional increments of NEO-SYNEPHRINE (10 mg or more) are added to the infusion bottle. The rate of flow is then adjusted until the desired blood pressure level is obtained. (In some cases, a more potent vasopressor, such as norepinephrine bitartrate, may be required.) Hypertension should be avoided. The blood pressure should be checked frequently. Headache and/or bradycardia may indicate hypertension. Arrhythmias are rare.

Spinal Anesthesia—Hypotension
Routine parenteral use of NEO-SYNEPHRINE has been recommended for the prophylaxis and treatment of hypotension during spinal anesthesia. It is best administered subcu-

taneously or intramuscularly three or four minutes before injection of the spinal anesthetic. The total requirement for high anesthetic levels is usually 3 mg, and for lower levels, 2 mg. For hypotensive emergencies during spinal anesthesia, NEO-SYNEPHRINE may be injected intravenously, using an initial dose of 0.2 mg. Any subsequent dose should not exceed the previous dose by more than 0.1 mg to 0.2 mg and no more than 0.5 mg should be administered in a single dose. To combat hypotension during spinal anesthesia in children, a dose of 0.5 mg to 1 mg per 25 pounds body weight, administered subcutaneously or intramuscularly, is recommended.

Prolongation of Spinal Anesthesia
The addition of 2 mg to 5 mg of NEO-SYNEPHRINE hydrochloride to the anesthetic solution increases the duration of motor block by as much as approximately 50 percent without any increase in the incidence of complications such as nausea, vomiting, or blood pressure disturbances.

Vasoconstrictor for Regional Analgesia
Concentrations about ten times those employed when epinephrine is used as a vasoconstrictor are recommended. The optimum strength is 1:20,000 (made by adding 1 mg of NEO-SYNEPHRINE hydrochloride to every 20 mL of local anesthetic solution). Some pressor responses can be expected when 2 mg or more are injected.

Paroxysmal Supraventricular Tachycardia
Rapid intravenous injection (within 20 to 30 seconds) is recommended; the initial dose should not exceed 0.5 mg, and subsequent doses, which are determined by the initial blood pressure response, should not exceed the preceding dose by more than 0.1 mg to 0.2 mg, and should never exceed 1 mg.

HOW SUPPLIED

Solution 1 percent
Each 1 mL contains 10 mg of NEO-SYNEPHRINE hydrochloride, 3.5 mg of sodium chloride, 4 mg of sodium citrate, 1 mg of citric acid monohydrate, and not more than 2 mg of sodium metabisulfite.

Uni-Nest™ ampuls of 1 mL, box of 25 (NDC 0024-1342-04).

CARPUJECT® Sterile Cartridge-Needle Unit, 10 mg/mL (1 mL fill in 2 mL cartridge), 22-gauge, 1¼ inch needle, dispensing box of 50 (NDC 0024-1340-02).

The air in all ampuls and Cartridge-Needle Units has been displaced by nitrogen gas.

Protect from light if removed from carton or dispensing bin.

NW-64-EE

NEO–SYNEPHRINE® Hydrochloride ℞
brand of phenylephrine hydrochloride
ophthalmic solution, USP
Vasoconstrictor and Mydriatic
SOLUTIONS 2.5% AND 10%
VISCOUS SOLUTION 10%

For Use in Ophthalmology

> **WARNING: PHYSICIANS SHOULD COMPLETELY FAMILIARIZE THEMSELVES WITH THE COMPLETE CONTENTS OF THIS LEAFLET BEFORE PRESCRIBING NEO-SYNEPHRINE.**

DESCRIPTION

NEO-SYNEPHRINE hydrochloride, brand of phenylephrine hydrochloride ophthalmic solution, is a sterile solution used as a vasoconstrictor and mydriatic for use in ophthalmology. NEO-SYNEPHRINE hydrochloride is a synthetic sympathomimetic compound structurally similar to epinephrine and ephedrine.

Phenylephrine hydrochloride is (–)-m-Hydroxy-α-[(methylamino)methyl] benzyl alcohol hydrochloride.

CLINICAL PHARMACOLOGY

NEO-SYNEPHRINE possesses predominantly α-adrenergic effects. In the eye, phenylephrine acts locally as a potent vasoconstrictor and mydriatic, by constricting ophthalmic blood vessels and the radial muscle of the iris.

The ophthalmologic usefulness of NEO-SYNEPHRINE hydrochloride is due to its rapid effect and moderately prolonged action, as well as to the fact that it produces no compensatory vasodilatation.

The action of different concentrations of ophthalmic solutions of NEO-SYNEPHRINE hydrochloride is shown in the following table:

Strength of solution (%)	Mydriasis		Paralysis of accommodation
	Maximal (minutes)	Recovery time (hours)	
2.5	15-60	3	trace
10	10-60	6	slight

Although rare, systemic absorption of sufficient quantities of phenylephrine may lead to systemic α-adrenergic effects, such as rise in blood pressure which may be accompanied by a reflex atropine-sensitive bradycardia.

INDICATIONS AND USAGE

NEO-SYNEPHRINE hydrochloride is recommended for use as a decongestant and vasoconstrictor and for pupil dilatation in uveitis (posterior synechiae), wide angle glaucoma, prior to surgery, refraction, ophthalmoscopic examination, and diagnostic procedures.

CONTRAINDICATIONS

Ophthalmic solutions of NEO-SYNEPHRINE hydrochloride are contraindicated in persons with narrow angle glaucoma (and in those individuals who are hypersensitive to NEO-SYNEPHRINE). NEO-SYNEPHRINE hydrochloride 10 percent ophthalmic solutions are contraindicated in infants and in patients with aneurysms.

WARNINGS

There have been rare reports associating the use of NEO-SYNEPHRINE 10 percent ophthalmic solutions with the development of serious cardiovascular reactions, including ventricular arrhythmias and myocardial infarctions. These episodes, some ending fatally, have usually occurred in elderly patients with preexisting cardiovascular diseases.

PRECAUTIONS

Exceeding recommended dosages or applying NEO-SYNEPHRINE hydrochloride ophthalmic solutions to the instrumented, traumatized, diseased or postsurgical eye or adnexa, or to patients with suppressed lacrimation, as during anesthesia, may result in the absorption of sufficient quantities of phenylephrine to produce a systemic vasopressor response.

A significant elevation in blood pressure is rare but has been reported following conjunctival instillation of recommended doses of NEO-SYNEPHRINE 10 percent ophthalmic solutions. Caution, therefore, should be exercised in administering the 10 percent solutions to children of low body weight, the elderly, and patients with insulin-dependent diabetes, hypertension, hyperthyroidism, generalized arteriosclerosis, or cardiovascular disease. The posttreatment blood pressure of these patients, and any patients who develop symptoms, should be carefully monitored.

Ordinarily, any mydriatic, including NEO-SYNEPHRINE hydrochloride, brand of phenylephrine hydrochloride ophthalmic solution, is contraindicated in patients with glaucoma, since it may occasionally raise intraocular pressure. However, when temporary dilatation of the pupil may free adhesions or when vasoconstriction of intrinsic vessels may lower intraocular tension, these advantages may temporarily outweigh the danger from coincident dilatation of the pupil.

Rebound miosis has been reported in older persons one day after receiving NEO-SYNEPHRINE hydrochloride ophthalmic solutions, and reinstillation of the drug produced a reduction in mydriasis. This may be of clinical importance in dilating the pupils of older subjects prior to retinal detachment or cataract surgery.

Due to a strong action of the drug on the dilator muscle, older individuals may also develop transient pigment floaters in the aqueous humor 30 to 45 minutes following the administration of NEO-SYNEPHRINE hydrochloride ophthalmic solutions. The appearance may be similar to anterior uveitis or to a microscopic hyphema.

To prevent pain, a drop of suitable topical anesthetic may be applied before using the 10 percent ophthalmic solution.

Drug Interaction: As with all other adrenergic drugs, when NEO-SYNEPHRINE 10 percent ophthalmic solutions or 2.5 percent ophthalmic solution is administered simultaneously with, or up to 21 days after, administration of monoamine oxidase (MAO) inhibitors, careful supervision and adjustment of dosages are required since exaggerated adrenergic effects may occur. The pressor response of adrenergic agents may also be potentiated by tricyclic antidepressants, propranolol, reserpine, guanethidine, methyldopa, and atropine-like drugs.

It has been reported that the concomitant use of NEO-SYNEPHRINE 10 percent ophthalmic solutions and systemic beta blockers has caused acute hypertension and, in one case, the rupture of a congenital cerebral aneurysm. NEO-SYNEPHRINE may potentiate the cardiovascular depressant effects of potent inhalation anesthetic agents.

Continued on next page

This product information was prepared in August, 1989. On these and other products of Winthrop Pharmaceuticals, detailed information may be obtained on a current basis by direct inquiry to the Professional Services Department, 90 Park Avenue, New York, NY 10016 (800) 446-6267.

Winthrop Pharm.—Cont.

Carcinogenesis, Mutagenesis, Impairment of Fertility: No long-term animal studies have been done to evaluate the potential of NEO-SYNEPHRINE in these areas.

Pregnancy Category C: Animal reproduction studies have not been conducted with NEO-SYNEPHRINE. It is also not known whether NEO-SYNEPHRINE can cause fetal harm when administered to a pregnant woman or can affect reproduction capacity. NEO-SYNEPHRINE should be given to a pregnant woman only if clearly needed.

Nursing Mothers: It is not known whether this drug is excreted in milk; many are. Caution should be exercised when NEO-SYNEPHRINE hydrochloride ophthalmic solution is administered to a nursing woman.

Pediatric Use: NEO-SYNEPHRINE hydrochloride 10 percent ophthalmic solutions are contraindicated in infants. (See CONTRAINDICATIONS.) For use in older children see DOSAGE AND ADMINISTRATION.

Exceeding recommended dosages or applying NEO-SYNEPHRINE hydrochloride ophthalmic solutions to the instrumented, traumatized, diseased or postsurgical eye or adnexa, or to patients with suppressed lacrimation, as during anesthesia, may result in the absorption of sufficient quantities of phenylephrine to produce a systemic vasopressor response.

The hypertensive effects of phenylephrine may be treated with an alpha-adrenergic blocking agent such as phentolamine mesylate, 5 mg to 10 mg intravenously, repeated as necessary.

The oral LD$_{50}$ of phenylephrine in the rat: 350 mg/kg, in the mouse: 120 mg/kg.

DOSAGE AND ADMINISTRATION

Prolonged exposure to air or strong light may cause oxidation and discoloration. Do not use if solution is brown or contains a precipitate.

Vasoconstriction and Pupil Dilatation

NEO-SYNEPHRINE hydrochloride 10 percent ophthalmic solutions are especially useful when rapid and powerful dilatation of the pupil and reduction of congestion in the capillary bed are desired. A drop of a suitable topical anesthetic may be applied, followed in a few minutes by 1 drop of the NEO-SYNEPHRINE hydrochloride 10 percent ophthalmic solution on the upper limbus. The anesthetic prevents stinging and consequent dilution of the solution by lacrimation. It may occasionally be necessary to repeat the instillation after one hour, again preceded by the use of the topical anesthetic.

Uveitis: Posterior Synechiae

NEO-SYNEPHRINE hydrochloride 10 percent ophthalmic solutions may be used in patients with uveitis when synechiae are present or may develop. The formation of synechiae may be prevented by the use of the 10 percent ophthalmic solutions and atropine to produce wide dilatation of the pupil. It should be emphasized, however, that the vasoconstrictor effect of NEO-SYNEPHRINE hydrochloride may be antagonistic to the increase of local blood flow in uveal infection.

To free recently formed posterior synechiae, 1 drop of the 10 percent ophthalmic solutions may be applied to the upper surface of the cornea. On the following day, treatment may be continued if necessary. In the interim, hot compresses should be applied for five or ten minutes three times a day, with 1 drop of a 1 or 2 percent solution of atropine sulfate before and after each series of compresses.

Glaucoma

In certain patients with glaucoma, temporary reduction of intraocular tension may be attained by producing vasoconstriction of the intraocular vessels; this may be accomplished by placing 1 drop of the 10 percent ophthalmic solutions on the upper surface of the cornea. This treatment may be repeated as often as necessary.

NEO-SYNEPHRINE hydrochloride, brand of phenylephrine hydrochloride ophthalmic solution, may be used with miotics in patients with wide angle glaucoma. It reduces the difficulties experienced by the patient because of the small field produced by miosis, and still it permits and often supports the effect of the miotic in lowering the intraocular pressure. Hence, there may be marked improvement in visual acuity after using NEO-SYNEPHRINE hydrochloride in conjunction with miotic drugs.

Surgery

When a short-acting mydriatic is needed for wide dilatation of the pupil before intraocular surgery, the 10 percent ophthalmic solutions or 2.5 percent ophthalmic solution may be applied topically from 30 to 60 minutes before the operation.

Refraction

Prior to determination of refractive errors, NEO-SYNEPHRINE hydrochloride 2.5 percent ophthalmic solution may be used effectively with homatropine hydrobromide, atropine sulfate, or a combination of homatropine and cocaine hydrochloride.

For *adults*, a drop of the preferred cycloplegic is placed in each eye, followed in five minutes by 1 drop of NEO-SYNEPHRINE hydrochloride 2.5 percent ophthalmic solution and in ten minutes by another drop of the cycloplegic. In 50 to 60 minutes, the eyes are ready for refraction.

For *children*, a drop of atropine sulfate 1 percent is placed in each eye, followed in 10 to 15 minutes by 1 drop of NEO-SYNEPHRINE hydrochloride 2.5 percent ophthalmic solution and in five to ten minutes by a second drop of atropine sulfate 1 percent. In one to two hours, the eyes are ready for refraction.

For a "one application method," NEO-SYNEPHRINE hydrochloride 2.5 percent ophthalmic solution may be combined with a cycloplegic to elicit synergistic action. The additive effect varies depending on the patient. Therefore, when using a "one application method," it may be desirable to increase the concentration of the cycloplegic.

Ophthalmoscopic Examination

One drop of NEO-SYNEPHRINE hydrochloride 2.5 percent ophthalmic solution is placed in each eye. Sufficient mydriasis to permit examination is produced in 15 to 30 minutes. Dilatation lasts from one to three hours.

Diagnostic Procedures

Provocative Test for Angle Block in Patients with Glaucoma: The 2.5 percent ophthalmic solution may be used as a provocative test when latent increased intraocular pressure is suspected. Tension is measured before application of NEO-SYNEPHRINE hydrochloride and again after dilatation. A 3 to 5 mm of mercury rise in pressure suggests the presence of angle block in patients with glaucoma; however, failure to obtain such a rise does not preclude the presence of glaucoma from other causes.

Shadow Test (Retinoscopy): When dilatation of the pupil without cycloplegic action is desired for the shadow test, the 2.5 percent ophthalmic solution may be used alone.

Blanching Test: One or 2 drops of the 2.5 percent ophthalmic solution should be applied to the injected eye. After five minutes, examine for perilimbal blanching. If blanching occurs, the congestion is superficial and probably does not indicate iritis.

HOW SUPPLIED

In Mono-Drop ® (plastic dropper) bottle:

Low surface tension solutions

2.5   percent ophthalmic solution — NEO-SYNEPHRINE hydrochloride, brand of phenylephrine hydrochloride ophthalmic solution, 2.5 percent in a sterile, isotonic, buffered, low surface tension vehicle with sodium phosphate, sodium biphosphate, boric acid, and, as antiseptic preservative, benzalkonium chloride, NF, 1:7500. The pH is adjusted with phosphoric acid or sodium hydroxide.

     Bottles of 15 mL (NDC 0024-1358-01)

10   percent ophthalmic solution — NEO-SYNEPHRINE hydrochloride 10 percent in a sterile, buffered, low surface tension vehicle with sodium phosphate, sodium biphosphate, and, as antiseptic preservative, benzalkonium chloride 1:10,000. The pH is adjusted with phosphoric acid or sodium hydroxide.

     Bottles of 5 mL (NDC 0024-1359-01)

Viscous solution

10   percent ophthalmic solution — NEO-SYNEPHRINE hydrochloride 10 percent in a sterile, buffered, viscous vehicle with sodium phosphate, sodium biphosphate, methylcellulose, and, as antiseptic preservative, benzalkonium chloride 1:10,000. The pH is adjusted with phosphoric acid or sodium hydroxide.

     Bottles of 5 mL (NDC 0024-1362-01)

NW-147-CC

NOVOCAIN®   ℞

brand of procaine hydrochloride injection, USP

DESCRIPTION

Procaine hydrochloride is benzoic acid, 4-amino-, 2-(diethylamino)ethyl ester, monohydrochloride, the ester of diethylaminoethanol and aminobenzoic acid.

It is a white crystalline, odorless powder that is freely soluble in water, but less soluble in alcohol.

HOW SUPPLIED

NOVOCAIN Solution 1 percent

Unit-Nest™, single-dose ampuls of 2 mL, box of 25 **NDC 0024-1381-25**

Single-dose ampuls of 6 mL, box of 50 **NDC** 0024-1381-05

Multiple-dose vials of 30 mL, box of 1 **NDC** 0024-1385-01

NOVOCAIN Solution 2 percent

Multiple-dose vials of 30 mL, box of 1 **NDC** 0024-1386-01

For complete prescribing information, see package insert or contact Professional Services Department.

NW-63-U

NOVOCAIN®   ℞

brand of procaine hydrochloride injection, USP

10% Solution for Spinal Anesthesia

DESCRIPTION

NOVOCAIN, brand of procaine hydrochloride, is benzoic acid, 4-amino-, 2-(diethylamino) ethyl ester, monohydrochloride, the ester of diethylaminoethanol and aminobenzoic acid.

It is a white crystalline, odorless powder that is freely soluble in water, but less soluble in alcohol. Each mL contains 100 mg procaine hydrochloride and 4 mg acetone sodium bisulfite as antioxidant. DO NOT USE SOLUTIONS IF CRYSTALS, CLOUDINESS, OR DISCOLORATION IS OBSERVED. EXAMINE SOLUTIONS CAREFULLY BEFORE USE. REAUTOCLAVING INCREASES LIKELIHOOD OF CRYSTAL FORMATION.

CLINICAL PHARMACOLOGY

NOVOCAIN stabilizes the neuronal membrane and prevents the initiation and transmission of nerve impulses, thereby effecting local anesthesia. NOVOCAIN lacks surface anesthetic activity. The onset of action is rapid (2 to 5 minutes) and the duration of action is relatively short (average 1 to 1½ hours), depending upon the anesthetic technique, the type of block, the concentration, and the individual patient.

NOVOCAIN is readily absorbed following parenteral administration and is rapidly hydrolyzed by plasma cholinesterase to aminobenzoic acid and diethylaminoethanol.

A vasoconstrictor may be added to the solution of NOVOCAIN to promote local hemostasis, delay systemic absorption, and increase duration of anesthesia.

INDICATIONS AND USAGE

NOVOCAIN is indicated for spinal anesthesia.

CONTRAINDICATIONS

Spinal anesthesia with NOVOCAIN is contraindicated in patients with generalized septicemia: sepsis at the proposed injection site; certain diseases of the cerebrospinal system, eg, meningitis, syphilis; and a known hypersensitivity to the drug, drugs of a similar chemical configuration, or aminobenzoic acid or its derivatives.

The decision as to whether or not spinal anesthesia should be used in an individual case should be made by the physician after weighing the advantages with the risks and possible complications.

WARNINGS

RESUSCITATIVE EQUIPMENT AND DRUGS SHOULD BE IMMEDIATELY AVAILABLE WHENEVER ANY LOCAL ANESTHETIC DRUG IS USED. Spinal anesthesia should only be administered by those qualified to do so.

Large doses of local anesthetics should not be used in patients with heart block.

Reactions resulting in fatality have occurred on rare occasions with the use of local anesthetics, even in the absence of a history of hypersensitivity.

Usage in Pregnancy. Safe use of NOVOCAIN has not been established with respect to adverse effects on fetal development. Careful consideration should be given to this fact before administering this drug to women of childbearing potential particularly during early pregnancy. This does not exclude the use of the drug at term for obstetrical analgesia.

Vasopressor agents (administered for the treatment of hypotension or added to the anesthetic solution for vasoconstriction) should be used with extreme caution in the presence of oxytocic drugs as they may produce severe, persistent hypertension with possible rupture of a cerebral blood vessel.

Solutions which contain a vasoconstrictor should be used with extreme caution in patients receiving drugs known to produce alterations in blood pressure (ie, monoamine oxidase inhibitors (MAOI), tricyclic antidepressants, phenothiazines, etc), as either severe sustained hypertension or hypotension may occur.

Local anesthetic procedures should be used with caution when there is inflammation and/or sepsis in the region of the proposed injection.

Contains acetone sodium bisulfite, a sulfite that may cause allergic-type reactions including anaphylactic symptoms and life-threatening or less severe asthmatic episodes in certain susceptible people. The overall prevalence of sulfite sensitivity in the general population is unknown and probably low. Sulfite sensitivity is seen more frequently in asthmatic than in nonasthmatic people.

PRECAUTIONS

Standard textbooks should be consulted for specific techniques and precautions for various spinal anesthetic procedures.

The safety and effectiveness of a spinal anesthetic depend upon proper dosage, correct technique, adequate precautions, and readiness for emergencies. The lowest dosage that results in effective anesthesia should be used to avoid high plasma levels and possible adverse effects. Tolerance varies with the status of the patient. Debilitated, elderly patients, or acutely ill patients should be given reduced doses commensurate with their weight and physical status. Reduced dosages are also indicated for obstetric delivery and patients with increased intra-abdominal pressure.

The decision whether or not to use spinal anesthesia in the following disease states depends on the physician's appraisal of the advantages as opposed to the risk: cardiovascular disease (ie, shock, hypertension, anemia, etc), pulmonary disease, renal impairment, metabolic or endocrine disorders, gastrointestinal disorders (ie, intestinal obstruction, peritonitis, etc), or complicated obstetrical deliveries.

NOVOCAIN SHOULD BE USED WITH CAUTION IN PATIENTS WITH KNOWN DRUG ALLERGIES AND SENSITIVITIES. A thorough history of the patient's prior experience with NOVOCAIN or other local anesthetics as well as concomitant or recent drug use should be taken (see CONTRAINDICATIONS). NOVOCAIN should not be used in any condition in which a sulfonamide drug is being employed since aminobenzoic acid inhibits the action of sulfonamides. Solutions containing a vasopressor should be used with caution in the presence of diseases which may adversely affect the cardiovascular system.

NOVOCAIN, brand of procaine hydrochloride injection, should be used with caution in patients with severe disturbances of cardiac rhythm, shock or heart block.

ADVERSE REACTIONS

Systemic adverse reactions involving the central nervous system and the cardiovascular system usually result from high plasma levels due to excessive dosage, rapid absorption, or inadvertent intravascular injection. In addition, use of inappropriate doses or techniques may result in extensive spinal blockade leading to hypotension and respiratory arrest.

A small number of reactions may result from hypersensitivity, idiosyncrasy, or diminished tolerance to normal dosage. *Excitatory CNS effects* (nervousness, dizziness, blurred vision, tremors) commonly represent the initial signs of local anesthetic systemic toxicity. However, these reactions may be very brief or absent in some patients in which case the first manifestation of toxicity may be drowsiness or convulsions merging into unconsciousness and respiratory arrest. *Cardiovascular system* reactions include depression of the myocardium, hypotension (or sometimes hypertension), bradycardia, and even cardiac arrest.

Allergic reactions are characterized by cutaneous lesions of delayed onset, or urticaria, edema, and other manifestations of allergy. The detection of sensitivity by skin testing is of limited value. As with other local anesthetics, hypersensitivity, idiosyncrasy and anaphylactoid reactions have occurred rarely. The reaction may be abrupt and severe and is not usually dose related.

The following adverse reactions may occur with spinal anesthesia: *Central Nervous System:* postspinal headache, meningismus, arachnoiditis, palsies, or spinal nerve paralysis. *Cardiovascular:* hypotension due to vasomotor paralysis and pooling of the blood in the venous bed. *Respiratory:* respiratory impairment or paralysis due to the level of anesthesia extending to the upper thoracic and cervical segments. *Gastrointestinal:* nausea and vomiting.

Treatment of Reactions. Toxic effects of local anesthetics require symptomatic treatment: there is no specific cure. The physician should be prepared to maintain an airway and to support ventilation with oxygen and assisted or controlled respiration as required. Supportive treatment of the cardiovascular system includes intravenous fluids and, when appropriate, vasopressors (preferably those that stimulate the myocardium, such as ephedrine). Convulsions may be controlled with oxygen and by the intravenous administration of diazepam or ultrashort-acting barbiturates or a short-acting muscle relaxant (succinylcholine). Intravenous anticonvulsant agents and muscle relaxants should only be administered by those familiar with their use and only when ventilation and oxygenation are assured. In spinal and epidural anesthesia, sympathetic blockade also occurs as a pharmacological reaction, resulting in peripheral vasodilation and often *hypotension*. The extent of the hypotension will usually depend on the number of dermatomes blocked. The blood pressure should therefore be monitored in the early phases of anesthesia. If hypotension occurs, it is readily controlled by vasoconstrictors administered either by the intramuscular or the intravenous route, the dosage of which would depend on the severity of the hypotension and the response to treatment.

DOSAGE AND ADMINISTRATION

As with all local anesthetics, the dose of NOVOCAIN, brand of procaine hydrochloride injection, varies and depends upon the area to be anesthetized, the vascularity of the tissues, the number of neuronal segments to be blocked, individual tolerance, and the technique of anesthesia. The lowest dose needed to provide effective anesthesia should be adminis-

tered. For specific techniques and procedures, refer to standard textbooks.
[See table above].
The diluent may be sterile normal saline, sterile distilled water, spinal fluid; and for hyperbaric technique, sterile dextrose solution.
The usual rate of injection is 1 mL per 5 seconds. Full anesthesia and fixation usually occur in 5 minutes.

STERILIZATION

The drug in intact ampuls is sterile. The preferred method of destroying bacteria on the exterior of ampuls before opening is heat sterilization (autoclaving). Immersion in antiseptic solution is not recommended.
Autoclave at 15-pound pressure, at 121°C (250°F), for 15 minutes. The diluent dextrose may show some brown discoloration due to caramelization.

HOW SUPPLIED

Uni-Nest™—ampuls of 2 mL (200 mg), box of 25 (NDC 0024-1384-25).
Protect solutions from light.
The air in the ampuls has been displaced by nitrogen gas.

NW 62-Q

PEDIACOF®   C ℞

DESCRIPTION

Each teaspoon (5 mL) contains:
Codeine phosphate, USP .... 5.0 mg
 (Warning: May be habit forming.)
Phenylephrine hydrochloride, USP .... 2.5 mg
Chlorpheniramine maleate, USP .... 0.75 mg
Potassium iodide, USP .... 75.0 mg
with sodium benzoate 0.2% as preservative and alcohol 5%.
Inactive Ingredients: Alcohol, Citric Acid, FD&C Red #40, Flavor, Glycerin, Liquid Glucose, Purified Water, Saccharin Sodium, Sodium Benzoate.

HOW SUPPLIED

Bottle of 16 fl oz (NDC 0024-1509-06)
Available on prescription only.
For complete prescribing information see package insert or contact Professional Services Department.

PW-295-K

---

pHisoDerm®   OTC

(See PDR For Nonprescription Drugs)

---

pHisoHex®   ℞
brand of hexachlorophene detergent cleanser

sudsing antibacterial soapless skin cleanser

DESCRIPTION

pHisoHex, brand of hexachlorophene detergent cleanser, is an antibacterial sudsing emulsion for topical administration. pHisoHex contains a colloidal dispersion of hexachlorophene 3% (w/w) in a stable emulsion consisting of entsufon sodium, petrolatum, lanolin cholesterols, methylcellulose, polyethylene glycol, polyethylene glycol monostearate, lauryl myristyl diethanolamide, sodium benzoate, and water. pH is adjusted with hydrochloric acid. Entsufon sodium is a synthetic detergent.
Chemically, hexachlorophene is Phenol, 2, 2'-methylenebis[3,4,6-trichloro-.

CLINICAL PHARMACOLOGY

pHisoHex is a bacteriostatic cleansing agent. It cleanses the skin thoroughly and has bacteriostatic action against staphylococci and other gram-positive bacteria. Cumulative antibacterial action develops with repeated use. Cleansing with alcohol or soaps containing alcohol removes the antibacterial residue.
Detectable blood levels of hexachlorophene following absorption through intact skin have been found in subjects who regularly scrubbed with hexachlorophene emulsion 3%. (See WARNINGS for additional information.)

pHisoHex has the same slight acidity as normal skin (pH value 5.0 to 6.0).

INDICATIONS AND USAGE

pHisoHex is indicated for use as a surgical scrub and a bacteriostatic skin cleanser. It may also be used to control an outbreak of gram-positive infection where other infection control procedures have been unsuccessful. Use only as long as necessary for infection control.

CONTRAINDICATIONS

pHisoHex should not be used on burned or denuded skin. It should not be used as an occlusive dressing, wet pack, or lotion.
It should not be used routinely for prophylactic total body bathing.
It should not be used as a vaginal pack or tampon, or on any mucous membranes.
pHisoHex should not be used on persons with sensitivity to any of its components. It should not be used on persons who have demonstrated primary light sensitivity to halogenated phenol derivatives because of the possibility of cross-sensitivity to hexachlorophene.

WARNINGS

RINSE THOROUGHLY AFTER EACH USE. Patients should be closely monitored and use should be immediately discontinued at the first sign of any of the symptoms described below.
Rapid absorption of hexachlorophene may occur with resultant toxic blood levels when preparations containing hexachlorophene are applied to skin lesions such as ichthyosis congenita, the dermatitis of Letterer-Siwe's syndrome, or other generalized dermatological conditions. Application to burns has also produced neurotoxicity and death.
PHISOHEX SHOULD BE DISCONTINUED PROMPTLY IF SIGNS OR SYMPTOMS OF CEREBRAL IRRITABILITY OCCUR.
Infants, especially premature infants or those with dermatoses, are particularly susceptible to hexachlorophene absorption. Systemic toxicity may be manifested by signs of stimulation (irritation) of the central nervous system, sometimes with convulsions.
Infants have developed dermatitis, irritability, generalized clonic muscular contractions and decerebrate rigidity following application of a 6 percent hexachlorophene powder. Examination of brainstems of those infants revealed vacuolization like that which can be produced in newborn experimental animals following repeated topical application of 3 percent hexachlorophene. Moreover, a study of histologic sections of premature infants who died of unrelated causes has shown a positive correlation between hexachlorophene baths and lesions in white matter of brains.

PRECAUTIONS

General—Avoid accidental contact of pHisoHex with the eyes.
If contact occurs, promptly rinse thoroughly with water. Periorbital skin or head application should be performed only before the patient, or eye, is anesthetized.
RINSE THOROUGHLY AFTER USE, especially from sensitive areas such as the scrotum and perineum.
pHisoHex is intended for external use only. If swallowed, pHisoHex is harmful, especially to infants and children.
pHisoHex should not be poured into measuring cups, medicine bottles, or similar containers since it may be mistaken for baby formula or other medications.
Carcinogenesis, Mutagenesis, Impairment of Fertility
Carcinogenicity studies in animals: Hexachlorophene was tested in one experiment in rats by oral administration; it had no carcinogenic effect.
Hexachlorophene was not mutagenic in *Salmonella typhimurium* and was negative in a dominant lethal assay in male

Continued on next page

This product information was prepared in August, 1989. On these and other products of Winthrop Pharmaceuticals, detailed information may be obtained on a current basis by direct inquiry to the Professional Services Department, 90 Park Avenue, New York, NY 10016 (800) 446-6267.

RECOMMENDED DOSAGE FOR SPINAL ANESTHESIA

| Extent of anesthesia | NOVOCAIN 10% Solution | | | |
	Volume of 10% Solution (mL)	Volume of Diluent (mL)	Total Dose (mg)	Site of Injection (lumbar interspace)
Perineum	0.5	0.5	50	4th
Perineum and lower extremities	1	1	100	3rd or 4th
Up to costal margin	2	1	200	2nd, 3rd or 4th

Winthrop Pharm.—Cont.

mice. Cytogenetic tests with cultured human lymphocytes were also negative.

Human data: No case reports or epidemiological studies were available.

Impairment of fertility: Topical exposure of neonatal rats to 3% hexachlorophene solution caused reduced fertility in 7-month-old males, due to inability to ejaculate.

Embryotoxicity and Teratogenicity

Placental transfer of hexachlorophene has been demonstrated in rats.

Hexachlorophene is embryotoxic and produces some teratogenic effects.

Pregnancy Category C

There are no adequate and well-controlled studies in pregnant women. Hexachlorophene should be used during pregnancy only if the potential benefit justifies potential risk to the fetus.

Hexachlorophene has been shown to be teratogenic and embryotoxic in rats when given by mouth or instilled into the vagina in large doses.

Administration of 500 mg/kg diet or 20 to 30 mg/kg bw/day by gavage to rats caused some malformations (angulated ribs, cleft palate, micro- and anophthalmia) and reduction in litter size.

Placental transfer and excretion in milk of hexachlorophene has been demonstrated in rats.

In another study, doses of up to 50 mg/kg diet failed to produce any effects in 3 generations of rats. Hexachlorophene did not interfere with reproduction in hamsters.

Nursing Mothers

It is not known whether this drug is excreted in human milk. Because many drugs are excreted in human milk and because of the potential for serious adverse reactions in nursing infants from hexachlorophene, a decision should be made whether to discontinue nursing or to discontinue the drug taking into account the importance of the drug to the mother.

Pediatric Use

pHisoHex, brand of hexachlorophene detergent cleanser, should not be used routinely for bathing infants. See **WARNINGS**. For premature infants: see **WARNINGS**.

ADVERSE REACTIONS

Adverse reactions to pHisoHex may include dermatitis and photosensitivity. Sensitivity to hexachlorophene is rare; however, persons who have developed photoallergy to similar compounds also may become sensitive to hexachlorophene.

In persons with highly sensitive skin the use of pHisoHex may at times produce a reaction characterized by redness and/or mild scaling or dryness, especially when it is combined with such mechanical factors as excessive rubbing or exposure to heat or cold.

OVERDOSAGE

The accidental ingestion of pHisoHex in amounts from 1 oz to 4 oz has caused anorexia, vomiting, abdominal cramps, diarrhea, dehydration, convulsions, hypotension, and shock, and in several reported instances, fatalities.

If patients are seen early, the stomach should be evacuated by emesis or gastric lavage. Olive oil or vegetable oil (60 mL or 2 fl oz) may then be given to delay absorption of hexachlorophene, followed by a saline cathartic to hasten removal. Treatment is symptomatic and supportive; intravenous fluids (5 percent dextrose in physiologic saline solution) may be given for dehydration. Any other electrolyte derangement should be corrected. If marked hypotension occurs, vasopressor therapy is indicated. Use of opiates may be considered if gastrointestinal symptoms (cramping, diarrhea) are severe. Scheduled medical or surgical procedures should be postponed until the patient's condition has been evaluated and stabilized.

DOSAGE AND ADMINISTRATION

Surgical Hand Scrub—

1. Wet hands and forearms with water. Apply approximately 5 mL of pHisoHex over the hands and rub into a copious lather by adding small amounts of water. Spread suds over hands and forearms and scrub well with a wet brush for 3 minutes. Pay particular attention to the nails and interdigital spaces. A separate nail cleaner may be used. *Rinse thoroughly* under running water.

2. Apply 5 mL of pHisoHex to hands again and scrub as above for another 3 minutes. *Rinse thoroughly* with running water and dry.

3. For repeat surgical scrubs during the day, scrub thoroughly with the same amount of pHisoHex for 3 minutes only. *Rinse thoroughly* with water and dry.

Bacteriostatic Cleansing—

Wet hands with water. Dispense approximately 5 mL of pHisoHex into the palm, work up a lather with water and apply to area to be cleansed.

Rinse thoroughly after each washing.

INFANT CARE: pHisoHex should not be used routinely for bathing infants. See **WARNINGS**.

PREMATURE INFANTS: See **WARNINGS**.

Use of baby skin products containing alcohol may decrease the antibacterial action of pHisoHex, brand of hexachlorophene detergent cleanser.

HOW SUPPLIED

pHisoHex is available in plastic squeeze bottle of 5 ounces (NDC 0024-1535-02) and 1 pint (NDC 0024-1535-06); in plastic bottle of 1 gallon (NDC 0024-1535-08) and 1/4 oz (8 mL) unit packets, box of 50 (NDC 0024-1535-05).

The following, specially constructed, refillable dispensers made with metals and plastics compatible with pHisoHex can also be supplied: 16 oz hand operated wall dispensers; 30 oz pedal operated wall dispensers; 30 oz pedal operated wall dispenser with stand; portable stand with two 30 oz pedal operated dispensers.

Prolonged direct exposure of pHisoHex to strong light may cause brownish surface discoloration but does not affect its antibacterial or detergent properties. Shaking will disperse the color. If pHisoHex is spilled or splashed on porous surfaces, rinse off to avoid discoloration.

> pHisoHex should not be dispensed from, or stored in, containers with ordinary metal parts. A special type of stainless steel must be used or undesirable discoloration of the product or oxidation of metal may occur. Specially designed dispensers for hospital or office use may be obtained through your local dealer.

Directions for Cleaning Dispensers: Before initial installation and use, run an antiseptic, such as an aqueous solution of benzalkonium chloride, NF, 1:500 to 1:750, or alcohol, through the working parts; rinse with sterile water. At weekly intervals thereafter, remove dispenser and pour off remainder of pHisoHex emulsion. Rinse empty dispenser with water. Run water through the working parts by operating the dispenser. Sanitize as described above. Rinse thoroughly with sterile water.

ANIMAL TOXICITY

The oral LD_{50} of hexachlorophene in male rats is 66 mg/kg bw, in females 56 mg/kg bw, and in weanling rats 120 mg/kg bw.

In suckling rats (10-days old), it is 9 mg/kg bw.

PW-61-FF

PLAQUENIL® Sulfate   ℞
brand of hydroxychloroquine sulfate tablets, USP

> **WARNING**
> PHYSICIANS SHOULD COMPLETELY FAMILIARIZE THEMSELVES WITH THE COMPLETE CONTENTS OF THIS LEAFLET BEFORE PRESCRIBING HYDROXY-CHLOROQUINE.

DESCRIPTION

The compound is a colorless crystalline solid, soluble in water to at least 20 percent; chemically the drug is 2-[[4-[(7-Chloro-4- quinolyl) amino] pentyl] ethylamino] ethanol sulfate (1:1).

Inactive Ingredients: Dibasic Calcium Phosphate, Magnesium Stearate, Starch.

ACTIONS

The drug possesses antimalarial actions and also exerts a beneficial effect in lupus erythematosus (chronic discoid or systemic) and acute or chronic rheumatoid arthritis. The precise mechanism of action is not known.

INDICATIONS

PLAQUENIL is indicated for the suppressive treatment and treatment of acute attacks of malaria due to *Plasmodium vivax*, *P. malariae*, *P. ovale*, and susceptible strains of *P. falciparum*. It is also indicated for the treatment of discoid and systemic lupus erythematosus, and rheumatoid arthritis.

CONTRAINDICATIONS

Use of this drug is contraindicated (1) in the presence of retinal or visual field changes attributable to any 4-aminoquinoline compound, (2) in patients with known hypersensitivity to 4-aminoquinoline compounds, and (3) for long-term therapy in children.

WARNINGS, General

PLAQUENIL is not effective against chloroquine-resistant strains of *P. falciparum*.

Children are especially sensitive to the 4-aminoquinoline compounds. A number of fatalities have been reported following the accidental ingestion of chloroquine, sometimes in relatively small doses (0.75 g or 1 g in one 3- year-old child). Patients should be strongly warned to keep these drugs out of the reach of children.

Use of PLAQUENIL in patients with psoriasis may precipitate a severe attack of psoriasis. When used in patients with porphyria the condition may be exacerbated. The preparation should not be used in these conditions unless in the judgment of the physician the benefit to the patient outweighs the possible hazard.

Usage in Pregnancy —Usage of this drug during pregnancy should be avoided except in the suppression or treatment of malaria when in the judgment of the physician the benefit outweighs the possible hazard. It should be noted that radioactively-tagged chloroquine administered intravenously to pregnant, pigmented CBA mice passed rapidly across the placenta. It accumulated selectively in the melanin structures of the fetal eyes and was retained in the ocular tissues for five months after the drug had been eliminated from the rest of the body.

PRECAUTIONS, General

Antimalarial compounds should be used with caution in patients with hepatic disease or alcoholism or in conjunction with known hepatotoxic drugs.

Periodic blood cell counts should be made if patients are given prolonged therapy. If any severe blood disorder appears which is not attributable to the disease under treatment, discontinuation of the drug should be considered. The drug should be administered with caution in patients having G-6-PD (glucose-6-phosphate dehydrogenase) deficiency.

OVERDOSAGE

The 4-aminoquinoline compounds are very rapidly and completely absorbed after ingestion, and in accidental overdosage, or rarely with lower doses in hypersensitive patients, toxic symptoms may occur within 30 minutes. These consist of headache, drowsiness, visual disturbances, cardiovascular collapse, and convulsions, followed by sudden and early respiratory and cardiac arrest. The electrocardiogram may reveal atrial standstill, nodal rhythm, prolonged intraventricular conduction time, and progressive bradycardia leading to ventricular fibrillation and/or arrest. Treatment is symptomatic and must be prompt with immediate evacuation of the stomach by emesis (at home, before transportation to the hospital) or gastric lavage until the stomach is completely emptied. If finely powdered, activated charcoal is introduced by the stomach tube, after lavage, and within 30 minutes after ingestion of the tablets, it may inhibit further intestinal absorption of the drug. To be effective, the dose of activated charcoal should be at least five times the estimated dose of hydroxychloroquine ingested. Convulsions, if present, should be controlled before attempting gastric lavage. If due to cerebral stimulation, cautious administration of an ultrashort-acting barbiturate may be tried but, if due to anoxia, it should be corrected by oxygen administration, artificial respiration or, in shock with hypotension, by vasopressor therapy. Because of the importance of supporting respiration, tracheal intubation or tracheostomy, followed by gastric lavage, may also be necessary. Exchange transfusions have been used to reduce the level of 4-aminoquinoline drug in the blood.

A patient who survives the acute phase and is asymptomatic should be closely observed for at least six hours. Fluids may be forced, and sufficient ammonium chloride (8 g daily in divided doses for adults) may be administered for a few days to acidify the urine to help promote urinary excretion in cases of both overdosage and sensitivity.

> **MALARIA**

ACTIONS

Like chloroquine phosphate, USP, PLAQUENIL sulfate is highly active against the erythrocytic forms of *P. vivax* and *malariae* and most strains of *P. falciparum* (but not the gametocytes of *P. falciparum*).

PLAQUENIL sulfate does not prevent relapses in patients with *vivax* or *malariae* malaria because it is not effective against exo-erythrocytic forms of the parasite, nor will it prevent *vivax* or *malariae* infection when administered as a prophylactic. It is highly effective as a suppressive agent in patients with *vivax* or *malariae* malaria, in terminating acute attacks, and significantly lengthening the interval between treatment and relapse. In patients with *falciparum* malaria, it abolishes the acute attack and effects complete cure of the infection, unless due to a resistant strain of *P. falciparum*.

INDICATIONS

PLAQUENIL sulfate, brand of hydroxychloroquine sulfate tablets, is indicated for the treatment of acute attacks and suppression of malaria.

WARNING

In recent years, it has been found that certain strains of *P. falciparum* have become resistant to 4-aminoquinoline compounds (including hydroxychloroquine) as shown by the fact that normally adequate doses have failed to prevent or cure clinical malaria or parasitemia. Treatment with quinine or other specific forms of therapy is therefore advised for patients infected with a resistant strain of parasites.

ADVERSE REACTIONS

Following the administration in doses adequate for the treatment of an acute malarial attack, mild and transient headache, dizziness, and gastrointestinal complaints (diarrhea, anorexia, nausea, abdominal cramps and, on rare occasions, vomiting) may occur.

DOSAGE AND ADMINISTRATION

One tablet of 200 mg of hydroxychloroquine sulfate is equivalent to 155 mg base.

Malaria: Suppression—*In adults,* 400 mg (=310 mg base) on exactly the same day of each week. *In infants and children,* the weekly suppressive dosage is 5 mg, calculated as base, per kg of body weight, but should not exceed the adult dose regardless of weight.

If circumstances permit, suppressive therapy should begin two weeks prior to exposure. However, failing this, in adults an initial double (loading) dose of 800 mg (= 620 mg base), or in children 10 mg base/kg may be taken in two divided doses, six hours apart. The suppressive therapy should be continued for eight weeks after leaving the endemic area.

Treatment of the acute attack—*In adults,* an initial dose of 800 mg (= 620 mg base) followed by 400 mg (= 310 mg base) in six to eight hours and 400 mg (310 mg base) on each of two consecutive days (total 2 g hydroxychloroquine sulfate or 1.55 g base). An alternative method, employing a single dose of 800 mg (= 620 mg base), has also proved effective.

The dosage for adults may also be calculated on the basis of body weight; this method is preferred for infants and children. A total dose representing 25 mg of base per kg of body weight is administered in three days, as follows:

First dose: 10 mg base per kg (but not exceeding a single dose of 620 mg base).

Second dose: 5 mg base per kg (but not exceeding a single dose of 310 mg base) 6 hours after first dose.

Third dose: 5 mg base per kg 18 hours after second dose.

Fourth dose: 5 mg base per kg 24 hours after third dose.

For radical cure of *vivax* and *malariae* malaria concomitant therapy with an 8-aminoquinoline compound is necessary.

LUPUS ERYTHEMATOSUS AND RHEUMATOID ARTHRITIS

INDICATIONS

PLAQUENIL is useful in patients with the following disorders who have not responded satisfactorily to drugs with less potential for serious side effects: lupus erythematosus (chronic discoid and systemic) and acute or chronic rheumatoid arthritis.

WARNINGS

PHYSICIANS SHOULD COMPLETELY FAMILIARIZE THEMSELVES WITH THE COMPLETE CONTENTS OF THIS LEAFLET BEFORE PRESCRIBING PLAQUENIL.

Irreversible retinal damage has been observed in some patients who had received long-term or high-dosage 4-aminoquinoline therapy for discoid and systemic lupus erythematosus, or rheumatoid arthritis. Retinopathy has been reported to be dose related.

When prolonged therapy with any antimalarial compound is contemplated, initial (base line) and periodic (every three months) ophthalmologic examinations (including visual acuity, expert slit-lamp, funduscopic, and visual field tests) should be performed.

If there is any indication of abnormality in the visual acuity, visual field, or retinal macular areas (such as pigmentary changes, loss of foveal reflex), or any visual symptoms (such as light flashes and streaks) which are not fully explainable by difficulties of accommodation or corneal opacities, the drug should be discontinued immediately and the patient closely observed for possible progression. Retinal changes (and visual disturbances) may progress even after cessation of therapy.

All patients on long-term therapy with this preparation should be questioned and examined periodically, including the testing of knee and ankle reflexes, to detect any evidence of muscular weakness. If weakness occurs, discontinue the drug.

In the treatment of rheumatoid arthritis, if objective improvement (such as reduced joint swelling, increased mobility) does not occur within six months, the drug should be discontinued. Safe use of the drug in the treatment of juvenile arthritis has not been established.

PRECAUTIONS

Dermatologic reactions to PLAQUENIL sulfate, brand of hydroxychloroquine sulfate tablets, may occur and, therefore, proper care should be exercised when it is administered to any patient receiving a drug with a significant tendency to produce dermatitis.

The methods recommended for early diagnosis of "chloroquine retinopathy" consist of (1) funduscopic examination of the macula for fine pigmentary disturbances or loss of the foveal reflex and (2) examination of the central visual field with a small red test object for pericentral or paracentral scotoma or determination of retinal thresholds to red. Any unexplained visual symptoms, such as light flashes or streaks should also be regarded with suspicion as possible manifestations of retinopathy.

If serious toxic symptoms occur from overdosage or sensitivity, it has been suggested that ammonium chloride (8 g daily in divided doses for adults) be administered orally three or four days a week for several months after therapy has been stopped, as acidification of the urine increases renal excretion of the 4-aminoquinoline compounds by 20 to 90 percent. However, caution must be exercised in patients with impaired renal function and/or metabolic acidosis.

ADVERSE REACTIONS

Not all of the following reactions have been observed with every 4-aminoquinoline compound during long-term therapy, but they have been reported with one or more and should be borne in mind when drugs of this class are administered. Adverse effects with different compounds vary in type and frequency.

CNS Reactions: Irritability, nervousness, emotional changes, nightmares, psychosis, headache, dizziness, vertigo, tinnitus, nystagmus, nerve deafness, convulsions, ataxia.

Neuromuscular Reactions: Extraocular muscle palsies, skeletal muscle weakness, absent or hypoactive deep tendon reflexes.

Ocular Reactions:

A. *Ciliary body:* Disturbance of accommodation with symptoms of blurred vision. This reaction is dose related and reversible with cessation of therapy.

B. *Cornea:* Transient edema, punctate to lineal opacities, decreased corneal sensitivity. The corneal changes, with or without accompanying symptoms (blurred vision, halos around lights, photophobia), are fairly common, but reversible. Corneal deposits may appear as early as three weeks following initiation of therapy.

The incidence of corneal changes and visual side effects appears to be considerably lower with hydroxychloroquine than with chloroquine.

C. *Retina:*

Macula: Edema, atrophy, abnormal pigmentation (mild pigment stippling to a "bull's-eye" appearance), loss of foveal reflex, increased macular recovery time following exposure to a bright light (photo-stress test), elevated retinal threshold to red light in macular, paramacular and peripheral retinal areas.

Other fundus changes include optic disc pallor and atrophy, attenuation of retinal arterioles, fine granular pigmentary disturbances in the peripheral retina and prominent choroidal patterns in advanced stage.

D. *Visual field defects:* pericentral or paracentral scotoma, central scotoma with decreased visual acuity, rarely field constriction.

The most common visual symptoms attributed to the retinopathy are: reading and seeing difficulties (words, letters, or parts of objects missing), photophobia, blurred distance vision, missing or blacked out areas in the central or peripheral visual field, light flashes and streaks.

Retinopathy appears to be dose related and has occurred within several months (rarely) to several years of daily therapy; a small number of cases have been reported several years after antimalarial drug therapy was discontinued. It has not been noted during prolonged use of weekly doses of the 4-aminoquinoline compounds for suppression of malaria. Patients with retinal changes may have visual symptoms or may be asymptomatic (with or without visual field changes). Rarely scotomatous vision or field defects may occur without obvious retinal change.

Retinopathy may progress even after the drug is discontinued. In a number of patients, early retinopathy (macular pigmentation sometimes with central field defects) diminished or regressed completely after therapy was discontinued. Paracentral scotoma to red targets (sometimes called "premaculopathy") is indicative of early retinal dysfunction which is usually reversible with cessation of therapy.

A small number of cases of retinal changes have been reported as occurring in patients who received only hydroxychloroquine. These usually consisted of alteration in retinal pigmentation which was detected on periodic ophthalmologic examination; visual field defects were also present in some instances. A case of delayed retinopathy has been reported with loss of vision starting one year after administration of hydroxychloroquine had been discontinued.

Dermatologic Reactions: Bleaching of hair, alopecia, pruritus, skin and mucosal pigmentation, skin eruptions (urticarial, morbilliform, lichenoid, maculopapular, purpuric, erythema annulare centrifugum and exfoliative dermatitis).

Hematologic Reactions: Various blood dyscrasias such as aplastic anemia, agranulocytosis, leukopenia, thrombocytopenia (hemolysis in individuals with glucose-6-phosphate dehydrogenase (G-6-PD) deficiency).

Gastrointestinal Reactions: Anorexia, nausea, vomiting, diarrhea, and abdominal cramps.

Miscellaneous Reactions: Weight loss, lassitude, exacerbation or precipitation of porphyria and nonlight-sensitive psoriasis.

DOSAGE AND ADMINISTRATION

One tablet of hydroxychloroquine sulfate, 200 mg, is equivalent to 155 mg base.

Lupus erythematosus—Initially, the average *adult* dose is 400 mg (=310 mg base) once or twice daily. This may be continued for several weeks or months, depending on the response of the patient. For prolonged maintenance therapy, a smaller dose, from 200 mg to 400 mg (=155 mg to 310 mg base) daily will frequently suffice.

The incidence of retinopathy has been reported to be higher when this maintenance dose is exceeded.

Rheumatoid arthritis—The compound is cumulative in action and will require several weeks to exert its beneficial therapeutic effects, whereas minor side effects may occur relatively early. Several months of therapy may be required before maximum effects can be obtained. If objective improvement (such as reduced joint swelling, increased mobility) does not occur within six months, the drug should be discontinued. Safe use of the drug in the treatment of juvenile rheumatoid arthritis has not been established.

Initial dosage—In *adults,* from 400 mg to 600 mg (=310 mg to 465 mg base) daily, each dose to be taken with a meal or a glass of milk. In a small percentage of patients, troublesome side effects may require temporary reduction of the initial dosage. Later (usually from five to ten days), the dose may gradually be increased to the optimum response level, often without return of side effects.

Maintenance dosage—When a good response is obtained (usually in four to twelve weeks), the dosage is reduced by 50 percent and continued at a usual maintenance level of 200 mg to 400 mg (=155 mg to 310 mg base) daily, each dose to be taken with a meal or a glass of milk. The incidence of retinopathy has been reported to be higher when this maintenance dose is exceeded.

Should a relapse occur after medication is withdrawn, therapy may be resumed or continued on an intermittent schedule if there are no ocular contraindications.

Corticosteroids and salicylates may be used in conjunction with this compound, and they can generally be decreased gradually in dosage or eliminated after the drug has been used for several weeks. When gradual reduction of steroid dosage is indicated, it may be done by reducing every four to five days the dose of cortisone by no more than from 5 mg to 15 mg; of hydrocortisone from 5 mg to 10 mg; of prednisolone and prednisone from 1 mg to 2.5 mg; of methylprednisolone and triamcinolone from 1 mg to 2 mg; and of dexamethasone from 0.25 mg to 0.5 mg.

HOW SUPPLIED

Tablets of 200 mg (equivalent to 155 mg of base), bottles of 100.

Distributed by Winthrop Pharmaceuticals
Division of Sterling Drug Inc.
New York, NY 10016
Manufactured by Sterling Pharmaceuticals Inc.
Barceloneta, Puerto Rico 00617
Shown in Product Identification Section, page 435

PW-306-R

PONTOCAINE® Hydrochloride   ℞
brand of tetracaine hydrochloride, USP

Prolonged Spinal Anesthesia

DESCRIPTION

Tetracaine hydrochloride is 2-(Dimethylamino)ethyl *p*-(butylamino) benzoate monohydrochloride. It is a white crystalline, odorless powder that is readily soluble in water, physiologic saline solution, and dextrose solution.

Tetracaine hydrochloride is a local anesthetic of the ester-linkage type, related to procaine.

PONTOCAINE hydrochloride is supplied in two forms for prolonged spinal anesthesia: Niphanoid® and 1% Solution.

NIPHANOID: A sterile, instantly soluble form consisting of a network of extremely fine, highly purified particles, resembling snow.

1% Solution: A sterile, isotonic, isobaric solution, each 1 mL containing 10 mg tetracaine hydrochloride, 6.7 mg sodium chloride, and not more than 2 mg acetone sodium bisul-

Continued on next page

This product information was prepared in August, 1989. On these and other products of Winthrop Pharmaceuticals, detailed information may be obtained on a current basis by direct inquiry to the Professional Services Department, 90 Park Avenue, New York, NY 10016 (800) 446-6267.

Winthrop Pharm.—Cont.

fite. The air in the ampuls has been displaced by nitrogen gas. The pH is 3.2 to 6.
These formulations do not contain preservatives.

CLINICAL PHARMACOLOGY
Parenteral administration of PONTOCAINE stabilizes the neuronal membrane and prevents initiation and transmission of nerve impulses thereby effecting local anesthesia. The onset of action is rapid, and the duration prolonged (up to two or three hours or longer of surgical anesthesia). PONTOCAINE is detoxified by plasma esterases to aminobenzoic acid and diethylaminoethanol.

INDICATIONS AND USAGE
PONTOCAINE is indicated for the production of spinal anesthesia for procedures requiring two to three hours.

CONTRAINDICATIONS
Spinal anesthesia with PONTOCAINE is contraindicated in patients with known hypersensitivity to tetracaine hydrochloride or to drugs of a similar chemical configuration (ester-type local anesthetics), or aminobenzoic acid or its derivatives; and in patients for whom spinal anesthesia as a technique is contraindicated.

The decision as to whether or not spinal anesthesia should be used for an individual patient should be made by the physician after weighing the advantages with the risks and possible complications. Contraindications to spinal anesthesia as a technique can be found in standard reference texts, and usually include generalized septicemia, infection at the site of injection, certain diseases of the cerebrospinal system, uncontrolled hypotension, etc.

WARNINGS
RESUSCITATIVE EQUIPMENT AND DRUGS SHOULD BE IMMEDIATELY AVAILABLE WHENEVER ANY LOCAL ANESTHETIC DRUG IS USED.
Large doses of local anesthetics should not be used in patients with heartblock.
Reactions resulting in fatality have occurred on rare occasions with the use of local anesthetics, even in the absence of a history of hypersensitivity.
Contains acetone sodium bisulfite, a sulfite that may cause allergic-type reactions including anaphylactic symptoms and life-threatening or less severe asthmatic episodes in certain susceptible people. The overall prevalence of sulfite sensitivity in the general population is unknown and probably low. Sulfite sensitivity is seen more frequently in asthmatic than in nonasthmatic people.

PRECAUTIONS
The safety and effectiveness of any spinal anesthetic depend upon proper dosage, correct technique, adequate precautions, and readiness for emergencies. The lowest dosage that results in effective anesthesia should be used to avoid high plasma levels and serious systemic side effects. Tolerance varies with the status of the patient; debilitated, elderly patients or acutely ill patients should be given reduced doses commensurate with their weight, age, and physical status. Reduced doses are also indicated for obstetric patients and those with increased intra-abdominal pressure.
Caution should be used in administering PONTOCAINE to patients with abnormal or reduced levels of plasma esterases.
Blood pressure should be frequently monitored during spinal anesthesia and hypotension immediately corrected.
Spinal anesthetics should be used with caution in patients with severe disturbances of cardiac rhythm, shock, or heartblock.
Drug Interactions: PONTOCAINE should not be used if the patient is being treated with a sulfonamide because aminobenzoic acid inhibits the action of sulfonamides.
Carcinogenesis, Mutagenesis, Impairment of Fertility: Long-term animal studies to evaluate carcinogenic potential and

reproduction studies in animals have not been performed. There is no evidence from human data that PONTOCAINE may be carcinogenic or that it impairs fertility.
Pregnancy Category C: Animal reproduction studies have not been conducted with PONTOCAINE. It is not known whether PONTOCAINE can cause fetal harm when administered to a pregnant woman or can affect reproduction capacity. PONTOCAINE should be given to a pregnant woman only if clearly needed and the potential benefits outweigh the risk.
Labor and Delivery: Vasopressor agents administered for the treatment of hypotension resulting from spinal anesthesia may result in severe persistent hypertension and/or rupture of cerebral blood vessels if oxytocic drugs have also been administered; therefore, vasopressors should be used with extreme caution in the presence of oxytocic drugs.
PONTOCAINE has a recognized use during labor and delivery; the effect of the drug on duration of labor, incidence of forceps delivery, status of the newborn, and later growth and development of the child have not been studied.
Nursing Mothers: It is not known whether PONTOCAINE is excreted in human milk; however, it is rapidly metabolized following absorption into the plasma. Because many drugs are excreted in human milk, caution should be exercised when PONTOCAINE, brand of tetracaine hydrochloride, is administered to a nursing woman.
Pediatric Use: Safety and effectiveness of PONTOCAINE in children have not been established.

ADVERSE REACTIONS
Systemic adverse reactions to PONTOCAINE are characteristic of those associated with other local anesthetics and can involve the central nervous system and the cardiovascular system. Systemic reactions usually result from high plasma levels due to excessive dosage, rapid absorption, or inadvertent intravascular injection.
A small number of reactions to PONTOCAINE may result from hypersensitivity, idiosyncrasy, or diminished tolerance to normal dosage.
Central nervous system effects are characterized by excitation or depression. The first manifestation may be nervousness, dizziness, blurred vision, or tremors, followed by drowsiness, convulsions, unconsciousness and possibly respiratory and cardiac arrest. Since excitement may be transient or absent, the first manifestation may be drowsiness, sometimes merging into unconsciousness and respiratory and cardiac arrest. Other central nervous system effects may be nausea, vomiting, chills, constriction of the pupils, or tinnitus.
Cardiovascular system reactions include depression of the myocardium, blood pressure changes (usually hypotension), and cardiac arrest.
Allergic reactions, which may be due to hypersensitivity, idiosyncrasy, or diminished tolerance, are characterized by cutaneous lesions (eg, urticaria), edema, and other manifestations of allergy. Detection of sensitivity by skin testing is of limited value. Severe allergic reactions including anaphylaxis have occurred rarely and are not usually dose-related.
Reactions Associated with Spinal Anesthesia Techniques:
Central Nervous System: post-spinal headache, meningismus, arachnoiditis, palsies, or spinal nerve paralysis. *Cardiovascular:* hypotension due to vasomotor paralysis and pooling of the blood in the venous bed. *Respiratory:* respiratory impairment or paralysis due to the level of anesthesia extending to the upper thoracic and cervical segments. *Gastrointestinal:* nausea and vomiting.
Treatment of Reactions: Toxic effects of local anesthetics require symptomatic treatment; there is no specific cure. **The most important measure is oxygenation of the patient by maintaining an airway and supporting ventilation.** Supportive treatment of the cardiovascular system includes intravenous fluids and, when appropriate, vasopressors (preferably those that stimulate the myocardium). Convulsions are usually controlled with adequate oxygenation alone but intravenous administration in small increments of a barbiturate (preferably an ultrashort-acting barbiturate such as

thiopental and thiamylal) or diazepam can be utilized. Intravenous barbiturates or anticonvulsant agents should only be administered by those familiar with their use and only if ventilation and oxygenation have first been assured. In spinal anesthesia, sympathetic blockade also occurs as a pharmacological action, resulting in peripheral vasodilation and often hypotension. The extent of the hypotension will usually depend on the number of dermatomes blocked. The blood pressure should therefore be monitored in the early phases of anesthesia. If hypotension occurs, it is readily controlled by vasoconstrictors administered either by the intramuscular or the intravenous route, the dosage of which would depend on the severity of the hypotension and the response to treatment.

DOSAGE AND ADMINISTRATION
As with all anesthetics, the dosage varies and depends upon the area to be anesthetized, the number of neuronal segments to be blocked, individual tolerance, and the technique of anesthesia. The lowest dosage needed to provide effective anesthesia should be administered. For specific techniques and procedures, refer to standard textbooks.
[See table below].
The extent and degree of spinal anesthesia depend upon dosage, specific gravity of the anesthetic solution, volume of solution used, force of the injection, level of puncture, position of the patient during and immediately after injection, etc.
When spinal fluid is added to either the NIPHANOID or solution, some turbidity results, the degree depending on the pH of the spinal fluid, the temperature of the solution during mixing, as well as the amount of drug and diluent employed. This cloudiness is due to the release of the *base* from the hydrochloride. Liberation of base (which is completed within the spinal canal) is held to be essential for satisfactory results with any spinal anesthetic.
The specific gravity of spinal fluid at 25°C/25°C varies under normal conditions from 1.0063 to 1.0075. A solution of the instantly soluble form (NIPHANOID) in spinal fluid has only a slightly greater specific gravity. The 1% concentration in saline solution has a specific gravity of 1.0060 to 1.0074 at 25°C/25°C.
A hyperbaric solution may be prepared by mixing equal volumes of the 1% Solution and Dextrose Solution 10% (which is available in ampuls of 3 mL).
If the NIPHANOID form is preferred, it is first dissolved in Dextrose Solution 10% in a ratio of 1 mL dextrose to 10 mg of the anesthetic. Further dilution is made with an equal volume of spinal fluid. The resulting solution now contains 5% dextrose with 5 mg of anesthetic agent per milliliter.
A hypobaric solution may be prepared by dissolving the NIPHANOID in Sterile Water for Injection, USP (1 mg per milliliter). The specific gravity of this solution is essentially the same as that of water, 1.000 at 25°C/25°C.
Examine ampuls carefully before use. Do not use solution if crystals, cloudiness, or discoloration is observed.
These formulations of tetracaine hydrochloride do not contain preservatives; therefore, unused portions should be discarded and the reconstituted NIPHANOID should be used immediately.

STERILIZATION OF AMPULS
The drug in intact ampuls is sterile. The preferred method of destroying bacteria on the exterior of ampuls before opening is heat sterilization (autoclaving). Immersion in antiseptic solution is not recommended.
Autoclave at 15-pound pressure, at 121°C (250°F), for 15 minutes. The NIPHANOID form may also be autoclaved in the same way but may lose its snowlike appearance and tend to adhere to the sides of the ampul. This may slightly decrease the rate at which the drug dissolves but does not interfere with its anesthetic potency.
Autoclaving increases likelihood of crystal formation. Unused autoclaved ampuls should be discarded. Under no circumstance should unused ampuls which have been autoclaved be returned to stock.

SUGGESTED DOSAGE FOR SPINAL ANESTHESIA

Extent of anesthesia	Using NIPHANOID			Using 1% Solution		
	Dose of NIPHANOID (mg)	Volume of spinal fluid (mL)	Dose of solution (mL)	Volume of spinal fluid (mL)	Site of injection (lumbar interspace)	
Perineum	5*	1	0.5 (=5 mg)*	0.5	4th	
Perineum and lower extremities	10	2	1 (=10 mg)	1	3d or 4th	
Up to costal margin	15 to 20†	3	1.5 to 2 (=15 mg to 20 mg)†	1.5 to 2	2d, 3d, or 4th	

*For vaginal delivery (saddle block), from 2 mg to 5 mg in dextrose.

† Doses exceeding 15 mg are rarely required and should be used only in exceptional cases. Inject solution at rate of about 1 mL per 5 seconds.

HOW SUPPLIED

Protect ampuls from light and store solution under refrigeration.

NIPHANOID (instantly soluble): Ampuls of 20 mg, box of 100.

NDC 0024-1577-06

Uni-Nest ™—1% isotonic isobaric solution: Ampuls of 2 mL, box of 25.

NDC 0024-1574-25

PW-56-Z

SULFAMYLON® Cream ℞
brand of mafenide acetate cream, USP

> **Topical Antibacterial Agent for Adjunctive Therapy in Second- and Third-Degree Burns**

DESCRIPTION

SULFAMYLON Cream is a soft, white, nonstaining, water-miscible, anti-infective cream for topical administration to burn wounds.

SULFAMYLON Cream spreads easily, and can be washed off readily with water. It has a slight acetic odor. Each gram of SULFAMYLON Cream contains mafenide acetate equivalent to 85 mg of the base. The cream vehicle consists of cetyl alcohol, stearyl alcohol, cetyl esters wax, polyoxyl 40 stearate, polyoxyl 8 stearate, glycerin, and water, with methylparaben, propylparaben, sodium metabisulfite, and edetate disodium as preservatives.

Chemically, mafenide acetate is α-Amino-*p*-toluenesulfonamide monoacetate.

CLINICAL PHARMACOLOGY

SULFAMYLON Cream, applied topically, produces a marked reduction in the bacterial population present in the avascular tissues of second- and third-degree burns. Reduction in bacterial growth after application of SULFAMYLON Cream has also been reported to permit spontaneous healing of deep partial-thickness burns, and thus prevent conversion of burn wounds from partial thickness to full thickness. It should be noted, however, that delayed eschar separation has occurred in some cases.

Absorption and Metabolism. Applied topically, SULFAMYLON Cream diffuses through devascularized areas, is absorbed, and rapidly converted to a metabolite (*p*-carboxybenzenesulfonamide) which is cleared through the kidneys. SULFAMYLON is active in the presence of pus and serum, and its activity is not altered by changes in the acidity of the environment.

Antibacterial Activity. SULFAMYLON exerts bacteriostatic action against many gram-negative and gram-positive organisms, including *Pseudomonas aeruginosa* and certain strains of anaerobes.

INDICATIONS AND USAGE

SULFAMYLON Cream is a topical agent indicated for adjunctive therapy of patients with second- and third-degree burns.

CONTRAINDICATIONS

SULFAMYLON is contraindicated in patients who are hypersensitive to it. It is not known whether there is cross sensitivity to other sulfonamides.

WARNINGS

Fatal hemolytic anemia with disseminated intravascular coagulation, presumably related to a glucose-6-phosphate dehydrogenase deficiency, has been reported following therapy with SULFAMYLON Cream.

Contains sodium metabisulfite, a sulfite that may cause allergic-type reactions including anaphylactic symptoms and life-threatening or less severe asthmatic episodes in certain susceptible people. The overall prevalence of sulfite sensitivity in the general population is unknown and probably low. Sulfite sensitivity is seen more frequently in asthmatic than in nonasthmatic people.

PRECAUTIONS

SULFAMYLON and its metabolite, *p*-carboxybenzenesulfonamide, inhibit carbonic anhydrase, which may result in metabolic acidosis, usually compensated by hyperventilation. In the presence of impaired renal function, high blood levels of SULFAMYLON and its metabolite may exaggerate the carbonic anhydrase inhibition. Therefore, close monitoring of acid-base balance is necessary, particularly in patients with extensive second-degree or partial thickness burns and in those with pulmonary or renal dysfunction. Some burn patients treated with SULFAMYLON Cream have also been reported to manifest an unexplained syndrome of marked hyperventilation with resulting respiratory alkalosis (slightly alkaline blood pH, low arterial pCO_2, and decreased total CO_2); change in arterial pO_2 is variable. The etiology and significance of these findings are unknown.

Mafenide acetate cream should be used with caution in burn patients with acute renal failure.

SULFAMYLON Cream should be administered with caution to patients with history of hypersensitivity to mafenide. It is not known whether there is cross sensitivity to other sulfonamides.

Fungal colonization in and below the eschar may occur concomitantly with reduction of bacterial growth in the burn wound. However, fungal dissemination through the infected burn wound is rare.

Carcinogenesis, Mutagenesis, Impairment of Fertility. No long-term animal studies have been performed to evaluate the drug's potential in these areas.

Pregnancy Category C. Animal reproduction studies have not been conducted with SULFAMYLON. It is also not known whether SULFAMYLON can cause fetal harm when administered to a pregnant woman or can affect reproduction capacity. Therefore, the preparation is not recommended for the treatment of women of childbearing potential, unless the burned area covers more than 20% of the total body surface, or the need for the therapeutic benefit of SULFAMYLON Cream is, in the physician's judgment, greater than the possible risk to the fetus.

Nursing Mothers. It is not known whether mafenide acetate is excreted in human milk. Because many drugs are excreted in human milk and because of the potential for serious adverse reaction in nursing infants from SULFAMYLON, a decision should be made whether to discontinue nursing or to discontinue the drug, taking into account the importance of the drug to the mother.

Pediatric Use. Same as for adults. (See DOSAGE AND ADMINISTRATION.)

ADVERSE REACTIONS

It is frequently difficult to distinguish between an adverse reaction to SULFAMYLON Cream and the effect of a severe burn. A single case of bone marrow depression and a single case of an acute attack of porphyria have been reported following therapy with SULFAMYLON Cream. Fatal hemolytic anemia with disseminated intravascular coagulation, presumably related to a glucose-6-phosphate dehydrogenase deficiency, has been reported following therapy with SULFAMYLON Cream.

Dermatologic: The most frequently reported reaction was pain on application or a burning sensation. Rare occurrences are excoriation of new skin, and bleeding of skin.

Allergic: Rash, itching, facial edema, swelling, hives, blisters, erythema, and eosinophilia.

Respiratory: Tachypnea or hyperventilation, decrease in arterial pCO_2.

Metabolic: Acidosis, increase in serum chloride.

Accidental ingestion of SULFAMYLON Cream has been reported to cause diarrhea.

DOSAGE AND ADMINISTRATION

Prompt institution of appropriate measures for controlling shock and pain is of prime importance. The burn wounds are then cleansed and debrided, and SULFAMYLON Cream, brand of mafenide acetate cream, is applied with a sterile gloved hand. Satisfactory results can be achieved with application of the cream once or twice daily, to a thickness of approximately $\frac{1}{16}$ inch; thicker application is not recommended. The burned areas should be covered with SULFAMYLON Cream at all times. Therefore, whenever necessary, the cream should be reapplied to any areas from which it has been removed (eg, by patient activity). The routine of administration can be accomplished in minimal time, since dressings usually are not required. If individual patient demands make them necessary, however, only a thin layer of dressing should be used.

When feasible, the patient should be bathed daily, to aid in debridement. A whirlpool bath is particularly helpful, but the patient may be bathed in bed or in a shower.

The duration of therapy with SULFAMYLON Cream depends on each patient's requirements. Treatment is usually continued until healing is progressing well or until the burn site is ready for grafting. *SULFAMYLON Cream should not be withdrawn from the therapeutic regimen while there is the possibility of infection.* However, if allergic manifestations occur during treatment with SULFAMYLON Cream, discontinuation of treatment should be considered.

If acidosis occurs and becomes difficult to control, particularly in patients with pulmonary dysfunction, discontinuing therapy with SULFAMYLON Cream for 24 to 48 hours while continuing fluid therapy may aid in restoring acid-base balance.

HOW SUPPLIED

Cans of 14.5 ounces (411 g)—NDC 0024-1884-09

Collapsible tubes of 4 ounces (113.4 g)

NDC 0024-1884-02

Collapsible tubes of 2 ounces (56.7 g)

NDC 0024-1884-01

SW-89-K

TALACEN® ℞
Pentazocine hydrochloride, USP,
equivalent to 25 mg base
and acetaminophen, USP, 650 mg

DESCRIPTION

TALACEN is a combination of pentazocine hydrochloride, USP, equivalent to 25 mg base and acetaminophen, USP, 650 mg.

Pentazocine is a member of the benzazocine series (also known as the benzomorphan series). Chemically, pentazocine is 1,2,3,4,5,6-hexahydro-6,11-dimethyl-3-(3-methyl-2-butenyl)-2,6-methano-3-benzazocin-8-ol, a white, crystalline substance soluble in acidic aqueous solutions.

Chemically, acetaminophen is Acetamide, *N*-(4-hydroxyphenyl).

Pentazocine is an analgesic and acetaminophen is an analgesic and antipyretic.

TALACEN is a pale blue, scored caplet for oral administration.

Inactive Ingredients: Colloidal Silicon Dioxide, FD&C Blue #1, Gelatin, Microcrystalline Cellulose, Potassium Sorbate, Pregelatinized Starch, Sodium Lauryl Sulfate, Sodium Metabisulfite, Sodium Starch Glycolate, Stearic Acid.

CLINICAL PHARMACOLOGY

TALACEN is an analgesic possessing antipyretic actions. Pentazocine is an analgesic with agonist/antagonist action which when administered orally is approximately equivalent on a mg for mg basis in analgesic effect to codeine. Acetaminophen is an analgesic and antipyretic.

Onset of significant analgesia with pentazocine usually occurs between 15 and 30 minutes after oral administration, and duration of action is usually three hours or longer. Onset and duration of action and the degree of pain relief are related both to dose and the severity of pretreatment pain. Pentazocine weakly antagonizes the analgesic effects of morphine, meperidine, and phenazocine; in addition, it produces incomplete reversal of cardiovascular, respiratory, and behavioral depression induced by morphine and meperidine. Pentazocine has about 1/50 the antagonistic activity of nalorphine. It also has sedative activity.

Pentazocine is well absorbed from the gastrointestinal tract. Plasma levels closely correspond to the onset, duration, and intensity of analgesia. The mean peak concentration in 24 normal volunteers was 1.7 hours (range 0.5 to 4 hours) after oral administration and the mean plasma elimination half-life was 3.6 hours (range 1.5 to 10 hours).

The action of pentazocine is terminated for the most part by biotransformation in the liver with some free pentazocine excreted in the urine. The products of the oxidation of the terminal methyl groups and glucuronide conjugates are excreted by the kidney. Elimination of approximately 60% of the total dose occurs within 24 hours. Pentazocine passes the placental barrier.

Onset of significant analgesic and antipyretic activity of acetaminophen when administered orally occurs within 30 minutes and is maximal at approximately $2\frac{1}{2}$ hours. The pharmacological mode of action of acetaminophen is unknown at this time.

Acetaminophen is rapidly and almost completely absorbed from the gastrointestinal tract. In 24 normal volunteers the mean peak plasma concentration was 1 hour (range 0.25 to 3 hours) after oral administration and the mean plasma elimination half-life was 2.8 hours (range 2 to 4 hours).

The effect of pentazocine on acetaminophen plasma protein binding or vice versa has not been established. For acetaminophen there is little or no plasma protein binding at normal therapeutic doses. When toxic doses of acetaminophen are ingested and drug plasma levels exceed 90 µg/mL, plasma binding may vary from 8% to 43%.

Acetaminophen is conjugated in the liver with glucuronic acid and to a lesser extent with sulfuric acid. Approximately 80% of acetaminophen is excreted in the urine after conjugation and about 3% is excreted unchanged. The drug is also conjugated to a lesser extent with cysteine and additionally metabolized by hydroxylation.

If TALACEN is taken every 4 hours over an extended period of time, accumulation of pentazocine and to a lesser extent, acetaminophen, may occur.

INDICATIONS AND USAGE

TALACEN is indicated for the relief of mild to moderate pain.

Continued on next page

This product information was prepared in August, 1989. On these and other products of Winthrop Pharmaceuticals, detailed information may be obtained on a current basis by direct inquiry to the Professional Services Department, 90 Park Avenue, New York, NY 10016 (800) 446-6267.

Winthrop Pharm.—Cont.

CONTRAINDICATIONS

TALACEN should not be administered to patients who are hypersensitive to either pentazocine or acetaminophen.

WARNINGS

Contains sodium metabisulfite, a sulfite that may cause allergic-type reactions including anaphylactic symptoms and life-threatening or less severe asthmatic episodes in certain susceptible people. The overall prevalence of sulfite sensitivity in the general population is unknown and probably low. Sulfite sensitivity is seen more frequently in asthmatic than in nonasthmatic people.

Head Injury and Increased Intracranial Pressure. As in the case of other potent analgesics, the potential of pentazocine for elevating cerebrospinal fluid pressure may be attributed to CO_2 retention due to the respiratory depressant effects of the drug. These effects may be markedly exaggerated in the presence of head injury, other intracranial lesions, or a preexisting increase in intracranial pressure. Furthermore, pentazocine can produce effects which may obscure the clinical course of patients with head injuries. In such patients, TALACEN must be used with extreme caution and only if its use is deemed essential.

Acute CNS Manifestations. Patients receiving therapeutic doses of pentazocine have experienced hallucinations (usually visual), disorientation, and confusion which have cleared spontaneously within a period of hours. The mechanism of this reaction is not known. Such patients should be closely observed and vital signs checked. If the drug is reinstituted, it should be done with caution since these acute CNS manifestations may recur.

There have been instances of psychological and physical dependence on parenteral pentazocine in patients with a history of drug abuse, and rarely, in patients without such a history. (See DRUG ABUSE AND DEPENDENCE.)

Due to the potential for increased CNS depressant effects, alcohol should be used with caution in patients who are currently receiving pentazocine.

Pentazocine may precipitate opioid abstinence symptoms in patients receiving courses of opiates for pain relief.

PRECAUTIONS

In prescribing TALACEN for chronic use, the physician should take precautions to avoid increases in dose by the patient.

Myocardial Infarction. As with all drugs, TALACEN should be used with caution in patients with myocardial infarction who have nausea or vomiting.

Certain Respiratory Conditions. Although respiratory depression has rarely been reported after oral administration of pentazocine, the drug should be administered with caution to patients with respiratory depression from any cause, severely limited respiratory reserve, severe bronchial asthma and other obstructive respiratory conditions, or cyanosis.

Impaired Renal or Hepatic Function. Decreased metabolism of the drug by the liver in extensive liver disease may predispose to accentuation of side effects. Although laboratory tests have not indicated that pentazocine causes or increases renal or hepatic impairment, the drug should be administered with caution to patients with such impairment. Since acetaminophen is metabolized by the liver, the question of the safety of its use in the presence of liver disease should be considered.

Biliary Surgery. Narcotic drug products are generally considered to elevate biliary tract pressure for varying periods following their administration. Some evidence suggests that pentazocine may differ from other marketed narcotics in this respect (ie, it causes little or no elevation in biliary tract pressures). The clinical significance of these findings, however, is not yet known.

CNS Effect. Caution should be used when TALACEN is administered to patients prone to seizures; seizures have occurred in a few such patients in association with the use of pentazocine although no cause and effect relationship has been established.

Information for Patients. Since sedation, dizziness, and occasional euphoria have been noted, ambulatory patients should be warned not to operate machinery, drive cars, or unnecessarily expose themselves to hazards. Pentazocine may cause physical and psychological dependence when taken alone and may have additive CNS depressant properties when taken in combination with alcohol or other CNS depressants.

Drug Interactions. Pentazocine is a mild narcotic antagonist. Some patients previously given narcotics, including methadone for the daily treatment of narcotic dependence, have experienced withdrawal symptoms after receiving pentazocine.

Carcinogenesis, Mutagenesis, Impairment of Fertility. Carcinogenesis, mutagenesis, and impairment of fertility studies have not been done with this combination product.

Pentazocine, when administered orally or parenterally, had no adverse effect on either the reproductive capabilities or the course of pregnancy in rabbits and rats. Embryotoxic effects on the fetuses were not shown.

The daily administration of 4 mg/kg to 20 mg/kg pentazocine subcutaneously to female rats during a 14 day pre-mating period and until the 13th day of pregnancy did not have any adverse effects on the fertility rate.

There is no evidence in long-term animal studies to demonstrate that pentazocine is carcinogenic.

Pregnancy Category C. Animal reproduction studies have not been conducted with TALACEN. It is also not known whether TALACEN can cause fetal harm when administered to pregnant women or can affect reproduction capacity. TALACEN should be given to pregnant women only if clearly needed. However, animal reproduction studies with pentazocine have not demonstrated teratogenic embryotoxic effects.

Nonteratogenic Effects. There has been no experience in this regard with the combination pentazocine and acetaminophen. However, there have been rare reports of possible abstinence syndromes in newborns after prolonged use of pentazocine during pregnancy.

Labor and Delivery. Patients receiving pentazocine during labor have experienced no adverse effects other than those that occur with commonly used analgesics. TALACEN should be used with caution in women delivering premature infants. The effect of TALACEN on the mother and fetus, the duration of labor or delivery, the possibility that forceps delivery or other intervention or resuscitation of the newborn may be necessary, or the effect of TALACEN, on the later growth, development, and functional maturation of the child are unknown at the present time.

Nursing Mothers. It is not known whether this drug is excreted in human milk. Because many drugs are excreted in human milk, caution should be exercised when TALACEN is administered to a nursing woman.

Pediatric Use. Safety and effectiveness in children below the age of 12 have not been established.

ADVERSE REACTIONS

Clinical experience with TALACEN has been insufficient to define all possible adverse reactions with this combination. However, reactions reported after oral administration of pentazocine hydrochloride in 50 mg dosage include *gastrointestinal:* nausea, vomiting, infrequently constipation; and rarely abdominal distress, anorexia, diarrhea. *CNS effects:* dizziness, lightheadedness, hallucinations, sedation, euphoria, headache, confusion, disorientation; infrequently weakness, disturbed dreams, insomnia, syncope, visual blurring and focusing difficulty, depression; and rarely tremor, irritability, excitement, tinnitus. *Autonomic:* sweating; infrequently flushing; and rarely chills. *Allergic:* infrequently rash; and rarely urticaria, edema of the face. *Cardiovascular:* infrequently decrease in blood pressure, tachycardia. *Hematologic:* rarely depression of white blood cells (especially granulocytes), which is usually reversible, moderate transient eosinophilia. *Other:* rarely respiratory depression, urinary retention, paresthesia, toxic epidermal necrolysis, and in one instance, an apparent anaphylactic reaction has been reported.

Numerous clinical studies have shown that acetaminophen, when taken in recommended doses, is relatively free of adverse effects in most age groups, even in the presence of a variety of disease states.

A few cases of hypersensitivity to acetaminophen have been reported, as manifested by skin rashes, thrombocytopenic purpura, rarely hemolytic anemia and agranulocytosis. Occasional individuals respond to ordinary doses with nausea and vomiting and diarrhea.

DRUG ABUSE AND DEPENDENCE

Controlled Substance. TALACEN is a Schedule IV controlled substance.

Abuse and Dependence. There have been some reports of dependence and of withdrawal symptoms with orally administered pentazocine. There have been recorded instances of psychological and physical dependence in patients using parenteral pentazocine. Abrupt discontinuance following the extended use of parenteral pentazocine has resulted in withdrawal symptoms. Patients with a history of drug dependence should be under closer supervision while receiving TALACEN. There have been rare reports of possible abstinence syndromes in newborns after prolonged use of pentazocine during pregnancy.

Some tolerance to the analgesic and subjective effects of pentazocine develops with frequent and repeated use.

Drug addicts who are given closely spaced doses of pentazocine (eg, 60 mg to 90 mg every 4 hours) develop physical dependence which is demonstrated by abrupt withdrawal or by administration of naloxone. The withdrawal symptoms exhibited after chronic doses of more than 500 mg of pentazocine per day have similar characteristics, but to a lesser degree, of opioid withdrawal and may be associated with drug seeking behavior.

OVERDOSAGE

Manifestations. Clinical experience with TALACEN has been insufficient to define the signs of overdosage with this product. It may be assumed that signs and symptoms of TALACEN overdose would be a combination of those observed with pentazocine overdose and acetaminophen overdose.

For pentazocine alone in single doses above 60 mg there have been reports of the occurrence of nalorphine-like psychotomimetic effects such as anxiety, nightmares, strange thoughts, and hallucinations. Marked respiratory depression associated with increased blood pressure and tachycardia have also resulted from excessive doses as have dizziness, nausea, vomiting, lethargy, and paresthesias. The respiratory depression is antagonized by naloxone (see *Treatment*).

In acute acetaminophen overdosage, dose-dependent, potentially fatal hepatic necrosis is the most serious adverse effect. Renal tubular necrosis, hypoglycemic coma, and thrombocytopenia may also occur.

In adults, a single dose of 10 g to 15 g (200 mg/kg to 250 mg/kg) of acetaminophen may cause hepatotoxicity. A dose of 25 g or more is potentially fatal. The potential seriousness of the intoxication may not be evident during the first two days of acute acetaminophen poisoning. During the first 24 hours, nausea, vomiting, anorexia, and abdominal pain occur. These may persist for a week or more. Liver injury may become evident the second day, initial signs being elevation of serum transaminase and lactic dehydrogenase activity, increased serum bilirubin concentration, and prolongation of prothrombin time. Serum albumin concentration and alkaline phosphatase activity may remain normal. The hepatotoxicity may lead to encephalopathy, coma, and death. Transient azotemia is evident in a majority of patients and acute renal failure occurs in some.

There have been reports of glycosuria and impaired glucose tolerance, but hypoglycemia may also occur. Metabolic acidosis and metabolic alkalosis have been reported. Cerebral edema and nonspecific myocardial depression have also been noted. Biopsy reveals centrolobular necrosis with sparing of the periportal area. The hepatic lesions are reversible over a period of weeks or months in nonfatal cases.

The severity of the liver injury can be determined by measurement of the plasma half-time of acetaminophen during the first day of acute poisoning. If the half-time exceeds 4 hours, hepatic necrosis is likely and if the half-time is greater than 12 hours, hepatic coma will probably occur. Only minimal liver damage has developed when the serum concentration was below 120 μg/mL at 12 hours after ingestion of the drug. If serum bilirubin concentration is greater than 4 mg/100 mL during the first 5 days, encephalopathy may occur.

The seven day oral LD_{50} value for TALACEN in mice is 3,570 mg/kg.

Treatment. Oxygen, intravenous fluids, vasopressors, and other supportive measures should be employed as indicated. Assisted or controlled ventilation should also be considered. For respiratory depression due to overdosage or unusual sensitivity to TALACEN, parenteral naloxone is a specific and effective antagonist.

The toxic effects of acetaminophen may be prevented or minimized by antidotal therapy with N-acetylcysteine. In order to obtain the best possible results, N-acetylcysteine should be administered within approximately 16 hours of ingestion of the overdose.

For complete prescribing information for the approved use of acetylcysteine in the treatment of acetaminophen overdose, see package insert for MUCOMYST® (acetylcysteine) Mead Johnson.

Vigorous supportive therapy is required in severe intoxication. Procedures to limit the continuing absorption of the drug must be readily performed since the hepatic injury is dose dependent and occurs early in the course of intoxication. Induction of vomiting or gastric lavage, followed by oral administration of activated charcoal should be done in all cases.

If hemodialysis can be initiated within the first 12 hours, it is advocated for patients with a plasma acetaminophen concentration exceeding 120 μg/mL at 4 hours after ingestion of the drug.

DOSAGE AND ADMINISTRATION

Adult. The usual adult dose is 1 tablet every 4 hours as needed for pain relief, up to a maximum of 6 tablets per day. The usual duration of therapy is dependent upon the condition being treated but in any case should be reviewed regularly by the physician. The effect of meals on the rate and extent of bioavailability of both pentazocine and acetaminophen has not been documented.

HOW SUPPLIED

Caplets®, pale blue, scored, each containing pentazocine hydrochloride equivalent to 25 mg base and acetaminophen 650 mg.

Bottles of 100 (NDC 0024-1937-04).

Unit Dose Dispenser Package of 250 (NDC 0024-1937-14), 10 sleeves of 25 CAPLETS each.
Distributed by
Winthrop Pharmaceuticals
Division of Sterling Drug Inc
New York, NY 10016
Manufactured by
Sterling Pharmaceuticals Inc
Barceloneta, Puerto Rico 00617
Shown in Product Identification Section, page 435
TW-262-J

TALWIN® Injection ℂⅣ ℞
brand of pentazocine lactate injection, USP
Analgesic for Parenteral Use

DESCRIPTION
TALWIN injection, brand of pentazocine lactate injection, is a member of the benzazocine series (also known as the benzomorphan series). Chemically, pentazocine lactate is 1, 2, 3, 4, 5, 6-hexahydro-6, 11-dimethyl-3-(3-methyl-2-butenyl)-2,6-methano-3- benzazocin-8-ol lactate, a white, crystalline substance soluble in acidic aqueous solutions.

CLINICAL PHARMACOLOGY
TALWIN is a potent analgesic and 30 mg is usually as effective an analgesic as morphine 10 mg or meperidine 75 mg to 100 mg; however, a few studies suggest the TALWIN to morphine ratio may range from 20 mg to 40 mg TALWIN to 10 mg morphine. The duration of analgesia may sometimes be less than that of morphine. Analgesia usually occurs within 15 to 20 minutes after intramuscular or subcutaneous injection and within 2 to 3 minutes after intravenous injection. TALWIN weakly antagonizes the analgesic effects of morphine, meperidine, and phenazocine; in addition, it produces incomplete reversal of cardiovascular, respiratory, and behavioral depression induced by morphine and meperidine. TALWIN has about 1/50 the antagonistic activity of nalorphine. It also has sedative activity.

INDICATIONS AND USAGE
For the relief of moderate to severe pain. TALWIN may also be used for preoperative or preanesthetic medication and as a supplement to surgical anesthesia.

CONTRAINDICATION
TALWIN should not be administered to patients who are hypersensitive to it.

WARNINGS
Drug Dependence. *Special care should be exercised in prescribing pentazocine for emotionally unstable patients and for those with a history of drug misuse. Such patients should be closely supervised when greater than 4 or 5 days of therapy is contemplated. There have been instances of psychological and physical dependence on TALWIN in patients with such a history and, rarely, in patients without such a history. Extended use of parenteral TALWIN may lead to physical or psychological dependence in some patients. When TALWIN is abruptly discontinued, withdrawal symptoms such as abdominal cramps, elevated temperature, rhinorrhea, restlessness, anxiety, and lacrimation may occur. However, even when these have occurred, discontinuance has been accomplished with minimal difficulty. In the rare patient in whom more than minor difficulty has been encountered, reinstitution of parenteral TALWIN with gradual withdrawal has ameliorated the patient's symptoms. Substituting methadone or other narcotics for TALWIN in the treatment of the pentazocine abstinence syndrome should be avoided. There have been rare reports of possible abstinence syndromes in newborns after prolonged use of TALWIN during pregnancy.*
In prescribing parenteral TALWIN for chronic use, particularly if the drug is to be self-administered, the physician should take precautions to avoid increases in dose and frequency of injection by the patient.
Just as with all medication, the oral form of TALWIN is preferable for chronic administration.
Tissue Damage at Injection Sites. Severe sclerosis of the skin, subcutaneous tissues, and underlying muscle have occurred at the injection sites of patients who have received multiple doses of pentazocine lactate. Constant rotation of injection sites is, therefore, essential. In addition, animal studies have demonstrated that TALWIN is tolerated less well subcutaneously than intramuscularly. (See DOSAGE AND ADMINISTRATION.)
Head Injury and Increased Intracranial Pressure. As in the case of other potent analgesics, the potential of TALWIN injection for elevating cerebrospinal fluid pressure may be attributed to CO_2 retention due to the respiratory depressant effects of the drug. These effects may be markedly exaggerated in the presence of head injury, other intracranial lesions, or a preexisting increase in intracranial pressure. Furthermore, TALWIN can produce effects which may obscure the clinical course of patients with head injuries. In such patients, TALWIN must be used with extreme caution and only if its use is deemed essential.
Usage in Pregnancy. Safe use of TALWIN during pregnancy (other than labor) has not been established. Animal reproduction studies have not demonstrated teratogenic or embryotoxic effects. However, TALWIN should be administered to pregnant patients (other than labor) only when, in the judgment of the physician, the potential benefits outweigh the possible hazards. Patients receiving TALWIN during labor have experienced no adverse effects other than those that occur with commonly used analgesics. TALWIN should be used with caution in women delivering premature infants.
Acute CNS Manifestations. Patients receiving therapeutic doses of pentazocine have experienced hallucinations (usually visual), disorientation, and confusion which have cleared spontaneously within a period of hours. The mechanism of this reaction is not known. Such patients should be closely observed and vital signs checked. If the drug is reinstituted, it should be done with caution since these acute CNS manifestations may recur.
Due to the potential for increased CNS depressant effects, alcohol should be used with caution in patients who are currently receiving pentazocine.
Usage in Children. Because clinical experience in children under twelve years of age is limited, the use of TALWIN in this age group is not recommended.
Ambulatory Patients. Since sedation, dizziness, and occasional euphoria have been noted, ambulatory patients should be warned not to operate machinery, drive cars, or unnecessarily expose themselves to hazards.
Myocardial Infarction. Caution should be exercised in the intravenous use of pentazocine for patients with acute myocardial infarction accompanied by hypertension or left ventricular failure. Data suggest that intravenous administration of pentazocine increases systemic and pulmonary arterial pressure and systemic vascular resistance in patients with acute myocardial infarction.
NOTE: Acetone sodium bisulfite, a sulfite that may cause allergic-type reactions including anaphylactic symptoms and life-threatening or less severe asthmatic episodes in certain susceptible people, is contained in both Carpuject® Sterile Cartridge-Needle Unit and multiple-dose vials. The overall prevalence of sulfite sensitivity in the general population is unknown and probably low. Sulfite sensitivity is seen more frequently in asthmatic than in nonasthmatic people.
The ampuls in the Uni-Amp® Pak and the Uni-Nest™ Pak do not contain acetone sodium bisulfite.

PRECAUTIONS
Certain Respiratory Conditions. The possibility that TALWIN may cause respiratory depression should be considered in treatment of patients with bronchial asthma. TALWIN injection, brand of pentazocine lactate injection, should be administered only with caution and in low dosage to patients with respiratory depression (eg, from other medication, uremia, or severe infection), severely limited respiratory reserve, obstructive respiratory conditions, or cyanosis.
Impaired Renal or Hepatic Function. Although laboratory tests have not indicated that TALWIN causes or increases renal or hepatic impairment, the drug should be administered with caution to patients with such impairment. Extensive liver disease appears to predispose to greater side effects (eg, marked apprehension, anxiety, dizziness, sleepiness) from the usual clinical dose, and may be the result of decreased metabolism of the drug by the liver.
Biliary Surgery. Narcotic drug products are generally considered to elevate biliary tract pressure for varying periods following their administration. Some evidence suggests that pentazocine may differ from other marketed narcotics in this respect (ie, it causes little or no elevation in biliary tract pressures). The clinical significance of these findings, however, is not yet known.
Patients Receiving Narcotics. TALWIN is a mild narcotic antagonist. Some patients previously given narcotics, including methadone for the daily treatment of narcotic dependence, have experienced withdrawal symptoms after receiving TALWIN.
CNS Effect. Caution should be used when TALWIN is administered to patients prone to seizures; seizures have occurred in a few such patients in association with the use of TALWIN although no cause and effect relationship has been established.
Use in Anesthesia. Concomitant use of CNS depressants with parenteral TALWIN may produce additive CNS depression. Adequate equipment and facilities should be available to identify and treat systemic emergencies should they occur.

ADVERSE REACTIONS
The most commonly occurring reactions are: nausea, dizziness or lightheadedness, vomiting, euphoria.
Dermatologic Reactions: Soft tissue induration, nodules, and cutaneous depression can occur at injection sites. Ulceration (sloughing) and severe sclerosis of the skin and subcutaneous tissues (and, rarely, underlying muscle) have been reported after multiple doses. Other reported dermatologic reactions include diaphoresis, sting on injection, flushed skin including plethora, dermatitis including pruritus.
Infrequently occurring reactions are—*respiratory:* respiratory depression, dyspnea, transient apnea in a small number of newborn infants whose mothers received TALWIN during labor; *cardiovascular:* circulatory depression, shock, hypertension; *CNS effects:* dizziness, lightheadedness, hallucinations, sedation, euphoria, headache, confusion, disorientation; infrequently weakness, disturbed dreams, insomnia, syncope, visual blurring and focusing difficulty, depression; and rarely tremor, irritability, excitement, tinnitus. *Gastrointestinal:* constipation, dry mouth; *other:* urinary retention, headache, paresthesia, alterations in rate or strength of uterine contractions during labor.
Rarely reported reactions include—*neuromuscular and psychiatric:* muscle tremor, insomnia, disorientation, hallucinations; *gastrointestinal:* taste alteration, diarrhea and cramps; *ophthalmic:* blurred vision, nystagmus, diplopia, miosis; *hematologic:* depression of white blood cells (especially granulocytes), which is usually reversible, moderate transient eosinophilia; *other:* tachycardia, weakness or faintness, chills, allergic reactions including edema of the face, toxic epidermal necrolysis.
See **Acute CNS Manifestations** and **Drug Dependence** under **WARNINGS.**

DOSAGE AND ADMINISTRATION
Adults, Excluding Patients in Labor. The recommended single parenteral dose is 30 mg by intramuscular, subcutaneous, or intravenous route. This may be repeated every 3 to 4 hours. Doses in excess of 30 mg intravenously or 60 mg intramuscularly or subcutaneously are not recommended. Total daily dosage should not exceed 360 mg.
The subcutaneous route of administration should be used only when necessary because of possible severe tissue damage at injection sites (see WARNINGS). When frequent injections are needed, the drug should be administered intramuscularly. In addition, constant rotation of injection sites (eg, the upper outer quadrants of the buttocks, mid-lateral aspects of the thighs, and the deltoid areas) is essential.
Patients in Labor. A single, intramuscular 30 mg dose has been most commonly administered. An intravenous 20 mg dose has given adequate pain relief to some patients in labor when contractions become regular, and this dose may be given two or three times at two-to three-hour intervals, as needed.
Children Under 12 Years of Age. Since clinical experience in children under twelve years of age is limited, the use of TALWIN in this age group is not recommended.
CAUTION. TALWIN should not be mixed in the same syringe with soluble barbiturates because precipitation will occur.

OVERDOSAGE
Manifestations: Clinical experience with TALWIN overdosage has been insufficient to define the signs of this condition.
Treatment: Oxygen, intravenous fluids, vasopressors, and other supportive measures should be employed as indicated. Assisted or controlled ventilation should also be considered. For respiratory depression due to overdosage or unusual sensitivity to TALWIN, brand of pentazocine lactate injection, parenteral naloxone is a specific and effective antagonist.

HOW SUPPLIED
UNI-AMP—Individual unit dose ampuls of 1 mL (30 mg) NDC 0024-1924-04, *1.5 mL (45 mg)* NDC 0024-1925-04, *and 2 mL (60 mg)* NDC 0024-1926-04 *in box of 25.*
UNI-NEST ampuls of 1 mL (30 mg) NDC 0024-1924-14 *and 2 mL (60 mg)* NDC 0024-1926-14 *in box of 25.*
Each 1 mL contains pentazocine lactate equivalent to 30 mg base and 2.8 mg sodium chloride, in Water for Injection.
CARPUJECT Sterile Cartridge-Needle Unit, *1 mL (30 mg)* NDC 0024-1917-02, *1.5 mL (45 mg)* NDC 0024-1918-02, *and 2 mL (60 mg)* NDC 0024-1919-02, all in 2 mL cartridges, box of 10. Each 1 mL contains pentazocine lactate equivalent to 30 mg base, 1 mg acetone sodium bisulfite, and 2.2 mg sodium chloride, in Water for Injection.
Multiple-dose vials of 10 mL NDC 0024-1916-01, box of 1. Each 1 mL contains pentazocine lactate equivalent to 30 mg base, 2 mg acetone sodium bisulfite, 1.5 mg sodium chloride, and 1 mg methylparaben as preservative, in Water for Injection.
The pH of TALWIN solutions is adjusted between 4 and 5 with lactic acid or sodium hydroxide. The air in the ampuls, vials, and Cartridge-Needle Units has been displaced by nitrogen gas.

TW-109-GG

Continued on next page

This product information was prepared in August, 1989. On these and other products of Winthrop Pharmaceuticals, detailed information may be obtained on a current basis by direct inquiry to the Professional Services Department, 90 Park Avenue, New York, NY 10016 (800) 446-6267.

Winthrop Pharm.—Cont.

TALWIN® Compound   Ⓒ ℞
brand of pentazocine hydrochloride
and aspirin tablets, USP

DESCRIPTION

TALWIN Compound is a combination of pentazocine hydrochloride, USP, equivalent to 12.5 mg base and aspirin, USP,
325 mg.

Pentazocine is a member of the benzazocine series (also
known as the benzomorphan series). Chemically, pentazocine is 1, 2, 3, 4, 5, 6 -hexahydro - 6, 11-dimethyl-3-(3-methyl-
2-butenyl)-2, 6-methano-3-benzazocin-8-ol, a white, crystalline substance soluble in acidic aqueous solutions.

Chemically, aspirin is Benzoic acid, 2-(acetyloxy)-;.

Inactive Ingredients: Magnesium Stearate, Microcrystalline Cellulose, Sodium Lauryl Sulfate, Starch.

CLINICAL PHARMACOLOGY

Pentazocine is a potent analgesic which when administered
orally is approximately equivalent, on a mg for mg basis, in
analgesic effect to codeine. Two Caplets® of TALWIN Compound when administered orally have the additive analgesic
effect equivalent to 25 mg of TALWIN plus 650 mg of aspirin.
TALWIN Compound provides the analgesic effects of pentazocine and the analgesic, anti-inflammatory, and antipyretic
actions of aspirin.

Onset of significant analgesia usually occurs between 15 and
30 minutes after oral administration, and duration of action
is usually three hours or longer. Onset and duration of action
and the degree of pain relief are related both to dose and the
severity of pretreatment pain. Pentazocine weakly antagonizes the analgesic effects of morphine, meperidine, and phenazocine; in addition, it produces incomplete reversal of cardiovascular, respiratory, and behavioral depression induced
by morphine and meperidine. Pentazocine has about $\frac{1}{50}$ the
antagonistic activity of nalorphine. It also has sedative activity.

INDICATION AND USAGE

For the relief of moderate pain

CONTRAINDICATIONS

TALWIN Compound should not be administered to patients
who are hypersensitive to either pentazocine or salicylates,
or in any situation where aspirin is contraindicated.

WARNINGS

*Drug Dependence. There have been instances of psychological
and physical dependence on parenteral pentazocine in patients
with a history of drug abuse, and rarely, in patients without
such a history. Abrupt discontinuance following the extended
use of parenteral pentazocine has resulted in withdrawal
symptoms. There have been a few reports of dependence and of
withdrawal symptoms with orally administered pentazocine.
Patients with a history of drug dependence should be under
close supervision while receiving TALWIN Compound orally.
There have been rare reports of possible abstinence syndromes
in newborns after prolonged use of pentazocine during pregnancy.*

*In prescribing TALWIN Compound for chronic use, the physi-
cian should take precautions to avoid increases in dose by the
patient and to prevent the use of the drug in anticipation of
pain rather than for the relief of pain.*

Head Injury and Increased Intracranial Pressure. The respiratory depressant effects of pentazocine and its potential for
elevating cerebrospinal fluid pressure may be markedly exaggerated in the presence of head injury, other intracranial
lesions, or a preexisting increase in intracranial pressure.
Furthermore, pentazocine can produce effects which may
obscure the clinical course of patients with head injuries. In
such patients, TALWIN Compound must be used with extreme caution and only if its use is deemed essential.

Usage in Pregnancy. Safe use of pentazocine during pregnancy (other than labor) has not been established. Animal
reproduction studies have not demonstrated teratogenic or
embryotoxic effects. However, TALWIN Compound should
be administered to pregnant patients (other than labor) only
when, in the judgment of the physician, the potential benefits outweigh the possible hazards. Patients receiving pentazocine during labor have experienced no adverse effects other
than those that occur with commonly used analgesics.
TALWIN Compound, brand of pentazocine hydrochloride
and aspirin tablets, should be used with caution in women
delivering premature infants.

Acute CNS Manifestations. Patients receiving therapeutic
doses of pentazocine have experienced hallucinations (usually visual), disorientation, and confusion which have
cleared spontaneously within a period of hours. The mechanism of this reaction is not known. Such patients should be
closely observed and vital signs checked. If the drug is reinstituted it should be done with caution since these acute CNS
manifestations may recur.

Due to the potential for increased CNS depressant effects,
alcohol should be used with caution in patients who are currently receiving pentazocine.

Usage in Children. Because clinical experience in children
under 12 years of age is limited, administration of TALWIN
Compound in this age group is not recommended.

Ambulatory Patients. Since sedation, dizziness, and occasional euphoria have been noted, ambulatory patients
should be warned not to operate machinery, drive cars, or
unnecessarily expose themselves to hazards.

Other. Because of its aspirin content, TALWIN Compound
should be used with caution in the presence of peptic ulcer, in
conjunction with anticoagulant therapy, or in any situation
where the effects of aspirin may be deleterious.

PRECAUTIONS

Certain Respiratory Conditions. Although respiratory depression has rarely been reported after oral administration of
pentazocine, TALWIN Compound, brand of pentazocine hydrochloride and aspirin tablets, should be administered with
caution to patients with respiratory depression from any
cause, severely limited respiratory reserve, severe bronchial
asthma and other obstructive respiratory conditions, or cyanosis.

Impaired Renal or Hepatic Function. Decreased metabolism of the drug by the liver in extensive liver disease may
predispose to accentuation of side effects. Although laboratory tests have not indicated that pentazocine causes or increases renal or hepatic impairment, TALWIN Compound
should be administered with caution to patients with such
impairment.

Myocardial Infarction. As with all drugs, TALWIN Compound should be used with caution in patients with myocardial infarction who have nausea or vomiting.

Biliary Surgery. Narcotic drug products are generally considered to elevate biliary tract pressure for varying periods
following administration. Some evidence suggests that pentazocine may differ in this respect (ie, it causes little or no
elevation in biliary tract pressures). The clinical significance
of these findings, however, is not yet known.

Patients Receiving Narcotics. Pentazocine is a mild narcotic
antagonist. Some patients previously given narcotics, including methadone for the daily treatment of narcotic dependence, have experienced withdrawal symptoms after receiving pentazocine.

CNS Effect. Caution should be used when pentazocine is
administered to patients prone to seizures. Seizures have
occurred in a few such patients in association with the use of
pentazocine although no cause and effect relationship has
been established.

ADVERSE REACTIONS

Reactions reported after oral administration of pentazocine
or TALWIN Compound include *gastrointestinal:* nausea,
vomiting; infrequently constipation; and rarely abdominal
distress, anorexia, diarrhea. *CNS Effects:* dizziness, lightheadedness, hallucinations, sedation, euphoria, headache,
confusion, disorientation; infrequently weakness, disturbed
dreams, insomnia, syncope, visual blurring and focusing
difficulty, depression; and rarely tremor, irritability, excitement, tinnitus. *Autonomic:* sweating; infrequently flushing;
and rarely chills. *Allergic:* infrequently rash; and rarely urticaria, edema of the face. *Cardiovascular:* infrequently decrease in blood pressure, tachycardia. *Hematologic:* rarely
depression of white blood cells (especially granulocytes),
which is usually reversible, moderate transient eosinophilia.
Other: rarely respiratory depression, urinary retention, paresthesia, toxic epidermal necrolysis.

DOSAGE AND ADMINISTRATION

Adults. The usual adult dose is 2 CAPLETS three or four
times a day.

Children Under 12 Years of Age. Since clinical experience in
children under 12 years of age is limited, administration of
TALWIN Compound in this age group is not recommended.

Duration of Therapy. Patients with chronic pain who receive
pentazocine orally for prolonged periods have only rarely
been reported to experience withdrawal symptoms when
administration was abruptly discontinued (see
WARNINGS). Tolerance to the analgesic effect of pentazocine has also been reported only rarely. Significant abnormalities of liver and kidney function tests have not been reported, even after prolonged administration of pentazocine.

OVERDOSAGE

Manifestations: Clinical experience with pentazocine overdosage has been insufficient to define the signs of this condition. Signs of salicylate overdosage include headache, dizziness, confusion, tinnitus, diaphoresis, thirst, nausea, vomiting, diarrhea, tachycardia, tachypnea, Kussmaul breathing,
convulsions, and coma. Death is usually from respiratory
failure.

Treatment: Treatment for overdosage of TALWIN Compound, brand of pentazocine hydrochloride and aspirin tablets, should include treatment for salicylate poisoning as
outlined in standard references.

Oxygen, intravenous fluids, vasopressors, and other supportive measures should be employed as indicated. Assisted or

controlled ventilation should also be considered. For respiratory depression due to overdosage or unusual sensitivity to
pentazocine, parenteral naloxone is a specific and effective
antagonist.

HOW SUPPLIED

CAPLETS, white, each containing pentazocine hydrochlo-
ride equivalent to 12.5 mg base and aspirin 325 mg.
Bottle of 100 (NDC 0024-1927-04).
Distributed by Winthrop Pharmaceuticals
Division of Sterling Drug Inc., New York, NY 10016
Manufactured by Sterling Pharmaceuticals Inc.
Barceloneta, Puerto Rico 00617

                                              TW-225-J(O)

TALWIN® Nx   Ⓒ ℞
brand of pentazocine and naloxone hydrochlorides tablets,
USP

Analgesic for Oral Use Only

> TALWIN® Nx is intended for oral use only. Severe,
> potentially lethal, reactions may result from misuse of
> TALWIN® Nx by injection either alone or in combina-
> tion with other substances. (See **DRUG ABUSE AND
> DEPENDENCE** section.)

DESCRIPTION

TALWIN Nx contains pentazocine hydrochloride, USP,
equivalent to 50 mg base and is a member of the benzazocine
series (also known as the benzomorphan series), and naloxone hydrochloride, USP, equivalent to 0.5 mg base.

TALWIN Nx is an analgesic for oral administration.

Chemically, pentazocine hydrochloride is 1,2,3,4,5,6-
Hexahydro -6,11 -dimethyl -3-(3-methyl-2-butenyl)-2, 6-me-
thano-3-benzazocin-8-ol hydrochloride, a white, crystalline
substance soluble in acidic aqueous solutions.

Chemically, naloxone hydrochloride is Morphinan-6-one,
4, 5-epoxy-3, 14-dihydroxy-17-(2-propenyl)-, hydrochloride,
(5α)-. It is a slightly off-white powder, and is soluble in water
and dilute acids.

Inactive Ingredients: Colloidal Silicon Dioxide, Dibasic Calcium Phosphate, D&C Yellow #10, FD&C Yellow #6, Magnesium Stearate, Microcrystalline Cellulose, Sodium Lauryl
Sulfate, Starch.

CLINICAL PHARMACOLOGY

Pentazocine is a potent analgesic which when administered
orally in a 50 mg dose appears equivalent in analgesic effect
to 60 mg (1 grain) of codeine. Onset of significant analgesia
usually occurs between 15 and 30 minutes after oral administration, and duration of action is usually three hours or
longer. Onset and duration of action and the degree of pain
relief are related both to dose and the severity of pretreatment pain. Pentazocine weakly antagonizes the analgesic
effects of morphine and meperidine; in addition, it produces
incomplete reversal of cardiovascular, respiratory, and behavioral depression induced by morphine and meperidine.
Pentazocine has about 1/50 the antagonistic activity of nalorphine. It also has sedative activity.

Pentazocine is well absorbed from the gastrointestinal tract.
Concentrations in plasma coincide closely with the onset,
duration, and intensity of analgesia; peak values occur 1 to 3
hours after oral administration. The half-life in plasma is 2
to 3 hours.

Pentazocine is metabolized in the liver and excreted primarily in the urine. Pentazocine passes into the fetal circulation.
Naloxone when administered orally at 0.5 mg has no pharmacologic activity. Naloxone hydrochloride administered
parenterally at the same dose is an effective antagonist to
pentazocine and a pure antagonist to narcotic analgesics.
TALWIN Nx is a potent analgesic when administered orally.
However, the presence of naloxone in TALWIN Nx will prevent the effect of pentazocine if the product is misused by
injection.

Studies in animals indicate that the presence of naloxone
does not affect pentazocine analgesia when the combination
is given orally. If the combination is given by injection the
action of pentazocine is neutralized.

INDICATIONS AND USAGE

> TALWIN® Nx is intended for oral use only. Severe,
> potentially lethal, reactions may result from misuse of
> TALWIN® Nx by injection either alone or in combina-
> tion with other substances. (See **DRUG ABUSE AND
> DEPENDENCE** section.)

TALWIN Nx is indicated for the relief of moderate to severe
pain.

TALWIN Nx is indicated for oral use only.

CONTRAINDICATIONS

TALWIN Nx should not be administered to patients who are hypersensitive to either pentazocine or naloxone.

WARNINGS

> TALWIN® Nx is intended for oral use only. Severe, potentially lethal, reactions may result from misuse of TALWIN® Nx by injection either alone or in combination with other substances. (See **DRUG ABUSE AND DEPENDENCE** section.)

Drug Dependence. Pentazocine can cause a physical and psychological dependence. (See **DRUG ABUSE AND DEPENDENCE.**)

Head Injury and Increased Intracranial Pressure. As in the case of other potent analgesics, the potential of pentazocine for elevating cerebrospinal fluid pressure may be attributed to CO_2 retention due to the respiratory depressant effects of the drug. These effects may be markedly exaggerated in the presence of head injury, other intracranial lesions, or a preexisting increase in intracranial pressure. Furthermore, pentazocine can produce effects which may obscure the clinical course of patients with head injuries. In such patients, pentazocine must be used wth extreme caution and only if its use is deemed essential.

Usage with Alcohol. Due to the potential for increased CNS depressant effects, alcohol should be used with caution in patients who are currently receiving pentazocine.

Patients Receiving Narcotics. Pentazocine is a mild narcotic antagonist. Some patients previously given narcotics, including methadone for the daily treatment of narcotic dependence, have experienced withdrawal symptoms after receiving pentazocine.

Certain Respiratory Conditions. Although respiratory depression has rarely been reported after oral administration of pentazocine, the drug should be administered with caution to patients with respiratory depression from any cause, severely limited respiratory reserve, severe bronchial asthma, and other obstructive respiratory conditions, or cyanosis.

Acute CNS Manifestations. Patients receiving therapeutic doses of pentazocine have experienced hallucinations (usually visual), disorientation, and confusion which have cleared spontaneously within a period of hours. The mechanism of this reaction is not known. Such patients should be very closely observed and vital signs checked. If the drug is reinstituted, it should be done with caution since these acute CNS manifestations may recur.

PRECAUTIONS

CNS Effect. Caution should be used when pentazocine is administered to patients prone to seizures; seizures have occurred in a few such patients in association with the use of pentazocine though no cause and effect relationship has been established.

Impaired Renal or Hepatic Function. Decreased metabolism of pentazocine by the liver in extensive liver disease may predispose to accentuation of side effects. Although laboratory tests have not indicated that pentazocine causes or increases renal or hepatic impairment, the drug should be administered with caution to patients with such impairment.

In prescribing pentazocine for long-term use, the physician should take precautions to avoid increases in dose by the patient.

Biliary Surgery. Narcotic drug products are generally considered to elevate biliary tract pressure for varying periods following their administration. Some evidence suggests that pentazocine may differ from other marketed narcotics in this respect (ie, it causes little or no elevation in biliary tract pressures). The clinical significance of these findings, however, is not yet known.

Information for Patients. Since sedation, dizziness, and occasional euphoria have been noted, ambulatory patients should be warned not to operate machinery, drive cars, or unnecessarily expose themselves to hazards. Pentazocine may cause physical and psychological dependence when taken alone and may have additive CNS depressant properties when taken in combination with alcohol or other CNS depressants.

Myocardial Infarction. As with all drugs, pentazocine should be used with caution in patients with myocardial infarction who have nausea or vomiting.

Drug Interactions. *Usage with Alcohol:* See **WARNINGS**.

Carcinogenesis, Mutagenesis, Impairment of Fertility. No long-term studies in animals to test for carcinogenesis have been performed with the components of TALWIN Nx, brand of pentazocine and naloxone hydrochlorides tablets.

Pregnancy Category C. Animal reproduction studies have not been conducted with TALWIN Nx. It is also not known whether TALWIN Nx can cause fetal harm when administered to pregnant women or can affect reproduction capacity. TALWIN Nx should be given to pregnant women only if clearly needed. However, animal reproduction studies with

pentazocine have not demonstrated teratogenic embryotoxic effects.

Labor and Delivery. Patients receiving pentazocine during labor have experienced no adverse effects other than those that occur with commonly used analgesics. TALWIN Nx should be used with caution in women delivering premature infants. The effect of TALWIN Nx on the mother and fetus, the duration of labor or delivery, the possibility that forceps delivery or other intervention or resuscitation of the newborn may be necessary, or the effect of TALWIN Nx on the later growth, development, and functional maturation of the child are unknown at the present time.

Nursing Mothers. It is not known whether this drug is excreted in human milk. Because many drugs are excreted in human milk, caution should be exercised when TALWIN Nx is administered to a nursing woman.

Pediatric Use. Safety and effectiveness in children below the age of 12 years have not been established.

ADVERSE REACTIONS

Cardiovascular: Hypotension, tachycardia, syncope.
Respiratory: Rarely, respiratory depression.
Acute CNS Manifestations: Patients receiving therapeutic doses of pentazocine have experienced hallucinations (usually visual), disorientation, and confusion which have cleared spontaneously within a period of hours. The mechanism of this reaction is not known. Such patients should be closely observed and vital signs checked. If the drug is reinstituted it should be done with caution since these acute CNS manifestations may recur.
Other CNS Effects: Dizziness, lightheadedness, hallucinations, sedation, euphoria, headache, confusion, disorientation; infrequently weakness, disturbed dreams, insomnia, syncope, visual blurring and focusing difficulty, depression; and rarely tremor, irritability, excitement, tinnitus.
Autonomic: Sweating; infrequently flushing; and rarely chills.
Gastrointestinal: Nausea, vomiting, constipation, diarrhea, anorexia, rarely abdominal distress.
Allergic: Edema of the face; dermatitis, including pruritus; flushed skin, including plethora; infrequently rash, and rarely urticaria.
Ophthalmic: Visual blurring and focusing difficulty.
Hematologic: Depression of white blood cells (especially granulocytes), which is usually reversible, moderate transient eosinophilia.
Other: Headache, chills, insomnia, weakness, urinary retention, paresthesia.

DRUG ABUSE AND DEPENDENCE

Controlled Substance. TALWIN Nx is a Schedule IV controlled substance.

There have been some reports of dependence and of withdrawal symptoms wth orally administered pentazocine. Patients with a history of drug dependence should be under close supervision while receiving pentazocine orally. There have been rare reports of possible abstinence syndromes in newborns after prolonged use of pentazocine during pregnancy.

There have been instances of psychological and physical dependence on parenteral pentazocine in patients with a history of drug abuse and rarely, in patients without such a history. Abrupt discontinuance following the extended use of parenteral pentazocine has resulted in withdrawal symptoms.

In prescribing pentazocine for chronic use, the physician should take precautions to avoid increases in dose by the patient.

The amount of naloxone present in TALWIN Nx (0.5 mg per tablet) has no action when taken orally and will not interfere with the pharmacologic action of pentazocine. However, this amount of naloxone given by injection has profound antagonistic action to narcotic analgesics.

Severe, even lethal, consequences may result from misuse of tablets by injection either alone or in combination with other substances, such as pulmonary emboli, vascular occlusion, ulceration and abscesses, and withdrawal symptoms in narcotic dependent individuals.

TALWIN Nx, brand of pentazocine and naloxone hydrochlorides tablets, contains an opioid antagonist, naloxone (0.5 mg). Naloxone is inactive when administered orally at this dose, and its inclusion in TALWIN Nx is intended to curb a form of misuse of oral pentazocine. Parenterally, naloxone is an active narcotic antagonist. Thus, TALWIN Nx has a lower potential for parenteral misuse than the previous oral pentazocine formulation TALWIN® 50, brand of pentazocine hydrochloride tablets, USP. However, it is still subject to patient misuse and abuse by the oral route.

OVERDOSAGE

Manifestations. Clinical experience of overdosage with this oral medication has been insufficient to define the signs of this condition.
Treatment. Oxygen, intravenous fluids, vasopressors, and other supportive measures should be employed as indicated. Assisted or controlled ventilation should also be considered. For respiratory depression due to overdosage or unusual

sensitivity to pentazocine, parenteral naloxone is a specific and effective antagonist.

DOSAGE AND ADMINISTRATION

> TALWIN® Nx is intended for oral use only. Severe, potentially lethal, reactions may result from misuse of TALWIN® Nx by injection either alone or in combination with other substances. (See **DRUG ABUSE AND DEPENDENCE** section.)

Adults. The usual initial adult dose is 1 tablet every three or four hours. This may be increased to 2 tablets when needed. Total daily dosage should not exceed 12 tablets. When anti-inflammatory or antipyretic effects are desired in addition to analgesia, aspirin can be administered concomitantly with this product.

Children Under 12 Years of Age. Since clinical experience in children under 12 years of age is limited, administration of this product in this age group is not recommended.

Duration of Therapy. Patients with chronic pain who receive TALWIN Nx orally for prolonged periods have only rarely been reported to experience withdrawal symptoms when administration was abruptly discontinued (see **WARNINGS**). Tolerance to the analgesic effect of pentazocine has also been reported only rarely. However, there is no long-term experience with the oral administration of TALWIN Nx.

HOW SUPPLIED

Tablets (oblong), yellow, scored, each containing pentazocine hydrochloride equivalent to 50 mg base and naloxone hydrochloride equivalent to 0.5 mg base.
Bottles of 100 (NDC 0024-1951-04).
Unit Dose Dispenser Package of 250 (NDC 0024-1951-24), 10 sleeves of 25 tablets each.

Distributed by
Winthrop Pharmaceuticals
Division of Sterling Drug Inc.
New York, NY 10016
Manufactured by
Sterling Pharmaceuticals Inc.
Barceloneta, Puerto Rico 00617
Shown in Product Identification Section, page 435
TW-267-H

TORNALATE®   ℞
(bitolterol mesylate)
Metered Dose Inhaler
Bronchodilator for Oral Inhalation

DESCRIPTION

TORNALATE (bitolterol mesylate) is the di-*p*-toluate ester of the β-adrenergic bronchodilator *N-t*-butylarterenol (colterol). It has a molecular weight of 557.7. Bitolterol mesylate is known chemically as 4-[2-[(1,1-dimethylethyl) amino]-1-hydroxyethyl]-1,2-phenylene 4-methylbenzoate (ester) methanesulfonate (salt).

TORNALATE (bitolterol mesylate), Metered Dose Inhaler, is a complete aerosol unit for oral inhalation. It consists of a plastic-coated bottle of ready-to-use aerosol solution and a detachable plastic mouthpiece with built-in nebulizer. The bottle contains 16.4 g (15 mL) of 0.8% bitolterol mesylate in a vehicle containing 38% alcohol (w/w), inert propellants (dichlorodifluoromethane and dichlorotetrafluoroethane), ascorbic acid, saccharin, and menthol.

Each bottle provides at least 300 actuations. Each actuation delivers a measured dose of 0.37 mg of bitolterol mesylate as a fine, even mist.

CLINICAL PHARMACOLOGY

TORNALATE (bitolterol mesylate) is administered as a prodrug which is hydrolyzed by esterases in tissue and blood to the active moiety colterol. TORNALATE administered as an inhaled aerosol, has a rapid (3 to 4 minutes) onset of bronchodilator activity. The duration of action with TORNALATE is at least 5 hours in most patients and 8 or more hours in 25% to 35% of patients, based on 15% or greater increase in forced expiratory volume in one second (FEV_1), as demonstrated in 3 month isoproterenol controlled multicenter trials. Based on mean maximal expiratory flow (MMEF) measurements, the duration of action is 6 to 7 hours. The duration of bronchodilator action with TORNALATE in these trials is longer than that seen with isoproterenol, especially in steroid-dependent patients. Duration of effect was reduced over time in steroid-dependent asthmatic patients where the du-

Continued on next page

This product information was prepared in August, 1989. On these and other products of Winthrop Pharmaceuticals, detailed information may be obtained on a current basis by direct inquiry to the Professional Services Department, 90 Park Avenue, New York, NY 10016 (800) 446-6267.

Winthrop Pharm.—Cont.

ration was 3.5 to 5 hours for FEV_1. The mean maximum increase in FEV_1 over baseline in the majority of patients was 39% to 42% and occurred by 30 to 60 minutes, similar to that seen in the isoproterenol group.

TORNALATE is a beta adrenergic agonist which has been shown by in vitro and in vivo pharmacological studies in animals to exert a preferential effect on $beta_2$ adrenergic receptors, such as those located in bronchial smooth muscle. However, controlled clinical trials in patients who were administered the drug have not revealed a preferential $beta_2$ adrenergic effect. At doses that produced long duration of bronchodilator activity (up to 8 hours in some patients) with a mean maximum bronchodilating effect of approximately 40% increase in FEV_1 (forced expiration volume in one second), a less than 10 beat per minute mean maximum increase in heart rate was seen. The effect on the heart rate was transient and similar to the increases seen in the isoproterenol treated patients in these studies.

Although blood levels of colterol formed by gradual release from the pro-drug (bitolterol) in the lungs are too low to be measured by currently available assay methods, data on disposition are available from oral studies in man. Following oral administration of 5.9 mg tritiated bitolterol mesylate to man, radioactivity measurements indicated mean maximum colterol concentration in blood of approximately 2.1 $\mu g/mL$ one hour after medication. Urinary excretion data indicate that 83 percent of the radioactivity of this oral dose was excreted within the first 24 hours. By 72 hours, 85.6 percent of the tritium had been excreted in the urine and 8.1 percent in the feces. Most of the radioactivity was excreted as conjugated colterol; free colterol accounted for 2.1 to 3.7 percent of the total radioactivity excreted in the urine. No intact bitolterol was detected in urine.

The pharmacologic effects of β-adrenergic drugs including TORNALATE (bitolterol mesylate) are attributable to stimulation of adenyl cyclase, the enzyme which catalyzes the conversion of adenosine triphosphate (ATP) to cyclic-3', 5'-adenosine monophosphate (c-AMP). Increased c-AMP levels are associated with relaxation of bronchial smooth muscle and with inhibition of release of mediators of immediate hypersensitivity.

In a six week clinical trial in which 24 asthmatic patients received TORNALATE and theophylline concurrently, improvement in pulmonary function was enhanced over that seen with either drug alone. No potentiation of side effects was observed, and 24-hour ECG recordings (Holter monitoring) indicated no greater degree of cardiac toxicity with TORNALATE alone or in combination with theophylline than that which occurred with theophylline alone.

TORNALATE did not adversely affect arterial oxygen tension in a blood-gas study in 24 asthmatic patients. However, a decrease in arterial oxygen tension has been reported with other adrenergic bronchodilators and could be anticipated to occur with TORNALATE as well.

In repetitive dosing studies, continued effectiveness was demonstrated throughout the 3 month period of treatment in the majority of patients. However, some overall decrease was observed in steroid dependent asthmatics.

INDICATIONS AND USAGE

TORNALATE (bitolterol mesylate) is indicated for both prophylactic and therapeutic use as a bronchodilator for bronchial asthma and for reversible bronchospasm. It may be used with or without concurrent theophylline and/or steroid therapy.

CONTRAINDICATIONS

TORNALATE (bitolterol mesylate) is contraindicated in patients who are hypersensitive to any of its ingredients.

WARNINGS

As with other β-adrenergic aerosols, TORNALATE (bitolterol mesylate) should not be used in excess. Use of aerosolized β-adrenergic drugs may have a deleterious cardiac effect. Paradoxical bronchoconstriction has been reported with administration of β-adrenergic agents. Immediate hypersensitivity (allergic) reactions can occur after the administration of TORNALATE. In such instances, the drug should be discontinued immediately and alternative therapy instituted.

PRECAUTIONS

General. As with all β-adrenergic stimulating agents, caution should be used when administering TORNALATE (bitolterol mesylate) to patients with cardiovascular disease such as ischemic heart disease or hypertension. Caution is also advised in patients with hyperthyroidism, diabetes mellitus, cardiac arrhythmias, convulsive disorders or unusual responsiveness to β-adrenergic agonists. Significant changes in systolic and diastolic blood pressure have been seen in individual patients and could be expected to occur in some patients after use of any β-adrenergic aerosol bronchodilator.

Information for Patients. The effects of TORNALATE may last up to eight hours or longer. It should not be used more often than recommended and the patient should not increase the number of inhalations or frequency of use without first asking the physician. If symptoms of asthma get worse, adverse reactions occur, or the patient does not respond to the usual dose, the patient should be instructed to contact the physician immediately. The patient should be advised to see the Illustrated Directions for Use.

Drug Interactions. Other sympathomimetic aerosol bronchodilators should not be used concomitantly with TORNALATE. If additional adrenergic drugs are to be administered by any route, they should be used with caution to avoid deleterious cardiovascular effects.

Carcinogenesis, Mutagenesis, and Impairment of Fertility. No tumorigenicity (and specifically no increase in leiomyomas) was observed in a two year oral study in Sprague-Dawley CD rats at doses of TORNALATE corresponding to 23 or 114 times the maximal daily human inhalational dose. TORNALATE was not tumorigenic in an 18 month oral study in Swiss-Webster mice at doses up to 568 times the maximal daily human inhalational dose. Ames Salmonella and mouse lymphoma mutation assays in vitro revealed no mutagenesis due to TORNALATE. Reproductive studies in male and female rats revealed no significant effects on fertility at doses of TORNALATE up to 364 times the maximal daily human inhalational dose.

Teratogenic Effects—Pregnancy Category C. No teratogenic effects were seen in rats and rabbits after oral doses of TORNALATE up to 557 times the maximal daily human inhalational dose and in mice after oral doses up to 284 times the maximal daily human inhalational dose.

When TORNALATE was injected subcutaneously into mice at doses of 2 mg/kg, 10 mg/kg, and 20 mg/kg (corresponding to 23, 114, and 227 times the maximal daily human inhalational dose) cleft palate incidences of 5.7 percent, 3.8 percent, and 3.3 percent (compared with 0.9 percent in controls) were found. Cleft palate induction with isoproterenol at 10 mg/kg SC as the positive control was 10.7 percent. Since no well-controlled studies in pregnant women are available, TORNALATE should be used during pregnancy only if the potential benefit justifies the potential risk to the fetus.

Nursing Mothers. It is not known whether TORNALATE is excreted in human milk. Because many drugs are excreted in human milk, caution should be exercised when TORNALATE is administered to a nursing woman.

Pediatric Use. Safety and effectiveness of TORNALATE in children 12 years of age or younger has not been established.

ADVERSE REACTIONS

The results of all clinical trials with TORNALATE (bitolterol mesylate) in 492 patients showed the following side effects:

CNS: Tremors (14%), nervousness (5%), headache (4%), dizziness (3%), lightheadedness (3%), insomnia (<1%), hyperkinesia (<1%).

Gastrointestinal: Nausea (3%).

Oro-Pharyngeal: Throat irritation (5%).

Cardiovascular: The overall incidence of cardiovascular effects was approximately 5% of patients and these effects included palpitations (approximately 3%), and chest discomfort (approximately 1%). Tachycardia was seen in less than 1%. Premature ventricular contractions and flushing were rarely seen.

Respiratory: Coughing (4%), bronchospasm (<1%), dyspnea (<1%), chest tightness (<1%).

Clinical relevance or relationship to administration of TORNALATE of rarely reported elevations of SGOT, decrease in platelets, decreases in WBC levels or proteinuria are not known.

In comparing the adverse reactions for bitolterol mesylate treated patients to those of isoproterenol treated patients, during three month clinical trials involving approximately 400 patients, the following moderate to severe reactions, as judged by the investigators, were reported for both steroid and non-steroid dependent patients. The table does not include mild reactions or those occurring only with the first dose.

PERCENT INCIDENCE OF MODERATE TO SEVERE ADVERSE REACTIONS

Reaction	Bitolterol N = 197	Isoproterenol N = 194
Central Nervous System		
Tremors	9.1%	1.5%
Nervousness	1.5%	1.0%
Headache	3.5%	6.1%
Dizziness	1.0%	1.5%
Insomnia	0.5%	0%
Cardiovascular		
Palpitations	1.5%	0%
PVC—Transient		
Increase	0.5%	0%
Chest Discomfort	0.5%	0%
Respiratory		
Cough	4.1%	1.0%
Bronchospasm	1.0%	0%
Dyspnea	1.0%	0%
Oro-Pharyngeal		
Throat Irritation	3.0%	3.1%
Gastrointestinal		
Nausea (Dyspepsia)	0.5%	0.5%

NOTE: In most patients, the total isoproterenol dosage was divided into three equally dosed inhalations, administered at three minute intervals. This procedure may have reduced the incidence of adverse reactions observed with isoproterenol.

OVERDOSAGE

Overdosage with TORNALATE (bitolterol mesylate) may be expected to result in exaggeration of those drug effects listed in the ADVERSE REACTIONS section. In such cases therapy with TORNALATE and all β-adrenergic stimulating drugs should be stopped, supportive therapy provided, and judicious use of a cardioselective β-adrenergic blocking agent should be considered bearing in mind the possibility that such agents can produce profound bronchospasm. As with all sympathomimetic aerosol medications, cardiac arrest and even death may be associated with abuse. The oral LD_{50} of TORNALATE in rats was greater than 5000 mg/kg and in mice greater than 6000 mg/kg.

DOSAGE AND ADMINISTRATION

The usual dose to relieve bronchospasm for adults and children over 12 years of age is two inhalations at an interval of at least one to three minutes followed by a third inhalation if needed. For prevention of bronchospasm, the usual dose is two inhalations every 8 hours. The dose of TORNALATE (bitolterol mesylate) should never exceed 3 inhalations every 6 hours or 2 inhalations every 4 hours. Medical consultation should be sought prior to an increase in the frequency of dosing because this may indicate a need for reevaluation of the patient's condition.

HOW SUPPLIED

TORNALATE (bitolterol mesylate), Metered Dose Inhaler, is supplied in 16.4 g (15 mL) self-contained aerosol units (NDC 0024-1060-01).
Refill of 16.4 g (15 mL) NDC 0024-1061-01.
Store at controlled room temperature between 15 °C and 30 °C (59 °F and 86 °F).
Distributed by Winthrop Pharmaceuticals
Division of Sterling Drug Inc. New York, NY 10016
Manufactured by Sterling Pharmaceuticals Inc.
Barceloneta, Puerto Rico 00617

TW 275-H

TRANCOPAL®   ℞
brand of chlormezanone
Nonhypnotic Antianxiety Agent

DESCRIPTION

TRANCOPAL, brand of chlormezanone, is [2-(p-Chlorophenyl)tetrahydro-3-methyl-4H-1, 3-thiazin-4-one 1, 1-dioxide], a white, virtually tasteless, crystalline powder with a solubility of less than 0.25 percent w/v in water.

Inactive Ingredients—Caplets® **100 mg:** Dibasic Calcium Phosphate, FD&C Yellow #6, Magnesium Stearate, Saccharin Sodium, Starch; CAPLETS **200 mg:** Dibasic Calcium Phosphate, D&C Yellow #10, FD&C Blue #1, Magnesium Stearate, Saccharin Sodium, Starch.

CLINICAL PHARMACOLOGY

TRANCOPAL improves the emotional state by allaying mild anxiety, usually without impairing clarity of consciousness. The relief of symptoms is often apparent in fifteen to thirty minutes after administration and may last up to six hours or longer.

INDICATIONS AND USAGE

TRANCOPAL is indicated for the treatment of mild anxiety and tension states.

The effectiveness of chlormezanone in long-term use, that is, more than 4 months, has not been assessed by systematic clinical studies. The physician should periodically reassess the usefulness of the drug for the individual patient.

CONTRAINDICATION

Contraindicated in patients with a history of a previous hypersensitivity reaction to chlormezanone.

WARNINGS

Should drowsiness occur, the dose should be reduced. As with other CNS-acting drugs, patients receiving chlormezanone should be warned against performing potentially hazardous tasks which require complete mental alertness, such as operating a motor vehicle or dangerous machinery. Patients should also be warned of the possible additive effects which may occur when the drug is taken with alcohol or other CNS-acting drugs.

Usage in Pregnancy. Safe use of this preparation in pregnancy or lactation has not been established, as no animal reproduction studies have been performed; therefore, use of the drug in pregnancy, lactation, or in women of childbearing age requires that the potential benefit of the drug be weighed against its possible hazards to the mother and fetus.

ADVERSE REACTIONS

Adverse effects reported to occur with TRANCOPAL include drowsiness, drug rash, dizziness, flushing, nausea, depression, edema, inability to void, weakness, excitement, tremor, confusion, and headache. Rare instances of erythema multiforme, Stevens-Johnson syndrome, and toxic epidermal necrolysis have been reported. Medication should be discontinued or modified as the case demands.

Jaundice, apparently of the cholestatic type, has been reported as occurring rarely during the use of chlormezanone, but was reversible on discontinuance of therapy.

OVERDOSAGE

Overdose with amounts as low as 7 grams has resulted in coma, hypotension, absence of reflexes, and flaccidity. Ingestion of higher doses may also result in alternation between coma and excitement.

DOSAGE AND ADMINISTRATION

The usual **adult** dosage is 200 mg orally three or four times daily but in some patients 100 mg may suffice. The dosage for **children from 5 to 12 years** is 50 mg to 100 mg three or four times daily. Since the effect of CNS-acting drugs varies, treatment, particularly in children, should begin with the lowest dosage which may be increased as needed.

HOW SUPPLIED

100 mg (peach colored, scored CAPLETS)
bottle of 100 (NDC 0024-1973-04)
200 mg (green colored, scored CAPLETS)
bottle of 100 (NDC 0024-1974-04)
bottle of 1000 (NDC 0024-1974-08)

Shown in Product Identification Section, page 435
TW 72-O

WINSTROL®   ℞
brand of stanozolol tablets, USP
For Oral Administration

DESCRIPTION

WINSTROL, brand of stanozolol tablets, is an anabolic steroid, a synthetic derivative of testosterone. Each tablet contains 2 mg of stanozolol. It is designated chemically as 17-methyl-$2'H$-5α-androst-2-eno[3,2-c]pyrazol-17β-ol.
Inactive Ingredients: Dibasic Calcium Phosphate, D&C Red #28, FD&C Red #40, Lactose, Magnesium Stearate, Starch.

CLINICAL PHARMACOLOGY

Anabolic steroids are synthetic derivatives of testosterone. Certain clinical effects and adverse reactions demonstrate the androgenic properties of this class of drugs. Complete dissociation of anabolic and androgenic effects has not been achieved. The actions of anabolic steroids are therefore similar to those of male sex hormones with the possibility of causing serious disturbances of growth and sexual development if given to young children. They suppress the gonadotropic functions of the pituitary and may exert a direct effect upon the testes.

WINSTROL has been found to increase low-density lipoproteins and decrease high-density lipoproteins. These changes are not associated with any increase in total cholesterol or triglyceride levels and revert to normal on discontinuation of treatment.

Hereditary angioedema (HAE) is an autosomal dominant disorder caused by a deficient or nonfunctional C1 esterase inhibitor (C1 INH) and clinically characterized by episodes of swelling of the face, extremities, genitalia, bowel wall, and upper respiratory tract.

In small scale clinical studies, stanozolol was effective in controlling the frequency and severity of attacks of angioedema and in increasing serum levels of C1 INH and C4. WINSTROL is not effective in stopping HAE attacks while they are under way. The effect of WINSTROL on increasing serum levels of C1 INH and C4 may be related to an increase in protein anabolism.

INDICATIONS AND USAGE

Hereditary Angioedema. WINSTROL is indicated prophylactically to decrease the frequency and severity of attacks of angioedema.

CONTRAINDICATIONS

The use of WINSTROL is contraindicated in the following:
1. Male patients with carcinoma of the breast, or with known or suspected carcinoma of the prostate.
2. Carcinoma of the breast in females with hypercalcemia; androgenic anabolic steroids may stimulate osteolytic resorption of bone.
3. Nephrosis or the nephrotic phase of nephritis.
4. WINSTROL can cause fetal harm when administered to a pregnant woman.

WINSTROL is contraindicated in women who are or may become pregnant. If this drug is used during pregnancy, or if the patient becomes pregnant while taking this drug, the patient should be apprised of the potential hazard to the fetus.

WARNINGS

PELIOSIS HEPATIS, A CONDITION IN WHICH LIVER AND SOMETIMES SPLENIC TISSUE IS REPLACED WITH BLOOD-FILLED CYSTS, HAS BEEN REPORTED IN PATIENTS RECEIVING ANDROGENIC ANABOLIC STEROID THERAPY. THESE CYSTS ARE SOMETIMES PRESENT WITH MINIMAL HEPATIC DYSFUNCTION, BUT AT OTHER TIMES THEY HAVE BEEN ASSOCIATED WITH LIVER FAILURE. THEY ARE OFTEN NOT RECOGNIZED UNTIL LIFE-THREATENING LIVER FAILURE OR INTRA-ABDOMINAL HEMORRHAGE DEVELOPS. WITHDRAWAL OF DRUG USUALLY RESULTS IN COMPLETE DISAPPEARANCE OF LESIONS.

LIVER CELL TUMORS ARE ALSO REPORTED. MOST OFTEN THESE TUMORS ARE BENIGN AND ANDROGEN-DEPENDENT, BUT FATAL MALIGNANT TUMORS HAVE BEEN REPORTED. WITHDRAWAL OF DRUG OFTEN RESULTS IN REGRESSION OR CESSATION OF PROGRESSION OF THE TUMOR. HOWEVER, HEPATIC TUMORS ASSOCIATED WITH ANDROGENS OR ANABOLIC STEROIDS ARE MUCH MORE VASCULAR THAN OTHER HEPATIC TUMORS AND MAY BE SILENT UNTIL LIFE-THREATENING INTRA-ABDOMINAL HEMORRHAGE DEVELOPS.

BLOOD LIPID CHANGES THAT ARE KNOWN TO BE ASSOCIATED WITH INCREASED RISK OF ATHEROSCLEROSIS ARE SEEN IN PATIENTS TREATED WITH ANDROGENS AND ANABOLIC STEROIDS. THESE CHANGES INCLUDE DECREASED HIGH-DENSITY LIPOPROTEIN AND SOMETIMES INCREASED LOW-DENSITY LIPOPROTEIN. THE CHANGES MAY BE VERY MARKED AND COULD HAVE A SERIOUS IMPACT ON THE RISK OF ATHEROSCLEROSIS AND CORONARY ARTERY DISEASE.

Cholestatic hepatitis and jaundice occur with 17-alpha-alkylated androgens at relatively low doses. If cholestatic hepatitis with jaundice appears, the anabolic steroid should be discontinued. If liver function tests become abnormal, the patient should be monitored closely and the etiology determined. Generally, the anabolic steroid should be discontinued although in cases of mild abnormalities, the physician may elect to follow the patient carefully at a reduced drug dosage.

In patients with breast cancer, anabolic steroid therapy may cause hypercalcemia by stimulating osteolysis. In this case, the drug should be discontinued.

Edema with or without congestive heart failure may be a serious complication in patients with preexisting cardiac, renal, or hepatic disease. Concomitant administration of adrenal cortical steroids or ACTH may add to the edema. Geriatric male patients treated with androgenic anabolic steroids may be at an increased risk for the development of prostatic hypertrophy and prostatic carcinoma.

In children, anabolic steroid treatment may accelerate bone maturation without producing compensatory gain in linear growth. This adverse effect may result in compromised adult stature. The younger the child, the greater the risk of compromising final mature height. The effect on bone maturation should be monitored by assessing bone age of the wrist and hand every six months.

Anabolic steroids have not been shown to enhance athletic ability.

PRECAUTIONS

General.
Anabolic steroids may cause suppression of clotting factors II, V, VII, and X, and an increase in prothrombin time. Women should be observed for signs of virilization (deepening of the voice, hirsutism, acne, and clitoromegaly). To prevent irreversible change, drug therapy must be discontinued, or the dosage significantly reduced when mild virilism is first detected. Such virilization is usual following androgenic anabolic steroid use at high doses. Some virilizing changes in women are irreversible even after prompt discontinuance of therapy and are not prevented by concomitant use of estrogens. Menstrual irregularities may also occur. The insulin or oral hypoglycemic dosage may need adjustment in diabetic patients who receive anabolic steroids.
Information for the Patient. The physician should instruct patients to report any of the following side effects of androgens:
Adult or Adolescent Males. Too frequent or persistent erections of the penis, appearance or aggravation of acne.

Women. Hoarseness, acne, changes in menstrual periods, or more hair on the face.
All Patients. Any nausea, vomiting, changes in skin color, or ankle swelling.
Laboratory Tests. Women with disseminated breast carcinoma should have frequent determination of urine and serum calcium levels during the course of androgenic anabolic steroid therapy (see WARNINGS).
Because of the hepatotoxicity associated with the use of 17-alpha-alkylated androgens, liver function tests should be obtained periodically.
Periodic (every 6 months) x-ray examinations of bone age should be made during treatment of prepubertal patients to determine the rate of bone maturation and the effects of androgenic anabolic steroid therapy on the epiphyseal centers.
In common with other anabolic steroids, WINSTROL, brand of stanozolol tablets, has been reported to lower the level of high-density lipoproteins and raise the level of low-density lipoproteins. These changes usually revert to normal on discontinuation of treatment. Increased low-density lipoproteins and decreased high-density lipoproteins are considered cardiovascular risk factors. Serum lipids and high-density lipoprotein cholesterol should be determined periodically. Hemoglobin and hematocrit should be checked periodically for polycythemia in patients who are receiving high doses of anabolic steroids.
Drug Interaction. Anabolic steroids may increase sensitivity to anticoagulants; therefore, dosage of an anticoagulant may have to be decreased in order to maintain the prothrombin time at the desired therapeutic level.
Drug/Laboratory Test Interferences. Therapy with androgenic anabolic steroids may decrease levels of thyroxine-binding globulin resulting in decreased total T_4 serum levels and increase resin uptake of T_3 and T_4. Free thyroid hormone levels remain unchanged and there is no clinical evidence of thyroid dysfunction.
Carcinogenesis, Mutagenesis, Impairment of Fertility. WINSTROL has not been tested in laboratory animals for carcinogenic or mutagenic effects. No tumorigenic or cancer-inducing properties of WINSTROL, brand of stanozolol tablets, were seen in one-year toxicity studies in rats.
WINSTROL administered orally (intragastrically) to pregnant rats at dosages of 2.5 mg/kg/day to 20 mg/kg/day increased the ano-genital distance in rat fetuses, indicative of a masculinizing effect. WINSTROL prevented pregnancy when given orally to rats from the 1st to the 21st day of gestation.
No teratogenic effects or congenital malformation were observed in offspring of rabbits given 0.5 mg/day, 1.0 mg/day, or 5.0 mg/day of WINSTROL from the 8th through the 16th day of pregnancy, nor were there any adverse effects on the course of pregnancy at these dose levels.
Liver cell tumors have been associated with prolonged use of androgenic anabolic steroids (see WARNINGS section).
Geriatric patients treated with anabolics may be at an increased risk for prostate hypertrophy and prostatic carcinoma.
Pregnancy Category X. See CONTRAINDICATIONS section.
Nursing Mothers. It is not known whether anabolic steroids are excreted in human milk. Many drugs are excreted in human milk and because of the potential for adverse reactions in nursing infants from WINSTROL, a decision should be made whether to discontinue nursing or discontinue the drug, taking into account the importance of the drug to the mother.
Pediatric Use. Anabolic agents may accelerate epiphyseal maturation more rapidly than linear growth in children, and the effect may continue for 6 months after the drug has been stopped. Therefore, therapy should be monitored by x-ray studies at 6 month intervals in order to avoid the risk of compromising the adult height. The safety and efficacy of WINSTROL in children with hereditary angioedema have not been established.

ADVERSE REACTIONS

Hepatic: Cholestatic jaundice with, rarely, hepatic necrosis and death. Hepatocellular neoplasms and peliosis hepatis have been reported in association with long-term androgenic-anabolic steroid therapy (see WARNINGS). Reversible changes in liver function tests also occur including increased bromsulphalein (BSP) retention and increases in serum bilirubin, glutamic oxaloacetic transaminase (SGOT), and alkaline phosphatase.
Genitourinary System: *In men. Prepubertal:* Phallic enlargement and increased frequency of erections.

Continued on next page

This product information was prepared in August, 1989. On these and other products of Winthrop Pharmaceuticals, detailed information may be obtained on a current basis by direct inquiry to the Professional Services Department, 90 Park Avenue, New York, NY 10016 (800) 446-6267.

Winthrop Pharm.—Cont.

Postpubertal: Inhibition of testicular function, testicular atrophy and oligospermia, impotence, chronic priapism, epididymitis and bladder irritability.
In women: Clitoral enlargement, menstrual irregularities.
In both sexes: Increased or decreased libido.
CNS: Habituation, excitation, insomnia, depression.
Gastrointestinal: Nausea, vomiting, diarrhea.
Hematologic: Bleeding in patients on concomitant anticoagulant therapy.
Breast: Gynecomastia.
Larynx: Deepening of the voice in women.
Hair: Hirsutism and male pattern baldness in women.
Skin: Acne (especially in women and prepubertal boys).
Skeletal: Premature closure of epiphyses in children (see PRECAUTIONS, **Pediatric Use**).
Fluid and Electrolytes: Edema, retention of serum electrolytes (sodium, chloride, potassium, phosphate, calcium).
Metabolic/Endocrine: Decreased glucose tolerance (see PRECAUTIONS), increased serum levels of low-density lipoproteins and decreased levels of high-density lipoproteins (see PRECAUTIONS, **Laboratory Tests**), increased creatine and creatinine excretion, increased serum levels of creatinine phosphokinase (CPK).

Some virilizing changes in women are irreversible even after prompt discontinuance of therapy and are not prevented by concomitant use of estrogens (see PRECAUTIONS).

DOSAGE AND ADMINISTRATION

The use of anabolic steroids may be associated with serious adverse reactions, many of which are dose related; therefore, patients should be placed on the lowest possible effective dose.
Hereditary Angioedema. The dosage requirements for continuous treatment of hereditary angioedema with WINSTROL should be individualized on the basis of the clinical response of the patient. It is recommended that the patient be started on 2 mg, three times a day. After a favorable initial response is obtained in terms of prevention of episodes of edematous attacks, the proper continuing dosage should be determined by decreasing the dosage at intervals of one to three months to a maintenance dosage of 2 mg a day. Some patients may be successfully managed on a 2 mg alternate day schedule. During the dose adjusting phase, close monitoring of the patient's response is indicated, particularly if the patient has a history of airway involvement.
The prophylactic dose of WINSTROL, brand of stanozolol tablets, to be used prior to dental extraction, or other traumatic or stressful situations has not been established and may be substantially larger.
Attacks of hereditary angioedema are generally infrequent in childhood and the risks from stanozolol administration are substantially increased. Therefore, long-term prophylactic therapy with this drug is generally not recommended in children, and should only be undertaken with due consideration of the benefits and risks involved (see PRECAUTIONS, **Pediatric Use**).

HOW SUPPLIED

Tablets of 2 mg, scored, bottle of 100 (NDC 0024-2253-04)
Distributed by Winthrop Pharmaceuticals
Division of Sterling Drug Inc
New York, NY 10016
Manufactured by Sterling Pharmaceuticals Inc
Barceloneta, Puerto Rico 00617
Shown in Product Identification Section, page 435

                                      WW 5-X

ZEPHIRAN® CHLORIDE   **OTC**
brand of benzalkonium chloride

(See PDR For Nonprescription Drugs)

Wyeth-Ayerst Laboratories
Division of American Home
Products Corporation
P.O. BOX 8299
PHILADELPHIA, PA 19101

Product Identification Codes

The following is a numerical list of National Drug Code (NDC) numbers with their corresponding product names for all oral solid dosage forms manufactured by Wyeth-Ayerst Laboratories.

Numerical Listing
Products Formerly of Wyeth Laboratories

Product Ident. Code	Product	
1	Equanil® (meprobamate) Tablet 400 mg.	℞
2	Equanil® (meprobamate) Tablet 200 mg.	℞
6	Serax® (oxazepam) Capsule 15 mg.	℞
13	Amphojel® [dried aluminum hydroxide gel (hydrated alumina)] Tablet 0.6 Gm. (10 gr.)	
19	Phenergan® (promethazine HCl) Tablet 12.5 mg.	
27	Phenergan® (promethazine HCl) Tablet 25 mg.	
28	Sparine® (promazine HCl) Tablet 50 mg.	
29	Sparine® (promazine HCl) Tablet 25 mg.	
51	Serax® (oxazepam) Capsule 10 mg.	℞
52	Serax® (oxazepam) Capsule 30 mg.	℞
53	Omnipen® (ampicillin) Capsule 250 mg.	
56	Ovral® (each tablet contains 0.5 mg. norgestrel with 0.05 mg. ethinyl estradiol) Tablet, white	
57	Unipen® [(nafcillin sodium) as the monohydrate] Capsule 250 mg.	
59	Pen·Vee® K (penicillin V potassium) Tablet 250 mg. (400,000 units)	
62	Ovrette® (norgestrel) Tablet	
64	Ativan® (lorazepam) Tablet 1 mg.	℞
65	Ativan® (lorazepam) Tablet 2 mg.	℞
71	Mazanor® (mazindol) Tablet 1 mg.	℞
73	Wytensin® (guanabenz acetate) Tablet 4 mg.	
74	Wytensin® (guanabenz acetate) Tablet 8 mg.	
75	Nordette-21® (each tablet contains 0.15 mg. levonorgestrel with 0.03 mg. ethinyl estradiol) Tablet	
78	Lo/Ovral® (each tablet contains 0.3 mg. norgestrel with 0.03 mg. ethinyl estradiol) Tablet, white	
81	Ativan® (lorazepam) Tablet 0.5 mg.	℞
85	Wygesic® (each tablet contains 65 mg. propoxyphene HCl, U.S.P., and 650 mg. acetaminophen, U.S.P.) Tablet	℞
91	Equagesic® (meprobamate with aspirin) Tablet	
119	Amphojel® [dried aluminum hydroxide gel (hydrated alumina)] Tablet 0.3 Gm. (5 gr.)	
165	Bicillin® (penicillin G benzathine) Tablet 200,000 units	
200	Sparine® (promazine HCl) Tablet 100 mg.	
227	Phenergan® (promethazine HCl) Tablet 50 mg.	
261	Mepergan® Fortis (meperidine HCl and promethazine HCl) Capsule	℞
268	Phenobarbital Tablet 30 mg. (½ gr.)	℞
308	Meperidine HCl Tablet USP 50 mg.	℞
309	Omnipen® (ampicillin) Capsule 500 mg.	
317	Serax® (oxazepam) Tablet 15 mg.	℞
320	Phenobarbital Tablet 60 mg. (1 gr.)	℞
326	Codeine Sulfate Tablet USP 30 mg. (½ gr.)	℞
360	Pathocil® (dicloxacillin sodium monohydrate) Capsule 250 mg.	
389	Tetracycline HCl Capsule USP 250 mg.	
390	Pen·Vee® K (penicillin V potassium) Tablet 500 mg. (800,000 units)	
434	Phenergan®-D (promethazine HCl with pseudoephedrine HCl) Tablet	
445	Ovral®-28 pink inert tablet	
464	Unipen® [(nafcillin sodium) as the monohydrate] Tablet 500 mg.	
471	Tetracycline HCl Capsule USP 500 mg.	
472	Basaljel® (dried basic aluminum carbonate gel) Capsule	
473	Basaljel® (dried basic aluminum carbonate gel) Tablet	
486	Nordette®-28, Lo/Ovral®-28 pink inert tablet	
559	Wymox® (amoxicillin) Capsule 250 mg.	
560	Wymox® (amoxicillin) Capsule 500 mg.	
576	Wyamycin®S (erythromycin stearate) Tablet, film coated, 250 mg.	
578	Wyamycin®S (erythromycin stearate) Tablet, film coated, 500 mg.	
593	Pathocil® (dicloxacillin sodium monohydrate) Capsule 500 mg.	
2511	Ovral®-28 Pilpak® (21 white tablets each containing 0.5 mg. norgestrel with 0.05 mg. ethinyl estradiol and 7 pink inert tablets)	
2514	Lo/Ovral®-28 Pilpak® (21 white tablets each containing 0.3 mg. norgestrel with 0.03 mg. ethinyl estradiol and 7 pink inert tablets)	
2533	Nordette®-28 Pilpak® (21 light-orange tablets each containing 0.15 mg. levonorgestrel with 0.03 mg ethinyl estradiol and 7 pink inert tablets)	
2535	Triphasil®-21 Tablets (levonorgestrel and ethinyl estradiol tablets—triphasic regimen)	
2536	Triphasil®-28 Tablets (levonorgestrel and ethinyl estradiol tablets—triphasic regimen)	
4125	Isordil® Tembids® Tablet 40 mg	
4126	Isordil® Sublingual Tablet 5 mg	
4130	Trecator®-SC, (ethionamide) Tablet 250 mg	
4132	Surmontil® (trimipramine) Capsule 25 mg	
4133	Surmontil® (trimipramine) Capsule 50 mg	
4139	Isordil® (isosorbide dinitrate) Sublingual Tablet 2.5 mg	
4140	Isordil® (isosorbide dinitrate) Tembids Capsule 40 mg	
4148	Cyclospasmol® (cyclandelate) Capsule 400 mg	
4152	Isordil® (isosorbide dinitrate) 5 Titradose Tablet 5 mg	
4153	Isordil® (isosorbide dinitrate) 10 Titradose Tablet 10 mg	
4154	Isordil® (isosorbide dinitrate) 20 Titradose Tablet 20 mg	
4158	Surmontil® (trimipramine) Capsule 100 mg	
4159	Isordil® (isosorbide dinitrate) 30 Titradose Tablet 30 mg	
4161	Isordil® (isosorbide dinitrate) Sublingual Tablet 10 mg	
4177	Sectral® (acebutolol) Capsule 200 mg	
4179	Sectral® (acebutolol) Capsule 400 mg	
4181	Orudis® (ketoprofen) Capsule 50 mg	
4186	Orudis® (ketoprofen) Capsule 25 mg	
4187	Orudis® (ketoprofen) Capsule 75 mg	
4188	Cordarone® (amiodarone) Tablet 200 mg	
4191	Synalgos®-DC (each capsule contains 16 mg. dihydrocodeine bitartrate, 356.4 mg. aspirin, and 30 mg. caffeine) Capsule	
4192	Isordil® (isosorbide dinitrate) 40 Titradose Tablet 40 mg	

Products Formerly of Ayerst Laboratories

Code	Product	
243	Atromid-S® (clofibrate) Capsule 500 mg.	
252	Mediatric® Capsule	℞
421	Inderal® (propranolol HCl) Tablet 10 mg.	
422	Inderal® (propranolol HCl) Tablet 20 mg.	
424	Inderal® (propranolol HCl) Tablet 40 mg.	
426	Inderal® (propranolol HCl) Tablet 60 mg.	
428	Inderal® (propranolol HCl) Tablet 80 mg.	
430	Mysoline® (primidone) Tablet 250 mg.	
431	Mysoline® (primidone) Tablet 50 mg.	
434	Grisactin® Ultra (griseofulvin, ultramicrosize) Tablet 125 mg.	
435	Grisactin® Ultra (griseofulvin, ultramicrosize) Tablet 250 mg.	
437	Grisactin® Ultra (griseofulvin, ultramicrosize) Tablet 330 mg.	
442	Grisactin® 125 (griseofulvin, microsize) Capsule 125 mg.	
443	Grisactin® 250 (griseofulvin, microsize) Capsule 250 mg.	
444	Grisactin® 500 (griseofulvin, microsize) Tablet 500 mg.	
455	Inderide® LA (each capsule contains 80 mg. Inderal® LA [propranolol HCl] and 50 mg. hydrochlorothiazide) Capsule	
457	Inderide® LA (each capsule contains 120 mg. Inderal® LA [propranolol HCl] and 50 mg. hydrochlorothiazide) Capsule	
459	Inderide® LA (each capsule contains 160 mg. Inderal® LA [propranolol HCl] and 50 mg. hydrochlorothiazide) Capsule	
470	Inderal® LA (propranolol HCl) Capsule 60 mg.	
471	Inderal® LA (propranolol HCl) Capsule 80 mg.	
473	Inderal® LA (propranolol HCl) Capsule 120 mg.	
479	Inderal® LA (propranolol HCl) Capsule 160 mg.	
484	Inderide® (each tablet contains 40 mg. Inderal® [propranolol HCl] and 25 mg. hydrochlorothiazide) Tablet	
488	Inderide® (each tablet contains 80 mg. Inderal® [propranolol HCl] and 25 mg. hydrochlorothiazide) Tablet	
702	Diucardin® (hydroflumethiazide) Tablet 50 mg.	
755	Plegine® (phendimetrazine tartrate) Tablet 35 mg.	℞
786	Thiosulfil® Forte (sulfamethazole) Tablet 500 mg.	
809	Antabuse® (disulfiram) Tablet 250 mg.	
810	Antabuse® (disulfiram) Tablet 500 mg.	
864	Premarin® (conjugated estrogens tablets, USP) Tablet 0.9 mg.	
865	Premarin® (conjugated estrogens tablets, USP) Tablet 2.5 mg.	
866	Premarin® (conjugated estrogens tablets, USP) Tablet 1.25 mg.	

867 Premarin® (conjugated estrogens tablets, USP) Tablet 0.625 mg.

868 Premarin® (conjugated estrogens tablets, USP) Tablet 0.3 mg.

878 Premarin® with Methyltestosterone (each tablet contains 0.625 mg. Premarin® [conjugated estrogens, USP] and 5 mg. methyltestosterone) Tablet

879 Premarin® with Methyltestosterone (each tablet contains 1.25 mg. Premarin® [conjugated estrogens, USP] and 10 mg. methyltestosterone) Tablet

880 PMB® 200 (each tablet contains 0.45 mg. Premarin® [conjugated estrogens, USP] and 200 mg. meprobamate) Tablet

881 PMB® 400 (each tablet contains 0.45 mg. Premarin® [conjugated estrogens, USP] and 400 mg. meprobamate) Tablet

894 Aygestin® (norethindrone acetate, USP) Tablet 5 mg.

896 Cycrin® (medroxyprogesterone acetate, USP) Tablet 10 mg.

ALUDROX® OTC
[al 'u-drox]
(alumina and magnesia)
ORAL SUSPENSION

COMPOSITION
Nonconstipating, noncathartic, effective and palatable antacid containing, in each 5 ml. teaspoonful of suspension, 307 mg. of aluminum hydroxide as a gel, and 103 mg. of magnesium hydroxide. The inactive ingredients present are artificial and natural flavors, benzoic acid, butylparaben, glycerin, hydroxypropyl methylcellulose, methylparaben, propylparaben, saccharin, simethicone, sorbitol solution, and water.

INDICATIONS
For the symptomatic relief of hyperacidity associated with the diagnosis of peptic ulcer, gastritis, peptic esophagitis, gastric hyperacidity, and hiatal hernia.

DOSAGE AND ADMINISTRATION
Two teaspoonfuls (10 ml.) of suspension every four hours, or as required. Suspension may be followed by a sip of water if desired. Ten ml. of ALUDROX suspension have the capacity to neutralize 24 mEq of acid.

WARNINGS
Patients are advised not to take more than 12 teaspoonfuls (60 ml) in a 24-hour period or use this maximum dosage for more than two weeks except under the advice and supervision of a physician. Pregnant women and nursing mothers are advised to seek the advice of a health professional before using this product.

DRUG INTERACTION PRECAUTIONS
This product must not be taken if the patient is presently taking a prescription antibiotic drug containing any form of tetracycline.

HOW SUPPLIED
Oral Suspension, bottles of 12 fluidounces.

AMPHOJEL® OTC
[am 'fo-jel]
(aluminum hydroxide gel)
SUSPENSION • TABLETS

COMPOSITION
Suspension—Each 5 ml. teaspoonful contains 320 mg. of aluminum hydroxide as a gel, and not more than 0.10 mEq of sodium. The inactive ingredients present are butylparaben, calcium benzoate, glycerin, hydroxypropyl methylcellulose, methylparaben, propylparaben, saccharin, simethicone, sorbitol solution, and water. *Tablets* contain a dried gel. The 0.3 Gm. (5 grain) strength is equivalent to about 1 teaspoonful of the suspension and the 0.6 Gm. (10 grain) strength is equivalent to about 2 teaspoonfuls. Each 0.3 Gm tablet contains 0.08 mEq of sodium and each 0.6 Gm tablet contains 0.13 mEq of sodium.

INDICATIONS
For the symptomatic relief of hyperacidity associated with the diagnosis of peptic ulcer, gastritis, peptic esophagitis, gastric hyperacidity, and hiatal hernia.

DOSAGE
Suspension—two teaspoonfuls followed by a sip of water if desired, five or six times daily, between meals and at bedtime. Two teaspoonfuls have the capacity to neutralize 20 mEq of acid. *Tablets*—Two tablets of the 0.3 Gm. strength, or one tablet of the 0.6 Gm. strength, five or six times daily between meals and at bedtime. Two tablets have the capacity to neutralize 16 mEq of acid.

WARNINGS
Patients are advised not to take more than 12 teaspoonfuls (60 ml) or twelve (12) 0.3 Gm tablets or six (6) 0.6 Gm tablets in a 24-hour period or use this maximum dosage for more than two weeks except under the advice and supervision of a physician. Pregnant women and nursing mothers are advised to seek the advice of a health professional before using this product.

PRECAUTION
May cause constipation.

DRUG INTERACTION PRECAUTIONS
This product must not be taken if the patient is presently taking a prescription antibiotic drug containing any form of tetracycline.

HOW SUPPLIED
Suspension—Peppermint flavored; without flavor—bottles of 12 fluidounces. *Tablets*—a convenient auxiliary dosage form—0.3 Gm. (5 gr.), bottles of 100; 0.6 Gm. (10 gr.), boxes of 100.

ANTABUSE® ℞
[an 'tah-būse]
Brand of disulfiram
In Alcoholism

CAUTION: Federal law prohibits dispensing without prescription.

> **WARNING**
> ANTABUSE should never be administered to a patient when he is in a state of alcohol intoxication, or without his full knowledge.
> The physician should instruct relatives accordingly.

DESCRIPTION
CHEMICAL NAME: bis(diethylthiocarbamoyl) disulfide
STRUCTURAL FORMULA:

ANTABUSE occurs as a white to off-white, odorless, and almost tasteless powder, soluble in water to the extent of about 20 mg in 100 mL, and in alcohol to the extent of about 3.8 g in 100 mL.
ANTABUSE contains these inactive ingredients:
Magnesium Aluminum Silicate
Magnesium Stearate, NF
Povidone, USP
Starch, NF

ACTION
ANTABUSE produces a sensitivity to alcohol which results in a highly unpleasant reaction when the patient under treatment ingests even small amounts of alcohol.
ANTABUSE blocks the oxidation of alcohol at the acetaldehyde stage. During alcohol metabolism following ANTABUSE intake, the concentration of acetaldehyde occurring in the blood may be 5- to 10-times higher than that found during metabolism of the same amount of alcohol alone.
Accumulation of acetaldehyde in the blood produces a complex of highly unpleasant symptoms referred to hereinafter as the ANTABUSE-alcohol reaction. This reaction, which is proportional to the dosage of both ANTABUSE and alcohol, will persist as long as alcohol is being metabolized. ANTABUSE does not appear to influence the rate of alcohol elimination from the body.
ANTABUSE is absorbed slowly from the gastrointestinal tract and eliminated slowly from the drug. One (or even two) weeks after a patient has taken his last dose of ANTABUSE, ingestion of alcohol may produce unpleasant symptoms. Prolonged administration of ANTABUSE does not produce tolerance; the longer a patient remains on therapy, the more exquisitely sensitive he becomes to alcohol.

INDICATION
ANTABUSE is an aid in the management of selected chronic alcoholic patients who want to remain in a state of enforced sobriety so that supportive and psychotherapeutic treatment may be applied to best advantage. (Used alone, without proper motivation and supportive therapy, ANTABUSE is not a cure for alcoholism, and it is unlikely that it will have more than a brief effect on the drinking pattern of the chronic alcoholic.)

CONTRAINDICATIONS
Patients who are receiving or have recently received metronidazole, paraldehyde, alcohol, or alcohol-containing preparations, eg, cough syrups, tonics and the like, should not be given ANTABUSE.
ANTABUSE is contraindicated in the presence of severe myocardial disease or coronary occlusion, psychoses, and hypersensitivity to disulfiram or to other thiuram derivatives used in pesticides and rubber vulcanization.

WARNINGS

> ANTABUSE should never be administered to a patient when he is in a state of alcohol intoxication, or without his full knowledge.
> The physician should instruct relatives accordingly.

The patient must be fully informed of the ANTABUSE-alcohol reaction. He must be strongly cautioned against surreptitious drinking while taking the drug and he must be fully aware of possible consequences. He should be warned to avoid alcohol in disguised form, ie, in sauces, vinegars, cough mixtures, and even aftershave lotions and back rubs. He should also be warned that reactions may occur with alcohol up to 14 days after ingesting ANTABUSE.
The ANTABUSE-ALCOHOL REACTION: ANTABUSE plus alcohol, even small amounts, produces flushing, throbbing in head and neck, throbbing headache, respiratory difficulty, nausea, copious vomiting, sweating, thirst, chest pain, palpitation, dyspnea, hyperventilation, tachycardia, hypotension, syncope, marked uneasiness, weakness, vertigo, blurred vision, and confusion. In severe reactions there may be respiratory depression, cardiovascular collapse, arrhythmias, myocardial infarction, acute congestive heart failure, unconsciousness, convulsions, and death.
The intensity of the reaction varies with each individual, but is generally proportional to the amounts of ANTABUSE and alcohol ingested. Mild reactions may occur in the sensitive individual when the blood alcohol concentration is increased to as little as 5- to 10- mg per 100 mL. Symptoms are fully developed at 50 mg per 100 mL and unconsciousness usually results when the blood alcohol level reaches 125 to 150 mg.
The duration of the reaction varies from 30 to 60 minutes, to several hours in the more severe cases, or as long as there is alcohol in the blood.

DRUG INTERACTIONS: Disulfiram appears to decrease the rate at which certain drugs are metabolized and therefore may increase the blood levels and the possibility of clinical toxicity of drugs given concomitantly.
DISULFIRAM SHOULD BE USED WITH CAUTION IN THOSE PATIENTS RECEIVING PHENYTOIN AND ITS CONGENERS, SINCE THE CONCOMITANT ADMINISTRATION OF THESE TWO DRUGS CAN LEAD TO PHENYTOIN INTOXICATION. PRIOR TO ADMINISTERING DISULFIRAM TO A PATIENT ON PHENYTOIN THERAPY, A BASELINE PHENYTOIN SERUM LEVEL SHOULD BE OBTAINED. SUBSEQUENT TO INITIATION OF DISULFIRAM THERAPY, SERUM LEVELS ON PHENYTOIN SHOULD BE DETERMINED ON DIFFERENT DAYS FOR EVIDENCE OF AN INCREASE, OR FOR A CONTINUING RISE IN LEVELS. INCREASED PHENYTOIN LEVELS SHOULD BE TREATED WITH APPROPRIATE DOSAGE ADJUSTMENT.
It may be necessary to adjust the dosage of oral anticoagulants upon beginning or stopping disulfiram, since disulfiram may prolong prothrombin time.
Patients taking isoniazid when disulfiram is given should be observed for the appearance of unsteady gait or marked changes in mental status; the disulfiram should be discontinued if such signs appear.
In rats, simultaneous ingestion of disulfiram and nitrite in the diet for 78 weeks has been reported to cause tumors, and it has been suggested that disulfiram may react with nitrites in the rat stomach to form a nitrosamine, which is tumorigenic. Disulfiram alone in the rats' diet did not lead to such tumors. The relevance of this finding to humans is not known at this time.
CONCOMITANT CONDITIONS: Because of the possibility of an accidental ANTABUSE-alcohol reaction, ANTABUSE should be used with extreme caution in patients with any of the following conditions: diabetes mellitus, hypothyroidism, epilepsy, cerebral damage, chronic and acute nephritis, hepatic cirrhosis or insufficiency.
USAGE IN PREGNANCY: The safe use of this drug in pregnancy has not been established. Therefore, ANTABUSE should be used during pregnancy only when, in the judgment of the physician, the probable benefits outweigh the possible risks.

PRECAUTIONS
Patients with a history of rubber contact dermatitis should be evaluated for hypersensitivity to thiuram derivatives before receiving ANTABUSE (see CONTRAINDICATIONS). It is suggested that every patient under treatment carry an Identification Card, stating that he is receiving ANTABUSE

Continued on next page

Wyeth-Ayerst—Cont.

and describing the symptoms most likely to occur as a result of the ANTABUSE-alcohol reaction. In addition, this card should indicate the physician or institution to be contacted in emergency. (Cards may be obtained from Wyeth-Ayerst Laboratories upon request.)

Alcoholism may accompany or be followed by dependence on narcotics or sedatives. Barbiturates and ANTABUSE have been administered concurrently without untoward effects; the possibility of initiating a new abuse should be considered. Baseline and follow-up transaminase tests (10–14 days) are suggested to detect any hepatic dysfunction that may result with ANTABUSE therapy. In addition, a complete blood count and a sequential multiple analysis-12 (SMA-12) test should be made every six months.

Patients taking ANTABUSE Tablets should not be exposed to ethylene dibromide or its vapors. This precaution is based on preliminary results of animal research currently in progress that suggest a toxic interaction between inhaled ethylene dibromide and ingested disulfiram resulting in a higher incidence of tumors and mortality in rats. A correlation between this finding and humans, however, has not been demonstrated.

ADVERSE REACTIONS
(See CONTRAINDICATIONS, WARNINGS, and PRECAUTIONS.)

OPTIC NEURITIS, PERIPHERAL NEURITIS, AND POLYNEURITIS MAY OCCUR FOLLOWING ADMINISTRATION OF ANTABUSE.

Multiple cases of both cholestatic and fulminant hepatitis have been reported to be associated with administration of ANTABUSE.

Occasional skin eruptions are, as a rule, readily controlled by concomitant administration of an antihistaminic drug.

In a small number of patients, a transient mild drowsiness, fatigability, impotence, headache, acneform eruptions, allergic dermatitis, or a metallic or garlic-like aftertaste may be experienced during the first two weeks of therapy. These complaints usually disappear spontaneously with the continuation of therapy, or with reduced dosage.

Psychotic reactions have been noted, attributable in most cases to high dosage, combined toxicity (with metronidazole or isoniazid), or to the unmasking of underlying psychoses in patients stressed by the withdrawal of alcohol.

DOSAGE AND ADMINISTRATION
ANTABUSE should never be administered until the patient has abstained from alcohol for at least 12 hours.

INITIAL DOSAGE SCHEDULE: In the first phase of treatment, a <u>maximum</u> of 500 mg daily is given in a single dose for one to two weeks. Although usually taken in the morning, ANTABUSE may be taken on retiring by patients who experience a sedative effect. Alternatively, to minimize, or eliminate, the sedative effect, dosage may be adjusted downward.

MAINTENANCE REGIMEN: The average maintenance dose is 250 mg daily (range, 125 to 500 mg); it should not exceed 500 mg daily.

NOTE: Occasionally patients, while seemingly on adequate maintenance doses of ANTABUSE, report that they are able to drink alcoholic beverages with impunity and without any symptomatology. All appearances to the contrary, such patients must be presumed to be disposing of their tablets in some manner without actually taking them. Until such patients have been observed reliably taking their daily ANTABUSE tablets (preferably crushed and well mixed with liquid), it cannot be concluded that ANTABUSE is ineffective.

DURATION OF THERAPY: The daily, uninterrupted administration of ANTABUSE must be continued until the patient is fully recovered socially and a basis for permanent self-control is established. Depending on the individual patient, maintenance therapy may be required for months, or even years.

TRIAL WITH ALCOHOL: During early experience with ANTABUSE, it was thought advisable for each patient to have at least one supervised alcohol-drug reaction. More recently, the test reaction has been largely abandoned. Furthermore, such a test reaction should never be administered to a patient over 50 years of age. A clear, detailed, and convincing description of the reaction is felt to be sufficient in most cases.

However, where a test reaction is deemed necessary, the suggested procedure is as follows:

After the first one to two weeks' therapy with 500 mg daily, a drink of 15 mL (½ oz) of 100 proof whiskey, or equivalent, is taken slowly. This test dose of alcoholic beverage may be repeated once only, so that the total dose does not exceed 30 mL (1 oz) of whiskey. Once a reaction develops, no more alcohol should be consumed. Such tests should be carried out only when the patient is hospitalized, or comparable supervision and facilities, including oxygen, are available.

MANAGEMENT OF ANTABUSE-ALCOHOL REACTION: In severe reactions, whether caused by an excessive test dose

or by the patient's unsupervised ingestion of alcohol, supportive measures to restore blood pressure and treat shock should be instituted. Other recommendations include: oxygen, carbogen (95% oxygen and 5% carbon dioxide), vitamin C intravenously in massive doses (1 g), and ephedrine sulfate. Antihistamines have also been used intravenously. Potassium levels should be monitored, particularly in patients on digitalis, since hypokalemia has been reported.

HOW SUPPLIED
ANTABUSE—Each tablet (scored) contains 250 mg disulfiram, in bottles of 100 (NDC 0046-0809-81)—Each tablet (scored) contains 500 mg disulfiram, in bottles of 50 (NDC 0046-0810-50) and 1,000 (NDC 0046-0810-91).

Shown in Product Identification Section, page 436

ANTIVENIN (CROTALIDAE)   ℞
[an ''te ven 'in]
POLYVALENT
(equine origin)

IMPORTANT
Pit viper bites may cause severe tissue damage or fatal envenomation, or both. The physician responsible for treatment of an envenomated patient should be familiar with the contents of this brochure and the pertinent medical literature concerning current concepts of first-aid and general supportive therapy as presented in the references listed at the end of this pamphlet.

COMPOSITION
Antivenin (Crotalidae) Polyvalent, Wyeth, is a refined and concentrated preparation of serum globulins obtained by fractionating blood from healthy horses immunized with the following venoms: *Crotalus adamanteus* (Eastern diamond rattlesnake), *C. atrox* (Western diamond rattlesnake), *C. durissus terrificus* (tropical rattlesnake, Cascabel), and *Bothrops atrox* ("Fer-de-lance"). Phenol, 0.25%, and thimerosal, 0.005%, are added as preservatives. The product is standardized by its ability to neutralize the lethal action of standard venoms by intravenous injection in mice.[1] Dried from the frozen state, the lyophilized serum has a moisture content of less than 1% and is soluble on addition of the diluent contained in each package (Bacteriostatic Water for Injection, USP, with preservative: 0.001% phenylmercuric nitrate).

Antivenin (Crotalidae) Polyvalent, Wyeth (hereinafter referred to as Antivenin) contains protective substances capable of neutralizing the toxic effects of venoms of crotalids (pit vipers) native to North, Central, and South America, including rattlesnakes (*Crotalus, Sistrurus*); copperhead and cottonmouth moccasins (*Agkistrodon*), including *A. halys* of Korea and Japan; the Fer-de-lance and other species of *Bothrops*; the tropical rattler (*Crotalus durissus* and similar species); the Cantil (*A. bilineatus*); and bushmaster (*Lachesis mutus*) of South and Central America.

INDICATION
Antivenin is indicated only for the treatment of envenomation caused by bites of those crotalids (pit vipers) specified in the immediately preceding paragraph.

PIT VIPER BITES AND ENVENOMATION
The symptoms, signs, and severity of snake-venom poisoning resulting from pit viper bites depend on many factors, including, but not limited to, the following variables: species, age, and size of the biting snake; the number and location of bite(s); the depth of venom deposit by the snake's fangs; the condition of the snake's fangs and venom glands; the length of time the snake "hangs on"; the age, general health, and size of the victim; the type and efficacy of any first-aid treatment rendered in an attempt to remove venom and how soon such treatment was applied. In any venomous snake bite, the actual amount of venom introduced into the victim is always an unknown. Even the type of clothing or leg-footwear through which the snake's fangs pass may affect the amount of venom delivered by the bite. Although most North American pit vipers tend to bite and introduce venom superficially, their fangs may get hung-up in the subcutaneous tissues during the biting act and can penetrate deeper tissues during the attempt to release the bitten part. In some bites the fangs may penetrate into muscle. In such cases, the usual local superficial manifestations of envenomation may not appear early in the course of poisoning. In bites by some species, systemic evidence of envenomation may be present in the absence of significant local manifestations. It may be difficult to determine the severity of envenomation during the first several hours after a pit viper bite and estimates of severity may need to be revised as poisoning progresses. It must be remembered, too, that not all pit viper bites result in envenomation. In approximately 20% of rattlesnake bites, the snake may not inject any venom. The local and systemic symptoms and signs of envenomation include the following:

LOCAL:
Fang puncture(s).
Swelling—edema is usually seen around the site of bite within five minutes. It may progress rapidly and involve the

entire extremity within an hour. More than 95% of all snakebites are inflicted on extremities.[2] Generally, however, edema spreads more slowly, usually over a period of 8 or more hours. Swelling is usually most severe following envenomation by the Eastern diamondback; less severe after bites by the Western diamondback, prairie, red, Pacific, Mojave, and blacktailed rattlers, the sidewinder and cottonmouth moccasins; least severe after bites by copperheads, massasaugas, and pygmy rattlers.

Ecchymosis and discoloration of the skin—often appear in the area of the bite within a few hours. Vesicles may form within a few hours and are usually present at 24 hours. Hemorrhagic blebs and petechiae are common. Necrosis may develop, necessitating amputation of an extremity or a portion thereof.

Pain—frequently a complaint of the victim beginning shortly after the bite by most pit vipers. Pain may be absent after bites by Mojave rattlers.

SYSTEMIC:
Weakness; faintness; nausea; sweating; numbness or tingling around the mouth, tongue, scalp, fingers, toes, site of bite; muscle fasciculations; hypotension; prolongation of bleeding and clotting times; hemoconcentration, early followed by a decrease in erythrocytes; thrombocytopenia; hematuria; proteinuria; vomiting, including hematemesis; melena; hemoptysis; epistaxis. In fatal poisoning, a frequent cause of death is associated with destruction of erythrocytes and changes in capillary permeability, especially of the pulmonary vascular system, leading to pulmonary edema; hemoconcentration usually occurs early, probably as a result of plasma loss secondary to vascular permeability; the hemoglobin may fall, and bleeding may occur throughout the body as early as 6 hours after the bite. Renal involvement is not uncommon. Mojave rattler venom may cause neuromuscular changes leading to respiratory failure.

An estimate of the severity of envenomation should be made as soon as possible and before any Antivenin is administered. The amount (volume) of the first dose of Antivenin is determined on this estimate of severity. Every symptom, sign, laboratory-test result, and any other pertinent information should be considered in estimating severity—local manifestations; systemic manifestations, including abnormal laboratory findings; species and size of the biting snake, if known; number and location of bite(s); size and health of the patient; type of first-aid treatment rendered; and interval between bite and arrival for treatment. Russell et al,[3] and Wingert and Wainschel[4] grade severity as follows:

No envenomation—no local or systemic manifestations.
Minimal envenomation—local swelling and other local changes; no systemic manifestations; normal laboratory findings.
Moderate envenomation—swelling progressing beyond the site of bite and one or more systemic manifestations; abnormal laboratory findings, for example, a fall in hematocrit or platelets.
Severe envenomation—marked local response, severe systemic manifestations and significant alteration in laboratory findings.

Parrish and Hayes,[5] McCollough and Gennaro,[6] and Watt and Gennaro[7] have used a Grade 0 (no envenomation) through Grade IV (very severe) classification of severity which was developed for the most part in treatment of envenomation by the Eastern diamondback and timber rattlers. This classification is more dependent on local manifestations, or the absence thereof, as the venoms of these species seem to be more consistent in inducing local tissue damage.

Any suspected envenomation should be treated as a medical emergency, and until careful observation provides clear evidence that envenomation has not occurred or is minimal, the following procedures are recommended:

Monitor vital signs at frequent intervals: Blood pressure, pulse, respiration.

Draw sufficient blood as soon as possible for baseline laboratory studies, including type and cross-match, CBC, hematocrit, platelet count, prothrombin time, clot retraction, bleeding and coagulation times, BUN, electrolytes, bilirubin. Some of these studies may need to be repeated at daily intervals, or less, depending on the severity of envenomation and the response to treatment. During the first 4 or 5 days of severe envenomations, hemoglobin, hematocrit, and platelet counts should be carried out several times a day.

Obtain urine samples at frequent intervals for analysis, with special attention to microscopic examination for presence of erythrocytes.

Chart fluid intake and urine output.

Measure and record the circumference of the bitten extremity just proximal to the bite and at one or more additional points each several inches closer to the trunk. Repeat measurements every 15-30 minutes to obtain information about progression of edema.

Have available and ready for immediate use: oxygen, resuscitation equipment including airway, tourniquet, epinephrine, injectable antihistaminic agents and corticosteroids.

Start an intravenous infusion in one or two extremities: one line to be used for supportive therapy, if needed, such as whole blood, plasma, packed red cells, specific clotting factors, platelet transfusion, plasma expanders; the other line to be used for administration of Antivenin and electrolytes. Carry out and interpret a skin test for horse-serum sensitivity. (See "Precautions" section below.)

DOSAGE AND ADMINISTRATION

Before administration, read "Precautions" and "Systemic Reactions" sections below. Since the possibility of a severe immediate reaction (anaphylaxis) exists whenever a horse-serum-containing product is administered, appropriate therapeutic agents, including a tourniquet, airway, oxygen, epinephrine, an injectable pressor amine, and corticosteroid, must be available and ready for immediate use. Constant attendance and observation of the patient for untoward reactions are mandatory when Antivenin is administered. Should any systemic reaction occur, administration should be discontinued immediately and appropriate treatment initiated.

The intravenous route of administration is preferred, and probably should always be used for moderate or severe envenomation. Intravenous administration is mandatory if venom-induced shock is present. To be most effective, Antivenin should be administered within 4 hours of the bite; it is less effective when given after 8 hours and may be of questionable value after 12 hours. However, it is recommended that Antivenin therapy be given in severe poisonings, even if 24 hours have elapsed since the time of the bite. It should be kept in mind that maximum blood levels of Antivenin may not be obtained for 8 or more hours after intramuscular administration.

For intravenous-drip use, prepare a 1:1 to 1:10 dilution of reconstituted Antivenin in Sodium Chloride Injection, USP, or 5% Dextrose Injection, USP. To avoid foaming, mix by gently swirling rather than shaking. Allow the initial 5 to 10 mL to infuse over a 3- to 5-minute period, with careful observation of the patient for evidence of untoward reaction. If no symptoms or signs of an immediate systemic reaction appear, continue the infusion with delivery at the maximum safe rate for intravenous fluid administration. The dilution of Antivenin to be used, the type of electrolyte solution used for dilution, and the rate of intravenous delivery of the diluted Antivenin must take into consideration the age, weight, and cardiac status of the patient; the severity of envenomation; the total amount and type of parenteral fluids it is anticipated will be given or are needed; and the interval between bite and initiation of specific therapy.

It is important to give as soon as possible the entire initial dose of Antivenin as based on the best estimate of the severity of envenomation at the time treatment is begun. The following initial doses are recommended:[3,4,8]

no envenomation—none
minimal envenomation—20-40 mL (contents of 2 to 4 vials)
moderate envenomation—50-90 mL (contents of 5 to 9 vials)
severe envenomation—100-150 mL or more (contents of 10 to 15 or more vials)

These recommended initial-dosage volumes are in general accord with those of others.[5-7,9]

The need for additional Antivenin must be based on the clinical response to the initial dose and continuing assessment of the severity of poisoning. If swelling continues to progress or if systemic symptoms or signs of envenomation increase in severity or if new manifestations appear, for example, fall in hematocrit or hypotension, administer an additional 10 to 50 mL (contents of 1 to 5 vials) intravenously.

Envenomation by large snakes in children or small adults requires larger doses of Antivenin. The amount administered to a child is not based on weight.

If Antivenin is given intramuscularly, it should be given into a large muscle mass, preferably the gluteal area, with care to avoid nerve trunks. Antivenin should never be injected into a finger or toe.

The effectiveness of corticosteroids in treatment of envenomation per se or venom shock is not resolved. Russell[3] and others[9,10] believe corticosteroids may mask the seriousness of hypovolemia in moderate or severe poisoning and have little, if any, effect on the local-tissue response to rattler venoms. Corticosteroids should not be given simultaneously with Antivenin on a routine basis or during the acute state of envenomation; however, their use may be necessary to treat immediate allergic reactions to Antivenin, and corticosteroids are the agents of choice for treating serious delayed reactions to Antivenin.

Snakes' mouths do not harbor *Clostridium tetani.* However, appropriate tetanus prophylaxis is indicated, since tetanus spores may be carried into the fang puncture wounds by dirt present on skin at time of bite or by nonsterile first-aid procedures.

A broad-spectrum antibiotic in adequate dosage is indicated if local tissue damage is evident.

Shock following envenomation is treated like shock resulting from hypovolemia from any cause, including administration of whole blood, plasma, albumin, or other plasma expanders, as indicated.

Aspirin or codeine is usually adequate for relieving pain. Sedation with phenobarbital or mild tranquilizers may be used if indicated, but not in the presence of respiratory failure.

The bitten extremity should not be packed in ice, and so-called "cryotherapy" is contraindicated.

Compartment syndromes may complicate pit viper envenomations, especially those caused by bites on the lower extremities. Prompt surgical consultation is indicated whenever a closed-compartment syndrome is suspected.[3,12]

Defibrination and disseminated intravascular coagulation (DIC) syndromes have been associated with envenomation caused by some pit vipers native to the United States, and appropriate therapy may be indicated.[3,9,10,13-17]

TECHNIC FOR RECONSTITUTING THE DRIED ANTIVENIN

Pry off the small metal disc in the cap over the diaphragms of the vials of Antivenin and diluent. Swab the exposed surface of the rubber diaphragms of both vials with an appropriate germicide. With a sterile 10 mL syringe and needle, withdraw the diluent (Bacteriostatic Water for Injection, USP, containing phenylmercuric nitrate 1:100,000) from the vial of diluent and inject it into the vial of Antivenin. Gentle agitation will hasten complete dissolution of the lyophilized Antivenin.

PRECAUTIONS

Before administration of any product prepared from horse serum, appropriate measures must be taken in an effort to detect the presence of dangerous sensitivity: (1) A careful review of the patient's history, including any report of (a) asthma, hay fever, urticaria, or other allergic manifestations; (b) allergic reactions upon exposure to horses; and (c) prior injections of horse serum. (2) A suitable test for detection of sensitivity. A skin test should be performed in every patient prior to administration, regardless of clinical history.

Skin test—Inject intracutaneously 0.02 to 0.03 mL of a 1:10 dilution of Normal Horse Serum or Antivenin. A control test on the opposite extremity, using Sodium Chloride Injection, USP, facilitates interpretation. Use of larger amounts for the skin-test dose increases the likelihood of false-positive reactions, and in the exquisitely sensitive patient, increases the risk of a systemic reaction from the skin-test dose. A 1:100 or greater dilution should be used for preliminary skin testing if the history suggests sensitivity. A positive reaction to a skin test occurs within five to thirty minutes and is manifested by a wheal with or without pseudopodia and surrounding erythema. In general, the shorter the interval between injection and the beginning of the skin reaction, the greater the sensitivity.

If the history is negative for allergy and the result of a skin test is negative, proceed with administration of Antivenin as outlined above. If the history is positive and a skin test is strongly positive, administration may be dangerous, especially if the positive sensitivity test is accompanied by systemic allergic manifestations. In such instances, the risk of administering Antivenin must be weighed against the risk of withholding it, keeping in mind that severe envenomation can be fatal. (See last paragraph of this section.)

A negative allergic history and absence of reaction to a properly applied skin test do not rule out the possibility of an immediate reaction. Also, a negative skin test has no bearing on whether or not delayed serum reactions (serum sickness) will occur after administration of the full dose.

If the history is negative, and the skin test is mildly or questionably positive, administer as follows to reduce the risk of a severe immediate systemic reaction: (a) Prepare, in separate sterile vials or syringes, 1:100 and 1:10 dilutions of Antivenin. (b) Allow at least 15 minutes between injections and proceed with the next dose if no reaction follows the previous dose. (c) Inject subcutaneously, using a tuberculin-type syringe, 0.1, 0.2, and 0.5 mL of the 1:100 dilution at 15-minute intervals; repeat with the 1:10 dilution, and finally undiluted Antivenin. (d) If a systemic reaction occurs after any injection, place a tourniquet proximal to the site of injections and administer an appropriate dose of epinephrine, 1:1000, proximal to the tourniquet or into another extremity. Wait at least 30 minutes before injecting another dose. The amount of the next dose should be the same as the last that did not evoke a reaction. (e) If no reaction occurs after 0.5 mL of undiluted Antivenin has been administered, switch to the intramuscular route and continue doubling the dose at 15-minute intervals until the entire dose has been injected intramuscularly or proceed to the intravenous route as described above under "Dosage and Administration."

Obviously, if the just-described schedule is used, 3 to 5 or more hours would be required to administer the initial dose suggested for a moderate or severe envenomation, and time is an important factor in neutralization of venom in a critically ill patient. Wingert and Wainschel[4] have described a procedure based on the experience of their group which they have used in some severely envenomated patients who have positive sensitivity tests: 50 to 100 mg of diphenhydramine hydrochloride is given intravenously, followed by slow intravenous infusion of diluted Antivenin for 15 to 20 minutes while carefully observing the patient for symptoms and signs of anaphylaxis; if anaphylaxis does not occur, Antivenin is continued, maintaining close observation of the patient. Patients who require Antivenin but develop signs of impending anaphylaxis in spite of this or the procedure described earlier present a difficult problem, and consultation should be sought.

SYSTEMIC REACTIONS

A. The immediate reaction (shock, anaphylaxis) usually occurs within 30 minutes. Symptoms and signs may develop before the needle is withdrawn and may include apprehension, flushing, itching, urticaria; edema of the face, tongue, and throat; cough, dyspnea, cyanosis, vomiting, and collapse.

B. Serum sickness usually occurs 5 to 24 days after administration. The incubation period may be less than 5 days, especially in those who have received horse-serum-containing preparations in the past. The usual symptoms and signs are malaise, fever, urticaria, lymphadenopathy, edema, arthralgia, nausea, and vomiting. Occasionally, neurological manifestations develop, such as meningismus or peripheral neuritis. Peripheral neuritis usually involves the shoulders and arms. Pain and muscle weakness are frequently present, and permanent atrophy may develop.

REFERENCES

1. GINGRICH, W. & HOHENADEL, J.: Standardization of polyvalent antivenin. "Venoms", edited by E. Buckley and N. Porges. Publication No. 44, Amer. Assoc. for the Advancement of Science, Washington, D.C., 1956, Pages 337–80.
2. PARRISH, H.: Incidence of treated snakebite in the United States. Pub. Hlth. Rep. 81:269, 1966.
3. RUSSELL, F., et al.: Snake venom poisoning in the United States. Experiences with 550 cases. JAMA 233:341, 1975. RUSSELL, F.: Venomous bites and stings: Poisonous snakes. In The Merck Manual of Diagnosis and Therapy, pp. 2450–2456, 14th Ed., 1982.
4. WINGERT, W. and WAINSCHEL, J.: Diagnosis and management of envenomation by poisonous snakes. South. Med. J. 68:1015, 1975.
5. PARRISH, H. & HAYES, R.: Hospital management of pit viper venenations. Clinical Toxicol. 3:501, 1970.
6. McCOLLOUGH, N. & GENNARO, J.: Diagnosis, symptoms, treatment and sequelae of envenomation by Crotalus adamanteus and Genus Agkistrodon. J. Florida Med. Assoc. 55:327, 1968.
7. WATT, C. & GENNARO, J.: Pit viper bites in South Georgia and North Florida. Tr. South. Surg. Assoc. 77:378, 1966.
8. MINTON, S.: Venom Diseases: Snakebite. In Textbook of Medicine, P. Beeson and W. McDermott (Eds.), pp. 88–92; Saunders, Philadelphia, 1975.
9. VAN MIEROP, L.: Snakebite symposium. J. Florida Med. Assoc. 63:101, 1976.
10. ARNOLD, R.: Treatment of snakebite. JAMA 236:1843, 1976; Controversies and hazards in the treatment of pit viper bites. South Med. J. 72:902, 1979.
11. Poisonous Snakes of the World. U.S. Government Printing Office, Washington, D.C., NAVMED, 1965.
12. GARFIN, S. et al.: Rattlesnake bites: Current concepts. Clin. Orthop. 140:50, 1979; Role of surgical decompression in treatment of rattlesnake bites. Surg. Forum 30:502, 1979.
13. VAN MIEROP, L. & KITCHENS, C.: Defibrination syndrome following bites by the Eastern diamondback rattlesnake. J. Florida Med. Assoc. 67:21, 1980.
14. HASIBA, U. et al.: DIC-like syndrome after envenomation by the snake, Crotalus horridus horridus. New Eng. J. Med. 292:505, 1975.
15. WEISS, H. et al.: Afibrinogenemia in man following the bite of a rattlesnake (Crotalus adamanteus). Am. J. Med. 47:625, 1969.
16. SIVAPRASAD, R. & CANTINI, E.: Western diamondback rattlesnake (Crotalus atrox) poisoning. Postgrad. Med. 71:223, 1982.
17. SABBACK, M. et al.: A study of the treatment of pit viper envenomization in 45 patients. J. Trauma 17:569, 1977.

HOW SUPPLIED

Each combination package contains one vacuum vial to yield 10 mL of serum—to be used immediately after reconstitution—(with preservatives: phenol 0.25% and thimerosal [mercury derivative] 0.005%). One vial containing 10 mL of Bacteriostatic Water for Injection, USP (with preservative: phenylmercuric nitrate 0.001%). One 1 mL vial of normal horse serum (diluted 1:10) as sensitivity testing material with preservatives: thimerosal (mercury derivative) 0.005% and phenol 0.35%. Not returnable.

ANTIVENIN (Micrurus fulvius)   ℞
[an "te ven 'in]
(equine origin)
North American Coral Snake Antivenin

COMPOSITION

Each combination package contains one vial of lyophilized Antivenin (Micrurus fulvius) with 0.25% phenol and 0.005%

Continued on next page

Wyeth-Ayerst—Cont.

thimerosal (mercury derivative) as preservatives (before lyophilization); one vial of diluent containing 10 ml. of Bacteriostatic Water for Injection, U.S.P., with phenylmercuric nitrate (1:100,000) as preservative.

HOW SUPPLIED

Combination packages as described (not returnable).
For prescribing information write to Professional Service, Wyeth-Ayerst Laboratories, Box 8299, Philadelphia, PA 19101, or contact your local Wyeth-Ayerst representative.

A.P.L.® ℞
Brand of chorionic gonadotropin for injection, USP
For Intramuscular Injection Only

CAUTION: Federal law prohibits dispensing without prescription.

DESCRIPTION

Human chorionic gonadotropin (HCG), a polypeptide hormone produced by the human placenta, is composed of an alpha and a beta subunit. The alpha subunit is essentially identical to the alpha subunits of the human pituitary gonadotropins, luteinizing hormone (LH) and follicle-stimulating hormone (FSH), as well as to the alpha subunit of human thyroid stimulating hormone (TSH). The beta subunits of these hormones differ in amino acid sequence.
A.P.L. (chorionic gonadotropin, USP) is a gonad-stimulating principle obtained from the urine of pregnant women. It is an amorphous powder prepared by cryodesiccation, and is freely soluble in water.

ACTIONS

The action of HCG is virtually identical to that of pituitary LH, although HCG appears to have a small degree of FSH activity as well. It stimulates production of gonadal steroid hormones by stimulating the interstitial cells (Leydig cells) of the testis to produce androgens and the corpus luteum of the ovary to produce progesterone. Androgen stimulation in the male leads to the development of secondary sex characteristics and may stimulate testicular descent when no anatomical impediment to descent is present. This descent is usually reversible when HCG is discontinued. During the normal menstrual cycle, LH participates with FSH in the development and maturation of the normal ovarian follicle, and the midcycle LH surge triggers ovulation. HCG can substitute for LH in this function.
During a normal pregnancy, HCG secreted by the placenta maintains the corpus luteum after LH secretion decreases, supporting continued secretion of estrogen and progesterone, and preventing menstruation. HCG HAS NO KNOWN EFFECT ON FAT MOBILIZATION, APPETITE OR SENSE OF HUNGER, OR BODY FAT DISTRIBUTION.

INDICATIONS

HCG HAS NOT BEEN DEMONSTRATED TO BE EFFECTIVE ADJUNCTIVE THERAPY IN THE TREATMENT OF OBESITY. THERE IS NO SUBSTANTIAL EVIDENCE THAT IT INCREASES WEIGHT LOSS BEYOND THAT RESULTING FROM CALORIC RESTRICTION, THAT IT CAUSES A MORE ATTRACTIVE OR "NORMAL" DISTRIBUTION OF FAT, OR THAT IT DECREASES THE HUNGER AND DISCOMFORT ASSOCIATED WITH CALORIE RESTRICTED DIETS.

1. Cryptorchidism not due to anatomic obstruction. In general, A.P.L. is thought to induce testicular descent in situations when descent would have occurred at puberty. A.P.L. thus may help to predict whether or not orchiopexy will be needed in the future. Although, in some cases, descent following A.P.L. administration is permanent, in most cases the response is temporary. Therapy is usually instituted between the ages of 4 and 9.
2. Selected cases of male hypogonadism secondary to pituitary failure.
3. Induction of ovulation and pregnancy in the anovulatory, infertile woman in whom the cause of anovulation is secondary and not due to ovarian failure, and who has been appropriately pretreated with human menotropins.

CONTRAINDICATIONS

Precocious puberty, prostatic carcinoma or other androgen-dependent neoplasia, prior allergic reaction to chorionic gonadotropin.

WARNINGS

HCG should be used in conjunction with human menopausal gonadotropins only by physicians experienced with infertility problems who are familiar with the criteria for patient selection, warnings, precautions, and adverse reactions described in the package insert for menotropins. The principal serious adverse reactions during this use are: (1) ovarian enlargement, ascites with or without

---

pain, and/or pleural effusion, (2) rupture of ovarian cysts with resultant hemoperitoneum, (3) multiple births, and (4) arterial thromboembolism.

PRECAUTIONS

Induction of androgen secretion by chorionic gonadotropin may induce precocious puberty in patients treated for cryptorchidism. If signs of precocious puberty occur, therapy should be discontinued.
Since androgens may cause fluid retention, chorionic gonadotropin should be used with caution in patients with epilepsy, migraine, asthma, cardiac or renal disease.

ADVERSE REACTIONS

Headache
Irritability
Restlessness
Depression
Tiredness
Edema
Precocious puberty
Gynecomastia
Pain at site of injection

DOSAGE AND ADMINISTRATION

There is a marked variance of opinion concerning the dosage regimens to be used. Therefore the regimen employed in any particular case will depend upon the indication for use, the age and weight of the patient, and the physician's preference. The following regimens have been advocated by various authorities.
Cryptorchidism: (Therapy is usually instituted between the ages of 4 and 9.)
  (1) 4,000 USP Units three times weekly for three weeks.
  (2) 5,000 USP Units every second day for four injections.
  (3) 15 injections of 500 to 1,000 USP Units over a period of six weeks.
  (4) 500 USP Units three times weekly for four to six weeks. If this course of treatment is not successful, another is begun one month later, giving 1,000 USP Units per injection.
Selected cases of male hypogonadism secondary to pituitary failure:
  (1) 500 to 1,000 USP Units three times a week for three weeks, followed by the same dose twice a week for three weeks.
  (2) 1,000 to 2,000 USP Units three times weekly.
  (3) 4,000 USP Units three times weekly for six to nine months, following which the dosage may be reduced to 2,000 USP Units three times weekly for an additional three months.
Induction of ovulation and pregnancy in the anovulatory, infertile woman in whom the cause of anovulation is secondary:
  5,000 to 10,000 USP Units one day following the last dose of menotropins.

HOW SUPPLIED

A.P.L. (Chorionic Gonadotropin for Injection, USP)
NDC 0046-0970-10 — Each package provides:
  (1) One vial containing 5,000 USP Units chorionic gonadotropin in dry form, and
  (2) One 10 mL ampul sterile diluent.
NDC 0046-0971-10 — Each package provides:
  (1) One vial containing 10,000 USP Units chorionic gonadotropin in dry form, and
  (2) One 10 mL ampul sterile diluent.
NDC 0046-0972-10 — Each package provides:
  (1) One vial containing 20,000 USP Units chorionic gonadotropin in dry form, and
  (2) One 10 mL ampul sterile diluent.
When reconstituted with 10 mL of accompanying sterile diluent, the resulting solutions also contain 2.0% benzyl alcohol, not more than 0.2% phenol, and the following concentrations of lactose: No. 970, 0.9%; No. 971, 1.8%; No. 972, 3.6%. The pH is adjusted with sodium hydroxide or hydrochloric acid.
MAY BE STORED FOR 30 DAYS IN A REFRIGERATOR AFTER RECONSTITUTION.

ATIVAN® © ℞
[*at'i-van*]
(lorazepam)
Injection

DESCRIPTION

Ativan (lorazepam) Injection, a benzodiazepine with antianxiety and sedative effects, is intended for intramuscular or intravenous route of administration. It has the chemical formula: 7-chloro-5-(o-chlorophenyl)-1,3-dihydro-3-hydroxy-2 H -1,4-benzodiazepin-2-one. The molecular weight is 321.2, and the C.A.S. No. is [846-49-1].
Lorazepam is a nearly white powder almost insoluble in water. Each mL of sterile injection contains either 2.0 or 4.0 mg of lorazepam, 0.18 mL polyethylene glycol 400 in propylene glycol with 2.0% benzyl alcohol as preservative.

CLINICAL PHARMACOLOGY

Intravenous or intramuscular administration of the recommended dose of 2 to 4 mg of Ativan (lorazepam) Injection to adult patients is followed by dose-related effects of sedation (sleepiness or drowsiness), relief of preoperative anxiety, and lack of recall of events related to the day of surgery in the majority of patients. The clinical sedation (sleepiness or drowsiness) thus noted is such that the majority of patients are able to respond to simple instructions whether they give the appearance of being awake or asleep. The lack of recall is relative rather than absolute, as determined under conditions of careful patient questioning and testing, using props designed to enhance recall. The majority of patients under these reinforced conditions had difficulty recalling perioperative events or recognizing props from before surgery. The lack of recall and recognition was optimum within 2 hours following intramuscular administration and 15 to 20 minutes after intravenous injection.
The intended effects of the recommended adult dose of lorazepam injection usually last 6 to 8 hours. In rare instances and where patients received greater than the recommended dose, excessive sleepiness and prolonged lack of recall were noted. As with other benzodiazepines, unsteadiness, enhanced sensitivity to CNS-depressant effects of ethyl alcohol and other drugs were noted in isolated and rare cases for greater than 24 hours.
Studies in healthy adult volunteers reveal that intravenous lorazepam in doses up to 3.5 mg/70 kg does not alter sensitivity to the respiratory stimulating effect of carbon dioxide and does not enhance the respiratory depressant effects of doses of meperidine up to 100 mg/70 kg (also determined by carbon dioxide challenge) as long as patients remain sufficiently awake to undergo testing. Upper airway obstruction has been observed in rare instances where the patient received greater than the recommended dose and was excessively sleepy and difficult to arouse. (See "Warnings" and "Adverse Reactions".)
Clinically employed doses of lorazepam injectable do not greatly affect the circulatory system in the supine position or employing a 70-degree tilt test. Doses of 8 mg to 10 mg of intravenous lorazepam (2 to 2½ times the maximum recommended dosage) will produce loss of lid reflexes within 15 minutes.
Studies in six (6) healthy young adults who received lorazepam injection and no other drugs revealed that visual tracking (the ability to keep a moving line centered) was impaired for a mean of eight (8) hours following administration of 4 mg of intramuscular lorazepam and four (4) hours following administration of 2 mg intramuscularly with considerable subject variation. Similar findings were noted with pentobarbital, 150 and 75 mg. Although this study showed that both lorazepam and pentobarbital interfered with eye-hand coordination, the data are insufficient to predict when it would be safe to operate a motor vehicle or engage in a hazardous occupation or sport.

PHARMACOKINETICS

Injectable Ativan (lorazepam) is readily absorbed when given intramuscularly. Peak plasma concentrations occur approximately 60 to 90 minutes following administration and appear to be dose-related, e.g., a 2.0 mg dose provides a level of approximately 20 ng/mL and a 4.0 mg dose approximately 40 ng/mL in plasma. The mean half-life of lorazepam is about 16 hours when given intravenously or intramuscularly. Ativan (lorazepam) is rapidly conjugated at the 3-hydroxyl group into its major metabolite, lorazepam glucuronide, which is then excreted in the urine. Lorazepam glucuronide has no demonstrable CNS activity in animals. When 5 mg of intravenous lorazepam was administered to volunteers once a day for four consecutive days, a steady state of free lorazepam was achieved by the second day (approximately 52 ng/mL of plasma three hours after the first dose and approximately 62 ng/mL three hours after each subsequent dose, one day apart). At clinically relevant concentrations, lorazepam is bound 85% to plasma proteins.

INDICATIONS AND USAGE

Ativan (lorazepam) Injection is indicated in adult patients for preanesthetic medication, producing sedation (sleepiness or drowsiness), relief of anxiety, and a decreased ability to recall events related to the day of surgery. It is most useful in those patients who are anxious about their surgical procedure and who would prefer to have diminished recall of the events of the day of surgery (see "Information for Patients").

CONTRAINDICATIONS

Ativan (lorazepam) Injection is contraindicated in patients with a known sensitivity to benzodiazepines or its vehicle (polyethylene glycol, propylene glycol, and benzyl alcohol) and in patients with acute narrow-angle glaucoma. The use of Ativan (lorazepam) Injection intra-arterially is contraindicated because, as with other injectable benzodiazepines, inadvertent intra-arterial injection may produce arteriospasm resulting in gangrene which may require amputation (see "Warnings").

WARNINGS

PRIOR TO INTRAVENOUS USE, ATIVAN INJECTION MUST BE DILUTED WITH AN EQUAL AMOUNT OF COMPATIBLE DILUENT (SEE "DOSAGE AND ADMINISTRATION"). INTRAVENOUS INJECTION SHOULD BE MADE SLOWLY AND WITH REPEATED ASPIRATION. CARE SHOULD BE TAKEN TO DETERMINE THAT ANY INJECTION WILL NOT BE INTRA-ARTERIAL AND THAT PERIVASCULAR EXTRAVASATION WILL NOT TAKE PLACE.

PARTIAL AIRWAY OBSTRUCTION MAY OCCUR IN HEAVILY SEDATED PATIENTS. INTRAVENOUS LORAZEPAM, WHEN GIVEN ALONE IN GREATER THAN THE RECOMMENDED DOSE, OR AT THE RECOMMENDED DOSE AND ACCOMPANIED BY OTHER DRUGS USED DURING THE ADMINISTRATION OF ANESTHESIA, MAY PRODUCE HEAVY SEDATION; THEREFORE, EQUIPMENT NECESSARY TO MAINTAIN A PATENT AIRWAY AND TO SUPPORT RESPIRATION/VENTILATION SHOULD BE AVAILABLE.

There is no evidence to support the use of lorazepam injection in coma, shock, or acute alcohol intoxication at this time. Since the liver is the most likely site of conjugation of lorazepam and since excretion of conjugated lorazepam (glucuronide) is a renal function, this drug is not recommended for use in patients with hepatic and/or renal *failure*. This does not preclude use of the drug in patients with mild-to-moderate hepatic or renal disease. When injectable lorazepam is selected for use in patients with mild-to-moderate hepatic or renal disease, the lowest effective dose should be considered since drug effect may be prolonged. Experience with other benzodiazepines and limited experience with parenteral lorazepam has demonstrated that tolerance to alcoholic beverages and other central-nervous-system depressants is diminished when used concomitantly.

As is true of similar CNS-acting drugs, patients receiving injectable lorazepam should not operate machinery or engage in hazardous occupations or drive a motor vehicle for a period of 24 to 48 hours. Impairment of performance may persist for greater intervals because of extremes of age, concomitant use of other drugs, stress of surgery, or the general condition of the patient.

Clinical trials have shown that patients over the age of 50 years may have a more profound and prolonged sedation with intravenous lorazepam. Ordinarily, an initial dose of 2 mg may be adequate unless a greater degree of lack of recall is desired.

As with all central-nervous-system depressant drugs, care should be exercised in patients given injectable lorazepam that premature ambulation may result in injury from falling.

There is no added beneficial effect to the addition of scopolamine to injectable lorazepam, and their combined effect may result in an increased incidence of sedation, hallucination, and irrational behavior.

PREGNANCY

ATIVAN (LORAZEPAM) MAY CAUSE FETAL DAMAGE WHEN ADMINISTERED TO PREGNANT WOMEN. An increased risk of congenital malformations associated with the use of minor tranquilizers (chlordiazepoxide, diazepam, and meprobamate) during the first trimester of pregnancy has been suggested in several studies. In humans, blood levels obtained from umbilical cord blood indicate placental transfer of lorazepam and lorazepam glucuronide.

Ativan Injection should not be used during pregnancy. There are insufficient data regarding obstetrical safety of parenteral lorazepam, including use in cesarean section. Such use, therefore, is not recommended.

Reproductive studies in animals were performed in mice, rats, and two strains of rabbits. Occasional anomalies (reduction of tarsals, tibia, metatarsals, malrotated limbs, gastroschisis, malformed skull, and microphthalmia) were seen in drug-treated rabbits without relationship to dosage. Although all of these anomalies were not present in the concurrent control group, they have been reported to occur randomly in historical controls. At doses of 40 mg/kg orally or 4 mg/kg intravenously and higher, there was evidence of fetal resorption and increased fetal loss in rabbits which was not seen at lower doses.

ENDOSCOPIC PROCEDURES

There are insufficient data to support the use of Ativan (lorazepam) Injection for outpatient endoscopic procedures. Inpatient endoscopic procedures require adequate recovery room observations.

Pharyngeal reflexes are not impaired when Ativan Injection is used for peroral endoscopic procedures; therefore, adequate topical or regional anesthesia is recommended to minimize reflex activity associated with such procedures.

PRECAUTIONS

GENERAL

The additive central-nervous-system effects of other drugs such as phenothiazines, narcotic analgesics, barbiturates, antidepressants, scopolamine, and monoamine-oxidase inhibitors should be borne in mind when these other drugs are used concomitantly with or during the period of recovery from Ativan (lorazepam) Injection. (See "Clinical Pharmacology" and "Warnings".)

Extreme care must be used in administering Ativan Injection to elderly patients, very ill patients, and to patients with limited pulmonary reserve because of the possibility that underventilation and/or hypoxic cardiac arrest may occur. Resuscitative equipment for ventilatory support should be readily available. (See "Warnings" and "Dosage and Administration".)

When lorazepam injection is used IV as the premedicant prior to regional or local anesthesia, the possibility of excessive sleepiness or drowsiness may interfere with patient cooperation to determine levels of anesthesia. This is most likely to occur when greater than 0.05 mg/kg is given and when narcotic analgesics are used concomitantly with the recommended dose. (See "Adverse Reactions".)

INFORMATION FOR PATIENTS

As appropriate, the patient should be informed of the pharmacological effects of the drug, such as sedation, relief of anxiety, and lack of recall, and the duration of these effects (about 8 hours), so that they may adequately perceive the risks as well as the benefits to be derived from its use.

Patients who receive Ativan Injection as a premedicant should be cautioned that driving an automobile or operating hazardous machinery, or engaging in a hazardous sport, should be delayed for 24 to 48 hours following the injection. Sedatives, tranquilizers, and narcotic analgesics may produce a more prolonged and profound effect when administered along with injectable Ativan. This effect may take the form of excessive sleepiness or drowsiness and, on rare occasions, interfere with recall and recognition of events of the day of surgery and the day after.

Getting out of bed unassisted may result in falling and injury if undertaken within 8 hours of receiving lorazepam injection. Alcoholic beverages should not be consumed for at least 24 to 48 hours after receiving lorazepam injectable due to the additive effects on central-nervous-system depression seen with benzodiazepines in general. Elderly patients should be told that Ativan (lorazepam) Injection may make them very sleepy for a period longer than six (6) to eight (8) hours following surgery.

LABORATORY TESTS

In clinical trials no laboratory test abnormalities were identified with either single or multiple doses of Ativan (lorazepam) Injection. These tests included: CBC, urinalysis, SGOT, SGPT, bilirubin, alkaline phosphatase, LDH, cholesterol, uric acid, BUN, glucose, calcium, phosphorus, and total proteins.

DRUG INTERACTIONS

Ativan (lorazepam) Injection, like other injectable benzodiazepines, produces depression of the central nervous system when administered with ethyl alcohol, phenothiazines, barbiturates, MAO inhibitors, and other antidepressants. When scopolamine is used concomitantly with injectable lorazepam, an increased incidence of sedation, hallucinations, and irrational behavior has been observed.

DRUG/LABORATORY TEST INTERACTIONS

No laboratory test abnormalities were identified when lorazepam was given alone or concomitantly with another drug, such as narcotic analgesics, inhalation anesthetics, scopolamine, atropine, and a variety of tranquilizing agents.

CARCINOGENESIS, MUTAGENESIS, IMPAIRMENT OF FERTILITY

No evidence of carcinogenic potential emerged in rats and mice during an 18-month study with oral lorazepam. No studies regarding mutagenesis have been performed. Preimplantation study in rats was performed with oral lorazepam at a 20 mg/kg dose and showed no impairment of fertility.

PREGNANCY

Pregnancy Category D; See "Warnings."

LABOR AND DELIVERY

There are insufficient data to support the use of Ativan (lorazepam) injection during labor and delivery, including cesarean section; therefore, its use in this situation is not recommended.

NURSING MOTHERS

Injectable lorazepam should not be administered to nursing mothers, because like other benzodiazepines, the possibility exists that lorazepam may be excreted in human milk and sedate the infant.

PEDIATRIC USE

There are insufficient data to support efficacy or make dosage recommendations for injectable lorazepam in patients less than 18 years of age; therefore, such use is not recommended.

ADVERSE REACTIONS

CENTRAL NERVOUS SYSTEM

The most frequent adverse effects seen with injectable lorazepam are an extension of the central-nervous-system depressant effects of the drug. The incidence varied from one study to another, depending on the dosage, route of administration, use of other central-nervous-system depressants, and the investigator's opinion concerning the degree and duration of desired sedation. Excessive sleepiness and drowsiness were the main side effects. This interfered with patient cooperation in approximately 6% (25/446) of patients undergoing regional anesthesia in that they were unable to assess levels of anesthesia in regional blocks or with caudal anesthesia. Patients over 50 years of age had a higher incidence of excessive sleepiness or drowsiness when compared with those under 50 (21/106 vs 24/245) when lorazepam was given intravenously (see "Dosage and Administration"). On rare occasion (3/1580) the patient was unable to give personal identification in the operating room on arrival, and one patient fell when attempting premature ambulation in the postoperative period.

Symptoms such as restlessness, confusion, depression, crying, sobbing, and delirium occurred in about 1.3% (20/1580). One patient injured himself by picking at his incision during the immediate postoperative period.

Hallucinations were present in about 1% (14/1580) of patients and were visual and self-limiting.

An occasional patient complained of dizziness, diplopia, and/or blurred vision. Depressed hearing was infrequently reported during the peak-effect period.

An occasional patient had a prolonged recovery room stay, either because of excessive sleepiness or because of some form of inappropriate behavior. The latter was seen most commonly when scopolamine was given concomitantly as a premedicant.

Limited information derived from patients who were discharged the day after receiving injectable lorazepam showed one patient complained of some unsteadiness of gait and a reduced ability to perform complex mental functions. Enhanced sensitivity to alcoholic beverages has been reported more than 24 hours after receiving injectable lorazepam, similar to experience with other benzodiazepines.

LOCAL EFFECTS

Intramuscular injection of lorazepam has resulted in pain at the injection site, a sensation of burning, or observed redness in the same area in a very variable incidence from one study to another. The overall incidence of pain and burning was about 17% (146/859) in the immediate postinjection period, and about 1.4% (12/859) at the 24-hour observation time. Reactions at the injection site (redness) occurred in approximately 2% (17/859) in the immediate postinjection period and were present 24 hours later in about 0.8% (7/859).

Intravenous administration of lorazepam resulted in painful responses in 13/771 patients or approximately 1.6% in the immediate postinjection period, and 24 hours later 4/771 patients or about 0.5% still complained of pain. Redness did not occur immediately following intravenous injection but was noted in 19/771 patients at the 24-hour observation period. This incidence is similar to that observed with an intravenous infusion before lorazepam is given.

CARDIOVASCULAR SYSTEM

Hypertension (0.1%) and hypotension (0.1%) have occasionally been observed after patients have received injectable lorazepam.

RESPIRATORY SYSTEM

Five patients (5/446) who underwent regional anesthesia were observed to have partial airway obstruction. This was believed due to excessive sleepiness at the time of the procedure and resulted in temporary underventilation. Immediate attention to the airway, employing the usual countermeasures, will usually suffice to manage this condition (see also "Clinical Pharmacology," "Warnings," and "Precautions").

OTHER ADVERSE EXPERIENCES

Skin rash, nausea, and vomiting have occasionally been noted in patients who have received injectable lorazepam combined with other drugs during anesthesia and surgery.

DRUG ABUSE AND DEPENDENCE

As with other benzodiazepines, Ativan (lorazepam) Injection has a low potential for abuse and may lead to limited dependence. Although there are no clinical data available for injectable lorazepam in this respect, physicians should be aware that repeated doses over a prolonged period of time may result in limited physical and psychological dependence.

OVERDOSAGE

Overdosage of benzodiazepines is usually manifested by varying degrees of central-nervous-system depression, ranging from drowsiness to coma. In mild cases symptoms include drowsiness, mental confusion, and lethargy. In more serious examples, symptoms may include ataxia, hypotonia, hypotension, hypnosis, stages one (1) to three (3) coma, and very rarely death.

Treatment of overdosage is mainly supportive until the drug is eliminated from the body. Vital signs and fluid balance should be carefully monitored. An adequate airway should be maintained and assisted respiration used as needed. With normally functioning kidneys, forced diuresis with intravenous fluids and electrolytes may accelerate elimination of benzodiazepines from the body. In addition, osmotic diuret-

Continued on next page

Wyeth-Ayerst—Cont.

ics, such as mannitol, may be effective as adjunctive measures. In more critical situations, renal dialysis and exchange blood transfusions may be indicated.

DOSAGE AND ADMINISTRATION

INTRAMUSCULAR INJECTION

For the designated indications as a premedicant, the usual recommended dose of lorazepam for intramuscular injection is 0.05 mg/kg up to a maximum of 4 mg. As with all premedicant drugs, the dose should be individualized. (See also "Clinical Pharmacology," "Warnings," "Precautions," and "Adverse Reactions.") Doses of other central-nervous-system depressant drugs should be ordinarily reduced. (See "Precautions.") *For optimum effect, measured as lack of recall, intramuscular lorazepam should be administered at least 2 hours before the anticipated operative procedure.* Narcotic analgesics should be administered at their usual preoperative time. There are insufficient data to support efficacy to make dosage recommendations for intramuscular lorazepam in patients less than 18 years of age; therefore, such use is not recommended.

INTRAVENOUS INJECTION

For the primary purpose of sedation and relief of anxiety, the usual recommended initial dose of lorazepam for intravenous injection is 2 mg total, or 0.02 mg/lb (0.044 mg/kg), whichever is smaller. This dose will suffice for sedating most adult patients, and should not ordinarily be exceeded in patients over 50 years of age. In those patients in whom a greater likelihood of lack of recall for perioperative events would be beneficial, larger doses as high as 0.05 mg/kg up to a total of 4 mg may be administered. (See "Clinical Pharmacology," "Warnings," "Precautions," and "Adverse Reactions.") Doses of other injectable central-nervous-system depressant drugs should ordinarily be reduced. (See "Precautions.") *For optimum effect, measured as lack of recall, intravenous lorazepam should be administered 15 to 20 minutes before the anticipated operative procedure.*

EQUIPMENT NECESSARY TO MAINTAIN A PATENT AIRWAY SHOULD BE IMMEDIATELY AVAILABLE PRIOR TO INTRAVENOUS ADMINISTRATION OF LORAZEPAM (see "Warnings").

There are insufficient data to support efficacy or make dosage recommendations for intravenous lorazepam in patients less than 18 years of age; therefore, such use is not recommended.

ADMINISTRATION

When given intramuscularly, Ativan Injection, undiluted, should be injected deep in the muscle mass.

Injectable Ativan (lorazepam) can be used with atropine sulfate, narcotic analgesics, other parenterally used analgesics, commonly used anesthetics, and muscle relaxants.

Immediately prior to intravenous use, Ativan (lorazepam) Injection must be diluted with an equal volume of compatible solution. When properly diluted the drug may be injected directly into a vein or into the tubing of an existing intravenous infusion. The rate of injection should not exceed 2.0 mg per minute.

Parenteral drug products should be inspected visually for particulate matter and discoloration prior to administration, whenever solution and container permit. Do not use if solution is discolored or contains a precipitate.

Ativan (lorazepam) Injection is compatible for dilution purposes with the following solutions: Sterile Water for Injection, USP; Sodium Chloride Injection, USP; 5% Dextrose Injection, USP.

HOW SUPPLIED

Ativan® (lorazepam) Injection, Wyeth®, is available in the following dosage strengths in TUBEX® Sterile Cartridge-Needle Units, 1 mL fill in 2 mL size (22 gauge × 1¼ inch needle), in cartons of 10 TUBEX:

2 mg per mL, NDC 0008-0581.
4 mg per mL, NDC 0008-0570.
For IM or IV injection.
Protect from light.
Keep in a refrigerator.

ALSO AVAILABLE

Ativam Injection is also available in the following dosage strengths in single-dose and multiple-dose vials:

2 mg per mL, NDC 0008-0581, 1 mL and 10 mL vials.
4 mg per mL, NDC 0008-0570, 1 mL and 10 mL vials.

DIRECTIONS FOR DILUTION FOR IV USE

To dilute, adhere to the following procedure:
For TUBEX—
1. Extrude the entire amount of air in the half-filled TUBEX.
2. Slowly aspirate the desired volume of diluent.
3. Pull back slightly on the plunger to provide additional mixing space.
4. Immediately mix contents thoroughly by gently inverting TUBEX repeatedly until a homogenous solution results.

Do not shake vigorously, as this will result in air entrapment.
For Vial—
Aspirate the desired amount of Ativan Injection into the syringe. Then proceed as described under TUBEX.

ATIVAN®   Ⓒ ℞
[at 'i-van]
(lorazepam)
Tablets

DESCRIPTION

Ativan (lorazepam), an antianxiety agent, has the chemical formula, 7-chloro-5-(o-chlorophenyl)-1,3-dihydro-3-hydroxy-2H-1,4-benzodiazepin-2-one.

It is a nearly white powder almost insoluble in water. Each Ativan (lorazepam) tablet, to be taken orally, contains 0.5 mg, 1 mg, or 2 mg of lorazepam. The inactive ingredients present are lactose and other ingredients.

CLINICAL PHARMACOLOGY

Studies in healthy volunteers show that in single high doses Ativan (lorazepam) has a tranquilizing action on the central nervous system with no appreciable effect on the respiratory or cardiovascular systems.

Ativan (lorazepam) is readily absorbed with an absolute bioavailability of 90 percent. Peak concentrations in plasma occur approximately 2 hours following administration. The peak plasma level of lorazepam from a 2 mg dose is approximately 20 mg/mL.

The mean half-life of unconjugated lorazepam in human plasma is about 12 hours and for its major metabolite, lorazepam glucuronide, about 18 hours. At clinically relevant concentrations, lorazepam is approximately 85% bound to plasma proteins. Ativan (lorazepam) is rapidly conjugated at its 3-hydroxy group into lorazepam glucuronide which is then excreted in the urine. Lorazepam glucuronide has no demonstrable CNS activity in animals.

The plasma levels of lorazepam are proportional to the dose given. There is no evidence of accumulation of lorazepam on administration up to six months.

Studies comparing young and elderly subjects have shown that the pharmacokinetics of lorazepam remain unaltered with advancing age.

INDICATIONS AND USAGE

Ativan (lorazepam) is indicated for the management of anxiety disorders or for the short-term relief of the symptoms of anxiety or anxiety associated with depressive symptoms. Anxiety or tension associated with the stress of everyday life usually does not require treatment with an anxiolytic.

The effectiveness of Ativan (lorazepam) in long-term use, that is, more than 4 months, has not been assessed by systematic clinical studies. The physician should periodically reassess the usefulness of the drug for the individual patient.

CONTRAINDICATIONS

Ativan (lorazepam) is contraindicated in patients with known sensitivity to the benzodiazepines or with acute narrow-angle glaucoma.

WARNINGS

Ativan (lorazepam) is not recommended for use in patients with a primary depressive disorder or psychosis. As with all patients on CNS-acting drugs, patients receiving lorazepam should be warned not to operate dangerous machinery or motor vehicles and that their tolerance for alcohol and other CNS depressants will be diminished.

PHYSICAL AND PSYCHOLOGICAL DEPENDENCE

Withdrawal symptoms, similar in character to those noted with barbiturates and alcohol (convulsions, tremor, abdominal and muscle cramps, vomiting, and sweating), have occurred following abrupt discontinuance of lorazepam. The more severe withdrawal symptoms have usually been limited to those patients who received excessive doses over an extended period of time. Generally milder withdrawal symptoms (e.g., dysphoria and insomnia) have been reported following abrupt discontinuance of benzodiazepines taken continuously at therapeutic levels for several months. Consequently, after extended therapy, abrupt discontinuation should generally be avoided and a gradual dosage-tapering schedule followed. Addiction-prone individuals (such as drug addicts or alcoholics) should be under careful surveillance when receiving lorazepam or other psychotropic agents because of the predisposition of such patients to habituation and dependence.

PRECAUTIONS

In patients with depression accompanying anxiety, a possibility for suicide should be borne in mind.

For elderly or debilitated patients, the initial daily dosage should not exceed 2 mg in order to avoid oversedation.

The usual precautions for treating patients with impaired renal or hepatic function should be observed.

In patients where gastrointestinal or cardiovascular disorders coexist with anxiety, it should be noted that lorazepam

---

has not been shown to be of significant benefit in treating the gastrointestinal or cardiovascular component.

Esophageal dilation occurred in rats treated with lorazepam for more than one year at 6 mg/kg/day. The no-effect dose was 1.25 mg/kg/day (approximately 6 times the maximum human therapeutic dose of 10 mg per day). The effect was reversible only when the treatment was withdrawn within two months of first observation of the phenomenon. The clinical significance of this is unknown. However, use of lorazepam for prolonged periods and in geriatric patients requires caution, and there should be frequent monitoring for symptoms of upper G.I. disease.

Safety and effectiveness of Ativan (lorazepam) in children of less than 12 years have not been established.

INFORMATION FOR PATIENTS

To assure the safe and effective use of Ativan (lorazepam), patients should be informed that, since benzodiazepines may produce psychological and physical dependence, it is advisable that they consult with their physician before either increasing the dose or abruptly discontinuing this drug.

ESSENTIAL LABORATORY TESTS: Some patients on Ativan (lorazepam) have developed leukopenia, and some have had elevations of LDH. As with other benzodiazepines, periodic blood counts and liver-function tests are recommended for patients on long-term therapy.

CLINICALLY SIGNIFICANT DRUG INTERACTIONS: The benzodiazepines, including Ativan (lorazepam), produce CNS depressant effects when administered with such medications as barbiturates or alcohol.

CARCINOGENESIS AND MUTAGENESIS: No evidence of carcinogenic potential emerged in rats during an 18-month study with Ativan (lorazepam). No studies regarding mutagenesis have been performed.

PREGNANCY: Reproductive studies in animals were performed in mice, rats, and two strains of rabbits. Occasional anomalies (reduction of tarsals, tibia, metatarsals, malrotated limbs, gastroschisis, malformed skull, and microphthalmia) were seen in drug-treated rabbits without relationship to dosage. Although all of these anomalies were not present in the concurrent control group, they have been reported to occur randomly in historical controls. At doses of 40 mg/kg and higher, there was evidence of fetal resorption and increased fetal loss in rabbits which was not seen at lower doses.

The clinical significance of the above findings is not known. However, an increased risk of congenital malformations associated with the use of minor tranquilizers (chlordiazepoxide, diazepam, and meprobamate) during the first trimester of pregnancy has been suggested in several studies. Because the use of these drugs is rarely a matter of urgency, the use of lorazepam during this period should almost always be avoided. The possibility that a woman of childbearing potential may be pregnant at the time of institution of therapy should be considered. Patients should be advised that if they become pregnant, they should communicate with their physician about the desirability of discontinuing the drug.

In humans, blood levels obtained from umbilical cord blood indicate placental transfer of lorazepam and lorazepam glucuronide.

NURSING MOTHERS: It is not known whether oral lorazepam is excreted in human milk like the other benzodiazepine tranquilizers. As a general rule, nursing should not be undertaken while a patient is on a drug, since many drugs are excreted in human milk.

ADVERSE REACTIONS

Adverse reactions, if they occur, are usually observed at the beginning of therapy and generally disappear on continued medication or upon decreasing the dose. In a sample of about 3,500 anxious patients, the most frequent adverse reaction to Ativan (lorazepam) is sedation (15.9%), followed by dizziness (6.9%), weakness (4.2%), and unsteadiness (3.4%). Less frequent adverse reactions are disorientation, depression, nausea, change in appetite, headache, sleep disturbance, agitation, dermatological symptoms, eye function disturbance, together with various gastrointestinal symptoms and autonomic manifestations. The incidence of sedation and unsteadiness increased with age.

Small decreases in blood pressure have been noted but are not clinically significant, probably being related to the relief of anxiety produced by Ativan (lorazepam).

Transient amnesia or memory impairment has been reported in association with the use of benzodiazepines.

OVERDOSAGE

In the management of overdosage with any drug, it should be borne in mind that multiple agents may have been taken. Manifestations of Ativan (lorazepam) overdosage include somnolence, confusion, and coma. Induced vomiting and/or gastric lavage should be undertaken, followed by general supportive care, monitoring of vital signs, and close observation of the patient. Hypotension, though unlikely, usually may be controlled with Levarterenol Bitartrate Injection, USP. The usefulness of dialysis has not been determined.

DOSAGE AND ADMINISTRATION

Ativan (lorazepam) is administered orally. For optimal results, dose, frequency of administration, and duration of therapy should be individualized according to patient response. To facilitate this, 0.5 mg, 1 mg, and 2 mg tablets are available.

The usual range is 2 to 6 mg/day given in divided doses, the largest dose being taken before bedtime, but the daily dosage may vary from 1 to 10 mg/day.

For anxiety, most patients require an initial dose of 2 to 3 mg/day given b.i.d. or t.i.d.

For insomnia due to anxiety or transient situational stress, a single daily dose of 2 to 4 mg may be given, usually at bedtime.

For elderly or debilitated patients, an initial dosage of 1 to 2 mg/day in divided doses is recommended, to be adjusted as needed and tolerated.

The dosage of Ativan (lorazepam) should be increased gradually when needed to help avoid adverse effects. When higher dosage is indicated, the evening dose should be increased before the daytime doses.

HOW SUPPLIED

Ativan® (lorazepam) Tablets, Wyeth®, are available in the following dosage strengths:

0.5 mg, NDC 0008-0081, white, five-sided tablet with a raised "A" on one side and "WYETH" and "81" on reverse side, in bottles of 100 and 500 tablets, in Redipak® cartons of 250 tablets (10 blister folders of 25), and in Redipak cartons of 100 tablets (10 blister strips of 10).

1 mg, NDC 0008-0064, white, five-sided tablet with a raised "A" on one side and "WYETH" and "64" on scored reverse side, in bottles of 100, 500, and 1000 tablets, in Redipak® cartons of 250 tablets (10 blister folders of 25), and in Redipak cartons of 100 tablets (10 blister strips of 10).

2 mg, NDC 0008-0065, white, five-sided tablet with a raised "A" on one side and "WYETH" and "65" on scored reverse side, in bottles of 100, 500, and 1000 tablets, in Redipak® cartons of 250 tablets (10 blister folders of 25), and in Redipak cartons of 100 tablets (10 blister strips of 10).

Store at controlled room temperature.

Keep bottles tightly closed.

Dispense in tight container.

The appearance of ATIVAN tablets is a registered trademark of Wyeth-Ayerst Laboratories.

Shown in Product Identification Section, page 436

ATROMID–S®

℞

[ă'trō-mid]

Brand of clofibrate capsules

Antilipidemic agent for reduction of elevated serum lipids

CAUTION: Federal law prohibits dispensing without prescription.

DESCRIPTION

ATROMID-S Capsules (clofibrate capsules) is ethyl 2-(p-chlorophenoxy)-2-methyl-propionate, an antilipidemic agent.

structural formula

Its molecular formula is $C_{12}H_{15}O_3Cl$, molecular weight 242.7, and boiling point 148°–150°C at 25 mm Hg. It is a stable, colorless to pale yellow liquid with a faint odor and characteristic taste, soluble in common solvents but not in water. Each ATROMID-S Capsule contains 500 mg clofibrate for oral administration.

ATROMID-S Capsules contain the following inactive ingredients: D&C Red No. 28, D&C Red No. 30, D&C Yellow No. 10, FD&C Blue No. 1, FD&C Red No. 3, FD&C Yellow No. 6, gelatin.

CLINICAL PHARMACOLOGY

ATROMID-S is an antilipidemic agent. It acts to lower elevated serum lipids by reducing the very low density lipoprotein fraction ($S_f20-400$) rich in triglycerides. Serum cholesterol may be decreased, particularly in those patients whose cholesterol elevation is due to the presence of IDL as a result of Type III hyperlipoproteinemia.

The mechanism of action has not been established definitively. Clofibrate may inhibit the hepatic release of lipoproteins (particularly VLDL), potentiate the action of lipoprotein lipase, and increase the fecal excretion of neutral sterols.

Between 95% and 99% of an oral dose of clofibrate is excreted in the urine as free and conjugated clofibric acid, thus the absorption of clofibrate is virtually complete. The half-life of clofibric acid in normal volunteers averages 18 to 22 hours (range 14 to 35 hours) but can vary by up to 7 hours in the same subject at different times. Clofibric acid is highly protein-bound (95% to 97%). In subjects undergoing continuous clofibrate treatment, 1 g q12h, plasma concentrations of clofibric acid range from 120 to 125 mcg/mL to an approximate peak of 200 mcg/mL.

Several investigators have observed in their studies that clofibrate may produce a decrease in cholesterol linoleate but an increase in palmitoleate and oleate, the latter being considered atherogenic in experimental animals. The significance of this finding is unknown at this time.

Reduction of triglycerides in some patients treated with clofibrate or certain of its clinically similar analogs may be associated with an increase in LDL cholesterol. Increase in LDL cholesterol has been observed in patients whose cholesterol is initially normal.

Animal studies suggest that clofibrate interrupts cholesterol biosynthesis prior to mevalonate formation.

INDICATIONS AND USAGE

The initial treatment of choice for hyperlipidemia is dietary therapy specific for the type of hyperlipidemia.[1] Excess body weight and alcoholic intake may be important factors in hypertriglyceridemia and should be addressed prior to any drug therapy. Physical exercise can be an important ancillary measure. Contributory diseases such as hypothyroidism or diabetes mellitus should be looked for and adequately treated. The use of drugs should be considered only when reasonable attempts have been made to obtain satisfactory results with non-drug methods. If the decision ultimately is to use drugs, the patient should be instructed that this does not reduce the importance of adhering to diet. Because ATROMID-S is associated with certain serious adverse findings reported in two large clinical trials (see WARNINGS), agents other than clofibrate may be more suitable for a particular patient.

ATROMID-S is indicated for Primary Dysbetalipoproteinemia (Type III hyperlipidemia) that does not respond adequately to diet.

ATROMID-S may be considered for the treatment of adult patients with very high serum triglyceride levels (Types IV and V hyperlipidemia) who present a risk of abdominal pain and pancreatitis and who do not respond adequately to a determined dietary effort to control them. Patients with triglyceride levels less than 750 mg per deciliter are not likely to present such risk.

ATROMID-S is not useful for the hypertriglyceridemia of Type I hyperlipidemia.

ATROMID-S has not been shown to be effective for prevention of coronary heart disease.

The biochemical response to ATROMID-S is variable, and it is not always possible to predict from the lipoprotein type or other factors which patients will obtain favorable results. LDL cholesterol, as well as triglycerides, should be rechecked during the first several months of therapy in order to detect rises in LDL cholesterol that often accompany fibric-acid-type drug-induced reductions in elevated triglycerides. It is essential that lipid levels be reassessed periodically and that the drug be discontinued in any patient in whom lipids do not show significant improvement.

CONTRAINDICATIONS

It is contraindicated in patients with clinically significant hepatic or renal dysfunction. Rhabdomyolysis and severe hyperkalemia have been reported in association with pre-existing renal insufficiency.

It is contraindicated in patients with primary biliary cirrhosis since it may raise the already elevated cholesterol in these cases.

It is contraindicated in patients with a known hypersensitivity to clofibrate.

It is contraindicated in nursing women (see PRECAUTIONS).

WARNINGS

In a large prospective study involving 5,000 patients in a clofibrate-treated group and 5,000 in a placebo-treated group followed for an average of five years on drug or placebo and one year beyond (the WHO study), there was a statistically significant 36% higher mortality due to noncardiovascular causes in the clofibrate-treated group than in a comparable placebo group. Half of this difference was due to malignancy; other causes of death included postcholecystectomy complications and pancreatitis.[2] In another prospective study involving 1,000 clofibrate- and 3,000 placebo-treated patients followed for an average of six years on drug or placebo (the Coronary Drug Project study), the noncardiovascular mortality rate, including that of malignancy, was not significantly different in the clofibrate- and placebo-treated groups.[3] This should not be interpreted to mean that clofibrate is not associated with an increased risk of noncardiovascular death, because the patients in the Coronary Drug Project were much older than those in the WHO study and they all had had a previous myocardial infarction, so that the deaths in the Coronary Drug Project were overwhelmingly due to cardiovascular causes, and it would have been very difficult to discern a clofibrate-associated risk of death due to noncardiovascular causes if it existed. Both studies demonstrated that clofibrate users have twice the risk of developing cholelithiasis and cholecystitis requiring surgery as do nonusers.

A potential benefit of clofibrate was, however, reported in the WHO study which involved patients with hypercholesterolemia and no history of myocardial infarction or angina pectoris. In this study, there was a statistically significant 25% decrease in subsequent nonfatal myocardial infarctions in the clofibrate-treated group when compared with the placebo group. There was no difference in incidence of fatal myocardial infarction in the two groups. If the study had been continued longer, had included diet, had been restricted to patients who had both hyperlipidemia and increased risk factors *and* who obtained significant clofibrate-induced reduction in serum lipids, it is possible that it may have shown a decrease in fatal myocardial infarctions. In the Coronary Drug Project study, which involved patients with or without hypercholesterolemia and/or hypertriglyceridemia and with a history of previous myocardial infarction, there was no significant difference in incidence of either nonfatal or fatal myocardial infarction between the clofibrate- and placebo-treated groups.[2]

As a result of these and other studies, the following can be stated:

1. Clofibrate, in general, causes a relatively modest reduction of serum cholesterol and a somewhat greater reduction of serum triglycerides. In Type III hyperlipidemia, however, substantial reductions of both cholesterol and triglycerides can occur with clofibrate use.

2. No study to date has shown a convincing reduction in incidence of *fatal* myocardial infarction.

3. A significantly increased incidence of cholelithiasis has been demonstrated consistently in clofibrate-treated groups, and an increase in morbidity from this complication and mortality from cholecystectomy must be anticipated during clofibrate treatment.

4. Several types of other undesirable events have been associated in a statistically significant way with clofibrate administration in the WHO or the Coronary Drug Project studies. There was an increase in incidence of noncardiovascular deaths reported in the WHO study. There was an increase in cardiac arrhythmias, intermittent claudication, and definite or suspected thromboembolic events, and angina reported in the Coronary Drug Project, which was not, however, reported in the WHO study.

5. Administration of clofibrate to mice and rats in long-term studies at eight times the human dose, and to rats at five times the human dose, resulted in a higher incidence of benign and malignant liver tumors than in controls. Lower doses were not included in these studies.

6. Administration of clofibrate to male monkeys at dosages of 2 to 6 times the human dose resulted in increases in mortality of 2- to 5-fold. As in the case of men in the WHO study, no specific cause of death was identified.

BECAUSE OF THE HEPATIC TUMORIGENICITY OF CLOFIBRATE IN RODENTS AND THE POSSIBLE INCREASED RISK OF MALIGNANCY ASSOCIATED WITH CLOFIBRATE IN THE HUMAN, AS WELL AS THE INCREASED RISK OF CHOLELITHIASIS, AND BECAUSE THERE IS NOT, TO DATE, SUBSTANTIAL EVIDENCE OF A BENEFICIAL EFFECT ON CARDIOVASCULAR MORTALITY FROM CLOFIBRATE, THIS DRUG SHOULD BE UTILIZED ONLY FOR THOSE PATIENTS DESCRIBED IN THE INDICATIONS SECTION, AND SHOULD BE DISCONTINUED IF SIGNIFICANT LIPID RESPONSE IS NOT OBTAINED.

Concomitant Anticoagulants

CAUTION SHOULD BE EXERCISED WHEN ANTICOAGULANTS ARE GIVEN IN CONJUNCTION WITH ATROMID-S. THE DOSAGE OF THE ANTICOAGULANT SHOULD BE REDUCED USUALLY BY ONE-HALF (DEPENDING ON THE INDIVIDUAL CASE) TO MAINTAIN THE PROTHROMBIN TIME AT THE DESIRED LEVEL TO PREVENT BLEEDING COMPLICATIONS. FREQUENT PROTHROMBIN DETERMINATIONS ARE ADVISABLE UNTIL IT HAS BEEN DEFINITELY DETERMINED THAT THE PROTHROMBIN LEVEL HAS BEEN STABILIZED.

Skeletal muscle:

Myalgia, myositis, and rhabdomyolysis with or without elevation of CPK have been associated with ATROMID-S therapy. Consideration should be given to withholding or discon-

Continued on next page

Wyeth-Ayerst—Cont.

tinuing drug therapy in any patient with a risk factor predisposing to the development of renal failure secondary to rhabdomyolysis, including: severe acute infection, hypotension, major surgery, trauma, severe metabolic, endocrine or electrolyte disorders and uncontrolled seizures.

ATROMID-S therapy should be discontinued if markedly elevated CPK levels occur or myositis is diagnosed.

Avoidance of Pregnancy

Strict birth control procedures must be exercised by women of childbearing potential. In patients who plan to become pregnant, clofibrate should be withdrawn several months before conception. Because of the possibility of pregnancy occurring despite birth control precautions in patients taking clofibrate, the possible benefits of the drug to the patient must be weighed against possible hazards to the fetus. (See Pregnancy section.)

PRECAUTIONS

General:

Before instituting therapy with clofibrate, attempts should be made to control serum lipids with appropriate dietary regimens, weight loss in obese patients, control of diabetes mellitus, etc.

Because of the long-term administration of a drug of this nature, adequate baseline studies should be performed to determine that the patient has significantly elevated serum lipid levels. Frequent determinations of serum lipids should be obtained during the first few months of ATROMID-S administration, and periodic determinations thereafter. The drug should be withdrawn after three months if response is inadequate. However, in the case of xanthoma tuberosum, the drug should be employed for longer periods (even up to one year) provided that there is a reduction in the size and/or number of the xanthomata.

Since cholelithiasis is a possible side effect of clofibrate therapy, appropriate diagnostic procedures should be performed if signs and symptoms related to disease of the biliary system should occur.

Clofibrate may produce "flu like" symptoms (muscular aching, soreness, cramping) associated with increased creatine kinase levels. The physician should differentiate this from actual viral and/or bacterial disease.

Use with caution in patients with peptic ulcer since reactivation has been reported. Whether this is drug-related is unknown.

Laboratory Tests:

Subsequent serum lipid determinations should be done to detect a paradoxical rise in serum cholesterol or triglyceride levels. Clofibrate will not alter the seasonal variations of serum cholesterol: peak elevations in midwinter and late summer and decreases in fall and spring. If the drug is discontinued, the patient should be continued on an appropriate hypolipidemic diet, and his serum lipids should be monitored until stabilized, as a rise in these values to or above the original baseline may occur.

During clofibrate therapy, frequent serum transaminase determinations and other liver function tests should be performed since the drug may produce abnormalities in these parameters. These effects are usually reversible when the drug is discontinued. Hepatic biopsies are usually within normal limits. If the hepatic function tests steadily rise or show excessive abnormalities, the drug should be withdrawn. Therefore, use with caution in those patients with a past history of jaundice or hepatic disease.

Complete blood counts should be done periodically since anemia, and more frequently, leukopenia have been reported in patients who have been taking clofibrate.

Drug Interactions:

Caution should be exercised when anticoagulants are given in conjunction with ATROMID-S. Usually, the dosage of the anticoagulant should be reduced by one-half (depending on the individual case) to maintain the prothrombin time at the desired level to prevent bleeding complications. Frequent prothrombin determinations are advisable until it has been determined definitely that the prothrombin level has been stabilized.

ATROMID-S may displace acidic drugs such as phenytoin or tolbutamide from their binding sites. Caution should be exercised when treating patients with either of these drugs or other highly protein-bound drugs and ATROMID-S. The hypoglycemic effect of tolbutamide has been reported to increase when ATROMID-S is given concurrently.

Carcinogenesis, Mutagenesis, Impairment of Fertility:

See WARNINGS section for information on carcinogenesis and mutagenesis.

Arrest of spermatogenesis has been seen in both dogs and monkeys at doses approximately 4 to 6 times the human therapeutic dose.

Pregnancy:

Teratogenic effects

Pregnancy Category C. Animal reproduction studies have not been conducted with ATROMID-S. It is also not known whether ATROMID-S can cause fetal harm when adminis-

tered to a pregnant woman or can affect reproductive capacity. However, animal reproduction studies with clofibrate plus androsterone showed increases in neonatal deaths and pup mortality during lactation.

Nursing Mothers:

ATROMID-S is contraindicated in lactating women since an active metabolite (CPIB) has been measured in breast milk.

Pediatric Use:

Safety and efficacy in children have not been established.

ADVERSE REACTIONS

The most common is nausea. Less frequently encountered gastrointestinal reactions are vomiting, loose stools, dyspepsia, flatulence, and abdominal distress. Reactions reported less often than gastrointestinal ones are headache, dizziness, and fatigue; muscle cramping, aching, and weakness; skin rash, urticaria, and pruritus; dry brittle hair, and alopecia. The following reported adverse reactions are listed alphabetically by systems:

Cardiovascular
  Increased or decreased angina
  Cardiac arrhythmias
  Both swelling and phlebitis at site of xanthomas
Dermatologic
  Allergic reactions including urticaria
  Skin rash
  Pruritus
  Dry skin and dry, brittle hair
  Alopecia
Gastrointestinal
  Gallstones
  Nausea
  Vomiting
  Diarrhea
  Gastrointestinal upset (bloating, flatulence, abdominal distress)
  Hepatomegaly (not associated with hepatotoxicity)
  Stomatitis and gastritis
Genitourinary
  Findings consistent with renal dysfunction as evidenced by dysuria, hematuria, proteinuria, decreased urine output. One patient's renal biopsy suggested "allergic reaction."
  Impotence and decreased libido
Hematologic
  Leukopenia
  Potentiation of anticoagulant effect
  Anemia
  Eosinophilia
  Agranulocytosis
Musculoskeletal
  Myalgia (muscle cramping, aching, weakness)
  "Flu-like" symptoms
  Myositis
  Rhabdomyolysis in the setting of pre-existing renal insufficiency
  Arthralgia
Neurologic
  Fatigue, weakness, drowsiness
  Dizziness
  Headache
Miscellaneous
  Weight gain
  Polyphagia
Laboratory Findings
  Abnormal liver function tests as evidenced by increased transaminase (SGOT and SGPT), BSP retention, and increased thymol turbidity
  Proteinuria
  Increased creatine phosphokinase
  Hyperkalemia in association with renal insufficiency and regular ambulatory peritoneal dialysis treatment

Reported adverse reactions whose direct relationship with the drug has not been established: peptic ulcer, gastrointestinal hemorrhage, rheumatoid arthritis, tremors, increased perspiration, systemic lupus erythematosus, blurred vision, gynecomastia, thrombocytopenic purpura.

OVERDOSAGE

While there has been no reported case of overdosage, should it occur, symptomatic supportive measures should be taken.

DOSAGE AND ADMINISTRATION

Initial: The recommended dosage for adults is 2 g daily in divided doses. Some patients may respond to a lower dosage.

Maintenance: Same as for initial dosage.

HOW SUPPLIED

ATROMID-S CAPSULES (clofibrate capsules)—Each orange, oblong, soft gelatin capsule contains 500 mg clofibrate, in bottles of 100 (NDC 0046-0243-81).

The appearance of these orange oblong soft gelatin capsules is a trademark of Ayerst Laboratories.

Store at room temperature (approximately 25° C). Avoid freezing and excessive heat.

REFERENCES

1. Coronary Risk Handbook (1973), American Heart Association.
2. Report from the Committee of Principal Investigators: A cooperative trial in the primary prevention of ischaemic heart disease using clofibrate, *Br Heart J* 40:1069, 1978.
3. The Coronary Drug Project Research Group: Clofibrate and niacin in coronary heart disease, *JAMA* 231:360, 1975.
Shown in Product Identification Section, page 436

AURALGAN®   ℞
[aw-răl´gan]
Otic Solution

CAUTION: Federal law prohibits dispensing without prescription.

DESCRIPTION

Each mL contains:

Antipyrine ....54.0 mg
Benzocaine ....14.0 mg
Glycerin dehydrated q.s. to ....1.0 mL
(contains not more than 0.6% moisture)
(also contains oxyquinoline sulfate)

TOPICAL DECONGESTANT AND ANALGESIC

AURALGAN is an otic solution containing antipyrine, benzocaine, and dehydrated glycerin. The solution congeals at 0° C (32° F), but returns to normal consistency, unchanged, at room temperature.

The structures of the components are:

antipyrine   benzocaine   glycerin

CLINICAL PHARMACOLOGY

AURALGAN combines the hygroscopic property of dehydrated glycerin with the analgesic action of antipyrine and benzocaine to relieve pressure, reduce inflammation and congestion, and alleviate pain and discomfort in acute otitis media.

AURALGAN does not blanch the tympanic membrane or mask the landmarks and, therefore, does not distort the otoscopic picture.

INDICATIONS AND USAGE

Acute otitis media of various etiologies
  — prompt relief of pain and reduction of inflammation in the congestive and serous stages
  — adjuvant therapy during systemic antibiotic administration for resolution of the infection

Because of the close anatomical relationship of the eustachian tube to the nasal cavity, otitis media is a frequent problem, especially in children in whom the tube is shorter, wider, and more horizontal than in adults.

Removal of cerumen
—facilitates the removal of excessive or impacted cerumen

CONTRAINDICATIONS

Hypersensitivity to any of the components or substances related to them.

Perforated tympanic membrane is considered a contraindication to the use of any medication in the external ear canal.

WARNINGS

Discontinue promptly if sensitization or irritation occurs.

PRECAUTIONS

Carcinogenesis, Mutagenesis, Impairment of Fertility:

No long-term studies in animals or humans have been conducted.

Pregnancy Category C: Animal reproduction studies have not been conducted with AURALGAN. It is also not known whether AURALGAN can cause fetal harm when administered to a pregnant woman, or can affect reproduction capacity. AURALGAN should be given to a pregnant woman only if clearly needed.

Nursing Mothers: It is not known whether this drug is excreted in human milk. Because many drugs are excreted in human milk, caution should be exercised when AURALGAN is administered to a nursing woman.

DOSAGE AND ADMINISTRATION

Acute otitis media: Instill AURALGAN permitting the solution to run along the wall of the canal until it is filled. Avoid touching the ear with dropper. Then moisten a cotton pledget with AURALGAN and insert into meatus. Repeat every one to two hours until pain and congestion are relieved.

Removal of cerumen

Before: Instill AURALGAN three times daily for two or three days to help detach cerumen from wall of canal and facilitate removal.

After: AURALGAN is useful for drying out the canal or relieving discomfort.

Before and after removal of cerumen, a cotton pledget moistened with AURALGAN should be inserted into the meatus following instillation.

NOTE: Do not rinse dropper after use. Replace dropper in bottle after each use. Hold dropper assembly by screw cap and, without compressing the rubber bulb, insert into drug container and screw down tightly.

Protect the solution from light and heat, and do not use it it is brown or contains a precipitate.

DISCARD THIS PRODUCT SIX MONTHS AFTER DROPPER IS FIRST PLACED IN THE DRUG SOLUTION.

HOW SUPPLIED

AURALGAN® Otic Solution, in package containing 10 mL bottle with separate dropper-screw cap attachment (NDC 0046-1000-10).

Store at room temperature (approximately 25° C).

AYGESTIN®   ℞

[ā-jĕs'tin]

Brand of norethindrone acetate tablets, USP

CAUTION: Federal law prohibits dispensing without prescription.

WARNING:

THE USE OF PROGESTATIONAL AGENTS DURING THE FIRST FOUR MONTHS OF PREGNANCY IS NOT RECOMMENDED.

Progestational agents have been used beginning with the first trimester of pregnancy in an attempt to prevent habitual abortion or treat threatened abortion. There is no adequate evidence that such use is effective and there is evidence of potential harm to the fetus when such drugs are given during the first four months of pregnancy. Furthermore, in the vast majority of women, the cause of abortion is a defective ovum, which progestational agents could not be expected to influence. In addition, the use of progestational agents with their uterine-relaxant properties, in patients with fertilized defective ova may cause a delay in spontaneous abortion. Therefore, the use of such drugs during the first four months of pregnancy is not recommended. Several reports suggest an association between intrauterine exposure to female sex hormones and congenital anomalies, including congenital heart defects and limb reduction defects.[1-5] One study[4] estimated a 4.7-fold increased risk of limb reduction defects in infants exposed in utero to sex hormones (oral contraceptives, hormone withdrawal tests for pregnancy, or attempted treatment for threatened abortion). Some of these exposures were very short and involved only a few days of treatment. The data suggest that the risk of limb reduction defects in exposed fetuses is somewhat less than 1 in 1,000 if the patient is exposed to AYGESTIN® (norethindrone acetate tablets, USP) during the first four months of pregnancy or if she becomes pregnant while taking this drug, she should be apprised of the potential risks to the fetus.

DESCRIPTION

AYGESTIN®

(norethindrone acetate tablets, USP)—

5 mg oral tablets.

AYGESTIN (17-hydroxy-19-nor-17α-pregn-4-en- 20-yn-3-one acetate), a synthetic, orally active progestin, is the acetic acid ester of norethindrone. It is a white, or creamy white, crystalline powder.

AYGESTIN Tablets contain the following inactive ingredients: lactose, magnesium stearate, and microcrystalline cellulose.

CLINICAL PHARMACOLOGY

Norethindrone acetate induces secretory changes in an estrogen-primed endometrium. It acts to inhibit the secretion of pituitary gonadotropins which, in turn, prevent follicular maturation and ovulation. On a weight basis it is twice as potent as norethindrone.

INDICATIONS AND USAGE

AYGESTIN is indicated for the treatment of secondary amenorrhea, endometriosis, and abnormal uterine bleeding due to hormonal imbalance in the absence of organic pathology such as submucous fibroids or uterine cancer.

CONTRAINDICATIONS

Thrombophlebitis, thromboembolic disorders, cerebral apoplexy, or a past history of these conditions

Markedly impaired liver function or liver disease

Known or suspected carcinoma of the breast

Undiagnosed vaginal bleeding

Missed abortion

As a diagnostic test for pregnancy

WARNINGS

1. Discontinue medication pending examination if there is a sudden partial or complete loss of vision, or if there is sudden onset of proptosis, diplopia, or migraine. If examination reveals papilledema or retinal vascular lesions, medication should be withdrawn.

2. Because of the occasional occurrence of thrombophlebitis and pulmonary embolism in patients taking progestogens, the physician should be alert to the earliest manifestations of the disease.

3. Masculinization of the female fetus has occurred when progestogens have been used in pregnant women.

PRECAUTIONS

A. General Precautions.

1. The pretreatment physical examination should include special reference to breasts and pelvic organs, as well as a Papanicolaou smear.

2. Because this drug may cause some degree of fluid retention, conditions which might be influenced by this factor, such as epilepsy, migraine, asthma, cardiac or renal dysfunctions, require careful observation.

3. In cases of breakthrough bleeding, as in all cases of irregular bleeding per vaginam, nonfunctional causes should be borne in mind. In cases of undiagnosed vaginal bleeding, adequate diagnostic measures are indicated.

4. Patients who have a history of psychic depression should be carefully observed and the drug discontinued if the depression recurs to a serious degree.

5. Any possible influence of prolonged progestogen therapy on pituitary, ovarian, adrenal, hepatic, or uterine functions awaits further study.

6. **Concomitant Use in Estrogen Replacement Therapy:** In postmenopausal estrogen replacement therapy, studies of the addition of a progestin for 7 or more days of a cycle of estrogen administration have reported a lowered incidence of endometrial hyperplasia. Morphological and biochemical studies of the endometrium suggest that 10 to 13 days of progestin are needed to provide maximal maturation of the endometrium and to eliminate any hyperplastic changes. Whether this will provide protection from endometrial carcinoma has not been clearly established. There are possible additional risks which may be associated with the inclusion of progestin in estrogen replacement regimens. Progestin therapy may have an adverse effect on lipid metabolism.

7. A decrease in glucose tolerance has been observed in a small percentage of patients on estrogen-progestogen combination drugs. The mechanism of this decrease is obscure. For this reason, diabetic patients should be carefully observed while receiving progestogen therapy.

8. The age of the patient constitutes no absolute limiting factor, although treatment with progestogens may mask the onset of the climacteric.

9. The pathologist should be advised of progestogen therapy when relevant specimens are submitted.

B. Information for the Patient. See text which appears after REFERENCES.

C. Carcinogenesis. Mutagenesis, and Impairment of Fertility. Some beagle dogs treated with medroxyprogesterone acetate developed mammary nodules. Although nodules occasionally appeared in control animals, they were intermittent in nature, whereas nodules in treated animals were larger and more numerous, and persisted. There is no general agreement as to whether the nodules are benign or malignant. Their significance with respect to humans has not been established.

D. Pregnancy Category X. See Boxed Warning.

E. Nursing Mothers. Detectable amounts of progestogens have been identified in the milk of mothers receiving them. The effect of this on the nursing infant has not been determined.

F. Pediatric Use. Safety and effectiveness in children have not been established.

ADVERSE REACTIONS

The following adverse reactions have been observed in women taking progestins:

breakthrough bleeding

spotting

change in menstrual flow

amenorrhea

edema

changes in weight (decreases, increases)

changes in cervical erosion and cervical secretions

cholestatic jaundice

rash (allergic) with and without pruritus

melasma or chloasma

mental depression

Progestins may alter the result of pregnanediol determinations. The following laboratory results may be altered by the concomitant use of estrogens with progestins:

hepatic function

coagulation tests—increase in prothrombin, factors VII, VIII, IX, and X

increase in PBI, BEI, and a decrease in T^3 uptake

metyrapone test

A statistically significant association has been demonstrated between use of estrogen-progestogen combination drugs and the following serious adverse reactions: thrombophlebitis, pulmonary embolism, and cerebral thrombosis and embolism. For this reason, patients on progestogen therapy should be carefully observed. Although available evidence is suggestive of an association, such a relationship has been neither confirmed nor refuted for the following serious adverse reactions:

Neuro-ocular lesions, eg, retinal thrombosis and optic neuritis.

The following adverse reactions have been observed in patients receiving estrogen-progestogen combination drugs.

1. Rise in blood pressure in susceptible individuals
2. Premenstrual-like syndrome
3. Changes in libido
4. Changes in appetite
5. Cystitis-like syndrome
6. Headache
7. Nervousness
8. Dizziness
9. Fatigue
10. Backache
11. Hirsutism
12. Loss of scalp hair
13. Erythema multiforme
14. Erythema nodosum
15. Hemorrhagic eruption
16. Itching

In view of these observations, patients on progestogen therapy should be carefully observed.

DOSAGE AND ADMINISTRATION

Therapy with AYGESTIN® must be adapted to the specific indications and therapeutic response of the individual patient. This dosage schedule assumes the interval between menses to be 28 days.

Secondary amenorrhea, abnormal uterine bleeding due to hormonal imbalance in the absence of organic pathology: 2.5 to 10 mg AYGESTIN may be given daily for from 5 to 10 days during the second half of the theoretical menstrual cycle to produce an optimum secretory transformation of an endometrium that has been adequately primed with either endogenous or exogenous estrogen.

Progestin withdrawal bleeding usually occurs within three to seven days after discontinuing AYGESTIN therapy. Patients with a past history of recurrent episodes of abnormal uterine bleeding may benefit from planned menstrual cycling with AYGESTIN.

Endometriosis:

Initial daily dosage of 5 mg AYGESTIN for two weeks. Dosage should be increased by 2.5 mg per day every two weeks until 15 mg per day of AYGESTIN is reached. Therapy may be held at this level for six to nine months or until annoying breakthrough bleeding demands temporary termination.

HOW SUPPLIED

Each scored AYGESTIN tablet contains 5 mg norethindrone acetate, USP, in bottles of 50 (NDC 0046-0894-50). Also in Cycle Packs of 10 (0046-0894-10).

PHYSICIAN REFERENCES

1. Gal I, Kirman B, Stern J: Hormonal pregnancy tests and congenital malformation. *Nature* 216 :83, 1967.
2. Levy EP, Cohen A, Fraser FC: Hormone treatment during pregnancy and congenital heart defects. *Lancet* 1 :611, 1973.
3. Nora JJ, Nora AH: Birth defects and oral contraceptives. *Lancet* 1 :941-942, 1973.
4. Janerich DT, Piper JM, Glebatis DM: Oral contraceptives and congenital limb-reduction defects. *N Engl J Med* 291 :697-700, 1974.
5. Heinonen OP, Slone D, Monson RR, et al: Cardiovascular birth defects and antenatal exposure to female sex hormones. *N Engl J Med* 296 :67-70, 1977.

INFORMATION FOR THE PATIENT

Your doctor has prescribed AYGESTIN® (norethindrone acetate tablets, USP), a progestin, for you. AYGESTIN is similar to the progesterone hormones naturally produced by

Continued on next page

Wyeth-Ayerst—Cont.

the body. Progestins are used to treat menstrual disorders and to test if the body is producing certain hormones.

WARNING

There is an increased risk of birth defects in children whose mothers take this drug during the first four months of pregnancy.

Progestins have been used as a test for pregnancy but such use is no longer considered safe because of possible damage to a developing baby. Also, more rapid methods for testing for pregnancy are now available.

These drugs have also been used to prevent miscarriage in the first few months of pregnancy. No adequate evidence is available to show that they are effective for this purpose and there is evidence of an increased risk of birth defects, such as heart or limb defects, if these drugs are taken during the first four months of pregnancy. Furthermore, most cases of early miscarriage are due to causes which could not be helped by these drugs.

The exact risk of taking these drugs early in pregnancy and having a baby with a birth defect is not known. However, one study found that babies born to women who had taken sex hormones (such as progesterone-like drugs) during the first three months of pregnancy were 4 to 5 times more likely to have abnormalities of the arms or legs than if their mothers had not taken such drugs. Some of these women had taken these drugs for only a few days. The chance that an infant whose mother had taken this drug will have this type of defect is about 1 in 1,000. If you take AYGESTIN (norethindrone acetate tablets, USP) and later find you were pregnant when you took it, be sure to discuss this with your doctor as soon as possible.

HOW SUPPLIED

AYGESTIN® (norethindrone acetate tablets, USP)—scored 5 mg tablets, in bottles of 50, for oral administration. Also available in Cycle Packs of 10.

Store at room temperature (approximately 25°C).

Shown in Product Identification Section, page 436

BASALJEL®   OTC
[bā´sel-jel]
(basic aluminum carbonate gel)
SUSPENSION • CAPSULES • SWALLOW TABLETS

COMPOSITION

Suspension—each 5 mL teaspoonful contains basic aluminum carbonate gel equivalent to 400 mg aluminum hydroxide. Inactive ingredients are artificial and natural flavors, butylparaben, calcium benzoate, glycerin, hydroxypropyl methylcellulose, methylparaben, mineral oil, propylparaben, saccharin, simethicone, sorbitol solution, and water. Capsule contains dried basic aluminum carbonate gel equivalent to 608 mg of dried aluminum hydroxide gel or 500 mg aluminum hydroxide. Inactive ingredients are D&C Yellow 10, FD&C Blue 1, FD&C Red 40, FD&C Yellow 6, gelatin, polacrilin potassium, polyethylene glycol, talc, and titanium dioxide. Tablet contains dried basic aluminum carbonate gel equivalent to 608 mg of dried aluminum hydroxide gel or 500 mg aluminum hydroxide. Inactive ingredients are cellulose, hydrogenated vegetable oil, magnesium stearate, polacrilin potassium, starch, and talc.

INDICATIONS

Symptomatic relief of hyperacidity associated with peptic ulcer, gastritis, peptic esophagitis, gastric hyperacidity, and hiatal hernia. For the treatment, control, or management of hyperphosphatemia, or for use with a low phosphate diet to prevent formation of phosphate urinary stones, through the reduction of phosphates in the serum and urine.

WARNINGS

No more than 24 tablets/capsules/teaspoonfuls of BASALJEL should be taken in a 24-hour period. Aluminum forms insoluble complexes with phosphate in the gastrointestinal tract, thus decreasing phosphate absorption. Prolonged use of aluminum-containing antacids by normophosphatemic patients may result in hypophosphatemia if phosphate intake is not adequate. In its more severe forms, hypophosphatemia can lead to anorexia, malaise, muscle weakness, and osteomalacia. A usually transient hypercalciuria of mild degree may be associated with the early weeks of therapy. Evidence suggests that elevated tissue aluminum levels have a role in development of the dialysis encephalopathy syndrome. A number of cases have been associated with elevated aluminum levels in the dialysate water. There is also evidence that small amounts of ingested aluminum are absorbed from the gastrointestinal tract, and it is likely that renal excretion of absorbed aluminum is impaired in renal failure. Prolonged use of aluminum-containing antacids in such patients may contribute to increased levels of aluminum. Pregnant women and nursing mothers are advised to

seek the advice of a health professional before using this product.

PRECAUTIONS

May cause constipation. Adequate fluid intake should be maintained in addition to the specific medical or surgical management indicated by the patient's condition.

DRUG INTERACTIONS

Alumina-containing antacids should not be used concomitantly with any form of tetracycline therapy.

DOSAGE AND ADMINISTRATION

Suspension—2 teaspoonfuls (10 mL) in water or fruit juice taken as often as every 2 hours up to 12 times daily. Two teaspoonfuls have the capacity to neutralize 23 mEq of acid. Capsules—2 capsules as often as every 2 hours up to 12 times daily. Two capsules have the capacity to neutralize 24 mEq of acid. Tablets—2 tablets as often as every 2 hours up to 12 times daily. Two tablets have the capacity to neutralize 25 mEq of acid.

Hyperphosphatemia: An initial dose of Basaljel equivalent to 1.0 gm aluminum hydroxide—2 capsules, 2 tablets, or 2.5 teaspoonfuls (12 mL) suspension—taken 3 to 4 times per day with meals (total daily dose 3–4 gm) is recommended. After therapy is initiated, Basaljel dosage should be adjusted to the minimum required amount by carefully monitoring dietary phosphate intake (patients should be instructed on maintaining a low phosphate diet) and measurement of serum phosphorus levels on a regular basis. Sodium content is: 0.13 mEq/5 mL for the suspension, 0.12 mEq per capsule, and 0.12 mEq per tablet.

HOW SUPPLIED

Suspension—bottles of 12 fluidounces; Capsules—bottles of 100 and 500; Tablets (scored)—bottles of 100.

BICILLIN® C-R   ℞
[bī-sil´in]
(penicillin G benzathine and penicillin G procaine suspension)
INJECTION

FOR DEEP INTRAMUSCULAR INJECTION ONLY

DESCRIPTION

Bicillin C-R (penicillin G benzathine and penicillin G procaine suspension), Wyeth, contains equal amounts of the benzathine and procaine salts of penicillin G. It is available for deep intramuscular injection.

Penicillin G benzathine is prepared by the reaction of dibenzylethylene diamine with two molecules of penicillin G. It is chemically designated as 3,3-dimethyl-7-oxo-6-(2-phenylacetamido)-4-thia-1-azabicyclo[3.2.0]heptane-2-carboxylic acid compound with N,N´-dibenzylethylenediamine(2:1), tetrahydrate. It occurs as a white, crystalline powder and is very slightly soluble in water and sparingly soluble in alcohol.

Penicillin G procaine, 3,3-dimethyl-7-oxo-6-(2-phenylacetamido)-4-thia-1-azabicyclo [3.2.0] heptane-2-carboxylic acid 2-(diethylamino)ethyl p-aminobenzoate compound(1:1) monohydrate, is an equimolar salt of procaine and penicillin G. It occurs as white crystals or a white, microcrystalline powder and is slightly soluble in water.

Bicillin C-R (penicillin G benzathine and penicillin G procaine suspension) contains in each mL the equivalent of 150,000 units of penicillin G as the benzathine salt and 150,000 units of penicillin G as the procaine salt in a stabilized aqueous suspension with sodium citrate buffer; and as w/v, approximately 0.5% lecithin, 0.55% carboxymethylcellulose, 0.55% povidone, 0.1% methylparaben, and 0.01% propylparaben.

Each disposable syringe (2 mL size) contains the equivalent of 1,200,000 units of penicillin G comprising: the equivalent of 600,000 units penicillin G as the benzathine salt and the equivalent of 600,000 units penicillin G as the procaine salt in a stabilized aqueous suspension with sodium citrate buffer; and as w/v, approximately 0.5% lecithin, 0.55% carboxymethylcellulose, 0.55% povidone, 0.1% methylparaben, and 0.01% propylparaben.

Each disposable syringe (4 mL size) contains the equivalent of 2,400,000 units of penicillin G comprising: the equivalent of 1,200,000 units of penicillin G as the benzathine salt and the equivalent of 1,200,000 units of penicillin G as the procaine salt in a stabilized aqueous suspension with sodium citrate buffer; and as w/v, approximately 0.5% lecithin, 0.55% carboxymethylcellulose, 0.55% povidone, 0.1% methylparaben, and 0.01% propylparaben.

Each TUBEX cartridge (1 mL size) contains the equivalent of 600,000 units of penicillin G comprising: the equivalent of 300,000 units penicillin G as the benzathine salt and the equivalent of 300,000 units penicillin G as the procaine salt in a stabilized aqueous suspension with sodium citrate buffer; and as w/v, approximately 0.5% lecithin, 0.55% carboxymethylcellulose, 0.55% povidone, 0.1% methylparaben, and 0.01% propylparaben.

Each TUBEX cartridge (2 mL size) contains the equivalent of 1,200,000 units of penicillin G comprising: the equivalent of 600,000 units of penicillin G as the benzathine salt and the equivalent of 600,000 units of penicillin G as the procaine salt in a stabilized aqueous suspension with sodium citrate buffer; and as w/v, approximately 0.5% lecithin, 0.55% carboxymethylcellulose, 0.55% povidone, 0.1% methylparaben, and 0.01% propylparaben.

Bicillin C-R suspension in the multiple-dose-vial formulation, disposable-syringe formulation, and the TUBEX formulation is viscous and opaque. Read "Contraindications," "Warnings," "Precautions," and "Dosage and Administration" sections prior to use.

CLINICAL PHARMACOLOGY

GENERAL

Penicillin G benzathine and penicillin G procaine have a low solubility and, thus, the drugs are slowly released from intramuscular injection sites. The drugs are hydrolyzed to penicillin G. This combination of hydrolysis and slow absorption results in blood serum levels much lower but more prolonged than other parenteral penicillins. Intramuscular administration of 600,000 units of Bicillin C-R in adults usually produces peak blood levels of 1.0 to 1.3 units per mL within 3 hours; this level falls to an average concentration of 0.32 units per mL at 12 hours, 0.19 units per mL at 24 hours, and 0.03 units per mL at seven days.

Intramuscular administration of 1,200,000 units of Bicillin C-R in adults usually produces peak blood levels of 2.1 to 2.6 units per mL within 3 hours; this level falls to an average concentration of 0.75 units per mL at 12 hours, 0.28 units per mL at 24 hours, and 0.04 units per mL at seven days.

Approximately 60% of penicillin G is bound to serum protein. The drug is distributed throughout the body tissues in widely varying amounts. Highest levels are found in the kidneys with lesser amounts in the liver, skin, and intestines. Penicillin G penetrates into all other tissues and the spinal fluid to a lesser degree. With normal kidney function, the drug is excreted rapidly by tubuler excretion. In neonates and young infants and in individuals with impaired kidney function, excretion is considerably delayed.

MICROBIOLOGY

Penicillin G exerts a bactericidal action against penicillin-susceptible microorganisms during the stage of active multiplication. It acts through the inhibition of biosynthesis of cell-wall mucopeptide. It is not active against the penicillinase-producing bacteria, which include many strains of staphylococci. The following *in-vitro* data are available, but their clinical significance is unknown. Penicillin G exerts high *in-vitro* activity against staphylococci (except penicillinase-producing strains), streptococci (Groups A, C, G, H, L, and M), and pneumococci. Other organisms susceptible to penicillin G are *Neisseria gonorrhoeae, Corynebacterium diphtheriae, Bacillus anthracis,* Clostridia species, *Actinomyces bovis, Streptobacillus moniliformis, Listeria monocytogenes,* and Leptospira species. *Treponema pallidum* is extremely susceptible to the bactericidal action of penicillin G. *Susceptibility Test:* If the Kirby-Bauer method of disc susceptibility is used, a 10-unit penicillin disc should give a zone greater than 28 mm when tested against a penicillin-sensitive bacterial strain.

INDICATIONS AND USAGE

This drug is indicated in the treatment of moderately severe infections due to penicillin-G-susceptible microorganisms that are susceptible to serum levels common to this particular dosage form. Therapy should be guided by bacteriological studies (including susceptibility testing) and by clinical response.

Bicillin C-R is indicated in the treatment of the following in children of all ages:

Moderately severe to severe infections of the upper-respiratory tract, scarlet fever, erysipelas, and skin and soft-tissue infections due to susceptible streptococci.

Note: Streptococci in Groups A, C, G, H, L, and M are very sensitive to penicillin G. Other groups, including Group D (enterococci), are resistant. Penicillin G sodium or potassium is recommended for streptococcal infections with bacteremia.

Moderately severe pneumonia and otitis media due to susceptible pneumococci.

Note: Severe pneumonia, empyema, bacteremia, pericarditis, meningitis, peritonitis, and arthritis of pneumococcal etiology are better treated with penicillin G sodium or potassium during the acute stage.

When high, sustained serum levels are required, penicillin G sodium or potassium, either IM or IV, should be used. This drug should not be used in the treatment of venereal diseases, including syphilis, gonorrhea, yaws, bejel, and pinta.

CONTRAINDICATIONS

A previous hypersensitivity reaction to any penicillin or to procaine is a contraindication.

Do not inject into or near an artery or nerve.

WARNINGS

The combination of penicillin G benzathine and penicillin G procaine should only be prescribed for the indications listed in this insert.

Serious and occasionally fatal hypersensitivity (anaphylactoid) reactions have been reported in patients on penicillin therapy. Although anaphylaxis is more frequent following parenteral therapy, it has occurred in patients on oral penicillins. These reactions are more apt to occur in individuals with a history of sensitivity to multiple allergens.

There are reports of patients with a history of penicillin hypersensitivity reactions who experienced severe hypersensitivity reactions when treated with a cephalosporin. Before therapy with a penicillin, careful inquiry should be made about previous hypersensitivity reactions to penicillins, cephalosporins, and other allergens. If an allergic reaction occurs, the drug should be discontinued and appropriate therapy should be instituted. Serious anaphylactoid reactions require immediate emergency treatment with epinephrine. Oxygen, intravenous steroids, airway management, including intubation, should also be administered as indicated.

Inadvertent intravascular administration, including inadvertent direct intraarterial injection or injection immediately adjacent to arteries, of Bicillin C-R and other penicillin preparations has resulted in severe neurovascular damage, including transverse myelitis with permanent paralysis, gangrene requiring amputation of digits and more proximal portions of extremities, and necrosis and sloughing at and surrounding the injection site. Such severe effects have been reported following injections into the buttock, thigh, and deltoid areas. Other serious complications of suspected intravascular administration which have been reported include immediate pallor, mottling or cyanosis of the extremity both distal and proximal to the injection site followed by bleb formation; severe edema requiring anterior and/or posterior compartment fasciotomy in the lower extremity. The above-described severe effects and complications have most often occurred in infants and small children. Prompt consultation with an appropriate specialist is indicated if any evidence of compromise of the blood supply occurs at, proximal to, or distal to the site of injection.[1-9] See "Contraindications," "Precautions," and "Dosage and Administration" sections. Quadriceps femoris fibrosis and atrophy have been reported following repeated intramuscular injections of penicillin preparations into the anterolateral thigh.

Injection into or near a nerve may result in permanent neurological damage.

PRECAUTIONS
GENERAL

Penicillin should be used with caution in individuals with histories of significant allergies and/or asthma.

Care should be taken to avoid intravenous or intraarterial administration, or injection into or near major peripheral nerves or blood vessels, since such injections may produce neurovascular damage. See "Contraindications," "Warnings," and "Dosage and Administration" sections.

A small percentage of patients are sensitive to procaine. If there is a history of sensitivity make the usual test: Inject intradermally 0.1 mL of a 1 to 2 percent procaine solution. Development of an erythema, wheal, flare, or eruption indicates procaine sensitivity. Sensitivity should be treated by the usual methods, including barbiturates, and procaine penicillin preparations should not be used. Antihistaminics appear beneficial in treatment of procaine reactions.

The use of antibiotics may result in overgrowth of nonsusceptible organisms. Constant observation of the patient is essential. If new infections due to bacteria or fungi appear during therapy, the drug should be discontinued and appropriate measures taken.

Whenever allergic reactions occur, penicillin should be withdrawn unless, in the opinion of the physician, the condition being treated is life-threatening and amenable only to penicillin therapy.

In prolonged therapy with penicillin, and particularly with high-dosage schedules, periodic evaluation of the renal and hematopoietic systems is recommended.

LABORATORY TESTS

In streptococcal infections, therapy must be sufficient to eliminate the organism; otherwise, the sequelae of streptococcal disease may occur. Cultures should be taken following completion of treatment to determine whether streptococci have been eradicated.

DRUG INTERACTIONS

Tetracycline, a bacteriostatic antibiotic, may antagonize the bactericidal effect of penicillin, and concurrent use of these drugs should be avoided.

Concurrent administration of penicillin and probenecid increases and prolongs serum penicillin levels by decreasing the apparent volume of distribution and slowing the rate of excretion by competitively inhibiting renal tubular secretion of penicillin.

PREGNANCY CATEGORY B

Reproduction studies performed in the mouse, rat, and rabbit have revealed no evidence of impaired fertility or harm to the fetus due to penicillin G. Human experience with the penicillins during pregnancy has not shown any positive evidence of adverse effects on the fetus. There are, however, no adequate and well-controlled studies in pregnant women showing conclusively that harmful effects of these drugs on the fetus can be excluded. Because animal reproduction studies are not always predictive of human response, this drug should be used during pregnancy only if clearly needed.

NURSING MOTHERS

Soluble penicillin G is excreted in breast milk. Caution should be exercised when penicillin G benzathine and penicillin G procaine are administered to a nursing woman.

CARCINOGENESIS, MUTAGENESIS, IMPAIRMENT OF FERTILITY

No long-term animal studies have been conducted with these drugs.

PEDIATRIC USE

See "Indications and Usage" and "Dosage and Administration."

ADVERSE REACTIONS

As with other penicillins, untoward reactions of the sensitivity phenomena are likely to occur, particularly in individuals who have previously demonstrated hypersensitivity to penicillins or in those with a hstory of allergy, asthma, hay fever, or urticaria.

The following have been reported with parenteral penicillin G:

General: Hypersensitivity reactions including the following: skin eruptions (maculopapular to exfoliative dermatitis), urticaria, laryngeal edema, fever, eosinophilia; other serum-sicknesslike reactions (including chills, fever, edema, arthralgia, and prostration); anaphylaxis. Note: Urticaria, other skin rashes, and serum-sicknesslike reactions may be controlled with antihistamines and, if necessary, systemic corticosteriods. Whenever such reactions occur, penicillin G should be discontinued unless, in the opinion of the physician, the condition being treated is life-threatening and amenable only to therapy with penicillin G. Serious anaphylactic reactions require the immediate use of epinephrine, oxygen, and intravenous steroids.

Hematologic: Hemolytic anemia, leukopenia, thrombocytopenia.

Neurologic: Neuropathy.

Urogenital: Nephropathy.

OVERDOSAGE

Penicillin in overdosage has the potential to cause neuromuscular hyperirritability or convulsive seizures.

DOSAGE AND ADMINISTRATION

Shake multiple-dose vial vigorously before withdrawing the desired dose.

Administer by DEEP, INTRAMUSCULAR INJECTION in the upper, outer quadrant of the buttock. In infants and small children, the midlateral aspect of the thigh may be preferable. When doses are repeated, vary the injection site.

When using the multiple-dose vial:

After selection of the proper site and insertion of the needle into the selected muscle, aspirate by pulling back on the plunger. While maintaining negative pressure for 2–3 seconds, carefully observe the neck of the syringe immediately proximal to the needle hub for appearance of blood or any discoloration. Blood or "typical blood color" may *not* be seen if a blood vessel has been entered—only a mixture of blood and Bicillin C-R. The appearance of any discoloration is reason to withdraw the needle and discard the syringe. If it is elected to inject at another site, a new syringe and needle should be used. If no blood or discoloration appears, inject the contents of the syringe slowly. Discontinue delivery of the dose if the subject complains of severe immediate pain at the injection site or if in infants and young children symptoms or signs occur suggesting onset of severe pain.

When using the TUBEX cartridge:

The Wyeth TUBEX cartridge for this product incorporates several features that are designed to facilitate the visualization of blood on aspiration if a blood vessel is inadvertently entered.

The design of this cartridge is such that blood which enters its needle will be quickly visualized as a red or dark-colored "spot." This "spot" will appear on the barrel of the glass cartridge immediately proximal to the blue hub. Prior to injection, in order to determine where this "spot" can be seen, the operator should first insert and secure the cartridge in the TUBEX syringe/injector in the usual fashion. The needle cover should then be partially removed to reveal a small yellow rectangle and the cartridge and syringe/injector held in one hand with the needle pointing away from the operator. If the 2 mL metal or plastic syringe is used, the glass cartridge should be rotated by turning the plunger of the syringe clockwise until the yellow rectangle is visualized. An imaginary straight line, drawn to extend the yellow rectangle to the shoulder of the glass cartridge, will point to the area on the cartridge where the "spot" can be visualized. If the 1 mL metal syringe is used, it will not be possible to continue to rotate the glass cartridge clockwise once it is properly engaged and fully threaded; it can, however, then be rotated counterclockwise as far as necessary to properly orient the yellow rectangle and locate the observation area. (In this same area in some cartridges, a dark spot may sometimes be visualized prior to injection. This is the proximal end of the needle and does not represent a foreign body in, or other abnormality of, the suspension.)

Thus, before the needle is inserted into the selected muscle, it is important for the operator to orient the yellow rectangle so that any blood which may enter after needle insertion and during aspiration can be visualized in the area on the cartridge where it will appear and not be obscured by any obstructions.

After selection of the proper site and insertion of the needle into the selected muscle, aspirate by pulling back on the plunger. While maintaining negative pressure for 2 to 3 seconds, carefully observe the barrel of the cartridge in the area previously identified (see above) for the appearance of a red or dark-colored "spot."

Blood or "typical blood color" may *not* be seen if a blood vessel has been entered—only a mixture of blood and Bicillin C-R. The appearance of *any* discoloration is reason to withdraw the needle and discard the glass TUBEX cartridge. If it is elected to inject at another site, a new cartridge should be used. If no blood or discoloration appears, inject the contents of the cartridge slowly. Discontinue delivery of the dose if the subject complains of severe immediate pain at the injection site or if, especially in infants and young children, symptoms or signs occur suggesting onset of severe pain.

Some TUBEX cartridges may contain a small air bubble which may be disregarded since it does not affect administration of the product. Because of the high concentration of suspended material in this product, the needle may be blocked if the injection is not made at a slow, steady rate.

When using the disposable syringe:

The Wyeth disposable syringe for this product incorporates several new features that are designed to facilitate its use. A single small indentation, or "dot," has been punched into the metal ring that surrounds the neck of the syringe near the base of the needle. It is important that this "dot" be placed in a position so that it can be easily visualized by the operator following the intramuscular insertion of the syringe needle.

After selection of the proper site and insertion of the needle into the selected muscle, aspirate by pulling back on the plunger. While maintaining negative pressure for 2 to 3 seconds, carefully observe the barrel of the syringe immediately proximal to the location of the "dot" for appearance of blood or any discoloration. Blood or "typical blood color" may *not* be seen if a blood vessel has been entered—only a mixture of blood and Bicillin C-R. The appearance of any discoloration is reason to withdraw the needle and discard the syringe. If it

Continued on next page

Wyeth-Ayerst—Cont.

is elected to inject at another site, a new syringe should be used. If no blood or discoloration appears, inject the contents of the syringe slowly. Discontinue delivery of the dose if the subject complains of severe immediate pain at the injection site or if in infants and young children symptoms or signs occur suggesting onset of severe pain.

Some disposable syringes may contain a small air bubble which may be disregarded, since it does not affect administration of the product.

Because of the high concentration of suspended material in this product, the needle may be blocked if the injection is not made at a slow, steady rate.

Streptococcal infections Group A—Infections of the upper-respiratory tract, skin and soft-tissue infections, scarlet fever, and erysipelas.

The following doses are recommended:

Adults and children over 60 lbs. in weight: 2,400,000 units.
Children from 30–60 lbs.: 900,000 units to 1,200,000 units.
Infants and children under 30 lbs.: 600,000 units.

NOTE: Treatment with the recommended dosage is usually given at a single session using multiple IM sites when indicated. An alternative dosage schedule may be used, giving one-half (½) the total dose on day 1 and one-half (½) on day 3. This will also insure the penicillinemia required over a 10-day period; however, this alternate schedule should be used only when the physician can be assured of the patient's cooperation.

Pneumococcal infections (except pneumococcal meningitis): 600,000 units in children and 1,200,000 units in adults, repeated every 2 or 3 days until the temperature is normal for 48 hours. Other forms of penicillin may be necessary for severe cases.

Parenteral drug products should be inspected visually for particulate matter and discoloration prior to administration whenever solution and container permit.

HOW SUPPLIED

300,000 units per mL—multiple-dose vials of 10 mL, NDC 0008-0176-01. *600,000 units per mL*—1 mL TUBEX® Sterile Cartridge-Needle Units (20 gauge × 1¼ inch needle) packages of 10, NDC 0008-0026-17; 2 mL TUBEX Sterile Cartridge-Needle Units (20 gauge × 1¼ inch needle) (1,200,000 units per TUBEX), packages of 10, NDC 0008-0026-16; 4 mL single-dose (2,400,000 units) disposable syringes (18 gauge × 2 inch needle), packages of 10, NDC 0008-0026-22.

Store in a refrigerator.
Keep from freezing.
Shake multiple-dose vials well before using.

REFERENCES

1. SHAW, E.: Transverse myelitis from injection of penicillin. *Am. J. Dis. Child.*, 111:548, 1966.
2. KNOWLES, J.: Accidental intra-arterial injection of penicillin. *Am. J. Dis. Child.*, 111:552, 1966.
3. DARBY, C., et al: Ischemia following an intragluteal injection of benzathine-procaine penicillin G mixture in a one-year-old boy. *Clin. Pediatrics*, 12:485, 1973.
4. BROWN, L. & NELSON, A.: Postinfectious intravascular thrombosis with gangrene. *Arch. Surg.*, 94:652, 1967.
5. BORENSTINE, J.: Transverse myelitis and penicillin (Correspondence). *Am. J. Dis. Child.*, 112:166, 1966.
6. ATKINSON, J.: Transverse myelopathy secondary to penicillin injection. *J. Pediatrics*, 75:867, 1969.
7. TALBERT, J. et al: Gangrene of the foot following intramuscular injection in the lateral thigh: A case report with recommendations for prevention. *J. Pediatrics*, 70:110, 1967.
8. FISHER, T.: Medicolegal affairs. *Canad. Med. Assoc. J.*, 112:395, 1975.
9. SCHANZER, H. et al: Accidental intraarterial injection of penicillin G. *JAMA*, 242:1289, 1979.

BICILLIN® C-R 900/300   ℞
[bī-sil'in]
(penicillin G benzathine and
penicillin G procaine suspension)
INJECTION

FOR DEEP INTRAMUSCULAR INJECTION ONLY

DESCRIPTION

Bicillin C-R 900/300 (penicillin G benzathine and penicillin G procaine suspension), Wyeth, contains the equivalent of 900,000 units of penicillin G as the benzathine and 300,000 units of penicillin G as the procaine salts. It is available for deep, intramuscular injection.

Penicillin G benzathine is prepared by the reaction of dibenzylethylene diamine with two molecules of penicillin G. It is chemically designated as 3,3-dimethyl-7-oxo-6-(2-phenylacetamido)-4-thia-1-azabicyclo [3.2.0] heptane-2-carboxylic acid compound with *N,N'*-dibenzylethylenediamine (2:1), tetrahydrate. It occurs as a white, crystalline powder and is very slightly soluble in water and sparingly soluble in alcohol.

Penicillin G procaine, 3,3-dimethyl-7-oxo-6-(2-phenylacetamido)-4-thia-1-azabicyclo [3.2.0] heptane-2-carboxylic acid compound with 2-(diethylamino)ethyl *p*-aminobenzoate compound (1:1) monohydrate, is an equimolar salt of procaine and penicillin G. It occurs as white crystals or a white, microcrystalline powder and is slightly soluble in water.

Each TUBEX® cartridge (2 mL size) contains 1,200,000 units of penicillin comprising: 900,000 units penicillin G benzathine and 300,000 units penicillin G procaine in a stabilized aqueous suspension with sodium citrate buffer; and as w/v, approximately 0.5% lecithin, 0.55% carboxymethylcellulose, 0.55% povidone, 0.1% methylparaben, and 0.01% propylparaben.

Bicillin C-R 900/300 suspension in the TUBEX formulation is viscous and opaque. Read "Contraindications," "Warnings," "Precautions," and "Dosage and Administration" sections prior to use.

CLINICAL PHARMACOLOGY

GENERAL

Penicillin G benzathine and penicillin G procaine have a low solubility and, thus, the drugs are slowly released from intramuscular injection sites. The drugs are hydrolyzed to penicillin G. This combination of hydrolysis and slow absorption results in blood serum levels much lower but more prolonged than other parenteral penicillins. Intramuscular administration of 1,200,000 units of Bicillin C-R 900/300 in patients weighing 100 to 140 lbs. usually produces average blood levels of 0.24 units/mL at 24 hours, 0.039 units/mL at 7 days, and 0.024 units/mL at 10 days.

Approximately 60% of penicillin G is bound to serum protein. The drug is distributed throughout the body tissues in widely varying amounts. Highest levels are found in the kidneys with lesser amounts in the liver, skin, and intestines. Penicillin G penetrates into all other tissues and the spinal fluid to a lesser degree. With normal kidney function, the drug is excreted rapidly by tubular excretion. In neonates and young infants and in individuals with impaired kidney function, excretion is considerably delayed.

MICROBIOLOGY

Penicillin G exerts a bactericidal action against penicillin-susceptible microorganisms during the stage of active multiplication. It acts through the inhibition of biosynthesis of cell-wall mucopeptide. It is not active against the penicillinase-producing bacteria, which include many strains of staphylococci.

The following *in-vitro* data are available, but their clinical significance is unknown. Penicillin G exerts high *in-vitro* activity against staphylococci (except penicillinase-producing strains), streptococci (Groups A, C, G, H, L, and M), and pneumococci. Other organisms susceptible to penicillin G are *Neisseria gonorrhoeae, Corynebacterium diphtheriae, Bacillus anthracis,* Clostridia species, *Actinomyces bovis, Streptobacillus moniliformis, Listeria monocytogenes,* and Leptospira species. *Treponema pallidum* is extremely susceptible to the bactericidal action of penicillin G.

Susceptibility Test: If the Kirby-Bauer method of disc susceptibility is used, a 10-unit penicillin disc should give a zone greater than 28 mm when tested against a penicillin-susceptible bacterial strain.

INDICATIONS AND USAGE

Bicillin C-R 900/300 is indicated in the treatment of infections as described below that are susceptible to serum levels characteristic of this particular dosage form. Therapy should be guided by bacteriological studies (including susceptibility testing) and by clinical response.

Bicillin C-R 900/300 is indicated in the treatment of the following in children of all ages:

Moderately severe to severe infections of the upper-respiratory tract, scarlet fever, erysipelas, and skin and soft-tissue infections due to susceptible streptococci.

Note: Streptococci in Groups A, C, G, H, L, and M are very susceptible to penicillin G. Other groups, including Group D (enterococci), are resistant. Penicillin G sodium or potassium is recommended for streptococcal infections with bacteremia.

Moderately severe pneumonia and otitis media due to susceptible pneumococci.

NOTE: Severe pneumonia, empyema, bacteremia, pericarditis, meningitis, peritonitis, and arthritis of pneumococcal etiology are better treated with penicillin G sodium or potassium during the acute stage.

When high, sustained serum levels are required, penicillin G sodium or potassium, either IM or IV, should be used. This drug should *not* be used in the treatment of venereal diseases, including syphilis, gonorrhea, yaws, bejel, and pinta.

CONTRAINDICATIONS

A previous hypersensitivity reaction to any penicillin or to procaine is a contraindication.

Do not inject into or near an artery or nerve.

WARNINGS

The combination of penicillin G benzathine and penicillin G procaine should only be prescribed for the indications listed in this insert.

Serious and occasionally fatal hypersensitivity (anaphylactoid) reactions have been reported in patients on penicillin therapy. Although anaphylaxis is more frequent following parenteral therapy, it has occurred in patients on oral penicillins. These reactions are more apt to occur in individuals with a history of sensitivity to multiple allergens.

There are reports of patients with a history of penicillin hypersensitivity reactions who experienced severe hypersensitivity reactions when treated with a cephalosporin. Before therapy with a penicillin, careful inquiry should be made about previous hypersensitivity reactions to penicillins, cephalosporins, and other allergens. If an allergic reaction occurs, the drug should be discontinued and appropriate therapy should be instituted. Serious anaphylactoid reactions require immediate emergency treatment with epinephrine. Oxygen, intravenous steroids, airway management, including intubation, should also be administered as indicated.

Inadvertent intravascular administration, including inadvertent direct intraarterial injection or injection immediately adjacent to arteries, of Bicillin C-R 900/300 and other penicillin preparations has resulted in severe neurovascular damage, including transverse myelitis with permanent paralysis, gangrene requiring amputation of digits and more proximal portions of extremities, and necrosis and sloughing at and surrounding the injection site. Such severe effects have been reported following injections into the buttock, thigh, and deltoid areas. Other serious complications of suspected intravascular administration which have been reported include immediate pallor, mottling or cyanosis of the extremity both distal and proximal to the injection site followed by bleb formation; severe edema requiring anterior and/or posterior compartment fasciotomy in the lower extremity. The above-described severe effects and complications have most often occurred in infants and small children. Prompt consultation with an appropriate specialist is indicated if any evidence of compromise of the blood supply occurs at, proximal to, or distal to the site of injection.[1-9] See "Contraindications," "Precautions," and "Dosage and Administration" sections.

Quadriceps femoris fibrosis and atrophy have been reported following repeated intramuscular injections of penicillin preparations into the anterolateral thigh.

Injection into or near a nerve may result in permanent neurological damage.

PRECAUTIONS

GENERAL

Penicillin should be used with caution in individuals with histories of significant allergies and/or asthma.

Care should be taken to avoid intravenous or intraarterial administration, or injection into or near major peripheral nerves or blood vessels, since such injections may produce neurovascular damage. See "Contraindications," "Warnings," and "Dosage and Administration" sections.

A small percentage of patients are sensitive to procaine. If there is a history of sensitivity make the usual test: Inject intradermally 0.1 mL of a 1 to 2 percent procaine solution. Development of an erythema, wheal, flare, or eruption indicates procaine sensitivity. Sensitivity should be treated by the usual methods, including barbiturates, and procaine penicillin preparations should not be used. Antihistaminics appear beneficial in treatment of procaine reactions.

The use of antibiotics may result in overgrowth of nonsusceptible organisms. Constant observation of the patient is essential. If new infections due to bacteria or fungi appear during therapy, the drug should be discontinued and appropriate measures taken.

Whenever allergic reactions occur, penicillin should be withdrawn unless, in the opinion of the physician, the condition being treated is life-threatening and amenable only to penicillin therapy.

In prolonged therapy with penicillin, and particularly with high-dosage schedules, periodic evaluation of the renal and hematopoietic systems is recommended.

LABORATORY TESTS

In streptococcal infections, therapy must be sufficient to eliminate the organism; otherwise, the sequelae of streptococcal disease may occur. Cultures should be taken following completion of treatment to determine whether streptococci have been eradicated.

DRUG INTERACTIONS

Tetracycline, a bacteriostatic antibiotic, may antagonize the bactericidal effect of penicillin, and concurrent use of these drugs should be avoided.

Concurrent administration of penicillin and probenecid increases and prolongs serum penicillin levels by decreasing the apparent volume of distribution and slowing the rate of excretion by competitively inhibiting renal tubular secretion of penicillin.

PREGNANCY CATEGORY B

Reproduction studies performed in the mouse, rat, and rabbit have revealed no evidence of impaired fertility or harm to the fetus due to penicillin G. Human experience with the penicillins during pregnancy has not shown any positive evidence of adverse effects on the fetus. There are, however, no adequate and well-controlled studies in pregnant women showing conclusively that harmful effects of these drugs on the fetus can be excluded. Because animal reproduction studies are not always predictive of human response, this drug should be used during pregnancy only if clearly needed.

NURSING MOTHERS

Soluble penicillin G is excreted in breast milk. Caution should be exercised when penicillin G benzathine and penicillin G procaine are administered to a nursing woman.

CARCINOGENESES, MUTAGENESIS, IMPAIRMENT OF FERTILITY

No long-term animal studies have been conducted with these drugs.

PEDIATRIC USE

See "Indications and Usage" and "Dosage and Administration."

ADVERSE REACTIONS

As with other penicillins, untoward reactions of the sensitivity phenomena are likely to occur, particularly in individuals who have previously demonstrated hypersensitivity to penicillins or in those with a history of allergy, asthma, hay fever, or urticaria.

The following have been reported with parenteral penicillin G:

General: Hypersensitivity reactions including the following: skin eruptions (maculopapular to exfoliative dermatitis), urticaria, laryngeal edema, fever, eosinophilia; other serum-sicknesslike reactions (including chills, fever, edema, arthralgia, and prostration); anaphylaxis. Note: Urticaria, other skin rashes, and serum-sicknesslike reactions may be controlled with antihistamines and, if necessary, systemic corticosteroids.

Whenever such reactions occur, penicillin G should be discontinued unless, in the opinion of the physician, the condition being treated is life-threatening and amenable only to therapy with penicillin G. Serious anaphylactic reactions require the immediate use of epinephrine, oxygen, and intravenous steroids.

Hematologic: Hemolytic anemia, leukopenia, thrombocytopenia.

Neurologic: Neuropathy.

Urogenital: Nephropathy.

OVERDOSAGE

Penicillin in overdosage has the potential to cause neuromuscular hyperirritability or convulsive seizures.

DOSAGE AND ADMINISTRATION

Administer by DEEP, INTRAMUSCULAR INJECTION in the upper, outer quadrant of the buttock. In infants and small children, the midlateral aspect of the thigh may be preferable. When doses are repeated, vary the injection site. The Wyeth TUBEX cartridge for this product incorporates several features that are designed to facilitate the visualization of blood on aspiration if a blood vessel is inadvertently entered.

The design of this cartridge is such that blood which enters its needle will be quickly visualized as a red or dark-colored "spot." This "spot" will appear on the barrel of the glass cartridge immediately proximal to the blue hub. Prior to injection, in order to determine where this "spot" can be seen, the operator should first insert and secure the cartridge in the TUBEX syringe/injector in the usual fashion. The needle cover should then be partially removed to reveal a small yellow rectangle and the cartridge and syringe/injector held in one hand with the needle pointing away from the operator. If the 2 mL metal or plastic syringe is used, the glass cartridge should be rotated by turning the plunger of the syringe clockwise until the yellow rectangle is visualized. An imaginary straight line, drawn to extend the yellow rectangle to the shoulder of the glass cartridge, will point to the area on the cartridge where the "spot" can be visualized. If the 1 mL metal syringe is used, it will not be possible to continue to rotate the glass cartridge clockwise once it is properly engaged and fully threaded; it can, however, then be rotated counterclockwise as far as necessary to properly orient the yellow rectangle and locate the observation area. (In this same area in some cartridges, a dark spot may sometimes be visualized prior to injection. This is the proximal end of the needle and does not represent a foreign body in, or other abnormality of, the suspension.)

Thus, before the needle is inserted into the selected muscle, it is important for the operator to orient the yellow rectangle so that any blood which may enter after needle insertion and during aspiration can be visualized in the area on the cartridge where it will appear and not be obscured by any obstructions.

After selection of the proper site and insertion of the needle into the selected muscle, aspirate by pulling back on the plunger. While maintaining negative pressure for 2 to 3 seconds, carefully observe the barrel of the cartridge in the area previously identified (see above) for the appearance of a red or dark-colored "spot."

Blood or "typical blood color" may not be seen if a blood vessel has been entered—only a mixture of blood and Bicillin C-R 900/300. The appearance of *any* discoloration is reason to withdraw the needle and discard the glass TUBEX cartridge. If it is elected to inject at another site, a new cartridge should be used. If no blood or discoloration appears, inject the contents of the cartridge slowly. Discontinue delivery of the dose if the subject complains of severe immediate pain at the injection site or if, especially in infants and young children, symptoms or signs occur suggesting onset of severe pain.

Some TUBEX cartridges may contain a small air bubble which may be disregarded since it does not affect administration of the product. Because of the high concentration of suspended material in this product, the needle may be blocked if the injection is not made at a slow, steady rate.

STREPTOCOCCAL INFECTIONS—Group A Infections of the upper respiratory tract, skin and soft-tissue infections, scarlet fever, and erysipelas:

A single injection of Bicillin C-R 900/300 is usually sufficient for the treatment of Group A streptococcal infections in children of all ages.

PNEUMOCOCCAL INFECTIONS (except pneumococcal meningitis): One TUBEX Bicillin C-R 900/300 repeated at 2- or 3-day intervals until the temperature is normal for 48 hours. Other forms of penicillin may be necessary for severe cases. Parenteral drug products should be inspected visually for particulate matter and discoloration prior to administration, whenever solution and container permit.

HOW SUPPLIED

Bicillin® C-R 900/300 (penicillin G benzathine and penicillin G procaine suspension), Wyeth®, is supplied in 2 mL size TUBEX® Sterile Cartridge-Needle Units (20 gauge × 1¼ inch needle) in packages of 10 TUBEX, as follows:

1,200,000 units per TUBEX, NDC 0008-0079.

Store in a refrigerator.

Keep from freezing.

REFERENCES

1. SHAW, E.: Transverse myelitis from injection of penicillin. *Am. J. Dis. Child.,* 111: 548, 1966.
2. KNOWLES, J.: Accidental intra-arterial injection of penicillin. *Am. J. Dis. Child.,* 111: 552, 1966.
3. DARBY, C., et al: Ischemia following an intragluteal injection of benzathine-procaine penicillin G mixture in a one-year-old boy. *Clin. Pediatrics,* 12: 485, 1973.
4. BROWN, L. & NELSON, A.: Postinfectious intravascular thrombosis with gangrene. *Arch. Surg.,* 94: 652, 1967.
5. BORENSTINE, J.: Transverse myelitis and penicillin (Correspondence). *Am. J. Dis. Child.,* 112: 166, 1966.
6. ATKINSON, J.: Transverse myelopathy secondary to penicillin injection. *J. Pediatrics,* 75: 867, 1969.
7. TALBERT, J. et al: Gangrene of the foot following intramuscular injection in the lateral thigh: A case report with recommendations for prevention. *J. Pediatrics, 70:* 110, 1967.
8. FISHER, T.: Medicolegal affairs. *Canad. Med. Assoc. J., 112:* 395, 1975.
9. SCHANZER, H. et al: Accidental intra-arterial injection of penicillin G. *JAMA, 242:* 1289, 1979.

BICILLIN® L-A   ℞

[bī-sil′in]

(sterile penicillin G benzathine suspension)

INJECTION

FOR DEEP INTRAMUSCULAR INJECTION ONLY

DESCRIPTION

Bicillin L-A (sterile penicillin G benzathine suspension), Wyeth, is prepared by the reaction of dibenzylethylene diamine with two molecules of penicillin G. It is chemically designated as 3,3-dimethyl-7-oxo-6-(2-phenylacetamido)-4-thia-1-azabicyclo[3.2.0]heptane-2-carboxylic acid compound with *N,N′*-dibenzylethylenediamine (2:1), tetrahydrate.

It is available for deep intramuscular injection. It contains sterile penicillin G benzathine in aqueous suspension with sodium citrate buffer and, as w/v, approximately 0.5% lecithin, 0.6% carboxymethylcellulose, 0.6% povidone, 0.1% methylparaben, and 0.01% propylparaben. It occurs as a white, crystalline powder and is very slightly soluble in water and sparingly soluble in alcohol.

Bicillin L-A suspension in the multiple-dose vial formulation, disposable syringe formulation and TUBEX formulation is viscous and opaque. The multiple-dose vial formulation contains the equivalent of 300,000 units per mL of penicillin G as the benzathine salt. The disposable syringe formulation is available in a 4 mL size containing the equivalent of 2,400,000 units of penicillin G as the benzathine salt. The TUBEX formulation is available in 1 mL and 2 mL TUBEX Sterile Cartridge-Needle Units containing the equivalent of 600,000 units and 1,200,000 units, respectively, of penicillin G as the benzathine salt. Read "Contraindications," "Warnings," "Precautions," and "Dosage and Administration" sections prior to use.

CLINICAL PHARMACOLOGY

GENERAL

Penicillin G benzathine has an extremely low solubility and, thus, the drug is slowly released from intramuscular injection sites. The drug is hydrolyzed to penicillin G. This combination of hydrolysis and slow absorption results in blood serum levels much lower but much more prolonged than other parenteral penicillins.

Intramuscular administration of 300,000 units of penicillin G benzathine in adults results in blood levels of 0.03 to 0.05 units per mL, which are maintained for 4 to 5 days. Similar blood levels may persist for 10 days following administration of 600,000 units and for 14 days following administration of 1,200,000 units. Blood concentrations of 0.003 units per mL may still be detectable 4 weeks following administration of 1,200,000 units.

Approximately 60% of penicillin G is bound to serum protein. The drug is distributed throughout the body tissues in widely varying amounts. Highest levels are found in the kidneys with lesser amounts in the liver, skin, and intestines. Penicillin G penetrates into all other tissues and the spinal fluid to a lesser degree. With normal kidney function, the drug is excreted rapidly by tubular excretion. In neonates and young infants and in individuals with impaired kidney function, excretion is considerably delayed.

MICROBIOLOGY

Penicillin G exerts a bactericidal action against penicillin-susceptible microorganisms during the stage of active multiplication. It acts through the inhibition of biosynthesis of cell-wall mucopeptide. It is not active against the penicillinase-producing bacteria, which include many strains of staphylococci.

The following *in-vitro* data are available, but their clinical significance is unknown. Penicillin G exerts high *in-vitro* activity against staphylococci (except penicillinase-producing strains); streptococci (Groups A, C, G, H, L, and M); and pneumococci. Other organisms susceptible to penicillin G are *Neisseria gonorrhoeae, Corynebacterium diphtheriae, Bacillus anthracis,* Clostridia species, *Actinomyces bovis, Streptobacillus moniliformis, Listeria monocytogenes,* and Leptospira species. *Treponema pallidum* is extremely susceptible to the bactericidal action of penicillin G.

Susceptibility Test: If the Kirby-Bauer method of disc susceptibility is used, a 20-unit penicillin disc should give a zone

Continued on next page

Wyeth-Ayerst—Cont.

greater than 28 mm when tested against a penicillin-susceptible bacterial strain.

INDICATIONS AND USAGE

Intramuscular penicillin G benzathine is indicated in the treatment of infections due to penicillin-G-sensitive microorganisms that are susceptible to the low and very prolonged serum levels common to this particular dosage form. Therapy should be guided by bacteriological studies (including sensitivity tests) and by clinical response.

The following infections will usually respond to adequate dosage of intramuscular penicillin G benzathine:

Mild-to-moderate infections of the upper respiratory tract due to susceptible streptococci.

Venereal infections—Syphilis, yaws, bejel, and pinta.

Medical Conditions in Which Penicillin G Benzathine Therapy Is Indicated as Prophylaxis: Rheumatic fever and/or chorea—Prophylaxis with penicillin G benzathine has proven effective in preventing recurrence of these conditions. It has also been used as follow-up prophylactic therapy for rheumatic heart disease and acute glomerulonephritis.

CONTRAINDICATIONS

A history of a previous hypersensitivity reaction to any of the penicillins is a contraindication.

Do not inject into or near an artery or nerve.

WARNINGS

Penicillin G benzathine should only be prescribed for the indications listed in this insert.

Serious and occasionally fatal hypersensitivity (anaphylactoid) reactions have been reported in patients on penicillin therapy. Although anaphylaxis is more frequent following parenteral therapy, it has occurred in patients on oral penicillins. These reactions are more apt to occur in individuals with a history of sensitivity to multiple allergens.

There are reports of patients with a history of penicillin hypersensitivity reactions who experienced severe hypersensitivity reactions when treated with a cephalosporin. Before therapy with a penicillin, careful inquiry should be made about previous hypersensitivity reactions to penicillins, cephalosporins, and other allergens. If an allergic reaction occurs, the drug should be discontinued and appropriate therapy should be instituted. Serious anaphylactoid reactions require immediate emergency treatment with epinephrine. Oxygen, intravenous steroids, airway management, including intubation, should also be administered as indicated.

Inadvertent intravascular administration, including inadvertent direct intraarterial injection or injection immediately adjacent to arteries, of Bicillin L-A and other penicillin preparations has resulted in severe neurovascular damage, including transverse myelitis with permanent paralysis, gangrene requiring amputation of digits and more proximal portions of extremities, and necrosis and sloughing at and surrounding the injection site. Such severe effects have been reported following injections into the buttock, thigh, and deltoid areas. Other serious complications of suspected intravascular administration which have been reported include immediate pallor, mottling or cyanosis of the extremity both distal and proximal to the injection site followed by bleb formation; severe edema requiring anterior and/or posterior compartment fasciotomy in the lower extremity. The above-described severe effects and complications have most often occurred in infants and small children. Prompt consultation with an appropriate specialist is indicated if any evidence of compromise of the blood supply occurs at, proximal to, or distal to the site of injection.[1-9] See "Contraindications," "Precautions," and "Dosage and Administration" sections.

Quadriceps femoris fibrosis and atrophy have been reported following repeated intramuscular injections of penicillin preparations into the anterolateral thigh.

Injection into or near a nerve may result in permanent neurological damage.

PRECAUTIONS

GENERAL

Penicillin should be used with caution in individuals with histories of significant allergies and/or asthma.

Care should be taken to avoid intravenous or intraarterial administration, or injection into or near major peripheral nerves or blood vessels, since such injection may produce neurovascular damage. See "Contraindications," "Warnings," and "Dosage and Administration" sections.

In streptococcal infections therapy must be sufficient to eliminate the organism; otherwise, the sequelae of streptococcal disease may occur. Cultures should be taken following completion of treatment to determine whether streptococci have been eradicated.

Prolonged use of antibiotics may promote the overgrowth of nonsusceptible organisms, including fungi. Should superinfection occur, appropriate measures should be taken.

LABORATORY TESTS

In streptococcal infections, therapy must be sufficient to eliminate the organism; otherwise, the sequelae of streptococcal disease may occur. Cultures should be taken following completion of treatment to determine whether streptococci have been eradicated.

DRUG INTERACTIONS

Tetracycline, a bacteriostatic antibiotic, may antagonize the bactericidal effect of penicillin, and concurrent use of these drugs should be avoided.

Concurrent administration of penicillin and probenecid increases and prolongs serum penicillin levels by decreasing the apparent volume of distribution and slowing the rate of excretion by competitively inhibiting renal tubular secretion of penicillin.

PREGNANCY CATEGORY B

Reproduction studies performed in the mouse, rat, and rabbit have revealed no evidence of impaired fertility or harm to the fetus due to penicillin G. Human experience with the penicillins during pregnancy has not shown any positive evidence of adverse effects on the fetus. There are, however, no adequate and well-controlled studies in pregnant women showing conclusively that harmful effects of these drugs on the fetus can be excluded. Because animal reproduction studies are not always predictive of human response, this drug should be used during pregnancy only if clearly needed.

NURSING MOTHERS

Soluble penicillin G is excreted in breast milk. Caution should be exercised when penicillin G benzathine is administered to a nursing woman.

CARCINOGENESIS, MUTAGENESIS, IMPAIRMENT OF FERTILITY

No long-term animal studies have been conducted with this drug.

PEDIATRIC USE

See "Indications and Usage" and "Dosage and Administration."

ADVERSE REACTIONS

As with other penicillins, untoward reactions of the sensitivity phenomena are likely to occur, particularly in individuals who have previously demonstrated hypersensitivity to penicillins or in those with a history of allergy, asthma, hay fever, or urticaria.

As with other treatments for syphilis, the Jarisch-Herxheimer reaction has been reported.

The following have been reported with parenteral penicillin G:

General: Hypersensitivity reactions including the following: skin eruptions (maculopapular to exfoliative dermatitis), urticaria, laryngeal edema, fever, eosinophilia; other serum-sicknesslike reactions (including chills, fever, edema, arthralgia, and prostration); anaphylaxis. Note: Urticaria, other skin rashes, and serum-sicknesslike reactions may be controlled with antihistamines and, if necessary, systemic corticosteroids.

Whenever such reactions occur, penicillin G should be discontinued unless, in the opinion of the physician, the condition being treated is life-threatening and amenable only to therapy with penicillin G.

Serious anaphylactic reactions require the immediate use of epinephrine, oxygen, and intravenous steroids.

Hematologic: Hemolytic anemia, leukopenia, thrombocytopenia.

Neurologic: Neuropathy.

Urogenital: Nephropathy.

OVERDOSAGE

Penicillin in overdosage has the potential to cause neuromuscular hyperirritability or convulsive seizures.

DOSAGE AND ADMINISTRATION

Administer by DEEP INTRAMUSCULAR INJECTION in the upper, outer quadrant of the buttock. In infants and small children, the midlateral aspect of the thigh may be preferable. When doses are repeated, vary the injection site.

When using the multiple-dose vial:

Shake multiple-dose vial vigorously before withdrawing the desired dose.

After selection of the proper site and insertion of the needle into the selected muscle, aspirate by pulling back on the plunger. While maintaining negative pressure for 2–3 seconds, carefully observe the neck of the syringe immediately proximal to the needle hub for appearance of blood or any discoloration. Blood or "typical blood color" may *not* be seen if a blood vessel has been entered—only a mixture of blood and Bicillin L-A. The appearance of any discoloration is reason to withdraw the needle and discard the syringe. If it is elected to inject at another site, a new syringe and needle should be used. If no blood or discoloration appears, inject the contents of the syringe slowly. Discontinue delivery of

the dose if the subject complains of severe immediate pain at the injection site or if in infants and young children symptoms or signs occur suggesting onset of severe pain.

When using the TUBEX cartridge:

The Wyeth TUBEX® cartridge for this product incorporates several features that are designed to facilitate the visualization of blood on aspiration if a blood vessel is inadvertently entered.

The design of this cartridge is such that blood which enters its needle will be quickly visualized as a red or dark-colored "spot." This "spot" will appear on the barrel of the glass cartridge immediately proximal to the blue hub. Prior to injection, in order to determine where this "spot" can be seen, the operator should first insert and secure the cartridge in the TUBEX syringe/injector in the usual fashion. The needle cover should then be partially removed to reveal a small yellow rectangle and the cartridge and syringe/injector held in one hand with the needle pointing away from the operator. If the 2 mL metal or plastic syringe is used, the glass cartridge should be rotated by turning the plunger of the syringe clockwise until the yellow rectangle is visualized. An imaginary straight line, drawn to extend the yellow rectangle to the shoulder of the glass cartridge, will point to the area on the cartridge where the "spot" can be visualized. If the 1 mL metal syringe is used, it will not be possible to continue to rotate the glass cartridge clockwise once it is properly engaged and fully threaded; it can, however, then be rotated counterclockwise as far as necessary to properly orient the yellow rectangle and locate the observation area. (In this same area in some cartridges, a dark spot may sometimes be visualized prior to injection. This is the proximal end of the needle and does not represent a foreign body in, or other abnormality of, the suspension.)

Thus, before the needle is inserted into the selected muscle, it is important for the operator to orient the yellow rectangle so that any blood which may enter after needle insertion and during aspiration can be visualized in the area on the cartridge where it will appear and not be obscured by any obstructions.

After selection of the proper site and insertion of the needle into the selected muscle, aspirate by pulling back on the plunger. While maintaining negative pressure for 2–3 seconds, carefully observe the barrel of the cartridge in the area previously identified (see above) for the appearance of a red or dark-colored "spot."

Blood or "typical blood color" may *not* be seen if a blood vessel has been entered—only a mixture of blood and Bicillin L-A. The appearance of *any* discoloration is reason to withdraw the needle and discard the glass TUBEX cartridge. If it is elected to inject at another site, a new cartridge should be used. If no blood or discoloration appears, inject the contents of the cartridge slowly. Discontinue delivery of the dose if the subject complains of severe immediate pain at the injection site or if, especially in infants and young children, symptoms or signs occur suggesting onset of severe pain.

Some TUBEX cartridges may contain a small air bubble which may be disregarded since it does not affect administration of the product.

Because of the high concentration of suspended material in this product, the needle may be blocked if the injection is not made at a slow, steady rate.

When using the disposable syringe:

The Wyeth disposable syringe for this product incorporates several new features that are designed to facilitate its use. A single small indentation, or "dot," has been punched into the metal or plastic ring that surrounds the neck of the syringe near the base of the needle. It is important that this "dot" be placed in a position so that it can be easily visualized by the operator following the intramuscular insertion of the syringe needle.

After selection of the proper site and insertion of the needle into the selected muscle, aspirate by pulling back on the plunger. While maintaining negative pressure for 2–3 seconds, carefully observe the barrel of the syringe immediately proximal to the location of the "dot" for appearance of blood or any discoloration. Blood or "typical blood color" may *not* be seen if a blood vessel has been entered—only a mixture of blood and Bicillin L-A. The appearance of any discoloration is reason to withdraw the needle and discard the syringe. If it is elected to inject at another site, a new syringe should be used. If no blood or discoloration appears, inject the contents of the syringe slowly. Discontinue delivery of the dose if the subject complains of severe immediate pain at the injection site or if in infants and young children symptoms or signs occur suggesting onset of severe pain.

STREPTOCOCCAL (GROUP A) UPPER-RESPIRATORY INFECTIONS (for example, pharyngitis)

Adults—a single injection of 1,200,000 units; older children—a single injection of 900,000 units; infants and children (under 60 lbs.)—300,000 to 600,000 units.

SYPHILIS

Primary, secondary, and latent—2,400,000 (1 dose). Late (tertiary and neurosyphilis)—2,400,000 at 7-day intervals for three doses.

Congenital—under 2 years of age: 50,000 units/kg/body weight; ages 2–12 years: adjust dosage based on adult dosage schedule.

YAWS, BEJEL, and PINTA—1,200,000 (1 injection).

PROPHYLAXIS—for rheumatic fever and glomerulonephritis.

Following an acute attack, penicillin G benzathine (parenteral) may be given in doses of 1,200,000 units once a month or 600,000 units every 2 weeks.

Some disposable syringes may contain a small air bubble which may be disregarded, since it does not affect administration of the product.

Because of the high concentration of suspended material in this product, the needle may be blocked if the injection is not made at a slow, steady rate.

Parenteral drug products should be inspected visually for particulate matter and discoloration prior to administration whenever solution and container permit.

HOW SUPPLIED

BICILLIN® L-A (sterile penicillin G benzathine suspension) Injection: *300,000 units per ml* —multiple-dose vials of 10 ml; *600,000 units per 1 ml* TUBEX® sterile cartridge-needle unit, packages of 10; *1,200,000 units per 2 ml* TUBEX, packages of 10; *2,400,000 units per 4 ml* disposable syringe, packages of 10.

Store in a refrigerator. Keep from freezing.
Shake disposable syringe well before using.

REFERENCES

1. SHAW, E.: Transverse myelitis from injection of penicillin. *Am. J. Dis. Child.,* 111: 548, 1966.
2. KNOWLES, J.: Accidental intra-arterial injection of penicillin. *Am. J. Dis. Child.,* 111: 552, 1966.
3. DARBY, C., et al: Ischemia following an intragluteal injection of benzathine-procaine penicillin G mixture in a one-year-old boy. *Clin. Pediatrics, 12:* 485, 1973.
4. BROWN, L. & NELSON, A.: Postinfectious intravascular thrombosis with gangrene. *Arch. Surg., 94:* 652, 1967.
5. BORENSTINE, J.: Transverse myelitis and penicillin (Correspondence). *Am. J. Dis. Child., 112:* 166, 1966.
6. ATKINSON, J.: Transverse myelopathy secondary to penicillin injection. *J. Pediatrics, 75:* 867, 1969.
7. TALBERT, J. et al: Gangrene of the foot following intramuscular injection in the lateral thigh: A case report with recommendations for prevention. *J. Pediatrics, 70:* 110, 1967.
8. FISHER, T.: Medicolegal affairs. *Canad. Med. Assoc. J., 112:* 395, 1975.
9. SCHANZER, H. et al: Accidental intra-arterial injection of penicillin G. *JAMA, 242:* 1289, 1979.

BIOLOGICALS

Each of Wyeth-Ayerst's biological products is listed separately in alphabetical order in Wyeth-Ayerst's Product Information Section.

For prescribing information on the products listed—and for which information is not provided—write to Professional Service, Wyeth-Ayerst Laboratories, P.O. Box 8299, Philadelphia, PA 19101, or contact your local Wyeth-Ayerst representative.

CEROSE–DM®   OTC
[*se-rōs´ DM*]
Cough/Cold Preparation with Dextromethorphan
Sugar Free ● Non-Narcotic

DESCRIPTION

Each teaspoonful (5 mL) contains 15 mg dextromethorphan hydrobromide, 4 mg chlorpheniramine maleate, and 10 mg phenylephrine hydrochloride. Alcohol 2.4%. The inactive ingredients present are artificial flavors, citric acid, edetate disodium, FD&C Yellow 6, glycerin, saccharin sodium, sodium benzoate, sodium citrate, sodium propionate, and water.

INDICATIONS

For the symptomatic control of cough due to colds.

DOSAGE AND ADMINISTRATION

Adults, and children 12 years and over, one to two teaspoonfuls 4 times daily. Children over 6 years, one teaspoonful 4 times daily. Children under 6, as directed by physician only.

CAUTION

Do not exceed recommended dosage. Individuals with high blood pressure, heart disease, diabetes, or thyroid disease should consult physician before using. If there is persistent cough or high fever which may indicate a serious condition, consult your physician. Drowsiness may occur; if so, do not drive or operate machinery or do not permit hazardous childhood activities.

WARNING

As with any drug, if you are pregnant or nursing a baby, seek the advice of a health professional before using this product. **Keep this and all drugs out of the reach of children. In case of accidental overdose, seek professional assistance or contact a Poison Control Center immediately.**

HOW SUPPLIED

Cerose-DM® is available in bottles of 4 fl. oz., cases of 12 bottles; and bottles of 1 pint.
Keep tightly closed below 77°F (25°C)

CERUBIDINE®   ℞
[*sĭ-rew "bĭ´dēan*]
(daunorubicin hydrochloride)
for Injection

> ### WARNINGS
>
> 1. Cerubidine must be given into a rapidly flowing intravenous infusion. It must *never* be given by the intramuscular or subcutaneous route. Severe local tissue necrosis will occur if there is extravasation during administration.
> 2. Myocardial toxicity manifested in its most severe form by potentially fatal congestive heart failure may be encountered when total cumulative dosage exceeds 550 mg/m^2 in adults, 300 mg/m^2 in children more than 2 years of age, or 10 mg/kg in children less than two years of age. This may occur either during therapy or several months after termination of therapy.
> 3. Severe myelosuppression occurs when used in therapeutic doses.
> 4. It is recommended that Cerubidine be administered only by physicians who are experienced in leukemia chemotherapy and in facilities with laboratory and supportive resources adequate to monitor drug tolerance and protect and maintain a patient compromised by drug toxicity. The physician and institution must be capable of responding rapidly and completely to severe hemorrhagic conditions and/or overwhelming infection.
> 5. Dosage should be reduced in patients with impaired hepatic or renal function.

DESCRIPTION

Cerubidine (daunorubicin hydrochloride) is the hydrochloride salt of an anthracycline cytotoxic antibiotic produced by a strain of *Streptomyces coeruleorubidus*. It is provided as a sterile reddish lyophilized powder in vials for intravenous administration only. Each vial contains 20 mg of base activity (21.4 mg as the hydrochloride salt) and 100 mg of mannitol. It is soluble in water when adequately agitated and produces a reddish solution. It has the following structural formula which may be described with the chemical name of 7-(3-amino-2, 3, 6-trideoxy-L-lyxohexosyloxy) -9-acetyl-7, 8, 9, 10-tetrahydro-6,9,11-trihydroxy-4-methoxy-5, 12-naphthacene-

quinone hydrochloride. Its empirical formula is $C_{27}H_{29}NO_{10}HCl$ with a molecular weight of 563.99. It is a hygroscopic crystalline powder. The pH of a 5 mg/mL aqueous solution is 4.5 to 6.5.

STRUCTURAL FORMULA

ACTION

Cerubidine inhibits the synthesis of nucleic acids; its effect on deoxyribonucleic acid is particularly rapid and marked. Cerubidine has antimitotic and cytotoxic activity although the precise mode of action is unknown. Cerubidine displays an immunosuppressive effect. It has been shown to inhibit the production of heterohemagglutinins in mice. *In vitro,* it inhibits blast-cell transformation of canine lymphocytes at 0.01 mcg/mL.

Cerubidine possesses a potent antitumor effect against a wide spectrum of animal tumors either grafted or spontaneous.

CLINICAL PHARMACOLOGY

Following intravenous injection of Cerubidine, plasma levels of daunorubicin decline rapidly, indicating rapid tissue uptake and concentration. Thereafter, plasma levels decline slowly with a half-life of 18.5 hours. By one hour after drug administration, the predominant plasma species is daunorubicinol, an active metabolite, which disappears with a half-life of 26.7 hours. Further metabolism via reduction cleavage of the glycosidic bond, 4-O demethylation, and conjugation with both sulfate and glucuronide have been demonstrated. Simple glycosidic cleavage of daunorubicin or daunorubicinol is not a significant metabolic pathway in man. Twenty-five percent of an administered dose of Cerubidine is eliminated in an active form by urinary excretion and an estimated 40% by biliary excretion.

There is no evidence that Cerubidine crosses the blood-brain barrier.

In the treatment of adult acute nonlymphocytic leukemia, Cerubidine, used as a single agent, has produced complete remission rates of 40 to 50%, and in combination with cytarabine, has produced complete remission rates of 53 to 65%.

The addition of Cerubidine to the two-drug induction regimen of vincristine-prednisone in the treatment of childhood acute lymphocytic leukemia does not increase the rate of complete remission. In children receiving identical CNS prophylaxis and maintenance therapy (without consolidation), there is prolongation of complete remission duration (statistically significant, p < 0.02) in those children induced with the three-drug (Cerubidine-vincristine-prednisone) regimen as compared to two drugs. There is no evidence of any impact of Cerubidine on the duration of complete remission when a consolidation (intensification) phase is employed as part of a total treatment program.

In adult acute lymphocytic leukemia, in contrast to childhood acute lymphocytic leukemia, Cerubidine during induction significantly increases the rate of complete remission, but not remission duration, compared to that obtained with vincristine, prednisone, and L-asparaginase alone. The use of Cerubidine in combination with vincristine, prednisone, and L-asparaginase has produced complete remission rates of 83% in contrast to a 47% remission in patients not receiving Cerubidine.

INDICATIONS AND USAGE

Cerubidine in combination with other approved anticancer drugs is indicated for remission induction in acute nonlymphocytic leukemia (myelogenous, monocytic, erythroid) of adults and for remission induction in acute lymphocytic leukemia of children and adults.

WARNINGS

BONE MARROW—Cerubidine is a potent bone marrow suppressant. Suppression will occur in all patients given a therapeutic dose of this drug. Therapy with Cerubidine should not be started in patients with preexisting drug-induced bone-marrow suppression unless the benefit from such treatment warrants the risk.

CARDIAC EFFECTS—Special attention must be given to the potential cardiac toxicity of Cerubidine, particularly in infants and children. Preexisting heart disease and previous therapy with doxorubicin are co-factors of increased risk of Cerubidine-induced cardiac toxicity and the benefit-to-risk ratio of Cerubidine therapy in such patients should be weighed before starting Cerubidine. In adults, at total cumulative doses less than 550 mg/m^2, acute congestive heart

Continued on next page

Wyeth-Ayerst—Cont.

failure is seldom encountered. However, rare instances of pericarditis-myocarditis, not dose-related, have been reported.

In adults, at cumulative doses exceeding 550 mg/m^2, there is an increased incidence of drug-induced congestive heart failure. Based on prior clinical experience with doxorubicin, this limit appears lower, namely 400 mg/m^2, in patients who received radiation therapy that encompassed the heart.[1]

In infants and children, there appears to be a greater susceptibility to anthracycline-induced cardiotoxicity compared to that in adults, which is more clearly dose-related. However, there is very little risk for children over two years of age in developing Cerubidine-related cardiotoxicity below a cumulative dose of 300 mg/m^2 [2-4] or in children less than two years of age (or < 0.5 m^2 body-surface area) below a cumulative dose of 10 mg/kg. In both children and adults, the total dose of Cerubidine administered should also take into account any previous or concomitant therapy with other potentially cardiotoxic agents or related compounds such as doxorubicin.

There is no absolutely reliable method of predicting the patients in whom acute congestive heart failure will develop as a result of the cardiac toxic effect of Cerubidine. However, certain changes in the electrocardiogram and a decrease in the systolic ejection fraction from pretreatment baseline may help to recognize those patients at greatest risk to develop congestive heart failure. On the basis of the electrocardiogram, a decrease equal to or greater than 30% in limb lead QRS voltage has been associated with a significant risk of drug-induced cardiomyopathy. Therefore, an electrocardiogram and/or determination of systolic ejection fraction should be performed before each course of Cerubidine. In the event that one or the other of these predictive parameters should occur, the benefit of continued therapy must be weighed against the risk of producing cardiac damage. Early clinical diagnosis of drug-induced congestive heart failure appears to be essential for successful treatment with digitalis, diuretics, sodium restriction, and bed rest.

EVALUATION OF HEPATIC AND RENAL FUNCTION— Significant hepatic or renal impairment can enhance the toxicity of the recommended doses of Cerubidine; therefore, prior to administration, evaluation of hepatic function and renal function using conventional clinical laboratory tests is recommended (see "Dosage and Administration").

PREGNANCY—Cerubidine may cause fetal harm when administered to a pregnant woman because of its teratogenic potential. An increased incidence of fetal abnormalities (parieto-occipital cranioschisis, umbilical hernias, or rachischisis) and abortions was reported in rabbits. Decreases in fetal birth weight and postdelivery growth rate were observed in mice. There are no adequate and well-controlled studies in pregnant women. If this drug is used during pregnancy, or if the patient becomes pregnant while taking this drug, the patient should be apprised of the potential hazard to the fetus. Women of childbearing potential should be advised to avoid becoming pregnant.

EXTRAVASATION AT INJECTION SITE—Extravasation of Cerubidine at the site of intravenous administration can cause severe local tissue necrosis.

PRECAUTIONS
Therapy with Cerubidine requires close patient observation and frequent complete blood-count determinations. Cardiac, renal, and hepatic function should be evaluated prior to each course of treatment.

Cerubidine may induce hyperuricemia secondary to rapid lysis of leukemic cells. As a precaution, allopurinol administration is usually begun prior to initiating antileukemic therapy. Blood uric acid levels should be monitored and appropriate therapy initiated in the event that hyperuricemia develops.

Appropriate measures must be taken to control any systemic infection before beginning therapy with Cerubidine.

Cerubidine may transiently impart a red coloration to the urine after administration, and patients should be advised to expect this.

CARCINOGENESIS, MUTAGENESIS, IMPAIRMENT OF FERTILITY
Cerubidine, when injected subcutaneously into mice, causes fibrosarcomas to develop at the injection site. When administered to mice orally or intraperitoneally, no carcinogenic effect was noted after 22 months of observation.

In male dogs at a daily dose of 0.25 mg/kg administered intravenously, testicular atrophy was noted at autopsy. Histologic examination revealed total aplasia of the spermatocyte series in the seminiferous tubules with complete aspermatogenesis.

PREGNANCY CATEGORY D. See "Warnings" section.

ADVERSE REACTIONS
Dose-limiting toxicity includes myelosuppression and cardiotoxicity (see Warnings). Other reactions include:

CUTANEOUS—Reversible alopecia occurs in most patients.

GASTROINTESTINAL—Acute nausea and vomiting occur but are usually mild. Antiemetic therapy may be of some help. Mucositis may occur three to seven days after administration. Diarrhea has occasionally been reported.

LOCAL—If extravasation occurs during administration, tissue necrosis can result at the site.

ACUTE REACTIONS—Rarely, anaphylactoid reaction, fever, chills, and skin rash can occur.

DOSAGE AND ADMINISTRATION
Parenteral drug products should be inspected visually for particulate matter and discoloration prior to administration, whenever solution and container permit.

PRINCIPLES—In order to eradicate the leukemic cells and induce a complete remission, a profound suppression of the bone marrow is usually required. Evaluation of both the peripheral blood and bone marrow are mandatory in the formulation of appropriate treatment plans.

It is recommended that the dosage of Cerubidine be reduced in instances of hepatic or renal impairment. For example, using serum bilirubin and serum creatinine as indicators of liver and kidney function, the following dose modifications are recommended:

Serum Bilirubin	Serum Creatinine	Recommended Dose
1.2 to 3.0 mg%		$^{3}/_{4}$ normal dose
> 3 mg%	>3 mg%	$^{1}/_{2}$ normal dose

REPRESENTATIVE DOSE SCHEDULES AND COMBINATION FOR THE APPROVED INDICATION OF REMISSION INDUCTION IN ADULT ACUTE NONLYMPHOCYTIC LEUKEMIA:

IN COMBINATION[6,7]—For patients under age 60, Cerubidine 45 mg/m^2/day IV on days 1, 2, 3 of the first course and on days 1, 2 of subsequent courses AND cytosine arabinoside 100 mg/m^2/day IV infusion daily for 7 days for the first course and for 5 days for subsequent courses.

For patients 60 years of age and above, Cerubidine 30 mg/m^2/day IV on days 1, 2, 3 of the first course and on days 1, 2 of subsequent courses AND cytosine arabinoside 100 mg/m^2/day IV infusion daily for 7 days for the first course and for 5 days for subsequent courses.[7] This Cerubidine dose-reduction is based on a single study and may not be appropriate if optimal supportive care is available.

The attainment of a normal-appearing bone marrow may require up to three courses of induction therapy. Evaluation of the bone marrow following recovery from the previous course of induction therapy determines whether a further course of induction treatment is required.

REPRESENTATIVE DOSE SCHEDULE AND COMBINATION FOR THE APPROVED INDICATION OF REMISSION INDUCTION IN PEDIATRIC ACUTE LYMPHOCYTIC LEUKEMIA:

IN COMBINATION—Cerubidine 25 mg/m^2 IV on day 1 every week, vincristine 1.5 mg/m^2 IV on day 1 every week, prednisone 40 mg/m^2 PO daily. Generally, a complete remission will be obtained within four such courses of therapy; however, if after four courses the patient is in partial remission, an additional one or, if necessary, two courses may be given in an effort to obtain a complete remission.

In children less than 2 years of age or below 0.5 m^2 body surface area, it has been recommended that the Cerubidine dosage calculation should be based on weight (1.0 mg/kg) instead of body surface area.[15]

REPRESENTATIVE DOSE SCHEDULES AND COMBINATION FOR THE APPROVED INDICATION OF REMISSION INDUCTION IN ADULT ACUTE LYMPHOCYTIC LEUKEMIA:

IN COMBINATION[8]—Cerubidine 45 mg/m^2/day IV on days 1, 2, and 3 AND vincristine 2 mg IV on days 1, 8, and 15; prednisone 40 mg/m^2/day PO on days 1 thru 22, then tapered between days 22 to 29; L-asparaginase 500 IU/kg/day × 10 days IV on days 22 thru 32.

The contents of a vial should be reconstituted with 4 mL of Sterile Water for Injection, USP, and agitated gently until the material has completely dissolved. The withdrawable vial contents provide 20 mg of daunorubicin activity, with 5 mg of daunorubicin activity per mL. The desired dose is withdrawn into a syringe containing 10 mL to 15 mL of normal saline and then injected into the tubing or sidearm of a rapidly flowing IV infusion of 5 percent glucose or normal saline solution. Cerubidine should not be administered mixed with other drugs or heparin. The reconstituted solution is stable for 24 hours at room temperature and 48 hours under refrigeration. It should be protected from exposure to sunlight. Procedures for proper handling and disposal of anticancer drugs should be considered. Several guidelines on this subject have been published.[9-14] There is no general agreement that all of the procedures recommended in the guidelines are necessary or appropriate.

HOW SUPPLIED
Cerubidine® (daunorubicin hydrochloride) for Injection, Wyeth®, is available in butyl-rubber-stoppered vials, each containing 20 mg of base activity (21.4 mg as the hydrochloride salt) and 100 mg of mannitol, as a sterile reddish lyophilized powder. When reconstituted with 4 mL of Sterile Water for Injection, USP, each mL contains 5 mg of daunorubicin activity. Each package contains 10 vials. NDC 0008-4155-01.

STORAGE
(+15° to +25° C).

REFERENCES
1. Gilladoga AC, Manuel C, Tan CTC, et al: The cardiotoxicity of Adriamycin and daunomycin in children. Cancer 37: 1070–1078, 1976.
2. Halzun JF, Wagner HR, Gaeta JF, et al: Daunorubicin cardiac toxicity in children with acute lymphocytic leukemia. Cancer 33: 545–554, 1974.
3. Von Hoff DD, Rozencweig M, Layard M, et al: Daunomycin-induced cardiotoxicity in children and adults: a review of 110 cases. Am J Med 62: 200–208, 1977.
4. Goorin AM, Borrow KM, Goldman A, et al: Congestive heart failure due to Adriamycin cardiotoxicity: its natural history in children. Cancer 47: 2810–2816, 1981.
5. Praga C, Bretta G, Vigo PL, et al: Adriamycin cardiotoxicity: A survey of 1273 patients. Cancer Treat Rep 63: 827–834, 1979.
6. Rai KR, Holland JF, Glidewell O, et al: Treatment of acute myelocytic leukemia: a study by Cancer and Leukemia Group B. Blood 58: 1203–1212, 1981.
7. Yates J, Glidewell O, Wiernik P, et al: Cytosine arabinoside with daunorubicin or Adriamycin for therapy of acute myelocytic leukemia: a CALGB study. Blood 60: 454–462, 1982.
8. Gottlieb AJ, Weinberg V, Ellison RR: Efficacy of daunorubicin in the therapy of adult acute lymphocytic leukemia: a prospective randomized trial by Cancer and Leukemia Group B. Blood 64: 267–274, 1984.
9. Recommendations for the Safe Handling of Parenteral Antineoplastic Drugs. NIH Publication No. 83-2621. For sale by the Superintendent of Documents, U.S. Government Printing Office, Washington, D.C. 20402.
10. AMA Council Report. Guidelines for Handling Parenteral Antineoplastics. JAMA, March 15, 1985.
11. National Study Commission on Cytotoxic Exposure—Recommendations for Handling Cytotoxic Agents. Available from Louis P. Jeffrey, Sc. D., Director of Pharmacy Services, Rhode Island Hospital, 593 Eddy Street, Providence, Rhode Island 02902.
12. Clinical Oncological Society of Australia: Guidelines and recommendations for safe handling of antineoplastic agents. Med J Australia 1 :426–428, 1983.
13. Jones RB, et al: Safe handling of chemotherapeutic agents: A report from the Mount Sinai Medical Center, Ca-A Cancer Journal for Clinicians Sept/Oct, 258–263, 1983.
14. American Society of Hospital Pharmacists technical assistance bulletin on handling cytotoxic drugs in hospitals. Am J Hosp Pharm 42 :131–137, 1985.
15. Sallan SE: Personal Communication, 1981.

Manufactured by RPS PROPHARM, France
by arrangement with RHONE-POULENC France
Distributed by WYETH-AYERST LABORATORIES INC., Philadelphia, PA 19101.

CHOLERA VACCINE, U.S.P.   ℞
[kol'er-ah vak'sēn]

DESCRIPTION
Each ml. contains 8 units each serotype antigen (Ogawa and Inaba). The preservative is 0.5% phenol.

HOW SUPPLIED
Vials of 1.5 mL. and 20 mL.
For prescribing information write to Professional Service, Wyeth-Ayerst Laboratories, Box 8299, Philadelphia, PA 19101, or contact your local Wyeth-Ayerst representative.

COLLYRIUM for FRESH EYES   OTC
[ko-lir'e-um]
A neutral borate solution
EYE WASH

DESCRIPTION
Soothing Collyrium Eye Wash for Fresh Eyes is specially formulated to soothe, refresh, and cleanse irritated eyes. Collyrium Eye Wash is a neutral borate solution that contains boric acid, sodium borate, thimerosal (not more than 0.002% as a preservative) and water.

INDICATIONS
Patients are advised of the following. Use Collyrium Eye Wash to cleanse the eye, loosen foreign material, air pollutants or chlorinated water.

RECOMMENDED USES

Home—For emergency flushing of foreign bodies or whenever a soothing eye rinse is necessary.
Hospitals, dispensaries and clinics—For emergency flushing of chemicals or foreign bodies from the eye.

DOSAGE AND ADMINISTRATION

Patients are advised of the following. Twist off sealed, tamper-resistant top and discard. Rinse eye cup with clean water immediately before and after each use. Avoid contamination of rim and inside surfaces of cup. Fill cup one-half full with Collyrium Eye Wash. Apply cup tightly to the affected eye to prevent escape of the liquid and tilt head backward. Open eyelid wide and rotate eyeball to thoroughly wash eye. Rinse cup with clean water after use and recap by twisting threaded eye cup on bottle.

WARNINGS

Patients are advised of the following. Do not use if solution changes color or becomes cloudy, or with a wetting solution for contact lenses or other eye care products containing polyvinyl alcohol. This product contains thimerosal (not more than 0.002% as a preservative). Do not use this product if you are sensitive to mercury.
To avoid contamination do not touch tip of container to any surface. Replace cap after using. If you experience eye pain, changes in vision, continued redness, irritation of the eye, or if the condition worsens or persists, consult a doctor. Obtain immediate medical treatment for all open wounds in or near the eyes.
Keep this and all medication out of the reach of children. Keep bottle tightly closed at Room Temperature, Approx. 77° F (25° C).

HOW SUPPLIED

Bottles of 6 FL. OZ. (177 mL) with eyecup.

COLLYRIUM FRESH™   OTC

[ko-lir'e-um]
Eye Drops
Lubricant • Redness Reliever

DESCRIPTION

Collyrium Fresh is a specially formulated sterile eye drop which can be used, up to 4 times daily, to relieve redness and discomfort due to minor eye irritations caused by dust, smoke, smog, swimming, or sun glare.
The active ingredients are tetrahydrozoline HCl (0.05%) and glycerin (1.0%). Other ingredients include benzalkonium chloride (0.01%) and edetate disodium (0.1%) as preservatives, boric acid, hydrochloric acid and sodium borate.

INDICATIONS

Patients are advised of the following. For the temporary relief of redness due to minor eye irritations or discomfort due to burning or exposure to wind or sun.

DOSAGE AND ADMINISTRATION

Patients are advised to tilt head back, gently pull down lower eyelid, and instill 1 to 2 drops in the affected eye(s). Then, the lower lid should be released, the eye closed and the eye rotated once or twice before opening. This procedure can be repeated up to four times daily, or as directed by a physician.

WARNINGS

Patients are advised of the following. Do not use if solution changes color or becomes cloudy. Remove contact lenses before using. If you have glaucoma, do not use this product except under the advice and supervision of a physician. Overuse of this product may produce increased redness of the eye. To avoid contamination, do not touch tip of container to any surface. Replace cap after using. If you experience eye pain, changes in vision, continued redness or irritation of the eye, or if the condition worsens or persists for more than 72 hours, discontinue use and consult a physician.
Keep this and all medication out of the reach of children. The product's carton should be retained for complete product information.
Keep bottle tightly closed at Room Temperature, Approx. 77° F (25° C).

HOW SUPPLIED

Bottles of 0.5 FL. OZ. (15 mL) with built-in eye dropper.

CORDARONE®   ℞

[kŏr'dă-rōn]
(amiodarone HCl)
Tablets

DESCRIPTION

Cordarone is a member of a new class of antiarrhythmic drugs with predominantly Class III (Vaughan Williams' classification) effects, available for oral administration as white, scored tablets containing 200 mg of amiodarone hydrochloride. The inactive ingredients present are colloidal silicon dioxide, lactose, magnesium stearate, povidone, and starch.

Cordarone is a benzofuran derivative: 2-butyl-3-benzofuranyl 4-[2-(diethylamino)-ethoxy]-3-5-diiodophenyl ketone, hydrochloride. It is not chemically related to any other available antiarrhythmic drug.
The structural formula is as follows:

$C_{25}H_{29}I_2NO_3 \cdot HCl$ Molecular Weight: 681.8

Amiodarone HCl is a white to cream-colored crystalline powder. It is slightly soluble in water, soluble in alcohol, and freely soluble in chloroform. It contains 37.3% iodine by weight.

CLINICAL PHARMACOLOGY

ELECTROPHYSIOLOGY/MECHANISMS OF ACTION

In animals, Cordarone is effective in the prevention or suppression of experimentally induced arrhythmias. The antiarrhythmic effect of Cordarone may be due to at least two major properties: 1) a prolongation of the myocardial cell-action potential duration and refractory period and 2) noncompetitive alpha- and beta-adrenergic inhibition.
Cordarone prolongs the duration of the action potential of all cardiac fibers while causing minimal reduction of dV/dt (maximal upstroke velocity of the action potential). The refractory period is prolonged in all cardiac tissues. Cordarone increases the cardiac refractory period without influencing resting membrane potential, except in automatic cells where the slope of the prepotential is reduced, generally reducing automaticity. These electrophysiologic effects are reflected in a decreased sinus rate of 15 to 20%, increased PR and QT intervals of about 10%, the development of U-waves, and changes in T-wave contour. These changes should not require discontinuation of Cordarone as they are evidence of its pharmacological action, although Cordarone can cause marked sinus bradycardia or sinus arrest and heart block. On rare occasions, QT prolongation has been associated with worsening of arrhythmia (see "Warnings").

HEMODYNAMICS

In animal studies and after intravenous administration in man, Cordarone relaxes vascular smooth muscle, reduces peripheral vascular resistance (afterload), and slightly increases cardiac index. After oral dosing, however, Cordarone produces no significant change in left ventricular ejection fraction (LVEF), even in patients with depressed LVEF. After acute intravenous dosing in man, Cordarone may have a mild negative inotropic effect.

PHARMACOKINETICS

Following oral administration in man, Cordarone is slowly and variably absorbed. The bioavailability of Cordarone is approximately 50%, but has varied between 35 and 65% in various studies. Maximum plasma concentrations are attained 3 to 7 hours after a single dose. Despite this, the onset of action may occur in 2 to 3 days, but more commonly takes 1 to 3 weeks, even with loading doses. Plasma concentrations with chronic dosing at 100 to 600 mg/day are approximately dose proportional, with a mean 0.5 mg/L increase for each 100 mg/day. These means, however, include considerable individual variability.
Cordarone has a very large but variable volume of distribution, averaging about 60 L/kg because of extensive accumulation in various sites, especially adipose tissue and highly perfused organs, such as the liver, lung, and spleen. One major metabolite of Cordarone, desethylamiodarone, has been identified in man. It accumulates to an even greater extent in almost all tissues. The pharmacological activity of this metabolite, however, is not known. During chronic treatment, the plasma ratio of metabolite to parent compound is approximately one.
The main route of elimination is via hepatic excretion into bile, and some enterohepatic recirculation may occur. However, its kinetics in patients with hepatic insufficiency have not been elucidated. Cordarone has a very low plasma clearance with negligible renal excretion, so that it does not appear necessary to modify the dose in patients with renal failure. In patients with renal impairment, the plasma concentration of Cordarone is not elevated. Neither Cordarone nor its metabolite is dialyzable.
In patients, following discontinuation of chronic oral therapy, Cordarone has been shown to have a biphasic elimination with an initial one-half reduction of plasma levels after 2.5 to 10 days. A much slower terminal plasma-elimination phase shows a half-life of the parent compound ranging from 26 to 107 days, with a mean of approximately 53 days and most patients in the 40- to 55-day range. In the absence of a

loading-dose period, steady-state plasma concentrations, at constant oral dosing, would therefore be reached between 130 and 535 days, with an average of 265 days. For the metabolite, the mean plasma-elimination half-life was approximately 61 days. These data probably reflect an initial elimination of the drug from well-perfused tissue (the 2.5- to 10-day half-life phase), followed by a terminal phase representing extremely slow elimination from poorly perfused tissue compartments such as fat.
The considerable intersubject variation in both phases of elimination, as well as uncertainty as to what compartment is critical to drug effect, requires attention to individual responses once arrhythmia control is achieved with loading doses because the correct maintenance dose is determined, in part, by the elimination rates. Daily maintenance doses of Cordarone should be based on individual patient requirements (see "Dosage and Administration").
Cordarone and its metabolite have a limited transplacental transfer of approximately 10 to 50%. The parent drug and its metabolite have been detected in breast milk.
Cordarone is highly protein-bound (approximately 96%). Although electrophysiologic effects, such as prolongation of QTc, can be seen within hours after a parenteral dose of Cordarone, effects on abnormal rhythms are not seen before 2 to 3 days and usually require 1 to 3 weeks, even when a loading dose is used. There may be a continued increase in effect for longer periods still. There is evidence that the time to effect is shorter when a loading-dose regimen is used. Consistent with the slow rate of elimination, antiarrhythmic effects persist for weeks or months after Cordarone is discontinued, but the time of recurrence is variable and unpredictable. In general, when the drug is resumed after recurrence of the arrhythmia, control is established relatively rapidly compared to the initial response, presumably because tissue stores were not wholly depleted at the time of recurrence.

PHARMACODYNAMICS

There is no well-established relationship of plasma concentration to effectiveness, but it does appear that concentrations much below 1 mg/L are often ineffective and that levels above 2.5 mg/L are generally not needed. Within individuals dose reductions and ensuing decreased plasma concentrations can result in loss of arrhythmia control. Plasma-concentration measurements can be used to identify patients whose levels are unusually low, and who might benefit from a dose increase, or unusually high, and who might have dosage reduction in the hope of minimizing side effects. Some observations have suggested a plasma concentration, dose, or dose/duration relationship for side effects such as pulmonary fibrosis, liver-enzyme elevations, corneal deposits and facial pigmentation, peripheral neuropathy, gastrointestinal and central nervous system effects.

MONITORING EFFECTIVENESS

Predicting the effectiveness of any antiarrhythmic agent in long-term prevention of recurrent ventricular tachycardia and ventricular fibrillation is difficult and controversial, with highly qualified investigators recommending use of ambulatory monitoring, programmed electrical stimulation with various stimulation regimens, or a combination of these, to assess response. There is no present consensus on many aspects of how best to assess effectiveness, but there is a reasonable consensus on some aspects:
1. If a patient with a history of cardiac arrest does not manifest a hemodynamically unstable arrhythmia during electrocardiographic monitoring prior to treatment, assessment of the effectiveness of Cordarone requires some provocative approach, either exercise or programmed electrical stimulation (PES).
2. Whether provocation is also needed in patients who do manifest their life-threatening arrhythmia spontaneously is not settled, but there are reasons to consider PES or other provocation in such patients. In the fraction of patients whose PES-inducible arrhythmia can be made noninducible by Cordarone (a fraction that has varied widely in various series from less than 10% to almost 40%, perhaps due to different stimulation criteria), the prognosis has been almost uniformly excellent, with very low recurrence (ventricular tachycardia or sudden death) rates. More controversial is the meaning of continued inducibility. There has been an impression that continued inducibility in Cordarone patients may not foretell a poor prognosis but, in fact, many observers have found greater recurrence rates in patients who remain inducible than in those who do not. A number of criteria have been proposed, however, for identifying patients who remain inducible but who seem likely nonetheless to do well on Cordarone. These criteria include increased difficulty of induction (more stimuli or more rapid stimuli), which has been reported to predict a lower rate of recurrence, and ability to tolerate the induced ventricular tachycardia without severe symptoms, a finding that has been reported to correlate with better survival but not with lower recurrence rates. While these criteria require confirmation and further study in general, *easier* inducibility or

Continued on next page

Wyeth-Ayerst—Cont.

poorer tolerance of the induced arrhythmia should suggest consideration of a need to revise treatment.

Several predictors of success not based on PES have also been suggested, including complete elimination of all non-sustained ventricular tachycardia on ambulatory monitoring and very low premature ventricular-beat rates (less than 1 VPB/1,000 normal beats).

While these issues remain unsettled for Cordarone, as for other agents, the prescriber of Cordarone should have access to (direct or through referral), and familiarity with, the full range of evaluatory procedures used in the care of patients with life-threatening arrhythmias.

It is difficult to describe the effectiveness rates of Cordarone, as these depend on the specific arrhythmia treated, the success criteria used, the underlying cardiac disease of the patient, the number of drugs tried before resorting to Cordarone, the duration of follow-up, the dose of Cordarone, the use of additional antiarrhythmic agents, and many other factors. As Cordarone has been studied principally in patients with refractory life-threatening ventricular arrhythmias, in whom drug therapy must be selected on the basis of response and cannot be assigned arbitrarily, randomized comparisons with other agents or placebo have not been possible. Reports of series of treated patients with a history of cardiac arrest and mean follow-up of one year or more have given mortality (due to arrhythmia) rates that were highly variable, ranging from less than 5% to over 30%, with most series in the range of 10 to 15%. Overall arrhythmia-recurrence rates (fatal and nonfatal) also were highly variable, as noted above, depended on response to PES and other measures, and depend on whether patients who do not seem to respond initially are included. In most cases, considering only patients who seemed to respond well enough to be placed on long-term treatment, recurrence rates have ranged from 20 to 40% in series with a mean follow-up of a year or more.

INDICATIONS AND USAGE

Because of its life-threatening side effects and the substantial management difficulties associated with its use (see "Warnings" below), Cordarone is indicated only for the treatment of the following documented, life-threatening recurrent ventricular arrhythmias when these have not responded to documented adequate doses of other available antiarrhythmics or when alternative agents could not be tolerated.

1. Recurrent ventricular fibrillation.
2. Recurrent hemodynamically unstable ventricular tachycardia.

As is the case for other antiarrhythmic agents, there is no evidence from controlled trials that the use of Cordarone favorably affects survival.

Cordarone should be used only by physicians familiar with and with access to (directly or through referral) the use of all available modalities for treating recurrent life-threatening ventricular arrhythmias, and who have access to appropriate monitoring facilities, including in-hospital and ambulatory continuous electrocardiographic monitoring and electrophysiologic techniques. Because of the life-threatening nature of the arrhythmias treated, potential interactions with prior therapy, and potential exacerbation of the arrhythmia, initiation of therapy with Cordarone should be carried out in the hospital.

CONTRAINDICATIONS

Cordarone is contraindicated in severe sinus-node dysfunction, causing marked sinus bradycardia; second- and third-degree atrioventricular block; and when episodes of bradycardia have caused syncope (except when used in conjunction with a pacemaker).

WARNINGS

Cordarone is intended for use only in patients with the indicated life-threatening arrhythmias because its use is accompanied by substantial toxicity.

Cordarone has several potentially fatal toxicities, the most important of which is pulmonary toxicity (interstitial pneumonitis/alveolitis) that has resulted in clinically manifest disease at rates as high as 10 to 15% in some series of patients with ventricular arrhythmias given doses around 400 mg/day, and as abnormal diffusion capacity without symptoms in a much higher percentage of patients. Pulmonary toxicity has been fatal about 10% of the time. Liver injury is common with Cordarone, but is usually mild and evidenced only by abnormal liver enzymes. Overt liver disease can occur, however, and has been fatal in a few cases. Like other antiarrhythmics, Cordarone can exacerbate the arrhythmia, e.g., by making the arrhythmia less well tolerated or more difficult to reverse. This has occurred in 2 to 5% of patients in various series, and significant heart block or sinus bradycardia has been seen in 2 to 5%. All

of these events should be manageable in the proper clinical setting in most cases. Although the frequency of such proarrhythmic events does not appear greater with Cordarone than with many other agents used in this population, the effects are prolonged when they occur.

Even in patients at high risk of arrhythmic death, in whom the toxicity of Cordarone is an acceptable risk, Cordarone poses major management problems that could be life-threatening in a population at risk of sudden death, so that every effort should be made to utilize alternative agents first.

The difficulty of using Cordarone effectively and safely itself poses a significant risk to patients. Patients with the indicated arrhythmias must be hospitalized while the loading dose of Cordarone is given, and a response generally requires at least one week, usually two or more. Because absorption and elimination are variable, maintenance-dose selection is difficult, and it is not unusual to require dosage decrease or discontinuation of treatment. In a retrospective survey of 192 patients with ventricular tachyarrhythmias, 84 required dose reduction and 18 required at least temporary discontinuation because of adverse effects, and several series have reported 15 to 20% overall frequencies of discontinuation due to adverse reactions. The time at which a previously controlled life-threatening arrhythmia will recur after discontinuation or dose adjustment is unpredictable, ranging from weeks to months. The patient is obviously at great risk during this time and may need prolonged hospitalization. Attempts to substitute other antiarrhythmic agents when Cordarone must be stopped will be made difficult by the gradually, but unpredictably, changing amiodarone body burden. A similar problem exists when Cordarone is not effective; it still poses the risk of an interaction with whatever subsequent treatment is tried.

PULMONARY TOXICITY

Cordarone causes a clinical syndrome of progressive dyspnea and cough accompanied by functional, radiographic, gallium-scan, and pathological data showing a pulmonary interstitial process, sometimes called alveolitis. The frequency of pulmonary toxicity has generally been low, varying from 2 to 7% in most published reports, but recent preliminary reports have found rates of 11 to 15% in patients treated for more than a year on average and there is evidence of increasing frequency with time and/or daily or cumulative dose. Although the syndrome is usually reversible when Cordarone is discontinued, with or without steroid therapy, fatalities have occurred in about 10% of cases. Any new respiratory symptom in a patient receiving Cordarone should suggest the possibility of pulmonary toxicity and lead to clinical and radiographic evaluation, with gallium-scan and pulmonary-function evaluation if needed. Particular care should be taken not to presume that such symptoms are related to cardiac failure. Again, diffusion capacity appears to be the pulmonary-function test most likely to show abnormality. Evidence of toxicity should lead, at a minimum, to dose reduction, and preferably to withdrawal of the drug to establish reversibility. In some cases rechallenge at a lower dose has not resulted in return of toxicity.

Periodic chest X rays and clinical evaluation (every 3 to 6 months) are recommended and baseline pulmonary-function tests, including diffusion capacity, should be obtained.

WORSENED ARRHYTHMIA

Cordarone, like other antiarrhythmics, can cause serious exacerbation of the presenting arrhythmia, a risk that may be enhanced by the presence of concomitant antiarrhythmics. Exacerbation has been reported in about 2 to 5% in most series, and has included new ventricular fibrillation, incessant ventricular tachycardia, increased resistance to cardioversion, and polymorphic ventricular tachycardia associated with QT prolongation (Torsade de Pointes).

In addition, Cordarone has caused symptomatic bradycardia or sinus arrest with suppression of escape foci in 2 to 4% of patients.

LIVER INJURY

Elevations of hepatic enzyme levels are seen frequently in patients exposed to Cordarone and in most cases are asymptomatic. If the increase exceeds three times normal, or doubles in a patient with an elevated baseline, discontinuation of Cordarone or dosage reduction should be considered. In a few cases in which biopsy has been done, the histology has resembled that of alcoholic hepatitis or cirrhosis. Hepatic failure has been a rare cause of death in patients treated with Cordarone.

PRECAUTIONS

CORNEAL MICRODEPOSITS; IMPAIRMENT OF VISION

Corneal microdeposits appear in the majority of adults treated with Cordarone. They are usually discernible only by slit-lamp examination, but give rise to symptoms such as visual halos or blurred vision in as many as 10% of patients. Corneal microdeposits are reversible upon reduction of dose

or termination of treatment. Asymptomatic microdeposits are not a reason to reduce dose or discontinue treatment.

PHOTOSENSITIVITY

Cordarone has induced photosensitization in about 10% of patients; some protection may be afforded by the use of sun-barrier creams or protective clothing. During long-term treatment, a blue-gray discoloration of the exposed skin may occur. The risk may be increased in patients of fair complexion or those with excessive sun exposure, and may be related to cumulative dose and duration of therapy.

THYROID ABNORMALITIES

Cordarone inhibits peripheral conversion of thyroxine (T_4) to triiodothyronine (T_3) and may cause increased thyroxine levels, decreased T_3 levels, and increased levels of inactive reverse T_3 (rT_3) in clinically euthyroid patients. It is also a potential source of large amounts of inorganic iodine. Because of its release of inorganic iodine, or perhaps for other reasons, Cordarone can cause either hypothyroidism or hyperthyroidism. Thyroid function should be monitored prior to treatment and periodically thereafter, particularly in elderly patients, and in any patient with a history of thyroid nodules, goiter, or other thyroid dysfunction. Because of the slow elimination of Cordarone and its metabolites, high plasma iodide levels, altered thyroid function, and abnormal thyroid function tests may persist for several weeks or even months following Cordarone withdrawal.

Hypothyroidism has been reported in 2 to 4% of patients in most series, but in 8 to 10% in some series. This condition may be identified by relevant clinical symptoms and particularly by elevated serum TSH levels. In some clinically hypothyroid amiodarone-treated patients, free thyroxine index values may be normal. Hypothyroidism is best managed by Cordarone dose reduction and/or thyroid hormone supplement. However, therapy must be individualized, and it may be necessary to discontinue Cordarone in some patients. Hyperthyroidism occurs in about 2% of patients receiving Cordarone, but the incidence may be higher among patients with prior inadequate dietary iodine intake. Cordarone-induced hyperthyroidism usually poses a greater hazard to the patient than hypothyroidism because of the possibility of arrhythmia breakthrough or aggravation. In fact, IF ANY NEW SIGNS OF ARRHYTHMIA APPEAR, THE POSSIBILITY OF HYPERTHYROIDISM SHOULD BE CONSIDERED. Hyperthyroidism is best identified by relevant clinical symptoms and signs, accompanied usually by abnormally elevated levels of serum T_3 RIA, and further elevations of serum T_4, and a subnormal serum TSH level (using a sufficiently sensitive TSH assay). The finding of a flat TSH response to TRH is confirmatory of hyperthyroidism and may be sought in equivocal cases. Since arrhythmia breakthroughs may accompany Cordarone-induced hyperthyroidism, aggressive medical treatment is indicated, including, if possible, dose reduction or withdrawal of Cordarone. The institution of antithyroid drugs, beta-adrenergic blockers and/or temporary corticosteroid therapy may be necessary. The action of antithyroid drugs may be especially delayed in amiodarone-induced thyrotoxicosis because of substantial quantities of preformed thyroid hormones stored in the gland. Radioactive iodine therapy is contraindicated because of the low radioiodine uptake associated with amiodarone-induced hyperthyroidism. Experience with thyroid surgery in this setting is extremely limited, and this form of therapy runs the theoretical risk of inducing thyroid storm. Cordarone-induced hyperthyroidism may be followed by a transient period of hypothyroidism.

HYPOTENSION POSTBYPASS

Rare occurrences of hypotension upon discontinuation of cardiopulmonary bypass during open-heart surgery in patients receiving Cordarone have been reported. The relationship of this event to Cordarone therapy is unknown.

LABORATORY TESTS

Elevations in liver enzymes (SGOT and SGPT) can occur. Liver enzymes in patients on relatively high maintenance doses should be monitored on a regular basis. Persistent significant elevations in the liver enzymes or hepatomegaly should alert the physician to consider reducing the maintenance dose of Cordarone or discontinuing therapy.

Cordarone alters the results of thyroid-function tests, causing an increase in serum T_4 and serum reverse T_3, and a decline in serum T_3 levels. Despite these biochemical changes, most patients remain clinically euthyroid.

DRUG INTERACTIONS

Although only a small number of drug-drug interactions with Cordarone have been explored formally, most of these have shown such an interaction. The potential for other interactions should be anticipated, particularly for drugs with potentially serious toxicity, such as other antiarrhythmics. If such drugs are needed, their dose should be reassessed and, where appropriate, plasma concentration measured.

In view of the long and variable half-life of Cordarone, potential for drug interactions exists not only with concomitant medication but also with drugs administered after discontinuation of Cordarone.

Digitalis

Administration of Cordarone to patients receiving digoxin therapy regularly results in an increase in the serum digoxin concentration that may reach toxic levels with resultant clinical toxicity. **On initiation of Cordarone, the need for digitalis therapy should be reviewed and the dose reduced by approximately 50% or discontinued.** If digitalis treatment is continued, serum levels should be closely monitored and patients observed for clinical evidence of toxicity. These precautions probably should apply to digitoxin administration as well.

Anticoagulants

Potentiation of warfarin-type anticoagulant response is almost always seen in patients receiving Cordarone and can result in serious or fatal bleeding. **The dose of the anticoagulant should be reduced by one-third to one-half, and prothrombin times should be monitored closely.**

Antiarrhythmic Agents

Other antiarrhythmic drugs, such as quinidine, procainamide, disopyramide, and phenytoin, have been used concurrently with Cordarone.

There have been case reports of increased steady-state levels of quinidine, procainamide, and phenytoin during concomitant therapy with Cordarone. In general, any added antiarrhythmic drug should be initiated at a lower than usual dose with careful monitoring.

In general, combination of Cordarone with other antiarrhythmic therapy should be reserved for patients with life-threatening ventricular arrhythmias who are incompletely responsive to a single agent or incompletely responsive to Cordarone. During transfer to Cordarone the dose levels of previously administered agents should be reduced by 30 to 50% several days after the addition of Cordarone, when arrhythmia suppression should be beginning. The continued need for the other antiarrhythmic agent should be reviewed after the effects of Cordarone have been established, and discontinuation ordinarily should be attempted. If the treatment is continued, these patients should be particularly carefully monitored for adverse effects, especially conduction disturbances and exacerbation of tachyarrhythmias, as Cordarone is continued. In Cordarone-treated patients who require additional antiarrhythmic therapy, the initial dose of such agents should be approximately half of the usual recommended dose.

Cordarone should be used with caution in patients receiving beta-blocking agents or calcium antagonists because of the possible potentiation of bradycardia, sinus arrest, or AV block; if necessary, Cordarone can continue to be used after insertion of a pacemaker in patients with severe bradycardia or sinus arrest.

[See table above].

ELECTROLYTE DISTURBANCES

Since antiarrhythmic drugs may be ineffective or may be arrhythmogenic in patients with hypokalemia, any potassium or magnesium deficiency should be corrected before instituting Cordarone therapy.

CARCINOGENESIS, MUTAGENESIS, IMPAIRMENT OF FERTILITY

Cordarone reduced fertility of male and female rats at a dose level of 90 mg/kg/day (8 × highest recommended human maintenance dose). Cordarone caused a statistically significant, dose-related increase in the incidence of thyroid tumors (follicular adenoma and/or carcinoma) in rats. The incidence of thyroid tumors was greater than control even at the lowest dose level of Cordarone tested, i.e., 5 mg/kg/day or approximately equal to ½ the highest recommended human maintenance dose. Mutagenicity studies (Ames, micronucleus, and lysogenic tests) with Cordarone were negative.

PREGNANCY: PREGNANCY CATEGORY C

Cordarone has been shown to be embryotoxic (increased fetal resorption and growth retardation) in the rat when given orally at a dose of 200 mg/kg/day (18 times the maximum recommended maintenance dose). Similar findings have been noted in one strain of mice at a dose of 5 mg/kg/day (approximately ½ the maximum recommended maintenance dose) and higher, but not in a second strain nor in the rabbit at doses up to 100 mg/kg/day (9 times the maximum recommended maintenance dose).

In general, Cordarone should be used during pregnancy only if the potential benefit to the mother justifies the unknown risk to the fetus.

LABOR AND DELIVERY

It is not known whether the use of Cordarone during labor or delivery has any immediate or delayed adverse effects. Preclinical studies in rodents have not shown any effect of Cordarone on the duration of gestation or on parturition.

NURSING MOTHERS

Cordarone is excreted in human milk, suggesting that breast-feeding could expose the nursing infant to a significant dose of the drug. Nursing offspring of lactating rats administered Cordarone have been shown to be less viable and have reduced body-weight gains. Therefore, when Cordarone therapy is indicated, the mother should be advised to discontinue nursing.

PEDIATRIC USE

The safety and effectiveness of Cordarone in children have not been established.

SUMMARY OF DRUG INTERACTIONS WITH CORDARONE

Concomitant Drug	Onset (days)	Interaction — Magnitude	Recommended Dose Reduction of Concomitant Drug
Warfarin	3 to 4	Increases prothrombin time by 100%	↓ ⅓ to ½
Digoxin	1	Increases serum concentration by 70%	↓ ½
Quinidine	2	Increases serum concentration by 33%	↓ ⅓ to ½ (or discontinue)
Procainamide	<7	Increases plasma concentration by 55%, NAPA* concentration by 33%	↓ ⅓ (or discontinue)

*NAPA = n-acetyl procainamide.

ADVERSE REACTIONS

Adverse reactions have been very common in virtually all series of patients treated with Cordarone for ventricular arrhythmias, with relatively large doses of drug (400 mg/day and above) occurring in about three-fourths of all patients and causing discontinuation in 7 to 18%. The most serious reactions are pulmonary toxicity, exacerbation of arrhythmia, and rare serious liver injury (see "Warnings"), but other adverse effects constitute important problems. They are often reversible with dose reduction and virtually always reversible with cessation of Cordarone treatment. Most of the adverse effects appear to become more frequent with continued treatment beyond six months, although rates appear to remain relatively constant beyond one year. The time and dose relationships of adverse effects are under continued study.

Neurologic problems are extremely common, occurring in 20 to 40% of patients and including malaise and fatigue, tremor and involuntary movements, poor coordination and gait, and peripheral neuropathy; they are rarely a reason to stop therapy and may respond to dose reductions.

Gastrointestinal complaints, most commonly nausea, vomiting, constipation, and anorexia, occur in about 25% of patients but rarely require discontinuation of drug. These commonly occur during high-dose administration (i.e., loading dose) and usually respond to dose reduction or divided doses. Asymptomatic corneal microdeposits are present in virtually all adult patients who have been on drug for more than 6 months. Some patients develop eye symptoms of halos, photophobia, and dry eyes. Vision is rarely affected and drug discontinuation is rarely needed.

Dermatological adverse reactions occur in about 15% of patients, with photosensitivity being most common (about 10%). Sunscreen and protection from sun exposure may be helpful, and drug discontinuation is not usually necessary. Prolonged exposure to Cordarone occasionally results in a blue-gray pigmentation. This is slowly and occasionally incompletely reversible on discontinuation of drug but is of cosmetic importance only.

Cardiovascular adverse reactions, other than exacerbation of the arrhythmias, include the uncommon occurrence of congestive heart failure (3%) and bradycardia. Bradycardia usually responds to dosage reduction but may require a pacemaker for control. CHF rarely requires drug discontinuation. Cardiac conduction abnormalities occur infrequently and are reversible on discontinuation of drug.

The following side-effect rates are based on a retrospective study of 241 patients treated for 2 to 1,515 days (mean 441.3 days).

The following side effects were reported in 10 to 33% of patients:

Gastrointestinal: Nausea and vomiting.

The following side effects were each reported in 4 to 9% of patients:

Dermatologic: Solar dermatitis/photosensitivity.

Neurologic: Malaise and fatigue, tremor/abnormal involuntary movements, lack of coordination, abnormal gait/ataxia, dizziness, paresthesias.

Gastrointestinal: Constipation, anorexia.

Ophthalmologic: Visual disturbances.

Hepatic: Abnormal liver-function tests.

Respiratory: Pulmonary inflammation or fibrosis.

The following side effects were each reported in 1 to 3% of patients:

Thyroid: Hypothyroidism, hyperthyroidism.

Neurologic: Decreased libido, insomnia, headache, sleep disturbances.

Cardiovascular: Congestive heart failure, cardiac arrhythmias, SA node dysfunction.

Gastrointestinal: Abdominal pain.

Hepatic: Nonspecific hepatic disorders.

Other: Flushing, abnormal taste and smell, edema, abnormal salivation, coagulation abnormalities.

The following side effects were each reported in less than 1% of patients:

Blue skin discoloration, rash, spontaneous ecchymosis, alopecia, hypotension, and cardiac conduction abnormalities.

Rare occurrences of hepatitis, cirrhosis, optic neuritis, epididymitis, vasculitis, pseudotumor cerebri, and thrombocytopenia have been reported in patients receiving Cordarone. The relationship of these events to Cordarone therapy has not been definitively established.

In surveys of almost 5,000 patients treated in open U.S. studies and in published reports of treatment with Cordarone, the adverse reactions most frequently requiring discontinuation of Cordarone included pulmonary infiltrates or fibrosis, paroxysmal ventricular tachycardia, congestive heart failure, and elevation of liver enzymes. Other symptoms causing discontinuations less often included visual disturbances, solar dermatitis, blue skin discoloration, hyperthyroidism and hypothyroidism.

OVERDOSAGE

There have been 3 reported cases of Cordarone overdose in which 3 to 8 grams were taken. There were no deaths or permanent sequelae. Animal studies indicate that Cordarone has a high oral LD_{50} (> 3,000 mg/kg).

In addition to general supportive measures, the patient's cardiac rhythm and blood pressure should be monitored, and if bradycardia ensues, a β-adrenergic agonist or a pacemaker may be used. Hypotension with inadequate tissue perfusion should be treated with positive inotropic and/or vasopressor agents. Neither Cordarone nor its metabolite is dialyzable.

DOSAGE AND ADMINISTRATION

BECAUSE OF THE UNIQUE PHARMACOKINETIC PROPERTIES, DIFFICULT DOSING SCHEDULE, AND SEVERITY OF THE SIDE EFFECTS IF PATIENTS ARE IMPROPERLY MONITORED, CORDARONE SHOULD BE ADMINISTERED ONLY BY PHYSICIANS WHO ARE EXPERIENCED IN THE TREATMENT OF LIFE-THREATENING ARRHYTHMIAS, WHO ARE THOROUGHLY FAMILIAR WITH THE RISKS AND BENEFITS OF CORDARONE THERAPY, AND WHO HAVE ACCESS TO LABORATORY FACILITIES CAPABLE OF ADEQUATELY MONITORING THE EFFECTIVENESS AND SIDE EFFECTS OF TREATMENT.

In order to insure that an antiarrhythmic effect will be observed without waiting several months, loading doses are required. A uniform, optimal dosage schedule for administration of Cordarone has not been determined. Individual patient titration is suggested according to the following guidelines.

For life-threatening ventricular arrhythmias, such as ventricular fibrillation or hemodynamically unstable ventricular tachycardia: Close monitoring of the patients is indicated during the loading phase, particularly until risk of recurrent ventricular tachycardia or fibrillation has abated. Because of the serious nature of the arrhythmia and the lack of predictable time course of effect, loading should be performed in a hospital setting. Loading doses of 800 to 1,600 mg/day are required for 1 to 3 weeks (occasionally longer) until initial therapeutic response occurs. (Administration of Cordarone in divided doses with meals is suggested for total daily doses of 1,000 mg or higher, or when gastrointestinal intolerance occurs.) If side effects become excessive, the dose should be reduced. Elimination of recurrence of ventricular fibrillation and tachycardia usually occurs within 1 to 3 weeks, along with reduction in complex and total ventricular ectopic beats.

Upon starting Cordarone therapy, an attempt should be made to gradually discontinue prior antiarrhythmic drugs (see section on "Drug Interactions"). When adequate arrhythmia control is achieved, or if side effects become prominent, Cordarone dose should be reduced to 600 to 800 mg/day for one month and then to the maintenance dose, usually 400 mg/day (see "Clinical Pharmacology"—"Monitoring Effectiveness"). Some patients may require larger maintenance doses, up to 600 mg/day, and some can be controlled on lower doses. Cordarone may be administered as a single daily dose, or in patients with severe gastrointestinal intolerance, as a b.i.d. dose. In each patient, the chronic maintenance dose should be determined according to antiarrhythmic effect as assessed by symptoms, Holter recordings, and/or programmed electrical stimulation and by patient tolerance. Plasma concentrations may be helpful in evaluating nonresponsiveness or unexpectedly severe toxicity (see "Clinical Pharmacology").

The lowest effective dose should be used to prevent the occurrence of side effects. In all instances, the physician must be guided by the severity of the individual patient's arrhythmia and response to therapy. When dosage adjustments are necessary, the patient should be closely monitored for an

Continued on next page

Wyeth-Ayerst—Cont.

extended period of time because of the long and variable half-life of Cordarone and the difficulty in predicting the time required to attain a new steady-state level of drug. Dosage suggestions are summarized below:
[See table below].

HOW SUPPLIED

Cordarone® (amiodarone HCl) Tablets, Wyeth®, are available in bottles of 60 tablets and in Redipak® cartons containing 100 tablets (10 blister strips of 10) as follows: 200 mg, NDC 0008-4188, round, convex, white to slightly cream-colored tablets, scored on one side and marked "WYETH" and "4188" on the reverse side.

Protect from light

Caution: Federal law prohibits dispensing without prescription.

Manufactured for
Wyeth-Ayerst Laboratories, Inc., Philadelphia, PA 19101
by Sanofi, S.A., Paris, France, by arrangement with
Sanofi Pharmaceuticals, Inc.
Shown in Product Identification Section, page 436

CYCRIN®   ℞

[sīc 'crĭn]

(medroxyprogesterone acetate tablets, USP)

CAUTION: Federal law prohibits dispensing without prescription.

> **WARNING**
> THE USE OF PROGESTATIONAL AGENTS DURING THE FIRST FOUR MONTHS OF PREGNANCY IS NOT RECOMMENDED.
> Progestational agents have been used, beginning with the first trimester of pregnancy, in an attempt to prevent habitual abortion or treat threatened abortion. There is no adequate evidence that such use is effective and there is evidence of potential harm to the fetus when such drugs are given during the first 4 months of pregnancy. Furthermore, in the vast majority of women, the cause of abortion is a defective ovum, which progestational agents could not be expected to influence. In addition, the use of progestational agents with their uterine-relaxant properties, in patients with fertilized defective ova may cause a delay in spontaneous abortion. Therefore, the use of such drugs during the first four months of pregnancy is not recommended. Several reports suggest an association between intrauterine exposure to female sex hormones and congenital anomalies, including congenital heart defects and limb reduction defects.[1-5] One study[4] estimated a 4.7-fold increased risk of limb reduction defects in infants exposed in utero to sex hormones (oral contraceptives, hormone withdrawal tests for pregnancy, or attempted treatment for threatened abortion). Some of these exposures were very short and involved only a few days of treatment. The data suggest that the risk of limb reduction defects in exposed fetuses is somewhat less than 1 in 1,000.
> If the patient is exposed to CYCRIN (medroxyprogesterone acetate tablets, USP) during the first 4 months of pregnancy, or if she becomes pregnant while taking this drug, she should be apprised of the potential risks to the fetus.

DESCRIPTION

CYCRIN Tablets contain medroxyprogesterone acetate, which is a derivative of progesterone. It is a white to off-white, odorless, crystalline powder, stable in air, melting between 200° and 210°C. It is freely soluble in chloroform, soluble in acetone and in dioxane, sparingly soluble in alcohol and in methanol, slightly soluble in ether and insoluble in water.
The chemical name for medroxyprogesterone acetate is Pregn-4-ene-3,20-dione, 17-(acetyloxy)-6-methyl-, (6α)-.
Its structural formula is:
[See Chemical Formula at top of next column].
CYCRIN is available in tablet form for oral administration. Each tablet contains 10 mg of medroxyprogesterone acetate and the following inactive ingredients: lactose, magnesium stearate, methylcellulose, microcrystalline cellulose, D&C Red No. 30, D&C Yellow No. 10, and talc.

CLINICAL PHARMACOLOGY

Medroxyprogesterone acetate, administered orally or parenterally in the recommended doses to women with adequate endogenous estrogen, transforms proliferative into secretory endometrium. Androgenic and anabolic effects have been noted, but the drug is apparently devoid of significant estrogenic activity. While parenterally administered medroxyprogesterone acetate inhibits gonadotropin production, which in turn prevents follicular maturation and ovulation, available data indicate that this does not occur when the usually recommended oral dosage is given as single daily doses.

INDICATIONS AND USAGE

Secondary amenorrhea; abnormal uterine bleeding due to hormonal imbalance in the absence of organic pathology, such as fibroids or uterine cancer.

CONTRAINDICATIONS

1. Thrombophlebitis, thromboembolic disorders, cerebral apoplexy, or patients with a past history of these conditions.
2. Liver dysfunction or disease.
3. Known or suspected malignancy of breast or genital organs.
4. Undiagnosed vaginal bleeding.
5. Missed abortion.
6. As a diagnostic test for pregnancy.
7. Known sensitivity to medroxyprogesterone acetate.

WARNINGS

1. The physician should be alert to the earliest manifestations of thrombotic disorders (thrombophlebitis, cerebrovascular disorders, pulmonary embolism, and retinal thrombosis). Should any of these occur or be suspected, the drug should be discontinued immediately.
2. Beagle dogs treated with medroxyprogesterone acetate developed mammary nodules, some of which were malignant. Although nodules occasionally appeared in control animals, they were intermittent in nature, whereas the nodules in the drug-treated animals were larger, more numerous, persistent, and there were some breast malignancies with metastases. Their significance with respect to humans has not been established.
3. Discontinue medication pending examination if there is sudden partial or complete loss of vision, or if there is a sudden onset of proptosis, diplopia, or migraine. If examination reveals papilledema or retinal vascular lesions, medication should be withdrawn.
4. Detectable amounts of progestin have been identified in the milk of mothers receiving the drug. The effect of this on the nursing infant has not been determined.
5. Usage in pregnancy is not recommended (see Boxed Warning).
6. Retrospective studies of morbidity and mortality in Great Britain and studies of morbidity in the United States have shown a statistically significant association between thrombophlebitis, pulmonary embolism, and cerebral thrombosis and embolism and the use of oral contraceptives.[6-9] The estimate of the relative risk of thromboembolism in the study by Vessey and Doll[8] was about sevenfold, while Sartwell and associates[9] in the United States found a relative risk of 4.4, meaning that the users are several times as likely to undergo thromboembolic disease without evident cause as nonusers. The U.S. study also indicated that the risk did not persist after discontinuation of administration, and that it was not enhanced by long, continued administration. The U.S. study was not designed to evaluate a difference between products.

PRECAUTIONS

1. The pretreatment physical examination should include special reference to breasts and pelvic organs, as well as a Papanicolaou smear.
2. Because progestogens may cause some degree of fluid retention, conditions which might be influenced by this factor, such as epilepsy, migraine, asthma, cardiac or renal dysfunction, require careful observation.
3. In cases of breakthrough bleeding, as in all cases of irregular bleeding per vaginum, nonfunctional causes should be borne in mind. In cases of undiagnosed vaginal bleeding, adequate diagnostic measures are indicated.
4. Patients who have a history of psychic depression should be carefully observed and the drug discontinued, if the depression recurs to a serious degree.
5. Any possible influence of prolonged progestin therapy on pituitary, ovarian, adrenal, hepatic, or uterine functions awaits further study.
6. A decrease in glucose tolerance has been observed in a small percentage of patients on estrogen-progestin combination drugs. The mechanism of this decrease is obscure. For this reason, diabetic patients should be carefully observed while receiving progestin therapy.
7. The age of the patient constitutes no absolute limiting factor, although treatment with progestins may mask the onset of the climacteric.
8. The pathologist should be advised of progestin therapy when relevant specimens are submitted.
9. Because of the occasional occurrence of thrombotic disorders (thrombophlebitis, pulmonary embolism, retinal thrombosis, and cerebrovascular disorders) in patients taking estrogen-progestin combinations, and since the mechanism is obsure, the physician should be alert to the earliest manifestation of these disorders.
10. *Concomitant Use in Estrogen Replacement Therapy:* In postmenopausal estrogen replacement therapy, studies of the addition of a progestin for 7 or more days of a cycle of estrogen administration have reported a lowered incidence of endometrial hyperplasia. Morphological and biochemical studies of the endometrium suggest that 10 to 13 days of progestin are needed to provide maturation of the endometrium and to eliminate any hyperplastic changes. Whether this will provide protection from endometrial carcinoma has not been clearly established. There are possible additional risks which may be associated with the inclusion of progestin in estrogen replacement regimens. The potential risks include adverse effects on carbohydrate and lipid metabolism. The dosage used may be important in minimizing these adverse effects.

Information for the Patient
See Patient Information at the end of insert.

ADVERSE REACTIONS

Pregnancy—(See Boxed Warning for possible adverse effects on the fetus.)
Breast—Breast tenderness or galactorrhea has been reported rarely.
Skin—Sensitivity reactions consisting of urticaria, pruritus, edema, and generalized rash have occurred in an occasional patient. Acne, alopecia, and hirsutism have been reported in a few cases.
Thromboembolic Phenomena—Thromboembolic phenomena, including thrombophlebitis and pulmonary embolism, have been reported.
The following adverse reactions have been observed in women taking progestins, including CYCRIN (medroxyprogesterone acetate tablets, USP):
breakthrough bleeding
spotting
change in menstrual flow
amenorrhea
edema
change in weight (increase or decrease)
change in cervical erosion and cervical secretions
cholestatic jaundice
anaphylactoid reactions and anaphylaxis
rash (allergic) with and without pruritus
mental depression
pyrexia
insomnia
nausea
somnolence
A statistically significant association has been demonstrated between use of estrogen-progestin combination drugs and the following serious adverse reactions: thrombophlebitis; pulmonary embolism; and cerebral thrombosis and embolism. For this reason patients on progestin therapy should be carefully observed.
Although available evidence is suggestive of an association, such a relationship has been neither confirmed nor refuted for the following serious adverse reactions:
neuro-ocular lesions, eg, retinal thrombosis, and optic neuritis.
The following adverse reactions have been observed in patients receiving estrogen-progestin combination drugs:
rise in blood pressure in susceptible individuals
premenstrual-like syndrome
changes in libido
changes in appetite
cystitis-like syndrome

	Loading Dose (Daily)	Adjustment and Maintenance Dose (Daily)	
Ventricular Arrhythmias	1 to 3 weeks	~1 month	usual maintenance
	800 to 1,600 mg	600 to 800 mg	400 mg

headache
nervousness
dizziness
fatigue
backache
hirsutism
loss of scalp hair
erythema multiforme
erythema nodosum
hemorrhagic eruption
itching

In view of these observations, patients on progestin therapy should be carefully observed.

The following laboratory results may be altered by the use of estrogen-progestin combination drugs:

Increased sulfobromophthalein retention and other hepatic-function tests.

Coagulation tests: increase in prothrombin factors VII, VIII, IX, and X.

Metyrapone test.

Pregnanediol determination

Thyroid function: increase in PBI, and butanol extractable protein-bound iodine and decrease in T^3 uptake values.

DOSAGE AND ADMINISTRATION

Secondary Amenorrhea—CYCRIN (medroxyprogesterone acetate tablets, USP) may be given in dosages of 5 mg to 10 mg daily for from 5 to 10 days. A dose for inducing an optimal secretory transformation of an endometrium that has been adequately primed with either endogenous or exogenous estrogen is 10 mg of CYCRIN Tablets daily for 10 days. In cases of secondary amenorrhea, therapy may be started at any time. Progestin withdrawal bleeding usually occurs within 3–7 days after discontinuing therapy with CYCRIN.

Abnormal Uterine Bleeding Due to Hormonal Imbalance in the Absence of Organic Pathology—Beginning on the calculated 16th or 21st day of the menstrual cycle, 5 to 10 mg of medroxyprogesterone tablets may be given daily for from 5 to 10 days. To produce an optimal secretory transformation of an endometrium that has been adequately primed with either endogenous or exogenous estrogen, 10 mg of medroxyprogesterone tablets daily for 10 days, beginning on the 16th day of the cycle, is suggested. Progestin withdrawal bleeding usually occurs within three to seven days after discontinuing therapy with CYCRIN. Patients with a past history of recurrent episodes of abnormal uterine bleeding may benefit from planned menstrual cycling with CYCRIN.

HOW SUPPLIED

CYCRIN® (medroxyprogesterone acetate tablets, USP) for oral administration.

Each oval-shaped, peach, scored tablet, debossed with two hexagonal "C"s and with "CYCRIN", contains 10 mg of medroxyprogesterone acetate, in bottles of 100 (NDC 0046-0896-81), and in Cycle Packs of 10 (NDC 0046-0896-10).

The appearance of these tablets is a registered trademark of Wyeth-Ayerst Laboratories.

Store at room temperature (approximately 25°C).

REFERENCES

1. Gal I, Kirman B, Stern J: Hormonal pregnancy tests and congenital malformation *Nature* 1967; 216:83.
2. Levy EP, Cohen A, Fraser FC: Hormone treatment during pregnancy and congenital heart defects. *Lancet* 1973; 1:611.
3. Nora JJ, Nora AH; Birth defects and oral contraceptives. *Lancet* 1973; 1:941-942.
4. Janerich DT, Piper JM, Glebatis DM: Oral contraceptives and congenital limb-reduction defects. *N Engl J Med* 1974; 291:697-700.
5. Heinonen OP, Slone D, Monson RR, *et al:* Cardiovascular birth defects and antenatal exposure to female sex hormones. *N Engl J Med* 1977; 296:67-70.
6. Royal College of General Practitioners: Oral contraception and thromboembolic disease. *J Coll Gen Pract* 1967; 13:267-279.
7. Inman WHW, Vessey MP: Investigation of deaths from pulmonary, coronary, and cerebral thrombosis and embolism in women of childbearing age. *Br Med J* 1968; 2:193-199.
8. Vessey MP, Doll R: Investigation of relation between use of oral contraceptives and thromboembolic disease. A further report. *Br Med J* 1969; 2:651-657.
9. Sartwell PE, Masi AT, Arthes FG, et al: Thromboembolism and oral contraceptives: An epidemiological case-control study. *Am J Epidemiol* 1969; 90:365-380.

PATIENT INFORMATION

CYCRIN Tablets contain medroxyprogesterone acetate, a progesterone. The information below is that which the U.S. Food and Drug Administration requires be provided for all patients taking progesterones. The information below relates only to the risk to the unborn child associated with the use of progesterones during pregnancy. For further information on the use, side effects, and other risks associated with this product, ask your doctor.

WARNING FOR WOMEN

There is an increased risk of birth defects in children whose mothers take this drug during the first 4 months of pregnancy.

Medroxyprogesterone acetate is similar to the progesterone hormones naturally produced by the body. Progesterone and progesterone-like drugs are used to treat menstrual disorders, to test if the body is producing certain hormones, and to treat some forms of cancer in women.

They have been used as a test for pregnancy but such use is no longer considered safe, because of possible damage to a developing baby. Also, more rapid methods for testing for pregnancy are now available.

These drugs have also been used to prevent miscarriage in the first few months of pregnancy. No adequate evidence is available to show that they are effective for this purpose. Furthermore, most cases of early miscarriage are due to causes which could not be helped by these drugs.

There is an increased risk of birth defects, such as heart or limb defects, if progesterone and progesterone-like drugs are taken during the first 4 months of pregnancy. The exact risk of taking this drug early in pregnancy and having a baby with a birth defect is not known. However, one study found that babies born to women who had taken sex hormones (such as progesterone-like drugs) during the first 3 months of pregnancy were 4 to 5 times more likely to have abnormalities of the arms or legs than if their mothers had not taken such drugs. Some of these women had taken these drugs for only a few days. The chance that an infant whose mother had taken this drug will have this type of defect is about 1 in 1,000.

If you take CYCRIN, and later find you were pregnant when you took it, be sure to discuss this with your doctor as soon as possible.

Shown in Product Identification Section, page 436

DIPHTHERIA AND TETANUS TOXOIDS ADSORBED   ℞
[dif-the 're-ah and tet 'ah-nus tok 'soids]
aluminum phosphate adsorbed
ULTRAFINED®
PEDIATRIC

DESCRIPTION

The diphtheria toxoid component is prepared by cultivating a suitable strain of *Corynebacterium diphtheriae* on a modified Mueller's casein hydrolysate medium (J. Immunology 37:103, 1939). The tetanus toxoid component is prepared by cultivating a suitable strain of *Clostridium tetani* on a protein-free semisynthetic medium (Appl. Microbiol. *10:* 146, 1962). Formaldehyde is used as the toxoiding (detoxifying) agent for both diphtheria and tetanus toxins. The final product contains no more than 0.02 percent free formaldehyde and contains 0.01 percent thimerosal (mercury derivative) as preservative.

The aluminum content of the final product does not exceed 0.85 mg per 0.5 mL dose.

During processing, hydrochloric acid and sodium hydroxide are used to adjust the pH. Sodium chloride is added to the finished product to control isotonicity.

HOW SUPPLIED

Vials of 5 mL., 0008-0338-02, and 0.5 mL TUBEX® Sterile Cartridge-Needle Units (25 gauge × ⅝ inch needle), packages of 10, 0008-0338-01.

For prescribing information write to Professional Service, Wyeth-Ayerst Laboratories, Box 8299, Philadelphia, PA 19101, or contact your local Wyeth-Ayerst representative.

DIUCARDIN®   ℞
[dī"ū-car'din]
Brand of Hydroflumethiazide Tablets, USP
A diuretic-antihypertensive agent

CAUTION: Federal law prohibits dispensing without prescription.

DESCRIPTION

DIUCARDIN® (hydroflumethiazide) is an oral thiazide (benzothiadiazide) diuretic-antihypertensive agent.

DIUCARDIN is available as 50 mg tablets for oral administration.

Chemical name: 3,4-Dihydro-6-(trifluoromethyl)-2H-1,2,4-benzothiadiazine-7-sulfonamide 1,1-dioxide.

Structural formula:

Hydroflumethiazide is an odorless white to cream colored, finely divided, crystalline powder. It has a melting point between 270° and 275° C. Hydroflumethiazide is freely soluble in acetone, soluble in alcohol, and slightly soluble in water.

The inactive ingredients contained in DIUCARDIN Tablets are: lactose, magnesium stearate, microcrystalline cellulose, povidone, and starch.

CLINICAL PHARMACOLOGY

Hydroflumethiazide is incompletely but fairly rapidly absorbed from the gastrointestinal tract. It appears to have a biphasic biological half-life with an estimated alpha-phase of about 2 hours and an estimated beta-phase of about 17 hours; it has a metabolite with a longer half-life, which is extensively bound to the red blood cells. Hydroflumethiazide is excreted in the urine; its metabolite has also been detected in the urine.

The mechanism of action results in an interference with the renal tubular mechanism of electrolyte reabsorption. At maximal therapeutic dosage all thiazides are approximately equal in their diuretic potency. The mechanism whereby thiazides function in the control of hypertension is unknown.

INDICATIONS AND USAGE

DIUCARDIN is indicated as adjunctive therapy in edema associated with congestive heart failure, hepatic cirrhosis and corticosteroid and estrogen therapy.

DIUCARDIN has also been found useful in edema due to various forms of renal dysfunction such as: nephrotic syndrome; acute glomerulonephritis; and chronic renal failure.

DIUCARDIN is indicated in the management of hypertension either as the sole therapeutic agent or to enhance the effect of other antihypertensive drugs in the more severe forms of hypertension.

Usage in Pregnancy: The routine use of diuretics in an otherwise healthy woman is inappropriate and exposes mother and fetus to unnecessary hazard. Diuretics do not prevent development of toxemia of pregnancy, and there is no satisfactory evidence that they are useful in the treatment of developed toxemia.

Edema during pregnancy may arise from pathological causes or from the physiologic and mechanical consequences of pregnancy. Thiazides are indicated in pregnancy when edema is due to pathologic causes just as they are in the absence of pregnancy (however, see WARNINGS, below). Dependent edema in pregnancy, resulting from restriction of venous return by the expanded uterus, is properly treated through elevation of the lower extremities and use of support hose. Use of diuretics to lower intravascular volume in this case is illogical and unnecessary. There is hypervolemia during normal pregnancy which is harmful to neither the fetus nor the mother (in absence of cardiovascular disease), but which is associated with edema, including generalized edema, in the majority of pregnant women. If this edema produces discomfort, increased recumbency will often provide relief. In rare instances, this edema may cause extreme discomfort which is not relieved by rest. In these cases, a short course of diuretics may provide relief and may be appropriate.

CONTRAINDICATIONS

Anuria.

Hypersensitivity to this or other sulfonamide-derived drugs.

WARNINGS

DIUCARDIN should be used with caution in severe renal disease. In patients with renal disease, thiazides may precipitate azotemia. Cumulative effects of the drug may develop in patients with impaired renal function.

Thiazides should be used with caution in patients with impaired hepatic function or progressive liver disease, since minor alterations of fluid and electrolyte balance may precipitate hepatic coma.

Thiazides may add to or potentiate the action of other antihypertensive drugs. Potentiation occurs with ganglionic or peripheral adrenergic blocking drugs.

Sensitivity reactions may occur in patients with a history of allergy or bronchial asthma.

The possibility of exacerbation or activation of systemic lupus erythematosus has been reported.

PRECAUTIONS

General:

All patients receiving thiazide therapy should be observed for clinical signs of fluid or electrolyte imbalance: namely, hyponatremia, hypochloremic alkalosis, and hypokalemia. Serum and urine electrolyte determinations are particularly important when the patient is vomiting excessively or receiving parenteral fluids. Medication such as digitalis may also influence serum electrolytes. Warning signs, irrespective of cause, are: dryness of mouth, thirst, weakness, lethargy, drowsiness, restlessness, muscle pains or cramps, muscular fatigue, hypotension, oliguria, tachycardia, and gastrointestinal disturbances such as nausea and vomiting.

Continued on next page

Wyeth-Ayerst—Cont.

Hypokalemia may develop with thiazides as with any other potent diuretic, especially with brisk diuresis, when severe cirrhosis is present, or during concomitant use of corticosteroids or ACTH.

Interference with adequate oral electrolyte intake will also contribute to hypokalemia.

Digitalis therapy may exaggerate metabolic effects of hypokalemia especially with reference to myocardial activity. Any chloride deficit is generally mild and usually does not require specific treatment except under extraordinary circumstances (as in liver disease or renal disease). Dilutional hyponatremia may occur in edematous patients in hot weather; appropriate therapy is water restriction, rather than administration of salt, except in rare instances when the hyponatremia is life-threatening. In actual salt depletion, appropriate replacement is the therapy of choice.

Hyperuricemia may occur or frank gout may be precipitated in certain patients receiving thiazide therapy.

Insulin requirements in diabetic patients may be increased, decreased, or unchanged. Latent diabetes mellitus may become manifested during thiazide administration.

Thiazide drugs may increase the responsiveness to tubocurarine.

The antihypertensive effects of the drug may be enhanced in the postsympathectomy patient.

Thiazides may decrease arterial responsiveness to norepinephrine. This diminution is not sufficient to preclude effectiveness of the pressor agent for therapeutic use.

If progressive renal impairment becomes evident, as indicated by a rising nonprotein nitrogen or blood urea nitrogen, a careful reappraisal of therapy is necessary with consideration given to withholding or discontinuing diuretic therapy. Thiazides may decrease serum PBI levels without signs of thyroid disturbance.

Lithium generally should not be given with diuretics because they reduce its renal clearance and increase the risk of lithium toxicity. Read circulars for lithium preparations before use of such concomitant therapy with DIUCARDIN.

Information for Patients—This medicine may cause a loss of potassium from your body. To help prevent this, your doctor may want you to:
- eat or drink foods that have a high potassium content (for example, orange or other citrus fruit juices), or
- take a potassium supplement, or
- take another medicine to help prevent the loss of the potassium in the first place.

It is very important to follow these directions. Also, it is important not to change your diet on your own. This is more important if you are already on a special diet (as for diabetes), or if you are taking a potassium supplement or a medicine to reduce potassium loss. Extra potassium may not be necessary and, in some cases, too much potassium could be harmful.

Check with your doctor if you become sick and have severe or continuing vomiting or diarrhea. These problems may cause you to lose additional water and potassium.

Caution: Diabetics—Thiazide diuretics may raise blood sugar levels. While you are using this medicine, be especially careful in testing for sugar in your urine. If you have any questions about this, check with your doctor.

A few people who take this medicine may become more sensitive to sunlight than they are normally. When you begin to take this medicine avoid too much sun or a sunlamp until you see how you react, especially if you tend to burn easily. If you have a severe reaction, check with your doctor.

For patients taking this medicine for high blood pressure:
- **Do not take other medicines unless they have been discussed with your doctor.**

This especially includes over-the-counter (nonprescription) medicines for appetite control, asthma, colds, cough, hay fever, or sinus.

Laboratory Tests—Periodic determination of serum electrolytes to detect possible electrolyte imbalance should be performed at appropriate intervals.

Drug Interactions—

Anticoagulants, oral

(effects may be decreased when used concurrently with thiazide diuretics; dosage adjustments may be necessary)

Antigout medications

(thiazide diuretics may raise the level of blood uric acid; dosage adjustment of antigout medications may be necessary to control hyperuricemia and gout)

Antihypertensive medications, other, especially diazoxide, or Preanesthetic and anesthetic agents used in surgery or Skeletal muscle relaxants, nondepolarizing, used in surgery

(effects may be potentiated when used concurrently with thiazide diuretics; dosage adjustments may be necessary)

Amphotericin B or Corticosteroids or Corticotropin (ACTH)

(concurrent use with thiazide diuretics may intensify electrolyte imbalance, particularly hypokalemia)

Cardiac glycosides

(concurrent use with thiazide diuretics may enhance the possibility of digitalis toxicity associated with hypokalemia)

Colestipol

(may inhibit gastrointestinal absorption of the thiazide diuretics; administration 1 hour before or 4 hours after colestipol is recommended)

Hypoglycemics

(thiazide diuretics may raise blood glucose levels; for adult-onset diabetics, dosage adjustment of hypoglycemic medications may be necessary during and after thiazide diuretic therapy; insulin requirements may be increased, decreased, or unchanged)

Lithium salts

(concurrent use with thiazide diuretics is not recommended, as they may provoke lithium toxicity because of reduced renal clearance)

Methenamine

(effectiveness may be decreased when used concurrently with thiazide diuretics because of alkalinization of the urine)

Diagnostic Interference—With expected physiologic effects

Blood and urine glucose levels (usually only in patients with a predisposition for glucose intolerance) and

Serum bilirubin levels (by displacement from albumin binding) and

Serum calcium levels (thiazide diuretics should be discontinued before parathyroid function tests are carried out) and

Serum uric acid levels (may be increased)

Serum magnesium, potassium, and sodium levels (may be decreased; serum magnesium levels may increase in uremic patients)

Serum protein-bound iodine (PBI) levels (may be decreased)

Carcinogenesis, Mutagenesis, Impairment of Fertility—No long-term studies in animals have been performed to evaluate carcinogenic or mutagenic potential or impairment of fertility.

Usage in Pregnancy—Pregnancy Category D:
Teratogenic Effects—DIUCARDIN can cause fetal harm when administered to a pregnant woman. These hazards include fetal or neonatal jaundice, thrombocytopenia, and possibly other adverse reactions which have occurred in the adult. If this drug is used in pregnancy, or if the patient becomes pregnant while taking this drug, the patient should be apprised of the potential hazard to the fetus.
Nonteratogenic Effects—Fetal or neonatal jaundice, thrombocytopenia, and possibly other adverse reactions which have occurred in the adult.
Nursing Mothers: Thiazides appear in breast milk. If use of the drug is deemed essential, the patient may consider stopping nursing.
Pediatric Use: Safety and effectiveness in children have not been established.

ADVERSE REACTIONS

The following adverse reactions have been observed, but there is not enough systematic collection of data to support an estimate of their frequency.

Gastrointestinal Systems: anorexia, gastric irritation, nausea, vomiting, cramping, diarrhea, constipation, jaundice (intrahepatic cholestatic jaundice), pancreatitis, sialadenitis
Central Nervous System: dizziness, vertigo, paresthesias, headache, xanthopsia
Hematologic: leukopenia, agranulocytosis, thrombocytopenia, aplastic anemia, hemolytic anemia
Cardiovascular: orthostatic hypotension (may be aggravated by alcohol, barbiturates, or narcotics)
Hypersensitivity: purpura, photosensitivity, rash, urticaria, necrotizing angiitis (vasculitis, cutaneous vasculitis), fever, respiratory distress including pneumonitis, anaphylactic reactions
Other: hyperglycemia, glycosuria, hyperuricemia, muscle spasm, weakness, restlessness, transient blurred vision
Whenever adverse reactions are moderate or severe, thiazide dosage should be reduced or therapy withdrawn.

OVERDOSAGE

Signs and Symptoms—Diuresis, lethargy progressing to coma with minimal cardiorespiratory depression and with or without significant serum electrolyte changes or dehydration; GI irritation; hypermotility; transient elevation in BUN level.
Treatment—Empty stomach by gastric lavage, taking care to avoid aspiration. Monitor serum electrolyte levels and renal function, and institute supportive measures, as required to maintain hydration, electrolyte balance, respiration, and cardiovascular and renal function. Treat GI effects symptomatically.

DIUCARDIN is slowly dialyzable.

DOSAGE AND ADMINISTRATION

Therapy should be individualized according to patient response. Use the smallest dosage necessary to maintain the required response.
The usual daily dosages for antihypertensive and diuretic effect are:

	Diuretic	Antihypertensive
Adult:	25 to 200 mg	50 to 100 mg

Dosage regimens using 25 mg DIUCARDIN may be adequate in some cases.
Dosage should not exceed 200 mg per day.
For Diuresis in the Adult:
Initial recommended dose is 50 mg once or twice a day. Daily maintenance dose may be as little as 25 mg or as much as 200 mg, depending on patient's response. With dosages in excess of 100 mg daily, it is generally preferable to administer DIUCARDIN in divided doses.
Many patients with edema respond to intermittent therapy, *i.e.*, administration on alternate days or on three to five days each week. With an intermittent schedule, excessive response and the resulting undesirable electrolyte imbalance are less likely to occur.
For Control of Hypertension in the Adult:
Usual starting dose is 50 mg twice daily. Dosage is increased or decreased according to the blood pressure response of the patient. Usual maintenance dose is 50 mg to 100 mg per day. Dosage should not exceed 200 mg per day.
Careful observations for changes in blood pressure must be made when this compound is used with other antihypertensive drugs, especially during initial therapy. The dosage of other agents must be reduced by at least 50 percent as soon as it is added to the regimen to prevent excessive drop in blood pressure. As the blood pressure falls under the potentiating effect of this agent, a further reduction in dosage, or even discontinuation, of other antihypertensive drugs may be necessary.

HOW SUPPLIED

DIUCARDIN—Each scored, white oval compressed tablet, inscribed "DIUCARDIN®50," contains 50 mg hydroflumethiazide, in bottles of 100 (NDC 0046-0702-81).
Store at room temperature (approximately 25° C).
Shown in Product Identification Section, page 436

EPITRATE®   ℞
[ĕp′i-trāt]
(epinephrine bitartrate
ophthalmic solution)

CAUTION: Federal law prohibits dispensing without prescription.

DESCRIPTION

EPITRATE (epinephrine bitartrate ophthalmic solution) is a sterile aqueous solution of levorotatory epinephrine bitartrate, 2% (equivalent to 1.1% base). Inactive ingredients include chlorobutanol (chloral derivative) 0.55%, sodium metabisulfite, sodium chloride, polyoxypropylene-polyoxyethylenediol, and disodium edetate. Epinephrine bitartrate is an adrenergic agent with the chemical name (-)-3,4,-Dihydroxy-α-[(methylamino) methyl] benzyl alcohol (+) tartrate (1:1) salt. It has a low surface tension.

HOW SUPPLIED

EPITRATE—ophthalmic solution of epinephrine bitartrate, 2% (equivalent to 1.1% base). Package containing 7.5 mL bottle with separate dropper-screw cap attachment (NDC 0046-1015-07).
For prescribing information write to Professional Service, Wyeth-Ayerst Laboratories, Box 8299, Philadelphia, PA 19101, or contact your local Wyeth-Ayerst representative.

EQUAGESIC®   ℂ ℞
[ek″wa-je′zik]
(meprobamate with aspirin)

DESCRIPTION

Each tablet of Equagesic contains 200 mg meprobamate and 325 mg aspirin. The inactive ingredients present are cellulose, D&C Yellow 10, FD&C Red 3, FD&C Yellow 6, hydrogenated vegetable oil, magnesium stearate, polacrilin potassium, and starch.

ACTIONS

Meprobamate is a carbamate derivative which has been shown (in animal and/or human studies) to have effects at multiple sites in the central nervous system, including the thalamus and limbic system.
Aspirin, acetylsalicylic acid, is a nonnarcotic analgesic with antipyretic and antiinflammatory properties.

INDICATIONS

As an adjunct in the short-term treatment of pain accompanied by tension and/or anxiety in patients with musculoskeletal disease. Clinical trials have demonstrated that in these situations relief of pain is somewhat greater than with aspirin alone.

The effectiveness of Equagesic in long-term use, that is, more than 4 months, has not been assessed by systematic clinical studies. The physician should periodically reassess the usefulness of the drug for the individual patient.

CONTRAINDICATIONS

ASPIRIN:

Allergic or idiosyncratic reactions to aspirin or related compounds.

MEPROBAMATE:

Acute intermittent porphyria and allergic or idiosyncratic reactions to meprobamate or related compounds, such as carisoprodol, mebutamate, or carbromal.

WARNINGS

ASPIRIN:

Salicylates should be used with extreme caution in patients with peptic ulcer, asthma, coagulation abnormalities, hypoprothrombinemia, vitamin K deficiency, or in those on anticoagulant therapy.

In rare instances, the use of aspirin in persons allergic to salicylates may result in life-threatening allergic episodes.

MEPROBAMATE:

DRUG DEPENDENCE: Physical dependence, psychological dependence, and abuse have occurred. Chronic intoxication from prolonged ingestion of, usually, greater-than-recommended doses is manifested by ataxia, slurred speech, and vertigo. Therefore, careful supervision of dose and amounts prescribed is advised, as well as avoidance of prolonged administration, especially for alcoholics and other patients with a known propensity for taking excessive quantities of drugs.

Sudden withdrawal of the drug after prolonged and excessive use may precipitate recurrence of preexisting symptoms such as anxiety, anorexia, or insomnia, or withdrawal reactions such as vomiting, ataxia, tremors, muscle twitching, confusional states, hallucinosis, and, rarely, convulsive seizures. Such seizures are more likely to occur in persons with central-nervous-system damage or preexistent or latent convulsive disorders. Onset of withdrawal symptoms occurs usually within 12 to 48 hours after discontinuation of meprobamate; symptoms usually cease within the next 12- to 48-hour period.

When excessive dosage has continued for weeks or months, dosage should be reduced gradually over a period of 1 to 2 weeks rather than abruptly stopped. Alternatively, a short-acting barbiturate may be substituted, then gradually withdrawn.

POTENTIALLY HAZARDOUS TASKS: Patients should be warned that meprobamate may impair the mental or physical abilities required for performance of potentially hazardous tasks, such as driving or operating machinery.

ADDITIVE EFFECTS: Since CNS-suppressant effects of meprobamate and alcohol or meprobamate and other psychotropic drugs may be additive, appropriate caution should be exercised with patients who take more than one of these agents simultaneously.

USAGE IN PREGNANCY AND LACTATION

An increased risk of congenital malformations associated with the use of minor tranquilizers (meprobamate, chlordiazepoxide, and diazepam) during the first trimester of pregnancy has been suggested in several studies. Because use of these drugs is rarely a matter of urgency, their use during this period should almost always be avoided. The possibility that a woman of childbearing potential may be pregnant at the time of institution of therapy should be considered. Patients should be advised that if they become pregnant during therapy or intend to become pregnant they should communicate with their physicians about the desirability of discontinuing the drug.

Meprobamate passes the placental barrier. It is present both in umbilical-cord blood at or near maternal plasma levels and in breast milk of lactating mothers at concentrations two to four times that of maternal plasma. When use of meprobamate is contemplated in breast-feeding patients, the drug's higher concentrations in breast milk as compared to maternal plasma levels should be considered.

USAGE IN CHILDREN: Preparations containing aspirin should be kept out of the reach of children. Equagesic (meprobamate with aspirin) is not recommended for patients 12 years of age and under.

PRECAUTIONS

ASPIRIN:

Salicylates antagonize the uricosuric activity of probenecid and sulfinpyrazone. Salicylates are reported to enhance the hypoglycemic effect of the sulfonylurea antidiabetic drugs.

MEPROBAMATE:

The lowest effective dose should be administered, particularly to elderly and/or debilitated patients, in order to preclude oversedation.

Meprobamate is metabolized in the liver and excreted by the kidney; to avoid its excess accumulation, caution should be exercised in the administration to patients with compromised liver or kidney function.

Meprobamate occasionally may precipitate seizures in epileptic patients.

The drug should be prescribed cautiously and in small quantities to patients with suicidal tendencies.

ADVERSE REACTIONS

ASPIRIN:

Aspirin may cause epigastric discomfort, nausea, and vomiting. Hypersensitivity reactions, including urticaria, angioneurotic edema, purpura, asthma, and anaphylaxis, may rarely occur.

Patients receiving large doses of salicylates may develop tinnitus.

MEPROBAMATE:

CENTRAL NERVOUS SYSTEM: Drowsiness, ataxia, dizziness, slurred speech, headache, vertigo, weakness, paresthesias, impairment of visual accommodation, euphoria, overstimulation, paradoxical excitement, fast EEG activity.

GASTROINTESTINAL: Nausea, vomiting, diarrhea.

CARDIOVASCULAR: Palpitation, tachycardia, various forms of arrhythmia, transient ECG changes, syncope, hypotensive crisis.

ALLERGIC OR IDIOSYNCRATIC: Milder reactions are characterized by an itchy, urticarial, or erythematous maculopapular rash which may be generalized or confined to the groin.

Other reactions have included leukopenia, acute nonthrombocytopenic purpura, petechiae, ecchymoses, eosinophilia, peripheral edema, adenopathy, fever, fixed drug eruption with cross-reaction to carisoprodol, and cross-sensitivity between meprobamate/mebutamate and meprobamate/carbromal.

More severe hypersensitivity reactions, rarely reported, include hyperpyrexia, chills, angioneurotic edema, bronchospasm, oliguria, and anuria. Also, anaphylaxis, exfoliative dermatitis, stomatitis, and proctitis. Stevens-Johnson syndrome and bullous dermatitis have occurred.

HEMATOLOGIC (SEE ALSO "ALLERGIC OR IDIOSYNCRATIC"): Agranulocytosis, aplastic anemia have been reported, although no causal relationship has been established, and thrombocytopenic purpura.

OTHER: Exacerbation of porphyric symptoms.

DOSAGE AND ADMINISTRATION

The usual dosage of Equagesic (meprobamate with aspirin) is one or two tablets, each tablet containing meprobamate, 200 mg, and aspirin, 325 mg, orally 3 to 4 times daily as needed for the relief of pain when tension or anxiety is present. Equagesic is not recommended for patients 12 years of age and under.

OVERDOSAGE

Treatment of overdose with Equagesic is essentially symptomatic and supportive. Any drug remaining in the stomach should be removed. Induction of vomiting or gastric lavage may be indicated. Activated charcoal may reduce absorption of both aspirin and meprobamate.

Overdosage with aspirin produces the usual symptoms and signs of salicylate intoxication. Observation and treatment should include management of hyperthermia, specific parenteral electrolyte therapy for ketoacidosis and dehydration, watching for evidence of hemorrhagic manifestations due to hypoprothrombinemia which, if it occurs, usually requires whole-blood transfusions.

Suicidal attempts with meprobamate have resulted in drowsiness, lethargy, stupor, ataxia, coma, shock, vasomotor and respiratory collapse. Some suicidal attempts have been fatal. The following data have been reported in the literature and from other sources. These data are not expected to correlate with each case (considering factors such as individual susceptibility and length of time from ingestion to treatment), but represent the usual ranges reported.

Acute simple overdose (meprobamate alone): Death has been reported with ingestion of as little as 12 grams meprobamate and survival with as much as 40 grams.

BLOOD LEVELS:

0.5 to 2.0 mg percent represents the usual blood-level range of meprobamate after therapeutic doses. The level may occasionally be as high as 3.0 mg percent.

3 to 10 mg percent usually corresponds to findings of mild-to-moderate symptoms of overdosage, such as stupor or light coma.

10 to 20 mg percent usually corresponds to deeper coma, requiring more intensive treatment. Some fatalities occur.

At levels greater than 20 mg percent, more fatalities than survivals can be expected.

Acute combined overdose (meprobamate with other psychotropic drugs or alcohol): Since effects can be additive, a history of ingestion of a low dose of meprobamate plus any of

these compounds (or of a relatively low blood or tissue level) cannot be used as a prognostic indicator.

In cases where excessive doses have been taken, sleep ensues rapidly and blood pressure, pulse, and respiratory rates are reduced to basal levels. Any drug remaining in the stomach should be removed and symptomatic treatment given. Should respiration or blood pressure become compromised, respiratory assistance, central-nervous-system stimulants, and pressor agents should be administered cautiously as indicated. Diuresis, osmotic (mannitol) diuresis, peritoneal dialysis, and hemodialysis have been used successfully in removing both aspirin and meprobamate. Alkalinization of the urine increases the excretion of salicylates. Careful monitoring of urinary output is necessary, and caution should be taken to avoid overhydration. Relapse and death, after initial recovery, have been attributed to incomplete gastric emptying and delayed absorption.

HOW SUPPLIED

Equagesic® (meprobamate with aspirin) Tablets, Wyeth®, 200 mg meprobamate and 325 mg aspirin, are available as follows:

NDC 0008-0091, pink and yellow, double-layer, round, scored tablet marked "WYETH" and "91", in bottles of 100 tablets.

Keep tightly closed.

Protect from light.

Dispense in light-resistant, tight container.

The appearance of EQUAGESIC tablets is a registered trademark of Wyeth-Ayerst Laboratories.

Shown in Product Identification Section, page 436

EQUANIL®   Ⓒ ℞

[*ek 'wah-nil*]

(meprobamate)

Tablets

DESCRIPTION

Meprobamate is a white powder with a characteristic odor and a bitter taste. It is slightly soluble in water, freely soluble in acetone and alcohol, and sparingly soluble in ether. Equanil tablets contain 200 mg or 400 mg meprobamate. The inactive ingredients present are lactose, methylcellulose, polacrilin potassium, and stearic acid.

HOW SUPPLIED

Equanil® (meprobamate) Tablets, Wyeth®, are available in the following dosage strengths:

200 mg, NDC 0008-0002, white, five-sided tablet marked "WYETH" and "2", in bottles of 100 tablets and in Redipak® Strip Pack cartons of 25 tablets.

400 mg, NDC 0008-0001, white, round, scored tablet marked "WYETH" and "1", in bottles of 100 and 500 tablets and in Redipak Strip Pack cartons of 25 tablets.

For prescribing information write to Professional Service, Wyeth-Ayerst Laboratories, Box 8299, Philadelphia, PA 19101, or contact your local Wyeth-Ayerst representative.

Shown in Product Identification Section, page 436

ESTRADURIN®   ℞

[*ĕs "tra-dū 'rin*]

Brand of polyestradiol phosphate

For Intramuscular Injection Only

CAUTION: Federal law prohibits dispensing without prescription.

DESCRIPTION

ESTRADURIN is a water-soluble, high molecular weight polyester of phosphoric acid and 17β-estradiol.

It is provided in a SECULE® containing 40 mg polyestradiol phosphate, 0.022 mg phenylmercuric nitrate, and 5.2 mg sodium phosphate. As solubilizing agents for the active ingredient, 25 mg niacinamide and 4 mg propylene glycol are also present. The pH is adjusted with sodium hydroxide. One 2 mL ampul of sterile diluent is also provided.

CLINICAL PHARMACOLOGY

Estrogens are important in the development and maintenance of the female reproductive system. In responsive tissues estrogens enter the cell and are transported into the nucleus.

In the male patient with androgenic hormone-dependent conditions, such as metastatic carcinoma of the prostate gland, estrogens counter the androgenic influence by competing for the receptor sites. As a result of treatment with estrogens, metastatic lesions in the bone may also show improvement.

Biologically active estradiol units are gradually split off from the large parent molecule, thus providing a continuous level of active estrogen over a prolonged period. The liberated estradiol is metabolized by the body in the same manner as the endogenous hormone. There is no depot effect at the site of injection—90 percent of injected dose leaves the bloodstream within 24 hours. Passive storage occurs in the reticu-

Continued on next page

Wyeth-Ayerst—Cont.

loendothelial system. As circulating levels of estradiol drop, more returns to the bloodstream from the site of storage for an even, continuous therapeutic effect. Increasing the dose acts to prolong the duration of pharmacologic action rather than to increase blood levels.

Metabolism and inactivation occur primarily in the liver. Some estrogens are excreted into the bile; however they are reabsorbed from the intestine and returned to the liver through the portal venous system. Water-soluble estrogen conjugates are strongly acidic and are ionized in body fluids, which favor excretion through the kidneys since tubular reabsorption is minimal.

INDICATION
ESTRADURIN (polyestradiol phosphate) is indicated in the treatment of prostatic carcinoma—palliative therapy of advanced disease.

CONTRAINDICATIONS
Estrogens should not be used in men with any of the following conditions:
1. Known or suspected cancer of the breast except in appropriately selected patients being treated for metastatic disease.
2. Known or suspected estrogen-dependent neoplasia.
3. Active thrombophlebitis or thromboembolic disorders.

WARNINGS
1. *Induction of malignant neoplasms.* Long-term, continuous administration of natural and synthetic estrogens in certain animal species increases the frequency of carcinomas of the breast, cervix, vagina, and liver.
2. *Gallbladder disease.* A recent study has reported a 2- to 3-fold increase in the risk of surgically confirmed gallbladder disease in women receiving postmenopausal estrogens,[1] similar to the 2-fold increase previously noted in users of oral contraceptives.[2,7a]
3. *Effects similar to those caused by estrogen-progestogen oral contraceptives.* There are several serious adverse effects of oral contraceptives. It has been shown that there is an increased risk of thrombosis in men receiving estrogens for prostatic cancer and women for postpartum breast engorgement.[3-6]
a. *Thromboembolic disease.* It is now well established that users of oral contraceptives have an increased risk of various thromboembolic and thrombotic vascular diseases, such as thrombophlebitis, pulmonary embolism, stroke, and myocardial infarction.[7-14] Cases of retinal thrombosis, mesenteric thrombosis, and optic neuritis have been reported in oral contraceptive users. There is evidence that the risk of several of these adverse reactions is related to the dose of the drug.[15,16] An increased risk of postsurgery thromboembolic complications has also been reported in users of oral contraceptives.[17,18] If feasible, estrogen should be discontinued at least 4 weeks before surgery of the type associated with an increased risk of thromboembolism, or during periods of prolonged immobilization.

Estrogens should not be used in persons with active thrombophlebitis or thromboembolic disorders. They should be used with caution in patients with cerebral vascular or coronary artery disease and only for those in whom estrogens are clearly indicated.

Large doses of estrogen (5 mg conjugated estrogens per day), comparable to those used to treat cancer of the prostate, have been shown in a large prospective clinical trial in men[19] to increase the risk of nonfatal myocardial infarction, pulmonary embolism and thrombophlebitis. When estrogen doses of this size are used, any of the thromboembolic and thrombotic adverse effects associated with oral contraceptive use should be considered a clear risk.
b. *Hepatic adenoma.* Benign hepatic adenomas appear to be associated with the use of oral contraceptives.[20-22] Although benign, and rare, these may rupture and may cause death through intra-abdominal hemorrhage. Such lesions have not yet been reported in association with other estrogen or progestogen preparations but should be considered in estrogen users having abdominal pain and tenderness, abdominal mass, or hypovolemic shock. Hepatocellular carcinoma has also been reported in women taking estrogen-containing oral contraceptives.[21] The relationship of this malignancy to these drugs is not known at this time.
c. *Elevated blood pressure.* Women using oral contraceptives sometimes experience increased blood pressure which, in most cases, returns to normal on discontinuing the drug. There is now a report that this may occur with use of estrogens in the menopause[23] and blood pressure should be monitored with estrogen use, especially if high doses are used.
d. *Glucose tolerance.* A worsening of glucose tolerance has been observed in a significant percentage of patients on estrogen-containing oral contraceptives. For this reason, diabetic patients should be carefully observed while receiving estrogen.
4. *Hypercalcemia.* Administration of estrogens may lead to severe hypercalcemia in patients with breast cancer and

bone metastases. If this occurs, the drug should be stopped and appropriate measures taken to reduce the serum calcium level.

PRECAUTIONS
1. A complete medical and family history should be taken prior to the initiation of any estrogen therapy. The pretreatment and periodic physical examinations should include special reference to blood pressure, breasts, abdomen, and pelvic organs. As a general rule, estrogen should not be prescribed for longer than one year without another physical examination being performed.
2. Fluid retention—Because estrogens may cause some degree of fluid retention, conditions which might be influenced by this factor such as asthma, epilepsy, migraine, and cardiac or renal dysfunction, require careful observation.
3. Certain patients may develop undesirable manifestations of excessive estrogenic stimulation, such as gynecomastia.
4. Oral contraceptives appear to be associated with an increased incidence of mental depression.[7a] Although it is not clear whether this is due to the estrogenic or progestogenic component of the contraceptive, patients with a history of depression should be carefully observed.
5. The pathologist should be advised of estrogen therapy when relevant specimens are submitted.
6. If jaundice develops in any patient receiving estrogen, the medication should be discontinued while the cause is investigated.
7. Estrogens may be poorly metabolized in patients with impaired liver function and they should be administered with caution in such patients.
8. Because estrogens influence the metabolism of calcium and phosphorus, they should be used with caution in patients with metabolic bone diseases that are associated with hypercalcemia or in patients with renal insufficiency.
9. Because of the effects of estrogens on epiphyseal closure, they should be used judiciously in young patients in whom bone growth is not complete.
10. Certain endocrine and liver function tests may be affected by estrogen-containing oral contraceptives. The following similar changes may be expected with larger doses of estrogen:
a. Increased sulfobromophthalein retention.
b. Increased prothrombin and factors VII, VIII, IX, and X; decreased antithrombin 3; increased norepinephrine-induced platelet aggregability.
c. Increased thyroid binding globulin (TBG) leading to increased circulating total thyroid hormone, as measured by PBI, T4 by column, or T4 by radioimmunoassay. Free T3 resin uptake is decreased, reflecting the elevated TBG; free T4 concentration is unaltered.
d. Impaired glucose tolerance.
e. Reduced response to metyrapone test.
f. Reduced serum folate concentration.
g. Increased serum triglyceride and phospholipid concentration.

ADVERSE REACTIONS
(See WARNINGS regarding induction of neoplasia, increased incidence of gallbladder disease, and adverse effects similar to those of oral contraceptives, including thromboembolism.) The following additional adverse reactions have been reported with estrogenic therapy, including oral contraceptives:
1. *Breasts:* Tenderness, enlargement, secretion.
2. *Gastrointestinal:* Nausea, vomiting; abdominal cramps, bloating; cholestatic jaundice.
3. *Skin:* Chloasma or melasma which may persist when drug is discontinued; erythema multiforme; erythema nodosum; hemorrhagic eruption; loss of scalp hair; hirsutism.
4. *Eyes:* Steepening of corneal curvature; intolerance to contact lenses.
5. *CNS:* Headache, migraine, dizziness; mental depression; chorea.
6. *Miscellaneous:* Increase or decrease in weight; reduced carbohydrate tolerance; aggravation of porphyria; edema; changes in libido.

ACUTE OVERDOSAGE
Numerous reports of ingestion of large doses of estrogen-containing oral contraceptives by young children indicate that acute serious ill effects do not occur. Overdosage of estrogen may cause nausea, and withdrawal bleeding may occur in females.

DOSAGE AND ADMINISTRATION
Inoperable progressing prostatic cancer—40 mg intramuscularly every two to four weeks or less frequently, depending on clinical response of the patient. If the response is not satisfactory doses up to 80 mg may be used. Experimental evidence indicates that increasing the dose primarily prolongs the duration of action, but the amount of estrogen available at any one time is not significantly increased. The dosage should be adjusted as indicated by careful observation of the patient.

Deep intramuscular injection only is recommended. (Initially, some patients may experience a burning sensation at site of injection. This is transitory, and it may not recur with subsequent injections, or may be obviated by concomitant administration of a local anesthetic.)

If a response to estrogen therapy is going to occur, it will be apparent within three months of the beginning of therapy. If it does occur, the hormone should be continued until the disease is again progressive. The hormone should then be stopped, and the patient may obtain another period of improvement known as "rebound regression." This occurs in 30% of the patients who show objective improvement on estrogens.

DIRECTIONS FOR USE
Reconstitution for use:
1. Introduce sterile diluent into SECULE, preferably with a 20 gauge needle affixed to a 5 mL syringe.
2. Swirl gently until a solution is effected. (DO NOT AGITATE VIOLENTLY.)
Stability: After reconstitution, if storage is desired, the solution should be kept at room temperature and away from direct light. Under these conditions the solution is stable for about 10 days, so long as cloudiness or evidence of a precipitate has not occurred.

HOW SUPPLIED
NDC 0046-0451-02—Each package provides:
1. One SECULE® containing 40 mg polyestradiol phosphate, 0.022 mg phenylmercuric nitrate, and 5.2 mg sodium phosphate. As solubilizing agents for the active ingredient, 25 mg niacinamide and 4 mg propylene glycol are also present. The pH is adjusted with sodium hydroxide.
2. One 2 mL ampul of sterile diluent.
ESTRADURIN (polyestradiol phosphate) is prepared by cryodesiccation.

PHYSICIAN REFERENCES
1. Boston Collaborative Drug Surveillance Program: N. Engl. J. Med. 290 :15–19, 1974.
2. Boston Collaborative Drug Surveillance Program: Lancet 1 :1399–1404, 1973.
3. Daniel, D. G., et al.: Lancet 2 :287–289, 1967.
4. The Veterans Administration Cooperative Urological Research Group: J. Urol. 98 :516–522, 1967.
5. Bailar, J. C.: Lancet 2 :560, 1967.
6. Blackard, C., et al.: Cancer 26 :249–256, 1970.
7. Royal College of General Practitioners: J. R. Coll. Gen. Pract. 13 :267–279, 1967.
7a. Royal College of General Practitioners: Oral Contraceptives and Health, New York, Pitman Corp., 1974.
8. Inman, W. H. W., et al.: Br. Med. J. 2 :193–199, 1968.
9. Vessey, M. P., et al.: Br. Med. J. 2 :651–657, 1969.
10. Sartwell, P. E., et al.: Am. J. Epidemiol. 90 :365–380, 1969.
11. Collaborative Group for the Study of Stroke in Young Women: N. Engl. J. Med. 288 :871–878, 1973.
12. Collaborative Group for the Study of Stroke in Young Women: J.A.M.A. 231 :718–722, 1975.
13. Mann, J. I., et al.: Br. Med. J. 2 :245–248, 1975.
14. Mann, J. I., et al.: Br. Med. J. 2 :241–245, 1975.
15. Inman, W. H. W., et al.: Br. Med. J. 2 :203–209, 1970.
16. Stolley, P. D., et al.: Am. J. Epidemiol. 102 :197–208, 1975.
17. Vessey, M. P., et al.: Br. Med. J. 3 :123–126, 1970.
18. Greene, G. R., et al.: Am. J. Public Health 62 :680–685, 1972.
19. Coronary Drug Project Research Group: J.A.M.A. 214 :1303–1313, 1970.
20. Baum, J., et al.: Lancet 2 :926–928, 1973.
21. Mays, E. T., et al.: J.A.M.A. 235 :730–732, 1976.
22. Edmondson, H. A., et al.: N. Engl. J. Med. 294 :470–472, 1976.
23. Pfeffer, R. I., et al.: Am. J. Epidemiol. 103 :445–456, 1976.
SECULE®—Trademark to designate a special vial containing an injectable preparation in dry form.

FACTREL® ℞
[făc-trĕl´]
(gonadorelin hydrochloride)
Synthetic Luteinizing Hormone Releasing Hormone (LH-RH)
DIAGNOSTIC USE ONLY

HOW SUPPLIED
LYOPHILIZED POWDER
in single-dose SECULE® vials containing 100 mcg (NDC 0046-0507-05) and 500 mcg (NDC 0046-0509-05) gonadorelin as the hydrochloride with 100 mg lactose, USP. Each SECULE® vial is accompanied by one ampul containing 2 mL sterile diluent of 2% benzyl alcohol in sterile water.
For full prescribing information turn to the Diagnostic Product Information section of this edition of the PDR.
Shown in Product Identification Section, page 436

FLUOTHANE®   ℞
[flū'o-thăn]
Brand of halothane, USP

CAUTION: Federal law prohibits dispensing without prescription.

DESCRIPTION

FLUOTHANE (halothane, USP) is supplied as a liquid and is vaporized for use as an inhalation anesthetic. It is 2-bromo-2-chloro-1, 1, 1-trifluoro-ethane and has the following structural formula:

$$F-\underset{\underset{F}{|}}{\overset{\overset{F}{|}}{C}}-\underset{\underset{H}{|}}{\overset{\overset{Br}{|}}{C}}-Cl$$

Halothane is miscible with alcohol, chloroform, ether, and other fat solvents.

The specific gravity is 1.872–1.877 at 20°C, and the boiling point (range) is 49°C–51°C at 760 mm Hg. The vapor pressure is 243 mm Hg at 20°C. The blood/gas coefficient is 2.5 at 37°C, and the olive oil/water coefficient is 220 at 37°C. Vapor concentrations within anesthetic range are nonirritating and have a pleasant odor. FLUOTHANE is nonflammable, and its vapors mixed with oxygen in proportions from 0.5 to 50% (v/v) are not explosive.

FLUOTHANE does not decompose in contact with warm soda lime. When moisture is present, the vapor attacks aluminum, brass, and lead, but not copper. Rubber, some plastics, and similar materials are soluble in FLUOTHANE; such materials will deteriorate rapidly in contact with FLUOTHANE vapor or liquid. Stability of FLUOTHANE is maintained by the addition of 0.01% thymol (w/w), up to 0.00025% ammonia (w/w).

CLINICAL PHARMACOLOGY

FLUOTHANE is an inhalation anesthetic. Induction and recovery are rapid and depth of anesthesia can be rapidly altered. FLUOTHANE progressively depresses respiration. There may be tachypnea with reduced tidal volume and alveolar ventilation. FLUOTHANE is not an irritant to the respiratory tract, and no increase in salivary or bronchial secretions ordinarily occurs. Pharyngeal and laryngeal reflexes are rapidly obtunded. It causes bronchodilation. Hypoxia, acidosis, or apnea may develop during deep anesthesia.

FLUOTHANE reduces the blood pressure, and frequently decreases the pulse rate. The greater the concentration of the drug, the more evident these changes become. Atropine may reverse the bradycardia. FLUOTHANE does not cause the release of catecholamines from adrenergic stores. FLUOTHANE also causes dilation of the vessels of the skin and skeletal muscles.

Cardiac arrhythmias may occur during FLUOTHANE anesthesia. These include nodal rhythm, AV dissociation, ventricular extrasystoles and asystole. FLUOTHANE sensitizes the myocardial conduction system to the action of epinephrine and norepinephrine, and the combination may cause serious cardiac arrhythmias. FLUOTHANE increases cerebral spinal fluid pressure. FLUOTHANE produces moderate muscular relaxation. Muscle relaxants are used as adjuncts in order to maintain lighter levels of anesthesia. FLUOTHANE augments the action of nondepolarizing relaxants and ganglionic-blocking agents. FLUOTHANE is a potent uterine relaxant.

The mechanism(s) whereby FLUOTHANE and other substances induce general anesthesia is unknown. FLUOTHANE is a very potent anesthetic in humans, with a minimum alveolar concentration (MAC) determined to be 0.64%. The MAC has been found to decrease with age (see MAC table in DOSAGE AND ADMINISTRATION).

INDICATIONS AND USAGE

FLUOTHANE (halothane, USP) is indicated for the induction and maintenance of general anesthesia.

CONTRAINDICATIONS

FLUOTHANE is not recommended for obstetrical anesthesia except when uterine relaxation is required.

WARNINGS

When previous exposure to FLUOTHANE was followed by unexplained hepatic dysfunction and/or jaundice, consideration should be given to the use of other agents.

PRECAUTIONS

General: FLUOTHANE should be used in vaporizers that permit a reasonable approximation of output, and preferably of the calibrated type. The vaporizer should be placed out of circuit in closed circuit rebreathing systems, otherwise overdosage is difficult to avoid. The patient should be closely observed for signs of overdosage, ie, depression of blood pressure, pulse rate, and ventilation, particularly during assisted or controlled ventilation.

FLUOTHANE increases cerebrospinal fluid pressure. Therefore, in patients with markedly raised intracranial pressure, if FLUOTHANE is indicated, administration should be preceded by measures ordinarily used to reduce cerebrospinal fluid pressure. Ventilation should be carefully assessed, and it may be necessary to assist or control ventilation to ensure adequate oxygenation and carbon dioxide removal.

In susceptible individuals, halothane anesthesia may trigger a skeletal muscle hypermetabolic state leading to a high oxygen demand and the clinical syndrome known as malignant hyperthermia. The syndrome includes nonspecific features such as muscle rigidity, tachycardia, tachypnea, cyanosis, arrhythmias, and unstable blood pressure. (It should also be noted that many of these nonspecific signs may appear with light anesthesia, acute hypoxia, etc.) An increase in overall metabolism may be reflected in an elevated temperature (which may rise rapidly early or late in the case, but usually is not the first sign of augmented metabolism) and an increased usage of the CO_2 absorption system (hot canister). PaO_2 and pH may decrease, and hyperkalemia and a base deficit may appear. Treatment includes discontinuance of triggering agents (eg, halothane), administration of intravenous dantrolene, and application of supportive therapy. Such therapy includes vigorous efforts to restore body temperature to normal, respiratory and circulatory support as indicated, and management of electrolyte-fluid-acid-base derangements. Renal failure may appear later, and urine flow should be sustained if possible. It should be noted that the syndrome of malignant hyperthermia secondary to halothane appears to be rare.

Information for Patients: When appropriate, as in some cases where discharge is anticipated soon after general anesthesia, patients should be cautioned not to drive automobiles, operate hazardous machinery or engage in hazardous sports for 24 hours or more (depending on the total dose of FLUOTHANE, condition of the patient and consideration given to other drugs administered after anesthesia).

Drug Interactions: Epinephrine or norepinephrine should be employed cautiously, if at all, during FLUOTHANE (halothane, USP) anesthesia since their simultaneous use may induce ventricular tachycardia or fibrillation.

Nondepolarizing relaxants and ganglionic-blocking agents should be administered cautiously, since their actions are augmented by FLUOTHANE (halothane, USP).

Clinical experience and animal experiments suggest that pancuronium should be given with caution to patients receiving chronic tricyclic antidepressant therapy who are anesthetized with halothane because severe ventricular arrhythmias may result from such usage.

Carcinogenesis, Mutagenesis, Impairment of Fertility: An 18-month inhalational carcinogenicity study of halothane at 0.05% in the mouse revealed no evidence of anesthetic-related carcinogenicity. This concentration is equivalent to 24 hours of 1% halothane.

Mutagenesis testing of halothane revealed both positive and negative results. In the rat, one-year exposure to trace concentrations of halothane (1 and 10 ppm) and nitrous oxide produced chromosomal damage to spermatogonia cells and bone marrow cells. Negative mutagenesis tests included: Ames bacterial assay, Chinese hamster lung fibroblast assay, sister chromatid exchange in Chinese hamster ovary cells, and human leukocyte culture assay.

Reproduction studies of halothane (10 ppm) and nitrous oxide in the rat caused decreased fertility. This trace concentration corresponds to 1/1000 the human maintenance dose.

Pregnancy:

Teratogenic Effects: Pregnancy Category C. Some studies have shown FLUOTHANE to be teratogenic, embryotoxic, and fetotoxic in the mouse, rat, hamster, and rabbit at subanesthetic and/or anesthetic concentrations. There are no adequate and well-controlled studies in pregnant women. FLUOTHANE should be used during pregnancy only if the potential benefit justifies the potential risk to the fetus.

Labor and Delivery: The uterine relaxation obtained with FLUOTHANE, unless carefully controlled, may fail to respond to ergot derivatives and oxytocic posterior pituitary extract.

Nursing Mothers: It is not known whether this drug is excreted in human milk. Because many drugs are excreted in human milk, caution should be exercised when FLUOTHANE is administered to a nursing woman.

Pediatric Use: Extensive clinical experience reveals that maintenance concentrations of halothane are generally higher in infants and children, and that maintenance requirements decrease with age. See MAC table, based upon age, in DOSAGE AND ADMINISTRATION.

ADVERSE REACTIONS

The following adverse reactions have been reported: mild, moderate and severe hepatic dysfunction (including hepatic necrosis); cardiac arrest, hypotension, respiratory arrest, cardiac arrhythmias, hyperpyrexia, shivering, nausea, and emesis.

OVERDOSAGE

In the event of overdosage, or what may appear to be overdosage, drug administration should be stopped, and assisted or controlled ventilation with pure oxygen initiated.

DOSAGE AND ADMINISTRATION

FLUOTHANE may be administered by the nonrebreathing technique, partial rebreathing, or closed technique. The induction dose varies from patient to patient, but is usually within the range of 0.5% to 3%. The maintenance dose varies from 0.5% to 1.5%.

FLUOTHANE may be administered with either oxygen or a mixture of oxygen and nitrous oxide.

FLUOTHANE should not be kept indefinitely in vaporizer bottles not specifically designed for its use. Thymol does not volatilize along with FLUOTHANE, and therefore accumulates in the vaporizer, and may, in time, impart a yellow color to the remaining liquid or to wicks in vaporizers. The development of such discoloration may be used as an indicator that the vaporizer should be drained and cleaned, and the discolored FLUOTHANE (halothane, USP) discarded. Accumulation of thymol may be removed by washing with diethyl ether. After cleaning a wick or vaporizer, make certain all the diethyl ether has been removed before reusing the equipment to avoid introducing ether into the system.

Because of the more rapid uptake of FLUOTHANE and the increased blood concentration required for anesthesia in younger patients, the minimum alveolar concentration (MAC)[1] values will decrease with age as follows:

Age	MAC %
Infants	1.08
3 yrs.	0.91
10 yrs.	0.87
15 yrs.	0.92
24 yrs.	0.84
42 yrs.	0.76
81 yrs.	0.64

HOW SUPPLIED

Unit packages of 125 mL (NDC 0046-3125-81) and 250 mL (NDC 0046-3125-82) of halothane, USP, stabilized with 0.01% thymol (w/w) and up to 0.00025% ammonia (w/w).

Handling and Storage: Store at room temperature (approximately 25°C) in a tight, closed container. Protect from light.

PHYSICIAN REFERENCE

1. Gregory, GA et al: *Anesthesiology* 1969; 30(5):488–491.

GRISACTIN®   ℞
[grĭz-ăc'tĭn]
brand of griseofulvin (microsize)

CAUTION: Federal law prohibits dispensing without prescription.

DESCRIPTION

Griseofulvin is an oral fungistatic antibiotic for the treatment of superficial mycoses. It is derived from a species of *Penicillium*.

GRISACTIN is produced by a special process that fractures griseofulvin particles into minute crystals of irregular shape offering a greater and more effective surface area for increased gastrointestinal absorption.

GRISACTIN Capsules and Tablets contain the following inactive ingredients:

—125 mg capsules: black iron oxide, D&C Yellow No. 10, FD&C Blue No. 2, FD&C Red No. 3, FD&C Red No. 40, FD&C Yellow No. 6, gelatin, lactose, talc, water.

—250 mg capsules: black iron oxide, D&C Yellow No. 10, FD&C Blue No. 2, FD&C Red No. 40, FD&C Yellow No. 6, gelatin, lactose, magnesium stearate, titanium dioxide, water.

—500 mg tablets: calcium carboxymethylcellulose, D&C Red No. 36, gelatin, magnesium stearate, starch.

ACTION

Griseofulvin is fungistatic with *in vitro* activity against various species of *Microsporum, Epidermophyton,* and *Trichophyton.* It has no effect on bacteria or on other genera of fungi. Griseofulvin is deposited in the keratin precursor cells and has a greater affinity for diseased tissue. The drug is tightly bound to the new keratin which becomes highly resistant to fungal invasions.

Griseofulvin absorption from the gastrointestinal tract varies considerably among individuals mainly because of insolubility of the drug in aqueous media of the upper G.I. tract. The peak serum level found in fasting adults given 0.5 g occurs at about four hours and ranges between 0.5 to 2.0 mcg/mL. The serum level may be increased by giving the drug with a meal with a high fat content.

INDICATIONS

Griseofulvin is indicated for the treatment of ringworm infections of the skin, hair, and nails, namely:

Tinea corporis
Tinea pedis
Tinea cruris

Continued on next page

Wyeth-Ayerst—Cont.

Tinea barbae
Tinea capitis
Tinea unguium (onychomycosis) when caused by one or more of the following genera of fungi:
Trichophyton rubrum
Trichophyton tonsurans
Trichophyton mentagrophytes
Trichophyton interdigitalis
Trichophyton verrucosum
Trichophyton megnini
Trichophyton gallinae
Trichophyton craateriform
Trichophyton sulphureum
Trichophyton schoenleini
Microsporum audouini
Microsporum canis
Microsporum gypseum
Epidermophyton floccosum.
NOTE: Prior to therapy, the type of fungi responsible for the infection should be identified.

The use of this drug is not justified in minor or trivial infections which will respond to topical agents alone.
Griseofulvin is *not* effective in the following:
Bacterial infections
Candidiasis (Moniliasis)
Histoplasmosis
Actinomycosis
Sporotrichosis
Chromoblastomycosis
Coccidioidomycosis
North American Blastomycosis
Cryptococcosis (Torulosis)
Tinea versicolor
Nocardiosis

CONTRAINDICATIONS
This drug is contraindicated in patients with porphyria, hepatocellular failure, and in individuals with a history of hypersensitivity to griseofulvin.

WARNINGS
Prophylactic Usage: Safety and efficacy of griseofulvin for prophylaxis of fungal infections has not been established.
Animal Toxicology: Chronic feeding of griseofulvin, at levels ranging from 0.5-2.5% of the diet, resulted in the development of liver tumors in several strains of mice, particularly males. Smaller particle sizes result in an enhanced effect. Lower oral dosage levels have not been tested. Subcutaneous administration of relatively small doses of griseofulvin, once a week, during the first three weeks of life has also been reported to induce hepatomata in mice. Although studies in other animal species have not yielded evidence of tumorigenicity, these studies were not of adequate design to form a basis for conclusions in this regard.
In subacute toxicity studies, orally administered griseofulvin produced hepatocellular necrosis in mice, but this has not been seen in other species. Disturbances in porphyrin metabolism have been reported in griseofulvin-treated laboratory animals. Griseofulvin has been reported to have a colchicine-like effect on mitosis and cocarcinogenicity with methylcholanthrene in cutaneous tumor induction in laboratory animals.
Usage in Pregnancy: The safety of this drug during pregnancy has not been established.
Animal Reproduction Studies: It has been reported in the literature that griseofulvin was found to be embryotoxic and teratogenic on oral administration to pregnant rats. Pups with abnormalities have been reported in the litters of a few bitches treated with griseofulvin. Additional animal reproduction studies are in progress.
Suppression of spermatogenesis has been reported to occur in rats, but investigation in man failed to confirm this.

PRECAUTIONS
Patients on prolonged therapy with any potent medication should be under close observation. Periodic monitoring of organ system function, including renal, hepatic, and hematopoietic, should be done.
Since griseofulvin is derived from species of *Penicillium*, the possibility of cross-sensitivity with penicillin exists; however, known penicillin-sensitive patients have been treated without difficulty.
Since a photosensitivity reaction is occasionally associated with griseofulvin therapy, patients should be warned to avoid exposure to intense natural or artificial sunlight. Lupus erythematosus, lupus-like syndromes, or exacerbation of existing lupus erythematosus have been reported in patients receiving griseofulvin.
Griseofulvin decreases the activity of warfarin-type anticoagulants so that patients receiving these drugs concomitantly may require dosage adjustment of the anticoagulant during and after griseofulvin therapy.

Barbiturates usually depress griseofulvin activity and concomitant administration may require a dosage adjustment of the antifungal agent.
The effect of alcohol may be potentiated by griseofulvin, producing such effects as tachycardia and flush.

ADVERSE REACTIONS
When adverse reactions occur, they are most commonly of the hypersensitivity type such as skin rashes, urticaria, and rarely, angioneurotic edema, and may necessitate withdrawal of therapy and appropriate countermeasures. Paresthesias of the hands and feet have been reported rarely after extended therapy. Other side effects reported occasionally are oral thrush, nausea, vomiting, epigastric distress, diarrhea, headache, fatigue, dizziness, insomnia, mental confusion, and impairment of performance of routine activities. Proteinuria and leukopenia have been reported rarely. Administration of the drug should be discontinued if granulocytopenia occurs.
When rare, serious reactions occur with griseofulvin, they are usually associated with high dosages, long periods of therapy, or both.

DOSAGE AND ADMINISTRATION
Accurate diagnosis of the infecting organism is essential. Identification should be made either by direct microscopic examination of a mounting of infected tissue in a solution of potassium hydroxide or by culture on an appropriate medium.
Medication must be continued until the infecting organism is completely eradicated as indicated by appropriate clinical or laboratory examination. Representative treatment periods are—*tinea capitis,* 4 to 6 weeks; *tinea corporis,* 2 to 4 weeks; *tinea pedis,* 4 to 8 weeks; *tinea unguium*—depending on rate of growth—fingernails, at least 4 months; toenails, at least 6 months.
General measures in regard to hygiene should be observed to control sources of infection or reinfection. Concomitant use of appropriate topical agents is usually required, particularly in treatment of *tinea pedis.* In some forms of athlete's foot, yeasts and bacteria may be involved as well as fungi. Griseofulvin will not eradicate the bacterial or monilial infection.
Adults: 0.5 g daily (125 mg q.i.d., 250 mg b.i.d., or 500 mg/day). Patients with less severe or extensive infections may require less, whereas those with widespread lesions may require a starting dose of 0.75 g to 1.0 g a day. This may be reduced gradually to 0.5 g or less after a response has been noted. In all cases, the dosage should be individualized.
Children: A dosage of 10 mg/kg daily is usually adequate (children from 30 to 50 lb, 125 mg to 250 mg daily; children over 50 lb, 250 mg to 500 mg daily, in divided doses). Dosage should be individualized, as with adults.
Clinical relapse will occur if the medication is not continued until the infecting organism is eradicated.

HOW SUPPLIED
GRISACTIN [griseofulvin (microsize)]—
GRISACTIN 125, each capsule contains 125 mg, in bottles of 100 (NDC 0046-0442-81).
GRISACTIN 250, each capsule contains 250 mg, in bottles of 100 (NDC 0046-0443-81) and 500 (NDC 0046-0443-85).
GRISACTIN 500, each tablet (scored) contains 500 mg, in bottles of 60 (NDC 0046-0444-60).
Store at room temperature (approximately 25℃).
Shown in Product Identification Section, page 436

GRISACTIN® Ultra   ℞
[*grĭz-ăc 'tĭn*]
(griseofulvin ultramicrosize)

CAUTION: Federal law prohibits dispensing without prescription.

DESCRIPTION
Griseofulvin is an oral fungistatic antibiotic for the treatment of superficial mycoses. It is derived from a species of *Penicillium.*
GRISACTIN Ultra tablets contain griseofulvin ultramicrosize in the following dosage strengths: 125 mg, 250 mg, and 330 mg.
GRISACTIN Ultra tablets contain the following inactive ingredients: lactose, magnesium stearate, microcrystalline cellulose, sodium starch glycolate.

ACTION
Griseofulvin is fungistatic with *in vitro* activity against various species of *Microsporum, Epidermophyton,* and *Trichophyton.* It has no effect on bacteria or on other genera of fungi.
Human Pharmacology: Following oral administration, griseofulvin is deposited in the keratin precursor cells and has a greater affinity for diseased tissue. The drug is tightly bound to the new keratin which becomes highly resistant to fungal invasions.
The efficiency of gastrointestinal absorption of ultramicrocrystalline griseofulvin is approximately one and one-half times that of the conventional microsize griseofulvin. This

factor permits the oral intake of two-thirds as much ultramicrocrystalline griseofulvin as the microsize form. However, there is currently no evidence that this lower dose confers any significant clinical difference with regard to safety and/or efficacy.

INDICATIONS
Griseofulvin is indicated for the treatment of ringworm infections of the skin, hair, and nails, namely:
Tinea corporis
Tinea pedis
Tinea cruris
Tinea barbae
Tinea capitis

Tinea unguium (onychomycosis) when caused by one or more of the following genera of fungi:

Trichophyton rubrum
Trichophyton tonsurans
Trichophyton mentagrophytes
Trichophyton interdigitalis
Trichophyton verrucosum
Trichophyton megnini
Trichophyton gallinae
Trichophyton craateriform
Trichophyton sulphureum
Trichophyton schoenleini
Microsporum audouini
Microsporum canis
Microsporum gypseum
Epidermophyton floccosum

NOTE: Prior to therapy, the type of fungi responsible for the infection should be identified.

The use of this drug is not justified in minor or trivial infections which will respond to topical agents alone.

Griseofulvin is *not* effective in the following:
Bacterial infections
Candidiasis (Moniliasis)
Histoplasmosis
Actinomycosis
Sporotrichosis
Chromoblastomycosis
Coccidioidomycosis
North American Blastomycosis
Cryptococcosis (Torulosis)
Tinea versicolor
Nocardiosis

CONTRAINDICATIONS
This drug is contraindicated in patients with porphyria, hepatocellular failure, and in individuals with a history of hypersensitivity to griseofulvin.

WARNINGS
Prophylactic Usage
Safety and efficacy of griseofulvin for prophylaxis of fungal infections has not been established.
Animal Toxicology
Chronic feeding of griseofulvin, at levels ranging from 0.5-2.5% of the diet, resulted in the development of liver tumors in several strains of mice, particularly males. Smaller particle sizes result in an enhanced effect. Lower oral dosage levels have not been tested. Subcutaneous administration of relatively small doses of griseofulvin, once a week, during the first three weeks of life has also been reported to induce hepatomata in mice. Although studies in other animal species have not yielded evidence of tumorigenicity, these studies were not of adequate design to form a basis for conclusions in this regard.
In subacute toxicity studies, orally administered griseofulvin produced hepatocellular necrosis in mice, but this has not been seen in other species. Disturbances in porphyrin metabolism have been reported in griseofulvin-treated laboratory animals. Griseofulvin has been reported to have a colchicine-like effect on mitosis and cocarcinogenicity with methylcholanthrene in cutaneous tumor induction in laboratory animals.
Usage in Pregnancy
The safety of this drug during pregnancy has not been established.
Animal Reproduction Studies
It has been reported in the literature that griseofulvin was found to be embryotoxic and teratogenic on oral administration to pregnant rats. Pups with abnormalities have been reported in the litters of a few bitches treated with griseofulvin. Additional animal reproduction studies are in progress.
Suppression of spermatogenesis has been reported to occur in rats, but investigation in man failed to confirm this.

PRECAUTIONS
Patients on prolonged therapy with any potent medication should be under close observation. Periodic monitoring of organ system function, including renal, hepatic, and hematopoietic, should be done.
Since griseofulvin is derived from species of *Penicillium,* the possibility of cross-sensitivity with penicillin exists; how-

ever, known penicillin-sensitive patients have been treated without difficulty.

Since a photosensitivity reaction is occasionally associated with griseofulvin therapy, patients should be warned to avoid exposure to intense natural or artificial sunlight.

Lupus erythematosus, lupus-like syndromes, or exacerbation of existing lupus erythematosus have been reported in patients receiving griseofulvin.

Griseofulvin decreases the activity of warfarin-type anticoagulants so that patients receiving these drugs concomitantly may require dosage adjustment of the anticoagulant during and after griseofulvin therapy.

Barbiturates usually depress griseofulvin activity and concomitant administration may require a dosage adjustment of the antifungal agent.

The effect of alcohol may be potentiated by griseofulvin, producing such effects as tachycardia and flush.

ADVERSE REACTIONS

When adverse reactions occur, they are most commonly of the hypersensitivity type such as skin rashes, urticaria, and rarely, angioneurotic edema, and may necessitate withdrawal of therapy and appropriate countermeasures. Paresthesias of the hands and feet have been reported rarely after extended therapy. Other side effects reported occasionally are oral thrush, nausea, vomiting, epigastric distress, diarrhea, headache, fatigue, dizziness, insomnia, mental confusion, and impairment of performance of routine activities. Proteinuria and leukopenia have been reported rarely. Administration of the drug should be discontinued if granulocytopenia occurs.

When rare, serious reactions occur with griseofulvin, they are usually associated with high dosages, long periods of therapy, or both.

DOSAGE AND ADMINISTRATION

Accurate diagnosis of the infecting organism is essential. Identification should be made either by direct microscopic examination of a mounting of infected tissue in a solution of potassium hydroxide or by culture on an appropriate medium.

Medication must be continued until the infecting organism is completely eradicated as indicated by appropriate clinical or laboratory examination. Representative treatment periods are—*tinea capitis*, 4 to 6 weeks; *tinea corporis*, 2 to 4 weeks; *tinea pedis*, 4 to 8 weeks; *tinea unguium*—depending on rate of growth—fingernails, at least 4 months; toenails, at least 6 months.

General measures in regard to hygiene should be observed to control sources of infection or reinfection. Concomitant use of appropriate topical agents is usually required, particularly in treatment of *tinea pedis*. In some forms of athlete's foot, yeasts and bacteria may be involved as well as fungi. Griseofulvin will not eradicate the bacterial or monilial infection.

Adults: Daily administration of 330 mg (as a single dose or in divided doses) will give a satisfactory response in most patients with *tinea corporis*, *tinea cruris*, and *tinea capitis*. For those fungal infections more difficult to eradicate such as *tinea pedis* and *tinea unguium*, a divided dose of 660 mg is recommended.

Children: Approximately 3.3 mg per pound of body weight per day of ultramicrosize griseofulvin is an effective dose for most children. On this basis the following dosage schedules are suggested:

Children weighing 35 to 50 lbs: 125 to 165 mg
Children weighing 50 to 75 lbs: 165 to 250 mg
Children weighing 75 lbs and over: 250 to 330 mg
Children 2 years of age and younger: dosage has not been established.

Clinical experience with griseofulvin in children with *tinea capitis* indicates that a single daily dose is effective. Clinical relapse will occur if the medication is not continued until the infecting organism is eradicated.

HOW SUPPLIED

GRISACTIN® Ultra tablets, 125 mg: white, square shaped, compressed tablets impressed with the trade name and dosage strength, in bottles of 100 (NDC 0046-0434-81).

GRISACTIN® Ultra tablets, 250 mg: white, square shaped, compressed tablets impressed with the trade name and dosage strength, in bottles of 100 (NDC 0046-0435-81).

GRISACTIN® Ultra tablets, 330 mg: scored, white, wide-oval shaped, compressed tablets impressed with the trade name and dosage strength, in bottles of 100 (NDC 0046-0437-81).

Store at room temperature (approximately 25° C).

Shown in Product Identification Section, page 436

HEPARIN   ℞
[*hep'ah-rin*]
Lock Flush Solution, USP

Heparin Lock Flush Solution is intended for maintenance of patency of intravenous injection devices only, and is not to be used for anticoagulant therapy.

DESCRIPTION

Wyeth's TUBEX® Heparin Lock Flush Solution, USP, is a sterile solution. Each mL contains either 10 or 100 USP units heparin sodium derived from porcine intestinal mucosa (standardized for use as an anticoagulant) in normal saline solution, and not more than 10 mg benzyl alcohol as a preservative.

The potency is determined by biological assay, using a USP reference standard based upon units of heparin activity per milligram.

Heparin is a heterogenous group of straight-chain anionic mucopolysaccharides, called glycosaminoglycans, having anticoagulant properties. Although others may be present, the main sugars occurring in heparin are: (1) α-L-iduronic acid 2-sulfate, (2) 2-deoxy-2-sulfamino-α-D-glucose 6-sulfate, (3) β-D-glucuronic acid, (4) 2-acetamido-2-deoxy-α-D-glucose, and (5) α-L-iduronic acid. These sugars are present in decreasing amounts, usually in the order (2) > (1) > (4) > (3) > (5), and are joined by glycosidic linkages, forming polymers of varying sizes. Heparin is strongly acidic because of its content of covalently linked sulfate and carboxylic acid groups. In heparin sodium, the acidic protons of the sulfate units are partially replaced by sodium ions.

STRUCTURE OF HEPARIN SODIUM (representative subunits):

CLINICAL PHARMACOLOGY

Heparin inhibits reactions that lead to the clotting of blood and the formation of fibrin clots both *in vitro* and *in vivo*. Heparin acts at multiple sites in the normal coagulation system. Small amounts of heparin in combination with antithrombin III (heparin cofactor) can inhibit thrombosis by inactivating activated Factor X and inhibiting the conversion of prothrombin to thrombin. Once active thrombosis has developed, larger amounts of heparin can inhibit further coagulation by inactivating thrombin and preventing the conversion of fibrinogen to fibrin. Heparin also prevents the formation of a stable fibrin clot by inhibiting the activation of the fibrin stabilizing factor.

Bleeding time is usually unaffected by heparin. Clotting time is prolonged by full therapeutic doses of heparin; in most cases, it is not measurably affected by low doses of heparin. Peak plasma levels of heparin are achieved 2 to 4 hours following subcutaneous administration, although there are considerable individual variations. Loglinear plots of heparin plasma concentrations with time, for a wide range of dose levels, are linear which suggests the absence of zero order processes. Liver and the reticulo-endothelial system are the sites of biotransformation. The biphasic elimination curve, a rapidly declining alpha phase ($t_{1/2} = 10$ min.), and after the age of 40 a slower beta phase, indicates uptake in organs. The absence of a relationship between anticoagulant half-life and concentration half-life may reflect factors such as protein binding of heparin.

Heparin does not have fibrinolytic activity; therefore, it will not lyse existing clots.

INDICATIONS AND USAGE

Heparin Lock Flush Solution, USP, is intended to maintain patency of an indwelling venipuncture device designed for intermittent injection or infusion therapy, or blood sampling. Heparin Lock Flush Solution, USP, may be used following initial placement of the device in the vein, after each injection of a medication, or after withdrawal of blood for laboratory tests.

Heparin Lock Flush Solution, USP, is not to be used for anticoagulant therapy.

Heparin may also be employed as an anticoagulant in blood transfusions, extracorporeal circulation, dialysis procedures, and in blood samples for laboratory purposes.

CONTRAINDICATIONS

Heparin sodium should not be used in patients with the following conditions:

Severe thrombocytopenia;

An uncontrollable active bleeding state (see "Warnings"), except when this is due to disseminated intravascular coagulation.

WARNINGS

Heparin is not intended for intramuscular use.

HYPERSENSITIVITY

Patients with documented hypersensitivity to heparin should be given the drug only in clearly life-threatening situations.

HEMORRHAGE

Hemorrhage can occur at virtually any site in patients receiving heparin. An unexplained fall in hematocrit, fall in blood pressure, or any other unexplained symptom should lead to serious consideration of a hemorrhagic event.

Heparin sodium should be used with extreme caution in disease states in which there is increased danger of hemorrhage. Some of the conditions in which increased danger of hemorrhage exists are:

Cardiovascular—Subacute bacterial endocarditis. Severe hypertension.

Surgical—During and immediately following (a) spinal tap or spinal anesthesia or (b) major surgery, especially involving the brain, spinal cord, or eye.

Hematologic—Conditions associated with increased bleeding tendencies, such as hemophilia, thrombocytopenia, and some vascular purpuras.

Gastrointestinal—Ulcerative lesions and continuous tube drainage of the stomach or small intestine.

Other—Menstruation, liver disease with impaired hemostasis.

THROMBOCYTOPENIA

Thrombocytopenia has been reported to occur in patients receiving heparin with a reported incidence of 0 to 30%. Mild thrombocytopenia (count greater than 100,000/mm³) may remain stable or reverse even if heparin is continued. However, thrombocytopenia of any degree should be monitored closely. If the count falls below 100,000/mm³ or if recurrent thrombosis develops (see "White-clot Syndrome," "Precautions"), the heparin product should be discontinued. If continued heparin therapy is essential, administration of heparin from a different organ source can be reinstituted with caution.

MISCELLANEOUS

This product contains benzyl alcohol as preservative. Benzyl alcohol has been reported to be associated with a fatal "Gasping Syndrome" in premature infants.

PRECAUTIONS

GENERAL

White-clot Syndrome

Rare patients on heparin may develop new thrombus formation in association with thrombocytopenia, resulting from irreversible aggregation of platelets induced by heparin, the so-called "white-clot syndrome." The process may lead to severe thromboembolic complications like skin necrosis, gangrene of the extremities, myocardial infarction, pulmonary embolism, and stroke. Therefore, heparin administration should be promptly discontinued if a patient develops new thrombosis in association with thrombocytopenia.

Heparin Resistance

Increased resistance to heparin is frequently encountered in fever, thrombosis, thrombophlebitis, infections with thrombosing tendencies, myocardial infarction, cancer, and in postsurgical patients.

Increased Risk in Older Women

A higher incidence of bleeding has been reported in women over 60 years of age.

LABORATORY TESTS

Periodic platelet counts, hematocrits, and tests for occult blood in stool are recommended during the entire course of heparin therapy, regardless of the route of administration (see "Dosage and Administration").

DRUG INTERACTIONS

Platelet Inhibitors

Drugs such as acetylsalicylic acid, dextran, phenylbutazone, ibuprofen, indomethacin, dipyridamole, hydroxychloroquine, and others that interfere with platelet-aggregation reactions (the main hemostatic defense of heparinized patients) may induce bleeding and should be used with caution in patients receiving heparin sodium.

Other Interactions

Digitalis, tetracyclines, nicotine, or antihistamines may partially counteract the anticoagulant action of heparin sodium.

CARCINOGENESIS, MUTAGENESIS, IMPAIRMENT OF FERTILITY

No long-term studies in animals have been performed to evaluate carcinogenic potential of heparin. Also, no reproduction studies in animals have been performed concerning mutagenesis or impairment of fertility.

Continued on next page

Wyeth-Ayerst—Cont.

PREGNANCY

Teratogenic Effects —Pregnancy Category C
Animal reproduction studies have not been conducted with heparin sodium. It is also not known whether heparin sodium can cause fetal harm when administered to a pregnant woman or can affect reproduction capacity. Heparin sodium should be given to a pregnant woman only if clearly needed.
Nonteratogenic Effects
Heparin does not cross the placental barrier.

NURSING MOTHERS

Heparin is not excreted in human milk.

ADVERSE REACTIONS

HEMORRHAGE

Hemorrhage is the chief complication that may result from heparin therapy (see "Warnings"). An overly prolonged clotting time or minor bleeding during therapy can usually be controlled by withdrawing the drug (see "Overdosage"). It should be appreciated that gastrointestinal- or urinary-tract bleeding during anticoagulant therapy may indicate the presence of an underlying occult lesion. Bleeding can occur at any site but certain specific hemorrhagic complications may be difficult to detect:

a. Adrenal hemorrhage, with resultant acute adrenal insufficiency, has occurred during anticoagulant therapy. Therefore, such treatment should be discontinued in patients who develop signs and symptoms of acute adrenal hemorrhage and insufficiency. Initiation of corrective therapy should not depend on laboratory confirmation of the diagnosis, since any delay in an acute situation may result in the patient's death.

b. Ovarian (corpus luteum) hemorrhage developed in a number of women of reproductive age receiving short- or long-term anticoagulant therapy. This complication, if unrecognized, may be fatal.

c. Retroperitoneal hemorrhage.

LOCAL IRRITATION

Local irritation, erythema, mild pain, hematoma, or ulceration may follow deep, subcutaneous (intrafat) injection of heparin sodium. These complications are much more common after intramuscular use, and such use is not recommended.

HYPERSENSITIVITY

Generalized hypersensitivity reactions have been reported, with chills, fever, and urticaria as the most usual manifestations, and asthma, rhinitis, lacrimation, headache, nausea and vomiting, and anaphylactoid reactions, including shock, occurring more rarely. Itching and burning, especially on the plantar side of the feet, may occur.

Thrombocytopenia has been reported to occur in patients receiving heparin with a reported incidence of 0 to 30%. While often mild and of no obvious clinical significance, such thrombocytopenia can be accompanied by severe thromboembolic complications, such as skin necrosis, gangrene of the extremities, myocardial infarction, pulmonary embolism, and stroke. (See "Warnings," "Precautions.")

Certain episodes of painful, ischemic and cyanosed limbs have in the past been attributed to allergic vasospastic reactions. Whether these are, in fact, identical to the thrombocytopenia-associated complications remains to be determined.

MISCELLANEOUS

Osteoporosis following long-term administration of high doses of heparin, cutaneous necrosis after systemic administration, suppression of aldosterone synthesis, delayed transient alopecia, priapism, and rebound hyperlipemia on discontinuation of heparin sodium have also been reported.

Significant elevations of aminotransferase (SGOT [S-AST] and SGPT [S-ALT]) levels have occurred in a high percentage of patients (and healthy subjects) who have received heparin.

OVERDOSAGE

SYMPTOMS

Bleeding is the chief sign of heparin overdosage. Nosebleeds, blood in urine, or tarry stools may be noted as the first sign of bleeding. Easy bruising or petechial formations may precede frank bleeding.

TREATMENT—Neutralization of Heparin Effect
When clinical circumstances (bleeding) require reversal of heparinization, protamine sulfate (1% solution) by slow infusion will neutralize heparin sodium. No more than 50 mg should be administered, very slowly, in any 10-minute period. Each mg of protamine sulfate neutralizes approximately 100 USP heparin units. The amount of protamine required decreases over time as heparin is metabolized. Although the metabolism of heparin is complex, it may, for the purpose of choosing a protamine dose, be assumed to have a half-life of about 1/2 hour after intravenous injection.

Administration of protamine sulfate can cause severe hypo- and anaphylactoid reactions. Because fatal reactions resembling anaphylaxis, have been reported, the

drug should be given only when resuscitation techniques and treatment of anaphylactoid shock are readily available.
For additional information consult the labeling of Protamine Sulfate Injection, USP, products.

DOSAGE AND ADMINISTRATION

Parenteral drug products should be inspected visually for particulate matter and discoloration prior to administration, whenever solution and container permit.
Slight discoloration does not alter potency.

MAINTENANCE OF PATENCY OF INTRAVENOUS DEVICES
To prevent clot formation in a heparin lock set or central venous catheter following its proper insertion, Heparin Lock Flush Solution, USP, is injected via the injection hub in a quantity sufficient to fill the entire device. This solution should be replaced each time the device is used. Aspirate before administering any solution via the device in order to confirm patency and location of needle or catheter tip. If the drug to be administered is incompatible with heparin, the entire device should be flushed with normal saline before and after the medication is administered; following the second saline flush, Heparin Lock Flush Solution, USP, may be reinstilled into the device. The device manufacturer's instructions should be consulted for specifics concerning its use. Usually this dilute heparin solution will maintain anticoagulation within the device for up to 4 hours.
NOTE: Since repeated injections of small doses of heparin can alter tests for activated partial thromboplastin time (APTT), a baseline value for APTT should be obtained prior to insertion of an intravenous device.
When heparin is added to an infusion solution for continuous intravenous administration, the container should be inverted at least six times to insure adequate mixing and prevent pooling of the heparin in the solution.

WITHDRAWAL OF BLOOD SAMPLES
Heparin Lock Flush Solution, USP, may also be used after each withdrawal of blood for laboratory tests. When heparin (or sodium chloride) would interfere with or alter the results of blood tests, the heparin solution should be cleared from the device by aspirating and discarding it before withdrawing the blood sample.

HOW SUPPLIED

Heparin Lock Flush Solution, USP, is supplied in TUBEX Sterile Cartridge-Needle Units which include 25 gauge $\times$ 5/8 inch needles.
Each 1 mL size TUBEX contains one of the following concentrations of heparin sodium, in packages of 50 TUBEX:
10 USP units per mL, NDC 0008-0523-01.
100 USP Units per mL, NDC 0008-0487-01.
Each 2.5 mL size TUBEX contains one of the following concentrations of heparin sodium, in packages of 50 TUBEX:
25 USP Units per TUBEX or 10 USP Units per mL, NDC 0008-0523-02.
250 USP Units per TUBEX or 100 USP Units per mL, NDC 0008-0487-03.
Do not freeze

HEPARIN FLUSH KITS
All TUBEX® Sterile Cartridge-Needle Units in the following packages include 25 gauge $\times$ 5/8 inch needles.
10 USP UNITS HEPARIN SODIUM PER ML
Each Unit of Use Kit contains:
NDC 0008-2528-01; one TUBEX (1 mL) Heparin Lock Flush Solution, USP; two TUBEX (2.5 mL each) Bacteriostatic Sodium Chloride Injection, USP; in packages of 50 Kits.
NDC 0008-2528-03; one TUBEX (1 mL) Heparin Lock Flush Solution, USP; two TUBEX (1 mL each) Bacteriostatic Sodium Chloride Injection, USP; in packages of 50 Kits.
100 USP UNITS HEPARIN SODIUM PER ML
Each Unit of Use Kit contains:
NDC 0008-2529-01; one TUBEX (1 mL) Heparin Lock Flush Solution, USP; two TUBEX (2.5 mL each) Bacteriostatic Sodium Chloride Injection, USP; in packages of 50 Kits.
NDC 0008-2529-03; one TUBEX (1 mL) Heparin Lock Flush Solution, USP; two TUBEX (1 mL each) Bacteriostatic Sodium Chloride Injection, USP; in packages of 50 Kits.
Do not freeze

HEPARIN   ℞

[*hep'ah-rin*]
Sodium Injection, USP

DESCRIPTION

Wyeth's TUBEX® Heparin Sodium Injection, USP, is a sterile solution. Each mL contains 1,000, 2,500, 5,000, 7,500, 10,000, 15,000, or 20,000 USP units heparin sodium, derived from porcine intestinal mucosa (standardized for use as an anticoagulant), in water for injection, and not more than 10 mg benzyl alcohol as a preservative.
The potency is determined by biological assay, using a USP reference standard based upon units of heparin activity per milligram.
Heparin is a heterogenous group of straight-chain anionic mucopolysaccharides, called glycosaminoglycans, having

anticoagulant properties. Although others may be present, the main sugars occurring in heparin are: (1) α-L-iduronic acid 2-sulfate, (2) 2-deoxy-2-sulfamino-α-D-glucose 6-sulfate, (3) β-D-glucuronic acid, (4) 2-acetamido-2-deoxy-α-D-glucose, and (5) α-L-iduronic acid. These sugars are present in decreasing amounts, usually in the order (2) > (1) > (4) > (3) > (5), and are joined by glycosidic linkages, forming polymers of varying sizes. Heparin is strongly acidic because of its content of covalently linked sulfate and carboxylic acid groups. In heparin sodium, the acidic protons of the sulfate units are partially replaced by sodium ions.
STRUCTURE OF HEPARIN SODIUM (representative subunits):

CLINICAL PHARMACOLOGY:

Heparin inhibits reactions that lead to the clotting of blood and the formation of fibrin clots both *in vitro* and *in vivo*. Heparin acts at multiple sites in the normal coagulation system. Small amounts of heparin in combination with antithrombin III (heparin cofactor) can inhibit thrombosis by inactivating activated Factor X and inhibiting the conversion of prothrombin to thrombin. Once active thrombosis has developed, larger amounts of heparin can inhibit further coagulation by inactivating thrombin and preventing the conversion of fibrinogen to fibrin. Heparin also prevents the formation of a stable fibrin clot by inhibiting the activation of the fibrin stabilizing factor.
Bleeding time is usually unaffected by heparin. Clotting time is prolonged by full therapeutic doses of heparin; in most cases it is not measurably affected by low doses of heparin. Peak plasma levels of heparin are achieved 2 to 4 hours following subcutaneous administration, although there are considerable individual variations. Loglinear plots of heparin plasma concentrations with time, for a wide range of dose levels, are linear which suggests the absence of zero order processes. Liver and the reticulo-endothelial system are the sites of biotransformation. The biphasic elimination curve, a rapidly declining alpha phase ($t_{1/2}$ = 10 min.), and after the age of 40 a slower beta phase, indicates uptake in organs. The absence of a relationship between anticoagulant half-life and concentration half-life may reflect factors such as protein binding of heparin.
Heparin does not have fibrinolytic activity; therefore, it will not lyse existing clots.

INDICATIONS AND USAGE

Heparin sodium injection is indicated for anticoagulant therapy in prophylaxis and treatment of venous thrombosis and its extension; in low-dose regimen for prevention of postoperative deep venous thrombosis and pulmonary embolism in patients undergoing major abdominothoracic surgery who are at risk of developing thromboembolic disease (see "Dosage and Administration"); for prophylaxis and treatment of pulmonary embolism; in atrial fibrillation with embolization; for diagnosis and treatment of acute and chronic consumptive coagulopathies (disseminated intravascular coagulation); for prevention of clotting in arterial and cardiac surgery; and for prophylaxis and treatment of peripheral arterial embolism.
Heparin may also be employed as an anticoagulant in blood transfusions, extracorporeal circulation, dialysis procedures, and in blood samples for laboratory purposes.

CONTRAINDICATIONS

Heparin sodium should not be used in patients:
with severe thrombocytopenia;
in whom suitable blood-coagulation tests—e.g., the whole-blood clotting time, partial thromboplastin time, etc.—cannot be performed at appropriate intervals (this contraindication refers to full-dose heparin; there is usually no need to monitor coagulation parameters in patients receiving low-dose heparin);
with an uncontrollable active bleeding state (see "Warnings"), except when this is due to disseminated intravascular coagulation.

WARNINGS

Heparin is not intended for intramuscular use.

HYPERSENSITIVITY

Patients with documented hypersensitivity to heparin should be given the drug only in clearly life-threatening situations.

HEMORRHAGE

Hemorrhage can occur at virtually any site in patients receiving heparin. An unexplained fall in hematocrit, fall in blood pressure, or any other unexplained symptom should lead to serious consideration of a hemorrhagic event.

Heparin sodium should be used with extreme caution in disease states in which there is increased danger of hemorrhage. Some of the conditions in which increased danger of hemorrhage exists are:

Cardiovascular—Subacute bacterial endocarditis. Severe hypertension.

Surgical—During and immediately following (a) spinal tap or spinal anesthesia or (b) major surgery, especially involving the brain, spinal cord, or eye.

Hematologic—Conditions associated with increased bleeding tendencies, such as hemophilia, thrombocytopenia, and some vascular purpuras.

Gastrointestinal—Ulcerative lesions and continuous tube drainage of the stomach or small intestine.

Other—Menstruation, liver disease with impaired hemostasis.

COAGULATION TESTING

When heparin sodium is administered in therapeutic amounts, its dosage should be regulated by frequent blood coagulation tests. If the coagulation test is unduly prolonged or if hemorrhage occurs, heparin sodium should be discontinued promptly (see "Overdosage").

THROMBOCYTOPENIA

Thrombocytopenia has been reported to occur in patients receiving heparin with a reported incidence of 0 to 30%. Mild thrombocytopenia (count greater than 100,000/mm³) may remain stable or reverse even if heparin is continued. However, thrombocytopenia of any degree should be monitored closely. If the count falls below 100,000/mm³ or if recurrent thrombosis develops (see "White-clot Syndrome," "Precautions"), the heparin product should be discontinued. If continued heparin therapy is essential, admistration of heparin from a different organ source can be reinstituted with caution.

MISCELLANEOUS

This product contains benzyl alcohol as preservative. Benzyl alcohol has been reported to be associated with a fatal "Gasping Syndrome" in premature infants.

PRECAUTIONS

GENERAL

White-clot Syndrome

Rare patients on heparin may develop new thrombus formation in association with thrombocytopenia, resulting from irreversible aggregation of platelets induced by heparin, the so-called "white-clot syndrome." The process may lead to severe thromboembolic complications like skin necrosis, gangrene of the extremities, myocardial infarction, pulmonary embolism, and stroke. Therefore, heparin administration should be promptly discontinued if a patient develops new thrombosis in association with thrombocytopenia.

Heparin Resistance

Increased resistance to heparin is frequently encountered in fever, thrombosis, thrombophlebitis, infections with thrombosing tendencies, myocardial infarction, cancer, and in postsurgical patients.

Increased Risk in Older Women

A higher incidence of bleeding has been reported in women over 60 years of age.

LABORATORY TESTS

Periodic platelet counts, hematocrits, and tests for occult blood in stool are recommended during the entire course of heparin therapy, regardless of the route of administration (see "Dosage and Administration").

DRUG INTERACTIONS

Oral Anticoagulants

Heparin sodium may prolong the one-stage prothrombin time. Therefore, when heparin sodium is given with dicumarol or warfarin sodium, a period of at least 5 hours after the last intravenous dose or 24 hours after the last subcutaneous dose should elapse before blood is drawn if a valid prothrombin time is to be continued.

Platelet Inhibitors

Drugs such as acetylsalicylic acid, dextran, phenylbutazone, ibuprofen, indomethacin, dipyridamole, hydroxychloroquine, and others that interfere with platelet-aggregation reactions (the main hemostatic defense of heparinized patients) may induce bleeding and should be used with caution in patients receiving heparin sodium.

Other Interactions

Digitalis, tetracyclines, nicotine, or antihistamines may partially counteract the anticoagulant action of heparin sodium.

DRUG/LABORATORY TEST INTERACTIONS

Hyperaminotransferasemia

Significant elevations of aminotransferase (SGOT [S-AST] and SGPT [S-ALT]) levels have occurred in a high percentage of patients (and healthy subjects) who have received heparin. Since aminotransferase determinations are important in the differential diagnosis of myocardial infarction, liver disease, and pulmonary emboli, rises that might be caused by drugs (like heparin) should be interpreted with caution.

CARCINOGENESIS, MUTAGENESIS, IMPAIRMENT OF FERTILITY

No long-term studies in animals have been performed to evaluate carcinogenic potential of heparin. Also, no reproduction studies in animals have been performed concerning mutagenesis or impairment of fertility.

PREGNANCY

Teratogenic Effects—Pregnancy Category C

Animal reproduction studies have not been conducted with heparin sodium. It is also not known whether heparin sodium can cause fetal harm when administered to a pregnant woman or can affect reproduction capacity. Heparin sodium should be given to a pregnant woman only if clearly needed.

Nonteratogenic Effects

Heparin does not cross the placental barrier.

NURSING MOTHERS

Heparin is not excreted in human milk.

PEDIATRIC USE

See "Dosage and Administration."

ADVERSE REACTIONS

HEMORRHAGE

Hemorrhage is the chief complication that may result from heparin therapy (see "Warnings").

An overly prolonged clotting time or minor bleeding during therapy can usually be controlled by withdrawing the drug (see "Overdosage"). It should be appreciated that gastrointestinal- or urinary-tract bleeding during anticoagulant therapy may indicate the presence of an underlying occult lesion. Bleeding can occur at any site but certain specific hemorrhagic complications may be difficult to detect:

a. Adrenal hemorrhage, with resultant acute adrenal insufficiency, has occurred during anticoagulant therapy. Therefore, such treatment should be discontinued in patients who develop signs and symptoms of acute adrenal hemorrhage and insufficiency. Initiation of corrective therapy should not depend on laboratory confirmation of the diagnosis, since any delay in an acute situation may result in the patient's death.

b. Ovarian (corpus luteum) hemorrhage developed in a number of women of reproductive age receiving short- or long-term anticoagulant therapy. This complication, if unrecognized, may be fatal.

c. Retroperitoneal hemorrhage.

LOCAL IRRITATION

Local irritation, erythema, mild pain, hematoma, or ulceration may follow deep, subcutaneous (intrafat) injection of heparin sodium. These complications are much more common after intramuscular use, and such use is not recommended.

HYPERSENSITIVITY

Generalized hypersensitivity reactions have been reported, with chills, fever, and urticaria as the most usual manifestations, and asthma, rhinitis, lacrimation, headache, nausea and vomiting, and anaphylactoid reactions, including shock, occurring more rarely. Itching and burning, especially on the plantar surface of the feet, may occur.

Thrombocytopenia has been reported to occur in patients receiving heparin with a reported incidence of 0 to 30%. While often mild and of no obvious clinical significance, such thrombocytopenia can be accompanied by severe thromboembolic complications, such as skin necrosis, gangrene of the extremities, myocardial infarction, pulmonary embolism, and stroke. (See "Warnings," "Precautions.")

Certain episodes of painful, ischemic and cyanosed limbs have in the past been attributed to allergic vasospastic reactions. Whether these are, in fact, identical to the thrombocytopenia-associated complications remains to be determined.

MISCELLANEOUS

Osteoporosis following long-term administration of high doses of heparin, cutaneous necrosis after systemic administration, suppression of aldosterone synthesis, delayed transient alopecia, priapism, and rebound hyperlipemia on discontinuation of heparin sodium have also been reported.

Significant elevations of aminotransferase (SGOT [S-AST] and SGPT [S-ALT]) levels have occurred in a high percentage of patients (and healthy subjects) who have received heparin.

OVERDOSAGE

SYMPTOMS

Bleeding is the chief sign of heparin overdosage. Nosebleeds, blood in urine, or tarry stools may be noted as the first sign of bleeding. Easy bruising or petechial formations may precede frank bleeding.

TREATMENT—Neutralization of Heparin Effect

When clinical circumstances (bleeding) require reversal of heparinization, protamine sulfate (1% solution) by slow infusion will neutralize heparin sodium. No more than 50 mg should be administered, very slowly, in any 10-minute period. Each mg of protamine sulfate neutralizes approximately 100 USP heparin units. The amount of protamine required decreases over time as heparin is metabolized. Although the metabolism of heparin is complex, it may, for the purpose of choosing a protamine dose, be assumed to have a half-life of about ½ hour after intravenous injection.

Administration of protamine sulfate can cause severe hypotensive and anaphylactoid reactions. Because fatal reactions, often resembling anaphylaxis, have been reported, the drug should be given only when resuscitation techniques and treatment of anaphylactoid shock are readily available.

For additional information consult the labeling of Protamine Sulfate Injection, USP, products.

DOSAGE AND ADMINISTRATION

Parenteral drug products should be inspected visually for particulate matter and discoloration prior to administration, whenever solution and container permit. Slight discoloration does not alter potency.

When heparin is added to an infusion solution for continuous intravenous administration, the container should be inverted at least six times to insure adequate mixing and prevent pooling of the heparin in the solution.

Heparin sodium is not effective by oral administration and should be given by intermittent intravenous injection, intravenous infusion, or deep, subcutaneous (intrafat, i.e., above the iliac crest or abdominal fat layer) injection. *The intramuscular route of administration should be avoided because of the frequent occurrence of hematoma at the injection site.*

The dosage of heparin sodium should be adjusted according to the patient's coagulation-test results. When heparin is given by continuous intravenous infusion, the coagulation time should be determined approximately every 4 hours in the early stages of treatment. When the drug is administered intermittently by intravenous injection, coagulation tests should be performed before each injection during the early stages of treatment and at appropriate intervals thereafter. Dosage is considered adequate when the activated partial thromboplastin time (APTT) is 1.5 to 2 times normal or when the whole-blood clotting time is elevated approximately 2.5 to 3 times the control value. After deep subcutaneous (intrafat) injections, tests for adequacy of dosage are best performed on samples drawn 4 to 6 hours after the injections. Periodic platelet counts, hematocrits, and tests for occult blood in stool are recommended during the entire course of heparin therapy, regardless of the route of administration.

CONVERTING TO ORAL ANTICOAGULANT

When an oral anticoagulant of the coumarin or similar type is to be begun in patients already receiving heparin sodium, baseline and subsequent tests of prothrombin activity must be determined at a time when heparin activity is too low to affect the prothrombin time. This is about 5 hours after the last IV bolus and 24 hours after the last subcutaneous dose. If continuous IV heparin infusion is used, prothrombin time can usually be measured at any time.

In converting from heparin to an oral anticoagulant, the dose of the oral anticoagulant should be the usual initial amount, and thereafter prothrombin time should be determined at the usual intervals. To ensure continuous anticoagulation, it is advisable to continue full heparin therapy for several days after the prothrombin time has reached the therapeutic range. Heparin therapy may then be discontinued without tapering.

THERAPEUTIC ANTICOAGULANT EFFECT WITH FULL-DOSE HEPARIN

Although dosage must be adjusted for the individual patient according to the results of suitable laboratory tests, the following dosage schedules may be used as guidelines:

[See table on next page].

PEDIATRIC USE

Follow recommendations of appropriate pediatric reference texts. In general, the following dosage schedule may be used as a guideline.

Initial Dose: 50 units/kg (IV, drip).

Maintenance Dose: 100 units/kg (IV, drip) every four hours, or 20,000 units/M²/24 hours continuously.

SURGERY OF THE HEART AND BLOOD VESSELS

Patients undergoing total body perfusion for open-heart surgery should receive an initial dose of not less than 150 units of heparin sodium per kilogram of body weight. Frequently, a dose of 300 units of heparin sodium per kilogram of body weight is used for procedures estimated to last less than 60 minutes; or 400 units per kilogram for those estimated to last longer than 60 minutes.

LOW-DOSE PROPHYLAXIS OF POSTOPERATIVE THROMBOEMBOLISM

A number of well-controlled clinical trials have demonstrated that low-dose heparin prophylaxis, given just prior to and after surgery, will reduce the incidence of postoperative deep-vein thrombosis in the legs, as measured by the l-125 fibrinogen technique and venography, and of clinical pulmonary embolism. The most widely used dosage has been 5,000 units 2 hours before surgery and 5,000 units every 8 to 12 hours thereafter for 7 days or until the patient is fully ambulatory, whichever is longer. The heparin is given by deep, subcutaneous injection in the arm or abdomen with a fine needle (25–26 gauge) to minimize tissue trauma. A concen-

Continued on next page

Wyeth-Ayerst—Cont.

trated solution of heparin sodium is recommended. Such prophylaxis should be reserved for patients over 40 undergoing major surgery. Patients with bleeding disorders, those having neurosurgery, spinal anesthesia, eye surgery, or potentially sanguineous operations should be excluded, as well as patients receiving oral anticoagulants or platelet-active drugs (see "Warnings"). The value of such prophylaxis in hip surgery has not been established. The possibility of increased bleeding during surgery or postoperatively should be borne in mind. If such bleeding occurs, discontinuance of heparin and neutralization with protamine sulfate is advisable. If clinical evidence of thromboembolism develops despite low-dose prophylaxis, full therapeutic doses of anticoagulants should be given unless contraindicated. All patients should be screened prior to heparinization to rule out bleeding disorders, and monitoring should be performed with appropriate coagulation tests just prior to surgery. Coagulation-test values should be normal or only slightly elevated. There is usually no need for daily monitoring of the effect of low-dose heparin in patients with normal coagulation parameters.

EXTRACORPOREAL DIALYSIS USE
Follow equipment manufacturer's operating directions carefully.

BLOOD TRANSFUSION
Addition of 400 to 600 USP units per 100 ml of whole blood. Usually, 7,500 USP units of heparin sodium are added to 100 mL of Sterile Sodium Chloride Injection (or 75,000 USP units per 1,000 mL of Sterile Sodium Chloride Injection) and mixed, and from this sterile solution, 6 to 8 mL is added per 100 mL of whole blood: Leukocyte counts should be performed on heparinized blood within two hours after addition of the heparin. Heparinized blood should not be used for iso-agglutinin, complement, erythrocyte fragility tests, or platelet counts.

LABORATORY SAMPLES
Addition of 70 to 150 units of heparin sodium per 10 to 20 mL sample of whole blood is usually employed to prevent coagulation of the sample. See comments under "Blood Transfusion."

HOW SUPPLIED
Heparin Sodium Injection, USP, is supplied in TUBEX® Sterile Cartridge-Needle Units.
Each 1 mL size TUBEX contains one of the following concentrations of heparin sodium:
1,000 USP Units per mL (22 gauge × 1¼ inch needle), NDC 0008-0275-01, in packages of 10 TUBEX.
2,500 USP Units per mL (25 gauge × ⅝ inch needle), NDC 0008-0482-01, in packages of 10 TUBEX.
5,000 USP Units per 0.5 mL (10,000 USP Units per mL) (25 gauge × ⅝ inch needle), NDC 0008-0277-02, in packages of 10 TUBEX.
5,000 USP Units per 0.5 mL (10,000 USP Units per mL) (25 gauge × ⅝ inch needle), NDC 0008-0277-03, in packages of 50 TUBEX.
5,000 USP Units per mL (25 gauge × ⅝ inch needle), NDC 0008-0278-02, in packages of 10 TUBEX.
7,500 USP Units per mL (25 gauge × ⅝ inch needle), NDC 0008-0293-01, in packages of 10 TUBEX.
10,000 USP Units per mL (25 gauge × ⅝ inch needle), NDC 0008-0277-01, in packages of 10 TUBEX.
20,000 USP Units per mL (25 gauge × ⅝ inch needle), NDC 0008-0276-01, in packages of 10 TUBEX.
Do not freeze

Method of Administration	Frequency	Recommended Dose [based on 150 lb (68 kg) patient]
Deep, Subcutaneous (Intrafat) Injection	Initial Dose	5,000 units by IV injection followed by 10,000–20,000 units of a concentrated solution, subcutaneously
A different site should be used for each injection to prevent the development of massive hematoma.	Every 8 hours (or) Every 12 hours	8,000–10,000 units of a concentrated solution 15,000–20,000 units of a concentrated solution
Intermittent, Intravenous Injection	Initial Dose	10,000 units, either undiluted or in 50–100 ml isotonic sodium chloride injection
	Every 4 to 6 hours	5,000–10,000 units, either undiluted or in 50–100 mL isotonic sodium chloride injection
Intravenous Infusion	Initial Dose	5,000 units by IV injection
	Continuous	20,000–40,000 units in 1,000 mL of isotonic sodium chloride solution for infusion/day

---

INDERAL®   ℞
[ĭn'der-al]
(propranolol hydrochloride)
TABLETS

CAUTION: Federal law prohibits dispensing without prescription.

DESCRIPTION
INDERAL (propranolol hydrochloride) is a synthetic beta-adrenergic receptor blocking agent chemically described as 1-(Isopropylamino)-3-(1-naphthyloxy)-2-propanol hydrochloride. Its structural formula is

$$O\ CH_2CHOHCH_2NHCH(CH_3)_2 \cdot HCl$$

Propranolol hydrochloride is a stable, white, crystalline solid which is readily soluble in water and ethanol. Its molecular weight is 295.81.
INDERAL is available as 10 mg, 20 mg, 40 mg, 60 mg, and 80 mg tablets for oral administration and as a 1 mg/mL sterile injectable solution for intravenous administration.
The inactive ingredients contained in INDERAL Tablets are: lactose, magnesium stearate, microcrystalline cellulose, and stearic acid. In addition, INDERAL 10 mg and 80 mg Tablets contain FD&C Yellow No. 6 and D&C Yellow No. 10; INDERAL 20 mg Tablets contain FD&C Blue No. 1; INDERAL 40 mg Tablets contain FD&C Blue No. 1, FD&C Yellow No. 6 and D&C Yellow No. 10; INDERAL 60 mg Tablets contain D&C Red No. 30.

CLINICAL PHARMACOLOGY
INDERAL is a nonselective beta-adrenergic receptor blocking agent possessing no other autonomic nervous system activity. It specifically competes with beta-adrenergic receptor stimulating agents for available receptor sites. When access to beta-receptor sites is blocked by INDERAL, the chronotropic, inotropic, and vasodilator responses to beta-adrenergic stimulation are decreased proportionately.
Propranolol is almost completely absorbed from the gastrointestinal tract, but a portion is immediately bound by the liver. Peak effect occurs in one to one and one-half hours. The biologic half-life is approximately four hours.
There is no simple correlation between dose or plasma level and therapeutic effect, and the dose-sensitivity range as observed in clinical practice is wide. The principal reason for this is that sympathetic tone varies widely between individuals. Since there is no reliable test to estimate sympathetic tone or to determine whether total beta blockade has been achieved, proper dosage requires titration.
The mechanism of the antihypertensive effect of INDERAL has not been established. Among the factors that may be involved in contributing to the antihypertensive action are (1) decreased cardiac output, (2) inhibition of renin release by the kidneys, and (3) diminution of tonic sympathetic nerve outflow from vasomotor centers in the brain. Although total peripheral resistance may increase initially, it readjusts to or below the pretreatment level with chronic use. Effects on plasma volume appear to be minor and somewhat variable. INDERAL has been shown to cause a small increase in serum potassium concentration when used in the treatment of hypertensive patients.
In angina pectoris, propranolol generally reduces the oxygen requirement of the heart at any given level of effort by blocking the catecholamine-induced increases in the heart rate, systolic blood pressure, and the velocity and extent of myocardial contraction. Propranolol may increase oxygen requirements by increasing left ventricular fiber length, end diastolic pressure, and systolic ejection period. The net physiologic effect of beta-adrenergic blockade is usually advantageous and is manifested during exercise by delayed onset of pain and increased work capacity.
Propranolol exerts its antiarrhythmic effects in concentrations associated with beta-adrenergic blockade and this appears to be its principal antiarrhythmic mechanism of action. In dosages greater than required for beta blockade, INDERAL also exerts a quinidine-like or anesthetic-like membrane action, which affects the cardiac action potential. The significance of the membrane action in the treatment of arrhythmias is uncertain.
The mechanism of the antimigraine effect of propranolol has not been established. Beta-adrenergic receptors have been demonstrated in the pial vessels of the brain.
The specific mechanism of INDERAL's antitremor effects has not been established, but beta-2 (noncardiac) receptors may be involved. A central effect is also possible. Clinical studies have demonstrated that INDERAL is of benefit in exaggerated physiological and essential (familial) tremor.
Beta-receptor blockade can be useful in conditions in which, because of pathologic or functional changes, sympathetic activity is detrimental to the patient. But there are also situations in which sympathetic stimulation is vital. For example, in patients with severely damaged hearts, adequate ventricular function is maintained by virtue of sympathetic drive, which should be preserved. In the presence of AV block greater than first degree, beta blockade may prevent the necessary facilitating effect of sympathetic activity on conduction. Beta blockade results in bronchial constriction by interfering with adrenergic bronchodilator activity, which should be preserved in patients subject to bronchospasm.
Propranolol is not significantly dialyzable.
The Beta-Blocker Heart Attack Trial (BHAT) was a National Heart, Lung and Blood Institute-sponsored multicenter, randomized, double-blind, placebo-controlled trial conducted in 31 U.S. centers (plus one in Canada) in 3,837 persons without history of severe congestive heart failure or presence of recent heart failure; certain conduction defects; angina since infarction, who had survived the acute phase of myocardial infarction. Propranolol was administered at either 60 or 80 mg t.i.d. based on blood levels achieved during an initial trial of 40 mg t.i.d. Therapy with INDERAL, begun 5-21 days following infarction, was shown to reduce overall mortality up to 39 months, the longest period of follow-up. This was primarily attributable to a reduction in cardiovascular mortality. The protective effect of INDERAL was consistent regardless of age, sex, or site of infarction. Compared with placebo, total mortality was reduced 39% at 12 months and 26% over an average follow-up period of 25 months. The Norwegian Multicenter Trial in which propranolol was administered at 40 mg q.i.d. gave overall results which support the findings in the BHAT.
Although the clinical trials used either t.i.d. or q.i.d. dosing, clinical, pharmacologic, and pharmacokinetic data provide a reasonable basis for concluding that b.i.d. dosing with propranolol should be adequate in the treatment of post-infarction patients.
CLINICAL: In the BHAT, patients on INDERAL were prescribed either 180 mg/day (82% of patients) or 240 mg/day (18% of patients). Patients were instructed to take the medication 3 times a day at mealtimes. This dosing schedule would result in an overnight dosing interval of 12 to 14 hours which is similar to the dosing interval for a b.i.d regimen. In addition, blood samples were drawn at various times and analyzed for propranolol. When the patients were grouped into tertiles based on the blood levels observed and the mortality in the upper and lower tertiles was compared, there was no evidence that blood levels affected mortality.
PHARMACOLOGIC: Studies in normal volunteers have shown that a 90 mg b.i.d. regimen maintains beta blockade at, or above, the minimum for 60 mg t.i.d. dosing for 24 hours even though differences occurred at two time intervals. At 10–12 hours after the first dose of the day, t.i.d. dosing gave more beta blockade than b.i.d. dosing; at 20–24 hours the trend of the relationship was reversed. These relationships were similar in direction to those observed for plasma propranolol levels. (See Pharmacokinetic.)
PHARMACOKINETIC: A bioavailability study in normal volunteers showed that the blood levels produced by 180 mg/day given b.i.d. are below those provided by the same daily dosage given t.i.d. at 10–12 hours after the first dose of the day, but above those of a t.i.d. regimen at 20–24 hours. However, the blood levels produced by b.i.d. dosing were always equivalent to or above the minimum for t.i.d. dosing throughout the 24 hours. In addition, the mean AUC on the fourth day for the b.i.d. regimen was about 17% greater than for the t.i.d. regimen (1,194 *vs.* 1,024 ng/mL·hr).

INDICATIONS AND USAGE
Hypertension
INDERAL is indicated in the management of hypertension. It may be used alone or used in combination with other anti-

hypertensive agents, particularly a thiazide diuretic. INDERAL is not indicated in the management of hypertensive emergencies.

Angina Pectoris Due to Coronary Atherosclerosis
INDERAL is indicated for the long-term management of patients with angina pectoris.

Cardiac Arrhythmias
1.) Supraventricular arrhythmias

a) Paroxysmal atrial tachycardias, particularly those arrhythmias induced by catecholamines or digitalis or associated with the Wolff-Parkinson-White syndrome. (See W-P-W under WARNINGS.)

b) Persistent sinus tachycardia which is noncompensatory and impairs the well-being of the patient.

c) Tachycardias and arrhythmias due to thyrotoxicosis when causing distress or increased hazard and when immediate effect is necessary as adjunctive, short-term (2–4 weeks) therapy.

May be used with, but not in place of, specific therapy. (See THYROTOXICOSIS under WARNINGS.)

d) Persistent atrial extrasystoles which impair the well-being of the patient and do not respond to conventional measures.

e) Atrial flutter and fibrillation when ventricular rate cannot be controlled by digitalis alone, or when digitalis is contraindicated.

2.) Ventricular tachycardias

Ventricular arrhythmias do not respond to propranolol as predictably as do the supraventricular arrhythmias.

a) Ventricular tachycardias

With the exception of those induced by catecholamines or digitalis, INDERAL is not the drug of first choice. In critical situations when cardioversion techniques or other drugs are not indicated or are not effective, INDERAL may be considered. If, after consideration of the risks involved, INDERAL is used, it should be given intravenously in low dosage and very slowly. (See DOSAGE AND ADMINISTRATION.) *Care in the administration of INDERAL with constant electrocardiographic monitoring is essential as the failing heart requires some sympathetic drive for maintenance of myocardial tone.*

b) Persistent premature ventricular extrasystoles which do not respond to conventional measures and impair the well-being of the patient.

3.) Tachyarrhythmias of digitalis intoxication

If digitalis-induced tachyarrhythmias persist following discontinuance of digitalis and correction of electrolyte abnormalities, they are usually reversible with *oral* INDERAL. Severe bradycardia may occur. (See OVERDOSAGE.)

Intravenous propranolol hydrochloride is reserved for life-threatening arrhythmias. Temporary maintenance with oral therapy may be indicated. (See DOSAGE AND ADMINISTRATION.)

4.) Resistant tachyarrhythmias due to excessive catecholamine action during anesthesia

Tachyarrhythmias due to excessive catecholamine action during anesthesia may sometimes arise because of release of endogenous catecholamines or administration of catecholamines. When usual measures fail in such arrhythmias, INDERAL may be given intravenously to abolish them. All general inhalation anesthetics produce some degree of myocardial depression. Therefore, when INDERAL is used to treat arrhythmias during anesthesia, it should be used with extreme caution and constant ECG and central venous pressure monitoring. (See WARNINGS.)

Myocardial Infarction
INDERAL is indicated to reduce cardiovascular mortality in patients who have survived the acute phase of myocardial infarction and are clinically stable.

Migraine
INDERAL is indicated for the prophylaxis of common migraine headache. The efficacy of propranolol in the treatment of a migraine attack that has started has not been established, and propranolol is not indicated for such use.

Essential Tremor
INDERAL is indicated in the management of familial or hereditary essential tremor. Familial or essential tremor consists of involuntary, rhythmic, oscillatory movements, usually limited to the upper limbs. It is absent at rest but occurs when the limb is held in a fixed posture or position against gravity and during active movement. INDERAL causes a reduction in the tremor amplitude but not in the tremor frequency. INDERAL is not indicated for the treatment of tremor associated with Parkinsonism.

Hypertrophic Subaortic Stenosis
INDERAL is useful in the management of hypertrophic subaortic stenosis, especially for treatment of exertional or other stress-induced angina, palpitations, and syncope. INDERAL also improves exercise performance. The effectiveness of propranolol hydrochloride in this disease appears to be due to a reduction of the elevated outflow pressure gradient, which is exacerbated by beta-receptor stimulation. Clinical improvement may be temporary.

Pheochromocytoma
After primary treatment with an alpha-adrenergic blocking agent has been instituted, INDERAL may be useful as *adjunctive* therapy if the control of tachycardia becomes necessary before or during surgery.

It is hazardous to use INDERAL unless alpha-adrenergic blocking drugs are already in use, since this would predispose to serious blood pressure elevation. Blocking only the peripheral dilator (beta) action of epinephrine leaves its constrictor (alpha) action unopposed.

In the event of hemorrhage or shock, there is a disadvantage in having both beta and alpha blockade since the combination prevents the increase in heart rate and peripheral vasoconstriction needed to maintain blood pressure.

With inoperable or metastatic pheochromocytoma, INDERAL may be useful as an adjunct to the management of symptoms due to excessive beta-receptor stimulation.

CONTRAINDICATIONS
INDERAL is contraindicated in 1) cardiogenic shock, 2) sinus bradycardia and greater than first degree block, 3) bronchial asthma, 4) congestive heart failure (see WARNINGS) unless the failure is secondary to a tachyarrhythmia treatable with INDERAL.

WARNINGS
CARDIAC FAILURE: Sympathetic stimulation may be a vital component supporting circulatory function in patients with congestive heart failure, and its inhibition by beta blockade may precipitate more severe failure. Although beta blockers should be avoided in overt congestive heart failure, if necessary, they can be used with close follow-up in patients with a history of failure who are well compensated and are receiving digitalis and diuretics. Beta-adrenergic blocking agents do not abolish the inotropic action of digitalis on heart muscle.

IN PATIENTS WITHOUT A HISTORY OF HEART FAILURE, continued use of beta blockers can, in some cases, lead to cardiac failure. Therefore, at the first sign or symptom of heart failure, the patient should be digitalized and/or treated with diuretics, and the response observed closely, or INDERAL should be discontinued (gradually, if possible).

IN PATIENTS WITH ANGINA PECTORIS, there have been reports of exacerbation of angina and, in some cases, myocardial infarction, following *abrupt* discontinuance of INDERAL therapy. Therefore, when discontinuance of INDERAL is planned the dosage should be gradually reduced over at least a few weeks and the patient should be cautioned against interruption or cessation of therapy without the physician's advice. If INDERAL therapy is interrupted and exacerbation of angina occurs, it usually is advisable to reinstitute INDERAL therapy and take other measures appropriate for the management of unstable angina pectoris. Since coronary artery disease may be unrecognized, it may be prudent to follow the above advice in patients considered at risk of having occult atherosclerotic heart disease who are given propranolol for other indications.

Nonallergic Bronchospasm (e.g., chronic bronchitis, emphysema)—PATIENTS WITH BRONCHOSPASTIC DISEASES SHOULD IN GENERAL NOT RECEIVE BETA BLOCKERS. INDERAL should be administered with caution since it may block bronchodilation produced by endogenous and exogenous catecholamine stimulation of beta receptors.

MAJOR SURGERY: The necessity or desirability of withdrawal of beta-blocking therapy prior to major surgery is controversial. It should be noted, however, that the impaired ability of the heart to respond to reflex adrenergic stimuli may augment the risks of general anesthesia and surgical procedures.

INDERAL, like other beta blockers, is a competitive inhibitor of beta-receptor agonists and its effects can be reversed by administration of such agents, e.g., dobutamine or isoproterenol. However, such patients may be subject to protracted severe hypotension. Difficulty in starting and maintaining the heartbeat has also been reported with beta blockers.

DIABETES AND HYPOGLYCEMIA: Beta blockers should be used with caution in diabetic patients if a beta-blocking agent is required. Beta blockers may mask tachycardia occurring with hypoglycemia, but other manifestations such as dizziness and sweating may not be significantly affected. Following insulin-induced hypoglycemia, propranolol may cause a delay in the recovery of blood glucose to normal levels.

THYROTOXICOSIS: Beta blockade may mask certain clinical signs of hyperthyroidism. Therefore, abrupt withdrawal of propranolol may be followed by an exacerbation of symptoms of hyperthyroidism, including thyroid storm. Propranolol may change thyroid-function tests, increasing T_4 and reverse T_3 and decreasing T_3.

IN PATIENTS WITH WOLFF-PARKINSON-WHITE SYNDROME, several cases have been reported in which, after propranolol, the tachycardia was replaced by a severe brady-

cardia requiring a demand pacemaker. In one case this resulted after an initial dose of 5 mg propranolol.

PRECAUTIONS
GENERAL: Propranolol should be used with caution in patients with impaired hepatic or renal function. INDERAL is not indicated for the treatment of hypertensive emergencies.

Beta-adrenoreceptor blockade can cause reduction of intraocular pressure. Patients should be told that INDERAL may interfere with the glaucoma screening test. Withdrawal may lead to a return of increased intraocular pressure.

CLINICAL LABORATORY TESTS: Elevated blood urea levels in patients with severe heart disease, elevated serum transaminase, alkaline phosphatase, lactate dehydrogenase.

DRUG INTERACTIONS: Patients receiving catecholamine-depleting drugs such as reserpine should be closely observed if INDERAL is administered. The added catecholamine-blocking action may produce an excessive reduction of resting sympathetic nervous activity, which may result in hypotension, marked bradycardia, vertigo, syncopal attacks, or orthostatic hypotension.

Caution should be exercised when patients receiving a beta blocker are administered a calcium-channel blocking drug, especially intravenous verapamil, for both agents may depress myocardial contractility or atrioventricular conduction. On rare occasions, the concomitant intravenous use of a beta blocker and verapamil has resulted in serious adverse reactions, especially in patients with severe cardiomyopathy, congestive heart failure or recent myocardial infarction.

Aluminum hydroxide gel greatly reduces intestinal absorption of propranolol.

Ethanol slows the rate of absorption of propranolol.

Phenytoin, phenobarbitone, and *rifampin* accelerate propranolol clearance.

Chlorpromazine, when used concomitantly with propranolol, results in increased plasma levels of both drugs.

Antipyrine and *lidocaine* have reduced clearance when used concomitantly with propranolol.

Thyroxine may result in a lower than expected T_3 concentration when used concomitantly with propranolol.

Cimetidine decreases the hepatic metabolism of propranolol, delaying elimination and increasing blood levels.

Theophylline clearance is reduced when used concomitantly with propranolol.

CARCINOGENESIS, MUTAGENESIS, IMPAIRMENT OF FERTILITY: Long-term studies in animals have been conducted to evaluate toxic effects and carcinogenic potential. In 18-month studies, in both rats and mice, employing doses up to 150 mg/kg/day, there was no evidence of significant drug-induced toxicity. There were no drug-related tumorigenic effects at any of the dosage levels. Reproductive studies in animals did not show any impairment of fertility that was attributable to the drug.

PREGNANCY: Pregnancy Category C: INDERAL has been shown to be embryotoxic in animal studies at doses about 10 times greater than the maximum recommended human dose.

There are no adequate and well-controlled studies in pregnant women. INDERAL should be used during pregnancy only if the potential benefit justifies the potential risk to the fetus.

NURSING MOTHERS: INDERAL is excreted in human milk. Caution should be exercised when INDERAL is administered to a nursing woman.

PEDIATRIC USE: High serum propranolol levels have been noted in patients with Down's syndrome (trisomy 21), suggesting that the bioavailability of propranolol may be increased in patients with this condition.

Evaluation of the effects of propranolol in children, relative to the drug's efficacy and safety, has not been as systematically performed as in adults. Information is available in the medical literature to allow fair estimates, and specific dosing information has been reasonably studied.

Cardiovascular diseases that are common to adults and children are generally as responsive to propranolol intervention in children as they are in adults. Adverse reactions are also similar; for example, bronchospasm and congestive heart failure related to propranolol therapy have been reported in children and occur through the same mechanisms as previously described in adults.

The normal echocardiogram evolves through a series of changes as the heart matures during growth and development in children. Should echocardiography be used to monitor propranolol therapy in children, the age-related changes in the echocardiogram need to be borne in mind.

ADVERSE REACTIONS
Most adverse effects have been mild and transient and have rarely required the withdrawal of therapy.

Cardiovascular: Bradycardia; congestive heart failure; intensification of AV block; hypotension; paresthesia of hands; thrombocytopenic purpura; arterial insufficiency, usually of the Raynaud type.

Continued on next page

Wyeth-Ayerst—Cont.

Central Nervous System: Light-headedness; mental depression manifested by insomnia, lassitude, weakness, fatigue; reversible mental depression progressing to catatonia; visual disturbances; hallucinations, vivid dreams, an acute reversible syndrome characterized by disorientation for time and place, short-term memory loss, emotional lability, slightly clouded sensorium, and decreased performance on neuropsychometrics. Total daily doses above 160 mg (when administered as divided doses of greater than 80 mg each) may be associated with an increased incidence of fatigue, lethargy, and vivid dreams.

Gastrointestinal: Nausea, vomiting, epigastric distress, abdominal cramping, diarrhea, constipation, mesenteric arterial thrombosis, ischemic colitis.

Allergic: Pharyngitis and agranulocytosis, erythematous rash, fever combined with aching and sore throat, laryngospasm, and respiratory distress.

Respiratory: Bronchospasm.

Hematologic: Agranulocytosis, nonthrombocytopenic purpura, thrombocytopenic purpura.

Auto-Immune: In extremely rare instances, systemic lupus erythematosus has been reported.

Miscellaneous: Alopecia, LE-like reactions, psoriasiform rashes, dry eyes, male impotence, and Peyronie's disease have been reported rarely. Oculomucocutaneous reactions involving the skin, serous membranes and conjunctivae reported for a beta blocker (practolol) have not been associated with propranolol.

DOSAGE AND ADMINISTRATION

The dosage range for INDERAL is different for each indication.

ORAL

HYPERTENSION—*Dosage must be individualized.*

The usual initial dosage is 40 mg INDERAL twice daily, whether used alone or added to a diuretic. Dosage may be increased gradually until adequate blood pressure control is achieved. The usual maintenance dosage is 120 mg to 240 mg per day. In some instances a dosage of 640 mg a day may be required. The time needed for full hypertensive response to a given dosage is variable and may range from a few days to several weeks.

While twice-daily dosing is effective and can maintain a reduction in blood pressure throughout the day, some patients, especially when lower doses are used, may experience a modest rise in blood pressure toward the end of the 12-hour dosing interval. This can be evaluated by measuring blood pressure near the end of the dosing interval to determine whether satisfactory control is being maintained throughout the day. If control is not adequate, a larger dose, or 3-times-daily therapy may achieve better control.

ANGINA PECTORIS—*Dosage must be individualized.*

Total daily doses of 80 mg to 320 mg, when administered orally, twice a day, three times a day, or four times a day, have been shown to increase exercise tolerance and to reduce ischemic changes in the ECG.

If treatment is to be discontinued, reduce dosage gradually over a period of several weeks. (See WARNINGS.)

ARRHYTHMIAS—10 mg to 30 mg three or four times daily, before meals and at bedtime.

MYOCARDIAL INFARCTION—The recommended daily dosage is 180 mg to 240 mg per day in divided doses. Although a t.i.d. regimen was used in the Beta-Blocker Heart Attack Trial and a q.i.d. regimen in the Norwegian Multicenter Trial, there is a reasonable basis for the use of either a t.i.d. or b.i.d. regimen (see CLINICAL PHARMACOLOGY). The effectiveness and safety of daily dosages greater than 240 mg for prevention of cardiac mortality have not been established. However, higher dosages may be needed to effectively treat coexisting diseases such as angina or hypertension (see above).

MIGRAINE—*Dosage must be individualized.*

The initial oral dose is 80 mg INDERAL daily in divided doses. The usual effective dose range is 160 mg to 240 mg per day. The dosage may be increased gradually to achieve optimum migraine prophylaxis.

If a satisfactory response is not obtained within four to six weeks after reaching the maximum dose, INDERAL therapy should be discontinued. It may be advisable to withdraw the drug gradually over a period of several weeks.

ESSENTIAL TREMOR—*Dosage must be individualized.*

The initial dosage is 40 mg INDERAL twice daily. Optimum reduction of essential tremor is usually achieved with a dose of 120 mg per day. Occasionally, it may be necessary to administer 240 mg to 320 mg per day.

HYPERTROPHIC SUBAORTIC STENOSIS—20 mg to 40 mg three or four times daily, before meals and at bedtime.

PHEOCHROMOCYTOMA—*Preoperatively*—60 mg daily in divided doses for three days prior to surgery, concomitantly with an alpha-adrenergic blocking agent.

—*Management of inoperable tumor*—30 mg daily in divided doses.

USE IN CHILDREN: Intravenous administration of INDERAL is not recommended in children. Oral dosage for treating hypertension requires individual titration, beginning with a 1.0 mg per kg (body weight) per day dosage regimen (ie, 0.5 mg per kg b.i.d.).

The usual pediatric dosage range is 2 mg to 4 mg per kg per day in two equally divided doses (i.e., 1.0 mg per kg b.i.d. to 2.0 mg per kg b.i.d.). Pediatric dosage calculated by weight (recommended) generally produces propranolol plasma levels in a therapeutic range similar to that in adults. On the other hand, pediatric doses calculated on the basis of body surface area (*not* recommended) usually result in plasma levels above the mean adult therapeutic range. Doses above 16 mg per kg per day should not be used in children.

If treatment with INDERAL is to be discontinued, a gradually decreasing dose titration over a 7- to 14-day period is necessary.

INTRAVENOUS

Parenteral drug products should be inspected visually for particulate matter and discoloration prior to administration, whenever solution and container permit.

Intravenous administration is reserved for life-threatening arrhythmias or those occurring under anesthesia. The usual dose is from 1 mg to 3 mg administered under careful monitoring, e.g., electrocardiographic, central venous pressure. The rate of administration should not exceed 1 mg (1 mL) per minute to diminish the possibility of lowering blood pressure and causing cardiac standstill. Sufficient time should be allowed for the drug to reach the site of action even when a slow circulation is present. If necessary, a second dose may be given after two minutes. Thereafter, additional drug should not be given in less than four hours. Additional INDERAL should not be given when the desired alteration in rate and/or rhythm is achieved.

Transference to oral therapy should be made as soon as possible.

The intravenous administration of INDERAL has not been evaluated adequately in the management of hypertensive emergencies.

OVERDOSAGE

INDERAL is not significantly dialyzable. In the event of overdosage or exaggerated response, the following measures should be employed:

General—If ingestion is or may have been recent, evacuate gastric contents, taking care to prevent pulmonary aspiration.

BRADYCARDIA—ADMINISTER ATROPINE (0.25 mg to 1.0 mg); IF THERE IS NO RESPONSE TO VAGAL BLOCKADE, ADMINISTER ISOPROTERENOL CAUTIOUSLY.

CARDIAC FAILURE—DIGITALIZATION AND DIURETICS.

HYPOTENSION—VASOPRESSORS, e.g., LEVARTERENOL OR EPINEPHRINE (THERE IS EVIDENCE THAT EPINEPHRINE IS THE DRUG OF CHOICE).

BRONCHOSPASM — ADMINISTER ISOPROTERENOL AND AMINOPHYLLINE.

HOW SUPPLIED

INDERAL

(propranolol hydrochloride)

TABLETS

INDERAL 10—Each hexagonal-shaped, orange, scored tablet, embossed with an "I" and imprinted with "INDERAL 10," contains 10 mg propranolol hydrochloride, in bottles of 100 (NDC 0046-0421-81); 1,000 (NDC 0046-0421-91); and 5,000 (NDC 0046-0421-95). Also in Unit Dose packages of 100 (NDC 0046-0421-99); and in Unit of Use packages of 60 (NDC 0046-0421-60); 90 (NDC 0046-0421-61); 100 (NDC 0046-0421-80); and 120 (NDC 0046-0421-62).

INDERAL 20—Each hexagonal-shaped, blue, scored tablet, embossed with an "I" and imprinted with "INDERAL 20", contains 20 mg propranolol hydrochloride, in bottles of 100 (NDC 0046-0422-81); 1,000 (NDC 0046-0422-91); and 5,000 (NDC 0046-0422-95). Also in Unit Dose packages of 100 (NDC 0046-0422-99); and in Unit of Use packages of 60 (NDC 0046-0422-60); 90 (NDC 0046-0422-61); 100 (NDC 0046-0422-80); and 120 (NDC 0046-0422-62).

INDERAL 40—Each hexagonal-shaped, green, scored tablet, embossed with an "I" and imprinted with "INDERAL 40," contains 40 mg propranolol hydrochloride, in bottles of 100 (NDC 0046-0424-81); 1,000 (NDC 0046-0424-91); and 5,000 (NDC 0046-0424-95). Also in Unit Dose packages of 100 (NDC 0046-0424-99); and in Unit of Use packages of 60 (NDC 0046-0424-60); 90 (NDC 0046-0424-61); 100 (NDC 0046-0424-80); and 120 (NDC 0046-0424-62).

INDERAL 60—Each hexagonal-shaped, pink, scored tablet, embossed with an "I" and imprinted with "INDERAL 60," contains 60 mg propranolol hydrochloride, in bottles of 100 (NDC 0046-0426-81) and 1,000 (NDC 0046-0426-91). Also in Unit Dose packages of 100 (NDC 0046-0426-99).

INDERAL 80 —Each hexagonal-shaped, yellow, scored tablet, embossed with an "I" and imprinted with "INDERAL 80", contains 80 mg propranolol hydrochloride, in bottles of 100 (NDC 0046-0428-81); 1,000 (NDC 0046-0428-91); and 5,000 (NDC 0046-0428-95). Also in Unit Dose packages of 100 (NDC 0046-0428-99); and in Unit of Use packages of 60

(NDC 0046-0428-60); 90 (NDC 0046-0428-61); 100 (NDC 0046-0428-80); and 120 (NDC 0046-0428-62).

The appearance of these tablets is a registered trademark of Wyeth-Ayerst Laboratories.

Store at room temperature (approximately 25℃).

INJECTABLE

—Each mL contains 1 mg of propranolol hydrochloride in Water for Injection. The pH is adjusted with citric acid. Supplied as: 1 mL ampuls in boxes of 10 (NDC 0046-3265-10).

Store at room temperature (approximately 25℃).

Shown in Product Identification Section, page 436

INDERAL® LA   ℞

[ĭn'der-al]

Brand of propranolol hydrochloride
(Long Acting Capsules)

CAUTION: Federal law prohibits dispensing without prescription.

DESCRIPTION

INDERAL (propranolol hydrochloride) is a synthetic beta-adrenergic receptor-blocking agent chemically described as 1-(Isopropylamino)-3-(1-naphthyloxy)-2-propanol hydrochloride. Its structural formula is

$$O\ CH_2CHOHCH_2NHCH(CH_3)_2 \cdot HCl$$

Propranolol hydrochloride is a stable, white, crystalline solid which is readily soluble in water and ethanol. Its molecular weight is 295.81.

INDERAL LA is formulated to provide a sustained release of propranolol hydrochloride. INDERAL LA is available as 60 mg, 80 mg, 120 mg, and 160 mg capsules.

INDERAL LA contains the following inactive ingredients: ethylcellulose, gelatin capsules, hydroxypropyl methylcellulose, microcrystalline cellulose, and titanium dioxide. In addition, INDERAL LA 60 mg Capsules contain FD&C Blue No. 1 and FD&C Red No. 3; INDERAL LA 80 mg and 120 mg Capsules contain FD&C Blue No. 1, FD&C Red No. 3, and D&C Red No. 28; INDERAL LA 160 mg Capsules contain FD&C Blue No. 1.

CLINICAL PHARMACOLOGY

INDERAL is a nonselective, beta-adrenergic receptor-blocking agent possessing no other autonomic nervous system activity. It specifically competes with beta-adrenergic receptor-stimulating agents for available receptor sites. When access to beta-receptor sites is blocked by INDERAL, the chronotropic, inotropic, and vasodilator responses to beta-adrenergic stimulation are decreased proportionally.

INDERAL LA Capsules (60, 80, 120, and 160 mg) release propranolol HCl at a controlled and predictable rate. Peak blood levels following dosing with INDERAL LA occur at about 6 hours, and the apparent plasma half-life is about 10 hours. When measured at steady state over a 24-hour period the areas under the propranolol plasma concentration-time curve (AUCs) for the capsules are approximately 60% to 65% of the AUCs for a comparable divided daily dose of INDERAL Tablets. The lower AUCs for the capsules are due to greater hepatic metabolism of propranolol, resulting from the slower rate of absorption of propranolol. Over a twenty-four (24) hour period, blood levels are fairly constant for about twelve (12) hours, then decline exponentially.

INDERAL LA should not be considered a simple mg-for-mg substitute for conventional propranolol and the blood levels achieved do not match (are lower than) those of two to four times daily dosing with the same dose. When changing to INDERAL LA from conventional propranolol, a possible need for retitration upwards should be considered, especially to maintain effectiveness at the end of the dosing interval. In most clinical settings, however, such as hypertension or angina where there is little correlation between plasma levels and clinical effect, INDERAL LA has been therapeutically equivalent to the same mg dose of conventional INDERAL as assessed by 24-hour effects on blood pressure and on 24-hour exercise responses of heart rate, systolic pressure, and rate pressure product. INDERAL LA can provide effective beta blockade for a 24-hour period.

The mechanism of the antihypertensive effect of INDERAL has not been established. Among the factors that may be involved in contributing to the antihypertensive action are: (1) decreased cardiac output, (2) inhibition of renin release by the kidneys, and (3) diminution of tonic sympathetic nerve outflow from vasomotor centers in the brain. Although total peripheral resistance may increase initially, it readjusts to or below the pretreatment level with chronic use. Effects on plasma volume appear to be minor and somewhat variable. INDERAL has been shown to cause a small increase in serum potassium concentration when used in the treatment of hypertensive patients.

In angina pectoris, propranolol generally reduces the oxygen requirement of the heart at any given level of effort by blocking the catecholamine-induced increases in the heart rate, systolic blood pressure, and the velocity and extent of myocardial contraction. Propranolol may increase oxygen requirements by increasing left ventricular fiber length, end diastolic pressure, and systolic ejection period. The net physiologic effect of beta-adrenergic blockade is usually advantageous and is manifested during exercise by delayed onset of pain and increased work capacity.

In dosages greater than required for beta blockade, INDERAL also exerts a quinidine-like or anesthetic-like membrane action which affects the cardiac action potential. The significance of the membrane action in the treatment of arrhythmias is uncertain.

The mechanism of the antimigraine effect of propranolol has not been established. Beta-adrenergic receptors have been demonstrated in the pial vessels of the brain.

Beta-receptor blockade can be useful in conditions in which, because of pathologic or functional changes, sympathetic activity is detrimental to the patient. But there are also situations in which sympathetic stimulation is vital. For example, in patients with severely damaged hearts, adequate ventricular function is maintained by virtue of sympathetic drive, which should be preserved. In the presence of AV block, greater than first degree, beta blockade may prevent the necessary facilitating effect of sympathetic activity on conduction. Beta blockade results in bronchial constriction by interfering with adrenergic bronchodilator activity, which should be preserved in patients subject to bronchospasm.

Propranolol is not significantly dialyzable.

INDICATIONS AND USAGE

Hypertension
INDERAL LA is indicated in the management of hypertension; it may be used alone or used in combination with other antihypertensive agents, particularly a thiazide diuretic. INDERAL LA is not indicated in the management of hypertensive emergencies.

Angina Pectoris Due to Coronary Atherosclerosis
INDERAL LA (propranolol HCl) is indicated for the long-term management of patients with angina pectoris.

Migraine
INDERAL LA is indicated for the prophylaxis of common migraine headache. The efficacy of propranolol in the treatment of a migraine attack that has started has not been established and propranolol is not indicated for such use.

Hypertrophic Subaortic Stenosis
INDERAL LA is useful in the management of hypertrophic subaortic stenosis, especially for treatment of exertional or other stress-induced angina, palpitations, and syncope. INDERAL LA also improves exercise performance. The effectiveness of propranolol hydrochloride in this disease appears to be due to a reduction of the elevated outflow pressure gradient which is exacerbated by beta-receptor stimulation. Clinical improvement may be temporary.

CONTRAINDICATIONS
INDERAL is contraindicated in 1) cardiogenic shock; 2) sinus bradycardia and greater than first-degree block; 3) bronchial asthma; 4) congestive heart failure (see WARNINGS), unless the failure is secondary to a tachyarrhythmia treatable with INDERAL.

WARNINGS
CARDIAC FAILURE: Sympathetic stimulation may be a vital component supporting circulatory function in patients with congestive heart failure, and its inhibition by beta blockade may precipitate more severe failure. Although beta blockers should be avoided in overt congestive heart failure, if necessary, they can be used with close follow-up in patients with a history of failure who are well compensated and are receiving digitalis and diuretics. Beta-adrenergic blocking agents do not abolish the inotropic action of digitalis on heart muscle.

IN PATIENTS WITHOUT A HISTORY OF HEART FAILURE, continued use of beta blockers can, in some cases, lead to cardiac failure. Therefore, at the first sign or symptom of heart failure, the patient should be digitalized and/or treated with diuretics, and the response observed closely, or INDERAL should be discontinued (gradually, if possible).

IN PATIENTS WITH ANGINA PECTORIS, there have been reports of exacerbation of angina and, in some cases, myocardial infarction, following *abrupt* discontinuance of INDERAL therapy. Therefore, when discontinuance of INDERAL is planned, the dosage should be gradually reduced over at least a few weeks, and the patient should be cautioned against interruption or cessation of therapy without the physician's advice. If INDERAL therapy is interrupted and exacerbation of angina occurs, it usually is advisable to reinstitute INDERAL therapy and take other measures appropri-

ate for the management of unstable angina pectoris. Since coronary artery disease may be unrecognized, it may be prudent to follow the above advice in patients considered at risk of having occult atherosclerotic heart disease who are given propranolol for other indications.

Nonallergic Bronchospasm (eg, chronic bronchitis, emphysema)—PATIENTS WITH BRONCHOSPASTIC DISEASES SHOULD IN GENERAL NOT RECEIVE BETA BLOCKERS. INDERAL should be administered with caution since it may block bronchodilation produced by endogenous and exogenous catecholamine stimulation of beta receptors.

MAJOR SURGERY: The necessity or desirability of withdrawal of beta-blocking therapy prior to major surgery is controversial. It should be noted, however, that the impaired ability of the heart to respond to reflex adrenergic stimuli may augment the risks of general anesthesia and surgical procedures.

INDERAL, like other beta blockers, is a competitive inhibitor of beta-receptor agonists and its effects can be reversed by administration of such agents, eg, dobutamine or isoproterenol. However, such patients may be subject to protracted severe hypotension. Difficulty in starting and maintaining the heartbeat has also been reported with beta blockers.

DIABETES AND HYPOGLYCEMIA: Beta blockers should be used with caution in diabetic patients if a beta-blocking agent is required. Beta blockers may mask tachycardia occurring with hypoglycemia, but other manifestations such as dizziness and sweating may not be significantly affected. Following insulin-induced hypoglycemia, propranolol may cause a delay in the recovery of blood glucose to normal levels.

THYROTOXICOSIS: Beta blockade may mask certain clinical signs of hyperthyroidism. Therefore, abrupt withdrawal of propranolol may be followed by an exacerbation of symptoms of hyperthyroidism, including thyroid storm. Propranolol may change thyroid function tests, increasing T_4 and reverse T_3, and decreasing T_3.

IN PATIENTS WITH WOLFF-PARKINSON-WHITE SYNDROME, several cases have been reported in which, after propranolol, the tachycardia was replaced by a severe bradycardia requiring a demand pacemaker. In one case this resulted after an initial dose of 5 mg propranolol.

PRECAUTIONS
GENERAL: Propranolol should be used with caution in patients with impaired hepatic or renal function. INDERAL (propranolol HCl) is not indicated for the treatment of hypertensive emergencies.

Beta-adrenoreceptor blockade can cause reduction of intraocular pressure. Patients should be told that INDERAL may interfere with the glaucoma screening test. Withdrawal may lead to a return of increased intraocular pressure.

CLINICAL LABORATORY TESTS: Elevated blood urea levels in patients with severe heart disease, elevated serum transaminase, alkaline phosphatase, lactate dehydrogenase.

DRUG INTERACTIONS: Patients receiving catecholamine-depleting drugs, such as reserpine, should be closely observed if INDERAL is administered. The added catecholamine-blocking action may produce an excessive reduction of resting sympathetic nervous activity, which may result in hypotension, marked bradycardia, vertigo, syncopal attacks, or orthostatic hypotension.

Caution should be exercised when patients receiving a beta blocker are administered a calcium-channel-blocking drug, especially intravenous verapamil, for both agents may depress myocardial contractility or atrioventricular conduction. On rare occasions, the concomitant intravenous use of a beta blocker and verapamil has resulted in serious adverse reactions, especially in patients with severe cardiomyopathy, congestive heart failure or recent myocardial infarction.

Aluminum hydroxide gel greatly reduces intestinal absorption of propranolol.

Ethanol slows the rate of absorption of propranolol.

Phenytoin, phenobarbitone, and *rifampin* accelerate propranolol clearance.

Chlorpromazine, when used concomitantly with propranolol, results in increased plasma levels of both drugs.

Antipyrine and *lidocaine* have reduced clearance when used concomitantly with propranolol.

Thyroxine may result in a lower than expected T_3 concentration when used concomitantly with propranolol.

Cimetidine decreases the hepatic metabolism of propranolol, delaying elimination and increasing blood levels.

Theophylline clearance is reduced when used concomitantly with propranolol.

CARCINOGENESIS, MUTAGENESIS, IMPAIRMENT OF FERTILITY: Long-term studies in animals have been conducted to evaluate toxic effects and carcinogenic potential. In 18-month studies, in both rats and mice, employing doses up to 150 mg/kg/day, there was no evidence of significant drug-induced toxicity. There were no drug-related tumorigenic effects at any of the dosage levels. Reproductive studies in animals did not show any impairment of fertility that was attributable to the drug.

PREGNANCY: Pregnancy Category C. INDERAL has been shown to be embryotoxic in animal studies at doses about 10 times greater than the maximal recommended human dose.

There are no adequate and well-controlled studies in pregnant women. INDERAL should be used during pregnancy only if the potential benefit justifies the potential risk to the fetus.

NURSING MOTHERS: INDERAL is excreted in human milk. Caution should be exercised when INDERAL (propranolol HCl) is administered to a nursing woman.

PEDIATRIC USE: Safety and effectiveness in children have not been established.

ADVERSE REACTIONS
Most adverse effects have been mild and transient and have rarely required the withdrawal of therapy.

Cardiovascular: Bradycardia; congestive heart failure; intensification of AV block; hypotension; paresthesia of hands; thrombocytopenic purpura; arterial insufficiency, usually of the Raynaud type.

Central Nervous System: Light-headedness, mental depression manifested by insomnia, lassitude, weakness, fatigue, reversible mental depression progressing to catatonia; visual disturbances; hallucinations; vivid dreams; an acute reversible syndrome characterized by disorientation for time and place, short-term memory loss, emotional lability, slightly clouded sensorium, and decreased performance on neuropsychometrics. For immediate formulations, fatigue, lethargy, and vivid dreams appear dose related.

Gastrointestinal: Nausea; vomiting; epigastric distress; abdominal cramping; diarrhea; constipation; mesenteric arterial thrombosis; ischemic colitis.

Allergic: Pharyngitis and agranulocytosis; erythematous rash; fever combined with aching and sore throat; laryngospasm and respiratory distress.

Respiratory: Bronchospasm.

Hematologic: Agranulocytosis, nonthrombocytopenic purpura, thrombocytopenic purpura.

Auto-Immune: In extremely rare instances, systemic lupus erythematosus has been reported.

Miscellaneous: Alopecia; LE-like reactions; psoriasiform rashes; dry eyes; male impotence; and Peyronie's disease have been reported rarely. Oculomucocutaneous reactions involving the skin, serous membranes and conjunctivae reported for a beta blocker (practolol) have not been associated with propranolol.

DOSAGE AND ADMINISTRATION
INDERAL LA provides propranolol hydrochloride in a sustained-release capsule for administration once daily. If patients are switched from INDERAL Tablets to INDERAL LA Capsules, care should be taken to assure that the desired therapeutic effect is maintained. INDERAL LA should not be considered a simple mg-for-mg substitute for INDERAL. INDERAL LA has different kinetics and produces lower blood levels. Retitration may be necessary especially to maintain effectiveness at the end of the 24-hour dosing interval.

HYPERTENSION—*Dosage must be individualized.* The usual initial dosage is 80 mg INDERAL LA once daily, whether used alone or added to a diuretic. The dosage may be increased to 120 mg once daily or higher, until adequate blood pressure control is achieved. The usual maintenance dosage is 120 to 160 mg once daily. In some instances a dosage of 640 mg may be required. The time needed for full hypertensive response to a given dosage is variable and may range from a few days to several weeks.

ANGINA PECTORIS—*Dosage must be individualized.* Starting with 80 mg INDERAL LA once daily, dosage should be gradually increased at three- to seven-day intervals until optimal response is obtained. Although individual patients may respond at any dosage level, the average optimal dosage appears to be 160 mg once daily. In angina pectoris, the value and safety of dosage exceeding 320 mg per day have not been established.

If treatment is to be discontinued, reduce dosage gradually over a period of a few weeks (see WARNINGS).

MIGRAINE—*Dosage must be individualized.* The initial oral dose is 80 mg INDERAL LA once daily. The usual effective dose range is 160-240 mg once daily. The dosage may be increased gradually to achieve optimal migraine prophylaxis. If a satisfactory response is not obtained within four to six weeks after reaching the maximal dose, INDERAL LA therapy should be discontinued. It may be advisable to withdraw the drug gradually over a period of several weeks.

HYPERTROPHIC SUBAORTIC STENOSIS—80–160 mg INDERAL LA once daily.

PEDIATRIC DOSAGE
At this time the data on the use of the drug in this age group are too limited to permit adequate directions for use.

Continued on next page

Wyeth-Ayerst—Cont.

OVERDOSAGE

INDERAL is not significantly dialyzable. In the event of overdosage or exaggerated response, the following measures should be employed:

GENERAL—If ingestion is or may have been recent, evacuate gastric contents, taking care to prevent pulmonary aspiration.

BRADYCARDIA—ADMINISTER ATROPINE (0.25 to 1.0 mg); IF THERE IS NO RESPONSE TO VAGAL BLOCKADE, ADMINISTER ISOPROTERENOL CAUTIOUSLY.

CARDIAC FAILURE—DIGITALIZATION AND DIURETICS.

HYPOTENSION—VASOPRESSORS, eg, LEVARTERENOL OR EPINEPHRINE (THERE IS EVIDENCE THAT EPINEPHRINE IS THE DRUG OF CHOICE).

BRONCHOSPASM—ADMINISTER ISOPROTERENOL AND AMINOPHYLLINE.

HOW SUPPLIED

INDERAL LA CAPSULES
(propranolol hydrochloride)

—Each white/light-blue capsule, identified by 3 narrow bands, 1 wide band, and "INDERAL LA 60," contains 60 mg of propranolol hydrochloride in bottles of 100 (NDC 0046-0470-81) and 1,000 (NDC 0046-0470-91). Also available in a Unit Dose package of 100 (NDC 0046-0470-99).

—Each light-blue capsule, identified by 3 narrow bands, 1 wide band, and "INDERAL LA 80," contains 80 mg of propranolol hydrochloride in bottles of 100 (NDC 0046-0471-81) and 1,000 (NDC 0046-0471-91). Also available in a Unit Dose package of 100 (NDC 0046-0471-99).

—Each light-blue/dark-blue capsule, identified by 3 narrow bands, 1 wide band, and "INDERAL LA 120," contains 120 mg of propranolol hydrochloride in bottles of 100 (NDC 0046-0473-81) and 1,000 (NDC 0046-0473-91). Also available in a Unit Dose package of 100 (NDC 0046-0473-99).

—Each dark-blue capsule, identified by 3 narrow bands, 1 wide band, and "INDERAL LA 160," contains 160 mg of propranolol hydrochloride in bottles of 100 (NDC 0046-0479-81) and 1,000 (NDC 0046-0479-91). Also available in a Unit Dose package of 100 (NDC 0046-0479-99).

The appearance of these capsules is a registered trademark of Wyeth-Ayerst Laboratories.

Store at room temperature (approximately 25° C). Protect from light and moisture.

Shown in Product Identification Section, page 436

INDERIDE®

℞

[ĭn 'de-rīde]
Propranolol hydrochloride
(INDERAL®) and hydrochlorothiazide

CAUTION: Federal law prohibits dispensing without prescription.

DESCRIPTION

INDERIDE Tablets for oral administration combine two antihypertensive agents: INDERAL (propranolol hydrochloride), a beta-adrenergic blocking agent, and hydrochlorothiazide, a thiazide diuretic-antihypertensive. INDERIDE 40/25 Tablets contain 40 mg propranolol hydrochloride and 25 mg hydrochlorothiazide; INDERIDE 80/25 Tablets contain 80 mg propranolol hydrochloride and 25 mg hydrochlorothiazide.

INDERAL (propranolol hydrochloride) is a synthetic beta-adrenergic receptor-blocking agent chemically described as 1-(Isopropylamino)-3-(1-naphthyloxy)-2-propanol hydrochloride. Its structural formula is:

Propranolol hydrochloride is a stable, white, crystalline solid which is readily soluble in water and ethanol. Its molecular weight is 295.81.

Hydrochlorothiazide is a white, or practically white, practically odorless, crystalline powder. It is slightly soluble in water freely soluble in sodium hydroxide solution; sparingly soluble in methanol; insoluble in ether, chloroform, benzene, and dilute mineral acids. Its chemical name is: 6-Chloro-3,4-dihydro-2H-1,2,4-benzothiadiazine-7-sulfonamide 1,1-dioxide. Its structural formula is:

[See Chemical Formula at top of next column].

The inactive ingredients contained in INDERIDE Tablets are lactose, magnesium stearate, microcrystalline cellulose, stearic acid, and yellow ferric oxide.

CLINICAL PHARMACOLOGY

Propranolol hydrochloride (INDERAL®):

Propranolol hydrochloride is a nonselective beta-adrenergic receptor blocking agent possessing no other autonomic nervous system activity. It specifically competes with beta-adrenergic receptor stimulating agents for available receptor sites. When access to beta-receptor sites is blocked by propranolol, the chronotropic, inotropic, and vasodilator responses to beta-adrenergic stimulation are decreased proportionately.

Propranolol is almost completely absorbed from the gastrointestinal tract, but a portion is immediately metabolized by the liver on its first pass through the portal circulation. Peak effect occurs in one to one-and-one-half hours. The biologic half-life is approximately four hours. Propranolol is not significantly dialyzable. There is no simple correlation between dose or plasma level and therapeutic effect, and the dose-sensitivity range, as observed in clinical practice, is wide. The principal reason for this is that sympathetic tone varies widely between individuals. Since there is no reliable test to estimate sympathetic tone or to determine whether total beta blockade has been achieved, proper dosage requires titration.

The mechanism of the antihypertensive effects of propranolol has not been established. Among the factors that may be involved are (1) decreased cardiac output, (2) inhibition of renin release by the kidneys, and (3) diminution of tonic sympathetic nerve outflow from vasomotor centers in the brain. Although total peripheral resistance may increase initially, it readjusts to, or below, the pretreatment level with chronic usage. Effects on plasma volume appear to be minor and somewhat variable. Propranolol has been shown to cause a small increase in serum potassium concentration when used in the treatment of hypertensive patients. Propranolol hydrochloride decreases heart rate, cardiac output, and blood pressure.

Beta-receptor blockade can be useful in conditions in which, because of pathologic or functional changes, sympathetic activity is detrimental to the patient. But there are also situations in which sympathetic stimulation is vital. For example, in patients with severely damaged hearts, adequate ventricular function is maintained by virtue of sympathetic drive, which should be preserved. In the presence of AV block greater than first degree, beta blockade may prevent the necessary facilitating effect of sympathetic activity on conduction. Beta blockade results in bronchial constriction by interfering with adrenergic bronchodilator activity, which should be preserved in patients subject to bronchospasm.

The proper objective of beta-blockade therapy is to decrease adverse sympathetic stimulation, but not to the degree that may impair necessary sympathetic support.

Hydrochlorothiazide:

Hydrochlorothiazide is a benzothiadiazine (thiazide) diuretic closely related to chlorothiazide. The mechanism of the antihypertensive effect of the thiazides is unknown. Thiazides do not affect normal blood pressure.

Thiazides affect the renal tubular mechanism of electrolyte reabsorption. At maximal therapeutic dosage, all thiazides are approximately equal in their diuretic potency.

Thiazides increase excretion of sodium and chloride in approximately equivalent amounts. Natriuresis causes a secondary loss of potassium and bicarbonate. Onset of diuretic action of hydrochlorothiazide occurs in 2 hours, and the peak effect in about 4 hours. Its action persists for approximately 6 to 12 hours. Thiazides are eliminated rapidly by the kidney.

INDICATIONS AND USAGE

INDERIDE is indicated in the management of hypertension.

This fixed combination is not indicated for initial therapy of hypertension. Hypertension requires therapy titrated to the individual patient. If the fixed combination represents the dosage so determined, its use may be more convenient in patient management.

CONTRAINDICATIONS

Propranolol hydrochloride (INDERAL®):

Propranolol is contraindicated in: 1) cardiogenic shock; 2) sinus bradycardia and greater than first-degree block; 3)

bronchial asthma; 4) congestive heart failure (see WARNINGS) unless the failure is secondary to a tachyarrhythmia with propranolol.

Hydrochlorothiazide:

Hydrochlorothiazide is contraindicated in patients with anuria or hypersensitivity to this or other sulfonamide-derived drugs.

WARNINGS

Propranolol hydrochloride (INDERAL®):

CARDIAC FAILURE: Sympathetic stimulation is a vital component supporting circulatory function in congestive heart failure, and inhibition with beta blockade always carries the potential hazard of further depressing myocardial contractility and precipitating cardiac failure. Propranolol acts selectively without abolishing the inotropic action of digitalis on the heart muscle (i.e., that of supporting the strength of myocardial contractions). In patients already receiving digitalis, the positive inotropic action of digitalis may be reduced by propranolol's negative inotropic effect. The effects of propranolol and digitalis are additive in depressing AV conduction.

PATIENTS WITHOUT A HISTORY OF HEART FAILURE: Continued depression of the myocardium over a period of time can, in some cases, lead to cardiac failure. In rare instances, this has been observed during propranolol therapy. Therefore, at the first sign or symptom of impending cardiac failure, patients should be fully digitalized and/or given additional diuretic, and the response observed closely: a) if cardiac failure continues, despite adequate digitalization and diuretic therapy, propranolol therapy should be withdrawn (gradually, if possible); b) if tachyarrhythmia is being controlled, patients should be maintained on combined therapy and the patient closely followed until threat of cardiac failure is over.

> ANGINA PECTORIS: There have been reports of exacerbation of angina and, in some cases, myocardial infarction following *abrupt* discontinuation of propranolol therapy. Therefore, when discontinuance of propranolol is planned, the dosage should be gradually reduced and the patient should be carefully monitored. In addition, when propranolol is prescribed for angina pectoris, the patient should be cautioned against interruption or cessation of therapy without the physician's advice. If propranolol therapy is interrupted and exacerbation of angina occurs, it usually is advisable to reinstitute propranolol therapy and take other measures appropriate for the management of unstable angina pectoris. Since coronary artery disease may be unrecognized, it may be prudent to follow the above advice in patients considered at risk of having occult atherosclerotic heart disease, who are given propranolol for other indications.

NONALLERGIC BRONCHOSPASM (e.g., chronic bronchitis, emphysema): PATIENTS WITH BRONCHOSPASTIC DISEASES SHOULD, IN GENERAL, NOT RECEIVE BETA BLOCKERS. Propranolol should be administered with caution since it may block bronchodilation produced by endogenous and exogenous catecholamine stimulation of beta receptors.

MAJOR SURGERY: The necessity or desirability of withdrawal of beta-blocking therapy prior to major surgery is controversial. It should be noted, however, that the impaired ability of the heart to respond to reflex adrenergic stimuli may augment the risks of general anesthesia and surgical procedures.

Propranolol, like other beta blockers, is a competitive inhibitor of beta-receptor agonists, and its effects can be reversed by administration of such agents, e.g., dobutamine or isoproterenol. However, such patients may be subject to protracted severe hypotension. Difficulty in starting and maintaining the heartbeat has also been reported with beta blockers.

DIABETES AND HYPOGLYCEMIA: Beta blockers should be used with caution in diabetic patients if a beta-blocking agent is required. Beta blockers may mask tachycardia occurring with hypoglycemia, but other manifestations such as dizziness and sweating may not be significantly affected. Following insulin-induced hypoglycemia, propranolol may cause a delay in the recovery of blood glucose to normal levels.

THYROTOXICOSIS: Beta blockade may mask certain clinical signs of hyperthyroidism. Therefore, abrupt withdrawal of propranolol may be followed by an exacerbation of symptoms of hyperthyroidism, including thyroid storm. Propranolol may change thyroid-function tests, increasing T_4 and reverse T_3, and decreasing T_3.

WOLFF-PARKINSON-WHITE SYNDROME: Several cases have been reported in which, after propranolol, the tachycardia was replaced by a severe bradycardia requiring a demand pacemaker. In one case this resulted after an initial dose of 5 mg propranolol.

Hydrochlorothiazide:

Thiazides should be used with caution in severe renal disease. In patients with renal disease, thiazides may precipitate azotemia. In patients with impaired renal function, cumulative effects of the drug may develop.

Thiazides should also be used with caution in patients with impaired hepatic function or progressive liver disease, since minor alterations of fluid and electrolyte balance may precipitate hepatic coma.

Thiazides may add to or potentiate the action of other antihypertensive drugs. Potentiation occurs with ganglionic or peripheral adrenergic-blocking drugs.

Sensitivity reactions may occur in patients with a history of allergy or bronchial asthma. The possibility of exacerbation or activation of systemic lupus erythematosus has been reported.

PRECAUTIONS
GENERAL
Propranolol hydrochloride (INDERAL®):
Propranolol should be used with caution in patients with impaired hepatic or renal function. INDERIDE is not indicated for the treatment of hypertensive emergencies.

Hydrochlorothiazide:
All patients receiving thiazide therapy should be observed for clinical signs of fluid or electrolyte imbalance, namely hyponatremia, hypochloremic alkalosis, and hypokalemia. Serum and urine electrolyte determinations are particularly important when the patient is vomiting excessively or receiving parenteral fluids. Medication such as digitalis may also influence serum electrolytes. Warning signs, irrespective of cause, are: dryness of mouth, thirst, weakness, lethargy, drowsiness, restlessness, muscle pains or cramps, muscular fatigue, hypotension, oliguria, tachycardia, and gastrointestinal disturbances such as nausea and vomiting.

Hypokalemia may develop, especially with brisk diuresis or when severe cirrhosis is present.

Interference with adequate oral electrolyte intake will also contribute to hypokalemia. Hypokalemia can sensitize or exaggerate the response of the heart to the toxic effects of digitalis (e.g., increased ventricular irritability).

Hypokalemia may be avoided or treated by use of potassium supplements or foods with a high potassium content.

Any chloride deficit is generally mild, and usually does not require specific treatment except under extraordinary circumstances (as in liver or renal disease). Dilutional hyponatremia may occur in edematous patients in hot weather; appropriate therapy is water restriction rather than administration of salt, except in rare instances when the hyponatremia is life-threatening. In actual salt depletion, appropriate replacement is the therapy of choice.

Hyperuricemia may occur or frank gout may be precipitated in certain patients receiving thiazide therapy.

Diabetes mellitus which has been latent may become manifest during thiazide administration.

The antihypertensive effects of the drug may be enhanced in the postsympathectomy patient.

If progressive renal impairment becomes evident, consider withholding or discontinuing diuretic therapy.

Calcium excretion is decreased by thiazides. Pathologic changes in the parathyroid gland with hypercalcemia and hypophosphatemia have been observed in a few patients on prolonged thiazide therapy. The common complications of hyperparathyroidism, such as renal lithiasis, bone resorption, and peptic ulceration, have not been seen.

INFORMATION FOR PATIENTS
Beta-adrenorecptor blockade can cause reduction of intraocular pressure. Patients should be told that INDERIDE may interfere with the glaucoma screening test. Withdrawal may lead to a return of increased intraocular pressure.

LABORATORY TESTS
Propranolol hydrochloride (INDERAL®):
Elevated blood urea levels in patients with severe heart disease, elevated serum transaminase, alkaline phosphatase, lactate dehydrogenase.

Hydrochlorothiazide:
Periodic determination of serum electrolytes to detect possible electrolyte imbalance should be performed at appropriate intervals.

DRUG/DRUG INTERACTIONS
Propranolol hydrochloride (INDERAL®):
Patients receiving catecholamine-depleting drugs such as reserpine should be closely observed if INDERIDE is administered. The added catecholamine-blocking action may produce an excessive reduction of resting sympathetic nervous activity, which may result in hypotension, marked bradycardia, vertigo, syncopal attacks, or orthostatic hypotension. Caution should be exercised when patients receiving a beta blocker are administered a calcium-channel blocking drug, especially intravenous verapamil, for both agents may depress myocardial contractility or atrioventricular conduction. On rare occasions, the concomitant intravenous use of a beta blocker and verapamil has resulted in serious adverse reactions, especially in patients with severe cardiomyopathy, congestive heart failure, or recent myocardial infarction. Blunting of the antihypertensive effect of beta-adrenoceptor blocking agents by nonsteroidal anti-inflammatory drugs has been reported.

Hypotension and coronary arrest have been reported with the concomitant use of propranolol and haloperidol.

Aluminum hydroxide gel greatly reduces intestinal absorption of propranolol.

Ethanol slows the rate of absorption of propranolol.

Phenytoin, phenobarbitone, and rifampin accelerate propranolol clearance.

Chlorpromazine, when used concomitantly with propranolol, results in increased plasma levels of both drugs.

Antipyrine and *lidocaine* have reduced clearance when used concomitantly with propranolol.

Thyroxine may result in a lower than expected T$_3$ concentration when used concomitantly with propranolol.

Cimetidine decreases the hepatic metabolism of propranolol, delaying elimination and increasing blood levels.

Theophylline clearance is reduced when used concomitantly with propranolol.

Hydrochlorothiazide:
Thiazide drugs may increase the responsiveness to tubocurarine.

Thiazides may decrease arterial responsiveness to norepinephrine. This diminution is not sufficient to preclude effectiveness of the pressor agent for therapeutic use.

Insulin requirements in diabetic patients may be increased, decreased, or unchanged.

Hypokalemia may develop during concomitant use of corticosteroids or ACTH.

DRUG/LABORATORY TEST INTERACTIONS
Hydrochlorothiazide:
Thiazides may decrease serum PBI levels without signs of thyroid disturbance.

Thiazides should be discontinued before carrying out tests for parathyroid function (see PRECAUTIONS—General).

CARCINOGENESIS, MUTAGENESIS, IMPAIRMENT OF FERTILITY
Propranolol hydrochloride (INDERAL®):
Long-term studies in animals have been conducted to evaluate toxic effects and carcinogenic potential. In 18-month studies in both rats and mice, employing doses up to 150 mg/kg/day, there was no evidence of significant drug-induced toxicity. There were no drug-related tumorigenic effects at any of the dosage levels. Reproductive studies in animals did not show any impairment of fertility that was attributable to the drug. Long-term studies in animals have not been conducted to evaluate the toxic effects and carcinogenic potential of INDERIDE.

Hydrochlorothiazide:
Hydrochlorothiazide is presently under study for carcinogenesis in rats and mice in the National Toxicology Research and Testing Program.

Hydrochlorothiazide was not mutagenic in *in vitro* Ames mutagenicity assays of *Salmonella typhimurium* strains TA 98, TA 100, TA 1535, TA 1537, and TA 1538 or in *in vivo* mutagenicity assays of mouse germinal-cell chromosomes and Chinese hamster bone-marrow-cell chromosomes. It was, however, mutagenic in inducing nondisjunction (96% frequency) in diploid strains of *Aspergillus nidulans.* Hydrochlorothiazide had no adverse effects on fertility in rats at a dose equivalent to the recommended maximum human dose and in mice at a dose equivalent to 25 times the recommended maximum human dose (4 mg/kg, assumed body weight of 50 kg).

PREGNANCY: Pregnancy Category C
Propranolol hydrochloride (INDERAL®):
Propranolol has been shown to be embryotoxic in animal studies at doses about 10 times greater than the maximum recommended human dose. There are no adequate and well-controlled studies in pregnant women. Propranolol should be used during pregnancy only if the potential benefit justifies the potential risk to the fetus.

Hydrochlorothiazide:
Thiazides cross the placental barrier and appear in cord blood. The use of thiazides in pregnant women requires that the anticipated benefit be weighed against possible hazards to the fetus. These hazards include fetal or neonatal jaundice, thrombocytopenia, and possibly other adverse reactions which have occurred in the adult.

Available information indicates that hydrochlorothiazide at doses as high as 330 times the recommended maximum human dose was not teratogenic in pregnant rats.

NURSING MOTHERS
Propranolol hydrochloride (INDERAL®):
Propranolol is excreted in human milk. Caution should be exercised when INDERIDE is administered to a nursing woman.

Hydrochlorothiazide:
Thiazides appear in breast milk. If the use of drug is deemed essential, the patient should stop nursing.

PEDIATRIC USE
Safety and effectiveness in children have not been established.

ADVERSE REACTIONS
The following adverse reactions have been observed, but there is not enough systematic collection of data to support an estimate of their frequency. Within each category, ad-

verse reactions are listed in decreasing order of severity. Although many side effects are mild and transient, some require discontinuation of therapy.

Propranolol hydrochloride (INDERAL®):
Cardiovascular: Congestive heart failure; hypotension; intensification of AV block; bradycardia; thrombocytopenic purpura; arterial insufficiency, usually of the Raynaud type; paresthesia of hands.

Central Nervous System: Reversible mental depression progressing to catatonia; mental depression manifested by insomnia, lassitude, weakness, fatigue; an acute reversible syndrome characterized by disorientation for time and place, short-term memory loss, emotional lability, slightly clouded sensorium, decreased performance on neuropsychometrics; hallucinations; visual disturbances; vivid dreams; lightheadedness. Total daily doses above 160 mg (when administered as divided doses of greater than 80 mg each) may be associated with an increased incidence of fatigue, lethargy, and vivid dreams.

Gastrointestinal: Mesenteric arterial thrombosis; ischemic colitis; nausea, vomiting, epigastric distress, abdominal cramping, diarrhea, constipation.

Allergic: Laryngospasm and respiratory distress; pharyngitis and agranulocytosis; fever combined with aching and sore throat; erythematous rash.

Respiratory: Bronchospasm.

Hematologic: Agranulcytosis; nonthrombocytopenic purpura; thrombocytopenic purpura.

Autoimmune: In extremely rare instances, systemic lupus erythematosus has been reported.

Miscellaneous: Male impotence. Alopecia, LE-like reactions, psoriasiform rashes, dry eyes, and Peyronie's disease have been reported rarely. Oculomucocutaneous reactions involving the skin, serous membranes, and conjunctivae reported for a beta blocker (practolol) have not been associated with propranolol.

Hydrochlorothiazide:
Cardiovascular: Orthostatic hypotension (may be aggravated by alcohol, barbiturates or narcotics).

Central Nervous System: Dizziness, vertigo, headache, xanthopsia, paresthesias.

Gastrointestinal: Pancreatitis; jaundice (intrahepatic cholestatic jaundice); sialadenitis; anorexia, nausea, vomiting, gastric irritation, cramping, diarrhea, constipation.

Hypersensitivity: Anaphylactic reactions; necrotizing angiitis (vasculitis, cutaneous vasculitis); respiratory distress including pneumonitis; fever; urticaria, rash, purpura, photosensitivity.

Hematologic: Aplastic anemia, agranulocytosis, leukopenia, thrombocytopenia.

Miscellaneous: Hyperglycemia, glycosuria; hyperuricemia; muscle spasm; weakness; restlessness; transient blurred vision.

Whenever adverse reactions are moderate or severe, thiazide dosage should be reduced or therapy withdrawn.

OVERDOSAGE
The propranolol hydrochloride component may cause bradycardia, cardiac failure, hypotension, or bronchospasm. Propranolol is not significantly dialyzable.

The hydrochlorothiazide component can be expected to cause diuresis. Lethargy of varying degree may appear and may progress to coma within a few hours, with minimal depression of respiration and cardiovascular function, and in the absence of significant serum electrolyte changes or dehydration. The mechanism of central nervous system depression with thiazide overdosage is unknown. Gastrointestinal irritation and hypermotility can occur, temporary elevation of BUN has been reported, and serum electrolyte changes could occur, especially in patients with impairment of renal function.

The oral LD$_{50}$ dosages in rats and mice for propranolol, hydrochlorothiazide, and combined propranolol/hydrochlorothiazide (40/25, 80/25) are 364 to 533 mg/kg, greater than 2,750 to 5,000 mg/kg, and 538 to 845 mg/kg, respectively.

TREATMENT
The following measures should be employed:

GENERAL—If ingestion is, or may have been, recent, evacuate gastric contents, taking care to prevent pulmonary aspiration.

BRADYCARDIA—Administer atropine (0.25 to 1.0 mg). If there is no response to vagal blockade, administer isoproterenol cautiously.

CARDIAC FAILURE—Digitalization and diuretics.

HYPOTENSION—Vasopressors, e.g., levarterenol or epinephrine.

BRONCHOSPASM—Administer isoproterenol and aminophylline.

STUPOR OR COMA—Administer supportive therapy as clinically warranted.

GASTROINTESTINAL EFFECTS—Though usually of short duration, these may require symptomatic treatment.

ABNORMALITIES IN BUN AND/OR SERUM ELECTROLYTES—Monitor serum electrolyte levels and renal

Continued on next page

Wyeth-Ayerst—Cont.

function; institute supportive measures as required individually to maintain hydration, electrolyte balance, respiration, and cardiovascular-renal function.

DOSAGE AND ADMINISTRATION

The dosage must be determined by individual titration. Hydrochlorothiazide can be given at doses of 25 to 100 mg per day when used alone, but in most patients, 50 mg exerts a maximal effect. The initial dose of propranolol is 80 mg daily, and it may be increased gradually until optimal blood pressure control is achieved. The usual effective dose when used alone is 160 to 480 mg per day.

One INDERIDE Tablet twice daily can be used to administer up to 160 mg of propranolol and 50 mg of hydrochlorothiazide. For doses of propranolol greater than 160 mg the combination products are not appropriate, because their use would lead to an excessive dose of the thiazide component.

When necessary, another antihypertensive agent may be added gradually beginning with 50 percent of the usual recommended starting dose to avoid an excessive fall in blood pressure.

HOW SUPPLIED

INDERIDE 40/25
—Each hexagonal-shaped, off-white, scored tablet, embossed with an "I" and imprinted with "INDERIDE 40/25," contains 40 mg propranolol hydrochloride (INDERAL®) and 25 mg hydrochlorothiazide, in bottles of 100 (NDC 0046-0484-81) and 1,000 (NDC 0046-0484-91). Also in Unit Dose packages of 100 (NDC 0046-0484-99).

INDERIDE 80/25
—Each hexagonal-shaped, off-white, scored tablet, embossed with an "I" and imprinted with "INDERIDE 80/25," contains 80 mg propranolol hydrochloride (INDERAL®) and 25 mg hydrochlorothiazide, in bottles of 100 (NDC 0046-0488-81) and 1,000 (NDC 0046-0488-91). Also in Unit Dose packages of 100 (NDC 0046-0488-99).

The appearance of these tablets is a registered trademark of Wyeth-Ayerst Laboratories.

Store at room temperature (approximately 25° C).
Dispense in well-closed, light-resistant containers.
Protect from moisture, freezing, and excessive heat.
Shown in Product Identification Section, page 436

INDERIDE® LA ℞

[*in 'de-rīde*]
Brand of propranolol hydrochloride
(INDERAL® LA) and hydrochlorothiazide
(Long Acting Capsules)

No. 455—Each INDERIDE® LA 80/50 Capsule contains:
Propranolol hydrochloride
(INDERAL® LA) .... 80 mg
Hydrochlorothiazide .... 50 mg
No. 457—Each INDERIDE® LA 120/50
Capsule contains:
Propranolol hydrochloride
(INDERAL® LA) .... 120 mg
Hydrochlorothiazide .... 50 mg
No. 459—Each INDERIDE® LA 160/50
Capsule contains:
Propranolol hydrochloride
(INDERAL® LA) ....160 mg
Hydrochlorothiazide .... 50 mg
CAUTION: Federal law prohibits dispensing without prescription.

DESCRIPTION

INDERIDE LA is indicated in the once-daily management of hypertension.

INDERIDE LA combines two antihypertensive agents: INDERAL (propranolol hydrochloride), a beta-adrenergic receptor-blocking agent, and hydrochlorothiazide, a thiazide diuretic-antihypertensive. INDERIDE LA is formulated to provide a sustained release of propranolol hydrochloride. Hydrochlorothiazide in INDERIDE LA exists in a conventional (not sustained-release) formulation.

INDERAL (propranolol hydrochloride) is a synthetic beta-adrenergic receptor-blocking agent chemically described as 1-(Isopropylamino)-3-(1-naphthyloxy)-2-propanol hydrochloride. Its structural formula is:

Propranolol hydrochloride is a stable, white, crystalline solid which is readily soluble in water and ethanol. Its molecular weight is 295.81.

Hydrochlorothiazide is a white, or practically white, practically odorless, crystalline powder. It is slightly soluble in

water; freely soluble in sodium hydroxide solution; sparingly soluble in methanol; insoluble in ether, chloroform, benzene, and dilute mineral acids. Its chemical name is 6-Chloro-3,4-dihydro-2H-1,2,4-benzothiadiazine-7-sulfonamide 1,1-dioxide. Its structural formula is:

INDERIDE LA contains the following inactive ingredients: calcium carbonate, ethylcellulose, gelatin capsules, hydroxypropyl methylcellulose, lactose, magnesium stearate, microcrystalline cellulose, sodium lauryl sulfate, sodium starch glycolate, titanium dioxide, and D&C Yellow No. 10. In addition, INDERIDE LA 80/50 mg and 120/50 mg Capsules contain D&C Red No. 33; INDERIDE LA 120/50 mg and 160/50 mg Capsules contain FD&C Blue No. 1 and FD&C Red No. 40.

CLINICAL PHARMACOLOGY

Propranolol hydrochloride (INDERAL®):
INDERAL is a nonselective, beta-adrenergic receptor-blocking agent possessing no other autonomic nervous system activity. It specifically competes with beta-adrenergic receptor-stimulating agents for available receptor sites. When access to beta-receptor sites is blocked by INDERAL, the chronotropic, inotropic, and vasodilator responses to beta-adrenergic stimulation are decreased proportionately.

INDERIDE LA Capsules (80/50, 120/50, and 160/50 mg) release propranolol hydrochloride at a controlled and predictable rate. Peak propranolol blood levels following dosing with INDERIDE LA occur at about 6 hours, and the apparent plasma half-life is about 10 hours. Over a 24-hour period, propranolol blood levels are fairly constant for about 12 hours, then decline exponentially. When measured at steady state over a 24-hour period, the areas under the propranolol plasma concentration-time curve (AUCs) for the capsules are approximately 60% to 65% of the AUCs for a comparable divided daily dose of INDERAL Tablets. The lower AUCs for the capsules are due to greater hepatic metabolism of propranolol resulting from the slower rate of absorption of propranolol.

INDERIDE LA should not be considered a simple mg-for-mg substitute for conventional INDERIDE Tablets, and the propranolol blood levels achieved do not match (are lower than) those of twice-daily dosing of INDERIDE Tablets with the same dose. When changing to INDERIDE LA from conventional INDERIDE Tablets, a possible need for retitration upwards should be considered.

The mechanism of the antihypertensive effect of propranolol has not been established. Among the factors that may be involved in contributing to the antihypertensive action are: (1) decreased cardiac output, (2) inhibition of renin release by the kidneys, and (3) diminution of tonic sympathetic nerve outflow from vasomotor centers in the brain.

Propranolol hydrochloride decreases heart rate, cardiac output, and blood pressure. Although total peripheral vascular resistance may increase initially, it readjusts to or below the pretreatment level with chronic usage. Effects on plasma volume appear to be minor and somewhat variable. INDERAL has been shown to cause a small increase in serum potassium concentration when used in the treatment of hypertensive patients.

Beta-receptor blockade is useful in conditions in which, because of pathologic or functional changes, sympathetic activity is excessive or inappropriate, and detrimental to the patient. But there are also situations in which sympathetic stimulation is vital. For example, in patients with severely damaged hearts, adequate ventricular function is maintained by virtue of sympathetic drive, which should be preserved. In the presence of AV block, beta blockade may prevent the necessary facilitating effect of sympathetic activity on conduction. Beta blockade results in bronchial constriction by interfering with adrenergic bronchodilator activity, which should be preserved in patients subject to bronchospasm.

The proper objective of beta-blockade therapy is to decrease adverse sympathetic stimulation, but not to the degree that may impair necessary sympathetic support.

Hydrochlorothiazide:
Hydrochlorothiazide is a benzothiadiazine (thiazide) diuretic closely related to chlorothiazide. The mechanism of the antihypertensive effect of the thiazides is unknown. Thiazides usually do not affect normal blood pressure.

Thiazides affect the renal tubular mechanism of electrolyte reabsorption. At maximal therapeutic dosage, all thiazides are approximately equal in their diuretic efficacy.

Thiazides increase excretion of sodium and chloride in approximately equivalent amounts. Natriuresis causes a secondary loss of potassium and bicarbonate.

Onset of diuretic action of thiazides occurs in 2 hours, and the peak effect in about 4 hours. Its action persists for approximately 6 to 12 hours. Thiazides are eliminated rapidly

by the kidney. The hydrochlorothiazide in INDERIDE LA is a conventional (not sustained-release) formulation.

INDICATIONS AND USAGE

INDERIDE LA is indicated in the management of hypertension.

This fixed-combination drug is not indicated for initial therapy of hypertension. Hypertension requires therapy titrated to the individual patient. If the fixed combination represents the dosage so determined, its use may be more convenient in patient management. The treatment of hypertension is not static, but must be reevaluated as conditions in each patient warrant.

CONTRAINDICATIONS

Propranolol hydrochloride (INDERAL®):
Propranolol is contraindicated in: 1) cardiogenic shock; 2) sinus bradycardia and greater than first-degree block; 3) bronchial asthma; 4) congestive heart failure (see WARNINGS), unless the failure is secondary to a tachyarrhythmia treatable with propranolol.

Hydrochlorothiazide:
Hydrochlorothiazide is contraindicated in patients with anuria or hypersensitivity to this or other sulfonamide-derived drugs.

WARNINGS

Propranolol hydrochloride (INDERAL®):
CARDIAC FAILURE: Sympathetic stimulation may be a vital component supporting circulatory function in patients with congestive heart failure, and its inhibition by beta blockade may precipitate more severe failure. Although beta blockers should be avoided in overt congestive heart failure, if necessary, they can be used with close follow-up in patients with a history of failure who are well compensated and are receiving digitalis and diuretics. Beta-adrenergic blocking agents do not abolish the inotropic action of digitalis on heart muscle.

IN PATIENTS WITHOUT A HISTORY OF HEART FAILURE, continued use of beta blockers can, in some cases, lead to cardiac failure. Therefore, at the first sign or symptom of heart failure, the patient should be digitalized and/or treated with diuretics, and the response observed closely, or propranolol should be discontinued (gradually, if possible).

IN PATIENTS WITH ANGINA PECTORIS, there have been reports of exacerbation of angina and, in some cases, myocardial infarction, following *abrupt* discontinuance of propranolol therapy. Therefore, when discontinuance of propranolol is planned, the dosage should be gradually reduced and the patient carefully monitored. In addition, when propranolol is prescribed for angina pectoris, the patient should be cautioned against interruption or cessation of therapy without the physician's advice. If propranolol therapy is interrupted and exacerbation of angina occurs, it usually is advisable to reinstitute propranolol therapy and take other measures appropriate for the management of unstable angina pectoris. Since coronary artery disease may be unrecognized, it may be prudent to follow the above advice in patients considered at risk of having occult atherosclerotic heart disease who are given propranolol for other indications.

THYROTOXICOSIS: Beta blockade may mask certain clinical signs of hyperthyroidism. Therefore, abrupt withdrawal of propranolol may be followed by an exacerbation of symptoms of hyperthyroidism, including thyroid storm. Propranolol does not distort thyroid function tests.

IN PATIENTS WITH WOLFF-PARKINSON-WHITE SYNDROME, several cases have been reported in which, after propranolol, the tachycardia was replaced by a severe bradycardia requiring a demand pacemaker. In one case this resulted after an initial dose of 5 mg propranolol.

MAJOR SURGERY: The necessity or desirability of withdrawal of beta-blocking therapy prior to major surgery is controversial. It should be noted, however, that the impaired ability of the heart to respond to reflex adrenergic stimuli may augment the risks of general anesthesia and surgical procedures.

Nonallergic Bronchospasm (eg, chronic bronchitis, emphysema)—PATIENTS WITH BRONCHOSPASTIC DISEASES SHOULD, IN GENERAL, NOT RECEIVE BETA BLOCKERS. INDERAL should be administered with caution since it may block bronchodilation produced by endogenous and exogenous catecholamine stimulation of beta receptors.

DIABETES AND HYPOGLYCEMIA: Beta-adrenergic blockade may prevent the appearance of certain premonitory signs and symptoms (pulse rate and pressure changes) of acute hypoglycemia in labile insulin-dependent diabetes. In these patients, it may be more difficult to adjust the dosage of insulin. Hypoglycemic attacks may be accompanied by a precipitous elevation of blood pressure.

Hydrochlorothiazide:

Thiazides should be used with caution in severe renal disease. In patients with renal disease, thiazides may precipitate azotemia. In patients with impaired renal function, cumulative effects of the drug may develop.

Thiazides should also be used with caution in patients with impaired hepatic function or progressive liver disease, since minor alterations of fluid and electrolyte balance may precipitate hepatic coma.

Thiazides may add to or potentiate the action of other antihypertensive drugs. Potentiation occurs with ganglionic or peripheral adrenergic-blocking drugs.

Sensitivity reactions may occur in patients with a history of allergy or bronchial asthma. The possibility of exacerbation or activation of systemic lupus erythematosus has been reported.

PRECAUTIONS

Propranolol hydrochloride (INDERAL®):

GENERAL: Propranolol should be used with caution in patients with impaired hepatic or renal function. Propranolol is not indicated for the treatment of hypertensive emergencies.

Beta-adrenoreceptor blockade can cause reduction of intraocular pressure. Patients should be told that propranolol may interfere with the glaucoma screening test. Withdrawal may lead to a return of increased intraocular pressure.

CLINICAL LABORATORY TESTS: Elevated blood urea levels in patients with severe heart disease, elevated serum transaminase, alkaline phosphatase, lactate dehydrogenase.

DRUG INTERACTIONS: Patients receiving catecholamine-depleting drugs, such as reserpine, should be closely observed if propranolol is administered. The added catecholamine-blocking action may produce an excessive reduction of resting sympathetic nervous activity, which may result in hypotension, marked bradycardia, vertigo, syncopal attacks, or orthostatic hypotension.

CARCINOGENESIS, MUTAGENESIS, IMPAIRMENT OF FERTILITY: Long-term studies in animals have been conducted to evaluate toxic effects and carcinogenic potential. In 18-month studies, in both rats and mice, employing doses up to 150 mg/kg/day, there was no evidence of significant drug-induced toxicity. There were no drug-related tumorigenic effects at any of the dosage levels. Reproductive studies in animals did not show any impairment of fertility that was attributable to the drug.

PREGNANCY: Pregnancy Category C. Propranolol has been shown to be embryotoxic in animal studies at doses about 10 times greater than the maximal recommended human dose. There are no adequate and well-controlled studies in pregnant women. Propranolol should be used during pregnancy only if the potential benefit justifies the potential risk to the fetus.

NURSING MOTHERS: Propranolol is excreted in human milk. Caution should be exercised when propranolol is administered to a nursing mother.

PEDIATRIC USE: Safety and effectiveness in children have not been established.

Hydrochlorothiazide:

GENERAL: Periodic determination of serum electrolytes to detect possible electrolyte imbalance should be performed at appropriate intervals.

All patients receiving thiazide therapy should be observed for clinical signs of fluid or electrolyte imbalance, namely: hyponatremia, hypochloremic alkalosis, and hypokalemia. Serum and urine electrolyte determinations are particularly important when the patient is vomiting excessively or receiving parenteral fluids. Medication such as digitalis may also influence serum electrolytes. Warning signs irrespective of cause are: Dryness of mouth, thirst, weakness, lethargy, drowsiness, restlessness, muscle pains or cramps, muscular fatigue, hypotension, oliguria, tachycardia, and gastrointestinal disturbances such as nausea and vomiting.

Hypokalemia may develop, especially with brisk diuresis, when severe cirrhosis is present or during concomitant use of corticosteroids or ACTH.

Interference with adequate oral electrolyte intake will also contribute to hypokalemia. Hypokalemia can sensitize or exaggerate the response of the heart to the toxic effect of digitalis (eg, increased ventricular irritability). Hypokalemia may be avoided or treated by use of potassium supplements, such as foods with a high potassium content.

Any chloride deficit is generally mild and usually does not require specific treatment, except under extraordinary circumstances (as in liver or renal disease). Dilutional hyponatremia may occur in edematous patients in hot weather; appropriate therapy is water restriction, rather than administration of salt, except in rare instances when the hyponatremia is life-threatening. In actual salt depletion, appropriate replacement is the therapy of choice.

Hyperuricemia may occur or frank gout may be precipitated in certain patients receiving thiazide therapy.

Insulin requirements in diabetic patients may be increased, decreased, or unchanged. Diabetes mellitus which has been latent may become manifest during thiazide administration.

If progressive renal impairment becomes evident, consider withholding or discontinuing diuretic therapy.

Thiazides may decrease serum PBI levels without signs of thyroid disturbance.

Calcium excretion is decreased by thiazides. Pathologic changes in the parathyroid gland with hypercalcemia and hypophosphatemia have been observed in a few patients on prolonged thiazide therapy. The common complications of hyperparathyroidism, such as renal lithiasis, bone resorption, and peptic ulceration have not been seen. Thiazides should be discontinued before carrying out tests for parathyroid function.

DRUG INTERACTIONS: Thiazide drugs may increase the responsiveness to tubocurarine.

The antihypertensive effects of thiazides may be enhanced in the postsympathectomy patient. Thiazides may decrease arterial responsiveness to norepinephrine. This diminution is not sufficient to preclude effectiveness of the pressor agent for therapeutic use.

PREGNANCY: Pregnancy Category C. Thiazides cross the placental barrier and appear in cord blood. The use of thiazides in pregnancy requires that the anticipated benefit be weighed against possible hazards to the fetus. These hazards include fetal or neonatal jaundice, thrombocytopenia, and possibly other adverse reactions which have occurred in the adult.

NURSING MOTHERS: Thiazides appear in human milk. If use of the drug is deemed essential, the patient should stop nursing.

PEDIATRIC USE: Safety and effectivenss in children have not been established.

ADVERSE REACTIONS

Propranolol hydrochloride (INDERAL®):

Most adverse effects have been mild and transient and have rarely required the withdrawal of therapy.

Cardiovascular: Bradycardia; congestive heart failure; intensification of AV block; hypotension; paresthesia of hands; thrombocytopenic purpura; arterial insufficiency, usually of the Raynaud type.

Central Nervous System: Lightheadedness; mental depression manifested by insomnia, lassitude, weakness, fatigue; reversible mental depression progressing to catatonia; visual disturbances; hallucinations; an acute reversible syndrome characterized by disorientation for time and place, short-term memory loss, emotional lability, slightly clouded sensorium, and decreased performance on neuropsychometrics.

Gastrointestinal: Nausea, vomiting, epigastric distress, abdominal cramping, diarrhea, constipation, mesenteric arterial thrombosis, ischemic colitis.

Allergic: Pharyngitis and agranulocytosis; erythematous rash; fever combined with aching and sore throat; laryngospasm and respiratory distress.

Respiratory: Bronchospasm.

Hematologic: Agranulocytosis; nonthrombocytopenic purpura, thrombocytopenic purpura.

Auto-Immune: In extremely rare instances, systemic lupus erythematosus has been reported.

Miscellaneous: Alopecia; LE-like reactions; psoriasiform rashes; dry eyes; male impotence; and Peyronie's disease have been reported rarely. Oculomucocutaneous reactions involving the skin, serous membrances, and conjunctivae reported for a beta blocker (practolol) have not been associated with propranolol.

Hydrochlorothiazide:

Gastrointestinal: Anorexia; gastric irritation, nausea, vomiting, cramping; diarrhea; constipation; jaundice (intrahepatic cholestatic jaundice); pancreatitis; sialadenitis.

Central Nervous System: Dizziness, vertigo; paresthesias; headache; xanthopsia.

Hematologic: Leukopenia; agranulocytosis; thrombocytopenia; aplastic anemia.

Cardiovascular: Orthostatic hypotension (may be aggravated by alcohol, barbiturates, or narcotics).

Hypersensitivity: Purpura; photosensitivity; rash; urticaria; necrotizing angiitis (vasculitis, cutaneous vasculitis); fever; respiratory distress, including pneumonitis; anaphylactic reactions.

Other: Hyperglycemia; glycosuria; hyperuricemia; muscle spasm; weakness; restlessness; transient blurred vision.

Whenever adverse reactions are moderate or severe, thiazide dosage should be reduced or therapy withdrawn.

DOSAGE AND ADMINISTRATION

The dosage must be determined by individual titration.

Hydrochlorothiazide can be given at doses of 25–100 mg per day when used alone, but in most patients, 50 mg exerts a maximal effect. The initial dose of propranolol is 80 mg daily, and it may be increased gradually until optimal blood pressure control is achieved. The usual effective dose, when used alone, is 160–480 mg per day.

One INDERIDE LA Capsule once-a-day can be used to administer up to 160 mg of propranolol and 50 mg of hydrochlorothiazide. For doses of propranolol greater than 160 mg, the combination products are not appropriate because their use would lead to an excessive dose of the thiazide component.

INDERIDE LA provides propranolol hydrochloride in a sustained-release form and hydrochlorothiazide in conventional formulation, for once-daily administration. If patients are switched from INDERIDE Tablets (or INDERAL plus hydrochlorothiazide) to INDERIDE LA, care should be taken to ensure that the desired therapeutic effect is maintained. INDERIDE LA should not be considered a mg-for-mg substitute for INDERIDE or INDERAL plus hydrochlorothiazide. INDERIDE LA has different kinetics and produces lower blood levels. Retitration may be necessary, especially to maintain effectiveness at the end of the 24-hour dosing interval.

When necessary, another antihypertensive agent may be added gradually, beginning with 50% of the usual recommended starting dose, to avoid an excessive fall in blood pressure.

OVERDOSAGE OR EXAGGERATED RESPONSE

The propranolol hydrochloride (INDERAL) component may cause bradycardia, cardiac failure, hypotension, or bronchospasm.

The hydrochlorothiazide component can be expected to cause diuresis. Lethargy of varying degree may appear and may progress to coma within a few hours, with minimal depression of respiration and cardiovascular function, and in the absence of significant serum electrolyte changes or dehydration. The mechanism of central nervous system depression with thiazide overdosage is unknown. Gastrointestinal irritation and hypermotility can occur; temporary elevation of BUN has been reported and serum electrolyte changes could occur, especially in patients with impairment of renal function.

TREATMENT

The following measures should be employed:

GENERAL—If ingestion is, or may have been, recent, evacuate gastric contents, taking care to prevent pulmonary aspiration.

BRADYCARDIA—Administer atropine (0.25–1.0 mg). If there is no response to vagal blockade, administer isoproterenol cautiously.

CARDIAC FAILURE—Digitalization and diuretics.

HYPOTENSION—Vasopressors, eg, levarterenol or epinephrine.

BRONCHOSPASM—Administer isoproterenol and aminophylline.

STUPOR OR COMA—Administer supportive therapy as clinically warranted.

GASTROINTESTINAL EFFECTS—Though usually of short duration, these may require symptomatic treatment.

ABNORMALITIES IN BUN AND/OR SERUM ELECTROLYTES—Monitor serum electrolyte levels and renal function; institute supportive measures, as required individually, to maintain hydration, electrolyte balance, respiration, and cardiovascular function.

HOW SUPPLIED

—Each beige capsule, identified by one wide band and 3 narrow bands, all in gold, and "INDERIDE LA 80/50," contains 80 mg of propranolol hydrochloride (INDERAL® LA) and 50 mg of hydrochlorothiazide, in bottles of 100 (NDC 0046-0455-81).

—Each beige/brown capsule, identified by one wide band and 3 narrow bands, all in gold, and "INDERIDE LA 120/50," contains 120 mg of propranolol hydrochloride (INDERAL® LA) and 50 mg of hydrochlorothiazide, in bottles of 100 (NDC 0046-0457-81).

—Each brown capsule, identified by one wide band and 3 narrow bands, all in gold, and "INDERIDE LA 160/50," contains 160 mg of propranolol hydrochloride (INDERAL® LA) and 50 mg of hydrochlorothiazide, in bottles of 100 (NDC 0046-0459-81).

The appearance of these capsules is a registered trademark of Wyeth-Ayerst Laboratories.

Store at room temperature (approximately 25° C).

Shown in Product Identification Section, page 436

INFLUENZA VIRUS   ℞
VACCINE, SUBVIRION TYPE
[*in "flu-en 'zah vi 'rus vak 'sēn sub vir 'ēon*]

The formulation of influenza virus vaccine for use during each season is established by the office of Biologics Research and Review, Food and Drug Administration. For current information about formulation, dosage and recommended use, consult product direction circular which can be obtained by writing Professional Service, Wyeth-Ayerst Laboratories, P.O. Box 8299, Philadelphia, PA 19101, or through your local Wyeth-Ayerst representative.

Continued on next page

Wyeth-Ayerst—Cont.

ISORDIL®   ℞

[ī'sore"dĭl]
(isosorbide dinitrate)
(1,4,3,6-dianhydro-sorbitol-2,5-dinitrate)

DESCRIPTION

Isosorbide dinitrate, an organic nitrate, is a vasodilator with effects on both arteries and veins. Isordil is available as 2.5 mg, 5 mg, and 10 mg Sublingual tablets; 5 mg, 10 mg, 20 mg, 30 mg, and 40 mg standard oral Titradose® tablets; and 40 mg controlled-release oral Tembids® capsules and tablets. Isordil Sublingual tablets contain 2.5 mg, 5 mg, or 10 mg isosorbide dinitrate. The inactive ingredients present are cellulose, lactose, magnesium stearate, and starch. The 2.5 mg dosage strength also contains D&C Yellow 10 and FD&C Yellow 6, and the 5 mg dosage strength also contains FD&C Red 3.
Isordil Titradose tablets contain 5 mg, 10 mg, 20 mg, 30 mg, or 40 mg isosorbide dinitrate. The inactive ingredients present are lactose, magnesium stearate, and other ingredients. The 5 mg, 20 mg, 30 mg, and 40 mg dosage strengths also contain the following: 5 mg—FD&C Red 3; 20 mg and 40 mg—D&C Yellow 10, FD&C Blue 1, and FD&C Yellow 6; 30 mg—FD&C Blue 1.
Isordil Tembids capsules contain 40 mg isosorbide dinitrate. The inactive ingredients present are confectioners sugar, starch, gelatin capsule, and other ingredients.
Isordil Tembids tablets contain 40 mg isosorbide dinitrate. The inactive ingredients present are D&C Yellow 10, FD&C Blue 1, FD&C Yellow 6, lactose, magnesium stearate, sodium silicoaluminate, talc, and other ingredients.
The chemical name for isosorbide dinitrate is 1,4,3,6-dianhydro-sorbitol-2,5-dinitrate, and compound has the following structural formula:

Molecular Weight 236.14

Isosorbide dinitrate is a white, crystalline, odorless compound which is stable in air and in solution, has a melting point of 70° C with an optical rotation of +134° (c = 1.0, alcohol, 20° C). Isosorbide dinitrate is freely soluble in organic solvents such as acetone, alcohol, and ether, but is only sparingly soluble in water.

CLINICAL PHARMACOLOGY

The principal pharmacological action of Isordil is relaxation of vascular smooth muscle, producing a vasodilatory effect on both peripheral arteries and veins, with predominant effects on the latter. Dilation of the postcapillary vessels, including large veins, promotes peripheral pooling of blood and decreases venous return to the heart, thereby reducing left-ventricular end-diastolic pressure (preload). Arteriolar relaxation reduces systemic vascular resistance and arterial pressure (afterload).
The mechanism by which Isordil relieves angina pectoris is not fully understood. Myocardial oxygen consumption or demand (as measured by the pressure-rate product, tension-time index, and stroke-work index) is decreased by both the arterial and venous effects of Isordil, and, presumably, a more favorable supply-demand ratio is achieved. While the large epicardial coronary arteries are also dilated by Isordil, the extent to which this contributes to relief of exertional angina is unclear.
Therapeutic doses of Isordil may reduce systolic, diastolic, and mean arterial blood pressures, especially in the upright posture. Effective coronary perfusion is usually maintained. The decrease in systemic blood pressure may result in reflex tachycardia, an effect which could unfavorably influence myocardial oxygen demand. Hemodynamic studies indicate that Isordil may reduce the abnormally elevated left ventricular end-diastolic and pulmonary capillary wedge pressures that occur during an acute episode of angina pectoris.
Isordil is metabolized by enzymatic denitration to the intermediate products, isosorbide-2-mononitrate and isosorbide-5-mononitrate. Both metabolites have biological activity, especially the 5-mononitrate which is also the principal metabolite. The liver is a principal site of metabolism, and oral isosorbide dinitrate is subject to a large first pass effect. The systemic clearance of the drug following intravenous infusion is about 3.4 liters/min. Since the clearance exceeds hepatic blood flow, considerable extrahepatic metabolism must also occur.
The average bioavailability of Isordil is 59 and 22 percent following sublingual and oral administration, respectively. The terminal half-life is about 20 minutes, 60 minutes, and 4

hours following IV, sublingual, and oral administration, respectively. The dependence of half-life on the route of administration is not understood. Over limited ranges of IV dosing, the pharmacokinetics of isosorbide dinitrate appear linear. However, both the 2- and 5-mononitrate metabolites have been shown to decrease the rate of disappearance of the dinitrate from the blood. The half-lives of isosorbide-5-mononitrate and isosorbide-2-mononitrate range from 4.0–5.6 and 1.5–3.1 hours, respectively.
The pharmacokinetics and/or bioavailability of isosorbide dinitrate during multiple dosing have not been well studied. Because the metabolites influence the clearance of isosorbide dinitrate, prediction of blood levels of parent compound or metabolites from single-dose studies is uncertain.

INDICATIONS AND USAGE

Isordil is indicated for the treatment and prevention of angina pectoris. Controlled clinical trials have demonstrated that the sublingual, immediate release, and controlled-release oral dosage forms of Isordil are effective in improving exercise tolerance in patients with angina pectoris. When single sublingual doses (5 mg) of isosorbide dinitrate were administered prophylactically to patients with angina pectoris in various clinical studies, duration of exercise until chest pain or fatigue was significantly improved for at least 45 minutes (and as long as 2 hours in some studies) following dosing. Similar studies after single oral (15 to 120 mg) and oral controlled-release (40 to 80 mg) doses of isosorbide dinitrate have shown significant improvement in exercise tolerance for up to 8 hours following dosing. The exercise electrocardiographic evidence suggests that improved exercise tolerance with Isordil is not at the expense of greater myocardial ischemia. All dosage forms of Isordil may therefore be used prophylactically to decrease frequency and severity of anginal attacks and can be expected to decrease the need for sublingual nitroglycerin.
The sublingual form of the drug is indicated for acute prophylaxis of angina pectoris when taken a few minutes before situations likely to provoke anginal attacks. Because of a slower onset of effect, the oral forms of Isordil are not indicated for acute prophylaxis.
In controlled clinical trials, sublingual isosorbide dinitrate was effective in relieving an acute attack of angina pectoris. Relief occurred with a mean time of 3.4 minutes compared to relief of angina with a mean time of 1.9 minutes following sublingual nitroglycerin. Because of the more rapid relief of chest pain with sublingual nitroglycerin, the use of sublingual isosorbide dinitrate for aborting an acute anginal attack should be limited to patients intolerant or unresponsive to sublingual nitroglycerin.

CONTRAINDICATIONS

Isosorbide dinitrate is contraindicated in patients who have shown purported hypersensitivity or idiosyncrasy to it or other nitrates or nitrites.

WARNINGS

The benefits of isosorbide dinitrate during the early days of an acute myocardial infarction have not been established. If one elects to use organic nitrates in early infarction, hemodynamic monitoring and frequent clinical assessment should be used because of the potential deleterious effects of hypotension.

PRECAUTIONS

General. Severe hypotensive response, particularly with upright posture, may occur with even small doses of isosorbide dinitrate. The drug should therefore be used with caution in subjects who may have blood volume depletion from diuretic therapy or in subjects who have low systolic blood pressure (e.g., below 90 mm Hg). Paradoxal bradycardia and increased angina pectoris may accompany nitrate-induced hypotension.
Nitrate therapy may aggravate the angina caused by hypertrophic cardiomyopathy. Tolerance to this drug and cross-tolerance to other nitrates and nitrites may occur.
Marked symptomatic, orthostatic hypotension has been reported when calcium channel blockers and organic nitrates were used in combination. Dose adjustment of either class of agents may be necessary.
Tolerance to the vascular and antianginal effects of isosorbide dinitrate or nitroglycerin has been demonstrated in clinical trials, experience through occupational exposure, and in isolated tissue experiments in the laboratory. The importance of tolerance to the appropriate use of isosorbide dinitrate in the management of patients with angina pectoris has not been determined. However, one clinical trial using treadmill exercise tolerance (as an endpoint) found an 8-hour duration of action of oral isosorbide dinitrate following the first dose (after a 2-week placebo washout) and only a 2-hour duration of effect of the same dose after 1 week of repetitive dosing at conventional dosing intervals. On the other hand, several trials have been able to differentiate isosorbide dinitrate from placebo after 4 weeks of therapy, and in open trials an effect seems detectable for as long as several months.

Tolerance clearly occurs in industrial workers continuously exposed to nitroglycerin. Moreover, physical dependence also occurs, since chest pain, acute myocardial infarction, and even sudden death have occurred during temporary withdrawal of nitroglycerin from the workers. In clinical trials in angina patients, there are reports of anginal attacks being more easily provoked and of rebound in the hemodynamic effects soon after nitrate withdrawal. The relative importance of these observations to the routine, clinical use of isosorbide dinitrate is not known. However, it seems prudent to gradually withdraw patients from isosorbide dinitrate when the therapy is being terminated, rather than stopping the drug abruptly.
Information for Patients. Headache may occur during initial therapy with isosorbide dinitrate. Headache is usually relieved by the use of standard headache remedies, or by lowering the dose, and tends to disappear after the first week or two of use.
Drug Interactions. Alcohol may enhance any marked sensitivity to the hypotensive effect of nitrates.
Isosorbide dinitrate acts directly on vascular smooth muscle; therefore, any other agent that depends on vascular smooth muscle as the final common path can be expected to have decreased or increased effect, depending on the agent.
Carcinogenesis, Mutagenesis, Impairment of Fertility. No long-term studies in animals have been performed to evaluate the carcinogenic potential of this drug. A modified two-litter reproduction study in rats fed isosorbide dinitrate at 25 or 100 mg/kg/day did not reveal any effects on fertility or gestation or any remarkable growth pathology in any parent or offspring fed isosorbide dinitrate as compared with rats fed a basal-controlled diet.
Pregnancy Category C. Isosorbide dinitrate has been shown to cause a dose-related increase in embryotoxicity (increase in mummified pups) in rabbits at oral doses 35 and 150 times the maximum recommended human daily dose. There are no adequate and well-controlled studies in pregnant women. Isosorbide dinitrate should be used during pregnancy only if the potential benefit justifies the potential risk to the fetus.
Nursing Mothers. It is not known whether this drug is excreted in human milk. Because many drugs are excreted in human milk, caution should be exercised when isosorbide dinitrate is administered to a nursing mother.
Pediatric Use. The safety and effectiveness of isosorbide dinitrate in children has not been established.

ADVERSE REACTIONS

Adverse reactions, particularly headache and hypotension, are dose related. In clinical trials at various doses, the following have been observed.
Headache is the most common adverse reaction and may be severe and persistent; reported incidence varies widely, apparently being dose-related, with an average occurrence of about 25%.
Cutaneous vasodilation with flushing may occur. Transient episodes of dizziness and weakness, as well as other signs of cerebral ischemia associated with postural hypotension, may occasionally develop (the incidence of reported symptomatic hypotension ranges from 2% to 36%). An occasional individual will exhibit marked sensitivity to the hypotensive effects of nitrates, and severe responses (nausea, vomiting, weakness, restlessness, pallor, perspiration, and collapse) may occur even with the usual therapeutic dose. Drug rash and-/or exfoliative dermatitis may occasionally occur. Nausea and vomiting appear to be uncommon.

OVERDOSAGE

Signs and Symptoms. These may include the following: a prompt fall in blood pressure, persistent and throbbing headache, vertigo, palpitation, visual disturbances, flushed and perspiring skin (later becoming cold and cyanotic), nausea and vomiting (possibly with colic and even bloody diarrhea), syncope (especially in the upright position), methemoglobinemia with cyanosis and anoxia, initial hyperpnea, dyspnea and slow breathing, slow pulse (dicrotic and intermittent), heart block, increased intracranial pressure with cerebral symptoms of confusion and moderate fever, paralysis and coma followed by clonic convulsions and possibly death due to circulatory collapse.
It is not known what dose of the drug is associated with symptoms of overdosing or what dose of the drug would be life-threatening. The acute oral LD50 of isosorbide dinitrate in rats was found to be approximately 1100 mg/kg of body weight. These animal experiments indicate that approximately 500 times the usual therapeutic dose would be required to produce such toxic symptoms in humans. It is not known whether the drug is dialyzable.
Treatment of Overdosage. Prompt removal of the ingested material by gastric lavage is reasonable but not documented to be useful. Keep the patient recumbent in a shock position and comfortably warm. Passive movements of the extremities may aid venous return. Administer oxygen and artificial respiration if necessary. If methemoglobinemia is present, administer methylene blue (1% solution), 1 to 2 mg/kg intravenously.

Methemoglobin. Case reports of clinically significant methemoglobinemia are rare at conventional doses of organic nitrates. The formation of methemoglobin is dose related, and in the case of genetic abnormalities of hemoglobin that favor methemoglobin formation, even conventional doses of organic nitrate could produce harmful concentrations of methemoglobin.

WARNING: Epinephrine is ineffective in reversing the severe hypotensive events associated with overdose. It and related compounds are contraindicated in this situation.

DOSAGE AND ADMINISTRATION

For the treatment of angina pectoris, the usual starting dose of sublingual Isordil is 2.5 to 5 mg.

Isordil should be titrated upward until angina is relieved or side effects limit the dose. In ambulatory patients, the magnitude of the incremental dose increase should be guided by measurements of standing blood pressure.

The initial dosage of sublingual Isordil for acute prophylactic therapy in angina pectoris patients is generally 5 or 10 mg every 2 to 3 hours. Adequate, controlled clinical studies demonstrating the effectiveness of chronic maintenance therapy with these dosage forms have not been reported.

For the treatment of chronic stable angina pectoris, the usual starting dose for immediate-release (swallowed) tablets is 5 to 20 mg; and for controlled release forms, 40 mg. For maintenance therapy, oral doses of 10 to 40 mg given every 6 hours or oral controlled-release doses of 40 to 80 mg given every 8 to 12 hours are generally recommended. The extent to which development of tolerance should modify the dosage program has not been defined. The oral controlled-release forms of Isordil should not be chewed.

HOW SUPPLIED

Isordil® (isosorbide dinitrate) Tablets, Wyeth®, are available as follows:
Sublingual, 2.5 mg, yellow tablets:
NDC 0008-4139-01, bottles of 100.
NDC 0008-4139-03, bottles of 500.
Sublingual, 5 mg, pink tablets:
NDC 0008-4126-01, bottles of 100.
NDC 0008-4126-03, bottles of 500.
Sublingual, 10 mg, white tablets:
NDC 0008-4161-01, bottles of 100.
Oral Titradose®, 5 mg, scored pink tablets:
NDC 0008-4152-01, bottles of 100.
NDC 0008-4152-02, bottles of 500.
NDC 0008-4152-03, bottles of 1000.
Oral Titradose, 10 mg, scored white tablets:
NDC 0008-4153-01, bottles of 100.
NDC 0008-4153-02, bottles of 500.
NDC 0008-4153-03, bottles of 1000.
Oral Titradose, 20 mg, scored green tablets:
NDC 0008-4154-01, bottles of 100.
NDC 0008-4154-02, bottles of 500.
Oral Titradose, 30 mg, scored blue tablets:
NDC 0008-4159-01, bottles of 100.
NDC 0008-4159-02, bottles of 500.
Oral Titradose, 40 mg, scored light-green tablets:
NDC 0008-4192-01, bottles of 100.
Tembids®, 40 mg, scored green controlled-release tablets:
NDC 0008-4125-01, bottles of 100.
NDC 0008-4125-02, bottles of 500.
NDC 0008-4125-03, bottles of 1000.

ALSO AVAILABLE

Redipak® Strip Pack cartons of 100 tablets (10 blister strips of 10) as follows:
Sublingual, 2.5 mg, NDC 0008-4139-05.
Sublingual, 5 mg, NDC 0008-4126-07.
Oral Titradose, 5 mg, NDC 0008-4152-05.
Oral Titradose, 10 mg, NDC 0008-4153-05.
Oral Titradose, 20 mg, NDC 0008-4154-05.
Oral Titradose, 30 mg, NDC 0008-4159-04.
Oral Titradose, 40 mg, NDC 0008-4192-04.
Isordil® (isosorbide dinitrate) Tembids® Capsules, Wyeth®, are available in 40 mg, controlled-release capsules (opaque, blue cap and colorless, transparent body):
NDC 0008-4140-01, bottles of 100.
NDC 0008-4140-02, bottles of 500.
US Pat. Nos. 3883647 and D224591 (Titradose®)
The appearances of Titradose® tablets and TEMBIDS® tablets and capsules are trademarks of Wyeth-Ayerst Laboratories.
Keep tightly closed.
Store at room temperature, approximately 25°C (77°F).
Shown in Product Identification Section, pages 436 & 437

LO/OVRAL® ℞
[lŏh-ōh´vral]
Tablets
(norgestrel and ethinyl estradiol tablets)

DESCRIPTION

Each LO/OVRAL® tablet contains 0.3 mg of norgestrel (dl-13-beta-ethyl-17-alpha-ethinyl-17-beta-hydroxygon-4-en-3-one), a totally synthetic progestogen, and 0.03 mg of ethinyl estradiol (19-nor-17α-pregna-1,3,5 (10)-trien-20-yne-3,17-diol). The inactive ingredients present are cellulose, lactose, magnesium stearate, and polacrilin potassium.

CLINICAL PHARMACOLOGY

Combination oral contraceptives act primarily through the mechanism of gonadotropin suppression due to the estrogenic and progestational activity of the ingredients. Although the primary mechanism of action is inhibition of ovulation, alterations in the genital tract, including changes in the cervical mucus (which increase the difficulty of sperm penetration) and the endometrium (which reduce the likelihood of implantation), may also contribute to contraceptive effectiveness.

INDICATIONS AND USAGE

LO/OVRAL is indicated for the prevention of pregnancy in women who elect to use oral contraceptives as a method of contraception. Oral contraceptives are highly effective. The pregnancy rate in women using conventional combination oral contraceptives (containing 35 mcg or more of ethinyl estradiol or 50 mcg or more of mestranol) is generally reported as less than one pregnancy per 100 woman-years of use. Slightly higher rates (somewhat more than 1 pregnancy per 100 woman-years of use) are reported for some combination products containing 35 mcg or less of ethinyl estradiol, and rates on the order of 3 pregnancies per 100 woman-years are reported for the progestogen-only oral contraceptives. These rates are derived from separate studies conducted by different investigators in several population groups and cannot be compared precisely. Furthermore, pregnancy rates tend to be lower as clinical studies are continued, possibly due to selective retention in the longer studies of those patients who accept the treatment regimen and do not discontinue as a result of adverse reactions, pregnancy, or other reasons.

In clinical trials with LO/OVRAL, 1,700 patients completed 22,489 cycles, and a total of two pregnancies were reported. This represents a pregnancy rate of 0.12 per 100 woman-years.

Table 1 gives ranges of pregnancy rates reported in the literature[1] for other means of contraception. The efficacy of these means of contraception (except the IUD) depends upon the degree of adherence to the method.

TABLE 1
PREGNANCIES PER 100 WOMAN-YEARS
IUD, less than 1–6; Diaphragm with spermicidal products (creams or jellies), 2–20; Condom, 3–36; Aerosol foams, 2–29; Jellies and creams, 4–36;
Periodic abstinence (rhythm) all types, less than 1–47:
1. Calendar method, 14–47;
2. Temperature method, 1–20;
3. Temperature method—intercourse only in postovulatory phase, less than 1–7;
4. Mucus method, 1–25;
No contraception, 60–80.

Dose-Related Risk of Thromboembolism from Oral Contraceptives: Two studies have shown a positive association between the dose of estrogens in oral contraceptives and the risk of thromboembolism.[2,3] For this reason, it is prudent and in keeping with good principles of therapeutics to minimize exposure to estrogen. The oral-contraceptive product prescribed for any given patient should be that product which contains the least amount of estrogen that is compatible with an acceptable pregnancy rate and patient acceptance. It is recommended that new acceptors of oral contraceptives be started on preparations containing 0.05 mg or less of estrogen.

CONTRAINDICATIONS

Oral contraceptives should not be used in women with any of the following conditions:
1. Thrombophlebitis or thromboembolic disorders.
2. A past history of deep-vein thrombophlebitis or thromboembolic disorders.
3. Cerebral-vascular or coronary-artery disease.
4. Known or suspected carcinoma of the breast.
5. Known or suspected estrogen-dependent neoplasia.
6. Undiagnosed abnormal genital bleeding.
7. Known or suspected pregnancy (see Warning No. 5).
8. Benign or malignant liver tumor which developed during the use of oral contraceptives or other estrogen-containing products.

WARNINGS

> **Cigarette smoking increases the risk of serious cardiovascular side effects from oral-contraceptive use. This risk increases with age and with heavy smoking (15 or more cigarettes per day) and is quite marked in women over 35 years of age. Women who use oral contraceptives should be strongly advised not to smoke.**

The use of oral contraceptives is associated with increased risk of several serious conditions, including thromboembolism, stroke, myocardial infarction, hepatic adenoma, gallbladder disease, hypertension. Prac-titioners prescribing oral contraceptives should be familiar with the following information relating to these risks.

1. *Thromboembolic Disorders and Other Vascular Problems:* An increased risk of thromboembolic and thrombotic disease associated with the use of oral contraceptives is well-established. Three principal studies in Great Britain[4-6] and three in the United States[7-10] have demonstrated an increased risk of fatal and nonfatal venous thromboembolism and stroke, both hemorrhagic and thrombotic. These studies estimate that users of oral contraceptives are 4 to 11 times more likely than nonusers to develop these diseases without evident cause (Table 2).

CEREBROVASCULAR DISORDERS
In a collaborative American study[9,10] of cerebrovascular disorders in women with and without predisposing causes, it was estimated that the risk of hemorrhagic stroke was 2.0 times greater in users than nonusers and the risk of thrombotic stroke was 4 to 9.5 times greater in users than in nonusers (Table 2).

TABLE 2
SUMMARY OF RELATIVE RISK OF THROMBOEMBOLIC DISORDERS AND OTHER VASCULAR PROBLEMS IN ORAL-CONTRACEPTIVE USERS COMPARED TO NONUSERS

	Relative risk, times greater
Idiopathic thromboembolic disease	4–11
Postsurgery thromboembolic complications	4–6
Thrombotic stroke	4–9.5
Hemorrhagic stroke	2
Myocardial infarction	2–12

MYOCARDIAL INFARCTION
An increased risk of myocardial infarction associated with the use of oral contraceptives has been reported,[11-13] confirming a previously suspected association. These studies, conducted in the United Kingdom, found, as expected, that the greater the number of underlying risk factors for coronary-artery disease (cigarette smoking, hypertension, hypercholesterolemia, obesity, diabetes, history of preeclamptic toxemia) the higher the risk of developing myocardial infarction, regardless of whether the patient was an oral-contraceptive user or not. Oral contraceptives, however, were found to be a clear additional risk factor.

In terms of relative risk, it has been estimated[52] that oral-contraceptive users who do not smoke (smoking is considered a major predisposing condition to myocardial infarction) are about twice as likely to have a fatal myocardial infarction as nonusers who do not smoke. Oral-contraceptive users who are also smokers have about a 5-fold increased risk of fatal infarction compared to users who do not smoke, but about a 10- to 12-fold increased risk compared to nonusers who do not smoke. Furthermore, the amount of smoking is also an important factor. In determining the importance of these relative risks, however, the baseline rates for various age groups, as shown in Table 3, must be given serious consideration. The importance of other predisposing conditions mentioned above in determining absolute and relative risks has not as yet been quantified; it is quite likely that the same synergistic action exists, but perhaps to a lesser extent.

TABLE 3
Estimated annual mortality rate per 100,000 women from myocardial infarction by use of oral contraceptives, smoking habits, and age (in years):

	Myocardial infarction			
	Women aged 30–39		Women aged 40–44	
Smoking habits	Users	Non-users	Users	Non-users
All smokers	10.2	2.6	62.0	15.9
Heavy*	13.0	5.1	78.7	31.3
Light	4.7	0.9	28.6	5.7
Nonsmokers	1.8	1.2	10.7	7.4
Smokers and nonsmokers	5.4	1.9	32.8	11.7

*Heavy smoker: 15 or more cigarettes per day.
From JAIN, A.K., *Studies in Family Planning,* 8:50, 1977

RISK OF DOSE
In an analysis of data derived from several national adverse-reaction reporting systems,[2] British investigators concluded that the risk of thromboembolism, including coronary thrombosis, is directly related to the dose of estrogen used in oral contraceptives. Preparations containing 100 mcg or more of estrogen were associated with a higher risk of thromboembolism than those containing 50–80 mcg of estrogen. Their analysis did suggest, however, that the quantity of estrogen may not be the sole factor involved. This finding has

Continued on next page

Wyeth-Ayerst—Cont.

been confirmed in the United States.[3] Careful epidemiological studies to determine the degree of thromboembolic risk associated with progestogen-only oral contraceptives have not been performed. Cases of thromboembolic disease have been reported in women using these products, and they should not be presumed to be free of excess risk.

ESTIMATE OF EXCESS MORTALITY FROM CIRCULATORY DISEASES

A large prospective study[53] carried out in the U.K. estimated the mortality rate per 100,000 women per year from diseases of the circulatory system for users and nonusers of oral contraceptives according to age, smoking habits, and duration of use. The overall excess death rate annually from circulatory diseases for oral-contraceptive users was estimated to be 20 per 100,000 (ages 15–34—5/100,000; ages 35–44—33/100,000; ages 45–49—140/100,000), the risk being concentrated in older women, in those with a long duration of use, and in cigarette smokers. It was not possible, however, to examine the interrelationships of age, smoking, and duration of use, nor to compare the effects of continuous vs. intermittent use. Although the study showed a 10-fold increase in death due to circulatory diseases in users for 5 or more years, all of these deaths occurred in women 35 or older. Until larger numbers of women under 35 with continuous use for 5 or more years are available, it is not possible to assess the magnitude of the relative risk for this younger age group. The available data from a variety of sources have been analyzed[14] to estimate the risk of death associated with various methods of contraception. The estimates of risk of death for each method include the combined risk of the contraceptive method (e.g., thromboembolic and thrombotic disease in the case of oral contraceptives) plus the risk attributable to pregnancy or abortion in the event of method failure. This latter risk varies with the effectiveness of the contraceptive method. The findings of this analysis are shown in the bar graph (Figure 1).[14] The study concluded that the mortality associated with all methods of birth control is low and below that associated with childbirth, with the exception of oral contraceptives in women over 40 who smoke. (The rates given for Pill only/smokers for each age group are for smokers as a class. For "heavy" smokers [more than 15 cigarettes a day], the rates given would be about double; for "light" smokers [less than 15 cigarettes a day], about 50 percent.) The lowest mortality is associated with the condom or diaphragm backed up by early abortion. The risk of thromboembolic and thrombotic disease associated with oral contraceptives increases with age after approximately age 30 and, for myocardial infarction, is further increased by hypertension, hypercholesterolemia, obesity, diabetes, or history of preeclamptic toxemia and especially by cigarette smoking.

Based on the data currently available, the following chart gives a gross estimate of the risk of death from circulatory disorders associated with the use of oral contraceptives:

SMOKING HABITS AND OTHER PREDISPOSING CONDITIONS— RISK ASSOCIATED WITH USE OF ORAL CONTRACEPTIVES

Age	Below 30	30–39	40+
Heavy smokers	C	B	A
Light smokers	D	C	B
Nonsmokers (no predisposing conditions)	D	C,D	C
Nonsmokers (other predisposing conditions)	C	C,B	B,A

A—Use associated with very high risk.
B—Use associated with high risk.
C—Use associated with moderate risk.
D—Use associated with low risk.

The physician and the patient should be alert to the earliest manifestations of thromboembolic and thrombotic disorders (e.g., thrombophlebitis, pulmonary embolism, cerebrovascular insufficiency, coronary occlusion, retinal thrombosis, and mesenteric thrombosis). Should any of these occur or be suspected, the drug should be discontinued immediately.

A four- to six-fold increased risk of postsurgery thromboembolic complications has been reported in oral-contraceptive users.[15,16] If feasible, oral contraceptives should be discontinued at least 4 weeks before surgery of a type associated with an increased risk of thromboembolism or prolonged immobilization.

[See figure next column]

PERSISTENCE OF RISK OF VASCULAR DISORDERS

Findings from one study in Great Britain involving cerebrovascular disease[54] and another study in the United States concerning myocardial infarction[55] suggest that an increased risk of these conditions in users of oral contracep-

Figure 1. Estimated annual number of deaths associated with control of fertility and no control per 100,000 nonsterile women, by regimen of control and age of woman.

Legend:
☐ No method
☒ Abortion only
▨ Pill only/ nonsmokers
☐ Pill only/ smokers
▨ IUDs only
▨ Traditional contraception only (diaphragm or condom)
■ Traditional contraception and abortion

tives persists after discontinuation of the oral contraceptive. In the British study, the risk of cerebrovascular disease remained elevated in former oral-contraceptive users for at least six years after discontinuation. In the U.S. study, an increased risk of myocardial infarction persisted for at least 9 years in women 40- to 49-years-old who had used oral contraceptives for five or more years. The findings in both these studies require confirmation since they are inconsistent with other published information.[9,11,13,56–60]

2. Ocular Lesions:

There have been reports of neuro-ocular lesions such as optic neuritis or retinal thrombosis associated with the use of oral contraceptives. Discontinue oral-contraceptive medication if there is unexplained, sudden or gradual, partial or complete loss of vision; onset of proptosis or diplopia; papilledema; or retinal-vascular lesions, and institute appropriate diagnostic and therapeutic measures.

3. Carcinoma:

Long-term continuous administration of either natural or synthetic estrogen in certain animal species increases the frequency of carcinoma of the breast, cervix, vagina, and liver. Certain synthetic progestogens, none currently contained in oral contraceptives, have been noted to increase the incidence of mammary nodules, benign and malignant, in dogs.

In humans, three case-control studies have reported an increased risk of endometrial carcinoma associated with the prolonged use of exogenous estrogen in postmenopausal women.[17–19] One publication[20] reported on the first 21 cases submitted by physicians to a registry of cases of adenocarcinoma of the endometrium in women under 40 on oral contraceptives. Of the cases found in women without predisposing risk factors for adenocarcinoma of the endometrium (e.g., irregular bleeding at the time oral contraceptives were first given, polycystic ovaries), nearly all occurred in women who had used a sequential oral contraceptive. These products are no longer marketed. No evidence has been reported suggesting an increased risk of endometrial cancer in users of conventional combination or progestogen-only oral contraceptives.

Several studies[8,21–24] have found no increase in breast cancer in women taking oral contraceptives or estrogens. One study,[25] however, while also noting no overall increased risk of breast cancer in women treated with oral contraceptives, found an excess risk in the subgroups of oral-contraceptive users with documented benign breast disease. A reduced occurrence of benign breast tumors in users of oral contraceptives has been well-documented.[8,21,25–27]

In summary, there is at present no confirmed evidence from human studies of an increased risk of cancer associated with oral contraceptives. Close clinical surveillance of all women taking oral contraceptives is, nevertheless, essential. In all cases of undiagnosed persistent or recurrent abnormal vaginal bleeding, appropriate diagnostic measures should be taken to rule out malignancy. Women with a strong family history of breast cancer or who have breast nodules, fibrocystic disease, or abnormal mammograms should be monitored with particular care if they elect to use oral contraceptives instead of other methods of contraception.

4. Hepatic Tumors:

Benign hepatic adenomas have been found to be associated with the use of oral contraceptives.[28–30,46] One study[46] showed that oral contraceptive formulations with high hormonal potency were associated with a higher risk than lower potency formulations. Although benign, hepatic adenomas may rupture and may cause death through intra-abdominal hemorrhage. This has been reported in short-term as well as long-term users of oral contraceptives. Two studies relate risk with duration of use of the contraceptive, the risk being much greater after 4 or more years of oral-contraceptive use.[30,46] While hepatic adenoma is a rare lesion, it should be considered in women presenting abdominal pain and tenderness, abdominal mass or shock. A few cases of hepatocellular carcinoma have been reported in women taking oral contraceptives. The relationship of these drugs to this type of malignancy is not known at this time.

5. Use in or Immediately Preceding Pregnancy, Birth Defects in Offspring, and Malignancy in Female Offspring:

The use of female sex hormones—both estrogenic and progestational agents—during early pregnancy may seriously damage the offspring. It has been shown that females exposed in utero to diethylstilbestrol, a nonsteroidal estrogen, have an increased risk of developing in later life a form of vaginal or cervical cancer that is ordinarily extremely rare.[31,32] This risk has been estimated to be of the order of 1 in 1,000 exposures or less.[33,47] Although there is no evidence at the present time that oral contraceptives further enhance the risk of developing this type of malignancy, such patients should be monitored with particular care if they elect to use oral contraceptives instead of other methods of contraception. Furthermore, a high percentage of such exposed women (from 30 to 90%) have been found to have epithelial changes of the vagina and cervix.[34–38] Although these changes are histologically benign, it is not known whether this condition is a precursor of vaginal malignancy. Male children so exposed may develop abnormalities of the urogenital tract.[48–50] Although similar data are not available with the use of other estrogens, it cannot be presumed that they would not induce similar changes.

An increased risk of congenital anomalies, including heart defects and limb defects, has been reported with the use of sex hormones, including oral contraceptives, in pregnancy.[39–42,51] One case-control study[42] has estimated a 4.7-fold increase in risk of limb-reduction defects in infants exposed in utero to sex hormones (oral contraceptives, hormonal withdrawal tests for pregnancy, or attempted treatment for threatened abortion). Some of these exposures were very short and involved only a few days of treatment. The data suggest that the risk of limb-reduction defects in exposed fetuses is somewhat less than one in 1,000 live births. In the past, female sex hormones have been used during pregnancy in an attempt to treat threatened or habitual abortion. There is considerable evidence that estrogens are ineffective for these indications, and there is no evidence from well-controlled studies that progestogens are effective for these uses.

There is some evidence that triploidy and possibly other types of polyploidy are increased among abortuses from women who become pregnant soon after ceasing oral contraceptives.[43] Embryos with these anomalies are virtually always aborted spontaneously. Whether there is an overall increase in spontaneous abortion of pregnancies conceived soon after stopping oral contraceptives is unknown. It is recommended that, for any patient who has missed two consecutive periods, pregnancy should be ruled out before continuing the contraceptive regimen. If the patient has not adhered to the prescribed schedule, the possibility of pregnancy should be considered at the time of the first missed period (or after 45 days from the last menstrual period if the progestogen-only oral contraceptives are used), and further use of oral contraceptives should be withheld until pregnancy has been ruled out. If pregnancy is confirmed, the patient should be apprised of the potential risks to the fetus, and the advisability of continuation of the pregnancy should be discussed in the light of these risks.

It is also recommended that women who discontinue oral contraceptives with the intent of becoming pregnant use an alternate form of contraception for a period of time before attempting to conceive. Many clinicians recommend 3 months, although no precise information is available on which to base this recommendation.

The administration of progestogen-only or progestogen-estrogen combinations to induce withdrawal bleeding should not be used as a test of pregnancy.

6. Gallbladder Disease:

Studies[8,23,26] report an increased risk of surgically confirmed gallbladder disease in users of oral contraceptives and estrogens. In one study, an increased risk appeared after 2 years of use and doubled after 4 or 5 years of use. In one of the other studies, an increased risk was apparent between 6 and 12 months of use.

7. Carbohydrate and Lipid Metabolic Effects:

A decrease in glucose tolerance has been observed in a significant percentage of patients on oral contraceptives. For this reason, prediabetic and diabetic patients should be carefully observed while receiving oral contraceptives.

An increase in triglycerides and total phospholipids has been observed in patients receiving oral contraceptives.[44] The clinical significance of this finding remains to be defined.

8. Elevated Blood Pressure:

An increase in blood pressure has been reported in patients receiving oral contraceptives.[26] In some women, hypertension may occur within a few months of beginning oral-contraceptive use. In the first year of use, the prevalence of women with hypertension is low in users and may be no higher than that of a comparable group of nonusers. The prevalence in users increases, however, with longer exposure, and in the fifth year of use is two-and-a-half to three times the reported prevalence in the first year. Age is also strongly correlated with the development of hypertension in oral-contraceptive users. Women who previously have had hypertension during pregnancy may be more likely to develop elevation of blood pressure when given oral contraceptives. Hypertension that develops as a result of taking oral contraceptives usually returns to normal after discontinuing the drug.

9. Headache:

The onset or exacerbation of migraine or development of headache of a new pattern which is recurrent, persistent, or severe, requires discontinuation of oral contraceptives and evaluation of the cause.

10. Bleeding Irregularities:

Breakthrough bleeding, spotting, and amenorrhea are frequent reasons for patients discontinuing oral contraceptives. In breakthrough bleeding, as in all cases of irregular bleeding from the vagina, nonfunctional causes should be borne in mind. In undiagnosed persistent or recurrent abnormal bleeding from the vagina, adequate diagnostic measures are indicated to rule out pregnancy or malignancy. If pathology has been excluded, time or a change to another formulation may solve the problem. Changing to an oral contraceptive with a higher estrogen content, while potentially useful in minimizing menstrual irregularity, should be done only if necessary, since this may increase the risk of thromboembolic disease.

Women with a past history of oligomenorrhea or secondary amenorrhea or young women without regular cycles may have a tendency to remain anovulatory or to become amenorrheic after discontinuation of oral contraceptives. Women with these preexisting problems should be advised of this possibility and encouraged to use other contraceptive methods. Post-use anovulation, possibly prolonged, may also occur in women without previous irregularities.

11. Ectopic Pregnancy:

Ectopic as well as intrauterine pregnancy may occur in contraceptive failures. However, in progestogen-only oral contraceptive failures, the ratio of ectopic to intrauterine pregnancies is higher than in women who are not receiving oral contraceptives, since the drugs are more effective in preventing intrauterine than ectopic pregnancies.

12. Breast-feeding:

Oral contraceptives given in the postpartum period may interfere with lactation. There may be a decrease in the quantity and quality of the breast milk. Furthermore, a small fraction of the hormonal agents in oral contraceptives has been identified in the milk of mothers receiving these drugs.[45] The effects, if any, on the breast-fed child have not been determined. If feasible, the use of oral contraceptives should be deferred until the infant has been weaned.

PRECAUTIONS

GENERAL

1. A complete medical and family history should be taken prior to initiation of oral contraceptives. The pretreatment and periodic physical examinations should include special reference to blood pressure, breasts, abdomen and pelvic organs, including Papanicolaou smear and relevant laboratory tests. As a general rule, oral contraceptives should not be prescribed for longer than 1 year without another physical examination being performed.

2. Under the influence of estrogen-progestogen preparations, preexisting uterine leiomyomata may increase in size.

3. Patients with a history of psychic depression should be carefully observed and the drug discontinued if depression recurs to a serious degree. Patients becoming significantly depressed while taking oral contraceptives should stop the medication and use an alternate method of contraception in an attempt to determine whether the symptom is drug-related.

4. Oral contraceptives may cause some degree of fluid retention. They should be prescribed with caution, and only with careful monitoring, in patients with conditions which might be aggravated by fluid retention, such as convulsive disorders, migraine syndrome, asthma, or cardiac or renal insufficiency.

5. Patients with a past history of jaundice during pregnancy have an increased risk of recurrence of jaundice while receiving oral-contraceptive therapy. If jaundice develops in any patient receiving such drugs, the medication should be discontinued.

6. Steroid hormones may be poorly metabolized in patients with impaired liver function and should be administered with caution in such patients.

7. Oral-contraceptive users may have disturbances in normal tryptophan metabolism which may result in a relative pyridoxine deficiency. The clinical significance of this is yet to be determined.

8. Serum folate levels may be depressed by oral-contraceptive therapy. Since the pregnant woman is predisposed to the development of folate deficiency and the incidence of folate deficiency increases with increasing gestation, it is possible that if a woman becomes pregnant shortly after stopping oral contraceptives, she may have a greater chance of developing folate deficiency and complications attributed to this deficiency.

9. The pathologist should be advised of oral-contraceptive therapy when relevant specimens are submitted.

10. Certain endocrine- and liver-function tests and blood components may be affected by estrogen-containing oral contraceptives:

a. Increased sulfobromophthalein retention.

b. Increased prothrombin and factors VII, VIII, IX, and X; decreased antithrombin 3; increased norepinephrine-induced platelet aggregability.

c. Increased thyroid-binding globulin (TBG) leading to increased circulating total-thyroid hormone, as measured by protein-bound iodine (PBI), T4 by column, or T4 by radioimmunoassay. Free T3 resin uptake is decreased, reflecting the elevated TBG; free T4 concentration is unaltered.

d. Decreased pregnanediol excretion.

e. Reduced response to metyrapone test.

INFORMATION FOR THE PATIENT

(See Patient Labeling Printed Below.)

DRUG INTERACTIONS

Reduced efficacy and increased incidence of breakthrough bleeding have been associated with concomitant use of rifampin. A similar association has been suggested with barbiturates, phenylbutazone, phenytoin sodium, ampicillin, and tetracycline.

CARCINOGENESIS

See Warnings section for information on the carcinogenic potential of oral contraceptives.

PREGNANCY

Pregnancy Category X. See Contraindications and Warnings.

NURSING MOTHERS

See Warnings.

ADVERSE REACTIONS

An increased risk of the following serious adverse reactions has been associated with the use of oral contraceptives (see Warnings):

> Thrombophlebitis.
> Pulmonary embolism.
> Coronary thrombosis.
> Cerebral thrombosis.
> Cerebral hemorrhage.
> Hypertension.
> Gallbladder disease.
> Benign hepatomas.
> Congenital anomalies.

There is evidence of an association between the following conditions and the use of oral contraceptives, although additional confirmatory studies are needed:

> Mesenteric thrombosis.
> Neuro-ocular lesions, e.g., retinal thrombosis and optic neuritis.

The following adverse reactions have been reported in patients receiving oral contraceptives and are believed to be drug-related:

> Nausea and/or vomiting, usually the most common adverse reactions, occur in approximately 10% or less of patients during the first cycle. Other reactions, as a general rule, are seen much less frequently or only occasionally.
> Gastrointestinal symptoms (such as abdominal cramps and bloating).
> Breakthrough bleeding.
> Spotting.
> Change in menstrual flow.
> Dysmenorrhea.
> Amenorrhea during and after treatment.

Temporary infertility after discontinuance of treatment.
Edema.
Chloasma or melasma which may persist.
Breast changes: tenderness, enlargement, and secretion.
Change in weight (increase or decrease).
Change in cervical erosion and cervical secretion.
Possible diminution in lactation when given immediately postpartum.
Cholestatic jaundice.
Migraine.
Increase in size of uterine leiomyomata.
Rash (allergic).
Mental depression.
Reduced tolerance to carbohydrates.
Vaginal candidiasis.
Change in corneal curvature (steepening).
Intolerance to contact lenses.

The following adverse reactions have been reported in users of oral contraceptives, and the association has been neither confirmed nor refuted:

> Premenstrual-like syndrome.
> Cataracts.
> Changes in libido.
> Chorea.
> Changes in appetite.
> Cystitis-like syndrome.
> Headache.
> Nervousness.
> Dizziness.
> Hirsutism.
> Loss of scalp hair.
> Erythema multiforme.
> Erythema nodosum.
> Hemorrhagic eruption.
> Vaginitis.
> Porphyria.
> Hemolytic uremic syndrome.

ACUTE OVERDOSE

Serious ill effects have not been reported following acute ingestion of large doses of oral contraceptives by young children. Overdosage may cause nausea, and withdrawal bleeding may occur in females.

DOSAGE AND ADMINISTRATION

To achieve maximum contraceptive effectiveness, LO/OVRAL must be taken exactly as directed and at intervals not exceeding 24 hours. The dosage of LO/OVRAL is one tablet daily for 21 consecutive days per menstrual cycle according to prescribed schedule. Tablets are then discontinued for 7 days (three weeks on, one week off).

It is recommended that LO/OVRAL tablets be taken at the same time each day, preferably after the evening meal or at bedtime.

During the first cycle of medication, the patient is instructed to take one LO/OVRAL tablet daily for twenty-one consecutive days beginning on day five of her menstrual cycle. (The first day of menstruation is day one.) The tablets are then discontinued for one week (7 days). Withdrawal bleeding should usually occur within three days following discontinuation of LO/OVRAL.

(If LO/OVRAL is first taken later than the fifth day of the first menstrual cycle of medication or postpartum, contraceptive reliance should not be placed on LO/OVRAL until after the first seven consecutive days of administration. The possibility of ovulation and conception prior to initiation of medication should be considered.) The patient begins her next and all subsequent 21-day courses of LO/OVRAL tablets on the same day of the week that she began her first course, following the same schedule: 21 days on—7 days off. She begins taking her tablets on the 8th day after discontinuance regardless of whether or not a menstrual period has occurred or is still in progress. Any time a new cycle of LO/OVRAL is started later than the 8th day the patient should be protected by another means of contraception until she has taken a tablet daily for seven consecutive days.

If spotting or breakthrough bleeding occurs, the patient is instructed to continue on the same regimen. This type of bleeding is usually transient and without significance; however, if the bleeding is persistent or prolonged, the patient is advised to consult her physician. Although the occurrence of pregnancy is highly unlikely if LO/OVRAL is taken according to directions, if withdrawal bleeding does not occur, the possibility of pregnancy must be considered. If the patient has not adhered to the prescribed schedule (missed one or more tablets or started taking them on a day later than she should have) the probability of pregnancy should be considered at the time of the first missed period and appropriate diagnostic measures taken before the medication is resumed. If the patient has adhered to the prescribed regimen and misses two consecutive periods, pregnancy should be ruled out before continuing the contraceptive regimen.

The patient should be instructed to take a missed tablet as soon as it is remembered. If two consecutive tablets are

Continued on next page

Wyeth-Ayerst—Cont.

missed they should both be taken as soon as remembered. The next tablet should be taken at the usual time.

Any time the patient misses one or two tablets she should also use another method of contraception until she has taken a tablet daily for seven consecutive days. If breakthrough bleeding occurs following missed tablets it will usually be transient and of no consequence. While there is little likelihood of ovulation occurring if only one or two tablets are missed, the possibility of ovulation increases with each successive day that scheduled tablets are missed. If three consecutive tablets are missed, all medication should be discontinued and the remainder of the package discarded. A new tablet cycle should be started on the 8th day after the last tablet was taken, and an alternate means of contraception should be prescribed during the seven days without tablets and until the patient has taken a tablet daily for seven consecutive days. In the nonlactating mother, LO/OVRAL may be prescribed in the postpartum period either immediately or at the first postpartum examination whether or not menstruation has resumed.

HOW SUPPLIED

LO/OVRAL® tablets (0.3 mg norgestrel and 0.03 mg ethinyl estradiol), Wyeth®, are available in packages of 6 PIL-PAK® dispensers with 21 tablets each as follows: NDC 0008-0078, white, round tablet marked "WYETH" and "78".

ALSO AVAILABLE

LO/OVRAL®-28 tablets in containers of 28 tablets, consisting of 21 white LO/OVRAL® tablets (0.3 mg norgestrel and 0.03 mg ethinyl estradiol) and 7 pink inert tablets.

REFERENCES

1. "Population Reports," Series H, Number 2, May 1974; Series I, Number 1, June 1974; Series B, Number 2, January 1975; Series H, Number 3, 1975; Series H, Number 4, January 1976 (published by the Population Information Program, The George Washington University Medical Center, 2001 S St. NW., Washington, D.C.).
2. Inman, W. H. W., Vessey, M. P., Westerholm, B., and Engelund, A., "Thromboembolic disease and the steroidal content of oral contraceptives. A report to the Committee on Safety of Drugs," Brit Med J 2 :203-209, 1970.
3. Stolley, P. D., Tonascia, J. A., Tockman, M. S., Sartwell, P. E., Rutledge, A. H., and Jacobs, M. P., "Thrombosis with low-estrogen oral contraceptives," Am J Epidemiol 102 :197-208, 1975.
4. Royal College of General Practitioners, "Oral contraception and thromboembolic disease," J Coll Gen Pract 13 :267-279, 1967.
5. Inman, W. H. W., and Vessey, M. P., "Investigation of deaths from pulmonary, coronary and cerebral thrombosis and embolism in women of childbearing age," Brit Med J 2 :193-199, 1968.
6. Vessey, M. P., and Doll, R., "Investigation of relation between use of oral contraceptives and thromboembolic disease. A further report," Brit Med J 2 :651-657, 1969.
7. Sartwell, P. E., Masi, A. T., Arthes, F. G., Greene, G. R., and Smith, H. E., "Thromboembolism and oral contraceptives: an epidemiological case control study," Am J Epidemiol 90 :365-380, 1969.
8. Boston Collaborative Drug Surveillance Program, "Oral contraceptives and venous thromboembolic disease, surgically confirmed gallbladder disease and breast tumors," Lancet 1 :1399-1404, 1973.
9. Collaborative Group for the Study of Stroke in Young Women, "Oral contraception and increased risk of cerebral ischemia or thrombosis," N Engl J Med 288 :871-878, 1973.
10. Collaborative Group for the Study of Stroke in Young Women, "Oral contraceptives and stroke in young women: associated risk factors," JAMA 231 :718-722, 1975.
11. Mann, J. I., and Inman, W. H. W., "Oral contraceptives and death from myocardial infarction," Brit Med J 2 :245-248, 1975.
12. Mann, J. I., Inman, W. H. W., and Thorogood, M., "Oral contraceptive use in older women and fatal myocardial infarction," Brit Med J 2 :445-447, 1976.
13. Mann, J. I., Vessey, M. P., Thorogood, M., and Doll, R., "Myocardial infarction in young women with special reference to oral contraceptive practice," Brit Med J 2 :241-245, 1975.
14. Tietze, C., "New Estimates of Mortality Associated with Fertility Control," Family Planning Perspectives, 9 :74-76, 1977.
15. Vessey, M. P., Doll, R., Fairbairn, A. S., and Glober, G., "Post-operative thromboembolism and the use of oral contraceptives," Brit Med J 3 :123-126, 1970.
16. Greene, G. R., Sartwell, P. E., "Oral contraceptive use in patients with thromboembolism following surgery, trauma, or infection," Am J Pub Health 62 :680-685, 1972.
17. Smith, D. C., Prentice, R., Thompson, D. J., and Herrmann, W. L., "Association of exogenous estrogen and endometrial carcinoma," N Engl J Med 293 :1164-1167, 1975.
18. Ziel, H. K., and Finkle, W. D., "Increased risk of endometrial carcinoma among users of conjugated estrogens," N Engl J Med 293 :1167-1170, 1975.
19. Mack, T. N., Pike, M. C., Henderson, B. E., Pfeffer, R. I., Gerkins, V. R., Arthur, M., and Brown, S. E., "Estrogens and endometrial cancer in a retirement community," N Engl J Med 294 :1262-1267, 1976.
20. Silverberg, S. G., and Makowski, E. L., "Endometrial carcinoma in young women taking oral contraceptive agents," Obstet Gynecol 46 :503-506, 1975.
21. Vessey, M. P., Doll, R., and Sutton, P. M., "Oral contraceptives and breast neoplasia: a retrospective study," Brit Med J 3 :719-724, 1972.
22. Vessey, M. P., Doll, R., and Jones K., "Oral contraceptives and breast cancer. Progress report of an epidemiological study," Lancet 1 :941-943, 1975.
23. Boston Collaborative Drug Surveillance Program, "Surgically confirmed gallbladder disease, venous thromboembolism and breast tumors in relation to postmenopausal estrogen therapy," N Engl J Med 290 :15-19, 1974.
24. Arthes, F. G., Sartwell, P. E., and Lewison, E. F., "The pill, estrogens, and the breast. Epidemiologic aspects," Cancer 28 :1391-1394, 1971.
25. Fasal, E., and Paffenbarger, R. S., "Oral contraceptives as related to cancer and benign lesions of the breast," J Natl Cancer Inst 55 :767-773, 1975.
26. Royal College of General Practitioners, "Oral Contraceptives and Health," London, Pitman, 1974.
27. Ory, H., Cole P., MacMahon, B., and Hoover, R., "Oral contraceptives and reduced risk of benign breast diseases," N Engl J Med 294 :419-422, 1976.
28. Baum, J., Holtz, F., Bookstein, J. J., and Klein, E. W., "Possible association between benign hepatomas and oral contraceptives," Lancet 2 :926-928, 1973.
29. Mays, E. T., Christopherson, W. M., Mahr, M. M., and Williams, H. C., "Hepatic changes in young women ingesting contraceptive steroids. Hepatic hemorrhage and primary hepatic tumors," JAMA 235 :730-732, 1976.
30. Edmondson, H. A., Henderson, B., and Benton, B., "Liver-cell adenomas associated with use of oral contraceptives," N Engl J Med 294 :470-472, 1976.
31. Herbst, A. L., Ulfedler, H., and Poskanzer, D. C., "Adenocarcinoma of the vagina," N Engl J Med 284 :878-881, 1971.
32. Greenwald, P., Barlow, J. J., Nasca, P. C., and Burnett, W., "Vaginal cancer after maternal treatment with synthetic estrogens," N Engl J Med 285 :390-392, 1971.
33. Lanier, A. P., Noller, K. L., Decker, D. G., Elveback, L., and Kurland, L. T., "Cancer and stilbestrol. A follow-up of 1719 persons exposed to estrogens in utero and born 1943-1959," Mayo Clin Pro 48 :793-799, 1973.
34. Herbst, A. L., Kurman, R. J., and Scully, R. E., "Vaginal and cervical abnormalities after exposure to stilbestrol in utero," Obstet Gynecol 40 :287-298, 1972.
35. Herbst, A. L., Robboy, S. J., Macdonald, G. J., and Scully, R. E., "The effects of local progesterone on stilbestrol-associated vaginal adenosis," Am J Obstet Gynecol 118 :607-615, 1974.
36. Herbst, A. L., Poskanzer, D. C., Robboy, S. J., Friedlander, L., and Scully, R. E., "Prenatal exposure to stilbestrol: a prospective comparison of exposed female offspring with unexposed controls," N Engl J Med 292 :334-339, 1975.
37. Stafl, A., Mattingly, R. F., Foley, D. V., Fetherston, W., "Clinical diagnosis of vaginal adenosis," Obstet Gynecol 43 :118-128, 1974.
38. Sherman, A. I., Goldrath, M., Berlin, A., Vakhariya, V., Banooni, F., Michaels, W., Goodman, P., and Brown, S., "Cervical-vaginal adenosis after in utero exposure to synthetic estrogens," Obstet Gynecol 44 :531-545, 1974.
39. Gal, I., Kirman, B., and Stern, J., "Hormone pregnancy tests and congenital malformation," Nature 216 :83, 1967.
40. Levy, E. P., Cohen, A., and Fraser, F. C., "Hormone treatment during pregnancy and congenital heart defects," Lancet 1 :611, 1973.
41. Nora, J. J., and Nora, A. H., "Birth defects and oral contraceptives," Lancet 1 :941-942, 1973.
42. Janerich, D. T., Piper, J. M., and Glebatis, D. M., "Oral contraceptives and congenital limb-reduction defects," N Engl J Med 291 :697-700, 1974.
43. Carr, D. H., "Chromosome studies in selected spontaneous abortions: I. Conception after oral contraceptives," Canad Med Assoc J 103 :343-348, 1970.
44. Wynn, V., Doar, J. W. H., and Mills, G. L., "Some effects of oral contraceptives on serum-lipid and lipoprotein levels," Lancet 2 :720-723, 1966.
45. Laumas, K. R., Malkani, P. K., Bhatnagar, S., and Laumas, V., "Radioactivity in the breast milk of lactating women after oral administration of 3 H-norethynodrel," Amer J Obstet Gynecol 98 :411-413, 1967.
46. Center for Disease Control, "Increased Risk of Hepatocellular Adenoma in Women with Long-term use of Oral Contraceptives," Morbidity and Mortality Weekly Report, 26 :293-294, 1977.
47. Herbst, A. L., Cole, P., Colton, T., Robboy, S. J., Scully, R. E., "Age-incidence and Risk of Diethylstilbestrol-related Clear Cell Adenocarcinoma of the Vagina and Cervix," Am. J. Obstet. Gynecol., 128 :43-50, 1977.
48. Bibbo, M., Al-Naqeeb, M., Baccarini, I., Gill, W., Newton, M., Sleeper, K. M., Sonek, M., Wied, G. L., "Follow-up Study of Male and Female Offspring of DES-treated Mothers. A Preliminary Report," Jour. of Repro. Med., 15 :29-32, 1975.
49. Gill, W. B., Schumacher, G. F. B., Bibbo, M., "Structural and Functional Abnormalities in the Sex Organs of Male Offspring of Mothers Treated with Diethylstilbestrol (DES)," Jour. of Repro. Med., 16 :147-153, 1976.
50. Henderson, B. E., Senton, B., Cosgrove, M., Baptista, J., Aldrich, J., Townsend, D., Hart, W., Mack, T., "Urogenital Tract Abnormalities in Sons of Women Treated with Diethylstilbestrol," Pediatrics, 58 :505-507, 1976.
51. Heinonen, O. P., Slone, D., Nonson, R. R., Hook, E. B., Shapiro, S., "Cardiovascular Birth Defects and Antenatal Exposure to Female Sex Hormones," N. Engl. J. Med., 296 :67-70, 1977.
52. Jain, A. K., "Mortality Risk Associated with the Use of Oral Contraceptives," Studies in Family Planning, 8 :50-54, 1977.
53. Beral, V., "Mortality Among Oral Contraceptive Users," Lancet, 2 :727-731, 1977.
54. Royal College of General Practitioners' Oral contraception study, "Incidence of arterial disease among oral contraceptive users," J Royal Col Gen Pract 33 :75-82, 1983.
55. Slone, D., Shapiro, S., Kaufman, D. W., Rosenberg, L., Miettinen, O., and Stolley, P., "Risk of myocardial infarction in relation to current and discontinued use of oral contraceptives," N Engl J Med 305 :420-424, 1981.
56. Inman, W.H.W., "Oral contraceptives and fatal subarachnoid haemorrhage," Brit Med J 2 :1468-1470, 1979.
57. Petitti, D. B., and Wingerd, J., "Use of oral contraceptives, cigarette smoking and risk of subarachnoid haemorrhage," Lancet 2 :234-236, 1978.
58. Thorogood, M., Adam, S. A., and Mann, J. I., "Fatal subarachnoid haemorrhage in young women: role of oral contraceptives," Brit Med J 283 :762, 1981.
59. Rosenberg, L., Hennekens, C.H., Rosner, B., Belanger, C., Rothman, K. J., and Speizer, F. E., "Oral contraceptive use in relation to nonfatal myocardial infarction," Am J Epidemiol 111 :59-66, 1980.
60. Adam, S. A., Thorogood, M., and Mann, J. I., "Oral contraception and myocardial infarction revisited: the effects of new preparations and prescribing patterns," Brit J Obstet Gynaecol 88 :838-845, 1981.

The patient labeling for oral-contraceptive drug products is set forth below:

Brief Summary Patient Package Insert

> Cigarette smoking increases the risk of serious adverse effects on the heart and blood vessels from oral-contraceptive use. This risk increases with age and with heavy smoking (15 or more cigarettes per day) and is quite marked in women over 35 years of age. Women who use oral contraceptives should not smoke.

Oral contraceptives taken as directed are about 99% effective in preventing pregnancy. (The mini-pill, however, is somewhat less effective.) Forgetting to take your pills increases the chance of pregnancy. Women who have or have had clotting disorders, cancer of the breast or sex organs, unexplained vaginal bleeding, a stroke, heart attack, angina pectoris, or who suspect they may be pregnant should not use oral contraceptives. Various drugs, such as some antibiotics, may also decrease the effectiveness of oral contraceptives. Most side effects of the pill are not serious. The most common side effects are nausea, vomiting, bleeding between menstrual periods, weight gain, and breast tenderness. However, proper use of oral contraceptives requires that they be taken under your doctor's continuous supervision, because they can be associated with serious side effects which may be fatal. Fortunately, these occur very infrequently. The serious side effects are:
1. Blood clots in the legs, lungs, brain, heart, or other organs, and hemorrhage into the brain due to bursting of a blood vessel. Certain of these effects may occur after pill use has been stopped.
2. Liver tumors, which may rupture and cause severe bleeding.
3. Birth defects if the pill is taken while you are pregnant.
4. High blood pressure.
5. Gallbladder disease.
The symptoms associated with these serious side effects are discussed in the detailed leaflet given you with your supply of pills. Notify your doctor if you notice any unusual physical disturbance while taking the pill.
The estrogen in oral contraceptives has been found to cause breast cancer and other cancers in certain animals. These findings suggest that oral contraceptives may also cause cancer in humans. However, studies to date in women taking currently marketed oral contraceptives have not confirmed that oral contraceptives cause cancer in humans.
The detailed leaflet describes more completely the benefits and risks of oral contraceptives. It also provides information on other forms of contraception. Read it carefully. If you have any questions, consult your doctor.

CAUTION

Oral contraceptives are of no value in the prevention or treatment of venereal disease.

DETAILED PATIENT LABELING

WHAT YOU SHOULD KNOW ABOUT ORAL CONTRACEPTIVES

Oral contraceptives ("the pill") are the most effective way (except for sterilization) to prevent pregnancy. They are also convenient and, for most women, free of serious or unpleasant side effects. Oral contraceptives must always be taken under the continuous supervision of a physician.

It is important that any woman who considers using an oral contraceptive understand the risks involved. Although the oral contraceptives have important advantages over other methods of contraception, they have certain risks that no other method has. Only you can decide whether the advantages are worth these risks. This leaflet will tell you about the most important risks. It will explain how you can help your doctor prescribe the pill as safely as possible by telling him about yourself and being alert for the earliest signs of trouble. And it will tell you how to use the pill properly, so that it will be as effective as possible. There is more detailed information available in the leaflet prepared for doctors. Your pharmacist can show you a copy; you may need your doctor's help in understanding parts of it.

WHO SHOULD NOT USE ORAL CONTRACEPTIVES

A. If you have any of the following conditions, you should not use the pill:
1. Clots in the legs or lungs.
2. Angina pectoris.
3. Known or suspected cancer of the breast or sex organs.
4. Unusual vaginal bleeding that has not yet been diagnosed.
5. Known or suspected pregnancy.

B. If you have had any of the following conditions, you should not use the pill:
1. Heart attack or stroke.
2. Clots in the legs or lungs.

> C. Cigarette smoking increases the risk of serious adverse effects on the heart and blood vessels from oral-contraceptive use. This risk increases with age and with heavy smoking (15 or more cigarettes per day) and is quite marked in women over 35 years of age. Women who use oral contraceptives should not smoke.

D. If you have scanty or irregular periods or are a young woman without a regular cycle, you should use another method of contraception because, if you use the pill, you may have difficulty becoming pregnant or may fail to have menstrual periods after discontinuing the pill.

DECIDING TO USE ORAL CONTRACEPTIVES

If you do not have any of the conditions listed above and are thinking about using oral contraceptives, to help you decide, you need information about the advantages and risks of oral contraceptives and of other contraceptive methods as well. This leaflet describes the advantages and risks of oral contraceptives. Except for sterilization, the IUD, and abortion, which have their own inherent risks, the only risks of other methods of contraception are those due to pregnancy should the method fail. Your doctor can answer questions you may have with respect to other methods of contraception. He can also answer any questions you may have after reading this leaflet on oral contraceptives.

1. What Oral Contraceptives Are and How They Work. Oral contraceptives are of two types. The most common, often simply called "the pill," is a combination of an estrogen and a progestogen, the two kinds of female hormones. The amount of estrogen and progestogen can vary, but the amount of estrogen is most important because both the effectiveness and some of the dangers of oral contraceptives are related to the amount of estrogen. This kind of oral contraceptive works principally by preventing release of an egg from the ovary. When the amount of estrogen is 50 micrograms or more, and the pill is taken as directed, oral contraceptives are more than 99% effective (i.e., there would be less than 1 pregnancy if 100 women used the pill for 1 year). Pills that contain 20 to 35 micrograms of estrogen vary slightly in effectiveness, ranging from 98% to more than 99% effective.

The second type of oral contraceptive, often called the "mini-pill," contains only a progestogen. It works in part by preventing release of an egg from the ovary but also by keeping sperm from reaching the egg and by making the uterus (womb) less receptive to any fertilized egg that reaches it. The mini-pill is less effective than the combination oral contraceptive, about 97% effective. In addition, the progestogen-only pill has a tendency to cause irregular bleeding which may be quite inconvenient, or cessation of bleeding entirely. The progestogen-only pill is used despite its lower effectiveness in the hope that it will prove not to have some of the serious side effects of the estrogen-containing pill (see below), but it is not yet certain that the mini-pill does in fact have fewer serious side effects. The discussion below, while based

mainly on information about the combination pills, should be considered to apply as well to the mini-pill.

2. Other Nonsurgical Ways to Prevent Pregnancy. As this leaflet will explain, oral contraceptives have several serious risks. Other methods of contraception have lesser risks or none at all. They are also less effective than oral contraceptives, but, used properly, may be effective enough for many women.

The following table gives reported pregnancy rates (the number of women out of 100 who would become pregnant in 1 year) for these methods.

PREGNANCIES PER 100 WOMEN PER YEAR

Intrauterine device (IUD), less than 1-6; Diaphragm with spermicidal products (creams or jellies), 2-20; Condom (rubber), 3-36; Aerosol foams, 2-29; Jellies and creams, 4-36; Periodic abstinence (rhythm) all types, less than 1-47:
1. Calendar method, 14-47;
2. Temperature method, 1-20;
3. Temperature method—intercourse only in postovulatory phase, less than 1-7;
4. Mucus method, 1-25;

No contraception, 60-80.

The figures (except for the IUD) vary widely because people differ in how well they use each method. Very faithful users of the various methods obtain very good results, except for users of the calendar method of periodic abstinence (rhythm). Except for the IUD, effective use of these methods requires somewhat more effort than simply taking a single pill every day, but it is an effort that many couples undertake successfully. Your doctor can tell you a great deal more about these methods of contraception.

3. The Dangers of Oral Contraceptives.

a. *Circulatory disorders (abnormal blood clotting and stroke due to hemorrhage).*

Blood clots (in various blood vessels of the body) are the most common of the serious side effects of oral contraceptives. A clot can result in a stroke (if the clot is in the brain), a heart attack (if the clot is in a blood vessel of the heart), or a pulmonary embolus (a clot which forms in the legs or pelvis, then breaks off and travels to the lungs). Any of these can be fatal. Clots also occur rarely in the blood vessels of the eye, resulting in blindness or impairment of vision in that eye. There is evidence that the risk of clotting increases with higher estrogen doses. It is therefore important to keep the dose of estrogen as low as possible, so long as the oral contraceptive used has an acceptable pregnancy rate and doesn't cause unacceptable changes in the menstrual pattern. Furthermore, cigarette smoking by oral-contraceptive users increases the risk of serious adverse effects on the heart and blood vessels. This risk increases with age and with heavy smoking (15 or more cigarettes per day) and begins to become quite marked in women over 35 years of age. For this reason, women who use oral contraceptives should not smoke.

The risk of abnormal clotting increases with age in both users and nonusers of oral contraceptives, but the increased risk from the contraceptive appears to be present at all ages. For oral-contraceptive users in general, it has been estimated that in women between the ages of 15 and 34 the risk of death due to a circulatory disorder is about 1 in 12,000 per year, whereas for nonusers the rate is about 1 in 50,000 per year. In the age group 35 to 44, the risk is estimated to be about 1 in 2,500 per year for oral-contraceptive users and about 1 in 10,000 per year for nonusers.

[See figure next column]

Even without the pill the risk of having a heart attack increases with age and is also increased by such heart attack risk factors as high blood pressure, high cholesterol, obesity, diabetes, and cigarette smoking. Without any risk factors present, the use of oral contraceptives alone may double the risk of heart attack. However, the combination of cigarette smoking, especially heavy smoking, and oral contraceptive use greatly increases the risk of heart attack. Oral-contraceptive users who smoke are about 5 times more likely to have a heart attack than users who do not smoke and about 10 times more likely to have a heart attack than nonusers who do not smoke. It has been estimated that users between the ages of 30 and 39 who smoke have about a 1 in 10,000 chance each year of having a fatal heart attack compared to about a 1 in 50,000 chance in users who do not smoke, and about a 1 in 100,000 chance in nonusers who do not smoke. In the age group 40 to 44, the risk is about 1 in 1,700 per year for users who smoke compared to about 1 in 10,000 for users who do not smoke and to about 1 in 14,000 per year for nonusers who do not smoke. Heavy smoking (about 15 cigarettes or more a day) further increases the risk. If you do not smoke and have none of the other heart attack risk factors described above, you will have a smaller risk than listed. If you have several heart attack risk factors, the risk may be considerably greater than listed. In addition to blood-clotting disorders, it has been estimated that women taking oral contraceptives are twice as likely as nonusers to have a stroke due to rupture of a blood vessel in the brain. There is evidence that patients who stop taking oral contraceptives after using them continuously for five or more years may continue to have an increased risk of stroke or heart attack for at least six to nine years after discontinuation.

Figure 1. Estimated annual number of deaths associated with control of fertility and no control per 100,000 nonsterile women, by regimen of control and age of woman.

b. *Formation of tumors.* Studies have found that when certain animals are given the female sex hormone, estrogen, which is an ingredient of oral contraceptives, continuously for long periods, cancers may develop in the breast, cervix, vagina, and liver.

These findings suggest that oral contraceptives may cause cancer in humans. However, studies to date in women taking currently marketed oral contraceptives have not confirmed that oral contraceptives cause cancer in humans. Several studies have found no increase in breast cancer in users, although one study suggested oral contraceptives might cause an increase in breast cancer in women who already have benign breast disease (e.g., cysts).

Women with a strong family history of breast cancer or who have breast nodules, fibrocystic disease, or abnormal mammograms or who were exposed to DES (diethylstilbestrol), an estrogen, during their mother's pregnancy must be followed very closely by their doctors if they choose to use oral contraceptives instead of another method of contraception. Many studies have shown that women taking oral contraceptives have less risk of getting benign breast disease than those who have not used oral contraceptives. Recently, strong evidence has emerged that estrogens (one component of oral contraceptives), when given for periods of more than one year to women after the menopause, increase the risk of cancer of the uterus (womb). There is also some evidence that a kind of oral contraceptive which is no longer marketed, the sequential oral contraceptive, may increase the risk of cancer of the uterus. There remains no evidence, however, that the oral contraceptives now available increase the risk of this cancer. Oral contraceptives do cause, although rarely, a benign (nonmalignant) tumor of the liver. These tumors do not spread, but they may rupture and cause internal bleeding, which may be fatal. A few cases of cancer of the liver have been reported in women using oral contraceptives, but it is not yet known whether the drug caused them.

c. *Dangers to a developing child if oral contraceptives are used in or immediately preceding pregnancy.* Oral contraceptives should not be taken by pregnant women because they may damage the developing child. An increased risk of birth defects, including heart defects and limb defects, has been associated with the use of sex hormones, including oral contraceptives, in pregnancy. In addition, the developing female child whose mother has received DES (diethylstilbestrol), an estrogen, during pregnancy has a risk of getting cancer of the vagina or cervix in her teens or young adulthood. This risk is estimated to be about 1 in 1,000 exposures or less. Abnormalities of the urinary and sex organs have been reported in

Continued on next page

Wyeth-Ayerst—Cont.

male offspring so exposed. It is possible that other estrogens, such as the estrogens in oral contraceptives, could have the same effect in the child if the mother takes them during pregnancy.

If you stop taking oral contraceptives to become pregnant, your doctor may recommend that you use another method of contraception for a short while. The reason for this is that there is evidence from studies in women who have had "miscarriages" soon after stopping the pill, that the lost fetuses are more likely to be abnormal. Whether there is an overall increase in "miscarriage" in women who become pregnant soon after stopping the pill as compared with women who do not use the pill is not known, but it is possible that there may be. If, however, you do become pregnant soon after stopping oral contraceptives, and do not have a miscarriage, there is no evidence that the baby has an increased risk of being abnormal.

d. *Gallbladder disease.* Women who use oral contraceptives have a greater risk than nonusers of having gallbladder disease requiring surgery. The increased risk may first appear within 1 year of use and may double after 4 or 5 years of use.

e. *Other side effects of oral contraceptives.* Some women using oral contraceptives experience unpleasant side effects that are not dangerous and are not likely to damage their health. Some of these may be temporary. Your breasts may feel tender, nausea and vomiting may occur, you may gain or lose weight, and your ankles may swell. A spotty darkening of the skin, particularly of the face, is possible and may persist. You may notice unexpected vaginal bleeding or changes in your menstrual period. Irregular bleeding is frequently seen when using the mini-pill or combination oral contraceptives containing less than 50 micrograms of estrogen. More serious side effects include worsening of migraine, asthma, epilepsy, and kidney or heart disease because of a tendency for water to be retained in the body when oral contraceptives are used. Other side effects are growth of preexisting fibroid tumors of the uterus; mental depression; and liver problems with jaundice (yellowing of the skin). Your doctor may find that levels of sugar and fatty substances in your blood are elevated; the long-term effects of these changes are not known. Some women develop high blood pressure while taking oral contraceptives, which ordinarily returns to the original levels when the oral contraceptive is stopped.

Other reactions, although not proved to be caused by oral contraceptives, are occasionally reported. These include more frequent urination and some discomfort when urinating, blood-cell breakdown with kidney failure, nervousness, dizziness, some loss of scalp hair, an increase in body hair, an increase or decrease in sex drive, appetite changes, cataracts, and a need for a change in contact lens prescription, or inability to use contact lenses.

After you stop using oral contraceptives, there may be a delay before you are able to become pregnant or before you resume having menstrual periods. This is especially true of women who had irregular menstrual cycles prior to the use of oral contraceptives. As discussed previously, your doctor may recommend that you wait a short while after stopping the pill before you try to become pregnant. During this time, use another form of contraception. You should consult your physician before resuming use of oral contraceptives after childbirth, especially if you plan to nurse your baby. Drugs in oral contraceptives are known to appear in the milk, and the long-range effect on infants is not known at this time. Furthermore, oral contraceptives may cause a decrease in your milk supply as well as in the quality of the milk.

4. Comparison of the Risks of Oral Contraceptives and Other Contraceptive Methods. The many studies on the risks and effectiveness of oral contraceptives and other methods of contraception have been analyzed to estimate the risk of death associated with various methods of contraception. This risk has two parts: (a) the risk of the method itself (e.g., the risk that oral contraceptives will cause death due to abnormal clotting), and (b) the risk of death due to pregnancy or abortion in the event the method fails. The results of this analysis are shown in the bar graph (Figure 1). The height of the bars is the number of deaths per 100,000 women each year. There are six sets of bars, each set referring to a specific age group of women. Within each set of bars, there is a single bar for each of the different contraceptive methods. For oral contraceptives, there are two bars—one for smokers and the other for nonsmokers. The analysis is based on present knowledge, and new information could, of course, alter it. The analysis shows that the risk of death from all methods of birth control is low and below that associated with childbirth, except for oral contraceptives in women over 40 who smoke. It shows that the lowest risk of death is associated with the condom or diaphragm (traditional contraception) backed up by early abortion in case of failure of the condom or diaphragm to prevent pregnancy. Also, at any age the risk of death (due to unexpected pregnancy) from the use of traditional contraception, even without a backup of abor-

tion, is generally the same as or less than that from use of oral contraceptives.

HOW TO USE ORAL CONTRACEPTIVES AS SAFELY AND EFFECTIVELY AS POSSIBLE, ONCE YOU HAVE DECIDED TO USE THEM

1. What to Tell your Doctor.

You can make use of the pill as safely as possible by telling your doctor if you have any of the following:

a. Conditions that mean you should not use oral contraceptives:

Clots in the legs or lungs.

Clots in the legs or lungs in the past.

A stroke, heart attack, or angina pectoris.

Known or suspected cancer of the breast or sex organs.

Unusual vaginal bleeding that has not yet been diagnosed.

Known or suspected pregnancy.

b. Conditions that your doctor will want to watch closely or which might cause him to suggest another method of contraception:

A family history of breast cancer.

Breast nodules, fibrocystic disease of the breast, or an abnormal mammogram.

Diabetes.	Heart or kidney
High blood	disease.
pressure.	Epilepsy.
High cholesterol.	Mental depression.
Cigarette smoking.	Fibroid tumors of the
Migraine	uterus.
headaches.	Gallbladder disease.

c. Once you are using oral contraceptives, you should be alert for signs of a serious adverse effect and call your doctor if they occur.

Sharp pain in the chest, coughing blood, or sudden shortness of breath (indicating possible clots in the lungs).

Pain in the calf (possible clot in the leg).

Crushing chest pain or heaviness (indicating possible heart attack).

Sudden severe headache or vomiting, dizziness or fainting, disturbance of vision or speech, or weakness or numbness in an arm or leg (indicating a possible stroke).

Sudden partial or complete loss of vision (indicating a possible clot in the eye).

Breast lumps (you should ask your doctor to show you how to examine your own breasts).

Severe pain in the abdomen (indicating a possible ruptured tumor of the liver).

Severe depression.

Yellowing of the skin (jaundice).

2. How to Take the Pill So That It is Most Effective.

Reduced effectiveness and an increased incidence of breakthrough bleeding have been associated with the use of oral contraceptives with antibiotics such as rifampin, ampicillin, and tetracycline or with certain other drugs such as barbiturates, phenylbutazone or phenytoin sodium. You should use an additional means of contraception during any cycle in which any of these drugs are taken.

To achieve maximum contraceptive effectiveness, oral contraceptives must be taken exactly as directed and at intervals not exceeding 24 hours. It is recommended that tablets be taken at the same time each day, preferably after the evening meal or at bedtime. Taking them on a definite schedule will decrease the chance of forgetting a tablet and also help keep the proper amount of medication in your system. See detailed instructions below for Nordette-21, Ovral® and Lo/Ovral®, Nordette-28, Ovral®-28 and Lo/Ovral®-28, and for Ovrette®.

NORDETTE®-21, OVRAL®, LO/OVRAL®

The dosage of Nordette-21, Ovral and Lo/Ovral is one tablet daily for 21 days in a row per menstrual cycle. Tablets are then discontinued for 7 days.

The basic schedule is 21 days on—7 days off.

During the first month, you should begin taking Nordette-21, Ovral or Lo/Ovral on Day 5 of your menstrual cycle whether or not you still have your period. (Day 1 is the first day of menstruation, even if it is almost midnight when you start.) Note: During your first month on Nordette-21, Ovral or Lo/Ovral, if you start taking tablets later than Day 5 of your menstrual cycle, you should protect yourself by also using another method of birth control until you have taken a tablet daily for seven consecutive days. Thereafter, if you follow directions carefully you will obtain the full contraceptive benefit. If you begin taking tablets later than the proper day, the possibility of ovulation and pregnancy occurring before beginning medication should be considered.

Take one tablet every day until you finish all 21 tablets. No tablets are then taken for one week (7 days). Your period will usually begin about three days after you take the last tablet. Don't be alarmed if the amount of bleeding is not the same as before. On the 8th day, start a new Pilpak®, even if you still have your period. If, for example, you took Nordette-21, Ovral or Lo/Ovral for the first time on a Tuesday, the 8th day will also be a Tuesday. Thus, you will always begin a new cycle on the same day of the week as long as you do not interrupt your original schedule. If you start taking tablets later than the 8th day, you should protect yourself by also using

another method of birth control until you have taken a tablet daily for seven days in a row.

NORDETTE®-28, OVRAL®-28, LO/OVRAL®-28

The dosage of Nordette-28, Ovral-28 and Lo/Ovral-28 is one white or light-orange active tablet daily for 21 consecutive days followed by one pink inactive tablet daily for 7 consecutive days. The basic schedule is 21 days on white or light-orange active tablets—7 days on pink inactive tablets. Always take all 21 white or light-orange tablets in each Pilpak before taking the pink tablets.

You should begin taking Nordette-28, Ovral-28 or Lo/Ovral-28 on the first Sunday after your menstrual period begins, whether or not you are still bleeding. If your period begins on a Sunday, take your first tablet that very same day. Your first white or light-orange tablet is marked with a large arrow and the word "Start". Note: During your first month on Nordette-28, Ovral-28 or Lo/Ovral-28, you should protect yourself by also using another method of birth control until you have taken a white or light-orange tablet daily for seven consecutive days. Thereafter, if you follow directions carefully, you will obtain the full contraceptive benefit. If you begin taking tablets later than the proper day, the possibility of ovulation and pregnancy occurring before beginning medication should be considered. Take one tablet every day until you finish all 21 white or light-orange tablets in a Pilpak, followed by all seven pink tablets. Your period will usually begin about three days after you take the last white or light-orange tablet, which will be during the time you are taking the pink tablets. Don't be alarmed if the amount of bleeding is not the same as before. The day after you have taken your last pink tablet, begin a new Pilpak of tablets (taking all 21 white or light-orange tablets first, just as you did before) so that you will take a tablet every day without interruption. The starting day for each new Pilpak will always be Sunday. If in any cycle you start tablets later than the proper day, you should also use another method of birth control until you have taken a white or light-orange tablet daily for 7 days in a row.

Spotting or Breakthrough Bleeding:

Spotting is slight staining between menstrual periods which may not even require a pad. Breakthrough bleeding is a flow much like a regular period, requiring sanitary protection. Spotting is more common than breakthrough bleeding, and both occur more often in the first few cycles than in later cycles. These types of bleeding are usually temporary and without significance. It is important to continue taking your pills on schedule. If the bleeding persists for more than a few days, consult your doctor.

Forgotten Pills:

Nordette-21, Ovral and Lo/Ovral each contain 21 active white or light-orange tablets per Pilpak. Nordette-28, Ovral-28 and Lo/Ovral-28 each contain 21 active white or light-orange tablets plus 7 pink inactive tablets per Pilpak.

The chance of becoming pregnant is probably quite small if you miss only one white or light-orange tablet in a cycle. Of course, with each additional one you skip, the chance increases. If you miss one or more pink tablets (Nordette-28, Ovral-28, Lo/Ovral-28) you are still protected against pregnancy as long as you begin taking your next white or light-orange tablet on the proper day. It is important to take a missed white or light-orange tablet as soon as it is remembered. If two consecutive white or light-orange tablets are missed they should both be taken as soon as remembered. The next tablet should then be taken at the usual time. Any time you miss one or two white or light-orange tablets, or begin a new Pilpak after the proper starting day, you should also use another method of birth control until you have taken a white or light-orange tablet daily for seven consecutive days. If breakthrough bleeding occurs following missed tablets, it will usually be temporary and of no consequence. While there is little likelihood of pregnancy occurring if only one or two white or light-orange tablets are missed, the possibility of pregnancy increases with each successive day that scheduled white or light-orange tablets are missed.

If you are taking Nordette-21, Ovral or Lo/Ovral and forget to take three white or light-orange tablets in a row, do not take them when you remember. Wait four more days—which makes a whole week without tablets. Then begin a new Pilpak on the 8th day after the last tablet was taken. During the seven days without tablets, and until you have taken a white or light-orange tablet daily for seven consecutive days, you should protect yourself from pregnancy by also using another method of birth control.

If you are taking Nordette-28, Ovral-28 or Lo/Ovral-28 and forget to take three white or light-orange tablets in a row, do not take them when you remember. Stop taking all medication until the first Sunday following the last missed tablet. Then, whether or not you have had your period, and even if you are still bleeding, start a new Pilpak. During the days without tablets, and until you have taken a white or light-orange tablet daily for seven consecutive days, you should protect yourself from pregnancy by also using another method of birth control.

OVRETTE®

Ovrette is administered on a continuous daily dosage schedule, one tablet each day, every day of the year. Take the first tablet on the first day of your menstrual period. Tablets should be taken at the same time every day, without interruption, whether bleeding occurs or not. If bleeding is prolonged (more than 8 days) or unusually heavy, you should contact your doctor.

Forgotten Pills:

The risk of pregnancy increases with each tablet missed. Therefore, it is very important that you take one tablet daily as directed. If you miss one tablet, take it as soon as you remember and also take your next tablet at the regular time. If you miss two tablets, take one of the missed tablets as soon as you remember, as well as your regular tablet for that day at the proper time. Furthermore, you should use another method of birth control in addition to taking Ovrette until you have taken fourteen days (2 weeks) of medication.

If more than two tablets have been missed, Ovrette should be discontinued immediately and another method of birth control used until the start of your next menstrual period. Then you may resume taking Ovrette.

At times there may be no menstrual period after a cycle of pills. Therefore, if you miss one menstrual period but have taken the pills *exactly as you were supposed to*, continue as usual into the next cycle. If you have not taken the pills correctly and miss a menstrual period, or if you are taking mini-pills and it is 45 days or more from the start of your last menstrual period, you may be pregnant and should stop taking oral contraceptives until your doctor determines whether or not you are pregnant. Until you can get to your doctor, use another form of contraception. If two consecutive menstrual periods are missed, you should stop taking pills until it is determined whether you are pregnant. If you do become pregnant while using oral contraceptives, you should discuss the risks to the developing child with your doctor.

3. Periodic Examination.

Your doctor will take a complete medical and family history before prescribing oral contraceptives. At that time and about once a year thereafter, he will generally examine your blood pressure, breasts, abdomen, and pelvic organs (including a Papanicolaou smear, i.e., test for cancer).

SUMMARY

Oral contraceptives are the most effective method, except sterilization, for preventing pregnancy. Other methods, when used conscientiously, are also very effective and have fewer risks. The serious risks of oral contraceptives are uncommon, and the "pill" is a very convenient method of preventing pregnancy.

If you have certain conditions or have had these conditions in the past, you should not use oral contraceptives, because the risk is too great. These conditions are listed in the leaflet. If you do not have these conditions, and decide to use the "pill", please read the leaflet carefully so that you can use the "pill" most safely and effectively.

Based on his or her assessment of your medical needs, your doctor has prescribed this drug for you. Do not give the drug to anyone else.

Shown in Product Identification Section, page 437

LO/OVRAL®-28   ℞
[lōh-oh 'vral-28]
Tablets
(norgestrel and ethinyl estradiol tablets)

DESCRIPTION

21 white LO/OVRAL® tablets, each containing 0.3 mg of norgestrel (dl -13-beta-ethyl-17-alpha-ethinyl-17-beta-hydroxygon-4-en-3-one), a totally synthetic progestogen, and 0.03 mg of ethinyl estradiol (19-nor-17α-pregna-1,3,5(10)-trien-20-yne-3,17-diol), and 7 pink inert tablets. The inactive ingredients present are cellulose, FD&C Red 3, lactose, magnesium stearate, and polacrilin potassium.

CLINICAL PHARMACOLOGY
See Lo/Ovral®.

INDICATIONS AND USAGE
See Lo/Ovral.
Dose-Related Risk of Thromboembolism from Oral Contraceptives: See Lo/Ovral.

CONTRAINDICATIONS
See Lo/Ovral.

WARNINGS
See Lo/Ovral.

PRECAUTIONS
See Lo/Ovral.
Information for the Patient: See Lo/Ovral.
Drug Interactions: See Lo/Ovral.
Carcinogenesis: See Lo/Ovral.
Pregnancy: See Lo/Ovral.
Nursing Mothers: See Lo/Ovral.

ADVERSE REACTIONS
See Lo/Ovral.

Acute Overdosage: See Lo/Ovral.

DOSAGE AND ADMINISTRATION

To achieve maximum contraceptive effectiveness, LO/OVRAL-28 must be taken exactly as directed and at intervals not exceeding 24 hours.

The dosage of LO/OVRAL-28 is one white tablet daily for 21 consecutive days followed by one pink inert tablet daily for 7 consecutive days according to prescribed schedule. It is recommended that tablets be taken at the same time each day, preferably after the evening meal or at bedtime.

During the first cycle of medication, the patient is instructed to begin taking LO/OVRAL-28 on the first Sunday after the onset of menstruation. If menstruation begins on a Sunday, the first tablet (white) is taken that day. One white tablet should be taken daily for 21 consecutive days followed by one pink inert tablet daily for 7 consecutive days. Withdrawal bleeding should usually occur within three days following discontinuation of white tablets.

During the first cycle, contraceptive reliance should not be placed on LO/OVRAL-28 until a white tablet has been taken daily for 7 consecutive days. The possibility of ovulation and conception prior to initiation of medication should be considered.

The patient begins her next and all subsequent 28-day courses of tablets on the same day of the week (Sunday) on which she began her first course, following the same schedule: 21 days on white tablets—7 days on pink inert tablets. If in any cycle the patient starts tablets later than the proper day, she should protect herself by using another method of birth control until she has taken a white tablet daily for 7 consecutive days.

If spotting or breakthrough bleeding occurs, the patient is instructed to continue on the same regimen. This type of bleeding is usually transient and without significance; however, if the bleeding is persistent or prolonged the patient is advised to consult her physician. Although the occurrence of pregnancy is highly unlikely if LO/OVRAL-28 is taken according to directions, if withdrawal bleeding does not occur, the possibility of pregnancy must be considered. If the patient has not adhered to the prescribed schedule (missed one or more tablets or started taking them on a day later than she should have) the probability of pregnancy should be considered at the time of the first missed period and appropriate diagnostic measures taken before the medication is resumed. If the patient has adhered to the prescribed regimen and misses two consecutive periods, pregnancy should be ruled out before continuing the contraceptive regimen.

The patient should be instructed to take a missed white tablet as soon as it is remembered. If two consecutive white tablets are missed they should both be taken as soon as remembered. The next tablet should be taken at the usual time. Any time the patient misses one or two white tablets, she should also use another method of contraception until she has taken a white tablet daily for seven consecutive days. If the patient misses one or more pink tablets she is still protected against pregnancy *provided* she begins taking white tablets again on the proper day.

If breakthrough bleeding occurs following missed white tablets it will usually be transient and of no consequence. While there is little likelihood of ovulation occurring if only one or two white tablets are missed, the possibility of ovulation increases with each successive day that scheduled white tablets are missed. (If three consecutive days white LO/OVRAL tablets are missed, all medication should be discontinued and the remainder of the 28-day package discarded. A new tablet cycle should be started on the first Sunday following the last missed tablet, and an alternate means of contraception should be prescribed during the days without tablets and until the patient has taken a white tablet daily for 7 consecutive days.) In the nonlactating mother, LO/OVRAL may be prescribed in the postpartum period either immediately or at the first postpartum examination whether or not menstruation has resumed.

HOW SUPPLIED

LO/OVRAL®-28 Tablets (0.3 mg norgestrel and 0.03 mg ethinyl estradiol), Wyeth®, are available in packages of 6 PILPAK® dispensers, each containing 28 tablets as follows: 21 active tablets, NDC 0008-0078, white, round tablet marked "WYETH" and "78".

7 inert tablets, NDC 0008-0486, pink, round tablet marked "WYETH" and "486".

REFERENCES
See Lo/Ovral.
Brief Summary Patient Package Insert: See Lo/Ovral.
DETAILED PATIENT LABELING: See Lo/Ovral.
Shown in Product Identification Section, page 437

MAZANOR®   ℞
[maz 'a-nor]
(mazindol)

DESCRIPTION

Mazanor (mazindol) is an imidazoisoindole anorectic agent. It is chemically designated as 5-p-chloro-phenyl-5-hydroxy-2,3-dihydro-5H-imidazo (2,1-a) isoindole, a tautomeric form of 2-[2'-(p-chlorobenzoyl) phenyl]-2-imidazoline. Mazanor tablets contain 1 mg mazindol. The inactive ingredients present are calcium sulfate, cellulose, lactose, magnesium stearate, povidone, and talc.

ACTIONS

Mazanor (mazindol), although an isoindole, has pharmacologic activity similar in many ways to the prototype drugs used in obesity, the amphetamines. Actions include central-nervous-system stimulation in humans and animals, as well as such amphetamine-like effects in animals as the production of stereotyped behavior. Animal experiments also suggest certain differences from phenethylamine anorectic drugs, e.g., amphetamine, with respect to site and mechanism of action; for example, mazindol appears to exert its primary effects on the limbic system. The significance of these differences for humans is uncertain. It does not cause brain norepinephrine depletion in animals; on the other hand, it does appear to inhibit storage-site uptake of norepinephrine as is suggested by its marked potentiation of the effect of exogenous norepinephrine on blood pressure in dogs (see "Warnings") and on smooth-muscle contraction *in vitro*. Tolerance has been demonstrated with all drugs of this class in which this phenomenon has been studied.

Drugs used in obesity are commonly known as "anorectics" or "anorexigenics." It has not been established, however, that the action of such drugs in treating obesity is exclusively one of appetite suppression. Other central nervous system actions or metabolic effects may be involved as well. Adult obese subjects, instructed in dietary management and treated with anorectic drugs, lose more weight on the average than those treated with placebo and diet, as determined in relatively short-term clinical trials.

The average magnitude of increased weight loss of drug-treated patients over placebo-treated patients in studies of anorectics in general is ordinarily only a fraction of a pound a week. The rate of weight loss is greatest in the first weeks of therapy for both drug and placebo subjects and tends to decrease in succeeding weeks.

The amount of weight loss associated with the use of Mazanor (mazindol), as with other anorectic drugs, varies from trial to trial, and the increased weight loss appears to be related in part to variables other than the drugs prescribed, such as the interaction between physician-investigator and the patient, the population treated, and the diet prescribed. The importance of non-drug factors in such weight loss has not been elucidated.

The natural history of obesity is measured in years, whereas, most studies cited are restricted to a few weeks' duration; thus, the total impact of drug-induced weight loss over that of diet alone must be considered clinically limited.

INDICATION

Mazanor (mazindol) is indicated in the management of exogenous obesity as a short-term (a few weeks) adjunct in a regimen of weight reduction based on caloric restriction. The limited usefulness of agents of this class (see "Actions") should be measured against possible risk factors inherent in their use, such as those described below.

CONTRAINDICATIONS

Glaucoma; hypersensitivity or idiosyncrasy to Mazanor (mazindol).
Agitated states.
Patients with a history of drug abuse.
During or within 14 days following the administration of monoamine oxidase inhibitors (hypertensive crises may result).

WARNINGS

Tolerance to the effect of many anorectic drugs may develop within a few weeks; if this occurs, the recommended dose should not be exceeded in an attempt to increase the effect; rather, the drug should be discontinued.

Mazanor (mazindol) may impair the ability of the patient to engage in potentially hazardous activities, such as operating machinery or driving a motor vehicle; the patient should therefore be cautioned accordingly.

DRUG INTERACTIONS

Mazanor (mazindol) may decrease the hypotensive effect of guanethidine; patients should be monitored accordingly.

Mazanor (mazindol) may markedly potentiate the pressor effect of exogenous catecholamines. If it should be necessary to give a pressor amine agent (e.g., levarterenol or isoproterenol) to a patient in shock (e.g., from a myocardial infarction) who has recently been taking Mazanor (mazindol), extreme care should be taken in monitoring blood pressure at fre-

Continued on next page

Wyeth-Ayerst—Cont.

quent intervals and initiating pressor therapy with a low initial dose and careful titration.

DRUG DEPENDENCE

Mazanor (mazindol) shares important pharmacologic properties with amphetamines. Amphetamines and related stimulant drugs have been extensively abused and can produce tolerance and severe psychologic dependence. In this regard, the manifestations of chronic overdosage or withdrawal of Mazanor (mazindol) have not been determined in humans. Abstinence effects have been observed in dogs after abrupt cessation for prolonged periods. There was some self-administration of the drug in monkeys. EEG studies and "liking" scores in human studies yielded equivocal results. While the abuse potential of Mazanor (mazindol) has not been further defined, the possibility of dependence should be kept in mind when evaluating the desirability of including Mazanor (mazindol) as part of a weight-reduction program.

USAGE IN PREGNANCY

Mazanor (mazindol) was studied in reproduction experiments in rats and rabbits, and an increase in neonatal mortality and a possible increased incidence of rib anomalies in rats were observed at relatively high doses. Although these studies have not indicated important adverse effects, use of mazindol by women who are or may become pregnant requires that the potential benefit be weighed against the possible hazard to mother and infant.

USAGE IN CHILDREN

Mazanor (mazindol) is not recommended for use in children under 12 years of age.

PRECAUTIONS

Insulin requirements in diabetes mellitus may be altered in association with the use of mazindol and the concomitant dietary regimen.

The least amount feasible should be prescribed or dispensed at one time in order to minimize the possibility of overdosage.

Use only with caution in hypertension with monitoring of blood pressure, since evidence is insufficient to rule out a possible adverse effect on blood pressure in some hypertensive patients. The drug is not recommended in severely hypertensive patients. The drug is not recommended for patients with symptomatic cardiovascular disease including arrhythmias.

ADVERSE REACTIONS

The most common adverse effects of Mazanor (mazindol) are: dry mouth, tachycardia, constipation, nervousness, and insomnia.

Cardiovascular: Palpitation, tachycardia.

Central Nervous System: Overstimulation, restlessness, dizziness, insomnia, dysphoria, tremor, headache, depression, drowsiness, weakness.

Gastrointestinal: Dryness of the mouth, unpleasant taste, diarrhea, constipation, nausea, other gastrointestinal disturbances.

Skin: Rash, excessive sweating, clamminess.

Endocrine: Impotence, changes in libido have rarely been observed with Mazanor (mazindol).

Eye: Treatment of dogs with high doses of Mazanor (mazindol) for long periods resulted in some corneal opacities, reversible on cessation of medication. No such effect has been observed in humans.

DOSAGE AND ADMINISTRATION

Usual dosage is 1 mg three times daily, one hour before meals, or 2 mg once daily, one hour before lunch. The lowest effective dose should be used. To determine the lowest effective dose, therapy with Mazanor may be initiated at 1 mg once a day, and adjusted to the need and response of the patient. Should G.I. discomfort occur, Mazanor may be taken with meals.

OVERDOSAGE

There are no data as yet on acute overdosage with Mazanor (mazindol) in humans.

Manifestations of acute overdosage with amphetamines and related substances include restlessness, tremor, rapid respiration, dizziness. Fatigue and depression may follow the stimulatory phase of overdosage. Cardiovascular effects include tachycardia, hypertension, and circulatory collapse. Gastrointestinal symptoms include nausea, vomiting, and abdominal cramps. While similar manifestations of overdosage may be seen with Mazanor (mazindol), their exact nature has yet to be determined. The management of acute intoxication is largely symptomatic. Data are not available on the treatment of acute intoxication with Mazanor (mazindol) by hemodialysis or peritoneal dialysis, but the substance is poorly soluble except at very acid pH.

HOW SUPPLIED

Mazanor® (mazindol) Tablets, Wyeth®, are available in the following dosage strength in bottles of 30 tablets:
1 mg, NDC 0008-0071, white, round, scored tablet marked "WYETH" and "71".

Keep bottles tightly closed.
Store below 25° C (77° F).
Dispense in tight containers.
Shown in Product Identification Section, page 437

MEDIATRIC®   © ℞
[mē″dē-ăt′rik]
Capsules

Each capsule contains:

Premarin®		
(Conjugated Estrogens, USP)	0.25	mg
Methyltestosterone	2.5	mg
Ascorbic acid (Vit. C)*	100.0	mg
Cyanocobalamin	2.5	mcg
Thiamine mononitrate	10.0	mg
Riboflavin	5.0	mg
Niacinamide	50.0	mg
Pyridoxine HCl	3.0	mg
Calc. pantothenate	20.0	mg
Dried ferrous sulfate	30.0	mg
Methamphetamine HCl	1.0	mg

*Provided as ascorbic acid, 70 mg, and as sodium ascorbate, 30 mg.

CAUTION: Federal law prohibits dispensing without prescription.

---

1. ESTROGENS HAVE BEEN REPORTED TO INCREASE THE RISK OF ENDOMETRIAL CARCINOMA.
Three independent case control studies have reported an increased risk of endometrial cancer in postmenopausal women exposed to exogenous estrogens for more than one year.[1-3] This risk was independent of the other known risk factors for endometrial cancer. These studies are further supported by the finding that incidence rates of endometrial cancer have increased sharply since 1969 in eight different areas of the United States with population-based cancer reporting systems, an increase which may be related to the rapidly expanding use of estrogens during the last decade.[4]

The three case control studies reported that the risk of endometrial cancer in estrogen users was about 4.5 to 13.9 times greater than in nonusers. The risk appears to depend on both duration of treatment[1] and on estrogen dose.[3] In view of these findings, when estrogens are used for the treatment of menopausal symptoms, the lowest dose that will control symptoms should be utilized and medication should be discontinued as soon as possible. When prolonged treatment is medically indicated, the patient should be reassessed on at least a semiannual basis to determine the need for continued therapy. Although the evidence must be considered preliminary, one study suggests that cyclic administration of low doses of estrogen may carry less risk than continuous administration[3]; it therefore appears prudent to utilize such a regimen.

Close clinical surveillance of all women taking estrogens is important. In all cases of undiagnosed persistent or recurring abnormal vaginal bleeding, adequate diagnostic measures should be undertaken to rule out malignancy.

There is no evidence at present that "natural" estrogens are more or less hazardous than "synthetic" estrogens at equiestrogenic doses.

2. ESTROGENS SHOULD NOT BE USED DURING PREGNANCY.
The use of female sex hormones, both estrogens and progestogens, during early pregnancy may seriously damage the offspring. It has been shown that females exposed in utero to diethylstilbestrol, a non-steroidal estrogen, have an increased risk of developing in later life a form of vaginal or cervical cancer that is ordinarily extremely rare.[5,6] This risk has been estimated as not greater than 4 per 1,000 exposures.[7] Furthermore, a high percentage of such exposed women (from 30% to 90%) have been found to have vaginal adenosis,[8-12] epithelial changes of the vagina and cervix. Although these changes are histologically benign, it is not known whether they are precursors of malignancy. Although similar data are not available with the use of other estrogens, it cannot be presumed they would not induce similar changes.

Several reports suggest an association between intrauterine exposure to female sex hormones and congenital anomalies, including congenital heart defects and limb reduction defects.[13-16] One case control study[16] estimated a 4.7-fold increased risk of limb reduction defects in infants exposed in utero to sex hormones (oral contraceptives, hormone withdrawal tests for pregnancy, or attempted treatment for threatened abortion). Some of these exposures were very short and involved only a few days of treatment. The data suggest that the risk of limb reduction defects in exposed fetuses is somewhat less than 1 per 1,000.

In the past, female sex hormones have been used during pregnancy in an attempt to treat threatened or habitual abortion. There is considerable evidence that estrogens are ineffective for these indications, and there is no evidence from well controlled studies that progestogens are effective for these uses.

If MEDIATRIC is used during pregnancy, or if the patient becomes pregnant while taking this drug, she should be apprised of the potential risks to the fetus, and the advisability of pregnancy continuation.

DESCRIPTION

MEDIATRIC provides estrogen and androgen in small doses, nutritional supplements, together with a mild antidepressant. Presented in soluble elastic capsules.

MEDIATRIC Capsules contain the following inactive ingredients: ethyl vanillin, FD&C Blue No. 1, FD&C Red No. 33, gelatin, lecithin, soybean oil, wax mixture.

ACTION

MEDIATRIC provides (1) *steroids* to help counteract declining gonadal hormone secretion, and as important regulators of metabolic processes; (2) *nutritional supplements* specially selected to meet the needs of the aged and aging patient, and to act as necessary catalysts for the maintenance of efficient enzyme systems; and (3) *a mild antidepressant* to impart a gentle emotional uplift.

INDICATION

For use in aging patients of both sexes.
MEDIATRIC HAS NOT BEEN SHOWN TO BE EFFECTIVE FOR ANY PURPOSE DURING PREGNANCY AND ITS USE MAY CAUSE SEVERE HARM TO THE FETUS (SEE BOXED WARNING).

CONTRAINDICATIONS

Estrogens should not be used in women (or men) with any of the following conditions:
1. Known or suspected cancer of the breast except in appropriately selected patients being treated for metastatic disease.
2. Known or suspected estrogen-dependent neoplasia.
3. Known or suspected pregnancy (See Boxed Warning).
4. Undiagnosed abnormal genital bleeding.
5. Active thrombophlebitis or thromboembolic disorders.
6. A past history of thrombophlebitis, thrombosis, or thromboembolic disorders associated with previous estrogen use (except when used in treatment of breast or prostatic malignancy).

Methyltestosterone should not be used in persons with any of the following conditions:
1. Known or suspected carcinoma of the prostate and in carcinoma of the male breast.
2. Severe liver damage.
3. Pregnancy or in breast-feeding mothers because of the possibility of masculinization of the female fetus or breast-fed infant.

WARNINGS

Associated with Estrogens
1. *Induction of malignant neoplasms.* Estrogens have been reported to increase the risk of endometrial carcinoma. (See Boxed Warning.) However, a large case-controlled study indicated no increase in risk of breast cancer in postmenopausal women.[18]
2. *Gallbladder disease.* A recent study has reported a 2- to 3-fold increase in the risk of surgically confirmed gallbladder disease in women receiving postmenopausal estrogens,[17] similar to the 2-fold increase previously noted in users of oral contraceptives.[19,24a]
3. *Effects similar to those caused by estrogen-progestogen oral contraceptives.* There are several serious adverse effects of oral contraceptives, most of which have not, up to now, been documented as consequences of postmenopausal estrogen therapy. This may reflect the comparatively low doses of estrogen used in postmenopausal women. It would be expected that the larger doses of estrogen used to treat prostatic or breast cancer or postpartum breast engorgement are more likely to result in these adverse effects, and, in fact, it has been shown that there is an increased risk of thrombosis in men receiving estrogens for prostatic cancer and women for postpartum breast engorgement.[20-23]
a. *Thromboembolic disease.* It is now well established that users of oral contraceptives have an increased risk of various thromboembolic and thrombotic vascular diseases, such as thrombophlebitis, pulmonary embolism, stroke, and myocardial infarction.[24-31] Cases of retinal thrombosis, mesenteric thrombosis, and optic neuritis have been reported in oral contraceptive users. There is evidence that the risk of several of these adverse reactions is related to the dose of the drug.[32,33] An increased risk of postsurgery thromboembolic complications has also been reported in users of oral contraceptives.[34,35] If feasible, estrogen should be discontinued at least 4 weeks before surgery of the type associated with an increased risk of thromboembolism, or during periods of prolonged immobilization.

While an increased rate of thromboembolic and thrombotic disease in postmenopausal users of estrogens has not been found,[17-24,25-36] this does not rule out the possibility that such an increase may be present or that subgroups of women who have underlying risk factors or who are receiving relatively large doses of estrogens may have increased risk. Therefore estrogens should not be used in persons with active thrombophlebitis or thromboembolic disorders, and they should not be used (except in treatment of malignancy) in persons with a history of such disorders in association with estrogen use. They should be used with caution in patients with cerebral vascular or coronary artery disease and only for those in whom estrogens are clearly indicated.

Large doses of estrogen (5 mg conjugated estrogens per day), comparable to those used to treat cancer of the prostate and breast, have been shown in a large prospective clinical trial in men[37] to increase the risk of nonfatal myocardial infarction, pulmonary embolism and thrombophlebitis. When estrogen doses of this size are used, any of the thromboembolic and thrombotic adverse effects associated with oral contraceptive use should be considered a clear risk.

b. *Hepatic adenoma.* Benign hepatic adenomas appear to be associated with the use of oral contraceptives.[38-40] Although benign, and rare, these may rupture and may cause death through intra-abdominal hemorrhage. Such lesions have not yet been reported in association with other estrogen or progestogen preparations but should be considered in estrogen users having abdominal pain and tenderness, abdominal mass, or hypovolemic shock. Hepatocellular carcinoma has also been reported in women taking estrogen-containing oral contraceptives.[39] The relationship of this malignancy to these drugs is not known at this time.

c. *Elevated blood pressure.* Women using oral contraceptives sometimes experience increased blood pressure which, in most cases, returns to normal on discontinuing the drug. There is now a report that this may occur with use of estrogens in the menopause[41] and blood pressure should be monitored with estrogen use, especially if high doses are used.

d. *Glucose tolerance.* A worsening of glucose tolerance has been observed in a significant percentage of patients on estrogen-containing oral contraceptives. For this reason, diabetic patients should be carefully observed while receiving estrogen.

4. *Hypercalcemia.* Administration of estrogens may lead to severe hypercalcemia in patients with breast cancer and bone metastases. If this occurs, the drug should be stopped and appropriate measures taken to reduce the serum calcium level.

Associated with Methyltestosterone

1. Female patients should be watched carefully for symptoms or signs of virilization such as hoarseness or deepening of the voice, oily skin, acne, hirsutism, enlarged clitoris, stimulation of libido, and menstrual irregularities. At the dosage necessary to achieve a tumor response, androgens will cause masculinization of a female, but occasionally a sensitive female may exhibit one or more of these signs on smaller doses. Some of these changes, such as voice changes, may be irreversible even after drug is stopped.

2. Cholestatic hepatitis with jaundice and altered liver function tests, such as increased BSP retention and rises in SGOT levels, have been reported with methyltestosterone. These changes appear to be related to dosage of the drug. Therefore, in the presence of any changes in liver function tests, the drug should be discontinued.

PRECAUTIONS

Associated with Estrogens

A. General Precautions.

1. A complete medical and family history should be taken prior to the initiation of any estrogen therapy. The pretreatment and periodic physical examinations should include special reference to blood pressure, breasts, abdomen, and pelvic organs, and should include a Papanicolaou smear. As a general rule, estrogen should not be prescribed for longer than one year without another physical examination being performed.

2. Fluid retention—Because estrogens may cause some degree of fluid retention, conditions which might be influenced by this factor such as asthma, epilepsy, migraine, and cardiac or renal dysfunction, require careful observation.

3. Certain patients may develop undesirable manifestations of excessive estrogenic stimulation, such as abnormal or excessive uterine bleeding, mastodynia, etc.

4. Oral contraceptives appear to be associated with an increased incidence of mental depression.[24a] Although it is not clear whether this is due to the estrogenic or progestogenic component of the contraceptive, patients with a history of depression should be carefully observed.

5. Preexisting uterine leiomyomata may increase in size during estrogen use.

6. The pathologist should be advised of estrogen therapy when relevant specimens are submitted.

7. Patients with a past history of jaundice during pregnancy have an increased risk of recurrence of jaundice while receiving estrogen-containing oral contraceptive therapy. If jaundice develops in any patient receiving estrogen, the medication should be discontinued while the cause is investigated.

8. Estrogens may be poorly metabolized in patients with impaired liver function and they should be administered with caution in such patients.

9. Because estrogens influence the metabolism of calcium and phosphorus, they should be used with caution in patients with metabolic bone diseases that are associated with hypercalcemia or in patients with renal insufficiency.

10. Because of the effects of estrogens on epiphyseal closure, they should be used judiciously in young patients in whom bone growth is not complete.

11. Certain endocrine and liver function tests may be affected by estrogen-containing oral contraceptives. The following similar changes may be expected with larger doses of estrogen:

a. Increased sulfobromophthalein retention.

b. Increased prothrombin and factors VII, VIII, IX, and X; decreased antithrombin 3; increased norepinephrine-induced platelet aggregability.

c. Increased thyroid binding globulin (TBG) leading to increased circulating total thyroid hormone, as measured by PBI, T4 by column, or T4 by radioimmunoassay. Free T3 resin uptake is decreased, reflecting the elevated TBG; free T4 concentration is unaltered.

d. Impaired glucose tolerance.

e. Decreased pregnanediol excretion.

f. Reduced response to metyrapone test.

g. Reduced serum folate concentration.

h. Increased serum triglyceride and phospholipid concentration.

Concomitant Progestin Use: The lowest effective dose appropriate for the specific indication should be utilized. Studies of the addition of a progestin for seven or more days of a cycle of estrogen administration have reported a lowered incidence of endometrial hyperplasia. Morphological and biochemical studies of the endometrium suggest that 10 to 13 days of progestin are needed to provide maximal maturation of the endometrium and to eliminate any hyperplastic changes. Whether this will provide protection from endometrial carcinoma has not been clearly established. There are possible additional risks which may be associated with the inclusion of progestin in estrogen-replacement regimens. The potential risks include adverse effects on carbohydrate and lipid metabolism. The choice of progestin and dosage may be important in minimizing these adverse effects.

B. Information for the Patient. See text which appears after the PHYSICIAN REFERENCES.

C. Pregnancy Category X. See CONTRAINDICATIONS and Boxed Warning.

D. Nursing Mothers. As a general principle, the administration of any drug to nursing mothers should be done only when clearly necessary since many drugs are excreted in human milk.

E. Mutagenesis and Carcinogenesis. Long-term continuous administration of natural and synthetic estrogens in certain animal species increases the frequency of carcinomas of the breast, cervix, vagina, and liver. However, in a large case-controlled study of postmenopausal women there was no increase in risk of breast cancer with the use of conjugated estrogens.[18]

Associated with Methyltestosterone

A. Prolonged dosage of androgen may result in sodium and fluid retention. This may present a problem, especially in patients with compromised cardiac reserve or renal disease.

B. If priapism or other signs of excessive sexual stimulation develop, discontinue therapy.

C. In the male, prolonged administration or excessive dosage may cause inhibition of testicular function, with resultant oligospermia and decrease in ejaculatory volume. Use cautiously in young boys to avoid possible premature epiphyseal closure or precocious sexual development.

D. Hypersensitivity and gynecomastia may occur rarely.

E. PBI may be decreased in patients taking androgens.

F. Hypercalcemia may occur. If this does occur, the drug should be discontinued.

ADVERSE REACTIONS

Associated with Estrogens

(See Warnings regarding induction of neoplasia, adverse effects on the fetus, increased incidence of gallbladder disease, and adverse effects similar to those of oral contraceptives, including thromboembolism.) The following additional adverse reactions have been reported with estrogenic therapy, including oral contraceptives:

1. *Genitourinary system:* Breakthrough bleeding, spotting, change in menstrual flow; dysmenorrhea; premenstrual-like syndrome; amenorrhea during and after treatment; increase in size of uterine fibromyomata; vaginal candidiasis; change in cervical erosion and in degree of cervical secretion; cystitis-like syndrome.

2. *Breasts:* Tenderness, enlargement, secretion.

3. *Gastrointestinal:* Nausea, vomiting; abdominal cramps, bloating; cholestatic jaundice.

4. *Skin:* Chloasma or melasma which may persist when drug is discontinued; erythema multiforme; erythema nodosum; hemorrhagic eruption; loss of scalp hair; hirsutism.

5. *Eyes:* Steepening of corneal curvature; intolerance to contact lenses.

6. *CNS:* Headache, migraine, dizziness; mental depression; chorea.

7. *Miscellaneous:* Increase or decrease in weight; reduced carbohydrate tolerance; aggravation of porphyria; edema; changes in libido.

Associated with Methyltestosterone

Cholestatic jaundice

Hypercalcemia, particularly in patients with metastatic breast carcinoma. This usually indicates progression of bone metastases.

Sodium and water retention

Priapism

Virilization in female patients

Hypersensitivity and gynecomastia

ACUTE OVERDOSAGE

Numerous reports of ingestion of large doses of estrogen-containing oral contraceptives by young children indicate that acute serious ill effects do not occur. Overdosage of estrogen may cause nausea, and withdrawal bleeding may occur in females.

DOSAGE AND ADMINISTRATION

Male and female—1 MEDIATRIC Capsule daily.

In the female: To avoid continuous stimulation of breast and uterus, cyclic therapy is recommended (3 week regimen with 1 week rest period—Withdrawal bleeding may occur during this 1 week rest period).

Treated patients with an intact uterus should be monitored closely for signs of endometrial cancer and appropriate diagnostic measures should be taken to rule out malignancy in the event of persistent or recurring abnormal vaginal bleeding.

In the male: A careful check should be made on the status of the prostate gland when therapy is given for protracted intervals.

HOW SUPPLIED

MEDIATRIC Capsules, in bottles of 100 (NDC 0046-0252-81).

PHYSICIAN REFERENCES

1. Ziel, H. K., *et al.*: N. Engl. J. Med. *293*:1167–1170, 1975.
2. Smith, D. C., *et al.*: N. Engl. J. Med. *293*:1164–1167, 1975.
3. Mack, T. M., *et al.*: N. Engl. J. Med. *294*:1262–1267, 1976.
4. Weiss, N. S., *et al.*: N. Engl. J. Med. *294*:1259–1262, 1976.
5. Herbst, A. L., *et al.*: N. Engl. J. Med. *284*:878–881, 1971.
6. Greenwald, P., *et al.*: N. Engl. J. Med. *285*:390–392, 1971.
7. Lanier, A., *et al.*: Mayo Clin. Proc. *48*:793–799, 1973.
8. Herbst, A., *et al.*: Obstet. Gynecol. *40*:287–298, 1972.
9. Herbst, A., *et al.*: Am. J. Obstet. Gynecol. *118*:607–615, 1974.
10. Herbst, A., *et al.*: N. Engl. J. Med. *292*:334–339, 1975.
11. Stafl, A., *et al.*: Obstet. Gynecol. *43*:118–128, 1974.
12. Sherman, A. I., *et al.*: Obstet. Gynecol. *44*:531–545, 1974.
13. Gal, I., *et al.*: Nature *216*:83, 1967.
14. Levy, E. P., *et al.*: Lancet *1*:611, 1973.
15. Nora, J., *et al.*: Lancet *1*:941–942, 1973.
16. Janerich, D. T., *et al.*: N. Engl. J. Med. *291*:697–700, 1974.
17. Boston Collaborative Drug Surveillance Program: N. Engl. J. Med. *290*:15–19, 1974.
18. Kaufman, D. W., *et al.*: J.A.M.A. 252:63–67, 1984.
19. Boston Collaborative Drug Surveillance Program: Lancet *1*:1399–1404, 1973.
20. Daniel, D. G., *et al.*: Lancet *2*:287–289, 1967.
21. The Veterans Administration Cooperative Urological Research Group: J. Urol. *98*:516–522, 1967.
22. Bailar, J. C.: Lancet *2*:560, 1967.
23. Blackard, C., *et al.*: Cancer *26*:249–256, 1970.
24. Royal College of General Practitioners: J. R. Coll. Gen. Pract. *13*:267–279, 1967.
24a. Royal College of General Practitioners: Oral Contraceptives and Health, New York, Pitman Corp., 1974.
25. Inman, W. H. W., *et al.*: Br. Med. J. *2*:193–199, 1968.
26. Vessey, M. P., *et al.*: Br. Med. J. *2*:651–657, 1969.
27. Sartwell, P. E., *et al.*: Am. J. Epidemiol. *90*:365–380, 1969.
28. Collaborative Group for the Study of Stroke in Young Women: N. Engl. J. Med. *288*:871–878, 1973.
29. Collaborative Group for the Study of Stroke in Young Women: J.A.M.A. *231*:718–722, 1975.
30. Mann, J. I., *et al.*: Br. Med. J. *2*:245–248, 1975.
31. Mann, J. I., *et al.*: Br. Med. J. *2*:241–245, 1975.
32. Inman, W. H. W., *et al.*: Br. Med. J. *2*:203–209, 1970.

Continued on next page

Wyeth-Ayerst—Cont.

33. Stolley, P. D., *et al.*: Am. J. Epidemiol. *102*:197–208, 1975.
34. Vessey, M. P., *et al.*: Br. Med. J. *3*:123–126, 1970.
35. Greene, G. R., *et al.*: Am. J. Public Health *62*:680–685, 1972.
36. Rosenberg, L., *et al.*: N. Engl. J. Med. *294*:1256–1259, 1976.
37. Coronary Drug Project Research Group: J.A.M.A. *214*:1303–1313, 1970.
38. Baum, J., *et al.*: Lancet *2*:926–928, 1973.
39. Mays, E. T., *et al.*: J.A.M.A. *235*:730–732, 1976.
40. Edmondson, H. A., *et al.*: N. Engl. J. Med. *294*:470–472, 1976.
41. Pfeffer, R. I., *et al.*: Am. J. Epidemiol. *103*:445–456, 1976.

INFORMATION FOR THE PATIENT

WHAT YOU SHOULD KNOW ABOUT ESTROGENS

Estrogens are female hormones produced by the ovaries. The ovaries make several different kinds of estrogens. In addition, scientists have been able to make a variety of synthetic estrogens. As far as we know, all these estrogens have similar properties and therefore much the same usefulness, side effects, and risks. This leaflet is intended to help you understand what estrogens are used for, the risks involved in their use, and how to use them as safely as possible.

This leaflet includes the most important information about estrogens, but not all the information. If you want to know more, you should ask your doctor for more information or you can ask your doctor or pharmacist to let you read the package insert prepared for the doctor.

USES OF ESTROGEN

THERE IS NO PROPER USE OF ESTROGENS IN A PREGNANT WOMAN.

Estrogens are prescribed by doctors for a number of purposes, including:

1. To provide estrogen during a period of adjustment when a woman's ovaries stop producing a majority of her estrogens, in order to prevent certain uncomfortable symptoms of estrogen deficiency. (With the menopause, which generally occurs between the ages of 45 and 55, women produce a much smaller amount of estrogens.)
2. To prevent symptoms of estrogen deficiency when a woman's ovaries have been removed surgically before the natural menopause.
3. To prevent pregnancy. (Estrogens are given along with a progestogen, another female hormone; these combinations are called oral contraceptives or birth control pills. Patient labeling is available to women taking oral contraceptives and they will not be discussed in this leaflet.)
4. To treat certain cancers in women and men.
5. To prevent painful swelling of the breasts after pregnancy in women who choose not to nurse their babies.

ESTROGENS IN THE MENOPAUSE

In the natural course of their lives, all women eventually experience a decrease in estrogen production. This usually occurs between ages 45 and 55 but may occur earlier or later. Sometimes the ovaries may need to be removed before natural menopause by an operation, producing a "surgical menopause."

When the amount of estrogen in the blood begins to decrease, many women may develop typical symptoms: feelings of warmth in the face, neck, and chest or sudden intense episodes of heat and sweating throughout the body (called "hot flashes" or "hot flushes"). These symptoms are sometimes very uncomfortable. Some women may also develop changes in the vagina (called "atrophic vaginitis") which cause discomfort, especially during and after intercourse.

Estrogens can be prescribed to treat these symptoms of the menopause. It is estimated that considerably more than half of all women undergoing the menopause have only mild symptoms or no symptoms at all and therefore do not need estrogens. Other women may need estrogens for a few months, while their bodies adjust to lower estrogen levels. Sometimes the need will be for periods longer than six months. In an attempt to avoid overstimulation of the uterus (womb), estrogens are usually given cyclically during each month of use, such as three weeks of pills followed by one week without pills.

Sometimes women experience nervous symptoms or depression during menopause. There is no evidence that estrogens are effective for such symptoms without associated vasomotor symptoms. In the absence of vasomotor symptoms, estrogens should not be used to treat nervous symptoms, although other treatment may be needed.

You may have heard that taking estrogens for long periods (years) after the menopause will keep your skin soft and supple and keep you feeling young. There is no evidence that this is so, however, and such long-term treatment carries important risks.

ESTROGENS TO PREVENT SWELLING OF THE BREASTS AFTER PREGNANCY

If you do not breast-feed your baby after delivery, your breasts may fill up with milk and become painful and engorged. This usually begins about 3 to 4 days after delivery and may last for a few days to up to a week or more. Sometimes the discomfort is severe, but usually it is not and can be controlled by pain-relieving drugs such as aspirin and by binding the breasts up tightly. Estrogens can be used to try to prevent the breasts from filling up. While this treatment is sometimes successful, in many cases the breasts fill up to some degree in spite of treatment. The dose of estrogens needed to prevent pain and swelling of the breasts is much larger than the dose needed to treat symptoms of the menopause and this may increase your chances of developing blood clots in the legs or lungs (see below). Therefore, it is important that you discuss the benefits and the risks of estrogen use with your doctor if you have decided not to breast-feed your baby.

THE DANGERS OF ESTROGENS

1. *Endometrial cancer.* There are reports that if estrogens are used in the postmenopausal period for more than a year, there is an increased risk of *endometrial cancer* (cancer of the lining of the uterus). Women taking estrogens have roughly 5 to 10 times as great a chance of getting this cancer as women who take no estrogens. To put this another way, while a postmenopausal woman not taking estrogens has 1 chance in 1,000 each year of getting endometrial cancer, a woman taking estrogens has 5 to 10 chances in 1,000 each year. For this reason *it is important to take estrogens only when they are really needed.*

The risk of this cancer is greater the longer estrogens are used and when larger doses are taken. Therefore you should not take more estrogen than your doctor prescribes. *It is important to take the lowest dose of estrogen that will control symptoms and to take it only as long as it is needed.* If estrogens are needed for longer periods of time, your doctor will want to reevaluate your need for estrogens at least every six months.

Women using estrogens should report any vaginal bleeding to their doctors; such bleeding may be of no importance, but it can be an early warning of endometrial cancer. If you have undiagnosed vaginal bleeding, you should not use estrogens until a diagnosis is made and you are certain there is no endometrial cancer.

NOTE: If you have had your uterus removed (total hysterectomy), there is no danger of developing endometrial cancer.

2. *Other possible cancers.* Estrogens can cause development of other tumors in animals, such as tumors of the breast, cervix, vagina, or liver, when given for a long time. At present there is no good evidence that women using estrogen in the menopause have an increased risk of such tumors, but there is no way yet to be sure they do not; and one study raises the possibility that use of estrogens in the menopause may increase the risk of breast cancer many years later. This is a further reason to use estrogens only when clearly needed. While you are taking estrogens, it is important that you go to your doctor at least once a year for a physical examination. Also, if members of your family have had breast cancer or if you have breast nodules or abnormal mammograms (breast x-rays), your doctor may wish to carry out more frequent examinations of your breasts.

3. *Gallbladder disease.* Women who use estrogens after menopause are more likely to develop gallbladder disease needing surgery than women who do not use estrogens. Birth control pills have a similar effect.

4. *Abnormal blood clotting.* Oral contraceptives increase the risk of blood clotting in various parts of the body. This can result in a stroke (if the clot is in the brain), a heart attack (clot in a blood vessel of the heart), or a pulmonary embolus (a clot which forms in the legs or pelvis, then breaks off and travels to the lungs). Any of these can be fatal.

At this time use of estrogens in the menopause is not known to cause such blood clotting, but this has not been fully studied and there could still prove to be such a risk. It is recommended that if you have had clotting in the legs or lungs or a heart attack or stroke while you were using estrogens or birth control pills, you should not use estrogens (unless they are being used to treat cancer of the breast or prostate). If you have had a stroke or heart attack or if you have angina pectoris, estrogens should be used with great caution and only if clearly needed (for example, if you have severe symptoms of the menopause).

The larger doses of estrogen used to prevent swelling of the breasts after pregnancy have been reported to cause clotting in the legs and lungs.

SPECIAL WARNING ABOUT PREGNANCY

You should not receive estrogen if you are pregnant. If this should occur, there is a greater than usual chance that the developing child will be born with a birth defect, although the possibility remains fairly small. A female child may have an increased risk of developing cancer of the vagina or cervix later in life (in the teens or twenties). Every possible effort should be made to avoid exposure to estrogens during pregnancy. If exposure occurs, see your doctor.

OTHER EFFECTS OF ESTROGENS

In addition to the serious known risks of estrogens described above, estrogens have the following side effects and potential risks:

1. *Nausea and vomiting.* The most common side effect of estrogen therapy is nausea. Vomiting is less common.
2. *Effects on breasts.* Estrogens may cause breast tenderness or enlargement and may cause the breasts to secrete a liquid. These effects are not dangerous.
3. *Effects on the uterus.* Estrogens may cause benign fibroid tumors of the uterus to get larger.
4. *Effects on liver.* Women taking oral contraceptives develop on rare occasions a tumor of the liver which can rupture and bleed into the abdomen and may cause death. So far, these tumors have not been reported in women using estrogens in the menopause, but you should report any swelling or unusual pain or tenderness in the abdomen to your doctor immediately.

Women with a past history of jaundice (yellowing of the skin and white parts of the eyes) may get jaundice again during estrogen use. If this occurs, stop taking estrogens and see your doctor.

5. *Other effects.* Estrogens may cause excess fluid to be retained in the body. This may make some conditions worse, such as asthma, epilepsy, migraine, heart disease, or kidney disease.

SUMMARY

Estrogens have important uses, but they have serious risks as well. You must decide, with your doctor, whether the risks are acceptable to you in view of the benefits of treatment. Except where your doctor has prescribed estrogens for use in special cases of cancer of the breast or prostate, you should not use estrogens if you have cancer of the breast or uterus, are pregnant, have undiagnosed abnormal vaginal bleeding, clotting in the legs or lungs, or have had a stroke, heart attack or angina, or clotting in the legs or lungs in the past while you were taking estrogens.

You can use estrogens as safely as possible by understanding that your doctor will require regular physical examinations while you are taking them and will try to discontinue the drug as soon as possible and use the smallest dose possible. Be alert for signs of trouble including:

1. Abnormal bleeding from the vagina.
2. Pains in the calves or chest or sudden shortness of breath, or coughing blood.
3. Severe headache, dizziness, faintness, or changes in vision.
4. Breast lumps (you should ask your doctor how to examine your own breasts).
5. Jaundice (yellowing of the skin).
6. Mental depression.

Your doctor has prescribed this drug for you and you alone. Do not give the drug to anyone else.

HOW SUPPLIED

MEDIATRIC®—provides estrogen and androgen in small doses, nutritional supplements, and a mild antidepressant. It is supplied as capsules.

Shown in Product Identification Section, page 437

MEPERGAN®   ⒸⒷ
[mep´er-gan]
(meperidine HCl and
promethazine HCl)
Injection

DESCRIPTION

This product is available in concentration providing 25 mg each of meperidine hydrochloride and promethazine hydrochloride per mL with 0.1 mg edetate disodium, 0.04 mg calcium chloride, and not more than 0.75 mg sodium formaldehyde sulfoxylate, 0.25 mg sodium metabisulfite, and 5 mg phenol with sodium acetate buffer.

ACTIONS

Meperidine hydrochloride is a narcotic analgesic with multiple actions qualitatively similar to those of morphine. Phenergan® (promethazine HCl) is a phenothiazine derivative that has several different pharmacologic properties including antihistaminic, sedative, and antiemetic actions.

INDICATIONS

As a preanesthetic medication when analgesia and sedation are indicated. As an adjunct to local and general anesthesia.

CONTRAINDICATIONS

Hypersensitivity to meperidine or promethazine.

Under no circumstances should Mepergan be given by intra-arterial injection, due to the likelihood of severe arteriospasm and the possibility of resultant gangrene (see "Warnings").

Mepergan should not be given by the subcutaneous route; evidence of chemical irritation has been noted, and necrotic lesions have resulted on rare occasions following subcutaneous injection. The preferred parenteral route of administration is by deep, intramuscular injection.

Meperidine is contraindicated in patients who are receiving monoamine-oxidase inhibitors (MAOI) or those who have received such agents within 14 days.

Therapeutic doses of meperidine have inconsistently precipitated unpredictable, severe, and occasionally fatal reactions in patients who have received such agents within 14 days. The mechanism of these reactions is unclear. Some have been characterized by coma, severe respiratory depression, cyanosis, and hypotension and have resembled the syndrome of acute narcotic overdose. In other reactions the predominant manifestations have been hyperexcitability, convulsions, tachycardia, hyperpyrexia, and hypertension. Although it is not known that other narcotics are free of the risk of such reactions, virtually all of the reported reactions have occurred with meperidine. If a narcotic is needed in such patients, a sensitivity test should be performed in which repeated, small, incremental doses of morphine are administered over the course of several hours while the patient's condition and vital signs are under careful observation. (Intravenous hydrocortisone or prednisolone have been used to treat severe reactions, with the addition of intravenous chlorpromazine in those cases exhibiting hypertension and hyperpyrexia. The usefulness and safety of narcotic antagonists in the treatment of these reactions is unknown.)

WARNINGS

Mepergan Injection contains sodium metabisulfite, a sulfite that may cause allergic-type reactions, including anaphylactic symptoms and life-threatening or less severe asthmatic episodes, in certain susceptible people. The overall prevalence of sulfite sensitivity in the general population is unknown and probably low. Sulfite sensitivity is seen more frequently in asthmatic than in nonasthmatic people.

Tolerance and Addiction Liability

Warning—may be habit forming

DRUG DEPENDENCE: Meperidine can produce drug dependence of the morphine type and therefore has the potential for being abused. Psychic dependence, physical dependence, and tolerance may develop upon repeated administration of meperidine, and it should be prescribed and administered with the same degree of caution appropriate to the use of morphine. Like other narcotics, meperidine is subject to the provisions of the Federal narcotic laws.

INTERACTION WITH OTHER CENTRAL NERVOUS SYSTEM DEPRESSANTS: Meperidine should be used with great caution and in reduced dosage in patients who are concurrently receiving other narcotic analgesics, general anesthetics, phenothiazines, other tranquilizers, sedative-hypnotics, tricyclic antidepressants, and other CNS depressants (including alcohol). Respiratory depression, hypotension, and profound sedation or coma may result.

The sedative action of promethazine hydrochloride is additive to the sedative effects of central nervous system depressants; therefore, agents such as alcohol, barbiturates, and narcotic analgesics should either be eliminated or given in reduced dosage in the presence of promethazine hydrochloride. When given concomitantly with promethazine hydrochloride, the dose of barbiturates should be reduced by at least one-half and the dose of analgesic depressants, such as morphine or meperidine, should be reduced by one-quarter to one-half.

HEAD INJURY AND INCREASED INTRACRANIAL PRESSURE: The respiratory-depressant effects of meperidine and its capacity to elevate cerebrospinal-fluid pressure may be markedly exaggerated in the presence of head injury, other intracranial lesions, or a preexisting increase in intracranial pressure. Furthermore, narcotics produce adverse reactions which may obscure the clinical course of patients with head injuries. In such patients, meperidine must be used with extreme caution and only if its use is deemed essential.

INADVERTENT INTRA-ARTERIAL INJECTION: Due to the close proximity of arteries and veins in the areas most commonly used for intravenous injection, extreme care should be exercised to avoid perivascular extravasation or inadvertent intra-arterial injection of Mepergan. Reports compatible with inadvertent intra-arterial injection suggest that pain, severe chemical irritation, severe spasm of distal vessels, and resultant gangrene requiring amputation is likely under such circumstances. Intravenous injection was intended in all the cases reported, but perivascular extravasation or arterial placement of the needle is now suspect. There is no proven successful management of this condition after it occurs, although sympathetic block and heparinization are commonly employed during the acute management because of the results of animal experiments with other arteriolar irritants. Aspiration of dark blood does not preclude intra-arterial needle placement, because blood is discolored upon contact with promethazine. Use of syringes with rigid plungers or of small bore needles might obscure typical arterial backflow if this is relied upon alone.

INTRAVENOUS USE: If necessary, meperidine may be given intravenously, but the injection should be given very slowly, preferably in the form of a diluted solution. Rapid intravenous injection of narcotic analgesics, including meperidine, increases the incidence of adverse reactions; severe respiratory depression, apnea, hypotension, peripheral circulatory collapse, and cardiac arrest have occurred. Meperidine should not be administered intravenously unless a narcotic antagonist and the facilities for assisted or controlled respiration are immediately available. When meperidine is given parenterally, especially intravenously, the patient should be lying down.

When used intravenously, Mepergan should be given at a rate not to exceed 1 mL (25 mg of each component) per minute. When administering any irritant drug intravenously, it is usually preferable to inject it through the tubing of an intravenous infusion set that is known to be functioning satisfactorily. In the event that a patient complains of pain during intended intravenous injection of Mepergan, the injection should immediately be stopped to provide for evaluation of possible arterial placement or perivascular extravasation.

ASTHMA AND OTHER RESPIRATORY CONDITIONS: Meperidine should be used with extreme caution in patients having an acute asthmatic attack, patients with chronic obstructive pulmonary disease or cor pulmonale, patients having a substantially decreased respiratory reserve, and patients with preexisting respiratory depression, hypoxia, or hypercapnia. In such patients, even usual therapeutic doses of narcotics may decrease respiratory drive while simultaneously increasing airway resistance to the point of apnea.

HYPOTENSIVE EFFECT: The administration of meperidine may result in severe hypotension in an individual whose ability to maintain his blood pressure has already been compromised by a depleted blood volume or concurrent administration of drugs such as the phenothiazines or certain anesthetics.

USAGE IN AMBULATORY PATIENTS: Meperidine may impair the mental and/or physical abilities required for the performance of potentially hazardous tasks, such as driving a car or operating machinery. The patient should be cautioned accordingly.

Meperidine, like other narcotics, may produce orthostatic hypotension in ambulatory patients.

USAGE IN PREGNANCY AND LACTATION: Meperidine should not be used in pregnant women prior to the labor period, unless in the judgment of the physician the potential benefits outweigh the possible hazards, because safe use in pregnancy prior to labor has not been established relative to possible adverse effects on fetal development.

When used as an obstetrical analgesic, meperidine crosses the placental barrier and can produce respiratory depression in the newborn; resuscitation may be required (see "Overdosage").

Meperidine appears in the milk of nursing mothers receiving the drug.

PRECAUTIONS

SUPRAVENTRICULAR TACHYCARDIAS: Meperidine should be used with caution in patients with atrial flutter and other supraventricular tachycardias because of a possible vagolytic action which may produce a significant increase in the ventricular response rate.

CONVULSIONS: Meperidine may aggravate preexisting convulsions in patients with convulsive disorders. If dosage is escalated substantially above recommended levels because of tolerance development, convulsions may occur in individuals without a history of convulsive disorders.

ACUTE ABDOMINAL CONDITIONS: The administration of meperidine or other narcotics may obscure the diagnosis or clinical course in patients with acute abdominal conditions.

SPECIAL-RISK PATIENTS: Meperidine should be given with caution, and the initial dose should be reduced in certain patients, such as the elderly or debilitated, and those with severe impairment of hepatic or renal function, hypothyroidism, Addison's disease, and prostatic hypertrophy or urethral stricture.

Antiemetics may mask the symptoms of an unrecognized disease and thereby interfere with diagnosis.

Patients in pain who have received inadequate or no analgesia have been noted to develop "athetoidlike" movements of the upper extremities following the parenteral administration of promethazine. These symptoms usually disappear upon adequate control of the pain.

Ambulatory patients should be cautioned against driving automobiles or operating dangerous machinery until it is known that they do not become drowsy or dizzy from promethazine hydrochloride therapy.

ADVERSE REACTIONS

The major hazards of meperidine, as with other narcotic analgesics, are respiratory depression and, to a lesser degree, circulatory depression; respiratory arrest, shock, and cardiac arrest have occurred.

The most frequently observed adverse reactions include light-headedness, dizziness, sedation, nausea, vomiting, and sweating. These effects seem to be more prominent in ambulatory patients and in those who are not experiencing severe pain. In such individuals, lower doses are advisable. Some adverse reactions in ambulatory patients may be alleviated if the patient lies down.

Other adverse reactions include:

CENTRAL NERVOUS SYSTEM: Euphoria, dysphoria, weakness, headache, agitation, tremor, uncoordinated muscle movements, transient hallucinations and disorientation, visual disturbances and, rarely, extrapyramidal reactions.

GASTROINTESTINAL: Dry mouth, constipation, biliary-tract spasm.

CARDIOVASCULAR: Flushing of the face, tachycardia, bradycardia, palpitation, faintness, syncope.

Cardiovascular effects from promethazine have been rare. Minor increases in blood pressure and occasional mild hypotension have been reported. Venous thrombosis at the injection site has been reported. Intra-arterial injection of Mepergan may result in gangrene of the affected extremity (see "Warnings").

GENITOURINARY: Urinary retention.

ALLERGIC: Pruritus, urticaria, other skin rashes, wheal and flare over the vein with IV injection.

Photosensitivity, although extremely rare, has been reported. Occurrence of photosensitivity may be a contraindication to further treatment with promethazine or related drugs.

OTHER: Pain at injection site; local tissue irritation, induration, and possible tissue necrosis, particularly when injection is repeated at same site; antidiuretic effect.

Patients may occasionally complain of autonomic reactions, such as dryness of the mouth, blurring of vision and, rarely, dizziness following the use of promethazine.

Very rare cases have been reported where patients receiving promethazine have developed leukopenia. In one instance agranulocytosis has been reported. In nearly every instance reported, other toxic agents known to have caused these conditions have been associated with the administration of promethazine.

DOSAGE AND ADMINISTRATION

Parenteral drug products should be inspected visually for particulate matter and discoloration prior to administration, whenever solution and container permit.

WARNING—BARBITURATES ARE NOT CHEMICALLY COMPATIBLE IN SOLUTION WITH MEPERGAN (MEPERIDINE HYDROCHLORIDE AND PROMETHAZINE HYDROCHLORIDE) AND SHOULD NOT BE MIXED IN THE SAME SYRINGE.

The TUBEX® Sterile Cartridge-Needle Unit is designed for single-dose use. VIALS should be used when required doses are fractions of a milliliter, as indicated below.

Mepergan is usually administered intramuscularly. However, in certain specific situations, the intravenous route may be employed. INADVERTENT INTRA-ARTERIAL INJECTION CAN RESULT IN GANGRENE OF THE AFFECTED EXTREMITY (see "Warnings"). SUBCUTANEOUS ADMINISTRATION IS CONTRAINDICATED, AS IT MAY RESULT IN TISSUE NECROSIS (see "Contraindications"). INJECTION INTO OR NEAR PERIPHERAL NERVES MAY RESULT IN PERMANENT NEUROLOGICAL DEFICIT.

When used intravenously, the rate should be not greater than 1 mL of Mepergan (25 mg of each component) per minute; it is preferable to inject through the tubing of an intravenous infusion set that is known to be functioning satisfactorily.

ADULT DOSE: 1 to 2 mL (25 to 50 mg of each component) per single injection, which can be repeated every 3 to 4 hours.

CHILDREN 12 YEARS OF AGE AND UNDER: 0.5 mg of each component per pound of body weight. The dosage may be repeated every 3 to 4 hours as necessary. For preanesthetic medication the usual adult dose is 2 mL (50 mg of each component) intramuscularly with or without appropriate atropinelike drug. Atropine sulfate, 0.3 to 0.4 mg, or scopolamine hydrobromide, 0.25 to 0.4 mg, in sterile solution may be mixed in the same syringe with Mepergan. Repeat doses of 50 mg or less of both promethazine and meperidine may be administered by either route at 3- to 4-hour intervals, as necessary. As an adjunct to local or general anesthesia, the usual dose is 2 mL (50 mg each of meperidine and promethazine).

OVERDOSAGE

SYMPTOMS: Serious overdose with meperidine is characterized by respiratory depression (a decrease in respiratory rate and/or tidal volume, Cheyne-Stokes respiration, cyanosis), extreme somnolence progressing to stupor or coma, skeletal muscle flaccidity, cold and clammy skin, and sometimes bradycardia and hypotension. In severe overdosage, particularly by the intravenous route, apnea, circulatory collapse, cardiac arrest, and death may occur.

TREATMENT: Primary attention should be given to the reestablishment of adequate respiratory exchange through provision of a patent airway and institution of assisted or controlled ventilation. The narcotic antagonist, naloxone

Continued on next page

Wyeth-Ayerst—Cont.

hydrochloride, is a specific antidote against respiratory depression which may result from overdosage or unusual sensitivity to narcotics, including meperidine. The usual initial adult dose of naloxone is 0.4 to 2.0 mg, administered intravenously. If the desired degree of counteraction and improvement in respiratory functions is not obtained, this dosage can be repeated at two- to three-minute intervals while resuscitation efforts continue. If 10 mg of naloxone have been administered without an improvement in the clinical situation, the diagnosis of MEPERGAN overdose should be questioned. An antagonist should not be administered in absence of clinically significant respiratory or cardiovascular depression. Oxygen, intravenous fluids, vasopressors, and other supportive measures should be employed as indicated.

NOTE: In an individual physically dependent on narcotics, the administration of the usual dose of a narcotic antagonist will precipitate an acute withdrawal syndrome. The severity of this syndrome will depend on the degree of physical dependence and the dose of antagonist administered. The use of narcotic antagonists in such individuals should be avoided if possible. If a narcotic antagonist must be used to treat serious respiratory depression in the physically dependent patient, the antagonist should be administered with extreme care and only one-tenth to one-fifth the usual initial dose administered.

Attempted suicides with promethazine have resulted in deep sedation, coma, rarely convulsions and cardiorespiratory symptoms compatible with the depth of sedation present. Extrapyramidal reactions may be treated with anticholinergic antiparkinson agents, diphenhydramine, or barbiturates.

If severe hypotension occurs, levarterenol or phenylephrine may be indicated. Epinephrine is probably best avoided, since it has been suggested that promethazine overdosage could produce a partial alpha-adrenergic blockade.

A paradoxical reaction, characterized by hyperexcitability and nightmares, has been reported in children receiving large single doses of promethazine.

HOW SUPPLIED

Mepergan® (meperidine HCl and promethazine HCl) Injection, Wyeth®, is supplied as follows:

NDC 0008-0234-1, in 10 mL vials, as single vials.

NDC 0008-0235-1, in TAMP-R-TEL® Tamper-Resistant packages of 10 TUBEX® Sterile Cartridge-Needle Units, 2 mL size (22 gauge × 1¼ inch needle).

Protect from light

Shown in Product Identification Section, page 437

MYSOLINE®   ℞

[mĭ'sō-lēn]

Brand of primidone

Anticonvulsant

CAUTION: Federal law prohibits dispensing without prescription.

DESCRIPTION

Chemical name: 5-ethyldihydro-5-phenyl-4,6 (1H, 5H) pyrimidine-dione

Structural formula:

MYSOLINE is a white, crystalline, highly stable substance, M.P. 279–284°C. It is poorly soluble in water (60 mg per 100 mL at 37°C) and in most organic solvents. It possesses no acidic properties, in contrast to its barbiturate analog.

MYSOLINE 50 mg Tablets contain these inactive ingredients: Gelatin, NF; Lactose, NF; Magnesium Stearate, NF; Polyethylene Glycol 8000, NF; Starch, NF.

MYSOLINE 250 mg Tablets contain these inactive ingredients: Gelatin, NF; Magnesium Stearate, NF; Polyethylene Glycol 8000, NF; Starch, NF.

MYSOLINE Suspension contains these inactive ingredients: Ammonia Solution, Diluted; Citric Acid, USP; D&C Yellow No. 10; FD&C Yellow No. 6; Magnesium Aluminum Silicate; Methylparaben, NF; Propylparaben, NF; Saccharin Sodium, NF; Sodium Alginate; Sodium Citrate; Sodium Hypochlorite Solution, USP; Sorbic Acid, NF; Sorbitan Monolaurate; Water, USP, Purified; Flavors.

ACTIONS

MYSOLINE raises electro- or chemoshock seizure thresholds or alters seizure patterns in experimental animals. The mechanism(s) of primidone's antiepileptic action is not known.

Primidone *per se* has anticonvulsant activity as do its two metabolites, phenobarbital and phenylethylmalonamide

(PEMA). In addition to its anticonvulsant activity, PEMA potentiates the anticonvulsant activity of phenobarbital in experimental animals.

INDICATIONS

MYSOLINE, used alone or concomitantly with other anticonvulsants, is indicated in the control of grand mal, psychomotor, and focal epileptic seizures. It may control grand mal seizures refractory to other anticonvulsant therapy.

CONTRAINDICATIONS

Primidone is contraindicated in: 1) patients with porphyria and 2) patients who are hypersensitive to phenobarbital (see ACTIONS).

WARNINGS

The abrupt withdrawal of anti-epileptic medication may precipitate status epilepticus.

The therapeutic efficacy of a dosage regimen takes several weeks before it can be assessed.

Usage in pregnancy: The effects of MYSOLINE in human pregnancy and nursing infants are unknown.

Recent reports suggest an association between the use of anticonvulsant drugs by women with epilepsy and an elevated incidence of birth defects in children born to these women. Data are more extensive with respect to diphenylhydantoin and phenobarbital, but these are also the most commonly prescribed anticonvulsants; less systematic or anecdotal reports suggest a possible similar association with the use of all known anticonvulsant drugs.

The reports suggesting an elevated incidence of birth defects in children of drug-treated epileptic women cannot be regarded as adequate to prove a definite cause and effect relationship. There are intrinsic methodologic problems in obtaining adequate data on drug teratogenicity in humans; the possibility also exists that other factors leading to birth defects, *eg,* genetic factors or the epileptic condition itself, may be more important than drug therapy. The majority of mothers on anticonvulsant medication deliver normal infants. It is important to note that anticonvulsant drugs should not be discontinued in patients in whom the drug is administered to prevent major seizures because of the strong possibility of precipitating status epilepticus with attendant hypoxia and threat to life. In individual cases where the severity and frequency of the seizure disorder are such that the removal of medication does not pose a serious threat to the patient, discontinuation of the drug may be considered prior to and during pregnancy, although it cannot be said with any confidence that even minor seizures do not pose some hazard to the developing embryo or fetus.

The prescribing physician will wish to weigh these considerations in treating or counseling epileptic women of childbearing potential.

Neonatal hemorrhage, with a coagulation defect resembling vitamin K deficiency, has been described in newborns whose mothers were taking primidone and other anticonvulsants. Pregnant women under anticonvulsant therapy should receive prophylactic vitamin K_1 therapy for one month prior to, and during, delivery.

PRECAUTIONS

The total daily dosage should not exceed 2 g. Since MYSOLINE therapy generally extends over prolonged periods, a complete blood count and a sequential multiple analysis-12 (SMA-12) test should be made every six months.

In nursing mothers: There is evidence that in mothers treated with primidone, the drug appears in the milk in substantial quantities. Since tests for the presence of primidone in biological fluids are too complex to be carried out in the average clinical laboratory, it is suggested that the presence of undue somnolence and drowsiness in nursing newborns of MYSOLINE-treated mothers be taken as an indication that nursing should be discontinued.

ADVERSE REACTIONS

The most frequently occurring early side effects are ataxia and vertigo. These tend to disappear with continued therapy, or with reduction of initial dosage. Occasionally, the following have been reported: nausea, anorexia, vomiting, fatigue, hyperirritability, emotional disturbances, sexual impotency, diplopia, nystagmus, drowsiness, and morbilliform skin eruptions. Occasionally, persistent or severe side effects may necessitate withdrawal of the drug. Megaloblastic anemia may occur as a rare idiosyncrasy to MYSOLINE and to other anticonvulsants. The anemia responds to folic acid without necessity of discontinuing medication.

DOSAGE AND ADMINISTRATION

Adult dosage: Patients 8 years of age and older who have received no previous treatment may be started on MYSOLINE according to the following regimen using either 50 mg or scored 250 mg MYSOLINE tablets.

Days 1–3: 100 to 125 mg at bedtime
Days 4–6: 100 to 125 mg bid
Days 7–9: 100 to 125 mg tid
Day 10-maintenance: 250 mg tid

For most adults and children 8 years of age and over, the usual maintenance dosage is three to four 250 mg

MYSOLINE tablets daily in divided doses (250 mg tid or qid). If required, an increase to five or six 250 mg tablets daily may be made but daily doses should not exceed 500 mg qid.

INITIAL: ADULTS AND CHILDREN OVER 8

KEY: · = 50 mg tablet   ● = 250 mg tablet

DAY	1	2	3	4	5	6
AM					··	
NOON						
PM	··	··	··	··	··	··

DAY	7	8	9	10	11	12
AM	··	··	··	●		
NOON	··	··	··	●	Adjust to	
PM	··	··	··	●	Maintenance	

Dosage should be individualized to provide maximum benefit. In some cases, serum blood level determinations of primidone may be necessary for optimal dosage adjustment. The clinically effective serum level for primidone is between 5–12 μg/mL.

In patients already receiving other anticonvulsants: MYSOLINE should be started at 100 to 125 mg at bedtime and gradually increased to maintenance level as the other drug is gradually decreased. This regimen should be continued until satisfactory dosage level is achieved for the combination, or the other medication is completely withdrawn. When therapy with MYSOLINE alone is the objective, the transition from concomitant therapy should not be completed in less than two weeks.

Pediatric dosage: For children under 8 years of age, the following regimen may be used:

Days 1–3:   50 mg at bedtime
Days 4–6:   50 mg bid
Days 7–9:   100 mg bid
Day 10-maintenance: 125 mg tid to 250 mg tid

For children under 8 years of age, the usual maintenance dosage is 125 to 250 mg three times daily or, 10–25 mg/kg/day in divided doses.

HOW SUPPLIED

MYSOLINE Tablets

Each tablet contains 250 mg of primidone (scored), in bottles of 100 (NDC 0046-0430-81) and 1,000 (NDC 0046-0430-91). Also in Unit Dose packages of 100 (NDC 0046-0430-99).

Each tablet contains 50 mg of primidone (scored), in bottles of 100 (NDC 0046-0431-81) and 500 (NDC 0046-0431-85).

MYSOLINE Suspension

Each 5 mL (teaspoonful) contains 250 mg of primidone, in bottles of 8 fluid ounces (NDC 0046-3850-08).

Shown in Product Identification Section, page 437

NORDETTE®–21   ℞

[nor-det '-21]

TABLETS

(levonorgestrel and ethinyl estradiol tablets)

DESCRIPTION

ORAL CONTRACEPTIVE

Each Nordette tablet contains 0.15 mg of levonorgestrel (d (-)-13 beta-ethyl-17-alpha-ethinyl-17-beta-hydroxygon-4-en-3-one), a totally synthetic progestogen, and 0.03 mg of ethinyl estradiol (19-nor-17α-pregna-1,3,5 (10)-trien-20-yne-3,17-diol). The inactive ingredients present are cellulose, FD&C Yellow 6, lactose, magnesium stearate, and polacrilin potassium.

CLINICAL PHARMACOLOGY

Combination oral contraceptives act primarily through the mechanism of gonadotropin suppression due to the estrogenic and progestational activity of the ingredients. Although the primary mechanism of action is inhibition of ovulation, alterations in the genital tract, including changes in the cervical mucus (which increase the difficulty of sperm penetration) and the endometrium (which reduce the likelihood of implantation), may also contribute to contraceptive effectiveness.

INDICATIONS AND USAGE

Nordette is indicated for the prevention of pregnancy in women who elect to use oral contraceptives as a method of contraception.

Oral contraceptives are highly effective. The pregnancy rate in women using conventional combination oral contraceptives (containing 35 mcg or more of ethinyl estradiol or 50 mcg or more of mestranol) is generally reported as less than one pregnancy per 100 woman-years of use. Slightly higher rates (somewhat more than 1 pregnancy per 100 woman-years of use) are reported for some combination products containing 35 mcg or less of ethinyl estradiol, and rates on the order of 3 pregnancies per 100 woman-years are reported for the progestogen-only oral contraceptives.

These rates are derived from separate studies conducted by different investigators in several population groups and cannot be compared precisely. Furthermore, pregnancy rates tend to be lower as clinical studies are continued, possibly due to selective retention in the longer studies of those patients who accept the treatment regimen and do not discontinue as a result of adverse reactions, pregnancy, or other reasons.

In clinical trials with Nordette, 1,084 patients completed 8,186 cycles, and a total of three pregnancies were reported. This represents a pregnancy rate of 0.48 per 100 woman-years.

Table 1 gives ranges of pregnancy rates reported in the literature[1] for other means of contraception. The efficacy of these means of contraception (except the IUD) depends upon the degree of adherence to the method.

TABLE 1
PREGNANCIES PER 100 WOMAN-YEARS
IUD, less than 1–6; Diaphragm with spermicidal products (creams or jellies), 2–20; Condom, 3–36; Aerosol foams, 2–29; Jellies and creams, 4–36;
Periodic abstinence (rhythm) all types, less than 1–47:
1. Calendar method, 14–47;
2. Temperature method, 1–20;
3. Temperature method—intercourse only in postovulatory phase, less than 1–7;
4. Mucus method, 1–25;
No contraception, 60–80.

Dose-Related Risk of Thromboembolism from Oral Contraceptives: Two studies have shown a positive association between the dose of estrogens in oral contraceptives and the risk of thromboembolism.[2,3] For this reason, it is prudent and in keeping with good principles of therapeutics to minimize exposure to estrogen. The oral-contraceptive product prescribed for any given patient should be that product which contains the least amount of estrogen that is compatible with an acceptable pregnancy rate and patient acceptance. It is recommended that new acceptors of oral contraceptives be started on preparations containing 0.05 mg or less of estrogen.

CONTRAINDICATIONS

Oral contraceptives should not be used in women with any of the following conditions:
1. Thrombophlebitis or thromboembolic disorders.
2. A past history of deep-vein thrombophlebitis or thromboembolic disorders.
3. Cerebral-vascular or coronary-artery disease.
4. Known or suspected carcinoma of the breast.
5. Known or suspected estrogen-dependent neoplasia.
6. Undiagnosed abnormal genital bleeding.
7. Known or suspected pregnancy (see Warning No. 5).
8. Benign or malignant liver tumor which developed during the use of oral contraceptives or other estrogen-containing products.

WARNINGS

> Cigarette smoking increases the risk of serious cardiovascular side effects from oral-contraceptive use. This risk increases with age and with heavy smoking (15 or more cigarettes per day) and is quite marked in women over 35 years of age. Women who use oral contraceptives should be strongly advised not to smoke.
>
> The use of oral contraceptives is associated with increased risk of several serious conditions, including thromboembolism, stroke, myocardial infarction, hepatic adenoma, gallbladder disease, hypertension. Practitioners prescribing oral contraceptives should be familiar with the following information relating to these risks.

1. *Thromboembolic Disorders and Other Vascular Problems:* An increased risk of thromboembolic and thrombotic disease associated with the use of oral contraceptives is well-established. Three principal studies in Great Britain[4-6] and three in the United States[7-10] have demonstrated an increased risk of fatal and nonfatal venous thromboembolism and stroke, both hemorrhagic and thrombotic. These studies estimate that users of oral contraceptives are 4 to 11 times more likely than nonusers to develop these diseases without evident cause (Table 2).

CEREBROVASCULAR DISORDERS
In a collaborative American study[9,10] of cerebrovascular disorders in women with and without predisposing causes, it was estimated that the risk of hemorrhagic stroke was 2.0 times greater in users than nonusers and the risk of thrombotic stroke was 4 to 9.5 times greater in users than in nonusers (Table 2).

TABLE 2
SUMMARY OF RELATIVE RISK OF THROMBOEMBOLIC DISORDERS AND OTHER VASCULAR PROBLEMS IN ORAL-CONTRACEPTIVE USERS COMPARED TO NONUSERS

	Relative risk, times greater
Idiopathic thromboembolic disease	4-11
Postsurgery thromboembolic complications	4-6
Thrombotic stroke	4-9.5
Hemorrhagic stroke	2
Myocardial infarction	2-12

MYOCARDIAL INFARCTION
An increased risk of myocardial infarction associated with the use of oral contraceptives has been reported,[11-13] confirming a previously suspected association. These studies, conducted in the United Kingdom, found, as expected, that the greater the number of underlying risk factors for coronary-artery disease (cigarette smoking, hypertension, hypercholesterolemia, obesity, diabetes, history of preeclamptic toxemia) the higher the risk of developing myocardial infarction, regardless of whether the patient was an oral-contraceptive user or not. Oral contraceptives, however, were found to be a clear additional risk factor.

In terms of relative risk, it has been estimated[52] that oral-contraceptive users who do not smoke (smoking is considered a major predisposing condition to myocardial infarction) are about twice as likely to have a fatal myocardial infarction as nonusers who do not smoke. Oral-contraceptive users who are also smokers have about a 5-fold increased risk of fatal infarction compared to users who do not smoke, but about a 10- to 12-fold increased risk compared to nonusers who do not smoke. Furthermore, the amount of smoking is also an important factor. In determining the importance of these relative risks, however, the baseline rates for various age groups, as shown in Table 3, must be given serious consideration. The importance of other predisposing conditions mentioned above in determining relative and absolute risks has not as yet been quantified; it is quite likely that the same synergistic action exists, but perhaps to a lesser extent.

TABLE 3
Estimated annual mortality rate per 100,000 women from myocardial infarction by use of oral contraceptives, smoking habits, and age (in years):
[See table next page]
RISK OF DOSE
In an analysis of data derived from several national adverse-reaction reporting systems,[2] British investigators concluded that the risk of thromboembolism, including coronary thrombosis, is directly related to the dose of estrogen used in oral contraceptives. Preparations containing 100 mcg or more of estrogen were associated with a higher risk of thromboembolism than those containing 50-80 mcg of estrogen. Their analysis did suggest, however, that the quantity of estrogen may not be the sole factor involved. This finding has been confirmed in the United States.[3] Careful epidemiological studies to determine the degree of thromboembolic risk associated with progestogen-only oral contraceptives have not been performed. Cases of thromboembolic disease have been reported in women using these products, and they should not be presumed to be free of excess risk.

ESTIMATE OF EXCESS MORTALITY FROM CIRCULATORY DISEASES
A large prospective study[53] carried out in the U.K. estimated the mortality rate per 100,000 women per year from diseases of the circulatory system for users and nonusers of oral contraceptives according to age, smoking habits, and duration of use. The overall excess death rate annually from circulatory diseases for oral-contraceptive users was estimated to be 20 per 100,000 (ages 15-34—5/100,000; ages 35-44—33/100,000; ages 45-49—140/100,000), the risk being concentrated in older women, in those with a long duration of use, and in cigarette smokers. It was not possible, however, to examine the interrelationships of age, smoking, and duration of use, nor to compare the effects of continuous vs. intermittent use. Although the study showed a 10-fold increase in death due to circulatory diseases in users for 5 or more years, all of these deaths occurred in women 35 or older. Until larger numbers of women under 35 with continuous use for 5 or more years are available, it is not possible to assess the magnitude of the relative risk for this younger age group.

The available data from a variety of sources have been analyzed[14] to estimate the risk of death associated with various methods of contraception. The estimates of risk of death for each method include the combined risk of the contraceptive method (e.g., thromboembolic and thrombotic disease in the case of oral contraceptives) plus the risk attributable to pregnancy or abortion in the event of method failure. This latter risk varies with the effectiveness of the contraceptive method. The findings of this analysis are shown in the bar graph (Figure 1).[14] The study concluded that the mortality associated with all methods of birth control is low and below that associated with childbirth, with the exception of oral contraceptives in women over 40 who smoke. (The rates given for Pill only/smokers for each age group are for smokers as a class. For "heavy" smokers [more than 15 cigarettes a day], the rates given would be about double; for "light" smokers [less than 15 cigarettes a day], about 50 percent.) The lowest mortality is associated with the condom or diaphragm backed up by early abortion. The risk of thromboem-

bolic and thrombotic disease associated with oral contraceptives increases with age after approximately age 30 and, for myocardial infarction, is further increased by hypertension, hypercholesterolemia, obesity, diabetes, or history of preeclamptic toxemia and especially by cigarette smoking. Based on the data currently available, the following chart gives a gross estimate of the risk of death from circulatory disorders associated with the use of oral contraceptives:
SMOKING HABITS AND OTHER PREDISPOSING CONDITIONS—RISK ASSOCIATED WITH USE OF ORAL CONTRACEPTIVES

Age	Below 30	30-39	40+
Heavy smokers	C	B	A
Light smokers	D	C	B
Nonsmokers (no predisposing conditions)	D	C,D	C
Nonsmokers (other predisposing conditions)	C	C,B	B,A

A—Use associated with very high risk.
B—Use associated with high risk.
C—Use associated with moderate risk.
D—Use associated with low risk.

The physician and the patient should be alert to the earliest manifestations of thromboembolic and thrombotic disorders (e.g., thrombophlebitis, pulmonary embolism, cerebrovascular insufficiency, coronary occlusion, retinal thrombosis, and mesenteric thrombosis). Should any of these occur or be suspected, the drug should be discontinued immediately.

A four- to six-fold increased risk of postsurgery thromboembolic complications has been reported in oral-contraceptive users.[15,16] If feasible, oral contraceptives should be discontinued at least 4 weeks before surgery of a type associated with an increased risk of thromboembolism or prolonged immobilization.

Figure 1. Estimated annual number of deaths associated with control of fertility and no control per 100,000 nonsterile women, by regimen of control and age of woman.

Legend:
- No method
- Abortion only
- Pill only/ nonsmokers
- Pill only/ smokers
- IUDs only
- Traditional contraception only (diaphragm or condom)
- Traditional contraception and abortion

PERSISTENCE OF RISK OF VASCULAR DISORDERS
Findings from one study in Great Britain involving cerebrovascular disease[56] and another study in the United States concerning myocardial infarction[57] suggest that an increased risk of these conditions in users of oral contraceptives persists after discontinuation of the oral contraceptive.

Continued on next page

Wyeth-Ayerst—Cont.

Smoking habits	Myocardial infarction			
	Women aged 30-39		Women aged 40-44	
	Users	Nonusers	Users	Nonusers
All smokers	10.2	2.6	62.0	15.9
Heavy*	13.0	5.1	78.7	31.3
Light	4.7	0.9	28.6	5.7
Nonsmokers	1.8	1.2	10.7	7.4
Smokers and nonsmokers	5.4	1.9	32.8	11.7

* Heavy smoker: 15 or more cigarettes per day.
From JAIN, A.K., *Studies in Family Planning*, 8:50, 1977.

In the British study, the risk of cerebrovascular disease remained elevated in former oral-contraceptive users for at least six years after discontinuation. In the U. S. study, an increased risk of myocardial infarction persisted for at least 9 years in women 40- to 49-years-old who had used oral contraceptives for five or more years. The findings in both these studies require confirmation since they are inconsistent with other published information.[9,11,13,58–62]

2. *Ocular Lesions:*
There have been reports of neuro-ocular lesions such as optic neuritis or retinal thrombosis associated with the use of oral contraceptives. Discontinue oral-contraceptive medication if there is unexplained, sudden or gradual, partial or complete loss of vision; onset of proptosis or diplopia; papilledema; or retinal-vascular lesions, and institute appropriate diagnostic and therapeutic measures.

3. *Carcinoma:*
Long-term continuous administration of either natural or synthetic estrogen in certain animal species increases the frequency of carcinoma of the breast, cervix, vagina, and liver. Certain synthetic progestogens, none currently contained in oral contraceptives, have been noted to increase the incidence of mammary nodules, benign and malignant, in dogs.
In humans, three case-control studies have reported an increased risk of endometrial carcinoma associated with the prolonged use of exogenous estrogen in postmenopausal women.[17–19] One publication[20] reported on the first 21 cases submitted by physicians to a registry of cases of adenocarcinoma of the endometrium in women under 40 on oral contraceptives. Of the cases found in women without predisposing risk factors for adenocarcinoma of the endometrium (e.g., irregular bleeding at the time oral contraceptives were first given, polycystic ovaries), nearly all occurred in women who had used a sequential oral contraceptive. These products are no longer marketed. No evidence has been reported suggesting an increased risk of endometrial cancer in users of conventional combination or progestogen-only oral contraceptives.
Several studies[8,21–24] have found no increase in breast cancer in women taking oral contraceptives or estrogens. One study,[25] however, while also noting no overall increased risk of breast cancer in women treated with oral contraceptives, found an excess risk in the subgroups of oral-contraceptive users with documented benign breast disease. A reduced occurrence of benign breast tumors in users of oral contraceptives has been well-documented.[8,21,25–27]
In summary, there is at present no confirmed evidence from human studies of an increased risk of cancer associated with oral contraceptives. Close clinical surveillance of all women taking oral contraceptives is, nevertheless, essential. In all cases of undiagnosed persistent or recurrent abnormal vaginal bleeding, appropriate diagnostic measures should be taken to rule out malignancy. Women with a strong family history of breast cancer or who have breast nodules, fibrocystic disease, or abnormal mammograms should be monitored with particular care if they elect to use oral contraceptives instead of other methods of contraception.

4. *Hepatic Tumors:*
Benign hepatic adenomas have been found to be associated with the use of oral contraceptives.[28–30,46] One study[46] showed that oral contraceptive formulations with high hormonal potency were associated with a higher risk than lower potency formulations. Although benign, hepatic adenomas may rupture and may cause death through intra-abdominal hemorrhage. This has been reported in short-term as well as long-term users of oral contraceptives. Two studies relate risk with duration of use of the contraceptive, the risk being much greater after 4 or more years of oral-contraceptive use.[30,46] While hepatic adenoma is a rare lesion, it should be considered in women presenting abdominal pain and tenderness, abdominal mass or shock. A few cases of hepatocellular carcinoma have been reported in women taking oral contraceptives. The relationship of these drugs to this type of malignancy is not known at this time.

5. *Use in or Immediately Preceding Pregnancy, Birth Defects in Offspring, and Malignancy in Female Offspring:*
The use of female sex hormones—both estrogenic and progestational agents—during early pregnancy may seriously damage the offspring. It has been shown that females exposed in utero to diethylstilbestrol, a nonsteroidal estrogen, have an increased risk of developing in later life a form of vaginal or cervical cancer that is ordinarily extremely rare.[31,32] This risk has been estimated to be of the order of 1 in 1,000 exposures or less.[33,47] Although there is no evidence at the present time that oral contraceptives further enhance the risk of developing this type of malignancy, such patients should be monitored with particular care if they elect to use oral contraceptives instead of other methods of contraception. Furthermore, a high percentage of such exposed women (from 30 to 90%) have been found to have epithelial changes of the vagina and cervix.[34–38] Although these changes are histologically benign, it is not known whether this condition is a precursor of vaginal malignancy. Male children so exposed may develop abnormalities of the urogenital tract.[48–50] Although similar data are not available with the use of other estrogens, it cannot be presumed that they would not induce similar changes.
An increased risk of congenital anomalies, including heart defects and limb defects, has been reported with the use of sex hormones, including oral contraceptives, in pregnancy.[39–42,51] One case-control study[42] has estimated a 4.7-fold increase in risk of limb-reduction defects in infants exposed in utero to sex hormones (oral contraceptives, hormonal withdrawal tests for pregnancy, or attempted treatment for threatened abortion). Some of these exposures were very short and involved only a few days of treatment. The data suggest that the risk of limb-reduction defects in exposed fetuses is somewhat less than one in 1,000 live births. In the past, female sex hormones have been used during pregnancy in an attempt to treat threatened or habitual abortion. There is considerable evidence that estrogens are ineffective for these indications, and there is no evidence from well-controlled studies that progestogens are effective for these uses.
There is some evidence that triploidy and possibly other types of polyploidy are increased among abortuses from women who become pregnant soon after ceasing oral contraceptives.[43] Embryos with these anomalies are virtually always aborted spontaneously. Whether there is an overall increase in spontaneous abortion of pregnancies conceived soon after stopping oral contraceptives is unknown. It is recommended that, for any patient who has missed two consecutive periods, pregnancy should be ruled out before continuing the contraceptive regimen. If the patient has not adhered to the prescribed schedule, the possibility of pregnancy should be considered at the time of the first missed period (or after 45 days from the last menstrual period if the progestogen-only oral contraceptives are used), and further use of oral contraceptives should be withheld until pregnancy has been ruled out. If pregnancy is confirmed, the patient should be apprised of the potential risks to the fetus, and the advisability of continuation of the pregnancy should be discussed in the light of these risks.
It is also recommended that women who discontinue oral contraceptives with the intent of becoming pregnant use an alternate form of contraception for a period of time before attempting to conceive. Many clinicians recommend 3 months, although no precise information is available on which to base this recommendation.
The administration of progestogen-only or progestogen-estrogen combinations to induce withdrawal bleeding should not be used as a test of pregnancy.

6. *Gallbladder Disease:*
Studies[8,23,26] report an increased risk of surgically confirmed gallbladder disease in users of oral contraceptives and estrogens. In one study, an increased risk appeared after 2 years of use and doubled after 4 or 5 years of use. In one of the other studies, an increased risk was apparent between 6 and 12 months of use.

7. *Carbohydrate and Lipid Metabolic Effects:*
A decrease in glucose tolerance has been observed in a significant percentage of patients on oral contraceptives. For this reason, prediabetic and diabetic patients should be carefully observed while receiving oral contraceptives.
An increase in triglycerides and total phospholipids has been observed in patients receiving oral contraceptives.[44] The clinical significance of this finding remains to be defined.

8. *Elevated Blood Pressure:*
An increase in blood pressure has been reported in patients receiving oral contraceptives.[26] In some women, hypertension may occur within a few months of beginning oral-contraceptive use. In the first year of use, the prevalence of women with hypertension is low in users and may be no higher than that of a comparable group of nonusers. The prevalence in users increases, however, with longer exposure, and in the fifth year of use is two-and-a-half to three times the reported prevalence in the first year. Age is also strongly correlated with the development of hypertension in oral-contraceptive users. Women who previously have had hypertension during pregnancy may be more likely to develop elevation of blood pressure when given oral contraceptives. Hypertension that develops as a result of taking oral contraceptives usually returns to normal after discontinuing the drug.

9. *Headache:*
The onset or exacerbation of migraine or development of headache of a new pattern which is recurrent, persistent, or severe, requires discontinuation of oral contraceptives and evaluation of the cause.

10. *Bleeding Irregularities:*
Breakthrough bleeding, spotting, and amenorrhea are frequent reasons for patients discontinuing oral contraceptives. In breakthrough bleeding, as in all cases of irregular bleeding from the vagina, nonfunctional causes should be borne in mind. In undiagnosed persistent or recurrent abnormal bleeding from the vagina, adequate diagnostic measures are indicated to rule out pregnancy or malignancy. If pathology has been excluded, time or a change to another formulation may solve the problem. Changing to an oral contraceptive with a higher estrogen content, while potentially useful in minimizing menstrual irregularity, should be done only if necessary, since this may increase the risk of thromboembolic disease.
Women with a past history of oligomenorrhea or secondary amenorrhea or young women without regular cycles may have a tendency to remain anovulatory or to become amenorrheic after discontinuation of oral contraceptives. Women with these preexisting problems should be advised of this possibility and encouraged to use other contraceptive methods. Post-use anovulation, possibly prolonged, may also occur in women without previous irregularities.

11. *Ectopic Pregnancy:*
Ectopic as well as intrauterine pregnancy may occur in contraceptive failures. However, in progestogen-only oral contraceptive failures, the ratio of ectopic to intrauterine pregnancies is higher than in women who are not receiving oral contraceptives, since the drugs are more effective in preventing intrauterine than ectopic pregnancies.

12. *Breast-feeding:*
Oral contraceptives given in the postpartum period may interfere with lactation. There may be a decrease in the quantity and quality of the breast milk. Furthermore, a small fraction of the hormonal agents in oral contraceptives has been identified in the milk of mothers receiving these drugs.[45,54,55] The effects, if any, on the breast-fed child have not been determined. If feasible, the use of oral contraceptives should be deferred until the infant has been weaned.

PRECAUTIONS
GENERAL
1. A complete medical and family history should be taken prior to initiation of oral contraceptives. The pretreatment and periodic physical examinations should include special reference to blood pressure, breasts, abdomen and pelvic organs, including Papanicolaou smear and relevant laboratory tests. As a general rule, oral contraceptives should not be prescribed for longer than 1 year without another physical examination being performed.
2. Under the influence of estrogen-progestogen preparations, preexisting uterine leiomyomata may increase in size.
3. Patients with a history of psychic depression should be carefully observed and the drug discontinued if depression recurs to a serious degree. Patients becoming significantly depressed while taking oral contraceptives should stop the medication and use an alternate method of contraception in an attempt to determine whether the symptom is drug-related.
4. Oral contraceptives may cause some degree of fluid retention. They should be prescribed with caution, and only with careful monitoring, in patients with conditions which might be aggravated by fluid retention, such as convulsive disorders, migraine syndrome, asthma, or cardiac or renal insufficiency.
5. Patients with a past history of jaundice during pregnancy have an increased risk of recurrence of jaundice while receiving oral-contraceptive therapy. If jaundice develops in any patient receiving such drugs, the medication should be discontinued.

6. Steroid hormones may be poorly metabolized in patients with impaired liver function and should be administered with caution in such patients.

7. Oral-contraceptive users may have disturbances in normal tryptophan metabolism which may result in a relative pyridoxine deficiency. The clinical significance of this is yet to be determined.

8. Serum folate levels may be depressed by oral-contraceptive therapy. Since the pregnant woman is predisposed to the development of folate deficiency and the incidence of folate deficiency increases with increasing gestation, it is possible that if a woman becomes pregnant shortly after stopping oral contraceptives, she may have a greater chance of developing folate deficiency and complications attributed to this deficiency.

INFORMATION FOR THE PATIENT
(See Patient Labeling which follows.)

LABORATORY TESTS
1. The pathologist should be advised of oral-contraceptive therapy when relevant specimens are submitted.
2. Certain endocrine- and liver-function tests and blood components may be affected by estrogen-containing oral contraceptives:
a. Increased sulfobromophthalein retention.
b. Increased prothrombin and factors VII, VIII, IX, and X; decreased antithrombin 3; increased norepinephrine-induced platelet aggregability.
c. Increased thyroid-binding globulin (TBG) leading to increased circulating total-thyroid hormone, as measured by protein-bound iodine (PBI), T4 by column, or T4 by radioimmunoassay. Free T3 resin uptake is decreased, reflecting the elevated TBG; free T4 concentration is unaltered.
d. Decreased pregnanediol excretion.
e. Reduced response to metyrapone test.

DRUG INTERACTIONS
Reduced efficacy and increased incidence of breakthrough bleeding have been associated with concomitant use of rifampin. A similar association has been suggested with barbiturates, phenylbutazone, phenytoin sodium, ampicillin, and tetracycline.

CARCINOGENESIS, MUTAGENESIS, IMPAIRMENT OF FERTILITY
See WARNINGS section #3, 4, and 5 for information on carcinogenesis, mutagenesis, and impairment of fertility.

PREGNANCY
Pregnancy Category X. See Contraindications and Warnings.

NURSING MOTHERS
See WARNINGS. Because of the potential for adverse reactions in nursing infants from oral-contraceptive tablets, a decision should be made whether to discontinue the drug, taking into account the importance of the drug to the mother.

ADVERSE REACTIONS
An increased risk of the following serious adverse reactions has been associated with the use of oral contraceptives (see Warnings):
    Thrombophlebitis.
    Pulmonary embolism.
    Coronary thrombosis.
    Cerebral thrombosis.
    Cerebral hemorrhage.
    Hypertension.
    Gallbladder disease.
    Benign hepatomas.
    Congenital anomalies.
There is evidence of an association between the following conditions and the use of oral contraceptives, although additional confirmatory studies are needed:
    Mesenteric thrombosis.
    Neuro-ocular lesions, e.g., retinal thrombosis and optic neuritis.
The following adverse reactions have been reported in patients receiving oral contraceptives and are believed to be drug-related:
    Nausea and/or vomiting, usually the most common adverse reactions, occur in approximately 10 percent or less of patients during the first cycle. Other reactions, as a general rule, are seen much less frequently or only occasionally.
    Gastrointestinal symptoms (such as abdominal cramps and bloating).
    Breakthrough bleeding.
    Spotting.
    Change in menstrual flow.
    Dysmenorrhea.
    Amenorrhea during and after treatment.
    Temporary infertility after discontinuance of treatment.
    Edema.
    Chloasma or melasma which may persist.
    Breast changes: tenderness, enlargement, and secretion.

    Change in weight (increase or decrease).
    Change in cervical erosion and cervical secretion.
    Possible diminution in lactation when given immediately postpartum.
    Cholestatic jaundice.
    Migraine.
    Increase in size of uterine leiomyomata.
    Rash (allergic).
    Mental depression.
    Reduced tolerance to carbohydrates.
    Vaginal candidiasis.
    Change in corneal curvature (steepening).
    Intolerance to contact lenses.
The following adverse reactions have been reported in users of oral contraceptives, and the association has been neither confirmed nor refuted:
    Premenstrual-like syndrome.
    Cataracts.
    Changes in libido.
    Chorea.
    Changes in appetite.
    Cystitis-like syndrome.
    Headache.
    Nervousness.
    Dizziness.
    Hirsutism.
    Loss of scalp hair.
    Erythema multiforme.
    Erythema nodosum.
    Hemorrhagic eruption.
    Vaginitis.
    Porphyria.
    Hemolytic uremic syndrome.

ACUTE OVERDOSE
Serious ill effects have not been reported following acute ingestion of large doses of oral contraceptives by young children. Overdosage may cause nausea, and withdrawal bleeding may occur in females.

DOSAGE AND ADMINISTRATION
To achieve maximum contraceptive effectiveness, Nordette-21 must be taken exactly as directed and at intervals not exceeding 24 hours. The dosage of Nordette-21 is one tablet daily for 21 consecutive days per menstrual cycle according to prescribed schedule. Tablets are then discontinued for 7 days (three weeks on, one week off). It is recommended that Nordette-21 tablets be taken at the same time each day, preferably after the evening meal or at bedtime.
During the first cycle of medication, the patient is instructed to take one Nordette-21 tablet daily for twenty-one consecutive days beginning on day five of her menstrual cycle. (The first day of menstruation is day one.) The tablets are then discontinued for one week (7 days). Withdrawal bleeding should usually occur within three days following discontinuation of Nordette-21.
(If Nordette-21 is first taken later than the fifth day of the first menstrual cycle of medication or postpartum, contraceptive reliance should not be placed on Nordette-21 until after the first seven consecutive days of administration. The possibility of ovulation and conception prior to initiation of medication should be considered.)
The patient begins her next and all subsequent 21-day courses of Nordette-21 tablets on the same day of the week that she began her first course, following the same schedule: 21 days on—7 days off. She begins taking her tablets on the 8th day after discontinuance regardless of whether or not a menstrual period has occurred or is still in progress. Any time a new cycle of Nordette-21 is started later than the 8th day the patient should be protected by another means of contraception until she has taken a tablet daily for seven consecutive days.
If spotting or breakthrough bleeding occurs, the patient is instructed to continue on the same regimen. This type of bleeding is usually transient and without significance; however, if the bleeding is persistent or prolonged the patient is advised to consult her physician. Although the occurrence of pregnancy is highly unlikely if Nordette-21 is taken according to directions, if withdrawal bleeding does not occur, the possibility of pregnancy must be considered. If the patient has not adhered to the prescribed schedule (missed one or more tablets or started taking them on a day later than she should have) the probability of pregnancy should be considered at the time of the first missed period and appropriate diagnostic measures taken before the medication is resumed. If the patient has adhered to the prescribed regimen and misses two consecutive periods, pregnancy should be ruled out before continuing the contraceptive regimen.
The patient should be instructed to take a missed tablet as soon as it is remembered. If two consecutive tablets are missed they should both be taken as soon as remembered. The next tablet should be taken at the usual time.
Any time the patient misses one or two tablets she should also use another method of contraception until she has taken a tablet daily for seven consecutive days. If breakthrough bleeding occurs following missed tablets it will usually be

transient and of no consequence. While there is little likelihood of ovulation occurring if only one or two tablets are missed, the possibility of ovulation increases with each successive day that scheduled tablets are missed. If three consecutive tablets are missed, all medication should be discontinued and the remainder of the package discarded. A new tablet cycle should be started on the 8th day after the last tablet was taken, and an alternate means of contraception should be prescribed during the seven days without tablets and until the patient has taken a tablet daily for seven consecutive days. In the nonlactating mother Nordette may be prescribed in the postpartum period either immediately or at the first postpartum examination whether or not menstruation has resumed.

HOW SUPPLIED
Nordette®-21 Tablets (0.15 mg levonorgestrel and 0.03 mg ethinyl estradiol tablets), Wyeth®, are available in 6 PIL-PAK® dispensers of 21 tablets each as follows: NDC 0008-0075, light-orange, round tablet marked "WYETH" and "75".

REFERENCES
1. "*Population Reports*," Series H, Number 2, May 1974; Series I, Number 1, June 1974; Series B, Number 2, January 1975; Series H, Number 3, 1975; Series H, Number 4, January 1976 (published by the Population Information Program, The George Washington University Medical Center, 2001 S St. NW., Washington, D.C.).
2. Inman, W. H. W., Vessey, M. P., Westerholm, B., and Engelund, A., "Thromboembolic disease and the steroidal content of oral contraceptives. A report to the Committee on Safety of Drugs," Brit Med J 2: 203-209, 1970.
3. Stolley, P. D., Tonascia, J. A., Tockman, M. S., Sartwell, P. E., Rutledge, A. H., and Jacobs, M. P., "Thrombosis with low-estrogen oral contraceptives," Am J Epidemiol 102: 197-208, 1975.
4. Royal College of General Practitioners, "Oral contraception and thromboembolic disease," J Coll Gen Pract 13: 267-279, 1967.
5. Inman, W. H. W., and Vessey, M. P., "Investigation of deaths from pulmonary, coronary and cerebral thrombosis and embolism in women of childbearing age," Brit Med J 2: 193-199, 1968.
6. Vessey, M. P., and Doll, R., "Investigation of relation between use of oral contraceptives and thromboembolic disease. A further report," Brit Med J 2: 651-657, 1969.
7. Sartwell, P. E., Masi, A. T., Arthes, F. G., Greene, G. R., and Smith, H. E., "Thromboembolism and oral contraceptives: an epidemiological case control study," Am J Epidemiol 90: 365-380, 1969.
8. Boston Collaborative Drug Surveillance Program, "Oral contraceptives and venous thromboembolic disease, surgically confirmed gallbladder disease and breast tumors," Lancet 1: 1399-1404, 1973.
9. Collaborative Group for the Study of Stroke in Young Women, "Oral contraception and increased risk of cerebral ischemia or thrombosis," N Engl J Med 288: 871-878, 1973.
10. Collaborative Group for the Study of Stroke in Young Women, "Oral contraceptives and stroke in young women: associated risk factors," JAMA 231: 718-722, 1975.
11. Mann, J. I., and Inman, W. H. W., "Oral contraceptives and death from myocardial infarction," Brit Med J 2: 245-248, 1975.
12. Mann, J. I., Inman, W. H. W., and Thorogood, M., "Oral contraceptive use in older women and fatal myocardial infarction," Brit Med J 2: 445-447, 1976.
13. Mann, J. I., Vessey, M. P., Thorogood, M., and Doll, R., "Myocardial infarction in young women with special reference to oral contraceptive practice," Brit Med J 2: 241-245, 1975.
14. Tietze, C., "New Estimates of Mortality Associated with Fertility Control," Family Planning Perspectives, 9: 74-76, 1977.
15. Vessey, M. P., Doll, R., Fairbairn, A. S., and Glober, G., "Post-operative thromboembolism and the use of oral contraceptives," Brit Med J 3: 123-126, 1970.
16. Greene, G. R., Sartwell, P. E., "Oral contraceptive use in patients with thromboembolism following surgery, trauma, or infection," Am J Pub Health 62: 680-685, 1972.
17. Smith, D. C., Prentice, R., Thompson, D. J., and Herrmann, W. L., "Association of exogenous estrogen and endometrial carcinoma," N Engl J Med 293: 1164-1167, 1975.
18. Ziel, H. K., and Finkle, W. D., "Increased risk of endometrial carcinoma among users of conjugated estrogens," N Engl J Med 293: 1167-1170, 1975.
19. Mack, T. N., Pike, M. C., Henderson, B. E., Pfeffer, R. I., Gerkins, V. R., Arthur, M., and Brown, S. E., "Estrogens and endometrial cancer in a retirement community," N Engl J Med 294: 1262-1267, 1976.
20. Silverberg, S. G., and Makowski, E. L., "Endometrial carcinoma in young women taking oral contraceptive agents," Obstet Gynecol 46: 503-506, 1975.

Continued on next page

Wyeth-Ayerst—Cont.

21. Vessey, M. P., Doll, R., and Sutton, P. M., "Oral contraceptives and breast neoplasia: a retrospective study," Brit Med J 3: 719-724, 1972.

22. Vessey, M. P., Doll, R., and Jones K., "Oral contraceptives and breast cancer. Progress report of an epidemiological study," Lancet 1: 941-943, 1975.

23. Boston Collaborative Drug Surveillance Program, "Surgically confirmed gallbladder disease, venous thromboembolism and breast tumors in relation to postmenopausal estrogen therapy," N Engl J Med 290: 15-19, 1974.

24. Arthes, F. G., Sartwell, P. E., and Lewison, E. F., "The pill, estrogens, and the breast. Epidemiologic aspects," Cancer 28: 1391-1394, 1971.

25. Fasal, E., and Paffenbarger, R. S., "Oral contraceptives as related to cancer and benign lesions of the breast," J Natl Cancer Inst 55: 767-773, 1975.

26. Royal College of General Practitioners, "Oral Contraceptives and Health," London, Pitman, 1974.

27. Ory, H., Cole, P., MacMahon, B., and Hoover, R., "Oral contraceptives and reduced risk of benign breast diseases," N Engl J Med 294: 419-422, 1976.

28. Baum, J., Holtz, F., Bookstein, J. J., and Klein, E. W., "Possible association between benign hepatomas and oral contraceptives," Lancet 2: 926-928, 1973.

29. Mays, E. T., Christopherson, W. M., Mahr, M. M., and Williams, H. C., "Hepatic changes in young women ingesting contraceptive steroids. Hepatic hemorrhage and primary hepatic tumors," JAMA 235: 730-732, 1976.

30. Edmondson, H. A., Henderson, B., and Benton, B., "Liver-cell adenomas associated with use of oral contraceptives," N Engl J Med 294: 470-472, 1976.

31. Herbst, A. L., Ulfedler, H., and Poskanzer, D. C., "Adenocarcinoma of the vagina," N Engl J Med 284: 878-881, 1971.

32. Greenwald, P., Barlow, J. J., Nasca, P. C., and Burnett, W., "Vaginal cancer after maternal treatment with synthetic estrogens," N Engl J Med 285: 390-392, 1971.

33. Lanier, A. P., Noller, K. L., Decker, D. G., Elveback, L., and Kurland, L. T., "Cancer and stilbestrol. A follow-up of 1719 persons exposed to estrogens in utero and born 1943-1959," Mayo Clin Pro 48: 793-799, 1973.

34. Herbst, A. L., Kurman, R. J., and Scully, R. E., "Vaginal and cervical abnormalities after exposure to stilbestrol in utero," Obstet Gynecol 40: 287-298, 1972.

35. Herbst, A. L. Robboy, S. J., Macdonald, G. J., and Scully, R. E., "The effects of local progesterone on stilbestrol-associated vaginal adenosis," Am J Obstet Gynecol 118: 607-615, 1974.

36. Herbst, A. L., Poskanzer, D. C., Robboy, S. J., Friedlander, L., and Scully, R. E., "Prenatal exposure to stilbestrol: a prospective comparison of exposed female offspring with unexposed controls," N Engl J Med 292: 334-339, 1975.

37. Stafl, A., Mattingly, R. F., Foley, D. V., Fetherston, W., "Clinical diagnosis of vaginal adenosis," Obstet Gynecol 43: 118-128, 1974.

38. Sherman, A. I., Goldrath, M., Berlin, A., Vakhariya, V., Banooni, F., Michaels, W., Goodman, P., and Brown S., "Cervical-vaginal adenosis after in utero exposure to synthetic estrogens," Obstet Gynecol 44: 531-545, 1974.

39. Gal, I., Kirman, B., and Stern, J., "Hormone pregnancy tests and congenital malformation," Nature 216: 83, 1967.

40. Levy, E. P., Cohen, A., and Fraser, F. C., "Hormone treatment during pregnancy and congenital heart defects," Lancet 1: 611, 1973.

41. Nora, J. J., and Nora, A. H., "Birth defects and oral contraceptives," Lancet 1: 941-942, 1973.

42. Janerich, D. T., Piper, J. M., and Glebatis, D. M., "Oral contraceptives and congenital limb-reduction defects," N Engl J Med 291: 697-700, 1974.

43. Carr, D. H., "Chromosome studies in selected spontaneous abortions: I. Conception after oral contraceptives," Canad Med Assoc J 103: 343-348, 1970.

44. Wynn, V., Doar, J. W. H., and Mills, G. L., "Some effects of oral contraceptives on serum-lipid and lipoprotein levels," Lancet 2: 720-723, 1966.

45. Laumas, K. R., Malkani, P. K., Bhatnagar, S., and Laumas, V., "Radioactivity in the breast milk of lactating women after oral administration of 3 H-norethynodrel," Amer J Obstet Gynecol 98: 411-413, 1967.

46. Center for Disease Control, "Increased Risk of Hepatocellular Adenoma in Women with Long-term use of Oral Contraceptives," Morbidity and Mortality Weekly Report, 26: 293-294, 1977.

47. Herbst, A. L., Cole, P., Colton, T., Robboy, S. J., Scully, R. E., "Age-incidence and Risk of Diethylstilbestrol-related Clear Cell Adenocarcinoma of the Vagina and Cervix," Am J Obstet Gynecol, 128: 43-50, 1977.

48. Bibbo, M., Al-Naqeeb, M., Baccarini, I., Gill, W., Newton, M., Sleeper, K. M., Sonek, M., Wied, G. L., "Follow-up Study of Male and Female Offspring of DES-treated Mothers. A Preliminary Report," J of Repro Med, 15: 29-32, 1975.

49. Gill, W. B., Schumacher, G. F. B., Bibbo, M., "Structural and Functional Abnormalities in the Sex Organs of Male

Offspring of Mothers Treated with Diethylstilbestrol (DES)," J of Repro Med, 16: 147-153, 1976.

50. Henderson, B. E., Senton, B., Cosgrove, M., Baptista, J., Aldrich, J., Townsend, D., Hart, W., Mack, T., "Urogenital Tract Abnormalities in Sons of Women Treated with Diethylstilbestrol," Pediatrics, 58: 505-507, 1976.

51. Heinonen, O. P., Slone, D., Nonson, R. R., Hook, E. B., Shapiro, S., "Cardiovascular Birth Defects and Antenatal Exposure to Female Sex Hormones," N Engl J Med 296: 67-70, 1977.

52. Jain, A. K., "Mortality Risk Associated with the Use of Oral Contraceptives," Studies in Family Planning 8: 50-54, 1977.

53. Beral, V., "Mortality Among Oral Contraceptive Users," Lancet, 2: 727-731, 1977.

54. Nilsson, S., Nygren, K., and Johansson, E., "Ethinyl Estradiol in Human Milk and Plasma after Oral Administration," Contraception 17: 131-139, 1978.

55. Nilsson, S., Nygren, K., and Johansson, E., "d-Norgestrel Concentrations in Maternal Plasma, Milk and Child Plasma During Administration of Oral Contraceptives to Nursing Women," Am J Obstet Gynecol, 129: 178, 1977.

56. Royal College of General Practitioners' Oral contraception study, "Incidence of arterial disease among oral contraceptive users," J Royal Col Gen Pract 33: 75-82, 1983.

57. Slone, D., Shapiro, S., Kaufman, D. W., Rosenberg, L., Miettinen, O., and Stolley, P., "Risk of myocardial infarction in relation to current and discontinued use of oral contraceptives," N Engl J Med 305: 420-424, 1981.

58. Inman, W.H.W., "Oral contraceptives and fatal subarachnoid haemorrhage," Brit Med J 2: 1468-1470, 1979.

59. Petitti, D. B., and Wingerd, J., "Use of oral contraceptives, cigarette smoking and risk of subarachnoid haemorrhage," Lancet 2: 234-236, 1978.

60. Thorogood, M., Adam, S. A., and Mann, J. I., "Fatal subarachnoid haemorrhage in young women: role of oral contraceptives," Brit Med J 283: 762, 1981.

61. Rosenberg, L., Hennekens, C. H., Rosner, B., Belanger, C., Rothman, K. J., and Speizer, F. E., "Oral contraceptive use in relation to nonfatal myocardial infarction," Am J Epidemiol 111: 59-66, 1980.

62. Adam, S. A., Thorogood, M., and Mann, J. I., "Oral contraception and myocardial infarction revisited: the effects of new preparations and prescribing patterns," Brit J Obstet Gynaecol 88: 838-845, 1981.

Brief Summary Patient Package Insert: See Lo/Ovral.
DETAILED PATIENT LABELING: See Lo/Ovral.

Shown in Product Identification Section, page 437

NORDETTE®-28   ℞
[nor-det'-28]
TABLETS
(levonorgestrel and ethinyl estradiol tablets)

DESCRIPTION
ORAL CONTRACEPTIVE
21 light-orange Nordette tablets, each containing 0.15 mg of levonorgestrel (d (-)-13 beta-ethyl -17-alpha-ethinyl-17-beta-hydroxygon-4-en-3-one), a totally synthetic progestogen, and 0.03 mg of ethinyl estradiol (19-nor-17α-pregna-1,3,5 (10)-trien-20-yne-3,17-diol), and 7 pink inert tablets. The inactive ingredients present are cellulose, FD&C Red 3, FD&C Yellow 6, lactose, magnesium stearate, and polacrilin potassium.

CLINICAL PHARMACOLOGY
See NORDETTE®-21

INDICATIONS AND USAGE
See NORDETTE-21
Dose-Related Risk of Thromboembolism from Oral Contraceptives: See NORDETTE-21

CONTRAINDICATIONS
See NORDETTE-21

WARNINGS
See NORDETTE-21

PRECAUTIONS
See NORDETTE-21

ADVERSE REACTIONS
See NORDETTE-21
Acute Overdosage: See NORDETTE-21

DOSAGE AND ADMINISTRATION
To achieve maximum contraceptive effectiveness, Nordette-28 must be taken exactly as directed and at intervals not exceeding 24 hours. The dosage of Nordette-28 is one light-orange tablet daily for 21 consecutive days, followed by one pink inert tablet daily for 7 consecutive days, according to prescribed schedule. It is recommended that tablets be taken at the same time each day, preferably after the evening meal or at bedtime.
During the first cycle of medication, the patient is instructed to begin taking Nordette-28 on the first Sunday after the onset of menstruation. If menstruation begins on a Sunday, the first tablet (light-orange) is taken that day. One light-

orange tablet should be taken daily for 21 consecutive days, followed by one pink inert tablet daily for 7 consecutive days. Withdrawal bleeding should usually occur within three days following discontinuation of light-orange tablets.
During the first cycle, contraceptive reliance should not be placed on Nordette-28 until a light-orange tablet has been taken daily for 7 consecutive days. The possibility of ovulation and conception prior to initiation of medication should be considered.
The patient begins her next and all subsequent 28-day courses of tablets on the same day of the week (Sunday) on which she began her first course, following the same schedule: 21 days on light-orange tablets—7 days on pink inert tablets. If in any cycle the patient starts tablets later than the proper day, she should protect herself by using another method of birth control until she has taken a light-orange tablet daily for 7 consecutive days.
If spotting or breakthrough bleeding occurs, the patient is instructed to continue on the same regimen. This type of bleeding is usually transient and without significance; however, if the bleeding is persistent or prolonged, the patient is advised to consult her physician. Although the occurrence of pregnancy is highly unlikely if Nordette-28 is taken according to directions, if withdrawal bleeding does not occur, the possibility of pregnancy must be considered. If the patient has not adhered to the prescribed schedule (missed one or more tablets or started taking them on a day later than she should have), the probability of pregnancy should be considered at the time of the first missed period and appropriate diagnostic measures taken before the medication is resumed. If the patient has adhered to the prescribed regimen and misses two consecutive periods, pregnancy should be ruled out before continuing the contraceptive regimen. The patient should be instructed to take a missed light-orange tablet as soon as it is remembered. If two consecutive light-orange tablets are missed, they should both be taken as soon as remembered. The next tablet should be taken at the usual time.
Any time the patient misses one or two light-orange tablets she should also use another method of contraception until she has taken a light-orange tablet daily for seven consecutive days. If the patient misses one or more pink tablets, she is still protected against pregnancy *provided* she begins taking light-orange tablets again on the proper day.
If breakthrough bleeding occurs following missed light-orange tablets, it will usually be transient and of no consequence. While there is little likelihood of ovulation occurring if only one or two light-orange tablets are missed, the possibility of ovulation increases with each successive day that scheduled light-orange tablets are missed. (If three consecutive light-orange Nordette tablets are missed, all medication should be discontinued and the remainder of the 28-day package discarded. A new tablet cycle should be started on the first Sunday following the last missed tablet, and an alternate means of contraception should be prescribed during the days without tablets and until the patient has taken a light-orange tablet daily for 7 consecutive days.) In the non-lactating mother, Nordette may be prescribed in the postpartum period either immediately or at the first postpartum examination whether or not menstruation has resumed.

HOW SUPPLIED
Nordette®-28 Tablets (0.15 mg levonorgestrel and 0.03 mg ethinyl estradiol tablets), Wyeth®, are available in 6 PIL-PAK® dispensers, each containing 28 tablets as follows:
21 active tablets, NDC 0008-2533, light-orange, round tablet marked "WYETH" and "75".
7 inert tablets, NDC 0008-0486, pink, round tablet marked "WYETH" and "486".

REFERENCES
See NORDETTE-21.
Brief Summary Patient Package Insert: See LO/OVRAL.
DETAILED PATIENT LABELING: See LO/OVRAL.

Shown in Product Identification Section, page 437

NURSOY®
[nur-soy]
Soy protein formula
READY-TO-FEED
CONCENTRATED LIQUID
POWDER

NURSOY® milk free formula is intended to meet the nutritional needs of infants and children who are not breast-fed and are allergic to cow's milk protein or intolerant to lactose. NURSOY Ready-to-Feed and Concentrated Liquid contain sucrose as their carbohydrate. NURSOY Powder contains corn syrup solids and sucrose as its carbohydrate. Professional advice should be followed.

INGREDIENTS
(in normal dilution supplying 20 calories per fluidounce): 87% water; 6.7% sucrose; 3.4% oleo, coconut, oleic (safflower) and soybean oils; 2.3% soy protein isolate; 0.10% potassium citrate; 0.09% monobasic sodium phosphate;

0.04% calcium carbonate; 0.04% dibasic calcium phosphate; 0.03% magnesium chloride; 0.03% calcium chloride; 0.03% soy lecithin; 0.03% calcium carrageenan; 0.03% calcium hydroxide; 0.03% l-methionine; 0.01% sodium chloride; 0.01% potassium bicarbonate; taurine; ferrous, zinc and cupric sulfates; L-carnitine; (68ppb) potassium iodide; ascorbic acid; choline chloride; alpha tocopheryl acetate; niacinamide; calcium pantothenate; riboflavin; vitamin A palmitate; thiamine hydrochloride; pyridoxine hydrochloride; beta-carotene; phytonadione; folic acid; biotin; cholecalciferol; cyanocobalamin. NURSOY Powder contains corn syrup solids and sucrose. NURSOY Ready-to-Feed and Concentrated Liquid contain only sucrose.

PROXIMATE ANALYSIS
at 20 calories per fluidounce
READY-TO-FEED, CONCENTRATED LIQUID and POWDER

	(W/V)
Protein	2.1%
Fat	3.6%
Carbohydrate	6.9%
Ash	0.35%
Water	87.0%
Crude fiber	not more than 0.01%
Calories/fl. oz.	20

Vitamins, Minerals: In normal dilution, each liter contains:

A	2,000	IU
D₃	400	IU
E	9.5	IU
K₁	100	mcg
C (ascorbic acid)	55	mg
B₁ (thiamine)	670	mcg
B₂ (riboflavin)	1000	mcg
B₆	420	mcg
B₁₂	2	mcg
Niacin	5000	mcg
Pantothenic acid	3000	mcg
Folic acid (folacin)	50	mcg
Choline	85	mg
Inositol	27	mg
Biotin	35	mcg
Calcium	600	mg
Phosphorus	420	mg
Sodium	200	mg
Potassium	700	mg
Chloride	375	mg
Magnesium	67	mg
Manganese	200	mcg
Iron	11.5	mg
Copper	470	mcg
Zinc	5	mg
Iodine	60	mcg

PREPARATION
Ready-to-Feed (32 fl. oz. cans of 20 calories per fluidounce formula)—shake can, open and pour into previously sterilized nursing bottle; attach nipple and feed. Cover opened can and immediately store in refrigerator. Use contents of can within 48 hours of opening.
Concentrated Liquid—For normal dilution supplying 20 calories per fluidounce, use equal amounts of Nursoy® liquid and cooled, previously boiled water. *Note: Prepared formula should be used within 24 hours.*
Powder—For normal dilution supplying 20 calories per fluidounce, add 1 scoop (8.9 grams or 1 standard tablespoonful) of NURSOY POWDER, packed and leveled, to 2 fluidounces of water. For larger amounts of formula, add ¼ standard measuring cup of powder (35.5 grams), packed and leveled, to 8 fluidounces (1 standard measuring cup) of water.

HOW SUPPLIED
Ready-to-Feed —presterilized and premixed, 32 fluidounce (1 quart) cans, cases of 6; *Concentrated Liquid* —13 fluidounce cans, cases of 24; *Powder*—1 pound cans, cases of 6.
Also available to hospitals only:
Ready-to-Feed 4 oz. disposable bottles (48 bottles/case) as part of the Wyeth Hospital Infant Feeding System.
Shown in Product Identification Section, page 437

OMNIPEN®
[om 'nĭ-pen]
(ampicillin)
CAPSULES

DESCRIPTION
Omnipen (ampicillin) is a semisynthetic penicillin derived from the basic penicillin nucleus, 6-amino-penicillanic acid. Omnipen capsules contain 250 mg or 500 mg ampicillin. The inactive ingredients present are D&C Red 22, D&C Red 28, FD&C Blue 1, gelatin, lactose, methylcellulose, stearic acid, and titanium dioxide.

HOW SUPPLIED
Omnipen® (ampicillin) Capsules, Wyeth®, contain 250 mg or 500 mg ampicillin anhydrous and are available as follows:

250 mg, NDC 0008-0053, violet and pink capsule marked "WYETH" and "53", in bottles of 500 capsules.
500 mg, NDC 0008-0309, violet and pink capsule marked "WYETH" and "309", in bottles of 100 and 500 capsules.
For prescribing information write to Professional Service, Wyeth-Ayerst Laboratories, Box 8299, Philadelphia, PA 19101, or contact your local Wyeth-Ayerst representative.
Shown in Product Identification Section, page 437

OMNIPEN®
[om 'nĭ-pen]
(ampicillin)
ORAL SUSPENSION

DESCRIPTION
Omnipen (ampicillin) is a semisynthetic penicillin derived from the basic penicillin nucleus, 6-amino-penicillanic acid. Omnipen for oral suspension is a powder which when reconstituted as directed yields a suspension of 125 mg or 250 mg ampicillin per 5 mL. The inactive ingredients present are artificial flavors, colloidal silicon dioxide, methylparaben, propylparaben, sodium benzoate, sodium citrate, sucrose, and water. Each dosage strength of suspension also contains the following:
125 mg per 5 mL—carboxymethylcellulose sodium FD&C Blue 1, FD&C Red 40, FD&C Yellow 6, and natural flavors; 250 mg per 5 mL—FD&C Red 3.

HOW SUPPLIED
Omnipen® (ampicillin) for Oral Suspension, Wyeth®, is available in the following dosage strengths as a powder, which when reconstituted as directed yields a palatable suspension:
125 mg per 5 mL, NDC 0008-0054, white powder in bottles to make 100 mL, 150 mL, or 200 mL of salmon-colored suspension.
250 mg per 5 mL, NDC 0008-0055, pink powder in bottles to make 100 mL, 150 mL, or 200 mL of pink suspension.
For prescribing information write to Professional Service, Wyeth-Ayerst Laboratories, Box 8299, Philadelphia, PA 19101, or contact your local Wyeth-Ayerst representative.

OMNIPEN®-N
[om 'nĭ-pen-N]
(ampicillin sodium)
INJECTION

HOW SUPPLIED
FOR PARENTERAL ADMINISTRATION
Conventional Vials (for intravenous or intramuscular use)
Supplied in packages of ten conventional vials in the following dosage strengths:
125 mg, NDC 0008-0315-07, equivalent to 125 mg ampicillin per vial.
250 mg, NDC 0008-0315-05, equivalent to 250 mg ampicillin per vial.
500 mg, NDC 0008-0315-06, equivalent to 500 mg ampicillin per vial.
1 gram, NDC 0008-0315-08, equivalent to 1 gram ampicillin per vial.
2 gram, NDC 0008-0315-10, equivalent to 2 gram ampicillin per vial.
FOR INTRAVENOUS USE ONLY
ADD-Vantage™ Vials
Supplied in packages of ten ADD-Vantage™ vials in the following dosage strengths:
500 mg, NDC 0008-0315-38, equivalent to 500 mg ampicillin per vial.
1 gram, NDC 0008-0315-40, equivalent to 1 gram ampicillin per vial.
2 gram, NDC 0008-0315-42, equivalent to 2 gram ampicillin per vial.
The ADD-Vantage Vials are only to be used with Abbott Laboratories' ADD-Vantage Flexible Diluent Container containing:
0.9% Sodium Chloride Injection, USP, 50 mL and 100 mL sizes.
5% Dextrose Injection, USP, 50 mL and 100 mL sizes.
Piggyback Vials
Supplied as single units in packages of ten piggyback vials in the following dosage strengths:
500 mg, NDC 0008-0315-28, equivalent to 500 mg ampicillin per vial.
1 gram, NDC 0008-0315-24, equivalent to 1 gram ampicillin per vial.
2 gram, NDC 0008-0315-26, equivalent to 2 gram ampicillin per vial.
Omnipen®-N (ampicillin sodium) for Injection, Wyeth®, in Pharmacy Bulk Packages of single vials is available in the following dosage strength:
10 gram, NDC 0008-0315-29, equivalent to 10 gram ampicillin per vial.

For prescribing information write to Professional Service, Wyeth-Ayerst Laboratories, Box 8299, Philadelphia, PA 19101, or contact your local Wyeth-Ayerst representative.

ORUDIS®   ℞
[ŏ "roo 'dĭs]
(ketoprofen)
Capsules

DESCRIPTION
Orudis (ketoprofen) is a nonsteroidal antiinflammatory drug. The chemical name for ketoprofen is 2-(3-benzoylphenyl)-propionic acid with the following structural formula:

Its empirical formula is $C_{16}H_{14}O_3$, with a molecular weight of 254.29.
Ketoprofen is a white or off-white, odorless, nonhygroscopic, fine to granular powder, melting at about 95°C. It is freely soluble in ethanol, chloroform, acetone, and ether; soluble in benzene and strong alkali, but practically insoluble in water at 20°C.
Orudis capsules contain 25 mg, 50 mg, or 75 mg of ketoprofen for oral administration. The inactive ingredients present are D&C Yellow 10, FD&C Blue 1, FD&C Yellow 6, gelatin, lactose, magnesium stearate, and titanium dioxide. The 25 mg dosage strength also contains FD&C Red 3.

CLINICAL PHARMACOLOGY
Orudis (ketoprofen) is a nonsteroidal antiinflammatory drug with analgesic and antipyretic properties.
The antiinflammatory, analgesic, and antipyretic properties of Orudis have been demonstrated in classical animal and *in vitro* test systems. In antiinflammatory models Orudis has been shown to have inhibitory effects on prostaglandin and leukotriene synthesis, to have antibradykinin activity, as well as to have lysosomal membrane-stabilizing action. However, its mode of action, like that of other nonsteroidal antiinflammatory drugs, is not fully understood.
Orudis is rapidly and completely absorbed from the gastrointestinal tract. Mean Orudis peak plasma levels are reached in 0.5 to 2 hours. The total absolute bioavailability of Orudis, as demonstrated by area under the plasma concentration-time curve (AUC), is approximately 90% for capsule formulations tested when compared to IV administration and is linear for 75 to 200 mg single doses. The plasma clearance of ketoprofen is approximately 0.08 L/kg/hr with a V_d of 0.1 L/kg after IV administration. The mean plasma elimination half-life of Orudis ranged from 2 to 4 hours in 14 pharmacokinetic studies which included 6 to 24 normal volunteers.
Following absorption, Orudis can be detected in plasma as the unchanged compound, hydroxylated metabolites and their respective glucuronides. There are no known active metabolites of Orudis. The drug is 99% bound to plasma proteins, mainly to the albumin fraction. Approximately 60% of an administered dose of Orudis is excreted in the urine primarily as the glucuronide metabolite in the first 24 hours. Enterohepatic recirculation of the drug has been postulated to account for the other 40% of the absorbed ketoprofen, although biliary levels have never been measured to confirm this.
Orudis has been shown to not induce drug-metabolizing enzymes.
Steady-state concentrations of Orudis are attained within 24 hours after commencing treatment.
When ketoprofen is administered with food, its total bioavailability (AUC) is not altered; however, the rate of absorption is slowed, resulting in delayed and reduced peak concentrations (C_{max}). Following a single 50 mg dose of Orudis while fasting, the mean C_{max} is 4.1 mg/L (at 1.1 hours); when administered after food, it decreases to 2.4 mg/L (at 2.0 hours).
To date, studies of the effects of age and renal-function impairment have been small, generally involving 5 to 8 subjects per group, but they indicate modest decrease in clearance in the elderly and in patients with impaired renal function. In normal elderly volunteers (mean age 73 years), the plasma and renal clearance and protein-binding were reduced while the V_d increased when compared to a younger normal population (mean age 27 years). (Plasma clearance and V_d were 0.05 L/kg/hr and 0.4 L/kg in elderly and 0.06 L/kg/hr and 0.3 L/kg in young subjects, respectively.) The mean half-life of Orudis in this normal geriatric population, as well as in a rheumatoid elderly population (mean age 64 years), was about 5 hours as compared to 3 hours in the younger population.

Continued on next page

Wyeth-Ayerst—Cont.

Patients with impaired renal function (mean age 44 years) also demonstrate decreases in plasma clearance (0.04 L/kg/hr) of drug, with the mean half-life increasing to about 3.5 hours.

For patients with alcoholic cirrhosis, no significant changes in the kinetic disposition of Orudis were observed relative to age-matched normal subjects; the plasma clearance of drug was 0.07 L/kg/hr) in both groups (N = 8 for each group) and total bioavailability was comparable. However, the protein unbound (biologically active) fraction was increased from 0.85% to 1.15%, probably due to hypoalbuminemia, and high variability was observed in the pharmacokinetics in cirrhotic patients. Therefore, these patients should be carefully monitored and daily doses kept at the minimum levels providing the desired therapeutic effect.

In healthy men, the average blood loss in stool, measured over a one-week period during administration of 200 mg per day of Orudis, was 50% lower than that resulting from administration of 3,900 mg per day of aspirin. In addition, a double-blind crossover trial using gastroscopy in 13 normal volunteers demonstrated fewer mucosal lesions with Orudis than aspirin.

The efficacy of Orudis has been demonstrated in patients with rheumatoid arthritis and osteoarthritis. Using standard assessment of therapeutic response, Orudis demonstrated effectiveness comparable to aspirin, ibuprofen, and indomethacin.

In studies in patients with rheumatoid arthritis, Orudis was administered in combination with gold salts, antimalarials, and/or corticosteroids with results comparable to those seen with the control nonsteroidal drugs.

The effectiveness of Orudis as a general purpose analgesic has been studied in standard pain models which have shown the effectiveness of doses of 25 to 150 mg. Doses of 25 mg were superior to placebo. Larger doses than 25 mg generally could not be shown significantly more effective but there was a tendency toward faster onset and greater duration of action with 50 mg and, in the case of dysmenorrhea, a significantly greater effect overall with 75 mg. Doses greater than 50 to 75 mg did not have increased analgesic effect.

INDICATIONS AND USAGE

Orudis is indicated for the acute or long-term treatment of the signs and symptoms of rheumatoid arthritis and osteoarthritis.

Orudis is indicated for the relief of mild-to-moderate pain. Orudis is also indicated for treatment of primary dysmenorrhea.

CONTRAINDICATIONS

Orudis is contraindicated in patients who have shown hypersensitivity to it. Orudis should not be given to patients in whom aspirin or other nonsteroidal antiinflammatory drugs induce asthma, urticaria, or other allergic-type reactions, because severe, rarely fatal, anaphylactic reactions to Orudis have been reported in such patients.

WARNINGS

RISK OF GI ULCERATION, BLEEDING, AND PERFORATION WITH NSAID THERAPY:

Serious gastrointestinal toxicity, such as bleeding, ulceration, and perforation, can occur at any time, with or without warning symptoms, in patients treated chronically with NSAID therapy. Athough minor upper-gastrointestinal problems, such as dyspepsia, are common, usually developing early in therapy, physicians should remain alert for ulceration and bleeding in patients treated chronically with NSAIDs even in the absence of previous GI-tract symptoms. In patients observed in clinical trials of several months to two years duration, symptomatic upper-GI ulcers, gross bleeding, or perforation appear to occur in approximately 1% of patients treated for 3 to 6 months, and in about 2–4% of patients treated for one year. Physicians should inform patients about the signs and/or symptoms of serious GI toxicity and what steps to take if they occur.

Studies to date have not identified any subset of patients not at risk of developing peptic ulceration and bleeding. Except for a prior history of serious GI events and other risk factors known to be associated with peptic ulcer disease, such as alcoholism, smoking, etc., no risk factors (e.g., age, sex) have been associated with increased risk. Elderly or debilitated patients seem to tolerate ulceration or bleeding less well than other individuals, and most spontaneous reports of fatal GI events are in this population. Studies to date are inconclusive concerning the relative risk of various NSAIDs in causing such reactions. High doses of any NSAID probably carry a greater risk of these reactions, although controlled clinical trials showing this do not exist in most cases. In considering the use of relatively large doses (within the recommended dosage range), sufficient benefit should be anticipated to offset the potential increased risk of GI toxicity.

GENERAL PRECAUTIONS

Orudis and other nonsteroidal antiinflammatory drugs cause nephritis in mice and rats associated with chronic administration. Cases of interstitial nephritis and nephrotic syndrome have been reported with Orudis since it has been marketed abroad.

A second form of renal toxicity has been seen in patients with conditions leading to a reduction in renal blood flow or blood volume, where renal prostaglandins have a supportive role in the maintenance of renal blood flow. In these patients administration of a nonsteroidal antiinflammatory drug results in a dose-dependent decrease in prostaglandin synthesis and, secondarily, in renal blood flow which may precipitate overt renal failure. Patients at greatest risk of this reaction are those with impaired renal function, heart failure, liver dysfunction, those taking diuretics, and the elderly. Discontinuation of nonsteroidal antiinflammatory drug therapy is typically followed by recovery to the pretreatment state.

Since ketoprofen is primarily eliminated by the kidneys and its pharmacokinetics are altered by renal failure (see "Clinical Pharmacology"), patients with significantly impaired renal function should be closely monitored, and a reduction of dosage should be anticipated to avoid accumulation of ketoprofen and/or its metabolites.

As with other nonsteroidal antiinflammatory drugs, borderline elevations of one or more liver-function tests may occur in up to 15% of patients. These abnormalities may progress, may remain essentially unchanged, or may disappear with continued therapy. The SGPT (ALT) test is probably the most sensitive indicator of liver dysfunction. Meaningful (3 times the upper limit of normal) elevations of SGPT or SGOT (AST) occurred in controlled clinical trials in less than 1% of patients. A patient with symptoms and/or signs suggesting liver dysfunction, or in whom an abnormal liver test has occurred, should be evaluated for evidence of the development of a more severe hepatic reaction while on therapy with ketoprofen. Serious hepatic reactions, including jaundice, have been reported from postmarketing experience with ketoprofen as well as with other nonsteroidal antiinflammatory drugs.

If steroid dosage is reduced or eliminated during therapy, it should be reduced slowly and the patients observed closely for any evidence of adverse effects, including adrenal insufficiency and exacerbation of symptoms of arthritis.

Anemia is commonly observed in rheumatoid arthritis and is sometimes aggravated by nonsteroidal antiinflammatory drugs, which may produce fluid retention or minor gastrointestinal blood loss in some patients. Therefore, patients with initial hemoglobin values of 10 g/dL or less who are to receive long-term therapy should have hemoglobin values determined frequently.

Peripheral edema has been observed in approximately 2% of patients taking ketoprofen. Therefore, as with other nonsteroidal antiinflammatory drugs, ketoprofen should be used with caution in patients with fluid retention, hypertension, or heart failure.

INFORMATION FOR PATIENTS

Orudis, like other drugs of its class, is not free of side effects. The side effects of these drugs can cause discomfort and, rarely, there are more serious side effects, such as gastrointestinal bleeding, which may result in hospitalization and even fatal outcomes.

NSAIDs (Nonsteroidal Anti-Inflammatory Drugs) are often essential agents in the management of arthritis and have a major role in the treatment of pain, but they also may be commonly employed for conditioins which are less serious. Physicians may wish to discuss with their patients the potential risks (see "Warnings", "Precautions," and "Adverse Reactions" sections) and likely benefits of NSAID treatment, particularly when the drugs are used for less serious conditions where treatment without NSAIDs may represent an acceptable alternative to both the patient and physician. Because aspirin causes an increase in the level of unbound ketoprofen, patients should be advised not to take aspirin while taking Orudis (see "Drug Interactions"). It is possible that minor adverse symptoms of gastric intolerance may be prevented by administering Orudis with antacids, food, or milk. Because antacids do not affect bioavailability (see "Drug Interactions") but food and milk do affect the rate but not the extent of absorption (see "Clinical Pharmacology"), physicians may want to make specific recommendations to patients about when they should take Orudis in relation to food and/or what patients should do if they experience minor GI symptoms associated with Orudis therapy.

LABORATORY TESTS

Because serious GI-tract ulceration and bleeding can occur without warning symptoms, physicians should follow chronically treated patients for the signs and symptoms of ulceration and bleeding and should inform them of the importance of this follow-up (see "Risk of GI Ulcerations, Bleeding, and Perforation with NSAID Therapy").

DRUG INTERACTIONS

The following drug interactions were studied with Orudis doses of 200 mg per day (50 mg q.i.d.). The possibility of in-

creased interaction should be kept in mind when Orudis doses greater than 50 mg as a single dose or 200 mg per day are used concomitantly with highly bound drugs.

1. *Antacids*
Concomitant administration of magnesium hydroxide and aluminum hydroxide does not interfere with the rate or extent of the absorption of ketoprofen.

2. *Aspirin*
Orudis does not alter aspirin absorption; however, in a study of 12 normal subjects, concurrent administration of aspirin decreased ketoprofen protein-binding and increased ketoprofen plasma clearance from 0.07 L/kg/hr without aspirin to 0.11 L/kg/hr with aspirin. The clinical significance of these changes has not been adequately studied. Therefore, concurrent use of aspirin and ketoprofen is not recommended.

3. *Diuretic*
Hydrochlorothiazide, given concomitantly with Orudis, produces a reduction in urinary potassium and chloride excretion compared to hydrochlorothiazide alone. Patients taking diuretics are at greater risk of developing renal failure secondary to a decrease in renal blood flow caused by prostaglandin inhibition (see "General Precautions").

4. *Digoxin*
In a study in 12 patients with congestive heart failure where Orudis and digoxin were concomitantly administered, Orudis did not alter the serum levels of digoxin.

5. *Warfarin*
In a short-term controlled study in 14 normal volunteers, Orudis did not significantly interfere with the effect of warfarin on prothrombin time. Bleeding from a number of sites may be a complication of warfarin treatment and GI bleeding a complication of Orudis treatment. Because prostaglandins play an important role in hemostasis and ketoprofen has an effect on platelet function as well (see "Blood Coagulation"), concurrent therapy with Orudis and warfarin requires close monitoring of patients on both drugs.

6. *Probenecid*
Probenecid increases both free and bound ketoprofen through reducing the plasma clearance of ketoprofen to about one-third, as well as decreasing its protein-binding. Therefore, the combination of Orudis and probenecid is not recommended.

7. *Methotrexate*
The coadministration of Orudis and methotrexate should be avoided because increased toxicity due to displacement of protein-bound methoxtrexate has been reported to occur when nonsteroidal antiinflammatory agents are administered simultaneously with methotrexate.

8. *Lithium*
Nonsteroidal antiinflammatory agents have been reported to increase steady-state plasma lithium levels. It is recommended that plasma lithium levels be monitored when Orudis is coadministered with lithium.

DRUG/LABORATORY TEST INTERACTIONS:
EFFECT ON BLOOD COAGULATION

Orudis decreases platelet adhesion and aggregation. Therefore, it can prolong bleeding time by approximately 3 to 4 minutes from baseline values. There is no significant change in platelet count, prothrombin time, partial thromboplastin time, or thrombin time.

CARCINOGENESIS, MUTAGENESIS, IMPAIRMENT OF FERTILITY

Chronic oral toxicity studies in mice (up to 32 mg/kg/day) did not indicate a carcinogenic potential for Orudis (maximum recommended human therapeutic dose for a 50 kg man is 6 mg/kg/day). A chronic oral toxicity study was also performed in rats (up to 12.5 mg/kg/day) with no statistically significant increase in any tumor type; however, this study was unacceptable because of poor survival. Orudis did not show mutagenic potential in the Ames Test. Orudis administered to male rats (up to 9 mg/kg/day) had no significant effect on reproductive performance or fertility. In female rats administered 6 or 9 mg/kg/day, a decrease in the number of implantation sites has been noted.

Abnormal spermatogenesis or inhibition of spermatogenesis developed in rats and dogs at high doses, and a decrease in the weight of the testes occurred in dogs and baboons at high doses.

TERATOGENIC EFFECTS: PREGNANCY CATEGORY B

In teratology studies Orudis administered to mice at doses up to 12 mg/kg/day and rats at doses up to 9 mg/kg/day, the approximate equivalent of 1.5 times the maximum recommended therapeutic dose in (a 50 kg) man, showed no teratogenic or embryotoxic effects. In separate studies in rabbits, maternally toxic doses were associated with embryotoxicity but not teratogenicity.

There are no adequate and well-controlled studies in pregnant women. Because animal teratology studies are not always predictive of the human response, Orudis should be used during pregnancy only if the potential benefit justifies the risk.

LABOR AND DELIVERY

The effects of Orudis on labor and delivery in pregnant women are unknown. Studies in rats have shown Orudis at doses of 6 mg/kg (approximately equal to the maximum recommended human dose) prolong pregnancy when given before the onset of labor. Because of the known effects of prostaglandin-inhibiting drugs on the fetal cardiovascular system (closure of ductus arteriosus), use of Orudis during late pregnancy should be avoided.

NURSING MOTHERS

In rats, Orudis at doses of 9 mg/kg (approximately 1.5 times the maximum human therapeutic dose) did not affect perinatal development. Upon administration to lactating dogs, the milk concentration of Orudis was found to be 4 to 5% of the plasma drug level. Data on secretion in human milk after ingestion of ketoprofen do not exist. As with other drugs that are excreted in milk, Orudis is not recommended for use in nursing mothers.

PEDIATRIC USE

Orudis is not recommended for use in children, because its safety and effectiveness have not been studied in children.

ADVERSE REACTIONS

The incidence of common adverse reactions (above 1%) was obtained from a population of 835 ketoprofen-treated patients in double-blind trials lasting from 4 to 54 weeks.

Minor gastrointestinal side effects predominated; upper gastrointestinal symptoms were more common than lower gastrointestinal symptoms. Peptic ulcer or GI bleeding occurred in controlled clinical trials in less than 1% of 1,076 patients; however, in open label continuation studies in 1,292 patients the rate was greater than 2%. The incidence of peptic ulceration in patients on NSAIDs is dependent on many risk factors including age, sex, smoking, alcohol use, diet, stress, concomitant drugs such as aspirin and corticoids, as well as the dose and duration of treatment with NSAIDs (see "Warnings"). These were followed in frequency by central nervous system side effects, such as headache, dizziness, or drowsiness. The incidence of some adverse reactions appears to be dose-related (see "Dosage and Administration"). Those rare adverse reactions (incidence less than 1%) were collected from foreign reports to manufacturers and regulatory agencies, publications, and U.S. clinical trials.

In double-blind trials, 233 ketoprofen-treated patients had fewer minor gastrointestinal complaints, tinnitus and hearing impairment, fluid retention, and minor abnormalities in liver-function tests than 228 aspirin-treated patients.

INCIDENCE GREATER THAN 1%
(PROBABLE CAUSAL RELATIONSHIP)

Digestive: Dyspepsia (11.5%)*, nausea*, abdominal pain*, diarrhea*, constipation*, flatulence*, anorexia, vomiting, stomatitis.

Central Nervous System: Headache*, dizziness, CNS inhibition (i.e., pooled reports of somnolence, malaise, depression, etc.) or excitation (i.e., insomnia, nervousness, dreams, etc.).*

Special Senses: Tinnitus, visual disturbance.

Skin and Appendages: Rash.

Urogenital: Impairment of renal function (edema, increased BUN)*, signs or symptoms of urinary-tract irritation.

*Side effects with incidence greater than 3%.

INCIDENCE LESS THAN 1%
(PROBABLE CAUSAL RELATIONSHIP)

Digestive: Appetite increased, dry mouth, eructation, gastritis, rectal hemorrhage, melena, fecal occult blood, salivation, peptic ulcer, gastrointestinal perforation, hematemesis, intestinal ulceration.

Central Nervous System: Amnesia, confusion, impotence, migraine, paresthesia, vertigo.

Special Senses: Conjunctivitis, conjunctivitis sicca, eye pain, hearing impairment, retinal hemorrhage and pigmentation change, taste perversion.

Skin and Appendages: Alopecia, eczema, pruritus, purpuric rash, sweating, urticaria, bullous rash, exfoliative dermatitis, photosensitivity, skin discoloration, onycholysis.

Body as a Whole: Chills, facial edema, infection, pain, allergic reaction, anaphylaxis.

Cardiovascular: Hypertension, palpitation, tachycardia, congestive heart failure, peripheral vascular disease, vasodilation.

Hemic: Hypocoagulability, agranulocytosis, anemia, hemolysis, purpura, thrombocytopenia.

Metabolic and Nutritional: Thirst, weight gain, weight loss, hepatic dysfunction, hyponatremia.

Musculoskeletal: Myalgia.

Respiratory: Dyspnea, hemoptysis, epistaxis, pharyngitis, rhinitis, bronchospasm, laryngeal edema.

Urogenital: Menometrorrhagia, hematuria, renal failure, interstitial nephritis, nephrotic syndrome.

INCIDENCE LESS THAN 1%
(CAUSAL RELATIONSHIP UNKNOWN)

The following rare adverse reactions, whose causal relationship to ketoprofen is uncertain, are being listed to serve as alerting information to the physician.

Digestive: Buccal necrosis, ulcerative colitis.

Central Nervous System: Dysphoria, hallucination, libido disturbance, nightmares, personality disorder.

Body as a Whole: Septicemia, shock.

Cardiovascular: Arrhythmias, myocardial infarction.

Endocrine: Diabetes mellitus (aggravated).

Metabolic and Nutritional: Jaundice.

Urogenital: Acute tubulopathy, gynecomastia.

OVERDOSAGE

The reports of overdosage with Orudis are rare. Of the 20 subjects reported in Great Britain (5 children, 14 adolescents or young adults, and 1 man 80-years-old), only 4 had mild symptoms (vomiting in 3, drowsiness in 1 child). The highest reported dose was 5,000 mg in the elderly man who displayed no symptoms.

Should a patient ingest a large number of capsules, the stomach should be emptied by gastric lavage or induction of vomiting and usual supportive measures employed. The drug is dialyzable; therefore, hemodialysis may be useful to remove circulating drug and to assist in case of renal failure.

DOSAGE AND ADMINISTRATION
RHEUMATOID ARTHRITIS AND OSTEOARTHRITIS

The recommended daily dose of Orudis is 150 to 300 mg, divided in three or four doses. The recommended starting dose is 75 mg three times or 50 mg four times a day. If minor side effects appear, they may disappear at a lower dose which may still have an adequate therapeutic effect. If well tolerated but not optimally effective, the dosage may be increased. Individual patients may show a better response to 300 mg daily as compared to 200 mg, although in well-controlled clinical studies patients on 300 mg did not show greater mean effectiveness. They did, however, show an increased frequency of upper- and lower-GI distress and headaches. It is of interest that women also had an increased frequency of these adverse effects compared to men. When treating patients with 300 mg a day, the physician should observe sufficient increased clinical benefit to offset potential increased risk. Dosages higher than 300 mg per day are not recommended because they have not been adequately studied. Relatively small people may need smaller doses.

Orudis is eliminated primarily by renal excretion; therefore, initial dosage should be reduced by $\frac{1}{2}$ to $\frac{1}{3}$ in patients with impaired renal function, including the elderly who normally have decreased renal function even with normal serum creatinine and/or BUN, because the lean body weight of older patients results in less creatinine formation.

Because hypoalbuminemia and reduced renal function both increase the fraction of free drug (biologically active form), patients who have both conditions may be at greater risk of adverse effects. Therefore, it is recommended that such patients also be started on lower doses and closely monitored. As with other nonsteroidal antiinflammatory drugs, the predominant adverse effects of ketoprofen are gastrointestinal. To attempt to minimize these effects, physicians may wish to prescribe that Orudis be taken with antacids, food, or milk. Although food affects the bioavailability of Orudis (see "Clinical Pharmacology"), in most of the clinical trials Orudis was taken with food or milk.

MILD-TO-MODERATE PAIN AND DYSMENORRHEA

The usual dose of Orudis recommended for mild-to-moderate pain and dysmenorrhea is 25 to 50 mg every 6 to 8 hours as necessary. A smaller dose should be utilized initially in small individuals, in debilitated or elderly patients, or in patients with renal or liver disease (see "Precautions"). A larger dose may be tried if the patient's response to a previous dose was less than satisfactory, but doses above 75 mg have not been shown to give added analgesia. Daily doses above 300 mg are not recommended because they have not been adequately studied. Because of its typical nonsteroidal antiinflammatory drug-side-effect profile, including as its principal adverse effect GI side effects (see "Warnings" and "Adverse Reactions"), higher doses of Orudis should be used with caution and patients receiving them observed carefully.

HOW SUPPLIED

Orudis® (ketoprofen) Capsules, Wyeth®, are available as follows:

25 mg, NDC 0008-4186, dark-green and red capsule marked "WYETH 4186" on one side and "ORUDIS 25" on the reverse side, in bottles of 100 capsules.

50 mg, NDC 0008-4181, dark-green and light-green capsule marked "WYETH 4181" on one side and "ORUDIS 50" on the reverse side, in bottles of 100 capsules.

75 mg, NDC 0008-4187, dark-green and white capsule marked "WYETH 4187" on one side and "ORUDIS 75" on the reverse side, in bottles of 100 and 500 capsules.

Keep tightly closed.

Dispense in tight container.

The appearance of these capsules is a trademark of Wyeth-Ayerst Laboratories.

Shown in Product Identification Section, page 437

OVRAL®   ℞
[oh´vral]
TABLETS
(norgestrel and ethinyl estradiol tablets)

DESCRIPTION

Each Ovral tablet contains 0.5 mg of norgestrel (*dl*-13-beta-ethyl-17-alpha-ethinyl -17- beta-hydroxygon -4- en -3- one),

a totally synthetic progestogen, and 0.05 mg of ethinyl estradiol (19-nor-17α-pregna-1,3,5 (10)-trien-20-yne-3,17-diol). The inactive ingredients present are cellulose, lactose, magnesium stearate, and polacrilin potassium.

CLINICAL PHARMACOLOGY

See LO/OVRAL®.

INDICATIONS AND USAGE

Ovral is indicated for the prevention of pregnancy in women who elect to use oral contraceptives as a method of contraception. Oral contraceptives are highly effective. The pregnancy rate in women using conventional combination oral contraceptives (containing 35 mcg or more of ethinyl estradiol or 50 mcg or more of mestranol) is generally reported as less than one pregnancy per 100 woman-years of use. Slightly higher rates (somewhat more than 1 pregnancy per 100 woman-years of use) are reported for some combination products containing 35 mcg or less of ethinyl estradiol, and rates on the order of 3 pregnancies per 100 woman-years are reported for the progestogen-only oral contraceptives.

These rates are derived from separate studies conducted by different investigators in several population groups and cannot be compared precisely. Furthermore, pregnancy rates tend to be lower as clinical studies are continued possibly due to selective retention in the longer studies of those patients who accept the treatment regimen and do not discontinue as a result of adverse reactions, pregnancy, or other reasons. In clinical trials with Ovral, 6,806 patients completed 127,872 cycles, and a total of 19 pregnancies were reported. This represents a pregnancy rate of 0.19 per 100 woman-years. All of the pregnancies reported in these trials were the result of patient failure.

Table 1 gives ranges of pregnancy rates reported in the literature[1] for other means of contraception. The efficacy of these means of contraception (except the IUD) depends upon the degree of adherence to the method.

TABLE 1
PREGNANCIES PER 100 WOMAN-YEARS
IUD, less than 1–6; Diaphragm with spermicidal products (creams or jellies), 2–20; Condom, 3–36; Aerosol foams, 2–29; Jellies and creams, 4–36;
Periodic abstinence (rhythm) all types, less than 1–47:
1. Calendar method, 14–47;
2. Temperature method, 1–20;
3. Temperature method—intercourse only in postovulatory phase, less than 1–7;
4. Mucus method, 1–25;

No contraception, 60–80.

Dose-Related Risk of Thromboembolism from Oral Contraceptives: See LO/OVRAL.

CONTRAINDICATIONS
See LO/OVRAL.

WARNINGS
See LO/OVRAL.

PRECAUTIONS
See LO/OVRAL.

INFORMATION FOR THE PATIENT
See LO/OVRAL.

DRUG INTERACTIONS
See LO/OVRAL.

CARCINOGENESIS
See LO/OVRAL.

PREGNANCY
See LO/OVRAL.

NURSING MOTHERS
See LO/OVRAL.

ADVERSE REACTIONS
See LO/OVRAL.

ACUTE OVERDOSE
See LO/OVRAL.

DOSAGE AND ADMINISTRATION

To achieve maximum contraceptive effectiveness, Ovral must be taken exactly as directed and at intervals not exceeding 24 hours. The dosage of Ovral is one tablet daily for 21 consecutive days per menstrual cycle according to prescribed schedule. Tablets are then discontinued for 7 days (three weeks on, one week off).

It is recommended that Ovral tablets be taken at the same time each day, preferably after the evening meal or at bedtime.

During the first cycle of medication, the patient is instructed to take one Ovral tablet daily for twenty-one consecutive days beginning on day five of her menstrual cycle. (The first day of menstruation is day one.) The tablets are then discontinued for one week (7 days). Withdrawal bleeding should usually occur within three days following discontinuation of Ovral. (If Ovral is first taken later than the fifth day of the

Continued on next page

Wyeth-Ayerst—Cont.

first menstrual cycle of medication or postpartum, contraceptive reliance should not be placed on Ovral until after the first seven consecutive days of administration. The possibility of ovulation and conception prior to initiation of medication should be considered.) The patient begins her next and all subsequent 21-day courses of Ovral tablets on the same day of the week that she began her first course, following the same schedule: 21 days on—7 days off.

She begins taking her tablets on the 8th day after discontinuance regardless of whether or not a menstrual period has occurred or is still in progress. Any time a new cycle of Ovral is started later than the 8th day, the patient should be protected by another means of contraception until she has taken a tablet daily for seven consecutive days.

If spotting or breakthrough bleeding occurs, the patient is instructed to continue on the same regimen. This type of bleeding is usually transient and without significance; however, if the bleeding is persistent or prolonged, the patient is advised to consult her physician. Although the occurrence of pregnancy is highly unlikely if Ovral is taken according to directions, if withdrawal bleeding does not occur, the possibility of pregnancy must be considered. If the patient has not adhered to the prescribed schedule (missed one or more tablets or started taking them on a day later than she should have) the probability of pregnancy should be considered at the time of the first missed period and appropriate diagnostic measures taken before the medication is resumed. If the patient has adhered to the prescribed regimen and misses two consecutive periods, pregnancy should be ruled out before continuing the contraceptive regimen.

The patient should be instructed to take a missed tablet as soon as it is remembered. If two consecutive tablets are missed, they should both be taken as soon as remembered. The next tablet should be taken at the usual time.

Any time the patient misses one or two tablets, she should also use another method of contraception until she has taken a tablet daily for seven consecutive days. If breakthrough bleeding occurs following missed tablets, it will usually be transient and of no consequence. While there is little likelihood of ovulation occurring if only one or two tablets are missed, the possibility of ovulation increases with each successive day that scheduled tablets are missed. If three consecutive tablets are missed, all medication should be discontinued and the remainder of the package discarded. A new tablet cycle should be started on the 8th day after the last tablet was taken, and an alternate means of contraception should be prescribed during the seven days without tablets and until the patient has taken a tablet daily for seven consecutive days. In the nonlactating mother, Ovral may be prescribed in the postpartum period either immediately or at the first postpartum examination whether or not menstruation has resumed.

HOW SUPPLIED

Ovral® Tablets (0.5 mg norgestrel and 0.05 mg ethyl estradiol), Wyeth®, are available in packages of 6 PILPAK® dispensers with 21 tablets each as follows: NDC 0008-0056, white, round tablet marked "WYETH" and "56".

REFERENCES
See LO/OVRAL.
Brief Summary Patient Package Insert: See LO/OVRAL.
DETAILED PATIENT LABELING: See LO/OVRAL.
Shown in Product Identification Section, page 437

OVRAL®-28 ℞
[oh 'vral-28]
Tablets
(norgestrel and ethinyl estradiol tablets)

DESCRIPTION

21 white Ovral tablets, each containing 0.5 mg of norgestrel (dl -13-beta-ethyl-17-alpha-ethinyl-17-beta-hydroxygon-4-en-3-one), a totally synthetic progestogen, and 0.05 mg of ethinyl estradiol (19-nor-17α-pregna-1,3,5 (10)-trien-20-yne-3,17-diol), and 7 pink inert tablets. The inactive ingredients present are cellulose, FD&C Red 3, lactose, magnesium stearate, and polacrilin potassium.

CLINICAL PHARMACOLOGY
See LO/OVRAL®.

INDICATIONS AND USAGE
See OVRAL®.
Dose-Related Risk of Thromboembolism from Oral Contraceptives: See LO/OVRAL.

CONTRAINDICATIONS
See LO/OVRAL.

WARNINGS
See LO/OVRAL.

PRECAUTIONS
See LO/OVRAL.

Information for the Patient: See LO/OVRAL.
Drug Interactions: See LO/OVRAL.
Carcinogenesis: See LO/OVRAL.
Pregnancy: See LO/OVRAL.
Nursing Mothers: See LO/OVRAL.

ADVERSE REACTIONS
See LO/OVRAL.

Acute Overdosage: See LO/OVRAL.

DOSAGE AND ADMINISTRATION

To achieve maximum contraceptive effectiveness, Ovral-28 must be taken exactly as directed and at intervals not exceeding 24 hours. The dosage of Ovral-28 is one white tablet daily for 21 consecutive days followed by one pink inert tablet for 7 consecutive days according to prescribed schedule. It is recommended that tablets be taken at the same time each day, preferably after the evening meal or at bedtime. During the first cycle of medication, the patient is instructed to begin taking Ovral-28 on the first Sunday after the onset of menstruation. If menstruation begins on a Sunday, the first tablet (white) is taken that day. One white tablet should be taken daily for 21 consecutive days followed by one pink inert tablet daily for 7 consecutive days. Withdrawal bleeding should usually occur within three days following discontinuation of white tablets.

During the first cycle, contraceptive reliance should not be placed on Ovral-28 until a white tablet has been taken daily for 7 consecutive days. The possibility of ovulation and conception prior to initiation of medication should be considered.

The patient begins her next and all subsequent 28-day courses of tablets on the same day of the week (Sunday) on which she began her first course, following the same schedule: 21 days on white tablets—7 days on pink inert tablets. If in any cycle the patient starts tablets later than the proper day, she should protect herself by using another method of birth control until she has taken a white tablet daily for 7 consecutive days.

If spotting or breakthrough bleeding occurs, the patient is instructed to continue on the same regimen. This type of bleeding is usually transient and without significance; however, if the bleeding is persistent or prolonged, the patient is advised to consult her physician. Although the occurrence of pregnancy is highly unlikely if Ovral-28 is taken according to directions, if withdrawal bleeding does not occur, the possibility of pregnancy must be considered. If the patient has not adhered to the prescribed schedule (missed one or more tablets or started taking them on a day later than she should have) the probability of pregnancy should be considered at the time of the first missed period and appropriate diagnostic measures taken before the medication is resumed. If the patient has adhered to the prescribed regimen and misses two consecutive periods, pregnancy should be ruled out before continuing the contraceptive regimen. The patient should be instructed to take a missed white tablet as soon as it is remembered. If two consecutive white tablets are missed they should both be taken as soon as remembered. The next tablet should be taken at the usual time.

Any time the patient misses one or two white tablets she should also use another method of contraception until she has taken a white tablet daily for seven consecutive days. If the patient misses one or more pink tablets she is still protected against pregnancy *provided* she begins taking white tablets again on the proper day.

If breakthrough bleeding occurs following missed white tablets, it will usually be transient and of no consequence. While there is little likelihood of ovulation occurring if only one or two white tablets are missed, the possibility of ovulation increases with each successive day that scheduled white tablets are missed. If three consecutive white Ovral tablets are missed, all medication should be discontinued and the remainder of the 28-day package discarded. A new tablet cycle should be started on the first Sunday following the last missed tablet, and an alternate means of contraception should be prescribed during the days without tablets and until the patient has taken a white tablet daily for 7 consecutive days. In the nonlactating mother, Ovral-28 may be prescribed in the postpartum period either immediately or at the first postpartum examination whether or not menstruation has resumed.

HOW SUPPLIED

Ovral®-28 Tablets (0.5 mg norgestrel and 0.05 mg ethinyl estradiol), Wyeth®, are available in packages of 6 PILPAK® dispensers, each containing 28 tablets as follows:
21 active tablets, NDC 0008-0056, white, round tablet marked "WYETH" and "56".
7 inert tablets, NDC 0008-0445, pink, round tablet marked "WYETH" and "445".

REFERENCES
See LO/OVRAL.
Brief Summary Patient Package Insert: See LO/OVRAL.
DETAILED PATIENT LABELING: See LO/OVRAL.
Shown in Product Identification Section, page 437

OVRETTE® ℞
[oh-vret ']
Tablets
(norgestrel tablets)

Each OVRETTE® tablet contains 0.075 mg of norgestrel (dl -13-beta-ethyl-17-alpha-ethinyl-17-beta-hydroxygon-4-en-3-one). The inactive ingredients present are cellulose, FD&C Yellow 5, lactose, magnesium stearate, and polacrilin potassium.

DESCRIPTION

Each OVRETTE tablet contains 0.075 mg of a single active steroid ingredient, norgestrel, a totally synthetic progestogen. The available data suggest that the d (-)enantiomeric form of norgestrel is the biologically active portion. This form amounts to 0.0375 mg per OVRETTE tablet.

CLINICAL PHARMACOLOGY

The primary mechanism through which OVRETTE prevents conception is not known, but progestogen-only contraceptives are known to alter the cervical mucus, exert a progestational effect on the endometrium, interfering with implantation, and, in some patients, suppress ovulation.

INDICATIONS AND USAGE

OVRETTE is indicated for the prevention of pregnancy in women who elect to use oral contraceptives as a method of contraception. Oral contraceptives are highly effective. The pregnancy rate in women using conventional combination oral contraceptives (containing 35 mcg or more of ethinyl estradiol or 50 mcg or more of mestranol) is generally reported as less than one pregnancy per 100 woman-years of use. Slightly higher rates (somewhat more than 1 pregnancy per 100 woman-years of use) are reported for some combination products containing 35 mcg or less of ethinyl estradiol, and rates on the order of 3 pregnancies per 100 woman-years are reported for the progestogen-only oral contraceptives. These rates are derived from separate studies conducted by different investigators in several population groups and cannot be compared precisely. Furthermore, pregnancy rates tend to be lower as clinical studies are continued, possibly due to selective retention in the longer studies of those patients who accept the treatment regimen and do not discontinue as a result of adverse reactions, pregnancy, or other reasons.

In clinical trials with OVRETTE, 2,752 patients completed 38,245 cycles, and a total of 78 pregnancies were reported. This represents a pregnancy rate of 2.45 per 100 woman-years. Approximately one-half of the pregnancies reported in these trials were due to method failure, and the other half were due to patient failure.

Table 1 gives ranges of pregnancy rates reported in the literature[1] for other means of contraception. The efficacy of these means of contraception (except the IUD) depends upon the degree of adherence to the method.

TABLE 1
PREGNANCIES PER 100 WOMAN-YEARS
IUD, less than 1–6; Diaphragm with spermicidal products (creams or jellies), 2–20; Condom, 3–36; Aerosol foams, 2–29; Jellies and creams, 4–36;
Periodic abstinence (rhythm) all types, less than 1–47:
1. Calendar method, 14–47;
2. Temperature method, 1–20;
3. Temperature method—intercourse only in postovulatory phase, less than 1–7;
4. Mucus method, 1–25;
No contraception, 60–80.

Dose-Related Risk of Thromboembolism from Oral Contraceptives: See LO/OVRAL®.

CONTRAINDICATIONS
See LO/OVRAL.

WARNINGS
See LO/OVRAL.

PRECAUTIONS
See LO/OVRAL.

INFORMATION FOR THE PATIENT
See LO/OVRAL.

DRUG INTERACTIONS
See LO/OVRAL.

CARCINOGENESIS
See LO/OVRAL.

PREGNANCY
See LO/OVRAL.

NURSING MOTHERS
See LO/OVRAL.

ADVERSE REACTIONS
See LO/OVRAL.

ACUTE OVERDOSE

See LO/OVRAL.

DOSAGE AND ADMINISTRATION

To achieve maximum contraceptive effectiveness, OVRETTE (norgestrel) must be taken exactly as directed and at intervals not exceeding 24 hours. OVRETTE is administered on a continuous daily dosage regimen starting on the first day of menstruation, i.e., one tablet each day, every day of the year.

Tablets should be taken at the same time each day and continued daily, without interruption, whether bleeding occurs or not. The patient should be advised that, if prolonged bleeding occurs, she should consult her physician. In the non-nursing mother, OVRETTE may be prescribed in the postpartum period either immediately or at the first postpartum examination whether or not menstruation has resumed.

The risk of pregnancy increases with each tablet missed. If the patient misses one tablet, she should be instructed to take it as soon as she remembers and to also take her next tablet at the regular time. If she misses two tablets, she should take one of the missed tablets as soon as she remembers, as well as taking her regular tablet for that day at the proper time. Furthermore, she should use a method of nonhormonal contraception in addition to taking OVRETTE until fourteen tablets have been taken. If more than 2 tablets have been missed, OVRETTE should be discontinued immediately and a method of nonhormonal contraception should be used until menses has appeared or pregnancy has been excluded. If menses does not appear within 45 days from the last period, a method of nonhormonal contraception should be substituted until the start of the next menstrual period or an appropriate diagnostic procedure is performed to rule out pregnancy.

HOW SUPPLIED

OVRETTE® tablets (0.075 mg norgestrel), Wyeth®, are available in packages of 6 PILPAK® dispensers with 28 tablets each as follows: NDC 0008-0062, yellow, round tablet marked "WYETH" and "62".

REFERENCES

See LO/OVRAL.

Brief Summary Patient Package Insert: See LO/OVRAL.
DETAILED PATIENT LABELING: See LO/OVRAL.

OXYTOCIN   ℞

[ok "se-to 'sin]
Injection, USP
(synthetic)

DESCRIPTION

Each mL of TUBEX® Oxytocin Injection sterile solution contains an oxytocic activity equivalent to 10 USP Posterior Pituitary Units, chlorobutanol (a chloroform derivative), 0.5%, as a preservative, and acetic acid to adjust pH (2.5 to 4.5). Wyeth Oxytocin is intended for IM or IV use. Oxytocin is a synthetic polypeptide; it occurs as a white powder and is soluble in water.

CLINICAL PHARMACOLOGY

The pharmacologic and clinical properties of oxytocin are identical with those of the naturally occurring oxytocin principle of the posterior lobe of the pituitary. Oxytocin exerts a selective action on the smooth musculature of the uterus, particularly toward the end of pregnancy, during labor, and immediately following delivery. Oxytocin stimulates rhythmic contractions of the uterus, increases the frequency of existing contractions, and raises the tone of the uterine musculature.

When given in appropriate doses during pregnancy, oxytocin is capable of eliciting graded increases in uterine motility from a moderate increase in the rate and force of spontaneous motor activity to sustained tetanic contraction. The sensitivity of the uterus to oxytocic activity increases progressively throughout pregnancy until term when it is maximal. Oxytocin is distributed throughout the extracellular fluid. Small amounts of this drug probably reach the fetal circulation. Oxytocin has a plasma half-life of about 3 to 5 minutes. Following parenteral administration, uterine response occurs within 3 to 5 minutes and persists for 2 to 3 hours. Its rapid removal from plasma is accomplished largely by the kidney and the liver. Only small amounts of oxytocin are excreted in the urine unchanged.

INDICATIONS AND USAGE

IMPORTANT NOTICE

Oxytocin is indicated for the medical rather than the elective induction of labor. Available data and information are inadequate to define the benefits-to-risks considerations in the use of the drug product for elective induction. Elective induction of labor is defined as the initiation of labor for convenience in an individual with a term pregnancy who is free of medical indications.

ANTEPARTUM: Oxytocin is indicated for the initiation or improvement of uterine contractions, where this is desirable and considered suitable for reasons of fetal or maternal concern, in order to achieve early vaginal delivery. It is indicated for (1) induction of labor in patients with a medical indication for the initiation of labor, such as Rh problems, maternal diabetes, preeclampsia at or near term, when delivery is in the best interest of mother and fetus or when membranes are prematurely ruptured and delivery is indicated; (2) stimulation or reinforcement of labor, as in selected cases of uterine inertia; (3) as adjunctive therapy in the management of incomplete or inevitable abortion. In the first trimester, curettage is generally considered primary therapy. In second trimester abortion, oxytocin infusion will often be successful in emptying the uterus. Other means of therapy, however, may be required in such cases.

POSTPARTUM: Oxytocin is indicated to produce uterine contractions during the third stage of labor and to control postpartum bleeding or hemorrhage.

CONTRAINDICATIONS

Oxytocin is contraindicated in any of the following conditions:

significant cephalopelvic disproportion;

unfavorable fetal positions or presentations which are undeliverable without conversion prior to delivery, e.g., transverse lies;

in obstetrical emergencies where the benefit-to-risk ratio for either the fetus or the mother favors surgical intervention;

in cases of fetal distress where delivery is not imminent;

hypertonic uterine patterns;

hypersensitivity to the drug.

Prolonged use in uterine inertia or severe toxemia is contraindicated.

Oxytocin should not be used in cases where vaginal delivery is not indicated, such as cord presentation or prolapse, total placenta previa, and vasa previa.

WARNINGS

Oxytocin, when given for induction or stimulation of labor, must be administered only by intravenous infusion (drip method) and with adequate medical supervision in a hospital.

PRECAUTIONS

GENERAL:

1. All patients receiving intravenous infusions of oxytocin must be under continuous observation by trained personnel with a thorough knowledge of the drug and qualified to identify complications. A physician qualified to manage any complications should be immediately available.

2. When properly administered, oxytocin should stimulate uterine contractions similar to those seen in normal labor. Overstimulation of the uterus by improper administration can be hazardous to both mother and fetus. Even with proper administration and adequate supervision, hypertonic contractions can occur in patients whose uteri are hypersensitive to oxytocin.

3. Except in unusual circumstances, oxytocin should not be administered in the following conditions: prematurity, borderline cephalopelvic disproportion, previous major surgery on the cervix or uterus, including cesarean section, overdistention of the uterus, grand multiparity, or invasive cervical carcinoma. Because of the variability of the combinations of factors which may be present in the conditions listed above, the definition of "unusual circumstances" must be left to the judgment of the physician. The decision can only be made by carefully weighing the potential benefits which oxytocin can provide in a given case against the rare occurrence of hypertonicity or tetanic spasm with this drug.

4. Maternal deaths due to hypertensive episodes, subarachnoid hemorrhage, rupture of the uterus, fetal deaths and permanent CNS or brain damage of the infant due to various causes have been reported to be associated with the use of parenteral oxytocic drugs for induction of labor or for augmentation in the first and second stages of labor.

5. Oxytocin has been shown to have an intrinsic antidiuretic effect, acting to increase water reabsorption from the glomerular filtrate. Consideration should, therefore, be given to the possibility of water intoxication, particularly when oxytocin is administered continuously by infusion and the patient is receiving fluids by mouth.

6. Oxytocin should be considered for use only in patients who have been carefully selected. Pelvic adequacy must be considered and maternal and fetal conditions thoroughly evaluated before use of the drug.

DRUG INTERACTIONS

Severe hypertension has been reported when oxytocin was given 3 to 4 hours following prophylactic administration of a vasoconstrictor in conjunction with caudal block anesthesia. Cyclopropane anesthesia may modify oxytocin's cardiovascular effects, so as to produce unexpected results such as hypotension. Maternal sinus bradycardia with abnormal atrioventricular rhythms has also been noted when oxytocin was used concomitantly with cyclopropane anesthesia.

CARCINOGENESIS, MUTAGENESIS, IMPAIRMENT OF FERTILITY

There are no animal or human studies on the carcinogenicity and mutagenicity of this drug, nor is there any information on its effect on fertility.

PREGNANCY

See "Indications and Usage."

Teratogenic Effects

Animal reproduction studies have not been conducted with oxytocin. There are no known indications for use in the first trimester of pregnancy other than in relation to spontaneous or induced abortion. Based on the wide experience with this drug and its chemical structure and pharmacological properties, it would not be expected to present a risk of fetal abnormalities when used as indicated.

Nonteratogenic Effects

See "Adverse Reactions" in the fetus or infant.

LABOR AND DELIVERY

See "Indications and Usage."

ADVERSE REACTIONS

The following adverse reactions have been reported in the mother:

Anaphylactic reaction
Postpartum hemorrhage
Cardiac arrhythmia
Fatal afibrinogenemia
Nausea
Vomiting
Premature ventricular contractions
Pelvic hematoma

Excessive dosage or hypersensitivity to the drug may result in uterine hypertonicity, spasm, tetanic contraction, or rupture of the uterus.

The possibility of increased blood loss and afibrinogenemia should be kept in mind when administering the drug.

Severe water intoxication with convulsions and coma has occurred, associated with a slow oxytocin infusion over a 24-hour period. Maternal death due to oxytocin-induced water intoxication has been reported.

The following adverse reactions have been reported in the fetus or infant:

(Due to induced uterine motility)
Bradycardia
Premature ventricular contractions and other arrhythmias
Permanent CNS or brain damage
Fetal death
(Due to use of oxytocin in the mother)
Low Apgar scores at five minutes
Neonatal jaundice
Neonatal retinal hemorrhage

OVERDOSAGE

Overdosage with oxytocin depends essentially on uterine hyperactivity whether or not due to hypersensitivity to this agent. Hyperstimulation with strong (hypertonic) or prolonged (tetanic) contractions, or a resting tone of 15 to 20 mmH$_2$O or more between contractions can lead to tumultuous labor, uterine rupture, cervical and vaginal lacerations, postpartum hemorrhage, utero-placental hypoperfusion, and variable deceleration of fetal heart, fetal hypoxia, hypercapnia or death. Water intoxication with convulsions, which is caused by the inherent antidiuretic effect of oxytocin, is a serious complication that may occur if large doses (40 to 50 milliunits/minute) are infused for long periods. Management consists of immediate discontinuation of oxytocin, and symptomatic and supportive therapy.

DOSAGE AND ADMINISTRATION

Parenteral drug products should be inspected visually for particulate matter and discoloration prior to administration, whenever solution and container permit.

Dosage of oxytocin is determined by uterine response. The following dosage information is based upon the various regimens and indications in general use.

A. INDUCTION OR STIMULATION OF LABOR

Intravenous infusion (drip method) is the only acceptable method of administration for the induction or stimulation of labor.

Accurate control of the rate of infusion flow is essential. An infusion pump or other such device and frequent monitoring of strength of contractions and fetal heart rate are necessary for the safe administration of oxytocin for the induction or stimulation of labor. If uterine contractions become too powerful, the infusion can be abruptly stopped, and oxytocic stimulation of the uterine musculature will soon wane.

1. An intravenous infusion of nonoxytocin-containing solution should be started. Physiologic electrolyte solution should be used except under unusual circumstances.

2. To prepare the usual solution for infusion, the contents of one 1-mL TUBEX® (10 units) is combined aseptically with 1,000 mL of nonhydrating diluent (physiologic electrolyte solution). The combined solution, rotated in the infusion bottle to insure thorough mixing, contains 10 mU/mL. Add the container with dilute oxytocic solution to the system through use of a constant infusion pump or other such device, to control accurately the rate of infusion.

Continued on next page

Wyeth-Ayerst—Cont.

3. The initial dose should be no more than 1–2 mU/min. The dose may be gradually increased in increments of no more than 1 to 2 mU/min. until a contraction pattern has been established which is similar to normal labor.

4. The fetal heart rate, resting uterine tone, and the frequency, duration, and force of contractions should be monitored.

5. The oxytocin infusion should be discontinued immediately in the event of uterine hyperactivity or fetal distress. Oxygen should be administered to the mother. The mother and the fetus must be evaluated by the responsible physician.

B. CONTROL OF POSTPARTUM UTERINE BLEEDING

1. Intravenous Infusion (Drip Method):

To control postpartum bleeding, 10 to 40 units of oxytocin may be added to 1,000 mL of a nonhydrating diluent (physiologic electrolyte solution) and run at a rate necessary to control uterine atony.

2. Intramuscular Administration:

1 mL (10 units) of oxytocin can be given after delivery of the placenta.

C. TREATMENT OF INCOMPLETE OR INEVITABLE ABORTION

Intravenous infusion with physiologic saline solution, 500 mL, or 5% dextrose in physiologic saline solution to which 10 units of oxytocin have been added should be infused at a rate of 20 to 40 drops per minute.

HOW SUPPLIED

Oxytocin Injection, USP (synthetic), 10 USP units in 1 mL TUBEX® Sterile Cartridge-Needle Unit (22 gauge × 1¼ inch needle), is supplied as follows:

NDC 0008-0406-01, package of 10 TUBEX.

Keep in a refrigerator; do not freeze.

When stored out of refrigeration at temperatures of up to 26° C (79° F), this product has exhibited acceptable data for a period not exceeding three (3) months.

PATHOCIL®   ℞

[*path 'o-sil*]
(dicloxacillin sodium monohydrate)
CAPSULES • ORAL SUSPENSION

DESCRIPTION

Dicloxacillin sodium monohydrate is an isoxazolyl penicillin which resists destruction by the enzyme penicillinase (beta-lactamase). It is the monohydrate sodium salt of 6-[3-(2, 6-Dichlorophenyl)-5-methyl-4-isoxazolecarboxamido]-3,3-dimethyl -7- oxo -4- thia-1-azabicyclo-[3.2.0] heptane-2-carboxylic acid.

Pathocil capsules contain 250 mg or 500 mg dicloxacillin sodium monohydrate. The inactive ingredients present are D&C Red 28, FD&C Blue 1, FD&C Red 40, gelatin, lactose, stearic acid, talc, and titanium dioxide.

Pathocil oral suspension is a powder which when reconstituted as directed yields a suspension with a concentration of 62.5 mg dicloxacillin sodium monohydrate per 5 mL. The inactive ingredients present are artificial and natural flavors, carboxymethylcellulose sodium, citric acid, colloidal silicon dioxide, edetate disodium, FD&C Red 3, saccharin sodium, sodium benzoate, sodium citrate, sucrose, and water.

HOW SUPPLIED

Pathocil® (dicloxacillin sodium monohydrate) Capsules, Wyeth®, are available in the following dosage strengths:

250 mg, NDC 0008-0360, purple and white capsule marked "WYETH" and "360", in bottles of 100 capsules.

500 mg, NDC 0008-0593, purple and white capsule marked "WYETH" and "593", in bottles of 50 capsules.

Keep bottles tightly closed.

Dispense in tight containers.

The appearance of Pathocil capsules is a registered trademark of Wyeth-Ayerst Laboratories.

Pathocil® (dicloxacillin sodium monohydrate) for Oral Suspension, Wyeth®, is available as a light-pink powder which when reconstituted as directed yields a palatable, pink suspension in the following dosage strength:

62.5 mg per 5 mL, NDC 0008-0361, in bottles to make 100 mL.

Shake well before using.

Keep bottles of suspension tightly closed.

After reconstitution store suspension in refrigerator. Discard any unused portion after two weeks.

Bibliography: A bibliography is available upon request.

For prescribing information write to Professional Service, Wyeth-Ayerst Laboratories, Box 8299, Philadelphia, PA 19101, or contact your local Wyeth-Ayerst representative.

Shown in Product Identification Section, page 437

PEN • VEE® K   ℞

[*pen-vee-kay*]
(penicillin V potassium)
TABLETS • FOR ORAL SOLUTION

DESCRIPTION

Penicillin V is the phenoxymethyl analog of penicillin G. Penicillin V potassium is the potassium salt of penicillin V. Pen·Vee K tablets contain 250 mg (400,000 units) or 500 mg (800,000 units) penicillin V potassium. The inactive ingredients present are carboxymethylcellulose sodium, magnesium stearate, and stearic acid. The 250 mg dosage strength also contains lactose.

Pen·Vee K for oral solution is a powder which when reconstituted as directed yields a suspension of 125 mg (200,000 units) or 250 mg (400,000 units) penicillin V potassium per 5 mL. The inactive ingredients present are artificial and natural flavors, citric acid, FD&C Red 40, saccharin sodium, sodium benzoate, sodium citrate, sodium propionate, sucrose, and water. The 250 mg per 5 mL dosage strength also contains edetate disodium and FD&C Yellow 6.

HOW SUPPLIED

Pen·Vee® K (penicillin V potassium) Tablets, Wyeth®, are available as white, round, scored tablets in the following dosage strengths:

250 mg (400,000 units), NDC 0008-0059, marked "WYETH" and "59", in bottles of 100 or 500 tablets, and in Redipak® cartons of 100 individually wrapped tablets.

500 mg (800,000 units), NDC 0008-0390, marked "WYETH" and "390", in bottles of 100 or 500 tablets, and in Redipak cartons of 100 individually wrapped tablets.

Keep tightly closed.

Dispense in tight container.

Pen·Vee® K (penicillin V potassium) for Oral Suspension, Wyeth®, is available as a powder which when reconstituted as directed yields a palatable solution in the following dosage strengths:

125 mg (200,000 units) per 5 mL, NDC 0008-0004, faint pink powder, in bottles to make 100 mL or 200 mL of red solution.

250 mg (400,000 units) per 5 mL, NDC 0008-0036, light peach-colored powder, in bottles to make 100 mL, 150 mL, or 200 mL of light-orange solution.

Keep tightly closed.

After reconstitution, solution must be stored in a refrigerator.

Discard any unused portion after 14 days.

For prescribing information write to Professional Service, Wyeth-Ayerst Laboratories, Box 8299, Philadelphia, PA 19101, or contact your local Wyeth-Ayerst representative.

Shown in Product Identification Section, page 437

PEPTAVLON®   ℞

[*pĕp-tăv 'lon*]
Brand of
pentagastrin
A diagnostic agent for
evaluation of gastric acid
secretory function.

HOW SUPPLIED

PEPTAVLON (pentagastrin)—In 2 mL ampuls. Each mL contains 0.25 mg (250 mcg) pentagastrin. Also contains 0.88% sodium chloride, and Water for Injection USP. The pH is adjusted with ammonium hydroxide and/or hydrochloric acid. Cartons of 10 (NDC 0046-3290-10).

REFRIGERATE AND PROTECT FROM LIGHT.

DO NOT USE IF DISCOLORED.

For full prescribing information turn to the Diagnostic Product Information section of this edition of the PDR.

PHENERGAN®   ℞

[*fen 'er-gan*]
(promethazine HCl)
INJECTION

DESCRIPTION

Promethazine HCl (10H-phenothiazine-10-ethanamine, N, N,α-trimethyl-, monohydrochloride).

Each mL of ampul contains either 25 or 50 mg promethazine hydrochloride with 0.1 mg edetate disodium, 0.04 mg calcium chloride, not more than 0.25 mg sodium metabisulfite and 5 mg phenol with sodium acetate-acetic acid buffer.

Each mL of TUBEX® Sterile Cartridge-Needle Unit contains either 25 or 50 mg promethazine hydrochloride with 0.1 mg edetate disodium, 0.04 mg calcium chloride, not more than 5 mg monothioglycerol and 5 mg phenol with sodium acetate-acetic acid buffer.

ACTIONS

Promethazine hydrochloride, a phenothiazine derivative, possesses antihistaminic, sedative, antimotion-sickness, antiemetic, and anticholinergic effects. The duration of action is generally from four to six hours. The major side reaction of this drug is sedation. As an antihistamine it acts by competitive antagonism, but does not block the release of histamine. It antagonizes in varying degrees most but not all of the pharmacological effects of histamine.

INDICATIONS

The injectable form of promethazine hydrochloride is indicated for the following conditions:

1. Amelioration of allergic reactions to blood or plasma.

2. In anaphylaxis as an adjunct to epinephrine and other standard measures after the acute symptoms have been controlled.

3. For other uncomplicated allergic conditions of the immediate type when oral therapy is impossible or contraindicated.

4. Active treatment of motion sickness.

5. Preoperative, postoperative, and obstetric (during labor) sedation.

6. Prevention and control of nausea and vomiting associated with certain types of anesthesia and surgery.

7. As an adjunct to analgesics for the control of postoperative pain.

8. For sedation and relief of apprehension and to produce light sleep from which the patient can be easily aroused.

9. Intravenously in special surgical situations, such as repeated bronchoscopy, ophthalmic surgery, and poor-risk patients, with reduced amounts of meperidine or other narcotic analgesic as an adjunct to anesthesia and analgesia.

CONTRAINDICATIONS

Promethazine is contraindicated in comatose states, in patients who have received large amounts of central-nervous-system depressants (alcohol, sedative hypnotics, including barbiturates, general anesthetics, narcotics, narcotic analgesics, tranquilizers, etc.), and in patients who have demonstrated an idiosyncrasy or hypersensitivity to promethazine. Under no circumstances should promethazine be given by intraarterial injection due to the likelihood of severe arteriospasm and the possibility of resultant gangrene (see "Warnings").

Phenergan injection should not be given by the subcutaneous route; evidence of chemical irritation has been noted, and necrotic lesions have resulted on rare occasions following subcutaneous injection. The preferred parenteral route of administration is by deep intramuscular injection.

WARNINGS

Phenergan Injection (ampuls only) contains sodium metabisulfite, a sulfite that may cause allergic-type reactions, including anaphylactic symptoms and life-threatening or less severe asthmatic episodes, in certain susceptible people. The overall prevalence of sulfite sensitivity in the general population is unknown and probably low. Sulfite sensitivity is seen more frequently in asthmatic than in nonasthmatic people.

Promethazine may impair the mental and/or physical abilities required for the performance of potentially hazardous tasks, such as driving a vehicle or operating machinery. The concomitant use of alcohol, sedative hypnotics (including barbiturates), general anesthetics, narcotics, narcotic analgesics, tranquilizers or other central-nervous-system depressants may have an additive sedative effect. Patients should be warned accordingly.

USAGE IN PREGNANCY: The safe use of promethazine has not been established with respect to the possible adverse effects upon fetal development. Therefore, the need for the use of this drug during pregnancy should be weighed against the possible but unknown hazards to the developing fetus.

USE IN CHILDREN: Excessively large dosages of antihistamines, including promethazine, in children may cause hallucinations, convulsions, and sudden death. In children who are acutely ill associated with dehydration, there is an increased susceptibility to dystonias with the use of promethazine hydrochloride injection.

CAUTION SHOULD BE EXERCISED WHEN ADMINISTERING PHENERGAN TO CHILDREN. ANTIEMETICS ARE NOT RECOMMENDED FOR TREATMENT OF UNCOMPLICATED VOMITING IN CHILDREN, AND THEIR USE SHOULD BE LIMITED TO PROLONGED VOMITING OF KNOWN ETIOLOGY. THE EXTRAPYRAMIDAL SYMPTOMS WHICH CAN OCCUR SECONDARY TO PHENERGAN ADMINISTRATION MAY BE CONFUSED WITH THE CNS SIGNS OF UNDIAGNOSED PRIMARY DISEASE, e.g., ENCEPHALOPATHY OR REYE'S SYNDROME. THE USE OF PHENERGAN SHOULD BE AVOIDED IN CHILDREN WHOSE SIGNS AND SYMPTOMS MAY SUGGEST REYE'S SYNDROME, OR OTHER HEPATIC DISEASES.

USE IN THE ELDERLY (APPROXIMATELY 60 YEARS OR OLDER): Since therapeutic requirements for sedative drugs tend to be less in elderly patients, the dosage of Phenergan should be reduced for these patients.

OTHER CONSIDERATIONS: Drugs having anticholinergic properties should be used with caution in patients with asthmatic attack, narrow-angle glaucoma, prostatic hypertrophy, stenosing peptic ulcer, pyloroduodenal obstruction, and bladder-neck obstruction.

Phenergan should be used with caution in patients with bone-marrow depression. Leukopenia and agranulocytosis have been reported, usually when Phenergan has been used in association with other known toxic agents.

INADVERTENT INTRAARTERIAL INJECTION: Due to the close proximity of arteries and veins in the areas most commonly used for intravenous injection, extreme care should be exercised to avoid perivascular extravasation or inadvertent intraarterial injection. Reports compatible with inadvertent intraarterial injection of promethazine, usually in conjunction with other drugs intended for intravenous use, suggest that pain, severe chemical irritation, severe spasm of distal vessels, and resultant gangrene requiring amputation are likely under such circumstances. Intravenous injection was intended in all the cases reported but perivascular extravasation or arterial placement of the needle is now suspect. There is no proven successful management of this condition after it occurs, although sympathetic block and heparinization are commonly employed during the acute management because of the results of animal experiments with other known arteriolar irritants. Aspiration of dark blood does not preclude intraarterial needle placement, because blood is discolored upon contact with promethazine. Use of syringes with rigid plungers or of small bore needles might obscure typical arterial backflow if this is relied upon alone.

When used intravenously, promethazine hydrochloride should be given in a concentration no greater than 25 mg per mL and at a rate not to exceed 25 mg per minute. When administering any irritant drug intravenously, it is usually preferable to inject it through the tubing of an intravenous infusion set that is known to be functioning satisfactorily. In the event that a patient complains of pain during intended intravenous injection of promethazine, the injection should immediately be stopped to provide for evaluation of possible arterial placement or perivascular extravasation.

PRECAUTIONS

Promethazine may significantly affect the actions of other drugs. It may increase, prolong, or intensify the sedative action of central-nervous-system depressants, such as alcohol, sedative hypnotics (including barbiturates), general anesthetics, narcotics, narcotic analgesics, tranquilizers, etc. When given concomitantly with promethazine hydrochloride, the dose of barbiturates should be reduced by at least one-half, and the dose of narcotics should be reduced by one-quarter to one-half. Dosage must be individualized. Excessive amounts of promethazine relative to a narcotic may lead to restlessness and motor hyperactivity in the patient with pain; these symptoms usually disappear with adequate control of the pain. Promethazine should be used cautiously in persons with cardiovascular disease or impairment of liver function.

Although reversal of the vasopressor effect of epinephrine has not been reported with promethazine, the possibility should be considered in case of promethazine overdose.

ADVERSE REACTIONS

CNS EFFECTS: Drowsiness is the most prominent CNS effect of this drug. Extrapyramidal reactions may occur with high doses; this is almost always responsive to a reduction in dosage. Other reported reactions include dizziness, lassitude, tinnitus, incoordination, fatigue, blurred vision, euphoria, diplopia, nervousness, insomnia, tremors, convulsive seizures, oculogyric crises, excitation, catatoniclike states, and hysteria.

CARDIOVASCULAR EFFECTS: Tachycardia, bradycardia, faintness, dizziness, and increases and decreases in blood pressure have been reported following the use of promethazine hydrochloride injection. Venous thrombosis at the injection site has been reported. INTRAARTERIAL INJECTION MAY RESULT IN GANGRENE OF THE AFFECTED EXTREMITY ("see Warnings").

GASTROINTESTINAL: Nausea and vomiting have been reported, usually in association with surgical procedures and combination drug therapy.

ALLERGIC REACTIONS: These include urticaria, dermatitis, asthma, and photosensitivity. Angioneurotic edema has been reported.

OTHER REPORTED REACTIONS: Leukopenia and agranulocytosis, usually when Phenergan has been used in association with other known toxic agents, have been reported. Thrombocytopenic purpura and jaundice of the obstructive type have been associated with the use of promethazine. The jaundice is usually reversible on discontinuation of the drug. Subcutaneous injection has resulted in tissue necrosis. Nasal stuffiness may occur. Dry mouth has been reported.

LABORATORY TESTS: The following laboratory tests may be affected in patients who are receiving therapy with promethazine hydrochloride:

Pregnancy Tests—Diagnostic pregnancy tests based on immunological reactions between HCG and anti-HCG may result in false-negative or false-positive interpretations.

Glucose Tolerance Test—An increase in glucose tolerance has been reported in patients receiving promethazine hydrochloride.

PARADOXICAL REACTIONS (OVERDOSAGE): Hyperexcitability and abnormal movements, which have been reported in children following a single administration of promethazine, may be manifestations of relative overdosage, in which case, consideration should be given to the discontinuation of the promethazine and to the use of other drugs. Respiratory depression, nightmares, delirium, and agitated behavior have also been reported in some of these patients.

DRUG INTERACTIONS

NARCOTICS AND BARBITURATES: The CNS-depressant effects of narcotics and barbiturates are additive with promethazine hydrochloride.

MONOAMINE OXIDASE INHIBITORS (MAOI): Drug interactions, including an increased incidence of extrapyramidal effects, have been reported when some MAOI and phenothiazines are used concomitantly. Although such a reaction has not been reported with promethazine, the possibility should be considered.

DOSAGE AND ADMINISTRATION

The preferred parenteral route of administration for promethazine hydrochloride is by deep intramuscular injection. The proper intravenous administration of this product is well tolerated, but use of this route is not without some hazard.

INADVERTENT INTRAARTERIAL INJECTION CAN RESULT IN GANGRENE OF THE AFFECTED EXTREMITY (see "Warnings"). SUBCUTANEOUS INJECTION IS CONTRAINDICATED, AS IT MAY RESULT IN TISSUE NECROSIS (see "Contraindications"). When used intravenously, promethazine hydrochloride should be given in concentration no greater than 25 mg/mL at a rate not to exceed 25 mg per minute; it is preferable to inject through the tubing of an intravenous infusion set that is known to be functioning satisfactorily.

ALLERGIC CONDITIONS: The average adult dose is 25 mg. This dose may be repeated within two hours if necessary, but continued therapy, if indicated, should be via the oral route as soon as existing circumstances permit. After initiation of treatment, dosage should be adjusted to the smallest amount adequate to relieve symptoms. The average adult dose for amelioration of allergic reactions to blood or plasma is 25 mg.

SEDATION: In hospitalized adult patients, nighttime sedation may be achieved by a dose of 25 to 50 mg of promethazine hydrochloride.

PRE- AND POSTOPERATIVE USE:

As an adjunct to pre- or postoperative medication, 25 to 50 mg of promethazine hydrochloride in adults may be combined with appropriately reduced doses of analgesics and atropinelike drugs as desired. Dosage of concomitant analgesic or hypnotic medication should be reduced accordingly.

NAUSEA AND VOMITING: For control of nausea and vomiting, the usual adult dose is 12.5 to 25 mg, not to be repeated more frequently than every four hours. When used for control of postoperative nausea and vomiting, the medication may be administered either intramuscularly or intravenously and dosage of analgesics and barbiturates reduced accordingly.

OBSTETRICS: Phenergan in doses of 50 mg will provide sedation and relieve apprehension in the early stages of labor. When labor is definitely established, 25 to 75 mg (average dose, 50 mg) promethazine hydrochloride may be given intramuscularly or intravenously with an appropriately reduced dose of any desired narcotic. Amnesic agents may be administered as necessary. If necessary, Phenergan with a reduced dose of analgesic may be repeated once or twice at four-hour intervals in the course of a normal labor. A maximum total dose of 100 mg of Phenergan may be administered during a 24-hour period to patients in labor.

CHILDREN: In children under the age of 12 years, the dosage should not exceed half that of the suggested adult dose. As an adjunct to premedication, the suggested dose is 0.5 mg per lb. of body weight in combination with an equal dose of narcotic or barbiturate and the appropriate dose of an atropinelike drug. Antiemetics should not be used in vomiting of unknown etiology in children.

MANAGEMENT OF OVERDOSAGE

Signs and symptoms of overdosage range from mild depression of the central nervous system and cardiovascular system, to profound hypotension, respiratory depression, and unconsciousness. Stimulation may be evident, especially in children and geriatric patients. Atropinelike signs and symptoms—dry mouth, fixed, dilated pupils, flushing, etc., as well as gastrointestinal symptoms, may occur. The treatment of overdosage is essentially symptomatic and supportive. Early gastric lavage may be beneficial if promethazine has been taken orally. Centrally acting emetics are of little use.

Avoid analeptics, which may cause convulsions. Severe hypotension usually responds to the administration of levarterenol or phenylephrine. EPINEPHRINE SHOULD NOT BE USED, since its use in a patient with partial adrenergic blockade may further lower the blood pressure. Extrapyramidal reactions may be treated with anticholinergic antiparkinson agents, diphenhydramine, or barbiturates. Additional measures include oxygen and intravenous fluids. Limited experience with dialysis indicates that it is not helpful.

HOW SUPPLIED

Phenergan® (promethazine HCl) Injection, Wyeth®, is available in packages of 25 ampules of 1 mL as follows:
25 mg per mL, NDC 0008-0063.
50 mg per mL, NDC 0008-0455.
Store at room temperature, approximately 25°C (77°F).
Protect from light.

ALSO AVAILABLE

Phenergan® (promethazine HCl) injection, Wyeth®, is also available in TUBEX® Sterile Cartridge-Needle Units, (22 gauge × 1¼ inch needle) in packages of 10 TUBEX (1 mL size), as follows:
25 mg per mL, NDC 0008-0416.
50 mg per mL, NDC 0008-0417.

PHENERGAN® ℞
[fen 'er-gan]
(promethazine HCl)
Syrup Plain and
PHENERGAN® ℞
(promethazine HCl)
Syrup Fortis

DESCRIPTION

Each teaspoon (5 mL) of Phenergan Syrup Plain contains 6.25 mg promethazine hydrochloride in a flavored syrup base with a pH between 4.7 and 5.2. Alcohol 7%. The inactive ingredients present are artificial and natural flavors, citric acid, D&C Red 33, D&C Yellow 10, FD&C Blue 1, FD&C Yellow 6, glycerin, saccharin sodium, sodium benzoate, sodium citrate, sodium propionate, water, and other ingredients.

Each teaspoonful (5 mL) of Phenergan Syrup Fortis contains 25 mg promethazine hydrochloride in a flavored syrup base with a pH between 5.0 and 5.5. Alcohol 1.5%. The inactive ingredients present are artificial and natural flavors, citric acid, saccharin sodium, sodium benzoate, sodium propionate, water, and other ingredients.

Promethazine hydrochloride is a racemic compound; the empirical formula is $C_{17}H_{20}N_2S \cdot HCl$ and its molecular weight is 320.88

Promethazine hydrochloride, a phenothiazine derivative, is designated chemically as N,N,α-trimethyl-10H-phenothiazine-10-ethanamine monohydrochloride with the following structural formula:

$$CH_2CH(CH_3)N(CH_3)_2$$

· HCl

Promethazine hydrochloride occurs as a white to faint yellow, practically odorless, crystalline powder which slowly oxidizes and turns blue on prolonged exposure to air. It is soluble in water and freely soluble in alcohol.

CLINICAL PHARMACOLOGY

Promethazine is a phenothiazine derivative which differs structurally from the antipsychotic phenothiazines by the presence of a branched side chain and no ring substitution. It is thought that this configuration is responsible for its relative lack (1/10 that of chlorpromazine) of dopaminergic (CNS) action.

Promethazine is an H_1 receptor blocking agent. In addition to its antihistaminic action, it provides clinically useful sedative and antiemetic effects. In therapeutic dosage, promethazine produces no significant effects on the cardiovascular system.

Promethazine is well absorbed from the gastrointestinal tract. Clinical effects are apparent within 20 minutes after oral administration and generally last four to six hours, although they may persist as long as 12 hours. Promethazine is metabolized by the liver to a variety of compounds; the sulfoxides of promethazine and N-demethylpromethazine are the predominant metabolites appearing in the urine.

INDICATIONS AND USAGE

Phenergan is useful for:
Perennial and seasonal allergic rhinitis.
Vasomotor rhinitis.
Allergic conjunctivitis due to inhalant allergens and foods.
Mild, uncomplicated allergic skin manifestations of urticaria and angioedema.

Continued on next page

Wyeth-Ayerst—Cont.

Amelioration of allergic reactions to blood or plasma.
Dermographism.
Anaphylactic reactions, as adjunctive therapy to epinephrine and other standard measures, after the acute manifestations have been controlled.
Preoperative, postoperative, or obstetric sedation.
Prevention and control of nausea and vomiting associated with certain types of anesthesia and surgery.
Therapy adjunctive to meperidine or other analgesics for control of postoperative pain.
Sedation in both children and adults, as well as relief of apprehension and production of light sleep from which the patient can be easily aroused.
Active and prophylactic treatment of motion sickness.
Antiemetic therapy in postoperative patients.

CONTRAINDICATIONS

Promethazine is contraindicated in individuals known to be hypersensitive or to have had an idiosyncratic reaction to promethazine or to other phenothiazines.
Antihistamines are contraindicated for use in the treatment of lower respiratory tract symptoms including asthma.

WARNINGS

Promethazine may cause marked drowsiness. Ambulatory patients should be cautioned against such activities as driving or operating dangerous machinery until it is known that they do not become drowsy or dizzy from promethazine therapy.
The sedative action of promethazine hydrochloride is additive to the sedative effects of central nervous system depressants; therefore, agents such as alcohol, narcotic analgesics, sedatives, hypnotics, and tranquilizers should either be eliminated or given in reduced dosage in the presence of promethazine hydrochloride. When given concomitantly with promethazine hydrochloride, the dose of barbiturates should be reduced by at least one-half, and the dose of analgesic depressants, such as morphine or meperidine, should be reduced by one-quarter to one-half.
Promethazine may lower seizure threshold. This should be taken into consideration when administering to persons with known seizure disorders or when giving in combination with narcotics or local anesthetics which may also affect seizure threshold.
Sedative drugs or CNS depressants should be avoided in patients with a history of sleep apnea.
Antihistamines should be used with caution in patients with narrow-angle glaucoma, stenosing peptic ulcer, pyloroduodenal obstruction, and urinary bladder obstruction due to symptomatic prostatic hypertrophy and narrowing of the bladder neck.
Administration of promethazine has been associated with reported cholestatic jaundice.

PRECAUTIONS

GENERAL

Promethazine should be used cautiously in persons with cardiovascular disease or with impairment of liver function.

INFORMATION FOR PATIENTS

Phenergan may cause marked drowsiness or impair the mental and/or physical abilities required for the performance of potentially hazardous tasks, such as driving a vehicle or operating machinery. Ambulatory patients should be told to avoid engaging in such activities until it is known that they do not become drowsy or dizzy from Phenergan therapy. Children should be supervised to avoid potential harm in bike riding or in other hazardous activities.
The concomitant use of alcohol or other central nervous system depressants, including narcotic analgesics, sedatives, hypnotics, and tranquilizers, may have an additive effect and should be avoided or their dosage reduced.
Patients should be advised to report any involuntary muscle movements or unusual sensitivity to sunlight.

DRUG INTERACTIONS

The sedative action of promethazine is additive to the sedative effects of other central nervous system depressants, including alcohol, narcotic analgesics, sedatives, hypnotics, tricyclic antidepressants, and tranquilizers; therefore, these agents should be avoided or administered in reduced dosage to patients receiving promethazine.

DRUG/LABORATORY TEST INTERACTIONS

The following laboratory tests may be affected in patients who are receiving therapy with promethazine hydrochloride:
Pregnancy Tests
Diagnostic pregnancy tests based on immunological reactions between HCG and anti-HCG may result in false-negative or false-positive interpretations.
Glucose Tolerance Test
An increase in blood glucose has been reported in patients receiving promethazine.

CARCINOGENESIS, MUTAGENESIS, IMPAIRMENT OF FERTILITY

Long-term animal studies have not been performed to assess the carcinogenic potential of promethazine, nor are there other animal or human data concerning carcinogenicity, mutagenicity, or impairment of fertility with this drug. Promethazine was nonmutagenic in the *Salmonella* test system of Ames.

PREGNANCY

Teratogenic Effects —Pregnancy Category C
Teratogenic effects have not been demonstrated in rat-feeding studies at doses of 6.25 and 12.5 mg/kg of promethazine. These doses are from approximately 2.1 to 4.2 times the maximum recommended total daily dose of promethazine for a 50-kg subject, depending upon the indication for which the drug is prescribed. Specific studies to test the action of the drug on parturition, lactation, and development of the animal neonate were not done, but a general preliminary study in rats indicated no effect on these parameters. Although antihistamines, including promethazine, have been found to produce fetal mortality in rodents, the pharmacological effects of histamine in the rodent do not parallel those in man. There are no adequate and well-controlled studies of promethazine in pregnant women. Phenergan should be used during pregnancy only if the potential benefit justifies the potential risk to the fetus.
Nonteratogenic Effects
Promethazine taken within two weeks of delivery may inhibit platelet aggregation in the newborn.

LABOR AND DELIVERY

Phenergan, in appropriate dosage form, may be used alone or as an adjunct to narcotic analgesics during labor and delivery. (See "Indications and Usage" and "Dosage and Administration.")
See also "Nonteratogenic Effects."

NURSING MOTHERS

It is not known whether promethazine is excreted in human milk. Caution should be exercised when promethazine is administered to a nursing woman.

PEDIATRIC USE

This product should not be used in children under 2 years of age because safety for such use has not been established.

ADVERSE REACTIONS

Nervous System —Sedation, sleepiness, occasional blurred vision, dryness of mouth, dizziness; rarely confusion, disorientation, and extrapyramidal symptoms such as oculogyric crisis, torticollis, and tongue protrusion (usually in association with parenteral injection or excessive dosage).
Cardiovascular —Increased or decreased blood pressure.
Dermatologic —Rash, rarely photosensitivity.
Hematologic —Rarely leukopenia, thrombocytopenia; agranulocytosis (1 case).
Gastrointestinal —Nausea and vomiting.

OVERDOSAGE

Signs and symptoms of overdosage with promethazine range from mild depression of the central nervous system and cardiovascular system to profound hypotension, respiratory depression, and unconsciousness.
Stimulation may be evident, especially in children and geriatric patients. Convulsions may rarely occur. A paradoxical reaction has been reported in children receiving single doses of 75 mg to 125 mg orally, characterized by hyperexcitability and nightmares.
Atropine-like signs and symptoms—dry mouth, fixed, dilated pupils, flushing, as well as gastrointestinal symptoms, may occur.

TREATMENT

Treatment of overdosage is essentially symptomatic and supportive. Only in cases of extreme overdosage or individual sensitivity do vital signs including respiration, pulse, blood pressure, temperature, and EKG need to be monitored. Activated charcoal orally or by lavage may be given, or sodium or magnesium sulfate orally as a cathartic. Attention should be given to the reestablishment of adequate respiratory exchange through provision of a patent airway and institution of assisted or controlled ventilation. Diazepam may be used to control convulsions. Acidosis and electrolyte losses should be corrected. Note that any depressant effects of promethazine are not reversed by naloxone. Avoid analeptics which may cause convulsions.
Severe hypotension usually responds to the administration of norepinephrine or phenylephrine. EPINEPHRINE SHOULD NOT BE USED, since its use in patients with partial adrenergic blockade may further lower the blood pressure.
Limited experience with dialysis indicates that it is not helpful.

DOSAGE AND ADMINISTRATION

ALLERGY

The average oral dose is 25 mg taken before retiring; however, 12.5 mg may be taken before meals and on retiring, if necessary. Children tolerate this product well. Single 25-mg doses at bedtime or 6.25 to 12.5 mg taken three times daily will usually suffice. After initiation of treatment in children

or adults, dosage should be adjusted to the smallest amount adequate to relieve symptoms.
Phenergan Rectal Suppositories may be used if the oral route is not feasible, but oral therapy should be resumed as soon as possible if continued therapy is indicated.
The administration of promethazine hydrochloride in 25-mg doses will control minor transfusion reactions of an allergic nature.

MOTION SICKNESS

The average adult dose is 25 mg taken twice daily. The initial dose should be taken one-half to one hour before anticipated travel and be repeated 8 to 12 hours later, if necessary. On succeeding days of travel, it is recommended that 25 mg be given on arising and again before the evening meal. For children, Phenergan Tablets, Syrup, or Rectal Suppositories, 12.5 to 25 mg, twice daily, may be administered.

NAUSEA AND VOMITING

The average effective dose of Phenergan for the active therapy of nausea and vomiting in children or adults is 25 mg. When oral medication cannot be tolerated, the dose should be given parenterally (cf. Phenergan Injection) or by rectal suppository. 12.5- to 25-mg doses may be repeated, as necessary, at 4- to 6-hour intervals.
For nausea and vomiting in children, the usual dose is 0.5 mg per pound of body weight, and the dose should be adjusted to the age and weight of the patient and the severity of the condition being treated.
For prophylaxis of nausea and vomiting, as during surgery and the postoperative period, the average dose is 25 mg repeated at 4- to 6-hour intervals, as necessary.

SEDATION

This product relieves apprehension and induces a quiet sleep from which the patient can be easily aroused. Administration of 12.5 to 25 mg Phenergan by the oral route or by rectal suppository at bedtime will provide sedation in children. Adults usually require 25 to 50 mg for nighttime, presurgical, or obstetrical sedation.

PRE- AND POSTOPERATIVE USE

Phenergan in 12.5- to 25-mg doses for children and 50-mg doses for adults the night before surgery relieves apprehension and produces a quiet sleep.
For preoperative medication children require doses of 0.5 mg per pound of body weight in combination with an equal dose of meperidine and the appropriate dose of an atropinelike drug.
Usual adult dosage is 50 mg Phenergan with an equal amount of meperidine and the required amount of a belladonna alkaloid.
Postoperative sedation and adjunctive use with analgesics may be obtained by the administration of 12.5 to 25 mg in children and 25- to 50-mg doses in adults.
Phenergan Syrup Plain and Phenergan Syrup Fortis are not recommended for children under 2 years of age.

HOW SUPPLIED

Phenergan® (promethazine HCl) Syrup Plain, Wyeth®, is a clear, green solution supplied as follows:
NDC 0008-0549-02, case of 24 bottles of 4 fl. oz. (118 mL).
NDC 0008-0549-03, bottle of 1 pint. (473 mL).
Phenergan® (promethazine HCl) Syrup Fortis, Wyeth®, is a clear, light straw-colored solution supplied as follows:
NDC 0008-0231-01, bottle of 1 pint (473 mL).
Keep bottles tightly closed.
Store at Room Temperature, between 15° C and 25° C (59° F and 77° F).
Protect from light.
Dispense in light-resistant, glass, tight containers.

PHENERGAN®   ℞
[fen 'er-gan]
(promethazine HCl)
TABLETS ●
SUPPOSITORIES

DESCRIPTION

Each tablet of Phenergan contains 12.5 mg, 25 mg, or 50 mg promethazine hydrochloride. The inactive ingredients present are lactose, magnesium stearate, and methylcellulose.
Each dosage strength also contains the following:
12.5 mg—FD&C Yellow 6 and saccharin sodium;
25 mg—saccharin sodium;
50 mg—FD&C Red 3 and FD&C Yellow 6.
Each rectal suppository of Phenergan contains 12.5 mg, 25 mg, or 50 mg promethazine hydrochloride with ascorbyl palmitate, silicon dioxide, white wax, and cocoa butter.
Promethazine hydrochloride is a racemic compound; the empirical formula is $C_{17}H_{20}N_2S \cdot HCl$ and its molecular weight is 320.88.
Promethazine hydrochloride, a phenothiazine derivative, is designated chemically as N,N,α-trimethyl-10H-phenothiazine-10-ethanamine monohydrochloride.
Promethazine hydrochloride occurs as a white to faint yellow, practically odorless, crystalline powder which slowly oxidizes and turns blue on prolonged exposure to air. It is soluble in water and freely soluble in alcohol.

CLINICAL PHARMACOLOGY

Promethazine is a phenothiazine derivative which differs structurally from the antipsychotic phenothiazines by the presence of a branched side chain and no ring substitution. It is thought that this configuration is responsible for its relative lack ($\frac{1}{10}$ that of chlorpromazine) of dopaminergic (CNS) action.

Promethazine is an H_1 receptor blocking agent. In addition to its antihistaminic action, it provides clinically useful sedative and antiemetic effects. In therapeutic dosage, promethazine produces no significant effects on the cardiovascular system.

Promethazine is well absorbed from the gastrointestinal tract. Clinical effects are apparent within 20 minutes after oral administration and generally last four to six hours, although they may persist as long as 12 hours. Promethazine is metabolized by the liver to a variety of compounds; the sulfoxides of promethazine and N-demethylpromethazine are the predominant metabolites appearing in the urine.

INDICATIONS AND USAGE

Phenergan, either orally or by suppository, is useful for:
Perennial and seasonal allergic rhinitis.
Vasomotor rhinitis.
Allergic conjunctivitis due to inhalant allergens and foods.
Mild, uncomplicated allergic skin manifestations of urticaria and angioedema.
Amelioration of allergic reactions to blood or plasma.
Dermographism.
Anaphylactic reactions, as adjunctive therapy to epinephrine and other standard measures, after the acute manifestations have been controlled.
Preoperative, postoperative, or obstetric sedation.
Prevention and control of nausea and vomiting associated with certain types of anesthesia and surgery.
Therapy adjunctive to meperidine or other analgesics for control of postoperative pain.
Sedation in both children and adults, as well as relief of apprehension and production of light sleep from which the patient can be easily aroused.
Active and prophylactic treatment of motion sickness.
Antiemetic therapy in postoperative patients.

CONTRAINDICATIONS

Promethazine is contraindicated in individuals known to be hypersensitive or to have had an idiosyncratic reaction to promethazine or to other phenothiazines.

Antihistamines are contraindicated for use in the treatment of lower respiratory tract symptoms including asthma.

WARNINGS

Promethazine may cause marked drowsiness. Ambulatory patients should be cautioned against such activities as driving or operating dangerous machinery until it is known that they do not become drowsy or dizzy from promethazine therapy.

The sedative action of promethazine hydrochloride is additive to the sedative effects of central nervous system depressants; therefore, agents such as alcohol, narcotic analgesics, sedatives, hypnotics, and tranquilizers should either be eliminated or given in reduced dosage in the presence of promethazine hydrochloride. When given concomitantly with promethazine hydrochloride, the dose of barbiturates should be reduced by at least one-half, and the dose of analgesic depressants, such as morphine or meperidine, should be reduced by one-quarter to one-half.

Promethazine may lower seizure threshold. This should be taken into consideration when administering to persons with known seizure disorders or when giving in combination with narcotics and local anesthetics which may also affect seizure threshold.

Sedative drugs or CNS depressants should be avoided in patients with a history of sleep apnea.

Antihistamines should be used with caution in patients with narrow-angle glaucoma, stenosing peptic ulcer, pyloroduodenal obstruction, and urinary bladder obstruction due to symptomatic prostatic hypertrophy and narrowing of the bladder neck.

Administration of promethazine has been associated with reported cholestatic jaundice.

PRECAUTIONS

GENERAL

Promethazine should be used cautiously in persons with cardiovascular disease or with impairment of liver function.

INFORMATION FOR PATIENTS

Phenergan may cause marked drowsiness or impair the mental and/or physical abilities required for the performance of potentially hazardous tasks, such as driving a vehicle or operating machinery. Ambulatory patients should be told to avoid engaging in such activities until it is known that they do not become drowsy or dizzy from Phenergan therapy. Children should be supervised to avoid potential harm in bike riding or in other hazardous activities.

The concomitant use of alcohol or other central nervous system depressants, including narcotic analgesics, sedatives, hypnotics, and tranquilizers, may have an additive effect and should be avoided or their dosage reduced.

Patients should be advised to report any involuntary muscle movements or unusual sensitivity to sunlight.

DRUG INTERACTIONS

The sedative action of promethazine is additive to the sedative effects of other central nervous system depressants, including alcohol, narcotic analgesics, sedatives, hypnotics, tricyclic antidepressants, and tranquilizers; therefore, these agents should be avoided or administered in reduced dosage to patients receiving promethazine.

DRUG/LABORATORY TEST INTERACTIONS

The following laboratory tests may be affected in patients who are receiving therapy with promethazine hydrochloride:

Pregnancy Tests

Diagnostic pregnancy tests based on immunological reactions between HCG and anti-HCG may result in false-negative or false-positive interpretations.

Glucose Tolerance Test

An increase in blood glucose has been reported in patients receiving promethazine.

CARCINOGENESIS, MUTAGENESIS, IMPAIRMENT OF FERTILITY

Long-term animal studies have not been performed to assess the carcinogenic potential of promethazine, nor are there other animal or human data concerning carcinogenicity, mutagenicity, or impairment of fertility with this drug. Promethazine was nonmutagenic in the *Salmonella* test system of Ames.

PREGNANCY

Teratogenic Effects —Pregnancy Category C

Teratogenic effects have not been demonstrated in rat-feeding studies at doses of 6.25 and 12.5 mg/kg of promethazine. These doses are from approximately 2.1 to 4.2 times the maximum recommended total daily dose of promethazine for a 50-kg subject, depending upon the indication for which the drug is prescribed. Specific studies to test the action of the drug on parturition, lactation, and development of the animal neonate were not done, but a general preliminary study in rats indicated no effect on these parameters. Although antihistamines, including promethazine, have been found to produce fetal mortality in rodents, the pharmacological effects of histamine in the rodent do not parallel those in man. There are no adequate and well-controlled studies of promethazine in pregnant women. Phenergan should be used during pregnancy only if the potential benefit justifies the potential risk to the fetus.

Nonteratogenic Effects

Promethazine taken within two weeks of delivery may inhibit platelet aggregation in the newborn.

LABOR AND DELIVERY

Phenergan, in appropriate dosage form, may be used alone or as an adjunct to narcotic analgesics during labor and delivery. (See "Indications and Usage" and "Dosage and Administration.")

See also "Nonteratogenic Effects."

NURSING MOTHERS

It is not known whether promethazine is excreted in human milk. Caution should be exercised when promethazine is administered to a nursing woman.

PEDIATRIC USE

This product should not be used in children under 2 years of age because safety for such use has not been established.

ADVERSE REACTIONS

Nervous System —Sedation, sleepiness, occasional blurred vision, dryness of mouth, dizziness; rarely confusion, disorientation, and extrapyramidal symptoms such as oculogyric crisis, torticollis, and tongue protrusion (usually in association with parenteral injection or excessive dosage).
Cardiovascular —Increased or decreased blood pressure.
Dermatologic —Rash, rarely photosensitivity.
Hematologic —Rarely leukopenia, thrombocytopenia; agranulocytosis (1 case).
Gastrointestinal —Nausea and vomiting.

OVERDOSAGE

Signs and symptoms of overdosage with promethazine range from mild depression of the central nervous system and cardiovascular system to profound hypotension, respiratory depression, and unconsciousness.

Stimulation may be evident, especially in children and geriatric patients. Convulsions may rarely occur. A paradoxical reaction has been reported in children receiving single doses of 75 mg to 125 mg orally, characterized by hyperexcitability and nightmares.

Atropinelike signs and symptoms—dry mouth, fixed, dilated pupils, flushing, as well as gastrointestinal symptoms, may occur.

TREATMENT

Treatment of overdosage is essentially symptomatic and supportive. Only in cases of extreme overdosage or individual sensitivity do vital signs, including respiration, pulse, blood pressure, temperature, and EKG, need to be monitored. Activated charcoal orally or by lavage may be given, or sodium or magnesium sulfate orally as a cathartic. Attention should be given to the reestablishment of adequate respiratory exchange through provision of a patent airway and institution of assisted or controlled ventilation. Diazepam may be used to control convulsions. Acidosis and electrolyte losses should be corrected. Note that any depressant effects of promethazine are not reversed by naloxone. Avoid analeptics which may cause convulsions.

Severe hypotension usually responds to the administration of norepinephrine or phenylephrine. EPINEPHRINE SHOULD NOT BE USED, since its use in patients with partial adrenergic blockade may further lower the blood pressure.

Limited experience with dialysis indicates that it is not helpful.

DOSAGE AND ADMINISTRATION

Allergy: The average oral dose is 25 mg taken before retiring; however, 12.5 mg may be taken before meals and on retiring, if necessary. Children tolerate this product well. Single 25-mg doses at bedtime or 6.25 to 12.5 mg taken three times daily will usually suffice. After initiation of treatment in children or adults, dosage should be adjusted to the smallest amount adequate to relieve symptoms. The administration of promethazine hydrochloride in 25-mg doses will control minor transfusion reactions of an allergic nature.

Motion Sickness: The average adult dose is 25 mg taken twice daily. The initial dose should be taken one-half to one hour before anticipated travel and be repeated 8 to 12 hours later, if necessary. On succeeding days of travel, it is recommended that 25 mg be given on arising and again before the evening meal. For children, Phenergan Tablets, Syrup, or Rectal Suppositories, 12.5 to 25 mg, twice daily, may be administered.

Nausea and Vomiting: The average effective dose of Phenergan for the active therapy of nausea and vomiting in children or adults is 25 mg. When oral medication cannot be tolerated, the dose should be given parenterally (cf. Phenergan Injection) or by rectal suppository. 12.5- to 25-mg doses may be repeated as necessary at 4- to 6-hour intervals. For nausea and vomiting in children, the usual dose is 0.5 mg per pound of body weight, and the dose should be adjusted to the age and weight of the patient and the severity of the condition being treated.

For prophylaxis of nausea and vomiting, as during surgery and the postoperative period, the average dose is 25 mg repeated at 4- to 6-hour intervals, as necessary.

Sedation: This product relieves apprehension and induces a quiet sleep from which the patient can be easily aroused. Administration of 12.5 to 25 mg Phenergan by the oral route or by rectal suppository at bedtime will provide sedation in children. Adults usually require 25 to 50 mg for nighttime, presurgical, or obstetrical sedation.

Pre- and Postoperative Use: Phenergan in 12.5- to 25-mg doses for children and 50-mg doses for adults the night before surgery relieves apprehension and produces a quiet sleep.

For preoperative medication children require doses of 0.5 mg per pound of body weight in combination with an equal dose of meperidine and the appropriate dose of an atropinelike drug.

Usual adult dosage is 50 mg Phenergan with an equal amount of meperidine and the required amount of a belladonna alkaloid.

Postoperative sedation and adjunctive use with analgesics may be obtained by the administration of 12.5 to 25 mg in children and 25- to 50-mg doses in adults.

Phenergan tablets and Phenergan suppositories are not recommended for children under 2 years of age.

HOW SUPPLIED

Phenergan® (promethazine HCl) Tablets, Wyeth®, are available as follows:

12.5 mg, orange tablet with "WYETH" on one side and "19" on the scored reverse side.
NDC 0008-0019-01, bottle of 100 tablets.
25 mg, white tablet with "WYETH" and "27" on one side and scored on the reverse side.
NDC 0008-0027-02, bottle of 100 tablets.
NDC 0008-0027-05, Redipak® carton of 100 tablets (10 blister strips of 10).
50 mg, pink tablet with "WYETH" on one side and "227" on the other side.
NDC 0008-0227-01, bottle of 100 tablets.
Keep tablets in tightly closed bottles.
Store at Room Temperature, between 15°C and 25°C (59°F and 77°F).
Protect from light.
Dispense in light-resistant, tight container.
Phenergan® (promethazine HCl) Suppositories, Wyeth®, are available as follows:
12.5 mg, ivory, cone-shaped suppository wrapped in copper-colored foil.

Continued on next page

Wyeth-Ayerst—Cont.

NDC 0008-0498-01, box of 12 suppositories.
25 mg, ivory, cone-shaped suppository wrapped in light-green foil.
NDC 0008-0212-01, box of 12 suppositories.
50 mg, ivory, torpedo-shaped suppository wrapped in light-green foil.
NDC 0008-0229-01, box of 12 suppositories.
Refrigerate suppositories.
Dispense in well-closed container.
Shown in Product Identification Section, page 437

PHENERGAN®   © ℞
[*fen'er-gan*]
with codeine
(Promethazine Hydrochloride and Codeine Phosphate) Syrup

DESCRIPTION
Each teaspoon (5 mL) of Phenergan with codeine contains 10 mg (1/6 grain) codeine phosphate (Warning—may be habit-forming) and 6.25 mg promethazine hydrochloride in a flavored syrup base with a pH between 4.7 and 5.2. Alcohol 7%. The inactive ingredients present are artificial and natural flavors, citric acid, D&C Red 33, FD&C Blue 1, FD&C Yellow 6, glycerine, saccharin sodium, sodium benzoate, sodium citrate, sodium propionate, water, and other ingredients.
Codeine is one of the naturally occurring phenanthrene alkaloids of opium derived from the opium poppy; it is classified pharmacologically as a narcotic analgesic. Codeine phosphate may be chemically named as (5α,6α)-7,8-didehydro-4, 5-epoxy-3-methoxy-17-methylmorphinan-6-ol phosphate (1:1) (salt) hemihydrate with the following structural formula:

The phosphate salt of codeine occurs as white, needle-shaped crystals or white crystalline powder. Codeine phosphate is freely soluble in water and slightly soluble in alcohol, with a molecular weight of 406.37. The empirical formula is $C_{18}H_{21}NO_3 \cdot H_3PO_4 \cdot \frac{1}{2}H_2O$, and the stereochemistry is 5α, 6α isomer as indicated in the structure.
Promethazine hydrochloride is a racemic compound; the empirical formula is $C_{17}H_{20}N_2S \cdot HCl$ and its molecular weight is 320.88.
Promethazine hydrochloride, a phenothiazine derivative, is designated chemically as N,N,α-trimethyl-10*H*-phenothiazine-10-ethanamine monohydrochloride with the following structural formula:

Promethazine hydrochloride occurs as a white to faint yellow, practically odorless, crystalline powder which slowly oxidizes and turns blue on prolonged exposure to air. It is soluble in water and freely soluble in alcohol.

CLINICAL PHARMACOLOGY
CODEINE
Narcotic analgesics, including codeine, exert their primary effects on the central nervous system and gastrointestinal tract. The analgesic effects of codeine are due to its central action; however, the precise sites of action have not been determined, and the mechanisms involved appear to be quite complex. Codeine resembles morphine both structurally and pharmacologically, but its actions at the doses of codeine used therapeutically are milder, with less sedation, respiratory depression, and gastrointestinal, urinary, and pupillary effects. Codeine produces an increase in biliary tract pressure, but less than morphine or meperidine. Codeine is less constipating than morphine.
Codeine has good antitussive activity, although less than that of morphine at equal doses. It is used in preference to morphine, because side effects are infrequent at the usual antitussive dose of codeine.
Codeine in oral therapeutic dosage does not usually exert major effects on the cardiovascular system.
Narcotic analgesics may cause nausea and vomiting by stimulating the chemoreceptor trigger zone (CTZ); however, they also depress the vomiting center, so that subsequent doses

are unlikely to produce vomiting. Nausea is minimal after usual oral doses of codeine.
Narcotic analgesics cause histamine release, which appears to be responsible for wheals or urticaria sometimes seen at the site of injection on parenteral administration. Histamine release may also produce dilation of cutaneous blood vessels, with resultant flushing of the face and neck, pruritus, and sweating.
Codeine and its salts are well absorbed following both oral and parenteral administration. Codeine is about 2/3 as effective orally as parenterally. Codeine is metabolized primarily in the liver by enzymes of the endoplasmic reticulum, where it undergoes O-demethylation, N-demethylation, and partial conjugation with glucuronic acid. The drug is excreted primarily in the urine, largely as inactive metabolites and small amounts of free and conjugated morphine. Negligible amounts of codeine and its metabolites are found in the feces. Following oral or subcutaneous administration of codeine, the onset of analgesia occurs within 15 to 30 minutes and lasts for four to six hours.
The cough-depressing action, in animal studies, was observed to occur 15 minutes after oral administration of codeine, peak action at 45 to 60 minutes after ingestion. The duration of action, which is dose-dependent, usually did not exceed 3 hours.
PROMETHAZINE
Promethazine is a phenothiazine derivative which differs structurally from the antipsychotic phenothiazines by the presence of a branched side chain and no ring substitution. It is thought that this configuration is responsible for its lack (1/10 that of chlorpromazine) of dopaminergic (CNS) action. Promethazine is an H_1 receptor blocking agent. In addition to its antihistaminic action, it provides clinically useful sedative and antiemetic effects. In therapeutic dosages, promethazine produces no significant effects on the cardiovascular system.
Promethazine is well absorbed from the gastrointestinal tract. Clinical effects are apparent within 20 minutes after oral administration and generally last four to six hours, although they may persist as long as 12 hours. Promethazine is metabolized by the liver to a variety of compounds; the sulfoxides of promethazine and N-demethylpromethazine are the predominant metabolites appearing in the urine.

INDICATIONS AND USAGE
Phenergan with codeine is indicated for the temporary relief of coughs and upper respiratory symptoms associated with allergy or the common cold.

CONTRAINDICATIONS
Codeine is contraindicated in patients with a known hypersensitivity to the drug.
Promethazine is contraindicated in individuals known to be hypersensitive or to have had an idiosyncratic reaction to promethazine or to other phenothiazines.
Antihistamines and codeine are both contraindicated for use in the treatment of lower respiratory tract symptoms, including asthma.

WARNINGS
CODEINE
Dosage of codeine SHOULD NOT BE INCREASED if cough fails to respond; an unresponsive cough should be reevaluated in 5 days or sooner for possible underlying pathology, such as foreign body or lower respiratory tract disease.
Codeine may cause or aggravate constipation.
Respiratory depression leading to arrest, coma, and death has occurred with the use of codeine antitussives in young children, particularly in the under-one-year infants whose ability to deactivate the drug is not fully developed.
Administration of codeine may be accompanied by histamine release and should be used with caution in atopic children.
Head Injury and Increased Intracranial Pressure
The respiratory-depressant effects of narcotic analgesics and their capacity to elevate cerebrospinal fluid pressure may be markedly exaggerated in the presence of head injury, intracranial lesions, or a preexisting increase in intracranial pressure. Narcotics may produce adverse reactions which may obscure the clinical course of patients with head injuries.
Asthma and Other Respiratory Conditions
Narcotic analgesics or cough suppressants, including codeine, should not be used in asthmatic patients (see "Contraindications"). Nor should they be used in acute febrile illness associated with productive cough or in chronic respiratory disease where interference with ability to clear the tracheobronchial tree of secretions would have a deleterious effect on the patient's respiratory function.
Hypotensive Effect
Codeine may produce orthostatic hypotension in ambulatory patients.
PROMETHAZINE
Promethazine may cause marked drowsiness. Ambulatory patients should be cautioned against such activities as driving or operating dangerous machinery until it is known that they do not become drowsy or dizzy from promethazine therapy.

The sedative action of promethazine hydrochloride is additive to the sedative effects of central nervous system depressants; therefore, agents such as alcohol, narcotic analgesics, sedatives, hypnotics, and tranquilizers should either be eliminated or given in reduced dosage in the presence of promethazine hydrochloride. When given concomitantly with promethazine hydrochloride, the dose of barbiturates should be reduced by at least one-half, and the dose of analgesic depressants, such as morphine or meperidine, should be reduced by one-quarter to one-half.
Promethazine may lower seizure threshold. This should be taken into consideration when administering to persons with known seizure disorders or when giving in combination with narcotics or local anesthetics which may also affect seizure threshold.
Sedative drugs or CNS depressants should be avoided in patients with a history of sleep apnea.
Antihistamines should be used with caution in patients with narrow-angle glaucoma, stenosing peptic ulcer, pyloroduodenal obstruction, and urinary bladder obstruction due to symptomatic prostatic hypertrophy and narrowing of the bladder neck.
Administration of promethazine has been associated with reported cholestatic jaundice.

PRECAUTIONS
Animal reproduction studies have not been conducted with the drug combination—promethazine and codeine. It is not known whether this drug combination can cause fetal harm when administered to a pregnant woman or can affect reproduction capacity. Phenergan with codeine should be given to a pregnant woman only if clearly needed.
GENERAL
Narcotic analgesics, including codeine, should be administered with caution and the initial dose reduced in patients with acute abdominal conditions, convulsive disorders, significant hepatic or renal impairment, fever, hypothyroidism, Addison's disease, ulcerative colitis, prostatic hypertrophy, in patients with recent gastrointestinal or urinary tract surgery, and in the very young or elderly or debilitated patients. Promethazine should be used cautiously in persons with cardiovascular disease or with impairment of liver function.
INFORMATION FOR PATIENTS
Phenergan with codeine may cause marked drowsiness or may impair the mental and/or physical abilities required for the performance of potentially hazardous tasks, such as driving a vehicle or operating machinery. Ambulatory patients should be told to avoid engaging in such activities until it is known that they do not become drowsy or dizzy from Phenergan with codeine therapy. Children should be supervised to avoid potential harm in bike riding or in other hazardous activities.
The concomitant use of alcohol or other central nervous system depressants, including narcotic analgesics, sedatives, hypnotics, and tranquilizers, may have an additive effect and should be avoided or their dosage reduced.
Patients should be advised to report any involuntary muscle movements or unusual sensitivity to sunlight.
Codeine, like other narcotic analgesics, may produce orthostatic hypotension in some ambulatory patients. Patients should be cautioned accordingly.
DRUG INTERACTIONS
CODEINE
In patients receiving MAO inhibitors, an initial small test dose is advisable to allow observation of any excessive narcotic effects or MAOI interaction.
PROMETHAZINE
The sedative action of promethazine is additive to the effects of other central nervous system depressants, including alcohol, narcotic analgesics, sedatives, hypnotics, tricyclic antidepressants, and tranquilizers; therefore, these agents should be avoided or administered in reduced dosage to patients receiving promethazine.
DRUG/LABORATORY TEST INTERACTIONS
Because narcotic analgesics may increase biliary tract pressure, with resultant increases in plasma amylase or lipase levels, determination of these enzyme levels may be unreliable for 24 hours after a narcotic analgesic has been given.
The following laboratory tests may be affected in patients who are receiving therapy with promethazine hydrochloride:
Pregnancy Tests
Diagnostic pregnancy tests based on immunological reactions between HCG and anti-HCG may result in false-negative or false-positive interpretations.
Glucose Tolerance Test
An increase in blood glucose has been reported in patients receiving promethazine.
CARCINOGENESIS, MUTAGENESIS, IMPAIRMENT OF FERTILITY
Long-term animal studies have not been performed to assess the carcinogenic potential of codeine or of promethazine, nor are there other animal or human data concerning carcinogenicity, mutagenicity, or impairment of fertility with these agents. Codeine has been reported to show no evidence of carcinogenicity or mutagenicity in a variety of test systems,

including the micronucleus and sperm abnormality assays and the *Salmonella* assay. Promethazine was nonmutagenic in the *Salmonella* test system of Ames.

PREGNANCY
Teratogenic Effects —Pregnancy Category C
CODEINE
A study in rats and rabbits reported no teratogenic effect of codeine administered during the period of organogenesis in doses ranging from 5 to 120 mg/kg. In the rat, doses at the 120-mg/kg level, in the toxic range for the adult animal, were associated with an increase in embryo resorption at the time of implantation. In another study a single 100-mg/kg dose of codeine administered to pregnant mice reportedly resulted in delayed ossification in the offspring.

There are no studies in humans, and the significance of these findings to humans, if any, is not known.

PROMETHAZINE
Teratogenic effects have not been demonstrated in rat-feeding studies at doses of 6.25 and 12.5 mg/kg of promethazine. These doses are 8.3 and 16.7 times the maximum recommended total daily dose of promethazine for a 50-kg subject. Specific studies to test the action of the drug on parturition, lactation, and development of the animal neonate were not done, but a general preliminary study in rats indicated no effect on these parameters. Although antihistamines, including promethazine, have been found to produce fetal mortality in rodents, the pharmacological effects of histamine in the rodent do not parallel those in man. There are no adequate and well-controlled studies of promethazine in pregnant women.

Phenergan with codeine should be used during pregnancy only if the potential benefit justifies the potential risk to the fetus.

Nonteratogenic Effects
Dependence has been reported in newborns whose mothers took opiates regularly during pregnancy. Withdrawal signs include irritability, excessive crying, tremors, hyperreflexia, fever, vomiting, and diarrhea. Signs usually appear during the first few days of life.

Promethazine taken within two weeks of delivery may inhibit platelet aggregation in the newborn.

LABOR AND DELIVERY
Narcotic analgesics cross the placental barrier. The closer to delivery and the larger the dose used, the greater the possibility of respiratory depression in the newborn. Narcotic analgesics should be avoided during labor if delivery of a premature infant is anticipated. If the mother has received narcotic analgesics during labor, newborn infants should be observed closely for signs of respiratory depression. Resuscitation may be required (see "Overdosage"). The effect of codeine, if any, on the later growth, development, and functional maturation of the child is unknown.

See also "Nonteratogenic Effects."

NURSING MOTHERS
Some studies, but not others, have reported detectable amounts of codeine in breast milk. The levels are probably not clinically significant after usual therapeutic dosage. The possibility of clinically important amounts being excreted in breast milk in individuals abusing codeine should be considered.

It is not known whether promethazine is excreted in human milk.

Caution should be exercised when Phenergan with codeine is administered to a nursing woman.

PEDIATRIC USE
This product should not be used in children under 2 years of age because safety for such use has not been established.

ADVERSE REACTIONS
CODEINE
*Nervous System —*CNS depression, particularly respiratory depression, and to a lesser extent circulatory depression; light-headedness, dizziness, sedation, euphoria, dysphoria, headache, transient hallucination, disorientation, visual disturbances, and convulsions.

*Cardiovascular —*Tachycardia, bradycardia, palpitation, faintness, syncope, orthostatic hypotension (common to narcotic analgesics).

*Gastrointestinal —*Nausea, vomiting, constipation, and biliary tract spasm. Patients with chronic ulcerative colitis may experience increased colonic motility; in patients with acute ulcerative colitis, toxic dilation has been reported.

*Genitourinary —*Oliguria, urinary retention; antidiuretic effect has been reported (common to narcotic analgesics).

*Allergic —*Infrequent pruritus, giant urticaria, angioneurotic edema, and laryngeal edema.

*Other —*Flushing of the face, sweating and pruritus (due to opiate-induced histamine release); weakness.

PROMETHAZINE
*Nervous System —*Sedation, sleepiness, occasional blurred vision, dryness of mouth, dizziness; rarely confusion, disorientation, and extrapyramidal symptoms such as oculogyric crisis, torticollis, and tongue protrusion (usually in association with parenteral injection or excessive dosage).

*Cardiovascular —*Increased or decreased blood pressure.
*Dermatologic —*Rash, rarely photosensitivity.
*Hematologic —*Rarely leukopenia, thrombocytopenia; agranulocytosis (1 case).
*Gastrointestinal —*Nausea and vomiting.

DRUG ABUSE AND DEPENDENCE
CONTROLLED SUBSTANCE
Phenergan with codeine is a Schedule V Controlled Substance.

ABUSE
Codeine is known to be subject to abuse; however, the abuse potential of oral codeine appears to be quite low. Even parenteral codeine does not appear to offer the psychic effects sought by addicts to the same degree as heroin or morphine. However, codeine must be administered only under close supervision to patients with a history of drug abuse or dependence.

DEPENDENCE
Psychological dependence, physical dependence, and tolerance are known to occur with codeine.

OVERDOSAGE
CODEINE
Serious overdose with codeine is characterized by respiratory depression (a decrease in respiratory rate and/or tidal volume, Cheyne-Stokes respiration, cyanosis), extreme somnolence progressing to stupor or coma, skeletal muscle flaccidity, cold and clammy skin, and sometimes bradycardia and hypotension. The triad of coma, pinpoint pupils, and respiratory depression is strongly suggestive of opiate poisoning. In severe overdosage, particularly by the intravenous route, apnea, circulatory collapse, cardiac arrest, and death may occur. Promethazine is additive to the depressant effects of codeine.

It is difficult to determine what constitutes a standard toxic or lethal dose. However, the lethal oral dose of codeine in an adult is reported to be in the range of 0.5 to 1.0 gram. Infants and children are believed to be relatively more sensitive to opiates on a body-weight basis. Elderly patients are also comparatively intolerant to opiates.

PROMETHAZINE
Signs and symptoms of overdosage with promethazine range from mild depression of the central nervous system and cardiovascular system to profound hypotension, respiratory depression, and unconsciousness.

Stimulation may be evident, especially in children and geriatric patients. Convulsions may rarely occur. A paradoxical reaction has been reported in children receiving single doses of 75 mg to 125 mg orally, characterized by hyperexcitability and nightmares.

Atropine-like signs and symptoms—dry mouth, fixed, dilated pupils, flushing, as well as gastrointestinal symptoms, may occur.

TREATMENT
The treatment of overdosage with Phenergan with codeine is essentially symptomatic and supportive. Only in cases of extreme overdosage or individual sensitivity do vital signs including respiration, pulse, blood pressure, temperature, and EKG need to be monitored. Activated charcoal orally or by lavage may be given, or sodium or magnesium sulfate orally as a cathartic. Attention should be given to the reestablishment of adequate respiratory exchange through provision of a patent airway and institution of assisted or controlled ventilation. The narcotic antagonist, naloxone hydrochloride, may be administered when significant respiratory depression occurs with Phenergan with codeine; any depressant effects of promethazine are not reversed with naloxone. Diazepam may be used to control convulsions. Avoid analeptics, which may cause convulsions. Acidosis and electrolyte losses should be corrected. A rise in temperature or pulmonary complications may signal the need for institution of antibiotic therapy.

Severe hypotension usually responds to the administration of norepinephrine or phenylephrine. EPINEPHRINE SHOULD NOT BE USED, since its use in a patient with partial adrenergic blockade may further lower the blood pressure.

Limited experience with dialysis indicates that it is not helpful.

Adults	1 teaspoon (5 mL) every 4 to 6 hours, not to exceed 30.0 mL in 24 hours.
Children 6 years to under 12 years	½ to 1 teaspoon (2.5 to 5 mL) every 4 to 6 hours, not to exceed 30.0 mL in 24 hours.
Children under 6 years (weight: 18 kg or 40 lbs)	¼ to ½ teaspoon (1.25 to 2.5 mL) every 4 to 6 hours, not to exceed 9.0 mL in 24 hours.
Children under 6 years (weight: 16 kg or 35 lbs)	¼ to ½ teaspoon (1.25 to 2.5 mL) every 4 to 6 hours, not to exceed 8.0 mL in 24 hours.
Children under 6 years (weight: 14 kg or 30 lbs)	¼ to ½ teaspoon (1.25 to 2.5 mL) every 4 to 6 hours, not to exceed 7.0 mL in 24 hours.
Children under 6 years (weight: 12 kg or 25 lbs)	¼ to ½ teaspoon (1.25 to 2.5 mL) every 4 to 6 hours, not to exceed 6.0 mL in 24 hours.

Phenergan with codeine is not recommended for children under 2 years of age.

DOSAGE AND ADMINISTRATION
The average effective dose is given in the following table: [See table above].

HOW SUPPLIED
Phenergan® with codeine, Wyeth®, is a clear, purple solution supplied as follows:
NDC 0008-0550-02, case of 24 bottles of 4 fl. oz. (118 mL).
NDC 0008-0550-03, bottle of 1 pint (473 mL).
Keep bottles tightly closed—Store at Room Temperature, between 15° C and 25° C (59° F and 77° F).
Protect from light.
Dispense in light-resistant, glass, tight containers.

PHENERGAN®　　　　　　　　　　　Ŗ
[fen 'er-gan]
with dextromethorphan

DESCRIPTION
Each teaspoon (5 mL) of Phenergan with dextromethorphan contains 6.25 mg promethazine hydrochloride and 15 mg dextromethorphan hydrobromide in a flavored syrup base with a pH between 4.7 and 5.2. Alcohol 7%. The inactive ingredients present are artificial and natural flavors, citric acid, D&C Yellow 10, FD&C Yellow 6, glycerin, saccharin sodium, sodium benzoate, sodium citrate, sodium propionate, water, and other ingredients.

Promethazine hydrochloride, a phenothiazine derivative, is designated chemically as N,N,α-trimethyl-$10H$-phenothiazine-10-ethanamine monohydrochloride with the following structural formula:

Promethazine hydrochloride occurs as a white to faint yellow, practically odorless, crystalline powder which slowly oxidizes and turns blue on prolonged exposure to air. It is soluble in water and freely soluble in alcohol.

Dextromethorphan hydrobromide is a salt of the methyl ether of the dextrorotatory isomer of levorphanol, a narcotic analgesic. It is chemically named as 3-methoxy-17-methyl-9α, 13α, 14α-morphinan hydrobromide monohydrate with the following structural formula:

Dextromethorphan hydrobromide occurs as white crystals sparingly soluble in water and freely soluble in alcohol.

CLINICAL PHARMACOLOGY
PROMETHAZINE
Promethazine is a phenothiazine derivative which differs structurally from the antipsychotic phenothiazines by the presence of a branched side chain and no ring substitution. It is thought that this configuration is responsible for its relative lack (1/10 that of chlorpromazine) of dopaminergic (CNS) action.

Promethazine is an H_1 receptor blocking agent. In addition to its antihistaminic action, it provides clinically useful sedative and antiemetic effects. In therapeutic dosages, promethazine produces no significant effects on the cardiovascular system.

Promethazine is well absorbed from the gastrointestinal tract. Clinical effects are apparent within 20 minutes after oral administration and generally last four to six hours, although they may persist as long as 12 hours. Promethazine is

Continued on next page

Wyeth-Ayerst—Cont.

metabolized by the liver to a variety of compounds; the sulfoxides of promethazine and N-demethylpromethazine are the predominant metabolites appearing in the urine.

DEXTROMETHORPHAN

Dextromethorphan is an antitussive agent and, unlike the isomeric levorphanol, it has no analgesic or addictive properties.

The drug acts centrally and elevates the threshold for coughing. It is about equal to codeine in depressing the cough reflex. In therapeutic dosage dextromethorphan does not inhibit ciliary activity.

Dextromethorphan is rapidly absorbed from the gastrointestinal tract and exerts its effect in 15 to 30 minutes. The duration of action after oral administration is approximately three to six hours. Dextromethorphan is metabolized primarily by liver enzymes undergoing O-demethylation, N-demethylation, and partial conjugation with glucuronic acid and sulfate. In humans, (+)-3-hydroxy-N-methylmorphinan, (+)-3-hydroxymorphinan, and traces of unmetabolized drug were found in urine after oral administration.

INDICATIONS AND USAGE

Phenergan with dextromethorphan is indicated for the temporary relief of coughs and upper respiratory symptoms associated with allergy or the common cold.

CONTRAINDICATIONS

Promethazine is contraindicated in individuals known to be hypersensitive or to have had an idiosyncratic reaction to promethazine or to other phenothiazines.

Antihistamines are contraindicated for use in the treatment of lower respiratory tract symptoms, including asthma.

Dextromethorphan should not be used in patients receiving a monoamine oxidase inhibitor (MAOl).

WARNINGS

PROMETHAZINE

Promethazine may cause marked drowsiness. Ambulatory patients should be cautioned against such activities as driving or operating dangerous machinery until it is known that they do not become drowsy or dizzy from promethazine therapy.

The sedative action of promethazine hydrochloride is additive to the sedative effects of central nervous system depressants; therefore, agents such as alcohol, narcotic analgesics, sedatives, hypnotics, and tranquilizers should either be eliminated or given in reduced dosage in the presence of promethazine hydrochloride. When given concomitantly with promethazine hydrochloride, the dose of barbiturates should be reduced by at least one-half, and the dose of analgesic depressants, such as morphine or meperidine, should be reduced by one-quarter to one-half.

Promethazine may lower seizure threshold. This should be taken into consideration when administering to persons with known seizure disorders or when giving in combination with narcotics or local anesthetics which may also affect seizure threshold.

Sedative drugs or CNS depressants should be avoided in patients with a history of sleep apnea.

Antihistamines should be used with caution in patients with narrow-angle glaucoma, stenosing peptic ulcer, pyloroduodenal obstruction, and urinary bladder obstruction due to symptomatic prostatic hypertrophy and narrowing of the bladder neck.

Administration of promethazine has been associated with reported cholestatic jaundice.

DEXTROMETHORPHAN

Administration of dextromethorphan may be accompanied by histamine release and should be used with caution in atopic children.

PRECAUTIONS

Animal reproduction studies have not been conducted with the drug combination—promethazine and dextromethorphan. It is not known whether this drug combination can cause fetal harm when administered to a pregnant woman or can affect reproduction capacity. Phenergan with dextromethorphan should be given to a pregnant woman only if clearly needed.

GENERAL

Promethazine should be used cautiously in persons with cardiovascular disease or with impairment of liver function. Dextromethorphan should be used with caution in sedated patients, in the debilitated, and in patients confined to the supine position.

INFORMATION FOR PATIENTS

Phenergan with dextromethorphan may cause marked drowsiness or impair the mental and/or physical abilities required for the performance of potentially hazardous tasks, such as driving a vehicle or operating machinery. Ambulatory patients should be told to avoid engaging in such activities until it is known that they do not become drowsy or dizzy from Phenergan with dextromethorphan therapy. Children

should be supervised to avoid potential harm in bike riding or in other hazardous activities.

The concomitant use of alcohol or other central nervous system depressants, including narcotic analgesics, sedatives, hypnotics, and tranquilizers, may have an additive effect and should be avoided or their dosage reduced.

Patients should be advised to report any involuntary muscle movements or unusual sensitivity to sunlight.

DRUG INTERACTIONS

The sedative action of promethazine is additive to the sedative effects of other central nervous system depressants, including alcohol, narcotic analgesics, sedatives, hypnotics, tricyclic antidepressants, and tranquilizers; therefore, these agents should be avoided or administered in reduced dosage to patients receiving promethazine.

DRUG/LABORATORY TEST INTERACTIONS

The following laboratory tests may be affected in patients who are receiving therapy with promethazine hydrochloride:

Pregnancy Tests

Diagnostic pregnancy tests based on immunological reactions between HCG and anti-HCG may result in false-negative or false-positive interpretations.

Glucose Tolerance Test

An increase in blood glucose has been reported in patients receiving promethazine.

CARCINOGENESIS, MUTAGENESIS, IMPAIRMENT OF FERTILITY

Long-term animal studies have not been performed to assess the carcinogenic potential of promethazine or of dextromethorphan. There are no animal or human data concerning the carcinogenicity, mutagenicity, or impairment of fertility with these drugs. Promethazine was nonmutagenic in the *Salmonella* test system of Ames.

PREGNANCY

Teratogenic Effects —Pregnancy Category C

Teratogenic effects have not been demonstrated in rat-feeding studies at doses of 6.25 and 12.5 mg/kg of promethazine. These doses are 8.3 and 16.7 times the maximum recommended total daily dose for a 50-kg subject. Specific studies to test the action of the drug on parturition, lactation, and development of the animal neonate were not done, but a general preliminary study in rats indicated no effect on these parameters. Although antihistamines, including promethazine, have been found to produce fetal mortality in rodents, the pharmacological effects of histamine in the rodent do not parallel those in man. There are no adequate and well-controlled studies of promethazine in pregnant women. Phenergan with dextromethorphan should be used during pregnancy only if the potential benefit justifies the potential risk to the fetus.

Nonteratogenic Effects

Promethazine taken within two weeks of delivery may inhibit platelet aggregation in the newborn.

LABOR AND DELIVERY

See "Nonteratogenic Effects."

NURSING MOTHERS

It is not known whether promethazine or dextromethorphan is excreted in human milk. Caution should be exercised when Phenergan with dextromethorphan is administered to a nursing woman.

PEDIATRIC USE

This product should not be used in children under 2 years of age because safety for that use has not been established.

ADVERSE REACTIONS

PROMETHAZINE

Nervous System —Sedation, sleepiness, occasional blurred vision, dryness of mouth, dizziness; rarely confusion, disorientation, and extrapyramidal symptoms such as oculogyric crisis, torticollis, and tongue protrusion (usually in association with parenteral injection or excessive dosage).

Cardiovascular —Increased or decreased blood pressure.

Dermatologic —Rash, rarely photosensitivity.

Hematologic —Rarely leukopenia, thrombocytopenia; agranulocytosis (1 case).

Gastrointestinal —Nausea and vomiting.

DEXTROMETHORPHAN

Dextromethorphan hydrobromide occasionally causes slight drowsiness, dizziness, and gastrointestinal disturbances.

DRUG ABUSE AND DEPENDENCE

According to the WHO Expert Committee on Drug Dependence, dextromethorphan could produce very slight psychic dependence but no physical dependence.

OVERDOSAGE

PROMETHAZINE

Signs and symptoms of overdosage with promethazine range from mild depression of the central nervous system and cardiovascular system to profound hypotension, respiratory depression, and unconsciousness.

Stimulation may be evident, especially in children and geriatric patients. Convulsions may rarely occur. A paradoxical reaction has been reported in children receiving single doses of 75 mg to 125 mg orally, characterized by hyperexcitability and nightmares.

Atropine-like signs and symptoms—dry mouth, fixed, dilated pupils, flushing, as well as gastrointestinal symptoms, may occur.

DEXTROMETHORPHAN

Dextromethorphan may produce central excitement and mental confusion. Very high doses may produce respiratory depression. One case of toxic psychosis (hyperactivity, marked visual and auditory hallucinations) after ingestion of a single dose of 20 tablets (300 mg) of dextromethorphan has been reported.

TREATMENT

Treatment of overdosage with Phenergan with dextromethorphan is essentially symptomatic and supportive. Only in cases of extreme overdosage or individual sensitivity do vital signs including respiration, pulse, blood pressure, temperature, and EKG need to be monitored. Activated charcoal orally or by lavage may be given, or sodium or magnesium sulfate orally as a cathartic. Attention should be given to the reestablishment of adequate respiratory exchange through provision of a patent airway and institution of assisted or controlled ventilation. Diazepam may be used to control convulsions. Acidosis and electrolyte losses should be corrected. The antidotal efficacy of narcotic antagonists to dextromethorphan has not been established; note that any of the depressant effects of promethazine are not reversed by naloxone. Avoid analeptics, which may cause convulsions.

Severe hypotension usually responds to the administration of norepinephrine or phenylephrine. EPINEPHRINE SHOULD NOT BE USED, since its use in a patient with partial adrenergic blockade may further lower the blood pressure.

Limited experience with dialysis indicates that it is not helpful.

DOSAGE AND ADMINISTRATION

The average effective dose for adults is one teaspoon (5 mL) every 4 to 6 hours, not to exceed 30.0 mL in 24 hours. For children 6 years to under 12 years of age, the dose is one-half to one teaspoon (2.5 to 5.0 mL) every 4 to 6 hours, not to exceed 20.0 mL in 24 hours. For children 2 years to under 6 years of age, the dose is one-quarter to one-half teaspoon (1.25 to 2.5 mL) every 4 to 6 hours, not to exceed 10.0 mL in 24 hours.

Phenergan with dextromethorphan is not recommended for children under 2 years of age.

HOW SUPPLIED

Phenergan® with dextromethorphan, Wyeth®, is a clear, yellow solution supplied as follows:

NDC 0008-0548-02, case of 24 bottles of 4 fl. oz.
NDC 0008-0548-06, case of 16 bottles of 6 fl. oz.
NDC 0008-0548-03, bottle of 1 pint.
NDC 0008-0548-04, bottle of 1 gallon.

Keep bottles tightly closed at Room Temperature, Approx. 25° C (77° F).

Protect from light.

Dispense in light-resistant, glass, tight containers.

PHENERGAN®–D   ℞

[fen 'er-gan-D]
(promethazine HCl and pseudoephedrine HCl)
Tablets

DESCRIPTION

Each Phenergan-D tablet contains 6.25 mg of promethazine hydrochloride and 60 mg of pseudoephedrine hydrochloride. The inactive ingredients present are cellulose, edetate disodium, FD&C Yellow 6, lactose, magnesium stearate, methylcellulose, and saccharin sodium. Phenergan-D has antihistaminic and nasal decongestant effects.

Promethazine hydrochloride, a phenothiazine derivative, is designated chemically as N,N,-trimethyl-10H-phenothiazine-10-ethanamine monohydrochloride with the following structural formula:

$$CH_2CH(CH_3)N(CH_3)_2$$

Promethazine hydrochloride occurs as a white to faint yellow, practically odorless, crystalline powder which slowly oxidizes and turns blue on prolonged exposure to air. It is soluble in water and freely soluble in alcohol.

Pseudoephedrine hydrochloride, a nasal decongestant, is designated chemically as [S-(R*,R*)]-α-[1-(methylamino)ethyl] benzenemethanol hydrochloride with the following structural formula:

Pseudoephedrine hydrochloride is the salt of a pharmacologically active stereoisomer of ephedrine. It occurs as fine white to off-white crystals or powder; it is sparingly soluble in water and freely soluble in alcohol.

CLINICAL PHARMACOLOGY
PROMETHAZINE
Promethazine is a phenothiazine derivative which differs structurally from the antipsychotic phenothiazines by the presence of a branched side chain and no ring substitution. It is thought that this configuration is responsible for its relative lack ($\frac{1}{10}$ that of chlorpromazine) of dopaminergic (CNS) action.

Promethazine is an H_1 receptor blocking agent. In addition to its antihistaminic action, it provides clinically useful sedative and antiemetic effects. In therapeutic dosages, promethazine produces no significant effects on the cardiovascular system. Promethazine is well absorbed from the gastrointestinal tract. Clinical effects are apparent within 20 minutes after oral administration and generally last 4 to 6 hours, although they may persist as long as 12 hours. Promethazine is metabolized by the liver to a variety of compounds; the sulfoxides of promethazine and N-demethylpromethazine are the predominant metabolites appearing in the urine.

PSEUDOEPHEDRINE
Pseudoephedrine acts as an indirect sympathomimetic agent by stimulating sympathetic (adrenergic) nerve endings to release norepinephrine. Norepinephrine in turn stimulates *alpha* and *beta* receptors throughout the body. The action of pseudoephedrine hydrochloride is apparently more specific for the blood vessels of the upper respiratory tract and less specific for the blood vessels of the systemic circulation. The vasoconstriction elicited at these sites results in the shrinkage of swollen tissues in the sinuses and nasal passages.

Pseudoephedrine is rapidly and almost completely absorbed from the gastrointestinal tract. Considerable variation in half-life has been observed (from about 4.5 to 10 hours), which is attributed to individual differences in absorption and excretion. Excretion rates are also altered by urine pH, increasing with acidification and decreasing with alkalinization. As a result, mean half-life falls to about 4 hours at pH 5 and increases to 12 to 13 hours at pH 8.

After administration of a 60-mg tablet, 87 to 96% of the pseudoephedrine is cleared from the body within 24 hours. The drug is distributed to body tissues and fluids, including fetal tissue, breast milk, and the central nervous system. About 55 to 75% of an administered dose is excreted unchanged in the urine; the remainder is apparently metabolized in the liver to inactive compounds by N-demethylation, parahydroxylation, and oxidative deamination.

INDICATIONS AND USAGE
Phenergan-D is indicated for the temporary relief of upper respiratory symptoms, including nasal congestion, associated with allergy or the common cold.

CONTRAINDICATIONS
Promethazine is contraindicated in individuals known to be hypersensitive or to have had an idiosyncratic reaction to promethazine or to other phenothiazines.

Antihistamines are contraindicated for use in the treatment of lower-respiratory-tract symptoms or asthma.

Sympathomimetic amines are contraindicated in patients with severe hypertension, severe coronary-artery disease, and in patients on monoamine-oxidase-inhibitor therapy (see "Drug Interactions").

Pseudoephedrine should not be used in patients known to be hypersensitive to sympathomimetic amines.

WARNINGS
PROMETHAZINE
Promethazine may cause marked drowsiness. Ambulatory patients should be cautioned against such activities as driving or operating dangerous machinery until it is known that they do not become drowsy or dizzy from promethazine therapy.

The sedative action of promethazine hydrochloride is additive to the sedative effects of central-nervous-system depressants; therefore, agents such as alcohol, narcotic analgesics, sedatives, hypnotics, and tranquilizers should either be eliminated or given in reduced dosage in the presence of promethazine hydrochloride. When given concomitantly with promethazine hydrochloride, the dose of barbiturates should be reduced by at least one-half, and the dose of analgesic depressants, such morphine or meperidine, should be reduced by one-quarter to one-half.

Promethazine may lower seizure threshold. This should be taken into consideration when administering to persons with known seizure disorders or when giving in combination with narcotics or local anesthetics which may also affect seizure threshold.

Sedative drugs or central-nervous-system depressants should be avoided in patients with a history of sleep apnea. Antihistamines should be used with caution in patients with narrow-angle glaucoma, stenosing peptic ulcer, pyloroduodenal obstruction, and urinary bladder obstruction due to symptomatic prostatic hypertrophy and narrowing of the bladder neck.

Administration of promethazine has been associated with reported cholestatic jaundice.

PSEUDOEPHEDRINE
Pseudoephedrine should be given with caution to patients with hypertension, diabetes mellitus, ischemic heart disease, increased intraocular pressure, and hyperthyroidism. Men with symptomatic benign prostatic hypertrophy can experience urinary retention when given oral nasal decongestants.

PRECAUTIONS
Animal reproduction studies have not been conducted with the drug combination—promethazine and pseudoephedrine. It is not known whether this drug combination can cause fetal harm when administered to a pregnant woman or can affect reproduction capacity. Phenergan-D should be given to a pregnant woman only if clearly needed.

GENERAL
Phenergan-D should be prescribed with caution for certain special-risk patients, such as the elderly or debilitated, and for those with severe impairment of liver function, respiratory impairment, cardiovascular disease, cardiac arrhythmias, history of bronchial asthma, prostatic hypertrophy, or urethral stricture, and in patients known to be taking other antitussive, antihistamine, or decongestant medications. Patients' self-medication habits should be investigated to determine their use of such medications.

INFORMATION FOR PATIENTS
Phenergan-D may cause marked drowsiness or impair the mental and/or physical abilities required for the performance of potentially hazardous tasks, such as driving a vehicle or operating machinery. Ambulatory patients should be told to avoid engaging in such activities until it is known that they do not become drowsy or dizzy from Phenergan-D therapy.

The concomitant use of alcohol or other central-nervous-system depressants, including narcotic analgesics, sedatives, hypnotics, and tranquilizers, may have an additive effect and should be avoided or their dosage reduced.

Patients should be advised to report any involuntary muscle movements or unusual sensitivity to sunlight.

DRUG INTERACTIONS
Promethazine
The sedative action of promethazine is additive to the sedative effects of other central-nervous-system depressants, including alcohol, narcotic analgesics, sedatives, hypnotics, tricyclic antidepressants, and tranquilizers; therefore, these agents should be avoided or administered in reduced dosage to patients receiving promethazine.

Pseudoephedrine
Monoamine-oxidase inhibitors increase the effect of pseudoephedrine. Sympathomimetics may reduce the antihypertensive effects of guanethidine, methyldopa, mecamylamine, and reserpine; therefore, these agents should be avoided (monoamine-oxidase inhibitors) or administered cautiously with close blood-pressure monitoring (guanethidine, methyldopa, etc.).

Because the renal elimination of pseudoephedrine is urinary-pH and urinary-flow dependent, the dose of pseudoephedrine should be adjusted during concurrent administration of urinary alkalizers or urinary acidifiers (see "Clinical Pharmacology").

DRUG/LABORATORY TEST INTERACTIONS
The following laboratory tests may be affected in patients who are receiving therapy with promethazine hydrochloride.

Pregnancy Tests—Diagnostic pregnancy tests based on immunological reactions between HCG and anti-HCG may result in false-negative or false-positive interpretations.

Glucose Tolerance Test—An increase in blood glucose has been reported in patients receiving promethazine.

CARCINOGENESIS, MUTAGENESIS, IMPAIRMENT OF FERTILITY
Promethazine
Long-term animal studies have not been performed to assess the carcinogenic potential of promethazine nor are there other animal or human data concerning carcinogenicity, mutagenicity, or impairment of fertility with these drugs. Promethazine was nonmutagenic in the *Salmonella* test system of Ames.

Pseudoephedrine
No adequate studies have been conducted in animals to determine whether pseudoephedrine has a potential for carcinogenesis, mutagenesis, or impairment of fertility.

PREGNANCY
TERATOGENIC EFFECTS—Pregnancy Category C
Promethazine
Teratogenic effects have not been demonstrated in rat-feeding studies at doses of 6.25 and 12.5 mg/kg of promethazine. These doses are 8.3 and 16.7 times the maximum recommended total daily dose of promethazine for a 50-kg subject. Specific studies to test the action of the drug on parturition, lactation, and development of the animal neonate were not done, but a general preliminary study in rats indicated no effect on these parameters. Although antihistamines, including promethazine, have been found to produce fetal mortality in rodents, the pharmacological effects of histamine in the rodent do not parallel those in man. There are no adequate and well-controlled studies of promethazine in pregnant women.

Pseudoephedrine
Teratogenic studies with pseudoephedrine were conducted in rats at doses up to 150 times the human dose with no evidence of teratogenic harm to the fetus. However, overt signs of toxicity were observed in the dams, which were also reflected in reduced average weight and length and rate of skeletal ossification in their fetuses.

Phenergan-D should be used during pregnancy only if the potential benefit justifies the potential risk to the fetus.

NONTERATOGENIC EFFECTS
Promethazine taken within two weeks of delivery may inhibit platelet aggregation in the newborn.

LABOR AND DELIVERY
Administration of sympathomimetic amines to patients in late pregnancy or labor may cause fetal anoxia or bradycardia by increasing contractility of the uterus and decreasing uterine blood flow.

NURSING MOTHERS
It is not known whether promethazine is excreted in human milk. Pseudoephedrine is excreted in breast milk in small amounts, but the significance of its effect on nursing infants is not known.

Because of the potential for serious adverse reactions from Phenergan-D in nursing infants, caution should be exercised when Phenergan-D is administered to a nursing woman.

PEDIATRIC USE
A pediatric dosage form is not available. Phenergan-D tablets are not recommended for use in children under 12 years of age.

USE IN THE ELDERLY (approximately 60 years or older)
The ingredients in Phenergan-D are more likely to cause adverse reactions in elderly than in younger patients.

ADVERSE REACTIONS
PROMETHAZINE
Nervous System —Sedation, sleepiness, occasional blurred vision, dryness of mouth, dizziness; rarely confusion, disorientation, and extrapyramidal symptoms, such as oculogyric crisis, torticollis, and tongue protrusion (usually in association with parenteral injection or excessive dosage).
Cardiovascular —Increased or decreased blood pressure.
Dermatologic —Rash, rarely photosensitivity.
Hematologic —Rarely leukopenia, thrombocytopenia; agranulocytosis (1 case).
Gastrointestinal —Nausea and vomiting.

PSEUDOEPHRINE
Nervous System —Dizziness, tenseness, restlessness, tremor, weakness, insomnia, hallucinations, convulsions, central-nervous-system depression, fear, anxiety, dry mouth.
Cardiovascular —Tachycardia, palpitations, arrhythmias, headache, pallor, cardiovascular collapse with hypotension.
Gastrointestinal —Nausea.
Respiratory —Respiratory difficulty.
Urinary —Dysuria.

OVERDOSAGE
PROMETHAZINE
Signs and symptoms of overdosage with promethazine range from mild depression of the central nervous system and cardiovascular system to profound hypotension, respiratory depression, and unconsciousness.

Stimulation may be evident, especially in children and geriatric patients. Convulsions may rarely occur. A paradoxical reaction has been reported in children receiving single doses of 75 mg to 125 mg orally, characterized by hyperexcitability and nightmares.

Atropinelike signs and symptoms—dry mouth, fixed dilated pupils, flushing, as well as gastrointestinal symptoms, may occur.

PSEUDOEPHEDRINE
Overdosage with pseudoephedrine can cause excessive central-nervous-system stimulation resulting in excitement, nervousness, anxiety, tremor, restlessness, and insomnia. Other effects include tachycardia, hypertension, pallor, mydriasis, hyperglycemia, and urinary retention. Severe overdosage may cause tachypnea or hyperpnea, hallucinations, convulsions, or delirium, but in some individuals there may be central-nervous-system depression with somnolence, stupor, or respiratory depression. Arrhythmias (including ventricular fibrillation) may lead to hypotension and circulatory collapse. Severe hypokalemia can occur, probably due to compartmental shift rather than depletion of potassium. No organ damage or significant metabolic derangement is associated with pseudoephedrine overdosage.

The toxic and lethal concentrations in human biologic fluids are not known. Excretion rates increase with urine acidification and decrease with alkalinization. Few reports of toxicity due to pseudoephedrine have been published, and no case of fatal overdosage is known.

Continued on next page

Wyeth-Ayerst—Cont.

TREATMENT

Treatment of overdosage with Phenergan-D is essentially symptomatic and supportive. In cases of extreme overdosage or individual sensitivity, vital signs, including respiration, pulse, blood pressure, temperature, and EKG, as well as electrolytes, need to be monitored. Therapy, if instituted within 4 hours of overdosage, is aimed at reducing further absorption of the drug.

In the conscious patient, vomiting should be induced even though it may have occurred spontaneously. If vomiting cannot be induced, gastric lavage is indicated. Adequate precautions must be taken to protect against aspiration. Charcoal slurry or other suitable agents should be instilled into the stomach after vomiting or lavage. Saline cathartics or milk of magnesia may be of additional benefit.

In the unconscious patient, attention should be given to the reestablishment of adequate respiratory exchange through provision of a patent airway and institution of assisted or controlled ventilation before attempting to evacuate the gastric contents.

Acidosis and electrolyte losses should be corrected. IV potassium should be given as indicated. Diazepam may be used to control convulsions. Note that any depressant effects of promethazine are not reversed by naloxone. Avoid analeptics which may cause convulsions. Severe hypotension usually responds to the administration of norepinephrine or phenylephrine. EPINEPHRINE SHOULD NOT BE USED, since its use in patients with partial adrenergic blockade may further lower blood pressure.

Pseudoephedrine is theoretically dialyzable, but the procedure has not been clinically established. Limited experience with dialysis with promethazine indicates that it is not helpful.

DOSAGE AND ADMINISTRATION

The recommended adult dose is one tablet every 4 hours to 6 hours, not to exceed 4 (four) tablets (25 mg promethazine hydrochloride and 240 mg pseudoephedrine hydrochloride) in 24 hours.

HOW SUPPLIED

Phenergan®-D (promethazine HCl and pseudoephedrine HCl) Tablets, Wyeth®, are available in bottles of 100: NDC 0008-0434, white and orange, double layer, round, scored tablet marked "WYETH" and "434".

Keep tightly closed at Room Temperature, Approx. 25°C (77°F).
Protect from light.
Dispense in light-resistant, tight container.
The appearance of these tablets is a trademark of Wyeth-Ayerst Laboratories.
Caution: Federal law prohibits dispensing without prescription.
Shown in Product Identification Section, page 437

PHENERGAN® VC   ℞
[fen 'er-gan]

DESCRIPTION

Each teaspoon (5 mL) of Phenergan VC contains 6.25 mg promethazine hydrochloride and 5 mg phenylephrine hydrochloride in a flavored syrup base with a pH between 4.7 and 5.2. Alcohol 7%. The inactive ingredients present are artificial and natural flavors, citric acid, FD&C Yellow 6, glycerin, saccharin sodium, sodium benzoate, sodium citrate, sodium propionate, water, and other ingredients.

Promethazine hydrochloride, a phenothiazine derivative, is designated chemically as N,N,α-trimethyl-10H-phenothiazine-10-ethanamine monohydrochloride with the following structural formula:

$$CH_2CH(CH_3)N(CH_3)_2$$

· HCl

Promethazine hydrochloride occurs as white to faint yellow, practically odorless, crystalline powder which slowly oxidizes and turns blue on prolonged exposure to air. It is soluble in water and freely soluble in alcohol.

Phenylephrine hydrochloride is a sympathomimetic amine salt. It may be chemically named as 3-hydroxy-α-[(methylamino)methyl]-benzenemethanol hydrochloride and has the following chemical formula:

$$CH_2NHCH_3 \cdot HCl$$

Phenylephrine hydrochloride occurs as white or nearly white crystals, having a bitter taste. It is freely soluble in water and alcohol. Phenylephrine hydrochloride is subject to oxidation and must be protected from light and air.

CLINICAL PHARMACOLOGY

PROMETHAZINE

Promethazine is a phenothiazine derivative which differs structurally from the antipsychotic phenothiazines by the presence of a branched side chain and no ring substitution. It is thought that this configuration is responsible for its relative lack (1/10 that of chlorpromazine) of dopaminergic (CNS) action.

Promethazine is an H_1 receptor blocking agent. In addition to its antihistaminic action, it provides clinically useful sedative and antiemetic effects. In therapeutic dosages, promethazine produces no significant effects on the cardiovascular system.

Promethazine is well absorbed from the gastrointestinal tract. Clinical effects are apparent within 20 minutes after oral administration and generally last four to six hours, although they may persist as long as 12 hours. Promethazine is metabolized by the liver to a variety of compounds; the sulfoxides of promethazine and N-demethylpromethazine are the predominant metabolites appearing in the urine.

PHENYLEPHRINE

Phenylephrine is a potent postsynaptic α-receptor agonist with little effect on β receptors of the heart. Phenylephrine has no effect on β-adrenergic receptors of the bronchi or peripheral blood vessels. A direct action at receptors accounts for the greater part of its effects, only a small part being due to its ability to release norepinephrine.

Therapeutic doses of phenylephrine mainly cause vasoconstriction. Phenylephrine increases resistance and, to a lesser extent, decreases capacitance of blood vessels. Total peripheral resistance is increased, resulting in increased systolic and diastolic blood pressure. Pulmonary arterial pressure is usually increased, and renal blood flow is usually decreased. Local vasoconstriction and hemostasis occur following topical application or infiltration of phenylephrine into tissues. The main effect of phenylephrine on the heart is bradycardia; it produces a positive inotropic effect on the myocardium in doses greater than those usually used therapeutically. Rarely, the drug may increase the irritability of the heart, causing arrhythmias. Cardiac output is decreased slightly. Phenylephrine increases the work of the heart by increasing peripheral arterial resistance.

Phenylephrine has a mild central stimulant effect.

Following oral administration or topical application of phenylephrine to the mucosa, constriction of blood vessels in the nasal mucosa relieves nasal congestion associated with allergy or head colds. Following oral administration, nasal decongestion may occur within 15 or 20 minutes and may persist for up to 4 hours.

Phenylephrine is irregularly absorbed from and readily metabolized in the gastrointestinal tract. Phenylephrine is metabolized in the liver and intestine by monoamine oxidase. The metabolites and their route and rate of excretion have not been identified. The pharmacologic action of phenylephrine is terminated at least partially by uptake of the drug into tissues.

INDICATIONS AND USAGE

Phenergan VC is indicated for the temporary relief of upper respiratory symptoms, including nasal congestion, associated with allergy or the common cold.

CONTRAINDICATIONS

Promethazine is contraindicated in individuals known to be hypersensitive or to have had an idiosyncratic reaction to promethazine or to other phenothiazines.

Antihistamines are contraindicated for use in the treatment of lower respiratory tract symptoms or asthma.

Phenylephrine is contraindicated in patients with hypertension or with peripheral vascular insufficiency (ischemia may result with risk of gangrene or thrombosis of compromised vascular beds). Phenylephrine should not be used in patients known to be hypersensitive to the drug or in those receiving a monoamine oxidase inhibitor (MAOI).

WARNINGS

PROMETHAZINE

Promethazine may cause marked drowsiness. Ambulatory patients should be cautioned against such activities as driving or operating dangerous machinery until it is known that they do not become drowsy or dizzy from promethazine therapy.

The sedative action of promethazine hydrochloride is additive to the sedative effects of central nervous system depressants; therefore, agents such as alcohol, narcotic analgesics, sedatives, hypnotics, and tranquilizers should either be eliminated or given in reduced dosage in the presence of promethazine hydrochloride. When given concomitantly with promethazine hydrochloride, the dose of barbiturates should be reduced by at least one-half, and the dose of analgesic depressants, such as morphine or meperidine, should be reduced by one-quarter to one-half.

Promethazine may lower seizure threshold. This should be taken into consideration when administering to persons with known seizure disorders or when giving in combination with narcotics or local anesthetics which may also affect seizure threshold.

Sedative drugs or CNS depressants should be avoided in patients with a history of sleep apnea.

Antihistamines should be used with caution in patients with narrow-angle glaucoma, stenosing peptic ulcer, pyloroduodenal obstruction, and urinary bladder obstruction due to symptomatic prostatic hypertrophy and narrowing of the bladder neck.

Administration of promethazine has been associated with reported cholestatic jaundice.

PHENYLEPHRINE

Because phenylephrine is an adrenergic agent, it should be given with caution to patients with thyroid diseases, diabetes mellitus, and heart diseases or those receiving tricyclic antidepressants.

Men with symptomatic, benign prostatic hypertrophy can experience urinary retention when given oral nasal decongestants.

Phenylephrine can cause a decrease in cardiac output, and extreme caution should be used when administering the drug, parenterally or orally, to patients with arteriosclerosis, to elderly individuals, and/or to patients with initially poor cerebral or coronary circulation.

Phenylephrine should be used with caution in patients taking diet preparations, such as amphetamines or phenylpropanolamine, because synergistic adrenergic effects could result in serious hypertensive response and possible stroke.

PRECAUTIONS

Animal reproduction studies have not been conducted with the drug combination—promethazine and phenylephrine. It is not known whether this drug combination can cause fetal harm when administered to a pregnant woman or can affect reproduction capacity. Phenergan VC should be given to a pregnant woman only if clearly needed.

GENERAL

Promethazine should be used cautiously in persons with cardiovascular disease or impairment of liver function.

Phenylephrine should be used with caution in patients with cardiovascular disease, particularly hypertension.

INFORMATION FOR PATIENTS

Phenergan VC may cause marked drowsiness or impair the mental and/or physical abilities required for the performance of potentially hazardous tasks, such as driving a vehicle or operating machinery. Ambulatory patients should be told to avoid engaging in such activities until it is known that they do not become drowsy or dizzy from Phenergan VC therapy. Children should be supervised to avoid potential harm in bike riding or other hazardous activities.

The concomitant use of alcohol or other central nervous system depressants, including narcotic analgesics, sedatives, hypnotics, and tranquilizers, may have an additive effect and should be avoided or their dosage reduced.

Patients should be advised to report any involuntary muscle movements or unusual sensitivity to sunlight.

DRUG INTERACTIONS

PROMETHAZINE

The sedative action of promethazine is additive to the sedative effects of other central nervous system depressants, including alcohol, narcotic analgesics, sedatives, hypnotics, tricyclic antidepressants, and tranquilizers; therefore, these agents should be avoided or administered in reduced dosage to patients receiving promethazine.

[See table on next page].

DRUG/LABORATORY TEST INTERACTIONS

The following laboratory tests may be affected in patients who are receiving therapy with promethazine hydrochloride:

Pregnancy Tests

Diagnostic pregnancy tests based on immunological reactions between HCG and anti-HCG may result in false-negative or false-positive interpretations.

Glucose Tolerance Test

An increase in blood glucose has been reported in patients receiving promethazine.

CARCINOGENESIS, MUTAGENESIS, IMPAIRMENT OF FERTILITY

PROMETHAZINE

Long-term animal studies have not been performed to assess the carcinogenic potential of promethazine, nor are there other animal or human data concerning carcinogenicity, mutagenicity, or impairment of fertility with this drug. Promethazine was nonmutagenic in the *Salmonella* test system of Ames.

PHENYLEPHRINE

A study which followed the development of cancer in 143,574 patients over a four-year period indicated that in 11,981 patients who received phenylephrine (systemic or topical), there was no statistically significant association between the drug and cancer at any or all sites.

Long-term animal studies have not been performed to assess the carcinogenic potential of phenylephrine, nor are there other animal or human data concerning mutagenicity.

A study of the effects of adrenergic drugs on ovum transport in rabbits indicated that treatment with phenylephrine did not alter incidence of pregnancy; the number of implantations was significantly reduced when high doses of the drug were used.

PREGNANCY
Teratogenic Effects—Pregnancy Category C
PROMETHAZINE
Teratogenic effects have not been demonstrated in rat-feeding studies at doses of 6.25 and 12.5 mg/kg of promethazine. These doses are 8.3 and 16.7 times the maximum recommended total daily dose of promethazine for a 50-kg subject. Specific studies to test the action of the drug on parturition, lactation, and development of the animal neonate were not done, but a general preliminary study in rats indicated no effect on these parameters. Although antihistamines, including promethazine, have been found to produce fetal mortality in rodents, the pharmacological effects of histamine in the rodent do not parallel those in man. There are no adequate and well-controlled studies of promethazine in pregnant women.

PHENYLEPHRINE
A study in rabbits indicated that continued moderate overexposure to phenylephrine (3 mg/day) during the second half of pregnancy (22nd day of gestation to delivery) may contribute to perinatal wastage, prematurity, premature labor, and possibly fetal anomalies; when phenylephrine (3 mg/day) was given to rabbits during the first half of pregnancy (3rd day after mating for seven days), a significant number gave birth to litters of low birth weight. Another study showed that phenylephrine was associated with anomalies of aortic arch and with ventricular septal defect in the chick embryo. Phenergan VC should be used during pregnancy only if the potential benefit justifies the potential risk to the fetus.
Nonteratogenic Effects
Promethazine taken within two weeks of delivery may inhibit platelet aggregation in the newborn.

LABOR AND DELIVERY
Administration of phenylephrine to patients in late pregnancy or labor may cause fetal anoxia or bradycardia by increasing contractility of the uterus and decreasing uterine blood flow.
See also "Nonteratogenic Effects."

NURSING MOTHERS
It is not known whether promethazine or phenylephrine is excreted in human milk.
Caution should be exercised when Phenergan VC is administered to a nursing woman.

PEDIATRIC USE
This product should not be used in children under 2 years of age because safety for such use has not been established.

ADVERSE REACTIONS
PROMETHAZINE
Nervous System—Sedation, sleepiness, occasional blurred vision, dryness of mouth, dizziness; rarely confusion, disorientation, and extrapyramidal symptoms such as oculogyric crisis, torticollis, and tongue protrusion (usually in association with parenteral injection or excessive dosage).
Cardiovascular—Increased or decreased blood pressure.
Dermatologic—Rash, rarely photosensitivity.
Hematologic—Rarely leukopenia, thrombocytopenia; agranulocytosis (1 case).
Gastrointestinal—Nausea and vomiting.
PHENYLEPHRINE
Nervous System—Restlessness, anxiety, nervousness, and dizziness.
Cardiovascular—Hypertension (see "Warnings").
Other—Precordial pain, respiratory distress, tremor, and weakness.

OVERDOSAGE
PROMETHAZINE
Signs and symptoms of overdosage with promethazine range from mild depression of the central nervous system and cardiovascular system to profound hypotension, respiratory depression, and unconsciousness.
Stimulation may be evident, especially in children and geriatric patients. Convulsions may rarely occur. A paradoxical reaction has been reported in children receiving single doses of 75 mg to 125 mg orally, characterized by hyperexcitability and nightmares.
Atropine-like signs and symptoms—dry mouth, fixed, dilated pupils, flushing, as well as gastrointestinal symptoms, may occur.
PHENYLEPHRINE
Signs and symptoms of overdosage with phenylephrine include hypertension, headache, convulsions, cerebral hemorrhage, and vomiting. Ventricular premature beats and short paroxysms of ventricular tachycardia may also occur. Headache may be a symptom of hypertension. Bradycardia may also be seen early in phenylephrine overdosage through stimulation of baroreceptors.

Drug	Effect
Phenylephrine with prior administration of monoamine oxidase inhibitors (MAOI).	Cardiac pressor response potentiated. May cause acute hypertensive crisis.
Phenylephrine with tricyclic antidepressants.	Pressor response increased.
Phenylephrine with ergot alkaloids.	Excessive rise in blood pressure.
Phenylephrine with bronchodilator sympathomimetic agents and with epinephrine or other sympathomimetics.	Tachycardia or other arrhythmias may occur.
Phenylephrine with prior administration of propranolol or other β-adrenergic blockers.	Cardiostimulating effects blocked.
Phenylephrine with atropine sulfate.	Reflex bradycardia blocked; pressor response enhanced.
Phenylephrine with prior administration of phentolamine or other α-adrenergic blockers.	Pressor response decreased.
Phenylephrine with diet preparations, such as amphetamines or phenylpropanolamine.	Synergistic adrenergic response.

TREATMENT
Treatment of overdosage with Phenergan VC is essentially symptomatic and supportive. Only in cases of extreme overdosage or individual sensitivity do vital signs including respiration, pulse, blood pressure, temperature, and EKG need to be monitored. Activated charcoal orally or by lavage may be given, or sodium or magnesium sulfate orally as a cathartic. Attention should be given to the reestablishment of adequate respiratory exchange through provision of a patent airway and institution of assisted or controlled ventilation. Diazepam may be used to control convulsions. Acidosis and electrolyte losses should be corrected. Note that any depressant effects of promethazine are not reversed by naloxone. Avoid analeptics which may cause convulsions.
Severe hypotension usually responds to the administration of norepinephrine or phenylephrine. EPINEPHRINE SHOULD NOT BE USED, since its use in patients with partial adrenergic blockade may further lower the blood pressure.
Limited experience with dialysis indicates that it is not helpful.

DOSAGE AND ADMINISTRATION
The recommended adult dose is one teaspoon (5 mL) every 4 to 6 hours, not to exceed 30.0 mL in 24 hours. For children 6 years to under 12 years of age, the dose is one-half to one teaspoon (2.5 to 5.0 mL) repeated at 4- to 6-hour intervals, not to exceed 30.0 mL in 24 hours. For children 2 years to under 6 years of age, the dose is one-quarter to one-half teaspoon (1.25 to 2.5 mL) every 4 to 6 hours.
Phenergan VC is not recommended for children under 2 years of age.

HOW SUPPLIED
Phenergan® VC, Wyeth®, is a clear, orange-yellow solution supplied as follows:
NDC 0008-0551-02, case of 24 bottles of 4 fl. oz.
NDC 0008-0551-06, case of 16 bottles of 6 fl. oz.
NDC 0008-0551-08, case of 12 bottles of 8 fl. oz.
NDC 0008-0551-03, bottle of 1 pint.
Keep bottles tightly closed below 25°C (77°F).
Protect from light.
Dispense in light-resistant, glass, tight containers.

PHENERGAN® VC   ©℞
[fen 'er-gan]
with codeine
(Promethazine Hydrochloride,
Phenylephrine Hydrochloride, and
Codeine Phosphate) Syrup

DESCRIPTION
Each teaspoon (5 mL) of Phenergan VC with codeine contains 10 mg (⅙ grain) codeine phosphate (Warning—may be habit-forming), 6.25 mg promethazine hydrochloride, and 5 mg phenylephrine hydrochloride in a flavored syrup base with a pH between 4.7 and 5.2. Alcohol 7%. The inactive ingredients present are artificial and natural flavors, citric acid, D&C Red 33, FD&C Yellow 6, glycerin, saccharin sodium, sodium benzoate, sodium citrate, sodium propionate, water, and other ingredients.
Codeine is one of the naturally occurring phenanthrene alkaloids of opium derived from the opium poppy; it is classified pharmacologically as a narcotic analgesic. Codeine phosphate may be chemically named as (5α,6α)-7,8-didehydro-4,5-epoxy-3-methoxy-17-methylmorphinan-6-ol phosphate (1:1) (salt) hemihydrate with the following structural formula:
[See Chemical Formula at top of next column].

PHENERGAN VC

The phosphate salt of codeine occurs as white, needle-shaped crystals or white crystalline powder. Codeine phosphate is freely soluble in water and slightly soluble in alcohol, with a molecular weight of 406.37. The empirical formula is $C_{18}H_{21}NO_3 \cdot H_3PO_4 \cdot \frac{1}{2}H_2O$, and the stereochemistry is 5α, 6α isomer as indicated in the structure.
Promethazine hydrochloride is a racemic compound; the empirical formula is $C_{17}H_{20}N_2S \cdot HCl$ and its molecular weight is 320.88.
Promethazine hydrochloride, a phenothiazine derivative, is designated chemically as N,N,α-trimethyl-10H-phenothiazine-10-ethanamine monohydrochloride with the following structural formula:

Promethazine hydrochloride occurs as a white to faint yellow, practically odorless, crystalline powder which slowly oxidizes and turns blue on prolonged exposure to air. It is soluble in water and freely soluble in alcohol.
Phenylephrine hydrochloride is a sympathomimetic amine salt. It may be chemically named as 3-hydroxy-α-[(methylamino)methyl]-benzenemethanol hydrochloride and has the following chemical formula:

Phenylephrine hydrochloride occurs as white or nearly white crystals, having a bitter taste. It is freely soluble in water and alcohol, with a molecular weight of 203.67. The empirical formula is $C_9H_{13}NO_2 \cdot HCl$, and the stereochemistry is R-isomer as indicated in the structure; Specific Rotation—between −42° and −47.5°. Phenylephrine hydrochloride is subject to oxidation and must be protected from light and air.

CLINICAL PHARMACOLOGY
CODEINE: Narcotic analgesics, including codeine, exert their primary effects on the central nervous system and gastrointestinal tract. The analgesic effects of codeine are due to its central action; however, the precise sites of action have not been determined, and the mechanisms involved appear to be quite complex. Codeine resembles morphine both structurally and pharmacologically, but its actions at the doses of codeine used therapeutically are milder, with less sedation, respiratory depression, and gastrointestinal, urinary, and pupillary effects. Codeine produces an increase in biliary tract pressure, but less than morphine or meperidine. Codeine is less constipating than morphine.

Continued on next page

Wyeth-Ayerst—Cont.

Codeine has good antitussive activity, although less than that of morphine at equal doses. It is used in preference to morphine, because side effects are infrequent at the usual antitussive dose of codeine.

Codeine in oral therapeutic dosage does not usually exert major effects on the cardiovascular system.

Narcotic analgesics may cause nausea and vomiting by stimulating the chemoreceptor trigger zone (CTZ); however, they also depress the vomiting center, so that subsequent doses are unlikely to produce vomiting. Nausea is minimal after usual oral doses of codeine.

Narcotic analgesics cause histamine release, which appears to be responsible for wheals or urticaria sometimes seen at the site of injection on parenteral administration. Histamine release may also produce dilation of cutaneous blood vessels, with resultant flushing of the face and neck, pruritus, and sweating.

Codeine and its salts are well absorbed following both oral and parenteral administration. Codeine is about ⅔ as effective orally as parenterally. Codeine is metabolized primarily in the liver by enzymes of the endoplasmic reticulum, where it undergoes O-demethylation, N-demethylation, and partial conjugation with glucuronic acid. The drug is excreted primarily in the urine, largely as inactive metabolites and small amounts of free and conjugated morphine. Negligible amounts of codeine and its metabolites are found in the feces. Following oral or subcutaneous administration of codeine, the onset of analgesia occurs within 15 to 30 minutes and lasts for four to six hours.

The cough-depressing action, in animal studies, was observed to occur 15 minutes after oral administration of codeine, peak action at 45 to 60 minutes after ingestion. The duration of action, which is dose-dependent, usually did not exceed 3 hours.

PROMETHAZINE: Promethazine is a phenothiazine derivative which differs structurally from the antipsychotic phenothiazines by the presence of a branched side chain and no ring substitution. It is thought that this configuration is responsible for its relative lack (1/10 that of chlorpromazine) of dopaminergic (CNS) action.

Promethazine is an H_1 receptor blocking agent. In addition to its antihistaminic action, it provides clinically useful sedative and antiemetic effects. In therapeutic dosages, promethazine produces no significant effects on the cardiovascular system.

Promethazine is well absorbed from the gastrointestinal tract. Clinical effects are apparent within 20 minutes after oral adminstration and generally last four to six hours, although they may persist as long as 12 hours. Promethazine is metabolized by the liver to a variety of compounds; the sulfoxides of promethazine and N-demethylpromethazine are the predominant metabolites appearing in the urine.

PHENYLEPHRINE: Phenylephrine is a potent postsynaptic α-receptor agonist with little effect on β receptors of the heart. Phenylephrine has no effect on β-adrenergic receptors of the bronchi or peripheral blood vessels. A direct action at receptors accounts for the greater part of its effects, only a small part being due to its ability to release norepinephrine.

Therapeutic doses of phenylephrine mainly cause vasoconstriction. Phenylephrine increases resistance and, to a lesser extent, decreases capacitance of blood vessels. Total peripheral resistance is increased, resulting in increased systolic and diastolic blood pressure. Pulmonary arterial pressure is usually increased, and renal blood flow is usually decreased. Local vasoconstriction and hemostasis occur following topical application or infiltration of phenylephrine into tissues. The main effect of phenylephrine on the heart is bradycardia; it produces a positive inotropic effect on the myocardium in doses greater than those usually used therapeutically. Rarely, the drug may increase the irritability of the heart, causing arrhythmias. Cardiac output is decreased slightly. Phenylephrine increases the work of the heart by increasing peripheral arterial resistance.

Phenylephrine has a mild central stimulant effect.

Following oral administration or topical application of phenylephrine to the mucosa, constriction of blood vessels in the nasal mucosa relieves nasal congestion associated with allergy or head colds. Following oral administration, nasal decongestion may occur within 15 or 20 minutes and may persist for up to 4 hours.

Phenylephrine is irregularly absorbed from and readily metabolized in the gastrointestinal tract. Phenylephrine is metabolized in the liver and intestine by monoamine oxidase. The metabolites and their route and rate of excretion have not been identified. The pharmacologic action of phenylephrine is terminated at least partially by uptake of the drug into tissues.

INDICATIONS AND USAGE

Phenergan VC with codeine is indicated for the temporary relief of coughs and upper respiratory symptoms, including nasal congestion, associated with allergy or the common cold.

CONTRAINDICATIONS

Codeine is contraindicated in patients with a known hypersensitivity to the drug.

Promethazine is contraindicated in individuals known to be hypersensitive or to have had an idiosyncratic reaction to promethazine or to other phenothiazines.

Phenylephrine is contraindicated in patients with hypertension or with peripheral vascular insufficiency (ischemia may result with risk of gangrene or thrombosis of compromised vascular beds). Phenylephrine should not be used in patients known to be hypersensitive to the drug or in those receiving a monoamine oxidase inhibitor (MAOI).

Antihistamines and codeine are both contraindicated for use in the treatment of lower respiratory tract symptoms, including asthma.

WARNINGS

CODEINE: Dosage of codeine SHOULD NOT BE INCREASED if cough fails to respond; an unresponsive cough should be reevaluated in 5 days or sooner for possible underlying pathology, such as foreign body or lower respiratory tract disease.

Codeine may cause or aggravate constipation.

Respiratory depression leading to arrest, coma, and death has occurred with the use of codeine antitussives in young children, particularly in the under-one-year infants whose ability to deactivate the drug is not fully developed.

Administration of codeine may be accompanied by histamine release and should be used with caution in atopic children.

Head Injury and Increased Intracranial Pressure

The respiratory-depressant effects of narcotic analgesics and their capacity to elevate cerebrospinal fluid pressure may be markedly exaggerated in the presence of head injury, intracranial lesions, or a preexisting increase in intracranial pressure. Narcotics may produce adverse reactions which may obscure the clinical course of patients with head injuries.

Asthma and Other Respiratory Conditions

Narcotic analgesics or cough suppressants, including codeine, should not be used in asthmatic patients (see "Contraindications"). Nor should they be used in acute febrile illness associated with productive cough or in chronic respiratory disease where interference with ability to clear the tracheobronchial tree of secretions would have a deleterious effect on the patient's respiratory function.

Hypotensive Effect

Codeine may produce orthostatic hypotension in ambulatory patients.

PROMETHAZINE: Promethazine may cause marked drowsiness. Ambulatory patients should be cautioned against such activities as driving or operating dangerous machinery until it is known that they do not become drowsy or dizzy from promethazine therapy.

The sedative action of promethazine hydrochloride is additive to the sedative effects of central nervous system depressants; therefore, agents such as alcohol, narcotic analgesics, sedatives, hypnotics, and tranquilizers should either be eliminated or given in reduced dosage in the presence of promethazine hydrochloride. When given concomitantly with promethazine hydrochloride, the dose of barbiturates should be reduced by at least one-half, and the dose of analgesic depressants, such as morphine or meperidine, should be reduced by one-quarter to one-half.

Promethazine may lower seizure threshold. This should be taken into consideration when administering to persons with known seizure disorders or when giving in combination with narcotics or local anesthetics which may also affect seizure threshold.

Sedative drugs or CNS depressants should be avoided in patients with a history of sleep apnea. Antihistamines should be used with caution in patients with narrow-angle glaucoma, stenosing peptic ulcer, pyloroduodenal obstruction, and urinary bladder obstruction due to symptomatic prostatic hypertrophy and narrowing of the bladder neck.

Administration of promethazine has been associated with reported cholestatic jaundice.

PHENYLEPHRINE: Because phenylephrine is an adrenergic agent, it should be given with caution to patients with thyroid diseases, diabetes mellitus, and heart diseases or those receiving tricyclic antidepressants.

Men with symptomatic, benign prostatic hypertrophy can experience urinary retention when given oral nasal decongestants.

Phenylephrine can cause a decrease in cardiac output, and extreme caution should be used when administering the drug, parenterally or orally, to patients with arteriosclerosis, to elderly individuals, and/or to patients with initially poor cerebral or coronary circulation.

Phenylephrine should be used with caution in patients taking diet preparations, such as amphetamines or phenylpropanolamine, because synergistic adrenergic effects could result in serious hypertensive response and possible stroke.

PRECAUTIONS

Animal reproduction studies have not been conducted with the drug combination—promethazine, phenylephrine, and codeine. It is not known whether this drug combination can cause fetal harm when administered to a pregnant woman or can affect reproduction capacity. Phenergan VC with codeine should be given to a pregnant woman only if clearly needed.

GENERAL

Narcotic analgesics, including codeine, should be administered with caution and the initial dose reduced in patients with acute abdominal conditions, convulsive disorders, significant hepatic or renal impairment, fever, hypothyroidism, Addison's disease, ulcerative colitis, prostatic hypertrophy, in patients with recent gastrointestinal or urinary tract surgery, and in the very young or elderly or debilitated patients. Promethazine should be used cautiously in persons with cardiovascular disease or with impairment of liver function. Phenylephrine should be used with caution in patients with cardiovascular disease, particularly hypertension.

INFORMATION FOR PATIENTS

Phenergan VC with codeine may cause marked drowsiness or impair the mental and/or physical abilities required for the performance of potentially hazardous tasks, such as driving a vehicle or operating machinery. Ambulatory patients should be told to avoid engaging in such activities until it is known that they do not become drowsy or dizzy from Phenergan VC with codeine therapy. Children should be supervised to avoid potential harm in bike riding or in other hazardous activities.

The concomitant use of alcohol or other central nervous system depressants, including narcotic analgesics, sedatives, hypnotics, and tranquilizers, may have an additive effect and should be avoided or their dosage reduced.

Patients should be advised to report any involuntary muscle movements or unusual sensitivity to sunlight.

Codeine, like other narcotic analgesics, may produce orthostatic hypotension in some ambulatory patients. Patients should be cautioned accordingly.

DRUG INTERACTIONS

CODEINE: In patients receiving MAO inhibitors, an initial small test dose is advisable to allow observation of any excessive narcotic effects or MAOI interaction.

PROMETHAZINE: The sedative action of promethazine is additive to the effects of other central nervous system depressants, including alcohol, narcotic analgesics, sedatives, hypnotics, tricyclic antidepressants, and tranquilizers; therefore, these agents should be avoided or administered in reduced dosage to patients receiving promethazine.

[See table on top next page].

DRUG/LABORATORY TEST INTERACTIONS

Because narcotic analgesics may increase biliary tract pressure, with resultant increases in plasma amylase or lipase levels, determination of these enzyme levels may be unreliable for 24 hours after a narcotic analgesic has been given. The following laboratory tests may be affected in patients who are receiving therapy with promethazine hydrochloride:

Pregnancy Tests

Diagnostic pregnancy tests based on immunological reactions between HCG and anti-HCG may result in false-negative or false-positive interpretations.

Glucose Tolerance Test

An increase in blood glucose has been reported in patients receiving promethazine.

CARCINOGENESIS, MUTAGENESIS, IMPAIRMENT OF FERTILITY

CODEINE AND PROMETHAZINE

Long-term animal studies have not been performed to assess the carcinogenic potential of codeine or of promethazine, nor are there other animal or human data concerning carcinogenicity, mutagenicity, or impairment of fertility with these agents. Codeine has been reported to show no evidence of carcinogenicity or mutagenicity in a variety of test systems, including the micronucleus and sperm abnormality assays and the *Salmonella* assay. Promethazine was nonmutagenic in the *Salmonella* test system of Ames.

PHENYLEPHRINE

A study which followed the development of cancer in 143,574 patients over a four-year period indicated that in 11,981 patients who received phenylephrine (systemic or topical), there was no statistically significant association between the drug and cancer at any or all sites.

Long-term animal studies have not been performed to assess the carcinogenic potential of phenylephrine, nor are there other animal or human data concerning mutagenicity.

A study of the effects of adrenergic drugs on ovum transport in rabbits indicated that treatment with phenylephrine did not alter incidence of pregnancy; the number of implantations was significantly reduced when high doses of the drug were used.

PREGNANCY

Teratogenic Effects —Pregnancy Category C

CODEINE: A study in rats and rabbits reported no teratogenic effect of codeine administered during the period of organogenesis in doses ranging from 5 to 120 mg/kg. In the rat, doses at the 120-mg/kg level, in the toxic range for the adult animal, were associated with an increase in embryo resorption at the time of implantation. In another study a single 100-mg/kg dose of codeine administered to pregnant mice reportedly resulted in delayed ossification in the offspring.

There are no studies in humans, and the significance of these findings to humans, if any, is not known.

PROMETHAZINE: Teratogenic effects have not been demonstrated in rat-feeding studies at doses of 6.25 and 12.5 mg/kg of promethazine. These doses are 8.3 and 16.7 times the maximum recommended total daily dose for a 50-kg subject. Specific studies to test the action of the drug on parturition, lactation, and development of the animal neonate were not done, but a general preliminary study in rats indicated no effect on these parameters. Although antihistamines, including promethazine, have been found to produce fetal mortality in rodents, the pharmacological effects of histamine in the rodent do not parallel those in man. There are no adequate and well-controlled studies of promethazine in pregnant women.

PHENYLEPHRINE: A study in rabbits indicated that continued moderate overexposure to phenylephrine (3 mg/day) during the second half of pregnancy (22nd day of gestation to delivery) may contribute to perinatal wastage, prematurity, premature labor, and possibly fetal anomalies; when phenylephrine (3 mg/day) was given to rabbits during the first half of pregnancy (3rd day after mating for seven days), a significant number gave birth to litters of low birth weight. Another study showed that phenylephrine was associated with anomalies of aortic arch and with ventricular septal defect in the chick embryo.

Phenergan VC with codeine should be used during pregnancy only if the potential benefit justifies the potential risk to the fetus.

Nonteratogenic Effects

Dependence has been reported in newborns whose mothers took opiates regularly during pregnancy. Withdrawal signs include irritability, excessive crying, tremors, hyperreflexia, fever, vomiting, and diarrhea. Signs usually appear during the first few days of life.

Promethazine taken within two weeks of delivery may inhibit platelet aggregation in the newborn.

LABOR AND DELIVERY

Narcotic analgesics cross the placental barrier. The closer to delivery and the larger the dose used, the greater the possibility of respiratory depression in the newborn. Narcotic analgesics should be avoided during labor if delivery of a premature infant is anticipated. If the mother has received narcotic analgesics during labor, newborn infants should be observed closely for signs of respiratory depression. Resuscitation may be required (see "Overdosage"). The effect of codeine, if any, on the later growth, development, and functional maturation of the child is unknown.

Administration of phenylephrine to patients in late pregnancy or labor may cause fetal anoxia or bradycardia by increasing contractility of the uterus and decreasing uterine blood flow.

See also "Nonteratogenic Effects."

NURSING MOTHERS

Some studies, but not others, have reported detectable amounts of codeine in breast milk. The levels are probably not clinically significant after usual therapeutic dosage. The possibility of clinically important amounts being excreted in breast milk in individuals abusing codeine should be considered.

It is not known whether either phenylephrine or promethazine is excreted in human milk.

Caution should be exercised when Phenergan VC with codeine is administered to a nursing woman.

PEDIATRIC USE

This product should not be used in children under 2 years of age because safety for such use has not been established.

ADVERSE REACTIONS

CODEINE

Nervous System —CNS depression, particularly respiratory depression, and to a lesser extent circulatory depression; light-headedness, dizziness, sedation, euphoria, dysphoria,

---

PHENERGAN VC WITH CODEINE

Drug	Effect
Phenylephrine with prior administration of monoamine oxidase inhibitors (MAOI).	Cardiac pressor response potentiated. May cause acute hypertensive crisis.
Phenylephrine with tricyclic antidepressants.	Pressor response increased.
Phenylephrine with ergot alkaloids.	Excessive rise in blood pressure.
Phenylephrine with bronchodilator sympathomimetic agents and with epinephrine or other sympathomimetics.	Tachycardia or other arrhythmias may occur.
Phenylephrine with prior administration of propranolol or other β-adrenergic blockers.	Cardiostimulating effects blocked.
Phenylephrine with atropine sulfate.	Reflex bradycardia blocked; pressor response enhanced.
Phenylephrine with prior administration of phentolamine or other α-adrenergic blockers.	Pressor response decreased.
Phenylephrine with diet preparations, such as amphetamines or phenylpropanolamine.	Synergistic adrenergic response.

---

headache, transient hallucination, disorientation, visual disturbances, and convulsions.

Cardiovascular —Tachycardia, bradycardia, palpitation, faintness, syncope, orthostatic hypotension (common to narcotic analgesics).

Gastrointestinal —Nausea, vomiting, constipation, and biliary tract spasm. Patients with chronic ulcerative colitis may experience increased colonic motility; in patients with acute ulcerative colitis, toxic dilation has been reported.

Genitourinary —Oliguria, urinary retention; antidiuretic effect has been reported (common to narcotic analgesics).

Allergic —Infrequent pruritus, giant urticaria, angioneurotic edema, and laryngeal edema.

Other —Flushing of the face, sweating and pruritus (due to opiate-induced histamine release); weakness.

PROMETHAZINE

Nervous System —Sedation, sleepiness, occasional blurred vision, dryness of mouth, dizziness; rarely confusion, disorientation, and extrapyramidal symptoms such as oculogyric crisis, torticollis, and tongue protrusion (usually in association with parenteral injection or excessive dosage).

Cardiovascular —Increased or decreased blood pressure.

Dermatologic —Rash, rarely photosensitivity.

Hematologic —Rarely leukopenia, thrombocytopenia; agranulocytosis (1 case).

Gastrointestinal —Nausea and vomiting.

PHENYLEPHRINE

Nervous System —Restlessness, anxiety, nervousness, and dizziness.

Cardiovascular —Hypertension (see "Warnings").

Other —Precordial pain, respiratory distress, tremor, and weakness.

DRUG ABUSE AND DEPENDENCE

CONTROLLED SUBSTANCE

Phenergan VC with codeine is a Schedule V Controlled Substance.

ABUSE

Codeine is known to be subject to abuse; however, the abuse potential of oral codeine appears to be quite low. Even parenteral codeine does not appear to offer the psychic effects sought by addicts to the same degree as heroin or morphine. However, codeine must be administered only under close supervision to patients with a history of drug abuse or dependence.

DEPENDENCE

Psychological dependence, physical dependence, and tolerance are known to occur with codeine.

OVERDOSAGE

CODEINE: Serious overdose with codeine is characterized by respiratory depression (a decrease in respiratory rate and/or tidal volume, Cheyne-Stokes respiration, cyanosis), extreme somnolence progressing to stupor or coma, skeletal muscle

---

flaccidity, cold and clammy skin, and sometimes bradycardia and hypotension. The triad of coma, pinpoint pupils, and respiratory depression is strongly suggestive of opiate poisoning. In severe overdosage, particularly by the intravenous route, apnea, circulatory collapse, cardiac arrest, and death may occur. Promethazine is additive to the depressant effects of codeine.

It is difficult to determine what constitutes a standard toxic or lethal dose. However, the lethal oral dose of codeine in an adult is reported to be in the range of 0.5 to 1.0 gram. Infants and children are believed to be relatively more sensitive to opiates on a body-weight basis. Elderly patients are also comparatively intolerant to opiates.

PROMETHAZINE: Signs and symptoms of overdosage with promethazine range from mild depression of the central nervous system and cardiovascular system to profound hypotension, respiratory depression, and unconsciousness.

Stimulation may be evident, especially in children and geriatric patients. Convulsions may rarely occur. A paradoxical reaction has been reported in children receiving single doses of 75 mg to 125 mg orally, characterized by hyperexcitability and nightmares.

Atropine-like signs and symptoms—dry mouth, fixed, dilated pupils, flushing, as well as gastrointestinal symptoms, may occur.

PHENYLEPHRINE: Signs and symptoms of overdosage with phenylephrine include hypertension, headache, convulsions, cerebral hemorrhage, and vomiting. Ventricular premature beats and short paroxysms of ventricular tachycardia may also occur. Headache may be a symptom of hypertension. Bradycardia may also be seen early in phenylephrine overdosage through stimulation of baroreceptors.

TREATMENT

Treatment of overdosage with Phenergan VC with codeine is essentially symptomatic and supportive. Only in cases of extreme overdosage or individual sensitivity do vital signs including respiration, pulse, blood pressure, temperature, and EKG need to be monitored. Activated charcoal orally or by lavage may be given, or sodium or magnesium sulfate orally as a cathartic. Attention should be given to the reestablishment of adequate respiratory exchange through provision of a patent airway and institution of assisted or controlled ventilation. The narcotic antagonist, naloxone hydrochloride, may be administered when significant respiratory depression occurs with Phenergan VC with codeine; any depressant effects of promethazine are not reversed by naloxone. Diazepam may be used to control convulsions. Avoid analeptics, which may cause convulsions. Acidosis and electrolyte losses should be corrected. A rise in temperature or pulmonary complications may signal the need for institution of antibiotic therapy.

Severe hypotension usually responds to the administration of norepinephrine or phenylephrine. EPINEPHRINE SHOULD NOT BE USED, since its use in a patient with partial adrenergic blockade may further lower the blood pressure.

Limited experience with dialysis indicates that it is not helpful.

DOSAGE AND ADMINISTRATION

The average effective dose is given in the following table:
[See table left]

HOW SUPPLIED

Phenergan® VC with codeine, Wyeth®, is a clear, reddish-orange solution supplied as follows:

PHENERGAN VC WITH CODEINE

Adults	1 teaspoon (5 mL) every 4 to 6 hours, not to exceed 30.0 mL in 24 hours.
Children 6 years to under 12 years	½ to 1 teaspoon (2.5 to 5 mL) every 4 to 6 hours, not to exceed 30.0 mL in 24 hours.
Children under 6 years (weight: 18 kg or 40 lbs)	¼ to ½ teaspoon (1.25 to 2.5 mL) every 4 to 6 hours, not to exceed 9.0 mL in 24 hours.
Children under 6 years (weight: 16 kg or 35 lbs)	¼ to ½ teaspoon (1.25 to 2.5 mL) every 4 to 6 hours, not to exceed 8.0 mL in 24 hours.
Children under 6 years (weight: 14 kg or 30 lbs)	¼ to ½ teaspoon (1.25 to 2.5 mL) every 4 to 6 hours, not to exceed 7.0 mL in 24 hours.
Children under 6 years (weight: 12 kg or 25 lbs)	¼ to ½ teaspoon (1.25 to 2.5 mL) every 4 to 6 hours, not to exceed 6.0 mL in 24 hours.

Phenergan VC with codeine is not recommended for children under 2 years of age.

Continued on next page

Wyeth-Ayerst—Cont.

NDC 0008-0552-02, case of 24 bottles of 4 fl. oz. (118 mL).
NDC 0008-0552-03, bottle of 1 pint (473 mL).
Keep bottles tightly closed—Stored at Room Temperature, between 15° C and 25° C (59° F and 77° F).
Protect from light.
Dispense in light-resistant, glass, tight containers.

PHOSPHOLINE IODIDE®   ℞

[fŏs 'fo-lĭn ĭ 'o-dīd]
(echothiophate iodide for ophthalmic solution)

HOW SUPPLIED

Each package contains sterile PHOSPHOLINE IODIDE (echothiophate iodide), sterile diluent, and dropper for dispensing 5 mL eyedrops of the strength indicated on the label. Four potencies are available:

NDC 0046-1062-05 .... 1.5 mg package
for 0.03%

White amorphous deposit on bottle walls. Aluminum crimp seal is blue.

NDC 0046-1064-05 .... 3.0 mg package
for 0.06%

White amorphous deposit on bottle walls. Aluminum crimp seal is red.

NDC 0046-1065-05 .... 6.25 mg package
for 0.125%

White amorphous deposit on bottle walls. Aluminum crimp seal is green.

NDC 0046-1066-05 .... 12.5 mg package
for 0.25%

White amorphous deposit on bottle walls. Aluminum crimp seal is yellow.

Handling and Storage:
Store at room temperature (approximately 25°C).
After reconstitution, keep eyedrops in refrigerator to obtain maximum useful life of 6 months. Room temperature is acceptable if drops will be used within a month.
Full prescribing information for this product appears in the PHYSICIANS' DESK REFERENCE for OPHTHALMOLOGY. Please refer to this book or, for prescribing information write to Professional Service, Wyeth-Ayerst Laboratories, Box 8299, Philadelphia, PA 19101, or contact your local Wyeth-Ayerst representative.

PLEGINE®   ©℞

[plĕj-ēn ']
Brand of phendimetrazine tartrate tablets
Anorexiant

CAUTION: Federal law prohibits dispensing without prescription.

DESCRIPTION

Chemical name: (+)-3,4-Dimethyl-2-phenylmorpholine Tartrate
Structural formula:

PLEGINE is the dextro isomer of phendimetrazine tartrate. Phendimetrazine tartrate is a white, odorless powder with a bitter taste. It is soluble in water, methanol, and ethanol. PLEGINE contains these inactive ingredients: D&C Yellow No. 10; FD&C Yellow No. 6; Lactose, NF; Magnesium Stearate; NF; Polyethylene Glycol 8000, NF.

ACTIONS

PLEGINE is a phenylalkylamine sympathomimetic with pharmacologic activity similar to the prototype drugs of this class used in obesity, the amphetamines. Actions include central nervous system (CNS) stimulation and elevation of blood pressure. Tachyphylaxis and tolerance have been demonstrated with all drugs of this class in which these phenomena have been looked for.
Drugs of this class used in obesity are commonly known as "anorectics" or "anorexigenics." It has not been established, however, that the action of such drugs in treating obesity is primarily one of appetite suppression. Other CNS actions, or metabolic effects, may be involved.
Adult obese subjects instructed in dietary management and treated with "anorectic" drugs, lose more weight on the average than those treated with placebo and diet, as determined in relatively short-term clinical trials.
The magnitude of increased weight loss of drug-treated patients over placebo-treated patients is only a fraction of a

pound a week. The rate of weight loss is greatest in the first weeks of therapy for both drug and placebo subjects and tends to decrease in succeeding weeks. The possible origins of the increased weight loss due to the various drug effects are not established. The amount of weight loss associated with use of an "anorectic" drug varies from trial to trial, and the increased weight loss appears to be related, in part, to variables other than the drug prescribed, such as the physician-investigator, the population treated, and the diet prescribed. Studies do not permit conclusions as to the relative importance of the drug and non-drug factors on weight loss.
The natural history of obesity is measured in years, whereas the studies cited are restricted to a few weeks' duration; thus, the total impact of drug-induced weight loss over that of diet alone must be considered clinically limited.

INDICATIONS

PLEGINE is indicated in the management of exogenous obesity as a short-term adjunct (a few weeks) in a regimen of weight reduction based on caloric restriction. The limited usefulness of agents of this class should be measured against possible risk factors inherent in their use (see ACTIONS).

CONTRAINDICATIONS

Known hypersensitivity or idiosyncratic reactions to sympathomimetics.
Advanced arteriosclerosis, symptomatic cardiovascular disease, moderate and severe hypertension, hyperthyroidism, glaucoma
Highly nervous or agitated patients
Patients with a history of drug abuse
Patients taking other CNS stimulants, including monamine oxidase inhibitors

WARNINGS

DRUG DEPENDENCE: PLEGINE is related chemically and pharmacologically to the amphetamines. Amphetamines and related stimulant drugs have extensively been abused, and the possibility of PLEGINE abuse should be kept in mind when evaluating the desirability of including a drug as part of a weight reduction program. Abuse of amphetamines and related drugs may be associated with intense psychological dependence and severe social dysfunction. There are reports of patients who have increased the dosage to many times that recommended. Abrupt cessation following prolonged high-dosage administration results in extreme fatigue and mental depression; changes are also noted on the sleep EEG. Manifestations of chronic intoxication with anorectic drugs include severe dermatoses, marked insomnia, irritability, hyperactivity, and personality changes. The most severe manifestation of chronic intoxication is psychosis, often clinically indistinguishable from schizophrenia.
Tolerance to the anorectic effect of PLEGINE develops within a few weeks. When this occurs, its use should be discontinued; the maximum recommended dose should not be exceeded.
Use of PLEGINE within 14 days following the administration of monamine oxidase inhibitors may result in a hypertensive crisis.
Abrupt cessation of administration following prolonged high dosage results in extreme fatigue and depression. Because of the effect on the central nervous system, PLEGINE may impair the patient's ability to engage in potentially hazardous activities such as operating machinery or driving a motor vehicle; the patient should therefore be cautioned accordingly.
Usage in Pregnancy: Safe use in pregnancy has not been established. Until more information is available, phendimetrazine tartrate should not be taken by women who are, or may become, pregnant unless, in the opinion of the physician, the potential benefits outweigh the possible hazards.
Usage in Children: PLEGINE is not recommended for use in children under 12 years of age.

PRECAUTIONS

Caution is to be exercised in prescribing PLEGINE for patients with even mild hypertension.
Insulin requirements in diabetes mellitus may be altered in association with the use of PLEGINE and the concomitant dietary regimen.
PLEGINE may decrease the hypotensive effect of guanethidine.
The least amount feasible should be prescribed or dispensed at one time in order to minimize the possibility of overdosage.

ADVERSE REACTIONS

Central Nervous System: Overstimulation, restlessness, insomnia, agitation, flushing, tremor, sweating, dizziness, headache, psychotic states, blurring of vision
Cardiovascular: Palpitation, tachycardia, elevated blood pressure
Gastrointestinal: Mouth dryness, nausea, diarrhea, constipation, stomach pain
Genitourinary: Urinary frequency, dysuria, changes in libido

DOSAGE AND ADMINISTRATION

Usual adult dosage: 1 tablet (35 mg) bid or tid, one hour before meals.
Dosage should be individualized to obtain an adequate response with the lowest effective dosage. In some cases, ½ tablet per dose may be adequate; dosage should not exceed 2 tablets tid.
Overdosage: Acute overdosage of phendimetrazine tartrate may manifest itself by the following signs and symptoms: unusual restlessness, confusion, belligerence, hallucinations, and panic states. Fatigue and depression usually follow the central stimulation. Cardiovascular effects include arrhythmias, hypertension, or hypotension and circulatory collapse. Gastrointestinal symptoms include nausea, vomiting, diarrhea, and abdominal cramps. Poisoning may result in convulsions, coma, and death.
The management of overdosage is largely symptomatic. It includes sedation with a barbiturate. If hypertension is marked, the use of a nitrate or rapid-acting alpha receptor-blocking agent should be considered. Experience with hemodialysis or peritoneal dialysis is inadequate to permit recommendations for its use.

HOW SUPPLIED

PLEGINE—Each scored tablet contains 35 mg phendimetrazine tartrate, in bottles of 100 (NDC 0046-0755-81) and 1,000 (NDC 0046-0755-91).
Shown in Product Identification Section, page 437

PMB® 200   ℞

Each tablet contains:
Premarin® (conjugated
estrogens, USP) ....0.45 mg
Meprobamate ....200.0 mg

PMB® 400

Each tablet contains:
Premarin® (conjugated
estrogens, USP) ....0.45 mg
Meprobamate ....400.0 mg

CAUTION: Federal law prohibits dispensing without prescription.

---

1. ESTROGENS HAVE BEEN REPORTED TO INCREASE THE RISK OF ENDOMETRIAL CARCINOMA. Three independent, case-controlled studies have reported an increased risk of endometrial cancer in post-menopausal women exposed to exogenous estrogens for more than one year.[1-3] This risk was independent of the other known risk factors for endometrial cancer. These studies are further supported by the finding that incidence rates of endometrial cancer have increased sharply since 1969 in eight different areas of the United States with population-based cancer reporting systems, an increase which may be related to the rapidly expanding use of estrogens during the last decade.[4]
The three case-controlled studies reported that the risk of endometrial cancer in estrogen users was about 4.5 to 13.9 times greater than in nonusers. The risk appears to depend on both duration of treatment[1] and on estrogen dose.[3] In view of these findings, when estrogens are used for the treatment of menopausal symptoms, the lowest dose that will control symptoms should be utilized and medication should be discontinued as soon as possible. When prolonged treatment is medically indicated, the patient should be reassessed, on at least a semi-annual basis to determine the need for continued therapy. Although the evidence must be considered preliminary, one study suggests that cyclic administration of low doses of estrogen may carry less risk than continuous administration.[3] It therefore appears prudent to utilize such a regimen.
Close clinical surveillance of all women taking estrogens is important. In all cases of undiagnosed persistent or recurring abnormal vaginal bleeding, adequate diagnostic measures should be undertaken to rule out malignancy.
There is no evidence at present that "natural" estrogens are more or less hazardous than "synthetic" estrogens at equi-estrogenic doses.
2. ESTROGENS SHOULD NOT BE USED DURING PREGNANCY.
The use of female sex hormones, both estrogens and progestogens, during early pregnancy may seriously damage the offspring. It has been shown that females exposed in utero to diethylstilbestrol, a nonsteroidal estrogen, have an increased risk of developing, in later life, a form of vaginal or cervical cancer that is ordinarily extremely rare.[5,6] This risk has been estimated as not greater than 4 per 1,000 exposures.[7] Furthermore, a high percentage of such exposed women (from 30% to 90%) have been found to have vaginal adenosis,[8-12]

epithelial changes of the vagina and cervix. Although these changes are histologically benign, it is not known whether they are precursors of malignancy. Although similar data are not available with the use of other estrogens, it cannot be presumed they would not induce similar changes.

Several reports suggest an association between intrauterine exposure to female sex hormones and congenital anomalies, including congenital heart defects and limb-reduction defects.[13-16] One case-controlled study[16] estimated a 4.7-fold increased risk of limb-reduction defects in infants exposed in utero to sex hormones (oral contraceptives, hormone withdrawal tests for pregnancy, or attempted treatment for threatened abortion). Some of these exposures were very short and involved only a few days of treatment. The data suggest that the risk of limb-reduction defects in exposed fetuses is somewhat less than 1 per 1,000.

In the past, female sex hormones have been used during pregnancy in an attempt to treat threatened or habitual abortion. There is considerable evidence that estrogens are ineffective for these indications, and there is no evidence from well-controlled studies that progestogens are effective for these uses.

If PMB is used during pregnancy, or if the patient becomes pregnant while taking this drug, she should be apprised of the potential risks to the fetus, and the advisability of pregnancy continuation.

3. THIS FIXED-COMBINATION DRUG IS NOT INDICATED FOR INITIAL THERAPY.

In cases where estrogen given alone has not alleviated anxiety and tension existing as part of the menopausal symptom complex, therapy may then consist of separate administration of estrogen and meprobamate in order to determine the appropriate dosage of each drug for the patient. If this fixed combination represents the dosage so determined, its use may be more convenient in patient management. The treatment of such patients is not static, but must be re-evaluated as conditions in each patient warrant.

DESCRIPTION

PMB is a combination of PREMARIN® (conjugated estrogens, USP) and meprobamate, a tranquilizing agent, in tablet form for oral administration.

PREMARIN (conjugated estrogens, USP) is a mixture of estrogens, obtained exclusively from natural sources, occurring as the sodium salts of water-soluble estrogen sulfates blended to represent the average composition of material derived from pregnant mares' urine. It contains estrone, equilin, and 17α-dihydroequilin, together with smaller amounts of 17α-estradiol, equilenin, and 17 α-dihydroequilenin as salts of their sulfate esters.

Meprobamate, USP, is the dicarbamic acid ester of 2-methyl-2-*n*-propyl-1,3-propanediol.

PMB 200: Each tablet contains 0.45 mg of PREMARIN® (conjugated estrogens, USP) and 200 mg Meprobamate, USP.

PMB 400: Each tablet contains 0.45 mg of PREMARIN® (conjugated estrogens, USP) and 400 mg Meprobamate, USP.

PMB Tablets contain the following inactive ingredients: calcium phosphate tribasic, calcium sulfate anhydrous, carnauba wax, lactose, magnesium stearate, methylcellulose, microcrystalline cellulose, pharmaceutical glaze, sucrose, talc, titanium dioxide.

—PMB 200 Tablets also contain: D&C Yellow No. 10, FD&C Blue No. 1, FD&C Yellow No. 6.

—PMB 400 Tablets also contain: FD&C Blue No. 2, FD&C Red No. 3.

CLINICAL PHARMACOLOGY

Estrogens are important in the development and maintenance of the female reproductive system and secondary sex characteristics. They promote growth and development of the vagina, uterus, and fallopian tubes, and enlargement of the breasts. Indirectly, they contribute to the shaping of the skeleton, maintenance of tone and elasticity of urogenital structures, changes in the epiphyses of the long bones that allow for the pubertal growth spurt and its termination, growth of axillary and pubic hair, and pigmentation of the nipples and genitals. Decline of estrogenic activity at the end of the menstrual cycle can bring on menstruation, although the cessation of progesterone secretion is the most important factor in the mature ovulatory cycle. However, in the preovulatory or nonovulatory cycle, estrogen is the primary determinant in the onset of menstruation. Estrogens also affect the release of pituitary gonadotropins.

The pharmacologic effects of conjugated estrogens are similar to those of endogenous estrogens. They are soluble in water and are well absorbed from the gastrointestinal tract. In responsive tissues (female genital organs, breasts, hypothalamus, pituitary) estrogens enter the cell and are transported into the nucleus. As a result of estrogen action, specific RNA and protein synthesis occurs.

Metabolism and inactivation occur primarily in the liver. Some estrogens are excreted into the bile; however, they are reabsorbed from the intestine and returned to the liver through the portal venous system. Water-soluble estrogen conjugates are strongly acidic and are ionized in body fluids, which favor excretion through the kidneys since tubular reabsorption is minimal.

Meprobamate is used clinically for the reduction of anxiety and tension. The precise mechanism(s) of its action is not known. It is well absorbed from the gastrointestinal tract and has a physiological half-life of about 10 hours. It is excreted in the urine primarily as hydroxymeprobamate and as a glucuronide.

The combination of PREMARIN with meprobamate as provided in PMB relieves the underlying estrogen deficiency and affords tranquilizing activity to ameliorate the anxiety and tension not due to estrogen deficiency.

INDICATIONS AND USAGE

For the treatment of moderate-to-severe vasomotor symptoms of the menopause when anxiety and tension are part of the symptom complex and only in those cases in which the use of estrogens alone has not resulted in alleviation of such symptoms.

PMB HAS NOT BEEN SHOWN TO BE EFFECTIVE FOR ANY PURPOSE DURING PREGNANCY AND ITS USE MAY CAUSE SEVERE HARM TO THE FETUS (SEE BOXED WARNING).

CONTRAINDICATIONS

Estrogens should not be used in women with any of the following conditions:

1. Known or suspected cancer of the breast except in appropriately selected patients being treated for metastatic disease.
2. Known or suspected estrogen-dependent neoplasia.
3. Known or suspected pregnancy (see Boxed Warning).
4. Undiagnosed abnormal genital bleeding.
5. Active thrombophlebitis or thromboembolic disorders.
6. A past history of thrombophlebitis, thrombosis, or thromboembolic disorders associated with previous estrogen use.

Meprobamate should not be used in patients with the following conditions:

1. A history of allergic or idiosyncratic reactions to meprobamate or related compounds such as carisoprodol, mebutamate, tybamate, or carbromal.
2. Acute intermittent porphyria.

WARNINGS

USAGE IN PREGNANCY AND LACTATION.

An increased risk of congenital malformations associated with the use of minor tranquilizers (meprobamate, chlordiazepoxide, and diazepam) during the first trimester of pregnancy has been suggested in several studies. Because use of these drugs is rarely a matter of urgency, their use during this period should almost always be avoided. The possibility that a woman of childbearing potential may be pregnant at the time of institution of therapy should be considered. Patients should be advised that if they become pregnant during therapy or intend to become pregnant they should communicate with their physicians about the desirability of discontinuing the drug.

Meprobamate passes the placental barrier. It is present both in umbilical cord blood at or near maternal plasma levels and in breast milk of lactating mothers at concentrations two to four times that of maternal plasma. When use of meprobamate is contemplated in breast-feeding patients, the drug's higher concentrations in breast milk as compared to maternal plasma levels should be considered.

Usage in Children—PMB is not intended for use in children.

Associated with Estrogen Administration:

1. *Induction of malignant neoplasms.* Estrogens have been reported to increase the risk of endometrial carcinoma. (See Boxed Warning.) However, a recent, large, case-controlled study indicated no increase in risk of breast cancer in postmenopausal women.[18]
2. *Gallbladder disease.* A recent study has reported a 2- to 3-fold increase in the risk of surgically confirmed gallbladder disease in women receiving postmenopausal estrogens,[17] similar to the 2-fold increase previously noted in users of oral contraceptives.[19,24a]
3. *Effects similar to those caused by estrogen-progestogen oral contraceptives.* There are several serious adverse effects of oral contraceptives, most of which have not, up to now, been documented as consequences of postmenopausal estrogen therapy. This may reflect the comparatively low doses of estrogen used in postmenopausal women. It would be expected that the larger doses of estrogen used to treat prostatic or breast cancer, or postpartum breast engorgement, are more likely to result in these adverse effects, and, in fact, it has been shown that there is an increased risk of thrombosis in men receiving estrogens for prostatic cancer and women for postpartum breast engorgement.[20-23]

a. *Thromboembolic disease.* It is now well established that users of oral contraceptives have an increased risk of various thromboembolic and thrombotic vascular diseases, such as thrombophlebitis, pulmonary embolism, stroke, and myocardial infarction.[24-31] Cases of retinal thrombosis, mesenteric thrombosis, and optic neuritis have been reported in oral-contraceptive users. There is evidence that the risk of several of these adverse reactions is related to the dose of the drug.[32,33] An increased risk of postsurgery thromboembolic complications has also been reported in users of oral-contraceptives.[34,35] If feasible, estrogen should be discontinued at least 4 weeks before surgery of the type associated with an increased risk of thromboembolism, or during periods of prolonged immobilization.

While an increased rate of thromboembolic and thrombotic disease in postmenopausal users of estrogens has not been found,[17-24,25-36] this does not rule out the possibility that such an increase may be present or that subgroups of women who have underlying risk factors or who are receiving relatively large doses of estrogens may have increased risk. Therefore estrogens should not be used in persons with active thrombophlebitis or thromboembolic disorders, and they should not be used (except in treatment of malignancy) in persons with a history of such disorders in association with estrogen use. They should be used with caution in patients with cerebral vascular or coronary artery disease and only for those in whom estrogens are clearly needed.

Large doses of estrogen (5 mg conjugated estrogens per day), comparable to those used to treat cancer of the prostate and breast, have been shown in a large prospective clinical trial in men[37] to increase the risk of nonfatal myocardial infarction, pulmonary embolism, and thrombophlebitis. When estrogen doses of this size are used, any of the thromboembolic and thrombotic adverse effects associated with oral contraceptive use should be considered a clear risk.

b. *Hepatic adenoma.* Benign hepatic adenomas appear to be associated with the use of oral contraceptives.[38-40] Although benign, and rare, these may rupture and may cause death through intra-abdominal hemorrhage. Such lesions have not yet been reported in association with other estrogen or progestogen preparations but should be considered in estrogen users having abdominal pain and tenderness, abdominal mass, or hypovolemic shock. Hepatocellular carcinoma has also been reported in women taking estrogen-containing oral contraceptives.[39] The relationship of this malignancy to these drugs is not known at this time.

c. *Elevated blood pressure.* Women using oral contraceptives sometimes experience increased blood pressure which, in most cases, returns to normal on discontinuing the drug. There is now a report that this may occur with use of estrogens in the menopause[41] and blood pressure should be monitored with estrogen use, especially if high doses are used.

d. *Glucose tolerance.* A worsening of glucose tolerance has been observed in a significant percentage of patients on estrogen-containing oral contraceptives. For this reason, diabetic patients should be carefully observed while receiving estrogen.

4. *Hypercalcemia.* Administration of estrogens may lead to severe hypercalcemia in patients with breast cancer and bone metastases. If this occurs, the drug should be stopped and appropriate measures taken to reduce the serum calcium level.

Associated with Meprobamate Administration:

1. *Drug Dependence*—Physical dependence, psychological dependence, and abuse have occurred. When chronic intoxication from prolonged use occurs, it usually involves ingestion of greater than recommended doses and is manifested by ataxia, slurred speech, and vertigo. Therefore, careful supervision of dose and amounts prescribed is advised, as well as avoidance of prolonged administration, especially for alcoholics and other patients with a known propensity for taking excessive quantities of drugs.

Sudden withdrawal of the drug after prolonged and excessive use may precipitate recurrence of pre-existing symptoms, such as anxiety, anorexia, or insomnia, or withdrawal reactions, such as vomiting, ataxia, tremors, muscle twitching, confusional states, hallucinosis, and, rarely, convulsive seizures. Such seizures are more likely to occur in persons with central nervous system damage or pre-existent or latent convulsive disorders. Onset of withdrawal symptoms occurs usually within 12 to 48 hours after discontinuation of meprobamate; symptoms usually cease within the next 12 to 48 hours.

When excessive dosage has continued for weeks or months, dosage should be reduced gradually over a period of one or two weeks rather than abruptly stopped. Alternatively, a short-acting barbiturate may be substituted, then gradually withdrawn.

2. *Potentially Hazardous Tasks*—Patients should be warned that this drug may impair the mental and/or physical abilities required for the performance of potentially hazardous tasks such as driving a motor vehicle or operating machinery.

3. *Additive Effects*—Since the effects of meprobamate and alcohol or meprobamate and other CNS depressants or psychotropic drugs may be additive, appropriate caution should

Continued on next page

Wyeth-Ayerst—Cont.

be exercised with patients who take more than one of these agents simultaneously.

PRECAUTIONS

A. General Precautions.

Associated with Estrogen:

1. A complete medical and family history should be taken prior to the initiation of any estrogen therapy. The pretreatment and periodic physical examinations should include special reference to blood pressure, breasts, abdomen, and pelvic organs, and should include a Papanicolaou smear. As a general rule, estrogen should not be prescribed for longer than one year without another physical examination being performed.

2. Fluid retention—Because estrogens may cause some degree of fluid retention, conditions which might be influenced by this factor such as asthma, epilepsy, migraine, and cardiac or renal dysfunction, require careful observation.

3. Certain patients may develop undesirable manifestations of excessive estrogenic stimulation, such as abnormal or excessive uterine bleeding, mastodynia, etc.

4. Prolonged administration of unopposed estrogen therapy has been reported to increase the risk of endometrial hyperplasia in some patients.

5. Oral contraceptives appear to be associated with an increased incidence of mental depression.[24a] Although it is not clear whether this is due to the estrogenic or progestogenic component of the contraceptive, patients with a history of depression should be carefully observed.

6. Pre-existing uterine leiomyomata may increase in size during estrogen use.

7. The pathologist should be advised of estrogen therapy when relevant specimens are submitted.

8. Patients with a past history of jaundice during pregnancy have an increased risk of recurrence of jaundice while receiving estrogen-containing oral contraceptive therapy. If jaundice develops in any patient receiving estrogen, the medication should be discontinued while the cause is investigated.

9. Estrogens may be poorly metabolized in patients with impaired liver function and should be administered with caution in such patients.

10. Because estrogens influence the metabolism of calcium and phosphorus, they should be used with caution in patients with metabolic bone diseases that are associated with hypercalcemia or in patients with renal insufficiency.

11. Because of the effects of estrogens on epiphyseal closure, they should be used judiciously in young patients in whom bone growth is not complete.

Concomitant Progestin Use: The lowest effective dose appropriate for the specific indication should be utilized. Studies of the addition of a progestin for 7 or more days of a cycle of estrogen administration have reported a lowered incidence of endometrial hyperplasia. Morphological and biochemical studies of the endometrium suggest that 10 to 13 days of progestin are needed to provide maximal maturation of the endometrium and to eliminate any hyperplastic changes. Whether this will provide protection from endometrial carcinoma has not been clearly established. There are possible additional risks which may be associated with the inclusion of progestin in estrogen replacement regimens. If concomitant progestin therapy is used, potential risks may include adverse effects on carbohydrate and lipid metabolism. The choice of progestin and dosage may be important in minimizing these adverse effects.

Associated with Meprobamate:

1. The lowest effective dose should be administered, particularly to debilitated patients, in order to preclude oversedation.

2. The possibility of suicide attempts should be considered and the least amount of drug feasible should be dispensed at any one time.

3. Meprobamate is metabolized in the liver and excreted by the kidney; to avoid its excess accumulation, caution should be exercised in administration to patients with compromised liver or kidney function.

4. Meprobamate occasionally may precipitate seizures in epileptic patients.

B. Information for Patients. (See text which appears after the PHYSICIAN REFERENCES.)

C. Drug/Laboratory Test Interactions: Certain endocrine and liver function tests may be affected by estrogen-containing oral contraceptives. The following similar changes may be expected with larger doses of estrogen.

a. Increased sulfobromophthalein retention.

b. Increased prothrombin and factors VII, VIII, IX, and X; decreased antithrombin 3; increased norephinephrine-induced platelet aggregability.

c. Increased thyroid binding globulin (TBG) leading to increased circulating total thyroid hormone, as measured by PBI, T_4 by column, or T_4 by radioimmunoassay. Free T_3 resin uptake is decreased, reflecting the elevated TBG; free T_4 concentration is unaltered.

d. Impaired glucose tolerance.

e. Decreased pregnanediol excretion.

f. Reduced response to metyrapone test.

g. Reduced serum folate concentration.

h. Increased serum triglyceride and phospholipid concentration.

D. Mutagenesis and Carcinogenesis. Long-term, continuous administration of natural and synthetic estrogens in certain animal species increases the frequency of carcinomas of the breast, cervix, vagina, and liver. However in a recent, large, case-controlled study of postmenopausal women, there was no increase in risk of breast cancer with use of conjugated estrogens.[18]

E. Pregnancy Category X. (See CONTRAINDICATIONS and Boxed Warning.)

F. Nursing Mothers. Because of the potential for serious adverse reactions in nursing infants from PMB, a decision should be made whether to discontinue nursing or to discontinue the drugs, taking into account the importance of the drug to the mother. (See WARNINGS section for information on use in pregnancy and lactation.)

G. Pediatric Use. Safety and effectiveness in children have not been established.

ADVERSE REACTIONS

Associated with Estrogen Administration

(See WARNINGS regarding induction of neoplasia, adverse effects on the fetus, increased incidence of gallbladder disease, and adverse effects similar to those of oral contraceptives, including thromboembolism.) The following additional adverse reactions have been reported with estrogenic therapy, including oral contraceptives:

1. *Genitourinary system:* Breakthrough bleeding, spotting, change in menstrual flow; dysmenorrhea; premenstrual-like syndrome; amenorrhea during and after treatment; increase in size of uterine fibromyomata; vaginal candidiasis; change in cervical erosion and in degree of cervical secretion; cystitis-like syndrome.

2. *Breasts:* Tenderness, enlargement, secretion.

3. *Gastrointestinal:* Nausea, vomiting; abdominal cramps, bloating; cholestatic jaundice.

4. *Skin:* Chloasma or melasma which may persist when drug is discontinued; erythema multiforme; erythema nodosum; hemorrhagic eruption; loss of scalp hair; hirsutism.

5. *Eyes:* Steepening of corneal curvature; intolerance to contact lenses.

6. *CNS:* Headache, migraine, dizziness; mental depression; chorea.

7. *Miscellaneous:* Increase or decrease in weight; reduced carbohydrate tolerance; aggravation of porphyria; edema; changes in libido.

The following have been reported with meprobamate therapy:

1. *Central Nervous System*—Drowsiness, ataxia, dizziness, slurred speech, headache, vertigo, weakness, paresthesias, impairment of visual accommodation, euphoria, overstimulation, paradoxical excitement, fast EEG activity.

2. *Gastrointestinal*—Nausea, vomiting, diarrhea.

3. *Cardiovascular*—Palpitations, tachycardia, various forms of arrhythmia, transient ECG changes, syncope; also, hypotensive crises (including one fatal case).

4. *Allergic or Idiosyncratic*—Allergic or idiosyncratic reactions are usually seen within the period of the first to fourth dose in patients having had no previous contact with the drug. Milder reactions are characterized by an itchy, urticarial, or erythematous maculopapular rash which may be generalized or confined to the groin. Other reactions have included leukopenia, acute nonthrombocytopenic purpura, petechiae, ecchymoses, eosinophilia, peripheral edema, adenopathy, fever, fixed drug eruption with cross reaction to carisoprodol, and cross sensitivity between meprobamate/mebutamate and meprobamate/carbromal.

More severe hypersensitivity reactions, rarely reported, include hyperpyrexia, chills, angioneurotic edema, bronchospasm, oliguria, and anuria. Also, anaphylaxis, erythema multiforme, exfoliative dermatitis, stomatitis, proctitis, Stevens-Johnson syndrome, and bullous dermatitis, including one fatal case of the latter, following administration of meprobamate in combination with prednisolone.

In case of allergic or idiosyncratic reactions to meprobamate, discontinue the drug and initiate appropriate symptomatic therapy, which may include epinephrine, antihistamines, and in severe cases corticosteroids. In evaluating possible allergic reactions, also consider allergy to excipients (information on excipients is available to physicians on request).

5. *Hematologic.* (See also *Allergic or Idiosyncratic.*) —Agranulocytosis and aplastic anemia have been reported, although no causal relationship has been established. These cases rarely were fatal. Rare cases of thrombocytopenic purpura have been reported.

6. *Other*—Exacerbation of porphyric symptoms.

OVERDOSAGE

Acute overdosage (estrogen alone):

Numerous reports of ingestion of large doses of estrogen-containing oral contraceptives by young children indicate

that acute serious ill effects do not occur. Overdosage of estrogen may cause nausea, and withdrawal bleeding may occur in females.

Acute simple overdosage (meprobamate alone): Death has been reported with ingestion of as little as 12 grams meprobamate and survival with as much as 40 grams.

Blood levels: 0.5—2.0 mg% represents the usual blood level range of meprobamate after therapeutic doses. The level may occasionally be as high as 3.0 mg%.

3—10 mg% usually corresponds to findings of mild-to-moderate symptoms of overdosage, such as stupor or light coma. 10—20 mg% usually corresponds to deeper coma, requiring more intensive treatment. Some fatalities occur.

At levels greater than 20 mg%, more fatalities than survivals can be expected.

Acute combined (alcohol or other CNS depressants or psychotropic drugs) Overdosage: Since effects can be additive, a history of ingestion of a low dose of meprobamate plus any of these compounds (or of a relatively low blood or tissue level) cannot be used as a prognostic indicator.

In cases where excessive doses have been taken, sleep ensues rapidly and blood pressure, pulse, and respiratory rates are reduced to basal levels. Any drug remaining in the stomach should be removed and symptomatic therapy given. Should respiration or blood pressure become compromised, respiratory assistance, central nervous system stimulants, and pressor agents should be administered cautiously as indicated. Meprobamate is metabolized in the liver and excreted by the kidney. Diuresis, osmotic (mannitol) diuresis, peritoneal dialysis, and hemodialysis have been used successfully. Careful monitoring of urinary output is necessary and caution should be taken to avoid overhydration. Relapse and death, after initial recovery, have been attributed to incomplete gastric emptying and delayed absorption. Meprobamate can be measured in biological fluids by two methods: colorimetric[42] and gas chromatographic.[43]

DOSAGE AND ADMINISTRATION

Given cyclically for short-term use only:

For the treatment of moderate-to-severe vasomotor symptoms of the menopause when anxiety and tension are part of the symptom complex and only in those cases in which the use of estrogens alone has not resulted in alleviation of such symptoms.

The lowest dose that will control symptoms should be chosen and medication should be discontinued as promptly as possible. The usual dosage of conjugated estrogen is 1.25 milligrams daily. The usual dosage of meprobamate is 1,200 to 1,600 milligrams daily.

Administration should be cyclic (eg, three weeks on and one week off).

Attempts to discontinue or taper medication should be made at three- to six-month intervals.

PMB® 200 & PMB® 400: The usual dosage is one tablet of either strength three times daily administered cyclically. Use of meprobamate during the rest period should be considered for those patients who may require continuing medication with tranquilizer. After the first few cycles of therapy, the patient's need for continuing the use of the meprobamate component should be re-evaluated.

Daily dosage should be adjusted to individual requirements. The daily dosage should not exceed 6 tablets of PMB 200 per day or 4 tablets of PMB 400 per day.

Treated patients with an intact uterus should be monitored closely for signs of endometrial cancer and appropriate diagnostic measures should be taken to rule out malignancy in the event of persistent or recurring abnormal vaginal bleeding.

HOW SUPPLIED

PMB® 200 [PREMARIN (conjugated estrogens, USP) with Meprobamate, USP] Tablets

Each oblong *green* tablet contains 0.45 mg PREMARIN and 200 mg meprobamate, in bottles of 60 (NDC 0046-0880-60).

PMB® 400 [PREMARIN (conjugated estrogens, USP) with Meprobamate, USP] Tablets

Each oblong *pink* tablet contains 0.45 mg PREMARIN and 400 mg meprobamate, in bottles of 60 (NDC 0046-0881-60).

The appearance of these tablets is a trademark of Wyeth-Ayerst Laboratories.

Store at room temperature (approximately 25°C).

PHYSICIAN REFERENCES

1. Ziel, H. K., *et al.*: N. Engl. J. Med. *293*:1167–1170, 1975.
2. Smith, D. C., *et al.*: N. Engl. J. Med. *293*:1164–1167, 1975.
3. Mack, T. M., *et al.*: N. Engl. J. Med. *294*:1262–1267, 1976.
4. Weiss, N. S., *et al.*: N. Engl. J. Med. *294*:1259–1262, 1976.
5. Herbst, A. L., *et al.*: N. Engl. J. Med. *284*:878–881, 1971.
6. Greenwald, P., *et al.*: N. Engl. J. Med. *285*:390–392, 1971.
7. Lanier, A., *et al.*: Mayo Clin. Proc. *48*:793–799, 1973.
8. Herbst, A., *et al.*: Obstet. Gynecol. *40*:287–298, 1972.
9. Herbst, A., *et al.*: Am. J. Obstet. Gynecol. *118*:607–615, 1974.

10. Herbst, A., *et al.*: N. Engl. J. Med. *292*:334–339, 1975.
11. Stafl, A., *et al.*: Obstet. Gynecol. *43*:118–128, 1974.
12. Sherman, A. I., *et al.*: Obstet. Gynecol. *44*:531–545, 1974.
13. Gal, I., *et al.*: Nature *216*:83, 1967.
14. Levy, E. P., *et al.*: Lancet *1*:611, 1973.
15. Nora, J., *et al.*: Lancet *1*:941–942, 1973.
16. Janerich, D. T., *et al.*: N. Engl. J. Med. *291*:697–700, 1974.
17. Boston Collaborative Drug Surveillance Program: N. Engl. J. Med. *290*:15–19, 1974.
18. Kaufman, D.W., *et al.*: J.A.M.A. *252*:63–67, 1984.
19. Boston Collaborative Drug Surveillance Program: Lancet *1*:1399–1404, 1973.
20. Daniel, D. G., *et al.*: Lancet *2*:287–289, 1967.
21. The Veterans Administration Cooperative Urological Research Group: J. Urol. *98*:516–522, 1967.
22. Bailar, J. C.: Lancet *2*:560, 1967.
23. Blackard, C., *et al.*: Cancer *26*:249–256, 1970.
24. Royal College of General Practitioners: J. R. Coll. Gen. Pract. *13*:267–279, 1967.
24a. Royal College of General Practitioners: Oral Contraceptives and Health, New York, Pitman Corp., 1974.
25. Inman, W. H. W., *et al.*: Br. Med. J. *2*:193–199, 1968.
26. Vessey, M. P., *et al.*: Br. Med. J. *2*:651–657, 1969.
27. Sartwell, P. E., *et al.*: Am. J. Epidemiol. *90*:365–380, 1969.
28. Collaborative Group for the Study of Stroke in Young Women: N. Engl. J. Med. *288*:871–878, 1973.
29. Collaborative Group for the Study of Stroke in Young Women: J.A.M.A. *231*:718–722, 1975.
30. Mann, J. I., *et al.*: Br. Med. J. *2*:245–248, 1975.
31. Mann, J. I., *et al.*: Br. Med. J. *2*:241–245, 1975.
32. Inman, W. H. W., *et al.*: Br. Med. J. *2*:203–209, 1970.
33. Stolley, P. D., *et al.*: Am. J. Epidemiol. *102*:197–208, 1975.
34. Vessey, M. P., *et al.*: Br. Med. J. *3*:123–126, 1970.
35. Greene, G. R., *et al.*: Am. J. Public Health *62*:680–685, 1972.
36. Rosenberg, L., *et al.*: N. Engl. J. Med. *294*:1256–1259, 1976.
37. Coronary Drug Project Research Group: J.A.M.A. *214*:1303–1313, 1970.
38. Baum, J., *et al.*: Lancet *2*:926–928, 1973.
39. Mays, E. T., *et al.*: J.A.M.A. *235*:730–732, 1976.
40. Edmondson, H. A., *et al.*: N. Engl. J. Med. *294*:470–472, 1976.
41. Pfeffer, R. I., *et al.*: Am. J. Epidemiol. *103*:445–456, 1976.
42. Hoffman, A. J., *et al.*: J. Am. Pharm. Assoc. *48*:740, 1959.
43. Douglas, J. F., *et al.*: Anal. Chem. *39*:956, 1967.

INFORMATION FOR THE PATIENT

WHAT YOU SHOULD KNOW ABOUT ESTROGENS

Estrogens are female hormones produced by the ovaries. The ovaries make several different kinds of estrogens. In addition, scientists have been able to make a variety of synthetic estrogens. As far as we know, all these estrogens have similar properties and, therefore, much the same usefulness, side effects, and risks. This leaflet is intended to help you understand what estrogens are used for, the risks involved in their use, and how to use them as safely as possible.

This leaflet includes the most important information about estrogens, but not all the information. If you want to know more, you should ask your doctor for more information, or you can ask your doctor or pharmacist to let you read the package insert prepared for the doctor.

USES OF ESTROGEN

THERE IS NO PROPER USE OF ESTROGENS IN A PREGNANT WOMAN

Estrogens are prescribed by doctors for a number of purposes, including:

1. To provide estrogen during a period of adjustment when a woman's ovaries stop producing a majority of her estrogens, in order to prevent certain uncomfortable symptoms of estrogen deficiency. (With the menopause, which generally occurs between the ages of 45 and 55, women produce a much smaller amount of estrogens.)
2. To prevent symptoms of estrogen deficiency when a woman's ovaries have been removed surgically before the natural menopause.
3. To prevent pregnancy. (Estrogens are given along with a progestogen, another female hormone; these combinations are called oral contraceptives, or birth control pills. Patient labeling is available to women taking oral contraceptives and they will not be discussed in this leaflet.)
4. To treat certain cancers in women and men.
5. To prevent painful swelling of the breasts after pregnancy in women who choose not to nurse their babies.

ESTROGENS IN THE MENOPAUSE

In the natural course of their lives, all women eventually experience a decrease in estrogen production. This usually occurs between ages 45 and 55, but may occur earlier or later. Sometimes the ovaries may need to be removed before

natural menopause by an operation, producing a "surgical menopause."

When the amount of estrogen in the blood begins to decrease, many women may develop typical symptoms: feelings of warmth in the face, neck, and chest or sudden intense episodes of heat and sweating throughout the body (called "hot flashes" or "hot flushes"). These symptoms are sometimes very uncomfortable. Some women may also develop changes in the vagina (called "atrophic vaginitis") that cause discomfort, especially during and after intercourse.

Estrogens can be prescribed to treat these symptoms of the menopause. It is estimated that considerably more than half of all women undergoing the menopause have only mild symptoms or no symptoms at all and therefore do not need estrogens. Other women may need estrogens for a few months, while their bodies adjust to lower estrogen levels. Sometimes the need will be for periods longer than six months. In an attempt to avoid overstimulation of the uterus (womb), estrogens are usually given cyclically during each month of use, such as three weeks of pills followed by one week without pills.

Sometimes women experience nervous symptoms or depression during menopause. There is no evidence that estrogens are effective for such symptoms without associated vasomotor symptoms. In the absence of vasomotor symptoms, estrogens should not be used to treat nervous symptoms, although other treatment may be needed.

You may have heard that taking estrogens for long periods (years) after the menopause will keep your skin soft and supple and keep you feeling young. There is no evidence that this is so, however, and such long-term treatment carries important risks.

ESTROGENS TO PREVENT SWELLING OF THE BREASTS AFTER PREGNANCY

If you do not breast-feed your baby after delivery, your breasts may fill up with milk and become painful and engorged. This usually begins about 3 to 4 days after delivery and may last for a few days to up to a week or more. Sometimes the discomfort is severe, but usually it is not and can be controlled by pain-relieving drugs such as aspirin and by binding the breasts up tightly. Estrogens can be used to try to prevent the breasts from filling up. While this treatment is sometimes successful, in many cases the breasts fill up to some degree in spite of treatment. The dose of estrogens needed to prevent pain and swelling of the breasts is much larger than the dose needed to treat symptoms of the menopause and this may increase your chances of developing blood clots in the legs or lungs (see below). Therefore, it is important that you discuss the benefits and the risks of estrogen use with your doctor if you have decided not to breast-feed your baby.

THE DANGERS OF ESTROGENS

1. *Endometrial cancer.* There are reports that if estrogens are used in the postmenopausal period for more than a year, there is an increased risk of *endometrial cancer* (cancer of the lining of the uterus). Women taking estrogens have roughly 5- to 10-times as great a chance of getting this cancer as women who take no estrogens. To put this another way, while a postmenopausal woman not taking estrogens has 1 chance in 1,000 each year of getting endometrial cancer, a woman taking estrogens has 5 to 10 chances in 1,000 each year. For this reason *it is important to take estrogens only when they are really needed.*

The risk of this cancer is greater the longer estrogens are used and when larger doses are taken. Therefore, you should not take more estrogen than your doctor prescribes. *It is important to take the lowest dose of estrogen that will control symptoms and to take it only as long as it is needed.* If estrogens are needed for longer periods of time, your doctor will want to re-evaluate your need for estrogens at least every six months.

Women using estrogens should report any vaginal bleeding to their doctors; such bleeding may be of no importance, but it can be an early warning of endometrial cancer. If you have undiagnosed vaginal bleeding, you should not use estrogens until a diagnosis is made and you are certain there is no endometrial cancer.

NOTE: If you have had your uterus removed (total hysterectomy), there is no danger of developing endometrial cancer.

2. *Other possible cancers.* Estrogens can cause development of other tumors in animals, such as tumors of the breast, cervix, vagina, or liver, when given for a long time. At present there is no good evidence that women using estrogen in the menopause have an increased risk of such tumors, but there is no way yet to be sure they do not; and one study raises the possibility that use of estrogens in the menopause may increase the risk of breast cancer many years later. This is a further reason to use estrogens only when clearly needed. While you are taking estrogens, it is important that you go to your doctor at least once a year for a physical examination. Also, if members of your family have had breast cancer or if you have breast nodules or abnormal mammo-

grams (breast x-rays), your doctor may wish to carry out more frequent examinations of your breasts.

3. *Gallbladder disease.* Women who use estrogens after menopause are more likely to develop gallbladder disease needing surgery then women who do not use estrogens. Birth control pills have a similar effect.

4. *Abnormal blood clotting.* Oral contraceptives increase the risk of blood clotting in various parts of the body. This can result in a stroke (if the clot is in the brain), a heart attack (clot in a blood vessel of the heart), or a pulmonary embolus (a clot which forms in the legs or pelvis, then breaks off and travels to the lungs). Any of these can be fatal.

At this time, use of estrogens in the menopause is not known to cause such blood clotting, but this has not been fully studied and there could still prove to be such a risk. It is recommended that if you have had clotting in the legs or lungs, or a heart attack or stroke while you were using estrogens or birth control pills, you should not use estrogens (unless they are being used to treat cancer of the breast or prostate). If you have had a stroke or heart attack, or if you have angina pectoris, estrogens should be used with great caution and only if clearly needed (for example, if you have severe symptoms of the menopause).

The larger doses of estrogen used to prevent swelling of the breasts after pregnancy have been reported to cause clotting in the legs and lungs.

SPECIAL WARNING ABOUT PREGNANCY

You should not receive estrogen if you are pregnant. If this should occur, there is a greater than usual chance that the developing child will be born with a birth defect, although the possibility remains fairly small. A female child may have an increased risk of developing cancer of the vagina or cervix later in life (in the teens or twenties). Every possible effort should be made to avoid exposure to estrogens during pregnancy. If exposure occurs, see your doctor.

OTHER EFFECTS OF ESTROGENS

In addition to the serious known risks of estrogens described above, estrogens have the following side effects and potential risks:

1. *Nausea and vomiting.* The most common side effect of estrogen therapy is nausea. Vomiting is less common.
2. *Effects on breasts.* Estrogens may cause breast tenderness or enlargement and may cause the breasts to secrete a liquid. These effects are not dangerous.
3. *Effects on the uterus.* Estrogens may cause benign fibroid tumors of the uterus to get larger.
4. *Effects on liver.* Women taking oral contraceptives develop, on rare occasions, a tumor of the liver which can rupture and bleed into the abdomen and may cause death. So far, these tumors have not been reported in women using estrogens in the menopause, but you should report any swelling or unusual pain or tenderness in the abdomen to your doctor immediately.

Women with a past history of jaundice (yellowing of the skin and white parts of the eyes) may get jaundice again during estrogen use. If this occurs, stop taking estrogens and see your doctor.

5. *Other effects.* Estrogens may cause excess fluids to be retained in the body. This may make some conditions worse, such as asthma, epilepsy, migraine, heart disease, or kidney disease.

SUMMARY

Estrogens have important uses, but they have serious risks as well. You must decide, with your doctor, whether the risks are acceptable to you in view of the benefits of treatment. Except where your doctor has prescribed estrogens for use in special cases of cancer of the breast or prostate, you should not use estrogens if you have cancer of the breast or uterus, are pregnant, have undiagnosed abnormal vaginal bleeding, clotting in the legs or lungs, or have had a stroke, heart attack or angina, or clotting in the legs or lungs in the past while you were taking estrogens.

You can use estrogens as safely as possible by understanding that your doctor will require regular physical examinations while you are taking them and will try to discontinue the drug as soon as possible and use the smallest dose possible. Be alert for signs of trouble including:

1. Abnormal bleeding from the vagina.
2. Pains in the calves or chest or sudden shortness of breath, or coughing blood.
3. Severe headache, dizziness, faintness, or changes in vision.
4. Breast lumps (you should ask your doctor how to examine your own breasts).
5. Jaundice (yellowing of the skin).
6. Mental depression.

Your doctor has prescribed this drug for you and you alone. Do not give the drug to anyone else.

Shown in Product Identification Section, page 437

Continued on next page

Wyeth-Ayerst—Cont.

PREMARIN® INTRAVENOUS   ℞

[prĕm 'a-rĭn]
Brand of conjugated estrogens, USP,
for Injection
Specially prepared for Intravenous &
Intramuscular use

CAUTION: Federal law prohibits dispensing without prescription.

---

1. ESTROGENS HAVE BEEN REPORTED TO IN-CREASE THE RISK OF ENDOMETRIAL CARCINOMA.

Three independent, case-controlled studies have reported an increased risk of endometrial cancer in postmenopausal women exposed to exogenous estrogens for more than one year.[1-3] This risk was independent of the other known risk factors for endometrial cancer. These studies are further supported by the finding that incidence rates of endometrial cancer have increased sharply since 1969 in eight different areas of the United States with population-based cancer-reporting systems, an increase which may be related to the rapidly expanding use of estrogens during the last decade.[4]

The three case-controlled studies reported that the risk of endometrial cancer in estrogen users was about 4.5 to 13.9 times greater than in nonusers. The risk appears to depend on both duration of treatment[1] and on estrogen dose.[3] In view of these findings, when estrogens are used for the treatment of menopausal symptoms, the lowest dose that will control symptoms should be utilized and medication should be discontinued as soon as possible. When prolonged treatment is medically indicated, the patient should be reassessed, on at least a semi-annual basis, to determine the need for continued therapy. Although the evidence must be considered preliminary, one study suggests that cyclic administration of low doses of estrogen may carry less risk than continuous administration.[3] It therefore appears prudent to utilize such a regimen.

Close clinical surveillance of all women taking estrogens is important. In all cases of undiagnosed persistent, or recurring abnormal vaginal bleeding, adequate diagnostic measures should be undertaken to rule out malignancy.

There is no evidence at present that "natural" estrogens are more or less hazardous than "synthetic" estrogens at equi-estrogenic doses.

2. ESTROGENS SHOULD NOT BE USED DURING PREGNANCY.

The use of female sex hormones, both estrogens and progestogens, during early pregnancy may seriously damage the offspring. It has been shown that females exposed in utero to diethylstilbestrol, a nonsteroidal estrogen, have an increased risk of developing, in later life, a form of vaginal or cervical cancer that is ordinarily extremely rare.[5,6] This risk has been estimated as not greater than 4 per 1,000 exposures.[7] Furthermore, a high percentage of such exposed women (from 30% to 90%) have been found to have vaginal adenosis,[8-12] epithelial changes of the vagina and cervix. Although these changes are histologically benign, it is not known whether they are precursors of malignancy. Although similar data are not available with the use of other estrogens, it cannot be presumed they would not induce similar changes.

Several reports suggest an association between intrauterine exposure to female sex hormones and congenital anomalies, including congenital heart defects and limb-reduction defects.[13-16] One case-controlled study[16] estimated a 4.7-fold increased risk of limb-reduction defects in infants exposed in utero to sex hormones (oral contraceptives, hormone withdrawal tests for pregnancy, or attempted treatment for threatened abortion). Some of these exposures were very short and involved only a few days of treatment. The data suggest that the risk of limb-reduction defects in exposed fetuses is somewhat less than 1 per 1,000.

In the past, female sex hormones have been used during pregnancy in an attempt to treat threatened or habitual abortion. There is considerable evidence that estrogens are ineffective for these indications, and there is no evidence from well-controlled studies that progestogens are effective for these uses.

If PREMARIN Intravenous (conjugated estrogens, USP, for injection) is used during pregnancy, or if the patient becomes pregnant while taking this drug, she should be apprised of the potential risks to the fetus, and the advisability of pregnancy continuation.

DESCRIPTION

Each Secule® vial contains 25 mg of conjugated estrogens, USP, in a sterile lyophilized cake which also contains lactose 200 mg, sodium citrate 12.5 mg and simethicone 0.2 mg. The pH is adjusted with sodium hydroxide or hydrochloric acid. A sterile diluent (5 mL) containing 2% benzyl alcohol in sterile water is provided for reconstitution. The reconstituted solution is suitable for intravenous or intramuscular injection.

PREMARIN (conjugated estrogens, USP) is a mixture of estrogens obtained exclusively from natural sources, occurring as the sodium salts of water-soluble estrogen sulfates blended to represent the average composition of material derived from pregnant mares' urine. It contains estrone, equilin, and 17 α-dihydroequilin, together with smaller amounts of 17 α-estradiol, equilenin, and 17 α-dihydroequilenin as salts of their sulfate esters.

CLINICAL PHARMACOLOGY

Estrogens are important in the development and maintenance of the female reproductive system and secondary sex characteristics. They promote growth and development of the vagina, uterus, and fallopian tubes, and enlargement of the breasts. Indirectly, they contribute to: the shaping of the skeleton, maintenance of tone and elasticity of urogenital structures, changes in the epiphyses of the long bones that allow for the pubertal growth spurt and its termination, growth of axillary and pubic hair, and pigmentation of the nipples and genitals. Decline of estrogenic activity at the end of the menstrual cycle can bring on menstruation, although the cessation of progesterone secretion is the most important factor in the mature ovulatory cycle. However, in the pre-ovulatory or nonovulatory cycle, estrogen is the primary determinant in the onset of menstruation. Estrogens also affect the release of pituitary gonadotropins.

The pharmacologic effects of conjugated estrogens are similar to those of endogenous estrogens. They are soluble in water and may be administered by intravenous or intramuscular injection.

In responsive tissues (female genital organs, breasts, hypothalamus, pituitary) estrogens enter the cell and are transported into the nucleus. As a result of estrogen action, specific RNA and protein synthesis occurs.

Metabolism and inactivation occur primarily in the liver. Some estrogens are excreted into the bile; however, they are reabsorbed from the intestine and returned to the liver through the portal venous system. Water-soluble estrogen conjugates are strongly acidic and, therefore, ionized in body fluids, which favor excretion through the kidneys since tubular reabsorption is minimal.

INDICATION

PREMARIN Intravenous (conjugated estrogens, USP, for injection) is indicated in the treatment of abnormal uterine bleeding due to hormonal imbalance in the absence of organic pathology.

CONTRAINDICATIONS

Estrogens should not be used in women with any of the following conditions:
1. Known or suspected cancer of the breast, except in appropriately selected patients being treated for metastatic disease.
2. Known or suspected estrogen-dependent neoplasia.
3. Known or suspected pregnancy (see Boxed Warning).
4. Undiagnosed abnormal genital bleeding.
5. Active thrombophlebitis or thromboembolic disorders.
6. A past history of thrombophlebitis, thrombosis, or thromboembolic disorders associated with previous estrogen use (except when used in treatment of breast malignancy).

WARNINGS

1. *Induction of malignant neoplasms.* Long-term, continuous administration of natural and synthetic estrogens in certain animal species increases the frequency of carcinomas of the breast, cervix, vagina, and liver. There are now reports that estrogens increase the risk of carcinoma of the endometrium in humans (see Boxed Warning).

At the present time there is no satisfactory evidence that estrogens given to postmenopausal women increase the risk of cancer of the breast,[17] although a recent long-term follow-up of a single physician's practice has raised this possibility.[18] Because of the animal data, there is a need for caution in prescribing estrogens for women with a strong family history of breast cancer, or who have breast nodules, fibrocystic disease, or abnormal mammograms.

2. *Gallbladder disease.* A recent study has reported a 2- to 3-fold increase in the risk of surgically confirmed gallbladder disease in women receiving postmenopausal estrogens,[17] similar to the 2-fold increase previously noted in users of oral contraceptives.[19,24a]

3. *Effects similar to those caused by estrogen-progestogen oral contraceptives.* There are several serious adverse effects of oral contraceptives, most of which have not, up to now, been documented as consequences of postmenopausal estrogen therapy. This may reflect the comparatively low doses of estrogen used in postmenopausal women. It would be ex-

---

pected that the larger doses of estrogen used to treat prostatic or breast cancer, or postpartum breast engorgement, are more likely to result in these adverse effects, and, in fact, it has been shown that there is an increased risk of thrombosis in men using estrogens for prostatic cancer and women for postpartum breast engorgement.[20-23]

a. *Thromboembolic disease.* It is now well established that users of oral contraceptives have an increased risk of various thromboembolic and thrombotic vascular diseases, such as thrombophlebitis, pulmonary embolism, stroke, and myocardial infarction.[24-31] Cases of retinal thrombosis, mesenteric thrombosis, and optic neuritis have been reported in oral-contraceptive users. There is evidence that the risk of several of these adverse reactions is related to the dose of the drug.[32,33] An increased risk of postsurgery thromboembolic complications has also been reported in users of oral contraceptives.[34,35] If feasible, estrogen should be discontinued at least 4 weeks before surgery of the type associated with an increased risk of thromboembolism, or during periods of prolonged immobilization.

While an increased rate of thromboembolic and thrombotic disease in postmenopausal users of estrogens has not been found,[17-24, 25-36] this does not rule out the possibility that such an increase may be present, or that subgroups of women who have underlying risk factors, or who are receiving relatively large doses of estrogens, may have increased risk. Therefore estrogens should not be used in persons with active thrombophlebitis or thromboembolic disorders, and they should not be used (except in treatment of malignancy) in persons with a history of such disorders in association with estrogen use. They should be used with caution in patients with cerebral vascular or coronary artery disease and only for those in whom estrogens are clearly needed.

Large doses of estrogen (5 mg conjugated estrogens per day), comparable to those used to treat cancer of the prostate and breast, have been shown in a large prospective clinical trial in men[37] to increase the risk of nonfatal myocardial infarction, pulmonary embolism, and thrombophlebitis. When estrogen doses of this size are used, any of the thromboembolic and thrombotic adverse effects associated with oral-contraceptive use should be considered a clear risk.

b. *Hepatic adenoma.* Benign hepatic adenomas appear to be associated with the use of oral contraceptives.[38-40] Although benign, and rare, these may rupture and may cause death through intra-abdominal hemorrhage. Such lesions have not yet been reported in association with other estrogen or progestogen preparations but should be considered in estrogen users having abdominal pain and tenderness, abdominal mass, or hypovolemic shock. Hepatocellular carcinoma has also been reported in women taking estrogen-containing oral contraceptives.[39] The relationship of this malignancy to these drugs is not known at this time.

c. *Elevated blood pressure.* Women using oral contraceptives sometimes experience increased blood pressure which, in most cases, returns to normal on discontinuing the drug. There is now a report that this may occur with use of estrogens in the menopause[41] and blood pressure should be monitored with estrogen use, especially if high doses are used.

d. *Glucose tolerance.* A worsening of glucose tolerance has been observed in a significant percentage of patients on estrogen-containing oral contraceptives. For this reason, diabetic patients should be carefully observed while receiving estrogen.

4. *Hypercalcemia.* Administration of estrogens may lead to severe hypercalcemia in patients with breast cancer and bone metastases. If this occurs, the drug should be stopped and appropriate measures taken to reduce the serum calcium level.

PRECAUTIONS

A. General Precautions.

1. A complete medical and family history should be taken prior to the initiation of any estrogen therapy. The pretreatment and periodic physical examinations should include special reference to blood pressure, breasts, abdomen, and pelvic organs, and should include a Papanicolaou smear. As a general rule, estrogen should not be prescribed for longer than one year without another physical examination being performed.

2. Fluid retention—Because estrogens may cause some degree of fluid retention, conditions which might be influenced by this factor such as asthma, epilepsy, migraine, and cardiac or renal dysfunction, require careful observation.

3. Certain patients may develop undesirable manifestations of excessive estrogenic stimulation, such as abnormal or excessive uterine bleeding, mastodynia, etc.

4. Oral contraceptives appear to be associated with an increased incidence of mental depression.[24a] Although it is not clear whether this is due to the estrogenic or progestogenic component of the contraceptive, patients with a history of depression should be carefully observed.

5. Pre-existing uterine leiomyomata may increase in size during estrogen use.

6. The pathologist should be advised of estrogen therapy when relevant specimens are submitted.

7. Patients with a past history of jaundice during pregnancy have an increased risk of recurrence of jaundice while receiving estrogen-containing oral contraceptive therapy. If jaundice develops in any patient receiving estrogen, the medication should be discontinued while the cause is investigated.

8. Estrogens may be poorly metabolized in patients with impaired liver function and they should be administered with caution in such patients.

9. Because estrogens influence the metabolism of calcium and phosphorus, they should be used with caution in patients with metabolic bone diseases that are associated with hypercalcemia or in patients with renal insufficiency.

10. Because of the effects of estrogens on epiphyseal closure, they should be used judiciously in young patients in whom bone growth is not yet complete.

11. Certain endocrine and liver function tests may be affected by estrogen-containing oral contraceptives. The following similar changes may be expected with larger doses of estrogen:

a. Increased sulfobromophthalein retention.

b. Increased prothrombin and factors VII, VIII, IX, and X; decreased antithrombin 3; increased norepinephrine-induced platelet aggregability.

c. Increased thyroid binding globulin (TBG) leading to increased circulating total thyroid hormone, as measured by PBI, T4 by column, or T4 by radioimmunoassay. Free T3 resin uptake is decreased, reflecting the elevated TBG; free T4 concentration is unaltered.

d. Impaired glucose tolerance.

e. Decreased pregnanediol excretion.

f. Reduced response to metyrapone test.

g. Reduced serum folate concentration.

h. Increased serum triglyceride and phospholipid concentration.

B. Information for the Patient. (See text which appears after the PHYSICIAN REFERENCES.)

C. Pregnancy Category X. (See CONTRAINDICATIONS and Boxed Warning.)

D. Nursing Mothers. As a general principle, the administration of any drug to nursing mothers should be done only when clearly necessary, since many drugs are excreted in human milk.

ADVERSE REACTIONS

(See WARNINGS regarding induction of neoplasia, adverse effects on the fetus, increased incidence of gallbladder disease, and adverse effects similar to those of oral contraceptives, including thromboembolism.) The following additional adverse reactions have been reported with estrogenic therapy, including oral contraceptives:

1. *Genitourinary system:* Breakthrough bleeding, spotting, change in menstrual flow; dysmenorrhea; premenstrual-like syndrome; amenorrhea during and after treatment; increase in size of uterine fibromyomata; vaginal candidiasis; change in cervical erosion and in degree of cervical secretion; cystitis-like syndrome.

2. *Breasts:* Tenderness, enlargement, secretion.

3. *Gastrointestinal:* Nausea, vomiting; abdominal cramps, bloating; cholestatic jaundice.

4. *Skin:* Chloasma or melasma which may persist when drug is discontinued; erythema multiforme; erythema nodosum; hemorrhagic eruption; loss of scalp hair; hirsutism.

5. *Eyes:* Steepening of corneal curvature; intolerance to contact lenses.

6. *CNS:* Headache, migraine, dizziness; mental depression; chorea.

7. *Miscellaneous:* Increase or decrease in weight; reduced carbohydrate tolerance; aggravation of porphyria; edema; changes in libido.

ACUTE OVERDOSAGE

Numerous reports of ingestion of large doses of estrogen-containing oral contraceptives by young children indicate that acute serious ill effects do not occur. Overdosage of estrogen may cause nausea, and withdrawal bleeding may occur in females.

DOSAGE AND ADMINISTRATION

Abnormal uterine bleeding due to hormonal imbalance: One 25 mg injection, intravenously or intramuscularly. Intravenous use is preferred since more rapid response can be expected from this mode of administration.

Repeat in 6 to 12 hours if necessary. The use of PREMARIN Intravenous (conjugated estrogens, USP, for injection) does not preclude the advisability of other appropriate measures. The usual precautionary measures governing intravenous administration should be adhered to. Injection should be made SLOWLY to obviate the occurrence of flushes.

Infusion of PREMARIN Intravenous (conjugated estrogens, USP, for injection) with other agents is not generally recommended. In emergencies, however, when an infusion has already been started, it may be expedient to make the injection into the tubing just distal to the infusion needle. If so used, compatibility of solutions must be considered.

Compatibility of solutions: PREMARIN Intravenous is compatible with normal saline, dextrose, and invert sugar solutions. IT IS NOT COMPATIBLE WITH PROTEIN HYDROLYSATE, ASCORBIC ACID, OR ANY SOLUTION WITH AN ACID pH.

Treated patients with an intact uterus should be monitored closely for signs of endometrial cancer, and appropriate diagnostic measures should be taken to rule out malignancy in the event of persistent or recurring abnormal vaginal bleeding.

DIRECTIONS FOR STORAGE AND RECONSTITUTION:

Storage before reconstitution: Store package in refrigerator, 2°–8°C (36°–46°F).

To reconstitute: First withdraw air from Secule® vial so as to facilitate introduction of sterile diluent. Then, flow the sterile diluent slowly against side of Secule® vial and agitate gently. DO NOT SHAKE VIOLENTLY.

Storage after reconstitution: It is common practice to utilize the reconstituted solution within a few hours. If it is necessary to keep the reconstituted solution for more than a few hours, store the reconstituted solution under refrigeration (2°–8°C). Under these conditions, the solution is stable for 60 days, and is suitable for use unless darkening or precipitation occurs.

HOW SUPPLIED

NDC 0046-0749-05—Each package provides: (1) One Secule® vial containing 25 mg of conjugated estrogens, USP, for injection (also lactose 200 mg, sodium citrate 12.5 mg, and simethicone 0.2 mg). The pH is adjusted with sodium hydroxide or hydrochloric acid. (2) One 5 mL ampul sterile diluent with 2% benzyl alcohol in sterile water. PREMARIN Intravenous (conjugated estrogens, USP, for injection) is prepared by cryodesiccation.

Secule®—Registered trademark to designate a vial containing an injectable preparation in dry form.

PHYSICIAN REFERENCES

1. Ziel, H. K., *et al.*: N. Engl. J. Med. *293* :1167–1170, 1975.
2. Smith, D. C., *et al.*: N. Engl. J. Med. *293* :1164–1167, 1975.
3. Mack, T. M., *et al.*: N. Engl. J. Med. *294* :1262–1267, 1976.
4. Weiss, N. S., *et al.*: N. Engl. J. Med. *294* :1259–1262, 1976.
5. Herbst, A. L., *et al.*: N. Engl. J. Med. *284* :878–881, 1971.
6. Greenwald, P., *et al.*: N. Engl. J. Med. *285* :390–392, 1971.
7. Lanier, A., *et al.*: Mayo Clin. Proc. *48* :793–799, 1973.
8. Herbst, A., *et al.*: Obstet. Gynecol. *40* :287–298, 1972.
9. Herbst, A., *et al.*: Am. J. Obstet. Gynecol. *118* :607–615, 1974.
10. Herbst, A., *et al.*: N. Engl. J. Med. *292* :334–339, 1975.
11. Stafl, A., *et al.*: Obstet. Gynecol. *43* :118–128, 1974.
12. Sherman, A. I., *et al.*: Obstet. Gynecol. *44* :531–545, 1974.
13. Gal, I., *et al.*: Nature *216* :83, 1967.
14. Levy, E. P., *et al.*: Lancet *1* :611, 1973.
15. Nora, J., *et al.*: Lancet *1* :941–942, 1973.
16. Janerich, D. T., *et al.*: N. Engl. J. Med. *291* :697–700, 1974.
17. Boston Collaborative Drug Surveillance Program: N. Engl. J. Med. *290* :15–19, 1974.
18. Hoover, R., *et al.*: N. Engl. J. Med. *295* :401–405, 1976.
19. Boston Collaborative Drug Surveillance Program: Lancet *1* :1399–1404, 1973.
20. Daniel, D. G., *et al.*: Lancet *2* :287–289, 1967.
21. The Veterans Administration Cooperative Urological Research Group: J. Urol. *98* :516–522, 1967.
22. Bailar, J. C.: Lancet *2* :560, 1967.
23. Blackard, C., *et al.*: Cancer *26* :249–256, 1970.
24. Royal College of General Practitioners: J. R. Coll. Gen. Pract. *13* :267–279, 1967.
24a. Royal College of General Practitioners: Oral Contraceptives and Health, New York, Pitman Corp., 1974.
25. Inman, W. H. W., *et al.*: Br. Med. J. *2* :193–199, 1968.
26. Vessey, M. P., *et al.*: Br. Med. J. *2* :651–657, 1969.
27. Sartwell, P. E., *et al.*: Am. J. Epidemiol. *90* :365–380, 1969.
28. Collaborative Group for the Study of Stroke in Young Women: N. Engl. J. Med. *288* :871–878, 1973.
29. Collaborative Group for the Study of Stroke in Young Women: J.A.M.A. *231* :718–722, 1975.
30. Mann, J. I., *et al.*: Br. Med. J. *2* :245–248, 1975.
31. Mann, J. I., *et al.*: Br. Med. J. *2* :241–245, 1975.
32. Inman, W. H. W., *et al.*: Br. Med. J. *2* :203–209, 1970.
33. Stolley, P. D., *et al.*: Am. J. Epidemiol. *102* :197–208, 1975.
34. Vessey, M. P., *et al.*: Br. Med. J. *3* :123–126, 1970.
35. Greene, G. R., *et al.*: Am. J. Public Health *62* :680–685, 1972.
36. Rosenberg, L., *et al.*: N. Engl. J. Med. *294* :1256–1259, 1976.
37. Coronary Drug Project Research Group: J.A.M.A. *214* :1303–1313, 1970.
38. Baum, J., *et al.*: Lancet *2* :926–928, 1973.
39. Mays, E. T., *et al.*: J.A.M.A. *235* :730–732, 1976.
40. Edmondson, H. A., *et al.*: N. Engl. J. Med. *294* :470–472, 1976.
41. Pfeffer, R. I., *et al.*: Am. J. Epidemiol. *103* :445–456, 1976.

INFORMATION FOR THE PATIENT

WHAT YOU SHOULD KNOW ABOUT ESTROGENS

Estrogens are female hormones produced by the ovaries. The ovaries make several different kinds of estrogens. In addition, scientists have been able to make a variety of synthetic estrogens. As far as we know, all these estrogens have similar properties and, therefore, much the same usefulness, side effects, and risks. This leaflet is intended to help you understand what estrogens are used for, the risks involved in their use, and how to use them as safely as possible.

This leaflet includes the most important information about estrogens, but not all the information. If you want to know more, you should ask your doctor for more information, or you can ask your doctor or pharmacist to let you read the package insert prepared for the doctor.

USES OF ESTROGEN

THERE IS NO PROPER USE OF ESTROGENS IN A PREGNANT WOMAN.

Estrogens are prescribed by doctors for a number of purposes, including:

1. To provide estrogen during a period of adjustment when a woman's ovaries stop producing a majority of her estrogens, in order to prevent certain uncomfortable symptoms of estrogen deficiency. (With the menopause, which generally occurs between the ages of 45 and 55, women produce a much smaller amount of estrogens.)

2. To prevent symptoms of estrogen deficiency when a woman's ovaries have been removed surgically before the natural menopause.

3. To prevent pregnancy. (Estrogens are given along with a progestogen, another female hormone; these combinations are called oral contraceptives, or birth control pills. Patient labeling is available to women taking oral contraceptives and they will not be discussed in this leaflet.)

4. To treat certain cancers in women and men.

5. To prevent painful swelling of the breasts after pregnancy in women who choose not to nurse their babies.

ESTROGENS IN THE MENOPAUSE

In the natural course of their lives, all women eventually experience a decrease in estrogen production. This usually occurs between ages 45 and 55, but may occur earlier or later. Sometimes the ovaries may need to be removed before natural menopause by an operation, producing a "surgical menopause."

When the amount of estrogen in the blood begins to decrease, many women may develop typical symptoms: feelings of warmth in the face, neck, and chest, or sudden intense episodes of heat and sweating throughout the body (called "hot flashes" or "hot flushes"). These symptoms are sometimes very uncomfortable. Some women may also develop changes in the vagina (called "atrophic vaginitis") that cause discomfort, especially during and after intercourse.

Estrogens can be prescribed to treat these symptoms of the menopause. It is estimated that considerably more than half of all women undergoing the menopause have only mild symptoms or no symptoms at all and, therefore, do not need estrogens. Other women may need estrogens for a few months, while their bodies adjust to lower estrogen levels. Sometimes the need will be for periods longer than six months. In an attempt to avoid overstimulation of the uterus (womb), estrogens are usually given cyclically during each month of use, such as three weeks of pills followed by one week without pills.

Sometimes women experience nervous symptoms or depression during menopause. There is no evidence that estrogens are effective for such symptoms without associated vasomotor symptoms. In the absence of vasomotor symptoms, estrogens should not be used to treat nervous symptoms, although other treatment may be needed.

You may have heard that taking estrogens for long periods (years) after the menopause will keep your skin soft and supple and keep you feeling young. There is no evidence that this is so, however, and such long-term treatment carries important risks.

ESTROGENS TO PREVENT SWELLING OF THE BREASTS AFTER PREGNANCY

If you do not breast-feed your baby after delivery, your breasts may fill up with milk and become painful and engorged. This usually begins about 3 to 4 days after delivery and may last for a few days to up to a week or more. Sometimes the discomfort is severe, but usually it is not and can be controlled by pain-relieving drugs such as aspirin and by binding the breasts up tightly. Estrogens can be used to try to prevent the breasts from filling up. While this treatment is sometimes successful, in many cases the breasts fill up to

Continued on next page

Wyeth-Ayerst—Cont.

some degree in spite of treatment. The dose of estrogens needed to prevent pain and swelling of the breasts is much larger than the dose needed to treat symptoms of the menopause and this may increase your chances of developing blood clots in the legs or lungs (see below). Therefore, it is important that you discuss the benefits and the risks of estrogen use with your doctor if you have decided not to breast-feed your baby.

THE DANGERS OF ESTROGENS

1. *Endometrial cancer.* There are reports that if estrogens are used in the postmenopausal period for more than a year, there is an increased risk of *endometrial cancer* (cancer of the lining of the uterus). Women taking estrogens have roughly 5- to 10-times as great a chance of getting this cancer as women who take no estrogens. To put this another way, while a postmenopausal woman not taking estrogens has 1 chance in 1,000 each year of getting endometrial cancer, a woman taking estrogens has 5 to 10 chances in 1,000 each year. For this reason *it is important to take estrogens only when they are really needed.*

The risk of this cancer is greater the longer estrogens are used and when larger doses are taken. Therefore, you should not take more estrogen than your doctor prescribes. *It is important to take the lowest dose of estrogen that will control symptoms and to take it only as long as it is needed.* If estrogens are needed for longer periods of time, your doctor will want to reevaluate your need for estrogens at least every six months.

Women using estrogens should report any vaginal bleeding to their doctors; such bleeding may be of no importance, but it can be an early warning of endometrial cancer. If you have undiagnosed vaginal bleeding, you should not use estrogens until a diagnosis is made and you are certain there is no endometrial cancer.

NOTE: If you have had your uterus removed (total hysterectomy), there is no danger of developing endometrial cancer.

2. *Other possible cancers.* Estrogens can cause development of other tumors in animals, such as tumors of the breast, cervix, vagina, or liver, when given for a long time. At present there is no good evidence that women using estrogen in the menopause have an increased risk of such tumors, but there is no way yet to be sure they do not; and one study raises the possibility that use of estrogens in the menopause may increase the risk of breast cancer many years later. This is a further reason to use estrogens only when clearly needed. While you are taking estrogens, it is important that you go to your doctor at least once a year for a physical examination. Also, if members of your family have had breast cancer, or if you have breast nodules, or abnormal mammograms (breast x-rays), your doctor may wish to carry out more frequent examinations of your breasts.

3. *Gallbladder disease.* Women who use estrogens after menopause are more likely to develop gallbladder disease needing surgery than women who do not use estrogens. Birth control pills have a similar effect.

4. *Abnormal blood clotting.* Oral contraceptives increase the risk of blood clotting in various parts of the body. This can result in a stroke (if the clot is in the brain), a heart attack (a clot in a blood vessel of the heart), or a pulmonary embolus (a clot which forms in the legs or pelvis, then breaks off and travels to the lungs). Any of these can be fatal.

At this time, use of estrogens in the menopause is not known to cause such blood clotting, but this has not been fully studied and there could still prove to be such a risk. It is recommended that if you have had clotting in the legs or lungs, or a heart attack or stroke, while you were using estrogens or birth control pills, you should not use estrogens (unless they are being used to treat cancer of the breast or prostate). If you have had a stroke or heart attack, or if you have angina pectoris, estrogens should be used with great caution and only if clearly needed (for example, if you have severe symptoms of the menopause).

The larger doses of estrogen used to prevent swelling of the breasts after pregnancy have been reported to cause clotting in the legs and lungs.

SPECIAL WARNING ABOUT PREGNANCY

You should not receive estrogen if you are pregnant. If this should occur, there is a greater than usual chance that the developing child will be born with a birth defect, although the possibility remains fairly small. A female child may have an increased risk of developing cancer of the vagina or cervix later in life (in the teens or twenties). Every possible effort should be made to avoid exposure to estrogens during pregnancy. If exposure occurs, see your doctor.

OTHER EFFECTS OF ESTROGENS

In addition to the serious known risks of estrogens described above, estrogens have the following side effects and potential risks:

1. *Nausea and vomiting.* The most common side effect of estrogen therapy is nausea. Vomiting is less common.

2. *Effects on breasts.* Estrogens may cause breast tenderness or enlargement and may cause the breasts to secrete a liquid. These effects are not dangerous.

3. *Effects on the uterus.* Estrogens may cause benign fibroid tumors of the uterus to get larger.

4. *Effects on liver.* Women taking oral contraceptives develop, on rare occasions, a tumor of the liver which can rupture and bleed into the abdomen and may cause death. So far, these tumors have not been reported in women using estrogens in the menopause, but you should report any swelling or unusual pain or tenderness in the abdomen to your doctor immediately.

Women with a past history of jaundice (yellowing of the skin and white parts of the eyes) may get jaundice again during estrogen use. If this occurs, stop taking estrogens and see your doctor.

5. *Other effects.* Estrogens may cause excess fluid to be retained in the body. This may make some conditions worse, such as asthma, epilepsy, migraine, heart disease, or kidney disease.

SUMMARY

Estrogens have important uses, but they have serious risks as well. You must decide, with your doctor, whether the risks are acceptable to you in view of the benefits of treatment. Except where your doctor has prescribed estrogens for use in special cases of cancer of the breast or prostate, you should not use estrogens if you have cancer of the breast or uterus, are pregnant, have undiagnosed abnormal vaginal bleeding, clotting in the legs or lungs, or have had a stroke, heart attack or angina, or clotting in the legs or lungs in the past while you were taking estrogens.

You can use estrogens as safely as possible by understanding that your doctor will require regular physical examinations while you are taking them, will try to discontinue the drug as soon as possible, and use the smallest dose possible. Be alert for signs of trouble including:

1. Abnormal bleeding from the vagina.
2. Pains in the calves or chest, or sudden shortness of breath, or coughing blood.
3. Severe headache, dizziness, faintness, or changes in vision.
4. Breast lumps (you should ask your doctor how to examine your own breasts).
5. Jaundice (yellowing of the skin).
6. Mental depression.

Your doctor has prescribed this drug for you and you alone. Do not give the drug to anyone else.

HOW SUPPLIED

PREMARIN® (conjugated estrogens tablets, USP) tablets for oral administration.

PREMARIN® VAGINAL CREAM—PREMARIN® in a nonliquefying base, designed for vaginal use.

PREMARIN® with METHYLTESTERONE—a combination of PREMARIN® and methyltestosterone (an androgen) in tablet form for oral administration.

PMB® 200, 400—a combination of PREMARIN® and meprobamate (a tranquilizing agent) in tablet form for oral administration.

PREMARIN® INTRAVENOUS—PREMARIN® specially prepared for intravenous and intramuscular use.

ESTROGENIC SUBSTANCE (estrone) in Aqueous Suspension—a sterile aqueous suspension of estrone, a short-acting estrogen, for intramuscular injection only.

PREMARIN®   ℞

[*prĕm ′a-rĭn*]
Conjugated estrogens tablets,
USP

CAUTION: Federal law prohibits dispensing without prescription.

---

1. ESTROGENS HAVE BEEN REPORTED TO INCREASE THE RISK OF ENDOMETRIAL CARCINOMA IN POSTMENOPAUSAL WOMEN.

Close clinical surveillance of all women taking estrogens is important. Adequate diagnostic measures, including endometrial sampling when indicated, should be undertaken to rule out malignancy in all cases of undiagnosed persistent or recurring abnormal vaginal bleeding. There is currently no evidence that "natural" estrogens are more or less hazardous than "synthetic" estrogens at equiestrogenic doses.

2. ESTROGENS SHOULD NOT BE USED DURING PREGNANCY.

Estrogen therapy during pregnancy is associated with an increased risk of congenital defects in the reproductive organs of the male and female fetus, an increased risk of vaginal adenosis, squamous-cell dysplasia of the uterine cervix, and vaginal cancer in the female later in life. The 1985 DES Task Force concluded that women who used DES during their pregnancies may subsequently experience an increased risk of breast cancer.

However, a causal relationship is still unproven, and the observed level of risk is similar to that for a number of other breast-cancer risk factors.

There is no indication for estrogen therapy during pregnancy. Estrogens are ineffective for the prevention or treatment of threatened or habitual abortion.

DESCRIPTION

PREMARIN (conjugated estrogens tablets, USP) for oral administration contains a mixture of estrogens obtained exclusively from natural sources, occurring as the sodium salts of water-soluble estrogen sulfates blended to represent the average composition of material derived from pregnant mares' urine. It contains estrone, equilin, and 17 α-dihydroequilin, together with smaller amounts of 17 α-estradiol, equilenin, and 17 α-dihydroequilenin as salts of their sulfate esters. Tablets for oral administration are available in 0.3 mg, 0.625 mg, 0.9 mg, 1.25 mg, and 2.5 mg strengths of conjugated estrogens.

PREMARIN Tablets contain the following inactive ingredients: calcium phosphate tribasic, calcium sulfate anhydrous, carnauba wax, glyceryl mono-oleate, lactose, magnesium stearate, methylcellulose, microcrystalline cellulose, pharmaceutical glaze, polyethylene glycol, stearic acid, sucrose, talc, titanium dioxide.

—0.3 mg tablets also contain: D&C Yellow No. 10, FD&C Blue No. 1, FD&C Yellow No. 6;

—0.625 mg tablets also contain: FD&C Blue No. 2, FD&C Red No. 3, FD&C Yellow No. 6;

—0.9 mg tablets also contain: D&C Red No. 6, D&C Red No. 7, polysorbate 20;

—1.25 mg tablets also contain: black iron oxide, D&C Yellow No. 10, FD&C Blue No. 1, FD&C Red No. 3, FD&C Yellow No. 6;

—2.5 mg tablets also contain: FD&C Blue No. 2, FD&C Red No. 3.

CLINICAL PHARMACOLOGY

Estrogens are important in the development and maintenance of the female reproductive system and secondary sex characteristics. They promote growth and development of the vagina, uterus, and fallopian tubes, and enlargement of the breasts. Indirectly, they contribute to the shaping of the skeleton, maintenance of tone and elasticity of urogenital structures, changes in the epiphyses of the long bones that allow for the pubertal growth spurt and its termination, growth of axillary and pubic hair, and pigmentation of the nipples and genitals. Decline of estrogenic activity at the end of the menstrual cycle can bring on menstruation, although the cessation of progesterone secretion is the most important factor in the mature ovulatory cycle. However, in the pre-ovulatory or nonovulatory cycle, estrogen is the primary determinant in the onset of menstruation. Estrogens also affect the release of pituitary gonadotropins.

The pharmacologic effects of conjugated estrogens are similar to those of endogenous estrogens. They are soluble in water and are well absorbed from the gastrointestinal tract. In responsive tissues (female genital organs, breasts, hypothalamus, pituitary) estrogens enter the cell and are transported into the nucleus. As a result of estrogen action, specific RNA and protein synthesis occurs.

Metabolism and inactivation occur primarily in the liver. Some estrogens are excreted into the bile; however, they are reabsorbed from the intestine and returned to the liver through the portal venous system. Water-soluble estrogen conjugates are strongly acidic and are ionized in body fluids, which favor excretion through the kidneys since tubular reabsorption is minimal.

INDICATIONS AND USAGE

PREMARIN (conjugated estrogens tablets, USP) is indicated in the treatment of:

1. Moderate to severe vasomotor symptoms associated with the menopause. There is no adequate evidence that estrogens are effective for nervous symptoms or depression which might occur during menopause and they should not be used to treat these conditions.
2. Atrophic vaginitis.
3. Atrophic urethritis.
4. Osteoporosis (loss of bone mass). The mainstays of prevention and management of osteoporosis are estrogen and calcium; exercise and nutrition may be important adjuncts. Estrogen replacement therapy is the most effective single modality for the prevention of osteoporosis in women. Estrogen reduces bone resorption and retards or halts postmenopausal bone loss. Case-controlled studies have shown an approximately 60-percent reduction in hip and wrist fractures in women whose estrogen replacement was begun within a few years of menopause. Studies also suggest that estrogen reduces the rate of vertebral fractures. Even when started as late as 6 years after menopause, estrogen prevents further loss of bone mass but does not restore it to premenopausal levels. The lowest effective dose for prevention and treatment of osteoporosis should be utilized. (See DOSAGE AND ADMINISTRATION.)

Woman are at higher risk than men because they have less bone mass, and for several years following natural or induced menopause, the rate of bone mass decline is accelerated. Early menopause is one of the strongest predictors for the development of osteoporosis. White women are at higher risk than black women, and white men are at higher risk than black men. Women who are underweight also have osteoporosis more often than overweight women. Cigarette smoking may be an additional factor in increasing risk. Calcium deficiency has been implicated in the pathogenesis of the disease. Therefore, when not contraindicated, it is recommended that postmenopausal women receive an elemental calcium intake of 1000 to 1500 mg/day.

Immobilization and prolonged bed rest produce rapid bone loss, while weight-bearing exercise has been shown both to reduce bone loss and to increase bone mass. The optimal type and amount of physical activity that would prevent osteoporosis have not been established.

5. Hypoestrogenism due to hypogonadism, castration, or primary ovarian failure.

6. Breast cancer (for palliation only) in appropriately selected women and men with metastatic disease.

7. Advanced androgen-dependent carcinoma of the prostate (for palliation only).

CONTRAINDICATIONS

Estrogens should not be used in women (or men) with any of the following conditions:

1. Known or suspected pregnancy (see Boxed Warning). Estrogen may cause fetal harm when administered to a pregnant woman.

2. Known or suspected cancer of the breast except in appropriately selected patients being treated for metastatic disease.

3. Known or suspected estrogen-dependent neoplasia.

4. Undiagnosed abnormal genital bleeding.

5. Active thrombophlebitis or thromboembolic disorders.

6. Women on estrogen replacement therapy have not been reported to have an increased risk of thrombophlebitis and/or thromboembolic disease. However, there is insufficient information regarding women who have had previous thromboembolic disease.

PREMARIN Tablets should not be used in patients hypersensitive to their ingredients.

WARNINGS

1. *Induction of malignant neoplasms.* Some studies have suggested a possible increased incidence of breast cancer in those women on estrogen therapy taking higher doses for prolonged periods of time. The majority of studies, however, have not shown an association with the usual doses used for estrogen replacement therapy. Women on this therapy should have regular breast examinations and should be instructed in breast self-examination. The reported endometrial cancer risk among estrogen users was about 4-fold or greater than in nonusers and appears dependent on duration of treatment and on estrogen dose. There is no significant increased risk associated with the use of estrogens for less than one year. The greatest risk appears associated with prolonged use—five years or more. In one study, persistence of risk was demonstrated for 10 years after cessation of estrogen treatment. In another study, a significant decrease in the incidence of endometrial cancer occurred six months after estrogen withdrawal.

Estrogen therapy during pregnancy is associated with an increased risk of fetal congenital reproductive-tract disorders. In females there is an increased risk of vaginal adenosis, squamous-cell dysplasia of the cervix, and cancer later in life; in the male, urogenital abnormalities. Although some of these changes are benign, it is not known whether they are precursors of malignancy.

2. *Gallbladder disease.* A recent study has reported a 2.5-fold increase in the risk of surgically confirmed gallbladder disease in women receiving postmenopausal estrogens.

3. *Cardiovascular disease.* Large doses of estrogen (5 mg conjugated estrogens per day), comparable to those used to treat cancer of the prostate and breast, have been shown in a large prospective clinical trial in men to increase the risk of nonfatal myocardial infarction, pulmonary embolism, and thrombophlebitis. It cannot necessarily be extrapolated from men to women. However, to avoid the theoretical cardiovascular risk caused by high estrogen doses, the doses for estrogen replacement therapy should not exceed the recommended dose.

4. *Elevated blood pressure.* There is no evidence that this may occur with use of estrogens in the menopause. However, blood pressure should be monitored with estrogen use, especially if high doses are used.

5. *Hypercalcemia.* Administration of estrogen may lead to severe hypercalcemia in patients with breast cancer and bone metastases. If this occurs, the drug should be stopped and appropriate measures taken to reduce the serum calcium level.

PRECAUTIONS

A. General.

1. *Addition of a progestin.* Studies of the addition of a progestin for seven or more days of a cycle of estrogen administration have reported a lowered incidence of endometrial hyperplasia. Morphological and biochemical studies of endometrium suggest that 10 to 13 days of progestin are needed to provide maximal maturation of the endometrium and to eliminate any hyperplastic changes. Whether this will provide protection from endometrial carcinoma has not been clearly established. There are possible additional risks which may be associated with the inclusion of progestin in estrogen replacement regimens. The potential risks include adverse effects on carbohydrate and lipid metabolism. The choice of progestin and dosage may be important in minimizing these adverse effects.

2. *Physical examination.* A complete medical and family history should be taken prior to the initiation of any estrogen therapy. The pretreatment and periodic physical examinations should include special reference to blood pressure, breasts, abdomen, and pelvic organs, and should include a Papanicolaou smear. As a general rule, estrogen should not be prescribed for longer than one year without another physical examination being performed.

3. *Fluid retention.* Because estrogens may cause some degree of fluid retention, conditions which might be influenced by this factor, such as asthma, epilepsy, migraine, and cardiac or renal dysfunction, require careful observation.

4. *Uterine bleeding and mastodynia.* Certain patients may develop undesirable manifestations of estrogenic stimulation, such as abnormal uterine bleeding and mastodynia.

5. *Uterine fibroids.* Preexisting uterine leiomyomata may increase in size during prolonged high-dose estrogen use.

6. *Impaired liver function.* Estrogens may be poorly metabolized in patients with impaired liver function and should be administered with caution.

7. *Hypercalcemia and renal insufficiency.* Prolonged use of estrogens can alter the metabolism of calcium and phosphorus. Estrogens should be used with caution in patients with metabolic bone disease.

B. Information for the Patient. See text of Patient Package Insert which appears after the HOW SUPPLIED section.

C. Laboratory Tests.

Clinical response at the smallest dose should generally be the guide to estrogen administration for relief of symptoms for those indications in which symptoms are observable. However, for prevention and treatment of osteoporosis see DOSAGE AND ADMINISTRATION section. Tests used to measure adequacy of estrogen replacement therapy include serum estrone and estradiol levels and suppression of serum gonadotrophin levels.

D. Drug/Laboratory Test Interactions.

Some of these drug/laboratory test interactions have been observed only with estrogen-progestin combinations (oral contraceptives):

1. Increased prothrombin and factors VII, VIII, IX, and X; decreased antithrombin 3; increased norepinephrine-induced platelet aggregability, decreased fibrinolysis.

2. Increased thyroid-binding globulin (TBG) leading to increased circulating total thyroid hormone, as measured by T_4 levels determined either by column or by radioimmunoassay. Free T_3 resin uptake is decreased, reflecting the elevated TBG; free T_4 concentration is unaltered.

3. Impaired glucose tolerance.

4. Reduced response to metyrapone test.

5. Reduced serum folate concentration.

E. Mutagenesis and Carcinogenesis. Long-term, continuous administration of natural and synthetic estrogens in certain animal species increases the frequency of carcinomas of the breast, cervix, vagina, and liver.

F. Pregnancy Category X. Estrogens should not be used during pregnancy. See CONTRAINDICATIONS and Boxed Warning.

G. Nursing Mothers. As a general principle, the administration of any drug to nursing mothers should be done only when clearly necessary since many drugs are excreted in human milk.

ADVERSE REACTIONS

(See WARNINGS regarding induction of neoplasia, adverse effects on the fetus, increased incidence of gallbladder disease.) The following additional adverse reactions have been reported with estrogenic therapy.

1. *Genitourinary system.* Changes in vaginal bleeding pattern and abnormal withdrawal bleeding or flow. Breakthrough bleeding, spotting. Increase in size of uterine fibromyomata. Vaginal candidiasis. Change in amount of cervical secretion.

2. *Breasts:* Tenderness, enlargement.

3. *Gastrointestinal:* Nausea, vomiting; abdominal cramps, bloating; cholestatic jaundice.

4. *Skin:* Chloasma or melasma that may persist when drug is discontinued; erythema multiforme; erythema nodosum; hemorrhagic eruption; loss of scalp hair; hirsutism.

5. *Eyes:* Steepening of corneal curvature; intolerance to contact lenses.

6. *CNS:* Headache, migraine, dizziness; mental depression; chorea.

7. *Miscellaneous:* Increase or decrease in weight; reduced carbohydrate tolerance; aggravation of porphyria; edema; changes in libido.

ACUTE OVERDOSAGE

Numerous reports of ingestion of large doses of estrogen-containing oral contraceptives by young children indicate that acute serious ill effects do not occur. Overdosage of estrogen may cause nausea and vomiting.

DOSAGE AND ADMINISTRATION

1. For treatment of moderate to severe vasomotor symptoms, atrophic vaginitis, and atrophic urethritis associated with the menopause. The lowest dose that will control symptoms should be chosen, and medication should be discontinued as promptly as possible.

Attempts to discontinue or taper medication should be made at 3-month to 6-month intervals.

Usual dosage ranges:

Vasomotor symptoms—1.25 mg daily. If the patient has not menstruated within the last two months or more, cyclic administration is started arbitrarily. If the patient is menstruating, cyclic (e.g., three weeks on and one week off) administration is started on day 5 of bleeding.

Atrophic vaginitis and Atrophic urethritis—0.3 mg to 1.25 mg or more daily, depending upon the tissue response of the individual patient. Administer cyclically.

2. Hypoestrogenism due to:

a. Female hypogonadism—2.5 mg to 7.5 mg daily, in divided doses for 20 days, followed by a rest period of 10 days' duration. If bleeding does not occur by the end of this period, the same dosage schedule is repeated. The number of courses of estrogen therapy necessary to produce bleeding may vary depending on the responsiveness of the endometrium.

If bleeding occurs before the end of the 10-day period, begin a 20-day estrogen-progestin cyclic regimen with PREMARIN, 2.5 mg to 7.5 mg daily in divided doses, for 20 days. During the last five days of estrogen therapy, give an oral progestin. If bleeding occurs before this regimen is concluded, therapy is discontinued and may be resumed on the fifth day of bleeding.

b. Female castration or primary ovarian failure— 1.25 mg daily, cyclically. Adjust dosage, upward or downward, according to severity of symptoms and response of the patient. For maintenance, adjust dosage to lowest level that will provide effective control.

3. Osteoporosis (loss of bone mass)—0.625 mg daily. Administration should be cyclic (e.g., three weeks on and one week off).

4. Advanced androgen-dependent carcinoma of the prostate, for palliation only—1.25 mg to 2.5 mg three times daily. The effectiveness of therapy can be judged by phosphatase determinations as well as by symptomatic improvement of the patient.

5. Breast cancer (for palliation only) in appropriately selected women and men with metastatic disease. Suggested dosage is 10 mg three times daily for a period of at least three months.

Treated patients with an intact uterus should be monitored closely for signs of endometrial cancer, and appropriate diagnostic measures should be taken to rule out malignancy in the event of persistent or recurring abnormal vaginal bleeding.

HOW SUPPLIED

PREMARIN® (conjugated estrogens tablets, USP)

—Each oval *purple* tablet contains 2.5 mg, in bottles of 100 (NDC 0046-0865-81) and 1,000 (NDC 0046-0865-91).

—Each oval *yellow* tablet contains 1.25 mg, in bottles of 100 (NDC 0046-0866-81); 1,000 (NDC 0046-0866-91); 5,000 (NDC 0046-0866-95); and Unit-Dose packages of 100 (NDC 0046-0866-99). Also in Cycle Packs of 25 (NDC 0046-0866-25).

—Each oval *white* tablet contains 0.9 mg, in bottles of 100 (NDC 0046-0864-81). Also in Cycle Packs of 25 (NDC 0046-0864-25).

—Each oval *maroon* tablet contains 0.625 mg, in bottles of 100 (NDC 0046-0867-81); 1,000 (NDC 0046-0867-91); 5,000 (NDC 0046-0867-95); and Unit-Dose packages of 100 (NDC 0046-0867-99). Also in Cycle Packs of 25 (NDC 0046-0867-25).

—Each oval *green* tablet contains 0.3 mg, in bottles of 100 (NDC 0046-0868-81) and 1,000 (NDC 0046-0868-91).

The appearance of these tablets is a trademark of Wyeth-Ayerst Laboratories.

Store at room temperature (approximately 25° C).

INFORMATION FOR THE PATIENT

This leaflet describes when and how to use estrogens and the risks of estrogen treatment.

Continued on next page

Wyeth-Ayerst—Cont.

ESTROGEN DRUGS

Estrogens have several important uses but also some risks. You must decide, with your doctor, whether the risks of estrogens are acceptable in view of their benefits. If you decide to start taking estrogens, check with your doctor to make sure you are using the lowest possible effective dose. The length of treatment with estrogens will depend upon the reason for use. This should also be discussed with your doctor.

USES OF ESTROGEN

To reduce menopausal symptoms. Estrogens are hormones produced by the ovaries. The decrease in the amount of estrogen that occurs in all women, usually between ages 45 and 55, causes the menopause. Sometimes the ovaries are removed by an operation, causing "surgical menopause." When the amount of estrogen begins to decrease, some women develop very uncomfortable symptoms, such as feelings of warmth in the face, neck and chest or sudden intense episodes of heat and sweating ("hot flashes"). The use of drugs containing estrogens can help the body adjust to lower estrogen levels.

Most women have none or only mild menopausal symptoms and do not need estrogens. Other women may need estrogens for a few months while their bodies adjust to lower estrogen levels. The majority of women do not need estrogen replacement for longer than six months for these symptoms.

To prevent brittle bones. After age 40, and especially after menopause, some women develop osteoporosis. This is a thinning of the bones that makes them weaker and more likely to break, often leading to fractures of vertebrae, hip, and wrist bones. Taking estrogens after the menopause slows down bone loss and may prevent bones from breaking. Eating foods that are high in calcium (such as milk products) or taking calcium supplements (1,000 to 1,500 milligrams per day) and certain types of exercise may also help prevent osteoporosis. Since estrogen use is associated with some risk, its use in the prevention of osteoporosis should be confined to women who appear to be susceptible to this condition. The following characteristics are often present in women who are likely to develop osteoporosis: white race, thinness, and cigarette smoking.

Women who had their menopause by the surgical removal of their ovaries at a relatively young age are good candidates for estrogen replacement therapy to prevent osteoporosis.

To treat certain types of abnormal uterine bleeding due to hormonal imbalance.

To treat atrophic vaginitis (itching, burning, dryness in or around the vagina) and *atrophic urethritis* (which may cause difficulty or burning on urination).

To treat certain cancers.

WHEN ESTROGENS SHOULD NOT BE USED

Estrogens should not be used:

During pregnancy. Although the possibility is fairly small, there is a greater risk of having a child born with a birth defect if you take estrogens during pregnancy. A male child may have an increased risk of developing abnormalities of the urinary system and sex organs. A female child may have an increased risk of developing cancer of the vagina or cervix in her teens or twenties. Estrogen is not effective in preventing miscarriage (abortion).

If you have had any heart or circulation problems. Estrogen therapy should be used only after consultation with your physician and only in recommended doses. Patients with a tendency for abnormal blood clotting should avoid estrogen use (see below).

If you have had cancer. Since estrogens increase the risk of certain cancers, you should not take estrogens if you have ever had cancer of the breast or uterus. In certain situations, your doctor may choose to use estrogen in the treatment of breast cancer.

When they are ineffective. Sometimes women experience nervous symptoms or depression during menopause. There is no evidence that estrogens are effective for such symptoms. You may have heard that taking estrogens for long periods (years) after menopause will keep your skin soft and supple and keep you feeling young. There is no evidence that this is so and such long-term treatment may carry serious risks.

DANGERS OF ESTROGENS

Cancer of the uterus. The risk of cancer of the uterus increases the longer estrogens are used and when larger doses are taken. One study showed that when estrogens are discontinued, this increased risk of cancer seems to fall off quickly. In another study, the persistence of risk was demonstrated for 10 years after stopping estrogen treatment. Because of this risk, *it is important to take the lowest dose of estrogen that will control your symptoms and to take it only as long as you need it.* There is a higher risk of cancer of the uterus if you are overweight, diabetic, or have high blood pressure.

If you have had your uterus removed (total hysterectomy), there is no danger of developing cancer of the uterus.

Cancer of the breast. The majority of studies have shown no association with the usual doses used for estrogen replacement therapy and breast cancer. Some studies have suggested a possible increased incidence of breast cancer in those women taking estrogens for prolonged periods of time and especially if higher doses are used.

Regular breast examinations by a health professional and self-examination are recommended for women receiving estrogen therapy, as they are for all women.

Gallbladder disease. Women who use estrogens after menopause are more likely to develop gallbladder disease needing surgery than women who do not use estrogens.

Abnormal blood clotting. Taking estrogens may increase the risk of blood clots. These clots can cause a stroke, heart attack or pulmonary embolus, any of which may be fatal.

SIDE EFFECTS

In addition to the risk listed above, the following side effects have been reported with estrogen use:

- Nausea and vomiting.
- Breast tenderness or enlargement.
- Enlargement of benign tumors of the uterus.
- Retention of excess fluid. This may make some conditions worsen, such as asthma, epilepsy, migraine, heart disease, or kidney disease.
- A spotty darkening of the skin, particularly on the face.

REDUCING RISK OF ESTROGEN USE

If you decide to take estrogens, you can reduce your risks by carefully monitoring your treatment.

See your doctor regularly. While you are taking estrogens, it is important that you visit your doctor at least once a year for a physical examination. If members of your family have had breast cancer or if you have ever had breast nodules or an abnormal mammogram (breast x-ray), you may need to have more frequent breast examinations.

Reevaluate your need for estrogens. You and your doctor should reevaluate your need for estrogens at least every six months.

Be alert for signs of trouble. Report these or any other unusual side effects to your doctor immediately:

- Abnormal bleeding from the vagina.
- Pains in the calves or chest, a sudden shortness of breath or coughing blood (indicating possible clots in the legs, heart, or lungs).
- Severe headache, dizziness, faintness, or changes in vision, indicating possible clots in the brain or eye.
- Breast lumps.
- Yellowing of the skin.
- Pain, swelling, or tenderness in the abdomen.

OTHER INFORMATION

Some physicians may choose to prescribe another hormonal drug to be used in association with estrogen treatment. These drugs, progestins, have been reported to lower the frequency of occurrence of a possible precancerous condition of the uterine lining. Whether this will provide protection from uterine cancer has not been clearly established. There are possible additional risks that may be associated with the inclusion of a progestin in estrogen treatment. The possible risks include unfavorable effects on blood fats and sugars. The choice of progestin and its dosage may be important in minimizing these effects.

Your doctor has prescribed this drug for you and you alone. Do not give the drug to anyone else.

If you will be taking calcium supplements as part of the treatment to help prevent osteoporosis, check with your doctor about the amounts recommended.

Keep this and all drugs out of the reach of children. In case of overdose, call your doctor, hospital, or poison control center immediately.

This leaflet provides the most important information about estrogens. If you want to read more, ask your doctor or pharmacist to let you read the professional labeling.

HOW SUPPLIED

PREMARIN® (conjugated estrogens tablets, USP)—tablets for oral administration.

    Each oval purple tablet contains 2.5 mg.
    Each oval yellow tablet contains 1.25 mg.
    Each oval white tablet contains 0.9 mg.
    Each oval maroon tablet contains 0.625 mg.
    Each oval green tablet contains 0.3 mg.

The appearance of these tablets is a trademark of Wyeth-Ayerst Laboratories.

Shown in Product Identification Section, page 436

PREMARIN®   ℞
[prĕm 'a-rin]
(CONJUGATED ESTROGENS)
VAGINAL CREAM
in a nonliquefying base

CAUTION: Federal law prohibits dispensing without prescription.

---

1. ESTROGENS HAVE BEEN REPORTED TO INCREASE THE RISK OF ENDOMETRIAL CARCINOMA.

Three independent, case-controlled studies have reported an increased risk of endometrial cancer in postmenopausal women exposed to exogenous estrogens for more than one year.[1–3] This risk was independent of the other known risk factors for endometrial cancer. These studies are further supported by the finding that incidence rates of endometrial cancer have increased sharply since 1969 in eight different areas of the United States with population-based cancer reporting systems, an increase which may be related to the rapidly expanding use of estrogens during the last decade.[4]

The three case-controlled studies reported that the risk of endometrial cancer in estrogen users was about 4.5 to 13.9 times greater than in nonusers. The risk appears to depend on both duration of treatment[1] and on estrogen dose.[3] In view of these findings, when estrogens are used for the treatment of menopausal symptoms, the lowest dose that will control symptoms should be utilized and medication should be discontinued as soon as possible. When prolonged treatment is medically indicated, the patient should be reassessed, on at least a semi-annual basis, to determine the need for continued therapy. Although the evidence must be considered preliminary, one study suggests that cyclic administration of low doses of estrogen may carry less risk than continuous administration.[3] It therefore appears prudent to utilize such a regimen.

Close clinical surveillance of all women taking estrogens is important. In all cases of undiagnosed persistent or recurring abnormal vaginal bleeding, adequate diagnostic measures should be undertaken to rule out malignancy.

There is no evidence at present that "natural" estrogens are more or less hazardous than "synthetic" estrogens at equi-estrogenic doses.

2. ESTROGENS SHOULD NOT BE USED DURING PREGNANCY.

The use of female sex hormones, both estrogens and progestogens, during early pregnancy may seriously damage the offspring. It has been shown that females exposed in utero to diethylstilbestrol, a nonsteroidal estrogen, have an increased risk of developing, in later life, a form of vaginal or cervical cancer that is ordinarily extremely rare.[5,6] This risk has been estimated as not greater than 4 per 1,000 exposures.[7] Furthermore, a high percentage of such exposed women (from 30% to 90%) have been found to have vaginal adenosis,[8–12] epithelial changes of the vagina and cervix. Although these changes are histologically benign, it is not known whether they are precursors of malignancy. Although similar data are not available with the use of other estrogens, it cannot be presumed they would not induce similar changes.

Several reports suggest an association between intrauterine exposure to female sex hormones and congenital anomalies, including congenital heart defects and limb reduction defects.[13–16] One case-controlled study[16] estimated a 4.7-fold increased risk of limb-reduction defects in infants exposed in utero to sex hormones (oral contraceptives, hormone withdrawal tests for pregnancy, or attempted treatment for threatened abortion). Some of these exposures were very short and involved only a few days of treatment. The data suggest that the risk of limb-reduction defects in exposed fetuses is somewhat less than 1 per 1,000.

In the past, female sex hormones have been used during pregnancy in an attempt to treat threatened or habitual abortion. There is considerable evidence that estrogens are ineffective for these indications, and there is no evidence from well-controlled studies that progestogens are effective for these uses.

If PREMARIN (conjugated estrogens) Vaginal Cream is used during pregnancy, or if the patient becomes pregnant while taking this drug, she should be apprised of the potential risks to the fetus, and the advisability of pregnancy continuation.

DESCRIPTION

Each gram of PREMARIN (conjugated estrogens) Vaginal Cream contains 0.625 mg conjugated estrogens. USP, in a nonliquefying base containing cetyl esters wax, cetyl alcohol, white wax, glyceryl monostearate, propylene glycol monostearate, methyl stearate, phenylethyl alcohol, sodium lauryl sulfate, glycerin, and mineral oil. PREMARIN Vaginal Cream is applied intravaginally.

PREMARIN (conjugated estrogens) is a mixture of estrogens obtained exclusively from natural sources, occurring as the sodium salts of water-soluble estrogen sulfates blended to represent the average composition of material derived from pregnant mares' urine. It contains estrone, equilin, and 17 α-dihydroequilin, together with smaller amounts of 17 α-estradiol, equilenin, and 17 α-dihydroequilenin as salts of their sulfate esters.

CLINICAL PHARMACOLOGY

Estrogens are important in the development and maintenance of the female reproductive system and secondary sex characteristics. They promote growth and development of the vagina, uterus, and fallopian tubes, and enlargement of the breasts. Indirectly, they contribute to the shaping of the skeleton, maintenance of tone and elasticity of urogenital structures, changes in the epiphyses of the long bones that allow for the pubertal growth spurt and its termination, growth of axillary and pubic hair, and pigmentation of the nipples and genitals. Decline of estrogenic activity at the end of the menstrual cycle can bring on menstruation, although the cessation of progesterone secretion is the most important factor in the mature ovulatory cycle. However, in the preovulatory or nonovulatory cycle, estrogen is the primary determinant in the onset of menstruation. Estrogens also affect the release of pituitary gonadotropins.

The pharmacologic effects of conjugated estrogens are similar to those of endogenous estrogens. They are soluble in water and may be absorbed from mucosal surfaces after local administration.

In responsive tissues (female genital organs, breasts, hypothalamus, pituitary) estrogens enter the cell and are transported into the nucleus. As a result of estrogen action, specific RNA and protein synthesis occurs.

Metabolism and inactivation occur primarily in the liver. Some estrogens are excreted into the bile; however, they are reabsorbed from the intestine and returned to the liver through the portal venous system. Water-soluble estrogen conjugates are strongly acidic and, therefore, ionized in body fluids, which favor excretion through the kidneys since tubular reabsorption is minimal.

INDICATIONS AND USAGE

PREMARIN (conjugated estrogens) Vaginal Cream is indicated in the treatment of atrophic vaginitis and kraurosis vulvae.

PREMARIN Vaginal Cream HAS NOT BEEN SHOWN TO BE EFFECTIVE FOR ANY PURPOSE DURING PREGNANCY AND ITS USE MAY CAUSE SEVERE HARM TO THE FETUS (SEE BOXED WARNING).

CONTRAINDICATIONS

Estrogens should not be used in women with any of the following conditions:

1. Known or suspected cancer of the breast except in appropriately selected patients being treated for metastatic disease.
2. Known or suspected estrogen-dependent neoplasia.
3. Known or suspected pregnancy (see Boxed Warning).
4. Undiagnosed abnormal genital bleeding.
5. Active thrombophlebitis or thromboembolic disorders.
6. A past history of thrombophlebitis, thrombosis, or thromboembolic disorders associated with previous estrogen use (except when used in treatment of breast malignancy).

PREMARIN Vaginal Cream should not be used in patients hypersensitive to its ingredients.

WARNINGS

1. *Induction of malignant neoplasms.* Long-term continuous administration of natural and synthetic estrogens in certain animal species increases the frequency of carcinomas of the breast, cervix, vagina, and liver. There are now reports that estrogens increase the risk of carcinoma of the endometrium in humans (see Boxed Warning).

At the present time there is no satisfactory evidence that estrogens given to postmenopausal women increase the risk of cancer of the breast,[17] although a recent long-term follow-up of a single physician's practice has raised this possibility.[18] Because of the animal data, there is a need for caution in prescribing estrogens for women with a strong family history of breast cancer or who have breast nodules, fibrocystic disease, or abnormal mammograms.

2. *Gallbladder disease.* A recent study has reported a 2- to 3-fold increase in the risk of surgically confirmed gallbladder disease in women receiving postmenopausal estrogens,[17] similar to the 2-fold increase previously noted in users of oral contraceptives.[19,24a]

3. *Effects similar to those caused by estrogen-progestogen oral contraceptives.* There are several serious adverse effects of oral contraceptives, most of which have not, up to now, been documented as consequences of postmenopausal estrogen therapy. This may reflect the comparatively low doses of estrogen used in postmenopausal women. It would be expected that the larger doses of estrogen used to treat prostatic or breast cancer, or postpartum breast engorgement, are more likely to result in these adverse effects, and, in fact, it has been shown that there is an increased risk of thrombosis in men receiving estrogens for prostatic cancer and women for postpartum breast engorgement.[20–23]

a. *Thromboembolic disease.* It is now well established that users of oral contraceptives have an increased risk of various thromboembolic and thrombotic vascular diseases, such as thrombophlebitis, pulmonary embolism, stroke, and myocar-

dial infarction.[24–31] Cases of retinal thrombosis, mesenteric thrombosis, and optic neuritis have been reported in oral-contraceptive users. There is evidence that the risk of several of these adverse reactions is related to the dose of the drug.[32,33] An increased risk of postsurgery thromboembolic complications has also been reported in users of oral contraceptives.[34,35] If feasible, estrogen should be discontinued at least 4 weeks before surgery of the type associated with an increased risk of thromboembolism, or during periods of prolonged immobilization.

While an increased rate of thromboembolic and thrombotic disease in postmenopausal users of estrogens has not been found,[17–24,25–36] this does not rule out the possibility that such an increase may be present or that subgroups of women who have underlying risk factors or who are receiving relatively large doses of estrogens may have increased risk. Therefore estrogens should not be used in persons with active thrombophlebitis or thromboembolic disorders, and they should not be used (except in treatment of malignancy) in persons with a history of such disorders in association with estrogen use. They should be used with caution in patients with cerebral vascular or coronary artery disease and only for those in whom estrogens are clearly needed.

Large doses of estrogen (5 mg conjugated estrogens per day), comparable to those used to treat cancer of the prostate and breast, have been shown in a large prospective clinical trial in men[37] to increase the risk of nonfatal myocardial infarction, pulmonary embolism, and thrombophlebitis. When estrogen doses of this size are used, any of the thromboembolic and thrombotic adverse effects associated with oral contraceptive use should be considered a clear risk.

b. *Hepatic adenoma.* Benign hepatic adenomas appear to be associated with the use of oral contraceptives.[38–40] Although benign and rare, these may rupture and may cause death through intra-abdominal hemorrhage. Such lesions have not yet been reported in association with other estrogen or progestogen preparations but should be considered in estrogen users having abdominal pain and tenderness, abdominal mass, or hypovolemic shock. Hepatocellular carcinoma has also been reported in women taking estrogen-containing oral contraceptives.[39] The relationship of this malignancy to these drugs is not known at this time.

c. *Elevated blood pressure.* Women using oral contraceptives sometimes experience increased blood pressure which, in most cases, returns to normal on discontinuing the drug. There is now a report that this may occur with use of estrogens in the menopause[41] and blood pressure should be monitored with estrogen use, especially if high doses are used.

d. *Glucose tolerance.* A worsening of glucose tolerance has been observed in a significant percentage of patients on estrogen-containing oral contraceptives. For this reason, diabetic patients should be carefully observed while receiving estrogens.

4. *Hypercalcemia.* Administration of estrogens may lead to severe hypercalcemia in patients with breast cancer and bone metastases. If this occurs, the drug should be stopped and appropriate measures taken to reduce the serum calcium level.

PRECAUTIONS

A. General Precautions.

1. A complete medical and family history should be taken prior to the initiation of any estrogen therapy. The pretreatment and periodic physical examinations should include special reference to blood pressure, breasts, abdomen, and pelvic organs, and should include a Papanicolaou smear. As a general rule, estrogen should not be prescribed for longer than one year without another physical examination being performed.

2. Fluid retention—Because estrogens may cause some degree of fluid retention, conditions which might be influenced by this factor such as asthma, epilepsy, migraine, and cardiac or renal dysfunction, require careful observation.

3. Certain patients may develop undesirable manifestations of excessive estrogenic stimulation, such as abnormal or excessive uterine bleeding, mastodynia, etc.

4. Prolonged administration of unopposed estrogen therapy has been reported to increase the risk of endometrial hyperplasia in some patients.

5. Oral contraceptives appear to be associated with an increased incidence of mental depression.[24a] Although it is not clear whether this is due to the estrogenic or progestogenic component of the contraceptive, patients with a history of depression should be carefully observed.

6. Preexisting uterine leiomyomata may increase in size during estrogen use.

7. The pathologist should be advised of estrogen therapy when relevant specimens are submitted.

8. Patients with a past history of jaundice during pregnancy have an increased risk of recurrence of jaundice while receiving estrogen-containing oral contraceptive therapy. If jaundice develops in any patient receiving estrogen, the medication should be discontinued while the cause is investigated.

9. Estrogens may be poorly metabolized in patients with impaired liver function and they should be administered with caution in such patients.

10. Because estrogens influence the metabolism of calcium and phosphorus, they should be used with caution in patients with metabolic bone diseases that are associated with hypercalcemia or in patients with renal insufficiency.

11. Because of the effects of estrogens on epiphyseal closure, they should be used judiciously in young patients in whom bone growth is not complete.

Concomitant Progestin Use: The lowest effective dose appropriate for the specific indication should be utilized. Studies of the addition of a progestin for 7 or more days of a cycle of estrogen administration have reported a lowered incidence of endometrial hyperplasia. Morphological and biochemical studies of the endometrium suggest that 10 to 13 days of progestin are needed to provide maximal maturation of the endometrium and to eliminate any hyperplastic changes. Whether this will provide protection from endometrial carcinoma has not been clearly established. There are possible additional risks which may be associated with the inclusion of progestin in estrogen replacement regimens. If concomitant progestin therapy is used, potential risks may include adverse effects on carbohydrate and lipid metabolism. The choice of progestin and dosage may be important in minimizing these adverse effects.

B. Information for Patients. (See text which appears after the PHYSICIAN REFERENCES.)

C. Drug/Laboratory Test Interactions. Certain endocrine and liver function tests may be affected by estrogen-containing oral contraceptives. The following similar changes may be expected with larger doses of estrogen:

a. Increased sulfobromophthalein retention.

b. Increased prothrombin and factors VII, VIII, IX, and X; decreased antithrombin 3; increased norepinephrine-induced platelet aggregability.

c. Increased thyroid binding globulin (TBG) leading to increased circulating total thyroid hormone, as measured by PBI, T4 by column, or T4 by radioimmunoassay. Free T3 resin uptake is decreased, reflecting the elevated TBG; free T4 concentration is unaltered.

d. Impaired glucose tolerance.

e. Decreased pregnanediol excretion.

f. Reduced response to metyrapone test.

g. Reduced serum folate concentration.

h. Increased serum triglyceride and phospholipid concentration.

D. Carcinogenesis, Mutagenesis, Impairment of Fertility. (See WARNINGS section for information on carcinogenesis.)

E. Pregnancy Category X. (See CONTRAINDICATIONS and Boxed Warning.)

F. Nursing Mothers. It is now known whether this drug is excreted in human milk. Because many drugs are excreted in human milk and because of the potential for serious adverse reactions in nursing infants from estrogens, a decision should be made whether to discontinue nursing or to discontinue the drug, taking into account the importance of the drug to the mother.

G. Pediatric Use. Safety and effectiveness in children have not been established.

ADVERSE REACTIONS

(See WARNINGS regarding induction of neoplasia, adverse effects on the fetus, increased incidence of gallbladder disease, and adverse effects similar to those of oral contraceptives, including thromboembolism.) The following additional adverse reactions have been reported with estrogenic therapy, including oral contraceptives.

1. *Genitourinary system:* Breakthrough bleeding, spotting, change in menstrual flow; dysmenorrhea; premenstrual-like syndrome; amenorrhea during and after treatment; increase in size of uterine fibromyomata; vaginal candidiasis; change in cervical erosion and in degree of cervical secretion; cystitis-like syndrome.

2. *Breasts:* Tenderness, enlargement, secretion.

3. *Gastrointestinal:* Nausea, vomiting; abdominal cramps, bloating; cholestatic jaundice.

4. *Skin:* Chloasma or melasma which may persist when drug is discontinued; erythema multiforme; erythema nodosum; hemorrhagic eruption; loss of scalp hair; hirsutism.

5. *Eyes:* Steepening of corneal curvature; intolerance to contact lenses.

6. *CNS:* Headache, migraine, dizziness; mental depression; chorea.

7. *Miscellaneous:* Increase or decrease in weight; reduced carbohydrate tolerance; aggravation of porphyria; edema; changes in libido.

OVERDOSAGE

Numerous reports of ingestion of large doses of estrogen-containing oral contraceptives by young children indicate that acute serious ill effects do not occur. Overdosage of es-

Continued on next page

Wyeth-Ayerst—Cont.

trogen may cause nausea, and withdrawal bleeding may occur in females.

DOSAGE AND ADMINISTRATION

Given cyclically for short-term use only:

For treatment of atrophic vaginitis, or kraurosis vulvae. The lowest dose that will control symptoms should be chosen and medication should be discontinued as promptly as possible.

Administration should be cyclic (e.g., three weeks on and one week off).

Attempts to discontinue or taper medication should be made at three- to six-month intervals.

Usual dosage range: 2 to 4 g (½ applicatorful to 1 applicatorful) daily, intravaginally, depending on the severity of the condition.

Instructions for use of applicator:
1. Remove cap from tube.
2. Puncture dispensing end of tube with plastic spike on cap.
3. Screw nozzle end of applicator onto tube.
4. Gently squeeze tube to force sufficient cream into the barrel to provide the prescribed dose.
5. Unscrew applicator from tube.
6. Lie on back with knees drawn up. To deliver medication, gently insert applicator deeply into vagina and press plunger downward to its original position.

TO CLEANSE: Pull plunger out from barrel. Wash with mild soap and warm water.

DO NOT BOIL OR USE HOT WATER.

Treated patients with an intact uterus should be monitored closely for signs of endometrial cancer, and appropriate diagnostic measures should be taken to rule out malignancy in the event of persistent or recurring abnormal vaginal bleeding.

HOW SUPPLIED

PREMARIN (conjugated estrogens) Vaginal Cream—Each gram contains 0.625 mg conjugated estrogens, USP. (Also contains cetyl esters wax, cetyl alcohol, white wax, glyceryl monostearate, propylene glycol monostearate, methyl stearate, phenylethyl alcohol, sodium lauryl sulfate, glycerin, and mineral oil.)

Combination package: Each contains Net Wt. 1½ oz (42.5 g) tube with one plastic applicator calibrated in 1 g increments to a maximum of 4 g (NDC 0046-0872-93).

Also Available—Refill package: Each contains Net Wt. 1½ oz (42.5 g) tube (NDC 0046-0872-01).

Store at room temperature (approximately 25° C).

PHYSICIAN REFERENCES

1. Ziel, H. K., *et al.*: N. Engl. J. Med. *293*:1167–1170, 1975.
2. Smith, D. C., *et al.*: N. Engl. J. Med. *293*:1164–1167, 1975.
3. Mack, T. M., *et al.*: N. Engl. J. Med *294*:1262–1267, 1976.
4. Weiss, N. S., *et al.*: N. Engl. J. Med. *294*:1259–1262, 1976.
5. Herbst, A. L., *et al.*: N. Engl. J. Med. *284*:878–881, 1971.
6. Greenwald, P., *et al.*: N. Engl. J. Med. *285*:390–392, 1971.
7. Lanier, A., *et al.*: Mayo Clin. Proc. *48*:793–799, 1973.
8. Herbst, A., *et al.*: Obstet. Gynecol. *40*:287–298, 1972.
9. Herbst, A., *et al.*: Am. J. Obstet. Gynecol. *118*:607–615, 1974.
10. Herbst, A., *et al.*: N. Engl. J. Med. *292*:334–339, 1975.
11. Stafl, A., *et al.*: Obstet. Gynecol. *43*:118–128, 1974.
12. Sherman, A. I., *et al.*: Obstet. Gynecol. *44*:531–545, 1974.
13. Gal, I., *et al.*: Nature *216*:83, 1967.
14. Levy, E. P., *et al.*: Lancet *1*:611, 1973.
15. Nora, J., *et al.*: Lancet *1*:941–942, 1973.
16. Janerich, D. T., *et al.*: N. Engl. J. Med. *291*:697–700, 1974.
17. Boston Collaborative Drug Surveillance Program: N. Engl. J. Med. *290*:15–19, 1974.
18. Hoover, R., *et al.*: N. Engl. J. Med. *295*:401–405, 1976.
19. Boston Collaborative Drug Surveillance Program: Lancet *1*:1399–1404, 1973.
20. Daniel, D. G., *et al.*: Lancet *2*:287–289, 1967.
21. The Veterans Administration Cooperative Urological Research Group: J. Urol. *98*:516–522, 1967.
22. Bailar, J. C.: Lancet *2*:560, 1967.
23. Blackard, C., *et al.*: Cancer *26*:249–256, 1970.
24. Royal College of General Practitioners: J. R. Coll. Gen. Pract. *13*:267–279, 1967.
24a. Royal College of General Practitioners: Oral Contraceptives and Health, New York, Pitman Corp., 1974.
25. Inman, W. H. W., *et al.*: Br. Med. J. *2*:193–199, 1968.
26. Vessey, M. P., *et al.*: Br. Med. J. *2*:651–657, 1969.
27. Sartwell, P. E., *et al.*: Am. J. Epidemiol. *90*:365–380, 1969.
28. Collaborative Group for the Study of Stroke in Young Women: N. Engl. J. Med. *288*:871–878, 1973.
29. Collaborative Group for the Study of Stroke in Young Women: J.A.M.A. *231*:718–722, 1975.
30. Mann, J. I., *et al.*: Br. Med. J. *2*:245–248, 1975.
31. Mann, J. I., *et al.*: Br. Med. J. *2*:241–245, 1975.
32. Inman, W. H. W., *et al.*: Br. Med. J. *2*:203–209, 1970.
33. Stolley, P. D., *et al.*: Am. J. Epidemiol. *102*:197–208, 1975.
34. Vessey, M. P., *et al.*: Br. Med. J. *3*:123–126, 1970.
35. Greene, G. R., *et al.*: Am. J. Public Health *62*:680–685, 1972.
36. Rosenberg, L., *et al.*: N. Engl. J. Med. *294*:1256–1259, 1976.
37. Coronary Drug Project Research Group: J.A.M.A. *214*:1303–1313, 1970.
38. Baum, J., *et al.*: Lancet *2*:926–928, 1973.
39. Mays, E. T., *et al.*: J.A.M.A. *235*:730–732, 1976.
40. Edmondson, H. A., *et al.*: N. Engl. J. Med. *294*:470–472, 1976.
41. Pfeffer, R. I., *et al.*: Am. J. Epidemiol. *103*:445–456, 1976.

INFORMATION FOR THE PATIENT
INSTRUCTIONS FOR USE OF PREMARIN®
(conjugated estrogens)
VAGINAL CREAM APPLICATOR:

1. Remove cap from tube.
2. Puncture dispensing end of tube with plastic spike on cap.
3. Screw nozzle end of applicator onto tube.
4. Gently squeeze tube to force sufficient cream into the barrel to provide the prescribed dose.
5. Unscrew applicator from tube.
6. Lie on back with knees drawn up. To deliver medication, gently insert applicator deeply into vagina and press plunger downward to its original position.

TO CLEANSE: Pull plunger out from barrel. Wash with mild soap and warm water.

DO NOT BOIL OR USE HOT WATER.

WHAT YOU SHOULD KNOW ABOUT ESTROGENS

Estrogens are female hormones produced by the ovaries. The ovaries make several different kinds of estrogens. In addition, scientists have been able to make a variety of synthetic estrogens. As far as we know, all these estrogens have similar properties and, therefore, much the same usefulness, side effects, and risks. This leaflet is intended to help you understand what estrogens are used for, the risks involved in their use, and how to use them as safely as possible.

This leaflet includes the most important information about estrogens, but not all the information. If you want to know more, you should ask your doctor for more information or you can ask your doctor or pharmacist to let you read the package insert prepared for the doctor.

USES OF ESTROGEN

THERE IS NO PROPER USE OF ESTROGENS IN A PREGNANT WOMAN.

Estrogens are prescribed by doctors for a number of purposes, including:

1. To provide estrogen during a period of adjustment when a woman's ovaries stop producing a majority of her estrogens, in order to prevent certain uncomfortable symptoms of estrogen deficiency. (With the menopause, which generally occurs between the ages of 45 and 55, women produce a much smaller amount of estrogens.)
2. To prevent symptoms of estrogen deficiency when a woman's ovaries have been removed surgically before the natural menopause.
3. To prevent pregnancy. (Estrogens are given along with a progestogen, another female hormone; these combinations are called oral contraceptives or birth control pills. Patient labeling is available to women taking oral contraceptives and they will not be discussed in this leaflet.)
4. To treat certain cancers in women and men.
5. To prevent painful swelling of the breasts after pregnancy in women who choose not to nurse their babies.

ESTROGENS IN THE MENOPAUSE

In the natural course of their lives, all women eventually experience a decrease in estrogen production. This usually occurs between ages 45 and 55 but may occur earlier or later. Sometimes the ovaries may need to be removed before natural menopause by an operation, producing a "surgical menopause."

When the amount of estrogen in the blood begins to decrease, many women may develop typical symptoms: feelings of warmth in the face, neck, and chest or sudden intense episodes of heat and sweating throughout the body (called "hot flashes" or "hot flushes"). These symptoms are sometimes very uncomfortable. Some women may also develop changes in the vagina (called "atrophic vaginitis") which cause discomfort, especially during and after intercourse.

Estrogens can be prescribed to treat these symptoms of the menopause. It is estimated that considerably more than half of all women undergoing the menopause have only mild symptoms or no symptoms at all and therefore do not need estrogens. Other women may need estrogens for a few months, while their bodies adjust to lower estrogen levels.

Sometimes the need will be for periods longer than six months. In an attempt to avoid overstimulation of the uterus (womb), estrogens are usually given cyclically during each month of use, such as three weeks of pills followed by one week without pills.

Sometimes women experience nervous symptoms or depression during menopause. There is no evidence that estrogens are effective for such symptoms without associated vasomotor symptoms. In the absence of vasomotor symptoms, estrogens should not be used to treat nervous symptoms, although other treatment may be needed.

You may have heard that taking estrogens for long periods (years) after the menopause will keep your skin soft and supple and keep you feeling young. There is no evidence that this is so, however, and such long-term treatment carries important risks.

ESTROGENS TO PREVENT SWELLING OF THE BREASTS AFTER PREGNANCY

If you do not breast-feed your baby after delivery, your breasts may fill up with milk and become painful and engorged. This usually begins about 3 to 4 days after delivery and may last for a few days to up to a week or more. Sometimes the discomfort is severe, but usually it is not and can be controlled by pain-relieving drugs such as aspirin and by binding the breasts up tightly. Estrogens can be used to try to prevent the breasts from filling up. While this treatment is sometimes successful, in many cases the breasts fill up to some degree in spite of treatment. The dose of estrogens needed to prevent pain and swelling of the breasts is much larger than the dose needed to treat symptoms of the menopause and this may increase your chances of developing blood clots in the legs or lungs (see below). Therefore, it is important that you discuss the benefits and the risks of estrogen use with your doctor if you have decided not to breast-feed your baby.

THE DANGERS OF ESTROGENS

1. *Endometrial cancer.* There are reports that if estrogens are used in the postmenopausal period for more than a year, there is an increased risk of *endometrial cancer* (cancer of the lining of the uterus). Women taking estrogens have roughly 5 to 10 times as great a chance of getting this cancer as women who take no estrogens. To put this another way, while a postmenopausal woman not taking estrogens has 1 chance in 1,000 each year of getting endometrial cancer, a woman taking estrogens has 5 to 10 chances in 1,000 each year. For this reason, *it is important to take estrogens only when they are really needed.*

The risk of this cancer is greater the longer estrogens are used and when larger doses are taken. Therefore, you should not take more estrogen than your doctor prescribes. *It is important to take the lowest dose of estrogen that will control symptoms and to take it only as long as it is needed.* If estrogens are needed for longer periods of time, your doctor will want to re-evaluate your need for estrogens at least every six months.

Women using estrogens should report any vaginal bleeding to their doctors; such bleeding may be of no importance, but it can be an early warning of endometrial cancer. If you have undiagnosed vaginal bleeding, you should not use estrogens until a diagnosis is made and you are certain there is no endometrial cancer.

NOTE: If you have had your uterus removed (total hysterectomy), there is no danger of developing endometrial cancer.

2. *Other possible cancers.* Estrogens can cause development of other tumors in animals, such as tumors of the breast, cervix, vagina, or liver, when given for a long time. At present there is no good evidence that women using estrogen in the menopause have an increased risk of such tumors, but there is no way yet to be sure they do not; and one study raises the possibility that use of estrogens in the menopause may increase the risk of breast cancer many years later. This is a further reason to use estrogens only when clearly needed. While you are taking estrogens, it is important that you go to your doctor at least once a year for a physical examination. Also, if members of your family have had breast cancer or if you have breast nodules or abnormal mammograms (breast x-rays), your doctor may wish to carry out more frequent examinations of your breasts.

3. *Gallbladder disease.* Women who use estrogens after menopause are more likely to develop gallbladder disease needing surgery than women who do not use estrogens. Birth control pills have a similar effect.

4. *Abnormal blood clotting.* Oral contraceptives increase the risk of blood clotting in various parts of the body. This can result in a stroke (if the clot is in the brain), a heart attack (a clot in a blood vessel of the heart), or a pulmonary embolus (a clot which forms in the legs or pelvis, then breaks off and travels to the lungs). Any of these can be fatal.

At this time use of estrogens in the menopause is not known to cause such blood clotting, but this has not been fully studied and there could still prove to be such a risk. It is recommended that if you have had clotting in the legs or lungs or a heart attack or stroke while you were using estrogens or birth control pills, you should not use estrogens (unless they are being used to treat cancer of the breast or prostate). If you have had a stroke or heart attack or if you have angina pectoris, estrogens should be used with great caution and only if clearly needed (for example, if you have severe symptoms of the menopause).

The larger doses of estrogen used to prevent swelling of the breasts after pregnancy have been reported to cause clotting in the legs and lungs.

SPECIAL WARNING ABOUT PREGNANCY

You should not receive estrogen if you are pregnant. If this should occur, there is a greater than usual chance that the developing child will be born with a birth defect, although the possibility remains fairly small. A female child may have an increased risk of developing cancer of the vagina or cervix later in life (in the teens or twenties). Every possible effort should be made to avoid exposure to estrogens during pregnancy. If exposure occurs, see your doctor.

OTHER EFFECTS OF ESTROGENS

In addition to the serious known risks of estrogens described above, estrogens have the following side effects and potential risks:

1. *Nausea and vomiting.* The most common side effect of estrogen therapy is nausea. Vomiting is less common.

2. *Effects on breasts.* Estrogens may cause breast tenderness or enlargement and may cause the breasts to secrete a liquid. These effects are not dangerous.

3. *Effects on the uterus.* Estrogens may cause benign fibroid tumors of the uterus to get larger.

4. *Effects on liver.* Women taking oral contraceptives develop, on rare occasions, a tumor of the liver which can rupture and bleed into the abdomen and may cause death. So far, these tumors have not been reported in women using estrogens in the menopause, but you should report any swelling or unusual pain or tenderness in the abdomen to your doctor immediately.

Women with a past history of jaundice (yellowing of the skin and white parts of the eyes) may get jaundice again during estrogen use. If this occurs, stop taking estrogens and see your doctor.

5. *Other effects.* Estrogens may cause excess fluid to be retained in the body. This may make some conditions worse, such as asthma, epilepsy, migraine, heart disease, or kidney disease.

SUMMARY

Estrogens have important uses, but they have serious risks as well. You must decide, with your doctor, whether the risks are acceptable to you in view of the benefits of treatment. Except where your doctor has prescribed estrogens for use in special cases of cancer of the breast or prostate, you should not use estrogens if you have cancer of the breast or uterus, are pregnant, have undiagnosed abnormal vaginal bleeding, clotting in the legs or lungs, or have had a stroke, heart attack or angina, or clotting in the legs or lungs in the past while you were taking estrogens.

You can use estrogens as safely as possible by understanding that your doctor will require regular physical examinations while you are taking them and will try to discontinue the drug as soon as possible and use the smallest dose possible. Be alert for signs of trouble including:

1. Abnormal bleeding from the vagina.

2. Pains in the calves or chest or sudden shortness of breath, or coughing blood.

3. Severe headache, dizziness, faintness, or changes in vision.

4. Breast lumps (you should ask your doctor how to examine your own breasts).

5. Jaundice (yellowing of the skin).

6. Mental depression.

Your doctor has prescribed this drug for you and you alone. Do not give the drug to anyone else.

HOW SUPPLIED

PREMARIN (conjugated estrogens) Vaginal Cream—Each gram contains 0.625 mg conjugated estrogens, USP. (Also contains cetyl esters wax, cetyl alcohol, white wax, glyceryl monostearate, propylene glycol monostearate, methyl stearate, phenylethyl alcohol, sodium lauryl sulfate, glycerin, and mineral oil.)

Combination package: Each contains Net Wt. 1½ oz (42.5 g) tube with one plastic applicator calibrated in 1 g increments to a maximum of 4 g (NDC 0046-0872-93).

Also Available—Refill package: Each contains Net Wt. 1½ oz (42.5 g) tube (NDC 0046-0872-01).

Store at room temperature (approximately 25° C).

Shown in Product Identification Section, page 437

PREMARIN®   ℞
[*prem'a-rin with meth"yl-tĕs-tŏs'ta-rōn*]
(conjugated estrogens, USP)
with METHYLTESTOSTERONE

No. 879—Each *yellow* tablet contains:
Premarin® (conjugated
  estrogens, USP) ....1.25 mg
Methyltestosterone ....10.0 mg
No. 878—Each *maroon* tablet contains:
Premarin® (conjugated
  estrogens, USP) ....0.625 mg
Methyltestosterone ....5.0 mg
CAUTION: Federal law prohibits dispensing without prescription.

---

1. ESTROGENS HAVE BEEN REPORTED TO INCREASE THE RISK OF ENDOMETRIAL CARCINOMA.
Three independent, case-controlled studies have reported an increased risk of endometrial cancer in postmenopausal women exposed to exogenous estrogens for more than one year.[1-3] This risk was independent of the other known risk factors for endometrial cancer. These studies are further supported by the finding that incidence rates of endometrial cancer have increased sharply since 1969 in eight different areas of the United States with population-based cancer reporting systems, an increase which may be related to the rapidly expanding use of estrogens during the last decade.[4]

The three case-controlled studies reported that the risk of endometrial cancer in estrogen users was about 4.5 to 13.9 times greater than in nonusers. The risk appears to depend on both duration of treatment[1] and on estrogen dose.[3] In view of these findings, when estrogens are used for the treatment of menopausal symptoms, the lowest dose that will control symptoms should be utilized and medication should be discontinued as soon as possible. When prolonged treatment is medically indicated, the patient should be reassessed on at least a semiannual basis to determine the need for continued therapy. Although the evidence must be considered preliminary, one study suggests that cyclic administration of low doses of estrogen may carry less risk than continuous administration.[3] It therefore appears prudent to utilize such a regimen.

Close clinical surveillance of all women taking estrogens is important. In all cases of undiagnosed persistent or recurring abnormal vaginal bleeding, adequate diagnostic measures should be undertaken to rule out malignancy.

There is no evidence at present that "natural" estrogens are more or less hazardous than "synthetic" estrogens at equiestrogenic doses.

2. ESTROGENS SHOULD NOT BE USED DURING PREGNANCY.
The use of female sex hormones, both estrogens and progestogens, during early pregnancy may seriously damage the offspring. It has been shown that females exposed in utero to diethylstilbestrol, a non-steroidal estrogen, have an increased risk of developing, in later life, a form of vaginal or cervical cancer that is ordinarily extremely rare.[5,6] This risk has been estimated as not greater than 4 per 1,000 exposures.[7] Furthermore, a high percentage of such exposed women (from 30% to 90%) have been found to have vaginal adenosis,[8-12] epithelial changes of the vagina and cervix. Although these changes are histologically benign, it is not known whether they are precursors of malignancy. Although similar data are not available with the use of other estrogens, it cannot be presumed they would not induce similar changes.

Several reports suggest an association between intrauterine exposure to female sex hormones and congenital anomalies, including congenital heart defects and limb reduction defects.[13-16] One case-controlled study[16] estimated a 4.7-fold increased risk of limb reduction defects in infants exposed in utero to sex hormones (oral contraceptives, hormone withdrawal tests for pregnancy, or attempted treatment for threatened abortion). Some of these exposures were very short and involved only a few days of treatment. The data suggest that the risk of limb reduction defects in exposed fetuses is somewhat less than 1 per 1,000.

In the past, female sex hormones have been used during pregnancy in an attempt to treat threatened or habitual abortion. There is considerable evidence that estrogens are ineffective for these indications, and there is no evidence from well-controlled studies that progestogens are effective for these uses.

If PREMARIN with METHYLTESTOSTERONE is used during pregnancy, or if the patient becomes pregnant while taking this drug, she should be apprised of the potential risks to the fetus, and the advisability of pregnancy continuation.

DESCRIPTION

PREMARIN with METHYLTESTOSTERONE is provided in tablets for oral administration.

PREMARIN (conjugated estrogens, USP) is a mixture of estrogens, obtained exclusively from natural sources, occurring as the sodium salts of water-soluble estrogen sulfates blended to represent the average composition of material derived from pregnant mares' urine. It contains estrone, equilin, and 17 α-dihydroequilin, together with smaller amounts of 17 α-estradiol, equilenin, and 17 α-dihydroequilenin as salts of their sulfate esters.

Methyltestosterone is an androgen.

Androgens are derivatives of cyclopentano-perhydrophenanthrene. Endogenous androgens are C-19 steroids with a side chain at C-17, and with two angular methyl groups. Testosterone is the primary endogenous androgen. Fluoxymesterone and methyltestosterone are synthetic derivatives of testosterone.

Methyltestosterone is a white to light-yellow crystalline substance that is virtually insoluble in water but soluble in organic solvents. It is stable in air but decomposes in light.

PREMARIN with METHYLTESTOSTERONE Tablets contain the following inactive ingredients: calcium phosphate tribasic, calcium sulfate anhydrous, carnauba wax, FD&C Blue No. 2, FD&C Yellow No. 6, glyceryl mono-oleate, guar gum, lactose, magnesium stearate, methylcellulose, microcrystalline cellulose, pharmaceutical glaze, polyethylene glycol, stearic acid, sucrose, titanium dioxide.

—0.625 mg PREMARIN with 5.0 mg methyltestosterone tablets also contain: FD&C Red No. 3.

—1.25 mg PREMARIN with 10.0 mg methyltestosterone tablets also contain: Black iron oxide, D&C Yellow No. 10, FD&C Red No. 40.

CLINICAL PHARMACOLOGY

Estrogens. Estrogens are important in the development and maintenance of the female reproductive system and secondary sex characteristics. They promote growth and development of the vagina, uterus, and fallopian tubes, and enlargement of the breasts. Indirectly, they contribute to the shaping of the skeleton, maintenance of tone and elasticity of urogenital structures, changes in the epiphyses of the long bones that allow for the pubertal growth spurt and its termination, growth of axillary and pubic hair, and pigmentation of the nipples and genitals. Decline of estrogenic activity at the end of the menstrual cycle can bring on menstruation, although the cessation of progesterone secretion is the most important factor in the mature ovulatory cycle. However, in the preovulatory or nonovulatory cycle, estrogen is the primary determinant in the onset of menstruation. Estrogens also affect the release of pituitary gonadotropins.

The pharmacologic effects of conjugated estrogens are similar to those of endogenous estrogens. They are soluble in water and are well absorbed from the gastrointestinal tract. In responsive tissues (female genital organs, breasts, hypothalamus, pituitary) estrogens enter the cell and are transported into the nucleus. As a result of estrogen action, specific RNA and protein synthesis occurs.

Estrogen Pharmacokinetics

Metabolism and inactivation occur primarily in the liver. Some estrogens are excreted into the bile; however, they are reabsorbed from the intestine and returned to the liver through the portal venous system. Water soluble estrogen conjugates are strongly acidic and are ionized in body fluids, which favor excretion through the kidneys since tubular reabsorption is minimal.

Androgens. Endogenous androgens are responsible for the normal growth and development of the male sex organs and for maintenance of secondary sex characteristics. These effects include the growth and maturation of prostate, seminal vesicles, penis, and scrotum; the development of male hair distribution, such as beard, pubic, chest, and axillary hair, laryngeal enlargement, vocal chord thickening, alterations in body musculature, and fat distribution. Drugs in this class also cause retention of nitrogen, sodium, potassium, phosphorus, and decreased urinary excretion of calcium. Androgens have been reported to increase protein anabolism and decrease protein catabolism. Nitrogen balance is improved only when there is sufficient intake of calories and protein.

Androgens are responsible for the growth spurt of adolescence and for the eventual termination of linear growth which is brought about by fusion of the epiphyseal growth centers. In children, exogenous androgens accelerate linear growth rates, but may cause a disproportionate advancement in bone maturation. Use over long periods may result in fusion of the epiphyseal growth centers and termination of growth process. Androgens have been reported to stimulate the production of red blood cells by enhancing the production of erythropoietic stimulating factor.

Androgen Pharmacokinetics

Testosterone given orally is metabolized by the gut and 44 percent is cleared by the liver in the first pass. Oral doses as high as 400 mg per day are needed to achieve clinically effec-

Continued on next page

Wyeth-Ayerst—Cont.

tive blood levels for full replacement therapy. The synthetic androgens (methyltestosterone and fluoxymesterone) are less extensively metabolized by the liver and have longer half-lives. They are more suitable than testosterone for oral administration. Testosterone in plasma is 98% bound to a specific testosterone-estradiol binding globulin, and about 2% is free. Generally, the amount of this sex-hormone-binding globulin in the plasma will determine the distribution of testosterone between free and bound forms, and the free testosterone concentration will determine its half-life.

About 90% of a dose of testosterone is excreted in the urine as glucuronic and sulfuric acid conjugates of testosterone and its metabolites; about 6% of a dose is excreted in the feces, mostly in the unconjugated form. Inactivation of testosterone occurs primarily in the liver. Testosterone is metabolized to various 17-keto steroids through two different pathways. There are considerable variations of the half-life of testosterone as reported in the literature, ranging from 10 to 100 minutes.

In many tissues the activity of testosterone appears to depend on reduction to dihydrotestosterone, which binds to cytosol receptor proteins. The steroid-receptor complex is transported to the nucleus where it initiates transcription events and cellular changes related to androgen action.

INDICATIONS

PREMARIN (conjugated estrogens, USP) with METHYL-TESTOSTERONE is indicated in the treatment of:

Moderate to severe *vasomotor* symptoms associated with the menopause in those patients not improved by estrogens alone. (There is no evidence that estrogens are effective for nervous symptoms or depression without associated vasomotor symptoms, and they should not be used to treat such conditions.)

PREMARIN with METHYLTESTOSTERONE HAS NOT BEEN SHOWN TO BE EFFECTIVE FOR ANY PURPOSE DURING PREGNANCY AND ITS USE MAY CAUSE SEVERE HARM TO THE FETUS (SEE BOXED WARNING).

CONTRAINDICATIONS

Estrogens should not be used in women with any of the following conditions:

1. Known or suspected cancer of the breast except in appropriately selected patients being treated for metastatic disease.
2. Known or suspected estrogen-dependent neoplasia.
3. Known or suspected pregnancy (see Boxed Warning).
4. Undiagnosed abnormal genital bleeding.
5. Active thrombophlebitis or thromboembolic disorders.
6. A past history of thrombophlebitis, thrombosis, or thromboembolic disorders associated with previous estrogen use (except when used in treatment of breast malignancy).

Methyltestosterone should not be used in:

1. The presence of severe liver damage.
2. Pregnancy and in breast-feeding mothers because of the possibility of masculinization of the female fetus or breast-fed infant.

WARNINGS

Associated with Estrogens

1. *Induction of malignant neoplasms.* Long-term continuous administration of natural and synthetic estrogens in certain animal species increases the frequency of carcinomas of the breast, cervix, vagina, and liver. There are now reports that estrogens increase the risk of carcinoma of the endometrium in humans. (See Boxed Warning.)

At the present time there is no satisfactory evidence that estrogens given to postmenopausal women increase the risk of cancer of the breast,[17] although a recent, long-term follow-up of a single physician's practice has raised this possibility.[18] Because of the animal data, there is a need for caution in prescribing estrogens for women with a strong family history of breast cancer or who have breast nodules, fibrocystic disease, or abnormal mammograms.

2. *Gallbladder disease.* A recent study has reported a 2- to 3-fold increase in the risk of surgically confirmed gallbladder disease in women receiving postmenopausal estrogens,[17] similar to the 2-fold increase previously noted in users of oral contraceptives.[19,24a]

3. *Effects similar to those caused by estrogen-progestogen oral contraceptives.* There are several serious adverse effects of oral contraceptives, most of which have not, up to now, been documented as consequences of postmenopausal estrogen therapy. This may reflect the comparatively low doses of estrogen used in postmenopausal women. It would be expected that the larger doses of estrogen used to treat prostatic or breast cancer or postpartum breast engorgement, are more likely to result in these adverse effects, and, in fact, it has been shown that there is an increased risk of thrombosis in men receiving estrogens for prostatic cancer and women for postpartum breast engorgement.[20–23]

a. *Thromboembolic disease.* It is now well established that users of oral contraceptives have an increased risk of various thromboembolic and thrombotic vascular diseases, such as thrombophlebitis, pulmonary embolism, stroke, and myocardial infarction.[24–31] Cases of retinal thrombosis, mesenteric thrombosis, and optic neuritis have been reported in oral contraceptive users. There is evidence that the risk of several of these adverse reactions is related to the dose of the drug.[32,33] An increased risk of postsurgery thromboembolic complications has also been reported in users of oral contraceptives.[34,35] If feasible, estrogen should be discontinued at least 4 weeks before surgery of the type associated with an increased risk of thromboembolism, or during periods of prolonged immobilization.

While an increased rate of thromboembolic and thrombotic disease in postmenopausal users of estrogens has not been found,[17–24,25–36] this does not rule out the possibility that such an increase may be present or that subgroups of women who have underlying risk factors or who are receiving relatively large doses of estrogens may have increased risk. Therefore estrogens should not be used in persons with active thrombophlebitis or thromboembolic disorders, and they should not be used (except in treatment of malignancy) in persons with a history of such disorders in association with estrogen use. They should be used with caution in patients with cerebral vascular or coronary artery disease and only for those in whom estrogens are clearly needed.

Large doses of estrogen (5 mg conjugated estrogens per day), comparable to those used to treat cancer of the prostate and breast, have been shown in a large prospective clinical trial in men[37] to increase the risk of nonfatal myocardial infarction, pulmonary embolism and thrombophlebitis. When estrogen doses of this size are used, any of the thromboembolic and thrombotic adverse effects associated with oral-contraceptive use should be considered a clear risk.

b. *Hepatic adenoma.* Benign hepatic adenomas appear to be associated with the use of oral contraceptives.[38–40] Although benign, and rare, these may rupture and may cause death through intra-abdominal hemorrhage. Such lesions have not yet been reported in association with other estrogen or progestogen preparations but should be considered in estrogen users having abdominal pain and tenderness, abdominal mass, or hypovolemic shock. Hepatocellular carcinoma has also been reported in women taking estrogen-containing oral contraceptives.[39] The relationship of this malignancy to these drugs is not known at this time.

c. *Elevated blood pressure.* Women using oral contraceptives sometimes experience increased blood pressure which, in most cases, returns to normal on discontinuing the drug. There is now a report that this may occur with use of estrogens in the menopause[41] and blood pressure should be monitored with estrogen use, especially if high doses are used.

d. *Glucose tolerance.* A worsening of glucose tolerance has been observed in a significant percentage of patients on estrogen-containing oral contraceptives. For this reason, diabetic patients should be carefully observed while receiving estrogen.

4. *Hypercalcemia.* Administration of estrogens may lead to severe hypercalcemia in patients with breast cancer and bone metastases. If this occurs, the drug should be stopped and appropriate measures taken to reduce the serum calcium level.

Associated with Methyltestosterone

In patients with breast cancer, androgen therapy may cause hypercalcemia by stimulating osteolysis. In this case, the drug should be discontinued.

Prolonged use of high doses of androgens has been associated with the development of peliosis hepatis and hepatic neoplasms including hepatocellular carcinoma. (See PRECAUTIONS—*Carcinogenesis*). Peliosis hepatis can be a life-threatening or fatal complication.

Cholestatic hepatitis and jaundice occur with 17-alpha-alkylandrogens at a relatively low dose. If cholestatic hepatitis with jaundice appears, or if liver function tests become abnormal, the androgen should be discontinued and the etiology should be determined. Drug-induced jaundice is reversible when the medication is discontinued.

Edema with or without heart failure may be a serious complication in patients with pre-existing cardiac, renal, or hepatic disease. In addition to discontinuation of the drug, diuretic therapy may be required.

PRECAUTIONS

Associated with Estrogens

A. General Precautions.

1. A complete medical and family history should be taken prior to the initiation of any estrogen therapy. The pretreatment and periodic physical examinations should include special reference to blood pressure, breasts, abdomen, and pelvic organs, and should include a Papanicolaou smear. As a general rule, estrogen should not be prescribed for longer than one year without another physical examination being performed.

2. Fluid retention—Because estrogens may cause some degree of fluid retention, conditions which might be influenced by this factor such as asthma, epilepsy, migraine, and cardiac or renal dysfunction, require careful observation.

3. Certain patients may develop undesirable manifestations of excessive estrogenic stimulation, such as abnormal or excessive uterine bleeding, mastodynia, etc.

4. Prolonged administration of unopposed estrogen therapy has been reported to increase the risk of endometrial hyperplasia in some patients.

5. Oral contraceptives appear to be associated with an increased incidence of mental depression.[24a] Although it is not clear whether this is due to the estrogenic or progestogenic component of the contraceptive, patients with a history of depression should be carefully observed.

6. Pre-existing uterine leiomyomata may increase in size during estrogen use.

7. The pathologist should be advised of estrogen therapy when relevant specimens are submitted.

8. Patients with a past history of jaundice during pregnancy have an increased risk of recurrence of jaundice while receiving estrogen-containing oral contraceptive therapy. If jaundice develops in any patient receiving estrogen, the medication should be discontinued while the cause is investigated.

9. Estrogens may be poorly metabolized in patients with impaired liver function and they should be administered with caution in such patients.

10. Because estrogens influence the metabolism of calcium and phosphorus, they should be used with caution in patients with metabolic bone diseases that are associated with hypercalcemia or in patients with renal insufficiency.

11. Because of the effects of estrogens on epiphyseal closure, they should be used judiciously in young patients in whom bone growth is not yet complete.

12. Certain endocrine and liver function tests may be affected by estrogen-containing oral contraceptives. The following similar changes may be expected with larger doses of estrogen.

a. Increased sulfobromophthalein retention.

b. Increased prothrombin and factors VII, VIII, IX, and X; decreased antithrombin 3; increased norepinephrine-induced platelet aggregability.

c. Increased thyroid binding globulin (TBG) leading to increased circulating total thyroid hormone, as measured by PBI, T4 by column, or T4 by radioimmunoassay. Free T3 resin uptake is decreased, reflecting the elevated TBG; free T4 concentration is unaltered.

d. Impaired glucose tolerance.

e. Decreased pregnanediol excretion.

f. Reduced response to metyrapone test.

g. Reduced serum folate concentration.

h. Increased serum triglyceride and phospholipid concentration.

Concomitant Progestin Use: The lowest effective dose appropiate for the specific indication should be utilized. Studies of the addition of a progestin for 7 or more days of a cycle of estrogen administration have reported a lowered incidence of endometrial hyperplasia. Morphological and biochemical studies of the endometrium suggest that 10 to 13 days of progestin are needed to provide maximal maturation of the endometrium and to eliminate any hyperplastic changes. Whether this will provide protection from endometrial carcinoma has not been clearly established. There are possible additional risks which may be associated with the inclusion of progestin in estrogen replacement regimens. If concomitant progestin therapy is used, potential risks may include adverse effects on carbohydrate and lipid metabolism. The choice of progestin and dosage may be important in minimizing these adverse effects.

B. Information for the Patient. (See text which appears after the PHYSICIAN REFERENCES.)

C. Pregnancy Category X. See CONTRAINDICATIONS and Boxed Warning.

D. Nursing Mothers. As a general principle, the administration of any drug to nursing mothers should be done only when clearly necessary since many drugs are excreted in human milk.

Associated with Methyltestosterone

A. General Precautions

1. Women should be observed for signs of virilization (deepening of the voice, hirsutism, acne, clitoromegaly, and menstrual irregularities). Discontinuation of drug therapy at the time of evidence of mild virilism is necessary to prevent irreversible virilization. Such virilization is usual following androgen use at high doses.

2. Prolonged dosage of androgen may result in sodium and fluid retention. This may present a problem, especially in patients with compromised cardiac reserve or renal disease.

3. Hypersensitivity may occur rarely.

4. PBI may be decreased in patients taking androgens.

5. Hypercalcemia may occur. If this does occur, the drug should be discontinued.

B. Information for the Patient

The physician should instruct patients to report any of the following side effects of androgens:

Women: Hoarseness, acne, changes in menstrual periods, or more hair on the face.

All Patients: Any nausea, vomiting, changes in skin color or ankle swelling.

C. Laboratory Tests

1. Women with disseminated breast carcinoma should have frequent determination of urine and serum calcium levels during the course of androgen therapy (See WARNINGS).

2. Because of the hepatotoxicity associated with the use of 17-alpha-alkylated androgens, liver function tests should be obtained periodically.

3. Hemoglobin and hematocrit should be checked periodically for polycythemia in patients who are receiving high doses of androgens.

D. Drug Interactions

1. *Anticoagulants* C-17 substituted derivatives of testosterone, such as methandrostenolone, have been reported to decrease the anticoagulant requirements of patients receiving oral anticoagulants. Patients receiving oral anticoagulant therapy require close monitoring, especially when androgens are started or stopped.

2. *Oxyphenbutazone.* Concurrent administration of oxyphenbutazone and androgens may result in elevated serum levels of oxyphenbutazone.

3. *Insulin.* In diabetic patients the metabolic effects of androgens may decrease blood glucose and insulin requirements.

E. Drug/Laboratory Test Interferences

Androgens may decrease levels of thyroxine-binding globulin, resulting in decreased T_4 serum levels and increased resin uptake of T_3 and T_4. Free thyroid hormone levels remain unchanged, however, and there is no clinical evidence of thyroid dysfunction.

F. Carcinogenesis

Animal Data. Testosterone has been tested by subcutaneous injection and implantation in mice and rats. The implant induced cervical-uterine tumors in mice, which metastasized in some cases. There is suggestive evidence that injection of testosterone into some strains of female mice increases their susceptibility to hepatoma. Testosterone is also known to increase the number of tumors and decrease the degree of differentiation of chemically induced carcinomas of the liver in rats.

Human Data. There are rare reports of hepatocellular carcinoma in patients receiving long-term therapy with androgens in high doses. Withdrawal of the drugs did not lead to regression of the tumors in all cases.

Geriatric patients treated with androgens may be at an increased risk for the development of prostatic hypertrophy and prostatic carcinoma.

G. Pregnancy

Teratogenic Effects. Pregnancy Category X (see CONTRAINDICATIONS).

H. Nursing Mothers

It is not known whether androgens are excreted in human milk. Because many drugs are excreted in human milk and because of the potential for serious adverse reactions in nursing infants from estrogens, a decision should be made whether to discontinue nursing or to discontinue the drug, taking into account the importance of the drug to the mother.

ADVERSE REACTIONS

Associated with Estrogens

(See WARNINGS regarding induction of neoplasia, adverse effects on the fetus, increased incidence of gallbladder disease, and adverse effects similar to those of oral contraceptives, including thromboembolism.) The following additional adverse reactions have been reported with estrogenic therapy, including oral contraceptives:

1. *Genitourinary system:* Breakthrough bleeding, spotting, change in menstrual flow; dysmenorrhea; premenstrual-like syndrome; amenorrhea during and after treatment; increase in size of uterine fibromyomata; vaginal candidiasis; change in cervical erosion and in degree of cervical secretion; cystitis-like syndrome.

2. *Breasts:* Tenderness, enlargement, secretion.

3. *Gastrointestinal:* Nausea, vomiting; abdominal cramps, bloating; cholestatic jaundice.

4. *Skin:* Chloasma or melasma which may persist when drug is discontinued; erythema multiforme; erythema nodosum; hemorrhagic eruption; loss of scalp hair; hirsutism.

5. *Eyes:* Steepening of corneal curvature; intolerance to contact lenses.

6. *CNS:* Headache, migraine, dizziness; mental depression; chorea.

7. *Miscellaneous:* Increase or decrease in weight; reduced carbohydrate tolerance; aggravation of porphyria; edema; changes in libido.

Associated with Methyltestosterone

A. Endocrine and Urogenital

1. *Female:* The most common side effects of androgen therapy are amenorrhea and other menstrual irregularities, inhibition of gonadotropin secretion, and virilization, including deepening of the voice and clitoral enlargement. The latter usually is not reversible after androgens are discontinued. When administered to a pregnant woman androgens cause virilization of external genitalia of the female fetus.

2. *Skin and Appendages:* Hirsutism, male pattern of baldness, and acne.

3. *Fluid and Electrolyte Disturbances:* Retention of sodium, chloride, water, potassium, calcium, and inorganic phosphates.

4. *Gastrointestinal:* Nausea, cholestatic jaundice, alterations in liver function test, rarely hepatocellular neoplasms, and peliosis hepatis (see WARNINGS).

5. *Hematologic:* Suppression of clotting factors II, V, VII, and X, bleeding in patients on concomitant anticoagulant therapy, and polycythemia.

6. *Nervous System:* Increased or decreased libido, headache, anxiety, depression, and generalized paresthesia.

7. *Metabolic:* Increased serum cholesterol.

8. *Miscellaneous:* Inflammation and pain at the site of intramuscular injection or subcutaneous implantation of testosterone-containing pellets, stomatitis with buccal preparations, and rarely anaphylactoid reactions.

ACUTE OVERDOSAGE

Numerous reports of ingestion of large doses of estrogen-containing oral contraceptives by young children indicate that acute serious ill effects do not occur. Overdosage of estrogens may cause nausea, and withdrawal bleeding may occur in females.

There have been no reports of acute overdosage with the androgens.

DOSAGE AND ADMINISTRATION

Given cyclically for short-term use only:

For treatment of moderate-to-severe *vasomotor* symptoms associated with the menopause in patients not improved by estrogen alone.

The lowest dose that will control symptoms should be chosen and medication should be discontinued as promptly as possible.

Administration should be cyclic (eg, three weeks on and one week off).

Attempts to discontinue or taper medication should be made at 3- to 6-month intervals.

Usual dosage range:

1.25 mg Conjugated Estrogens, USP, and 10.0 mg Methyltestosterone (1 yellow tablet, No. 879, or 2 maroon tablets, No. 878), daily and cyclically.

Treated patients with an intact uterus should be monitored closely for signs of endometrial cancer and appropriate diagnostic measures should be taken to rule out malignancy in the event of persistent or recurring abnormal vaginal bleeding.

HOW SUPPLIED

PREMARIN (conjugated estrogens, USP) with Methyltestosterone Tablets

—Each round *yellow* tablet contains 1.25 mg PREMARIN and 10.0 mg Methyltestosterone, in bottles of 100 (NDC 0046-0879-81).

—Each round *maroon* tablet contains 0.625 mg PREMARIN and 5.0 mg Methyltestosterone, in bottles of 100 (NDC 0046-0878-81).

The appearance of these tablets is a trademark of Wyeth-Ayerst Laboratories.

Store at room temperature (approximately 25° C).

PHYSICIAN REFERENCES

1. Ziel, H. K., et al.: N. Engl. J. Med. 293:1167–1170, 1975.
2. Smith, D. C., et al.: N. Engl. J. Med. 293:1164–1167, 1975.
3. Mack, T. M., et al.: N. Engl. J. Med. 294:1262–1267, 1976.
4. Weiss, N. S., et al.: N. Engl. J. Med. 294:1259–1262, 1976.
5. Herbst, A. L., et al.: N. Engl. J. Med. 284:878–881, 1971.
6. Greenwald, P., et al.: N. Engl. J. Med. 285:390–392, 1971.
7. Lanier, A., et al.: Mayo Clin. Proc. 48:793–799, 1973.
8. Herbst, A., et al.: Obstet. Gynecol. 40:287–298, 1972.
9. Herbst, A., et al.: Am. J. Obstet. Gynecol. 118:607–615, 1974.
10. Herbst, A., et al.: N. Engl. J. Med. 292:334–339, 1975.
11. Stafl, A., et al.: Obstet. Gynecol. 43:118–128, 1974.
12. Sherman, A. I., et al.: Obstet. Gynecol. 44:531–545, 1974.
13. Gal, I., et al.: Nature 216:83, 1967.
14. Levy, E. P., et al.: Lancet 1:611, 1973.
15. Nora, J., et al.: Lancet 1:941–942, 1973.
16. Janerich, D. T., et al.: N. Engl. J. Med. 291:697–700, 1974.
17. Boston Collaborative Drug Surveillance Program: N. Engl. J. Med. 290:15–19, 1974.
18. Hoover, R., et al.: N. Engl. J. Med. 295:401–405, 1976.
19. Boston Collaborative Drug Surveillance Program: Lancet 1:1399–1404, 1973.
20. Daniel, D. G., et al.: Lancet 2:287–289, 1967.
21. The Veterans Administration Cooperative Urological Research Group: J. Urol. 98:516–522, 1967.
22. Bailar, J. C.: Lancet 2:560, 1967.
23. Blackard, C., et al.: Cancer 26:249–256, 1970.
24. Royal College of General Practitioners: J. R. Coll. Gen. Pract. 13:267–279, 1967.
24a. Royal College of General Practitioners: Oral Contraceptives and Health, New York, Pitman Corp., 1974.
25. Inman, W. H. W., et al.: Br. Med. J. 2:193–199, 1968.
26. Vessey, M. P., et al.: Br. Med. J. 2:651–657, 1969.
27. Sartwell, P. E., et al.: Am. J. Epidemiol. 90:365–380, 1969.
28. Collaborative Group for the Study of Stroke in Young Women: N. Engl. J. Med. 288:871–878, 1973.
29. Collaborative Group for the Study of Stroke in Young Women: J.A.M.A. 231:718–722, 1975.
30. Mann, J. I., et al.: Br. Med. J. 2:245–248, 1975.
31. Mann, J. I., et al.: Br. Med. J. 2:241–245, 1975.
32. Inman, W. H. W., et al.: Br. Med. J. 2:203–209, 1970.
33. Stolley, P. D., et al.: Am. J. Epidemiol. 102:197–208, 1975.
34. Vessey, M. P., et al.: Br. Med. J. 3:123–126, 1970.
35. Greene, G. R., et al.: Am. J. Public Health 62:680–685, 1972.
36. Rosenberg, L., et al.: N. Engl. J. Med. 294:1256–1259, 1976.
37. Coronary Drug Project Research Group: J.A.M.A. 214:1303–1313, 1970.
38. Baum, J., et al.: Lancet 2:926–928, 1973.
39. Mays, E. T., et al.: J.A.M.A. 235:730–732, 1976.
40. Edmondson, H. A., et al.: N. Engl. J. Med. 294:470–472, 1976.
41. Pfeffer, R. I., et al.: Am. J. Epidemiol. 103:445–456, 1976.

Androgen references available upon request.

INFORMATION FOR THE PATIENT

WHAT YOU SHOULD KNOW ABOUT ESTROGENS

Estrogens are female hormones produced by the ovaries. The ovaries make several different kinds of estrogens. In addition, scientists have been able to make a variety of synthetic estrogens. As far as we know, all these estrogens have similar properties and, therefore, much the same usefulness, side effects, and risks. This leaflet is intended to help you understand what estrogens are used for, the risks involved in their use, and how to use them as safely as possible.

This leaflet includes the most important information about estrogens, but not all the information. If you want to know more, you should ask your doctor for more information or you can ask your doctor or pharmacist to let you read the package insert prepared for the doctor.

USES OF ESTROGEN

THERE IS NO PROPER USE OF ESTROGENS IN A PREGNANT WOMAN.

Estrogens are prescribed by doctors for a number of purposes, including:

1. To provide estrogen during a period of adjustment when a woman's ovaries stop producing a majority of her estrogens, in order to prevent certain uncomfortable symptoms of estrogen deficiency. (With the menopause, which generally occurs between the ages of 45 and 55, women produce a much smaller amount of estrogens.)

2. To prevent symptoms of estrogen deficiency when a woman's ovaries have been removed surgically before the natural menopause.

3. To prevent pregnancy. (Estrogens are given along with a progestogen, another female hormone; these combinations are called oral contraceptives or birth control pills. Patient labeling is available to women taking oral contraceptives and they will not be discussed in this leaflet.)

4. To treat certain cancers in women and men.

5. To prevent painful swelling of the breasts after pregnancy in women who choose not to nurse their babies.

ESTROGENS IN THE MENOPAUSE

In the natural course of their lives, all women eventually experience a decrease in estrogen production. This usually occurs between ages 45 and 55, but may occur earlier or later. Sometimes the ovaries may need to be removed before natural menopause by an operation, producing a "surgical menopause."

When the amount of estrogen in the blood begins to decrease, many women may develop typical symptoms: feelings of warmth in the face, neck, and chest or sudden intense episodes of heat and sweating throughout the body (called "hot flashes" or "hot flushes"). These symptoms are sometimes very uncomfortable. Some women may also develop changes in the vagina (called "atrophic vaginitis") that cause discomfort, especially during and after intercourse.

Estrogens can be prescribed to treat these symptoms of the menopause. It is estimated that considerably more than half of all women undergoing the menopause have only mild symptoms or no symptoms at all and, therefore, do not need estrogens. Other women may need estrogens for a few months, while their bodies adjust to lower estrogen levels. Sometimes the need will be for periods longer than six

Continued on next page

Wyeth-Ayerst—Cont.

months. In an attempt to avoid overstimulation of the uterus (womb), estrogens are usually given cyclically during each month of use, such as three weeks of pills followed by one week without pills.

Sometimes women experience nervous symptoms or depression during menopause. There is no evidence that estrogens are effective for such symptoms without associated vasomotor symptoms. In the absence of vasomotor symptoms, estrogens should not be used to treat nervous symptoms, although other treatment may be needed.

You may have heard that taking estrogens for long periods (years) after the menopause will keep your skin soft and supple and keep you feeling young. There is no evidence that this is so, however, and such long-term treatment carries important risks.

ESTROGENS TO PREVENT SWELLING OF THE BREASTS AFTER PREGNANCY

If you do not breast-feed your baby after delivery, your breasts may fill up with milk and become painful and engorged. This usually begins about 3 to 4 days after delivery and may last for a few days to up to a week or more. Sometimes the discomfort is severe, but usually it is not and can be controlled by pain-relieving drugs such as aspirin and by binding the breasts up tightly. Estrogens can be used to try to prevent the breasts from filling up. While this treatment is sometimes successful, in many cases the breasts fill up to some degree in spite of treatment. The dose of estrogens needed to prevent pain and swelling of the breasts is much larger than the dose needed to treat symptoms of the menopause and this may increase your chances of developing blood clots in the legs or lungs (see below). Therefore, it is important that you discuss the benefits and the risks of estrogen use with your doctor if you have decided not to breast-feed your baby.

THE DANGERS OF ESTROGENS

1. *Endometrial cancer.* There are reports that if estrogens are used in the postmenopausal period for more than a year, there is an increased risk of *endometrial cancer* (cancer of the lining of the uterus). Women taking estrogens have roughly 5- to 10-times as great a chance of getting this cancer as women who take no estrogens. To put this another way, while a postmenopausal woman not taking estrogens has 1 chance in 1,000 each year of getting endometrial cancer, a woman taking estrogens has 5 to 10 chances in 1,000 each year. For this reason *it is important to take estrogens only when they are really needed.*

The risk of this cancer is greater the longer estrogens are used and when larger doses are taken. Therefore you should not take more estrogen than your doctor prescribes. *It is important to take the lowest dose of estrogen that will control symptoms and to take it only as long as it is needed.* If estrogens are needed for longer periods of time, your doctor will want to reevaluate your need for estrogens at least every six months.

Women using estrogens should report any vaginal bleeding to their doctors; such bleeding may be of no importance, but it can be an early warning of endometrical cancer. If you have undiagnosed vaginal bleeding, you should not use estrogens until a diagnosis is made and you are certain there is no endometrial cancer.

NOTE: If you have had your uterus removed (total hysterectomy), there is no danger of developing endometrial cancer.

2. *Other possible cancers.* Estrogens can cause development of other tumors in animals, such as tumors of the breast, cervix, vagina, or liver, when given for a long time. At present there is no good evidence that women using estrogen in the menopause have an increased risk of such tumors, but there is no way yet to be sure they do not; and one study raises the possibility that use of estrogens in the menopause may increase the risk of breast cancer many years later. This is a further reason to use estrogens only when clearly needed. While you are taking estrogens, it is important that you go to your doctor at least once a year for a physical examination. Also, if members of your family have had breast cancer or if you have breast nodules or abnormal mammograms (breast x-rays), your doctor may wish to carry out more frequent examinations of your breasts.

3. *Gallbladder disease.* Women who use estrogens after menopause are more likely to develop gallbladder disease needing surgery than women who do not use estrogens. Birth control pills have a similar effect.

4. *Abnormal blood clotting.* Oral contraceptives increase the risk of blood clotting in various parts of the body. This can result in a stroke (if the clot is in the brain), a heart attack (if the clot is in a blood vessel of the heart), or a pulmonary embolus (a clot which forms in the legs or pelvis, then breaks off and travels to the lungs). Any of these can be fatal.

At this time, use of estrogens in the menopause is not known to cause such blood clotting, but this has not been fully studied and there could still prove to be such a risk. It is recommended that if you have had clotting in the legs or lungs or a heart attack or stroke while you were using estrogens or birth control pills, you should not use estrogens (unless they are being used to treat cancer of the breast or prostate). If you have had a stroke or heart attack, or if you have angina pectoris, estrogens should be used with great caution and only if clearly needed (for example, if you have severe symptoms of the menopause).

The larger doses of estrogen used to prevent swelling of the breasts after pregnancy have been reported to cause clotting in the legs and lungs.

SPECIAL WARNING ABOUT PREGNANCY

You should not receive estrogen if you are pregnant. If this should occur, there is a greater than usual chance that the developing child will be born with a birth defect, although the possibility remains fairly small. A female child may have an increased risk of developing cancer of the vagina or cervix later in life (in the teens or twenties). Every possible effort should be made to avoid exposure to estrogens during pregnancy. If exposure occurs, see your doctor.

OTHER EFFECTS OF ESTROGENS

In addition to the serious known risks of estrogens described above, estrogens have the following side effects and potential risks:

1. *Nausea and vomiting.* The most common side effect of estrogen therapy is nausea. Vomiting is less common.

2. *Effects on breasts.* Estrogens may cause breast tenderness or enlargement and may cause the breasts to secrete a liquid. These effects are not dangerous.

3. *Effects on the uterus.* Estrogens may cause benign fibroid tumors of the uterus to get larger.

4. *Effects on liver.* Women taking oral contraceptives develop, on rare occasions, a tumor of the liver which can rupture and bleed into the abdomen and may cause death. So far, these tumors have not been reported in women using estrogens in the menopause, but you should report any swelling or unusual pain or tenderness in the abdomen to your doctor immediately.

Women with a past history of jaundice (yellowing of the skin and white parts of the eyes) may get jaundice again during estrogen use. If this occurs, stop taking estrogens and see your doctor.

5. *Other effects.* Estrogens may cause excess fluid to be retained in the body. This may make some conditions worse, such as asthma, epilepsy, migraine, heart disease, or kidney disease.

SUMMARY

Estrogens have important uses, but they have serious risks as well. You must decide, with your doctor, whether the risks are acceptable to you in view of the benefits of treatment. Except where your doctor has prescribed estrogens for use in special cases of cancer of the breast or prostate, you should not use estrogens if you have cancer of the breast or uterus, are pregnant, have undiagnosed abnormal vaginal bleeding, clotting in the legs or lungs, or have had a stroke, heart attack or angina, or clotting in the legs or lungs in the past while you were taking estrogens.

You can use estrogens as safely as possible by understanding that your doctor will require physical examinations while you are taking them and will try to discontinue the drug as soon as possible and use the smallest dose possible. Be alert for signs of trouble including:

1. Abnormal bleeding from the vagina.
2. Pains in the calves or chest or sudden shortness of breath, or coughing blood.
3. Severe headache, dizziness, faintness, or changes in vision.
4. Breast lumps (you should ask your doctor how to examine your own breasts).
5. Jaundice (yellowing of the skin).
6. Mental depression.

Your doctor has prescribed this drug for you and you alone. Do not give the drug to anyone else.

HOW SUPPLIED

PREMARIN® (conjugated estrogens tablets, USP)—tablets for oral administration.

Each oval *purple* tablet contains 2.5 mg
Each oval *yellow* tablet contains 1.25 mg
Each oval *white* tablet contains 0.9 mg
Each oval *maroon* tablet contains 0.625 mg
Each oval *green* tablet contains 0.3 mg

PREMARIN® with METHYLTESTOSTERONE—a combination of PREMARIN and methyltestosterone (an androgen) in tablet form for oral administration.

Each round *yellow* tablet contains 1.25 mg PREMARIN and 10.0 mg methyltestosterone
Each round *maroon* tablet contains 0.625 mg PREMARIN and 5 mg methyltestosterone

PMB® 200, 400—a combination of PREMARIN® and meprobamate (a tranquilizing agent) in tablet form for oral administration.

Each oblong *green* tablet contains 0.45 mg PREMARIN and 200 mg meprobamate
Each oblong *pink* tablet contains 0.45 mg PREMARIN and 400 mg meprobamate

The appearance of these tablets is a trademark of Wyeth-Ayerst Laboratories.

PREMARIN® VAGINAL CREAM—PREMARIN® in a nonliquefying base, designed for vaginal use.
PREMARIN® INTRAVENOUS—PREMARIN® specially prepared for intravenous and intramuscular use.
ESTROGENIC SUBSTANCE (estrone) in Aqueous Suspension—a sterile aqueous suspension of estrone, a short-acting estrogen, for intramuscular injection only.

Shown in Product Identification Section, page 437

PROTOPAM® CHLORIDE   ℞
[prō"tō-pam klaw'rīde]
Brand of pralidoxime chloride

CAUTION: Federal law prohibits dispensing without prescription.

DESCRIPTION

PROTOPAM CHLORIDE is a cholinesterase reactivator. Chemically, it is 2-formyl-1-methylpyridinium chloride oxime (pyridine-2-aldoxime methochloride), and has the generic name pralidoxime chloride. It has also been referred to as 2-PAM Chloride.
The chemical structure is:

PROTOPAM CHLORIDE occurs as a white, nonhygroscopic, crystalline powder which is soluble in water to the extent of 1 g in less than 1 mL.

The specific activity of the drug resides in the 2-formyl-1-methylpyridinium ion and is independent of the particular salt employed.

PROTOPAM CHLORIDE Tablets contain the following inactive ingredients: citric acid, magnesium stearate, methylcellulose, and microcrystalline cellulose.

ACTIONS

The principal action of PROTOPAM is to reactivate cholinesterase (mainly outside of the central nervous system) which has been inactivated by phosphorylation due to an organophosphate pesticide or related compound. The destruction of accumulated acetylcholine can then proceed and neuromuscular junctions will again function normally. PROTOPAM also slows the process of "aging" of phosphorylated cholinesterase to a non-reactivatable form, and detoxifies certain organophosphates by direct chemical reaction. The drug has its most critical effect in relieving paralysis of the muscles of respiration. Because PROTOPAM is less effective in relieving depression of the respiratory center, atropine is always required concomitantly to block the effect of accumulated acetylcholine at this site. PROTOPAM relieves muscarinic signs and symptoms, salivation, bronchospasm, etc., but this action is relatively unimportant since atropine is adequate for this purpose.

PROTOPAM antagonizes the effects on the neuromuscular junction of the carbamate anticholinesterases, neostigmine, pyridostigmine and ambenonium, used in the treatment of myasthenia gravis. However, it is not nearly as effective as an antidote to these drugs as it is to the organophosphates. PROTOPAM (pralidoxime) is distributed throughout the extracellular water; it is not bound to plasma protein. The drug is rapidly excreted in the urine partly unchanged, and partly as a metabolite produced by the liver. Consequently, PROTOPAM is relatively short acting and repeated doses may be needed, especially where there is any evidence of continuing absorption of the poison.

INDICATIONS

PROTOPAM is indicated as an antidote: (1) in the treatment of poisoning due to those pesticides and chemicals of the organophosphate class which have anticholinesterase activity, and (2) in the control of overdosage by anticholinesterase drugs used in the treatment of myasthenia gravis.

WARNINGS

Use of PROTOPAM should always be under supervision of the subject's personal physician or of the medical department of his employer.

PROTOPAM is not effective in the treatment of poisoning due to phosphorus, inorganic phosphates or organophosphates not having anticholinesterase activity.

Until further information is available, no recommendation is made as to the use of PROTOPAM in intoxication by pesticides of the carbamate class.

PRECAUTIONS

PROTOPAM has been very well tolerated in most cases, but it must be remembered that the desperate condition of the organophosphate-poisoned patient will generally mask such minor signs and symptoms as have been noted in normal subjects.

Intravenous administration of PROTOPAM should be carried out slowly and, preferably, by infusion, since certain side effects, such as tachycardia, laryngospasm, and muscle rigidity, have been attributed in a few cases to a too rapid rate of injection. (See DOSAGE AND ADMINISTRATION.) Because PROTOPAM is excreted in the urine, a decrease in renal function will result in increased blood levels of the drug. Thus, the dosage of PROTOPAM should be reduced in the presence of renal insufficiency.

PROTOPAM should be used with great caution in treating organophosphate overdosage in cases of myasthenia gravis since it may precipitate a myasthenic crisis.

The following precautions should be kept in mind in the treatment of anticholinesterase poisoning, although they do not bear directly on the use of PROTOPAM (pralidoxime): since barbiturates are potentiated by the anticholinesterases, they should be used cautiously in the treatment of convulsions; morphine, theophylline, aminophylline, succinylcholine, reserpine, and phenothiazine-type tranquilizers should be avoided in patients with organophosphate poisoning.

ADVERSE REACTIONS

Dizziness, blurred vision, diplopia and impaired accommodation, headache, drowsiness, nausea, tachycardia, hyperventilation, and muscular weakness have been reported after the use of PROTOPAM, but it is very difficult to differentiate the toxic effects produced by atropine or the organophosphate compounds from those of the drug. When atropine and PROTOPAM are used together, the signs of atropinization may occur earlier than might be expected when atropine is used alone. This is especially true if the total dose of atropine has been large and the administration of PROTOPAM has been delayed. Excitement and manic behavior immediately following recovery of consciousness have been reported in several cases. However, similar behavior has occurred in cases of organophosphate poisoning that were not treated with PROTOPAM.

DOSAGE AND ADMINISTRATION

Organophosphate poisoning

Initial measures should include removal of secretions, maintenance of a patent airway and, if necessary, artificial ventilation.

In the absence of cyanosis, atropine should be given intravenously in doses of 2 to 4 mg; where cyanosis is present, this dose of atropine should be given intramuscularly while simultaneously initiating measures for improving ventilation. Atropine administration should be repeated at 5 to 10 minute intervals until signs of atropine toxicity appear. Some degree of atropinization should be maintained for at least 48 hours.

PROTOPAM administration should be started at the same time as atropine.

In adults, inject an initial dose of 1 to 2 g of PROTOPAM, preferably as an infusion in 100 mL of saline, over a 15 to 30 minute period. If this is not practicable or if pulmonary edema is present, the dose should be given slowly by intravenous injection as a 5 percent solution in water over not less than five minutes. After about an hour, a second dose of 1 to 2 g will be indicated if muscle weakness has not been relieved. Additional doses may be given cautiously if muscle weakness persists. If intravenous administration is not feasible, intramuscular or subcutaneous injection should be used. *In children,* the dose should be 20 to 40 mg per kg.

Treatment will be most effective if given within a few hours after poisoning has occurred. Usually, little will be accomplished if the drug is first administered more than 48 hours after exposure, but in severe poisoning, it is, nevertheless, indicated since occasionally patients have responded after such an interval.

In severe cases, especially after ingestion of the poison, it may be desirable to monitor the effect of therapy electrocardiographically because of the possibility of heart block due to the anticholinesterase. Where the poison has been ingested, it is particularly important to take into account the likelihood of continuing absorption from the lower bowel since this constitutes new exposure. In such cases, additional doses of PROTOPAM (pralidoxime) may be needed every three to eight hours. In effect, the patient should be "titrated" with PROTOPAM as long as signs of poisoning recur.

In the absence of severe gastrointestinal symptoms, resulting from the anticholinesterase intoxication, PROTOPAM may be administered orally in doses of 1 to 3 g (2 to 6 tablets) every five hours. As in all cases of organophosphate poisoning, care should be taken to keep the patient under observation for at least 24 hours.

If convulsions interfere with respiration, sodium thiopental (2.5 percent solution) may be given intravenously with care.

Anticholinesterase overdosage

As an antagonist to such anticholinesterases as neostigmine, pyridostigmine, and ambenonium, which are used in the treatment of myasthenia gravis, PROTOPAM may be given in a dosage of 1 to 2 g intravenously followed by increments of 250 mg every five minutes.

OVERDOSAGE

Artificial respiration and other supportive therapy should be administered as needed.

HOW SUPPLIED

NDC 0046-0375-98—*Emergency Kit:* This contains one 20 mL vial of 1 g of sterile PROTOPAM CHLORIDE (pralidoxime chloride) white to off white porous cake*; one 20 mL ampul of sterile diluent without preservatives (consisting of sterile water); sterile, disposable 20 mL syringe; needle; alcohol swab. This is a single dose kit for intravenous administration. Intramuscular or subcutaneous injection may be used when intravenous injection is not feasible.

NDC 0046-0374-06—*Hospital Package:* This contains six 20 mL vials of 1 g each of sterile PROTOPAM CHLORIDE (pralidoxime chloride) white to off white porous cake*, without diluent or syringe. Solution may be prepared by adding 20 mL of Sterile Water for Injection, USP, or sterile diluent as provided in Emergency Kit (NDC 0046-0375-98). These are single dose vials for intravenous injection or for intravenous infusion after further dilution with physiologic saline. Intramuscular or subcutaneous injection may be used when intravenous injection is not feasible.

*When necessary, either 1N hydrochloric acid or 1N sodium hydroxide may be added during processing to adjust the pH.

PROTOPAM CHLORIDE for Injection is prepared by cryodesiccation.

A FULL DISCUSSION OF THE ACTIONS AND USES OF PROTOPAM (PRALIDOXIME) IS GIVEN IN A PROFESSIONAL BROCHURE WHICH IS AVAILABLE FROM WYETH-AYERST LABORATORIES ON REQUEST.

ANIMAL PHARMACOLOGY AND TOXICOLOGY

The following table lists chemical and trade or generic names of pesticides, chemicals, and drugs against which PROTOPAM (usually administered in conjunction with atropine) has been found to have antidotal activity on the basis of animal experiments. All compounds listed are organophosphates having anticholinesterase activity. A great many additional substances are in industrial use but have been omitted because of lack of specific information.

AAT—see PARATHION

AFLIX®—see FORMOTHION

ALKRON®—see PARATHION

AMERICAN CYANAMID 3422—see PARATHION

AMITON—diethyl -S- (2-diethyl-aminoethyl) phosphorothiolate

ANTHIO®—see FORMOTHION

APHAMITE—see PARATHION

ARMIN—ethyl-4-nitrophenyl-ethylphosphonate

AZINPHOS-METHYL—dimethyl-S- (4-oxo-1, 2, 3, -benzotriazin-3 (4 H) -ylmethyl) phosphorodithioate

AZODRIN—dimethyl phosphate of 3-hydroxy-N-methyl-cis-crotonamide

BAYER 16259—see ETHYL GUTHION

BAYER 19639—see DISULFOTON

BAYER 25141— diethyl-4-methyl-sulfinylphenylphosphorothionate

BAYER 29493—see FENTHION

BAYER L13/59—see TRICHLOROFON

BAYER E605—see PARATHION

BAYTEX®—see FENTHION

CHIPMAN R6199—see AMITON

COMPOUND 3422—see PARATHION

COMPOUND 4049—see MALATHION

COMPOUND 4072— 2-chloro-1-(2,4-dichlorophenyl) vinyl diethyl-phosphate

CO-RAL®—see COUMAPHOS

COROTHION—see PARATHION

COUMAPHOS—3-chloro -4- methyl coumarin-7-yl-diethyl-phosphorothionate

DBD —see AZINPHOS-METHYL

DDVP—see DICHLORVOS

DELNAV—see DIOXATHION

DEMETON—Mixture of SYSTOX® and ISOSYSTOX®

DEMETON-S—see ISOSYSTOX®

DFP—see ISOFLUROPHATE

DIAZINON— diethyl-(2-isopropyl-4-methyl-6-pyrimidyl) phosphorothionate

DICHLORVOS—dimethyl-2, 2-dichloro vinyl phosphate

DIETHYL-p-NITROPHENYL-PHOSPHORO THIONATE—see PARATHION

DIETHYL -p- NITROPHENYL - THIONO PHOSPHATE— see PARATHION

DIOXATHION—2,3-p-dioxanedithio-S, S-bis (O,O-diethyl phosphorodithioate)

DIPTEREX®—see TRICHLOROFON

DISULFOTON—diethyl -S- (2-ethylthioethyl) phosphorodithiate

DISYSTON®—see DISULFOTON

DITHIOSYSTOX—see DISULFOTON

DNTP—see PARATHION

DPP—see PARATHION

DSDP—see AMITON

DYFLOS—see DFP

DYLOX®—see TRICHLOROFON

E 600—see PARAOXON

E 601—see METHYL PARATHION

E 605—see PARATHION

E 1059—see SYSTOX

ECHOTHIOPHATE IODIDE —diethoxyphosphinylthiocholine iodide

EKATIN®—see MORPHOTHION

ENDOTHION— 2-(dimethoxyphosphinylthiomethyl)-5-methoxy-4-pyrone

ENT 15108—see PARATHION

ENTEX®—see FENTHION

EPN— ethyl-4-nitrophenyl-phenylphosphonothionate

ETHION—O,O,O',O'-tetraethyl-S,S'-methylene-bis-phosphoro dithioate

ETHYL GUSATHION—see ETHYL GUTHION

ETHYLGUTHION® —diethyl-S-(4-oxo-1,2,3,-benzotriazinyl-3-methyl) phosphorodithioate

ETILON—see PARATHION

FENTHION—dimethyl-(4-methylthio-3-tolyl) phosphorothionate

FLOROPRYL®—see DFP

FOLIDOL®—see PARATHION

FORMOTHION—dimethyl-S-(N-formyl-N-methylcarbamylmethyl) phosphorodithioate

Continued on next page

Wyeth-Ayerst—Cont.

G 24480—see DIAZINON

GB—see SARIN

GENITHION—see PARATHION

GUSATHION®—see AZINPHOSMETHYL

GUTHION®—see AZINPHOSMETHYL

HETP—see TEPP

I-ARMIN—isopropyl-4-nitro-phenyl methylphosphonate

ISOFLUROPHATE— diisopropyl-phosphorofluoridate

ISOSYSTOX®— diethyl-S-(2-ethylmercapto-ethyl)-phosphorothiolate

LEBACYD®—see FENTHION

MACKOTHION—see PARATHION

MALATHION— dimethyl-S-(1, 2-dicarbethoxyethyl)-phosphorodithioate

MALATHON—see MALATHION

M-ARMIN—ethyl-4-nitrophenyl methylphosphonate

MECARBAM— 0,0-dimethyl-S-(N-ethoxycarbonyl-N-methyl carbamoylmethyl) phosphorodithioate

METACIDE—see METHYL PARATHION

METASYSTOX®—see METHYL DEMETON

METASYSTOX I®—dimethyl-2-ethyl-mercaptoethylphosphorothiolate

METASYSTOX R®—see OXYDEMETONMETHYL

METHYL DEMETON—mixture of dimethyl(2-ethylmercapto-ethyl) phosphorothionate and dimethyl-S-(2-ethylmercapto-ethyl) phosphorothiolate

METHYL PARATHION— dimethyl-(4-nitrophenyl) phosphorothionate

MEVINPHOS— 1-carbomethoxy-1-propen-2-yl-dimethyl-phosphate

MINTACOL®—see PARAOXON

ML 97—see PHOSPHAMIDON

MORPHOTHION— dimethyl-S-2-keto-2-(N-morpholyl ethyl-phosphorodithioate

NEGUVON®—see TRICHLOROFON

NIRAN®—see PARATHION

NITROSTIGMINE—see PARATHION

O, O-DIETHYL -O- p-NITRO-PHENYL PHOSPHOROTHI-OATE—see PARATHION

O, O-DIETHYL -O- p-NITRO-PHENYLTHIO PHOSPHATE —see PARATHION

OR 1191—see PHOSPHAMIDON

OS 1836—see VINYLPHOS

OXYDEMETONMETHYL—dimethyl-S-2-(ethylsulfinyl) ethyl phosphorothiolate

PARAOXON—diethyl (4-nitro-phenyl) phosphate.

PARATHION—diethyl (4-nitro-phenyl) phosphorothionate

PENPHOS—see PARATHION

PHENCAPTON—diethyl-S-(2, 5-dichlorophenylmercapto-methyl) phosphorodithioate

PHOSDRIN®—see MEVINPHOS

PHOS-KIL—see PARATHION

PHOSPHAMIDON—1-chloro -1- diethylcarbamoyl -1- propen -2- yl-dimethylphosphate

PHOSPHOLINE IODIDE®—see echothiophate iodide

PHOSPHOROTHIOIC ACID, 0,0-DIETHYL-0-p-NITRO-PHENYL ESTER—see PARATHION

PLANTHION—see PARATHION

QUELETOX—see FENTHION

RHODIATOX®—see PARATHION

RUELENE®— 4-tert-butyl-2-chlorophenyl-methyl-N-methyl-phosphoroamidate

SARIN— isopropyl - methylphos - phonofluoridate

SHELL OS 1836—see VINYLPHOS

SHELL 2046—see MEVINPHOS

SNP—see PARATHION

SOMAN—pinacolyl - methyl - phosphonofluoridate

SYSTOX®—diethyl - (2-ethyl-mercaptoethyl) phosphorothionate

TEP—see TEPP

TEPP—tetraethylpyro phosphate

THIOPHOS®—see PARATHION

TIGUVON—see FENTHION

TRICHLOROFON—dimethyl-1-hydroxy-2,2,2-trichloro ethylphosphonate

VAPONA®—see DICHLORVOS

VAPOPHOS—see PARATHION

VINYLPHOS—diethyl -2- chloro-vinylphosphate

PROTOPAM CHLORIDE appears to be ineffective, or marginally effective, against poisoning by:
CIODRIN® (alpha-methylbenzyl-3-[dimethoxyphosphinyl-oxy]-cis-crotonate)
DIMEFOX (tetramethylphosphorodiamidic fluoride)
DIMETHOATE (dimethyl-S-[N-methylcarbamoylmethyl]-phosphorodithioate)
METHYL DIAZINON (dimethyl-[2-isopropyl-4-methyl-pyrimidyl]-phosphorothionate)
METHYL PHENCAPTON (dimethyl-S- [2, 5-dichloro-phenylmercaptomethyl] phosphorodithioate)
PHORATE (diethyl -S- ethylmercaptomethylphosphorodi-thioate)
SCHRADAN (octamethylpyrophosphoramide)
WEPSYN® (5-amino-1-[bis-(dimethylamino)phosphinyl]-3-phenyl-1,2,4-triazole)
The use of PROTOPAM CHLORIDE should, nevertheless, be considered in any life-threatening situation resulting from poisoning by these compounds, since the limited and arbitrary conditions of pharmacologic screening do not always accurately reflect the usefulness of PROTOPAM in the clinical situation.

CLINICAL STUDIES
The use of PROTOPAM (pralidoxime) has been reported in the treatment of human cases of poisoning by the following substances:
Azodrin
Diazinon
Dichlorvos (DDVP) with chlordane
Disulfoton
EPN
Isoflurophate
Malathion
Metasystox I® and Fenthion
Methyl demeton
Methyl parathion
Mevinphos
Parathion
Parathion and Mevinphos
Phosphamidon
Sarin
Systox®
TEPP
Of these cases, over 100 were due to parathion, about a dozen each to malathion, diazinon, and mevinphos, and a few to each of the other compounds.

REFERENCES
A.M.A. Council on Drugs: New Drugs, Chicago, American Medical Association, 1967, pp. 546-8.
Calesnick, B., Christensen, J. A., and Richter, M.: Human toxicity of various oximes, Arch. Environ. Health 15:599 (Nov.) 1967.
Durham, W. F., and Hayes, W.J.: Organic phosphorus poisoning and its therapy, Arch. Environ. Health 5:21 (July) 1962.
Ellin, R. I., and Wills, J. H.: Oximes antagonistic to inhibitors of cholinesterase, Part I, J. Pharm. Sci. 53:995 (Sept) 1964; ibid. Part II, 1143 (Oct.).
Hayes, W.J.: Parathion poisoning and its treatment, J.A.M.A. 192:49 (Apr. 5) 1965.
Jager, B. V., and Stagg, G .N.: Toxicity of diacetyl monoxime and of pyridine-2-aldoxime methiodide in man, Bull. Johns Hopkins Hosp. 102:203 (Apr.) 1958.
Jager, B.V., Stagg, G .N., Green N., and Jager, L.: Studies on distribution and disappearance of pyridine-2-aldoxime methiodide (PAM) and of diacetyl monoxime (DAM) in man and in experimental animals, Bull. Johns Hopkins Hosp. 102:225 (May) 1958.
Quinby, G. E.: Further therapeutic experience with pralidoximes in organic phosphorus poisoning, J.A.M.A. 187:114 (Jan. 18) 1964.

RESOL®   OTC
[ree 'sol]
Oral Electrolyte Rehydration and Maintenance Solution

RESOL® is intended for replacement and maintenance of water and electrolytes in diarrhea with mild to moderate dehydration in children older than one week. RESOL is ready to feed and presterilized, and water should not be added. Sterilized nipples should be used.

INGREDIENTS
Water, glucose, sodium chloride, potassium citrate, citric acid, disodium phosphate, magnesium chloride, calcium chloride, and sodium citrate.

PROXIMATE ANALYSIS
One liter supplies 80 calories.

	mEq/liter	Approximate mEq/8 fl. oz. (237 mL)
Sodium	50	12
Potassium	20	4.7
Calcium	4	0.95
Magnesium	4	0.95
Chloride	50	12
Citrate	34	8.0
Phosphate (HPO_4^{-2})	5	1.2
	gram/liter	
Glucose	20	
	mOsm/kg H_2O	
Osmolality	269	

HOW SUPPLIED
Ready to feed—presterilized, 8 fluidounce bottles, cartons of 6 bottles (Hospital Package only); ready-to-feed—presterilized, 32 fluidounce cartons, cases of 6 cartons.
Shown in Product Identification Section, page 437

SECTRAL®   ℞
[sek 'tral]
(acebutolol hydrochloride)
Capsules

DESCRIPTION
Sectral® (acebutolol HCl) is a selective, hydrophilic beta-adrenoreceptor blocking agent with mild intrinsic sympathomimetic activity for use in treating patients with hypertension and ventricular arrhythmias. It is marketed in capsule form for oral administration. Sectral capsules are provided in two dosage strengths which contain 200 or 400 mg of acebutolol as the hydrochloride salt. The inactive ingredients present are D&C Red 22, FD&C Blue 1, FD&C Yellow 6, gelatin, povidone, starch, stearic acid, and titanium dioxide. The 200 mg dosage strength also contains D&C Red 28 and the 400 mg dosage strength also contains FD&C Red 40.
Acebutolol HCl has the following structural formula:

$C_{18}H_{28}N_2O_4 \cdot HCl$ M.W. 372.9

Acebutolol HCl is a white or slightly off-white powder freely soluble in water, and less soluble in alcohol. Chemically it is defined as Butanamide, N-[3-acetyl-4-[2-hydroxy-3-[(1-methylethyl)amino]propoxy]phenyl]-, (±)- or (±)-3'-Acetyl-4'-[2-hydroxy -3- (isopropylamino) propoxy] butyranilide.

CLINICAL PHARMACOLOGY

Sectral is a cardioselective, β -adrenoreceptor blocking agent, which possesses mild intrinsic sympathomimetic activity (ISA) in its therapeutically effective dose range.

PHARMACODYNAMICS

β_1-cardioselectivity has been demonstrated in experimental animal studies. In anesthetized dogs and cats, Sectral is more potent in antagonizing isoproterenol-induced tachycardia (β_1) than in antagonizing isoproterenol-induced vasodilatation (β_2). In guinea pigs and cats, it is more potent in antagonizing this tachycardia than in antagonizing isoproterenol-induced bronchodilatation (β_2). ISA of Sectral has been demonstrated in catecholamine-depleted rats by tachycardia induced by intravenous administration of this agent. A membrane-stabilizing effect has been detected in animals, but only with high concentrations of Sectral.

Clinical studies have demonstrated β_1-blocking activity at the recommended doses by: a) reduction in the resting heart rate and decrease in exercise-induced tachycardia; b) reduction in cardiac output at rest and after exercise; c) reduction of systolic and diastolic blood pressures at rest and postexercise; d) inhibition of isoproterenol-induced tachycardia.

The β_1-selectivity of Sectral has also been demonstrated on the basis of the following vascular and bronchial effects:

Vascular Effects: Sectral has less antagonistic effects on peripheral vascular β_2-receptors at rest and after epinephrine stimulation than nonselective β-antagonists.

Bronchial Effects: In single-dose studies in asthmatics examining effects of various beta-blockers on pulmonary function, low doses of acebutolol produce less evidence of bronchoconstriction and less reduction of beta$_2$ agonist, bronchodilating effects, than nonselective agents like propranolol but more than atenolol.

ISA has been observed with Sectral in man, as shown by a slightly smaller (about 3 beats per minute) decrease in resting heart rate when compared to equivalent β-blocking doses of propranolol, metoprolol or atenolol. Chronic therapy with Sectral induced no significant alteration in the blood lipid profile.

Sectral has been shown to delay AV conduction time and to increase the refractoriness of the AV node without significantly affecting sinus node recovery time, atrial refractory period, or the HV conduction time. The membrane-stabilizing effect of Sectral is not manifest at the doses used clinically.

Significant reductions in resting and exercise heart rates and systolic blood pressures have been observed 1.5 hours after Sectral administration with maximal effects occurring between 3 and 8 hours postdosing in normal volunteers. Sectral has demonstrated a significant effect on exercise-induced tachycardia 24 to 30 hours after drug administration.

There are significant correlations between plasma levels of acebutolol and both the reduction in resting heart rate and the percent of β-blockade of exercise-induced tachycardia. The antihypertensive effect of Sectral has been shown in double-blind controlled studies to be superior to placebo and similar to propranolol and hydrochlorothiazide. In addition, patients responding to Sectral administered twice daily had a similar response whether the dosage regimen was changed to once daily administration or continued on a b.i.d. regimen. Most patients responded to 400 to 800 mg per day in divided doses.

The antiarrhythmic effect of Sectral was compared with placebo, propranolol, and quinidine. Compared with placebo, Sectral significantly reduced mean total ventricular ectopic beats (VEB), paired VEB, multiform VEB, R-on-T beats, and ventricular tachycardia (VT). Both Sectral and propranolol significantly reduced mean total and paired VEB and VT. Sectral and quinidine significantly reduced resting total and complex VEB; the antiarrhythmic efficacy of Sectral was also observed during exercise.

PHARMACOKINETICS AND METABOLISM

Sectral is well absorbed from the GI tract. It is subject to extensive first-pass hepatic biotransformation, with an absolute bioavailability of approximately 40% for the parent compound. The major metabolite, an N-acetyl derivative (diacetolol), is pharmacologically active. This metabolite is equipotent to Sectral and in cats is more cardioselective than Sectral; therefore, this first-pass phenomenon does not attenuate the therapeutic effect of Sectral. Food intake does not have a significant effect on the area under the plasma concentration-time curve (AUC) of Sectral although the rate of absorption and peak concentration decreased slightly.

The plasma elimination half-life of Sectral is approximately 3 to 4 hours, while that of its metabolite, diacetolol, is 8 to 13 hours. The time to reach peak concentration for Sectral is 2.5 hours and for diacetolol, after oral administration of Sectral, 3.5 hours.

Within the single oral dose range of 200 to 400 mg, the kinetics are dose proportional. However, this linearity is not seen at higher doses, probably due to saturation of hepatic biotransformation sites. In addition, after multiple dosing the lack of linearity is also seen by AUC increases of approximately 100% as compared to single oral dosing. Elimination via renal excretion is approximately 30% to 40% and by nonrenal mechanisms 50% to 60%, which includes excretion into the bile and direct passage through the intestinal wall. Sectral has a low binding affinity for plasma proteins (about 26%). Sectral and its metabolite, diacetolol, are relatively hydrophilic and, therefore, only minimal quantities have been detected in the cerebrospinal fluid (CSF).

Drug interaction studies with tolbutamide and warfarin indicated no influence on the therapeutic effects of these compounds. Digoxin and hydrochlorothiazide plasma levels were not affected by concomitant Sectral administration. The kinetics of Sectral were not significantly altered by concomitant administration of hydrochlorothiazide, hydralazine, sulfinpyrazone, or oral contraceptives.

In patients with renal impairment, there is no effect on the elimination half-life of Sectral, but there is decreased elimination of the metabolite, diacetolol, resulting in a two- to three-fold increase in its half-life. For this reason, the drug should be administered with caution in patients with renal insufficiency (see "Precautions"). Sectral and its major metabolite are dialyzable.

Sectral crosses the placental barrier, and is secreted in breast milk.

In geriatric patients, the bioavailability of Sectral and its metabolite is increased, approximately two-fold, probably due to decreases in the first-pass metabolism and renal function in the elderly.

INDICATIONS AND USAGE

HYPERTENSION: Sectral is indicated for the management of hypertension in adults. It may be used alone or in combination with other antihypertensive agents, especially thiazide-type diuretics.

VENTRICULAR ARRHYTHMIAS: Sectral is indicated in the management of ventricular premature beats; it reduces the total number of premature beats, as well as the number of paired and multiform ventricular ectopic beats, and R-on-T beats.

CONTRAINDICATIONS

Sectral is contraindicated in: 1) persistently severe bradycardia; 2) second- and third-degree heart block; 3) overt cardiac failure; and 4) cardiogenic shock. (See "WARNINGS.")

WARNINGS

CARDIAC FAILURE: Sympathetic stimulation may be essential for support of the circulation in individuals with diminished myocardial contractility, and its inhibition by β-adrenergic receptor blockade may precipitate more severe failure. Although β-blockers should be avoided in overt cardiac failure, Sectral can be used with caution in patients with a history of heart failure who are controlled with digitalis and/or diuretics. Both digitalis and Sectral impair AV conduction. If cardiac failure persists, therapy with Sectral should be withdrawn.

IN PATIENTS WITHOUT A HISTORY OF CARDIAC FAILURE: In patients with aortic or mitral valve disease or compromised left ventricular function, continued depression of the myocardium with β-blocking agents over a period of time may lead to cardiac failure. At the first signs of failure, patients should be digitalized and/or be given a diuretic and the response observed closely. If cardiac failure continues despite adequate digitalization and/or diuretic, Sectral therapy should be withdrawn.

EXACERBATION OF ISCHEMIC HEART DISEASE FOLLOWING ABRUPT WITHDRAWAL: Following abrupt cessation of therapy with certain β-blocking agents in patients with coronary artery disease, exacerbation of angina pectoris and, in some cases, myocardial infarction and death have been reported. Therefore, such patients should be cautioned against interruption of therapy without a physician's advice. Even in the absence of overt ischemic heart disease, when discontinuation of Sectral is planned, the patient should be carefully observed, and should be advised to limit physical activity to a minimum while Sectral is gradually withdrawn over a period of about two weeks. (If therapy with an alternative β-blocker is desired, the patient may be transferred directly to comparable doses of another agent without interruption of β-blocking therapy.) If an exacerbation of angina pectoris occurs, antianginal therapy should be restarted immediately in full doses and the patient hospitalized until his condition stabilizes.

PERIPHERAL VASCULAR DISEASE: Treatment with β-antagonists reduces cardiac output and can precipitate or aggravate the symptoms of arterial insufficiency in patients with peripheral or mesenteric vascular disease. Caution should be exercised with such patients, and they should be observed closely for evidence of progression of arterial obstruction.

BRONCHOSPASTIC DISEASES: PATIENTS WITH BRONCHOSPASTIC DISEASE SHOULD, IN GENERAL, NOT RECEIVE A β-BLOCKER. Because of its relative β_1-selectivity, however, low doses of Sectral may be used with caution in patients with bronchospastic disease who do not respond to, or who cannot tolerate, alternative treatment. Since β_1-selectivity is not absolute and is dose-dependent, the lowest possible dose of Sectral should be used initially, preferably in divided doses to avoid the higher plasma levels associated with the longer dose-interval. A bronchodilator, such as a theophylline or a β_2-stimulant, should be made available in advance with instructions concerning its use.

ANESTHESIA AND MAJOR SURGERY: The necessity, or desirability, of withdrawal of a β-blocking therapy prior to major surgery is controversial. β-adrenergic receptor blockade impairs the ability of the heart to respond to β-adrenergically mediated reflex stimuli. While this might be of benefit in preventing arrhythmic response, the risk of excessive myocardial depression during general anesthesia may be enhanced and difficulty in restarting and maintaining the heart beat has been reported with beta-blockers. If treatment is continued, particular care should be taken when using anesthetic agents which depress the myocardium, such as ether, cyclopropane and trichlorethylene, and it is prudent to use the lowest possible dose of Sectral. Sectral, like other β-blockers, is a competitive inhibitor of β-receptor agonists, and its effect on the heart can be reversed by cautious administration of such agents (e.g., dobutamine or isoproterenol—see "Overdose").

Manifestations of excessive vagal tone (e.g., profound bradycardia, hypotension) may be corrected with atropine 1 to 3 mg IV in divided doses.

DIABETES AND HYPOGLYCEMIA: β-blockers may potentiate insulin-induced hypoglycemia and mask some of its manifestations such as tachycardia; however, dizziness and sweating are usually not significantly affected. Diabetic patients should be warned of the possibility of masked hypoglycemia.

THYROTOXICOSIS: β-adrenergic blockade may mask certain clinical signs (tachycardia) of hyperthyroidism. Abrupt withdrawal of β-blockade may precipitate a thyroid storm; therefore, patients suspected of developing thyrotoxicosis from whom Sectral therapy is to be withdrawn should be monitored closely.

PRECAUTIONS

IMPAIRED RENAL OR HEPATIC FUNCTION: Studies on the effect of acebutolol in patients with renal insufficiency have not been performed in the U.S. Foreign published experience shows that acebutolol has been used successfully in chronic renal insufficiency. Acebutolol is excreted through the G.I. tract, but the active metabolite, diacetolol, is eliminated predominantly by the kidney. There is a linear relationship between renal clearance of diacetolol and creatinine clearance. Therefore, the daily dose of acebutolol should be reduced by 50% when the creatinine clearance is less than 50 mL/min and by 75% when it is less than 25 mL/min. Sectral should be used cautiously in patients with impaired hepatic function.

Sectral has been used successfully and without problems in elderly patients in the U.S. clinical trials without specific adjustment of dosage. However, elderly patients may require lower maintenance doses because the bioavailability of both Sectral and its metabolite are approximately doubled in this age group.

INFORMATION FOR PATIENTS: Patients, especially those with evidence of coronary artery disease, should be warned against interruption or discontinuation of Sectral therapy without a physician's supervision. Although cardiac failure rarely occurs in properly selected patients, those being treated with β-adrenergic blocking agents should be advised to consult a physician if they develop signs or symptoms suggestive of impending CHF, or unexplained respiratory symptoms.

Patients should also be warned of possible severe hypertensive reactions from concomitant use of α-adrenergic stimulants such as the nasal decongestants commonly used in OTC cold preparations and nasal drops.

CLINICAL LABORATORY FINDINGS: Sectral, like other β-blockers, has been associated with the development of antinuclear antibodies (ANA). In prospective clinical trials, patients receiving Sectral had a dose-dependent increase in the development of positive ANA titers and the overall incidence was higher than that observed with propranolol. Symptoms (generally persistent arthralgias and myalgias) related to this laboratory abnormality were infrequent (less than 1% with both drugs). Symptoms and ANA titers were reversible upon discontinuation of treatment.

DRUG INTERACTIONS: Catecholamine-depleting drugs, such as reserpine, may have an additive effect when given with β-blocking agents. Patients treated with Sectral plus catecholamine depletors should, therefore, be observed closely for evidence of marked bradycardia or hypotension which may present as vertigo, syncope/presyncope, or orthostatic changes in blood pressure without compensatory tachycardia. Exaggerated hypertensive responses have been reported from the combined use of β-adrenergic antagonists and α-adrenergic stimulants, including those contained in

Continued on next page

Wyeth-Ayerst—Cont.

proprietary cold remedies and vasoconstrictive nasal drops. Patients receiving β-blockers should be warned of this potential hazard. No significant interactions with digoxin, hydrochlorothiazide, hydralazine, sulfinpyrazone, oral contraceptives, tolbutamide, or warfarin have been observed.

CARCINOGENESIS, MUTAGENESIS, IMPAIRMENT OF FERTILITY: Chronic oral toxicity studies in rats and mice, employing dose levels as high as 300 mg/kg/day, which is equivalent to 15 times the maximum recommended (60 kg) human dose, did not indicate a carcinogenic potential for Sectral. Diacetolol, the major metabolite of Sectral in man, was without carcinogenic potential in rats when tested at doses as high as 1800 mg/kg/day. Sectral and diacetolol were also shown to be devoid of mutagenic potential in the Ames Test. Sectral, administered orally to two generations of male and female rats at doses of up to 240 mg/kg/day (equivalent to 12 times the maximum recommended therapeutic dose in a 60-kg human) and diacetolol, administered to two generations of male and female rats at doses of up to 1000 mg/kg/day, had no significant impact on reproductive performance or fertility.

PREGNANCY
TERATOGENIC EFFECTS:
Pregnancy Category B: Reproduction studies have been performed with Sectral in rats (up to 630 mg/kg/day) and rabbits (up to 135 mg/kg/day). These doses are equivalent to approximately 31.5 and 6.8 times the maximum recommended therapeutic dose in a 60-kg human, respectively. The compound was not teratogenic in either species. In the rabbit, however, doses of 135 mg/kg/day caused slight fetal growth retardation; this effect was considered to be a result of maternal toxicity, as evidenced by reduced food intake, a lowered rate of body weight gain, and mortality. Studies have also been performed in these species with diacetolol (at doses of up to 450 mg/kg/day in rabbits and up to 1800 mg/kg/day in rats.) Other than a significant elevation in postimplantation loss with 450 mg/kg/day diacetolol, a level at which food consumption and body weight gain were reduced in rabbit dams and a nonstatistically significant increase in incidence of bilateral cataract in rat fetuses from dams treated with 1800 mg/kg/day diacetolol, there was no evidence of harm to the fetus. There are no adequate and well-controlled trials in pregnant women. Because animal teratology studies are not always predictive of the human response, Sectral should be used during pregnancy only if the potential benefit justifies the risk to the fetus.

Nonteratogenic Effects:
Studies in humans have shown that both acebutolol and diacetolol cross the placenta. Neonates of mothers who have received acebutolol during pregnancy had reduced birth weight, decreased blood pressure, and decreased heart rate. In the newborn the elimination half-life of acebutolol was 6 to 14 hours, while the half-life of diacetolol was 24 to 30 hours for the first 24 hours after birth, followed by a half-life of 12 to 16 hours. Adequate facilities for monitoring these infants at birth should be available.

Labor and Delivery: The effect of Sectral on labor and delivery in pregnant women is unknown. Studies in animals have not shown any effect of Sectral on the usual course of labor and delivery.

Nursing Mothers: Acebutolol and diacetolol also appear in breast milk with a milk:plasma ratio of 7.1 and 12.2, respectively. Use in nursing mothers is not recommended.

Pediatric Use: Safety and effectiveness in children have not been established.

ADVERSE REACTIONS

Sectral is well tolerated in properly selected patients. Most adverse reactions have been mild, not required discontinuation of therapy, and tended to decrease as duration of treatment increases.

The following table shows the frequency of treatment-related side effects derived from controlled clinical trials in patients with hypertension, angina pectoris, and arrhythmia. These patients received Sectral, propranolol, or hydrochlorothiazide as monotherapy, or placebo.
[See table below].

The following selected (potentially important) side effects were seen in up to 2% of Sectral patients:
Cardiovascular: hypotension, bradycardia, heart failure.
Central Nervous System: anxiety, hyper/hypoesthesia, impotence.
Dermatological: pruritus.
Gastrointestinal: vomiting, abdominal pain.
Genitourinary: dysuria, nocturia.
Musculoskeletal: back pain, joint pain.
Respiratory: pharyngitis, wheezing.
Special Senses: conjunctivitis, dry eye, eye pain.
The incidence of drug-related adverse effects (volunteered and solicited) according to Sectral dose is shown below. (Data from 266 hypertensive patients treated for 3 months on a constant dose.)

Body System	400 mg/day (N = 132)	800 mg/day (N = 63)	1200 mg/day (N = 71)
Cardiovascular	5%	2%	1%
Gastrointestinal	3%	3%	7%
Musculoskeletal	2%	3%	4%
Central Nervous System	9%	13%	17%
Respiratory	1%	5%	6%
Skin	1%	2%	1%
Special Senses	2%	2%	6%
Genitourinary	2%	3%	1%

POTENTIAL ADVERSE EFFECTS

In addition, certain adverse effects not listed above have been reported with other β-blocking agents and should also be considered as potential adverse effects of Sectral.
Central Nervous System: Reversible mental depression progressing to catatonia (an acute syndrome characterized by disorientation for time and place), short-term memory loss,

emotional lability, slightly clouded sensorium, and decreased performance (neuropsychometrics).
Cardiovascular: Intensification of AV block (see "Contraindications").
Allergic: Erythematous rash, fever combined with aching and sore throat, laryngospasm, and respiratory distress.
Hematologic: Agranulocytosis, nonthrombocytopenic, and thrombocytopenic purpura.
Gastrointestinal: Mesenteric arterial thrombosis and ischemic colitis.
Miscellaneous: Reversible alopecia and Peyronie's disease. The oculomucocutaneous syndrome associated with the β-blocker practolol has not been reported with Sectral during investigational use and extensive foreign clinical experience.

OVERDOSAGE

No specific information on emergency treatment of overdosage is available for Sectral. However, overdosage with other β-blocking agents has been accompanied by extreme bradycardia, advanced atrioventricular block, intraventricular conduction defects, hypotension, severe congestive heart failure, seizures, and in susceptible patients, bronchospasm and hypoglycemia. Although specific information on the emergency treatment of Sectral overdose is not available, on the basis of the pharmacological actions and the observations in treating overdoses with other β-blockers, the following general measures should be considered:
1. Empty stomach by emesis or lavage.
2. Bradycardia: IV atropine (1 to 3 mg in divided doses). If antivagal response is inadequate, administer isoproterenol cautiously since larger than usual doses of isoproterenol may be required.
3. Persistent hypotension in spite of correction of bradycardia: Administer vasopressor (e.g., epinephrine, levarterenol, dopamine, or dobutamine) with frequent monitoring of blood pressure and pulse rate.
4. Bronchospasm: A theophylline derivative, such as aminophylline and/or parenteral β₂-stimulant, such as terbutaline.
5. Cardiac failure: Digitalize the patient and/or administer a diuretic. It has been reported that glucagon is useful in this situation.
Sectral is dialyzable.

DOSAGE AND ADMINISTRATION

HYPERTENSION: The initial dosage of Sectral in uncomplicated mild-to-moderate hypertension is 400 mg. This can be given as a single daily dose, but in occasional patients twice daily dosing (200 mg b.i.d.) may be required for adequate 24-hour blood-pressure control. An optimal response is usually achieved with dosages of 400 to 800 mg per day, although some patients have been maintained on as little as 200 mg per day. Patients with more severe hypertension or who have demonstrated inadequate control may respond to a total of 1200 mg daily (administered b.i.d.), or to the addition of a second antihypertensive agent. Beta-1 selectivity diminishes as dosage is increased.
VENTRICULAR ARRHYTHMIA: The usual initial dose of Sectral is 400 mg daily given as 200 mg b.i.d. Dosage should be increased gradually until an optimal clinical response is obtained, generally at 600 to 1200 mg per day. If treatment is to be discontinued, the dosage should be reduced gradually over a period of about two weeks.
USE IN OLDER PATIENTS: Older patients have an approximately 2-fold increase in bioavailability and may require lower maintenance doses. Doses above 800 mg/day should be avoided in the elderly.

HOW SUPPLIED

Sectral® (acebutolol HCl), Wyeth®, is available in the following dosage strengths:
200 mg, opaque purple and orange capsule marked "WYETH 4177" and "Sectral 200"
NDC 0008-4177-01, in bottles of 100 capsules.
NDC 0008-4177-04, in Redipak® cartons of 100 capsules (10 blister strips of 10).
400 mg, opaque brown and orange capsule marked "WYETH 4179" and "Sectral 400"
NDC 0008-4179-01, in bottles of 100 capsules.
Keep at Room Temperature, Approx. 25° C (77° F).
The appearance of these capsules is a trademark of Wyeth-Ayerst Laboratories.

by arrangement with RHONE-POULENC France

Shown in Product Identification Section, page 437

SERAX®   Ⓒ ℞
[ser 'aks]
(oxazepam)
CAPSULES ● TABLETS

DESCRIPTION

Serax is the first of a chemically new series of compounds, the 3-hydroxybenzodiazepinones. A new therapeutic agent providing versatility and flexibility in control of common emotional disturbances, this product exerts prompt action in

TOTAL VOLUNTEERED AND ELICITED (U.S. STUDIES)

Body System/ Adverse Reaction	SECTRAL (N = 1002) %	Propranolol (N = 424) %	Hydrochloro- thiazide (N = 178) %	Placebo (N = 314) %
Cardiovascular				
Chest Pain	2	4	4	1
Edema	2	2	4	1
Central Nervous System				
Depression	2	1	3	1
Dizziness	6	7	12	2
Fatigue	11	17	10	4
Headache	6	9	13	4
Insomnia	3	6	5	1
Abnormal dreams	2	3	0	1
Dermatologic				
Rash	2	2	4	1
Gastrointestinal				
Constipation	4	2	7	0
Diarrhea	4	5	5	1
Dyspepsia	4	6	3	1
Flatulence	3	4	7	1
Nausea	4	6	3	0
Genitourinary				
Micturition (frequency)	3	1	9	<1
Musculoskeletal				
Arthralgia	2	1	3	2
Myalgia	2	1	4	0
Respiratory				
Cough	1	1	2	0
Dyspnea	4	6	4	2
Rhinitis	2	1	4	<1
Special Senses				
Abnormal Vision	2	2	3	0

a wide variety of disorders associated with anxiety, tension, agitation, and irritability, and anxiety associated with depression. In tolerance and toxicity studies on several animal species, this product reveals significantly greater safety factors than related compounds (chlordiazepoxide and diazepam) and manifests a wide separation of effective doses and doses inducing side effects.

Serax capsules contain 10 mg, 15 mg, or 30 mg oxazepam. The inactive ingredients present are gelatin, lactose, titanium dioxide, and other ingredients. Each dosage strength also contains the following:

10 mg—D&C Red 22, D&C Red 28, and FD&C Blue 1;
15 mg—FD&C Red 40 and FD&C Yellow 6;
30 mg—D&C Red 28, FD&C Red 40, and FD&C Blue 1.

Serax tablets contain 15 mg oxazepam. The inactive ingredients present are FD&C Yellow 5, lactose, magnesium stearate, methylcellulose, and polacrilin potassium.

Serax is 7 chloro-1,3,-dihydro-3-hydroxy-5-phenyl-$2H$-1,4-benzodiazepin-2-one, a white crystalline powder with a molecular weight of 286.7.

CLINICAL PHARMACOLOGY

Pharmacokinetic testing in twelve volunteers demonstrated that when given as a single 30 mg dose, the capsule, tablet, and suspension were equivalent in extent of absorption. For the capsule and tablet, peak plasma levels averaged 450 ng/mL and were observed to occur about 3 hours after dosing. The mean elimination half-life for oxazepam was approximately 8.2 hours (range 5.7 to 10.9 hours).

This product has a single, major inactive metabolite in man, a glucuronide excreted in the urine.

ANIMAL PHARMACOLOGY AND TOXICOLOGY

In mice, SERAX exerts an anticonvulsant (anti-Metrazol®) activity at 50 percent effective doses of about 0.6 mg/kg orally. (Such anticonvulsant activity of benzodiazepines correlates with their tranquilizing properties.) To produce ataxia (rotabar test) and sedation (abolition of spontaneous motor activity), the 50 percent effective doses of this product are greater than 5 mg/kg orally. Thus, about ten times the therapeutic (anticonvulsant) dose must be given before ataxia ensues, indicating a wide separation of effective doses and doses inducing side effects.

In evaluation of antianxiety activity of compounds, conflict behavioral tests in rats differentiate continuous response for food in the presence of anxiety-provoking stress (shock) from drug-induced motor incoordination. This product shows significant separation of doses required to relieve anxiety and doses producing sedation or ataxia. Ataxia-producing doses exceed those of related CNS-acting drugs.

Acute oral LD$_{50}$ in mice is greater than 5000 mg/kg, compared to 800 mg/kg for a related compound (chlordiazepoxide).

Subacute toxicity studies in dogs for four weeks at 480 mg/kg daily showed no specific changes; at 960 mg/kg two out of eight died with evidence of circulatory collapse. This wide margin of safety is significant compared to chlordiazepoxide HCl, which showed nonspecific changes in six dogs at 80 mg/kg. On chlordiazepoxide, two out of six died with evidence of circulatory collapse at 127 mg/kg, and six out of six died at 200 mg/kg daily. Chronic toxicity studies of Serax in dogs at 120 mg/kg/day for 52 weeks produced no toxic manifestation.

Fatty metamorphosis of the liver has been noted in six-week toxicity studies in rats given this product at 0.5% of the diet. Such accumulations of fat are considered reversible as there is no liver necrosis or fibrosis.

Breeding studies in rats through two successive litters did not produce fetal abnormality.

Oxazepam has not been adequately evaluated for mutagenic activity.

In a carcinogenicity study, oxazepam was administered with diet to rats for two years. Male rats receiving 30 times the maximum human dose showed a statistical increase, when compared to controls, in benign thyroid follicular cell tumors, testicular interstitial cell adenomas, and prostatic adenomas. An earlier published study reported that mice fed dietary dosages of 35 or 100 times the human daily dose of oxazepam for 9 months developed a dose-related increase in liver adenomas.[1] In an independent analysis of some of the microscopic slides from this mouse study several of these tumors were classified as liver carcinomas. At this time, there is no evidence that clinical use of oxazepam is associated with tumors.

INDICATIONS

SERAX (oxazepam) is indicated for the management of anxiety disorders or for the short-term relief of the symptoms of anxiety. Anxiety or tension associated with the stress of everyday life usually does not require treatment with an anxiolytic.

Anxiety associated with depression is also responsive to SERAX (oxazepam) therapy.

This product has been found particularly useful in the management of anxiety, tension, agitation, and irritability in older patients.

SERAX (oxazepam)
USUAL DOSE

Mild-to-moderate anxiety, with associated tension, irritability, agitation, or related symptoms of functional origin or secondary to organic disease.	10 to 15 mg, 3 or 4 times daily
Severe anxiety syndromes, agitation, or anxiety associated with depression.	15 to 30 mg, 3 or 4 times daily
Older patients with anxiety, tension, irritability, and agitation.	Initial dosage: 10 mg, 3 times daily. If necessary, increase cautiously to 15 mg, 3 or 4 times daily
Alcoholics with acute inebriation, tremulousness, or anxiety on withdrawal.	15 to 30 mg, 3 or 4 times daily

Alcoholics with acute tremulousness, inebriation, or with anxiety associated with alcohol withdrawal are responsive to therapy.

The effectiveness of SERAX in long-term use, that is, more than 4 months, has not been assessed by systematic clinical studies. The physician should reassess periodically the usefulness of the drug for the individual patient.

CONTRAINDICATIONS

History of previous hypersensitivity reaction to oxazepam. Oxazepam is not indicated in psychoses.

WARNINGS

As with other CNS-acting drugs, patients should be cautioned against driving automobiles or operating dangerous machinery until it is known that they do not become drowsy or dizzy on oxazepam therapy.

Patients should be warned that the effects of alcohol or other CNS-depressant drugs may be additive to those of Serax, possibly requiring adjustment of dosage or elimination of such agents.

PHYSICAL AND PSYCHOLOGICAL DEPENDENCE

Withdrawal symptoms, similar in character to those noted with barbiturates and alcohol (convulsions, tremor, abdominal and muscle cramps, vomiting, and sweating), have occurred following abrupt discontinuance of oxazepam. The more severe withdrawal symptoms have usually been limited to those patients who received excessive doses over an extended period of time. Generally milder withdrawal symptoms (e.g., dysphoria and insomnia) have been reported following abrupt discontinuance of benzodiazepines taken continuously at therapeutic levels for several months. Consequently, after extended therapy, abrupt discontinuation should generally be avoided and a gradual dosage-tapering schedule followed. Addiction-prone individuals (such as drug addicts or alcoholics) should be under careful surveillance when receiving oxazepam or other psychotropic agents because of the predisposition of such patients to habituation and dependence.

USE IN PREGNANCY

An increased risk of congenital malformations associated with the use of minor tranquilizers (chlordiazepoxide, diazepam, and meprobamate) during the first trimester of pregnancy has been suggested in several studies. Serax, a benzodiazepine derivative, has not been studied adequately to determine whether it, too, may be associated with an increased risk of fetal abnormality. Because use of these drugs is rarely a matter of urgency, their use during this period should almost always be avoided. The possibility that a woman of childbearing potential may be pregnant at the time of institution of therapy should be considered. Patients should be advised that if they become pregnant during therapy or intend to become pregnant they should communicate with their physician about the desirability of discontinuing the drug.

PRECAUTIONS

Although hypotension has occurred only rarely, oxazepam should be administered with caution to patients in whom a drop in blood pressure might lead to cardiac complications. This is particularly true in the elderly patient.

SERAX 15 mg tablets, *but none of the other available dosage forms of this product,* contain FD&C Yellow No. 5 (tartrazine) which may cause allergic-type reactions (including bronchial asthma) in certain susceptible individuals. Although the overall incidence of FD&C Yellow No. 5 (tartrazine) sensitivity in the general population is low, it is frequently seen in patients who also have aspirin hypersensitivity.

INFORMATION FOR PATIENTS

To assure the safe and effective use of Serax (oxazepam), patients should be informed that, since benzodiazepines may produce psychological and physical dependence, it is advisable that they consult with their physician before either increasing the dose or abruptly discontinuing this drug.

ADVERSE REACTIONS

The necessity for discontinuation of therapy due to undesirable effects has been rare. Transient mild drowsiness is commonly seen in the first few days of therapy. If it persists, the dosage should be reduced. In few instances, dizziness, vertigo, headache, and rarely syncope have occurred either alone or together with drowsiness. Mild paradoxical reactions, i.e., excitement, stimulation of affect, have been reported in psychiatric patients; these reactions may be secondary to relief of anxiety and usually appear in the first two weeks of therapy.

Other side effects occurring during oxazepam therapy include rare instances of minor diffuse skin rashes—morbilliform, urticarial and maculopapular—nausea, lethargy, edema, slurred speech, tremor, and altered libido. Such side effects have been infrequent and are generally controlled with reduction of dosage.

Although rare, leukopenia and hepatic dysfunction including jaundice have been reported during therapy. Periodic blood counts and liver-function tests are advisable.

Ataxia with oxazepam has been reported in rare instances and does not appear to be specifically related to dose or age.

Although the following side reactions have not as yet been reported with oxazepam, they have occurred with related compounds (chlordiazepoxide and diazepam): paradoxical excitation with severe rage reactions, hallucinations, menstrual irregularities, change in EEG pattern, blood dyscrasias including agranulocytosis, blurred vision, diplopia, incontinence, stupor, disorientation, fever, and euphoria.

Transient amnesia or memory impairment has been reported in association with the use of benzodiazepines.

DOSAGE AND ADMINISTRATION

Because of the flexibility of this product and the range of emotional disturbances responsive to it, dosage should be individualized for maximum beneficial effects.

[See table above].

This product is not indicated in children under 6 years of age. Absolute dosage for children 6–12 years of age is not established.

HOW SUPPLIED

Serax® (oxazepam) Capsules and Tablets, Wyeth® are available in the following dosage strengths:

10 mg, NDC 0008-0051, white and pink capsule banded with Wyeth logo and marked "SERAX", "10", and "51", in bottles of 100 and 500 capsules, in Redipak® cartons of 250 capsules (10 blister folders of 25), and in Redipak cartons of 100 capsules (10 blister strips of 10).

15 mg, NDC 0008-0006, white and red capsule banded with Wyeth logo and marked "SERAX", "15", and "6", in bottles of 100 and 500 capsules, in Redipak® cartons of 250 capsules (10 blister folders of 25) and in Redipak® cartons of 100 capsules (10 blister strips of 10).

30 mg. NDC 0008-0052, white and maroon capsule banded with Wyeth logo and marked "SERAX", "30", and "52", in bottles of 100 and 500 capsules, in Redipak® cartons of 250 capsules (10 blister folders of 25) and in Redipak® cartons of 100 capsules (10 blister strips of 10).

15 mg, NDC 0008-0317, yellow, five-sided tablet with a raised "S" and a "15" on one side and "WYETH" and "317" on reverse side, in bottles of 100 tablets.

The appearance of SERAX capsules and tablets is a trademark of Wyeth-Ayerst Laboratories.

Keep bottles tightly closed.

Dispense in tight containers.

REFERENCE

1. FOX, KA.; LAHCEN, R.B.: Liver-cell Adenomas and Peliosis Hepatis in Mice Associated with Oxazepam. Res. Commun. Chem. Pathol. Pharmacol. 8:481–488, 1974.

Shown in Product Identification Section, pages 437 & 438

Continued on next page

Wyeth-Ayerst—Cont.

SMA®
[ess-em-ay]
Iron fortified
infant formula
READY–TO–FEED
CONCENTRATED LIQUID
POWDER

Breast milk is the preferred feeding for newborns. Infant formula is intended to replace or supplement breast milk when breast feeding is not possible or is insufficient, or when mothers elect not to breast feed.

Good maternal nutrition is important for the preparation and maintenance of breast feeding. Extensive or prolonged use of partial bottle feeding, before breast feeding has been well established, could make breast feeding difficult to maintain. A decision not to breast feed could be difficult to reverse.

Professional advice should be followed on all matters of infant feeding. Infant formula should always be prepared and used as directed. Unnecessary or improper use of infant formula could present a health hazard. Social and financial implications should be considered when selecting the method of infant feeding.

SMA® is unique among prepared formulas for its physiologic fat blend, whey-dominated protein composition, amino acid pattern, mineral content and inclusion of beta-carotene. SMA, utilizing a hybridized safflower (oleic) oil, became the first infant formula offering fat and calcium absorption equal to that of human milk, with a physiologic level of linoleic acid. Thus, the fat blend in SMA provides a ready source of energy, helps protect infants against neonatal tetany and produces a ratio of vitamin E to polyunsaturated fatty acids (linoleic acid) more than adequate to prevent hemolytic anemia and yields a serum lipid profile comparable to the breast fed infant.

By combining reduced minerals whey with skimmed cow's milk, SMA reduces the protein content to fall within the range of human milk, adjusts the whey-protein to casein ratio to that of human milk, and subsequently reduces the mineral content to a physiologic level.

The resultant 60:40 whey-protein to casein ratio provides protein nutrition superior to a casein-dominated formula. In addition, the essential amino acids, including cystine, are present in amounts close to those of human milk. So the protein in SMA is of high biologic value.

The physiologic mineral content makes possible a low renal solute load which helps protect the functionally immature infant kidney, increases expendable water reserves and helps protect against dehydration.

Use of lactose as the carbohydrate results in a physiologic stool flora and a low stool pH, decreasing the incidence of perianal dermatitis.

INGREDIENTS

SMA® Concentrated Liquid or Ready-to-Feed. Water; nonfat milk; reduced minerals whey; oleo, coconut, oleic (safflower), and soybean oils; lactose; soy lecithin; taurine; calcium carrageenan. *Minerals:* Potassium bicarbonate; calcium chloride and citrate; potassium chloride; sodium citrate; ferrous sulfate; sodium bicarbonate; zinc, cupric, and manganese sulfates. *Vitamins:* Ascorbic acid, alpha tocopheryl acetate, niacinamide, vitamin A palmitate, calcium pantothenate, thiamine hydrochloride, riboflavin, pyridoxine hydrochloride, beta-carotene, folic acid, phytonadione, cholecalciferol, biotin, cyanocobalamin.

SMA® Powder. Reduced minerals whey; oleo, coconut, oleic (safflower) and soybean oils; nonfat milk; lactose; soy lecithin; taurine. *Minerals:* Calcium chloride; sodium bicarbonate; calcium hydroxide; ferrous sulfate; potassium hydroxide and bicarbonate; potassium chloride; zinc, cupric, and manganese sulfates. *Vitamins:* Ascorbic acid, alpha tocopheryl acetate, niacinamide, vitamin A palmitate, calcium pantothenate, thiamine hydrochloride, riboflavin, pyridoxine hydrochloride, betacarotene, folic acid, phytonadione, activated 7-dehydrocholesterol, biotin, cyanocobalamin.

PROXIMATE ANALYSIS
at 20 calories per fluidounce
READY-TO-FEED, POWDER, and CONCENTRATED LIQUID:

	(w/v)
Fat	3.6%
Carbohydrate	7.2%
Protein	1.5%
60% Lactalbumin (whey protein)	0.9%
40% Casein	0.6%
Ash	0.25%
Crude Fiber	None
Total Solids	12.6%
Calories/fl. oz.	20

Vitamins, Minerals: In normal dilution, each liter contains:

A	2000 IU
D_3	400 IU
E	9.5 IU
K_1	55 mcg
C (ascorbic acid)	55 mg
B_1 (thiamine)	670 mcg
B_2 (riboflavin)	1000 mcg
B_6 (pyroxidine hydrochloride)	420 mcg
B_{12}	1.3 mcg
Niacin	5000 mcg
Pantothenic Acid	2100 mcg
Folic Acid (folacin)	50 mcg
Choline	100 mg
Biotin	15 mcg
Calcium	420 mg
Phosphorus	280 mg
Sodium	150 mg
Potassium	560 mg
Chloride	375 mg
Magnesium	45 mg
Manganese	150 mcg
Iron	12 mg
Copper	470 mcg
Zinc	5 mg
Iodine	60 mcg

PREPARATION

Ready-to-Feed (8 and 32 fl. oz. cans of 20 calories per fluidounce formula)—shake can, open and pour into previously sterilized nursing bottle; attach nipple and feed. Cover opened can and immediately store in refrigerator. Use contents of can within 48 hours of opening.

Powder—(1 pound can)—For normal dilution supplying 20 calories per fluidounce, use 1 scoop (or 1 standard tablespoonful) of powder, packed and leveled, to 2 fluidounces of cooled, previously boiled water. For larger amount of formula, use ¼ standard measuring cup of powder, packed and leveled, to 8 fluidounces (1 cup) of water. Three of these portions make 26 fluidounces of formula.

Concentrated Liquid—For normal dilution supplying 20 calories per fluidounce, use equal amounts of SMA liquid and cooled, previously boiled water.

Note: Prepared formula should be used within 24 hours.

HOW SUPPLIED

Ready-to-Feed—presterilized and premixed, 32 fluidounce (1 quart) cans, cases of 6; 8 fluidounce cans, cases of 24 (4 carriers of 6 cans). *Powder*—1 pound cans with measuring scoop, cases of 6. *Concentrated Liquid* — 13 fluidounce cans, cases of 24.

For Hospital Nursery Use—an infant feeding system which provides premixed, presterilized, ready-to-feed items, thus saving space, time and equipment. It eliminates washing, measuring, mixing, sterilizing, refrigerating and heating. The system is offered in a choice of two forms:

1. Prefilled and presterilized 4 oz. glass bottles for which sterile nipple assemblies are available, to be attached before feeding. These units may be used again after resterilizing or may be discarded, as desired.
2. The E-Z NURSER® (single unit nurser), also prefilled and presterilized, consists of a 4 oz. glass bottle with sterile nipple already attached; the entire unit is designed to be discarded after use.

The following items are supplied in both the forms described above:

SMA® Ready-to-Feed	
13 calories/oz.	48 bottles of 4 fl. oz.
20 calories/oz.	48 bottles of 4 fl. oz.
24 calories/oz.	48 bottles of 4 fl. oz.
27 calories/oz.	48 bottles of 4 fl. oz.
SMA® lo-iron Ready-to-Feed	
13 calories/oz.	48 bottles of 4 fl. oz.
20 calories/oz.	48 bottles of 4 fl. oz.
24 calories/oz.	48 bottles of 4 fl. oz.
"preemie" SMA® Ready-to-Feed	
24 calories/oz.	48 bottles of 4 fl. oz.
(Not available in the E-Z NURSER®)	
Distilled Water	48 bottles of 4 fl. oz.
Glucose, 5% in Distilled	
Water, 6 calories/oz.	48 bottles of 4 fl. oz.
Glucose, 10% in Distilled	
Water, 12 calories/oz.	48 bottles of 4 fl. oz.
NURSOY® (soy protein formula)	
20 calories/oz.	48 bottles of 4 fl. oz.
(Not available in the E-Z NURSER®)	

Supplied in 8 oz. bottles, to which sterile nipple assemblies must be attached before feeding, are the following:

SMA® Ready-to-Feed	
20 calories/oz.	24 bottles of 8 fl. oz.
Oral Electrolyte Solution	24 bottles of 8 fl. oz.
Distilled Water	24 bottles of 8 fl. oz.

NIPPLE ASSEMBLIES—presterilized, for both premature and term infants, single-hole and cross-cut, suitable for use with all ready-to-feed products requiring them, cartons of 288 nipple units. Single-hole, cross cut and orthodontic nipples.

ACCUFEED™, Wyeth Graduated Nursers—presterilized, disposable nursers (60 ml capacity) for accurately measured feedings, packages of 200.

Also Available: SMA® lo-iron. For those who appreciate the particular advantages of SMA®, the infant formula closest in composition nutritionally to mother's milk, but who sometimes need or wish to recommend a formula that does not contain a high level of iron, now there is SMA lo-iron with all the benefits of regular SMA but with a reduced level of iron of 1.4 mg per quart. Infants should receive supplemental dietary iron from an outside source to meet daily requirements.

Concentrated Liquid, 13 fl. oz. cans, cases of 24. Powder, 1 pound cans with measuring scoop, cases of 6. Ready-to-Feed, 32 fl. oz. cans, cases of 6.

Preparation of the standard 20 calories per fluidounce formula of SMA lo-iron is the same as SMA iron fortified given above.

Shown in Product Identification Section, page 437

SURMONTIL®
[sir'mon "til]
(trimipramine maleate)
Capsules

℞

DESCRIPTION

Surmontil (trimipramine maleate) is 5-(3-dimethylamino-2-methylpropyl)-10,11-dihydro-5H-dibenz (b,f) azepine acid maleate (racemic form).

MOLECULAR FORMULA: $C_{20}H_{26}N_2 \cdot C_4H_4O_4$

MOLECULAR WEIGHT: 410.5

Surmontil capsules contain trimipramine maleate equivalent to 25 mg, 50 mg, or 100 mg of trimipramine as the base. The inactive ingredients present are FD&C Blue 1, gelatin, lactose, magnesium stearate, and titanium dioxide. The 25 mg dosage strength also contains D&C Yellow 10 and FD&C Yellow 6; the 50 mg dosage strength also contains D&C Red 28, FD&C Red 40, and FD&C Yellow 6.

Trimipramine maleate is prepared as a racemic mixture which can be resolved into levorotatory and dextrorotatory isomers. The asymmetric center responsible for optical isomerism is marked in the formula by an asterisk. Trimipramine maleate is an almost odorless, white or slightly cream-colored, crystalline substance, melting at 140–144°C. It is very slightly soluble in ether and water, is slightly soluble in ethyl alcohol and acetone, and freely soluble in chloroform and methanol at 20°C.

CLINICAL PHARMACOLOGY

Surmontil is an antidepressant with an anxiety-reducing sedative component to its action. The mode of action of Surmontil on the central nervous system is not known. However, unlike amphetamine-type compounds it does not act primarily by stimulation of the central nervous system. It does not act by inhibition of the monoamine oxidase system.

INDICATIONS

Surmontil is indicated for the relief of symptoms of depression. Endogenous depression is more likely to be alleviated than other depressive states. In studies with neurotic outpatients, the drug appeared to be equivalent to amitriptyline in the less-depressed patients but somewhat less effective than amitriptyline in the more severely depressed patients. In hospitalized depressed patients, trimipramine and imipramine were equally effective in relieving depression.

CONTRAINDICATIONS

Surmontil is contraindicated in cases of known hypersensitivity to the drug. The possibility of cross-sensitivity to other dibenzazepine compounds should be kept in mind. Surmontil should not be given in conjunction with drugs of the monoamine oxidase inhibitor class (e.g., tranylcypromine, isocarboxazid or phenelzine sulfate). The concomitant use of monoamine oxidase inhibitors (MAOI) and tricyclic compounds similar to Surmontil has caused severe hyperpyretic reactions, convulsive crises, and death in some patients. At least two weeks should elapse after cessation of therapy with MAOI before instituting therapy with Surmontil. Initial dosage should be low and increased gradually with caution and careful observation of the patient. The drug is contraindicated during the acute recovery period after a myocardial infarction.

WARNINGS

Use in Children—This drug is not recommended for use in children, since safety and effectiveness in the pediatric age group have not been established.

General Consideration for Use—Extreme caution should be used when this drug is given to patients with any evidence of cardiovascular disease because of the possibility of conduction defects, arrhythmias, myocardial infarction, strokes, and tachycardia.

Caution is advised in patients with increased intraocular pressure, history of urinary retention, or history of narrow-angle glaucoma because of the drug's anticholinergic properties; hyperthyroid patients or those on thyroid medication because of the possibility of cardiovascular toxicity; patients with a history of seizure disorder, because this drug has been shown to lower the seizure threshold; patients receiving guanethidine or similar agents, since Surmontil may block the pharmacologic effects of these drugs.

Since the drug may impair the mental and/or physical abilities required for the performance of potentially hazardous tasks, such as operating an automobile or machinery, the patient should be cautioned accordingly.

PRECAUTIONS

The possibility of suicide is inherent in any severely depressed patient and persists until a significant remission occurs. When a patient with a serious suicidal potential is not hospitalized, the prescription should be for the smallest amount feasible.

In schizophrenic patients activation of the psychosis may occur and require reduction of dosage or the addition of a major tranquilizer to the therapeutic regime.

Manic or hypomanic episodes may occur in some patients, in particular those with cyclic-type disorders. In some cases therapy with Surmontil must be discontinued until the episode is relieved, after which therapy may be reinstituted at lower dosages if still required.

Concurrent administration of Surmontil and electroshock therapy may increase the hazards of therapy. Such treatment should be limited to those patients for whom it is essential. When possible, discontinue the drug for several days prior to elective surgery.

There is evidence that cimetidine inhibits the elimination of tricyclic antidepressants. Downward adjustment of Surmontil dosage may be required if cimetidine therapy is initiated: upward adjustment if cimetidine therapy is discontinued.

Patients should be warned that the concomitant use of alcoholic beverages may be associated with exaggerated effects. It has been reported that tricyclic antidepressants can potentiate the effects of catecholamines. Similarly, atropinelike effects may be more pronounced in patients receiving anticholinergic therapy. Therefore, particular care should be exercised when it is necessary to administer tricyclic antidepressants with sympathomimetic amines, local decongestants, local anesthetics containing epinephrine, atropine or drugs with an anticholinergic effect. In resistant cases of depression in adults, a dose of 2.5 mg/kg/day may have to be exceeded. If a higher dose is needed, ECG monitoring should be maintained during the initiation of therapy and at appropriate intervals during stabilization of dose.

Usage in Pregnancy—Pregnancy Category C. Surmontil has shown evidence of embryo-toxicity and/or increased incidence of major anomalies in rats or rabbits at doses 20 times the human dose. There are no adequate and well-controlled studies in pregnant women. Surmontil should be used during pregnancy only if the potential benefit justifies the potential risk to the fetus.

Semen studies in man (four schizophrenics and nine normal volunteers) revealed no significant changes in sperm morphology. It is recognized that drugs having a parasympathetic effect, including tricyclic antidepressants, may alter the ejaculatory response.

Chronic animal studies showed occasional evidence of degeneration of seminiferous tubules at the highest dose of 60 mg/kg/day.

Surmontil should be used with caution in patients with impaired liver function.

Chronic animal studies showed occasional occurrence of hepatic congestion, fatty infiltration, or increased serum liver enzymes at the highest dose of 60 mg/kg/day.

Both elevation and lowering of blood sugar have been reported with tricyclic antidepressants.

ADVERSE REACTIONS

Note: The pharmacological similarities among the tricyclic antidepressants require that each of the reactions be considered when Surmontil is administered. Some of the adverse reactions included in this listing have not in fact been reported with Surmontil.

Cardiovascular—Hypotension, hypertension, tachycardia, palpitation, myocardial infarction, arrhythmias, heart block, stroke.

Psychiatric—Confusional states (especially the elderly) with hallucinations, disorientation, delusions; anxiety, restlessness, agitation; insomnia and nightmares; hypomania; exacerbation of psychosis.

Neurological—Numbness, tingling, paresthesias of extremities; incoordination, ataxia, tremors, peripheral neuropathy; extrapyramidal symptoms; seizures, alterations in EEG patterns; tinnitus; syndrome of inappropriate ADH (antidiuretic hormone) secretion.

Anticholinergic—Dry mouth and, rarely, associated sublingual adenitis; blurred vision, disturbances of accommodation, mydriasis, constipation, paralytic ileus; urinary retention, delayed micturition, dilation of the urinary tract.

Allergic—Skin rash, petechiae, urticaria, itching, photosensitization, edema of face and tongue.

Hematologic—Bone-marrow depression including agranulocytosis, eosinophilia; purpura; thrombocytopenia. Leukocyte and differential counts should be performed in any patient who develops fever and sore throat during therapy; the drug should be discontinued if there is evidence of pathological neutrophil depression.

Gastrointestinal—Nausea and vomiting, anorexia, epigastric distress, diarrhea, peculiar taste, stomatitis, abdominal cramps, black tongue.

Endocrine—Gynecomastia in the male; breast enlargement and galactorrhea in the female; increased or decreased libido, impotence; testicular swelling; elevation or depression of blood-sugar levels.

Other—Jaundice (simulating obstructive); altered liver function; weight gain or loss; perspiration; flushing; urinary frequency; drowsiness, dizziness, weakness, and fatigue; headache; parotid swelling; alopecia.

Withdrawal Symptoms—Though not indicative of addiction, abrupt cessation of treatment after prolonged therapy may produce nausea, headache, and malaise.

DOSAGE AND ADMINISTRATION

Dosage should be initiated at a low level and increased gradually, noting carefully the clinical response and any evidence of intolerance.

Lower dosages are recommended for elderly patients and adolescents. Lower dosages are also recommended for outpatients as compared to hospitalized patients who will be under close supervision. It is not possible to prescribe a single dosage schedule of Surmontil that will be therapeutically effective in all patients. The physical psychodynamic factors contributing to depressive symptomatology are very complex; spontaneous remissions or exacerbations of depressive symptoms may occur with or without drug therapy. Consequently, the recommended dosage regimens are furnished as a guide which may be modified by factors such as the age of the patient, chronicity and severity of the disease, medical condition of the patient, and degree of psychotherapeutic support. Most antidepressant drugs have a lag period of ten days to four weeks before a therapeutic response is noted. Increasing the dose will not shorten this period but rather increase the incidence of adverse reactions.

Usual Adult Dose:

Outpatients and Office Patients—Initially, 75 mg/day in divided doses, increased to 150 mg/day. Dosages over 200 mg/day are not recommended. Maintenance therapy is in the range of 50 to 150 mg/day. For convenient therapy and to facilitate patient compliance, the total dosage requirement may be given at bedtime.

Hospitalized Patients—Initially, 100 mg/day in divided doses. This may be increased gradually in a few days to 200 mg/day, depending upon individual response and tolerance. If improvement does not occur in 2 to 3 weeks, the dose may be increased to the maximum recommended dose of 250 to 300 mg/day.

Adolescent and Geriatric Patients—Initially, a dose of 50 mg/day is recommended, with gradual increments up to 100 mg/day, depending upon patient response and tolerance.

Maintenance—Following remission, maintenance medication may be required for a longer period of time, at the lowest dose that will maintain remission. Maintenance therapy is preferably administered as a single dose at bedtime. To minimize relapse, maintenance therapy should be continued for about three months.

OVERDOSAGE

Signs and Symptoms—The response of the patient to toxic overdosage of tricyclic antidepressants may vary in severity and is conditioned by factors such as age, amount ingested, amount absorbed, interval between ingestion and start of treatment. Surmontil is not recommended for infants or young children. Should accidental ingestion occur in any amount, it should be regarded as serious and potentially fatal.

CNS abnormalities may include drowsiness, stupor, coma, ataxia, restlessness, agitation, hyperactive reflexes, muscle rigidity, athetoid and choreiform movements, and convulsions. Cardiac abnormalities may include arrhythmia, tachycardia, ECG evidence of impaired conduction, and signs of congestive heart failure. Other symptoms may include respiratory depression, cyanosis, hypotension, shock, vomiting, hyperpyrexia, mydriasis, and diaphoresis.

Treatment is supportive and symptomatic as no specific antidote is known. Depending upon need the following measures can be considered:

1. Surmontil is not recommended for use in infants and children. Hospitalization with continuous cardiac monitoring for up to 4 days is recommended for children who have ingested Surmontil in any amount. This is based on the reported greater sensitivity of children to acute overdosage with tricyclic antidepressants.

2. Blood and urine levels may not reflect the severity of the poisoning and are mostly of diagnostic value.

3. CNS involvement, respiratory depression, or cardiac arrhythmia can occur suddenly; hospitalization and close observation are necessary, even when the amount ingested is thought to be small or initial toxicity appears slight. Patients with any alteration of ECG should have continuous cardiac monitoring for at least 72 hours and be observed until well after the cardiac status has returned to normal; relapses may occur after apparent recovery.

4. The slow intravenous administration of physostigmine salicylate has been reported to reverse most of the cardiovascular and CNS effects of overdosage with tricyclic antidepressants. In adults, 1 to 3 mg has been reported to be effective. In children, start with 0.5 mg and repeat at 5-minute intervals to determine the minimum effective dose; do not exceed 2.0 mg. Avoid rapid injection, to reduce the possibility of physostigmine-induced convulsions. Because of the short duration of action of physostigmine, it may be necessary to repeat doses at 30- to 60-minute intervals as necessary.

5. In the alert patient, empty the stomach rapidly by induced emesis, followed by lavage. In the obtunded patient, secure the airway with a cuffed endotracheal tube before beginning lavage (do not induce emesis). Instillation of activated-charcoal slurry may help reduce absorption of trimipramine.

6. Minimize external stimulation to reduce the tendency to convulsions. If anticonvulsants are necessary, diazepam, short-acting barbiturates, paraldehyde, or methocarbamol may be useful. Do not use barbiturates if MAO inhibitors have been taken recently.

7. Maintain adequate respiratory exchange. Do not use respiratory stimulants.

8. Shock should be treated with supportive measures, such as intravenous fluids, oxygen, and corticosteroids. Digitalis may increase conduction abnormalities and further irritate an already sensitized myocardium. If congestive heart failure necessitates rapid digitalization, particular care must be exercised.

9. Hyperpyrexia should be controlled by whatever external means available, including ice packs and cooling sponge baths if necessary.

10. Hemodialysis, peritoneal dialysis, exchange transfusions, and forced diuresis have been generally reported as ineffective in tricyclic poisoning.

HOW SUPPLIED

Surmontil® (trimipramine maleate) Capsules, Wyeth®, are available in the following dosage strengths:

25 mg, NDC 0008-4132, opaque blue and yellow capsule marked "WYETH" and "4132", in bottles of 100 capsules and in Redipak® cartons of 100 capsules (10 blister strips of 10).

50 mg, NDC 0008-4133, opaque blue and orange capsule marked "WYETH" and "4133", in bottles of 100 capsules and in Redipak cartons of 100 capsules (10 blister strips of 10).

100 mg, NDC 0008-4158, opaque blue and white capsule marked "WYETH" and "4158", in bottles of 100 capsules.

Keep tightly closed.

Dispense in tight container.

The appearance of these capsules is a trademark of Wyeth-Ayerst Laboratories.

by arrangement with RHONE-POULENC France

Shown in Product Identification Section, page 438

SYNALGOS®-DC

[*sĭn ′al ″gōs*]
Capsules

DESCRIPTION

Each Synalgos-DC capsule contains 16 mg drocode (dihydrocodeine) bitartrate (Warning—may be habit-forming), 356.4 mg aspirin, and 30 mg caffeine.

The inactive ingredients present are alginic acid, cellulose, D&C Red 28, FD&C Blue 1, gelatin, iron oxides, stearic acid, and titanium dioxide.

ACTIONS

Dihydrocodeine is a semisynthetic narcotic analgesic, related to codeine, with multiple actions qualitatively similar to those of codeine; the most prominent of these involve the central nervous system and organs with smooth-muscle components. The principal action of therapeutic value is analgesia.

Synalgos-DC also contains the non-narcotic antipyretic-analgesic, aspirin.

Continued on next page

Wyeth-Ayerst—Cont.

INDICATIONS
For the relief of moderate to moderately severe pain.

CONTRAINDICATIONS
Hypersensitivity to dihydrocodeine, codeine, or aspirin.

WARNINGS
Salicylates should be used with extreme caution in the presence of peptic ulcer or coagulation abnormalities.

Drug Dependence: Dihydrocodeine can produce drug dependence of the codeine type and therefore has the potential of being abused. Psychic dependence, physical dependence, and tolerance may develop upon repeated administration of dihydrocodeine, and it should be prescribed and administered with the same degree of caution appropriate to the use of other oral narcotic-containing medications.

Like other narcotic-containing medications, dihydrocodeine is subject to the provisions of the Federal Controlled Substances Act.

Usage in Ambulatory Patients: Dihydrocodeine may impair the mental and/or physical abilities required for the performance of potentially hazardous tasks, such as driving a car or operating machinery. The patient using Synalgos-DC should be cautioned accordingly.

Interactions with Other Central Nervous System Depressants: Patients receiving other narcotic analgesics, general anesthetics, tranquilizers, sedative-hypnotics, or other CNS depressants (including alcohol) concomitantly with Synalgos-DC may exhibit an additive CNS depression. When such combined therapy is contemplated, the dose of one or both agents should be reduced.

Usage in Pregnancy: Reproduction studies have not been performed in animals. There is no adequate information on whether this drug may affect fertility in human males and females or has a teratogenic potential or other adverse effect on the fetus.

Usage in Children: Preparations containing aspirin should be kept out of the reach of children. Synalgos-DC is not recommended for patients 12 years of age and under. Since there is no experience in children who have received this drug, safety and efficacy in children have not been established.

PRECAUTIONS
Synalgos-DC should be given with caution to certain patients, such as the elderly or debilitated.

ADVERSE REACTIONS
The most frequently observed reactions include light-headedness, dizziness, drowsiness, sedation, nausea, vomiting, constipation, pruritus, and skin reactions.

DOSAGE AND ADMINISTRATION
Dosage should be adjusted according to the severity of the pain and the response of the patient. Synalgos-DC is given orally. The usual adult dose is two capsules every 4 hours as needed for pain.

DRUG INTERACTIONS
The CNS-depressant effects of Synalgos-DC may be additive with that of other CNS depressants.
See "Warnings."
Aspirin may enhance the effects of anticoagulants and inhibit the uricosuric effects of uricosuric agents.

HOW SUPPLIED
Synalgos®-DC Capsules, Wyeth®, are supplied in bottles of 100 and 500 capsules as follows:
NDC 0008-4191, blue and gray capsule marked "WYETH" and "4191".
Store below 25°C (77°F).
Keep tightly closed.
Dispense in tight containers.
Shown in Product Identification Section, page 438

TETANUS AND DIPHTHERIA TOXOIDS ADSORBED for Adult Use ℞
[tet 'ah-nus and dif-the 're-ah tok 'soids]
aluminum phosphate adsorbed
ULTRAFINED®

DESCRIPTION
The diphtheria toxoid component is prepared by cultivating a suitable strain of *Corynebacterium diphtheriae* on a modified Mueller's casein hydrolysate medium (J. Immunology 37: 103, 1939). The tetanus toxoid component is prepared by cultivating a suitable strain of *Clostridium tetani* on a protein-free semisynthetic medium (Appl. Microbiol. 10: 146, 1962). Formaldehyde is used as the toxoiding (detoxifying) agent for both diphtheria and tetanus toxins. The final product contains 0.02 percent free formaldehyde and contains 0.01 percent thimerosal (mercury derivative) as preservative. Each dose (0.5 mL) contains the same amount of purified tetanus toxoid that is in an individual dose of Tetanus Toxoid Adsorbed, Aluminum Phosphate Adsorbed, Ultrafined, Wyeth. In addition, each dose contains no more than 2 Lf of purified diphtheria toxoid. The aluminum content of the final product does not exceed 0.85 mg per 0.5 mL dose. During processing hydrochloric acid and sodium hydroxide are used to adjust the pH. Sodium chloride is added to the finished product to control isotonicity.

HOW SUPPLIED
Tetanus and Diphtheria Toxoids Adsorbed **for Adult Use**, Aluminum Phosphate Adsorbed, Ultrafined®, is available in vials of 5 mL and 0.5 mL TUBEX® Sterile Cartridge-Needle Units (25 gauge × ⅝ inch needle) packaged in cartons of 10 TUBEX, NDC 0008-0341.
For prescribing information write to Professional Service, Wyeth-Ayerst Laboratories, Box 8299, Philadelphia, PA 19101, or contact your local Wyeth-Ayerst representative.

TETANUS TOXOID ℞
[tet 'ahnus tok 'soid]
fluid, purified
ULTRAFINED®

DESCRIPTION
Tetanus Toxoid, fluid, is prepared by growing a suitable strain of *Clostridium tetani* on a protein-free semisynthetic medium (Appl. Microbiol. 10: 146, 1962). Formaldehyde is used as the toxoiding (detoxifying) agent for tetanus toxin. The final product contains no more than 0.02% free formaldehyde and contains 0.01% thimerosal (mercury derivative) as preservative.

Tetanus toxoid is refined by methods perfected in the Wyeth Institute for Medical Research. These methods eliminate at least 97% of the nontoxoid nitrogen. During processing, hydrochloric acid and sodium hydroxide are used to adjust the pH. Sodium chloride is added to the finished product to control isotonicity.

HOW SUPPLIED
Tetanus Toxoid, fluid, purified, Ultrafined®, Wyeth®, NDC 0008-0340, is available in vials of 7.5 mL and in 0.5 mL TUBEX® Sterile Cartridge-Needle Units (25 gauge × ⅝ inch needle), packaged in boxes of 10 TUBEX.
For prescribing information write to Professional Service, Wyeth-Ayerst Laboratories, Box 8299, Philadelphia, PA 19101, or contact your local Wyeth-Ayerst representative.

TETANUS TOXOID ADSORBED ℞
[tet 'ah-nus tok 'soid]
aluminum phosphate adsorbed,
ULTRAFINED®

DESCRIPTION
TETANUS TOXOID ADSORBED, Aluminum Phosphate Adsorbed, Wyeth, is prepared by growing a suitable strain of Cl. tetani on a protein-free, semisynthetic medium (Appl. Microbiol. 10: 146, 1962). Formaldehyde is used as the toxoiding (detoxifying) agent for tetanus toxin. The final product contains no more than 0.02% free formaldehyde and contains 0.01% thimerosal (mercury derivative) as preservative. TETANUS TOXOID ADSORBED, Wyeth, is refined by methods which eliminate at least 97% of the nontoxoid nitrogen. Adsorption of purified antigens on an optimal quantity of aluminum phosphate, a mineral adjuvant, prolongs and enhances the antigenic properties by retarding the rate of absorption. The aluminum content of the final product does not exceed 0.85 mg per 0.5 mL dose. During processing, hydrochloric acid and sodium hydroxide are used to adjust the pH. Sodium chloride is added to the finished product to control isotonicity.

HOW SUPPLIED
Vials of 5 mL.; and 0.5-mL. TUBEX ® Sterile Cartridge-Needle Units, packages of 10.
For prescribing information write to Professional Service, Wyeth-Ayerst Laboratories, Box 8299, Philadelphia, PA 19101, or contact your local Wyeth-Ayerst representative.

THIOSULFIL® Forte ℞
[thī "o-sul 'fil fawrta]
(sulfamethizole 500 mg)

CAUTION: Federal law prohibits dispensing without prescription.

DESCRIPTION
THIOSULFIL Forte is an antibacterial sulfonamide available in tablet form for oral administration.
Chemical name: N′-(5-methyl-1,3,4-thiadiazol-2-yl) sulfanilamide.
Structural formula:
[See Chemical Formula at top of next column].
Sulfamethizole is a 5-membered heterocyclic sulfanilamide, occurring as a white or light buff-colored crystalline powder. Solubility in water is dependent upon the pH (1 g/5 mL at pH

7.5; 1 g/4000 mL at pH 6.5). It is soluble in alcohol, and practically insoluble in benzene.
THIOSULFIL Forte Tablets contain the following inactive ingredients: gelatin, magnesium stearate, microcrystalline cellulose, starch.

CLINICAL PHARMACOLOGY
Mechanism of sulfonamide bacteriostatic action: The primary mechanism of bacteriostatic action by THIOSULFIL Forte is the same as that of most sulfonamides. By competing with the precursor para-aminobenzoic acid, sulfonamides inhibit bacterial synthesis of folic (pteroylglutamic) acid which is required for bacterial growth. Resistant strains are capable of utilizing folic acid precursors or preformed folic acid.

Antibacterial spectrum: The antibacterial spectrum of all sulfonamides is similar. *In vitro* sensitivity of bacteria to sulfonamides does not always reflect *in vivo* sensitivity. Therefore, efficacy must be carefully evaluated with bacteriologic and clinical responses in the individual patient. (See WARNINGS.)

Factors determining efficacy: Efficacy of antimicrobial therapy is dependent upon a number of factors including the *in vivo* sensitivity of the involved organisms, the concentration of the drug required for bacteriostasis, and the achievable concentration of the sulfonamide at the desired site of action.

Because of the very rapid renal clearance of sulfamethizole, the blood levels attained are low, and accumulation of the drug in tissues outside the urinary tract is very limited. Therefore, sulfamethizole is not appropriate for treatment of systemic infections such as nocardiosis or for local lesions outside the urinary tract such as chancroid and trachoma. However, its low degree of acetylation and its rapid renal clearance permit high concentrations of active sulfamethizole to occur in the urinary tract, making it especially applicable for the treatment of infections of this tract. In addition, the possibility of crystalluria is minimized because of the high solubility of the drug in urine.

Approximately 95% of a given dose of sulfamethizole is not metabolized; less than 5% is acetylated. As a consequence, almost all of a given dose of THIOSULFIL Forte is present in its active form in the body.

Approximately 80% of an administered dose is recoverable within eight hours; approximately 98% is cleared within 15 to 24 hours. Sulfamethizole is cleared by the kidney at a rate only 10% to 20% lower than that for creatinine.

Blood concentrations: Following a single 2 g dose of sulfamethizole, peak total drug levels in whole blood are in the range of 6 mg %, the levels fall to about 50% in four hours, and are negligible at eight hours. Approximately the same concentrations are found in children following a single dose of 100 mg/kg.

Urine concentrations: The following average values of free drug in mg/mL were found after a single 4 g dose of sulfamethizole:

0 to 2 hours—	7.01
2 to 4 " —	10.97
4 to 6 " —	5.93
6 to 10 " —	1.09
10 to 24 " —	0.31

Following a single 2 g dose, the following average concentrations of total drug in mg/mL of urine were found:

0 to 4 hours—	5.15
4 to 8 " —	1.8
8 to 12 " —	0.4
16 to 24 " —	0.1

Following a single 1 g dose of sulfamethizole, the average concentration of total drug during the first 3.5 hours was 2.9 mg/mL.

Solubility in urine: Sulfamethizole is highly soluble in urine. The solubilities of free and acetylated drug in buffered urine at 37° C at various pH's, in mg/mL, are given below:

pH	free	acetylated
4.5	108	33
5.3	220	.....
5.6	480	278
6.0	729	310
6.5	5,650	380
7.0	8,250	1,500
7.5	54,000	.....

INDICATIONS AND USAGE
THIOSULFIL Forte is indicated in the treatment of urinary tract infections (primarily pyelonephritis, pyelitis, and cystitis) in the absence of obstructive uropathy or foreign bodies, when these infections are caused by susceptible strains of the following organisms: *Escherichia coli, Klebsiella-Enterobacter, Staphylococcus aureus, Proteus mirabilis,* and *Proteus vulgaris.*

Important note, *In vitro* sulfonamide sensitivity tests are not always reliable. The test must be carefully coordinated with bacteriologic and clinical reponse. When the patient is already taking sulfonamides, follow-up cultures should have aminobenzoic acid added to the culture media.

Currently, the increasing frequency of resistant organisms is a limitation of the usefulness of antibacterial agents, including the sulfonamides, especially in the treatment of recurrent and complicated urinary tract infections.

Wide variation in blood levels may result with identical doses. Blood levels should be measured in patients receiving sulfonamides for serious infections. Free sulfonamide blood levels of 5–15 mg per 100 mL may be considered therapeutically effective for most infections, with blood levels of 12–15 mg per 100 mL optimal for serious infections; 20 mg per 100 mL should be the maximum total sulfonamide level, as adverse reactions occur more frequently above this level.

CONTRAINDICATIONS

Sulfonamides should not be used in patients hypersensitive to sulfa drugs. They should not be used in infants less than two months of age, in pregnancy at term, and during the nursing period because sulfonamides cross the placenta and are excreted in breast milk and may cause kernicterus.

WARNINGS

Deaths associated with the administration of sulfonamides have been reported from hypersensitivity reactions, agranulocytosis, aplastic anemia, and other blood dyscrasias. The occurrence of sore throat, fever, pallor, purpura, or jaundice during sulfonamide administration may be an early indication of serious blood dyscrasias.

PRECAUTIONS

General : The usual precautions used in sulfonamide therapy should be observed, including the maintenance of an adequate fluid intake. Sulfonamides should be used with caution in patients with impairment of hepatic or renal function, severe allergy or bronchial asthma, and in patients with glucose-6-phosphate dehydrogenase deficiency since sulfas may cause hemolysis in this latter group.

Information for the Patient: Adequate fluid intake should be maintained while taking THIOSULFIL Forte. Patients should drink a full 8 oz. glass of water with each dose of THIOSULFIL Forte and drink additional fluids at frequent intervals throughout the day.

Patients should immediately report any adverse side effects to their physician.

Laboratory Tests: Frequent blood counts and renal function tests should be carried out during sulfonamide treatment, especially during prolonged administration. Microscopic urinalyses should be done once a week when a patient is treated for longer than two weeks. Urine cultures should be made to confirm eradication of bacteriuria.

Drug Interactions: The most important interactions between the sulfonamides and other drugs involve those with oral anticoagulants, the sulfonylurea hypoglycemic agents, and the hydantoin anticonvulsants. In each case, sulfonamides can potentiate the effects of the other drug. Dosage adjustments may have to be made when these drugs are given concomitantly. Cross sensitivity may exist with these agents. PABA and certain local anesthetics such as procaine that are esters of PABA, antagonize the effects of sulfonamides and therefore decrease their effectiveness.

An insoluble precipitate may form in acidic urine when sulfamethizole is used concomitantly with methenamine mandelate.

Tolbutamide, diphenylhydantoin, phenytoin, and warfarin may have prolonged half-lives when administered with sulfamethizole.

Carcinogenesis, Mutagenesis, Impairment of Fertility : Rats appear to be especially susceptible to the goitrogenic effects of sulfonamides, and long-term administration has produced thyroid malignancies in the species.

No long-term fertility or mutagenicity studies have been conducted in animals or humans.

Pregnancy: Teratogenic Effects, Pregnancy Category C.

Usage in Pregnancy: The safe use of sulfonamides in pregnancy has not been established. The teratogenicity potential of most sulfonamides has not been thoroughly investigated in either animals or humans. However, a significant increase in the incidence of cleft palate and other bony abnormalities of offspring has been observed when sulfonamides of the short-, intermediate-, and long-acting types were given to pregnant rats and mice at high oral doses (7 to 25 times the human dose).

THIOSULFIL Forte should be used during pregnancy only if the potential benefit justifies the potential risk to the fetus.

Nursing Mothers: THIOSULFIL Forte is contraindicated in pregnant women and nursing mothers. Sulfonamides cross the placenta and are excreted in breast milk to a significant degree. Because of the potential for serious adverse reactions in nursing infants from sulfonamides, a decision should be made whether to discontinue nursing or to discontinue the drug, taking into account the importance of the drug to the mother. See CONTRAINDICATIONS.

Pediatric Use: Sulfamethizole is not indicated for use in infants less than two months old. See CONTRAINDICATIONS and DOSAGE AND ADMINISTRATION.

ADVERSE REACTIONS

Blood dyscrasias: Agranulocytosis, aplastic anemia, thrombocytopenia, leukopenia, hemolytic anemia, purpura, hypoprothrombinemia, and methemoglobinemia.

Allergic reactions: Drug fever, erythema multiforme (Stevens-Johnson syndrome), generalized skin eruptions, epidermal necrolysis, urticaria, serum sickness, pruritus, exfoliative dermatitis, anaphylactoid reactions, periorbital edema, conjunctival and scleral injection, photosensitization, arthralgia, and allergic myocarditis.

Gastrointestinal reactions: Nausea, emesis, abdominal pains, hepatitis, diarrhea, anorexia, pancreatitis, and stomatitis.

CNS reactions: Headache, peripheral neuritis, mental depression, convulsions, ataxia, hallucinations, tinnitus, vertigo, and insomnia.

Renal: Crystalluria, toxic nephrosis with oliguria and anuria.

Miscellaneous reactions: Chills, periarteritis nodosum, and LE phenomenon.

The sulfonamides bear certain chemical similarities to some goitrogens, diuretics (acetazolamide and the thiazides), and oral hypoglycemic agents. Goiter production, diuresis, and hypoglycemia have occurred rarely in patients receiving sulfonamides. Cross-sensitivity may exist with these agents. (See PRECAUTIONS: Carcinogenesis, Mutagenesis, Impairment of Fertility.)

OVERDOSAGE

The maximum tolerated single dose of sulfa drug has not been established. Sulfamethoxazole has been given in single doses up to 2000 mg. The acute signs and symptoms associated with sulfonamide overdose include anorexia, nausea, colicky abdominal pain, vertigo, headache, drowsiness and unconsciousness. Pyrexia, hematuria and crystalluria have been reported. Blood dyscrasias and jaundice are late manifestations of overdosing.

General treatment of overdose for sulfonamides includes induction of emesis and gastric lavage. Urine output should be maintained by either oral or I.V. fluid administration in patients with normal renal function. Renal function with appropriate blood chemistries including electrolytes should be monitored closely in the acute period. Hematologic parameters should be followed over the next 10 days to two weeks after the overdose ingestion. Methemoglobinuria can be acutely reversed with intravenous 1% methylene blue. Sulfamethizole is only minimally dialyzable by hemodialysis and is not dialyzable by peritoneal dialysis. Other supportive measures should be instituted appropriate to signs and symptoms.

DOSAGE AND ADMINISTRATION

Usual dosage: *Adults:* 500 mg to 1 g, three or four times daily.

Children and infants (over 2 months of age): 30 to 45 mg/kg/24 hours, divided into 4 doses.

HOW SUPPLIED

THIOSULFIL Forte—Each white, biconvex, scored, oval tablet contains sulfamethizole 500 mg (scored), in bottles of 100 (NDC 0046-0786-81).

Store at room temperature (approximately 25° C.)

Shown in Product Identification Section, page 438

TRECATOR®-SC   ℞

[*trek "ă 'tōre*]
(ethionamide)
Sugar-Coated Tablets

DESCRIPTION

Ethionamide is a yellow crystalline substance that is practically insoluble in water. It has a faint-to-moderate sulfide odor and is stable at all ordinary temperatures and levels of humidity.

Trecator-SC tablets contain 250 mg ethionamide. The inactive ingredients present are acacia, calcium carbonate, confectioners sugar, FD&C Red 3, FD&C Yellow 6, gelatin, lactose, magnesium stearate, methylcellulose, pharmaceutical glaze, polacrilin potassium, sucrose, talc, and titanium dioxide.

Trecator has the following structural formula:

ACTION

Bacteriostatic against *Mycobacterium tuberculosis.*

INDICATIONS

Failure after adequate treatment with primary drugs (i.e., isoniazid, streptomycin, aminosalicylic acid) in any form of active tuberculosis. Ethionamide should only be given with other effective antituberculous agents.

CONTRAINDICATIONS

Severe hypersensitivity.
Severe hepatic damage.

WARNING

USE IN PREGNANCY: Teratogenic effects have been demonstrated in animals (rabbits, rats) receiving doses in excess of those recommended in humans. Use of the drug should be avoided during pregnancy or in women of childbearing potential unless the benefits outweigh its possible hazard.

USE IN CHILDREN: Optimum dosage for children has not been established. This, however, does not preclude use of the drug when its use is crucial to therapy.

PRECAUTIONS

Pretreatment examinations should include *in vitro* susceptibility tests of recent cultures of *M. tuberculosis* from the patient as measured against ethionamide and the usual primary antituberculous drugs.

Determinations of serum transaminase (SGOT, SGPT) should be made prior to and every 2 to 4 weeks during therapy.

In patients with diabetes mellitus, management may be more difficult and hepatitis occurs more frequently.

Ethionamide may intensify the adverse effects of the other antituberculous drugs administered concomitantly. Convulsions have been reported, and special care should be taken, particularly when ethionamide is administered with cycloserine.

ADVERSE REACTIONS

The most common side effect is gastrointestinal intolerance. Other adverse effects similar to those seen with isoniazid have been reported: peripheral neuritis, optic neuritis, psychic disturbances (including mental depression), postural hypotension, skin rashes, thrombocytopenia, pellagralike syndrome, jaundice and/or hepatitis, increased difficulty in management of diabetes mellitus, stomatitis, gynecomastia, and impotence.

DOSAGE AND ADMINISTRATION

Ethionamide should be administered with at least one other effective antituberculous drug.

Average Adult Dose: 0.5 gram to 1.0 gram/day in divided doses.

Concomitant administration of pyridoxine is recommended.

HOW SUPPLIED

Trecator®-SC (ethionamide) Tablets, Wyeth®, are supplied in bottles of 100 tablets as follows:

250 mg, NDC 0008-4130, orange, sugar-coated tablet marked "WYETH" and "4130".

Keep tightly closed
Dispense in tight container.

TRIPHASIL®-21   ℞

[*tri-fa 'sil*]
Tablets
(levonorgestrel and ethinyl estradiol tablets—triphasic regimen)

DESCRIPTION

Each Triphasil cycle of 21 tablets consists of three different drug phases as follows: Phase 1 comprised of 6 brown tablets, each containing 0.050 mg of levonorgestrel (d(-)-13 beta-ethyl-17-alpha-ethinyl-17-beta-hydroxygon-4-en-3-one), a totally synthetic progestogen, and 0.030 mg of ethinyl estradiol (19-nor-17α-pregna-1,3,5(10)-trien-20-yne-3,17-diol); phase 2 comprised of 5 white tablets, each containing 0.075 mg levonorgestrel and 0.040 mg ethinyl estradiol; and phase 3 comprised of 10 light-yellow tablets, each containing 0.125 mg levonorgestrel and 0.030 mg ethinyl estradiol. The inactive ingredients present are calcium carbonate, glycerin, iron oxides, lactose, magnesium stearate, methylparaben, polyethylene glycol, povidone, propylparaben, sodium benzoate, starch, sucrose, talc, and titanium dioxide.

Levonorgestrel

Continued on next page

Wyeth-Ayerst—Cont.

Ethinyl Estradiol

CLINICAL PHARMACOLOGY

Combination oral contraceptives act primarily through the mechanism of gonadotropin suppression due to the estrogenic and progestational activity of the ingredients. Although the primary mechanism of action is inhibition of ovulation, alterations in the genital tract, including changes in the cervical mucus (which increase the difficulty of sperm penetration) and the endometrium (which reduce the likelihood of implantation), may also contribute to contraceptive effectiveness.

INDICATIONS AND USAGE

Triphasil-21 Tablets are indicated for the prevention of pregnancy in women who elect to use oral contraceptives as a method of contraception.

Oral contraceptives are highly effective. The pregnancy rate in women using conventional combination oral contraceptives (containing 35 mcg or more of ethinyl estradiol or 50 mcg or more of mestranol) is generally reported as less than one pregnancy per 100 woman-years of use. Slightly higher rates (somewhat more than 1 pregnancy per 100 woman-years of use) are reported for some combination products containing 35 mcg or less of ethinyl estradiol, and rates on the order of 3 pregnancies per 100 woman-years are reported for the progestogen-only oral contraceptives.

These rates are derived from separate studies conducted by different investigators in several population groups and cannot be compared precisely. Furthermore, pregnancy rates tend to be lower as clinical studies are continued, possibly due to selective retention in the longer studies of those patients who accept the treatment regimen and do not discontinue as a result of adverse reactions, pregnancy, or other reasons.

In clinical trials with Triphasil Tablets, 3,546 patients completed 35,036 cycles, and a total of nine pregnancies were reported. This represents a pregnancy rate of 0.33 per 100 woman-years. When used as directed, two pregnancies resulted for a corrected pregnancy rate of 0.07 per 100 woman-years.

Table 1 gives ranges of pregnancy rates reported in the literature[1] for other means of contraception. The efficacy of these means of contraception (except the IUD) depends upon the degree of adherence to the method.

TABLE 1
PREGNANCIES PER 100 WOMAN-YEARS
IUD, less than 1–6; Diaphragm with spermicidal products (creams or jellies), 2–20; Condom, 3–36; Aerosol foams, 2–29; Jellies and creams, 4–36;
Periodic abstinence (rhythm) all types, less than 1–47:
1. Calendar method, 14–47;
2. Temperature method, 1–20;
3. Temperature method—intercourse only in postovulatory phase, less than 1–7;
4. Mucus method, 1–25;
No contraception, 60–80.

Dose-Related Risk of Thromboembolism from Oral Contraceptives: Two studies have shown a positive association between the dose of estrogens in oral contraceptives and the risk of thromboembolism.[2,3] For this reason, it is prudent and in keeping with good principles of therapeutics to minimize exposure to estrogen. The oral-contraceptive product prescribed for any given patient should be that product which contains the least amount of estrogen that is compatible with an acceptable pregnancy rate and patient acceptance. It is recommended that new acceptors of oral contraceptives be started on preparations containing 0.05 mg or less of estrogen.

CONTRAINDICATIONS

Oral contraceptives should not be used in women with any of the following conditions:
1. Thrombophlebitis or thromboembolic disorders.
2. A past history of deep-vein thrombophlebitis or thromboembolic disorders.
3. Cerebral-vascular or coronary-artery disease.
4. Known or suspected carcinoma of the breast.
5. Known or suspected estrogen-dependent neoplasia.
6. Undiagnosed abnormal genital bleeding.
7. Known or suspected pregnancy (see Warning No. 5).
8. Benign or malignant liver tumor which developed during the use of oral contraceptives or other estrogen-containing products.

WARNINGS

> Cigarette smoking increases the risk of serious cardiovascular side effects from oral-contraceptive use. This risk increases with age and with heavy smoking (15 or more cigarettes per day) and is quite marked in women over 35 years of age. Women who use oral contraceptives should be strongly advised not to smoke.

The use of oral contraceptives is associated with increased risk of several serious conditions, including thromboembolism, stroke, myocardial infarction, hepatic adenoma, gallbladder disease, hypertension. Practitioners prescribing oral contraceptives should be familiar with the following information relating to these risks.

1. *Thromboembolic Disorders and Other Vascular Problems:* An increased risk of thromboembolic and thrombotic disease associated with the use of oral contraceptives is well-established. Three principal studies in Great Britain[4–6] and three in the United States[7–10] have demonstrated an increased risk of fatal and nonfatal venous thromboembolism and stroke, both hemorrhagic and thrombotic. These studies estimate that users of oral contraceptives are 4 to 11 times more likely than nonusers to develop these diseases without evident cause (Table 2).

CEREBROVASCULAR DISORDERS
In a collaborative American study[9,10] of cerebrovascular disorders in women with and without predisposing causes, it was estimated that the risk of hemorrhagic stroke was 2.0 times greater in users than nonusers and the risk of thrombotic stroke was 4 to 9.5 times greater in users than in nonusers (Table 2).

TABLE 2
SUMMARY OF RELATIVE RISK OF THROMBOEMBOLIC DISORDERS AND OTHER VASCULAR PROBLEMS IN ORAL-CONTRACEPTIVE USERS COMPARED TO NONUSERS

	Relative risk, times greater
Idiopathic thromboembolic disease	4–11
Postsurgery thromboembolic complications	4–6
Thrombotic stroke	4–9.5
Hemorrhagic stroke	2
Myocardial infarction	2–12

MYOCARDIAL INFARCTION
An increased risk of myocardial infarction associated with the use of oral contraceptives has been reported,[11–13] confirming a previously suspected association. These studies, conducted in the United Kingdom, found, as expected, that the greater the number of underlying risk factors for coronary-artery disease (cigarette smoking, hypertension, hypercholesterolemia, obesity, diabetes, history of preeclamptic toxemia) the higher the risk of developing myocardial infarction, regardless of whether the patient was an oral-contraceptive user or not. Oral contraceptives, however, were found to be a clear additional risk factor.

In terms of relative risk, it has been estimated[52] that oral-contraceptive users who do not smoke (smoking is considered a major predisposing condition to myocardial infarction) are about twice as likely to have a fatal myocardial infarction as nonusers who do not smoke. Oral-contraceptive users who are also smokers have about a 5-fold increased risk of fatal infarction compared to users who do not smoke, but about a 10- to 12-fold increased risk compared to nonusers who do not smoke. Furthermore, the amount of smoking is also an important factor. In determining the importance of these relative risks, however, the baseline rates for various age groups, as shown in Table 3, must be given serious consideration. The importance of other predisposing conditions mentioned above in determining relative and absolute risks has not as yet been quantified; it is quite likely that the same synergistic action exists, but perhaps to a lesser extent.

TABLE 3
Estimated annual mortality rate per 100,000 women from myocardial infarction by use of oral contraceptives, smoking habits, and age (in years):

	Myocardial infarction			
	Women aged 30–39		Women aged 40–44	
Smoking habits	Users	Non-users	Users	Non-users
All smokers	10.2	2.6	62.0	15.9
Heavy*	13.0	5.1	78.7	31.3
Light	4.7	0.9	28.6	5.7
Nonsmokers	1.8	1.2	10.7	7.4
Smokers and nonsmokers	5.4	1.9	32.8	11.7

*Heavy smoker: 15 or more cigarettes per day.

From JAIN, A.K., *Studies in Family Planning, 8*:50, 1977

RISK OF DOSE

In an analysis of data derived from several national adverse-reaction reporting systems,[2] British investigators concluded that the risk of thromboembolism, including coronary thrombosis, is directly related to the dose of estrogen used in oral contraceptives. Preparations containing 100 mcg or more of estrogen were associated with a higher risk of thromboembolism than those containing 50–80 mcg of estrogen. Their analysis did suggest, however, that the quantity of estrogen may not be the sole factor involved. This finding has been confirmed in the United States.[3] Careful epidemiological studies to determine the degree of thromboembolic risk associated with progestogen-only oral contraceptives have not been performed. Cases of thromboembolic disease have been reported in women using these products, and they should not be presumed to be free of excess risk.

ESTIMATE OF EXCESS MORTALITY FROM CIRCULATORY DISEASES

A large prospective study[53] carried out in the U.K. estimated the mortality rate per 100,000 women per year from diseases of the circulatory system for users and nonusers of oral contraceptives according to age, smoking habits, and duration of use. The overall excess death rate annually from circulatory diseases for oral-contraceptive users was estimated to be 20 per 100,000 (ages 15-34—5/100,000; ages 35-44—33/100,000; ages 45-49—140/100,000), the risk being concentrated in older women, in those with a long duration of use, and in cigarette smokers. It was not possible, however, to examine the interrelationships of age, smoking, and duration of use, nor to compare the effects of continuous vs. intermittent use. Although the study showed a 10-fold increase in death due to circulatory diseases in users for 5 or more years, all of these deaths occurred in women 35 or older. Until larger numbers of women under 35 with continuous use for 5 or more years are available, it is not possible to assess the magnitude of the relative risk for this younger age group. The available data from a variety of sources have been analyzed[14] to estimate the risk of death associated with various methods of contraception. The estimates of risk of death for each method include the combined risk of the contraceptive method (e.g., thromboembolic and thrombotic disease in the case of oral contraceptives) plus the risk attributable to pregnancy or abortion in the event of method failure. This latter risk varies with the effectiveness of the contraceptive method. The findings of this analysis are shown in the bar graph (Figure 1).[14] The study concluded that the mortality associated with all methods of birth control is low and below that associated with childbirth, with the exception of oral contraceptives in women over 40 who smoke. (The rates given for Pill only/smokers for each age group are for smokers as a class. For "heavy" smokers [more than 15 cigarettes a day], the rates given would be about double; for "light" smokers [less than 15 cigarettes a day], about 50 percent.) The lowest mortality is associated with the condom or diaphragm backed up by early abortion. The risk of thromboembolic and thrombotic disease associated with oral contraceptives increases with age after approximately age 30 and, for myocardial infarction, is further increased by hypertension, hypercholesterolemia, obesity, diabetes, or history of preeclamptic toxemia and especially by cigarette smoking.

Based on the data currently available, the following chart gives a gross estimate of the risk of death from circulatory disorders associated with the use of oral contraceptives:

SMOKING HABITS AND OTHER PREDISPOSING CONDITIONS—RISK ASSOCIATED WITH USE OF ORAL CONTRACEPTIVES

Age	Below 30	30–39	40+
Heavy smokers	C	B	A
Light smokers	D	C	B
Nonsmokers (no predisposing conditions)	D	C,D	C
Nonsmokers (other predisposing conditions)	C	C,B	B,A

A—Use associated with very high risk.
B—Use associated with high risk.
C—Use associated with moderate risk.
D—Use associated with low risk.

The physician and the patient should be alert to the earliest manifestations of thromboembolic and thrombotic disorders (e.g., thrombophlebitis, pulmonary embolism, cerebrovascular insufficiency, coronary occlusion, retinal thrombosis, and mesenteric thrombosis). Should any of these occur or be suspected, the drug should be discontinued immediately.

A four- to six-fold increased risk of postsurgery thromboembolic complications has been reported in oral-contraceptive users.[15,16] If feasible, oral contraceptives should be discontinued at least 4 weeks before surgery of a type associated with an increased risk of thromboembolism or prolonged immobilization.

Figure 1. Estimated annual number of deaths associated with control of fertility and no control per 100,000 nonsterile women, by regimen of control and age of woman.

Regimen of control

☐ No method   ☒ Abortion only   ▨ Pill only/ nonsmokers   ▨ Pill only/ smokers

☒ IUDs only   ▧ Traditional contraception only (diaphragm or condom)   ■ Traditional contraception and abortion

PERSISTENCE OF RISK OF VASCULAR DISORDERS

Findings from one study in Great Britain involving cerebrovascular disease[54] and another study in the United States concerning myocardial infarction[55] suggest that an increased risk of these conditions in users of oral contraceptives persists after discontinuation of the oral contraceptive. In the British study, the risk of cerebrovascular disease remained elevated in former oral-contraceptive users for at least six years after discontinuation. In the U.S. study, an increased risk of myocardial infarction persisted for at least 9 years in women 40- to 49-years-old who had used oral contraceptives for five or more years. The findings in both these studies require confirmation since they are inconsistent with other published information.[9,11,13,56– 60]

2. Ocular Lesions:

There have been reports of neuro-ocular lesions such as optic neuritis or retinal thrombosis associated with the use of oral contraceptives. Discontinue oral-contraceptive medication if there is unexplained, sudden or gradual, partial or complete loss of vision; onset of proptosis or diplopia; papilledema; or retinal-vascular lesions, and institute appropriate diagnostic and therapeutic measures.

3. Carcinoma:

Long-term continuous administration of either natural or synthetic estrogen in certain animal species increases the frequency of carcinoma of the breast, cervix, vagina, and liver. Certain synthetic progestogens, none currently contained in oral contraceptives, have been noted to increase the incidence of mammary nodules, benign and malignant, in dogs.

In humans, three case-control studies have reported an increased risk of endometrial carcinoma associated with the prolonged use of exogenous estrogen in postmenopausal women.[17–19] One publication[20] reported on the first 21 cases submitted by physicians to a registry of cases of adenocarcinoma of the endometrium in women under 40 on oral contraceptives. Of the cases found in women without predisposing risk factors for adenocarcinoma of the endometrium (e.g., irregular bleeding at the time oral contraceptives were first given, polycystic ovaries), nearly all occurred in women who had used a sequential oral contraceptive. These products are no longer marketed. No evidence has been reported suggesting an increased risk of endometrial cancer in users of conventional combination or progestogen-only oral contraceptives.

Several studies[8,21–24] have found no increase in breast cancer in women taking oral contraceptives or estrogens. One study,[25] however, while also noting no overall increased risk of breast cancer in women treated with oral contraceptives,

found an excess risk in the subgroups of oral-contraceptive users with documented benign breast disease. A reduced occurrence of benign breast tumors in users of oral contraceptives has been well-documented.[8,21,25– 27]

In summary, there is at present no confirmed evidence from human studies of an increased risk of cancer associated with oral contraceptives. Close clinical surveillance of all women taking oral contraceptives is, nevertheless, essential. In all cases of undiagnosed persistent or recurrent abnormal vaginal bleeding, appropriate diagnostic measures should be taken to rule out malignancy. Women with a strong family history of breast cancer or who have breast nodules, fibrocystic disease, or abnormal mammograms should be monitored with particular care if they elect to use oral contraceptives instead of other methods of contraception.

4. Hepatic Tumors:

Benign hepatic adenomas have been found to be associated with the use of oral contraceptives.[28–30,46] One study[46] showed that oral contraceptive formulations with high hormonal potency were associated with a higher risk than lower potency formulations. Although benign, hepatic adenomas may rupture and may cause death through intra-abdominal hemorrhage. This has been reported in short-term as well as long-term users of oral contraceptives. Two studies relate risk with duration of use of the contraceptive, the risk being much greater after 4 or more years of oral-contraceptive use.[30,46] While hepatic adenoma is a rare lesion, it should be considered in women presenting abdominal pain and tenderness, abdominal mass or shock. A few cases of hepatocellular carcinoma have been reported in women taking oral contraceptives. The relationship of these drugs to this type of malignancy is not known at this time.

5. Use in or Immediately Preceding Pregnancy, Birth Defects in Offspring, and Malignancy in Female Offspring:

The use of female sex hormones—both estrogenic and progestational agents—during early pregnancy may seriously damage the offspring. It has been shown that females exposed in utero to diethylstilbestrol, a nonsteroidal estrogen, have an increased risk of developing in later life a form of vaginal or cervical cancer that is ordinarily extremely rare.[31,32] This risk has been estimated to be of the order of 1 in 1,000 exposures or less.[33,47] Although there is no evidence at the present time that oral contraceptives further enhance the risk of developing this type of malignancy, such patients should be monitored with particular care if they elect to use oral contraceptives instead of other methods of contraception. Furthermore, a high percentage of such exposed women (from 30 to 90%) have been found to have epithelial changes of the vagina and cervix.[34–38] Although these changes are histologically benign, it is not known whether this condition is a precursor of vaginal malignancy. Male children so exposed may develop abnormalities of the urogenital tract.[48–50] Although similar data are not available with the use of other estrogens, it cannot be presumed that they would not induce similar changes.

An increased risk of congenital anomalies, including heart defects and limb defects, has been reported with the use of sex hormones, including oral contraceptives, in pregnancy.[39–42,51] One case-control study[42] has estimated a 4.7-fold increase in risk of limb-reduction defects in infants exposed in utero to sex hormones (oral contraceptives, hormonal withdrawal tests for pregnancy, or attempted treatment for threatened abortion). Some of these exposures were very short and involved only a few days of treatment. The data suggest that the risk of limb-reduction defects in exposed fetuses is somewhat less than one in 1,000 live births.

In the past, female sex hormones have been used during pregnancy in an attempt to treat threatened or habitual abortion. There is considerable evidence that estrogens are ineffective for these indications, and there is no evidence from well-controlled studies that progestogens are effective for these uses.

There is some evidence that triploidy and possibly other types of polyploidy are increased among abortuses from women who become pregnant soon after ceasing oral contraceptives.[43] Embryos with these anomalies are virtually always aborted spontaneously. Whether there is an overall increase in spontaneous abortion of pregnancies conceived soon after stopping oral contraceptives is unknown. It is recommended that, for any patient who has missed two consecutive periods, pregnancy should be ruled out before continuing the contraceptive regimen. If the patient has not adhered to the prescribed schedule, the possibility of pregnancy should be considered at the time of the first missed period (or after 45 days from the last menstrual period if the progestogen-only oral contraceptives are used), and further use of oral contraceptives should be withheld until pregnancy has been ruled out. If pregnancy is confirmed, the patient should be apprised of the potential risks to the fetus, and the advisability of continuation of the pregnancy should be discussed in the light of these risks.

It is also recommended that women who discontinue oral contraceptives with the intent of becoming pregnant use an alternate form of contraception for a period of time before attempting to conceive. Many clinicians recommend 3

months, although no precise information is available on which to base this recommendation.

The administration of progestogen-only or progestogen-estrogen combinations to induce withdrawal bleeding should not be used as a test of pregnancy.

6. Gallbladder Disease:

Studies[8,23,26] report an increased risk of surgically confirmed gallbladder disease in users of oral contraceptives and estrogens. In one study, an increased risk appeared after 2 years of use and doubled after 4 or 5 years of use. In one of the other studies, an increased risk was apparent between 6 and 12 months of use.

7. Carbohydrate and Lipid Metabolic Effects:

A decrease in glucose tolerance has been observed in a significant percentage of patients on oral contraceptives. For this reason, prediabetic and diabetic patients should be carefully observed while receiving oral contraceptives.

An increase in triglycerides and total phospholipids has been observed in patients receiving oral contraceptives.[44] Three studies[61,62,63] have been performed with the Triphasil Tablets (Levonorgestrel and Ethinyl Estradiol Tablets—Triphasic Regimen) formulation and no significant alterations in lipid metabolism were noted with the exception of a slight increase in triglyceride levels in one study.[62] The clinical significance of these findings remains to be defined.

8. Elevated Blood Pressure:

An increase in blood pressure has been reported in patients receiving oral contraceptives.[26] In some women, hypertension may occur within a few months of beginning oral-contraceptive use. In the first year of use, the prevalence of women with hypertension is low in users and may be no higher than that of a comparable group of nonusers. The prevalence in users increases, however, with longer exposure, and in the fifth year of use is two-and-a-half to three times the reported prevalence in the first year. Age is also strongly correlated with the development of hypertension in oral-contraceptive users. Women who previously have had hypertension during pregnancy may be more likely to develop elevation of blood pressure when given oral contraceptives. Hypertension that develops as a result of taking oral contraceptives usually returns to normal after discontinuing the drug.

9. Headache:

The onset or exacerbation of migraine or development of headache of a new pattern which is recurrent, persistent, or severe, requires discontinuation of oral contraceptives and evaluation of the cause.

10. Bleeding Irregularities:

Breakthrough bleeding, spotting, and amenorrhea are frequent reasons for patients discontinuing oral contraceptives. In breakthrough bleeding, as in all cases of irregular bleeding from the vagina, nonfunctional causes should be borne in mind. In undiagnosed persistent or recurrent abnormal bleeding from the vagina, adequate diagnostic measures are indicated to rule out pregnancy or malignancy. If pathology has been excluded, time or a change to another formulation may solve the problem. Changing to an oral contraceptive with a higher estrogen content, while potentially useful in minimizing menstrual irregularity, should be done only if necessary, since this may increase the risk of thromboembolic disease.

Women with a past history of oligomenorrhea or secondary amenorrhea or young women without regular cycles may have a tendency to remain anovulatory or to become amenorrheic after discontinuation of oral contraceptives. Women with these preexisting problems should be advised of this possibility and encouraged to use other contraceptive methods. Post-use anovulation, possibly prolonged, may also occur in women without previous irregularities.

11. Ectopic Pregnancy:

Ectopic as well as intrauterine pregnancy may occur in contraceptive failures. However, in progestogen-only oral contraceptive failures, the ratio of ectopic to intrauterine pregnancies is higher than in women who are not receiving oral contraceptives, since the drugs are more effective in preventing intrauterine than ectopic pregnancies.

12. Breast-feeding:

Oral contraceptives given in the postpartum period may interfere with lactation. There may be a decrease in the quantity and quality of the breast milk. Furthermore, a small fraction of the hormonal agents in oral contraceptives has been identified in the milk of mothers receiving these drugs.[45,64,65] The effects, if any, on the breast-fed child have not been determined. If feasible, the use of oral contraceptives should be deferred until the infant has been weaned.

PRECAUTIONS

GENERAL

1. A complete medical and family history should be taken prior to initiation of oral contraceptives. The pretreatment and periodic physical examinations should include special reference to blood pressure, breasts, abdomen and pelvic organs, including Papanicolaou smear and relevant laboratory tests. As a general rule, oral contraceptives should not

Continued on next page

Wyeth-Ayerst—Cont.

be prescribed for longer than 1 year without another physical examination and PAP smear being performed.

2. Under the influence of estrogen-progestogen preparations, preexisting uterine leiomyomata may increase in size.

3. Patients with a history of psychic depression should be carefully observed and the drug discontinued if depression recurs to a serious degree.

Patients becoming significantly depressed while taking oral contraceptives should stop the medication and use an alternate method of contraception in an attempt to determine whether the symptom is drug-related.

4. Oral contraceptives may cause some degree of fluid retention. They should be prescribed with caution, and only with careful monitoring, in patients with conditions which might be aggravated by fluid retention, such as convulsive disorders, migraine syndrome, asthma, or cardiac or renal insufficiency.

5. Patients with a past history of jaundice during pregnancy have an increased risk of recurrence of jaundice while receiving oral-contraceptive therapy. If jaundice develops in any patient receiving such drugs, the medication should be discontinued.

6. Steroid hormones may be poorly metabolized in patients with impaired liver function and should be administered with caution in such patients.

7. Oral-contraceptive users may have disturbances in normal tryptophan metabolism which may result in a relative pyridoxine deficiency. The clinical significance of this is yet to be determined.

8. Serum folate levels may be depressed by oral-contraceptive therapy. Since the pregnant woman is predisposed to the development of folate deficiency and the incidence of folate deficiency increases with increasing gestation, it is possible that if a woman becomes pregnant shortly after stopping oral contraceptives, she may have a greater chance of developing folate deficiency and complications attributed to this deficiency.

9. The pathologist should be advised of oral-contraceptive therapy when relevant specimens are submitted.

10. Certain endocrine- and liver-function tests and blood components may be affected by estrogen-containing oral contraceptives:

a. Increased sulfobromophthalein retention.

b. Increased prothrombin and factors VII, VIII, IX, and X; decreased antithrombin 3; increased norepinephrine-induced platelet aggregability.

c. Increased thyroid-binding globulin (TBG) leading to increased circulating total-thyroid hormone, as measured by protein-bound iodine (PBI), T4 by column, or T4 by radioimmunoassay. Free T3 resin uptake is decreased, reflecting the elevated TBG; free T4 concentration is unaltered.

d. Decreased pregnanediol excretion.

e. Reduced response to metyrapone test.

INFORMATION FOR THE PATIENT
(See patient labeling which follows.)

DRUG INTERACTIONS
Reduced efficacy and increased incidence of breakthrough bleeding have been associated with concomitant use of rifampin. A similar association has been suggested with barbiturates, phenylbutazone, phenytoin sodium, ampicillin, and tetracycline.

CARCINOGENESIS
See "Warnings" section for information on the carcinogenic potential of oral contraceptives.

PREGNANCY
Pregnancy Category X. See "Contraindications" and "Warnings."

NURSING MOTHERS
See "Warnings."

ADVERSE REACTIONS
An increased risk of the following serious adverse reactions has been associated with the use of oral contraceptives (see "Warnings"):
   Thrombophlebitis.
   Pulmonary embolism.
   Coronary thrombosis.
   Cerebral thrombosis.
   Cerebral hemorrhage.
   Hypertension.
   Gallbladder disease.
   Benign hepatomas.
   Congenital anomalies.
There is evidence of an association between the following conditions and the use of oral contraceptives, although additional confirmatory studies are needed:
   Mesenteric thrombosis.
   Neuro-ocular lesions, e.g., retinal thrombosis and optic neuritis.

The following adverse reactions have been reported in patients receiving oral contraceptives and are believed to be drug-related:
   Nausea and/or vomiting, usually the most common adverse reactions, occur in approximately 10% or less of patients during the first cycle. Other reactions, as a general rule, are seen much less frequently or only occasionally.
   Gastrointestinal symptoms (such as abdominal cramps and bloating).
   Breakthrough bleeding.
   Spotting.
   Change in menstrual flow.
   Dysmenorrhea.
   Amenorrhea during and after treatment.
   Temporary infertility after discontinuance of treatment.
   Edema.
   Chloasma or melasma which may persist.
   Breast changes: tenderness, enlargement, and secretion.
   Change in weight (increase or decrease).
   Change in cervical erosion and cervical secretion.
   Possible diminution in lactation when given immediately postpartum.
   Cholestatic jaundice.
   Migraine.
   Increase in size of uterine leiomyomata.
   Rash (allergic).
   Mental depression.
   Reduced tolerance to carbohydrates.
   Vaginal candidiasis.
   Change in corneal curvature (steepening).
   Intolerance to contact lenses.
The following adverse reactions have been reported in users of oral contraceptives, and the association has been neither confirmed nor refuted:
   Premenstrual-like syndrome.
   Cataracts.
   Changes in libido.
   Chorea.
   Changes in appetite.
   Cystitis-like syndrome.
   Headache.
   Nervousness.
   Dizziness.
   Hirsutism.
   Loss of scalp hair.
   Erythema multiforme.
   Erythema nodosum.
   Hemorrhagic eruption.
   Vaginitis.
   Porphyria.
   Hemolytic uremic syndrome.

ACUTE OVERDOSE
Serious ill effects have not been reported following acute ingestion of large doses of oral contraceptives by young children. Overdosage may cause nausea, and withdrawal bleeding may occur in females.

DOSAGE AND ADMINISTRATION
To achieve maximum contraceptive effectiveness, Triphasil-21 Tablets (Levonorgestrel and Ethinyl Estradiol Tablets—Triphasic Regimen) must be taken exactly as directed and at intervals not exceeding 24 hours. Triphasil-21 Tablets are a three-phase preparation. The dosage of Triphasil-21 Tablets is **one tablet daily** for 21 consecutive days per menstrual cycle in the following order: 6 brown tablets (phase 1), followed by 5 white tablets (phase 2), and then followed by the last 10 light-yellow tablets (phase 3), according to the prescribed schedule. Tablets are then discontinued for 7 days (three weeks on, one week off).

It is recommended that Triphasil-21 Tablets be taken at the same time each day, preferably after the evening meal or at bedtime. During the first cycle of medication, the patient should be instructed to take one Triphasil-21 Tablet daily in the order of 6 brown, 5 white and, finally, 10 light-yellow tablets for twenty-one (21) consecutive days, beginning on day one (1) of her menstrual cycle. (The first day of menstruation is day one.) The tablets are then discontinued for one week (7 days). Withdrawal bleeding usually occurs within 3 days following discontinuation of Triphasil-21 Tablets. (If Triphasil-21 Tablets are first taken later than the first day of the first menstrual cycle of medication or postpartum, contraceptive reliance should not be placed on Triphasil-21 Tablets until after the first 7 consecutive days of administration. The possibility of ovulation and conception prior to initiation of medication should be considered.)

When switching from another oral contraceptive, Triphasil-21 Tablets should be started on the first day of bleeding following the last tablet taken of the previous oral contraceptive.

The patient begins her next and all subsequent 21-day courses of Triphasil-21 Tablets on the same day of the week that she began her first course, following the same schedule: 21 days on—7 days off. She begins taking her brown tablets on the 8th day after discontinuance regardless of whether or not a menstrual period has occurred or is still in progress. Any time the next cycle of Triphasil-21 Tablets are started later than the 8th day, the patient should be protected by another means of contraception until she has taken a tablet daily for seven consecutive days.

If spotting or breakthrough bleeding occurs, the patient is instructed to continue on the same regimen. This type of bleeding is usually transient and without significance; however, if the bleeding is persistent or prolonged, the patient is advised to consult her physician. Although the occurrence of pregnancy is highly unlikely if Triphasil-21 Tablets are taken according to directions, if withdrawal bleeding does not occur, the possibility of pregnancy must be considered. If the patient has not adhered to the prescribed schedule (missed one or more tablets or started taking them on a day later than she should have), the probability of pregnancy should be considered at the time of the first missed period and appropriate diagnostic measures taken before the medication is resumed. If the patient has adhered to the prescribed regimen and misses two consecutive periods, pregnancy should be ruled out before continuing the contraceptive regimen.

The patient should be instructed to take a missed tablet as soon as it is remembered. If two consecutive tablets are missed they should both be taken as soon as remembered. The next tablet should be taken at the usual time.

Any time the patient misses one or two tablets she should also use another method of contraception until she has taken a tablet daily for seven consecutive days. If breakthrough bleeding occurs following missed tablets it will usually be transient and of no consequence. While there is little likelihood of ovulation occurring if only one or two tablets are missed, the possibility of ovulation increases with each successive day that scheduled tablets are missed. If three consecutive tablets are missed, all medication should be discontinued and the remainder of the package discarded. A new package of Triphasil-21 Tablets should be started on the first day of the patient's next bleed after the last tablet was taken. An alternate means of contraception should be prescribed during the days without tablets and continued until the patient has taken a tablet daily for seven consecutive days. In the nonlactating mother, Triphasil-21 Tablets may be prescribed in the postpartum period either immediately or at the first postpartum examination whether or not menstruation has resumed.

HOW SUPPLIED
Triphasil®-21 Tablets (Levonorgestrel and Ethinyl Estradiol Tablets—Triphasic Regimen), Wyeth®, NDC 0008-2535, are available in packages of 3 compacts, and in packages of 6 compact refills; packages of 12 Pilpak® dispensers are also available for clinic use only. Each cycle contains 21 coated tablets as follows:

NDC 0008-0641, six brown tablets, each containing 0.050 mg levonorgestrel and 0.030 mg ethinyl estradiol;

NDC 0008-0642, five white tablets, each containing 0.075 mg levonorgestrel and 0.040 mg ethinyl estradiol; and

NDC 0008-0643, ten light-yellow tablets, each containing 0.125 mg levonorgestrel and 0.030 mg ethinyl estradiol.

REFERENCES

1. "*Population Reports,*" Series H, Number 2, May 1974; Series I, Number 1, June 1974; Series B, Number 2, January 1975; Series H, Number 3, 1975; Series H, Number 4, January 1976 (published by the Population Information Program, The George Washington University Medical Center, 2001 S St. NW., Washington, D.C.).

2. Inman, W. H. W., Vessey, M. P., Westerholm, B., and Engelund, A., "Thromboembolic disease and the steroidal content of oral contraceptives. A report to the Committee on Safety of Drugs," Brit Med J *2* :203–209, 1970.

3. Stolley, P. D., Tonascia, J. A., Tockman, M. S., Sartwell, P. E., Rutledge, A. H., and Jacobs, M. P., "Thrombosis with low-estrogen oral contraceptives," Am J Epidemiol *102* :197–208, 1975.

4. Royal College of General Practitioners, "Oral contraception and thromboembolic disease," J Coll Gen Pract *13* :267–279, 1967.

5. Inman, W. H. W., and Vessey, M. P., "Investigation of deaths from pulmonary, coronary and cerebral thrombosis and embolism in women of childbearing age," Brit Med J *2* :193–199, 1968.

6. Vessey, M. P., and Doll, R., "Investigation of relation between use of oral contraceptives and thromboembolic disease. A further report," Brit Med J *2* :651–657, 1969.

7. Sartwell, P. E., Masi, A. T., Arthes, F. G., Greene, G. R., and Smith, H. E., "Thromboembolism and oral contraceptives: an epidemiological case control study," Am J Epidemiol *90* :365–380, 1969.

8. Boston Collaborative Drug Surveillance Program, "Oral contraceptives and venous thromboembolic disease, surgically confirmed gallbladder disease and breast tumors," Lancet *1* :1399–1404, 1973.

9. Collaborative Group for the Study of Stroke in Young Women, "Oral contraception and increased risk of cerebral ischemia or thrombosis," N Engl J Med *288* :871–878, 1973.

10. Collaborative Group for the Study of Stroke in Young Women, "Oral contraceptives and stroke in young women: associated risk factors," JAMA 231 :718–722, 1975.

11. Mann, J. I., and Inman, W. H. W., "Oral contraceptives and death from myocardial infarction," Brit Med J 2 :245–248, 1975.

12. Mann, J. I., Inman, W. H. W., and Thorogood, M., "Oral contraceptive use in older women and fatal myocardial infarction," Brit Med J 2 :445–447, 1976.

13. Mann, J. I., Vessey, M. P., Thorogood, M., and Doll, R., "Myocardial infarction in young women with special reference to oral contraceptive practice," Brit Med J 2 :241–245, 1975.

14. Tietze, C., "New Estimates of Mortality Associated with Fertility Control," Family Planning Perspectives, 9 :74–76, 1977.

15. Vessey, M. P., Doll, R., Fairbairn, A. S., and Glober, G., "Post-operative thromboembolism and the use of oral contraceptives," Brit Med J 3 :123–126, 1970.

16. Greene, G. R., and Sartwell, P. E., "Oral contraceptive use in patients with thromboembolism following surgery, trauma, or infection," Am J Pub Health 62 :680–685, 1972.

17. Smith, D. C., Prentice, R., Thompson, D. J., and Herrmann, W. L., "Association of exogenous estrogen and endometrial carcinoma," N Engl J Med 293 :1164–1167, 1975.

18. Ziel, H. K., and Finkle, W. D., "Increased risk of endometrial carcinoma among users of conjugated estrogens," N Engl J Med 293 :1167–1170, 1975.

19. Mack, T. N., Pike, M. C., Henderson, B. E., Pfeffer, R. I., Gerkins, V. R., Arthur, M., and Brown, S. E., "Estrogens and endometrial cancer in a retirement community," N Engl J Med 294 :1262–1267, 1976.

20. Silverberg, S. G., and Makowski, E. L., "Endometrial carcinoma in young women taking oral contraceptive agents," Obstet Gynecol 46 :503–506, 1975.

21. Vessey, M. P., Doll, R., and Sutton, P. M., "Oral contraceptives and breast neoplasia: a retrospective study," Brit Med J 3 :719–724, 1972.

22. Vessey, M. P., Doll, R., and Jones K., "Oral contraceptives and breast cancer. Progress report of an epidemiological study," Lancet 1 :941–943, 1975.

23. Boston Collaborative Drug Surveillance Program, "Surgically confirmed gallbladder disease, venous thromboembolism and breast tumors in relation to postmenopausal estrogen therapy," N Engl J Med 290 :15–19, 1974.

24. Arthes, F. G., Sartwell, P. E., and Lewison, E. F., "The pill, estrogens, and the breast. Epidemiologic aspects," Cancer 28 :1391–1394, 1971.

25. Fasal, E., and Paffenbarger, R. S., "Oral contraceptives as related to cancer and benign lesions of the breast," J Natl Cancer Inst 55 :767–773, 1975.

26. Royal College of General Practitioners, "Oral Contraceptives and Health," London, Pitman, 1974.

27. Ory, H., Cole P., MacMahon, B., and Hoover, R., "Oral contraceptives and reduced risk of benign breast diseases," N Engl J Med 294 :419–422, 1976.

28. Baum, J., Holtz, F., Bookstein, J. J., and Klein, E. W., "Possible association between benign hepatomas and oral contraceptives," Lancet 2 :926–928, 1973.

29. Mays, E. T., Christopherson, W. M., Mahr, M. M., and Williams, H. C., "Hepatic changes in young women ingesting contraceptive steroids. Hepatic hemorrhage and primary hepatic tumors," JAMA 235 :730–732, 1976.

30. Edmondson, H. A., Henderson, B., and Benton, B., "Liver-cell adenomas associated with use of oral contraceptives," N Engl J Med 294 :470–472, 1976.

31. Herbst, A. L., Ulfedler, H., and Poskanzer, D. C., "Adenocarcinoma of the vagina," N Engl J Med 284 :878–881, 1971.

32. Greenwald, P., Barlow, J. J., Nasca, P. C., and Burnett, W., "Vaginal cancer after maternal treatment with synthetic estrogens," N Engl J Med 285 :390–392, 1971.

33. Lanier, A. P., Noller, K. L., Decker, D. G., Elveback, L., and Kurland, L. T., "Cancer and stilbestrol. A follow-up of 1719 persons exposed to estrogens in utero and born 1943–1959," Mayo Clin Pro 48 :793–799, 1973.

34. Herbst, A. L., Kurman, R. J., and Scully, R. E., "Vaginal and cervical abnormalities after exposure to stilbestrol in utero," Obstet Gynecol 40 :287–298, 1972.

35. Herbst, A. L., Robboy, S. J., Macdonald, G. J., and Scully, R. E., "The effects of local progesterone on stilbestrol-associated vaginal adenosis," Am J Obstet Gynecol 118 :607–615, 1974.

36. Herbst, A. L., Poskanzer, D. C., Robboy, S. J., Friedlander, L., and Scully, R. E., "Prenatal exposure to stilbestrol: a prospective comparison of exposed female offspring with unexposed controls," N Engl J Med 292 :334–339, 1975.

37. Stafl, A., Mattingly, R. F., Foley, D. V., Fetherston, W., "Clinical diagnosis of vaginal adenosis," Obstet Gynecol 43 :118–128, 1974.

38. Sherman, A. I., Goldrath, M., Berlin, A., Vakhariya, V., Banooni, F., Michaels, W., Goodman, P., and Brown, S., "Cervical-vaginal adenosis after in utero exposure to synthetic estrogens," Obstet Gynecol 44 :531–545, 1974.

39. Gal, I., Kirman, B., and Stern, J., "Hormone pregnancy tests and congenital malformation," Nature 216 :83, 1967.

40. Levy, E. P., Cohen, A., and Fraser, F. C., "Hormone treatment during pregnancy and congenital heart defects," Lancet 1 :611, 1973.

41. Nora, J. J., and Nora, A. H., "Birth defects and oral contraceptives," Lancet 1 :941–942, 1973.

42. Janerich, D. T., Piper, J. M., and Glebatis, D. M., "Oral contraceptives and congenital limb-reduction defects," N Engl J Med 291 :697–700, 1974.

43. Carr, D. H., "Chromosome studies in selected spontaneous abortions: I. Conception after oral contraceptives," Canad Med Assoc J 103 :343–348, 1970.

44. Wynn, V., Doar, J. W. H., and Mills, G. L., "Some effects of oral contraceptives on serum-lipid and lipoprotein levels," Lancet 2 :720–723, 1966.

45. Laumas, K. R., Malkani, P. K., Bhatnagar, S., and Laumas, V., "Radioactivity in the breast milk of lactating women after oral administration of 3 H-norethynodrel," Am J Obstet Gynecol 98 :411–413, 1967.

46. Center for Disease Control, "Increased Risk of Hepatocellular Adenoma in Women with Long-term use of Oral Contraceptives," Morbidity and Mortality Weekly Report, 26 :293–294, 1977.

47. Herbst, A. L., Cole, P., Colton, T., Robboy, S. J., and Scully, R. E., "Age-incidence and Risk of Diethylstilbestrol-related Clear Cell Adenocarcinoma of the Vagina and Cervix," Am J Obstet Gynecol 128 :43–50, 1977.

48. Bibbo, M., Al-Naqeeb, M., Baccarini, I., Gill, W., Newton, M., Sleeper, K. M., Sonek, M., and Wied, G. L., "Follow-up Study of Male and Female Offspring of DES-treated Mothers. A Preliminary Report," J of Repro Med 15 :29–32, 1975.

49. Gill, W. B., Schumacher, G. F. B., and Bibbo, M., "Structural and Functional Abnormalities in the Sex Organs of Male Offspring of Mothers Treated with Diethylstilbestrol (DES)," J of Repro Med 16 :147–153, 1976.

50. Henderson, B. E., Senton, B., Cosgrove, M., Baptista, J., Aldrich, J., Townsend, D., Hart, W., and Mack, T., "Urogenital Tract Abnormalities in Sons of Women Treated with Diethylstilbestrol," Pediatrics, 58 :505–507, 1976.

51. Heinonen, O. P., Slone, D., Nonson, R. R., Hook, E. B., and Shapiro, S., "Cardiovascular Birth Defects and Antenatal Exposure to Female Sex Hormones," N Engl J Med 296 :67–70, 1977.

52. Jain, A. K., "Mortality Risk Associated with the Use of Oral Contraceptives," Studies in Family Planning, 8 :50–54, 1977.

53. Beral, V., "Mortality Among Oral Contraceptive Users," Lancet, 2 :727–731, 1977.

54. Royal College of General Practitioners' Oral contraception study, "Incidence of arterial disease among oral contraceptive users," J Royal Col Gen Pract 33 :75–82, 1983.

55. Slone, D., Shapiro, S., Kaufman, D. W., Rosenberg, L., Miettinen, O., and Stolley, P., "Risk of myocardial infarction in relation to current and discontinued use of oral contraceptives," N Engl J Med 305 :420–424, 1981.

56. Inman, W.H.W., "Oral contraceptives and fatal subarachnoid haemorrhage," Brit Med J 2 :1468–1470, 1979.

57. Petitti, D. B., and Wingerd, J., "Use of oral contraceptives, cigarette smoking and risk of subarachnoid haemorrhage," Lancet 2 :234–236, 1978.

58. Thorogood, M., Adam, S. A., and Mann, J. I., "Fatal subarachnoid haemorrhage in young women: role of oral contraceptives," Brit Med J 283 :762, 1981.

59. Rosenberg, L., Hennekens, C.H., Rosner, B., Belanger, C., Rothman, K. J., and Speizer, F. E., "Oral contraceptive use in relation to nonfatal myocardial infarction," Am J Epidemiol 111 :59–66, 1980.

60. Adam, S. A., Thorogood, M., and Mann, J. I., "Oral contraception and myocardial infarction revisited: the effects of new preparations and prescribing patterns," Brit J Obstet Gynaecol 88 :838–845, 1981.

61. Data on file.

62. Briggs, M. H., "Implications and assessment of metabolic effects of oral contraceptives." New considerations in oral contraception. Proceedings of an international symposium, Catholic University-Leuven, Leuven, Belgium. September, 1981 Ed. I. Brosens.

63. Vermeulen, A., and Thiery, M., "Metabolic effects of the triphasic oral contraceptive Trigynon®." Contraception 26 :505–513, 1982.

64. Nilsson, S., Nygren, K., and Johansson, E., "Ethinyl Estradiol in Human Milk and Plasma after Oral Administration." Contraception 17 :131–139, 1978.

65. Nilsson, S., Nygren, K., and Johansson, E., "d-Norgestrel Concentrations in Maternal Plasma, Milk, and Child Plasma During Administration of Oral Contraceptives to Nursing Women." Am J Obstet Gynecol 129 :178, 1977.

The patient labeling for oral-contraceptive drug products is set forth below:

Brief Summary Patient Package Insert

> Cigarette smoking increases the risk of serious adverse effects on the heart and blood vessels from oral-contraceptive use. This risk increases with age and with heavy smoking (15 or more cigarettes per day) and is quite marked in women over 35 years of age. Women who use oral contraceptives should not smoke.

Oral contraceptives taken as directed are about 99% effective in preventing pregnancy. (The mini-pill, however, is somewhat less effective.) Forgetting to take your pills increases the chance of pregnancy. Women who have or have had clotting disorders, cancer of the breast or sex organs, unexplained vaginal bleeding, a stroke, heart attack, angina pectoris, or who suspect they may be pregnant should not use oral contraceptives. Various drugs, such as some antibiotics, may also decrease the effectiveness of oral contraceptives. Most side effects of the pill are not serious. The most common side effects are nausea, vomiting, bleeding between menstrual periods, weight gain, and breast tenderness. However, proper use of oral contraceptives requires that they be taken under your doctor's continuous supervision, because they can be associated with serious side effects which may be fatal. Fortunately, these occur very infrequently. The serious side effects are:

1. Blood clots in the legs, lungs, brain, heart, or other organs, and hemorrhage into the brain due to bursting of a blood vessel. Certain of these effects may occur after pill use has been stopped.
2. Liver tumors, which may rupture and cause severe bleeding.
3. Birth defects if the pill is taken while you are pregnant.
4. High blood pressure.
5. Gallbladder disease.

The symptoms associated with these serious side effects are discussed in the detailed leaflet given you with your supply of pills. Notify your doctor if you notice any unusual physical disturbance while taking the pill.

The estrogen in oral contraceptives has been found to cause breast cancer and other cancers in certain animals. These findings suggest that oral contraceptives may also cause cancer in humans. However, studies to date in women taking currently marketed oral contraceptives have not confirmed that oral contraceptives cause cancer in humans.

The detailed leaflet describes more completely the benefits and risks of oral contraceptives. It also provides information on other forms of contraception. Read it carefully. If you have any questions, consult your doctor.

CAUTION

Oral contraceptives are of no value in the prevention or treatment of venereal disease.

DETAILED PATIENT LABELING

WHAT YOU SHOULD KNOW ABOUT ORAL CONTRACEPTIVES

Oral contraceptives ("the pill") are the most effective way (except for sterilization) to prevent pregnancy. They are also convenient and, for most women, free of serious or unpleasant side effects. Oral contraceptives must always be taken under the continuous supervision of a physician.

It is important that any woman who considers using an oral contraceptive understand the risks involved. Although the oral contraceptives have important advantages over other methods of contraception, they have certain risks that no other method has. Only you can decide whether the advantages are worth these risks. This leaflet will tell you about the most important risks. It will explain how you can help your doctor prescribe the pill as safely as possible by telling him about yourself and being alert for the earliest signs of trouble. And it will tell you how to use the pill properly, so that it will be as effective as possible. There is more detailed information available in the leaflet prepared for doctors. Your pharmacist can show you a copy; you may need your doctor's help in understanding parts of it.

WHO SHOULD NOT USE ORAL CONTRACEPTIVES

A. If you have any of the following conditions, you should not use the pill:

1. Clots in the legs or lungs.
2. Angina pectoris.
3. Known or suspected cancer of the breast or sex organs.
4. Unusual vaginal bleeding that has not yet been diagnosed.
5. Known or suspected pregnancy.

B. If you have had any of the following conditions, you should not use the pill:

1. Heart attack or stroke.
2. Clots in the legs or lungs.

> C. Cigarette smoking increases the risk of serious adverse effects on the heart and blood vessels from oral-contraceptive use. This risk increases with age and with heavy smoking (15 or more cigarettes per day) and is quite marked in women over 35 years of age. Women who use oral contraceptives should not smoke.

D. If you have scanty or irregular periods or are a young woman without a regular cycle, you should use another method of contraception because, if you use the pill, you may

Continued on next page

Wyeth-Ayerst—Cont.

have difficulty becoming pregnant or may fail to have menstrual periods after discontinuing the pill.

DECIDING TO USE ORAL CONTRACEPTIVES

If you do not have any of the conditions listed above and are thinking about using oral contraceptives, to help you decide, you need information about the advantages and risks of oral contraceptives and of other contraceptive methods as well. This leaflet describes the advantages and risks of oral contraceptives. Except for sterilization, the IUD, and abortion, which have their own inherent risks, the only risks of other methods of contraception are those due to pregnancy should the method fail. Your doctor can answer questions you may have with respect to other methods of contraception. He can also answer any questions you may have after reading this leaflet on oral contraceptives.

1. What Oral Contraceptives Are and How They Work. Oral contraceptives are of two types. The most common, often simply called "the pill," is a combination of an estrogen and a progestogen, the two kinds of female hormones. The amount of estrogen and progestogen can vary, but the amount of estrogen is most important because both the effectiveness and some of the dangers of oral contraceptives are related to the amount of estrogen. This kind of oral contraceptive works principally by preventing release of an egg from the ovary. When the amount of estrogen is 50 micrograms or more, and the pill is taken as directed, oral contraceptives are more than 99% effective (i.e., there would be less than 1 pregnancy if 100 women used the pill for 1 year). Pills that contain 20 to 35 micrograms of estrogen vary slightly in effectiveness, ranging from 98% to more than 99% effective.

The second type of oral contraceptive, often called the "mini-pill," contains only a progestogen. It works in part by preventing release of an egg from the ovary but also by keeping sperm from reaching the egg and by making the uterus (womb) less receptive to any fertilized egg that reaches it. The mini-pill is less effective than the combination oral contraceptive, about 97% effective. In addition, the progestogen-only pill has a tendency to cause irregular bleeding which may be quite inconvenient, or cessation of bleeding entirely. The progestogen-only pill is used despite its lower effectiveness in the hope that it will prove not to have some of the serious side effects of the estrogen-containing pill (see below), but it is not yet certain that the mini-pill does in fact have fewer serious side effects. The discussion below, while based mainly on information about the combination pills, should be considered to apply as well to the mini-pill.

2. Other Nonsurgical Ways to Prevent Pregnancy. As this leaflet will explain, oral contraceptives have several serious risks. Other methods of contraception have lesser risks or none at all. They are also less effective than oral contraceptives, but, used properly, may be effective enough for many women.

The following table gives reported pregnancy rates (the number of women out of 100 who would become pregnant in 1 year) for these methods.

PREGNANCIES PER 100 WOMEN PER YEAR

Intrauterine device (IUD), less than 1–6; Diaphragm with spermicidal products (creams or jellies), 2–20; Condom (rubber), 3–36; Aerosol foams, 2–29; Jellies and creams, 4–36; Periodic abstinence (rhythm) all types, less than 1–47:

1. Calendar method, 14–47;
2. Temperature method, 1–20;
3. Temperature method—intercourse only in postovulatory phase, less than 1–7;
4. Mucus method, 1–25;

No contraception, 60–80.

The figures (except for the IUD) vary widely because people differ in how well they use each method. Very faithful users of the various methods obtain very good results, except for users of the calendar method of periodic abstinence (rhythm). Except for the IUD, effective use of these methods requires somewhat more effort than simply taking a single pill every day, but it is an effort that many couples undertake successfully. Your doctor can tell you a great deal more about these methods of contraception.

3. The Dangers of Oral Contraceptives.

a. *Circulatory disorders (abnormal blood clotting and stroke due to hemorrhage).* Blood clots (in various blood vessels of the body) are the most common of the serious side effects of oral contraceptives. A clot can result in a stroke (if the clot is in the brain), a heart attack (if the clot is in a blood vessel of the heart), or a pulmonary embolus (a clot which forms in the legs or pelvis, then breaks off and travels to the lungs). Any of these can be fatal. Clots also occur rarely in the blood vessels of the eye, resulting in blindness or impairment of vision in that eye. There is evidence that the risk of clotting increases with higher estrogen doses. It is therefore important to keep the dose of estrogen as low as possible, so long as the oral contraceptive used has an acceptable pregnancy rate and doesn't cause unacceptable changes in the menstrual pattern. Furthermore, cigarette smoking by oral-contraceptive users increases the risk of serious adverse effects on the heart and blood vessels. This risk increases with age and with heavy smoking (15 or more cigarettes per day) and begins to become quite marked in women over 35 years of age. For this reason, women who use oral contraceptives should not smoke.

The risk of abnormal clotting increases with age in both users and nonusers of oral contraceptives, but the increased risk from the contraceptive appears to be present at all ages. For oral-contraceptive users in general, it has been estimated that in women between the ages of 15 and 34 the risk of death due to a circulatory disorder is about 1 in 12,000 per year, whereas for nonusers the risk is about 1 in 50,000 per year. In the age group 35 to 44, the risk is estimated to be about 1 in 2,500 per year for oral-contraceptive users and about 1 in 10,000 per year for nonusers.

Even without the pill, the risk of having a heart attack increases with age and is also increased by such heart attack risk factors as high blood pressure, high cholesterol, obesity, diabetes, and cigarette smoking. Without any risk factors present, the use of oral contraceptives alone may double the risk of heart attack. However, the combination of cigarette smoking, especially heavy smoking, and oral contraceptive use greatly increases the risk of heart attack. Oral-contraceptive users who smoke are about 5 times more likely to have a heart attack than users who do not smoke and about 10 times more likely to have a heart attack than nonusers who do not smoke. It has been estimated that users between the ages of 30 and 39 who smoke have about a 1 in 10,000 chance each year of having a fatal heart attack compared to about a 1 in 50,000 chance in users who do not smoke, and about a 1 in 100,000 chance in nonusers who do not smoke. In the age group 40 to 44, the risk is about 1 in 1,700 per year for users who smoke compared to about 1 in 10,000 for users who do not smoke and to about 1 in 14,000 per year for nonusers who do not smoke. Heavy smoking (about 15 cigarettes or more a day) further increases the risk. If you do not smoke and have none of the other heart attack risk factors described above, you will have a smaller risk than listed. If you have several heart attack risk factors, the risk may be considerably greater than listed.

In addition to blood-clotting disorders, it has been estimated that women taking oral contraceptives are twice as likely as nonusers to have a stroke due to rupture of a blood vessel in the brain. There is evidence that patients who stop taking oral contraceptives after using them continuously for five or more years may continue to have an increased risk of stroke or heart attack for at least six to nine years after discontinuation.

b. *Formation of tumors.* Studies have found that when certain animals are given the female sex hormone, estrogen, which is an ingredient of oral contraceptives, continuously for long periods, cancers may develop in the breast, cervix, vagina, and liver.

These findings suggest that oral contraceptives may cause cancer in humans. However, studies to date in women taking currently marketed oral contraceptives have not confirmed that oral contraceptives cause cancer in humans. Several studies have found no increase in breast cancer in users, although one study suggested oral contraceptives might cause an increase in breast cancer in women who already have benign breast disease (e.g., cysts).

Women with a strong family history of breast cancer or who have breast nodules, fibrocystic disease, or abnormal mammograms or who were exposed to DES (diethylstilbestrol), an estrogen, during their mother's pregnancy must be followed very closely by their doctors if they choose to use oral contraceptives instead of another method of contraception. Many studies have shown that women taking oral contraceptives have less risk of getting benign breast disease than those who have not used oral contraceptives. Recently, strong evidence has emerged that estrogens (one component of oral contraceptives), when given for periods of more than one year to women after the menopause, increase the risk of cancer of the uterus (womb). There is also some evidence that a kind of oral contraceptive which is no longer marketed, the sequential oral contraceptive, may increase the risk of cancer of the uterus. There remains no evidence, however, that the oral contraceptives now available increase the risk of this cancer. Oral contraceptives do cause, although rarely, a benign (nonmalignant) tumor of the liver. These tumors do not spread, but they may rupture and cause internal bleeding, which may be fatal. A few cases of cancer of the liver have been reported in women using oral contraceptives, but it is not yet known whether the drug caused them.

c. *Dangers to a developing child if oral contraceptives are used in or immediately preceding pregnancy.* Oral contraceptives should not be taken by pregnant women because they may damage the developing child. An increased risk of birth defects, including heart defects and limb defects, has been associated with the use of sex hormones, including oral contraceptives, in pregnancy. In addition, the developing female child whose mother has received DES (diethylstilbestrol), an estrogen, during pregnancy has a risk of getting cancer of the vagina or cervix in her teens or young adulthood. This risk is estimated to be about 1 in 1,000 exposures or less. Abnormalities of the urinary and sex organs have been reported in male offspring so exposed. It is possible that other estrogens, such as the estrogens in oral contraceptives, could have the same effect in the child if the mother takes them during pregnancy.

If you stop taking oral contraceptives to become pregnant, your doctor may recommend that you use another method of contraception for a short while. The reason for this is that there is evidence from studies in women who have had "miscarriages" soon after stopping the pill, that the lost fetuses are more likely to be abnormal. Whether there is an overall increase in "miscarriage" in women who become pregnant soon after stopping the pill as compared with women who do not use the pill is not known, but it is possible that there may be. If, however, you do become pregnant soon after stopping oral contraceptives, and do not have a miscarriage, there is no evidence that the baby has an increased risk of being abnormal.

d. *Gallbladder disease.* Women who use oral contraceptives have a greater risk than nonusers of having gallbladder disease requiring surgery. The increased risk may first appear within 1 year of use and may double after 4 or 5 years of use.

e. *Other side effects of oral contraceptives.* Some women using oral contraceptives experience unpleasant side effects that are not dangerous and are not likely to damage their health. Some of these may be temporary. Your breasts may feel tender, nausea and vomiting may occur, you may gain or lose weight, and your ankles may swell. A spotty darkening of the skin, particularly of the face, is possible and may persist. You may notice unexpected vaginal bleeding or changes in your menstrual period. Irregular bleeding is frequently seen when using the mini-pill or combination oral contraceptives containing less than 50 micrograms of estrogen.

More serious side effects include worsening of migraine, asthma, epilepsy, and kidney or heart disease because of a tendency for water to be retained in the body when oral contraceptives are used.

Other side effects are growth of preexisting fibroid tumors of the uterus; mental depression, and liver problems with jaundice (yellowing of the skin). Your doctor may find that levels of sugar and fatty substances in your blood are elevated; the long-term effects of these changes are not known. Some women develop high blood pressure while taking oral contraceptives, which ordinarily returns to the original levels when the oral contraceptive is stopped.

Other reactions, although not proved to be caused by oral contraceptives, are occasionally reported. These include more frequent urination and some discomfort when urinating, blood cell breakdown with kidney failure, nervousness, dizziness, some loss of scalp hair, an increase in body hair, an increase or decrease in sex drive, appetite changes, cataracts, and a need for a change in contact lens prescription, or inability to use contact lenses.

After you stop using oral contraceptives, there may be a delay before you are able to become pregnant or before you resume having menstrual periods. This is especially true of women who had irregular menstrual cycles prior to the use of oral contraceptives. As discussed previously, your doctor may recommend that you wait a short while after stopping the pill before you try to become pregnant. During this time, use another form of contraception. You should consult your physician before resuming use of oral contraceptives after childbirth, especially if you plan to nurse your baby. Drugs in oral contraceptives are known to appear in the milk, and the long-range effect on infants is not known at this time. Furthermore, oral contraceptives may cause a decrease in your milk supply as well as in the quality of the milk.

4. Comparison of the Risks of Oral Contraceptives and Other Contraceptive Methods. The many studies on the risks and effectiveness of oral contraceptives and other methods of contraception have been analyzed to estimate the risk of death associated with various methods of contraception. This risk has two parts: (a) the risk of the method itself (e.g., the risk that oral contraceptives will cause death due to abnormal clotting), and (b) the risk of death due to pregnancy or abortion in the event the method fails. The results of this analysis are shown in the bar graph (Figure 1). The height of the bars is the number of deaths per 100,000 women each year. There are six sets of bars, each set referring to a specific age group of women. Within each set of bars, there is a single bar for each of the different contraceptive methods. For oral contraceptives, there are two bars—one for smokers and the other for nonsmokers. The analysis is based on present knowledge, and new information could, of course, alter it. The analysis shows that the risk of death from all methods of birth control is low and below that associated with childbirth, except for oral contraceptives in women over 40 who smoke. It shows that the lowest risk of death is associated with the condom or diaphragm (traditional contraception) backed up by early abortion in case of failure of the condom or diaphragm to prevent pregnancy. Also, at any age the risk of death (due to unexpected pregnancy) from the use of traditional contraception, even without a backup of abortion, is generally the same as or less than that from use of oral contraceptives.

HOW TO USE ORAL CONTRACEPTIVES AS SAFELY AND EFFECTIVELY AS POSSIBLE, ONCE YOU HAVE DECIDED TO USE THEM

1. What to Tell your Doctor.

You can make use of the pill as safely as possible by telling your doctor if you have any of the following:

a. Conditions that mean you should not use oral contraceptives:

Clots in the legs or lungs.

Clots in the legs or lungs in the past.

A stroke, heart attack, or angina pectoris.

Known or suspected cancer of the breast or sex organs.

Unusual vaginal bleeding that has not yet been diagnosed.

Known or suspected pregnancy.

b. Conditions that your doctor will want to watch closely or which might cause him to suggest another method of contraception:

A family history of breast cancer.

Breast nodules, fibrocystic disease of the breast, or an abnormal mammogram.

Diabetes.	Heart or kidney disease.
High blood pressure.	Epilepsy.
High cholesterol.	Mental depression.
Cigarette smoking.	Fibroid tumors of the uterus.
Migraine headaches.	Gallbladder disease.

c. Once you are using oral contraceptives, you should be alert for signs of a serious adverse effect and call your doctor if they occur.

Sharp pain in the chest, coughing blood, or sudden shortness of breath (indicating possible clots in the lungs).

Figure 1. Estimated annual number of deaths associated with control of fertility and no control per 100,000 nonsterile women, by regimen of control and age of woman.

Pain in the calf (possible clot in the leg).

Crushing chest pain or heaviness (indicating possible heart attack).

Sudden severe headache or vomiting, dizziness or fainting, disturbance of vision or speech, or weakness or numbness in an arm or leg (indicating a possible stroke).

Sudden partial or complete loss of vision (indicating a possible clot in the eye).

Breast lumps (you should ask your doctor to show you how to examine your own breasts).

Severe pain in the abdomen (indicating a possible ruptured tumor of the liver).

Severe depression.

Yellowing of the skin (jaundice).

2. How to Take the Pill So That It is Most Effective.

Reduced effectiveness and an increased incidence of breakthrough bleeding have been associated with the use of oral contraceptives with antibiotics such as rifampin, ampicillin, and tetracycline or with certain other drugs such as barbiturates, phenylbutazone or phenytoin sodium. You should use an additional means of contraception during any cycle in which any of these drugs are taken.

To achieve maximum contraceptive effectiveness, oral contraceptives must be taken exactly as directed and at intervals not exceeding 24 hours. It is recommended that tablets be taken at the same time each day, preferably after the evening meal or at bedtime. Taking them on a definite schedule will decrease the chance of forgetting a tablet and also help keep the proper amount of medication in your system. See detailed instructions below for Triphasil-21 Tablets (Levonorgestrel and Ethinyl Estradiol Tablets—Triphasic Regimen) and Triphasil-28 Tablets (Levonorgestrel and Ethinyl Estradiol Tablets—Triphasic Regimen)

For specific instructions on **how to use your particular package,** refer to the Brief Summary Patient Package insert provided with your pill package.

TRIPHASIL®-21 TABLETS (LEVONORGESTREL AND ETHINYL ESTRADIOL TABLETS—TRIPHASIC REGIMEN)

Triphasil is a three-phased contraceptive, different from the usual same-dose-every-day combination oral contraceptive. Triphasil-21 Tablets contain 21 active pills divided among 6 brown pills, 5 white pills, and 10 light-yellow pills in each package.

The dosage of Triphasil-21 Tablets is **one pill daily** for 21 days in a row in your menstrual cycle beginning with the first brown pill, continuing through the white pills and finishing the cycle with the light-yellow pills, **in that order.** Pills are then discontinued for 7 days. The basic schedule is 21 days on—7 days off.

In the first month, you should begin taking Triphasil-21 Tablets on day one (1) of your menstrual cycle, which is the first day of your menstruation regardless of the amount of bleeding or spotting. (Day 1 is the first day of menstruation, even if it is almost midnight when you start.) Note: During the first month on Triphasil-21 Tablets, if you start taking pills later than day 1 of your menstrual cycle, you should protect yourself by also using another method of birth control until you have taken a pill daily for seven days in a row (6 brown pills followed by 1 white pill). Thereafter, if you follow directions carefully you will obtain the full contraceptive benefit. If you begin taking pills later than the proper day, the possibility of ovulation and pregnancy occurring before or during the taking of the brown pills should be considered.

Take one pill every day until you finish all 21 pills. No pills are then taken for one week (7 days). Your period will usually begin about three days after you take the last light-yellow pill. Don't be alarmed if the amount of bleeding is not the same as before. On the 8th day, start with a brown pill from a new package, even if you still have your period. If, for example, you took Triphasil-21 Tablets for the first time on a Tuesday, the 8th day will also be a Tuesday. **If you have taken the pills as directed,** you will begin the next cycle on the same day of the week. If you start taking pills later than the 8th day, you should protect yourself by also using another method of birth control until you have taken a pill daily for seven days in a row.

When switching from another oral contraceptive, Triphasil-21 Tablets should be started on the first day of bleeding following the last pill taken of the previous oral contraceptive.

TRIPHASIL®-28 TABLETS (LEVONORGESTREL AND ETHINYL ESTRADIOL TABLETS—TRIPHASIC REGIMEN)

Triphasil is a three-phased contraceptive, different from the usual same-dose-every-day combination oral contraceptive. Triphasil-28 Tablets contain active pills divided among 6 brown pills, 5 white pills, and 10 light-yellow pills plus 7 light-green inactive pills per package.

The dosage of Triphasil-28 Tablets is one active pill daily for 21 days in a row beginning with the 6 brown pills, followed by the 5 white pills, followed by the 10 light-yellow pills, and then one of the 7 light-green inactive pills daily for the next 7 days, **in that order,** for a total of 28 days or 4 weeks. The basic schedule is 21 days on active pills (brown, white, and light-yellow)—7 days on light-green inactive pills. Always take all of the 21 active pills (brown, white, and light-yellow) in each package before taking the light-green pills.

When you start your **first** cycle of Triphasil-28 Tablets, you should begin taking your pills on the **first** day of your next menstrual period, regardless of the day of the week or the amount of the bleeding or spotting. Note: During the first month on Triphasil-28 Tablets, if you start taking pills later than day 1 of your menstrual cycle, you should protect yourself by also using another method of birth control until you have taken a pill daily for seven days in a row (6 brown pills followed by 1 white pill). Thereafter, if you follow directions carefully you should obtain the full contraceptive benefit. If you begin taking pills later than the proper day, the possibility of ovulation and pregnancy occurring before or during the taking of the brown pills should be considered. Take one pill every day until you finish all 6 brown, 5 white, and 10 light-yellow pills in a package followed by all 7 light-green pills. Your period will usually begin about three days after you take the last light-yellow pill, which will be during the

time you are taking the light-green pills. Don't be alarmed if the amount of bleeding is not the same as before.

The day after you have taken your last light-green pill, begin a new package of pills (first taking the 6 brown, then the 5 white, and then the 10 light-yellow pills one a day just as you did before) so that you will take a pill every day without interruption. **If you have taken the pills as directed,** the starting day for each new package will always be the same day as in the previous cycle. When switching from another oral contraceptive, Triphasil-28 Tablets should be started on the first day of bleeding following the last pill taken of the previous oral contraceptive.

Spotting or Breakthrough Bleeding:

Spotting is slight staining between menstrual periods which may not even require a pad. Breakthrough bleeding is a flow much like a regular period, requiring sanitary protection. Spotting is more common than breakthrough bleeding, and both occur more often in the first few cycles than in later cycles. These types of bleeding are usually temporary and without significance. It is important to continue taking your pills on schedule. If the bleeding persists for more than a few days, consult your doctor.

MISSED PILLS

There is a chance of becoming pregnant if you miss one brown, white, or light-yellow pill, and that chance increases with each additional brown, white, or light-yellow pill missed. If you miss any one of these pills, it is important it be taken as soon as remembered. If you miss any two of these pills consecutively, it is important both be taken as soon as remembered. The next pill should then be taken at the usual time. Any time you miss one or two brown, white, or light-yellow pills, **or begin a new package later than directed,** you should also use another method of birth control until you have taken a brown, white, or light-yellow pill daily for seven consecutive days. If you miss one or more light-green inactive pills (Triphasil-28 Tablets only), you are still protected against pregnancy **provided** you begin taking your next brown pill on the proper day. If breakthrough bleeding occurs following missed pills, it will usually be temporary and of no consequence.

If you forget to take brown, white, or light-yellow pills three days in a row, do not take them when you remember but stop the medication and discard the package. Begin a new package, as directed above, on the first day of bleeding of your next period. During the days without pills, and until you have taken 6 brown and a white pill daily for seven consecutive days, you should protect yourself from pregnancy by also using another method of birth control.

At times there may be no menstrual period after a cycle of pills. Therefore, if you miss one menstrual period but have taken the pills **exactly as you were supposed to,** continue as usual into the next cycle. If you have not taken the pills correctly and miss a menstrual period, you may be pregnant and should stop taking oral contraceptives until your doctor determines whether or not you are pregnant. Until you can get to your doctor, use another form of contraception. If two consecutive menstrual periods are missed, you should stop taking pills until it is determined whether you are pregnant. If you do become pregnant while using oral contraceptives, you should discuss the risks to the developing child with your doctor.

3. Periodic Examination.

Your doctor will take a complete medical and family history before prescribing oral contraceptives. At that time and about once a year thereafter, he will generally examine your blood pressure, breasts, abdomen, and pelvic organs (including a Papanicolaou smear, i.e., test for cancer).

SUMMARY

Oral contraceptives are the most effective method, except sterilization, for preventing pregnancy. Other methods when used conscientiously, are also very effective and have fewer risks. The serious risks of oral contraceptives are uncommon, and the "pill" is a very convenient method of preventing pregnancy. If you have certain conditions or have had these conditions in the past, you should not use oral contraceptives, because the risk is too great. These conditions are listed in the leaflet. If you do not have these conditions, and decide to use the "pill", please read the leaflet carefully so that you can use the "pill" most safely and effectively. Based on his or her assessment of your medical needs, your doctor has prescribed this drug for you. Do not give the drug to anyone else.

Shown in Product Identification Section, page 438

Continued on next page

Wyeth-Ayerst—Cont.

TRIPHASIL®-28   R

[tri-fa'sil]
Tablets
(levonorgestrel and ethinyl estradiol tablets—triphasic regimen)

DESCRIPTION

Each Triphasil cycle of 28 tablets consists of three different drug phases as follows: Phase 1 comprised of 6 brown tablets, each containing 0.050 mg of levonorgestrel (d(-)-13-beta-ethyl-17-alpha-ethinyl-17-beta-hydroxygon-4-en-3-one), a totally synthetic progestogen, and 0.030 mg of ethinyl estradiol (19-nor-17α-pregna-1,3,5(10)-trien-20-yne-3,17-diol); phase 2 comprised of 5 white tablets, each containing 0.075 mg levonorgestrel and 0.040 mg ethinyl estradiol; and phase 3 comprised of 10 light-yellow tablets, each containing 0.125 mg levonorgestrel and 0.030 mg ethinyl estradiol; then followed by 7 light-green inert tablets. The inactive ingredients present are calcium carbonate, cellulose, FD&C Blue 1, glycerin, iron oxides, lactose, magnesium stearate, methylparaben, polyethylene glycol, povidone, propylparaben, sodium benzoate, starch, sucrose, talc, and titanium dioxide.

Levonorgestrel

Ethinyl Estradiol

CLINICAL PHARMACOLOGY
See Triphasil®-21.

INDICATIONS AND USAGE
See Triphasil-21.

Dose-Related Risk of Thromboembolism from Oral Contraceptives: See Triphasil-21.

CONTRAINDICATIONS
See Triphasil-21.

WARNINGS
See Triphasil-21.

PRECAUTIONS
See Triphasil-21.

INFORMATION FOR THE PATIENT
See Triphasil-21.

DRUG INTERACTIONS
See Triphasil-21.

CARCINOGENESIS
See Triphasil-21.

PREGNANCY
See Triphasil-21.

NURSING MOTHERS
See Triphasil-21.

ADVERSE REACTIONS
See Triphasil-21.

ACUTE OVERDOSE
See Triphasil-21.

DOSAGE AND ADMINISTRATION

To achieve maximum contraceptive effectiveness, Triphasil-28 Tablets (Levonorgestrel and Ethinyl Estradiol Tablets—Triphasic Regimen) must be taken exactly as directed and at intervals not exceeding 24 hours. Triphasil-28 Tablets are a three-phase preparation plus 7 inert tablets. The dosage of Triphasil-28 Tablets is **one tablet daily** for 28 consecutive days per menstrual cycle in the following order: 6 brown tablets (phase 1), followed by 5 white tablets (phase 2), followed by 10 light-yellow tablets (phase 3), plus 7 light-green inert tablets, according to the prescribed schedule.

It is recommended that Triphasil-28 tablets be taken at the same time each day, preferably after the evening meal or at bedtime. During the first cycle of medication, the patient should be instructed to take one Triphasil-28 Tablet daily in the order of 6 brown, 5 white, 10 light-yellow tablets, and then 7 light-green inert tablets for twenty-eight (28) consecutive days, beginning on day one (1) of her menstrual cycle.

(The first day of menstruation is day one.) Withdrawal bleeding usually occurs within 3 days following the last light-yellow tablet. (If Triphasil-28 Tablets are first taken later than the first day of the first menstrual cycle of medication or postpartum, contraceptive reliance should not be placed on Triphasil-28 Tablets until after the first 7 consecutive days of administration. The possibility of ovulation and conception prior to initiation of medication should be considered.)

When switching from another oral contraceptive, Triphasil-28 Tablets should be started on the first day of bleeding following the last tablet taken of the previous oral contraceptive.

The patient begins her next and all subsequent 28-day courses of Triphasil-28 Tablets on the same day of the week that she began her first course, following the same schedule. She begins taking her brown tablets on the next day after ingestion of the last light-green tablet, regardless of whether or not a menstrual period has occurred or is still in progress. Any time a subsequent cycle of Triphasil-28 Tablets is started later than the next day, the patient should be protected by another means of contraception until she has taken a tablet daily for seven consecutive days.

If spotting or breakthrough bleeding occurs, the patient is instructed to continue on the same regimen. This type of bleeding is usually transient and without significance; however, if the bleeding is persistent or prolonged, the patient is advised to consult her physician. Although the occurrence of pregnancy is highly unlikely if Triphasil-28 Tablets are taken according to directions, if withdrawal bleeding does not occur, the possibility of pregnancy must be considered. If the patient has not adhered to the prescribed schedule (missed one or more tablets or started taking them on a day later than she should have), the probability of pregnancy should be considered at the time of the first missed period and appropriate diagnostic measures taken before the medication is resumed. If the patient has adhered to the prescribed regimen and misses two consecutive periods, pregnancy should be ruled out before continuing the contraceptive regimen.

The patient should be instructed to take a missed brown, white, or light-yellow tablet as soon as it is remembered. If two consecutive brown, white, or light-yellow tablets are missed they should both be taken as soon as remembered. The next tablet should be taken at the usual time.

Any time the patient misses one or two brown, white, or light-yellow tablets, she should also use another method of contraception until she has taken a brown, white, or light-yellow tablet daily for seven consecutive days. If the patient misses one or more light-green tablets, she is still protected against pregnancy provided she begins taking brown tablets again on the proper day. If breakthrough bleeding occurs following missed brown, white, or light-yellow tablets, it will usually be transient and of no consequence.

While there is little likelihood of ovulation occurring if only one or two brown, white, or light-yellow tablets are missed, the possibility of ovulation increases with each successive day that scheduled tablets are missed. If three consecutive brown, white, or light-yellow tablets are missed, all medication should be discontinued and the remainder of the package discarded. A new package of Triphasil-28 Tablets should be started on the first day of the patient's next bleed after the last tablet was taken. An alternate means of contraception should be prescribed during the days without tablets and continued until the patient has taken a tablet daily for seven consecutive days. In the nonlactating mother, Triphasil-28 Tablets may be prescribed in the postpartum period either immediately or at the first postpartum examination whether or not menstruation has resumed.

HOW SUPPLIED

Triphasil®-28 Tablets (Levonorgestrel and Ethinyl Estradiol Tablets—Triphasic Regimen), Wyeth®, NDC 0008-2536, are available in packages of 3 compacts, and in packages of 6 compact refills; packages of 12 Pilpak® dispensers are also available for clinic use only. Each cycle contains 28 coated tablets as follows:
NDC 0008-0641, six brown tablets, each containing 0.050 mg levonorgestrel and 0.030 mg ethinyl estradiol;
NDC 0008-0642, five white to off-white tablets, each containing 0.075 mg levonorgestrel and 0.040 mg ethinyl estradiol;
NDC 0008-0643, ten light-yellow tablets, each containing 0.125 mg levonorgestrel and 0.030 mg ethinyl estradiol; and
NDC 0008-0650, seven light-green inert tablets.

REFERENCES
See Triphasil-21.

Brief Summary Patient Package Insert: See Triphasil-21.

CAUTION
See Triphasil-21.

DETAILED PATIENT LABELING: See Triphasil-21.

Shown in Product Identification Section, page 438

TUBEX® Closed Injection System
[tū'beks]

The TUBEX® closed injection system delivers injectable medication in accurately machine-measured doses with each sterile, prefilled cartridge-needle unit permanently identified up to the moment of injection. Precisely calibrated single-use cartridge-needle units eliminate cross contamination and minimize dosage errors. Super-sharp, siliconized needles minimize penetration pressure. Medication is easily delivered via the sturdy, stainless TUBEX hypodermic syringe, the Tubex Fast-Trak® syringe, or the TUBEX Injector.

TUBEX sterile cartridge-needle units are ready for instant use, fit easily into the physician's bag, and are readily stored and inventoried in the office.

TAMP-R-TEL® (tamper-resistant package) — a clear, sturdy plastic package for all TUBEX narcotics and barbiturates — adds a new dimension to the handling and record keeping of these controlled drugs. In TAMP-R-TEL, each TUBEX sterile cartridge-needle unit is locked into an individual slot within the package by its own end-lock tab, which is easily broken to release the unit for use. Once the end-lock tab is broken, it is almost impossible to replace it. TAMP-R-TEL thus enhances package integrity, discourages pilferage and facilitates "at a glance" drug count.

The following products are currently available in TUBEX closed injection system. *For prescribing information on products listed write to Professional Service, Wyeth-Ayerst Laboratories, P.O. Box 8299, Philadelphia, PA 19101, or contact your local Wyeth-Ayerst representative.*

Product and Needle Size Units Per Pkg	NDC 0008-
NARCOTICS in TAMP-R-TEL® (tamper-resistant package)	
CODEINE PHOSPHATE, USP Ⓒ●	
30 mg (½ gr.) (25 G × ⅝″)	
10—1 mL	0608-01
60 mg (1 gr.) (25 G × ⅝″)	
10—1 mL	0609-01
HYDROMORPHONE HYDROCHLORIDE, USP Ⓒ●	
1 mg (1/60 gr.) (25 G × ⅝″)	
10—1 mL fill in 2 mL	0387-01
1 mg (1/60 gr.) (22 G × 1¼″)	
10—1 mL fill in 2 mL	0387-03
2 mg (1/30 gr.) (25 G × ⅝″)	
10—1 mL fill in 2 mL	0295-02
2 mg (1/30 gr.) (22 G × 1¼″)	
10—1 mL fill in 2 mL	0295-01
3 mg (1/20 gr.) (25 G × ⅝″)	
10—1 mL fill in 2 mL	0388-01
4 mg (1/15 gr.) (25 G × ⅝″)	
10—1 mL fill in 2 mL	0296-02
4 mg (1/15 gr.) (22 G × 1¼″)	
10—1 mL fill in 2 mL	0296-01
MEPERGAN® (Meperidine HCl and Promethazine HCl) 25 mg each/mL Ⓒ●	
(22 G × 1¼″)	
10—2 mL	0235-01
MEPERIDINE HYDROCHLORIDE, USP Ⓒ●	
25 mg (22 G × 1¼″)	
10—1 mL fill in 2 mL	0601-02
50 mg (22 G × 1¼″)	
10—1 mL fill in 2 mL	0602-02
75 mg (22 G × 1¼″)	
10—1 mL fill in 2 mL	0605-02
100 mg (22 G × 1¼″)	
10—1 mL fill in 2 mL	0613-02
MORPHINE SULFATE, USP Ⓒ●	
2 mg (1/30 gr.) (25 G × ⅝″)	
10—1 mL	0649-01
4 mg (1/15 gr.) (25 G × ⅝″)	
10—1 mL	0653-01
8 mg (1/8 gr.) (25 G × ⅝″)	
10—1 mL fill in 2 mL	0655-01
8 mg (1/8 gr.) (22 G × 1¼″)	
10—1 mL fill in 2 mL	0655-03

10 mg (1/6 gr.) (25 G × ⅝″)
10—1 mL fill in 2 mL   0656-02

10 mg (1/6 gr.) (22 G × 1¼″)
10—1 mL fill in 2 mL   0656-01

15 mg (¼ gr.) (25 G × ⅝″)
10—1 mL fill in 2 mL   0657-02

15 mg (¼ gr.) (22 G × 1¼″)
10—1 mL fill in 2 mL   0657-01

BARBITURATES in TAMP-R-TEL®
PENTOBARBITAL SODIUM, USP Ⓒ•
100 mg (1½ gr.) (22 G × 1¼″)
10—2 mL   0303-02

PHENOBARBITAL SODIUM, USP Ⓒ
30 mg (½ gr.) (22 G × 1¼″)
10—1 mL   0499-01

60 mg (1 gr.) (22 G × 1¼″)
10—1 mL   0457-01

130 mg (2 gr.) (22 G × 1¼″)
10—1 mL   0304-01

SECOBARBITAL SODIUM, USP Ⓒ•
100 mg (1½ gr.) (22 G × 1¼″)
10—1 mL   0305-02

• Narcotic order blank required.

ANTIBIOTICS
BICILLIN® C-R (Penicillin G Benzathine and Penicillin G Procaine Suspension) 300,000 U each/mL
600,000 U (20 G × 1¼″)
10—1 mL   0026-17

1,200,000 U (20 G × 1¼″)
10—2 mL   0026-16

2,400,000 U (18 G × 2″)
10—4 mL   0026-22
(disposable syringe)

BICILLIN C-R 900/300
(900,000 units Penicillin G Benzathine and 300,000 units Penicillin G Procaine in suspension)
1,200,000 U (20 G × 1¼″)
10—2 mL   0079-01

BICILLIN LONG-ACTING (Sterile Penicillin G Benzathine Suspension)
600,000 U (20 G × 1¼″)
10—1 mL   0021-08

1,200,000 U (20 G × 1¼″)
10—2 mL   0021-07

2,400,000 U (18 G × 2″)
10—4 mL   0021-12
(disposable syringe)

WYCILLIN® (Sterile Penicillin G Procaine Suspension)
600,000 U (20 G × 1¼″)
10—1 mL   0018-10

1,200,000 U (20 G × 1¼″)
10—2 mL   0018-08

2,400,000 U (18 G × 2″)
10—4 mL   0018-12
(disposable syringe)

WYCILLIN Injection and PROBENECID Tablets
(Sterile Penicillin G Procaine Suspension and Probenecid Tablets)
2,400,000 U (18 G × 2″)
4 mL   2517-01
(package contains two disposable syringes and two 0.5 gram Probenecid tablets, USP)

BIOLOGICALS
DIPHTHERIA and TETANUS TOXOIDS ADSORBED (PEDIATRIC)
(25 G × ⅝″)
10—0.5 mL   0338-01

INFLUENZA VIRUS VACCINE
(purified subvirion)
1988-1989 Formula
(25 G × ⅝″)
10—0.5 mL   0699-02

TETANUS and DIPHTHERIA TOXOIDS ADSORBED for Adult Use
(25 G × ⅝″)
10—0.5 mL   0341-01

TETANUS TOXOID ADSORBED
(25 G × ⅝″)
10—0.5 mL   0339-01

TETANUS TOXOID FLUID
(25 G × ⅝″)
10—0.5 mL   0340-01

VITAMINS
CYANOCOBALAMIN, USP
100 mcg (22 G × 1¼″)
10—1 mL   0265-01

1,000 mcg (25 G × ⅝″)
10—1 mL   0264-03

1,000 mcg (22 G × 1¼″)
10—1 mL   0264-01

THIAMINE HYDROCHLORIDE, USP
100 mg (22 G × 1¼″)
10—1 mL fill in 2 mL   0302-01

CARDIOVASCULAR AGENTS
DIGOXIN, USP
0.25 mg (22 G × 1¼″)
10—1 mL   0480-02

0.5 mg (22 G × 1¼″)
10—2 mL   0480-01

EPINEPHRINE, USP (1:1000)
(25 G × ⅝″)
10—1 mL   0263-01

HEPARIN SODIUM, USP
1,000 USP units (22 G × 1¼″)
10—1 mL   0275-01

2,500 USP units (25 G × ⅝″)
10—1 mL   0482-01

5,000 USP units (25 G × ⅝″)
10—0.5 mL   0277-02

5,000 USP units (25 g × ⅝″)
50—0.5 mL   0277-03

5,000 USP units (25 G × ⅝″)
10—0.5 mL   0278-02

7,500 USP units (25 G × ⅝″)
10—1 mL   0293-01

10,000 USP units (25 G × ⅝″)
10—1 mL   0277-01

20,000 USP units (25 G × ⅝″)
10—1 mL   0276-01

SPECIAL AGENTS
ATIVAN® (Lorazepam) Ⓒ
2 mg/mL (22 G × 1¼″)
10—1 mL fill in 2 mL   0581-02

4 mg/mL (22 G × 1¼″)
10—1 mL fill in 2 mL   0570-02

DIMENHYDRINATE, USP
50 mg (22 G × 1¼″)
10—1 mL   0485-01

DIPHENHYDRAMINE HYDROCHLORIDE, USP
50 mg (22 G × 1¼″)
10—1 mL   0384-01

CVC HEPARIN FLUSH KITS
25 USP units
(25 G × ⅝″)
30 Kits   2528-02
Each Unit of Use Kit contains:
One 2.5 mL size (25 G × ⅝″) TUBEX Heparin Lock Flush Solution, USP, 10 USP units per mL and two 2.5 mL size (25 G × ⅝″) TUBEX Bacteriostatic Sodium Chloride Injection, USP.

250 USP units
(25 G × ⅝″)
30 Kits   2529-02
Each Unit of Use Kit contains:
One 2.5 mL size (25 G × ⅝″) TUBEX Heparin Lock Flush Solution, USP, 100 USP units per mL and two 2.5 mL size (25 G × ⅝″) TUBEX Bacteriostatic Sodium Chloride Injection, USP.

HEPARIN FLUSH KITS
10 USP units
(25 G × ⅝″)
50 Kits   2528-01
Each Unit of Use Kit contains:
One 1 mL size (25 G × ⅝″) TUBEX Heparin Lock Flush Solution, USP, 10 USP units per mL and two 2.5 mL size (25 G × ⅝″) TUBEX Bacteriostatic Sodium Chloride Injection, USP.

100 USP units
(25 G × ⅝″)
50 Kits   2529-01
Each Unit of Use Kit contains:
One 1 mL size (25 G × ⅝″) TUBEX Heparin Lock Flush Solution, USP, 100 USP units per mL and two 2.5 mL size (25 G × ⅝″) TUBEX Bacteriostatic Sodium Chloride Injection, USP.

HEPARIN FLUSH 1 mL KITS
10 USP units
(25 G × ⅝″)
50 Kits   2528-03
Each Unit of Use Kit contains:
One 1 mL size (25 G × ⅝″) TUBEX Heparin Lock Flush Solution, USP, 10 USP units per mL and two 1 mL size (25 G × ⅝″) TUBEX Bacteriostatic Sodium Chloride Injection, USP.

100 USP units
(25 G × ⅝″)
50 Kits   2529-03
Each Unit of Use Kit contains:
One 1 mL size (25 G × ⅝″) TUBEX Heparin Lock Flush Solution, USP, 100 USP units per mL and two 1 mL size (25 G × ⅝″) TUBEX Bacteriostatic Sodium Chloride Injection, USP.

HEPARIN LOCK FLUSH Solution, USP
10 USP units per mL (25 G × ⅝″)
50—1 mL   0523-01

100 USP units per mL (25 G × ⅝″)
50—1 mL   0487-01

10 USP units per mL—25 USP units per TUBEX
(25 G × ⅝″)
50—2.5 mL   0523-02

100 USP units per mL—250 USP units per TUBEX
(25 G × ⅝″)
50—2.5 mL   0487-03

OXYTOCIN, USP (Synthetic)
10 USP units (22 G × 1¼″)
10—1 mL   0406-01

PHENERGAN® (Promethazine HCl)
25 mg (22 G × 1¼″)
10—1 mL   0416-01

50 mg (22 G × 1¼″)
10—1 mL   0417-01

PROCHLORPERAZINE EDISYLATE, USP
5 mg (22 G × 1¼″)
10—1 mL   0542-01

10 mg (22 G × 1¼″)
10—2 mL   0542-02

SODIUM CHLORIDE, USP (Bacteriostatic)
(25 G × ⅝″)
50—1 mL   0333-08

(22 G × 1¼″)
50—2.5 mL   0333-05

(25 G × ⅝″)
50—2.5 mL   0333-02

SPARINE® (Promazine HCl)
50 mg (22 G × 1¼″)
10—1 mL   0236-01

TUBEX, EMPTY, STERILE CARTRIDGE-NEEDLE UNITS
(22 G × 1¼″)
50—2 mL   9103-03

Shown in Product Identification Section, page 436

Continued on next page

Wyeth-Ayerst—Cont.

Wyeth®
TUBEX® Injector
DIRECTIONS FOR USE

Ribbed Collar

Plunger Rod   Plunger   TUBEX® Sterile
                         Cartridge-Needle Unit

NOTE: The TUBEX® Injector is reusable; do not discard.
To load the TUBEX® Injector
1. Turn the ribbed collar to the "OPEN" position until it stops.

CLOSE   OPEN

2. Hold the Injector with the open end up and fully insert the TUBEX® Sterile Cartridge-Needle Unit.
Firmly tighten the ribbed collar in the direction of the "CLOSE" arrow.

CLOSE

3. Thread the plunger rod into the plunger of the TUBEX® Sterile Cartridge-Needle Unit until slight resistance is felt.

The Injector is now ready for use in the usual manner.

To administer
Method of administration is the same as with conventional syringe. Remove needle cover by grasping it securely; twist and pull. Introduce needle into patient, aspirate by pulling back slightly on the plunger, and inject.

To remove the empty TUBEX® Cartridge-Needle Unit
1. Do not recap the needle. Disengage the plunger rod.

2. Hold the Injector, needle down, over a needle disposal container and loosen the ribbed collar. TUBEX® Cartridge-Needle Unit will drop into the container.

OPEN

Discard the needle cover.
Used TUBEX® Cartridge-Needle units should not be employed for successive injections or as multiple-dose containers. They are intended to be used only once and discarded.
NOTE: Any graduated markings on TUBEX® Sterile Cartridge-Needle Units are to be used only as a guide in mixing, withdrawing, or administering measured doses.
Wyeth-Ayerst does not recommend and will not accept responsibility for the use of any cartridge-needle unit other than TUBEX® in the TUBEX® Injector.

Fast-Trak® Syringe
QUICK-LOADING
1 and 2 mL size

DIRECTIONS FOR USE
NOTE: The TUBEX Fast-Trak Syringe is reusable: do not discard after use.
To load the TUBEX Fast-Trak Syringe

1. With plunger rod fully withdrawn, insert TUBEX Sterile Cartridge-Needle Unit, needle end first, into the barrel. Rotate the cartridge clockwise to engage the threads on the needle hub with the threads at front end of syringe (a clicking sound will be heard when fully engaged).

2. After engaging the TUBEX cartridge in the TUBEX Fast-Trak Syringe, hold the syringe barrel with one hand and thread the plunger rod to the rubber plunger by gently rotating the plunger rod. Both ends of the TUBEX Sterile Cartridge-Needle Unit should be fully, but lightly, engaged.
To maintain sterility, leave rubber needle sheath in place until just before use.

To administer
Method of administration is the same as with conventional syringe. Remove rubber sheath by grasping securely at the tip and pulling firmly. Do not discard sheath. Introduce needle into patient, aspirate by pulling back slightly on the plunger, and inject.

To remove the empty TUBEX Cartridge-Needle Unit

Place sheath on a flat level surface with opening facing the operator. Do not hold or touch sheath with hand. Hold syringe in one hand and insert needle into the opening of the sheath. Lift the sheath onto the needle with a sweeping motion of the syringe. Bring syringe into a vertical (needle-up) position, allowing the sheath to drop over needle. Then carefully pull down on the proximal (open) end of the sheath to fully cover the needle base.[1]

Unscrew and withdraw the plunger rod. Rotate cartridge counterclockwise to disengage at front end of syringe. Remove the used TUBEX Cartridge-Needle Unit and discard in an efficient needle-disposal system.
Used TUBEX Cartridge-Needle Units should not be employed for successive injections or as multiple-dose containers. They are intended to be used only once and discarded.
NOTE: Any graduated markings on TUBEX Sterile Cartridge-Needle Units are to be used only as a guide in mixing, withdrawing, or administering measured doses.
Wyeth-Ayerst does not recommend and will not accept any responsibility for the use of any cartridge-needle unit other than TUBEX® in the TUBEX® Fast-Trak® Syringe.
Reference
1. GREEN, S. T.: Avoiding needle sticks. Lancet *1(8489):* 1096, 1986.

TUBEX®
Metal Syringe
QUICK-LOADING
1 and 2 mL size

DIRECTIONS FOR USE
To load the METAL TUBEX Hypodermic Syringe

1. Grasp barrel of syringe in one hand. With the other hand, pull back firmly on plunger and swing the entire handle-section downward so that it locks at right angle to the barrel.

2. Insert TUBEX Sterile Cartridge-Needle Unit, needle end first, into the barrel. Engage needle hub by rotating it clockwise in the threads at front end of syringe.

3. Swing plunger back into place and attach end to the threaded shaft of the piston. Hold the syringe barrel with one hand and rotate plunger until both ends of TUBEX Sterile Cartridge-Needle Unit are fully, but lightly, en-

gaged. To maintain sterility, leave the rubber sheath in place until just before use.

To administer

Method of administration is the same as with conventional syringe. Remove rubber sheath by grasping securely at the tip and pulling firmly. Do not discard sheath. Introduce needle into patient, aspirate by pulling back slightly on the plunger, and inject.

To remove the empty TUBEX Cartridge-Needle Unit

Place sheath on a flat level surface with opening facing the operator. Do not hold or touch sheath with hand. Hold syringe in one hand and insert needle into the opening of the sheath. Lift the sheath onto the needle with a sweeping motion of the syringe. Bring syringe into a vertical (needle-up) position, allowing the sheath to drop over needle. Then carefully pull down on the proximal (open) end of the sheath to fully cover the needle base.[1]

Disengage plunger from piston by rotating counterclockwise, and open syringe as in step number 1. Do not pull plunger back before disengaging or syringe will jam.

Rotate TUBEX Cartridge-Needle Unit counterclockwise to disengage at front end of syringe, remove from syringe, and discard in an efficient needle-disposal system.

To adapt 2 mL syring to 1 ml TUBEX

The 2 mL syringe can be used for a 1 mL TUBEX. Engage both ends of TUBEX and push the slide through so the number "1" appears. After use, the syringe automatically resets itself for 2 mL TUBEX.

Used TUBEX Cartridge-Needle Units should not be employed for successive injections or as multiple-dose containers. They are intended to be used only once and discarded. NOTE: Any graduated markings on TUBEX Sterile Cartridge-Needle Units are to be used only as a guide in mixing, withdrawing, or administering measured doses.

Wyeth-Ayerst does not recommend and will not accept any responsibility for the use of any cartridge-needle unit other than TUBEX® in the TUBEX® Syringe.

Reference
1. GREEN, S. T.: Avoiding needle sticks. Lancet *1(8489):* 1096, 1986.

TYPHOID VACCINE, USP   ℞

[*ti 'foid vak 'sēn*]

DESCRIPTION

Typhoid Vaccine, USP, Wyeth, is a saline suspension containing not more than 1000 million Salmonella typhosa (Ty-2-strain) organisms per ml. After growing on veal infusion agar (containing 0.5 percent sodium chloride, 2 percent peptone, and 5 percent agar), the bacteria are washed off the medium, suspended in buffered sodium chloride injection, and killed by a combination of phenol and heat. Phenol (0.5 percent) is added to the final vaccine as preservative. Typhoid Vaccine, USP, Wyeth, is tested for safety, potency, and purity and standardized according to F.D.A. Additional Standards for Bacterial Vaccines, 21 C.F.R. 620.10-620.15.

HOW SUPPLIED

Typhoid Vaccine, USP, Wyeth is supplied in vials of 5 ml and 10 ml, each containing 8 units per ml.

For prescribing information write to Professional Service, Wyeth-Ayerst Laboratories, Box 8299, Philadelphia, PA 19101, or contact your local Wyeth-Ayerst representative.

UNIPEN®   ℞

[*ū 'ni-pen*]

(nafcillin sodium) as the monohydrate
INJECTION • CAPSULES • POWDER
FOR ORAL SOLUTION • TABLETS

DESCRIPTION

UNIPEN (nafcillin sodium) is a semisynthetic penicillin developed by Wyeth research. Although primarily designed as an antistaphylococcal penicillin, in limited clinical trials it has been shown to be effective in the treatment of infections caused by pneumococci and Group A beta-hemolytic streptococci. Because of this wide gram-positive spectrum, this product is particularly suitable for *Initial Therapy* in severe or potentially severe infections before definitive culture results are known and in which staphylococci are suspected.

This product is readily soluble and can be conveniently administered in both oral and parenteral dosage forms. It is resistant to inactivation by staphylococcal penicillinase. Following intramuscular administration in humans, it rapidly appears in the plasma, penetrates body tissues in high concentration, and diffuses well into pleural, pericardial, and synovial fluids.

Unipen capsules contain 250 mg nafcillin sodium as the monohydrate. The inactive ingredients present are calcium carbonate, D&C Yellow 10, FD&C Blue 1, FD&C Yellow 6, gelatin, mineral oil, and titanium dioxide.

Unipen tablets contain 500 mg nafcillin sodium as the monohydrate. The inactive ingredients present are calcium carbonate, cellulose, hydroxypropyl methylcellulose, lactose, magnesium stearate, polacrilin potassium, starch, and talc.

Unipen for oral suspension is a powder which when reconstituted as directed yields a suspension of 250 mg nafcillin sodium per 5 mL. The inactive ingredients present are artificial and natural flavors, citric acid, edetate disodium, FD&C Red 40, FD&C Yellow 6, saccharin sodium, sodium benzoate, sodium citrate, sodium propionate, sucrose, and water.

Unipen injection is available in vial sizes of 500 mg, 1 gram, and 2 gram nafcillin sodium as the monohydrate. When reconstituted as directed each vial contains, respectively, 2 mL, 4 mL, or 8 mL of solution. Each mL contains nafcillin sodium equivalent to 250 mg nafcillin buffered with 10 mg sodium citrate.

NOTE: Unipen contains 2.9 milliequivalents of sodium per gram of nafcillin as the sodium salt.

MICROBIOLOGY

UNIPEN is a bactericidal penicillin which has shown activity *in vitro* against both penicillin-G-sensitive and penicillin-G-resistant strains of *Staphylococcus aureus* as well as against pneumococcus, beta-hemolytic streptococcus, and alpha streptococcus (viridans).

In experimental mouse infections induced with pneumococci, beta-hemolytic streptococci, and both penicillin-G-susceptible and penicillin-G-resistant strains of *Staph. aureus*, nafcillin sodium was compared with methicillin and oxacillin. Regardless of the route of drug administration (intramuscular or oral), nafcillin sodium was consistently and significantly more effective than the other two penicillins.

The fate of a penicillin-G-resistant strain of *Staph. aureus* was determined in the kidneys of mice treated with penicillin G, methicillin, and nafcillin sodium. Animals injected with the nafcillin sodium showed negative cultures after the fourteenth day, whereas positive kidney cultures were obtained during the entire 28-day period from mice treated with penicillin G and methicillin.

PHARMACOLOGY

UNIPEN is relatively nontoxic for animals. The acute LD50 of this product by oral administration in rats and mice was greater than 5 g/kg; by intramuscular administration in rats, 2800 mg/kg; by intraperitoneal administration in rats, 1240 mg/kg; and by intravenous administration in mice, 1140 mg/kg. The intraperitoneal LD50 in dogs is 600 mg/kg. Animal studies indicated that local tissue responses following intramuscular administration of 25% solutions were minimal and resembled those of penicillin G rather than methicillin.

Animal studies indicate that antibacterial amounts are concentrated in the bile, kidney, lung, heart, spleen, and liver. Eighty-four percent of an intravenously administered dose can be recovered by biliary cannulation and 13 percent by renal excretion in 24 hours. High and prolonged tissue levels can be demonstrated by both biological activity assays and C[14] distribution patterns.

At comparable dosage, intramuscular absorption of this product is nearly equivalent to that of intramuscular methicillin, and oral absorption to that of oral oxacillin. Blood concentrations may be tripled by the concurrent use of probenecid. Clinical studies with nafcillin sodium monohydrate in infants under three days of age and prematures have revealed higher blood levels and slower rates of urinary excretion than in older children and adults.

Studies of the effect of this product on reproduction in rats and rabbits have been completed and reveal no fetal or ma-

ternal abnormalities. These studies include the observation of the effects of administration of the drug before conception and continuously through weaning (one generation).

Disc Susceptibility Tests: Quantitative methods that require measurement of zone diameters give the most precise estimates of antibiotic susceptibility. One such procedure* has been recommended for use with discs for testing susceptibility to penicillinase-resistant penicillin-class antibiotics. Interpretations correlate diameters on the disc test with MIC values for penicillinase-resistant penicillins. With this procedure, a report from the laboratory of "susceptible" indicates that the infecting organism is likely to respond to therapy. A report of "resistant" indicates that the infecting organism is not likely to respond to therapy. A report of "intermediate susceptibility" suggests that the organism would be susceptible if high dosage is used, or if the infection is confined to tissues and fluids (e.g., urine) in which high antibiotic levels are attained.

*Bauer, A.W., Kirby, W.M.M., Sherris, J.C., and Turck, M.: Antibiotic Testing by a Standardized Single-Discs Method, Am. J. Clin. Pathol., *45* :493, 1966; Standardized Disc Susceptibility Test, FEDERAL REGISTER *37* :20527-29, 1972.

INDICATIONS

Although the principal indication for nafcillin sodium is in the treatment of infections due to penicillinase-producing staphylococci, it may be used to initiate therapy in such patients in whom a staphylococcal infection is suspected. (See Important Note below.)

Bacteriologic studies to determine the causative organisms and their sensitivity to nafcillin sodium should be performed.

In serious, life-threatening infections, oral preparations of the penicillinase-resistant penicillins should not be relied on for initial therapy.

IMPORTANT NOTE

When it is judged necessary that treatment be initiated before definitive culture and sensitivity results are known, the choice of nafcillin sodium should take into consideration the fact that it has been shown to be effective only in the treatment of infections caused by pneumococci, Group A beta-hemolytic streptococci, and penicillin-G-resistant and penicillin-G-sensitive staphylococci. If the bacteriology report later indicates the infection is due to an organism other than a penicillin-G-resistant staphylococcus sensitive to nafcillin sodium, the physician is advised to continue therapy with a drug other than nafcillin sodium or any other penicillinase-resistant, semisynthetic penicillin.

Recent studies have reported that the percentage of staphylococcal isolates resistant to penicillin G outside the hospital is increasing, approximating the high percentage of resistant staphylococcal isolates found in the hospital. For this reason, it is recommended that penicillinase-resistant penicillin be used as initial therapy for any suspected staphylococcal infection until culture and sensitivity results are known.

Methicillin is a compound that acts through a mechanism similar to that of nafcillin sodium against penicillin-G-resistant staphylococci. Strains of staphylococci resistant to methicillin have existed in nature, and it is known that the number of these strains reported has been increasing. Such strains of staphylococci have been capable of producing serious disease, in some instances resulting in fatality. Because of this there is concern that widespread use of the penicillinase-resistant penicillins may result in the appearance of an increasing number of staphylococcal strains which are resistant to these penicillins.

Methicillin-resistant strains are almost always resistant to all other penicillinase-resistant penicillins (cross-resistance with cephalosporin derivatives also occurs frequently). Resistance to any penicillinase-resistant penicillin should be interpreted as evidence of clinical resistance to all, in spite of the fact that minor variations in *in vitro* sensitivity may be encountered when more than one penicillinase-resistant penicillin is tested against the same strain of staphylococcus.

CONTRAINDICATIONS

A history of allergic reaction to any of the penicillins is a contraindication.

WARNINGS

Serious and occasionally fatal hypersensitivity (anaphylactoid) reactions have been reported in patients on penicillin therapy. Although anaphylaxis is more frequent following parenteral therapy, it has occurred in patients on oral penicillins. These reactions are more apt to occur in individuals with a history of sensitivity to multiple allergens.

There have been reports of individuals with a history of penicillin hypersensitivity reactions who have experienced severe hypersensitivity reactions when treated with a cephalosporin. Before therapy with a penicillin, careful inquiry should be made concerning previous hypersensitivity reactions to penicillins, cephalosporins, and other allergens. If an

Continued on next page

Wyeth-Ayerst—Cont.

allergic reaction occurs, appropriate therapy should be instituted, and discontinuation of nafcillin therapy considered. The usual agents (antihistamines, pressor amines, corticosteroids) should be readily available.

Unipen injection should be used with caution when administered by the intravenous route because of the possibility of thrombophlebitis. To help minimize the risk of thrombophlebitis, it is important to administer Unipen through the tubing of an intravenous infusion set that is known to be functioning satisfactorily and to administer it in recommended concentrations (see "Dosage and Administration"). Caution should also be exercised to avoid extravasation, since under such circumstances chemical irritation of perivascular tissues may be severe. Reports of injuries following extravasation have included ulceration, tissue necrosis, sloughing, and gangrene which, in some cases, required surgical debridement and skin grafting. In the event that a patient complains of pain during intravenous infusion of Unipen, the infusion should immediately be stopped to provide for evaluation of possible thrombophlebitis or perivascular extravasation.

PRECAUTIONS

As with any potent drug, periodic assessment of organ-system function, including renal, hepatic, and hematopoietic, should be made during prolonged therapy.

The possibility of bacterial and fungal overgrowth should be kept in mind during long-term therapy. If overgrowth of resistant organisms occurs, appropriate measures should be taken.

The oral route of administration should not be relied upon in patients with severe illness, or with nausea, vomiting, gastric dilatation, cardiospasm, or intestinal hypermotility. Safety for use in pregnancy has not been established.

ADVERSE REACTIONS

Reactions to nafcillin sodium have been infrequent and mild in nature. As with other penicillins, the possibility of an anaphylactic reaction or serum-sickness like reactions should be considered. A careful history should be taken. Patients with histories of hay fever, asthma, urticaria, or previous sensitivity to penicillin are more likely to react adversely.

Transient leukopenia, neutropenia with evidence of granulocytopenia or thrombocytopenia are infrequent and usually associated with prolonged therapy with high doses of penicillin. These alterations have been noted to return to normal after cessation of therapy.

The few reactions associated with the intramuscular use of nafcillin sodium have been skin rash, pruritus, and possible drug fever. As with other penicillins, reactions from oral use of the drug have included nausea, vomiting, diarrhea, urticaria, and pruritus.

DOSAGE AND ADMINISTRATION

Parenteral drug products should be inspected visually for particulate matter and discoloration prior to administration, whenever solution and container permit.

It is recommended that parenteral therapy be used initially in severe infections. The patient should be placed on oral therapy with this product as soon as the clinical condition warrants. Very severe infections may require very high doses.

Intravenous Route: 500 mg every 4 hours; double the dose if necessary in very severe infections.

The required amount of drug should be diluted in 15 to 30 mL of Sterile Water for Injection, USP, or Sodium Chloride Injection, USP, and injected over a 5- to 10-minute period. This may be accomplished through the tubing of an intravenous infusion if desirable.

To add nafcillin sodium to an intravenous solution, reconstitute the vials as directed under "How Supplied"—"For Parenteral Administration." Add the reconstituted vial contents immediately to the intravenous solution or within 8 hours following reconstitution if the vials are kept at room temperature (25° C) or within 48 hours following reconstitution if the vials are kept at refrigeration (2°-8° C).

Stability studies on nafcillin sodium at concentrations of 2 mg/mL to 40 mg/mL in the following intravenous solutions indicate the drug will lose less than 10% activity at room temperature (70° F) or, if kept under refrigeration, during the time period stipulated:

STABILITY OF	ROOM TEMPERATURE	REFRIGERATED
Sterile Water for Injection	24 hours	96 hours
Isotonic sodium chloride	24 hours	96 hours
5% dextrose in water	24 hours	96 hours
5% dextrose in 0.4% sodium chloride solution	24 hours	96 hours
Ringer's solution	24 hours	96 hours
M/6 sodium lactate solution	24 hours	96 hours

Discard any unused portions of intravenous solutions after 24 hours if kept at room temperature or after 96 hours if kept under refrigeration.

Only those solutions listed above should be used for the intravenous infusion of Unipen (nafcillin sodium). The concentration of the antibiotic should fall within the range of 2 to 40 mg/mL. The drug concentrate and the rate and volume of the infusion should be adjusted so that the total dose of nafcillin is administered before the drug loses its stability in the solution in use.

There is no clinical experience available on the use of this agent in neonates or infants for this route of administration. This route of administration should be used for relatively short-term therapy (24 to 48 hours) because of the occasional occurrence of thrombophlebitis, particularly in elderly patients.

This route of administration requires care be taken not to allow perivascular extravasation (see "Warnings").

PIGGYBACK UNITS (for Intravenous Drip Use)

As diluents, use the following solutions: Sterile Water for Injection, Isotonic Sodium Chloride, 5% dextrose in water, 5% dextrose in 0.4% sodium chloride solution, Ringer's solution, or M/6 sodium lactate solution.

1-GRAM BOTTLE:

Add a minimum of 49 mL diluent and shake well. If lower concentrations are desired, the solution could be further diluted with up to a total of 99 mL of diluent.

Amount of Diluent	Concentration of Solution
49 mL	20 mg/mL
99 mL	10 mg/mL

2-GRAM BOTTLE:

Add a minimum of 49 mL diluent and shake well. If lower concentrations are desired, the solution could be further diluted with up to a total of 99 mL of diluent.

Amount of Diluent	Concentration of Solution
49 mL	40 mg/mL
99 mL	20 mg/mL

The resulting solutions may then be administered alone or with the intravenous solutions listed above. Discard unused solution after 24 hours at room temperature (70°F) or 96 hours if kept under refrigeration. Administer piggyback through an IV tubing very slowly (at least 30 to 60 minutes) to avoid vein irritation.

At times it may be desired to use the contents of the piggyback bottles for addition to large-volume IV fluids. In this case the entire vial contents should be dissolved in not less than 25 mL of Sterile Water for Injection. Use the resulting concentration within 24 hours when kept at room temperature or within 96 hours when kept under refrigeration.

TEN-GRAM BOTTLE

Add 94 mL Sterile Water for Injection, USP, or Sodium Chloride Injection, USP, and shake well. For ease of reconstitution, the amount of diluent should be added in two portions; the first portion should not exceed 25 mL. Shake gently after each addition and before using. The final concentration will be approximately 100 mg/mL. After reconstitution, use within 8 hours if kept at room temperature or within 48 hours if kept under refrigeration.

The closure shall be penetrated only one time after reconstitution with a suitable sterile transfer device or dispensing set which allows measured dispensing of the contents. The Pharmacy Bulk Package is to be used only in a suitable work area, such as a laminar flow hood (or an equivalent clean-air compounding area).

IV INFUSION

The recommended dosage should be withdrawn from the stock solution and further diluted with water or saline to a maximum concentration of 40 mg/mL or less. The solution thus diluted will remain stable for 24 hours at room temperature or 96 hours under refrigeration. Any unused portion of the above-mentioned solutions must be discarded after the time periods specified above.

Caution: Administer slowly by intravenous route over a period of at least 30 to 60 minutes to avoid vein irritation.

ADD-Vantage™ VIALS—500 mg, 1 gram, and 2 gram. Unipen® (nafcillin sodium) in the ADD-Vantage system is intended as a single dose for intravenous administration after dilution with the ADD-Vantage Flexible Diluent Container containing 50 mL or 100 mL of 0.9% Sodium Chloride Injection, USP, or 5% Dextrose, USP. See "Instructions for Use of the Add-Vantage Vial."

Stability studies on reconstituted Unipen at concentrations of 5 mg/mL to 40 mg/mL in the ADD-Vantage system's various intravenous solutions indicate that the drug will lose less than 10% activity at room temperature (70°F) during the time period stated:

Intravenous Solutions	Room Temperature
0.9% Sodium Chloride Inj.	24 hours
5% Dextrose Inj.	24 hours

CAUTION: Administer slowly by intravenous route over a period of at least 20 minutes. More rapid administration may result in convulsive seizures.

CONVENTIONAL VIALS—500 mg, 1 gram, and 2 gram.

Intramuscular Route: 500 mg every 6 hours in adults; decrease the interval to 4 hours if necessary in severe infections. In infants and children, a dose of 25 mg/kg (about 12 mg/lb) twice daily is usually adequate.

For neonates, 10 mg/kg is recommended twice daily.

To reconstitute see directions and table below.

The clear solution should be administered by deep intragluteal injection immediately after reconstitution. After reconstitution, keep refrigerated (2°-8° C) and use within 7 days, keep at room temperature (25° C) and use within 3 days, or keep frozen (−20° C) for up to 3 months.

Oral Route: In adults a dose of 250 to 500 mg every 4 to 6 hours is sufficient for mild-to-moderate infections. In severe infections 1 gram every 4 to 6 hours may be necessary.

In children, streptococcal pharyngitis cases have responded to a dosage of 250 mg t.i.d. Beta-hemolytic streptococcal infections should be treated for at least ten days to prevent development of acute rheumatic fever or glomerulonephritis.

Children and infants with scarlet fever and pneumonia should receive 25 mg/kg/day in four divided doses. For staphylococcal infections, 50 mg/kg/day in four divided doses is recommended. For neonates, 10 mg/kg three to four times daily is recommended. If inadequate, resort to parenteral UNIPEN® (nafcillin sodium, Wyeth).

To reconstitute the powder for oral solution, add the water in two separate portions. Shake well after each addition. After reconstitution the solution must be refrigerated. Discard any unused portion after 7 days.

HOW SUPPLIED
FOR ORAL ADMINISTRATION

Capsules

Supplied as capsules containing nafcillin sodium, as the monohydrate, equivalent to 250 mg nafcillin buffered with calcium carbonate as follows:

NDC 0008-0057, green and yellow capsule marked "WYETH" and "57", in bottles of 100 capsules.

Keep tightly closed.

Dispense in tight container.

The appearance of these capsules is a trademark of Wyeth-Ayerst Laboratories.

Tablets

Supplied as tablets containing nafcillin sodium as the monohydrate, equivalent to 500 mg nafcillin buffered with calcium carbonate, as follows:

NDC 0008-0464, white, capsule-shaped, scored, film-coated tablet marked "WYETH" and "464", in bottles of 50 tablets.

Keep tightly closed.

Protect from light.

Dispense in light-resistant, tight container.

Oral Solution

Supplied as a powder for oral solution as follows. When reconstituted with water, each 5 mL will contain nafcillin sodium equivalent to 250 mg nafcillin.

NDC 0008-0513, white powder in bottles to make 100 mL of solution.

Keep tightly closed.

FOR PARENTERAL ADMINISTRATION

Conventional Vials (for intravenous or intramuscular use)

Supplied in vial sizes of 500 mg, 1 gram, and 2 gram nafcillin sodium as the monohydrate, buffered with 40 mg sodium citrate per gram, as follows:

NDC 0008-0751, in packages of 10 vials.

When reconstituted as recommended (see table below) with Sterile Water for Injection, USP, Sodium Chloride Injection, USP, Bacteriostatic Water for Injection, USP (TUBEX®), or Bacteriostatic Water for Injection, USP, with parabens or with benzyl alcohol, each vial contains, respectively, 2 mL, 4 mL, or 8 mL of solution. Each mL contains nafcillin sodium equivalent to 250 mg nafcillin, buffered with 10 mg sodium citrate.

Vial Size	Amount of Diluent	Nafcillin Sodium Solution
500 mg	1.7 mL	2 mL
1 gram	3.4 mL	4 mL
2 gram	6.8 mL	8 mL

FOR INTRAVENOUS USE ONLY

ADD-Vantage™ Vials

Supplied in vial sizes of 500 mg, 1 gram, and 2 gram nafcillin sodium as the monohydrate, buffered with 40 mg sodium citrate per gram, as follows:

NDC 0008-0751, in packages of 10 ADD-Vantage Vials.

The ADD-Vantage Vials are only to be used with Abbott Laboratories' ADD-Vantage Flexible Diluent Container containing:

0.9% Sodium Chloride Injection, USP, 50 mL and 100 mL sizes.

5% Dextrose Injection, USP, 50 mL and 100 mL sizes.

Piggyback Units

Supplied in single units equivalent to 1 gram or 2 gram nafcillin per unit, buffered with 40 mg sodium citrate per gram, as follows:

NDC 0008-0751, in packages of 10 PIGGYBACK vials.

Bulk Vial (for IV stock solution only)

Supplied in vial size of 10 gram nafcillin per vial, buffered with 40 mg sodium citrate per gram, as follows:

NDC 0008-0751, as single vials.

Shake vial well after adding diluent and before using.

Use solution within 8 hours if kept at room temperature or 48 hours if kept under refrigeration.

Caution: Federal law prohibits dispensing without prescription.

BIBLIOGRAPHY

A bibliography is available upon request.

Shown in Product Identification Section, page 438

WYAMYCIN® S   ℞

[*wi-a-mi'sin*]

Film-coated Tablets

(erythromycin stearate)

DESCRIPTION

Wyamycin S (erythromycin stearate) is produced by a strain of *Streptomyces erythraeus* and belongs to the macrolide group of antibiotics. It is basic and readily forms salts with acids. The base, the stearate salt, and the esters are poorly soluble in water and are suitable for oral administration. Each film-coated tablet contains 250 mg or 500 mg erythromycin as erythromycin stearate, USP. The inactive ingredients present are acacia, diacetylated monoglycerides, ethylcellulose, FD&C Red 3, hydroxypropyl methylcellulose, magnesium stearate, povidone, sodium citrate, and sodium starch glycolate.

HOW SUPPLIED

Wyamycin® S (erythromycin stearate) Tablets, Wyeth®, containing the equivalent of 250 mg or 500 mg erythromycin, are available as follows:

250 mg, NDC 0008-0576, pink, round, film-coated tablet marked "WYETH" and "576", in bottles of 100 and 500 tablets.

500 mg, NDC 0008-0578, pink, elliptical, film-coated tablet marked "WYETH" and "578", in bottles of 100 tablets.

Keep tightly closed.

Protect from light and moisture.

Dispense in light-resistant, tight container.

For prescribing information write to Professional Service, Wyeth-Ayerst Laboratories, Box 8299, Philadelphia, PA 19101, or contact your local Wyeth-Ayerst representative.

Shown in Product Identification Section, page 438

WYANOIDS® Relief Factor   OTC

[*wi'a-noids*]

Hemorrhoidal Suppositories

DESCRIPTION

Active ingredients: Live Yeast Cell Derivative, Supplying 2,000 units Skin Respiratory Factor Per Ounce of Cocoa Butter Suppository Base and Shark Liver Oil 3%. Inactive Ingredients: Beeswax Glycerin, Phenylmercuric Nitrate 1:10,000 (as a preservative), Polyethylene Glycol 600 Dilaurate.

INDICATIONS

To help shrink swelling of hemorrhoidal tissues and provide prompt, temporary relief from pain and itching.

USUAL DOSAGE

Patients are advised to use one suppository up to five times daily, especially in the morning, at night, and after bowel movements, or as directed by a physician.

DIRECTIONS

Remove wrapper and insert one suppository rectally using gentle pressure. Frequent application and lubrication with Wyanoids® Relief Factor provide continual therapy which will lead to more rapid improvement of rectal conditions.

CAUTION

In case of bleeding or if the condition persists, the patient should consult a physician. Keep this and all medications out of the reach of children. Do not store above 80° F.

HOW SUPPLIED

Boxes of 12 and 24.

Shown in Product Identification Section, page 438

WYCILLIN®   ℞

[*wi-sil'in*]

(sterile penicillin G procaine suspension)

INJECTION

FOR DEEP INTRAMUSCULAR INJECTION ONLY

DESCRIPTION

This product is designed to provide a stable aqueous suspension of sterile penicillin G procaine, ready for immediate use. This eliminates the necessity for addition of any diluent, required for the usual dry formulation of injectable penicillin.

Each TUBEX® Sterile Cartridge-Needle Unit, Wyeth, 1,200,000 units (2 mL size) or 600,000 units (1 mL size) or disposable syringe, 2,400,000 units (4 mL size), contains penicillin G procaine in a stabilized aqueous suspension with sodium citrate buffer; and as w/v, approximately 0.5% lecithin, 0.5% carboxymethylcellulose, 0.5% povidone, 0.1% methylparaben, and 0.01% propylparaben.

Each TUBEX 300,000 units (1 mL size), contains penicillin G procaine in a stabilized aqueous suspension with sodium citrate buffer; and as w/v, approximately 0.3% lecithin, 0.9% carboxymethylcellulose, 0.9% povidone, 0.14% methylparaben, and 0.015% propylparaben.

Each syringe, 2,400,000 units (4 mL size), contains penicillin G procaine in a stabilized aqueous suspension with sodium citrate buffer; and as w/v, approximately 0.5% lecithin, 0.5% carboxymethylcellulose, 0.5% povidone, 0.1% methylparaben, and 0.01% propylparaben.

Wycillin (sterile penicillin G procaine suspension) must be stored in a refrigerator. Keep from freezing. This will prevent deterioration and assure that no significant loss of potency occurs within the expiration date.

Wycillin suspension in the TUBEX and disposable syringe formulations is viscous and opaque. Read "Contraindications," "Warnings," "Precautions," and "Dosage and Administration" sections prior to use.

ACTIONS AND PHARMACOLOGY

Penicillin G exerts a bactericidal action against penicillin-sensitive microorganisms during the stage of active multiplication. It acts through the inhibition of biosynthesis of cell-wall mucopeptide. It is not active against the penicillinase-producing bacteria, which include many strains of staphylococci. Penicillin G exerts high *in vitro* activity against staphylococci (except penicillinase-producing strains), streptococci (Groups A, C, G, H, L, and M), and pneumococci. Other organisms sensitive to penicillin G are *Neisseria gonorrhoeae, Corynebacterium diphtheriae, Bacillus anthracis,* Clostridia, *Actinomyces bovis, Streptobacillus moniliformis, Listeria monocytogenes,* and Leptospira. *Treponema pallidum* is extremely sensitive to the bactericidal action of penicillin G.

Sensitivity Plate Testing: If the Kirby-Bauer method of disc sensitivity is used, a 10-unit penicillin disc should give a zone greater than 28 mm when tested against a penicillin-sensitive bacterial strain.

Penicillin G procaine is an equimolecular compound of procaine and penicillin G, administered intramuscularly as a suspension. It dissolves slowly at the site of injection, giving a plateau type of blood level at about 4 hours which falls slowly over a period of the next 15 to 20 hours.

Approximately 60% of penicillin G is bound to serum protein. The drug is distributed throughout the body tissues in widely varying amounts. Highest levels are found in the kidneys with lesser amounts in the liver, skin, and intestines. Penicillin G penetrates into all other tissues to a lesser degree with a very small level found in the cerebrospinal fluid. With normal kidney function, the drug is excreted rapidly by tubular excretion. In neonates and young infants and in individuals with impaired kidney functions, excretion is considerably delayed. Approximately 60 to 90 percent of a dose of parenteral penicillin G is excreted in the urine within 24 to 36 hours.

INDICATIONS

Penicillin G procaine is indicated in the treatment of moderately severe infections due to penicillin-G-sensitive microorganisms that are sensitive to the low and persistent serum levels common to this particular dosage form. Therapy should be guided by bacteriological studies (including sensitivity tests) and by clinical response.

NOTE: When high, sustained serum levels are required, aqueous penicillin G, either IM or IV, should be used.

The following infections will usually respond to adequate dosages of intramuscular penicillin G procaine:

Streptococcal infections (Group A—without bacteremia). Moderately severe to severe infections of the upper respiratory tract, skin and soft-tissue infections, scarlet fever, and erysipelas.

NOTE: Streptococci in Groups A, C, G, H, L, and M are very sensitive to penicillin G. Other groups, including Group D (enterococcus), are resistant. Aqueous penicillin is recommended for streptococcal infections with bacteremia.

Pneumococcal infections. Moderately severe infections of the respiratory tract.

NOTE: Severe pneumonia, empyema, bacteremia, pericarditis, meningitis, peritonitis, and arthritis of pneumococcal etiology are better treated with aqueous penicillin G during the acute stage.

Staphylococcal infections—penicillin-G-sensitive. Moderately severe infections of the skin and soft tissues.

NOTE: Reports indicate an increasing number of strains of staphylococci resistant to penicillin G, emphasizing the need for culture and sensitivity studies in treating suspected staphylococcal infections.

Indicated surgical procedures should be performed.

Fusospirochetosis (Vincent's gingivitis and pharyngitis). Moderately severe infections of the oropharynx respond to therapy with penicillin G procaine.

NOTE: Necessary dental care should be accomplished in infections involving the gum tissue.

Treponema pallidum (syphilis); all stages.

N. gonorrhoeae; acute and chronic (without bacteremia).

Yaws, Bejel, Pinta.

C. diphtheriae —penicillin G procaine as an adjunct to antitoxin for prevention of the carrier stage.

Anthrax.

Streptobacillus moniliformis and *Spirillum minus* infections (rat-bite fever).

Erysipeloid.

Subacute bacterial endocarditis (Group A streptococcus), only in extremely sensitive infections.

Although no controlled clinical efficacy studies have been conducted, aqueous crystalline penicillin G for injection and penicillin G procaine suspension have been suggested by the American Heart Association and the American Dental Association for use as part of a combined parenteral-oral regimen for prophylaxis against bacterial endocarditis in patients who have congenital heart disease or rheumatic or other acquired valvular heart disease when they undergo dental procedures and surgical procedures of the upper respiratory tract.[1]

Since it may happen that *alpha*-hemolytic streptococci relatively resistant to penicillin may be found when patients are receiving continuous oral penicillin for secondary prevention of rheumatic fever, prophylactic agents other than penicillin may be chosen for these patients and prescribed in addition to their continuous rheumatic fever prophylactic regimen.

NOTE: When selecting antibiotics for the prevention of bacterial endocarditis, the physician or dentist should read the full joint statement of the American Heart Association and the American Dental Association.[1]

CONTRAINDICATIONS

A previous hypersensitivity reaction to any penicillin is a contraindication.

Do not inject into or near an artery or nerve.

WARNINGS

Serious and occasionally fatal hypersensitivity (anaphylactoid) reactions have been reported in patients on penicillin therapy.

Serious anaphylactoid reactions require immediate emergency treatment with epinephrine. Oxygen and intravenous corticosteroids should also be administered as indicated.

Although anaphylaxis is more frequent following parenteral therapy, it has occurred in patients on oral penicillins. These reactions are more apt to occur in individuals with a history of sensitivity to multiple allergens.

There have been well-documented reports of individuals with a history of penicillin hypersensitivity reactions who have experienced severe hypersensitivity reactions when treated with a cephalosporin. Before therapy with a penicillin, careful inquiry should be made concerning previous hypersensitivity reactions to penicillins, cephalosporins, and other allergens. If an allergic reaction occurs, the drug should be discontinued and the patient treated with the usual agents, e.g., pressor amines, antihistamines, and corticosteroids.

Immediate toxic reactions to procaine may occur in some individuals, particularly when a large single dose is administered in the treatment of gonorrhea (4.8 million units). These reactions may be manifested by mental disturbances, including anxiety, confusion, agitation, depression, weakness, seizures, hallucinations, combativeness, and expressed "fear of impending death." The reactions noted in carefully controlled studies occurred in approximately one in 500 patients treated for gonorrhea. Reactions are transient, lasting from 15 to 30 minutes.

Inadvertent intravascular administration, including inadvertent direct intra-arterial injection or injection immediately adjacent to arteries, of Wycillin and other penicillin preparations has resulted in severe neurovascular damage, including transverse myelitis with permanent paralysis, gangrene requiring amputation of digits and more proximal portions of extremities, and necrosis and sloughing at and surrounding the injection site. Such severe effects have been reported following injections into the buttock, thigh, and

Continued on next page

Wyeth-Ayerst—Cont.

deltoid areas. Other serious complications of suspected intra-vascular administration which have been reported include immediate pallor, mottling or cyanosis of the extremity both distal and proximal to the injection site followed by bleb formation; severe edema requiring anterior and/or posterior compartment fasciotomy in the lower extremity. The above described severe effects and complications have most often occurred in infants and small children. Prompt consultation with an appropriate specialist is indicated if any evidence of compromise of the blood supply occurs at, proximal to, or distal to the site of injection.[2-10] See "Contraindications," "Precautions," and "Dosage and Administration" sections. Quadriceps femoris fibrosis and atrophy have been reported following repeated intramuscular injections of penicillin preparations into the anterolateral thigh.

Injection into or near a nerve may result in permanent neurological damage.

PRECAUTIONS

Penicillin should be used with caution in individuals with histories of significant allergies and/or asthma.

Care should be taken to avoid intravenous or intraarterial administration, or injection into or near major peripheral nerves or blood vessels, since such injections may produce neurovascular damage. See "Contraindications," "Warnings," and "Dosage and Administration" sections.

In suspected staphylococcal infections, proper laboratory studies, including sensitivity tests, should be performed.

A small percentage of patients are sensitive to procaine. If there is a history of sensitivity, make the usual test: Inject intradermally 0.1 mL of a 1 to 2 percent procaine solution. Development of an erythema, wheal, flare, or eruption indicates procaine sensitivity. Sensitivity should be treated by the usual methods, including barbiturates, and procaine penicillin preparations should not be used. Antihistaminics appear beneficial in treatment of procaine reactions.

The use of antibiotics may result in overgrowth of nonsusceptible organisms. Constant observation of the patient is essential. If new infections due to bacteria or fungi appear during therapy, the drug should be discontinued and appropriate measures taken.

Whenever allergic reactions occur, penicillin should be withdrawn unless, in the opinion of the physician, the condition being treated is life-threatening and amenable only to penicillin therapy.

In prolonged therapy with penicillin, and particularly with high-dosage schedules, periodic evaluation of the renal and hematopoietic systems is recommended.

When treating gonococcal infections in which primary or secondary syphilis may be suspected, proper diagnostic procedures, including dark-field examinations, should be done. In all cases in which concomitant syphilis is suspected, monthly serological tests should be made for at least four months.

ADVERSE REACTIONS

Penicillin is a substance of low toxicity but does possess a significant index of sensitization. The following hypersensitivity reactions associated with use of penicillin have been reported: Skin rashes, ranging from maculopapular eruptions to exfoliative dermatitis; urticaria; serum-sicknesslike reactions, including chills, fever, edema, arthralgia, and prostration. Severe and often fatal anaphylaxis has been reported (see "Warnings"). As with other treatments for syphilis, the Jarisch-Herxheimer reaction has been reported. Procaine toxicity manifestations have been reported (see "Warnings"). Although procaine hypersensitivity reactions have not been reported with this drug, there are patients who are sensitive to procaine (see "Precautions").

DOSAGE AND ADMINISTRATION

Parenteral drug products should be inspected visually for particulate matter and discoloration prior to administration, whenever solution and container permit.

Penicillin G procaine (aqueous) is for intramuscular injection only.

Administer by DEEP, INTRAMUSCULAR INJECTION in the upper, outer quadrant of the buttock. In infants and small children, the midlateral aspect of the thigh may be preferable. When doses are repeated, vary the injection site.

When using the TUBEX cartridge:

The Wyeth TUBEX cartridge for this product incorporates several features that are designed to facilitate the visualization of blood on aspiration if a blood vessel is inadvertently entered.

The design of this cartridge is such that blood which enters its needle will be quickly visualized as a red or dark-colored "spot." This "spot" will appear on the barrel of the glass cartridge immediately proximal to the blue hub. Prior to injection, in order to determine where this "spot" can be seen, the operator should first insert and secure the cartridge in the TUBEX syringe/injector in the usual fashion. The needle cover should then be partially removed to reveal a small yellow rectangle and the cartridge and syringe/injector held in one hand with the needle pointing away from the operator. If the 2 mL metal or plastic syringe is used, the glass cartridge should be rotated by turning the plunger of the syringe clockwise until the yellow rectangle is visualized. An imaginary straight line, drawn to extend the yellow rectangle to the shoulder of the glass cartridge, will point to the area on the cartridge where the "spot" can be visualized. If the 1 mL metal syringe is used, it will not be possible to continue to rotate the glass cartridge clockwise once it is properly engaged and fully threaded; it can, however, then be rotated counterclockwise as far as necessary to properly orient the yellow rectangle and locate the observation area. (In this same area in some cartridges, a dark spot may sometimes be visualized prior to injection. This is the proximal end of the needle and does not represent a foreign body in, or other abnormality of, the suspension.)

Thus, before the needle is inserted into the selected muscle, it is important for the operator to orient the yellow rectangle so that any blood which may enter after needle insertion and during aspiration can be visualized in the area on the cartridge where it will appear and not be obscured by any obstructions.

After selection of the proper site and insertion of the needle into the selected muscle, aspirate by pulling back on the plunger. While maintaining negative pressure for 2 to 3 seconds, carefully observe the barrel of the cartridge in the area previously identified (see above) for the appearance of a red or dark-colored "spot."

Blood or "typical blood color" may not be seen if a blood vessel has been entered—only a mixture of blood and Wycillin. The appearance of *any* discoloration is reason to withdraw the needle and discard the glass TUBEX cartridge. If it is elected to inject at another site, a new cartridge should be used. If no blood or discoloration appears, inject the contents of the cartridge slowly. Discontinue delivery of the dose if the subject complains of severe immediate pain at the injection site or if, especially in infants and young children, symptoms or signs occur suggesting onset of severe pain.

Some TUBEX cartridges may contain a small air bubble which may be disregarded, since it does not affect administration of the product.

Because of the high concentration of suspended material in this product, the needle may be blocked if the injection is not made at a slow, steady rate.

When using the disposable syringe:

The Wyeth disposable syringe for this product incorporates several new features that are designed to facilitate its use. A single small indentation, or "dot", has been punched into the metal ring that surrounds the neck of the syringe near the base of the needle. It is important that this "dot" be placed in a position so that it can be easily visualized by the operator following the intramuscular insertion of the syringe needle.

After selection of the proper site and insertion of the needle into the selected muscle, aspirate by pulling back on the plunger. While maintaining negative pressure for 2 to 3 seconds, carefully observe the barrel of the syringe immediately proximal to the location of the "dot" for appearance of blood or any discoloration. Blood or "typical blood color" may *not* be seen if a blood vessel has been entered—only a mixture of blood and Wycillin. The appearance of any discoloration is

reason to withdraw the needle and discard the syringe. If it is elected to inject at another site, a new syringe should be used. If no blood or discoloration appears, inject the contents of the syringe slowly. Discontinue delivery of the dose if the subject complains of severe immediate pain at the injection site or if in infants and young children symptoms or signs occur suggesting onset of severe pain.

Pneumonia (pneumococcal), moderately severe (uncomplicated): 600,000–1,000,000 units daily.

Streptococcal infections (Group A), moderately severe to severe tonsillitis, erysipelas, scarlet fever, upper respiratory tract, skin and soft tissue: 600,000–1,000,000 units daily for 10-day minimum.

Staphylococcal infections, moderately severe to severe: 600,000–1,000,000 units daily.

In pneumonia, streptococcal (Group A) and staphylococcal infections in children under 60 pounds: 300,000 units daily.

Bacterial endocarditis (Group A streptococci) only in extremely sensitive infections: 600,000–1,000,000 units daily.

For prophylaxis against bacterial endocarditis[1] in patients with congenital heart disease or rheumatic or other acquired valvular heart disease when undergoing dental procedures or surgical procedures of the upper respiratory tract, use a combined parenteral-oral regimen. One million units of aqueous crystalline penicillin G (30,000 units/kg in children) intramuscularly mixed with 600,000 units penicillin G procaine (600,000 units for children) should be given one-half to one hour before the procedure. Oral penicillin V (phenoxymethyl penicillin), 500 mg for adults or 250 mg for children less than 60 lbs., should be given every 6 hours for 8 doses. Doses for children should not exceed recommendations for adults for a single dose or for a 24-hour period.

Syphilis—

Primary, secondary, and latent with a negative spinal fluid in adults and children over 12 years of age: 600,000 units daily for 8 days—total 4,800,000 units.

Late (tertiary, neurosyphilis, and latent syphilis with positive spinal-fluid examination or no spinal-fluid examination): 600,000 units daily for 10 to 15 days—total 6 to 9 million units.

Congenital syphilis under 70-lb. body weight: 10,000 units/kg/day for 10 days.

Yaws, Bejel, and Pinta: Treatment as syphilis in corresponding stage of disease.

Although some isolates of *Neisseria gonorrhoeae* have decreased susceptibility to penicillin, this inherent resistance is relative, not absolute, and penicillin in large doses remains the drug of choice for these strains. Strains producing penicillinase, however, are resistant to penicillin G, and a drug other than penicillin G should be used. Physicians are cautioned not to use less than the recommended doses.

GONORRHEAL INFECTIONS (UNCOMPLICATED)—MEN OR WOMEN: Aqueous penicillin G procaine, 4.8 million units intramuscularly, divided into at least two doses and injected at different sites at one visit, together with 1 gram of oral probenecid, preferably given just before the injection.

NOTE: Treatment of severe complications of gonorrhea should be individualized, using large amounts of short-acting penicillin. Gonorrheal endocarditis should be treated intensively with aqueous penicillin G. Prophylactic or epidemiologic treatment for gonorrhea (male and female) is accomplished with the same treatment schedules as for the uncomplicated gonorrhea.

Retreatment

The National Center for Disease Control, Venereal Disease Branch, U.S. Department of Health, Education and Welfare, Atlanta, Georgia, recommends:

Test of cure procedures at approximately 7 to 14 days after therapy. In the male, a gram-stained smear is adequate if positive; otherwise, a culture specimen should be obtained from the anterior urethra. In the female, culture specimens should be obtained from both the endocervical and anal canal sites.

Retreatment in the male is indicated if the urethral discharge persists for three or more days following initial therapy and the smear or culture remains positive. Follow-up treatment consists of 4,800,000 units of aqueous penicillin G procaine intramuscularly, divided in two injection sites at a single visit.

In uncomplicated gonorrhea in the female, retreatment is indicated if follow-up cervical or rectal cultures remain positive for *N. gonorrhoeae*. Follow-up treatment consists of 4,800,000 units of aqueous penicillin G procaine daily on two successive days.

SYPHILIS: All gonorrhea patients should have a serologic test for syphilis at the time of diagnosis. Patients with gonorrhea who also have syphilis should be given additional treatment appropriate to the stage of syphilis.

Diphtheria — adjunctive therapy with antitoxin: 300,000 to 600,000 units daily.

Diphtheria carrier state: 300,000 units daily for 10 days.

Anthrax-cutaneous: 600,000 to 1,000,000 units/day.

Vincent's infection (fusospirochetosis): 600,000 to 1,000,000 units/day.

Erysipeloid: 600,000 to 1,000,000 units/day.
Streptobacillus moniliformis and *Spirillum minus* (rat-bite fever): 600,000 to 1,000,000 units/day.

HOW SUPPLIED

Wycillin® (sterile penicillin G procaine suspension), Wyeth®, is available in packages of 10 TUBEX Sterile Cartridge-Needle Units (20 gauge × 1¼ inch needle), NDC 0008-0018, as follows: 1 mL size, 600,000 units per TUBEX; and 2 mL size, 1,200,000 units per TUBEX; and in 4 mL size single-dose disposable syringe (18 gauge × 2 inch needle), 2,400,000 units, in packages of 10 disposable syringes.
Store in a refrigerator.
Keep from freezing.

REFERENCES

1. American Heart Association: Prevention of bacterial endocarditis. *Circulation,* 56: 139A-143A, 1977.
2. SHAW, E.: Transverse myelitis from injection of penicillin. *Am. J. Dis. Child.,* 11: 548, 1966.
3. KNOWLES, J.: Accidental intra-arterial injection of penicillin. *Am. J. Dis. Child.,* 111: 552, 1966.
4. DARBY, C., et al: Ischemia following an intragluteal injection of benzathine-procaine penicillin G mixture in a one-year-old boy. *Clin. Pediatrics,* 12: 485, 1973.
5. BROWN, L. & NELSON, A.: Postinfectious intravascular thrombosis with gangrene. *Arch. Surg.,* 94: 652, 1967.
6. BORENSTINE, J.: Transverse myelitis and penicillin (Correspondence). *Am. J. Dis. Child.,* 112: 166, 1966.
7. ATKINSON, J.: Transverse myelopathy secondary to penicillin injection. *J. Pediatrics,* 75: 867, 1969.
8. TALBERT, J. et al: Gangrene of the foot following intramuscular injection in the lateral thigh: A case report with recommendations for prevention. *J. Pediatrics,* 70: 110, 1967.
9. FISHER, T.: Medicolegal affairs. *Canad. Med. Assoc. J.,* 112: 395, 1975.
10. SCHANZER, H. et al: Accidental intra-arterial injection of penicillin G. *JAMA,* 242: 1289, 1979.

WYCILLIN® and PROBENECID   ℞

[wi-sil'in and pro-ben'is-id]
(sterile penicillin G procaine suspension and probenecid tablets)
Disposable Syringe and Tablets
Wycillin is for deep IM injection only.

DESCRIPTION

The Wycillin disposable syringe is designed to provide a stable aqueous suspension of sterile penicillin G procaine, ready for immediate use. This eliminates the necessity for addition of any diluent, required for the usual dry formulation of injectable penicillin.
Each syringe, 2,400,000 units (4 mL size), contains penicillin G procaine in a stabilized aqueous suspension with sodium citrate buffer; and as w/v, approximately 0.5% lecithin, 0.5% carboxymethylcellulose, 0.5% povidone, 0.1% methylparaben, and 0.01% propylparaben.
Wycillin must be stored in a refrigerator. Keep from freezing. This will prevent deterioration and assure that no significant loss of potency occurs within the expiration date.
Probenecid is a uricosuric and renal tubular-blocking agent. Probenecid tablets contain 0.5 gram probenecid. The inactive ingredients present are calcium stearate, D&C Yellow 10, gelatin, hydroxypropyl methylcellulose, iron oxide, magnesium carbonate, polyethylene glycol, starch, talc, and titanium dioxide.
Wycillin suspension in the disposable syringe formulation is viscous and opaque. Read "Contraindications," "Warnings," "Precautions," and "Dosage and Administration" sections prior to use.

ACTIONS AND PHARMACOLOGY

Penicillin G exerts a bactericidal action against penicillin-sensitive microorganisms during the stage of active multiplication. It acts through the inhibition of biosynthesis of cell-wall mucopeptide. It is not active against the penicillinase-producing bacteria, which include many strains of staphylococci. *Neisseria gonorrhoeae* are included among the various organisms which are sensitive to penicillin G. Penicillin G procaine is an equimolecular salt of procaine and penicillin G, administered intramuscularly as a suspension. It dissolves slowly at the site of injection, giving a plateau type of blood level at about 4 hours which falls slowly over a period of the next 15 to 20 hours. Approximately 60% to 90% of a dose of penicillin G is excreted in the urine within 24 to 36 hours.
Approximately 60% of penicillin G is bound to serum protein. The drug is distributed throughout the body tissues in widely varying amounts, with highest levels found in the kidneys and lesser amounts in the liver, skin, and intestines. Penicillin G penetrates into all other tissues to a lesser degree, with a very small level found in the cerebrospinal fluid. With normal kidney function the drug is excreted rapidly by tubular excretion. In neonates and young infants and in individuals with impaired kidney function, excretion is considerably delayed.

Probenecid inhibits the tubular reabsorption of urate, thus increasing the urinary excretion of uric acid and decreasing serum uric acid levels. It also inhibits the tubular excretion of penicillin and usually increases penicillin plasma levels, regardless of the route by which the antibiotic is given. A 2-fold to 4-fold elevation has been demonstrated for various penicillins. Probenecid does not influence plasma concentrations of salicylates, nor the excretion of streptomycin, chloramphenicol, chlortetracycline, oxytetracycline, or neomycin.

INDICATIONS

Wycillin and Probenecid is indicated for the single-dose treatment of uncomplicated (without bacteremia) urethral, cervical, rectal, or pharyngeal infections caused by *Neisseria gonorrhoeae* (gonorrhea) in men and women.
Susceptibility studies should be performed when recurrent infections or resistant strains are encountered. Urethritis and the presence of gram-negative diplococci in urethral smears are strong presumptive evidence of gonorrhea. Culture or fluorescent antibody studies will confirm the diagnosis. Therapy may be instituted prior to obtaining results of susceptibility testing.

CONTRAINDICATIONS

A history of a previous hypersensitivity reaction to any of the penicillins or to Probenecid is a contraindication.
Probenecid is not recommended in persons with known blood dyscrasias or uric acid kidney stones or during an acute attack of gout. It is not recommended in conjunction with penicillin G procaine suspension in the presence of known renal impairment.
Do not inject into or near an artery or nerve.

WARNINGS

PENICILLIN G PROCAINE: Serious and occasionally fatal hypersensitivity (anaphylactoid) reactions have been reported in patients on penicillin therapy. Serious anaphylactoid reactions require immediate emergency treatment with epinephrine. Oxygen and intravenous corticosteroids should also be administered as indicated. Although anaphylaxis is more frequent following parenteral therapy, it has occurred in patients on oral penicillins. These reactions are more apt to occur in individuals with a history of sensitivity to multiple allergens.
There have been well-documented reports of individuals with a history of penicillin-hypersensitivity reactions who have experienced severe hypersensitivity reactions when treated with a cephalosporin. Before therapy with a penicillin, careful inquiry should be made concerning previous hypersensitivity reactions to penicillins, cephalosporins, and other allergens. If an allergic reaction occurs, the drug should be discontinued and the patient treated with the usual agents, e.g., pressor amines, antihistamines, and corticosteroids.
Immediate toxic reactions to procaine may occur in some individuals, particularly when a large single dose is administered in the treatment of gonorrhea (4.8 million units). These reactions may be manifested by mental disturbances, including anxiety, confusion, agitation, depression, weakness, seizures, hallucinations, combativeness, and expressed "fear of impending death." The reactions noted in carefully controlled studies occurred in approximately one in 500 patients treated for gonorrhea. Reactions are transient, lasting from 15 to 30 minutes.
Inadvertent intravascular administration, including inadvertent direct intraarterial injection or injection immediately adjacent to arteries, of Wycillin and other penicillin preparations has resulted in severe neurovascular damage, including transverse myelitis with permanent paralysis, gangrene requiring amputation of digits and more proximal portions of extremities, and necrosis and sloughing at and surrounding the injection site. Such severe effects have been reported following injections into the buttock, thigh, and deltoid areas. Other serious complications of suspected intravascular administration which have been reported include immediate pallor, mottling or cyanosis of the extremity both distal and proximal to the injection site followed by bleb formation; severe edema requiring anterior and/or posterior compartment fasciotomy in the lower extremity. The above-described severe effects and complications have most often occurred in infants and small children. Prompt consultation with an appropriate specialist is indicated if any evidence of compromise of the blood supply occurs at, proximal to, or distal to the site of injection.[1-9] See "Contraindications," "Precautions," and "Dosage and Administration" sections.
Quadriceps femoris fibrosis and atrophy have been reported following repeated intramuscular injections of penicillin preparations into the anterolateral thigh.
Injection into or near a nerve may result in permanent neurological damage.
PROBENECID: Exacerbation of gout following therapy with Probenecid may occur; in such cases colchicine therapy is advisable.
In patients on Probenecid, the use of salicylates in either small or large doses is not recommended because it antagonizes the uricosuric action of Probenecid. Patients on Pro-

benecid who require a mild analgesic agent should receive acetaminophen rather than salicylates, even in small doses.
USAGE IN PREGNANCY: The safety of these drugs for use in pregnancy has not been established.

PRECAUTIONS

PENICILLIN G PROCAINE: When treating gonococcal infections in which primary or secondary syphilis may be suspected, proper diagnostic procedures, including dark-field examinations, should be done. In all cases in which concomitant syphilis is suspected, monthly serological tests should be made for at least four months. Patients with gonorrhea, who also have syphilis, should be given additional appropriate parenteral penicillin treatment.
Penicillin should be used with caution in individuals with histories of significant allergies and/or asthma. When administering Wycillin, care should be taken to avoid intravenous or intra-arterial administration, or injection into or near major peripheral nerves or blood vessels, since such injections may produce neurovascular damage. See "Contraindications," "Warnings," and "Dosage and Administration" sections.
A small percentage of patients are sensitive to procaine. If there is a history of sensitivity, make the usual test: Inject intradermally 0.1 mL of a 1- to 2-percent procaine solution. Development of an erythema, wheal, flare, or eruption indicates procaine sensitivity. Sensitivity should be treated by the usual methods, including barbiturates, and procaine penicillin preparations should not be used. Antihistaminics appear beneficial in treatment of procaine reactions.
PROBENECID: Use Probenecid with caution in patients with a history of peptic ulcer. A reducing substance may appear in the urine of patients receiving Probenecid. Although this disappears with discontinuance of therapy, a false diagnosis of glycosuria may be made because of a false-positive Benedict's test.

ADVERSE REACTIONS

WYCILLIN: Penicillin is a substance of low toxicity but does possess a significant index of sensitization. The following hypersensitivity reactions associated with use of penicillin have been reported: skin rashes, ranging from maculopapular eruptions to exfoliative dermatitis; urticaria; serum-sickness like reactions, including chills, fever, edema, arthralgia, and prostration. Severe and often fatal anaphylaxis has been reported (see "Warnings"). As with other treatments for syphilis, the Jarisch-Herxheimer reaction has been reported.
Procaine toxicity manifestations have been reported (see "Warnings"). Although procaine hypersensitivity reactions have not been reported with this drug, there are patients who are sensitive to procaine (see "Precautions").
PROBENECID: The following are the principal adverse reactions which have been reported as associated with the use of Probenecid, generally with more prolonged or repeated administration: Hypersensitivity reactions (including anaphylaxis), nephrotic syndrome, hepatic necrosis, aplastic anemia; also other anemias, including hemolytic anemia related to genetic deficiency of glucose-6-phosphate dehydrogenase.

DOSAGE AND ADMINISTRATION

Parenteral drug products should be inspected visually for particulate matter and discoloration prior to administration, whenever solution and container permit.
Penicillin G procaine (aqueous) is for intramuscular injection only.
Administer by DEEP INTRAMUSCULAR INJECTION in the upper, outer quadrant of the buttock. When doses are repeated, vary the injection site.
The Wyeth disposable syringe for this product incorporates several new features that are designed to facilitate its use. A single small indentation, or "dot", has been punched into the metal ring that surrounds the neck of the syringe near the base of the needle. It is important that this "dot" be placed in a position so that it can be easily visualized by the operator following the intramuscular insertion of the syringe needle.
After selection of the proper site and insertion of the needle into the selected muscle, aspirate by pulling back on the plunger. While maintaining negative pressure for 2 to 3 seconds, carefully observe the barrel of the syringe immediately proximal to the location of the "dot" for appearance of blood or any discoloration. Blood or "typical blood color" may *not* be seen if a blood vessel has been entered—only a mixture of blood and Wycillin. The appearance of any discoloration is reason to withdraw the needle and discard the syringe. If it is elected to inject at another site, a new syringe should be used. If no blood or discoloration appears, inject the contents of the syringe slowly. Discontinue delivery of the dose if the subject complains of severe immediate pain at the injection site or if in infants and young children symptoms or signs occur suggesting onset of severe pain.
Although some isolates of *Neisseria gonorrhoeae* have decreased susceptibility to penicillin, this inherent resistance is relative, not absolute, and penicillin in large doses remains

Continued on next page

Wyeth-Ayerst—Cont.

the drug of choice for these strains. Strains producing penicillinase, however, are resistant to penicillin G, and a drug other than penicillin G should be used.

GONORRHEAL INFECTIONS (UNCOMPLICATED) MEN OR WOMEN: Aqueous penicillin G procaine, 4.8 million units intramuscularly, divided into at least two doses and injected at different sites at one visit, together with 1 gram (2 tablets, 0.5 gram each) of Probenecid orally, given just before the injections. Physicians are cautioned to use no less than the recommended dosages.

NOTE: Treatment of severe complications of gonorrhea should be individualized, using large amounts of short-acting penicillin. Gonorrheal endocarditis should be treated intensively with aqueous penicillin G. Prophylactic or epidemiologic treatment for gonorrhea (male and female) is accomplished with the same treatment schedules as for the uncomplicated gonorrhea.

RETREATMENT: The National Center for Disease Control, Venereal Disease Branch, U.S. Department of Health, Education and Welfare, Atlanta, Georgia, recommends: Test of cure procedures at approximately 7 to 14 days after therapy. In the male, a gram-stained smear is adequate if positive; otherwise, a culture specimen should be obtained from the anterior urethra. In the female, culture specimens should be obtained from both the endocervical and anal canal sites.

Retreatment in the male is indicated if the urethral discharge persists for three or more days following initial therapy and the smear or culture remains positive. Follow-up treatment consists of 4,800,000 units of aqueous penicillin G procaine, intramuscular, divided in two injection sites at a single visit.

In uncomplicated gonorrhea in the female, retreatment is indicated if follow-up cervical or rectal cultures remain positive for *N. gonorrhoeae*. Follow-up treatment consists of 4,800,000 units of aqueous penicillin G procaine daily on two successive days.

SYPHILIS: All gonorrhea patients should have a serologic test for syphilis at the time of diagnosis. Patients with gonorrhea who also have syphilis should be given additional treatment appropriate to the stage of syphilis.

HOW SUPPLIED

Wycillin® (sterile penicillin G procaine suspension) Injection and Probenecid Tablets is supplied as a combination package, NDC 0008-2517, containing the following:

Two disposable syringes of Wycillin (2,400,000 units each), 4 mL size (18 gauge × 2 inch needle), and

Two tablets Probenecid, Benemid® (0.5 gram each).

Store in a refrigerator—Keep from freezing.

Wycillin® Disposable Syringes manufactured by **Wyeth-Ayerst Laboratories Inc.**, Philadelphia, PA 19101

Probenecid Tablets (Benemid®) manufactured by **Merck, Sharp and Dohme**, Division of Merck & Co., West Point, PA 19486

REFERENCES

1. SHAW, E.: Transverse myelitis from injection of penicillin. *Am. J. Dis. Child.*, 111: 548, 1966.
2. KNOWLES, J.: Accidental intra-arterial injection of penicillin. *Am. J. Dis. Child.*, 111: 552, 1966.
3. DARBY, C., et al: Ischemia following an intragluteal injection of benzathine-procaine penicillin G mixture in a one-year-old boy. *Clin. Pediatrics*, 12: 485, 1973.
4. BROWN, L. & NELSON, A.: Postinfectious intravascular thrombosis with gangrene. *Arch. Surg.*, 94: 652, 1967.
5. BORENSTINE, J.: Transverse myelitis and penicillin (Correspondence). *Am. J. Dis. Child.*, 112: 166, 1966.
6. ATKINSON, J.: Transverse myelopathy secondary to penicillin injection. *J. Pediatrics*, 75: 867, 1969.
7. TALBERT, J. et al: Gangrene of the foot following intramuscular injection in the lateral thigh: A case report with recommendations for prevention. *J. Pediatrics*, 70: 110, 1967.
8. FISHER, T.: Medicolegal affairs. *Canad. Med. Assoc. J.*, 112: 395, 1975.
9. SCHANZER, H. et al: Accidental intra-arterial injection of penicillin G. *JAMA*, 242: 1289, 1979.

WYDASE®   ℞

[wi-dās]

(hyaluronidase)

DESCRIPTION

Wydase, a protein enzyme, is a preparation of highly purified bovine testicular hyaluronidase. The exact chemical structure of this enzyme is unknown. Wydase is available in two dosage forms:

WYDASE LYOPHILIZED

Hyaluronidase, dehydrated in the frozen state under high vacuum, with lactose and thimerosal (mercury derivative), is supplied as a sterile, white, odorless, amorphous solid and is to be reconstituted with Sodium Chloride Injection, USP,

before use, usually in the proportion of one mL per 150 USP units of hyaluronidase (Wydase Lyophilized).

Each vial of 1,500 USP units contains 1.0 mg thimerosal (mercury derivative), added as a preservative, and 13.3 mg lactose. Each vial of 150 USP units contains 0.075 mg thimerosal (mercury derivative), added as a preservative, and 2.66 mg lactose.

WYDASE STABILIZED SOLUTION

A hyaluronidase injection solution ready for use, colorless and odorless, containing 150 USP units of hyaluronidase per mL with 8.5 mg sodium chloride, 1 mg edetate disodium, 0.4 mg calcium chloride, monobasic sodium phosphate buffer, and not more than 0.1 mg thimerosal (mercury derivative). The USP and the NF hyaluronidase units are the equivalent to the turbidity-reducing (TR) unit and to the International Unit.

HOW SUPPLIED

Wydase®, Lyophilized, Wyeth®, is supplied as follows:
150 USP (TR) units of hyaluronidase
NDC 0008-0121-01, 1 mL vial, as single vials.
1,500 USP (TR) units of hyaluronidase
NDC 0008-0149-01, 10 mL vial, as single vials.
Not Recommended for IV Use.
Keep at controlled room temperature in a dry place. Sterile reconstituted solution may be stored below 30°C (86°F) for two weeks without significant loss of potency.
Wydase®, Stabilized Solution, Wyeth®, is supplied as follows:
150 USP (TR) units of hyaluronidase per mL
NDC 0008-0170-01, 1 mL vial, as single vials.
NCD 0008-0170-02, 10 mL vial, as single vials.
Not Recommended for IV Use.
Must be refrigerated.
Do not use if solution is discolored or contains a precipitate.
For prescribing information write to Professional Service, Wyeth-Ayerst Laboratories, Box 8299, Philadelphia, PA 19101, or contact your local Wyeth-Ayerst representative.

WYGESIC®   ⒸⅣ ℞

[wi-je'zik]

(propoxyphene HCl and acetaminophen)
Tablets

DESCRIPTION

Wygesic tablets contain 65 mg propoxyphene HCl and 650 mg acetaminophen. The inactive ingredients present are cellulose, D&C Yellow 10, FD&C Blue 1, FD&C Yellow 6, hydrogenated vegetable oil, hydroxypropyl cellulose, hydroxypropyl methylcellulose, methylcellulose, polacrilin potassium, and titanium dioxide.

Propoxyphene hydrochloride is an odorless white crystalline powder with a bitter taste. It is freely soluble in water. Chemically, it is [S-(R*,S*)]-α[2-(dimethylamino)-1-methylethyl]-α-phenylbenzeneethanol, propanoate (ester), hydrochloride, which can be represented by the following structural formula:

$$\text{(CH}_3\text{)}_2\text{NCH}_2-\overset{\overset{\text{CH}_3}{|}}{\underset{\underset{\text{H}}{|}}{C}}-\overset{\overset{\text{O}}{\overset{||}{\text{OCC}_2\text{H}_5}}}{\underset{|}{C}}-\text{CH}_2 \cdot \text{HCl}$$

Acetaminophen is a white, crystalline powder, possessing a slightly bitter taste. It is soluble in boiling water and freely soluble in alcohol. Chemically, it is N-Acetyl-p-aminophenol, which can be presented by the following structural formula:

$$\text{HO}-\!\!\!\bigcirc\!\!\!-\text{NHCOCH}_3$$

CLINICAL PHARMACOLOGY

Propoxyphene is a centrally acting narcotic analgesic agent. Equimolar doses of propoxyphene hydrochloride provide similar plasma concentrations. Following administration of 65, 130, or 195 mg of propoxyphene hydrochloride, the bioavailability of propoxyphene is equivalent to that of 100, 200, or 300 mg respectively of propoxyphene napsylate. Peak plasma concentrations of propoxyphene are reached in 2 to 2½ hours. After a 65 mg oral dose of propoxyphene hydrochloride, peak plasma levels of 0.05 to 0.1 mcg/mL are achieved.

Repeated doses of propoxyphene at 6-hour intervals lead to increasing plasma concentrations, with a plateau after the ninth dose at 48 hours.

Propoxyphene is metabolized in the liver to yield norpropoxyphene. Propoxyphene has a half-life of 6 to 12 hours, whereas that of norpropoxyphene is 30 to 36 hours.

Norpropoxyphene has substantially less central nervous system depressant effect than propoxyphene, but a greater local anesthetic effect, which is similar to that of amitriptyline and antiarrhythmic agents, such as lidocaine and quinidine.

In animal studies in which propoxyphene and norpropoxyphene were continuously infused in large amounts, intracardiac conduction time (P-R and QRS intervals) was prolonged. Any intracardiac conduction delay attributable to high concentrations of norpropoxyphene may be of relatively long duration.

ACTIONS

Propoxyphene is a mild narcotic analgesic structurally related to methadone.

The combination of propoxyphene and acetaminophen produces greater analgesia than that produced by either propoxyphene or acetaminophen administered alone.

INDICATIONS

These products are indicated for the relief of mild-to-moderate pain, either when pain is present alone or when it is accompanied by fever.

CONTRAINDICATIONS

Hypersensitivity to propoxyphene or to acetaminophen.

WARNINGS

Do not prescribe propoxyphene for patients who are suicidal or addiction-prone.

Prescribe propoxyphene with caution for patients taking tranquilizers or antidepressant drugs and patients who use alcohol in excess.

Tell your patients not to exceed the recommended dose and to limit their intake of alcohol.

Propoxyphene products in excessive doses, either alone or in combination with other CNS depressants, including alcohol, are a major cause of drug-related deaths. Fatalities within the first hour of overdosage are not uncommon. In a survey of deaths due to overdosage conducted in 1975, in approximately 20% of the fatal cases, death occurred within the first hour (5% occurred within 15 minutes). Propoxyphene should not be taken in doses higher than those recommended by the physician. The judicious prescribing of propoxyphene is essential to the safe use of this drug. With patients who are depressed or suicidal, consideration should be given to the use of nonnarcotic analgesics. Patients should be cautioned about the concomitant use of propoxyphene products and alcohol because of potentially serious CNS-additive effects of these agents. Because of its added depressant effects, propoxyphene should be prescribed with caution for those patients whose medical condition requires the concomitant administration of sedatives, tranquilizers, muscle relaxants, antidepressants, or other CNS-depressant drugs. Patients should be advised of the additive depressant effects of these combinations.

Many of the propoxyphene-related deaths have occurred in patients with previous histories of emotional disturbances or suicidal ideation or attempts as well as histories of misuse of tranquilizers, alcohol, and other CNS-active drugs. Some deaths have occurred as a consequence of the accidental ingestion of excessive quantities of propoxyphene alone or in combination with other drugs. Patients taking propoxyphene should be warned not to exceed the dosage recommended by the physician.

DRUG DEPENDENCE: Propoxyphene, when taken in higher-than-recommended doses over long periods of time, can produce drug dependence characterized by psychic dependence and, less frequently, physical dependence and tolerance. Propoxyphene will only partially suppress the withdrawal syndrome in individuals physically dependent on morphine or other narcotics. The abuse liability of propoxyphene is qualitatively similar to that of codeine although quantitatively less, and propoxyphene should be prescribed with the same degree of caution appropriate to the use of codeine.

USAGE IN AMBULATORY PATIENTS: Propoxyphene may impair the mental and/or physical abilities required for the performance of potentially hazardous tasks, such as driving a car or operating machinery. The patient should be cautioned accordingly.

PRECAUTIONS

GENERAL:

Propoxyphene should be administered with caution to patients with hepatic or renal impairment since higher serum concentrations or delayed elimination may occur.

DRUG INTERACTIONS: The CNS-depressant effect of propoxyphene is additive with that of other CNS depressants, including alcohol.

As is the case with many medicinal agents, propoxyphene may slow the metabolism of a concomitantly administered drug. Should this occur, the higher serum concentrations of that drug may result in increased pharmacologic or adverse effects of that drug. Such occurrences have been reported when propoxyphene was administered to patients on antidepressants, anticonvulsants, or warfarin-like drugs.

USAGE IN PREGNANCY: Safe use in pregnancy has not been established relative to possible adverse effects on fetal development. Instances of withdrawal symptoms in the neonate have been reported following usage during pregnancy. Therefore, propoxyphene should not be used in pregnant women unless, in the judgment of the physician, the potential benefits outweigh the possible hazards.

USAGE IN NURSING MOTHERS: Low levels of propoxyphene have been detected in human milk. In postpartum studies involving nursing mothers who were given propoxyphene, no adverse effects were noted in infants receiving mother's milk.

USAGE IN CHILDREN: Propoxyphene is not recommended for use in children, because documented clinical experience has been insufficient to establish safety and a suitable dosage regimen in the pediatric age group.

Patient Information is available for this product. See text following "How Supplied" section below.

ADVERSE REACTIONS

In a survey conducted in hospitalized patients, less than 1% of patients taking propoxyphene hydrochloride at recommended doses experienced side effects. The most frequently reported have been dizziness, sedation, nausea, and vomiting. Some of these adverse reactions may be alleviated if the patient lies down.

Other adverse reactions include constipation, abdominal pain, skin rashes, light-headedness, headache, weakness, euphoria, dysphoria, and minor visual disturbances.

Liver dysfunction has been reported in association with both active components of propoxyphene and acetaminophen tablets.

Propoxyphene therapy has been associated with abnormal liver-function tests and, more rarely, with instances of reversible jaundice.

Hepatic necrosis may result from acute overdoses of acetaminophen (see Management of Overdosage). In chronic ethanol abusers, this has been reported rarely with short-term use of acetaminophen doses of 2.5 to 10 g/day. Fatalities have occurred.

MANAGEMENT OF OVERDOSAGE

In all cases of suspected overdosage, call your regional Poison Control Center to obtain the most up-to-date information about the treatment of overdosage. This recommendation is made because, in general, information regarding the treatment of overdosage may change more rapidly than do package inserts.

Initial consideration should be given to the management of the CNS effects of propoxyphene overdosage. Resuscitative measures should be initiated promptly.

SYMPTOMS OF PROPOXYPHENE OVERDOSAGE: The manifestations of acute overdosage with propoxyphene are those of narcotic overdosage. The patient is usually somnolent, but may be stuporous or comatose and convulsing. Respiratory depression is characteristic. The ventilatory rate and/or tidal volume is decreased, which results in cyanosis and hypoxia. Pupils, initially pinpoint, may become dilated as hypoxia increases. Cheyne-Stokes respiration and apnea may occur. Blood pressure and heart rate are usually normal initially, but blood pressure falls and cardiac performance deteriorates, which ultimately results in pulmonary edema and circulatory collapse unless the respiratory depression is corrected and adequate ventilation is restored promptly. Cardiac arrhythmias and conduction delay may be present. A combined respiratory-metabolic acidosis occurs, owing to retained CO_2 (hypercapnea) and to lactic acid formed during anaerobic glycolysis. Acidosis may be severe if large amounts of salicylates have also been ingested. Death may occur.

TREATMENT OF PROPOXYPHENE OVERDOSAGE: Attention should be directed first to establishing a patent airway and to restoring ventilation. Mechanically assisted ventilation, with or without oxygen, may be required, and positive-pressure respiration may be desirable if pulmonary edema is present.

The narcotic antagonist naloxone will markedly reduce the degree of respiratory depression, and 0.4 to 2 mg should be administered promptly, preferably intravenously. If the desired degree of counteraction with improvement in respiratory function is not obtained, naloxone should be repeated at 2- to 3-minute intervals. The duration of action of the antagonist may be brief. If no response is observed after 10 mg of naloxone have been administered, the diagnosis of propoxyphene toxicity should be questioned. Naloxone may also be administered by continuous intravenous infusion.

TREATMENT OF PROPOXYPHENE OVERDOSAGE IN CHILDREN:

The usual initial dose of naloxone in children is 0.01 mg/kg body weight given intravenously. If this dose does not result in the desired degree of clinical improvement, a subsequent increased dose of 0.1 mg/kg body weight may be administered. If an IV route of administration is not available, naloxone may be administered IM or subcutaneously in divided doses. If necessary, naloxone can be diluted with sterile water for injection.

Blood gases, pH, and electrolytes should be monitored in order that acidosis and any electrolyte disturbance present may be corrected promptly. Acidosis, hypoxia, and generalized CNS depression predispose to the development of cardiac arrhythmias. Ventricular fibrillation or cardiac arrest may occur and necessitate the full complement of cardiopulmonary resuscitation (CPR) measures. Respiratory acidosis rapidly subsides as ventilation is restored and hypercapnea eliminated, but lactic acidosis may require intravenous bicarbonate for prompt correction.

Electrocardiographic monitoring is essential. Prompt correction of hypoxia, acidosis, and electrolyte disturbance (when present) will help prevent these cardiac complications and will increase the effectiveness of agents administered to restore normal cardiac function.

In addition to the use of a narcotic antagonist, the patient may require careful titration with an anticonvulsant to control convulsions. Analeptic drugs (for example, caffeine or amphetamine) should not be used because of their tendency to precipitate convulsions.

General supportive measures, in addition to oxygen, include, when necessary, intravenous fluids, vasopressor-inotropic compounds, and, when infection is likely, anti-infective agents. Gastric lavage may be useful, and activated charcoal can adsorb a significant amount of ingested propoxyphene. Dialysis is of little value in poisoning due to propoxyphene. Efforts should be made to determine whether other agents, such as alcohol, barbiturates, tranquilizers, or other CNS depressants, were also ingested, since these increase CNS depression as well as cause specific toxic effects.

SYMPTOMS OF ACETAMINOPHEN OVERDOSAGE: Shortly after oral ingestion of an overdosage of acetaminophen and for the next 24 hours, anorexia, nausea, vomiting, and abdominal pain have been noted. The patient may then present no symptoms, but evidence of liver dysfunction may be apparent during the next 24 to 48 hours, with elevated serum transaminase and lactic dehydrogenase levels, an increase in serum bilirubin concentrations, and a prolonged prothrombin time. Death from hepatic failure may result 3 to 7 days after overdosage.

Acute renal failure may accompany the hepatic dysfunction and has been noted in patients who do not exhibit signs of fulminant hepatic failure. Typically, renal impairment is more apparent 6 to 9 days after ingestion of the overdose.

TREATMENT OF ACETAMINOPHEN OVERDOSAGE: Acetaminophen in massive overdosage may cause hepatic toxicity in some patients. In case of suspected overdose, you may wish to call your regional poison center for assistance in diagnosis and for directions in the use of N-acetylcysteine as an antidote.

In adults, hepatic toxicity has rarely been reported with acute overdoses of less than 10 g and fatalities with less than 15 g.

Importantly, young children seem to be more resistant than adults to the hepatotoxic effect of an acetaminophen overdose. Despite this, the measures outlined below should be initiated in any adult or child suspected of having ingested an acetaminophen overdose. Clinical and laboratory evidence of hepatic toxicity may not be apparent until 48 to 72 hours postingestion. Early symptoms following a potentially hepatotoxic overdose may include: nausea, vomiting, diaphoresis, and general malaise.

The stomach should be emptied promptly by lavage or by induction of emesis with syrup of ipecac. Patients' estimates of the quantity of a drug ingested are notoriously unreliable. Therefore, if an acetaminophen overdose is suspected, a serum acetaminophen assay should be obtained as early as possible, but no sooner than four hours following ingestion. Liver-function studies should be obtained initially and repeated at 24-hour intervals.

The antidote, N-acetylcysteine, should be administered as early as possible, preferably within 16 hours of the overdose ingestion for optimal results, but in any case, within 24 hours. Following recovery, there are no residual, structural or functional hepatic abnormalities.

DOSAGE AND ADMINISTRATION

The product is given orally. The usual dose is 65 mg propoxyphene HCl and 650 mg acetaminophen every 4 hours as needed for pain. The maximum recommended dose of propoxyphene HCl is 390 mg per day.

Consideration should be given to a reduced total daily dosage in patients with hepatic or renal impairment.

HOW SUPPLIED

Wygesic® (propoxyphene HCl and acetaminophen) Tablets, Wyeth®, 65 mg propoxyphene and 650 mg acetaminophen, are available as follows:

NDC 0008-0085, green, capsule-shaped, scored, film-coated tablet marked "WYETH" and "85", in bottles of 100 and 500 tablets, and in REDIPAK® cartons of 100 tablets (10 blister strips of 10).

Keep tightly closed.

Protect from light.

Dispense in light-resistant, tight container.

PATIENT INFORMATION

Summary

Products containing propoxyphene are used to relieve pain. LIMIT YOUR INTAKE OF ALCOHOL WHILE TAKING THIS DRUG. Make sure your doctor knows if you are taking tranquilizers, sleep aids, antidepressants, antihistamines, or any other drugs that make you sleepy. Combining propoxyphene with alcohol or these drugs in excessive doses in dangerous.

Use care while driving a car or using machines until you see how the drug affects you, because propoxyphene can make you sleepy. Do not take more of the drug than your doctor prescribed. Dependence has occurred when patients have taken propoxyphene for a long period of time at doses greater than recommended.

The rest of this leaflet gives you more information about propoxyphene. Please read it and keep it for further use.

Uses for Propoxyphene

Products containing propoxyphene are used for the relief of mild to moderate pain. Products which contain propoxyphene plus aspirin or acetaminophen are prescribed for the relief of pain or pain associated with fever.

Before taking Propoxyphene

Make sure your doctor knows if you have ever had an allergic reaction to propoxyphene, aspirin, or acetaminophen. Some forms of propoxyphene products contain aspirin to help relieve the pain. Your doctor should be advised if you have a history of ulcers or if you are taking an anticoagulant ("blood thinner"). The aspirin may irritate the stomach lining and may cause bleeding, particularly if an ulcer is present. Also, bleeding may occur if you are taking an anticoagulant. In small groups of people, aspirin may cause an asthma attack. If you are one of these people, be sure your drug does not contain aspirin.

The effect of propoxyphene in children under 12 has not been studied. Therefore, use of the drug in this age group is not recommended.

Also, due to the possible association between aspirin and Reye's Syndrome, those propoxyphene products containing aspirin should not be given to children, including teenagers, with chicken pox or flu unless prescribed by a physician.

How to take Propoxyphene

Follow your doctor's directions exactly. Do not increase the amount you take without your doctor's approval. If you miss a dose of the drug, do not take twice as much the next time.

Pregnancy

Do not take propoxyphene during pregnancy unless your doctor knows you are pregnant and specifically recommends its use. Cases of temporary dependence in the newborn have occurred when the mother has taken propoxyphene consistently in the weeks before delivery. As a general principle, no drug should be taken during pregnancy unless it is clearly necessary.

General Caution

Heavy use of alcohol with propoxyphene is hazardous and may lead to overdosage symptoms (see "Overdosage" below); THEREFORE, LIMIT YOUR INTAKE OF ALCOHOL WHILE TAKING PROPOXYPHENE.

Combinations of excessive doses of propoxyphene, alcohol, and tranquilizers are dangerous. Make sure your doctor knows if you are taking tranquilizers, sleep aids, antidepressant drugs, antihistamines, or any other drugs that make you sleepy. The use of these drugs with propoxyphene increases their sedative effects and may lead to overdosage symptoms, including death (see "Overdosage" below).

Propoxyphene may cause drowsiness or impair your mental and/or physical abilities; therefore, use caution when driving a vehicle or operating dangerous machinery. DO NOT perform any hazardous task until you have seen your response to this drug.

Propoxyphene may increase the concentration in the body of medications such as anticoagulants ("blood thinners"), antidepressants, or drugs used for epilepsy. The result may be excessive or adverse effects of these medications. Make sure your doctor knows if you are taking any of these medications.

Dependence

You can become dependent on propoxyphene if you take it in higher than recommended doses over a long period of time. Dependence is a feeling of need for the drug and a feeling that you cannot perform normally without it.

Continued on next page

Wyeth-Ayerst—Cont.

Overdosage

An overdosage of propoxyphene, alone or in combination with other drugs, including alcohol, may cause weakness, difficulty in breathing, confusion, anxiety, and more severe drowsiness and dizziness. Extreme overdosage may lead to unconsciousness and death.

If the propoxyphene product contains acetaminophen, the overdosage symptoms include nausea, vomiting, lack of appetite, and abdominal pain. Liver damage may occur.

In any suspected overdosage situation, contact your doctor or nearest hospital emergency room. GET EMERGENCY HELP IMMEDIATELY.

KEEP THIS AND ALL DRUGS OUT OF THE REACH OF CHILDREN.

Possible Side Effects

When propoxyphene is taken as directed, side effects are infrequent. Among those reported are drowsiness, dizziness, nausea, and vomiting. If these effects occur, it may help if you lie down and rest.

Less frequently reported side effects are constipation, abdominal pain, skin rashes, light-headedness, headache, weakness, minor visual disturbances, and feelings of elation or discomfort.

If side effects occur and concern you, contact your doctor.

Other Information

The safe and effective use of propoxyphene depends on your taking it exactly as directed. This drug has been prescribed specifically for you and your present condition. Do not give this drug to others who may have similar symptoms. Do not use it for any other reason.

If you would like more information about propoxyphene, ask your doctor or pharmacist. They have a more technical leaflet (professional labeling) you may read.

Shown in Product Identification Section, page 438

WYMOX®　℞

[wi 'moks]
(amoxicillin)
Capsules and Oral Suspension

DESCRIPTION

Wymox (amoxicillin) is a semisynthetic penicillin, an analog of ampicillin, with a broad spectrum of bactericidal activity against many gram-positive and gram-negative microorganisms. Chemically, it is D-(-)-a-amino-p-hydroxybenzyl penicillin trihydrate.

Wymox (amoxicillin) capsules contain 250 mg or 500 mg amoxicillin as the trihydrate. The inactive ingredients present are colloidal silicon dioxide, D&C Yellow 10, FD&C Blue 1, gelatin, iron oxide, magnesium stearate, sodium lauryl sulfate, and titanium dioxide.

Wymox (amoxicillin) oral suspension is a powder which when reconstituted as directed yields a suspension of either 125 mg or 250 mg amoxicillin trihydrate per 5 mL. The inactive ingredients present are artificial flavors, carboxymethylcellulose sodium, cellulose, citric acid, FD&C Red 3, mannitol, sodium citrate, sucrose, and water.

HOW SUPPLIED

Wymox® (amoxicillin) Capsules, Wyeth®, contain 250 mg or 500 mg amoxicillin as the trihydrate and are supplied as follows:

250 mg, NDC 0008-0559, grey and green capsule marked "WYETH" and "559", in bottles of 100 and 500 capsules.

500 mg, NDC 0008-0560, grey and green capsule marked "WYETH" and "560", in bottles of 50 and 500 capsules.

Wymox® (amoxicillin) Oral Suspension, Wyeth®, is available as a pink powder which when reconstituted as directed yields a palatable, pink suspension of amoxicillin trihydrate in the following dosage strengths:

125 mg per 5 mL, NDC 0008-0557, in bottles to make 100 mL or 150 mL.

250 mg per 5 mL, NDC 0008-0558, in bottles to make 80 mL, 100 mL, or 150 mL.

For prescribing information write to Professional Service, Wyeth-Ayerst Laboratories, Box 8299, Philadelphia, PA 19101, or contact your local Wyeth-Ayerst representative.

Shown in Product Identification Section, page 438

WYTENSIN®　℞

[wi-ten 'sin]
(guanabenz acetate)

DESCRIPTION

Wytensin (guanabenz acetate), an antihypertensive agent for oral administration, is an aminoguanidine derivative, 2,6-dichlorobenzylideneaminoguanidine acetate, and its structural formula is:

[See Chemical Formula at top of next column].

It is an odorless, white to off-white, crystalline substance, sparingly soluble in water and soluble in alcohol, with a mo-

lecular weight of 291.14. Each tablet of Wytensin is equivalent to 4 mg or 8 mg of free guanabenz base. The inactive ingredients present are cellulose, iron oxide, lactose, and magnesium stearate. The 8 mg dosage strength also contains FD&C Blue 2.

Wytensin is available as 4 mg or 8 mg tablets for oral administration.

CLINICAL PHARMACOLOGY

Wytensin is an orally active central alpha-2 adrenergic agonist. Its antihypertensive action appears to be mediated via stimulation of central alpha adrenergic receptors, resulting in a decrease of sympathetic outflow from the brain at the bulbar level to the peripheral circulatory system.

PHARMACOKINETICS

In human studies, about 75% of an orally administered dose of Wytensin is absorbed and metabolized with less than 1% of unchanged drug recovered from the urine. Peak plasma concentrations of unchanged drug occur between two and five hours after a single oral dose. The average half-life for Wytensin is about 6 hours. The site or sites of metabolism of Wytensin have not been determined. The effect of meals on the absorption of Wytensin has not been studied.

PHARMACODYNAMICS

The onset of the antihypertensive action of Wytensin begins within 60 minutes after a single oral dose and reaches a peak effect within two to four hours. The effect of an acute single dose is reduced appreciably six to eight hours after administration, and blood pressure approaches baseline values within 12 hours of administration.

The acute antihypertensive effect of Wytensin occurs without major changes in peripheral resistance, but its chronic effect appears to be a decrease in peripheral resistance. A decrease in blood pressure is seen in both the supine and standing positions without alterations of normal postural mechanisms, so that postural hypotension has not been observed. Wytensin decreases pulse rate by about 5 beats per minute. Cardiac output and left ventricular ejection fraction are unchanged during long-term therapy.

In clinical trials, Wytensin, given orally to hypertensive patients, effectively controlled blood pressure without any significant effect on glomerular filtration rate, renal blood flow, body fluid volume or body weight. Wytensin given parenterally to dogs has produced a natriuresis. Similarly, hypertensive subjects, 24 hours after salt loading, have shown a decrease in blood pressure and a natriuresis (5% to 240% increase in sodium excretion) following a single oral dose of Wytensin. After seven consecutive days of administration and effective blood-pressure control, no significant change on glomerular filtration rate, renal blood flow, or body weight was observed. However, in clinical trials of six to thirty months duration, hypertensive patients with effective blood-pressure control by Wytensin lost one to four pounds of body weight. The mechanism of this weight loss has not been established. Tolerance to the antihypertensive effect of Wytensin has not been observed.

During long-term administration of Wytensin, there is a small decrease in serum cholesterol and total triglycerides without any change in the high-density lipoprotein fraction. Plasma norepinephrine, serum dopamine beta-hydroxylase and plasma renin activity are decreased during chronic administration of Wytensin. No changes in serum electrolytes, uric acid, blood-urea nitrogen, calcium, or glucose have been observed.

Wytensin and hydrochlorothiazide have been shown to have at least partially additive effects in patients not responding adequately to either drug alone.

INDICATIONS AND USAGE

Wytensin (guanabenz acetate) is indicated in the treatment of hypertension. It may be employed alone or in combination with a thiazide diuretic.

CONTRAINDICATION

Wytensin is contraindicated in patients with a known sensitivity to the drug.

PRECAUTIONS

1. Sedation: Wytensin causes sedation or drowsiness in a large fraction of patients. When Wytensin is used with centrally active depressants, such as phenothiazines, barbiturates, and benzodiazepines, the potential for additive sedative effects should be considered.

2. Patients with vascular insufficiency: Wytensin, like other antihypertensive agents, should be used with caution in patients with severe coronary insufficiency, recent myocardial infarction, cerebrovascular disease, or severe hepatic or renal failure.

3. Rebound: Sudden cessation of therapy with central alpha agonists like Wytensin may rarely result in "overshoot"

hypertension and more commonly produces an increase in serum catecholamines and subjective symptomatology.

4. Patients with hepatic impairment: The disposition of orally administered Wytensin is altered in patients with alcohol-induced liver disease. Mean plasma concentrations of Wytensin were higher in these patients than in healthy subjects. The clinical significance of this finding is unknown. However, careful monitoring of blood pressure is suggested when Wytensin is administered to patients with hypertension and coexisting chronic hepatic dysfunction.

5. Patients with renal impairment: The disposition of orally administered Wytensin is altered modestly in patients with renal impairment. Wytensin's half-life is prolonged and clearance decreased, more so in patients on hemodialysis. The clinical significance of these findings is unknown. Careful monitoring of blood pressure during Wytensin dose titration is suggested in patients with coexisting hypertension and renal impairment.

INFORMATION FOR PATIENTS

Patients who receive Wytensin should be advised to exercise caution when operating dangerous machinery or driving motor vehicles until it is determined that they do not become drowsy or dizzy from the medication. Patients should be warned that their tolerance for alcohol and other CNS depressants may be diminished. Patients should be advised not to discontinue therapy abruptly.

LABORATORY TESTS

In clinical trials, no clinically significant laboratory-test abnormalities were identified during either acute or chronic therapy with Wytensin. Tests carried out included CBC, urinalysis, electrolytes, SGOT, bilirubin, alkaline phosphatase, uric acid, BUN, creatinine, glucose, calcium, phosphorus, total protein, and Coombs' test. During long-term administration of Wytensin, there was a small decrease in serum cholesterol and total triglycerides without any change in the high-density lipoprotein fraction. In rare instances an occasional nonprogressive increase in liver enzymes has been observed. However, no clinical evidence of hepatic disease has been found.

DRUG INTERACTIONS

Wytensin has not been demonstrated to cause any drug interactions when administered with other drugs, such as digitalis, diuretics, analgesics, anxiolytics, and antiinflammatory or antiinfective agents, in clinical trials. However, the potential for increased sedation when Wytensin is administered concomitantly with CNS-depressant drugs should be noted.

DRUG/LABORATORY TEST INTERACTIONS

No laboratory-test abnormalities were identified with the use of Wytensin.

CARCINOGENESIS, MUTAGENESIS, IMPAIRMENT OF FERTILITY

No evidence of carcinogenic potential emerged in rats during a two-year oral study with Wytensin at doses up to 9.5 mg/kg/day, i.e., about 10 times the maximum recommended human dose. In the Salmonella microsome mutagenicity (Ames) test system, Wytensin at 200-500 mcg per plate or at 30-50 mcg/mL in suspension gave dose-related increases in the number of mutants in one (TA 1537) of five *Salmonella typhimurium* strains with or without inclusion of rat liver microsomes. No mutagenic activity was seen at doses up to those which inhibit growth in the eukaryotic microorganism, *Schizosaccharomyces pombe,* or in Chinese hamster ovary cells at doses up to those which were lethal to the cells in culture. In another eukaryotic system, *Saccharomyces cerevisiae,* Wytensin produced no activity in an assay measuring induction of repairable DNA damage. Reproductive studies showed a decreased pregnancy rate in rats administered high oral doses (9.6 mg/kg) of Wytensin, suggesting an impairment of fertility. The fertility of treated males (9.6 mg/kg) may also have been affected, as suggested by the decreased pregnancy rate of their mates, even though the females received Wytensin only during the last third of pregnancy.

PREGNANCY

Pregnancy Category C

WYTENSIN MAY HAVE ADVERSE EFFECTS ON THE FETUS WHEN ADMINISTERED TO PREGNANT WOMEN. A teratology study in mice has indicated a possible increase in skeletal abnormalities when Wytensin is given orally at doses of 3 to 6 times the maximum recommended human dose of 1.0 mg/kg. These abnormalities, principally costal and vertebral, were not noted in similar studies in rats and rabbits. However, increased fetal loss has been observed after oral Wytensin administration to pregnant rats (14 mg/kg) and rabbits (20 mg/kg). Reproductive studies of Wytensin in rats have shown slightly decreased live-birth indices, decreased fetal survival rate, and decreased pup body weight at oral doses of 6.4 and 9.6 mg/kg. There are no adequate, well-controlled studies in pregnant women. Wytensin should be used during pregnancy only if the potential benefit justifies the potential risk to the fetus.

NURSING MOTHERS

Because no information is available on the excretion of Wytensin in human milk, it should not be administered to nursing mothers.

PEDIATRIC USE
The safety and effectiveness of Wytensin in children less than 12 years of age have not been demonstrated. Therefore, its use in this age group cannot be recommended at this time.

ADVERSE REACTIONS
The incidence of adverse effects has been ascertained from controlled clinical studies conducted in the United States and is based on data from 859 patients who received Wytensin for up to 3 years. There is some evidence that the side effects are dose-related.

The following table shows the incidence of adverse effects occurring in at least 5% of patients in a study comparing Wytensin (guanabenz acetate) to placebo, at a starting dose of 8 mg b.i.d.

Adverse Effect	Placebo (%) n=102	Wytensin (%) n=109
Dry mouth	7	28
Drowsiness or sedation	12	39
Dizziness	7	17
Weakness	7	10
Headache	6	5

In other controlled clinical trials at the starting dose of 16 mg/day in 476 patients, the incidence of dry mouth was slightly higher (38%) and that of dizziness was slightly lower (12%), but the incidence of the most frequent adverse effects was similar to the placebo-controlled trial. Although these side effects were not serious, they led to discontinuation of treatment about 15% of the time. In more recent studies using an initial dose of 8 mg/day in 274 patients, the incidence of drowsiness or sedation was lower, about 20%.

Other adverse effects were reported during clinical trials with Wytensin but are not clearly distinguishable from placebo effects and occurred with a frequency of 3% or less:
Cardiovascular—chest pain, edema, arrhythmias, palpitations.
Gastrointestinal—nausea, epigastric pain, diarrhea, vomiting, constipation, abdominal discomfort.
Central nervous system—anxiety, ataxia, depression, sleep disturbances.
ENT disorders—nasal congestion.
Eye disorders—blurring of vision.
Musculoskeletal—aches in extremities, muscle aches.
Respiratory—dyspnea.
Dermatologic—rash, pruritus.
Urogenital—urinary frequency, disturbances of sexual function (decreased libido, impotence).
Other—gynecomastia, taste disorders.

DRUG ABUSE AND DEPENDENCE
No reported dependence or abuse has been associated with the administration of Wytensin.

OVERDOSAGE
Accidental ingestion of Wytensin caused hypotension, somnolence, lethargy, irritability, miosis, and bradycardia in two children aged one and three years. Gastric lavage and administration of pressor substances, fluids, and oral activated charcoal resulted in complete and uneventful recovery within 12 hours in both patients.

Since experience with accidental overdosage is limited, the suggested treatment is mainly supportive while the drug is being eliminated from the body and until the patient is no longer symptomatic. Vital signs and fluid balance should be carefully monitored. An adequate airway should be maintained and, if indicated, assisted respiration instituted. There are no data available on the dialyzability of Wytensin.

DOSAGE AND ADMINISTRATION
Dosage with Wytensin should be individualized. A starting dose of 4 mg twice a day is recommended, whether Wytensin is used alone or with a thiazide diuretic. Dosage may be increased in increments of 4 to 8 mg per day every one to two weeks, depending on the patient's response. The maximum dose studied to date has been 32 mg twice daily, but doses as high as this are rarely needed.

HOW SUPPLIED
Wytensin® (guanabenz acetate) Tablets, Wyeth®, are available in the following dosage strengths:
4 mg, NDC 0008-0073, orange, five-sided tablet with a raised "W" and a "4" under the "W" on one side and "WYETH 73" on reverse side, in bottles of 100 and 500 tablets and in Redipak® cartons of 100 tablets (10 blister strips of 10).
8 mg, NDC 0008-0074, gray, five-sided tablet with a raised "W" and an "8" under the "W" on one side and "WYETH 74" on scored reverse side, in bottles of 100 tablets.
The appearance of these tablets is a trademark of Wyeth-Ayerst Laboratories.
Keep tightly closed.
Dispense in tight containers.
Protect from light.
Shown in Product Identification Section, page 438

EDUCATIONAL MATERIAL

Films—Slides—Videos
The Wyeth-Ayerst Audiovisual Catalog, listing films, audiovisual, and slide programs available through the Wyeth-Ayerst Film Library or on loan through the local Wyeth-Ayerst representative, can be obtained by writing Professional Service, Wyeth-Ayerst Laboratories, Box 8299, Philadelphia, PA 19101.

Young Pharmaceuticals Inc.
1840 BERLIN TURNPIKE
WETHERSFIELD, CT 06109

PHARMACREME™   OTC
[far'ma-krēm]
Emollient Topical Vehicle and Diluent

DESCRIPTION
PHARMACREME™ is a hydrophilic cream vehicle consisting of Stearic acid, Isopropyl myristate, Polyoxyl 40 Stearate, Stearyl alcohol, Xanthan gum, Sorbic acid, Butylated hydroxytoluene and Purified water. Diazolidinyl urea added as a preservative.
PHARMACREME™ provides topical moisturizing actions and is a versatile vehicle and diluent for selected dermatologic additives. This non-ionic formula contains no fragrances, parabens or Propylene glycol which may irritate sensitive skin.

WARNINGS
Extemporaneous formulations of PHARMACREME™ should be considered to share in the full range of Warnings, Precautions, Contraindications and Adverse Reactions of all additives.
Laboratory and clinical evaluations necessary to determine the safety and efficacy of the preparations resulting from the addition of any ingredients to PHARMACREME™ have not been conducted. Young Pharmaceuticals Inc. makes no claims regarding the safety and efficacy of extemporaneously prepared products.

PRECAUTIONS
General
For external use only. Keep away from eyes. In case of eye contact, rinse eye thoroughly with water and consult physician. Keep out of reach of children.

HOW SUPPLIED
20 grams in plastic jars. The jar is filled to approximately ½ capacity to accommodate the addition of selected dermatologic additives. A plastic spatula is also provided to facilitate product preparation and application (NDC 52185-950-20).
PHARMACREME™ is also supplied 480 grams in plastic jars for larger compounding requirements. The jar is filled to approximately ½ capacity to accommodate the addition of selected dermatologic additives (NDC 52185-950-48).
Store below 80°F (27°C).
For additional information, call Young Pharmaceuticals Inc. Laboratory Services Department toll-free at 1-800-874-9686. In Connecticut, call (203) 529-7919 collect.

Discontinued Products

Listed below are products discontinued by manufacturers this past year. Please check the Product Name Index to determine if marketing has been assumed by another manufacturer.

Abbott Laboratories

Eutonyl Filmtab
Gemonil
Tral

Adams Laboratories, Inc.

Deconsal Capsules 100s

Alpha Therapeutic Corporation

Profilate Heat-Treated

Burroughs Wellcome Company

Fluorouracil
Wellcovorin Injection

Central Pharmaceuticals, Inc.

Pavacen Capsules
Synophylate Elixir

Elkins-Sinn, Inc.

Cefazolin
Gentamicin Sulfate Plastic
   Bags
Hydrocortisone
Methylprednisolone

Everett Laboratories, Inc.

Dipimol Tablets, 25 mg,
   50 mg, 75 mg
Florvite + Iron Drops .5 mg
   (now 0.25 mg)
Fumide Tablets 20 mg &
   40 mg
Ibuprofen 400 mg, 600 mg,
   800 mg
PreNatal + Iron 1 mg
   Tablets
Tusso DM Syrup

Knoll Pharmaceuticals

Isoptin Syringes

Merck Sharp & Dohme

Redisol Injectable
   (cyanocobalamin, MSD)

Pfizer Laboratories

Antiminth Oral Suspension
Sustaire

Reed & Carnrick

Phazyme-PB Tablets

Savage Laboratories

Trymex Cream & Ointment

Sclavo, Inc.

Antirabies Serum
Cholera Vaccine
Diphtheria Toxoid
   Adsorbed Pediatric

G.D. Searle & Co.

Aminophylline Injection
Anavar

Smith Kline &French Laboratories

Hispril (brand of diphenyl-
   pyraline)
Paredrine 1% (brand of hy-
   droxyamphetamine hy-
   drobromide) with Boric
   Acid, Ophthalmic Solu-
   tion

E.R. Squibb & Sons Inc.

Proto-Chol (Natural Fish
   Oils)

Syntex Laboratories, Inc.

Norinyl 1 + 80 Tablets
   (norethindrone and mestranol)
Norinyl 2 mg Tablets
   (norethindrone and mestranol)

SECTION 7
Diagnostic Product Information

Products described in PHYSICIANS' DESK REFERENCE® which have official package circulars must be in full compliance with Food & Drug Administration regulations pertaining to labeling for prescription drugs. These regulations require that for PDR copy, "indications, effects, dosages, routes, methods, and frequency and duration of administration, and any relevant warnings, hazards, contraindications, side effects, and precautions" must be the *"same in language and emphasis"* as the approved labeling for the product. FDA regards the words *"same in language and emphasis"* as requiring VERBATIM use of the approved labeling providing such information. Furthermore, information in the approved labeling that is emphasized by the use of type set in a box or in capitals, bold face, or italics must also be given the same emphasis in PDR. For products which do not have official package circulars, the Publisher emphasized to manufacturers the necessity of describing such products comprehensively so that physicians would have access to all information essential for intelligent and informed prescribing. In organizing and presenting the material in PHYSICIANS' DESK REFERENCE, the Publisher is providing all the information made available to PDR by manufacturers.

This edition of PHYSICIANS' DESK REFERENCE contains the latest product information available at press-time. During the year, however, new and revised information about the products described herein may be furnished us. This information will be published in the PDR Supplement. Therefore, before prescribing or administering any product described in the following pages, you should first consult the PDR Supplement.

In presenting the following material to the medical profession, the Publisher is not necessarily advocating the use of any product listed.

Boehringer Mannheim Diagnostics

Division of Boehringer Mannheim Corporation
9115 HAGUE ROAD
INDIANAPOLIS, IN 46250

CHEMSTRIP bG®

[kim'strip bee-jee']

BLOOD GLUCOSE TEST

Test Strips for
Semi-Quantitative Determination
of Glucose in Whole Blood

SUMMARY AND EXPLANATION

CHEMSTRIP bG Test Strip is a sensitive and specific test strip which facilitates accurate semi-quantitative determination of blood glucose within 2 minutes.

CHEMSTRIP bG Test Strips have 2 separate test zones whose different reagent concentrations optimize sensitivity and colorimetric accuracy of semi-quantitative values from 20 mg/dL to 800 mg/dL. A wide range of test values permits wide use of CHEMSTRIP bG Strips for clinical monitoring of diabetes mellitus, and in home blood glucose monitoring programs. When used with an Accu-Chek® II and Accu-Chek® IIm Blood Glucose Monitors, Chemstrip bG Test Strips (Cat. No. 00502, 00508 only) are also intended for use in monitoring glucose values in neonates who have been diagnosed by conventional means.

SPECIMEN COLLECTION AND PREPARATION

The Chemstrip bG strip is highly specific when used with fresh capillary blood. Both test pads are specific for D-glucose in whole blood and nonreactive to fructose, lactose, galactose, and pentose sugars. Reducing substances such as uric acid and ascorbic acid (when occurring at normal blood concentrations) do not interfere with this procedure, nor does therapy with heparin, EDTA or the usual plasma expanders. Therapy with dopamine at the therapeutic blood concentration of .01 mg/dL, or methyldopa at .01–.35 mg/dL, does not inhibit the reaction of the strips. Above 200 mg/dL glucose, extremes in hematocrits can affect results. Elevated hematocrits in the greater than 55%–80% range can lower glucose results by as much as 15%, while very low hematocrits (below 35%) can increase the glucose results by as much as 10%. Caution is advised for the interpretation of neonate glucose values below 50 mg/dL. Do not use preservatives that contain fluoride.

PROCEDURE FOR *IN VITRO* DIAGNOSTIC USE

Two-minute test procedure requires only 3 steps: (1) Place a single large drop of whole blood on the reagent area to cover both test zones completely. (2) After 60 seconds, wipe off all of the blood with a dry white cotton or rayon ball. **Do not use water;** unlike other strips, CHEMSTRIP bG Strips need no washing. (3) After another 60 seconds, read test results by comparing test-zone colors with the vial label's color values for 20, 40, 80, 120, 180, and 240 mg/dL. (For colors **darker** than those for 240 mg/dL, wait an extra minute before reading 400 or 800 mg/dL.) The 8 distinct, precalibrated color values facilitate reproducible reading and permit practical estimation of intermediate values.

HOW SUPPLIED

Nonbreakable vials of test strips, moisture protected by drying agents in vial cap. Vials of 25 strips for visual reading, Cat. No. 00501.
Vials of 50 strips for Accu-Chek® bG Blood Glucose Monitor, Cat. No. 00503.
Vials of 50 or 100 strips for Accu-Chek II Monitor, Cat. No. 00502, 00508.
Complete self-testing system also available. Kit includes 25 test strips, lancets, cotton balls, alcohol wipes, illustrated "How-to-Use" card and diabetic information guide. Cat. No. 00505.

TRACER bG™ TEST STRIPS

The Tracer bG Test Strip, used as directed with the Tracer™ and Tracer II Blood Glucose Monitors, will accurately measure blood glucose values. The strip changes color as it reacts to glucose in a drop of blood, and the Tracer and Tracer II monitors measure this color change. The blood glucose level is then displayed by the monitor. Tracer bG Test Strip utilizes one reagent pad that requires less blood than many other test strips.

HOW SUPPLIED

Vials of 50 for use with Tracer and Tracer II Blood Glucose Monitors, Cat. No. 00535.
ORDERING / PRICING / TECHNICAL INFORMATION CALL (800) 858-8072.

CHEMSTRIP®

[kim' strip]

URINE TESTING STRIPS

Dip-and-Read Test Strips for
Nitrite, pH, Protein, Glucose, Ketones,
Urobilinogen, Bilirubin, Blood, and Leukocytes
in Urine

SUMMARY AND EXPLANATION

The CHEMSTRIP urine test strip is uniquely constructed of an inert plastic strip to which a nylon mesh bonds, without glue, 1 to 9 reagent-impregnated paper pads for determination of nitrite, pH, protein, glucose, ketones, urobilinogen, bilirubin, blood, and leukocytes in urine. The nylon mesh holds the reagent pad in place, protects it, and promotes rapid and even urine diffusion into the test area. To prevent the "run-over" phenomenon, certain reagent pads also have an inert absorbent paper between the reagent paper pads and the plastic strip.

[See table below for CHEMSTRIP test parameters.]

SPECIMEN COLLECTION AND PREPARATION

CHEMSTRIP urine test strips may be used on any freshly voided urine specimen or on urines collected under special conditions, such as first-morning specimens and postprandial urine specimens. The urine must be collected in a clean container and should be tested as soon as possible after collection (do not centrifuge). It is of particular importance to use fresh urine to obtain the best results with the test for urine bilirubin due to the instability of bilirubin when exposed to room temperatures and strong light. If testing cannot be performed within an hour after collection, the sample specimen should be immediately refrigerated between 2 and 8° C. Return the sample to room temperature prior to testing. Mix specimen thoroughly before use.
FOR *IN VITRO* DIAGNOSTIC USE.

PROCEDURE

For convenience, all values on the test strips may be read at 60 seconds (during the second minute) after immersion in the urine. Color changes occurring more than 2 minutes after strip immersion are not of diagnostic value. Color changes that occur only along the edge of the test strip should be ignored. Careful removal of excess urine should eliminate this effect.
The CHEMSTRIP test strips do not require any calibration. The color blocks on the test vial label are created by the use of precise standards during an unique manufacturing process.

PRICING/TECHNICAL INFORMATION

(800) 858-8072.

Helena Laboratories

1530 LINDBERGH DRIVE
P.O. BOX 752
BEAUMONT, TX 77704

COLOSCREEN SELF-TEST (CS-T™)

Fecal Occult Blood Test

DESCRIPTION

ColoScreen Self-Test (CS-T™) is a simple, sanitary, one-step test for the detection of occult blood in the stool. No stool sample collection or color development reagents are needed. The patient simply places a test pad in the toilet, watches for a color change and records the results. No dietary fruit or vegetable restrictions are necessary. Red meat and vitamin C dietary restrictions should be followed.

ORDER INFORMATION

CS-T Office Packs contain an instruction sheet for the physician and 25 or 50 patient kits. Each patient kit consists of 3 CS-T test pads, instructions for the patient, and a reply card for return of results to the physician.

CS-T™ 50 Patient Kit Office Pack	Cat. No. 5176
CS-T™ 25 Patient Kit Office Pack	Cat. No. 5170

COLOSCREEN

Fecal Occult Blood Test

DESCRIPTION

ColoScreen is the standard guaiac slide test for the detection of occult blood in the stool. The patient smears a small fecal sample on the slide and then returns the slide to the physician's office or lab for testing. ColoScreen is identical in specificity and sensitivity to Hemoccult® (a registered trademark of SmithKline Diagnostics, Inc.). As with other guaiac slide tests, certain fruits and vegetables, red meats and vitamin C should be restricted from the diet.

ORDER INFORMATION

ColoScreen Kits contain all materials necessary for complete testing, including developer and instructions. (Lab packs are also available in cartons of 1000 tests.)

ColoScreen III Office Pack	**Cat. No. 5071**
100 Patient Kits (300 Tests). Each patient kit consists of one ColoScreen triple slide with monitors and applicators in a mail-back envelope printed with instructions for the patient.	
ColoScreen Lab Pack	**Cat. No. 5072**
100 Single Slides with Monitors (100 Tests)	
ColoScreen III Lab Pack	**Cat. No. 5082**
34 Triple Slides with Monitors (102 Tests)	
ColoScreen Tape	**Cat. No. 5079**
2 Rolls (100 Tests/Roll) with perforated Segments and Monitors	

Products are cross-indexed by
generic and chemical names
in the
YELLOW SECTION

Chemstrip Test Parameters

	Nitrite	Blood	Protein	Glucose	Ketones	Urobilinogen	Bilirubin	pH	Leukocytes	Catalog No.	Strips Per Vial
CHEMSTRIP® 9	X	X	X	X	X	X	X	X	X	417109	100
CHEMSTRIP® 8		X	X	X	X	X	X	X	X	417117	100
CHEMSTRIP® 7		X	X	X	X		X	X	X	417126	100
CHEMSTRIP® 6		X	X	X	X			X	X	417135	100
CHEMSTRIP® 2GP			X	X						200743	100
CHEMSTRIP® uGK				X	X					00513 or 00514	100 or 50
CHEMSTRIP® K					X					00515 or 00516	100 or 25
CHEMSTRIP® uG				X						00511	100
CHEMSTRIP® 2LN	X								X	417152	100
CHEMSTRIP® 4 the OB™		X	X	X						417144	100

Hoechst-Roussel Pharmaceuticals Inc.
SOMERVILLE, NJ 08876-1258

RELEFACT® TRH   ℞
(protirelin)
Injection IV

DESCRIPTION
Chemically, Relefact® TRH (protirelin) is identified as 5-oxo-L-prolyl-L-histidyl-L-proline amide. It is a synthetic tripeptide which is believed to be structurally identical with the naturally-occurring thyrotropin-releasing hormone produced by the hypothalamus.
The structural formula is:

Relefact TRH is supplied as 1 mL ampuls. Each ampul contains 500 mcg protirelin in a sterile non-pyrogenic isotonic saline solution having a pH of approximately 6.5. In addition, each ampul contains sodium chloride, 9.0 mg, Water for Injection, and hydrochloric acid as needed to adjust pH. Relefact TRH is intended for intravenous administration.

CLINICAL PHARMACOLOGY
Pharmacologically, Relefact TRH increases the release of the thyroid stimulating hormone (TSH) from the anterior pituitary. Prolactin release is also increased. It has recently been observed that approximately 65% of acromegalic patients tested respond with a rise in circulating growth hormone levels; the clinical significance is as yet not clear. Following intravenous administration, the mean plasma half-life of protirelin in normal subjects is approximately five minutes. TSH levels rise rapidly and reach a peak at 20 to 30 minutes. The decline in TSH levels takes place more slowly, approaching baseline levels after approximately three hours.

INDICATIONS AND USAGE
Relefact® TRH (protirelin) is indicated as an adjunctive agent in the diagnostic assessment of thyroid function. As an adjunct to other diagnostic procedures, testing with Relefact TRH may yield useful information in patients with pituitary or hypothalamic dysfunction.
Relefact TRH is indicated as an adjunct to evaluate the effectiveness of thyrotropin suppression with a particular dose of T4 in patients with nodular or diffuse goitre. A normal TSH baseline value and a minimal difference between the 30 minute and baseline response to Relefact TRH injection would indicate adequate suppression of the pituitary secretion of TSH.
Relefact TRH may be used, adjunctively, for adjustment of thyroid hormone dosage given to patients with primary hypothyroidism. A normal or slightly blunted TSH response, thirty minutes following Relefact TRH injection, would indicate adequate replacement therapy.

WARNINGS
Transient changes in blood pressure, either increases or decreases, frequently occur immediately following administration of Relefact TRH (protirelin). Blood pressure should therefore be measured before Relefact TRH is administered and at frequent intervals during the first 15 minutes after its administration.
Increases in systolic pressure (usually less than 30 mm Hg) and/or increases in diastolic pressure (usually less than 20 mm Hg) have been observed more frequently than decreases in pressure. These changes have not ordinarily persisted for more than 15 minutes nor have they required therapy. More severe degrees of hypertension or hypotension with or without syncope have been reported in a few patients. To minimize the incidence and/or severity of hypotension, the patient should be supine before, during, and after Relefact TRH administration. If a clinically important change in blood pressure occurs, monitoring of blood pressure should be continued until it returns to baseline levels.
Relefact® TRH (protirelin) should not be administered to patients in whom marked, rapid changes in blood pressure would be dangerous unless the potential benefit clearly outweighs the potential risk.

PRECAUTIONS
Thyroid hormones reduce the TSH response to Relefact TRH. Accordingly, patients in whom Relefact TRH is to be used diagnostically should be taken off liothyronine (T3) approximately seven days prior to testing and should be taken off thyroid medications containing levothyroxine (T4),

e.g., desiccated thyroid, thyroglobulin, or liatrix, at least 14 days before testing. Hormone therapy is NOT to be discontinued when the test is used to evaluate the effectiveness of thyroid suppression with a particular dose of T4 in patients with nodular or diffuse goitre, or for adjustment of thyroid hormone dosage given to patients with primary hypothyroidism. Chronic administration of levodopa has been reported to inhibit the TSH response to Relefact TRH.
It is not advisable to withdraw maintenance doses of adrenocortical drugs used in the therapy of known hypopituitarism. Several published reports have shown that prolonged treatment with glucocorticoids at physiologic doses has no significant effect on the TSH response to thyrotropin releasing hormone, but that the administration of pharmacologic doses of steroids reduces the TSH response.
Therapeutic doses of acetylsalicylic acid (2 to 3.6 g/day) have been reported to inhibit the TSH response to protirelin. The ingestion of acetylsalicylic acid caused the peak level of TSH to decrease approximately 30% as compared to values obtained without acetylsalicylic acid administration. In both cases, the TSH peak occurred 30 minutes post-administration of protirelin.
Pregnancy: Reproduction studies have been performed in rats and rabbits. At doses 1½ and 6 times the human dose, there was an increase in the number of resorption sites in the pregnant rabbit. There are no studies in pregnant women which bear on the safety of Relefact® TRH (protirelin) for the human fetus. Relefact TRH should be used in pregnant women only when clearly needed.

ADVERSE REACTIONS
Side effects have been reported in about 50% of the patients tested with Relefact TRH. Generally, the side effects are minor, have occurred promptly, and have persisted for only a few minutes following injection.
Cardiovascular reactions:
Marked changes in blood pressure, including both hypertension and hypotension with or without syncope, have been reported in a small number of patients.
Endocrine reaction: Breast enlargement and leakage in lactating women for up to two or three days.
Other reactions:
Headaches, sometimes severe, and transient amaurosis in patients with pituitary tumors.
Rarely, convulsions may occur in patients with predisposing conditions, e.g. epilepsy, brain damage.
Nausea; urge to urinate; flushed sensation; lightheadedness; bad taste; abdominal discomfort; and dry mouth. Less frequently reported were: anxiety; sweating; tightness in the throat; pressure in the chest; tingling sensation; and drowsiness.
Pituitary apoplexy requiring acute neurosurgical intervention has been reported infrequently for patients with pituitary macroadenomas following the acute administration of protirelin (TRH) injection in the setting of combined anterior pituitary function testing in conjunction with LHRH and insulin.

DOSAGE AND ADMINISTRATION
Relefact TRH is intended for intravenous administration with the patient in the supine position. The drug is administered as a bolus over a period of 15 to 30 seconds, with the patient remaining supine until all scheduled postinjection blood samples have been taken. Blood pressure should be measured before Relefact TRH is administered and at frequent intervals during the first 15 minutes thereafter (see **Warnings**).
Dosage: Adults: 500 mcg. Doses between 200 and 500 mcg have been used. 500 mcg is considered the optimum dose to give the maximum response in the greatest number of pa-

tients. Doses greater than 500 mcg are unlikely to elicit a greater TSH response.
Children age 6 to 16 years: 7 mcg/kg body weight up to a dose of 500 mcg.
Infants and children up to 6 years: Experience is limited in this age group; doses of 7 mcg/kg have been administered. One blood sample for TSH assay should be drawn immediately prior to the injection of Relefact® TRH (protirelin), and a second sample should be obtained 30 minutes after injection.
The TSH response to Relefact TRH is reduced by repetitive administration of the drug. Accordingly, if the Relefact TRH test is repeated, an interval of seven days before testing is recommended.
Elevated serum lipids may interfere with the TSH assay. Thus, fasting (except in patients with hypopituitarism) or a low-fat meal is recommended prior to the test.

INTERPRETATION OF TEST RESULTS
Interpretation of the TSH response to Relefact TRH requires an understanding of thyroid-pituitary-hypothalamic physiology and knowledge of the clinical status of the individual patient.
Because the TSH test results may vary with the laboratory, the physician should be familiar with the TSH assay method used and the normal range for the laboratory performing the assay.
TSH response 30 minutes after Relefact TRH administration in normal subjects and in patients with hyperthyroidism and hypothyroidism are presented in Figure 1. The diagnoses were established prior to the administration of Relefact TRH on the basis of the clinical history, physical examination, and the results of other thyroid and/or pituitary function tests.
Among the normal euthyroid subjects, women and children were found to have higher levels of TSH at 30 minutes than men. Among the patients with hyperthyroidism or primary (thyroidal), secondary (pituitary), or tertiary (hypothalamic) hypothyroidism, no significant differences in TSH levels by age or sex were found.
[See table above].
Normal: Baseline TSH levels of less than 10 micro-units/mL (μU/mL) were observed in 97% of euthyroid normal subjects tested. Thirty minutes after Relefact® TRH (protirelin), the serum TSH increased by 2.0 μU/mL or more in 95% of euthyroid subjects.
Hyperthyroidism: All hyperthyroid patients tested had baseline TSH levels of less than 10 μU/mL and a rise of less than 2 μU/mL 30 minutes after Relefact TRH.
Primary (thyroidal) hypothyroidism: The diagnosis of primary hypothyroidism is frequently supported by finding clearly elevated baseline TSH levels; 93% of patients tested had levels above 10 μU/mL. Relefact TRH administration to these patients generally would not be expected to yield additional useful information. Ninety-four percent of patients with primary hypothyroidism given Relefact TRH in clinical trials responded with a rise in TSH of 2.0 μU/mL or greater, since this response is also found in normal subjects. Relefact TRH testing does not differentiate primary hypothyroidism from normal.

Figure 1
Mean ± One Standard Deviation of TSH Levels (μU/mL)
Observed at Baseline and 30 Minutes After Relefact® TRH (protirelin)

Number of Patients	Condition	
73	Euthyroid Women	
111	Euthyroid Men	
56	Secondary Hypothyroid (pituitary)	
21	Tertiary Hypothyroid (hypothalamic)	
75	Hyperthyroid	

Baseline
30 Minutes

Continued on next page

Hoechst-Roussel—Cont.

Table 1
Characterization Based on
Serum TSH Levels at
Baseline and 30 Minutes after Relefact TRH

	Baseline Serum TSH (μU/mL)	Change of Serum TSH (μU/mL) at 30 minutes
Euthyroidism (normal thyroid function)	10 or less (usually 6 or less: 20% have < 1.5 μU/mL)	2 or more (usually 6 to 30)
Hyperthyroidism	10 or less (usually 4 or less)	less than 2
Primary Hypothyroidism (thyroidal)	more than 10 (usually 15 to 100)	2 or more (usually 20 or more)
Secondary Hypothyroidism (pituitary)	10 or less (usually 6 or less)	less than 2 (59%) 2 to 50 (41%)
Tertiary Hypothyroidism (hypothalamic)	10 or less (often less than 2)	2 or more

Secondary (pituitary) and tertiary (hypothalamic) hypothyroidism: In the presence of clinical and other laboratory evidence of hypothyroidism, the finding of a baseline TSH level less than 10 μU/mL should suggest secondary or tertiary hypothyroidism. In this situation, a response to Relefact® TRH (protirelin) of less than 2 μU/mL suggests secondary hypothyroidism since this response was observed in about 60% of patients with secondary hypothyroidism and approximately 5% of patients with tertiary hypothyroidism. A TSH response to Relefact TRH greater than 2 μU/mL is not helpful in differentiating between secondary and tertiary hypothyroidism since this response was noted in about 40% of the former and about 95% of the latter.

Establishing the diagnosis of secondary or tertiary hypothyroidism requires a careful history and physical examination along with appropriate tests of anterior pituitary and/or target gland function. The Relefact TRH test should not be used as the only laboratory determinant for establishing these diagnoses.

HOW SUPPLIED

As 1 mL ampuls - boxes of 5 (NDC 0039-0081-08). Each mL contains Relefact TRH 0.50 mg (500 mcg), sodium chloride 9.0 mg for isotonicity, and hydrochloric acid for pH adjustment.

* RELEFACT® REG TM HOECHST AG
781000-6/86

Lederle Biologicals
A Division of American Cyanamid Co.
ONE CYANAMID PLAZA
WAYNE, NJ 07470

TUBERCULIN, OLD, TINE TEST®   ℞
[to-ber-cu-lin]

DESCRIPTION

The Tuberculin, Old, TINE TEST is a sterile, simple, multiple-puncture, disposable intradermal test device for the detection of tuberculin reactivity. These convenient devices are especially useful in mass tuberculosis screening programs. Each test unit consists of a stainless steel disc attached to a plastic handle. Projecting from the disc are four triangular-shaped prongs (tines) which are 2 mm long and approximately 4 mm apart. The tines have been mechanically dipped in a solution of Old Tuberculin, containing 7% Acacia (Gum Arabic) and 8.5% lactose as stabilizers, and then dried. The entire unit has been sterilized by Colbalt 60 irradiation. No preservative has been added. The unit is disposable and there is no need for syringes, needles, and other equipment necessary for the standard intradermal tests.

Tuberculin, Old, TINE TEST units have been standardized by clinical evaluation in human subjects to give reactions equivalent to or more potent than 5 T.U.* of standard old tuberculin administered intradermally in the Mantoux test. However, all multiple puncture-type devices must be regarded as screening tools and other appropriate diagnostic procedures such as the Mantoux test should be utilized for retesting reactors.

*US (International) tuberculin units.

CLINICAL PHARMACOLOGY

Tuberculin deposited in the skin of tuberculin reactive individuals reacts with sensitized lymphocytes to effect the release of mediators of cellular hypersensitivity. Some of these indicators (eg, skin reactive factor) induce an inflammatory response in the skin causing the edema and erythema characteristic of a "positive" reaction.[1,2]

INDICATIONS AND USAGE

Tuberculin, Old, TINE TEST is indicated to detect tuberculin-sensitive individuals. TINE TEST units are also useful in programs to determine priorities for additional testing (ie, chest X-rays) and in epidemiological surveys to identify those areas having high levels of infection.

In clinical studies covering various geographical areas of the US and all age groups, with a total of 30,588 test subjects, there were 911 (4%) false positive reactors among 26,236 subjects who were Mantoux negative, and 342 (8%) false negative reactors among 4,352 subjects who were Mantoux positive.

The frequency of repeated tuberculin tests depends on the risk of exposure of the child and on the prevalence of tuberculosis in the population group. For the pediatrician's office or outpatient clinic, an annual or biennial tuberculin test, unless local circumstances clearly indicate otherwise, is appropriate. The initial test should be done at the time of, or preceding, the measles immunization.[3] The repeated testing of uninfected individuals does not sensitize to tuberculin. Among individuals with waning sensitivity to homologous or heterologous mycobacterial antigens, however, the stimulus of a tuberculin test may "boost" or increase the size of the reaction to a second test, even causing an apparent development of sensitivity in some cases.[4]

Tuberculin testing should be done with caution in individuals with active tuberculosis (see **PRECAUTIONS**).

CONTRAINDICATIONS

There are no known contraindications for use of Tuberculin, Old, TINE TEST. See **PRECAUTIONS** section for information regarding special care to be exercised for safe and effective use.

WARNINGS

There are no known serious adverse reactions or potential safety hazards associated with the use of Tuberculin, Old, TINE TEST. However, as with the use of any biological product, the possibility of anaphylactic reaction should be considered. See **PRECAUTIONS** section for information regarding special care to be exercised for safe and effective use.

PRECAUTIONS

Tuberculin testing should be done with caution in individuals with active tuberculosis. Although activation of quiescent lesions is rare, if a patient has a history of occurrence of vesiculation and necrosis with a previous tuberculin test by any method, tuberculin testing should be avoided.

Although clinical allergy to acacia is very rare, this product contains some acacia as stabilizer and should be used with caution in patients with known allergy to this component. In this instance remedial measures for anaphylactoid reactions, including epinephrine injection (1:1000), must be available for immediate use.

Reactivity to the test may be suppressed in patients who are receiving corticosteroids or immunosuppressive agents, or those who have recently been vaccinated with live virus vaccines such as measles, mumps, rubella, polio, etc.

With a positive reaction further diagnostic procedures must be considered. These may include X-ray of the chest, microbiologic examinations of sputa and other specimens, and confirmation of the positive TINE TEST reaction (except vesiculation reactions) using the Mantoux method. In general, the TINE TEST does not need to be repeated.

Antituberculous chemotherapy should not be instituted solely on the basis of a single positive TINE TEST.

When vesiculation occurs, the reaction is to be interpreted as strongly positive and a repeat test by the Mantoux method must not be attempted. Similar or more severe vesiculation with or without necrosis is likely to occur.

Pregnancy Category C. Animal reproduction studies have not been conducted with Tuberculin, Old, TINE TEST. It is also not known whether Tuberculin, Old, TINE TEST can cause fetal harm when administered to a pregnant woman or can affect reproduction capacity. Tuberculin, Old, TINE TEST should be given to a pregnant woman only if clearly needed.

During pregnancy, known positive reactors may demonstrate a negative response to a Tuberculin TINE TEST.

Tuberculin, Old, TINE TEST units must never be reused.

ADVERSE REACTIONS

Vesiculation (positive reaction), ulceration, or necrosis may occur at the test site in highly sensitive persons. Pain, pruritus, and discomfort at the test site may be relieved by cold packs or by topical glucocorticoid ointment or cream. Transient bleeding may be observed at a puncture site and is of no significance.

DOSAGE AND ADMINISTRATION

Tuberculin, Old, TINE TEST UNITS have been standardized by clinical evaluation in human subjects to give reactions equivalent to or more potent than 5 T.U.* of standard old

*US (International) tuberculin units.

tuberculin administered intradermally in the Mantoux test. However, all multiple puncture-type devices must be regarded as screening tools and other appropriate diagnostic procedures such as the Mantoux test should be utilized for retesting reactors.

The volar surface of the upper one-third of the forearm, over a muscle belly, is the preferred site. Hairy areas, and areas without adequate subcutaneous tissue, eg, concavities over a tendon or bone should be avoided.

Alcohol, acetone, ether, or soap and water may be used to cleanse the skin. The area must be clean and thoroughly dry before application of the Tuberculin, Old, TINE TEST.

Expose the four coated tines by removing the protective cap while holding the plastic handle. Grasp the patient's forearm firmly, since the sharp momentary sting may cause the patient to jerk his or her arm, resulting in scratching. Stretch the skin of the forearm tightly and apply the disc with the other hand. **Hold at least one second.** Release tension grip on forearm. Withdraw tine unit.

Sufficient pressure should be exerted so that the four puncture sites, and circular depression of the skin from the plastic base are visible.

Local care of the skin is not necessary.

Tuberculin, Old, TINE TEST unit must never be reused.

Reading Reactions. Tests should be read at 48 to 72 hours. Vesiculation or the extent of induration are the determining factors; erythema without induration is of no significance. Readings should be made in good light with the forearm slightly flexed. The size of the induration in millimeters should be determined by inspection, measuring, and palpation with gentle finger stroking. Identification of the application site is usually easy because of the distinct four-point pattern. The diameter of the largest single reaction around one of the puncture sites should be measured. With pronounced reactions, the areas of induration around the puncture sites may coalesce.

Interpretation:

Positive Reactions

A. Vesiculation. If vesiculation is present, the test may be interpreted as positive, in which case the management of the patient is the same as that for one classified as positive to the Mantoux test.[5]

B. Induration, 2mm or greater. The test may be interpreted as positive but further diagnostic procedures must be considered. These may include X-ray of the chest, microbiologic examination of sputa and other specimens, and confirmation of the positive TINE TEST reaction using the Mantoux Method.

Negative Reaction. Induration less than 2 mm. With a negative reaction there is no need for retesting unless the person is a contact of a patient with tuberculosis or there is clinical evidence suggestive of the disease.[5]

Descriptive literature illustrating typical reactions is available upon request.

HOW SUPPLIED

Tuberculin, Old, TINE TEST is supplied as follows:
    NDC 0005-2722-25   25 individual tests
    NDC 0005-2722-28   100 individual tests
    NDC 0005-2722-34   250 individual tests
Military Depot: NSN 6505-00-890-1534—25 tests
STORE AT CONTROLLED ROOM TEMPERATURE 15–30°C (59–86°F). DO NOT REFRIGERATE.

REFERENCES

1. Comstock, CW, et al: The tuberculin skin test, *Am Rev Respir Dis* 1981;124:356–363.
2. Burrows W: *Immunity and Hypersensitivity: Textbook of Microbiology* 1979, 369–424.
3. Report of the Committee on the Control of Infectious Diseases. American Academy of Pediatrics, 1977.
4. Comstock, CW, et al: The tuberculin skin test, *Am Rev Respir Dis* 1971;104:769–775.
5. Committee on Diagnostic Skin Testing of the American Thoracic Society: The Tuberculin Test (rev). New York, American Lung Association, 1974.

LEDERLE LABORATORIES DIVISION
American Cyanamid Company
Pearl River, NY 10965   Rev. 6/87
                             21081

TINE TEST® PPD   ℞
[tine test]
Tuberculin, Purified Protein Derivative

DESCRIPTION

THE Tuberculin, Purified Protein Derivative TINE TEST PPD is a sterile, simple, multiple-puncture, disposable intradermal test device for the detection of tuberculin reactivity. These convenient devices are especially useful in mass tuberculosis screening programs.

Each test unit consists of a stainless steel disc attached to a light blue plastic handle. Projecting from the disc are four triangular-shaped prongs (tines) which are 2 mm long and approximately 4 mm apart. The tines have been mechanically dipped into a concentrated solution of PPD. The PPD concentrate is prepared by the Seibert Process[1,2] and is stabilized with 7% acacia (gum Arabic), 30% dextrose, and 5% glycerol. The glycerol also acts as a humectant preventing the film on the tines from becoming brittle-dry. The final PPD concentrate is standardized against U.S. Standard PPD. The tines are dipped into concentrated PPD, capped and sterilized with ethylene oxide. No preservative has been added. The TINE TEST (PPD) unit is disposable, and there is no need for syringes, needles, and other equipment necessary for the standard intradermal tests.

The Tine Test (PPD) units have been standardized by clinical evaluation in human subjects to give reactions equivalent to or more potent than 5 T.U.* of standard PPD administered intradermally in the Mantoux test. However, all multiple puncture-type devices must be regarded as screening tools and other appropriate diagnostic procedures such as the Mantoux test should be utilized for retesting reactors.

* U.S. (International) tuberculin units.

CLINICAL PHARMACOLOGY

Tuberculin deposited in the skin of tuberculin reactive individuals reacts with sensitized lymphocytes to effect the release of mediators of cellular hypersensitivity. Some of these indicators (eg, skin reactive factor) induce an inflammatory response in the skin causing the edema and erythema characteristic of a "positive" reaction.[3,4]

INDICATIONS AND USAGE

Tuberculin, Purified Protein Derivative TINE TEST PPD is indicated to detect tuberculin-sensitive individuals. TINE TEST units are also useful in programs to determine priorities for additional testing (ie, chest X-rays) and in epidemiological surveys to identify those areas having high levels of infection.

Data obtained from clinical studies with a total of 3,062 volunteer subjects (males and females), ranging in age from 4 to 96 years, of which 47.5% (1,443) were Mantoux positive, clearly demonstrates that TINE TEST PPD, when used as a screening test to determine tuberculin reactivity is associated with very little, if any, adverse reactivity. Other than the skin test reaction itself, slight vesiculation and slight ulceration were the only adverse experiences reported. The slight to mild vesiculation was equally divided between the two tests (TINE TEST, 54/3062, 1.78%, and PPD-T Mantoux, 55/3062, 1.81%). The slight ulceration observed with one subject at 72 hours was associated with the TINE TEST site. Of the subjects classified as positive or intermediate by PPD-T Mantoux, 93.8% were classified similarly with the TINE TEST. The results of the clinical trials revealed a 72-hour false positive rate of 10.9% and a false negative rate of 6.2%. In clinical studies of more than 1,800 PPD-S Mantoux positive subjects only 6.3% gave negative TINE TEST PPD reactions at 72 hours; of more than 1,900 TINE TEST PPD positive tests, less than 11% gave negative Mantoux results.

The frequency of repeated tuberculin tests depends on risk of exposure of the child and on the prevalence of tuberculosis in the population group. For the pediatrician's office or outpatient clinic, an annual or biennial tuberculin test, unless local circumstances clearly indicate otherwise, is appropriate. The initial test should be done at the time of, or preceding, the measles immunization.[5] The repeated testing of uninfected individuals does not sensitize to tuberculin. Among individuals with waning sensitivity to homologous or heterologous mycobacterial antigens, however, the stimulus of a tuberculin test may "boost" or increase the size of the reaction to a second test, even causing an apparent development of sensitivity in some cases.[6]

Tuberculin testing should be done with caution in individuals with active tuberculosis. (See **PRECAUTIONS**.)

CONTRAINDICATIONS

There are no known contraindications for use of Tuberculin, Purified Protein Derivative TINE TEST PPD. See **PRECAUTIONS** section for information regarding special care to be exercised for safe and effective use.

WARNINGS

There are no known serious adverse reactions or potential safety hazards associated with the use of Tuberculin, Purified, Protein Derivative TINE TEST PPD. However, as with the use of any biological product, the possibility of anaphylactic reaction should be considered. See **PRECAUTIONS** section for information regarding special care to be exercised for safe and effective use.

PRECAUTIONS

Tuberculin testing should be done with caution in individuals with active tuberculosis. However, activation of quiescent lesions is rare. If a patient has a history of occurrence of vesiculation and necrosis with a previous tuberculin test by any method, tuberculin testing should be avoided.

Although clinical allergy to acacia is very rare, this product contains some acacia as stabilizer and should be used with caution in patients with known allergy to this component. In these instances remedial measures for anaphylactoid reac-

tions, including epinephrine injection (1:1000), must be available for immediate use.

Reactivity to the test may be suppressed in patients who are receiving corticosteroids or immunosuppressive agents, or those who have recently been vaccinated with live virus vaccines such as measles, mumps, rubella, polio, etc.

With a positive reaction further diagnostic procedures must be considered. These may include X-ray of the chest, microbiologic examinations of sputa and other specimens, and confirmation of the positive TINE TEST reaction (except vesiculation reactions) using the Mantoux method. In general, the TINE TEST does not need to be repeated.

Antituberculous chemotherapy should not be instituted solely on the basis of a single positive TINE TEST.

When vesiculation occurs, the reaction is to be interpreted as strongly positive and a repeat test by the Mantoux method must not be attempted. Similar or more severe vesiculation with or without necrosis is likely to occur.

Pregnancy Category C: Animal reproduction studies have not been conducted with Tuberculin, Purified Protein Derivative TINE TEST PPD. It is also not known whether Tuberculin, Purified Protein Derivative (PPD) TINE TEST can cause fetal harm when administered to a pregnant woman or can affect reproduction capacity. Tuberculin, Purified Protein Derivative TINE TEST PPD should be given to a pregnant woman only if clearly needed.

During pregnancy, known positive reactors may demonstrate a negative response to a Tuberculin TINE TEST PPD. Tuberculin, Purified Protein Derivative TINE TEST PPD units must never be reused.

ADVERSE REACTIONS

Vesiculation (positive reaction), ulceration, or necrosis may occur at the test site in highly sensitive persons. Pain, pruritus, and discomfort at the test site may be relieved by cold packs or by topical glucocorticoid ointment or cream. Transient bleeding may be observed at a puncture site and is of no significance.

DOSAGE AND ADMINISTRATION

Tuberculin, (PPD) TEST Units have been standardized by clinical evaluation in human subjects to give reactions equivalent to or more potent than 5 T.U.* of standard PPD administered intradermally in the Mantoux test. However, all multiple puncture-type devices must be regarded as screening tools and other appropriate diagnostic procedures such as the Mantoux test should be utilized for retesting reactors.

The volar surface of the upper one-third of the forearm, over a muscle belly, is the preferred site. Hairy areas, and areas without adequate subcutaneous tissue, eg, concavities over a tendon or bone should be avoided.

* U.S. (International) tuberculin units.

Alcohol, acetone, ether, or soap and water may be used to cleanse the skin. The area must be clean and thoroughly dry before application of the TINE TEST PPD.

Expose the four coated tines by removing the protective cap while holding the plastic handle. Grasp the patient's forearm firmly, since the sharp momentary sting may cause the patient to jerk his or her arm, resulting in scratching. Stretch the skin of the forearm tightly and apply the disc with the other hand. **Hold at least one second.** Release tension grip on forearm. Withdraw tine unit.

Sufficient pressure should be exerted so that the four puncture sites, and circular depression of the skin from the plastic base are visible.

Local care of the skin is not necessary.

Tuberculin, Purified Protein Derivative TINE TEST PPD Unit **must never be reused.**

Reading Reactions: Tests should be read at 48 to 72 hours. Vesiculation or the extent of induration are the determining factors; erythema without induration is of no significance. Readings should be made in good light with the forearm slightly flexed. The size of the induration in millimeters should be determined by inspection, measuring, and palpation with gentle finger stroking. Identification of the application site is usually easy because of the distinct four-point pattern. The diameter of the largest single reaction around one of the puncture sites should be measured. With pronounced reactions, the areas of induration around the puncture sites may coalesce.

INTERPRETATION

Positive Reactions:

A. Vesiculation. If vesiculation is present, the test may be interpreted as positive, in which case the management of the patient is the same as that for one classified as positive to the Mantoux Test.[7]

B. Induration, 2mm or greater. The test may be interpreted as positive but further diagnostic procedures must be considered. These may include X-ray of the chest, microbiologic examination of sputa and other specimens, and confirmation of the positive TINE TEST reaction using the Mantoux Method.

Negative Reaction:

Induration less than 2mm. With a negative reaction there is no need for retesting unless the person is a contact of a

patient with tuberculosis or there is clinical evidence suggestive of the disease.[7]

Descriptive literature illustrating typical reactions is available upon request.

HOW SUPPLIED

Tuberculin, Purified Protein Derivative TINE TEST PPD is supplied as follows:

NDC 0005-2720-25   25 individual tests
NDC 0005-2720-28   100 individual tests
STORE AT CONTROLLED ROOM TEMPERATURE 15–30°C (59°–86°F). DO NOT REFRIGERATE.

REFERENCES

1. Seibert, FB: Isolation and Properties of Purified Protein Derivative of Tuberculin. *Am Rev Tuberc*, 1934;30:713.
2. Seibert, FB, Glenn, JF: Tuberculin Purified Protein Derivative—Preparation and Analysis of a Large Quantity for Standard. *Am Rev Tuberc* 1941;44:9.
3. Comstock, CW, et al: The Tuberculin Skin Test, *Amer Rev Respiratory Dis* 1981;124:356–363.
4. Burrows, W: Immunity and Hypersensitivity: Textbook of Microbiology 1982, 369–424.
5. Report of the Committee on the Control of Infectious Diseases. American Academy of Pediatrics, 1977.
6. Comstock, GW, et al: The Tuberculin Skin Test, *Amer Rev Respiratory Dis* 1971;104(5):769–775.
7. Committee on Diagnostic Skin Testing of the American Thoracic Society, The Tuberculin Test (Revised 1974). New York, American Lung Association, 1974.

LEDERLE LABORATORIES DIVISION
American Cyanamid Company
Pearl River, NY 10965   Rev. 6/87
                             21079

Eli Lilly and Company
LILLY CORPORATE CENTER
INDIANAPOLIS, IN 46285

TES-TAPE®   OTC
[tĕs'tāp]
(glucose enzymatic test strip)
USP

For In Vitro Diagnostic Use in Testing for the Presence and Semiquantitative Measurement of Glucose in Human Urine

Tes-Tape has been used since 1956, when Dr. A. S. Keston described the novel idea of using 2 enzymes simultaneously to test for glucose and Dr. J. P. Comer published data on the specificity and accuracy of Tes-Tape for the semiquantitative analysis of urine glucose.

During the development and testing of this urine test method, Tes-Tape was found to be an accurate and reliable semiquantitative method for determining urine glucose. To date, relatively few instances of faulty results have occurred with the use of Tes-Tape. Problems associated with the product are usually due to improper techniques, exposure of the tape to adverse conditions, or drugs that have an inhibitory effect on the enzyme reaction. Considerable data may be found in the published scientific documents.

Tes-Tape is impregnated with the enzymes glucose oxidase and peroxidase and an oxidizable substrate, orthotolidine. When the tape is dipped into urine containing glucose, the glucose oxidase catalyzes the reaction of the glucose in the urine with oxygen from the air to form gluconic acid and hydrogen peroxide. The enzyme peroxidase (from horseradish) then catalyzes the reaction of hydrogen peroxide and orthotolidine, forming a blue color. With the addition of a yellow dye (FDC Yellow No. 5) to the paper, the possible color range of the test is extended from yellow to light green to deep blue. If no glucose is present, the tape maintains its yellow color.

Reactive Ingredient	Approximate Amount per 1.5 Inches of Tape
Glucose oxidase	3.78 units
Horseradish peroxidase	2.82 PZ units
O-tolidine	0.136 mg

Nonreactive ingredients include filter paper, FDC Yellow No. 5 coloring, buffers, stabilizers, and wetting agents.

For in vitro diagnostic use. Store below 86°F (30°C). Protect from high humidity and light.

Do not use if the tape becomes dark yellow or yellowish-brown or if a 2% reading is not obtained when the reliability is tested, as described under the heading **IMPORTANT**.

The urine should be collected in a container free of chemicals and glucose.

If the freshly voided specimen is not to be tested within 4 hours, it should be refrigerated.

Drugs that are known to have an inhibitory effect on the enzyme reactions include ascorbic acid (vitamin C), dipyrone,

Continued on next page

Lilly—Cont.

gentisic acid (a metabolite of aspirin), homogentisic acid (present in alkaptonuria), levodopa, meralluride injection, and methyldopa. The inhibiting effect is notable on the dipped part of the tape, but accurate readings may be obtained by observing the narrow band of color at the junction of the dry and wet portions. A separation of glucose from the inhibitory substances occurs as the urine travels along the dry portion of the tape. Ingestion of more than 1.5 g of ascorbic acid may produce urine with inhibitory action on Tes-Tape due to acidity.

Specimens for storage or shipment should be refrigerated or preserved with up to 0.37% formaldehyde.

All materials are provided for the test; these include dispenser, tape, and color chart.

Results on the color chart are expressed in percent of glucose (urine sugar) and by a corresponding arbitrary system of 0, +, + +, + + +, + + + +, representing 0, $\frac{1}{10}$, $\frac{1}{4}$, $\frac{1}{2}$, 2 (or more) % of glucose respectively.

When testing, do not place the tape on the lavatory or on paper or allow moistened portion to contact fingers. Contamination of the tape by glucose from other sources (eg, perspiration, tears, and saliva) or with a residue of chlorine from lavatory cleansing agents can cause false-positive results. Patients who are receiving high doses of ascorbic acid or whose urine contains dipyrone, meralluride, homogentisic acid, gentisic acid, levodopa, or methyldopa should read only the very narrow band of color in the moist portion of the tape above the level to which it was dipped into the specimen. Very high doses of ascorbic acid may cause a false-negative test despite taking the above precaution. (Urinary levels of ascorbic acid in excess of 0.1% are necessary to block the test completely. This concentration is most likely to appear within 3 to 7 hours after a single dose of 1.5 g or more.) Penicillin, cephalosporin, and aminoglycoside antibiotics have not been shown to adversely influence Tes-Tape accuracy in measuring urine glucose levels.

Normal urine should test 0% with Tes-Tape. Persons using Tes-Tape for a screening test should report all values above 0% to their physician. Diabetic urine values in the range of the color chart should also be recorded and reported to the patient's physician. Measured values of 2% should be reported as 2% or more.

The overall semiquantitative accuracy of Tes-Tape originally reported in 1956 on 1,000 determinations was 96%. This was confirmed in 1973 on 14,000 determinations over a 2-year period. These data were obtained by taking urine samples containing concentrations of glucose at each measurable increment on the color chart. The color chart provided is based on the average color perception of many observers. Patients who have difficulty in differentiating color should seek the advice of their physician before using Tes-Tape. Numerous other clinical and laboratory studies have shown that Tes-Tape is accurate in qualitative and semiquantitative determinations of urine sugar. Tes-Tape is specific for glucose in urine sugar testing. Contamination of the tape or urine receptacle with glucose from other sources (eg, perspiration, tears, and saliva) or with a residue of chlorine from cleansing agents, have produced false-positive results for glucose. False high values can also be obtained if Tes-Tape is exposed to peroxide-containing detergents. When Tes-Tape is exposed to these detergents (ie, inadequately rinsed urine specimen containers cleansed with these detergents), the peroxides in the detergent can oxidize the dye in the enzyme strip, producing a false-positive reaction. Except for the instances mentioned above, there are no known clinical situations in which a false-positive test for glucose occurs with Tes-Tape. The sensitivity of Tes-Tape is such that it will react with concentrations of 0.05% glucose or more. Trace reactions, shown by the development of a very light yellow-green color, may be observed with less than this amount of glucose.

After opening plastic wrapper, use tape within 4 months. It must be used prior to expiration date.

IMPORTANT

The reliability of a roll of Tes-Tape may easily be checked by dipping a piece into a properly prepared glucose solution.* The tape should be removed immediately, as one would when testing a urine specimen. After 2 minutes have elapsed, the reading obtained when the tape is compared with the color chart should be approximately + + + + (2%). If such a reading is not obtained, the tape has apparently deteriorated and should not be used.

Measurements for the amount of glucose present (semiquantitative) should not be made after 2 minutes because the colors gradually change as the tape dries. Screening tests for

---

*If a properly prepared glucose solution is not available, any nationally known *sugar (glucose)-containing* beverage from a freshly opened bottle or can is satisfactory. (Diet cola beverages would not be satisfactory.)

---

the presence of glucose (qualitative) in urine may be made for several hours after the tape has dried.

The patient should consult the package insert in regard to Procedure, What to Do If Tape Breaks, and a record chart for urine sugar tests with Tes-Tape.

HOW SUPPLIED

M-73, Tes-Tape® (Glucose Enzymatic Test Strip, USP), dispenser package, approximately 100 tests, in single packages. (NDC 0002-2344-41) [020288]

Merieux Institute, Inc.
P. O. BOX 523980
MIAMI, FL 33152-3980

MULTITEST CMI® ℞
[mul 'ti-test]
(Skin Test Antigens for Cellular Hypersensitivity)

NDC 50361-780-80

DESCRIPTION
Skin Test Antigens for Cellular Hypersensitivity, MULTITEST CMI® is a disposable, plastic applicator consisting of eight sterile test heads preloaded with the following seven delayed hypersensitivity skin test antigens and glycerin negative control for precutaneous administration: Tetanus Toxoid Antigen, Diphtheria Toxoid Antigen, Streptococcus Antigen, Old Tuberculin, Candida Antigen, Trichophyton Antigen, and Proteus Antigen.

MULTITEST CMI® provides a quick, convenient and uniform procedure for delayed cutaneous hypersensitivity testing.

Supplied in box of 10 individual cartons containing one preloaded MULTITEST CMI® per carton.

TUBERCULIN, MONO-VACC® ℞
TEST (O.T.)
[tu-ber'ku-lin mon'ō-vak]
(old tuberculin)
Multiple Puncture Device

NDC 50361-770-40   25 tests per box
Supplied in plastic tamper proof box of 25 tests per box; test reading cards in English, Spanish, Vietnamese and Chinese are also available.

Parke-Davis
DIVISION OF WARNER-LAMBERT COMPANY
201 TABOR ROAD
MORRIS PLAINS, NEW JERSEY 07950

APLISOL® ℞
[ă'plĭ-sŏl "]
(Tuberculin Purified Protein Derivative, Diluted
[Stabilized Solution])

DESCRIPTION
Aplisol (tuberculin PPD, diluted) is a sterile aqueous solution of a purified protein fraction for intradermal administration as an aid in the diagnosis of tuberculosis. The solution is stabilized with polysorbate (Tween) 80, buffered with potassium and sodium phosphates and contains approximately 0.35% phenol as a preservative.

The product is clinically equivalent in potency to the standard PPD-S* (5 TU** per 0.1 ml) of the U.S. Public Health Service, National Center for Disease Control, and is ready for immediate use without further dilution. This product meets all applicable standards.

CLINICAL PHARMACOLOGY
The purified protein fraction is isolated from culture filtrates of human type strains of *Mycobacterium tuberculosis* by the method of F.B. Seibert.[1,2] This product is made from a single master lot (No. 924994) to eliminate lot to lot variation inherent in manufacturing.

The 5 TU dose of Tuberculin PPD intradermally (Mantoux) is recommended as the standard tuberculin test, and Tuberculin PPD is recommended by the American Lung Association as an aid in the detection of infection with *Mycobacterium tuberculosis*.

Reactions to the Mantoux test are interpreted on the basis of a quantitative measurement of the response to a specific dose (5 TU PPD-S or equivalent) of Tuberculin PPD. Other dosages are regarded as having no demonstrable usefulness in ordinary practice.[3] Accordingly, Aplisol is available in only one potency (5 TU equivalent) and the use of this potency only is recommended. The selection of 5 TU as the test dose is based upon data indicating that (1) the 5 TU dose gives measurable reactions in over 95 percent of the known tuberculous infected; (2) doses larger than 5 TU might elicit reac-

---

tions not caused by tuberculosis infection; and (3) nonreactors to doses considerably less than 5 TU are not accepted as negative but are retested with a stronger dose.[3]

INDICATIONS AND USAGE
Tuberculin PPD is recommended by the American Lung Association as an aid in the detection of infection with *Mycobacterium tuberculosis*. The standard tuberculin test recommended employs the intradermal (Mantoux) test using a 5 TU dose of tuberculin PPD.[3] The 0.1 ml test dose of Aplisol (tuberculin PPD, diluted) is equivalent to the 5 TU dose recommended as clinically established and standardized with PPD-S.

CONTRAINDICATIONS
None known.

WARNINGS
Tuberculin should not be administered to known tuberculin-positive reactors because of the severity of reactions (e.g., vesiculation, ulceration or necrosis) that may occur at the test site in very highly sensitive individuals.

Avoid injecting tuberculin subcutaneously. If this occurs, no local reaction develops, but a general febrile reaction and/or acute inflammation around old tuberculous lesions may occur in highly sensitive individuals.

PRECAUTIONS
General
A separate heat sterilized syringe and needle, or a sterile disposable unit, should be used for each individual patient to prevent possible transmission of homologous serum hepatitis virus and other infectious agents from one person to another.

Syringes that have previously been used with histoplasmin, blastomycin and other antigens should not be used for tuberculin.

As with any biological product, epinephrine should be immediately available in case an anaphylactoid or acute hypersensitivity reaction occurs.

Pregnancy
Teratogenic effects: Pregnancy Category C. Animal reproduction studies have not been conducted with Aplisol. It is also not known whether Aplisol can cause fetal harm when administered to a pregnant woman or can affect the reproduction capacity. Aplisol should be given to a pregnant woman only if clearly needed.

However, the risk of unrecognized tuberculosis and the close postpartum contact between a mother with active disease and an infant leaves the infant in grave danger of tuberculosis and complications such as tuberculous meningitis. Although there have been not been reported any adverse effects upon the fetus recognized as being due to tuberculosis skin testing, the prescribing physician will want to consider if the potential benefits outweigh the possible risks for performing the tuberculin test on a pregnant woman or woman of childbearing age, particularly in certain high risk populations.

ADVERSE REACTIONS
In highly sensitive individuals, strongly positive reactions including vesiculation, ulceration or necrosis may occur at the test site. Cold packs or topical steroid preparations may be employed for symptomatic relief of the associated pain, pruritus, and discomfort.

Strongly positive test reactions may result in scarring at the test site.

Immediate erythematous or other reactions may occur at the injection site. The reason(s) for these infrequent occurrences are presently unknown.

DOSAGE AND ADMINISTRATION
Standard Method (Mantoux Test)
The Mantoux test is performed by intradermally injecting with a syringe and needle exactly 0.1 ml of tuberculin PPD, diluted. The result is read 48 to 72 hours later and induration only is considered in interpreting the test. The standard test is performed as follows:

1. The site of the test is usually the flexor or dorsal surface of the forearm about 4″ below the elbow. Other skin sites may be used, but the flexor surface of the forearm is preferred.
2. The skin at the injection site is cleansed with 70% alcohol and allowed to dry.
3. The test material is administered with a tuberculin syringe (0.5 or 1.0 ml) fitted with a short (½″) 26 or 27 gauge needle.
4. The syringe and needle should be of a sterile disposable, single use type or should have been sterilized by autoclaving, boiling or by the use of dry heat. A separate sterile unit should be used for each person tested.
5. The diaphragm of the vial-stopper should be wiped with 70% alcohol.
6. The needle is inserted through the stopper diaphragm of the inverted vial. Exactly 0.1 ml is filled into the syringe, with care being taken to exclude air bubbles and to maintain the lumen of the needle filled.

7. The point of the needle is inserted into the most superficial layers of the skin with the needle bevel pointing upward. As the tuberculin solution is injected, a pale bleb 6 to 10 mm in size ($\frac{3}{8}''$) will rise over the point of the needle. This is quickly absorbed and no dressing is required.

In the event the injection is delivered subcutaneously (ie, no bleb will form), or if a significant part of the dose leaks from the injection site, the test should be repeated immediately at another site at least 5 cm (2″) removed.

Aplisol vials should be inspected visually for particulate matter and discoloration prior to administration.

The Mantoux test is the standard of comparison for all other tuberculin tests.

Aplisol is a stabilized solution of Tuberculin PPD. Data indicate that Aplisol is stable when prefilled into syringes and stored in a refrigerator for up to 30 days.

However, the practice of storing such prefilled syringes is not recommended as good practice because of the increased potential for contamination.

Interpretation of Tuberculin Reaction

Readings of Mantoux reactions should be made during the period from 48 to 72 hours after the injection. Induration only should be considered in interpreting the test. The diameter of induration should be measured transversely to the long axis of the forearm and recorded in millimeters. Erythema of less than 10 mm should be disregarded. If the area of erythema is greater than 10 mm and induration is absent the injection may have been made too deeply and retesting is indicated.

Reactions should be interpreted as follows:

Positive—Induration measuring 10 mm or more. This indicates hypersensitivity to tuberculoprotein and should be interpreted as positive for past or present infection with *M. tuberculosis*.

Doubtful—Induration measuring 5 to 9 mm. Retesting is indicated using a different site of injection. Evaluation to rule out cross-reaction from other mycobacterial infection should be considered.

Negative—Induration of less than 5 mm. This indicates a lack of hypersensitivity to tuberculoprotein and tuberculous infection is highly unlikely.

It should be noted that reactivity to tuberculin may be depressed or suppressed for as long as four weeks by viral infections, live virus vaccines (i.e., measles, smallpox, polio, rubella and mumps), or by the administration of corticosteroids. Malnutrition may also have a similar effect. When of diagnostic importance, a negative test should be accepted as proof that hypersensitivity is absent only after normal reactivity to nonspecific irritants has been demonstrated. A primary injection of tuberculin may possibly have a boosting effect on subsequent tuberculin reactions.

A child who is known to have been exposed to a tuberculous adult must not be adjudged free of infection until he has a negative tuberculin reaction at least ten weeks after contact with the tuberculous person has ceased.[4]

A positive tuberculin reaction does not necessarily signify the presence of active disease. Further diagnostic procedures should be carried out before a diagnosis of tuberculosis is made. A small percentage of responders may not have been infected with *M. tuberculosis* but by some other mycobacterium.

HOW SUPPLIED

N 0071-4525-03 (Bio. 1525)
1 ml (10 tests)—rubber-diaphragm-capped vial
N 0071-4525-08 (Bio. 1607)
5 ml (50 tests)—rubber-diaphragm-capped vial
This product should be stored at 2° to 8°C (36° to 46°F), and protected from light.

REFERENCES

1. Seibert, F.B.: Am. Rev. Tuberc. 30:713, 1934.
2. Seibert, F.B., and Glenn, J.T.: Am. Rev. Tuberc. 44:9, 1941.
3. Diagnostic Standards and Classification of Tuberculosis and Other Mycobacterial Diseases, American Lung Association, New York, 1974.
4. Sewell, E.M., O'Hare, D., and Kendig, E.L., Jr.: The Tuberculin Test, Pediatrics, Vol. 54, No. 5, Nov. 1974.

* PPD-S (No. 49608) World Health Organization International PPD-Tuberculin Standard (PPD-S is a dried powder from which WHO and U.S. Standard tuberculin solutions are made.)
** U.S. Tuberculin Unit

4525G033

APLITEST®
[ă'plĭ-tĕst″]
Tuberculin Purified Protein Derivative
Multiple-Puncture Device

℞

DESCRIPTION

Aplitest (tuberculin PPD) is a sterile, single-use, multiple-puncture type device for percutaneous administration for use in determining the tuberculin sensitivity status of individuals. Aplitest, a diagnostic aid, has been clinically compared with 5 US Tuberculin Units of PPD-S administered intradermally.

These disposable devices are useful in mass tuberculosis screening programs. The product packaging facilitates the use of Aplitest units for testing of individual patients in office, ward, or clinic settings.

Each Aplitest unit consists of a cylindrical plastic holder bearing four equally spaced stainless steel tines at one end. The tines have been coated by dipping in a solution of tuberculin PPD and dried. The tuberculin solution applied to the tines is buffered with potassium and sodium phosphates and contains approximately 0.5% phenol as a preservative. The narrow (tine-bearing) end of each unit fits into a protective cap to protect the tines and maintain their sterility.

The purified tuberculin protein fraction is isolated from culture filtrates of human-type strains of *Mycobacterium tuberculosis* by the method of F.B. Seibert.[1,2] Purified tuberculin protein solution is prepared from a single master lot (No. 975302) to eliminate lot to lot variation.

CLINICAL PHARMACOLOGY

Tuberculin deposited in the skin of tuberculin-reactive individuals reacts with sensitized lymphocytes to effect the release of mediators of cellular hypersensitivity. Some of these mediators, eg, skin reactive factor, induce an inflammatory response to the skin, causing the induration characteristic of a "positive" or "significant" reaction.

Aplitest has been standardized by clinical studies in human subjects against 5 TU* of PPD-S administered intradermally by the Mantoux test, and guidelines relating response to the two treatments have been formulated. (See "Interpretation of Response" section.)

INDICATIONS AND USAGE

Aplitest is indicated to detect tuberculin-sensitive individuals. Aplitest units are also useful in programs to establish priorities for additional testing (ie, chest x-rays) and in epidemiological surveys to identify areas with high levels of infection.

All multiple-puncture type devices should be regarded as screening tools, and appropriate diagnostic procedures (eg, Mantoux test with tuberculin PPD diluted, Aplisol®) should be employed for retesting "doubtful" reactors.

Regular periodic (annual or biennial)[3] testing of tuberculin-negative persons is recommended and is especially valuable because the conversion of an individual from negative to positive is highly indicative of recent tuberculosis infection. Repeated testing of the uninfected individual does not sensitize to tuberculin. In persons with waning sensitivity to homologous or heterologous mycobacterial antigens, however, the stimulus of a tuberculin test may "boost" or increase the size of reaction to a second test, even causing an apparent development of sensitivity in some instances.

CONTRAINDICATIONS

None known.

WARNINGS

Tuberculin should not be administered to known tuberculin-positive reactors because of the severity of reactions (eg, vesiculation, ulceration or necrosis) that may occur at the test site in very highly sensitive individuals.

As with any biological product, epinephrine should be immediately available in case an anaphylactoid or acute hypersensitivity reaction occurs.

PRECAUTIONS

General: A separate, sterile unit must be used for each individual patient and disposed of after use.

Sensitivity may decrease or disappear temporarily during or immediately following severe febrile illness, measles, and other exanthemas, live virus vaccination, sarcoidosis, overwhelming miliary or pulmonary tuberculosis, and the administration of corticosteroids or immunosuppressive drugs. Severe malnutrition may also have a similar effect.

A positive tuberculin reaction does not necessarily signify the presence of active disease. Further diagnostic procedures should be carried out before a diagnosis of tuberculosis is made.

Simultaneous application of two or more multiple-puncture devices is not recommended. The response of an individual to a single multiple-puncture device may be altered by the simultaneous administration of additional tuberculin tests (multiple-puncture or Mantoux).[4]

Pregnancy: Teratogenic effects: Pregnancy Category C. Animal reproduction studies have not been conducted with Aplitest. It is also not known whether Aplitest can cause fetal harm when administered to a pregnant woman or can affect reproduction capacity. Aplitest should be given to a pregnant woman only if clearly needed.

However, the risk of unrecognized tuberculosis and the close postpartum contact between a mother with active disease and an infant leaves the infant in grave danger of tuberculosis and complications such as tuberculous meningitis. Although there have not been reported any adverse effects upon the fetus recognized as being due to tuberculosis skin testing, the prescribing physician will want to consider if the potential benefits outweigh the possible risks for performing the tuberculin test on a pregnant woman or a woman of childbearing age, particularly in certain high risk populations.

ADVERSE REACTIONS

In highly sensitive individuals, strongly positive reactions, including vesiculation, ulceration or necrosis, may occur at the test site. Cold packs or topical steroid preparations may be employed for symptomatic relief of the associated pain, pruritus and discomfort.

Strongly positive test reactions may result in scarring at the test site.

Minimal bleeding may be experienced at a puncture site. This occurs infrequently and does not affect the interpretation of the test.

DOSAGE AND ADMINISTRATION

Each Aplitest unit provides for the intradermal administration of one test-dose of tuberculin PPD.

Method of Application

1. The preferred site of the test is the flexor surface of the forearm about 4 inches below the elbow. Other suitable skin sites, such as the dorsal surface of the forearm, may be used. Areas without adequate subcutaneous tissue, such as over a tendon, should be avoided.
2. The skin at the test site should be cleaned with 70% alcohol, or other suitable agent, and allowed to dry thoroughly.
3. To expose the four impregnated tines, grasp the device and twist to break the perforated label seal.
4. Grasp the patient's forearm firmly to stretch the skin taut at the test site and to prevent any jerking motion of the arm that could cause scratching with the tines.
5. Apply the Aplitest unit firmly and without twisting to the test area for approximately one second. Sufficient pressure should be exerted to assure that all four tines have penetrated the skin of the test area.
6. Dispose of used units in a manner to avoid accidents. Do not reuse.

Interpretation of Response

Selection of the appropriate criteria for interpretation of response to the tuberculin PPD Aplitest should be made in accordance with the objectives of the specific testing program and with consideration of the history and clinical status of the individuals.

Reading of reactions should be made during the period from 48 to 72 hours after application of Aplitest and should be conducted under good lighting conditions. Induration only should be considered in interpreting the test. Erythema should be disregarded. The diameter of the induration of the greatest response at any of the four puncture points should be determined by visual inspection and palpation. If there is coalescence of reaction, the largest diameter of coalescent induration should be measured and recorded.

The American Thoracic Society recommends that all multiple-puncture tuberculin skin test devices be interpreted as follows: If vesiculation is present, the test may be interpreted as positive. If vesiculation is not present, induration of 2 mm or more is considered as a doubtful reaction and a Mantoux test for diagnostic evaluation should be given. Decisions concerning management should be based on the reaction to the Mantoux test and relevant diagnostic criteria. Induration of less than 2 mm and/or erythema of any size is a negative test and there is no need for retesting.[5]

In clinical studies with Aplitest, it has been determined that coalescence of the induration around two or more puncture sites corresponds more than 90% of the time to 10 mm or more of induration in the same individual tested by Mantoux test at the 5 TU level with PPD-S.†

Thus, the following criteria of interpretation have been established.

1. Vesiculation—Positive Reaction
The test should be interpreted as positive and the management of the subject is the same as that for one classified as positive by Mantoux test.

2. Coalescence of induration from two or more puncture points—Doubtful Reaction
A subject with a coalescent reaction may be considered for Mantoux retest. However, more than 90% of the time this reaction was equivalent to a reaction of 10 mm or more of induration with PPD-S (5 TU) administered by Mantoux test.[6] Other criteria, such as contact with tuberculosis patients and case history, should be considered to determine the likelihood that such a reaction is considered positive.

3. 2 mm or more of induration without coalescence—Doubtful Reaction

Continued on next page

This product information was prepared in August, 1989. On these and other Parke-Davis Products, information may be obtained by addressing PARKE-DAVIS, Division of Warner-Lambert Company, Morris Plains, New Jersey 07950.

Parke-Davis—Cont.

Reactions of this size range reflect sensitivity that can result from infection with either atypical mycobacteria or *M tuberculosis;* hence, they are classified as doubtful.

A standard Mantoux test should be done on all subjects in this group. Management should be based on the reaction to the Mantoux test, as well as other clinical considerations.

4. Less than 2 mm of induration—Negative Reaction

There is no need for retesting unless the individual is in contact with a case of tuberculosis or there is clinical evidence suggestive of the disease.

HOW SUPPLIED

N 0071-4589-13 (Bio. 1590) 25-test package. Twenty-five individually capped Aplitest units in a dispensing package. Aplitest (tuberculin PPD, multiple-puncture device) units should be stored at no warmer than 30°C (86°F).

REFERENCES

1. Seibert, F.B.: Am. Rev. Tuberc. 30:713, 1934.
2. Seibert, F.B., and Glenn J.T.: Am. Rev. Tuberc. 44:9, 1941.
3. Report of the Committee on Infectious Diseases, American Academy of Pediatrics, 1982.
4. Rosenthal, S.R., and Libby, J.E.P.: Bull. Wld. Hlth. Org. 23:689, 1960.
5. Diagnostic Standards and Classification of Tuberculosis and Other Mycobacterial Diseases, American Lung Association, 1974.
6. Unpublished data from Warner-Lambert Co. available upon request.

---

* U.S. (International) tuberculin units.
† Purified Protein Derivative (Seibert). Lot No. 49608, the standard adopted by the World Health Organization in 1952 as International PPD Tuberculin and used to prepare the official U.S. Public Health Service 5 TU solution of tuberculin for skin testing known as PPD-S.

                                             4589G022

Savage Laboratories
a division of Altana Inc.
60 BAYLIS ROAD
MELVILLE, NY 11747

ETHIODOL®   ℞
[ĕ-thī'ō'dŏl]
(brand of ethiodized oil injection)

DESCRIPTION

Ethiodol, brand of ethiodized oil, is a sterile injectable radioopaque diagnostic agent for use in hysterosalpingography and lymphography. It contains 37% iodine (475 mg/ml) organically combined with ethyl esters of fatty acids (primarily as ethyl monoiodostearate and ethyl diiodostearate) of poppyseed oil. Stabilized with poppyseed oil, 1%. The precise structure of Ethiodol is unknown at this time. Ethiodol is a straw to amber colored, oil fluid, which because of simplified molecular structure, possesses a greatly reduced viscosity (1.280 specific gravity at 15°C yields viscosity of 0.5 to 1.0 poise). This high fluidity provides a new flexibility for radiographic exploration.

HOW SUPPLIED

Ethiodol® (brand of ethiodized oil for injection) is supplied in a box of two 10 ml ampules, NDC 0281-7062-37.

Products are
listed alphabetically
in the
PINK SECTION.

Sclavo Inc.
5 MANSARD COURT
WAYNE, NJ 07470

SclavoTest®–PPD   ℞
Tuberculin Purified Protein Derivative (PPD)
Multiple Puncture Device

COMPOSITION/DESCRIPTION

SclavoTest-PPD is a sterile multiple-puncture device containing a tuberculin PPD used for the identification of individuals who have a delayed hypersensitivity to tuberculin. SclavoTest-PPD is an easy-to-use, self-contained, unit-dose disposable system which minimizes waste and can be stored at room temperature. No needles, syringes, or vials are needed.

The SclavoTest-PPD device is composed of a plastic handle with four sharp stainless steel points to which has been affixed and dried a tuberculin PPD solution. The retracted points are projected, after the device is placed upon the skin, by gentle pressure applied through a spring inside the handle. SclavoTest-PPD is stored at room temperature until the moment of use in a hermetically sealed unit-dose blister pack, which is designed to impede the passage of moisture and maintain sterility.

ADVERSE REACTIONS

Vesication, occasionally necrosis, ulceration.

HOW SUPPLIED

20 or 250 units individually blister-sealed in strips of 1.

Winthrop Pharmaceuticals
90 PARK AVENUE
NEW YORK, NY 10016

OMNIPAQUE® 140 180 240 300 350   ℞
INJECTION (IOHEXOL)
Section I—Intrathecal
Section II—Intravascular

DESCRIPTION

Iohexol, *N,N'*-Bis(2,3-dihydroxypropyl)-5-[*N*-(2,3-dihydroxypropyl)-acetamido]-2,4,6-triiodoisophthalamide, is a nonionic, water-soluble radiographic contrast medium with a molecular weight of 821.14 (iodine content 46.36%). In aqueous solution each triiodinated molecule remains undissociated.

OMNIPAQUE is provided as a sterile, pyrogen-free, colorless to pale yellow solution, in the following iodine concentrations: 140, 180, 240, 300, and 350 mgI/mL. OMNIPAQUE 140 contains 302 mg of iohexol equivalent to 140 mg of organic iodine per mL; OMNIPAQUE 180 contains 388 mg of iohexol equivalent to 180 mg of organic iodine per mL; OMNIPAQUE 240 contains 518 mg of iohexol equivalent to 240 mg of organic iodine per mL; OMNIPAQUE 300 contains 647 mg of iohexol equivalent to 300 mg of organic iodine per mL; and OMNIPAQUE 350 contains 755 mg of iohexol equivalent to 350 mg of organic iodine per mL. Each milliliter of iohexol solution contains 1.21 mg tromethamine and 0.1 mg edetate calcium disodium with the pH adjusted between 6.8 and 7.7 with hydrochloric acid or sodium hydroxide. All solutions are sterilized by autoclaving and contain no preservatives. Unused portions must be discarded. Iohexol solution is sensitive to light and therefore should be protected from exposure.

The five available concentrations have the following physical properties:
[See table below].

OMNIPAQUE 140, OMNIPAQUE 180, OMNIPAQUE 240, OMNIPAQUE 300, and OMNIPAQUE 350 have osmolalities from approximately 1.1 to 3.0 times that of plasma (285 mOsm/kg water) or cerebrospinal fluid (301 mOsm/kg water) as shown in the above table and are hypertonic under conditions of use.

CLINICAL PHARMACOLOGY—Intrathecal

Iohexol is absorbed from cerebrospinal fluid (CSF) into the bloodstream and is eliminated by renal excretion. No significant metabolism, deiodination, or biotransformation occurs. In five adult patients receiving 16 to 18 milliliters of iohexol (180 mgI/mL) by lumbar intrathecal injection, approximately 88 (73.1–98.2) percent of the injected dose was excreted in the urine within the first 24 hours after administration. The renal and body clearances were 99 (47–137) milliliters per minute and 109 (52–138) milliliters per minute. The mean maximal plasma concentration was 119 (72–177) micrograms of iohexol per milliliter and occurred after 3.8 (2–6) hours. The volume of distribution was 557 (350–849) milliliters per kilogram. In one patient with a large spinal cord tumor, excretion was delayed (67 percent of the dose appeared in the urine within the first 24 hours) with no difference in the total overall recovery in the urine after 48 hours. The delay in excretion appeared to be related to a decrease in the rate of transfer of iohexol from the cerebrospinal fluid to the blood (plasma maximal concentration was approximately 30 micrograms/mL).

The initial concentration and volume of the medium, in conjunction with appropriate patient manipulation and the volume of CSF into which the medium is placed, will determine the extent of the diagnostic contrast that can be achieved.

Following intrathecal injection in conventional radiography, OMNIPAQUE 180, OMNIPAQUE 240, and OMNIPAQUE 300 will continue to provide good diagnostic contrast for at least 30 minutes. Slow diffusion of iohexol takes place throughout the CSF with subsequent absorption into the bloodstream. Once in the systemic circulation, iohexol displays little tendency to bind to serum or plasma proteins. At approximately 1 hour following injection, contrast of diagnostic quality will no longer be available for conventional myelography. If computerized tomographic (CT) myelography is to follow, consideration should be given to a delay of several hours to allow the degree of contrast to decrease.

After administration into the lumbar subarachnoid space, computerized tomography shows the presence of contrast medium in the thoracic region in about 1 hour, in the cervical region in about 2 hours, and in the basal cisterns in 3 to 4 hours.

In patients with renal impairment, depending on the degree of impairment, prolonged plasma iohexol levels may be anticipated due to decreased renal elimination.

INDICATIONS AND USAGE—Intrathecal

OMNIPAQUE 180, OMNIPAQUE 240, and OMNIPAQUE 300 are indicated for intrathecal administration in adults including myelography (lumbar, thoracic, cervical, total columnar) and in contrast enhancement for computerized tomography (myelography, cisternography, ventriculography).

CONTRAINDICATIONS—Intrathecal

OMNIPAQUE should not be administered to patients with a known hypersensitivity to iohexol.

Myelography should not be performed in the presence of significant local or systemic infection where bacteremia is likely.

Intrathecal administration of corticosteroids with OMNIPAQUE (iohexol) is contraindicated.

Because of the possibility of overdosage, immediate repeat myelography in the event of technical failure is contraindicated (see DOSAGE AND ADMINISTRATION).

WARNINGS—General

If grossly bloody CSF is encountered, the possible benefits of a myelographic procedure should be considered in terms of the risk to the patient.

Caution is advised in patients with a history of epilepsy, severe cardiovascular disease, chronic alcoholism, or multiple sclerosis.

Elderly patients may present a greater risk following myelography. The need for the procedure in these patients should be evaluated carefully. Special attention must be paid to dose and concentration of the medium, hydration, and technique used.

Patients who are receiving anticonvulsants should be maintained on this therapy. Should a seizure occur, intravenous diazepam or phenobarbital sodium is recommended. In patients with a history of seizure activity who are not on anticonvulsant therapy, premedication with barbiturates should be considered.

Prophylactic anticonvulsant treatment with barbiturates should be considered in patients with evidence of inadvertent intracranial entry of a large or concentrated bolus of the contrast medium since there may be an increased risk of seizure in such cases.

Drugs which lower the seizure threshold, especially phenothiazine derivatives, including those used for their antihistamine properties, are not recommended for use with OMNIPAQUE. Others include MAO inhibitors, tricyclic antidepressants, CNS stimulants, and psychoactive drugs

---

Concentration (mgI/mL)	Osmolality* (mOsm/kg water)	Osmolarity (mOsm/L)	Absolute Viscosity (cp) 20°C	Absolute Viscosity (cp) 37°C	Specific Gravity 37°C
140	322	273	2.3	1.5	1.164
180	408	331	3.1	2.0	1.209
240	520	391	5.8	3.4	1.280
300	672	465	11.8	6.3	1.349
350	844	541	20.4	10.4	1.406

*By vapor-pressure osmometry.

described as analeptics, major tranquilizers, or antipsychotic drugs. While the contributory role of these medications has not been established, the use of such drugs should be based on physician evaluation of potential benefits and potential risks. Physicians have discontinued these agents at least 48 hours before and for at least 24 hours postprocedure. Care is required in patient management to prevent inadvertent intracranial entry of a large dose or concentrated bolus of the medium. Also, effort should be directed to avoid rapid dispersion of the medium causing inadvertent rise to intracranial levels (eg, by active patient movement). Direct intracisternal or ventricular administration for standard radiography (not CT) is not recommended.

In most reported cases of major motor seizures with nonionic myelographic media, one or more of the following factors were present. Therefore avoid:

- Deviations from recommended procedure or in myelographic management.
- Use in patients with a history of epilepsy.
- Overdosage.
- Intracranial entry of a bolus or premature diffusion of a high concentration of the medium.
- Medication with neuroleptic drugs or phenothiazine antinauseants.
- Failure to maintain elevation of the head during the procedure, on the stretcher, or in bed.
- Excessive and particularly active patient movement or straining.

PRECAUTIONS—General

Diagnostic procedures which involve the use of radiopaque diagnostic agents should be carried out under the direction of personnel with the prerequisite training and with a thorough knowledge of the particular procedure to be performed. Appropriate facilities should be available for coping with any complication of the procedure, as well as for emergency treatment of severe reactions to the contrast agent itself. After parenteral administration of a radiopaque agent, competent personnel and emergency facilities should be available for at least 30 to 60 minutes since severe delayed reactions have occurred. (See ADVERSE REACTIONS.)

Preparatory dehydration is dangerous and may contribute to acute renal failure in patients with advanced vascular disease, diabetic patients, and in susceptible nondiabetic patients (often elderly with preexisting renal disease). Dehydration in these patients seems to be enhanced by the osmotic diuretic action of contrast agents. *Patients should be well hydrated prior to and following administration of any contrast medium, including iohexol.*

The possibility of a reaction, including serious, life-threatening, fatal, anaphylactoid or cardiovascular reactions, should always be considered (see ADVERSE REACTIONS). Therefore, it is of utmost importance that a course of action be carefully planned in advance for the immediate treatment of serious reactions, and that adequate and appropriate facilities and personnel be readily available in case of any reaction.

The possibility of an idiosyncratic reaction in susceptible patients should always be considered (see ADVERSE REACTIONS). The susceptible population includes, but is not limited to, patients with a history of a previous reaction to contrast media, patients with a known sensitivity to iodine per se, and patients with a known clinical hypersensitivity: bronchial asthma, hay fever, and food allergies.

The occurrence of severe idiosyncratic reactions has prompted the use of several pretesting methods. However, pretesting cannot be relied upon to predict severe reactions and may itself be hazardous for the patient. It is suggested that a thorough medical history with emphasis on allergy and hypersensitivity, prior to the injection of any contrast media, may be more accurate than pretesting in predicting potential adverse reactions.

A positive history of allergies or hypersensitivity does not arbitrarily contraindicate the use of a contrast agent where a diagnostic procedure is thought essential, but caution should be exercised (see ADVERSE REACTIONS). Premedication with antihistamines or corticosteroids to avoid or minimize possible allergic reactions in such patients should be considered. Recent reports indicate that such pretreatment does not prevent serious life-threatening reactions, but may reduce both their incidence and severity.

In patients with severe renal insufficiency or failure, compensatory biliary excretion of the drug is anticipated to occur, with a slow clearance into the bile. Patients with hepatorenal insufficiency should not be examined unless the possibility of benefit clearly outweighs the additional risk.

Administration of contrast media should be performed by qualified personnel familiar with the procedure and appropriate patient management (see PATIENT MANAGEMENT). Sterile technique must be used with any spinal puncture.

When OMNIPAQUE (iohexol) is to be injected using plastic disposable syringes, the contrast medium should be drawn into the syringe and used immediately.

If nondisposable equipment is used, scrupulous care should be taken to prevent residual contamination with traces of cleansing agents.

Parenteral products should be inspected visually for particulate matter and discoloration prior to administration. If particulate matter or discoloration is present, do not use.

Repeat Procedures: If in the clinical judgment of the physician sequential or repeat examinations are required, a suitable interval of time between administrations should be observed to allow for normal clearance of the drug from the body (see DOSAGE AND ADMINISTRATION and CLINICAL PHARMACOLOGY).

Information for Patients

Patients receiving injectable radiopaque diagnostic agents should be instructed to:

1. Inform your physician if you are pregnant (see CLINICAL PHARMACOLOGY).
2. Inform your physician if you are diabetic or if you have multiple myeloma, pheochromocytoma, homozygous sickle cell disease or known thyroid disorder (see WARNINGS).
3. Inform your physician if you are allergic to any drugs, food, or if you had any reactions to previous injections of dyes used for x-ray procedures (see PRECAUTIONS—General).
4. Inform your physician about any other medications you are currently taking, including nonprescription drugs, before you are administered this drug.

Drug Interactions

Drugs which lower seizure threshold, especially phenothiazine derivatives including those used for their antihistaminic or antinauseant properties, are not recommended for use with OMNIPAQUE 180, OMNIPAQUE 240, or OMNIPAQUE 300. Others include monoamine oxidase (MAO) inhibitors, tricyclic antidepressants, CNS stimulants, psychoactive drugs described as analeptics, major tranquilizers, or antipsychotic drugs. Such medications should be discontinued at least 48 hours before myelography, should not be used for the control of nausea or vomiting during or after myelography, and should not be resumed for at least 24 hours postprocedure. In nonelective procedures in patients on these drugs, consider prophylactic use of anticonvulsants.

Carcinogensis, Mutagenesis, Impairment of Fertility

No long-term animal studies have been performed to evaluate carcinogenic potential, mutagenesis, or whether OMNIPAQUE (iohexol) can affect fertility in men or women.

Pregnancy Category B

Reproduction studies have been performed in rats and rabbits with up to 100 times the recommended human dose. No evidence of impaired fertility or harm to the fetus has been demonstrated due to OMNIPAQUE. There are, however, no studies in pregnant women. Because animal reproduction studies are not always predictive of human response, this drug should be used during pregnancy only if clearly needed.

Nursing Mothers

It is not known to what extent iohexol is excreted in human milk. However, many injectable contrast agents are excreted unchanged in human milk. Although it has not been established that serious adverse reactions occur in nursing infants, caution should be exercised when intravascular contrast media are administered to nursing women. Bottle feedings may be substituted for breast feedings for 24 hours following administration of OMNIPAQUE.

Pediatric Use

Safety and effectiveness in children have not been established.

ADVERSE REACTIONS—Intrathecal

The most frequently reported adverse reactions with OMNIPAQUE 180, OMNIPAQUE 240, and OMNIPAQUE 300 are headache, mild to moderate pain including backache, neckache and stiffness, nausea, and vomiting. These reactions usually occur 1 to 10 hours after injection, and almost all occur within 24 hours. They are usually mild to moderate in degree, lasting for a few hours, and usually disappearing within 24 hours. Rarely, headaches may be severe or persist for days. Headache is often accompanied by nausea and vomiting and tends to be more frequent and persistent in patients not optimally hydrated.

Transient alterations in vital signs may occur and their significance must be assessed on an individual basis. Those reactions reported in clinical studies with OMNIPAQUE are listed below in decreasing order of occurrence, based on clinical studies of 1531 patients.

Headaches: The most frequently occurring adverse reaction following myelography has been headache, with an incidence of approximately 18%. Headache may be caused by either a direct effect of the contrast medium or by CSF leakage at the dural puncture site. However, in managing the patient, it is considered more important to minimize intracranial entry of contrast medium by postural management than attempting to control possible CSF leakage (see PATIENT MANAGEMENT).

Pain: Mild to moderate pain including backache, neckache and stiffness, and neuralgia occurred following injection with an incidence of about 8%.

Nausea and Vomiting: Nausea was reported with an incidence of about 6%, and vomiting about 3% (see PATIENT MANAGEMENT). Maintaining normal hydration is very important. The use of phenothiazine antinauseants is not recommended. (See WARNINGS—General.) Reassurance to the patient that the nausea will clear usually is all that is required.

Dizziness: Transient dizziness was reported in about 2% of the patients.

Other Reactions: Other reactions occurring with an individual incidence of less than 0.1% included: feeling of heaviness, hypotension, hypertonia, sensation of heat, sweating, vertigo, loss of appetite, drowsiness, hypertension, photophobia, tinnitus, neuralgia, paresthesia, difficulty in micturition, and neurological changes. All were transient and mild with no clinical sequelae.

General Adverse Reactions to Contrast Media

Physicians should remain alert for the occurrence of adverse effects in addition to those discussed above, particularly the following reactions which have been reported in the literature for other nonionic, water-soluble myelographic media, and rarely with iohexol. These have included, but are not limited to, convulsion, aseptic and bacterial meningitis, and CNS and other neurological disturbances.

An aseptic meningitis syndrome has been reported rarely (less than 0.01%). It was usually preceded by pronounced headaches, nausea and vomiting. Onset usually occurred about 12 to 18 hours postprocedure. Prominent features were meningismus, fever, sometimes with oculomotor signs and mental confusion. Lumbar puncture revealed a high white cell count, high protein content often with a low glucose level and with absence of organisms. The condition usually started to clear spontaneously about 10 hours after onset, with complete recovery over 2 to 3 days.

Allergy or Idiosyncrasy: Chills, fever, profuse diaphoresis, pruritus, urticaria, nasal congestion, dyspnea, and a case of Guillain-Barré syndrome.

CNS Irritation: Mild and transitory perceptual aberrations such as hallucinations, depersonalization, amnesia, hostility, amblyopia, diplopia, photophobia, psychosis, insomnia, anxiety, depression, hyperesthesia, visual or auditory or speech disturbances, confusion and disorientation. In addition, malaise, weakness, convulsion, EEG changes, meningismus, hyperreflexia or areflexia, hypertonia or flaccidity, hemiplegia, paralysis, quadriplegia, restlessness, tremor, echoacousia, echolalia, asterixis, and dysphasia have occurred.

Profound mental disturbances have also rarely been reported. They have usually consisted of various forms and degrees of aphasia, mental confusion, or disorientation. The onset is usually at 8 to 10 hours and lasts for about 24 hours, without aftereffects. However, occasionally they have been manifest as apprehension, agitation, or progressive withdrawal in several instances to the point of somnolence, stupor, and coma. In a few cases these have been accompanied by transitory hearing loss or other auditory symptoms and visual disturbances (believed subjective or delusional), including unilateral or bilateral loss of vision which may last for hours. In one case, persistent cortical loss of vision has been reported in association with convulsions. Ventricular block has been reported; amnesia of varying degrees may be present for the reaction event.

Rarely, persistent though transitory weakness in the leg or ocular muscles has been reported.

Peripheral neuropathies have been rare and transitory. They include sensory and/or motor or nerve root disturbances, myelitis, persistent leg muscle pain or weakness, 6th nerve palsy, or cauda equina syndrome. Muscle cramps, fasciculation or myoclonia, spinal convulsion, or spasticity is unusual and has responded promptly to a small intravenous dose of diazepam.

In general, the reactions which are known to occur upon parenteral administration of iodinated contrast agents are possible with any nonionic agent. Approximately 95 percent of adverse reactions accompanying the use of water-soluble contrast agents are mild to moderate in degree. However, severe, life-threatening, anaphylactoid and fatal reactions, mostly of cardiovascular origin, have occurred.

Adverse reactions to injectable contrast media fall into two categories: chemotoxic reactions and idiosyncratic reactions. Chemotoxic reactions result from the physicochemical properties of the contrast media, the dose, and speed of injection. All hemodynamic disturbances and injuries to organs or vessels perfused by the contrast medium are included in this category.

Continued on next page

This product information was prepared in August, 1989. On these and other products of Winthrop Pharmaceuticals, detailed information may be obtained on a current basis by direct inquiry to the Professional Services Department, 90 Park Avenue, New York, NY 10016 (800) 446-6267.

Winthrop Pharm.—Cont.

Idiosyncratic reactions include all other reactions. They occur more frequently in patients 20 to 40 years old. Idiosyncratic reactions may or may not be dependent on the amount of dose injected, the speed of injection, and the radiographic procedure. Idiosyncratic reactions are subdivided into minor, intermediate, and severe. The minor reactions are self-limited and of short duration; the severe reactions are life-threatening and treatment is urgent and mandatory.

The reported incidence of adverse reactions to contrast media in patients with a history of allergy is twice that of the general population. Patients with a history of previous reactions to a contrast medium are three times more susceptible than other patients. However, sensitivity to contrast media does not appear to increase with repeated examinations. Most adverse reactions to injectable contrast media appear within 1 to 3 minutes after the start of injection, but delayed reactions may occur.

OVERDOSAGE

Clinical consequences of overdosage with OMNIPAQUE (iohexol) have not been reported. However, based on experience with other nonionic myelographic media, physicians should be alert to a potential increase in frequency and severity of CNS-mediated reactions. Even use of a recommended dose can produce effects tantamount to overdosage, if incorrect management of the patient during or immediately following the procedure permits inadvertent early intracranial entry of a large portion of the medium.

The intracisternal LD_{50} value of OMNIPAQUE (in grams of iodine per kilogram body weight) is greater than 2.0 in mice.

DOSAGE AND ADMINISTRATION—Intrathecal

The volume and concentration of OMNIPAQUE 180, OMNIPAQUE 240, or OMNIPAQUE 300 to be administered will depend on the degree and extent of contrast required in the area(s) under examination and on the equipment and technique employed.

OMNIPAQUE 180 at a concentration of 180 mgI/mL, OMNIPAQUE 240 at a concentration of 240 mgI/mL, or OMNIPAQUE 300 at a concentration of 300 mgI/mL is recommended for the examination of the lumbar, thoracic, and cervical regions in adults by lumbar or direct cervical injection and is slightly hypertonic to CSF.

A total dose of 3060 mg iodine or a concentration of 300 mgI/mL should not be exceeded in a single myelographic examination. This is based on clinical trial evaluation to date in the United States. As in all diagnostic procedures, the minimum volume and dose to produce adequate visualization should be used. Most procedures do not require either maximum dose or concentration.

Anesthesia is not necessary. Premedication sedatives or tranquilizers are usually not needed (see PRECAUTIONS). Patients should be well hydrated prior to and following contrast administration. Seizure-prone patients should be maintained on anticonvulsant medication.

Many radiopaque contrast agents are incompatible in vitro with some antihistamines and many other drugs; therefore, concurrent drugs should not be physically admixed with contrast agents.

Rate of Injection: To avoid excessive mixing with CSF and consequent dilution of contrast, injection should be made slowly over 1 to 2 minutes.

Depending on the estimated volume of contrast medium which may be required for the procedure a small amount of CSF may be removed to minimize distention of the subarachnoid spaces.

The lumbar or cervical puncture needle may be removed immediately following injection since it is not necessary to remove OMNIPAQUE (iohexol) after injection into the subarachnoid space.

The usual recommended total doses for use in lumbar, thoracic, cervical, and total columnar myelography are 1.2 gI to 3.06 gI as follows:

[See table below].

Withdrawal of contrast agents from their containers should be accomplished under aseptic conditions with sterile syringes. Spinal puncture must always be performed under sterile conditions.

Parenteral products should be inspected visually for particulate matter or discoloration prior to administration. If particulate matter or discoloration is present, do not use.

Repeat Procedures: If in the clinical judgment of the physician sequential or repeat examinations are required, a suitable interval of time between administrations should be observed to allow for normal clearance of the drug from the body. An interval of at least 48 hours should be allowed before repeat examination; however, whenever possible, 5 to 7 days is recommended.

PATIENT MANAGEMENT—Intrathecal

Suggestions for Usual Patient Management

Good patient management should be exercised at all times to minimize the potential for procedurally related complications.

Preprocedure
- Discontinuance of neuroleptic drugs (including phenothiazines, eg, chlorpromazine, prochlorperazine, and promethazine) at least 48 hours beforehand should be considered.
- Maintain normal diet up to 2 hours before procedure.
- Ensure hydration—fluids up to procedure.

During Procedure
- Use minimum dose and concentration required for satisfactory contrast (see DOSAGE AND ADMINISTRATION).
- In all positioning techniques keep the patient's head elevated above highest level of spine.
- Do not lower head of table more than 15° in moving contrast medium cranially.
- In patients with excessive lordosis, consider lateral position for injection and movement of the medium cephalad.
- Inject slowly (over 1 to 2 minutes) to avoid excessive mixing.
- To maintain as a bolus, move medium to distal area very slowly. Use fluoroscopic monitoring.
- Avoid intracranial entry of a mass.
- Avoid early and high cephalad dispersion of the medium.
- Avoid abrupt or active patient movement to minimize excessive mixing of medium with CSF. Instruct patient to remain passive. Move patient slowly and only as necessary.

Postprocedure
- Raise head of stretcher to at least 30° before moving patient onto it.
- Movement onto and off the stretcher should be done slowly with the patient completely passive, maintaining head-up position.
- Before moving patient onto bed, raise head of bed 30° to 45°.
- Advise patient to remain still in bed, in a sitting or semisitting position, especially in the first few hours.
- Maintain close observation for at least 12 hours after myelogram.
- Obtain visitors' cooperation in keeping the patient quiet and in head-up position, especially in first few hours.

- Encourage oral fluids. Diet as tolerated.
- If nausea or vomiting occurs, do not use phenothiazine antinauseants. Persistent nausea and vomiting will result in dehydration. Therefore, prompt consideration of replacement by intravenous fluids is recommended.

Alternative Postprocedure Method
- Recent evidence with nonionic, water-soluble contrast media suggests that maintaining the patient postmyelography in an upright position (via wheelchair or ambulation) may help minimize adverse effects. The upright position may help to delay upward dispersion of the medium and to maximize the spinal arachnoid absorption.

HOW SUPPLIED

OMNIPAQUE 180
Vials of 10 mL, 180 mgI/mL, boxes of 10 (NDC 0024-1411-10)
Vials of 20 mL, 180 mgI/mL, boxes of 10 (NDC 0024-1411-20)
OMNIPAQUE 240
Vials of 10 mL, 240 mgI/mL, boxes of 10 (NDC 0024-1412-10)
Vials of 20 mL, 240 mgI/mL, boxes of 10 (NDC 0024-1412-20)
OMNIPAQUE 300
Vials of 10 mL, 300 mgI/mL, boxes of 10 (NDC 0024-1413-10)
MYELO-KIT® containing: One 10 mL sterile vial of OMNIPAQUE 180, 180 mgI/mL, in REDI-UNIT™, and one sterile myelogram tray, boxes of 5 (NDC 0024-1415-05)
MYELO-KIT containing: One 20 mL sterile vial of OMNIPAQUE 180, 180 mgI/mL, in REDI-UNIT, and one sterile myelogram tray, boxes of 5 (NDC 0024-1415-06)
MYELO-KIT containing: One 10 mL sterile vial of OMNIPAQUE 240, 240 mgI/mL, in REDI-UNIT and one sterile myelogram tray, boxes of 5 (NDC 0024-1416-05)
REDI-UNIT containing: One sterile 10 mL vial of OMNIPAQUE 180, 180 mgI/mL, boxes of 5 (NDC 0024-1411-07)
REDI-UNIT containing: One sterile 20 mL vial of OMNIPAQUE 180, 180 mgI/mL, boxes of 5 (NDC 0024-1411-08)
REDI-UNIT containing: One sterile 10 mL vial of OMNIPAQUE 240, 240 mgI/mL, boxes of 5 (NDC 0024-1412-07)
Storage: Protect vials of OMNIPAQUE (iohexol) from strong daylight and direct exposure to sunlight. Do not freeze. Store at 59°F to 86°F (15°C to 30°C).

SECTION II

CLINICAL PHARMACOLOGY—Intravascular/Body Cavities

Following intravascular injection, iohexol is distributed in the extracellular fluid compartment and is excreted unchanged by glomerular filtration. It will opacify those vessels in the path of flow of the contrast medium permitting radiographic visualization of the internal structures until significant hemodilution occurs.

Approximately 90% or more of the injected dose is excreted within the first 24 hours, with the peak urine concentrations occurring in the first hour after administration. Plasma and urine iohexol levels indicate that the iohexol body clearance is due primarily to renal clearance. An increase in the dose from 500 mgI/kg to 1500 mgI/kg does not significantly alter the clearance of the drug. The following pharmacokinetic values were observed following the intravenous administration of iohexol (between 500 mgI/kg to 1500 mgI/kg) to 16 adult human subjects: renal clearance—120 (86-162) mL/min; total body clearance—131 (98-165) mL/min; and volume of distribution—165 (108-219) mL/kg.

Renal accumulation is sufficiently rapid that the period of maximal opacification of the renal passages may begin as early as 1 minute after intravenous injection. Urograms become apparent in about 1 to 3 minutes with optimal contrast occurring between 5 to 15 minutes. In nephropathic conditions, particularly when excretory capacity has been altered, the rate of excretion may vary unpredictably, and opacification may be delayed after injection. Severe renal impairment may result in a lack of diagnostic opacification of the collecting system and, depending on the degree of renal impairment, prolonged plasma iohexol levels may be anticipated. In these patients, as well as in infants with immature kidneys, the route of excretion through the gallbladder and into the small intestine may increase.

Iohexol displays a low affinity for serum or plasma proteins and is poorly bound to serum albumin. No significant metabolism, deiodination or biotransformation occurs.

OMNIPAQUE (iohexol) probably crosses the placental barrier in humans by simple diffusion. It is not known to what extent iohexol is excreted in human milk.

Animal studies indicate that iohexol does not cross an intact blood-brain barrier to any significant extent following intravascular administration.

OMNIPAQUE enhances computed tomographic imaging through augmentation of radiographic efficiency. The degree of density enhancement is directly related to the iodine content in an administered dose; peak iodine blood levels occur immediately following rapid intravenous injection. Blood levels fall rapidly within 5 to 10 minutes and the vascular compartment half-life is approximately 20 minutes. This can be accounted for by the dilution in the vascular and

Procedure	Formulations	Concentration (mgI/mL)	Volume (mL)	Dose (gI)
Lumbar Myelography (via lumbar injection)	OMNIPAQUE 180	180	10–17	1.8–3.06
	OMNIPAQUE 240	240	7–12.5	1.7–3.0
Thoracic Myelography (via lumbar or cervical injection)	OMNIPAQUE 240	240	6–12.5	1.7–3.0
	OMNIPAQUE 300	300	6–10	1.8–3.0
Cervical Myelography (via lumbar injection)	OMNIPAQUE 240	240	6–12.5	1.4–3.0
	OMNIPAQUE 300	300	6–10	1.8–3.0
Cervical Myelography (via C1-2 injection)	OMNIPAQUE 180	180	7–10	1.3–1.8
	OMNIPAQUE 240	240	6–12.5	1.4–3.0
	OMNIPAQUE 300	300	4–10	1.2–3.0
Total Columnar Myelography (via lumbar injection)	OMNIPAQUE 240	240	6–12.5	1.4–3.0
	OMNIPAQUE 300	300	6–10	1.8–3.0

extravascular fluid compartments which causes an initial sharp fall in plasma concentration. Equilibration with the extracellular compartments is reached in about ten minutes; thereafter, the fall becomes exponential.

The pharmacokinetics of iohexol in both normal and abnormal tissue have been shown to be variable. Contrast enhancement appears to be greatest immediately after bolus administration (15 seconds to 120 seconds). Thus, greatest enhancement may be detected by a series of consecutive two-to-three second scans performed within 30 to 90 seconds after injection (ie, dynamic computed tomographic imaging). Utilization of a continuous scanning technique (ie, dynamic CT scanning) may improve enhancement and diagnostic assessment of tumor and other lesions such as abscess, occasionally revealing unsuspected or more extensive disease. For example, a cyst may be distinguished from a vascularized solid lesion when precontrast and enhanced scans are compared; the nonperfused mass shows unchanged x-ray absorption (CT number). A vascularized lesion is characterized by an increase in CT number in the few minutes after a bolus of intravascular contrast agent; it may be malignant, benign, or normal tissue, but would probably not be a cyst, hematoma, or other nonvascular lesion.

Because unenhanced scanning may provide adequate diagnostic information in the individual patient, the decision to employ contrast enhancement, which may be associated with risk and increased radiation exposure, should be based upon a careful evaluation of clinical, other radiological, and unenhanced CT findings.

CT SCANNING OF THE HEAD

In contrast enhanced computed tomographic head imaging, OMNIPAQUE does not accumulate in normal brain tissue due to the presence of the normal blood-brain barrier. The increase in x-ray absorption in normal brain is due to the presence of contrast agent within the blood pool. A break in the blood-brain barrier such as occurs in malignant tumors of the brain allows for the accumulation of contrast medium within the interstitial tissue of the tumor. Adjacent normal brain tissue does not contain the contrast medium.

Maximum contrast enhancement in tissue frequently occurs after peak blood iodine levels are reached. A delay in maximum contrast enhancement can occur. Diagnostic contrast enhanced images of the brain have been obtained up to 1 hour after intravenous bolus administration. This delay suggests that radiographic contrast enhancement is at least in part dependent on the accumulation of iodine containing medium within the lesion and outside the blood pool, although the mechanism by which this occurs is not clear. The radiographic enhancement of nontumoral lesions, such as arteriovenous malformations and aneurysms, is probably dependent on the iodine content of the circulating blood pool. In patients where the blood-brain barrier is known or suspected to be disrupted, the use of any radiographic contrast medium must be assessed on an individual risk to benefit basis. However, compared to ionic media, nonionic media are less toxic to the central nervous system.

CT SCANNING OF THE BODY

In contrast enhanced computed tomographic body imaging (nonneural tissue), OMNIPAQUE diffuses rapidly from the vascular into the extravascular space. Increase in x-ray absorption is related to blood flow, concentration of the contrast medium, and extraction of the contrast medium by interstitial tissue of tumors since no barrier exists. Contrast enhancement is thus due to the relative differences in extravascular diffusion between normal and abnormal tissue, quite different from that in the brain.

BODY CAVITY IMAGING

Visualization of joint spaces, the uterus, fallopian tubes, peritoneal herniations, pancreas, pancreatic and bile ducts can be accomplished by direct injection of contrast medium into the region to be studied. The use of appropriate iodine concentrations assures diagnostic density. For most body cavities, the injected OMNIPAQUE is absorbed into the surrounding tissue and eliminated by the kidneys and bowel as previously described. Examinations of the uterus involve the immediate drainage of contrast medium from the cavity upon the conclusion of radiographic procedures.

INDICATIONS AND USAGE, General—Intravascular/Body Cavities

OMNIPAQUE 350 is indicated in adults for angiocardiography (ventriculography, selective coronary arteriography), aortography including studies of the aortic root, aortic arch, ascending aorta, abdominal aorta and its branches, contrast enhancement for computed tomographic head and body imaging, intravenous digital subtraction angiography of the head, neck, abdominal, renal and peripheral vessels, peripheral arteriography, excretory urography, and arthrography.

OMNIPAQUE 350 is indicated in children for angiocardiography (ventriculography, pulmonary arteriography, and venography; studies of the collateral arteries and aortography, including studies of the aortic root, aortic arch, ascending and descending aorta).

OMNIPAQUE 300 is indicated in adults for aortography including studies of the aortic arch, abdominal aorta and its branches, contrast enhancement for computed tomographic head and body imaging, cerebral arteriography, peripheral venography (phlebography), excretory urography, arthrography, and hysterosalpingography.

OMNIPAQUE 300 is indicated in children for angiocardiography (ventriculography) and for urography (including voiding cystourethrography).

OMNIPAQUE 240 is indicated in adults for contrast enhancement for computed tomographic head imaging, and peripheral venography (phlebography), arthrography, endoscopic retrograde pancreatography and cholangiopancreatography, herniography, and hysterosalpingography.

OMNIPAQUE 140 is indicated in adults for intra-arterial digital subtraction angiography of the head, neck, abdominal, renal and peripheral vessels.

CONTRAINDICATIONS

OMNIPAQUE (iohexol) should not be administered to patients with a known hypersensitivity to iohexol.

WARNINGS—General

Nonionic iodinated contrast media inhibit blood coagulation, in vitro, less than ionic contrast media. Clotting has been reported when blood remains in contact with syringes containing nonionic contrast media.

Serious, rarely fatal, thromboembolic events causing myocardial infarction and stroke have been reported during angiographic procedures with both ionic and nonionic contrast media. Therefore, meticulous intravascular administration technique is necessary, particularly during angiographic procedures, to minimize thromboembolic events. Numerous factors, including length of procedure, catheter and syringe material, underlying disease state, and concomitant medications may contribute to the development of thromboembolic events. For these reasons, meticulous angiographic techniques are recommended including close attention to guidewire and catheter manipulation, use of manifold systems and/or three-way stopcocks, frequent catheter flushing with heparinized saline solutions and minimizing the length of the procedure. The use of plastic syringes in place of glass syringes has been reported to decrease but not eliminate the likelihood of in vitro clotting.

OMNIPAQUE should be used with extreme care in patients with severe functional disturbances of the liver and kidneys, severe thyrotoxicosis, or myelomatosis. Diabetics with a serum creatinine level above 3 mg/dL should not be examined unless the possible benefits of the examination clearly outweigh the additional risk. OMNIPAQUE (iohexol) is not recommended for use in patients with anuria.

Radiopaque contrast agents are potentially hazardous in patients with multiple myeloma or other paraproteinemia, particularly in those with therapeutically resistant anuria. Although neither the contrast agent nor dehydration has separately proven to be the cause of anuria in myeloma, it has been speculated that the combination of both may be causative factors. The risk in myelomatous patients is not a contraindication; however, special precautions are necessary. Partial dehydration in the preparation of these patients prior to injection is not recommended since this may predispose the patient to precipitation of the myeloma protein in the renal tubules. No form of therapy, including dialysis, has been successful in reversing the effect. Myeloma, which occurs most commonly in persons over age 40, should be considered before instituting intravascular administration of contrast agents.

Ionic contrast media, when injected intravenously or intraarterially, may promote sickling in individuals who are homozygous for sickle cell disease.

Administration of radiopaque materials to patients known or suspected of having pheochromocytoma should be performed with extreme caution. If, in the opinion of the physician, the possible benefits of such procedures outweigh the considered risks, the procedures may be performed; however, the amount of radiopaque medium injected should be kept to an absolute minimum. The patient's blood pressure should be assessed throughout the procedure and measures for the treatment of hypertensive crisis should be readily available. Reports of thyroid storm following the use of iodinated, ionic radiopaque contrast media in patients with hyperthyroidism or with an autonomously functioning thyroid nodule suggest that this additional risk be evaluated in such patients before use of any contrast medium.

Urography should be performed with caution in patients with severely impaired renal function and patients with combined renal and hepatic disease.

PRECAUTIONS—General

Diagnostic procedures which involve the use of radiopaque diagnostic agents should be carried out under the direction of personnel with the prerequisite training and with a thorough knowledge of the particular procedure to be performed.

Appropriate facilities should be available for coping with any complication of the procedure, as well as for emergency treatment of severe reactions to the contrast agent itself. After parenteral administration of a radiopaque agent, competent personnel and emergency facilities should be available for at least 30 to 60 minutes since severe delayed reactions have occurred (see ADVERSE REACTIONS: Intravascular—General).

Preparatory dehydration is dangerous and may contribute to acute renal failure in patients with advanced vascular disease, diabetic patients, and in susceptible nondiabetic patients (often elderly with preexisting renal disease), infants and small children. Dehydration in these patients seems to be enhanced by the osmotic diuretic action of urographic agents. It is believed that overnight fluid restriction prior to excretory urography generally does not provide better visualization in normal patients. *Patients should be well hydrated prior to and following administration of any contrast medium, including iohexol.*

Acute renal failure has been reported in diabetic patients with diabetic nephropathy and in susceptible nondiabetic patients (often elderly with preexisting renal disease) following excretory urography. Therefore, careful consideration of the potential risks should be given before performing this radiographic procedure in these patients.

Immediately following surgery, excretory urography should be used with caution in renal transplant recipients.

The possibility of a reaction, including serious, life-threatening, fatal, anaphylactoid or cardiovascular reactions should always be considered (see ADVERSE REACTIONS: Intravascular—General). It is of utmost importance that a course of action be carefully planned in advance for immediate treatment of serious reactions, and that adequate and appropriate personnel be readily available in case of any reaction.

The possibility of an idiosyncratic reaction in susceptible patients should always be considered (see ADVERSE REACTIONS: Intravascular—General). The susceptible population includes, but is not limited to, patients with a history of a previous reaction to contrast media, patients with a known sensitivity to iodine per se, and patients with a known clinical hypersensitivity: bronchial asthma, hay fever, and food allergies.

The occurrence of severe idiosyncratic reactions has prompted the use of several pretesting methods. However, pretesting cannot be relied upon to predict severe reactions and may itself be hazardous for the patient. It is suggested that a thorough medical history with emphasis on allergy and hypersensitivity, prior to the injection of any contrast media, may be more accurate than pretesting in predicting potential adverse reactions.

A positive history of allergies or hypersensitivity does not arbitrarily contraindicate the use of a contrast agent where a diagnostic procedure is thought essential, but caution should be exercised (see ADVERSE REACTIONS: Intravascular—General). Premedication with antihistamines or corticosteroids to avoid or minimize possible allergic reactions in such patients should be considered and administered using separate syringes. Recent reports indicate that such pretreatment does not prevent serious life-threatening reactions, but may reduce both their incidence and severity.

Even though the osmolality of OMNIPAQUE is low compared to diatrizoate- or iothalamate-based ionic agents of comparable iodine concentration, the potential transitory increase in the circulatory osmotic load in patients with congestive heart failure requires caution during injection. These patients should be observed for several hours following the procedure to detect delayed hemodynamic disturbances.

General anesthesia may be indicated in the performance of some procedures in selected adult patients; however, a higher incidence of adverse reactions has been reported in these patients, and may be attributable to the inability of the patient to identify untoward symptoms, or to the hypotensive effect of anesthesia which can reduce cardiac output and increase the duration of exposure to the contrast agent.

Angiography should be avoided whenever possible in patients with homocystinuria, because of the risk of inducing thrombosis and embolism.

In angiographic procedures, the possibility of dislodging plaques or damaging or perforating the vessel wall should be borne in mind during the catheter manipulations and contrast medium injection. Test injections to ensure proper catheter placement are recommended.

Selective coronary arteriography should be performed only in those patients in whom the expected benefits outweigh the potential risk. The inherent risks of angiocardiography in patients with chronic pulmonary emphysema must be weighed against the necessity for performing this procedure.

When OMNIPAQUE (iohexol) is to be injected using plastic disposable syringes, the contrast medium should be drawn into the syringe and used immediately.

Continued on next page

This product information was prepared in August, 1989. On these and other products of Winthrop Pharmaceuticals, detailed information may be obtained on a current basis by direct inquiry to the Professional Services Department, 90 Park Avenue, New York, NY 10016 (800) 446-6267.

Winthrop Pharm.—Cont.

If nondisposable equipment is used, scrupulous care should be taken to prevent residual contamination with traces of cleansing agents.

Parenteral products should be inspected visually for particulate matter and discoloration prior to administration. If particulate matter or discoloration is present, do not use.

Information for Patients

Patients receiving injectable radiopaque diagnostic agents should be instructed to:

1. Inform your physician if you are pregnant (see CLINICAL PHARMACOLOGY—Intravascular/Body Cavities).
2. Inform your physician if you are diabetic or if you have multiple myeloma, pheochromocytoma, homozygous sickle cell disease, or known thyroid disorder (see WARNINGS).
3. Inform your physician if you are allergic to any drugs, food, or if you had any reactions to previous injections of dyes used for x-ray procedures (see PRECAUTIONS—General).
4. Inform your physician about any other medications you are currently taking, including nonprescription drugs, before you are administered this drug.

Drug/Laboratory Test Interaction

If iodine-containing isotopes are to be administered for the diagnosis of thyroid disease, the iodine-binding capacity of thyroid tissue may be reduced for up to 2 weeks after contrast medium administration. Thyroid function tests which do not depend on iodine estimation, eg, T_3 resin uptake or direct thyroxine assays, are not affected.

Many radiopaque contrast agents are incompatible in vitro with some antihistamines and many other drugs; therefore, no other pharmaceuticals should be admixed with contrast agents.

Carcinogenesis, Mutagenesis, Impairment of Fertility

No long-term animal studies have been performed to evaluate carcinogenic potential, mutagenesis, or whether OMNIPAQUE (iohexol) can affect fertility in men or women.

Pregnancy Category B

Reproduction studies have been performed in rats and rabbits with up to 100 times the recommended human dose. No evidence of impaired fertility or harm to the fetus has been demonstrated due to OMNIPAQUE. There are, however,no studies in pregnant women. Because animal reproduction studies are not always predictive of human response, this drug should be used during pregnancy only if clearly needed.

Nursing Mothers

It is not known to what extent iohexol is excreted in human milk. However, many injectable contrast agents are excreted unchanged in human milk. Although it has not been established that serious adverse reactions occur in nursing infants, caution should be exercised when intravascular contrast media are administered to nursing women. Bottle feedings may be substituted for breast feedings for 24 hours following administration of OMNIPAQUE.

Pediatric Use (Indicated for Angiocardiography and Urography)

Pediatric patients at higher risk of experiencing adverse events during contrast medium administration may include those having asthma, a sensitivity to medication and/or allergens, congestive heart failure, a serum creatinine greater than 1.5 mg/dL or those less than 12 months of age.

ADVERSE REACTIONS: Intravascular—General

Adverse reactions following the use of OMNIPAQUE 140, OMNIPAQUE 240, OMNIPAQUE 300, and OMNIPAQUE 350 are usually of mild to moderate severity. However, serious, life-threatening and fatal reactions, mostly of cardiovascular origin, have been associated with the administration of iodine-containing contrast media, including OMNIPAQUE. The injection of contrast media is frequently associated with the sensation of warmth and pain, especially in peripheral angiography; pain and warmth are less frequent and less severe with OMNIPAQUE than with many contrast media.

Cardiovascular System: Arrhythmias including PVCs and PACs (2%), angina/chest pain (1%), and hypotension (0.7%). Others including cardiac failure, asystole, bradycardia, tachycardia, and vasovagal reaction were reported with an individual incidence of 0.3% or less. In controlled clinical trials involving 1400 patients, one fatality occurred. A cause and effect relationship between this death and iohexol has not been established.

Nervous System: Vertigo (including dizziness and lightheadedness) (0.6%), pain (3%), photomas (2%), headache (2%), and taste perversion (1%). Others including anxiety, blurred vision, fever, motor and speech dysfunction, convulsion, paresthesia, somnolence, stiff neck, hemiparesis, syncope, transient ischemic attack, cerebral infarction, and nystagmus were reported, with an individual incidence of 0.4% or less.

Respiratory System: Dyspnea, rhinitis, coughing, and laryngitis, with an individual incidence of 0.2% or less.

Gastrointestinal System: Nausea (2%) and vomiting (0.7%). Others including diarrhea, dyspepsia, and dry mouth were reported, with an individual incidence of less than 0.1%.

Skin and Appendages: Urticaria (0.3%), purpura (0.1%), abscess (0.1%), and pruritus (0.1%).

Individual adverse reactions which occurred to a significantly greater extent for a specific procedure are listed under that indication.

Pediatrics

In controlled clinical trials involving 324 patients for pediatric angiocardiography and urography, adverse reactions following the use of OMNIPAQUE 300 and OMNIPAQUE 350 were generally less frequent than with adults.

Cardiovascular System: Ventricular tachycardia (0.6%), 2:1 heart block (0.6%), hypertension (0.3%), and anemia (0.3%).

Nervous System: Pain (0.6%), fever (0.6%), and convulsion (0.3%).

Respiratory System: Congestion (0.3%) and apnea (0.3%).

Gastrointestinal System: Nausea (1%), hypoglycemia (0.3%), and vomiting (2%).

Skin and Appendages: Rash (0.3%).

ADVERSE REACTIONS: Body Cavities—General

Cardiovascular System: Hypertension (0.4%).

Nervous System: Pain (29%), headache (0.4%), somnolence (0.8%), fever (0.4%), dizziness (0.4%), muscle weakness, burning and unwell feeling, each with an individual incidence of 0.4%.

Respiratory System: None.

Gastrointestinal System: Nausea (0.4%), vomiting (0.4%), diarrhea (0.8%), flatulence (1%), and pressure (0.4%).

Skin and Appendages: Hematoma injection site (0.4%), swelling (26%), heat (8%).

Individual adverse reactions which occurred to a significantly greater extent for a specific procedure are listed under that indication.

General Adverse Reactions to Contrast Media

Physicians should remain alert for the occurrence of adverse effects in addition to those discussed above.

The following reactions have been reported after administration of other intravascular iodinated contrast media, and rarely with iohexol. *Reactions due to technique:* hematomas and ecchymoses. *Hemodynamic reactions:* vein cramp and thrombophlebitis following intravenous injection. *Cardiovascular reactions:* rare cases of cardiac arrhythmias, reflex tachycardia, chest pain, cyanosis, hypertension, hypotension, peripheral vasodilatation, shock, and cardiac arrest. *Renal reactions:* occasionally, transient proteinuria, and rarely, oliguria or anuria. *Allergic reactions:* asthmatic attacks, nasal and conjunctival symptoms, dermal reactions such as urticaria with or without pruritus, as well as pleomorphic rashes, sneezing and lacrimation and, rarely, anaphylactic reactions. Rare fatalities have occurred, due to this or unknown causes. *Signs and symptoms related to the respiratory system:* pulmonary or laryngeal edema, bronchospasm, dyspnea; *or to the nervous system:* restlessness, tremors, convulsions. *Other reactions:* flushing, pain, warmth, metallic taste, nausea, vomiting, anxiety, headache, confusion, pallor, weakness, sweating, localized areas of edema, especially facial cramps, neutropenia, and dizziness. Rarely, immediate or delayed rigors can occur, sometimes accompanied by hyperpyrexia. Infrequently, "iodism" (salivary gland swelling) from organic iodinated compounds appears two days after exposure and subsides by the sixth day.

In general, the reactions which are known to occur upon parenteral administration of iodinated contrast agents are possible with any nonionic agent. Approximately 95 percent of adverse reactions accompanying the use of water-soluble intravascularly administered contrast agents are mild to moderate in degree. However, severe, life-threatening anaphylactoid reactions, mostly of cardiovascular origin, have occurred. Reported incidences of death range from 6.6 per 1 million (0.00066 percent) to 1 in 10 000 (0.01 percent). Most deaths occur during injection or 5 to 10 minutes later; the main feature being cardiac arrest with cardiovascular disease as the main aggravating factor. Isolated reports of hypotensive collapse and shock are found in the literature. The incidence of shock is estimated to be 1 out of 20 000 (0.005 percent) patients.

Adverse reactions to injectable contrast media fall into two categories: chemotoxic reactions and idiosyncratic reactions. Chemotoxic reactions result from the physicochemical properties of the contrast media, the dose, and speed of injection. All hemodynamic disturbances and injuries to organs or vessels perfused by the contrast medium are included in this category.

Idiosyncratic reactions include all other reactions. They occur more frequently in patients 20 to 40 years old. Idiosyncratic reactions may or may not be dependent on the amount of dose injected, the speed of injection, and the radiographic procedure. Idiosyncratic reactions are subdivided into minor, intermediate, and severe. The minor reactions are self-limited and of short duration; the severe reactions are life-threatening and treatment is urgent and mandatory.

The reported incidence of adverse reactions to contrast media in patients with a history of allergy are twice that of the general population. Patients with a history of previous reactions to a contrast medium are three times more susceptible than other patients. However, sensitivity to contrast media does not appear to increase with repeated examinations. Most adverse reactions to injectable contrast media appear within 1 to 3 minutes after the start of injection, but delayed reactions may occur.

Regardless of the contrast agent employed, the overall estimated incidence of serious adverse reactions is higher with angiocardiography than with other procedures. Cardiac decompensation, serious arrhythmias, angina pectoris, or myocardial ischemia or infarction may occur during angiocardiography and left ventriculography. Electrocardiographic and hemodynamic abnormalities occur less frequently with OMNIPAQUE than with diatrizoate meglumine and diatrizoate sodium injection.

OVERDOSAGE

Overdosage may occur. The adverse effects of overdosage are life-threatening and affect mainly the pulmonary and cardiovascular systems. The symptoms included: cyanosis, bradycardia, acidosis, pulmonary hemorrhage, convulsions, coma, and cardiac arrest. Treatment of an overdosage is directed toward the support of all vital functions, and prompt institution of symptomatic therapy.

The intravenous LD_{50} values of OMNIPAQUE (iohexol) (in grams of iodine per kilogram body weight) are 24.2 in mice and 15.0 in rats.

DOSAGE AND ADMINISTRATION—General

As with all radiopaque contrast agents, the lowest dose of OMNIPAQUE necessary to obtain adequate visualization should be used. A lower dose may reduce the possibility of an adverse reaction. Most procedures do not require use of either the maximum volume or the highest concentration of OMNIPAQUE. The combination of volume and concentration of OMNIPAQUE (iohexol) to be used should be carefully individualized accounting for factors such as age, body weight, size of the vessel and the rate of blood flow within the vessel. Other factors such as anticipated pathology, degree and extent of opacification required, structure(s) or area to be examined, disease processes affecting the patient, and equipment and technique to be employed should be considered.

Sterile technique must be used in all vascular injections involving contrast media.

Withdrawal of contrast agents from their containers should be accomplished under aseptic conditions with sterile equipment. Sterile techniques must be used with any invasive procedure.

If nondisposable equipment is used, scrupulous care should be taken to prevent residual contamination with traces of cleansing agents.

It may be desirable that solutions of radiopaque diagnostic agents be used at body temperature when injected.

Parenteral products should be inspected visually for particulate matter and discoloration prior to administration whenever solution and container permit. Solutions of OMNIPAQUE should be used only if clear and within the normal colorless to pale yellow range. If particulate matter or discoloration is present, do not use.

INDIVIDUAL INDICATIONS AND USAGE

ANGIOCARDIOGRAPHY

Pharmacology—Hemodynamic Changes

OMNIPAQUE 350 at a concentration of 350 mgI/mL is indicated in adults for angiocardiography (ventriculography, aortic root injections, and selective coronary arteriography). OMNIPAQUE 350 at a concentration of 350 mgI/mL is indicated in children for angiocardiography (ventriculography, pulmonary arteriography, and venography, and studies of collateral arteries).

OMNIPAQUE 300 at a concentration of 300 mgI/mL is indicated in children for angiocardiography (ventriculography).

After both ventricular and coronary injection, decreases in systolic pressure were less pronounced and returned to baseline values earlier with OMNIPAQUE 350 than with diatrizoate meglumine and diatrizoate sodium injection.

OMNIPAQUE 350 produced less Q-T interval prolongation than seen with diatrizoate meglumine and diatrizoate sodium injection.

In children, after injection of all sites, but particularly following ventricular and pulmonary artery injections, decreases in both systolic and diastolic intravascular pressure were significantly less pronounced with OMNIPAQUE 350 than with diatrizoate meglumine and diatrizoate sodium injection. In children, OMNIPAQUE 350 produced significantly less shortening of the R-R interval than seen with diatrizoate meglumine and diatrizoate sodium injection.

If repeat injections are made in rapid succession, all these changes are likely to be more pronounced. (See DOSAGE AND ADMINISTRATION.)

Precautions: During administration of large doses of OMNIPAQUE 350, continuous monitoring of vital signs is desirable. Caution is advised in the administration of large volumes to patients with incipient heart failure because of the possibility of aggravating the preexisting condition. Hypotension should be corrected promptly since it may induce serious arrhythmias.

Special care regarding dosage should be observed in patients with right ventricular failure, pulmonary hypertension, or stenotic pulmonary vascular beds because of the hemodynamic changes which may occur after injection into the right heart outflow tract. (See PRECAUTIONS—General.) Pediatric patients at higher risk of experiencing adverse events during contrast medium administration may include those having asthma, a sensitivity to medication and/or allergens, congestive heart failure, a serum creatinine greater than 1.5 mg/dL or those less than 12 months of age.

Adverse Reactions: Cardiovascular system reactions in angiocardiography included angina (8%), hypotension (2.5%), bradycardia (1.0%), and tachycardia (1.0%). (See ADVERSE REACTIONS: Intravascular—General.)

Dosage and Administration: The individual dose or volume is determined by the size of the structure to be visualized, the anticipated degree of hemodilution, and valvular competence. Weight is a minor consideration in adults, but must be considered in infants and young children. The volume of each individual injection is a more important consideration than the total dosage used. When large individual volumes are administered, as in ventriculography and aortography, it has been suggested that several minutes be permitted to elapse between each injection to allow for subsidence of possible hemodynamic disturbances.

The recommended single injection volume of OMNIPAQUE 350 for angiocardiographic procedures in adults and the recommended single injection volumes of OMNIPAQUE 350 and OMNIPAQUE 300 for angiographic procedures in children are as follows:

Ventriculography

Adults: The usual adult volume for a single injection is 40 mL with a range of 30 mL to 60 mL. This may be repeated as necessary. When combined with selective coronary arteriography, the total administered volume should not exceed 250 mL (87.5 gI).

Pediatrics: The usual single injection dose of OMNIPAQUE 350 is 1.25 mL/kg of body weight with a range of 1.0 mL/kg to 1.5 mL/kg. For OMNIPAQUE 300 the usual single injection dose is 1.75 mL/kg with a range of 1.5 mL/kg to 2.0 mL/kg. When multiple injections are given, the total administered dose should not exceed 5 mL/kg up to a total volume of 250 mL of OMNIPAQUE 350 or up to a total volume of 291 mL of OMNIPAQUE 300.

Selective Coronary Arteriography

The usual adult volume for right or left coronary arteriography is 5 mL (range 3 mL to 14 mL) per injection.

Aortic Root and Arch Study When Used Alone

The usual adult single injection volume is 50 mL, with a range of 20 mL to 75 mL.

Pulmonary Angiography

Pediatrics: The usual single injection dose is 1.0 mL/kg of OMNIPAQUE 350.

Combined Angiocardiographic Procedures

Multiple Procedures

Adults: The visualization of multiple vascular systems and target organs is possible during a single radiographic examination of the patient.

Large doses of OMNIPAQUE 350 were well tolerated in angiographic procedures requiring multiple injections.

The maximum total volume for multiple procedures should not exceed 250 mL of 350 mgI/mL (87.5 gI).

Pediatrics: Visualization of multiple vascular systems and target organs is possible during a single radiographic examination of the patient.

The maximum total dose for multiple injection procedures should not exceed 5.0 mL/kg up to a total volume of 250 mL of OMNIPAQUE 350 or 6.0 mL/kg up to a total volume of 291 mL of OMNIPAQUE 300.

AORTOGRAPHY

OMNIPAQUE 300 at a concentration of 300 mgI/mL or OMNIPAQUE (iohexol) 350 at a concentration of 350 mgI/mL is indicated in adults for use in aortography including aortic arch studies, ascending aorta, and abdominal aorta and its branches.

OMNIPAQUE 350 at a concentration of 350 mgI/mL is indicated in children for use in aortography including studies of the aortic root, aortic arch, ascending and descending aorta.

Precautions: Under conditions of slowed aortic circulation there is an increased likelihood for aortography to cause muscle spasm. Occasional serious neurologic complications, including paraplegia, have also been reported in patients with aortoiliac obstruction, femoral artery obstruction, abdominal compression, hypotension, hypertension, spinal anesthesia, and injection of vasopressors to increase contrast. In these patients the concentration, volume, and number of repeat injections of the medium should be maintained at a minimum with appropriate intervals between injections. The position of the patient and catheter tip should be carefully monitored.

Entry of a large aortic dose into the renal artery may cause, even in the absence of symptoms, albuminuria, hematuria, and an elevated creatinine and urea nitrogen. Rapid and complete return of function usually follows. (See PRECAUTIONS—General.)

Adverse Reactions: See ADVERSE REACTIONS: Intravascular—General and ADVERSE REACTIONS—ANGIOCARDIOGRAPHY.

Dosage and Administration:

Adults: The usual adult volume as a single injection is 50 mL to 80 mL, repeated if indicated, but not to exceed a total volume which contains 87.5 gI.

Pediatrics: The usual single injection dose is 1.0 mL/kg of OMNIPAQUE 350 and should not exceed 5.0 mL/kg up to a total volume of 250 mL of OMNIPAQUE 350.

CEREBRAL ARTERIOGRAPHY

OMNIPAQUE 300 at a concentration of 300 mgI/mL is indicated in adults for use in cerebral arteriography.

The degree of pain and flushing as the result of the use of OMNIPAQUE 300 in cerebral arteriography is less than that seen with comparable injections of many contrast media.

In cerebral arteriography, patients should be appropriately prepared consistent with existing or suspected disease states.

Precautions: Cerebral arteriography should be undertaken with extreme care with special caution in elderly patients, patients in poor physical condition, advanced arteriosclerosis, severe arterial hypertension, recent cerebral embolism or thrombosis, and cardiac decompensation.

Since the contrast medium is given by rapid injection, the patient should be monitored for possible untoward reactions. (See PRECAUTIONS—General.)

Adverse Reactions: Cerebral arteriography with water-soluble contrast media has been associated with temporary neurologic complications including seizures, drowsiness, transient paresis, and mild disturbances in vision such as photomas of 1-second or less duration.

Central nervous system reactions in cerebral arteriography included photomas (15%), headache (5.5%), and pain (4.5%). (See ADVERSE REACTIONS: Intravascular—General.)

Dosage and Administration: OMNIPAQUE 300 is recommended for cerebral arteriography at the following volumes: common carotid artery (6 mL to 12 mL), internal carotid artery (8 mL to 10 mL), external carotid artery (6 mL to 9 mL), and vertebral artery (6 mL to 20 mL).

CONTRAST ENHANCED COMPUTED TOMOGRAPHY

OMNIPAQUE 240 at a concentration of 240 mgI/mL, OMNIPAQUE 300 at a concentration of 300 mgI/mL, and OMNIPAQUE 350 at a concentration of 350 mgI/mL are indicated in adults for use in intravenous contrast enhanced computed tomographic head and body imaging by rapid injection or infusion technique.

CT SCANNING OF THE HEAD

OMNIPAQUE may be used to redefine diagnostic precision in areas of the brain which may not otherwise have been satisfactorily visualized.

Tumors

OMNIPAQUE (iohexol) may be useful to investigate the presence and extent of certain malignancies such as: gliomas including malignant gliomas, glioblastomas, astrocytomas, oligodendrogliomas and gangliomas, ependymomas, medulloblastomas, meningiomas, neuromas, pinealomas, pituitary adenomas, carniopharyngiomas, germinomas and metastatic lesions. The usefulness of contrast enhancement for the investigation of the retrobulbar lesion and in cases of low grade or infiltrative glioma has not been demonstrated. In calcified lesions, there is less likelihood of enhancement. Following therapy, tumors may show decreased or no enhancement. The opacification of the inferior vermis following contrast media administration has resulted in false-positive diagnosis in a number of otherwise normal studies.

Nonneoplastic Conditions

OMNIPAQUE may be beneficial in the image enhancement of nonneoplastic lesions. Cerebral infarctions of recent onset may be better visualized with contrast enhancement, while some infarctions are obscured if contrast medium is used. The use of iodinated contrast media results in enhancement in about 60 percent of cerebral infarctions studied from one to four weeks from the onset of symptoms.

Sites of active infection may also be enhanced following contrast medium administration.

Arteriovenous malformations and aneurysms will show contrast enhancement. For these vascular lesions the enhancement is probably dependent on the iodine content of the circulating blood pool. Hematomas and intraparenchymal bleeders seldom demonstrate contrast enhancement. However, in cases of intraparenchymal clot, for which there is no obvious clinical explanation, contrast media administration may be helpful in ruling out the possibility of associated arteriovenous malformation.

CT SCANNING OF THE BODY

OMNIPAQUE (iohexol) may be useful for enhancement of computed tomographic images for detection and evaluation of lesions in the liver, pancreas, kidneys, aorta, mediastinum, pelvis, abdominal cavity, and retroperitoneal space. Enhancement of computed tomography with OMNIPAQUE may be of benefit in establishing diagnoses of certain lesions in these sites with greater assurance than is possible with CT alone. In other cases, the contrast agent may allow visualization of lesions not seen with CT alone (ie, tumor extension) or may help to define suspicious lesions seen with unenhanced CT (ie, pancreatic cyst).

Precautions: See PRECAUTIONS—General.

Adverse Reactions: Immediately following intravascular injection of contrast medium, a transient sensation of mild warmth is not unusual. Warmth is less frequent with OMNIPAQUE than with ionic media. (See ADVERSE REACTIONS: Intravascular—General.)

Dosage and Administration: The concentration and volume required will depend on the equipment and imaging technique used.

OMNIPAQUE Injection (Iohexol)

The dosage recommended for use in contrast enhanced computed tomography is as follows:

Head Imaging by Injection:	70 mL to 150 mL (21 to 45 gI) of OMNIPAQUE 300 (300 mgI/mL) 80 mL (28 gI) of OMNIPAQUE 350 (350 mgI/mL)
Head Imaging by Infusion:	120 mL to 250 mL (29 to 60 gI) of OMNIPAQUE 240 (240 mgI/mL)
Body Imaging by Injection:	50 mL to 200 mL (15 to 60 gI) of OMNIPAQUE 300 (300 mgI/mL) 60 mL to 100 mL (21 to 35 gI) of OMNIPAQUE 350 (350 mgI/mL)

DIGITAL SUBTRACTION ANGIOGRAPHY

Intravenous Administration

OMNIPAQUE 350 at a concentration of 350 mgI/mL is indicated in adults for use in intravenous digital subtraction angiography (I.V. DSA) of the vessels of the head, neck, and abdominal, renal and peripheral vessels.

Arteriograms of diagnostic quality can be obtained following the intravenous administration of contrast media employing digital subtraction and computer imaging enhancement techniques. The intravenous route of administration using these techniques has the advantage of being less invasive than the corresponding selective catheter placement of medium. The dose is administered into a peripheral vein, the superior vena cava or right atrium, usually by mechanical injection although sometimes by rapid manual injection. The technique has been used to visualize the ventricles, aorta and most of its larger branches, including the carotids, cerebrals, vertebrals, renal, celiac, mesenterics, and the major peripheral vessels of the limbs. Radiographic visualization of these structures is possible until significant hemodilution occurs.

OMNIPAQUE 350 can be injected intravenously as a rapid bolus to provide arterial visualization using digital subtraction radiography. Preprocedural medications are not considered necessary. OMNIPAQUE 350 has provided diagnostic arterial radiographs in about 95% of patients. In some cases, poor arterial visualization has been attributed to patient movement. OMNIPAQUE 350 is very well tolerated in the vascular system. Patient discomfort (general sensation of heat and/or pain) following injection is less than with various other contrast media.

Precautions: Since the contrast medium is usually administered mechanically under high pressure, rupture of smaller peripheral veins can occur. It has been suggested that this can be avoided by using an intravenous catheter threaded proximally beyond larger tributaries or, in the case of the antecubital vein, into the superior vena cava. Sometimes the femoral vein is used. (See PRECAUTIONS—General.)

Adverse Reactions: Cardiovascular system reactions in digital arteriography included transient PVCs (16%) and PACs (6.5%). (See ADVERSE REACTIONS: Intravascular—General.)

Dosage and Administration: The usual injection volume of OMNIPAQUE 350 for the intravenous digital technique is 30 mL to 50 mL of a 350 mgI/mL solution. This is administered as a bolus at 7.5 to 30 mL/second using a pressure injector. The volume and rate of injection will depend primarily on the type of equipment and technique used.

Frequently three or more injections may be required, up to a total volume not to exceed 250 mL (87.5 gI).

Intra-arterial Administration

OMNIPAQUE 140 at a concentration of 140 mgI/mL is indicated for use in intra-arterial digital subtraction angiography of head, neck, abdominal, renal and peripheral vessels. The intra-arterial route of administration has the advantages of allowing a lower total dose of contrast agent since there is less hemodilution than with the intravenous route of

Continued on next page

This product information was prepared in August, 1989. On these and other products of Winthrop Pharmaceuticals, detailed information may be obtained on a current basis by direct inquiry to the Professional Services Department, 90 Park Avenue, New York, NY 10016 (800) 446-6267.

Winthrop Pharm.—Cont.

administration. Patients with poor cardiac output would be expected to have better contrast enhancement following intra-arterial administration as compared with intravenous administration. A higher concentration of contrast agent may be needed to facilitate catheter placement under fluoroscopic control.

Precautions: High pressure intra-arterial injections may cause the rupture of smaller peripheral arteries. (See PRECAUTIONS—General.)

Adverse Reactions: Central nervous system reactions in intra-arterial digital angiography include transient ischemia attacks (1.6%) and cerebral infarctions (1.6%). These occurred in high risk patients having a cerebral examination and the relationship to the contrast medium was uncertain. (See ADVERSE REACTIONS—General.) Headache occurred in 6.3% of the patients, all of whom were having cerebral examinations.

Dosage and Administration: Mechanical or hand injection can be used to administer one or more bolus intra-arterial injections of OMNIPAQUE 140. The volume and rate of injection will depend on the type of equipment, technique used, and the vascular area to be visualized. The following volumes and rates of injection have been used with OMNIPAQUE 140.

Arteries	Volume/ Injection (mL)	Rate of Injection (mL/sec)
Aorta	20–45	8–20
Carotid	5–10	3–6
Femoral	9–20	3–6
Vertebral	4–10	2–8
Renal	6–12	3–6
Other Branches of the Aorta (includes subclavian, axillary, innominate and iliac)	8–25	3–10

PERIPHERAL ANGIOGRAPHY

OMNIPAQUE (iohexol) 300 at a concentration of 300 mgI/mL or OMNIPAQUE 350 at a concentration of 350 mgI/mL is indicated in adults for use in peripheral arteriography. OMNIPAQUE 240 at a concentration of 240 mgI/mL or OMNIPAQUE 300 at a concentration of 300 mgI/mL is indicated in adults for use in peripheral venography.

Sedative medication may be employed prior to use. Anesthesia is not considered necessary.

Patient discomfort during and immediately following injection is substantially less than that following injection of various other contrast media. Moderate to severe discomfort is very unusual.

Precautions: Pulsation should be present in the artery to be injected. In thromboangiitis obliterans, or ascending infection associated with severe ischemia, angiography should be performed with extreme caution, if at all. (See PRECAUTIONS—General.)

Adverse Reactions: A transient sensation of mild warmth is usual, immediately following injection. This has not interfered with the procedure.

In phlebography the incidence of leg pain was 21%. This usually was mild and lasted a short time after injection. (See ADVERSE REACTIONS: Intravascular—General.)

Dosage and Administration: The volume required will depend on the size, flow rate, and disease state of the injected vessel and on the size and condition of the patient, as well as the imaging technique used.

The dosage recommended for use in peripheral angiography is as follows:

Aortofemoral runoffs:
20 mL to 70 mL of OMNIPAQUE 350 (350 mgI/mL)
30 mL to 90 mL of OMNIPAQUE 300 (300 mgI/mL)

Selective arteriograms (femoral/iliac):
10 mL to 30 mL of OMNIPAQUE 350 (350 mgI/mL)
10 mL to 60 mL of OMNIPAQUE 300 (300 mgI/mL)

Venography (per leg):
20 mL to 150 mL of OMNIPAQUE 240 (240 mgI/mL)
40 mL to 100 mL of OMNIPAQUE 300 (300 mgI/mL)

EXCRETORY UROGRAPHY

OMNIPAQUE (iohexol) 300 at a concentration of 300 mgI/mL or OMNIPAQUE 350 at a concentration of 350 mgI/mL is indicated for use in adults in excretory urography to provide diagnostic contrast of the urinary tract.

OMNIPAQUE 300 at a concentration of 300 mgI/mL is indicated in children for excretory urography, including voiding cystourethrography (VCU).

For pharmacokinetics of excretion in adults, see CLINICAL PHARMACOLOGY—INTRAVASCULAR/Body Cavities.

Precautions: Preparatory dehydration is not recommended in the elderly, infants, young children, diabetic, or azotemic patients, or in patients with suspected myelomatosis.

Pediatric patients at higher risk of experiencing adverse events during contrast medium administration may include those having asthma, a sensitivity to medication and/or allergens, congestive heart failure, a serum creatinine greater than 1.5 mg/dL or those less than 12 months of age.

Since the VCU procedure requires instrumentation, special precautions should be observed in those patients known to have an acute urinary tract infection. Filling of the bladder should be done at a steady rate, exercising caution to avoid excessive pressure. Sterile procedures are essential.

Since there is a possibility of temporary suppression of urine formation, it is recommended that a suitable interval elapse before excretory urography is repeated, especially in patients with unilateral or bilateral reduction in renal function. (See PRECAUTIONS—General.)

Adverse Reactions: See ADVERSE REACTIONS: Intravascular—General.

Dosage and Administration: *Adults:* OMNIPAQUE 300 and OMNIPAQUE 350 at dosages from 200 mgI/kg body weight to 350 mgI/kg body weight have produced diagnostic opacification of the excretory system in patients with normal renal function.

Pediatrics

Excretory Urography

OMNIPAQUE 300 at doses of 0.5 mL/kg to 3.0 mL/kg of body weight has produced diagnostic opacification of the excretory tract. The usual dose for children is 1.0 mL/kg to 1.5 mL/kg. Dosage for infants and children should be administered in proportion to age and body weight. The total administered dose should not exceed 3 mL/kg.

Voiding Cystourethrography (VCU)

OMNIPAQUE 300 at a concentration of 300 mgI/mL may be diluted, utilizing aseptic technique, with Sterile Water for Injection to a concentration of 50 mgI/mL to 100 mgI/mL for voiding cystourethrography. The concentration may vary depending upon the patient's size and age and also with the technique and equipment used. Sufficient volume of contrast medium should be administered to adequately fill the bladder. The usual volume ranges from 50 mL to 300 mL of OMNIPAQUE at a concentration of 100 mgI/mL and 50 mL to 600 mL of OMNIPAQUE at a concentration of 50 mgI/mL. OMNIPAQUE 300 may be diluted with Sterile Water for Injection as indicated in the table below:

To Achieve	Add	
A Final Concentration (mgI/mL) of	Per 100 mL of OMNIPAQUE 300 Sterile Water for Injection, USP (mL)	Volume of Final Solution (mL)
100	200	300
90	233	333
80	275	375
70	330	430
60	400	500
50	500	600

ARTHROGRAPHY

OMNIPAQUE 240 at a concentration of 240 mgI/mL or OMNIPAQUE 300 at a concentration of 300 mgI/mL or OMNIPAQUE 350 at a concentration of 350 mgI/mL is indicated in radiography of the knee joint in adults, and OMNIPAQUE 300 at a concentration of 300 mgI/mL is indicated in radiography of the shoulder joint in adults. Arthrography may be helpful in the diagnosis of posttraumatic or degenerative joint diseases, synovial rupture, the visualization of communicating bursae or cysts, and in meniscography.

Precautions: See PRECAUTIONS—General.

Strict aseptic technique is required to prevent infection. Fluoroscopic control should be used to ensure proper needle placement, prevent extracapsular injection, and prevent dilution of contrast medium. Undue pressure should not be exerted during injection.

Adverse Reactions: Injection of OMNIPAQUE into the joint is associated with transient discomfort, ie, pain, swelling. However, delayed, severe or persistent discomfort may occur occasionally. Severe pain may often result from undue use of pressure or the injection of large volumes. Joint swelling after injection is less with OMNIPAQUE than with high osmolar ionic contrast medium. These types of reactions are generally procedurally dependent and of greater frequency when double-contrast technique is employed.

Reactions in arthrography included pain (36%), swelling sensation (58%), heat sensation (8%), and muscle weakness (0.4%).

Skin and appendages reaction included hematoma injection site (1%). (See ADVERSE REACTIONS: Body Cavities—General.)

Dosage and Administration: Arthrography is usually performed under local anesthesia. The amount of OMNIPAQUE (iohexol) injected is dependent on the size of the joint to be examined and the technique employed. Lower volumes of contrast medium are usually injected when dou-

ble-contrast examinations using 30 mL to 100 mL of air are performed.

The following concentrations and volumes are recommended for normal adult knee and shoulder joints but should serve as guidelines since joints may require more or less contrast medium for optimal visualization.

KNEE

OMNIPAQUE 240	5 mL to 15 mL
OMNIPAQUE 300	5 mL to 15 mL
OMNIPAQUE 350	5 mL to 10 mL

SHOULDER

OMNIPAQUE 300	10 mL

Passive or active manipulation is used to disperse the medium throughout the joint space.

ENDOSCOPIC RETROGRADE PANCREATOGRAPHY (ERP)/ENDOSCOPIC RETROGRADE CHOLANGIOPANCREATOGRAPHY (ERCP)

OMNIPAQUE 240 at a concentration of 240 mgI/mL is indicated in adults for use in ERP/ERCP.

Precautions: See PRECAUTIONS—General.

Adverse Reactions: Injection of OMNIPAQUE in ERP ERCP is associated with transient pain. However, delayed, severe or persistent pain may occur and can persist for 24 hours. The cause of the pain may be due as much to the procedure itself as to the contrast medium injected, therefore, attention should be paid to the injection pressure and total volume injected to minimize disruptive distention of the ducts examined.

Cardiovascular adverse reactions included hypertension (1%).

Central nervous system adverse reactions included pain (17%), somnolence (1%), and burning (1%). (See ADVERSE REACTIONS: Body Cavities—General.)

Gastrointestinal adverse reactions included vomiting, diarrhea, and pressure, each with an individual incidence of 1%.

Dosage and Administration: The recommended dose of OMNIPAQUE 240 at a concentration of 240 mgI/mL is 10 mL to 50 mL but may vary depending on individual anatomy and/or disease state.

HYSTEROSALPINGOGRAPHY

OMNIPAQUE 240 at a concentration of 240 mgI/mL or OMNIPAQUE 300 at a concentration of 300 mgI/mL is indicated in radiography of the internal group of adult female reproductive organs; ovaries, fallopian tubes, uterus, and vagina. Hysterosalpingography is utilized as a diagnostic and therapeutic modality in the treatment of infertility and other abnormal gynecological conditions.

Contraindications: The procedure should not be performed during the menstrual period or when menstrual flow is imminent, nor should it be performed when infection is present in any portion of the genital tract, including the external genitalia. The procedure is also contraindicated for pregnant women or for those in whom pregnancy is suspected. Its use is not advised for 6 months after termination of pregnancy or 30 days after conization or curettage.

Precautions: In patients with carcinoma or in those in whom the condition is suspected, caution should be exercised to avoid possible spreading of the lesion by the procedure.

Adverse Reactions: Injection of OMNIPAQUE in hysterosalpingography is associated with immediate but transient pain. The cause of the pain may be due as much to the procedure itself as to the contrast medium injected, therefore attention should be paid to the injection pressure and volume instilled to avoid disruptive distention of the uterus and fallopian tubes. Fluoroscopic monitoring is recommended.

Central nervous system adverse reactions included pain (49%), somnolence, and fever each with an individual incidence of 3%.

Gastrointestinal adverse reactions included nausea (3%). (See ADVERSE REACTIONS: Body Cavities—General.)

Dosage and Administration: The recommended dosage of OMNIPAQUE 240 is 15 mL to 20 mL and of OMNIPAQUE 300 is 15 mL to 20 mL but will vary depending on individual anatomy and/or disease state.

HERNIOGRAPHY

OMNIPAQUE 240 at a concentration of 240 mgI/mL is indicated in adults for use in herniography.

Precautions: See PRECAUTIONS—General.

Adverse Reactions: Central nervous system adverse reactions included pain (7%), headache (3%), and unwell feeling (3%).

Gastrointestinal system adverse reactions included diarrhea (3%) and flatulence (10%). (See ADVERSE REACTIONS: Body Cavities—General.)

Dosage and Administration: The recommended dosage of OMNIPAQUE 240 is 50 mL but may vary depending on individual anatomy and/or disease state.

HOW SUPPLIED

OMNIPAQUE 140
Vials of 50 mL, 140 mgI/mL, boxes of 10
(NDC 0024-1401-50)
OMNIPAQUE 240
Vials of 10 mL, 240 mgI/mL, boxes of 10
(NDC 0024-1412-10)

Vials of 20 mL, 240 mgI/mL, boxes of 10
(NDC 0024-1412-20)
Vials of 50 mL, 240 mgI/mL, boxes of 10
(NDC 0024-1412-50)
100 mL fill in 100 mL bottle with hanger, 240 mgI/mL,
boxes of 10 (NDC 0024-1412-60)
150 mL fill in 200 mL bottle with hanger, 240 mgI/mL,
boxes of 10 (NDC 0024-1412-49)
200 mL fill in 200 mL bottle with hanger, 240 mgI/mL,
boxes of 10, with 10 infusion sets, (NDC 0024-1412-04)
OMNIPAQUE 300
Vials of 10 mL, 300 mgI/mL, boxes of 10
(NDC 0024-1413-10)
Vials of 30 mL, 300 mgI/mL, boxes of 10
(NDC 0024-1413-30)
Vials of 50 mL, 300 mgI/mL, boxes of 10
(NDC 0024-1413-50)
100 mL fill in 100 mL bottle with hanger, 300 mgI/mL,
boxes of 10 (NDC 0024-1413-60)
150 mL fill in 200 mL bottle with hanger, 300 mgI/mL,
boxes of 10, with 10 infusion sets, (NDC 0024-1413-70)
OMNIPAQUE 350
Vials of 50 mL, 350 mgI/mL, boxes of 10
(NDC 0024-1414-50)
100 mL fill in 100 mL bottle with hanger, 350 mgI/mL,
boxes of 10 (NDC 0024-1414-60)
150 mL fill in 200 mL bottle with hanger, 350 mgI/mL,
boxes of 10 (NDC 0024-1414-03)
200 mL fill in 200 mL bottle with hanger, 350 mgI/mL,
boxes of 10 (NDC 0024-1414-04)

Storage: Protect vials and bottles of OMNIPAQUE (iohexol) from strong daylight and direct exposure to sunlight. Do not freeze. Store at 59°F to 86°F (15°C to 30°C).

Distributed by Winthrop Pharmaceuticals
Division of Sterling Drug Inc.
New York, NY 10016
Manufactured by Sterling Pharmaceuticals Inc.
Barceloneta, Puerto Rico 00617

OW-107 P

Wyeth-Ayerst Laboratories
Division of American Home
Products Corporation
P.O. BOX 8299
PHILADELPHIA, PA 19101

FACTREL®   ℞
[fāc 'trel]
(gonadorelin hydrochloride)
Synthetic Luteinizing Hormone Releasing
Hormone (LH-RH)
DIAGNOSTIC USE ONLY

CAUTION: Federal law prohibits dispensing without prescription.

DESCRIPTION
An agent for use in evaluating hypothalamic-pituitary gonadotropic function. FACTREL (gonadorelin hydrochloride) injectable is available as a sterile lyophilized powder for reconstitution and administration by subcutaneous or intravenous routes.
Chemical Name: 5-oxo-L-prolyl-L-histidyl-L-tryptophyl-L-seryl -L- tyrosyl-glycyl -L- leucyl-L-arginyl-L-prolyl glycinamide hydrochloride
[See table above right]
FACTREL is $C_{55}H_{75}N_{17}O_{13}HCl$, as the mono- or dihydrochloride, or their mixture. The gonadorelin base has a molecular weight of 1182.33. It is a white powder, soluble in alcohol and water, hygroscopic and moisture-sensitive, and stable at room temperature. The synthetic decapeptide, FACTREL, has a chemical composition and structure identical to the natural hormone, identified from porcine or ovine hypothalami.
Each SECULE® vial of FACTREL contains 100 or 500 mcg gonadorelin as the hydrochloride, with 100 mg lactose, USP. Each ampul of sterile diluent contains 2% benzyl alcohol in sterile water.

CLINICAL PHARMACOLOGY
FACTREL has been shown to have gonadotropin-releasing effects upon the anterior pituitary. The range for normal baseline LH levels, as determined from the literature, is 5–25 mIU/mL in postpubertal males, and postpubertal and premenopausal females. The standard used is the Second International Reference Preparation—HMC. This range may not correspond in each laboratory performing the assay since the concentration of LH in normal individuals varies with different assay methods. The normal responses to FACTREL analyzed from the results of clinical studies included:
(1) LH peak (mIU/mL)
(highest LH value post-FACTREL administration)
(2) Maximum LH increase (mIU/mL)
(peak LH value—LH baseline value)

Structural Formula:

(3) LH percent response
$$\frac{\text{peak LH—baseline LH}}{\text{baseline LH}} \times 100\%$$
(4) Time to peak (minutes)
(time required to reach LH peak value)
Normal adult subjects were shown to have these LH responses following FACTREL administration by subcutaneous or intravenous routes.

I. MALE ADULTS:
A) Subcutaneous Administration
The results are based on 18 tests in males between the ages of 18–42 years, inclusive:
(1) LH peak: mean 60.3 ± 26.2 mIU/mL
100% ≥ 24.0 mIU/mL
90% ≥ 32.8 mIU/mL
(2) Maximum LH increase: mean 46.7 ± 20.8 mIU/mL
100% ≥ 12.3 mIU/mL
90% ≥ 20.9 mIU/mL
(3) LH percent response: mean 437 ± 243% range: 66–1853%
90% ≥ 188%
(4) Time to peak: mean 34 ± 13 min.
B) Intravenous Administration
The results are based on 26 tests in males between the ages of 19–58 years, inclusive:
(1) LH peak: mean 63.8 ± 40.3 mIU/mL
100% ≥ 12.6 mIU/mL
90% ≥ 26.0 mIU/mL
(2) Maximum LH increase: mean 51.3 ± 35.2 mIU/mL
100% ≥ 7.4 mIU/mL
90% ≥ 14.8 mIU/mL
(3) LH percent response: mean 481 ± 184% range: 67–2139%
90% ≥ 142%
(4) Time to peak: mean 27 ± 14 min.
In males older than 50 years, the LH baseline and peak levels tend to be higher; however, the maximum LH increases do not differ in regard to age.

II. FEMALE ADULTS:
A) Subcutaneous Administration
The results are based on 38 tests in females between the ages of 19–36 years, inclusive:
(1) LH peak: mean 67.9 ± 27.5 mIU/mL
100% ≥ 12.5 mIU/mL
90% ≥ 39.0 mIU/mL
(2) Maximum LH increase: mean 52.8 ± 26.4 mIU/mL
100% ≥ 7.5 mIU/mL
90% ≥ 23.8 mIU/mL
(3) LH percent response: mean 374 ± 221% range: 108–981%
90% ≥ 185%
(4) Time to peak: mean 71.5 ± 49.6 min.
B) Intravenous Administration
The results are based on 31 tests in females between the ages of 20–35 years inclusive:
(1) LH peak: mean 57.6 ± 36.7 mIU/mL
100% ≥ 20.0 mIU/mL
90% ≥ 24.6 mIU/mL
(2) Maximum LH increase: mean 44.5 ± 31.8 mIU/mL
100% ≥ 7.5 mIU/mL
90% ≥ 16.2 mIU/mL
(3) LH percent response: mean 356 ± 282% range: 60–1300%
90% ≥ 142%
(4) Time to peak: mean 36 ± 24 min.
The FACTREL tests on which the normal female responses are based were performed in the early follicular phase of the menstrual cycle (Days 1–7).
In menopausal and postmenopausal females, the baseline LH levels are elevated and the maximum LH increases are exaggerated when compared with the premenopausal levels.

Patients with clinically diagnosed or suspected pituitary and/or hypothalamic dysfunction were often shown to have subnormal or no LH responses following FACTREL administration. For example, in clinical tests of 6 patients with known postpubertal panhypopituitarism, and 11 patients with Prader-Willi syndrome, 100% showed subnormal responses or no rise in LH. Subnormal responses to the FACTREL test also were observed in 21 (95%) of 22 patients with prepubertal panhypopituitarism. In 19 patients with Sheehan's syndrome, 16 (84%) had a subnormal response. In the FACTREL test in 44 patients with Kallmann's syndrome, 33 (77%) had subnormal LH responses.

INDICATIONS AND USAGE
FACTREL as a single injection is indicated for evaluating the functional capacity and response of the gonadotropes of the anterior pituitary. This single-injection test does not measure pituitary gonadotropic reserve for which more prolonged or repeated administration may be required. The LH response is useful in testing patients with suspected gonadotropin deficiency, whether due to the hypothalamus alone or in combination with anterior pituitary failure. FACTREL is also indicated for evaluating residual gonadotropic function of the pituitary following removal of a pituitary tumor by surgery and/or irradiation. In clinical studies to date, however, the single-injection test has not been useful in differentiating pituitary disorders from hypothalamic disorders. The FACTREL test can be performed concomitantly with other post-treatment evaluations.
The results of the FACTREL test complement the clinical examination and other laboratory tests used to confirm or substantiate hypogonadotropic hypogonadism.
In cases where there is a normal response, it indicates the presence of functional pituitary gonadotropes. The single-injection test does not measure pituitary gonadotropic reserve.

CONTRAINDICATIONS
Hypersensitivity to gonadorelin hydrochloride or any of the components.

PRECAUTIONS
Although allergic and hypersensitivity reactions have been observed with other polypeptide hormones, and rarely with multiple doses of FACTREL, to date no such reactions have been reported following the administration of a single 100 mcg dose of FACTREL.
Antibody formation has been reported rarely after chronic administration of large doses of FACTREL.
The FACTREL test should be conducted in the absence of other drugs which directly affect the pituitary secretion of the gonadotropins. These would include a variety of preparations which contain androgens, estrogens, progestins, or glucocorticoids. The gonadotropin levels may be transiently elevated by spironolactone, minimally elevated by levodopa, and suppressed by oral contraceptives and digoxin. The response to FACTREL may be blunted by phenothiazines and dopamine antagonists which cause a rise in prolactin.
Pregnancy Category B. Reproduction studies have been performed in mice, rats, and rabbits at doses up to 50 times the human dose, and have revealed no evidence of harm to the fetus due to FACTREL. There are, however, no adequate and well-controlled studies in pregnant women. Because animal reproduction studies are not always predictive of human response, this drug should be used during pregnancy only if clearly needed.
Appropriate precautions should be taken because the effects of LH-RH on the fetus and developing offspring have not been adequately evaluated. Repetitive, high doses of FACTREL may cause luteolysis and inhibition of spermatogenesis.

ADVERSE REACTIONS
Systemic complaints such as headaches, nausea, lightheadedness, abdominal discomfort, and flushing have been re-

Continued on next page

Wyeth-Ayerst—Cont.

ported rarely following administration of 100 mcg of FACTREL. Local swelling, occasionally with pain and pruritus, at the injection site may occur if FACTREL is administered subcutaneously. Local and generalized skin rash have been noted after chronic subcutaneous administration. Rare instances of hypersensitivity reaction (bronchospasm, tachycardia, flushing, urticaria, induration at injection site) and one case of anaphylactic reaction have been reported following multiple-dose administration.

OVERDOSAGE

FACTREL has been administered parenterally in doses up to 3 mg bid for 28 days without any signs or symptoms of overdosage. In case of overdosage or idiosyncrasy, symptomatic treatment should be administered as required.

DOSAGE AND ADMINISTRATION

Adults: 100 mcg dose, subcutaneously or intravenously. In females for whom the phase of the menstrual cycle can be established, the test should be performed in the early follicular phase (Days 1–7).

TEST METHODOLOGY

To determine the status of the gonadotropin secretory capacity of the anterior pituitary, a test procedure requiring seven venous blood samples for LH is recommended.

PROCEDURE:

1. Venous blood samples should be drawn at -15 minutes and immediately prior to FACTREL administration. The LH baseline is obtained by averaging the LH values of the two samples.
2. Administer a bolus of 100 mcg of FACTREL subcutaneously or intravenously.
3. Draw venous blood samples at 15, 30, 45, 60, and 120 minutes after administration.
4. Blood samples should be handled as recommended by the laboratory that will determine the LH content. It must be emphasized that the reliability of the test is directly related to the inter-assay and intra-assay reliability of the laboratory performing the assay.

INTERPRETATION OF TEST RESULTS

Interpretation of the LH response to FACTREL requires an understanding of the hypothalamic-pituitary physiology, knowledge of the clinical status of the individual patient, and familiarity with the normal ranges and the standards used in the laboratory performing the LH assays.

Figures 1 through 4 represent the LH response curves after FACTREL administration in normal subjects. The normal LH response curves were established between the 10th percentile (B line) and 90th percentile (A line) of all LH responses in normal subjects analyzed from the results of clinical studies. LH values are reported in units of mIU/mL and time is displayed in minutes. Individual patient responses should be plotted on the appropriate curve. A subnormal response in patients is defined as three or more LH values which fall below the B line of the normal LH response curve. In cases where there is a blunted or borderline response, the FACTREL test should be repeated.

Fig. 1
Normal Male LH Response After FACTREL 100 mcg,
Subcutaneous Administration 10th and 90th percentiles.

Fig. 2:
Normal Male LH Response After FACTREL 100 mcg,
Intravenous Administration 10th and 90th percentiles.

Fig. 3:
Normal Female LH Response After FACTREL 100 mcg,
Subcutaneous Administration 10th and 90th percentiles.

Fig. 4:
Normal Female LH Response After FACTREL 100 mcg,
Intravenous Administration 10th and 90th percentiles.

The FACTREL test complements the clinical assessment of patients with a variety of endocrine disorders involving the hypothalamic-pituitary axis. In cases where there is a normal response, it indicates the presence of functional pituitary gonadotropes. The single-injection test does not determine the pathophysiological cause for the subnormal response and does not measure pituitary gonadotropic reserve.

HOW SUPPLIED

LYOPHILIZED POWDER—
in single-dose SECULE® vials containing 100 mcg (NDC 0046-0507-05) and 500 mcg (NDC 0046-0509-05) gonadorelin as the hydrochloride with 100 mg lactose, USP. Each SECULE® vial is accompanied by one ampul containing 2 mL sterile diluent of 2% benzyl alcohol in sterile water.

DIRECTIONS

Store at room temperature (approximately 25°C).
Reconstitute <u>100</u> mcg SECULE® vial with <u>1.0</u> mL of the accompanying sterile diluent.
Reconstitute <u>500</u> mcg SECULE® vial with <u>2.0</u> mL of the accompanying sterile diluent.
Prepare solution immediately before use.
After reconstitution, store at room temperature and use within 1 day.
Discard unused reconstituted solution and diluent.
Diagnostic Method of Use Patent 3,947,569
Shown in Product Identification Section, page 436

PEPTAVLON®   ℞
[pĕp-tăv'lon]
Brand of
pentagastrin
A diagnostic agent for
evaluation of gastric
acid secretory function.

CAUTION: Federal law prohibits dispensing without prescription.

DESCRIPTION

Chemical name: N-t-butyloxycarbonyl-B-alanyl-L-tryptophyl-L-methionyl-L-aspartyl-L-phenylalanyl amide.
Structural formula:

Pentagastrin is a synthetic pentapeptide containing the carboxyl terminal tetrapeptide, the active portion found in all natural gastrins. Pentagastrin is a colorless crystalline solid. It is soluble in dimethylformamide and dimethylsulfoxide; it is almost insoluble in water, ethanol, ether, benzene, chloroform, and ethyl acetate.

ACTIONS

PEPTAVLON (pentagastrin) contains the C-terminal tetrapeptide responsible for the actions of the natural gastrins

and, therefore, acts as a physiologic gastric acid secretagogue. The recommended dose of 6 mcg/kg subcutaneously produces a peak acid output which is reproducible when used in the same individual.

PEPTAVLON stimulates gastric acid secretion approximately ten minutes after subcutaneous injection, with peak responses occurring in most cases twenty to thirty minutes after administration. Duration of activity is usually between sixty and eighty minutes.

INDICATIONS

PEPTAVLON is used as a diagnostic agent to evaluate gastric acid secretory function. It is useful in testing for:
Anacidity:—as a diagnostic aid in patients with suspected pernicious anemia, atrophic gastritis, or gastric carcinoma.
Hypersecretion:—as a diagnostic aid in patients with suspected duodenal ulcer or postoperative stomal ulcer, and for the diagnosis of Zollinger-Ellison tumor.
PEPTAVLON (pentagastrin) is also useful in determining the adequacy of acid-reducing operations for peptic ulcer.

CONTRAINDICATIONS

Hypersensitivity or idiosyncrasy to pentagastrin.

WARNINGS

Use in Pregnancy—The use of pentagastrin in pregnancy has NOT been studied, and the benefit of administration of the drug must be weighed against any possible risk to the mother and/or fetus.
Use in Children—There are insufficient data to recommend the use of, or establish a dosage, in children.

****

In amounts in excess of the recommended dose, pentagastrin may cause inhibition of gastric acid secretion.

PRECAUTIONS

Use with caution in patients with pancreatic, hepatic, or biliary disease. Like gastrin, pentagastrin could, in some cases, have the physiologic effect of stimulating pancreatic enzyme and bicarbonate secretion, as well as biliary flow.

ADVERSE REACTIONS

Pentagastrin causes fewer and less severe cardiovascular and other adverse reactions than histamine or betazole. The majority of reactions to pentagastrin are related to the gastrointestinal tract.
The following reactions associated with the use of pentagastrin have been reported.
Gastrointestinal: Abdominal pain, desire to defecate, nausea, vomiting, borborygmi, blood-tinged mucus
Cardiovascular: Flushing, tachycardia
Central Nervous System: Dizziness, faintness or light-headedness, drowsiness, sinking feeling, transient blurring of vision, tiredness, headache
Allergic and Hypersensitivity Reactions: May occur in some patients.
Miscellaneous: Shortness of breath, heavy sensation in arms and legs, tingling in fingers, chills, sweating, generalized burning sensation, warmth, pain at site of injection, bile in collected specimens

DOSAGE AND ADMINISTRATION

Adults: 6 mcg/kg subcutaneously. Effect begins in about ten minutes; peak response usually occurs in twenty to thirty minutes. (For discussion of the test and explicit directions, consult Baron, JH: Gastric Function Tests, in Wastell, C: *Chronic Duodenal Ulcer,* New York, Appleton-Century-Crofts, 1972, pp 82–114.)
Note: Data are inadequate to recommend the use of, or establish a dosage, in children.

OVERDOSAGE

In case of overdosage or idiosyncrasy, symptomatic treatment should be administered as required.

HOW SUPPLIED

PEPTAVLON (pentagastrin)—In 2 mL ampuls. Each mL contains 0.25 mg (250 mcg) pentagastrin. Also contains 0.88% sodium chloride, and Water for Injection, USP. The pH is adjusted with ammonium hydroxide and/or hydrochloric acid. Cartons of 10 (NDC 0046-3290-10).
Refrigerate and protect from light.
Do not use if discolored.

CLINICAL STUDIES

Gastric Acid Secretion: Peak gastric output in mEq/hr caused by subcutaneous injection of 6 mcg/kg pentagastrin does not differ significantly from that caused by the standard subcutaneous injection of the histamine acid phosphate dose used in the augmented histamine test (40 mcg/kg). For example, in 25 normal volunteers, pentagastrin produced an average peak acid output of 28.4 mEq/hr compared with 24.7 mEq/hr by histamine. In 45 patients with duodenal ulcer, or suspected duodenal ulcer, pentagastrin produced an average peak gastric acid output of 39.7 mEq/hr, compared with 33.7 mEq/hr by histamine. In 18 patients with gastric ulcer, or suspected gastric ulcer, pentagastrin produced an average peak acid output of 17.4 mEq/hr, compared with 19.4 mEq/hr by histamine. The overall mean for peak acid secretion by pentagastrin was 24.8 mEq/hr, compared with 22.6 mEq/hr by histamine. No biochemical abnormality which might indicate specific organ toxicity has been encountered following the administration of pentagastrin.

GUIDE TO MANAGEMENT OF DRUG OVERDOSE

Prepared by:
Eric G. Comstock, M.D.
and
Eugene V. Boisaubin, M.D.
Department of Medicine
Baylor College of Medicine
Houston, Texas

INTRODUCTION: The following discussion is designed for use in adult patients. In the pediatric age group, general principles apply, but the volumes of fluid or suggested medication must be adjusted for body size. Symptomatic and supportive care is the basis for treatment of drug overdose. All other approaches are secondary. Procedures directed toward the offending substance, such as the performance of gastric lavage or the administration of a specific pharmacologic antagonist, should be undertaken only after adequate vital function has been assured. Procedures to facilitate excretion of toxic substances, such as peritoneal or extracorporeal dialysis and forced diuresis are required infrequently, and should never be relied upon as the primary approach to treatment. For sedative, hypnotic, and tranquilizer drugs, alone or in combination, supportive care is sufficient as outlined in the following discussion.

INITIAL ASSESSMENT: If the patient is symptomatic, determine the adequacy of respiration and cardiac function and note reflex activity, such as pupillary, corneal, gag and deep tendon. If vital function is compromised, or consciousness is impaired, proceed immediately to supportive measures.

THE ASYMPTOMATIC PATIENT: The drug overdosed patient may be asymptomatic because he has not ingested a sufficient dose of the drugs, or because a sufficient quantity has not yet been absorbed to produce symptoms. After the ingestion of a life threatening quantity of drugs, symptoms may be delayed as long as six hours, although ordinarily symptoms are manifested within thirty (30) minutes to two (2) hours. Ingestion of alcohol simultaneously with drugs may shorten the time for symptoms to appear. Vomiting should be induced only during the asymptomatic interval. If significant central nervous system depression intervenes between the administration of emetic and the occurrence of vomiting, then the airway should be protected by insertion of a cuffed endotracheal tube. Fluids must be forced orally to obtain satisfactory results from any effort to induce vomiting. An alternate approach to the asymptomatic patient alleged to have ingested drugs, is the administration by mouth of a slurry of no less than 100 grams of activated charcoal powder (USP) in water. Gastric lavage with a large caliber tube (34 French) may be performed in the asymptomatic patient. Any patient whose consciousness is impaired to the point where a cuffed endotracheal tube will be tolerated should be intubated prior to the performance of gastric lavage.

THE SYMPTOMATIC PATIENT: If the patient is symptomatic all treatment procedures directed toward the toxic substance are secondary to the support of vital function. If the patient is in coma, attention to respiratory support and cardiac function should proceed immediately.

RESPIRATORY SUPPORT: Examine the mouth. Remove all foreign material including dentures. Position the head so that respiration is not sonorous and so that regurgitated stomach contents are not readily aspirated. If respiration is not present, provide ventilation by mouth-to-mouth, ambu bag, or positive pressure respirator until the patient is adequately oxygenated. Insert an oropharyngeal airway and suction excess secretions while preparing to insert an endotracheal tube. A cuffed endotracheal tube should be inserted and inflated. Bronchial suction should be administered to clear mucus and foreign material. Determine that the chest is being inflated symmetrically and that breath sounds are audible bilaterally. After the acute emergency, determine placement of the endotracheal tube by x-ray. Monitor adequacy of ventilation using arterial blood gases.

IV ACCESS AND CARDIAC FUNCTION: While one member of the treatment team is assuring adequate ventilation, a second member of the team should be assuring adequate IV access by insertion of an 18 gauge venous catheter and initiation of IV fluid administration such as Ringers Lactate or $\frac{1}{2}$ normal saline at a maintenance rate in adults of 150 ml. per hour. Since hypotension from sedative drug intoxication results from relative hypovolemia complicated frequently by dehydration, the rate of intravenous infusion should be increased to 10-20 cc per minute if the systolic pressure is under 80 mm of mercury. Placing the patient in the Trendelenburg position may quickly correct small to moderate degrees of hypotension. A central venous pressure catheter or a Swan-Ganz catheter is required if the continuous high rate infusion reaches one (1) liter within one hour or if the positive fluid balance exceeds two (2) liters during the first two hours. Intermittent monitoring of central venous pressure should continue throughout the period of intensive supportive care. A baseline electrocardiogram should be obtained as soon as vital functions have been supported. The appearance of conduction defects should lead to suspicion of drugs with direct cardiac effects, such as the tricyclic antidepressants. In uncomplicated sedative drug overdose, the central venous pressure will be under ten centimeters of water and will not change appreciably with high volume fluid infusion. If the central venous pressure increases abruptly in excess of five centimeters of water, or if the CVP exceeds 16 centimeters of water, high rate fluid infusion should be stopped pending evaluation of cardiac status. Adequate tissue perfusion is obtained with a systolic pressure in the range of 80 to 100 milliliters of mercury. A systolic pressure higher than this is required only in the patient with pre-existing hypertension. The formation of urine is an indication that tissue perfusion is adequate.

URINARY CATHETERIZATION: An in-dwelling urinary catheter should be inserted early in the course of treatment of any unconscious drug overdose patient. Upon insertion of the catheter, the volume of residual urine should be measured and the specimen should be saved separately for urinalysis including specific gravity, labeled for drug analysis, and sent to the laboratory to be retained for 24 hours. Recording of urine output hourly is necessary to maintain fluid balance records. Abrupt cessation of urine output most frequently is due to an obstructed catheter, but deserves immediate appraisal. Anuria for a period in excess of one hour should lead to reduction of high rate intravascular volume infusion until cardiac and renal status has been reappraised. Failure to achieve adequate urinary output after initial emptying of the bladder may reflect uncompensated dehydration and relative hypovolemia, each of which must be corrected before balanced fluid intake and output plus insensible loss can be achieved. The immediate or automatic use of diuretics at this stage only aggravates the basic defect and may result in intractable hypotension. Addition of vasopressor drugs at this stage may precipitate renal failure. Electrolyte solutions as transient volume expanders are preferred to whole blood or plasma to avoid congestive heart failure when normal vascular tone is re-established. A positive fluid balance of 2 to 4 liters may be required before fluid intake and output are in equilibrium. As vascular tone returns, urine output may increase abruptly exceeding one liter per hour. Profound diuresis may precede recurrence of deep tendon reflexes and heralds reduction in CNS depression.

GASTRIC LAVAGE: Gastric lavage should be performed only after vital function has been determined to be adequate or procedures for support have been implemented. Gastric lavage should be undertaken only after a cuffed endotracheal tube is protecting the airway. If corrosive substances are thought to have been ingested, lavage should not be performed until examination demonstrates there is no destruction of the mucous membranes of the mouth or of the esophagus as determined by esophagoscopy. Gastric lavage should be performed if the ingestion of drugs is estimated to have been within the preceding six hours. If there are no audible bowel sounds, gastric lavage should be performed regardless of the time lapse between ingestion and treatment. A 34 French lavage tube should be used. Smaller tubes do not permit sufficiently rapid fluid flow to remove particulate material. Gastric contents should be aspirated prior to lavage and saved in the event subsequent laboratory analysis is required. In an adult, lavage should be performed in cyles of 300 to 500 milliliters of fluid instilled over one to two minutes, left in place for about one minute, and drained by gravity over a period of approximately three to four minutes. If these time intervals cannot be maintained, then the lavage system is defective. The total fluid volume to be used in lavage should be three liters beyond that volume required to obtain a clear return. Lavage may be performed with tap water or normal saline solution.

ACTIVATED CHARCOAL: Powdered activated charcoal effectively adsorbs the vast majority of drugs, thereby limiting their bio-availability. One hundred (100) grams of activated charcoal suspended in six ounces of water should be instilled through the lavage tube after initial gastric aspiration and prior to lavage. The activated charcoal forms an effective barrier between any remaining particulate material and the gastrointestinal mucosa. Drugs adsorbed on activated charcoal are not desorbed to any practical extent in the lower intestinal tract. When an enteroenteric circulation of the active drug exists, excess activated charcoal in the intestine effectively prevents reabsorption thereby facilitating excretion. This appears effective with the tricyclic antidepressants and the cardiac glycosides. Activated charcoal is not effective with cyanide or small electrolytes such as sodium, potassium or mineral acids or bases.

SPECIFIC ANTIDOTES: Specific antidotal substances effective in the treatment of drug overdose are few. They should be used only with specific indications and never should be used prophyllactically or in quantities sufficient to return the comatose patient to consciousness. They should be used only to improve adequacy of vital function and never be relied upon to the exclusion of supportive care. When specific antidotes are used, special attention must be given to duration of action of the antidote as compared with the duration of action of the primary drug. Release of a patient after administration of a relatively short acting antidote may result in serious compromise of clinical status after the patient has been released from medical care.

AVOID UNNECESSARY DRUGS: Central nervous system depression and coma should be treated by the supportive means described above and should not be treated by central nervous system stimulant drugs. Shortening of coma with CNS stimulant drugs may result in hyperpyrexia and convulsions which otherwise might be avoided. Hypotension resulting from sedative or tranquilizer drug overdose is due to relative hypovolemia properly corrected by increasing the intravascular volume. Vaso-

pressor drugs are not helpful and should be avoided. Body temperature outside of the normal range should be controlled by heat exchangers which warm or cool the body mechanically. Anti-pyretic drugs should be avoided. Anti-pyretic drugs in overdose cause hyperpyrexia. Alkaline diuresis is effective in removing phenobarbital and barbital, but only rarely is it an essential part of treatment of overdose due to these drugs. Except for salicylate, the risk benefit ratio of forced diuresis in the treatment of other drugs does not favor its use. Diuretic drugs should not be used routinely in the treatment of drug overdose.

CONTINUING CARE: Coma from sedative drug intoxication may persist for many days. Total apnea for five days and an isoelectric electroencephalogram for intervals up to 36 hours have been recorded with drug overdose patients who have survived without apparent neurologic sequelae. Continuing care should be provided in a medical intensive care unit with monitoring of temperature, blood pressure, pulse, respiratory rate, tidal volume, electrocardiogram, central venous pressure, fluid balance, electrolytes, and arterial blood gases with appropriate compensatory treatment of abnormalities. Intensive respiratory care should include frequent tracheal suction, and repositioning, and frequent chest x-rays. Endotracheal tubes should be changed under supervision of a critical care specialist. Tracheostomy should be performed only for surgical indications. Carefully attentive continuous nursing care is essential.

COMPLICATIONS: Aspiration pneumonia and subsequent infection is the most commonly occuring complication of coma secondary to drug overdose. Treatment consists of vigorous tracheal suction and antibiotic coverage. Interstitial edema is common in profound coma and usually represents increased capillary permeability rather than overhydration. Parenteral steroids may be helpful in this situation. Always be mindful that the patient may have sustained traumatic injury especially to the head, so be watchful for lateralizing neurologic signs.

TOXICOLOGIC ANALYSIS: Any ingested material, initial gastric aspirate, and the first catheterized urine specimen all should be saved and labeled for laboratory examination with instructions to hold at least twenty-four (24) hours prior to discarding. Analysis of these fluids for drugs occasionally will change fundamental approach to treatment. Frequently multiple drugs are involved. Interpretation of quantitative findings is extremely difficult and usually is helpful only to follow the clearance of substances from the body. Previous drug use may result in tolerance which prevents meaningful interpretation of absolute concentrations. Instructions for management of specific drugs identified should be consulted once symptomatic and supportive care is under way.

CHARCOAL HEMOPERFUSION: During the past decade interest has increased in the insertion of innert adsorbent material into the blood stream of poisoned patients to improve clearance of the toxic substance. The most popular current technique utilizes adsorbent hemoperfusion cartridges containing activated charcoal. Extremely high clearance occurs of virtually all commonly ingested intoxicants and several life-saving case reports utilizing this procedure have appeared. Despite the theoretical virtues of this new technique there are problems associated with its use. First, aggressive but simpler comprehensive supportive management as outlined above has already reduced mortality of even severely intoxicated hospitalized patients to 2% or less. Side effects may occur and include hypotension, thrombocytopenia and the complications of systemic heparinization. The system requires additional skilled personnel and concern with the hemoperfusion technique may distract attention from the more proven supportive measures. Hemoperfusion may have a role in select, severely poisoned patients where supportive therapy is insufficient, but it is not currently recommended for routine use.